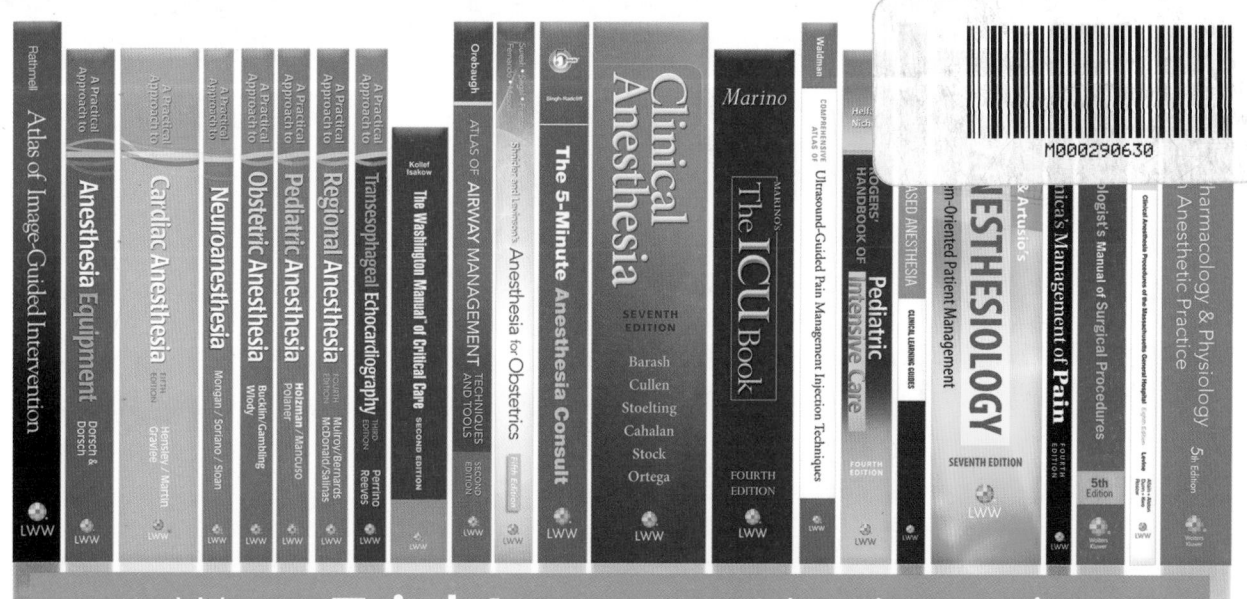

Want **Trial Access** to Lippincott's LWW Health Library: Anesthesiology Collection?

M000290630

Try the brand New ***LWW Health Library: Anesthesiology Collection***, **free for 30 days**. **Search** across the **newest editions** of over **20 gold-standard titles** in an **easy-to-use portal** on your **computer**, **tablet**, or **smartphone**.

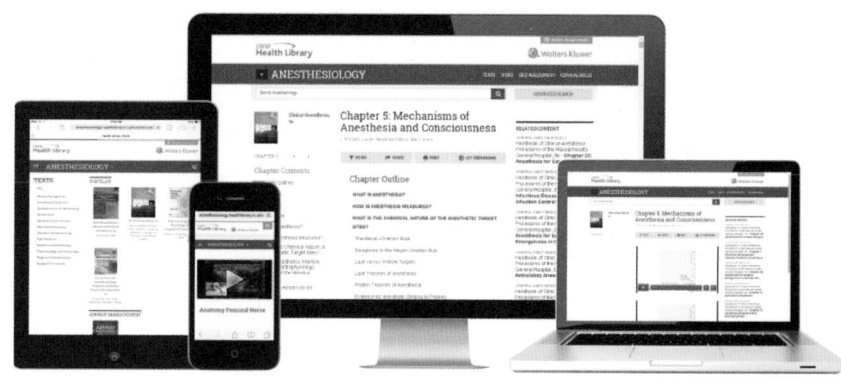

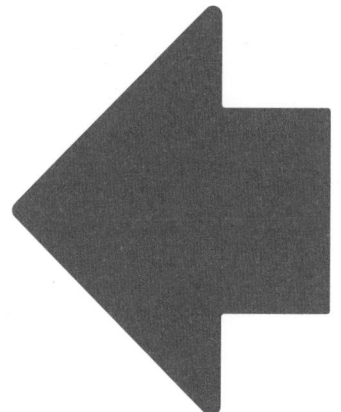

Go to
http://lwwhealthlibrary.com/anesthesiology
and enter the access code on the adjoining page to start your free 30-day trial!

Note: The same code will activate both the enhanced ebook and the 30 day trial of the LWW Health Library

Wolters Kluwer · **LWW** Health Library

ROGERS' TEXTBOOK OF PEDIATRIC INTENSIVE CARE

Hülya Bayir, MD
Professor
Department of Critical Care Medicine
Department of Environmental and
    Occupational Health
Director of Research
Pediatric Critical Care Medicine
Associate Director
Center for Free Radical and
    Antioxidant Health
Safar Center for Resuscitation
    Research
University of Pittsburgh
Pittsburgh, Pennsylvania

Michael J. Bell, MD
Professor
Critical Care Medicine
Neurological Surgery and Pediatrics
Director
Pediatric Neurotrauma Center
Director
Pediatric Neurocritical Care
Associate Director
Safar Center for Resuscitation
    Research
University of Pittsburgh School of
    Medicine
Pittsburgh, Pennsylvania

Kimberly S. Bennett, MD, MPH
Associate Professor
Pediatric Critical Care
University of Colorado School of
    Medicine
Aurora Colorado

**Robert A. Berg, MD, FAAP,
FCCM, FAHA**
Russell Raphaely Endowed Chair
Division Chief
Critical Care Medicine
Children's Hospital of Philadelphia
Professor of Anesthesia and Critical
    Care Medicine
Professor of Pediatrics
Perelman School of Medicine at the
    University of Pennsylvania
Philadelphia, Pennsylvania

Rachel P. Berger, MD, MPH
Associate Professor
Department of Pediatrics
Associate Director
Safar Center for Resuscitation
    Research
University of Pittsburgh School of
    Medicine
Division Chief
Child Advocacy Center
Children's Hospital of Pittsburgh
Pittsburgh, Pennsylvania

Ivor D. Berkowitz, MBBCh, MD
Associate Professor
Department of Anesthesiology and
    Critical Care Medicine
Clinical Director
Johns Hopkins University School of
    Medicine
Baltimore, Maryland

Monica Bhatia, MD
Associate Professor of Pediatrics
Columbia University Medical Center
Director
Pediatric Stem Cell Transplantation
    Program
Columbia University Medical Center
New York, New York

Katherine V. Biagas, MD
Associate Professor of Pediatrics
Department of Pediatrics
Columbia University Medical Center
New York, New York

**Michael T. Bigham, MD, FAAP,
FCCM**
Medical Director of Critical Care
    Transport
Assistant Director of Patient Safety
Division of Pediatric Critical Care
Akron Children's Hospital
Associate Professor of Pediatrics
Northeast Ohio Medical University
Akron, Ohio

Clifford W. Bogue, MD
Professor and Interim Chair
Department of Pediatrics
Yale School of Medicine
New Haven, Connecticut

**Christopher P. Bonafide, MD,
MSCE**
Assistant Professor of Pediatrics
Department of Pediatrics
Perelman School of Medicine at the
    University of Pennsylvania
Division of General Pediatrics
Children's Hospital of Philadelphia
Philadelphia, Pennsylvania

Geoffrey J. Bond, MBBS
Assistant Professor
Department of Surgery
University of Pittsburgh
Pediatric Transplant Surgery/Pediatric
    General Thoracic Surgery
Children's Hospital of Pittsburgh at
    UPMC
Pittsburgh, Pennsylvania

Desmond Bohn, MB, FRCPC
Department of Critical Care Medicine
The Hospital for Sick Children
Professor of Anesthesia and Pediatrics
The University of Toronto
Toronto, Canada

**Glendaliz Bosques, MD,
FAAPMR**
Department of Physical Medicine and
    Rehabilitation
Chair
Pediatric and Rehabilitation Medicine
University of Texas–Health Science
    Center at Houston
Houston, Texas

Rebecca Hulett Bowling, MD
Assistant Professor
Mallinkrodt Institute of Radiology
Washington University
Staff Radiologist
Department of Pediatric Radiology
St. Louis Children's Hospital
St. Louis, Missouri

Kenneth M. Brady, MD
Associate Professor
Departments of Anesthesiology and
    Pediatrics
Texas Children's Hospital
Houston, Texas

Patrick W. Brady, MD, MSc
Assistant Professor
Department of Pediatrics
University of Cincinnati College of
    Medicine
Attending Physician
Division of Hospital Medicine
Cincinnati Children's Hospital Medical
    Center
Cincinnati, Ohio

**Richard J. Brilli, MD, FAAP,
FCCM**
Professor
Pediatrics
Division of Pediatric Critical Care
    Medicine
The Ohio State University College of
    Medicine
Chief Medical Officer
Nationwide Children's Hospital
Columbus, Ohio

Ronald A. Bronicki, MD
Associate Professor
Department of Pediatrics
Baylor College of Medicine
Associate Medical Director
Cardiac Intensive Care Unit
Department of Pediatrics
Texas Children's Hospital
Houston, Texas

Kate L. Brown, MRCPCH, MPH
Consultant
Cardiac Intensive Care Unit
Great Ormond Street Hospital for
    Children
Institute for Cardiovascular Science
University College London
London, United Kingdom

CONTRIBUTORS

Nicholas S. Abend, MD
Assistant Professor of Neurology
  and Pediatrics
Department of Neurology and
  Pediatrics
Children's Hospital of Philadelphia
Perelman School of Medicine at the
  University of Pennsylvania
Philadelphia, Pennsylvania

Mateo Aboy, PhD
Professor
Department of Electronics Engineering
  and Technology
Oregon Institute of Technology
Portland, Oregon

**Alice D. Ackerman, MD, MBA,
FAAP, FCCM**
Professor and Chair
Department of Pediatrics
Virginia Tech Carilion School of
  Medicine
Chair and Chief Pediatric Officer
Carilion Clinic Children's Hospital
Roanoke, Virigina

Iki Adachi, MD
Associate Surgeon
Congenital Heart Surgery
Co-Director
Mechanical Support
Texas Children's Hospital
Assistant Professor
Michael E. DeBakey
Department of Surgery and Pediatrics
Baylor College of Medicine
Houston, Texas

**P. David Adelson, MD, FACS,
FAAP**
Director
Diane and Bruce Halle Endowed Chair
  in Pediatric Neurosciences
Chief
Pediatric Neurosurgery
Barrow Neurological Institute at
  Phoenix Children's Hospital
Professor and Chief Neurological
  Surgery
Department of Child Health
University of Arizona College of
  Medicine–Phoenix

Adjunct Professor
Ira A. Fulton School of Biological and
  Health Systems Engineering
Arizona State University
Phoenix, Arizona

Rachel S. Agbeko, FRCPCH, PhD
Consultant Paediatric Intensivist
Great North Children's Hospital
  at the Royal Victoria Infirmary
London, United Kingdom

Jeffrey B. Anderson, MD
Associate Professor
Department of Pediatrics
Chief Quality Officer
The Heart Center
Division of Pediatric Cardiology
Cincinnati Children's Hospital
  Medical Center
Cincinnati, Ohio

Linda Aponte-Patel, MD, FAAP
Assistant Professor of Pediatrics
Columbia University Medical
  Center
Division of Pediatric Critical Care
  Medicine Department of Pediatrics
Columbia University College of
  Physicians and Surgeons
New York, New York

**Andrew C. Argent, MBBCh,
MMed (Paediatrics), MD,
FCPaeds (SA)**
Professor
Medical Director Paediatric
  Intensive Care
University of Cape Town and Red
  Cross War Memorial Children's
  Hospital
Cape Town, South Africa

John H. Arnold, MD
Professor
Department of Anesthesia (Pediatrics)
Harvard Medical School
Senior Associate
Anesthesia and Critical Care
Medical Director
Respiratory Care/ECMO
Children's Hospital
Boston, Massachusetts

Stephen Ashwal, MD
Distinguished Professor
Department of Pediatrics
Loma Linda University School of
  Medicine
Attending Physician
Department of Pediatrics
Division of Child Neurology
Loma Linda Children's Hospital
Loma Linda, California

Swapnil S. Bagade, MD
Fellow
Mallinkrodt Institute of Radiology
Washington University
Fellow
Department of Pediatric Radiology
St. Louis Children's Hospital
St. Louis, Missouri

John Scott Baird, MS, MD
Associate Professor of Pediatrics
Columbia University Medical Center
Columbia University
New York, New York

Adnan M. Bakar, MD
Assistant Professor of Pediatrics
Section Head
Pediatric Cardiac Critical Care
Cohen Children's Medical Center of
  New York
New Hyde Park, New York

Kenneth J. Banasiak, MD, MS
Pediatrician
Division of Pediatric Critical Care
Connecticut Children's Medical Center
Hartford, Connecticut

**Arun Bansal, MD, MRCPCH,
MAMS**
Additional Professor
Department of Pediatrics
Advance Pediatric Centre
Postgraduate Institute of Medical
  Education & Research
Chandigarh, India

Aarti Bavare, MD, MPH
Assistant Professor of Pediatrics
Baylor College of Medicine
Houston, Texas

INTRODUCTION

The fifth edition of the *Rogers' Textbook of Pediatric Intensive Care* represents both the continuity of the text and the continued evolution of the editors, authors, and contents of the book.

With this edition, Hal Shaffner of Johns Hopkins joins David G. Nichols as coeditor of the textbook. These are welcome changes, as are the addition of many new authors and many new topics that reflect the rapid advancements in our field.

The essence of a textbook is that it is relevant over decades only if it evolves as the field that it covers evolves and changes. This relevance continues in the fifth edition of the *Rogers' Textbook of Pediatric Intensive Care* and will, I am confident, continue to do so in the decades ahead.

Mark C. Rogers, MD

DEDICATION

"In memory of Dorothy Gene "Dottie" Lappe, RN, MSN [May 10, 1954–December 22, 2009]
PICU nurse manager, author, editor, and friend."

Acquisitions Editor: Keith Donnellan
Product Development Editor: Nicole Dernoski
Editorial Assistant: Kathryn Leyendecker
Senior Production Project Manager: Alicia Jackson
Design Coordinator: Joan Wendt
Manufacturing Coordinator: Beth Welsh
Marketing Manager: Dan Dressler
Prepress Vendor: S4Carlisle Publishing Services

5th edition

Printed in China
Library of Congress Cataloging-in-Publication Data

Rogers' textbook of pediatric intensive care / editors, David G. Nichols and Donald H. Shaffner ; section editors, Andrew C. Argent [and 25 others]. — Fifth edition.
    p. ; cm.
  Textbook of pediatric intensive care
  Includes bibliographical references and index.
  ISBN 978-1-4511-7662-9 (alk. paper)
  I. Nichols, David G. (David Gregory), 1951- , editor. II. Shaffner, Donald H., editor. III. Title: Textbook of pediatric intensive care.
  [DNLM: 1. Infant. 2. Intensive Care. 3. Child. WS 366]
  RJ370
  618.92'0028—dc23   2015016445

ROGERS' TEXTBOOK OF PEDIATRIC INTENSIVE CARE FIFTH EDITION

Editors

David G. Nichols, MD, MBA

Professor of Anesthesiology and Critical Care
   Medicine and Pediatrics
Johns Hopkins University School of Medicine
   (on leave)
Baltimore, Maryland
President and CEO
The American Board of Pediatrics
Chapel Hill, North Carolina

Donald H. Shaffner, MD

Associate Professor
Departments of Anesthesiology and Critical Care Medicine
   and Pediatrics
Director
Division of Pediatric Anesthesiology and Critical Care
   Medicine
Johns Hopkins University School of Medicine
Baltimore, Maryland

Section Editors

Andrew C. Argent, MBBCh, MMed, MD, FCPaeds

John H. Arnold, MD

Katherine V. Biagas, MD

Desmond Bohn, MB, FRCPC

Jeffrey P. Burns, MD, MPH

Joseph A. Carcillo, MD, FCCM

Paul A. Checchia, MD, FCCM, FACC

Heidi J. Dalton, MD

Steve Davis, MD, MMM

Jennifer G. Duncan, MD

Mark W. Hall, MD

Niranjan "Tex" Kissoon, MD, FRCP(C), FAAP, FCCM, FACPE

Patrick M. Kochanek, MD, MCCM

Jacques Lacroix, MD, FRCPC

Graeme MacLaren, MBBS, FCICM, FCCM

Nilesh M. Mehta, MD

Vinay M. Nadkarni, MD, MS

Charles L. Schleien, MD, MBA

Sunit C. Singhi, MBBS, MD, FIAP, FAMS, FISCCM, FICCM, FCCM

Bo Sun, MD

Robert C. Tasker, MA, MD, MBBS, DCH, FRCPCH, FRCP, FHEA, AM, MD

Joseph D. Tobias, MD

Hans-Dieter Volk, MD

Randall C. Wetzel, MBBS, MBM, FRCS, LRCP, FAAP, FCCM

Hector R. Wong, MD

Myron Yaster, MD

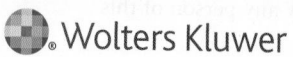 Wolters Kluwer

Philadelphia • Baltimore • New York • London
Buenos Aires • Hong Kong • Sydney • Tokyo

Richard J. Czosek, MD
Associate Professor
Department of Pediatrics
The Heart Center
Division of Pediatric Cardiology
Cincinnati Children's Hospital
  Medical Center
Cincinnati, Ohio

Mary K. Dahmer, PhD
Division of Pediatric Critical Care
  Medicine
Department of Pediatrics and
  Communicable Diseases
University of Michigan
Ann Arbor, Michigan

Heidi J. Dalton, MD
Professor of Child Health
University of Arizona College of
  Medicine/Phoenix
Phoenix, Arizona

Sally L. Davidson Ward, MD
Chief
Division of Pediatric Pulmonology and
  Sleep Medicine
Associate Professor of Pediatrics
Children's Hospital Los Angeles
Keck School of Medicine of the
  University of Southern California
Los Angeles, California

Steve Davis, MD, MMM
Pediatric Critical Care Medicine
Cleveland Clinic Children's
  Administration
Chief Operating Officer
Hillcrest Hospital
Cleveland, Ohio

J. Michael Dean, MD, MBA
HA and Edna Presidential Professor of
  Pediatrics
Vice Chairman for Research
Department of Pediatrics
Chief
Division of Pediatric Critical Care
University of Utah School of Medicine
Salt Lake City, Utah

Allan de Caen, MD, FRCP
Clinical Professor/Pediatric Intensivist
Pediatric Critical Care Medicine
Edmonton Clinic Health Academy—
  University of Alberta
Stollery Children's Hospital
Edmonton
Alberta, Canada

Artur F. Delgado, PhD
Chief of Pediatric Intensive Care Unit
Department of Pediatrics
University Federal de São Paulo
São Paulo, Brazil

Denis J. Devictor, MD, PhD
Assistance Publique-Hopitaux de Paris
Paris SUD University
Pediatric Intensive Care Unit
Hopital de Bicetre le Kremlin Bicetre
Paris, France

Troy E. Dominguez, MD
Consultant
Cardiac Intensive Care Unit
Great Ormond Street Hospital for
  Children
NHS Foundation Trust
London, United Kingdom

Aaron J. Donoghue, MD, MSCE
Associate Professor of Pediatrics and
  Critical Care Medicine
Perelman School of Medicine at the
  University of Pennsylvania
Emergency Medicine
Children's Hospital of Philadelphia
Philadelphia, Pennsylvania

Lesley Doughty, MD
Associate Professor
Critical Care Medicine
Cincinnati Children's Hospital Medical
  Center
Cincinnati, Ohio

Laurence Ducharme-Crevier, MD
Pediatric Intensivist
Department of Pediatrics
CHU Sainte-Justine
Montreal, Quebec, Canada

Jonathan P. Duff, MD, Med, FRCPC
Associate Professor
Department of Pediatrics
University of Alberta
Edmonton, Alberta, Canada

Trevor Duke, MD, FRACP, FJFICM
Director & Associate Professor
Department of Pediatrics
University of Melbourne
Royal Children's Hospital
Parkville
Parkville, Victoria, Australia

Jennifer G. Duncan, MD
Assistant Professor
Program Director
Critical Care Fellowship
Department of Pediatrics
Washington University School of
  Medicine
Seattle, Washington

Genevieve Du Pont-Thibodeau, MD
Pediatric Intensivist
Department of Pediatrics
CHU Sainte-Justine
Montreal, Quebec, Canada

R. Blaine Easley, MD
Fellowship Director
Pediatric Anesthesiology
Division Director
Anesthesiology Critical Care
Texas Children's Hospital
Houston, Texas

Janeth C. Ejike, MBBS, FAAP
Associate Professor
Department of Pediatrics
Loma Linda University
Loma Linda, California

Conrad L. Epting, MD, FAAP
Assistant Professor of Pediatrics
Department of Pediatrics
Northwestern University Feinberg
  School of Medicine
Attending Physician
Division of Pediatric Critical Care
Ann and Robert H. Lurie Children's
  Hospital of Chicago
Chicago, Illinois

Maria Cristina Esperanza, MD
Associate Chief
Division of Pediatric Critical Care
  Medicine
North Shore LIJ Health System
Cohen Children's Medical Center of
  New York
New Hyde Park, New York

Ori Eyal, MD
Assistant Professor
Sackler Faculty of Medicine
Tel Aviv University
Clinical Director
Department of Pediatric Endocrinology
Tel Aviv Medical Center
Tel Aviv, Israel

Tracy B. Fausnight, MD
Associate Professor
Department of Pediatrics
Penn State College of Medicine
Division Chief
Division of Allergy and Immunology
Department of Pediatrics
Penn State Hershey Children's Hospital
Hershey, Pennsylvania

Edward Vincent S. Faustino, MD, MHS
Associate Professor of Pediatrics
Yale School of Medicine
New Haven, Connecticut

Kathryn A. Felmet, MD
Department of Pediatrics
Division of Pediatric Critical Care
  Medicine
Oregon Health and Science University
Portland, Oregon

Werther Brunow de Carvalho, MD
Full Professor of Intensive Care/
   Neonatology
Department of Pediatrics
Federal University of São Paulo
São Paulo, Brazil

Jeffrey P. Burns, MD, MPH
Chief and Shapiro Chair of Critical
   Care Medicine
Department of Anesthesiology,
   Perioperative, and Pain Medicine
Boston Children's Hospital and
   Harvard Medical School
Boston, Massachusetts

Warwick W. Butt, MD
Director
Intensive Care
Royal Children's Hospital
Associate Professor
Department of Paediatrics
University of Melbourne
Group Leader
Clinical Sciences Theme
Murdoch Children's Research Institute
Melbourne, Australia

James D. Campbell, MD, MS
Department of Pediatrics
Center for Vaccine Development
University of Maryland School of
   Medicine
Baltimore, Maryland

Michael F. Canarie, MD
Clinical Instructor
Department of Pediatrics
Yale University School of Medicine
New Haven, Connecticut

G. Patricia Cantwell, MD, FCCM
Professor & Chief
Pediatric Critical Care Medicine
Department of Pediatrics
University of Miami Miller School of
   Medicine
Holtz Children's Hospital
Miami, Florida

Joseph A. Carcillo, MD, FCCM
Associate Professor
Critical Care Medicine & Pediatrics
Children's Hospital of Pittsburgh
University of Pittsburgh Medical
   Center
Pittsburgh, Pennsylvania

Todd Carpenter, MD
Associate Professor of Pediatrics
Section of Pediatric Critical Care
University of Colorado School of
   Medicine
Aurora, Colorado

Elena Cavazzoni, MB, ChB, PhD, FCICM
Staff Specialist
Paediatric Intensive Care Unit
Children's Hospital at Westmead
Sydney, Australia

Dominic Cave, MBBS, FRCPC
Medical Director
Pediatric Cardiac Intensive Care
Stollery Children's Hospital
Associate Clinical Professor
Department of Anesthesiology and Pain
   Management
Associate Clinical Professor
Department of Pediatrics
University of Alberta
Edmonton
Alberta, Canada

Paul A. Checchia, MD, FCCM, FACC
Director
Cardiovascular Intensive Care Unit
Professor of Pediatrics
Sections of Critical Care Medicine and
   Cardiology
Texas Children's Hospital
Baylor College of Medicine
Houston, Texas

Ira M. Cheifetz, MD, FCCM, FAARC
Professor of Pediatrics
Chief
Pediatric Critical Care Medicine
Director
Pediatric Critical Care Services
DUHS
Duke Children's Hospital
Durham, North Carolina

Nataliya Chorny, MD
Assistant Professor
Hofstra North Shore-LIJ School of
   Medicine
Attending Physician
Department of Pediatric Nephrology
Cohen Children's Medical Center
New Hyde Park, New York

Wendy K. Chung, MD, PhD
Associate Professor of Pediatrics and
   Medicine
Columbia University
New York, New York

Robert S. B. Clark, MD
Professor
Critical Care Medicine and Pediatrics
University of Pittsburgh School of
   Medicine
Chief
Pediatric Critical Care Medicine
Critical Care Medicine
Children's Hospital of Pittsburgh of
   UPMC
Pittsburgh, Pennsylvania

Erin Coletti
Undergraduate Student in Biology
Harriet L. Wilkes Honors College of
   Florida Atlantic University
Jupiter, Florida

Steven A. Conrad, MD, PhD, MCCM
Professor of Emergency Medicine
Internal Medicine and Pediatrics
Louisiana State University Health
   Sciences Center
Director
Extracorporeal Life Support
   Program
University Health System
Shreveport, Louisiana

Arthur Cooper, MD, MS
Professor of Surgery
Columbia University College of
   Physicians and Surgeons
Director of Trauma & Pediatric
   Surgical Services
Harlem Hospital Center
New York, New York

Fernando F. Corrales-Medina, MD
Pediatrics Hematology/Oncology
   Fellow
Department of Pediatrics
UT/MD Anderson Cancer Center
Houston, Texas

Jose A. Cortes, MD
Assistant Professor
Department of Pediatrics
The University of Texas
MD Anderson Cancer Center
MD Anderson Children's Cancer
   Hospital
Houston, Texas

John M. Costello, MD, MPH
Associate Professor of Pediatrics
Department of Pediatrics
Northwestern University Feinberg
   School of Medicine
Director
Inpatient Cardiology
Medical Director
Regenstein Cardiac Care Unit
Ann and Robert H. Lurie Children's
   Hospital of Chicago
Chicago, Illinois

Jason W. Custer, MD
Assistant Professor of Pediatrics
Division of Pediatric Critical Care
University of Maryland School of
   Medicine
Baltimore, Maryland

Jeffrey R. Fineman, MD
Professor of Pediatrics
Investigator
Cardiovascular Research Institute
UCSF Benioff Children's Hospital
San Francisco, California

Ericka L. Fink, MD, MS
Associate Professor
Division of Pediatric Critical Care
    Medicine
Children's Hospital of Pittsburgh of
    UPMC
Pittsburgh, Pennsylvania

Douglas S. Fishman, MD
Director
Gastrointestinal Endoscopy
Texas Children's Hospital
Associate Professor of Pediatrics
Baylor College of Medicine
Houston, Texas

Julie C. Fitzgerald, MD, PhD
Assistant Professor
Department of Anesthesia and Critical
    Care Medicine
Perelman School of Medicine at the
    University of Pennsylvania
Children's Hospital of Philadelphia
Philadelphia, Pennsylvania

George L. Foltin, MD
Department of Pediatrics
SUNY Downstate Medical Center
Brooklyn, New York

**Marcelo Cunio Machado
Fonseca, MD, MSc**
Department of Pediatrics
University Federal deSão Paulo
São Paulo, Brazil

**Jim Fortenberry, MD, FCCM,
FAAP**
Pediatrician in Chief
Children's Healthcare of Atlanta
Professor of Pediatric Critical Care
Emory University School of Medicine
Atlanta, Georgia

Alain Fraisse, MD, PhD
Consultant and Director
Paediatric Cardiology Service
Royal Brompton Hospital
London, United Kingdom

Charles D. Fraser, Jr, MD, FACS
Surgeon-in-Chief
Texas Children's Hospital
Professor of Pediatrics and Surgery
Baylor College of Medicine
Houston, Texas

**Philippe S. Friedlich, MD, MS
Epi, MBA**
Professor of Clinical Pediatrics &
    Surgery
Keck School of Medicine of the
University of Southern California
Interim Center Director & Division
    Chief
Center f or Fetal and Neonatal
    Medicine
USC Division of Neonatal Medicine
Department of Pediatrics
Children's Hospital Los Angeles
Los Angeles, California

James J. Gallagher, MD, FACS
Assistant Professor
Department of Surgery
Weill Cornell Medical College
New York, New York

Cynthia Gauger, MD
Division of Pediatric Hematology and
    Oncology
Nemours Children's Specialty Care
Jacksonville, Florida

**Jonathan Gillis, MB, BS, PhD,
FRACP, FCICM**
Clinical Associate Professor
Department of Paediatrics and Child
    Health
University of Sydney
New South Wales, Australia

**Brahm Goldstein, MD, MCR,
FAAP, FCCM**
Professor of Pediatrics
University of Medicine and Dentistry
    of New Jersey
Robert Wood Johnson Medical School
New Brunswick, New Jersey

Salvatore R. Goodwin, MD
Department of Anesthesiology
Office of the Vice President Quality
    and Safety
Nemours Children's Specialty Care
Associate Professor of Anesthesiology
Mayo Clinic
Jacksonville, Florida

Alan S. Graham, MD
Pediatric Critical Care
Cardon Children's Medical Center
Mesa, Arizona

Robert J. Graham, MD
Associate in Division of Critical Care
Director
Critical Care Anesthesia
Perioperative Extension (CAPE) and
    Home Ventilation Program
Department of Anesthesiology,
    Perioperative, and Pain Medicine
Boston Children's Hospital
Boston, Massachusetts

David Grant, MBChB, MRCPCH
Consultant in Paediatric Intensive Care
Director
Bristol Paediatric Simulation
    Programme
University Hospitals Bristol
Bristol, United Kingdom

Bruce M. Greenwald, MD
Professor of Clinical Pediatrics
Department of Pediatrics
Weill Cornell Medical College
New York, New York

**Anne-Marie Guerguerian, MD,
PhD, FRCPC, FAAP**
Departments of Critical Care &
    Paediatrics
The Hospital for Sick Children and
    Research Institute
University of Toronto
Toronto, Ontario, Canada

Gabriel G. Haddad, MD
Distinguished Professor of Pediatrics
    and Neuroscience
Chairman
Department of Pediatrics
University of California
Physician-in-Chief and Chief Scientific
    Officer
Rady Children's Hospital
San Diego, California

Mark W. Hall, MD, FCCM
Critical Care Medicine
Nationwide Children's Hospital
Columbus, Ohio

E. Scott Halstead, MD, PhD
Assistant Professor of Pediatrics
Pennsylvania State University College
    of Medicine
Hershey, Pennsylvania

Donna S. Hamel, RCP
Assistant Director
Clinical Trial Operations
Duke Clinical Research Unit
Duke University Medical Center
Durham, North Carolina

Yong Y. Han, MD
Assistant Professor
Department of Pediatrics
University of Missouri-Kansas City
    School of Medicine
Department of Critical Care Medicine
Children's Mercy Hospital
Kansas City, Missouri

George E. Hardart, MD, MPH
Associate Professor
Department of Pediatrics
Columbia University
Associate Attending Physician
Department of Pediatrics
Children's Hospital of New York
New York, New York

William G. Harmon, MD
Associate Professor of Pediatrics
Director
Pediatric Critical Care Services
University of Virginia Children's
    Hospital
Charlottesville, Virginia

Z. Leah Harris, MD
Division Director
Pediatric Critical Care Medicine
Posy and John Krehbiel Professor of
    Critical Care Medicine
Professor
Department of Pediatrics
Northwestern University Feinberg
    School of Medicine
Ann & Robert H. Lurie Children's
    Hospital of Chicago
Chicago, Illinois

Silvia M. Hartmann, MD
Assistant Professor
Pediatric Critical Care Medicine
Seattle Children's Hospital/University
    of Washington
Seattle, Washington

Abeer Hassoun, MD
Assistant Professor of Clinical Pediatrics
Department of Pediatrics
Columbia University
Attending Physician
Department of Pediatrics
Children's Hospital of New York
New York, New York

Masanori Hayashi, MD
Johns Hopkins University
Baltimore, Maryland

**Mary Fran Hazinski, RN, MSN,
FAAN, FAHA, FERC**
Professor
Vanderbilt University School of
    Nursing Clinical Nurse Specialist
Monroe Carrell Jr. Children's Hospital
    at Vanderbilt
Nashville, Tennessee

Gregory P. Heldt, MD
Professor of Pediatrics
University of California
San Diego, California

Mark J. Heulitt
Professor of Pediatrics
Physiology and Biophysics College of
    Medicine
University of Arkansas for Medical
    Sciences
Little Rock, Arkansas

Siew Yen Ho, MD
Imperial College
National Heart & Lung Institute
London, United Kingdom

Julien I. Hoffman, MD
Professor Emeritus of Pediatrics
Medical Center at UCSF
San Francisco, California

Aparna Hoskote, MRCP, MD
Consultant in Cardiac Intensive Care
    & ECMO
Honorary Senior Lecturer in University
    College London
Institute of Child Health
Great Ormond Street Hospital for
    Children
NHS Foundation Trust
London, United Kingdom

**Joy D. Howell, MD, FAAP,
FCCM**
Associate Professor of Clinical
    Pediatrics
Pediatric Critical Care Medicine
Fellowship Director
Weill Cornell Medical College
Department of Pediatrics
New York, New York

Winston W. Huh, MD
Associate Professor
Division of Pediatrics
The University of Texas MD Anderson
    Cancer Center
Houston, Texas

**Elizabeth A. Hunt, MD,
MPH, PhD**
Drs. David S. and Marilyn M.
    Zamierowski Director
Johns Hopkins Medicine Simulation
    Center
Associate Professor
Departments of Anesthesiology &
    Critical Care Medicine
Pediatrics and Division of Health
    Informatics
John Hopkins University School of
    Medicine
Baltimore, Maryland

Tomas Iölster, MD
Associate Professor
Department of Pediatrics
Hospital Universitario Austral Pilar
Buenos Aires, Argentina

Narayan Prabhu Iyer, MBBS, MD
Attending Neonatalogist
Children's Hospital Los Angeles
Los Angeles, California

Ronald Jaffe, MB, BCh
Professor of Pathology
Department of Pathology
University of Pittsburgh School
    of Medicine
Pathologist
Department of Pediatric Pathology
Children's Hospital of Pittsburgh
Pittsburgh, Pennsylvania

**M. Jayashree, MD, DNB
Pediatrics**
Additional Professor
Department of Pediatrics
Advanced Pediatrics Centre
Postgraduate Institute of Medical
    Education and Research
Chandigarh, India

Larry W. Jenkins, PhD
Professor
Safari Center
University of Pittsburgh
Pittsburgh, Pennsylvania

Lulu Jin, PharmD, BCPS
Pediatric Clinical Pharmacist
UCSF Benioff Children's Hospital
Assistant Clinical Professor
UCSF School of Pharmacy
San Francisco, California

Sachin S. Jogal, MD
Assistant Professor of Pediatrics
Division of Pediatric Hematology/
    Oncology/BMT
Medical College of Wisconsin
Milwaukee, Wisconsin

Khaliah Johnson, MD
Assistant Professor
Pediatrics
Emory University
Atlanta, Georgia

Cintia Johnston, MD
Department de Medicina e Pediatria
University Federal de São Paulo
São Paulo, Brazil

Philippe Jouvet, MD, PhD
Full Professor
Director of the Pediatric Intensive Care
    Unit
Department of Pediatrics
CHU Sainte-Justine
Montreal, Quebec, Canada

Sushil K. Kabra, MD, DNB
Professor
Department of Pediatrics
All India Institute of Medical Sciences
New Delhi, India

Siripen Kalayanarooj, MD
Professor
Queen Sirikit National Institute of
    Child Health
College of Medicine
Rangsit University
Bangkok, Thailand

Rebecca Johnson Kameny, MD
Adjunct Assistant Professor
Pediatric Critical Care
University of California
San Francisco, California

Oliver Karam, MD, MSc
Associate Professor
Attending Physician
Pediatric Critical Care Unit
Geneva University Hospital
Department of Pediatrics
Geneva University
Geneva, Switzerland

Ann Karimova, MD
Consultant in Cardiac Intensive Care
    and ECMO
Honorary Senior Lecturer in University
    College London
Institue of Child Health
Great Ormond Street Hospital for
    Children
NHS Foundation Trust
London, United Kingdom

Todd J. Karsies, MD
Clinical Assistant Professor of
    Pediatrics
Pediatric Critical Care
The Ohio State University College of
    Medicine/Nationwide Children's
    Hospital
Columbus, Ohio

Thomas G. Keens, MD
Professor of Pediatrics
Physiology and Biophysics
Keck School of Medicine of the
    University of Southern California
Division of Pediatric Pulmonology and
    Sleep Medicine
Children's Hospital Los Angeles
Los Angeles, California

Andrea Kelly, MD
Pediatric Endocrinology
Children's Hospital of Philadelphia
Assistant Professor of Pediatrics
Perelman School of Medicine at the
    University of Pennsylvania
Philadelphia, Pennsylvania

Praveen Khilnani, MD, FCCM
Department of Pediatrics
Indraprastha Apollo Hospital
New Delhi, India

**Apichai Khongphatthanayothin,
MD, MPPM**
Chief of Pediatric Cardiology
Bangkok Heart Hospital
Professor of Pediatrics
Faculty of Medicine
Chulalongkorn University
Bangkok, Thailand
Professor of Clinical Pediatrics
LAC-USC Medical Center
Keck School of Medicine of the
    University of Southern California
Los Angeles, California

Fenella Kirkham, FRCPCH
Paediatric Neurology
University Hospital Southampton
Southampton, Hampshire
United Kingdom

**Niranjan "Tex" Kissoon, MD,
RCP(C), FAAP, FCCM, FACPE**
Vice President
Medical Affairs
BC Children's Hospital and Sunny Hill
    Health Centre for Children
Professor—Global Child Health
University of British Columbia and BC
    Children's Hospital
Vancouver, British Columbia, Canada

Nigel J. Klein, MB, BS, BSc, PhD
Professor of Infection and Immunity
UCL Institute of Child Health
London, United Kingdom

Monica E. Kleinman, MD
Associate Professor of Anesthesia
    (Pediatrics)
Division of Critical Care Medicine
Department of Anesthesia
Boston Children's Hospital
Harvard Medical School
Boston, Massachusetts

Timothy K. Knilans, MD
Professor
Department of Pediatrics
The Heart Center
Division of Pediatric Cardiology
Cincinnati Children's Hospital Medical
    Center
Cincinnati, Ohio

**Patrick M. Kochanek, MD,
MCCM**
Ake N. Grenvik Professor of Critical
    Care Medicine
Professor and Vice Chairman
Department of Critical Care Medicine
Professor of Anesthesiology
Pediatrics
Bioengineering, and Clinical and
    Translational Science
Director
Safar Center for Resuscitation Research
University of Pittsburgh School of
    Medicine
Pittsburgh, Pennsylvania

Nikoleta S. Kolovos, MD
Associate Professor of Pediatrics
Division of Pediatric Critical Care
    Medicine
Washington University in St. Louis
    School of Medicine
Quality and Outcomes Physician
BJC Healthcare
St. Louis, Missouri

Karen L. Kotloff, MD
Professor
Department of Pediatrics
University of Maryland School of
    Medicine
Baltimore, Maryland

Megan E. Kramer, PhD
Neuropsychologist
Department of Neuropsychology
Kennedy Krieger Institute
Baltimore, Maryland

Sapna R. Kudchadkar, MD
Assistant Professor
Anesthesiology and Critical Care
    Medicine and Pediatrics
Johns Hopkins University School of
    Medicine
Baltimore, Maryland

Sheila S. Kun, RN, MS
Keck School of Medicine of the
    University of Southern California
Division of Pediatric Pulmonology
Children's Hospital Los Angeles
Los Angeles, California

Jacques Lacroix, MD, FRCPC
Professor
Department of Pediatrics
Universite de Montreal
CHU Sainte-Justine
Montreal, Quebec, Canada

Patricia Lago, MD, PhD
Associate Professor of Pediatrics at
    Federal University of Ciencias da
    Saude de Porto Alegre
Pediatric Intensivist
Hospital de Clinicas de Porto Alegre
Porto Alegre, Brazil

Professor Dr. Jos M. Latour
Professor in Clinical Nursing
Plymouth University
Faculty of Health, Education
    and Society
School of Nursing and Midwifery
Plymouth, United Kingdom

Miriam K. Laufer, MD
Associate Professor
Department of Pediatrics
Center for Vaccine Development
University of Maryland School
    of Medicine
Baltimore, Maryland

Matthew B. Laurens, MD, MPH
Associate Professor
Department of Pediatrics
University of Maryland School of
    Medicine
Baltimore, Maryland

Jan Hau Lee, MBBS, MRCPCH
Consultant
Children's Intensive Care Unit
Department of Paediatric
  Subspecialties
KK Women's and Children's
  Hospital
Adjunct Assistant Professor
Duke-NUS Graduate School of
  Medicine
Singapore, Singapore

Heitor Pons Leite, MD
Affiliate Professor
Department of Pediatrics
Federal University of São Paulo
São Paulo, Brazil

Daniel J. Licht, MD
Associate Professor of Neurology
  and Pediatrics
Division of Neurology
Children's Hospital of Philadelphia
Perelman School of Medicine at the
  University of Pennsylvania
Philadelphia, Pennsylvania

Fangming Lin, MD, PhD
Division of Pediatric Nephrology
Department of Pediatrics
Columbia University College of
  Physicians and Surgeons
New York, New York

Rakesh Lodha, MD
Additional Professor
Department of Pediatrics
All India Institute of Medical
  Sciences
New Delhi, India

David M. Loeb, MD, PhD
Assistant Professor
Oncology & Pediatrics
Johns Hopkins University
Bunting Blaustein Cancer Research
  Building
Baltimore, Maryland

Laura L. Loftis, MD, MS, FAAP
Associate Professor
Department of Pediatrics & Medical
  Ethics
Baylor College of Medicine
Pediatric Critical Care Medicine
Texas Children's Hospital
Houston, Texas

Anne Lortie, MD, FRCPc
Professor Agrege de clinique
Neurologie
Department of Pediatrics
Faculty of Medicine
CHU Sainte-Justine
Montreal, Quebec, Canada

Naomi L.C. Luban, MD
Director of the E.J. Miller Blood Donor
  Center
Division of Laboratory Medicine
Children's National Medical Center
Vice Chair of Academic Affairs
Department of Pediatrics
George Washington University School
  of Medicine and Health Sciences
Washington, District of Columbia

Graeme MacLaren, MBBS, FCICM, FCCM
Paediatric ICU
Royal Children's Hospital
Melbourne, Australia
Director
Cardiothoracic Intensive Care
National University Hospital
Singapore, Singapore

Mioara D. Manole, MD
Assistant Professor of Pediatrics
Division of Emergency Medicine
Department of Pediatrics
University of Pittsburgh School of
  Medicine
Children's Hospital of Pittsburgh
Pittsburgh, Pennsylvania

Bruno Maranda, MD, MSc
Investigator, Mother & Child Axis
Centre de recherche de CHUS
Medical Geneticist
Centre Hospitalier Universitaire
  de Sherbrooke
Director of Department of Genetics
Assistant Professor
Department of Pediatrics
Division of Genetics
Faculty of Medicine and Health
  Sciences
Universite de Sherbrooke
Sherbrooke, Quebec, Canada

James P. Marcin, MD, MPH
Professor
Pediatric Critical Care
Department of Pediatrics
UC Davis Children's Hospital
Sacramento, California

Bradley S. Marino, MD, MPP, MSCE
Staff Cardiac Intensivist
Cardiac Intensive Care Unit
Cincinnati Children's Hospital Medical
  Center
Cincinnati, Ohio

M. Michele Mariscalco, MD
Professor
Department of Pediatrics
Regional Dean
University of Illinois College of
  Medicine at Urbana–Champaign
Urbana, Illinois

Barry P. Markovitz, MD, MPH
Professor
Department of Anesthesiology and
  Pediatrics
Keck School of Medicine of the
  University of Southern California
Director
Critical Care Medicine
Department of Anesthesiology &
  Critical Care Medicine
Children's Hospital Los Angeles
Los Angeles, California

Dolly Martin, AS
Data Coordinator and Analyst
Department of Transplantation
  Surgery
Children's Hospital of Pittsburgh/
  Thomas E. Starzl Transplantation
  Institute
UPMC Liver Cancer Center
Pittsburgh, Pennsylvania

Mudit Mathur, MD, FAAP, FCCP
Associate Professor of Pediatrics
Division of Pediatric Critical Care
Loma Linda University Children's
  Hospital
Loma Linda, California

Riza C. Mauricio, MD
Pediatric ICU Nurse Practitioner
Department of Pediatrics
Children's Hospital of MD Anderson
  Cancer Center
Houston, Texas

Patrick O'Neal Maynord, MD
Assistant Professor of Pediatrics
Division of Critical Care Medicine
Department of Pediatrics
Vanderbilt University School of
  Medicine
Monroe Carell Jr Children's Hospital
  at Vanderbilt
Nashville, Tennessee

George V. Mazariegos, MD
Professor
Department of Surgery and Critical
  Care Medicine
University of Pittsburgh School of
  Medicine
Chief
Department of Pediatric
  Transplantation
Department of Surgery
Children's Hospital of Pittsburgh of
  UPMC
Pittsburgh, Pennsylvania

Jennifer A. McArthur, DO
Associate Professor of Pediatrics
Division of Critical Care Medicine
Medical College of Wisconsin
Milwaukee, Wisconsin

Mary E. McBride, MD
Assistant Professor of Pediatrics
Department of Pediatrics
Northwestern University Feinberg
  School of Medicine
Attending Physician
Division of Cardiology
Ann and Robert H. Lurie Children's
  Hospital of Chicago
Chicago, Illinois

Craig D. McClain, MD, MPH
Senior Associate in Perioperative
  Anesthesia
Boston Children's Hospital
Assistant Professor of Anaesthesia
Harvard Medical School
Boston, Massachusetts

Michael C. McCrory, MD, MS
Assistant Professor
Departments of Anesthesiology and
  Pediatrics
Wake Forest University School of
  Medicine
Winston-Salem, North Carolina

John K. McGuire, MD
Associate Professor
Department of Pediatrics
Associate Division Chief
Pediatric Critical Care Medicine
University of Washington School
  of Medicine
Seattle Children's Hospital
Seattle, Washington

**Michael L. McManus, MD,
MPH**
Senior Associate
Department of Anesthesiology,
  Perioperative, and Pain Medicine
Division of Critical Care
Boston Children's Hospital and
  Harvard Medical School
Boston, Massachusetts

Kathleen L. Meert, MD
Chief
Pediatric Critical Care Medicine
Children's Hospital of Michigan
Professor of Pediatrics
Wayne State University
Detroit, Michigan

Nilesh M. Mehta, MD
Associate Professor of Anaesthesia
Harvard Medical School
Director
Critical Care Nutrition
Associate Medical Director
Critical Care Medicine
Department of Anesthesiology,
  Perioperative, and Pain
  Medicine
Boston Children's Hospital
Boston, Massachusetts

Rodrigo Mejia, MD, FCCM
Professor
Deputy Division Head
Director
Pediatric Critical Care
Division of Pediatrics
The University of Texas MD Anderson
  Cancer Center
Division of Pediatrics
Houston, Texas

Jessica Mesman, RN, PhD
Associate Professor
Department of Technology and Society
  Studies
Maastricht University
Maastricht, The Netherlands

David J. Michelson, MD
Assistant Professor of Pediatrics and
  Neurology
Loma Linda University School of
  Medicine
Loma Linda, California

Sabina Mir, MD
Assistant Professor of Pediatrics
Division of Gastroenterology
University of North Carolina School
  of Medicine
Chapel Hill, North Carolina

**Katsuyuki Miyasaka, MD,
PhD, FAAP**
Professor of Perianesthesia Nursing
  and Perioperative Center
St. Luke's International University
  and Hospital
Tokyo, Japan

Vinai Modem, MBBS, MS
Assistant Professor
Department of Pediatrics
Divisions of Critical Care and Nephrology
University of Texas Southwestern
  Medical Center
Dallas, Texas

Vicki L. Montgomery, MD, FCCM
Chief
Division of Pediatric Critical Care
  Medicine
University of Louisville
Chief
Division of Women and Children's
  CARE Innovation
Norton Healthcare
Louisville, Kentucky

Wynne E. Morrison, MD, MBE
Attending Physician
Critical Care and Palliative Care
Children's Hospital of Philadelphia
Associate Professor
Department of Anesthesiology and
  Critical Care
Perelman School of Medicine at the
  University of Pennsylvania
Philadelphia, Pennsylvania

M. Michele Moss, MD
Professor and Vice Chairman of
  Clinical Services
Department of Pediatrics
University of Arkansas for Medical
  Sciences
Little Rock, Arkansas

Jennifer A. Muszynski, MD
Assistant Professor of Pediatrics
Division of Critical Care Medicine
The Ohio State University College of
  Medicine
Nationwide Children's Hospital
Columbus, Ohio

Simon Nadel, FRCP
Adjunct Professor of Paediatric
  Intensive Care
St. Mary's Hospital and Imperial
  College Healthcare NHS Trust
London, United Kingdom

Vinay M. Nadkarni, MD, MS
Endowed Chair
Pediatric Critical Care Medicine
Departments of Anesthesia, Critical
  Care & Pediatrics
Perelman School of Medicine at the
  University of Pennsylvania
Department of Anesthesia and
  Critical Care
Children's Hospital of Philadelphia
Philadelphia, Pennsylvania

**Thomas A. Nakagawa, MD,
FAAP, FCCM**
Professor
Anesthesiology of Pediatrics
Department of Anesthesiology
Wake Forest University School of
  Medicine
Section Head
Pediatric Critical Care
Director
Pediatric Critical Care and Respiratory
  Care
Wake Forest Baptist Health
Brenner Children's Hospital
Winston-Salem, North Carolina

Michael A. Nares, MD
Assistant Professor of Clinical
  Pediatrics
Department of Pediatrics
Miller School of Medicine
University of Miami
Pediatric Critical Care
Holtz Children's Hospital
Miami, Florida

David P. Nelson, MD
Professor of Pediatrics
Director
Cardiac Intensive Care
The Heart Institute at Cincinnati
  Children's Hospital
Cincinnati, Ohio

Kristen L. Nelson McMillan, MD
Assistant Professor
Pediatric Critical Care Medicine
Department of Anesthesiology/Critical
    Care Medicine
Johns Hopkins University School of
    Medicine
Baltimore, Maryland

David G. Nichols, MD, MBA
Professor of Anesthesiology and
    Critical Care Medicine and
    Pediatrics
Johns Hopkins University School of
    Medicine (on leave)
Baltimore, Maryland
President and CEO
The American Board of Pediatrics
Chapel Hill, North Carolina

Matt Norvell, MDiv
Pediatric Chaplain
Johns Hopkins Children's Center
Baltimore, Maryland

Samuel Nurko, MD
Director
Center for Motility and Functional
    Gastrointestinal Disorders
Boston Children's Hospital
Boston, Massachusetts

Sharon E. Oberfield, MD
Professor of Pediatrics
Department of Pediatrics
Columbia University
Director
Division of Pediatric Endocrinology,
    Diabetes & Metabolism
Columbia University Medical
    Center
New York, New York

**George Ofori-Amanfo, MD,
ChB, FACC**
Associate Professor of Pediatrics
Duke University
Durham, North Carolina

Peter Oishi, MD
Associate Professor of Pediatrics
Pediatric Critical Care Medicine
University of California
UCSF Benioff Children's Hospital
San Francisco, California

Regina Okhuysen, MD
Associate Professor
Department of Pediatrics
University of Texas MD Anderson
    Cancer Center
Attending Physician
PICU, Pediatric Critical Care
    Medicine
MD Anderson's Children's Cancer
    Hospital
Houston, Texas

Richard A. Orr, MD, FCCM
Professor
Critical Care Medicine and Pediatrics
University of Pittsburgh School of
    Medicine
Children's Hospital of Pittsburgh
Pittsburgh, Pennsylvania

John Pappachan, MD
Senior Lecturer in Paediatric Intensive
    Care
University Hospital Southampton
NHS Foundation Trust
NIHR Southampton Respiratory
    Biomedical Research Unit
Southampton, United Kingdom

Robert I. Parker, MD
Professor
Pediatric Hematology/Oncology
Department of Pediatrics
Stony Brook University School of
    Medicine
Stony Brook, New York

Christopher S. Parshuram, MD
Physician Critical Care Program
Senior Scientist Child Health
    Evaluative Sciences
The Research Institute
Department of Critical Care
    Medicine
Hospital for Sick Children
Associate Professor Paediatrics
Critical Care, Health Policy,
    Management & Evaluation
Faculty
Center for Patient Safety
University of Toronto
Toronto, Canada

Mark J. Peters, MD
Professor of Paediatric Intensive
    Care
UCL Institute of Child Health
    and Honorary Consultant
    Intensivist
Great Ormond Street Hospital NHS
    Trust Foundation
London, United Kingdom

Frank S. Pidcock, MD
Associate Professor
Department of Physical Medicine
    and Rehabilitation
Johns Hopkins University School
    of Medicine
Kennedy Krieger Institute
Baltimore, Maryland

Matthew Pitt, MD, FRCP
Consultant Clinical Neurophysiologist
Department of Clinical
    Neurophysiology
Great Ormond Street Hospital NHS
    Foundation Trust
London, United Kingdom

**Jefferson Pedro Piva, MD,
MSc, PhD**
Full Professor of Pediatrics
School of Medicine
Universidade Federal deo Rio Grande
    do Sul (UFRGS)-Brazil
Director of Pediatric Emergency and
    Critical Care Department
UTI pediatrica—Hospital de Clinicas
    de Porto Alegre
Porto Alegre, Brazil

Murray M. Pollack, MD
Chair
Department of Child Health
University of Arizona College of
    Medicine–Phoenix
Chief Academic Officer
Phoenix Children's Hospital
Phoenix, Arizona

Steven Pon, MD
Associate Professor of Clinical
    Pediatrics
Pediatric Critical Care Medicine
Department of Pediatrics
Weill Cornell Medical College
Medical Director
Pediatric Intensive Care Unit
New York Presbyterian Hospital
New York, New York

Renee M. Potera, MD
Instructor
Department of Pediatrics
University of Texas Southwestern
    Medical Center
Dallas, Texas

Frank L. Powell, PhD
Chief
Division of Physiology
Professor
Department of Medicine
University of California
La Jolla
San Diego, California

Suzanne V. Prestwich, MD
Medical Director of Inpatient
    Pediatric Rehabilitation Unit
Kennedy Krieger Institute
Department of Pediatrics
Johns Hopkins University School
    of Medicine
Baltimore, Maryland

Jack F. Price, MD
Pediatric Cardiology
Department of Pediatrics
Baylor College of Medicine
Texas Children's Hospital
Houston, Texas

Michael Quasney, MD, PhD
Division of Pediatric Critical Care
    Medicine
Department of Pediatrics and
    Communicable Diseases
University of Michigan
Ann Arbor, Michigan

Elizabeth L. Raab, MD, MPH
Attending Neonatologist
Pediatrix Medical Group, Inc
Huntington Memorial Hospital
Pasadena, California

Surender Rajasekaran, MD, MPH
Pediatric Intensivist
Helen DeVos Children's Hospital
Grand Rapids, Michigan

Rangasamy Ramanathan, MBBS, MD
Professor of Pediatrics
Division Chief
Division of Neonatal Medicine
LAC + USC Medical Center
Director
NPM Fellowship Program and NICU
Associate Center Director
Center for Neonatal Medicine–CHLA
Keck School of Medicine of the
    University of Southern California
Los Angeles, California

Courtney D. Ranallo, MD
Pediatric Critical Care-PICU
Oklahoma University Medicine
Oklahoma City, Oklahoma

Suchitra Ranjit, MD
Senior Consultant
Pediatric Intensive Care
Apollo Hospitals
Chennai, India

Chitra Ravishankar, MD
Attending Cardiologist
Staff Cardiologist
Cardiac Intensive Care Unit
Associate Director
Cardiology Fellowship Training
    Program
Children's Hospital of Philadelphia
Assistant Professor of Pediatrics
Perelman School of Medicine at the
    University of Pennsylvania
Philadelphia, Pennsylvania

Nidra I. Rodriguez, MD
Associate Professor
Department of Pediatrics
The University of Texas HSC
MD Anderson Cancer Center and
    Children's Memorial Hermal Hospital
Gulf States Hemophilia Treatment
    Center
Houston, Texas

Antonio Rodríguez-Núñez, MD, PhD
Pediatric Emergency and Critical
    Care Division
Pediatric Area
Hospital Clinico Universitario de
    Santiago de Compostela
Unidad de Cuidados Intensivos
    Pediatricos
Santiago de Compostela, Spain

Lewis H. Romer, MD
Professor
Department of Anesthesiology/Critical
    Care Medicine
Johns Hopkins University School of
    Medicine
Baltimore, Maryland

Susan R. Rose, MD, Med
Professor of Pediatrics and
    Endocrinology
Cincinnati Children's Hospital Medical
    Center and University of Cincinnati
    School of Medicine
Cincinnati, Ohio

Michael A. Rosen, MA, PhD
Associate Professor of Anesthesiology
    and Critical Care Medicine
Johns Hopkins University School of
    Medicine
Baltimore, Maryland

Joseph W. Rossano, MD
Pediatric Cardiology
Department of Pediatrics
Children's Hospital of Philadelphia
Perelman School of Medicine at the
    University of Pennsylvania
Philadelphia, Pennsylvania

Eitan Rubinstein, MD
Center for Motility and Functional
    Gastrointestinal Disorders
Children's Hospital Boston
Boston, Massachusetts

Jeffrey A. Rudolph, MD
Assistant Professor
Department of Pediatrics
University of Pittsburgh
Director
Intestinal Care and Rehabilitation
Department of Pediatrics
Children's Hospital of Pittsburgh of
    UPMC
Pittsburgh, Pennsylvania

Ricardo D. Russo, MD
Chief of Pediatric Surgery
Co-Director of Fetal Surgery Program
Department of Pediatrics
Hospital Universitario Austral Pilar
Buenos Aires, Argentina

Monique M. Ryan, MD
Paediatric Neurologist
Children's Neuroscience Centre
Research Fellow
Murdoch Children's Research Institute
Royal Children's Hospital
Parkville, Victoria, Australia

Melissa J. Sacco, MD
Assistant Professor
Department of Pediatrics
Division of Pediatric Critical Care
University of Virginia Health System
Charlottesville, Virginia

Cristina L. Sadowsky, MD
Clinical Director
International center for Spinal Cord
    Injury
Kennedy Krieger Institute
Assistant Professor
Physical Medicine and Rehabilitation
Johns Hopkins University School of
    Medicine
Baltimore, Maryland

Sanju S. Samuel, MD
Assistant Professor
Department of Pediatrics
University of Texas MD Anderson
    Cancer Center
Pediatric Intensive Care Physician
Pediatric Intensive Care Unit
MD Anderson Children's Cancer
    Hospital
Houston, Texas

Naveen Sankhyan, MD, DM
Pediatric Neurology Unit
Department of Pediatrics
Advanced Pediatrics Centre
Postgraduate Institute of Medical
    Education and Research
Chandigarh, India

Smarika Sapkota, MD
Resident Physician
Department of Internal Medicine
Marcy Catholic Medical Center
Aldan, Pennsylvania

Cheryl L. Sargel, PharmD
Clinical Pharmacy Specialist—Critical
    Care Medicine
Department of Pharmacy
Nationwide Children's Hospital
Columbus, Ohio

Stephen M. Schexnayder, MD, FAAP, FACP, FCCM
Professor and Vice Chairman
Department of Pediatrics College of
    Medicine
University of Arkansas for Medical
    Sciences
Arkansas Children's Hospital
Little Rock, Arkansas

Charles L. Schleien, MD, MBA
Philip Lanzkowsky Chairman of
    Pediatrics
Hofstra North Shore-LIJ School of
    Medicine
Cohen Children's Medical Center of
    New York
New Hyde Park, New York

James Schneider, MD
Assistant Professor
Department of Pediatrics
Hofstra North Shore-LIJ School of
    Medicine
Cohen Children's Medical Center of
    New York
New Hyde Park, New York

Eduardo J. Schnitzler, MD
Associate Professor
Department of Pediatrics
Hospital Universitario Austral Pilar
Buenos Aires, Argentina

Jennifer J. Schuette, MD, MS
Attending Physician
Cardiac Intensive Care Unit
Fellowship Director
Pediatric Critical Care Medicine
Children's National Health System
Assistant Professor of Pediatrics
George Washington University School
    of Medicine and Health Sciences
Washington, District of Columbia

Scott C. Schultz, MD
Instructor
Kennedy Krieger Institute
Johns Hopkins University School of
    Medicine
Baltimore, Maryland

**Steven M. Schwartz, MD,
FRCPC, FAHA**
Professor of Paediatrics
Senior Associate Scientist
Head
Division of Cardiac Critical Care
    Medicine
Norine Rose Chair in Cardiovascular
    Sciences
The Labatt Family Heart Centre
Departments of Critical Care Medicine
    and Paediatrics
University of Toronto
Toronto, Canada

Istvan Seri, MD, PhD, HonD
Professor of Pediatrics
Weill Cornell Medical College
Professor of Pediatrics (Adjunct)
Keck School of Medicine of the
    University of Southern California
Director
Sidra Neonatology Center of
    Excellence
Chief
Division of Neonatology

Vice Chair of Faculty Development
Department of Pediatrics
Sidra Medical and Research Center
Doha, Qatar

Christine B. Sethna, MD, EdM
Division Director
Pediatric Nephrology
Cohen Children's Medical Center
    of New York
Assistant Professor
Hofstra North Shore-LIJ School of
    Medicine
New Hyde Park, New York

Donald H. Shaffner, MD
Associate Professor
Departments of Anesthesiology
    and Critical Care Medicine and
    Pediatrics
Director
Division of Pediatric Anesthesiology
    and Critical Care Medicine
Johns Hopkins University School
    of Medicine
Baltimore, Maryland

**Thomas P. Shanley, MD,
FCCM**
Ferrantino Professor of Pediatrics
Associate Dean for Clinical and
    Translational Research
Michigan Institute for Clinical &
    Health Research
University of Michigan Medical
    School
Ann Arbor, Michigan

**Lara S. Shekerdemian, MB ChB,
MD, MHA, FRACP**
Professor and Vice Chair of Clinical
    Affairs
Diagnostic Imaging of the
Baylor College of Medicine
Chief of Critical Care
Texas Children's Hospital
Houston, Texas

Naoki Shimizu, MD, PhD
Chief
Department of Paedtric Emergency &
    Critical Care Medicine
Tokyo Metropolitan Children's
    Medical Centre
Tokyo, Japan

Peter Silver MD, MBA, FCCM
Chief
Pediatric Critical Care Medicine
Steven and Alexandra Cohen
    Children's Medical Center of
    New York
Hofstra North Shore-LIJ School
    of Medicine
New Hyde Park, New York

Dennis W. Simon, MD
Assistant Professor of Critical Care
    Medicine and Pediatrics
Children's Hospital of Pittsburgh of
    UPMC
University of Pittsburgh School of
    Medicine
Pittsburgh, Pennsylvania

**Shari Simone, DNP, CPNP-AC,
FCCM**
Senior NP Clinical Program Manager
Women & Children's Services
University of Maryland Medical Center
Baltimore, Maryland

Rakesh Sindhi, MD
Professor
Department of Surgery
University of Pittsburgh
Surgeon
Department of Pediatric Abdominal
    Transplant
Children's Hospital of Pittsburgh of
    UPMC
Pittsburgh, Pennsylvania

**Pratibha D. Singhi, MD, FIAP,
FAMS**
Chief
Pediatric Neurology and Neuro
    Development
Advanced Pediatrics Centre
Post Graduate Institute of Medical
    Education and Research
Chandigarh, India

**Sunit C. Singhi, MBBS, MD,
FIAP, FAMS, FISCCM, FICCM,
FCCM**
Head
Department of Pediatrics & Advanced
    Pediatrics Centre
Postgraduate Institute of Medical
    Education and Research
Chandigarh, India

Ruchi Sinha, MBChB, MRCPCH
Consultant Paediatric Intensivist
Paediatric Intensive Care
St. Mary's Hospital
Imperial College Healthcare NHS Trust
London, United Kingdom

Peter W. Skippen, MBBS, JFICM
Clinical investigator
Division of Pediatric Critical Care
Department of Pediatrics
BC Children's Hospital
Vancouver, British Columbia, Canada

Zdenek Slavik, MD, FRCPCH
Royal Brompton & Harefield NHS
    Trust
Royal Brompton Hospital
London, United Kingdom

Anthony D. Slonim, MD, DrPH
University of Medicine and Dentistry
of New Jersey
New Jersey Medical School
Professor
Department of Medicine
Pediatrics
Community Health, and Preventive
Medicine
Newark, New Jersey
Executive Vice President/Chief Medical
Officer
Barnabas Health
West Orange, New Jersey

Arthur J. Smerling, MD
Medical Director Cardiac Critical Care
Department of Pediatrics and
Anesthesiology Columbia University
New York, New York

Kyle A. Soltys, MD
Assistant Professor of Surgery
Department of Surgery
University of Pittsburgh
Surgeon
Pediatric Abdominal Transplant
Children's Hospital of Pittsburgh of
UPMC
Pittsburgh, Pennsylvania

F. Meridith Sonnett, MD, FAAP, FACEP
Chief
Division of Pediatric Emergency
Medicine
New York Presbyterian Morgan
Stanley Children's Hospital
Associate Professor of Pediatrics
Columbia University Medical Center
Columbia College of Physicians and
Surgeons
New York, New York

David S. Spar, MD
Assistant Professor
Department of Pediatrics
Pediatric cardiologist
The Heart Center
Division of Pediatric Cardiology
Cincinnati Children's Hospital Medical
Center
Cincinnati, Ohio

Neil C. Spenceley, MB, ChB, MRCPCH
Lead Clinician/Patient Safety Fellow
Paediatric Critical Care
Royal Hospital for Sick Children
Glasgow, Scotland

Kevin B. Spicer, MD, PhD, MPH
Paediatric Consultant (Infectious
Diseases)
Pietermaritzburg Metropolitan
Hospitals Complex
Department of Health: KwaZulu-Natal
Pietermaritzburg, South Africa

Philip C. Spinella, MD, FCCM
Associate Professor of Pediatrics
Division of Critical Care Medicine
Director
Critical Care Translational Research
Program
Washington University School of
Medicine
St. Louis, Missouri

Kurt R. Stenmark, MD
Professor of Pediatrics and Medicine
Division Head
Pediatric Critical Care Medicine
Director
Developmental Lung Biology and
Cardiovascular Pulmonary Research
Laboratories
University of Colorado Denver
Aurora, Colorado

John P. Straumanis, MD, FAAP, FCCM
Chief Medical Officer
Vice President of Medical Affairs
University of Maryland Rehabilitation
& Orthopaedic Institute
Clinical Assistant Professor
University of Maryland Medical
School
Baltimore, Maryland

Kevin J. Sullivan, MD
Assistant Professor
Deptartment of Anesthesiology &
Critical Care
Nemours Children's Specialty Care/
Mayo School of Medicine
Jacksonville, Florida

Clifford M. Takemoto, MD
Associate Professor
Division of Pediatric Hematology
Johns Hopkins School of Medicine
Baltimore, Maryland

Robert F. Tamburro, MD
Penn State Hershey Pediatric Critical
Care Medicine
Hershey, Pennsylvania

Robert C. Tasker, MA, MD (Cantab), MBBS (Lond), DCH, FRCPCH, FRCP, FHEA (UK), AM (Harvard), MD (MA)
Professor of Neurology
Professor of Anaesthesia (Pediatrics)
Harvard Medical School
Chair in Neurocritical Care
Senior Associate Staff Physician
Department of Neurology
Department of Anesthesiology,
Perioperative, and Pain Medicine
Division of Critical Care Medicine
Boston Children's Hospital
Boston, Massachusetts

Neal J. Thomas, MS, MSc
Professor of Pediatrics and Public
Health Sciences
Division of Pediatric Critical Care
Medicine
Penn State Hershey Children's
Hospital
The Pennsylvania State University
College of Medicine
Hershey, Pennsylvania

Jill S. Thomas, MSN, CRNP
Pediatric Critical Care Nurse
Practitioner
Division of Pediatric Critical Care
Medicine
Baltimore, Maryland

James A. Thomas, MD
Professor
Department of Pediatrics
Critical Care Medicine
Baylor College of Medicine/Texas
Children's Hospital
Houston, Texas

James Tibballs, MBBS, MD, FANZCA, FCICM, FACLM
Associate Professor
Departments of Paediatrics &
Pharmacology
University of Melbourne
Deputy Director
Paediatric Intensive Care Unit
Royal Children's Hospital
Melbourne, Australia

Pierre Tissieres, MD, PhD
Director
Pediatric Intensive Care and Neonatal
Medicine
Paris South University Hospitals
Le Kremlin Bicetre
Paris, France

Joseph D. Tobias, MD
Chairman
Department of Anesthesiology &
Pain Medicine
Nationwide Children's Hospital
Professor of Anesthesiology &
Pediatrics
The Ohio State University
Columbus, Ohio

Melissa K. Trovato, MD
Assistant Professor
Department of Physical Medicine
and Rehabilitation
Johns Hopkins School of Medicine
Faculty
Pediatric Rehabilitation
Kennedy Krieger Institute
Baltimore, Maryland

Meredith G. van der Velden, MD
Department of Anesthesiology,
    Perioperative, and Pain Medicine
Division of Critical Care Medicine
Boston Children's Hospital
Instructor in Aensthesia
Harvard Medical School
Boston, Massachusetts

Edwin van der Voort, MD
Retired
Pediatric Critical Care
Pediatrician
Rotterdam, The Netherlands

Colin B. Van Orman, MD
Professor (Clinical) Pediatrics and
    Neurology
University of Utah
Salt Lake City, Utah

Shekhar T. Venkataraman, MD
Professor
Department of Critical Care Medicine
    and Pediatrics
University of Pittsburgh School of
    Medicine
Pittsburgh, Pennsylvania

Kathleen M. Ventre, MD
Assistant Professor
Department of Pediatrics/Critical Care
    Medicine
University of Colorado
Attending Physician
Department of Pediatrics/Critical Care
    Medicine
Children's Hospital of Colorado
Aurora, Colorado

Hans-Dieter Volk, MD
BCRT and IMI
Charité – University Medicine
Belrin, Germany

**Steven A. Webber, MBChB
(Hons), MRCP**
James C. Overall Professor and
    Chair
Department of Pediatrics
Vanderbilt University School of
    Medicine
Monroe Carell Jr. Children's Hospital
    at Vanderbilt
Nashville, Tennessee

Stuart A. Weinzimer, MD
Associate Professor
Department of Pediatrics
Yale University School of Medicine
New Haven, Connecticut

Richard S. Weisman, PharmD
Associate Dean for Admissions and
    Professor of Pediatrics
University of Miami Miller School
    of Medicine
Director
Florida Poison Control–Miami
Miami, Florida

Scott L. Weiss, MD, MSCE
Assistant Professor of Anesthesia
Critical Care, and Pediatrics
Department of Anesthesiology and
    Critical Care Medicine
Children's Hospital of Philadelphia
Philadelphia, Pennsylvania

David L. Wessel, MD
Executive Vice President
Chief Medical Officer for Hospital and
    Specialty Services
Ikaria Distinguished Professor of
    Critical Care Medicine
Division of Critical Care Medicine
Children's National Medical Center
Children's National Health System
Professor of Anesthesiology and
    Critical Care Medicine and
    Pediatrics
George Washington University School
    of Medicine and Health Sciences
Washington, District of Columbia

**Randall C. Wetzel, MBBS, MBM,
FRCS, LRCP, FAAP, FCCM**
Professor of Pediatrics and
    Anesthesiology
Keck School of Medicine of the
    University of Southern California
Chair
Anesthesiology Critical Care Medicine
Children's Hospital Los Angeles
Los Angeles, California

Derek S. Wheeler, MD, MMM
Associate Professor of Clinical
    Pediatrics
Associate Chair
Clinical Affairs
University of Cincinnati College of
    Medicine
Associate Chief of Staff
Division of Critical Care Medicine
Cincinnati Children's Hospital Medical
    Center
Cincinnati, Ohio

Michael Wilhelm, MD
Assistant Professor of Pediatrics
Department of Pediatrics
Division of Critical Care
University of Wisconsin
Madison, Wisconsin

**Kenneth D. Winkel, MBBS,
BMedSci, PhD**
Senior Research Fellow
Department of Pharmacology and
    Therapeutics
University of Melbourne
Victoria, Australia

Gerhard K. Wolf, MD
Associate in Critical Care Medicine
Pediatric Medical Director
Boston MedFlight
Assistant Professor of Anaesthesia
Division of Critical Care
Boston Children's Hospital
Boston, Massachusetts

Jennifer E. Wolford, DO, MPH
Assistant Professor
Department of Pediatrics
University of Pittsburgh School of
    Medicine
Pittsburgh, Pennsylvania

Edward C.C. Wong, MD
Director of Hematology
Associate Director of Transfusion
    Medicine
Center for Cancer and Blood
    Disorders
Division of Laboratory Medicine
Children's National Medical Center
Children's National Health System
Sheikh Zayed Campus for Advanced
    Children's Medicine
Associate Professor of Pediatrics and
    Pathology
George Washington University
    School of Medicine and Health
    Sciences
Washington, District of Columbia

Hector R. Wong, MD
Director
Division of Critical Care Medicine
Cincinnati Children's Hospital Medical
    Center
Cincinnati Children's Research
    Foundation
Professor of Pediatrics
Department of Pediatrics
University of Cincinnati College of
    Medicine
Cincinnati, Ohio

Heather Woods Barthel
Director
Legislative and Intergovernmental
    Affairs
Maryland Department of the
    Environment
Baltimore, Maryland

Robert P. Woroniecki, MD, MS
Chief
Division of Pediatric Nephrology and
Hypertension
Associate Professor of Clinical
Pediatrics
Director
Pediatric Residency Scholarly Activity
Program
SUNY School of Medicine
Stony Brook Children's Hospital
Stony Brook, New York

Angela T. Wratney, MD, MHSc
Attending Physician
Pediatric Critical Care
Children's National Medical Center
Assistant Professor
Department of Pediatrics
George Washington University School
of Medicine and Health Sciences
Washington, District of Columbia

Myron Yaster, MD
Richard J. Traystman Professor
Departments of Anesthesiology
Critical Care Medicine and Pediatrics
Johns Hopkins University School of
Medicine
Baltimore, Maryland

Roger W. Yurt, MD
Johnson & Johnson Professor and
Vice Chairman
Department of Surgery
Chief
Division of Burns, Critical Care, and
Trauma
New York Presbyterian Weill Medical
Center
New York, New York

**David Anthony Zideman,
LVO, QHP(C), BSc, MBBS,
FRCA, FRCP, FIMC, FERC**
Consultant
Department of Anaesthetics
Hammersmith Hospital
Imperial College Healthcare
NHS Trust
London, United Kingdom

Basilia Zingarelli, MD, PhD
Professor
Department of Pediatrics
University of Cincinnati College of
Medicine
Cincinnati Children's Hospital Medical
Center
Cincinnati, Ohio

Athena F. Zuppa, MD, MSCE
Assistant Professor
Department of Anesthesia and Critical
Care Medicine
Children's Hospital of Philadelphia
Philadelphia, Pennsylvania

■ PREFACE

The fifth anniversary of the *Rogers' Textbook* is a cause for celebration on many levels. As outlined more fully in Dr. Donald H. Shaffner's preface, this edition summarizes the many new areas that encompass modern pediatric critical care medicine as well as the great progress in understanding and managing critical illness in children. The combined efforts of so many pediatric intensivists, nurses, and other professionals have produced better outcomes all over the world for children in sepsis, congenital heart disease, cardiac arrest, and multiple organ failure, just to name a few areas. We also celebrate the leaders in our field who regularly come together as section editors and authors to distill the latest evidence into a coherent picture designed to facilitate bedside care and learning by a new generation of professionals devoted to caring for very sick children.

The 25 years since Dr. Rogers first asked me to write a chapter and edit a section have been filled with gratitude toward so many, but let me single out three groups: fellows, patients (and their parents), and my own family. The fellows have taught me much more than I taught them by challenging me to confront what I did not know and find better answers. The resilience of a sick child surrounded by a loving family has encouraged me beyond measure about the possibilities in life. Finally, my family (and especially my wife, Mayme) has been so patient in giving up the nights and weekends needed to see a major book through to completion. I know my family is not unique, so I say a big thank-you to all the families of all the authors and editors.

May the collective efforts of the fifth-edition team help sick children and their caregivers all over the world.

David G. Nichols, MD, MBA
Editor in Chief

The fifth edition of the *Rogers' Textbook of Pediatric Intensive Care* offers the pediatric critical care clinician several new enhancements. There is the increased visual appeal that the addition of color brings to the figures and headings throughout the text. Each chapter begins with a "key point" summary which is hyperlinked to the related section of text so that the reader can quickly focus on specific topics of interest. In addition, the authors have highlighted the best available evidence (randomized controlled trials, systematic reviews, or evidenced-based guidelines) for each topic, which are likely to be of high interest to the reader.

The fifth edition marks over 25 years of the *Rogers' Textbook of Pediatric Intensive Care*, and it is remarkable to look back at the stunning improvements in the understanding, treatments, technologies, and outcomes of critical illness in children. An explosion of publications reflects this growth of the field. This edition addresses the new areas and seeks to distill the knowledge into a practical and evidence-based approach to the sick child. Fifteen new chapters have been added and all existing chapters have been thoroughly updated and rewritten. New topics that appear as chapters include Learning from the Data—Discovery Informatics for Critically Ill Children (Chapter 12), Integrating Palliative Care and Critical Care (Chapter 13), Rapid Response Systems (Chapter 29), Noninvasive Ventilation (added to the Inhaled Gases chapter) (Chapter 39), Electrodiagnostic Techniques in Neuromuscular Disease (Chapter 52), Neurosurgical and Neuroradiologic Critical Care (Chapter 60), Abusive Head Trauma (Chapter 62), Pulmonary Hypertension (Chapter 80), Dengue and Other Viral Hemorrhagic Fevers (includes Ebola) (Chapter 89), Secretory and Motility Issues of the Gastrointestinal Tract (Chapter 98), Gastrointestinal Bleeding (Chapter 99), Abdominal Compartment Syndrome (Chapter 100), Diagnostic Imaging of the Abdomen (Chapter 102), and an appendix of Pediatric Critical Care Formulas. Combined chapters that have been split to increase dedicated coverage include Professionalism and Leadership in Pediatric Critical Care (Chapter 3) and Simulation Training and Team Dynamics (Chapter 4); Injury from Chemical, Biologic, Radiologic, and Nuclear Agents (Bioterrorism) (Chapter 33) and Mass Casualty Events (Chapter 34); and Acute Kidney Injury (Chapter 110) and Chronic Kidney Disease, Dialysis, and Renal Transplantation (Chapter 111).

The current edition of the *Roger's Textbook* continues to provide comprehensive coverage of the fundamental science of pediatric critical care, extending from the macro level of organ system interactions to the micro level of molecular physiology and the genetics that steer it. The global emphasis of the textbook continues as worldwide issues become increasingly relevant through continued growth in travel and communication. As well, there is the continued intent to provide a textbook that has appeal for all levels of pediatric critical care practitioners.

The significance of the *Roger's Textbook* is due to the foresight and effort of the people behind it. The *Textbook of Pediatric Intensive Care* began with Mark C. Rogers, the first director of pediatric critical care at Johns Hopkins. He was a great visionary and one of the fathers of modern pediatric critical care medicine. David G. Nichols, one of the finest teachers in pediatric critical care and recipient of this year's Society of Critical Care Medicine Master Educator Award, has built on the tradition and stature of the textbook through the current edition. David has assembled a terrifically impressive collection of section editors who are leaders in this field and who heavily contributed to the planning and production of this textbook through their help in establishing goals and objectives and in recruiting (or retaining) authors. The most important contribution to this textbook comes from the authors, amassed from prestigious institutions around the world, subject experts as recognized by their peers and other leaders, and who provide their valuable time and effort to educate and update those of us lucky enough to be involved in providing care to critically ill children.

On a personal note, I am humbled and honored to be able to participate as a book editor with this impressive collection of dedicated experts. Dr. Rogers greatly contributed to my career, and I still revere the copy of the original *Textbook of Pediatric Intensive Care* that was personally delivered by Dr. Rogers and contained the hand-written inscription "To Hal Shaffner, with best wishes for a bright career in Pediatric Intensive Care, Mark C. Rogers 7-1-88." David G. Nichols continues to be the role model of an educator and clinician held by me and any of those lucky enough to have trained under him. His expertise and guidance made the effort needed for this textbook more than worthwhile. My coworkers and I are grateful to both men as they continue to be involved in the program at Johns Hopkins and continue to influence and inspire young clinicians who chose pediatric critical care as their life's endeavor.

It is difficult to express how impressed I am by the group of section editors who provided (and continue to provide) their efforts and guidance in the production of this edition, and they have my heartfelt gratitude. I am also sincerely grateful to the authors who were willing to contribute their effort to this textbook; they are an amazing collection of writers that range from young stars under the tutelage of skilled experts to deans of major universities and who, despite their other workloads, provided new, or updated existing, chapters. Others who deserve recognition are the staff and leaders from Wolters Kluwer Health who were extremely helpful and supportive and include Nicole Dernoski, Robyn Alvarez, Keith Donnellan, and Brian Brown. Finally, I am extremely lucky for, and grateful to, my wife and children, *Teresa, Laura, Ryan and Chloe*, who were incredibly supportive of and patient with the time and efforts required during the production of this important textbook.

Donald H. Shaffner, MD
Co-Editor in Chief
Baltimore, Maryland

CONTENTS

PART ONE ▪ CRITICAL CARE INTEGRATION

SECTION I ▪ INTRODUCTION TO THE PRACTICE OF PEDIATRIC CRITICAL CARE

SECTION II ▪ PROFESSIONALISM, LEADERSHIP, AND SYSTEMS-BASED PRACTICE

PART THREE ◼ CRITICAL CARE ORGAN SYSTEMS

SECTION VIII ■ RENAL, ENDOCRINE, AND METABOLIC DISORDERS

SECTION IX ■ ONCOLOGIC AND HEMATOLOGIC DISORDERS

                 Monica Bhatia and Katherine V. Biagas

Chapter 118 Coagulation Issues in the PICU   1946
                 Robert I. Parker and David G Nichols

Chapter 119 Sickle Cell Disease   1977
                 *Kevin J. Sullivan, Erin Coletti, Salvatore R. Goodwin, Cynthia Gauger,
                 and Niranjan "Tex" Kissoon*

                 Appendix   A1
                 Index   I1

A SELECTED GLOSSARY OF ABBREVIATIONS

^{131}I-MIBG	iodine-131 metaiodobenzylguanidine
^{153}Sm-EDTMP	samarium-153 ethylene diamine tetramethylene phosphonate
2,3-DPG	2,3-diphosphoglycerate
3-D	three dimensional
5-HT	serotonin
AA	arachidonic acid
AAC	amino acid chromatography
AACT	American Academy of Clinical Toxicology
AAMC	American Association of Medical Colleges
AAP	American Academy of Pediatrics
ABC	airway, breathing, and circulation
ABCD	amphotericin B colloidal dispersion
ABG	arterial blood gas
ABI	acquired brain injury
ABLC	amphotericin B lipid complex
ABP	American Board of Pediatrics
AC	adenylate cyclase
AC	alternating current
ACA	asphyxial cardiac arrest
ACCM	American College of Critical Care Medicine
ACCP	American College of Chest Physicians
ACD	anticoagulant citrate dextrose
ACE	angiotensin-converting enzyme
ACEI	angiotensin-converting enzyme inhibitor
ACGME	Accreditation Council for Graduate Medical Education
ACS	American College of Surgeons
ACS	abdominal compartment syndrome
ACS	acute chest syndrome
ACT	activated clotting time
ACT	activated coagulation time
ACTH	adrenocorticotropic hormone
AD	autonomic dysreflexia
AD	autosomal dominant
ADA	adenosine deaminase
ADC	apparent diffusion coefficient
ADEM	acute disseminated encephalomyelitis
ADH	antidiuretic hormone
ADMA	asymmetric dimethylarginine
ADP	adenosine diphosphate
AED	automated external defibrillator
AEDs	antiepileptic drugs
AEIMSE	acute encephalopathy with inflammation-mediated status epilepticus
AFB	acid-fast bacilli
AFP	acute flaccid paralysis
AG	aminoglycoside
AG	anion gap
aGVHD	acute GVHD
AHA	American Heart Association
AHRQ	Agency for Healthcare Research and Quality
AHT	abusive head trauma
AI	artificial intelligence
AICDA	activation-induced cytidine deaminase
AIDP	acute inflammatory demyelinating polyneuropathy
AIDS	acquired immune deficiency syndrome
AIF	apoptosis-inducing factor
AIMG	autoimmune myasthenia gravis
AIP	acute intermittent porphyria
AIS	arterial ischemic stroke
AIS	ASIA Impairment Scale
AKI	acute kidney injury
AKIN	Acute Kidney Injury Network
ALA	α-linolenic acid
ALARA	as low as reasonably achievable
ALC	absolute lymphocyte count
ALF	acute liver failure
ALI	acute lung injury
ALK-1	activin receptor–like kinase 1
ALL	acute lymphoblastic leukemia
AlloHCT	allogeneic stem-cell transplantation
ALPS	autoimmune lymphoproliferative syndrome
ALS	advanced life support
ALT	alanine aminotransferase
ALT	alanine transaminase
ALTE	apparent life-threatening event
AMAN	acute motor axonal neuropathy
AML	acute myelogenous leukemia
AML	acute myeloid leukemia
AMPA	α-amino-3-hydroxy-5-methyl-4-isoxazolepropionic acid
AMR	antibody-mediated rejection
AMSAN	acute motor and sensory axonal neuropathy
AMV	avoidance of mechanical ventilation
ANC	absolute neutrophil count
ANCA	anti-neutrophil cytoplasmic antibody
AND	allow natural death
ANF	atrial natriuretic factor
ANOVA	analysis of variance
ANP	A-type natriuretic peptide
AOD	atlanto-occipital dislocation
AP	acute pancreatitis
AP-1	activator protein-1
APACHE	Acute Physiology and Chronic Health Evaluation
APC	activated protein C
APC	antigen-presenting cell
APECED	autoimmune polyendocrinopathy–candidiasis–ectodermal dystrophy
APL	acute promyelocytic leukemia
aPL	antiphospholipid antibodies

APML	acute promyelocytic leukemia		BiPAP	biphasic level positive airway pressure
APNs	advanced-practice nurses		BIS	bispectral index
APP	abdominal perfusion pressure		BLS	bare lymphocyte syndrome
APRV	airway-pressure-release ventilation		BLS	basic life support
APS	antiphospholipid antibody syndrome		BM	bone marrow
aPTT	activated partial thromboplastin time		BMD	bone mineral density
AQP	aquaporin		BMDI	bedside medical device interface
AR	acetate Ringer's solution		BMI	body mass index
AR	autosomal recessive		BMPR-II	bone morphogenetic factor receptor type-II
ARB	angiotensin receptor blocker		BMT	bone marrow transplant
ARDS	acute respiratory distress syndrome		BMT	bone marrow transplantation
ARF	acute renal failure		BNP	brain natriuretic peptide
ARF	acute respiratory failure		BNP	B-type natriuretic peptide
ARIMA	autoregressive integrated moving average		BO	bronchiolitis obliterans
ARR	absolute risk reduction		BOOP	bronchiolitis obliterans with organizing pneumonia
ART	antiretroviral therapy		BOS	bronchiolitis obliterans syndrome
ARVC	arrhythmogenic right ventricular cardiomyopathy		BP	blood pressure
AS	aortic valve stenosis		BPD	bronchopulmonary dysplasia
ASC	apoptosis-associated speck-like CARD-containing protein		BPEG	British Pacing and Electrophysiology Group
ASD	atrial septal defect		BPI	bactericidal/permeability-increasing
ASFA	American Society for Apheresis		BPNA	Bereaved Parent Needs Assessment
ASIA	American Spinal Injury Association		BSA	body surface area
ASSC	acute splenic sequestration crisis		BSAER	brainstem auditory-evoked responses
AST	aspartate aminotransferase		BSL	biosafety level
ASVD	atrioventricular septal defect		BSSL	bile salt–stimulated lipase
ATC	automatic tube compensation		BTK	Bruton tyrosine kinase
ATG	antithymocyte globulin		BTPS	body temperate and pressure saturated
AT-III	antithrombin III		BUN	blood urea nitrogen
ATLS	Advanced Trauma Life Support		BURP	backward, upward, and rightward push
ATN	acute tubular necrosis		BVVL	Brown–Vialetto–Van Laere
ATP	adenosine triphosphate		CA	cardiac arrest
ATRA	all-*trans* retinoic acid		CA-MRSA	community-acquired methicillin-resistant *Staphylococcus aureus*
AUC	area under the curve		CAD	caspase-activated deoxyribonuclease
AutoHCT	autologous stem-cell transplantation		CAD	C-terminal activation domain
AV	arteriovenous		C-AMB	conventional amphotericin B
AV	atrioventricular		cAMP	cyclic adenosine monophosphate
AVDGlu	arterial-venous difference of glucose		CAMTS	Commission on Accreditation of Medical Transport Systems
AVDo$_2$	arterial-venous difference of oxygen		Cao$_2$	arterial oxygen content
AVM	arteriovenous malformation		CAP	community-acquired pneumonia
AVNRT	AV nodal reentrant tachycardia		CAR	coxsackie adenovirus receptor
AVP	arginine vasopressin		CARS	compensatory anti-inflammatory response syndrome
AVRT	atrioventricular reciprocating tachycardia		CASQ2	Calsequestrin-2
AVSD	atrioventricular septal defect		CASR	calcium-sensing receptor
BA	biliary atresia		CAT	computed axial tomography
BAFF	B lymphocyte–activating factor		CAUTI	catheter-associated urinary tract infection
BAL	British anti-Lewisite		CAVH	continuous arteriovenous hemofiltration
BAL	bronchoalveolar fluid		CB	cord blood
BAL	bronchoalveolar lavage		CBC	complete blood count
BALF	bronchoalveolar lavage fluid		CBF	cerebral blood flow
B-ALL	Burkitt lymphoma/leukemia		CBRN	chemical, biologic, radiologic, and nuclear
BBB	blood–brain barrier		CBT	cognitive-based therapy
BBGD	biotin-responsive basal ganglia disease		CBV	cerebral blood volume
BCAA	branched-chain amino acid		CC	choledochal cyst
BCG	Bacille Calmette–Guerin		CCB	calcium channel blocker
BDNF	brain-derived neurotrophic factor		CCHF	Crimean–Congo hemorrhagic fever
BEC	bronchial epithelial cell		CCHS	congenital central hypoventilation
bHLH	basic helix–loop–helix			
BIG	botulism immune globulin			
BIP	bleomycin-induced pneumonitis			
BiPAP	bi-level positive airway pressure			

	syndrome
CCI	corrected count increment
CCKb	type B cholecystokinin receptor
CD	cluster of differentiation
CD	Crohn disease
CDC	Centers for Disease Control and Prevention
CDDS	computerized diagnostic decision support
CDG	carbohydrate-deficient glycoprotein
CDH	congenital diaphragmatic hernia
CDP	continuous distending pressure
CDSR	Cochrane Database of Systematic Reviews
cEEG	continuous electroencephalography
CF	cystic fibrosis
CFH	Complement Factor H
CFR	case fatality rate
CFTR	cystic fibrosis transmembrane conductance regulator
CFU	colony-forming unit
CGD	chronic granulomatous disease
cGMP	$3'$-$5'$-cyclic guanosine monophosphate
cGVHD	chronic GVHD
CHAT	choline acetyltransferase
CHCA	Child Health Corporation of America
CHD	congenital heart disease
CHILD	Children's Health and Human Resources Interagency Leadership on Disasters
CHIME	Collaborative Home Infant Monitoring Evaluation
ChIP	chromatin immunoprecipitation assay
CHP	capillary hydrostatic pressure
CI	cardiac index
CI	confidence interval
CICU	cardiac intensive care unit
CID	combined immunodeficiency
CIM	critical illness myopathy
CINM	critical illness neuromyopathy
CIP	critical illness polyneuropathy
CIPO	chronic intestinal pseudo-obstruction
CKD	chronic kidney disease
CL	clearance
CLABSI	central line–associated bloodstream infection
CMAP	compound muscle action potentials
CML	chronic myelogenous leukemia
CMO	corticosterone methyloxidase
CMP	comprehensive metabolic panel
CMR	cardiac magnetic resonance imaging
CMRg	cerebral metabolic rate for glucose
CMRGlu	cerebral metabolic rate for glucose
$CMRO_2$	cerebral metabolic rate for oxygen
CMS	Center for Medicare and Medicaid Services
CMS	congenital myasthenic syndrome
CMT 1	Charcot–Marie–Tooth disease type 1
CMV	cytomegalovirus
CN	cranial nerve
CNL	clinical nurse leader
CNP	C-type natriuretic peptide
CNS	central nervous system
CNV	copy number variants
CO	carbon monoxide
CO	cardiac output

CO_2	carbon dioxide
CoA	coenzyme A
COAT	Children's Orientation and Amnesia Test
CoBaTrICE	Competency-Based Training programme in Intensive Care Medicine for Europe
COBRA	Consolidated Omnibus Budget Reconciliation Act
COHb	Carboxyhemoglobin
COMT	catechol-O-methyltransferase
COPD	chronic obstructive pulmonary disease
COPE	Creating Opportunities for Parent Empowerment
COX	cyclooxygenase
COX-2	cyclooxygenase-2
CP	cancer procoagulant
CPAM	congenital pulmonary airway malformation
CPAP	continuous positive airway pressure
CPB	cardiopulmonary bypass
CPCCRN	Collaborative Pediatric Critical Care Research Network
CPD	citrate phosphate dextrose
CPFA	coupled plasma filtration and adsorption
CPK	creatine phosphokinase
CPM	central pontine myelinolysis
CPOE	computerized physician order entry
CPP	cerebral perfusion pressure
	coronary perfusion pressure
CPR	cardiopulmonary resuscitation
CPS	Child Protective Service
CPT	Current Procedural Terminology
CPVT	catecholaminergic polymorphic VT
CQI	continuous quality improvement
CRBSI	catheter-related bloodstream infection
CREB	cAMP response element–binding protein
CRF	chronic respiratory failure
CRH	corticotropin-releasing hormone
CRIB	Clinical Risk Index for Babies
CRISIS	critical illness stress-induced immune suppression
CRP	C-reactive protein
CRRT	continuous renal replacement therapy
CRS	Congressional Research Service
CRT	capillary refill time
CRT	cardiac resynchronization therapy
CSE	convulsive status epilepticus
CSF	cerebrospinal fluid
CSI	chemical-shift imaging
CSL	Commonwealth Serum Laboratories
CSW	cerebral salt wasting
CSWS	cerebral salt-wasting syndrome
CT	computed tomography
CTE	chronic traumatic encephalopathy
CTG	cytosine–thymine–guanine
CTL	cytotoxic T lymphocyte
CTV	CT venography
CTX	ciguatoxin
CV	conventional ventilation
CVA	cerebrovascular accident
CVC	central venous catheter
CVD	cerebrovascular disorder
CVID	common variable immunodeficiency
CVL	central venous lines

CVP	central venous pressure		DVT	deep vein thrombosis
CVVH	continuous venovenous hemofiltration		DWI	diffusion-weighted imaging
CVVHD	continuous venovenous hemodialysis		DXA	dual-energy x-ray absorptiometry
CVVHDF	continuous venovenous hemodiafiltration		EA	esophageal atresia
CVVP	continuous venovenous plasmafiltration		EAA	excitatory amino acid
CXR	x-ray film of chest		EAPCCT	European Association of Poisons Centres and Clinical Toxicologists
CyanoHb	cyanohemoglobin		EAT	ectopic atrial tachycardia
DA	duodenal atresia		EBER	Epstein–Barr virus encoded small RNAs
DAG	diacylglycerol		EBM	evidence-based medicine
DAH	diffuse alveolar hemorrhage		EBV	Epstein–Barr virus
DAMP	damage-associated molecular pattern		EBV	estimated blood volume
DAMP	danger-associated molecular pattern		ECC	extracorporeal circulation
DBD	donation after brain death		ECD	ethylene cysteine diethyl ester
DBDD	donation after brain determination of death		ECE	endothelin-converting enzyme
			ECF	extracellular fluid
DBP	diastolic blood pressure		ECG	electrocardiogram
DC	dendritic cell		ECHO	economic, clinical, and humanistic outcomes
DC	direct current			
DCC	data coordinating center		ECL	enteric-chromaffin–like cells
DCD	donation after cardiac or circulatory death		ECLS	extracorporeal life support
			ECM	extracellular matrix
DCDD	donation after cardiac or circulatory determination of death		ECMO	extracorporeal membrane oxygenation
			ECOST	extracorporeal organ support therapy
DCM	dilated cardiomyopathy		ECPR	extracorporeal cardiopulmonary resuscitation
DCR	damage-control resuscitation			
DCT	distal convoluted tubule		ECS	electrocerebral silence
DDAVP	1-desamino-8-D-arginine vasopressin		ECT	electroconvulsive therapy
DENV	dengue virus		ED	emergency department
DEPOSE	Design, Equipment, Procedures, Operators, Supplies and materials, and Environment		EDCF	endothelial-derived constrictor factor
			EDH	epidural hematoma
			EDHF	endothelial-derived hyperpolarizing factor
DF	dengue fever		EDP	end-diastolic pressure
DGS	DiGeorge syndrome		EDPVR	end-diastolic pressure–volume relationship
DHA	dihydroartemisinin			
DHA	docosahexaenoic acid		EDS	expanded dengue syndrome
DHEA	dehydroepiandrosterone		EDTA	ethylenediaminetetraacetic acid
DHEA-S	dehydroepiandrosterone sulfate		EDV	end-diastolic volume
DHF	dengue hemorrhagic fever		EE	energy expenditure
DI	diabetes insipidus		EEE	eastern equine encephalitis
DIC	disseminated intravascular coagulation		EEG	electroencephalography/ electroencephalogram
DISC	death-inducing signaling complex			
DKA	diabetic ketoacidosis		EELV	end-expiratory lung volume
DL	decompressive laparotomy		EF	ejection fraction
DMD	Duchenne muscular dystrophy		EGDT	early goal-directed therapy
DMG	donor management goal		EGF	epidermal growth factor
DMSO	dimethyl sulfoxide		EHR	electronic health record
DNA	deoxyribonucleic acid		EIA	enzyme immunoassay
DNAR	do not attempt resuscitation		EIAD	extended-interval aminoglycoside dosing
DNI	do not intubate		EIP	end-inspiratory pressure
DNR	do not resuscitate		ELANE	elastase-neutrophil expressed
Do_2	oxygen delivery		ELBW	extremely low birth weight
DORV	double outlet right ventricle		ELISA	enzyme-linked immunosorbent assay
dPAP	diastolic pulmonary arterial pressure		ELSO	Extracorporeal Life Support Organization
DPI	dry-powder inhalers		EMG	electromyography
DPPC	dipalmitoylphosphatidylcholine		EMS	emergency medical service
DS	duodenal stenosis		EMSC	EMS for children
DSA	donor-specific antibody		EMT	epithelial–mesenchymal transdifferentiation
DSD	Dejerine–Sottas disease			
DSS	decision support system		EMTALA	Emergency Medical Transportation and Labor Act
DSS	dengue shock syndrome			
DTH	delayed-type hypersensitivity		EN	enteral nutrition
DTO	diluted tincture of opium		ENA	epithelial-derived neutrophil attractant
DTPA	diethylene triamine-pentaacetic acid			

ENA-78	epithelial-derived neutrophil-activating peptide-78
ENaC	epithelial sodium channel
eNOS	endothelial nitric oxide synthase
ENS	enteric nervous system
EPA	eicosapentaenoic acid
EPOCH	Evaluating Processes of Care & the Outcomes of Children in Hospital
ER	endoplasmic reticulum
ERA	endothelin receptor antagonist
ERCP	endoscopic retrograde cholangiopancreatography/ cholangiopancreatogram
ERK 1/2	extracellular signal–regulated kinase 1 and 2
ERK	extracellular receptor kinase
ERK	extracellular signal–regulated kinase
ESA	erythropoiesis-stimulating agent
ESICM	European Society of Intensive Care Medicine
ESLD	end-stage liver disease
ESPVR	end-systolic pressure–volume relationship
ESR	erythrocyte sedimentation rate
ESRD	end-stage renal disease
EST	endoscopic sclerotherapy
ET	endothelin
ET 1	endothelin-1
ETC	electron transport chain
ETCO$_2$	end-tidal carbon dioxide
ETI	endotracheal intubation
ETL	extract, transform, and load
ETT	endotracheal tube
EUA	emergency use authorization
EVD	Ebola virus disease
EVL	endoscopic variceal ligation
EVLW	extravascular lung water
EWS	early warning score
FA	fractional anisotropy
FACS	fluorescent-activated cell sorting
FACT	Foundation for Accreditation of Cellular Therapies
FAD	flavin adenine dinucleotide
FAOD	fatty acid oxidation disorder
FAs	fatty acids
FAST	focused abdominal sonography for trauma
FAST	focused assessment by sonography in trauma
FBG	fibrinogen
FDA	U.S. Food and Drug Administration
FDP	fructose-1,6-diphosphatase
FEAST	Fluid Expansion as Supportive Therapy
FEMA	Federal Emergency Management Agency
FeNO	fraction of exhaled nitric oxide
FFM	fat-free mass
FFP	fresh frozen plasma
FGF-10	fibroblast growth factor 10
FIO$_2$	fractional inspired oxygen
FIRES	fever-induced refractory epileptic encephalopathy in school-aged children
FLAIR	fluid-attenuated inversion recovery

FMEA	Failure Modes and Effects Analysis
FMN	flavin mononucleotide
FN	false negative
FN	fever and neutropenia
FP	false positive
FRC	functional residual capacity
FS	fractional shortening
FSGS	focal segmental glomerulosclerosis
FSM	Frequency Sequence Mining
G6PD	glucose-6-phosphate dehydrogenase
GA	gestational age
GABA	γ-aminobutyric acid
GAS	group A *Streptococcus*
GBM	glioblastoma multiforme
GBS	Guillain–Barré syndrome
GC	glucocorticoids
GCP	granulocyte chemotactic peptide
GCS	Glasgow Coma Scale
GCS	Glasgow Coma Score
GCSE	generalized convulsive status epilepticus
GCSF	granulocyte colony-stimulating factor
GDP	guanosine diphosphate
GEE	generalized estimating equation
GER	gastroesophageal reflux
GERD	gastroesophageal reflux disease
GFR	glomerular filtration rate
GGT	gamma glutamyl-transférase
GH	growth hormone
GHB	γ-hydroxybutyrate
GI	gastrointestinal
GLA	γ-linoleic acid
GLP-1	glucagon-like peptide-1
GLUT	glucose transporter protein
GM-CSF	granulocyte–macrophage colony-stimulating factor
GOS E-Peds	Glasgow Outcome Scale Extended for Pediatrics
GP	glycoprotein
GRE	gradient-recalled echo
GRO	growth-related oncogene
GRP	gastrin-releasing peptide
GS	glutamine synthetase
GSD	glycogen storage disorder
GSH	glutathione
GSSG	glutathione disulfide
GTP	guanosine triphosphate
GVHD	graft-versus-host disease
GVL	graft versus leukemia
GWAS	genome-wide association study
GWTG	Get with the Guidelines
HA	hemagglutinin
HA	hyaluronic acid
HAART	highly active antiretroviral therapy
HAE	hereditary angioedema
HAI	healthcare-associated infection
HALF-PINT	Heart And Lung Failure—Pediatric INsulin Titration Trial
HAS	human albumin solution
HAT	human African trypanosomiasis
HAV	hepatitis A virus
Hb	hemoglobin
HbF	fetal Hb

HBO	hyperbaric oxygen			Administration
HbS	sickle hemoglobin		HRT	hormone replacement therapy
HbSC	hemoglobin S hemoglobin C disease		HSCT	hematopoietic stem-cell transplantation
HBV	hepatitis B virus		HSE	heat shock element
HCAP	healthcare-associated pneumonia		HSE	herpes simplex encephalitis
HCDM	human cell differentiation molecule		HSF	heat shock factor
HC-II	heparin cofactor II		HSM	hepatosplenomegaly
HCM	hypertrophic cardiomyopathy		HSP	heat shock protein
HCT	hematopoietic cell transplantation		HSV	herpes simplex virus
HCV	hepatitis C virus		HTIG	human tetanus immunoglobulin
HD	Hirschsprung disease		HTLV	human T-cell lymphotrophic virus
HDEI	high-dose extended interval		HUS	hemolytic uremic syndrome
HE	hepatic encephalopathy		IAA	interruption of the aortic arch
HFE	human factors engineering		IAH	intra-abdominal hypertension
HFI	hereditary fructose intolerance		IAHS	infection-associated hemophagocytic
HFJV	high-frequency jet ventilation			syndrome
HFNC	high-flow nasal cannula		IAP	intra-abdominal pressure
HFOV	high-frequency oscillatory ventilation		IART	intra-atrial reentrant tachycardia
HFRS	hemorrhagic fever with renal syndrome		IASP	International Association for the Study of
HFV	high-frequency ventilation			Pain
HGF	hepatocyte growth factor		IBD	inflammatory bowel disease
HHNS	hyperglycemic hyperosmolar nonketotic		IBW	ideal body weight
	syndrome		IC	indirect calorimetry
HHS	hyperglycemic hyperosmolar syndrome		ICA	internal carotid artery
HHT	hereditary hemorrhagic telangiectasia		ICAM	intercellular adhesion molecule
HHV	human herpesvirus		ICC	interstitial cells of Cajal
HHV-6	human herpes virus type 6		ICD	implantable cardioverter-defibrillator
HI	hemagglutination inhibition		ICD	implanted cardiodefibrillator
Hib	*Haemophilus influenzae* type b		ICD	International Classification of Diseases
HIE	health information exchange		ICF	International Classification of
HIE	hypoxic–ischemic encephalopathy			Functioning, Disability, and Health
HIES	hyper-IgE syndrome		ICF	intracellular fluid
HIF	hypoxia-inducible factor		ICH	intracerebral hemorrhage
HIGM	hyper-IgM		ICOS	inducible T-cell costimulator
HIT	heparin-induced thrombocytopenia		ICP	intracranial pressure
HITECH	Health Information Technology for		ICU	intensive care unit
	Economic and Clinical Health		ICUAW	ICU-acquired weakness
HIV	human immunodeficiency virus		IDDM	insulin-dependent diabetes mellitus
HLA	human leukocyte antibody		IDE	Investigational Device Exemption
HLA	human leukocyte antigen		IDMS	isotope dilution mass spectrometry
HLAs	histocompatibility leukocyte antigens		IEM	inborn errors of metabolism
HLH	hemophagocytic lymphohistiocytosis		IF	intrinsic factor
HLHS	hypoplastic left heart syndrome		IFN	interferon
HME	heat moisture exchange		IG	immunoglobulin
HMGB	high-mobility group box		IGF	insulin-like growth factor
HMGB1	high-mobility group box 1		IgG	immunoglobulin G
HMPAO	hexamethylpropylene-amineoxime		IGHMBP2	immunoglobulin mu-binding protein 2
HMV	home mechanical ventilation		IgM	immunoglobulin M
HO	heme oxygenase		IGT	impaired gastrointestinal transit
HOPE	HIV Organ Policy Equity		IHD	intermittent hemodialysis
HPA	hypothalamic–pituitary axis		IHHS	idiopathic hemiconvulsive-hemiplegia
HPA	hypothalamic–pituitary–adrenal			syndrome
HPAH	heritable pulmonary arterial hypertension		IKK	inhibitor of κB kinase
HPCs	Hematopoietic progenitor cells		IL	interleukin
HPE	homeostatic peripheral expansion		IL-1	interleukin-1
HPS	hantavirus pulmonary syndrome		IL-2	interleukin-2
HPS	hypertrophic pyloric stenosis		IL-2R	interleukin-2 receptor
HR	hazard ratio		IM	intramuscular
HR	heart rate		IM	intramuscularly
HR	human resource		IMCI	Integrated Management of Childhood
HRE	hypoxia response element			Illness
HRSA	Health Resources and Services		IMV	intermittent mandatory ventilation

IND	investigational new drug
iNO	inhaled nitric oxide
iNOS	inducible nitric oxide synthase
INR	international normalized ratio
INSURE	intubate-surfactant-extubate
INTERMACS	Interagency Registry for Mechanically Assisted Circulatory Support
IO	intraosseous
IOI	IO infusion
IOM	Institute of Medicine
IP	ischemic preconditioning
IP3	inositol 1,4,5-triphosphate
IPA	invasive pulmonary aspergillosis
IPAF	ICE protease–activating factor
IPAH	idiopathic pulmonary arterial hypertension
IPEX	immune deficiency, polyendocrinopathy, X-linked
IPS	idiopathic pulmonary syndrome
IPSSW	International Pediatric Simulation Symposium and Workshops
IQR	interquartile range
IRAK	IL-1 receptor–associated kinase
ISHLT	International Society for Heart and Lung Transplantation
ISS	injury severity score
ITP	idiopathic thrombocytopenic purpura
ITP	immune thrombocytopenia
ITP	immune thrombocytopenic purpura
ITP	intrathoracic pressure
IU	indexed unit
IV	intravenous
IVA	isovaleric acidemia
IVC	inferior vena cava
IVIG	intravenous immunoglobulin
IVS	intact ventricular septum
JE	Japanese encephalitis
JET	junctional ectopic tachycardia
JMML	juvenile myelomonocytic leukemia
JNK	c-Jun amino-terminal kinase
KGF	keratinocyte growth factor
KID	Kids' Inpatient Database
KIM	kidney injury molecule
KSA	knowledge, skills, and attitudes
LAD	leukocyte adhesion deficiency
L-AMB	liposomal amphotericin B
LAP	left atrial pressure
LBP	LPS-binding protein
LBW	low birth weight
LCMRg	local cerebral metabolic rate for glucose
LCMV	lymphocytic choriomeningitis virus
LCOS	low cardiac output syndrome
LCTs	long-chain triglycerides
LDH	lactate dehydrogenase
LEI	lipid emulsion infusion
LFA	leukocyte functional antigen
LFGNR	lactose-fermenting gram-negative rod
LFT	liver function test
LGMD	limb-girdle muscular dystrophy
LHR	lung–head ratio
LHV	left hepatic vein
LIP	lower inflection point
LIP	lymphoid interstitial pneumonitis

LMA	laryngeal mask airway
LMWH	low-molecular-weight heparin
LODS	Logistic Organ Dysfunction Score
LOE	level of evidence
LOS	length of stay
LP	lumbar puncture
LPS	lipopolysaccharide
LQTS	long QT syndrome
LR	lactate Ringer's solution
LRR	leucine-rich repeat
LSD	lysergic acid diethylamide
LT	leukotriene
LTD	long-term depression
LTP	long-term potentiation
LTs	liver transplantations
LV	left ventricle
LVNC	left-ventricular noncompaction cardiomyopathy
LVOT	left-ventricular outflow tract
LVPWT	left-ventricular posterior wall thickness
MAC	membrane attack complex
MAC	minimum alveolar concentration
MAC	*Mycobacterium avium* complex
MALDI-TOF	matrix-assisted laser desorption ionization-time of flight
MAO	monoamine oxidase
MAOI	monoamine oxidase inhibitor
MAP	mean airway pressure
MAP	mean arterial pressure
MAP	multidisciplinary action plan
MAPK	mitogen-activated protein kinase
MARS	molecular absorbent recirculating system
MAS	macrophage activation syndrome
MAS	meconium aspiration syndrome
MASP	MBL-activated serine protease
MAT	multifocal atrial tachycardia
MBL	mannan-binding lectin
MBL	mannose-binding lectin
MBP	mean blood pressure
MBP	myelin basic protein
MCA	middle cerebral artery
MCD	multiple carboxylase deficiency
MCE	mass casualty event
MCHB	Maternal and Child Health Bureau
MCHC	mean corpuscular Hb concentration
MCP-1	monocyte chemoattractant protein 1
MCS	mechanical circulatory support
MCTs	medium-chain triglycerides
MDA	methylenedioxyamphetamine
MDGs	Millennium Development Goals
MDI	Mental Developmental Index
MDI	metered-dose inhaler
MDMA	3,4-methylenedioxymethylamphetamine
MELAS	mitochondrial encephalopathy, lactic acidosis, and stroke
MELD	Model for End-Stage Liver Disease
MERIT	Medical Emergency Response and Intervention Trial
MERRF	mitochondrial encephalopathy with ragged red fibers
MERS	Middle East respiratory syndrome
MERS-CoV	Middle East respiratory syndrome coronavirus

MET	medical emergency team
MetHb	methemoglobin
MG	myasthenia gravis
MGSA	melanocyte growth-stimulating activity
MH	malignant hyperthermia
MHC	major histocompatibility complex
MHC	myosin heavy chain
MHLS	malignant hyperthermia-like syndrome
MI	myocardial ischemia
MIC	minimum inhibitory concentration
MIF	migration inhibitory factor
MIP	macrophage inflammatory peptide
MKP-1	mitogen-activated protein kinase phosphatase-1
ML	machine learning
MLC	myosin light chain
MLCK	MLC kinase
MLT	microlaryngeal tracheal
MM	mucous membrane
MMA	methylmalonic acidemia
MMC	migrating myoelectric complex
MMF	mycophenolate mofetil
MMP	matrix metalloproteinase
MOC	Maintenance of Certification
MODS	Multiple Organ Dysfunction Score
MODS	multiple organ dysfunction syndrome
MOF	multiple organ failure
MONA	morphine, oxygen, nitroglycerin, aspirin
MOOSE	meta-analysis of observational studies in epidemiology
MOSF	multiple organ system failure
MP	metalloproteinase
MPA	main pulmonary artery
mPAP	mean pulmonary artery pressure
MR	magnetic resonance
MRA	magnetic resonance angiography
MRCP	magnetic resonance cholangiopancreatography
MRI	magnetic resonance imaging
MRP1	multidrug resistance–associated protein 1
MRS	magnetic resonance spectroscopy
MRS	MR spectroscopy
MRSA	methicillin-resistant *Staphylococcus aureus*
MRV	magnetic resonance venography/venogram
MS	multiple sclerosis
MSAF	meconium-stained amniotic fluid
MSC	mesenchymal stem cell
MSCC	malignant spinal cord compression
MSOF	multiple system organ failure
MSSA	methicillin-sensitive *Staphylococcus aureus*
MSUD	maple syrup urine disease
mtNOS	mitochondrial nitric oxidase synthase
MTP	massive transfusion protocol
MUAC	mid–upper arm circumference
MuSK	muscle-specific kinase
MV	measles virus
MV	mechanical ventilation
MVCs	motor vehicle collisions
MYPT	myosin phosphatase
NA	neuraminidase
NAA	*N*-acetyl aspartate

NAC	*N*-acetylcysteine
NACHRI	National Association of Children's Hospitals and Related Institutions
NAD	nicotinamide adenine dinucleotide
NAD	N-terminal activation domain
NADP	nicotinamide adenine dinucleotide phosphate
NAG	*N*-acetyl-β-glucosaminidase
NAIT	neonatal alloimmune thrombocytopenia
NAPQI	*N*-acetyl-*p*-benzoquinone-imine
NAS	Neonatal Abstinence Scoring
NASPE	North American Society of Pacing and Electrophysiology
NAVA	neurally adjusted ventilatory assist
NBW	normal birth weight
NCC	neurocysticercosis
NCHS	National Center for Health Statistics
NCPAP	nasal continuous positive airway pressure
NCS	nerve conduction study
NCSE	nonconvulsive status epilepticus
NDMV	neutrophil-derived microvesicle
NEC	necrotizing enterocolitis
NEI	neuroendocrine immune
NEMO	nuclear factor-κB essential modulator
NET	neutrophil extracellular traps
NF	nuclear factor
NF-κB	nuclear factor-κB
NG	nasogastric
NGAL	neutrophil gelatinase–associated lipocalin
NGF	nerve growth factor
NHSN	National Health & Safety Network
NI	neuraminidase inhibitor
NI	nosocomial infection
NICE	UK National Institute for Health and Clinical Excellence
NICHD	National Institute for Child Health and Human Development
NICU	neonatal intensive care unit
NIF	negative inspiratory force
NIH	National Institutes of Health
NIHSS	National Institutes of Health Stroke Scale
NINOS	Neonatal Inhaled Nitric Oxide Study Group
NIPPV	noninvasive positive-pressure ventilation
NIRS	near-infrared spectroscopy
NIV	noninvasive ventilation
NK	natural killer
NLF	neonatal liver failure
NLFGNR	non–lactose-fermenting gram-negative rods
NLR	NOD-like receptor
NLRP3	NOD-like receptor protein 3
NMB	neuromuscular blocking
NMBA	neuromuscular blocking agent
NMD	neuromuscular disease
NMDA	*N*-methyl-ᴅ-aspartate
NMDAR	NMDA receptor
NMJ	neuromuscular junction
NMS	neuroleptic malignant syndrome
NNIS	National Nosocomial Infections Surveillance
nNOS	neuronal nitric oxide synthase
NNRTI	nonnucleoside reverse transcriptase

	inhibitor
NNT	number needed to treat
NO	nitric oxide
NO_2	nitrogen dioxide
NOD	nucleotide-binding oligomerization domain
NOMID	neonatal onset multisystem inflammatory disease
NORSE	new-onset RSE
NOS	nitric oxide synthase
NPA	nasopharyngeal airway
NPO	nil per os
NPPV	noninvasive positive-pressure ventilation
NPs	nurse practitioners
NPV	negative predictive value
NPV	negative-pressure ventilator
NRP	Neonatal Resuscitation Program
NRTI	nucleoside reverse transcriptase inhibitor
NS	normal saline
NSAID	nonsteroidal anti-inflammatory drug
NSE	neuron-specific enolase
NSS	normal saline solution
NTM	nontuberculous *Mycobacterium*
NTR	neurotrophin receptor
NTS	nucleus tractus solitarius
NYHA	New York Heart Association
OAC	organic acid chromatography
OBWS	Opioid and Benzodiazepine Withdrawal Score
ODD	oxygen-dependent degradation domain
OER	oxygen extraction ratio
OGIB	obscure GI bleeding
OHCAs	out-of-hospital cardiac arrests
OI	oxygenation index
OM	oral mucositis
ONOO	peroxynitrite
OP	organophosphate
OPA	oropharyngeal airway
OPO	organ procurement organization
OPS	Observational Pain Scale
OPS	orthogonal polarization spectral
OPTN	Organ Procurement and Transplantation Network
OR	odds ratio
OR	operating room
OSA	obstructive sleep apnea
OSAS	obstructive sleep apnea syndrome
OTC	ornithine transcarbamylase
PA	propionic aciduria
PA	pulmonary atresia
PAC	premature atrial complex
PAC	pulmonary artery catheter
$PaCO_2$	partial pressure of carbon dioxide
PAE	postantibiotic effect
PAED	Paediatric Anesthesia Emergence Delirium Scale
PAF	platelet-activating factor
PAFR	platelet-activating factor receptor
PAH	pulmonary arterial hypertension
PAI	plasminogen activator inhibitor
PAI-1	platelet activator inhibitor-1
PALF	pediatric acute liver failure
PALISI	Pediatric Acute Lung Injury and Sepsis Investigators
PALS	Pediatric Advanced Life Support
PAMP	pathogen-associated molecular pattern
PaO_2	partial pressure of oxygen
PAOP	pulmonary artery occlusion pressure
PAP	pulmonary arterial pressure
PAPVC	partial anomalous pulmonary venous connection
PAR	protease-activated receptor
PARP	poly(ADP-ribose) polymerase
PARP-1	poly(ADP-ribose) polymerase-1
PAS	Per-ARNT-Sim
PAs	physician assistants
PAS	platelet additive solution
PATD	pulmonary artery thermodilution
PAV	proportional assist ventilation
PAWP	pulmonary arterial wedge pressure
PBB	protected bronchial brush
PBC	pre-Botzinger complex
PBMC	peripheral blood monocyte
PbO_2	pressure of brain tissue oxygen
PBP	penicillin-binding protein
PBSCT	peripheral blood stem-cell transplant
$Pbto_2$	pressure of brain tissue oxygen
PC	phosphatidylcholine
PC	pressure control
PCA	patient-controlled analgesia
pCAM-ICU	pediatric Confusion Assessment Method-ICU
PCCTSDP	Pediatric Critical Care and Trauma Scientist Development Program
PCD	programmed cell death
PCH	pulmonary capillary hemangiomatosis
PCMR	Pediatric Cardiomyopathy Registry
PCP	phencyclidine
PCP	*Pneumocystis jiroveci (carinii)* pneumonia
PCP	*Pneumocystis* pneumonia
PCPC	pediatric cerebral performance category
PCR	polymerase chain reaction
PCT	procalcitonin
PCT	proximal convoluted tubule
PCWP	pulmonary capillary wedge pressure
PD	peritoneal dialysis
PD	pharmacodynamics
PDA	patent ductus arteriosus
PDE	phosphodiesterase
PDE5	phosphodiesterase type-5
PDH	pyruvate dehydrogenase
PDRP	peritoneal dialysis-related peritonitis
PDVI	Pediatric Dengue Vaccine Initiative
PE	phenytoin equivalent
PEA	pulseless electrical activity
PECAM	platelet–endothelial cell adhesion molecule
PECARN	Pediatric Emergency Care Applied Research Network
PEEP	positive end-expiratory pressure
PEFR	peak expiratory flow rate
PEG-ES	polyethylene glycol electrolyte solution
PEGFR	platelet-derived growth factor receptor
PELD	Pediatric end-stage liver disease

PELOD	pediatric logistic organ dysfunction
PEMOD	pediatric multiple organ dysfunction
PEP	postexposure prophylaxis
PERDS	peri-engraftment respiratory distress syndrome
PET	partial exchange transfusion
PET	positron emission tomography
PEWS	Paediatric Early Warning Score
PFI	peripheral perfusion (flow) index
PFO	patent foramen ovale
PFT	pulmonary function testing
PGE	prostaglandin
PGE1	prostaglandin E1
PGIS	prostacyclin synthase
PH	pulmonary hypertension
PHIS	Pediatric Health Information System
PHTS	Pediatric Heart Transplant Study
PI	pneumatosis intestinalis
PI	protease inhibitor
PI3K	phosphatidylinositol-3-kinase
PI3K	phosphoinositide 3-kinase
PIB	pressure-immobilization bandage
PICC	peripherally inserted central catheter
PiCCO	pulse index contour cardiac output
PICU	pediatric intensive care unit
PID	pelvic inflammatory disease
PIE	pulmonary interstitial emphysema
PIM	Pediatric Index of Mortality
PIP	peak inspiratory pressure
PJP	*Pneumocystis jiroveci* pneumonia
PJRT	permanent form of junctional reciprocating tachycardia
PK	pharmacokinetics
PKA	protein kinase A
PKB	protein kinase B
PKC	protein kinase C
PLA	phospholipases A
PLADO	PLAtelet DOse
PLC	Phospholipase C
PLED	periodic lateralized epileptiform discharge
PLRP2	pancreatic lipase–related protein-2
PMA	postmenstrual age
PMN	polymorphonuclear cell
PMNL	polymorphonuclear leukocyte
P-MODS	Pediatric Multiple Organ Dysfunction Score
PMV	prolonged mechanical ventilation
PN	parenteral nutrition
PNC	platelet neutrophil complex
PNP	polynucleotide phosphorylase
PNS	peripheral nervous system
POC	point of care
POMC	proopiomelanocortin
POPC	Pediatric Overall Performance Category
POPE	postobstructive pulmonary edema
POR	P450 oxidoreductase
POS	probability of survival
PPACA	Patient Protections and Affordable Care Act
PPAR	peroxisome proliferator-activated receptor
PPD	purified protein derivative
PPE	personal protective equipment

PPHN	persistent pulmonary hypertension of the newborn
PPI	proton-pump inhibitor
PPV	positive predictive value
PPV	positive-pressure ventilation
PRBC	packed red blood cell
PRES	posterior-reversible encephalopathy syndrome
PRIMACORP	prophylactic intravenous use of milrinone after cardiac operation in pediatrics
PRIS	Pediatric Research in Inpatient Settings
PRIS	propofol-related infusion syndrome
PRISM	Pediatric Risk of Mortality
PROTEKT	PROphylaxis of ThromboEmbolism in Kids
PRR	pattern recognition receptor
PRSW	preload-recruitable stroke work
PRTH	pituitary resistance to thyroid hormone
PRVC	pressure-regulated volume control
PSV	pressure-support ventilation
PT	prothrombin time
PTA	posttraumatic amnesia
PTC	percutaneous transhepatic cholangiography
PTE	posttraumatic epilepsy
PTH	parathyroid hormone
PTHrP	parathyroid hormone–related peptide
PTL	pancreatic colipase-dependent triglyceride lipase
PTLD	posttransplant lymphoproliferative disorder
PTS	posttraumatic seizure
PTSD	posttraumatic stress disorder
PTT	partial thromboplastin time
PTT	Pediatric Triage Tape
PUD	peptic ulcer disease
PUFA	polyunsaturated fatty acid
PV	pressure–volume
PVC	premature ventricular complex
pVHL	von Hippel–Lindau protein
PVOD	pulmonary veno-occlusive disease
PVR	peripheral vascular resistance
PVR	pulmonary vascular resistance
PVRI	pulmonary vascular resistive index
PYY	peptide YY
QI	quality improvement
qPCR	quantitative PCR
QUOROM	Quality of Reporting of Meta-Analyses
RA	retinoic acid
RA	right atrium
RAAS	renin–angiotensin–aldosterone system
RACK1	receptor of activated protein C kinase
RANK	receptor activator of nuclear factor κB
RAR	retinoic acid receptor
RASS	Richmond Agitation–Sedation Scale
RBC	red blood cell
RBF	renal blood flow
RBRVS	Resource-Based Relative Value Scale
RCH	Royal Children's Hospital
RCM	restrictive cardiomyopathy
RCP	respiratory care practitioner
RCT	randomized controlled trial
RDD	radioactive dispersal device

RDP	random donor platelet	SBAR	Situation, Background, Assessment, and Recommendation
RDS	respiratory distress syndrome	SBDS	Shwachman–Bodian–Diamond syndrome
REE	resting energy expenditure	SBFT	small-bowel follow-through
REM	rapid eye movement	SBP	spontaneous bacterial peritonitis
RESOLVE	resolution of organ failure in pediatric patients with severe sepsis	SBS	State Behavioral Scale
RevMan	Review Manager	SBTT	simulation-based team training
RFR	replacement fluid rate	SC	sieving coefficient
RHAMM	receptor for hyaluronic acid–mediated motility	SCA	sickle cell anemia
		SCCLD	sickle cell chronic lung disease
RHIOs	Regional Health Information Organizations	SCCM	Society of Critical Care Medicine
		SCD	sickle cell disease
RHV	right hepatic vein	SCD	spinal cord dysfunction
RIFLE	risk, injury, failure, loss, and end-stage renal disease	SCD	sudden cardiac death
		SCFAs	short-chain fatty acids
RING	Resolving Infection in Neutropenia with Granulocytes	SCI	spinal cord injury
		SCID	severe combined immunodeficiency disease
RIPC	remote ischemic preconditioning	SCIWORA	spinal cord injury without radiographic abnormality
RLR	RIG-I-like receptor		
RNS	reactive nitrogen species	SCN	severe congenital neutropenia
ROC	receiver operating characteristic	SCT	sickle cell trait
ROK	Rho A/Rho kinase	SCUF	slow continuous ultrafiltration
ROM	range of motion	SD	standard deviation
RONS	reactive oxygen and nitrogen species	SDD	selective digestive decontamination
ROP	retinopathy of prematurity	SDF-1	stromal-derived factor 1
ROS	reactive oxygen species	SDH	subdural hemorrhage
ROSC	return of spontaneous circulation	SE	sleep efficiency
RPLS	reversible posterior leukoencephalopathy syndrome	SE	spin echo
		SE	status epilepticus
RQ	respiratory quotient	SEARO	Southeast Asian Region Office
RR	relative risk	SEM	standard error of the mean
RR	risk ratio	SFEMG	single muscle fiber needle EMG
RR	respiratory rate	SGLT	sodium/glucose cotransporters or linked transporters
RRR	relative risk reduction		
RRS	rapid response system	SIADH	syndrome of inappropriate secretion antidiuretic hormone
RRT	renal replacement therapy		
RSE	refractory status epilepticus	SIDS	sudden infant death syndrome
RSI	rapid sequence intubation	SIMV	synchronized intermittent mandatory ventilation
RSV	respiratory syncytial virus		
RT	reverse transcriptase	Si-PAP	synchronized inspiratory positive airway pressure
RTA	road traffic accident		
RTH	resistance to thyroid hormone	SIRS	systemic inflammatory response syndrome
rTPA	recombinant tissue plasminogen activator	SL	sleep latency
RT-PCR	reverse transcription polymerase chain reaction	SLE	systemic lupus erythematosus
		SLOS	Smith–Lemli–Optiz syndrome
RV	rhinovirus	SLP	seizure-like phenomenon
RV	right ventricle	SMA	spinal muscular atrophy
RVOT	right ventricular outflow tract	SMA	superior mesenteric artery
RVOTO	right ventricular outflow tract obstruction	SMARD	spinal muscular atrophy with respiratory distress
RVSP	right ventricular systolic pressure		
RXR	retinoid x receptor	SMRs	standardized mortality ratios
RYR2	ryanodine receptor 2	SMS	superior mediastinal syndrome
S1P	sphingosine-1-phosphate	SMV	superior mesenteric vein
SA	sinoatrial	SNAP	Score for Neonatal Acute Physiology
SA	surface area	SNAP	sensory nerve action potential
SAH	subarachnoid hemorrhage	SNARE	soluble N-ethylmaleimide-sensitive factor attachment protein receptor
SAM	surface-active material		
SAP	signaling lymphocyte activation molecule–associated protein	SND	sinus node dysfunction
		SNP	single nucleotide polymorphism
SARS	severe acute respiratory syndrome	SNP	sodium nitroprusside
SAVE	Secondary Assessment of Victim Endpoint	SNS	sympathetic nervous system
SAX	symbolic aggregate approximation		

SOC	store-operated calcium		TBI	traumatic brain injury
SOD	superoxide dismutase		TBM	tubercular meningitis
SOFA	Sequential Organ Failure Assessment		TBSA	total-body surface area
SOI	severity of illness		TBWD	total-body water distribution
SOJIA	systemic onset juvenile idiopathic arthritis		TCA	tricarboxylic acid
SOS	sinusoidal obstructive syndrome		TCA	tricyclic antidepressant
SOS	Sophia Observation withdrawal Symptoms scale		TCD	transcranial Doppler
SP	surfactant protein		TCDB	Traumatic Coma Databank
SPECS	safe pediatric euglycemia after cardiac surgery		Td	diphtheria toxoid
			TD	tumefactive demyelination
SPECT	single-photon emission computed tomography		TDF	tenofovir disoproxil fumarate
			TdP	torsades de pointes
SPLIT	Studies in Pediatric Liver Transplantation		TEC	transient erythrocytopenia of childhood
SPRR	shortest ventricular preexcited RR interval		TEE	transesophageal echocardiography
SRBD	sleep-related breathing disorder		TEF	tracheoesophageal fistula
SS	serotonin syndrome		TF	tissue factor
SSEP	somatosensory evoked potential		TFPI	tissue factor pathway inhibitor
SSPE	subacute sclerosing panencephalitis		TGA	transposition of the great artery
SSRI	selective serotonin reuptake inhibitor		TGC	tight glycemic control
SSSI	skin and skin structure infection		TGF	transforming growth factor
START	simple treatment and rapid transport		THAPCA	Therapeutic Hypothermia after Pediatric Cardiac Arrest
StimSFEMG	stimulation SFEMG		TIA	transient ischemic attack
STPD	standard temperature and pressure and dry		TIMP	tissue inhibitors of metalloproteinase
			TIPS	transjugular intrahepatic portosystemic shunt
STSS	streptococcal TSS			
SulfHb	sulfhemoglobin		TIR	toll/IL-1R
SUPPORT	Surfactant Positive Airway Pressure and Pulse Oximetry Trial		TISS	Therapeutic Intervention Scoring System
			TKIs	tyrosine kinase inhibitors
SV	stroke volume		TLC	total lung capacity
SVAD	systemic VAD		TLR	toll-like receptor
SVC	superior vena cava		TLS	tumor lysis syndrome
SVDK	snake venom detection kit		TM	tympanic membrane
SVI	stroke volume index		TMP	transmembrane pressure
Svo_2	central venous oxygen saturation		TMP-SMX	trimethoprim–sulfamethoxazole
SVR	systemic vascular resistance		TMP-SMZ	trimethoprim–sulfamethoxazole
SVS	slit ventricle syndrome		TN	true negative
SVT	supraventricular tachycardia		TNF	tumor necrosis factor
SVV	stroke volume variability		TNF-α	tumor necrosis factor-α
SWI	susceptibility-weighted imaging		TOF	tetralogy of Fallot
SWS	slow-wave sleep		TOR	target of rapamycin
TA	truncus arteriosus		TP	true positive
TAC	temporary abdominal closure		tPA	tissue plasminogen activator
TACI	transmembrane activator and calcium modulator and cyclophilin ligand interactor		TPE	total plasma exchange
			TPN	total parenteral nutrition
			TPT	technetium-99m pertechnetate
TAG	triacylglycerol		TQS	Tetanus Quick Stick
TAH	total artificial heart		TR	thyroid hormone receptor
TAI	traumatic axonal injury		TR	tricuspid valve regurgitation
TAL	thick ascending limb		TRAF	TNF receptor–associated factor
TALH	thick ascending limb of the loop of Henle		TRAP	Transport Risk Assessment in Pediatrics
TAMOF	thrombocytopenia-associated multiple organ failure		TRE	thyroid hormone response element
			TRH	thyrotropin-releasing hormone
TAP	transporter-associated antigen-processing protein		TRICC	transfusion requirements in critical care
			TRIM	transfusion-related immune modulation
TAPS	Transfusion Alternatives Preoperatively in Sickle Cell Disease		TRP	tubular reabsorption of phosphate
			TRPC	transient receptor potential channel
TAPVC	total anomalous pulmonary venous connection		TRV	tricuspid regurgitation velocity
			TSH	thyroid-stimulating hormone
TB	tuberculosis		TSS	toxic shock syndrome
TBG	thyroxine-binding globulin		TST	total sleep time
TBI	total-body irradiation		TT	thrombin time

TTN	transient tachypnea of the newborn	VILI	ventilator-induced lung injury
TTP	thrombotic thrombocytopenic purpura	VLA	very late activation antigen
TV	tricuspid valve	VLA	very late antigen
TXA2	thromboxane A2	VLBW	very low birth weight
UAC	umbilical arterial catheter	VLPO	ventrolateral preoptic
UAGA	Uniform Anatomical Gift Act	VNTR	variable number of tandem repeat
UC	ulcerative colitis	Vo_2	total-body oxygen consumption
UC	umbilical cord	VOC	vaso-occlusive crisis
UD	unusual manifestation of dengue	VOD	veno-occlusive disease
UFH	unfractionated heparin	VP	ventriculoperitoneal
UFR	ultrafiltration rate	VPS	Virtual PICU Systems
UGI	upper GI	VRE	vancomycin-resistant enterococci
UGT	uridine glucuronosyltransferase	VS	volume support
UIMA	Unstructured Information Management Architecture	VSD	ventricular septal defect
		VT	ventricular tachycardia
UIP	upper inflection point	VTE	venous thromboembolism
UNG	uracil DNA glycosylase	VV	venovenous
UNOS	United Network for Organ Sharing	vWF	von Willebrand factor
UNSAFE	Unrecognized Situation Awareness Failure Events	VZIG	varicella-zoster immune globulin
		VZV	varicella-zoster virus
UOP	urine output	WAS	Wiskott–Aldrich syndrome
u-PA	urokinase-type plasminogen activator	WASP	WAS protein
URAP	unidirectional retrograde accessory pathway	WAT-1	Withdrawal Assessment Tool-Version 1
		WB	whole blood
URI	upper respiratory infection	WBC	white blood cell
US	ultrasound	WBC	white blood count
UTP	uridine triphosphate	WBGT	wet-bulb globe temperature
UVC	umbilical venous catheter	WGAP	Working Group on Abdominal Problems
VA	veno-arterial	WHO	World Health Organization
VAD	ventricular assist device	WNND	West Nile neuroinvasive disease
VAE	ventilator-associated event	WNV	West Nile virus
VAP	ventilator-associated pneumonia	WOB	work of breathing
VAT	ventilator-associated tracheitis	WPW	Wolff–Parkinson–White syndrome
VAV	venoarteriovenous	WSACS	World Society of Abdominal Compartment Syndrome
VC	vital capacity		
VC	volume control	WTC	World Trade Center
VCAM	vascular cell adhesion molecule	XDH	xanthine dehydrogenase
Vd	volume of distribution	XLA	X-linked agammaglobulinemia
VDJ	Variable Diverse Joining	XLP	X-linked lymphoproliferative disease
VDRs	vitamin D receptors	XO	xanthine oxidase
VEGF	vascular endothelial growth factor	XOR	xanthine oxidoreductase
VF	ventricular fibrillation	ZO	zonula occludens

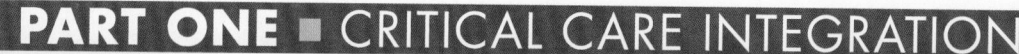

PART ONE ■ CRITICAL CARE INTEGRATION

CHAPTER 1 ■ PEDIATRIC INTENSIVE CARE: A GLOBAL PERSPECTIVE

TREVOR DUKE, NIRANJAN "TEX" KISSOON, AND EDWIN VAN DER VOORT

KEY POINTS

1. The development of pediatric intensive care services should take account of the level of preventive and basic curative treatment that are available to all children in that country, and the national and subnational mortality rates. It should also be based on an understanding of disease epidemiology in that country or region.

2. Dramatic reductions in child mortality and overall improvements in child health have occurred in high-income and many transitional economies, but within many developing countries, inequity in child health outcomes remains vast. The causes of inequity are poverty and its consequences, such as low education, poor access to quality health services, and inadequate attention to human rights.

3. Pneumonia, diarrhea, malaria, and injuries are consistently the leading causes of deaths in children outside the neonatal period, and preterm complications, birth asphyxia and neonatal sepsis, are consistently the commonest causes of neonatal deaths. Worldwide, the rates for some diseases are falling dramatically because of better disease control programs.

4. Most of the care of seriously ill children in the least-developed countries is provided by nurses, paramedical workers, and nonspecialist doctors in rural or remote hospitals or overcrowded urban hospitals.

5. In developing and transitional countries, pediatric intensive care specialists have the potential to improve the management of seriously ill children throughout their country, by providing training for staff in smaller hospitals and by encouraging the building of effective emergency health systems for children.

6. In the countries with limited resources, the provision of publicly funded intensive care that will benefit only a few has to be weighed against the greater needs of many.

7. Outside North America, Europe, Australia, and New Zealand, there are over 60 countries that have under-5 mortality rates <30 per 1000 live births, where intensive care services are likely to have a substantial impact on child survival at a population level.

8. Innovations in intensive care in developing countries should focus on simpler, safer, and cheaper technology, and this has the potential to influence the way intensive care is practiced worldwide.

9. In the next decade, children with chronic health conditions will be greater users of the intensive care services in developing countries. This changing epidemiology needs to be considered in planning and prioritizing services, and in considering the ethical dimensions of intensive care.

INTRODUCTION

In the last 100 years, there have been dramatic reductions in child mortality and overall improvements in child health in Western countries. These have resulted from economic development, public health interventions, better nutrition, maternal health, immunization, education, and advances in health technology and curative care. Child mortality rates fell from over 100 per 1000 live births in the United Kingdom, North America, Australia, New Zealand, Japan, Scandinavian countries, and Western Europe at the end of the 19th century, to <10 per 1000 live births at the beginning of the 21st century.

Pediatric intensive care played a small but significant role in these remarkable outcomes, although the majority of reductions in child mortality occurred long before the first use of prolonged per-laryngeal intubation of infants using polyvinyl chloride tubes in the early 1960s; the event that allowed children to be mechanically ventilated for prolonged periods of time without tracheostomy, and allowed pediatric intensive care units (PICUs) to develop (1). In 1960–1964, the under-5 mortality rate of 21 countries in Europe, North America, Australasia, and Asia that would go on to develop modern PICUs was 29 per 1000 live births (interquartile range: 24–34). By 2011, the under-5 mortality rate for these countries was 4.2 per 1000 live births (interquartile range: 3.4–4.7) (2).

Perspective

Despite these advances in rich countries, 90% of the world's children, the majority of whom live in developing countries and in poorer areas in countries with mixed economies, have not shared in this remarkable prosperity and progress. The World Health Organization (WHO) estimates that in 2010 and 2011 6.9–7.6 million children died each year; >95% of these deaths occurred in developing countries (2–4). **Figure 1.1** shows the distribution of child mortality globally in 2000; the majority of these under-5 deaths were in sub-Saharan Africa and South Asia. In 2011, 68 countries still had child mortality rates >40 per 1000 live births; 48 in Africa, 14 in Asia, 3 in the Pacific, and 1 each in the Middle East, Latin America, and the Caribbean (2). Twenty-three countries—all in sub-Saharan Africa—had mortality rates of >100 per 1000 live births.

For most children throughout the world, access to intensive care is nonexistent, and access to even basic healthcare is a

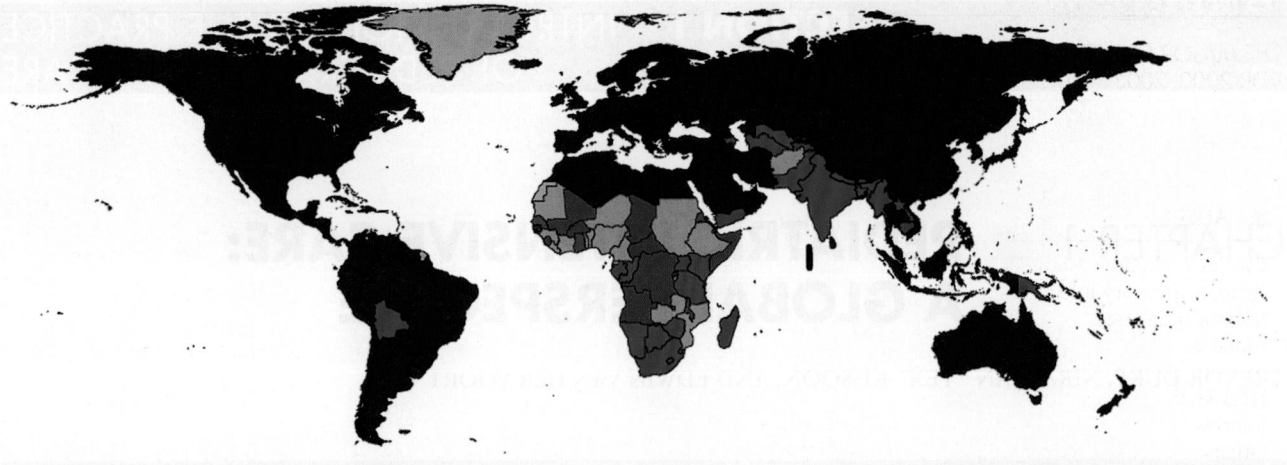

Under-five mortality rate (deaths per 1,000 live births)

■ Less than 40   ■ 100–149   ■ Data not available

■ 40–99   ■ 150 or more

Note: Data for Sudan refer to the country as it was constituted in 2010, before South Sudan seceded on 9 July 2011.

FIGURE 1.1. Children in Southern Asia and Sub-Saharan Africa face a higher risk of dying before their fifth birthday. (From You D, Jones G, Wardlaw T; for United Nations Inter-agency Group for Child Mortality Estimation. *Levels & Trends in Child Mortality: Report 2011*. United Nations Children's Fund, 2011, New york.)

challenge. Even in many transitional economies, access to intensive care is so expensive that it is only for the richer classes and can drive less wealthy families into poverty. Most of the care of seriously ill children in the least-developed countries is provided by nurses, paramedical workers, and nonspecialist doctors in rural or remote hospitals or overcrowded urban hospitals. In most such hospitals, resources are inadequate, there is poor access to evidence and information, and there is little ongoing professional development or staff training (5,6). These basic deficiencies affect the lives of millions of children each year and are the background to any consideration of the appropriate role of intensive care.

In an ideal world, good quality intensive care would be available to all children worldwide. However, in the countries with limited resources, the provision of intensive care that will only benefit a few has to be weighed against the greater needs of many. Attending to less costly but vitally important basic healthcare needs reduces global inequity and may decrease the need for intensive care resources. An examination of causes of global childhood mortality underlines this point.

CAUSES OF GLOBAL CHILD MORTALITY

The major causes of deaths in children under 5 years of age globally are listed in **Table 1.1** (7). Pneumonia, diarrhea, malaria, and injuries are consistently the leading causes of deaths in children outside the neonatal period, and preterm complications, birth asphyxia and neonatal sepsis, are consistently the commonest causes of neonatal deaths. The proportions are region-specific, with skewed distribution in the Africa region. For example, 94% and 89% of the world's malaria and HIV/AIDS deaths occur in Africa. Worldwide, the rates for some diseases are falling dramatically because of better disease control programs. For example, there has been a comprehensive approach to malaria control, including a change

to artemisinin-based drug treatment, rapid diagnostic tests, indoor residual insecticide spraying, and research into malaria vaccines. However, the largest impact on malaria morbidity and mortality has occurred from widespread distribution of insecticide-treated mosquito nets. Malaria cases are falling in at least 25 endemic countries in 5 WHO regions. In 22 of these countries, the number of reported cases fell by 50% or more between 2000 and 2006–2007.

More than 50% of children who die in developing countries have moderate or severe malnutrition, and malnutrition is implicated in deaths from diarrhea (61%), malaria (57%), pneumonia (52%), and measles (45%). Nearly three-fourths of the world's malnourished children live in 10 countries, and >99% live in developing countries. While children often present with a single condition (e.g., acute respiratory infection), those who are most likely to die will often have experienced several other infections in recent months, have more than one infection currently (e.g., pneumonia and diarrhea, or pneumonia and malaria), and have malnutrition with micronutrient (such as iron, zinc, or vitamin A) deficiency (**Fig. 1.2**). In the first decade of this century, child death rates continued to decline such that >2 million fewer children died in 2011 than in 2000. (4)

THE WORLD HEALTH ORGANIZATION'S APPROACH TO GLOBAL CHILD MORTALITY

In 2003, the *Lancet* published a series on child survival, outlining the evidence for effectiveness of interventions in reducing child mortality. Twenty-three interventions (15 preventive and 8 curative) aimed at the commonest causes of child mortality had high-grade evidence for effectiveness, that is, large randomized trials or systematic reviews (8). These interventions were selected for being low cost and having the potential for implementation at near-universal scale

TABLE 1.1

THE MAJOR CAUSES OF DEATHS IN CHILDREN UNDER 5 YEARS OF AGE GLOBALLY, WITH ESTIMATES FOR 2000–2003 AND 2010

■ CAUSE	■ NO OF DEATHS (THOUSANDS) IN 2000–2003	■ % OF TOTAL ANNUAL GLOBAL DEATHS IN 2000–2003	■ NO OF DEATHS (THOUSANDS) IN 2010	■ % OF TOTAL ANNUAL GLOBAL DEATHS IN 2010
Causes in children 1 mo – 5 y	6685	63	4369	59
Acute respiratory infections	2027	19	1071	14
Diarrheal diseases	1762	17	751	10
Malaria	853	8	564	8
Measles	395	4	114	2
HIV/AIDS	321	3	159	2
Injuries	305	3	354	5
Others	1022	10	1356	18
Neonatal causes	3910	37	3072	41
Preterm birth	1083	10	1078	15
Severe infection	1016	10	718	10
Birth asphyxia	894	8	717	10
Congenital anomalies	294	3	270	4
Neonatal tetanus	257	2	58	1
Diarrheal diseases	108	1	50	1
Others	258	2	181	2
Total	10,595		7400	

2000–2003 data: From World Health Organization. Statistical annex. World Health Report 2005—Make every mother and child count; 2005:190. http://www.who.int/whr/2005/en/; 2010 data: Adapted from Liu L, Johnson HL, Cousens S, et al. Global, regional, and national causes of child mortality: An updated systematic review for 2010 with time trends since 2000. *Lancet* 2012;379(9832):2151–61.

in low-income countries. Some interventions protect against deaths from many causes, for example, breast-feeding protects against deaths from diarrhea, pneumonia, and neonatal sepsis; insecticide-treated materials (bed nets, sheets, etc.) protect against deaths from malaria and anemia and also reduce deaths from preterm delivery. However, with the exception of breast-feeding (estimated global coverage of 90%), global coverage of basic interventions for reducing child deaths from common conditions is low. The WHO/UNICEF Child Survival Strategy aims for the universal implementation of a basic package of interventions, along with advocacy for better health financing, and a better political environment for child survival. The United Nations Millennium Development Goals (MDGs) contain benchmarks and targets for countries in reducing child mortality rates, with most countries aiming for a two-thirds reduction in under-5 mortality from the national figure in 1990, by 2015 (9). That time is fast approaching, and now there is a need to see beyond 2015 and set targets beyond the MDGs.

A part of the Child Survival Strategy is integrated case management. To promote a comprehensive model of care for the sick child, WHO developed the Integrated Management of Childhood Illness (IMCI) in 1995. IMCI focuses on primary health workers managing the most important causes of childhood illness, including identification and treatment of children with multiple pathologies. Evaluation of IMCI in Bangladesh and Tanzania showed improvements in the quality of case management and reductions in mortality in some studies, although a direct causation was not established. Over 90 countries adopted the strategy, albeit often in pilot projects or in fragmented and relatively resource-intensive ways that have been difficult to sustain in many countries (10,11).

There is a need for better linking of community health worker programs for recognition of serious illness with early treatment, communication with and transport to rural, district

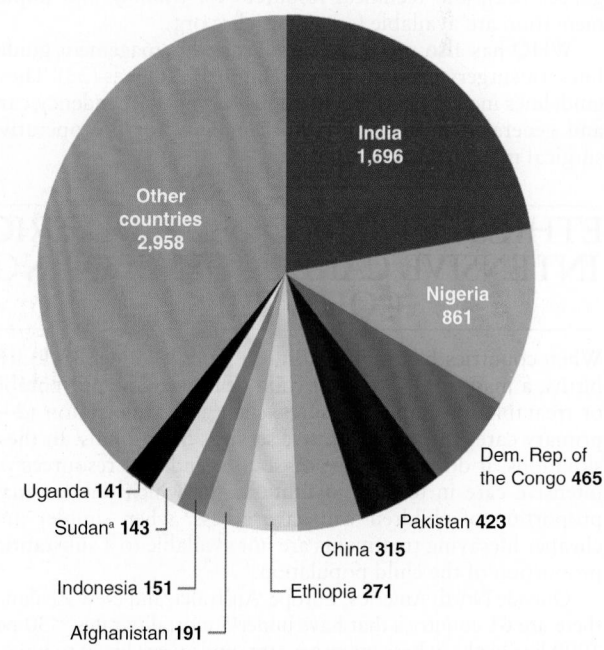

Number of under-five deaths, by country, 2010 (thousands)

India 1,696 · Nigeria 861 · Dem. Rep. of the Congo 465 · Pakistan 423 · China 315 · Ethiopia 271 · Afghanistan 191 · Indonesia 151 · Sudan[a] 143 · Uganda 141 · Other countries 2,958

a. Data refer to Sudan as it was constituted in 2010, before South Sudan seceded on 9 July 2011.

FIGURE 1.2. Half of under-5 deaths occur in just five countries. (From You D, Jones G, Wardlaw T; for United Nations Inter-agency Group for Child Mortality Estimation. *Levels & Trends in Child Mortality: Report 2011.* United Nations Children's Fund, 2011, New York.)

and provincial hospitals. Many children die before getting to a hospital or arrive too late to be saved.

IMPROVING THE QUALITY OF HOSPITAL CARE FOR CHILDREN

Rural, district, or small provincial hospitals play essential roles in preventing child morbidity and mortality. It has been estimated that well-run district hospitals may prevent up to 44% of child deaths that would otherwise occur in the absence of any hospital. Yet, in developing countries, these hospitals are generally understaffed, underresourced, and have little or no ongoing staff education; sick children are usually cared for by general nurses and nonspecialist doctors, who are not specifically trained in the care of seriously ill children. In recognizing these needs, WHO has produced complimentary guidelines on pediatric care for district or provincial hospitals, contained in the Pocket Book of Hospital Care for Children (12). These guidelines include treatment recommendations for the most important causes of child mortality and emphasize that diagnosis and drug treatment are not sufficient for optimal care of the seriously ill child. The Hospital Care for Children guidelines emphasize that triage, emergency care, supportive care (including oxygen, nutrition, and safe administration of IV fluids), monitoring, discharge planning, and follow-up are also essential. These processes of care were found to be deficient in audits of practice in many developing and transitional countries (13–15). There is now increasing evidence that triage and emergency care (16), standardized management of severe malnutrition (17–19), severe pneumonia (20), and neonatal conditions (21) can reduce in-hospital mortality. The WHO Pocket Book of Hospital Care for Children has been applied to varying degrees in 98 low- and middle-income countries, including 50 countries with under-5 childhood mortality rates >40 deaths per 1000 live births (22). It is available in 17 languages (22), and technical resources for training and implementation are available (see www.ichrc.org).

WHO has also produced standardized management guidelines for surgery in countries with limited resources (23). These guidelines include recommendations for high-dependency care and general intensive care with capability for postoperative surgical management of children.

ETHICS OF PROVIDING PEDIATRIC INTENSIVE CARE IN DEVELOPING COUNTRIES

When countries have child mortality rates >30 per 1000 live births, a major proportion of child deaths will be preventable or treatable by simple measures, such as immunization (24), primary care, and basic curative services in hospitals. In these situations, it does not make sense to spend vast resources on intensive care in tertiary institutions for which only a small proportion of children will have access, when simpler and cheaper lifesaving treatments are not available to a substantial proportion of the child population.

Outside North America, Europe, Australia, and New Zealand, there are 61 countries that have under-5 mortality rates <30 per 1000 live births, where intensive care services are likely to have a substantial impact on child survival at a population level.

It is important to note that child mortality rates are not evenly distributed; within most countries, there are regions or districts with higher mortality and others with lower mortality than the national average. The factors behind such uneven distribution of mortality include poverty, lack of access to services, minority groups, and geographical isolation.

An ethical approach to intensive care is therefore problematic. Is it appropriate to provide intensive care to children in middle-class urban areas that have low child mortality, when children in remote rural areas or urban slums do not have access to basic health interventions? Ethical considerations are not constrained by national boundaries, although practical decisions of resource distribution invariably are. Should a child in a rich Western country receive surgery for hypoplastic left heart syndrome when children in poor developing countries have no access to surgery for simple cardiac anomalies such as a ventricular septal defect, or even to antibiotics when they have pneumonia? To a large extent, questions of equity of access and disparity between countries are tempered by practical realities. If children in Western countries were *not* offered palliative surgery for complex cardiac disease, this would not mean that children in developing countries would necessarily be more likely to receive surgery for cardiac defects with better prognoses. These ethical dilemmas will remain while there is income inequity and extreme poverty in the world, but can be partly addressed by greater global cooperation and collaboration between child health institutions, and greater generosity by rich governments in the provision of overseas development aid.

Following the principles of equity, countries should ensure that highly cost-effective health interventions that will reduce mortality are available to *all* children, *before* funding intensive care services. Evidence of extremely high mortality rates and low occupancy rates (because of inability to pay) in adult ICUs in very poor countries emphasizes the limited value of intensive care services in these settings to population health (25).

Some authors have argued for defining a minimum level of care that, based on the nation's resources, must be available for all children, in accordance with the principle of distributive justice (26). In India, for example, it has been suggested that oxygen, intravenous access, fluid resuscitation, antibiotics, and noninvasive application of continuous positive airway pressure (CPAP) in a clean environment be considered the minimum level of intensive care support that should be made available to all children (26). In South Africa, the HIV epidemic has placed a large burden on pediatric intensive care (27,28) and raised complex ethical issues. In the past, authors have suggested a utilitarian approach whereby it is ethically defensible to refuse to ventilate children with severe HIV-associated pneumonia if the resources for doing so were redirected toward programs aimed at preventing mother-to-child transmission (29). Such decisions can never be made in isolation, but rather only after consideration of issues of justice and broader health policies.

There are good practical and ethical arguments for providing selective and limited postoperative intensive care services even where national or regional mortality rates are high. Many patients who have undergone surgery die for want of appropriate supportive care, including mechanical ventilation or close monitoring in the first 24 postoperative hours. The WHO suggests that facilities for intensive care should be available in any hospital where surgery and anesthesia are performed, and has published standards for ICUs in large referral hospitals, district/provincial hospitals, and small hospitals in developing countries (23). These standards outline conditions that should be able to be managed, procedures that should be able to be performed, and personnel, drugs, and equipment that are necessary. Where mechanical ventilation is available, there is a good basis for providing intensive care for a few selected other nonsurgical conditions also, particularly neuromuscular paralysis after snakebite, which is time-limited and likely to result in a good outcome if appropriate supportive care is provided.

Intensive care brings major dilemmas in expectations of survival and extent of treatment. In developing countries, parents often have more conservative attitudes toward withdrawal of life support than treating clinicians, who, in general, have a more utilitarian attitude to resource allocation, with emphasis on avoidance of significant handicap (30). Limitation of treatment is the most commonly reported mode of death in developing country PICUs, and active withdrawal is not widely practiced (31). These have not only ethical but also resource implications and need to be considered when planning pediatric intensive care services for areas with limited human, technical, and financial resources.

An equitable pediatric intensive care service is one for which the indication for admission is the severity of illness and the likelihood of a good outcome; that admission or access to treatment is not limited by inability to pay, and where the provision of that care does not adversely affect the healthcare that can be provided for other children. In developing countries, serious childhood illness is a major economic burden on many families, especially if the care of their child is provided away from their community. The need to cease work and, pay for transport, and admission and prolonged expensive treatment costs can lead to a cycle of poverty and poor health that affects the entire family.

EXPERIENCES OF PEDIATRIC INTENSIVE CARE IN TRANSITIONAL OR MIXED ECONOMIES

Transitional countries in Asia and the Americas, and in South Africa, where there is a wide range of economic and health development, have introduced pediatric intensive care services in the last two decades. Limiting factors to quality of care that were identified in South America included inadequate interdepartmental organization, lack of treatment protocols, too few pediatric intensivists, inferior equipment, lack of qualified technicians, and lack of training and recognition of pediatric intensive care nurses (32). A standard of quality in the PICU was proposed; the highest priorities were training and certification of intensive care specialists, nurses and residents, administration, supervision, protocol development, and equipment upgrading.

The development of pediatric intensive care has also been well documented in Malaysia (33,34). In Kuala Lumpur, introduction of 24-hour staffing by critical care physicians reduced the case-mix–adjusted mortality. Each of these structural and organizational issues was considered to be far more important than invasive hemodynamic monitoring, or costly drugs and equipment.

Nosocomial sepsis is an ever present danger in PICUs and has been a feature of pediatric and neonatal ICUs in developing countries (35–39). Strictly applied evidence-based antibiotic policies, hand washing, and other infection-control procedures are vital to ensure patient safety and should be the cornerstones of intensive care. However, studies have shown that it is difficult to directly implement and sustain Western guidelines for prevention of nosocomial infections in PICUs in developing countries, but that adapted, locally appropriate guidelines should be further studied, and the importance of institutional commitment to rational antibiotic prescribing, and infection-control and microbiology services should be emphasized (40,41).

Models of pediatric intensive care in developing and industrialized countries designed to minimize risk should include the use of safe and simple procedures for appropriate periods, particular attention to drug prescribing and selection of appropriate aims and modes of therapy, including noninvasive methods (42).

Regionalization or Decentralization

There is strong evidence from Western countries that centralization of pediatric intensive care services results in lower mortality than decentralized or fragmented services (43). However, there are several prerequisites for centralized services, including transportation to a tertiary hospital from peripheral facilities and appropriate pretransport management (44). In many developing countries, roads are poor, appropriate vehicles are often not available, and fuel costs are prohibitive (45). Families may be required to pay for fuel costs or a transportation fee, another impediment to access. If transportation is not freely available, pediatric intensive care will not fulfill the principle of equity, because it will not be accessible to a large proportion of the population. Furthermore, children from remote areas may die in transit as their families attempt to make their own ways to hospitals.

Appropriate pretransport management requires good communication infrastructure and, for peripheral hospitals in many countries, improved quality of basic emergency care. Both should be addressed before or in parallel with the development of pediatric intensive care services.

In Malaysia, the outcome for children transferred from community hospitals by nonspecialized transport was no different from those directly admitted to the PICU from within the tertiary institution (46), but this did not take account of critically ill children who never reached the tertiary center. In the same country, the outcome from major trauma managed in district hospitals is significantly worse than major trauma in adults and children managed in tertiary centers. This emphasizes the benefit of centralized management of acute severe illness when this is possible, *and* the importance of improving the quality of care in district hospitals, regardless of whether care is regionalized or decentralized (47). Planning for intensive care should take into consideration the entire spectrum of services necessary to care for the critically ill (48), including prehospital resuscitation, transport, and subspecialty support services.

Making Technology Simpler, Safer, and Cheaper

In the last 10 years, there have been innovations in technology that can make intensive care simpler and less expensive. Particular problems, such as limited and expensive oxygen supplies, are leading to trials of new technologies, for example, a high-flow oxygen concentrator that can deliver bubble-CPAP over a range of fraction of inspired oxygen. This is low cost, easy to use, noninvasive, and independent of cylinder oxygen or medical air. Cheaper pulse oximeters have made oximetry more widely available in operating rooms and increasingly in children's wards (49,50). These innovations have helped make high-dependency services feasible, at <5% of the cost of Western ICUs, which are largely built around expensive electronic mechanical ventilators.

NEONATAL MORTALITY

More than one-third of all under-5 deaths occur in the first month of life (**Table 1.1**), and the majority of neonatal deaths occur in the first few days after birth. Most of the 3 million annual neonatal deaths occur in socioeconomic deprivation in developing countries. Programs to improve neonatal survival are focusing on supervised clean deliveries, essential care of the newborn (early breast-feeding, skin-to-skin warmth), steroids for preterm labor, antibiotics for premature rupture of membranes, maternal tetanus toxoid to prevent neonatal tetanus, prevention of mother-to-child transmission of HIV, and identification of sick neonates requiring referral to hospitals.

Recently, the WHO has produced guidelines for the management of seriously ill neonates in hospitals in developing countries (12). Hospital care for seriously ill neonates should focus first on high-dependency level care; this will include evidence-based antibiotic prescribing, prevention of nosocomial infections, enteral nutrition, safe use of oxygen and intravenous fluids, staff training, and audit and management (21). Where staff resources are limited, involving mothers in high-dependency care has been shown to be highly effective (51). When these interventions are being done optimally, the introduction of bubble-CPAP may be the most effective initial approach to ventilatory support (52). There are many reports of neonatal intensive care in developing countries (53–55) and debate about regionalization of care (56), but these are beyond the scope of this chapter.

As neonatal mortality falls, resources need to be available to deal with the increased morbidity that will occur in survivors. Such morbidities include malnutrition, chronic lung disease, and neurological disease among survivors of prematurity. These have implications for pediatric services, including intensive care.

THE ROLE OF PEDIATRIC INTENSIVE CARE IN COMPLEX EMERGENCIES

Complex emergencies are identified as acute situations in which there is excess mortality (>1 death per 10,000 population per day). They may be due to natural (e.g., earthquake, floods, tsunami) or unnatural (war, famine) disasters, or both. Complex emergencies are dynamic, with variable durations of emergency, recovery, resettlement, rehabilitation, and development phases. After the initial disaster, high mortality rates are usually due to diarrheal disease (including cholera and dysentery), measles, malaria, meningococcal disease, tuberculosis, neonatal causes, trauma, malnutrition, and micronutrient deficiency (57). The United Nations High Commission for Refugees estimates that such circumstances affect up to 10 million people per year.

Many factors impede the delivery of healthcare in such situations, including lack of human resources and referral services, security constraints, poor supervision and coordination, and failure of integration with local health services or transition to a sustainable health system (58). In addition, lack of evidence-based, locally adapted guidelines limit the effectiveness of healthcare in these situations, and contribute to the chaos (57). The earliest priorities in complex emergencies will be management of the initial casualties, for which good emergency care systems and trauma management are vital (59), and intensive care, especially for postoperative management, is optimal. After the immediate emergency phase, addressing high mortality rates in complex emergencies will be through public health measures and developing basic services. The establishment of tent-hospital ICUs in complex emergencies in developing countries has not worked effectively. This has often been done by well-meaning hospitals or universities from unaffected Western countries. Services arrive too late to benefit immediate casualties, staff from Western countries are not experienced in the context, they rotate for brief periods of time, and by the time services are established, the care is predominantly provided to surviving children in the population who have chronic illnesses rather than illness or injury related to the emergency.

CONCLUSIONS AND FUTURE DIRECTIONS

The development of pediatric intensive care services should take account of the level of preventive and basic curative treatment that are available to all children in that country, and the national and subnational mortality rates. It should also be based on an understanding of disease epidemiology in that country or region. Preexisting conditions for pediatric intensive care are good vaccine services, accessible quality primary and first referral level care, under-5 mortality rates <30 per 1000 live births, availability of transportation, and sufficient human resources. Some form of intensive care, with capacity for management of children after surgery, should be available in any hospital where surgery and anesthesia are performed. Innovations in intensive care in developing countries should focus on simpler, safer, and cheaper technology, and this has the potential to influence the way intensive care is practiced worldwide.

Hospitals should be recognized by governments and communities as core social institutions. The quality of care provided in hospitals, and the nature of interactions among health systems, patients, and their families have major consequences for child health, human rights, poverty alleviation, and development, as well as for child survival. In developing and transitional countries, pediatric intensive care specialists have the potential to improve the management of seriously ill children throughout their country, by providing training for staff in smaller hospitals, and by encouraging the building of effective emergency health systems for children, as well as by providing high quality clinical care in tertiary settings where there is a PICU.

References

1. Shann FA, Duncan AW, Brandstater B. Prolonged per-laryngeal endotracheal intubation in children: 40 years on. *Anesth Intens Care* 2006;31(6):663–6.
2. Lozano R, Wang H, Foreman KJ, et al. Progress towards Millennium Development Goals 4 and 5 on maternal child mortality: An updated systematic analysis. *Lancet* 2011;378:1139–65.
3. Liu L, Johnson HL, Cousens S, et al. Global, regional, and national causes of child mortality: An updated systematic review for 2010 with time trends since 2000. *Lancet* 2012;379(9832):2151–61.
4. UNICEF. *Committing to Child Survival: A Promise Renewed.* New York, NY: United Nations Children's Fund, 2012.
5. Duke T. Clinical care for seriously ill children in district hospitals: A global public health issue. *Lancet* 2004;363:1922–3.
6. Duke T, Tamburlini G; Paediatric Quality Care Group. Improving the quality of paediatric care in peripheral hospitals in developing countries. *Arch Dis Child* 2003;88(7):563–5.
7. World Health Organization. Statistical annex. World Health Report 2005—Make every mother and child count; 2005:190. http://www.who.int/whr/2005/en/.
8. Jones G, Steketee RW, Black RE, et al; Bellagio Child Survival Study Group. How many child deaths can we prevent this year? *Lancet* 2003;362:65–71.
9. The World Bank Group. Millennium development goals; 2004. http://www.developmentgoals.org/Child_Mortality.htm. Accessed April 2006.
10. Chopra M, Binkin NJ, Mason E, et al. Integrated management of childhood illness: What have we learned and how can it be improved? *Arch Dis Child* 2012;97(4):350–4.
11. Duke T. Child survival and IMCI: In need of sustained global support. *Lancet* 2009;374(361):362.
12. World Health Organization. *Hospital Care for Children: Guidelines for the Management of Common Illnesses with Limited*

Resources. Geneva, Switzerland: WHO, 2005. http//www.who.int/child-adolescent-health/publications/CHILD_HEALTH/PB.htm and www.ichrc.org.

13. Nolan T, Angos P, Cunha AJLA, et al. Quality of hospital care for seriously ill children in less developed countries. *Lancet* 2001;357:106–10.

14. English M, Esamai F, Wasunna A, et al. Assessment of inpatient paediatric care in first referral level hospitals in 13 districts in Kenya. *Lancet* 2004;363:1948–53.

15. Duke T, Keshishiyan E, Kuttumuratova A, et al. The quality of hospital care for children in Kazakhstan, Republic of Moldova and Russia. *Lancet* 2006;367:919–25.

16. Molyneux E, Ahmad S, Robertson A. Improved triage and emergency care for children reduces inpatient mortality in a resource-constrained setting. *Bull World Health Organ* 2006;84(314):319.

17. Ahmed T, Ali M, Ullah MM, et al. Mortality in severely malnourished children with diarrhoea and use of a standardised management protocol. *Lancet* 2001;353(9168):1912–22.

18. Wilkinson D, Scrace M, Boyd N. Reduction in in-hospital mortality of children with malnutrition. *J Trop Pediatr* 1996;42:114–5.

19. Puoane T, Sanders D, Chopra M, et al. Evaluating the clinical management of severely malnourished children—A study of two rural district hospitals. *South Africa Med J* 2001;91(2):137–41.

20. Duke T, Frank D, Mgone J. Hypoxaemia in children with severe pneumonia in Papua New Guinea. *Int J TB Lung Dis* 2000;5(6):511–9.

21. Duke T, Willie L, Mgone JM. The effect of introduction of minimal standards of neonatal care on in-hospital mortality. *PNG Med J* 2000;43(1–2):127–36.

22. Li MY, Kelly J, Subhi R, et al. Global use of the WHO pocket book of hospital care for children: A systematic survey. *Paediatr Int Child Health* 2012;33(1):4–17.

23. World Health Organization. *Anaesthetic Infrastructure and Supplies. Surgical Care at the District Hospital*. 1st ed. Geneva, Switzerland: WHO, 2003:15-1–15-12.

24. Victora CG, Wagstaff A, Schellenberg JA, et al. Applying an equity lens to child health and mortality: More of the same is not enough. *Lancet* 2003;362(9379):233–41.

25. Ouédraogo N, Niakara A, Simpore A, et al. Intensive care in Africa: A report of the first two years of activity of the intensive care unit of Ouagadougou national hospital (Burkina Faso). *Sante* 2002;12(4):375–82.

26. Sarnaik AP, Daphtary K, Sarnaik AA. Ethical issues in paediatric intensive care in developing countries: Combining Western technology and Eastern wisdom. *Indian J Pediatr* 2005;72(4):339–42.

27. Zar HJ, Apolles P, Argent A, et al. The etiology and outcome of pneumonia in human immunodeficiency virus-infected children admitted to intensive care in a developing country. *Pediatr Crit Care Med* 2001;2(2):108–12.

28. Jeena PM, Wesley AG, Coovadia HM. Admission patterns and outcomes in a paediatric intensive care unit in South Africa over a 25-year period (1971–1995). *Intensive Care Med* 2006;25(1):88–94.

29. Jeena PM, McNally LM, Stobie M, et al. Challenges in the provision of ICU services to HIV infected children in resource poor settings: A South African case study. *J Med Ethics* 2005;31:226–30.

30. Wainer S, Khuzwayo H. Attitudes of mothers, doctors, and nurses towards neonatal intensive care in a developing society. *Pediatrics* 1993;91(6):1171–5.

31. Goh AY-T, Lum LC, Chan PW, et al. Withdrawal and limitation of life support in paediatric intensive care. *Arch Dis Child* 1999;80(5):424–8.

32. Garcia PC. International standard of quality in the paediatric intensive care unit: A model for paediatric intensive care units in South America. *Crit Care Med* 1993;9(suppl):S409–10.

33. Goh AY-T, Lum LC, Chan PW. Paediatric intensive care in Kuala Lumpur, Malaysia: A developing subspecialty. *J Trop Pediatr* 1999;45(6):362–4.

34. Goh AY-T, Lum LC, Abdel-Latif ME. Impact of 24 hour critical care physician staffing on case-mix adjusted mortality in paediatric intensive care. *Lancet* 2006;357:445–6.

35. Jeena P, Thompson E, Nchabeleng M, et al. Emergence of multi-drug resistant *Acinetobacter anitratus* species in neonatal and paediatric intensive care units in a developing country: Concerns about antimicrobial policies. *Ann Trop Paediatr* 2001;21(3):245–51.

36. Musoke RN, Revathi G. Emergence of multidrug-resistant gram-negative organisms in a neonatal unit and the therapeutic implications. *J Trop Paediatr* 2000;46(2):86–91.

37. Khuri-Bulos NA, Shennak M, Agabi S, et al. Nosocomial infections in the intensive care units at a university hospital in a developing country: Comparison with National Nosocomial Infections Surveillance intensive care unit rates. *Am J Infect Control* 1999;27(6):547–52.

38. Merchant M, Karnad DR, Kanbur AA. Incidence of nosocomial infections in a medical intensive care unit and general medical ward in a public hospital in Bombay, India. *J Hosp Infect* 2006;39(2):143–8.

39. Morrow BM, Argent A. Ventilator-associated pneumonia in a paediatric intensive care unit in a developing country with high HIV prevalence. *J Paediatr Child Health* 2009;45(3):104–11.

40. Rhinehart E, Goldmann DA, O'Rourke EJ. Adaptation of the Centers for Disease Control guidelines for the prevention of nosocomial infection in a pediatric intensive care unit in Jakarta, Indonesia. *Am J Med* 1991;91(3B):213S–20S.

41. Berg DE, Hershow RC, Ramirez CA, et al. Control of nosocomial infections in an intensive care unit in Guatamala City. *Clin Infect Dis* 1995;32(9):953–8.

42. Frey B, Argent A. Safe paediatric intensive care. Part 1: Does more medical care lead to improved outcomes? *Intensive Care Med* 2004;30(6):1041–6.

43. Pearson G, Shann F, Barry P, et al. Should paediatric intensive care be centralised? Trent verses Victoria. *Lancet* 1997;349:1213–7.

44. Goh AY-T, Abdel-Latif ME. Transport of critically ill children in a resource-limited setting: Alternatives to a specialized retrieval team. *Intensive Care Med* 2004;30:339.

45. Duke T. Transport of seriously ill children: A neglected global issue. *Intensive Care Med* 2003;29:1414–6.

46. Goh AY-T, Abdel-Latif ME-A, Lum LC-S, et al. Outcome of children with different accessibility to tertiary pediatric intensive care in a developing country—A prospective cohort study. *Intensive Care Med* 2003;29:97–102.

47. Sethi D, Aljunid S, Saperi SB, et al. Comparison of the effectiveness of major trauma services provided by tertiary and secondary hospitals in Malaysia. *J Trauma* 2002;53(508):516.

48. Kissoon N. Child with absent vital signs. *Indian J Pediatr* 2001;68(273):278.

49. Duke T, Subhi R, Peel D, et al. Pulse oximetry: Technology to reduce child mortality in developing countries. *Ann Trop Paediatr* 2009;29(3):165–75.

50. Thoms GMM, McHugh GA, O'Sullivan E. The global oximetry initiative. *Anaesthesia* 2009;62(suppl 1):75–7.

51. Arif MA, Arif K. Low birthweight babies in the third world: Maternal nursing versus professional nursing care. *J Trop Pediatr* 2006;45:278–80.

52. Koyamaibole L, Kado J, Qovu JD, et al. An evaluation of bubble-CPAP in a neonatal unit in a developing country: Effective respiratory support that can be applied by nurses. *J Trop Pediatr* 2006;52(4):249–53.

53. Trotman H, Barton M. The impact of the establishment of a neonatal intensive care unit on the outcome of very low birthweight infants at the University Hospital of the West Indies. *West Indian Med J* 2005;54(5):297–301.

54. Grupo Colaborativo Neocosur. Very-low-birth-weight infant outcomes in 11 South American NICUs. *J Perinatol* 2003;22(1):2–7.

55. Singh M, Deorari AL, Paul VK, et al. Three-year experience with neonatal ventilation from a tertiary care hospital in Delhi. *Indian Pediatr* 1993;30(6):783–9.

56. Paul VK, Singh M. Regionalized perinatal care in developing countries. *Semin Neonatol* 2004;9(2):117–24.

57. Moss WJ, Ramakrishnan M, Storms D, et al. Child health in complex emergencies. *Bull World Health Organ* 2006;84(58):64.

58. Burkle FM Jr, Argent A, Kissoon N, et al. The reality of pediatric emergency mass critical care in the developing world. *Pediatr Crit Care Med* 2011;12:S169–79.

59. Goosen J, Mock C, Quansah R. Preparing and responding to mass casualties in the developing world. *Int J Inj Contr Saf Promot* 2005;12(2):115–7.

CHAPTER 2 ■ IMPACT OF PEDIATRIC CRITICAL CARE ON THE FAMILY, COMMUNITY, AND SOCIETY

LEWIS H. ROMER, DAVID G. NICHOLS, JESSICA MESMAN, HEATHER WOODS BARTHEL, MATT NORVELL, MELISSA J. SACCO, KHALIAH JOHNSON, AND JOS M. LATOUR

KEY POINTS

1 PICU care involves multiple interfaces with the child, family, and community.

2 The model of family-centered care includes the specific context and needs of the family in the care plan.

3 Shared goals and wishes for the good of the child, and the use of templated approaches for conflict resolution can energize successful building of a therapeutic alliance between the child's family and their PICU providers.

4 Early planning for disposition and special needs, including counseling, teaching, and training, is required to optimally provide for care beyond the PICU.

5 Posttraumatic stress disorder is a widely pervasive sequel of critical care that requires early intervention and long-term follow-up.

6 Skillful direction of care in the terminal scenario requires the empathetic anticipation of the needs of family and staff, and well-planned bereavement follow-up care.

7 Individualized approaches to self-care may help providers increase effectiveness and longevity on the job.

8 PICU practice offers the opportunity, beyond the walls of the hospital, for patient advocacy to decrease the incidence of childhood disease and injury.

Circumstances that bring children and their families to the PICU often involve crises that summon the attention of extended families and have ripple effects throughout their communities. Care of the critically ill child therefore has a high **1** impact on families and entire communities. As a consequence, the PICU care team has the opportunity to make a positive impact on a wide range of individuals with diverse backgrounds and perspectives both within and outside the walls of the PICU.

The goals of this chapter include the enhancement of sensitivity, efficiency, and effectiveness in the PICU professional's interactions with the families that they serve. The major focus points are the initial establishment of a working relationship; management of disability, death, and bereavement; provider self-care; and the PICU practitioner's advocacy of child health and safety.

PATIENT- AND FAMILY-CENTERED CARE

The admission of a critically ill child to the PICU involves caring not only for the child, but also for the parents, siblings, grandparents, and significant others. This patient- and family-centered care is now recognized worldwide and has become standard practice in the PICU. The needs of parents may vary by country (or even within a single community) on account of ethnic, social, cultural, or personal differences. Knowledge of both specific parental needs and past parental experiences in a PICU environment is crucial for healthcare workers to set common goals for the process of guiding the parents through the intensive-care period and beyond.

The philosophy of patient- and family-centered care has recently gained reinforcement from politicians, insurance carriers, and patient advocacy groups, but practice styles and parent satisfaction still vary widely (1–3). The American Academy of Pediatrics considers the provision of patient- and family-centered care to be a professional responsibility of the pediatrician (1).

Family Structure and Function

Effective patient- and family-centered care requires the provider team to understand the family's structure and level of functioning. The traditional definition of the family as a two-parent unit in which the mother is the caretaker of the children and the household and the father is the breadwinner has given way to a wide array of family structures.

These changing and diverse aspects of family life increase the need for healthcare workers to understand the family structure of each child admitted to a PICU. Nursing and medical personnel usually initiate this assessment, which is often carried further by social workers, play therapists, and members of the pastoral care team. The initial family assessment includes current marital relationship(s), parental roles, other important persons (e.g., grandparent, clergy), communication and coping patterns, religious background, cultural values, and factors that identify this child as unique (e.g., only child, only son, only daughter, youngest, or eldest). Knowledge of a family's coping style and modes of function provides essential insights for multidisciplinary, psychosocial intervention for the child and family throughout the hospital admission period (4,5). Each family's values, norms, behaviors, and attitudes will heavily influence parental coping with critical illness regardless of the family structure.

11

Dimensions of Patient- and Family-Centered Care

The PICU care team should manage patient- and family-centered care in a structured manner, while considering the dimensions that affect care. There are six dimensions of comprehensive family-centered care related to the roles of the professionals and the parents (**Table 2.1**) (6). Similarly, the Institute for Patient- and Family-Centered Care promotes nine tenets of patient- and family-centered care (http://www.ipfcc. org), which can be grouped into these dimensions.

❷ *Respect for the child and family* is an essential goal of patient- and family-centered care. This dimension addresses *equity* in healthcare. Racial and ethnic disparities in PICU admissions and outcomes of various critical illnesses have been well documented (7). While the causes of disparities may be multifactorial, implicit or explicit bias in care is considered an avoidable cause and unethical. Avoidable inequalities of care are termed *health inequities*, the elimination of which is a declared goal of the World Health Organization 2009 World Health Assembly. Disparities in access to care and quality of service may arise from differences in insurance coverage, economic means, language and cultural barriers, geography, or internecine conflict. PICUs should regularly measure access, care processes, and outcomes by demographic group and socioeconomic status. If differences are found, the care team should search for and eliminate all avoidable causes of inequity as part of routine quality improvement in the PICU.

Providing *information and education* to parents is a dimension that builds a basis for collaboration in the care of the critically ill child. Effective and understandable communication between parents and professionals decreases parental stress and anxiety and fosters trust (see below).

Coordination of care in a PICU entails collaboration with other departments, such as the emergency room and the pediatric wards. A PICU is a transitional unit, with frequent admissions and discharges from and to other locations within the medical center. The PICU team must carefully coordinate transfers to precisely address multiple facets of care, such as the basic daily care plan, diagnostic tests, procedures, and consultations (8). For parents, the continuity of these processes becomes visible only when communications from the professionals are timely, accurate, and linked to a schedule.

TABLE 2.1

SIX DIMENSIONS OF FAMILY-CENTERED CARE

Respect for the child and family	Respect for multicultural and diversity issues, such as race, ethnicity, rituals, norms, values, beliefs, and socioeconomics
Information and education	Communication and teaching in an understandable language
Coordination of care	Timely and accurate coordination of care within a single unit and between units
Physical support	Prevention of suffering from pain and discomfort
Emotional support	Support that facilitates the family's emotional and spiritual needs
Involvement of parents	An open and flexible organization that facilitates parental participation in decision making and care based on the needs of child and family

Parents are concerned about *pain and the provision of comfort measures* for their child. Incomplete communication about painful procedures or pain control may increase parental stress. The explanation and transparent use of validated pain and comfort assessment instruments can improve the recovery of the critically ill child and the well-being of the parent (9). Child life therapists are effective allies in this effort and can also teach nonpharmacologic pain-management strategies to children and parents.

Emotional support to parents hinges upon recognition of the traumatic stress symptoms that are common among parents in the PICU (10). Parent educational and support programs may be valuable in the PICU for both short- and long-term improvement of parents' mental health. Although identification of parental stress and coping strategies in the PICU has been studied extensively, effective interventions to reduce stress are limited in scope. An effective example is the Creating Opportunities for Parent Empowerment (COPE) program, which uses educational media about the emotions and behaviors of sick children to improve the psychosocial outcomes of critically ill children and their mothers (11,12). This educational–behavioral intervention may decrease the incidence of posttraumatic stress disorder (PTSD) among mothers 1 year after PICU admission of their child.

The *involvement of parents* in PICU care is widely incorporated in concepts of best practice. Several policies may foster parental involvement, including open visiting hours, parental participation in decision making, and parental presence during invasive procedures, medical rounds, and resuscitation (13,14). The American Academy of Critical Care Medicine has developed evidence-based clinical practice guidelines for the support of patients and their families during ICU care that address each of these considerations (15). Visiting policies for the PICU vary worldwide—units in the United States and northern Europe trend toward more open policies, whereas other parts of the world have more restrictions (16,17). The physical layout of the PICU has a substantial impact on this issue, as privacy and parental presence on rounds are more easily accommodated in units with single-patient rooms. Advocates for parental involvement in medical rounds have debunked several myths regarding this practice (18). Studies indicating that parental presence during PICU rounds does not affect the length or teaching quality of the rounds support this practice (19). Additionally, a survey study showed that only 5% of the 98 parents that were interviewed regarding parent involvement in medical rounds had concerns about compromised privacy (20).

Resuscitations present challenging circumstances, and the support and incorporation of parental presence at the bedside during resuscitation remains a controversial issue (21,22). The majority of the relevant literature does show beneficial outcomes that have led to positive statements on family presence during resuscitation from both American and European critical care practice associations (15,23).

Communication Skills and the Therapeutic Alliance

The goal of patient- and family-centered care is to forge a collaborative relationship based on mutual respect and open communication between the healthcare professionals and the parents—*the therapeutic alliance*. The foundation of this alliance rests on empathic communication and a consensus that the best interest of the child is of fundamental importance. The therapeutic alliance must acknowledge the parental priorities of empathic communication and proximity to their child (4,24–26). Parents experience predictable

TABLE 2.2

A TEMPLATE FOR COMMUNICATION WITH FAMILIES IN CRISIS

Setting	Introduce self and provide your role. Ask parents preferred method of address.
Perception	Learn parents' perception of situation.
Invitation	Invite parents to set the agenda for the encounter.
Knowledge	Learn the parents' goals of care for each issue they identified while setting their agenda.
	Disseminate appropriate medical explanation in easy-to-understand terms.
Empathy	Express in words and deeds.
	Words: Verbalize understanding, acknowledge emotions.
	Deeds: Attentive eye contact, therapeutic touch, receptive body language.
Summary	Use goals of care to summarize the encounter.
	Close the encounter with identified provider deliverables and a plan to return to update the family on these deliverables.

From Baile WF, Buckman R, Lenzi R, et al. SPIKES-A six-step protocol for delivering bad news: Application to the patient with cancer. *Oncologist* 2000;5:302–11.

moments of heightened anxiety during admission, discharge, or unexpected changes in condition where clear communication becomes especially important (5,27,28). The therapeutic alliance provides a shared context for the team–family communications that are essential to care (29). It is also a framework for additional conflict-resolution and consensus-building measures.

The "SPIKES" model is an approach to difficult conversations that provides a consistent and reassuring framework for providers and families alike (30) (**Table 2.2**). This template incorporates six components: Setting, Perception, Invitation, Knowledge, Empathy, and Summary—a formulaic approach that has been deemed effective for families in crisis (31). The first goal in a difficult encounter is establishing the roles of participants. Introducing one's self and identifying one's provider role orients families. Many families prefer the use of their names rather than being addressed as the generic "Mom" or "Dad" and expect providers to introduce themselves (32). Asking the family whether "this is a good time to talk" gives them some control over the encounter. The next two steps involve determining the family's perception of their child's health: inviting the family to share their chief concerns and goals for the encounter by both asking for their input and using active listening techniques. This will generate insights into the level of understanding and cues for effective vocabulary that may be used for the next step—the knowledge exchange. This is when providers seek to discover the family's specific concerns, correct misconceptions, and establish mutual goals. Empathetic expression, gestures, and body language can help align the care team with the family. Summarizing the discussion, highlighting major issues, and setting a time frame for follow-up are all essential ingredients for assuring families that they have been heard. These conversations are most effective when accomplished and documented within 24–48 hours of the PICU admission (33). **Table 2.3** outlines the strategies necessary for consistent conversations with families to

TABLE 2.3

STRATEGIES FOR RESOLUTION OF TEAM–FAMILY CONFLICT

■ SOURCES OF CONFLICT	■ STRATEGIES FOR RESOLUTION
Uncertainty regarding reversibility of condition and potential for improvement	Determine parents' understanding of likelihood that care will influence outcome.
Suboptimal communication or multiple sources of care-provider input	Provide support, data, and perspective.
	Encourage questions.
	Conduct family and team meetings.
	Incorporate major consultants' input into family meeting.
	Provide unified message from a single care provider.
Parental concerns over invasive monitoring and/or therapy	Explain downside of avoiding monitoring or therapy.
	Explain the need to balance multiple risks in the quest for optimal long-term outcome.
	Explore sources of parental anxiety.
Setbacks or complications in the child's clinical course	Focus on long view and the fact that inconsistent progress is typical of a complex PICU course.
	Explain time-limited trials of new therapies.
	Obtain subspecialty consultation.
Feelings of powerlessness	Emphasize parents' role on the care team.
	Clarify parental expectations regarding their role in decision making.
	Reassure parents regarding the essential role of parental love, support, and encouragement.
Concerns regarding pain	Ensure parental involvement in pain score assessments and patient-, parent-, or nurse-controlled analgesia.
Fear regarding possible death of the child	Validate risk of death and provide context.
	Explain aspects of integrative view of multisystem management—care of the whole child.
	Encourage parents to articulate their personal and family experiences with loss.

TABLE 2.4

PARENTAL NEEDS IN THE PICU

Knowing how the child is treated
Being with the child
Feeling that hope exists
Participating in the care
Unrestricted visiting
Receiving honest answers from the healthcare team
Receiving understandable information
Receiving daily information
Having a place to rest near the PICU
Receiving empathy from professionals

cement a working therapeutic alliance. **Table 2.4** emphasizes the broader context of parental needs that should frame all discussions.

Parental Satisfaction Surveys and Quality Improvement

Integrating patient and parent perspectives in quality and performance indicators is one of the recent trends in healthcare, and this has made parent satisfaction a focus of clinical study in the PICU setting. The development of a methodologically reliable and valid parent satisfaction questionnaire requires a multidisciplinary approach that incorporates parental input (34,35). The implementation of such an instrument may improve collaboration between parents and healthcare professionals. The 7-item Family-Centered Care Scale focuses on parental satisfaction with family-centered care by the nursing team (36). The "EMPATHIC" series focuses on parental satisfaction with family-centered care by the entire PICU care team. It consists of comprehensive questionnaires of varying length and focus that provide both objective metrics and qualitative data, including stories of in-depth parental experiences during PICU admissions (37–39). The shortened 30-item survey can direct and define interventions for quality improvement (**Table 2.5**).

RECOVERY AND REINTEGRATION AFTER CRITICAL ILLNESS

The challenges for the child and family may continue following discharge if the child has a chronic illness or was left with sequelae after their PICU stay. These challenges are often physical, psychosocial, educational, and financial in nature. The PICU team should prepare the family for the reintegration of the child into family and community life.

Discharge Planning

The overarching goal of discharge planning is to empower parents to manage the ongoing recovery of their child with skill and confidence. A traditional view of discharge planning has presented the parents with an integrated set of instructions (for disposition, medications, medical equipment, diet, and medical follow-up) only at the time of discharge from the hospital (40). However, a randomized controlled trial by Melnyk et al. (41) showed that discharge planning beginning as soon as the child is *admitted* to the PICU is far more likely

TABLE 2.5

THE EMPATHIC-30 PARENTAL SATISFACTION QUESTIONNAIRE

Score range: 1–6 (1 = certainly no; 6 = certainly yes)

Information

1. We had daily talks about our child's care and treatment with the doctors.
2. We had daily talks about our child's care and treatment with the nurses.
3. The doctor clearly informed us about the consequences of our child's treatment.
4. We received clear information about the examinations and tests.
5. We received understandable information about the effects of the drugs.

Care and Treatment

6. The doctors and nurses worked closely together.
7. We were well prepared for our child's discharge by the doctors.
8. We were well prepared for our child's discharge by the nurses.
9. The team was alert to the prevention and treatment of pain in our child.
10. Our child's comfort was taken into account by the doctors.
11. Our child's comfort was taken into account by the nurses.
12. Every day we knew who was responsible for our child, regarding the doctors.
13. Every day we knew who was responsible for our child, regarding the nurses.

Organization

14. The team worked efficiently.
15. The IC unit could easily be reached by telephone.
16. There was enough space around our child's bed.
17. The IC unit was clean.
18. Noise in the IC unit was muffled as well as possible.

Parent Participation

19. During our stay, the staff regularly asked for our experiences.
20. We were actively involved in decision making on care and treatment of our child.
21. We were encouraged to stay close to our child.
22. We had confidence in the doctors.
23. We had confidence in the nurses.
24. Even during intensive procedures, we could always stay close to our child.

Professional Attitude

25. We received sympathy from the doctors.
26. We received sympathy from the nurses.
27. The team worked hygienically.
28. The team respected the privacy of our child and of us.
29. The team showed respect for our child and for us.
30. At admission we felt welcome.

From Latour JM, Duivenvoorden HJ, Tibboel D, et al. The shortened Empowerment of Parents in The Intensive Care 30 questionnaire adequately measured parent satisfaction in pediatric intensive care units. *J Clin Epidemiol* 2013;66:1045–50.

to mitigate the significant psychological risks to parent and child associated with critical illness. An effective intervention program included the following elements:

- Phase I (6–16 hours after *admission* to PICU)
  - Audiotaped and written information on the range of behaviors exhibited by young children during and after hospitalization.

- A directed program for involvement in the child's physical and emotional care while in the PICU.
- Phase II ("booster intervention" upon transfer to general medical ward)
  - Review of audiotaped and written information received at PICU admission.
  - Completion of a parent–child workbook involving puppet play, therapeutic medical play, and discussion of a book about a young child who successfully manages a stressful hospitalization.
- Phase III (a scripted telephone call 2–3 days after hospital discharge)
  - Reinforce information on typical child emotion and behavior after critical illness.
  - Discuss positive parental coping mechanisms.
  - Encouragement to continue workbook activities.

Table 2.6 lists other major objectives of discharge planning.

TABLE 2.6

DISCHARGE PLANNING OBJECTIVES

Determine best practical disposition (rehabilitation hospital vs. home).

Help parents gain access to insurance programs and other financial services for children with chronic illnesses.

Ensure that parents are trained in cardiopulmonary resuscitation and the use of relevant medical technology.

Arrange for home nursing.

Arrange for a medical technology company to service medical equipment in the home.

Instruct parents on discharge medications, and work with physician staff to simplify the medication list where possible.

Connect the parents with support and patient advocacy groups.

Give the family a realistic understanding of the challenges they face.

Spread hope and optimism to the child and family.

Physical Aspects of Recovery and Reintegration

At the most basic level, the child returning home after a prolonged PICU stay has several physical needs. Critical illness, mechanical ventilation, and prolonged immobilization contribute to ICU-acquired weakness secondary to critical illness polyneuropathy or myopathy (42). (See also Chapter 53.) In addition to good nutrition, family members can provide physical therapy, which serves both to improve mobility and strength and to provide an opportunity for bonding and renewing alliances with the child. Conversely, data from adult studies (43) suggest that caregiver dysfunction in mood or physical health delays strength recovery, thus underscoring the importance of the parental empowerment and psychological preparation program described above.

Newborns and infants may be malnourished after a prolonged PICU stay but usually recover by 6 months after discharge (44). With proper attention to nutritional support during the PICU stay, older children generally avoid malnutrition. Nevertheless, parents require very specific instructions on proper diet for the returning child. When possible, oral feeding should be encouraged because it also provides an opportunity for parent–child bonding. Tube feedings to maintain adequate caloric intake may be required in some children, especially those with severe neurologic disability. Conversely,

a small subset of patients with morbid obesity and upper airway obstruction requires caloric restriction as part of their discharge plan.

Technologic Aspects of Recovery and Reintegration

Numerous technologic devices now support care in the home. These devices range from mechanical ventilators to feeding tubes, dialysis machines, infusion pumps, and monitoring devices. In addition, many children have implanted devices (defibrillators, ventriculoperitoneal shunts, etc.). Most devices have achieved a remarkable safety record and are clearly beneficial in extending the lives of chronically ill children outside of the hospital (45,46). Parents need to understand the technology and its use with their child, know how to troubleshoot problems, and have adequate backup supplies and an alternate power source. A home safety inspection for reliable power, phone communication, and transportation is considered mandatory before the discharge of a technology-dependent child. Adequate preparation in these areas will maximize both the safety of the child and the psychological health of the parents.

Most families develop rather astounding mastery of the technical details. The far greater challenge is to adapt to the disruption of "normal" family life that occurs during the care of technology-dependent children. Alarms ring. Interventions must be performed on schedule. Changes in the child's condition require urgent parental attention. These realities will inevitably stress the normal rhythm of family life. Parental sleep deprivation often results (47). If families are to manage a technology-dependent child at home, parents and medical professionals must devise a reasonable care schedule that includes family members, supported by visiting nurses and other medical professionals. If families cannot cope, the physician should assist the family in defining a care plan that allows for care in another venue. Options include a children's home, a medical day care facility, or a pediatric chronic care hospital. The availability and specific services of each of these options will vary widely by country and region.

Psychological Aspects of Recovery and Reintegration—The Child

A short visit to the doctor may frighten a child. A prolonged stay in a PICU marked by organ failure, invasive procedures, and separation from family and familiar surroundings may lead to lasting neuropsychiatric damage in the form of PTSD. There has been general recognition that the *Diagnostic and Statistical Manual of Mental Disorders (DSM-IV and DSM-V)* definitions of PTSD do not accommodate the behavioral and developmental characteristics of children (48). Therefore, Scheeringa et al. (49) have proposed an alternative algorithm for the diagnosis of PTSD in children (**Table 2.7**).

PTSD is a clinical syndrome following extreme traumatic stress that is accompanied by fear, agitation, recurrent intrusive thoughts, avoidance of stimuli associated with the trauma (or generalized withdrawal), and persistent physiologic arousal for >1 month after the traumatic event. If symptoms occur within 1 month after the traumatic event, they are labeled "acute stress disorder" and predict later PTSD. Although estimates vary, a systematic review of the literature suggests that PTSD is highly prevalent (10%–28%) among children who have experienced critical illness (50).

Studies are divided on whether the severity of the critical illness or the number of invasive procedures is associated with PTSD; however, pre–critical illness behavioral or

TABLE 2.7

DSM-IV CRITERIA FOR PTSD SHOWING ALTERNATIVE ALGORITHM CHANGES

■ DIAGNOSTIC CRITERIA FOR POST-TRAUMATIC STRESS DISORDER

A. The person has been exposed to a traumatic event in which the following were present:

1. The person experienced, witnessed, or was confronted with an event or events that involved actual or threatened death or serious injury, or a threat to the physical integrity of self or others (no change from *DSM-IV*).

B. The traumatic event is persistently reexperienced in one (or more) of the following ways:

1. Recurrent and intrusive distressing recollections of the event, including images, thoughts, or perceptions. *Note: In young children, repetitive play or repetitive behaviors may occur in which themes or aspects of the trauma are expressed. Furthermore, recollections may appear not to be distressing in young children.*
2. Recurrent distressing dreams of the event. *Note: In children, there may be frightening dreams without recognizable content.*
3. Acting or feeling as if the traumatic event was recurring (includes a sense of reliving the experience, illusions, hallucinations, and dissociative flashback episodes, including those that occur on awakening or when intoxicated). *Note: In young children, trauma-specific reenactment may occur.*
4. Intense psychological distress at exposure to internal or external cues that symbolize or resemble an aspect of the traumatic event.
5. Physiological reactivity on exposure to internal or external cues that symbolize or resemble an aspect of the traumatic event.

C. Persistent avoidance of stimuli associated with the trauma and numbing of responsiveness (not present before the trauma), as indicated by one or more of the following:

1. Efforts to avoid thoughts, feelings, or conversations associated with the trauma.
2. Efforts to avoid activities, places, or people that arouse recollections of the trauma.
3. Inability to recall an important aspect of the trauma.
4. Markedly diminished interest or participation in significant activities. *Note: In young children, this may be manifest as constriction in play.*
5. Feeling of detachment or estrangement from others (e.g., unable to have loving feelings). *Note: In young children, this may be manifest as social withdrawal.*
6. Restricted range of affect.
7. Sense of foreshortened future (e.g., does not expect to have a career, marriage, children, or a normal life span).

D. Persistent symptoms of increased arousal (not present before the trauma), as indicated by two (or more) of the following:

1. Difficulty falling or staying asleep.
2. Irritability, outbursts of anger, or *extreme temper tantrums in young children.*
3. Difficulty concentrating.
4. Hypervigilance.
5. Exaggerated startle response.

E. Duration of the disturbance (symptoms in Criteria B, C, and D) is more than 1 month.

F. The disturbance causes clinically significant distress or impairment in social, occupational, or other important areas of functioning.

Note: Criteria specific to children are in italics. Please also see the *DSM-V* modifications to this approach in paragraph 3, page 9 of the following web document: http://www.dsm5.org/Documents/changes from dsm-iv-tr to dsm-5.pdf.
From Scheeringa MS, Zeanah CH, Cohen JA. PTSD in children and adolescents: Toward an empirically based algorithma. *Depress Anxiety* 2011;28:770–82.

developmental problems as well as a parental psychiatric diagnosis appear to be associated with an increased risk of PTSD after critical illness (50). The origins of this disorder are not fully understood because it may occur even among children who appear to have been adequately sedated for invasive procedures. Yet the consequences of PTSD are quite clear in the form of diminished intellectual and social functioning, heightened parental stress, and even decreased immunocompetence (51).

Given the prevalence and destructive impact of PTSD, the authors recommend that every child and parent who has endured a prolonged critical illness undergo screening for this disorder (**Table 2.7**). If a diagnosis of PTSD is established, a simple explanation and demystification of the symptomatology opens the door for cognitive and pharmacologic therapy for the child and/or parents. The primary care physician and appropriate school officials should also be alerted. A Cochrane database systematic review of psychological therapies for childhood PTSD secondary to various etiologies (domestic violence, sexual assault, motor vehicle trauma, etc.) found

cognitive-based therapy (CBT) to be effective within 1 month of completing therapy, with lasting benefit for up to 1 year after therapy (52). Although some guidelines have suggested combination CBT and pharmacotherapy (usually with an SSRI), the evidence to date is insufficient to conclude that combination therapy is superior to CBT alone (53).

Psychological Aspects of Recovery and Reintegration—The Family

Even in the absence of a formal diagnosis of PTSD, the parents and siblings experience stress as they attempt to reintegrate the now chronically ill child after a PICU stay. Carnevale et al. identified six principal themes of this stress: (a) the reality of overwhelming parental responsibility, (b) the intense desire for a "normal" family life that seems no longer attainable, (c) confrontation with the outside world that seems to devalue the life of the chronically ill child, (d) social isolation, (e) uncertainty about the child's (or sibling's) feelings, and (f) a sense of unfairness and helplessness in the face of a moral order that allows child and family suffering. Despite the complex tensions produced by these feelings, most families also report a sense of enrichment by the presence of the injured or chronically ill child who is so demanding of their care (54).

The management of stress begins in the hospital with an explanation about the nature of the stress and reassurance that their response is common and expected under the circumstances. The next steps involve teaching parents about the behaviors and emotions that their child may display after hospitalization, and fostering parental involvement in the child's physical and emotional care, services that may be provided or augmented by child life therapists. Formal stress-management techniques may also be associated with reduced depression and stress among parents (41). Healthcare professionals should also ensure that attention is directed toward fostering optimal functioning of the entire family unit (55).

The financial burdens associated with the care of a PICU survivor may also be substantial if the child is left with chronic disability. Adequate health insurance is a tremendous help for these families, but out-of-pocket finances are still necessary for care, as indicated by the greater financial burden that low-income families assume even after controlling for insurance status (56). In the United States and in some European countries, most families with a ventilator-dependent child can receive at least 8 hours of in-home nursing assistance per day if federal support programs are utilized properly. A social worker or other medical professional knowledgeable in federal assistance programs for children with chronic disabilities should counsel the parents.

Reintegration into the Community

The return to school exemplifies the milestone of reintegration into the community for the child. Parents must educate teachers, the principal, and the school nurse about medications, medical equipment, behavior patterns, and special needs. Equally important is the parent's role as a relentless advocate for the child to receive the specialized services necessary to enhance the chances for learning and social adaptation. The primary care pediatrician must support the parents in this advocacy role, serve as a resource for the school in the individual child's case, and generally provide guidance on the proper nurturing of the disabled child within the school system.

PREPARING FOR AND RESPONDING TO DEATH

To cope with the death of their child, parents need support from their relatives, friends, and the involved staff members. The staff, in turn, should have well-established policies, procedures, and role clarity for end-of-life care that is sensitive to the social, cultural, and other unique circumstances of each family.

Anticipating Loss

Unexpected death shortly after admission complicates the supportive role of the PICU team as they struggle to care for a shattered family in shock. It is helpful if one team member stays with the parents to explain the course of events and to outline necessary medical and legal procedures. In a case of suspected *child abuse*, parents have not only lost their child but have also become part of a police investigation. (See also

Chapter 62.) Even in this challenging situation, PICU caregivers must strive to remain supportive to parents, while providing appropriate medical information to child protective authorities and the police. If emotions threaten to overwhelm the PICU team attending the death of a child abuse victim, it may be useful for specific team members to focus on parental support, while others interface with government authorities.

When death is expected, the staff has the opportunity to prepare parents for the process of dying. Although one may recognize similar patterns of grief and distress in families of different backgrounds, each situation requires an individual approach. Each parent must be allowed a role in the end-of-life care of the dying child. The PICU team helps parents develop their roles by listening, understanding, and helping them to interpret the unfolding events. Resolution of any disagreements between the care team and the family over end-of-life care may benefit from support by a third party, such as a social worker or family advocate.

Parents should be prepared for the changing appearance of the child, including gasping and other potential responses of the dying body. Great care should be taken to ensure that symptoms around the end of life are adequately managed and that the child's overall comfort level is optimized. The appearance of a dying child may provoke not only grief, but also fear, alarm, and even revulsion among some family members, and staff should be prepared for a variety of family member responses.

The family should be given advice on pragmatic issues, such as access to external support networks, funeral arrangements, death registration, and postmortem examination. Informing family is crucial, but other details are equally important. The staff must seek out insights into the specific questions, wishes, fears, and expectations that parents might have. Some parents want to take their child home before dying or initiate religious or spiritual rituals. These requests may require planning and communication with other parties or authorities.

Cultural Context of Death and Dying

Death in the PICU, regardless of the mode, occurs within a specific sociocultural context. Modern technology has multiplied the possible pathways to the end of a child's life in a PICU. Potential pathways include death despite active treatment, brain death, limitation of critical care (nontreatment), and active withdrawal of life support. Goh et al. (57) stress the fact that limitation of critical care as a common mode of death is based on a Western ethical frame of justification and may therefore be inappropriate for people with other cultural backgrounds. Increasing cultural diversity in most societies makes it important to take these cultural differences into account. (For an extensive discussion on the implications of cultural differences in end-of-life care, see Appendix D, pp. 509–552, of the Institute of Medicine publication *When Children Die* (58)). Factors in planning for the mode of death extend beyond medical considerations and include the family's social relations, religion, and other responsibilities, as well as the previous personal experiences of the physicians—each of these factors may explain some of the various modes of death chosen within the context of Western medicine (57). The death of a child in a PICU in Anglo-Saxon–influenced countries is the outcome of decision making that includes a deliberative process in which the parents participate. In the more Greek/Latin-influenced part of Europe, most children in the PICU may die despite active treatment (59). In Europe, clinicians do not give away the final authority over withdrawal of life support (60). In Islamic culture, withdrawal of life support may not be an option. At the other end of the spectrum, the Dutch parliament recently passed a law specifically allowing various categories of physician-assisted dying for children above 12 years of age (61). Despite these evident differences, every parent is unique and acts accordingly, sometimes in ways that are contrary to specific cultural attitudes. Collaboration between the PICU team and a hospital chaplain or local faith leaders may improve the recognition and support of needs that are specific to families' cultural, religious, and individual needs.

Decision Making and End-of-Life Care

The physician usually initiates the discussion regarding discontinuation of treatment; however, parents may consider this possibility even before the physician raises the issue (62). The choice between withdrawal and limitation of life support is not always clear for parents or clinicians. Although at this juncture some parents defer to physicians, they must live with the ultimate decision for years to come as they try to make the best choice they can, given their life experience (63). Therefore, involvement of families in this decision-making process should be encouraged but not demanded.

To be able to participate effectively in the decision-making process, parents must be well informed about their child's condition, level of discomfort, prognosis, and available treatments and their consequences. Parental assessment of the child's physical and emotional suffering plays an important role in the decision about the continuation of life support (62). It should be clear for parents that palliative care, with its focus on prevention and relief of physical and emotional suffering, is a major part of the overall care policy throughout the remainder of the child's life and that it does not necessarily preclude cure-directed or life-prolonging care (64).

Practice patterns regarding the involvement of the child in the decision-making process vary widely and depend on the child's age, level of understanding, and physical condition. Where possible, children should be informed about their condition, and their wishes should be respected.

Nurses are often the team members who are most involved in the care of the child and the support of the parents throughout the PICU stay. They instruct the family about their child's treatment, show them around the PICU, inform them in everyday language about the child's condition, and function as their touchstones. Despite the primacy of this relationship, many studies show that bedside nurses are underrepresented in decision-making meetings (64).

A Presence during Death and Dying

The presence of important individuals during the dying process may add meaning and comfort to a grieving family. Some parents try to preserve the relationship with their dying child by being present and by touching and talking to their child. Meert et al. (65) stress that a spiritual element is associated with the efforts of parents to stay connected with their child. Memories of specific events, such as holding the child on their lap, or tangible mementoes can be considered in the search for meaning and the need to be connected that ensue over the months following the death of a child. Other related imperatives include the parents' acceptance of the child's death and their perception that care of their child has been given with compassion and respect and that the ultimate trust invested in the care team has been upheld.

Ideally, families should be offered a "family advocate"— someone separate from the PICU team whose sole function is to comfort and advocate on behalf of the family. The parents might prefer the presence of a pastoral care provider as their advocate, especially when rituals such as praying and reading sacred texts are vital elements that strengthen the family

through hope and faith. The PICU team should know the parents' religious affiliation and avoid misunderstandings by first checking to determine whether specific pastoral care is desired. The care team should be sensitive to conflicting needs between parents, especially in cases of divorce and blended families. Often a sympathetic explanation or interpretation of the conflicting needs followed by a renewed focus on the child may avoid unnecessary friction between the parents.

In cases in which it is age appropriate, sibling involvement in end-of-life care is an important part of their bereavement process. Their grief and their capability to help or understand should not be dismissed. However, young children are not always able to comprehend the situation or to interpret the intense grief of their parents, and it is essential to regularly re-evaluate their emotional and intellectual capacity to deal with the situation. The involvement of child life therapists can often help children of varied ages and developmental levels cope with their own grief and loss and that of surrounding family members.

During the process of dying, the staff carefully tries to deal with the needs of children and their families. The family tries to cope with their situation by finding meaning in what is happening and by living day to day (64). Through a constant redefinition of the situation they are confronting, parents try to prepare for death and, at the same time, preserve their relationship with their child. Involvement of family in the end-of-life care of their child is a way to endorse the parental roles as child's original caregiver, provider of love, and decision maker (66). Marginalization of parents during the process of care will result in feelings of helplessness. Preservation of the child–parent relationship is an important parental coping mechanism, and fathers and mothers may exhibit different types of coping mechanisms. If one parent (often the father) withdraws when he knows his child is dying, the reasons should be explored and an opportunity provided for the inclusion of the withdrawn parent in the planning of care. Care team members' open admissions of sorrow for the loss can be helpful for parents, as they allow parents to perceive that their child is special (67).

Coping Strategies

The emotional bond between parent and child lingers after a child's death. Staff members aid parents in coping with their loss by helping them toward the recognition that strengthening the emotional bond with their child helps them to integrate the loss. After their child's death, parents are allowed to spend as much time alone with their child as they wish and bid farewell in quietude. In addition to privacy, social and religious rituals may be important parts of the bereavement process. Physical care, such as touching, bathing, and dressing their child after death, may be an important part of the bereavement process. Such contact after their child has died may reduce parents' sense of guilt and improve their self-worth. These activities can act as a corridor for the (nursing) staff in their effort to help parents with their grief. Mementoes, such as a foot- or handprint or a lock of hair, may be offered as tangible links to the child during the grieving process and beyond (68). Overall, these postmortem practices may be very helpful to families, but it is important to note that they are not universally accepted by all ethnic groups.

Follow-up Meetings—Moments of Reflection

Follow-up meetings are crucial to help parents deal with the loss of their child. They are equally important for parents who lose a child suddenly and for those for whom the child's death was expected. Bereavement meetings offer the opportunity for reflection on the death of the child in several

TABLE 2.8

KEY POINTS IN COMMUNICATION WITH BEREAVED FAMILIES

1. Use open-ended questions, for example, "How has the death affected you?"
2. Emphasize support and encouragement and practical problem solving.
3. Prepare for strong, often volatile, reactions that may be directed at you.
4. Understand that well-intended questions such as "Surely you're feeling better today?" can be counterproductive.
5. Show genuine concern and caring without being patronizing, avoid comments such as "You should be getting over this by now."
6. Referral to others if the care provider's personal needs threaten to interfere with the process.
7. Stay nonjudgmental as attempts to explain the loss will usually be met with resentment or rejection.
8. Avoid suggestions that they have to feel better "for the sake of others."
9. Acknowledge the gravity of the situation for the person.
10. Nurture hope by normalizing the process, and reinforce expectation that loss will be accommodated and that the pain will subside.

Love AW. Progress in understanding grief, complicated grief, and caring for the bereaved. *Contemp Nurse* 2007;27:73–83.

ways, and Cook et al. (69) propose some key elements to be included in them. The staff can explain in more detail what has happened on the basis of all of the available information. The parents can use this meeting to express their concerns and ask for clarification—it is important to remember that they are carrying around their own questions and dissonant memories. The intensivist should allow enough time (often several weeks) before the follow-up meeting in order for the staff to collect relevant information (including postmortem results when available) and for families to reflect on what has happened. A visit to the PICU where the child died can be a crucial element of the follow-up and helpful in the grieving process but must be done on a voluntary basis only. Follow-up meetings are specifically aimed at a form of retrospection that allows parents to move on with their lives. Table 2.8 presents the key points in the syntax of caring for the bereaved.

Bereavement and the Supportive Network

Factors such as the family of origin, family structure, other recent losses, and financial and vocational impact of hospitalizations are all important modulators of the grieving process. Strobe and Schut's Dual Process Model provides a helpful illustration of the ways individuals may vacillate between focusing on the loss and focusing on the future path to restoration after the loss (70).

It is important to ensure that adequate support is available beyond what is provided by the PICU team. Indeed, some investigators express their concern about the dominance of staff members as the primary support network during the process of dying (62). They stress the need for families to maintain and strengthen their private support network. It is also advisable to facilitate the involvement of other support networks, such as hospital or community bereavement support counselors or support groups, religious communities, and palliative care programs in order to establish continuity of care after death.

GRIEF EXPERIENCES OF PICU STAFF

Staff members will experience a wide range of emotions while caring for a dying child. When a child's stay in the PICU lasts several months, the emotional bonding process may cause staff members to identify with the parents (71). Caring for a chronically ill child frequently leads to a high level of attachment. Strong emotional engagement does not always distort professional judgment—it may cause staff to better relate to families' responses. Nor is emotional detachment always a virtue, given that it can blind people's awareness of suffering and lead to medical decisions that are insensitive to parents' needs. Furthermore, parents understand the genuine emotional expressions of staff as supportive, which helps them in their process of grief.

Considering the high level of involvement of PICU staff in the dying process and their exposure to many deaths, careful attention to their grief experience is also necessary. More than casual and occasional support from colleagues, family, and friends is needed to help staff through these cases. A study of the grief experiences of PICU nurses describes how the intensity and duration of their grief are related to personal experiences, to their relationships with the child and the family, and to their individual perceptions of professional responsibility and personal mortality (72,73). High levels of attachment to the child and/or the family affect the depth and duration of feelings of sadness. More experienced nurses feel less overwhelmed by their feelings of sadness and anger than do their less experienced colleagues. Ideal notions about why a child should die, in what way, and with what type of involvement from the PICU staff may clash painfully with the reality of the situation. Some argue that such situations of dissonance have a strong effect on grief responses (73). Personal grief is an ongoing learning process, and more experienced colleagues can play a supportive role in this process. To cope with their own feelings of grief, some PICU nurses share their feelings with colleagues, whereas others prefer a more private sphere in which to express their sadness. Other coping strategies are self-nurturing, maintaining a balance between involvement and detachment while the child is dying, and seeking closure of the relationship with the family after the child has died.

BURNOUT AND SELF-CARE IN THE PEDIATRIC ICU

The formidable nature of working in a PICU may impact the emotional and physical experiences of healthcare providers. One commonly encountered result of intensive care is burnout—a state in which providers develop a defensive response to prolonged or repetitive exposure to demanding events that cause psychological strain (74). Compassion fatigue, primary and secondary traumatization, and posttraumatic stress are processes that may also be experienced by clinicians in pediatric critical care, and each of these can have an impact on productivity, quality of care, and overall personal well-being (75,76).

Self-care can be defined as exercises or practices that promote wellness and the ability to maintain balance between the input and output of energy in one's personal and professional life (77). PICU clinicians will likely benefit from both collegial and individual pursuit of self-care. Regular peer group, or "debriefing," meetings after difficult scenarios can serve as an important source of support for the maintenance of morale, overall health, and emotional well-being of PICU staff by

TABLE 2.9

SELF-CARE STRATEGIES

Physical	Emotional/Cognitive
Stretching	Giving oneself permission to cry
Regular exercise	Writing
Breathing techniques	Having time alone
Regular medical check-ups	Talking through feelings
Massage	Silence
Hot baths/showers	Meditation
Regular sleep	Making time for "play" (gardening, dance, travel, cooking, etc.)

Relational	Spiritual
Connecting with family/friends	Spending time in nature
Time with children	Prayer
Setting appropriate boundaries	Attending worship service
Communicating in the face of conflict	Reading sacred scripture
	Listening to or making music

From Jones SH. A self-care plan for hospice workers. *Am J Hosp Palliat Care* 2005;22:125–8.

validating the shared unique bond of operating in a strenuous and high-stress environment (78). On the individual level, experienced clinicians have described a variety of effective strategies (including mindfulness techniques, leisure activity, quality time with family, and psychotherapy (79)). Personalized self-care plans allow professionals to monitor their own feelings and behaviors, set appropriate limits, and find meaning in the practice of medicine by implementing customized collages of techniques that bring stress relief and renewal to their lives. While **Table 2.9** includes a variety of self-care components, the most important principles here are the identification of approaches that work best for the individual and a commitment to practicing them regularly.

THE ROLE OF THE PEDIATRIC CRITICAL CARE PROFESSIONAL IN SOCIETY

The PICU provides willing observers with a unique window on society; themes and patterns of childhood illness and injury can be indicators of the effects of public policy. Despite these insights, the pressures of patient care, institutional and academic responsibilities, and professional development leave little time in the work life of the critical care practitioner for the pursuit of child advocacy. Moreover, most healthcare professionals are not conversant with the process and bureaucracy of legislative bodies and human-service delivery systems. These realities are powerful supporters of the status quo. However, strategies for the reduction of preventable disease and injury are essential elements of our commitment to the improvement of child health and safety. Furthermore, each publicly visible effort that the pediatric critical care community makes in this regard has the potential to inspire the next generation of PICU professionals and child health advocates. Society entrusts pediatric critical care providers with the care of its sickest children. An extension of that trust is the confidence that caring professionals will act on opportunities for responsible citizenship by working toward the overall improvement of child health and safety.

CONCLUSIONS AND FUTURE DIRECTIONS

Recent research into the impact of the PICU has yielded important indicators of difficulty with communication and adaptation in the PICU environment. The next step includes the development and testing of benchmarks and programs that can be used to improve the management of PICU stressors for both families and PICU staff. Reduction in the incidence of psychosocial sequelae for our patients may require the development of multidisciplinary PICU follow-up programs. The challenge of PTSD should be addressed similarly through integrated strategies for the prevention, early detection, and treatment of graded severities of this disorder. Specific data are needed regarding the association of PTSD with specific sedative and analgesic strategies during invasive procedures in the PICU (80).

PICU care at the end of life could be improved by developing the broad implementation of training and team building for care providers, using real-time interaction with standardized patients (81). These efforts must encompass the entire family of PICU professionals, including all practitioner- and student-level frontline personnel: physicians, nurses, respiratory therapists, extracorporeal membrane oxygenation specialists, social workers, psychologists, and pastoral care providers. Careful attention to provider self-care can strengthen team effectiveness at all levels.

Finally, a coordinated and broadly based effort is necessary to more effectively and immediately channel awareness of pressing child health–related issues into public policy.

ACKNOWLEDGMENT

The authors thank Drs. Jason Custer, Jamie Schwartz, and Hal Shaffner for helpful discussions.

References

1. Committee on Hospital Care and Institute for Patient- and Family-Centered Care. Patient- and family-centered care and the pediatrician's role. *Pediatrics* 2012;129:394–404.
2. Latour JM. Is family-centred care in critical care units that difficult? A view from Europe. *Nurs Crit Care* 2005;10:51–3.
3. Latour JM, Haines C. Families in the ICU: Do we truly consider their needs, experiences and satisfaction? *Nurs Crit Care* 2007; 12:173–4.
4. Atkins E, Colville G, John M. A "biopsychosocial" model for recovery: A grounded theory study of families' journeys after a paediatric intensive care admission. *Intensive Crit Care Nurs* 2012;28:133–40.
5. Colville G, Darkins J, Hesketh J, et al. The impact on parents of a child's admission to intensive care: Integration of qualitative findings from a cross-sectional study. *Intensive Crit Care Nurs* 2009;25:72–9.
6. Latour JM, van Goudoever JB, Hazelzet JA. Parent satisfaction in the pediatric ICU. *Pediatr Clin North Am* 2008;55:779–90, xii–xiii.
7. Turner D, Simpson P, Li SH, et al. Racial disparities in pediatric intensive care unit admissions. *South Med J* 2011;104:640–6.
8. Vats A, Goin KH, Villarreal MC, et al. The impact of a lean rounding process in a pediatric intensive care unit. *Crit Care Med* 2012;40:608–17.
9. Ista E, van Dijk M, van Achterberg T. Do implementation strategies increase adherence to pain assessment in hospitals? A systematic review. *Int J Nurs Stud* 2013;50:552–68.
10. Colville G, Cream P. Post-traumatic growth in parents after a child's admission to intensive care: Maybe Nietzsche was right? *Intensive Care Med* 2009;35:919–23.

11. Melnyk BM, Feinstein NF. Reducing hospital expenditures with the COPE (Creating Opportunities for Parent Empowerment) program for parents and premature infants: An analysis of direct healthcare neonatal intensive care unit costs and savings. *Nurs Adm Q* 2009;33:32–7.

12. Melnyk BM, Crean HF, Feinstein NF, et al. Testing the theoretical framework of the COPE program for mothers of critically ill children: An integrative model of young children's post-hospital adjustment behaviors. *J Pediatr Psychol* 2007;32:463–74.

13. Eggly S, Meert KL. Parental inclusion in pediatric intensive care rounds: How does it fit with patient- and family-centered care? *Pediatr Crit Care Med* 2011;12:684–5.

14. Ladak LA, Premji SS, Amanullah MM, et al. Family-centered rounds in Pakistani pediatric intensive care settings: Non-randomized pre- and post-study design. *Int J Nurs Stud* 2013;50:717–26.

15. Davidson JE, Powers K, Hedayat KM, et al. Clinical practice guidelines for support of the family in the patient-centered intensive care unit: American College of Critical Care Medicine Task Force 2004–2005. *Crit Care Med* 2007;35:605–22.

16. Giannini A. Visiting policies and family presence in ICU: A matter for legislation? *Intensive Care Med* 2013;39:161.

17. Giannini A, Miccinesi G. Parental presence and visiting policies in Italian pediatric intensive care units: A national survey. *Pediatr Crit Care Med* 2011;12:e46–50.

18. McPherson G, Jefferson R, Kissoon N, et al. Toward the inclusion of parents on pediatric critical care unit rounds. *Pediatr Crit Care Med* 2011;12:e255–61.

19. Phipps LM, Bartke CN, Spear DA, et al. Assessment of parental presence during bedside pediatric intensive care unit rounds: Effect on duration, teaching, and privacy. *Pediatr Crit Care Med* 2007;8:220–4.

20. Aronson PL, Yau J, Helfaer MA, et al. Impact of family presence during pediatric intensive care unit rounds on the family and medical team. *Pediatrics* 2009;124:1119–25.

21. Dingeman RS, Mitchell EA, Meyer EC, et al. Parent presence during complex invasive procedures and cardiopulmonary resuscitation: A systematic review of the literature. *Pediatrics* 2007;120:842–54.

22. Porter J, Cooper SJ, Sellick K. Attitudes, implementation and practice of family presence during resuscitation (FPDR): A quantitative literature review. *Int Emerg Nurs* 2013;21:26–34.

23. Fulbrook P, Latour J, Albarran J, et al. The presence of family members during cardiopulmonary resuscitation: European Federation of Critical Care Nursing Associations, European Society of Paediatric and Neonatal Intensive Care and European Society of Cardiology Council on Cardiovascular Nursing and Allied Professions Joint Position Statement. *Eur J Cardiovasc Nurs* 2007;6:255–8.

24. Farrell MF, Frost C. The most important needs of parents of critically ill children: Parents' perceptions. *Intensive Crit Care Nurs* 1992;8:130–9.

25. Fisher MD. Identified needs of parents in a pediatric intensive care unit. *Crit Care Nurse* 1994;14:82–90.

26. Scott LD. Perceived needs of parents of critically ill children. *J Soc Pediatr Nurs: JSPN* 1998;3:4–12.

27. Colville GA, Gracey D. Mothers' recollections of the paediatric intensive care unit: Associations with psychopathology and views on follow up. *Intensive Crit Care Nurs* 2006;22:49–55.

28. Latour JM, van Goudoever JB, Schuurman BE, et al. A qualitative study exploring the experiences of parents of children admitted to seven Dutch pediatric intensive care units. *Intensive Care Med* 2011;37:319–25.

29. Studdert DM, Burns JP, Mello MM, et al. Nature of conflict in the care of pediatric intensive care patients with prolonged stay. *Pediatrics* 2003;112:553–8.

30. Baile WF, Buckman R, Lenzi R, et al. SPIKES-A six-step protocol for delivering bad news: Application to the patient with cancer. *Oncologist* 2000;5:302–11.

31. Orioles A, Miller VA, Kersun LS, et al. "To be a phenomenal doctor you have to be the whole package": Physicians' interpersonal behaviors during difficult conversations in pediatrics. *J Palliat Med* 2013;16:929–33.

32. Amer A, Fischer H. "Don't call me 'mom'": How parents want to be greeted by their pediatrician. *Clin Pediatr* 2009;48:720–22.

33. Walter JK, Benneyworth BD, Housey M, et al. The factors associated with high-quality communication for critically ill children. *Pediatrics* 2013;131(suppl 1):S90–5.

34. Latour JM, van Goudoever JB, Duivenvoorden HJ, et al. Perceptions of parents on satisfaction with care in the pediatric intensive care unit: The EMPATHIC study. *Intensive Care Med* 2009;35:1082–9.

35. Latour JM, Hazelzet JA, Duivenvoorden HJ, et al. Perceptions of parents, nurses, and physicians on neonatal intensive care practices. *J Pediatr* 2010;157:215–20.e3.

36. Curley MA, Hunsberger M, Harris SK. Psychometric evaluation of the family-centered care scale for pediatric acute care nursing. *Nurs Res* 2013;62:160–8.

37. Latour JM, Duivenvoorden HJ, Tibboel D, et al. The shortened Empowerment of PArents in THe Intensive Care 30 questionnaire adequately measured parent satisfaction in pediatric intensive care units. *J Clin Epidemiol* 2013;66:1045–50.

38. Latour JM, van Goudoever JB, Duivenvoorden HJ, et al. Construction and psychometric testing of the EMPATHIC questionnaire measuring parent satisfaction in the pediatric intensive care unit. *Intensive Care Med* 2011;37:310–18.

39. Latour JM, Duivenvoorden HJ, Hazelzet JA, et al. Development and validation of a neonatal intensive care parent satisfaction instrument. *Pediatr Crit Care Med* 2012;13:554–9.

40. Rahi JS, Manaras I, Tuomainen H, et al. Meeting the needs of parents around the time of diagnosis of disability among their children: Evaluation of a novel program for information, support, and liaison by key workers. *Pediatrics* 2004;114:e477–82.

41. Melnyk BM, Alpert-Gillis L, Feinstein NF, et al. Creating opportunities for parent empowerment: Program effects on the mental health/coping outcomes of critically ill young children and their mothers. *Pediatrics* 2004;113:e597–607.

42. Bolton CF. Neuromuscular manifestations of critical illness. *Muscle Nerve* 2005;32:140–63.

43. Batt J, dos Santos CC, Cameron JI, et al. Intensive care unit-acquired weakness: Clinical phenotypes and molecular mechanisms. *Am J Respir Crit Care Med* 2013;187:238–46.

44. Hulst J, Joosten K, Zimmermann L, et al. Malnutrition in critically ill children: From admission to 6 months after discharge. *Clin Nutr* 2004;23:223–32.

45. Amin RS, Fitton CM. Tracheostomy and home ventilation in children. *Semin Neonatol* 2003;8:127–35.

46. Srinivasan S, Doty SM, White TR, et al. Frequency, causes, and outcome of home ventilator failure. *Chest* 1998;114:1363–7.

47. Heaton J, Noyes J, Sloper P, et al. Families' experiences of caring for technology-dependent children: A temporal perspective. *Health Soc Care Community* 2005;13:441–50.

48. Scheeringa MS, Myers L, Putnam FW, et al. Diagnosing PTSD in early childhood: An empirical assessment of four approaches. *J Traum Stress* 2012;25:359–67.

49. Scheeringa MS, Zeanah CH, Cohen JA. PTSD in children and adolescents: Toward an empirically based algorithma. *Depress Anxiety* 2011;28:770–82.

50. Davydow DS, Richardson LP, Zatzick DF, et al. Psychiatric morbidity in pediatric critical illness survivors: A comprehensive review of the literature. *Arch Pediatr Adolesc Med* 2010;164:377–85.

51. Surtees P, Wainwright N, Day N, et al. Adverse experience in childhood as a developmental risk factor for altered immune status in adulthood. *Int J Behav Med* 2003;10:251–68.

52. Gillies D, Taylor F, Gray C, et al. Psychological therapies for the treatment of post-traumatic stress disorder in children and adolescents. *Cochrane Database Syst Rev* 2012;12:CD006726.

53. Hetrick SE, Purcell R, Garner B, et al. Combined pharmacotherapy and psychological therapies for post traumatic stress disorder (PTSD). *Cochrane Database Syst Rev.* 2010 Jul 7;(7):CD007316. doi: 10.1002/14651858.CD007316.pub2.

54. Carnevale FA, Alexander E, Davis M, et al. Daily living with distress and enrichment: The moral experience of families with ventilator-assisted children at home. *Pediatrics* 2006;117:e48–60.

55. Raina P, O'Donnell M, Rosenbaum P, et al. The health and well-being of caregivers of children with cerebral palsy. *Pediatrics* 2005;115:e626–36.

56. Newacheck PW, Inkelas M, Kim SE. Health services use and health care expenditures for children with disabilities. *Pediatrics* 2004;114:79–85.

57. Goh AY, Lum LC, Chan PW, et al. Withdrawal and limitation of life support in paediatric intensive care. *Arch Dis Child* 1999;80:424–8.

58. Koenig BA, Davies E. *Cultural Dimensions of Care at Life's End for Children and Their Families in When Children Die: Improving Palliative and End-of-Life Care for Children and Their Families.* Washington, DC: IOM, 2004.

59. Devictor DJ, Nguyen DT. Forgoing life-sustaining treatments in children: A comparison between Northern and Southern European pediatric intensive care units. *Pediatr Crit Care Med* 2004;5:211–15.

60. Devictor DJ, Latour JM, and the EURYDICE II study group. Forgoing life support: How the decision is made in European pediatric intensive care units. *Intensive Care Med* 2011;37(11):1881–7.

61. Vrakking AM, van der Heide A, Arts WF, et al. Medical end-of-life decisions for children in the Netherlands. *Arch Pediatr Adolesc Med* 2005;159:802–9.

62. Meyer EC, Burns JP, Griffith JL, et al. Parental perspectives on end-of-life care in the pediatric intensive care unit. *Crit Care Med* 2002;30:226–31.

63. Hinds PS, Oakes LL, Hicks J, et al. "Trying to be a good parent" as defined by interviews with parents who made phase I, terminal care, and resuscitation decisions for their children. *J Clin Oncol Official J Am Soc Clin Oncol* 2009;27:5979–85.

64. Field M, Behrman RE. *When Children Die: Improving Palliative and End-of-Life Care for Children and Their Families.* Washington, DC: IOM, 2004.

65. Meert KL, Thurston CS, Briller SH. The spiritual needs of parents at the time of their child's death in the pediatric intensive care unit and during bereavement: A qualitative study. *Pediatr Crit Care Med* 2005;6:420–7.

66. Meyer EC, Ritholz MD, Burns JP, et al. Improving the quality of end-of-life care in the pediatric intensive care unit: Parents' priorities and recommendations. *Pediatrics* 2006;117:649–57.

67. Johnson AH. Death in the PICU: Caring for the "other" families. *J Pediatr Nurs* 1997;12:273–7.

68. Lipton H, Coleman M. Bereavement practice guidelines for health care professionals in the emergency department. *Int J Emerg Ment Health* 2000;2:19–31.

69. Cook P, White DK, Ross-Russell RI. Bereavement support following sudden and unexpected death: Guidelines for care. *Arch Dis Child* 2002;87:36–8.

70. Stroebe M, Schut H. The dual process model of coping with bereavement: A decade on. *Omega* (Westport) 2010;61:273–89.

71. Peebles-Kleiger MJ. Pediatric and neonatal intensive care hospitalization as traumatic stressor: Implications for intervention. *Bull Menninger Clin* 2000;64:257–80.

72. Papadatou D. A proposed model of health professionals' grieving process. *Omega* 2000;41:59–77.

73. Rashotte J. Dwelling with stories that haunt us: Building a meaningful nursing practice. *Nurs Inq* 2005;12:34–42.

74. Meldrum H. Exemplary physicians' strategies for avoiding burnout. *Health Care Manag* 2010;29:324–31.

75. Khamisa N, Peltzer K, Oldenburg B. Burnout in relation to specific contributing factors and health outcomes among nurses: A systematic review. *Int J Environ Res Public Health* 2013;10: 2214–40.

76. Meadors P, Lamson A, Swanson M, et al. Secondary traumatization in pediatric healthcare providers: Compassion fatigue, burnout, and secondary traumatic stress. *Omega* (Westport) 2009;60: 103–28.

77. Jones SH. A self-care plan for hospice workers. *Am J Hosp Palliat Care* 2005;22:125–8.

78. Eagle S, Creel A, Alexandrov A. The effect of facilitated peer support sessions on burnout and grief management among health care providers in pediatric intensive care units: A pilot study. *J Palliat Med* 2012;15:1178–80.

79. Zwack J, Schweitzer J. If every fifth physician is affected by burnout, what about the other four? Resilience strategies of experienced physicians. *Acad Med* 2013;88:382–9.

80. Rennick JE, Morin I, Kim D, et al. Identifying children at high risk for psychological sequelae after pediatric intensive care unit hospitalization. *Pediatr Crit Care Med* 2004;5:358–63.

81. Serwint JR. The use of standardized patients in pediatric residency training in palliative care: Anatomy of a standardized patient case scenario. *J Palliat Med* 2002;5:146–53.

CHAPTER 3 ■ PROFESSIONALISM AND LEADERSHIP IN PEDIATRIC CRITICAL CARE

VINAY M. NADKARNI AND ALICE D. ACKERMAN

KEY POINTS

1. Although the notion of the medical professional originated with Hippocrates in the 4th century BCE, it has evolved over the succeeding centuries.
2. Many "prescriptions" for professional physician behavior are available.
3. These prescriptions relate to "core competencies," including: patient care, practice-based learning and improvement, interpersonal communication skills, professionalism, and systems-based practice.
4. Teaching professionalism demands attention to both the overt and covert curricula and may be most effectively approached through reflective learning.
5. Simulation is a useful approach to teach needed skills, assess competencies, and enhance professionalism.
6. Leadership skills can be learned.

The goals of this chapter are to address several important concepts of professionalism and leadership that are important for an effective, ethical, and rewarding pediatric critical care practice. Interdisciplinary education and practice are both desirable and essential, and cultural context affects what is acceptable and desirable in professional conduct. For the practical focus of this chapter, we will describe aspects of professionalism and leadership most pertinent to physicians from North America and Europe. Professionalism and leadership are core competencies with measurable milestones that should be addressed in cognitive and psychomotor training and the practice of intensivists worldwide.

PROFESSIONALISM

Historical Background

Origins of Professionalism

The Western approach to professionalism has its origin with Hippocrates in the 4th century, BCE. The Hippocratic Oath states a commitment to the best interests of the patient, honors the teachers and mentors of the medical profession, and speaks to the ethics and morals of the physician, in the context of medical practice. It addresses the importance of patient confidentiality and trust. This oath has guided our expectations of Western physicians' ethical and moral behavior for over 2000 years. However, the specific relevance and application of the Hippocratic principles applied to modern issues (e.g., health information portability protection, medical euthanasia, organ recovery) are complex, and thus "code of professional conduct" committees have become commonplace in medical schools and hospitals, to review and enforce good clinical and professional conduct.

Evolution of Professionalism in the 20th Century to Current Practice

Starting in the mid-1900s, the tenets of professionalism became more society-norm based than individually focused. Modern society expects that the members of a profession be specifically trained, demonstrate competency, and have a mechanism to ensure maintenance of competency throughout medical practice. Most societies allow the profession to be largely self-regulating and develop professional guidelines for education, performance, and discipline. In exchange, society generally accords members of the profession high stature and respect.

Over time, changes in society and medical systems have led to concerns about the self-regulated medical profession, and specifically the behavior of individual members of the profession. External pressures from rising healthcare costs, the stress of changing mechanisms of physician documentation and reimbursement, and increased reliance on complex technology have affected perceptions of what constitutes appropriate professional behavior.

Guidelines and standards for most accreditation councils of graduate medical education require that professionalism be taught to residents and fellows (1,2). In the USA, standards for maintenance of certification (MOC) of the American Board of Pediatrics (ABP) require evidence of ongoing professional behavior in its diplomats (3). Other requirements for MOC in the USA include excellence in patient care, evidence of practice-based learning and improvement, evaluation of interpersonal and communication skills, demonstration of the understanding of the components of systems-based practice and satisfactory completion of the traditional standardized secure examination.

Professionalism and the "Core Competencies"

In 2003, the Institute of Medicine (IOM) (4) recommended that modern medical professionals should provide patient-centered care, work in interdisciplinary teams, employ evidence-based principles, apply quality-improvement methodologies, and utilize informatics in the practice of medicine. These five noncognitive concepts were adapted by graduate medical training and oversight committees into five "core competencies": patient care, practice-based learning and improvement, interpersonal communication skills, professionalism, and systems-based practice (1). The relationship between the core competencies and medical professionalism was addressed (5,6) in a summit of North American and European medical societies, resulting in a call to action. Ten elements of professionalism were chartered (**Table 3.1**) that guide the ethical principles of supporting patient welfare, patient autonomy, and social justice. However, a roadmap to reach the proposed optimal state of medical professionalism was not explicit in the charter. Concurrently, the Royal College of Paediatrics and Child Health (United Kingdom) (7) published a statement specific to the professional duties and responsibilities of pediatricians. The Royal College identified actions and behaviors that could cause loss of professional license registration. Specific examples of unacceptable behavior are provided, in each of eight major areas: (a) professional competence, (b) ensuring appropriate access to care, (c) maintenance of good medical practice, (d) teaching, training, appraising, and assessing, (e) relationships with patients (e.g., consent, confidentiality, trust, communication), (f) dealing with problems in professional practice (conduct and performance of colleagues, complaints, and malpractice insurance), (g) working with colleagues (treating colleagues fairly, working in and leading teams, arranging coverage, accepting appointments, sharing information, delegation and referral), and (h) "probity," which deals with personal conflicts of interest including research, personal health, and financial interests (7).

The *Competency-based Training* programme in *Intensive Care Medicine for Europe* (CoBaTrICE) collaboration published a list of competencies expected of adult intensive care physicians that are based on consensus that was developed over a 3-year period. Professionalism was one of the 12 "domains," weighted heavily in importance by the majority of the participants. Within the professionalism domain, CoBaTrICE includes the following three competencies: (a) communication skills, (b) professional relationships with patients, relatives, and members of the health care team, and (c) "self-governance" (8). Surveys of trainees and of patients and their families confirmed the importance of maintaining these professionalism attributes throughout everyday practice (9,10).

Personal Attributes of the Medical Professional. These descriptions of professionalism place a great deal of emphasis on the outward (measurable or observable) conduct of the physician, but pay little attention to the intrinsic attributes that identify a physician as a true professional. The American Association of Medical Colleges (AAMC) has determined that the medical professional in today's society should be knowledgeable, skillful, altruistic, and dutiful. To this end, the AAMC has encouraged schools of medicine to incorporate teaching of professional attitudes and behaviors into their curricula (11). Recommendations by others add qualities such as compassion, integrity, fidelity, and self-effacement as important in the "good" doctor (12). G. Luke Larkin, who writes about how to model and mentor students in professionalism, suggests that we first map virtues and vices in professional practice. He has identified "four valences" of professional behavior in the order of best to worst: ideal, desired, unacceptable, and egregious (13). For example, ideal behaviors would include showing altruism toward others and having humility regarding one's own achievements. Desired behaviors would be acting in the best interest of the patient and arriving on time for work. On the negative side of the spectrum, unprofessional behaviors would include arriving late or breaching confidentiality, while egregious behaviors would include lying, falsifying medical records, and engaging in substance abuse.

Teaching Professionalism

Once we understand what actions, behaviors, and attributes are consistent with professionalism, the next question becomes: "How do we teach this?" The answer is both simple and complex. The most important aspect of learning to act as a professional appears to be having the appropriate role models (11,12); despite this we must find a way to help our students and trainees understand the relationship between such ideal attributes as altruism and the behaviors—good and bad—that they observe daily at patients' bedsides. Many health education schools have developed courses on professionalism and humanism (14–16). Trainees arrive with a personal identity formed since birth. Each individual's journey from layperson

TABLE 3.1

COMMITMENTS OF THE MEDICAL PROFESSIONAL

■ COMMITMENT	■ EXAMPLES
Professional competence	Engage in lifelong learning; maintain necessary skills for self and team; ensure that all members of the profession remain competent
Honesty with patients	Inform patients truthfully; acknowledge errors
Patient confidentiality	This may not be possible if patient poses a risk to society.
Maintaining appropriate relationships with patients	Includes the avoidance of sexual relationships, using patients for financial gain, etc.
Improve quality of care	At both an individual and systems-wide level, participate in mechanisms that encourage continuous improvement in care delivery
Improve access to care	Promote public health, preventive medicine, and patient advocacy; eliminate discrimination within physician's own system of practice
Ensure just distribution of resources	Provide cost-effective care; use evidence-based guidelines
Further scientific knowledge	Uphold scientific standards; promote research; create new knowledge; ensure its integrity
Manage conflicts of interest	Full disclosure
Professional responsibilities	Work collaboratively with others; discipline those who fail to uphold professional standards; develop new standards and train new members appropriately

Adapted from Medical Professionalism Project. Medical professionalism in the new millennium: A physician charter. *Ann Intern Med* 2002;136:243–6.

to skilled professional is unique and is affected by "who they are" at the beginning and later by "who they wish to become." Recent consensus leaders recommend that ethics and humanities-based knowledge, skills, and conduct that promote professionalism should be taught with accountability, flexibility, and the premise that all these traits are essential to the formation of a modern professional health care provider (16).

Gaps Between Ideal Behavior and Reality. Students learn in the clinical setting by observing the behavior of many individuals with whom they interact. It is not just the wise professor, who embodies all of the desired virtues of the physician, who will affect those most likely to be influenced. Rather, it appears that students are most influenced by those with whom they spend the most time. In fact, both positive attitude and cynicism are commonly taught and learned from peers (11,12,15). Critical care clinicians should stay centered on the core values of the medical profession as we care for patients and educate trainees. Professional schools and hospital systems, while indicating that they desire faculty to exhibit professional behavior and serve as role models for trainees, rarely reward outstanding clinician-teacher role models as well or as overtly as they reward the successful research scientists (13,17). The gap between what we say we desire and what we reward must be addressed, if medicine truly wishes to make professionalism a reality and to establish meaningful role models.

Impact of Burnout on Professional Behavior. Many health care professionals suffer from burnout (a syndrome of emotional exhaustion, depersonalization, and low personal esteem), and this can easily be transmitted to the trainees and colleagues with whom they work. Burnout is recognized as a major problem among residents, fellows, and attending physicians (18–20). Burnout among internal medicine residents was associated with self-reported unprofessional behavior (21). Critical care units are stressful places; black humor and disdain for the patient occur on occasion. The risk of unintentionally teaching unprofessional behavior through our actions is increased under these circumstances (22–25).

Reflective Learning. To overcome the challenges and tension between "overt" and "covert" curricula in medical education that pertain to professionalism (26), a "reflective learning" approach has been advocated (12). In this way, we improve our ability to recognize, acknowledge, and reflect on our behavior when it deviates from optimal. Constructive reflection may prevent cynicism. As we become more reflective, we can acquire stories that pertain to the emotional issues in response to our involvement with patients and their situations.

A specific approach, termed "narrative-based professionalism," presents the opportunity to rectify the tension between tacit and explicit values (12,27,28), such as between altruism and self-interest. In this scheme, young professionals are immersed in a wide array of narratives or stories that help to develop role modeling, self-awareness, narrative competence, and community service. In addition, many graduate medical education organizations offer resources to teach and assess professionalism, including 360-degree evaluations (2,29–31).

Professionalism Training Using Simulation-Based Methodology

As scientific and regulatory bodies seek to ensure that physicians are *intentionally* trained in and competent in key aspects of professionalism, we cannot assume that traditional training ensures professionalism competence. The aviation, defense, and nuclear energy industries have a history of success in safety and skill-based performance improvement using simulation training. In 1999, the IOM specifically called for the establishment of interdisciplinary team-training programs that incorporate efficient training methods, including simulation (32). Thus, interest has dramatically increased in identifying innovative mechanisms (such as simulation) to enhance traditional training methods and to measure the effectiveness of those methods.

Simulation training has the potential to contribute to professionalism through a variety of mechanisms. First, flat-screen, manikin-based, or standardized simulation can be accomplished without "practicing on" or "harming" real patients. Procedural training using simulation offers one good example, transforming a "see one, do one, teach one" philosophy to deliberate manikin practice. A growing number of published controlled trials demonstrate that physicians randomized to training programs that utilize simulation perform "better" (defined variably as faster completion of surgery, fewer errors made during a procedure, etc.) than those trained through usual programs (including laparoscopic surgery (33–35), vascular catheterizations (36–39), and early airway management) (40–44). An example of a pediatric critical care procedure that could be practiced prior to performing on a live patient is the placement of a central venous catheter. A new fellow could practice the myriad steps involved in successfully performing this procedure from beginning to end, including the steps that require communication with others. The trainee could rehearse attitudes, behaviors, and skills necessary to obtain informed consent, address family presence for the procedure, establish a sterile field, use ultrasound guidance to identify the vessel, practice the Seldinger technique, secure and dress the catheter, and document the procedure in the medical record. Increasing evidence demonstrates that simulation can shorten the time to competence and increase the likelihood that, when a physician is performing a procedure on a patient for the first time, the patient is safer than if the physician did not have simulation training.

Another important way in which simulation can be used to enhance professionalism is through various exercises focused on improving communication. Standardized patients can be used with multidisciplinary intensive care teams to practice talking to families about issues such as delivering bad news, discussion of brain death, and approaching the family about organ donation (45–47). Such interventions are associated with increased organ donation rates, presumably due to more effective communication. Other training scenarios that involve standardized patients to enhance communication with real patients or families include: obtaining consent, discussion of withdrawal of care, request for autopsy, disclosure of errors, and delivering an apology.

Simulation can be used to diagnose and address deficiencies in team management of critical care issues. Mock codes have been used to identify deficiencies in the management of simulated pediatric trauma victims in the trauma bay and of simulated medical emergencies (44,48–56). These interdisciplinary exercises are a powerful means of observing team dynamics and assessing complex issues, such as leadership, communication, and adherence to important protocols (e.g., the American Heart Association's Basic, Pediatric, and Advanced Life Support algorithms).

Simulation can also be used to help assess competency (57–61). Although validation of application of simulation evaluation to certification or accreditation has only been applied in selected circumstances, formative and summative assessments of clinician adherence to accepted protocols and time critical interventions is possible. For example, programs can create scenarios with a high-fidelity simulator to test whether participants achieve time critical interventions for management challenges of cardiopulmonary arrest, foreign body airway obstruction, septic shock, or traumatic brain injury (62,63). Deviation from clinical protocols can be identified and addressed to improve protocol understanding and compliance and to employ a "train-to-success" approach.

LEADERSHIP

Leadership is one aspect of professionalism that can be improved with coaching, guided reflection, and a simulation-based approach. Fellows entering pediatric critical care and pediatric anesthesiology training demonstrated limited knowledge and understanding of the meaning and importance of the core competencies (64). Attempted curriculum development for systems-based practice, professionalism, and communication skills revealed that (a) although trainees were willing to try to learn the material, they were not willing to devote much time to it, and (b) faculty members found it difficult to prepare and deliver the competencies within the existing structure.

Other institutions are developing similar programs to address the competencies and help their trainees and faculty to develop stronger leadership skills (64–67). Such training differs from the standard "professional development" courses traditionally offered at professional schools, which focus on competency in research and teaching methods and preparation for promotion. Although important for success within professional school hierarchy, this traditional training may not be sufficient to improve communication, clinical outcomes or to develop the kind of skills necessary to prepare clinicians to lead the diverse and rapidly changing subspecialty of pediatric critical care into the future.

What Is a Leader?

The definition of a leader can be complex. Most simply, a leader is a person who "gets things done." Whether in the clinical ICU or administrative meeting room, leadership skills are important, to empower ourselves, others, and ensure a better future for our profession.

Health care accreditation organizations have established guidelines and standards that pertain to demonstration of leadership skills in hospitals (68). Most requirements are based on understanding of the relationship between demonstrated leadership and the provision of quality health care, with an emphasis on patient safety. The medical staff of the hospital is identified as one of three components of hospital leadership, the other two being the governing body (e.g., the board of directors) and the management. Medical staff must become intimately involved with developing the mission and vision of the institution, participate in developing safety and quality goals, and become involved in all facets of financially accountable care. The medical staff is expected to be knowledgeable about the population served by the institution, about applicable laws and regulations, and about their own individual and shared responsibilities and accountabilities.

Hospitals are responsible for orienting the medical staff leaders to these areas. In addition, each institution is expected to provide training for all leaders in conflict management, cognitive bias, systems-based practice, team structure and function, evidence-based decision making, and development of mutual respect between disciplines. Each hospital is expected to monitor the effectiveness of its leadership groups and to engage outside expertise (consultants) if adequate expertise does not reside within the institution for training and performance of the leadership tasks. Other valuable skills include effective communication and conflict management.

Leadership Training

Leadership training teaches individuals multiple skills, including time management, effective communication, program development, visioning, and team development and leadership.

Participants are helped to understand their "leadership style" through a number of possible mechanisms. Much of current leadership training is based on the development of what has been termed "emotional intelligence" by Daniel Goleman, a noted leader in executive development (69–71). Emotional intelligence is composed of four fundamental components: self-awareness, self-management, social awareness, and social skill. Each of these areas contains specific competencies to be developed. Different styles of leadership emphasize different patterns of emotional intelligence and, therefore, competencies. Because competencies can be taught and learned, it follows that effective leaders can be developed.

Most pediatric critical care fellows and junior faculty report that they have not received any formal training in management or leadership. They feel particularly unprepared to handle stress, manage conflict (within their own team or with other groups), manage time, and evaluate team performance (72–74). Leadership training is therefore clearly needed.

Leadership training exists in many forms and may be accessed in a variety of ways. Readers are encouraged to seek training at the local level when available. Numerous Web-based programs are also available, many through society MOC programs, such as the American Academy of Pediatrics (AAP), Pediatric Leadership Alliance, the American College of Physician Executives, and the American Medical Association. Emphasis is placed upon learning and practicing communication skills, identification and management of cognitive bias, management of conflict, dealing with disruptive physician behavior, time management, stress management, and conflict resolution (75–77).

Practicing Leadership Through Management of Interdisciplinary Teams

To achieve a positive change in the medical society requires the physician to be both a "team player" and a "team leader." Learning to work as part of an interdisciplinary team may be difficult for the physician, who is traditionally taught to function alone and assume individual responsibility. The fact that the interdisciplinary team is proving to be the best method to ensure that patients receive coordinated, appropriate care is recognized by practitioners of primary care, internal medicine, geriatrics, and other specialties. In an interdisciplinary team, members from various disciplines coordinate their efforts, communicating with each other directly, for the benefit of the patient and to achieve optimal patient outcomes (78). Pediatric critical care has long embraced the notion of the interdisciplinary health care team. In forming a highly effective team, it is necessary that the leader establish both the urgency and the direction of the team. Expectations should be clear. Our challenge now is to leverage our teams into highly functional teams that achieve time critical interventions in an efficient, effective, and patient-/family-friendly manner. Team dynamics and function are covered in Chapter 4.

CONCLUSIONS AND FUTURE DIRECTIONS

Professionalism deserves emphasis in today's medicine both in clinical care and in the classroom. Although the optimal methods to teach and evaluate professionalism are constantly improving and being refined, the use of role modeling, simulation, and leadership training remain valuable approaches to this important undertaking.

Leadership development and training is essential to enhance professional development, improve patient care, and to engage in systems-based practice. These core competencies are key components of the increased focus on credentialing, certification, MOC, and competency-based training. Leadership can be learned. Effective means of teaching leadership techniques have been developed in many businesses and industries, and are being adapted to medicine.

References

1. Holt KD, Miller RS, Nasca TJ. Residency programs' evaluations of the competencies: Data provided to the ACGME about types of assessments used by programs. *J Grad Med Educ* 2010;2(4):649–55. doi: 10.4300/JGME-02-04-30.
2. ACGME. Advancing education in medical professionalism. An educational resource from the ACGME outcome project: Accreditation Council for Graduate Medical Education, 2004.
3. Miles PV. Maintenance of certification: The role of the American Board of Pediatrics in improving children's health care. *Pediatr Clin North Am.* 2009 Aug;56(4):987-94. doi: 10.1016/j.pcl.2009.05.010.
4. Greiner AC, Knebel E. *Health Professions Education: A Bridge to Quality.* Washington, DC: National Academies Press, 2003.
5. Medical Professionalism Project. Medical professionalism in the new millennium: A physicians' charter. *Ann Intern Med* 2002;136:243–6.
6. Medical Professionalism Project. Medical professionalism in the new millennium: A physicians' charter. *Lancet* 2002;359(9305):520-2.
7. Royal College of Paediatrics. *Good Medical Practice in Paediatrics and Child Health: Duties and Responsibilities of Paediatricians.* London, UK: Royal College of Paediatrics and Child Health, 2002. http://www.rcpch.ac.uk/sites/default/files/asset_library/Publications/G/GMP.pdf
8. CoBaTrICE. Development of core competencies for an international training programme in intensive care medicine. *Intensive Care Med* Berlin, : Springer-Verlag, 2006.
9. van Mook WN, de Grave WS, Gorter SL, et al. Fellows' in intensive care medicine views on professionalism and how they learn it. *Intensive Care Med* 2010;36:296–303.
10. Bion J, Rothen HU. Models for intensive care training. A European perspective. *Am J Respir Crit Care Med* 2014;189:256–62.
11. Inui TS. *A Flag in the Wind: Educating for Professionalism in Medicine.* Washington, DC: Association of American Medical Colleges, 2003.
12. Coulehan J. Viewpoint: Today's professionalism: Engaging the mind but not the heart. *Acad Med* 2005;80:892–8.
13. Larkin GL. Mapping, modeling and mentoring: Charting a course for professionalism in graduate medical education. *Camb Q Healthc Ethics* 2003;12:167–77.
14. Al-Eraky MM. Twelve tips for teaching medical professionalism at all levels of medical education [published online ahead of print on March 17, 2015]. *Med Teach*:1–8.
15. Cruess RL, Cruess SR, Boudreau JD, et al. A schematic representation of the professional identity formation and socialization of medical students and residents: A guide for medical educators [published online ahead of print on March 17, 2015]. *Acad Med.*
16. Doukas DJ, Kirch DG, Brigham TP, et al. Transforming educational accountability in medical ethics and humanities education toward professionalism [published online ahead of print on December 23, 2014]. *Acad Med.*
17. Dickinson H, Ham C, Snelling I, et al. Medical leadership arrangements in English healthcare organisations: Findings from a national survey and case studies of NHS trusts. *Health Serv Manage Res* 2013;26:119–25.
18. Chen SM, McMurray A. "Burnout" in intensive care nurses. *J Nurs Res* 2001;9:152–64.
19. Levi BH, Thomas NJ, Green MJ, et al. Jading in the pediatric intensive care unit: Implications for healthcare providers of medically complex children. *Pediatr Crit Care Med* 2004;5:275–7.
20. Meier DE, Back AL, Morrison RS. The inner life of physicians and care of the seriously ill. *JAMA* 2001;286:3007–14.
21. Shanafelt TD, Bradley KA, Wipf JE, et al. Burnout and self-reported patient care in an internal medicine residency program. *Ann Intern Med* 2002;136:358–67.
22. Gauthier T, Meyer RM, Grefe D, et al. An on-the-job mindfulness-based intervention for pediatric ICU nurses: A pilot. *J Pediatr Nurs* 2015;30:402–9.
23. Gazelle G, Liebschutz JM, Riess H. Physician burnout: Coaching a way out. *J Gen Intern Med* 2015;30(4):508–13.
24. Guntupalli KK, Wachtel S, Mallampati A, et al. Burnout in the intensive care unit professionals. *Indian J Crit Care Med* 2014;18:139–43.
25. Meyer RM, Li A, Klaristenfeld J, et al. Pediatric novice nurses: Examining compassion fatigue as a mediator between stress exposure and compassion satisfaction, burnout and job satisfaction. *J Pediatr Nurs* 2015;30:174–83.
26. Connelly JE. The other side of professionalism: Doctor to doctor. *Camb Q Healthc Ethics* 2003;12:178–83.
27. Arntfield SL, Slesar K, Dickson J, et al. Narrative medicine as a means of training medical students toward residency competencies. *Patient Educ Couns* 2013;91:280–6.
28. Quaintance JL, Arnold L, Thompson GS. What students learn about professionalism from faculty stories: An "appreciative inquiry" approach. *Acad Med* 2010;85:118–23.
29. Lanken PN, Novack DH, Daetwyler C, et al. Efficacy of an internet-based learning module and small-group debriefing on trainees' attitudes and communication skills toward patients with substance use disorders: Results of a cluster randomized controlled trial. *Acad Med* 2015;90:345–54.
30. Fromme HB, Whicker SA, Paik S, et al. Pediatric resident-as-teacher curricula: A national survey of existing programs and future needs. *J Grad Med Educ* 2011;3:168–75.
31. Varga-Atkins T, Dangerfield P, Brigden D. Developing professionalism through the use of wikis: A study with first-year undergraduate medical students. *Med Teach* 2010;32:824–9.
32. Kohn L. To err is human: An interview with the Institute of Medicine's Linda Kohn. *Jt Comm J Qual Improv* 2000;26:227–34.
33. Ekkelenkamp VE, Koch AD, de Man RA, et al. Training and competence assessment in GI endoscopy: A systematic review [published online ahead of print on January 30, 2015]. *Gut.*
34. Stefanidis D, Gardner C, Paige JT, et al. Multicenter longitudinal assessment of resident technical skills. *Am J Surg* 2015;209(1):120–5.
35. Steigerwald SN, Park J, Hardy KM, et al. Does laparoscopic simulation predict intraoperative performance? A comparison between the fundaments of laparoscopic surgery and Lap VR evaluation metrics. *Am J Surg* 2015;209(1):34–9.
36. Thomas SM, Burch W, Kuehnle SE, et al. Simulation training for pediatric residents on central venous catheter placement: A pilot study. *Pediatr Crit Care Med* 2013;14(9):e416–e423.
37. Barsuk JH, Cohen ER, Potts S, et al. Dissemination of a simulation-based mastery learning intervention reduces central line-associated bloodstream infections. *BMJ Qual Saf* 2014;23(9):749–56.
38. Barsuk JH, Cohen ER, McGaghie WC, et al. Long-term retention of central venous catheter insertion skills after simulation-based mastery learning. *Acad Med* 2010;85(10, suppl):S9–S12.
39. Cohen ER, Feinglass J, Barsuk JH, et al. Cost savings from reduced catheter-related bloodstream infection after simulation-based education for residents in a medical intensive care unit. *Simul Healthc* 2010;5(2):98–102.
40. Chaer R, Derubertis B, Lin S, et al. Simulation improves resident performance in catheter-based intervention: Results of a randomized, controlled study. *Ann Surg* 2006;244:343–52.
41. Grantcharov T, Kristiansen V, Bendix J, et al. Randomized clinical trial of virtual reality simulation for laparoscopic skills training. *Br J Surg* 2004;91:146–50.
42. Mayo P, Hackney J, Mueck J, et al. Achieving house staff competence in emergency airway management: Results of a teaching

program using a computerized patient simulator. *Crit Care Med* 2004;32:2422–7.

43. Sharara-Chami R, Taher S, Kaddoum R, et al. Simulation training in endotracheal intubation in a pediatric residency. *Middle East J Anaesthesiol* 2014;22(5):477–85.

44. Mills DM, Williams DC, Dobson JV. Simulation training as a mechanism for procedural and resuscitation education for pediatric residents: A systematic review. *Hosp Pediatr* 2013;3(2):167–76.

45. Williams M. Interdisciplinary experiential training for end-of-life care and organ donation. National Consent Conference on Organ Donation; April 2003; Orlando, FL.

46. Taniguchi M, Furukawa H, Kawai T, et al. Establishment of educational program for multiorgan procurement from deceased donors. *Transplant Proc* 2014;46(4):1071–3.

47. Bramstedt KA, Moolla A, Rehfield PL. Use of standardized patients to teach medical students about living organ donation. *Prog Transpl* 2012;22(1):86–90.

48. DeVita M, Schaefer J, Lutz J, et al. Improving medical emergency team (MET) performance using a novel curriculum and a computerized human patient simulator. *Qual Saf Health Care* 2005;14:326–31.

49. Hunt E, Hohenhaus S, Luo X, et al. Simulation of pediatric trauma stabilization in 35 North Carolina emergency departments: Identification of targets for performance improvement. *Pediatrics* 2006;117:641–8.

50. Cheng A, Brown LL, Duff JP, et al. Improving cardiopulmonary resuscitation with a CPR feedback device and refresher simulations (CPR CARES study): A randomized clinical trial. *JAMA Pediatr* 2015;169(2):137–44.

51. Hunt EA, Cruz-Eng H, Bradshaw JH, et al. A novel approach to life support training using "action-linked phrases." *Resuscitation* 2014;86C:1–5.

52. Sullivan NJ, Duval-Arnold J, Twilley M, et al. Simulation exercise to improve retention of cardiopulmonary resuscitation priorities for in-hospital cardiac arrests: A randomized controlled trial. *Resuscitation* 2014;86C:6–13.

53. Su L, Spaeder MC, Jones MB, et al. Implementation of an extracorporeal cardiopulmonary resuscitation simulation program reduces extracorporeal cardiopulmonary resuscitation times in real patients. *Pediatr Crit Care Med* 2014;15(9):856–60.

54. Blackwood J, Duff JP, Nettel-Aguirre A, et al. Does teaching crisis resource management skills improve resuscitation performance in pediatric residents? *Pediatr Crit Care Med* 2014;15(4):e168–e174.

55. Hunt EA, Duval-Arnould JM, Nelson-McMillan KL, et al. Pediatric resident resuscitation skills improve after "rapid cycle deliberate practice" training. *Resuscitation* 2014;85(7):945–51.

56. Mills DM, Wu CL, Williams DC, et al. High-fidelity simulation enhances pediatric residents' retention, knowledge, procedural proficiency, group resuscitation performance, and experience in pediatric resuscitation. *Hosp Pediatr* 2013;3(3):266–75.

57. Qayumi K, Pachev G, Zheng B, et al. Status of simulation in health care education: An international survey. *Adv Med Educ Pract* 2014;5:457–67.

58. Unterman A, Achiron A, Gat I, et al. A novel simulation-based training program to improve clinical teaching and mentoring skills. *Isr Med Assoc J* 2014;16(3):184–90.

59. Ben-Gal G, Weiss EI, Gafni N, et al. Testing manual dexterity using a virtual reality simulator: Reliability and validity. *Eur J Dent Educ* 2013;17(3):138–42.

60. Berkenstadt H, Ben-Menachem E, Dach R, et al. Deficits in the provision of cardiopulmonary resuscitation during simulated obstetric crises: Results from the Israeli Board of Anesthesiologists. *Anesth Analg* 2012;115(5):1122–6.

61. Holmboe E, Rizzolo MA, Sachdeva AK, et al. Simulated-based assessment and the regulation of healthcare professionals. *Simul Healthc* 2011;(6, suppl):S58–S62.

62. Cheng A, Grant V, Auerbach M. Using simulation to improve patient safety: Dawn of a new era [published online ahead of print on March 9, 2015]. *JAMA Pediatr*.

63. Auerbach M, Roney L, Aysseh A, et al. In situ pediatric trauma simulation: Assessing the impact and feasibility of an interdisciplinary pediatric in situ trauma care quality improvement simulation program. *Pediatr Emerg Care* 2014;30(12):884–91.

64. Lattore P, Wetzel RC, Yanofsky SD. Professionalism, interpersonal communications, and leadership in anesthesiology. Annual Meeting of the Association of University Anesthesiologists and Anesthesia Education Foundation; 2006; Tuscon, Arizona.

65. Coolen EH, Draaisma JM, den Hamer S, et al. Leading teams during simulated pediatric emergencies: A pilot study. *Adv Med Educ Pract* 2015;6:19–26.

66. Nicksa GA, Anderson C, Fidler R, et al. Innovative approach using interprofessional simulation to educate surgical residents in technical and nontechnical skills in high-risk clinical scenarios. *JAMA Surg* 2015;150(3):201–7.

67. Stringfellow TD, Rohrer RM, Loewenthal L, et al. Defining the structure of undergraduate medical leadership and management teaching and assessment in the UK [published online ahead of print on October 10, 2014]. *Med Teach*:1–8.

68. Hakim A. JCAHO standards up the ante for leadership. *Physician Exec* 2006;32:30–3.

69. Goleman D. Leadership that gets results. *Harv Bus Rev* 2000:78–90.

70. Tyczkowski B, Vandenhouten C, Reilly J, et al. Emotional intelligence (EI) and nursing leadership styles among nurse managers. *Nurs Adm Q* 2015;39(2):172–80.

71. Hammerly ME, Harmon L, Schwaitzberg SD. Good to great: Using 360-degree feedback to improve physician emotional intelligence. *J Healthc Manag* 2014;59(5):354–65.

72. Stockwell DC, Pollack MM, Turenne WM, et al. Leadership and management training of pediatric intensivists: How do we gain our skills? *Pediatr Crit Care Med* 2005;6:665–70.

73. Walsh K. Emotional intelligence of medical residents: Further work is required. *Acta Med Iran* 2015;53(3):198.

74. Olson K, Kemper KJ, Mahan JD. What factors promote resilience and protect against burnout in first-year pediatric and medicine-pediatric residents [published online ahead of print on February 18, 2015]. *J Evid Based Complementary Altern Med*.

75. Byrne A, Tanesini A. Instilling new habits: Addressing implicit bias in healthcare professionals [published online ahead of print on March 15, 2015]. *Adv Health Sci Educ Theory Pract*.

76. Park CS, Stojiljkovic L, Milicic B, et al. Training induces cognitive bias: The case of a simulation-based emergency airway curriculum. *Simul Healthc* 2014;9(2):85–93.

77. Minehart RD, Rudolph J, Pian-Smith MC, et al. Improving faculty feedback to resident trainees during a simulated case: A randomized, controlled trial of an educational intervention. *Anesthesiology* 2014;120(1):160–71.

78. Hall P, Weaver L. Interdisciplinary education and teamwork: A long and winding road. *Med Educ* 2001;35:867–75.

CHAPTER 4 ■ SIMULATION TRAINING AND TEAM DYNAMICS

ELIZABETH A. HUNT, DAVID GRANT, AND MICHAEL ROSEN

KEY POINTS

1. Healthcare Education has evolved from an apprentice model of "see one, do one, teach one" to a model that prioritizes patient safety and the expectation that a learner will "practice on plastic first".
2. Simulation training refers to a technique, not a technology and should incorporate educational best practices and evolving evidence on the most effective ways to leverage this technique.
3. Pediatric critical care practitioners work as teams and thus should train as teams. Simulation is an effective methodology to teach teamwork dynamics.

Children admitted to a PICU are, by definition, critically ill and in the most vulnerable of situations. They deserve excellent clinical care in order to optimize their outcomes. It has become clear that the use of simulation can bring training for both novice and expert clinicians to a new level. We can improve patient safety and the quality of care we deliver by utilizing simulation resources for healthcare providers. Simulation is engaging, and follows adult learning theory, and educational research continues to inform strategies to optimize its impact. In addition, simulation can be used not only merely to train novice clinicians how to perform procedures but also to train them to communicate compassionately and to train all levels and disciplines of providers to work as teams. Teamwork is a fundamental and integral feature of pediatric critical care. This chapter reviews the historical and theoretical background to simulation, key concepts fundamental to successful simulation training and teamwork training in critical care.

SIMULATION TRAINING

Simulation has become a growing component of educational and research strategies in healthcare over the past two decades. One reflection of this is the number of simulation centers dedicated to housing simulated clinical spaces, equipment, and personnel to support these endeavors (see **Fig. 4.1**) (1). The exponential curve on this graph reminds us that healthcare simulation is a relatively new field, and best practices are currently being defined and refined. This rapid growth is also reflected in the development and membership of simulation societies and conferences that foster networking and sharing of new developments. An important example in the field of pediatrics is the International Pediatric Simulation Society who in 2014 celebrated their sixth annual meeting, that is, International Pediatric Simulation Symposium and Workshops (IPSSW).

It is interesting that after hundreds (or really thousands) of years of rarely using surrogates (actors, manikins) in education in medicine, nursing, and allied health, there has been such a paradigm shift. It raises the question of why simulation is now considered such an important component element of the healthcare curriculum.

One of the first major shifts in medical education paradigms occurred with the Flexner Report of 1910. After a detailed examination of the curriculum, facilities, finances, faculty, and clinical resources of medical schools in the United States, Abraham Flexner made a detailed report to the sponsoring Carnegie Foundation that included insightful observations that remain relevant today. He observed: "On the pedagogic side, modern medicine, like all scientific teaching, is characterized by activity. The student no longer merely watches, listens, memorizes; he *does*." He continued, "An education in medicine nowadays involves both learning and learning how; the student cannot effectively know, unless he knows how." "Out and out didactic treatment is hopelessly antiquated; . . . The lecture indeed continues of limited use." Ironically, much of his reference was to the "active learning" in the basic science (Anatomy and Chemistry) laboratories. He strongly felt these subjects were better learned in an active manner (dissecting rather than reading from an Anatomy atlas). He highlighted that the success of a medical curriculum is integrally linked to the relationship between a medical school and its hospital and clinic population. He emphasized medical schools, most specifically Johns Hopkins University School of Medicine (Baltimore, MD), that moved their students from the classroom and basic science laboratories after 2 years into the clinical environment, as defining best practices in medical education (2). Subsequently, this became the model of the modern medical school that stood for another century.

Sir William Osler (3) has been quoted as having said, "He who studies medicine without books sails an uncharted sea, but he who studies medicine without patients does not go to sea at all." These two men stressed that one must get out of the classroom to truly learn medicine, or more specifically "to learn how." The apprentice model ruled healthcare education for the next 100 years, didactic knowledge gained in the classroom followed by intense bedside experiences, where the skills of taking a history, listening to patients, conducting a physical

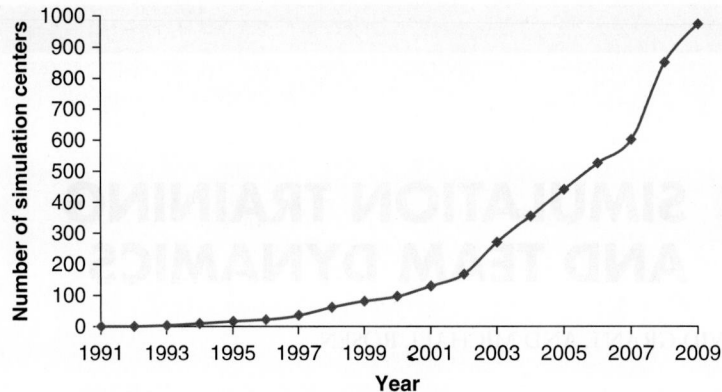

FIGURE 4.1. Growth of medical simulation centers in the United States, 1991–2009. (Plot and data analysis by Emma Baillargeon and Joseph T. Samosky, Simulation and Medical Technology R & D Center, University of Pittsburgh. Data derived from Worldwide Simulation Centre Database, Bristol Medical Simulation Centre, Bristol, UK. From Sherwin J. More than make believe: The power and promise of simulation. *Biomed Instrum Technol* 2012;46(4):254–63.)

exam, and performing procedures were learned by first watching senior clinicians before attempting. In fact, Osler was known for examining his patient's microbiology specimens and conducting his own autopsies so that he understood every aspect of his patient's diseases. Learning at the bedside, on patients, was the norm and bedside teaching revered.

The learning during this period is accurately reflected by a phrase that was common at the time: "see one, do one, teach one" (4). There was no expectation that students would learn clinical skills in a laboratory, prior to performing them on actual patients. While there are clearly reports of leading edge, iconic human patient simulators being developed and utilized in medical education in the 1960s and 1970s, very few simulators were developed for healthcare education prior to the 21st century, partially due to low demand (5). In marked contrast, the airline and aeronautic industries were developing sophisticated simulators to intensely train pilots and flight teams *prior* to flying actual planes in an attempt to avoid catastrophic errors (6).

In 1999, the Institute of Medicine released a report entitled "To Err is Human: Building a Safer Healthcare System." The report estimated that 98,000 patients died each year within U.S. hospitals secondary to errors (7). The fact that medical errors were a leading cause of death sent shock waves through the medical system. This was part of a cascade of international literature that highlighted problems with healthcare systems and called for higher quality of care and attention to patient safety. One of the causes of errors emphasized was fatigue; that physician trainees were working >100 hours per week contributed to errors. This resulted in regulatory requirements to limit physician trainee work hours. As a result, trainees were protected from excessively long workweeks, but the reduction in patient care and follow-up limited the educational experience these duties provided. In addition to less time for patient care, other changes in the education of healthcare trainees in the last decade include a concerted effort to make medical care more transparent and more patient- and family-centered as well as a progressive expectancy to disclose errors, to allow family presence during critical events, to respect requests for senior clinician involvement in procedures, etc. All of this translates to a sea of change in terms of how we educate our healthcare trainees.

The factors described above aligned in a manner analogous to what Gladwell (8) referred to as The Tipping Point, "that magic moment when an idea, trend, or social behavior crosses a threshold, tips, and spreads like wildfire." Simulation

is spreading like wildfire through healthcare, and pediatrics in particular. In another of his works entitled "Outliers: The Story of Success," Gladwell refers to seminal work by Anders Ericsson where he methodically analyzed what it takes to become a world-class expert in a field, that is, chess, athletics, music, etc. He is widely quoted as demonstrating that it takes 10,000 hours of practice at one's specialty to become a true expert (9,10). However, Ericsson clearly states that "practice" is not sufficient; it is "deliberate practice" that is the key. In healthcare, the physician who is seeing patients day to day is not in deliberate practice, that is, "game time" is more effective if performance is analyzed, feedback given, and that time used to implement feedback and improve performance. A key ingredient to success is a coach who is invested in, and cares about, their students' success, observes them, gives specific feedback on performance with tips targeted at addressing deficiencies, and provides practice that deliberately focuses on narrowing identified gaps. Simulation can be used to provide "deliberate practice" and debriefing with direct feedback, important tools to improve healthcare education and training.

Weinstock et al. (11) described why simulation is relevant for those who care for children, and coined the phrase the "pediatric training paradox." In addition to the factors listed above, the relative rarity of high stakes, high-risk events such as cardiac arrest or difficult airway management in children results in less "hands-on" practice of procedures and teamwork that are made more difficult by the small size, limited space for a team around the patient and heightened emotions related to the vulnerable population. We encounter the problem of very difficult procedures, which require the most amount of practice for proficiency, are the least available to practice. Simulation has the potential to provide a student with efficient practice of rare events despite decreased trainee hours, low incidence, or seasonality of disease. If we acknowledge that simulation has become an important tool in our educational toolbox for pediatric critical care medicine, we can address how to best approach and optimize its use (**Table 4.1**).

Reflecting on Flexner's words, "An education in medicine nowadays involves both learning and learning how," we find similarity in work that psychologist George Miller proposed in 1990 for *assessing* clinical competence using what is now referred to as Miller's Pyramid. This pyramid has four levels; at the base rather than "learning and learning how" Miller (12) uses the language "knows" and "knows how," followed by "shows how" and "does" (see **Fig. 4.2**). This is our ultimate

TABLE 4.1

TYPES OF SIMULATION—EXAMPLES FROM PEDIATRIC CRITICAL CARE

■ TYPE OF SIMULATION	■ EXAMPLES FROM PEDIATRIC CRITICAL CARE PRACTICE
Standardized patients	Training toward effective and compassionate communication: end-of-life discussions, autopsy, organ donation, obtaining consent, disclosure of errors, offering apologies, and HIV exposure
High-technology mannequin	Team training: cardiopulmonary resuscitation, difficult airway scenarios, shock management, elevated intracranial pressure management
Virtual reality	Bronchoscopy, endoscopy, endovascular procedures
Partial task trainer	Airway trainers: bag-valve-mask ventilation and nasal and oral–tracheal intubation, central-line chests, lumbar puncture trainers, and arterial-line trainers
Screen-based microsimulation	Advanced cardiac life support, trauma management, and critical care scenarios

goal, that our frontline clinicians can demonstrate the required knowledge and skills through answers on Multiple Choice Questions tests, in physical demonstration in a safe setting (simulated clinical environment), and ultimately at the bedside (the top of Miller's Pyramid). This pyramid emphasizes the importance of hands-on, experiential learning in which the learner demonstrates to the teacher that they have mastered the appropriate skills and knowledge. Another important paradigm for evaluating the effectiveness of a training program is Kirkpatrick's (13) four steps, or "levels," first proposed in the 1950s and subsequently refined. The four levels Reaction, Learning, Behavior, and Results are used as a progressive chain of evidence on the effectiveness of a training program (see **Fig. 4.3**) (14). Ultimately, we should target our educational and training programs to the top of Miller's Pyramid (the learner is able to perform what was taught in a clinical environment) and Kirkpatrick's Results level (assessment of whether the training program improves clinical outcomes).

Donald Schön, in his book *Educating the Reflective Practitioner*, states "Professional education should be redesigned to combine the teaching of applied science with coaching in the artistry of reflection-in-action." This statement emphasizes the role of the educator in guiding the student through the process of continual critical evaluation of their own performance by "coaching" them during their active learning experience (15).

We have reviewed the rationale and underlying goals of simulation training and will now focus on the essential elements for designing simulation curriculum. One of the most important principles is that the students involved in healthcare simulation are adult learners, and teaching adults is different from teaching children. Malcolm Knowles popularized the term andragogy, originally introduced by the German professor Alexander Knapp. Knowles initially defined andragogy as "the art and science of helping adults learn," and pedagogy as "the art and science of teaching children." However, he felt this was too simplistic and ultimately saw them as two ends of a spectrum of educational approaches that extends from those used for learners who are dependent on the teacher for direction and priorities to learners that are self-directed. He realized that both the age of the learner as well as the content being taught might influence the learner's needs (16). Knowles et al. (17) describe six key components of andragogy (see **Fig. 4.4**). These factors should be explicitly considered when developing curriculum for adult learners in order to deliver material in the most engaging and motivating approach.

Another helpful concept to consider when developing simulation-based curriculum is David Kolb's "Experiential Learning Cycle." Kolb (18) described four phases of this cycle: (1) concrete experience, (2) observation and experience,

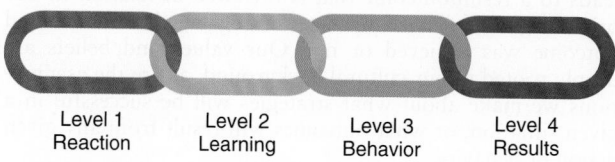

| Level 1 Reaction | Level 2 Learning | Level 3 Behavior | Level 4 Results |

Level 1: Reaction

To what degree participants react favorably to the training

Level 2: Learning

To what degree participants acquire the intended knowledge, skills, attitudes, confidence and commitment based on their participation in a training event

Level 3: Behavior

To what degree participants apply what they learned during training when they are back on the job

Level 4: Results

To what degree targeted outcomes occur as a result of the training event and subsequent reinforcement

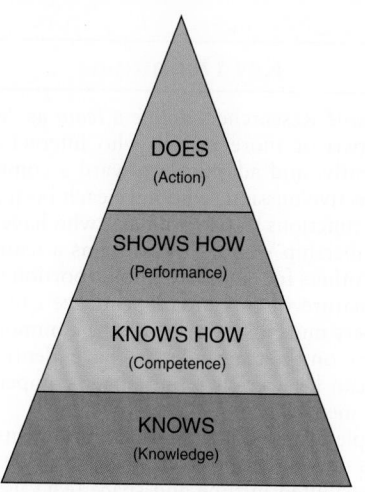

FIGURE 4.2. Miller's Pyramid—Assessment of clinical skills. (From Miller GE. The assessment of clinical skills/competence/performance. *Acad Med* 1990:S63–7.)

FIGURE 4.3. The Kirkpatrick model. http://www.kirkpatrickpartners.com/OurPhilosophy/TheKirkpatrickModel/tabid/302/Default.aspx

1. The Learner's need to know
2. Self concept of the learner
3. Prior experience of the learner
4. Readiness to learn
5. Orientation to learn
6. Motivation to learn

FIGURE 4.4. Six principles of andragogy to be considered when teaching adult learners per Knowles. (From Knowles MS, Holton EF, Swanson RA. *The Adult Learner—The Definitive Classic in Adult Education and Human Resource Development*. Oxford, England: Elsevier, 2011.)

(3) forming abstract concepts, and (4) testing in new situations. Simulation methodology fits into this cycle very well: participation in an immersive simulation exercise is the concrete experience (phase 1) followed by facilitated debriefing to discuss the observations (phase 2), during which the learner forms ideas and hypotheses on ways to improve their performance (phase 3), and then, ideally, they have the opportunity to test out their theory, trying to incorporate the feedback they received during the debriefing by participating in another simulation (phase 4), and the cycle begins again.

The pivotal part of the "Experiential Learning Cycle" as it relates to simulation is the facilitated debriefing. In the debriefing, understanding the learner's interpretation of events will assist with the reflection on their performance. Several models of debriefing in healthcare have been described. The educational goals of these models determine the optimal methodology for implementation.

Argyris and Schön (19) described two pathways of learning from experience: single-loop and double-loop learning. Both are valid methods when applied to the correct settings.

Constructivist theory postulates that humans actively construct personal realities and create their own representational models of the world. Based on this theory, Argyris and Schön introduced the concept of theories of action. They described theories of action as the mental maps (governing variables) that guide our actions. The implementation of our actions leads to a result/outcome that is reviewed in relation to our original goal; followed by determining whether the desired outcome was achieved or not. Our values and beliefs are deeply rooted in our cultural background, as are the assumptions we make about what strategies will be successful in a given situation, or what outcomes will result from any given action or behavior.

During single-loop learning, the learner connects an action with a result, and if, upon review, the result is not the desired outcome, they implement a different approach to achieve their goal. The key here is that the goals, values, plans, and rules that governed their actions remain unquestioned. Single-loop learning is particularly relevant for novice learners and is facilitated through deliberate practice and coaching. An example of single-loop learning with focused feedback and deliberate practice to achieve a level of competency is a method referred to as "Rapid Cycle Deliberate Practice" (20).

During double-loop learning, the learner evaluates their mental maps (governing variables) that guided their actions. During this process, they reevaluate their goals, values, and beliefs. This involves a more sophisticated way of engaging with their experience, and this is where the debriefing facilitator plays a central role. The richness of this learning is in its potential to affect many actions rather than just those observed through changing the learner's mental maps. The most common debriefing methodology to facilitate double-loop learning incorporates advocacy inquiry techniques (21).

TEAMWORK DYNAMICS

Modern healthcare delivery is complex and relies on the coordination of inputs from increasingly diversified care providers, staff members, patients, and family members. Managing this complexity requires a shift from thinking exclusively about individual expertise and competence to a broader perspective including the interdependencies and interactions between multiple experts. Also, this shift needs to extend to an understanding of the diversity expertise involved in effective patient care and the respect for input from other staff and nonclinical experts. Converging evidence indicates that failures of leadership, teamwork, and communication contribute to a large proportion of the preventable patient harm (22). Communication failures are causal or contributing factors in a large proportion of sentinel events (incidents of severe and lasting patient harm or death) (23). In the hospital, cross-sectional surveys indicate that people's perceptions of teamwork within and between units (a culture of safety) account for up to 25% of the variance in preventable harms (24).

These general findings are borne out in the critical care literature as well. An observational study revealed that 37% of the errors in the ICU involved breakdowns in verbal communication between physicians and nurses, a finding all the more striking in that communication comprised only 2% of the activities observed (25). Pronovost and colleagues replicated this finding in a multicenter review of incident reports from 23 ICUs over the period of 1 year. Specifically, they found that teamwork-related failures were critical factors in 32% of incidents (26). Conversely, positive teamwork is associated with lower lengths of stay, lower incidents of periventricular/intraventricular hemorrhage or periventricular leukomalacia, and reduced likelihood of mortality and readmission (27–29).

This expansion of focus from individual to team expertise is supported by academic and educational entities (Interprofessional Education Collaborative Expert Panel, 2011) (7,30). Consequently, both researchers and practitioners focus on teamwork as a core strategy for improving safety and quality of patient care. The growth in peer-reviewed scientific literature pertaining to teamwork in healthcare has accelerated over the past decade, in line with trends discussed above for simulation in healthcare (31). To summarize this growing literature, we provide a review of definitions, competencies, and improvement strategies with an emphasis on simulation-based team training (SBTT).

Key Definitions

What is a team? Researchers define a *team* as "a distinguishable set of two or more people who interact dynamically, interdependently, and adaptively toward a common and valued goal/objective/mission, who have each been assigned specific roles or functions to perform, and who have a limited life span of membership" (32). To qualify as a team, individuals must rely on others for completing some portion of their work, though the nature of this interdependence can vary greatly. Team members must also work to some common ends. However, everyone on the team may not have identical goals, and therefore it can be necessary to manage competing priorities among team members.

The complexity of critical care environments complicates applying the above definition of a team. Critical care teams are often distributed in time and space (e.g., using asynchronous technology, to communicate "different time, different place" tools that do not provide real time communication) and have highly permeable boundaries with shifting membership (e.g., frequent rotation of shifts, the temporary involvement of consultants). These team configurations pose severe challenges to continuity of care and effective communication and create the opportunity for multiple types of communication failures: (a) system failures (i.e., communication channels do not exist), (b) message failures (i.e., communication channels exist, but information is omitted or not transmitted in a timely, complete, or accurate manner), and (c) reception failure (i.e., communication channels exist and information is transmitted, but transmission is dismissed or misinterpreted by receiver) (33).

What are team performance and team effectiveness? Team performance comprises *task work* (the components of an individual's job that are not interdependent with other team members) and *teamwork* (the aspects of performance involving exchanges with other team members). Teamwork encompasses a wide range of interaction processes, including communication, cooperation, coordination, cognition (i.e., the collective knowledge and shared understanding among team members), conflict resolution, and coaching (i.e., developmental feedback provided to team members). This broad range of processes can be grouped into action (i.e., things the team does while performing a specific task), transition (i.e., things the team does while preparing for or reflecting on a performance episode), and interpersonal (i.e., things team members do to manage relationships on the team) processes (34). *Team effectiveness* is valuebased judgment of the products of the team's work relative to predetermined criteria of success, typically including efficiency, accuracy, safety, and team learning (i.e., has the team improved its ability to work together in the future?), and viability (i.e., an affective outcome relating to team relationships and indicating whether or not team members want to work together in the future).

Teamwork Competencies in Critical Care

In order to develop systems to improve skill in a given domain, it is necessary to define effective performance and determine what competencies underlie that performance. Teamwork competencies are the knowledge, skills, and attitudes (KSAs) that underlie effective team performance (i.e., what do people need to know, do, and value or feel in order to be effective team members?). Currently, there is no standard or universally accepted model of teamwork competencies for healthcare in general or for critical care medicine specifically. Building a competency model for teamwork can involve both top-down and bottom-up strategies (35).

Top-down strategies for developing competencies use the preexisting consensus models of teamwork for a given specialty or task situation as well as the existing general science of teams. For example, the general science of teams provides insights from decades of empirical and theoretical work-defining mechanisms of effective teamwork (36). Additionally, many professional societies are defining teamwork-related competencies for their fields, and the Interprofessional Education Collaborative (a joint venture between the American Association of Medical Colleges, American Dental Education Association, American Association of Colleges of Pharmacy, American Association of Colleges of Nursing, American Association of Colleges of Osteopathic Medicine, and the Association of Schools of Public Health) has advanced a highlevel four-domain model of interprofessional competency, including values and ethics of interprofessional practice, roles and responsibilities, interprofessional communication, and teams and teamwork (30). Past reviews of teamwork training programs in healthcare indicate that the most commonly trained skills include communication, situational awareness, leadership, role clarity, and coordination (37,38).

Bottom-up strategies for developing competency models involve using the existing empirical evidence for a specific work domain or task as well as task analysis techniques to define what aspects are most important for a given situation or set of tasks. A recent review of teamwork research in critical care revealed communication, leadership, collaboration, and team climate/culture as the most frequently researched constructs (39). However, consistent use of terminology and clarity of constructs is a challenge that needs to be addressed in future work. As with the general teamwork literature and the simulation-based teamwork training literature, the language used to define teamwork is loose and frequently the same labels are used for different aspects of team performance (40).

Improvement Strategies

Three main strategies are used to improve teamwork in healthcare: work redesign, structured communication tools, and team training (41). Growing evidence supports the effectiveness of each of these interventions; however, they are frequently combined into multifactorial interventions, a strategy that is likely to be most effective (37,42). A combination such as work redesign and structured communication tools provides embedded support in the work environment to encourage the transfer of teamwork skills developed in training (43).

Work redesign approaches target teamwork inputs such as the task and team structure, work processes, or the physical environment in order to facilitate more effective or reliable interactions. For example, including pharmacists on multidisciplinary rounds reduces prescribing errors (44). This intervention targets team structure by changing team composition (i.e., who is on the team?) to ensure that the team has access to the most detailed and up-to-date information about medications. Other potential areas targeted by work redesign initiatives are staff scheduling, information technology, the physical layout of a unit, and work processes or policies. For time-sensitive emergencies, examples of work redesign include choreographing and scripting specific team interactions during traumas, cardiac arrests, or difficult airway situations.

Structured communication tools aim to improve the reliability of critical team interactions. Predictably occurring critical team interactions are identified and scripted to some extent to promote reliability of the process. Preoperative briefings, postoperative debriefings, and patient handoffs are some of the most widely used and evaluated structured communication tools (45). Specifically, in critical care environments, the daily goals form is a structured communication tool designed to facilitate the development of a clear and common understanding of patient care priorities (26). Additionally, structured verbal scripts such as the two-challenge rule (i.e., setting expectations for assertiveness and escalation of unresolved safety issues) and "red flag" words (i.e., a controlled vocabulary that helps staff members communicate efficiently) are commonly implemented (46). In the Johns Hopkins Hospital, a recent development to facilitate team functioning of the Pediatric Rapid Response Team is a structured script for the pharmacists. There are four questions to be asked sequentially: "Who is the team leader?" "What is the child's weight?" "Is there a working IV?" and "What algorithm are we in?" During simulations and subsequent clinical situations, these simple questions have been noted to not only help the pharmacist perform his or her assigned tasks but also trigger positive and productive team communication and interactions. Similarly, choreographing positions of team members during traumas and cardiac arrests provides structure to the interactions, which optimizes the process and outcomes of time-sensitive critical events.

Team training encompasses content (i.e., the teamwork competencies addressed above), tools (e.g., performance measures, task analysis techniques), and delivery methods (i.e., information-, demonstration-, and practice-based methods) that all together comprise an instructional strategy for building effective teams (35). A variety of approaches have been used to train teams, and the emerging evidence indicates that these interventions are effective across the full range of training evaluation criteria: learner reactions (i.e., people have positive reactions to the training and believe that it will be useful in their practice), learning (i.e., people acquire the targeted knowledge and skills), transfer (i.e., teamwork behaviors change on the job), and results (i.e., improvements in teamwork are associated with improvements in other outcomes of value such as efficiency, safety, and patient outcomes) (31).

Simulation-Based Team Training

3 Structured, guided practice and developmental feedback are critical for building individual expertise. The same is true of teamwork expertise. While many factors are known to influence learning outcomes of SBTT, we focus here on four interrelated components: simulator fidelity, scenarios, performance measurement, and feedback.

Simulator Fidelity

2 Simulation is an instructional strategy, not a technology. A wide variety of simulators (i.e., some representation of a component of the task or task environment) can be used for training teams. The degree to which these simulators accurately mimic what they are simulating is referred to as the fidelity of the simulator. The relationship between simulator fidelity and learning outcomes has been studied for decades and found to be highly nuanced (47). However, research clearly distinguishes between the physical fidelity of the simulator (i.e., the degree to which the simulator accurately replicates audio, visual, and tactile cues of the "real thing") and functional or cognitive fidelity (i.e., the degree to which the simulator requires the learner to use the same performance processes as they would in the "real thing") (48). The cognitive or functional fidelity of a simulator plays a much more central role in learning than physical fidelity. For example, in a multicenter study of pediatric resuscitations, Cheng et al. (49) found that there was no significant impact of simulator fidelity on learning outcomes. It is imperative that we recognize that in the Cheng study the "child" was in cardiac arrest and thus did not require the simulator to simulate the features of an awake and interacting human being with associated physical signs. If the scenario learning objectives required the use of more nuanced physical cues, the simulator would likely require higher levels of physical fidelity. In line with this evidence, Rudolph et al. (50) suggest focusing on three aspects of fidelity (emotional, conceptual, and technical) to ensure high levels of learner engagement and their sense of realism. The specific learning objectives of a given curriculum will define which of these three aspects of fidelity is the most important to effectively teach a given objective.

Simulation Scenarios

To be effective, practice-based learning opportunities need to be structured (51). In SBTT, the *scenario is the curriculum* (52). It determines whether or not learners will have an opportunity to practice targeted behaviors or not. Consequently, scenario design should be driven by the specific learning objectives (i.e., what teamwork knowledge, skills, or attitudes is the training attempting to build?). Event-based methods are a general instructional design approach for developing practice-based learning opportunities used widely in military, aviation, and healthcare domains (53,54). In this approach, learning objectives are used to define scenario events (i.e., changes in simulated patient physiology, behaviors of confederates acting in the scenario) and targeted responses (i.e., what should effective teams do in response to these events?).

Learning objectives typically include a combination of teamwork skills and technical skills (cognitive or procedural), though the "medical knowledge" elements of the scenario serve mainly as mechanisms to create stressors that place learners on the edge of their learning curve. The two most common techniques used for designing team training scenarios are as follows: (a) Titration of complexity, where the complexity of a simulated clinical event is titrated (gradually increased) to place the learner on the edge of the learning curve. This can be done preemptively (scripted) or dynamically during the simulated clinical event. (b) Teamwork-specific design, where technique involves specific incorporation of teamwork elements. The flow and progression of the scenario directed through introducing confederate actors as team members or family members, and/or controlling the simulated clinical environment through providing or withholding key resources, which should trigger teamwork issues. For example, in a cardiac resuscitation scenario, a confederate actor in the scenario could be performing chest compressions and purposely slow the rate of compressions to be significantly below the rate prescribed by the standard resuscitation guidelines. This creates an opportunity for team members to recognize this performance decrement (i.e., situation monitoring) and to adapt (i.e., leadership behaviors of delegation). Similarly, a team-based procedural simulation might involve a physician confederate performing placement of a central venous catheter and intentionally contaminating the guide wire, with a desired response of the nurse participant noticing this infectious risk and speaking up to point out the infraction and offering a clean wire and set of gloves. Ideally, the nurse would have several opportunities to practice speaking up until he or she felt comfortable doing so to increasing the likelihood of transferring this important teamwork skill into actual clinical practice. These clinical "events" define the basic structure and flow of the scenario and ensure that it will provide opportunities for learners to practice targeted competencies.

Measuring Performance

Measurement is important to evaluate the effectiveness of a training initiative as well as for assisting with systematic developmental feedback. There are two general methods available for measuring team performance: survey and observation. Each of these approaches has strengths and weaknesses. Self-report survey measures are well suited for capturing inherently subjective aspects of teamwork such as attitudes (e.g., mutual trust, collective efficacy). Observational methods are well suited to capture behavioral components of teamwork while avoiding well-known biases in self-ratings of performance (55). An increasing number of general observational tools and tools built for specific specialty areas are available in the literature (56). However, scenarios built using the event-based method described above translate into measurement protocols. Specifically, scenario events are treated as scale items (i.e., an opportunity to demonstrate a specific component of teamwork), and an observer rates whether or not (or the degree to which) team members exhibit the targeted behaviors. These performance checklists or rating forms are scenario specific, but they flow directly from learning objectives and are useful for driving process-oriented, developmental feedback.

Providing Feedback

Educational feedback is the most important feature of simulation-based learning (57). In team training, this feedback most frequently comes in the form of facilitated team debriefs. Team debriefs are powerful tools for improvement, with meta-analysis indicating that team debriefs can improve performance by as much as 20% (58). Conversely, team members' skills can fail to develop at all without debriefing (59). Practice alone is insufficient. Reflection and feedback are necessary components of learning from practice. However, team debriefs can be harmful if implemented poorly (e.g., team members learn the "wrong lessons") (60). Evidence-based best practices in team debriefing are still emerging, but commonly recommended features of an effective team debrief include establishing a safe learning environment, focusing on teamwork process (and not just task outcomes), diagnosing the team's performance (i.e., seeking to understand why the team performed the way it did), and using a structured approach to ensure consistency and alignment with learning objectives. For example, a multicenter study on pediatric resuscitation found that the use of a script to facilitate debriefing significantly improved knowledge and leadership behaviors in teams when compared with those randomized to an unstructured debrief condition (49).

While debriefing has clearly been recognized as an essential element for an effective simulation, no clear "best" method of debriefing has emerged. In fact, just as one should carefully choose what elements of fidelity are necessary for a given learning objective, similarly, the debriefing approach should be chosen to match the learning objective. A description of different approaches to debriefing is beyond the scope of this chapter, but includes approaches focused on understanding the learners' frame of reference and improving their critical thinking ("Advocacy Inquiry"), approaches focused on direct feedback with multiple opportunities to "try again" in order to master specific skills and teamwork skills ("Rapid Cycle Deliberate Practice") or a hybrid of debriefing styles that are thoughtfully chosen to fit the learning objectives (20,21).

CONCLUSIONS AND FUTURE DIRECTIONS

Simulation training and teamwork dynamics are both fundamental to pediatric critical care and inextricably intertwined. The historical and theoretical framework provides a backdrop to substantiate why we must diligently incorporate both into our future training curricula in order to optimize the care we provide to critically ill children, increasing the impact we will make by ultimately saving more lives.

References

1. Sherwin J. More than make believe: The power and promise of simulation. *Biomed Instrum Technol* 2012;46(4):254–63.
2. http://www.carnegiefoundation.org/sites/default/files/elibrary/Carnegie_Flexner_Report.pdf. Accessed May 8, 2014.
3. http://www.oslersymposia.org/about-Sir-William-Osler.html. Accessed May 8, 2014.
4. Rodriguez-Paz JM, Kennedy M, Salas E, et al. Beyond "see one, do one, teach one": Toward a different training paradigm. *Postgrad Med J* 2009;85(1003):244–9.
5. Hunt EA, Nelson KL, Shilkofski NA. Simulation in medicine: Addressing patient safety and improving the interface between healthcare providers and medical technology. *Biomed Instrum Technol* 2006;40(5):399–404.
6. Helmreich RL, Merritt AC, Wilhelm JA. The evolution of crew resource management training in commercial aviation. *Int J Aviat Psychol* 1999;9:19–32.
7. Kohn L, Corrigan J, Donaldson M. *To Err Is Human: Building a Safer Health System*. Washington, DC: The National Academies Press, 1999.
8. http://gladwell.com/the-tipping-point/. Accessed May 11, 2014.
9. Gladwell M. *Outliers: The Story of Success*. New York, NY: Little, Brown and Company, 2008.
10. Ericsson KA, Krampe RT, Tesch-Romer C. The role of deliberate practice in the acquisition of expert performance. *Psych Rev* 1993;100(3):363–406.
11. Weinstock PH, Kappus LJ, Kleinman ME, et al. Toward a new paradigm in hospital-based pediatric education: The development of an onsite simulator program. *Pediatr Crit Care Med* 2005;6(6):635–41.
12. Miller GE. The assessment of clinical skills/competence/performance. *Acad Med* 1990 Sep;65(9 Suppl):S63–7.
13. Kirkpatrick DL. Techniques for evaluating training programs. *J ASTD* 1959;11:1–13.
14. Kirkpatrick DL. *Evaluating Training Programs: The Four Levels*. San Francisco, CA: Berrett-Koehler, 1994.
15. Schön DA. *Educating the Reflective Practitioner*. San Francisco, CA: Jossey-Bass, 1987.
16. Knowles MS. *The Modern Practice of Adult Education: From Pedagogy to Andragogy—Revised and Updated*. Englewood Cliffs, NJ: Prentice Hall/Cambridge, 1988.
17. Knowles MS, Holton EF, Swanson RA. *The Adult Learner—The Definitive Classic in Adult Education and Human Resource Development*. Oxford, England: Elsevier, 2011.
18. Kolb DA. *Experiential Learning: Experience as the Source of Learning and Development*. Englewood Cliffs, NJ: Prentice Hall, 1984.
19. Argyris C, Schön DA. *Theory in Practice: Increasing Professional Effectiveness*. San Francisco, CA: Jossey Bass, 1974.
20. Hunt EA, Duval-Arnould JM, Nelson-McMillan KL, et al. Pediatric resident resuscitation skills improve after "rapid cycle deliberate practice" training. *Resuscitation* 2014;85(7):945–51.
21. Rudolph JW, Simon R, Dufresne RL, et al. There's no such thing as "nonjudgmental" debriefing: A theory and method for debriefing with good judgment. *Simul Healthc* 2006;1(1):49–55.
22. Pham JC, Aswani MS, Rosen M, et al. Reducing medical errors and adverse events. *Ann Rev Med* 2012;63:447–463.
23. The Joint Commission (2014). Sentinel event data: Root causes by event type. http://www.jointcommission.org/assets/1/18/Root_Causes_by_Event_Type_2004-2Q2013.pdf. Accessed June 4, 2014.
24. Mardon RE, Khanna K, Sorra J, et al. Exploring relationships between hospital patient safety culture and adverse events. *J Patient Saf* 2010;6(4):226–32.
25. Donchin Y, Gopher D, Olin M, et al. A look into the nature and causes of human errors in the intensive care unit. *Crit Care Med* 1995;23(2):294–300.
26. Pronovost PJ, Thompson DA, Holzmueller CG, et al. Toward learning from patient safety reporting systems. *J Crit Care* 2006;21(4):305–15.
27. Shortell SM, Zimmerman JE, Rousseau DM, et al. The performance of intensive care units: Does good management make a difference? *Med Care* 1995;32(5):508–25.
28. Pollack MM, Koch MA. Association of outcomes with organizational characteristics of neonatal intensive care units*. *Crit Care Med* 2003;31(6):1620–9.
29. Baggs JG, Schmitt MH, Mushlin AI, et al. Association between nurse-physician collaboration and patient outcomes in three intensive care units. *Crit Care Med* 1999;27(9):1991–8.
30. I. E. C. Core competencies for interprofessional collaborative practice: Report of an expert panel. Interprofessional Education Collaborative Expert Panel, 2011.

31. Weaver SJ, Dy SM, Rosen MA. Team-training in healthcare: A narrative synthesis of the literature. *BMJ Qual Saf* 2014;23(5):359–72.

32. Salas E, Dickinson TL, Converse SA, et al. Toward an understanding of team performance and training. In: Sezey RW, Salas E, eds. *Teams: Their Training and Performance*. Norwood, NJ: Ablex, 1992.

33. Dayton E, Henriksen K. Communication failure: Basic components, contributing factors, and the call for structure. *Jt Comm J Qual Patient Saf* 2007;33(1):34–47.

34. LePine JA, Piccolo RF, Jackson CL, et al. A meta-analysis of teamwork processes: Tests of a multidimensional model and relationships with team effectiveness criteria. *Personnel Psych* 2008;61(2):273–307.

35. Rosen MA, Salas E, Tannenbaum SI, et al. Simulation-based team training in healthcare: Designing scenarios, measuring performance, and providing feedback. In: Carayon P, ed. *Handbook of Human Factors and Ergonomics in Health Care and Patient Safety*. 2nd ed. New York, NY: Routledge, 2012:573–94.

36. Salas E, Rosen MA, Burke CS, et al. The wisdom of collectives in organizations: An update of the teamwork competencies. In: Salas E, Goodwin GF, Burke CS, eds. *Team Effectiveness in Complex Organizations: Cross-Disciplinary Perspectives and Approaches*. New York, NY: Routledge, 2009:39–79.

37. Weaver SJ, Lyons R, DiazGranados D, et al. The anatomy of health care team training and the state of practice: A critical review. *Acad Med* 2010;85(11):1746–60.

38. Rabøl LL, Østergaard D, Mogensen T. Outcomes of classroom-based team training interventions for multiprofessional hospital staff. A systematic review. *Qual Saf Health Care* 2010;19(6):e27.

39. Dietz AS, Pronovost PJ, Benson KN, et al. A systematic review of behavioural marker systems in healthcare: what do we know about their attributes, validity and application? *BMJ Qual Saf.* 2014 Aug 25.

40. Nestel D, Walker K, Simon R, et al. Nontechnical skills: An inaccurate and unhelpful descriptor? *Simul Healthc* 2011;6(1):2–3.

41. Buljac-Samardzic M, Dekker-van Doorn CM, van Wijngaarden JD et al. Interventions to improve team effectiveness: A systematic review. *Health Policy* 2010;94(3):183–95.

42. Salas E, Rosen MA. Building high reliability teams: Progress and some reflections on teamwork training. *BMJ Qual Saf* 2013;22(5):369–73.

43. Salas E, King HB, Rosen MA. Improving teamwork and safety: Toward a practical systems approach, a commentary on Deneckere et al. *Soc Sci Med* 2012;75(6):986–9.

44. Leape LL, Cullen DJ, Clapp MD, et al. Pharmacist participation on physician rounds and adverse drug events in the intensive care unit. *JAMA* 1999;282(3):267–70.

45. Haynes AB, Weiser TG, Berry WR, et al. A surgical safety checklist to reduce morbidity and mortality in a global population. *N Engl J Med* 2009;360(5):491–9.

46. Pian-Smith MC, Simon R, Minehart RD, et al. Teaching residents the two-challenge rule: A simulation-based approach to improve education and patient safety. *Simul Healthc* 2009;4(2):84–91.

47. Hays RT, Singer MJ. *Simulation fidelity in training system design: Bridging the gap between reality and training.* New York, NY: Springer-Verlag, 1989.

48. Curtis MT, DiazGranados D, Feldman M. Judicious use of simulation technology in continuing medical education. *J Contin Educ Health Prof* 2012;32(4):255–60.

49. Cheng A, Hunt EA, Donoghue A, et al; EXPRESS Investigators. Examining pediatric resuscitation education using simulation and scripted debriefing: A multicenter randomized trial. *JAMA Pediatr* 2013;167(6):528–36.

50. Rudolph J, Simon R, Raemer D. Which reality matters? Questions in the path to high engagement in healthcare simulation. *Simul Healthc* 2007;2(3):161–3.

51. Kirschner PA, Sweller J, Clark RE. Why minimal guidance during instruction does not work: An analysis of the failure of constructivist, discovery, problem-based, experiential, and inquiry-based teaching. *Educ Psychol* 2006;41(2):75–86.

52. Salas E, Priest HA, Wilson KA, et al. Scenario-based training: Improving military mission performance and adaptability. In: Adler AB, Castro CA, Britt TW, eds. *Military life: The Psychology of Serving in Peace and Combat.* Westport, CT: Praeger Security International, 2006:32–53.

53. Fowlkes J, Dwyer DJ, Oser RL, et al. Event-based approach to training (EBAT). *Int J Aviat Psychol* 1998;8(3):209–21.

54. Rosen MA, Salas E, Wu TS, et al. Promoting teamwork: An event-based approach to simulation-based teamwork training for emergency medicine residents. *Acad Emerg Med* 2008;15(11):1190–8.

55. Davis DA, Mazmanian PE, Fordis M, et al. Accuracy of physician self-assessment compared with observed measures of competence: A systematic review. *JAMA* 2006;296(9):1094–102.

56. Dietz AS, Pronovost PJ, Benson KN, et al. A systematic review of behavioural marker systems in healthcare: what do we know about their attributes, validity and application? *BMJ Qual Saf.* 2014 Aug 25.

57. Issenberg SB, Mcgaghie WC, Petrusa ER, et al. Features and uses of high-fidelity medical simulations that lead to effective learning: A BEME systematic review. *Med Teach* 2005;27(1):10–28.

58. Tannenbaum SI, Cerasoli CP. Do team and individual debriefs enhance performance? A meta-analysis. *Hum Factors* 2013;55(1):231–45.

59. Savoldelli GL, Naik VN, Park J, et al. Value of debriefing during simulated crisis management: Oral versus video-assisted oral feedback. *Anaesthesiology* 2006;105(2):279–85.

60. Rall M, Manser T, Howard SK. Key elements of debriefing for simulator training. *Eur J Anaesthesiol* 2000;17:516–7.

CHAPTER 5 ■ PICU ORGANIZATION AND PHYSICAL DESIGN

M. MICHELE MOSS AND SHARI SIMONE

KEY POINTS

1 Seriously and critically ill and injured pediatric patients are best cared for in PICUs separate from adult or neonatal ICUs.

2 Because of the uneven distribution of resources, the regionalization of PICUs is often recommended.

3 Optimal care is provided by a multidisciplinary team that includes physicians, nurses, respiratory therapists, pharmacists, and others.

4 Various staffing patterns exist, depending on acuity of patients in the PICU and availability of support staff.

5 PICU design should be multidisciplinary and includes members of the healthcare team, architects, engineers, hospital administration, and family.

PICU HISTORY

1 Optimal care for the unique needs of the seriously ill pediatric patient occurs best in an ICU specifically designed for children and separate from adult or neonatal facilities. During the 1970s, as technology advanced in the care of critically ill patients, healthcare professionals recognized that specialized units were needed for this specific group of patients. The first recognized ICU was developed in the 1950s, in Copenhagen, Denmark (1), with the primary purpose of caring for victims of the poliomyelitis epidemic (2). In the United States, ICUs for predominantly adult patients were developed in the 1960s; shortly thereafter, the earliest NICUs were formed (1).

The first PICU in the United States was opened in 1967 at Children's Hospital of Philadelphia by Dr. John Downes (1). PICUs initially developed as free-standing units within hospitals during the late 1960s and early 1970s but were mostly found in large, metropolitan areas at large, free-standing children's hospitals or within large, usually university-affiliated medical centers. During the 1980s, PICUs proliferated to essentially all free-standing children's hospitals. The mean number of PICU beds per pediatric population in the United States in 2001 was 1:18,542 (3). Currently, the Society for Critical Care Medicine lists the United States as having 337 PICUs with ~4044 beds, and over 1500 neonatal intensive care units with ~20,000 beds (http://www.sccm.org/Communications/Pages/CriticalCareStats.aspx).

The development of PICUs in Europe predated the US experience, with the first PICU being founded at Children's Hospital in Goteborg, Sweden, in the 1950s in response to the poliomyelitis epidemic that also resulted in the formation of the ICU in Copenhagen (2). PICUs proliferated in Europe as in the United States, with most being located within large multidisciplinary hospitals. For example, by 2000, Spain had 34 PICUs, all linked to the Public Health System (4). All were combined medical and surgical units, and 12 were combined pediatric and neonatal units.

Developing countries have a wide range of models and types of facilities to care for critically ill children depending on the financial resources available to the country. However, spurred by the Millennium Development Goals, the Global Sepsis Initiative, and other international and local projects, the last decade has witnessed significant progress in advancing pediatric intensive care to the developing world.

REGIONALIZATION OF PEDIATRIC CRITICAL CARE SERVICES

The resources required to support the demanding staffing and highly technical needs of critically ill and injured pediatric patients are often unevenly proportioned due to multiple factors, including population disparities, geographic limitations and financial constraints. Regionalization is defined in a statement from the AAP (5) as "a process for organizing resources within a geographic region to ensure access to medical care within a level appropriate to a patient's needs." In Pediatrics, regionalization of critical care services was developed initially for NICUs, such that the more critical and complex neonates were transported and cared for in those NICUs with the most sophisticated equipment and broader support staff. This concept spread with the advent of PICUs in the 1970s. Considering the relatively few critical or potentially unstable children with illness or injuries as compared to adults, and the broader range of diseases and injuries, the concept of regionalization makes even more sense for the pediatric population. Government or financial entities can mandate regionalization, but more commonly, regionalization has developed due to geographic constraints and well-developed referral patterns.

2 Studies (6,7) have supported the concept of regionalization (often called *centralization* in Europe) with their demonstration of better patient outcomes. A study that compared risk-adjusted mortality in a centralized pediatric intensive care system in Australia with a no centralized system in England, where children were often cared for in adult ICUs, found twice the mortality rate in the noncentralized system (8). Regionalization or centralization was supported by a study that showed an inverse relationship between the volume of PICU patients and the risk-adjusted mortality (or length of stay) (9). Regionalization has also been supported for pediatric cardiac surgery where there is less mortality in centers with the highest volumes (10,11).

In the United States, there continues to be wide variability in access of pediatric patients to specialized pediatric emergency and critical care. Due to concern about disaster preparedness for children, data were developed evaluating proximity of children to a PICU (12). In the United States, 81.5% of the pediatric population live within 50 miles of a PICU (as of 2008). However, there is state-by-state variability with some states having essentially all children within 50 miles of a PICU and others as little as 10% of the population living within that radius. A recent study utilized a telephone survey of 5% of the almost 5000 emergency departments listed in the National Emergency Department Inventory to evaluate resource availability for emergency pediatric services as recommended by the joint guidelines on care of children in the emergency department (13,14). In that study, only 11% of emergency departments were located in facilities that had a PICU suggesting that the majority of children needing higher-level care would have to be transported to a facility with the capability of delivering PICU care.

In the United States, three geographic models of regionalization have been described (15). The first are regions composed of large geographic areas, as seen in largely rural settings, with only one or two large urban centers that are able to support a high-level PICU. Such examples are found mostly in the western and southern states such as New Mexico or Arkansas. In this model, the geographic area is large but often not highly populated, so that few critically ill children are spread over large distances. The transport of patients to the appropriate PICU requires preparation and well-developed transport services.

The second model is a large geographic area that is both rural and suburban, with multiple urban centers capable of housing an upper-level PICU. Often, considerable overlap of services is found in these areas, such that referral patterns may not be the most geographically logical. "Competition" for patients may exist in these areas, and financial referral patterns are often seen. Illinois is an example of a state that has urban, suburban, and large rural areas and multiple PICUs.

The third type of geographic referral area is seen in the more populated eastern states. This model is a relatively small geographic area with a large population and, frequently, multiple PICUs. New York City is an example. Rather than geographic area, the local referral patterns and financial constraints define regionalization.

Regionalization of pediatric critical care includes both the PICU and the continuum of services from prehospital care, hospital-based emergency care, intensive care, and specialized services to rehabilitation services. Even the prehospital education components of injury prevention, recognition of serious and critical illness and injury, and accessing the total healthcare system available are parts of this continuum. Emergency medical services for children are also part of this continuum and have been studied and supported by grants from Maternal and Child Health. In 1993, the Institute of Medicine recognized the importance of the development of this pediatric continuum in its report *Emergency Medical Services for Children*, which argued that "society has a special obligation to address the needs of children" (16). Often, pediatric services are buried within adult services, and adequate training and experience are lacking for caregivers to deliver optimal care to children. Evidence suggests that there is better quality of care for pediatric patients in PICUs rather than adult ICUs (17). Training for prehospital and primary hospital caregivers is crucial to provide the best care and outcomes for children. Safe and efficient transport (again, with adequate training of the caregivers) to

higher levels of care must also be provided for a system to be appropriate.

The state of California had early experience in the regionalization of pediatric critical care services. In 1981, the Pediatric Intensive Care Network of Northern and Central California was formed by the medical directors of the 10 PICUs that existed at that time (15). They undertook a study that examined pediatric intensive care resources and, from that, developed a model of regionalization. An extensive effort was undertaken to outline where patients who "could benefit from PICU intervention" were receiving their care. During the study in 1984, 3889 patients were admitted to one of the existing PICUs, with a 5.8% rate of death and an average length of stay of 4.9 days (15). During the same period, 3066 patients, ranging in age from 7 days to 18 years, were admitted to community hospitals that did not have designated PICUs. Due to a marked discrepancy in the severity of illness, the PICUs had a higher rate of death than did the community hospitals. Using this data and with a grant from the Division of Maternal and Child Health of the Department of Health and Human Services, a model for regionalization in northern California was developed. A networking process among the PICUs in the region resulted in cooperative data collection, educational programs, and development and review of statewide standards for PICUs (15).

Countries outside of the United States have also struggled with the issues surrounding regionalization. Sweden undertook the task of centralizing pediatric cardiac surgery from four centers to two during the 1990s, resulting in a reduction in mortality rate from 9.5% to 1.9% over a 5-year period (18). The need for regionalization of pediatric care in India was recognized in an editorial in *Indian Pediatrics* that called for development of a four-tier system that would provide low-cost interventions and technology to children throughout the country and not just in the high-population and higher-income areas (19). The author proposed that caregivers able to recognize the need for urgent referral and access to oxygen, intravenous/intraosseous fluids, and antibiotics would be available at primary health centers throughout the country. Level 1 hospitals would be able to handle serious pediatric illness, whereas Level 2 hospitals would have small, 4- to 6-bed PICUs that would function as Level 2 PICUs, according to guidelines for PICUs developed in India. Level 3 hospitals would be major teaching institutions located in each state and would have a tertiary PICU capable of state-of-the-art pediatric critical care. Embedded in the mission of these tertiary PICUs would be education of physicians, nurses, and healthcare workers, as well as research. A strong transport system would have to be developed throughout the country to address the need to move patients along the levels of care (19).

PICU POPULATION

Patients admitted to PICUs represent a broad range of age groups and disease states. Generally, NICUs admit newborns who have complications of prematurity or delivery or who have congenital anatomic defects. PICUs admit patients from the neonatal period through adolescence. Additionally, because patients with chronic "pediatric" diseases are now living into adulthood, many of those critically ill patients are cared for in PICUs.

Admission Criteria

Admission criteria for PICUs have been defined by the Society for Critical Care Medicine and the AAP (20). In general, admission to a PICU requires acute respiratory, neurologic, or hemodynamic instability; some other specific organ dysfunction; or the imminent risk of instability. Often, the patients are postoperative patients who are at risk for respiratory or hemodynamic instability or specific organ dysfunction. Usually, patients require specific technologic intervention that can only be performed in an intensive care setting with its increased nursing staff. In the United States, most patients cared for in PICUs in 2001 (3) were medical, with approximately one-third being surgical and another 10% being cardiac medical or cardiac surgical patients. In developing countries with limited resources, the admission criterion for a PICU is often the need for mechanical ventilation. Other types of intensive care, such as dialysis or close monitoring of vital signs in unstable patients, may occur outside the PICU, if at all.

Adults with Childhood-Onset Chronic Conditions

In 2008, of the 70 PICUs participating in the Virtual Pediatric Intensive Care Unit Systems database, 13.5% of admissions were aged 15–18 years and 2.7% were greater than 19 years (21). The most common diagnoses in the older age group admitted to PICUs were congenital cardiac abnormalities, generalized developmental delay, and epilepsy. Acute lung injury and respiratory distress syndrome were also represented. PICUs with higher patient volumes were more likely to admit patients greater than 19 years old. When comparing the adult group to the older adolescent group, the adults have poorer functionality as measured by the pediatric overall performance category and the pediatric cerebral performance category scores. Additionally, the adult patients had a 126% higher incidence of PICU mortality than the adolescent group. In a subgroup analysis adjusting for secondary diagnoses and the Pediatric Index of Mortality 2 score, adults aged 20–29 years had a greater than two times odds of PICU mortality and the adults aged >30 years had greater that three times odds of PICU mortality. The diminished functionality on admission and the higher mortality is consistent with the presence of chronic conditions in the adults. Although not clearly studied, the reasons for adults being admitted to PICUs may include a lack of resources and expertise in adult ICUs with conditions such as congenital heart disease, lack of preparation by the patient's medical home to transition care, and lack of adult providers with experience, training, and comfort in caring for patients with childhood-onset chronic diseases or conditions.

Pediatric Cardiac- and Other Specialty ICUs

Specialized PICUs have been developed in areas with large referral bases, such as pediatric cardiac ICUs, pediatric burn ICUs, and more recently pediatric neurointensive care units. Cardiac ICUs have been proliferating since the mid-1990s, although several large programs have had dedicated cardiac ICUs since the 1980s. Currently, most pediatric cardiac centers with high surgical volume, defined as greater than 300 cases per year, have geographically distinct pediatric cardiac ICUs. One perceived advantage of the separate pediatric cardiac ICU is that the staff training and experience are focused on cardiac medical and postoperative issues, allowing for more standardized practice and efficient care. Because the technology required to support these patients becomes increasingly complex with the proliferation of mechanical support devices and complex pharmacologic strategies, additional, extensive staff training is required.

The cardiac ICU patient management team is composed of nurses; respiratory therapists; mid-level practitioners, such as advanced-practice nurses (APNs) or physician assistants (PAs); and physicians, including intensivists, pediatric cardiologists,

pediatric cardiovascular surgeons, and pediatric cardiac anesthesiologists. Residents in pediatrics and cardiac surgery and fellows in critical care and cardiology play varying roles in these cardiac ICUs. The intensive care patient management is generally led by pediatric intensivists, pediatric cardiologists with intensive care experience, pediatric cardiac anesthesiologists, or physicians dually trained and board certified in pediatric critical care and cardiology. Currently, postgraduate fellowship programs exist that are generally 1 year in length and provide additional training in pediatric cardiac intensive care after completing training in pediatric intensive care and/or pediatric cardiology. These programs are not recognized by the Accreditation Council for Graduate Medical Education (ACGME) at this time, and board certification or special competency is not currently available in the discipline of pediatric cardiac intensive care.

Specialized PICUs are less common outside of the United States and Europe, mostly because of limited resources. Pediatric burn patients in Russia, for example, are referred to the national burn hospital but are admitted to the general PICU (22).

PICU PERSONNEL AND STAFFING MODELS

❸ Optimal care for seriously ill and injured pediatric patients requires coordinated multidisciplinary care by physicians, nurses, respiratory therapists, and others, including pharmacists, child-life specialists, social workers, chaplains, nutritionists, and physical, occupational, and speech therapists. Pediatric intensivists should coordinate patient care among the pediatric medical and surgical subspecialists, physicians in training, and primary care physicians.

The development of the discipline of pediatric critical care medicine paralleled the development of PICUs. Care of the critically ill adult patient initially focused on organ-specific failure, and care was provided by a specialist; for example, a pulmonologist cared for patients with respiratory failure, or a cardiologist managed patients with acute cardiac conditions. With the advent of neonatal intensive care, a new model of care developed. Premature and other seriously ill newborns were cared for by pediatricians who oversaw the complete patient, recognizing that all of the organs were at risk during critical illness. The model of the neonatologist was then translated into the pediatric intensivist model.

Intensivist Credentialing and Certification

The pediatric intensivist oversees the "total" patient, with training in both specific organ failure and the interaction of whole-body systems. Training programs in pediatric critical care management initially developed from anesthesiology training programs and ultimately from pediatric training programs. Early on, anesthesiologists applied their intraoperative experience in caring for the whole patient with the need for extensive monitoring to the intensive care environment. Pediatricians, emulating both the anesthesiology and the neonatology model, progressed to the current pediatric intensivist model.

In 1985, the American Board of Pediatrics (ABP) led the recognition for the pediatric critical care medicine subspecialty and offered the first board exam in 1987. The first accreditation of postgraduate fellowship programs followed in 1990, with recognition by the Residency Review Committee of the ACGME. Nursing also recognized pediatric critical care as a special entity. In 1986, the American Association of Critical Care Nurses offered a certification program in pediatric critical care and, in 1999, a program for clinical nurse specialists in pediatric critical care.

Currently, certification by the ABP for pediatric intensivists requires completion of 3 years of pediatric residency training with certification by the ABP in general pediatrics, and completion of 3 years of pediatric critical care fellowship training in an ACGME-approved training program. Pediatric anesthesiologists and pediatric surgeons can earn a certificate of Special Competency in Critical Care. Certification by the ABP is time-limited, and the practitioner must enter into the Maintenance of Certification (MOC) process. MOC is a 10-year cycle structured around 4 parts that evaluate the 6 core competencies defined by the ACGME (www.abp.org). The four parts include Professional Standing as noted by maintaining medical license, Lifelong Learning and Self-Assessment, Cognitive Expertise—secure exam, and Performance in Practice. Successful passing of the secure exam is required only once every 10-year cycle. In both Part 2 Lifelong Learning and Part 4 Performance in Practice, points are earned through activities approved by the ABP. A total of 100 points must be earned every 5 years in the MOC cycle with 40 points in each of Part 2 and Part 4 and the other 20 points in either Part 2 or 4 activities. Lifelong Learning activities include ABP-guided literature reviews, online educational modules such as the AAP PREP ICU, or various educational courses approved by the ABP such as the Society of Critical Care Medicine Pediatric Board Review. Performance in Practice activities include meaningful participation in quality improvement activities approved by the ABP. Some are activities that can be personally performed on a physician's own patient data through web-based improvement modules. Institutions that have received Multi-Specialty Portfolio Program status from ABP may designate MOC credit for physicians participating in institutional quality improvement projects. Many such activities are through quality improvement collaboratives such as the Children's Hospital Association PICU Central Line Associated Blood Stream Infection Prevention Collaborative.

Worldwide certification in intensive care, and particularly pediatric intensive care, is varied and often not available. For some countries, intensive care is certified through specialty boards such as internal medicine or surgery. In Spain, Switzerland, Australia, New Zealand, and Hong Kong, for example, critical care is a primary specialty with separate certification (23). Training requirements vary throughout the world. Because of this variability and despite some similarities in curricula, a process was undertaken by the *competency-based training program in intensive care medicine in Europe* collaboration to develop core competencies for an international training program in adult critical care. This collaboration is composed of physicians from Europe, Asia, North America, South America, and Africa and is supported by various organizations, including the European Society of Intensive Care Medicine and the Society of Critical Care Medicine. Currently, no process is underway for an international training program in pediatric critical care. In many locations, physicians who practice in PICUs are pediatricians with special interest in intensive care who have been unable to train in an organized training program.

In addition to the expanding workload in PICUs due to pharmacologic and technologic advances, pediatric intensivists have a variety of other work-related activities. Because most PICUs are associated with pediatric and/or pediatric critical care training programs, most pediatric intensivists have teaching commitments for a variety of audiences, including residents, critical care fellows, nursing staff, and other medical caregivers. Additionally, many pediatric intensivists are members of an academic faculty, which means they also have research and administrative responsibilities such as medical direction of code teams, medical emergency teams, and transport systems. The clinical arena for the pediatric intensivist has broadened to include coordinating sedation programs for patients who need procedures outside of the operating room and participating in palliative care programs. In addition, due to the multidisciplinary roles in the PICU, pediatric intensivists actively participate in hospital and university committees. The 2003 Future of Pediatric Education II Survey of Sections project (24) revealed that, overall, pediatric intensivists devote ~15% time to teaching across all age groups. Younger intensivists (<40 years old) spend 14% of their time in research, whereas intensivists 40–49 years of age spend 10%, and those ≥50 years old spend 7%. Intensivists who are >50 years old spend ~20% of their time on administrative duties as compared to intensivists who are <40 years old, who spend on average ~12% of their time on administrative duties.

Physician Staffing Models

Multiple staffing models exist for PICUs throughout the world. In the United States, most PICUs are staffed by ABP-certified or ABP-eligible pediatric intensivists (3). From 1995 to 2001, the number of PICUs staffed by pediatric intensivists rose from ~90% to 94% (3). Intensivists provide care through different staffing patterns, and most frequently, the intensivists are the primary physicians or they co-attend with a medical or surgical specialty service. In another model, intensivists serve as primary attendings on a small number of patients but consultants on all PICU patients. In the United States, pediatric intensivists control most PICU admissions. Patient coverage in the PICU frequently involves residents or fellows in addition to the pediatric intensivists.

The effect of training programs on mortality has been shown to vary. One study suggested a higher risk of mortality when PICUs were staffed by residents alone and a much lower risk when staffed by intensive care fellows (25). Larger PICUs in the United States, more commonly than smaller units, have 24-hour, in-house, attending-level coverage, with as many as 40% of those with >20 beds having attending-level, in-house coverage. A study in Malaysia showed that having pediatric intensivists in-house around the clock rather than only during the day, with the night time covered by general pediatricians, lowered standardized mortality ratios and decreased lengths of stay (26).

The Pediatric Hospitalist and the PICU

An alternative medical staffing model gaining popularity in the United States and Canada is a collaborative intensivist-hospitalist model and/or the inclusion of hospitalists providing overnight care (27–31). Since its introduction in 1996, the hospitalist role has been largely responsible for filling clinical gaps in the care of hospitalized patients and is currently the fastest-growing specialty in the United States (32). The Society of Hospital Care defines the hospitalist as "the physician whose primary focus is the general medical care of hospitalized patients." The hospitalist's activities include patient care, teaching, research, and leadership related to hospitalized care (www.hospitalmedicine.org). However, the range of practice areas and clinical responsibilities of the hospitalist varies substantially depending on the individual needs of institutions. Freed et al (33) conducted the largest national survey of hospitalist program directors to date ($n = 112$) examining the characteristics of the pediatric hospitalist workforce. Forty-eight percent of hospitalists were identified as working in teaching hospitals. The majority of hospitals surveyed employed hospitalists with board certification in pediatrics (82%), and some with medicine-pediatric (15%), critical care (7%), or emergency care (2%) training. Only 20 hospitals (18%) reported employing hospitalists in PICUs and only 33% of hospitals reported measuring any clinical outcomes associated with hospitalist care, thus limiting data to demonstrate the impact of the role.

The rapid proliferation of hospitalists in all inpatient practice areas including pediatrics lead to early policy and curriculum development. The American Academy of Pediatrics laid the ground work by publishing in 2005 guiding principles for pediatric hospitalist programs. Also in 2005, the Society of Hospital Medicine created a Pediatric Core Curriculum Taskforce to initiate the development of pediatric hospital medicine core competencies. This comprehensive blueprint endorsed by the American Academy of Pediatrics and Academic Pediatric Association serves as a foundation for the development of curricula and a guide for standardization of training practice (34). In addition to inpatient clinical competencies, an emphasis on systems of care competencies and the role of the hospitalist in leading organizational improvement initiatives was incorporated to meet increasing demands to improve individual patient outcomes and improve performance of healthcare systems. However, as fellowship training programs in pediatric hospital medicine have only recently emerged, standardization in requirements and training has yet to be defined (35,36).

Early outcome data suggest benefits of the hospitalist role in pediatric settings including the PICU. Tenner et al (30,37–39) conducted a retrospective review one year after implementation of the hospitalist role in the PICU to determine the impact on mortality outcomes. The researchers compared the survival of patients in a teaching hospital cared for by residents and hospitalists after-hours without an intensivist in house. The findings revealed improved survival with hospitalists suggesting improved quality of care with more experienced physicians. The most notable study is a systematic review conducted by Landrigan et al. (37) to determine the effects of pediatric hospitalist models on outcomes. Although limited data were available on quality of patient care provided, reductions in hospital costs and length of stay were seen in the hospitalist models when compared to traditional models. Currently, minimal data supporting the role of the pediatric hospitalist in the PICU exist, but as physician shortages increase worldwide, opportunities exist to demonstrate the contributions of this group of physicians in improving clinical processes of care outcomes.

PICU Nurses

Pediatric critical care nurses provide unique contributions to the delivery of care for medically unstable and vulnerable infants and children. The critical care nurse performs continuous, vigilant, compassionate care that is based on the needs and characteristics of the patient and family and that allows for ongoing physiologic patient assessments, implementation and evaluation of responses to the treatment plan, and assessment and development of plans to meet the needs of the family. An essential skill of the critical care nurse is the ability to effectively communicate with all members of the healthcare team and maintain ongoing dialogue to ensure rapid responses to changes in the child's condition.

The current nurse shortage and an aging nurse workforce is a common experience worldwide and has created unique challenges in providing comprehensive care that optimizes patient outcomes. Nursing leadership has been challenged to develop innovative staffing and nursing care models to maintain a high quality of care. Adequate nurse staffing is critical to the delivery of quality patient care and directly influences the rate of preventable adverse events (40–42). In a study of unplanned estuations in a children's hospital PICU in the United States, a patient-to-nurse ratio of 1:1 was significantly associated with a decrease in unplanned extubations (43). Not surprising, the presence of the nurse at the patient's bedside is essential to ensure patient safety.

A study conducted in Hong Kong found that 51% of incidents were detected by direct observation versus 27% by monitor detection (44). The investigators concluded that, despite advances in technology, there was no substitute for the expertise of the nurse providing direct patient care.

Nurse-to-patient ratios in ICUs are primarily based on patient census and acuity and may range from 1:3 to 2:1 (45). However, other factors must be considered in determining staffing needs, including the level of experience of the nurses who are providing the care, available technology, unit layout, and support staff. In addition, because the condition of critically ill children can rapidly change, maintaining flexibility in nursing staff is imperative.

Critical care nursing organizations such as the American Association of Critical Care Nurses, the Australian College of Critical Care Nurses, and the British Association of Critical Care Nurses have developed ICU nursing workforce position statements that outline nurse staffing standards based on best-practice evidence; these statements are available at their respective websites. In addition, the World Federation of Critical Care Nurses, an organization comprising over 35 critical care nursing associations, has developed minimum workforce requirements that can be adapted to meet the nursing staff and system requirements of a particular country or jurisdiction (46).

Nursing Care-Delivery Models

Nursing care-delivery models continue to evolve with the changing critical care environment; these models include an emphasis on the patient–family relationship, customer-focused behaviors, process improvement, safety, and achieving high-quality clinical and behavioral outcomes. Since 1990, the Magnet Nursing Services Recognition Program for Excellence in Nursing Services of the American Nurses Credentialing Center has honored national and international organizations that demonstrate excellence in nursing practice with Magnet status. Magnet hospitals have demonstrated higher-than-average nurse recruitment and retention rates, as well as other indicators of quality (47). One important component evaluated is the effective use of a patient care-delivery model that promotes nursing responsibility, authority, and autonomy and one in which best practices are utilized. Nursing departments are charged to shape a patient care-delivery model that fits the individual organization's core values and to design a structural framework that will help to operationalize those values through the delivery of quality patient care. Recent studies have reported improved patient outcomes within hospital environments that support professional nursing practice (48,49).

Expanded nursing roles have also been developed in response to changes in the healthcare system. In the United States, the role of nursing case management has greatly impacted discharge planning of medically complex patients. In other nations, similar specialist roles (i.e., liaison nurses) have been created to streamline ICU transitional care and reduce the impact and potential complications associated with transferring patients within the healthcare system (50).

Nursing Leadership

Effective nursing leadership has been shown to be a key component in the retention of hospital nurses (51). The leadership characteristics of the nurse manager greatly affect the work environment of critical care nurses. Therefore, desirable qualifications of the nurse manager include substantial pediatric expertise and completion of a master's degree in nursing administration. The nurse manager must have a vision for the unit, the skills and expertise to lead the team, the trust of employees, and ongoing dialogue with the PICU team.

Other nursing leadership roles that may have differing titles but similar functions around the world include clinical nurse specialists and critical care nurse consultants. The qualifications required for these advanced-practice nursing roles include a master's degree in nursing and extensive expertise in pediatric critical care. The clinical nurse specialist in the United States and Canada incorporates the roles of expert clinician, consultant, educator, and researcher. The roles of the nurse consultant in the UK parallel those of the clinical nurse specialist in the United States and Canada, with the addition of functioning as a transformational leader who influences both organizational and educational development (52).

The Clinical Nurse Leader (CNL), unlike the clinical nurse specialist role, is a generalist nursing role currently only offered in the United States. The development of this role was in response to the Institute of Medicine's recommendations to improve healthcare systems and capability of frontline healthcare staff (53,54). The CNL role was designed to address the need for nursing leadership to improve the quality of healthcare systems while controlling costs (55). As the CNL is a relatively new role, the impact of this position has yet to be determined. However, early findings suggest the addition of the CNL to the nursing staff mix, which improves outcomes and a potential solution in meeting clinical nurse leadership needs internationally (56–58).

Nursing Professional Development

The professional development of the nursing staff in the PICU is the responsibility of experienced staff members, unit educators, mentors, and APNs, including a clinical nurse specialist. The pediatric clinical nurse specialist or similar advanced-practice nurse ideally coordinates the process. Staff education begins with a didactic and clinical orientation program that provides a foundation for novice nurses to safely care for critically ill children. In addition, designing a professional development program that outlines a realistic advancement plan and identifies those strategies necessary to achieve goals is an important responsibility of the PICU leadership team. Benner's model of knowledge and skill acquisition is a useful framework for identifying how a nurse progresses from novice to expert practitioner (59). The characteristics of each of these levels of clinical expertise can be incorporated to meet the educational needs and promote successful advancement of the individual.

As the novice staff nurse gains expertise, the professional development plan should specify the education, mentoring, and skill acquisition required to prepare the novice to take on additional roles. Examples include charge nurse responsibilities, arrest team member, transport team member, trauma team member, ECMO team member, preceptor for newly hired nurses, and mentor for nurses following orientation. Other important requirements to ensure mastery of skills include completion of pediatric advanced life support provider certification, ongoing emergency simulation exercises, and an annual review of high-risk, low-volume therapies and patient-specific core competencies. Obtaining pediatric critical care nursing certification is now considered the criterion standard of practice (60,61). The critical care registered nurse certification distinguishes nurses who have obtained an advanced body of knowledge necessary to care for critically ill patients.

Participation in ongoing educational programs specific to pediatric critical care is essential for nurses to build on previously acquired knowledge and skills. Continuing nursing education requirements are broadly defined by state nursing legislation, regulations, and professional organizations. Nursing education programs span the spectrum from unit-based in-services, hospital workshops, local seminars, and regional conferences, to national and international nursing conferences. All provide unique opportunities for nurses to expand knowledge and skills, exchange ideas, network, identify best practices from other institutions, and share information with the healthcare team.

The nursing staff is also responsible for participating in those unit functions necessary to support and improve the delivery of quality patient care. Activities include, but are not limited to, quality improvement programs; the development of policies, procedures, standards of care, critical pathways, and guidelines; and the evaluation of practice outcomes.

Nurse Practitioners and Physician Assistants

Nurse practitioners (NPs) and PAs have become integral members of the PICU multidisciplinary team, primarily in the United States. The emergence of these roles in the PICU environment was largely a result of pediatric residency curriculum changes combined with increasing PICU demands (62–64). In July 2003, all residency programs in the United States were subject to the ACGME's new restriction in duty hours. PICU resources have been further impacted by the aging nurse workforce and the increasing complexity of patient care, coupled with the demands for improved patient and PICU outcomes. These changes have propelled modifications in traditional physician staffing patterns and have led to the addition of NPs, PAs, and most recently hospitalists to provide continuity and quality care to critically ill children (65,66). As duty-hour standards for residents in the United States continue to change, restructuring workflow in the PICU will likely require a greater utilization of nonphysician providers to ensure patient safety and maintain quality-of-care outcomes (66,67).

Various PICU collaborative practice models have been reported in which physicians, in combination with NPs and/or PAs, collectively use knowledge and skill sets to enhance patient care (62–64,68–71). In university-affiliated teaching hospitals, the traditional medical team of intensivists, fellows, and residents now includes NPs and PAs. Examples of patient care models in large PICUs include staffing two complete teams, one composed of residents and the other composed of NPs; a combined team of residents and NPs; a combined team of residents, PAs, and NPs; or a team of only NPs. Separate NP and resident teams allow faculty to provide education that is directed toward the specific needs of the group. For example, educational rounds for rotating residents may include a discussion of the evidence-based management for patients with status asthmaticus. In comparison, educational rounds for seasoned NPs may include a discussion on evidence-based therapies for acute respiratory failure when conventional management fails. Tailoring educational needs and clinical skills may result in improved satisfaction for NPs and rotating residents. However, teams composed of residents, NPs, and/or PAs provide unique leadership and mentoring opportunities for practitioners. Staffing patterns in smaller PICUs include various combinations of residents, NPs, and PAs. The team composition affects the distribution of responsibilities given to NPs and PAs, but in general, the primary focus involves managing a daily caseload of patients and often supplementing the 24-hour on-call coverage previously filled by residents and fellows. In centers without fellowship programs, NPs play a greater role in supervising resident teams. In community hospitals, the numbers of NPs and PAs in critical care are substantially greater, because more positions are required to provide daily 24-hour coverage.

Since the emergence of pediatric acute care and critical care NP programs during the early 1990s, the number of NPs in the PICU has increased exponentially. The differences and similarities between NPs and PAs are listed in **Table 5.1**. The educational preparation and clinical expertise of NPs and PAs differ; therefore, the clinicians' contributions to the delivery of care in the PICU are unique. PICU NPs are nurses who typically have some pediatric nursing experience and have completed a graduate program with a pediatric acute care or critical care

TABLE 5.1

SCOPE OF PRACTICE OF NURSE PRACTITIONERS AND PHYSICIAN ASSISTANTS

■ RESPONSIBILITIES	■ NURSE PRACTITIONERS	■ PHYSICIAN ASSISTANTS
Patient management		
Assessment	Comprehensive and problem-specific model of care	Problem-specific model of care
Diagnosis and treatment	Diagnosis rendered independently with awareness of the entire system and the patient's response to illness	Diagnosis rendered under direct supervision of physician
Procedures	Proficient to perform procedures to support/monitor patient condition, treat acute problems, or prevent complications independently by practice agreement	Proficient to perform procedures under direction of physician
Prescription and documentation	Full prescriptive authority, independent documentation	Requires co-signature for prescription and documentation of practice
Education		
Patient education	Promotes health maintenance	Provides health education specific to medical treatment plan
Staff mentoring	Mentors nurses, nurse practitioners, residents, and students	Mentors physician assistants, residents, and medical students
Consultant	Serves as a consultant for variety of nursing care issues	May participate in unit-specific activities
	Participates on hospital committees as advanced nurse practitioner representative	Primary role is direct patient management
	Participates in development of policies/standards/competencies for pediatric critical care	
Research	Advances pediatric nursing knowledge by contributing to evidence-based practice	May participate in research in a variety of roles
System management	Advanced nursing skills promote system evaluation and efforts to improve care delivery	No specific training in this area, but impacts care system

emphasis; some may have completed a pediatric primary care program. However, the advanced-practice education of the NP in the United States is currently undergoing considerable curriculum redesign as there is a concerted movement to transition advanced-practice programs to a doctorate degree by 2015 (72). The Doctor of Nursing Practice is a clinical degree that is intended to prepare the NP or other APN to assume practice leadership roles.

In comparison, PAs complete 2 years of college courses in basic science and behavioral sciences before entering a PA program that averages 26 months and consists of an intense curriculum with both clinical and didactic components. PAs are educated in the medical model, which is designed to complement physician training. They often have previous healthcare experience as emergency medical technicians or paramedics.

Published reports describe the NP and PA scope of practice and the debate surrounding best-practice models in the PICU setting (63,64,68–75). Two national surveys that describe the functions of pediatric and adult critical and acute practitioners demonstrate that the NP provides aspects of care that are reflective of advanced-practice nursing in addition to direct patient management responsibilities (64,76). Global responsibilities include providing comprehensive patient management combined with consultation, education, research, quality improvement, and leadership activities.

In contrast to the NP role, the PA philosophical basis mimics the medical model and is disease focused. PAs are licensed to practice medicine with physician supervision. In the PICU setting, PAs perform direct patient management, including conducting physical exams, diagnosing and treating patients, ordering and interpreting tests, and performing duties that require advanced technical skills. Few publications exist on the role of the PA in pediatric critical care (63). However, the literature describes the success of the PA in specialty care settings and adult intensive care units (72,77,78).

The first study to examine the use of NPs and PAs in pediatric critical care surveyed medical directors of PICUs in the

United States and found that 62.8% of responding institutions employed NPs or PAs (79). The physician respondents reported a skill level of NPs and PAs that was comparable to second- or third-year residents. Since this early study, there has been increasing evidence supporting the positive effect of NP and PA care on patient and system outcomes in critical care settings worldwide. Kleinpell et al (63,72,75,80–87) conducted a systematic review to assess the impact and outcomes of the NP and PA in critical care. Only 31 studies were found, of which 29 were adult and 2 neonatal. Although the data are limited, the evidence demonstrates that the integration of NPs and PAs in critical care positively impacts outcomes including decreasing lengths of stay, decreasing costs of care, decreasing adverse complications, enhancing communication and collaboration, parental and staff satisfaction, and continuity of care (63,82,87). Similar findings were found in a recent international review of the impact of NPs in critical care (83).

Because most nations of the world are experiencing rising healthcare costs and a shortage of healthcare providers, the need for alternative healthcare practitioners has resulted in the development of NP and PA roles in primary care settings since the early 1990s (88). These roles have expanded substantially in acute care areas but continue to evolve in pediatric critical care. As there are currently no international NP practice standards, international colleagues may gain insight by examining the successes and mistakes of the United States, because the advanced-practice issues faced in role development and implementation, including educational standards, credentialing, licensure, titling, prescribing medications, liability, and reimbursement, are common to all.

Respiratory Therapists

Respiratory therapists are an integral part of the bedside care of the pediatric intensive care patient. Respiratory disease in most PICUs is the most common diagnosis, and the impairment of respiratory function complicates many other diseases. In addition to their expertise in mechanical ventilators, respiratory therapists provide pulmonary treatments, including inhaled medications, and they should be trained in pediatric modalities of aerosol delivery and mechanical ventilation. For all levels of PICUs, the American College of Critical Care Medicine of the SCCM recommends that an in-house respiratory therapist who is experienced in pediatric respiratory failure be available at all times (89). Frequently, respiratory therapists have expanded duties, including sampling and running blood gas and other bedside laboratories, participating in patient transport both intra- and interfacility, and participating in extracorporeal membrane oxygenation support. Their participation in the care of the PICU patient is crucial for optimal outcomes. In many countries outside the United States, appropriately trained bedside nurses may provide a function similar to the respiratory therapist.

Other Ancillary Personnel

Multiple other personnel are required for the best care of the PICU patient. Pharmacists are an integral part of the PICU team. A satellite pharmacy should be close to the PICU; in lieu of that, a system must be available to allow immediate dispensing of medications. Additionally, the presence of a clinical pharmacologist helps in the management of patients with complex medication regimens and variable pharmacokinetics. Nutritionists, physical therapists, occupational therapists, speech therapists, and social workers also play significant roles in the care of the PICU patient; consequently, they should have training in pediatric environments. Child life and play therapists also have an important role in helping patients and their families to adjust to critical illness. Chaplains and bereavement teams can also be instrumental in assisting a family to cope with the death of their child.

PHYSICAL DESIGN

Environment of Care

❺ When designing a PICU, several aspects must be taken into account, including regulations from oversight institutions such as government agencies and the Joint Commission, available physical space and location, expertise and needs of the PICU personnel, and pediatric patient- and family-centered concepts. The American College of Critical Care Medicine published revised guidelines for ICU design in 2012 (86,90). As in PICU patient care, a multidisciplinary approach was suggested that involves ICU leaders, including the nurse manager, medical director, architects, engineering staff, information technology specialists, and hospital administration. Additionally, family, interior designers, nursing staff, physician staff, respiratory therapy staff, and others involved in patient care should be asked for design input. Clinical members of the design team need to become familiar with specific regulations in order to better understand design limitations.

The American College of Critical Care Medicine also included the environment of care as an important component to patient- and family-centered care in their Clinical Practice Guidelines for Support of the Family in the Patient-Centered ICU. The environment of care has been shown in multiple studies to have an impact on patient outcome. In addition to the design affecting infection control and improving patient outcomes by limiting spread of infections, it can affect other aspects of the patient experience.

According to the ACCM Guidelines for Intensive Care Unit Design, "the goal of the design is to create a healing environment" (86,90). Evidence exists in multiple areas for the improved outcomes based on good design. In *A Review of the Research Literature on Evidence-based Healthcare Design*, Ulrich et al. (91) found evidence of improved outcomes through environmental measures in the following three areas: improved patient safety, improved "other patient" outcomes, and improved staff outcomes. The area of patient safety with the most evidence of improvement based on design is in the area of infection control. The design measures recommended at a baseline for decreasing healthcare-acquired infections included the following:

- Effective air quality control measures. This is especially important during construction or remodeling to prevent airborne infections.
- Locating alcohol-based hand-rub dispensers in accessible areas particularly at the bedside.
- Choosing coverings for the floor, millwork, and furniture that are easy to clean.
- Installation of appropriate water system including proper temperature, pressure, and drainage with maintenance of the system that includes routine cleaning of point-of-use fixtures.
- Provide single bedrooms to decrease patient-to-patient transmission, reduce airborne infection transmission, and to aid in effective, appropriate cleaning.

In addition to decreasing infection risk, design can impact other safety issues including decreased medical errors by better workflow, improved lighting, and decreased noise. Reducing fall risk, which is more important in elderly populations, can also be impacted by improved design, and reduction of pain is another patient outcome that has been associated with improved design—using nature as a distraction by direct visualization through windows or through photographs. Quality of sleep has been shown to have an effect on patient outcomes in the PICU and can be improved by better acoustic and lighting design (92). The ICU environment can also improve staff outcomes such as decreased injuries using lift systems (which has become more important in pediatrics due to the obesity epidemic), decreased stress through noise control and improved lighting, and increased staff effectiveness through more efficient unit configuration.

Unit Architectural Design

Individual Rooms

Initially, PICUs were of large, ward-type designs. Today, the recommendation is for individual rooms designed in such a way that the risk of infection is decreased, the staff can adequately visualize the patient and monitors, and the patient and family can have privacy. Although the minimum recommended area for pediatric patients is 250 ft^2 (~23 m^2) per bed space (87), each room must be large enough to comfortably accommodate the patient's bed, increasingly complex types and amount of medical equipment, computer equipment, and power and vacuum sources. Because of the importance of family presence in the care of pediatric patients in the PICU setting, larger rooms are being designed to accommodate sleeping and private spaces for parents. In addition to the ability of the room to accommodate all the necessary functions performed in the room, the design of the room must allow flexibility depending on the patient age, size, and medical condition. **Figure 5.1** shows a schematic of technology-enabled single ICU room (93).

Infection is spread by both direct-contact and airborne routes; having separate rooms for each bed space in the PICU minimizes direct-contact spread. Sinks placed in easily accessible areas for hand washing also decrease infection spread by

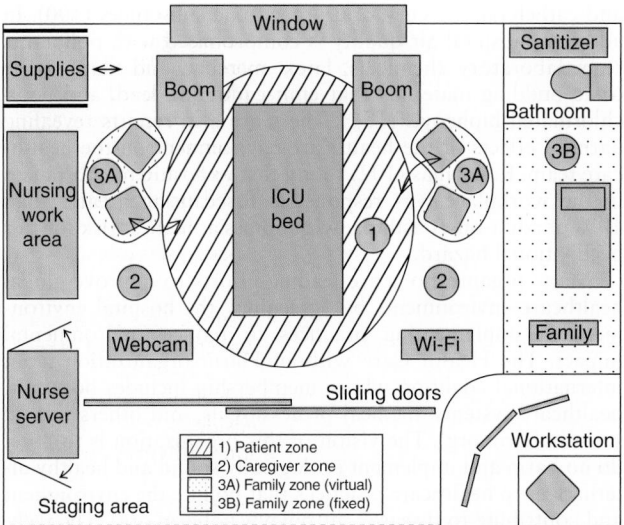

Supplies ↔
Window
Boom   Boom
Sanitizer
Bathroom
Nursing work area
3A   3A   3B
ICU bed   1
2   2
Family
Webcam   Wi-Fi
Nurse server
Sliding doors
Workstation
Staging area

1) Patient zone
2) Caregiver zone
3A) Family zone (virtual)
3B) Family zone (fixed)

FIGURE 5.1. A schematic drawing of a modern, technology-enabled ICU room divided into a patient zone, a parent/family zone, and a nursing zone. Natural light enters through a window on one side and sliding doors open to a staging area on the other. Mobile articulating arms (booms) may hold monitors, pumps, ventilators, and other high-technology equipment.(Reproduced with permission from Halpern NA. Innovative designs for the smart ICU. *Chest* 2014;145:646–58.)

direct contact. But perhaps more important is locating multiple alcohol-based hand rubs around the bedside and at the entrance/exit of each room. Individual rooms can have specific air-flow patterns to prevent infection. Patients who are immunocompromised should be in rooms with positive air flow, i.e., the air in the room is sent out and not pulled in. Patients with potentially communicable diseases, including being colonized with resistant organisms, should be in rooms in which the air is pulled in and not sent out. Some systems allow the flow patterns to be changed depending on the type of patient in the room. A low room ventilation rate defined as "room air changes per hour" is associated with increased airborne transmission (91,94). Other forms of ventilation have been shown to decrease infection such as laminar air flow, which is high-efficiency particulate air–filtered air blown into a room at a given rate.

Spread of infection by contact is the more common form of transmission. Contact can be direct from person to person spread or indirect from an environmental surface. Hand hygiene is the most important prevention strategy for either direct or indirect spread. Handwashing compliance can be improved using design features such as adequate number and accessibility of handwashing facilities and alcohol-based hand gels and the use of automated technology for both. Decreasing surface contamination can be improved by choosing surfaces that are easy to clean. In general, carpet is difficult to clean and therefore undesirable in PICUs; however, it does offer advantages in noise control, decreasing fall risk and improving family comfort. Waterborne infection is less common but can occur.

Noise

ICUs of all types can be noisy environments because of the amount of equipment, alarms, and staff necessary for patient care and safety. Excessive noise has been shown to have a negative effect on patients, as noted by decreased oxygen saturations, decreased sleep, and increased blood pressure and

heart rate (95). Ambient noise levels in hospitals may run as high as 45–70 dB; the World Health Organization recommendation is that ambient noise levels should not exceed 35 dB (96). The multiple hard surfaces (e.g., floors and cabinetry) in hospitals and ICUs can accentuate noise levels. The use of high-performance sound-absorbing materials for floor coverings and ceilings can abate the noise level, while maintaining easy cleaning and infection control. Materials should not only absorb sound, but also decrease reverberation of noise.

Lighting

Lighting has also been shown to impact patient outcome. Most studies, which have evaluated adult patients, have shown that patients who are exposed to natural sunlight have decreased lengths of stay and improved mental status (95). According to the ACCM Guidelines, there should not be less than one window per patient bed area (86,90). Some guidelines also recommend that the level of lighting for patient rooms not exceed 30 fc (foot candles), with the ability to dim the level to as low as 6.5 fc at night (97). Adequate lighting must be available for charting and for emergencies and procedures, thereby requiring lighting systems with multiple types of lights.

Electrical and Communication Requirements

Each room or bed space must have ample electrical power, oxygen, compressed air, and vacuum outlets. Electrical outlets and vacuum outlets should be placed at the head of the bed and 36 in (1 m) above ground for easy access. Other outlets may be necessary in other parts of the room. The electrical power to the PICU should be delivered by a feeder separate from other parts of the hospital. Additionally, power should be connected to an emergency power source.

The PICU should have adequate hard-wire support, so that computers can be placed at each bedside, charting area, and other workspaces. Wireless connection to the Internet should be available in the PICU for both staff and families. Each PICU should have an area for viewing digital radiographs, CT and MRI scans, and ultrasound studies. Telemedicine units are present in many PICUs allowing remote access to other ICUs, emergency departments, or transport vehicles.

Intercommunication systems that link the patient rooms, workstations, physician office/call room, conference rooms, and staff lounge should be present in the PICU (86,90). Multiple phone lines with multiple extensions are needed. Telephones should be equipped with soft-toned ringers to help control noise. In the event of power failure or damage to standard telephone lines, the PICU should have access to emergency telephone systems. Many PICUs are now utilizing personal tracking devices instead of overhead paging systems to improve efficiency and noise control. Previously there was concern that cellular devices affected medical equipment in the PICU, especially the mechanical ventilator but that has been shown not to be true (98).

Emergency Power

The emergency power source for the hospital should be safe from the effects of potential disaster situations. For example, emergency generators should not be in the basement of a hospital if the area is at any risk of flooding (99). Life-support equipment, such as extracorporeal membrane oxygenation circuits or mechanical ventilators, should be on outlets that are connected to emergency generator power, whereas other less critical pieces of equipment may be connected to outlets not supported during power shortages. Water must be available in each room for handwashing and other uses. If hemodialysis is to be performed at the bedside, the water source must be certified.

Central Areas

Central areas should have adequate visualization of the patient rooms and adequate desk space for all caregivers, including nurses, physicians, respiratory therapists, consultants, social workers, pharmacists, and others. A centralized monitoring system should be nearby. The workflow within the unit must be studied to adequately design these clinical support zones.

Storage

In addition to the centralized charting and monitor areas, storage for emergency equipment and ventilators must be within the unit. Each unit should have "dirty" and "clean" utility areas as well as food and formula preparation areas. A satellite pharmacy is best for the PICU; in lieu of that, medication storage and preparation areas, with refrigeration and locked areas as indicated, should be available.

Family and Caregiver Areas

In addition to the patient rooms, the overall PICU should be designed to allow for optimal patient care and support for the caregivers. The unit should have an entry primarily for family and visitors that can be controlled for security. Another entry should be available for patient transport and medical personnel.

Further family-support areas (in addition to family space within the patient's room) are important. They should have a waiting room with seating for approximately two family members per patient. Waiting areas can include nourishment-support areas with refrigerators and microwaves, laundry support, access to telephones, and diversions, such as television, video games, and aquariums. Lockers for safe storage of the family's personal belongings should be provided. Private areas for conferences between medical caregivers, social workers, and family should be available. A private area for lactation equipment should also be available.

Additional Considerations

Other age-appropriate toys that are easily disinfected can be provided as needed. The functional design of the unit may also accommodate pet visitation if it is available. An easily readable clock should be in each patient room. Twenty-four–hour atomic clocks are easily seen and can help to decrease time variability on documentation.

Green Environment

Supporting sustainable healthy work environments without compromising patient safety has become an important responsibility of our professional practice as mounting evidence reveals the negative impact of the healthcare industry on the environment. Currently, the healthcare industry generates more than 2 million tons of waste per year and releases environmental pollutants from incinerators burning medical wastes made of polyvinylchloride plastics (i.e., flexible intravenous tubing

and catheters), mercury, and other toxic substances (100). In addition, hospital air quality is compromised with pollutants from laboratory chemicals, latex, mercury, and many other toxic building materials that emit cadmium, lead, and polychlorinated biphenyls (101). There are also reports revealing harmful effects of the healthcare environment on the healthcare team. Kogevinas (102) found that exposure to substances in the workplace was responsible for causing greater than 10% of adult-onset asthma, with nurses at highest risk for this occupational hazard.

Many organizations are leading efforts to improve global healthcare environments by "greening" the hospital environment or implementing practices to reduce environmental impact. The Health Care without Harm organization is an international coalition whose membership includes hospitals, healthcare systems, medical professionals, and others (http://www.noharm.org). The vision of this organization is to "first do no harm and implement ecologically sound and healthy alternatives to healthcare practices that pollute the environment and contribute to disease" (http:www.noharm.org). The website has many resources including a green guide for healthcare, which is a toolkit that can be used to assist healthcare institutions in greening the workplace. In addition, The U.S. Green Building Council has developed the Leadership in Energy and Environmental Design certification, which includes standards in healthy and sustainable building design, construction, and operations for health care (http://www.usgbc.org).

Grassroots efforts to "go green" within hospitals begins with creating a multidisciplinary "Green Team" and "Green Team" champions within individual units to raise environmental awareness and lead green indicatives (103,104). There are many opportunities to reduce environmental impact in the intensive care setting without affecting patient safety and these efforts demonstrate to the public the organization's commitment to the health of the greater community. Table 5.2 outlines some important best greening practices and examples that can be easily adopted in PICUs to promote reducing, reusing, and recycling efforts (103,104).

CONCLUSIONS AND FUTURE DIRECTIONS

Seriously ill pediatric patients are best cared for in ICUs designed for them, and the physical design of the facility and personnel organization are integral components of PICUs. In the United States, pediatric intensive care resources are regionalized into three models: large geographic areas that encompass rural areas, rural and suburban areas, and small geographic areas that house large populations. Healthcare providers in the PICU include multidisciplinary teams of intensivists, hospitalists, other physicians, NPs, PAs, nurses, pharmacists, therapists, and others. These health professionals provide a care-delivery model focused on beneficial clinical and behavioral outcomes, patient–family relationships, and safety. Government and accreditation agencies regulate PICU physical design, including room design, noise level, and lighting and electrical requirements. Evidence suggests that the current model of pediatric intensive care provides high-quality healthcare to a vulnerable patient population.

Because of the aging and limited workforce, the future of the field is challenged by the need for more physicians, nurses, mid-level practitioners, and other healthcare providers who are specialized in pediatric intensive care. As technology becomes more complicated, both staffing and unit design must adjust to meet the needs of the newer technologies. Additionally, the focus of the PICU, both in design and in treatment, must continue to be the patients and their families.

TABLE 5.2

IMPLEMENTING GREEN BEST PRACTICES IN THE PICU

■ GREEN BEST PRACTICES	■ EXAMPLES
Reduce use of toxic materials, i.e., mercury, PVC, DEHP, cleaning materials, flame retardants, and pesticides	Purchase PVC- and DEHP-free products when possible. DEHP is a chemical that provides flexibility to many items such as intravenous tubing and bags, feeding tubes Use mercury-free equipment (i.e., use digital thermometers)
Increase use of proper waste management	Reduce red bag (medical) waste by removing from individual rooms and placing in central areas (increases proper use of red bag receptacles)
Increase recycling and reuse	Use reusable sharp containers Display and label bins to recycle items such as alkaline batteries, intravenous fluid bags and tubing Paper shredder on unit Recycle or reuse equipment (work with vendors or reuse for educational purposes) Recycle plastic, bottles, and cans in staff lounge and family waiting areas
Purchase energy star products	Purchase products with recycled content Purchase only environmentally green (EPEAT) labeled electronics (i.e., computers, monitors)
Decrease unnecessary use	Eliminate unnecessary paper copies, or only use double-sided Display all meeting agendas and educational content electronically Reduce purchase of kits/trays with unneeded or extra supplies Turn off lights in empty rooms and bed spaces Turn off idle computers in offices

PVC, polyvinylchloride; DEHP, di(2-ethylhexyl)phthalate; EPEAT, Electronic Product Environmental Assessment Tool.

References

1. Downes JJ. The historical evolution, current status, and prospective development of pediatric critical care. *Crit Care Clin* 1992;8(1):1–22.
2. Lassen HC. A preliminary report on the 1952 epidemic of poliomyelitis in Copenhagen with special reference to the treatment of acute respiratory insufficiency. *Lancet* 1953;1(1):37–41.
3. Randolph AG, Gonzales CA, Cortellini L, et al. Growth of pediatric intensive care units in the United States from 1995 to 2001. *J Pediatr* 2004;144:792–8.
4. López-Herce J, Sancho L, Martinó JM. Study of paediatric intensive care units in Spain. *Intensive Care Med* 2000;26:62–8.
5. American Academy of Pediatrics, Committee on Pediatric Emergency Medicine and American College of Critical Care Medicine and Society of Critical Care Medicine, Pediatric Section, Task Force on Regionalization of Pediatric Critical Care. Consensus report for regionalization of services for critically ill or injured children. *Pediatrics* 2000;105(1):152–5.
6. Richardson DK, Reed K, Cutler C, et al. Perinatal regionalization versus hospital competition: The Hartford example. *Pediatrics* 1995;96:417–23.
7. West JG, Cales RH, Gazzaniga AB. Impact of regionalization. The Orange County experience. *Arch Surg* 1983;118(6):740–4.
8. Pearson G, Shann F, Barry P, et al. Should paediatric intensive care be centralized? Trent versus Victoria. *Lancet* 1997;349(9060):1213–7.
9. Tilford JM, Simpson PM, Green JW, et al. Volume-outcome relationships in pediatric intensive care units. *Pediatrics* 2000;106(2):289–94.
10. Jenkins KJ, Newburger JW, Lock JE, et al. In-hospital mortality for surgical repair of congenital heart defects: Preliminary observations of variation by hospital caseload. *Pediatrics* 1995;95(3):323–30.
11. Hornick CP, He X, Jacobs JP, et al. Relative impact of surgeon and center volume on early mortality after the Norwood operation. *Ann Thorac Surg* 2012;93:1992–7.
12. Brantley MD, Lu H, Barfield WD, et al. Mapping US pediatric hospitals and subspecialty critical care for public health preparedness and disaster response, 2008. *Disaster Med Public Health Prep* 2012;6(2):117–25.
13. Sullivan AF, Rudders SA, Gonsalves AL, et al. National survey of pediatric services available in US emergency departments. *Int J Emerg Med* 2013;6:13.
14. American Academy of Pediatrics, Committee on Hospital Care and Section on Critical Care and Society of Critical Care Medicine, Pediatric Section Admission Criteria Task Force. Guidelines for developing admission and discharge policies for the pediatric intensive care unit. *Pediatrics* 1999;103(4):840–2.
15. Yeh TS. Regionalization of pediatric critical care. *Crit Care Clin* 1992;8(1):23–35.
16. Durch JS, Lohr KN. *Emergency Medical Services for Children.* Washington, DC: National Academy Press, 1993.
17. Cogo PE, Poole D, Codazzi D, et al. Outcome of children admitted to adult intensive care units in Italy between 2003 and 2007. *Intensive Care Med* 2010;36(8):1403–9.
18. Lundstrom NR, Berggren H, Björkhem G, et al. Centralization of pediatric heart surgery in Sweden. *Pediatr Cardiol* 2000;21:353–7.
19. Govil YC. Pediatric intensive care in India: Time for introspection and intensification. *Indian Pediatr* 2006;43:675–6.
20. American Academy of Pediatrics, Policy Statement Guiding Principles for Pediatric Hospitalist Programs. *Pediatrics* 2005;115:1101–2.
21. Edward JD, Houtrow AJ, Vasilevskis EE, et al. Multi-institutional profile of adults admitted to pediatric intensive care units. *JAMA Pediatr* 2013:167(5):436–43.
22. DiCarlo JV, Zaitseva TA, Khodateleva TV, et al. Comparative assessment of pediatric intensive care in Moscow, the Russian Federation: A prospective, multicenter study. *Crit Care Med* 1996;24(8):1403–7.
23. Besso J, Bhagwanjee S, Takezawa J, et al. A global view of education and training in critical care medicine. *Crit Care Clin* 2006;22:539–46.
24. Anderson MR, Jewett EA, Cull WL, et al. Practice of pediatric critical care medicine: Results of the future of Pediatric Education II Survey of Sections project. *Pediatr Crit Care Med* 2003;4(4):412–7.

25. Pollack MM, Cuerdon TC, Getson PR. Pediatric intensive care units: Results of a national survey. *Crit Care Med* 1993;21(4):607–14.

26. Goh AY-T, Lum LC-S, Abdel-Latif ME-A. Impact of 24-hour critical care physician staffing on case-mix-adjusted mortality in paediatric intensive care. *Lancet* 2001;357:445–6.

27. Baudendister TE, Wachter RM. The evolution of the hospitalist movement in the USA. *Clin Med JRCPL* 2002;2:327–30.

28. Beck CA, Parkin PC, Freedman JN. Pediatric hospitalist medicine: An overview and a perspective from Toronto, Canada. *Clin Pediatr* 2008;47(6):546–8.

29. Oshimvra J, Sperring J, Bauer BD, et al. Inpatient management within pediatric residency programs: Work restrictions and the evolving role of the pediatric hospitalist. *J Hosp Med* 2012;7(4):299–303.

30. Wachter RM, Goldman L. The hospitalist movement 5 years later. *JAMA* 2002;287:487–94.

31. Fischer ES. Pediatric hospital medicine: Historical perspectives, inspired future. *Curr Probl Pediatr Adolesc Health Care* 2012;42:107–112.

32. Wachter RM, Goldman L. The emerging role of hospitalists in the American health care system. *N Engl J Med* 1996;335:514–7.

33. Freed GL, Brzoznowski K, Neighbors K, et al. Characteristics of the Pediatric Hospitalist workforce: It's role and work environment. *Pediatrics* 2007;120:33–9.

34. Stucky ER, Maniscalco J, Ottolini MC, et al. The Pediatric Hospital Medicine Core Competencies Supplement: A Framework for Curriculum Development by the Society of Hospital Medicine with acknowledgement to pediatric hospitalists from the American Academy of Pediatrics and the Academic Pediatric Association. *J Hosp Med* 2010;5(suppl 2):1–114.

35. Freed GL, Dunham KM. Characteristics of Pediatric Hospitalist Medicine fellowships and training programs. *J Hosp Med* 2009;4(37):157–63.

36. Landrigan CP, Srivastavia R. Pediatric hospitalists. *Arch Pediatr Adolesc Med* 2010;166(8):696–9.

37. Landrigan CP, Conway PH, Edwards S, et al. Pediatric hospitalists: A systematic review of the literature. *Pediatrics* 2006;117(5): 1736–44.

38. Boyd J, Sammaddar K, Parra-Roide L, et al. Comparison of outcome measures for a traditional pediatric faculty service and nonfaculty hospitalist services in a community teaching hospital. *Pediatrics* 2006;118(4):1327–31.

39. Tenner PA, Dibrell H, Taylor RP. Improved survival with hospitalists in a pediatric intensive care unit. *Crit Care Med* 2003; 31(3):847–52.

40. Needleman J, Buerhaus P, Mattke S, et al. Nurse-staffing levels and the quality of care in hospitals. *N Engl J Med* 2002;346:1715–21.

41. Potter P, Barr N, McSweeney M, et al. Identifying nurse staffing and patient outcome relationships: A guide for change in care delivery. *Nurs Econ* 2003;21:158–66.

42. Kane RL, Shamliyan TA, Mueller C, et al. The association of registered nurse staffing levels and patient outcomes: Systematic review and meta-analysis. *Med Care* 2007;45(12):1195–204.

43. Marcin JP, Rutan E, Rapetti PM, et al. Nurse staffing and unplanned extubation in the pediatric intensive care unit. *Pediatr Crit Care Med* 2005;6:254–7.

44. Buckley T, Short T, Rowbottom Y, et al. Critical incident reporting in the intensive care unit. *Anaesthesia* 1997;52(5):403–9.

45. Odetola FO, Clark, SJ, Freed GL, et al. A national survey of pediatric critical care resources in the United States. *Pediatrics* 2005;115:382–6.

46. World Federation of Critical Care Nurses. http://wfccn.org/wp-content/uploads/workforce. Accessed September 15, 2012.

47. Aiken LH, Havens DS, Sloane DM. The Magnet Nursing Services Recognition® program: A comparison of two groups of magnet hospitals. *Am J Nurs* 2000;100(3):26–30.

48. Allen DE, Vitale-Nolen RA. Patient care delivery model improves nurse job satisfaction. *J Contin Educ Nurs* 2005;36:277–82.

49. Foley BJ, Kee CC, Minick P, et al. Characteristics of nurses and hospital work environments that foster satisfaction and clinical expertise. *J Nurs Adm* 2002;5:273–81.

50. Chaboyer W, Foster MM, Kendall E. The intensive care unit liaison nurse: Towards a clear role description. *Intensive Crit Care Nurs* 2004;20(2):77–86.

51. Boyle DK, Bott MJ, Hansen HE, et al. Managers' leadership and critical care nurses' intent to stay. *Am J Crit Care* 1999;8:361–71.

52. Davidson JE, Powers K, Hedayat KM, et al. American College of Critical Care Medicine Task Force 2004–2005, Society of Critical Care Medicine. Clinical practice guidelines for support of the family in the patient-centered ICU. *Crit Care Med* 2007;35(2):605–22.

53. Institute of Medicine (IOM). *Health Professions Education: A Bridge to Quality.* Washington, DC: National Academy Press, 2001.

54. Institute of Medicine (IOM). *Crossing the Quality Chasm.* Washington, DC: National Academy Press, 2003.

55. Baernholdt M, Cottingham S. The clinical nurse leader—new nursing role with global implications. *Int Nurs Rev* 2011;58:74–8.

56. Hix C, McKeon L, Walters S. Clinical nurse leader impact on clinical microsystems outcomes. *J Nurs Adm* 2009;39(2):71–6.

57. Rosseter R. A new role for nurses: making room for clinical nurse leaders. *Jt Comm Perspect* 2009;9(8):5–7.

58. Stanley JM, Gannon J, Gabuat J, et al. The clinical nurse leader: A catalyst for improving quality and patient safety. *J Nurs Manag* 2008;16(5):614-22.

59. Gatley EP. From novice to expert: The use of intuitive knowledge as a basis for district nurse education. *Nurse Educ Today* 1992;12(2):81–7.

60. Fleischman RK, Meyer L, Watson C. Best practices in creating a culture of certification. *AACN Adv Crit Care* 2011;22(1):33–49.

61. American Association of Critical Care Nurses, American College of Chest Physicians, American Thoracic Society & Society of Critical Care Medicine. *Critical Care Workforce Position Statement.* 2001. http://www.aacn.org/wd/practice/docs/public policy/critical_care_workforce_position_statement.pdf. Accessed September 15, 2012.

62. Derengowski SL, Irving SY, Koogle PV, et al. Defining the role of the pediatric critical care nurse practitioner in a tertiary care center. *Crit Care Med* 2000;28(7):2626–30.

63. Mathur M, Rampersad A, Howard K, et al. Physician assistants as physician extenders in the pediatric intensive care unit setting—a 5-year experience. *Pediatr Crit Care Med* 2005;6(1):14–9.

64. Verger JT, Marcoux KK, Madden MA, et al. Nurse practitioners in pediatric critical care: Results of a national survey. *AACN Clin Issues* 2005;16(3):396–408.

65. Nasca TJ, Day SH, Amis ES. The new recommendations on duty hours from the ACGME Task Force. *N Engl J Med* 2010:363:e3.

66. Typpo KV, Tcharmtchi MH, Thomas EJ, et al. Impact of resident duty hour limits on safety in the intensive care unit: A national survey of pediatric and neonatal intensivists. *Pediatr Crit Care Med* 2012;13(5):578–582.

67. Pastores SM, O'Connor M, Kleinpell RM, et al. The Accreditation Council for Graduate Medical Education resident duty hour new standards: History, changes, and impact on staffing of intensive care units. *Crit Care Med* 2011;39(11):2540.

68. Delametter GL. Advanced practice nursing and the role of the pediatric critical care nurse practitioner. *Crit Care Nurs Q* 1999;21(4):16–22.

69. Martin SA. The pediatric critical care nurse practitioner: Evolution and impact. *Pediatr Nurs* 1999;25(5):505–17.

70. Molitor-Kirsch S, Thompson L, Milonovich L. The changing face of critical care medicine. *AACN Clin Issues* 2005;16(2):172–7.

71. Cramer CL, Orlowski JP, DeNicola LK. Pediatric intensivist extenders in the pediatric ICU. *Pediatr Clin North Am* 2008;55(3): 687–708.

72. American Association of Colleges of Nursing. *AACN Position Statement on the Practice Doctorate in Nursing.* October, 2004. http://www.aacn.nche.edu/publications/position/DNPpositionstatement.pdf. Accessed September 15, 2012.

73. Gershengorn HB, Johnson MP, Factor P. The use of nonphysician providers in adult intensive care units. *Am J Respir Crit Care Med* 2012:185:600.

74. American Academy of Pediatrics, Committee on Pediatric Workforce. Scope of practice issues in the delivery of pediatric health care. *Pediatrics* 2003;111(2):426–35.

75. Druss BG, Marcus SC, Olfson M, et al. Trends in care by nonphysician clinicians in the United States. *N Engl J Med* 2003;348(2):130–7.

76. Kleinpell R, Gawlinski A. Assessing outcomes in advanced practice nursing practice: The use of quality indicators and evidence-based practice. *AACN Clin Issues* 2005;16(1):43–57.

77. Carzoli RP, Martinez-Cruz M, Cuevas LL, et al. Comparison of neonatal nurse practitioners, physician assistants, and residents in the neonatal intensive care unit. *Arch Pediatr Adolesc Med* 1994;148:1271–6.

78. Ottley RG, Agbontaen JX, Wilkow BR. The hospitalist PA: An emerging opportunity. *JAAPA* 2000;13(11):21–8.

79. DeNicola L, Kleid D, Brink L, et al. Use of pediatric physician extenders in pediatric and neonatal intensive care units. *Crit Care Med* 1994;22(11):1856–64.

80. Rudy EB, Davidson LJ, Daly B, et al. Care activities and outcomes of patients cared for by acute care nurse practitioners, physician assistants, and resident physicians: A comparison. *Am J Crit Care* 1998;7(4):267–81.

81. Oswanski MF, Sharma OP, Shekhar SR. Comparative review of use of physician assistants in a level I trauma center. *Am Surg* 2004;70(3):272–9.

82. Christmas AB, Reynolds J, Hodges S, et al. Physician extenders impact trauma systems. *J Trauma* 2005;58(5):917–20.

83. Fry M. Literature review of the impact of nurse practitioners in critical care services. *Nurs Crit Care* 2011;16(2):58–66.

84. Meyer SC, Miers LJ. Effect of cardiovascular surgeon and acute care nurse practitioner collaboration on postoperative outcomes. *AACN Clin Issues* 2005;16:149–58.

85. Reynolds EW, Bricker JT. Nonphysician clinicians in the neonatal intensive care unit: Meeting the needs of our smallest patients. *Pediatrics* 2007;63:128–34.

86. Thourani VH, Miller JI. Physician's assistants in cardiothoracic surgery: A 30-year experience in a university center. *Ann Thorac Surg* 2006;81:195–99.

87. Kleinpell RM, Ely E, Grabenkort R. Nurse practitioners and physician assistants in the intensive care unit: An evidence-based review. *Crit Care Med* 2008;36(10):2888–97.

88. Pearson A, Peels S. Advanced practice in nursing: International perspective. *Int J Nurs Pract* 2002;8(2):S1–S4.

89. Rosenberg DI, Moss MM. American College of Critical Care Medicine of the Society of Critical Care Medicine. Guidelines and levels of care for pediatric intensive care units. *Pediatrics* 2004;114(4):1114–25.

90. Thompson DR, Hamilton DK, Cadenhead CD, et al. American College of Critical Care Medicine Guidelines for ICU Design. *Crit Care Med* 2012:40(5):1586–600.

91. Ulrich RS, Zimring C, Zhu X, et al. A review of the research literature on evidence-based healthcare design. *HERD* 2008;1(3):61–125.

92. Al-Samsam RH, Cullen P. Sleep and adverse environmental factors in sedated mechanically ventilated pediatric intensive care patients. *Pediatr Crit Care Med* 2005;6(5):562–567.

93. Halpern NA. Innovative designs for the smart ICU. *Chest* 2014;145:646–58.

94. Jiang SP, Huang LW, Chen XL, et al. Ventilation of wards and nosocomial outbreak of severe acute respiratory syndrome among healthcare workers. *Chin Med J (Engl)* 2003;116(9):1293–7.

95. Ulrich R, Quan X, Zimring C, et al. The role of the physical environment in the hospital of the 21st century: A once-in-a-lifetime opportunity. http://www.rwjf.org/publications/otherlist.jsp. Accessed August 29, 2006.

96. British Association of Critical Care Nurses. Critical Care Networks-National Nurse Leads. Royal College of Nursing Critical Care Forum. Standards for Nursing Staffing in Critical Care Units. 2010. http://www.ics.ac.uk/professional/standards_and_guidelines/baccn_standards_for_nurse_staffing_in_critical_care. Accessed September 15, 2012.

97. Society of Hospital Medicine. Definition of Hospitalist. http://www.hospitalmedicine.org/AM/Template.cfm?Section=Hospitalist_Definition&Template=/cm/HTML_display.CFM&ContentID=24835. Accessed October 1, 2012.

98. Tri JL, Severson RP, Firl AR, et al. Cellular telephone interference with medical equipment. *Mayo Clin Proc* 2005;80:1286–90.

99. Perrin K. A first for this century: Closing and reopening of a children's hospital during a disaster. *Pediatrics* 2006;117(5):381–5.

100. Minnema L. Medicine gears up for a code green: Doctors, hospitals put environment on their charts. *The Washinton Post* 2008:HE05.

101. Roberts G, Guenther R. Environmentally responsible hospitals. In Marberry SO, ed. *Improving Health Care with Better Building Design*. Chicago: Health Administration Press, 2006.

102. Kogevinas M. Exposure to substances in the workplace and new-onset asthma: An international prospective population-based study (ECRHS-II). *Lancet* 2007;370:336–341.

103. Pate MFD. It is easy being green: Greening the pediatric intensive care unit. *AACN Adv Crit Care* 2012;23(1):18–23.

104. Chapman M, Chapman A. Greening critical care. *Crit Care* 2011;15(2):302.

CHAPTER 6 ■ PRACTICE MANAGEMENT: THE BUSINESS OF PEDIATRIC CRITICAL CARE

MEREDITH G. VAN DER VELDEN AND JEFFREY P. BURNS

KEY POINTS

1 Understanding the business of critical care medicine is essential for critical care practitioners.

2 Practice leaders and members should be responsible for understanding traditional human resource functions as well as other personnel management issues including recruitment, hiring, credentialing, performance evaluations, mentoring and retention.

3 Critical care medicine is a significant contributor of healthcare costs.

4 Provider billing occurs separately from hospital billing in the United States.

5 Determining hospital costs and reimbursement is complicated but important to understand to highlight opportunities for revenue enhancement and cost containment.

6 Physicians bill professional fees as CPT codes that are linked to diagnoses based on ICD codes.

7 There are both revenue- and non-revenue-based productivity measures that can be used to measure physician productivity.

---

1 When the primary purpose of one's clinical role is to deliver care to a critically ill or injured child, consideration of administrative affairs associated with delivering the care can be difficult. However, whether one's pediatric critical care affiliation is with a large academic group or a small private practice, both short- and long-term attentions to these details are vital. Knowledge of the nonmedical aspects of the field will allow those practicing the trade to determine its landscape and direction (1). This is true not only for those in the role of managing the practice but also for all involved in its delivery. For those in academic environments, these agendas need to be reconciled with obligations to provide teaching, research, and other academic pursuits. Furthermore, consideration of the administrative aspects of the career is often missing from critical care training and occasionally at odds with what is taught (2).

Although ICUs are invariably part of larger departments and organizations, they still can be considered as businesses, in and of themselves, and consequently should be accountable for the relevant aspects of business operations (3). This may include managing finances, business strategy, marketing, and customer relations (4). How can you ensure the costs incurred for delivery of your services will be paid for and allow your practice to continue to operate and grow? How do you prepare for anticipated changes in the field and workforce? How do you make sure you attract, develop, and retain the right members of your group?

Although the answers to these questions and a comprehensive review of the business of pediatric critical care are beyond the scope of this chapter, we will offer some insight to the field and address the topics of personnel management (human resources [HR]), finance, and productivity and performance. Information technology, leadership, and organizational structure are also pertinent to the business of practice and are covered in other chapters.

PERSONNEL MANAGEMENT (HUMAN RESOURCES)

Personnel management, or HR, typically pertains to activities **2** related to the management of those employed by the business. While much of this is covered through standard administrative practices by hospital (or group) HR organizations, we contend that for physician faculty, the responsibility of these functions often belongs to the practice leadership and members themselves. This is particularly accurate when the functions of HR are considered beyond the typical administration (e.g., payroll, credentialing) to include activities that promote faculty development to align with the strategy of the business (the delivery of high-quality pediatric critical care medicine) (5). Functions covered under this agenda include recruiting, hiring, maintaining credentials, evaluating performance, training, mentoring, guiding advancement, and retention. As mentioned earlier, many of these will be shared responsibilities between hospital or practice administrative parties, faculty leadership, and the individual faculty. However, as the balance of responsibility will be variably shifted among these parties based on practice location and type, it is increasingly important for all to understand the landscape of this administrative domain.

There is generally a compulsion to relieve the physicians and their leadership of the full burden of responsibility for these duties as they may have little to no training or experience to complete them. While appreciation of, and participation in, such activities is essential, we cannot stress enough the importance of working with personnel with background in areas such as business administration, accounting, and data analytics and management. Furthermore, much of the activities mentioned earlier will fall under the responsibility of group leadership rather than the physicians themselves. While traditional concepts of leadership are addressed in other chapters,

50

the functions addressed here may be considered to fall under the role of manager (2).

Practice Membership

It is self-evident that critical care medicine practices are composed of critical care medicine physicians. Consideration of the recruitment, hiring, and retention of these physicians will customarily be led by the group's manager and will predictably require collaboration with the hospital (or larger physician group) to ensure compliance with relevant legal matters (4). Recruitment and hiring are often based on a number of factors dependent on the type and location of practice and must include consideration of direct and indirect compensation. Once hired, physician members must maintain relevant licensing, credentialing, and malpractice coverage based on their responsibilities within the practice. In addition, these concerns would also pertain to trainees working with the practice.

Communication and Cohesiveness

Because of the nature of critical care practice, it can be challenging for physician members to find a time and place to communicate and remain cohesive about important business and clinical matters. These matters may include, but are not limited to, changes in unit and hospital policies, patient safety and event review, finances, and quality improvement initiatives and data review. Regardless of the challenge it presents, it is imperative for groups to ensure these important topics are addressed and all appropriate practice members remain accountable. Traditional forums such as faculty meetings and retreats are examples of means of disseminating vital information. However, based on the obstacles mentioned earlier, innovative ways of ensuring communication and cohesiveness should be entertained.

Development and Retention

Within any practice, academic or not, attention to the development and retention of its members is essential. Physician members need to be supported in their growth both clinically and in the other roles they may have. In the academic setting, mentorship, as a form of "development," may include roles such as teacher, advisor, role model, and coach (6). Good mentorship has been associated with job satisfaction as well as a variety of physician productivity measures (7). Faculty development and mentorship may include support for additional education and training as well as travel expenses for relevant meetings and conferences both nationally and internationally. With adequate mentorship and development, physician members should be primed for advancement in their roles and/or academic promotion. Furthermore, satisfaction and growth will assuredly lead to retention in the practice.

Finally, professional development includes feedback and evaluation, which should be distinguished from physician productivity measures and comparative performance (discussed later). Professional feedback and evaluation, for the purpose of individual improvement, is designed with the goal of improving one's effectiveness in the expectations set for one's roles. Feedback in this form may come solely from the manager or preferably in the form of comprehensive, multisource feedback, as in a 360-degree assessment, including input from peers, self, other healthcare professionals, trainees, and patients (8). This feedback should be repeated on a recurring basis, with goals for improvement outlined and updated on review.

FINANCE

❸ The overall cost of health care in the United States is higher than anywhere else in the world and has been the source of much national attention. This is no less true for critical care medicine, which contributes to a significant percentage of these healthcare costs (9–11). These critical care expenses continue to grow despite decreases in acute hospital expenditures overall (9). Since Medicare is the single largest payer to hospitals and reimbursement for intensive care in the population covered by Medicare is poor (12), cost containment in the ICU has received significant attention both by hospitals focused on their bottom line and from funding agencies (10). While pediatric critical care medicine is unlikely to garner the attention of our adult counterparts, we remain an expensive endeavor (13) and should similarly focus attention on evaluation of our cost and effectiveness. This need for providing cost containment along with valuable care is increasingly pressing as evolving models of reimbursement tie payment for services with quality and outcome (14). Now, more than ever, as described by Michael Porter and Lee (15), health care is being called upon to deliver value—high-quality care with proven outcomes at the lowest possible cost. While discussions of quality will be considered briefly below with regard to physician productivity as well as more comprehensively in other chapters, we will discuss the basics of financing critical care here.

As is true of any business, without profitability, medical care practices, hospital-based and otherwise, cannot continue; therefore, attention to the bottom line is paramount (1,3). In simple finance terms, a business's profitability is a result of the revenues generated minus the expenses incurred (16). Plainly stated, profitability will increase by enhancing revenue, decreasing costs, or both. While a complete description of the details of this balance sheet for pediatric critical care services is complicated and beyond the scope of this chapter, we will briefly discuss some basic sources of expense and revenue at the practice level as well as give an overview of hospital costs and billing followed by a more in-depth tutorial on physician billing.

It is important to note that revenue and expenses for pediatric critical care services will differ based on hospital size and type. Sources of revenue generation primarily center on billing fees for provision of clinical services. It is important to distinguish professional charges and hospital charges. Physicians bill professional fees as Current Procedural Terminology (CPT) codes linked to diagnoses based on International Classification of Diseases (ICD) codes (17). Additional sources of revenue may come from the provision of clinical services outside of the ICU such as coverage of intermediate care and sedation services, direct hospital support, research and grant funding, remuneration for administrative and teaching roles, and philanthropic gifts. Expenses of the practice may include physician salaries, fringe benefits, insurance coverage, space and capital, salaries for intensivists in training, and administrative support (3).

Hospital Costs and Billing

Defining hospital costs for critical care is complex (12) but can be generally divided into fixed and variable costs. Fixed costs are those that can be attributed to the operations of delivering critical care and do not vary based on patients. Examples of fixed costs include hospital staffing (salaries), ICU equipment, and maintenance costs. Variable costs are those associated with individual patients and include things such as medications and disposable equipment. Fixed costs comprise the majority of hospital costs and are therefore, the target of many cost reduction strategies (18).

④ Currently in the United States, provider billing (discussed subsequently) occurs separately from hospital billing. Hospitals are reimbursed for services by payers (government, private insurance, self-pay, etc.) based on a number of established reimbursement schemes. Examples of these schemes include a fixed level of reimbursement based on the patient's diagnosis or surgical procedure without reimbursement for actual treatments, "per diem" payments where hospitals are reimbursed for each day a patient is in the hospital, and fee-for-service reimbursement where each activity performed on a patient (e.g., test, procedure, medication) is reimbursed separately (18).

As would be expected to sustain profitability and growth, even in a nonprofit institution, these charges submitted for critical care must exceed the costs (19). In spite of this, reimbursement for intensive care is often not greater than or ⑤ equal to the cost (12) and therefore, may threaten a healthy balance sheet. This has led hospitals to use cost shifting, which attempts to make up hospital costs lost from payers who reimburse poorly, such as the government, to those who reimburse well, such as private payers (20).

Attempts at revenue enhancement are complicated and will vary based on the institution and the population it serves. Regardless of type, these may include common measures such as optimizing reimbursement through billing and coding procedures. Novel approaches, such as one by Bekes et al. (21), describe critical care as a "product line" and suggest development of a business plan to allow for new ways to enhance profitability of critical care services. On the basis of the incredible complexity of the ICU environment, attempts to unravel which interventions will lead to reduction in costs can be challenging (18). The use of newer schemes that incorporate quality and outcome into the equation makes the overall assessment even more complicated.

The Framework for Professional Reimbursement in the United States

Unlike pediatric critical care practitioners in many other countries with a national health service where a single-payer system predominates, the United States, even with the passage of the Affordable Care Act, continues to have a combination of private and public healthcare financing. In order to accurately describe and convey the precise and peculiar language that defines and determines the authoritative reimbursement rules, the authors have chosen to directly quote the federal code where applicable. The authoritative federal code quoted in this section on reimbursement can be found at http://www.cms.gov/Outreach-and-Education/Medicare-Learning-Network-MLN/MLNMattersArticles/downloads/mm5993.pdf or in pages 65–77 of the document at http://www.cms.gov/Regulations-and-Guidance/Guidance/Manuals/downloads/clm104c12.pdf (22).

Resource-Based Relative Value Scale

As documented by the Centers for Medicare and Medicaid Services (CMS), in 1992 Medicare significantly changed the way it paid for physicians' services. Instead of basing payments on charges, the federal government established a standardized physician payment schedule based on a resource-based relative value scale (RBRVS). In the RBRVS system, payments for services are determined by the resource costs needed to provide them. The cost of providing each service is divided into three components: physician work, practice expense, and professional liability insurance. Payments are also adjusted for geographical differences in resource costs.

The physician work component accounts, on average, for nearly half of the total relative value for each service. The factors used to determine physician work include the time it takes to perform the service; the technical skill and physical effort; the required mental effort and judgment; and the stress due to the potential risk to the patient. The physician work relative values are updated each year to account for changes in medical practice as determined by the CPT process. Also, the legislation enacting the RBRVS requires the CMS to review the whole scale at least every 5 years.

Current Procedural Terminology

Annual updates to the physician work relative values are based on recommendations from a committee involving the American Medical Association and national medical specialty societies to make recommendations to CMS on the relative values to be assigned to new or revised codes in CPT. The purpose of CPT is to provide a uniform language that accurately describes medical, surgical, and diagnostic services, and thereby serves as an effective means for reliable nationwide communication among physicians, other healthcare providers, patients, and third parties such as public and private health insurance programs. The uniform language is also applicable to medical education and research by providing a useful basis for local, regional, and national utilization comparisons (23).

Definition of Critical Care Services

Definition. The currently accepted CPT terminology states that, "Critical care is defined as a physician's (or physicians') direct delivery of medical care for a critically ill or critically injured patient. A critical illness or injury acutely impairs one or more vital organ systems such that there is a high probability of imminent or life threatening deterioration in the patient's condition."

Location. Whether the context meets the CMS definition of critical care service is not dependent on the location where the service is provided, but rather on whether the patient context "involves high complexity decision making to assess, manipulate, and support vital system functions to treat single, or multiple, vital organ system failure; and/or to prevent further life threatening deterioration of the patient's condition." Similarly, CMS describes examples of patients who may not satisfy Medicare medical necessity criteria for critical care payment, such as "Patients admitted to a critical care unit because no other hospital beds were available; Patients admitted to a critical care unit for close nursing observation and/or frequent monitoring of vital signs (e.g., drug toxicity or overdose); or Patients admitted to a critical care unit because hospital rules require certain treatments (e.g., insulin infusions) to be administered in the critical care unit."

Full Attention of the Physician. CMS emphasizes that the physician must be devoting full attention to the specific patient to submit for critical care services: "The duration of critical care services that physicians should report is the time you actually spend evaluating, managing, and providing the critically ill, or injured, patient's care. Be aware that during this time, you cannot provide services to any other patient, but rather must devote your full attention to this particular critically ill patient. This time must be spent at the patient's immediate bedside or elsewhere on the floor, or unit, so long as you are immediately available to the patient. For example, time spent reviewing laboratory test results or discussing the critically ill patient's care with other medical staff in the unit or at the nursing station on the floor would be reported as critical care, even when it does not occur at the bedside; if this time represents your full attention to the management of the critically ill/injured patient. Time spent off the unit or floor where the critically ill/injured patient is located (i.e., telephone calls, whether taken at home, in the office, or elsewhere in the hospital) floor may not be reported as critical care time because the physician is not immediately available to the patient."

Qualified Nonphysician Practitioners. Critical care services that can be submitted by nonphysician practitioners for payment "when these services meet the above critical care services definition and requirements" and are "within the scope of practice and licensure requirements for the State in which they practice and provide the services" and "meet the collaboration, physician supervision requirements, and billing requirements."

Postoperative Critical Care. Preoperative and/or postoperative critical care services provided "may be paid if the patient is critically ill and requires the full attention of the physician; and the critical care is unrelated to the specific anatomic injury or general surgical procedure performed. Such patients may meet the definition of being critically ill and criteria for conditions where there is a high probability of imminent or life threatening deterioration in the patient's condition. In order for these services to be paid, two reporting requirements must be met. Codes 99291–99292 and modifier –25 (significant, separately identifiable evaluation and management services by the same physician on the day of the procedure) must be used, and documentation identifying that the critical care was unrelated to the specific anatomic injury or general surgical procedure performed must be submitted."

Family Discussions. Time involved with family members or other surrogate decision makers, "whether to obtain a history or to discuss treatment options may be counted toward critical care time when these specific criteria are met: The patient is unable or incompetent to participate in giving a history and/or making treatment decisions; and the discussion is necessary for determining treatment decisions. Telephone calls to family members and or surrogate decision makers may be counted toward critical care time, only if they meet the same criteria no other family discussions (no matter how lengthy) may be additionally counted toward critical care."

Teaching Physicians. A teaching physician, to bill for critical care services, must meet the requirements for critical care described earlier. "For procedure codes determined on the basis of time, such as critical care, the teaching physician must be present for the entire period of time for which the claim is submitted. For example, payment will be made for 35 minutes of critical care services only if the teaching physician is present for the full 35 minutes. Time spent teaching may *not* be counted

toward critical care time." Nor, can the teaching physician bill, as critical care or other time-based services, for time spent by the resident (in the teaching physician's absence). Only time that the teaching physician spends with the patient (or that the attending and resident spend together with the patient) can be counted toward critical care time. "A combination of the teaching physician's documentation and the resident's documentation may support critical care services. Provided that all requirements for critical care services are met, the teaching physician documentation may be the resident's documentation for specific patient history, physical findings, and medical assessment."

Time-Based Critical Care Services

For a critically ill patient 6 years of age and older, time-based codes apply (**Table 6.1**). Time counted toward critical care services (**Table 6.2**) "may be continuous clock time or intermittent in aggregated time increments (e.g., 50 minutes of continuous clock time or five 10-minute blocks of time spread over a given calendar date). Only one physician may bill for critical care services during any one single period of time even if more than one physician is providing care to a critically ill patient. For each medical encounter, the physician's progress notes must document the total time that critical care services are provided."

TABLE 6.1

CPT CODES FOR TIME-BASED CRITICAL CARE SERVICES

■ TOTAL DURATION OF CRITICAL CARE (min)	■ APPROPRIATE CPT CODE
<30	99232 or 99233 or other appropriate E/M codes
30–74	99291 × 1
75–104	99291 × 1 and 99292 × 1
105–134	99291 × 1 and 99292 × 2
135–164	99291 × 1 and 99292 × 3
165–194	99291 × 1 and 99292 × 4
194 or longer	99291–99292 as appropriate (per the above illustrations)

TABLE 6.2

TIME-BASED CRITICAL CARE SERVICES

■ SERVICES ALLOWED	■ SERVICES NOT ALLOWED
Time spent on floor/unit in the care of a critically ill or injured patient	Time spent in activities that does not directly contribute to the care of a critically ill or injured patient
Time spent at the patient's bedside	Time spent on indirect care, such as phone calls taken at home, office, or elsewhere in hospital (not immediately available to the patient)
Time spent on floor/unit engaging in work directly relating to the patient	Time spent providing care to other patients, either in critical care unit or elsewhere
Time spent on floor/unit discussing patient's care with other staff	Time spent with residents on rounds or other venues discussing the patient
Time spent on floor/unit documenting the performance of specific services, clinical findings, and orders	Time spent performing procedures not bundled in critical care services
Time spent on floor/unit with family or surrogate decision makers when the discussion bears directly on the medical decision making because patient is unable to participate	Time spent with family members or other surrogate decision makes when patient is competent to make medical decisions

Procedures Included in Time-Based Critical Care CPT Codes.

According to the current CMS rules, "The following services when performed on the day a physician bills for critical care, are included in the critical care service, and should not be reported separately:

- The interpretation of cardiac output measurements
- Chest x-rays, professional component
- Blood draw for specimen; blood gases, and information data stored in computers (e.g., ECGs, blood pressures, hematologic data)
- Gastric intubation
- Pulse oximetry
- Temporary transcutaneous pacing
- Ventilator management
- Vascular access procedures

Medicare Part B under the physician fee schedule does not pay for ventilator management services in addition to an E/M service (e.g., critical care services, CPT codes 99291–99292) on the same day for the patient even when the E/M service is billed with CPT modifier –25. No other procedure codes are bundled into the critical care services. Therefore, other medically necessary procedure codes may be billed separately."

Separately Billable Procedures Not Included in Time-Based Critical Care CPT Codes.

Procedures that can be added to the 99291–99292 CPT codes using the "CPT –25 modifier" include all of the following:

- CPR (92950) (while being performed)
- Endotracheal intubation (31500)
- Central line placement (36555, 36556)
- Intraosseous placement (36680)
- Tube thoracostomy (32551)
- Temporary transvenous pacemaker (33210)
- Electrocardiogram—routine ECG with at least 12 leads; interpretation and report only (93010)
- Elective electrical cardioversion (92960).

Bundled CPT Codes for Neonatal and Pediatric Critical Care Services

Neonatal and pediatric critical care services are covered when a newborn, infant, or child (up through 5 years of age) is critically ill or injured (as defined in CPT) and direct personal management by a physician is required. With very few exceptions, all services that the physician provides are covered under a single, age-based, bundled code (99468–99476, **Table 6.3**). These

TABLE 6.3

CPT CODES FOR NEONATAL AND PEDIATRIC CRITICAL CARE SERVICES

■ AGE AND CONTEXT	■ APPROPRIATE CPT CODE
Initial neonatal critical care, per day, 28 d of age or younger	99468
Subsequent neonatal critical care, per day, 28 d of age or younger	99469
Initial pediatric critical care, per day, 29 d through 24 mo	99471
Subsequent pediatric critical care, per day, 29 d through 24 mo	99472
Initial pediatric critical care, per day, 2 through 5 y	99475
Subsequent pediatric critical care, per day, 2 through 5 y	99476

codes must be reported by a single provider and encompass all critical care services delivered to the child on one calendar day and cannot be billed twice by two different providers on the same day (24). The specific CPT definition states: "Neonatal and Pediatric Critical Care involves the management, monitoring, and treatment of the patient, including:

- Enteral and parenteral nutritional maintenance
- Metabolic and hematologic maintenance
- Respiratory, pharmacologic control of the circulatory system
- Parent/family counseling
- Case management services
- Personal direct supervision of the healthcare team in the performance of cognitive and procedural activities."

Separately Billable Procedures Not Included in the Bundled Neonatal and Pediatric Critical Care CPT Codes.

Neonatal and pediatric CPT codes bundle all the usual critical care services with the following exceptions that can be separately submitted as a critical care service:

- Exchange transfusion (36450)
- Planned tracheostomy (31600)
- Bronchoscopy (31622)
- Thoracentesis, with insertion of tube (32421, 32422)
- Cardiopulmonary resuscitation (92950).

Time-Based Pediatric CPT Codes.

Pediatric critical care can be billed in a time-based or non-time-based manner. Paradoxically, some of the documentation requirements for these time-based (noncritical care) codes are more detailed. For example, subsequent hospital care (CPT codes 99231–99233), per day, for the evaluation and management of a patient, requires at least two of three key components (a detailed interval history, a detailed examination, or medical decision making of high complexity). Counseling and/or coordination of care with other physicians, other qualified healthcare professionals, or agencies are provided consistent with the nature of the problem(s) and the patient's and/or family's needs. Usually, the patient is unstable or has developed a significant complication or a significant new problem. A 99231 code is used when the patient is stable, recovering, or improving. Typically, 15 minutes are spent at the bedside and on the patient's hospital floor or unit. A 99232 code is used when the patient is responding inadequately to therapy or has developed a minor complication. Typically, 25 minutes are spent at the bedside and on the patient's hospital floor or unit. A 99233 code is used when the patient is unstable or has developed a significant complication or a significant new problem. Typically, 35 minutes are spent at the bedside and on the patient's hospital floor or unit.

Documentation, Coding, and Compliance

In addition to communicating important aspects of patient care, documentation is essential for compliance with billing for patient care services. As described above, professional charges are entered utilizing CPT codes. These charges are linked to ICD-9 codes based on the patient's diagnosis (17), the 10th version of which is on the horizon. It is essential for both sets of codes to be backed by the appropriate documentation. Compliance with this process falls under the scope of Program Integrity (PI) and is essential not only for proper reimbursement but for the avoidance of fraud, abuse, and waste (25).

As proper documentation and coding are imperative for the reasons stated above, many hospitals have established Clinical Documentation Improvement (CDI) programs to enhance the quality of documentation and coding within the institution. These programs may include education of physician providers with accountability for compliance and the training of clinical documentation specialists to review documentation, work with physician providers, and implement practices that support the improvement of documentation (26).

PRODUCTIVITY AND PERFORMANCE

7 Measurement of productivity is essential to any business model, including health care. These measures are customarily focused on revenue generation; however, we will mention non-revenue-based options as well.

Revenue-Based Productivity

Most physician productivity is tracked according to revenue generated. While metrics such as number of patients cared for or amount billed may be considered, they both have serious limitations with regard to their ability to truly assess productivity. The solution to this dilemma of assessing clinical productivity in clinical practice has been resolved with the use of relative value unit or RVU.

As described earlier in reference to professional billing, the RBRVS assigns an RVU to every CPT code that is billed. A component of that RVU is attributed to physician work and is meant to be reflective of the complexity and difficulty of the service. This "work RVU" can be used to calculate an individual physician's productivity.

To accomplish this, the work RVUs of an individual practitioner can be calculated for a time period and then benchmarked internally or through external organizations based on characteristics of the work environment. They are then adjusted to consider the fraction of one's full-time equivalent (FTE) that should be devoted to clinical productivity. The results of these analyses can be used to compare productivity among physicians within a practice group. Thoughtful attention to how benchmarking is accomplished and comparisons are made is crucial to avoid misleading comparisons (3).

Non-Revenue-Based Productivity

Since the landmark Institute of Medicine (IOM) reports were published (27,28), quality improvement activities have become central to healthcare delivery. As called upon in these reports, evolving pay-for-performance models of reimbursement look to align reimbursement with the delivery of quality care (14). This indirect effect on financial productivity begs the consideration of quality measures as a potential for tracking physician productivity. In the Donabedian model, the focus is on process measures (physician patient interactions) to drive good outcomes (29). In this model, the potential increase in profitability due to decreased costs associated with poor quality of care would be used for tracking physician productivity in the ICU.

Another non-revenue assessment of physician performance that could be considered is the 360-degree evaluation. As mentioned before, these include feedback from multiple sources, including nursing staff, physician peers, patients, and self, and may lead to improved performance and professional development (8). Other measures of productivity can include goals based on other roles the faculty member may have, including leadership, teaching, grant support, or academic productivity.

CONCLUSIONS AND FUTURE DIRECTIONS

The business of critical care medicine is becoming increasingly more important as the costs of doing business are rising both absolutely and relatively. Understanding financial and other administrative aspects of the practice is essential to maintaining control of its existence, direction, and growth potential. This will become increasingly important as the business and quality improvement worlds merge with the changes in the landscape of healthcare delivery and payment. Both ICUs and providers will be held accountable for their value. Teaching the business of critical care medicine should be a priority of critical care training programs going forward.

References

1. Matthews M Jr. Medicine as a business. *Mt Sinai J Med* 2004;71:225–30.
2. Fritts HW Jr. *On Leading a Clinical Department: A Guide for Physicians.* Baltimore: The Johns Hopkins University Press, 1997.
3. Schleien CL. The pediatric intensive care unit business model. *Pediatr Clin North Am* 2013;60:593–604.
4. Running a Business. http://www.sba.gov/category/navigation-structure/starting-managing-business/managing-business/running-business
5. Ulrich D. A new mandate for human resources. *Harv Bus Rev* 1998;76:123–34.
6. Tobin MJ. Mentoring: Seven roles and some specifics. *Am J Respir Crit Care Med* 2004;170:114–7.
7. Reid MB, Misky GJ, Harrison RA, et al. Mentorship, productivity, and promotion among academic hospitalists. *J Gen Intern Med* 2012;27:23–7.
8. Dubinsky I, Jennings K, Greengarten M, et al. 360-degree physician performance assessment. *Healthc Q* 2010;13:71–6.
9. Pastores SM, Dakwar J, Halpern NA. Costs of critical care medicine. *Crit Care Clin* 2012;28:1–10, v.
10. Chalfin DB, Cohen IL, Lambrinos J. The economics and cost-effectiveness of critical care medicine. *Intensive Care Med* 1995;21:952–61.
11. Pittoni GM, Scatto A. Economics and outcome in the intensive care unit. *Curr Opin Anaesthesiol* 2009;22:232–6.
12. Cooper LM, Linde-Zwirble WT. Medicare intensive care unit use: Analysis of incidence, cost, and payment. *Crit Care Med* 2004;32:2247–53.
13. Chalom R, Raphaely RC, Costarino AT Jr. Hospital costs of pediatric intensive care. *Crit Care Med* 1999;27:2079–85.
14. Christianson JB, Knutson DJ, Mazze RS. Physician pay-for-performance. Implementation and research issues. *J Gen Intern Med* 2006;21(suppl 2):S9–S13.
15. Porter ME, Lee TH. The strategy that will fix health care. *Harv Bus Rev* 2013;91:1–19.
16. Stauffer D. The key financial statements. *HBR Guide to Finance Basics for Managers.* Boston, MA: Harvard Business Press Books, 2012:9–39.
17. Buck CJ. *ICD-9-CM for Physicians, Volumes 1 & 2.* St. Louis, MO: Elsevier Saunders, 2013.
18. Wunsch H, Gershengorn H, Scales DC. Economics of ICU organization and management. *Crit Care Clin* 2012;28:25–37, v.
19. Finkler SA. The distinction between cost and charges. *Ann Intern Med* 1982;96:102–9.
20. Dowless RM. The health care cost-shifting debate: Could both sides be right? *J Health Care Finance* 2007;34:64–71.
21. Bekes CE, Dellinger RP, Brooks D, et al. Critical care medicine as a distinct product line with substantial financial profitability: The role of business planning. *Crit Care Med* 2004;32:1207–14.
22. MLN Matters Number: 5993. http://www.cms.gov/Outreach-and-Education/Medicare-Learning-Network-MLN/MLNMattersArticles/downloads/mm5993.pdf. http://www.cms.gov/Regulations-and-Guidance/Guidance/Manuals/downloads/clm104c12.pdf

23. About CPT®. http://www.ama-assn.org/ama/pub/physician-resources/solutions-managing-your-practice/coding-billing-insurance/cpt/about-cpt.page?

24. Lesnick BL. Bundled babies and bundled billing: How to properly use the new pediatric critical care codes. *Chest* 2010;137:701–4.

25. Agrawal S, Tarzy B, Hunt L, et al. Expanding physician education in health care fraud and program integrity. *Acad Med* 2013;88:1081–7.

26. AHRQ Quality Indicators Toolkit: Documentation and Coding for Patient Safety Indicators. http://www.ahrq.gov/professionals/systems/hospital/qitoolkit/b4_documentationcoding.pdf

27. Institute of Medicine (US) - Committee on Quality of Health Care in America. *To Err is Human: Building a Safer Health System*. In: Kohn LT, Corrigan JM, Donaldson MS, eds. Washington, DC: National Academies Press, 2000.

28. Institute of Medicine (US) - Committee on Quality of Health Care in America. *Crossing the Quality Chasm: A New Health System for the 21st Century*. Washington, DC: National Academies Press, 2001.

29. Curtis JR, Cook DJ, Wall RJ, et al. Intensive care unit quality improvement: A "how-to" guide for the interdisciplinary team. *Crit Care Med* 2006;34:211–8.

WYNNE E. MORRISON, ELIZABETH A. HUNT, J. MICHAEL DEAN, AND ANNE-MARIE GUERGUERIAN

KEY POINTS

Study Design

1. Defining a clear, detailed, answerable research question is the first step in beginning a project.
2. Involving experts in methods of study design and statistical analysis during the early planning phases of a study will save much wasted effort.
3. A well-designed randomized controlled trial (RCT) is the gold standard of comparative trials, but is resource intensive and may not be possible in some situations.
4. Observational study designs (case-control or cohort studies) can be very helpful if their limitations are understood.
5. Systematic review and meta-analysis cannot improve the quality of the data from the individual trials included.
6. Qualitative research includes a variety of observational and exploratory techniques. Methods in these studies should be just as rigorous as in quantitative studies.

Statistical Analysis

7. Computers are an invaluable tool for performing statistical analyses, but they cannot determine if the right question has been asked or if the appropriate test has been used.
8. The type of statistical test chosen depends on the type of data, distribution of the data, total number of subjects, number of groups involved, number of measurements per subject, whether measurements are made over time, and what question is asked.
9. Visually inspecting patterns in the data before running any statistical test is necessary and will help in choosing the appropriate test.
10. Investigators choose the amount of risk of reaching a wrong conclusion that they are willing to accept. Cutoffs, such as an α level of 0.05, are arbitrary and established by convention.
11. Confidence intervals are more informative tools with which to describe the precision of an estimate, rather than believing that a p value will provide a definitive yes/no answer.
12. Trials that are either far too large or far too small are both wasteful and potentially unethical if subjects are exposed to unnecessary risks. Proper planning using available information before beginning the trial can sometimes prevent these errors.

Research in pediatric critical care is necessary in order to bring therapies that are safe, innovative, and tailored to their developmental biology to the bedside of critically ill children. It is important to examine the dogma of usual clinical practice and to determine which therapies are appropriate to adapt from adults to children. Sixty years ago, the highest possible oxygen concentrations were presumed to be best for sick neonates (1). Now the toxic effects of this approach are well recognized. Similarly, much of our vigorously defended current standard of care will someday fall by the wayside as we continue to study and learn from past errors.

Performing research during critical illness requires adapting methods and approaches because of the variety of disease states, patient's ages and developmental differences, and the relative rarity of one generally accepted approach to treatment. The risk of mortality of most conditions affecting critically ill children is relatively lower than in adults admitted to intensive care, which can make extrapolating results from adult studies using mortality outcomes problematic. In addition, research in the PICU by definition involves vulnerable subjects and families, which leads to special ethical and regulatory requirements.

The scope of this chapter does not allow us to discuss in detail all topics important to clinical research and is intended to serve as an introduction to basic principles. We focus predominantly on core concepts of clinical trial design and statistical analysis rather than basic science or translational research, although many of the statistical methods can apply to all types of research. Also, we do not address the ethics or regulation of research, monitoring of trials, or database management and, instead, focus on basic methods in clinical trial design and statistical analysis. This brief overview is in no way a substitute for collaboration with experts in statistics and trial design, and many common mistakes and much wasted effort can be avoided by the involvement of those with appropriate expertise in the earliest planning phases of a study.

STUDY DESIGN

Defining the Research Question

The first step of a study is to define the research question. A well-constructed question will delineate the important components of a study. There is a difference between asking "Does insulin use in the PICU reduce mortality?" and asking "Does targeted glucose control with an insulin infusion versus placebo reduce 30-day mortality in PICU patients younger than 18 years who are mechanically ventilated or receiving vasoactive infusions?" In the latter question, it is clear that the *study subjects* are children who are ventilated or on vasoactive infusions. The *study site* is the PICU. The *intervention* is glucose control with an insulin infusion. The *alternative* is placebo. Both groups will receive *standard therapy*. The *outcome* of interest is 30-day mortality. A precise question also helps determine to which groups of patients your results are applicable.

The question should explicitly state the *primary outcome measure* also called the *dependent variable*—the variable that is dependent on the intervention. It should also contain the primary *independent variable* being studied. This will be something to which the subjects are exposed, either experimentally, as during a *randomized controlled trial* (RCT), or as part of their usual daily life or medical care, as during an observational *cohort study*. The independent variable is also referred to as the *exposure variable* and may be a potential risk factor or an intervention.

The Research Team

A clinician-scientist will usually undertake a study with a clinical research team, similar to the core personnel of a laboratory for a preclinical investigator. Meinert emphasizes the importance of explicitly assigning tasks to members of the research team at the beginning of a study (2). One should consider inviting a methodologist, such as an epidemiologist or someone trained in study design to be on the team. Whereas the clinician-scientist will have clinical expertise about the topic in the context of critical illness, the methodologist can address study design, power calculations, and issues related to limiting bias during the design phase of the study (**Table 7.1**) (3).

Someone with biostatistics training should be consulted early to ensure that data collection and the database format facilitate analysis and enable the answering of the defined research question. The data set collected should be as parsimonious as possible, focusing closely on variables required to answer the study question and avoiding variables that do not help in answering the question. Excessive data collection without a planned purpose will take time, be distracting, and may diminish the overall quality of data collection. One may

be tempted to overstate conclusions if the extra data are not related to the original hypothesis. Additionally, research assistants serve an integral role on a research team, but they must be properly trained. It is a shame to discover that, after 100 or 200 chart reviews, they have been using the wrong definition for your primary outcome measure!

Choosing a Study Design

Once the research question is clear, the best possible design to answer it should be selected. The investigator should ask, "If I had unlimited resources, how would I design my study to have the best chance of answering the question?" and then balance this ideal with a study design that can be feasibly conducted using available resources. Possible resource limitations that may ultimately affect the study design include the availability of subjects with the exposure or outcome of interest, resources (money, people, space), and time. Each study design has specific limitations and potential biases (**Table 7.1**) that can be anticipated and perhaps minimized.

Observational versus Experimental Studies

Studies are either observational or experimental. *Observational studies* observe nature as is, with no manipulation or interventions. Investigators note whether subjects were exposed to the independent variable of interest and whether they developed the outcome of interest; however, the investigator does not control if the subject is exposed to the independent variable or putative risk factor (4). In any study, other factors associated with the dependent variable should be identified, especially those that may serve as *confounders* or *interact* with the exposure of interest (see **Table 7.1**) (3). A limitation of observational studies is the uncertainty of whether the association between the independent and dependent variables was because of the relationship of interest or because of unmeasured exposures (5). Examples of observational study designs include case-control studies, pre-post interventional studies, and cohort studies (5).

In an *experimental study*, the investigator controls which study group the patient will join. Ideally, enrollment into a

TABLE 7.1

DEFINITIONS

Bias—Deviation of results or inferences from the truth, or processes leading to such deviation. Any trend in the collection, analysis, interpretation, publication, or review of data that can lead to conclusions that are systematically different from the truth (3).
Confounder—A situation in which a measure of the effect of an exposure or risk is distorted because of the association of exposure with other factor(s) that influence the outcome of the study (3).
Interaction—Differences in the effects of one or more factors according to the level of the remaining factor(s), also called *effect modification* (3).
Equipoise—A state of genuine uncertainty about the benefits or harms that may result from each of two or more regimens. A state of equipoise is an indication for a randomized controlled trial because there are no ethical concerns about one regimen being better for a particular patient (3).
Stratified randomization—A randomization procedure in which strata are identified and subjects randomly allocated within each (3).
Masked/blinded study—A study in which observer(s) and/or subjects are kept ignorant of the group to which the subjects are assigned, as in the experiment, or of the population from which the subjects come, as in the nonexperimental study. The intent of keeping subjects and/or investigators masked/blinded (i.e., unaware of knowledge that might introduce bias) is to eliminate the effect of such biases (3).
Quasi-experiment—A situation in which the investigator lacks full control over the allocation and/or timing of intervention but nonetheless conducts the study as if it were an experiment, allocating subjects to groups (3).
Misclassification—The erroneous classification of an individual, a value, or an attribute into a category other than that to which it should be assigned. The probability of misclassification may be the same in all study groups (nondifferential misclassification) or may vary between groups (differential misclassification) (3).
Publication bias—A delay in publication or nonpublication of studies with small treatment effects or negative results (87–89).

particular study arm is by random assignment. If any other factor, such as age, sex, socioeconomic status, or severity of disease, influences the chances that a subject will be assigned to a particular study arm, the study arms will not be equivalent in all respects. One will be less sure that associations between the independent and dependent variables are *because* of the independent variable as opposed to the factor that influenced group assignment. For example, in a pre-post intervention trial, the period in which a subject was enrolled dictates his study group and intervention, which makes it an observational study. Differences between groups could be due to the independent variable of interest or due to other factors that varied between the periods.

Rothman and Greenland state that the "ideal experiment would create a set of circumstances across which only one factor affecting the outcome of interest would vary," that is, the independent variable of interest (4). The impossible ideal would be to enroll a group of subjects, observe their baseline characteristics, and then observe how many of the subjects develop the outcome of interest when exposed to a placebo. The next key step would be to go back in time and enroll the *same* group of subjects into the other study arm so that differences in baseline characteristics could not be a factor and then have every single aspect of their treatment be identical, except they would be treated with the study intervention rather than placebo.

The idea of having an imaginary study group that is identical in every way to a placebo group except for the independent variable of interest is counter to fact, and thus we refer to this argument as the *counterfactual* (4,6). Although the counterfactual state cannot be achieved, clinical investigators should always be aware of this limitation and attempt to conduct the best study that gives the most reliable estimate of the isolated effect of the independent variable of interest.

❸ Randomized Controlled Trial

An RCT is considered the highest quality prospective experimental clinical study type and the closest design to the counterfactual ideal. Random allocation of the intervention attempts to minimize *selection bias* and achieve study groups that are otherwise as similar as possible (5). If, for example, one study group is older than the other, and older subjects are more likely to develop the outcome of interest, then the true relationship between the independent and dependent variables may be obscured. In this case, age either may act as a confounder or may interact with the exposure variable. In either case, randomization provides the highest likelihood of ensuring an equal balance of known and unknown confounders between the study groups.

Multiple quality issues must be considered to achieve a well-designed and conducted RCT, the first issue being the randomization process. Mechanisms such as the use of random digit tables, opaque envelopes, and central data centers exist to ensure that assignment *remains* completely random and to prevent manipulation of the process. Imagine that a clinician believes that an intervention is effective and would prefer that particularly sick patients get the intervention rather than placebo (which suggests an ethical problem with *equipoise* going into the study) (see **Table 7.1**). If the physician is able to hold the envelopes up to light and sort through them to identify one in the desired group, the process is no longer random. A truly concealed allocation process provides the best possible chance of balancing known and unknown confounders between the study groups.

An issue to consider with a statistician during the design phase is whether randomization should be stratified or blocked. Consider the implications if older children are known to have a higher likelihood of a bad outcome than are infants for a particular disease and, by chance, most of the older children in a study are randomized to the placebo arm and most of the infants are randomized to the intervention arm. If the results show that those in the placebo arm do worse than those in the intervention arm, it will be difficult to discern whether this difference is because of the intervention or because of the age difference of the study groups. This situation can be avoided by performing *stratified randomization* at the beginning of the study to ensure that the age distribution between the study groups will be as similar as possible (see **Table 7.1**) (3).

Block randomization is a means to ensure that an equal number of patients will be in each study arm at the end of prespecified enrollment periods or blocks. This process is especially valuable when conducting a relatively small study. For example, if a sample size calculation reveals the need to enroll 20 patients in a study but, due to chance, 18 of the patients were randomized to intervention and 2 to placebo, the question at hand would not be answered. If patients had been randomized into blocks of 4, investigators would know that for every 4 patients enrolled, 2 would be in the intervention arm and 2 would be in the placebo arm, and that, ultimately, 10 patients would be in the intervention arm and 10 in the study arm. A downside to block randomization is that, if the process is transparent, a clinician may be able to predict to which arm the next subject would be enrolled and thus have the potential to manipulate the randomization process. This shortcoming can be overcome by varying the size of the blocks in a random order so that it is no longer predictable at which point the blocks become even.

Another important feature of a controlled trial is *blinding* or *masking* (see **Table 7.1**) (2,3). The purpose of blinding is to attempt to eliminate or reduce the chances that a subject will be treated differently or evaluated differently merely because of the study group to which he has been assigned. Language referring to blinding—single, double, and the like—is not used consistently. However, groups that may be blinded to maintain validity of the study include (a) study subjects, (b) clinicians who are treating the study subjects, (c) investigators who are assessing whether or not the subject developed the outcome of interest, and (d) statisticians who are performing analysis of the results. The consensus is that, to maintain the highest likelihood that study results will remain valid, it is best to blind the first three groups; however, debate continues regarding whether the statistician should be blinded and most agree that members of the Data and Safety Monitoring Board should not be (7).

High-quality studies include a proper power calculation based on the primary outcome during the design phase and proper maintenance of group assignment, including attention to attrition, crossovers, adherence, and contamination (5). If the study groups become incomparable for any reason, it is no longer certain that an association seen between the intervention and the outcome of interest is because of the intervention, although statistical methods, such as multivariate regression analysis, can sometimes be used to account for known confounders. A well-conducted, prospective, blinded RCT is the closest to the counterfactual experiment possible and thus provides the highest chance of obtaining valid and reliable results.

Although an RCT may be the ideal evaluation of an intervention, this study design may not be feasible or ethical. RCTs are expensive in terms of cost, number of patients, and time required to obtain a valid answer. For some questions (e.g., diagnostic test evaluation), they are not appropriate. Also, ethically, subjects cannot be randomized to study interventions or placebos that are believed to be harmful. In circumstances where an intervention cannot be introduced without inadvertently changing care practices across the intensive care unit (the *Hawthorne effect*), the study design best suited may be a *cluster randomized trial.* In cluster randomized trials, a group (or place) is randomized rather than an individual subject. To prevent the Hawthorne effect (by introducing an intervention which may change practice), the randomization may be the intensive care unit and not the individual subject. For cases in which an RCT is not appropriate, the highest quality nonrandomized controlled trial or observational study method possible should be chosen (8).

Nonrandomized Controlled Trials

Not all experimental clinical studies are RCTs. As long as the investigator is able to assign the study group to which an individual will be enrolled, the study is still considered experimental. However, some refer to studies in which factors other than randomization influence the study arm to which a subject is assigned as *quasi-experimental* (3,4). The lack of true randomization introduces possible bias.

❹ Observational Studies

We will briefly review several types of observational studies. Being familiar with the strengths and limitations of each one allows the researcher to make the best choice of study design possible.

Case Report

A *case report* is an account of an interesting observation in a single patient and can be a valuable addition to the literature. Examples of useful case reports would be those that inform the medical community about a new pathogen, genetic variant, procedure, or medication. The problem with case reports is that they may lead the reader to conclude causality when none exists. For example, if an author reports that he performed a new procedure and the patient recovered, we will never know if the patient would also have recovered *without* the procedure. The counterfactual cannot occur, so it is prudent to be wary of drawing conclusions, particularly regarding causal relationships, from a single case report.

Case Series

A *case series* is a report of a number of patients with a similar presentation, diagnostic test, therapeutic maneuver, or outcome. Valid conclusions are more likely to be drawn from a case series if the reported cases represent consecutive cases or a random sampling of all cases. If all cases of a particular disease are identified, valuable statistics can be calculated, such as the *case fatality rate,* which is the proportion of patients with a disease who die from that disease (3). Also, details regarding the demographics of cases can be reported. Although valuable lessons can be learned from the experience of others, definitive conclusions regarding the observations are impossible because no control group is provided for comparison. Subjects included in a case series may be prospectively or retrospectively identified.

A prospective case series of consecutive patients treated with an intervention is often used to illustrate local practice (9) or to bring a large group of patients together into a central data repository such as a registry for a relatively rare condition. Examples are the Extracorporeal Life Support Organization (ELSO) registry which is a voluntary case series of patients supported with extracorporeal membrane oxygenation (10,11) and the Get with the Guidelines (GWTG) cardiopulmonary arrest registry in pediatric in-hospital patients (12). Investigators can report interesting information using the denominator of a series of patients; however, without controls, they cannot definitively assess an intervention. The information gleaned from case series can be informative and can help to provide preliminary statistics useful for designing future studies, such as planning enrollment rates or power calculations, but these reports provide little evidence that a particular treatment is more effective than another.

Case-Control Study

Some observational studies utilize a control population and move closer to the counterfactual ideal by including a comparison group. In a *case-control study,* an investigator compares patients who have the outcome of interest (cases) to those who do not (controls) and measures any significant difference in the proportion of each who were exposed to the independent variable of interest. The beauty of the case-control study is that it is a very efficient study design in that it can be completed in a relatively short period and few study personnel are needed. Thus, it is relatively inexpensive to perform.

The key component of case-control studies is that cases are identified before controls. The number of cases can be the most important limiting resource. Increasing the number of cases is the most effective method of increasing the power of the study; thus, financial and personnel resources should be directed at identifying as many additional cases as possible. It is also possible to increase the power of a study by choosing more than one control per case. Depending on the limitations set on the type of control for the study, it would theoretically be possible to choose an unlimited number of controls per case. However, expenses in terms of both time and money are associated with each enrollment; thus, a point of diminishing return is reached. It is generally accepted that enrolling more than four controls per case does not significantly improve power (5,13). Using a larger number of controls makes sense only when minimal excess resources are expended (e.g., secondary analysis of data from a database).

Case-control studies are ideal in two scenarios. The first situation occurs when the study must be completed in a short time, such as during a suspected toxic exposure leading to a number of ICU admissions. The other situation is for the study of rare diseases. If an investigator tries to conduct an RCT or cohort study for a rare disease or outcome of interest, a great deal of time and money would have to be expended, perhaps enrolling thousands of patients, in an effort to enlist a sufficient number of cases for analysis. However, if a registry of cases of the rare disease exists, a case-control study could capitalize on such a resource.

Potential problems are associated with case-control studies. It is possible that controls are actually latent cases not yet identified or that those identified as exposed were not actually exposed. Either type of error would be referred to as *misclassification* (**Table 7.1**) (3). Such an *information bias* can affect the validity of the conclusions. Another limitation of case-control studies is that they cannot demonstrate *temporality.* Data on both cases and controls are gathered at the same time (*cross-sectional*), so that it is generally difficult to prove that the subject was first exposed to the putative risk factor and subsequently developed the outcome of interest. Conclusions about causality will be much stronger if investigators develop methods to assess the timing of exposure in relation to when the disease or outcome of interest developed.

Another potential misclassification problem is *recall bias.* Once cases and controls are identified, the investigator attempts to ascertain whether the subjects were "exposed." A risk exists that patients who have developed a disease have been considering how they did so and are more likely to recall that they have been exposed. Such differences in recall would tend to overestimate the effect of the exposure on the likelihood of developing the outcome. Finally, when cases and controls are chosen rather than being randomly sampled from the source population, the possibility of *selection bias* exists.

Because randomization is not an option, confounders must be dealt with during either the design or analysis phases of the study. During the design phase, *matching* can be used to try to force patients to have similar baseline characteristics. Care must be taken to avoid matching on the exposures being studied because such matching will preclude analysis. If matching occurs on any variable, an appropriate matched analysis must be performed (4), and consulting a statistician is strongly advised. An alternative to matching is to perform stratified analysis at the end of the study or use regression to adjust for confounders.

Pre-Post Intervention Study

A pre-post intervention study uses historical controls. Data are collected on a patient population prior to a change in practice, and these are compared with data collected after the change in practice. Ideally, the study is designed before the intervention or change in practice is in place. Data should be collected on potential confounding variables, including severity of illness indices and therapies that might affect outcomes. It is important to keep other components of care as similar as possible. Unfortunately, any changes in practice over time, including improved care due to experience of the healthcare team, will make the groups less comparable. A common problem occurs when data collection for the postintervention period are prospective, while those for the preintervention period are retrospective. Retrospective data collection is often less detailed and less reliable.

Cohort Study

To study potentially harmful exposures for which randomization would be unethical, a *cohort* study may be the best option. For a cohort study, patients are enrolled and information is collected on exposures and outcomes. Some of the exposures will be the focus of the study, and others will be potential confounders. The participants are then followed over time and observed to see who will develop the outcome. The relationship between the independent and dependent variables can be studied in patients who begin the study free of the outcome of interest by comparing those who are not exposed and others who are either (a) naturally exposed or (b) choose to be exposed. Because the subjects begin disease free, the disease incidence rate for the exposed group can ultimately be compared to that for the unexposed group; this is the *relative risk.*

A well-conducted prospective cohort study is generally considered the strongest type of observational study. In terms of being able to make causal inferences, its main strength is demonstration of *temporality.* If the subjects are disease free upon enrollment, it can at least be demonstrated that the exposure came before the outcome, which is a necessary but not sufficient component for proving causality.

Unfortunately, prospective cohort studies are very resource intensive, including time, money, and subjects. Efficiency can be increased by performing a *retrospective cohort*, which entails going back in time, collecting data on a defined population, and determining whether each subject subsequently developed the outcome of interest. Although data will be collected on as many known confounders as possible, it will not be possible to collect data on *unknown* confounders.

❺ Systematic Reviews and Meta-Analysis

Synthesizing data in the form of a review that incorporates new knowledge within a larger body of available evidence has been part of healthcare research and education for more than a century. Traditional reviews or overviews are *narrative reviews,* which usually contain noncomprehensive synthesis of data, nonsystematic searching and evaluation of the literature, and expert opinion, without specific attention to the research design of the published studies. These sometimes include simple methods to summarize findings across studies. *Systematic reviews* use a preestablished methodology to comprehensively select, describe, and summarize a body of research. They are prepared using a systematic approach, incorporated into a protocol, and detailed in a methods section. Like most experimental designs, systematic reviews specifically intend to minimize bias and random errors (14,15).

A systematic review may or may not contain a *meta-analysis.* A meta-analysis is a statistical analysis designed to synthesize the data from two or more *independent* studies toward answering a specific research question. A systematic review should respond to uncertainty surrounding a research or clinical question; for example, when many studies have shown small effects, when larger trials may be impossible to perform, when studies have apparently conflicting results, when a clinical practice is not supported by empirical evidence, or when the importance of the evidence is not appreciated. Systematic reviews may justify pursuing (or not) a clinical trial and help to avoid pitfalls in designing a new trial.

The quality of studies examined in a systematic review determines the quality of the review. Biases in the original studies will not disappear, and the validity of results will not improve in a systematic review. Heterogeneity between studies limits the ability to produce valid summaries when combining studies. Systematic reviews attempt to minimize *selection bias* by adopting a systematic, unbiased method to include or exclude studies. However, as published data are usually relied upon, *publication bias* (see **Table 7.1**) is unavoidable.

A systematic review should be approached like any well-designed experiment. The Quality of Reporting of Meta-Analyses (QUOROM) (16,17) and Meta-Analysis of Observational Studies in Epidemiology (MOOSE) (18) groups have produced recommendations for the reporting of systematic reviews and meta-analyses; others offer specific approaches, methods, and templates, such as the Cochrane Collaboration Systematic Reviews (16,19). These guidelines are intended to strengthen and homogenize the quality and reporting of systematic reviews. There are suggested methods to perform systematic reviews of different study designs, such as randomized trials (16), observational studies (18), diagnostic studies, and prognostic studies (20). In-depth analyses should include both an assessment of the quality of the studies and a quantitative assessment of the data. Omitting the qualitative assessment may lead to a cookbook approach that fails to identify important sources of bias or heterogeneity between studies; determining the minimal acceptable methodologic quality a priori maintains the quality of the review.

The methods used to locate studies should be well described, including search terms used, databases searched (e.g., Medline, Embase, Psychinfo, Cochrane), whether references were hand searched, and if a reference was the result of a personal communication with experts. Final eligibility of studies should be determined by more than one team member, with processes for maintaining a log of included and excluded studies and resolving disagreements. A checklist should be developed to determine which studies meet inclusion criteria; quality scales for inclusion have been developed by several authors (15,19,21–24).

Data presentation and a meta-analysis require choosing a common summary statistic and units of measurement because the individual studies may not have reported the treatment effect in the same format. *Summary plots* can illustrate trends, differences, and commonalities between studies. *Forrest plots* (**Fig. 7.1**) help investigators to compare the treatment effect and relative weight of each study in the overall analysis. Other methods (e.g., *sensitivity analyses*) can be used to detect an overwhelming effect of one study on the combined analysis. The assistance of an experienced methodologist is essential in choosing a valid summary statistic and computing a combined treatment effect. Meta-analysis can legitimately proceed (14) if the individual studies are not qualitatively or quantitatively heterogeneous. Software is available—some at no cost, such as Review Manager (RevMan) from Cochrane, and some commercially—for performing meta-analyses.

Qualitative Research

The term *qualitative research* is generally used to describe a group of techniques that have been adapted from the social sciences and applied to healthcare. The research is often exploratory and observational and typically deals more with the cultural aspects of medicine and the personal experience of healthcare providers, patients, and families. Qualitative studies are not necessarily subject to randomization or the experimental method of altering one variable while keeping all others stable because the complexity of the real world does not usually allow such control (25); such studies are often described as *inductive* rather than *deductive*. Yet, this very fact allows examination of those issues and questions that do not lend themselves to interventional trial design; quantitative and qualitative methods should, therefore, be complementary and each implemented where appropriate to the research question (26).

A variety of techniques can fall under the label "qualitative." Examples include in-depth interviews, focus groups, textual analysis, or observation of behaviors. Recent qualitative studies in pediatric critical care demonstrate how such methods can be used to explore complex topics. Meert et al. (27) interviewed parents regarding their spiritual needs following a child's death. They describe themes that recur in the interviews, such as a need to maintain a connection with the child during the illness and after death. Although the information obtained is not easily amenable to statistical comparisons, it is still useful to practitioners who are trying to understand the family's experience. Another study used focus groups to explore parent and healthcare worker opinions regarding an exception from informed consent for an RCT of therapeutic hypothermia following pediatric cardiac arrest (28), illustrating that a thorough exploration of a research question may require a combination of qualitative and quantitative methods.

A well-done qualitative analysis is just as rigorous as any study (29). A well-formulated research question, clear methods, and an assessment of validity and reliability are essential. Not all results will be generalizable, but the population should be described well enough that it is apparent when they are not. Standard methods include using multiple investigators to code themes so that their results can be compared and "member checking" by taking results back to interviewees or group attendees to confirm if the formal description adequately reflects their experience. Sample size is often not determined a priori; rather, data collection continues until no new themes are identified (*thematic saturation*) (30).

Comparative Effectiveness Research

Recently in the United States, there has been an increased funding focus on *comparative effectiveness research*. The definition can include trial designs of many different types discussed above, from observational studies to randomized interventions (31). These types of studies have in common the

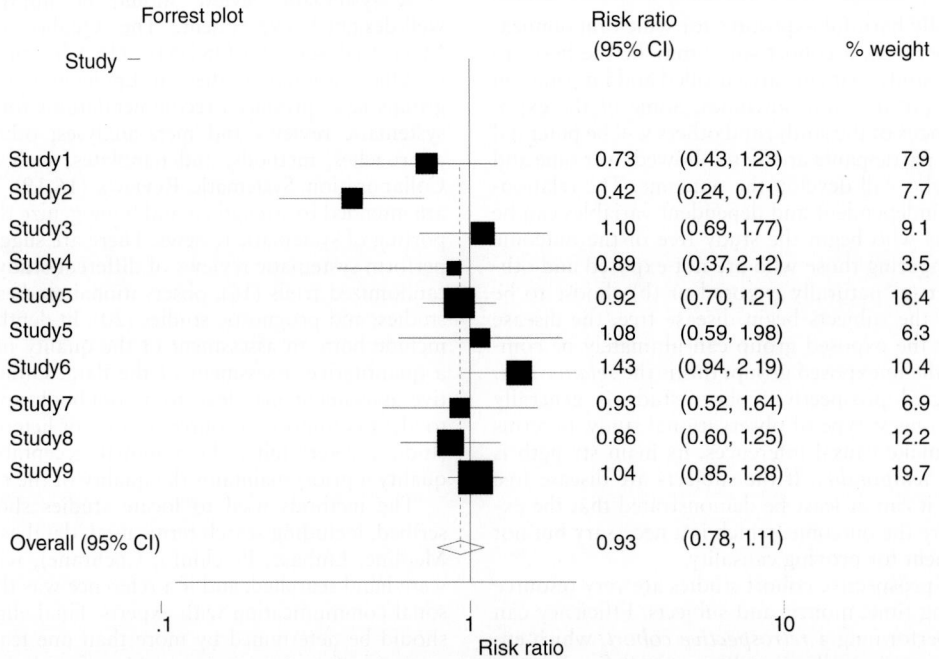

FIGURE 7.1. A Forrest plot visually compares studies in a meta-analysis. Studies with greater patient numbers have larger boxes, and the precision of the confidence intervals is represented by the length of the horizontal bars. Positive and negative effects are indicated by whether the central point of the line falls to the left or right of the vertical bar. The confidence intervals for the risk ratio for almost all the studies shown here include 1, as does the overall estimate, leading to an acceptance of the null hypothesis of no treatment effect.

attempt to "to prevent, diagnose, treat, and monitor a clinical condition, or to improve the delivery of care" (32), with the ultimate goal of minimizing variability in practice and identifying interventions with the most advantageous benefit-to-cost ratio. Many of these studies will rely on data from large administrative databases that have an inherent risk of bias, but may be used to refine questions for interventional studies or attempt to answer questions that cannot be addressed by randomized controlled experiments. The subsequent interventional studies themselves (e.g., assessments of goal-directed therapies, guidelines, or monitoring practices at the bedside) could also fall into this category of research.

STATISTICAL ANALYSIS

7 ## Introduction

Statistics is a science of probability, not certainty. For any clinician who is either performing research or hoping to apply the results of research in the care of patients, it is important to understand what conclusions can be drawn from statistical tests, what the limitations are, and what common mistakes investigators make in the analysis and presentation of data. Although computerized software packages can perform the calculations required for most statistical analyses, computers are unable to judge the accuracy, validity, or importance of the data they are given. Computers will faithfully provide an answer, even when asked the wrong question. Both a clinician's insight into the problem and a statistician's input into choosing an appropriate test are invaluable. The following is a brief primer on statistical methods, from a clinician's perspective, with a focus more on vocabulary, context, and concepts than on equations.

Sample vs. Population

The first step on the road to learning statistics is a familiarity with the language. Methods generally involve collecting and analyzing information on a *sample* of a population and making inferences about the population as a whole. *Population* does not necessarily imply individuals; examples of populations could be "all children younger than 2 years with traumatic brain injury," "all academic medical centers in the United States," etc. Whether a sample is chosen appropriately will have a tremendous effect on whether the results can be meaningfully interpreted (33). For example, a proven intervention for inpatients at an academic center (those at the severe end of the disease spectrum) may not be applicable to outpatients with the same disease. The difference between population and sample statistics leads to the confusing habit of having two symbols for most summary statistics; for example, s^2 and σ^2 for the sample and population variance, respectively.

8 ## Types of Data

Different tests are appropriate for different types of data (7). *Nominal* or *categorical* variables fall into categories without a specific order (e.g., race, car color, blood type). A *dichotomous* or *binary* variable has only two categories (e.g., gender, mortality). Summary statistics for categorical variables are usually expressed as proportions; "30% female" makes more sense than an "average" gender. An *ordinal* variable is a categorical variable that is ranked (e.g., grade in school, Glasgow outcome scale). These are all *discrete* variables, meaning that gaps exist between possible values (e.g., the Glasgow outcome scale does not include a score of 2.6).

For a *continuous* variable, any value can be taken along a scale with infinite possible values (e.g., weight). Some technically discrete variables can be statistically treated as if they are continuous if a sufficient number of possible ranked values exist (e.g., Pediatric Risk of Mortality score).

Descriptive Statistics

The *distribution* of a variable refers to a frequency plot in which the data fall. Several summary statistics can be applied to a distribution. It is good practice to develop the habit of looking at data graphically rather than relying solely on summary statistics to describe the data; surprising patterns can emerge. Statistics that somehow describe the "middle" of the data are called *measures of central tendency*. The *mode* is the most common value of the variable. A bimodal distribution has two "most common" values. The *median* is the middle value when the values are ranked. The *mean* (average) is the sum of the values divided by the number of measurements.

The dispersion or variability of data should also be described. A *range* is simply the difference between the largest and smallest values. A *percentile* refers to the value in the data that is larger than a given percentage of observations when they are ranked. Thus, the 90th percentile would be the observation larger than 90% of observations. The 50th percentile is the same as the median. *Quartile* refers to dividing the data into quarters—with the lowest quartile, therefore, being all observations below the 25th percentile. The interquartile range (IQR) is the difference between the 25th and 75th percentiles and contains the middle 50% of data.

The *variance* (s^2) is one way to describe variability in a sample. It measures how much individual observations differ from the mean by adding the squares of each of those differences and dividing by the degrees of freedom ($n-1$). A greater variance means more values in the sample fall far from the mean and may make an investigator less certain that the mean represents the true population mean. The *standard deviation* is the square root of the variance, which is a more intuitively meaningful number because the units are the same as the original observations (e.g., years rather than years²).

The *standard error of the mean* (SEM) is sometimes confused with the standard deviation (SD). If a sample of "n" randomly selected observations is repeatedly taken from a population, the SEM is the variability of the *means* of those repeated samples. It is obtained by dividing the SD by the square root of the sample size (n). The SD should be used when describing the variability of a sample; the SEM, instead, is a description of the precision of an estimate of the population mean. The SEM is always smaller than the SD, and authors sometimes make their data appear less variable than they truly are by inappropriately presenting the SEM rather than the SD when simply describing the sample.

Normal Distribution

Continuous data in nature often tend to take the shape of a *normal distribution*, which is a typical bell-shaped curve (**Fig. 7.2**), in which the mean, mode, and median are the same and the frequency of each value decreases the farther away it is from that mean. The distribution is symmetric above and below the mean and is predictable (95% of observations are within 1.96 standard deviations of the mean). Many physiologic variables behave in a somewhat normal fashion; for example, an "average" blood pressure is far more common than an extremely high or low one. Some statistical tests (e.g., Student's t test; analysis of variance, ANOVA) assume that a continuous outcome variable follows a fairly normal distribution. A distribution is

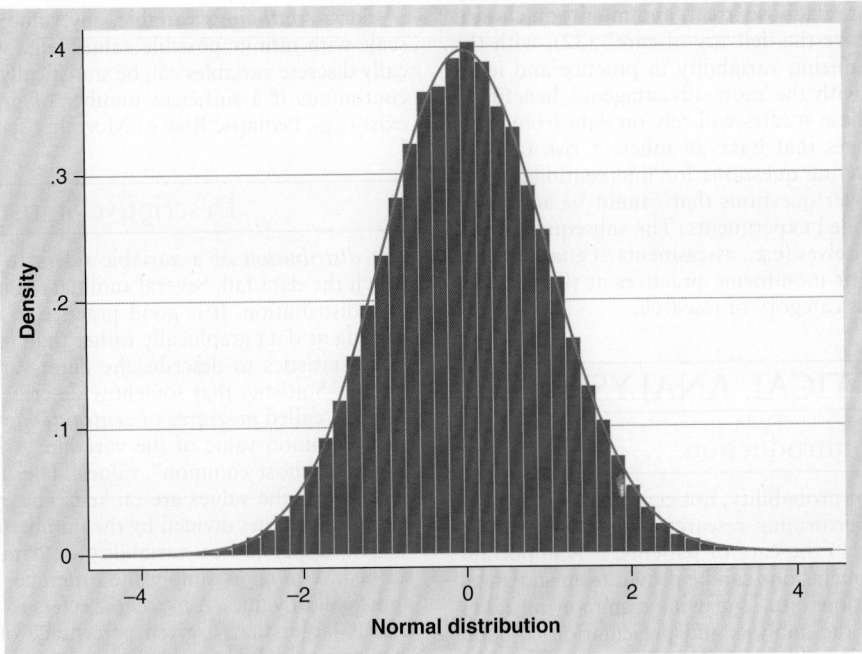

FIGURE 7.2. Standard normal distribution. The mean is both the most common value and the median. The distribution is symmetric on either side of the mean, with more extreme values becoming progressively less frequent.

skewed when the values are not symmetric around the mean (**Fig. 7.3**). A median and IQR are better descriptors of highly skewed data than are the mean and the SD. Extreme outliers will pull the mean in their direction but have little effect on the median, as the outlier only counts as a "high" or "low" value in choosing a median rather than contributing numerically to the calculation (34). For example, if a billionaire moved into my neighborhood, the mean income would increase dramatically; in contrast, the median would change minimally, if at all.

Skewed Data and Transformation

What if the data are not normally distributed? A possible solution is to *transform* the data so that it appears normal. Probably the most commonly used transformation is a logarithmic

transformation, as it tends to take data that are highly positively skewed and pull the extreme values closer to the center (**Fig. 7.4**) (35). Each value is replaced with the log of the value, and the statistical test is run on the transformed data. Many other transformations can be used, from square or cube roots, to reciprocals, to some combination of the above. In some ways, transforming data seems like cheating, but it is usually a valid solution that has the advantage of mathematically preserving the relationships of the original data. One caveat is that it is important to present results in the original units, which will make more intuitive sense than "log-days," for instance. Nonparametric tests (tests designed for non-normally distributed data; discussed later) are another option; nonparametric tests, however, lose some of the information contained in the original data because each value gets converted to a rank rather than simply having a mathematical function applied to transform it.

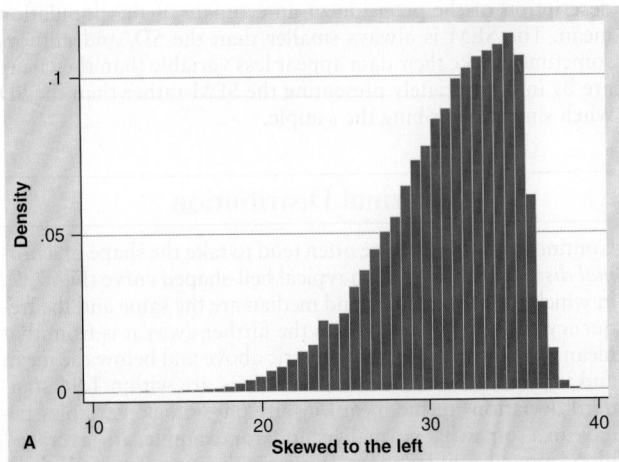

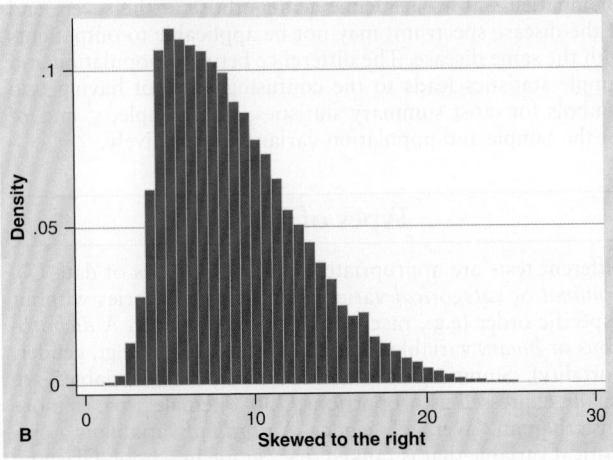

FIGURE 7.3. Skewness. A distribution that is skewed to the left has outliers that are much smaller than the median, which will pull the mean lower than the median. A distribution that is skewed to the right has outliers that are much higher than the median, pulling the mean up.

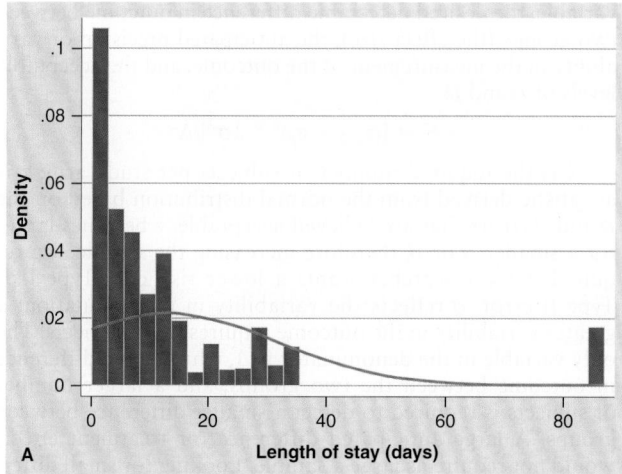
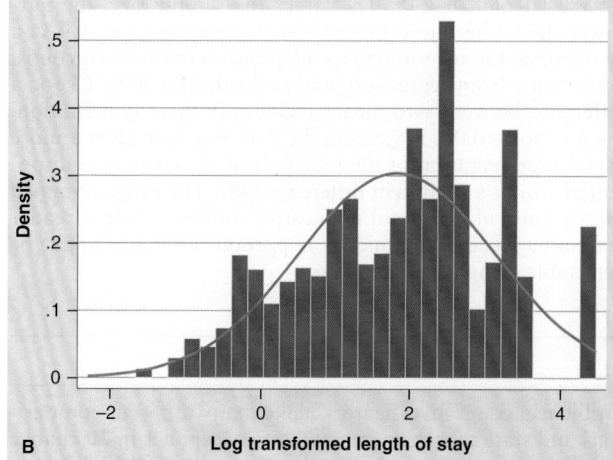

FIGURE 7.4. Data transformation. (A) Length of stay (usually highly skewed to the right) of children admitted to a PICU over 1 year. (B) A natural log transformation often helps right-skewed data to better approximate a normal distribution in order to fulfill the mathematical assumptions of this probability distribution.

Confidence Intervals and Hypothesis Testing

Hypothesis Testing

Hypothesis testing refers to using statistics to either accept or reject a hypothesis; it is never possible to *prove* a hypothesis, only accept or reject it to some degree of certainty. The *null hypothesis* is the assumption that no difference exists between the result and the true population parameter (or, when comparing two samples, that no difference exists between them). The *alternative hypothesis* is that a difference really exists. *Equivalency* trials are becoming more common, however, in which the null hypothesis is actually that a difference *does* exist between groups.

It is possible to be wrong when you accept or reject a hypothesis. Two types of errors exist:

■ Type I error [alpha error (α), false positive]: The null hypothesis is incorrectly rejected (e.g., it is concluded that two therapies are different when really they are the same).

■ Type II error [beta error (β), false negative]: The null hypothesis is incorrectly accepted (e.g., no difference is found between two therapies when in reality a difference does exist).

Investigators decide what level of α and β error they are willing to accept. The α level is typically set at 0.05 (meaning a 5%, or 1-in-20 chance of a Type I error) and the β level is often set at 0.1 to 0.2. In general, the less willing one is to mistakenly accept the null hypothesis, the more one must be willing to mistakenly reject it. The only way to decrease the chances of both an α and β error is to increase the sample size (see discussion on power analysis and sample size calculation later in the chapter).

The "0.05" α cutoff is familiar to clinicians as the most commonly accepted level of *statistical significance*. The *p value* was originally developed by Fisher during the 1920s as a scale for assessing strength of evidence, and it was not intended to provide a definitive "accept" or "reject"; it is defined as the *probability*, under the assumption of no true difference (i.e., the null hypothesis is correct), of obtaining—due to chance alone—a result equal to or more extreme than the one seen. As often used today, the null hypothesis (no difference demonstrated) is accepted if $p \geq 0.05$ and the null

hypothesis (difference demonstrated) is rejected if $p < 0.05$. Many different statistical tests can generate a p value. The cutoff is arbitrary; some conclusions may be drawn from $p = 0.07$ (most commonly "a larger study is indicated!"), and $p = 0.001$ is more convincing than $p = 0.04$. Presenting exact p values, which computers make possible, is more useful than stating only a range.

A p value reflects only the strength of the data used to compute it; it does not take into account any prior evidence (other studies, lab data, physiologic reasoning) that might affect interpretation of the data. *Bayesian* theory refers to using the results of any study to adjust the *pre-test probability* of a certain belief, rather than drawing potentially incorrect conclusions by making each study stand completely on its own (36,37).

It is also important not to confuse statistical significance with *clinical importance*. Especially in trials employing large numbers, it is possible to find a statistically significant result in which the magnitude of the difference shown is so small that it is really not relevant in the real world. The same thing can happen when the outcome chosen is not important in the long run. This type of mistake does not fall into the realm of Type I or Type II error because the mathematical/statistical conclusions are perfectly valid, but it is a mistake nonetheless. A hypothetical example would be enrolling 2000 patients in a trial of vitamin E for bronchiolitis and showing that the average oxygen saturation in the intervention versus control group was 95% versus 94%, with $p = 0.02$. Regardless of the p value, this difference is nothing to get excited about.

Confidence Intervals

Many statisticians and investigators are uncomfortable with the "yes/no" results obtained with typical hypothesis testing and feel that confidence intervals are a much more informative way to present data. A *95% confidence interval* (CI) is the mathematical corollary of a p value of 0.05. As an example, if investigators decided to study platelet counts in the PICU and, after evaluating 50 patients, found that the mean platelet count was 242, with a 95% CI range of 206–277, they would be 95% certain that the true population value (mean platelet count for *all* similar children) fell within that range. After evaluating 500 children, they found a mean of 236, with a 95% CI of 226–245. The larger the sample size, the narrower the CI becomes (the estimate is more precise). CIs can be obtained for any estimate: a difference between two groups, odds ratios from regression, and so forth. If a 95% CI for a difference between two means includes 0, then by definition, the p is not <0.05. Presenting the data this way gives a more useful representation of the precision of the estimate and potential size of a treatment difference (38). The range obtained can be particularly useful in negative studies to help a reader determine whether a clinically important difference might be detectable using larger numbers.

Multiple Comparisons

Problems arise if investigators make many different comparisons and state that they are willing to accept a 1 in 20 chance of a Type I error for each. It makes sense that, if 100 different comparisons are made, a statistically significant result (in this case, a false positive) would be found, on average, in five of them by chance alone. The overall risk of a Type I error may become unacceptably high. A particular problem occurs in *data dredging* or extensive subgroup analysis, in which investigators examine large amounts of data looking for significant relationships that were not anticipated a priori—inevitably, significant but erroneous results will be found (39). Statistical methods exist, such as the *Bonferroni procedure*, which adjust for multiple comparisons by setting a more stringent α cutoff for each comparison to decrease the overall risk of error. Of course, being too strict can increase the chance of missing important relationships. The same reasoning applies to the practice of setting a lower p value for stopping a trial early due to an *interim analysis*. Examining the data too often increases the chance of making a Type I error, so that such analyses should be planned prospectively in such a way that the risks are understood. An extreme example of this mistake would be an investigator who keeps adding 5 more patients to the study until the desired answer is statistically significant (which is almost certain to occur, by chance, at some point) and then stops enrollment, guaranteeing he gets the answer he wants.

⑫ Power Analysis and Sample Size Calculations

Choosing an appropriate sample size is essential to good study design (40). A study that is too large wastes time and resources and unnecessarily exposes too many patients to the risks of randomization by continuing to assign patients to placebo or treatment groups when a therapy could have been proven helpful/harmful/useless at an earlier point. A study that is too small fails to conclusively answer a question and is also ultimately wasteful. Sample size and power calculations are always, however, approximations (7).

The *power* of a study is defined as 1 minus β, or 100% minus the risk of making a Type II error. Thus, a study with 80% power accepts a Type II error of 0.2; a study with 90% power accepts a β of 0.1. Equations for sample size calculations vary, depending on what type of outcome is chosen (e.g., continuous vs. dichotomous data) and what type of statistical analysis is planned (e.g., univariate comparisons vs. multiple regression vs. survival analysis). An example of a specific calculation (for comparing means from two groups with equal variances and equal numbers of subjects in each group) is useful to show what information may be used for a typical calculation. The key items an investigator needs to estimate a sample size for a comparative trial are the type of outcome

variable, the desired detectable difference in outcome between two groups (the effect size), the anticipated precision or variability in the measurement of the outcome, and the acceptable levels of α and β:

$$N = [(z_{\alpha/2} + z_\beta)^2 * 2\sigma^2]/\Delta^2$$

N is the required number of subjects per study arm; z is a statistic derived from the normal distribution based on the α and β errors that are believed acceptable. z becomes larger for a smaller α or β, therefore increasing the sample size required if the researcher wants a lower risk of a Type I or Type II error. σ reflects the variability in the population; a greater variability in the outcome requires more subjects. The only variable in the denominator is Δ, which is the difference in outcome between the two groups, and a larger number of subjects is required to detect a smaller difference between groups. A large anticipated difference (or treatment effect) would not require as large a sample. Looking for small differences requires very large numbers. The equations do not account for dropouts or study logistical issues; these problems should be anticipated, and they often increase the enrollment goal by 10%–30%.

Some information, such as the precision or variability in the outcome to be measured, may not be reliably known before beginning the study. Investigators often obtain this information from published studies in similar patient populations, from their own pilot data, or by making an educated guess.

In attempting to design a feasible study, investigators may use various strategies to try to decrease the required sample size, some of which are more legitimate than others (41). Accepting a slightly higher risk of a Type I or Type II error or anticipating a greater treatment effect may be reasonable if the trade-offs are well understood. Choosing a more common surrogate end point (e.g., ventilator-free days rather than mortality) may allow for a smaller study, but care must be taken to ensure that clinically relevant outcomes are still considered. If possible, using a more precise outcome and minimizing variability is helpful.

Using a "1-tailed" versus "2-tailed" α will greatly decrease the required numbers, but is usually not appropriate (42). Using a "2-tailed" or "2-sided" test means understanding that the intervention could either improve or worsen the outcome—it is hardly ever the case that one can be certain that the effect will only be in one direction (the above equation includes "$\alpha/2$," assuming a 2-tailed α).

Sensitivity and Specificity

Sensitivity and specificity are important in evaluating diagnostic tests (43), but similar concepts can apply when considering the association of a certain risk factor with a disease. The best way to remember the definitions is to visualize them on a 2 × 2 table:

	DISEASE	
	Present	Absent
TEST		
Positive	TP	FP
Negative	FN	TN

Columns represent the true disease state or the best approximation—a *gold standard* test. Rows represent the test being evaluated. TP refers to true positive, FP refers to false positive, FN refers to false negative, and TN refers to true negative. Sensitivity and specificity are obtained by adding down columns. *Sensitivity* is the probability that a test is positive given that the disease is truly present: TP/(TP + FN). *Specificity* is the probability that the test is negative given that the disease is truly absent: TN/(TN + FP). In the clinical situation, it is usually not known beforehand if the disease is present or not; therefore, *predictive values* (the rows) are relevant, rather than sensitivity and specificity. If a test is positive, the *positive predictive value* is the probability that the disease is really present: PPV = TP/(TP + FP). Conversely, if a test is negative, the *negative predictive value* is the probability that the disease is truly absent: NPV = TN/(TN + FN). The problem with the PPV and NPV is that these values vary with the prevalence of disease.

As an example, suppose investigators develop a rapid bedside test for respiratory syncytial virus (RSV), and they evaluate house staff use of the test one winter in 138 infants who present with lower respiratory tract symptoms. Their 2 × 2 table comparing the new test to the gold standard respiratory syncytial virus direct fluorescent antibody shows:

DISEASE

TEST	Present	Absent	
Positive	61	5	66
Negative	6	66	72
	67	71	138

The sensitivity of the test is, therefore, 61/67 (91%), and the specificity is 66/71 (93%). The PPV is 61/66 (92%), and the NPV is 66/72 (92%). The disease *prevalence* in this case is 67/138 (49%). The investigators are excited and decide to put the test into clinical use. They train the incoming interns in July by having them try the test on all patients admitted that month, regardless of the presenting symptoms. The prevalence

of the disease has changed dramatically—only 1% of 1,000 patients admitted have RSV. The table now looks as follows:

DISEASE

TEST	Present	Absent	
Positive	9	69	78
Negative	1	921	922
	10	990	1000

Although the sensitivity and specificity are not affected by prevalence, the PPV is now 9/78 (12%) and the NPV is 921/922 (99.9%), and false positives now outnumber true positives. This example illustrates the same point stressed in the earlier discussion of Bayesian analysis—that knowledge of the pretest probability of disease before performing the test (or study!) will inevitably affect interpretation of the results. This is a frequently encountered problem when an attempt is made to adapt a test or therapy proven useful in one population to a population in which it has not been evaluated.

When a continuous variable is being evaluated as a diagnostic test, a balance between sensitivity and specificity must be achieved in setting a cutoff point for diagnosing a disease. As an example, consider two hypothetical overlapping curves along the range of serum calcium levels for patients with and without hyperparathyroidism (**Fig. 7.5**). If serum calcium level were used as a diagnostic test for this disease, setting a lower cutoff (e.g., 9 mg/dL) would be an overly sensitive test. Most patients with the disease would have a positive test, but many without would as well. Setting a higher cutoff (e.g., 12 mg/dL) would conversely be overly specific. This method would render very few false positives, but many potential cases (true positives) would be missed. Choosing a different, more *accurate* test (i.e., one with less overlap between the two curves) would be the only way to improve both sensitivity and specificity.

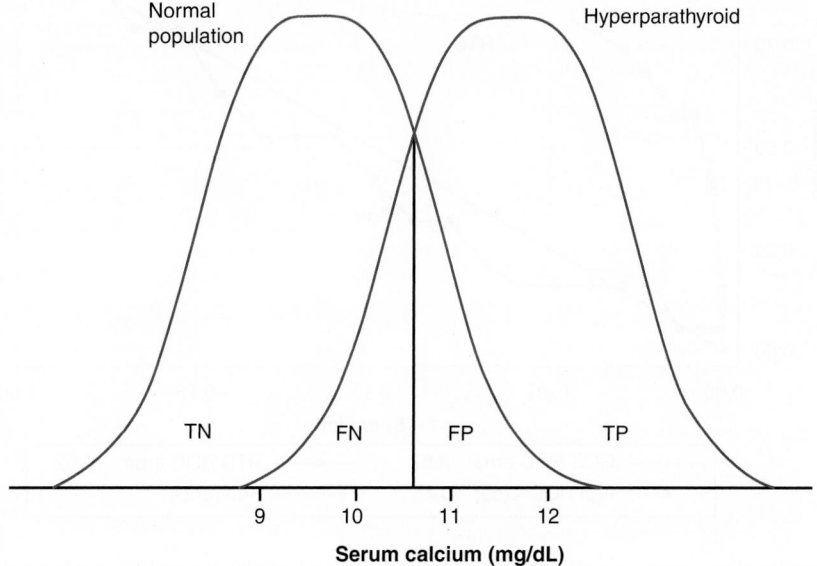

FIGURE 7.5. Overlapping curves of calcium values in normal and hyperparathyroid patients illustrate tradeoffs in sensitivity and specificity, with varying cutoff points for what is considered an "abnormal" test. TN, true negative; FN, false negative; FP, false positive; TP, true positive.

Receiver Operating Characteristic Curves

Receiver operating characteristic (ROC) curves are often presented when comparing the performance of diagnostic tests, risk factors, or scales to predict dichotomous outcomes (**Fig. 7.6**). The curve is obtained by plotting **sensitivity** on the y-axis versus **1 − specificity** (1 minus specificity, highest specificity at origin, least specificity at right end of axis) on the x-axis for various cutoff points of a diagnostic test. The *area under the curve* (AUC) is calculated as a measure of the discriminatory power of the test. A perfect test (sensitivity and specificity of 100% at all points) would be a right angle, with the apex at the upper left corner, and it would have an AUC of 1.0. A test no better than chance would fall on the diagonal line and have an AUC of 0.5 (see **Chapter 10**). The best cutoff point for the diagnostic test falls at the point along the curve closest to the upper left corner.

Figure 7.6 illustrates the use of the Glasgow Coma Scale (GCS), revised trauma score (RTS), and age as predictors of mortality in more than 11,000 patients with traumatic brain injury. GCS appears to be the best predictor (AUC = 0.87) versus RTS (AUC = 0.82). Age is no better than chance, with an AUC = 0.45, despite the fact that younger age was a highly significant predictor of greater mortality (not shown); it is still a very poor *discriminatory* test for giving a "cutoff" point. Additionally, even though GCS is the best predictor of the three, its best cutoff point reaches a sensitivity of 75% and specificity of 90%, making it not very useful as a diagnostic test. The example also illustrates that, when evaluating a potential diagnostic test, it does not necessarily help to say "a statistically significant difference in GCS is observed between survivors and non-survivors" because doing so begins with the result and looks backward. Rather, the predictive power of different cutoff points should be examined, such as by using an ROC curve, to determine sensitivity and specificity, and it should be determined if the test performs adequately with a given prevalence of disease (5).

Specific Statistical Tests

The following is a brief overview of several statistical tests that provides some guidance on choosing the correct test to use; more detailed references and software are available for guidance on performing each test (44–47). The list is not exhaustive, but it presents some of the most commonly encountered methods. The choice of test depends on the type of outcome to be analyzed, number of different groups to be compared, size of the sample, variability of data, and nature of the question.

Student's *t* test

Student's *t* test can be used to compare means of continuous data. The formulae vary based on whether the test is paired and whether variances are equal, but all generate a "*t* statistic," which is compared with a standard curve or table to generate a *p* value; in other words, the proportion of time that a difference as extreme as the one seen or greater would occur by chance alone. It is possible to compare a single mean with a population parameter (i.e., normal value) or to compare *two* means. If the two values are related (e.g., before and after measurement on the same patient), it is necessary to use a *paired t* test. The curve used to determine the *p* value depends on the degrees of freedom, so that a larger sample results in a narrower curve and, hence, a lower *p* value. One of the assumptions of the *t* test is that the continuous outcome follows a roughly normal distribution; large numbers allow for some deviation from this requirement.

Analysis of Variance

The ANOVA is used to compare the mean of a continuous outcome from *more than two groups*. This tool is useful when comparing several groups to avoid starting with repeated

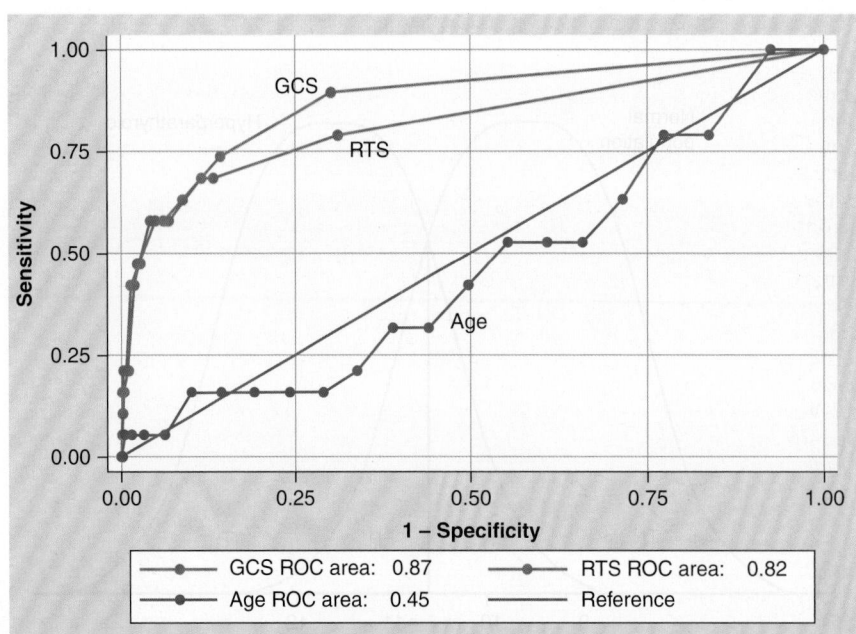

FIGURE 7.6. Receiver operating characteristic curve, evaluating Glasgow Coma Scale (GCS), Revised Trauma Score (RTS), and age as predictors of mortality.

t tests between pairs of groups, which can lead to the problem of multiple comparisons. ANOVA examines the variability in the observations between the groups and compares this with the variability within the groups. Significantly more variability "between" than "within" the groups suggests that a real difference exists between them. ANOVA generates a *variance ratio* or *F statistic* from the ratio of between and within group sums of squared deviations from the mean, adjusted for the degrees of freedom. Standard tables then provide the risk that such a difference could be seen by chance.

Like the *t* test, ANOVA assumes that the outcome is roughly normally distributed, with greater deviations from normality allowed as the numbers get larger. Other assumptions are that the groups have fairly equal variances. A very important assumption is that the values are independent of each other; classical ANOVA analysis cannot be used to compare multiple measurements on single individuals.

One-way ANOVA refers to models with only one independent variable. An example would be a study of time that physicians spend talking with families based on the families' educational levels (time would be the continuous outcome; educational level—high school, college, graduate school—would be the categorical independent variable). *Two-way ANOVA* refers to an analysis with two factors as independent variables. An example might be looking at the effect of race and gender on blood pressure. *Repeated-measures ANOVA* is the counterpart of the paired *t* test and is used when the measurements are somehow connected, such as a series of measurements on individual patients.

Nonparametric Tests

What should be done if an investigator wants to compare the means of two or more groups, and the outcome is not even close to normally distributed? The first step is to see if a transformation will work (see the earlier discussion). If not, it is possible to use a *nonparametric test*. Nonparametric tests make no assumptions about the distribution of data and are typically appropriate in the same cases in which a median should be used rather than a mean as a descriptive statistic. The most common method is to replace the actual values in the data with *ranks* so that, instead of comparing actual blood pressure measurements, for example, the difference in blood pressure between two groups is decided on the basis of whether the higher values are predominantly in one group and the lower values are in the other. Ranking solves the problem of highly skewed or variable data and extreme outliers because a value that is far out of range of all the others becomes simply the "highest" value. The problem is that some of the information contained in the original data is lost by converting it to ranks (i.e., the fact that extreme outliers exist might actually be important to your results). The nonparametric equivalents of paired and unpaired *t* tests are the *Wilcoxon rank sum* and the *Mann-Whitney U*, respectively. The *Kruskal-Wallis test*, the nonparametric equivalent of ANOVA, is used for comparing medians of more than two groups. The *Friedman test* is the nonparametric equivalent of two-way or repeated measures ANOVA.

Chi-Squared and Fisher's Exact Test

The chi-squared (χ^2) test is used to compare *counts* or *proportions* obtained with nominal or categorical data. Data of this sort are often presented in 2 × 2 (or 2 × 3, etc.) *contingency tables*. As a hypothetical example, comparison of mortality among male and female infants born at 23 weeks' gestation might appear as follows.

	Died	Survived
Male	53 (56%)	42 (44%)
Female	34 (41%)	48 (59%)
Total	87 (49%)	90 (51%)

The χ^2 statistic is calculated by comparing the observed to expected values in each cell (the expected value would be that obtained if the percentage of males and females who died was exactly the same). The formula is:

$$\text{Chi squared} = \sum \frac{(O - E)^2}{E}$$

with "O" being the observed value in a cell and "E" being the expected value in that cell if the percentages were exactly the same as the overall percentages. Each difference between observed and expected is squared, then divided by the expected value, and then the results of that calculation for each cell are summed. For the top left cell in the above example, the equation would yield $(53 - 47)^2 / 47$, since 47 is the number of male deaths that would be expected if the deaths of males exactly corresponded to the percentage of overall deaths. Each cell is calculated similarly and added together. The result is then compared with a χ^2 table for the appropriate degrees of freedom (larger values of this statistic indicate a greater deviation from expected results) to yield a percentage of time that such a result would be obtained by chance alone. The χ^2, as opposed to a *t* test, can also be used for more than two groups. *McNemar's test* is the equivalent of χ^2 for paired data. Using a *kappa* statistic is an example of applying a similar analysis of observed and expected values to evaluate agreement between two observers, or *interrater reliability*.

The χ^2 approximation runs into difficulty when small numbers are expected. Any time that the expected frequency for a cell is ≤5, it is better to use *Fisher's exact* test. Fisher's exact test can also be used with larger numbers; however, the calculations are far more laborious than they are for the χ^2 test (which is, of course, made less of a problem with computers).

Correlation

Correlation is one way to examine a relationship between two variables. *Pearson's correlation coefficient (r)* (also known as *sample correlation coefficient* or *product–moment correlation coefficient*) evaluates a linear relationship between two continuous variables. The result obtained is a number somewhere between −1 and 1. A result of $r = 1.0$ would indicate a perfect positive correlation, $r = 0$ would be no correlation (or no relationship between the variables), and $r = -1.0$ would be a perfect negative correlation. In real life, such absolute numbers are rarely obtained. Because the test can detect only *linear* relationships, it is important to examine data to ensure that other, nonlinear, relationships are not missed (**Fig. 7.7**). A visual observation also helps to detect outliers that may pull the slope of the line in their direction. As is the case with most statistical tests, even a very strong relationship indicates an association

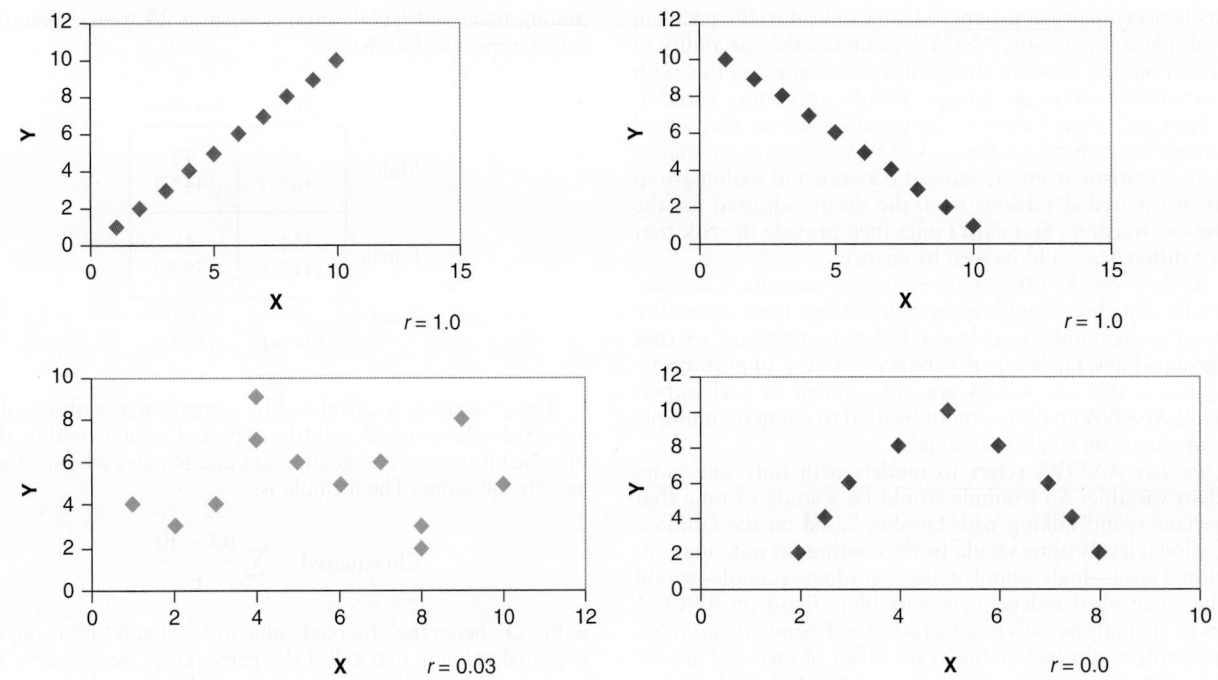

FIGURE 7.7. Pearson's correlation coefficient (r) is shown for each of the above graphs, with perfect linear relationships shown with $r = 1.0$ and $r = -1.0$ and almost no relationship shown with $r = 0.03$. The bottom right graph illustrates that the test is sensitive only to linear relationships; $r = 0$, which would imply no relationship, but it is obvious from looking at the data that a relationship actually exists between x and y.

only, and not causality. Confidence intervals or a p value can accompany the correlation coefficient and give an idea of the estimate's precision. For a curve of a similar shape (and hence similar r), a greater number of measurements results in a lower p value. Yet, if a significant p value is obtained, but the correlation coefficient shows only a weak relationship (e.g., $r = 0.1$, $p < 0.01$), the low p value should not be interpreted as an important finding—only a weak relationship has been demonstrated. Pearson's assumes that the data are fairly normally distributed. The nonparametric equivalent is *Spearman's rho* (ρ).

The square of the correlation coefficient (r^2) is called the *coefficient of determination* and is an indication of the extent to which the variability in the y variable is explained by variability in the x variable. Values for r^2 ranges from 0 to 1 and becomes much more meaningful when used in the context of multiple regression.

Regression

As opposed to correlation, in which the x and y variables are basically interchangeable, regression is a technique that involves *predicting* an outcome variable on the basis of one or more other variables (48–51). The *predictor variable* can also be known as the *explanatory variable* or *independent variable*. The *outcome variable* can also be called the *response variable* or *dependent variable*. Whereas in correlation both variables must be continuous, in regression, it is possible to have other variable types (dichotomous, categorical) as predictors. Although the terms *prediction* and *predictor* are commonly used, any relationship between predictor and outcome variables cannot be proven causative, but merely statistically associated. A full discussion of regression is far beyond the scope of this chapter.

Linear regression is used when the outcome variable is a continuous measurement, such that the predictive equation is mathematically the equation of a line:

$$y = a + b_1 x_1 + b_2 x_2 \ldots + e$$

where

  y = outcome variable
  x = predictor variable(s)
  a = y-intercept, or value of y when $x = 0$ (often not a meaningful number)
  b = change in y for each unit change in x (often called the *coefficient, beta, β,* or *slope*)
  e = error (variability in y not accounted for by the equation = *residual*)

Simple linear regression refers to a model with one predictor variable; *multiple linear regression* means that more than one predictor is present. A simple regression model can be visualized graphically (**Fig. 7.8**). The computer estimates the coefficient for the variable (i.e., slope of the line) by finding the line that minimizes the total distance of each individual point from that line. The *residual* value is the difference between the actual value (the point) and the predicted value (the line) from the equation. *Residual analysis* examines patterns found in the residuals; a random scatter about the line provides reassurance that the model has a good fit. An equation with multiple predictors cannot be visualized; statistically, a "line" is generated with a coefficient for each predictor variable that yields the best prediction of the outcome variable. Such an analysis can be used to *adjust* for possible *confounders* or other variables that are anticipated to affect the outcome of interest. For example, in the example shown in **Figure 7.8**, gender or race might be entered into the equation used to predict weight from age. Another frequently used technique is to adjust for a severity of illness measure (see **Chapter 10**) when assessing the impact of a variable of interest on an outcome. Any coefficient derived can be tested for statistical significance (generating a p value or 95% CI for the true value of the coefficient). For linear regression, a 95% CI that includes 0 would be equivalent to a p value >0.05. In the simple regression model shown in the graph (sometimes called *univariate* analysis), each increase in age by 1 year is associated with a 4.4-kg increase in weight (95% CI, 3.9–5; $p < 0.0005$). As seen in this example, an

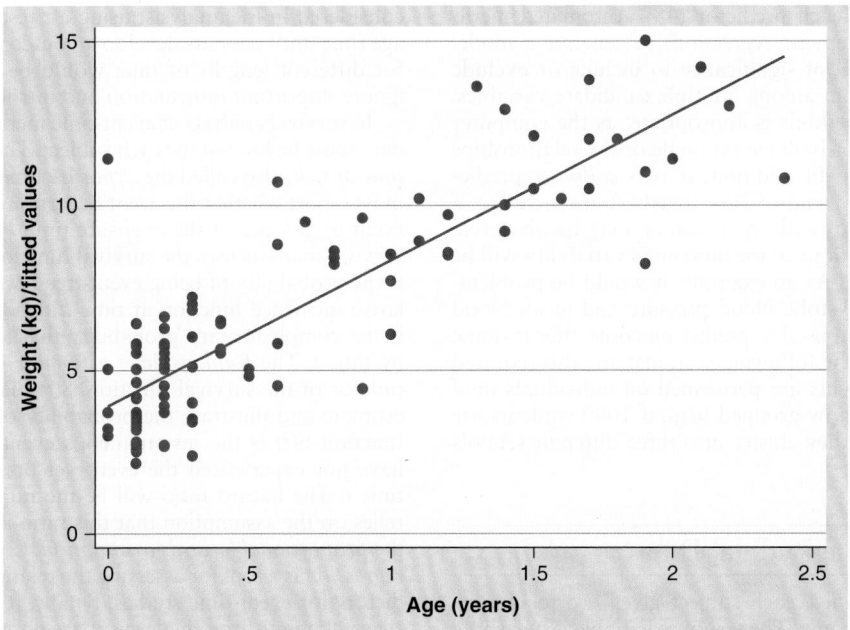

FIGURE 7.8. A scatterplot of age and weight of children <2.5 years of age on admission to a PICU. The line represents the *best fit* line determined by a regression equation generated to predict weight from age. *Residuals* are the distances between the predicted weight (*the line*) and each actual weight (*individual points*).

equation derived from one population should not be applied to a dissimilar group, as such a rapid yearly increase in weight would not be expected in teenagers.

When presenting regression data, it is important to report how the variables have been defined. In the example, the coefficient would be different if age had been entered in months rather than in years. In addition, if gender were entered into the equation, stating that the coefficient for gender is "+0.2 kg" makes no sense, unless the readers know that gender has been coded as 0 for females and 1 for males (in which case males would, on average, weigh 0.2 kg more than females *of the same age* in this data set). The value for r^2 is similar to the coefficient of determination mentioned under correlation. It is an indicator of the amount of variability in the outcome variable that is accounted for by the variability in all the predictors. r^2 will usually increase, even if only slightly, for every variable added to the model; the goal is to achieve a model that is as *parsimonious* as possible, meaning that it has a reasonably high r^2 with the fewest possible predictors.

Logistic regression is a similar technique that is used when the outcome is dichotomous, such as survival or mortality. Many investigators will present results of a logistic regression

analysis as an *odds ratio* (OR) rather than give the coefficients from the equation. The OR is defined as the odds of the outcome event occurring (with the predictor variable present) divided by the odds of it occurring if the predictor is absent (for continuous or ordinal predictors, the ratio is the increase in odds for each unit increase in the predictor). **Table 7.2** presents ORs for predicting death in patients who were admitted to a PICU after trauma, based on a regression equation including the gender, age, and whether the injury was in a motor vehicle crash. In this example, which includes only three predictors in the equation, gender appears to have no significant effect on mortality, as the 95% CI for the OR includes 1 (0.92–1.21). Increasing age is significantly associated with a lower risk of death (OR, 0.96; 95% CI, 0.95–0.97 for each increase in age by 1 year), and having a motor vehicle crash as the mechanism of injury increases the odds of mortality (OR, 1.8; 95% CI, 1.61–2.13).

Pitfalls of regression include trying to fit too many variables into an equation when the numbers are relatively small—called *overfitting*. Sample size calculations are possible but more complicated. A general rule of thumb is that 10 times as many subjects must be included as predictor variables. For logistic regression, more than 10 *outcome events* (e.g., deaths)

TABLE 7.2

ODDS RATIOS FOR DEATH AMONG CHILDREN ADMITTED TO A PICU FOLLOWING TRAUMA

	ODDS RATIO	95% CONFIDENCE INTERVAL	*p* VALUE
Sex (0 = M, 1 = F)	1.06	0.93–1.21	0.391
Age (years)	0.96	0.95–0.97	<0.001
MVC (0 = No, 1 = Yes)	1.80	1.61–2.13	<0.001

MVC, motor vehicle crash.

must be included for each predictor (48). Automated methods also exist (e.g., stepwise regression) to generate a model by using a cutoff level of significance to include or exclude predictor variables from among multiple candidate variables. Caution with these methods is appropriate, as the computer has no appreciation for biologic rationale or the relationships between the variables. In addition, if two *collinear* predictor variables (i.e., they tend to vary together) are included, a meaningful relationship with the outcome may be obscured, as significant contributions to the outcome's variability will be divided between them. As an example, it would be problematic to include both systolic blood pressure and mean blood pressure in an equation used to predict outcome after trauma. Special methods (see the following sections) are also required if repeated measurements are performed on individuals or if the subjects are somehow grouped (e.g., if 1000 students are studied, the fact that they cluster into three different schools must be considered).

Longitudinal Data

In *cross-sectional studies*, each subject gives rise to one response or a single outcome. The response variable is measured once or is an irreversible end point (e.g., death from acute respiratory distress syndrome). In *longitudinal studies*, the investigator examines a sample of subjects over time. When the response of interest involves not only whether or not the event occurs once, but more importantly, the interval of time between a baseline landmark and when the event occurs (i.e., the *time to the event*), methods collectively known as *survival analysis* are used to analyze the results. When the response or outcome of interest is measured in the same subject repeatedly over time (e.g., seizures, blood pressure, oxygen index, serum sodium), a different approach using *longitudinal data analysis methods* should be used (52–54). Because repeated measurements in individual or related subjects are correlated, this correlation must be taken into account to avoid making erroneous estimates. The simplest example of a continuous outcome measured twice (e.g., blood pressure before and after an intervention) can be compared using a paired *t* test. More than two measurements warrant different methods. The type of outcome (continuous, dichotomous, or counts) determines the type of longitudinal analysis method.

Multivariate analysis of variance (MANOVA) can be used when multiple dependent as well as multiple independent variables exist. This method can also be used to compare groups over time; however, the intervals of time must be weighted equally. To examine an outcome measured repeatedly over time using several predictor variables, more complex techniques of longitudinal analysis, called *generalized estimating equations* (GEE) or mixed random effects model, are required (55). These methods can also be used to account for *clustering* within certain subgroups.

Survival Analysis

Survival analysis methods relate to the analysis of data for which the *time to an event* (e.g., time to death, time to graft failure, time to extubation, time to developing an infection, time to wean off extracorporeal membrane oxygenation) is the outcome of interest; the term *survival time* is often used whether the event is death or not. Event-time methods take into account *censoring*, which refers to the possibility that some subjects will not experience the event of interest by the end of the observation period. Censoring also occurs when some subjects are followed for different periods of time than others, or lost to follow-up entirely. These data must be considered in the analysis; using a *t* test to compare the average time until patients develop an outcome if they are followed for different lengths of time would be incorrect as it would ignore important information and introduce bias.

In survival analysis or event-time methods, two fundamental data must be known for each subject. The first is the interval of *time at risk*, also called the *exposure* time. The second indicator must report whether the event occurs or if censoring occurs (no event by the end of the exposure time). The basic notation for survival analysis uses the survival function at time t, $S(t)$, which is the probability of being event-free beyond time t. The cumulative incidence function at time t, denoted as $F(t) = 1 - S(t)$, is the complementary probability that the event has occurred by time t. The *Kaplan-Meier estimator* is a nonparametric estimator of the survival function, $S(t)$ that can be computed to estimate and illustrate the probability of survival. The hazard function $h(t)$ is the instantaneous event rate of subjects who have not experienced the event yet or who have survived to time t. The hazard ratio will be the ratio of two hazards and relies on the assumption that this ratio is constant over time—the *proportional hazards assumption. Cox proportional hazard regression* is a tool for assessing the relationship of multiple predictors for event-time studies. Finally, if more than two exclusive end points for a single event are possible (e.g., in congenital heart disease repair, there could be survival with reoperation, survival after one operation, or death), different methods must be used, such as competing risks analysis methods (56).

A hypothetical data set that evaluates central line–related infections in jugular compared with femoral lines can illustrate the Kaplan-Meier estimator, which uses the series of conditional probabilities for each subject of being infection free on day $t + 1$ if the subject was infection free on day t (**Table 7.3** and **Fig. 7.9**). The log-rank test allows a comparison of both curves by setting the null hypothesis of no difference between curves at all follow-up times and the alternative that the curves differ at one or more times. The aim is to compare the probability of being event free (infection free) at time t between groups. The calculations take into account both whether an infection occurred and whether the patient was discharged (censored) without having to exclude patients because their follow-up period was short.

REPORTING RESULTS

Standards for preparing, analyzing, and reporting research results exist. Multidisciplinary research teams, including methodologists such as biostatisticians, epidemiologists, and clinical trialists, improve the quality of the design and analysis and should be involved in the preparation of the results and their interpretation to minimize bias in the inferences and interpretation of the evidence. Certain organizations and journals have proposed guidelines to improve the quality of the reporting of RCTs (57) or surveys (58) that are useful for investigators (20). Although pediatric critical care investigators cannot be expert in all domains of the analysis, as principal investigators or coinvestigators, they remain responsible for the preparation of the manuscripts and of the message disseminated by the reports.

COLLABORATIVE RESEARCH NETWORKS

Critical care has improved drastically for children over the past three decades, and research that aims at altered mortality or morbidity has become more difficult to accomplish within single-center settings. This is because adverse outcomes have

TABLE 7.3

HYPOTHETICAL DATA FOR CENTRAL LINE INFECTIONS IN TWO GROUPS OF 10 CHILDREN AFTER CARDIAC SURGERY WITH FEMORAL VERSUS JUGULAR LINES

■ LINE INSERTED	■ TIME DAY OF FOLLOW-UP	■ NUMBER AT RISK (N_I)	■ NUMBER INFECTED (Y_I)	■ NUMBER CENSORED: TRANSFERRED FROM ICU	■ CONDITIONAL PROBABILITY OF BEING FREE OF INFECTION ($N_I - Y_I)/N_I$	■ SURVIVAL FUNCTION: KAPLAN-MEIER ESTIMATOR OF THE PROBABILITY OF BEING FREE OF INFECTION
Jugular	1	10	0	0	$(10 - 0)/10 = 1$	1
	2	10	0	0	$(10 - 0)/10 = 1$	$1 \times 1 = 1$
	3	10	1	1	$(10 - 1)/10 = 0.9$	$0.9 \times 1 = 0.9$
	4	8	0	0	$(8 - 0)/8 = 1$	$1 \times 0.9 = 0.9$
	5	8	2	0	$(8 - 2)/8 = 0.75$	$0.75 \times 0.9 = 0.675$
	6	6	1	1	$(6 - 1)/6 = 0.83$	$0.83 \times 0.675 = 0.56$
	7	4	1	0	$(4 - 1)/4 = 0.75$	$0.75 \times 0.56 = 0.42$
	8	3	1	0	$(3 - 1)/3 = 0.66$	$0.66 \times 0.42 = 0.27$
	9	2	1	1	$(2 - 1)/2 = 0.5$	$0.5 \times 0.27 = 0.13$
	10	1	0	0	$(1 - 0)/1 = 1$	$1 \times 0.13 = 0.13$
Femoral	1	10	1	0	$(10 - 1)/10 = 0.9$	0.9
	2	9	2	0	$(9 - 2)/9 = 0.78$	$0.78 \times 0.9 = 0.69$
	3	7	1	1	$(7 - 1)/7 = 0.85$	$0.85 \times 0.69 = 0.59$
	4	5	3	0	$(5 - 3)/5 = 0.4$	$0.4 \times 0.59 = 0.236$
	5	2	1	0	$(2 - 1)/2 = 0.5$	$0.5 \times 0.236 = 0.12$
	6	1	1	0	$(1 - 1)/1 = 0$	$0 \times 0.12 = 0$
	7	None				
	8	None				
	9	None				
	10	None				

Numbers of infections, as well as number of children transferred (censored), are noted. Those who have been discharged are no longer followed for infections; therefore, the conditional probability of being infection free at each time period is based only on those children who have neither failed (infection) nor been censored (transferred).

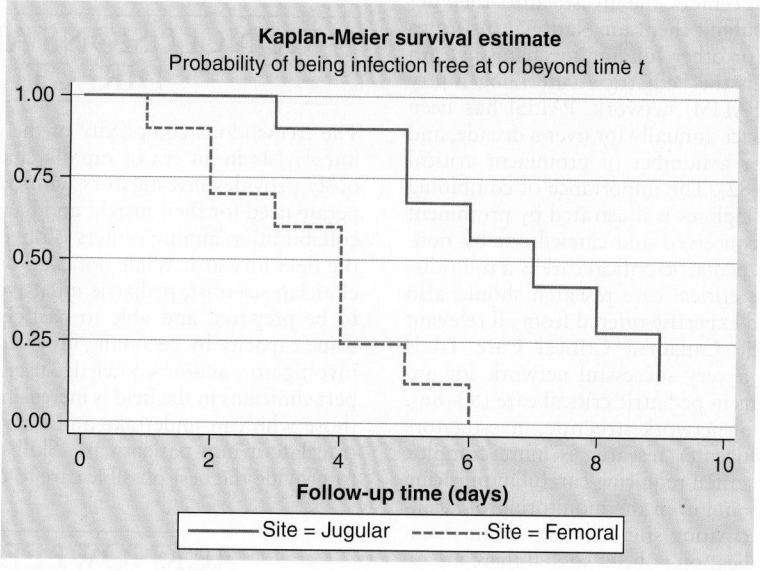

Kaplan-Meier survival estimate
Probability of being infection free at or beyond time *t*

FIGURE 7.9. Plot of the Kaplan-Meier estimate of the survival function, S(*t*), of the probability of being infection free by time, *t*, from the example shown in **Table 7.3**. On visual inspection, the probability of being infection free at a given time seems greater in the group with jugular lines. Formal statistical testing with the log rank test provides a *p* value of 0.002.

decreased in frequency, lowering the rate of occurrence of the events often used to power studies (such as mortality). Thus, it has become very difficult to accomplish research concerning disorders that intensivists might consider common, such as acute lung injury, or therapies that are clearly common, such as mechanical ventilation. For these reasons, collaborative research involving multiple institutions, as well as multiple intellectual disciplines, will become increasingly important for accomplishing successful clinical research in the future.

Networks may be prospectively funded to conceive scientific concepts, develop protocols, and implement studies; one example is the *Eunice Kennedy Shriver* National Institute for Child Health and Human Development (NICHD) Collaborative Pediatric Critical Care Research Network (CPCCRN). In this model, investigators and their centers compete to become members of the CPCCRN. The CPCCRN Steering Committee develops and implements studies using preallocated protocol research funds. CPCCRN receives strong and direct scientific leadership from NICHD scientists. Examples of CPCCRN studies include the critical illness stress-induced immune suppression (CRISIS) Prevention Trial (59,60) as well as the Therapeutic Hypothermia after Pediatric Cardiac Arrest (THAPCA) Trials (61–64), which are being conducted in collaboration with another federally funded network, the Pediatric Emergency Care Applied Research Network (PECARN). PECARN is funded by the Health Resources and Services Administration (HRSA) Maternal and Child Health Bureau (MCHB) Emergency Medical Services for Children (EMSC) Program.

CPCCRN also includes a designated data coordinating center (DCC), which provides efficiency because individual project investigators do not have to identify a DCC for individual projects, and information systems are identical between network projects. This lowers the cost of training research coordinators. Theoretically, networks such as CPCCRN develop into very efficient platforms for carrying out multicenter clinical research, but there is usually a 3–5 year (or more) ramp-up period as the investigators develop their initial research protocols. Following this initial ramp-up period, these types of networks generally publish 10–25 (or more) manuscripts per year.

An alternative mechanism is one that lacks prospective infrastructure funding, involves interested investigators meeting for scientific discourse, with consideration of new projects at these meetings. When projects generate sufficient interest from a sufficient number of centers, the investigators then develop their protocols and submit them for National Institutes of Health (NIH) funding (or other funding mechanisms). An example of this approach is the Pediatric Acute Lung Injury and Sepsis Investigators (PALISI) network. PALISI has been quite successful, meeting twice annually for over a decade, and obtaining NIH funding for a number of prominent critical care research projects (65–82). The importance of combining expertise from multiple disciplines is illustrated by prominent PALISI studies that were conceived and carried out by non-physicians (65–73). Just as pediatric critical care is a multidisciplinary clinical endeavor, critical care research should also benefit from the talents and expertise offered from all relevant intellectual disciplines. The Canadian Critical Care Trials Group has similarly been a very successful network in answering important questions in pediatric critical care (83–86).

Regardless of the type of network structure, investigators should be aware that multicenter research is more complex than single-center research, often requiring careful monitoring of data entry, data quality, and even the monitoring of scientific integrity at each participating site. It is important to establish authorship and publication policies so that there are no misunderstandings about the order of authors, criteria for authorship participation, and accountability for writing responsibilities. Most networks have eventually written very detailed publication procedures to prevent potentially traumatic and emotional angst when a paper is published and a participant feels slighted by nonauthorship.

RESEARCH TRAINING AND FUNDING

Incorporating research, clinical or basic, into the busy clinical career of a critical care physician requires significant dedication and investment of resources. Fellows and junior faculty need to seriously consider the importance of research for their own careers, and for those who desire to make research a significant component of their career, it is important to recognize the need to focus on research training and preparation. By making the early investment, the feasibility of life-long extramural research funding is greatly enhanced. It may be necessary to devote at least 75% of one's early career to research training and development in order to have long-term success.

The National Institutes of Health (NIH) provides the largest amount of funding for research, and the standard grant mechanism is a research project grant, called the R01. Competition for these research grants is intense, and in order to enable young physician scientists to be able to compete successfully for these types of grants, the NIH has a variety of training grant mechanisms that are focused on physicians. These include the K08 (basic science) and K23 (patient-oriented) mechanisms, which are mentored physician scientist awards. Junior faculty who are interested in research careers should seriously consider competing for one of these K mechanisms. These grants provide up to 5 years of funding and provide an opportunity to obtain didactic scientific training while carrying out a research project that will prepare the young scientist to successfully obtain later R01 grant funding.

The NIH also funds K12 training programs that are generally associated with individual institutions. The Pediatric Critical Care and Trauma Scientist Development Program (PCCTSDP) is a unique K12 program that is *not* based at a single institution, but is administered on behalf of the fields of pediatric critical care and pediatric trauma surgery. In its 10th year, the PCCTSDP has funded nearly 30 scholars, who have then been able to subsequently obtain their own K08 or K23 awards, and a number are now competing successfully for R01 NIH grants.

CONCLUSIONS AND FUTURE DIRECTIONS

The tremendous complexity of the care provided by pediatric intensivists in an era of rapidly changing technology continuously provides investigators with fruitful questions and a desperate need for their insight and hard work. The importance of collaboration among centers is obvious and necessary to move the field forward. While not everyone is expected to become a clinician scientist, pediatric intensive care physicians will want to be prepared and able to participate in clinical research in some capacity by becoming involved as a site collaborator, site investigator, and/or knowledge user. Just as the demand for expert clinicians in the field is increasing, the need will increase for those who can undertake and interpret complex research and translate it into patient care. Skill in both arenas is necessary to provide the best possible care to children and their families.

ACKNOWLEDGMENT

The authors would like to acknowledge the debt owed to the faculty of the Johns Hopkins Bloomberg School of Public Health, particularly Scott Zeger, PhD, Marie Diener-West,

PhD, Leon Gordis, MD, DrPH, and Steven Goodman, MD, PhD, on whose lectures and class notes we relied heavily for the content of this chapter.

References

1. Silverman WA. A cautionary tale about supplemental oxygen: The albatross of neonatal medicine. *Pediatrics* 2004;113(2):394–6.
2. Meinert CL, Tonascia S. *Clinical Trials: Design, Conduct, and Analysis.* New York, NY: Oxford University Press, 1986.
3. Last JM. *International Epidemiological Association: A Dictionary of Epidemiology.* 4th ed. New York, NY: Oxford University Press, 2001.
4. Rothman KJ, Greenland S. *Modern Epidemiology.* 2nd ed. Philadelphia, PA: Lippincott-Raven, 1998.
5. Gordis L. *Epidemiology.* Philadelphia, PA: Saunders, 2009.
6. Newman SC. *Biostatistical Methods in Epidemiology.* New York, NY: John Wiley & Sons, 2001.
7. Piantadosi S. *Clinical Trials: A Methodologic Perspective.* 2nd ed. Hoboken, NJ: Wiley-Interscience, 2005.
8. Evaluating processes of care and the outcomes of children in hospital (EPOCH): A cluster randomized trial of the bedside paediatric early warning system. http://clinicaltrials.gov/ct2/show/NCT01260831?term=bedside+pews&rank=2.
9. Berkenbosch JW, Grueber RE, Graff GR, et al. Patterns of helium-oxygen (heliox) usage in the critical care environment. *J Intensive Care Med* 2004;19(6):335–44.
10. Zabrocki LA, Brogan TV, Statler KD, et al. Extracorporeal membrane oxygenation for pediatric respiratory failure: Survival and predictors of mortality. *Crit Care Med* 2011;39(2):364–70.
11. Rollins MD, Hubbard A, Zabrocki L, et al. Extracorporeal membrane oxygenation cannulation trends for pediatric respiratory failure and central nervous system injury. *J Pediatr Surg* 2012;47(1):68–75.
12. Ortmann L, Prodhan P, Gossett J, et al. Outcomes after in-hospital cardiac arrest in children with cardiac disease: A report from get with the guidelines-resuscitation. *Circulation* 2011;124(21):2329–37.
13. Szklo M, Nieto FJ. *Epidemiology: Beyond the Basics.* Sudbury, MA: Jones and Bartlett, 2004.
14. Egger M, Smith GD, Altman DG. *Systematic Reviews in Health Care: Meta-analysis in Context.* 2nd ed. London: BMJ, 2001.
15. Juni P, Altman DG, Egger M. Systematic reviews in health care: Assessing the quality of controlled clinical trials. *BMJ* 2001;323(7303):42–6.
16. Moher D, Cook DJ, Eastwood S, et al. Improving the quality of reports of meta-analyses of randomised controlled trials: The QUOROM statement. Quality of Reporting of Meta-analyses. *Lancet* 1999;354(9193):1896–900.
17. Shea B, Moher D, Graham I, et al. A comparison of the quality of Cochrane reviews and systematic reviews published in paper-based journals. *Eval Health Prof* 2002;25(1):116–29.
18. Stroup DF, Berlin JA, Morton SC, et al. Meta-analysis of observational studies in epidemiology: A proposal for reporting. Meta-analysis of Observational Studies in Epidemiology (MOOSE) group. *JAMA* 2000;283(15):2008–12.
19. Moher D, Jadad AR, Tugwell P. Assessing the quality of randomized controlled trials. Current issues and future directions. *Int J Technol Assess Health Care* 1996;12(2):195–208.
20. Simera I, Moher D, Hoey J, et al. A catalogue of reporting guidelines for health research. *Eur J Clin Invest* 2010;40(1):35–53.
21. Dickersin K, Berlin JA. Meta-analysis: State-of-the-science. *Epidemiol Rev* 1992;14:154–76.
22. Jadad AR, McQuay HJ. Meta-analyses to evaluate analgesic interventions: A systematic qualitative review of their methodology. *J Clin Epidemiol* 1996;49(2):235–43.
23. Khan KS, Daya S, Jadad A. The importance of quality of primary studies in producing unbiased systematic reviews. *Arch Intern Med* 1996;156(6):661–6.
24. Schulz KF, Chalmers I, Hayes RJ, et al. Empirical evidence of bias. Dimensions of methodological quality associated with estimates of treatment effects in controlled trials. *JAMA* 1995;273(5):408–12.
25. Pope C, Mays N. Opening the black box: An encounter in the corridors of health services research. *BMJ* 1993;306(6873):315–8.
26. Feudtner C. How qualitative studies can improve the quality of clinical studies. *J Pediatr Gastroenterol Nutr* 2013;57(3):267–8.
27. Meert KL, Thurston CS, Briller SH. The spiritual needs of parents at the time of their child's death in the pediatric intensive care unit and during bereavement: A qualitative study. *Pediatr Crit Care Med* 2005;6(4):420–7.
28. Morris MC, Nadkarni VM, Ward FR, et al. Exception from informed consent for pediatric resuscitation research: Community consultation for a trial of brain cooling after in-hospital cardiac arrest. *Pediatrics* 2004;114(3):776–81.
29. Green J, Britten N. Qualitative research and evidence based medicine. *BMJ* 1998;316(7139):1230–2.
30. Sandelowski M. Sample size in qualitative research. *Res Nurs Health* 1995;18(2):179–83.
31. Golub RM, Fontanarosa PB. Comparative effectiveness research: Relative successes. *JAMA* 2012;307(15):1643–5.
32. Initial National Priorities for Comparative Effectiveness Research. Committee on Comparative Effectiveness Research Prioritization, Board on Health Care Services, Institute of Medicine of the National Academies. Washington, DC: The National Academies Press, 2009. http://www.iom.edu/reports/2009/comparativeeffectivenessresearchpriorities.aspx.
33. Moye LA, Deswal A. Perils of the random experiment. *Am J Ther* 2003;10(2):112–21.
34. Altman DG, Bland JM. Detecting skewness from summary information. *BMJ* 1996;313(7066):1200.
35. Keene ON. The log transformation is special. *Stat Med* 1995;14(8):811–9.
36. Goodman SN. Introduction to Bayesian methods I: Measuring the strength of evidence. *Clin Trials* 2005;2(4):282–90; discussion 301–284, 364–278.
37. Goodman SN, Sladky JT. A Bayesian approach to randomized controlled trials in children utilizing information from adults: The case of Guillain-Barre syndrome. *Clin Trials* 2005;2(4):305–10; discussion 364–78.
38. Young KD, Lewis RJ. What is confidence? Part 1: The use and interpretation of confidence intervals. *Ann Emerg Med* 1997;30(3):307–10.
39. Lagakos SW. The challenge of subgroup analyses—Reporting without distorting. *N Engl J Med* 2006;354(16):1667–9.
40. Lachin JM. Introduction to sample size determination and power analysis for clinical trials. *Control Clin Trials* 1981;2(2):93–113.
41. Scales DC, Rubenfeld GD. Estimating sample size in critical care clinical trials. *J Crit Care* 2005;20(1):6–11.
42. Guidance for Industry: E9 Statistical Principles for Clinical Trials. U.S. Department of Health and Human Services Food and Drug Administration, Center for Drug Evaluation and Research and Center for biologics Evaluation and Research. Rockville, MD: 1998. http://www.fda.gov/downloads/drugs/guidancecomplianceregulatoryinformation/guidances/ucm073137.pdf.
43. Pepe MS. *The Statistical Evaluation of Medical Tests for Classification and Prediction.* 1st ed. New York, NY: Oxford University Press, 2003.
44. Dawson B, Trapp RG. *Basic & Clinical Biostatistics.* 4th ed. New York, NY: Lange Medical Books/McGraw-Hill, Medical Pub. Division, 2004.
45. Hassard TH. *Understanding Biostatistics.* St. Louis, MO: Mosby Year Book,1991.
46. Myers JL, Well A. *Research Design and Statistical Analysis.* 2nd ed. Mahwah, NJ: Lawrence Erlbaum Associates, 2003.
47. Rosner B. *Fundamentals of Biostatistics.* 6th ed. Belmont, CA: Thomson-Brooks/Cole, 2006.

48. Concato J, Feinstein AR, Holford TR. The risk of determining risk with multivariable models. *Ann Intern Med* 1993;118(3):201–10.

49. Hosmer DW, Lemeshow S. *Applied Logistic Regression.* 2nd ed. New York, NY: Wiley, 2000.

50. Kleinbaum DG, Kleinbaum DG. *Applied Regression Analysis and Other Multivariable Methods.* 3rd ed. Pacific Grove, CA: Duxbury Press, 1998.

51. Vittinghoff E. *Regression Methods in Biostatistics: Linear, Logistic, Survival, and Repeated Measures Models.* New York, NY: Springer; 2005.

52. Twisk JWR. *Applied Longitudinal Data Analysis for Epidemiology: A Practical Guide.* New York, NY: Cambridge University Press, 2003.

53. Zeger SL, Liang KY. Longitudinal data analysis for discrete and continuous outcomes. *Biometrics* 1986;42(1):121–30.

54. Zeger SL, Liang KY, Albert PS. Models for longitudinal data: A generalized estimating equation approach. *Biometrics* 1988;44(4):1049–60.

55. Diggle P, Diggle P. *Analysis of Longitudinal Data.* 2nd ed. New York, NY: Oxford University Press, 2002.

56. Amark KM, Karamlou T, O'Carroll A, et al. Independent factors associated with mortality, reintervention, and achievement of complete repair in children with pulmonary atresia with ventricular septal defect. *J Am Coll Cardiol* 2006;47(7):1448–56.

57. Begg C, Cho M, Eastwood S, et al. Improving the quality of reporting of randomized controlled trials. The CONSORT statement. *JAMA* 1996;276(8):637–9.

58. Kelley K, Clark B, Brown V, et al. Good practice in the conduct and reporting of survey research. *Int J Qual Health Care* 2003;15(3):261–6.

59. Carcillo J, Holubkov R, Dean JM, et al. Rationale and design of the pediatric critical illness stress-induced immune suppression (CRISIS) prevention trial. *JPEN J Parenter Enteral Nutr* 2009; 33(4):368–74.

60. Carcillo JA, Dean JM, Holubkov R, et al. The randomized comparative pediatric critical illness stress-induced immune suppression (CRISIS) prevention trial. *Ped Crit Car Med* 2012; 13(2):165–73.

61. Meert KL, Donaldson A, Nadkarni V, et al. Multicenter cohort study of in-hospital pediatric cardiac arrest. *Ped Crit Car Med* 2009;10(5):544–53.

62. Moler FW, Donaldson AE, Meert K, et al. Multicenter cohort study of out-of-hospital pediatric cardiac arrest. *Crit Care Med* 2011;39(1):141–9.

63. Moler FW, Meert K, Donaldson AE, et al. In-hospital versus out-of-hospital pediatric cardiac arrest: A multicenter cohort study. *Crit Care Med* 2009;37(7):2259–67.

64. Pemberton VL, Browning B, Webster A, et al. Therapeutic hypothermia after pediatric cardiac arrest trials: The vanguard phase experience and implications for other trials. *Ped Crit Car Med* 2013;14(1):19–26.

65. Grant MJ, Scoppettuolo LA, Wypij D, et al. Prospective evaluation of sedation-related adverse events in pediatric patients ventilated for acute respiratory failure. *Crit Care Med* 2012;40(4):1317–23.

66. Grant MJ, Balas MC, Curley MA. Defining sedation-related adverse events in the pediatric intensive care unit. *Heart Lung* 2013;42(3):171–6.

67. Curley MA. Prone positioning of patients with acute respiratory distress syndrome: A systematic review. *Am J Crit Care* 1999; 8(6):397–405.

68. Curley MA, Arnold JH, Thompson JE, et al. Clinical trial design—Effect of prone positioning on clinical outcomes in infants and children with acute respiratory distress syndrome. *J Crit Care* 2006;21(1):23–32; discussion 32–27.

69. Curley MA, Fackler JC. Weaning from mechanical ventilation: Patterns in young children recovering from acute hypoxemic respiratory failure. *Am J Crit Care* 1998;7(5):335–45.

70. Curley MA, Hibberd PL, Fineman LD, et al. Effect of prone positioning on clinical outcomes in children with acute lung injury: A randomized controlled trial. *JAMA* 2005;294(2):229–37.

71. Curley MA, Razmus IS, Roberts KE, et al. Predicting pressure ulcer risk in pediatric patients: The Braden Q Scale. *Nurs Res* 2003;52(1):22–33.

72. Curley MA, Thompson JE, Arnold JH. The effects of early and repeated prone positioning in pediatric patients with acute lung injury. *Chest* 2000;118(1):156–63.

73. Curley MA, Zimmerman JJ. Alternative outcome measures for pediatric clinical sepsis trials. *Ped Crit Car Med* 2005;6(suppl 3):S150–6.

74. Randolph AG. The unique challenges of enrolling patients into multiple clinical trials. *Crit Care Med* 2009;37(suppl 1):S107–11.

75. Randolph AG, Clemmer TP, East TD, et al. Evaluation of compliance with a computerized protocol: Weaning from mechanical ventilator support using pressure support. *Comput Methods Programs Biomed* 1998;57(3):201–15.

76. Randolph AG, Lacroix J. Randomized clinical trials in pediatric critical care: Rarely done but desperately needed. *Ped Crit Car Med* 2002;3(2):102–6.

77. Randolph AG, Vaughn F, Sullivan R, et al. Critically ill children during the 2009–2010 influenza pandemic in the United States. *Pediatrics* 2011;128(6):e1450–8.

78. Randolph AG, Wypij D, Venkataraman ST, et al. Effect of mechanical ventilator weaning protocols on respiratory outcomes in infants and children: A randomized controlled trial. *JAMA* 2002;288(20):2561–8.

79. Agus MS, Steil GM, Wypij D, et al. Tight glycemic control versus standard care after pediatric cardiac surgery. *N Engl J Med* 2012;367(13):1208–19.

80. Willson DF, Thomas NJ, Markovitz BP, et al. Effect of exogenous surfactant (calfactant) in pediatric acute lung injury: A randomized controlled trial. *JAMA* 2005;293(4):470–6.

81. Willson DF, Chess PR, Notter RH. Surfactant for pediatric acute lung injury. *Pediatr Clin North Am* 2008;55(3):545–75, ix.

82. Dahmer MK, Randolph A, Vitali S, et al. Genetic polymorphisms in sepsis. *Ped Crit Car Med* 2005;6(suppl 3):S61–73.

83. Hutchison JS, Ward RE, Lacroix J, et al. Hypothermia therapy after traumatic brain injury in children. *N Engl J Med* 2008; 358(23):2447–56.

84. Lacroix J, Hebert PC, Hutchison JS, et al. Transfusion strategies for patients in pediatric intensive care units. *N Engl J Med* 2007;356(16):1609–19.

85. Jouvet P, Hutchison J, Pinto R, et al. Critical illness in children with *influenza* A/pH1N1 2009 infection in Canada. *Ped Crit Car Med* 2010;11(5):603–9.

86. Hutchison J, Ward R, Lacroix J, et al. Hypothermia pediatric head injury trial: The value of a pretrial clinical evaluation phase. *Dev Neurosci* 2006;28(4–5):291–301.

87. Dickersin K. The existence of publication bias and risk factors for its occurrence. *JAMA* 1990;263(10):1385–9.

88. Goldstein B, Nadel S, Peters M, et al. ENHANCE: Results of a global open-label trial of drotrecogin alfa (activated) in children with severe sepsis. *Pediatr Crit Care Med* 2006;7(3):200–11.

89. Peters JL, Sutton AJ, Jones DR, et al. Comparison of two methods to detect publication bias in meta-analysis. *JAMA* 2006; 295(6):676–80.

CHAPTER 8 ■ EVIDENCE-BASED MEDICINE

BARRY P. MARKOVITZ AND KATHLEEN L. MEERT

CASE SCENARIOS

Case 1

A 5-year-old boy is admitted to the PICU following an unintentional hanging injury. He was found apneic and bradycardic after an indeterminate time period. His mother, a pediatric ER nurse, administered rescue breaths; his heart rate improved, and spontaneous, irregular respirations ensued. Emergency medical services (EMS) arrived shortly thereafter, intubated his trachea, and initiated manual ventilation. He arrives in the PICU with stable hemodynamics, but still unconscious. The parents ask if anything can be done to improve their son's chance of a favorable neurologic recovery. They specifically mention hearing that hypothermia may be useful in this situation.

Case 2

A 6-month-old girl is being treated in the PICU for pneumococcal sepsis. She is on full mechanical ventilatory support and requires dopamine and epinephrine to maintain a satisfactory blood pressure, despite aggressive fluid resuscitation. The medical student on the service, having just completed an adult ICU rotation, asks if her adrenal function has been evaluated. She states that, in adults, adrenal insufficiency in septic shock portends a very poor outcome. An adrenocorticotropic hormone stimulation test is performed using 250 mcg corticotropin. The patient's serum cortisol concentration increases from 15 mcg/dL at baseline to 20 mcg/dL 60 minutes after receiving corticotropin. What does this mean?

Case 3

A 7-year-old, developmentally delayed boy is admitted to the PICU with aspiration pneumonitis. He is tachypneic with labored breathing, anxious but alert. On a nonrebreather face mask, his oxygen saturations are 90%. His chest radiograph demonstrates diffuse airspace disease. With his progressive course, preparations are made to intubate and initiate mechanical ventilation. The parents ask if any other means of respiratory support is available so that invasive ventilation can be avoided.

INTRODUCTION

As intensivists in our PICUs, we are faced with the above situations and questions daily. How would such questions be addressed at the time of the first edition of this textbook? We would have relied on a combination of our experience, discussions with colleagues, textbooks, or memory of a study in the medical literature. In this "classic" paradigm, few qualms were expressed about our reliance on unsystematic, anecdotal observations to draw conclusions. We believed that a thorough grounding in pathophysiology should usually enable us to determine the proper management of patients and that common sense was sufficient to adequately evaluate new therapies and diagnostic tests. Guidelines could be developed on the basis of the "expertise" of content knowledge and clinical experience. This approach was not considered "anti-intellectual." Indeed, the more experience one had, the more wisdom one acquired, and great respect has always been (and should always be) afforded to the wise among us. However, the learning curve associated with gaining such wisdom was gradual and protracted.

Beginning formally in 1992, the paradigm shifted. Guyatt et al. coined the term *evidence-based medicine* (EBM) and formed the Evidence-Based Medicine Working Group (1). EBM "is the conscientious, explicit, and judicious use of current best evidence in making decisions about the care of individual patients" (2). EBM involves the integration of this evidence with clinical experience and each patient's preferences and values. Instinct, experience, knowledge of disease mechanisms, and common sense are necessary but insufficient to properly evaluate and apply new therapies, diagnostic modalities, or prediction tools. Rules of evidence interpretation must be learned to practice EBM; the rules were developed and disseminated during more than a decade of publishing in the *Journal of the American Medical Association (JAMA)* in what has become the living handbook of EBM: *The Users' Guides to the Medical Literature* (3). Now available in print (4,5) and on the Web (including an interactive textbook) (6), these guides outline core methods for the critical appraisal of evidence (Step 3 below).

Five steps are involved in the EBM approach to patient care:

1. Framing the sometimes nebulous need for information into a structured "clinical question."
2. Tracking down the available evidence to answer the question through a focused search of the medical literature.
3. Critically appraising the evidence identified for its validity (degree of freedom from bias), results (magnitude of effect), and applicability to the patient.
4. Integrating the appraised evidence with our experience and the patient's unique situation and values.
5. Self-appraising of our effectiveness in steps 1–4.

EBM's roots extend into the 1980s, when the science of clinical epidemiology was codified by Sackett et al. (7) at McMaster University in Hamilton, Ontario. Their landmark text, *Clinical Epidemiology: A Basic Science for Clinical Medicine*, published in 1985, described the quantitative tools that would become the "acronym soup" of EBM: RR (relative risk), RRR (relative risk reduction), NNT (number needed to treat), etc. From just two citations in the National Library of Medicine's PubMed (MEDLINE) in 1992 to 87,703 in 2013, EBM has grown to a worldwide phenomenon, to the extent that the basic paradigm is now rarely questioned. Although many now espouse its value, in assessing its impact, it is difficult to submit EBM to the same rigorous methodology that it requires of the questions that it is used to answer. Furthermore, EBM has several clear limitations.

Some critiques can be answered readily:

- EBM has been pejoratively labeled "cookbook medicine." EBM explicitly calls for the integration of the uniqueness of each patient—both their pathophysiology and their values—in determining how to apply evidence from clinical research.
- EBM has been maligned as a tool of administrators determined to cut costs by refusing to pay for therapies not "proven effective" by EBM standards. EBM, however, is just as likely to proffer support for very expensive interventions as it is for low-cost care.

EBM engenders more troublesome questions. Despite a huge increase in the publication of well-designed and clinically meaningful research studies over the past several decades, many questions remain for which valid evidence simply does not exist. In our field of pediatric critical care in particular, it has been difficult to conduct the type of definitive, randomized, controlled trials that should form our evidence base.

Two suggested solutions are: (a) This deficiency can often be addressed by careful consideration of trials in other populations, such as neonates or adults, and (b) this reality should, and indeed has, spurred our community to aggressively form networks and seek funding to conduct the multicentered trials necessary to address this void.

Another concern, given the often hectic nature of our practice, asks how one should find the time to create clinical questions, search for trials, properly and critically appraise them, and apply them judiciously to our patient care—in "real time?" The criticism has been leveled, therefore, that EBM is an "ivory tower" exercise that is unrealistic to expect busy practitioners to consistently undertake. This criticism is also not easily deflected because practicing EBM "by the book" does require additional time. Two answers to this concern are: (a) Many of our patients have similar conditions, so that once we learn the "correct" answers to our clinical questions, we need not reinvent the wheel with each subsequent patient (although we must remain attuned to possible changes from new research findings), and (b) "shortcuts" do exist, such as tapping into preappraised sources of evidence, so that all that needs to be critically considered is the applicability of the evidence to each individual patient (see "Secondary Evidence Sources").

GETTING STARTED: THE CLINICAL QUESTION

The first step in the EBM approach to obtain focused evidence involves creating a structured "clinical question," which usually takes the "PICO" format: *Population, Intervention, Comparison* (if applicable), and *Outcomes*. Thus, a well-designed clinical question for our first case scenario might read: In children with acute hypoxic-ischemic encephalopathy (population), does hypothermia (intervention), compared with standard supportive care (comparison), reduce mortality and improve neurologic recovery (outcome)? A poorly phrased clinical question for this case might read "What is the role of hypothermia in the PICU?" or "Is hypothermia neuroprotective?" These make for nice (nonsystematic) review article titles, but their lack of focus leads us on an unnecessarily inefficient literature search. The importance of focus and the need for efficiency will be clear shortly.

TYPES OF EVIDENCE

Before we begin to search for evidence to answer our questions, we must clearly define the types of evidence available. Although several classification schemes could be considered, we will simply refer to the evidence sources as "primary" or "secondary."

Primary evidence refers to individual, or original, clinical research trials that report the findings of therapeutic intervention studies, tests of new diagnostic technology or prediction tools, and the like. These original trials form the base of an evidence pyramid (**Fig. 8.1**). They are the foundation of whether and how we can and/or should draw conclusions about the validity, results, and applicability of the best available evidence from clinical research. The pure EBM paradigm has the modern clinician searching for, identifying, and then critically appraising an original research study to decide the best care for his patient.

In many cases, however, trials are not particularly well designed or executed, leaving serious validity questions. Ultimately, if a trial is truly so potentially biased that we should not trust the results (which should be discernible from a critical appraisal of the trial), the results should not influence

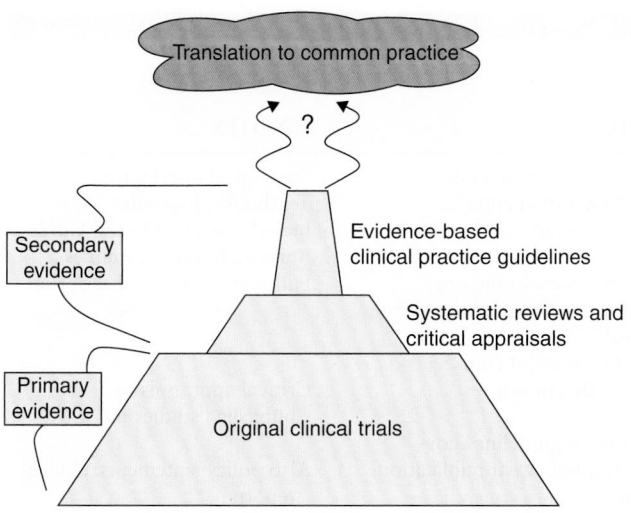

FIGURE 8.1. The evidence pyramid.

us in either direction. However, other problems are associated with using original trials in the practice of EBM.

Sometimes clinical trials have too few subjects to detect a treatment difference (inadequate "power"); such "negative" trials also do not help our decision making because they do not rule in or out a significant treatment effect. In addition, several trials may be published on a given question, and reading, appraising, and integrating them all would clearly constitute an improbable bedside exercise. What is the solution to these issues?

Secondary evidence sources include preappraised evidence, systematic reviews, and evidence-based clinical practice guidelines. The busy clinician may not need to perform a rigorous critical appraisal of a primary research paper if such an appraisal has already been performed and published. In our field, for example, since 1997, the PedsCCM Evidence-based Journal Club has posted hundreds of critical appraisals of relevant studies, all easily accessible on the PedsCCM Web site (PedsCCM.org). Many other such "journal clubs" exist on the Web and serve as one of the "shortcuts" to practicing EBM.

Systematic reviews represent the next and even more valuable level of secondary evidence, depending on the question at hand. A systematic review, unlike a typical general topic review, is focused on a defined clinical question and follows a rigorous (and reproducible) methodology in searching for, including and excluding, assessing, and summarizing original clinical trials. A systematic review would (or should) almost certainly never be entitled "Myocarditis in 2006: A Review." However, an overview (synonymous term for systematic review) could well carry the title: "Immunoglobulin Therapy for Myocarditis: A Systematic Review." When specific quantitative analysis is undertaken to pool the results of numerous trials in a systematic review, it constitutes a *meta-analysis*. All meta-analyses are systematic reviews, but the converse is not necessarily the case. In a properly completed systematic review, a large amount of evidence is filtered, appraised, and summarized.

The third and highest level of secondary evidence can be found as evidence-based *clinical practice guidelines*. Organizations, hospitals, and government agencies may have already undertaken a full evidence-based review of a clinical question and appraised and synthesized the results as a practice guideline. The strength of the recommendations flows from the strength of the evidence. Inconsistent systems have been used to grade evidence and recommendations, but it is hoped that a more consistent toolset will be adopted in time (8).

To add yet another level, *users' guides* are also available for systematic reviews (9) and clinical practice guidelines to enable us to appraise secondary evidence sources (10,11).

SEARCHING FOR THE EVIDENCE

MEDLINE from the National Library of Medicine is the premiere database of citations and abstracts of the biomedical literature and is freely available online via PubMed (**Table 8.1** provides a list of resources and URLs). The built-in EBM filters, accessible from the "clinical queries" link, are particularly helpful for focusing searches in this huge database. These filters allow very focused searching for study type (e.g., therapy, diagnosis, etc.) as well as the ability to set the search to be very sensitive or more specific. Limits are easily defined to find results based on systematic reviews, age groups, and other search criteria. PubMed's LinkOut service provides direct links from the abstracts to a manuscript's full-text version, usually on the publisher's Web site. (Accessing the full-text version often requires a personal or institutional subscription to the journal.)

The *Cochrane Collaboration* is an international organization dedicated to producing and maintaining a database of systematic reviews on virtually every aspect of healthcare. The Cochrane Database of Systematic Reviews (CDSR) is its primary product and should be part of the repertoire of all EBM practitioners. Although the CDSR is now indexed in MEDLINE, a personal or institutional subscription is necessary to access the full reviews.

Evidence-based clinical practice guidelines can be found via MEDLINE searches if they have been published in cited journals. Organizations, such as the Society of Critical Care Medicine and the American Academy of Pediatrics offer their guidelines freely online. The National Guideline Clearinghouse is a valuable service of the US Department of Health and Human Services.

An increasing number of hybrid subscription products can be found online that offer a range of evidence types, obscuring the boundary between primary and secondary sources. MEDLINE can also be searched from proprietary interfaces, such as those provided by OVID. These subscription products offer many other features, including full-text journal and textbook access, as well as the ability to search across different types of resources. Many also offer unique EBM filter tools, similar to the "clinical queries" feature of PubMed noted earlier. Focused and succinct, evidence-based topic summaries can also be found in Clinical Evidence and UpToDate Online.

APPRAISING AND APPLYING THE EVIDENCE

The core exercise of EBM is the critical appraisal of evidence, and the handbook (some would say "bible") of critical appraisal is the *JAMA* series noted earlier: *The Users' Guides to the Medical Literature*. Although different evidence types require different specific criteria, all can be organized into three major questions: Is the study valid? What are the results? Are the results applicable to my patient? Let us address the three case scenarios presented at the beginning of the chapter as exercises in formulating clinical questions, searching for, appraising, and applying the evidence.

Therapy Article Appraisal

In Case 1, to respond to the parents' question regarding the use of hypothermia in their son with nonintentional hanging

TABLE 8.1

DATABASES AND EBM RESOURCES ON THE WORLD WIDE WEB

■ RESOURCE TYPE	■ NAME	■ URL	■ NOTES
MEDLINE	PubMed	http://www.pubmed.gov	See clinical queries tool
	OVID*	http://www.ovid.com/	Textbooks, Journals
Users' guides to the medical literature	JAMAevidence*	http://www.jamaevidence.com	Includes original Users' Guides and additional resources
Systematic reviews	Cochrane Collaboration	http://www.cochrane.org	Full-text requires subscription
Evidence-based reviews	Clinical evidence*	http://www.clinicalevidence.bmj.com/	
	UptoDate*	http://www.utdol.com	
EB Journal Club	PedsCCM EBJC	http://pedsccm.org	Critical appraisals of published studies in CCM
Clinical practice guidelines	National Guideline Clearinghouse	http://www.guidelines.gov	
	American Academy of Pediatrics	http://aappolicy.aappublications.org/	Also policy statements, clinical reports
	Society of Critical Care Medicine/ American College of Critical Care Medicine	http://www.sccm.org	
Search tools/ directories	Google Scholar	http://scholar.google.com	Extensive database/search tool
	Trip	http://www.tripdatabase.com	
Diagnostic decision support	Isabel*	http://www.isabelhealthcare.com	Web and mobile versions
	Dxplain®	http://dxplain.org	
EBM tools/ calculators	WWWeb Epidemiology and EBM Sources	http://www.vetmed.wsu.edu/courses-jmgay/EpiLinks.htm	Very comprehensive resource list
	StatSoft Textbook	http://www.statsoft.com/textbook	Online extensive statistics textbook
	Centre for Evidence-Based Medicine Toronto	http://ktclearinghouse.ca/cebm/practise/ca/calculators/statscalc	EBM calculator and critical appraisal tips Explanations and calculators
Online EBM tutorial	Introduction to EBM	http://guides.mclibrary.duke.edu/ebmtutorial	From Duke University and UNC–Chapel Hill

*Subscription (institutional or personal) required.

injury, the following focused clinical question would be formulated: In children with hypoxic-ischemic encephalopathy, does hypothermia improve outcome? A MEDLINE search using the key words "hypothermia" and "hypoxic-ischemic encephalopathy," limiting the search to randomized, controlled trials, produced seven studies, all conducted in neonates. Retrieving and reviewing the most recent trial, "Whole-Body Hypothermia for Neonates with Hypoxic-Ischemic Encephalopathy," published by the NICHD Neonatal Research Network (12), showed that the objective of the study was to determine whether whole-body cooling initiated before 6 hours of age and continued for 72 hours in term infants with moderate-to-severe encephalopathy would reduce death or disability at 18–22 months of age, as compared with usual care. As outlined in the *Users' Guides to the Medical Literature* series, you undertake a critical appraisal of this study. The three major steps of the appraisal are (a) determining the study's validity, (b) summarizing the results, and (c) determining the applicability of the results to your patient.

Are the Results of the Study Valid?

Validity is a measure of how well the results of a study represent the true magnitude and direction of the treatment's effect, free from a number of potential sources of bias. For example, many factors in addition to total body cooling are likely to influence the outcome of patients with hypoxic-ischemic encephalopathy. For the study results to be valid, the study must be designed in such a way as to prevent these other factors from confounding patient outcomes in a systematic way.

Several questions can be asked to help assess the validity of the hypothermia trial (13):

Was the Assignment of Patients to Treatments Randomized?
Random assignment to treatment and control groups makes it more likely that factors known to influence outcome (e.g., severity of illness) and unknown factors will be evenly distributed between the two groups at the start of the trial. Infants enrolled in the hypothermia study were randomly assigned to whole-body cooling to 33.5°C for 72 hours or normothermia.

Were All Patients Who Entered the Trial Properly Accounted for and Attributed at Its Conclusion?
Follow-up was achieved in all patients in the hypothermia group (100%) and in all but three of the patients in the normothermia group (96.5%). Patients lost to follow-up may have different outcomes than do those remaining in a trial. For example, if patients lost to follow-up in the normothermia group failed to keep their appointments because they had recovered completely, and if these patients were dropped from the analysis, the lack of follow-up would cause the normothermia group to appear to have a worse outcome than if the lost patients had been included. Keeping patients in the groups to which they were randomized, rather than excluding those who were noncompliant with therapy or lost to follow-up, is referred to as an *intention-to-treat analysis*.

Were Patients, Health Workers, and Study Personnel Blind to Treatment?
Blinding helps to prevent researchers' opinions about the experimental treatment from influencing their assessment of patient outcomes. In the hypothermia trial,

caregivers were not blinded, but those who assessed patient outcomes were unaware of the group assignments.

Were the Groups Similar at the Start of the Trial? As mentioned, many factors other than the experimental therapy can influence patient outcomes. Ideally, these other factors should be similar between groups at the start of the trial. Randomization helps to ensure a balance of baseline patient characteristics between groups in large clinical trials. However, if specific patient characteristics are known or suspected to be important confounding variables, the investigators should demonstrate that the treatment and control groups were similar with respect to these variables. In the hypothermia trial, both groups were similar in such baseline characteristics as age, sex, weight, and severity of illness.

Aside from the Experimental Intervention, Were the Groups Treated Equally? Cointerventions may also confound patient outcomes. In some trials, explicit treatment protocols for major cointerventions are employed. Major cointerventions and their use should at least be described. Particularly in nonblinded studies, the differential use of cointerventions between groups can confound results. In the hypothermia trial, infants in the two groups received the same monitoring of vital signs and surveillance for organ dysfunction. Protocols for the use of oxygen, mechanical ventilation, sedation, and other treatments were not explicitly mentioned.

What Were the Results?

An excellent review of how to evaluate results is available from Guyatt et al. (14).

How Large Was the Treatment Effect? Death or moderate-to-severe disability occurred in 45 of 102 (44%) infants in the hypothermia group, compared with 64 of 103 (62%) in the control group. Dichotomous outcomes (i.e., survived vs. died) can be best described in terms of the *absolute risk reduction* (ARR), *relative risk* (RR), *relative risk reduction* (RRR), and *number needed to treat* (NNT). ARR is the arithmetic difference in rates of poor outcomes between the treatment and control groups. In this study, the ARR is 62% − 44%, or 18%. RR can otherwise be defined as the ratio of risk between treated group: control group; here, the RR is 44/62, or 0.71. RRR is the proportional reduction in the rates of bad outcomes between treatment and control groups. In the study under consideration, the RRR is (62 − 44)/62, or 0.29. The NNT is the number of patients who need to be treated to achieve one additional favorable outcome; NNT is calculated as 1/ARR. Here, the NNT is 1/0.18, or 6 (the NNT is, by convention, typically rounded up to the next whole number). An advantage of ARR and NNT is that these metrics take into account the prevalence rate in untreated patients, whereas RR and RRR do not. For example, if death or disability occurred in 4.4% of hypothermia-treated patients and in 6.2% of controls, the RR and RRR would remain as 0.71 and 0.29, respectively. However, ARR would be markedly decreased to 6.2% − 4.4%, or 1.8%, and NNT would increase to 60.

How Precise Was the Estimate of the Treatment Effect? The magnitude of the treatment effect reported in a study is really an estimate of the true effect based on the sample of patients included in the trial. *Confidence intervals* (CIs) help us to evaluate how precise that estimate is. In the hypothermia trial, the 95% CI for ARR for death or disability is 4%–31%. The true ARR may be as low as 4% or as high as 31%, but we can be 95% sure that the true value for ARR lies within this range. The 95% CIs for RR, RRR, and NNT are 0.54–0.95, 0.05–0.46, and 3–22, respectively. Although these ranges are rather wide, indicating a lack of precision, the lower 95% CI of the ARR is greater than zero, enabling us to conclude that a

"statistically significant" difference exists in rates of poor outcomes between the two groups. We must then decide whether such a small difference is worth the burden of therapy. It may seem "worth it" to treat as few as 3 infants with hypothermia to prevent one poor outcome, but is it still "worth it" if we must treat 22 infants?

Will the Results Help Me in Caring for My Patient?

Can the Results be Applied to My Patient Care? Patients to whom we intend to apply the results of a trial should be similar to the patients included in the trial. We must consider how similar the boy with nonintentional hanging injury is to the patients enrolled in the hypothermia study. Study patients were infants of at least 36 weeks' gestational age, <6 hours old, with severe acidosis or perinatal complications, who underwent resuscitation at birth and who had moderate-to-severe encephalopathy. Our patient is older, and the mechanism of injury is different. Whether the results can be applied to our patient is unknown.

Were All Clinically Important Outcomes Considered? Many clinical trials only evaluate physiologic markers as outcomes. Unless strong evidence supports the use of such markers as good surrogates for the outcomes that are important to patients, families, and physicians (e.g., mortality, disability), such studies should be viewed with caution. The medical literature is replete with examples of how a particular therapy was shown to improve a physiologic marker, only to be later shown to increase morbidity or mortality. In the hypothermia trial, several secondary outcomes were considered, including disabling cerebral palsy, blindness, and hearing impairment. Applying a neuroprotective strategy may be associated with a risk of reducing mortality while increasing the number of survivors with disabilities. However, both mortality and disabilities tended to decrease in hypothermia-treated infants.

Are the Likely Treatment Benefits Worth the Potential Harms and Costs? This question takes into consideration not only the risks and benefits of therapy, but also the patient's and family's preferences and values. In the hypothermia trial, infants who received the therapy had better outcomes, whereas the incidence of serious adverse events was similar between groups. However, because the applicability of these findings to our patient is unknown, treatment with hypothermia may or may not be indicated.

Scenario Resolution

On the basis of a review of this valid and meaningful randomized, controlled trial, the boy undergoes total body cooling in the PICU. Because a question remains regarding the applicability of the results to this patient, the practitioner should explain to the parents that cooling may or may not improve the boy's chance of survival or reduce disabilities.

Prediction Article Appraisal

Regarding the case of the 6-month-old girl with pneumococcal sepsis (Case 2), the physician is unsure of how to answer the medical student's question and asks her to look up the answer and present it to the team. The physician helps the student to formulate the following focused clinical question: Does adrenal insufficiency predict mortality in children with septic shock? The student, pressed for time, goes directly to PedsCCM.org to try to find an existing critical appraisal on the topic (15). Using the search term "adrenal insufficiency," she finds two articles that have been reviewed. She downloads the article that includes "children" in the title and presents it to the group. The article, "Absolute and Relative Adrenal Insufficiency in Children with Septic Shock" by Pizarro et al. (16), aims to evaluate the incidence of adrenal insufficiency and determine the relationship between adrenal function, the development of catecholamine-resistant septic shock, and outcome in children.

Are the Results of the Study Valid?

Prognosis refers to the possible outcomes of a disease and their frequency. Prognostic factors are patient characteristics such as symptoms, signs, or laboratory tests that can be used to predict outcome. Combinations of prognostic factors, or prediction tools, can be developed to categorize heterogeneous groups of patients into different levels of risk for a specified outcome. In the septic shock study by Pizarro et al., several factors, including corticotropin response, are evaluated as potential predictors of two outcomes—the development of catecholamine-resistant shock and mortality. To assess the validity of a prediction tool, the following questions must be answered (17):

Was a Representative Group of Patients Completely Followed up? Prediction tools may perform well in one population and poorly in another. Therefore, the population studied must be representative of the target population to which the tool will be applied. Consecutive or random inclusion of patients helps to prevent selection bias. The septic shock study included 57 children consecutively admitted to the PICU who met criteria established by the American College of Critical Care Medicine (ACCM) for the diagnosis of septic shock. All patients were followed until death or PICU discharge. Such complete follow-up is important because if patients lost to follow-up have a better or worse outcome than other study patients, the prediction tool may not perform as well when applied in another population.

Were All Potential Predictors Included? Investigators must decide which variables to test as potential predictors of an outcome. In general, the more relevant the variables included, the more likely a satisfactory prediction tool will result. In the septic shock study, patients were categorized into four groups on the basis of their baseline cortisol level and response to corticotropin as follows: (a) absolute adrenal insufficiency (baseline cortisol <20 mcg/dL, with increase ≤9 mcg/dL), (b) relative adrenal insufficiency (baseline cortisol ≥20 mcg/dL with increase ≤9 mcg/dL), (c) adequate adrenal response with elevated baseline cortisol (baseline cortisol ≥20 mcg/dL, with increase >9 mcg/dL), and (d) adequate adrenal response without elevated baseline cortisol (baseline cortisol <20 mcg/dL, with increase >9 mcg/dL). Patients were also categorized into three groups on the basis of their need for cardiovascular support: (a) fluid-responsive shock, (b) fluid-refractory dopamine/dobutamine-responsive shock, and (c) catecholamine-resistant shock. Other potential predictors assessed were the presence of chronic disease and multiple organ failure.

Did the Investigators Test the Independent Contribution of Each Predictor Variable? Clinical variables are often correlated with each other. To show that a variable is an independent predictor of outcome, its predictive power must remain when other potential predictors are taken into consideration. For example, the presence of catecholamine-resistant shock was associated with death when evaluated as a single variable using univariate statistics. However, when chronic disease, multiple organ failure, and catecholamine-resistant shock were evaluated using multiple regression analysis, catecholamine resistance was no longer a significant predictor of mortality. The independence of a predictor variable is a function of the set of variables with which it is being evaluated. For example, catecholamine resistance might be an independent predictor of mortality if evaluated as part of a completely different set of variables.

Were Outcome Variables Clearly and Objectively Defined? For patient outcomes to be reliably assessed, outcomes should be clearly and objectively defined. Also, knowledge of the presence or absence of predictors in individual patients may lead to bias in the assessment of outcomes. In the septic shock study, two outcomes were considered. The first outcome, catecholamine-resistant shock, was defined using ACCM criteria. The second outcome, mortality, was obvious and objective. Clinicians were blinded to the results of the corticotropin stimulation test until after study completion.

What Are the Results?

Prediction tools with a few easily assessed predictor variables that place patients into clear outcome categories are most useful.

What Are the Prediction Tools? Two prediction tools were reported. First, corticotropin response (≤9 mcg/dL) and multiple organ failure independently predicted catecholamine-resistant shock. Second, chronic illness and multiple organ failure independently predicted mortality. Importantly, corticotropin response did not predict mortality on univariate or multivariate testing.

How Well Does the Model Categorize Patients into Different Levels of Risk? The four categories of adrenal response placed patients into four categories of risk for catecholamine-resistant shock. Of those patients with absolute adrenal insufficiency, 100% had catecholamine-resistant shock. Of those with relative adrenal insufficiency, 80% had catecholamine-resistant shock. Of those with adequate adrenal response and elevated baseline cortisol, 60% had catecholamine-resistant shock. Of those with adequate adrenal response without elevated baseline cortisol, 30% had catecholamine-resistant shock. When patients with absolute and relative adrenal insufficiency were combined (corticotropin response ≤9 mcg/dL) and compared with those having adequate response (>9 mcg/dL), the RR of catecholamine-resistant shock was 1.88 (95% CI, 1.26–2.79).

Patients with absolute and relative adrenal insufficiency tended to have higher mortality (50% and 53%, respectively), compared with those having adequate adrenal response, with or without elevated baseline cortisol (33% and 24%, respectively); however, the relationship was not significant. The RR of death for patients with adrenal insufficiency compared with those having adequate adrenal response was 1.72 (95% CI, 0.97–3.06).

What Is the Confidence Level in the Estimates of Risk? The precision of the estimates of relative risk are again reflected in the CIs. The relative risk of developing catecholamine-resistant shock for septic patients with adrenal insufficiency may be as low as 1.26 or as high as 2.79, on the basis of a 95% CI. The RR of death for patients with adrenal insufficiency may be as low as 0.97 or as high as 3.06. Of note, a CI for relative risk that includes 1 indicates that no statistically significant difference in outcome between groups is observed. Given that the lower limit of the CI for mortality is <1 in this sample, confirmation of the study's findings in another sample of pediatric patients with septic shock appears warranted before widespread application of these findings in clinical practice.

Can You Apply the Prediction Tool in Your Patient Care?

Does the Tool Maintain Its Predictive Power in a New Sample of Patients? Prediction tools are derived using one sample of patients and, ideally, are tested in another sample. If the prediction tool maintains its accuracy in the new sample, confidence in the tool's usefulness increases. In the septic shock study, the predictors were not tested in a new sample of patients, leaving uncertainty in the tool's validity.

Are Your Patients Similar to Those Used in Deriving and Validating the Tool? If the patient populations used to derive and validate the prediction tool differ greatly from your patient population, the tool may not perform well in your patients. For example, chronic disease was present in 74% of patients in the septic shock study, with the most frequent diagnoses being malignancy (16%), hepatic failure (14%), and neurologic illness (11%). Therefore, the prediction tool may not perform well for the previously healthy pediatric patient presenting with septic shock.

Does the Tool Improve Your Clinical Decisions? Prediction tools are most useful if they can be shown to improve decision making beyond clinician judgment. The septic shock study provides evidence that adrenal insufficiency is common in children with septic shock (i.e., 44% of patients) and that it is associated with catecholamine-resistant shock. Whether hydrocortisone replacement will reduce catecholamine-resistant shock or mortality in septic patients cannot be answered from this study.

Scenario Resolution

The patient has catecholamine-resistant shock and absolute adrenal insufficiency on the basis of the definitions used in this study. On the basis of the literature review, the physician suspects that her chance of mortality is high. Therapy is initiated with hydrocortisone, with uncertainty as to whether it will improve her outcome. Practicing EBM at the bedside does not always result in definitive answers. Clinicians must continue to incorporate pathophysiology and clinical experience into the decisions they make.

Systematic Review Appraisal

In the case of the 7-year-old, developmentally delayed boy with respiratory failure (Case 3), the following focused clinical question can be formulated: In children with hypoxemic respiratory failure, does noninvasive ventilation (compared with invasive ventilation) result in improved outcomes? A PubMed search, using the key words "noninvasive ventilation" and "acute hypoxemic respiratory failure," produces 47 articles on the subject. Rather than reviewing all of the articles, the search strategy is limited to include "reviews" only. The limit setting for "meta-analysis" on PubMed is occasionally too restrictive and will not include all systematic reviews. The article by Keenan et al. (18), "Does noninvasive positive-pressure ventilation improve outcome in acute hypoxemic respiratory failure? A systematic review" is chosen. The objective of the article is to systematically review the randomized, controlled trials of patients with acute hypoxemic respiratory failure unrelated to cardiogenic pulmonary edema, to determine the effect of the addition of noninvasive positive-pressure ventilation (NPPV) to standard therapy on endotracheal intubation, ICU and hospital lengths of stay, and mortality. A critical appraisal of the review is undertaken that assesses the validity, results, and applicability in a manner similar to the therapy and prediction appraisals described earlier (3) and notes the direct parallel of these questions to similar assessments of primary trials.

Are the Results of the Overview Valid?

Did the Overview Address a Focused Clinical Question? The objective of a systematic review should be clearly stated so that the reader can know whether the review is applicable to the clinical question he is trying to answer. As demonstrated by the Keenan review, study objectives are often best stated in terms of the relationship between an exposure (i.e., NPPV), and one or more outcomes (i.e., endotracheal intubation, ICU days, hospital days, and mortality) in a specific population (i.e., patients with noncardiogenic acute hypoxemic respiratory failure).

Were the Criteria Used to Select Articles for Inclusion Appropriate? The criteria used to select articles for inclusion in an evidence-based review should be explicitly described, analogous to the inclusion and exclusion criteria for patients in a primary clinical trial. Criteria for including trials in a review may include the exposures, outcomes, patients, and methodologic standards for each individual trial. Defining the inclusion criteria helps to prevent investigators from choosing studies that support their own opinions. In the NPPV review, selection criteria were well suited to answer the clinical question. Selection criteria were (a) comparison of NPPV and standard therapy to standard therapy alone; (b) outcomes of need for endotracheal intubation, length of ICU and hospital stay, and mortality; (c) study populations comprised mostly patients with acute hypoxemic respiratory failure not associated with cardiogenic pulmonary edema or chronic obstructive pulmonary disease (COPD) and not requiring immediate ventilator support; and (d) randomized, controlled trials.

Is It Unlikely that Important Relevant Studies Were Missed? Searching several bibliographic databases and reference lists of identified articles and using personal communications are ways to ensure that relevant studies are not missed in a review. US physicians should appreciate that a minority of biomedical publications are cited in MEDLINE and that high-quality trials from around the world (not cited in MEDLINE) are rapidly increasing in volume. Personal communications with investigators in the field of inquiry can help to identify published trials that may otherwise have been missed, as well as studies that are still in press or otherwise unpublished. The analogy to primary clinical trials here is the recruitment strategy. For example, just as using a convenience sample of patients (i.e., only those admitted between 9 a.m. and 5 p.m.) may bias a primary study, searching only for published trials in MEDLINE may bias a systematic review. In the NPPV review, the authors searched MEDLINE, EMBASE, and the Cochrane Library. They searched abstracts from key professional meetings, reference lists from all identified studies, and contacted the first-named authors of some studies to help identify studies not otherwise retrieved by their search strategy.

Was the Validity of the Included Studies Appraised? It is important to know whether or not the individual studies included in the review are of good quality. If the individual studies are not valid, confidence in the overall results of the review should be limited. Validity of the individual studies can be assessed by asking questions similar to those described earlier for therapy and prediction tools. The parallel between appraising systematic reviews and primary clinical trials here is obvious but more complex. No standards exist by which individual trials in a systematic review are measured, which leads to a varying quality of trials included in most reviews. In the NPPV review, the authors appraised the individual trials using 11 validity criteria. These included randomization, concealment, blinding, patient selection, comparability of groups at baseline, treatment protocols, confounders, cointerventions, outcome definitions, extent of follow-up, and intention-to-treat analysis.

Were Assessments of Studies Reproducible? Authors of reviews must make many decisions, such as which trials to include, how valid the trials are, and what data to abstract from them. Knowing that these types of decisions were made independently by more than one author, and that they were agreed upon, increases our confidence in the results. The parallel issue here to the clinical trial is whether the clinical trial reported reproducibility of assessments between observers who made subjective measurements (i.e., radiographic assessments). Clinical trials often report agreement coefficients, such as kappa (κ) scores, or mention independent assessors and agreement by consensus. In the NPPV review, data abstractions and validity assessments were performed by two of the authors independently and in duplicate. Differences in opinion were resolved by consensus or by consulting a third investigator.

Were the Results Similar from Study to Study?

We would have greater confidence in the results of a systematic review if we knew that the individual studies included in the review showed treatment effects that were all going in the same direction. In other words, if each of the individual studies showed a treatment benefit, we would have more confidence than if some studies showed benefit and others did not. Lack of consistency between studies can be due to differences in exposures, outcomes, patients, study design, or chance alone. Statistical tests of homogeneity tell us whether differences in results between studies are likely due to chance or other study factors. In the NPPV review, significant heterogeneity between studies (differences likely not due to chance) was demonstrated for the effect of NPPV on endotracheal intubation rates. Statistically significant heterogeneity was not demonstrated for the other outcomes assessed. However, Keenan et al. suspected that clinically important heterogeneity was present, on the basis of visual inspection and comparison of the plotted ARRs and CIs for each of the studies. Differences between studies were attributed primarily to differences in the study populations. It is important to regard quantitative results (i.e., meta-analyses) with suspicion if significant heterogeneity is identified. It may not be appropriate to combine such trials.

What Are the Results?

What Are the Overall Results of the Overview?

A systematic review attempts to provide an overall average effect of a therapy, prediction tool, or other exposure. The overall results are considered in the same way that the results from individual studies are considered. Systematic reviews should present results using summary measures that clearly show the clinical importance of the result. For example, for systematic reviews of a therapy, these measures would include ARRs, RRs, and NNTs. Some authors may weight individual studies included in the review according to their sample size or validity, with larger, more valid studies contributing more weight to the overall result. In the NPPV review, 763 studies were identified in the initial search. Of these, eight randomized, controlled trials with a total of 366 patients met the authors' inclusion criteria. Six of the trials included patients with COPD or cardiogenic pulmonary edema; however, the authors were able to obtain patient-specific data on patients without these diagnoses. Overall, NPPV was associated with a significantly lower rate of endotracheal intubation than standard therapy (ARR, 23%; 95% CI, 10% to 35%), a reduction in ICU length of stay (1.9 days; 95% CI, 1 to 2.9 days), an increase in length of hospital stay (2.8 days; 95% CI, 0.9 to 4.7 days), and a reduction in ICU mortality (ARR, 17%; 95% CI, 8% to 26%), with a trend toward lower hospital mortality (ARR, 10%; 95% CI, −7% to 27%). Subgroup analyses of trials that excluded patients with COPD or cardiogenic pulmonary edema showed similar results.

How Precise Were the Results?

CIs can be calculated to demonstrate the range of the average treatment effect across studies. In the NPPV study, the 95% CIs for the ARR for endotracheal intubation and ICU mortality are relatively wide; however, their lower limits still represent important clinical effects (i.e., ARR of 8% for ICU mortality). The 95% CI for ARR for hospital mortality includes zero, suggesting that hospital mortality may increase or decrease with the use of NPPV.

Will the Results Help Me in Caring for My Patients?

Can the Results Be Applied to My Patient Care?

An advantage of systematic reviews is that they typically include large numbers of patients with diverse clinical characteristics. If the results of individual studies included in the review are consistent, it is more likely that the overall results of the review will be applicable to your patient. However, in the NPPV study, we found important heterogeneity in the results between studies, probably due to differences in patient populations. For example, of the eight trials included in the review, two focused on immunocompromised patients, one on surgical patients after lung resection, one on community-acquired pneumonia, one on postextubation respiratory failure, and three on more diverse groups of patients. Also, all of the study patients were adults. Therefore, any application of the results to our patient should proceed with caution.

Were All Clinically Important Outcomes Considered?

Although focused systematic reviews, like focused clinical trials, are more likely to demonstrate valid results, important clinical outcomes should not be ignored. In the NPPV study, such outcomes as cost, complications, and patients' comfort and sedation requirements were not considered.

Are the Benefits Worth the Costs and Potential Harm?

Valid overviews can provide strong evidence regarding the effect of a therapy or other exposure on patient outcomes. In the NPPV study, however, a determination of overall benefit is difficult to make because of heterogeneity between included studies and the lack of information on such outcomes as complications and cost. Heterogeneity between studies suggests that specific populations may derive benefit from the application of NPPV, whereas others may not. When deciding to apply a therapy, clinicians must take patient and family preferences and concerns into consideration.

Scenario Resolution

On the basis of critical appraisal, it is explained to the parents that the risks and benefits of NPPV in children with aspiration pneumonitis are not known. The parents request that NPPV be tried because they are unsure as to whether endotracheal intubation is in the best interest of their child in light of his severe developmental delay. NPPV is instituted, and the boy's oxygen saturations increase to 98%. The physician and the parents then discuss options for care and decide on a further course of action should the boy's condition deteriorate.

BRINGING IT ALL TOGETHER

EBM is part of mainstream healthcare. The skills involved are core competencies for postgraduate medical training, as part of "practice-based learning" (19). Subspecialty residents (fellows) in pediatric critical care medicine training programs across the country (and internationally) are submitting critical appraisals to the PedsCCM Evidence-based Journal Club, in part, to fulfill these requirements. The challenge, then, is the consistent practice of EBM in the PICU over time.

Some challenges to practicing EBM in the PICU in real time have already been addressed. In addition to some of the solutions offered, the staff of each PICU—physicians and nurses—should consider a regular process of reviewing evidence with the goal of creating local evidence-based policies and procedures for sets of conditions for which national or international guidelines do not exist, thus accomplishing three objectives: (a) establishment (or reaffirmation) of the multidisciplinary approach to patient care in the PICU, (b) engagement of all the key stakeholders in the PICU in the EBM process, and (c) establishment of a growing local library of care protocols and pathways to optimize consistency across providers. Although it has been difficult to prove in pediatric critical care, consistency of care in virtually every other aspect of healthcare has been shown to be synonymous with improved quality of care. This process may also serve to address the little-discussed fifth step of EBM—self-appraisal of effectiveness in practicing EBM.

Other "holes" in the EBM paradigm have no easy solutions. What if multiple primary studies exist with no systematic review to combine (if appropriate) the results? What happens when a large randomized, controlled trial is published that contradicts findings of an existing systematic review? How, exactly, should we apply the results of studies in adults to children? There are no pat answers to these difficult questions. We are left, ultimately, with recognizing EBM for what it truly is—a set of tools to supplement our clinical skills. EBM cannot and should not replace clinical judgment. It is not a cookbook to be blindly followed. Like any tool, sometimes it is very useful, and sometimes it is not.

CONCLUSIONS AND FUTURE DIRECTIONS

EBM requires ready access to evidence. It is almost quaint to read the early *Users' Guides to the Medical Literature*, which describe residents going to the medical library to search MEDLINE and photocopy studies from print journals. Computing power and networking capabilities have advanced exponentially in a decade. The tools to enable the practice of "point-of-care" EBM are already here. Modern PICUs have Internet-enabled wired or wireless workstations at the patient's bedside to enable direct database searching. Primary and secondary evidence sources can be accessed around the clock. Mobile devices are in nearly every physician's pocket, and all these resources are literally now in the palm of our hands. Limitations to evidence are no longer physical, but temporal. It still takes precious time to search, read, appraise, and apply evidence. Perhaps someday in the not-too-distant future, we will be able to make a call from our cell phones and have the evidence downloaded directly to our cerebrums, as "Trinity" does when she "learns" to fly a military helicopter with just a brief fluttering of her eyelids in the 1999 motion picture *The Matrix*. Until such time, EBM's role is much like Morpheus' guiding of Neo in the same movie: It can show us the door, but we have to walk through it.

References

1. Evidence-Based Medicine Working Group. Evidence-based medicine. A new approach to teaching the practice of medicine. *JAMA* 1992;268(17):2420–5.
2. Sackett DL, Rosenberg WM, Gray JA, et al. Evidence based medicine: What it is and what it isn't. *Br Med J* 1996;312(7023):71–2.
3. Oxman AD, Sackett DL, Guyatt GH; for the Evidence-Based Medicine Working Group. Users' guides to the medical literature: I. How to get started. *JAMA* 1993;270(17):2093–5.
4. Guyatt G, Rennie D, Meade MO, et al., eds. *Users' Guides to the Medical Literature: Essentials of Evidence-Based Practice.* 2nd ed. New York, NY: McGraw Hill, 2008.
5. Straus SE, Richardson WS, Glaszioù P, et al., eds. *Evidence-Based Medicine: How to Practice and Teach EBM.* London, UK: Elsevier, 2005.
6. JAMAevidence. http://www.jamaevidence.com. Accessed August 11, 2013.
7. Sackett DL, Haynes RB, Tugwell P, eds. *Clinical Epidemiology: A Basic Science for Clinical Medicine.* Boston, MA: Little Brown, 1985.
8. Atkins D, Best D, Briss PA, et al; GRADE Working Group. Grading quality of evidence and strength of recommendations. *Br Med J* 2004;328(7454):1490.
9. Oxman AD, Cook DJ, Guyatt GH; for the Evidence-Based Medicine Working Group. Users' guides to the medical literature: VI. How to use an overview. *JAMA* 1994;272(17):1367–71.
10. Hayward RSA, Wilson MC, Tunis SR, et al. Users' guides to the medical literature: VIII. How to use clinical practice guidelines A. Are the recommendations valid? *JAMA* 1995;274(7):570–4.
11. Wilson MC, Hayward RSA, Tunis SR, et al. Users' guides to the medical literature. VIII. How to use clinical practice guidelines B. What are the recommendations and will they help you in caring for your patients? *JAMA* 1995;274(20):1630–2.
12. Shankaran S, Laptook AR, Ehrenkranz RA, et al; for the NICHHD Neonatal Research Network. Whole-body hypothermia for neonates with hypoxic-ischemic encephalopathy. *N Engl J Med* 2005;353:1574–84.
13. Guyatt GH, Sackett DL, Cook DJ; for the Evidence-Based Medicine Working Group. Users' guides to the medical literature: II. How to use an article about therapy or prevention. A. Are the results of the study valid? *JAMA* 1993;270:2598–601.
14. Guyatt GH, Sackett DL, Cook DJ; for the Evidence-Based Medicine Working Group. Users' guides to the medical literature: II. How to use an article about therapy or prevention. B. What were the results and will they help me in caring for my patients? *JAMA* 1994;271:59–63.
15. The PedsCCM Evidence-Based Journal Club. http://pedsccm.org. Accessed February 14, 2006.
16. Pizarro CF, Troster EJ, Damiani D, et al. Absolute and relative adrenal insufficiency in children with septic shock. *Crit Care Med* 2005;33:855–9.
17. Randolph AG, Guyatt GH, Calvin JE, et al. Evidenced Based Medicine in Critical Care Group. Understanding articles describing clinical prediction tools. *Crit Care Med* 1998;26:1603–12.
18. Keenan SP, Sinuff T, Cook DJ, et al. Does noninvasive positive pressure ventilation improve outcome in acute hypoxemic respiratory failure? A systematic review. *Crit Care Med* 2004;32:2516–23.
19. Accreditation Council for Graduate Medical Education. Common Program Requirements. (*Pediatrics*, February 2004). http://www.acgme.org/acgmeweb/Portals/0/dh_dutyhoursCommonPR07012007.pdf. Accessed August 11, 2013.

CHAPTER 9 ■ QUALITY IMPROVEMENT, PATIENT SAFETY, AND MEDICAL ERROR

ANDREW C. ARGENT AND VICKI L. MONTGOMERY

KEY POINTS

1 Medical error is associated with high morbidity, mortality, and costs.

2 Patient safety is defined as the avoidance, prevention, and amelioration of adverse outcomes or injuries that stem from the processes of healthcare.

3 Improvement of quality of care and patient safety requires an understanding of factors within the PICU environment that may contribute to the occurrence of adverse events.

4 Both actual and potential adverse events must be documented in a systematic way and considered in their full context to allow the development of realistic and appropriate responses to limit further problems.

5 Institutions must develop structured and appropriate responses to adverse events to ensure that the harmful effects are minimized and that future problems are averted.

6 Most legal systems require that the facts regarding adverse events should be honestly and fully presented to the family and individuals affected.

7 Changes in legal definitions of "reasonable care" may potentially affect the way in which institutions are held liable for adverse events that occur.

Historically, intensivists have been committed to improving the quality of care provided to their patients, but PICUs across the world still have substantial "room to improve" in terms of patient safety and freedom from adverse events (1). A number of processes can contribute to the ultimate goal of improving outcomes for patients admitted to the PICU, including defining the goals and standards to be achieved in conjunction with the resources available; addressing the issues associated with provision of safe care (or avoiding harm); responding appropriately to potential or actual adverse events; monitoring the standards, processes, and outcomes of pediatric intensive care; learning from the available data; developing and implementing strategies to improve delivery of quality care; evaluating the initiatives; and reiterating the process. However, the underpinning challenge is to create an environment that is constantly focused on ensuring that patients receive safe and effective care despite the challenges of this complex setting (1).

The object of this chapter is to provide the pediatric intensivist with (a) an overview of patient safety, including common definitions; (b) an approach to continuous quality improvement, working within teams and systems; (c) principles of human factors engineering; and a discussion of practical responses to, and legal implications of, adverse events in the PICU.

Since the 1960s, attention has been focused on the fact that quality of healthcare delivery can be improved by understanding the processes of providing care and by applying principles that have been developed in other industries to improve quality (2). In the 1990s, authors started to focus on errors in medicine and helped to develop an understanding of factors that contribute to adverse events in healthcare (3). During the same period, a number of publications started to identify the extent of adverse events in healthcare and the possible ramifications in terms of human life and costs, with 44,000–98,000 Americans dying each year as a result of medical error and costs associated with preventable adverse events in healthcare being estimated **1** at $17 billion. At the beginning of the 21st century, a number

of landmark reports were published, such as the Institute of Medicine's (IOM) "To Err is Human: Building a Safer Health System" (4) and the United Kingdom National Health Service's "An Organization with a Memory" (5). These publications and similar reports in Australia prompted an escalation in patient safety initiatives at local and national levels in many countries throughout the world. The public developed an unprecedented awareness of medical error and the harm that might be experienced as a result of entering the healthcare system.

The true scope of morbidity related to medical error, particularly in infants and children, is unknown. Error rates in hospitalized children have been estimated to range from 1.81 to 2.96 per 100 discharges (6). While the incidence of error in the PICU is unknown, most reports suggest that more errors, particularly medication errors, occur in the PICU than in any other location in the hospital. Agarwal et al. (7) performed a multicenter retrospective study using a PICU-specific trigger tool and found that 62% of PICU patients had at least one adverse event for a rate of 28.6 adverse events per 100 patient-days. The rate for adverse drug events in this population was 4.9 per 100 patient-days (7). There is much room for improving safety. However, before the risk of error in the PICU can be reduced, the language of patient safety must be understood and a deeper understanding must be developed of the principles of systems analysis, work models, and other problem-solving tools and skills frequently used in other industries to minimize risks of adverse events.

DEFINITIONS

The National Patient Safety Foundation defines *patient safety* as the avoidance, prevention, and amelioration of adverse outcomes or injuries stemming from the processes of health-**2** care (8). The IOM defines patient safety simply as "freedom from accidental injury" (4). Although other definitions exist, this simple definition is the essence of a long-standing tenet of medical care that originated with Hippocrates: "First do no harm." Patients expect to receive healthcare without experiencing preventable harm.

An *adverse event* is an unintended event that occurs during medical care that is not directly related to the underlying condition of the patient (4). Some adverse events result in harm. Not all adverse events result from errors (a patient with no known drug allergies develops urticaria while receiving penicillin), while others are considered preventable and result from medical error (a patient with a penicillin allergy receives ampicillin and develops anaphylaxis).

Medical error is the failure of a planned action to be completed as intended (sometimes referred to as *an error in execution*) or the use of a wrong plan to achieve an aim (sometimes referred to as *an error of planning*) (3,4). An example of an error in execution is intubating the esophagus when the intent was to intubate the trachea and failing to recognize the malposition. Failure to perform a procedure according to policy is another example. Treating a patient with *Enterobacter* pneumonia with a drug that only covers Gram-positive organisms illustrates an error of planning.

Reason (3), a noted expert on human factors and error, further categorizes medical error into narrower categories that are important to understand the role that humans have in causing an error and to guide the development of strategies to prevent the error from occurring in the future. Slips and lapses are errors in execution. A *slip* is an observable action that deviates from what was planned (the wrong drug is programmed into an IV pump or ordered from a drop-down menu), while a *lapse* represents a memory failure (a nurse placing a nasogastric tube fails to follow all of the steps of the policy, and placement in the trachea is unrecognized until respiratory distress develops). A *mistake* is a knowledge-based failure: A plan is carried out correctly, but the planned action was wrong for the situation. *Active errors* (also referred to as *sharp-end errors*) typically occur in a patient care area by a frontline provider, and the effect is almost immediately apparent. *Latent errors* (also referred to as *blunt errors*) are usually system-based problems and may relate to poor design, incorrect installation, look-alike packaging, sound-alike names, faulty maintenance, and bad management decisions. Latent errors are usually more difficult to identify than active errors and may have occurred days, weeks, months, or years before the accident. These errors are typically hard to recognize and may be hidden within the structure of the organization, the computer program, or care process. Workers in healthcare frequently develop "*work arounds*" for these remote system problems, which leads to generalized acceptance that the "work around" is normal. However, fully investigating and uncovering latent errors is more likely to result in the development of a better system than is focusing on active errors.

Work models provide a conceptual framework for investigating events and processes so that all contributing factors are evaluated. Many versions exist. The PDCA cycle, Plan–Do–Check–Act (or -Adjust), is one that is commonly used. The DEPOSE (Design, Equipment, Procedures, Operators, Supplies and materials, and Environment) (4) model provides a guide for investigation of events. The premise of work models is that an organized, systematic approach to event investigation results in reliable data that can be used to develop a new system.

A *system* is "a set of interdependent human and nonhuman elements interacting to achieve a common aim" (4). A system can be a unit or department within a hospital, an entire hospital, or many hospitals. Systems can be simple (linear) or complex, loosely or tightly coupled, and isolated or overlapping with other systems. Healthcare is considered a complex, tightly coupled system. In the PICU, the system elements include the people (patients, healthcare providers, environmental services, visitors, etc.), equipment (monitors, devices, computers, and other communication tools), environment (lighting, noise, lack of standardization, high acuity, staffing), and decision making (complex, multiple data sources, frequent interruptions).

The process of improving healthcare is generally referred to as *continuous quality improvement* (CQI), which is a continual process of reviewing and improving the practices and procedures associated with providing goods or services (9). CQI programs may evaluate structure, process, or outcome, either as independent components of the CQI process or, more commonly, all simultaneously, as considerable overlap exists between the components and quality of care. Structure is essentially the people, the physical layout, management, and equipment. Factors such as adequate staffing for patient acuity levels, the right equipment at the right time, and involvement of an intensivist in the care of all critically ill patients are examples of structures influencing quality. Processes refer to how care is delivered: are policies routinely followed, are evidence-based medicine guidelines routinely followed, does transfer of patients occur in an organized manner? Outcomes summarize the effectiveness of care, including adverse events. Common outcome measures include risk-adjusted mortality, hospital-acquired infections, and adverse medication errors. In healthcare, CQI should lead to improved patient safety and better outcomes (9,10). However, because many physicians and other healthcare professionals lack formal training in CQI and related concepts (the use of work models, human factors engineering, and understanding systems), progress has been slow compared with that in non-healthcare industries.

MEDICAL ERROR: HUMAN ERROR AND SYSTEMS

Rarely does medical error result from a healthcare worker intentionally inflicting harm to a patient. More commonly, medical error results when the healthcare worker fails to perform perfectly (active errors) and the system does not have adequate redundancy or layers to prevent the error from reaching the patient. Reason's book, *Human Error*, provides an easy-to-read, in-depth discussion of human error (3). In it, he examines the etiologies of human errors and the factors necessary for developing processes to minimize the risk that human error will result in harm. After all, active errors will *always* occur because of limitations inherent to humans, which include the impact of emotions, perceptions, stress, fatigue, cognition, and the environment on performance and decision-making abilities. Stated another way, error occurs when cognitive processes converge with three other elements: nature of the task and its environmental circumstances, the mechanisms that govern performance, and the nature of the individual who produced the failure (3). Thus, reduction and elimination of medical error in the PICU must take into account these elements as well as other principles of systems analysis and event investigation.

The healthcare system, whether referring to a single ICU, hospital, state, or nation, is a complex, tightly coupled system. The components of a complex system interact with many other components in both predictable and unexpected ways, are specialized and interdependent, and serve multiple functions. A fundamental problem of complex systems is that it is difficult for anyone to predict the outcomes of events within that system (10). Tightly coupled systems have no buffer between actions and are more difficult to change than loosely coupled systems. In tightly coupled systems, one action quickly gives rise to other actions such that it is nearly impossible to recognize failure or intercede and prevent the failure from reaching a patient. The "Swiss Cheese Model" described by Reason (3) is a conceptual framework for thinking about error prevention in complex systems. In this model, each layer has associated potential failures that represent "holes" in the layers. When multiple holes line up, the downstream effect is that failure happens. In the case of patient care, a medical error occurs. However, complex, tightly coupled systems can be made safer, as demonstrated by successes in aviation and nuclear energy industries. Within medicine, the specialty of Anesthesiology has been successful in improving patient safety. Characteristics of safe, complex systems include simplification when possible, standardization of processes, redundancy and backup, many checks and balances, and automation whenever possible so that error does not result in an inferior product or service—or in the case of healthcare, patient harm. Unfortunately, healthcare has developed as individual pieces rather than a cohesive system. Device and technology manufacturers, the pharmaceutical industry, and the competition for patients contribute to the complexity of the system, particularly in the area of standardization. It is common in pediatric intensive care to have multiple brands of IV infusion devices, ventilators, monitors, and central-line products within the same unit.

Clearly, safety is not the responsibility of a single person, device, or department within a system, but rather the product of the interactions of components of the system (4). Implementation of checklists has clearly improved outcomes in surgery (11,12) despite some resistance. Significant successes have been demonstrated in projects to standardize care (as an example, using "bundles of care" that standardize the procedures that must be followed on all patients) and address problems such as central-line sepsis (13), ventilator-associated pneumonia (14), and unexpected extubation in ventilated patients (15).

Various pressures drive the processes within healthcare (and other) environments. Pressures such as financial concerns and need for increased patient turnover may work against patient safety (10). As expressed in Rasmussen's dynamic safety model (16), system operating points may be pushed toward unacceptable limits by economic and workload pressures. While systems remain within the acceptable safety range, adverse events are unlikely, but the closer the systems come to the margins, higher the risk of adverse events increases (often with very little warning). As these pressures increase in hospital systems, it is important to understand how factors such as operating close to capacity may increase the risks of errors and accidents (17) even in environments that are well managed, efficient, and highly effective (10).

There is increasing awareness of the characteristics that are present in "high-reliability organizations" (1,18) (organizations which achieve safety despite significant inherent risks in their operations, e.g., aircraft carriers or nuclear power plants). These organizations are able to not only decrease predicted risks but also anticipate and respond to unexpected events. It is a characteristic of these organizations that they are "mindfully organized" (1), with features such as preoccupation with failure (a capacity to constantly review problems with their systems); sensitivity to operations (an ongoing focus on what is actually happening within the organization and how that aligns with organizational goals); reluctance to discount threats (an ability to address all of the available information without discounting the implications of that information); deference to expertise (the organization and its members defer to expertise rather than to authority structure—as an example, parents in the PICU may be the experts on the implications of their child's specific behaviors); and commitment to resilience (although standardization of work with appropriate guidelines and protocols may be useful, these organizations are also committed to responding effectively and rapidly to changing and unexpected situations, calling on all the experience and insight of the full team).

THE PICU ENVIRONMENT

Complexity of the Environment

The physical and psychological milieu of the PICU contributes to the risk of medical error. The daily staffing, patient acuity, and census may significantly or unexpectedly change. To make the best decisions possible for patients, much data, multiple assessments, and the opinions from physician and nonphysician caregivers must be analyzed in a quick, organized manner. Decision making is complex and involves interpreting multiple pieces of data in a short amount of time in an environment that may require multitasking. Frequently, patient care must be triaged, as it is impossible to be at the bedside of more than one patient at a time. Intensivists routinely discuss death, withdrawal or limitation of care, and life-altering consequences of the critical illness or injury with parents and other family members. Intensivists must have a working knowledge of many types and brands of equipment. The environment is noisy, full of distractions, and lacks standardization and ergonomic design. It is rare for a task to progress to completion without at least one interruption. All of these characteristics contribute to the complexity of the PICU environment and have the potential to negatively impact patient safety.

Impact of the PICU Environment on Human Error

Understanding how we interact with our environment is essential to developing processes and systems that improve safety in the PICU. The study of the interactions between humans, the tools they use, and the environment in which they live and work is referred to as *human factors engineering* (4,19). Evaluating human factors to provide insight into where and why systems or processes break down has been applied in other industries for years. For example, investigation of aviation accidents demonstrated that take-offs and landings are the times of highest risk during flight. The concept of the "sterile" cockpit developed because factors contributing to human error, such as stress, authority gradients, and distractions, were identified as playing a role in crash investigations. During take-offs and landings, a detailed checklist is used, and conversation related to only these activities is allowed. Distractions are minimized, and roles are well defined.

Human performance is influenced by psychological limits of the individual, their training and education, knowledge, fatigue, communication, and perceptions. In the PICU, the high acuity of illness, constant exposure to death and grieving parents, fatigue, inappropriate staffing (numbers and skill set), an ever-changing body of knowledge, lack of equipment standardization, multiple simultaneous demands, and the use of many interventions associated with narrow therapeutic windows all affect human performance. A commentary published by the Agency for Healthcare Research and Quality in 2005 highlights the impact of working conditions (such as interruptions and keeping pace with the changing needs of patients) on the clinical decision-making abilities of nurses (20). A study by Grayson and Potter (21) found that errors tend to occur within 30 minutes after sudden changes in patient needs in an environment that is dominated by distractions and interruptions. In the PICU environment, where patient status and census are constantly changing and multitasking is normal, it is easy to understand why ICUs are among the most error-prone areas in hospitals. Overall, compared with other industries, 0little is known about human factors and the ICU environment, but recent studies related to increased workload, fatigue, and emotional stress clearly demonstrate the influence of human factors on patient (and healthcare provider) safety (22–28).

Workload and Fatigue

It is clear from the sleep literature that acute and chronic sleep deprivation negatively impact performance and place sleep-deprived practitioners at risk for personal injury, mood disturbances, and stress-related illnesses (20,29). The extent to which fatigue-related errors actually contribute to patient harm is largely unknown, although fatigue is often identified as a factor in the root-cause analysis investigation of events. Sleep research conducted in laboratory and clinical settings suggests that fatigue significantly impairs performance of healthcare providers.

Cumulative sleepiness, mood disturbance, and psychomotor vigilance performance decreases during a week of sleep restricted to 4–5 hours per night (30). Interns made significantly more serious medical and diagnostic errors during the critical care rotation when the schedule (traditional) included "call every third night" and extended (>24 hours) shifts (26). In another study that uses a similar design, interns who were working a traditional schedule had more attentional failures during the night (27). Although increasing data describe the benefit of decreasing sleep deprivation and fatigue, the increased number of patient handovers has become a new source of error. As staff changes occur, with handover of information from one group of caregivers to another, valuable patient information may not be communicated. New strategies for improving teamwork and access to patient information are necessary to minimize the occurrence of handover-related errors.

Unfortunately, many physicians underappreciate the effect of fatigue and stress on performance and do not perceive that inadequate rest or stressful situations contribute to medical error. These attitudes differ substantially from those in other industries. A direct comparison of the aviation industry to medicine regarding the attitudes and perceptions toward teamwork, stress, fatigue, and error showed that, compared to pilots, physicians underplay the importance of fatigue and workload on error (31). When trained observers rated the function of the team, the aviation team routinely received standard or higher ratings (85% of the time, a standard or higher rating was assigned) compared to surgical, anesthetic, and surgical–anesthetic teams (30%–50%, of the time, a poor to minimal rating was assigned). The aviation industry has had considerable success in improving passenger safety, largely because of advances in addressing fatigue, stress, and need for teamwork.

The need for adequate rest and appropriate staffing levels is also important for nurses (32,33). Lower patient-to-nurse staffing ratios (fewer patients assigned to one nurse) have been associated with a lower risk of adverse events, such as urinary tract infections and decubitus ulcers (25,32). Having nurses at the bedside with the appropriate skill set (education and training) and adequate rest is also important for outcomes (24,25,28,32). ICU nurses complete many tasks during a shift, and the higher their patient's acuity, the more tasks a nurse must complete during a shift. These tasks include direct patient care; documentation; and discussions with physicians, therapists, and families. It is unknown how many actions can be completed by one nurse in the ICU environment before the risk of error increases. Pediatric intensivists, particularly those who function as medical directors, should advocate for appropriate staffing levels, orientation, ongoing education, and rewards for staff nurses.

Communication

Effective communication is another area that is essential to improving safety. Communication between all members of the healthcare team is crucial to safe patient handovers. The Joint Commission for the Accreditation of Hospitals and Other Organizations (JCAHO) has noted that poor communication is a factor in the majority of sentinel events. The 2006 JCAHO national patient-safety goals include several requirements for improving communication throughout the hospital.

Patients in the PICU move throughout the hospital to have specialized procedures and diagnostic testing, and providers from multiple disciplines enter the PICU to care for these patients. In an ideal system, information should flow easily between all team members without regard to professional stature, seniority, discipline, expertise, or authority. Patient data should be available, legible, timely, and complete. A specific structure for sharing patient information, particularly at the time of patient handovers, facilitates good communication, as has been demonstrated by the use of daily goals (34). For critically ill infants and children, communication is fundamental to ensuring that patients receive appropriate care whether the handover is between nurses or physicians either in the PICU, in other areas of the hospital, or in the transport of the patient from one facility to another.

The ideal communication system is difficult to achieve in healthcare in view of authority gradients, time and physical restraints, technology limitations, and a perception that teamwork is not essential to good patient outcomes. The negative impact of authority gradients on safety was first noted in the aviation industry. Investigation of events demonstrated that effective communication between pilots and copilots was negatively impacted if a significant difference existed in their experience, perceived expertise, or authority. Authority gradients affect the ability of the lower-ranking person to voice concern and the ability of the higher-ranking person to accept and act upon the concern. The concept of authority gradients was introduced to medicine in the 2000 IOM report (35). The traditional hierarchical approach to patient care in medicine hinders effective and timely communication between attending physicians and trainees, physicians and nurses, and administration and staff. A technique called SBAR (Situation, Background, Assessment, and Recommendation) has been introduced to the healthcare field as a method by which to improve communication between team members and to overcome perceived and real restrictions related to hierarchy. This technique provides the healthcare worker with a framework for communicating a concern about a patient or situation and empowers the worker to move up the authority gradient if the concern is not addressed in a professional or timely manner. Another communication tool, "PASS the BATON," developed by the Defense Department to comply with a JCAHO patient safety goal, provides structure for transferring patient care from one individual to another regardless of the disciplines involved. The acronym provides prompts for relaying Patient data, such as name, age, sex, and location; Assessment, such as chief complaint, vital signs, active problems, signs and symptoms; Situation, which includes current status and circumstances; Safety concerns, including critical lab values and reports, allergies; Background, which includes pertinent past medical history and current medications; Actions, including what has been done and what needs to be done; Timing of care-related activities, including urgent matters and prioritization; Ownership (nurse, physician, therapist) of specific care issues; and Next, which details anticipated changes in condition and any plans or contingency plans to manage changes.

Fundamentally excellent communication can happen only within environments where there are high levels of trust between all members of the team.

ERROR PREVENTION: SAFETY CULTURE, REPORTING, SYSTEMS ANALYSIS, CQI, AND TECHNOLOGY

If the ICU environment is a complex system with ample opportunity for medical error to occur, how does the intensivist develop a safer PICU? Conceptually, intensivists should facilitate development of an environment that allows investigation of actual and averted (near-miss) events and that learns from errors. Four subcultures are necessary for supporting an environment in which learning from errors is embraced: reporting, just, flexible, and learning (36). In a *reporting culture*, members of the staff are actively engaged in reporting accidents and near misses. Various assurances exist that reporting of events is not handled in a punitive manner. The aviation industry has had great success with creating and maintaining a reporting culture. In a *just culture*, safeguards exist that allow the identification of individuals who repeatedly fail to follow policies or who act with malicious intent, while protecting those who report errors and near misses. The willingness and competence to correctly interpret safety data, form correct conclusions, and implement new processes describe features of a *learning culture*. Perhaps the most difficult culture to develop is that of flexibility. In a *flexible culture*, individuals must be willing to move between a traditional, hierarchical structure to a flatter, professional structure, so that individuals with expertise in an area may investigate and design solutions.

To identify ways to improve patient safety in the PICU, an error-reporting system(s) must exist. Identification of adverse events is the only way to know that issues exist. Types of reporting systems include voluntary reporting, mandatory reporting, concurrent surveillance, automated surveillance, and chart review (37). Automated and concurrent surveillance methods generally detect more events than does voluntary self-reporting. Automated surveillance is ideal for detecting events that require antidotes or specific laboratory monitoring (e.g., an order for naloxone triggers a concurrent review of a patient's record to evaluate for error). Concurrent surveillance is more suited for identifying errors manifested by changes in signs and symptoms (37).

Voluntary and mandatory reporting systems of actual events generally underdetect error and are, by definition, reactionary, as a report is generated after an event has occurred. Historically, many barriers have impeded the reporting of errors in medicine. These barriers include the negative emotional impact that disclosure has on the person (people) involved, risk of disclosure on medical malpractice, and risk of job or other punitive acts. To maximize the effectiveness of self-reporting systems, leaders must avoid blaming the involved staff for the error and demonstrate that reports generate changes in practice. Successful reporting systems are user friendly and readily accessible. Allowing anonymous reporting also improves reporting rates and helps to foster the concept of a "just culture." Some institutions choose to start with the reporting of averted or near-miss events, as actual patient harm does not occur in these instances and the individuals involved perceive less threat to self. Identifying averted errors is a proactive, rather than reactive, approach to improving patient safety because events that could lead to patient harm are evaluated before actual harm occurs. Once an area of concern is identified, the process must be scrutinized so that each component is identified and evaluated for its contribution to the event. Applying work-model principles is integral to beginning and completing the process in a manner that leads to adequate safeguards for preventing an error from reaching a patient. If only the most obvious link to the error is recognized, the same error will likely occur again, as other aspects of the process that contributed to the original event are not recognized. The trialing and redesigning phases help to ensure that the final product is a good solution and provides a clearly defined end point to the project.

When an event occurs or an opportunity to improve safety is prospectively identified, a team is assembled to design a new process. The team should include representation from any area or service that had a role in the care of the patient. Inclusion of the appropriate personnel helps to ensure that a thorough planning stage occurs. Once the team is assembled, the existing process should be diagrammed so that each component is articulated, and personnel not on the team interviewed. These steps will provide the basis for identifying where failure is likely to occur, developing an alternative process, trialing the new process, evaluating the new process, and redesigning as needed. Essentially, these steps encompass the basis of systems analysis, human factors engineering, and CQI. Pronovost et al. (38) detailed how to apply processes for improving patient safety in an ICU by describing an incident that occurred in an adult ICU, how it was investigated, and the steps that were taken to prevent it from happening again.

Various work models exist that provide a template for ensuring a logical, thoughtful, and inclusive process for revising a current process or developing a new one. A frequently used work model is "Plan–Do–Check–Act" (4). Using a work model is key to fully appreciating the successes and limitations of the current process, identifying why error occurred, and developing an alternative system that eliminates current limitations and has minimal risk of introducing new sources of error.

Minimizing the risk of new error or evaluating current processes for sources of error can be accomplished by an organized approach to evaluating where failure may occur and the significance if the error occurs. A commonly used failure analysis tool is "Failure Modes and Effects Analysis (FMEA)." In performing an analysis with FMEA, a specific procedure and tool are used to identify possible failures of a product or service and to determine the frequency and impact of the failure. Information about this tool and how to use it can be found at several Web sites (39). The information learned from an FMEA may provide valuable data for designing a safer process, as failures are anticipated and solutions for preventing failures from causing patient harm are built into the process. However, there are potential problems with implementation of this process in the health system (40).

Intensivists function within teams on a daily basis, but few have formal training in leading teams and understanding how teams function. Additional reading and training on these topics, especially for those who aspire to leadership roles in the ICU, should be obtained. In a study that distributed the Intensive Care Unit Management Attitudes Questionnaire, which was adapted from the Flight Management Attitudes Questionnaire, to 226 physicians and 324 nurses from ICUs in six hospitals, physician members of teams perceived the function of the team differently than other members of the team (31,41). In general, the physicians rated the quality of collaboration and communication much higher than the nurses did. Unfortunately, this finding is not unique to this study. Physicians tend to perceive teamwork and communication as being better than do the non-physician members of the team. This discrepancy contributes to the slower progress in safety initiatives in medicine compared with other industries and to the disconnect that occurs between physicians and nurses in the daily care of patients.

Preexisting attitudes, whether held by physician or non-physician staff, can lead to failure of even the best-investigated and designed projects. Introducing change and providing education is fundamental to success. Such strategies as mass mailings of educational materials or conducting conferences are least likely to effect changes in physician practice. Multiple small sessions, individualized audits and feedback, informal and formal sessions directed by local opinion leaders, and frequent reminders and prompts (preprinted order sets, pop-up windows) are all necessary to bring success to project implementation and long-term sustainability.

Introduction of new technology in the PICU should undergo the same scrutiny that other processes do. That is, the technology should be assessed for potential advances in care as well as potential failures to maximize the successes and minimize the risk of failures. Prior to purchase and implementation, a detailed process for use and a sound educational program are essential to achieve success with the new technology. Also, assessment of the technology should include assignment of value, as technology is usually a significant financial investment for a hospital. Value can be demonstrated in a variety of ways, including showing savings, improved market advantage, improved efficiency, improved customer satisfaction, and improved patient safety.

On the surface, it seems intuitive that technology should contribute to advances in patient safety (42). The rapidly expanding body of knowledge to be mastered, the need to simultaneously monitor many parameters of patient status, the multiple team members involved in a patient's care, and the complexity of the system are reasons that technology could be beneficial. Information technology can facilitate better communication by allowing on-site and remote access to patient records and providing a foundation for patient handovers. Access to reference materials, policies, evidence-based medicine guidelines, and databases is easier and wider with modern technology than it has been at any time in the history of medicine.

In addition, information technology has allowed the introduction of computerized physician order entry (CPOE) and clinical decision support systems. The use of CPOE combined with clinical decision support has led to decreases in some types of medication errors, particularly those related to calculations, prescribing drugs for which the patient has an allergy, and ordering drugs contraindicated based on organ dysfunction or drug–drug interactions. The use of forcing functions—automatic prompts that appear when preprogrammed rules are violated—are known to decrease errors and improve compliance with treatment guidelines. Monitoring trends in vital signs and laboratory data by computer programs can provide early warning to staff about worrisome patient changes and allow appropriate interventions before an adverse event occurs. "Smart pump" technology is another application that is aimed at decreasing the number of errors related to continuous drug infusions. These pumps allow selection of a drug from a library. During the pump-programming phase, prompts and alarms help to minimize the risk of the wrong drug dose being entered.

Although advances in technology have decreased the frequency of error in some areas, other types of error have not been reduced, and new types of error have been introduced. Selection of the wrong drug during CPOE and ignoring forcing functions or alerts because too many appear are actions that demonstrate that technology can contribute to error. Selection of the wrong patient can also occur during CPOE, so that medications are ordered on the wrong patient. Increases in mortality and adverse drug events have been reported post-implementation of CPOE programs. Development of computer programs by independent vendors or practitioners has led to new communication problems. The lack of standardization or "talk" between proprietary programs limits the sharing of patient information that may lead to duplication of work (physician enters a drug, but the CPOE program does not interface with the pharmacy program, requiring the drug order to be entered a second time). Most computerized systems have not resulted in decreases in documentation time. Physicians and other providers now spend more time interfacing with various types of technology. This increase in time spent on technology has led to decreased time for direct contact with patients and families and dissatisfaction among practitioners. The lack of integration of the various programs within hospitals, between hospitals, and between inpatient and outpatient facilities is another source of error and frustration.

Despite some of the limitations that still exist, decreasing medical error in the PICU is achievable. Sincen 2000, the results from several studies performed in PICUs have shown that decreases in medical error can occur with or without the introduction of new technology. The use of work models

allowed investigators at two institutions to decrease the rate of unplanned extubations (15,43). A study conducted by one of the groups illustrated the application of CQI methodology to reduce an event that was associated with patient harm (43). In their PICU, a multidisciplinary team was formed to evaluate unplanned extubations using the institution's CQI model of "Plan–Do–Check–Act." The team reviewed all unplanned extubation events to identify areas in which the care of intubated patients could be altered. Inadequate sedation and an unorganized approach to weaning and extubating patients were identified as factors that contributed to unplanned extubations. In the "Do–Check–Act" phases, processes were added and refined to address these factors, and the incidence of unplanned extubations decreased.

Both of these studies demonstrate important principles for embarking on CQI projects –relevance, feasibility, and lack of controversy. The project must have relevance to the unit. If the unit has a very low incidence of unplanned extubations but a high incidence of catheter-related bloodstream infections, the staff is more likely to become vested in a project to decrease catheter-related infections than in one to decrease unplanned extubations. The project must be feasible—a key aspect when introducing CQI. It is much easier to change culture and develop a cohesive team if early projects have short timelines and achieve success. Early CQI activities are also beneficial if noncontroversial projects are chosen. The development of guidelines and pathways is another strategy by which to apply CQI to improve or standardize a procedure or practice. The team should understand that CQI is not a fast process. The project to reduce unplanned extubations described above occurred over several years. The time invested allows the team to study the process and develop solutions that are likely to improve the process with minimal risk of introducing new sources of error.

Many of the above approaches rely on the fundamental assumption that it is possible to break down all systems into components that can be fully understood. In fact, many aspects of medical systems behave as complex systems where it is not always possible to predict the effect of changes or events within the system (10). As systems of care become ever more complex, it is essential that managers grapple with the understanding of systems rather than a collection of components. One consequence of complex systems is that it may be impossible for individuals to predict the consequences of particular actions or plans, and this is an extremely important issue when adverse events are examined within a legal framework which attempts to attribute blame.

MEDICAL ERROR AND THE PICU ENVIRONMENT

The IOM's report "Crossing the Quality Chasm" (20,44) recommended six aims for improvement: safety, effectiveness, equity, timeliness, patient centeredness, and efficiency. These aims may be used as a framework for specific areas of intervention to advance quality of care in the PICU (45) (**Table 9.1**).

Intensive care is provided within the wider environment of hospitals and healthcare systems. The aims are applicable to the healthcare system in its entirety, as well as within the particular context of the PICU, but achievement of the aims in the larger environment may be dependent on the achievement of the aims in areas such as the PICU.

A number of studies have clearly demonstrated that specific organizational structures for pediatric critical care within a healthcare system are associated with better outcomes (46). It is also useful to evaluate the specific activities within the PICU in terms of the aims described above.

TABLE 9.1

SPECIFIC AREAS OF INTERVENTION TO ADVANCE QUALITY OF CARE IN PICU

■ AIMS FOR IMPROVEMENT	■ CATEGORIES AND DEFINITIONS	■ POTENTIAL MONITORING AND INTERVENTION
Patient safety	Diagnostic errors	Autopsies
		Morbidity and mortality discussions
	Treatment errors, including Medication errors	Regular review of prescriptions and drug administration by pharmacy staff
	Nosocomial infections	Monitoring of nosocomial infections in the PICU
	Procedures	Monitoring of incidents such as accidental extubation, complications of vascular access
	Prevention	Ensuring that preventative policies are clear-cut and regularly implemented
Effectiveness	Evidence-based practice based on sound research evidence	Implementation of clinical guidelines where possible and focus on collection of appropriate data to inform decisions
Equity	Access to appropriate care for all regardless of factors such as race, ethnicity, financial status, and gender	Regular review of patient population and identification of disparities in care between various groupings of people
Timeliness	Timely provision of care and information	Monitoring of time taken for care and intervention
	Timely transmission of information	Focus on optimal transmission of information between members of the PICU team
Patient centeredness		Use of validated surveys of families
Efficiency	Efficient and cost-effective utilization of resources	Cost per patient
		Severity of illness and acuity of care scoring
	Appropriate planning of intensive and high care bed numbers	Monitoring of "nonintensive care" activities

From Slonim AD, Pollack MM. Integrating the Institute of Medicine's six quality aims into pediatric critical care: Relevance and applications. *Pediatr Crit Care Med* 2005;6(3):264–9.

QUALITY MANAGEMENT AND RESOURCE ALLOCATION

It is clear from the above discussion that resources must be allocated to the process of quality management and that a linkage exists between the overall resources available to a PICU and the standards that can realistically be achieved in that unit. In all contexts, the need exists for definition of the standards and goals of treatment to be offered in the PICU, reasonable allocation of resources, appropriate management of those resources, accountability for the use of those resources, and ongoing feedback to the stakeholders.

Fundamental to the process of setting the standards and goals of therapy is involvement of all the stakeholders, including patients and families, healthcare workers, hospital managers, and funders of health services. Failure to involve all stakeholders almost inevitably leads to problems of communication and failure of clinical services as documented in the enquiry into pediatric cardiac services in Bristol, United Kingdom (47).

Both the process of setting standards and goals and that of resource allocation inevitably require the use of rationing. *Rationing* refers to process of allocating scarce resources and is different from to of eliminating waste, optimizing expenditures and withholding inappropriate therapy. Rationing itself may happen at a number of levels, including at the bedside (clinician making a decision about whether to admit a child or not), at the institutional level (managers allocating resources to the PICU), and at higher levels (national or provincial allocation of health budgets). It is frequently done implicitly, but ideally should be done explicitly, with accountability for

the decisions taken. Rationing includes the process of making rational, defensible, and ethical decisions about *which beneficial interventions to withhold* from which patientsz so that *resources can be allocated toward other (possibly more) beneficial activities.*

Although it may be difficult to establish a system for fair allocation of resources (48), the concept of accountability for reasonableness (A4R) is one model that facilitates the process (49). The A4R concept includes the following:

Relevance—decisions should be made on the basis of reasons that are relevant under the circumstances.
Publicity—decisions and the processes by which they are reached should be transparent and publicly available.
Revision—opportunities should be available to alter those decisions in the light of further information or argument.
Enforcement—either voluntary or public regulation of the process should be possible to ensure that the first three conditions are actually met.

Others have described rationing resources on the basis of concepts such as **autonomy, utility,** and **equity** (50).

Ideally, therapy and interventions offered in the PICU should be evidence based (although data are limited in many situations), and measurement of the standards and goals that are achieved should be required to provide motivation or justification to the resources allocated to the services. Stakeholders should agree both on the treatment to be offered in the PICU and on the measurable standards and goals of the service. As described above, these measurements must be relevant to the clinical service, accurate, reproducible, and doable. It is particularly important that measured outcomes are relevant to all healthcare services—not just to the PICU (e.g., measuring the overall outcome of congenital heart disease in a region and measuring the postoperative mortality of pediatric cardiac surgery may differ considerably). The processes of measuring risk-adjusted morbidity and mortality are relevant to this process and are discussed in detail in Chapter 7.

The body of evidence from adult intensive care on the outcomes of triage decisions made by intensivists is increasing (51). Intrinsic to this literature is the fact that the quality of intensive care services cannot be fully assessed solely from data on patients admitted to the ICU. It is essential to collect and appropriately interpret data regarding the outcomes of patients who were either refused or not offered admission to the ICU.

In the light of current concerns about the possibility of large outbreaks of communicable disease, or of large numbers of casualties from disasters of other kinds, the potential for expansion of current intensive care services to deal with such events should also be considered. This marker of resource allocation has rarely been considered until very recently (52–54). The legal standing of admission and discharge criteria for the PICU has rarely been challenged, but it is likely that courts would sympathetically view criteria that have been established using the A4R principles.

LEGAL ISSUES AND QUALITY CONTROL IN THE PICU

The legal issues that relate to the practice of pediatric intensive care vary throughout the world. However, a number of themes are common to most systems: the recognition of criminal intent; negligence and malpractice; identification of "truth"; issues related to compensation of anyone who suffers an adverse event while in the PICU, and the use of the legal system to enforce quality of healthcare.

It is generally agreed that the vast majority of healthcare workers do not harbor criminal intent toward their patients; however, rare incidents have been reported in which nurses or doctors have set out to harm patients, and such instances must be guarded against.

Most legal processes are designed to apportion blame and appropriate retribution. In addition, compensation may be provided to victims of adverse events and their families. A variety of systems exist throughout the world, including approaches such as no-fault compensation, tort (or allocation of blame) litigation, availability of mediators, structured settlements, capped awards, and open disclosure. The particular system applicable has significant implications for legal processes. In Scandinavian countries, where most healthcare needs are automatically covered by the state, claims for compensation are significantly reduced. In the United States, compensation is provided by the tort system, but the process is expensive (in one estimate as much as 54 cents per dollar spent on compensation went into administrative costs (55)) and a number of studies have shown that the system serves only a tiny proportion of people who have been harmed (56).

Ideally, information that is required for allocation of blame and assessment of damages (i.e., data that can be used in the legal process) should be separate from information required for improvement and development of healthcare services (which should be confidential and legally privileged). Unfortunately, few countries in the world allow such a separation (56).

Negligence has been defined as a failure to maintain the standard expected of a reasonably careful and knowledgeable practitioner acting in a similar situation (57). In many countries, the standard is that of "current practice." Recently, courts in the United States have moved away from this definition of standard care to a "reasonableness test," and this may happen with regard to adoption of new technology (57), clinical practice guidelines, and informed consent. In the area of new technology, the test entails an evaluation of the costs and benefits of specific technology, particularly regarding patient safety. Guidelines for clinical practice that are authoritative and evidence based can also be used as criteria for evaluation of negligence, and this has implications for healthcare providers and for the organizations that establish clinical practice guidelines. In many countries, guidelines for clinical practice are increasingly being provided at the national level. Finally, regarding consent for procedures, some courts have held that fully informed consent includes provision of information about the location of recognized centers of care for the particular conditions involved. The Bristol Royal infirmary enquiry also highlighted the need for parents to be given full information and appropriate length of time in which to make decisions about consent for major surgical interventions (47).

It is clear that litigation will more likely ensue when families have a sense that they have not received full information about an event. Some families have even made it clear that their reason for litigation was to discover the "truth." Much litigation could be avoided if full and appropriate information were provided to families by the team responsible for the care of their child. In fact, evidence suggests that courts in a number of countries believe that doctors particularly have a positive legal duty to inform the patient and his/her family of the facts surrounding an error (58).

Recommendations for appropriate response in the event of the occurrence of an adverse event have been reviewed (59) and include the following:

1. Managing the patient and his/her family. Ensure that the problem is dealt with and that any further threats to patient safety are eliminated. Inform the patient and the family that a problem has occurred. The exact timing of this process will depend on the condition of the child and the family, but should ideally occur within a maximum of 24 hours from the event. The most senior person available at the time should do the informing, and the physician responsible for the patient's care should also be informed immediately and personally speak with the family as soon as possible. The process should include providing information about what happened, accepting responsibility, apologizing for the event, and advising what has been done to prevent further adverse events. Follow-up meetings to provide information should be scheduled as appropriate and should be attended by appropriate representatives from the hospital management. Support for the patient and the family (including attention to billing issues) must be provided. It seems that early discussion of possible compensation is appropriate and helpful.

2. Ensure that PICU personnel involved in the adverse event receive appropriate support, adequate time to recover from the effects of the incident, and ongoing support in dealing with the process. Clearly, this requires established training programs and support systems. If the primary care provider is not able to function normally and effectively, a replacement must be found (and the family must be informed of the change).

3. Ensure that everything possible is done to preserve the evidence and information that may be required to understand exactly what happened. The lengths taken must relate to the severity of the episode (or near miss). In some circumstances, it may be appropriate to seal the area in which the incident took place until it has been fully evaluated.

4. The process used to investigate the incident and provide clarity it must be established and come into action immediately. The sooner the process is enacted, the more effective it is likely to be. In constituting the group of people who will undertake the investigation, it is advisable to involve those who have an understanding of the clinical context, functioning of PICU systems, implications of the event for the patient and the family, and potential financial and other implications of the event; they should also have independence from the personal aspects of the problems.
5. All aspects of this process should be appropriately and carefully documented.
6. The events should be reported to the appropriate authorities within the hospital and health system.

The available evidence suggests that, at least in the United States, the above process is associated with reduced litigation and associated costs, reduced claims for compensation, and significant improvements in relationships between healthcare systems and patients. However, it also appears that rather than the occurrence of an adverse event, or an adverse event due to negligence, the severity of the patient's disability is more likely to determine the size of the payment to the plaintiff (60).

There is agreement from many countries that physicians have an ethical obligation to disclose adverse events to the families who are affected by these events (61–63). There is evidence that most parents (irrespective of background) expect disclosure if adverse events affecting their children occur (not as many expect disclosure if the events were "near-miss" events with no specific harm) (64). However, there is also evidence that specific training is required to prepare physicians and healthcare workers for appropriate disclosure (approach, timing, content, etc.) (65).

CONCLUSIONS AND FUTURE DIRECTIONS

Much can be done to improve the quality of care of patients in pediatric intensive care and to reduce the risks of adverse events and errors. The quality of care that can be provided in a particular situation is limited by the resources that are available, but resources should always be allocated to the specific task of identifying areas of concern and developing ways of improving care. It is essential that comprehensive team- and systems-based approaches are employed to improve care and limit errors. Ongoing measurement and assessment of systems is an essential component of quality improvement.

Legal systems can be developed to aid in improving the quality of medical care, although current systems in many parts of the world are particularly expensive and relatively ineffective in improving the quality of care.

If adverse events occur, there is a moral responsibility for healthcare workers to disclose the information regarding that event to the family, but many healthcare workers will benefit from specific training in how best to do that.

References

1. Niedner MF, Muething SE, Sutcliffe KM. The high-reliability pediatric intensive care unit. *Pediatr Clin North Am* 2013;60(3):563–80.
2. Donabedian A. Quality assessment and monitoring. Retrospect and prospect. *Eval Health Prof* 1983;6(3):363–75.
3. Reason J. *Human Error.* Cambridge, UK: Cambridge University Press, 1990.
4. Kohn LT, Corrigan JM, Donaldson, MS, eds. *To Err is Human: Building a Safer Health System.* Washington, DC: National Academy Press, 2000.
5. Donaldson L. *An Organisation with a Memory: Report of an Expert Group on Learning from Adverse Events in the NHS Chaired by the Chief Medical Officer.* London, England: The Stationery Office, 2000.
6. Slonim AD, LaFleur BJ, Ahmed W, et al. Hospital-reported medical errors in children. *Pediatrics* 2003;111(3):617–21.
7. Agarwal S, Classen D, Larsen G, et al. Prevalence of adverse events in pediatric intensive care units in the United States. *Pediatr Crit Care Med* 2010;11(5):568–78.
8. Cooper JB, Gaba DM, Liang B, et al. The National Patient Safety Foundation agenda for research and development in patient safety. *MedGenMed* 2000;2(3). E38
9. Counte MA, Meurer S. Issues in the assessment of continuous quality improvement implementation in health care organizations. *Int J Qual Health Care* 2001;13(3):197–207.
10. Dekker S. *Drift into Failure: From Hunting Broken Components to Understanding Complex Systems.* Surrey, England: Ashgate Publishing, 2011.
11. Haynes AB, Weiser TG, Berry WR, et al. A surgical safety checklist to reduce morbidity and mortality in a global population. *N Engl J Med* 2009;360(5):491–9.
12. Weiser TG, Haynes AB, Dziekan G, et al. Effect of a 19-item surgical safety checklist during urgent operations in a global patient population. *Ann Surg* 2010;251(5):976–80.
13. Pronovost PJ, Marsteller JA, Goeschel CA. Preventing bloodstream infections: A measurable national success story in quality improvement. *Health Aff* 2011;30(4):628–34.
14. Bigham MT, Amato R, Bondurrant P, et al. Ventilator-associated pneumonia in the pediatric intensive care unit: Characterizing the problem and implementing a sustainable solution. *J Pediatr* 2009;154(4):582–7.e2.
15. Popernack ML, Thomas NJ, Lucking SE. Decreasing unplanned extubations: Utilization of the Penn State Children's Hospital Sedation Algorithm. *Pediatr Crit Care Med* 2004;5(1):58–62.
16. Rasmussen J. Risk Management in a dynamic society a modelling problem. *Saf Sci* 1997;27(2):183–213.
17. Cook R, Rasmussen J. "Going solid": A model of system dynamics and consequences for patient safety. *Qual Saf Health Care* 2005;14(2):130–4.
18. Weick KE, Sutcliffe KM. *Managing the Unexpected: Assuring High Performance in an Age of Complexity.* San Francisco, CA: Jossey Bass, 2001.
19. Weinger MB, Pantiskas C, Wiklund ME, et al. Incorporating human factors into the design of medical devices. *JAMA* 1998;280(17):1484.
20. Hughes RG, Clancy CM. Working conditions that support patient safety. *J Nurs Care Qual* 2005;20(4):289–92.
21. Grayson DB, Potter P. Do transient working conditions trigger medical errors? In: Henriksen KB, Marks ES, Lewin DI, eds. *Advances in Patient Safety: From Research to Implementation. Vol 1, Research Findings.* Rockville, MD: Agency for Healthcare Research and Quality, 2005:53–64. AHRQ publication 05-0021-1.
22. Aiken LH, Clarke SP, Sloane DM, et al. Hospital nurse staffing and patient mortality, nurse burnout, and job dissatisfaction. *JAMA* 2002;288(16):1987–93.
23. Bartel P, Offermeier W, Smith F, et al. Attention and working memory in resident anaesthetists after night duty: Group and individual effects. *Occup Environ Med* 2004;61(2):167–70.
24. Blegen MA, Goode CJ, Reed L. Nurse staffing and patient outcomes. *Nurs Res* 1998;47(1):43–50.
25. Blegen MA, Vaughn T. A multisite study of nurse staffing and patient occurrences. *Nurs Econ* 1998;16(4):196–203.
26. Landrigan CP, Rothschild JM, Cronin JW, et al. Effect of reducing interns' work hours on serious medical errors in intensive care units. *N Engl J Med* 2004;351(18):1838–48.

27. Lockley SW, Cronin JW, Evans EE, et al. Effect of reducing interns' weekly work hours on sleep and attentional failures. *N Engl J Med* 2004;351(18):1829–37.

28. Rogers AE, Hwang WT, Scott LD, et al. The working hours of hospital staff nurses and patient safety. *Health Affairs* 2004;23(4):202–12.

29. Van Drogen HPA, Dinges DF. Circadian rhythms in fatigue, alertness, and performance. In: Kryger MH, Roth T, Dement WC, eds. *Principles and Practice of Sleep Medicine*. 3rd ed. Philadelphia, PA: W.B. Saunders, 2000:391–9.

30. Dinges DF, Pack F, Williams K, et al. Cumulative sleepiness, mood disturbance, and psychomotor vigilance performance decrements during a week of sleep restricted to 4–5 hours per night. *Sleep* 1997;20(4):267–77.

31. Sexton JB, Thomas EJ, Helmreich RL. Error, stress, and teamwork in medicine and aviation: Cross sectional surveys. *BMJ* 2000;320(7237):745–9.

32. Lankshear AJ, Sheldon TA, Maynard A. Nurse staffing and healthcare outcomes: A systematic review of the international research evidence. *Adv Nurs Sci* 2005;28(2):163–74.

33. Sochalski J. Is more better? The relationship between nurse staffing and the quality of nursing care in hospitals. *Med Care* 2004;42(2 suppl):II67–73.

34. Pronovost P, Berenholtz S, Dorman T, et al. Improving communication in the ICU using daily goals. *J Crit Care* 2003;18(2):71–5.

35. Kohn LT, Corrigan JM, Donaldson MS, eds. *To Err is Human: Building a Safer Health System*. Washington, DC: The National Academies Press, 2000.

36. Ruchlin HS, Dubbs NL, Callahan MA. The role of leadership in instilling a culture of safety: Lessons from the literature. *J Healthc Manage* 2004;49(1):47–58; discussion 9.

37. Aspden P, Corrigan JM, Wolcott J, eds et al. *Patient Safety: Achieving a New Standard for Care*. Washington, DC: The National Academies Press, 2004.

38. Pronovost PJ, Wu AW, Sexton JB. Acute decompensation after removing a central line: Practical approaches to increasing safety in the intensive care unit. *Ann Int Med* 2004;140(12):1025–33.

39. Failure Mode Effects Analysis (FMEA) ASQ; The material can be accessed at: http://asq.org/learn-about-quality/process-analysis-tools/overview/fmea.html (accessed on 9th September 2014).

40. Shebl NA, Franklin BD, Barber N. Failure mode and effects analysis outputs: Are they valid? *BMC Health Services Res* 2012;12:150.

41. Thomas EJ, Sexton JB, Helmreich RL. Discrepant attitudes about teamwork among critical care nurses and physicians. *Crit Care Med* 2003;31(3):956–9.

42. Bates DW, Gawande AA. Improving safety with information technology. *N Engl J Med* 2003;348(25):2526–34.

43. Sadowski R, Dechert RE, Bandy KP, et al. Continuous quality improvement: Reducing unplanned extubations in a pediatric intensive care unit. *Pediatrics* 2004;114(3):628–32.

44. Committee on Quality of Health Care in America IoMUS. *Crossing the Quality Chasm: A New Health System for the 21st Century*. Washington, DC: National Academies Press, 2001.

45. Slonim AD, Pollack MM. Integrating the Institute of Medicine's six quality aims into pediatric critical care: Relevance and applications. *Pediatr Crit Care Med* 2005;6(3):264–9.

46. Pearson G, Shann F, Barry P, et al. Should paediatric intensive care be centralised? Trent versus Victoria. *Lancet* 1997;349(9060):1213–7.

47. Department of Health, Bristol Royal Infirmary Inquiry. *Learning from Bristol: The Report of the Public Inquiry into Children's Heart Surgery at the Bristol Royal Infirmary 1984–1995 (Command Paper: CM 5207)*. London, England: Stationery Office, 2001.

48. Argent AC, Ahrens J, Morrow BM, et al. Pediatric intensive care in South Africa: An account of making optimum use of limited resources at the Red Cross War Memorial Children's Hospital*. *Pediatr Crit Care Med* 2014;15(1):7–14.

49. Daniels N, Sabin J. The ethics of accountability in managed care reform. *Health Aff* 1998;17(5):50–64.

50. Cook D, Giacomini M. The sound of silence: Rationing resources for critically ill patients. *Crit Care* 1999;3(1):R1–3.

51. Joynt GM, Gomersall CD. Is 'more' always 'better'? Moving towards optimal utilization and of high dependency and intensive care beds by selecting the right patients for admission. *Anaesth Intensive Care* 2006;34(4):423–5.

52. Gomersall CD, Tai DY, Loo S, et al. Expanding ICU facilities in an epidemic: Recommendations based on experience from the SARS epidemic in Hong Kong and Singapore. *Intensive Care Med* 2006;32(7):1004–13.

53. Antommaria AH, Powell T, Miller JE, et al. Ethical issues in pediatric emergency mass critical care. *Pediatr Crit Care Med* 2011;12(6 suppl):S163–8.

54. Burkle FM Jr, Argent AC, Kissoon N. The reality of pediatric emergency mass critical care in the developing world. *Pediatr Crit Care Med* 2011;12(6 suppl):S169–79.

55. Studdert DM, Mello MM, Gawande AA, et al. Claims, errors, and compensation payments in medical malpractice litigation. *N Engl J Med* 2006;354(19):2024–33.

56. Runciman WB, Merry AF, Tito F. Error, blame, and the law in health care—An antipodean perspective. *Ann Intern Med* 2003;138(12):974–9.

57. Mello MM, Studdert DM, Brennan TA. The Leapfrog standards: Ready to jump from marketplace to courtroom? *Health Aff* 2003;22(2):46–59.

58. Hebert PC, Levin AV, Robertson G. Bioethics for clinicians: 23. Disclosure of medical error. *CMAJ* 2001;164(4):509–13.

59. Errors MCftpom. *When Things Go Wrong: Responding to Adverse Events: A Consensus Statement of the Harvard Hospitals*, 2006, published by the Massachusetts Coalition for the Prevention of Medical Errors..

60. Brennan TA, Sox CM, Burstin HR. Relation between negligent adverse events and the outcomes of medical-malpractice litigation. *N Engl J Med* 1996;335(26):1963–7.

61. Cole AP, Block L, Wu AW. On higher ground: Ethical reasoning and its relationship with error disclosure. *BMJ Qual Saf* 2013;22(7):580–5.

62. Parker M. A fair dinkum duty of open disclosure following medical error. *J Law Med* 2012;20(1):35–43.

63. Detsky AS, Baerlocher MO, Wu AW. Admitting mistakes: Ethics says yes, instinct says no. *CMAJ* 2013;185(5):448.

64. Matlow AG, Moody L, Laxer R, et al. Disclosure of medical error to parents and paediatric patients: Assessment of parents' attitudes and influencing factors. *Arch Dis Child* 2010;95(4):286–90.

65. Petronio S, Torke A, Bosslet G, et al. Disclosing medical mistakes: A communication management plan for physicians. *Permanente J* 2013;17(2):73–9.

CHAPTER 10 ■ SEVERITY-OF-ILLNESS MEASUREMENT: FOUNDATIONS, PRINCIPLES, AND APPLICATIONS

ANTHONY D. SLONIM, JAMES P. MARCIN, AND MURRAY M. POLLACK

KEY POINTS

1 Severity-of-illness scores can be used to better understand the clinical performance and resource allocation of providers caring for populations, to provide guidance for quality improvement activities, and to adjust for case mix differences in clinical research and comparative benchmarking.

2 Specific severity-of-illness scoring systems for critically ill children have been available for decades and perform well at the group level in predicting outcomes.

3 Epidemiologic and statistical principles are fundamental to the design, validation, and application of severity-of-illness scoring systems.

4 Standardized ratios can be used for outcomes of mortality, length of stay, infection rates, and other quality outcomes

to determine statistically significant differences of actual performance from expected.

5 Standardized ratios are created by dividing the observed outcomes rates by the expected. A value <1 indicates performance that is better than expected, whereas a value >1 indicates performance that is worse than expected.

6 Newly developed severity-of-illness scoring systems require validation to assure that they accurately predict and discriminate on the outcome of interest in other populations.

7 As medical care changes, scoring systems require recalibration to assure that they remain contemporary indicators for adjusting case mix.

8 Severity-of-illness scores assist in population stratification based on disease burden.

Severity-of-illness (SOI) measurement provides an objective assessment of disease burden so that meaningful comparisons among and between patient populations with respect to outcomes can be achieved. SOI measurement uses factors internal to the patient such as age, chronic condition, disease burden, and derangements in physiologic status (**Fig. 10.1**). In addition, many SOI measurement systems also account for factors that are external to the patient such as the application of specific treatments and therapies (**Fig. 10.1**). A well-constructed SOI index provides an effective method for integrating physiology, diagnosis, interventions, and outcomes into an objective and quantifiable measure of risk that can be used to compare clinical approaches, to enhance quality, and to perform clinical

1 research across populations of critically ill children (**Fig. 10.1**). When complemented by objective physician assessments, estimates of outcomes may be enhanced.

HISTORICAL PERSPECTIVE

Early History

Long before the discipline of critical care medicine was conceptualized and applied to children in the 1970s, there was attention to improving the quality of medical care. Nearly a century ago, Dr. Ernest Amory Codman began evaluating the long-term outcomes of patients a year after discharge to determine the benefits provided by their medical care (1). Dr. Codman's work provided a historical context for medical providers and healthcare institutions to use data and measurement to evaluate their performance against standards of patient care. His

appreciation of the significance of both the stage of disease and the issue of comorbidity when evaluating outcomes contributed to his place in the history of SOI measurement (1).

Increasingly, the need for simple, accurate, and reliable measures of patient acuity was recognized. In the 1950s, Dr. Virginia Apgar (2) advanced a newborn screening tool that remains clinically relevant 60 years after its development. Dr. Avedis Donabedian (3,4) discussed the objective elements of the physician–patient relationship as a foundation for the assessment of the quality of medical care. He defined medical quality and proposed scientific approaches for gathering data, assuring their validity, attending to bias, and evaluating outcomes (3,4). There followed a series of disease-specific severity measures for adults, which included the Glasgow Coma Score (5), the Ranson Criteria for acute pancreatitis (6), and Child's classification for acute liver disease (7,8).

Applicable to the intensive care unit (ICU), the Clinical Classification Scoring System categorized the scope of a patient's anticipated clinical needs from routine ward care (Category 1) to frequent physician and nursing assessments and therapeutic interventions (Category 4). The subsequent Therapeutic Intervention Scoring System (TISS) score represented the concept that as patients become sicker they receive more therapies such as mechanical ventilation or vasoactive agent infusions; thus, the number and sophistication of therapies serve as a surrogate for SOI (9).

A series of generic ICU severity scores developed as SOI measurement matured in the early 1980s. These SOI scores incorporated physiologic derangements as the basis for illness severity and were agnostic to disease states or organ system. These SOI systems maintained the premise of being objective,

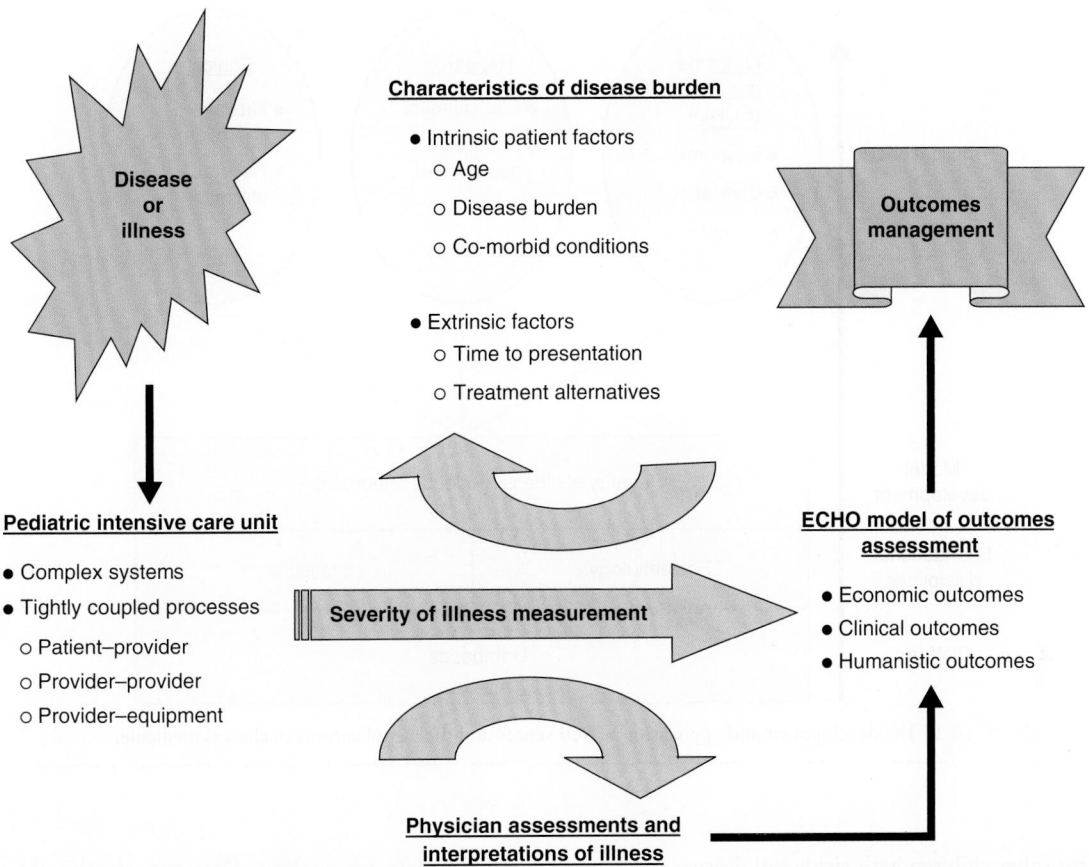

FIGURE 10.1. A model for demonstrating the relationships between the objective measures of disease burden, the complex and potentially dangerous processes of the ICU, and the iterative assessments of physicians that determine a patient's SOI and their relationships to outcomes. One purpose for appropriately measuring and assessing outcomes is that they can be managed so that clinical care is improved.

accurate, and simple to use to compare cohorts of patients. Their development was intended to identify patients who were most likely to benefit from the high intensity and costly care of the ICU. The Acute Physiology and Chronic Health Evaluation System (APACHE) was a generic adult critical care SOI measurement tool that underwent several revisions (10). Generic pediatric tools, including the Pediatric Risk of Mortality (PRISM) and Pediatric Index of Mortality (PIM), became similarly well known and have continued worldwide utilization with revised algorithms known as PRISM III and PIM II, respectively (11–14). Similar systems, the Score for Neonatal Acute Physiology (SNAP) and the Clinical Risk Index for Babies (CRIB), have been used to assess the severity of newborns (15,16).

In the early 1990s, managed care became an important concept for reducing healthcare costs. Concerns about healthcare quality led to new and innovative techniques for measuring the outcomes associated with healthcare delivery in a variety of settings, including the ICU. Outcomes represent the end result of the healthcare experience (**Fig. 10.1**). Once appropriate outcomes are identified and accurately measured, they can be managed and improved through the application of clinical standards and guidelines that incorporate evidence-based best practices (**Fig. 10.1**). The fundamental principle that allowed the comparison of illness severity across patient populations remained an evolving scientific discipline.

This approach provided the ability to compare organ system involvement, as a measure of severity, across patient populations. The premise lies in the concept of an association between the number of organ systems that failed and the SOI and perhaps death. The Sequential Organ Failure Assessment (SOFA) and Multi-organ System Failure (MOSF) scores for adults were designed to assist with comparing SOI based on organ system failures (17–19). In pediatric patients, the Pediatric Logistic Organ Dysfunction (PELOD) Score and Pediatric Multiple Organ Dysfunction Score (P-MODS) helped to advance this effort (20–22).

FOUNDATIONS

Physicians expend considerable effort during their education and training learning how to assess the severity and burden of disease. Traditional approaches include learning how to assess patient symptoms, how to objectively measure clinical dysfunction, and how to appropriately use diagnostic tests and radiologic procedures in their clinical decision making (**Fig. 10.1**). Physicians interpret this information and conceptualize a disease pattern based on what they have learned and previously experienced (**Fig. 10.1**).

This approach enables physicians to compare a current case and its disease burden to their mental library of similar cases and to prognosticate potential outcomes based on their subjective assessment of similarities and differences between the two cases (**Fig. 10.1**). For example, a patient with sickle cell disease who presents with chest pain, hypoxemia, and pulmonary infiltrates fits a pattern that can be easily recognized as acute chest syndrome. The physician understands, based

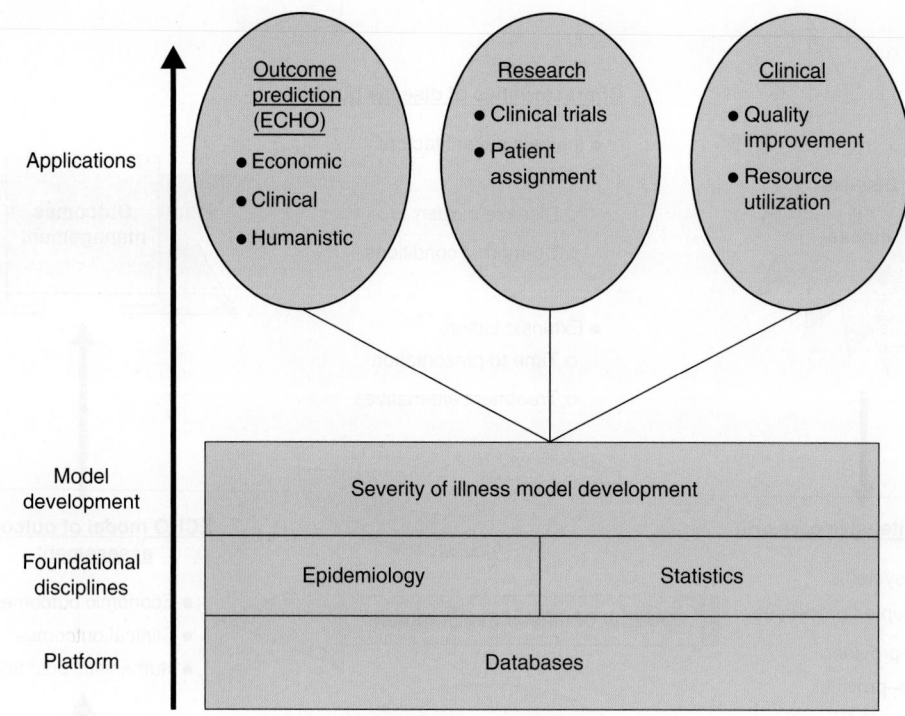

FIGURE 10.2. The development and application of SOI scores and their applications in clinical medicine.

on caring for other children with sickle cell disease and acute chest syndrome, that some of these children develop respiratory failure and that many will recover, although a few will die.

Unfortunately, the physician's assessment alone often lacks objectivity, is unable to integrate the numerous inputs of the assessment, and can be biased because of experience, ignorance, recent events, or human elements like fatigue (23). In addition, the complex care delivered to critically ill children in the ICU depends on tightly integrated and coordinated processes and systems of care to achieve outstanding outcomes (**Fig. 10.1**) (24). These process factors, and their potential failures, are often not considered by physicians in generating the range of potential outcomes. These outcomes are influenced by professional expertise and the ability to apply sound scientific principles and therapies to a heterogeneous population of patients with diverse diseases and conditions.

A well-constructed SOI measure uses effectively linked, objective measures to overcome subjective biases, guide appropriate interventions, and track disease progression over time for a given population of patients (**Fig. 10.1**). In addition, SOI measures can help to level-set different patient groups and target subgroups that will benefit most from intervention. Databases provide a major platform upon which the foundational disciplines of epidemiology and statistics can be applied objectively in the design and application of SOI measures (**Fig. 10.2**). Once developed and validated, the SOI measure can be used for a variety of applications to enhance clinical care (**Fig. 10.2**).

Databases

To effectively compare patient populations, one must understand the characteristics of the population under study. The greatest contribution to improving population analysis has been the availability of desktop computing. Databases and patient registries have revolutionized the ability to collect and organize data for analysis. Data can also be obtained from electronic health records, abstracted discharge records, disease registries, insurance claims, and patient-related outcomes surveys. Prior to using these data sources, one should consider the validity of the data. Coding errors, nonclinical abstractors, reporting bias, problems linking patient encounters or substantiating diagnoses, and truncation of the comorbid conditions can limit the characterization of the severity for that encounter. The database's accuracy can be measured through a reabstraction process that correlates the accuracy of a sample of charts to the database.

Epidemiology

The discipline of epidemiology is an important foundational discipline for SOI assessment. Epidemiology is focused on the occurrence and pattern of health events in populations. Epidemiologic practice uses data, study designs, and statistical techniques to better understand risk factors as predictors of a specific disease or outcome so that prevention, treatment, or improvement strategies might be applied. In the context of epidemiology, SOI measurement is especially important because it allows for meaningful comparisons of populations and subgroups. It is essential to verify that the populations under comparison are objectively similar so that the differences in outcome are appropriately attributed to extrinsic events outside of the population.

Standardized Ratios

One important epidemiologic tool that has been frequently used in critical care severity assessment is the use of the standardized ratios (25). The standardized ratio is the ratio of the observed to expected outcome where the expected estimate is derived from that outcome in a similar population under similar circumstances.

Standardized ratios have previously been used for the measurement of ICU mortality and length of stay (LOS) because of their importance as measures of ICU quality and efficiency (25–27). Additional standardized ratios have been used for infection rates and other outcomes of importance to ICU providers such as the use of central venous catheters (e.g., standardized catheter ratio) (28,29).

The interpretation of a standardized ratio is the same regardless of the outcome being investigated. If the ratio of observed to expected cases equals 1, this implies that the observed outcomes equal those of the expected given a similar population for comparison. If the ratio is >1, then there is a higher observed rate than expected, and if the ratio is <1, then there is a lower observed rate than expected (26). Standardized ratios can be used with statistical parameters such as confidence intervals or p values to help interpret whether statistically significant different outcomes have occurred.

Statistics

Statistics for Model Development

The statistical methods for SOI development have become relatively routine. Usually, a systematic investigation of individual variables is followed by a process to determine the most effective combination of these variables into a prediction model. In univariate analysis, the contribution of each variable or each variable range is tested for its relationship to the outcome without considering the effects of other variables. Multivariable analysis is the current statistical standard for both variable selection and the determination of the relative weights or variable coefficients in a prediction model. Often, variables that are statistically significant in the univariate analysis or that are considered important in the model are combined in the multivariable model.

Multivariable logistic regression is most often utilized for dichotomous outcomes including survival and death, multivariable linear regression analysis is most often utilized for continuous variables such as LOS, and multivariable linear analysis or quadratic discriminant function analysis is most often used for categorical outcomes such as diagnoses (30). The coefficients for the independent variables may be converted into the scoring system.

Care must be taken when developing a score or risk prediction model using multivariate analyses to avoid "overfitting," or the creation of a model that is fitted to idiosyncrasies (noise) of the data. This is most likely to occur when the number of variables included in the analysis or in the score is relatively large compared to the size of the database. A common rule suggests that there be at least 10 outcome events (e.g., deaths) per independent variable included in the analysis (more stringent) or prediction rule (less stringent). Data reduction techniques, including deleting variables known to have high measurement error, principal components analysis, deriving summary indexes, and variable clustering have been described to avoid overfitting.

Model Development and Performance

Model development depends on attention to methodological standards. The first step for the development of a generalized SOI measure is to assure that the sample population for development is representative of populations that will use the measure, but include some heterogeneity. The use of very specific sample populations for SOI model development (e.g., isolated cardiac surgery, blunt trauma) may limit the generalizability of the developed model. Second, and perhaps the most important step, is to clearly define an outcome (dependent variable) that is common, relevant, definable, and measurable. The most commonly measured PICU outcomes are mortality, organ dysfunction, LOS, and functional outcome. The next step is to identify the predictor (independent) variables. To minimize observation bias, data elements used to create a score should be selected a priori and collected blinded from the outcome. The variables' definitions need to be clear, and the frequency of measurement and periodicity need to be specified. The final set of predictor variables and their relative weights or importance are determined from candidate variables by a combination of expert opinion and statistical analyses. For example, in selecting predictor variables for a mortality prediction score, variables such as blood pressure, heart rate, mental status, and diagnosis should be seriously considered because expert opinion determines their importance. These predictor variables must be not only available but also reliably measured.

Model Reliability

Reliability may be assessed in two ways: a measurement that one observer obtains for a predictor variable is remeasured by the same person (intraobserver reliability), or it is remeasured by a different person (interobserver reliability). There are different statistical measures of reliability, depending on whether the variable is nominal (kappa statistic), ordinal (weighted kappa statistic), or continuous (intraclass correlation coefficient). An example of a potentially unreliable variable is the Po_2/Fio_2 ratio because the actual or tracheal Fio_2 when delivered by face mask is only an estimate, and children frequently do not have their face masks appropriately situated to reliably estimate the Fio_2.

Model Validation

The SOI models also require validation to assure that they can accurately predict the outcome of interest. Internal validation, or validation of the score in population subset(s) from which the score was derived, is usually performed first because poor internal validation often predicts a model's failure to validate to an external data set. There are three common methods for internal validation: data-splitting, cross-validation, and bootstrapping.

In data-splitting, a random portion of the sample is used for the model development (training set) and the remainder is used for the model validation (validation set). Cross-validation is repeated data-splitting, generating many training and validation data sets. This technique is superior to data-splitting for small data sets. Bootstrapping involves testing the performance of the model on a large number of samples randomly drawn from the original data set, with replacement (data are not removed with each sampling and are available to be resampled from the original sample/data set).

Ideally, the score should be validated in an independent (external) data set. Validation of the measure using an independent data set adds to the measure's validity and is the ultimate test whether the measure can be used for other populations. However, when the scoring system is being used to assess an issue such as "quality of care," there is no assurance that the external data set will have the identical quality of care as the data set used for model development.

Score Performance: Discrimination and Calibration

For scoring systems that predict a threshold for a dichotomous outcome (e.g., survival, death), important measures of performance are the sensitivity, specificity, and positive and negative predictive values. For scoring systems that predict a probability or continuous outcomes (e.g., risk of death), important measures of a score's performance are discrimination and calibration.

Discrimination, or the ability of a model to distinguish between outcome groups, is most often assessed by the area under the receiver operator characteristic curve (ROC). This measure is commonly referred to as the "area under the curve" (AUC) or "C-statistic." The AUC is a measure of how well a model separates those predicted to experience the outcome from those predicted not to experience the outcome (31). The AUC for the most recent PRISM score approximates 0.90 in most data sets. For example, if one places all the PRISM mortality predictions of survivors in one bucket and all the PRISM mortality predictions of non-survivors in another bucket, 90% of the time, a randomly selected mortality prediction among non-survivors would be higher than a randomly selected mortality prediction among survivors. Chance performance results in an AUC of 0.5. While satisfactory performance is considered an AUC > 0.7, most outcome prediction models should have an AUC > 0.8.

The calibration of a model is a comparison of the number of predicted outcomes to the number of actual outcomes for a range of prediction intervals. For example, one would expect that among patients with an average predicted mortality of 20%, this cohort of patients would experience an actual mortality rate close to 20%. The most accepted method for measuring calibration is the goodness-of-fit statistic proposed by Hosmer and Lemeshow (32). While the calibration of a scoring system is necessary in the data used to develop the score, deviations from calibration in independent data sets are more difficult to evaluate. Often, deviations from predicted values are expected in independent data sets because of real differences between performances of the independent data set and the reference data set from which the model was developed. As medical care changes, scoring systems require recalibration to assure that they remain contemporary indicators for adjusting case mix.

PRINCIPLES FOR APPLYING SEVERITY-OF-ILLNESS MEASUREMENT

The degree to which healthcare services deliver the intended outcomes is a measure of quality. When evaluating the effect of healthcare interventions for populations based on the inputs of the care, patient populations need to be appropriately stratified to assure similar comparisons based on disease burden. This stratification is accomplished by applying SOI instruments that can adjust the characteristics of the population and allow for appropriate comparisons. Not all SOI tools will be calibrated equally across all outcomes, and it is important to recognize that a particular measure, while useful for one outcome, may not be similarly fit to predict other outcomes in the same patient cohort. Nonetheless, a full range of patient outcome categories is important to entertain when discussing SOI measurement.

Outcomes

For the purposes of SOI measurement, outcome variables need to be objective and clearly defined. While there are a number of outcome models available, the major categories of economic, clinical, and humanistic outcomes (ECHO) make the ECHO model of outcomes research applicable and highly relevant to the ICU (Fig. 10.1) (33).

Economic Outcomes

Economic outcomes are widely available and useful in helping to understand the costs of care. LOS and costs are resource outcomes with economic implications that are commonly

measured. The LOS is a difficult variable to understand even with appropriate SOI adjustment. The LOS is a heavily skewed variable and outliers for LOS may only partially be predicted by illness severity (34). In addition, the LOS is a major driver of the total costs of healthcare. Direct medical costs include expenses such as medication or ventilator use. Nonmedical costs include overhead expenses for linens or electricity required to provide care. Indirect costs such as those incurred to improve efficiency also contribute to economic outcomes. Severity-adjusted LOS and readmission rates are endorsed as quality measures for PICU patients (35).

Clinical Outcomes

The two major categories of clinical outcomes are vitality and quality. Vitality outcomes, survival or death, have been the primary clinical outcome measures used in ICUs and are a well-accepted and endorsed measure of quality of care for PICUs (35). They occur with sufficient frequency, are well defined, and are clearly important. Quality outcomes deal with the performance or process of care and include adverse events and a variety of morbidities such as nosocomial infection, surgical complications, and medication errors. Functional status and disability can be considered within the context of quality outcomes. The currently available SOI measures were not designed to predict functional status or morbidity, only mortality.

Humanistic Outcomes

Humanistic outcomes focus on the impact of the disease or condition on functionality and health status, including disability and quality of life. Recent developments in predicting and assessing functional status at PICU discharge based on SOI at PICU admission are likely to advance outcome prediction as new SOI measurement tools are developed (36). The patient's and family's perceptions of these outcomes are important for determining how they may interpret risk–benefit profiles of care. Patient satisfaction is an example of a humanistic outcome.

APPLICATIONS

The rationale for developing SOI models is to compare the disease burden in different populations so that appropriate adjustments can be made when the outcomes of these populations are analyzed. The applications and uses for SOI models fall into several major categories, including quality improvement, clinical research, and outcomes management.

Quality Assurance, Improvement, and Management

Quality has been defined as the degree to which healthcare outcomes for individuals and populations are consistent with best practices and personal choice. Until relatively recently, quality has not been well understood. A seminal effort within the last decade defined the six components of healthcare quality as safety, effectiveness, efficiency, timeliness, equity, and patient centeredness (37). This rubric has helped to provide clarity and stood the test of time in terms of what healthcare quality means and the outcome categories in which quality could be measured.

Quality Assurance

Once clinicians began to understand what was meant by quality, they began to appreciate that there was quality work that they "have to do" and quality work that they "want to do." In terms of the 'have to do' quality work, this usually falls into the category of regulatory and compliance issues. In delivering healthcare, clinicians must follow the law and must subscribe to the regulations from the Joint Commission and the Centers for Medicare and Medicaid Services (CMS) as fundamental elements of assuring healthcare quality. This approach, often known as quality assurance, because it relies heavily on auditing a list of standards and regulations, is insufficient if the highest levels of clinical care will be achieved for patients.

Quality Improvement

The components for advancing patient care quality are the things that clinicians understand as fundamental to improving care in the PICU. These activities include avoiding medication errors, reducing hospital-associated infection rates, and minimizing complications of care, including ventilator-associated pneumonia and procedural complications. To effectively perform this work, clinicians need data and an understanding of process analysis. Only then, can quality improvement proceed. However, when comparing the rates of events across populations, SOI measurement becomes important. There is no surprise that children who are admitted sicker will tend to have longer lengths of stay, which creates more opportunities for adverse events to occur. The SOI models can help to assure that comparisons across patient populations are appropriate so that quality improvement work can proceed with valid data considerations.

Quality Management

Quality management becomes important when clinicians compare different approaches across comparable populations. This is known as benchmarking. Maximizing economic, clinical, and humanistic outcomes by comparing performance to best practices and then using similar treatment protocols and pathways can assist in assuring that patients achieve their full potential after a disease or illness. When investigating economic outcomes, like LOS, ventilator days, and costs per case, the term *utilization management* is often used. When comparing rates of adverse clinical outcomes, like medication errors, procedural complications, and hospital-acquired infections, the term *patient safety* is applied because the patient was harmed by care that was intended to help him or her. Finally, when measures of disability and morbidity are compared, the term *quality of life* is often used. Regardless of the type of outcome, all of these approaches require that SOI measurement be used to appropriately compare performance and control for population differences so that these different outcomes are appreciated.

Clinical Research

Clinical research is another important application for SOI measurement. Epidemiologic studies on the risk and outcome of disease rely on having comparable cases and controls. In non-concurrent, cohort studies, also known as database research, this is particularly important. However, assignment to different treatment arms in clinical trials can also be performed with the use of severity scores, particularly those that focus on specific diseases and their outcomes.

Future Directions: Population Management, Allocating Care, and Healthcare Reform

Recent efforts in healthcare reform were accomplished through the Patient Protections and Affordable Care Act (PPACA) and have increased the focus on improving outcomes of care. These primarily include improving healthcare quality and reducing cost. A major component of this legislation requires that populations are compared across these outcomes. Tools that allow the comparison of the SOI, both in the ICU and in the general population, are essential for assuring fair and equitable comparisons and scorekeeping over time at the population level. One of the important discussions that have already emerged in this work is how to allocate scarce resources like ICU care when patients may not be sick enough to require ICU care or might be too sick to benefit from it. These conversations about resource allocation have been discussed before and led to new and innovative methods of measuring SOI in the 1980s and 1990s. These new developments are likely to continue to advance innovative efforts of estimating disease burden and outcome in populations of patients, and SOI scoring systems will once again be at the center of the conversation.

SUMMARY

Adjusting for SOI measurement is important when measuring outcomes to assure that patient populations are appropriately compared. Confidence in the predictive ability of the SOI score depends on the quality, reliability, and validity of the data that are used to create it. Numerous factors related to the patient, including their diagnoses and the care provided, need to be incorporated into comparative scores to provide realistic predictive models of outcomes. These efforts, when performed successfully, provide an opportunity to use these scores across populations to compare provider performance on quality and resource use, to assign patients for clinical research trials, and to stratify patients for treatment protocols, and to research factors influencing patient outcomes. With time, more sophisticated techniques and larger databases may allow the application of these scores for prognostication on individual patients and for additional ICU outcomes like quality of life.

FUTURE DIRECTIONS

Despite the value provided by current SOI scoring systems, there are a number of unique opportunities that could continue to enhance their utility in pediatric critical care medicine. First, model performance depends on its ability to predict uncommon outcomes such as mortality in samples with low mortality rates. As computerization improves and managing larger data sets becomes easier, analytic techniques beyond the current approaches may allow for better and more sophisticated prediction models. Second, models of the future need to be more "dynamic." A mechanism that incorporates clinician input, in real time, to adapt the predictions provided by the static data sets used to create the SOI score could improve user acceptance and aid in clinical care. Finally, most of the ICU severity scores have focused on the outcome of mortality. Additional morbidity and quality-of-life outcomes are important focal points that need to be included as SOI measurement improves.

References

1. Neuhauser D. Heroes and martyrs of quality and safety. Ernest Amory Codman MD. *Qual Saf Health Care* 2002;11:104–105.
2. Apgar V. A proposal for a new method of evaluation of the newborn infant. *Anesth Analg* 1953;32:260–7.
3. Donabedian A. Evaluating the quality of medical care. *Milbank Mem Fund Q* 1966;44(suppl):166–206.
4. Donabedian A. *Explorations in Quality Assessment and Monitoring: The Definition of Quality and Approaches to Its Assessment.* Ann Arbor, MI: Health Administration Press, 1980.

5. Teasdale G, Jennett B. Assessment of coma and impaired consciousness. *Lancet* 1974;304:81–4.

6. Ranson JH, Rifkind KM, Roses DF, et al. Prognostic signs and the role of operative management in acute pancreatitis. *Surg Gynecol Obstet* 1974;139:69–81.

7. Pugh RNH, Murray-Lyon IM, Dawson JL, et al. Transection of the esophagus for bleeding esophageal varices. *Br J Surg* 1973; 60:646–54.

8. Child CG, Turcotte JG. Surgery and portal hypertension. In: Child CG, ed. *The Liver and Portal Hypertension*. Philadelphia, PA: Saunders, 1964:50–64.

9. Cullen DJ, Civetta JM, Briggs BA, et al. Therapeutic intervention scoring system: A method for quantitative comparison of patient care. *Crit Care Med* 1974;2:57–60.

10. Knaus WA, Draper EA, Wagner DP, et al. APACHE: Acute physiology and chronic health evaluation: A physiologically based classification system. *Crit Care Med* 1981;9:591–95.

11. Pollack MM, Ruttimann UE, Getson PR. Pediatric risk of mortality (PRISM) score. *Crit Care Med* 1988;16:1110–6.

12. Pollack MM, Patel KM, Ruttimann UE. PRISM III: An updated pediatric risk of mortality score. *Crit Care Med* 1996;24:743–52.

13. Shann F, Pearson G, Slater A, et al. Paediatric index of mortality (PIM): A mortality prediction model for children in intensive care. *Intensive Care Med* 1997;23:201–7.

14. Slater A, Shann F, Pearson G. PIM2: A revised version of the paediatric index of mortality. *Intensive Care Med* 2003;29:278–85.

15. The International Neonatal Network. The CRIB (clinical risk index for babies) score: A tool for assessing initial neonatal risk and comparing performance of neonatal intensive care units. *Lancet* 1993;342:193–8.

16. Richardson DK, Gray JE, McCormick MC, et al. Score for neonatal acute physiology: A physiologic severity index for neonatal intensive care. *Pediatrics* 1993;91:617–23.

17. Vincent JL, Moreno R, Takala J, et al. The SOFA (sepsis-related organ failure assessment) score to describe organ dysfunction/failure. On behalf of the Working Group on Sepsis-Related Problems of the European Society of Intensive Care Medicine. *Intensive Care Med* 1996;22:707–10.

18. Knaus WA, Draper EA, Wagner DP, et al. Prognosis in acute organ system failure. *Ann Surg* 1985;202:685–93.

19. Wilkinson JD, Pollack MM, Ruttimann UE, et al. Outcome of pediatric patients with multiple organ system failure. *Crit Care Med* 1986;14:271–4.

20. Graciano AL, Balko JA, Rahn DS, et al. The pediatric multiple organ dysfunction score (P-MODS): Development and validation of an objective scale to measure the severity of multiple organ dysfunction in critically ill children. *Crit Care Med* 2005;33:1484–91.

21. Leteurtre S, Martinot A, Duhamel A, et al. Validation of the paediatric logistic organ dysfunction (PELOD) score: Prospective, observational, multicentre study. *Lancet* 2003;236:192–7.

22. Leteurtre S, Duhamel A, Frandbastien B, et al. Paediatric logistic organ dysfunction (PELOD) score. *Lancet* 2003;367:897.

23. Marcin JP, Pollack MM, Patel KM, et al. Prognostication and certainty in the pediatric intensive care unit. *Pediatrics* 1999;104:868–73.

24. Slonim AD, Pollack MM. Integrating the Institute of Medicine's six quality aims into pediatric critical care: Relevance and applications. *Pediatr Crit Care Med* 2005;6:264–9.

25. Teres D, Lemeshow S. Using severity measures to describe high performance intensive care units. *Crit Care Clinics* 1993;9:543–74.

26. Pollack MM. Prediction of outcome. In: Fuhrman BP, Zimmerman JJ, eds. *Pediatric Critical Care*. 2nd ed. Saint Louis, MO: Mosby, 1998.

27. Teres D, Lemeshow S. Severity of illness modeling and potential applications. In: Rippe JM, Irwin RS, Fink MP, et al., eds. *Intensive Care Medicine*. 3rd ed. Boston, MA: Little Brown, 1996.

28. Maugat S, Joly C, L'hériteau F, et al. Standardized incidence ratio: A risk index for catheter-related infection surveillance in intensive care units (REACAT network) in Northern France. *Rev Epidemiol Sante Publique* 2005;53:39–46.

29. Sehgal AR, Silver MR, Covinsky KE, et al. Use of standardized ratios to examine variability in hemodialysis vascular access across facilities. *Am J Kidney Dis* 2000;35:275–81.

30. Hand DJ. Statistical methods in diagnosis. *Stat Methods Med Res* 1992;1:49–67.

31. Hosmer DW, Lemeshow S. *Applied Logistic Regression*. New York, NY: John Wiley and Sons, 1988.

32. Hosmer DW, Hosmer T, LeCessie S, et al. A comparison of goodness of fit tests for the logistic regression model. *Stat Med* 1997;16:965–80.

33. Gunter MJ. The role of the ECHO model in outcomes research and clinical practice improvement. *Am J Manag Care* 1999; 5(4 suppl):S217–24.

34. Marcin JP, Slonim AD, Pollack MM, et al. Long-stay patients in the pediatric intensive care unit. *Crit Care Med* 2001;29:652–7.

35. NQF Endorses Pulmonary and Critical Care Measures http://www.qualityforum.org/News_And_Resources/Press_Releases/2012/NQF_Endorses_Pulmonary_and_Critical_Care_Measures.aspx. Accessed on September 30, 2012.

36. Pollack MM, Holubkov R, Glass P, et al. Functional status scale: New pediatric outcome measure. *Pediatrics* 2009;124:e18–28.

37. Institute of Medicine, Committee on Quality of Health Care in America. *Crossing the Quality Chasm: A New Health System for the 21st Century*. Washington, DC: National Academy Press, 2001.

CHAPTER 11 ■ COMMUNICATION AND INFORMATION TECHNOLOGY IN THE PICU

STEVEN PON AND BARRY P. MARKOVITZ

KEY POINTS

1 Information technology promises many benefits but is not without limitations and pitfalls. Physicians must learn about these to develop realistic expectations, maximize benefit, ensure patient safety, and avoid potentially catastrophic perils.

2 Potential and real benefits of the electronic health record (EHR) include improved quality of care, cost savings, higher productivity, and easier aggregation and analysis of health data. Specific benefits include providing rapid access to integrated clinical data and extant medical knowledge, improving communication and adherence to clinical guidelines, and decreasing some medical errors. The EHR can also facilitate research, education, quality improvement, outcomes assessment, and strategic planning.

3 While electronic prescribing can reduce certain types of medication errors, it can also increase the rates of other errors and facilitate new types of errors. The medical information space is vastly more complicated than is often appreciated, and EHR software programs are enormously complex. Implementation requires tremendous effort by both clinicians and technical specialists to configure these systems according to the specific needs of an institution and in ways that will enhance care rather than impede it. Technology does not simply replace paper; it also reengineers care—deliberately or not.

4 Clinical decision support systems (DSSs) help clinicians make better decisions by providing timely, relevant information or by otherwise improving cognitive performance. Passive systems are activated when clinicians request help such as reference material, automated calculations, or data review. Active systems include alerts and reminders that are triggered by preprogrammed rules governing specific circumstances. Clinical DSS seems most effective when reminders are generated automatically, but this may result in "alert overload," a real and significant problem.

5 Human–machine interfaces designed to enhance cognitive performance can be viewed as decision support, particularly for the data-intense critical care unit. More attention must be devoted to developing information-priority, task-specific, and hypothesis-driven displays. Well-designed displays can significantly reduce task load and time to task completion while reducing errors of cognition.

6 Telemedicine can be used to ensure equitable access to expert medical care in remote and underserved areas, provide remote patient and provider education, reduce travel requirements, improve patient care, and reduce costs. The application of telemedicine in ICUs can allow off-site intensivists to monitor and care for more ICU patients than is possible with direct, hands-on care. Telemedicine has been implemented with fixed cameras and microphones in patient rooms and remote connections to monitors and the electronic medical record, but other implementations use mobile robots. It is also possible to implement it inexpensively with a mobile computer configured with a Web cam or even by staff members armed with a smartphone.

7 Smartphones can change the way we practice medicine. The applications most likely to be used in the ICU are disease diagnosis, drug reference, and medical calculator applications. These applications make smartphones useful tools in the practice of evidence-based medicine at the point of care.

8 Rapidly developing new technologies can help physicians better communicate, detect trouble, diagnose problems, provide more effective and efficient care, and conduct research. Knowledge of these technologies may allow physicians to take better advantage of them.

Medicine is an information service. For most physicians in general and pediatric intensivists in particular, information technology has changed the way medicine is practiced. To say that we are living in the midst of a technologic revolution is neither hyperbole nor cliché. Consider that the typewriter, slide projector, and *Index Medicus* are now dusty, obsolete relics. Consider that smartphones, the Internet, and personal computers are technologies that barely existed 10, 20, and 30 years ago, respectively. Consider the pace of change involving once novel technologies that are now ubiquitous and no longer bear mentioning on these pages. Specifically, there will be no discussion of electronic mail, personal digital assistants, security passwords, or the "magic" of the Internet. However, there will be new topics, including algorithms, smartphones, artificial intelligence, and "big data." Embrace the revolution.

THE ELECTRONIC HEALTH RECORD

Information technology will rescue healthcare from inefficiency and waste and will prevent its practitioners from drowning in an ever-expanding ocean of information and complexity. At least, that is the hope of its many proponents. From its 2001 report, *Crossing the Quality Chasm* (1), to its 2012 report, *Best Care at Lower Cost* (2), the Institute of Medicine (IOM) has documented its faith in information technology to improve quality and efficiency. This conviction also helped prompt the federal government to pass the 2009 Health Information Technology for Economic and Clinical Health (HITECH) Act designed to hasten adoption of electronic health records (EHRs) (3).

In the decade between the two IOM reports, some of the promise has been realized but much remains to be done. Potential and real benefits of the EHRs include improved quality of care, cost savings, and higher productivity. The EHRs can also facilitate research, education, quality improvement, outcomes assessment, and strategic planning. Some of the benefits touted by early research have been criticized for being results of highly customized systems built and designed by a dedicated crew of medical informatics enthusiasts, leaving the remainder of us to struggle with commercial products that may not mesh well with the way we work (4). Nonetheless, recent data suggest that having an EHR with specific, key functions is associated with high-quality hospitals (5,6), fewer complications, lower mortality rates, and lower costs (7).

The three principal functions of such a database, like any database, are data acquisition, data access, and data storage.

Data Acquisition

The complete EHR acquires data from a wide variety of sources. One of the significant challenges to any implementation of an EHR is engineering the various interfaces between it and the host of systems that feed it data, maintaining those interfaces, creating contingencies for the inevitable downtimes, and planning for the eventual upgrading and replacement of component systems.

In the ICU, data originating from bedside devices, such as cardiopulmonary monitors, ventilators, and intravenous infusion pumps, represent critical elements of the patient care record. Manual transcription of these data into the EHR is associated with inefficiency and error. Technology is currently available to connect devices to the EHR through *bedside medical device interfaces* (BMDIs). BMDIs allow properly formatted data from a medical device to flow into and update the patient's EHR. One of the challenges in BMDI relates to the diversity of medical devices and EHRs, making it impractical for most vendors to directly connect. Often, biomedical device integration systems are required to extract, read, interpret, and forward data to the EHR in order for it to be useful.

The capture of textual information, such as progress notes, nursing assessments, or even radiology reports, presents particular challenges for several reasons. Text is generally entered via a keyboard, but human transcription and voice recognition software transcription are available. Semiautomated text entry with menu systems feeding structured and unstructured forms have met with some success. Although these solutions do not have the same expressivity of free text, they lend themselves to the capture of text as data. Collecting data better allows for future analysis, but this method tends to be rigid, generally requires more time to collect, and can make documenting the unusual almost impossible. It can be a significant source of frustration for the clinician. The decision to pursue data rather than text requires an institutional commitment to the philosophy that data are more valuable and are worth the difficulties they can present. An as yet untested strategy is to allow free text entries but to apply natural language processing to extract from it data for analysis. Recognizing that most medical information is in the form of notes, researchers at

the IBM Watson Research Center are collaborating with academic centers to develop means of mining these data using the Unstructured Information Management Architecture (UIMA) used in Watson, the Jeopardy champion (8,9). (See the section on Artificial Intelligence.)

Several mechanisms have been developed to make note writing less onerous. These include preformed templates, macros to import information from other parts of the chart, automatic acronym expansion, and copying of all or part of other notes and pasting on to a new document. While many notes written with these shortcuts are verbose, redundant, and filled with jargon, the worst offense is the perpetuation of inaccuracies. A brief statement in the Office of Inspector General 2013 Work Plan noting the increased frequency of "identical documentation across services" in EHRs will receive increased scrutiny (10). Promises to review documentation practices associated with improper payments have caused many institutions to set policies and develop programs to warn their practitioners against the practice of "*cloned notes.*"

Data Access

An ideal computerized patient record should be available when and where it is needed. However, databases with sensitive information must be controlled to prevent unauthorized use or alteration. These systems must satisfy five requirements: access control, authentication, confidentiality, integrity, and attribution/nonrepudiation. *Access control* means that only authorized persons are allowed access for authorized uses. *Authentication* refers to confirmation that a person granted access is, in fact, who he or she purports to be. *Confidentiality* prevents unauthorized disclosure of information. *Integrity* ensures that information content remains unalterable except under authorized circumstances. *Attribution/nonrepudiation* means that all actions taken (access, data entry, and data modification) are all reliably traceable.

The system should be capable of providing a full, seamless view of the patient over time and across points of care. Views should be configurable so that a given user's information needs and workflow can be accommodated. Both detailed and summary views that juxtapose relevant data allow the clinician to acquire the information required to optimize expedient decision making. Displays should be configured to highlight key information while suppressing clutter but making all pertinent data readily accessible. Dynamic linkages should exist between the computerized patient record and supporting functions such as expert systems, clinical pathways, protocols, policies, reference material, and the medical literature.

Data Storage

Databases must be stored in safe and secure locations with contingencies for every kind of emergency. They must be backed up periodically to ensure against data loss, with the copies stored in remote locations to further guard against catastrophe. Developing and maintaining a strategy for seamless backup and recovery are imperative with an EHR.

Once stored, the data should retain an indelible time stamp. Although the data can be modified, both the original and the revised versions should be maintained with appropriate time stamping. Appropriate safeguards must ensure database integrity so that its pieces do not lose their links and that the data are not subject to unauthorized modification. Supplanting the paper record with the EHR as the official medical record requires thoughtful consideration of the limitations of paper printouts in being able to reflect accurately the electronic record. Sanctioned hard copies of the patient record will be necessary for sharing with other healthcare institutions or with the legal system. This may become particularly important as systems are retired after serial upgrades.

The patient database can also support many areas of research, education, decision support, and external reporting. Thus, data in aggregate can be accessed by administration, finance, quality assurance, and research personnel. A clinical database is optimized to retrieve data on individual patients. Queries run directly on these databases can compromise their performance, making them intolerably slow for clinical work. For this reason, patient data are typically copied to a data warehouse, a database designed to support data analysis across patients. Unlike the database used for patient care that must be kept up to date, the data warehouse can be more static, requiring update much less frequently. Often, data in a warehouse are aggregated from multiple sources and require a process known as "extract, transform, and load" (ETL) where the data are extracted from multiple sources, transformed to fit operational needs, and loaded on to the target database. This target database is typically specially designed to hold disparate types of data, including radiographic images and scanned documents. It should be noted that combining data sets from disparate hospitals or even within hospitals is not a trivial undertaking. The semantic structure, nomenclature, and programming aspects make combination of the patient-level data difficult. Although there is a common standard for medical data (HL-7), standards to facilitate data aggregation and analysis are unfortunately sparse. Subsets of a data warehouse that are structured to support a single department or function are considered "data marts." These subsets are designed to perform periodic analyses or to produce standard reports run repeatedly, such as monthly financial statements or quality measures.

Computerized Physician Order Entry

Perhaps the greatest benefits offered by information technology lie in the safety advantages of computerized physician order entry (CPOE). Numerous studies seem to confirm this benefit, some of which report significant reduction of medication errors (11,12) and "almost a complete elimination" of medication errors even with commercial products (13–15). The impact on adverse drug events was less marked but still positive (13–15).

While most of the single-site observational studies cited earlier suggest a benefit, many do not distinguish error severity. The minor errors are often reported to decrease the most (16). Other studies are even less positive, showing either little benefit (17,18) or an unexpected increase in mortality (19). While the ultimate conclusions of many studies seem to depend more on the author than on the specific aspects of information technology being studied (11,12,18,20–23), the discrepant results point to the possibility that the specifics of the implementation process could be a decisive factor that determines success or failure (15).

Other authors point out that while electronic prescribing reduces certain types of medication errors, it can also increase the rates of other errors and facilitate new types of errors (21,24,25). Transcription errors are the most commonly cited errors that are eliminated by CPOE (26). There are reports of increases in the rate of duplicate orders or failure to discontinue medications because of problems with the human interface (16). Other errors include orders that are written in the open chart of one patient mistaken for those of another. New types of errors include "juxtaposition errors" where clinicians intending to select one item select a different but nearby item within a long, dense pick list displayed in a small font. Inflexible data input can result in misinterpretation of orders

because important data can be misplaced or not found. Other aspects of the EHR can contribute to creating other kinds of new errors. Fragmentation of data displays can prevent coherent views of information or might induce physicians to write duplicate orders if the original order is not visible. Interface issues can lead to the misdirection of data to the wrong patient's chart. Transfers of the patient that are not coordinated with the electronic transfer of the chart may result in missed care or care delivered to the wrong patient (27).

Promises and Limitations

EHRs promise improved patient care (7,28). Potential benefits of information technology include providing rapid access to integrated clinical data and extant medical knowledge, eliminating illegibility, improving communication, and issuing applicable reminders and checks for appropriate medical actions (29).

A number of studies show that information technology can provide various benefits, including increasing adherence to guidelines (particularly in the outpatient arena) and decreasing some medication errors (26,30). However, the majority of these studies come from a very small number of institutions with homegrown clinical information systems that were developed by devoted groups of clinicians (31). Few studies show that the commercially available systems confer similar benefits, and even if they do, it is unclear that their success can be migrated from one implementation to another (16,17,32). In fact, any benefit may be outweighed by new problems introduced by the systems themselves. In effect, one set of problems may be traded for another (33,34).

Despite considerable progress, the sentiment expressed by G. Octo Barnett in 1966 is often echoed today: "It is frustrating to meet with repeated disappointments when the objectives are superficially so simple" (35). The medical information space is vastly more complicated than it seems at first. EHR software programs are enormously complex. Implementation currently requires tremendous effort by both clinicians and technical specialists to configure these systems according to the specific needs of an institution and in ways that will enhance care rather than impede it. An often unappreciated complicating factor is that the technology does not simply replace paper; it also reengineers care—deliberately or not.

Numerous other unintended consequences result from implementing an EHR, including creation of new kinds of errors, increase in work for clinicians, untoward alteration of workflow and change in communication patterns, increase in system demands, continuation of the persistence of paper use, and fostering of potential overdependence on the technology (21,24,36–39) (Table 11.1).

Human Factors Engineering

Human factors engineering (HFE) is the multidisciplinary field at the intersection of cognitive science and computer science that studies the interactions between humans and technology. Its principles can be used to help evaluate and refine the design of systems, software, environments, training, and personnel management. Some human factors principles may seem self-evident but can be overlooked when not approached systematically. Developers must understand the users, undertake detailed task analyses, and assess computer-supported cooperative work—the study of how people work within organizations and how technology affects them and their work (40,41).

Information technology does not directly impact patient safety; it affects the entire system of patient care and only indirectly produces conditions that are safer or more hazardous.

TABLE 11.1

UNINTENDED ADVERSE CONSEQUENCES RELATED TO CPOE

■ EFFECT	■ EXAMPLES
New kinds of errors	■ Juxtaposition errors in which clinicians mistakenly select an item among a long list of similar items displayed in a small font ■ Entering orders or notes on the wrong patient because a distant patient's chart is open at the bedside ■ Missed doses of phenobarbital or methadone because of rigidly enforced regulations for controlled substances to limit duration of treatment
Increased work for clinicians	■ Excessive alerts that interrupt thought processes and add cognitive work, sometimes resulting in errors ■ Requiring physicians to select precise timing schedules for medications, a function formerly performed by nurses ■ Prolonged log in processes or poorly designed interfaces that require complex navigation to commonly used functions ■ Loss of notes or orders in progress due to interface crashes or inopportune automatic time-outs and log-offs ■ Requiring structured documentation, while enhancing completeness and facilitating future data analysis, sometimes forces clinicians to find ways to fit round pegs into square holes ■ Arcane naming conventions without sufficient synonyms or search capabilities can force clinicians to spend inordinate amounts of time entering the correct order ■ Increasing cognitive work because the data required to solve a specific problem is recorded in different parts of the chart, requiring the clinician remember data while navigating the chart
Unfavorable alteration of workflow	■ Medications prepared for patients expected to arrive emergently can no longer be ordered through a CPOE system that requires the patient to be formally admitted in the system ■ Computerized orders bypass the nurse who used to "pick up" the order before it was sent to pharmacy and who would know that a medication in pill form could not be administered via a nasogastric tube or who could readjust the dosing schedule ■ Orders can be written remotely while bypassing the bedside nurse, sometimes resulting in scheduling conflicts
Untoward changes in communication	■ Users assume that the right person will see relevant information just because it went into the system, producing an "illusion of communication" ■ Consultants may write a note after seeing a patient but may edit their recommendations after leaving the unit and the primary team may not recognize that the document had been revised ■ Clinicians spend more time interacting with the system rather than with each other ■ Because all or some portion of a note can be copied from one document and pasted on to another, notes become repetitive and voluminous, sometimes perpetuating erroneous text verbatim ■ Automatic transcription of data such as laboratory results or vital signs often bypasses cognition, something that does not happen when data are transcribed by hand
High system demands and frequent changes	■ Frequent "upgrades" of hardware and software ensure the system will never be static or stable ■ Ongoing changes to the system requires careful testing and ongoing training ■ Some configuration changes requested by one group may also adversely affect other users in unexpected ways
Persistence of paper	■ Increase in paper towel consumption because it is used as scrap paper to record vital signs to be entered later ■ Reports for handoffs and medication administration may be routinely printed and discarded at the end of shift ■ Printed records used for communication with entities outside of the institution such as rehabilitation centers or the legal system may not accurately reflect the more complex electronic record
Overdependence on technology	■ Breakdown in the delivery of care as a direct result of EHR down time ■ Advice from a clinical decision support may, under certain circumstances, be incorrect and lead to a medication error ■ Overreliance on clinical alerts can lead to an erroneous medication order assumed to be correct because no alert was triggered

Human factors engineering can improve safety by enhancing the cognitive performance of the healthcare providers (42) (Table 11.2).

Interface design can significantly affect cognitive performance. Interfaces should be simple and consistent, with important data highlighted, such as the patient name or weight. "*Progressive disclosure*" means that commonly used and important functions should be presented first and in a logical order, whereas infrequently used functions should be hidden but available. Minimizing "human memory load" can be accomplished by displaying all relevant information together. Potential user errors should be anticipated, and easy error recovery should be designed into the system. Error messages should be informative and could include advice about error

TABLE 11.2

WAYS AN EHR MIGHT AFFECT COGNITIVE PERFORMANCE

■ IMPROVE	■ REDUCE
■ Improve legibility and accessibility	■ Decrease efficiency with poorly designed interfaces, slow start up, and log-in processes
■ Increase availability of problem lists or allergy lists that were often lost in the paper record	■ Bury relevant data among the irrelevant
■ Improve completeness of documentation	■ Encourage excessively long notes with copy and paste functions
■ Reduce delays in receiving results of diagnostic tests	■ Encourage documentation without cognition with automatic data dumps into notes
■ Automatically collate and sort relevant data	
■ Reduce fragmentation of the medical record	■ Increase work by introducing additional steps that were previously performed by others
■ Automatically flag abnormal results	
■ Increase availability of references	■ Increase confusion with distracting alerts

recovery. Feedback should be provided to acknowledge user actions, particularly when the system appears frozen. Given the chaotic healthcare environment, the interface should also be designed to forgive interruptions, allow work to be saved and tasks to be resumed at a later time.

Implementation

Implementation of an EHR system requires an investment of additional staff, hardware, software, and an expanded network infrastructure. For large hospital networks, the costs can be exorbitant (43).

The specific needs of the institution must be examined, particularly with regard to the existing technology and practices. The process should be viewed as an opportunity to enhance care by reengineering healthcare delivery rather than simply to replace the paper record (44,45).

Ensuring that the EHR satisfies every need involves considerable planning, designing, and testing. Even well-designed, off-the-shelf EHR systems satisfy only 80% of the complex requirements of any multi-practitioner organization. The remainder must be either adapted from other content or created from scratch. Substantial "expert" direction from teams of physicians, nurses, other allied healthcare providers, and medical records and financial staff is required to assist in developing the design and implementation of all EHRs (46). If clinicians abdicate their responsibility in participating in this tedious process, they are virtually ensuring that the resulting system will fail to satisfy their needs. Physician acceptance and participation can be enhanced by acknowledging the importance of physicians in the process, training them early and often, frequently and routinely eliciting their feedback, and demonstrating responsiveness to their needs and concerns.

User satisfaction is an important predictor of system success. Satisfaction is enhanced when the systems are designed with the users' needs and preferences in mind. Peers who serve as advocates for their groups during development and subsequently teach other users generally increase acceptance of the systems. Ease of use, rapid response times, flexibility, customizability, mobile workstations, implementation of effective

decision support tools, access to reference information, and adequate training and support are all important factors in enhancing both user satisfaction and system success (47).

DECISION SUPPORT

Clinical Decision Support in the EHR

Decision support is an interactive system designed to help clinicians make better decisions by providing timely, relevant information or by otherwise improving cognitive performance. Decision support systems (DSSs) can be passive or active. Passive systems do not trigger themselves and are activated when clinicians request help. Such assistance can come as reference material, automated calculations, or data review. Active systems include alerts and reminders that are triggered by preprogrammed rules governing specific circumstances, as when an order for penicillin in a patient who is allergic to it can invoke a displayed warning. Safety improvements secondary to CPOE systems are extended with the development and implementation of integrated clinical DSSs (12,31).

An effective DSS must have accurate data, a reliable knowledge base, and a good inference mechanism. The knowledge base can include information regarding risks, costs, disease states, clinical and laboratory findings, and clinical guidelines. The inference engine determines how and when to apply the appropriate knowledge while carefully minimizing disruptions of workflow (48,49).

DSSs can also help clinicians make better choices of medications (20,50) or laboratory tests (20,26) and thereby reduce costs (20). Clinical decision support designed to impact specific aspects of care such as adherence to clinical guidelines for specific diseases (51), administration of preventive care (52), or optimizing drug ordering (50,52) has been shown to improve quality and sometimes to reduce costs, but few studies show any benefit on patient outcomes (52). Compliance with evidence-based guidelines can be increased by incorporating these guidelines into treatment protocols (53). Use of automated reminders based on clinical practice guidelines, computer-assisted diagnosis or management, and evidence-based medicine can improve the effectiveness of medical care (27).

While our understanding of the complex interactions of clinical DSSs is limited, they seem most effective when reminders are generated automatically rather than by requiring users to ask for advice (54). Systems that advise users about existing therapies by adjusting the dose or by recommending laboratory testing seem to be particularly effective (54). Nonetheless, the safety benefits of these tools are not always clear (16), and at least one study reports that the majority of providers prefer that the drug interaction alerts be turned off to reduce "alert overload" (49).

A recent survey of commercially available EHRs revealed that not all had the full range of clinical decision support tools (55), and careful evaluation of these tools should play a role in deciding which product to purchase and implement.

Interfaces and Dashboards

Human–machine interfaces, when designed to enhance cognitive performance, can be viewed as a less active but no less important method of decision support.

Clinical information overload and medical record data inaccessibility plague clinicians everywhere, but most particularly in the ICU. The relevant data is often buried deep among volumes of the irrelevant. In the ICU, an estimated 25% of the clinical data in EHRs are never used, while 33% are used more than 50% of the time on admission (56).

Information in the electronic medical record is often organized by how it is collected rather than how the clinician uses it. Vital signs are collected by nurses on one flow sheet while the record of administered medications are placed somewhere else. Similarly, laboratory data and radiology reports are collected in separate sections of the record. Clinicians trying to answer a specific clinical question, such as why their patient is tachycardic, would typically have to hunt through multiple displays to answer that question. Each step of this hunt increases the cognitive load and ultimately makes it more difficult to provide accurate decisions in a timely fashion.

5 More attention must be devoted to developing information-priority, task-specific, and hypothesis-driven displays. Well-designed displays can significantly reduce task load, time to task completion, and errors of cognition (56–59).

In the ICU, the ability to retrieve detailed data from physiologic monitors in a synchronized fashion is important for real-time problem solving. This capability can help the physician determine the precise sequence of events and ascertain the cause of clinical events, something not easily done with only hourly vital signs recorded by the bedside nurse. Integrating these data and displaying them on a "dashboard" may improve staff efficiency, accelerate decision making, streamline workflow, and reduce oversights and errors in clinical practice (60).

The concept of real-time surveillance of important clinical data can also be applied across patients to an entire unit. Displaying critical data may help clinicians identify problems early while providing "situational awareness" for the staff (61).

Algorithms

Physiologic data may be able to predict the course of a patient's illness and may be able to identify the deteriorating patient before traditional assessments can (62–66). This premise underlies a growing area of research (and entrepreneurship (65,66)) made possible by the growing ability to collect large volumes of synchronized physiologic data from multiple bedside monitors. New technologies are also making it possible to process this data in real time. It is the processed data that might identify predictable patterns that the raw data cannot.

While the specifics of each algorithm and how it is derived are well beyond the scope of this chapter, this is an area of research that is particularly relevant to pediatric critical care medicine and certainly bears watching.

Diagnostic Decision Support

Since the IOM's report in 2001 suggesting nearly 100,000 people die in the United States every year because of medical errors, countless studies, projects, dollars, and lives have been dedicated to reducing such mistakes (1). Much of this effort is based on the presumption that patients are harmed by errors in treatment, but in fact, there is evidence that the most harmful types of medical error are related to missed or delayed diagnosis.

Diagnosis errors are much harder to study than medication errors, since they are rarely charted or tracked. A recent review of malpractice claims in the United States over a 25-year period found that the highest percentage of claims were related to diagnosis errors and that these resulted in the most harm and the highest monetary damages awarded (67). Similarly, autopsy studies consistently reveal a significant number of patients die in the hospital with undiagnosed and potentially treatable conditions (68). How physicians make

diagnostic errors has been studied, and this purely cognitive process is susceptible to several pitfalls (69–71). The most common flaw seen across the studies is *anchoring*, or premature closure. This occurs as the physician latches on to one diagnosis, closing his or her mind too quickly to consider alternatives. Data supporting this diagnosis are incorporated, while data that do not support the diagnosis are ignored. If computer decision support tools can help prevent therapeutic errors, can *computerized diagnostic decision support* (CDDS) help prevent diagnostic errors?

A recent analysis by Bond et al. (72) evaluated four commercially available diagnostic decision support programs that met their criteria for creating differential diagnosis lists, enabling entry of multiple symptoms or signs, indicating critical diagnoses (or ranking them) and were available via a hospital or personal subscription. The two most robust systems were DXPlain (Massachusetts General Hospital) and Isabel (Isabel Healthcare Inc.). DXPlain utilizes an iterative process of questioning the user, allowing more data entry (including negative findings) and rank ordering its lists to suggest the most likely diagnoses. Isabel is the only system that allows natural language entry of multiple signs, symptoms, or laboratory/radiologic findings at once, and the diagnosis lists are not ranked, though critical "do not miss" diagnoses are flagged. DXPlain, only available via institutional subscription, has links to disease definitions and to PubMed and Google searches. Isabel, available by individual or institutional subscription, links each diagnosis to a range of resources depending on the institution's access, such as to UpToDate. Graber and Matthew (73) evaluated Isabel by challenging it with 50 case reports from the *New England Journal of Medicine*, and the correct diagnosis was displayed 96% of the time. A true interventional study testing the value of CDDS has not yet been undertaken. If such tools only help keep the physician's mind open to other possibilities and prevent premature closure, they will likely prove valuable in the clinical workflow. And to minimize workflow disruption, Isabel is working with EHR vendors to have elements of the EHR trigger differential diagnosis lists automatically.

Artificial Intelligence

While there has been some success in applying artificial intelligence to support diagnosis, the technology has not been enthusiastically embraced by medical practitioners (74). However, there may be a breakthrough on the horizon that will change the game.

In February of 2011, the IBM system known as Watson won the Jeopardy! Grand Challenge. Using natural language processing, hypothesis generation, and evidence-based machine learning, Watson is able to access and assess vast amounts of unstructured data to answer questions, even those with subtle cues in double meanings, puns, and rhymes.

Watson is not just an advanced search engine with a vast database; it can process 60 million pages of text per second and apply what it learns (65,75). Using UIMA, it can read textbooks, journal articles, and evidence-based clinical guidelines and has access to that knowledge to answer clinical questions. It can also read patient charts both to apply prior knowledge to evaluate those charts and to create new knowledge through the analysis of thousands or even millions of charts (9). In its first commercial application (developed by a collaboration of IBM, Memorial Sloan–Kettering Cancer Center, and WellPoint insurance company), it provides advanced clinical decision support for oncologists and tools to assist nurses in the insurance authorization process (76). Whether this strategy will prove to be a commercial success or not, more applications of this technology are likely in our future.

COMMUNICATION

Telemedicine

Telemedicine is defined as "the use of electronic information and telecommunication technologies to support long-distance clinical healthcare, patient and professional health-related education, public health, and health administration" (77). It can ensure equitable access to expert medical care in remote and underserved areas, provide remote patient and provider education, reduce travel requirements, improve patient care, and reduce costs, and improve collaboration in areas outside of direct patient care.

Full-time intensivist coverage in ICUs seems to result in significant reductions in mortality, lengths of stay, and resource utilization (78,79). However, the national shortage of intensivists and their high cost are barriers that preclude some hospitals from providing such services. The application of telemedicine in ICUs can partially overcome these barriers by allowing off-site intensivists to monitor and care for more ICU patients than is possible with direct, hands-on care. Although remote ICU care via telemedicine cannot replace on-site care, it can supplement existing care by raising the level of expert physician coverage. In some cases, telemedicine can even allow pediatric patients to safely receive care in a local adult ICU if they cannot be safely transported to a distant pediatric ICU (80,81).

Despite early systematic reviews of telemedicine that showed mixed or negative results (82,83), there is mounting support for this technology particularly in the ICU or other, similar high-acuity settings. These studies show that the use of telemedicine technologies can result in higher quality of care, more efficient resource use, improved cost-effectiveness, and higher satisfaction among patients, parents, and remote providers (84–87).

In many settings, telemedicine is implemented by fixed cameras and microphones in patient rooms and remote connections to monitors and the electronic medical record (85–87), but there are reports of the use of mobile robots that roam from bedside to bedside (88). Telemedicine can also be implemented inexpensively with a mobile computer configured with a Web cam and wireless connection (89) or by staff members who use a smartphone.

Smartphones

Just as personal computers and the Internet spurred revolutionary changes, smartphones can change the way we practice medicine. While there are applications and peripherals that help patients manage chronic disease, measure blood pressure, monitor blood glucose, or record electrocardiograms (65,90), the applications most likely to be used in the ICU are disease diagnosis, drug reference, and medical calculator applications. These applications make smartphones useful tools in the practice of evidence-based medicine at the point of care (91).

Since most smartphones are configured with a camera, they provide a higher degree of functionality than other wireless phones that can bring telecommunications to the bedside. There are at least two series that describe the use of smartphones to transmit radiographic images to neurosurgical referral centers (92,93). It is but a small leap to suggest that smartphones can provide ad hoc video telemedicine to any bedside at any hour without the expense of the original, hard-wired systems.

MEDICAL KNOWLEDGE BASES

The vast amount of medical information that clinicians require to practice evidence-based medicine can only reasonably be managed by networked, searchable, and linked medical knowledge bases. Online search engines, accessible with natural language queries unfettered by complex rule-based search terminology requirements, give practitioners unprecedented access to medical information.

Resources available for free access online include classical original medical literature citations, such as via the National Library of Medicine's PubMed site. Powerful and focused results are now possible without understanding the difference between MeSH (Medical Subject Headings) terms and keywords. Abstracts are presented, and if the full-text paper is online anywhere, PubMed provides a direct link. More and more publishers and journals are opening (at least) their archived editions older than 6–12 months to free access on the Internet. PubMed itself is a large repository of freely available manuscripts from a wide range of journals.

Also online are pharmaceutical databases, medical calculators, textbooks, image libraries, and evidence-based reviews and guidelines, though not all are necessarily freely available. For physicians in academic medical centers, contractual arrangements between universities or hospitals and publishing cooperatives enable apparently free access to the end user if the resource is accessed from within the institution's network. Many publishers also allow free access to users in developing countries, potentially revolutionizing education and communication in even remote corners of the world.

THE INTERNET AND THE PATIENT

Not only does the Internet give ready access to the medical literature to clinicians, it also gives it to patients. This is what Eric Topol (94) calls "Medical Gutenberg," the democratization of medical information.

Some of the Web sites aimed at patients are reliable and understandable, and others are not (95). In 2006, 30% of surveyed health professionals reported that 80% of their patients were Web informed, and 63% of professionals recommended a Web site to their patients for more information (96). These numbers are most certainly higher now. The Internet can also allow access to online support groups that can reduce the feelings of isolation and can direct patients to resources of which they would otherwise be unaware (95).

The Internet can also afford patients access to consumer information on health plans, participating providers, eligibility for procedures, and covered drugs in a formulary (2,97). Some information regarding cost, outcomes, and value associated with hospitals, practices, or individual physicians can be collected and made available through information technology. Access to practical, usable, and transparent information may help improve the value of care as patients approach healthcare as consumers (98).

The increasingly frustrated consumer of healthcare uses the Internet to acquire information to manage his or her own health. Purveyors of electronic health are providing health information, decision support, and Web-based tools to navigate the healthcare system and insurance plans while perhaps influencing patterns of healthcare consumption (97).

Spurred by the HITECH legislation, the development of patient portals gives patients unprecedented access to their medical records. Clinicians consider valuable the patient's ability to review and comment on data in his or her EHR as it may increase accuracy of those data (99). For many of these portals, a delay is imposed between test result and release of that data to allow the patient's physician time to review the results and to contact the patient to discuss the meaning of those results. While intended to limit the panic that some patients may experience when the implications of certain results are initially unclear, many programs are reducing this imposed delay, perhaps encouraging physicians to address those results in an even timelier fashion.

Through patient portals connected to their EHRs, patients can communicate with their physician, obtain medical advice, or receive customized health education and disease management information (97). These portals can decrease the number of office visits or telephone contacts, readily allow for changes in the medication regimens, and better adherence to treatment (100). At least one healthcare system implemented electronic visits through these portals to substitute for some types of office visits (101). Personal health records, whether they are independently managed by patient themselves, hosted by insurance companies or by the healthcare systems to which they belong, are empowering patients to control their health information, though there may be some serious concerns over privacy and security (102).

RESEARCH AND QUALITY DATABASES

With more patient information being collected in electronic form, opportunities to exploit these data abound. In the past, the only way to aggregate relevant data was to develop stand-alone systems such as the Virtual PICU Systems (VPS). This system was developed by a collaboration of the National Association of Children's Hospitals and Related Institutions (NACHRI), the National Outcomes Center located at Milwaukee Children's Hospital and Medical System, and the Virtual PICU (funded by the Children's Hospital Los Angeles and the L.K. Whittier Foundation). It was specifically designed to understand pediatric critical care, the distribution of demographics, diagnoses and outcomes, and to form a basis for clinical research, quality improvement, and comparative data analysis exploring outcomes. The personnel entering the data are specifically trained, and the data entered is monitored for quality. The scope and implementation of the VPS has yielded an unprecedented pediatric critical care database of over 300,000 anonymized records that allows for the ongoing recalibration of severity scoring systems and for informing national research projects (103).

While the VPS was specifically designed for its purpose, there are a number of administrative databases that are available for research. These include the Pediatric Health Information System produced by the Child Health Corporation of America (CHCA, which in 2011 merged with NACHRI to form the Children's Hospital Association), Healthcare Cost and Utilization Project databases sponsored by the Agency for Healthcare Research and Quality, and Thomson's National Pediatric Discharge Database. Because these databases are not designed specifically for research, they have their drawbacks. The advantage of these databases lies in the sheer number of cases, significantly increasing the power of any studies. A collaboration of CHCA, the Pediatric Research in Inpatient Settings (PRIS) network, and the University of Utah Biomedical Informatics Core is developing an enhanced Pediatric Health Information System (PHIS) database that integrates clinical data into a common repository called PHIS+ (104).

In addition to the existing databases, there are even more on the horizon. The Health Data Initiative of the Department of Health and Human Services promises to release government-held anonymous health-related data. Private insurers, through the Health Care Cost Institute, promise to do the same for privately held data (105).

Yet another approach lies in the development of the health information exchange (HIE) that allows for sharing of healthcare information electronically across organizations and is a specific implementation of "*interoperability*," the ability of systems to work with one another. Formal organizations, governmental or independent or partnerships of public and private, are emerging to allow for HIE. The 2009 HITECH legislation provided for grants designed to develop Regional Health Information Organizations (RHIOs) (2). The potential benefits of these exchanges include increasing the availability of data on patients who have care delivered by different organizations. Through these exchanges an emergency department can access data from the outpatient health records from the numerous specialists who follow a patient with a complicated medical history, and a rehabilitation facility can access data from a patient's recent hospitalization. There is some evidence that HIE can reduce diagnostic imaging and improve adherence to evidence-based guidelines (106).

The term "big data" applies to most of these databases. Big data has four dimensions: volume, velocity, variety, and veracity. By definition, the data are produced in large volumes at high velocity with a wide variety of data types, but the veracity of the data can be highly variable. The use of big data is made possible by the increasingly powerful tools available to manage it, including high-speed processors, high-capacity and low-latency memory, and clever programs. In addition, mechanisms by which personal identifiers are stripped from the data are more robust and can safeguard individual privacy.

With clinical data collected electronically at every encounter, there are data sets yet to be tapped that are even bigger than those described earlier. Collecting and using these big data to produce the science and evidence to further improve care would support the "continuously learning healthcare system" described in the IOM's report *Best Care at Lower Cost* (2). While there are impediments to using these data based on concerns about ensuring privacy, the information captured at the point of care is a central asset of the healthcare delivery system that can improve the system's effectiveness and efficiency (107,108).

CONCLUSIONS AND FUTURE DIRECTIONS

Medicine is an information service, and critical care is perhaps the most information-intensive medical subspecialty. It is no accident that many intensivists have a particular interest in information technology, but every practitioner would be more effective if he or she possessed the skills to better manage the flow of information. Furthermore, as physician leaders focusing on information technology, intensivists can lead the way in creating a safer environment for all patients. Understanding the limitations and pitfalls of the technology and exercising caution as the EHR is implemented and upgraded is of paramount importance for success.

Technology to help us communicate, to support our decisions, and to help us learn to be more effective and efficient continues to change and improve. Awareness of these new technologies allows clinicians to take better advantage of them.

Information technology greatly enhances our lives and our work. It profoundly augments what we know and the speed with which we know it. Both our patients and we are better because of it.

Though powerful, information technology is no panacea. For us to reap the benefits without suffering the pitfalls that this technology brings, we must approach it intelligently and wisely—at least until the artificial intelligence exceeds our own.

References

1. Institute of Medicine, Committee on Quality of Health Care in America. *Crossing the Quality Chasm: A New Health System for the 21st Century*. Washington, DC: National Academy Press, 2001. http://www.nap.edu/openbook.php?record_id=10027&page=R1. Accessed March 27, 2014.

2. Institute of Medicine, Committee on Quality of Health Care in America. *Best Care at Lower Cost: The Path to Continuously Learning Health Care in America*. Washington, DC: The National Academies Press, 2012. http://www.nap.edu/openbook.php?record_id=13444. Accessed March 27, 2014.

3. Blumenthal D. Stimulating the adoption of health information technology. *N Engl J Med* 2009;360:1477–9.

4. Bitton A, Flier LA, Jha AK. Health information technology in the era of care delivery reform: To what end? *JAMA* 2012;307:2593–4.

5. Elnahal SM, Joynt KE, Bristol SJ, et al. Electronic health record functions differ between best and worst hospitals. *Am J Manag Care* 2011;17:e121–47.

6. Restuccia JD, Cohen AB, Horwitt JN, et al. Hospital implementation of health information technology and quality of care: Are they related? *BMC Med Inform Decis Mak* 2012;12:109.

7. Amarasingham R, Plantinga L, Diener-West M, et al. Clinical information technologies and inpatient outcomes: A multiple hospital study. *Arch Intern Med* 2009;169:108–14.

8. Chute CG, Pathak J, Savova GK, et al. The SHARPn project on secondary use of Electronic Medical Record data: Progress, plans, and possibilities. *AMIA Annu Symp Proc* 2011;2011:248–56.

9. Keim B. Paging Dr. Watson. Artificial intelligence as a prescription for health care. *Wired Science* 2012. http://www.wired.com/wiredscience/2012/10/watson-for-medicine/. Accessed February 27, 2013.

10. Fiscal Year 2013 HHS OIG Work Plan. *Office of Inspector General, U.S. Department of Health & Human Services*. http://oig.hhs.gov/reports-and-publications/archives/workplan/2013/Work-Plan-2013.pdf. Accessed June 20, 2013.

11. Bates DW, Leape LL, Cullen DJ, et al. Effect of computerized physician order entry and a team intervention on prevention of serious medication errors. *JAMA* 1998;280:1311–6.

12. Bates DW, Teich JM, Lee J, et al. The impact of computerized physician order entry on medication error prevention. *J Am Med Inform Assoc* 1999;6:313–21.

13. King WJ, Paice N, Rangrej J, et al. The effect of computerized physician order entry on medication errors and adverse drug events in pediatric inpatients. *Pediatrics* 2003;112:506–9.

14. Potts AL, Barr FE, Gregory DF, et al. Computerized physician order entry and medication errors in a pediatric critical care unit. *Pediatrics* 2004;113:59–63.

15. Van Rosse F, Maat B, Rademaker CMA, et al. The effect of computerized physician order entry on medication prescription errors and clinical outcome in pediatric and intensive care: A systematic review. *Pediatrics* 2009;123:1184–90.

16. Reckmann MH, Westbrook JI, Koh Y, et al. Does computerized provider order entry reduce prescribing errors for hospital inpatients? A systematic review. *J Am Med Inform Assoc* 2009;16:613–23.

17. Weir CR, Staggers N, Phansalkar S. The state of the evidence for computerized provider order entry: A systematic review and analysis of the quality of the literature. *Int J Med Inform* 2009;78:365–74.

18. Walsh KE, Landrigan CP, Adams WG, et al. Effect of computer order entry on prevention of serious medication errors in hospitalized children. *Pediatrics* 2008;121:e421–7.

19. Han YY, Carcillo JA, Venkataraman ST, et al. Unexpected increased mortality after implementation of a commercially sold computerized physician order entry system. *Pediatrics* 2005;116:1506–12.

20. Bates DW, Pappius EM, Kuperman GJ, et al. Measuring and improving quality using information systems. *Stud Health Technol Inform* 1998;52(pt 2):814–8.

21. Walsh KE, Adams WG, Bauchner H, et al. Medication errors related to computerized order entry for children. *Pediatrics* 2006;118:1872–9.

22. Karsh B-T, Weinger MB, Abbott PA, et al. Health information technology: Fallacies and sober realities. *J Am Med Inform Assoc* 2010;17:617–23.

23. Karsh B-T, Holden RJ, Alper SJ, et al. A human factors engineering paradigm for patient safety: Designing to support the performance of the healthcare professional. *Qual Saf Health Care* 2006;15(suppl 1):i59–65.

24. Koppel R, Metlay JP, Cohen A, et al. Role of computerized physician order entry systems in facilitating medication errors. *JAMA* 2005;293:1197–203.

25. Turchin A, Shubina M, Goldberg S. Unexpected effects of unintended consequences: EMR prescription discrepancies and hemorrhage in patients on warfarin. *AMIA Annu Symp Proc* 2011;2011:1412–7.

26. Mekhjian HS, Kumar RR, Kuehn L, et al. Immediate benefits realized following implementation of physician order entry at an academic medical center. *J Am Med Inform Assoc* 2002;9:529–39.

27. Pon S, Markovitz B, Weigle C, et al. Information technology in critical care. In: Fuhrman BP, Zimmerman JJ, eds. *Pediatric Critical Care: Expert Consult Premium*. Philadelphia, PA: Elsevier Health Sciences, 2011:75–91.

28. Amarasingham R, Pronovost PJ, Diener-West M, et al. Measuring clinical information technology in the ICU setting: Application in a quality improvement collaborative. *J Am Med Inform Assoc* 2007;14:288–94.

29. Dick RS, Steen EB, Detmer DE, et al. *The Computer-Based Patient Record: An Essential Technology for Health Care*. Rev. ed. Washington, DC: The National Academies Press, 1997.

30. Bates DW, Cohen M, Leape LL, et al. Reducing the frequency of errors in medicine using information technology. *J Am Med Inform Assoc* 2001;8:299–308.

31. Kaushal R, Shojania KG, Bates DW. Effects of computerized physician order entry and clinical decision support systems on medication safety: A systematic review. *Arch Intern Med* 2003;163:1409.

32. Niazkhani Z, Pirnejad H, Berg M, et al. The impact of computerized provider order entry systems on inpatient clinical workflow: A literature review. *J Am Med Inform Assoc* 2009;16:539–49.

33. Aarts J, Koppel R. Implementation of computerized physician order entry in seven countries. *Health Aff (Millwood)* 2009;28:404–14.

34. Chaudhry B, Wang J, Wu S, et al. Systematic review: Impact of health information technology on quality, efficiency, and costs of medical care. *Ann Intern Med* 2006;144:742–52.

35. Barnett GO. Report to the National Institutes of Health Division of Research Grants Computer Research Study Section on computer applications in medical communication and information retrieval systems as related to the improvement of patient care and the medical record—September 26, 1966. *J Am Med Inform Assoc* 2006;13:127–35; discussion 136–7.

36. Ash JS, Berg M, Coiera E. Some unintended consequences of information technology in health care: The nature of patient care information system-related errors. *J Am Med Inform Assoc* 2004;11:104–12.

37. Ash JS, Sittig DF, Dykstra RH, et al. Categorizing the unintended sociotechnical consequences of computerized provider order entry. *Int J Med Inform* 2007;76(suppl 1):S21–7.

38. Ash JS, Sittig DF, Dykstra R, et al. The unintended consequences of computerized provider order entry: Findings from a mixed methods exploration. *Int J Med Inform* 2009;78:S69–76.

39. Campbell EM, Sittig DF, Ash JS, et al. Types of unintended consequences related to computerized provider order entry. *J Am Med Inform Assoc* 2006;13:547–56.

40. Harrison MI, Koppel R, Bar-Lev S. Unintended consequences of information technologies in health care—An interactive socio-technical analysis. *J Am Med Inform Assoc* 2007;14:542–9.

41. Saathoff A. Human factors considerations relevant to CPOE implementations. *J Healthc Inf Manag* 2005;19:71–8.

42. Holden RJ. Cognitive performance-altering effects of electronic medical records: An application of the human factors paradigm for patient safety. *Cogn Technol Work* 2011;13:11–29.

43. Kuperman GJ, Gibson RF. Computer physician order entry: Benefits, costs, and issues. *Ann Intern Med* 2003;139:31–9.

44. Scott T, Rundall TG, Vogt TM, et al. *Implementing an Electronic Medical Record System: Successes, Failures, Lessons.* Oxford, England: Radcliffe Publishing, 2007.

45. Ash JS, Stavri PZ, Kuperman GJ. A consensus statement on considerations for a successful CPOE implementation. *J Am Med Inform Assoc* 2003;10:229–34.

46. Schulman J, Kuperman GJ, Kharbanda A, et al. Discovering how to think about a hospital patient information system by struggling to evaluate it: A committee's journal. *J Am Med Inform Assoc* 2007;14:537–41.

47. Johnson CM, Johnson TR, Zhang J. A user-centered framework for redesigning health care interfaces. *J Biomed Inform* 2005;38:75–87.

48. Mack EH, Wheeler DS, Embi PJ. Clinical decision support systems in the pediatric intensive care unit. *Pediatr Crit Care Med* 2009;10:23–8.

49. Van der Sijs H, Aarts J, van Gelder T, et al. Turning off frequently overridden drug alerts: Limited opportunities for doing it safely. *J Am Med Inform Assoc* 2008;15:439–48.

50. Evans RS, Pestotnik SL, Classen DC, et al. A computer-assisted management program for antibiotics and other antiinfective agents. *N Engl J Med* 1998;338:232–8.

51. Durieux P, Nizard R, Ravaud P, et al. A clinical decision support system for prevention of venous thromboembolism: Effect on physician behavior. *JAMA* 2000;283:2816–21.

52. Jaspers MWM, Smeulers M, Vermeulen H, et al. Effects of clinical decision-support systems on practitioner performance and patient outcomes: A synthesis of high-quality systematic review findings. *J Am Med Inform Assoc* 2011;18:327–34.

53. Hesdorffer DC, Ghajar J, Iacono L. Predictors of compliance with the evidence-based guidelines for traumatic brain injury care: A survey of United States trauma centers. *J Trauma* 2002;52:1202–9.

54. Pearson S-A, Moxey A, Robertson J, et al. Do computerised clinical decision support systems for prescribing change practice? A systematic review of the literature (1990–2007). *BMC Health Serv Res* 2009;9:154.

55. Wright A, Sittig DF, Ash JS, et al. Clinical decision support capabilities of commercially-available clinical information systems. *J Am Med Inform Assoc* 2009;16:637–44.

56. Pickering BW, Gajic O, Ahmed A, et al. Data utilization for medical decision making at the time of patient admission to ICU. *Crit Care Med* 2013;41:1502–10.

57. Ahmed A, Chandra S, Herasevich V, et al. The effect of two different electronic health record user interfaces on intensive care provider task load, errors of cognition, and performance. *Crit Care Med* 2011;39:1626–34.

58. Heldt T, Long B, Verghese GC, et al. Integrating data, models, and reasoning in critical care. *Conf Proc IEEE Eng Med Biol Soc* 2006;1:350–3.

59. Martich GD. Paradise by the dashboard light. *Crit Care Med* 2013;41:1586–7.

60. Egan M. Clinical dashboards: Impact on workflow, care quality, and patient safety. *Crit Care Nurs Q* 2006;29:354–61.

61. O'Neill AE, Miranda D. The right tools can help critical care nurses save more lives. *Crit Care Nurs Q* 2006;29:275–81.

62. Ahmad S, Tejuja A, Newman KD, et al. Clinical review: A review and analysis of heart rate variability and the diagnosis and prognosis of infection. *Crit Care* 2009;13:232.

63. Dosani M, Lim J, Yang P, et al. Clinical evaluation of algorithms for context-sensitive physiological monitoring in children. *Br J Anaesth* 2009;102:686–91.

64. Ansermino JM, Daniels JP, Hewgill RT, et al. An evaluation of a novel software tool for detecting changes in physiological monitoring. *Anesth Analg* 2009;108:873–80.

65. Cohn J. The robot will see you now. *The Atlantic.* 2013. http://www.theatlantic.com/magazine/archive/2013/03/the-robot-will-see-you-now/309216/. Accessed February 27, 2013.

66. Young S. Algorithms in the ICU. *MIT Technology Review.* 2013. http://www.technologyreview.com/news/515461/machine-learning-and-risk-prediction-in-the-icu/. Accessed July 1, 2013.

67. Saber Tehrani AS, Lee H, Mathews SC, et al. 25-Year summary of US malpractice claims for diagnostic errors 1986–2010: An analysis from the National Practitioner Data Bank. *BMJ Qual Saf* 2013;22:672–80.

68. Winters B, Custer J, Galvagno SM Jr, et al. Diagnostic errors in the intensive care unit: A systematic review of autopsy studies. *BMJ Qual Saf* 2012;21:894–902.

69. Graber ML, Franklin N, Gordon R. Diagnostic error in internal medicine. *Arch Intern Med* 2005;165:1493–9.

70. Ogdie AR, Reilly JB, Pang WG, et al. Seen through their eyes: Residents' reflections on the cognitive and contextual components of diagnostic errors in medicine. *Acad Med* 2012;87:1361–7.

71. Groopman J. *How Doctors Think.* New York, NY: Houghton Mifflin Harcourt, 2008.

72. Bond WF, Schwartz LM, Weaver KR, et al. Differential diagnosis generators: An evaluation of currently available computer programs. *J Gen Intern Med* 2012;27:213–9.

73. Graber ML, Mathew A. Performance of a web-based clinical diagnosis support system for internists. *J Gen Intern Med* 2008;23(suppl 1):37–40.

74. Ramesh AN, Kambhampati C, Monson JRT, et al. Artificial intelligence in medicine. *Ann R Coll Surg Engl* 2004;86:334–8.

75. Cerrato P. IBM Watson finally graduates medical school. *Informationweek* 2012. http://www.informationweek.com/healthcare/clinical-systems/ibm-watson-finally-graduates-medical-sch/24000 9562. Accessed June 22, 2013.

76. Terry K. IBM Watson helps doctors fight cancer. *Informationweek* 2013. http://www.informationweek.com/healthcare/clinical-systems/ibm-watson-helps-doctors-fight-cancer/240148236. Accessed June 22, 2013.

77. The Office for the Advancement of Telehealth. Telehealth. *Health Resources and Services Administration, Rural Health.* http://www.hrsa.gov/ruralhealth/about/telehealth/telehealth.html. Accessed September 17, 2012.

78. Hanson CW 3rd, Deutschman CS, Anderson HL III, et al. Effects of an organized critical care service on outcomes and resource utilization: A cohort study. *Crit Care Med* 1999;27:270–4.

79. Pronovost PJ, Angus DC, Dorman T, et al. Physician staffing patterns and clinical outcomes in critically ill patients: A systematic review. *JAMA* 2002;288:2151–62.

80. Marcin JP, Nesbitt TS, Kallas HJ, et al. Use of telemedicine to provide pediatric critical care inpatient consultations to underserved rural Northern California. *J Pediatr* 2004;144:375–80.

81. Marcin JP, Schepps DE, Page KA, et al. The use of telemedicine to provide pediatric critical care consultations to pediatric trauma patients admitted to a remote trauma intensive care unit: A preliminary report. *Pediatr Crit Care Med* 2004;5:251–6.

82. Currell R, Urquhart C, Wainwright P, et al. Telemedicine versus face to face patient care: Effects on professional practice and health care outcomes. *Cochrane Database Syst Rev* 2000; CD002098.

83. Whitten PS, Mair FS, Haycox A, et al. Systematic review of cost effectiveness studies of telemedicine interventions. *BMJ* 2002;324:1434–7.

84. Marcin JP. Telemedicine in the pediatric intensive care unit. *Pediatr Clin North Am* 2013;60:581–92.

85. Breslow MJ, Rosenfeld BA, Doerfler M, et al. Effect of a multiple-site intensive care unit telemedicine program on clinical and economic outcomes: An alternative paradigm for intensivist staffing. *Crit Care Med* 2004;32:31–8.

86. Thomas EJ, Lucke JF, Wueste L, et al. Association of telemedicine for remote monitoring of intensive care patients with mortality, complications, and length of stay. *JAMA* 2009;302:2671–78.

87. Young LB, Chan PS, Lu X, et al. Impact of telemedicine intensive care unit coverage on patient outcomes: A systematic review and meta-analysis. *Arch Intern Med* 2011;171:498–506.

88. Garingo A, Friedlich P, Tesoriero L, et al. The use of mobile robotic telemedicine technology in the neonatal intensive care unit. *J Perinatol* 2012;32:55–63.

89. Yager PH, Cummings BM, Whalen MJ, et al. Nighttime telecommunication between remote staff intensivists and bedside personnel in a pediatric intensive care unit: A retrospective study. *Crit Care Med* 2012;40:2700–3.

90. Wac K. Smartphone as a personal, pervasive health informatics services platform: Literature review. *Yearb Med Inform* 2012;7:83–93.

91. Mosa ASM, Yoo I, Sheets L. A systematic review of healthcare applications for smartphones. *BMC Med Inform Decis Mak* 2012;12:67.

92. Bullard TB, Rosenberg MS, Ladde J, et al. Digital images taken with a mobile phone can assist in the triage of neurosurgical patients to a level 1 trauma centre. *J Telemed Telecare* 2013;19:80–3.

93. Waran V, Selladurai BM, Bahuri NFA, et al. Teleconferencing using multimedia messaging service (MMS) for long-range consultation of patients with neurosurgical problems in an acute situation. *J Trauma* 2008;64:362–5; discussion 365.

94. Topol EJ. Topol on why medical Gutenberg is important for clinicians. *Medscape* 2013. http://www.medscape.com/viewarticle/778828?src=ptalk&wnl_edit_specol=16823EY. Accessed March 27, 2014.

95. Cain MM, Sarasohn-Kahn J, Wayne JC. Health e-people: The online consumer experience. *California HealthCare Foundation* 2000. http://www.chcf.org/publications/2000/08/health-epeople-the-online-consumer-experience. Accessed September 20, 2012.

96. Podichetty VK, Booher J, Whitfield M, et al. Assessment of internet use and effects among healthcare professionals: A cross sectional survey. *Postgrad Med J* 2006;82:274–9.

97. Goldsmith J. The Internet and managed care: A new wave of innovation. *Health Aff (Millwood)* 2000;19:42–56.

98. Yong PL, Saunders RS, Olsen L; for Institute of Medicine (US) Roundtable on Evidence-Based Medicine. *The Healthcare Imperative: Lowering Costs and Improving Outcomes: Workshop Series Summary.* Washington, DC: The National Academies Press, 2010. http://www.nap.edu/openbook.php?record_id=12750. Accessed March 27, 2014.

99. Siteman E, Businger A, Gandhi T, et al. Clinicians recognize value of patient review of their electronic health record data. *AMIA Annu Symp Proc* 2006;2006:1101.

100. Ammenwerth E, Schnell-Inderst P, Hoerbst A. Patient empowerment by electronic health records: First results of a systematic review on the benefit of patient portals. *Stud Health Technol Inform* 2011;165:63–7.

101. Walters B, Barnard D, Paris S. "Patient portals" and "e-visits". *J Ambul Care Manage* 2006;29:222–4.

102. Paton C, Hansen M, Fernandez-Luque L, et al. Self-tracking, social media and personal health records for patient empowered self-care. Contribution of the IMIA Social Media Working Group. *Yearb Med Inform* 2012;7:16–24.

103. Wetzel RC. The virtual pediatric intensive care unit. Practice in the new millennium. *Pediatr Clin North Am* 2001;48:795–814.

104. Narus SP, Srivastava R, Gouripeddi R, et al. Federating clinical data from six pediatric hospitals: Process and initial results from the PHIS+ consortium. *AMIA Annu Symp Proc* 2011;2011:994–1003.

105. Fineberg HV. A successful and sustainable health system—How to get there from here. *N Engl J Med* 2012;366:1020–7.

106. Bailey JE, Wan JY, Mabry LM, et al. Does health information exchange reduce unnecessary neuroimaging and improve quality of headache care in the emergency department? *J Gen Intern Med* 2013;28:176–83. http://www.ncbi.nlm.nih.gov/pubmed/22648609. Accessed September 21, 2012.

107. Murdoch TB, Detsky AS. The inevitable application of big data to health care. *JAMA* 2013;309:1351–2.

108. Larson EB. Building trust in the power of "big data" research to serve the public good. *JAMA* 2013;309:2443–4.

CHAPTER 12 ■ LEARNING FROM THE DATA—DISCOVERY INFORMATICS FOR CRITICALLY ILL CHILDREN

RANDALL C. WETZEL

KEY POINTS

1 Meaningful use of digital data

2 The importance of "Big Data" in healthcare—discovery informatics using clinical data

3 The challenge of data management in the PICU

4 Learning from the data—knowledge discovery

5 The Virtual PICU

6 Use of clinical data registries for research

7 Challenges to learning from the data—computer engineering and architecture

8 Use of artificial intelligence for data analysis

The collection, analysis, interpretation, and application of data from myriad medical transactions occurring during healthcare processes will improve healthcare and patients' outcomes in the next decade more than the biomedical sciences have in the last century (1,2). At the moment, this hope is perhaps more hype than reality; however, the promise is being realized daily in pediatric critical care medicine. Since the beginning of medicine we have been exhorted to pay attention to the patient's data, to examine the evidence of disease, and to learn from our practice. This has not changed—what is changing is the information technology revolution that will radically assist our ability to do this and thus improve the care we provide our patients through what the National Science Foundation calls *Discovery Informatics* (3).

MEANINGFUL USE OF MEDICAL DATA—CAPTURE, INGEST, CURATE, ANALYZE, AND LEARN

Building on a growing awareness of the importance of information technology in healthcare signaled by the 2009 Health Information Technology for Economic and Clinical Health (HITECH) Act, Medicare and Medicaid Electronic Health Records (EHR) Incentive Programs now provide financial incentives for the "meaningful use" of certified EHR technology to improve patient care. To receive an EHR incentive payment, providers must show that they are "meaningfully using" their EHRs by meeting thresholds for a number of objectives. Centers for Medicare & Medicaid Services (CMS) has established the objectives for "meaningful use" that eligible professionals, eligible hospitals, and critical access hospitals must meet to receive an incentive payment. The enthusiasm of the federal government for the installation, adoption, and use of information technology for healthcare is evident by CMS's commitment of 27 billion dollars for the

meaningful use initiative. Nevertheless, there is a problem: "right now computational and biomedical research travel largely on uncoordinated parallel tracks" (4). Since 2000 the National Institute of Health (NIH) and National Library of Medicine (NLM) have launched scores of initiatives to bring the fruits of computation to healthcare such as the **Biomedical Information Science and Technology Initiative (BISTI), which** bridges all NIH institutes (www.bisti.nih.gov). "People might make an algorithmic advance that will eventually have some impact in biomedical research but it's not a coordinated effort. . . . The two fields speak different languages, so it's really tough to translate state of the art developments in computer science, artificial intelligence (AI) and math into things that will be useful in biomedical research" (4). Although this is a necessary first step, the meaningful use of complex healthcare data will require more than just installing EHRs.

Healthcare generates massive amounts of data. We have continuously captured clinical data, laboratory results, mountains of clinician notes (doctors, nurses, social workers, etc.), business information, diagnostic coding, therapeutic data, and even outcomes data. In addition, to this great volume of data, there is obviously great variety in the data collected and increasingly stored, and the data come at us with great velocity—overwhelming our human data management systems. We all suspect that these data have great value and they also have the quality of veracity—that is, they tell us what has occurred around patient care process, often in great detail. These five v's, volume, velocity, variety, value, and veracity, attributes of medical data, are the same as those frequently used to describe so-called 'Big Data.' Big Data can be loosely described as massive amounts of data that pose new and overwhelming challenges for "traditional" data management and computational approaches. The challenge of Big Data, in turn, has led to innovative developments in acquiring, curating, storing, and analyzing very large amounts of continuously streaming data – such as we increasingly see in healthcare (5,6).

114

Big Data is all around us. Each engine of the jet flying from Los Angeles to New York generates 10 TB of data every 30 minutes. In 2013 Internet data, mostly user-contributed, will account for 1000 exabytes (an exabyte is a unit of information equal to one quintillion [10^{12}] bytes). Open weather data collected by the National Oceanic and Atmospheric Association have an annual estimated value of $10 billion. Every day we create 2.5 quintillion bytes of data. Ninety percent of the data in the world today have been created in the past 2 years. Google receives 2 million search requests *every minute*, and responds to these requests with innovative machine learning (ML) search technologies. Every industry has benefited from the capture and analysis of Big Data often in real time. The recent America's cup victory by the Oracle Team USA was powered by real-time Big Data analytics analyzing gigabytes of data per hour during and after each race. Formula 1 motor racing has become a Big Data–driven exercise, informing drivers in real time, organizing pit stops, and redesigning and rebuilding the race cars (Peter van Mannan's Ted talk: https://www.ted.com/talks/peter_van_manen_how_can_formula_1_racing_help_babies, to understand this and how it is being applied in neonatal critical care.)

Like these sports, our specialty is time constrained, valuable, high-risk, mission critical, requires teamwork, and is very complex. Yet the care we deliver in our ICUs continues to be driven by what the human eye sees, the ear hears, and the brain analyzes. Although our brains are superior analytic and pattern recognition biologic entities, the data upon which they act are often limited and often dependent on human attention and recall, and influenced by memory, bias, prejudice, exhaustion, distraction, and other systematic sources of human error. All of this is based on our practice experience, and we revere the ability to recall clinical experience and combine these actual experiences into clinical anecdotes upon which we base a significant amount of our practice. Unfortunately, recall is our problem; practice is long, but memory short.

> "Discovery Informatics focuses on computing advances aimed at identifying scientific discovery processes that require knowledge assimilation and reasoning and applying principles of intelligent computing and information systems in order to understand, automate, improve and innovate any aspect of those processes."
>
> *Yolanda Gil, NSF workshop on Discovery Informatics (3)*

Fortunately, we are living in the revolutionary era of Big Data. Many segments of our economy have been radically transformed by collecting, analyzing, and learning from large amounts of data captured during their normal production processes. Whether this is used to improve manufacturing, to enhance the value of social media, to provide marketing advantages or for national security reasons, Big Data and its analysis are currently all the rage and are here to stay. In research, a recent *Nature* editorial commented: "Researchers need to adapt their institutions and practices in response to torrents of new data—and need to complement smart science with smart searching" (7). This adaptation is urgent in healthcare. Perhaps the last great domain waiting to benefit from the acquisition and analysis of Big Data is healthcare—although this is rapidly changing. Recently, the Human Genome Project in the 1990s has done for healthcare Big Data research what President Kennedy's commitment to go to the moon in 1963 did for computer science.

At its heart, analysis of Big Data is about discovering new knowledge and therefore about learning. It can inform us about quality improvement, process improvement, process efficiency, safety, and product reliability, and can reveal

insights about how best to manage our patients—surely the most important topics in healthcare today. We need to both improve and accelerate the data, to predictive modeling, to therapeutic action cycle to achieve the dual goals of improving care while bringing down costs. This approach will improve not just our clinical care but also many aspects of the practice of intensive care medicine (**Fig. 12.1**).

Surely we can bring to bear an information technology "cognitive prosthesis" to enhance our skills and ensure that what actually happens to our patients is accurately recalled and analyzed. These captured data, detailing medical interactions and their outcomes, can be used to enhance and expand our experience. Furthermore, the amount of information in our ICUs has burgeoned. When care was informed by looking at paper flow sheets of a few vital signs recorded every 15 minutes, human ability to analyze these sparse data was not strained. Now critical care requires the interpretation of multiple waveforms, combined with blood gases, laboratory results, MRIs, and the data streaming from our observational armamentarium of what is occurring within our patients. It is daunting. Additionally, that may be only 1 of 20 patients who are critically ill in an ICU. Engineers would consider the data management of a single ICU a streaming terabyte problem. Yet our practice has changed little, while the world around us has been transformed by Big Data analytics. Add to this the often quoted realization pointed out by Miller in 1956: "The span of absolute judgment and the span of immediate memory impose severe limitations on the amount of information that humans are able to receive, process, and remember." This has been referred to as the *Magic Number 7* (8). The observation that we are limited to managing only seven continuous data streams at a time suggests that managing hundreds of simultaneous data streams from scores of patients is not merely a daunting (if not impossible) task but one that might be expected to be rife with error, missed information, poor safety, poor quality, little time to reflect on patient care issues, frustration, and bad outcomes.

In this setting of streams of data telling us how our patients are responding, intensivists must not only consume and process these data but also take into account what we are doing to our patients. There are myriad transactional occurrences for every child in the ICU every hour from drips, to ventilators, to drug infusions and injections, sedation, paralysis, antibiotics dialysis, and the results of all of the interventions. These transactions occur during the continuous collection of physiologic data from critically ill children. The intensivist is expected to not only observe but also analyze and act on this information for the benefit of our patients. In this sea of data, what is a clinician to do? How can he or she avoid drowning in the continuous barrage of voluminous, variable, high-velocity data and instead learn from it to guide practice-the care of our next patient? This is essentially the informatics challenge to which many industries have risen, and that healthcare is just discovering. Finally, we must also learn from these data. This is called practice-based learning or evidence-based healthcare (2). Appropriate data management will allow us to continuously learn from routinely collected healthcare data (9).

Thankfully, we live in a connected, computationally sophisticated world (**Fig. 12.2**). There is little new about the call to observe and learn from our patients; after all, Hippocrates exhorted us to carefully collect and record the evidence about patients and their illnesses, and to learn from that data to help our future patients. In fact, healthcare is based on the careful observation of patients and how they respond to our interventions—these all form natural experiments from which we can learn. In fact, failure to learn from our practice and experience is an unethical failure of our responsibility to our next patient. Yet in our ICUs, we have done literally millions of experiments, captured and perhaps even observed the data—but then

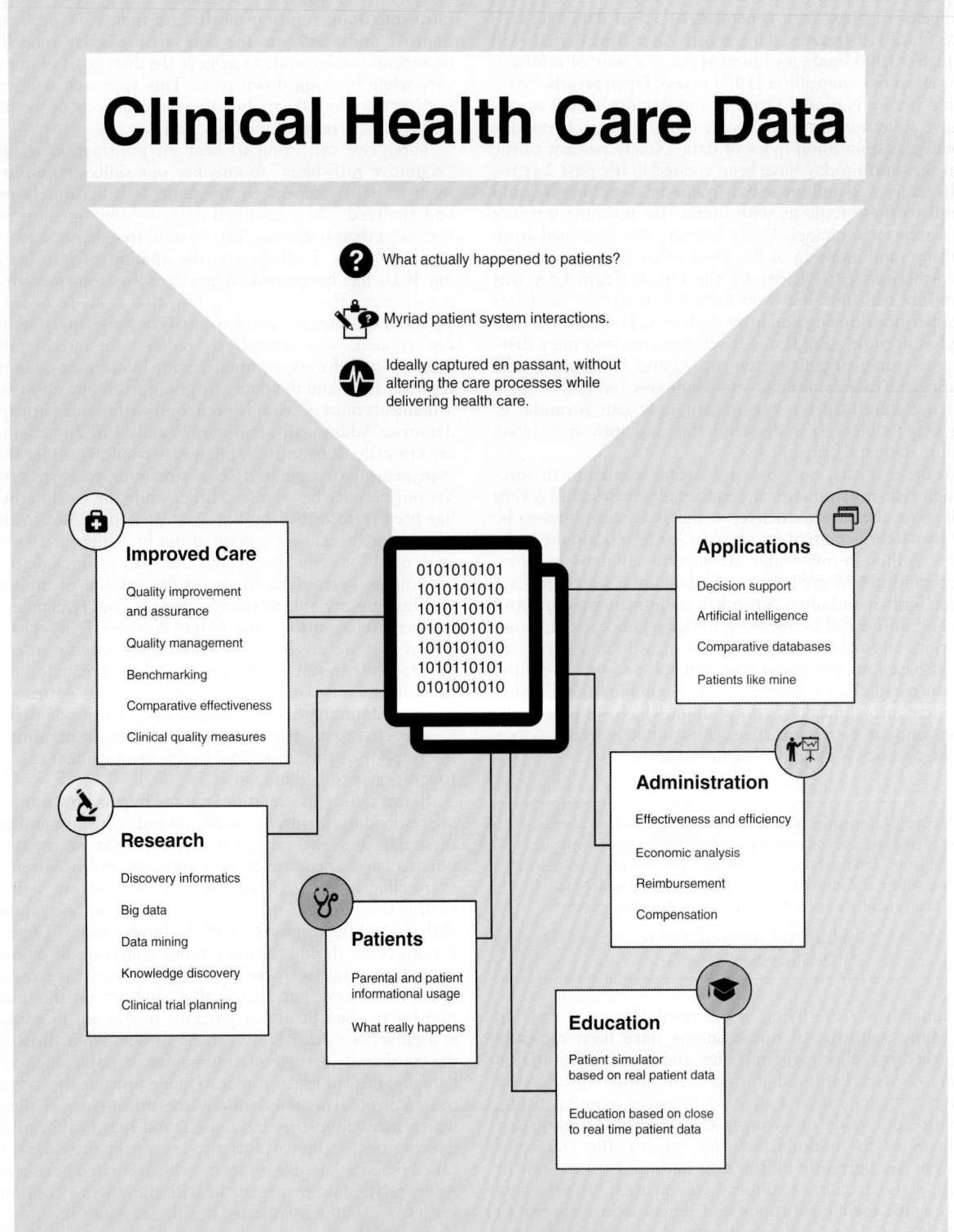

Clinical Health Care Data

? What actually happened to patients?

? Myriad patient system interactions.

Ideally captured en passant, without altering the care processes while delivering health care.

0101010101
1010101010
1010110101
0101001010
1010101010
1010110101
0101001010

Improved Care

Quality improvement and assurance

Quality management

Benchmarking

Comparative effectiveness

Clinical quality measures

Applications

Decision support

Artificial intelligence

Comparative databases

Patients like mine

Research

Discovery informatics

Big data

Data mining

Knowledge discovery

Clinical trial planning

Administration

Effectiveness and efficiency

Economic analysis

Reimbursement

Compensation

Patients

Parental and patient informational usage

What really happens

Education

Patient simulator based on real patient data

Education based on close to real time patient data

FIGURE 12.1. This figure shows the potential of gathering and analyzing Big Data in multiple critical areas of critical care. There is probably no area, that will not be enhanced by the critical application of Big Data analytics.

thrown it away, not subjected it to analysis, and failed to learn from it. Until recently, with the advent of the EHR, accessing large amounts of detailed clinical data has been extremely difficult. But we live in a different world. What is new is the informatics era in which we live that enables us to do this in an increasingly effective fashion.

So how do we learn from the data generated in terabyte quantities as we practice every day? There are many ways to learn: experientially, didactically, interactively, and, yes, in healthcare, anecdotally—by our practice and experience—often dependent on our recall. Yet we have come to mistrust the anecdote, and for good reasons based to some extent on

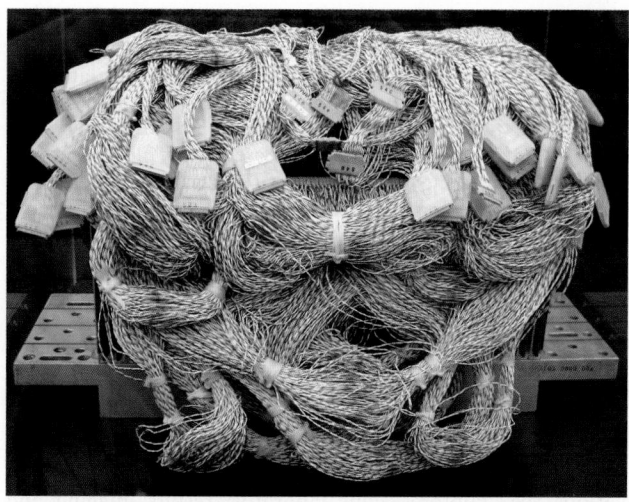

FIGURE 12.2. In 1995, the epitome of computational excellence was Seymour Cray's computer made up of "Cray bricks," each weighing over 20 pounds and approximately 2 cubic feet in size, connected by thousands of wires and cabled to multiple output devices, filling a room. Data had to be manually input. Who could have imagined that 20 years later a supercomputer smaller than a textbook would be economical enough to be given to school students and, what's more, it would connect to the sum of mankind's knowledge, without cables? Think about the i-PAD with which the 2-year-old child interacts with its world.

the failure of human recall. Instead, we have relied on experimental testing and the powerful research tool of falsification of hypothesis—so-called evidence-based medicine. The "evidence" is that derived from carefully controlled clinical trials or well-designed observational studies. These are increasingly hard to perform, expensive, and often unable to be performed owing to the lack of clinical equipoise; and although valid, results may lack external validity and only poorly inform what we can do for our next patient (is my patient like these patients?), and require internal validity and exacting experimental test statistics. This tool has served medicine well. Nevertheless, not surprisingly, intensivists frequently lament that only a minority of our practice is evidence based and that the majority of our practice is unexamined, resulting in idiosyncratic, diverse, and often contradictory management of equivalent patients by multiple intensivists across many ICUs. Clearly, there are large parts of intensive care that require further knowledge discovery to determine optimal therapies and best practices and to improve outcomes.

Research is the discovery of new knowledge, the recognition of new relationships, and the understanding of fundamental processes. For thousands of years of human existence, new knowledge was discovered empirically—by observation and deduction, relying on the accurate collection of data from which conclusions could be drawn. If the observations were "true," then the deductions were true. These provided experimental proofs. Yet our human ability to maintain and manage sufficient data, and recall it accurately without bias is limited, and thus this limited the power of deduction to move us forward as rapidly as the new inductive method of science. Falsification of hypothesis was a way to know what was *not true*, and if we failed experimentally to falsify the null hypothesis, the hypothesis was upheld—at least until it too fell to the sword of disproof. This is a very powerful experimental technique at the heart of the scientific method that has revolutionized healthcare. Demonstrate once with good experimental design that a therapy is of no value, and it falls out of use. Failure to support the null hypothesis—there is no difference

between a drug and a placebo—and the drug is adopted. But this too is now failing. And we live in a different world.

It is now possible to precisely capture myriad observations of what happens to our patients. Of course, in our postmodern age, we are highly skeptical of "truth." Nevertheless, we daily base our practice, treat our patients, and observe their outcomes on the basis of what is recorded at the bedside, reported from the laboratory or imaged. These data are all recorded, captured, and available for observation of what happened in the natural experiments that occur during the healthcare process. We have treated millions of critically ill children, yet failed to learn from the majority of the data in an organized, rational fashion. This is immoral and has got to stop. Using the same informatics tools available throughout other industries—used to make race cars faster, market products better, understand population behaviors, weather patterns, and more—medicine can learn from the thousands of patient healthcare interactions that occur every day (1,2,5,6).

Now that we can capture large volumes of high-variety, high-velocity, and high-value clinical data can we learn from it? The implications for scientific discovery are fundamental. The old style of discovery was to identify a medical problem, ask answerable questions (pose a disprovable hypothesis), collect data, and answer the questions. The Big Data way is to identify collected, valid data, identify questions from the data, mine the data, and answer the questions. This is a major scientific paradigm shift. Nevertheless, it will only produce value when rigorously executed and controlled and statistically supported. It is the experimental rigor in data utilization that frees anecdote (stories from which we learn) from error. Practice guided by accurate, multiple, serial anecdotes based on healthcare data is evidence-based medicine and provides a source of knowledge learned from the observations around the care we provide. How do we get there?

In 1997, the Virtual PICU (VPICU; www.picu.net) was founded by a group of pediatric intensivists with the mission to create a common information space for the caregivers providing critical care for children and their families (10). Since that time, information technologies enabling distance learning, telemedicine, quality improvement, and data analysis have been explored. A principal goal has always been to learn from the data generated around caring for critically ill children and to share that knowledge. A spin-off of the VPICU is an independent company owned by two children's hospitals and the Children's Hospital Association called VPS, LLC (www.myvps.org). The mission of VPS is to inform intensivists about their practice and how it compares with the practice of others around the country. Currently, more than 130 ICUs have contributed data about all of their PICU admissions for

---

VPICU Vision

We will create a common information space for the international community of care givers providing critical care for children. Every critically ill child will have access to the Virtual PICU which will provide the essential information required to optimize their outcome

---

more than 700,000 critically ill children. All of those data is severity of illness adjusted (PIM, PRISM, PELOD), and all of the data is captured by trained data collectors, validated, confirmed by VPS, and available for comparative reporting and research. More than 100 research papers have been published using this data repository. Hundreds of hospital QA projects have been supported, and we now have a better understanding of how critical care is practiced for children in the United States (11).

VPS is not unique. There are other data registries that have collected both data from patients in other areas of healthcare (12). These can largely be divided into clinical, administrative, and research database types, depending on their original purpose—although all may serve the goal of improving healthcare for patients. These databases provide a rich source of potentially new knowledge to improve healthcare. Recently, Lauer and D'Agostino described "The Randomized Registry Trial the Next Disruptive Technology in Clinical Research?" They observed (13):

"Today we can no longer afford to undertake randomized effectiveness trials that cost tens or hundreds of millions of dollars. But today we also have registries and other powerful digital platforms. Today it may be possible to design and conduct megatrials with what we have: bigger data and smaller budgets. Yet we must also recognize and acknowledge the daunting challenges that diverse groups of researchers and stakeholders must overcome to get there."

This description clearly recognizes the value of the data from the care process that have already been collected.

An example of such a trial in pediatric critical care is that of Gupta et al. (14), comparing high-frequency oscillatory ventilation (HFOV) with conventional ventilation (CV) in acute respiratory failure (ARF) in children retrospectively by analyzing prospectively collected VPS data. It demonstrated the utility of such methodology in a pediatric critical care population. Using an advanced statistical technique called propensity score matching, they were able to compare the efficacy of HFOV in 889 children with CV having matched both populations in more than 50 dimensions of data, including severity of illness. Although the patients were not classically randomized to treatment groups, the use of clinical decisions about ventilation by many intensivists from multiple (98) different ICUs, for patients who were rigorously matched to those who did not receive HFOV, presented a reasonable argument for matched populations given alternative therapies in which to compare outcomes. The results demonstrated that children receiving HFOV had significantly increased length of ventilation, increased length of ICU stay, and increased mortality with standardized mortality ratios (SMRs, actual/expected deaths) compared with the conventionally treated group. The SMR was >2 for the HFOV group and <0.75 for the conventional group. These results in pediatric critical care ARF based on nearly 900 episodes of HFOV represent the largest report of the efficacy of HFOV in children. It is a study that would be prohibitively expensive to design and perform prospectively and must be considered when choosing oscillatory ventilation in children with ARF in the future.

Another application of Big Data analytics was reported by Berry et al. (15) performing a retrospective cohort analysis to provide a longitudinal, multi-institutional study demonstrating the growing population and concentration of chronically ill children in large freestanding children's hospitals. This study involved 28 hospitals and more than 2 million hospital admissions, and used the Pediatric Health Information System (PHIS) managed database by the Children's Hospital Association containing administratively collected data.

Numerous other such trials, using already collected, high-quality clinical data, are underway, and as pointed out by Lauer and D'Agostino (13): "Because the registry trial is inexpensive, investigators can enroll large numbers of patients, thus offering clinicians insights that are potentially based on a representative sample, a real-world population created from consecutively enrolled registry patients." In other words, results learned from the evidence of what actually happened in the clinical setting. Gupta et al. (14) reported, "Further studies using large clinical databases may provide evidence of efficacy (or lack thereof) for other commonly used therapeutic interventions in critical care that may be difficult to study with classic prospective randomized controlled trials due to expense, logistics, and clinical balance." Use of such databases for comparative effectiveness research may, in the future, shorten the discovery cycle, decrease the cost of discovery, and guide us in improving outcomes for critically ill patients. In another study using propensity score matching and a clinical database, Kothari and coworkers (16) reported that the treatment of hypotension with pressors in critically ill adults decreased both the duration and the severity of hypotension but (paradoxically) significantly increased ICU length of stay, serum creatinine, and in-hospital mortality. Taken together, these reports demonstrate that large datasets gleaned from clinical records have important information for our practice of critical care.

These examples illustrate the utility of analyzing data that have been previously collected. To truly benefit from Big Data analytics in healthcare, it is necessary to capture the observations, the symptoms, signs, laboratory results, imaging, and other tests (not to mention the increasing ability to genetically define our patients' makeup) and learn how to best analyze the millions of details from thousands of patients and derive new knowledge about patient care. This has the potential to decrease the time to discovery and inform clinical decisions creating true learning organizations based on analysis of accurately captured clinical data. Of course, the advent of digital data from our monitors captured by our EHRs makes this tantalizingly possible (5).

It is now possible to truly consider:

- Automated, electronic data collection from the care process.
- Data analysis including data clustering and data mining.
- Effectiveness research among scores of ICUs with thousands of patients.
- Date-driven analysis and decision support.
- Care based on 10,000s of similar previous patients and their outcomes for the next patient.

All of these would be based on observations from clinical transactions of what actually happened—clinical evidence-based practice. This will require capturing (extracting) data from various clinical sources, transforming the data into analyzable data products, analyzing complex medical data using both classic and advanced analytic techniques including ML and AI, and finally making the information and knowledge learned from the clinical data available to guide the care of the next patient in the ICU through both education and decision support.

There are many barriers to such data acquisition. To bring data together from disparate clinical databases, which are often idiosyncratic to a given hospital, of uncertain and idiosyncratic semantic architecture, and trapped in proprietary data systems (vendor lock), for analysis and research is an extremely challenging task. Although, these pose many challenging problems, they are not insurmountable. We have previously described an architectural schema to enable the retrieval of clinical data from disparate data sources and prepare useful multiple clinical data products that can serve research, quality improvement, and decision support needs (Fig. 12.3) (17,18). Acquiring data from clinical systems requires informatics skills and computer engineers and is not trivial. Vendors of EHR systems do not readily share their data in a format useful for further analysis. Clinicians and hospital administrators do not value such use of clinical data. Of course, access to medical data with all of the moral, ethical, and legal issues around privacy, HIPAA, and the necessary requirement to protect confidential private health information are important considerations. Technological solutions to all of these issues are available; however, governance of the data and data security

Participating Hospital

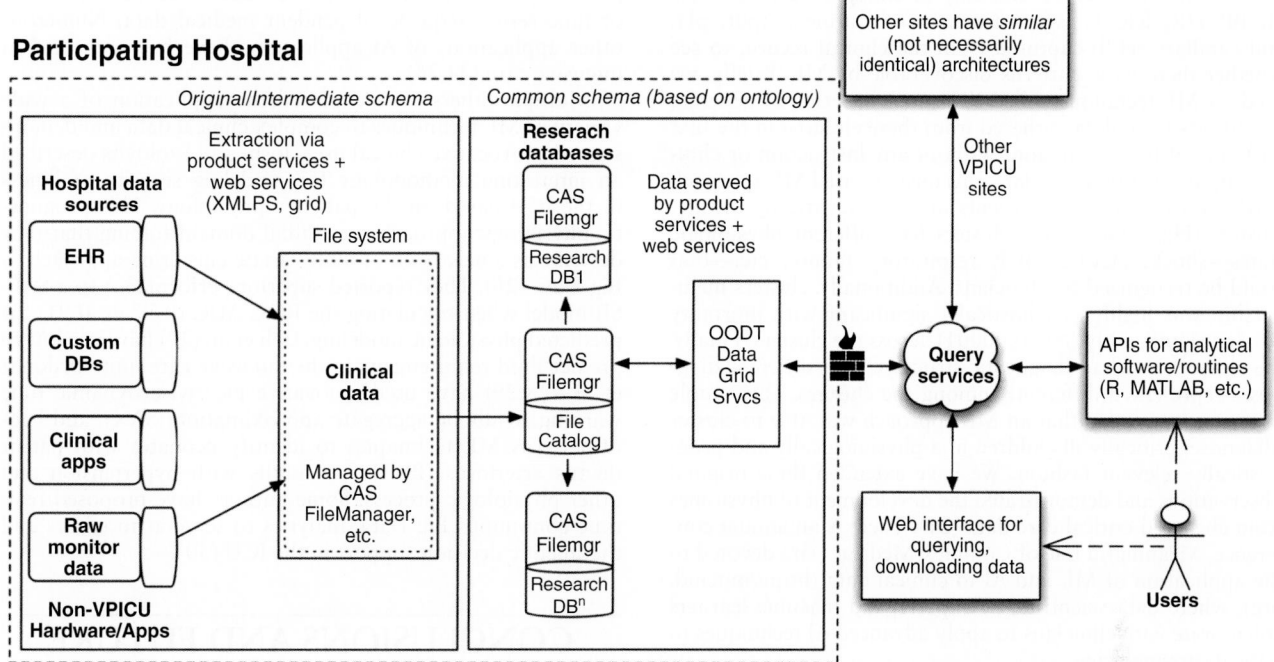

FIGURE 12.3. A proposed architectural schema for extracting clinical data from multiple disparate data sources on the left, extraction, loading and transformation of data occur to result in a clinical data file system that is unique to the institution. From this common data schema data can be exported to multiple common scheme data bases for various uses including reporting, research and export of data. A common open source Apache software firm data grid (OODT) serves as the architectural infrastructure. Outside of the hospital firewall query services permit data use in a federated structure. This process 'de-links' clinical, idiosyncratic production data from research and other use data requests in a rapidly accessible common structure (18).

must remain foremost. The VPICU has assembled a granular database of more than 12,000 PICU admissions suitable for data mining, and the Massachusetts Institute of Technology (MIT) project MIMIC (Multiparameter Intelligent Monitoring in Intensive Care; http://physionet.org/mimic2/index.shtml) has long made physiologic datasets available for investigator analysis. Many investigators are committed to acquiring large amounts of clinical critical care data for future analysis (5).

Once the data are acquired, what can be done with them? It seems axiomatic as Chen et al. (1) state: "Data from the EHR offers us a chance to re-examine and improve the value of critical care." The data from the EHR healthcare data are unique. Apart from the privacy issues, the data come in many varieties (normally distributed; nonnormally distributed; dichotomous; categorical; descriptive; patient notes; and radiology, cardiology, and pathology reports). All of these different data formats require differing analytic approaches—although solutions for all forms exist from natural language processing to pattern recognition. Greater understanding of how to manage and analyze large volumes of clinical data supports the inevitable application of Big Data to critical care (6).

Artificial Intelligence

More than 20 years ago, Miksch (19) called for the application of data-driven AI for decision support in ICUs. In 1992, Szolovits (20) at MIT defined three aims of knowledge-based care in healthcare:

1. "To develop expert computer programs for clinical use, making possible the inexpensive dissemination of the best medical expertise…

2. To formalize medical expertise to enable physicians to understand better what they know and give them a systematic structure for teaching…

3. To test AI theories in a real-world domain and further improve AI application…"

Since that time, numerous other uses and techniques have expanded the value of gathering and analyzing medical data. Most of these analytic techniques are statistically based, and there has been tremendous improvement in analytic techniques to statistically analyze complex medical data. *ML* is a domain of AI that enables a statistical approach to learning from data that are based on data representation—large amounts of, in this case, clinical data and the ability to generalize observations to future data sets. In a way, this is similar to internal and external validity. This approach often relies on building predictive models describing what happens to populations of patients that can be used to describe relationships, even causality, and to model what may happen to given patients. We have grown skeptical of earlier attempts to model mortality, severity of illness and outcomes for individual patients, with just reason; however, newer approaches using AI are demonstrating the ability to guide patient care. It is probable that ML can generate models from the known data that represent the data in a reproducible, reliable fashion (internally valid) and create models that are model generalizable to other patients (external validity) and that can be tested on data sets different from those used to derive the model.

ML focuses on prediction from a training data set of what will happen in a test data set, and is thus perhaps analogous to our use of logistic regression analysis to "predict" mortality in ICU populations as with PIM and PRISM. ML uses more sophisticated statistical techniques than hitherto. This also forms the basis for providing an ability to learn from complex clinical data. An example of such learning from data follows.

We examined 11,000 critically ill children's clinical signs (T, BP, HR, RR, Glasgow Coma Score, urine output, pH, and capillary refill) captured from the clinical record, to see whether there were patterns discoverable by ML. Briefly, we used an ML technique called K-means clustering to generate 30 clusters from data gathered from these children in the first 24 hours of ICU admission. Without any instruction or clinician input other than the data, this unsupervised ML approach was able to resolve the patients into 30 statistically distinct clusters (**Fig. 12.4**). These clusters had different physiologic states—shock, elevated ICP, respiratory failure, etc.—that could be recognized by clinicians. Additionally, clusters membership was highly prognostically significant with mortality varying significantly ($p < 0.00001$) across the clusters. Finally, the clusters also had diagnostic structure with different diagnoses represented differently among the clusters. This simple experiment revealed that an ML approach was able to cluster (diagnose) critically ill children in a physiologically and prognostically relevant fashion. We have extended these original observations and demonstrated the development of physiomes from clustered critical care data (21). There is an annual conference, Meaningful Use of Complex Medical Data devoted to the application of ML and AI to clinical data (http://mucmd.org), where data scientists, AI experts, and machine learners collaborate with clinicians to apply advanced AI techniques to critical care medicine.

Other investigators have successfully used ML approaches to the mining of clinical data. This can be a difficult process owing to the time dependence, sequence alignment and complexity, sparseness, and *missingness* of medical data. Analyzing Big Data to ultimately drive medical decision making and derive new information from the data to guide future therapy is tantalizingly close. In an interesting paper in 2000 by Kapadia et al. (22), a Markovian ML technique was able to accurately model PICU length of stay. One approach to mining time sequence data is Frequency Sequence Mining (FSM) used in many domains, but the nature of health data complicates its application. Perer and Wang (23) of the IBM Watson Research Center have described a way of combining this approach with computer-generated data visualization to facilitate medical data exploration, which is promising for sorting clinical phenotypes and following complex patients. We have described another ML approach using a kernel-based framework for learning from PICU time series observations, which was subsequently able to predict mortality and classify patients in similar

physiologic groups. This approach addressed the challenges of time series, sequence-dependent medical data. Numerous other applications of AI applications have been reported in intensive care (24,25).

Multiple others have explored the application of a wide variety of ML techniques to complex clinical data and demonstrated provocative clinical uses. Joshi and Szolovits described an interesting methodology for modeling severity of illness in the ICU based on the patient's physiology. This prognostic physiology approach uses radial domain folding that they describe as a new form of multivariate clustering approach to Big Data (26). They reported superior performance to a SAP-SII model when calculating the ROC AUC (0.77 vs. 0.91) for predicted physiologic modeling. Celi et al. (27) have used AI to predict fluid requirements in the intensive care unit. Ordonez et al. (28,29) have used innovative piecewise dynamic time warping, symbolic aggregate approximation (SAX), and bag-of-patterns ML techniques to identify neonates with patent ductus arteriosus (PDA) and adults with hypertension and other physiologic process. Some authors have proposed real-time continuous Big Data analytics to serve as monitors and therapeutic decision support in the ICU (30).

CONCLUSIONS AND FUTURE DIRECTIONS

Discovery informatics applied to critical care data has great potential to improve the care we provide critically ill children. Understanding this potential and becoming familiar with new scientific techniques to learn from the data will challenge pediatric intensivists in the very near future. The application of Big Data in critical care will make personalized intensive care available for critically ill children.

References

1. Chen L, Kennedy E, Sales A, et al. Use of health IT for higher-value critical care. *N Engl J Med* 2013;368(7):594–97.
2. Horvitz E. From data to predictions and decision: Enabling evidence-based healthcare. Computing Community Consortium Version 6, September 16, 2010:1–11.
3. Gil Y, Hirsh H. Final report on 2012 NSF Workshop on Discovery Informatics. National Science Foundation Workshop (report, August 2012). www.discoveryinfomaticsinitiative.org/diw2012.
4. Miller K. Bringing the fruits of computation to bear on human health: It's a tough job but the NIH has to do it. *Biomed Comp Rev* 2009;1–11Vol. 5(2).
5. Celi LA, Mark RG, Stone DJ, et al. "Big data" in the intensive care unit. *Am J Respir Crit Care Med* 2013;187(11):1157–66.
6. Murdoch TB, Detsky AB. The inevitable application of big data to health care. *JAMA* 2013;309(13):1351–52.
7. Editorial Community Cleverness Required. *Nature* 2008;455:1.
8. Miller G. The magical number seven, plus or minus two: Some limits on our capacity for processing information. *Psychol Rev* 1956;63(2):81–97.
9. Okun S, McGray D, Stang P, et al. Making the case for continuous leaning from routinely collected data. Discussion papers. Washington, DC: Institute of Medicine, 2013. http://www.iom.edu/meanningthecase.
10. Wetzel RC. The virtual pediatric intensive care unit. Practice in the new millennium. *Pediatr Clin North Am* 2001;48(3):795–814.
11. Rice TB, Sachedeva R, Wetzel RC. Are all ICUs the same? *Pediatr Anesth* 2011;21(7):787–93. doi:10.1111/j.1460-9592.2011.03595.x.
12. Jeffries HE, LaRovere JM, Rice TB, et al. Databases for assessing the outcomes of the treatment of patients with

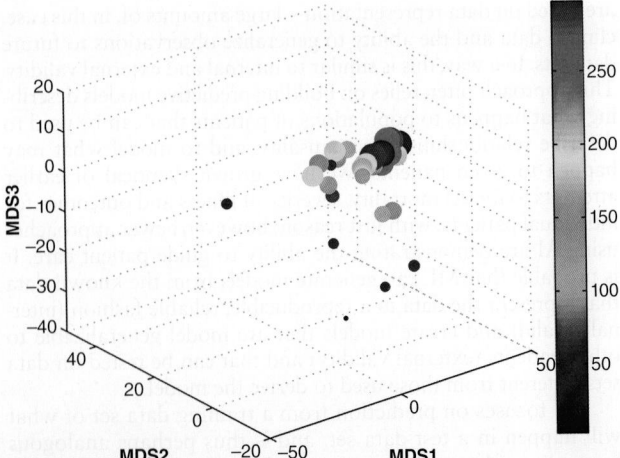

FIGURE 12.4. This figure represents clusters distributed in multidimensional space. Axis labels represent dimensions of the data, and cluster size and color represent numbers of patients per cluster.

congenital and pediatric cardiac disease—The perspective of critical care. *Cardiol Young* 2008;18(suppl 2):130–6. doi:10.1017/S1047951108002886.

13. Lauer MS, D'Agostino RB. The randomized registry trial—The next disruptive technology in clinical research? *N Eng J Med* 2013;369:1579–81.

14. Gupta T, Green JW, Tang X, et al. Comparison of high-frequency oscillatory ventilation and conventional mechanical ventilation in pediatric respiratory failure. *JAMA Pediatr* 2014;168(3):243–9. doi:10.1001/Jamapediatrics.2013.4463.

15. Berry JG, Hall M, Hall DE, et al. Inpatient growth and resource use in 28 children's hospitals. *JAMA* 2013;167(2):170–7. doi:10.1001/jamapedaitrics.2013-432.

16. Lee J, Kothari R, Ladapo JA, et al. Interrogating a clinical database to study treatment of hypotension in the critically ill. *BMJ Open* 2012;2(3). pii:e000916.

17. Crichton D, Mattmann C, Wetzel R, et al. An open-source, grid-based software framework for management and sharing of pediatric intensive care unit data. *J Crit Care* 2010;26(2):e13–14.

18. Hart AF, Kale D, Mattmann CA, et al. An informatics architecture for the Virtual Pediatric Intensive Care Unit. In Proceedings of the 26th IEEE International Symposium on Computer-Based Medical Systems (CBMS), 2011;1–6. doi:10.1109/CBMS.2011.5999031.

19. Miksch S. Artificial intelligence for decision support: Needs, possibilities, and limitations in ICU. In: Proceedings of the10th Postgraduate Course in Critical Care Medicine A.P.I.C.E.'95, 1995:1–11. Springer.

20. Szolovits P. Artificial intelligence and medicine. In: Szolovitz P, ed. *Artificial Intelligence in Medicine*. Boulder, CO: Westview Press, 1992.

21. Marlin BM, Robinder GK, Kale D, et al. Unsupervised pattern discover in electronic health care data using probabilistic clustering models. In: IHI'12, January 28–30, 2012.

22. Kapadia AS, Chan W, Sachdeva R, et al. Predicting duration of stay in a pediatric intensive care unit: A Markovian approach. *Eur J Operation Res* 2000;124:353–9.

23. Perer A, Wang F. Frequence: Interactive mining and visualization of temporal frequent event sequences. In: IUI'14, February 24–27, 2014, Haifa, Israel. New York, NY: ACM. http://dx.doi.org/10.1145/2557500.2557508.

24. Lasko TA, Denny JC, Levy MA. *Computational Phenotype Discovery Using Unsupervised Feature Learning over Noisy, Sparse, and Irregular Clinical Data*. PLoS ONE. 2013 Jun;8(6):e66341.

25. Hanson WC, Marshall B. Artificial intelligence application in the intensive care unit. *Crit Care Med* 2001;29(2):427–35.

26. Joshi R, Szolovits P. *Prognostic Physiology: Modeling Patient Severity in Intensive Care Units Using Radial Domain Folding*. National Institute of Biomedical Imaging and Bioengineering (NIBIB), NIH;2RO1 EB001659,2012.

27. Celi LA, Hinske CL, Altervoitza G, et al. An artificial intelligence tool to predict fluid requirement in the intensive care unit: A proof-of-concept study. *Crit Care* 2008;12:R151. doi:10.1186/cc7140.

28. Using Modified Multivariate Bag-of-Words Models to Classify Physiological Data Ordonez, P. T. Armstrong, T. Oates, T. Fackler, Data Mining Workshops (ICDMW), 2011 IEEE 11th International Conference on 10.1109/ICDMW.2011.174 Publication Year: 2011, Page(s): 534–539 IEEE CONFERENCE PUBLICATIONS.

29. Ordóñez, Patricia, Tom Armstrong, Tim Oates, and Jim Fackler. "Classification of patients using novel multivariate time series representations of physiological data." In *Machine Learning and Applications and Workshops (ICMLA), 2011 10th International Conference on*, vol. 2, pp. 172–179. IEEE, 2011.

30. Blount M, Ebling MR, Eklund MJ, et al. Real-time analysis for intensive care. *IEEE Eng Med Biol Mag*, 2010;29(2):110–8. doi:10.1109/MEMB.2010.936454

CHAPTER 13 ■ INTEGRATING PALLIATIVE CARE AND CRITICAL CARE

WYNNE E. MORRISON, PATRICIA LAGO, JEFFERSON PEDRO PIVA, AND KATHLEEN L. MEERT

KEY POINTS

1 Currently, the majority of children who die do so in hospitals and many in ICUs. Skill in symptom management and compassionate care of patients and families at the end of a child's life are therefore core competencies of pediatric critical care. Collaboration with consultative palliative care teams and home hospice services may be helpful in the care of some patients.

2 Pharmacologic management of symptoms at the end of life is appropriate and important. Appropriately titrated doses are ethically justifiable and should rarely hasten death. Opioids and sedatives may both be helpful.

3 Withholding or withdrawing ICU interventions such as cardiopulmonary resuscitation and mechanical ventilation is often indicated at the end of life. It is important to manage symptoms appropriately when doing so and communicate with families in a supportive fashion regarding such decisions.

4 At the time of a child's death, families report a need to remain close to their child and for honest and clear information from the team. Families may have cultural or religious traditions, which are important to them at this time, and the team should assess such needs on an individual basis. Most families appreciate follow-up from the medical team after a child's death.

5 Caring for dying children and their families can be both distressing and rewarding for the medical team. Good communication regarding the plan of care is essential and should involve the multidisciplinary staff as well as consultants.

6 Pediatric palliative care is a rapidly growing specialty that involves the care of many children with potentially life-limiting illnesses, not just those who are dying. Systems of care, training, and reimbursement should continue to be developed in order to allow access to such support for children and families worldwide.

More than 40,000 children die every year in the United States and more than 10 million children worldwide (1,2). Estimates of how many of these children die in intensive care units vary widely by country, but in most reports the majority of pediatric deaths occur in the hospital (3–7). Caring for dying children and supporting their families is therefore a common experience for pediatric intensivists and a core competency of pediatric critical care. Necessary skills include the support of family decision making, navigation of the ethical issues involved, management of the application and removal of technologic support, intensive management of pain and other symptoms at the end of life, and care for the family during and after a death. Pediatric palliative care has been defined as "an active approach to the care of children and young people with life-limiting conditions, embracing physical, emotional, social and spiritual elements through death and beyond" (4). Because of the location of many pediatric deaths, it is often the ICU team who provides much of this care.

In addition to caring for children who are clearly dying, pediatric intensivists will also manage complex care for many children living with chronic conditions. As supportive technologies have improved over the past several decades, many children are living with conditions that would have been universally fatal in the past (7–11). Examples include congenital heart disease, chronic lung disease of prematurity, and genetic disorders that lead to severe neuromuscular weakness, metabolic abnormalities, or developmental disabilities. The proportion of pediatric critical care patients with such conditions is increasing over time even as mortality rates are falling (9,12).

These children may have an impaired level of functioning at baseline with episodic deterioration leading to recurrent ICU admissions. In such cases, parents may need help navigating how aggressive to be with potentially life-saving technology, especially if concerns arise that such technology only prolongs suffering or a poor quality of life. It is important to focus on quality of life and management of pain and suffering whether curative, life-prolonging, or palliate care continues.

End-of-life care in pediatrics differs in significant ways from what typically occurs in adult medicine. For adult patients, hospice referrals often occur only in the last few days or weeks of life (13). For many pediatric illnesses, life expectancy and developmental prognosis are often uncertain, and pediatric palliative care teams frequently follow patients for months or even years following referral (14). It can certainly be useful for palliative care teams to meet patients earlier in the course of illness so that they can build a relationship before a child's condition deteriorates (15,16). In addition, evidence is beginning to emerge from adult studies that earlier palliative care referral may not only improve the quality of life of patients with a terminal illness, but also actually prolong life (17). Unfortunately, there are not enough resources available to allow all children and families facing a potentially life-limiting illness to be followed by specialized pediatric palliative care teams. Such teams may not exist in all institutions or all countries, and even when they do it may not be possible for them to meet and care for all pediatric patients who are or may be dying. It is therefore necessary for pediatric intensivists to be skilled and knowledgeable at providing "primary" pediatric palliative care while being aware of what "specialty" services are available at their particular institution when needed.

LOCATION OF DEATH

The majority of deaths in the pediatric ICU follow a decision to withdraw or withhold life-sustaining treatment rather than failed resuscitative efforts, although there is variation by country and region. In North America and the United Kingdom, withdrawal of treatment precedes more than half of pediatric ICU deaths, while authors from Europe and Brazil have reported that the proportion at their centers is below 50% (18–28). A recent multi-institutional study in the United States reported that out of 1,263 pediatric deaths, 12% of the children died despite ongoing interventions, 23% of children were declared dead by neurologic criteria, and 65% had do not attempt resuscitation (DNAR) orders initiated or had therapies withdrawn (29).

For patients whose death is anticipated, a question may arise about whether it is appropriate for the patient to remain in the ICU or be transferred elsewhere. Many factors may affect this decision. It could be important to consider how quickly the patient is anticipated to die following the discontinuation of technological or pharmacologic support, whether the patient is well known by a service in the hospital other than the ICU, how complicated the care might be for a team outside of the ICU, and whether the family is comforted or distressed by being in the ICU. The parents of many oncology patients, for instance, might prefer to have their child return to an oncology floor for the last few days of life if the care can be managed there, as they often have a long-term relationship with the physicians and nurses on the ward. Yet for a patient who is expected to live for only a few hours at most following an extubation, it would not be appropriate to transfer care to a new team who does not know the patient or family. Some relevant factors such as the availability of a private space for the family to be with the patient or the amount of noise in a given unit may vary by institution.

Another question that may arise involves when it is appropriate for a patient with a DNAR order to be admitted to the ICU. Even when procedures such as intubation and resuscitation are not desired, there are still many reasons that a patient might benefit from being in an ICU. An example could be a family who has decided that they do not want their child with a severe neuromuscular disorder to undergo another prolonged intubation and ICU stay for a respiratory decompensation, but would be willing to have a time-limited trial of vigorous pulmonary toilet and noninvasive ventilation to see if there is a rapid turnaround. It is also possible that some medications necessary to manage refractory symptoms at the end of life (e.g., ketamine for severe pain, octreotide for bowel obstruction) are only available in the ICU. In addition, intensive attention to pain and symptom management may require a nurse-to-patient ratio that is available only in the ICU.

It is usually appropriate to prepare a family that there is uncertainty about the exact timing of death following removal of therapies or a decision not to escalate. Plans can be put in place based on a best estimate, with an acknowledgement that the plan would need to be altered for an unexpectedly rapid or slow deterioration. A family may lose trust in the medical team if they expect death to occur within seconds of an extubation but the child breathes spontaneously for days to weeks. Avoiding overly precise statements can be accomplished by using ranges and phrases such as "I expect he could breathe for minutes to hours" or "We often see children who remain in this state for days to weeks before death." Some families can actually find comfort in knowing that they are not choosing

the time of death in deciding to remove a ventilator—the medical team and the family are simply deciding to remove technology that is no longer helpful; the patient, disease process, or a higher power (if the family speaks in those terms) will determine what happens next.

HOME AND HOSPICE SUPPORT

For many families, being at home in familiar surroundings with their child at the time of death can be a great source of comfort. For others, the thought of being at home is terrifying and they are more comfortable remaining in the hospital with the full support of the medical team. There is no one place that is right for every patient. While studies have shown that more pediatric patients are using home hospice services over time (30,31), many ICU patients have clinical instability or a need for minute-to-minute nursing interventions that make a transfer to home unfeasible. Often, those children for whom a transfer home is considered are the patients who survive for several days following the withdrawal of technology, or for whom decisions are made not to escalate after arrival in the ICU.

Occasionally, a family feels strongly that they would prefer their child to die at home and asks if it is possible to transfer home for withdrawal of life-prolonging interventions there. Organizing a compassionate extubation or discontinuation of infusions in the home takes planning and preparation (32,33). Merely arranging for a transport team is insufficient. Appropriate supports need to be in place to continue to care for the patient and treat pain or dyspnea if the patient survives for some time. Hospice agencies are skilled at providing such support in the home setting and should be involved in the planning phases.

One of the first modern hospices was founded in the late 1960s in London by Dame Cicely Saunders, a nurse who subsequently pursued degrees in both medicine and social work in order to better advocate for comfort and dignity for dying patients (34). Her efforts led to a worldwide movement to improve care of the dying. In the United States, hospices are independent agencies structured to be compliant with Medicare guidelines (35,36). Although there are hospice agencies dedicated specifically to the care of children in some large urban areas, most care predominantly for adults. Many will consider caring for children if a pediatric medical team works with them to offer advice or co-manage. Hospices are dedicated to providing comfort and psychosocial support to patients with life-limiting illnesses. This care is often provided in the home, by a team of nurses who are on call 24 hours a day to come to the home in order to help a family assess symptoms or manage a change in status. Hospices do not provide "shift" nursing care for a patient who has long-term, minute-to-minute needs in the home, but can often provide "continuous care" for up to 72 hours for a patient who is actively deteriorating. Many of the agencies also have inpatient beds in hospitals or in their own facilities, which can be used when a family needs respite or when a patient's needs cannot be met in the home. Hospices are also invaluable in managing the logistics of having a patient at home, can arrange for the delivery of medications and equipment, can help a family maintain a "nonmedical" atmosphere, and can provide a mechanism for allowing death to be declared in the home. In addition to the team of nurses, hospices have a physician medical director, social worker, a chaplain, a bereavement support team, and the ability to provide some hours of assistance from nurse's aides or volunteers. Even when a patient is expected to live for only a few hours following a transfer home from the ICU, having hospice involved for this sort of follow-up support can be important for a family. In regions or countries where structured home care systems are less available, a primary physician or hospital team may need to be much more closely involved to transfer an ICU patient home, and it may not be possible to do so. There is wide variability in the development of hospice and palliative care services by country (31,37,38), and many economically developing nations do have robust systems in place. Challenges to providing such care in much of the developing world include inadequate infrastructures, extremely impoverished patients, restrictions on opioid prescribing, and few educational opportunities for healthcare staff (3).

Medicare regulations in the United States require that a physician certify a patient's disease process has a typical life expectancy of less than 6 months in order to qualify for the hospice benefit. Pediatric patients are not usually covered by Medicare, but hospice agencies typically still require that such a form be completed for every patient. Because the trajectory of disease processes are much more difficult to predict for children, parents may need to be warned (or reassured) that providing such a certification is not an accurate prediction of life expectancy for an individual patient.

Concurrent care refers to the concept of providing hospice support to patients while they are simultaneously receiving ongoing curative or life-prolonging therapy (39). A quandary often arises when patients or families wish to pursue ongoing treatments such as experimental cancer therapies but would also prefer to remain home as much as possible rather than being hospitalized. Referral to hospice is often the best way of supporting the latter goal, but in the past this benefit was usually unavailable to patients who wanted ongoing disease-directed treatments. Recent legislation requires that state programs support concurrent care for children (40), and most private insurers have followed by adding this benefit. It is not always clear, however, when timing of hospice referral is appropriate for children (39).

PALLIATIVE CARE TEAMS

Palliative care teams are distinct from hospices. These hospital-based clinical teams focus on pain and symptom management, and psychosocial and decision-making support for patients with potentially life-limiting illnesses and their families. Many of these teams work closely with hospices to help assure smooth transitions of care between inpatient and outpatient teams, but not all patients followed by palliative care teams are enrolled in hospice (14). Pediatric-specific teams are not available in all institutions, but the numbers are increasing (41).

Palliative care teams certainly do not need to be involved in the care of every patient who dies in an ICU. Managing pain and symptoms, navigating difficult decisions with a family, withdrawing life-sustaining technologies, and handling the logistics of a death should be core competencies for any ICU team regardless of whether a palliative care team is available. A consultative palliative care team may be most useful when a transition to home or a prolonged survival beyond the ICU stay might be anticipated, when focused expertise on difficult symptoms is needed, or when significant time devoted to helping a family make decisions becomes necessary. Most palliative care teams also have a strong multidisciplinary focus, with possible team members including physicians, nurses, social workers, chaplains, psychologists, therapists, and bereavement coordinators who can continue to support families following a child's death.

PAIN AND SYMPTOM MANAGEMENT

The medications used to treat pain and symptoms at the end of life are common tools in the armamentarium of any intensivist. When goals of care shift to comfort rather than life prolongation, medications may be titrated and escalated differently than in other patients in the ICU. Clinicians are sometimes concerned that medications administered to treat suffering may hasten death (42). The *principle of double effect* (see also Chapter 15) justifies using medications to treat suffering when necessary even if a patient's respiratory effort is compromised (43). In typical practice, it is rarely necessary to invoke this argument as both neonatal and adult studies have suggested that doses of medications used are not associated with time to death (44,45). If doses are titrated on the basis of symptoms (often a 20% increase in a dose or infusion for mild symptoms or a 50% increase for severe symptoms (46)), then symptom control should usually occur before respiratory depression (47). In end-of-life care, it is particularly important to recognize that there is no "ceiling" on the doses of medications that can be used, particularly for patients who may have become tolerant to medication effects over time. If the patient is still in pain or is dyspneic, the dose can be increased, rapidly if needed. For patients who may go home with hospice, it is important to coordinate with the agency regarding which medications are available to them for home use.

Analgesics

Opioids are a mainstay of treating both pain and dyspnea (48). These agents work via central nervous system μ-receptors to provide analgesia and euphoria, with potential side effects of respiratory depression, constipation, nausea, itching, and urinary retention. When using these agents, it is important to anticipate side effects and prevent them if possible (e.g., a bowel regimen). Morphine is a commonly available and inexpensive medication that comes in both short-acting and long-acting preparations. It can lead to a release of histamine, which can worsen itching, and when used in high doses can lead to hyperalgesia or myoclonus (46). Changing agents may be helpful in these circumstances. Hydromorphone and oxycodone may be useful alternatives, and sometimes rotation between agents improves pain relief and decreases side effects (49). It is usually best to avoid using codeine and meperidine. Codeine tends to cause nausea out of proportion to its degree of pain relief, and it is ineffective in up to 10% of the population who are slow metabolizers to its active form. When meperidine is used in high doses, the metabolite normeperidine can accumulate, which can lead to seizures.

Fentanyl is often used in ICUs because it is fast acting and lipophilic and acts directly rather than through metabolites. However, fentanyl and the other fast-acting synthetic opioids (e.g., remifentanil, sufentanil) are less commonly used at the end of life because of expense and the rapid development of tolerance. There is little advantage to its short duration of action in these circumstances, but it may be useful in the transdermal (patch) form when medication administration is difficult by other routes.

Methadone differs from the other narcotics in that it has a very long half-life and also has additional effects at the n-methyl-D-aspartate (NMDA) receptor (50,51). The NMDA effects can be beneficial in achieving pain control when other agents are becoming ineffective and may offer additional help for neuropathic pain (52). Because of its long half-life, the drug may accumulate days after it is initiated. Close monitoring for side effects such as mental status changes and familiarity with dose titration are both important. Methadone can also prolong the QT interval (53), so screening electrocardiograms should be performed when starting it. Other medications that can have this side effect should be avoided. Ketamine is a nonopioid dissociative anesthetic which also works via the NMDA receptor and can therefore be a useful adjunct when opioids are not working. At high doses, it has the potential to cause disturbing hallucinations.

Nebulized opioids have been studied for a proposed ability to relieve dyspnea with fewer systemic side effects (54), with most controlled trials showing little added benefit. In the ICU, most patients have intravenous access and there may be little reason to avoid systemic administration, but inhaled agents could be tried on a case-by-case basis.

Sedatives

Just as many ICU patients require sedation in order to tolerate ICU interventions and monitoring, many patients at the end of life require sedation for the management of symptoms. Low doses can often be used as an adjunct to relieve anxiety and allow for better pain control. Higher doses that diminish awareness may be necessary for intractable symptoms. *Terminal sedation*, or titration of medications to the point of unconsciousness at the end of life, is often discussed as a point of potential ethical controversy, yet *palliative sedation* may be a better descriptor (55,56). In the ICU, sedation to unconsciousness merely represents one end of the spectrum of medication use that may be necessary for otherwise uncontrollable symptoms.

Benzodiazepines are the most common sedative used at the end of life (57), with intravenous dosing (either intermittently or by infusion) as the usual route in the ICU. Barbiturates are sometimes also used, but usually only when the goal is to diminish awareness. Other agents typically used for deep sedation or anesthesia, such as propofol or dexmedetomidine, are rarely necessary but could be used to treat intractable suffering when other medications have failed.

Medications that do not treat suffering but have a sole intent of hastening death should be avoided. Professional organizations have issued guidelines recommending against the use of neuromuscular blocking agents at the time of ventilator withdrawal (58,59). Although a patient may appear "peaceful" if unable to move, neuromuscular blockade may make it impossible for the medical team to detect pain or dyspnea. In cases where ventilator withdrawal is being considered or discussed, infusions of neuromuscular blockers should be transitioned to an intermittent dosing regimen to avoid accumulation of drug that would take a significant amount of time to clear and a delay in being able to remove a ventilator.

NONPHARMACOLOGIC ADJUNCTS

For most ICU patients, intravenous opioids and benzodiazepines will be the mainstay of symptom management. For patients who may have some awareness of their environment, attention to their surroundings can also help. Music, dimming the lights, encouraging parents to hold a child, or providing familiar objects can all be helpful (48). Supplemental oxygen should be used if it seems to improve comfort, but is not necessary for hypoxemia if the patient is not distressed by it. Noninvasive ventilation is sometimes used following extubation, often for those patients who are chronically maintained on it at home or who are expected to potentially survive. If a decision has been made that the patient will not be reintubated, then the team should also choose a reasonable maximum pressure that will be used noninvasively to avoid escalating to high-enough pressures to cause discomfort.

LIMITATIONS ON ICU INTERVENTIONS

In cases where a disease process has been determined to be irreversible, or the burdens of continuing invasive interventions offer little prospect of benefit in either survival or quality of life, a patient's authorized decision maker and the medical team may decide that it is time to either limit further escalation of invasive therapies or to remove some interventions that are already in place. Goals may shift over time, and often many conversations between a family and clinicians are necessary to reach consensus on what goals are achievable and how to best reach them (21,22,60–62). It is important for a team to work closely with a family to make sure that medically appropriate choices are being offered and to give a family time to understand the situation and trajectory of illness. Many factors could influence what goals are appropriate, including the likelihood of recovery from the illness or injury, length of time spent in the ICU, baseline level of functioning or quality of life, frequency of ICU admissions, whether interventions are causing pain and suffering, and the values of the patient and family. Resource availability for ongoing ICU or long-term support of the child may be a factor in some areas.

Attention to the language used in discussing withdrawal is important so that a family is not left believing that they "gave up" on their child or "pulled the plug." The clinician should avoid saying that the plan is to "withdraw care" (because "care" will always be provided, whether an invasive treatment plan is in place or not), and focusing on comfort should never be phrased as "doing nothing." Similarly, it is unfair to a family for the ICU team to ask "Do you want us to do everything for your child?" (63–65) as many will rapidly default to saying yes to "everything" since it sounds like what one should do. Many families need reassurance from the physician that a focus on comfort can be what is best for their child and that they are good parents making loving decisions (66).

DNAR Orders

DNAR orders (formerly DNR orders) are unique in medicine in that they specify therapies or interventions that will *not* be performed (67,68). They exist because the default assumption is that emergency interventions such as cardiopulmonary resuscitation (CPR) and intubation should be provided, unless a thoughtful decision has been made that they would not be beneficial or desired. The lay public may have an unrealistic expectation of how successful resuscitative efforts are likely to be (69), so a clinician should educate a patient and family about what benefits might be anticipated in that patient's situation. Some centers are changing the terminology to "allow natural death" (AND) orders rather than DNAR as a way to focus on the positive aspects rather than on what will not be provided (70–72).

In discussing DNAR orders with families, it is better to focus on overall goals (e.g., providing comfort, time at home, extending life, providing time to see if a situation can improve, gaining time for extended family to arrive, etc.) rather than running through a checklist of what interventions will or will not be provided. The clinician can then decide what interventions make sense in light of the goals (73–75). Not all DNAR orders are the same—in some cases it makes sense to avoid CPR and defibrillation, but to consider intubation and mechanical ventilation. In other cases, it may be best to forego CPR, intubation, vasoactive medications, antibiotics, and almost all other interventions other than those focused on treating pain and suffering. There are also some interventions (e.g., extracorporeal support, dialysis) that a team decides not to offer because they would not help, without necessarily needing an explicit order or family discussion to avoid them. For some families, it is easier to consider avoiding *new* interventions but continuing those that are already in place for some time. Although ethically there is little difference between withdrawing a therapy versus not starting it in the first place (see Chapter 15), nonescalation may cause less emotional distress.

Occasionally, a patient with a DNAR and/or do not intubate (DNI) order may benefit from an operative procedure that is being considered to either treat symptoms or prolong life, but with no plans for long-term mechanical supports. If such a patient is going to the operating room, it is very important for proactive discussions to occur between the surgeon, anesthesiologist, ICU team and family to make sure that all are comfortable with a plan to either rescind or continue a DNAR order in the perioperative period (76). Again, keeping goals in mind is the first priority. It might make sense to revoke the DNI portion of the order for a few days around a procedure, but reassess if things do not go as expected. Some families may prefer that CPR not be performed even in this setting, but the surgical and anesthesiology teams have to be comfortable with this plan since the surgical procedure or anesthetic provided could potentially be the cause of an arrest.

Discontinuing Mechanical Ventilation

Decisions regarding how to discontinue ICU interventions may be case specific but should always focus on how to best minimize the suffering of the child. *Removing a ventilator* is a relatively common procedure at the end of life, so there are several important steps to keep in mind.

A very important first step is to prepare the family for what will happen. They should understand that the team will be there with them to continually assess and treat discomfort. They should be told what to expect their child to look like—discussing the possibility of color changes and irregular or noisy breathing. If at all possible, the room should be prepared to give them privacy and a peaceful environment. Helping a family hold their child or lie in bed with their child before, during, or after extubation is important. As discussed above, clinicians should avoid predicting exactly when a child will die following an extubation, but reassure the family that they can be with their child throughout the process. In addition, it is important to notify the appropriate organ procurement organization affiliated with the institution for any anticipated death so an assessment can be made before withdrawal about whether the patient could be an organ or tissue donor following death. Although traditionally most organ donors are patients declared dead by neurologic criteria, many institutions do have protocols in place for organ donation after a circulatory determination of death. Attempting such a donation may only be possible if a fairly rapid death is anticipated following the removal of the ventilator (typically less than one hour) and usually changes the location where the withdrawal will happen (77) (see Chapter 16).

Before discontinuing a ventilator, it is also important to assess a patient's comfort and level of awareness. Although removing an endotracheal tube may improve comfort, it is also possible that there will be increased dyspnea afterward. Additional doses of medication or infusions should be prepared and readily available, and escalating medications before the extubation is important if the clinician anticipates distress. The clinician may want to decrease the ventilatory support before extubation to see if the patient shows signs of respiratory distress to allow anticipatory dosing. Stopping other interventions, such as vasoactive infusions, before extubation can facilitate an assessment of whether death is anticipated quickly. Institutional checklists or protocols for discontinuing interventions at the end of life may be helpful to staff (78).

SUPPORT OF THE FAMILY

Support of the family is an essential component of care for the critically ill or dying child (79). Parents are the natural caregivers of their children (80). Parents routinely provide, protect and advocate for their children and maintain authority over many aspects of their children's lives. The authority bestowed on parents promotes family integrity, ensures availability of an identifiable decision maker, and acknowledges the role parents play in shaping their children's development. However, during critical illness, many of parents' caregiving roles and responsibilities are transferred to health professionals because of the complex and specialized care required. Alteration of parental role has been identified as the greatest source of stress among parents whose children are hospitalized in ICUs (81–84). Helping parents to "be the parents" in the face of their child's life-threatening illness requires an understanding of parents' needs and a team of health professionals and environment of care that acknowledges and supports these needs. Supporting the parental role has the potential to improve quality of care for the child as well as long-term outcomes for parents and families.

Parents' needs during a child's critical illness and death are often shaped by the ways parents define themselves. For many parents, "being a parent" is a key part of their personal identity. Parents typically seek to maintain relationship with their critically ill child before, during, and even after death through physical proximity, words, and symbols (85,86). Physical proximity includes the need to touch, hold, and be present with the child. In a study of parental satisfaction with end-of-life care in the pediatric ICU, 65% of parents were with their child at the time of death, none of whom regretted being present. Of the 35% who were not present at the time of death, 63% later regretted not being there (87). For many parents, regrets evolved from the lost opportunity to say good bye. Mementos such as a lock of hair, handprint or blanket serve as tangible symbols of the child's life. Mementos not only bring comfort to parents at the time of death but also anchor parents' memories to help them stay connected to their child during bereavement (85,86).

Part of "being a parent" is making decisions for the child, and parents have a need for their authority in decision making to be respected (85). In daily life, parents make many decisions for their children such as what to eat, what to wear, when to sleep, and what activities to engage in at home or school. However, children may have interests independent of their families, and parents' authority in decision making is not absolute (80,88). Shared decision making is the primary decision-making model recommended for use during critical illness (62,89,90). When employed in the ICU, both parents and health professionals are asked to discuss options, share views, and reach consensus on a plan of action that is in the best interest of the child. A recent study on parents' decision-making preferences in ICUs suggests that most parents prefer their role in decision making to be shared with their doctor or to have significant autonomy in the final decision (91). In some cultures, families may not expect or desire to play an active role in decision making, and clinicians should be willing to take on more responsibility for determining the best course of action when a family prefers they do so (7,23,92–94). It is also appropriate for the physician to be more directive in cases where the outcome is more certain, and most families will appreciate such help (95,96). In cases where it is clear that the child is terminally ill, the physician should help a family understand that there are other things they can do to help their child (provide comfort, being present, making sure their child knows he/she is loved) that do not involve escalating uncomfortable and ultimately nonbeneficial ICU interventions.

Cultural, religious, and family traditions also contribute to parents' sense of identity and continuity as they are faced with the critical illness and death of their child (85,86,97). Parents have a need for their beliefs, values, customs, and traditions to be respected. Staff should assess and accommodate, to the extent possible, the cultural and religious preferences of parents when providing end-of-life care in the ICU. Parents may request specific practices such as prayer, rituals, or sacred readings, which may be accomplished by hospital chaplains or members of the parents' religious community. Staff should remember that parents can be easily offended by unwanted cultural or religious practices that are imposed upon them. Awareness of parents' beliefs and traditions can help health professionals prepare for difficult interactions with families such as discussions of poor prognoses, limitations of care, organ donation, and autopsy (18,98–106). Sensitivity to parents' beliefs and traditions can help parents develop greater trust in health professionals and thereby foster a sense of calmness and hope during end-of-life situations rather than fear and despair.

Parents have a need for personal and professional support during their child's critical illness and death (85). Personal support usually comes from family and friends and professional support from hospital staff. However, these types of support often overlap especially for parents whose child has a prolonged ICU stay. Parents may rely on family and friends to assist with activities of daily living (e.g., groceries, laundry, and mail) as well as for short periods of respite from their ill child's bedside. Professional support is expert care that can guide parents throughout their child's illness and death. Professional support includes both the emotional support needed to get through the crisis as well as the instrumental support needed to deal with the paperwork, rules, and logistics of the hospital system. Many diverse professionals work in ICUs, and parents sometimes have difficulty discerning their various roles. Parents need to perceive a sense of teamwork among the professionals caring for their child; failure to do so contributes to parents' distress (107).

Attributes of professional support desired by parents include compassion, trust, honest communication, and respect for their child's personhood (85). Compassion is often perceived by parents through comforting words and small acts of kindness offered by staff (e.g., glass of water, chair, facial tissues). Trust develops when parents perceive that they can rely on the advice and actions of health professionals and that the care provided is in the best interest of their child. For some parents, establishing rapport is an important aspect of building trust. Honest communication is sharing information with parents in ways that do not mislead or prevent full understanding (60,92,107,108). Although it may be difficult for parents to learn of a child's poor prognosis, withholding such information may lead to false hope and distrust (109). Honest disclosure of information should be communicated with compassion. Respect for the child's personhood requires staff to recognize the child as human and as having social worth. Respect for personhood can often be accomplished through simple acts such as acknowledging the child by name and gender.

Parents' needs are also shaped by the built environment of the ICU and the ways in which it is used (83,85,110). ICUs are high-tech, fast-paced settings designed for continuous observation of patients. Parents are often keenly aware of the environment surrounding their child's death and parents whose children have died in an ICU have described the need for greater privacy, creation of a sacred atmosphere, enough time and various types of facility support. Privacy in the ICU setting may be difficult to achieve as it involves seclusion from the sight, sound, or presence of others. However, parents often need to be by themselves, alone with family or alone with their dying child. Many parents want their child's death to be treated as a sacred time. Parents appreciate the staff's efforts to create a private and reverent atmosphere by closing doors or blinds, turning down alarms, speaking softly, and playing music. Parents also have a need for adequate time to make

decisions, gather family, and grieve in the presence of their child's body. Other environmental needs described by parents near the time of their child's death in the ICU include the need for open visitation and adequate space to accommodate family and friends, and facilities for personal care such as showers, lockers, and a place to sleep near their child.

Attention to helping siblings understand and cope can be invaluable for a family struggling with a child's critical illness (111). Parents may wonder how to answer another child's questions about the illness and whether to allow young children to visit their ill or dying sibling. Many institutions employ psychologists, social workers, or child life specialists who can help families navigate these concerns and prepare children for what they might see in an ICU. Siblings may also benefit from having playrooms available in a hospital, and support groups can be helpful for older children (92,112,113).

After a child's death, many parents desire continued contact from staff and feel a sense of abandonment when such contact does not occur (85,114–116). Parents often appreciate sympathy cards, emails, telephone calls, and visits from staff and perceive these as signs of extended caring (117). Some parents want a follow-up meeting with the ICU physician and staff who cared for their child to gain additional information, emotional support, and provide feedback on their hospital experiences (118). Topics that parents most often want to discuss during follow-up meetings include the chronology of events leading to ICU admission and death, cause of death, treatment, autopsy, genetic risk, medical documents, withdrawal of life support, ways to help others, and avenues for bereavement support. Although a few reports have described physicians' experiences meeting with parents after their child's death (119–121), the extent to which follow-up meetings improve bereaved parents' outcomes has not been empirically studied.

Assessing parents' needs can be challenging especially during unfamiliar crisis situations when parents may not fully realize what their needs are. Several instruments for measuring the needs of family members of hospitalized patients exist; however, few have been used to evaluate the needs of parents whose children die in the ICU (122). Recently, the *Bereaved Parent Needs Assessment* (BPNA) was developed to assess parents' needs around the time of their child's death in the ICU and the extent to which parents perceive their needs as met (123). Quantitative tools such as the BPNA can be used to identify specific areas of parental need within and across ICUs for which supportive interventions can be developed.

MULTIDISCIPLINARY APPROACH AND SUPPORT OF THE STAFF

A collaborative approach across many different disciplines is critical to providing effective end-of-life care in the ICU (124–126). Bedside nurses can be important advocates for patients and families (127,128), and including them in family meetings helps the whole team provide a consistent message about prognosis and plans. It is important to make sure the whole ICU team, including physicians, nurses, therapists, psychosocial support staff and trainees, understands the current goals of therapy and has a chance to ask questions or express discomfort with a plan. The inclusion of primary physicians and long-term subspecialists in the conversation may help both the family and team (92). Educational programs for staff about end-of-life care can be very helpful (119,129–133).

While caring for a dying child and supporting a family through a difficult time can bring professional satisfaction for many clinicians, staff can also experience significant emotional distress at losing a patient, dealing with conflict, or providing interventions that may cause suffering (134–136). Team awareness that staff may need support or structured debriefings are one way to give all members of the team a chance to learn how to handle such challenges in their professional lives and hopefully prevent burnout (135,137–139).

BROADER PERSPECTIVE AND THE FUTURE

Pediatric palliative care is a relatively new subspecialty, but compassionate and skillful end-of-life care has been provided by pediatric ICU teams for decades, and the tenets of good palliative care are also core competencies of good critical care (140). Training programs, systems of care, and home support services should be expanded so that all children and families can have the option of focusing on a dying child's comfort or being home when doing so is appropriate and feasible (3,4,93,141). Providing quality end-of-life care and developing systems of reimbursement for such patient-centered care should be a global public health priority (3,37,142–145). Research initiatives examining symptom-management strategies, outcomes, and resource availability can also help extend quality end-of-life care to many patients for whom it is currently unavailable (11,18,22). In pediatrics, such efforts will likely require collaborative networks since experience at any single center is limited (146). Pediatric intensivists, as they are often highly experienced at helping children and families navigate such difficult situations, should be involved in any such efforts. In clinical care, advocacy, and research, it is important to focus on everything that we can do to help critically ill children and their families, even when curing a disease or saving a life is not possible.

References

1. Hamilton BE, Hoyert DL, Martin JA, et al. Annual summary of vital statistics: 2010–2011. *Pediatrics* 2013;131(3):548–58.
2. Global Health Observatory Data Repository. http://apps.who.int/gho/data/?theme=main
3. Crozier F, Hancock LE. Pediatric palliative care: Beyond the end of life. *Pediatr Nurs* 2012;38(4):198–203, 227; quiz 204.
4. Hain R, Heckford E, McCulloch R. Paediatric palliative medicine in the UK: Past, present, future. *Arch Dis Child* 2012;97(4):381–4.
5. Feudtner C, Connor SR. Epidemiology and health services research. In: Carter BS, Levetown M, eds. *Palliative Care for Infants, Children, and Adolescents: A Practical Handbook*. Baltimore, MD: Johns Hopkins University Press, 2004:399.
6. Feudtner C, Christakis DA, Zimmerman FJ, et al. Characteristics of deaths occurring in children's hospitals: Implications for supportive care services. *Pediatrics* 2002;109(5):887–93.
7. Carter BS, Howenstein M, Gilmer MJ, et al. Circumstances surrounding the deaths of hospitalized children: Opportunities for pediatric palliative care. *Pediatrics* 2004;114(3):e361–6.
8. Edwards JD, Houtrow AJ, Vasilevskis EE, et al. Chronic conditions among children admitted to U.S. pediatric intensive care units: Their prevalence and impact on risk for mortality and prolonged length of stay. *Crit Care Med* 2012;40(7):2196–203.
9. Namachivayam P, Shann F, Shekerdemian L, et al. Three decades of pediatric intensive care: Who was admitted, what happened in intensive care, and what happened afterward. *Pediatr Crit Care Med* 2010;11(5):549–55.
10. Piva JP, Schnitzler E, Garcia PC, et al. The burden of paediatric intensive care: A South American perspective. *Paediatr Respir Rev* 2005;6(3):160–5.
11. Lago P, Piva JP. Pediatric palliative care in Brazil. In: Knapp C, Madden V, Fowler-Kerry S, eds. *Pediatric Palliative Care: Global Perspectives*. New York, NY: Springer Dordrecht, 2010:417–30.
12. Miller RL, Gebremariam A, Odetola FO. Pediatric high-impact conditions in the United States: Retrospective analysis of hospitalizations and associated resource use. *BMC Pediatr* 2012;12:61.
13. Miller SC, Weitzen S, Kinzbrunner B. Factors associated with the high prevalence of short hospice stays. *J Palliat Med* 2003;6(5):725–36.
14. Feudtner C, Kang TI, Hexem KR, et al. Pediatric palliative care patients: A prospective multicenter cohort study. *Pediatrics* 2011;127(6):1094–101.
15. Rapoport A, Beaune L, Weingarten K, et al. Living life to the fullest: Early integration of palliative care into the lives of children with chronic complex conditions. *Curr Pediatr Rev* 2012;8(2):152–65.
16. Mack JW, Wolfe J. Early integration of pediatric palliative care: For some children, palliative care starts at diagnosis. *Curr Opin Pediatr* 2006;18(1):10–4.
17. Temel JS, Greer JA, Muzikansky A, et al. Early palliative care for patients with metastatic non-small-cell lung cancer. *N Engl J Med* 2010;363(8):733–42.
18. Devictor DJ, Nguyen DT. Forgoing life-sustaining treatments in children: A comparison between Northern and Southern European pediatric intensive care units. *Pediatr Crit Care Med* 2004;5(3):211–15.
19. Devictor DJ, Latour JM. Forgoing life support: How the decision is made in European pediatric intensive care units. *Intensive Care Med* 2011;37(11):1881–7.
20. Zawistowski CA, DeVita MA. A descriptive study of children dying in the pediatric intensive care unit after withdrawal of life-sustaining treatment. *Pediatr Crit Care Med* 2004;5(3):216–23.
21. Kipper DJ, Piva JP, Garcia PC, et al. Evolution of the medical practices and modes of death on pediatric intensive care units in southern Brazil. *Pediatr Crit Care Meds* 2005;6(3):258–63.
22. Devictor D, Latour JM, Tissieres P. Forgoing life-sustaining or death-prolonging therapy in the pediatric ICU. *Pediatr Clin North Am* 2008;55(3):791–804, xiii.
23. Lago PM, Piva J, Garcia PC, et al. End-of-life practices in seven Brazilian pediatric intensive care units. *Pediatr Crit Care Med* 2008;9(1):26–31.
24. Lantos JD, Berger AC, Zucker AR. Do-not-resuscitate orders in a children's hospital. *Crit Care Med* 1993;21(1):52–5.
25. Mink RB, Pollack MM. Resuscitation and withdrawal of therapy in pediatric intensive care. *Pediatrics* 1992;89(5):961–3.
26. Vernon DD, Dean JM, Timmons OD, et al. Modes of death in the pediatric intensive care unit: Withdrawal and limitation of supportive care. *Crit Care Med* 1993;21(11):1798–802.
27. Levetown M, Pollack MM, Cuerdon TT, et al. Limitations and withdrawals of medical intervention in pediatric critical care. *JAMA* 1994;272(16):1271–5.
28. Randolph AG, Zollo MB, Egger MJ, et al. Variability in physician opinion on limiting pediatric life support. *Pediatrics* 1999;103(4):e46.
29. Lee KJ, Tieves K, Scanlon MC. Alterations in end-of-life support in the pediatric intensive care unit. *Pediatrics* 2010;126(4):e859–64.
30. Feudtner C, Feinstein JA, Satchell M, et al. Shifting place of death among children with complex chronic conditions in the United States, 1989–2003. *JAMA* 2007;297(24):2725–32.
31. Feudtner C, Hexem KR, Rourke MT. Epidemiology and the care of children with complex conditions. In: Wolfe J, Hinds PS, Sourkes BM, eds. *Textbook of Interdisciplinary Pediatric Palliative Care*. Philadelphia, PA: Elsevier, 2011:7–18.
32. Needle JS. Home extubation by a pediatric critical care team: Providing a compassionate death outside the pediatric intensive care unit. *Pediatr Crit Care Med* 2010;11(3):401–3.
33. Zwerdling T, Hamann KC, Kon AA. Home pediatric compassionate extubation: Bridging intensive and palliative care. *Am J Hosp Palliat Care* 2006;23(3):224–8.
34. The History of Hospice. http://www.nationalhospicefoundation.org/i4a/pages/index.cfm?pageid=218.

35. Hoyer T. A history of the Medicare hospice benefit. *Hosp J* 1998; 13(1–2):61–9.

36. Connor SR. U.S. hospice benefits. *J Pain Symptom Manage* 2009; 38(1):105–9.

37. Singer PA, Bowman KW. Quality end-of-life care: A global perspective. *BMC Palliat Care* 2002;1(1):4.

38. Knapp C, Madden V, Fowler-Kerry S. *Pediatric Palliative Care: Global Perspectives.* New York, NY: Springer Dordrecht, 2010.

39. Miller EG, Laragione G, Kang TI, et al. Concurrent care for the medically complex child: Lessons of implementation. *J Palliat Med* 2012;15(11):1281–3.

40. The Patient Protection and Affordable Care Act. Washington, DC: U.S. Government Printing Office, 2010.

41. Kang TI, Feudtner C. Advances in pediatric palliative medicine in the United States. *Prog Palliat Care* 2012;20(6):331–6.

42. Sprung CL, Ledoux D, Bulow HH, et al. Relieving suffering or intentionally hastening death: Where do you draw the line? *Crit Care Med* 2008;36(1):8–13.

43. Truog RD, Brock DW, White DB. Should patients receive general anesthesia prior to extubation at the end of life? *Crit Care Med* 2012;40(2):631–3.

44. Chan JD, Treece PD, Engelberg RA, et al. Narcotic and benzodiazepine use after withdrawal of life support: Association with time to death? *Chest* 2004;126(1):286–93.

45. Wall SN, Partridge JC. Death in the intensive care nursery: Physician practice of withdrawing and withholding life support. *Pediatrics* 1997;99(1):64–70.

46. Zernikow B, Michel E, Craig F, et al. Pediatric palliative care: Use of opioids for the management of pain. *Paediatr Drugs* 2009;11(2):129–151.

47. Morrison W. Titration of medication and the management of suffering at the end of life. *Virtual Mentor* 2012;14(10):780–3.

48. Friedrichsdorf SJ, Kang TI. The management of pain in children with life-limiting illnesses. *Pediatr Clin North Am* 2007; 54(5):645–72.

49. Nalamachu SR. Opioid rotation in clinical practice. *Adv Ther* 2012;29(10):849–63.

50. Friedrichsdorf SJ, Nugent AP. Management of neuropathic pain in children with cancer. *Curr Opin Support Palliat Care* 2013;7(2):131–8.

51. Friedrichsdorf SJ. Pain management in children with advanced cancer and during end-of-life care. *Pediatr Hematol Oncol* 2010;27(4):257–61.

52. Mercadante S. Switching methadone: A 10-year experience of 345 patients in an acute palliative care unit. *Pain Med* 2012;13(3):399–404.

53. Reddy S, Hui D, El Osta B, et al. The effect of oral methadone on the QTc interval in advanced cancer patients: A prospective pilot study. *J Palliat Med* 2010;13(1):33–8.

54. Ullrich CK, Mayer OH. Assessment and management of fatigue and dyspnea in pediatric palliative care. *Pediatr Clin North Am* 2007;54(5):735–56.

55. de Graeff A, Dean M. Palliative sedation therapy in the last weeks of life: A literature review and recommendations for standards. *J Palliat Med* 2007;10(1):67–85.

56. Claessens P, Menten J, Schotsmans P, et al. Palliative sedation: A review of the research literature. *J Pain Symptom Manage* 2008;36(3):310–33.

57. Wusthoff CJ, Shellhaas RA, Licht DJ. Management of common neurologic symptoms in pediatric palliative care: Seizures, agitation, and spasticity. *Pediatr Clin North Am* 2007;54(5): 709–33.

58. American Academy of Pediatrics Committee on Bioethics: Guidelines on foregoing life-sustaining medical treatment. *Pediatrics* 1994;93(3):532–6.

59. Truog RD, Cist AF, Brackett SE, et al. Recommendations for end-of-life care in the intensive care unit: The Ethics Committee of the Society of Critical Care Medicine. *Crit Care Med* 2001;29(12):2332–48.

60. Meyer EC, Ritholz MD, Burns JP, et al. Improving the quality of end-of-life care in the pediatric intensive care unit: Parents' priorities and recommendations. *Pediatrics* 2006;117(3):649–57.

61. Oberender F, Tibballs J. Withdrawal of life-support in paediatric intensive care—a study of time intervals between discussion, decision and death. *BMC Pediatr* 2011;11:39.

62. Kon AA. The shared decision-making continuum. *JAMA* 2010;304(8):9034.

63. Quill TE, Arnold R, Back AL. Discussing treatment preferences with patients who want "everything". *Ann Intern Med* 2009;151(5):345–9.

64. Feudtner C, Morrison W. The darkening veil of "do everything". *Arch Pediatr Adolesc Med* 2012;166(8):694–5.

65. Feudtner C, Munson D, Morrison W. Framing permission for halting or continuing life-extending therapies. *Virtual Mentor* 2008;10(8):506–10.

66. Hinds PS, Oakes LL, Hicks J, et al. "Trying to be a good parent" as defined by interviews with parents who made phase I, terminal care, and resuscitation decisions for their children. *J Clin Oncol* 2009;27(35):5979–85.

67. Morrison W, Berkowitz I. Do not attempt resuscitation orders in pediatrics. *Pediatr Clin North Am* 2007;54(5):757–71.

68. Burns JP, Edwards J, Johnson J, et al. Do-not-resuscitate order after 25 years. *Crit Care Med* 2003;31(5):1543–50.

69. Diem SJ, Lantos JD, Tulsky JA. Cardiopulmonary resuscitation on television. Miracles and misinformation. *N Engl J Med* 1996;334(24):1578–82.

70. Cohen RW. A tale of two conversations. *Hastings Cent Rep* 2004;34(3):49.

71. Knox C, Vereb JA. Allow natural death: A more humane approach to discussing end-of-life directives. *J Emerg Nurs* 2005, 31(6):560–1.

72. Schlairet MC, Cohen RW. Allow-natural-death (AND) orders: Legal, ethical, and practical considerations. *HEC Forum* 2013;25(2):161–71.

73. Feudtner C. The breadth of hopes. *N Engl J Med* 2009;361 (24):2306–7.

74. Tulsky JA. Beyond advance directives: Importance of communication skills at the end of life. *JAMA* 2005;294(3):359–65.

75. Sulmasy DP, Snyder L. Substituted interests and best judgments: An integrated model of surrogate decision making. *JAMA* 2010;304(17):1946–7.

76. Fallat ME, Deshpande JK. Do-not-resuscitate orders for pediatric patients who require anesthesia and surgery. *Pediatrics* 2004;114(6):1686–92.

77. Antommaria AH, Trotochaud K, Kinlaw K, et al. Policies on donation after cardiac death at children's hospitals: A mixed-methods analysis of variation. *JAMA* 2009;301(18):1902–8.

78. Munson D. Withdrawal of mechanical ventilation in pediatric and neonatal intensive care units. *Pediatr Clin North Am* 2007;54(5):773–85.

79. Field MJ, Behrman RE, eds. *When Children Die: Improving Palliative and End-of-Life Care for Children and their Families.* Washington, DC: National Academy Press, 2003.

80. Fleischman AR, Nolan K, Dubler NN, et al. Caring for gravely ill children. *Pediatrics* 1994;94(4 pt 1):433–9.

81. Kirschbaum MS. Needs of parents of critically ill children. *Dimens Crit Care Nurs* 1990;9(6):344–52.

82. Board R, Ryan-Wenger N. Long-term effects of pediatric intensive care unit hospitalization on families with young children. *Heart Lung* 2002;31(1):53–66.

83. Smith AB, Hefley GC, Anand KJ. Parent bed spaces in the PICU: Effect on parental stress. *Pediatr Nurs* 2007;33(3):215–21.

84. Macdonald ME, Liben S, Carnevale FA, et al. An office or a bedroom? Challenges for family-centered care in the pediatric intensive care unit. *J Child Health Care* 2012;16(3):237–49.

85. Meert KL, Briller SH, Schim SM, et al. Examining the needs of bereaved parents in the pediatric intensive care unit: A qualitative study. *Death Stud* 2009;33(8):712–40.

86. Meert KL, Thurston CS, Briller SH. The spiritual needs of parents at the time of their child's death in the pediatric intensive care unit and during bereavement: A qualitative study. *Pediatr Crit Care Med* 2005;6(4):420–7.

87. Meert KL, Thurston CS, Sarnaik AP. End-of-life decision-making and satisfaction with care: Parental perspectives. *Pediatr Crit Care Med* 2000;1(2):179–85.

88. Morrison W, Feudtner C. The contested territory of medical decision-making for children. In: Ravistsky V, Fiester A, Caplan A, eds. *Penn Center Guide to Bioethics*. New York, NY: Springer, 2009.

89. Davidson JE, Powers K, Hedayat KM, et al. Clinical practice guidelines for support of the family in the patient-centered intensive care unit: American College of Critical Care Medicine Task Force 2004–2005. *Crit Care Med* 2007;35(2):605–22.

90. Elwyn G, Frosch D, Thomson R, et al. Shared decision making: A model for clinical practice. *J Gen Intern Med* 2012;27(10):1361–7.

91. Madrigal VN, Carroll KW, Hexem KR, et al. Parental decision-making preferences in the pediatric intensive care unit. *Crit Care Med* 2012;40(10):2876–82.

92. Meyer EC, Burns JP, Griffith JL, et al. Parental perspectives on end-of-life care in the pediatric intensive care unit. *Crit Care Med* 2002;30(1):226–31.

93. Rodriguez-Arias D, Moutel G, Aulisio MP, et al. Advance directives and the family: French and American perspectives. *Clin Ethics* 2007;2(3):139–45.

94. Smith AK, Sudore RL, Perez-Stable EJ. Palliative care for Latino patients and their families: Whenever we prayed, she wept. *JAMA* 2009;301(10):1047–57, E1041.

95. Clark JD, Dudzinski DM. The culture of dysthanasia: Attempting CPR in terminally ill children. *Pediatrics* 2013;131(3):572–80.

96. Morrison WE. "Is that all you got?". *J Palliat Med* 2010; 13(11):1384–5.

97. Lanctot D, Morrison W, Kock KD, et al. Spiritual dimensions. In: Carter BS, Levetown M, Friebert SE, eds. *Palliative Care for Infants, Children, and Adolescents: A Practical Handbook*. 2nd ed. Baltimore, MD: Johns Hopkins University Press, 2011:227–43.

98. Firth S. End-of-life: A Hindu view. *Lancet* 2005;366(9486):682–6.

99. Sachedina A. End-of-life: The Islamic view. *Lancet* 2005;366 (9487):774–9.

100. Dorff EN. End-of-life: Jewish perspectives. *Lancet* 2005;366 (9488):862–5.

101. Keown D. End of life: The Buddhist view. *Lancet* 2005;366 (9489):952–5.

102. Engelhardt HT Jr, Iltis AS. End-of-life: The traditional Christian view. *Lancet* 2005;366(9490):1045–9.

103. Markwell H. End-of-life: A catholic view. *Lancet* 2005; 366(9491):1132–5.

104. Baggini J, Pym M. End of life: The humanist view. *Lancet* 2005; 366(9492):1235–7.

105. Baggs JG, Norton SA, Schmitt MH, et al. Intensive care unit cultures and end-of-life decision making. *J Crit Care* 2007; 22(2):159–68.

106. Steinberg SM. Cultural and religious aspects of palliative care. *Int J Crit Illn Inj Sci* 2011;1(2):154–6.

107. Meert KL, Eggly S, Pollack M, et al. Parents' perspectives on physician-parent communication near the time of a child's death in the pediatric intensive care unit. *Pediatr Crit Care Med* 2008;9(1):2–7.

108. Levetown M. Communicating with children and families: From everyday interactions to skill in conveying distressing information. *Pediatrics* 2008;121(5):e1441–60.

109. Fallowfield LJ, Jenkins VA, Beveridge HA. Truth may hurt but deceit hurts more: Communication in palliative care. *Palliat Med* 2002;16(4):297–303.

110. Meert KL, Briller SH, Schim SM, et al. Exploring parents' environmental needs at the time of a child's death in the pediatric intensive care unit. *Pediatr Crit Care Med* 2008;9(6):623–8.

111. Muriel AC, Case C, Sourkes BM. Children's voices: The experience of patients and their siblings. In: Wolfe J, Hinds PS, Sourkes BM, eds. *Textbook of Interdisciplinary Pediatric Palliative Care*. Philadelphia, PA: Elsevier, 2011.

112. Contro N, Larson J, Scofield S, et al. Family perspectives on the quality of pediatric palliative care. *Arch Pediatr Adolesc Med* 2002;156(1):14–9.

113. Children and the death of a sibling. In: Corr CA, ed. *Handbook of Childhood Death and Bereavement*. New York, NY: Springer, 1996:149–64.

114. Back AL, Young JP, McCown E, et al. Abandonment at the end of life from patient, caregiver, nurse, and physician perspectives: Loss of continuity and lack of closure. *Arch Intern Med* 2009;169(5):474–9.

115. Han PK, Arnold RM. Palliative care services, patient abandonment, and the scope of physicians' responsibilities in end-of-life care. *J Palliat Med* 2005;8(6):1238–45.

116. Quill TE, Cassel CK. Nonabandonment: A central obligation for physicians. *Ann Intern Med* 1995;122(5):368–74.

117. Macdonald ME, Liben S, Carnevale FA, et al. Parental perspectives on hospital staff members' acts of kindness and commemoration after a child's death. *Pediatrics* 2005;116(4):884–90.

118. Meert KL, Eggly S, Pollack M, et al. Parents' perspectives regarding a physician-parent conference after their child's death in the pediatric intensive care unit. *J Pediatr* 2007;151(1):50–5, e51–2.

119. Meert KL, Eggly S, Berger J, et al. Physicians' experiences and perspectives regarding follow-up meetings with parents after a child's death in the pediatric intensive care unit. *Pediatr Crit Care Med* 2011;12(2):e64–8.

120. Stein J, Peles-Borz A, Buchval I, et al. The bereavement visit in pediatric oncology. *J Clin Oncol* 2006;24(22):3705–7.

121. Cook P, White DK, Ross-Russell RI. Bereavement support following sudden and unexpected death: Guidelines for care. *Arch Dis Child* 2002;87(1):36–8.

122. Meert KL, Schim SM, Briller SH. Parental bereavement needs in the pediatric intensive care unit: Review of available measures. *J Palliat Med* 2011;14(8):951–64.

123. Meert KL, Templin TN, Michelson KN, et al. The Bereaved Parent Needs Assessment: A new instrument to assess the needs of parents whose children died in the pediatric intensive care unit. *Crit Care Med* 2012;40(11):3050–7.

124. Baker JN, Hinds PS, Spunt SL, et al. Integration of palliative care practices into the ongoing care of children with cancer: Individualized care planning and coordination. *Pediatr Clin North Am* 2008;55(1):223–50.

125. Truog RD, Meyer EC, Burns JP. Toward interventions to improve end-of-life care in the pediatric intensive care unit. *Crit Care Med* 2006;34(11 suppl):S373–9.

126. Lago PM, Devictor D, Piva JP, et al. End-of-life care in children: The Brazilian and the international perspectives. *J Pediatr (Rio J)* 2007;83(2 suppl):S109–16.

127. Brien IO, Duffy A, Shea EO. Medical futility in children's nursing: Making end-of-life decisions. *Br J Nurs* 2010;19(6):352–6.

128. Copnell B. Death in the pediatric ICU: Caring for children and families at the end of life. *Crit Care Nurs Clin North Am* 2005;17(4):349–60.

129. Ferrell BR, Virani R, Grant M, et al. Evaluation of the end-of-life nursing education consortium undergraduate faculty training program. *J Palliat Med* 2005;8(1):107–14.

130. Roberts KE, Boyle LA. End-of-life education in the pediatric intensive care unit. *Crit Care Nurse* 2005;25(1):51–7.

131. Hough CL, Hudson LD, Salud A, et al. Death rounds: End-of-life discussions among medical residents in the intensive care unit. *J Crit Care* 2005;20(1):20–5.

132. Bagatell R, Meyer R, Herron S, et al. When children die: A seminar series for pediatric residents. *Pediatrics* 2002;110(2 pt 1):348–53.

133. Serwint JR, Rutherford LE, Hutton N, et al. "I learned that no death is routine": Description of a death and bereavement seminar for pediatrics residents. *Acad Med* 2002, 77(4):278–84.

134. Jellinek MS, Todres ID, Catlin EA, et al. Pediatric intensive care training: Confronting the dark side. *Crit Care Med* 1993;21(5):775–9.

135. Rushton CH, Reder E, Hall B, et al. Interdisciplinary interventions to improve pediatric palliative care and reduce health care professional suffering. *J Palliat Med* 2006;9(4):922–33.

136. Ruppe MD, Feudtner C, Hexem KR, et al. Family factors affect clinician attitudes in pediatric end-of-life decision making: A randomized vignette study. *J Pain Symptom Manage* 2013;45(5):832–40.

137. Keene EA, Hutton N, Hall B, et al. Bereavement debriefing sessions: An intervention to support health care professionals in managing their grief after the death of a patient. *Pediatr Nurs* 2010;36(4):185–9; quiz 190.

138. Bateman ST, Dixon R, Trozzi M. The wrap-up: A unique forum to support pediatric residents when faced with the death of a child. *J Palliat Med* 2012;15(12):1329–34.

139. Serwint JR. One method of coping: Resident debriefing after the death of a patient. *J Pediatr* 2004;145(2):229–34.

140. Clarke EB, Curtis JR, Luce JM, et al. Quality indicators for end-of-life care in the intensive care unit. *Crit Care Med* 2003;31(9):2255–62.

141. Wolff J, Robert R, Sommerer A, et al. Impact of a pediatric palliative care program. *Pediatr Blood Cancer* 2010;54(2):279–83.

142. Knapp C, Woodworth L, Wright M, et al. Pediatric palliative care provision around the world: A systematic review. *Pediatr Blood Cancer* 2011;57(3):361–8.

143. Lamas D, Rosenbaum L. Painful inequities—palliative care in developing countries. *N Engl J Med* 2012;366(3):199–201.

144. Brennan F. Palliative care as an international human right. *J Pain Symptom Manage* 2007;33(5):494–9.

145. Marston J, Germ RM, Granera Lopez DJ, et al. Children's hospice and palliative care worldwide. In: Armstrong-Dailey A, Zarbock S, eds. *Hospice Care for Children*. New York, NY: Oxford University Press, 2009:365–77.

146. Willson DF, Dean JM, Meert KL, et al. Collaborative pediatric critical care research network: Looking back and moving forward. *Pediatr Crit Care Med* 2010;11(1):1–6.

147. Bioethical Issues in Pediatrics: Pediatric Palliative Care. *Pediatrics* February 2014, 133(S1).

CHAPTER 14 ■ PAIN AND SEDATION MANAGEMENT

SAPNA R. KUDCHADKAR, R. BLAINE EASLEY, KENNETH M. BRADY, AND MYRON YASTER

We must all die. But that I can save (a person) from days of torture, that is what I feel as my great and ever new privilege. Pain is a more terrible lord of mankind than even death itself.

Albert Schweitzer

KEY POINTS

1. The PICU poses unique challenges for pain and sedation management. Hospitalization in general, and admission to the PICU in particular, are frightening and painful experiences to children and their families.

2. The goals of pain and sedation management in the PICU are to provide a child with anxiolysis and comfort while maintaining safety, promoting sleep, and preventing delirium.

3. Infants and children may be unable to describe their pain or their subjective experiences. Pain assessment and management are interdependent, and it is important to delineate accurate data about the location and intensity of pain, as well as the effectiveness of measures used to alleviate or abolish it.

4. Optimal sedation management involves measuring a child's level of sedation at regular intervals and to use these measures to avoid oversedation or undersedation as both have the potential to produce morbidity and mortality.

5. Given the complex team framework of staff who provide and manage sedation, the use of a streamlined sedation assessment tool is necessary to facilitate consistent communication and optimal therapy. The most commonly used sedation assessment tools are the State Behavioral Scale and the COMFORT Scale.

6. Very few studies have evaluated the pharmacokinetic and pharmacodynamic properties of analgesic and sedative drugs in critically ill patients. Most of the recommendations in this chapter are based on experience and best practice, rather than evidence-based medicine.

7. Opioids bind G-protein–coupled receptors and regulate transmembrane signaling. The most commonly used opioids in pain management are μ agonists, which include morphine, meperidine, methadone, codeine, oxycodone, and the fentanyls. All of the μ-opioid agonists have similar pharmacodynamic effects at equianalgesic doses, including analgesia, respiratory depression, sedation, nausea and vomiting, pruritus, constipation, miosis, tolerance, and physical dependence.

8. Although fentanyl is the least sedating of the opioids, it is the most commonly used analgesic for procedures and

pain control in the PICU. It is short-acting following single doses (redistribution), but can be long-acting ("context-sensitive half-life") following infusions.

9. Local anesthetics are beneficial for the treatment of procedure-related pain. They reversibly block conduction of neural impulses along central and peripheral nerve pathways.

10. The systemic toxic effects of local anesthetics are determined by the total dose delivered, protein binding, rapidity of absorption into the blood, and the site of injection. Bupivacaine toxicity is the most dangerous and can lead to cardiac arrest and death.

11. Most sedatives, specifically benzodiazepines, chloral hydrate, propofol, and the barbiturates, have no analgesic properties.

12. The benzodiazepines are potent amnestics, hypnotics, and skeletal muscle relaxants.

13. Benzodiazepine withdrawal symptoms are similar to alcohol withdrawal (delirium tremens).

14. Long-term neuromuscular blockade, which has no analgesic or sedating qualities, should be reserved for clinical scenarios in which sedation and analgesia are adequate and immobility is necessary to facilitate recovery from the child's illness.

15. It is imperative that the level of neuromuscular blockade is constantly monitored to prevent prolonged blockade and critical illness myopathy.

16. The interplay between sedation, sleep, and delirium is an important consideration in the comprehensive management of the critically ill child. Many of the drugs used for sedation and analgesia have deleterious effects on sleep, which can lead to a vicious cycle of increased sedation and analgesic needs and finally, delirium.

17. Delirium is known to increase morbidity and mortality in critically ill patients, and validated screening tools are available to screen for this important entity.

18. Behavioral interventions such as noise minimization and light optimization to maintain the day–night cycle are instrumental for preventing sleep disturbances and delirium.

The treatment and alleviation of pain is a basic human right that exists regardless of age (1). Indeed, all of the nerve pathways essential for the transmission and perception of pain are present and functioning by 24 weeks of gestation (2). Failure to provide analgesia for pain to newborn animals and human newborns results in "rewiring" the nerve pathways responsible for pain transmission in the dorsal horn of the spinal cord and results in increased pain perception for *future* painful insults (3).

The PICU poses unique challenges for pain and sedation management. Hospitalization in general, and admission to the PICU in particular, are frightening and painful experiences to children and their families. Pain in the PICU can be the result of the primary illness, trauma or the disease process, or the result of medical interventions. In addition, pain can be exacerbated by emotional distress and anxiety, two common components of the PICU stay. This distress may be the result of separation from one's parents and family, being surrounded by unfamiliar people, sleep loss and fragmentation, and the fear of pain, loss of control, or even death (4). Thus, not only is pain control imperative in the critically ill but so too is the need for sedation. Nonpharmacologic measures such as open communication, reassurance, parental presence, sleep hygiene, and psychological interventions are helpful and essential in basic management. Nevertheless, many critically ill children need pharmacologically induced sedation to facilitate mechanical ventilation, invasive procedures, and treatment of multi–organ system dysfunction. Regardless of the methods used, the goals of sedation in the PICU are to provide a child with anxiolysis and comfort while maintaining safety to prevent inadvertent removal of invasive instrumentation such as endotracheal tubes and vascular access devices.

Fortunately, there is an increased interest in pain and sedation research and in the development of pediatric pain services, primarily under the direction of pediatric anesthesiologists. Pain service teams provide the pain management for acute, postoperative, terminal, neuropathic, and chronic pain. In this chapter, we have tried to consolidate in a comprehensive manner some of the recent advances in pain and sedation management in an attempt to provide a better understanding of how to manage pain and sedation in the critically ill child.

PAIN AND SEDATION ASSESSMENT

Pain Assessment

The International Association for the Study of Pain (IASP) defines pain as "an unpleasant and emotional experience associated with actual or potential tissue damage, or described in terms of such damage." Pain is a subjective experience, and infants and children may be unable to describe their pain or their subjective experiences. This has led many to conclude incorrectly that children do not experience pain in the same way that adults do. It is becoming increasingly clear that the child's perspective of pain is an indispensable facet of pediatric pain management and an essential element in the specialized study of childhood pain. Pain assessment and management are interdependent and require accurate data about the location and intensity of pain, as well as the effectiveness of the measures being used to alleviate or abolish it.

Instruments currently exist to measure and assess pain in children of all ages, although few have been validated for patients admitted to the PICU. The most commonly used instruments measure the quality and intensity of pain and

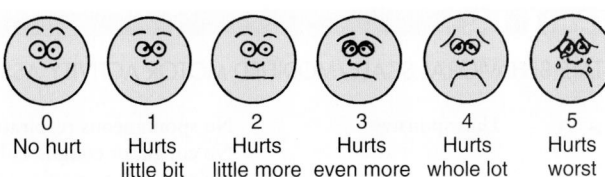

FIGURE 14.1. Six-Face Pain Scale for use with children.

are "self-report measures" that make use of pictures or word descriptors to describe pain. Pain intensity or severity can be measured in children as young as 3 years by using either the Oucher Scale, a two-part scale with a vertical numerical scale (0–100) on one side and six photographs of a young child on the other, or a visual analogue scale, a 10-cm line with a smiling face on one end and a distraught, crying face on the other. Because of its simplicity, the authors primarily use a simplified Six-Face Pain Scale originally developed by Dr. Donna Wong and modified by others (Fig. 14.1) (5). Obviously, self-report measures are impossible to use in intubated, sedated, and paralyzed patients.

In infants and newborns, pain has been assessed by measuring physiologic responses to a nociceptive stimulus, such as blood pressure and heart rate (HR) changes (Observational Pain Scale [OPS]) or by measuring levels of adrenal stress hormones (6). Scales that rely on physiologic parameters can be misleading in an ICU setting, where alterations in vital signs can occur that are unrelated to the level of sedation. Additionally, patients with cardiovascular dysfunction requiring vasoactive medications may not develop tachycardia and hypertension, despite severe agitation or pain. Alternatively, behavioral approaches have utilized facial expression, body movements, and the intensity and quality of crying as indices of response to nociceptive stimuli.

Sedation Assessment

Sedation of the critically ill child is not one-size-fits-all, it requires titration to effect. Thus, it is imperative to measure a child's level of sedation at regular intervals and use these measures to guide and titrate therapy to avoid oversedation or undersedation, both of which have the potential to produce morbidity and mortality. Given the complex team framework of nurses, residents, nurse practitioners, fellows, respiratory therapists, and attendings who provide and manage sedation, the use of a streamlined sedation assessment tool is necessary to facilitate consistent communication and optimal therapy.

In the PICU, the most commonly used sedation assessment tools validated for use in critically ill, mechanically ventilated children are the State Behavioral Scale (SBS) and the COMFORT Scale (7). The SBS was designed and validated in 2006 to define the sedation–agitation continuum in critically ill infants and children to guide goal-directed therapy (8) (Table 14.1). A single digit bipolar numeric from −3 to +2 provides a descriptor of the level of sedation using a patient's response to voice, gentle touch, and noxious stimuli such as suctioning. In contrast, the COMFORT Scale (Table 14.2) relies on the measurement of five behavioral variables (alertness, facial tension, muscle tone, agitation, and movement) and three physiologic variables (HR, respiration, and blood pressure). A modified COMFORT Scale that eliminates physiologic parameters has also been developed (9,10).

Although not validated in critically ill children, other scoring systems used commonly in adult ICUs include the

TABLE 14.1

STATE BEHAVIORAL SCALE/MODIFIED MOTOR ACTIVITY ASSESSMENT SCALE

>−3	Unresponsive	No spontaneous respiratory effort No cough, or coughs only with suctioning No response to noxious stimuli Unable to pay attention to care provider Does not distress with any procedure (including noxious) Does not move
−2	Responsive only to noxious stimuli[a]	Spontaneous yet supported breathing Coughs with suctioning/repositioning Responds to noxious stimuli Unable to pay attention to care provider Will distress with a noxious procedure Does not move/occasional movement of limbs or shifting of position
−1	Responsive to touch or name	Spontaneous but ineffective nonsupported breaths Coughs with suctioning/repositioning Responds to touch/voice Able to pay attention but drifts off after stimulation Distresses with procedures Able to calm with comforting touch or voice when stimulus is removed Occasional movement of limbs or shifting of position
0	Calm and cooperative	Spontaneous and effective breathing Coughs when repositioned/occasional spontaneous cough Responds to voice/no external stimulus is required to elicit response Spontaneously pays attention to care provider Distresses with procedures Able to calm with comforting touch or voice when stimulus is removed Occasional movement of limbs or shifting of position/increased movement (restless, squirming)
+1	Restless and cooperative	Spontaneous effective breathing/having difficulty breathing with ventilator Occasional spontaneous cough Responds to voice/no external stimulus is required to elicit response Drifts off/spontaneously pays attention to care provider Intermittently unsafe Does not consistently calm, despite 5-min attempt/unable to console Increased movement (restless, squirming)
+2	Agitated	May have difficulty breathing with ventilator Coughing spontaneously No external stimulus required to elicit response Spontaneously pays attention to care provider Unsafe (biting endotracheal tube, pulling at catheters, cannot be left alone) Unable to console Increased movement (restless, squirming, or thrashing side-to-side, kicking legs)

[a]Noxious stimuli, endotracheal tube suctioning, or 5 s of nail bed pressure. From Curley MA, Harris SK, Fraser KA, et al. State Behavioral Scale: A sedation assessment instrument for infants and young children supported on mechanical ventilation. *Pediatr Crit Care Med* 2006;7:107–14, with permission.

Richmond Agitation–Sedation Scale (RASS), the Sedation–Agitation Scale, and the Ramsay Sedation Scale (11). A unique component of the RASS is the integration of duration of eye contact following verbal stimulation as a part of the assessment (12). This is important because this metric incorporates both components of consciousness—arousal and content of thought (13). The Sedation–Agitation Scale eliminates the use of physiologic parameters and utilizes visual assessment of the patient's comfort, on a scale of 1–7 (14). Similarly, the Ramsay Sedation Scale score categorizes sedation at six different levels based on the observation of the patient but also includes a tactile stimulus provided to the patient, in this case a glabellar tap (15).

The desire for objective measurements has led many to advocate the use of bispectral index (BIS) monitoring as a means of assessing the depth of sedation without the need for stimulating the patient or relying on physiologic parameters. First developed for use in adults undergoing isoflurane general anesthesia, the BIS monitor uses an algorithmic analysis of the electroencephalogram (EEG) to provide a single, dimensionless number to guide titration of anesthetic agents. The number is determined from three primary factors, including the frequency of the electroencephalographic waves, the synchronization of low and high frequency information, and the percentage of time in burst suppression. The depth of sedation/anesthesia is displayed numerically, ranging from 0 to 100, with 40–60 being a suitable level of surgical anesthesia. Its use has spread to patients of all ages who are undergoing moderate sedation to general anesthesia utilizing intravenous sedatives and hypnotics. Given that the algorithm of the BIS monitor is derived from adult EEG data and the EEG of children changes as the brain matures, it remains controversial whether BIS can

TABLE 14.2

COMFORT SCALE

■ ALERTNESS		■ CALMNESS/AGITATION		■ RESPIRATORY RESPONSE		■ PHYSICAL MOVEMENT	
Deeply asleep	1	Calm	1	No coughing and no spontaneous respiration	1	No spontaneous movement	1
Lightly asleep	2	Slightly anxious	2	Spontaneous respiration minimal response to vent	2	Occasional slight movement	2
Drowsy	3	Anxious	3	Occasional cough or resistance to vent	3	Frequent, slight movement	3
Fully awake and alert	4	Very anxious	4	Actively breathes against vent or coughs regularly	4	Vigorous movement, extremities only	4
Hyper-alert	5	Panicky	5	Fights vent, coughing, or choking	5	Vigorous movement, including torso and head	5

■ MEAN ARTERIAL BLOOD PRESSURE		■ HEART RATE		■ MUSCLE TONE		■ FACIAL TENSION	
Any observation LO	1	Any observation LO	1	Totally relaxed, no tone	1	Facial muscles totally relaxed	1
All six observations within baseline range	2	All six observations within baseline range	2	Reduced tone	2	Facial muscle tone normal, no tension evident	2
One to three of six observations HI	3	One to three of six observations HI	3	Normal tone	3	Tension evident in some facial muscles	3
Four to five of six observations HI	4	Four to five of six observations HI	4	Increased tone with flexion of fingers and toes	4	Tension evident throughout facial muscles	4
All six observations HI	5	All six observations HI	5	Extreme rigidity and flexion of fingers and toes	5	Facial muscles contorted and grimacing	5

Review the medical record for heart rate and blood pressure data recorded over the 24-h period prior to initial COMFORT score determination. Using the following data and equations, calculate the baseline range limits (e.g., HI, LO), and record where appropriate.

Heart Rate:

1. Range of Normal Values

Age (y)	Rate (beats/min)
0–1	120–180
>1–2	100–130
>2–4	90–120
>4–8	80–110
>8	70–100

2. Study Limit Calculations
   Observed baseline heart rate = lowest heart rate within the range of normal values charted over the 24-h period preceding observation #1 =_____
   LO limit heart rate = Observed baseline − (Observed baseline × 0.15) =_____
   HI limit heart rate = Observed baseline + (Observed baseline × 0.15) =_____

Mean arterial pressure (MAP):

1. Range of Normal Values

Age (y)	Pressure (mm Hg)
0–1	47–82
>1–5	60–90
>5–7	60–93
>7–10	67–100
>10–12	68–102
>12–14	72–107

2. Study Limit Calculations
   Observed Baseline MAP = lowest MAP within the range of normal values charted over the 24-h period preceding observation #1 =_____

   LO limit MAP = Observed baseline − (Observed baseline × 0.15) =_____
   HI limit MAP = Observed baseline + (Observed baseline × 0.15) =_____

Adapted from Ambuel B, Hamlett KW, Marx CM, et al. Assessing distress in pediatric intensive care environments: The COMFORT scale. *J Pediatr Psychol* 1992;17:95–109.

be generalized to infants and children in the operating room and ICU settings (16,17).

Although formal guidelines for critically ill children do not exist, the Society of Critical Care Medicine advocates for goal-directed delivery of psychoactive medications in critically ill adults (18). Therefore, it is plausible to assume that children (especially those undergoing active neurocognitive development) would benefit from the same emphasis on the utilization of sedation assessment tools that can be translated across time and a multidisciplinary team of care providers. It is essential to optimize pain and sedation management through consistent use of the available validated tools for the PICU to strike a balance between comfort and safety. Failure to provide adequate pain and sedation can be devastating and lead to posttraumatic stress disorder, while oversedation can lead to rapid development of tolerance, excessive drug delivery, sleep disturbances, and delirium.

PAIN AND SEDATION MANAGEMENT—GENERAL PRINCIPLES

Physiologic Changes Affecting Pharmacokinetics in the Critically Ill Patient

Unfortunately, very few studies have evaluated the pharmacokinetic and pharmacodynamic properties of drugs in critically ill patients. Most studies are performed using healthy adult volunteers or adult patients in a stable phase of a chronic disease. These data are then extrapolated to infants, children, adolescents, and to both adult and pediatric critically ill patients. To help remedy this situation, the U.S. Food and Drug Administration has mandated pediatric pharmacokinetic and pharmacodynamic studies in all new drugs that enter the marketplace. Unfortunately, studies performed in healthy patients may offer little insight into how these drugs perform in the critically ill, who often have significant hemodynamic alterations and organ dysfunction, which may significantly alter drug absorption, transport, metabolism, and excretion of drugs.

Absorption

In healthy patients, the enteral route of drug administration is most common and is the most widely studied. Drainage of intestinal blood flow into the portal system presents the drug to the liver for metabolism before the drug can be distributed throughout the body. This leads to the first-pass effect seen with many oral drugs, that is, much of the absorbed drug is taken directly to the liver via the portal circulation and is rapidly metabolized and "lost" before it ever reaches the systemic circulation. Alteration of venous blood flow such that it bypasses the liver could result in significantly higher serum drug levels after oral absorption and lead to clinical sequelae. Absorption from the gastrointestinal (GI) tract may be reduced in ICU patients for several reasons, including altered GI motility and peristalsis, reduced gut function and absorptive surface area, reduced GI blood flow, and physical removal of drug by nasogastric (NG) suctioning. On the other hand, as a patient's overall condition improves, gut function also improves, and the enteral route may be considered as a viable route of drug administration.

Parenteral drug administration through intravenous access is most common in the critically ill ICU patient. Intramuscular, transdermal, and SQ injections are rarely used in the critically ill because drug absorption from muscle or through skin or subcutaneous tissue may be decreased because of decreased tissue perfusion and decreased movement of drug through edematous tissue. However, as patients improve, the transdermal route (e.g., fentanyl, clonidine) may become useful, particularly when IV access becomes a severe problem.

Distribution

As described in Chapter 22, distribution describes the transportation and movement of a drug throughout the body. Several factors associated with critical illness have the potential to affect the distribution of drugs in the body. Poor perfusion is often a factor that limits distribution of a drug to its target tissue. Altered receptor binding as a result of edema, malnutrition, uremic toxins, and downregulation will also change the amount of drug attached to tissue. Many analgesic drugs are transported through the body attached to the serum proteins albumin and gamma globulin. The extent of protein binding varies considerably among analgesic drugs, from 7% for codeine to 93% for sufentanil. This may decrease in critical illness, causing elevated free levels of drug and possible toxicity. Additionally, third spacing of fluid may result in additional volume into which the drug can distribute.

Metabolism and Elimination

The liver is the major route for drug metabolism and detoxification for a wide variety of analgesic and sedative drugs. Most are lipid-soluble compounds; this lipid solubility enhances their passage through the blood–brain barrier and also preselects the liver as the organ of elimination, as renal physiology requires drugs to be water soluble to be filtered and excreted. Some degree of hepatic dysfunction is present in many critically ill patients and may result in reduced drug clearance; therefore, the clinician must expect unpredictable metabolism and elimination of drugs and must monitor for therapeutic outcomes and possible adverse effects. Most, but not all, drugs are metabolized in a two-part process, the goal of which is to change fat-soluble, active, unexcretable drugs into water-soluble, inactive drugs that can be excreted in the bile or by the kidneys (Fig. 14.2). The first, or phase I metabolism, commonly involves the cytochrome P450 (CYP) system. The metabolites of these reactions may be less active or highly reactive and even toxic. The phase I metabolite is then metabolized further by a phase II enzyme that conjugates it with a glucuronide, a sulfide group, an amino acid, or a glutathione (Fig. 14.2). Some drugs are metabolized directly by phase II enzymes (e.g., morphine). A third metabolic pathway is becoming increasingly important, namely, metabolism by blood and tissue esterases. These enzymes are ubiquitous and are found in large supply in the blood and elsewhere. Drugs that are metabolized by esterases such as remifentanil are unlikely to be affected by disease.

Most pain and sedation medications used in the critically ill are metabolized by phase I or phase II reactions in the liver. In general, the metabolism of opioid analgesics is very effective and is limited more by blood flow to the liver than by the inherent ability of the hepatocyte enzymes. The cytochrome P450 microenzyme system is significantly altered in critical illness, decreasing phase I oxidative metabolism. One of the P450 enzymes, cytochrome P450 2D6 is subject to genetic polymorphism and does not function in 10% of the population even in normal conditions. This enzyme metabolizes codeine to morphine. In patients who lack a functioning cytochrome P450 2D6, either genetically or because of liver disease, codeine will be a poor or ineffective analgesic. In addition to the reduction in the cytochrome P450 enzyme system, phase II conjugation pathways such as glucuronidation may also be impaired in ICU patients, particularly if the liver is subjected to low blood flow, hypoxia, and/or stress. Chronic liver disease

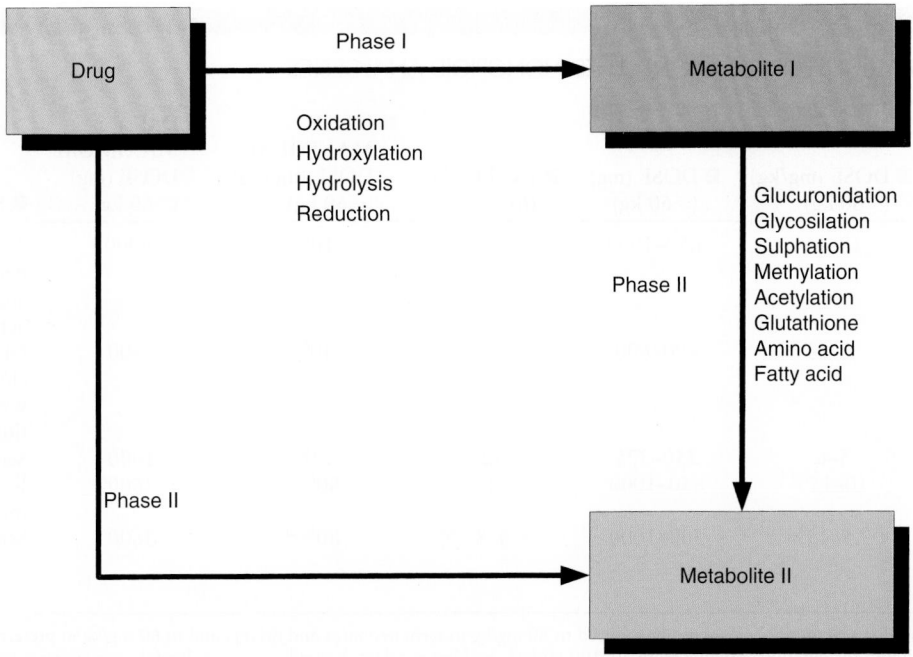

FIGURE 14.2. The two-part process by which most drugs are metabolized, the goal of which is to change fat-soluble, active, unexcretable drugs into water-soluble, inactive drugs that can be excreted in the bile or by the kidneys.

appears selectively to impair oxidative pathways while leaving glucuronidation intact.

The kidneys are responsible for clearing both the parent drug and metabolites produced by the liver. In renal failure, both the parent drug and metabolites may accumulate and result in toxicity (see section Morphine).

ANALGESICS IN THE PICU

The basic principles of pain management—listening to the child and their family, utilizing pain scores to guide management, optimizing sleep, and the rapid delivery of analgesics when they are needed—are the building blocks of pain management in not just the critically ill but all patients. What is often different and surprising is the enormous variation in dosing and the rapid development of tolerance in the critically ill and very young. Practitioners generally use what is needed and titrate medications to effect. Furthermore, a multimodal approach to therapy is advocated, in which different families of drugs as well as cognitive and alternative approaches (music therapy, light touch, etc.) are utilized from the initiation of therapy. In the next sections, the pharmacology, pharmacokinetics, and special issues unique to the use of analgesics and sedative drugs in critically ill children will be reviewed.

Analgesics with Antipyretic Activity or Nonopioid ("Weaker") Analgesics

The "weaker" or "milder" analgesics with antipyretic activity, of which acetaminophen (paracetamol), salicylate (aspirin), ibuprofen, naproxen, and diclofenac are the classic examples, comprise a heterogeneous group of nonsteroidal anti-inflammatory drugs (NSAIDs) and nonopioid analgesics (Table 14.3). They provide pain relief primarily by blocking peripheral and central prostaglandin production through the inhibition of cyclooxygenase types I, II, and III. These analgesic

agents are administered enterally via the oral or, on occasion, the rectal route and are particularly useful for inflammatory, bony, or rheumatic pain. Parenterally administered NSAIDs, such as ketorolac, are available for use in children in whom the oral or rectal routes of administration are not possible. Unfortunately, regardless of dose, the nonopioid analgesics reach a "ceiling effect" above which pain cannot be relieved by these drugs alone. Indeed, because of this, these weaker analgesics are often administered in oral combination forms with opioids such as codeine, oxycodone, or hydrocodone. Of note, in 2012, the U.S. Food and Drug Administration issued a strong warning against the use of codeine-containing products to manage pain in children post-tonsillectomy and/or adenoidectomy because of concerns about children who are "ultrarapid metabolizers" and have increased conversion to morphine and risk of overdose and death.

Aspirin, one of the oldest and most effective nonopioid analgesics, has been largely abandoned in pediatric practice because of its possible role in Reye syndrome, its effects on platelet function, and its gastric irritant properties. Despite these problems, choline-magnesium trisalicylate, a unique aspirin-like compound that does not bind to platelets, is increasingly being used in the management of postoperative pain and in children with cancer. It is convenient for pediatric use because of its availability in both a liquid and tablet form and it can be administered either twice a day or every 6 hours.

The most commonly used nonopioid analgesic in pediatric practice remains acetaminophen (paracetamol). Unlike aspirin and the NSAIDs, acetaminophen works primarily centrally (COX III) and has minimal, if any, anti-inflammatory activity. When administered in recommended doses, acetaminophen is extremely safe and has very few serious side effects. It is an antipyretic, and like all enterally administered NSAIDs, it takes about 30 minutes to provide effective analgesia. Several investigators have reported that acetaminophen should be administered rectally in significantly higher doses than previous recommendations suggested (19). There are many clinical scenarios in which oral or rectal acetaminophen may not be an

TABLE 14.3

ORAL DOSING GUIDELINES FOR COMMONLY USED NONOPIOID ANALGESICS

■ DRUG	■ DOSE (mg/kg) (<60 kg)	■ DOSE (mg) (>60 kg)	■ INTERVAL (h)	■ DAILY MAXIMUM DOSE (mg/kg) (<60 kg)	■ DAILY MAXIMUM DOSE (mg) (>60 kg)	■ SIDE EFFECTS
Acetaminophen	10–15[a]	650–1000	4	100[a]	4000	Toxic doses—hepatotoxicity; lacks anti-inflammatory activity
Ibuprofen	5–10	400–600[c]	6	40[b,c]	2400[c]	GI irritation, bronchospasm, interferes with platelet function, hematuria
Naproxen	5–6[c]	250–375[c]	12	24[b,c]	1000[c]	See ibuprofen
Aspirin[d]	10–15[c,d]	650–1000[c]	4	80[b,c,d]	3600[c]	Reye syndrome,[d] see ibuprofen
Choline Mg Tri-Salicylate[e] (Trilisate)	7.5–15[b,c]	500–1000[c]	4–8	80[b,c,d]	3600[c]	See aspirin

[a]Maximum daily doses for acetaminophen should be reduced to 80 mg/kg in term neonates and infants and to 60 mg/kg in preterm neonates. Supplied in multiple liquid formulations ranging from 20–100 mg/mL, making accidental overdosage easy. Rectal suppositories are available, dosing 25–40 mg/kg every 6 h.
[b]Dosing guidelines for neonates and infants have not been established.
[c]Higher doses may be used in selected cases for treatment of rheumatologic conditions in children.
[d]Aspirin carries a risk of provoking Reye syndrome in infants and children. If other analgesics are available, aspirin use should be restricted to indications in which antiplatelet or anti-inflammatory effect is required, rather than as a routine analgesic or antipyretic in neonates, infants, or children. Dosing guidelines for aspirin in neonates have not been established.
[e]Aspirin-like compound that does not affect platelet adhesiveness or aggregation
Adapted from Berde CB, Sethna NF. Analgesics for the treatment of pain in children. N Engl J Med 2002;347:1094–103.

option for the critically ill child. Intravenous acetaminophen and its prodrug, paracetamol, have been widely available in Europe for many years, and it was approved by the U.S. Food and Drug Administration in 2010. It has been studied in a variety of postoperative settings among children and adults, and although it has been shown to be safe and efficacious, these data have not demonstrated any significant clinical benefit with regards to analgesia over enteral formulations (20). There is a paucity of data with regards to its relative benefit as an antipyretic, and it is not recommended as a replacement for enteral acetaminophen unless this route cannot be utilized. Intravenous acetaminophen is administered over 15 minutes as an infusion and provides effective analgesia in ~15 minutes. Given its high drug cost and high volume of administration (which may be a concern in critically ill children with fluid overload), its main use is in children who cannot receive drugs either orally or rectally. It is also a good option for a patient with contraindications to other intravenous nonopioid analgesics or antipyretics, such as NSAIDs. Regardless of route of delivery, the daily maximum acetaminophen dose in the preterm, term, and older child is 60, 80, 90 mg/kg, respectively (Table 14.3).

Opioid Analgesics

The beneficial psychological and physiologic effects of opium as well as its toxicity and potential for addiction and abuse have been well known to physicians and the public for centuries. As a result, many physicians through the ages have underutilized opium when treating patients in pain because of their fear that their patients would be harmed by its use.

In the pediatric critical care setting, opioid analgesics play a very important role in the multimodal management of pain and sedation in critically ill children.

Opioid Receptors

Over the past 30 years, multiple opioid receptors and subtypes have been identified and classified. An understanding of the complex nature and organization of these multiple opioid receptors is essential for an adequate understanding of the response to, and control of, pain. In the central nervous system, there are four primary opioid receptor types, designated μ (for morphine), κ, δ, and σ. Recently, the μ, κ, and δ receptors have been cloned and have yielded invaluable information on receptor structure and function (21).

The differentiation of agonists and antagonists is fundamental to pharmacology. The intrinsic activity of a drug defines the ability of the drug–receptor complex to initiate a pharmacologic effect. Drugs that produce less than a maximal response have a lowered intrinsic activity and are called partial agonists. Partial agonists also have antagonistic properties, because by binding the receptor site, they block access of full agonists to the receptor site. Morphine and related opiates are μ agonists, and drugs that block the effects of opiates at the μ receptor, such as naloxone, are designated antagonists.

The μ, κ, and δ receptors are unique but produce analgesia primarily by inhibiting synaptic transmission in the central nervous system and in the myenteric plexus. They are usually found on the presynaptic nerve terminal and decrease the release of excitatory neurotransmitters from terminals carrying nociceptive stimuli. As a result, neurons are hyperpolarized, which suppresses spontaneous discharge and evoked responses.

DRUG SELECTION

The opioids most commonly used in the management of pain are μ agonists (Table 14.4). These include morphine,

TABLE 14.4

OPIOID ANALGESIC INITIAL DOSAGE GUIDELINES

	Equianalgesic Dose (MG)		Usual Starting IV (SC) Doses and Intervals		Parenteral/ Oral ratio	Usual Starting Oral Doses and Intervals	
DRUG	**IV, IM, SC**	**ORAL**[b]	**<50 kg**	**>50 kg**		**<50 kg**	**>50 kg**
Fentanyl	0.1	NA[b]	**Bolus:** 0.5–1 μg/kg every 0.5–2 h **Infusion:** 0.5–2 μg/kg/h	**Bolus:** 25–50 μg every 1–2 h **Infusion:** 25–100 μg/h	NA	NA	NA
Hydrocodone	NA	10–20	NA	NA	NA		5–10 mg every 3–4 h[a]
Hydromorphone	1.5–2	3–5[c]	**Bolus:** 0.02 mg/kg every 0.5–2 h **Infusion:** 0.004 mg/kg/h	**Bolus:** 1 mg every 0.5–2 h **Infusion:** 0.3 mg/h	1:2 1:4[c]	0.1 mg/kg every 3–4 h 0.03–0.08 mg/kg every 3–4 h	2–4 mg every 3–4 h
Methadone	10	10–20	**Bolus:** 0.1 mg/kg every 4–8 h	5–10 mg every 4–8 h	1:2	0.2 mg/kg every 4–8 h	10 mg every 4–8 h
Morphine	10	30–50	**Bolus:** 0.1 mg/kg every 0.5–2 h **Infusion:** 0.025 mg/kg/h	**Bolus:** 5–10 mg every 0.5–2 h **Infusion:** 2 mg/h	1:3 chronic 1:5 single	**Immediate Release:** 0.3 mg/kg every 3–4 h **Sustained Release:** 20–35 kg: 10–15 mg every 8–12 h 35–50 kg: 15–30 mg every 8–12	**Immediate Release:** 15–20 mg every 3–4 h **Sustained Release:** 30–45 mg every 8–12 h
Oxycodone	NA	10–20	NA	NA	NA	0.1 mg/kg every 3–4 h	5–10 mg every 3–4 h[a,d]

[a]Commercial preparations are often combined with acetaminophen or ibuprofen; must be converted to morphine by CYP2D6 for analgesic effect.
[b]Oral transmucosal form available (Actiq): dose 10–15 μg/kg.
[c]The equianalgesic oral dose and parenteral/oral dose ratios are not well established.
[d]A sustained-release preparation is available.
Adapted from Berde CB, Sethna NF. Analgesics for the treatment of pain in children. *N Engl J Med* 2002;347:1094–103.

meperidine, methadone, codeine, oxycodone, and the fentanyls. In the PICU, fentanyl and morphine are the most commonly utilized opioids (7). Neither codeine nor meperidine should be used because of associated complications and unpredictable effects. Mixed agonist–antagonist drugs act as agonists or partial agonists at one receptor and antagonists at another receptor. These include pentazocine, butorphanol, and nalbuphine; these are agonists or partial agonists at the κ and δ receptors and antagonists or partial agonists at the μ receptor. These drugs are increasingly being used as well as low-dose naloxone to tame or prevent some opioid-induced side effects such as pruritus and nausea (22). Buprenorphine is considered a partial agonist at the μ and κ receptors and may have a role in the prevention or treatment of opioid dependence.

At equianalgesic doses, the pharmacodynamic effects of all the μ opioid agonists are similar and include analgesia, respiratory depression, sedation, nausea and vomiting, pruritus, constipation, miosis, tolerance, and physical dependence (Table 14.4). While the opioids may cause some sedation, they are not amnestic agents, and in the PICU, they are often coadministered with anxiolytic and amnestic medications such as benzodiazepines (midazolam, diazepam, and lorazepam) or ketamine. The choice of which opioid to use in the PICU may be determined by differences in pharmacokinetic, pharmacodynamic, and physiochemical properties, all of which may affect the latency, potency, and duration of analgesic action. Often, drug selection is based on pharmacokinetic parameters such as half-life. With the opioids, the terminal or β phase half-life alone is not an appropriate measure for drug selection, because the onset and duration of effect with a single dose may have more to do with distribution and redistribution of the drug into and out of the brain than with elimination half-life. Opioid distribution into the brain is based partially on the lipid solubility of the drug. The more lipid-soluble the drug the faster is its penetration into the brain and the quicker the response. Fentanyl, for example, a very lipid-soluble drug, has a rapid onset and short duration of action following a single bolus dose because of the rapid redistribution of drug out of the brain, not because of a short elimination half-life. Continuous long-term opioid administration may be associated with the accumulation of the drug in fat tissue. As a result, duration of action may be affected more by the redistribution of drug out of fat tissue than by the elimination half-life.

Morphine

Morphine is the gold standard μ agonist and can be administered in the critically ill patient using the IV, epidural, intrathecal, oral, IM, and rectal routes, for both analgesia and sedation. It is a moderately potent opioid and is commonly administered intravenously in doses of 0.1 mg/kg for acute pain management (Table 14.4). Indeed, this dose must be modified based on patient age and disease state. In order to minimize the complications associated with intravenous opioid administration, it is always recommended to *titrate the dose at the bedside* until the desired level of analgesia is achieved. When administered by the oral route, morphine has an IV:oral dose ratio of approximately 1:3. This ratio reflects the high first-pass effect rather than the extent of absorption, which is nearly 100%. In healthy children, the terminal elimination half-life ($t_{1/2}$) is 2–3 hours. Peak effect occurs within 20 minutes, with a duration of action of 2–7 hours following IV administration. Morphine is less lipid soluble than fentanyl, so it has a slower onset of action and a longer duration, as well as a smaller volume of distribution.

Morphine is primarily glucuronidated into two forms: an inactive form, morphine-3-glucuronide, and an active form, morphine-6-glucuronide. Both glucuronides are excreted by the kidney. In patients with renal failure or with reduced glomerular filtration rates (e.g., neonates), the morphine 6-glucuronide can accumulate and cause toxic side effects, including respiratory depression. This is important to consider not only when prescribing morphine but also when administering other opioids that are metabolized into morphine (e.g., methadone and codeine).

Many disease states common in ICU patients may alter the metabolism and elimination of morphine. Severe cirrhosis, septic shock, and renal failure decrease the clearance of morphine and its metabolites, resulting in prolonged duration and possible toxicity. Although glucuronidation is thought to be less affected in liver cirrhosis, the clearance of morphine is decreased and oral bioavailability increased. The consequence of reduced drug metabolism is the risk of accumulation in the body, especially with repeated administration. Lower doses or longer administration intervals should be used to minimize this risk.

Fentanyl(s)

Because of its rapid onset (usually <1 minute) and brief duration of action (30–45 minutes), fentanyl has become a favored analgesic for short procedures, such as bone marrow aspirations, fracture reductions, suturing lacerations, and endoscopy and dental procedures, as well as for patients admitted to the PICU. Fentanyl is ~100 times more potent than morphine and is largely devoid of hypnotic or sedative activity (Table 14.4). Sufentanil is a potent fentanyl derivative and is ~10 times more potent than fentanyl. Alfentanil is approximately 5–10 less potent than fentanyl and has an extremely short duration of action, usually less than 15–20 minutes. Remifentanil is a μ-opioid receptor agonist with unique pharmacokinetic properties. It is ~10 times more potent than fentanyl and must be given by continuous intravenous infusion because it has an extremely short half-life (23).

Fentanyl is considered to be the most hemodynamically stable opioid and has become the opioid of choice for critically ill patients (7). Nevertheless, the principles of careful monitoring and titration to effect also apply to fentanyl, particularly in the hypovolemic patient. Furthermore, in addition to its ability to block the systemic and pulmonary hemodynamic responses to pain, fentanyl also prevents the biochemical and endocrine stress (catabolic) response to painful stimuli that may be so detrimental in the critically ill patient. Fentanyl does have some serious side effects, namely, the development of glottic and chest wall rigidity following rapid infusions of ≥5 μg/kg and the development of bradycardia. The etiology of the glottic and chest wall rigidity is unclear, but its implications are not, namely, it may make ventilation difficult or impossible. Chest wall rigidity can be treated with either neuromuscular relaxants or naloxone.

Like morphine, fentanyl is primarily glucuronidated into inactive forms that are excreted by the kidney. It is highly lipid soluble and is rapidly distributed to tissues that are well perfused, such as the brain and the heart. Normally, the effect of a single dose of fentanyl is terminated by rapid redistribution to inactive tissue sites such as fat, skeletal muscles, and lung, rather than by elimination. This rapid redistribution produces a dramatic decline in the plasma concentration of the drug. In this manner, its very short duration of action is very much akin to other drugs whose action is terminated by redistribution such as thiopental. However, following multiple or large doses of fentanyl (e.g., when it is used as a primary anesthetic agent or when used in high dose or lengthy continuous infusions), prolongation of effect will occur, because elimination and not distribution will determine the duration of effect. Indeed, it is now clear that the duration of drug action for many drugs is not solely the function of clearance or terminal elimination half-life but rather reflects the complex interaction of drug elimination, drug absorption, and rate constants for drug transfer to and from sites of action ("effect sites"). The term "context-sensitive half-life" refers to the time for drug concentration at idealized effect sites to decrease in half. The context-sensitive half-life for fentanyl increases dramatically when it is administered by continuous infusion (24). In newborns receiving fentanyl infusions for >36 hours, the context-sensitive half-life was >9 hours following cessation of the infusion (25). Even single doses of fentanyl may have prolonged effects in the newborn, particularly those neonates with abnormal or decreased liver blood flow following acute illness or abdominal surgery. Additionally, certain conditions that may raise intra-abdominal pressure may further decrease liver blood flow by shunting blood away from the liver via the still-patent ductus venosus.

Fentanyl, sufentanil, alfentanil, and remifentanil are highly lipophilic drugs that rapidly penetrate all membranes including the blood–brain barrier. Following an intravenous bolus, fentanyl is rapidly eliminated from plasma as the result of its extensive uptake by body tissues. The fentanyls are highly bound to α_1-acid glycoproteins in the plasma, which are reduced in the newborn.

The pharmacokinetics of remifentanil is unique and is characterized by small volumes, rapid clearances, and low variability compared to other intravenous anesthetic drugs. The drug has a rapid onset of action (half-time for equilibration between blood and the effect compartment is 1.3 minutes) and a short context-sensitive half-life (3–5 minutes). The latter property is attributable to hydrolytic metabolism of the compound by nonspecific tissue and plasma esterases. The pharmacokinetics of remifentanil suggests that within 10 minutes of starting an infusion, remifentanil will nearly reach steady state; therefore, changing the infusion rate will produce rapid changes in drug effect. The rapid metabolism of remifentanil and its small volume of distribution mean that remifentanil will not accumulate. Discontinuing the drug rapidly terminates its effects regardless of how long it was being administered. Finally, the primary metabolite has little biologic activity making it safe even in patients with renal disease.

Fentanyl is metabolized by the liver to inactive metabolites, which are eliminated by the kidney. Compared to morphine, fentanyl has a larger volume of distribution, slower clearance, and a longer terminal half-life of ~8 hours. While renal failure does not significantly alter the pharmacokinetics and pharmacodynamics of fentanyl in most patients, a few studies have demonstrated increases in the volume of distribution and elimination half-life in critically ill patients with renal failure receiving continuous fentanyl infusions. A study in renal failure patients who received kidney transplants found a decrease in fentanyl clearance associated with prolonged ventilatory depression (26).

Metabolism of fentanyl is determined primarily by liver perfusion. Diseases associated with decreased liver blood flow, such as cardiac failure, may decrease the clearance of fentanyl. Long-term continuous infusions of fentanyl may result in a prolonged elimination $t_{1/2}$ and duration of action as a result of drug accumulation in peripheral tissues. Administering fentanyl by continuous infusion requires frequent titration, as the terminal $t_{1/2}$ may be as long as 16 hours in this setting. Unlike morphine, fentanyl is not associated with mast cell histamine release and may be preferred in patients susceptible to the cardiovascular effects of morphine.

Hydromorphone

Hydromorphone, a derivative of morphine, is an opioid with appreciable selectivity for μ-opioid receptors. It is noted for

its rapid onset and 4–6-hour duration of action. It differs from its parent compound morphine, in that it is 5 times more potent and 10 times more lipid soluble and does not have an active metabolite (Table 14.4). Its elimination half-life is 3–4 hours and, like morphine and meperidine, shows very wide intraindividual pharmacokinetic variability. Hydromorphone is less sedating than morphine and is thought by many to be associated with fewer systemic side effects. Indeed, it is often used as an alternative to morphine in IV patient-controlled analgesia (PCA) or when the latter produces too much sedation, nausea, or itching. Additionally, hydromorphone is receiving renewed attention as an alternative to morphine for treatment of prolonged cancer-related pain because it can be prepared in more concentrated aqueous solutions than morphine. Hydromorphone is effective when administered intravenously, subcutaneously, epidurally, and orally. The intravenous route of administration is the most commonly used technique in the ICU, and dosing guidelines are included in Table 14.4.

Methadone

Previously considered as a drug to treat or wean opioid-addicted or -dependent patients, methadone is increasingly being used for postoperative pain relief and for the treatment of intractable pain. It is noted for its slow elimination, very long duration of effective analgesia, and high oral bioavailability (Table 14.4). Methadone is metabolized extremely slowly and has a very prolonged duration of action partly because its principal metabolite is morphine. The elimination half-life of methadone averages 19 hours and clearance averages 5.4 mL/min/kg in children 1–18 years of age.

Methadone has the longest elimination half-life of any of the commonly available opiates and may provide 12–36 hours of analgesia following a single intravenous or oral dose. From a pharmacokinetic standpoint, children are indistinguishable from young adults. Because a single dose of methadone can achieve and sustain a high drug plasma level, it is a convenient way to provide prolonged analgesia without requiring an intramuscular injection. Indeed, when administered either orally or intravenously, it may be viewed as an alternative to the use of continuous intravenous opioid infusions. The influence of pathophysiology on the pharmacokinetics and pharmacodynamics of methadone is unknown primarily because its use as an analgesic is a relatively recent phenomenon. Dosing decisions in the very young and in patients with various end-organ diseases must be made conservatively.

It has become more common to utilize methadone to wean patients who have become physically dependent to opioids following prolonged analgesic therapy. When used to treat dependence and withdrawal symptoms, clonidine or dexmedetomidine, both α_2 agonists, can be concomitantly administered to significantly reduce withdrawal symptomatology. Finally, because methadone is extremely well absorbed from the GI tract and has a bioavailability of 80%–90%, it is extremely easy to convert intravenous dosing regimens to oral ones. Recently the conversion dose of morphine to methadone has been challenged. Traditionally, it has been thought that the ratio of morphine to methadone was approximately 1:1; it now appears that it is closer to 1:0.25 or even 1:0.1. Underestimating methadone's potency substantially increases the risk of potential life-threatening toxicity. Methadone may provide analgesia even when patients become tolerant to other opioids. This is sometimes referred to as "incomplete cross-tolerance." Incomplete cross-tolerance for methadone may be due, in part, to its antagonist actions at the N-methyl-D-aspartate (NMDA) receptor.

Patient- and Surrogate (Parent, Nurse)-Controlled Analgesia

Because of the enormous individual variations in pain perception and opioid metabolism, fixed doses and time intervals make little sense. Based on the pharmacokinetics of the opioids, it should be clear that intravenous boluses of morphine may need to be given at intervals of 1–2 hours in order to avoid marked fluctuations in plasma drug levels. Continuous intravenous infusions can provide steady analgesic levels and are preferable to intramuscular injections. Continuous infusions have been used with great safety and effectiveness in children and are commonly used in the PICU. Table 14.5 lists common opioid infusion regimens. However, they are not a panacea, because the perception and intensity of pain are not constant. For example, a postoperative patient may be very comfortable resting in bed and may require little adjustment in pain management. This same patient may experience excruciating pain when coughing, or voiding, or getting out of bed. Thus, rational pain management requires some form of titration to effect, whenever any opioid is administered. In order to give patients (in some cases parents and nurses) some measure of control over their (their child's) pain therapy, demand analgesia or PCA devices have been developed. These are microprocessor-driven pumps with a button that the patient (or surrogate) presses to self-administer a small dose of opioid.

PCA devices allow patients to administer small amounts of an analgesic whenever they feel a need for more pain relief. The dosage of opioid, number of boluses per hour, and the time interval between boluses (the "lock-out period") are programmed into the equipment by the pain service physician to allow maximum patient flexibility and sense of control with minimal risk of overdosage. Generally, because older patients know that if they have severe pain they can obtain relief immediately, many prefer dosing regimens that result in mild-to-moderate pain in exchange for fewer side effects such as nausea or pruritus. The most commonly prescribed opioids for IV PCA are morphine, hydromorphone, and fentanyl.

The PCA pump computer stores within its memory how many boluses the patient has received as well as how many attempts the patient has made at administering boluses. This allows the physician to evaluate how well the patient understands the use of the pump and provides information to program the pump more efficiently. Many PCA pumps allow low "background" continuous infusions in addition to self-administered boluses. A continuous background infusion is particularly useful at night to prevent the patient awakening in pain. Yet, it also increases the potential for overdosage (27). Although the adult literature on pain does not support the use of continuous background infusions, it has been the authors' experience that continuous infusions are beneficial for both the patient and physicians (fewer phone calls, problems, etc.). Another major benefit to the use of PCA in the PICU setting is the potential decrease in line breaks to administer boluses of opioid when compared to a continuous infusion by a PCA pump.

PCA requires a patient with the developmental level, manual dexterity, and the strength necessary to operate the pump. Thus, it was initially limited to adolescents and teenagers, but the lower age limit in whom this treatment modality can be used continues to fall. In fact, it has been observed that any child able to play computerized games can operate a PCA pump (age 5–6 years). Allowing surrogates such as parents or nurses to initiate a PCA bolus is very controversial. Some centers empower nurses and parents to initiate PCA boluses and use this technology in children less than even a year of age. The incidence of common opioid-induced side effects is similar to that observed in older patients. Interestingly, respiratory depression is very rare, but does occur, reinforcing the need for close monitoring and established nursing protocols. Disadvantages to PCA include its increased costs, patient age limitations, and the systematic (physician, nursing, and pharmacy) obstacles (protocols, education, storage arrangements) that must be overcome prior to its implementation. Contraindications include inability to push the bolus button (weakness, arm restraints), inability to understand how to use the machine, and a patient's desire not to assume responsibility for his/her own care.

Preventing Opioid-Induced Side Effects

Regardless of method of administration, all opioids produce unwanted side effects, such as pruritus, nausea, vomiting, constipation, urinary retention, cognitive impairment,

TABLE 14.5

COMMON OPIOID INFUSION RATES IN THE PICU

■ AGENT	■ LOAD/P.R.N.	■ INFUSION RANGE	■ COMMENTS
Fentanyl	1 μg/kg	1–5 μg/kg/h	Extensive clinical experience Relatively stable hemodynamic effects Blunts the stress response Pharmacology similar to morphine after prolonged infusion (>18 h)
Morphine	0.05–0.1 mg/kg	0.05–0.1 mg/kg/h	Inexpensive Extensive clinical experience Histamine release and venodilation may cause hypotension
Hydromorphone	0.015 mg/kg	10–15 μg/kg/h	Fewer opioid-induced side effects such as pruritus and histamine release More expensive than morphine
Remifentanil	0.5–1 μg/kg	0.1–0.5 μg/kg/min	Short duration of infusion Rapid development of tolerance Esterase metabolism rapid breakdown and no analgesia after 10 min Expensive

These are suggested boluses and initiation ranges, and their effect must be titrated for each patient to the appropriate level of analgesia. p.r.n., as needed.

tolerance, and dependence. Indeed, many patients suffer needlessly because they would rather experience pain than these opioid-induced side effects. In a randomized controlled clinical trial, it was demonstrated that low-dose naloxone infusions (0.25 μg/kg/h) can significantly reduce opioid-induced side effects without affecting opioid-induced analgesia (22). This study has changed our practice and led to further research to delineate the optimal dose (28).

LOCAL ANESTHETICS

Local anesthetics are drugs that reversibly block conduction of neural impulses along central and peripheral nerve pathways. To be effective, local anesthetics must be physically deposited, usually by needles or by indwelling catheters, in the immediate vicinity of the nerves to be blocked. In this way, local anesthetics are unlike virtually all other drugs used in modern medicine, which, regardless of their means of entry into the body, are delivered to their site of action by a carrier, namely, the blood. Removal of local anesthetics from the neural tissue results in spontaneous and complete return of nerve conduction with no evidence of structural damage to nerve fibers as a result of the drug's effects.

Procedure-related pain is the pain that is inflicted on patients in the course of their medical or surgical treatment. It is also among the most difficult forms of pain to deal with by both the patient experiencing it and the healthcare professionals who inflict it. Examples of procedure-related pain include insertion of an arterial or intravenous catheter (e.g., routine percutaneous intravenous access or cardiac catheterization), bone marrow aspiration, thoracostomy tube placement, lumbar puncture, dressing changes, and repair of minor surgical wounds (traumatic lacerations or deliberate incisions, e.g., prior to a cutdown for venous access). It can be easy to minimize the need for preventing and treating procedure-related pain when dealing with children because they can be physically restrained, may not be routinely asked if they are in pain, and are usually unable to withdraw their consent. Fortunately, the appropriate use of local anesthesia can abolish much of this pain.

Because regional anesthesia produces profound analgesia with minimal physiologic alterations, it is increasingly being used in children as a component of intra- and postoperative pain management, posttraumatic pain management, and for pain that is difficult to treat with systemic narcotics. For example, children who cannot tolerate opioids because of opioid-induced ventilatory depression or who have become tolerant to the analgesic effects of opioids can be completely pain-free with the use of local anesthetic techniques. Prolonged analgesia can also be provided by administering local anesthetic agents continuously through indwelling catheters placed in the epidural, intrathecal, intercostal, intrapleural, or other spaces. Thanks to these myriad benefits, and because of our ability to overcome many of the technical difficulties that limited the use of local anesthetics in the past, local anesthetics and regional anesthetic techniques have become an essential component in the armamentarium of managing childhood pain. Thus, an understanding of the effects and uses of local anesthetics may be extremely helpful to intensive care physicians.

Pharmacology and Pharmacokinetics of Local Anesthetics

Structure–Activity Relationships

All local anesthetics share a common chemical structure as tertiary amines and weak bases, composed of a lipophilic and a hydrophilic portion that are separated by a hydrocarbon chain. The lipophilic portion is essential for the drug's anesthetic activity, linked to its carbon chain by either an amide (–CONH–) or an ester (–COO–) bond. The nature of this linkage is the basis for classifying the two major classes of local anesthetic agents used in clinical practice—esters and amides (Table 14.6). The final component of the molecule, the hydrophilic end, is a tertiary amine that confers the properties of a weak base as well as its water solubility. Modifying the chemical structure of the local anesthetic molecule alters its intrinsic anesthetic potency, duration of action, rate of biodegradation, protein binding, and intrinsic toxicity. For example, adding a butyl group to the hydrophilic end of mepivacaine produces bupivacaine, a drug that is 35 times more lipid soluble and is 3–4 times more potent than the parent molecule. Additionally, this simple addition also yields a molecule that has a greater degree of protein binding and a longer duration of action. Metabolism and biodegradation can also be affected by simple changes to the basic local anesthetic molecular structure. Adding a chlorine molecule to the lipophilic end of procaine produces chloroprocaine, a molecule that is hydrolyzed by serum cholinesterase 4 times faster than its parent molecule, procaine. This rapid hydrolysis limits chloroprocaine's duration of action and systemic toxicity.

TABLE 14.6

MAXIMUM LOCAL ANESTHETIC DOSING GUIDELINES

■ DRUG	■ DOSE (mg/kg) WITHOUT EPINEPHRINE	■ DOSE (mg/kg) WITH EPINEPHRINE	■ DURATION (h)	■ CONTRAINDICATIONS	■ COMMENTS
Bupivacaine[a]	2	3	3–6		Reduce dose by 50% in neonates
Chloroprocaine[b]	8	10	1	Plasma cholinesterase deficiency	Short-acting, rapid metabolism; useful in neonates and patients with seizures or liver disease
Lidocaine	5	7	1		
Ropivacaine	2	3	3–6		Less cardiotoxicity than bupivacaine

[a] When given by epidural continuous infusion: 0.2–0.4 mg/kg/h.
[b] In neonatal epidural continuous infusion: 10–15 mg/kg/h. Ropivacine, a stereoselective enantioner is less toxic than bupivacine (28).

Several local anesthetics, such as bupivacaine, ropivacaine, and mepivacaine, exist in left (S or L)- and right (D or R)-handed configurations, which may vary their pharmacokinetics, pharmacodynamics, and most importantly their toxicity. Thus, an increasingly important feature in new local anesthetic drug development is the development of stereoselective enantiomers, which are presumed to be less toxic than racemic mixtures. In fact, ropivacaine, a local anesthetic recently introduced into practice as a safer alternative to bupivacaine (see what follows), has been developed as a pure left enantiomer.

Local anesthetics are weak bases that exist in equilibrium between the neutral (B) and protonated charged (BH$^+$) forms. Local anesthetics can inhibit Na$^+$ channels in both the ionized and nonionized forms. To reach the sodium channel, the local anesthetic must cross the nerve membrane and it is primarily the nonionized (base) form of the drug that can do this. How much drug is available to cross the nerve membrane depends on the pK_a of the drug and the pH of the fluid surrounding the nerve. Thus, these agents predominantly exist in the ionized (cationic) form in biologic fluids at physiologic pH. The lower the pK_a of a drug, the more nonionized drug is available to cross the nerve membrane at physiologic pH. For example, 28% of lidocaine exists in the base (nonionized) form at pH 7.4 compared to only 2.5% for chloroprocaine because the pK_a of these drugs are 7.9 and 9.0, respectively. Acidosis and hypercarbia in the environment in which a local anesthetic is injected will further increase the ionized fraction of local anesthetics, explaining the poor analgesia that results when local anesthetics are infiltrated into infected or ischemic tissues.

The minimum concentration of local anesthetic necessary to block impulse conduction along a given nerve fiber is called the C_m. A variety of factors affect C_m, including fiber size and degree of myelination of the nerve to be blocked, pH, local calcium concentration, and the rate at which a nerve is stimulated. Each local anesthetic has a unique C_m, which reflects the differing potencies of each drug. Relatively unmyelinated fibers, such as the Aδ and C fibers carry nociceptive information and have a lower C_m than heavily myelinated fibers that control muscle contraction. Because of the lower C_m, less local anesthetic is necessary to block the transmission of pain than is necessary to produce muscle paralysis; therefore, one can block pain sensation and avoid motor blockade by using dilute concentrations of local anesthetics. This is sometimes referred to as "differential nerve block." In fact, concentrated local anesthetic solutions (e.g., 2% lidocaine vs. 1.0%) increase the quality of sensory blockade only minimally. On the other hand, a concentrated local anesthetic will increase the incidence of motor blockade and systemic toxicity! To minimize this, concentrated solutions of local anesthetics can be diluted with preservative-free normal saline.

Other factors also influence the quality and duration of a nerve block, such as the addition of a vasoconstrictor to the anesthetic mixture, the use of mixtures of local anesthetics, and the site of drug administration. Vasoconstrictors, particularly epinephrine, are frequently added to local anesthetic solutions. Epinephrine decreases the rate of vascular absorption of local anesthetic from the site of administration, thereby increasing the time the local anesthetic is in contact with nerve fibers, particularly for drugs that are poorly lipid soluble such as lidocaine. This lengthens the duration of sensory blockade for lidocaine by almost 50% and decreases peak plasma local anesthetic concentrations by a third. More lipid-soluble agents such as bupivacaine, ropivacaine, and etidocaine are less affected by the addition of epinephrine.

By causing local vasoconstriction, epinephrine also reduces bleeding at sites of injury. Interestingly, epinephrine also improves the intensity of anesthesia and increases the effectiveness of dilute concentration of local anesthetics. Epinephrine-containing solutions should never be injected into areas supplied by end arteries, such as the penis or digit, as it may lead to tissue ischemia or necrosis. Epinephrine is often added to local anesthetic solutions in concentrations of 5–10 μg/mL (1:200,000–100,000). Higher epinephrine concentrations offer no advantage in further reducing peak plasma local anesthetic concentrations and may, in fact, produce adverse systemic hemodynamic effects.

The systemic toxic effects of local anesthetics are determined by the total dose of drug administered, protein binding, the rapidity of absorption into the blood, and the site of injection. Toxicity primarily occurs by unintended intravenous administration or by accumulation of excessive amounts of drug administered either by repeated bolus dosing or by continuous infusion. This belies the idea of accepted "maximum" doses of these drugs, since even small fractions of the accepted "maximum" dosages of local anesthetics will produce toxic systemic effects if the local anesthetic is injected intra-arterially, intravenously, or into any highly vascular location (**Table 14.6**). In general, peak absorption of local anesthetic is dependent on the site of the block because the site of injection influences the rate of plasma uptake by the vascularity of the tissues. The order of absorption from highest to lowest is as follows: intercostal, intrapleural, intratracheal > caudal/epidural > brachial plexus > distal peripheral > subcutaneous > fat. Bupivacaine toxicity is the most feared because the electrical asystole it produces has been refractory to treatment and often resulted in death. Some patients have been saved from bupivacaine-induced cardiac arrest by being placed on cardiopulmonary bypass. Recently, intravenous intralipid, acting as a sponge or sink to "soak up" bupivacaine, has been used successfully (29).

Lidocaine is the only local anesthetic that is used intravenously. Intravenous lidocaine is commonly used as an antiarrhythmic and as method of treating neuropathic pain. Lidocaine is beneficial in the treatment of neuropathic pain states by blocking conduction of sodium channels in peripheral and central neurons, and thereby dampening peripheral nociceptor sensitization and, ultimately, central nervous system hyperexcitability. An oral capsule form of lidocaine, mexiletine, is available and is commonly used in the treatment of arrhythmias and neuropathic pain that is alleviated by intravenous lidocaine. Topical lidocaine, available as a patch, is also a promising method of treating neuropathic pain.

EPIDURAL ANESTHESIA/ANALGESIA

The epidural space lies between the spinal dura mater and the spinal periosteum (the ligamentum flavum) and contains arteries and veins, exiting nerves, and fat. The upper limit of the space is the foramen magnum and the lower limit is the sacrococcygeal ligament. Deposition of local anesthetics, and/or opioids, α_2 agonists (clonidine), midazolam, steroids, and/or ketamine can be used to palliate acute pain and is most commonly used in pediatrics for the management of postoperative pain as well as traumatic pain. Additionally, this technique is useful in treating cancer or sickle cell vaso-occlusive crisis-related pain of the abdomen, pelvis, or lower extremities, and ischemic or vascular insufficiency pain of the lower extremities (purpura fulminans). Dermatomal distribution of drugs deposited in the epidural space is very much dependent on the site of entry into the epidural space. Thus, the level of entry into the space describes the block whether it is caudal (sacrococcygeal ligament), lumbar, or thoracic. Short-term (<4 days) nontunneled and long-term (weeks to months) tunneled epidural catheters can be easily inserted for prolonged analgesia (30). In infants and young children, the caudal approach to the epidural space is the easiest and most common. Indeed, in young infants and children, catheters can be thread from the sacrococcygeal ligament to the thorax and can provide analgesia to the chest. The volume, or coverage, of the epidural catheter is dictated by both the location of the tip of the catheter and the volume of material maintained in the epidural space. This volume of anesthetic (and often other agents) bathes the spinal cord and nerve roots creating a dermatomal distribution of anesthesia and/or analgesia.

Assessment of the dermatomal blockade is important, but limited primarily to children >5 years of age who are verbal and can differentiate between the various sensations of cold, touch, and pinprick. With the pinprick, the patient is asked to discriminate between sharp or dull sensation. Generalized patient comfort is perhaps the best assessment. Additional bedside evaluation should include inspection of the site of the epidural insertion under a transparent dressing; any evidence of redness or leakage of fluid should be reported to the service supporting the perioperative epidural usage. Only experienced individuals should remove the epidural catheter.

Complications from epidural catheterization are rare. In adults, hypotension is the most often noted complication during bolus dosing and the higher thoracic level blocks increases the risk for these events. However, in children <8 years of age, hypotension is extremely rare even with higher level blocks. However, like adults, if hypotension does occur, it is often related to sympathetic blockade or systemic absorption of local anesthetic into the blood stream. Aside from the potential for local anesthetic toxicity from continuous infusions into the epidural space, or direct intravascular injection, other reported complications are urinary retention, site infection, chemical meningitis, and inadvertent spinal anesthesia. Epidural insertion is contraindicated in patients with coagulation disorders and if there is an infection at the intended site of insertion.

Local Anesthetic Dosage for Epidural Analgesia

Bupivacaine and lidocaine are the most commonly used agents for epidural analgesia. There are many techniques to facilitate the initiation and maintenance of epidural anesthesia and analgesia. In neonates and infants, we prefer to use lidocaine because it is less toxic and, unlike bupivacaine, plasma lidocaine levels can be measured and can be used to guide therapy.

Adjuvants Used in Epidural Analgesia

In addition to local anesthetics, additional agents have been added to regional and neuraxial blocks to augment the properties of duration and intensity of analgesia. The most common and effective adjuvants are opioids and the α_2 agonist clonidine. Less commonly used adjuvants include ketamine, midazolam, and steroids. Unlike local anesthetics that are primarily active on the spinal cord and nerve roots, both opioids and α_2 agonists have a substantial amount of systemic absorption and central activity that are perhaps greater than their local effect. These central effects are perhaps their most important site of action and are also the source of complications that the PICU clinician should recognize when evaluating patients with epidural analgesia that may contain these agents.

Regardless of the opioid used in the epidural space, a regular system of monitoring for respiratory depression is required. Clinical signs that predict impending respiratory depression include somnolence, small pupils, and small tidal volumes. We also use and recommend oxygen saturation monitoring in all patients with opioids in the epidural space, particularly in the first 24 hours of instituting therapy. Adverse (or desired) effects of α_2 agonists include somnolence, sedation, and hypotension.

SEDATIVES IN THE PICU

While the treatment of pain with analgesics due to invasive instrumentation such as the endotracheal tube is imperative, most children in the PICU require some level of sedation to decrease the anxiety and fear that are associated with admission to the ICU and critical illness. One of the most important roles of the PICU care provider is to identify the ideal level of sedation on the awake–coma continuum to prevent inadvertent removal of lifesaving devices while providing adequate anxiolysis and minimizing exposure to psychoactive medications. This underlines the importance of goal-directed therapy using sedation scoring/assessment tools. The sedation needs of a critically ill child may constantly be changing—a child with severe Acute Respiratory Distress Syndrome (ARDS) may require complete immobilization with amnesia because of life-threatening hypoxia and the need to control mechanical ventilation, while the same child may benefit from minimal sedation to promote rehabilitation and spontaneous ventilation with an endotracheal tube in place days later. Assessing a child's sedation needs at regular intervals is key to decreasing the length of mechanical ventilation and days in the ICU.

Anxiety and fear, along with a sense of helplessness and lack of sleep, will potentiate pain and, if left untreated, can lead to delirium and psychosis in critically ill patients. With the exception of dexmedetomidine, which is known to induce a natural, sleep-like state, the sedatives traditionally used in the PICU are known to decrease restorative sleep (31). ICU delirium is a well-described phenomenon in adult patients and has recently been demonstrated to be a significant morbidity for critically ill children in the PICU (32–34). Furthermore, the failure to provide adequate sedation, analgesia, and amnesia can lead to the development of posttraumatic stress syndrome, particularly in children who are in the ICU because to a traumatic event such as a severe burn or motor vehicle collision (35). Both sleep disturbances and delirium in the PICU are discussed in detail at the end of this chapter.

Sedation for patients requiring prolonged immobility may last for days or even weeks (**Table 14.7**). Alternatively, sedation for painful or nonpainful procedures may be brief, lasting less than 30–60 minutes. Indeed, procedural sedation is an increasingly important function of the ICU and its staff. Because of their airway, monitoring, and rescue skills, in many institutions, the intensivist provides pediatric procedural sedation for not only critically ill patients but also for healthy children undergoing scheduled procedures such as diagnostic imaging studies, bone marrow aspirations, and endoscopy. In choosing a technique for procedural sedation, it is first essential to clearly identify the goals of the sedation plan and to differentiate between sedation and analgesia. Not all procedures or clinical situations demand both, and there is commonly a greater need for one more than the other.

Procedural sedation exists across a continuum varying from a state of wakefulness, to anxiolysis, to moderate sedation ("conscious sedation"), to deep sedation, to general anesthesia. The drugs chosen and the underlying condition of the patient may make this transition more or less likely, and individual variations in drug response are not always predictable. Thus, physicians must always be prepared for the common possibility that the patient may pass into a greater depth of sedation than initially planned and be able to manage the consequences.

Benzodiazepines

The benzodiazepines comprise a family of drugs that are the most important sedative/hypnotic/anxiolytic drugs currently

TABLE 14.7

COMMON INITIATION RANGES FOR SEDATIVE INFUSIONS IN THE PICU

■ AGENT	■ LOAD/P.R.N.	■ INFUSION RANGE	■ COMMENTS
Midazolam	0.05–0.1 mg/kg	0.05–0.1 mg/kg/h	Commonly used sedative Extensive clinical experience Metabolism via cytochrome P450
Lorazepam	0.05–0.1 mg/kg	0.025–0.05 mg/kg/h	Less clinical experience Polyethylene glycol preservative; watch for osmolar gap and acidosis Metabolized via glucuronyl transferase Maximum p.r.n. dose, 2 mg
Pentobarbital	0.5–1 mg/kg	1–2 mg/kg/h	Negative inotropic effect Can monitor levels
Propofol	2–3 mg/kg	75–250 μg/kg/min	Rapid emergence Short procedural sedation only! Contraindicated for prolonged infusions in children secondary to lethal propofol infusion syndrome
Dexmedetomidine	0.3–1 μg/kg	0.25–0.7 μg/kg/h	Adverse bradycardia and hypotension during loading Limited clinical experience in children
Ketamine	1–2 mg/kg	1–2 mg/kg/h	Increased heart rate and blood pressure secondary to catecholamine release; bronchodilator May need supplemental benzodiazepine and antisialagogue

These are suggested boluses and initiation ranges, and their effect must be titrated for each patient to the appropriate level of sedation.

used in clinical practice. Diazepam, midazolam, triazolam, and lorazepam are members of this family (Table 14.8). These drugs are extremely potent amnestics, anticonvulsants, sedatives, hypnotics, and skeletal muscle relaxants and are effective whether given parenterally or enterally. *They have no analgesic properties.* They work by augmenting γ-aminobutyric acid (GABA) and glycine transmission. Binding of a benzodiazepine to its receptor on the α subunit of the GABA transmembrane receptor facilitates the binding of GABA to the β subunit (shifts the dose response to the left) and allows extracellular chloride to enter into a cell. This causes membrane hyperpolarization and resistance to neuronal excitation and results in sedation, anxiolysis, muscle relaxation, and anticonvulsant activity. Alternatively, the binding of an antagonist, such as flumazenil, does not alter GABA synaptic transmission efficiency, but competitively blocks the actions of agonist agents.

Within the central nervous system, the benzodiazepines reduce cerebral metabolism and blood flow. They alter consciousness along a dose-dependent continuum ranging from

anxiolysis to general anesthesia but do not produce normal sleep; indeed, they interfere with normal sleep architecture by decreasing slow-wave sleep, the most restorative component of natural sleep (31). The benzodiazepines are potent anticonvulsants and impair the acquisition of new information ("anterograde amnesia") without affecting previously stored information ("retrograde amnesia"). The latter attribute is quite useful to the intensivist because there are many situations in which a patient is too hemodynamically unstable to adequately sedate (e.g., cardioversion, intubation). Benzodiazepines provide intense anterograde amnesia and can prevent a patient from remembering a painful or unpleasant procedure. Although they provide the benefits of amnesia, anxiolysis, and sedation desired for the mechanically ventilated child, one major disadvantage is an increased risk of delirium with prolonged administration (36–38).

Benzodiazepines produce dose-dependent depression of breathing and affect both the ventilatory responses to hypoxia and hypercapnia. In small doses, the benzodiazepines

TABLE 14.8

COMMONLY USED BENZODIAZEPINES

■ GENERIC	■ BRAND	■ HOW SUPPLIED		■ ACTIVE METABOLITE	■ EQUIPOTENT IV DOSE (mg/kg)
Diazepam	Valium	Parenteral: Tablet: Oral solution:	5 mg/mL 2, 5, 10 mg 1, 5 mg/mL	Yes	0.1–0.2
Lorazepam	Ativan	Parenteral: Tablet: Oral solution:	2, 4 mg/mL 0.5, 1, 2 mg 2 mg/mL	No	0.03–0.05
Midazolam	Versed	Parenteral: Oral solution:	1, 5 mg/mL 2 mg/mL	Yes	0.05–0.1
Oxazepam	Serax	Tablet: Capsule:	15 mg 10, 15, 30 mg	No	NA
Triazolam	Halcion	Tablet:	0.125, 0.25 mg	No	NA

minimally affect minute ventilation. In higher doses, however, they can blunt or abolish the respiratory responses to both hypercarbia and hypoxia. Drug-induced respiratory depression is quantified by the ventilatory response to inhaled or rebreathed CO_2 (**Fig. 14.3**) (39). The depressant drug may either reduce the slope of the CO_2 response curve or shift the x-intercept to the right. A reduced slope implies a diminished ventilatory response at any given arterial $PaCO_2$ level. The x-intercept of the curve, known as the apneic threshold, indicates relative position of the curve and is defined as that $PaCO_2$ required to stimulate spontaneous respiration. The benzodiazepines produce hypoventilation primarily by decreasing tidal volume. This is manifested by a reduction of the slope of the CO_2 response curve without a change in the x-intercept (**Fig. 14.3**). The depressant effect of the benzodiazepines begins within 1–4 minutes of an intravenous injection and lasts for at least 30 minutes.

The benzodiazepine-induced decrease in the ventilatory response to hypoxia is particularly dangerous, since the hypoxic drive is the "backup" system in the control of ventilation. Drug-induced hypoventilation rapidly decreases alveolar and arterial oxygen saturation. In unmedicated persons, the hypoxic ventilatory drive provides some protection from hypoventilation-induced hypoxia. If both the hypoxic and hypercarbic drive to breath are blunted or blocked by the benzodiazepines, apnea and death may result from their use. Furthermore, the respiratory depression seen with the benzodiazepines is potentiated with the concomitant administration of any opioid. Thus, a reduction in the dose of both drugs is required when these drugs are administered together and underscores the need for very close observation and monitoring of patients who receive these drugs. The risk of using these drugs may be significantly increased in children with chronic CO_2 retention, less than 1–2 months of age, chronically dependent on the hypoxic drive to ventilate, and who are receiving opioids concomitantly. Finally, the respiratory depression produced by the benzodiazepine agonists can be antagonized by flumazenil.

The benzodiazepines produce variable cardiovascular effects. They reduce both preload and afterload; arterial blood pressure and cardiac output are minimally affected. However, in the presence of hypovolemia or catecholamine depletion,

the benzodiazepines, like virtually all other sedatives, may produce significant hypotension, and must, therefore, be administered with great caution, particularly if administered by a rapid bolus injection. Benzodiazepines significantly affect blood pressure and cardiac output when combined with opioids and are therefore more dangerous when combined than when either is given alone. Interestingly, diazepam has been reported to decrease coronary vascular resistance and has a nitroglycerine-like effect. Midazolam, on the other hand, decreases coronary sinus blood flow and myocardial oxygen consumption but does not change coronary vascular resistance.

The use of continuous infusions versus intermittent dosing of benzodiazepines is debatable. The advantages of continuous infusions, namely, stable blood levels and clinical effects without "peaks and valleys," may be counterbalanced by an increased risk for drug accumulation and more rapid development of tolerance. Interestingly, the use of continuous infusions in post–cardiac surgical patients has resulted in depression of cardiac output by >20% (40). In general, the use of continuous infusions is most common when shorter-acting agents like midazolam are used (7). Long-term infusions and altered metabolism secondary to illness increase the risk for drug accumulation and modified pharmacokinetics even when short-half-life drugs are used. Longer-acting agents (e.g., lorazepam, diazepam) may be less likely to induce tolerance, allow sedation to be interrupted for patient evaluation, and are often significantly cheaper than continuous infusions (41).

Diazepam

At one time the most commonly used benzodiazepine, diazepam has been largely replaced in clinical practice by midazolam and lorazepam (7). Data are limited on the use of diazepam in the ICU setting. It is poorly water soluble, and the vehicle for parenteral administration contains several organic solvents, such as propylene glycol and sodium benzoate, both of which are toxic in the newborn. Its poor water solubility makes absorption from an intramuscular site erratic and incomplete. Thus, the oral or intravenous route of administration is preferred. Unfortunately, even the intravenous route is problematic because diazepam can be painful when administered intravenously and can cause thrombophlebitis. Following absorption, diazepam is very slowly N-demethylated in the liver into two active metabolites: des-methyl diazepam and oxazepam. The presence of these active metabolites explains, in part, the very long duration of action of diazepam and why it has largely been replaced by midazolam. On the other hand, the prolonged sedation may be a desired effect in patients who require extended sedation.

Dosage and Route of Administration

Diazepam is an effective sedative, anxiolytic, and amnestic when administered orally, rectally, or intravenously. When administered intravenously, 0.05–0.1 mg/kg, it rapidly allays anxiety and apprehension and can be titrated to effect. Additionally, this same dose can be used as an anticonvulsant to temporarily stop seizure activity. The oral dose is two to three times the intravenous dose and takes 30–90 minutes to produce similar hypnotic effects.

Midazolam

Midazolam is a water-soluble benzodiazepine that is four times more potent than diazepam and is well absorbed via intramuscular, oral, rectal, or transmucosal routes of administration. Unlike diazepam, midazolam can be administered

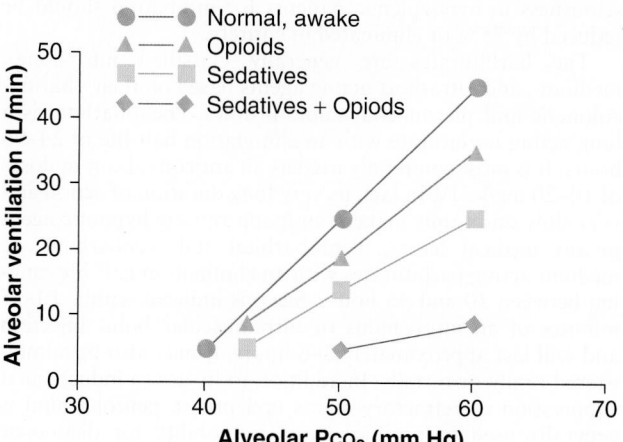

FIGURE 14.3. The relationship between ventilation and CO_2 is represented by a family of curves. Each curve has two parameters (an intercept and slope). Sedatives and opioids shift the position and slope to the right. The combination of drugs produces the most profound effects. (From Yaster M, Nichols DG, Deshpande JK, et al. Midazolam-fentanyl intravenous sedation in children: Case report of respiratory arrest. *Pediatrics* 1990;86:463–7, with permission.)

intravenously and rarely causes thrombophlebitis. Although manufactured as an acid to make it water soluble at physiologic pH, midazolam becomes highly lipophilic and rapidly crosses the blood–brain barrier to gain access to the benzodiazepine receptors in the central nervous system. This accounts for its dramatic clinical effect. It has a relatively large volume of distribution, short elimination half-life, high clearance, and is hydroxylated in the liver into inactive metabolites. It is characterized by rapid onset, short duration of action following a single parenteral dose, and by little accumulation following repeated or continuous infusion dosing. When administered enterally, usually for procedural sedation, <50% of the administered dose is bioavailable because of extraction by the liver ("first pass").

Dosage and Route of Administration

When used for sedation prior to procedures or as a premedication, midazolam can be administered intravenously (0.05–0.1 mg/kg), intramuscularly (0.1 mg/kg), rectally (0.3–1.0 mg/kg), orally (0.5–1.0 mg/kg; maximum dose 20 mg), or nasally (0.2 mg/kg). Obviously, intravenous administration produces the most rapid onset of effect and, therefore, must be titrated with continuous cardiorespiratory monitoring. It also produces the shortest duration of effect. When administered rectally, midazolam takes ~10 minutes to produce its effect, whereas when administered orally, it takes 20–30 minutes to achieve adequate sedation.

Midazolam is commonly administered in the ICU by continuous intravenous infusion for prolonged sedation (7). Tolerance and dependence will develop to prolonged midazolam infusions, and, if stopped suddenly, will result in severe withdrawal symptoms. Benzodiazepine withdrawal symptoms are similar to alcohol withdrawal symptoms ("delirium tremens") and will occur when cumulative midazolam dosing exceeds 60 mg/kg (42). Clonidine, administered orally or transdermally, or dexmedetomidine administered intravenously may ameliorate many of these withdrawal symptoms. Alternatively, patients should be weaned slowly by gradually tapering the dosage, rather than abrupt discontinuance of these drugs.

Lorazepam

Lorazepam is a relatively inexpensive, water-soluble benzodiazepine, which is recommended in adult guidelines for long-term sedation. High-grade evidence suggests lorazepam infusions, when compared to midazolam, require fewer dosage adjustments, require less time to achieve adequate sedation, and provide more predictability for awakening times and time to extubation compared to midazolam (7,43). The duration of action of lorazepam (2–4 hours) is longer than that of midazolam, allowing intermittent administration. Unlike midazolam, lorazepam is metabolized by glucuronyl transferase, and not by the cytochrome P450 system. Thus, it is less affected by liver disease and by other drugs that are metabolized by the P450 system, such as anticonvulsants, rifampin, and cimetidine. Additionally, lorazepam has no active metabolites. As with all benzodiazepines, tolerance develops with its use, and abrupt cessation results in symptoms of withdrawal (42).

Dosage and Route of Administration

Lorazepam is an effective sedative, anxiolytic, and amnestic when administered orally or intravenously. When administered intravenously, 0.05–0.1 mg/kg (maximum dose 2 mg), it rapidly allays anxiety and apprehension and should be titrated to effect. Additionally, this same dose can be used

as an anticonvulsant to stop seizure activity. The oral dose is two times the intravenous dose and is often used to wean benzodiazepine-dependent patients slowly.

Barbiturates

Largely utilized to induce coma in children with refractory seizures, barbiturates are neither anxiolytics nor analgesics. They globally depress the central nervous system to various degrees and produce effects ranging from sedation to general anesthesia in a dose-dependent manner. When dealing with patients in pain, caution must be exercised in the use of barbiturates because, in small dose, they increase the perception of pain and cause excitement rather than sedation ("antanalgesia"). However, when barbiturates are given in doses that are high enough to produce general anesthesia, pain perception, in addition to consciousness is obliterated. Thus, a dose-dependent continuum of central nervous system effects exists following barbiturate administration. At lower doses, barbiturates produce sleep and, at higher doses, they produce general anesthesia. Infrequently, barbiturates produce an idiosyncratic, hyperkinetic reaction in children characterized by agitation, incoherence, disorientation, and tantrums. All but methohexital are potent anticonvulsants and can be used acutely and chronically for this purpose. Additionally, they reduce cerebral blood flow and cerebral metabolism and are often used for this purpose following head injury in the ICU. However, these drugs are of no prophylactic value in preventing or minimizing secondary brain injury in patients with elevated intracranial pressure. Indeed, the use of barbiturate-induced coma for this purpose has not been shown to improve survival or neurologic recovery.

The barbiturates have significant effects on the cardiovascular system. They must be given with great caution in hemodynamically unstable patients. All of the barbiturates directly depress the myocardium and the arterial vascular tone, both of which can cause significant hypotension. If the baroreceptor compensatory system is intact, hypotension results in a reflex tachycardia that may help restore blood pressure. When barbiturates are given to patients with minimal compensatory reserves, such as patients who are catecholamine- or volume-depleted, profound hypotension and even cardiac arrest can occur. Indeed, the dose barbiturates used to induce unconsciousness in hypovolemic patients for intubation should be reduced by 75% or eliminated in entirety.

The barbiturates are generally classified into long-, medium-, and ultrashort-acting agents based on their pharmacokinetic and pharmacodynamic profiles. Phenobarbital is a long-acting barbiturate with an elimination half-life of 24–96 hours. It is most commonly used as an anticonvulsant in doses of 10–20 mg/kg IV. In fact, its very long duration of action and very slow onset time make it an inappropriate hypnotic agent in any medical setting. Pentobarbital and secobarbital are medium-acting barbiturates with an elimination half-life ranging between 20 and 45 hours. Sleep is induced within 10–15 minutes of an intravenous or intramuscular bolus injection and will last approximately 2–6 hours. It may also be administered orally or rectally. In addition to its use to induce burst suppression in refractory status epilepticus, pentobarbital is generally used to produce sleep, immobility for diagnostic imaging studies, and long-lasting sedation and is administered as 2–6 mg/kg IM or 1–3 mg/kg IV, with a maximum dose of 150 mg. Intravenous thiopental (now no longer produced in the United States), 4–7 mg/kg IV, and methohexital, 1–2 mg/kg IV, are ultrashort-acting agents (i.e., they produce unconsciousness for <10 minutes) despite having elimination half-lives of 4–24 hours. Recovery from the effects of intravenous thiopental and methohexital is determined by redistribution from the brain to other body tissue compartments. This has very important clinical implications. If, for example, thiopental is given by repeated intermittent doses or by a prolonged intravenous infusion (e.g., in head trauma), prolongation of effect will occur, because elimination and not distribution will determine the duration of the drug's effect.

Propofol

Propofol, a 2,6-diisopropylphenol, is an alkylphenol intravenous general anesthetic widely used in the operating room and in adult ICUs. It is unrelated to other general anesthetics and is formulated as a 1% (10 mg/mL) solution in 10% soybean oil, 2.25% glycerol, and 1.2% egg phosphatide. The drug's rapid onset of action, its dose-proportional sedative/anesthetic effects, and its rapid dissipation of clinical effects after discontinuing drug administration are responsible for its widespread acceptance as a general anesthetic, and for its potential use as a sedative to facilitate mechanical ventilation in critically ill patients in the ICU. Propofol, like barbiturates and other general anesthetics, appears to bind to the γ-aminobutyric acid (GABA) receptor, namely, the A subunit (GABA-A), which potentiates GABA-mediated synaptic inhibition within the central nervous system.

The pharmacokinetics of propofol after bolus doses or following continuous infusions has been studied extensively in healthy children and adults. The drug's disposition profile is best characterized by a three-compartment pharmacokinetic model (44). After intravenous administration, propofol rapidly distributes from the central compartment (blood) into two additional compartments: a larger, rapidly equilibrating compartment and an enormous, slowly equilibrating third compartment. Clearance from the central compartment is very rapid, exceeding total hepatic blood flow, and results in rapid recovery of consciousness. It is the rapid clearance from the central compartment rather than metabolism that is responsible for its short duration of effect. Propofol undergoes hepatic metabolism by conjugation and the resultant water-soluble compounds are excreted in the kidney. Complete elimination from the body may take many hours or even days despite minimal blood concentrations.

Although their actions are similar, propofol is chemically unrelated to the barbiturates. Like the barbiturates, it has negative inotropic properties and is a potent vasodilator. It is a rapidly acting sedative/amnestic agent without analgesic properties that also allows rapid recovery. Indeed, because of its rapid onset, rapid recovery time, and lack of active metabolites, it has largely replaced thiopental as the most commonly used intravenous general anesthetic induction agent in the operating room. Additionally, it is commonly given by infusion, in combination with short-lived opioids like fentanyl, to produce general anesthesia for short procedures like bronchoscopy and endoscopy. In the PICU, it is used to produce unconsciousness prior to intubation and in the adult ICU to produce prolonged, continuous sedation and to treat refractory status epilepticus. The latter effect is interesting because at low doses propofol may actually be proconvulsant and propofol administration has been associated with abnormal, myoclonic movements often referred to as seizure-like phenomenon (SLP). Propofol is manufactured in a lipid emulsion derived from egg whites. This causes pain on injection and makes the solution an ideal culture media for bacterial growth. The pain on injection can be prevented by pretreatment with IV lidocaine, fentanyl, or ketamine. The risk of bacterial contamination of the solution can be prevented by meticulous aseptic technique. Once a vial is opened the unused content should be disposed of promptly and not saved for later use. If an infusion is being used, the syringe and tubing should be dated, timed, and changed every 6 hours.

Unlike the operating room, in which propofol is given to relatively healthy patients for periods ranging from minutes to hours, patients in the ICU are by definition critically ill and may receive propofol for days. Because of this, insignificant effects during anesthesia become very important in the critically ill. Indeed, there have been many reports of unexpected fatal metabolic acidosis in critically ill children being sedated for prolonged periods with propofol, known as the propofol infusion syndrome (also propofol-related infusion syndrome) (45,46). There is also emerging evidence that propofol infusion syndrome is not limited to children, with a multitude of case reports in the adult ICU literature (47). A multifactorial disease with high mortality, propofol infusion syndrome is likely a result of the key pathogenetic mechanism of imbalance between energy demand and utilization. The syndrome may include metabolic acidosis, hyperlipidemia, hyperkalemia, rhabdomyolysis, subsequent renal failure, hepatomegaly, and cardiac dysrhythmias that may lead to cardiac failure. High doses of propofol in combination with exogenous catecholamines appear to be triggering factors (48). Given these data and available alternatives for sedation, it is recommended to avoid prolonged (>6 hour) propofol infusions in critically ill children.

Dosing and Route of Administration

When given in the ICU to induce deep sedation/general anesthesia for intubation or other painful procedures like cardioversion, 2–3 mg/kg of propofol is often given by IV push. Because of the effects of myocardial depression and decrease in systemic vascular resistance, caution must be taken when giving this drug in this way to already compromised children, and lower doses may be adequate to induce general anesthesia—titration is the key. If sustained procedural sedation is desired for a PICU patient, an infusion of undiluted propofol can be given at 50–100 µg/kg/min. Healthy children usually tolerate 150–250 µg/kg/min for deep sedation. This infusion rate is titrated up and down based on the level of procedural stimulation. At the conclusion of the procedure, the infusion can be stopped suddenly or titrated down in anticipation of its end. Return to preprocedural state of consciousness is rapid and dependent on dose and duration of the propofol infusion.

INHALATIONAL ANESTHETICS

Inhalational anesthetic agents are commonly used in the operating room to provide general anesthesia (amnesia, immobility, loss of consciousness, and analgesia) for surgery. Although their mechanism of action is unknown, general vapor anesthetics are predictable, have a rapid onset and emergence, and are easily titratable to effect. These features are appealing for use in the ICU. However, costs, variability in clinician and nursing credentialing and comfort with this class of drug, and the logistical issues of administering a volatile anesthetic gas for extended periods of time in the ICU have prevented their widespread use. Usage in the PICU is most often for sedation failures, detoxification following prolonged use of other sedatives and opioids, and in the treatment of status asthmaticus.

Isoflurane

Although all of the volatile general anesthetic agents have been used in the PICU, we will focus our discussion on isoflurane because it is the oldest, cheapest, and most commonly used. Isoflurane is a halogenated ether compound that when vaporized has a pungent odor that may irritate the airway and induce laryngospasm and bronchospasm in patients who are not anesthetized. In contrast, sevoflurane has a less offensive aroma and can be used to induce general anesthesia in non-anesthetized patients. The airway irritation produced by isoflurane can be prevented by administration only after general anesthesia with an IV medication or sevoflurane inhalation. Both agents are useful bronchodilators once general anesthesia is induced. Isoflurane, like all volatile general anesthetics, has a very narrow therapeutic index; the end-tidal concentration required to produce general anesthesia is 1.2%, and the potentially lethal end-tidal concentration is 4%. The drug is dispensed via a vaporizer that converts liquid isoflurane into a gas and can be adjusted to vary the concentration of volatile anesthetic that the patient breathes. Unlike N_2O, anesthetic doses of the volatile anesthetics do not significantly lower the fraction of inspired oxygen.

For the intensivist, an understanding of the primary physiologic effects of the vapor anesthetics is essential. Isoflurane is a negative inotrope and vasodilator, and increasing its concentration (and anesthetic depth) produces a progressive myocardial depression and peripheral vasodilation. This results in hypotension and a compensatory increase in HR. Volatile anesthetics are also potent respiratory depressants and decrease minute ventilation by >30%. They primarily do this by decreasing tidal volume and by altering the respiratory centers hypoxic and hypercarbic drive to breathe. And yet, patients breathing spontaneously on a vapor anesthetic appear to be tachypneic with respiratory rates as high as 40 breaths/minute. This increase in respiratory rate is an ineffective compensation for the decrease in tidal volume that these drugs produce. Indeed, anesthetized patients breathing spontaneously will have end-tidal CO_2 levels in the mid-50-mm-Hg range. Finally, once general anesthesia is induced (airway reflexes are blunted), isoflurane like the other vapor anesthetics are potent bronchodilators. Many patients in status asthmaticus who are unresponsive to other treatment will improve rapidly ("break") when anesthetized with isoflurane (49,50).

Isoflurane causes a decrease in cerebral metabolic rate and increases in cerebral blood flow, cerebral vasodilation, and possibly intracranial pressure (though this is blunted with hyperventilation). This uncoupling of cerebral metabolic rate to cerebral blood flow increases the risk of the use of isoflurane in patients with increased intracranial pressure. Finally, isoflurane is a potent anticonvulsant and is occasionally used in the treatment of refractory status epilepticus.

When used in isolation, the sedative effects from isoflurane can be observed at exhaled concentrations of 0.3%–1%, while analgesic and general anesthetic effects usually require concentrations of 1%–1.2%. These effects occur at lower concentrations when the patient is also being exposed to other sedating medications. It is important to note that the longer the gas is inhaled, the more volatile agent will be distributed and stored in fat-soluble compartments. Thus, the duration of agent administration and the size of the patient are important factors in achieving adequate sedation, analgesia, and anesthesia and also in wake up and recovery.

In addition to concerns with volatile anesthetic usage in altered intracranial compliance, volatile agents are contraindicated in those patients with a history of malignant hyperthermia (MH) or who are at risk of developing MH such as patients with core myopathies. Additionally, like N_2O, the use of isoflurane is limited by institutional and nursing credentialing, availability of specialized delivery and monitoring equipment, and the ability to scavenge exhaled gas.

Ketamine

Structurally related to phencyclidine (PCP), ketamine is an NMDA antagonist that produces an altered state of consciousness (dissociation), amnesia, and analgesia (51). Ketamine is most commonly manufactured as a racemic mixture containing both chiral S(+) and R(−) enantiomers. These stereoisomers have different anesthetic potencies (4:1, respectively) but have similar kinetics and are both metabolized by hepatic N-methylation to norketamine, which is further metabolized by hydroxylation and ultimately excreted in the urine. Because the pharmacokinetics of ketamine relies on both hepatic metabolism and renal excretion, its duration of action and dose effect will be altered in many critically ill patients.

Pharmacokinetic data in pediatric patients are limited. Hartvig et al. described ketamine and norketamine elimination in postoperative cardiac patients and found that their elimination half-lives were 3.1 hours and 6 hours, respectively (52). Although tolerance has been reported, there are no clinical reports of dependence or withdrawal following ketamine administration. The minimal respiratory depressant effects and relatively stable hemodynamics associated with its use make this an appealing drug for procedural sedation in the PICU.

In addition to its binding to the NMDA receptor, ketamine causes an increase in catecholamine release and cholinergic receptor stimulation. This results in bronchodilation and an increase in systemic vascular resistance, HR, and cardiac output. Thus, ketamine is often used in asthmatic patients as well as in hemodynamically unstable patients or patients with congenital heart disease (53). Nevertheless, it is important to realize that ketamine is actually a negative inotrope and it is this catecholamine release that helps support blood pressure. This relationship is important when ketamine is administered to patients who are catecholamine depleted, because in these patients, ketamine can cause profound hypotension and shock. Other adverse effects of ketamine include hallucinations, myoclonic movements, and excessive salivation. The hallucinations that are a result of ketamine administration may increase the risk of ICU delirium even after cessation of administration and decrease in drug levels. Ketamine also raises cerebral blood flow and cerebral oxygen consumption. Nevertheless, recent systematic reviews of the literature suggest that ketamine does not increase IntraCranial Pressure (ICP) in ventilated, sedated patients with severe traumatic brain injury (53a). Because of the psychomotor agitation, vocalization, and salivation, coadministration of glycopyrrolate or atropine and midazolam helps to reduce these symptoms and recall.

Other adverse effects remain controversial and include the occurrence of apnea in infants, a possible increased incidence of laryngospasm, lowering of the seizure threshold, and elevation of intracranial pressure. These are infrequent events, but should be considered by the practitioner. Certainly they emphasize the need for strict fasting guidelines, careful monitoring during and after usage, and preparation for additional or alternative agents to be available in case adverse events occur.

Dosage and Route of Administration

Ketamine can be administered for procedural sedation by nasal, oral, intravenous, and intramuscular routes with good results. With intravenous administration, onset of action and recovery are relatively rapid (1–2 minutes and 30–60 minutes, respectively) but can be quite variable. Further, when given in rapid IV doses of 2 mg/kg, ketamine induces general anesthesia and can be used for rapid sequence inductions (RSIs). Like other IV agents, ketamine can be titrated for sedation in aliquots of 0.5–1 mg/kg every 2–3 minutes until an adequate level of sedation/analgesia is achieved. Intramuscular administration can be used if intravenous access is unavailable. Typically IM dosing is 3–5 mg/kg for sedation and 5–7 mg/kg for general anesthesia equivalent. The IM delivery can include ketamine (3–5 mg/kg), midazolam (0.1 mg/kg), and atropine (0.01 mg/kg) in one syringe to avoid multiple needle sticks. Similarly, it can be given orally as ketamine (5 mg/kg), coadministered with midazolam (0.5–1 mg/kg) and atropine (0.02 mg/kg). For patients requiring nonprocedural sedation, ketamine infusions have been used with mixed success. Typically, a loading dose of 1–2 mg/kg is followed by a continuous infusion ranging between 1 and 4 mg/kg/h. Issues of delirium, tolerance, and withdrawal symptoms have been raised following prolonged infusions, and patients should be closely monitored following discontinuation of prolonged ketamine exposure.

α_2-ADRENERGIC AGONISTS IN SEDATION AND PAIN MANAGEMENT

α_2 agonists exert their effects by activating α_2-adrenergic receptors throughout the body. Three subtypes of this G-protein–coupled receptor have been characterized. The α_{2A} adrenoreceptor mediates sedation, sleep, analgesia, and sympatholysis, whereas the α_{2B} adrenoreceptor mediates vasoconstriction, antishivering, and endogenous analgesia. The α_{2C} receptor has been linked to learning, neuroprotection, and sympatholysis (54,55). Despite these effects on learning, the α_2 agonists have virtually no amnestic properties. Both clonidine and dexmedetomidine belong to the imidazoline class of α_2-adrenergic agonists. Drugs from this class have a variety of physiologic effects on the heart, brain, lungs, kidneys, and on hormonal regulation. They are used clinically for their antihypertensive and sedative/analgesic effects. Indeed, in the ICU, a bolus dose of an α_2 adrenoreceptor agonist can result in hypotension and bradycardia, particularly in volume-depleted patients (see what follows).

Clonidine

Clonidine is an imidazole α_2 agonist that binds to α_2:α_1 receptors in a ratio of 200:1. Clonidine is moderately lipid soluble and is almost completely absorbed following an oral dose. Peak serum levels occur at 1–3 hours and in as little as 15–20 minutes following epidural or spinal administration. Because of its large volume of distribution, clonidine has a long elimination half-life of 12–24 hours. It has little, if any, ventilatory depressant effects and best achieves analgesia when it is administered epidurally. Sedation, sleep, and the treatment of withdrawal symptomatology (from opioids, benzodiazepines, etc.) are the result of activation of α_2 receptors in the locus ceruleus. α_2 receptors, when centrally stimulated, prevent the presynaptic release of norepinephrine in the sympathetic nervous system ("negative feedback loop") and account for clonidine's antihypertensive effects. Of note, the rebound hypertension seen with abrupt discontinuation of clonidine is thought to be from removal of the central inhibition of sympathetic activity. Interestingly, direct action on peripheral α_2 receptors results in peripheral vasoconstriction. Finally, adult studies have demonstrated clonidine to be an effective antishivering drug. The mechanism of this effect is thought to be through central thermoregulatory inhibition rather than peripherally on the muscles thermogenic activity.

Because of its bioavailability, clonidine can be administered by almost every route. It can be given subcutaneously, orally, intravenously, transdermally, intranasally, and rectally. For

sedation in the PICU and operating rooms, oral sedative doses of 2–5 μg/kg are given every 4–6 hours. This dose of the oral (neuraxial or crushed tablets) solution has also been given rectally. When given intranasally, the neuraxial solution should be used at the same dose. In patients with prolonged opioid and benzodiazepine exposure, clonidine patches (release rates of 100, 200, or 300 μg/day; total content 2.5, 5.0, and 7.5 mg; size 3.5, 7.0, and 10.5 cm^2) are frequently used. Typically, we start with the lower-dose patch of 100 μg (release rate, 4 μg/h) and titrate up over 3–4 days. For treatment of shivering, an IV dose of 1.5 μg/kg can be given. Unfortunately, the IV solution is not available in the United States. Though the concerns over rebound hypertension from clonidine are always present, we have been able to stop clonidine after 3–4 days of use without problem. If using a patch, we will typically step down over 2 to 3 weeks, once weaning from other agents has been completed.

Dexmedetomidine

Dexmedetomidine was approved by the U.S. Food and Drug Administration in 1999 for sedation in adults whose airways were intubated in the ICU and in 2008 for sedation for surgical or medication procedures in adults without intubated airways outside the ICU. Currently, dexmedetomidine is not approved for use in children in any country (56). As an off-label medication, dexmedetomidine has been administered as an adjunct to anesthesia (general and regional) in and out of the operating rooms for both surgical and medical procedures in children and for sedation in the PICU. Perhaps its widest application in children has been for procedural sedation in radiology because dexmedetomidine uniquely provides sedation and analgesia without significant respiratory depression (57,58). In the past decade, the clinical applications of dexmedetomidine have been expanding with reports of its use as a premedication before anesthesia, as an adjunctive drug intraoperatively and postoperatively, to attenuate emergence complications including delirium, shivering, and pain in the perioperative period and for sedation, analgesia, hemodynamic management, and airway management in the ICU.

As discussed elsewhere in this chapter, critically ill patients exhibit severe sleep deprivation with virtually complete disruption of sleep architecture. Although there are many reasons for this including excessive noise and lighting, the very drugs used to produce sedation in the ICU, namely the benzodiazepines and opioids, negatively affect sleep architecture (31). Dexmedetomidine is pivotally different. The α_2-adrenoceptor agonists acting in the locus ceruleus directly affect the ventrolateral preoptic (VLPO) nucleus in the anterior hypothalamus which controls normal sleep through the release of GABA, serotonin, orexin, and histamine (**Fig. 14.4**). Thus, dexmedetomidine inhibits norepinephrine release in the VLPO and induces a state that is most similar to natural sleep when compared to all other available sedatives. The ability of dexmedetomidine to produce this natural sleep not only may have profound effects through sleep promotion but may play a role in preventing ICU delirium and psychosis (7). Finally, these central effects in the locus ceruleus may also be responsible for the prevention and treatment of opioid and benzodiazepine drug withdrawal syndromes.

Pharmacokinetics in Children

A limited number of studies have investigated the pharmacokinetics of dexmedetomidine in children. Much like adults, when administered IV, 93% of the dexmedetomidine is protein bound in children with a rapid (α phase) redistribution half-life is ~7 minutes, clearance is ~15 mL/kg/min, and the terminal (β phase) elimination half-life is ~2 hours (56,59,60).

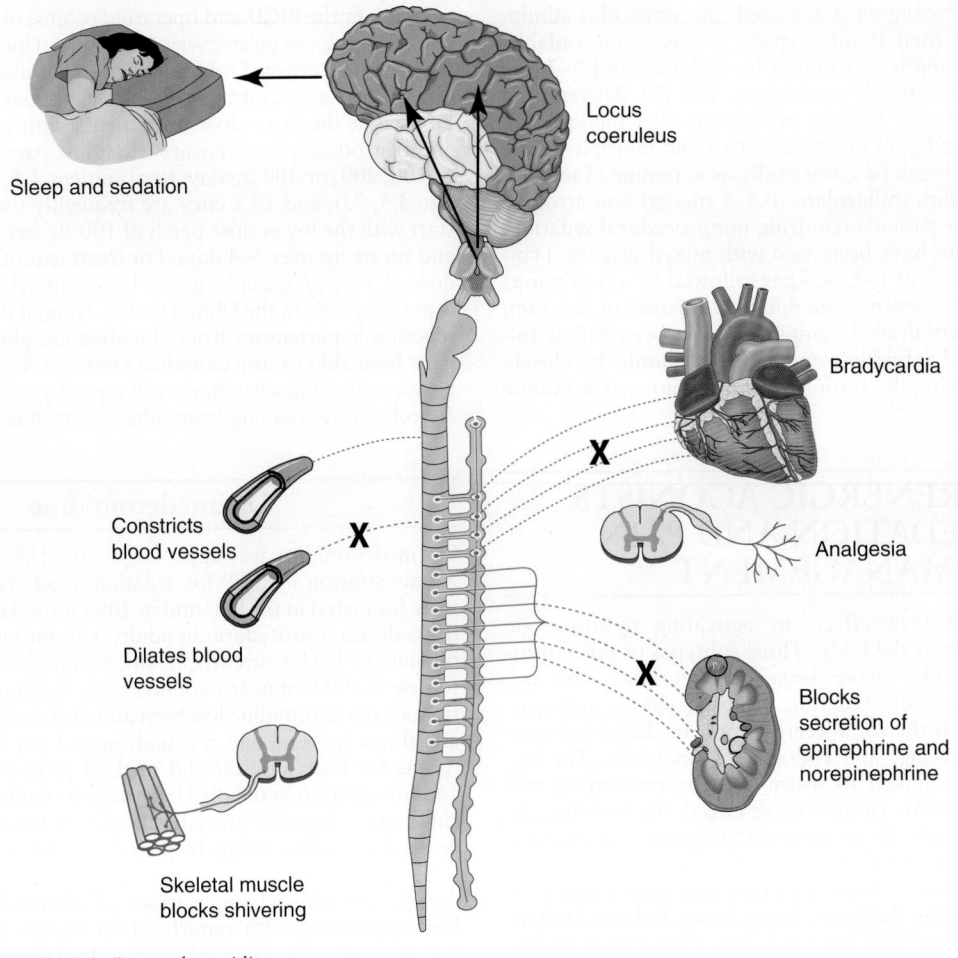

FIGURE 14.4. Dexmedetomidine.

Physiologic Effects

Aside from its hypnotic and analgesic effects, perhaps the most important physiologic effects of dexmedetomidine to the intensivist are its cardiovascular effects. As discussed earlier, the cardiovascular effects of dexmedetomidine are mediated via adrenoreceptors in both the central and peripheral nervous systems (**Fig. 14.4**). In children, large bolus doses of dexmedetomidine cause peripheral vasoconstriction, which may lead to transient systemic hypertension, whereas low doses cause central sympatholysis, which can lead to systemic hypotension (56,60). If an initial loading dose of dexmedetomidine is not administered or if the loading dose is infused slowly (i.e., over 10 minutes), the severity of the hypotension after dexmedetomidine is attenuated. In such cases, systolic blood pressure decreases up to 30% from baseline (56). In healthy children, the severity of the hypotension varies directly with the dose of dexmedetomidine. When a loading dose between 0.5 and 1 μg/kg dexmedetomidine is administered over ~10 minutes as the sole sedative, systolic blood pressure decreases as the dose increases, reaching a maximum decrease of 30% from baseline at 1 μg/kg (56,60). Larger doses of dexmedetomidine, 2–3 μg/kg/h, cause more profound decreases in systolic blood pressure (with a 24% incidence of hypotension) as the dose increases, particularly in young infants (56,61). HR also decreases up to 30% from awake measurements after an initial loading dose of dexmedetomidine, 0.5–1 μg/kg, over 10 minutes in children. These HR responses were not attenuated by pretreating the children with IV glycopyrrolate (5 μg/kg) (56). Interestingly, HR does not decrease after a loading dose of the combination

ketamine (2 mg/kg) and dexmedetomidine (1 μg/kg), followed by an infusion of dexmedetomidine (2 μg/kg/h and then 1 μg/kg/h) (62). Children who developed bradycardia maintained their systolic blood pressure within normal limits. As a result, the authors did not believe that the slow HRs posed a substantive threat to the children and, therefore, did not treat them. However, if bradycardia occurs in the presence of marked hypotension, then aggressive intervention is recommended to prevent end-organ ischemic damage. Such intervention should include but is not limited to stopping the dexmedetomidine infusion, stimulating the child with verbal and tactile stimulation, and perhaps the administration of β agonists and/or inotropes. Caution should be exercised when administering anticholinergics to treat isolated dexmedetomidine-associated bradycardia in children.

In addition to cardiovascular effects, anecdotal evidence suggests that long-term use of dexmedetomidine infusions (>48 hours) can result in physiologic tolerance, withdrawal, and possibly adrenal insufficiency (63–65). Given the increased prevalence of dexmedetomidine use as well as a trend of increased duration of use in the PICU setting, these long-term effects warrant study through prospective research designs.

THE CHALLENGING PATIENT

Infants and children who require prolonged (days to weeks) sedation and immobility often require prodigious amounts of sedation. As drugs and dosing requirements escalate over time, the challenge of finding an alternative and safe sedation strategy becomes a paramount issue in medical management. Often with infants and children, these challenging patients require a collaborative approach and no formulaic solution will work for every patient. Certainly early consultation with a pediatric pain specialist is warranted. Often, parental anxiety and fears contribute to the difficulties in providing a level of comfort that is safe for the patient but allows for autonomy of the family. When concern for harm is great (i.e., surgical wound is compromised, airway is unstable), then patient safety must become paramount. Developing an organized and systematic plan will help to inform nursing, surgeons, and staff what will be the next approach if the problems of analgesia and sedation continue. Certainly, the addition of paralytic agents and/or general anesthesia with isoflurane are options (see sections Inhalational Anesthetics and Neuromuscular Blockade). However, prior to instituting these solutions, other drug combinations and timing of medications can be pursued. Often, standing doses of medications need to be altered on a timed, around-the-clock basis, (a) to provide new agents to help keep the agitated patient calm, but (b) to prevent the adverse effects of stacking analgesics and sedatives and creating negative cardiorespiratory effects. Alternative sedatives are listed in **Table 14.9**. Though difficult-to-sedate patients are a frequent problem in the PICU, clear communication with family and staff, and emphasis on a goal-directed, team solution to the problem will address many of the issues that an improved and rationale pharmacologic approach to sedation cannot.

Neuromuscular Blockade

The principal pharmacologic effect of neuromuscular blocking agents (NMBAs) is to interrupt the transmission of nerve impulses to the neuromuscular junction. *These drugs have no analgesic or sedative properties and must always be administered after adequate sedation has been achieved.* However, the clinical need for immobility in mechanically ventilated children occasionally necessitates neuromuscular blockade. Based on their mechanism of action these drugs can be divided into two types: depolarizing (mimic the action of acetylcholine) and nondepolarizing (competitively block the actions of acetylcholine) agents. These drugs can also be subdivided into short (succinylcholine, mivacurium)-, intermediate (atracurium, vecuronium, rocuronium, cisatracurium)-, and long (pancuronium, doxacurium, pipecuronium)-acting drugs (**Table 14.10**). The onset of neuromuscular blockade is more rapid and less intense at the laryngeal muscles (vocal cords) than at the peripheral muscles. Further, the diaphragm is the muscle most resistant to paralysis; indeed, twice the dose is required to paralyze the diaphragm than is needed to paralyze the adductor pollicis muscle. NMBAs are large, highly charged, water-soluble particles at physiologic pH. Thus, they are limited to the extracellular volume and cannot cross the blood–brain barrier, placenta, or GI epithelium. Therefore, these drugs have no CNS or analgesic effects, cannot be given orally, and when given to pregnant women do not affect the fetus.

The principal use of NMBAs in the ICU is to provide paralysis to facilitate tracheal intubation and to improve the conditions needed to mechanically ventilate patients or to keep patients immobile. The choice of drug is influenced by the speed of onset, duration of action, method of excretion (kidney, liver, or plasma), and the drug's side effect profile. The fastest paralytic agent is succinylcholine; it achieves total paralysis in less than a minute and has a very brief duration of action (3–5 minutes), making it an ideal agent for rapid sequence inductions in patients without contraindications to succinylcholine. The only nondepolarizing agent that comes close to the onset time of succinylcholine-induced paralysis is rocuronium. Rocuronium takes 1–2 minutes to achieve paralysis but has a duration of action that is significantly longer than that of succinylcholine (45–90 minutes). Regardless of the drug used to achieve paralysis, the degree of neuromuscular blockade is best evaluated by monitoring the evoked

TABLE 14.9

ALTERNATIVE SEDATIVE AGENTS IN THE PICU

DRUG	DOSE (mg/kg)	ROUTE	INTERVAL (h)	COMMENTS
Diphenhydramine	0.5–1	PO, IV, IM	4–6	Antihistamine; provides sedation and is antipruritic and antiemetic Adverse effects include dry mouth, tachycardia, and respiratory depression
Butorphanol	0.01–0.02	IV	4–6	Mixed opioid agonist/antagonist; risk of reversing analgesic effects of μ-agonist opioids
	0.05	PO		Weak analgesic with minimal respiratory depressive effects
Promethazine	0.5–1	IV, PO, PR, IM	6–8	Phenothiazine commonly used as an antiemetic Risk of causing extrapyramidal reactions and neuroleptic malignant syndrome
Haloperidol	0.01–0.02	IV, IM	8–12	Antipsychotic; can have dystonic reactions and neuroleptic malignant syndrome
	0.1–0.2	PO		Not for p.r.n. use
Chloral hydrate	50–100	PO, PR	24	Aliphatic alcohol, unknown mechanism of action Not to be used repetitively or in prolonged fashion Unpredictable onset and duration of sedative effects GI irritant No analgesic effects
Clonidine	0.002–0.005	PO	4–6	α2 adrenergic agonist Possible hypotension Potentiates sedative/analgesic effects of other agents Available in transcutaneous patches of 0.1, 0.2, 0.3 mg, which are changed every 7 d

TABLE 14.10

COMPARATIVE PHARMACOLOGY OF NONDEPOLARIZING NEUROMUSCULAR BLOCKING DRUGS

■ DRUG	■ ED95 (mg/kg)	■ INTUBATING DOSE (mg/kg)	■ ONSET TO MAXIMUM TWITCH DEPRESSION (min)	■ DURATION TO RETURN TO 25% CONTROL TWITCH HEIGHT (min)	■ DURATION TO RETURN TO TRAIN OF FOUR >0.9 (min)	■ CONTINUOUS INFUSION (μg/kg/min)
Pancuronium	0.05	0.1	3–5	60–90	120–220	NA
Vecuronium	0.05	0.1	3–5	20–35	50–80	1
Rocuronium	0.3	0.6–1.2	1–2	20–35	50–80	3–10
Cis-atracurium	0.05	0.1	3–5	20–35	60–90	0.4–4

skeletal responses produced by an electrical stimulus delivered percutaneously to the ulnar or facial nerves by a peripheral nerve stimulator.

Succinylcholine

The only depolarizing agent in current use is succinylcholine. Succinylcholine mimics acetylcholine in its structure, binding to the acetylcholine receptor at the motor end plate in a noncompetitive fashion, resulting in depolarization. This is manifest in older children and adults by a phase of muscular fasciculation. Muscle fasciculations increase intragastric, intraocular, and intracranial pressure. They may also be associated with the development of the myalgias that are common after succinylcholine administration. Interestingly, children under the age of 4 years may not fasciculate. The resolution of the brief phase muscle fasciculation heralds the onset of a short period of profound neuromuscular paralysis as succinylcholine continues to occupy the receptor. Succinylcholine subsequently diffuses off the receptor and is metabolized by plasma and hepatic pseudocholinesterase. Newborn infants are relatively resistant to the effects of succinylcholine when dose requirements are compared with adults on an mg/kg basis. This is probably due to their increased volume of distribution. In fact, the neonate requires about twice as much succinylcholine (2 mg/kg) as does the adult (1 mg/kg) to facilitate tracheal intubation.

Redistribution and metabolism of succinylcholine determine the duration of its neuromuscular blockade. Despite a lower plasma concentration of pseudocholinesterase in infancy, the redistribution of succinylcholine from a relatively small muscle mass to a large extracellular fluid compartment quickly terminates the neuromuscular blocking effects. With prolonged or repeated exposure to succinylcholine, the membrane repolarizes but remains refractory to subsequent depolarization by acetylcholine. A so-called phase II block results, the clinical characteristics of which resemble a nondepolarizing block. The exact mechanism of this block has not been elucidated.

The neuromuscular blockade following succinylcholine can be prolonged if the patient has an abnormal, genetically derived variant of pseudocholinesterase. The diagnosis of this disorder relies on clinical history of prolonged neuromuscular blockade following standard doses of succinylcholine and may be substantiated by assaying the plasma pseudocholinesterase inhibition by dibucaine. A positive family history is supportive evidence for the diagnosis. Management should consist of controlled ventilation with sedation until the block spontaneously dissipates. Although the administration of blood or plasma has been advocated for the treatment of this disorder, it cannot be recommended because of the inherent risks involved with this

approach. Hepatic dysfunction, hypermagnesemia, and pregnancy are also associated with a prolonged block following succinylcholine administration.

Because a variety of side effects accompanies the administration of succinylcholine, its use must be carefully considered in the context of each situation. Side effects include life-threatening hyperkalemia (potassium concentrations >10 mEq/L) in patients with muscular dystrophy, acute denervation injury leading to skeletal muscle atrophy (e.g., spinal cord trauma), demyelinating diseases, and following third-degree unhealed burns. Interestingly, succinylcholine produces a rise in potassium (0.5 mEq/L) even in normal patients. Additional side effects of succinylcholine include severe bradycardia and other dysrhythmias, myalgia, myoglobinuria, increased gastric, intraocular, and intracranial pressure, and sustained skeletal muscle contractions, particularly of the masseter muscles. It is also a profound trigger of MH in susceptible patients. Because of the risk of giving succinylcholine to males with undiagnosed muscular dystrophy, the U.S. Food and Drug Administration has issued a black-box warning concerning its use. Indeed, because of the myriad problems associated with this drug, most pediatric anesthesiologists no longer use this drug for routine (nonrapid sequence) intubation.

Finally, succinylcholine stimulates all cholinergic autonomic receptors: nicotinic receptors of both sympathetic and parasympathetic ganglia and muscarinic receptors in the sinus node of the heart. This results in a negative inotropic and chronotropic effects following an initial dose. In children, in whom the parasympathetic tone predominates, severe bradycardia and even sinus arrest may occur. The bradycardia occurs with greater frequency and severity following a second dose of succinylcholine in older children and adults. It *can* be effectively prevented by pretreatment with atropine (0.02 mg/kg, minimum dose 0.15 mg) or glycopyrrolate (0.01 mg/kg).

Nondepolarizing Neuromuscular Blocking Drugs

Nondepolarizing muscle relaxants are either aminosteroidal (rocuronium, vecuronium, and pancuronium) or benzylisoquinolinium (atracurium, mivacurium, cisatracurium, and doxacurium) compounds. These drugs competitively occupy the postsynaptic nicotinic acetylcholine receptor without causing a change in the configuration of the receptor. Occupancy of 65% of these receptors by nondepolarizing muscle relaxants does not produce any evidence of weakness or paralysis. Neuromuscular transmission falls when 80% of the receptors are occupied. Interestingly, when 95% of receptors are occupied, patients cannot swallow, cough, or protect their airways but can achieve normal tidal volumes and even vital capacity breaths. Because of this, it is wise to monitor weakness and recovery with blockade monitors. Indeed, prolonged use in the ICU may result in muscular weakness on recovery ("critical illness myopathy"), and there are some data to suggest that there may be an increased risk of myopathy with prolonged administration of aminosteroidal compounds, particularly with concomitant steroid therapy (66). Choosing a nondepolarizing muscle relaxant is based on differences in onset time, duration of action, method of metabolism and excretion (kidney vs. liver vs. plasma), and cardiovascular side effect profile. Nondepolarizing muscle relaxants exert cardiovascular effects via blockade of cardiac muscarinic receptors (e.g., pancuronium produces tachycardia).

Several drugs and events and medical conditions unrelated to drug therapy may enhance the neuromuscular block produced by nondepolarizing muscle relaxants. These include the concomitant use of aminoglycoside antibiotics, volatile anesthetic agents, high-dose furosemide, magnesium and lithium therapy; and cyclosporine. Hypercarbia and hypothermia potentiate the neuromuscular blockade produced by nondepolarizing muscle relaxants. The former is particularly pernicious; with muscle weakness, one breathes less, which produces hypercarbia, which, in turn, potentiates the paralysis, weakening the diaphragm and the cycle repeats. Finally, burn injuries and female gender also are associated with enhanced neuromuscular blockade.

Anticholinesterase Drugs—Reversal of Paralysis

Anticholinesterase drugs such as neostigmine (0.07 mg/kg), edrophonium (0.5–1 mg/kg), and pyridostigmine (0.2 mg/kg) are often administered to antagonize the paralysis produced by nondepolarizing muscle relaxants. Neostigmine has the most favorable risk–benefit profile and is used most commonly. These drugs inhibit acetylcholinesterase, which is normally responsible for the rapid hydrolysis of acetylcholine into choline and acetic acid at the neuromuscular junction. The inhibition of acetylcholine hydrolysis by the esterase allows more acetylcholine to be available at the neuromuscular junction and thereby return of muscle function. It also allows more acetylcholine to be available at muscarinic and nicotinic acetylcholine receptors and thereby produce bradycardia, salivation, miosis, and hyperperistalsis as well as the desired return of neuromuscular function. Thus, whenever giving an anticholinesterase to reverse nondepolarizing muscle relaxants, one must always preadminister an anticholinergic such as atropine (0.02 mg/kg, minimum dose 0.15 mg) or glycopyrrolate (0.01 mg/kg), to prevent adverse muscarinic effects such as bradycardia and hypersalivation.

The presence of residual neuromuscular blockade can be evaluated by using a peripheral nerve stimulator. The poles of the stimulator are placed over the peripheral nerve, usually the ulnar nerve at the wrist or elbow, and an impulse is applied. The twitch response of the adductor pollicis and flexor digitorum muscles to specific types of electrical stimulation gives clues to the presence or absence of blockade. The nondepolarizing neuromuscular blockade is characterized by (a) decreased contraction to a single impulse; (b) unsustained response to tetanic stimulation of 50 Hz at 2.5 seconds; (c) diminution of the fourth twitch response compared with the first twitch response, of >70% following four 2-Hz stimuli (train of four); (d) facilitation of the contractile response following tetanic stimulation; and (e) antagonism by acetylcholinesterase inhibitors. Abolition of the fourth twitch response of the train of four correlates with a 75% reduction

in standard twitch tension. It must be remembered, however, that the magnitude and duration of the impulse influence the twitch response and that twitch response is not altered until >75% of the receptors are blocked. On the other hand, abolition of all four twitches on a train of four corresponds to 95% receptor blockade.

WEANING OF OPIOIDS/SEDATIVES

Dependence and Prevention of Withdrawal

Tolerance and *physical dependence* with repeated opioid and sedative administration are common phenomenon in the PICU. The most studied and characteristic features are described in all μ-opioid agonists. *Tolerance* is the development of a need to increase the dose of an opioid or benzodiazepine agonist to achieve the same analgesic or sedative effect previously achieved with a lower dose. Tolerance to the analgesic effects of opioids usually develops following 10–21 days of morphine administration. On the other hand, patients rarely develop tolerance to the constipating effects of opioids. Additionally, cross-tolerance develops between all of the μ-opioid agonists. However, this is rarely complete, so opioid rotation, that is, changing from one opioid to another, can be helpful in preventing a continuous escalation in analgesic dosing. When it is necessary to switch, careful consideration must be given to the choice of opioid, dose, and degree of cross-tolerance. Indeed, when switching opioids in tolerant patients, we conservatively underestimate the equianalgesic dosing by a factor of 2.

Physical dependence, sometimes referred to as "neuroadaptation," is caused by repeated administration of an opioid, which necessitates the continued administration of the drug to prevent the appearance of a withdrawal or abstinence syndrome that is characteristic for that particular drug. It usually occurs after 2–3 weeks of morphine administration, but may occur after only just a few days of therapy. Very young infants treated with very-high-dose fentanyl infusions following surgical repair of congenital heart disease and/or who required extracorporeal membrane oxygenation (ECMO) have been identified to be at particular risk.

When physical dependence has been established, sudden discontinuation of an opioid or benzodiazepine agonist produces a *withdrawal* syndrome within 24 hours of drug cessation. Symptoms reach their peak within 72 hours and include abdominal cramps, vomiting, diarrhea, tachycardia, hypertension, diaphoresis, restlessness, insomnia, movement disorders, reversible neurologic abnormalities, and seizures. Clinical and experimental data suggest that the duration of receptor occupancy is an important factor in the development of tolerance and dependence. Thus, continuous infusions may produce tolerance more rapidly than intermittent therapy (67,68). This is particularly true for fentanyl. Fentanyl is a potent, rapidly acting, lipophilic opioid that is frequently used for procedure-related pain (e.g., dressing changes, laceration repair) and for pain management in critically ill children. Tolerance and dependence *predictably* develops following only 5–10 days (2.5 mg/kg total fentanyl dose) of continuous fentanyl infusions. Nevertheless, prolonged therapy (>10 days) even by intermittent bolus administration should be *expected* to produce opioid dependence.

Withdrawal Scales and Weaning Strategies

In the PICU, opioid, benzodiazepine, and α agonist withdrawal are common iatrogenic complications of the necessary analgesic and sedative strategies used to care for critically ill children.

Just as the judicious monitoring and administration of these agents correlate with improved care, appropriate assessment tools to recognize and treat withdrawal symptoms must be utilized, as well as strategies developed to effectively wean those patients who are at risk to have withdrawal symptoms.

Withdrawal/Abstinence Scales for Infants and Children in the PICU

In the neonatal ICU (NICU), withdrawal scores were originally developed to care for infants born to drug-addicted mothers. Neonatal, like adult, opioid withdrawal is a disorder characterized by generalized irritability, respiratory distress, GI distress, autonomic overactivity, and even, seizures. Similar symptoms and degree of severity are seen in iatrogenic abstinence from opioids and are less well described but attributable to other sedatives/analgesics like benzodiazepines.

The most commonly used and recommended tool for quantifying the severity of withdrawal in neonates in the United States is the modified Neonatal Abstinence Scoring System (NAS). The American Academy of Pediatrics (AAP) committee of drug usage reviewed and updated this issue and published their recommendation in 2012 (69). The modified NAS assigns a total score based on the observation of 21 items relating to signs of neonatal withdrawal at regular intervals (69). Of note, the NAS has not been validated in infants with iatrogenic, ex-utero exposure to opioids and benzodiazepines. The AAP consensus statement includes that each institution should adopt an abstinence scoring method to measure the severity of withdrawal. They advocated for nonpharmacologic supportive measures including minimizing environmental stimuli, promoting sleep, and optimizing nutrition as the initial approach to therapy. They felt the evidence indicated that abstinence scoring provides a consistent means of quantifying signs of psychomotor behavior, and correlating these scores with severity of withdrawal is necessary to provide the best decision about the institution of pharmacologic therapy. Further, the study section suggested that the evidence for a combined approach including individualized clinical assessment would be more objective and allow a quantitative strategy to increasing or decreasing dosing, since an optimal threshold score for abstinence assessment instruments is not known. In a major change from the 1998 guidelines, the AAP concluded that when pharmacologic treatment is chosen, they support the use of oral morphine solution and methadone, based on limited evidence from controlled trials. They also suggested that oral clonidine may be effective as either a primary or adjunctive therapy, but were clear that further study is needed. Whereas the 1998 recommendations advocated for diluted tincture of opium (DTO) as a first-line therapy, the recent revision raises concern about the 25-fold higher concentration of morphine in DTO when compared to oral morphine solutions, increasing the risk of drug error and overdose.

Despite clear, evidence-based recommendations from the AAP, the management of the newborn with psychomotor behavior consistent with withdrawal varies widely. Sarkar and Donn (70) recently published a survey of neonatal withdrawal treatment. They found inconsistent policies, scale utilization, and treatment regimens between institutions and individual physicians. These results reflect similar findings of earlier studies and reemphasize the disparity between the published evidence/recommendations supporting the use of withdrawal scoring and current clinical practice for neonatal withdrawal treatment.

As mentioned, neonatal assessment tools for withdrawal continue to be applied to infants and children beyond the newborn period despite the lack of validation for use in this age range. Reflecting an increase in the use of sedatives and analgesics for sedation in neonates requiring mechanical ventilation and invasive interventions after birth in the NICU, the 2012 AAP recommendations included a section on acquired opioid and benzodiazepine dependency (69). They emphasized the challenges of management of opioid and benzodiazepine withdrawal due to overlap in symptomatology when both classes of medications are being administered concurrently, and a paucity of data in the neonatal population. Their recommendations for prevention and management in the neonate exposed to opioids and benzodiazepines after birth include establishing a threshold for cumulative opioid and benzodiazepine exposure to anticipate the need for a weaning protocol (69). Careful continuing clinical assessment is recommended as the basis for weaning, and they determine that 80% of neonates can be successfully weaned from methadone in 5–10 days. With regards to benzodiazepines, intravenous benzodiazepines can be converted to oral lorazepam, and the time for weaning is likely proportional to the duration of exposure to intravenous benzodiazepines. Finally, the AAP study section advises that there is no evidence to support the initiation of clonidine, chloral hydrate, or continuous intravenous naloxone during therapy with continuous opioid infusions to decrease the severity or likelihood of withdrawal (69).

Over the last decade, we have seen the development and validation of new assessment tools for withdrawal in infants and children in the PICU setting. In 2004, Franck et al. (71) investigated the use of an adapted neonatal assessment tool to older children, the "Opioid and Benzodiazepine Withdrawal Score (OBWS)," which provided preliminary data on the use of a withdrawal assessment tool targeted for children in the ICU setting. Their group then went on to develop an assessment tool utilizing 19 symptoms of withdrawal adapted from the OBWS, the Withdrawal Assessment Tool-Version 1 (WAT-1). The WAT-1 assessment consisted of four components: (a) a review of the patient's record for the past 12 hours, (b) direct observation of the patient for 2 minutes, (c) patient assessment during a progressive stimulated exam routinely performed to assess level of consciousness at the beginning of each 12-hour shift, and (d) assessment of poststimulus recovery (8,72). Studies demonstrated a strong correlation between WAT-1 scores and nurses' clinical judgment of withdrawal symptoms, in addition to predictive validity suggested by correlations with cumulative opioid exposure before weaning, days of weaning, and length of therapy. They followed this with a study of the WAT-1's generalizability and validity in children initially supported on mechanical ventilation and confirmed that the tool has good psychometric properties, excellent feasibility, and is a generalizable when used to evaluate clinically relevant withdrawal in the PICU setting (73). Children with WAT-1 scores ≥3 were more likely to have higher total cumulative opioid exposure prior to weaning, longer duration of opioid therapy before weaning, and longer duration of weaning when compared to children with WAT-1 scores <3 (73). The WAT-1 has been an extremely useful and feasible tool for assessing clinically relevant withdrawal in the PICU.

The Sophia Observation withdrawal Symptoms scale (SOS) was developed in 2009 as a result of studying co-occurrences of withdrawal symptoms in critically ill children, with a goal of identifying the signs and symptoms that are essential for a valid withdrawal assessment tool (74) (Table 14.11). In a follow-up study, it was determined that the SOS and WAT-1 have similar sensitivity and specificity, although the SOS may be a better tool for benzodiazepine withdrawal, as it includes the benzodiazepine-specific withdrawal symptoms of grimacing, inconsolable crying, and hallucinations (75). The high negative predictive value was contrasted by the low positive predictive value, which was attributed to overlap between withdrawal symptoms and symptoms of pain, distress, and delirium.

TABLE 14.11

OPIOID AND BENZODIAZEPINE TAPERING GUIDELINES

If opioids or benzodiazepines have been in use for 3–5 d, consider the following:
1. Initiate withdrawal assessment tool every 4–6 h and continue for 1–2 d after cessation of all opioids/sedatives.
2. Reduce opioid/benzodiazepine administration by 20% of pre taper dose every day.
3. If withdrawal symptoms develop, stop weaning for 24 h.
4. If withdrawal symptoms/scores do not improve or worsen:
   a. Increase opioid/benzodiazepine to previous dose.
   b. Consider adding clonidine, especially if symptoms do not improve.
   c. Consult pain service.

If opioids or benzodiazepines in use >10 d, consider the following options:
1. Follow above guidelines.
2. Reduce opioid/benzodiazepine slowly. Perform a reduction of 10% of pretapered dose every day. If patient is on multiple agents, alternate between agents for reduction, effectively reducing each agent every other day.
3. If withdrawal symptoms develop, stop weaning for 24 h.
4. If withdrawal symptoms/scores do not improve or worsen:
   a. Increase last agent weaned to previous dose.
   b. Add or increase clonidine.
   c. Consult pain service.

Adapted from Franck LS, Naughton I, Winter I. Opioid and benzodiazepine withdrawal symptoms in paediatric intensive care patients. *Intensive Crit Care Nurs* 2004; 20:344–51.

Weaning Strategies in Infants and Children with Critical Illness

Tolerance and physical dependence are the consequence of duration and quantity of opioids and sedatives utilized in the ICU. As discussed earlier, tolerance will develop following opioid and benzodiazepine use to some degree following 3–5 days of usage. When the risk for withdrawal symptoms is increased, it is recommended to wean patients from their opioids and sedatives rather than abruptly stopping therapy (76). We believe that this is a more appropriate clinical strategy than one designed to treat the symptoms of withdrawal and is akin to the therapeutic strategy used in weaning patients from other drugs (e.g., steroids) where abrupt cessation can be catastrophic. Shorter intervals of exposure facilitate more aggressive weaning strategies, while duration of exposure for >10 days is a more cautious weaning strategy (Tables 14.11 and 14.12).

To simplify the weaning process, we make every effort to convert the patient from intravenous to oral therapy and from continuous infusions to intermittent bolus therapy. This makes the care of the patient significantly easier and allows for the final tapering and weaning to be accomplished in an outpatient setting. In most cases, the same opioid can be used in weaning that was used therapeutically. For practical reasons though, it may be necessary to change from one opioid to another because of ease of administration, duration of action, and ability to taper the dose.

On changing from one opioid to another, equianalgesic dosing is mandatory. Additionally, in order to avoid over- or underdosing when converting from one drug to another, we recommend being conservative and titrating the dosage downward to achieve the desired clinical effect. Furthermore, the calculated conversion should be given for 24–48 hours before any attempt at weaning is made. Once this is accomplished, we administer the drugs on a 6-hour (morphine) or 12-hour (methadone) around-the-clock basis and weaning is begun. The patient's drug regimen is decreased by 10%–20% of the original total opioid dose a day. When the lowest doses are reached, usually in 5–7 days, the interval of drug dosing is increased from every 6 hours to every 8 or 12 hours, to once a day. Therapy is then stopped completely. We believe

that this schedule should be strictly adhered to. If symptoms of withdrawal develop, we treat these symptoms with clonidine 2–4 mg/kg every 4–6 hours on an as-needed basis. The α_2 adrenergic agents prevent or mitigate the occurrence of drug withdrawal syndrome symptomatology regardless of the drug causing addiction or dependence. We have used clonidine and dexmedetomidine in treating infants born to drug-addicted mothers as well as in patients who have become opioid dependent secondary to pain and sedation therapy. There is some evidence to support the use of dexmedetomidine to prevent withdrawal symptoms in patients dependent on opioids and sedatives (77,78). We suspect that this will become an important weapon in our arsenal in the future.

SLEEP IN THE PICU

Sleep and the restorative effects of normal sleep are essential in all humans. A variety of factors prevent sleep in critically ill patients, and these sleep disturbances may have the most profound effect on children who are undergoing active neurocognitive development (Fig. 14.5) (4). Aside from the direct effects on the brain, normal sleep–wake homeostasis is important for multiple organ systems, including the cardiac, respiratory, GI, and immunologic systems, in addition to playing a major role in thermoregulation and prevention of the catabolic state—integral when a child is recovering from critical illness (31). Patients in the ICU are subjected to constant light, noise, rounds, visitors, anxious family, pain, procedures, blood sampling, and more often than not, an endotracheal tube. Children are frightened by the machines in the ICU and may misinterpret staff conversations heard from around the bed as well. Furthermore, many of the drugs that produce sedation interfere with normal sleep architecture and thereby paradoxically increase the need for more sedation (4,31). Table 14.13 presents several common ICU medications and their effects on sleep parameters (31).

A recent systematic review of the literature surrounding sleep in the PICU demonstrated only nine studies, four from the same randomized controlled trial, which have investigated the quality of sleep in critically ill children. Only half of these

TABLE 14.12

CONVERSION STRATEGIES FOR WEANING FROM COMMONLY USED SEDATIVES AND ANALGESICS

Benzodiazepines (IV midazolam to oral lorazepam):
1. Calculate the total daily dose being provided to the patient by infusion and any additional daily "as-needed doses" of midazolam.
2. Calculate the total midazolam dose (in mg) and divide by 8. Result will be the milligrams of lorazepam to be given orally per day. This lorazepam amount should be divided and dosed every 4–6 h.
3. After the second oral lorazepam dose, reduce the midazolam infusion by 50%.
4. After the third oral lorazepam dose, reduce the midazolam infusion by 50%.
5. After the fourth lorazepam dose, discontinue IV midazolam.

Opioid (IV fentanyl to oral methadone):
1. Calculate the total daily dose being provided to the patient by infusion and any additional daily "as-needed doses" of fentanyl.
2. Calculate the total fentanyl dose (in mg). Because of the off-setting effects of bioavailability, potency, and half-life, an equivalent oral methadone dose can be administered. Divide this methadone dose every 12 h.
3. After the second oral methadone dose, reduce the fentanyl infusion by 50%.
4. After the third oral methadone dose, reduce the fentanyl infusion by 50%.
5. After the fourth oral methadone dose, discontinue IV fentanyl.
6. Over next 24 h, rescue doses of morphine (0.05 mg/kg IV or oral) are provided for withdrawal symptoms. The total morphine dose administered is calculated and added to the total daily methadone dose. This new total daily methadone dose is divided and dosed every 12 h for the next day.
7. Repeat step 6 until a stable methadone dose is achieved.

Barbiturate (IV pentobarbital to oral phenobarbital):
1. Stop the pentobarbital infusion and convert to IV phenobarbital as follows:

Pentobarbital Infusion (mg/kg/h)	Phenobarbital loading dose (mg/kg)
1–2	8
2–3	15
3–4	20

2. Six hours later, administer half of the loading dose of phenobarbital IV over 1 h.
3. Six hours later, infuse second half of phenobarbital loading dose over 1 h.
4. Six hours later, administer first maintenance phenobarbital dose (1/3 of initial loading dose) IV and repeat every 12 h.
5. If evidence of withdrawal is observed during this conversion, provide additional maintenance dose of phenobarbital IV and continue IV dosing every 12 h.
6. After a 24-h period of maintenance IV phenobarbital, with minimal or no withdrawal symptoms, and no additional doses of phenobarbital, change to oral phenobarbital at same 12-h interval.
7. Maintenance oral phenobarbital dosing is then weaned 10%–20% every week from the preweaning dosage.

Adapted from Tobias JD. Tolerance, withdrawal, and physical dependency after long-term sedation and analgesia of children in the pediatric intensive care unit. *Crit Care Med* 2000;28:2122–32.

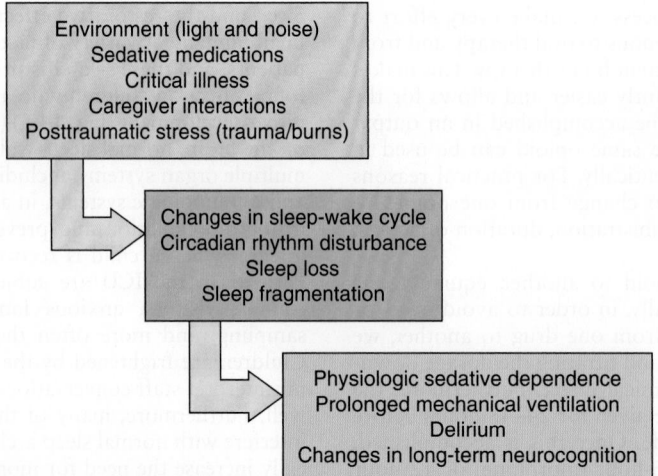

FIGURE 14.5. Proposed causal pathway for changes in sleep behavior as a modulator of outcomes in critically ill children. (From Kudchadkar SR, Aljohani OA, Punjabi NM. Sleep of critically ill children in the pediatric intensive care unit: A systematic review. *Sleep Med Rev* 2014;18(2):103–10.)

TABLE 14.13

COMMON ICU MEDICATIONS AND THEIR EFFECT ON SLEEP

■ MEDICATION	■ EFFECT ON SLEEP	■ POSSIBLE MECHANISM
Sedative/Hypnotic		
Benzodiazepines	↑TST, ↓SWS, ↓REM, ↓W	GABA (type A) receptor stimulation
Propofol	↑TST, ↓W, ↓SL	GABA (type A) receptor stimulation
Dexmedetomidine	↑SWS, ↓SL, ↓REM	α_2 agonist
Analgesics		
Opioids	↑W, ↓TST, ↓SWS, ↓REM	μ receptor stimulation
NSAIDs	↓TST, ↓SE	Prostaglandin synthesis inhibition
Antipsychotics		
Typical (haloperidol)	↑SE, ↓W, ↓SL	
Atypical (olanzapine)	↑SE, ↑TST, ↑SWS, ↓W, ↓SL	
Antidepressants		
Tricyclics	↑TST, ↓W, ↓REM	Anticholinergic and α_1 receptor stimulation
SSRI	↑W, ↓TST, ↓SE, ↓REM	Increased serotonin activity
Cardiovascular Agents		
Epinephrine/norepinephrine	↓SWS, ↓REM	α_1 receptor stimulation
Dopamine	Insomnia, ↓SWS, ↓REM	D_2 receptor stimulation
β blockers	Insomnia, nightmares, ↓REM	CNS β blockade
Clonidine	↓REM	Central α_2 agonist
Amiodarone	Nightmares	Unknown
Anticonvulsants		
Barbiturates	↑TST, ↓W, ↓SL, ↓REM	
Carbamazepines	↑SWS, ↓SL, ↓REM	
Gabapentin	↑TST, ↑REM, ↑SWS, ↓W	
Phenytoin	↑Sleep fragmentation	
Valproic acid	↑TST, ↓W	
Other		
Steroids	Insomnia, ↓REM, ↓SWS	Reduced melatonin secretion
Aminophylline	↑W, ↓TST, ↓REM, ↓SE, ↓SWS	CNS stimulation/activity
Quinolones	Insomnia	GABA type A inhibitor

NSAIDs, nonsteroidal anti-inflammatory drugs; SSRI, selective serotonin reuptake inhibitor; TST, total sleep time; SWS, slow-wave sleep; SE, sleep efficiency; REM, rapid eye movement; W, wakefulness; SL, sleep latency.
From Kudchadkar S, Sterni L, Yaster M, et al. Sleep in the intensive care unit. *Contemp Crit Care* 2009;7:1–12.

utilized polysomnography, the gold standard for evaluating sleep architecture, while the rest utilized subjective observational tools. These studies universally demonstrated significant sleep fragmentation and decreases in slow-wave sleep, the most restorative aspect of sleep and an integral component of cognitive maturation during childhood and adolescence. Our recent work has shown that sleep promotion is not a priority in the PICU culture, despite increasing evidence in the adult literature that sleep loss and fragmentation in the critically ill increase the risk of ICU delirium, an important risk factor for increased morbidity and mortality (7). Although there are proven, inexpensive, and noninvasive modalities such as eye masks, earplugs, lighting protocols, and noise reduction protocols to decrease sleep interruptions during nighttime hours, such methods are rarely used in adult and pediatric ICU settings (7).

Light levels are central to maintaining circadian rhythmicity during a child's critical illness. Exposure to natural light during the daytime and minimizing nighttime light exposure are integral for hormonal regulation to optimize the sleep–wake cycle, specifically playing a role in melatonin release. Few PICUs employ noise reduction strategies to target WHO-recommended levels (<30 dBA Leq for day and nighttime), and the current literature demonstrates that ICU noise levels are often >50 dBA regardless of the time of day, with several intermittent peaks to >80 dBA (79). It is clear that the complex interplay between sedation and sleep warrants further research.

DELIRIUM IN THE PICU

Pediatric delirium is becoming increasingly recognized as an important diagnostic entity in the care and management of critically ill children. Delirium is characterized by an acute onset and fluctuating course with reduced awareness, impairments in attention, and changes in cognition (memory deficits, language disturbances, hallucinations), all in combination with a pathophysiologic cause (80). The causes of delirium are summarized by the I WATCH DEATH acronym (**Fig. 14.6**) (81). There are three subtypes: hypoactive, hyperactive, and mixed delirium. Unfortunately, child psychiatrists are often only consulted in cases of obvious hyperactive delirium, whereas cases of hypoactive and mixed delirium may be missed owing to a lack of active surveillance. As demonstrated by a large body of literature in the adult ICU, delirium is associated with worse functional outcomes, increased hospital length of stay, morbidity, and mortality (82).

ICU delirium is caused by a combination of factors including the patient's premorbid condition (attitude toward illness, age, and defense mechanisms), psychological disturbances, the environment (frightening atmosphere, unusual and disturbing sounds, lack of windows, deprivation of day–night cycles, etc.), and sleep loss and fragmentation. The primary risk factors for adults and children are very similar, with the most common pediatric risk factors being infection, drug withdrawal, and young age. In addition, children who are receiving

Differential Diagnosis for Delirium: I WATCH DEATH

Infectious

Withdrawal (opioids, barbiturates, benzodiazepines)

Acute metabolic disorder (electrolyte abnormalities, renal failure)

Trauma

CNS pathology

Hypoxia

Deficiencies (thiamine, folate, Vitamin B12)

Endocrinopathies

Acute vascular (vasculitis, shock)

Toxins

Heavy metals

FIGURE 14.6. Differential diagnosis for delirium: I WATCH DEATH.

polypharmacy for sedation and analgesia while being mechanically ventilated are also at increased risk. Delirium in the ICU is usually multifactorial, and benzodiazepines have been shown to be a strong independent risk factor (36).

Diagnosis of delirium in critically ill children can be particularly challenging due to different levels of development as well as effects of critical illness and interventions (i.e., the endotracheal tube) on the ability to communicate with family and care providers. Nevertheless, the consequences of undiagnosed delirium can be catastrophic on several levels. Hyperactive delirium can compromise the safety of the patient due to autoextubation and removal of lines. Delirium causes neurometabolic stress that is detrimental to recovery from critical illness. In addition to being a traumatic experience for family members witnessing their child with delirium, 33% of children who experience unrecognized delirium will go on to have

posttraumatic stress syndrome (83). Children with delirium in the hospital setting are often misdiagnosed owing to a lack of diagnostic criteria that are updated for the pediatric population. The importance of effective and efficient bedside testing, direct involvement of PICU care providers, and longitudinal assessment are critical to timely diagnosis and treatment of delirium in critically ill children.

Although knowledge about the importance of delirium diagnosis and treatment in the PICU continues to grow, instruments for delirium assessment have been validated and described in the literature. The pediatric Confusion Assessment Method-ICU (pCAM-ICU) was adapted from the adult version (CAM-ICU) for children >5 years of age, and can be used for children who are intubated (**Fig. 14.7**) (84). The visual attention component of the CAM-ICU was modified with images adapted to children, and the logical thinking questions were modified to be developmentally appropriate. One of the hallmarks of this and other tools is the importance of consistent and streamlined sedation assessment. Although the pCAM-ICU is a useful instrument for older children, there remains a gap in delirium assessment tools for perhaps some of the most challenging patients to diagnose—infants and toddlers. Schieveld and colleagues have proposed a diagnostic algorithm that incorporates the RASS for sedation assessment followed by rating with the Paediatric Anesthesia Emergence Delirium Scale (PAED) (**Fig. 14.8**) (80a,85). Combined with the opinion of the caregiver, these assessments lead to decisions about management, including identification of somatic and pharmacologic etiologies, ruling out reasons for discomfort, and evaluation of patient from a psychosocial standpoint.

The single most important component of delirium treatment in all patients is to first identify the underlying cause. Once this has been addressed, delirium treatment in children is composed of two interventions: nonpharmacologic environmental

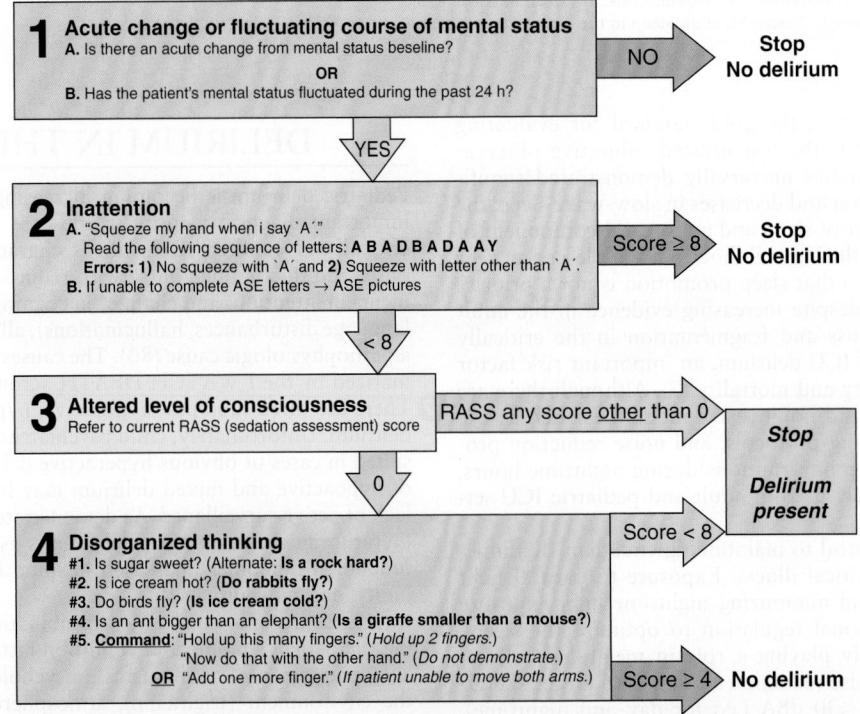

FIGURE 14.7. Pediatric Confusion Assessment Method for the ICU (pCAM-ICU). Positive features 1 and 2 with any positive feature 3 or 4 confirm the diagnosis of delirium. The pCAM-ICU can also be performed with the State Behavioral Scale (SBS). RASS, Richmond Agitation–Sedation Scale. (From Smith HA, Boyd J, Fuchs DC, et al. Diagnosing delirium in critically ill children: Validity and reliability of the Pediatric Confusion Assessment Method for the Intensive Care Unit. *Crit Care Med* 2011;39:150–7.)

1. The child makes eye contact with the caregiver.
2. The child's actions are purposeful.
3. The child is aware of his/her surroundings.
4. The child is restless.
5. The child is inconsolable.

Items 1, 2, and 3 are reversed scored as follows: 4 = not at all, 3 = just a little, 2 = quite a bit, 1 = very much, 0 = extremely. Items 4 and 5 are scored as follows: 0 = not at all, 1 = just a little, 2 = quite a bit, 3 = very much, 4 = extremely. The scores of each item were summed to obtain a total Pediatric Anesthesia Emergence Delirium (PAED) scale score. The degree of emergence delirium increased deirecly with the total score.

FIGURE 14.8. The Pediatric Anesthesia Emergence Delirium Scale. (From Sikich N, Lerman J. Development and psychometric evaluation of the pediatric anesthesia emergence delirium scale. *Anesthesiology* 2004;100:1138–45.)

(psychosocial) interventions and pharmacologic interventions (antipsychotics). Nonpharmacologic interventions described in the adult literature include sleep hygiene promotion with exposure to sunlight during the daytime and noise reduction and light minimization at night, increasing mobility, orienting the patient to time of day and location regularly, and stimulating activities during the daytime. These can all be easily adapted to children in the PICU. Pharmacologic treatment includes haloperidol and atypical antipsychotics, and should be introduced with the close consultation of a pediatric neuropsychiatrist, given the complexity of the critically ill patient and concomitant medications (34,86).

It must be emphasized that one of the most difficult scenarios for the pediatric intensivist is differentiating withdrawal from delirium. The courses can be very similar, and a prolonged and unusually severe presentation of withdrawal, without correlated medications changes, should present a high index of suspicion for delirium. Once again, the key is addressing the underlying cause of agitation for which withdrawal or delirium may be on the differential.

CONCLUSIONS AND FUTURE DIRECTIONS

We have attempted to consolidate in a comprehensive manner much of the available information on pain and sedation management in critically ill children. All children, even the newborn and critically ill require analgesia for pain and for painful procedures. Unrelieved pain interferes with sleep, leads to fatigue and a sense of helplessness, and may result in increased morbidity and/or mortality. Sedation practices in critically ill patients have been shown to alter duration of mechanical ventilation, length of hospital stay, and incidence of delirium. Understanding the complex interplay between sedation, analgesia, and sleep is imperative for the pediatric intensivist to optimize a child's care during critical illness. The driving force and ultimate goal of comfort must be emphasized to improve the quality of the lives of these children. If these issues are left unaddressed, they undermine part of our fundamental humanity and role as healers and physicians.

References

1. Schechter NL, Berde CB, Yaster M. *Pain in Infants, Children, and Adolescents.* 2nd ed. Philadelphia, PA: Lippincott Williams & Wilkins, 2003.
2. Lee SJ, Ralston HJ, Drey EA, et al. Fetal pain: A systematic multidisciplinary review of the evidence. *JAMA* 2005;294:947–54.
3. Taddio A, Katz J, Ilersich AL, et al. Effect of neonatal circumcision on pain response during subsequent routine vaccination. *Lancet* 1997;349:599–603.
4. Kudchadkar SR, Yaster M, Punjabi NM. Sedation, Sleep Promotion, and Delirium Screening Practices in the Care of Mechanically Ventilated Children: A wake-up call for the pediatric critical care community. *Crit Care Med* 2014:42(7):1592–600.
5. Spagrud LJ, Piira T, Von Baeyer CL. Children's self-report of pain intensity. *Am J Nurs* 2003;103:62–4.
6. Franck LS, Miaskowski C. Measurement of neonatal responses to painful stimuli: A research review. *J Pain Symptom Manage* 1997; 14:343–78.
7. Kudchadkar SR, Yaster M, Punjabi NM. Sedation, Sleep Promotion, and Delirium Screening Practices in the Care of Mechanically Ventilated Children: A wake-up call for the pediatric critical care community. *Critical Care Medicine,* July 2014 42(7):1592–600.
8. Curley MA, Harris SK, Fraser KA, et al. State Behavioral Scale: A sedation assessment instrument for infants and young children supported on mechanical ventilation. *Pediatr Crit Care Med* 2006;7:107–14.
9. Ista E, van Dijk M, Tibboel D, et al. Assessment of sedation levels in pediatric intensive care patients can be improved by using the COMFORT "behavior" scale. *Pediatr Crit Care Med* 2005;6:58–63.
10. Ambuel B, Hamlett KW, Marx CM, et al. Assessing distress in pediatric intensive care environments: The COMFORT Scale. *J Pediatr Psychol* 1992;17:95–109.
11. Sessler CN, Gosnell MS, Grap MJ, et al. The Richmond Agitation-Sedation Scale: Validity and reliability in adult intensive care unit patients. *Am J Respir Crit Care Med* 2002;166:1338–44.
12. Ely EW, Truman B, Shintani A, et al. Monitoring sedation status over time in ICU patients: Reliability and validity of the Richmond Agitation-Sedation Scale (RASS). *JAMA* 2003;289:2983–91.
13. Plum F, Posner JB. *The Diagnosis of Stupor and Coma.* 3rd ed. Philadelphia, PA: F. A. Davis, 1980.
14. Riker RR, Fraser GL, Simmons LE, et al. Validating the Sedation-Agitation Scale with the bispectral index and visual analog scale in adult ICU patients after cardiac surgery. *Intensive Care Med* 2001;27:853–8.
15. Ramsay MA. Measuring level of sedation in the intensive care unit. *JAMA* 2000;284:441–2.
16. Kim HS, Oh AY, Kim CS, et al. Correlation of bispectral index with end-tidal sevoflurane concentration and age in infants and children. *Br J Anaesth* 2005;95:362–6.
17. Malviya S, Voepel-Lewis T, Tait AR, et al. Effect of age and sedative agent on the accuracy of bispectral index in detecting depth of sedation in children. *Pediatrics* 2007;120:e461–70.
18. Barr J, Fraser GL, Puntillo K, et al. Clinical practice guidelines for the management of pain, agitation, and delirium in adult patients in the intensive care unit. *Crit Care Med* 2013;41:263–306.
19. Birmingham PK, Tobin MJ, Henthorn TK, et al. Twenty-four-hour pharmacokinetics of rectal acetaminophen in children: An old drug with new recommendations. *Anesthesiology* 1997;87: 244–52.
20. Zuppa AF, Hammer GB, Barrett JS, et al. Safety and population pharmacokinetic analysis of intravenous acetaminophen in neonates, infants, children, and adolescents with pain or fever. *J Pediatr pharmacol Ther* 2011;16:246–61.
21. Raynor K, Kong H, Chen Y, et al. Pharmacological characterization of the cloned kappa-, delta-, and mu-opioid receptors. *Mol Pharmacol* 1994;45:330–4.
22. Maxwell LG, Kaufmann SC, Bitzer S, et al. The effects of a small-dose naloxone infusion on opioid-induced side effects and analgesia in children and adolescents treated with intravenous patient-controlled analgesia: A double-blind, prospective, randomized, controlled study. *Anesth Analg* 2005;100:953–8.
23. Glass PS, Gan TJ, Howell S. A review of the pharmacokinetics and pharmacodynamics of remifentanil. *Anesth Analg* 1999;89: S7–14.

24. Hughes MA, Glass PS, Jacobs JR. Context-sensitive half-time in multicompartment pharmacokinetic models for intravenous anesthetic drugs. *Anesthesiology* 1992;76:334–41.

25. Santeiro ML, Christie J, Stromquist C, et al. Pharmacokinetics of continuous infusion fentanyl in newborns. *J Perinatol* 1997;17:135–9.

26. Koehntop DE, Rodman JH. Fentanyl pharmacokinetics in patients undergoing renal transplantation. *Pharmacotherapy* 1997;17:746–52.

27. Monitto CL, Greenberg RS, Kost-Byerly S, et al. The safety and efficacy of parent-/nurse-controlled analgesia in patients less than six years of age. *Anesth Analg* 2000;91:573–9.

28. Monitto CL, Kost-Byerly S, White E, et al. The optimal dose of prophylactic intravenous naloxone in ameliorating opioid-induced side effects in children receiving intravenous patient-controlled analgesia morphine for moderate to severe pain: A dose finding study. *Anesth Analg* 2011;113:834–42.

29. Weinberg GL, Ripper R, Murphy P, et al. Lipid infusion accelerates removal of bupivacaine and recovery from bupivacaine toxicity in the isolated rat heart. *Reg Anesth Pain Med* 2006;31:296–303.

30. Aram L, Krane EJ, Kozloski LJ, et al. Tunneled epidural catheters for prolonged analgesia in pediatric patients. *Anesth Analg* 2001;92:1432–8.

31. Kudchadkar S, Sterni L, Yaster M, et al. Sleep in the intensive care unit. *Contemp Crit Care* 2009;7:1–12.

32. Schieveld JN, Lousberg R, Berghmans E, et al. Pediatric illness severity measures predict delirium in a pediatric intensive care unit. *Crit Care Med* 2008;36:1933–6.

33. Pandharipande P, Ely EW. Sedative and analgesic medications: Risk factors for delirium and sleep disturbances in the critically ill. *Crit Care Clin* 2006;22:313–27.

34. Schieveld JN, Leroy PL, van Os J, et al. Pediatric delirium in critical illness: Phenomenology, clinical correlates and treatment response in 40 cases in the pediatric intensive care unit. *Intensive Care Med* 2007;33:1033–40.

35. Stoddard FJ, Ronfeldt H, Kagan J, et al. Young burned children: The course of acute stress and physiological and behavioral responses. *Am J Psychiatry* 2006;163:1084–90.

36. Pandharipande P, Shintani A, Peterson J, et al. Lorazepam is an independent risk factor for transitioning to delirium in intensive care unit patients. *Anesthesiology* 2006;104:21–6.

37. Ji F, Li Z, Nguyen H, et al. Perioperative dexmedetomidine improves outcomes of cardiac surgery. *Circulation* 2013;127:1576–84.

38. Pandharipande PP, Pun BT, Herr DL, et al. Effect of sedation with dexmedetomidine vs lorazepam on acute brain dysfunction in mechanically ventilated patients: The MENDS randomized controlled trial. *JAMA* 2007;298:2644–53.

39. Yaster M, Nichols DG, Deshpande JK, et al. Midazolam-fentanyl intravenous sedation in children: Case report of respiratory arrest. *Pediatrics* 1990;86:463–7.

40. Silvasi DL, Rosen DA, Rosen KR. Continuous intravenous midazolam infusion for sedation in the pediatric intensive care unit. *Anesth Analg* 1988;67:286–8.

41. Lugo RA, Chester EA, Cash J, et al. A cost analysis of enterally administered lorazepam in the pediatric intensive care unit. *Crit Care Med* 1999;27:417–21.

42. Dominguez KD, Crowley MR, Coleman DM, et al. Withdrawal from lorazepam in critically ill children. *Ann Pharmacother* 2006;40:1035–9.

43. Jacobi J, Fraser GL, Coursin DB, et al. Clinical practice guidelines for the sustained use of sedatives and analgesics in the critically ill adult. *Crit Care Med* 2002;30:119–41.

44. Schuttler J, Ihmsen H. Population pharmacokinetics of propofol: A multicenter study. *Anesthesiology* 2000;92:727–38.

45. Cray SH, Robinson BH, Cox PN. Lactic acidemia and bradyarrhythmia in a child sedated with propofol. *Crit Care Med* 1998;26:2087–92.

46. Bray RJ. The propofol infusion syndrome in infants and children: Can we predict the risk? *Curr Opin Anaesthesiol* 2002;15:339–42.

47. Orsini J, Nadkarni A, Chen J, et al. Propofol infusion syndrome: Case report and literature review. *Am J Health Syst Pharm* 2009;66:908–15.

48. Vasile B, Rasulo F, Candiani A, et al. The pathophysiology of propofol infusion syndrome: A simple name for a complex syndrome. *Intensive Care Med* 2003;29:1417–25.

49. Shankar V, Churchwell KB, Deshpande JK. Isoflurane therapy for severe refractory status asthmaticus in children. *Intensive Care Med* 2006;32:927–33.

50. Wheeler DS, Clapp CR, Ponaman ML, et al. Isoflurane therapy for status asthmaticus in children: A case series and protocol. *Pediatr Crit Care Med* 2000;1:55–9.

51. White PF, Way WL, Trevor AJ. Ketamine—Its pharmacology and therapeutic uses. *Anesthesiology* 1982;56:119–36.

52. Hartvig P, Larsson E, Joachimsson PO. Postoperative analgesia and sedation following pediatric cardiac surgery using a constant infusion of ketamine. *J Cardiothorac Vasc Anesth* 1993;7:148–53.

53. Jat KR, Chawla D. Ketamine for management of acute exacerbations of asthma in children. *Cochrane Database Syst Rev* 2012;11:CD009293.

53a. Zeiler FA, Teitelbaum J, West M, Gillman LM. The ketamine effect on intracranial pressure in nontraumatic neurological illness. *Journal of Critical Care.* In press

54. Sanders RD, Maze M. Alpha2-adrenoceptor agonists. *Curr Opin Investig Drugs* 2007;8:25–33.

55. Sallinen J, Link RE, Haapalinna A, et al. Genetic alteration of alpha 2C-adrenoceptor expression in mice: Influence on locomotor, hypothermic, and neurochemical effects of dexmedetomidine, a subtype-nonselective alpha 2-adrenoceptor agonist. *Mol Pharmacol* 1997;51:36–46.

56. Mason KP, Lerman J. Review article: Dexmedetomidine in children: Current knowledge and future applications. *Anesth Analg* 2011;113:1129–42.

57. Sanders RD, Maze M. Alpha 2-agonists and other sedatives and amnestics. In: Evers AS, Maze M, Kharasch ED, eds. *Anesthetic Pharmacology: Basic Principles and Clinical Practice.* 2nd ed. Cambridge, England: Cambridge University Press, 2011:478–92.

58. Belleville JP, Ward DS, Bloor BC, et al. Effects of intravenous dexmedetomidine in humans. I. Sedation, ventilation, and metabolic rate. *Anesthesiology* 1992;77:1125–33.

59. Potts AL, Anderson BJ, Warman GR, et al. Dexmedetomidine pharmacokinetics in pediatric intensive care—A pooled analysis. *Paediatr Anaesth* 2009;19:1119–29.

60. Petroz GC, Sikich N, James M, et al. A phase I, two-center study of the pharmacokinetics and pharmacodynamics of dexmedetomidine in children. *Anesthesiology* 2006;105:1098–110.

61. Wong J, Steil GM, Curtis M, et al. Cardiovascular effects of dexmedetomidine sedation in children. *Anesth Analg* 2012;114:193–9.

62. Mason KP, Zurakowski D, Zgleszewski SE, et al. High dose dexmedetomidine as the sole sedative for pediatric MRI. *Paediatr Anaesth* 2008;18:403–11.

63. Weber MD, Thammasitboon S, Rosen DA. Acute discontinuation syndrome from dexmedetomidine after protracted use in a pediatric patient. *Paediatr Anaesth* 2008;18:87–8.

64. Darnell C, Steiner J, Szmuk P, et al. Withdrawal from multiple sedative agent therapy in an infant: Is dexmedetomidine the cause or the cure? *Pediatr Crit Care Med* 2010;11:e1–3.

65. Tucker EW, Cooke DW, Kudchadkar SR, et al. Dexmedetomidine infusion associated with transient adrenal insufficiency in a pediatric patient: A case report. *Case Rep Pediatr* 2013;2013:207907.

66. Watling SM, Dasta JF. Prolonged paralysis in intensive care unit patients after the use of neuromuscular blocking agents: A review of the literature. *Crit Care Med* 1994;22:884–93.

67. Katz R, Kelly HW, Hsi A. Prospective study on the occurrence of withdrawal in critically ill children who receive fentanyl by continuous infusion. *Crit Care Med* 1994;22:763–7.

68. Anand KJ, Clark AE, Willson DF, et al. Opioid analgesia in mechanically ventilated children: Results from the multicenter measuring opioid tolerance induced by fentanyl study. *Pediatr Crit Care Med* 2013;14:27–36.

69. Hudak ML, Tan RC; Committee on Drugs; Committee on Fetus and Newborn; American Academy of Pediatrics. Neonatal drug withdrawal. *Pediatrics* 2012;129:e540–60.

70. Sarkar S, Donn SM. Management of neonatal abstinence syndrome in neonatal intensive care units: A national survey. *J Perinatol* 2006;26:15–7.

71. Franck LS, Naughton I, Winter I. Opioid and benzodiazepine withdrawal symptoms in paediatric intensive care patients. *Intensive Crit Care Nurs* 2004;20:344–51.

72. Franck LS, Harris SK, Soetenga DJ, et al. The Withdrawal Assessment Tool-1 (WAT-1): An assessment instrument for monitoring opioid and benzodiazepine withdrawal symptoms in pediatric patients. *Pediatr Crit Care Med* 2008;9:573–80.

73. Franck LS, Scoppettuolo LA, Wypij D, et al. Validity and generalizability of the Withdrawal Assessment Tool-1 (WAT-1) for monitoring iatrogenic withdrawal syndrome in pediatric patients. *Pain* 2012;153:142–8.

74. Ista E, van Dijk M, de Hoog M, et al. Construction of the Sophia Observation withdrawal Symptoms-scale (SOS) for critically ill children. *Intensive Care Med* 2009;35:1075–81.

75. Ista E, de Hoog M, Tibboel D, et al. Psychometric Evaluation of the Sophia Observation Withdrawal Symptoms scale in critically ill children. *Pediatr Crit Care Med* 2013;14:761–9.

76. Yaster M, Kost-Byerly S, Berde C, et al. The management of opioid and benzodiazepine dependence in infants, children, and adolescents. *Pediatrics* 1996;98:135–40.

77. Finkel JC, Johnson YJ, Quezado ZM. The use of dexmedetomidine to facilitate acute discontinuation of opioids after cardiac transplantation in children. *Crit Care Med* 2005;33:2110–2.

78. Tobias JD. Dexmedetomidine to treat opioid withdrawal in infants following prolonged sedation in the pediatric ICU. *J Opioid Manag* 2006;2:201–5.

79. Busch-Vishniac IJ, West JE, Barnhill C, et al. Noise levels in Johns Hopkins Hospital. *J Acoust Soc Am* 2005;118:3629–45.

80. Creten C, Van Der Zwaan S, Blankespoor RJ, et al. Pediatric delirium in the pediatric intensive care unit: A systematic review and an update on key issues and research questions. *Minerva Anestesiol* 2011;77:1099–107.

80a. Janssen NJ, Tan EY, Staal M, et al. On the utility of diagnostic instruments for pediatric delirium in critical illness: an evaluation of the Pediatric Anesthesia Emergence Delirium Scale, the Delirium Rating Scale 88, and the Delirium Rating Scale-Revised R-98. *Intensive Care Medicine* 2011;37:1331–7.

81. Wise MG, Rundell JR. *The American Psychiatric Publishing Textbook of Consultation-Liaison Psychiatry: Psychiatry in the Medically Ill*. 2nd ed. Washington, DC: American Psychiatric Publishing, 2002.

82. Inouye SK, Rushing JT, Foreman MD, et al. Does delirium contribute to poor hospital outcomes? A three-site epidemiologic study. *J Gen Intern Med* 1998;13:234–42.

83. Colville G, Kerry S, Pierce C. Children's factual and delusional memories of intensive care. *Am J Respir Crit Care Med* 2008;177:976–82.

84. Smith HA, Boyd J, Fuchs DC, et al. Diagnosing delirium in critically ill children: Validity and reliability of the Pediatric Confusion Assessment Method for the Intensive Care Unit. *Crit Care Med* 2011;39:150–7.

85. Sikich N, Lerman J. Development and psychometric evaluation of the pediatric anesthesia emergence delirium scale. *Anesthesiology* 2004;100:1138–45.

86. Silver GH, Kearney JA, Kutko MC, et al. Infant delirium in pediatric critical care settings. *Am J Psychiatry* 2010;167:1172–7.

CHAPTER 15 ■ ETHICS

GEORGE E. HARDART AND DENIS J. DEVICTOR

KEY POINTS

1 Knowledge of ethical theory is necessary to construct coherent justifications for dilemmas in clinical decision making. Foundational ethical theories include those based on consequences, such as *utilitarianism*, and those based on duties, such as *Kantianism*.

2 Legal considerations provide a general framework for decision making but rarely provide a definitive answer to complex ethical questions. The law typically represents the floor, and not the ceiling, of standards of morality.

3 Informed consent is a process, not an event, and it has four key requirements: competency, disclosure, understanding, and voluntariness.

4 Competency involves the capacity to *understand* the therapy in question, *consider* the risks and benefits, *decide* on a course of action, and *appreciate* the consequences of the choice.

5 The two main standards for *surrogate decision making* are the *substituted judgment standard* (choosing what the patient would have chosen, if still competent) and the *best-interests standard* (choosing what seems to be objectively best for the patient). The former is used for patients who were once competent and who expressed preferences, while the latter is used for patients who have never been competent, including children.

6 Clinicians should refrain from speaking about withdrawal of care. While treatments may be withdrawn, *care is never withdrawn*. Care may be redirected from a focus on cure to a focus on comfort.

7 Distinguishing between treatments that are *ordinary* and those that are *extraordinary* is rarely helpful, as determina-

tion of whether to withdraw a treatment should be made based on the balance of benefits and burdens, as perceived by the patient, rather than on any particular feature of the treatment itself (e.g., ECMO (extracorporeal membrane oxygenation) may be "ordinary" in one context and "extraordinary" in another).

8 While clinicians are generally more comfortable *withholding* a treatment (e.g., tracheal intubation) than *withdrawing* it, better decisions are made if these events are seen as equivalent, for example, allowing patients to receive trials of therapy with the understanding that the treatment may be withdrawn later if it is not sufficiently beneficial.

9 Sedatives and analgesics should be administered to dying patients, even if they hasten the patient's death, as long as they are *titrated* to the level of the patient's distress and are administered with the *intention* of relieving the patient's pain and suffering, not with the intention of causing death.

10 Clinicians should be cautious when judging medical treatments to be futile, as these decisions are rarely based entirely on medical factors and usually involve value judgments. Determinations of futility should only be made in the context of a *carefully defined procedure* that assures due process for the patient and his or her family.

11 *Neuromuscular blocking agents* should never be administered at the end of life to patients who have not been receiving them for therapeutic purposes. When life support is withdrawn from patients who are therapeutically paralyzed, the paralytic effects should generally be allowed to wear off before life support is withdrawn.

Today's practicing pediatric intensivist is likely to face ethically challenging situations with regularity. The climate of the PICU is charged with forces that cause such situations to occur with much greater frequency than in general medical practice. These forces include the availability, power, and cost of life-sustaining technology, the fast pace and inherent uncertainty of treatment decisions, the common occurrence of end-of-life decisions and care, and the subtleties of surrogate decision making for children, particularly as they approach the age where they can begin to decide for themselves.

This chapter begins with an introduction to the history of medical ethics and an overview of the ethical theories that are useful in understanding and framing moral dilemmas, followed by a discussion of informed consent and surrogate decision making. Mastery of these essential concepts is perhaps the most important tool for effectively managing ethically challenging situations. Finally, the chapter includes a comprehensive section on end-of-life care in the PICU. Since one of the most important duties of the pediatric intensivist is to assist patients and families through the dying process, a thorough understanding of this complex issue is required for all who teach and practice pediatric critical care.

THE FOUNDATION OF MEDICAL ETHICS

The terms "ethics" and "morality" are often used interchangeably, but most philosophers draw a subtle distinction between the two. *Morality* consists of social norms of behavior and often varies dramatically between cultures. The discipline of *ethics*, on the other hand, involves the development of philosophic reasons for or against a set of moral judgments. Usually, the latter effort attempts to articulate and justify principles that form the foundation for rules of conduct and decision making in the face of competing moral claims.

Medical ethics is the discipline devoted to the identification, analysis, and resolution of value-based problems that arise in the care of patients. It is a special kind of ethics only insofar as it relates to the peculiar dilemmas that arise in medicine, not because it embodies or appeals to some special moral principles or methodology. The term "bioethics" is often used interchangeably with "medical ethics," although the former has a slightly broader meaning, including ethical problems that arise outside of the area of medicine (e.g., issues surrounding research on animals). In summary, the practice of medical ethics seeks to identify and resolve competing moral claims among patients, their families, healthcare professionals, healthcare institutions, and society at large.

The Development of Medical Ethics

Concern for ethical issues in medicine dates back at least to the time of Hippocrates. Nevertheless, until the middle of the 20th century, little additional thought was given to the unique problems that arise in the context of clinical practice and medical research. The revelations of the Nazi atrocities after World War II led to the reaffirmation of the importance of ethics in medicine and research and were directly responsible for the formulation of codes of ethics pertaining to research on human subjects (e.g., the Nuremberg Code in the late 1940s, followed by the Declaration of Helsinki in 1964).

In the decades following World War II, the development of antibiotics, vaccines, and effective diagnostic therapeutic technologies transformed medicine from a profession that focused on caring to one that focused on curing. The expectations of physicians and patients have grown considerably; yet, medical advances have brought with them ethical dilemmas that increasingly find their way into public and professional consciousness.

Publication of a 1962 *LIFE* magazine article entitled "They Decide Who Lives, Who Dies" presented such an event. The article described the efforts of a committee of ordinary citizens, not physicians, in Seattle who were charged with the task of allocating access to hemodialysis therapy (then a scarce resource) for critically ill patients who would die without it. The committee disbanded itself after it realized that its selection process was influenced by its own middle-class values rather than by an objectively fair allocation procedure. Public—and then Congressional—dismay at the reality of scarce but effective medical technology led to the 1973 passage of the end-stage renal disease program. Under this legislation, the Federal Medicare Program assumed responsibility for anyone in need of chronic dialysis, regardless of socioeconomic status. Like many federal initiatives in the 1960s and 1970s, this program has proven to be far more costly than initially expected and serves as a lasting illustration of the pitfalls inherent with using governmental assurances of payment as a means for solving problems of medical scarcity (1).

The medical profession's attention to these issues was further heightened by a 1973 article in the *New England Journal of Medicine* that described the decision by physicians and parents to withhold treatment from 43 critically ill infants in the neonatal ICU at Yale–New Haven Hospital (2). This account was among the first to bring attention to the fact that medical technology had reached a point at which the decision to end life had to be made deliberately by physicians and families.

Perhaps no event captured public and professional attention to these difficult issues more than the 1976 New Jersey Supreme Court decision on Karen Ann Quinlan. On the night of April 15, 1973, this 21-year-old woman experienced a respiratory arrest that left her in a persistent vegetative state. Her father petitioned the court for authority to be named as her guardian and for permission to discontinue the ventilator. His request was opposed by her doctors, the hospital, and the prosecutors for the local county and the state of New Jersey. The New Jersey Supreme Court ruled that the patient had a constitutional "right to privacy" to be removed from the ventilator if the family, the physicians, and the hospital ethics committee agreed. Despite the prevailing opinion of her doctors, she did not die when removed from the ventilator, but lived for almost another decade. This was the first of many cases that helped to shape our current views about the withdrawal of life-sustaining treatments.

Overview of Ethical Theories

Broadly speaking, two ethical theories—*utilitarianism* and *deontology* (or *Kantianism*)—have dominated Western intellectual tradition. Both theories attempt to provide a set of "first principles" for approaching ethical conflict. More recently, a number of alternative theories—some ancient and some new—have emerged as useful tools for analyzing complex ethical decisions. Perhaps the best known of these has come to be known as *principlism*, but several other theories offer unique and powerful perspectives and will be described in this section.

The Utilitarian and Deontological Theories

English philosophers Jeremy Bentham and John Stuart Mill developed the utilitarian philosophy in the 18th and 19th centuries. *Utilitarianism* is rooted in the thesis that an action or practice is right (when compared to any alternative action or practice) if it leads to the greatest possible balance of good consequences or the least possible balance of bad consequences in the world as a whole. According to this view, moral codes and traditions are designed to promote human welfare by maximizing benefits and minimizing harm.

The other dominant ethical theory, *deontology*, was heavily influenced by the writings of the philosopher Immanuel Kant. According to this approach, consequence is rejected as the first principle; Kant argued that actions should be guided by generalizable moral obligations or duties, regardless of consequences.

The ongoing debate about euthanasia illustrates the differences between these approaches. Utilitarians may argue, for example, that when a terminally ill patient requests to be killed, the consequences of complying with that request are favorable for everyone concerned. The patient's desires are satisfied, the physician can rest assured that the act was in the patient's best interest (as defined by the patient), and even society may benefit by not incurring the expenses associated with a prolonged dying process. Deontologists, on the other hand, feel that the prohibition against killing should stop us from taking the life of another, regardless of the consequences. Under this approach, euthanasia is always wrong, even if we are convinced that carrying it out does not harm anyone's interest. Some deontologists base their beliefs on a religious perspective (the Ten Commandments are a typical list of deontological principles), whereas others derive a set of duties and obligations by theoretical analysis. Even utilitarians often agree that rules have an important place in ethics, if only because of the inherent difficulties involved in predicting the consequences of our actions. To use the euthanasia example again, a deontologist might argue that even though performing euthanasia does not *appear* to harm anyone's interest, the *long-term* consequences of permitting this act might be diminishment of our respect for human life and possible eventual erosion of the core values of the medical profession. This argument would be a reason to oppose euthanasia, even by the utilitarian standard.

Principlism

In reality, few people are pure deontologists or consequentialists. Most of us blend these two perspectives (as well as others) in our reasoning about ethical issues. In the search for practical guidance to moral dilemmas, therefore, leading ethical theorists over the last 30 years have turned instead to a "principles approach" to moral reasoning. For example, in what is widely regarded as a classic textbook on modern medical ethics, Tom Beauchamp and James Childress advocate four principles on which to base ethical analysis: respect for autonomy (self-determination), beneficence (doing good), non-maleficence (avoiding harm), and justice (fair distribution) (3). When faced with a moral dilemma, one's task is to identify the relevant ethical principles that bear on the case, which will suggest a set of rules that are pertinent to the situation. From these rules, one should be able to discern the proper judgment regarding the particular case.

The problem with this approach is that, because more than one principle may have bearing on any given case, conflicting rules and judgments may be the fruit of deliberation. As principlism does not rank the four principles in order of priority, this approach falls short of comprehensively resolving many ethical dilemmas that arise in clinical practice. Nevertheless, a principles approach is often very useful for identifying the most salient ethical issues that arise in challenging clinical scenarios.

Other Ethical Theories

Virtue-based ethics represent perhaps the most ancient medical ethical theory, and they dominated Eastern and Western medical ethics until the 20th century. While now overshadowed by the language of principles, duties, and rights, virtue ethics is reemerging as an important approach to thinking about moral issues in medicine (4). The basic premise of virtue ethics is that the character and motives of moral agents, such as physicians, matter greatly. Fidelity, truthfulness, compassion, justice, temperance, integrity, and fortitude are some of the moral virtues that are highly valued in physicians. Proponents of virtue ethics do not argue that this theory could replace or make unnecessary rules and principles: in a pluralistic society such as ours, minimum expectations must be established, and even the most virtuous person is capable of performing wrong actions. Conversely, a role for virtue in practice is made apparent through the recognition that it is not difficult for doctors to evade a set of rules if they are intent on doing so. Finally, a virtue ethics approach may be particularly valuable when conflicts among principles arise; moral virtues can play a role in guiding the balancing of principles and arriving at morally acceptable resolutions.

Proponents of "case-based reasoning," or casuistic analysis, argue that a principles-based approach is too indeterminate and abstract to be of much help with real-life dilemmas (5). They advocate instead for the use of "paradigmatic cases," that is, real cases about which a consensus currently exists. As new cases arise, they are analyzed in terms of the ways that they are similar to, or different from, the paradigmatic cases, a method referred to as "moral triangulation." For example, since the "Baby Doe" episode in 1984, general agreement exists in medicine, law, and ethics that babies with Down syndrome and correctable surgical anomalies should undergo surgical repair of their conditions and not be allowed to die from them. Similarly, general agreement also prescribes that babies with Trisomy 13 or 18 who have potentially lethal congenital defects need not be offered life-prolonging therapies, but may ethically be treated with only comfort care. When faced with the problem of how to treat a newborn with congenital anomalies intermediate between those of trisomy 21 and 13/18, a proponent of the case-based approach might attempt to address the question by first exploring the ways in which the child is more like an infant with Down syndrome or more like an infant with trisomy 13/18. In combination with such factors as the severity of the defects and the preferences of the family, this approach would attempt to "triangulate" toward the most reasonable solution.

An alternative theory that has arisen from the feminist movement is an approach based on the primacy of "caring" (6). In its more radical form, this perspective minimizes the importance of ethical theory and principles and seeks resolutions to difficult cases that best preserve the relationships involved. As opposed to a principles-based approach, this perspective is less concerned with maintaining internal consistency and the observance of formal rules. When confronted with a case about whether to allow a small child to donate a kidney to a sibling, for example, a proponent of the "caring" approach would ask which of the alternative options would best promote the well-being of the relationships between the family and others involved.

Finally, a perspective that has developed within the fields of literature and the humanities focuses on the value of "narrative (7)." Unlike the terse case histories that tend to be favored in the busy hospital setting, this approach emphasizes the importance of understanding cases in all of their detail and complexity. Rather than attempting to "shrink" cases to their essential elements and then applying a specific "rule" or "principle," the proponent of the narrative approach will insist that only by analyzing cases in all of their richness and texture can we hope to arrive at solutions that are sufficiently nuanced and sophisticated. Indeed, this approach hearkens back to the admonitions of many of the great medical clinicians who emphasized the overriding importance of careful history taking. These giants of medicine would undoubtedly be just as critical of our overreliance on invasive technology and imaging studies as the proponent of narrative is critical of "principles."

Applications and Limitations of Theories

It can be safely stated that no single "correct" ethical theory exists. When subjected to intense analytic scrutiny, all ethical theories have shortcomings and imperfections. The descriptions of the major ethical theories offered in this section are not intended to serve as a menu from which the readers should choose their favorite theory and apply it in their clinical practice. Rather, it is likely that knowledge of all of these ethical theories will enhance moral decision making as it occurs at the bedside. It may be that, in discussions of rationing, utilitarian arguments are most appropriate for framing the issues, whereas in intrafamilial conflicts about treatment choices, it is possible that feminist ethics reasoning will be most helpful in resolving a dilemma. Finally, it should be noted that, more often than not, application of each of these theories to individual cases would ultimately lead to similar moral conclusions; such convergence serves to strengthen our moral judgments.

Ethics and the Law

Physicians generally have one of two attitudes toward the law. Either they claim to be unconcerned about legal precedent and only interested in practicing "good medicine," or they are fearful of making any decision or taking any action without first learning whether it is "legal." Both extreme views could lead to naïve or imprudent decisions about difficult ethical dilemmas in clinical practice.

First, when considering legal precedents in ethical decision making, it is important to keep in mind that no single, monolithic statement can be made about the "law" in most ethical controversies. The body of law that supports the American legal system is actually the product of many factors. For example, legislative mandates or court decisions in one state do not hold as precedent or law in any other state. Superimposed on state law and legislation is the federal system with its own jurisdictions, which can also disagree concerning key points.

Second, while both ethics and the law are concerned with identifying which actions are acceptable within a given society, they remain fundamentally distinct. Acting in accordance with the law is no guarantee that one is acting ethically, as emphasized by the Nuremberg Court in evaluating the actions of the Nazi concentration camp guards. Law, as it relates to morality, usually represents the minimum requirements regarding moral duties and rights for a given society. Law represents the floor, and not the ceiling, for standards about morality.

ESSENTIAL ELEMENTS OF MEDICAL DECISION MAKING

3

Informed Consent

Although the practice of obtaining informed consent is second nature to today's physicians, many view it as a burden imposed by lawyers. Viewed this way, the communication process is reduced to the physician's effort to avoid a lawsuit. A more constructive mindset is that the informed consent process can actually help strengthen and improve the communication in the physician–patient relationship. As noted by Gutheil and colleagues (8):

> Informed consent is not an empty gesture toward liability reduction, but an interaction between physician and patient, a dialogue intended not only to satisfy their legal requirements, but to do more as well. The real clinical opportunity offered by informed consent is that of transforming uncertainty from a threat into the very basis on which an alliance can be formed.

From this perspective, it becomes clear that an understanding and appreciation of the role of informed consent are central to sound and ethical medical practice.

Many people are surprised that the idea that the patient should be the primary source of decision-making power in the physician–patient relationship is a very recent development, at least in historic terms. Dating from the age of Hippocrates until the very recent past, most decisions were the sole prerogative of the physician. This approach to medical care can no longer be justified, however, as it fails to respect the fundamental importance of the patient's values and goals by placing the clinician's value structure ahead of that of the patient. The ascendancy of respect for patient autonomy and the right to self-determination have become paramount only in the last several decades, yet the roots of this transformation are much deeper. The philosophic and ethical basis for self-determination can be found among the medieval and Renaissance thinkers, who so greatly influenced the framers of the American Constitution and Bill of Rights. Philosophers such as John Locke, Edmund Burke, and Immanuel Kant, among others, articulated the intellectual foundation for the notion that it is not the state but the individual who is sovereign. In its modern form, informed consent must satisfy four requirements: competency, disclosure, understanding, and voluntariness.

4

Competency

A competent individual has the capacity to *understand* the therapy in question, *consider* the risks and benefits, *decide* on a course of action, and *appreciate* the consequences of the choice (9). While adults are generally presumed to be legally competent, children are considered incompetent in the United States until the age of 18 or 21, depending on the jurisdiction. In both ethics and law, however, this arbitrary age cutoff is overly simplistic. Two major exceptions deserve mention. "Emancipated minors" are deemed to be competent on the basis of legal definitions, whereas "mature minors" are competent on the basis of a judicial decision in a particular case. For example, many states define emancipated minors as those who are pregnant or a parent, those serving in the armed forces, or

those living independent of guardians. Alternatively, minors who are not emancipated may nevertheless be deemed competent by a judge to make medical decisions on their own, which may occur, for example, when a judge determines that a minor's Jehovah's Witness religious beliefs are sufficiently mature and considered that the patient may legally refuse blood products, despite the wishes of his or her parents or caregivers.

Although physicians implicitly assess their patient's competence during virtually all of their encounters, questions of competence typically arise when the patient's behavior is unusual, when "clearly beneficial" treatment is refused, or when decisions with serious consequences (such as end-of-life decisions) are being made. When faced with such questions, it is sometimes helpful to draw a distinction between competence and decision-making capacity. A thorough evaluation can determine that a patient who was formerly granted the legal presumption of competence has been incapacitated by medical illness or mental disorder and has forfeited his or her decision-making authority. Conversely, it is possible to have decision-making capacity—the ability to understand medical information, reason about risks and benefits, appreciate consequences, and make stable choices—but still be considered legally incompetent. This point is most strikingly displayed in the case of adolescents.

The legal age of majority is an oversimplification of the maturational and developmental process in children. Children as young as 6 or 7 years are often able to have reasoned opinions about certain aspects of their care, and most adolescents have views and perspectives that deserve serious consideration. The fact that parents must give legal consent for medical treatments performed on minor children does not mean that the opinions of the children and adolescents should be considered irrelevant or ignored. In 1995, the Committee on Bioethics of the American Academy of Pediatrics issued a statement that advocated a dramatic broadening of the authority ceded to minor patients in medical decision making (10). In this statement, they recommended that, for older school-aged children (e.g., 9–12 years old), physicians should seek the patient's assent for proposed tests and treatments in developmentally appropriate situations, such as an orthopedic device to manage scoliosis in an 11-year-old. However, they did note that "in situations in which the patient will have to receive medical care despite his or her objection, the patient should be told that fact and should not be deceived." For adolescent patients (e.g., 14–17 years old) the committee encouraged physicians to obtain informed consent for a broad range of tests and treatments provided the patient has decisional capacity and law permits it. They did, however, encourage parental involvement in such cases. These recommendations have proven to be controversial in theory and challenging to implement in practice. It has been argued that these recommendations go too far and that it is ultimately in the best interest of minor patients that parents retain final decision-making authority (11).

Disclosure

The concept of disclosure (of information) has been, and remains, a central component of the doctrine of informed consent. The question of what constitutes "sufficient information" to ensure a truly informed consent has been addressed by the courts. Until recently the accepted practice held physicians to the *professional standard*, which required physicians to disclose only that information which would be customarily disclosed by their colleagues. However, in the pivotal 1972 case of *Canterbury v. Spence*, the Federal Appeals Court in Washington, DC, established the *reasonable person standard*, which holds that the degree of disclosure should be determined by the information that a reasonable person (or reasonable group of persons, such as a jury) would require to make a decision regarding medical therapy.

Understanding

The inclusion of understanding in the definition of informed consent addresses one of the historic concerns about disclosure as the sole determinant of informed consent. One can easily imagine situations in which understanding does not occur despite a *competent* decision maker and full *disclosure* of information. If the physician uses excessive medical jargon or the patient is ignorant of "basic" medical concepts, then understanding is unlikely. Similarly, because of the effects of illness or the stress of an illness in a loved one, a patient or family member may not "hear" what is said, in which case understanding is not achieved. How can the physician ensure that the decision maker fully understands the nature, implications, and extent of the therapy under consideration? The answer is that the physician cannot *guarantee* complete understanding but has an obligation to try to establish an adequate level of understanding for the decision at hand. This shifts the paradigm of informed consent away from a one-sided disclosure of information by the physician to a two-way communication process, whereby the physician and decision maker ask questions of each other and learn about one another. Misconceptions are exposed, pockets of ignorance are addressed, and trust is established. Through this process, understanding is maximized.

Voluntariness

An action is voluntary when it is free from the coercive and manipulative influences of others. Coercive influences are those for which the weight of the influence is derived from a credible threat, such as when revocation of privileges is used to "encourage" prisoners to consent to medical research. Influences may be manipulative if a physician takes advantage of the unequal distribution of information and knowledge in the physician–patient relationship to "nonpersuasively" influence the outcome of a decision. Such influences may be subtle or blatant, ranging from the withholding or de-emphasizing of information that might affect the patient's decision to outright lying in deliberations with patients. However, the obligation to avoid coercion and manipulation does not alleviate the professional obligation to exert *persuasive* influence over patients when one course of action is clearly indicated, through the use of persistent and rational argument (e.g., when a competent patient refuses to undergo an appendectomy for simple appendicitis).

Exceptions to Informed Consent

Several exceptions to informed consent have traditionally been recognized. The first, and least controversial, is the emergency exception, which allows a physician to treat a patient when significant harm is imminent, when the patient is incapable of consenting, and when no surrogate is immediately available.

More controversial is the therapeutic privilege exception. Under this exception, physicians may forgo attempts to obtain informed consent when they believe that the patient will experience more harm than benefit from the disclosure. Recently, the tendency in law and ethics has been to constrain this exception because it assumes that the physician knows what is best for the patient. This assumption violates the general view that patients themselves provide the most reliable information about what is in their best interest; it also ignores a body of empirical evidence that indicates that physicians systematically underestimate the desire of patients to know their diagnosis and to be involved in decision making (12).

The use of placebos is a tempting application of the therapeutic privilege exception that is almost always unjustified. For example, the secret administration of a placebo rather than an active agent to a patient with substance abuse problems may be thought to be justified as being in the patient's best interests in overcoming addiction, but the loss of trust that occurs when the patient realizes that he or she has been tricked almost always leads to more harm than good.

Finally, the "waiver" exception arises when patients choose to relinquish decisional authority to the physician. While the legitimacy of waivers is generally accepted, some do express concern that widespread use of waivers would have a negative effect on the general practice of informed consent.

Proxy Decision Making

Proxy, or surrogate, decision makers must make medical decisions for patients who are incompetent. The justification for proxy decisions depends on whether the patient was formerly competent or never competent. For formerly competent patients, decisions are based on the principle of respect for autonomy, just as for competent patients. However, in the case of never-competent patients who have, therefore, never been autonomous decision makers, decisions must be justified through appeal to the principles of beneficence (the provision of benefits) and nonmaleficence (the avoidance of harm) that direct proxies to choose the course that is "best" for the patient.

The Substituted Judgment Standard

The formulation for decision making when the patient was formerly competent is called *substituted judgment*. Under this approach, proxies are asked to discern the course of action that is most consistent with the patient's long-standing wishes, beliefs, values, and life goals. In other words, an attempt is made to preserve the patient's autonomy by reconstructing, as precisely as possible, his or her subjective beliefs. While this approach is sound in theory, it becomes difficult and imprecise when put into practice. Is the surrogate close enough to the patient to truly reconstruct his or her values and preferences? Did the patient discuss these preferences frankly, or is the surrogate merely imagining what the patient would have wanted? Is the decision partially based on the surrogate's own interests in the outcome of the decision, or solely on the patient's interests?

Despite its shortcomings, however, the substituted judgment standard remains the accepted approach for formerly competent patients. Some have proposed that this approach be abandoned in favor of others that address its shortcomings, such as approaches that provide better approximations of the patient's preferences (e.g., advanced directives) and those that rely on more objective criteria for decisions (e.g., the best-interests standard).

The Best-Interests Standard

If patients have never expressed preferences, beliefs, and values, it naturally follows that they cannot be used as a basis for proxy decision making. Such is the case for never-competent persons, such as young children and mentally retarded adults. In these cases in which subjective information is unavailable, more objective strategies must be utilized to make medical decisions on their behalf. The best-interests standard asks decision makers to perform an analysis of the benefits and burdens of a medical situation and arrive at the decision that maximizes the benefit-to-burden ratio for the patient. This standard, while being the age-old modus operandi for parental decision making, also faces many hurdles in application. While in its ideal state it is an objective criterion, in practice it is open to value judgments on many levels. The personal preferences of the decision maker, which theoretically should not be considered in the benefit-versus-burden analysis, may enter into the decision about whether the life is "meaningful" or is "worth living." Additionally, the "social worth" of the patient and the burdens of the patient on the family and society may slip into the benefit-versus-burden analysis.

Although some believe that these challenges in implementation of the best-interests standard are obstacles to overcome, others believe that they are evidence that the best-interests standard is fundamentally flawed. As will be discussed more fully in the section Family Interests in Medical Decision Making, it may be that the best-interests standard fails to properly account for the role of the parent in medical decision making for children and other never-competent individuals. Ross (13) has argued for a standard of constrained parental autonomy, asserting that beyond a minimum threshold of care obligated for each child, parents should be free to make decisions based on a variety of interests, not just those of the child in question.

Advance Directives

In response to the shortcomings of proxy decision making, advance directives that attempt to preserve the patient's subjective values during times of legal incompetence have been developed. The ideal advance directive would be readily available in emergencies, frequently updated to reflect a person's current preferences and values, broad enough to be useful in a multitude of situations, and specific enough to provide clear guidance in decision making.

Most states now have legislation that recognizes the legality of certain advanced directives. Written and oral instructions, often called "living wills," contain treatment directives to be followed if and when a patient becomes incapable of making treatment decisions. These documents have been criticized as being too ambiguous in many critical decisions, as no one could possibly anticipate every potential occurrence.

The healthcare durable power of attorney has emerged as an increasingly popular and available alternative to living wills. Unlike living wills, which specify treatment decisions in advance, the healthcare proxy establishes a decision-making process. Healthcare proxy laws permit patients to delegate the authority for their medical treatment decisions to a person of their choosing in the event of incapacity. Under these circumstances, many of the theoretical problems with proxy decision making evaporate, but this also is not an ideal solution. Family members often know little about the patient's treatment preferences (14). Further, there is variability regarding how patients expect proxies to approach decisions for them: some expect proxies to strictly follow their treatment preferences, while others prefer that proxies consider family burden when making decisions (15). The Patient Self-Determination Act, passed by Congress in 1991, requires that all Medicare/Medicaid-participating institutions inform patients of their rights to formulate advance directives upon admission.

SPECIAL TOPICS IN MEDICAL DECISION MAKING

Religious Beliefs in the Decision-Making Process

While the courts have acknowledged the virtually unlimited right of competent adults to refuse medical treatment, they have been much more protective of children. The threshold for overriding parents' wishes depends on an objective assessment of the risks to the child. In general, if the circumstances do not involve life-threatening choices or certain risks of substantial harm to the child, the physician is obligated to respect the decisions of the parents, even when the physician strongly disagrees with the choice. In some jurisdictions, for example, parents are permitted the right to refuse standard immunizations for religious reasons.

However, as the threat to the child increases and the benefits of treatment are more certain, actions to override parental choices are not only legally supported, but, in most jurisdictions, required. Numerous court opinions have upheld the notion, first articulated in the 1944 case of *Prince* v. *Massachusetts*, that a parent may make a martyr of himself because of religious convictions, "but he is not free to make a martyr of his child." In numerous decisions since then, courts have upheld the right of physicians to override parental refusal of transfusions or other accepted therapy when a child's life is at risk. Court-ordered blood transfusions for the children of Jehovah's Witness parents have become perhaps the best-known and most frequent example of this type of judicial involvement.

Uncertainty

Physicians (and patients, as well) virtually never make decisions without some degree of uncertainty. Decisions are based on probabilities, intuition, clinical experience, and medical knowledge. Even the most "scientific" of these, medical knowledge, can rarely be said to be certain. The knowledge of medicine is based on information derived from experiments, and these experiments are based on probabilistic estimates of their chances of revealing "truth." In other words, physicians are constantly making decisions based on a less-than-ideal amount of information and cannot predict with certainty the consequences of their decisions. Given that uncertainty is an essential part of decision making for physicians, the degree of uncertainty will vary from decision to decision, as will the magnitude of the consequences of those decisions. Over 50 years ago, Renée Fox (16) identified three sources of uncertainty in physician practice: (a) insufficient mastery of available knowledge, (b) limitations of available knowledge, and (c) physician difficulty in distinguishing personal ignorance from limitations in available knowledge.

With regard to decisions involving life and death in the PICU, uncertainty is frequently high and the consequences extreme. Despite uncertainty, however, decisions must be made, and physicians respond in different ways. While many of their responses are predictable and understandable, one noteworthy tendency is reluctance on the part of physicians to disclose uncertainty to the patient and family and, sometimes, to disregard altogether the uncertainty in the decision-making process. In fact, Fox observed that as physicians moved from theoretical discussions about uncertain decisions to actual clinical encounters, their disregard for any element of uncertainty became highly pervasive. This disregard for uncertainty frequently is translated into certainty about the proper course of action when discussing the situation with the patient and family. While this aura of certainty may have positive effects (maintaining trust in the physician–patient relationship, avoidance of stress within the patient and family, timeliness of decisions, etc.), it has been argued that this "mask of infallibility" also serves to maintain professional control over decision making and to exclude the patient and family from meaningful participation in the decision-making process (17).

Rationing

American society is acutely aware that the financial costs of the US healthcare system are staggering, and this reality is naturally transmitted to clinicians who feel a sense of duty to use healthcare dollars efficiently in treating patients. This pressure is intensified by the prevalence of managed care organizations that routinely track the money that clinicians spend in treating patients and frequently equate good performance with low cost. Ethical issues are raised by the possibility that bedside physicians might "microallocate" resources (i.e., refrain from providing potentially beneficial treatment based on monetary cost or other limitations). Traditionally, physicians have had fiduciary relationships with their patients that obligate them to serve the patient's health interests without compromise. This traditional approach has come under increasing attack as financial pressures on physicians and hospitals have mounted.

In allocating *absolutely* scarce resources, such as ICU beds, physicians have long been responsible for triaging the recipient of the resource, based on need, ability to benefit, or the principle of "first come, first served." On the other hand, a healthcare budget represents a *relatively* scarce resource; if the patient, insurance company, or society was willing to pay the price, then the treatment could be provided. Until recently, physicians have considered it unethical to deny patients any treatment that is only relatively scarce (i.e., to deny a treatment on purely financial grounds). As we increasingly acknowledge that the healthcare budget is not infinite, however, this old dichotomy is breaking down. While clinicians and ethicists have long been exploring ways to ration financial resources, in an open and equitable manner, society and the federal government have now vigorously joined the debate. This new development is not without its critics, who hold that doctors must uncompromisingly make the welfare of their individual patients their primary objective. Critics further argue that, while healthcare costs to the nation are high, resources in this country are plentiful, and it is a fiction to suppose that the money saved through cheaper medical care would be diverted to nobler purposes in society. More likely, those dollars will go toward the profit margin of an institution or toward a societal expenditure with no relationship to healthcare. To quote Marcia Angell (18), "Doctors should continue to care for each patient unstintingly, even while they join with other citizens to devise a more efficient and just health care system."

Family Interests in Medical Decision Making

Surrogate decision makers are usually family members or others with close, intimate relationships to the patient that give the surrogates' decisions legitimacy, because presumably they know the patient's preferences very well and are motivated by close emotional ties to act in the patient's best interest. Paradoxically, one of the main criticisms of proxy decision making is that family members may be *too close* to act as proxies and may make decisions based on their own lives and interests and not truly on those of the patient and that the broad range of acceptable options available to proxies will make detection of these conflicts very difficult. Others feel that this is an oversimplified conception of the physician–patient relationship that does not acknowledge the complexity of family relationships and the interdependency of individual and family interests. For example, imagine a young woman who is a loving mother, sister, and daughter. It is extremely unlikely that she would make any important decision, such as taking a new job in a different city, without considering how the decision would impact her family. It is argued that this woman would obviously want family interests considered in her important healthcare decisions, and that to think of this as a conflict of interest, with herself and her family as adversaries, would be inaccurate and a disservice to all involved (19). Supporting this view, a study of adult intensivists, pediatric intensivists, and neonatologists found that a majority of all three groups believed that family interests are legitimate considerations in medical decision making and that the physician–patient relationship is not exclusive (20).

The parent–child relationship represents a very special type of surrogate decision-making role. Traditionally, the

parent–child relationship is one of the few situations in which the state grants authority to one individual over another. Furthermore, unlike the state, parents are not bound by the best-interests criterion when dealing with their children. For example, consider such common parental decisions as placing children in daycare or in the hands of a teenage babysitter, or requiring them to do household chores. It would be difficult to argue that exposing children to the countless microbes in daycare or to an inexperienced caregiver is strictly in their best interests. Despite this, parents daily make decisions such as these for their children. Such decisions—and parental authority in general—are justified by an appeal to family welfare and character, recognizing that children, as family members, have certain responsibilities to the family. Thus, in our society and law, the greatest latitude is given to parents in making healthcare decisions for their minor children. Significantly less leeway is given to families in deciding for adult family members, and when the state is called on to decide, it must strictly adhere to the best-interests standard.

ESSENTIAL ELEMENTS OF END-OF-LIFE CARE

The Goals of Care

Approximately 50,000 children die in the United States each year; 20%–25% of these deaths occur in the PICU. These statistics, coupled with the fact that the death of a child is always extraordinarily tragic, highlight the critical role that pediatric intensivists play in end-of-life care. In this section, issues pertaining to the dying process in the PICU and the healthcare team's role in that process will be addressed. These issues have the most relevance for those patients whose goals of care have been redirected from life-sustaining, curative goals to comfort-ensuring goals, usually patients with terminal illnesses or other conditions for which the benefits of further life-sustaining therapy are in question (e.g., neurologically devastated patients).

Implicit in the phrase "redirecting the goals of care" is that care is never withdrawn from a patient, only life-sustaining treatment. While this is arguably a semantic point, studies have shown that physicians spend less time caring for patients with do-not-resuscitate (DNR) orders than they spend caring for patients without them (21). Indeed, the withdrawal of care is one of the greatest fears of patients and families in these situations. Thinking in terms of the goals of care for an individual patient can aid the physician in discussions with the healthcare team and the family when making or revising a management plan.

Delivering Bad News

Effective communication is particularly important when dealing with critically ill patients and their families. Unfortunately, doctors receive limited training in communicating with patients. Studies show that patients, families, nurses, social workers, and chaplains often complain of the brevity and poor choice of words doctors use in these settings (22). While the approach to each meeting in which bad news is conveyed must be individualized, several strategies may prove helpful for the pediatric intensivist:

a. *Prepare in advance.* Know who will be in the meeting and their relationship to the patient before entering the room. Anticipate questions and prepare answers that will be clear, direct, and understandable to the family.
b. *Have everyone seated.* Studies have shown that families like to be seated near the door when receiving bad news so as to reduce the feeling of being trapped. Do not stand

during the conversation. Families find this particularly offensive, and it has been shown that people consistently think the doctor spent less time with them when the physician was standing during the conversation.

c. *Introduce yourself and all of your colleagues by title and name.* Although many families cannot remember anyone's name after hearing tragic news, they appreciate the personal connection that the formal introduction establishes.

d. *Avoid jargon.* Doctors and nurses easily slip into the jargon associated with the intensive care culture, but these loose terms only confuse families or lead to misconceptions that can be difficult to resolve.

e. *Talk less.* Studies show that family satisfaction with meetings is inversely correlated to the percentage of time occupied by physician speech (23). Avoid opening meetings with a long monolog. Use the beginning of meetings to determine the family's level of understanding, specific areas of concern, and desire for information.

f. *Show compassion.* Although most physicians believe that they show appropriate compassion, families consistently believe the opposite after they receive bad news. Many want to hear an expression of sorrow by the healthcare team as an affirmation of their grief. They also wish to be allowed time to talk and express their feelings.

g. *Avoid distractions.* To the extent possible, physicians should establish a therapeutic environment in which to share the sensitive information. They should leave pagers outside the room, position someone near the door to avoid interruptions, ensure follow-up, both immediately and in the following days and weeks with appropriate counselors (24).

The manner in which difficult news is conveyed can leave a lasting impression; physicians, especially critical care physicians, would be well served to master the above skills as well as they do some of the more technical aspects of practice.

Do-Not-Resuscitate Orders

Until 1976, no hospital in the United States publicly acknowledged that they provided care that was not intended to prolong and preserve life. In that year, both the Massachusetts General Hospital and Boston's Beth Israel Hospital acknowledged their use of DNR orders in the *New England Journal of Medicine.* Since that time, DNR orders have become commonplace; in fact, the Joint Commission now requires that hospitals have DNR policies. While they are ubiquitous, DNR orders and policies are not without problems in theory and implementation.

For example, the name itself implies that the choice is whether to resuscitate or not, implying that resuscitation is possible, but will not be attempted. For many dying patients, the outcomes from resuscitation are dismal. This problem has been reinforced on television and in the movies, where high rates of successful resuscitation have generated false expectations among the public at large (25). For these reasons, many hospitals have adopted a new terminology, referring instead to "do-not-attempt-resuscitation" (DNAR). This conveys to families that even if resuscitation is attempted, the results may be uncertain at best. In addition, DNR orders are often vague and open to interpretation, leaving substantial opportunity for miscommunication and error. Such difficulties in implementation have led to the development of novel approaches to DNR policies, such as procedure-specific DNR policies and goal-directed DNR orders.

Finally, DNR orders are unique in that they focus exclusively on what will not be done, rather than what will be done.

In this sense, they address only a small fraction of the issues that arise in the care of seriously ill patients. As such, patients with DNR orders often feel that their caregivers have abandoned them. Indeed, as previously mentioned, studies have shown that physicians do, in fact, spend less time caring for patients who have DNR orders. This is unfortunate, as patients with DNR orders often need more attention in the form of aggressive palliative care than do patients who are not imminently dying. Many hospitals now recognize this adverse effect of DNR orders and have responded with the development of palliative care services that focus on what can be done for the dying patient, rather than what will be withheld.

Forgoing Life-Sustaining Treatments

The rights of patients or their surrogates to refuse or remove unwanted medical treatment, even if such a decision involves life-sustaining therapy, have been supported by the US Supreme Court, a special Presidential Commission, and in policy statements by the American Medical Association, the Society for Critical Care Medicine, and the American Thoracic Society.

In discussions about whether or not to provide life-sustaining therapies, several issues arise commonly, including the distinction between ordinary and extraordinary treatments, the distinction between withholding a treatment and withdrawing a treatment, the appropriate role of sedatives and analgesics in the care of the dying, and whether artificial nutrition and hydration ("tube" feedings) may ever be forgone. These issues are discussed in what follows.

The Ordinary–Extraordinary Distinction

One of the most commonly used justifications for withholding "high-tech" therapy from patients is the belief that "extraordinary" treatments are not ethically mandatory. For example, one study showed that 74% of physicians and nurses think that the ordinary–extraordinary distinction is helpful in resolving ethical dilemmas (26). Although this terminology is still used in the writings of some religious traditions, clinicians should understand that the distinction between ordinary and extraordinary treatments is not considered to be helpful when attempting to reason through the ethical aspects of difficult decisions. According to the prevailing interpretation of the distinction, ordinary treatments are morally required, whereas extraordinary treatments are morally optional. However, this is essentially a circular argument, as it claims that ordinary treatments are morally required because they are ordinary and extraordinary treatments are morally optional because they are extraordinary.

In one study, pediatricians were asked about their views on repair of duodenal atresia in healthy babies and in babies with Down syndrome (27). Most pediatricians said that duodenal atresia was an "ordinary" procedure in the case of healthy infants, but an "extraordinary" procedure in the case of babies with Down syndrome. In that the procedure was the same in each case, the use of the terms "ordinary" and "extraordinary" served to mask the ethical judgments that were being made about the nature of the clinical condition.

A much more legitimate and useful approach to thinking about whether a procedure is ethically required is to inquire about the balance of the benefits versus the burdens for a particular procedure in a particular patient. In other words, rather than relying on such terminology as ordinary and extraordinary to decide whether a treatment should be offered, it should be considered whether the proposed benefits exceed the burdens. If, for example, a child with a malignancy is very unlikely to survive even with the administration of highly toxic chemotherapy, then the burdens of that therapy clearly exceed the benefits. On the other hand, physicians and society now generally agree that the benefits of repairing duodenal atresia in patients with Down syndrome exceed the burdens, and thus the procedure is morally required.

8 The Withholding/Withdrawing Distinction

Is there a difference between stopping a treatment once it is started and not starting it in the first place? In other words, is there an ethical difference between deciding not to intubate a patient because we do not think that he or she will recover, and extubating a patient who has failed to recover despite a period of ventilation? Surveys have repeatedly shown that physicians believe a difference does exist. For example, one study reported that 66% of physicians and nurses discern an ethical difference between withdrawing and withholding a treatment, and nearly half agreed with the statement "there is an emerging consensus . . . that withdrawing a treatment is ethically different from withholding or not starting it" (28). In another survey of 360 attending physicians, house staff, and medical students, 73% felt that withdrawing is different from withholding (29). These reports indicate that physicians are much more comfortable in withholding treatments than in withdrawing them.

It is interesting that this strong opinion reported among clinicians is strikingly at odds with the prevailing view among ethicists and lawyers. Legal scholars and ethicists have been quite consistent in expressing the opinion that doctors should not differentiate between decisions to withhold or withdraw medical treatments. In the landmark *Cruzan* case, for example, justices from the US Supreme Court wrote that doctors should consider decisions to withhold and withdraw as equivalent to ensure that patients receive adequate trials of therapy. A typical example occurs in the delivery room, when the viability of premature babies is often difficult to assess in the moments immediately following birth. The Supreme Court's decision implies that physicians should deal with this uncertainty by proceeding with resuscitation, but that they should be willing to withdraw the life-sustaining treatment if, after a trial of therapy, further support is no longer justified. Despite these opinions from law and philosophy, clinicians persist in believing that these two actions are differentiated. Part of the reason is clearly psychological. Physicians feel more responsible for the death of a patient when it results from the withdrawal of a therapy than they do when it results from the withholding of a therapy. This psychological distinction is important and cannot be made to disappear by legal or philosophic reasoning, no matter how persuasive. Nevertheless, when confronted with these situations, physicians should consider the perspectives from law and philosophy, as in many cases adoption of these views will lead to better clinical decision making.

Medical Nutrition and Hydration

Should techniques for providing medical nutrition and hydration (IV fluids, parenteral nutrition, tube feedings, etc.) be considered medical treatments? If so, can they then be ethically withdrawn by the same process and criteria that are used for other types of medical treatment? In other words, if it is ethically acceptable to withdraw a ventilator from a terminally ill patient, is it also ethically acceptable to withdraw medically provided nutrition and hydration? (Note that this question does not propose withholding oral feedings from patients who wants to eat or drink.) A gradually emerging consensus in both law and ethics answers these questions in the affirmative (30). A large number of court decisions, including the decision in the above-mentioned *Cruzan* case, concluded that medically-provided nutrition and hydration should be considered medical treatments and that patients or their surrogates should have

the right to refuse them. The decision of whether or not to administer this therapy should be based on the same criteria outlined above for other treatments, that is, an analysis of the balance between the benefits and burdens of providing the therapy. This consensus was recently challenged in the highly publicized case of Terry Schiavo, a 41-year-old woman in a persistent vegetative state whose husband and parents were locked in a decade-long legal duel over the husband's decision as legal surrogate to withdraw medical nutrition and hydration from his wife. Despite her parents' attempts—through the courts, the political process, and involvement of the national media—to stop the withdrawal of nutrition and hydration, the courts consistently decided in favor of the husband as legal surrogate, and she died after withdrawal of nutrition and hydration in March 2005. While this case did not seriously challenge the legal status of medical nutrition and hydration as medical interventions that can be refused or withdrawn, it did expose a public rift in the moral acceptance of this practice (31).

Many clinicians have been reluctant to accept the withdrawal of medical nutrition and hydration, at least in part because "feeding" seems to be such a basic and fundamental aspect of the care they provide to their patients. In the terminology of the distinction discussed earlier, it seems so "ordinary." However, this provides yet another example of the inadequacies of the ordinary–extraordinary distinction, as for certain patients, particularly those who are permanently unconscious or imminently dying, medically administered feedings can no longer provide any benefit.

Pediatricians have been particularly slow to acknowledge this emerging consensus (32) for several reasons. First, prognoses are often more uncertain in children, given their remarkable ability to recover from injury. Second, even normal newborns need assistance with feedings, so pediatricians are less likely to see artificial feedings as a "medical" treatment. Third, whereas the hospice experience shows that refusal of food and water is frequently seen in elderly patients who are dying a natural death, the death of a child is never a "natural" event, and caregivers are reluctant to accept it with apparent passivity. Nevertheless, the principles that have evolved in governing the administration or withdrawal of medically provided feedings in adults are equally applicable in children, and no reason is justifiable to treat the pediatric population differently.

9 Sedatives and Analgesics in the Care of the Dying

Physicians who care for patients in a PICU will be called on to discontinue life support from dying patients. In these tragic circumstances, the question then becomes how best to manage the patient during the dying process. Some erroneously believe that no sedatives or analgesics should be given in these situations based on their belief that it is important both ethically and legally that the patient die from his underlying disease, without any contribution from the respiratory or cardiac depression that are frequent side effects of these medications.

The reluctance of many physicians to aggressively treat the pain and suffering experienced by the terminally ill has been one of the most powerful forces driving the movement in favor of euthanasia and physician-assisted suicide. Individuals who have watched loved ones die without adequate pain relief have spearheaded this movement with the belief that patients should have the opportunity to commit suicide if their suffering is unbearable, particularly when physicians seem unwilling to do whatever is necessary to control the suffering. This unwillingness on the part of the physician is unfortunate, particularly as nothing in the law, ethics, or any of the major religious traditions precludes physicians from aggressively treating the pain and suffering of the terminally ill, even when such treatment may hasten a patient's demise. Nevertheless, it has been shown that as many as 40% of doctors and nurses give inadequate pain medication, most often out of fear of hastening a patient's death (26).

The ethical principle that is relevant to this question is the doctrine of double effect, originally developed within the Catholic tradition but now widely acknowledged in other religious traditions, as well as in law and philosophy. The doctrine states that when an action has two effects, one of which is inherently good and the other inherently bad, it can be justified if certain conditions are met (**Fig. 15.1**). For example, the administration of morphine to a dying patient produces both a good effect (relief of pain and suffering) and the potential for a bad effect (hastening the patient's death through respiratory depression). The conditions that must be satisfied in order for the action to be justified are as follows:

a. *The action in itself must be good or, at least, morally indifferent.* (Administration of the morphine itself is morally indifferent.)

b. *The agent must intend only the good effect and not the evil effect. The evil effect is foreseen, not intended. It is allowed, not sought.* (In the case of administering morphine to a terminally ill patient, the physician must intend only the relief of the patient's pain and suffering. Respiratory depression and the potential for an earlier death is a foreseen complication, but is not sought.)

c. *The evil effect cannot be a means to the good effect.* (If the physician administers a bolus of potassium chloride instead of morphine, this condition would be violated. By administering potassium chloride, the evil effect [death] becomes the means to the good effect [relief from suffering]. By contrast, morphine does not depend on the side effect of death to effectively relieve pain.)

d. *The good intended must outweigh the evil permitted.* In the case of an imminently dying patient, the benefit of pain relief clearly outweighs the risk of death. This would not be true if the patient were not terminally ill. For example, if an otherwise healthy patient was given so much morphine for pain control that he developed serious respiratory depression, he should be placed on a ventilator and not allowed to die.

In summary, despite the beliefs of many clinicians, no moral, legal, or religious reasons justify withholding adequate pain relief from dying patients. Pain and suffering should always be adequately treated, even if the treatment results in a foreseen but unintended hastening of death.

What is the difference between currently accepted practice and the performance of euthanasia? The key difference lies in the *intention* of the physician. As long as the physician's intention is treatment of the patient's pain and suffering, the administration of analgesics and sedatives is noncontroversial. When the physician's intention is to kill the patient, then the line between accepted practice and euthanasia has been crossed.

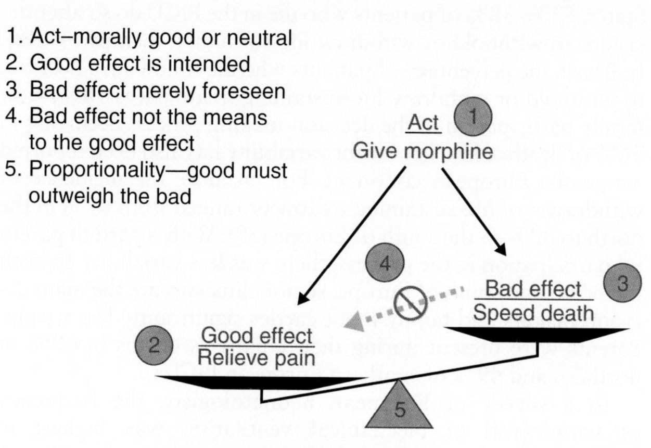

SPECIAL TOPICS IN END-OF-LIFE CARE

Futility

The extra*ordinary* advances in life-sustaining therapies that have developed in the last few decades have spawned a new type of ethical conflict between physicians and families over decisions to continue or forgo life-support therapy. Intensivists can expect to face situations in which they believe that further treatment for a given patient is "futile," while the patient's family feels strongly that the treatment must continue. In fact, over 80% of ICU physicians reported having withdrawn support from patients on the grounds of futility, and at least sometimes this was done over the objections of the family (33). The potential for these conflicts has led to the development of approaches to the problem of futility that seek to resolve conflicts between physicians and families and justify difficult decisions in these troublesome cases.

The earliest approach to the futility debate was to attempt to define futility. These definitions largely rely on either quantitative or qualitative criteria. Quantitative definitions attempt to attach "hard" statistical prognostications to treatment decisions. For example, Schneiderman et al. (34) suggested that if "in the last 100 cases a medical treatment has been useless, [physicians] should regard that treatment as futile." Qualitative definitions attempt to identify specific clinical outcomes (such as the persistent vegetative state), in which life-sustaining treatments would not provide benefit and, therefore, should not be offered. Ultimately, attempts to resolve futility disputes through the use of definitions were not successful, as it was recognized that the conflict in such cases does not typically revolve around the medical facts, statistics, and definitions of the case; instead, the crux of the dispute is almost always a conflict of values and a disagreement over whether or not the treatment in question is "worth it."

More recently, "fair process"–based approaches to futility have been developed and advocated by hospitals and by the American Medical Association in a 1999 report (35), and in 1999, Texas became the first state to enact a law that establishes a statewide fair process approach to futility cases based this report. One Texas hospital reported 47 futility consultations over a 2-year period. In 43 of these cases, the ethics committee agreed that further treatment was futile, and in 37 of these, the families agreed to withdrawal of life-sustaining treatment. In 6 cases, however, the families disagreed with the determination of futility. In 3 cases, the families agreed within a few days, in 2 cases the patients died during the 10-day waiting period mandated by the legislation, and in 1 case, the patient died awaiting transfer to an alternate provider, who had agreed to provide treatment (36).

While this legislation and other procedural approaches do give weight to the subjective determination by the patient or the patient's surrogate of what constitutes a worthwhile outcome, they also clearly allow for the possibility that the process will result in a unilateral decision by the institution to not offer the treatment in question. Such approaches, if they are to be successful, must honor the value system of the patient and family, protect the integrity of the medical professionals involved, and function in an open and fair manner that maximizes the chances for an acceptable resolution. The elements of such a procedural approach appear in **Table 15.1**.

1. Act–morally good or neutral
2. Good effect is intended
3. Bad effect merely foreseen
4. Bad effect not the means to the good effect
5. Proportionality—good must outweigh the bad

FIGURE 15.1. The doctrine of double effect.

TABLE 15.1

KEY ELEMENTS OF A HOSPITAL POLICY ON POTENTIALLY FUTILE TREATMENT

Hospital policy should be "bilateral," addressing overtreatment by both clinicians and families.
- Families can request a consult if they believe clinicians are demanding "overtreatment."
- Clinicians can request a consult when they believe families are demanding "overtreatment."

Efforts to achieve resolution with the patient and family must be clearly documented, emphasizing that limiting the use of life-sustaining treatments will not lead to abandonment.

If sustained and repeated efforts fail, the case is referred to the institutional Ethics Advisory Committee.

Three-phase consultation process:
- Phase 1: Meeting with Committee and clinical team. The purpose is to present the medical perspective on the case.
- Phase 2: Meeting with Committee and the patient or family. The purpose is so that the patient or family can "tell their story."
- Phase 3: The Committee meets alone. The purpose is to make a determination of whether further use of life-sustaining treatment is inappropriate or harmful.

If the Committee supports the caregivers' assessment, then four options should be considered:
- Clinicians may pursue further attempts at consensus with the patient or surrogate, but only when clear avenues for negotiation exist that have not already been explored.
- Clinicians may attempt to transfer care to another physician within the hospital or to another hospital, which serves as a check on the system and provides evidence of community consensus.
- The hospital administration could seek a judicial resolution to the conflict, on grounds that the patient's surrogate is not acting in the patient's best interest.
- The hospital administration could sanction the unilateral forgoing or removal of life-sustaining treatments. Such action should occur only after informing the patient or surrogate decision maker of the plan and only after giving them sufficient opportunity to seek alternate medical care, legal advice, and, possibly, judicial involvement, if desired.

The Use of Neuromuscular Blocking Agents during Withdrawal of Life Support

As outlined in the section Sedatives and Analgesics in the Care of the Dying, the use of opioids, benzodiazepines, and even barbiturates is justified if intended to alleviate the patient's suffering during the dying process. Neuromuscular blocking agents (NMBAs) cannot serve this purpose, as they have no analgesic, anxiolytic, or sedative effect; their sole effect is chemical paralysis. The use of these agents may even serve to mask the presence of treatable suffering, less likely to be diagnosed owing to lack of patient communication and movement. Nevertheless, it has been reported that anywhere from 6% to 12% of intensive care physicians have used NMBAs during withdrawal of life support. Although some justify the use of these drugs as useful in reducing the suffering experienced by family members who witness agonal movements, the Ethics Committee of the Society of Critical Care Medicine recommends that these drugs not be used during withdrawal of life support, stating that "the best way to relieve their suffering is by reassuring them of the patient's comfort through the use of adequate sedation and analgesia (37)." Consequently, the best course of action is to ensure the absence of pharmacologic paralysis before withdrawal of ventilator support.

A rare but difficult dilemma can arise when the pharmacologic effects of the NMBAs are not reversible (due to overdosage or renal/hepatic failure) for days or weeks. Under these unusual circumstances, it may be permissible to proceed with ventilator withdrawal provided that (a) it is highly certain that the patient cannot survive without the ventilator, (b) the patient's comfort is carefully managed with sufficient dosages of sedatives and analgesics, and (c) it is determined that the benefits of waiting for the return of neuromuscular function (e.g., interaction with family members before death) do not outweigh the burdens (37).

International Perspectives on End-of-life Care

Important international differences exist in end-of-life practices in the ICU (38–42). As might be expected, marked variability in end-of-life practice is seen around the world, but it is interesting that a substantial amount of variability is also seen within countries (43). Variability has been documented in all aspects of decision making, including the range of acceptable practices, the decision-making participants, and the frequency of limitations of life-sustaining therapies.

Perhaps the most salient international differences in end-of-life care relate to questions of decision-making participation and authority. Fundamental differences in end-of-life decision making for competent and formerly competent adults have been well documented across country and culture. For instance, French physicians—not parents—have a dominant role in medical decisions for children. The justification for this practice is that French intensivists believe that parental autonomy in intensive care is an illusion, as parents do not possess the knowledge or experience necessary to make truly informed decisions. Further, French pediatric intensivists believe that this practice protects parents from the responsibility and guilt of making tragic decisions for their child (44). This paternalistic attitude is firmly contested by North American intensivists (45,46).

Substantial variability has also been reported among countries regarding decisions to forgo life support. In the United States, 53%–58% of patients who die in the PICU do so after decisions to withhold or withdraw life-sustaining therapy (47,48). In Brazil, the percentage of patients who die following a decision to withhold or withdraw life-sustaining treatment is 18%, with family participation in the decision-making process occurring in 36% of deaths (43). Significant variability has also been reported across the European continent. For instance, the incidence of withdrawal of life-sustaining treatment ranged from 47% in the north to 30% in the south of Europe (39). With regard to parental participation in the process, there was less variability. In both the north and south of Europe, senior clinicians are the main decision makers and family input carries significantly less weight. Parents were present during their children's deaths in 69% of northern and 49% of southern European PICUs.

In a survey of European neonatologists, the frequency of withdrawal of mechanical ventilation was highest in the Netherlands, the United Kingdom, and Sweden; it was intermediate in France and Germany and lowest in Spain and Italy (38). Physicians more likely to agree with ideas consistent with preserving life at all costs were from Hungary, Estonia, Lithuania, and Italy, while those more likely to agree with statements that quality of life must be taken into account were from the United Kingdom, the Netherlands, and Sweden.

With regard to end-of-life issues, the ethical climate in Europe appears to be evolving. The European Commission has ruled that the patient has the right to self-determination, including the right to refuse unwanted therapies. Recently, laws pertaining to patient rights have also been adopted in France and Belgium; they explicitly state that doctors must respect the refusal of treatment expressed by a competent patient, even if his or her life is threatened.

While it is easy to document differences between countries, it is more difficult to explain them. Diverse cultural, religious, philosophic, legal, and professional attitudes may be involved. European cultures are not static or homogeneous. Even within a particular ethnic group, significant differences may exist, depending on the country of residence, gender, age, education, social circumstances, generation, and assimilation into the host society (49). For example, significant differences have been found in end-of-life decision-making styles between Japanese living in Japan and Japanese-speaking and English-speaking Japanese Americans in California. (50).

In many Western countries, national and supranational legal authorities have begun debating the issue, and quality care at the end of life is recognized as a global problem for public health and health systems (28). The international community has begun the process of measuring, analyzing, and debating the differences between cultures and countries with regard to end-of-life treatment, as it is recognized that studying international practices may lead to opportunities to improve the quality of end-of-life care across borders. A convergence of opinion about good practice appears to be developing among professional societies in Europe and in the United States (49). End-of-life issues are becoming an essential topic at international congresses, and international consensus meetings have been organized on the subject (49). This emerging international dialogue will likely lead to a deeper understanding of, and appreciation for, the many differences found in the practice of end-of-life care and—it is hoped—to incremental improvement in the field.

SUMMARY AND FUTURE DIRECTIONS

Medical ethics is a relatively young area of active inquiry and research. Most of the early work has been done in North America and Western Europe and has been based on the philosophic methods that have been dominant in those cultures. While beneficial in the sense of bringing many previously taboo subjects to light for vigorous discussion and debate, this Western focus has resulted in a disproportionate emphasis on a narrow range of intellectual and cultural background. Increasingly, globalization is changing the fundamental fabric of social practices throughout the world, and medicine is at the heart of this evolution. Over the next decades, we can anticipate research that will provide empirical descriptions of how bioethical dilemmas are managed in different countries and cultures, and we will benefit from the input of other philosophic, religious, and intellectual perspectives as we grapple with these exceedingly difficult and important aspects of the practice of pediatric critical care medicine.

References

1. Iglehart JK. The American health care system. The end-stage renal disease program. N Engl J Med 1993;328:366–71.
2. Duff RS, Campbell AG. Moral and ethical dilemmas in the special-care nursery. N Engl J Med 1973;289:890–4.
3. Beauchamp TL, Childress JF. Principles of Biomedical Ethics. 5th ed. New York, NY: Oxford University Press, 2001.
4. Pellegrino ED, Thomasma DC. The Virtues in Medical Practice. New York, NY: Oxford University Press, 1993.
5. Jonsen AR, Toulmin S. The Abuse of Casuistry. Los Angeles: University of California Press, 1988.
6. Carse AL. The "voice of care": Implications for bioethical education. J Med Philos 1991;16:5–28.
7. Coles R. The Call of Stories: Teaching and the Moral Imagination. Boston, MA: Houghton Mifflin, 1989.
8. Gutheil TG, Bursztajn H, Brodsky A. Malpractice prevention through the sharing of uncertainty. Informed consent and the therapeutic alliance. N Engl J Med 1984;311:49–51.
9. Appelbaum PS, Grisso T. Assessing patients' capacities to consent to treatment. N Engl J Med 1988;319:1635–8.
10. Informed consent, parental permission, and assent in pediatric practice. Committee on Bioethics, American Academy of Pediatrics. Pediatrics 1995;95:314–7.
11. Ross LF. Health care decision making by children. Is it in their best interest? Hastings Cent Rep 1997;27:41–5.
12. Annas GJ. Informed consent, cancer, and truth in prognosis. N Engl J Med 1994;330:223–5.
13. Ross LF. Children, Families and Healthcare Decision-Making. Oxford, UK: Clarendon Press, 1998.
14. Shalowitz D, Garrett-Mayer E, Wendler D. The accuracy of surrogate decision-makers: A systematic review. Arch Intern Med 2006;166:493–7.
15. Berger JT, DeRenzo EG, Schwartz J. Surrogate decision making: Reconciling ethical theory and clinical practice. Ann Intern Med 2008;149:48–53.
16. Fox, R. "Training for Uncertainty" in The Student Physician. eds. R. Merton, G. Reader, and P. Kendall. Cambridge, Harvard University Press. (1957) page 207.
17. Katz J. Why doctors don't disclose uncertainty. Hastings Cent Rep 1984;14:35–44.
18. Angell M. The doctor as double agent. Kennedy Inst Ethics J 1993;3:279–86.
19. Hardwig J. What about the family? Hastings Cent Rep 1990;20:5–10.
20. Hardart GE, Truog RD. Attitudes and preferences of intensivists regarding the role of family interests in medical decision making for incompetent patients. Crit Care Med 2003;31:1895–900.
21. Wray NP, Friedland JA, Ashton CM, et al. Characteristics of house staff work rounds on two academic general medicine services. J Med Educ. 1986;61:893–900.
22. Greenberg LW, Jewett LS, Gluck RS, et al. Giving information for a life-threatening diagnosis. Parents' and oncologists' perceptions. Am J Dis Child 1984;138:649–53.
23. McDonagh JR, Elliott TB, Engelberg RA, et al. Family satisfaction with family conferences about end-of-life care in the intensive care unit: Increased proportion of family speech is associated with increased satisfaction. Crit Care Med 2004;32:1484–8.
24. Sharp MC, Strauss RP, Lorch SC. Communicating medical bad news: Parents' experiences and preferences. J Pediatr 1992;121:539–46.
25. Diem SJ, Lantos JD, Tulsky JA. Cardiopulmonary resuscitation on television. Miracles and misinformation. N Engl J Med 1996;334:1578–82.
26. Solomon MZ, O'Donnell L, Jennings B, et al. Decisions near the end of life: Professional views on life-sustaining treatments. Am J Public Health 1993;83:14–23.
27. Shaw A, Randolph JG, Manard B. Ethical issues in pediatric surgery: A national survey of pediatricians and pediatric surgeons. Pediatrics 1977;60:588–99.
28. Singer PA, Bowman KW. Quality end-of-life care: A global perspective. BMC Palliat Care 2002;1:4.
29. Caralis PV, Hammond JS. Attitudes of medical students, housestaff, and faculty physicians toward euthanasia and termination of life-sustaining treatment. Crit Care Med 1992;20:683–90.

30. McCann RM, Hall WJ, Groth-Juncker A. Comfort care for terminally ill patients. The appropriate use of nutrition and hydration. *JAMA* 1994;272:1263–6.

31. Quill TE. Terri Schiavo—A tragedy compounded. *N Engl J Med* 2005;352:1630–3.

32. Frader J. Forgoing life-sustaining food and water: Newborns. In: Lynn J, ed. *By No Extraordinary Means: The Choice to Forgo Life-Sustaining Food and Water.* Bloomington: Indiana University Press, 1989:180–5.

33. Asch DA, Hansen-Flaschen J, Lanken PN. Decisions to limit or continue life-sustaining treatment by critical care physicians in the United States: Conflicts between physicians' practices and patients' wishes. *Am J Respir Crit Care Med* 1995;151:288–92.

34. Schneiderman LJ, Jecker NS, Jonsen AR. Medical futility: Its meaning and ethical implications. *Ann Intern Med* 1990;112:949–54.

35. Medical futility in end-of-life care: Report of the Council on Ethical and Judicial Affairs. *JAMA* 1999;281:937–41.

36. Fine RL, Mayo TW. Resolution of futility by due process: Early experience with the Texas Advance Directives Act. *Ann Intern Med* 2003;138:743–6.

37. Truog RD, Cist AF, Brackett SE, et al. Recommendations for end-of-life care in the intensive care unit: The Ethics Committee of the Society of Critical Care Medicine. *Crit Care Med* 2001;29:2332–48.

38. Cuttini M, Nadai M, Kaminski M, et al. End-of-life decisions in neonatal intensive care: Physicians' self-reported practices in seven European countries. EURONIC Study Group. *Lancet* 2000;355:2112–8.

39. Devictor DJ, Nguyen DT. Forgoing life-sustaining treatments in children: A comparison between Northern and Southern European pediatric intensive care units. *Pediatr Crit Care Med* 2004;5:211–5.

40. Sprung CL, Eidelman LA. Worldwide similarities and differences in the foregoing of life-sustaining treatments. *Intensive Care Med* 1996;22:1003–5.

41. Vincent JL. Forgoing life support in western European intensive care units: The results of an ethical questionnaire. *Crit Care Med* 1999;27:1626–33.

42. Yaguchi A, Truog RD, Curtis JR, et al. International differences in end-of-life attitudes in the intensive care unit: Results of a survey. *Arch Intern Med* 2005;165:1970–5.

43. Kipper DJ, Piva JP, Garcia PC, et al. Evolution of the medical practices and modes of death on pediatric intensive care units in southern Brazil. *Pediatr Crit Care Med* 2005;6:258–63.

44. Devictor DJ, Nguyen DT. Forgoing life-sustaining treatments: How the decision is made in French pediatric intensive care units. *Crit Care Med* 2001;29:1356–9.

45. Frader JE. Forgoing life support across borders: Who decides and why? *Pediatr Crit Care Med* 2004;5:289–90.

46. Hoehn KS, Nelson RM. Parents should not be excluded from decisions to forgo life-sustaining treatments! *Crit Care Med* 2001;29:1480–1.

47. Burns JP, Mitchell C, Outwater KM, et al. End-of-life care in the pediatric intensive care unit after the forgoing of life-sustaining treatment. *Crit Care Med* 2000;28:3060–6.

48. Vernon DD, Dean JM, Timmons OD, et al. Modes of death in the pediatric intensive care unit: Withdrawal and limitation of supportive care. *Crit Care Med* 1993;21:1798–802.

49. Carlet J, Thijs LG, Antonelli M, et al. Challenges in end-of-life care in the ICU. Statement of the 5th International Consensus Conference in Critical Care: Brussels, Belgium, April 2003. *Intensive Care Med* 2004;30:770–84.

50. Matsumura S, Bito S, Liu H, et al. Acculturation of attitudes toward end-of-life care: A cross-cultural survey of Japanese Americans and Japanese. *J Gen Intern Med* 2002;17:531–9.

CHAPTER 16 ■ ORGAN DONATION

KRISTEN L. NELSON MCMILLAN, THOMAS A. NAKAGAWA, AND IVOR D. BERKOWITZ

KEY POINTS

1. Options for organ donation include donation after brain death (DBD), donation after cardiac or circulatory death (DCD), and living donation.

2. The demand for organs currently far exceeds the available supply for several reasons. Approximately 50% of family members currently refuse to give consent for organ donation from their deceased loved ones. Other reasons include the failure to identify eligible donors and failure to give families the option of donation.

3. Request for organ donation should be a collaborative process between the ICU team and the organ procurement organization (OPO) ensuring the family is approached in a professional and compassionate manner to inform the family of the death of their loved one and request donation.

4. The option of donation should be preserved for all patients.

5. In cases of DCD, the decision to withdraw life-sustaining medical therapies must always have been made prior to discussing organ donation.

6. Relatively few absolute contraindications exist to rule out organ donation, and often these absolutes become relative based on the individual recipient.

7. Many OPOs and ICUs utilize standardized donor management protocols.

8. Donor management of the brain-dead patient requires a change in goals of care from cerebral-protective strategies to organ-donor–supportive strategies.

9. Several hemodynamic changes occur in brain-dead patients that may ultimately affect the potential transplantability of organs.

10. Brainstem ischemia results in uncontrolled sympathetic stimulation commonly referred to as "catecholamine storm," which ultimately results in catecholamine depletion and hemodynamic collapse from myocardial dysfunction and poor vascular tone. As many as 25% of potential donors are lost due to this hemodynamic instability.

11. Hypotension is the most common problem encountered by physicians who care for pediatric organ donors; it can be caused by vasodilation, hypovolemia (due to diuretic use, diabetes insipidus [DI], osmotic diuresis, and hypothermia), and myocardial dysfunction.

12. Optimal central venous pressure (CVP) for managing brain-dead organ donors is often between 8 and 10 mm Hg.

13. Myocardial dysfunction is multifactorial and may be due to altered loading conditions, ischemia, acidosis, hypoxia, and massive cytokine release, which results in a systemic inflammatory state and abnormal function of the hypothalamic–pituitary axis resulting in pituitary hormone depletion.

14. Dopamine has been the vasopressor most commonly used in pediatric organ donors, because renal and splanchnic blood flow can often be maintained at levels <10 $\mu g/$kg min.

15. The vasoconstriction associated with α-adrenergic agents, such as phenylephrine, epinephrine, and norepinephrine, must be taken into account, because perfusion to organs may be compromised, particularly the kidneys, liver, and heart.

16. Vasopressin acts synergistically with catecholamines and may result in a much-reduced requirement for catecholamines.

17. Intractable hypotension should raise the suspicion of hormone deficiency, and replacement with thyroid hormone and corticosteroids should be strongly considered.

18. Currently, most transplant centers and OPOs routinely administer T_3 or T_4, in addition to methylprednisolone, vasopressin, and, often, insulin to brain-dead donors to improve or prevent the deterioration in myocardial function and restore normal physiologic parameters.

19. Potential donor lungs may be compromised by neurogenic pulmonary edema, pneumonia, and the systemic inflammatory response associated with brain death.

20. A Pao_2 of >300 mm Hg on 100% oxygen or a Pao_2-to-Fio_2 ratio ≥300 mm Hg often signifies lung viability for transplantation.

21. Hypernatremia in the brain-dead donor due to hypertonic saline administration, DI, or osmotic diuresis can adversely affect potentially transplantable organs, especially the liver.

22. The treatment of DI often includes vasopressin supplementation. 1-Desamino-8-D-arginine vasopressin (DDAVP) can be used as an agent to control DI in the hemodynamically stable patient. In the initial phase of management until urine output can be effectively controlled with vasopressin, fluid replacement may be necessary to prevent dehydration. The longer half-life of DDAVP is of concern for some surgeons.

23. Severely brain-injured patients may frequently develop a significant disseminated intravascular consumptive coagulopathy, which may result from the release of thromboplastin and tissue plasminogen from injured and necrotic brain tissue.

Since the first successful organ transplant >50 years ago, organ donation has saved several hundred thousand lives. In 2012 alone, >28,000 solid organs were transplanted in the United States, with an average of 76 organs being transplanted each day (Organ Procurement and Transplantation Network [OPTN] data). 1760 of these transplants were performed in pediatric patients. To date, over 25,000 pediatric donors <18 years of age have donated over 70,000 organs allowing other children to live longer and better-quality lives (OPTN data as of August 5, 2013).

Kidneys, heart, liver, lungs, intestine, and pancreas are transplantable solid organs. Depending on the organ referenced, solid organs can be donated following brain death (donation after brain determination of death [DBDD or DBD]), donation after cardiac or circulatory determination of death (DCDD or DCD), or living donation. Currently, most transplanted organs come from deceased donors who have been declared brain-dead. However, an increasing number of organs are being obtained by living donation and from DCD donors. Indeed, in 2001, for the first time in transplant history, the number of living donors exceeded the number of deceased donors (http://organdonor.gov/legislation/timeline.html). Furthermore, the number of organs recovered from DCD donors continues to increase annually.

A marked imbalance continues to exist between the demand for transplantable organs and the supply of organs for transplantation. As of 2013, almost 120,000 people are awaiting a needed organ transplant for end-organ failure. Of these candidates, almost 2200 are <18 years of age. For patients <18 years old, the greatest number of patients are waiting for a kidney, followed by children waiting for liver, and heart transplantation. Unfortunately, an average of almost 17 people die per day while on the waiting list to receive an organ (OPTN data). A significant number of transplant candidates, including children, are also removed from the waiting list because their condition worsens to a point where they are too ill to receive a transplant (OPTN data). In fact, children <1 year of age have the highest death rate waiting for a needed organ (OPTN data). Specific challenges exist for pediatric donors and transplant candidates. Parents and guardians must act as surrogate decision makers without benefit of being guided by the donor's wishes. Additionally, organ availability, the need to match the size of the donor organ to the size of the recipient, and technically challenging procedures in smaller patients create unique challenges for children. Whereas most organs must be transplanted intact, necessitating close size matching, liver and lungs can be transplanted into smaller children as a segment of a larger organ, thereby increasing transplantation options. Recent data show that despite fewer pediatric donors, more organs are being recovered and transplanted in children. Children are also receiving more organs from pediatric donors although the majority of organs recovered from pediatric donors are still transplanted into adults. Fortunately, over the past 10 years, waiting list mortality has decreased dramatically for children (1).

Perhaps the most important factor accounting for the widening gap between the demand for organs and their supply is the failure to obtain consent for organ donation from families of potential organ donors. Consent rates vary widely among geographic areas of the country and racial groups. While >75% of Americans view organ donation as a positive way to help others, <50% of eligible donor families who are asked about donation consent to allowing their loved become a donor. Contributing factors associated with this discrepancy between what individuals say they would do and how families really decide include hospital experiences, difficulty understanding death, unrecognized donor potential from hospital staff, and racial barriers.

A family's hospital experience substantially influences whether they consent for organ donation from a deceased family member. Families who refuse consent are less satisfied with their hospital experiences, especially with the quality of care received by their loved ones, than are families who chose donation. Families are also less satisfied with end-of-life care and the donation process. These families are less likely to believe that they had adequate time and privacy to decide about donation (2,3). The unrecognized donor potential of brain-dead individuals is another one of the primary reasons consent rates are low. Families of brain-dead eligible donors may not be given the option of donation, either because potentially eligible donors are not identified or because consent for donation is not requested. Donation may also be requested at an inappropriate time and by an inappropriate requestor. Families who decline donation are also less likely to have a clear understanding of brain death (2,3). Families approached early before they understand their loved one has died decline consent because they do not understand that their loved one has died. Indeed, a majority of these family members believed that a brain-dead person would recover. On the other hand, donor families were much more likely to understand the concept of brain death and were satisfied with the care received by their loved ones and with the process of request. A wide variation in consent rates is also found among transplant centers across the country, with some centers obtaining consent as often as 90% of the time. Additionally, race, level of education, and prejudice may contribute to the perception that some families may not be interested in donation. For example, the families of eligible brain-dead African American donors are less likely to consent to donation than Caucasian families (2,3).

A coordinated approach for families facing end-of-life issues with a loved one should be emphasized to provide a positive hospital experience. Several prominent organizations and government departments, including but not limited to the Institute of Medicine (IOM), the Department of Health and Human Services, and the United Network for Organ Sharing (UNOS), have realized that changes can be made affecting the process of organ donation and end-of-life care to maximize the number of organs recovered and subsequently transplanted, while ensuring comfort to the donors and their families (4–6). These systems changes necessary to save the lives of those on the waiting list require collaboration with all involved organizations and healthcare employees—including the pediatric intensivists, who will play a pivotal role.

HISTORY OF ORGAN DONATION

The first successful organ transplant took place in Boston in 1954 when a kidney was transplanted from one identical twin to the other twin. Over the next 15 years, other organs were successfully procured from non–heart-beating organ donors and transplanted into nonrelated individuals. As transplant techniques and technology improved, so did the interest in easily identifying those patients who were in need of a transplant. In 1968, the Southeast Organ Procurement Foundation was formed as an organization for transplant professionals. This was followed by implementation of the first computer-based organ matching system, known as the UNOS in 1977. UNOS became an independent nonprofit organization in 1984 and received the first federal contract to operate the OPTN. This contract is still held by UNOS today. Members of the OPTN include transplant hospitals and organ procurement organizations (OPOs). OPOs are nonprofit organizations responsible for coordinating the process of organ and tissue donation. Additionally, OPOs work closely with the donor and donor family, transplant hospitals, and potential transplant recipients in an effort to ensure that the organ donation process is maximized and that all involved parties are emotionally and ethically comfortable with the process.

The Uniform Anatomical Gift Act (UAGA) also expanded public awareness for the need for organ donors in 1968. The UAGA gave individuals who are ≥18 years of age the right to donate organs and tissues. The UAGA remains operative in all states in the United States. The wish to donate organs is expressed by individuals on a donor card, driver's license, or donor registry.

ORGAN DONATION AFTER BRAIN DEATH

In 1967, the first organ transplantation from a brain-dead patient occurred, and several age-old ethical issues related to the declaration of death again received national attention. The Harvard criteria for brain death were published in 1968 and subsequently modified by professional societies as technology and knowledge in this field increased (7,8).

Brain death refers to complete and irreversible cessation of brain function, and its declaration is a topic of complex medical, legal, ethical, and religious importance (see Chapter 67).

By the 1980s, determination of death by brain-death criteria was accepted in all states in the United States, including the District of Columbia. In 1987, a task force consisting of representatives from the American Academy of Pediatrics (AAP) and the American Academy of Neurology, as well as representatives from several other professional medical and legal societies, proposed guidelines for the determination of brain death in children in the United States (9). These pediatric brain death guidelines were revised in 2012 (7,8).

Currently, most recovered organs for transplantation come from brain-dead donors, although living donation and DCD donation constitute a significantly increasing proportion of organs available for transplantation. Mandatory seat belt laws and other safety initiatives, such as helmet laws, have resulted in a reduction in the number of individuals who sustain severe head injuries during motor vehicle accidents. Furthermore, improvement in the management of severely brain-injured patients has played an important role in decreasing the number of brain-dead donors. This is in great part because of pediatric intensivists and specialized critical care teams that have made a significant impact in morbidity and mortality for all age groups. Currently, about 55% of all brain-dead children become organ donors (10). Because some organs cannot be transplanted from living donors, and the number of people awaiting an organ transplant continues to significantly outweigh the number of donors, DCD and other sources of organ donation (including neonatal donation) continue to be explored as a means to increase the pool of organ donors (11,12).

Process

Donation is a process that begins when a critically ill or injured patient is identified as a potential donor with early recognition of potential death and a timely referral to the OPO. Clinical triggers alerting the OPO of a possible donor are essential for a timely referral to occur and prevent a rushed approach to donation. Appropriate time is needed to determine if the patient is a potential donor followed by extensive testing to determine suitability and placement of organs recovered for transplantation. Efficient time management is essential, because delays exceeding 72 hours (from time of brain death to aortic cross-clamp) have been associated with poorer outcomes in organ function posttransplant. In addition to identifying a potential donor, determination of death must be made in a timely and efficient manner. The patient must be continually monitored and medically supported until death has been declared or withdrawal of medical therapies occurs. A continuum of care will exist if the family agrees to donation. During this crucial period following death until organs are recovered, the medical management of the potential pediatric organ donor requires knowledge of the physiologic derangements associated with this patient population. The donation process relies on all caregivers working to support the potential donor and family through end-of-life issues. This process is essential to maximize organ recovery from a limited population of patients.

Several ethical issues exist regarding the process of organ donation. It is important to understand these issues, because the intensivist plays a vital role in the identification of donors, in family discussions concerning organ donation consent, and in the management of organ donors and potential transplant recipients.

The ethical framework for organ donation in the United States is based on two primary principles. The first is the "dead donor rule," which explicitly states that organ removal must not be the proximate cause of death. The dead donor rule applies to both brain-dead and DCD donors. Second is the principle of autonomy, as it is applied to the potential donor and the family. The patient or the wishes of the patient's family regarding donation when the patient does not have a donor designation must be honored. The implication of this principle is that every family must be asked about their loved one's wishes—including the wishes of the parents when a minor is involved. Indeed, US legislation now mandates that patients' families be asked about organ and tissue donation at the time death occurs. The decision to donate is made in conjunction with the medical team, not by the medical team. Medical staff may no longer make subjective judgments as to which families they believe will consent to organ donation. All families must be approached in a systematic fashion that allows families the option of donation. The option for organ donation should be made available to every family. It should be the expectation that the family will be approached in a professional, compassionate manner that allows for open discussion during the most difficult, agonizing time in their lives. The AAP supports organ donation and the role of the OPO and medical team in this process (5,8).

Based on these principles, physicians and the healthcare team can be faced with complex issues caring for profoundly brain-injured children who might progress to brain death (13). The physician and healthcare team must provide the best medical care for their patients. This includes discussing the likelihood and even reality of progression to neurologic devastation with a hopeless prognosis, and even the progression to brain death. This same team of care providers must also refer such patients to the OPO in a timely manner. Increasingly, US society is exposed by public media to the issues and concepts of brain death. Nevertheless, brain death is poorly understood by not only the lay public but also the medical community (3,5). In fact, the majority of lay people believe death occurs when cardiac arrest occurs. It is very difficult for a family to believe that their child is dead when the child is warm to the touch, the cardiorespiratory monitor displays a heartbeat, the chest moves with each ventilator breath, and urine collects in the bladder catheter tubing. It is the responsibility of the pediatric intensivist caring for a neurologically devastated patient who might progress to brain death to educate the family about death. Emphasis should be placed on the death of the person, not the death of an organ. Additionally, the intensivist and healthcare team should guide the family through end-of-life issues ensuring that the patient and family are well cared for and supported during this difficult time.

The second responsibility of the physician and healthcare team, in an attempt to maximize the likelihood of organ donation, is to make an early referral to the regional OPO if progression to death appears likely. This process enables the OPO to begin the process of determining transplant eligibility. Many ICUs in the United States use clinical triggers developed in conjunction with the OPO to allow early referral to occur. A Glasgow Coma Scale score of 3–5, discussions about withdrawal of medical therapies, de-escalation of medical treatment, or resuscitation status are common triggers used by OPOs (4).

Dealing with the grieving family of a previously healthy child who is now dying can be an emotionally difficult and wrenching experience for caretakers. The medical team may harbor feelings of guilt and failure of not being able to save the life of a critically injured child. These feelings may be compounded when the caretakers are placed in the trying ethical situation of caring for a potential organ donor and a possible transplant recipient, a situation that may arise in multidisciplinary ICUs. On the other hand, caregivers can see the benefits of transplantation as organ function is restored in a patient with end-organ failure. Additionally, donation plays an important role in the healing process for grieving families knowing that some good came from the death of their loved one (2,14,15).

After the determination of brain death, this information should be conveyed to the family in a compassionate, yet clear and decisive fashion to explain that the child has died. Brain death is a medical term. Communication with families should be clear and concise using simple terms so that parents and family members understand that their child has died. Although no national law for brain death exists, it is important to clarify for the family that once death has been declared, their child meets legal criteria for death. Families may become confused or angry if discussions regarding withdrawal of support or medical therapies are entertained after declaring death. It should be made clear that once death has occurred, continuation of medical therapies, including ventilator support, is no longer an option unless organ donation is planned (2,3).

Appropriate timing regarding discussions related to consent for donation and who discusses those issues with the family are important considerations for successful donation to occur. Previous recommendations suggested separating the request for organ donation from discussions about death. This process of "decoupling" continues to occur in many ICUs and can be accomplished by a subsequent meeting with the family at which point organ donation and other postdeath issues (request for autopsy and funeral information) can be discussed. However, we continue to learn that children and their families are different. One study found that timing of the first request relative to discussions of brain death did not influence the decision to donate organs, and consent for donation was more likely when parents had sufficient time to discuss this issue (3).

Another often-raised concern is who should discuss the issue of donation with the family—the child's physician, who has an established clinical relationship with the family, or the OPO representative, who is a complete stranger to them (15). In 1998, the US Health Care Financing Administration, now the Centers for Medicare and Medicaid services, changed the Federal Conditions of Participation, mandating that hospitals notify their local OPO when a patient's death is "imminent" so that families can be approached and the option of organ and tissue donation can be discussed. The legislation was aimed at increasing rates of organ donation. Physicians perceived this as excluding them from the care and counseling of their patients, especially during such a devastating time for their patients' families. The Conditions of Participation were subsequently revised and clarified; they now require collaboration between the hospital and the OPO staff and suggest that, ideally, the OPO and hospital together decide how and by whom the family will be approached. Organ donor consent rates are highest when the families are approached jointly by members of the healthcare team and the OPO. Many parents may prefer discussions regarding donation with the pediatric intensivist or a member of the healthcare team they have come to trust, rather than just the OPO coordinator (2,16,17). This concept is vastly different from the traditional approach of the OPO coordinator requesting consent, which occurs in many adult ICUs. Additionally, family-initiated donation is becoming more common (16,18). Medical teams should be prepared to discuss donation issues with the family along with the OPO representative in these instances. A collaborative team approach has

been adopted by many institutions when discussing donation with families. This practice is encouraged in the US Department of Health and Human Services Organ Donation Collaborative final report on best practices (4,6).

Best practices promote coordinated efforts between OPO coordinators and medical professionals to improve consent rates while assisting families with end-of-life care issues. Family support from patient advocates, social workers, nurses, and physicians must remain a priority both during the dying process and after the declaration of death, when the child remains in the PICU before going to the operating room for organ removal (15). Involvement of palliative care teams has also been identified as another resource to assist the ICU team and parents, and families facing end-of-life issues with their child.

ORGAN DONATION AFTER CIRCULATORY DEATH

Organ donation from patients who have experienced "cardiac death" commonly referred to as the non–heart-beating organ donor or donation after cardiac death determination (DCD) actually began in the 1960s. DCD is the foundation of modern organ recovery preceding the practice of donation following brain death. Technologies and advancement of intensive care medicine that appeared during the 1950s and 1960s, particularly mechanical ventilation and inotropic support, meant that many patients without neurologic function and who would have died were able to be resuscitated and kept alive. It was realized that such severely brain-injured patients often progressed to brain death and that intensive care management of these brain-dead patients allowed for adequate perfusion of organs (kidney, liver, heart, lungs, intestine, and pancreas) for potential organ procurement. The improved quality of organs recovered from brain-dead donors led to a significant reduction in interest in DCD organ recovery.

Resurgence of interest in DCD occurred in 1997, with the Executive Summary of the IOM on "Non–Heart-Beating Organ Transplantation: Medical and Ethical Issues in Procurement." This report was prompted by the imbalance between the number of potential organ donors and the number of those awaiting transplantation, and reflected an effort to explore other options to expand the donor pool (11). The expression of family autonomy in demanding that institutions abide by their wishes to donate the organs of their neurologically devastated but not brain-dead family members also stimulated medical institutions to develop policies for DCD donation. "Organ donation after cardiac or circulatory death" has currently replaced the phrase "non–heart-beating organ donation" used in the initial IOM report and is discussed in detail in the 2006 IOM report as well (11,12,19). DCD refers to the donation of organs (usually kidneys and, less frequently, liver, pancreas, and lungs) from organ donors who have been declared dead on the basis of cardiorespiratory criteria; that is, a documented cessation of both cardiac and respiratory function. Cardiac transplantation, while rare, has occurred using organs from DCD donors (16,20–22).

Two main categories of DCD have been subsequently described: (a) uncontrolled DCD and (b) controlled DCD. In uncontrolled DCD, known formerly as Maastricht type II organ donor, death is declared after attempted resuscitation. This most often occurs in an emergency department. Organs, usually only kidneys, are rapidly removed for transplantation after determination of death. This mode of organ recovery was the primary way cadaveric organs were obtained before 1968, when brain death was defined and began to be accepted as a legal definition of death. Uncontrolled DCD donation is currently not practiced in the United States, although it is used as a mode of obtaining donor organs in other countries in which DBD and controlled DCD are not widely accepted (21,22). The single uncontrolled DCD study in the United States unfortunately failed to recruit any patients (23). Controlled DCD, formerly known as Maastricht type III, is, on the other hand, becoming an increasingly common mode for obtaining organs for donation and will be the mode of DCD donation referred to in the remainder of this chapter.

DCD remains a highly charged topic with ethical challenges for some in the medical community (11,12,18,19,22). Many of the ethical concerns related to DCD surround the exact timing of death for the donor and potential violation of the dead donor rule. The dead donor rule is based on ethical standards that govern the recovery and transplantation of organs. The dead donor rules state that (a) vital organs should be taken only from dead patients and (b) living patients should not be killed for or by organ procurement. Additionally, lack of a standardization to determine death in this group of patients has contributed to some of the ethical concerns with this type of donation (11,12,18,19,22). A detailed discussion about these controversies is beyond the scope of this chapter, but it is important to note that DCD donation has been extensively reviewed by many medical oversight committees and national organizations, including the AAP (5,20,21,22,24). The AAP also recognizes these ethical challenges, which are outlined in an ethical considerations publication (5).

Candidates

Patients who may qualify as DCD donors are those for whom the decision has been made to withdraw life-sustaining therapy (mechanical ventilation and vasopressor support). Most of the children who undergo DCD have sustained a profound, irreversible neurologic injury (head injury, hypoxic ischemic encephalopathy, or stroke), but do not meet the criteria for brain death. Some children may have other single-organ, noncerebral neurologic disease, or life-threatening medical problems from which they will not recover, such as respiratory failure secondary to progressive spinal muscular atrophy or dependence on extracorporeal membrane oxygenation for irreversible cardiac or respiratory failure.

Process

The decision to withdraw medical therapy is based on consideration of the patient's and surrogate's wishes, the prognosis, the burden and benefits of continued therapy, issues of futility of future medical treatment, and goals of care. This decision to withdraw life-sustaining medical therapies must be made completely independent to the discussion regarding organ donation. This ensures the absence of any coercion and appearance or perception that the healthcare team is withdrawing life-sustaining therapy and hastening death to obtain organs. This sequence of events during the process of any donation can potentially present ethical challenges for the staff in a multidisciplinary ICU. Staff who may be caring for potential organ recipient may also be responsible for the care of children who may become organ donors. Indeed, some intensivists, in an effort to avoid the perception that life-sustaining therapy has been withdrawn to obtain organs, feel the care of the dying child and the discussion about organ donation should not be carried out by the same physician who might be involved with the care of an organ recipient. Involving other physicians to participate in this process may be logistically difficult. Palliative care physicians and teams may be of benefit in these situations. To further ensure the integrity of the DCD process, some institutions have mandated a formal ethics committee

consultation. To address these ethical issues, the IOM published criteria that should be followed by hospitals that desire to implement DCD. All OPOs should discuss the option of DCD with local hospitals, healthcare professionals, and the community, and a protocol should be in place for DCD to occur. Importantly, organ procurement must not hasten death, and the entire process of donation should focus on ensuring that the patient and family are comfortable as they face end-of-life issues (4,20).

Prior to approaching the family about any type of organ donation opportunity, the local OPO must be notified, and the child should be evaluated for donor suitability. It is devastating for a family to be approached for organ donation and to give consent only later to discover that the child is not an appropriate donor candidate.

The process of controlled DCD differs in some important ways from DBD. These differences must be carefully explained to the donor's family. The withdrawal of life-sustaining therapies from a DCD donor involves the cessation of vasopressors and mechanical ventilation, through either disconnecting the ventilator or extubation. This process can occur in the ICU, the operating room, or an adjacent holding room. Withdrawal in the ICU requires transport time to the operating room, which can prolong organ ischemia and must be taken into consideration for DCD. However, the location of the withdrawal of medical therapies should ensure the comfort of the donor and the family. Family members, if they desire, should be permitted to remain with the patient until the onset of mechanical asystole (pulselessness or loss of pulse pressure) occurs. The family will be escorted out of the operating suite or the patient will be separated from the family and taken to the operating suite where preparation begins for organ recovery. Death is declared, usually after an interval of 2–5 minutes of observation to ensure that autoresuscitation (return of spontaneous circulation) does not occur. Death is declared following this observation period, and organ recovery can be initiated. Regardless of the location of withdrawal of life-sustaining therapy, support for the family must continue to be provided by the ICU medical team, family advocates, clergy, and other support staff. Appropriate comfort care and symptom management must remain a priority for the dying patient. Most extrarenal organs successfully recovered for transplantation are from DCD donors who had relatively short warm ischemic times.

Implicit in DCD is the necessity to accurately determine death prior to organ recovery (the "dead donor" rule). The determination of death by cardiorespiratory criteria necessitates determination of *irreversible cessation* of cardiorespiratory function (21,22,24). Cessation of respiratory function is determined by the absence of breathing. Cessation of circulatory activity is determined by the absence of antegrade circulation (mechanical asystole). Electrical activity of the heart is needed to generate contractile activity required for the heart to generate circulation. Detecting electrical activity of the heart is not an indication of contractility. Electrical activity may persist in the absence of circulation. The absence of circulation as a result of a lack of ventricular ejection can be demonstrated by the absence of pulsatility on an arterial waveform tracing or by echocardiographic Doppler flow study. Although the 1997 IOM report suggested that asystole be present, the definitive criteria for death is absent circulation, documented by lack of cardiac ejection resulting in antegrade flow. The issue of "irreversibility" in the definition of cardiorespiratory criteria for death of the DCD donor is addressed by closely monitoring the patient for a period of time to ensure that autoresuscitation does not occur. Autoresuscitation is the phenomenon of spontaneous restoration of circulation following a period of absent circulation. The Society of Critical Care Medicine has recommended that "at least 2 minutes of observation is required and >5 minutes is not recommended (21)." Most institutions use a

5-minute observation period with documented absence of circulation (6,20). If the patient autoresuscitates, the observation time starts again and requires a period of 2–5 minutes from that point to determine death.

Another issue that must be explained to donor families is the maximal time window for natural death to occur after withdrawal of life-supporting therapies. Most transplant centers will only accept organs from a DCD donor if the patient dies within 1 hour following discontinuation of life-sustaining therapies. Most centers will only accept a liver from a DCD donor if death occurs within 30 minutes. Longer time periods exceeding 60 minutes may be considered for kidney donation. It must be explained to the family that if death does not ensue within the established time period, their loved one will be returned to the ICU or other patient care area for continuation of comfort care.

To avoid creating false hope for families that their loved one will become an organ donor, the option of DCD should only be offered for patients who, in the best judgment of their physicians, will die within the specified time period following discontinuation of life-sustaining therapies. It is often difficult to ascertain with complete certainty that this will occur. Investigators at the University of Wisconsin developed an adult scoring system that assists in predicting the likelihood that potential DCD donor will die within 60–120 minutes following withdrawal of life-sustaining therapies; other groups have modified this tool for neurocritical care patients (25). This evaluation tool is based on the patient's age, body mass index, oxygen saturation level, level of spontaneous ventilation, requirement and dosage of vasopressors, and mechanical ventilation indices. Based on the Wisconsin tool, an accurate prediction of death within 1–2 hours after extubation was achieved in >90% of patients (26). UNOS has also developed a set of criteria to aid in identifying those patients who may become DCD candidates. A recent publication outlined the development of a bedside tool to predict time to death after withdrawal of life-sustaining therapies in children (27). This predictive tool for pediatric patients provides the bedside caregiver with information that seems to predict time to death fairly accurately in 87% of the patient studied.

The administration of drugs to the DCD organ donor that can potentially reduce ischemia–reperfusion injury to the transplanted organs has generated some ethical concern in the medical community. Clinical and experimental evidence supports the use of premortem administration of heparin for its protective effect on vascular endothelium and preventing thrombosis in the donor organs. Administration of heparin does improve the function of organs removed from DCD donors. Phentolamine, an α-blocker vasodilator, is also used by some OPOs to improve the quality of the donated organs. The ethical concern surrounding the administration of these drugs is that no benefit accrues to the donor. Some believe that these drugs may be harmful and perhaps even hasten death of the donor by causing bleeding or hypotension, in the case of heparin and phentolamine, respectively. A recent consensus report of a national conference on DCD extensively reviewed available literature and stated that no evidence exists that heparin causes bleeding of a magnitude that will hasten death after the withdrawal of life-sustaining therapy. It is recommended that heparin be administered to the organ donor following withdrawal but only after consent for administration has been obtained from the family. The indications for the use of phentolamine and antioxidants (e.g., N-acetyl cysteine and vitamin E) are not clear, and their use varies by individual OPO and hospital DCD policies (22,24).

The organization of DCD requires extensive coordination that may take as long as 24–48 hours. This waiting period can be difficult for any family. The process must be carefully and sensitively explained to families so that they can understand and prepare for donation to occur.

Organs that have been successfully transplanted after DCD donation include kidneys, livers, pancreata, lungs, and even hearts in a few cases. DCD heart transplants have been performed under a clinical trial, and there were no late deaths for these patients as of 2008 (16).

As many potential DCD candidates have significant neurologic injury but do not meet criteria for brain death, OPO representatives will often discuss and consent for both DBD and DCD, in the event that the patient progresses to brain death during the period of evaluation.

EVALUATION OF DONOR ELIGIBILITY

No tests specific to organ donation, such as viral serologic tests or tissue typing, should be obtained from a patient prior to obtaining family consent for donation; this applies in cases of both DBD and DCD. Once consent has been obtained, serologic evaluation includes testing for human immunodeficiency virus (HIV), human T-cell lymphotrophic virus (HTLV), venereal disease (VDRL test), cytomegalovirus (CMV), as well as hepatitis B core antibody, hepatitis B surface antigen, and hepatitis C antibody. Liver and renal function tests are usually already available. Blood, urine, and sputum cultures should be obtained from each potential donor.

Two-dimensional echocardiography is helpful to assess intra-cardiac filling and contractility and can be performed serially to reevaluate the effects of management. Bronchoscopy is often required to assess anatomic variations and injuries to each lung. Other evaluations and laboratory tests to be performed can be found in the UNOS Critical Pathway for the Pediatric Organ Donor (https://www.unos.org/docs/Critical_Pathway_Pediatric.pdf).

Contraindications to Organ Donation

Relatively few absolute contraindications exist to organ donation. The ultimate decision concerning whether an organ should be recovered for transplantation rests with the OPO medical director and transplant surgeon. Most OPOs will consider the following conditions as contraindications to organ donation:

- Active CMV infection
- Rabies
- Active West Nile virus infection
- Uncontrolled metastatic cancer
- Prion protein illness (Creutzfeldt–Jakob disease)
- Acute disseminated tuberculosis

HIV, hepatitis C, and hepatitis B are now only relative contraindications because of programs allowing seropositive organ donation to seropositive recipients.

Presumed organ damage or ischemia is the most common contraindication for donation. The decision on organ suitability is based on information gathered by the OPO and intensive care team, as well as visual inspection of the organ at the time of procurement. The surgeon and the transplant team must decide if the risks to the potential recipient of continuing to wait for a transplant outweigh the risks of transplantation with a "less-than-ideal" organ. This approach has been encompassed in one of the "best practice" principles adopted by organized groups of transplant hospitals and OPOs (known collectively as organ transplant breakthrough collaboratives) and is known as the "rule-in" philosophy: "Refer and evaluate every donor, every time," regardless of the medical status of the donor (4,6,28). The importance of this philosophy is based on a less-than-ideal organ may prevent death or provide a bridge to a better organ for a patient who may not survive until an ideal organ becomes available. The goals of the collaboratives are discussed later in this chapter.

Infections

Untreated, overwhelming sepsis usually precludes organ donation, but bacteremia and fungemia are not absolute contraindications. Although aggressive treatment of infections is critical in donors, recipient outcomes do not significantly differ between infected and noninfected donors. Furthermore, organ donation can often proceed with treatment of bacterial sepsis and bacterial meningitis after 24 hours of appropriate antibiotics.

Potential organ donors infected with hepatitis B or C may be eligible to donate organs to those individuals infected with the same virus. Patients with HIV infection are living longer lives due to the efficacy of protease inhibitors. However, transplantation from HIV-positive donors is currently contraindicated, although the HIV Organ Policy Equity (HOPE) Act bill was passed in the full Senate and House of Representatives. This bill would allow organ transplantation from HIV-positive donors to HIV-positive recipients and possibly result in an additional 1000 organs for those on the waiting list. Regardless, all patients should be referred to the OPO for discussion with the transplant team to determine suitability for donation.

The CMV status of the donor and recipient is extremely important. The risk of infection in the immunosuppressed recipient is high. Those patients with a negative CMV status can become infected with CMV if they receive an organ from a CMV-positive donor. Ganciclovir prophylaxis of CMV-negative recipients who receive organs from CMV-positive donors has greatly reduced the morbidity and mortality associated with CMV infection in these patients.

Malignancies

Most active malignancies represent a contraindication to donation. There are exceptions, such as some low-grade brain tumors and nonmelanomatous skin cancer. The malignancies most frequently encountered in the pediatric patient are leukemia, lymphoma, and often high-grade brain tumors. These malignancies create a barrier to donation because they have a potential high rate of recurrence in recipients. However, candidates with brain tumors without metastasis may be eligible to donate organs. Controversy exists regarding the "safe" period of cancer-free time (remission or cure) that potential donors must demonstrate before becoming eligible donors.

Medical Examiner Cases

Annually, nearly 200 potential deceased donors are prevented from donating viable organs by coroners or medical examiners. These denials for donation translate into a loss of several hundred potential organs for transplantation. Due in part to the growing organ waiting list and the shortage of organs, as well as to the heroic efforts of the organ transplant breakthrough collaboratives, the National Association of Medical Examiners has adopted a goal of "zero denials" for potential donor cases referred to them (29).

Even though many pediatric patients who die from causes with legal implications, such as motor vehicle accidents or child abuse, must be referred to the medical examiner for autopsy, donation can successfully occur in these cases. An autopsy does not preclude organ donation. Visual inspection of the body and organs, complemented by medical photography by the medical examiner, who can potentially even be present

in the operating room prior to organ removal, provides sufficient legal evidence. Close cooperation between forensic investigators, treating physicians, the transplant team, and the OPO can facilitate organ recovery in these cases and decrease denials for donation.

PHYSIOLOGIC CONSIDERATIONS AND MEDICAL MANAGEMENT OF THE PEDIATRIC ORGAN DONOR

Physicians caring for eligible organ donors following brain death must work together as a team with the OPO coordinator, ICU nurses, respiratory therapists, clergy, social workers, family advocates, and medical examiners (in some cases) to optimize therapy and maintain the viability of potential donor organs. Many OPOs and ICUs utilize standardized donor management protocols. These protocols have been adopted from the UNOS Critical Pathway for the Organ Donor. Separate pathways exist for adult (27) and pediatric donors (https://www.unos.org/docs/Critical_Pathway_Pediatric.pdf).

General

To effectively manage pediatric organ donors, an intensivist must be able to anticipate and recognize the multitude of physiologic derangements that occur during severe brain injury and progression to brain death (**Figs. 16.1** and **16.2**).

Hemodynamic changes occur in brain-dead patients that ultimately affect the potential suitability of transplantable organs. The severity of these changes is related to the time course of progression of the brain injury. More rapid increases in elevated intracranial pressure (ICP) and subsequent brain death often result in more extensive pathophysiologic changes (30,31).

Although the physiologic changes that occur with brain death have been extensively studied, the interactions and mechanisms that underlie this process remain incompletely understood. The classic studies from Novitzky and colleagues in the 1980s used a baboon model of brain death. These studies have provided important information about this complex physiologic process. In these experimental animal models, as progressive elevation of ICP developed prior to brain death, cerebral ischemia occurred in a craniocaudal direction. Brainstem ischemia resulted in vagal activation with resultant bradycardia. As the ischemia progressed involving the pons, the well-described Cushing response occurred with hypertension (due to sympathetic stimulation) and bradycardia (due to continued vagal stimulation). Progressive ischemia of the vagal nucleus in the medulla oblongata resulted in cessation of function with uncontrolled sympathetic stimulation commonly referred to as "catecholamine storm" (17,30,32,33). The catecholamine storm is a period of intense vasoconstriction, systemic hypertension, tachycardia, and resultant tissue ischemia. An increase in pulmonary vascular resistance can occur as well. The duration and severity of this catecholamine storm varies and may be related to how rapidly brain death progresses. Pituitary hormone depletion often accompanies this storm, associated with ischemia of the anterior and posterior pituitary.

At a cellular level, elevated catecholamine levels lead to activation of second-messenger systems. This results in accumulation of intracellular calcium. Elevated intracellular calcium activates proteases, lipases, endonucleases, oxygen reactive species, and free radicals, which culminates in mitochondrial dysfunction, DNA injury, and cell death, thus affecting cells in all organs. The loss of high-energy phosphates upon cell

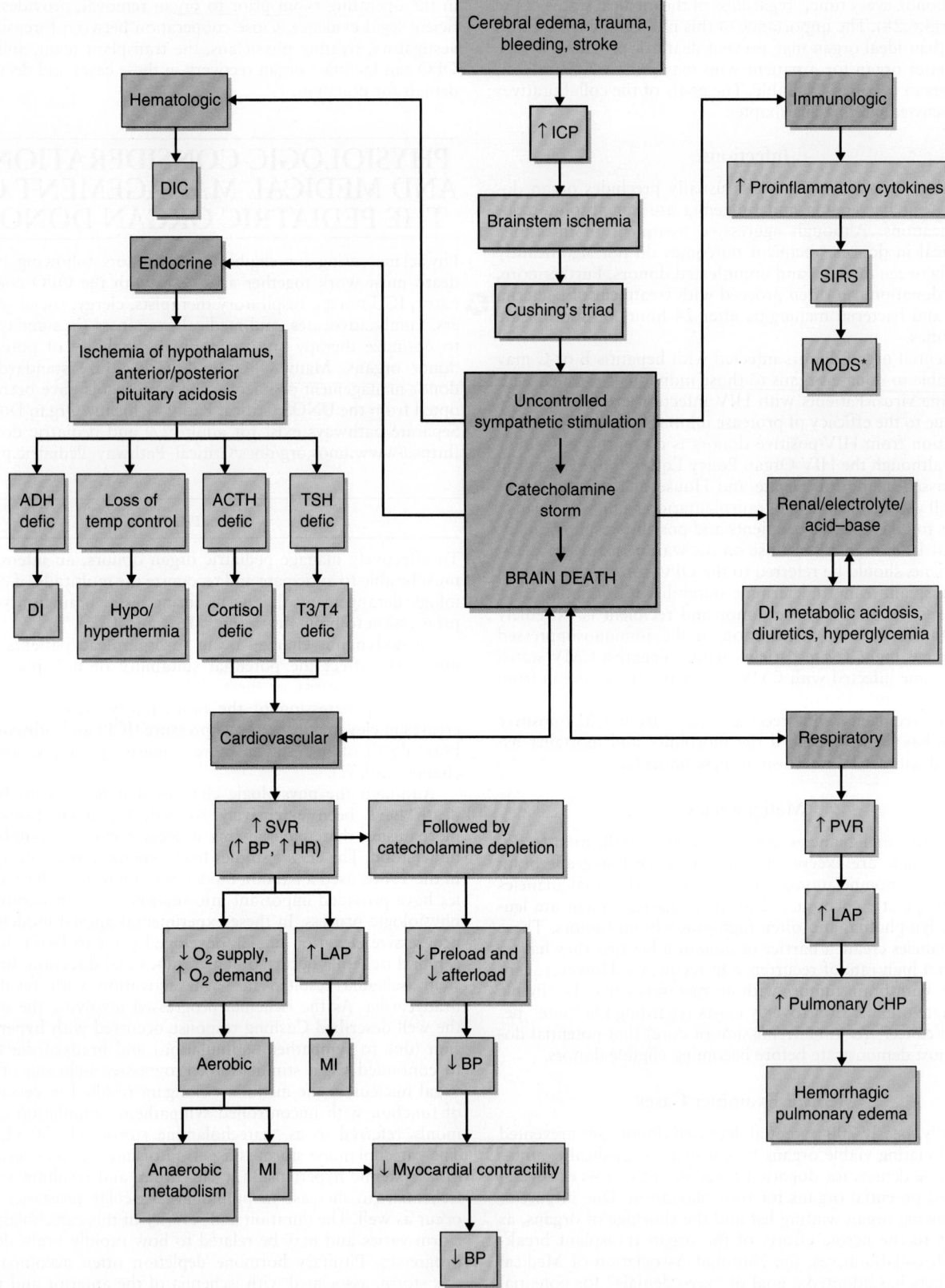

FIGURE 16.1. Physiologic events associated with brain death. Brain death has physiologic consequences for multiple organ systems that translate to complex medical management. DIC, disseminated intravascular coagulopathy;
MODS, multiple organ dysfunction syndrome; ACTH, adrenocorticotropic hormone; ADH, antidiuretic hormone;
BP, blood pressure; HR, heart rate; LAP, left atrial pressure; MI, myocardial ischemia; PVR, peripheral vascular
resistance; CHP, capillary hydrostatic pressure. *The systemic inflammatory response elicited by brain death may
ultimately contribute to organ dysfunction in the heart, lungs, kidneys, and liver.

A. Cardiovascular, Fluid/Electrolyte, and Hematologic Abnormalities
1. Assess blood pressure, heart rate, peripheral perfusion, urine output
2. Maintain normothermia
3. Obtain labs (CMP with Mg, Phos, CBC, PT/INR, PTT, FBG, ABG, cardiac enzymes)
4. Hemodynamic, fluid resuscitation, and hematologic goals

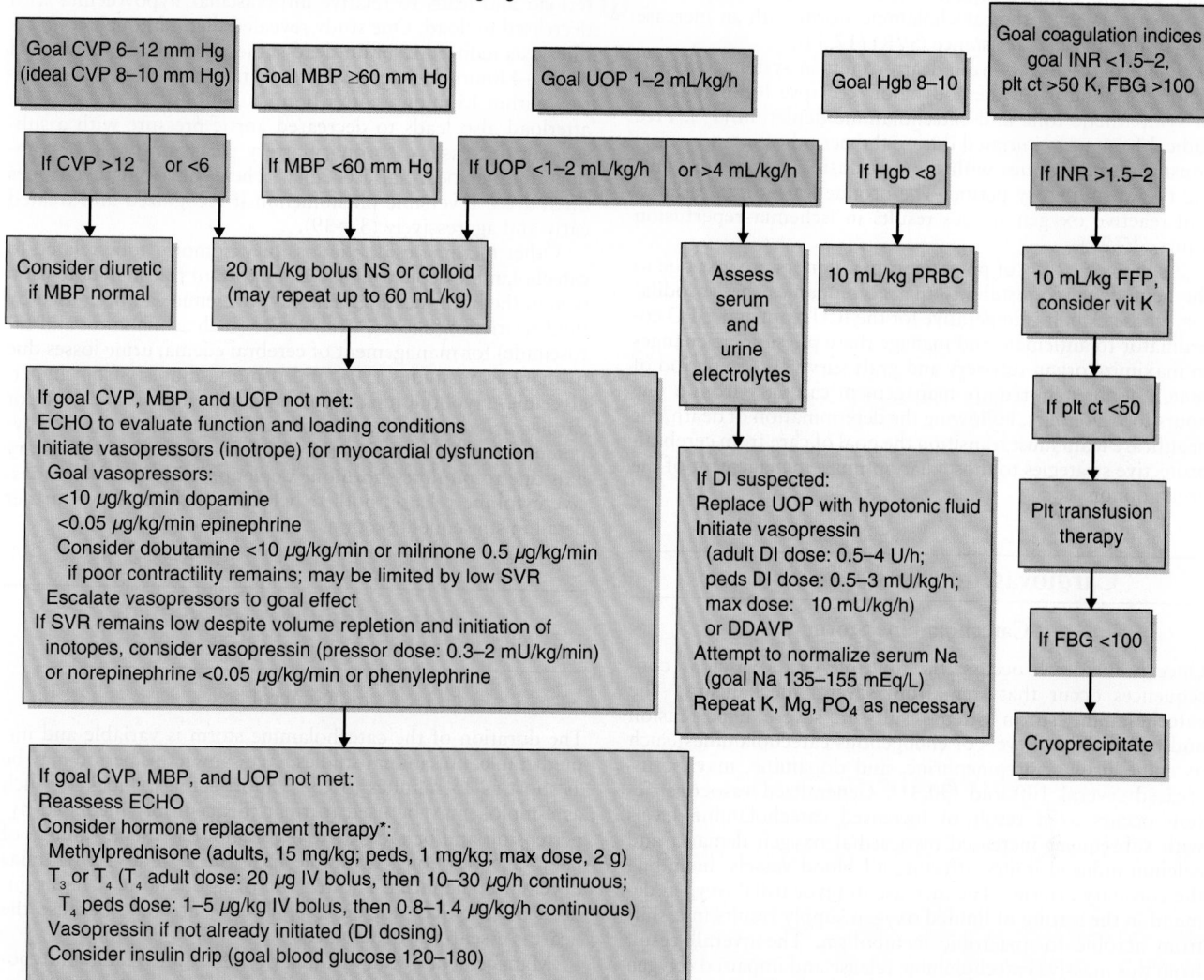

B. Respiratory Abnormality (multifactorial)
1. Mechanical ventilation goals
    a. FIO_2 40%
    b. PEEP 5 cm H_2O
    c. Peak inspiratory pressure or plateau pressure <30–35 mm Hg
    d. Tidal volume (if volume control) 8–10 mL/kg; 6–8 mL/kg if ARDS
    e. Normal pH and $PaCO_2$
    f. PaO_2 >100 or sats >95%, $PaO_2{:}FIO_2$ ratio >300
2. Evaluate anatomy, injury, infection with bronchoscopy and serial chest x-ray if needed
    a. Obtain sputum for Gram stain, culture
3. Hypoxia or other injury (contusion, edema, pneumonia)
    a. Mechanical ventilation adjustment (i.e., increase FIO_2, PEEP)
    b. Consider diuretics if pulmonary edema noted if MBP normal, especially if CVP >8
    c. Consider methylprednisone if not previously administered
    d. Consider naloxone 8 mg IV

FIGURE 16.2. The management of the potential pediatric organ donor is often complex and involves frequent reassessment and adjustments in care. Management of these patients should be done in conjunction with the local OPO. CMP, comprehensive metabolic panel; UOP, urine output; CVP, central venous pressure; Hgb, hemoglobin; INR, international normalized ratio; plt, platelet; FBG, fibrinogen; MBP, mean blood pressure; NS, normal saline; PRBC, packed red blood cells; FFP, frozen fresh plasma; DDAVP, 1-deamino-8-D-arginine vasopressin; ARDS, acute respiratory distress syndrome; PEEP, positive end-expiratory pressure. *Some institutions and OPOs may institute HRT earlier.

death results in decreased production of adenosine triphosphate (ATP). Without the necessary energy provided by ATP for ion channel regulation, the sarcoplasmic reticulum cannot take up or release cytosolic calcium, perpetuating the intracellular calcium–induced injury. This calcium-related injury occurs at the peak of the catecholamine storm with an increase in systemic vascular resistance (SVR) (17,33).

The progression to brain death results in systemic vasodilation, culminating in hemodynamic collapse following loss of sympathetic tone and catecholamine depletion (17). Free radical formation initiated during the period of intense vasoconstriction continues with the reperfusion that occurs during this vasodilatory period. The production of free radicals and reactive oxygen species results in ischemia–reperfusion injury (17,27).

As many as 25% of potential organ donors are lost due to the hemodynamic instability that accompanies this vasodilatory phase (10). It is imperative for the ICU team and OPO coordinator to anticipate and manage these physiologic changes to maximize organ recovery and graft survival. The period of time a donor may require management can vary from a few hours to >24 hours. Following the determination of death, the healthcare team must transition the goal of care from cerebral-protective strategies to those that optimize management of the organ donor.

Cardiovascular Pathophysiology

Catecholamine Storm

Once brain death occurs, the multiple cardiovascular consequences occur that stem from several mechanisms. The catecholamine storm often results in severe hypertension and tachycardia. Levels of endogenous catecholamines, such as epinephrine, norepinephrine, and dopamine, may be increased several 100-fold (30,31). Generalized vasoconstriction occurs as a result of increased catecholamine levels with subsequent increased myocardial oxygen demand and calcium-induced injury affecting all blood vessels, including the coronary arteries. The increase in myocardial oxygen demand in the setting of limited oxygen supply results in a shift from aerobic to anaerobic metabolism. The overall result from this massive catecholamine release and impaired oxygen balance is subendocardial ischemia, which may be reflected by electrocardiographic changes. Ischemic changes are predominantly seen in the left ventricle, resulting in decreased left ventricular cardiac output (CO), despite the increase in contractility induced by the catecholamine storm (34). At the point of maximal SVR, an imbalance in CO occurs with right ventricular CO now exceeding left ventricular CO. The effect of this imbalance is an accumulation of blood in the lungs resulting in significant elevation of left atrial pressure that temporarily exceeds mean pulmonary artery pressure. This contributes to the formation of neurogenic pulmonary edema (discussed later) (35). Subendocardial ischemia affects the papillary muscles resulting in mitral insufficiency and further increases left atrial pressure.

Although the shift to anaerobic metabolism is in large part due to significant ischemia with lack of energy stores, it may also be due in part to relative thyroid deficiency, which is discussed in more detail later. The final result of this shift to anaerobic metabolism often manifests as decreased contractility, usually within a few hours after brain death has occurred (30,34).

Cardiac arrhythmias may also occur due to necrosis of the conduction system or an irritable myocardium as a result of ischemia during the catecholamine storm. Bradyarrhythmias and supraventricular and ventricular arrhythmias have all been documented (30,31,34).

Generalized Vasodilation

Hypotension is the most common problem encountered by physicians caring for pediatric organ donors. Loss of sympathetic vasomotor tone results in a dramatic decrease in afterload and leads to relative intravascular hypovolemia with decreased preload. One study revealed that, although contractility was reduced in brain-dead subjects, this event developed over 3–4 hours despite the decrease in SVR or afterload occurring within 15 minutes after brain death (36). The decrease in afterload also leads to decreased aortic pressure with a subsequent decrease in coronary artery perfusion pressure compounding myocardial ischemia. These physiologic changes often are a reversible phenomenon if recognized and treated early and aggressively (37–39).

Other factors beside the loss of vasomotor tone related to catecholamine depletion play an important role in hypotension seen in the brain-dead patient. Hypovolemia can be caused by fluid restriction, the use of diuretics (such as mannitol and furosemide) for management of cerebral edema, urine losses due to diabetes insipidus (DI), and osmotic diuresis from hyperglycemia. Hypothermia, occurring after either brain death or cardiac arrest, may also induce a diuresis. Other causes of hypotension include dysfunction of the hypothalamic–pituitary axis due to pituitary hormone depletion and potentially massive cytokine release, both of which are discussed in further detail in subsequent sections.

Evaluation and Management of Cardiovascular Abnormalities

General

The duration of the catecholamine storm is variable and unpredictable, but animal studies have shown this period may be as short as 15 minutes (30,34). Short-acting β-blockers, such as esmolol, may be used to treat this centrally mediated hypertension and/or tachycardia. Esmolol has the advantage of being a continuous, titratable infusion. If bradyarrhythmias develop, epinephrine is often the drug of choice. The brain-dead patient may not be responsive to atropine because the heart is essentially denervated.

Management of the vasodilatory phase and resultant hypotension requires aggressive medical management to restore circulating volume and maintain CO (Table 16.1). Initial therapy consists of restoring intravascular volume followed, if necessary, by vasopressor therapy. In many instances, volume and vasopressor therapy are instituted simultaneously. Assessment and maintenance of adequate intravascular volume can be difficult in brain-dead patients. Central venous pressure (CVP) measurement can provide helpful information. Optimal CVP is often between 8 and 10 mm Hg. Higher CVP measurements have been associated with increases in the arterial–alveolar gradient and hypoxia that can potentially affect the recovery and transplantability of lungs from the organ donor (37,40). On the other hand, a CVP of <8 mm Hg may adversely affect recovery and graft function of liver and kidneys, which require higher arterial pressures for adequate perfusion (9).

Even in cases of poor myocardial contractility, volume infusion is often initially indicated, because the decreased contractility may be secondary to diminished preload. CVP monitoring and serial ECHOs may be helpful to evaluate preload, afterload, and contractility. The choice of fluids for intravascular volume expansion includes isotonic crystalloid solutions (normal saline) or colloid solutions (5% albumin). Packed red blood cell transfusions may be indicated if the hematocrit is <25%–30% and the donor is hemodynamically unstable, or <21% if hemodynamically stable. Use of synthetic colloids

TABLE 16.1

TREATMENT CHOICES FOR MAINTAINING MEAN ARTERIAL PRESSURE IN THE PEDIATRIC ORGAN DONOR

■ HEMODYNAMICALLY STABLE	■ HEMODYNAMICALLY UNSTABLE
Methylprednisolone	Volume loading with crystalloid or colloid
Levothyroxine or T_3	Inotropic support (dopamine, epinephrine, phenylephrine, norepinephrine)
Desmopressin or vasopressin	Methylprednisolone
	Levothyroxine or T_3
	Desmopressin or vasopressin

should be avoided since these agents may precipitate or exacerbate renal insufficiency (9,41) and hypoglycemia.

If hypotension persists despite volume replacement, evaluation of cardiac function and initiation of inotropic therapy are indicated. ECHO is the best clinically available method for imaging a potential heart donor and may be performed at the bedside by either transthoracic or transesophageal routes. If ventricular ejection fraction is <45%, or if regional wall motion abnormalities are seen, aggressive cardiac resuscitation may be needed before such a heart is suitable for transplantation. Correction of alterations in preload, afterload, and factors, such as acidosis, hypoxia, hypercarbia, electrolyte abnormalities, anemia, dehydration, and/or overhydration, are essential. Correcting these factors may improve myocardial performance and suitability for transplantation (25,37). Most acute deaths following cardiac transplantation in the recipient are caused by right ventricular failure as a result of elevated pulmonary vascular resistance or decreased contractility of the donor graft. Treatment of impaired contractility in the donor may improve right ventricular failure and prolong the graft life in the recipient. An electrocardiogram should also be obtained in the cardiac assessment to determine potential myocardial injury. Serial ECHOs should be performed to evaluate improvement in cardiac function as treatment progresses and correction of the above-mentioned adverse conditions is reversed. In a study performed by the California Transplant Donor Network, 16 donor patients whose hearts had been declined by regional transplant centers based on initial ECHO findings underwent repeat ECHOs after optimizing loading and metabolic conditions, including infusion of IV steroids within 10 hours after the initial cardiac ECHO. Improvement in left ventricular ejection fraction was noted on follow-up ECHO, and 12 of the 16 donor hearts were successfully transplanted. Survival rate was 92% at an average follow-up of 16 months (25).

Vasopressors

The use of vasopressor agents to maintain blood pressure and improve cardiac function in organ donors is often required after adequate intravascular volume replacement (Table 16.2). Vasopressor use is indicated if myocardial dysfunction is present, or to increase SVR in cases of severe vasodilation. Dopamine has been the vasopressor most commonly used in pediatric organ donors, because renal and splanchnic blood flow can often be maintained at dosages of <10 μg/kg/min.

TABLE 16.2

PEDIATRIC DONOR MANAGEMENT ALGORITHM FOR HEMODYNAMIC SUPPORT

■ HEMODYNAMIC SUPPORT		BLOOD PRESSURE	
		■ SYSTOLIC	■ DIASTOLIC
■ Normalization of blood pressure	Neonate	60–90	35–60
■ Systolic BP (SBP) appropriate for age	Infants (6 mo)	80–95	50–65
■ Normal SBP = 80 × 2 (age in years)	Toddler (2 y)	85–100	50–65
■ Note: Lower SBP may be acceptable if biomarkers,	School age (7 y)	90–115	60–70
such as lactate, are normal	Adolescent (15 y)	110–130	65–80
■ CVP < 12 (if measured)			
■ Dopamine < 10 μg/kg/min			
■ Normal serum lactate			

■ OXYGENATION AND VENTILATION	■ FLUIDS AND ELECTROLYTES	
■ Maintain Pao_2 >100 mm Hg	Serum Na	130–150 mEq/L
■ Fio_2 0.40	Serum K	3.0–5.0 mEq/L
■ Normalize $Paco_2$ 35–45 mm Hg	Serum glucose	60–150 mEq/L
■ Arterial pH 7.30–7.45	Ionized Ca	0.8–1.2 mmol/L
■ Tidal volumes 8–10 mL/kg		(if decreased cardiac contractility,
■ PEEP 5 cm H_2O		aim for level 1.2)

■ THERMAL REGULATION
Core body temperature 36°C–38°C

Adapted from Nakagawa TA. http://www.natco1.org/Professional-Development/documents/NATCOpeddonormanagementguidelines.pdf

Low-dose epinephrine or norepinephrine (≤ 0.05 μg/kg/min) may be instituted as second-line inotropes. Catecholamines and dopamine appear to have immunomodulating effects that may help blunt the inflammatory response associated with brain death and may improve kidney graft function (27,42).

Another case-controlled study of kidney transplant recipients found a significant decrease in rejection and increase in graft survival in donors who were treated with catecholamines, compared with those who were not (27). Catecholamines have also been shown to downregulate adhesion molecules, which may at least partially explain some of the positive effects seen with catecholamine administration. Adhesion molecules are postulated to play an important adverse role in recipient rejection of transplanted organs. However, administration of exogenous catecholamines with both α- and β-agonist action (such as dopamine, epinephrine, and norepinephrine) may further deplete myocardial ATP stores and downregulate β-receptors. This may adversely affect posttransplant cardiac function in the recipient (32,42). Norepinephrine use in the donor has been shown to be associated with increased post–renal transplant acute tubular necrosis and continued dialysis requirements in recipients. Norepinephrine has also been associated with reduced myocardial function after cardiac transplantation, but its use does not appear to compromise transplanted livers (43,44). In contrast, epinephrine in modest doses has been shown in animal models to maintain renal perfusion while simultaneously improving cardiac function.

Patients who have experienced significant or prolonged hypotension, hypoxia, and/or ischemia are at particular risk for myocardial dysfunction that may require additional inotropic therapy. Dobutamine, a pure β-agonist, may be needed in such cases. However, peripheral vasodilation may limit its use in these patients due to diminished SVR. Furthermore, β-receptor downregulation may occur in these patients making dobutamine less effective. Although evidence for use is lacking, milrinone, a phosphodiesterase inhibitor, may be instituted in cases where dobutamine is not tolerated but cardiac dysfunction exists. This inodilator is more commonly used in pediatric patients with myocardial dysfunction.

The prolonged use of catecholamine vasopressor agents, especially in high doses, has been inconsistently associated with poor or delayed organ function and survival precluding the viability of some organs for transplantation. Transplant centers often consider a donor heart to be unsuitable for transplantation if the vasopressor requirement is significant. However, a retrospective study (in over 2400 transplanted kidneys) that evaluated the effect of donor catecholamine use on graft survival revealed a beneficial effect of donor catecholamine administration on the 4-year renal graft survival ($>75\%$) (42).

Despite volume replacement and inotropic therapy, some patients may continue to have hypotension associated with severe vasodilation and reduced SVR. Agents with pure α-agonist function, such as phenylephrine or norepinephrine, may be required in such cases. However, the vasoconstriction associated with α-adrenergic agents may compromise the perfusion of potential donor organs, particularly the kidneys, liver, and heart. Lower doses of vasopressors may be used if biomarkers, such as serum lactate and systemic venous oxygenation, indicate adequate CO and perfusion to tissues.

The use of vasopressin in the setting of hemodynamic instability associated with vasodilation and low SVR has received increased attention. Vasopressin is used to control DI through its effect on the V_1 receptor in the brain-dead organ donor. Vasopressin stimulation of the V_2 receptor causes vasoconstrictor effects. A defect in the baroreceptor reflex-mediated secretion of vasopressin from the posterior pituitary results in brain-dead patients developing exquisite sensitivity to the vasoconstrictive effects of vasopressin, even without the presence of DI. The attraction of vasopressin as a pressor lies in its ability to act synergistically with catecholamines, often resulting in a much-reduced need for catecholamines (45,46). In a retrospective review of critically ill children undergoing evaluation for brain death and potential organ recovery, those children who had been treated with vasopressin were seven times more likely to be weaned from α-agonist vasopressors, compared to age-matched controls. Furthermore, graft function of transplanted livers, kidneys, and hearts was acceptable and not sufficiently different in the vasopressin-treated group (47). Good graft function in transplanted livers, kidneys, and hearts has also been shown in a randomized, controlled study of vasopressin versus saline (45). The usual pediatric vasopressor dose range of vasopressin is 0.3–2 mU/kg/min (0.0003–0.002 U/kg/min) as an IV infusion. Improved management of the potential donor is resulting in more organs being recovered and transplanted (2). Despite the significant deficiency of available organs, if a donor does require high doses of vasopressors, organs may still be considered for transplantation, albeit at a potentially higher risk for delayed graft function and failure in the recipient. The ultimate decision to accept or reject an organ for transplantation rests with the OPO and transplant surgeon.

Hormone Replacement Therapy

Since most brain-dead donors develop hemodynamic instability, it is important to evaluate donor suitability in terms of potential for successful organ resuscitation and subsequent donation, as opposed to simply relying on the initial assessment of organ function alone. Once significant intravascular volume has been restored and hypotension persists despite aggressive use of inotropes and vasopressors, pituitary hormone depletion should be suspected. The loss of an intact hypothalamic–pituitary neuroendocrine axis may result in cardiovascular derangements, temperature instability, and fluid and electrolyte disturbances due to deficiency of hypothalamic and pituitary hormones. Deficiency of adrenocorticotropic hormone and thyroid-stimulating hormone (TSH), in particular, will produce cortisol and thyroid hormone deficiency, respectively, both of which can play important roles in hemodynamic stability. Indications of hormone deficiency include signs of myocardial dysfunction as these hormones are normally involved in maintaining myocardial contractility and basal metabolic rate. Intractable hypotension despite increasing vasopressor doses should raise the suspicion of hormone deficiency, and replacement with thyroid hormone and corticosteroids should be strongly considered. Many transplant centers and OPOs routinely administer triiodothyronine (T_3) or thyroxine (T_4) in addition to steroids (methylprednisolone), vasopressin, and, often, insulin to stable and unstable brain-dead donors. In a classic study, hormone replacement therapy (HRT) consisting of T_3, cortisol, and insulin was evaluated in brain-dead donors compared with those who did not receive replacement therapy. The hormone-replacement group had a significant decrease in vasopressor requirement, with an increase in mean arterial blood pressure and CO, compared with the nontreated group (17,36,47). In another study, investigators evaluated 150 potential adult multiorgan donors, of which 35% (52 patients) were initially deemed unacceptable donors based on vasopressor requirements that averaged the equivalent of 25 μg of dopamine per kg/min and mean arterial blood pressures <55 mm Hg. After the institution of methylprednisolone, vasopressin, T_3, and insulin combined with glucose as necessary, organs from $>80\%$ of these patients were successfully retrieved and transplanted, despite the significant vasopressor support and other altered hemodynamic parameters (48).

HRT has been associated with an increased number of organs recovered from donors (3,30,31,49). There are no published studies available in children; however, one unpublished abstract retrospectively reviewed 1903 pediatric donors who received hormonal replacement therapy compared against other pediatric donors who received no hormonal replacement therapy. In this study, hormonal replacement therapy was associated with significantly increased odds of having the liver and at least one kidney and lung transplanted (29). There was no significant increase in the odds of the heart being transplanted. The greatest benefit of HRT in donor management may in fact be improved graft function following transplantation (37,39,50). A retrospective study of the effects of HRT using methylprednisolone, vasopressin, and/or T_3 or T_4 administered to brain-dead donors compared with those who did not receive hormone replacement showed that 1-month organ recipient graft survival in the triple hormone replacement group was significantly increased and early graft dysfunction was decreased (51). However, other studies dealing with adults revealed no beneficial effect to the donor or recipient (36,50,52).

It is hoped that ongoing clinical trials in this area will clarify the use of hormone replacement in brain-dead donors, specifically in children. Despite these observations, many OPOs continue the use of hormonal replacement therapy as a routine part of donor management. Commonly used agents and doses for hormonal resuscitation in pediatric donors are listed in **Table 16.3**.

Respiratory Pathophysiology

The greatest discrepancy between supply and demand in organ donation is for lungs, with only 7%–22% of potential lung donors deemed suitable for donation. Furthermore, >30% of the lungs deemed potentially suitable are not transplanted due to brain-death–associated lung injury, which includes neurogenic pulmonary edema and a profound systemic inflammatory response associated with cytokine and thromboxane release and adhesion molecule upregulation (53–55).

Brain-dead patients may develop neurogenic pulmonary edema, requiring significant mechanical ventilation support using high ventilator settings. The mechanisms responsible for neurogenic pulmonary edema include vasoconstriction resulting in elevated SVR associated with the catecholamine storm. This intense vasoconstriction results in a large volume shift of blood away from the peripheral circulation toward the central circulation. Increased central circulation affects preload and ultimately an increase in left atrial pressure with subsequent increased pulmonary capillary hydrostatic pressure culminating in hemorrhagic pulmonary edema. Concomitantly, increased capillary permeability occurs due to the local release of norepinephrine and neuropeptide Y during the catecholamine surge (35).

Other causes of respiratory insufficiency may result from direct injury due to pulmonary contusions, mucus plugging, pulmonary microemboli, aspiration or aggressive fluid resuscitative efforts required for the hemodynamic instability that follows herniation. Some area of the lung may not be effectively perfused resulting in ventilation–perfusion defects. This ventilation–perfusion alteration occurs following catecholamine depletion (53). Lung injury in the donor is common and is the main reason for the inability to recover this organ for transplantation.

Evaluation and Management of Respiratory Abnormalities

Pulmonary management of the donor is crucial to optimize oxygenation and ventilation allowing the best possible chance of recovering not only lungs, but other organs for transplantation. Every effort should be made to preserve lung function using lung-protective ventilation strategies. Smaller children may be intubated with an uncuffed endotracheal tube (ETT). A cuffed ETT should be placed in all potential donors to minimize the risk of aspiration (23,35,47). The primary goal is to prevent any secretions from entering the lungs. Balloon cuff pressure becomes irrelevant since lung recovery will not include the trachea. The head of the bed should be elevated to 30 degrees, and oral care with chlorhexidine should be used to reduce the chance of any ventilator-associated infection. Routine turning and pulmonary toilet are essential to prevent

TABLE 16.3

PHARMACOLOGIC AGENTS USED FOR HORMONAL RESUSCITATION THERAPY

■ DRUG	■ DOSE	■ ROUTE	■ COMMENTS
Desmopressin (DDAVP)	0.5 μg/h	IV	$t_{1/2}$ life 75–120 min Titrate to decrease UOP to 3–4 mL/kg/h May be beneficial with an ongoing coagulopathy
Vasopressin (Pitressin)	0.5–1 mU/kg/h	IV	$t_{1/2}$ life 10–35 min Titrate to decrease UOP to 3–4 mL/kg/h
Treatment of diabetes insipidus should consist of pharmacologic management to decrease but not completely stop UOP. Replacement of UOP with ¼ or ½ NS can be used in conjunction with these agents to maintain serum Na levels between 130 and 150 mEq/L			
Levothyroxine (Synthroid)	0.8–1.4 μg/kg/h	IV	Bolus dose 1–5 μg/kg can be administered Infants and smaller children require a larger bolus and infusion dose
Triiodothyronine (T_3)	0.05–0.2 μg/kg/h	IV	Bolus dose 1–2 μg/kg can be administered
Methylprednisolone (Solu-Medrol)	20–30 mg/kg	IV	Dose may be repeated in 8–12 h Fluid retention Glucose intolerance
Insulin	0.05–0.1 U/kg/h	IV	Titrate to control blood glucose levels to 60–150 mg/dL Monitor for hypoglycemia
Hormonal replacement therapy should be considered early in the course of donor management. Use of hormonal replacement therapy may allow weaning of inotropic support and assist with metabolic stability			

Adapted from Nakagawa TA. http://www.natco1.org/Professional-Development/documents/NATCOpeddonormanagementguidelines.pdf

atelectasis. In smaller children, prone position may be beneficial to maintain optimal ventilation–perfusion matching.

High ventilatory pressures may initially be required to maintain adequate minute ventilation in the patient with traumatic brain injury. These patients may require mild hyperventilation to assist with treatment of intracranial hypertension. Additionally, high levels of positive end-expiratory pressure (PEEP) may be required to maintain oxygenation and prevent atelectasis. With progression to brain death and reduced cerebral metabolism, carbon dioxide production becomes minimal. Minute ventilation will need to be greatly reduced in these patients to normalize $PaCO_2$ and correct or prevent a respiratory alkalosis. Reduction in minute ventilation should allow lowering of ventilatory pressures thus helping preserve viable lung tissue for potential transplantation. Common mechanical ventilation goals implemented by OPOs exist, but no conclusive evidence supports these ventilation parameters. To address this issue, a multicentered, randomized, controlled study conducted to determine the optimal protective ventilatory strategies in organ donors was stopped prematurely due to funding. Results revealed that a lung-protective strategy using tidal volumes of 6–8 mL/kg, PEEP of 8–10 cm H_2O with use of CPAP for apnea tests and a closed ventilation circuit for airway suctioning increased the number of eligible and transplanted lungs compared with a conventional strategy (31). This is consistent with acute respiratory distress syndrome (ARDS) and acute lung injury (ALI) research showing benefits with low-tidal volume strategies. Additionally, the use of higher tidal volumes may play a role in the exacerbation of inflammatory lung injury. However, many OPO ventilation management guidelines still use 8–10 mL/kg tidal volume strategies with intermittent recruitment maneuvers. For volume-ventilated patients, if a difference of >10 cm H_2O exists between the peak and plateau pressures, increased airway resistance may be the problem. Pulmonary toilet and use of bronchodilators may improve this issue. If the difference is <10 cm H_2O, decreased compliance may be the problem. Treatment of the underlying disease process is essential to diminish the potential for barotrauma. If peak pressures remain high, switching to pressure ventilation, which is used commonly in pediatric patients, may be appropriate. For pressure-ventilated patients, peak inspiratory pressure, which represents the peak airway pressure, should ideally be maintained at <30–35 cm H_2O. PEEP should continue to allow lung expansion to be maintained at or above functional residual capacity to prevent atelectasis. Maintaining oxygen saturations of at least 92%–95% and a PaO_2 of at least 100 mm Hg using ≤40% oxygen should be a target donor management goal (DMG). High concentrations of inspired oxygen diminish the alveolar nitrogen content and result in "resorption atelectasis." This can create or worsen ventilation–perfusion defects with resultant hypoxemia (23,47). Maneuvers to decrease resistance or increase compliance may improve lung function allowing for potential organ recovery. However, if the pulmonary abnormality cannot be reversed, the lungs will not be suitable for transplantation. In such cases, altering mechanical ventilation settings to provide lower tidal volumes or lower peak inspiratory pressures may still preserve the viability of other organs by diminishing the systemic inflammatory response associated with high ventilating pressures.

A tracheal Gram stain and aspirate should be obtained to identify any potential infectious process. Serial chest radiographs may be required as surveillance for the development of infiltrates, atelectasis, and pneumothoraces. A unilateral infiltrate does not exclude the possibility of donation. Bronchoscopy may also be required to evaluate the airway for secretions and aspirated contents to obtain respiratory cultures. Tracheal cultures obtained from the ETT may not always reflect lower-airway flora. Antibiotic coverage in recipients of a transplanted lung should be based on positive cultures and sensitivities obtained from the donor during bronchoscopy. For the donor, aggressive pulmonary toilet, frequent suctioning, repositioning, and chest physiotherapy, when appropriate, are vital to maintaining suitability of the lungs for transplantation.

A bolus dose of IV methylprednisolone (usual dose: 15 mg/kg in adults, 15–30 mg/kg in children) given to the brain-dead donor is often used to decrease the systemic inflammatory effect in the donor. Steroids use in the donor may also assist with immunosuppression and potentially decrease the possibility of rejection following lung transplantation. Steroid administration may also result in better oxygenation and graft function, especially when administered early following brain death (54). Steroids also have been shown to stabilize pulmonary function, reduce lung water accumulation, and increase lung recovery from donors (54,56).

Little supportive data exist for the use of naloxone to preserve lung function in the donor. Some investigators have advocated for the use of a bolus dose of naloxone administered as a component of lung management strategy. The precise mechanism of naloxone's action in this role is unknown, but free radical scavenging has been proposed (57).

An oxygen challenge test is often performed to assess lung function and transplantability. The lowest possible level of PEEP is used for the test, often 4–5 mm Hg, and the inspired oxygen is then increased to 100%. Following a 5- to 10-min period for equilibrium, an arterial blood gas is obtained. A PaO_2 on 100% oxygen or a PaO_2-to-FiO_2 ratio ≥300 mm Hg is often used as a marker of lung viability for transplantation (23). Although the use of high ventilator settings to improve this ratio may increase lung transplantability, preliminary evidence suggests that such settings may increase the systemic inflammatory response in the liver, kidneys, and heart, potentially diminishing their transplantability.

Immune System Pathophysiology

The process of brain death is associated with signs of the systemic inflammatory response syndrome (SIRS) (increased secretion of proinflammatory cytokines, chemokines, and adhesion molecules) affecting most organs (Chapter 67) (58). Additionally, free radical formation associated with brain death causes increased production of nuclear factor-κB resulting in the release of acute phase cytokines, such as tumor necrosis factor (TNF)-α and interleukin (IL)-2 (28,55,58). Some of these cytokines may contribute to cell apoptosis, vasodilation, and increased vessel capacitance. This cascade exacerbates the injury associated with the catecholamine surge and subsequent hypotension (58).

The increased levels of inflammatory cytokines and adhesion molecules have been associated with impaired graft survival of organs from brain-dead individuals when compared with donated organs from non–brain-dead donors. Not only brain death but also its initiating insults (e.g., trauma and cardiac arrest) contribute to the SIRS. Finally, ischemia and reperfusion of transplanted organs that are uniformly present in organ transplantation generate reactive oxygenation species and aggravate the previously initiated inflammation (58).

Brain death contributes to the SIRS via the release of inflammatory mediators from ischemic and traumatized brain. The catecholamine storm associated with brain injury induces intense vasoconstriction, alters aerobic to anaerobic metabolism, changes shear stress across endothelial cells, and increases stress hormones, which also contribute to SIRS. Experimental studies have produced conflicting results in the relationship between brain death and organ inflammation. Although the exact mechanisms associated with the inflammatory cytokine release are not completely understood, it appears that a hemodynamic mechanism is at least partially responsible. In animal studies in which fluid resuscitation prevented hypotension after brain death, inflammation was absent in the heart, liver, and kidneys. In a rat model of brain death, serum pretreatment of the animals with phentolamine, an α-adrenergic antagonist, prevented the hypertensive crisis seen with the catecholamine surge, resulting in lower serum levels of levels of IL-1β and TNF-α and better oxygenation (58). Clinical studies consistently demonstrate an association between brain death and inflammation of donor heart, liver, and lungs, but the relationship is less clear as regards renal inflammation. Furthermore, treatment of the hypotension with norepinephrine following catecholamine depletion also decreased serum cytokine levels (55).

Evaluation and Management of Inflammation

Anti-inflammatory treatment of the brain-dead donor has been a frustrating exercise. Steroids have been shown to decrease the systemic inflammatory response presumably because of the decrease in cytokine production. In a prospective study of cytokine expression in both living and brain-dead donors, cytokine levels were significantly increased in brain-dead donors compared with the living donor controls. In contrast, the brain-dead donors who were given steroids prior to harvesting had cytokine levels comparable with the living donors (55,58). However, several early studies demonstrated that steroid treatment of the brain-dead donor did not result in improved graft function. Follette et al. demonstrated that there was an increase in suitable lungs for transplantation and improved function posttransplantation in steroid-treated brain-dead lung donors (54). The recommendation for steroid dosing is included in **Table 16.3.**

Endocrine Pathophysiology

Diabetes Insipidus

DI is due to destruction of the posterior pituitary and results in central antidiuretic hormone deficiency. It is a common endocrinologic complication encountered in severely brain-injured and particularly in brain-dead patients. However, DI does not develop in all patients. The development of DI should, in fact, alert the physician that brain death may be developing. DI results from the inability of the kidney tubules to reabsorb water in the absence of antidiuretic hormone. Left untreated, this condition may lead to severe dehydration, hypernatremia, and hypotension with eventual cardiovascular collapse.

Evaluation and Management of Diabetes Insipidus. Clinical signs of DI include polyuria, a urine osmolarity often <200 mOsm/L, and hypernatremia, often with a serum sodium >150 mEq/L. The treatment of DI often includes pharmacologic treatment with vasopressin and fluid replacement for excessive volume loss. Vasopressin can be instituted as a continuous infusion with a usual starting dose of 0.5 mU/kg/h. This agent can be titrated based on urine output (UOP), which can be profound in DI. Titration of continuous vasopressin therapy may occur as frequently as every 10 minutes until the desired effect is achieved, usually with a decrease in urine output in the range of 2–4 mL/kg/h. If the desired output is not achieved, the rate of the vasopressin infusion may be doubled, usually up to 2–4 mU/kg/h. By titrating in this way, one preserves renal function and avoids volume overload and metabolic abnormalities, such as hyponatremia and hyperkalemia. The current suggested maximum pediatric dose for DI is 10 mU/kg/h; however, larger doses have been used to control DI.

Vasopressin acts on V_1 and V_2 vasopressin receptors to stimulate contraction of smooth muscle. It is important to remember that vasopressin possesses vasoconstrictive properties, especially at higher doses. This vasoconstriction may lead to increased vasomotor tone and hypertension, potentially impairing perfusion to other organs. The use of vasopressin can reduce the need for inotropic support. Desmopressin acetate, on the other hand, is essentially devoid of vasopressor effects. It is more specific for the V_2 vasopressin receptor. On a weight per weight basis, this agent is more potent than vasopressin in controlling urine output. However, it has a longer half-life, which can make titration of this agent difficult (12). Desmopressin can be administered by continuous IV infusion at 0.5 μg/h and titrated to control urine output (50,51,59). This agent may be beneficial in cases where hypotension is not an issue. The overall goal of pharmacologic treatment for DI is to reduce and not to stop urine output.

In many cases of brain-dead patients with DI, fluid administration is necessary to replace excessive fluid loss and resultant dehydration until urine output can be effectively controlled with vasopressin or desmopressin administration. This process can be particularly harmful in brain-dead patients who already often have diminished preload from a variety of other sources, as previously described (35,59). Urine output can, in fact, be as high as 10 mL/kg/h, such that rapid dehydration with hypotension and cardiovascular collapse can develop. Fluid replacement is essential in the stabilization of these patients. If the patient is volume depleted, fluid resuscitation with isotonic fluids should occur. Fluid replacement for excessive urine output once the patient is euvolemic is usually in the form of hypotonic IV fluids, often 0.25%–0.5% normal saline, in an attempt to match the ongoing hypotonic urine losses. Glucose-containing replacement IV fluids should be avoided, because hyperglycemia will result in further urine loss through an osmotic diuresis. Frequent assessment of vascular volume, electrolyte measurements, and hemodynamic status is imperative in patients with DI to prevent dehydration, as well as overhydration and possible hyponatremia (52). Once urine output of 2–4 mL/kg/h has been achieved, fluid replacement can be discontinued to prevent overhydration and edema. Other electrolyte abnormalities that often accompany DI are due to polyuria and include hypokalemia, hypocalcemia, hypophosphatemia, and hypomagnesemia.

Adrenal Dysfunction

Adrenocorticotropic hormone deficiency may occur in brain-dead patients secondary to anterior pituitary necrosis, with consequent adrenal dysfunction and low cortisol levels. Altered steroid production may contribute to myocardial dysfunction (52). A relative adrenal insufficiency has been described in trauma and critically ill patients; this may result in higher requirements for vasopressors. However, the data supporting cortisol replacement therapy in brain-dead patients have not been well studied, but most OPO donor management protocols utilize steroids dose, usually in the form of methylprednisolone, in addition to the other HRT previously discussed. Steroids may decrease the systemic inflammatory response effect and reduce the need for vasopressor support (54). The potential benefit of hydrocortisone and other steroids may lie in their ability to alter adrenergic receptors and regulate vascular tone by increasing sensitivity to catecholamines. Large bolus IV doses of methylprednisolone 15–30 mg/kg are often used.

Thyroid Dysfunction

Thyroid deficiency may follow brain death and may result in a shift toward anaerobic metabolism, exacerbating hemodynamic instability and resulting in elevated serum lactate levels (17). The normal physiologic effects of thyroid hormone are likely due to T_3, of which 80% is formed in peripheral nonthyroid tissue by conversion from T_4. The remaining percentage of T_3 is released from the thyroid gland itself. Low T_3 and T_4 with normal TSH levels and elevated reverse T_3 levels are often noted in critically ill adults and children, often representing the "sick euthyroid" state. Three stages of "sick euthyroid" state have been described in critical illness, and these may represent a progression in severity. Initially, with critical illness, T_3 levels may be decreased, with an increase in reverse T_3 levels, while the remainder of thyroid testing is normal. As the illness becomes more severe or prolonged, T_4 levels may decrease. The most severe form of "sick euthyroid" state is represented by a concomitant decrease in TSH. The use of certain vasopressors, such as dopamine and possibly dobutamine, aggravates the sick euthyroid syndrome by decreasing the secretion of TSH from the pituitary. This effect would presumably be minimal in brain-dead patients because of pituitary necrosis.

Evaluation and Management of Thyroid Dysfunction. Thyroid hormone replacement has been studied in critical illness, including following cardiopulmonary bypass, as well as in brain-dead donors. The studies have produced varied results, and more definitive studies are necessary.

However, in brain-dead donors, supplementation of T_3 or T_4 may result in improved myocardial function and lower vasopressor requirements, with improved blood pressure and CO. A shift back to aerobic metabolism may also occur, with improved organ perfusion and a decrease in lactic acidosis. Levothyroxine (Synthroid) and T_3 are the two intravenous thyroid agents available for administration. T_3 is used in some centers for HRT; however, the cost of this medication may be prohibitive.

Most data on the replacement of thyroid hormone are in the adult transplantation literature. Data on this topic in pediatric brain-dead donors are limited. The effects of T_4 infusion alone on vasopressor support in brain-dead children were retrospectively evaluated. T_4 administration was associated with decreased vasopressor requirements in such children, after adjusting for steroid use, fluid status, and baseline vasopressor need prior to T_4 administration (31). The usual adult bolus dose of T_4 is 20 μg IV, followed by a continuous infusion of 10 μg/h IV; in children, the bolus dose is 1–5 μg/kg, with a continuous infusion of 0.8–1.4 μg/kg/h (13,50).

Hyperglycemia and Insulin

Hyperglycemia occurs frequently in brain-dead patients. The catecholamine surge that occurs with brain death invariably contributes to this hyperglycemia. Additionally, reduced cerebral glucose metabolism in a dying or dead brain may be a factor as well. During acute illness, elevated glucose levels represent an appropriate physiologic response to stress, supplying the brain and other organs with the energy necessary for increased metabolic demands. Catecholamines are known to result in insulin resistance, thus inhibiting glucose uptake. If the physiologic stress is not reduced or removed, hyperglycemia continues. The adverse effects of hyperglycemia and the mechanisms responsible for these effects in critically ill adults continue to be intensely studied. In a prospective, randomized, controlled study of critically ill patients in a surgical ICU who were treated with either conventional or intensive insulin therapy, in addition to other positive findings, the need for vasopressors decreased in the intensively treated group (60). Controlled studies should be conducted in brain-dead donors to determine if a similar response to glucose management occurs in this patient population.

Complications associated with hyperglycemia in brain-dead donors include an osmotic diuresis, which further exacerbates the hemodynamic instability associated with catecholamine depletion. An insulin infusion to maintain serum glucose levels in the range of 80–180 mg/dL should reduce the osmotic load and prevent the osmotic diuresis associated with hyperglycemia. Furthermore, studies have shown that hyperglycemia in brain-dead organ donors may impair subsequent liver (47) and pancreatic function in transplant recipients (61). However, hyperglycemia is not usually thought to be due to primary endocrine insufficiency and should not be used as a marker of pancreatic function. Hyperglycemia also induces the formation of oxygen radicals thereby producing an inflammatory effect (49). The exact consequences of hyperglycemia on recipient organ function have yet to be elucidated. Importantly, hypoglycemia or excessive hyperglycemia should be avoided.

Temperature Instability

Temperature instability is often one of the first clinical signs that neurologic injury has progressed to brain death. This lack of temperature control and subsequent poikilothermia is ultimately due to loss of hypothalamic–pituitary function controlling thermoregulatory response. Hyperthermia may initially be noted as a result of vasoconstriction associated with the catecholamine surge. This is followed by hypothermia as intense vasodilation occurs. The large surface area-to-mass ratio contributes to the child's predisposition for heat loss. Vasoconstriction of the peripheral blood vessels occurs in an attempt to reduce this heat loss. Additionally, the ability to shiver is lost once brain death occurs, thereby preventing heat generation. Thyroid hormone deficiency also exacerbates the lack of thermoregulatory control.

Complications of hypothermia may develop in the brain-dead donor and include a "cold-induced diuresis"; coagulopathy, resulting in an increased risk of bleeding and thrombosis; and neutrophil dysfunction, potentially predisposing the donor to infection. In addition, hypothermia shifts the hemoglobin oxygen dissociation curve to the left, further decreasing the supply of oxygen to tissues and exacerbating the metabolic acidosis that often develops from the vasoconstriction associated with hypothermia.

Management of Thermoregulatory Abnormalities. To maintain the body temperature of the brain-dead organ donor, environmental temperature can be increased and measures to limit heat loss provided. Radiant or convective warmers, thermal mattresses, heated inspired gases, and warm IV fluids can be used to maintain body temperature. Ideally, core body temperature should be maintained within the normal range. Thyroid hormone replacement may also improve temperature regulation.

Renal, Electrolyte, and Acid–Base Disorders

Several metabolic derangements frequently develop in the critically ill patient and are often exacerbated when brain death occurs. Hypernatremia that accompanies brain death is multifactorial. Often caused by DI, hypernatremia can also be caused by the use of hypertonic saline and diuretics to manage elevated ICP. Unfortunately, hypernatremia can adversely affect potentially transplantable organs, especially the liver. One study examined the effect of donor serum sodium concentration on postoperative function of liver transplant recipients. This study demonstrated that a serum sodium value >155 mEq/L adversely affected graft survival and was an independent predictor of early graft loss in the recipient (13,44).

Metabolic acidosis may also occur due to numerous factors, such as myocardial dysfunction, low CO, renal insufficiency, and hypothermia. Evaluation and treatment of the underlying cause of acidosis is vital to maintenance of organ suitability for transplantation. Hyperkalemia associated with metabolic acidosis may predispose to arrhythmias in an already irritable myocardium. Hyperkalemia may also be due in part to the hyperglycemia that frequently accompanies brain death. With appropriate treatment of hyperglycemia, potassium levels should be routinely monitored as potassium begins to enter the cells.

Several other electrolyte abnormalities may occur that include hypokalemia, hypophosphatemia, hypocalcemia, and hypomagnesemia, all of which may contribute to myocardial dysfunction and should be appropriately monitored and supplemented.

Coagulopathy

Severely brain-injured patients may frequently develop a significant disseminated intravascular consumptive coagulopathy, which may result from release of thromboplastin and tissue plasminogen from injured and necrotic brain tissue (35). Aggressive fluid resuscitation with colloid, crystalloid, and blood products may result in dilution of platelets and circulating clotting factors. Additionally, the use of synthetic starches has been associated with a coagulopathy. Hypothermia can also cause or exacerbate a coagulopathy and increase platelet aggregation. The platelet count should be maintained at ≥50,000, while fibrinogen should be at least 100 mg/dL. This is especially important in the few hours prior to organ recovery. Coagulopathy should be corrected with fresh frozen plasma, cryoprecipitate, and platelets, as necessary. Use of thrombotic agents should be avoided to prevent clotting of graft tissue.

ORGAN RECOVERY AND SURVIVAL RATES

Currently about 3.5 organs from each brain-dead donor are transplanted. 1.85 organs for DCD donors are transplanted, as there are fewer organs that can be recovered by this mode of donation. Management of the brain-dead donor clearly impacts the quality and number of organs available for recovery and transplantation. Meeting specific DMGs, such as minimal inotropic use, normalization of blood pressure, oxygenation and ventilation parameters, correction of electrolyte disturbances, and controlling fluid balance, improve chances of organ recovery and graft function posttransplant (6,50). Achieving DMGs in children has also shown similar results. In an unpublished study of 148 pediatric brain-dead donors reviewed over a 5 year period, when DMGs were met, 3.37 organs were transplanted per donor (6). Pediatric DMGs are listed in **Table 16.2**.

Recipient survival is highest in those who have received an organ through living donation. Kidneys obtained from DCD donors demonstrate graft survival rates at 1, 5, and 10 years comparable with those organs obtained from DBD (41). There is a slightly increased rate of delayed graft function from DCD kidneys (13,62). Improvements in patient selection, management, immunosuppression, and recovery processes have improved graft function in the recipients of kidneys from DCD donors. Livers obtained from DCD donors often have higher rates of graft failure, compared with those obtained from DBD donors (13,62). However, in one series of liver transplants obtained through controlled DCD, 100% recipient and organ survival at an average of 18 months was observed. No events of primary nonfunction were reported, but 75% of recipients developed acute rejection at some point during this follow-up.

All episodes of rejection responded to steroid administration, and no episodes of chronic rejection occurred (24). An analysis of OPTN data revealed that, when low-risk recipients receive low-risk DCD livers, defined by warm ischemia time of <30 minutes and cold ischemia time of <10 hours, the graft survival rates are comparable with those obtained from DBD donors (24). Another review of the UNOS database revealed that at least 1000 organs transplanted per year in the United States are recovered from brain-dead donors who received CPR prior to death declaration and that graft survival of transplanted organs was not significantly different from those who did not require CPR. Due to the collaborative efforts of the organ donation movement, the period from 1995 to 2010 has seen 206 children receive transplantation after DCD versus 20,677 after DBD (63).

CONCLUSIONS AND FUTURE DIRECTIONS

Several prominent healthcare and governmental organizations have realized the urgent need for improvement in the organ donor process, extending from how team members approach donors and their families to the management of the organ donor after consent has been obtained. The IOM issued a follow-up report in May 2006 that called for improvements in the current system of organ procurement. This report highlights the efforts of the Health Resources and Services Administration in the formation of a series of organ donation breakthrough collaboratives (19). The first collaborative was convened in April 2003 and involved 95 hospitals and OPOs, although no children's hospitals were included. In the second collaborative, launched in 2004, 11 children's hospitals participated in an effort to help focus on pediatric organ donation "best practices." The goal of these collaboratives was to create a systematic national program to spread these accepted "best practices" of the organ procurement process to the nation's largest hospitals in order to achieve organ donation rates >75% and 3.75 organs transplanted per standard criteria donor. To date, participating hospitals have achieved major increases in *conversion rates*, the term applied to consent for organ donation, which has also led to increases of organs recovered and transplanted at a national level (4,6,28). Sustaining this level of success is imperative to continue to recover more organs for transplantation.

Education regarding best practices for discussions with families about organ donation, timely identification and referral of appropriate patients to OPOs, and aggressive organ donor management are all key factors to ensure that the highest quality care is provided to organ donors so that their gift of organ donation can improve the life of potential recipients. Such education should begin in medical school and continue to be emphasized on a recurring basis. There are few curriculums that educate providers in this critical area. With the continued joint efforts of the ICU staff, the OPO members involved in the management of potential organ donors, and additional initiatives to spread "best practices" and promote public awareness, it is hoped that many more waiting recipients will receive a lifesaving transplant that improves their quality of life. Preserving the option for donation is imperative for all families to minimize lost opportunities for donation that results in deaths of patients on the national waiting list.

ACKNOWLEDGMENT

Regarding all OPTN data, this work was supported in part by Health Resources and Services Administration contract 231-00-0115. The content is the responsibility of the authors alone and does not necessarily reflect the views or policies of the Department of Health and Human Services, nor does mention of trade names, commercial products, or organizations imply endorsement by the US Government.

References

1. *2005 Annual Report of the U.S. Organ Procurement and Transplantation Network and the Scientific Registry of Transplant Recipients: Transplant Data 1994–2004.* Rockville, MD: Department of Health and Human Services, Health Resources and Services Administration, Healthcare Systems Bureau, Division of Transplantation; Richmond, VA: United Network for Organ Sharing; Ann Arbor, MI: University Renal Research and Education Association, 2005.

2. Siminoff LA, Mercer MB, Arnold R. Families' understanding of brain death. *Prog Transplant* 2003;13:218–24.

3. Siminoff LA, Gordon N, Hewlett J, et al. Factors influencing families' consent for donation of solid organs for transplantation. *JAMA* 2001;286:71–7.

4. Bratton SL, Kolovos NS, Roach ES, et al. Pediatric organ transplantation needs: Organ donation best practices. *Arch Pediatr Adolesc Med* 2006;160:468–72.

5. Committee on Hospital Care, Section on Surgery, and Section on Critical Care. Policy Statement—Pediatric organ donation and transplantation. *Pediatrics* 2010;125:822–8.

6. Organ Donation Breakthrough Collaborative. Best practices evaluation final report. http://www.lewin.com/~/media/lewin/site_sections/publications/organdonationbreakthroughcollaborative.pdf. Accessed September 1, 2006.

7. Task Force for the Determination of Brain Death in Children. Guidelines for the determination of brain death in children. *Neurology* 1987;37:1077–8.

8. Nakagawa TA, Ashwal S, Mathur M, et al.; Society of Critical Care Medicine, Section on Critical Care, and Section on Neurology of the American Academy of Pediatrics; Child Neurology Society. Clinical report—Guidelines for the determination of brain death in infants and children: An update of the 1987 task force recommendations. *Pediatrics* 2011;128(3):e720–40.

9. Brockmann JG, Vaidya A, Reddy S, et al. Retrieval of abdominal organs for transplantation. *Br J Surg* 2006;93:133–46.

10. Sheehy E, Conrad SL, Brigham LE, et al. Estimating the number of potential organ donors in the United States. *N Engl J Med* 2003;349:667–74.

11. Institute of Medicine; National Academy of Sciences. *Non-Heart-Beating Organ Transplantation: Medical and Ethical Issues in Procurement.* Washington, DC: National Academy Press, 1997.

12. Institute of Medicine. *Non-Heart-Beating Organ Transplantation: Practice and Protocols.* Washington, DC: National Academy Press, 2000.

13. Shemie SD, Ross H, Pagliarello J, et al. Organ donor management in Canada: Recommendations of the forum on medical management to optimize organ potential. *CMAJ* 2006;174:S13–30.

14. Truog RD, Christ G, Browning DM, et al. Sudden traumatic death in children: "We did everything, but your child didn't survive." *JAMA* 2006;295:2646–54.

15. Williams MA, Lipsett PA, Rushton CH, et al. The physician's role in discussing organ donation with families. *Crit Care Med* 2003;31:1568–73.

16. Boucek MM, Mashburn C, Dunn SM, et al. Pediatric heart transplant after declaration of cardiocirculatory death. *N Engl J Med* 2008;359:709–14.

17. Novitzky D, Cooper DK, Morrell D, et al. Brain death, triiodothyronine depletion, and inhibition of oxidative phosphorylation: Relevance to management of organ donors. *Transplant Proc* 1987;19:4110–11.

18. Carcillo JA, Orr R, Bell M, et al. A call for public disclosure and moratorium on donation after cardiac death in children. *Pediatr Crit Care Med* 2010;11(5):641–2.

19. Institute of Medicine. *Organ Donation: Opportunities for Action.* Washington, DC: National Academy Press, 2006. http://www.nap.edu/catalog/11643.html. Accessed February 8, 2007.

20. Antommaria AHM, Trotochaud K, Kinlaw K, et al. Policies on donation after cardiac death at Children's Hospitals: A mixed-methods analysis of variation. *JAMA* 2009;301(18):1902–8.

21. Ethics Committee, American College of Critical Care Medicine; Society of Critical Care Medicine. Recommendation for non-heart-beating organ donation. A position paper by the ethics committee, American College of Critical Care Medicine, Society of Critical Care Medicine. *Crit Care Med* 2001;29:1826–31.

22. Gries CJ, White DB, Truog RD, et al.; American Thoracic Society Health Policy Committee. An official American Thoracic Society/International Society for Heart and Lung Transplantation/Society of Critical Care Medicine/Association of Organ and Procurement Organizations/United Network of Organ Sharing Statement: Ethical and policy considerations in organ donation after circulatory determination of death. *Am J Respir Crit Care Med* 2013;188(1):103–9.

23. Mascia L, Bosma K, Pasero D, et al. Ventilatory and hemodynamic management of potential organ donors: An observational survey. *Crit Care Med* 2006;34:321–7.

24. Bernat JL, D'Alessandro AM, Port FK, et al. Report of a national conference on donation after cardiac death. *Am J Transplant* 2006;6:281–91.

25. Rosendale JD, Kauffman HM, McBride MA, et al. Hormonal resuscitation yields more transplanted hearts with improved early function. *Transplantation* 2003;75:1336–41.

26. Lewis J, Peltier J, Nelson H, et al. Development of the University of Wisconsin donation after cardiac death evaluation tool. *Prog Transplant* 2003;13:265–73.

27. Schnuelle P, Lorenz D, Mueller A, et al. Donor catecholamine use reduces acute allograft rejection and improves graft survival after cadaveric renal transplantation. *Kidney Int* 1999;56:738–46.

28. Metzger RA, Taylor GJ, McGaw LJ, et al. Research to practice: A national consensus conference. *Prog Transplant* 2005;15(4):379–84.

29. Shafer TJ, Schkade LL, Evans RW, et al. Cardiocirculatory effects of acutely increased intracranial pressure and subsequent brain death. *Eur J Cardiothorac Surg* 1995;9:360–72.

30. Smith M. Physiologic changes during brain stem death—Lessons for management of the organ donor. *J Heart Lung Transplant* 2004;23:S217–22.

31. Szabo G. Physiologic changes after brain death. *J Heart Lung Transplant* 2004;23:S223–6.

32. Novitzky D. Detrimental effects of brain death on the potential organ donor. *Transplant Proc* 1997;29:3770–2.

33. Pratschke J, Tullius SG, Neuhaus P. Brain death associated ischemia/reperfusion injury. *Ann Transplant* 2004;9:78–80.

34. Sebening C, Hagl C, Szabo G, et al. Cardiocirculatory effects of acutely increased intracranial pressure and subsequent brain death. *Eur J Cardiothorac Surg* 1995;9:360–72.

35. Lutz-Dettinger N, de Jaeger A, Kerremans I. Care of the potential pediatric organ donor. *Pediatr Clin North Am* 2001;48:715–49.

36. Powner DJ, Hernandez M. A review of thyroid hormone administration during adult donor care. *Prog Transplant* 2005;15:202–7.

37. Wheeldon DR, Potter CD, Oduro A, et al. Transforming the "unacceptable" donor: Outcomes from the adoption of a standardized donor management technique. *J Heart Lung Transplant* 1995;14:734–42.

38. Zaroff JG, Babcock WD, Shiboski SC, et al. Temporal changes in left ventricular systolic function in heart donors: Results of serial echocardiography. *J Heart Lung Transplant* 2003;22:383–8.

39. Zuppa AF, Nadkarni V, Davis L, et al. The effect of a thyroid hormone infusion on vasopressor support in critically ill children with cessation of neurologic function. *Crit Care Med* 2004;32:2318–22.

40. Pilcher DV, Scheinkestel CD, Snell GI, et al. High central venous pressure is associated with prolonged mechanical ventilation and increased mortality after lung transplantation. *J Thorac Cardiovasc Surg* 2005;129:912–8.

41. Alonso A, Fernandez-Rivera C, Villaverde P, et al. Renal transplantation from non-heart-beating donors: A single-center 10-year experience. *Transplant Proc* 2005;37:3658–60.

42. Schnuelle P, Berger S, deBoer J, et al. Effects of catecholamine application to brain-dead donors on graft survival in solid organ transplantation. *Transplantation* 2001;72:455–63.

43. Mateo R, Cho Y, Singh G, et al. Risk factors for graft survival after liver transplantation from donation after cardiac death donors: An analysis of OPTN/UNOS data. *Am J Transplant* 2006;6(4):791–6.

44. Totsuka E, Fung U, Hakamada K, et al. Analysis of clinical variables of donors and recipients with respect to short-term graft outcome in human liver transplantation. *Transplant Proc* 2004;36:2215–8.

45. Katz K, Lawler J, Wax J, et al. Vasopressin pressor effects in critically ill children during evaluation for brain death and organ recovery. *Resuscitation* 2000;47:33–40.

46. Pennefather SH, Bullock RE, Mantle D, et al. Use of low dose arginine vasopressin to support brain-dead organ donors. *Transplantation* 1995;59:58–62.

47. Novitzky D. Donor management: State of the art. *Transplant Proc* 1997;29:3773–5.

48. Shore PM, Huang R, Roy L, Darnell C, Grein H, Robertson T, Thompson L. Development of a bedside tool to predict time to death after withdrawal of life-sustaining therapies in infants and children. *PCCM* 2012;13(4):415–22.

49. Singer P, Shapiro H, Cohen J. Brain death and organ damage: The modulating effects of nutrition. *Transplantation* 2005;80:1363–8.

50. Wood KE, Becker BN, McCartney JG, et al. Care of the potential organ donor. *N Engl J Med* 2004;351:2730–9.

51. Rosendale JD, Chabalewski FL, McBride MA, et al. Increased transplanted organs from the use of a standardized donor management protocol. *Am J Transplant* 2002;2:761–8.

52. Wise-Faberowski L, Soriano SG, Ferrari L, et al. Perioperative management of diabetes insipidus in children. *J Neurosurg Anesthesiol* 2004;16(3):220–5.

53. Avlonitis VS, Wigfield CH, Kirby JA, et al. The hemodynamic mechanisms of lung injury and systemic inflammatory response following brain death in the transplant donor. *Am J Transplant* 2005;5:684–93.

54. Follette DM, Rudich SM, Babcock WD. Improved oxygenation and increased lung donor recovery with high-dose steroid administration after brain death. *J Heart Lung Transplant* 1998;17:423–9.

55. Kuecuek O, Mantouvalou L, Klemz R, et al. Significant reduction of proinflammatory cytokines by treatment of the brain-dead donor. *Transplant Proc* 2005;37:387–8.

56. Matuschak GM. Optimizing ventilatory support of the potential organ donor during evolving brain death: Maximizing lung availability for transplantation. *Crit Care Med* 2006;34:548–9.

57. Markham L, Moncure M, Webster P, et al. Improvement in pulmonary function following administration of naloxone in brain dead patients. *Transplantation* 2006;82:439–40.

58. Land WG. The role of postischemic reperfusion injury and other nonantigen-dependent inflammatory pathways in transplantation. *Transplantation* 2005;79:505–14.

59. Lugo N, Silver P, Nimkoff L, et al. Diagnosis and management algorithm of acute onset of central diabetes insipidus in critically ill children. *J Pediatr Endocrinol Metab* 1997;10(6):633–9.

60. van den Berghe G, Wouters P, Weekers F, et al. Intensive insulin therapy in the critically ill patients. *N Engl J Med* 2001;345:1359–67.

61. Powner DJ. Donor care before pancreatic tissue transplantation. *Prog Transplant* 2005;15:129–36.

62. Scientific Registry of Transplant Recipients. People living with a functioning graft at year end by organ, 1995–2005. http://www.ustransplant.org/. Accessed August 1, 2013.

63. Yoo PS, Olthoff KM, Abt PL. Donation after cardiac death in pediatric organ transplantation. *Curr Opin Organ Transplant* 2011;16:483–8.

CHAPTER 17 ■ REHABILITATION

MELISSA K. TROVATO, GLENDALIZ BOSQUES, ROBERT J. GRAHAM, MEGAN E. KRAMER, FRANK S. PIDCOCK, SUZANNE V. PRESTWICH, CRISTINA L. SADOWSKY, AND SCOTT C. SCHULTZ

KEY POINTS

Basic Concepts of Rehabilitation

1 A physiatrist should be consulted early in the course of the illness.
2 Palliative care and rehabilitation are not mutually exclusive.

Prevention and Treatment of Clinical Complications

3 Positioning is important for the prevention of contractures and decubitus ulcers.
4 Prolonged bed rest negatively impacts multiple systems.
5 Bowel and bladder programs should be initiated in the PICU.

Psychological Issues

6 Children hospitalized in the intensive care setting are at risk for acute distress and adverse psychological symptoms.
7 Factors specific to the injury/illness, child and family, and the PICU environment all appear to play a role in a child's risk for poor psychological outcome.

8 Early identification of children at risk and the provision of developmentally appropriate and family-inclusive interventions are essential.

Rehabilitation of Specific Critical Illnesses

9 Children with acquired brain injury or spinal cord injury (SCI) often have related dysfunction in multiple other systems.
10 Agitation is a natural phase of recovery from traumatic brain injury (TBI).
11 High cervical SCI is frequently associated with TBI.
12 Patients with SCI at T6 and above are at risk for autonomic dysreflexia.

Rehabilitation and Weaning from Prolonged Mechanical Ventilation

13 Weaning from respiratory support may be the last and most protracted aspect of rehabilitation.

The rehabilitation needs of a child with critical illness may not be apparent or may be difficult to prioritize while a child is receiving intensive care. As medical care advances, children are increasingly surviving severe injuries and illnesses. The survival of a critical illness may be associated with acquired disability of either a transient or a permanent nature. Following the onset of disability, rehabilitation services help to maximize the function of children in their home, school, and community. Topics discussed in this chapter include (a) basic concepts of rehabilitation, (b) the importance of early rehabilitation, (c) prevention and treatment of clinical complications, and (d) the rehabilitation treatment and management of specific illnesses.

BASIC CONCEPTS OF REHABILITATION

Rehabilitation is the process of maximizing function and independence in an individual with a disability. The World Health Organization's International Classification of Functioning, Disability, and Health (ICF) provides structure for discussing the sequelae of disease based on an individual's function at

the levels of impairment, activity, and participation (1). *Impairment* is defined as a disturbance at the organ level (e.g., muscle weakness or contracture), *limitation in activity* is a disturbance at the person level (e.g., the inability to walk), and *limitation in participation* (e.g., a wheelchair user's inability to attend a school in a nonaccessible building) involves how an individual interacts with his/her community and society. Rehabilitation professionals evaluate an individual's function at the impairment, activity, and participation levels and subsequently design a program of care to maximize the child's participation at home, at school, and in the community.

Rehabilitation in the PICU

Consultation with the rehabilitation team early during a hospitalization allows for monitoring for secondary impairments while maximizing preventive efforts, ensures the appropriate advancement of rehabilitation treatments as soon as the child is medically ready, and facilitates discharge planning.

The rehabilitation team is led by a *physiatrist* who is a physician specializing in physical medicine and rehabilitation.

196

Physiatrists are trained in a broad range of medical and functional problems that are associated with illness and injury. Training includes a minimum of 4 years of a postdoctoral residency, comprising 1 year of internship and 3 years of specialty training. A pediatric physiatrist may have also completed a pediatric residency and/or pediatric rehabilitation fellowship. While a child is in the PICU, the physiatrist serves as a link between the rehabilitation and PICU teams; the physiatrist's role includes monitoring the child's medical status and initiating appropriate rehabilitation services when appropriate, as well as coordinating the rehabilitative care program. The rehabilitation team may be composed of physical therapists, occupational therapists, speech and language pathologists, as well as psychologists and therapeutic recreation specialists, depending on the institution. Ideally, the rehabilitation and PICU teams work together to prevent complications of bed rest, such as contractures, so that when a child is ready for more aggressive rehabilitation services, secondary impairments that might impede functional progress have been limited or prevented.

PALLIATIVE CARE AND REHABILITATION

2 Rehabilitation and palliative care are not mutually exclusive. Palliative care "seeks to prevent or relieve the physical and emotional distress produced by a life-threatening medical condition or its treatment, to help patients with such conditions and their families live as normally as possible" (2). Palliative care is not limited to those children who are thought to be in the active process of dying. With increased focus on delivering palliative care services to an expanded group of children, attention should be directed not only to symptom management but also toward maintaining function and age-appropriate independence.

Ideally, rehabilitation focuses on preserving and maximizing skills to prevent or slow the progression of disability. As the child's disease progresses, rehabilitative efforts build on previously learned strategies to mitigate symptoms of weakness and fatigue by making environmental modifications and introducing compensatory measures and assistive devices so that the child can maintain independence as long as possible. Rehabilitation strategies also focus on family and caregiver education—teaching strategies that will ease the burden of care. Thus, palliative care services and rehabilitation services aim to "add life to the child's years, not simply years to the child's life" (3).

REHABILITATION CONTINUUM OF CARE

The ideal characteristics of a rehabilitation system include (a) adjacency to an acute medical center (enabling close cooperation between the acute care and rehabilitation teams); (b) continuity of rehabilitation care throughout the acute and rehabilitation hospitalizations; (c) a full complement of rehabilitation professionals and services available to meet the needs of the patients, working together as a coordinated, interdisciplinary team with common goals; (d) specialized expertise for specialized problems (such as cognitive and behavioral rehabilitation for patients with brain injury or intense motor therapy for patients with spinal cord injury [SCI]); (e) early transfers to the rehabilitation setting, where certain problems (e.g., agitation in a patient with brain injury) are better managed by an experienced interdisciplinary team; (f) a continuum of services flexibly provided in a range of environments to best meet the individual needs of the children and their families; and (g) resources to facilitate and optimize community/school reintegration.

Related to the principle that "specialized populations require specialized programs," children and adolescents are best served by specialized pediatric rehabilitation programs, thereby ensuring the provision of essential components of care, including (a) expertise in the rehabilitation of children, taking into account the growth and development of the child; (b) developmentally appropriate treatments and environment; (c) a family-centered approach; and (d) attention to the education of the child as well as the reintegration of that child into the educational system. Concerning accreditation of rehabilitation programs, the Commission on Accreditation of Rehabilitation Facilities has clinically relevant accreditation guidelines that help ensure that a program meets standards specific for pediatric rehabilitation, as well as for subspecialty programs, such as for brain injury. The family-centered approach recognizes the child and the family as the most important and unchanging members of the rehabilitation team. Not only is the family actively involved in defining the rehabilitation goals for the child, but it also partners in the child's medical and rehabilitation care.

Ideally, a rehabilitation system should allow for the delivery of the appropriate intensity and type of rehabilitation in the most efficacious and least restrictive setting. At times it is often most efficacious for patients to learn new skills and strategies in the actual environment in which they will need to perform. Consequently, although an acute inpatient rehabilitation program that can provide constant medical and nursing care and intense rehabilitation may be the best place for the initial rehabilitation, an alternate setting might be the best way to complete the rehabilitation. The rehabilitation system at the Johns Hopkins/Kennedy Krieger Institute provides such a flexible continuum, with an acute rehabilitation umbrella that includes an inpatient hospital unit, a day hospital (also licensed as a school), and an in-the-home/community program—all of which have dedicated interdisciplinary teams—as well as appropriate outpatient services. This system provides rehabilitation in the setting that best matches the patient's needs and abilities as well as the family's resources.

The last and arguably most important step in rehabilitation is community reintegration and, for children, school reentry. The assistance that the child will need to facilitate the transition from rehabilitation to the educational system will vary based on the disability. The need for assistance can range from problem solving with regard to architectural barriers for a student with orthopedic impairments to developing an entirely new educational placement to accommodate the cognitive, behavioral, and motor impairments of a child with brain injury. In facilitating this process, it is important to know that, as required by law, all students are guaranteed free access to state-of-the-art public education that is individualized to meet their needs in the least restrictive setting (4).

PREVENTION AND TREATMENT OF CLINICAL COMPLICATIONS

Effects of Inactivity and Bed Rest

Many anatomic and physiologic changes are known to occur within the musculoskeletal, cardiovascular, and pulmonary systems in response to bed rest, including diminished muscle mass, decreased muscle strength, muscle shortening, osteoporosis, and cardiovascular and pulmonary deconditioning (5). In addition, inactivity puts the skin at risk for breakdown.

Musculoskeletal Complications

Bed rest results in generalized atrophy that is more prominent in those muscles that provide antigravity strength, such as the gastrocnemius–soleus. During strict bed rest, muscle strength is reduced by up to 15% of baseline strength per week; a plateau in loss of function is reached at 25%–40% of baseline strength. It may take 2–3 weeks to recover strength lost during 1 week of bed rest. Stretching of a muscle during periods of inactivity may reduce atrophy and maintain contractile properties by holding the muscle in a lengthened position and slowing the formation of noncontractile proteins (6). Stretching will also prevent muscle shortening or contracture formation.

Musculoskeletal contractures and peripheral nerve injuries are insidious, potentially debilitating, and preventable complications of immobility in the intensive care setting. Disease-related changes in muscle tone, limb restraints, and awkward positions are factors that predispose the pediatric patient in the PICU to these problems. Protracted abnormal limb and joint position in the absence of active movements can rapidly progress to muscle contractures and limitation in joint range of motion (ROM), especially noted in the ankles, knees, and hips, but possibly involving any area. A goal of early rehabilitation intervention in the PICU is to preserve ROM in weight-bearing joints in the lower extremity for ambulation and in the manipulative joints of the upper extremity for self-care and fine motor activities.

The mainstay of treatment to prevent muscle contractures is ROM exercises. Acceptable parameters for performing these movements should be established in conjunction with the PICU staff. Factors that may limit the ability to perform ROM exercises include increased intracranial pressure, skin grafts across joints, wound dressings, intravascular lines or endotracheal tubes, and hemodynamic instability.

Plastic splints designed to hold a joint in an antideformity position are commonly used to provide a static stretch of muscles that cross joints to minimize the development of muscle contractures. The ankles and wrists are the most common joints on which these splints are used. The splints hold the joints as close to the neutral anatomic position as possible. Skin breakdown caused by unrelieved pressure is a complication of these splints. They require careful application and consistent skin checks to ensure that decubitus ulcers do not form, which is especially important if the patient is insensate or unable to communicate discomfort or pain.

Peripheral nerves such as peroneal and ulnar nerves are at high risk for nerve impingement due to their exposure at the knee and elbow, respectively. The brachial plexus is susceptible to stretch injury from interventions that require wide adduction or external rotation of the shoulders. Although critical illness polyneuropathy or myopathy may also cause limb weakness in the PICU setting, it is important to consider a mononeuropathy as the cause of weakness.

Bed rest also results in reduced bone mineral density. Stimulation to bones from weight bearing, gravity, and muscle activity are necessary to maintain adequate bone health, and these forces are significantly diminished during bed rest. Disuse osteopenia is typically noted in the subperiosteal region of the bones. Bone density can decrease by 40% after 12 weeks of bed rest, resulting in osteoporosis (7). Bone resorption during immobility can result in symptomatic hypercalcemia, particularly in adolescent males following trauma (8).

Cardiovascular Complications

Inactivity caused by critical illness has serious implications for the resting cardiovascular system. Venous and arterial thromboembolism related to invasive catheters, stasis, and hypercoagulable states are discussed later in this chapter and should be considered during all phases of illness. Independent of acute events, alterations in cardiac dynamics and vasomotor tone occur as a result of prolonged bed rest. Changes in renal perfusion, sympathetic nervous system dysfunction, atrial stretch receptors, electrolyte imbalances, iatrogenic fluid restriction, and diuretic administration can alter intravascular volume homeostasis through fluctuations in the renin–angiotensin–aldosterone system, antidiuretic hormone, and atrial naturetic peptide. Relative degrees of anemia can also occur as a result of blood loss, chronic illness, and nutritional depletion. While resting, cardiac output may not change significantly, and baseline heart rate may increase to compensate for decreased stroke volume. Capacity to respond to stress, exercise, and even a simple change to an upright position may be limited. Bed rest in otherwise healthy individuals can potentiate orthostatic hypotension in a matter of weeks owing to impaired vasomotor response and change in vascular capacitance. Several weeks of therapy may be required for the body to redevelop compensatory responses to change in positioning. Prevention of (and early treatment for) cardiovascular deconditioning may include early mobilization, compression stockings, ROM exercises, isometric and/or isotonic strengthening exercises, upright positioning in bed, and gradual reintroduction of standing. Assistance by a therapist and use of safety equipment are crucial to prevent secondary complications, including trauma or syncopal events.

Children and young adults with congenital structural heart disease, pulmonary hypertension, or acquired heart disease (myocarditis or cardiomyopathy) require special rehabilitation consideration. Collaboration between postcritical care providers (i.e., physician, nursing, and therapist) and the primary cardiologist is crucial. Anatomy, postsurgical considerations (e.g., artificial valves, conduits, shunts, and thrombosis risks), arrhythmia potential, and potential manifestation of decompensation should be reviewed explicitly. Physiologic and functional goals may differ from those of patients without underlying cardiac disease. A plan for routine monitoring as well as specific follow-up evaluation (cardiology clinic visits, electrocardiography, chest radiography, echocardiography, Holter monitoring, cardiac MRI, or cardiac catheterization) should be discussed. Cardiopulmonary interactions should also be considered as part of respiratory evaluation and determination of weaning potential.

Pulmonary Complications

While many pediatric patients present with primary lung impairment from infection, parapneumonic processes, trauma, or inhalational injury, there are numerous mechanisms of indirect respiratory injury and dysfunction. Orthopedic and neuromuscular perturbations related to disuse, neurologic conditions (e.g., Guillain–Barré), postsurgical changes in abdominal–thoracic mechanics, pain, nutritional depletion, neuromuscular blockade, and steroid-related myopathy can all contribute to weakness of the diaphragm, intercostal and abdominal muscles, and impaired respiratory mechanics (9). Resulting changes in respiratory function may include reductions in tidal volume, minute volume, vital capacity, and maximum voluntary ventilation. Impaired secretion clearance may result in persistent atelectasis and risk of secondary pneumonia. Volitional recruitment with incentive spirometry, or assisted recruitment via positive pressure therapy, will aid in reconditioning and lung expansion. Chest physiotherapy through manual or automated percussion, cough assist/insufflation–exsufflation devices, and correct positioning are important preventive measures. If noninvasive ventilation continues, skin integrity at mask and head gear interface should be assessed regularly; pressure ulcerations serve as an additional nidus for invasive infections as well as a caloric burden for wound healing. Bedside monitoring of forced vital capacity and negative inspiratory force may be implemented, where appropriate and tolerated, and facilitate weaning or advancement of interventions.

Acknowledging aerodigestive issues is crucial. While potentiated in patients with central nervous system injury or bulbar impairment, micro- and macro-aspiration can result in profound or chronic pulmonary compromise in any critically ill and deconditioned child. Route of feeding, timing of therapies around feeding, positioning, administration of antiemetics, limiting impact of aerophagia, and weaning of sedatives are all important considerations. Early consultation with speech–language/feeding specialist may dictate the need for radiology, swallowing studies, or salivagrams. On rare occasion, laryngoscopy may be required to assess vocal cord function.

An understanding of cardiopulmonary interactions for the individual patient is also necessary. Myocardial dysfunction may result in pulmonary congestion or secondary effusion. Suboptimal pulmonary recruitment may lead to higher pulmonary vascular resistance, impaired CO_2 clearance, and right ventricular strain. Management of fluid and diuretic therapy, lung recruitment strategies, and vasoactive therapies may require a multidisciplinary approach.

Population-specific needs should also be considered. Patients with underlying neuromuscular conditions (muscular dystrophy or spinal muscular atrophy) will have limited respiratory capacity at baseline. Acute illness or perioperative needs may compound these issues, and attention to applicable guidelines may be warranted (10–12). Immunocompromised patients will be vulnerable to unusual pathogens and require more aggressive screening as well as aggressive secretion clearance and early administration of broad-spectrum antimicrobial agents. Children and young adults with cystic fibrosis or other parenchymal (restrictive, obstructive, or obliterative) pulmonary disease may be at risk for pneumothoraces, hemoptysis, reactive airway exacerbations, or complications of drug-resistant bacterial infection. Coordination with primary care teams is important for these populations.

Decubitus Ulcers

Immobility may lead to skin integrity concerns resulting in pressure or decubitus ulcers through bony prominences and other pressure-dependent surfaces. Approximately 27% of patients may develop a pressure ulcer when admitted to PICU (13). Decubitus ulcers occur not just because of unrelieved pressure but also because of friction, shearing, moisture (incontinence), and increased body temperature.

Risk assessment is essential for the identification of potential modifiable risks which could be targeted during the admission, in addition to identifying additional preventive strategies and their efficacy. Since malnourishment and inadequate protein intake may place children at increased risk for skin breakdown (14), a nutritional evaluation may be of value in order to optimize the patient's status.

The most common sites for the development of decubitus ulcers are usually the sacro-coccygeal region, heels, and the ankle malleoli (15). In younger children (<36 months), the scalp in the occipital area may be at an increased risk of pressure and breakdown due to the difference in head size (16).

Prevention is vital in the management of pressure ulcers. Nursing should be aware of the risk assessment tools available and deliver interventions, such as repositioning, adequate transfer techniques to diminish shearing and friction, and should provide pressure-relieving surfaces (gel pads or pillows), when necessary. The amount of time a patient spends in a specific position with unrelieved pressure is the highest contributing factor to the development of pressure ulcers. Therefore, the patient should be turned every 2 hours to minimize this risk. Providers should carefully look for erythema, blanching, or ulceration. The presence of blisters, bruising, or bogginess should also be noted. If the child is hemodynamically unstable, a pressure-relieving surface such as a specialty and continuous and reactive low-pressure mattress and bed may decrease the incidence of decubiti (17). Proper management when a pressure ulcer develops includes the alleviation of pressure to the area, optimization of nutritional status, and provision of appropriate wound care.

Venous Thrombosis

Pediatric venous thromboembolisms (VTEs) are associated with an increased risk of morbidity and mortality (18). The risks for thromboembolism have been historically described in the literature as Virchow's triad, which include hypercoagulable state, circulatory stasis, and endothelial injury. There have been reports that the incidence of VTEs has increased 10-fold in the past 20 years. This increase has been reported specifically in children admitted to tertiary care settings (19,20). The current hypothesis is that this increase is due to improved survival in the critically ill child, increased use of central catheters, and an increased rate of detection of thrombi. A high index of suspicion is specifically important for children with paralysis and infants because VTE can be clinically silent. Sometimes the only physical finding is a vascular catheter with sluggish blood return (21).

Historically, the use of routine Doppler screening has not been cost-effective in the pediatric population (22). Recent studies have shown a decrease in the incidence, morbidity, and mortality related to VTEs for patients in the PICU with the use of risk stratification strategies and early detection and management. This includes the use of screening ultrasound evaluations for assessment of high-risk patients (23).

Risk stratification is highly recommended for prevention of VTEs. Multiple studies have reported risk factors associated with the development of VTEs that include immobility, the presence of a central venous catheter, SCI, complex lower extremity fractures, thrombophilia, infection, and malignancy. Prepubertal children may be at a low risk for the development of VTEs. For children in whom there is a concern, there may be benefit from mechanical prophylaxis with the use of sequential pneumatic compression and early ambulation. Children who are postpubertal (or older than 13 years), who are immobile, and who have one additional risk factor may be classified as "High Risk" (21,24–26). If no risk of bleeding is identified, these patients may benefit from both sequential pneumatic compression and pharmacologic prophylaxis with unfractionated or low-molecular-weight heparin. The use of an indwelling subcutaneous catheter, or Insuflon, should be considered for administration to diminish discomfort associated with injections. Diagnosis may be confirmed with compression ultrasonography of the affected extremity.

PSYCHOLOGICAL FACTORS SURROUNDING INTENSIVE CARE ADMISSIONS

Children who survive critical illnesses are at risk for psychological sequelae following PICU hospitalization. This can include psychiatric morbidity, such as acute stress disorder, posttraumatic stress disorder (PTSD), depressive symptoms, functional limitations, and diminished quality of life. Children and their families are often exposed to traumatic events in the PICU both personally and via secondary exposure to other patients and families. Negative psychological sequelae in children can also develop weeks to months after discharge, potentially impacting children's rehabilitation and recovery from their illness or injury. While there is growing awareness of the importance of identifying children who are at risk for poor psychological outcomes and providing appropriate intervention, there is limited research to address these concerns.

Children may experience acute periods of confusion or disorientation, and exhibit delusions, illusions, or hallucinations in the PICU. Formerly called "ICU syndrome" or "ICU psychosis," the term *delirium* is now used to describe an acute state of brain dysfunction in children or adults in a critical care setting (27). The causes of delirium symptoms include direct effects of the injury or illness, medication effects, and environmental factors. The atypical sensory environment in the PICU environment can produce or exacerbate cognitive and psychiatric symptoms. Children are exposed to unfamiliar situations and procedures and may experience either sensory overload or deprivation due to the lights and sounds of the machines, combined with the lack of movement and relative monotony of the environmental stimuli. Perhaps most important is the effect of sleep disruption or deprivation due to the medical condition, pain, constant light, noise, and frequent nursing care activities (27,28). Prevention and treatment of delirium in the PICU is an emerging area of concern, as studies suggest that critical illness is associated with neurocognitive and functional impairments in children and adults (27).

Children in the PICU are at significant risk for development of PTSD due to trauma exposure and subsequent experiences of fear and hopelessness. The reported incidence of PTSD varies with some indication of a higher rate of PTSD among children in the PICU versus the general wards (29). Recent reviews suggest risk factors for developing PTSD following PICU admission and include illness severity, length of PICU stay, number of invasive procedures, parental emotional distress, and symptoms of posttraumatic stress (29,30).

There are several ways to lessen the impact of the PICU environment and potential for distress in children with critical illnesses. Providing frequent orientation to time, day, and place, as well as implementation of a normal day/night routine can reduce the potential for disorientation (28). Managing pain and facilitating sleep have also been effective (27). When possible, providing familiar objects and child-friendly stimuli, reducing social isolation, and allowing frequent visits from family members can reduce anxiety in the PICU environment. Therapeutic touch provided by parents or nurses has been shown to reduce stress and provide comfort (28). Studies have demonstrated the positive impact on the child and parent when the parent is present and frequently participates in the child's cares (31). Staff should be vigilant for acute symptoms of distress in children and their families and should identify when additional intervention is needed (32). Psychologists provide behavioral coping strategies, provide supportive psychological intervention to patients and their families to improve coping and adjustment, and facilitate positive interactions between families and staff members. In general, it is recommended that medical staff communicate with children using age-appropriate language and involve them in care (28). Child life specialists deliver reassurance and explain medical procedures in a developmentally appropriate manner to provide children with a sense of control and safety. Social workers also support families in the management of stressors related to having a child hospitalized in the PICU and help facilitate access to resources outside of the hospital.

REHABILITATION OF SPECIFIC CRITICAL ILLNESSES

Acquired Brain Injury

Acquired brain injury (ABI) has many etiologies, including trauma, infection, hypoxia, ischemia, genetic and metabolic disorders, tumors, and vascular abnormalities. Trauma is the most common etiology of ABI. Approximately 1.7 million individuals each year suffer traumatic brain injuries (TBIs) in the United States (33). In children under 14 years of age, an estimated 475,000 children suffer from TBI each year (34). In children 17 years of age and younger, the overall rate of hospitalizations for TBI in the United States was 70 per 100,000 (35).

Classification of Severity of Injury

There are two major ways to classify the severity of a TBI: Glasgow Coma Scale (GCS) and duration of posttraumatic amnesia (PTA). GCS assesses eye opening (scored from 1 to 4), verbal response (1 to 5), and motor response (1 to 6) within the first 24 hours after injury. The scores from motor response, verbal response, and eye opening are added together, with higher scores indicating a less severe brain injury. The lowest GCS score is 3 and the highest score is 15. Scores of 8 or below indicate a severe TBI, scores 9–12 indicate a moderate TBI, and scores 13–15 indicate a mild TBI. With a score below 8 one is said to be comatose (36). Duration of PTA is also used to classify brain injury severity. Duration of PTA includes the length of time in coma and the time after coma it takes to remember events and store new memories. The Children's Orientation and Amnesia Test (COAT) is a widely used tool to assess PTA. In mild TBI, duration of PTA is less than 1 hour. In moderate TBI, duration of PTA is between 1 hour and 1 day. In severe TBI, duration of PTA is greater than 1 day (37). It is important to recognize that PTA criteria can stand alone when classifying severity of injury.

Medical Issues after Acquired Brain Injury

Central autonomic dysfunction can manifest as hypertension, tachycardia, hyperthermia, tachypnea, hypertonia, or decerebrate posturing in the very severely injured. This condition is associated with dysfunction of the thalamus or hypothalamus and the connections to the cortical, subcortical, and brainstem areas that mediate autonomic functions. Bromocriptine has been shown to help the hyperthermic symptoms (38). Propranolol has been shown to help the hemodynamic changes (39).

Nutrition/Gastrointestinal: The delivery of adequate enteral nutrition may be complicated by early feeding intolerance due to altered gastric motility, gastroesophageal reflux, and dysphagia. A feeding tube may be indicated to provide adequate nutrition. Constipation needs to be monitored, and stool softeners may need to be incorporated into the bowel regimen.

Neurologic: Posttraumatic seizures are classified as immediate (within the first 24 hours), early (within the first week), or late (after the first week). Immediate posttraumatic seizures do not have significant prognostic utility. Risk of posttraumatic epilepsy increases with increasing severity of injury (0.5% for mild, 1.2% for moderate, and 10% for severe TBI) and with certain types of injuries (e.g., skull fracture and contusion with subdural hematoma) (40). Anticonvulsant prophylaxis with phenytoin (Dilantin) has been shown to be efficacious only for the first week postinjury (41). Posttraumatic hydrocephalus is most commonly a result of cerebral atrophy (hydrocephalus ex vacuo), but progressive hydrocephalus must be ruled out. The risk of hydrocephalus increases with longer duration of coma, increased age, and decompressive craniotomy (42). Cranial neuropathies may also occur. The cranial nerves most commonly involved are the olfactory, facial, and vestibulocochlear nerves. Agitation is a natural phase of recovery from ABI. It typically is self-limiting. Generally, sedating medications should be avoided, and environment modifications should be implemented first. A low-stimulus environment can help with agitation. The use of a floor bed can also be helpful and may eliminate the need for restraints. Bladder incontinence is common after a brain injury, usually due to detrusor hyperreflexia. Timed voids are helpful.

Endocrine: Endocrine abnormalities include the syndrome of inappropriate antidiuretic hormone secretion, diabetes insipidus, and cerebral salt wasting. Examination of serum sodium, serum osmolality, urine osmolality, and urine specific gravity help to distinguish these and to guide the appropriate treatment.

Prognostic Factors and Outcome after Acquired Brain Injury

Aspects important to consider in predicting recovery include etiology of injury, severity of injury, age at injury, premorbid concerns/deficits, family function, and access to resources (43). An increased incidence of premorbid learning and behavioral problems is seen among children with TBI. The majority of children can be expected to make considerable neurologic recovery; however, there are subsets of individuals with poorer prognosis, for example, individuals with an anoxic brain injury (such as those that occur with near-drowning or prolonged cardiac arrest) (44). Secondary injuries can also impact prognosis. Children with mild TBI can experience physical, cognitive, emotional, and sleep symptoms following injury which typically resolve over days to weeks. Children with moderate and severe TBI are at greater risk for experiencing more persistent neurobehavioral and cognitive changes (40,45,46). Many children with TBI require significant modifications and supports for their cognitive and behavioral difficulties in order to participate successfully in their home, school, and community settings. Plasticity of the young brain with focal injuries will aid in the recovery of these impairments. Unlike an adult, a child under 5–8 years of age with a new left middle cerebral artery stroke associated with aphasia can be expected to recover a significant amount of speech and language.

After TBI, children's deficits are related to the location and severity of their injury (45). Of note, the full extent of diffuse axonal injury may not be appreciated on clinical CT or MRI. Focal contusions are most common in the frontal and temporal lobes and can result in cognitive and behavioral deficits. Common neuropsychological sequelae of TBI include impairments in memory, attention, processing speed, expressive and receptive language (including aphasia), executive functioning, visuospatial skills, and academic skills. Novel behavioral and psychiatric disorders are common after TBI; problems stemming from disinhibition, such as secondary attention deficit hyperactivity disorder, are most notable (40,45,46).

Behavioral and cognitive impairments are seen as the most problematic for patients with TBI and their families, however, motor impairments occur and their effects should not be minimized. Even for those who have a good recovery, motor speed and high-level coordination are usually diminished. For the smaller subset of patients with continuing severe motor disabilities, impairments include disorders of tone, balance, coordination, ataxia, and tremors. These impairments are usually associated with deep injuries to the basal ganglia, thalamus, brainstem, and cerebellar outflow tracts.

Recovery and Rehabilitation after Acquired Brain Injury

As a general rule, most of the recovery after ABI occurs within the first year, and the majority of that recovery usually occurs within the first 3–6 months. However, it is important to recognize that spontaneous recovery is known to occur years after injury. With therapeutic intervention, improvements can occur despite a level of function that has been stable for years.

Cognitive and behavioral recovery after TBI occurs in a relatively predictable manner, as described by the Rancho Los Amigos Scale of Cognitive Functioning (**Table 17.1**), which helps staff and families understand the expected progression

TABLE 17.1

RANCHO LOS AMIGOS SCALE OF COGNITIVE FUNCTIONING

■ LEVEL	■ CLINICAL DESCRIPTION
Level I	No response
Level II	Generalized response
Level III	Localized response
Level IV	Confused, agitated response
Level V	Confused, nonagitated response
Level VI	Confused, appropriate response
Level VII	Automatic, appropriate response
Level VIII	Purposeful, appropriate response

of recovery. Behavioral and environmental guidelines should be provided as appropriate for the child's stage of recovery to minimize agitation. The basic goal is to reduce sensory overload (which is difficult in the PICU), yet at the same time provide enough familiar sensory input so that the patient can be as oriented as possible. Manipulating the environment and schedule to allow for distinction between day and night and promoting appropriate sleep are beneficial.

Rehabilitation after the PICU

The need for continuing brain injury rehabilitation will be determined by the number, type, and severity of impairments that affect the child's ability to communicate, perform activities of daily living (ADLs), and ambulate. As a general rule, acute, intense, interdisciplinary rehabilitation is justifiable if the patient has multiple impairments and will benefit from a minimum of 3 hours of therapy per day. It is the obligation of the acute medical system to identify these functional impairments and the need for rehabilitation and to make certain that appropriate rehabilitation services are arranged.

Acquired Spinal Cord Injuries

In children, spinal cord dysfunction (SCD) may be the result of any of multiple etiologies, including trauma, infection, a tumor, a vascular event, an autoimmune processes, or an iatrogenic cause (i.e., spine stabilization or reconstruction, epidural or spinal injections). Of the approximately 11,000 new traumatic SCIs that occur yearly in the United States, 6% occur in children younger than 16 years and 27% occur in individuals younger than 21 (47). Based on unique anatomic and biomechanical differences in the cervical spine between younger and older children, different patterns of traumatic SCI are seen in children aged 0–8 years and those aged 9–19 years. In young children, neural damage can occur even without radiographic (x-ray, CT) evidence of spinal column injury. This phenomenon is termed SCI without radiographic abnormality (SCIWORA), and is presumed to occur secondary to an increased elasticity of the spine that results in transient subluxation of the spinal column and causes the cord to stretch. In children, a latent period from 30 minutes to 4 days between injury and onset of paralysis has been reported after SCIWORA. After major trauma in young children, any worsening on serial neurologic examination should prompt efforts to rule out spinal cord lesion. MRI techniques are helpful for detailing soft-tissue injury in 65% of children with SCIWORA and may reveal abnormalities that include rupture of anterior or posterior longitudinal ligaments, endplate fractures, intradisk abnormalities, and spinal cord changes ranging from edema or hemorrhage to complete transection (48).

Acute intervention to treat the SCI itself is limited. In May 2008, the Consortium for Spinal Cord Medicine published clinical practice guidelines for management of adults suffering from acute SCI (49). Administration of methylprednisolone has been advocated in adults within the first 8 hours after injury, but the controversies surrounding the medical risks of steroid administration (increased gastric ulceration, increased number of infections, etc.) versus the neurologic benefits resulting from the treatment and the fact that the intervention was not specifically studied in children under 13 years of age allow for individualized decision of care. Very little evidence regarding the effectiveness of hypothermia in traumatic SCI exists. Spine immobilization is important in limiting further injury. Younger children (under the age of 8) have proportionally larger heads, necessitating thoracic elevation or/and occipital recess to prevent flexion of the head and neck and to best align the cervical spine during spine immobilization. The need for, and timing of, surgical intervention depends on the type of injury and neurologic findings (50). Acute SCI, particularly higher cervical injury, is frequently associated with TBI; so assessment and documentation of TBI in the form of loss of consciousness and PTA is recommended (49).

Medical Issues after Spinal Cord Injuries

A systematic approach to medical management of children with SCI in the PICU is advocated. *Respiratory*: The primary respiratory dysfunction in children with SCI is restrictive respiratory insufficiency induced by muscle paralysis. A smaller obstructive component exists in children with high cervical injuries owing to unbalanced vagal nerve activity, predisposing to airway hyperreactivity. Patients with C1 to C3 injury are usually dependent on mechanical ventilation. During initial hospitalization, pneumococcal vaccine should be given to children >2 years of age with respiratory dysfunction, and influenza vaccination should be administered yearly to children who are >6 months (51).

Cardiovascular: VTE occurs in 1.1% of children 13 years or younger with SCI, compared with 4.4% among those 14–19 years old (52). Recommendations for prophylaxis and treatment for VTE in children over the age of 14 with SCI are similar to those in adults (53,49); because of the low incidence of VTE in children <14 years, case-by-case consideration of the actual risk is advised (52).

Autonomic dysreflexia (AD), a phenomenon unique to persons with injury at T6 level or above, manifests with sweating, facial flushing, headaches, piloerection, and hypertension (hypertension that can result in cerebral hemorrhage). The mechanism for AD is postulated to be an accumulation of substance P and a deficiency of inhibitory neurotransmitters (e.g., norepinephrine, GABA, 5HT) below the level of injury, with resultant supersensitivity of spinal α- and peripheral adrenoreceptors. The carotid sinus and aortic arch baroreceptors are less sensitive to very high or very low blood pressure values (<60 or >160 mm Hg), thus limiting their ability to respond during AD. The treatment of AD is symptomatic. The patient should be positioned upright, thus producing an orthostatic decrease in blood pressure. The precipitating factor should be identified and removed. Lower urinary tract irritants account for 75%–85% of AD episodes and anorectal stimulation for 13%–19%; thus, the bladder should be catheterized or indwelling catheter should be checked for dysfunction and/or replaced, and the bowel program should be performed using lidocaine gel to prevent noxious stimuli. Other gastrointestinal (GI) factors (i.e., ileus, stress ulcer, cholecystitis), cutaneous stimuli (wounds, bunched clothing/bed sheets, etc.), trauma (bruises, cuts), fractures (occult or diagnosed), and deep venous thrombosis should also be considered. For individuals who present with high blood pressure and do not respond to conservative measures, the use of antihypertensive medications with rapid onset and short half-life (e.g., nitroglycerin SL/paste/IV, clonidine PO, hydralazine IV) should be considered.

Fever: Differential diagnoses include infection, VTE, pressure ulcer, and heterotopic ossification/myositis ossificans (periarticular bone-like formation in the muscle tissue that occurs below neurologic injury level, most commonly in the hips, knees, elbows, and shoulders). In 8%–11% of hospitalized adolescents and adults with SCI, no etiology for fever is found, and the fever is presumed to be secondary to thermoregulatory abnormalities (54).

Gastrointestinal: The early establishment of a bowel regimen that ensures complete and regular emptying is important. Stool softeners, rectal stimulation, and laxatives are the mainstays of therapy. Initiation of GI prophylaxis with H_2 blockers is advocated owing to high incidence of stress ulcer formation.

Hypercalcemia: Hypercalcemia of immobility can occur in 10%–23% of individuals with SCI, mostly adolescents and young males (8). The elevation in calcium can occur as early as 2 weeks following the SCI, but is most common 4–8 weeks after injury. Management includes hydration, furosemide, and biphosphonates, such as pamidronate.

Genitourinary: Genitourinary system manifestations in the acute phase consist mainly of urinary retention secondary to nervous system dysfunction and urinary tract infections related to bladder instrumentation. In the PICU, rapidly transitioning from the use of an indwelling device to a program of intermittent catheterization will limit infection.

Derma: In a patient with neurologic deficits, skin ulcerations or pressure sores can occur after only 1–2 hours of immobilization on a backboard. Proper positioning and frequent position changes, along with the use of pressure-relieving materials and devices, are the mainstays of skin care in individuals with limited mobility and insensate skin.

Soft Tissue and Joints: Soft tissue and joint contractures are frequent complications in children with SCI. ROM can be preserved by starting early and aggressive rehabilitation and by using adequate splinting.

Muscular: Within 1 month of SCI, muscle fiber cross-sectional area declines and muscle fibers are smaller, have less contractile protein, produce lower peak contractile forces, and have decreased resistance to fatigue. Stretching and strength training of the spared muscles during bed rest prevent atrophy and the loss of strength and contractile proteins. Electric neuromuscular stimulation of the paralyzed muscles may provide similar benefits (55).

Prognostic Factors and Outcome after Spinal Cord Injury

Clinicians should avoid extremes of offering false hope or frank pessimism when talking with patients with SCI and their families. Most who survive SCI do not experience complete severance of their spinal cords. An accurate neurologic examination aids in predicting recovery; however, any prognostication should be made cautiously early after injury, because spinal shock and other confounding variables (very young age, difficulty following instructions, head injury, mechanical ventilation, intoxication, severe multiple injuries) may interfere with the neurologic examination (56). Patients with MRI findings of hemorrhage or extensive segments of edema will have less motor recovery in comparison with patients with small, nonhemorrhagic lesions, although MRI itself is not as accurate a predictor as the physical examination (57). The most utilized neurologic assessment in SCI is based on the International Standards for Neurological Classification of SCI (American Spinal Injury Association [ASIA] Impairment Scale [AIS]) and, if confounders are carefully considered, it is the best tool for early prognostication. An accurate classification of impairment after SCI requires thorough understanding of the standards of AIS and careful neurologic examination. Details of the examination and scoring method can be found in the booklet that describes the standards (58). Elements of ASIA standard assessment consist of manual strength testing of 10 key muscles and sensory function assessment (light touch and pinprick) in 28 dermatomes on each side of the body.

The AIS consists of five grades of impairment: A, complete; B, sensory incomplete; C and D, motor incomplete; and E, normal motor and sensory functions. Determining precise motor level and injury severity is highly correlated with functional recovery in adults (57). Because young children (under 6 years of age) often cannot follow instructions to cooperate with the rigorous testing of the ASIA examination, this examination may not be as useful for prognostication, and clinical judgment should be exercised in interpreting a child's function (59). Prognosis may be more accurate if based on ASIA examination 72 hours after the acute injury rather than on the initial emergency room evaluation (56). If the child is in spinal shock, the examination should be repeated once the child emerges from spinal shock. Various criteria have been used to indicate resolution of spinal shock, with the return of bulbocavernosus reflex (segmental spinal reflex supplied by the S3–S4 sacral nerves) as the most commonly accepted clinical sign (60). Caution should be exercised when the AIS terminology of "completeness" of injury is discussed with the family. "Complete injury," AIS-A, indicates lack of sacral sparing, but does not necessarily indicate lack of function below the level of injury and does not mean that no axons cross the injury site. Conversion from complete to incomplete SCI has been reported as late as 2.5 years after injury in adults (57). In all SCI patients, the occurrence of conversion from complete to incomplete has been reported from 4.1% to 25.3%, with the rate of distal motor function recovery from 2.5% to 15.5% (60). Because the timing of initial classification of completeness in these studies varies from 1 day to several months after injury, and due to methodological differences, it is difficult to interpret this literature.

The majority of neurologic recovery in complete SCI occurs during the first 6–9 months (56). Studies have shown that considerable potential for recovery of the damaged human spinal cord continues for years after injury. In patients with complete tetraplegia, every motor level regained has significant functional implications and correlates with self-care function. Patients with injuries at C1 to C4 who are classified as AIS-A are dependent for self-care and transfers and are independent with power wheelchair mobility with specialized controls; those with functional levels of C8 to T1 are independent in activities of daily living, transfers, and bed mobility, and are able to use a manual wheelchair. Studies of adults revealed that those with complete tetraplegia typically gain an additional motor level in the upper extremity within 1 year after injury. Those with complete paraplegia rarely demonstrate change in neurologic level between 1 month and 1 year postinjury. Patients with complete SCI rarely walk, although those with incomplete injuries have a more favorable prognosis for community ambulation (56). The neurologic outcome of patients with SCIWORA is considered to be even better (61).

Rehabilitation after Spinal Cord Injury

Consultation from a pediatric physiatrist and rehabilitation services will provide a baseline motor–sensory and functional assessment, initiate a rehabilitation plan, help to outline prognosis, and facilitate transition from an intensive care setting to a rehabilitation phase that is focused on recovery and maximizing function of the injured child. Physical and occupational therapy will provide assistance with positioning and bracing, introduce exercises, and begin mobilization and functional training. Appropriate positioning is indicated to prevent skin breakdown, compression neuropathy, contractures, and increased spasticity. Patients with high cervical cord injuries benefit from speech pathology evaluation and therapy to assist with communication (augmentative technology, speaking valves) and with evaluation of the swallowing mechanism. For ventilator-dependent patients, the ability to direct others in how to assist them is important.

Amputations

Trauma is the leading cause of amputation in childhood, with etiologies varying depending on the region of the country and the age of the child (62). Traumatic amputations are twice as frequent as disease-related amputations, which are typically due to either tumor or infection. A single limb is involved in more than 90% of cases of pediatric amputation. Multiple limb involvement secondary to autoamputation is most commonly seen in cases that result from septic emboli, purpura fulminans, or disseminated intravascular coagulopathy.

During the acute postamputation period, rehabilitation goals include pain control, positioning to prevent loss of ROM, maintenance of strength and flexibility, and emotional support. In addition to adequate analgesic intervention, a skin desensitization program that consists of gentle tapping, massage, and soft tissue and scar mobilization can be an important part of treatment for phantom sensations and phantom pain (63).

Positioning the residual limb to prevent the development of flexion contractures is critical, especially in lower limb amputations, when walking with a prosthesis is usually the ultimate goal. Common contractures that must be avoided include hip flexion, hip adduction, hip external rotation, and knee flexion. Procedures and positions to prevent these complications include lying with the hip positioned neutrally or in extension (often aided by prone positioning), facilitating neutral rotation of the leg at the hip, and early ambulation. Positions to avoid include propping the residual limb with pillows, prolonged sitting, and lying with the leg positioned in flexion, adduction, and external rotation. In upper limb amputations, mobilization exercises for the shoulder and scapulae should be performed to prevent contracture formation that would limit the ability to move an upper limb prosthesis through space. A consult by the physical medicine and rehabilitation team may be beneficial to help with prosthesis prescription, recommendations about residual limb preparation, and family counseling regarding anticipated progress with functional use of the prosthetic limb.

As the patient's condition improves, attention should be given to the child's potential to develop psychological and social adjustment problems. This process begins in the PICU by assessing family interactions, temperament, coping style, and planning skills. Medical social workers play an instrumental role in helping families to obtain supportive community services. Psychosocial intervention may be as important as optimal wound healing and residual limb care with regard to the long-term function of the child and family. Successful reintegration into the community and school will in part depend on self-esteem, motivation, and family support. It is not too early to start addressing these issues in the PICU.

Rehabilitation Care for Critically Ill Children with Burns

The rehabilitation management of burns in the PICU focuses on the prevention of secondary complications that impair function following medical stabilization. Early rehabilitation goals include prevention of predictable deformities and secondary injuries through a program of positioning and splinting plus

ROM exercises. Another early priority should be to establish a long-term relationship between the patient and family and the rehabilitation team to facilitate continuation of, and compliance with, therapies after discharge from the PICU (64).

Even in the early phase of burn treatment, general positioning guidelines within the constraints required for graft healing and fluid management have an important role in decreasing contractures and subsequent deformity. Unfortunately, the position of comfort may not be the optimal position to prevent contractures. Guidelines for positioning based on the area of the burn (Table 17.2) should be posted, reviewed, and adjusted by the burn therapists and communicated to the nursing staff on a daily basis (65).

In preambulatory infants, the development of lower extremity contractures can adversely affect the development of walking ability. Positioning in prone, if tolerated, can prevent hip flexion contractures, and the use of knee immobilizers is helpful for decreasing knee flexion contractures. The frequency and duration of specialized positioning are determined by the patient's medical needs, ability to tolerate the interventions, and skin integrity. In sedated, immobile patients, a pressure-relieving mattress or overlay should be used in combination with repositioning and turning at least every 2 hours to prevent skin breakdown from unrelieved pressure. Proper positioning can also help in the control of edema. The elevation of hands and feet for edema control should be instituted during the first 72 hours following a burn injury.

Splints provide a static stretch in a desired position over time and are a useful addition to the positioning program. Splinting should be instituted when skin tightness is noticed or preemptively in cases of large body surface burns that involve the neck, axilla, hands, or feet (65). Flexion deformities of the neck can be minimized with the judicious use of thermoplastic neck splints and positioning in slight neck extension if the patient is unable to tolerate a neck collar. Ankle plantar flexion contractures commonly develop with prolonged bed rest and should be treated with the use of an ankle splint that blocks plantar flexion. Careful application of these splints, with attention to pressure points at the heel and metatarsal heads, is necessary so that skin breakdown does not occur in these areas.

During the acute period of treatment for a severe burn injury, ROM exercises may be limited by the requirements for immobilization during the process of skin grafting. However, if joints are not moved through their ROM for a prolonged period, contraction of joint capsules and shortening of tendon

and muscles that cross joints can occur rapidly. Therefore, clear communication between therapists and physicians as to when it is appropriate to perform ROM exercises is an integral part of ensuring optimal results from the grafting procedures. ROM exercises should generally occur during twice-a-day therapy sessions that are coordinated with the PICU staff's routines and schedules. Ideally, these sessions should be scheduled during times of planned analgesia or anesthesia to allow more aggressive joint movements. Often, it is practical to schedule ROM exercises during dressing changes so that stretching can occur once bulky dressings have been removed. Therapists should set a goal of moving all joints through a full ROM while paying attention to factors (including anxiety, wound status, extremity perfusion, and security of the patient's airway and vascular access devices) that may concurrently compromise the patient's medical stability (64).

The rehabilitation interventions just described can also decrease the risk of secondary neurologic and skin injuries associated with prolonged immobility. Although fairly common, weakness and sensory deficits due to peripheral neuropathies unrelated to direct burn injury are easily overlooked, particularly in a critically ill child (66). Although a generalized peripheral neuropathy syndrome is the neuromuscular abnormality most frequently diagnosed in association with burn injuries, localized neuropathies due to compression or stretch injuries also occur. Focal neuropathies may be prevented through meticulous attention to proper positioning, splint checks for appropriate fit, and skin checks for early sign of pressure damage.

REHABILITATION AND WEANING FROM PROLONGED MECHANICAL VENTILATION

Pulmonary rehabilitation begins in the acute care setting and must be approached as part of a multidisciplinary model in the context of the individual child's short- and long-term goals of care. *Prolonged mechanical ventilation* (PMV) has been defined as the need for mechanical ventilation for greater than 21 days for at least 6 hours per day (67,68). This definition, however, traditionally pertained to transtracheal support and the adult population. The need for flexibility in the pediatric population reflects a number of factors including: (a) heterogeneous conditions necessitating chronic, mechanical respiratory supports (i.e., congenital abnormalities, acute lung injury, airway

TABLE 17.2

POSITIONING THE PEDIATRIC BURN PATIENT

■ AREA OF BURN	■ CONTRACTURE RISK	■ CONTRACTURE PREVENTION
Anterior neck	Flexion	Extension, no pillows
Anterior axilla	Shoulder adduction	90-degree adduction with neutral rotation
Posterior axilla	Shoulder extension	Shoulder flexion
Elbow/forearm	Flexion/pronation	Elbow extended, forearm supinated
Wrists	Flexion	15–20-degree extension
Metacarpophalangeals	Hyperextension	70–90-degree flexion
Interphalangeals	Flexion	Full extension
Palmar burn	Finger flexion, thumb opposition	All joints full extension, thumb radially adducted
Chest	Lateral/anterior flexion	Straight, no lateral or anterior flexion
Hips	Flexion, adduction, external rotation	Extension, 10-degree adduction, neural rotation
Knees	Flexion	Extension
Ankles	Plantar flexion	90-degree dorsiflexion

Adapted from Taggart P, Haining R. Rehabilitation of burn injuries. In: Molnar GE, Alexander MA, eds. *Pediatric Rehabilitation*. 3rd ed. Philadelphia, PA: Hanley & Belfus, 1999:351–64.

anomalies, neuromuscular disease, acquired neurologic injury, and other conditions) (69,70); (b) absence of consensus for tracheostomy placement in the pediatric acute care setting; and (c) the expanding range of noninvasive support options (i.e., BiPAP, cough assist/insufflation–exsufflation devices, automated chest percussion, high-flow nasal cannula devices, and a range of pediatric interfaces). It is often helpful to recalibrate providers (whether nursing, physician, respiratory, or other therapists), the patient, and their family to a different paradigm and slower tempo when managing acute respiratory failure versus pulmonary rehabilitation.

Providers must consider physiologic, functional, and psychosocial factors when developing and implementing a pulmonary rehabilitation plan (69,71). Rigorous assessment may include gas exchange measures with routine pulse oximetry, transcutaneous CO_2 measurement, end-tidal CO_2, and correlative blood gases (the latter is helpful at the outset), pulmonary function testing, radiographic assessment, weight gain or loss trends, endurance and strength measures, and, potentially, polysomnography to assess for nocturnal variation. Allowance should be made for growth and developmental considerations, quality of life, disease trajectory, family preferences, functional capacity, and ability to facilitate transition to the community setting. If a tracheostomy tube is in place, routine airway assessment is required to gauge mucosal integrity, appropriate tube size and positioning, and determination of dynamic or fixed suprastomal and subglottic obstruction. It is worth noting that complete weaning of respiratory supports, removal of tracheostomy, discontinuation of noninvasive measures, elimination of oxygen, and monitoring devices may not be feasible or desirable for some patients and their respective families.

In the multidisciplinary context, weaning from respiratory support may be the last and most protracted aspect of rehabilitation. As previously noted, cardiopulmonary interactions and aerodigestive issues must be considered. Use of mechanical support will also minimize physiologic workload, permitting the patient to recover from a nutritional perspective while expending calories for maximal effort during physical and occupational therapies. Close collaboration with speech and language therapists will facilitate oral feeding and speaking (if safe and feasible). Ventilators can be an impediment to mobility; hence nocturnal support may be maintained once a daytime therapy threshold and capacity is reached. Ultimately, a patient- and family-driven weaning plan devised with the care team will be the most successful, addressing medical, psychological, and pragmatic needs. In order for the patient to transition home on support, extensive planning, education, supports, outreach to community providers, school arrangements, and follow-up with primary care and specialty providers are required (72).

CONCLUSIONS AND FUTURE DIRECTIONS

Children admitted to the PICU for a variety of diagnoses and mechanisms of injury can benefit from rehabilitation services. A rehabilitation consult by a physiatrist is best sought early in the course of treatment so that appropriate interventions, such as positioning and splinting, may be initiated to prevent muscle shortening, contractures, and other problems. Preventing complications when possible will make for a smoother recovery and, possibly, shorter rehabilitation course. Rehabilitation services not only are appropriate for children who are expected to recover but may also be useful in cases in which palliative care is the goal. Acute rehabilitation stays can help with family adjustment and training in caring for the child's needs and appropriate use of equipment prior

to discharge home. Currently, intensivists and physiatrists are collaborating to examine various PICU interventions to understand their impact on long-term outcomes, such as neurologic recovery following ABI or SCI. Future efforts could be directed toward optimizing rehabilitation interventions to decrease such sequelae of critical illness as complications of prolonged bed rest.

References

1. World Health Organization. *International Classification of Functioning, Disability, and Health (ICF)*. Geneva, Switzerland: World Health Organization, 2001.
2. Field MJ, Behrman BE, eds. *When Children Die: Improving Palliative and End-of-Life Care for Children and Their Families*. Washington, DC: National Academic Press, 2003.
3. American Academy of Pediatrics. Committee on Bioethics and Committee on Hospital Care. Palliative care for children. *Pediatrics* 2000;106(2):351–7.
4. Savage R. Identification, classification, and placement issues for students with traumatic brain injuries. *J Head Trauma Rehabil* 1991;6:1–9.
5. Halar EM, Bell K. Immobility and inactivity: Physiological and functional changes, prevention and treatment. In: DeLisa JA, Gans BM, Walsh NE, et al., eds. *Physical Medicine and Rehabilitation: Principles and Practice*. 4th ed. Vol 2. Philadelphia, PA: Lippincott Williams & Wilkins, 2005:1447–67.
6. Herbert RD, Balnave RJ. The effect of position of immobilization on resting length, resting stiffness, and weight of the soleus muscle of the rabbit. *J Orthop Res* 1993;11(3):358–66.
7. Minare P. Immobilization osteoporosis: A review. *Clin Rheumatol* 1989;8:95–103.
8. Maynard FM. Immobilization hypercalcemia following spinal cord injury. *Arch Phys Med Rehabil* 1986;67:41–4.
9. Levine S, Nguyen T, Taylor N, et al. Rapid disuse atrophy of diaphragm fibers in mechanically ventilated humans. *N Engl J Med* 2008;358(13):1327–35.
10. Birnkrant DJ, Panitch HB, Benditt JO, et al. American College of Chest Physicians consensus statement on the respiratory and related management of patients with Duchenne muscular dystrophy undergoing anesthesia or sedation. *Chest* 2007;132(6):1977–86.
11. Finder JD, Birnkrant D, Carl J, et al. Respiratory care of the patient with Duchenne muscular dystrophy: ATS consensus statement. *Am J Respir Crit Care Med* 2004;170(4):456–65.
12. Schroth MK. Special considerations in the respiratory management of spinal muscular atrophy. *Pediatrics* 2009;123(suppl 4):S245–9.
13. Curley MA, Quigley SM, Lin M. Pressure ulcers in pediatric intensive care: Incidence and associated factors. *Pediatr Crit Care Med* 2003;4(3):284–90.
14. Rodriguez-Key M, Alonzi A. Nutrition, skin integrity, and pressure ulcer healing in chronically ill children: An overview. *Ostomy Wound Manage* 2007;53(6):56–8,60,62,passim.
15. Groeneveld A, Anderson M, Allen S, et al. The prevalence of pressure ulcers in a tertiary care pediatric and adult hospital. *J Wound Ostomy Continence Nurs* 2004;31(3):108–20;quiz 121–2.
16. Butler CT. Pediatric skin care: Guidelines for assessment, prevention, and treatment. *Pediatr Nurs* 2006;32(5):443–50.
17. Garcia-Molina P, Balaguer-López E, Torra I Bou JE, et al. A prospective, longitudinal study to assess use of continuous and reactive low-pressure mattresses to reduce pressure ulcer incidence in a pediatric intensive care unit. *Ostomy Wound Manage* 2012;58(7):32–9.
18. Andrew M, David M, Adams M, et al. Venous thromboembolic complications (VTE) in children: First analyses of the Canadian Registry of VTE. *Blood* 1994;83:1251–7.
19. Kerlin BA. Current and future management of pediatric venous thromboembolism. *Am J Hematol* 2012;87(suppl 1):S68–74.

20. Raffini L, Huang YS, Witmer C, et al. Dramatic increase in venous thromboembolism in children's hospitals in the United States from 2001 to 2007. *Pediatrics* 2009;124(4):1001–8.

21. van Ommen CH, Heijboer H, Büller HR, et al. Venous thromboembolism in childhood: A prospective two-year registry in The Netherlands. *J Pediatr* 2001;139(5):676–81.

22. Rohrer MJ, Cutler BS, MacDougall E, et al. A prospective study of the incidence of deep venous thrombosis in hospitalized children. *J Vasc Surg* 1996;24:46–50.

23. Hanson SJ, Punzalan RC, Arca MJ, et al. Effectiveness of clinical guidelines for deep vein thrombosis prophylaxis in reducing the incidence of venous thromboembolism in critically ill children after trauma. *J Trauma Acute Care Surg* 2012;72(5):1292–7.

24. Kenet G, Nowak-Gottl U. Venous thromboembolism in neonates and children. *Best Pract Res Clin Haematol* 2012;25(3):333–44.

25. Raffini L, Trimarchi T, Beliveau J, et al. Thromboprophylaxis in a pediatric hospital: A patient-safety and quality-improvement initiative. *Pediatrics* 2011;127(5):e1326–32.

26. Sharathkumar AA, Mahajerin A, Heidt L, et al. Risk-prediction tool for identifying hospitalized children with a predisposition for development of venous thromboembolism: Peds-Clot clinical Decision Rule. *J Thromb Haemost* 2012;10(7):1326–34.

27. Smith HA, Fuchs DC, Pandharipande PP, et al. Delirium: An emerging frontier in the management of critically ill children. *Crit Care Clin* 2009;25(3):593–614.

28. Baker C. Preventing ICU syndrome in children. *Paediatric Nurs* 2004;16(10):32–5.

29. Nelson LP, Gold JI. Posttraumatic stress disorder in children and their parents following admission to the pediatric intensive care unit: A review. *Pediatr Crit Care Med* 2012;13(3):338–47.

30. Brosbe MS, Hoefling K, Faust J. Predicting posttraumatic stress following pediatric injury: A systematic review. *J Pediatr Psychol* 2011;36(6):718–29.

31. Melnyk BM, Alpert-Gillis L, Feinstein NF, et al. Creating opportunities for parent empowerment: Program effects on the mental health/coping outcomes of critically ill young children and their mothers. *Pediatrics* 2004;113(6):e597–607.

32. Kazak AE, Kassam-Adams N, Schneider S, et al. (2006). An integrative model of pediatric medical traumatic stress. *J Pediatr Psychol* 2006;31(4):343–55.

33. Faul M, Xu L, Wald MM, et al. *Traumatic Brain Injury in the United States: Emergency Department Visits, Hospitalizations, and Deaths*. Atlanta, GA: Centers for Disease Control and Prevention, National Center for Injury Prevention and Control, 2010.

34. Langlois JA, Rutland-Brown W, Wald MM. The epidemiology and impact of traumatic brain injury: A brief overview. *J Head Trauma Rehab* 2006;21(5):375–8.

35. Schneier AJ, Shields BJ, Hostetler SG, et al. Incidence of pediatric traumatic brain injury and associated hospital resource utilization in the United States. *Pediatrics* 2006;118(2):483–92.

36. Chung CY, Chen CL, Cheng PT, et al. Critical score of Glasgow Come Scale for pediatric traumatic brain injury. *Pediatr Neurol* 2006;34(5):379–87.

37. Wilson JT, Teasdale GM, Hadley DM, et al. Post-traumatic amnesia: Still a valuable yardstick. *J Neurol Neurosurg Psych* 1994;57(2):198–201.

38. Russo RN, O'Flahery S. Bromocriptine for the management of autonomic dysfunction after severe traumatic brain injury. *J Pediatr Child Health* 2000;36(3):283–5.

39. Meythaler JM, Stinson AM. Fever of central origin in traumatic brain injury controlled with propranolol. *Arch Phys Med Rehabil* 1994;75(7):816–8.

40. Jaffe KM, Polissar NL, Fay GC, et al. Recovery trends over three years following pediatric traumatic brain injury. *Arch Phys Med Rehabil* 1995;76:17–26.

41. Temkin NJ, Dikmen SS, Wilensky AJ, et al. A randomized, double-blind study of phenytoin for the prevention of post-traumatic seizures. *N Engl J Med* 1993;323:497–502.

42. Mazzini L, Campini R, Angelino E, et al. Post-traumatic hydrocephalus: A clinical, neuroradiologic and neuropsychologic assessment of long-term outcome. *Arch Phys Med Rehabil* 2003;84:1637–41.

43. Jiang J, Gao G, Wei-Ping L, et al. Early indicators of prognosis in 846 cases of severe traumatic brain injury. *J Neurotrauma* 2002;19(7):869–74.

44. Kriel RL, Krach LE, Luxenberg MG, et al. Outcome of severe anoxic/ischemic brain injury in children. *Pediatr Neurol* 1994;10(3):207–12.

45. Fay GC, Jaffe KM, Polissar NL, et al. Outcome of pediatric traumatic brain injury at three years: A cohort study. *Arch Phys Med Rehabil* 1994;75(7):733–41.

46. Schwartz L, Taylor HG, Drotar D, et al. Long-term behavior problems following pediatric traumatic brain injury: Prevalence, predictors, and correlates. *J Pediatr Psychol* 2003;28(4):251–63.

47. 2011 NSCISC Annual Statistical Report. *National Spinal Cord Injury Statistical Center, University of Alabama at Birmingham*. http://www.nscisc.uab.edu/reports.aspx.

48. Pang D. Spinal cord injury without radiographic abnormalities in children, two decades later. *Neurosurgery* 2004;55(6):1325–43.

49. Consortium for Spinal Cord Medicine. Early acute management in adults with spinal cord injury: A clinical practice guideline for health-care professionals. *J Spinal Cord Med* 2008;31(4):403–79.

50. Parent S, Mac-Thiong JM, Roy-Beaudry M, et al. Spinal cord injury in the pediatric population: A systematic review of the literature. *J Neurotrauma* 2011;28(8):1515–24.

51. Waites KB, Canupp KC, Edwards K, et al. Immunogenicity of pneumococcal vaccine in persons with spinal cord injury. *Arch Phys Med Rehabil* 1998;79(12):1504–9.

52. Jones T, Ugalde V, Franks P, et al. Venous thromboembolism after spinal cord injury: Incidence, time course and associated risk factors in 16,240 adults and children. *Arch Phys Med Rehabil* 2005;86:2240–7.

53. Consortium for Spinal Cord Medicine. Prevention of thromboembolism in spinal cord injury. *J Spinal Cord Med* 1997;20:259–83.

54. Beraldo PS, Neves EG, Alves CM, et al. Pyrexia in hospitalized spinal cord injury patients. *Paraplegia* 1993;31(3):186–91.

55. Karatzanos E, Gerovasili V, Zervakis D, et al. Electrical muscle stimulation: An effective form of exercise and early mobilization to preserve muscle strength in critically ill patients. *Crit Care Res Pract* 2012;2012:432752.

56. Burns AS, Ditunno JF. Establishing prognosis and maximizing functional outcomes after spinal cord injury. *Spine* 2001;26(24S):S137–45.

57. Kirshblum SC, O'Connor KC. Predicting neurologic recovery in traumatic cervical spinal cord injury. *Arch Phys Med Rehabil* 1998;79:1456–66.

58. American Spinal Injury Association. *International Standards for Neurological Classification of SCI*. Rev. 2011. Atlanta, GA: American Spinal Injury Association, 2011.

59. Mulcahey MJ, Gaughan JP, Chafetz RS, et al. Interrater reliability of the international standards for neurological classification of spinal cord injury in youths with chronic spinal cord injury. *Arch Phys Med Rehabil* 2011;92(8):1264–9.

60. Fisher CG, Noonan VK, Smith DE, et al. Motor recovery, functional status, and health-related quality of life in patients with complete spinal cord injuries. *Spine* 2005;30(19):2200–7.

61. Neva MH, Roeder CP, Felder U, et al. Neurological outcome, working capacity and prognostic factors of patients with SCI-WORA. *Spinal Cord* 2012;50:78–80.

62. Gaebler-Spira D, Uellendahl J. Pediatric limb deficiencies. In: Molnar GA, Alexander MA, eds. *Pediatric Rehabilitation*. 3rd ed. Philadelphia, PA: Hanley & Belfus; 1999:331–50.

63. Esquenazi A. Upper limb amputee rehabilitation and prosthetic restoration. In: Braddom RL, ed. *Physical Medicine & Rehabilitation*. 1st ed. Philadelphia, PA: W.B. Saunders, 1996:275–88.

64. Sheridan RL. Burn Rehabilitation. *eMedicine*. http://www.emedicine.com/pmr/topic163.htm. Accessed July 18, 2006.

65. Taggart P, Haining R. Rehabilitation of burn injuries. In: Molnar GE, Alexander MA, eds. *Pediatric Rehabilitation*. 3rd ed. Philadelphia, PA: Hanley & Belfus, 1999:351–64.

66. Helm PA, Pandian G, Heck E. Neuromuscular problems in the burn patient: Cause and prevention. *Arch Phys Med Rehabil* 1985;66:451–53.

67. MacIntyre NR, Cook DJ, Ely EW Jr, et al. Evidence-based guidelines for weaning and discontinuing ventilatory support: A collective task force facilitated by the American College of Chest Physicians; the American Association for Respiratory Care; and the American College of Critical Care Medicine. *Chest* 2001;120(6 suppl):375S–95S.

68. MacIntyre NR, Epstein SK, Carson S, et al. Management of patients requiring prolonged mechanical ventilation: Report of a NAMDRC consensus conference. *Chest* 2005;128(6):3937–54.

69. Ceriana P, Carlucci A, Navalesi P, et al. Weaning from tracheotomy in long-term mechanically ventilated patients: Feasibility of a decisional flowchart and clinical outcome. *Intens Care Med* 2003;29(5):845–8.

70. Graham RJ, Fleegler EW, Robinson WM. Chronic ventilator need in the community: A 2005 pediatric census of Massachusetts. *Pediatrics* 2007;119(6):e1280–7.

71. O'Brien JE, Birnkrant DJ, Dumas HM, et al. Weaning children from mechanical ventilation in a post-acute care setting. *Pediatr Rehabil* 2006;9(4):365–72.

72. Panitch HB, Downes JJ, Kennedy JS, et al. Guidelines for home care of children with chronic respiratory insufficiency. *Pediatr Pulmonol* 1996;21(1):52–6.

CHAPTER 18 ■ OMICS AND CRITICAL CARE

MARY K. DAHMER AND MICHAEL QUASNEY

KEY POINTS

❶ "Omic" approaches may provide better insight into highly complex diseases, such as sepsis, trauma, and other illnesses with multiorgan dysfunction that could result in improved diagnostic tests and novel therapies.

❷ Genomics is the study of the structure and function of DNA within cells. Genomics includes efforts to determine nucleotide sequences, to fine-scale map genes, and to analyze interactions between loci that occur within the genome.

❸ Variants that alter protein levels or function are partially responsible for genetically determined variation in our physical characteristics, physiology, and personality traits. Genetic variability also explains some of the variability in disease susceptibility, disease severity, and response to treatment that is observed in patient populations.

❹ Epigenetics is the study of heritable changes in gene activity and expression that are not dependent on changes in the gene sequence, and epigenomics is the study of the global epigenetic signature in a cell or tissue.

❺ The transcriptome refers to all RNAs produced in the cell, including messenger RNA, ribosomal RNA, and transfer RNA in addition to noncoding RNAs, such as microRNAs (miRNAs). The majority of research on the transcriptome has focused on examining gene expression profiles in different disease states or following various treatments.

Specifically, these studies have examined gene expression or repression in various conditions, such as sepsis or acute respiratory distress syndrome.

❻ Genome-wide expression profiling in children with septic shock has been instrumental in providing a better understanding of the molecular biology of sepsis.

❼ In critical illnesses, miRNAs have been examined as potential biomarkers of diseases, such as sepsis, traumatic brain injury, and cardiac arrest, and may be useful in understanding mechanisms of disease.

❽ Proteomic studies have been performed in several processes relevant to critical care, including sepsis, acute lung injury, trauma, burns, acute kidney injury, and traumatic brain injury.

❾ Critical illnesses and injury are accompanied by severe metabolic changes. Another "omics" approach that has clinical applications in critical care is metabolomics, which commonly uses mass spectrometry or high-resolution nuclear magnetic resonance to characterize and quantify small molecules generated from cellular metabolic activity.

❿ In conclusion, the recent development of new "omic" technologies has provided new tools for examining the "global" molecular response to critical illness and injury that occurs in children.

Humans are complex and dynamic organisms. Their biology is often difficult to predict, especially in times of severe stress that commonly occur with critical illness and injury. Biomedical research has taken the reductionist approach to understanding the individual parts of organisms to better predict the behavior of the organism in entirety. Over the last several years, the development of high-throughput techniques has permitted characterization of intracellular and extracellular environments at the molecular and biochemical levels. Analysis of high-throughput data relies on bioinformatics and computational modeling and allows for a system-wide approach that focuses on complex interactions, which are particularly relevant to the field of critical care. These advances have rapidly expanded our understanding of complex disease processes and altered the vision of how medicine will be practiced in the future. Furthermore, these technologies have helped to foster the idea of personalized or individualized medicine, whereby patients will be treated with medical therapies customized to the individual rather than with standard therapies specific to the disease. These technological advances are making inroads into the pediatric intensive care unit. They provide a better understanding of the pathophysiology of diseases, such as sepsis and acute respiratory distress syndrome (ARDS), and may potentially be used to stratify patients and to discover new biomarkers that will help determine risk factors and prognosis.

This chapter will describe these new techniques and how they are used to study critical illness and injury.

OMICS

Novel large-scale and data-rich technologies have been developed to examine various fields of biology including genomics, transcriptomics, proteomics, and metabolomics. These new approaches have had a dramatic impact on our understanding of various biological processes and have revealed complex interactions among them. Integration of the analyses of these datasets to gain insights that may not be revealed by analyzing them individually has gained widespread interest and is beginning to impact a number of medical disciplines including critical illness.

Omics refers to approaches that globally assess a specific class of biological molecules in a cell, tissue, or biological fluid. For example, genomics refers to the study of the structure and function of the entire genome, which is composed of all DNAs within a cell. Likewise, study of the transcriptome (RNA transcripts in cells or tissues), proteome (proteins in cells or tissues), and metabolome (small metabolites in cells, tissues or bodily fluids) give rise to the fields of transcriptomics, proteomics, and metabolomics. In addition, epigenomics is the study of global epigenetic changes in cells or tissues. High-throughput, high-dimensional study of the genome, transcriptome, proteome, metabolome, and epigenome has produced a massive amount of interconnecting data from many biological systems and processes. However, the sheer volume and complexity of these data make analyses and interpretation extremely challenging. Increasingly sophisticated bioinformatics tools and computational analyses are required to perform studies using **❶** these technologies. These "omic" approaches may provide better insight into highly complex diseases, such as sepsis, trauma, and other illnesses with multiorgan dysfunction that could result in improved diagnostic tests and novel therapies. In the following sections, these various "omics" disciplines will be discussed in relation to critical illness and injury.

GENOMICS

❷ Genomics is the study of the structure and function of DNA within cells. Genomics includes efforts to determine nucleotide sequences, to conduct fine-scale genetic mapping, and to analyze interactions between loci that occur within the genome. The key technology driving genomics is high-throughput DNA sequencing combined with bioinformatics to analyze the large volumes of data. High-throughput DNA sequencing technology facilitated the sequencing of the entire human genome, in addition to the genomes of many other organisms. These data revealed that many sites in the human genome are variable and there are numerous differences in DNA sequences between individuals.

The most frequent type of genetic variation is a single nucleotide polymorphism (SNP) that results from a nucleotide substitution. Variations may also arise from insertions or deletions of DNA fragments or from the presence of a variable number of tandem repeats (VNTRs) of short, repetitive DNA sequences. In some individuals, the differences in sequence are large (>1 kilobase), resulting in alterations in DNA copy number. Such variants are called copy number variants (CNVs). CNVs are relatively common in human genomes and contribute significantly to human genetic variation. Given that individuals have two copies of each gene, an individual is either heterozygous or homozygous for one or the other variant whether it is an SNP, VNTR, or CNV.

Variants do not necessarily affect the expression or the function of the gene product, particularly when they occur in a noncoding region of the gene that is not involved in regulating messenger RNA (mRNA) transcription from a DNA template or in mRNA processing or stability. Variants resulting from large changes in coding regions are likely to affect the protein product; however, many SNPs in the coding region do not affect gene function or stability if the encoded amino acid remains the same (a silent substitution) or if the amino acid substitution does not affect protein stability or function. There are instances where genetic variants, including SNPs, affect protein expression (by altering noncoding regulatory regions of the gene) or function (by altering the amino acid sequence), but not all such changes are necessarily deleterious. In many instances, genetic variants explain the variation in protein levels observed in the general population. Variants that alter protein levels or function are partially responsible **❸** for genetically determined variation in our physical characteristics, physiology, and personality traits. Genetic variability also explains some of the variability in disease susceptibility, disease severity, and response to treatment that is observed in patient populations.

Genotyping to identify specific variants in a particular gene is commonplace for diagnosing genetic disorders in the clinical setting. Nearly all genotyping techniques utilize polymerase chain reaction (PCR) to amplify a DNA fragment that contains the site of interest. For amplification, PCR uses small pieces of DNA, termed primers, which are complementary to the regions that flank the site of interest. Early techniques identified genotypes based on the size of the PCR product (insertions or deletions, VNTRs, SNPs present in restriction enzyme recognition sites) or by using allele-specific hybridization approaches, such as allele-specific PCR or hybridization with labeled allele-specific oligonucleotide probes. Genotyping is now routinely performed as a single-site assay or by genotyping hundreds to millions of SNPs using custom-made arrays or arrays that probe for SNPs from across the entire genome (genome-wide SNP arrays). These techniques are more amenable to high-throughput technology. Genome-wide SNP arrays are used for genome-wide association studies (GWASs), which examine millions of SNPs simultaneously to determine whether any are associated with specific diseases.

Next-generation sequencing technologies are commonplace (1), partly due to a reduction in the cost of DNA sequencing. Using this technique, DNA is randomly fragmented and ligated to common adaptor sequences to form a library. The library is hybridized to an array platform of millions of spatially fixed PCR fragments that are complementary to the DNA fragments. Given that the array contains multiple PCR fragments that are complementary to a DNA library fragment, millions of short DNA reads are produced in a highly efficient manner. Following enzyme-driven biochemistry and imaging-based data processing, short reads are mapped to a source genome to generate a sequence read. Recent advances in DNA sequencing technologies, combined with reduced cost, make sequencing the human genome much less expensive and make it realistic to use this technology to identify novel genetic variants.

The technologies described above have been used to examine the influence of genetic variation on the susceptibility to, and outcomes of, various diseases relevant to critical care. This information may allow physicians to identify children who are at greatest risk for poor outcomes, allowing for modified monitoring strategies in the intensive care unit or novel therapies. Several genes that harbor genetic variations associated with the severity of sepsis or acute lung injury (ALI) in critically ill populations have been described (**Tables 18.1** and **18.2**). One example is the cystic fibrosis transmembrane conductance regulator (*CFTR*) gene, which codes for a chloride channel protein expressed on epithelial cells in bronchi, bronchioles, and alveoli (2–5). Influx of fluid into the alveoli following increased permeability of the alveolar-capillary barrier is one of the hallmarks of ARDS (6), and the ability to clear fluid rapidly is associated with improved outcome (7). The clearance of alveolar fluid occurs through active ion transport (8), and CFTR has a role in both cyclic adenosine monophosphate–stimulated fluid absorption and modulation of the epithelial sodium channel (2,3,9). *CFTR* contains 27 exons that are spliced together to give mature CFTR mRNA. Alternatively spliced transcripts are relatively common, and levels of CFTR protein and activity vary between individuals (10). Mutations in the *CFTR* gene cause cystic fibrosis (CF), a disease characterized by progressive injury to the lungs (11). Interestingly, *in vitro* and *ex vivo* studies suggest that CFTR deficiency results in a dysregulated inflammatory response (12–17) and promotes lipopolysaccharide (LPS)-induced lung injury in mice (15,18), suggesting that CFTR has immune modulatory activity.

In addition to the relatively rare variants that affect CFTR function, two common polymorphisms affect the function of CFTR. One polymorphism is the $(TG)_mT_n$ variable repeat region located in intron 8. Both *in vitro* and *in vivo* studies show an association between either a higher number of TG repeats and/or a lower number of Ts with an increased proportion of mRNA transcripts deficient in exon 9 (19–23). Mechanistic studies also reveal that different alleles at the $(TG)_mT_n$

TABLE 18.1

GENETIC POLYMORPHISMS ASSOCIATED WITH SEPSIS

■ GENE	■ POLYMORPHISM[a]	■ CONSEQUENCE OF POLYMORPHISM	■ REFERENCE
ACE	Insertion/deletion (I/D)	DD associated with increased serum and tissue levels; associated with more severe meningococcal disease; DD associated with decreased risk of sepsis	144,145
BPI	+545 G/C rs4358188 (+645 A/G, Lys216Glu)	Increased risk of gram - sepsis and mortality	146
CD14	−1145 G/A rs7524551 (−159 C/T)	Association with CD14 expression, MODS, and sepsis Association with CD14 levels, MODS, sepsis, mortality, and gram - infections	147–152
FCγRIIa	rs1801274 (H131R)	Associated with decreased affinity to IgG_2 and opsonization; associated with increased risk of meningococcal and septic shock	153–157
HSPA1L	rs2227956 (−2437 C/T)	Associated with increased cytokine levels and liver failure but not sepsis-related morbidity	158–160
HSPA1B	(−1538 G/A)	Associated with increased cytokine levels and liver failure but not sepsis-related morbidity	158–160
HSP70-2	rs1061581 (+1267 G/A)	An allele associated with septic shock in adults with CAP	161
IL-1β and IL-1$_{RA}$	rs16944 (−511 T/C) Variable 86-bp repeat −1470 G/C rs1143627 (−31 C/T)	−511 allele associated with increased survival of meningococcemia; combination of IL-1β and IL-1$_{RA}$ alleles associated with decreased survival	162–165
IL-6	rs4800795 (−174 G/C) rs1800796 (−572 G/C)	Associated with increased IL-6 levels and risk of sepsis and severity of sepsis	166
IL-10	rs1800896 (−1082 G/A) rs1800871 (−819 C/T) rs1800872 (−592 C/A)	GCC haplotype associated with increased levels; associated with sepsis and some variations associated with mortality	167–170
LBP	rs1780616 (−1978 C/T) rs5741812 (−921 A/T) rs2232571 (−836 C/T) rs1780617 (−763 A/G) rs2232618 (26877 T/C Phe436Leu)	Severe sepsis for four SNP haplotype CATA; serum LBP increased and mortality for −836 C/T; Phe436Leu associated with sepsis in trauma cohort	171–173
TNF-β and LT-α	rs1800629 (−308 G/A) rs361525 (−238 G/A) Many others rs909253 (LT-α+252 G/A)	Associated with increased TNF-α levels; associated with increased mortality in sepsis and bacteremia	174–201
MBL	rs11003125 (−550 G/C) rs7096206 (−221 G/C) rs5030737 (Arg$_{52}$Cys C/T) rs1800450 (Gly$_{54}$Asp G/A) rs1800451 (Gly$_{57}$Glu G/A)	−221 associated with MBL levels, sepsis, but not to mortality; structural variants associated with decreased levels and activity and increased risk of infection and severity of disease	149,202–207
ND1	rs1599988 (m4216 T/C)	Associated with decreased NADH dehydrogenase 1 activity	208,209
PAI-1	4G/5G	4G associated with increased levels; associated with septic shock and DIC in meningococcal disease	210–215
Protein C	rs1799808 (−1654 C/T) rs1799809 (−1641 G/A) rs2069912 (673 T/C)	CA haplotype (−1654 and −1641) and C allele associated with increased mortality in Asian populations; CG haplotype associated with more severe meningococcal disease in Caucasians	216–218
TIMP-1	rs4898 (372 T/C)	Associated with higher levels of TIMP-1 and higher 30-day mortality	219
TLR1	rs5743551 (−7202 A/G)	Associated with greater immune response, higher mortality, and worse organ function	220,221
TLR2	−16933 A/T rs1895830 (−15607 A/G) rs3804099 (597 C/T) 2029 C/T (Arg677Trp) rs5743708 (2257 A/G, Arg753Gln)	Associated with gram + sepsis but not survival Associated with cytokine expression Associated with cytokine expression, MODS, and morbidity Associated with mycobacterial infections Associated with increased severe bacterial infections, increased sepsis in African Americans	149,198, 222–227

■ GENE	■ POLYMORPHISM[a]	■ CONSEQUENCE OF POLYMORPHISM	■ REFERENCE
TLR4	−2242 T/C rs4986790 (Asp299Gly) Thr399Ile	Associated with increased cytokine expression, sepsis-related morbidity, and MODS; gram - bacteremia; associated with increased risk of sepsis and mortality	150,190,226, 228,229
VEGF	rs3025039 (936 C/T)	Associated with development of AKI in patients with severe sepsis	230

[a]Terminology used for the various polymorphisms are the ones most commonly used in the literature and may refer to the nucleotide position, amino acid position, or name of the allele. This table is representative of polymorphisms examined in sepsis, but does not include all such polymorphisms. ACE, angiotensin-converting enzyme; BPI, bactericidal permeability increasing protein; MODS, multiorgan dysfunction syndrome; Ig, immunoglobulin; HSP, heat shock protein; CAP, community-acquired pneumonia; IL-1$_{RA}$, interleukin 1 receptor antagonist (GCC haplotype of the IL-10 promoter is defined by three single-site polymorphisms at −1082, −819, and −592); LBP, lipopolysaccharide-binding protein; TNF, tumor necrosis factor; LT, lymphotoxin; MBL, mannose-binding lectin; PAI, plasminogen activator inhibitor; DIC, disseminated intravascular coagulation; TIMP, tissue inhibitor of matrix metalloproteinase; TLR, Toll-like receptor; VEGF, vascular endothelial growth factor.

TABLE 18.2

GENETIC POLYMORPHISMS ASSOCIATED WITH ALI

■ GENE	■ POLYMORPHISM[a]	■ CONSEQUENCE OF POLYMORPHISM	■ REFERENCE
ACE	Insertion/deletion	D/D associated with increased serum and tissue levels; associated with development of ALI	231–233
ANGPT2	rs2959811 rs2515475 rs1868554	Associated with variable plasma levels of angiopoietin-2 and development of ALI in adults with trauma	234,235
CFTR	(TG)$_m$T$_n$	More TGs or fewer Ts associated with more skipping of exon 9 and, therefore, less CFTR; associated with more severe lung injury in African American children with CAP	30
F5	rs6025 (Arg506Gln)	Associated with decreased mortality in Caucasian adults with ARDS	236
FAS	rs17447140 (−11341 A/T) rs2147420 (9325 G/A) rs2234978 (21541 C/T) rs1051070 (22484 A/T)	Haplotype associated with increased FAS mRNA in response to LPS and risk of ALI but not mortality	237
FTL	rs905238 rs918546 rs2230267	Frequency of SNPs higher in adult cohort with ARDS	238
HMOX2	rs1362626 rs2404579 rs2270366 rs1051308 rs7702	Frequency of specific genotypes and haplotypes lower in adults with ARDS	238
IL-1$_{RA}$	rs4251961 variable 86-bp repeat	Associated with variable levels of IL-1$_{RA}$ and VNTR associated with risk of severe lung injury in children	239,240
IL-6	rs4800795 (−174 G/C) Several others	Associated with variable levels of IL-6 and haplotype associated with increased susceptibility to ARDS in adults	241–244
IRAK3	rs10506481	Associated with increased risk of ARDS in adults with sepsis	245
MBL2	rs1800451	Associated with lower levels of MBL and more severe sepsis and sepsis-induced ARDS	246–248
MIF	rs2070767 rs755622	Haplotypes associated with sepsis and ALI and both European-descent and African-descent populations	249
MYLK	rs9840993 rs4678047 rs28497577	Individual SNPs as well as haplotypes associated with increased risk of ALI especially in African American population	250,251
NFE2L2 (Nrf2)	rs1754059 (−617 C/A)	A allele reduces activity of gene promoter and was associated with ALI in trauma patients	252
NFKBIA	rs3138053 (−881 A/G) rs2233406 (−826 C/T) rs2233409 (−297 C/T)	GTC haplotype is associated with ARDS	253
NQO1	rs689455 (−1221 A/C)	C allele associated with decreased transcription and lower incidence of ALI in trauma patients	254

(continued)

TABLE 18.2 (*continued*)

■ GENE	■ POLYMORPHISM[a]	■ CONSEQUENCE OF POLYMORPHISM	■ REFERENCE
PAI-1	4G/5G	4G associated with increased levels; associated with increased mortality in ALI	214
PBEF1	rs41496055	Associated with decreased transcription of PBEF and higher risk of ALI in adults with sepsis	64
PLAU	rs1916341 rs2227562 rs2227564 rs2227566 rs2227571 rs4065	CGCCCC haplotype associated with 60-day mortality and ventilator-free days but not risk for developing ALI in adults with sepsis	255
PPFIA1	rs471931	Associated with ALI in adults using GWAS	31
SFTPB	rs1130866 (+1580 C/A)	Associated with development of ALI and worse lung injury; allele may impact glycosylation and processing of protein	256
SOD3	rs1007991 rs8192291 rs2695232 rs2855262	GCCT haplotype associated with decreased ALI in adults with sepsis and lower mortality	257
TLR1	rs5743551 (−7202 A/G)	Associated with sepsis-induced ALI and mortality in adults	220
TNF-α	rs1800629 (−308 G/A)	A allele is associated with increased level of production and with mortality in patients with ARDS	258
VEGF	rs833061 (−460 C/T) rs2010963 (+405 C/G) rs3025039 (+936 C/T)	Specific genotypes and haplotypes associated with lower levels of VEGF and higher mortality in ARDS	259,260

[a]Terminology used for the various polymorphisms are the ones most commonly used in the literature and may refer to the nucleotide position, amino acid position, or name of the allele. This table is representative of polymorphisms examined in ALI but may not include all such polymorphisms. ACE, angiotensin-converting enzyme; ALI, acute lung injury; ANGPT2, angiopoietin-2; CFTR, cystic fibrosis transmembrane conductance regulator; F5, factor V Leiden; FTL, ferritin light chain; HMOX2, heme oxygenase 2; IL-1$_{RA}$, interleukin 1 receptor antagonist; IL-6, interleukin 6; IRAK3, interleukin-1 receptor-associated kinase 3; MBL, mannose-binding lectin; MIF, macrophage migration inhibitory factor; MYLK, myosin light chain kinase; NFE2L2, nuclear factor (erythroid-derived)-like 2; NFKBIA, nuclear factor kappa B inhibitor alpha; NQO1, NADPH quinone oxidoreductase 1; PAI-1, plasminogen activator inhibitor 1; PBEF1, pre-B-cell colony-enhancing factor 1; PLAU, plasminogen activator urokinase; PPFIA 1, protein tyrosine phosphatase receptor type F polypeptide-interacting protein alpha-1; SFTPB, surfactant protein B; SOD, superoxide dismutase; TLR1, Toll-like receptor 1; TNF, tumor necrosis factor; VEGF, vascular endothelial growth factor.

site affect exon 9 skipping owing to differences in the binding affinity of splicing regulatory proteins (24,25). Exon 9 is essential for CFTR function given that, together with exons 10–12, it encodes the first nucleotide-binding domain, and mRNA transcripts without exon 9 do not produce functional CFTR (26–28). In healthy individuals, 5%–90% of CFTR transcripts are missing exon 9 (29), suggesting that CFTR activity in healthy individuals varies greatly. Although CFTR activity may be reduced to <5% of normal in CF, other variants that have less profound effects on CFTR may still increase the risk of other lung diseases (11). We examined the $(TG)_mT_n$ alleles in a cohort of children with community-acquired pneumonia (CAP). African American children with CAP who have $(TG)_mT_n$ alleles associated with increased exon 9 skipping are more likely to require mechanical ventilation and to develop ARDS (30). These data suggest that less functional CFTR may contribute to more severe lung injury and that the genetic makeup of the host may contribute to an increased risk for ARDS.

GWAS has been used to identify SNPs associated with the development of ARDS in adult trauma patients (31). In addition to validating previously identified SNPs, this study revealed a novel association between ARDS and a variant in *PPFIA1*, a gene that codes for the liprin-α protein (32). Liprin-α affects the localization of β$_1$-integrins (33), which are involved in the pathogenesis of ARDS, through interactions with the extracellular matrix that result in altered cell adhesion and lung vascular permeability (34,35). In addition to providing a better understanding of the pathophysiology of ARDS, GWAS may also help identify novel genes that could serve as potential therapeutic targets.

EPIGENOMICS

Epigenetics is the study of heritable changes in gene activity and expression that are not dependent on changes in the gene sequence, and epigenomics is the study of the global epigenetic signature in a cell or tissue. Many epigenetic changes are the result of covalent modifications in DNA or histone proteins around which DNA wraps. These covalent modifications play an important role in regulating gene expression in diverse biological processes, particularly in embryogenesis, development (36), and memory formation (37,38). Covalent modifications include DNA methylation and phosphorylation, acetylation, and methylation of histone proteins (**Fig. 18.1**). Certain epigenetic modifications regulate gene expression by relaxing chromatin, making DNA more accessible to transcription factors and regulatory proteins (**Fig. 18.2**), resulting in increased transcription. Other epigenetic modifications result in compacted chromatin and reduced transcription.

Various techniques have been used to study the epigenome. Bisulfite sequencing is commonly used to examine DNA methylation. In this process, unmethylated cytosines are modified by bisulfite treatment and deaminated to uracil. Following PCR to amplify the DNA region to be sequenced, the methylated cytosines are preserved while the unmethylated cytosines are converted to uracils. The methylation patterns can then be analyzed by comparing cytosines to uracils in the sequencing reaction. Another technique for examining DNA methylation is to precipitate the methylated DNA using antibodies specific to methylated DNA or methyl-binding domain proteins (39).

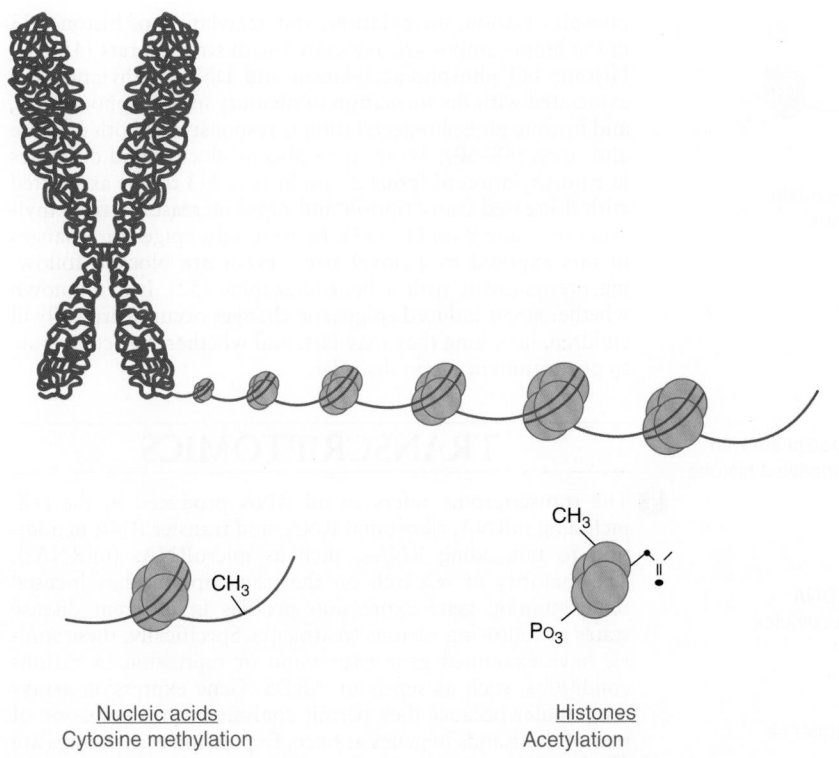

FIGURE 18.1. Chromatin structure and epigenetic modifications. DNA helix is wrapped around histone proteins. Epigenetic modifications include methylation of cytosines in the DNA strand and histone protein methylation and phosphorylation.

Nucleic acids
Cytosine methylation

Histones
Acetylation
Phosphorylation
Methylation

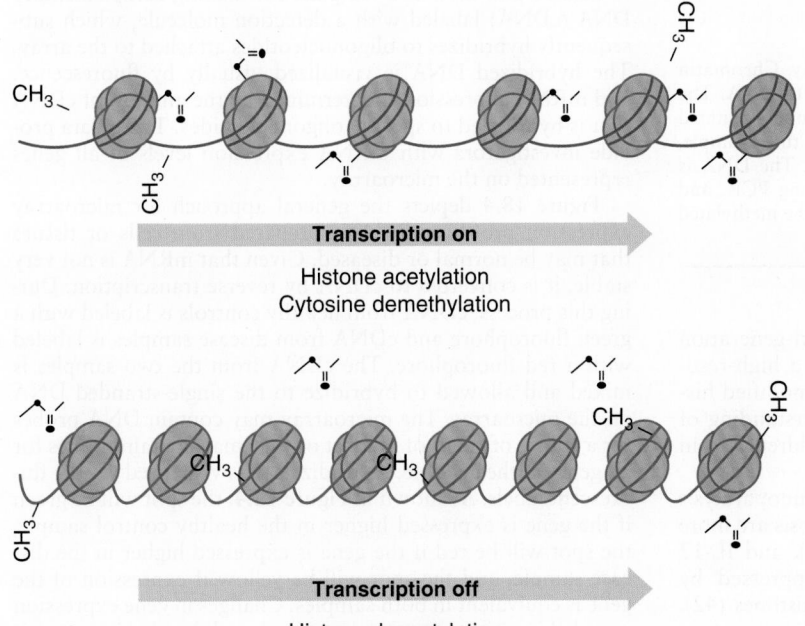

Transcription on

Histone acetylation
Cytosine demethylation

Transcription off

Histone deacetylation
Cytosine methylation

FIGURE 18.2. Epigenetic regulation of gene expression. Transcription of specific genes is upregulated following acetylation of histone proteins and demethylation of cytosines that induce chromatin relaxation. Gene expression is suppressed following histone deacetylation and cytosine methylation that result in chromatin compaction.

These techniques allow researchers to analyze genome-wide methylation patterns by microarray or other sequencing platforms. Regions of interest identified by these methods are confirmed using bisulfite treatment and sequencing as described above.

Chromatin immunoprecipitation assay (ChIP) has been used to study epigenetic modifications of histone proteins near specific DNA sequences, such as promoter regions (**Fig. 18.3**). In this technique, chromatin (the DNA and histone complex found in chromosomes) is fixed with formaldehyde to covalently bind DNA to histones. Following DNA fragmentation, epigenetically modified histones attached to fragmented DNA are immunoprecipitated using antibodies against the modified histones. For example, **Figure 18.3** depicts antibody binding a methylated histone protein. When examining genome-wide epigenetic changes, the DNA is extracted from the precipitated DNA:histone complex and sequenced or hybridized to a microarray to determine DNA sequences that are closest to the

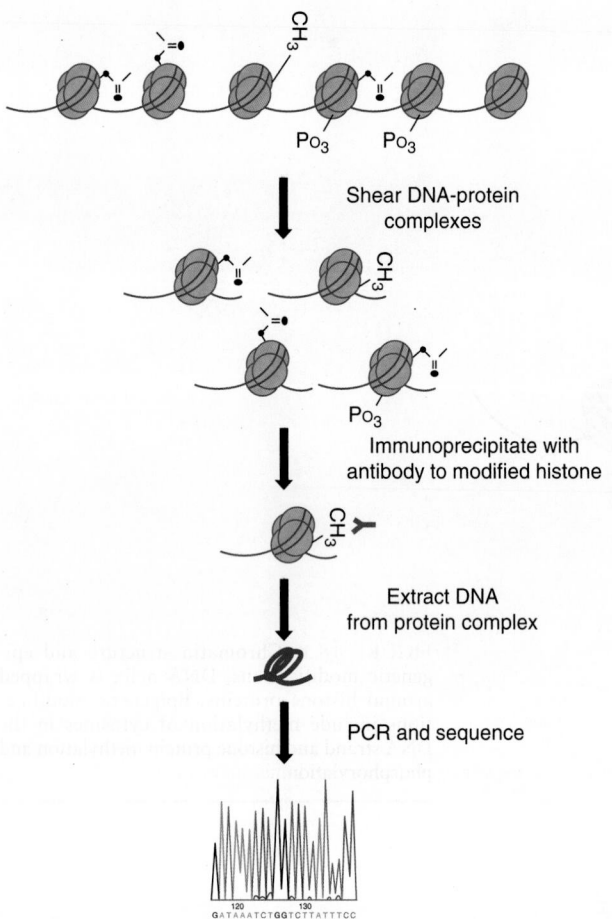

Shear DNA-protein complexes

Immunoprecipitate with antibody to modified histone

Extract DNA from protein complex

PCR and sequence

GATAAATCTGGTCTTATTTCC

FIGURE 18.3. Chromatin immunoprecipitation assay. Chromatin is treated with formaldehyde to fix histone proteins to DNA. The chromatin is then sheared into small pieces and immunoprecipitated with antibodies directed against modified histones. In this example, the antibody is directed against methylated histones. The DNA is extracted from the immunoprecipitate, amplified using PCR, and sequenced to identify DNA sequences associated with the methylated histones.

modified histones. Newer techniques using next-generation sequencing combined with ChIP assays provide a high-resolution, genome-wide analysis of DNA linked to modified histones. These technologies will improve our understanding of regulation of gene expression in critically ill children and in the pathophysiology of critical illness.

Epigenetics appears to play a role in the immunoparalysis that occurs in critical illness. Mice that survive sepsis are more susceptible to a secondary fungal challenge (40), and IL-12 production is significantly and persistently suppressed by dendritic cells (41) via epigenetic alterations to histones (42). Epigenetic changes were examined after cardiopulmonary bypass (CPB) in a small group of pediatric patients, and data revealed histone modifications in the IL-10 promoter that are associated with increased IL-10 expression (an anti-inflammatory cytokine), immunosuppression, and an increased risk of developing a postoperative infection (43). Similar epigenetic signatures are found on circulating monocytes in other populations of critically ill children (Shanley and Cornell, personal communication October, 2013).

Stress appears to trigger epigenetic modifications in the brain (44), particularly in the hippocampus that is prone to structural, functional, and neurogenic changes in response to stress and trauma. Acetylation of histone H4 and phosphorylation, methylation, and acetylation of histone H3 in the hippocampus are associated with stress in rats (45–47). Histone H3 phospho-acetylation and DNA methylation are associated with the formation of memory in the hippocampus, and histone phospho-acetylation is responsive to both exercise and stress (48–50). Acute stress also produces rapid decreases in trimethylation of lysine 27 on histone H3 that is associated with decreased transcription and rapid increases in trimethylation of lysine 9 on H3 (51). Interestingly, epigenetic changes in rats exposed to a novel stress event are blocked following pretreatment with a benzodiazapine (52). It is unknown whether stress-induced epigenetic changes occur in critically ill children, how long they may last, and whether they contribute to posttraumatic stress disorder.

TRANSCRIPTOMICS

The transcriptome refers to all RNA produced in the cell, including mRNA, ribosomal RNA, and transfer RNA in addition to noncoding RNAs, such as microRNAs (miRNAs). The majority of research on the transcriptome has focused on examining gene expression profiles in different disease states or following various treatments. Specifically, these studies have examined gene expression or repression in various conditions, such as sepsis or ARDS. Gene expression arrays are popular because they permit analysis of the expression of tens of thousands of genes at once. Expression microarrays are platforms, consisting of a glass slide, nylon membrane, or silicon chip, to which thousands of specific single-stranded oligonucleotides representing short sequences from all the genes in the genome attach. The mRNA from cells or tissues of interest is isolated and used as a template for making complementary DNA (cDNA) labeled with a detection molecule, which subsequently hybridizes to oligonucleotides attached to the array. The hybridized DNA is visualized, usually by fluorescence, and mRNA expression is determined by the amount of cDNA that is hybridized to specific oligonucleotides. These data provide investigators with mRNA expression levels of all genes represented on the microarray.

Figure 18.4 depicts the general approach for microarray expression profiling. RNA is prepared from cells or tissues that may be normal or diseased. Given that mRNA is not very stable, it is converted to cDNA by reverse transcription. During this process, cDNA from healthy controls is labeled with a green fluorophore and cDNA from disease samples is labeled with a red fluorophore. The cDNA from the two samples is mixed and allowed to hybridize to the single-stranded DNA on the microarray. The microarray may contain DNA probes for a subset of genes of interest or they may contain probes for all genes in the genome. Hybridization is visualized via the fluorescent labels. As shown in Figure 18.4, the spot will be green if the gene is expressed higher in the healthy control sample, the spot will be red if the gene is expressed higher in the disease sample, and the spot will be yellow if expression of the gene is equivalent in both samples. Changes in gene expression revealed by microarray are commonly validated using quantitative PCR. In addition, an increase in mRNA does not always translate into an increase in protein. Consequently, it is also useful to confirm that changes in gene expression correlate to changes in protein expression.

Examination of the transcriptome has occurred in several areas related to critical care (53–55). For example, the use of transcription arrays in cell-culture models of infection demonstrated differential responses of LPS, tumor necrosis factor-α (TNF-α), and stretch in alveolar epithelial cells (56). Gene expression profiles of leukocytes in mouse models of sepsis, traumatic injury, or thermal injury demonstrated that the majority of the leukocyte mRNAs expressed were unique to

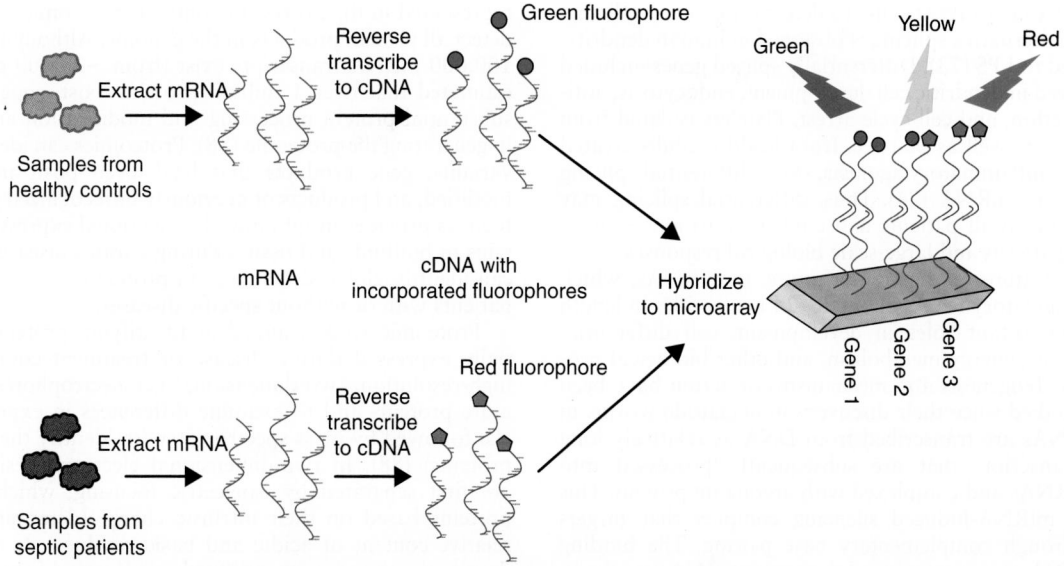

FIGURE 18.4. Expression profiling of cells from normal healthy controls or septic patients using a DNA microarray. mRNA is purified from normal and diseased cells, converted to cDNA using reverse transcriptase, and labeled with nucleotides that fluoresce either green *(circles)* or red *(pentagons)*. The cDNA samples are mixed and hybridized to a DNA microarray composed of single-stranded oligonucleotides from genes of interest attached to specific spots on the array. If a gene is expressed only in normal tissue, the spot on the array will fluoresce green *(gene 1)*. If a gene is expressed only in diseased tissues, it will fluoresce red *(gene 3)*. If a gene is expressed in both normal and diseased tissue, it will fluoresce yellow *(gene 2)*. In this example, *genes 1* and *3* are differentially expressed in normal and diseased cells, with *gene 1* expressed only in normal cells and *gene 3* expressed only in diseased cells. *Gene 2* is expressed in samples obtained from both cell types.

the type of injury (57). However, several mRNAs were upregulated or downregulated similarly in all three injuries, suggesting that there is a common transcriptional response to injury regardless of the inciting stimulus. In an animal model of mild traumatic brain injury, microarrays have revealed significant differential regulation of genes involved in neuroprotection, inflammation, nerve repair, and epithelial differentiation (58). Similarly, cultured microglial cells show expression patterns that are dependent on the duration of a pulse of pressure that simulates blast-induced traumatic brain injury (59). Organ-specific transcriptional responses have also been shown in animal models of sepsis (60,61). This animal model has increased mRNA expression of proinflammatory and anti-inflammatory cytokines, antiproteases, antioxidants, cytokine receptor antagonists, tissue and vascular permeability factors, and apoptotic factors. LPS-induced (62) and nickel-induced (63) mouse models of lung injury have increased expression of a large number of inflammatory genes and transforming growth factor-β.

In a study of critically ill patients, gene expression has been examined in cells in bronchoalveolar fluid (BAL) using microarrays. Results demonstrated elevated expression of pre-B-cell colony-enhancing factor in BAL fluid from adults with ARDS (64). In critically ill patients undergoing CPB, which is associated with a profound systemic inflammatory response, expression microarrays have been used to examine leukocyte transcript levels. Quantitative changes were observed in several mRNA transcripts, including MAP4K1, an activator of proinflammatory and pro-apoptotic pathways (65). In adults with blunt trauma, expression microarray analysis of whole blood leukocytes revealed altered expression of >80% of the leukocyte transcriptome (66), with simultaneous activation of genes involved in innate immunity and the inflammatory response and suppression of genes involved in adaptive immunity. These observations support the paradigm that prolonged immune

suppression following critical illness may contribute to organ dysfunction and poor outcomes. Rather than attempting to suppress the excessive proinflammatory response as attempted in earlier sepsis clinical trials, restoring the adaptive immune response may be a more rational option.

Genome-wide expression profiling in children with septic shock has been instrumental in providing a better understanding of the molecular biology of sepsis. Increased expression of genes involved with innate immunity, and decreased expression of genes involved in adaptive immunity have been observed in this population (67). In addition, three subclasses of differentially regulated genes are found in children with sepsis. With further refinement and using only 100 class-defining genes, gene expression mosaics could be easily differentiated by clinicians who lack formal expression array training, allowing them to identify subclasses of sepsis in children that correlate with varying degrees of mortality (68). Altered expressions of genes involved in matrix metallopeptidase-8, glucocorticoid receptor signaling, and zinc homeostasis are associated with greater severity of illness and mortality (53,67–69). Collectively, these studies demonstrate that gene expression microarray analyses of the transcriptome have yielded important insights into critical illness in both children and adults.

Transcriptome studies have also revealed that alterations in levels of alternative splicing and splice variants are important in human disease (70–72). During the generation of the mature mRNA transcript, the primary mRNA is spliced to remove the noncoding sequences. This process involves a large number of splicing factors that constitute the spliceosome in addition to specific nucleotide sequences near intron/exon junctions that identify proper splicing sites. There can be variation in whether introns are excised, resulting in different mRNA transcripts and potentially varying protein isoforms with altered function. The relevance of splice variants in critical illness and injury is unclear, but several examples suggest that differential splicing may occur. Using arrays specific to detect differential splicing, widespread alternative splicing is observed in human dendritic cells exposed to LPS (73). Differentially spliced genes included those involved in dendritic cell development, endocytosis, antigen presentation, and cell-cycle arrest. Platelets isolated from septic adults, as well as platelets from healthy adults treated with various inflammatory agonists, show differential splicing of tissue factor mRNA (74). Thus, differential splicing may occur in critically ill patients and contribute to altered gene expression patterns and large-scale biological responses.

Another feature of the transcriptome is miRNAs, which are small, regulatory RNAs about 20–24 nucleotides in length that play important roles in development, cell differentiation, apoptosis, energy metabolism, and other biological processes. Their biogenesis and mechanisms of action have been intensely studied since their discovery in nematode worms in 1993. miRNAs are transcribed from DNA as relatively long primary transcripts that are subsequently processed into smaller miRNAs and complexed with argonaute protein. This creates an miRNA-induced silencing complex that targets mRNAs through complementary base pairing. The binding of the miRNA–argonaute complex to target RNAs results in decreased mRNA processing, stability, and translation. A key to understanding the effect of miRNA on expression is to identify the target mRNA that it regulates. One way to accomplish this is to isolate total RNA from a model in which the miRNA is overexpressed or underexpressed, and perform microarray to identify genes that are differentially expressed. Analysis of these data will reveal genes that are regulated by the miRNA.

7 In critical illnesses, miRNAs have been examined as potential biomarkers of diseases, such as sepsis (75–78), traumatic brain injury (79), and cardiac arrest (80), and may be useful in understanding mechanisms of disease. In a rat model of sepsis, several hepatic miRNAs are differentially expressed but return to baseline level following activated protein C treatment, suggesting that activated protein C may alter gene expression via an miRNA pathway (81). In primary human monocytes, the anti-inflammatory cytokine IL-10 inhibits expression of TNF-α, IL-6, and the p40 subunit of IL-12 via miRNA-187 (82). miRNAs are also differentially regulated in acute kidney injury (AKI) (83), and some miRNAs serve as predictors of mortality in adults with AKI (84). Urinary miRNA-494 levels are 60-fold higher in patients with AKI compared with normal controls, and miRNA-494 may influence renal injury via inhibition of activating transcription factor 3 (ATF3) (85). Overexpression of miRNA-494 in a mouse model of AKI attenuates ATF3 levels, leading to increased expression of inflammatory mediators. Of interest, some circulating miRNAs are not removed by hemodialysis (86). Thus, miRNAs need to be considered when examining the impact of critical illness on the regulation of gene expression and the transcriptome.

PROTEOMICS

Proteomics is the large-scale study of the proteome, which is all proteins in a cell or tissue. The proteome differs between cell types and tissues because each expresses a unique set of proteins. The proteome of a particular cell or tissue can also change during differentiation, development of disease, and response to extracellular signals or drugs. Proteomics aims to study global differences in protein populations, including alterations in protein levels, posttranslational modifications, and protein–protein interactions. The proteome is a particularly important area of study because mRNA levels do not always correlate with levels of the corresponding protein product (87), highlighting an important disadvantage when study is limited to the transcriptome. In addition, transcriptional arrays typically only measure mRNA transcripts of *known* genes that are

represented in the arrays. In contrast, proteomics attempts to detect all protein products in the genome. Although more than 100,000 mRNA transcripts exist (from ~23,000 genes), it is estimated that over 1 million proteins exist, suggesting that substantial protein processing and modification are involved in generating the proteome (88). Proteomics can identify splice variants, gene products that have been posttranslationally modified, and products of previously unrecognized genes. Proteomics provides insight into the functional expression of proteins in biofluids and tissues during various disease states and can identify global differences in protein expression between patients with or without specific diseases.

Proteomic studies aimed at identifying proteins differentially expressed during disease or treatment commonly use high-resolution, two-dimensional gel electrophoresis (to separate proteins and to examine differences in expression levels) followed by mass spectrometry (to identify the individual proteins) (88). In two-dimensional electrophoresis, proteins are first separated by isoelectric focusing, which separates proteins based on their intrinsic charge (determined by the relative content of acidic and basic residues). In the second dimension, the proteins are further separated based on mass. Proteins are then visualized and quantified by staining. Mass spectrometry is then used to identify proteins of interest, which are commonly differentially expressed when comparing normal versus diseased samples. For mass spectrometry, the region of the gel containing the protein of interest is removed, digested with trypsin protease, and the mass of each peptide is determined. Matrix-assisted laser desorption ionization-time of flight (MALDI-TOF) mass spectrometry is ideal because it is sensitive, accurate, and automated for high-throughput uses. To identify the proteins, the peptide mass map generated by mass spectrometry is used to search a database that contains the predicted proteins of all identified genes and the predicted mass of all proteolytic peptide products of these genes. Other types of mass spectrometry are available if the proteins cannot be identified using MALDI-TOF mass spectrometry. Owing to the diversity of physical characteristics of proteins and limitations of the current technology, studying the proteome is more challenging than studying gene sequences or mRNA expression. There is great interest in and effort aimed at developing new techniques that will make it less complicated to use proteomics to study disease.

Proteomic approaches are used to characterize changes in the proteome associated with cancer development and prognosis (i.e. biomarkers). In addition, proteomic approaches are useful for identifying novel drug targets and for evaluating both mechanism of action and toxicity of new drugs. There are differences in the proteome of BAL fluid from patients with various lung diseases (89–91), and in the proteome of alveolar macrophages during different stages of disease progression or following exposure to various agents (92). Newer techniques allow for examination of subsets of the proteome. For example, investigators can study the global phosphoproteome, which are all phosphorylated proteins. The importance of this technique is emphasized by the role of protein phosphorylation in the regulation of numerous biological processes (93,94). Recent studies have examined the phosphoproteome of plasma, serum (95–97), and BAL fluid (98).

8 Proteomic studies have been performed in several processes relevant to critical care, including sepsis (54,99–106), ALI (107–111), trauma (112,113), burns (114,115), AKI (116), and traumatic brain injury (117–121). These data have identified several proteins that provide accurate diagnostic and prognostic information and may provide additional insight into the pathophysiology of disease. In addition, there are variations in the proteome in sepsis patients of varying ages. For example, in neonates with early-onset sepsis, neutrophil defensin-1 and defensin-2 and S100A12 (calgranulin C) and

S100A8 (calgranulin A) can help diagnose early-onset sepsis (122–125). Proteins involved in inflammation, acute-phase response, and lipid metabolism were also identified in neonatal early- and late-onset sepsis using proteomic approaches (126). Similar proteomic patterns occur in adults but also include proteins involved in oxidative stress, complement, and coagulation (106,127).

Proteomic techniques have also been used to study continuous renal replacement therapy (CRRT). CRRT is used for treating sepsis and acute renal failure and may modulate the effects of proteins and metabolites by removing them from the circulation. However, it is unclear which proteins and metabolites are modulated. In septic patients, a proteomic approach identified several proteins whose serum measurements are altered by CRRT (128). For example, CD5 antigen-like precursor, which plays an important role in regulating the innate and adaptive immune systems, is decreased and isoform 2 of ubiquitin-activating enzyme E1-like protein 2 is increased in septic patients undergoing CRRT. Ubiquitin-like posttranslational modification of proteins may alter various immune regulators, but the specific role of the ubiquitin-activating enzyme is not well characterized. However, one can appreciate how this approach may provide insight into both the pathophysiology of sepsis and novel targets for therapy.

Proteomic techniques used to analyze plasma from patients with severe burns have revealed significant alterations in the plasma protein profile, particularly in proteins involved in the inflammatory and hypermetabolic response to burn injury. In addition, nearly 50 proteins appear to be novel, burn-associated proteins that are involved in immune response, inflammation, cell adhesion and movement, metabolic response, and antioxidant response (129).

METABOLOMICS

9 Critical illnesses and injury are accompanied by severe metabolic changes. Another "omics" approach that has clinical applications in critical care is metabolomics, which commonly uses mass spectrometry or high-resolution nuclear magnetic resonance to characterize and quantify small molecules generated from cellular metabolic activity. The value of metabolomics resides in its ability to identify and quantify changes in metabolites reflecting specific pathways that are altered in the disease state. Metabolomics may provide useful information in the intensive care unit because critical illness and injury often cause significant disruptions in biochemical homeostasis. Metabolomics has been applied to a number of critical care–relevant disease states, including sepsis (130–132), ALI (133), trauma (134,135), meningitis (136), and rabies (137). The identified metabolites may be used as potential biomarkers to aid in earlier diagnosis or differentiation of disease. For example, mass spectroscopy of serum samples reveals that acylcarnitines and glycerophosphatidylcholines are significantly higher in adults with sepsis compared to adults with systemic inflammatory response syndrome (SIRS), thereby allowing differentiation of patients with noninfectious SIRS versus sepsis (131). In critically ill adults, metabolomics has been used to identify novel biomarkers of sepsis-induced ARDS (133) and to differentiate patients with SIRS from those with multiple organ dysfunction (134). Temporal changes in metabolites may also serve as indices of progression of disease or response to therapy. In addition, metabolomics may provide insight into the biochemical processes involved in critical illnesses and may help identify novel biomarkers that will lend themselves to rapid, point-of-care testing. For example, metabolomic studies of children with septic shock revealed associations between specific metabolite profiles and poor outcomes (132).

Another potential use of metabolomics is demonstrated by the observation that quinolinate, a potent agonist of the N-methyl-D-aspartate (NMDA) receptor that promotes excitotoxic damage in the brain (138), is elevated in the cerebral spinal fluid of patients with rabies. The Milwaukee protocol (139), which has been used to successfully treat patients with rabies, uses ketamine, an inhibitor of quinolinate-mediated stimulation of the NMDA receptor (140), to sedate rabies patients. A rabies survivor treated according to the Milwaukee protocol had decreased quinolinate in Cerberospinal fluid following ketamine treatment. Thus, these studies provide a deeper understanding of the pathophysiology of rabies and may help identify novel therapies for targeting metabolic pathways.

Metabolomics can also be used for evaluating resuscitative efforts by providing understanding of the cellular and subcellular milieu. Current indices of resuscitation may indicate a normal physiology, but they may not accurately reflect hypoperfusion. Metabolomic evaluation of plasma and serum samples provides a view of the metabolic functions of various organs at a cellular and subcellular level and gives clinicians another tool for examining the efficacy of resuscitation.

BIOINFORMATICS

Critical illness and injury invoke complex, nonlinear responses in inflammation and coagulation. Responses to biological stress involve a cascade of events mediated by numerous cell types and produce changes in many molecules, including proteins, nucleic acids, lipids, free radicals, and small metabolites. This biocomplexity is further increased by multiple feedback loops, multiscale emergent properties, and nonintuitive, paradoxical behavior (141,142). Because of the vast number of "participants," various bioinformatics tools and statistical tests are needed to perform system-wide analyses. Bioinformatics is the discipline that integrates computer science, mathematics, and statistics to help analyze and bring meaning to large datasets.

Analytical tools have been developed over the years to help analyze the large datasets that are the product of high-throughput technologies. Analytic tools include freely available bioinformatics initiatives, such as Gene Ontology, that groups genes and gene products into functional categories. The National Center for Biotechnology Information (http://www.ncbi.nlm.nih.gov/guide/all/#tools) has an extensive list of links to free tools that aid researchers in analyzing large datasets of biomolecules. Various statistical tests have been refined for use in analyzing high-throughput datasets. For example, principal components analysis is used to reduce data complexity and to identify global trends and associations. In metabolomics research, recent statistical innovations that incorporate quantitative molecular descriptors for each metabolite have improved disease signatures (143). Thus, while new technologies have resulted in an explosion of data, they have also created unique challenges for researchers in analyses and interpretation.

CONCLUSIONS AND FUTURE DIRECTIONS

10 In conclusion, the recent development of new "omic" technologies has provided new tools for examining the "global" molecular response to critical illness and injury that occurs in children. These tools have allowed researchers to examine individual variability in susceptibility to and outcome of critical illness and injury in addition to response to therapies.

These studies will also provide insight into the pathogenesis of critical illnesses and potentially guide the development of new treatment strategies.

SUMMARY

- New techniques developed in the "omic" fields provide a better understanding of the pathophysiology of critical illnesses and response to severe stress.
- Individual variation may influence susceptibility to and outcome of illnesses common in the pediatric intensive care unit in addition to therapeutic response.

References

1. Shendure J, Ji H. Next-generation DNA sequencing. *Nat Biotechnol* 2008;26(10):1135–45.
2. Fang X, Fukuda N, Barbry P, et al. Novel role for CFTR in fluid absorption from the distal airspaces of the lung. *J Gen Physiol* 2002;119(2):199–207.
3. Fang X, Song Y, Hirsch J, et al. Contribution of CFTR to apical-basolateral fluid transport in cultured human alveolar epithelial type II cells. *Am J Physiol Lung Cell Mol Physiol* 2006;290(2):L242–9.
4. Nagel G, Szellas T, Riordan JR, et al. Non-specific activation of the epithelial sodium channel by the CFTR chloride channel. *EMBO Rep* 2001;2(3):249–54.
5. Reddy MM, Light MJ, Quinton PM. Activation of the epithelial Na+ channel (ENaC) requires CFTR Cl- channel function. *Nature* 1999;402(6759):301–4.
6. Ware LB, Matthay MA. The acute respiratory distress syndrome. *N Engl J Med* 2000;342(18):1334–49.
7. Matthay MA. Alveolar fluid clearance in patients with ARDS: Does it make a difference? *Chest* 2002;122(6 suppl): 340S–343S.
8. Matthay MA, Robriquet L, Fang X. Alveolar epithelium: Role in lung fluid balance and acute lung injury. *Proc Am Thorac Soc* 2005;2(3):206–13.
9. Regnier A, Dannhoffer L, Blouquit-Laye S, et al. Expression of cystic fibrosis transmembrane conductance regulator in the human distal lung. *Hum Pathol* 2008;39(3):368–76.
10. Bremer S, Hoof T, Wilke M, et al. Quantitative expression patterns of multidrug-resistance P-glycoprotein (MDR1) and differentially spliced cystic-fibrosis transmembrane-conductance regulator mRNA transcripts in human epithelia. *Eur J Biochem* 1992;206(1):137–49.
11. Davis PB. Cystic fibrosis since 1938. *Am J Respir Crit Care Med* 2006;173(5):475–82.
12. Hunter MJ, Treharne KJ, Winter AK, et al. Expression of wild-type CFTR suppresses NF-kappaB-driven inflammatory signaling. *PLoS One* 2010;5(7):e11598.
13. Tirouvanziam R, de Bentzmann S, Hubeau C, et al. Inflammation and infection in naive human cystic fibrosis airway grafts. *Am J Respir Cell Mol Biol* 2000;23(2):121–7.
14. Vandivier RW, Richens TR, Horstmann SA, et al. Dysfunctional cystic fibrosis transmembrane conductance regulator inhibits phagocytosis of apoptotic cells with proinflammatory consequences. *Am J Physiol Lung Cell Mol Physiol* 2009;297(4):L677–86.
15. Vij N, Mazur S, Zeitlin PL. CFTR is a negative regulator of NFkappaB mediated innate immune response. *PLoS One* 2009;4(2):e4664.
16. Weber AJ, Soong G, Bryan R, et al. Activation of NF-kappaB in airway epithelial cells is dependent on CFTR trafficking and Cl- channel function. *Am J Physiol Lung Cell Mol Physiol* 2001;281(1):L71–8.
17. Mueller C, Braag SA, Keeler A, et al. Lack of cystic fibrosis transmembrane conductance regulator in CD3+ lymphocytes leads to aberrant cytokine secretion and hyperinflammatory adaptive immune responses. *Am J Respir Cell Mol Biol* 2011;44(6):922–9.
18. Su X, Looney MR, Su HE, et al. Role of CFTR expressed by neutrophils in modulating acute lung inflammation and injury in mice. *Inflamm Res* 2011;60(7):619–32.
19. Chu CS, Trapnell BC, Curristin S, et al. Genetic basis of variable exon 9 skipping in cystic fibrosis transmembrane conductance regulator mRNA. *Nat Genet* 1993;3(2):151–6.
20. Chu CS, Trapnell BC, Murtagh JJ Jr, et al. Variable deletion of exon 9 coding sequences in cystic fibrosis transmembrane conductance regulator gene mRNA transcripts in normal bronchial epithelium. *EMBO J* 1991;10(6):1355–63.
21. Cuppens H, Lin W, Jaspers M, et al. Polyvariant mutant cystic fibrosis transmembrane conductance regulator genes. The polymorphic (Tg)m locus explains the partial penetrance of the T5 polymorphism as a disease mutation. *J Clin Invest* 1998;101(2):487–96.
22. Pagani F, Buratti E, Stuani C, et al. Missense, nonsense, and neutral mutations define juxtaposed regulatory elements of splicing in cystic fibrosis transmembrane regulator exon 9. *J Biol Chem* 2003;278(29):26580–8.
23. Niksic M, Romano M, Buratti E, et al. Functional analysis of cis-acting elements regulating the alternative splicing of human CFTR exon 9. *Hum Mol Genet* 1999;8(13):2339–49.
24. Buratti E, Baralle FE. Characterization and functional implications of the RNA binding properties of nuclear factor TDP-43, a novel splicing regulator of CFTR exon 9. *J Biol Chem* 2001;276(39):36337–43.
25. Dujardin G, Buratti E, Charlet-Berguerand N, et al. CELF proteins regulate CFTR pre-mRNA splicing: Essential role of the divergent domain of ETR-3. *Nucleic Acids Res* 2010;38(20):7273–85.
26. Strong TV, Wilkinson DJ, Mansoura MK, et al. Expression of an abundant alternatively spliced form of the cystic fibrosis transmembrane conductance regulator (CFTR) gene is not associated with a cAMP-activated chloride conductance. *Hum Mol Genet* 1993;2(3):225–30.
27. Delaney SJ, Rich DP, Thomson SA, et al. Cystic fibrosis transmembrane conductance regulator splice variants are not conserved and fail to produce chloride channels. *Nat Genet* 1993;4(4):426–31.
28. Gregory RJ, Rich DP, Cheng SH, et al. Maturation and function of cystic fibrosis transmembrane conductance regulator variants bearing mutations in putative nucleotide-binding domains 1 and 2. *Mol Cell Biol* 1991;11(8):3886–93.
29. Chu CS, Trapnell BC, Curristin SM, et al. Extensive posttranscriptional deletion of the coding sequences for part of nucleotide-binding fold 1 in respiratory epithelial mRNA transcripts of the cystic fibrosis transmembrane conductance regulator gene is not associated with the clinical manifestations of cystic fibrosis. *J Clin Invest* 1992;90(3):785–90.
30. Baughn JM, Quasney MW, Simpson P, et al. Association of cystic fibrosis transmembrane conductance regulator gene variants with acute lung injury in African American children with pneumonia*. *Crit Care Med* 2012;40(11):3042–9.
31. Christie JD, Wurfel MM, Feng R, et al. Genome wide association identifies PPFIA1 as a candidate gene for acute lung injury risk following major trauma. *PLoS One* 2012;7(1):e28268.
32. Serra-Pages C, Medley QG, Tang M, et al. Liprins, a family of LAR transmembrane protein-tyrosine phosphatase-interacting proteins. *J Biol Chem* 1998;273(25):15611–20.
33. Asperti C, Pettinato E, de Curtis I. Liprin-alpha1 affects the distribution of low-affinity beta1 integrins and stabilizes their permanence at the cell surface. *Exp Cell Res* 2010;316(6):915–26.
34. Reutershan J, Ley K. Bench-to-bedside review: Acute respiratory distress syndrome—how neutrophils migrate into the lung. *Crit Care* 2004;8(6):453–61.

35. Crosby LM, Waters CM. Epithelial repair mechanisms in the lung. *Am J Physiol Lung Cell Mol Physiol* 2010;298(6):L715–31.

36. Sassone-Corsi P. Unique chromatin remodeling and transcriptional regulation in spermatogenesis. *Science* 2002;296(5576):2176–8.

37. Guo JU, Ma DK, Mo H, et al. Neuronal activity modifies the DNA methylation landscape in the adult brain. *Nat Neurosci* 2011;14(10):1345–51.

38. Chwang WB, Arthur JS, Schumacher A, et al. The nuclear kinase mitogen- and stress-activated protein kinase 1 regulates hippocampal chromatin remodeling in memory formation. *J Neurosci* 2007;27(46):12732–42.

39. Thu KL, Vucic EA, Kennett JY, et al. Methylated DNA immunoprecipitation. *J Vis Exp* 2009;(23). doi:10.3791/935.

40. Benjamim CF, Hogaboam CM, Lukacs NW, et al. Septic mice are susceptible to pulmonary aspergillosis. *Am J Pathol* 2003;163(6):2605–17.

41. Wen H, Hogaboam CM, Gauldie J, et al. Severe sepsis exacerbates cell-mediated immunity in the lung due to an altered dendritic cell cytokine profile. *Am J Pathol* 2006;168(6):1940–50.

42. Wen H, Dou Y, Hogaboam CM, et al. Epigenetic regulation of dendritic cell-derived interleukin-12 facilitates immunosuppression after a severe innate immune response. *Blood* 2008;111(4):1797–804.

43. Cornell TT, Sun L, Hall MW, et al. Clinical implications and molecular mechanisms of immunoparalysis after cardiopulmonary bypass. *J Thorac Cardiovasc Surg* 2012;143(5):1160–1166.e1.

44. McEwen BS, Eiland L, Hunter RG, et al. Stress and anxiety: Structural plasticity and epigenetic regulation as a consequence of stress. *Neuropharmacology* 2012;62(1):3–12.

45. Tsankova NM, Berton O, Renthal W, et al. Sustained hippocampal chromatin regulation in a mouse model of depression and antidepressant action. *Nat Neurosci* 2006;9(4):519–25.

46. Bilang-Bleuel A, Ulbricht S, Chandramohan Y, et al. Psychological stress increases histone H3 phosphorylation in adult dentate gyrus granule neurons: Involvement in a glucocorticoid receptor-dependent behavioural response. *Eur J Neurosci* 2005;22(7):1691–700.

47. Chandramohan Y, Droste SK, Reul JM. Novelty stress induces phospho-acetylation of histone H3 in rat dentate gyrus granule neurons through coincident signalling via the N-methyl-D-aspartate receptor and the glucocorticoid receptor: Relevance for c-fos induction. *J Neurochem* 2007;101(3):815–28.

48. Collins A, Hill LE, Chandramohan Y, et al. Exercise improves cognitive responses to psychological stress through enhancement of epigenetic mechanisms and gene expression in the dentate gyrus. *PLoS One* 2009;4(1):e4330.

49. Miller CA, Sweatt JD. Covalent modification of DNA regulates memory formation. *Neuron* 2007;53(6):857–69.

50. Reul JM, Hesketh SA, Collins A, et al. Epigenetic mechanisms in the dentate gyrus act as a molecular switch in hippocampus-associated memory formation. *Epigenetics* 2009;4(7):434–9.

51. Hunter RG, McCarthy KJ, Milne TA, et al. Regulation of hippocampal H3 histone methylation by acute and chronic stress. *Proc Natl Acad Sci U S A* 2009;106(49):20912–7.

52. Papadopoulos A, Chandramohan Y, Collins A, et al. GABAergic control of novelty stress-responsive epigenetic and gene expression mechanisms in the rat dentate gyrus. *Eur Neuropsychopharmacol* 2011;21(4):316–24.

53. Wong HR, Cvijanovich N, Allen GL, et al. Genomic expression profiling across the pediatric systemic inflammatory response syndrome, sepsis, and septic shock spectrum. *Crit Care Med* 2009;37(5):1558–66.

54. Skibsted S, Bhasin MK, Aird WC, et al. Bench-to-bedside review: Future novel diagnostics for sepsis—a systems biology approach. *Crit Care* 2013;17(5):231.

55. Wong HR. Clinical review: Sepsis and septic shock—the potential of gene arrays. *Crit Care* 2012;16(1):204.

56. dos Santos CC, Han B, Andrade CF, et al. DNA microarray analysis of gene expression in alveolar epithelial cells in response to TNFalpha, LPS, and cyclic stretch. *Physiol Genomics* 2004;19(3):331–42.

57. Brownstein BH, Logvinenko T, Lederer JA, et al. Commonality and differences in leukocyte gene expression patterns among three models of inflammation and injury. *Physiol Genomics* 2006;24(3):298–309.

58. Colak T, Cine N, Bamac B, et al. Microarray-based gene expression analysis of an animal model for closed head injury. *Injury* 2012;43(8):1264–70.

59. Kane MJ, Angoa-Perez M, Francescutti DM, et al. Altered gene expression in cultured microglia in response to simulated blast overpressure: Possible role of pulse duration. *Neurosci Lett* 2012;522(1):47–51.

60. Chinnaiyan AM, Huber-Lang M, Kumar-Sinha C, et al. Molecular signatures of sepsis: Multiorgan gene expression profiles of systemic inflammation. *Am J Pathol* 2001;159(4):1199–209.

61. Cobb JP, Laramie JM, Stormo GD, et al. Sepsis gene expression profiling: Murine splenic compared with hepatic responses determined by using complementary DNA microarrays. *Crit Care Med* 2002;30(12):2711–21.

62. Jeyaseelan S, Chu HW, Young SK, et al. Transcriptional profiling of lipopolysaccharide-induced acute lung injury. *Infect Immun* 2004;72(12):7247–56.

63. Wesselkamper SC, Case LM, Henning LN, et al. Gene expression changes during the development of acute lung injury: Role of transforming growth factor beta. *Am J Respir Crit Care Med* 2005;172(11):1399–411.

64. Ye SQ, Simon BA, Maloney JP, et al. Pre-B-cell colony-enhancing factor as a potential novel biomarker in acute lung injury. *Am J Respir Crit Care Med* 2005;171(4):361–70.

65. Seeburger J, Hoffmann J, Wendel HP, et al. Gene expression changes in leukocytes during cardiopulmonary bypass are dependent on circuit coating. *Circulation* 2005;112(9 suppl):I224–8.

66. Xiao W, Mindrinos MN, Seok J, et al. A genomic storm in critically injured humans. *J Exp Med* 2011;208(13):2581–90.

67. Wong HR, Cvijanovich N, Lin R, et al. Identification of pediatric septic shock subclasses based on genome-wide expression profiling. *BMC Med* 2009;7:34.

68. Wong HR, Cvijanovich NZ, Allen GL, et al. Validation of a gene expression-based subclassification strategy for pediatric septic shock. *Crit Care Med* 2011;39(11):2511–7.

69. Wong HR, Shanley TP, Sakthivel B, et al. Genome-level expression profiles in pediatric septic shock indicate a role for altered zinc homeostasis in poor outcome. *Physiol Genomics* 2007;30(2):146–55.

70. Brett D, Pospisil H, Valcarcel J, et al. Alternative splicing and genome complexity. *Nat Genet* 2002;30(1):29–30.

71. Dutertre M, Sanchez G, Barbier J, et al. The emerging role of pre-messenger RNA splicing in stress responses: Sending alternative messages and silent messengers. *RNA Biol* 2011;8(5):740–7.

72. Tang JY, Lee JC, Hou MF, et al. Alternative splicing for diseases, cancers, drugs, and databases. *ScientificWorldJournal* 2013;2013:703568.

73. Rodrigues R, Grosso AR, Moita L. Genome-wide analysis of alternative splicing during dendritic cell response to a bacterial challenge. *PLoS One* 2013;8(4):e61975.

74. Rondina MT, Schwertz H, Harris ES, et al. The septic milieu triggers expression of spliced tissue factor mRNA in human platelets. *J Thromb Haemost* 2011;9(4):748–58.

75. Vasilescu C, Rossi S, Shimizu M, et al. MicroRNA fingerprints identify miR-150 as a plasma prognostic marker in patients with sepsis. *PLoS One* 2009;4(10):e7405.

76. Wang HJ, Zhang PJ, Chen WJ, et al. Four serum microRNAs identified as diagnostic biomarkers of sepsis. *J Trauma Acute Care Surg* 2012;73(4):850–4.

77. Wang H, Zhang P, Chen W, et al. Serum microRNA signatures identified by Solexa sequencing predict sepsis patients' mortality: A prospective observational study. *PLoS One* 2012;7(6):e38885.

78. Wang H, Meng K, Chen W, et al. Serum miR-574-5p: A prognostic predictor of sepsis patients. *Shock* 2012;37(3):263–7.

79. Redell JB, Moore AN, Ward NH III, et al. Human traumatic brain injury alters plasma microRNA levels. *J Neurotrauma* 2010;27(12):2147–56.

80. Stammet P, Goretti E, Vausort M, et al. Circulating microRNAs after cardiac arrest. *Crit Care Med* 2012;40(12):3209–14.

81. Moore CC, McKillop IH, Huynh T. MicroRNA expression following activated protein C treatment during septic shock. *J Surg Res* 2013;182(1):116–26.

82. Rossato M, Curtale G, Tamassia N, et al. IL-10-induced microRNA-187 negatively regulates TNF-alpha, IL-6, and IL-12p40 production in TLR4-stimulated monocytes. *Proc Natl Acad Sci U S A* 2012;109(45):E3101–10.

83. Saikumar J, Hoffmann D, Kim TM, et al. Expression, circulation, and excretion profile of microRNA-21, -155, and -18a following acute kidney injury. *Toxicol Sci* 2012;129(2):256–67.

84. Lorenzen JM, Kielstein JT, Hafer C, et al. Circulating miR-210 predicts survival in critically ill patients with acute kidney injury. *Clin J Am Soc Nephrol* 2011;6(7):1540–6.

85. Lan YF, Chen HH, Lai PF, et al. MicroRNA-494 reduces ATF3 expression and promotes AKI. *J Am Soc Nephrol* 2012;23(12):2012–23.

86. Martino F, Lorenzen J, Schmidt J, et al. Circulating microRNAs are not eliminated by hemodialysis. *PLoS One* 2012;7(6):e38269.

87. Pradet-Balade B, Boulme F, Beug H, et al. Translation control: Bridging the gap between genomics and proteomics? *Trends Biochem Sci* 2001;26(4):225–9.

88. Stults JT, Arnott D. Proteomics. *Methods Enzymol* 2005;402:245–89.

89. Bowler RP, Duda B, Chan ED, et al. Proteomic analysis of pulmonary edema fluid and plasma in patients with acute lung injury. *Am J Physiol Lung Cell Mol Physiol* 2004;286(6):L1095–104.

90. Wattiez R, Falmagne P. Proteomics of bronchoalveolar lavage fluid. *J Chromatogr B Analyt Technol Biomed Life Sci* 2005;815(1–2):169–78.

91. Wu J, Kobayashi M, Sousa EA, et al. Differential proteomic analysis of bronchoalveolar lavage fluid in asthmatics following segmental antigen challenge. *Mol Cell Proteomics* 2005;4(9):1251–64.

92. Wu HM, Jin M, Marsh CB. Toward functional proteomics of alveolar macrophages. *Am J Physiol Lung Cell Mol Physiol* 2005;288(4):L585–95.

93. Grimsrud PA, Swaney DL, Wenger CD, et al. Phosphoproteomics for the masses. *ACS Chem Biol* 2010;5(1):105–19.

94. Eyrich B, Sickmann A, Zahedi RP. Catch me if you can: Mass spectrometry-based phosphoproteomics and quantification strategies. *Proteomics* 2011;11(4):554–70.

95. Carrascal M, Gay M, Ovelleiro D, et al. Characterization of the human plasma phosphoproteome using linear ion trap mass spectrometry and multiple search engines. *J Proteome Res* 2010;9(2):876–84.

96. Zhou W, Ross MM, Tessitore A, et al. An initial characterization of the serum phosphoproteome. *J Proteome Res* 2009;8(12):5523–31.

97. Garbis SD, Roumeliotis TI, Tyritzis SI, et al. A novel multidimensional protein identification technology approach combining protein size exclusion prefractionation, peptide zwitterion-ion hydrophilic interaction chromatography, and nano-ultraperformance RP chromatography/nESI-MS2 for the in-depth analysis of the serum proteome and phosphoproteome: Application to clinical sera derived from humans with benign prostate hyperplasia. *Anal Chem* 2011;83(3):708–18.

98. Giorgianni F, Mileo V, Desiderio DM, et al. Characterization of the phosphoproteome in human bronchoalveolar lavage fluid. *Int J Proteomics* 2012;2012:460261.

99. Hinkelbein J, Kalenka A, Schubert C, et al. Proteome and metabolome alterations in heart and liver indicate compromised energy production during sepsis. *Protein Pept Lett* 2010;17(1):18–31.

100. Ng PC, Ang IL, Chiu RW, et al. Host-response biomarkers for diagnosis of late-onset septicemia and necrotizing enterocolitis in preterm infants. *J Clin Invest* 2010;120(8):2989–3000.

101. Ling XB, Mellins ED, Sylvester KG, et al. Urine peptidomics for clinical biomarker discovery. *Adv Clin Chem* 2010;51:181–213.

102. Siqueira-Batista R, Mendonca AF, Gomes AP, et al. Proteomic updates on sepsis. *Rev Assoc Med Bras* 2012;58(3):376–82.

103. Su L, Zhou R, Liu C, et al. Urinary proteomics analysis for sepsis biomarkers with iTRAQ labeling and two-dimensional liquid chromatography-tandem mass spectrometry. *J Trauma Acute Care Surg* 2013;74(3):940–5.

104. Sylvester KG, Ling XB, Liu GY, et al. Urine protein biomarkers for the diagnosis and prognosis of necrotizing enterocolitis in infants. *J Pediatr* 2014;164(3):607–12.

105. Cao Z, Robinson RA. The role of proteomics in understanding biological mechanisms of sepsis. *Proteomics Clin Appl* 2013;8(1–2):35–52.

106. Cao Z, Yende S, Kellum JA, et al. Proteomics reveals age-related differences in the host immune response to sepsis. *J Proteome Res* 2014;13(2):422–32.

107. de Torre C, Ying SX, Munson PJ, et al. Proteomic analysis of inflammatory biomarkers in bronchoalveolar lavage. *Proteomics* 2006;6(13):3949–57.

108. Schnapp LM, Donohoe S, Chen J, et al. Mining the acute respiratory distress syndrome proteome: Identification of the insulin-like growth factor (IGF)/IGF-binding protein-3 pathway in acute lung injury. *Am J Pathol* 2006;169(1):86–95.

109. Chang DW, Hayashi S, Gharib SA, et al. Proteomic and computational analysis of bronchoalveolar proteins during the course of the acute respiratory distress syndrome. *Am J Respir Crit Care Med* 2008;178(7):701–9.

110. Gharib SA, Nguyen E, Altemeier WA, et al. Of mice and men: Comparative proteomics of bronchoalveolar fluid. *Eur Respir J* 2010;35(6):1388–95.

111. Poon TC, Pang RT, Chan KC, et al. Proteomic analysis reveals platelet factor 4 and beta-thromboglobulin as prognostic markers in severe acute respiratory syndrome. *Electrophoresis* 2012;33(12):1894–900.

112. Boutte AM, Yao C, Kobeissy F, et al. Proteomic analysis and brain-specific systems biology in a rodent model of penetrating ballistic-like brain injury. *Electrophoresis* 2012;33(24):3693–704.

113. Zhou JY, Krovvidi RK, Gao Y, et al. Trauma-associated human neutrophil alterations revealed by comparative proteomics profiling. *Proteomics Clin Appl* 2013;7(7–8):571–83.

114. Finnerty CC, Jeschke MG, Qian WJ, et al. Determination of burn patient outcome by large-scale quantitative discovery proteomics. *Crit Care Med* 2013;41(6):1421–34.

115. Finnerty CC, Ju H, Spratt H, et al. Proteomics improves the prediction of burns mortality: Results from regression spline modeling. *Clin Transl Sci* 2012;5(3):243–9.

116. Bihorac A, Baslanti TO, Cuenca AG, et al. Acute kidney injury is associated with early cytokine changes after trauma. *J Trauma Acute Care Surg* 2013;74(4):1005–13.

117. Agoston DV, Gyorgy A, Eidelman O, et al. Proteomic biomarkers for blast neurotrauma: Targeting cerebral edema, inflammation, and neuronal death cascades. *J Neurotrauma* 2009;26(6):901–11.

118. Svetlov SI, Larner SF, Kirk DR, et al. Biomarkers of blast-induced neurotrauma: Profiling molecular and cellular mechanisms of blast brain injury. *J Neurotrauma* 2009;26(6):913–21.

119. Van Boven RW, Harrington GS, Hackney DB, et al. Advances in neuroimaging of traumatic brain injury and posttraumatic stress disorder. *J Rehabil Res Dev* 2009;46(6):717–57.

120. Kovesdi E, Luckl J, Bukovics P, et al. Update on protein biomarkers in traumatic brain injury with emphasis on clinical use in adults and pediatrics. *Acta Neurochir (Wien)* 2010;152(1):1–17.

121. Guingab-Cagmat JD, Cagmat EB, Hayes RL, et al. Integration of proteomics, bioinformatics, and systems biology in traumatic brain injury biomarker discovery. *Front Neurol* 2013;4:61.

122. Buhimschi IA, Christner R, Buhimschi CS. Proteomic biomarker analysis of amniotic fluid for identification of intra-amniotic inflammation. *BJOG* 2005;112(2):173–81.

123. Buhimschi CS, Bhandari V, Hamar BD, et al. Proteomic profiling of the amniotic fluid to detect inflammation, infection, and neonatal sepsis. *PLoS Med* 2007;4(1):e18.

124. Buhimschi CS, Buhimschi IA, Abdel-Razeq S, et al. Proteomic biomarkers of intra-amniotic inflammation: Relationship with funisitis and early-onset sepsis in the premature neonate. *Pediatr Res* 2007;61(3):318–24.

125. Buhimschi IA, Zhao G, Funai EF, et al. Proteomic profiling of urine identifies specific fragments of SERPINA1 and albumin as biomarkers of preeclampsia. *Am J Obstet Gynecol* 2008;199(5):551.e1–16.

126. Buhimschi CS, Bhandari V, Dulay AT, et al. Proteomics mapping of cord blood identifies haptoglobin "switch-on" pattern as biomarker of early-onset neonatal sepsis in preterm newborns. *PLoS One* 2011;6(10):e26111.

127. Qian WJ, Jacobs JM, Camp DG II, et al. Comparative proteome analyses of human plasma following in vivo lipopolysaccharide administration using multidimensional separations coupled with tandem mass spectrometry. *Proteomics* 2005;5(2):572–84.

128. Gong Y, Chen N, Wang FQ, et al. Serum proteome alteration of severe sepsis in the treatment of continuous renal replacement therapy. *Nephrol Dial Transplant* 2009;24(10):3108–14.

129. Qian WJ, Petritis BO, Kaushal A, et al. Plasma proteome response to severe burn injury revealed by 18O-labeled "universal" reference-based quantitative proteomics. *J Proteome Res* 2010;9(9):4779–89.

130. Izquierdo-García J, Nin N, Ruíz-Cabello J, et al. A metabolomic approach for diagnosis of experimental sepsis. *Intensive Care Med* 2011;37(12):2023–32.

131. Schmerler D, Neugebauer S, Ludewig K, et al. Targeted metabolomics for discrimination of systemic inflammatory disorders in critically ill patients. *J Lipid Res* 2012;53(7):1369–75.

132. Mickiewicz B, Vogel HJ, Wong HR, et al. Metabolomics as a novel approach for early diagnosis of pediatric septic shock and its mortality. *Am J Respir Crit Care Med* 2013;187(9):967–76.

133. Stringer KA, Serkova NJ, Karnovsky A, et al. Metabolic consequences of sepsis-induced acute lung injury revealed by plasma (1)H-nuclear magnetic resonance quantitative metabolomics and computational analysis. *Am J Physiol Lung Cell Mol Physiol* 2011;300(1):L4–11.

134. Mao H, Wang H, Wang B, et al. Systemic metabolic changes of traumatic critically ill patients revealed by an NMR-based metabonomic approach. *J Proteome Res* 2009;8(12):5423–30.

135. Cohen M, Serkova NJ, Wiener-Kronish J, et al. 1H-NMR-based metabolic signatures of clinical outcomes in trauma patients—beyond lactate and base deficit. *J Trauma* 2010;69:31–40.

136. Coen M, O'Sullivan M, Bubb WA, et al. Proton nuclear magnetic resonance-based metabonomics for rapid diagnosis of meningitis and ventriculitis. *Clin Infect Dis* 2005;41(11):1582–90.

137. O'Sullivan A, Willoughby RE, Mishchuk D, et al. Metabolomics of cerebrospinal fluid from humans treated for rabies. *J Proteome Res* 2013;12(1):481–90.

138. Stone T. Neuropharmacology of quinolinic and kynurenic acids. *Pharmacol Rev* 1993;45:309–79.

139. Willoughby RE Jr, Tieves KS, Hoffman GM, et al. Survival after treatment of rabies with induction of coma. *N Engl J Med* 2005;352(24):2508–14.

140. Keilhoff G, Wolf G, Stastny F. Effects of MK-801, ketamine and alaptide on quinolinate models in the maturing hippocampus. *Neuroscience* 1991;42(2):379–85.

141. Csete ME, Doyle JC. Reverse engineering of biological complexity. *Science* 2002;295(5560):1664–9.

142. Kitano H. Systems biology: A brief overview. *Science* 2002;295(5560):1662–4.

143. Zhu H, Luo M. Chemical structure informing statistical hypothesis testing in metabolomics. *Bioinformatics* 2014;30(4):514–22.

144. Harding D, Baines PB, Brull D, et al. Severity of meningococcal disease in children and the angiotensin-converting enzyme insertion/deletion polymorphism. *Am J Respir Crit Care Med* 2002;165(8):1103–6.

145. Cogulu O, Onay H, Uzunkaya D, et al. Role of angiotensin-converting enzyme gene polymorphisms in children with sepsis and septic shock. *Pediatr Int* 2008;50(4):477–80.

146. Michalek J, Svetlikova P, Fedora M, et al. Bactericidal permeability increasing protein gene variants in children with sepsis. *Intensive Care Med* 2007;33(12):2158–64.

147. Baldini M, Lohman IC, Halonen M, et al. A polymorphism* in the 5' flanking region of the CD14 gene is associated with circulating soluble CD14 levels and with total serum immunoglobulin E. *Am J Respir Cell Mol Biol* 1999;20(5):976–83.

148. Gibot S, Cariou A, Drouet L, et al. Association between a genomic polymorphism within the CD14 locus and septic shock susceptibility and mortality rate. *Crit Care Med* 2002;30(5):969–73.

149. Sutherland AM, Walley KR, Russell JA. Polymorphisms in CD14, mannose-binding lectin, and Toll-like receptor-2 are associated with increased prevalence of infection in critically ill adults. *Crit Care Med* 2005;33(3):638–44.

150. Barber RC, Chang LY, Arnoldo BD, et al. Innate immunity SNPs are associated with risk for severe sepsis after burn injury. *Clin Med Res* 2006;4(4):250–5.

151. Barber RC, Aragaki CC, Chang LY, et al. CD14-159 C allele is associated with increased risk of mortality after burn injury. *Shock* 2007;27(3):232–7.

152. Gu W, Dong H, Jiang DP, et al. Functional significance of CD14 promoter polymorphisms and their clinical relevance in a Chinese Han population. *Crit Care Med* 2008;36(8):2274–80.

153. Bredius RG, Derkx BH, Fijen CA, et al. Fc gamma receptor IIa (CD32) polymorphism in fulminant meningococcal septic shock in children. *J Infect Dis* 1994;170(4):848–53.

154. Platonov AE, Kuijper EJ, Vershinina IV, et al. Meningococcal disease and polymorphism of FcγRIIa (CD32) in late complement component-deficient individuals. *Clin Exp Immunol* 1998;111(1):97–101.

155. Platonov AE, Shipulin GA, Vershinina IV, et al. Association of human Fc gamma RIIa (CD32) polymorphism with susceptibility to and severity of meningococcal disease. *Clin Infect Dis* 1998;27(4):746–50.

156. Domingo P, Muniz-Diaz E, Baraldes MA, et al. Associations between Fc gamma receptor IIA polymorphisms and the risk and prognosis of meningococcal disease. *Am J Med* 2002;112(1):19–25.

157. van Sorge NM, van der Pol WL, van de Winkel JG. FcgammaR polymorphisms: Implications for function, disease susceptibility and immunotherapy. *Tissue Antigens* 2003;61(3):189–202.

158. Schroeder S, Reck M, Hoeft A, et al. Analysis of two human leukocyte antigen-linked polymorphic heat shock protein 70 genes in patients with severe sepsis. *Crit Care Med* 1999;27(7):1265–70.

159. Schroder O, Schulte KM, Ostermann P, et al. Heat shock protein 70 genotypes HSPA1B and HSPA1L influence cytokine concentrations and interfere with outcome after major injury. *Crit Care Med* 2003;31(1):73–9.

160. Bowers DJ, Calvano JE, Alvarez SM, et al. Polymorphisms of heat shock protein-70 (HSPA1B and HSPA1L loci) do not influence infection or outcome risk in critically ill surgical patients. *Shock* 2006;25(2):117–22.

161. Waterer GW, ElBahlawan L, Quasney MW, et al. Heat shock protein 70-2 +1267 AA homozygotes have an increased risk of septic shock in adults with community-acquired pneumonia. *Crit Care Med* 2003;31(5):1367–72.

162. Read RC, Cannings C, Naylor SC, et al. Variation within genes encoding interleukin-1 and the interleukin-1 receptor antagonist influence the severity of meningococcal disease. *Ann Intern Med* 2003;138(7):534–41.

163. Endler G, Marculescu R, Starkl P, et al. Polymorphisms in the interleukin-1 gene cluster in children and young adults with systemic meningococcemia. *Clin Chem* 2006;52(3):511–4.

164. Brouwer MC, de Gans J, Heckenberg SG, et al. Host genetic susceptibility to pneumococcal and meningococcal disease: A systematic review and meta-analysis. *Lancet Infect Dis* 2009;9(1):31–44.

165. Wen AQ, Gu W, Wang J, et al. Clinical relevance of IL-1beta promoter polymorphisms (-1470, -511, and -31) in patients with major trauma. *Shock* 2010;33(6):576–82.

166. Michalek J, Svetlikova P, Fedora M, et al. Interleukin-6 gene variants and the risk of sepsis development in children. *Hum Immunol* 2007;68(9):756–60.

167. Wattanathum A, Manocha S, Groshaus H, et al. Interleukin-10 haplotype associated with increased mortality in critically ill patients with sepsis from pneumonia but not in patients with extrapulmonary sepsis. *Chest* 2005;128(3):1690–8.

168. Stanilova SA, Miteva LD, Karakolev ZT, et al. Interleukin-10-1082 promoter polymorphism in association with cytokine production and sepsis susceptibility. *Intensive Care Med* 2006;32(2):260–6.

169. Zeng L, Gu W, Chen K, et al. Clinical relevance of the interleukin 10 promoter polymorphisms in Chinese Han patients with major trauma: Genetic association studies. *Crit Care* 2009;13(6):R188.

170. Accardo Palumbo A, Forte GI, Pileri D, et al. Analysis of IL-6, IL-10 and IL-17 genetic polymorphisms as risk factors for sepsis development in burned patients. *Burns* 2012;38(2):208–13.

171. Chien JW, Boeckh MJ, Hansen JA, et al. Lipopolysaccharide binding protein promoter variants influence the risk for Gram-negative bacteremia and mortality after allogeneic hematopoietic cell transplantation. *Blood* 2008;111(4):2462–9.

172. Flores C, Perez-Mendez L, Maca-Meyer N, et al. A common haplotype of the LBP gene predisposes to severe sepsis. *Crit Care Med* 2009;37(10):2759–66.

173. Zeng L, Gu W, Zhang AQ, et al. A functional variant of lipopolysaccharide binding protein predisposes to sepsis and organ dysfunction in patients with major trauma. *Ann Surg* 2012;255(1):147–57.

174. Stuber F, Udalova IA, Book M, et al. -308 tumor necrosis factor (TNF) polymorphism is not associated with survival in severe sepsis and is unrelated to lipopolysaccharide inducibility of the human TNF promoter. *J Inflamm* 1995;46(1):42–50.

175. Dumon K, Rossbach C, Harms B, et al. Tumor necrosis factor-alpha (TNF-alpha) gene polymorphism in surgical intensive care patients with SIRS [in German]. *Langenbecks Arch Chir Suppl Kongressbd* 1998;115(suppl I):387–90.

176. Mira JP, Cariou A, Grall F, et al. Association of TNF2, a TNF-alpha promoter polymorphism, with septic shock susceptibility and mortality: A multicenter study. *JAMA* 1999;282(6):561–8.

177. Nuntayanuwat S, Dharakul T, Chaowagul W, et al. Polymorphism in the promoter region of tumor necrosis factor-alpha gene is associated with severe meliodosis. *Hum Immunol* 1999;60(10):979–83.

178. Tang GJ, Huang SL, Yien HW, et al. Tumor necrosis factor gene polymorphism and septic shock in surgical infection. *Crit Care Med* 2000;28(8):2733–6.

179. Appoloni O, Dupont E, Vandercruys M, et al. Association of tumor necrosis factor-2 allele with plasma tumor necrosis factor-alpha levels and mortality from septic shock. *Am J Med* 2001;110(6):486–8.

180. Waterer GW, Quasney MW, Cantor RM, et al. Septic shock and respiratory failure in community-acquired pneumonia have different TNF polymorphism associations. *Am J Respir Crit Care Med* 2001;163(7):1599–604.

181. Majetschak M, Obertacke U, Schade FU, et al. Tumor necrosis factor gene polymorphisms, leukocyte function, and sepsis susceptibility in blunt trauma patients. *Clin Diagn Lab Immunol* 2002;9(6):1205–11.

182. McArthur JA, Zhang Q, Quasney MW. Association between the A/A genotype at the lymphotoxin-alpha+250 site and increased mortality in children with positive blood cultures. *Pediatr Crit Care Med* 2002;3(4):341–4.

183. O'Keefe GE, Hybki DL, Munford RS. The G—>A single nucleotide polymorphism at the -308 position in the tumor necrosis factor-alpha promoter increases the risk for severe sepsis after trauma. *J Trauma* 2002;52(5):817–25; discussion 825–6.

184. Calvano JE, Um JY, Agnese DM, et al. Influence of the TNF-alpha and TNF-beta polymorphisms upon infectious risk and outcome in surgical intensive care patients. *Surg Infect (Larchmt)* 2003;4(2):163–9.

185. Gallagher PM, Lowe G, Fitzgerald T, et al. Association of IL-10 polymorphism with severity of illness in community acquired pneumonia. *Thorax* 2003;58(2):154–6.

186. Schaaf BM, Boehmke F, Esnaashari H, et al. Pneumococcal septic shock is associated with the interleukin-10-1082 gene promoter polymorphism. *Am J Respir Crit Care Med* 2003;168(4):476–80.

187. Treszl A, Kocsis I, Szathmari M, et al. Genetic variants of TNF-[FC12]a, IL-1beta, IL-4 receptor [FC12]a-chain, IL-6 and IL-10 genes are not risk factors for sepsis in low-birth-weight infants. *Biol Neonate* 2003;83(4):241–5.

188. Zhang D, Li J, Jiang ZW, et al. Association of two polymorphisms of tumor necrosis factor gene with acute severe pancreatitis. *J Surg Res* 2003;112(2):138–43.

189. Zhang DL, Li JS, Jiang ZW, et al. Association of two polymorphisms of tumor necrosis factor gene with acute biliary pancreatitis. *World J Gastroenterol* 2003;9(4):824–8.

190. Barber RC, Aragaki CC, Rivera-Chavez FA, et al. TLR4 and TNF-alpha polymorphisms are associated with an increased risk for severe sepsis following burn injury. *J Med Genet* 2004;41(11):808–13.

191. Gordon AC, Lagan AL, Aganna E, et al. TNF and TNFR polymorphisms in severe sepsis and septic shock: A prospective multicentre study. *Genes Immun* 2004;5(8):631–40.

192. Jaber BL, Rao M, Guo D, et al. Cytokine gene promoter polymorphisms and mortality in acute renal failure. *Cytokine* 2004;25(5):212–9.

193. Nakada TA, Hirasawa H, Oda S, et al. Influence of toll-like receptor 4, CD14, tumor necrosis factor, and interleukine-10 gene polymorphisms on clinical outcome in Japanese critically ill patients. *J Surg Res* 2005;129(2):322–8.

194. Watanabe E, Hirasawa H, Oda S, et al. Extremely high interleukin-6 blood levels and outcome in the critically ill are associated with tumor necrosis factor- and interleukin-1-related gene polymorphisms. *Crit Care Med* 2005;33(1):89–97; discussion 242–3.

195. Garnacho-Montero J, Aldabo-Pallas T, Garnacho-Montero C, et al. Timing of adequate antibiotic therapy is a greater determinant of outcome than are TNF and IL-10 polymorphisms in patients with sepsis. *Crit Care* 2006;10(4):R111.

196. Sipahi T, Pocan H, Akar N. Effect of various genetic polymorphisms on the incidence and outcome of severe sepsis. *Clin Appl Thromb Hemost* 2006;12(1):47–54.

197. Jessen KM, Lindboe SB, Petersen AL, et al. Common TNF-alpha, IL-1 beta, PAI-1, uPA, CD14 and TLR4 polymorphisms are not associated with disease severity or outcome from Gram negative sepsis. *BMC Infect Dis* 2007;7:108.

198. McDaniel DO, Hamilton J, Brock M, et al. Molecular analysis of inflammatory markers in trauma patients at risk of postinjury complications. *J Trauma* 2007;63(1):147–57; discussion 157–8.

199. Menges T, Konig IR, Hossain H, et al. Sepsis syndrome and death in trauma patients are associated with variation in the gene encoding tumor necrosis factor. *Crit Care Med* 2008;36(5):1456–62, e1–6.

200. Teuffel O, Ethier MC, Beyene J, et al. Association between tumor necrosis factor-alpha promoter -308 A/G polymorphism and susceptibility to sepsis and sepsis mortality: A systematic review and meta-analysis. *Crit Care Med* 2010;38(1):276–82.

201. Song Z, Song Y, Yin J, et al. Genetic variation in the TNF gene is associated with susceptibility to severe sepsis, but not with mortality. *PLoS One* 2013;7(9):e46113.

202. Hibberd ML, Sumiya M, Summerfield JA, et al. Association of variants of the gene for mannose-binding lectin with susceptibility to meningococcal disease. Meningococcal Research Group. *Lancet* 1999;353(9158):1049–53.

203. Koch A, Melbye M, Sorensen P, et al. Acute respiratory tract infections and mannose-binding lectin insufficiency during early childhood. *JAMA* 2001;285(10):1316–21.

204. Arcaroli J, Fessler MB, Abraham E. Genetic polymorphisms and sepsis. *Shock* 2005;24(4):300–12.

205. Huh JW, Song K, Yum JS, et al. Association of mannose-binding lectin-2 genotype and serum levels with prognosis of sepsis. *Crit Care* 2009;13(6):R176.

206. Garnacho-Montero J, Garcia-Cabrera E, Jimenez-Alvarez R, et al. Genetic variants of the MBL2 gene are associated with mortality in pneumococcal sepsis. *Diagn Microbiol Infect Dis* 2012;73(1):39–44.

207. Ozkan H, Koksal N, Cetinkaya M, et al. Serum mannose-binding lectin (MBL) gene polymorphism and low MBL levels are associated with neonatal sepsis and pneumonia. *J Perinatol* 2012;32(3):210–7.

208. Gomez R, O'Keeffe T, Chang LY, et al. Association of mitochondrial allele 4216C with increased risk for complicated sepsis and death after traumatic injury. *J Trauma* 2009;66(3):850–7; discussion 857–8.

209. Huebinger RM, Gomez R, McGee D, et al. Association of mitochondrial allele 4216C with increased risk for sepsis-related organ dysfunction and shock after burn injury. *Shock* 2010;33(1):19–23.

210. Haralambous E, Hibberd ML, Hermans PW, et al. Role of functional plasminogen-activator-inhibitor-1 4G/5G promoter polymorphism in susceptibility, severity, and outcome of meningococcal disease in Caucasian children. *Crit Care Med* 2003;31(12):2788–93.

211. Geishofer G, Binder A, Muller M, et al. 4G/5G promoter polymorphism in the plasminogen-activator-inhibitor-1 gene in children with systemic meningococcaemia. *Eur J Pediatr* 2005;164(8):486–90.

212. Binder A, Endler G, Muller M, et al. 4G4G genotype of the plasminogen activator inhibitor-1 promoter polymorphism associates with disseminated intravascular coagulation in children with systemic meningococcemia. *J Thromb Haemost* 2007;5(10):2049–54.

213. Garcia-Segarra G, Espinosa G, Tassies D, et al. Increased mortality in septic shock with the 4G/4G genotype of plasminogen activator inhibitor 1 in patients of white descent. *Intensive Care Med* 2007;33(8):1354–62.

214. Sapru A, Hansen H, Ajayi T, et al. 4G/5G polymorphism of plasminogen activator inhibitor-1 gene is associated with mortality in intensive care unit patients with severe pneumonia. *Anesthesiology* 2009;110(5):1086–91.

215. Madach K, Aladzsity I, Szilagyi A, et al. 4G/5G polymorphism of PAI-1 gene is associated with multiple organ dysfunction and septic shock in pneumonia induced severe sepsis: Prospective, observational, genetic study. *Crit Care* 2010;14(2):R79.

216. Binder A, Endler G, Rieger S, et al. Protein C promoter polymorphisms associate with sepsis in children with systemic meningococcemia. *Hum Genet* 2007;122(2):183–90.

217. Chen QX, Wu SJ, Wang HH, et al. Protein C -1641A/-1654C haplotype is associated with organ dysfunction and the fatal outcome of severe sepsis in Chinese Han population. *Hum Genet* 2008;123(3):281–7.

218. Russell JA, Wellman H, Walley KR. Protein C rs2069912 C allele is associated with increased mortality from severe sepsis in North Americans of East Asian ancestry. *Hum Genet* 2008;123(6):661–3.

219. Lorente L, Martin MM, Plasencia F, et al. The 372 T/C genetic polymorphism of TIMP-1 is associated with serum levels of TIMP-1 and survival in patients with severe sepsis. *Crit Care* 2013;17(3):R94.

220. Wurfel MM, Gordon AC, Holden TD, et al. Toll-like receptor 1 polymorphisms affect innate immune responses and outcomes in sepsis. *Am J Respir Crit Care Med* 2008;178(7):710–20.

221. Thompson CM, Holden TD, Rona G, et al. Toll-like receptor 1 polymorphisms and associated outcomes in sepsis after traumatic injury: A Candidate Gene Association Study. *Ann Surg* 2014;259(1):179–85.

222. Lorenz E, Mira JP, Cornish KL, et al. A novel polymorphism in the toll-like receptor 2 gene and its potential association with staphylococcal infection. *Infect Immun* 2000;68(11):6398–401.

223. Kang TJ, Chae GT. Detection of Toll-like receptor 2 (TLR2) mutation in the lepromatous leprosy patients. *FEMS Immunol Med Microbiol* 2001;31(1):53–8.

224. Moore CE, Segal S, Berendt AR, et al. Lack of association between Toll-like receptor 2 polymorphisms and susceptibility to severe disease caused by *Staphylococcus aureus*. *Clin Diagn Lab Immunol* 2004;11(6):1194–7.

225. Thuong NT, Hawn TR, Thwaites GE, et al. A polymorphism in human TLR2 is associated with increased susceptibility to tuberculous meningitis. *Genes Immun* 2007;8(5):422–8.

226. Chen K, Wang YT, Gu W, et al. Functional significance of the Toll-like receptor 4 promoter gene polymorphisms in the Chinese Han population. *Crit Care Med* 2010;38(5):1292–9.

227. Chen KH, Gu W, Zeng L, et al. Identification of haplotype tag SNPs within the entire TLR2 gene and their clinical relevance in patients with major trauma. *Shock* 2011;35(1):35–41.

228. Lorenz E, Mira JP, Frees KL, et al. Relevance of mutations in the TLR4 receptor in patients with gram-negative septic shock. *Arch Intern Med* 2002;162(9):1028–32.

229. Shalhub S, Junker CE, Imahara SD, et al. Variation in the TLR4 gene influences the risk of organ failure and shock posttrauma: A cohort study. *J Trauma* 2009;66(1):115–22; discussion 122–3.

230. Cardinal-Fernandez P, Ferruelo A, El-Assar M, et al. Genetic predisposition to acute kidney injury induced by severe sepsis. *J Crit Care* 2013;28(4):365–70.

231. Marshall RP, Webb S, Bellingan GJ, et al. Angiotensin converting enzyme insertion/deletion polymorphism is associated with susceptibility and outcome in acute respiratory distress syndrome. *Am J Respir Crit Care Med* 2002;166(5):646–50.

232. Jerng JS, Yu CJ, Wang HC, et al. Polymorphism of the angiotensin-converting enzyme gene affects the outcome of acute respiratory distress syndrome. *Crit Care Med* 2006;34(4):1001–6.

233. Adamzik M, Frey U, Sixt S, et al. ACE I/D but not AGT (-6)A/G polymorphism is a risk factor for mortality in ARDS. *Eur Respir J* 2007;29(3):482–8.

234. Su L, Zhai R, Sheu CC, et al. Genetic variants in the angiopoietin-2 gene are associated with increased risk of ARDS. *Intensive Care Med* 2009;35(6):1024–30.

235. Meyer NJ, Li M, Feng R, et al. ANGPT2 genetic variant is associated with trauma-associated acute lung injury and altered plasma angiopoietin-2 isoform ratio. *Am J Respir Crit Care Med* 2011;183(10):1344–53.

236. Adamzik M, Frey UH, Riemann K, et al. Factor V Leiden mutation is associated with improved 30-day survival in patients with acute respiratory distress syndrome. *Crit Care Med* 2008;36(6):1776–9.

237. Glavan BJ, Holden TD, Goss CH, et al. Genetic variation in the FAS gene and associations with acute lung injury. *Am J Respir Crit Care Med* 2011;183(3):356–63.

238. Lagan AL, Quinlan GJ, Mumby S, et al. Variation in iron homeostasis genes between patients with ARDS and healthy control subjects. *Chest* 2008;133(6):1302–11.

239. Patwari PP, O'Cain P, Goodman DM, et al. Interleukin-1 receptor antagonist intron 2 VNTR polymorphism and respiratory failure in children with community acquired pneumonia. *Pediatr Crit Care Med* 2008;9:553–9.

240. Reiner AP, Wurfel MM, Lange LA, et al. Polymorphisms of the IL1-receptor antagonist gene (IL1RN) are associated with

multiple markers of systemic inflammation. *Arterioscler Thromb Vasc Biol* 2008;28(7):1407–12.

241. Marshall RP, Webb S, Hill MR, et al. Genetic polymorphisms associated with susceptibility and outcome in ARDS. *Chest* 2002;121(3 suppl):68S–69S.

242. Nonas SA, Finigan JH, Gao L, et al. Functional genomic insights into acute lung injury: Role of ventilators and mechanical stress. *Proc Am Thorac Soc* 2005;2(3):188–94.

243. Sutherland AM, Walley KR, Manocha S, et al. The association of interleukin 6 haplotype clades with mortality in critically ill adults. *Arch Intern Med* 2005;165(1):75–82.

244. Flores C, Ma SF, Maresso K, et al. IL6 gene-wide haplotype is associated with susceptibility to acute lung injury. *Transl Res* 2008;152(1):11–7.

245. Pino-Yanes M, Ma SF, Sun X, et al. Interleukin-1 receptor-associated kinase 3 gene associates with susceptibility to acute lung injury. *Am J Respir Cell Mol Biol* 2010;45(4):740–5.

246. Ip WK, Chan KH, Law HK, et al. Mannose-binding lectin in severe acute respiratory syndrome coronavirus infection. *J Infect Dis* 2005;191(10):1697–704.

247. Gong MN, Zhou W, Williams PL, et al. Polymorphisms in the mannose binding lectin-2 gene and acute respiratory distress syndrome. *Crit Care Med* 2007;35(1):48–56.

248. Garcia-Laorden MI, Sole-Violan J, Rodriguez de Castro F, et al. Mannose-binding lectin and mannose-binding lectin-associated serine protease 2 in susceptibility, severity, and outcome of pneumonia in adults. *J Allergy Clin Immunol* 2008;122(2):368–74, 374.e1–2.

249. Gao L, Flores C, Fan-Ma S, et al. Macrophage migration inhibitory factor in acute lung injury: Expression, biomarker, and associations. *Transl Res* 2007;150(1):18–29.

250. Gao L, Grant A, Halder I, et al. Novel polymorphisms in the myosin light chain kinase gene confer risk for acute lung injury. *Am J Respir Cell Mol Biol* 2006;34(4):487–95.

251. Christie JD, Ma SF, Aplenc R, et al. Variation in the myosin light chain kinase gene is associated with development of acute lung injury after major trauma. *Crit Care Med* 2008;36(10):2794–800.

252. Marzec JM, Christie JD, Reddy SP, et al. Functional polymorphisms in the transcription factor NRF2 in humans increase the risk of acute lung injury. *Faseb J* 2007;21(9):2237–46.

253. Zhai R, Zhou W, Gong MN, et al. Inhibitor kappaB-alpha haplotype GTC is associated with susceptibility to acute respiratory distress syndrome in Caucasians. *Crit Care Med* 2007;35(3):893–8.

254. Reddy AJ, Christie JD, Aplenc R, et al. Association of human NAD(P)H:quinone oxidoreductase 1 (NQO1) polymorphism with development of acute lung injury. *J Cell Mol Med* 2009; 13(8B):1784–91.

255. Arcaroli J, Sankoff J, Liu N, et al. Association between urokinase haplotypes and outcome from infection-associated acute lung injury. *Intensive Care Med* 2008;34(2):300–7.

256. Dahmer MK, O'Cain P, Patwari PP, et al. The influence of genetic variation in surfactant protein B on severe lung injury in black children. *Crit Care Med* 2011;39(5):1138–44.

257. Arcaroli JJ, Hokanson JE, Abraham E, et al. Extracellular superoxide dismutase haplotypes are associated with acute lung injury and mortality. *Am J Respir Crit Care Med* 2009;179(2): 105–12.

258. Gong MN, Zhou W, Williams PL, et al. -308GA and TNFB polymorphisms in acute respiratory distress syndrome. *Eur Respir J* 2005;26(3):382–9.

259. Medford AR, Keen LJ, Bidwell JL, et al. Vascular endothelial growth factor gene polymorphism and acute respiratory distress syndrome. *Thorax* 2005;60(3):244–8.

260. Zhai R, Gong MN, Zhou W, et al. Genotypes and haplotypes of the VEGF gene are associated with higher mortality and lower VEGF plasma levels in patients with ARDS. *Thorax* 2007;62(8):718–22.

CHAPTER 19 ■ INNATE IMMUNITY AND INFLAMMATION

JAMES A. THOMAS

KEY POINTS

① Innate immunity refers to the cells, subcellular elements, and molecules that protect the host from spread of infection and tissue damage.

② Innate immune function is essential for host survival, and its sophistication acknowledges the complexity of diverse evolutionary pressures facing the mammalian genome.

③ The acute inflammatory response demonstrates innate immunity at work.

④ Microbial molecules that activate innate immunity are better understood than endogenous injury signals.

⑤ Current understanding of host injury–sensing mechanisms, while growing, remains limited.

⑥ The ability to prevent or successfully manage devastating problems treated in the ICU, including severe sepsis, acute respiratory distress syndrome, disseminated intravascular coagulation, and multiple organ dysfunction, will depend on successful decoding of the regulation of the innate immune response.

INTRODUCTION AND HISTORICAL BACKGROUND

To understand inflammation is, in some respects, to grasp the breadth of human disease. Necrotizing enterocolitis in premature neonates stressed by cold, infection, or formula feeding; bronchiolitis in infants with respiratory syncytial virus infections; and reperfusion injury in children after cardiac arrest or cardiopulmonary bypass are all characterized by intense local responses in affected tissues and sometimes activation of a highly catabolic systemic cascade that affects the entire host. Different injuries provoke distinct manifestations of the inflammatory response. A complex host can generate many more reactions (foreign body, granulomatous, suppurative, hypersensitivity, immune complex, and toxic or septic shock) than one with a simpler genome. While a comprehensive categorization of different inflammatory processes exceeds the scope of this chapter, the following sections outline some elements of an ancient system that has evolved to protect the host from insults to its integrity, innate immunity.

The survival of a species depends on its ability to perpetuate itself. To accomplish this, members must succeed at three fundamental activities. First, they must generate adequate nutrition to reach reproductive age. In the process of growing and maturing, they must also avoid becoming another organism's food source. Finally, organisms must ensure passage of the species' genetic information to the next generation.

The struggle to achieve these ends is fraught with danger. During the course of activities to survive and reproduce, organisms encounter agents that compromise their physical integrity and threaten their self-propagation. Gravity can hurl bodies from trees during food foraging, and bacteria can gain access to the warm, humid, and nutrient-rich subepithelium via abrasions or puncture wounds. Most major injuries or infections, such as those treated in modern ICUs, would be nonsurvivable without antibiotics, antiseptic surgery, and modern nursing care. To maintain a competitive advantage and survive minor to moderate threats, however, most species have evolved a repertoire of behavioral and physiologic responses to help them avoid or defend themselves against threats to their integrity. These countermeasures include mechanisms to limit secondary injury or microbial dissemination, if an initial attack succeeds and primary (epithelial) defenses are breached. After containing a threat, additional mechanisms modulate the intensity of the reaction and commence repairing the damage occasioned by the insult. Defects that impair any of these responses hamper the host's survival chances.

The aggregate of early physiologic responses that detect and respond to injury is loosely referred to as innate immunity, while the inflammatory response represents innate immunity at work. This chapter summarizes the history of our evolving understanding of host defense and inflammation. It then defines major concepts associated with innate immunity and the inflammatory response. Subsequent sections review current thinking about the nature of injury signals, the acute cellular and systemic responses to injury, and their regulation and overall impact.

History of Knowledge of Inflammation and Innate Immunity

The concept of innate immunity is more modern than the notion of inflammation (1–5). Early Mesopotamian caregivers were familiar with the signs and symptoms of inflammation, but as an early codifier of medical knowledge, Hippocrates (460–377 BC) receives credit for both documenting the early vocabulary associated with the inflammatory response and recognizing it as a prerequisite for the healing process.

The Roman encyclopedist, Aulus Cornelius Celsus (~35–50 BC) is the second ancient Westerner whose contribution to the study of inflammation survives. In his treatise, *De Medicina*, he coined the initial four cardinal signs of inflammation: calor (heat), dolor (pain), tumor (swelling), and rubor (redness or erythema). The fifth sign *functio laesa* (dysfunction of inflamed organs) was attributed to the Greek physician Galen of Pergamon (129–200 AD), whose writings dominated Western medical thought until the European Renaissance. According to some scholars, Galen's influence over the practice of medicine in Europe stifled observation and empiricism, and that medieval Muslim physicians in Spain, North Africa, and the Middle East contributed more to the understanding and treatment of inflammation than their European counterparts during this period.

Beutler identifies two threads in what we would now call the history of inflammation research. The first focuses on characterizing what is sensed or what triggers the inflammatory response. Before Koch promulgated his postulates, investigators attempted to purify toxins from putrid meat to better understand why the same process in a patient's injured leg triggered gangrene, shock, and death. These studies ultimately gave way to the isolation and characterization of microbial toxins, such as lipopolysaccharide, peptidoglycan, and lipoteichoic acid.

The second line of inquiry concentrated on describing the response to infection and invasion. The Scottish surgeon, John Hunter (1728–1793) first recognized leukocytes at the site of inflammation and was one of the first to describe the inflammatory response as a form of host defense and not a disease process. Moreover, as light microscopy improved in the 18th and 19th centuries, investigators such as Dutrochet, Virchow, Waller, and Addison described inflammatory leukocyte morphology, loose association with the vessel wall, firm adherence to the vessel wall, and extravasation of leukocytes beyond the vessel wall. Cohnheim detailed the stepwise events of leukocyte rolling, adhesion, and diapedesis and speculated that changes in vascular wall properties promoted this process. Schultze's descriptions of different leukocyte morphologies preceded Elie Metchnikov's observations of phagocytosis in macrophages and granulocytes that led to the formulation of his cellular theory of immunity in 1884. Paul Erlich's identification and analysis of antibodies and complement gave rise to the concept of humoral immunity and opened the era of functional studies that have characterized subsequent studies of immunity and inflammation.

Since the early 20th century, efforts to unravel the *adaptive immune response* eclipsed the study of innate immunity. Description of the first genetic defect underlying chronic granulomatous disease in the 1960s; isolation and characterization of cytokines, receptors, and signaling molecules critical to inflammation; recognition that adaptive immunity depends on innate immunity to function; and the information windfall from the Human Genome Project, have all helped fuel resurgent interest in understanding the depth and complexity of innate immunity.

Recognition of the relationship between inflammation and the neuroendocrine system has coalesced more recently than our comprehension of the roles of leukocytes, soluble mediators, and the vascular system. Investigation into the stress response has also highlighted the importance and interdependence of the central nervous system (CNS) and the hypothalamic–pituitary axis (HPA) in preparing complex hosts to defend themselves against different threats.

DEFINITIONS AND GENERAL CONCEPTS

Innate Immunity

As Beutler (6) observes, "it is sometimes difficult to decide where the innate immune system ends and the rest of the host begins." The statement reflects the difficulty inherent in trying to distinguish one physiologic system from another in an organism that functions as an integrated whole. Although the host's innate response to injury or infection employs specialized cells and macromolecules to defend itself, any body tissue may become infected, traumatized, or deprived of blood flow. Tissues considered "nonimmune" must be able to detect and respond to an insult and have evolved different mechanisms (e.g., near-universal Toll-like receptor [TLR] expression, or interleukin-6 [IL-6] *trans*-signaling) to meet this challenge (7,8).

Defining the limits of the innate immune system may be futile, but characterizing core features and functions of innate immunity is possible. First, it is old, much older than adaptive (lymphocyte-based) immunity. In fact, it most likely developed in parallel with early metazoans >600 million years ago (9). Moreover, elements of immunity shared by plants, invertebrates, and vertebrates alike, such as intracellular kinases (critical to disease resistance and pathogen recognition), are older than components found only in vertebrates. Second, like the nervous system with which it is tightly linked, innate immunity has both afferent and efferent limbs, suggesting the two systems may have evolved from a common ancestral system to sense threats and respond (6). Third, the cellular receptors for sensing invasion or injury are encoded in the germ line of the host, signifying that (a) they have evolved to recognize something essential and therefore invariant in either microbes or host, and (b) they can be mobilized quickly.

Three essential functions of innate immunity deserve mention, but only two will be discussed further. Pathogen or injury recognition is the first and most important of these. Without this ability, the host is immunologically blind to the threats surrounding it. The second function of innate immunity is to respond to the threat. Doing so effectively requires mechanisms to assess the magnitude, localization, and type of insult, and to match, coordinate, and regulate the response to that threat. Finally, and as an integral component of its response to microbial invasion, innate immunity instructs and focuses the adaptive immune response to the identity of the invader, and provides additional information about the preferred adaptive effector response (B cell– vs. T cell–mediated) (10). The adaptive immune response is discussed in subsequent chapters.

What, then, is innate immunity? The term refers to the cells, subcellular elements, and molecules that act to eliminate invading pathogens and limit the spread of tissue damage. The cells involved include leukocytes, particularly polymorphonuclear (PMN) cells (neutrophils, basophils, and eosinophils), mast cells, and mononuclear phagocytes (monocytes, tissue macrophages, and dendritic cells), but also lymphocytes, natural killer (NK) cells, neurons, and neuroendocrine cells. Platelets are the major subcellular elements and are essential to coagulation. Molecular mediators of innate immunity range from major antimicrobial proteins (complement, defensins, cathelicidins, lysozyme, and lactoferrin) to pro- and anti-inflammatory cytokines and chemokines (tumor necrosis factor TNF-α, IFN-α, IFN-β, IL-1β, IL-8, IL-6, IFN-γ, and IL-10) and to neurotransmitters involved in neurogenic inflammation (substance P, calcitonin gene–related peptide, epinephrine, and serotonin). The remainder of the chapter outlines how some of these components cooperate to protect the host following injury.

Adaptive Immunity

In contrast to the notion of a preset responsiveness inherent in innate immunity, adaptive immunity denotes the ability to vary an immune response depending on the received stimulus. The existence of this adaptability implies two additional qualities: the capacity to distinguish among different stimuli and a preexisting pool of effectors capable of responding to almost any molecular motif. The nearly unlimited repertoire of lymphocytes, generated by somatic recombination and hypermutation of the genes that code for their antigen receptors, arises from the interaction between innate immune cells (antigen-presenting cells) and lymphocytes (T helper cells). Although adaptive immunity is a more recent and restricted system of host defense than innate immunity, it remains dependent on its evolutionary predecessor for proper function (10).

Inflammation

Defining inflammation is complex because it comes in many guises. A peritonsillar abscess and necrotizing bacterial pneumonia, lupus nephritis and acute tubular necrosis leading to renal failure, and the cerebral responses to trauma and viral encephalitis are all inflammatory diseases. These reactions share elements in common, but also have unique aspects to them that are determined by the injury itself, the tissue(s) involved, and the overall state of the host at the time of insult. The inflammatory response, broadly defined, is:

> A localized reaction, that can be elicited by microbial invasion or sterile tissue injury, which serves to destroy, dilute, or sequester both the injurious agent and injured tissue and to initiate the healing process.

An intact inflammatory response is essential for host survival, performing at least three critical functions. First it prevents disease extension. Through a variety of strategies, including extravasation of serum proteins, migration of leukocyte effectors, and local thrombosis, innate immunity contains invading microbes and delineates boundaries between viable and nonviable tissue. Second, the response is critical for the development of adaptive immunity against infectious organisms. Its "adjuvant effect" on antigen presentation to T cells results in their response to the antigen as an invader. Finally, control and resolution of the inflammatory response promotes eventual healing, with a combination of regeneration, remodeling, and scarring.

Several general concepts about inflammation deserve mention. First, when it functions appropriately, the inflammatory response is a localized phenomenon. The reaction may either occur within a microscopic domain, such as a Ghon complex within a lymph node, or occupy an entire body cavity, as occurs during peritonitis. Though the extent of the response is much broader in the second example, the host has evolved measures to contain inflammatory mediators within the focus, and prevent their systemic spillover (11). A second, related idea is that generalized activation of even a single component of the inflammatory response can be lethal to the host. A ruptured appendix, for example, may trigger pulmonary endothelial activation, neutrophil influx into remote alveoli and the development of acute respiratory distress syndrome (ARDS), a nonsurvivable condition without intensive care. The third notion is that the acute inflammatory response is invariant and stereotyped. While there is considerable variability in extent and intensity of the reaction depending on the degree of insult, in general the host's innate immunity will use the same mechanisms and kinetics to sense and respond to repeated injuries.

Inflammation is also an integrated biological response, the overall control of which is still poorly understood. Distinctions between soluble or humoral components, cellular mediators, and the neuroendocrine systems represent attempts to tease out components of an interdependent reaction pattern, closely related to the stress response that has evolved over billions of years. Most attempts at comprehensive descriptions of the host response to infection and injury remain phenomenological, and only recently have investigators applied a more system-oriented approach to try understanding of aspects of innate immunity (e.g., the monocyte-phagocyte system or neutrophil biology) (12–15).

Finally, different schemata have evolved to categorize inflammation. We distinguish between acute, subacute, and chronic inflammation to group inflammatory responses according to onset and duration. Effector mechanisms based on pathological description of an inflammatory lesion (neutrophilic infiltrative, caseating, necrotizing, histiocytic) provide another basis for distinction. We also describe inflammatory responses based on the inciting injury mechanisms, such as infectious, immune complex, trauma, hypoxic–ischemic, though these descriptors provide little insight into the type of specific inflammatory response they trigger.

Essential Elements of a Host Defense System

A host response to insult must accomplish a minimum of five functions. It must first **detect** a threat and determine whether tissue injury or microbial invasion has occurred. Second, an effective system must be able to **alert** the appropriate effectors, both local and distant from the lesion. These sensing and alerting functions constitute the afferent limb of the response. Third, in the efferent arm, an effective system must **contain** the injury or infection, minimizing the chances that microbes, the contents of necrotic cells, or the toxic endogenous mediators elaborated at the site of inflammation spill into the blood and lymph or spread throughout natural cavities or along tissue planes. Fourth, the response should **eliminate** the invading organism and/or damaged or dead tissue. Fifth, it must be able to **cycle off** and initiate the healing process. Vertebrates have also evolved the ability to prevent productive reinfection via lymphocyte-mediated immunological memory, a sixth function absent in most other multicellular organisms. Innate immunity is critical to each of these functions, but it collaborates with adaptive immunity in eliminating some pathogens and in the generation of a memory response.

The necessary components of a host defense system must subserve the five functions outlined above, possessing, at minimum, three capabilities. The first is an injury-sensing apparatus. Without the ability to sense damage to its integrity, the host cannot engage in responses to prevent further injury and repair the primary injury. Second, such a system must be able to initiate local protective responses and recruit distant support to reinforce the local response. Finally, it must incorporate controls that modulate the type, intensity, and timing of responses. Following consideration of the nature of injury signals, the remainder of the chapter examines how the mammalian host protects itself against infections and other injuries.

INJURY SIGNALS

The term "injury signal" carries inherent ambiguity. It can signify either a stimulus causing injury or a marker of tissue injury or invasion. The following discussion refers to the second meaning, the indicator of possible damage. It is also convenient to distinguish between primary and secondary injury signals. *Primary injury signals* are generated or liberated by an insult that threatens the host. They can be molecules or forces (such as bacterial endotoxin, products of necrotic cell death, or thermal injury) that in turn generate endogenous, *secondary injury signals* (e.g., cytokines or neurotransmitters) that extend, amplify, propagate or terminate primary injury signals. This section focuses on the nature and identity of primary injury signals, while the subsequent two sections examine secondary injury signals.

Background

In *Lives of the Cell*, Lewis Thomas commented on the symbolic importance of injury sensing, hinting at the existence of an injury language.

> It is the information carried by the bacteria that we cannot abide. The gram-negative [sic] bacteria are the best examples of this. They display lipopolysaccharide endotoxin (LPS) in their walls, and these macromolecules are read by our tissues as the very worst of bad news. When we sense lipopolysaccharide, we are likely to turn on every defense at our disposal.. There is nothing intrinsically poisonous about endotoxin, but it must look awful, or feel awful, when sensed by cells. (16)

Early attempts to understand illness recognized the association between rotting or putrefaction and its toxic effects on different hosts (5). By the mid-19th century, investigators had begun to isolate activities from dead bacteria that could sicken animals immunized against infection with them, suggesting that an inanimate property of a formerly live organism encoded a threat. Subsequent work on lymphocyte recognition of pathogens led Burnet, Lederburg, and others to propose a dichotomous antigen-sensing system in which lymphocytes that sensed self-antigens were suppressed, whereas those that recognized nonself persisted (17,18). Limitation of this "either-or" code and the acknowledgement that effective vaccines required inflammation-causing adjuvants to ensure specific immunity prompted Janeway to propose that innate immunity recognized invariant attributes specific to classes of pathogens ("pathogen-associated molecular patterns," PAMPs) via a germ line–encoded sensory system ("pattern recognition receptors," PRRs) (19). This "stranger theory" failed to account for certain phenomena, such as autoimmunity and the temporary tolerance of the pregnant female to the foreign fetus within her body. Matzinger (20) later articulated the "danger theory," which proposed that the threat or presence of injury determined responsiveness more than the foreignness of the stimulus. Though this theory fails to account for certain realities of the innate immune response, it does highlight the role of tissue damage in initiating the inflammatory response (21).

Current Knowledge

Despite knowledge about the major injury mechanisms and their consequences, information about the molecular character of the injury signals they generate has emerged more slowly. The consequences of physical/mechanical (burn/scald, temperature extreme, electrical, radiation, atmospheric pressure), toxic (metabolic poison, free radical), ischemia–reperfusion, autoimmune, or infectious injuries have been extensively documented in clinical and experimental literatures. Many of these injuries can cause extensive tissue destruction, which in itself can pose a threat to survival through secondary injury such as exsanguinating hemorrhage, unconsciousness, airway obstruction, or critical organ dysfunction (e.g., status epilepticus, myocardial depression, renal failure). With the exception of microbial invasion and infection, however, the molecular identities of primary signals produced by these injuries have been more difficult to characterize, though considerable progress has occurred in the last two decades.

So what, precisely, is known about primary injury signals, what is suspected and what remains, at this time speculative? First, many injury signals from bacteria, fungi, and viruses have been isolated and chemically characterized. Although Janeway referred to them as "patterns," they are, above all, molecules or domains within molecules (6), and they belong to most major macromolecular classes, including carbohydrates, lipids, nucleic acids, proteins, as well as compound macromolecules such as glycolipids, lipopeptides, and glycoproteins. LPS, for example, is a complex, phosphorylated glycolipid that composes ~75% of the outer leaflet of the outer membrane of Gram-negative bacteria. Although different species have varying patterns of LPS acylation and glycosylation, the lipid A moiety activates the innate immune system (22,23).

Second, the presence of these molecules alone does not by itself represent a threat to the host. Facultative anaerobic Gram-negative commensal species in the human GI and respiratory tracts synthesize similar hexacylated, lipid A–containing lipid-containing poly- and oligosaccharides, putative "mucosal" LPSs that are best recognized by the CD-14/TLR4/MD2 receptor apparatus. Their presence in the oropharynx or intestine does not trigger an ongoing inflammatory response, and in fact some evidence exists to suggest that their presence actually protects the host (R.S. Munford, personal communication, 2006). Moreover, as will be discussed briefly, appearance of one or a few of these microbial products outside of the their usual domains does not trigger a full-blown injury response, but rather indicates a possible threat and initiates a preparative or priming response that can be escalated should the host encounter additional evidence of microbial injury or tissue destruction (14).

Third, as discussed in the following section, the mammalian injury-sensing system depends on both redundancy and complexity to generate a repertoire of effector responses. For example, different signals from very different organisms or injuries activate overlapping, sometimes identical, signaling pathways. Molecules from viruses, Gram-negative and Gram-positive bacteria, and fungi activate the TLR/IL-1 signaling pathway and NF-κB transcription factor and lead to similar cellular responses, such as cytokine and chemokine production, and cell surface marker changes. Moreover, the same injury molecule can elicit different responses, depending on how it is presented. Flagellin (bacterial filament protein) in the extracellular space activates TLR5 and NF-κB and TNF-α secretion, while its intracellular injection into a host macrophage by a microbial Type III secretion system triggers the ICE protease-activating factor (IPAF) inflammasome and massive IL-1β and IL-18 release (14).

The existence of primary injury signals of endogenous origin has been postulated, but their exact identity has been more difficult to document, in part because of the difficulty in conducting experiments free of contaminating endotoxin (24). A few molecules of host origin, however, appear to qualify as such. The most convincing demonstration to date of an endogenous primary injury signal has been the biochemical purification of a low-molecular-weight activity from dying cells that augments an adaptive immune response. Investigators identified uric acid as the signal and demonstrated its biological activity as an injury signal occurred when its concentration approached crystal formation, suggesting that a phase transition from soluble to insoluble (as monosodium urate crystals in the extracellular space) leads to cellular uptake, activation of caspase-1, and IL-1β release (25,26).

Extracellular matrix (ECM) degradation products may also function as primary injury signals. Separate groups identified the immunostimulatory potential of soluble hyaluronic acid (HA) fragments, the breakdown products of solid-phase polymeric HA (27,28), later demonstrating TLR4- and TLR2-dependent signal transduction (29). Thus, alterations to the ECM, normally immunologically silent, precipitated by injury may convert this and other macromolecules, such as biglycan and heparin sulfate, into injury signals (24).

Additional candidate primary injury signals include the chromatin-associated protein HMGB1 (high-mobility group box 1 protein) and extracellular ATP. The former is an ancient DNA-binding protein that stabilizes nucleosomes and functions as an activating transcription factor. More recent studies demonstrate that its secretion from activated macrophages and dendritic cells, interaction with the RAGE receptor (*receptor for advanced glycation end products*), and localized inflammation confers a cytokine function on it. However, demonstration of its release from necrotic and pyroptotic cells and TLR2- and TLR4-dependent initiation of an innate immune response also suggests a role as primary injury signal (30,31).

ATP released from necrotic and pyroptotic cells accumulates in the extracellular space following tissue injury and is a potent marker of tissue injury. Signaling through the low-affinity $P2X_7$ extracellular receptor and pannexin leads to potassium efflux and triggers assembly of one or more inflammasomes (see below) in innate immune cells. It is a key factor in critical caspase-1-dependent responses, including pyroptosis and the processing and release of mature IL-1β and IL-18. Macrophages stimulated by LPS, for example, accumulate large amounts of intracellular pro-IL-1β, and pro-IL-18, but a second signal in the form of ATP acting on the $P2X_7$ receptor is required to activate caspase-1, which cleaves the procytokines and leads to their massive release of mature cytokine (32).

Summary

Although present knowledge of microbial molecules that trigger innate immune responses exceeds current understanding of endogenous injury signals, much remains to be learned about both. For example, in 18 short years, we understand the essential outline of how ligands activating the TLRs trigger a massive reprogramming of cellular gene expression through the NF-κB transcription factor, and have mapped many of those ligand–receptor interactions. Signal concentration matters as well, though less is known about how the host has evolved different thresholds for sensing different signals, and what those thresholds imply for subsequent responses. Picogram quantities of LPS trigger TNF-α production, while milligram amounts of uric acid, at least locally, are required for its crystallization to an activating form in physiologic solutions. Finally, the identity, characterization, and classification of novel injury signals may uncover unexpected strategies used by the host to distinguish normal homeostasis from a threat, some of which may represent minute deviations from the range of normal concentration or activity. For example, the mammalian equivalent of the plant "guard hypothesis," in which intracellular sentinels targeted by viral proteins are under the surveillance of proteins that can detect viral modifications and mount a resistance response when these changes are detected, has yet to be described in mammalian innate immunity.

CELLULAR RECOGNITION AND RESPONSE TO INJURY SIGNALS

Characteristics of an Injury-Sensing Apparatus

5 The first required component of a defense system, an injury-sensing apparatus, must meet several conditions to protect the host. It must be widely distributed, with components either present or rapidly inducible in all tissues. Second, the sensory machinery must be tuned to the appropriate sensitivity, with activation thresholds that reflect the potential threat to the host. High sensitivity favors early detection at low injury burden, but lower sensitivity may be appropriate to prevent excessive reactivity to "background noise," such as low levels of microbial products translocated from the GI tract.

A third characteristic, that injury sensors be promiscuous (capable of detecting more than a single signal), is neither required nor universal, but would maximize genetic economy. TLR2, for example, senses lipoteichoic acid, porins, and lipo-arabinomannan in bacteria, zymosan and phospholipomannan in fungi, tGPI-mutin in trypanosomes, and measles virus hemagglutinin protein (33). This ability to recognize more than one activator, particularly when coupled with the ability to associate with different family members (e.g., when TLR2 and TLR6 combine to detect lipoteichoic acid), provides the host with an extended recognition spectrum from a limited number of genes.

A final, required feature of the host sensory apparatus is the sequestration of sensors from signals in the uninjured state. Nature accomplishes this separation through different strategies. Epithelial barriers, for example, constitute the most effective means of partitioning microbial invaders and their sensors, but plasma membranes accomplish the same purpose at a cellular level, particularly if intracellular molecules signal cellular injury when released. Breakdown products of ECM, prevalent in some rheumatic diseases may also be recognized as injury, while the polymeric forms are immunologically inert (21,28,29). The rationale for this sequestration requirement is obvious. Either signal and sensor in continuous contact would maintain the system in a state of constant activation, or the organism would have developed a damping mechanism ("tolerance") to render it insensitive to real injury or infection.

Current Knowledge

Mammalian hosts have evolved multiple means of recognizing injury, depending on the type, location, and severity. Pyogenic extracellular bacteria and herpes viruses can kill the undefended host, albeit by different mechanisms. In fact, the distinct strategies employed by mammals result from eons of coexisting with commensal bacteria and viruses, keeping them at bay or quiescent and quickly containing them following the breaching of barriers. Opportunistic infections occur when commensals and nonpathogenic organisms exploit a host with impaired immune surveillance or responsiveness, while pathogens have evolved mechanisms to circumvent intact defenses.

Cataloging all injury sensors and their signal transducers exceeds the scope of this chapter. Some sensing systems represent "generic" recognition strategies capable of sensing injuries caused by a range of insults, whereas others detect insults due to a specific mechanism. Sensor systems based on the ancient leucine-rich repeat (LRR) include the TLRs and the NACHT-LRRs (including the nucleotide-binding oligomerization domain [NODs] and NACCHT-, LRR-pyrin domain [PYD]-containing proteins [NALPs]). Other, C-type lectin receptors recognize different bacterial carbohydrate structures, as well as some Gram-negative outer membrane proteins. RIG-I-like receptors (RLRs) are RNA helicases that recognize viral RNA and RNA injected into different host cell cytoplasm and help trigger an antiviral response. Proteinase-activated receptors constitute a fourth family of receptors activated by cellular injury and tissue damage that may link the innate immune and nervous systems in the inflammatory response. Periodic publication of excellent reviews provides frequent updates on these and other mammalian sensing systems (5,34–36). Examples of mechanism-specific injury sensors include the family of prolyl hydroxylases that sense cellular hypoxia (37) and the RIG-I RNA helicase sensor of double-stranded viral RNA (38).

Toll-Like Receptors as a Prototypical Component of an Injury-Sensing System

Though first described in the late 1990s, the TLRs, their intracellular signal transduction pathways, and the cellular responses that their activation triggers have taken center stage in innate immunity research and the links between innate and adaptive immune responses. This interest in TLR function owes itself to the fact that this family of receptors and signal transducers constitute a highly evolved sensing system capable of detecting a broad range of molecules, endogenous and exogenous. Conservation of elements of this system (LRRs, immunity-associated kinases, and so forth) across kingdoms, not just species, suggests that these motifs represent a common strategy for different hosts forged in the evolutionary crucible. The following paragraphs review core features of this system, discuss both the general principles of sensing and response and higher order complexities of detecting and initiating cellular responses to injury, and ultimately highlight what remains unknown and challenges current investigators. Several excellent review articles are published each year on our growing understanding of TLR recognition and signaling (5,34,39), so readers are referred to these for more detailed descriptions.

TLR/IL-1R Superfamily. The first TLR discovered was the *Drosophila* protein Toll. Later, sequencing of RNA expressed in multiple mouse and human tissues and public deposition of these sequences led to the recognition of other receptors resembling Toll (40). Humans express 11 TLR family members. Their basic structure consists of an ectodomain composed of LRRs differing in number and organization. The structure of these ectodomains distinguishes one TLR from another and confers on each its recognition specificity. In the case of TLR4, the major endotoxin sensor, MD2 is also associated with the ectodomain and is required for endotoxin recognition. The intracellular domain, common to both TLR and the IL-1 receptor subfamilies, is composed of a Toll/IL-1R (TIR) domain. Across different receptors amino acid similarity ranges from 20% to 30%, but in conserved regions the similarity is higher. This intracellular domain engages the intracellular signaling apparatus (**Fig. 19.1**) (39,41).

TLRs are expressed differentially within cells such as macrophages. Some TLRs are present on the plasma membrane and respond to ligands in the extracellular space. This is true for TLR1, TLR2, TLR4, TLR5, and TLR6. Other TLRs (3,7–9) are expressed within the endosomal compartment and detect ligands that have either been taken up by the cell or somehow managed to gain entry and wind up in the endosomes (34).

Activation of TLRs triggers intracellular signal transduction. As depicted in the accompanying figure (**Fig. 19.2**) (34), receptor engagement induces assembly of multiprotein receptor complexes through protein domain interactions, phosphorylation, and displacement of proteins from different subcellular compartments. Where the TLR signal goes next depends very much on what else the cell is "seeing" and which TLR is seeing it. MyD88 (or TRIF in the case of TLR3 and some TLR4 activations), a dual-domain adaptor protein, is recruited to the activated receptor complex through TIR:TIR domain interactions. Then, MyD88 or TRIF activates signaling cascades that culminate in NF-κB (see below) and AP-1 activation to prepare a coordinated local and systemic inflammatory response, or a type 1 interferon response, critical to early host antiviral defenses. For a more comprehensive map of the TLR signaling network, please consult the work of Oda and Kitano (42).

Cellular Responses

Cellular responses to injury signals fall into two broad categories: genomic and nongenomic. Genomic responses refer to those reactions that involve changes in gene expression. They can be either upregulatory or suppressive, promoting gene transcription and translation or inhibiting them. Many signals, if not most, that indicate the presence of cellular injury involve activation of the transcription factor NF-κB, making this molecule a central regulator of the inflammatory response.

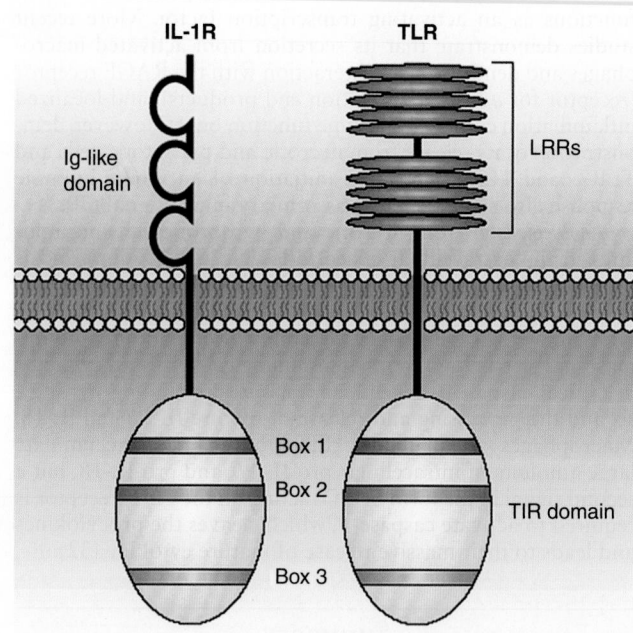

FIGURE 19.1. Humans express 11 TLRs. Their basic structure consists of an ectodomain composed of LRRs and an intracellular domain, common to both TLR and the IL-1 receptor subfamilies, containing a TIR domain. The structure and organization of the LRRs within these ectodomains differ in number and organization for each TLR and confer recognition specificity on each. Ig, immunoglobulin.

Nongenomic responses involve activation of constitutively synthesized molecules (see inflammasome section below) or release of preformed effector stores such as the retrograde release of substance P from C-fibers (afferent sensory nerves involved in nociception).

Nuclear Factor-κB and Genomic Responses to Injury. Although originally identified in activated B cells and believed to be a regulator of immunoglobulin expression, NF-κB orchestrates many aspects of the inflammatory response. NF-κB actually consists of 10 related genes that encode transcription factors or their inhibitors, constituting a system of proinflammatory responsiveness. Interaction of these dimers with the inhibitor proteins of the IκB family prevents DNA binding of the transcription factors with the promoter sequences of NF-κB-responsive genes. Detection of an injury signal, either primary (via TLRs, NLRs, or other receptors) or secondary (through proinflammatory cytokine receptors), triggers degradation of the IκB proteins, freeing the transcription factors to interact with the promoters of responsive genes. There are, in reality, two distinct NF-κB pathways. The pathway described above, called the *canonical pathway*, is responsible for regulating the inflammatory response, including proliferation and apoptosis of lymphoid cells involved in this response. The second, the *noncanonical pathway* belongs more appropriately to the realm of adaptive immunity, as it is responsible for development of the lymphoid organs necessary for appropriate antigen processing, presentation, and mounting of the adaptive immune response (43,44).

When activated, NF-κB influences the expression of over 500 genes involved in the inflammatory response. Examination of these genes reveals a map of the inflammatory response to injury and infection (see http://bioinfo.lifl.fr/NF-KB/ for a current tally of target genes). Genes regulated by NF-κB belong to several categories, essential to initiation, regulation, or termination of the inflammatory response. Genes promoting the local inflammatory response include those specifying

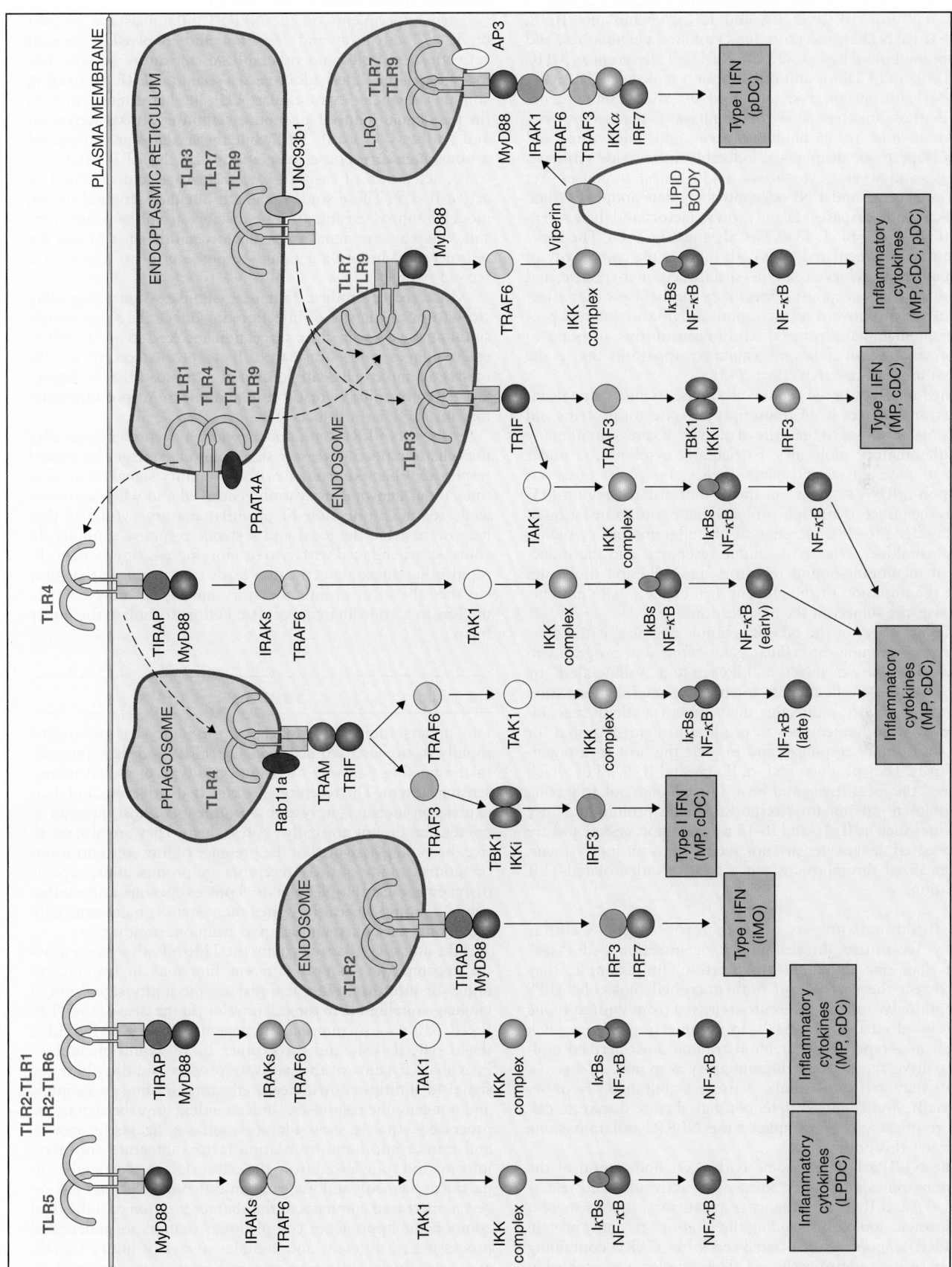

FIGURE 19.2. TLR/IL-1R signal transduction.

231

other transcription factors (interferon regulatory factors, Jun B, Bcl3, c-myb, c-myc, and glucocorticoid receptor); cytokines (IL-1, TNF-α, MIP-1, IFN-γ, and IL-2); chemokines (IL-8, MCP-1, RANTES); receptors for cytokines, chemokines, and membrane-bound ligands (TLR2, NOD2, TNF receptor, MHC II, CD40, and CD86); and cell adhesion molecules (ICAM-1, VCAM-1, fibronectin, P-selectin, and DC-SIGN). Other genes include those involved in the acute phase (C-reactive protein, serum amyloid A, LPS-binding protein, and β-defensins) and stress (superoxide dismutases, inducible nitric oxide synthase, COX-2, and several cytochrome p450 genes) responses. Yet additional genes under NF-κB control regulate apoptosis (Bax, Fas, Bcl-2, and caspase-11) and growth factors and their receptors (FGF-8, IGFBP-1, EPO, G-CSF, and VEGF-C). The sheer range of genes regulated by NF-κB hints at the complexity of mechanisms to achieve cell type–specific, context-specific, and stimulus-specific responses. Specificity mechanisms that affect NF-κB activity, govern transcription on NF-κB-regulated promoters, and radiate from NF-κB dimer isoforms all point to the presence of an elaborate regulatory apparatus that is the current focus of research efforts (43).

The final steps in the genomic response to injury signals involve translation of RNA transcripts into effector proteins and transport or release to their site of activity. Expression of many proinflammatory molecules, particularly cytokines, is under translational control, and many of these molecules possess a common mRNA sequence in the 3′-untranslated region (45) that is the target of multiple proteins that permit translation of the message (46–48). Secretion of proinflammatory cytokines and chemokines, release of soluble receptors, and the induction of membrane-bound receptors and adhesion molecules mark the initiation of the efferent arm of the innate immune response, the subject of the next section.

The net effect of the NF-κB genomic response is the massive reprogramming of cellular gene expression programs to prepare for injury or infection. Likened to a "yellow alert" by some (14), these cells prepare for possible microbial invasion or spreading injury, redirecting their protein synthesis machinery away from homeostasis to produce proteins required for both local injury responses and to alert the host to a potential threat. They produce TNF-α, IL-12, and IL-6, all of which "prime" the local tissue and host, but fall short of triggering a full-blown inflammatory response. Potent proinflammatory cytokines such as IL-1β and IL-18 remain unprocessed and are not released, leukocytes are not recruited to an injury focus, and localized thrombosis is not activated with isolated TLR activation.

The Inflammasome as an Integrator of the Cellular Injury Response. In real injury or infection cells "see" more than one signal. In an infection, for example, they may detect the presence of both microbial molecules (LPS or peptidoglycan) and molecules released from injured tissue (mitochondrial DNA or ATP). In noninfectious injury, such as ischemia–reperfusion or blunt trauma, host-derived molecules drive the ensuing inflammatory response. Moreover, signals may arrive at cellular sensors simultaneously or sequentially, and timing differences may dictate disparate cellular responses. The example of the NLRP3 inflammasome illustrates this point.

The NLRP3 inflammasome is the best understood of the inflammasomes and is best known for activating and releasing IL-1β and IL-18 from inactive precursors. It consists of a multiprotein complex, including the Nod-like receptor protein 3 (NLRP3), apoptosis-associated speck-like CARD-containing protein (ASC) and pro-caspase-1. The complex is assembled in response to a number of different injury signals, such as silica, extracellular ATP, and monosodium urate crystals, among others. Once assembled, the complex cleaves pro-caspase-1, an

inactive cysteine protease into its active form, whereupon it begins to cleave available substrate (49).

Early experiments on the NLRP3 inflammasome focused on IL-1β activation and secretion and involved sequential activation of TLRs and other NF-κB-activating stimuli, followed by (hours later) addition of a second, NLRP3-activating stimulus, such as extracellular ATP. In these initial studies, the first signal induced a genomic response (NF-κB activation and synthesis of pro-IL-1β), while the second signal triggered a nongenomic response (assembly of the NLRP3 inflammasome, activation of caspase-1, and cleavage and secretion of active IL-1β). These studies, though not their original intent, modeled injury sensing at some distance from the original insult, whereby one signal arrived before another, permitting the sensor cell to mount a genomic response prior to receipt of a second signal.

More recent studies, that may simulate injury signaling close to or at the site of infection, introduce the same signals simultaneously or in close succession and lead to a very different cellular response. Instead of IL-1β production, these cells undergo a rapid cell death known as pyroptosis that is characterized by membrane disruption and release of proinflammatory intracellular products (50).

Thus, the NLRP3 inflammasome may represent one way the cell attempts to integrate signals into a coherent biological response. When confronted with two injury signals spaced in time, inflammasome activation is delayed and when activated leads to the production of proinflammatory cytokines that help orchestrate the local and systemic response to injury. In contrast, when faced with two or more signals simultaneously, rapid inflammasome activation leads to a response that may enhance the local proinflammatory milieu, but may contribute less to a coordinated, regulated effort to isolate the injury focus.

Summary

Our understanding of how cells sense injury has progressed rapidly in the last two decades. The TLRs and their intracellular signaling pathway constitute one type of global injury-sensing system. The receptors are widely distributed, and their expression increases in response to threats to host integrity in tissues that do not normally express them. They are also sensitive, becoming activated in the presence of low concentrations of agonist. Many of these receptors are promiscuous, capable of recognizing multiple signals, both exogenous and endogenous. Finally, in healthy states the system is quiescent, with signal and sensor remaining apart from one another.

Like any surveillance system, the TLR-NF-κB sensing module accomplishes several different functions in response to injury or infection. First, it translates the injury signal into a language intelligible to the cell interior (in the case of the TLR/IL-1R pathway, a common language used by 10 of 11 TLRs, the IL-1R, IL-18R and three other IL-1R family members). Proximal elements of the pathway process and distribute the signal to multiple downstream effectors, leading to genomic and nongenomic responses. Understanding how the signals are processed—that is, how adaptors, kinases, ligases, proteases, and transcription and translation factors integrate and parse information transferred from the cell surface, endosomal compartment, cytosol, and nucleus—in different cell types has received increased emphasis as the characterization of individual components approaches completion. Attempts to understand processing of different and complex arrays of injury signals, as occurs during infection and real injury, are beginning to embrace complex system-based concepts that describe cells' (and indeed entire organisms') response by difficult-to-predict, emergent properties.

LOCAL RESPONSE AND ALERTING HOST DEFENSE

Once sentinel cells have detected injury or microbial invasion, they unleash a response with the goal of containing the insult and eliminating invading microbes and injured and dying cells. The host must engage both local tissue and systemic components to accomplish these dual objectives, the latter to muster distant resources (e.g., mobilize marginated neutrophils, produce acute phase reactants) and support the local response. Through cytokine, chemokine, and antimicrobial peptide production and action; neuroendocrine system activation; localized endothelial cell changes; leukocyte influx into the injured tissue; and the acute phase response, the host attempts to neutralize the threat to its integrity and restore homeostasis.

Because even the basic inflammatory response is so complex, the following summary selects only a few details, and although they are important, it is by no means comprehensive. The synopsis also outlines the acute local injury and neutrophil influx responses to bacterial tissue invasion or localized tissue necrosis (e.g., following ischemia). This reaction depicts the earliest activation of innate immunity. Chronic inflammatory responses, as occur with some pathogens or in chronic inflammatory states such as autoimmunity, use analogous localization mechanisms but differ in recruited cell type and involvement of adaptive immunity.

Requirements for Effective Injury Response

Once injury has occurred and been detected, the host begins to respond. The host defense system must marshal both local and distant resources to confront the threat. Tissue adjacent to the microbial invasion site commences the containment and elimination of damaged tissue or invading microorganisms while recruiting additional support to the site of injury from more remote sources. In the afferent arm, the host translates the primary injury signals, detected by specialized sensor cells, into a language intelligible to all host cells. This translation function alerts uninjured but at-risk cells in the vicinity of the injury and amplifies the original injury signal. Finally, communication networks distribute the signal to more distant sites critical to supporting and coordinating the integrated inflammatory response (e.g., CNS, liver). The efferent arm exercises two distinct functions. First, it directs effectors to the site of injury. Neurogenic inflammation, cytokine production, altered local endothelium, and chemokine gradients promote leukocyte arrival at the injury site and prime them to enact their assigned inflammatory actions. This vectorial component is essential to proper localization of the injury response. Failure to localize correctly, or indiscriminate activation of inflammatory functions away from infectious foci or injury sites, may underlie certain parainfectious syndromes such as ARDS, severe sepsis, macrophage activation syndrome, or DIC (3). The second function carried out by the efferent limb of a host defense system concentrates the inflammatory response to a limited area while ensuring containment of invading microorganisms and toxic inflammatory products to that site. Balance between potent local proinflammatory effectors and systemic anti-inflammatory mediators is essential to this circumscription function (11).

Local Response

An effective local response accomplishes four objectives. It first ensures placement of effectors at the injury site. Since effectors range in size from small molecules and proteins to large leukocytes, the local response utilizes different mechanisms to achieve this first goal. The local reaction also contains microbial invasion and limits the impact of necrotic cell death on both adjacent and distant tissues. Failure to do so would result in systemic spread of pathogens and toxic substances that could destabilize the host. As containment is accomplished, the local response also cleans up the detritus of injury. This includes both contained microbes and dead and dying host cells. Finally, the local inflammatory response initiates the healing process. Depending on the affected tissue and the injury mechanism, healing may involve regeneration, scarring, or a combination of the two. Healing will not be discussed further.

Three general processes are critical during an acute inflammatory response. First, the initial injury signal undergoes local amplification. That process involves spreading an intelligible alarm and generating injury location information. The second process involves alteration of the local vasculature to permit soluble and cellular effectors in the bloodstream to leave the vascular space and prevent microbes and toxins from entering the circulation. Lastly, leukocytes migrate from the vascular space to the injury site in a regulated process that destroys invaders and infected cells, scavenges injured and dying tissue, and promotes an adaptive immune response to infections. The following section examines aspects of these processes in greater detail.

Local Amplification of Injury Signal

Specialization poses interesting problems for the host. Tissues evolved to enact particular functions (e.g., gas exchange, blood circulation, or solute excretion) often lack other capacities. Many specialized cell types either lack or exhibit deficiencies in the ability to sense injury. TLR protein expression, both scattered and nonubiquitous, illustrates this point. When a tissue is threatened at one site, however, the host must have a means to alert surrounding cells and engage their participation in mounting a protective response. At least two systems exist in mammals to perform this essential function. The first consists of different systems of soluble mediators collectively referred to as cytokines, while the second utilizes the peripheral nervous system.

Cytokines. Cytokines refer to soluble proteins or glycoproteins made by cells to affect the behavior of other cells (51). They are usually produced in response to a stimulus (as opposed to constitutively), act over a short distance, and are distinguished from hormones and growth factors on the basis of arbitrary criteria, though properties and functions often overlap. Some cytokines are pleiotropic, and others exhibit narrow spectra of targets and effects. Various schemata have been used to classify families of cytokines. The discussion below will focus on two categories of cytokines: the primary proinflammatory cytokines and the granulocyte-attracting chemokines.

The Proinflammatory Cytokines: TNF-α and IL-1β. Shortly after local injury or microbial invasion, specialized injury-sensing cells produce and release both TNF-α and IL-1β. Though structurally unrelated and recognized by different receptors, the expression of these two cytokines is under similar control and they elicit overlapping biological effects. Transcription of both messenger RNAs is regulated by NF-κB, and a shared AU-rich region in the 3′-untranslated region, common to many proinflammatory molecules, controls message translation. Secretion of these cytokines, however, follows distinct pathways. TNF-α is synthesized as a precursor, membrane-anchored secretory protein. A dedicated pathway targets trimeric pro-TNF-α to a recycling endosome, and triggers its cleavage and extracellular release by its processing enzyme, TACE, following membrane fusion (52). Following a nonclassical secretory route, pro-IL-1β and its processing protease, caspase-1, are both targeted to specialized secretory lysosomes. Extracellular ATP or other signals then provide a second stimulus that triggers cleavage of the procytokine to mature IL-1β and its secretion via exocytosis (see previous inflammasome section).

Secreted cytokine binds to ubiquitous cognate receptors, triggering activation of NF-κB and other key intracellular inflammatory mediators. These molecules lead, in turn, to the production and release of additional molecules that activate local endothelium, serve as chemoattractants, and begin to cycle off the acute proinflammatory response.

The net effect of TNF and IL-1β action is threefold. First, these cytokines convert a cryptic injury signal into a language shared by most host cells. Second, they spread the alarm to a greater number of cells in the area of injury. This propagation function amplifies the original injury signal by inducing more cells to contribute to the local inflammatory response. Third, this initial proinflammatory cytokine response provides the host with positional information about the site of injury. The intensity of the response is highest closest to the primary injury or invasion site. Chemokine concentrations are highest nearer the center of injury, diminishing in a radial fashion. Endothelial activation is also more intense in vessels closer to the infection or site of necrosis than in more distant ones.

ELR+ CXC Chemokines. Chemokines are cytokines that exert chemotactic functions. There are ~50 chemokines, belonging to at least four families, classified according to molecular structure, although both families and individual molecules exhibit redundant functions (53). The CXC chemokines contain two cysteine residues separated by a variable residue at their amino terminus. These molecules are further subdivided according to the presence (ELR+) or absence (ELR−) of tripeptide motif. The ELR+ CXC chemokines are considered the primary neutrophil chemoattractants, with IL-8 (or CXCL8, according to newer nomenclature) representing the prototype. These molecules interact with two cognate receptors (CXCR1 and CXCR2) with similar biological effects. Synthesis of the ELR+ CXC chemokines occurs in response to proinflammatory stimuli, as a result of direct infection (e.g., LPS), injury (e.g., hypoxic–ischemic injury), or primary cytokine (TNF-α or IL-1β) stimulation.

Through an overlapping, multistep process, IL-8 and other ELR+ CXC chemokines enable the movement of neutrophils out of the vascular space to the site of inflammation. Initial interaction between IL-8 and CXCR1 and 2 may occur as neutrophils rolling along the endothelium arrest, allowing high-avidity interactions between ligand and receptor (54). IL-8 forms a gradient, mediated in part by immobilization on basement membrane proteins, with highest concentrations at the site of inflammation that decrease with distance from the primary focus. Neutrophils migrate down the chemokine gradient from lower to higher concentration, becoming more activated as they approach the site of infection or injury.

Thus, the CXC ELR+ chemokines, as well as other inducible chemokines, enact three essential functions for the acute local response. First, they provide positional information to cellular effectors migrating to the inflammatory focus. Because the concentration gradient is continuous, these molecules also map out the route to the site. Finally, they gradually arm the leukocyte, enhancing its level of activation as the effector cell approaches the center of maximal injury. This latter function maximizes destructive potential where appropriate and minimizes the chances of damage to uninjured tissue.

Neurogenic Inflammation. The term "neurogenic inflammation" refers to a specific reaction to infection or injury mediated by the peripheral nervous system. Primary sensory nerve fibers, can be activated by both endogenous and exogenous stimuli, many of which act through the polyvalent receptor channel TRPV1. Following activation by a number of different proinflammatory stimuli, these fibers not only relay the signal centrally (an afferent function) but also carry out antidromic (efferent) transmission. Following local injury, narrow-diameter, unmyelinated C-fibers in close proximity to, or in membrane contact with, innate immune cells (especially mast cells) release neuropeptides (in particular, substance P and calcitonin gene–related peptide). These neuropeptides, in turn, act on local immune cells, nerves, endothelium, and vascular smooth muscle to elicit many effects, including the cardinal signs of inflammation (55). Substance P, for example, promotes vasodilation, plasma extravasation, leukocyte activation, and adhesion molecule expression on endothelium (4) and leads to enhanced sensitization to painful stimuli (hyperalgesia). Most known inducers or enhancers of neurogenic inflammation are endogenous (bradykinin, glutamate, PGE2, nerve growth factor, and acetylcholine), raising the question of whether this represents an amplification step only. However, heat, ATP, and hydrogen ions can also trigger this response, and other primary stimuli may yet be identified. Moreover, the sympathetic nervous system promotes neurogenic inflammation, as sympathectomy abrogates this reaction (e.g., protective effect of prior brachial plexus injury (56)), and increased sympathetic activity in certain arthritis models is associated with more severe joint destruction (57).

Localized Vascular Response

The vasculature plays a critical role in the acute, and subacute, response to infection and injury. It routes both plasma, which contains potent antibacterial and proinflammatory proteins, and nonresident cells, principally different types of leukocytes, close to the site of insult. An effective inflammatory response, therefore, maximizes delivery of these soluble and cellular components to the injury neighborhood (providing for both increased flux and correct localization) and facilitates extravasation of these mediators, while at the same time preventing systemic spread of toxins or microbes from the focus.

Vasodilation and Increased Permeability. Different types of injury (e.g., ischemia–reperfusion, bacterial invasion, blunt trauma) provoke similar initial responses. Whether sensed directly, by the presence of class-identifying molecules, or indirectly, by the presence of tissue damage, the challenge provokes an initial response that involves release of preformed mediators. Histamine, serotonin (from mast cells), and substance P (from sensory neurons) collaborate to induce local arteriolar vasodilatation, giving rise to hyperemia in the vicinity of the injury. These substances, together with others that potentiate further release of these primary mediators (e.g., bradykinin, tryptase, vasoactive intestinal peptide, and PGE$_2$), trigger formation of reversible gaps between endothelial cells that lead to increased vascular permeability, transudation, and angiogenic edema. The wheal–flare reaction seen with urticaria or dermographism illustrates this early response even in the absence of any significant injury, but more damage is accompanied by a cellular infiltrate that develops later.

Vasodilation promotes bulk movement of blood components to the region of an injury or microbial invasion, while increased permeability permits translocation of soluble effectors out of the vascular space. The net effect of these combined processes is threefold. First, they facilitate targeting of antimicrobial and proinflammatory molecules to the site of injury or invasion. Second, increased bulk fluid delivery to the focus dilutes and neutralizes toxic mediators to help minimize secondary tissue damage. Finally, increased interstitial fluid increases lymphatic flow, which irrigates the focus and facilitates development of the adaptive immune response to pathogens in the wound site by delivering antigens to draining lymph nodes.

Endothelial Activation. The arteriovenous vasculature is not, as the above might imply, simply a conduit for blood components. It provides essential information about the location and intensity of an injury, serves as a portal for the cellular infiltrate of inflammation, and regulates its own role in this response. The endothelium, however, in concert with the peripheral nervous system, confers this important additional functionality on the blood vessels. Although the endothelium has multiple functions during the inflammatory response, this section touches on two.

Leukocyte Recruitment. The histologic hallmark of inflammation is the presence of leukocytes at the injury site or infection focus. While most leukocytes carry out continuous surveillance while trafficking from the arteriovenous vasculature through the tissue to the lymphatic vascular system before returning to blood, a few, usually of monocytic lineage, take up residence in specific tissues. Following different acute insults, however, neutrophils rapidly congregate in large numbers at the site of injury, in a directed, nonrandom fashion. Activated endothelium in the vicinity of injured tissues furnishes both information regarding the location of the inflammatory focus to leukocytes patrolling the vascular space as well as the means to initiate migration out of the vessel to the injury site.

After microbial invasion or other tissue damage, the postcapillary venules become the principal site of leukocyte extravasation. Two critical forces determine the efficiency with which this process occurs. The first is the relatively low shear stress (force exerted by flowing blood along the vessel wall that opposes the tendency to adhere to the vessel wall) compared to vessels on the arteriolar side of the microcirculation. The second is the expression of molecules on the activated endothelial cell surface that promote leukocyte adherence and help these cells resist the shear stress of blood flow, help reduce their profile, and facilitate their migration out of the vessel.

Endothelial activation is a complex process. Multiple factors influence the degree of activation. The intensity of the injury itself or the pathogen load is a primary determinant of activation. More extensive local tissue damage, higher bacterial or viral load, and higher local primary cytokine (particularly IL-1β and TNF-α, but also IFN-γ) concentration increase the intensity of the endothelial response in the region of injury. Localized shear stress, uninjured stromal cells (e.g., smooth muscle cells and fibroblasts), and even the ECM further modulate endothelial activation. One of the principal responses of activated endothelium is adhesion molecule and chemokine expression. Upregulation of selectins and VCAM-1 help "tether" circulating neutrophils, after which they "roll," "crawl," and come to a halt ("arrest"), becoming tightly adherent to the activated endothelium. ICAM-1 and endothelial surface-associated chemokines, such as MCP-1, interact with the arrested leukocyte triggering integrin signaling within the PMN, subsequent flattening, "crawling" to a transendothelial migration site, and then transendothelial migration of the leukocyte out of the vascular space into the adjacent tissue (58). From there, the neutrophils begin their migration down changing chemokine gradients through the tissue to the injury site (see Extravascular Migration below).

Thrombosis. Coagulation and inflammation are closely linked, though the detailed knowledge of this relationship is still emerging. In fact, the systems that protect against hemorrhage and microbial dissemination may have evolved from a common ancestral strategy that accomplished both. In the horseshoe crab, bacterial invasion precipitates a localized response involving hemolymph coagulation and hemocyte agglutination that immobilizes the invader and prevents systemic spread prior to engulfment or killing (59). This *Limulus* coagulation response forms the basis for current endotoxin detection

tests. Both inflammation and coagulation influence each other. In general, local inflammation tends to downregulate natural anticoagulant systems, favoring thrombosis, while processes that skew the balance of pro- and anticoagulation forces toward antithrombosis and fibrinolysis have anti-inflammatory effects (60).

Coagulation is a surface-associated phenomenon. Under normal circumstances, the apical surface of the vascular endothelium possesses anticoagulant properties that discourage thrombus formation. Tissue injury or infection, however, can either disrupt endothelial continuity or induce changes in the endothelial surface that favor thrombus formation. Direct injury to the vessel exposes the soluble components of the extrinsic coagulation cascade to tissue factor expressed on monocytes, smooth muscle cells, and fibroblasts, triggering a proteolytic sequence resulting in thrombin formation. Thrombin in turn exerts both procoagulant functions (fibrin formation, platelet shape change, activator release, and aggregation) and proinflammatory effects (vasoconstriction and cytokine production). Thrombosis can also occur within the vascular space with an intact epithelium. Though less well understood, intravascular coagulation can also occur in the setting of both localized and systemic inflammation. Factors favoring the occurrence of intravascular coagulation include increase in negatively charged membrane surfaces (e.g., increased circulating microvesicles), downregulation of the natural anticoagulant, activated protein C (through decreases in thrombomodulin and the endothelial cell protein C receptor), and neutrophil-mediated endothelial cell damage (converting the endothelium into a procoagulant surface).

The net effect of thrombosis is threefold. First, as in the horseshoe crab, it isolates an area of injury, preventing blood flow into or out of the affected zone. Containment achieves two ends. It prevents nutrient delivery to the site. Oxygen deprivation seals the fate of most host cells in the immediate vicinity of injury or invasion, but it may prevent viral replication or intracellular bacterial survival (by killing the parasitized host cell), and even extracellular aerobic pathogen survival. Confinement also protects against systemic microbial spread or dissemination of the toxic products of tissue damage. Second, thrombosis delimits a zone of nonviability. Other cells in the vicinity remain at risk (see below), but those deprived of blood flow constitute the tissue lost to the primary injury. Third, thrombosis is also an intrinsic signal of host injury. By altering local hemodynamics and amplifying proinflammatory stimuli, both directly and indirectly, this process contributes additional information about the location, size, and severity of the threat to the host.

Leukocyte Effector Response

Leukocytes enact different effector programs depending on their lineage and the insult they respond to. Neutrophils perform distinct functions from T lymphocytes, and even neutrophils will respond differently to tissue injured by hypoxic–ischemic injury or microbial invasion. The effector response involves arriving at the correct site, carrying out the appropriate host defense reactions, and providing for resolution of one phase of the response and initiating the subsequent phase. An overview of neutrophil function in acute inflammation follows. Macrophage and lymphocyte recruitment and activity are also essential to resolving an acute inflammatory response, but space precludes a discussion of their roles in this response.

Extravascular Migration. Following transendothelial migration, neutrophils must traverse the tissue to the injury focus. This process involves three essential elements. First, the neutrophils must be able to sense chemoattractant concentration differences in the extracellular milieu. They must then use those gradients to orient (polarize) the cell to head toward higher concentrations. Finally, they must be able to physically displace themselves through the tissue.

Neutrophils actually sense at least two broad categories of chemoattractants: intermediary and end target. Molecules such as the ELR+ CXC chemokines, produced as a result of the primary injury or infection or during the initial amplification phase, belong to the former class. Chemotactic bacterial products (such as formyl-Met-Leu-Phe or the complement component C5a generated at the site of infection) constitute end-target chemoattractants. Moreover, neutrophils exhibit a preferential response to the latter class of molecule; given a choice between the two classes of agents, regardless of the concentration of either, neutrophils will respond preferentially to those agents generated at the site of infection. This hierarchical responsiveness is attributable to the intracellular signaling pathway triggered by each, with intermediary chemokines acting through phosphatidylinositol-3-kinase pathway and end-target molecules activating the p38 MAPK pathway (61).

Movement of neutrophils through the tissues depends on transient adhesive interactions between integrin superfamily members and ligands composing the ECM (e.g., collagen, laminin, fibronectin, and tenascin). In this role, leukocyte integrins act as both (a) anchoring proteins, providing physical interaction between ECM proteins (through binding of their ectodomains) and intracellular cytoskeletal molecules (via the cytoplasmic domains), and (b) signal transducers, communicating binding and release information, together with signals to enhance the neutrophil's activation state as it approaches the injury site. The β1-integrin family mediates these interactions and coordinates locomotion through the ECM, though the migration process requires more than integrin–ECM interactions (58).

Effector Responses. As they approach the injured site, neutrophils undergo progressive activation, such that by arrival, they are fully primed to carry out the appropriate effector function. Actual effector responses are determined by what the neutrophils encounter at the site and involve a combination of release and activation of preformed mediators (e.g., granule proteins/peptides and reactive oxygen species) with new gene expression.

The presence of bacteria at the injury site may or may not prompt phagocytosis. When bacteria cannot be phagocytosed, the neutrophil releases antimicrobial and proteolytic proteins and generates reactive oxygen species, resulting in bacterial and tissue destruction. Microbial engulfment, in contrast, triggers granule content release into the phagosome and generation of reactive oxygen species to destroy the ingested bacteria, as well as a two-stage genomic response involving upregulation and downregulation of genes. In the first wave, cytokines and chemokines are expressed that recruit and activate macrophages and lymphocytes, and support wound healing. Following this first surge of new gene expression, a second response ensues with upregulation of proapoptotic genes and downregulation of receptors for different inflammatory mediators and injury-sensing proteins (cytokines, chemokines, immunoglobulins, and TLRs). Neutrophils then undergo apoptosis and are ingested by macrophages, marking entrance into the resolution phase of the acute inflammatory response (13).

Neutrophils recruited to sterile injury sites exhibit a similar initial proinflammatory genomic response, but in the absence of phagocytosis, express antiapoptotic genes and prolong the period of neutrophil protection against infection (13). Less is known about the genomic response of neutrophils responding to sites with significant necrotic tissue damage.

Alerting Host Defense

While much of the local inflammatory response outlined in the preceding section is tissue-autonomous (i.e., triggered by the involved tissues themselves), when the insult is significant enough, it triggers a supporting systemic response that overlaps with the host's reaction to fearful situations. Signs of systemic responses may include fever, hypothalamic–pituitary–adrenocortical axis and hypothalamic–adrenomedullary–autonomic nervous system activation, and acute phase protein production. Defining thresholds for activation of these responses is difficult because they vary depending on the ground state of the host at the time of injury or infection. Two generalizations about the intact response, however, bear mention. First, while this response supports the local inflammatory process, its net impact on the host appears to be anti-inflammatory, making the host temporarily less reactive to inflammatory and infectious stimuli (11). Second, proper activation and modulation requires coordination between both hardwired and soluble components. Because space limitations preclude a complete discussion, the following paragraphs will focus on two critical intermediaries that alert the host to a localized threat to its integrity: the peripheral nervous system and the cytokine IL-6.

Peripheral Nervous System

The peripheral nervous system refers to the network of nerves that either resides entirely within non-CNS tissue or originates or terminates in the CNS but with the principal function of carrying signals to or from the visceral organs or somatic tissues. These nerves contain a variety of different fibers. As alluded to above, they may be afferent or efferent, and may subserve either somatic or autonomic functions. In alerting the host to local injury or infection, the afferent component of both somatic and autonomic nerves enacts an essential function.

Infections or injuries to the viscera activate afferent neurons that form part of the vagus nerve. When stimulated, these afferent fibers signal to neurons with connections throughout the CNS, including the hypothalamus and cortex. The host responds by increasing its thermal balance point (fever), local cytokine production in the CNS, and secretion of pituitary hormones (ACTH and MSH) that support the host's ability to handle the stress of visceral injury or infection, including behaviors such as the fight–flight response, and maintenance of an anti-inflammatory milieu. If the insult is noxious enough, the host may sense pain referred to the body wall represented by the area of sensory cortex activated by the autonomic afferent signals (e.g., periumbilical region during appendicitis, left shoulder, neck, and jaw with myocardial ischemia). Acute vagotomy, in contrast, attenuates the ability of experimental animals to mount a fever when injected intraperitoneally with LPS, even though they produce higher TNF-α and IL-1β concentrations. Vagotomized humans, so treated because of severe peptic ulcer disease (believed to be precipitated by stress), do not, however, appear to have deficient responses to visceral infections or injuries, suggesting the existence of redundant systems to alert the host to threats within body cavities.

Injuries to the limbs and body wall (soma) activate peripheral sensory fibers that transmit an array of complex information about the insult to the CNS, and trigger efferent responses that further behaviors and physiologic responses to separate from noxious stimuli (withdrawal) and support the local inflammatory response to the injury or infection, including many of those referred to in the preceding paragraph.

Interleukin-6

IL-6 is the best studied soluble activator of a systemic response to local injury or infection. It is synthesized in response to primary injury signals (e.g., LPS and other microbial products) and secondary amplifiers (TNF-α and IL-1β). Unlike these primary and secondary signals, which appear in the circulation only following massive or overwhelming insult, IL-6 represents a convenient, if nonspecific, marker of localized inflammation. While this cytokine exhibits marked pleiotropy, only two functions will be highlighted here: pyrogen and acute phase response activator.

First, IL-6 links the inflammatory focus to the CNS, effecting changes in host physiology and behavior to confront the challenge posed by the insult. Clinically, the most notable effect of IL-6 on the CNS is its role in the febrile response, though it also modulates activation of the HPA. In its function as a "pyrogenic cytokine," it enters the circulation via lymphatic and hematogenous routes following release from tissue-based and extravasated leukocytes, and endothelium. As it circulates through the vasculature of the CNS, it interacts with specialized neurons (the circumventricular organ system) that sample the circulating milieu. Elevated serum IL-6 concentrations induce prostaglandin E2 synthesis within these neurons and secretion in the hypothalamus, leading to the febrile response. This response in humans involves not only redistributing the circulation away from the periphery until the higher temperature is reached but also behavioral changes such as huddling in smaller species.

IL-6 serves as a critical bridge between the site of inflammation and the liver, the second major organ supporting the innate immune response to infection and injury. It constitutes the most important soluble trigger of the acute phase response, a complex stereotyped reprogramming of hepatic protein synthesis. Elevated IL-6 levels stimulate synthesis of proteins to support the host response. C-reactive protein, a pentraxin with potent antimicrobial and anti-inflammatory properties, mannose-binding protein, and serum amyloid P represent three acute phase proteins whose expression IL-6 upregulates. IL-6 also suppresses the synthesis of other proteins, such as albumin and haptoglobin as part of this hepatic genomic response.

REGULATION AND OUTCOME OF INFLAMMATION

Any system that detects and responds to injury to the host must be regulated. Failure to control and ultimately terminate an inflammatory reaction would result in a self-perpetuating, destructive spiral. Unfortunately, relatively little is known about higher order regulation of the innate immune response. Three categories of controls can be envisioned. In the first, an effective host defense system must regulate the **type** of response. Mobilization of NK cells to eliminate a staphylococcal skin infection would be wasteful, but failure to do so in hepatitis C infection could be lethal to the host. Knowledge of how the host recruits the right kinds of cells to different injuries is fragmented and confusing, especially given the overlapping cellular and receptor targets for different cytokines (gp130-mediated signaling) and chemokines (e.g., CXCR1 and 2) and hierarchical relationships among different chemoattractant molecules.

The second type of control regulates the **intensity** of a response according to the threat imposed by the insult. Generation of an exuberant pyogenic reaction with extensive distal thrombosis resulting in autoamputation would be excessive for a pyonychia, but might be more appropriate in an ascending fasciitis. In the case of neutrophil recruitment, activation state increases with proximity to the inflammatory focus, stemming

in part from increasing chemoattractant concentrations. Less is known, however, about how the host determines how many neutrophils are enough to accomplish the specific task (a form of polling) and regulates their arrival (an executive function).

Finally, the responses, no matter what type or intensity, should have a beginning, middle, and an end. Therefore, the third type of control involves **phasing**. IL-6-*trans*-signaling, in which the balance between IL-6, its soluble receptor, and the receptor antagonist soluble gp130 determines the biological response, exemplifies an elegant, self-regulating system that both promotes and suppresses IL-6 function at the inflammatory focus (8,62).

Systems biology approaches that account for multiple inputs and extreme complexity will ultimately shed more light on these regulatory issues than reductionist methods characteristic of the molecular biology era. Moreover, development of new therapies targeting the inflammatory response will depend on a more complete understanding of its regulation (15,63).

Outcome of Inflammation: Demarcation of Three Domains

The injury itself and the host's response establish an ongoing dialectic. Until its resolution, this exchange defines three domains within any host. These domains are both anatomic and functional. At the site of injury or microbial invasion and radiating outward, some tissue and function are irretrievably lost (**Fig. 19.3**, domain 1). The extent of this domain is determined solely by the magnitude of the primary injury. Factors affecting the magnitude of the initial insult include time (e.g., duration of ischemia), force (energy of impact, speed of body, or projectile), or virulence or infectivity of microbe. Beyond this core of destruction lies a field of tissue at risk for loss (domain 2). The loss of at-risk tissue (domain 2-to-1 transition) is referred to clinically as "secondary injury." The concept of at-risk tissue is analogous to a "watershed area" or "penumbra" in ischemic or traumatic neurologic injuries. Similarly, the idea of a functional domain 2 is encompassed by the notion of "stunned" or "hibernating" myocardium. Multiple factors determine the proportion of tissue or function that is ultimately lost, or preserved, including the magnitude of primary injury, genetic background of host influencing the injury response, nongenetic modifiers of the host response (e.g., nutrition, immunosuppression), and exogenous interventions. Most therapeutic interventions, and their side effects, target the remaining three factors with the goal of preventing

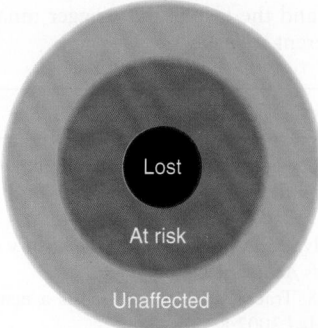

FIGURE 19.3. Outcome of inflammation: Demarcation of three domains. The size or mass of each domain will be determined by the magnitude of the injury and the host's response to it. The response itself can be appropriate, insufficient, or excessive and lead, in the latter two circumstances, to additional tissue damage or loss of function.

or minimizing secondary injury, and many aim to modulate the inflammatory response.

Outside the vulnerable area resides tissue unaffected by the injury (domain 3). The accompanying figure (**Fig. 19.3**) depicts these domains graphically, though it fails to capture the dynamic tension at the interfaces between these domains. Necrotizing pneumonia, characterized by the microbial invasion site and necrotic center surrounded by alveolar, airway, and supporting tissue vulnerable to progressive invasive disease flanked by functionally normal lung, illustrates this concept clinically. The size or mass of each domain will be determined by the magnitude of the injury and the host's response to it, which can be either insufficient or excessive and lead, in either instance, to additional damage.

Organ function and host survival depend on sufficient domain 3 mass to maintain homeostasis. In general, loss of between 75% and 90% of functional tissue (e.g., nephrons, cardiac myocytes) exceeds an organ's capacity to compensate and results in overt organ failure. Occasionally, this loss of function is transient, suggesting the existence of either poorly functioning at-risk tissue that recovers and restores organ function, rejoining domain 3, or significant regenerative capacity. If, however, organ function fails to return, host survival is threatened. In this scenario, organ transplantation often constitutes the best, though still suboptimal, solution to restore the lost function of certain organs. Replacement therapy (e.g., insulin use for endocrine pancreatic failure) represents an alternative when the lost function is relatively simple to mimic.

CONCLUSIONS AND FUTURE DIRECTIONS

To conclude this introduction to innate immunity and inflammation, a few key points about this system deserve to be highlighted. First, innate immunity is essential to survival; without it, the host would fall victim to even the commensal organisms residing on mucosal surfaces or the skin. Second, though often characterized as "primitive," especially in comparison to adaptive immunity, it too exhibits tremendous complexity and is tightly integrated with multiple nonimmune systems in the host (vascular, neuroendocrine). Despite its complexity, however, it really evolved to respond to small or moderate injuries. Severe insults, such as massive trauma or overwhelming septicemia, condition treated in ICUs throughout the world, may trigger widespread activation of innate immunity, but rather than protecting the host, this activation usually worsens the host's condition, causing ARDS, shock, and DIC. Finally, therapeutic manipulation of this response will ultimately depend on much more detailed knowledge of the interactions between hosts and the insults that trigger innate immune responses in different tissues.

References

1. Ley K. History of inflammation research. In: Ley K, ed. *Physiology of Inflammation*. New York, NY: Oxford University Press, 2001:1–10.
2. Rocha E, Silva M. A brief survey of the history of inflammation. 1978. *Agents Actions* 1994;43:86–90.
3. Munford RS, Tracey KJ. Is severe sepsis a neuroendocrine disease? *Mol Med* 2002;8:437–42.
4. Schaible HG, Del Rosso A, Matucci-Cerinic M. Neurogenic aspects of inflammation. *Rheum Dis Clin North Am* 2005;31:77–101, ix.
5. Beutler BA. TLRs and innate immunity. *Blood* 2009;113:1399–407.
6. Beutler B. Innate immunity: An overview. *Mol Immunol* 2004;40:845–59.
7. Casanova JL, Abel L, Quintana-Murci L. Human TLRs and IL-1Rs in host defense: Natural insights from evolutionary, epidemiological, and clinical genetics. *Annu Rev Immunol* 2011;29:447–91.
8. Rose-John S. IL-6 trans-signaling via the soluble IL-6 receptor: Importance for the pro-inflammatory activities of IL-6. *Int J Biol Sci* 2012;8:1237–47.
9. Beck G, Habicht G. Immunity and the invertebrates. *Sci Am* 1996;275(5):60–6.
10. Iwasaki A, Medzhitov R. Regulation of adaptive immunity by the innate immune system. *Science* 2010;327:291–5.
11. Munford RS, Pugin J. Normal responses to injury prevent systemic inflammation and can be immunosuppressive. *Am J Respir Crit Care Med* 2001;163:316–21.
12. Hume DA. The mononuclear phagocyte system. *Curr Opin Immunol* 2006;18:49–53.
13. Theilgaard-Monch K, Porse BT, Borregaard N. Systems biology of neutrophil differentiation and immune response. *Curr Opin Immunol* 2006;18:54–60.
14. Zak DE, Aderem A. Systems biology of innate immunity. *Immunol Rev* 2009;227:264–82.
15. Aderem A, Smith KD. A systems approach to dissecting immunity and inflammation. *Semin Immunol* 2004;16:55–67.
16. Thomas L. *The Lives of a Cell: Notes of a Biology Watcher*. New York, NY: The Viking Press, 1974.
17. Burnet FM. *The Clonal Selection Theory of Acquired Immunity*. Cambridge, MA: Cambridge University Press, 1959.
18. Lederberg J. Genes and antibodies: Do antigens bear instructions for antibody specificity or de they select cell lines that arise by mutation? *Science* 1959;129:1649–53.
19. Janeway CA Jr. Approaching the asymptote? Evolution and revolution in immunology. *Cold Spring Harb Symp Quant Biol* 1989;54(pt 1):1–13.
20. Matzinger P. Tolerance, danger, and the extended family. *Annu Rev Immunol* 1994;12:991–1045.
21. Pradeu T, Cooper EL. The danger theory: 20 years later. *Front Immunol* 2012;3:287.
22. Rietschel ET, Westphal O. Endotoxin: Historical perspectives. In: Brade H, Opal SM, Vogel SN, et al, eds. *Endotoxin in Health and Disease*. New York, NY: Marcel Dekker, 1999:1–30.
23. Vaara M. Lipopolysaccharide and the permeability of the bacterial outer membrane. In: Brade H, Opal SM, Vogel SN, et al, eds. *Endotoxin in Health and Disease*. New York, NY: Marcel Dekker, 1999:31–8.
24. Erridge C. Endogenous ligands of TLR2 and TLR4: Agonists or assistants? *J Leukocyte Biol* 2010;87:989–99.
25. Shi Y, Evans JE, Rock KL. Molecular identification of a danger signal that alerts the immune system to dying cells. *Nature* 2003;425:516–21.
26. Shi Y. Caught red-handed: Uric acid is an agent of inflammation. *J Clin Invest* 2010;120:1809–11.
27. Noble PW, McKee CM, Cowman M, et al. Hyaluronan fragments activate an NF-kappa B/I-kappa B alpha autoregulatory loop in murine macrophages. *J Exp Med* 1996;183:2373–8.
28. Termeer CC, Hennies J, Voith U, et al. Oligosaccharides of hyaluronan are potent activators of dendritic cells. *J Immunol* 2000;165:1863–70.
29. Jiang D, Liang J, Noble PW. Hyaluronan as an immune regulator in human diseases. *Physiol Rev* 2011;91:221–64.
30. Lotze MT, Tracey KJ. High-mobility group box 1 protein (HMGB1): Nuclear weapon in the immune arsenal. *Nat Rev Immunol* 2005;5:331–42.
31. Klune JR, Dhupar R, Cardinal J, et al. HMGB1: Endogenous danger signaling. *Mol Med* 2008;14:476–84.
32. Davis BK, Wen H, Ting JP. The inflammasome NLRs in immunity, inflammation, and associated diseases. *Annu Rev Immunol* 2011;29:707–35.
33. Akira S, Uematsu S, Takeuchi O. Pathogen recognition and innate immunity. *Cell* 2006;124:783–801.

34. Kawai T, Akira S. Toll-like receptors and their crosstalk with other innate receptors in infection and immunity. *Immunity* 2011;34:637–50.

35. Elinav E, Strowig T, Henao-Mejia J, et al. Regulation of the anti-microbial response by NLR proteins. *Immunity* 2011;34:665–79.

36. Loo YM, Gale M Jr. Immune signaling by RIG-I-like receptors. *Immunity* 2011;34:680–92.

37. Greer SN, Metcalf JL, Wang Y, et al. The updated biology of hypoxia-inducible factor. *EMBO J* 2012;31:2448–60.

38. Aoshi T, Koyama S, Kobiyama K, et al. Innate and adaptive immune responses to viral infection and vaccination. *Curr Opin Virol* 2011;1:226–32.

39. O'Neill LA, Golenbock D, Bowie AG. The history of Toll-like receptors—Redefining innate immunity. *Nat Rev Immunol* 2013;13:453–60.

40. Rock FL, Hardiman G, Timans JC, et al. A family of human receptors structurally related to Drosophila Toll. *Proc Natl Acad Sci U S A* 1998;95:588–93.

41. Akira S, Takeda K. Toll-like receptor signalling. *Nat Rev Immunol* 2004;4:499–511.

42. Oda K, Kitano K. A comprehensive map of the toll-like receptor signaling network. *Mol Syst Biol* 2006;2:E1–20.

43. Hoffmann A, Baltimore D. Circuitry of nuclear factor kappaB signaling. *Immunol Rev* 2006;210:171–86.

44. Hayden MS, Ghosh S. NF-kappaB, the first quarter-century: Remarkable progress and outstanding questions. *Genes Dev* 2012;26:203–34.

45. Caput D, Beutler B, Hartog K, et al. Identification of a common nucleotide sequence in the 3'-untranslated region of mRNA molecules specifying inflammatory mediators. *Proc Natl Acad Sci U S A* 1986;83:1670–4.

46. Gueydan C, Droogmans L, Chalon P, et al. Identification of TIAR as a protein binding to the translational regulatory AU-rich element of tumor necrosis factor alpha mRNA. *J Biol Chem* 1999;274:2322–6.

47. Lewis T, Gueydan C, Huez G, et al. Mapping of a minimal AU-rich sequence required for lipopolysaccharide-induced binding of a 55-kDa protein on tumor necrosis factor-alpha mRNA. *J Biol Chem* 1998;273:13781–6.

48. Gueydan C, Houzet L, Marchant A, et al. Engagement of tumor necrosis factor mRNA by an endotoxin-inducible cytoplasmic protein. *Mol Med* 1996;2:479–88.

49. Lamkanfi M, Dixit VM. 2014. Mechanisms and functions of inflammasomes. *Cell* 157:1013–22.

50. Lin KM, Hu W, Troutman TD, et al. IRAK-1 bypasses priming and directly links TLRs to rapid NLRP3 inflammasome activation. *Proc Natl Acad Sci U S A* 2014;111:775–80.

51. Klein J, Václav H. *Immunology*. Malden, MA: Blackwell Science, 722.

52. Sedger LM, McDermott MF. TNF and TNF-receptors: From mediators of cell death and inflammation to therapeutic giants—Past, present and future. *Cytokine Growth Factor Rev* 2014;25(4):453–72.

53. Mantovani A. The chemokine system: Redundancy for robust outputs. *Immunol Today* 1999;20:254–7.

54. Bizzarri C, Beccari AR, Bertini R, et al. ELR(+) CXC chemokines and their receptors (CXC chemokine receptor 1 and CXC chemokine receptor 2) as new therapeutic targets. *Pharmacol Ther* 2006;112(1):139–49.

55. Bodkin JV, Fernandes ES. TRPV1 and SP: Key elements for sepsis outcome? *Br J Pharmacol* 2013;170:1279–92.

56. Willis TM, Hopp RJ, Romero JR, et al. The protective effect of brachial plexus palsy in purpura fulminans. *Pediatr Neurol* 2001;24:379–81.

57. Black PH. Stress and the inflammatory response: A review of neurogenic inflammation. *Brain Behav Immun* 2002;16:622–53.

58. Pick R, Brechtefeld D, Walzog B. Intraluminal crawling versus interstitial neutrophil migration during inflammation. *Mol Immunol* 2013;55:70–5.

59. Iwanaga S. The molecular basis of innate immunity in the horseshoe crab. *Curr Opin Immunol* 2002;14:87–95.

60. Esmon CT. Inflammation and the activated protein C anticoagulant pathway. *Semin Thromb Hemost* 2006;32(suppl 1):49–60.

61. Phillipson M, Kubes P. The neutrophil in vascular inflammation. *Nature Med* 2011;17:1381–90.

62. Jones SA. Directing transition from innate to acquired immunity: Defining a role for IL-6. *J Immunol* 2005;175:3463–8.

63. Vodovotz Y, An G. Systems biology and inflammation. *Methods Mol Biol* 2010;662:181–201.

CHAPTER 20 ■ CELLULAR ADAPTATIONS TO STRESS

DEREK S. WHEELER AND HECTOR R. WONG

KEY POINTS
---

1 The heat shock response and heat shock proteins provide protection against a broad variety of cellular stresses and injuries.

2 The heat shock response and heat shock proteins are potent modulators of inflammation-associated signal transduction.

3 Heme oxygenase plays a broad range of cytoprotective roles, and a large portion of this protective effect seems to be mediated by carbon monoxide, which is a primary end product of heme oxygenase–mediated degradation of heme.

4 Extracellular heat shock proteins have emerged as important signaling molecules in innate immunity and other cellular processes.

5 Ischemic preconditioning describes a specific form of cellular adaptation whereby brief periods of nonlethal ischemia confer cellular resistance to subsequent and otherwise lethal periods of ischemia.

6 Hypoxic preconditioning is a similar concept to that of ischemic preconditioning, but it is specific to hypoxic conditions, rather than ischemia.

7 Hypoxia inducible factor (HIF) is a key molecule in cellular adaptations to hypoxia.

8 Endotoxin tolerance describes an intriguing adaptation whereby cellular exposure to low levels of endotoxin reprograms the cellular response to subsequent exposure to higher levels of endotoxin.

9 The clinical significance of endotoxin tolerance to clinical medicine and innate immunity remains unclear at the present time.

10 Reactive oxygen species (ROS) are inevitably derived from the requisite use of oxygen by aerobic organisms, and excessive amounts of ROS can lead to oxidative cellular and tissue injury.

11 The major antioxidant mechanisms that serve to protect against these ROS include superoxide dismutase, catalase, glutathione peroxidase, thioredoxin, and thioredoxin reductase.

12 Epigenetics refers to heritable changes in gene expression patterns that are not related to direct changes to the DNA sequence of a given gene.

13 Epigenetic modifications are increasingly being described for immunity- and inflammation-related genes and may have important functional consequences for recovery from critical illness.

Biologic stress is a common phenomenon in virtually all forms of critical illness and stems either from the disease process itself or from therapies used in the ICU. Common examples of biologic stress in the ICU include hypoxia and ischemia associated with various disease processes, oxidant stress with therapeutic oxygen administration, and mechanical stress with positive pressure ventilation. While some therapeutic strategies in the ICU are directly targeted at these stressors, most therapeutic strategies are fundamentally supportive. As such, many forms of therapy in the ICU provide time and a platform to allow for endogenous cellular stress adaptations to take place. Success or failure of these cellular responses is critical to the eventual development of organ failure, and consequently to patient outcome.

All cells respond to stress through the activation of primitive, evolutionarily conserved genetic programs that maintain homeostasis and assure cell survival (**Fig. 20.1**). *Stress adaptation*, which is known in the literature by a myriad of terms (tolerance, desensitization, conditioning, and reprogramming), is a common paradigm found throughout nature. In stress adaptation, a primary exposure of a cell or organism to a stressful stimulus (e.g., heat, ischemia, hypoxia, endotoxin) results in an adaptive response that allows the cell or organism to better withstand a second exposure to the same stressor. *Cross-tolerance* is a related adaptive response, in which primary exposure to a stressful stimulus leads to an adaptive response whereby the cell or organism is resistant to a subsequent stress that is different from the initial stress (i.e., exposure to heat stress leading to resistance to hypoxia). Several examples of stress adaptation are well described and are discussed in detail in this chapter, including the heat shock response, ischemic preconditioning (IP), and endotoxin tolerance.

It is imperative that physicians caring for critically ill and injured children possess an understanding of these concepts, as an understanding of stress adaptation is necessary to recognize the current limits of supportive care and to make progress in research endeavors and novel therapeutic strategies. The goal of this chapter is to introduce some fundamental concepts of how cells adapt (or maladapt) to stress. Generalized adaptive responses to various cell stressors will be reviewed, followed by a brief discussion of the more commonly implicated mediators of these responses.

THE HEAT SHOCK RESPONSE

The heat shock response was first described over four decades ago in common fruit flies exposed to increased environmental temperature. What was once an obscure observation of questionable biologic relevance has now evolved into a fundamental tenet of how cells adapt, in response to, and survive a broad **1** variety of biologic stresses (1–3). The heat shock response is

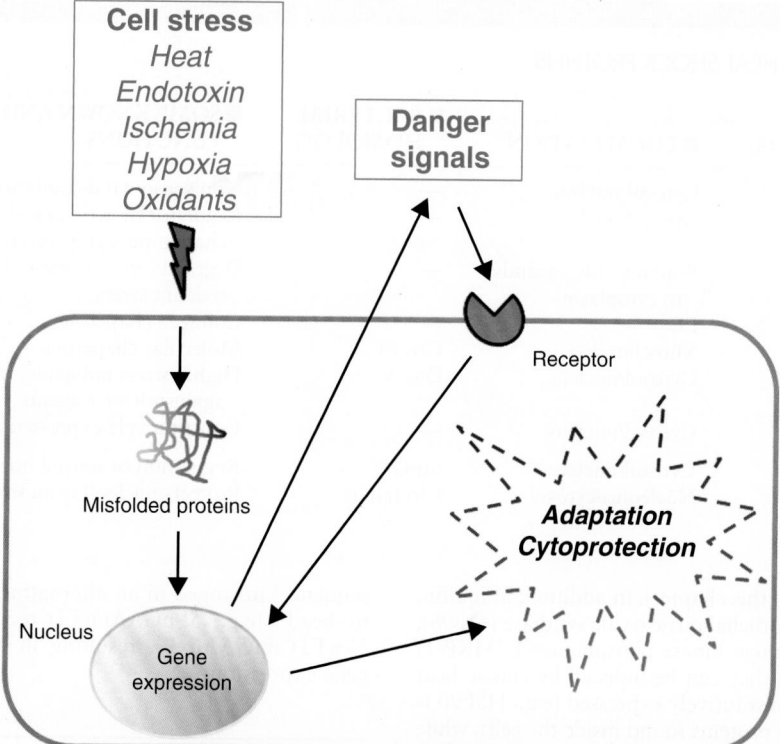

FIGURE 20.1. Simplified representation of the basic mechanisms of cellular adaptation. Exposure to stress (e.g., heat, endotoxin, ischemia, hypoxia, oxygen radicals, etc.) results in perturbations of the intracellular milieu (e.g., stress-induced misfolding of intracellular proteins) that trigger new gene expression and/or the release of danger signals that activate stress responses via receptor-mediated signal transduction. In either case, the reprograming of gene expression allows for cellular adaptations to stress and cytoprotection.

characterized by the rapid expression of a unique group of proteins known collectively as *heat shock proteins* (HSPs), when a cell or organism is exposed to environmental stress. The structure, mode of regulation, and function of HSPs are highly conserved among different species, and HSPs have been identified in virtually all eukaryotic and prokaryotic species examined. While classically described as a response to heat stress (hence the term *heat shock response*), HSPs can be induced by a wide variety of nonthermal stressors and pharmacologic agents (**Table 20.1**). For this reason, the terms "stress response" and "stress proteins" may be descriptors that are more appropriate. Many of these stimuli are relevant to the critically ill patient, and it is now well established that critically ill patients readily express HSPs (i.e., mounting a heat shock response) (4–7). Moreover, and, particularly germane to pediatric critical care medicine, the experimental literature suggests that younger animals have a greater capacity to express HSPs than older animals (8). Indeed, the loss of the ability to generate a stress response may contribute to the aging process (9,10).

HSPs comprise a large family of proteins that are found in virtually every cellular compartment, including the nucleus, cytoplasm, and mitochondria (**Table 20.2**). HSPs also exist in the extracellular compartment, and these extracellular HSPs are highly active biologically (see in what follows). By convention, HSPs are classified according to their molecular mass (e.g., HSP25 represents the 25 kDa family of HSPs) and range in molecular mass from 7 to 110 kDa (e.g., HSP25, HSP32, HSP47, HSP60, HSP70, HSP90, and HSP110). Some HSPs have additional functions that are not related to heat shock, though they are still classified as HSPs. For example, the enzyme heme oxygenase (HO) is also known as HSP32

TABLE 20.1

INDUCERS OF THE STRESS RESPONSE

■ TYPE OF STRESS	■ AGENT
Environmental	Temperature
	Heavy metals
	Ethanol
	Oxygen radicals
Metabolic	Hyperosmolality
	Glucose starvation
	Tunicamycin
	Calcium ionophores
	Amino acid analogs
Clinical	Ischemia/reperfusion
	Shock
	Anoxia
	Endotoxin
Pharmacologic	Sodium arsenite
	Herbimycin A
	Geldanamycin
	Prostaglandin A1
	Dexamethasone
	Aspirin
	Nonsteroidal anti-inflammatory drugs
	Pyrrolidine dithiocarbamate
	Diethyldithiocarbamate
	Bimoclomol
	Serine protease inhibitors
	Curcumin
	Geranylgeranylacetone

TABLE 20.2

THE MAJOR FAMILIES OF HEAT SHOCK PROTEINS

■ NAME	■ SIZE (KDA)	■ LOCALIZATION	■ BACTERIAL HOMOLOG	■ SOME KNOWN AND POSSIBLE FUNCTIONS
Ubiquitin	8	Cytosol/nucleus	—	Nonlysosomal degradation pathways
HSP 27	27	Cytosol/nucleus	—	Regulator of actin cytoskeleton; molecular chaperone; cytoprotection
HO	32	Bound to ER, extends to cytoplasm	—	Degradation of heme to bilirubin; resistance to oxidant stress
HSP 47	47	ER	—	Collagen chaperone
HSP 60	60	Mitochondria	Gro EL	Molecular chaperone
HSP 70	72	Cytosol/nucleus	Dna K	Highly stress inducible; involved in cytoprotection against diverse agents
	73	Cytosol/nucleus	—	Constitutively expressed chaperone
HSP 90	90	Cytosol/nucleus	htpG	Regulation of steroid hormone activity
HSP 110	110	Nucleolus/cytosol	Clp family	Protects nucleoli from stress

(discussed in detail later in this chapter). In addition, ubiquitin, inhibitor of κB (IκB), endothelial nitric oxide synthase (eNOS), and mitogen-activated protein kinase phosphatase-1 (MKP-1) are listed as HSPs in that they can be induced by classic heat shock. Many HSPs are constitutively expressed (e.g., HSP90 is one of the most abundant proteins found inside the cell), while others are rapidly and highly expressed in response to cellular stress. Among the latter, HSP72 is one of the more well-studied inducible HSPs in the context of cellular adaptations to stress and consequent protection against cellular injury (see in what follows).

Regulation of the Heat Shock Response

Cells respond to stressful stimuli (e.g., heat shock) by increasing HSP gene expression in proportion to the severity of the stress—a temperature threshold of 4°C–8°C above the normal growing temperature is required for induction of HSP expression (3). The cellular "sensor" for heat stress appears to be alterations of protein structure; heat stress leads to protein unfolding, and it is the intracellular accumulation of unfolded proteins, rather than temperature per se, that directly activates the heat shock response. Accordingly, the same response can be activated by any stimulus that generates intracellular accumulation of unfolded proteins (e.g., oxidant stress, ischemia, and heavy metals). Experimental support for this mechanism is shown by the fact that microinjection of denatured proteins into cells results in the upregulation of HSP expression.

A family of transcription factors, known as *heat shock factors* (HSFs), regulates HSP gene expression (3). Three HSFs are present in humans (HSF1, -2, and -4), of which HSF1 appears to be the most important stress-inducible HSF. The HSFs are characterized by a highly conserved amino-terminal, helix-turn-helix DNA binding domain, and a carboxy-terminal transactivation domain. HSF1 is present as a constitutively phosphorylated monomer during the resting, unstressed state. HSP70, a product of HSF1 activation, associates with HSF1 via protein–protein interaction and retains HSF1 in the cytoplasm, in an inactive, monomeric form. In response to heat shock, HSP70 disassociates from HSF1 and allows HSF1 trimerization, and these HSF1 trimers rapidly translocate into the nucleus. While trimerization is sufficient for DNA binding, transactivation requires inducible serine phosphorylation. HSF1 binds to *heat shock elements* (HSEs) within the promoter regions of HSP genes, defined by a tandem repeat of the pentamer nGAAn ("n" denoting a less conserved

sequence) arranged in an alternating orientation either "head to head" (e.g., 5'-nGAAnnTTCn-3') or "tail to tail" (e.g., 5'-nTTCnnGAAn-3'), resulting in the upregulation of HSP gene expression.

Heat Shock Proteins, HSP72, and Cytoprotection

The most well-known biologic function of HSPs is their ability to serve as molecular chaperones (1,2). In this role, HSPs serve to fold, transport, and stabilize intracellular proteins. Since many forms of cellular injury lead to misfolding of intracellular proteins and to defects of intracellular protein processing and trafficking, the molecular chaperone properties of HSPs are thought to play a major role in the mechanisms by which the heat shock response confers protection in such diverse forms of cellular injury. Experimentally, the heat shock response can be induced either by thermal stress or through pharmacologic induction. In either case, it is well established that induction of the heat shock response confers protection in various animal models of critical illness, including septic shock, acute lung injury, oxidant stress, and ischemia–reperfusion injury (11,12). That HSP72 plays a major role in cytoprotection is evident by studies in which HSP72 is overexpressed genetically, and the experimental animals are afforded similar protection to that seen by induction of HSP72 through thermal stress or pharmacologic induction. For example, adenovirus-mediated transfer of the HSP72 gene to the lung epithelium confers protection in an animal model of acute lung injury (13).

The Heat Shock Response and Inflammation

Another mechanism by which the heat shock response confers cytoprotection is through its ability to modulate cellular proinflammatory responses. Numerous studies have demonstrated that induction of the heat shock response inhibits subsequent production of cytokines, chemokines, and nitric oxide (NO) when cells are exposed to proinflammatory stimuli. This has been demonstrated in both in vitro and *in vivo* experimental models. One major mechanism by which the heat shock response inhibits cellular proinflammatory responses is through inhibition of the nuclear factor-κB (NF-κB) signal transduction pathway (14). NF-κB is a transcription factor that regulates the expression of many genes involved in inflammation (see Chapter 19). Heat shock–mediated inhibition of the NF-κB pathway involves inhibition of IκB kinase and increased de novo expression of the endogenous NF-κB inhibitory protein, IκBα. These inhibitory effects of heat shock on cellular proinflammatory responses and the NF-κB pathway appear to be relatively specific, rather than a global downregulation of cellular function and gene expression. Furthermore, genome-level studies indicate that the mononuclear cell response to heat stress is highly divergent compared with the mononuclear cell response to endotoxin (15).

Heme Oxygenase

The visible transformation of a common bruise is an ancient colorimetric reaction that is dependent upon the enzyme HO. HO is the first and rate-limiting step in the degradation of heme (purple hue) to biliverdin (green hue), and finally to bilirubin (yellow hue) (**Fig. 20.2**). Three known isoforms of HO exist: HO-1, -2, and -3. In the context of cellular adaptation to stress, HO-1 appears to be the most relevant isoform. HO-1 is identical to HSP32 and is highly inducible by a variety of cellular stressors and stimuli, including heme, NO, cytokines, heavy metals, hyperoxia, hypoxia, endotoxin, heavy metals, and heat shock (16).

HO-1 activity is present in virtually all organs. The importance of HO-1 in human health and disease was recently demonstrated by the description of a 6-year-old boy with complete HO-1 deficiency (17). This patient's clinical condition was characterized by severe growth retardation, hemolytic anemia, tissue iron deposits, widespread evidence of endothelial cell damage, and increased susceptibility to oxidant injury. These findings are remarkably similar to the phenotype commonly observed in HO-1 null mice.

In vitro studies involving gene transfection or gene transfer approaches have provided clear evidence that HO-1 confers cytoprotection (16,18). For example, overexpression of HO-1 conferred protection against oxygen toxicity, hemoglobin toxicity, tumor necrosis factor (TNF)-α–mediated apoptosis, and *Pseudomonas*-mediated cellular injury and apoptosis. Experiments in animal models, involving either pharmacologic induction of HO-1 or genetic overexpression of HO-1, confirm that HO-1 confers cytoprotection in vivo. Induction of HO-1, by intravenous hemoglobin administration, protected rats against the lethal effects of endotoxemia. Lung epithelial overexpression of HO-1, via an adenovirus vector, conferred protection in rats exposed to hyperoxia; cardiac-specific overexpression conferred protection in a murine model of ischemia. There is also interest in HO-1–mediated cytoprotection in the field of transplant biology. In a cardiac xenograft transplantation model, increased expression of HO-1 improved graft survival.

The by-products of HO enzymatic activity include carbon monoxide (CO), bilirubin, and ferritin (**Fig. 20.2**), and each of these by-products has been postulated to play a role in cytoprotection. Ferritin is known to protect against oxidant stress, and bilirubin can function as a potent antioxidant. The most recent work in the field implicates CO-related cell signaling as the key component of HO-1–mediated cytoprotection (19–21). For example, HO-1–derived CO appears to play an important role in the host defense to severe infection in a murine model of polymicrobial sepsis (22). CO shares a variety of properties with NO, including neurotransmission, regulation of vascular tone, and activation of soluble guanylate cyclase. The reported biologic effects of CO include potent anti-inflammatory effects (via the mitogen-activated protein kinase [MAPK] pathway), anti-apoptotic effects, and antioxidant effects. In vivo administration of low concentrations of inhaled CO protected rats against hyperoxia-mediated acute lung injury, and administration of exogenous CO to cardiac tissue protected the tissue against ischemia–reperfusion injury following transplantation. Several experimental studies have confirmed these initial results, demonstrating that CO inhalation or pharmacologic administration of CO-releasing drugs is cytoprotective in several different animal models of sepsis and acute lung injury (23,24). These studies are particularly intriguing because the amount of CO administered in these experiments is within the range administered to patients undergoing lung diffusion scans. Unfortunately, a recent study in nonhuman primates showed that the doses of inhalational CO that produced anti-inflammatory effects also resulted in relatively high and potentially toxic levels of carboxyhemoglobin (CO-Hb) levels (>30%) (25). However, the anti-inflammatory effects of CO were recently examined in a randomized, double-blind, placebo-controlled, two-way crossover trial in which healthy volunteers were injected with a 2 ng/kg dose of lipopolysaccharide (LPS). Inhalation of 500 ppm CO versus air had no effect on the inflammatory cytokine production, though no adverse side effects were observed (CO-Hb levels increased to as high as 7%) (26). Conversely, inhalation of CO by patients with stable Chronic Obstructive Pulmonary Disease (COPD) at doses of 100–125 ppm for 2 hours/day for 4 days was effective in improving lung inflammation and function (27). Clearly, further studies are required. In addition, as yet there have been no clinical trials of CO-releasing agents in humans.

Extracellular Heat Shock Proteins

HSPs have been classically regarded as exclusively *intracellular* proteins. Studies over the last decade, however, clearly illustrate that HSPs can also exist in the *extracellular* compartment.

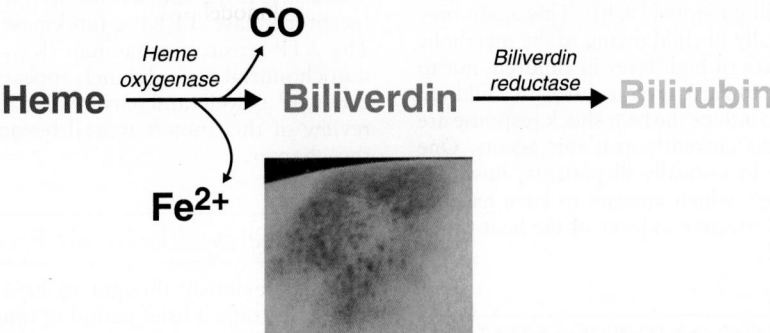

FIGURE 20.2. HO-mediated degradation of heme. HO degrades heme to biliverdin and concomitantly generates CO and iron (Fe). Biliverdin is subsequently converted to bilirubin via biliverdin reductase. The respective colorimetric reactions that coincide with the generation of these heme degradation products are readily evident in the various hues of a common bruise.

For example, adult patients suffering from major trauma have increased serum levels of HSP72 (4). Critically ill children with septic shock also have increased serum levels of HSP72, and the absolute levels are much higher than that reported for critically ill adult patients following multisystem trauma (5). The latter may be reflective of an increased capacity of children to express HSPs compared with adults, consistent with the experimental literature previously mentioned.

Whether increased levels of extracellular HSPs represent active release/secretion of HSPs or a nonspecific release of HSPs from dying cells remains to be determined. Current evidence indicates that both processes are operative (28). Regardless of how HSPs enter the extracellular compartment, emerging evidence indicates that extracellular HSPs are biologically active. For example, HSP72 has been demonstrated to activate proinflammatory and antibacterial responses in macrophages (28–32). In this context, extracellular HSPs are said to serve as "danger signals" for the innate immune system.

The biologic role, if any, of extracellular HSPs in critical illness remains to be defined and is currently an active area of investigation. It is possible that extracellular HSPs are simply an epiphenomenon of illness severity reflecting induction of the heat shock response in critically ill patients. The experimental data mentioned earlier, however, indicate that extracellular HSPs are capable of modulating the innate immune system, and this biologic effect is of obvious potential significance to the critically ill patient. The difficulty of elucidating this significance is highlighted by the observations that increased extracellular HSPs correlate with improved survival in adult patients with trauma (4), but correlate with illness severity and mortality in children with septic shock (5). In addition, a recently developed multi–biomarker-based risk model to predict outcome in children with septic shock includes HSP72 as one of the major decision rules, with increased HSP72 serum concentrations being an indicator of increased mortality risk (33). Finally, there are now multiple studies in critically ill patients with diverse conditions that have shown a significant correlation between extracellular HSP72 levels and increased morbidity and mortality (34–38).

The Heat Shock Response as a Therapeutic Strategy

Recognizing that induction of the heat shock response confers broad cytoprotection against diverse forms of cellular injury has generated interest in developing clinically feasible strategies to safely induce the heat shock response (1). Deliberate induction of hyperthermia is not likely to be feasible given the metabolic consequences of severe hyperthermia in critically ill patients. A related concept is the controversial topic of not treating fever in critically ill patients (39,40). This again may not be feasible in the critically ill child owing to the metabolic and neurologic consequences of high fever in children, not to mention societal attitudes toward fever control in children. Pharmacologic strategies to induce the heat shock response are hampered by toxicity of the currently available agents. One agent that shows promise in critically ill patients, however, is the amino acid glutamine, which appears to have feasibility as a relatively safe and effective inducer of the heat shock response in humans (41,42).

ISCHEMIC PRECONDITIONING

The phenomenon of IP, in which multiple, brief ischemic episodes (i.e., preconditioning) protect the heart from a subsequent sustained ischemic insult, was first described in a canine model of myocardial ischemia produced by coronary occlusion in 1986 (43). Four cycles of brief (5 minutes) ischemia prior to a more prolonged period of ischemia (40 minutes) reduced infarct size by nearly 75% (**Fig. 20.3**A and B). Since that time, IP has been shown to reduce the infarct size in every species tested, and both in vitro data involving cardiomyocytes and clinical data from small case series suggest that IP is cytoprotective in humans as well (44,45). IP is more readily recognized in the clinical setting in the context of the acute coronary syndrome, in which patients who have at least one episode of prodromal angina are somewhat protected from a subsequent, more severe episode of myocardial ischemia (i.e., "the cardiac warm-up phenomenon").

While the mechanism(s) underlying IP have not been fully elucidated, there appears to be both an early ("classical" IP) and a late ("delayed" IP) phase to the cytoprotective response (44,45). For example, cytoprotection appears within minutes of the preconditioning stimulus and lasts only 2–3 hours (early phase or first window of protection), though tissue protection later reappears 24 hours after the preconditioning stimulus (late phase or second window of protection). Classic IP depends mainly upon activation of ion channels and/or post-translational modification of preexisting cellular proteins, which makes intuitive sense given the rapidity with which this response occurs. On the other hand, delayed preconditioning involves the simultaneous activation of multiple stress-responsive genes and de novo synthesis of several proteins (including ion channel proteins, receptor proteins, enzymes, and molecular chaperones such as the HSPs discussed earlier), which ultimately results in the development of a cytoprotective phenotype. While IP was first described in the heart, preconditioning has also been described in the liver, kidney, lung, intestine, and brain (46–48). Finally, preconditioning is not confined to one organ, but can also limit infarct size in remote, non-preconditioned organs (so-called *remote ischemic preconditioning [RIPC]*).

Classical Ischemic Preconditioning

Adenosine appears to play a major role as both a trigger and an effector of classic IP. As discussed in Chapter 21, ischemia leads to the rapid degradation of ATP to adenosine, which then accumulates in the ischemic tissue. In addition to adenosine, several other potential mediators of classic IP are released by the ischemic myocardium, including bradykinin, norepinephrine, opioids, and reactive oxygen species (ROS). Adenosine appears to mediate classic IP via stimulation of adenosine receptor subtypes A_1 and A_3, thereby activating cytoprotective pathways involving protein kinase C (PKC) (especially the isoform PKC-ε), phosphatidylinositol-3-kinase (PI3K), and several MAPKs, including extracellular receptor kinase (ERK), c-Jun kinase (JNK), and p38 MAPK. The ATP-sensitive potassium (K_{ATP}) channel, especially the mitochondrial K_{ATP} channel, appears to play a crucial role in classic IP as well (and may involve HSP27), though a detailed review of this subject is well beyond the intended scope of this chapter.

Delayed Ischemic Preconditioning

IP was previously thought to be a transient phenomenon, lasting for only a brief period of time after the initial preconditioning stress. Subsequent studies have now shown, however, that the cytoprotective response reappears 24 hours later (44). While not as robust as the earlier phase of cytoprotection, this second window of protection lasts up to 72 hours. This distinctive time-course strongly suggests that

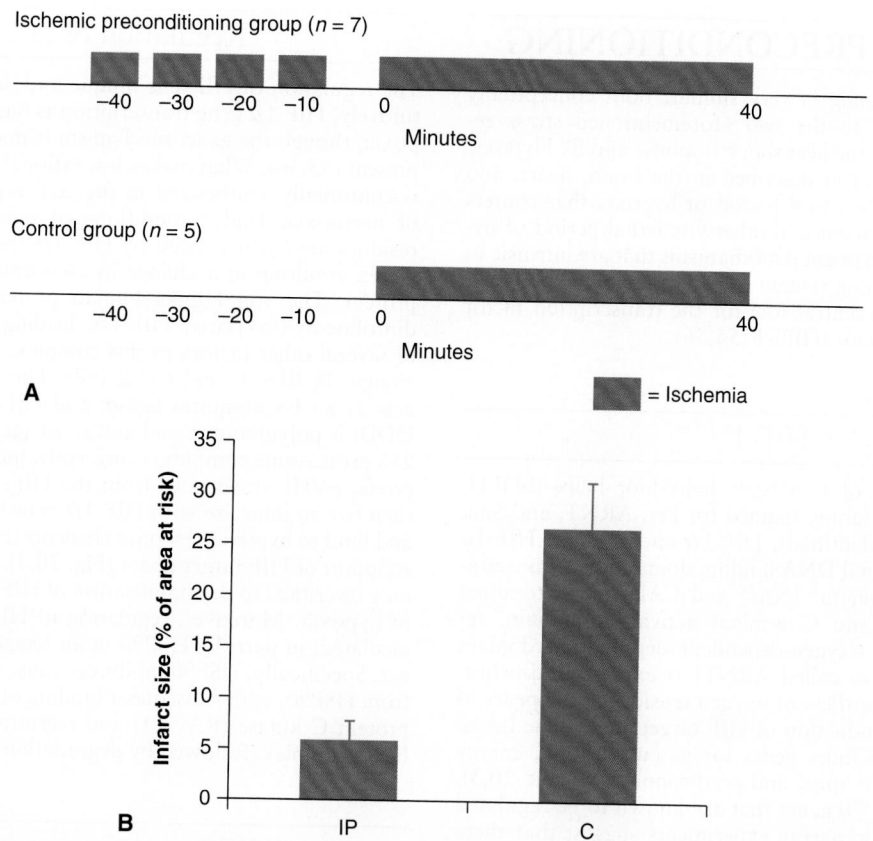

FIGURE 20.3. Experimental protocol used in the landmark study by Murry et al. (43). **A:** In the IP group, dogs ($n = 7$) were exposed to four 5-minute cycles of myocardial ischemia (produced by temporary coronary occlusion) followed by 5 minutes of reperfusion prior to a sustained 40-minute period of myocardial ischemia. Longer episodes of IP (i.e., 10-minute cycles) were associated with excessive mortality. Animals in the control (C) group ($n = 5$) were exposed to the sustained 40-minute period of myocardial ischemia alone. The animals were sacrificed at 4 days, and infarct size was measured. **B:** Infarct size (expressed as the percentage of the area at risk) was reduced by approximately 75% in the IP group compared with the C group ($p < 0.05$).

delayed IP is mediated, at least in part, by upregulation of gene expression and the subsequent synthesis of new proteins. While classic IP and delayed IP share several key features (especially the agents that trigger the cytoprotective response, e.g., adenosine, bradykinin, opioids, and norepinephrine), endogenous protection via NO appears to play an important role as a trigger of delayed IP. Activation of several stress-responsive signal transduction pathways converges upon the transcription factor, NF-κB, resulting in upregulation of gene expression of various stress-responsive, cytoprotective proteins, including superoxide dismutase (SOD), inducible nitric oxide synthase (iNOS), cyclooxygenase-2 (COX-2), aldose reductase, and HSP. K_{ATP} channels are also potentially involved in delayed IP, though the mechanisms are not well understood.

Ischemic Preconditioning as a Therapeutic Strategy

The clinical correlate of IP, the so-called "cardiac work-up phenomenon," has been shown to have a protective effect in patients who progress to acute coronary syndrome (49). The cytoprotective effect appears to diminish significantly if more than 24 hours lapses between prodromal angina and myocardial infarction. Similarly, patients who experience a

transient ischemic attack (TIA) during the week prior to a stroke have a more favorable recovery. These epidemiologic studies, with the wealth of experimental and animal data, clearly support the application of the general concept of IP in the clinical setting. However, making the transition from the bench to the bedside has been slow and difficult. Pharmacologic preconditioning (e.g., targeting the adenosine receptor or K_{ATP} channel) in patients undergoing coronary angioplasty has produced encouraging results. Classic or pharmacologic preconditioning has been used in several small clinical trials in patients undergoing cardiothoracic surgery (e.g., coronary artery bypass grafting, cardiopulmonary bypass, lung resection surgery), hepatic surgery (especially liver resection and liver transplantation), and vascular surgery. There have now been several clinical studies using a technique called RIPC, in which several brief periods of limb ischemia (induced by inflating a blood pressure cuff) are performed prior to a planned procedure (e.g., cardiac surgery, angioplasty, vascular surgery, etc.). A meta-analysis of 17 clinical trials suggested that RIPC is associated with improved serologic markers of ischemia–reperfusion injury, though larger clinical studies need to be performed (50). More germane to the present discussion, there have been several small studies testing the effects of RIPC in children undergoing cardiac surgery (51–54). Importantly, these trials are limited by patient heterogeneity (53) and by differences in timing of the RIPC (54), making comparison difficult.

HYPOXIC PRECONDITIONING

Hypoxic preconditioning is very similar, both conceptually and mechanistically, to the two aforementioned stress responses, for example, the heat shock response and IP. Hypoxic preconditioning has been described in the brain, heart, and other tissues, and refers to a period of hypoxia that confers tolerance on a subsequent and otherwise lethal period of hypoxia. While the fundamental mechanisms that are intrinsic to hypoxic preconditioning remain to be elucidated, experimental studies suggest a central role for the transcription factor *hypoxia inducible factor* (HIF)-1 (55,56).

HIF-1

HIF-1 is composed of two basic helix-loop-helix (bHLH) proteins of the PAS family (named for Per, ARNT, and Sim, the first members identified), HIF-1α and HIF-1β. HIF-1α contains an N-terminal DNA binding domain, two transcriptional activating domains (NAD and CAD, for N-terminal activation domain and C-terminal activation domain, respectively), and an oxygen-dependent degradation domain (ODD). HIF-1β (also called ARNT) is expressed constitutively in all cells regardless of oxygen tension, but appears to be essential to the induction of HIF target genes. The list of HIF target genes includes genes for vascularization, energy metabolism, vascular tone, and erythropoiesis (**Table 20.3**). There are now over 70 genes that are known to be regulated by HIF-1α (57). Microarray experiments suggest that there are many, many more genes that are likely to be regulated by hypoxia.

TABLE 20.3

HIF TARGET GENES

Genes Involved in Vascularization
VEGF
VEGF receptor FLT-1

Genes Involved in Energy Metabolism
Aldolase
Enolase I
Glucose transporter 1
Glucose transporter 3
Glyceraldehyde phosphate dehydrogenase
Hexokinase
Insulin-like growth factor
Lactate dehydrogenase
Phosphofructokinase
Phosphoglycerate kinase
Pyruvate kinase

Genes Involved in Regulation of Vascular Tone
α_{1B}-adrenergic receptor
Endothelin-1
Nitric oxide synthase (NOS-2; inducible isoform of NOS)

Genes Involved in Regulation of Iron Metabolism and Erythropoiesis
Erythropoeitin
HO-1
Transferrin
Transferrin receptor

Regulation of HIF-1

The regulation of HIF-1 is unique and deserves mention. Intuitively, HIF-1α gene transcription is highly inducible by hypoxia, though the exact mechanism is not well understood at present (55,56). What makes less rational sense is that HIF-1α is continually synthesized in the cell, even under conditions of normoxia. Under conditions of normoxia, two proline residues are hydroxylated by HIF-1α–specific prolyl hydroxylases, resulting in a change in conformation of the HIF-1α protein. The von Hippel–Lindau protein (pVHL) binds to diproline-hydroxylated HIF-1α, leading to the recruitment of several other factors to this complex, including elongin C, elongin B, Rbx 1, and Cul-2 (58). This multimeric complex acts as an E3 ubiquitin ligase, and HIF-1α (specifically, the ODD) is polyubiquitinated and subsequently degraded by the 26S proteasome complex. Conversely, under conditions of hypoxia, pVHL dissociates from the HIF-1α protein, which is then free to dimerize with HIF-1β, translocate to the nucleus, and bind to hypoxia response elements (HREs) to induce transcription of HIF target genes (**Fig. 20.4**). Importantly, HSP90 may be critical to the stabilization of HIF-1α under conditions of hypoxia. Moreover, regulation of HIF-1α stability is also mediated, in part, by HSP90 in an oxygen-independent manner. Specifically, HSP90 inhibitors cause the release of HIF-1α from HSP90, with subsequent binding of receptor of activated protein C kinase (RACK1) and recruitment of the ubiquitin ligase complex, followed by degradation of HIF-1α (57).

HIF-1 and Cytoprotection

The biologic importance of HIF-1 has been established in transgenic mice with targeted deletions of either HIF-1α or HIF-1β (55,56). For example, mice homozygous for deletions of either subunit (HIF-1α −/− or HIF-1β −/−) die during embryogenesis secondary to insufficient vascular development. In contrast, heterozygote mice (HIF-1α +/−) appear to develop normally. When exposed to hypoxia, however, these animals have impairment of the classical responses and adaptations to hypoxia.

The cytoprotective properties of HIF-1 relate primarily to the HIF-1–dependent target genes that allow for adaptation to hypoxia. For example, induction of the HIF-1–dependent erythropoietin gene expression leads to increased production of red blood cells, thereby increasing the oxygen carrying capacity of blood to compensate for hypoxia. This type of cytoprotective response is particularly important, for example, in children with cyanotic heart disease. Another example involves the HIF-1–dependent vascular endothelial growth factor (VEGF) gene expression, which is a critical growth factor for the development of blood vessels. In tissues subjected to ischemia, such as the myocardium, expression of VEGF promotes the development of neovascularization as a potential means of increasing blood flow to the ischemic tissue. Yet another role for HIF-1 involves HIF-1–dependent expression of iNOS (discussed in what follows) and IP of the myocardium.

While the heat shock response and classic IP allow for more immediate forms of cytoprotection, the cytoprotective responses and adaptations associated with hypoxic preconditioning and HIF-1 activation are comparatively slower to develop and allow for longer term adaptation. In addition, some of the responses induced by HIF-1 activation can be maladaptive/pathologic depending on the duration of activation (59,60). For example, HIF-1 activation is thought to play a role in the development of pulmonary hypertension in the setting of chronic hypoxia. Thus, a greater understanding of HIF-1 regulation and activity will be necessary in order to manipulate HIF-1 activity as a therapeutic option.

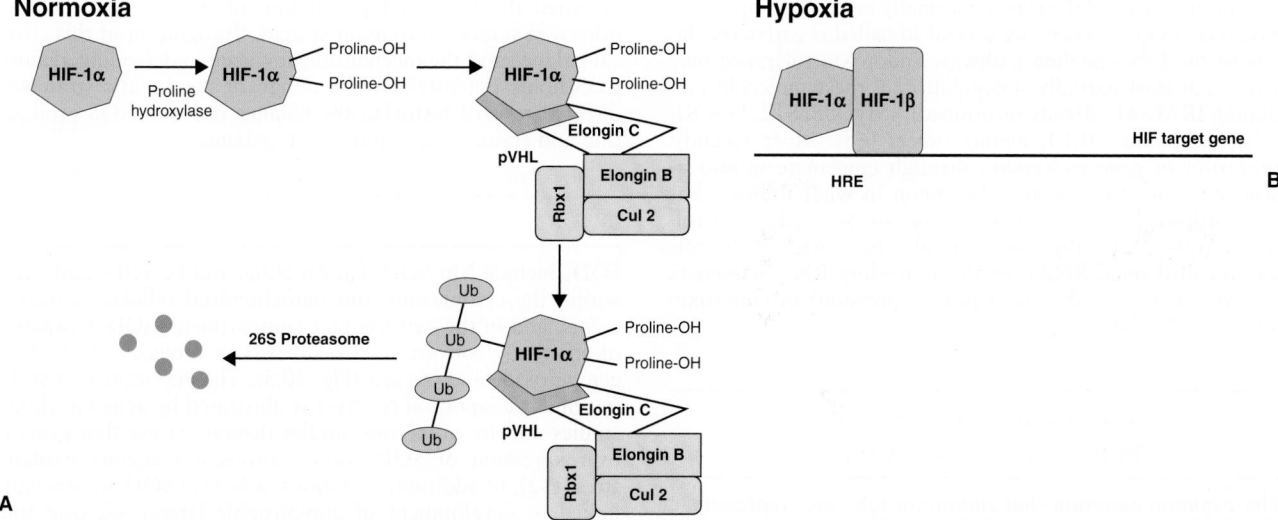

FIGURE 20.4. Regulation of HIF-1. **A:** Under conditions of normoxia, HIF-1α associates with the pVHL and forms a complex resulting in its polyubiquitination and degradation by the 26S proteasome. **B:** Under conditions of hypoxia, HIF-1α dissociates from pVHL and combines with HIF-1β to translocate to the nucleus, where it upregulates HIF target genes.

HIF-2

HIF-2 is another member of the HIF family of transcription factors that consists of a heterodimer with an oxygen labile subunit (HIF-2α) and the constitutive HIF-1β subunit. HIF-2α shares about 48% of the amino acid sequence and protein structure with HIF-1α, though the two transcription factors have distinct target genes and mechanisms of regulation. For example, HSP70 is involved in HIF-1α, but not HIF-2α regulation (61). Importantly, HIF-1α may be more important during short periods (2–24 hours) of severe hypoxia or anoxia (<0.1% O_2), while HIF-2α is more important during more prolonged periods (48–72 hours) of moderate hypoxia (<5% O_2) (62). In this sense, HIF-1α may "turn on" gene expression of hypoxia response genes during acute hypoxia, while HIF-2α may do the same in conditions of chronic hypoxia (63). This has been termed the "HIF switch" and remains to be further elucidated (64). The clinical significance of HIF-2 also requires further study.

ENDOTOXIN TOLERANCE

LPS, or endotoxin, a membrane glycolipid of gram-negative bacteria, is a potent inducer of proinflammatory gene expression. In keeping with the concept of stress adaptation and the tolerance paradigm, primary exposure of a cell or organism to LPS (preconditioning) produces a change in phenotype whereby a second exposure to LPS produces a minimal response. For example, LPS administration produces fever, tachycardia, tachypnea, and hemodynamic instability (i.e., the systemic inflammatory response syndrome [SIRS]) in laboratory animals, while a second dose of LPS produces minimal response. Similarly, LPS induces a dramatic increase in TNF-α gene expression in human peripheral blood monocytes (PBMC), though a second exposure produces a markedly attenuated response with decreased TNF-α gene expression.

Molecular Mechanisms of Endotoxin Tolerance

While the basic concept has been known for decades, the fundamental mechanisms occurring at the molecular level that

lead to endotoxin tolerance remain to be elucidated (65–68). Two distinct phases are historically described: *early* or *classic endotoxin tolerance* and *late endotoxin tolerance* (note the similarities to early or classic IP and delayed IP described earlier). Early or classic endotoxin tolerance is transient (generally lasting <72 hours following preconditioning) and is nonspecific, in that endotoxin derived from one bacterial species can induce tolerance to endotoxin derived from yet another bacterial species. Classic endotoxin tolerance occurs independently of antibody formation. Conversely, late tolerance (>72 hours following preconditioning) is type-specific (i.e., specific to endotoxin derived from a particular bacterial species) and antibody-dependent. The remainder of the present discussion will focus on classic endotoxin tolerance.

An in-depth, conceptual understanding of normal LPS signaling is essential before discussing the purported mechanistic basis of endotoxin tolerance. As discussed in Chapter 19, LPS binding to its receptor complex (TLR4/CD14/MD2) is facilitated by LPS-binding protein (LBP), triggering a cascade of events that culminates in the recruitment of the myeloid differentiation adapter protein (MyD8) and the IL-1 receptor–associated kinase (IRAK) to this complex. IRAK undergoes autophosphorylation and recruits the additional adapter protein, TNF receptor–associated factor (TRAF) 6, which then phosphorylates and activates an upstream, heterotrimeric member of the NF-κB pathway, the IκB protein kinase complex (IκK-α, -β, and -γ, which is also called NEMO), resulting in the phosphorylation of IκBα. Once phosphorylated, IκBα is targeted for poly-ubiquitination and degradation by the 26S proteasome. Degradation of IκBα unmasks the nuclear localization sequence of the p50 subunit, and nuclear translocation of NF-κB occurs. NF-κB then binds to the NF-κB consensus sequence to initiate transcription of a number of key proinflammatory-related genes.

One potentially attractive mechanism of endotoxin tolerance is downregulation of cell surface expression of individual components of the LPS receptor complex (e.g., TLR4, CD14, MB-2). Conflicting data from both in vitro and in vivo studies indicate that this mechanism is unlikely. Rather, alterations in the intracellular components of the LPS signal transduction appear more likely, including decreased expression of IRAK-1 (perhaps with the concomitant upregulation of its inhibitor, IRAK-M), increased expression of IκBα, or alteration of the normal components of NF-κB (i.e., shift from the p65/p50 heterodimer toward the transcriptionally inactive p50/p50 homodimer) (65,66). There are several so-called negative regulators of the LPS signaling pathway. Endotoxin tolerance may involve, at least partially, upregulation of these molecules, including IRAK-M (already mentioned), sMyD88, ST2, SOCS1, SHIP, A20, and MKP1, among others (68). More recently, alteration of gene expression through epigenetic modification of chromatin (see also discussion in what follows) has been proposed as a potential mechanism for endotoxin tolerance (69–72). Finally, there may also be a mechanistic role for so-called microRNAs (small, noncoding RNA sequences involved in the regulation of gene expression) in endotoxin tolerance (73,74).

Does Endotoxin Tolerance Have Clinical Relevance?

The common assertion that endotoxin tolerance represents a global downregulation of proinflammatory gene expression is perhaps incomplete and not entirely accurate. For example, while TNF-α production is significantly diminished in tolerant cells, as well as tolerant animals, production of other proinflammatory cytokines such as IL-1β and IL-6 may be increased, decreased, or unchanged. Several studies have noted that PBMC isolated from both children and adults with SIRS (secondary to surgery, trauma, cardiopulmonary bypass, cardiac arrest and resuscitation, etc.) and septic shock show strikingly similar alterations in intracellular signal transduction pathways that are consistent with the endotoxin tolerance phenotype (66). For example, impaired–LPS-stimulated ex vivo cytokine production has been demonstrated in leukocytes obtained from patients with sepsis and trauma, and low levels of LPS-stimulated ex vivo cytokine production from these patients have been associated with poor clinical outcome. This response is commonly referred to as *immunoparalysis*. However, from a conceptual standpoint, immunoparalysis appears to be strikingly different from classic endotoxin tolerance in one regard. Early studies suggested that preconditioning macrophages and mononuclear cells with small doses of LPS (i.e., classic endotoxin tolerance) resulted in both (a) a diminished proinflammatory response to a subsequent dose of LPS and (b) *increased* phagocytosis and resistance to bacterial infection (the latter not being consistent with the concept of immunoparalysis). Endotoxin tolerance, therefore, may not necessarily equate with immunoparalysis (75–80). Additional studies are necessary to shed further insight into the potential clinical relevance of endotoxin tolerance.

ANTIOXIDANT SYSTEMS

Oxidant Stress

While the use of oxygen is requisite for aerobic organisms, this process inevitably leads to the production of ROS, including hydrogen peroxide, superoxide anion, hydroxyl radicals, NO, and peroxynitrite. When produced in large amounts, ROS can cause excessive oxidant stress leading to cellular and tissue injury. ROS-mediated cellular and tissue injury involves damage to genomic and mitochondrial DNA, lipid peroxidation, and protein modification. In addition, cell death secondary to oxidant stress can occur from either necrosis or apoptosis.

Potent antioxidant systems have evolved to counterbalance the normal production of ROS that occurs during many cellular processes, as well as the excessive amounts of ROS that can occur during pathologic states (81). Despite this elegant counter-regulatory system, ROS can lead to cellular injury either when a component of the antioxidant system is defective

or when the high-level production of ROS overwhelms an otherwise intact antioxidant system. Recognition of this critical balance and the mechanisms involved in defending against ROS holds potential for the design of therapeutic strategies directed toward restoring the balance between ROS production and endogenous antioxidant systems.

Superoxide Dismutases

SODs include Mn-SOD, Cu/Zn-SOD, and Fe-SOD, and exist within the cytoplasmic and mitochondrial cellular compartments, and in the extracellular compartment. SOD is capable of efficiently converting two superoxide molecules to hydrogen peroxide and oxygen (**Fig. 20.5**). The importance of SOD in cellular adaptation to stress is illustrated by gene knockout studies and by numerous studies demonstrating that genetic overexpression of SOD confers protection against oxidant stress (82). In addition, mutations of human SOD are strongly linked to development of amyotrophic lateral sclerosis and are likely be operative in certain critically ill patients. Unfortunately, pharmacologic strategies to augment SOD activity have not been successful to date despite showing tremendous promise in the preclinical setting.

Catalase and Glutathione Peroxidase

Catalases are synergistic with SOD by converting hydrogen peroxide to water and oxygen (**Fig. 20.5**). By lowering intracellular levels of hydrogen peroxide, catalases can also prevent formation of hydroxyl radicals that could occur via the Fenton reaction (**Fig. 20.5**). Glutathione (GSH) peroxidases consist of at least four isoforms in mammals and are widely distributed in many tissues. Similar to catalases, all members of the GSH peroxidases can convert hydrogen peroxide to water by using glutathione as a substrate.

Thioredoxin

Thioredoxin and thioredoxin reductase serve as another major antioxidant mechanism in mammals (83). In conjunction with NADPH, thioredoxin reductase leads to the reduction of the

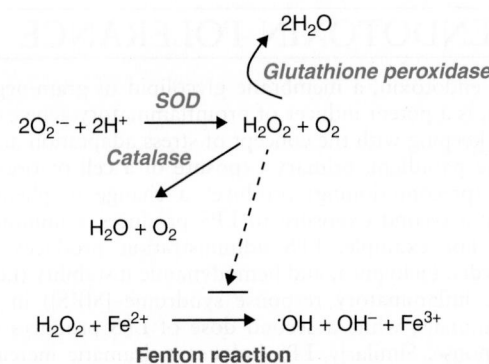

FIGURE 20.5. Schematic depicting the activities of SOD, catalase, and glutathione peroxidase. SOD converts two molecules of superoxide anion to hydrogen peroxide and water. The hydrogen peroxide produced from this reaction can be further reduced by either catalase or glutathione peroxidase. Catalase converts hydrogen peroxide to oxygen and water. Glutathione peroxidase converts hydrogen peroxide to two molecules of water using glutathione as a substrate. In addition, the reduction of hydrogen peroxide by catalase and glutathione peroxidase decreases the participation of hydrogen peroxide in the Fenton reaction, which can lead to the formation of hydroxyl radicals.

active disulfide site of thioredoxin. Thioredoxin, in turn, can broadly function as a protein disulfide reductant. In addition, the thioredoxin system provides an efficient mechanism for the regeneration of various low-molecular-weight antioxidants such as vitamin E, vitamin C, selenium-related compounds, lipoic acid, and ubiquinones. Interestingly, children with meningococcal septic shock have low plasma thioredoxin levels during both the acute and the convalescent phases of disease (84).

EPIGENETICS

Epigenetic modifications represent another fundamental, and long-lasting, cellular adaptation to stress. Epigenetics refers to heritable changes in gene expression patterns that are not related to direct changes to the DNA sequence of a given gene (85). The epigenetic mechanisms that regulate gene expression include chemical modifications of DNA (typically methylation), posttranslational modifications of histones (typically acetylation, methylation, and/or phosphorylation), and micro-RNAs that regulate gene expression by binding specific mRNA molecules and targeting them for degradation. A key concept of epigenetic-mediated gene regulation is that the epigenetic modifications can be "inherited" (i.e., passed on to daughter cells) and can therefore lead to long-lasting effects on gene expression.

An example of epigenetic regulation of gene expression is provided in **Figure 20.6**. Nucleosomes are the basic unit of DNA packaging into chromatin and chromosomes. A nucleosome consists of DNA segments wound around an octamer of histone proteins. The histone proteins can be modified by the addition, or removal, of methyl or acetyl groups to specific amino acids. These histone modifications can, in turn, alter DNA conformation and consequently alter the ability of transcription factors to bind DNA promoter regions and regulate gene expression. In the example provided in **Figure 20.6**, the addition of three methyl groups to lysine 27 of histone subunit H3 leads to a

prohibitive DNA confirmation that does not allow transcription factor binding to the gene promoter, thus suppressing gene expression. Alternatively, the addition of three methyl groups to lysine 4 of histone subunit H3 leads to a permissive DNA confirmation that allows transcription factor binding to the gene promoter, thus rendering the gene as being inducible.

An active area of research, in the area of cellular adaptation (or maladaptation) to stress, surrounds the epigenetic regulation of immunity- and inflammation-related gene expression (86). For example, the phenomenon of endotoxin tolerance discussed earlier is mediated, in part, by epigenetic mechanisms involving histone, chromatin, and DNA modifications (70,71,87,88). In addition, production of some cytokines and chemokines by immune cells challenged with endotoxin appears to be partially dependent on epigenetic mechanisms (89,90). From a potential therapeutic standpoint, a recent study demonstrated that the administration of a compound that mimics acetylated histones disrupts chromatin complexes related to inflammatory responses in macrophages and confers protection in rodent models of sepsis (91).

An evolving paradigm in the sepsis field surrounds the concept of altered adaptive immunity and immune suppression (92). Additionally, it is now well established that patients that recover from various forms of critical illness, sepsis in particular, are at increased risk of death for several years after discharge from the ICU (93–95). Evolving experimental data indicate that sepsis induces epigenetic changes in dendritic cells and lymphocytes that render the host immune deficient for a remarkably long period of time after the initial sepsis challenge (96–98). Additionally, genome-wide expression studies in children with septic shock demonstrated differential expression of a group of genes corresponding to gene networks involved in transcriptional repression and epigenetic regulation, in parallel with suppression of adaptive immunity genes (99). Thus, it is possible that our future approach to the recovering critically ill patient will need to take into consideration the epigenetic impact of critical illness.

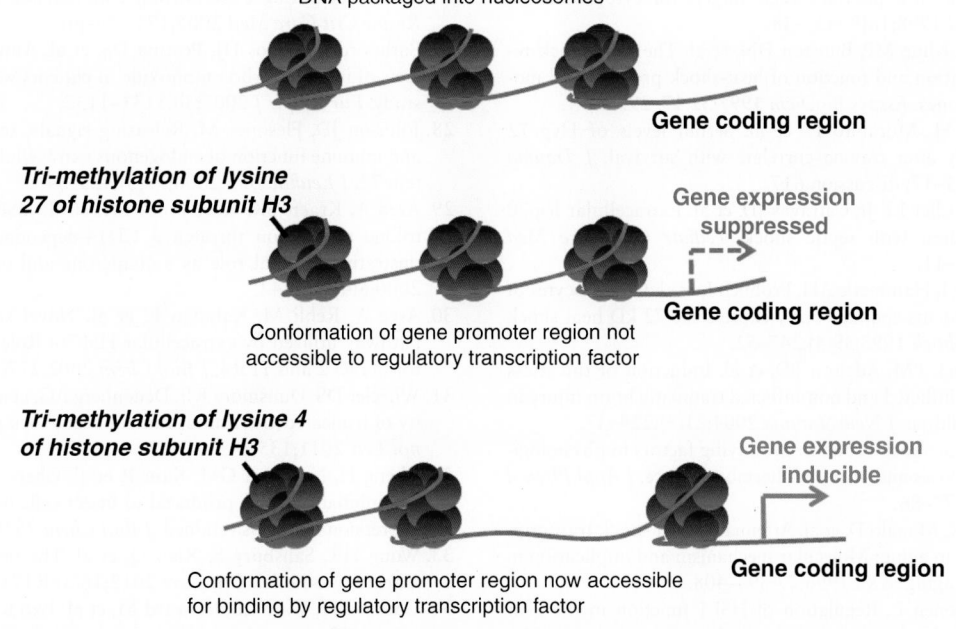

FIGURE 20.6. Schematic example of epigenetic regulation of gene expression. The upper panel illustrates the basic packaging of DNA into nucleosomes by winding around histone cores. The middle panel illustrates that the addition of three methyl groups to lysine 27 of histone subunit H3 leads to a DNA confirmation that does not allow for transcription factor binding to the gene promoter region, thus repressing gene expression. The bottom panel illustrates that the addition of three methyl groups to lysine 4 of histone subunit H3 leads to a DNA confirmation that allows transcription factor binding to the gene promoter region, thus facilitating gene expression.

CONCLUSIONS AND FUTURE DIRECTIONS

In this chapter, we have described a broad range of cellular adaptations to stress. The adaptations range from broad responses that confer generalized cytoprotection (e.g., the heat shock response) to responses limited toward specific forms of cellular stress (e.g., antioxidant responses to oxidative stress) and to potentially maladaptive responses leading to immune suppression (e.g., epigenetic modifications of immunity-related genes). The importance of these adaptations in the clinical care of critically ill children cannot be overstated. Much of critical care–related intervention is directed at organ support. In effect, much of this organ support provides a platform and a time frame to allow cellular stress adaptations to become operative. It is through these responses, then, that many critically ill children ultimately recover from a given illness or injury. Conversely, inadequate adaptations or failure to adapt can lead to organ failure and death despite optimal organ support.

An important challenge in the field is to devise safe therapeutic strategies to manipulate and/or enhance these adaptations for the benefit of our patients. By understanding the molecular mechanisms that allow for adaptations, the field will be better positioned to meet this challenge. The evolution and development of novel pharmacologic agents, molecular-based strategies, and even gene-based therapy collectively hold the potential to effectively manipulate and harness these forms of cellular adaptation as a therapeutic strategy that goes well beyond organ support.

References

1. Westerheide SD, Morimoto RI. Heat shock response modulators as therapeutic tools for diseases of protein conformation. *J Biol Chem* 2005;280(39):33097–100.
2. Morimoto RI, Santoro MG. Stress-inducible responses and heat shock proteins: New pharmacologic targets for cytoprotection. *Nat Biotechnol* 1998;16(9):833–38.
3. Morimoto RI, Kline MP, Bimston DN, et al. The heat-shock response: Regulation and function of heat-shock proteins and molecular chaperones. *Essays Biochem* 1997;32:17–29.
4. Pittet JF, Lee H, Morabito D, et al. Serum levels of Hsp 72 measured early after trauma correlate with survival. *J Trauma* 2002;52(4):611–17; discussion 617.
5. Wheeler DS, Fisher LE Jr, Catravas JD, et al. Extracellular hsp70 levels in children with septic shock. *Pediatr Crit Care Med* 2005;6(3):308–11.
6. Kindas-Mugge I, Hammerle AH, Frohlich I, et al. Granulocytes of critically ill patients spontaneously express the 72 kD heat shock protein. *Circ Shock* 1993;39(4):247–52.
7. Lai Y, Kochanek PM, Adelson PD, et al. Induction of the stress response after inflicted and non-inflicted traumatic brain injury in infants and children. *J Neurotrauma* 2004;21(3):229–37.
8. Kregel KC. Heat shock proteins: Modifying factors in physiological stress responses and acquired thermotolerance. *J Appl Physiol* 2002;92(5):2177–86.
9. Liu AY, Lee YK, Manalo D, et al. Attenuated heat shock transcriptional respone in aging: Molecular mechanism and implication in the biology of aging. *EXS* 1996;77:393–408.
10. Anckar J, Sistonen L. Regulation of HSF1 function in the heat stress response: Implications in aging and disease. *Annu Rev Biochem* 2011;80:1089–115.
11. Wong HR. Potential protective role of the heat shock response in sepsis. *New Horiz* 1998;6(2):194–200.
12. Wheeler DS, Wong HR. Heat shock response and acute lung injury. *Free Radic Biol Med* 2007;42(1):1–14.
13. Weiss YG, Maloyan A, Tazelaar J, et al. Adenoviral transfer of HSP-70 into pulmonary epithelium ameliorates experimental acute respiratory distress syndrome. *J Clin Invest* 2002;110(6):801–6.
14. Malhotra V, Wong HR. Interactions between the heat shock response and the nuclear factor-kappa B signaling pathway. *Crit Care Med* 2002;30(1 suppl):S89–95.
15. Wong HR, Odoms K, Sakthivel B. Divergence of canonical danger signals: The genome-level expression patterns of human mononuclear cells subjected to heat shock or lipopolysaccharide. *BMC Immunol* 2008;9:24.
16. Morse D, Choi AM. Heme oxygenase-1: From bench to bedside. *Am J Respir Crit Care Med* 2005;172(6):660–70.
17. Yachie A, Niida Y, Wada T, et al. Oxidative stress causes enhanced endothelial cell injury in human heme oxygenase-1 deficiency. *J Clin Invest* 1999;103(1):129–35.
18. Otterbein LE, Choi AM. Heme oxygenase: Colors of defense against cellular stress. *Am J Physiol Lung Cell Mol Physiol* 2000;279(6):L1029–37.
19. Ryter SW, Otterbein LE, Morse D, et al. Heme oxygenase/carbon monoxide signaling pathways: Regulation and functional significance. *Mol Cell Biochem* 2002;234–235(1–2):249–63.
20. Choi AM, Otterbein LE. Emerging role of carbon monoxide in physiologic and pathophysiologic states. *Antioxid Redox Signal* 2002;4(2):227–28.
21. Kim HP, Ryter SW, Choi AM. CO as a cellular signaling molecule. *Annu Rev Pharmacol Toxicol* 2006;6:411–49.
22. Chung SW, Liu X, Macias AA, et al. Heme oxygenase-1-derived carbon monoxide enhances the host defense response to microbial sepsis in mice. *J Clin Invest* 2008;118:239–47.
23. Ryter SW, Choi AM. Heme oxygenase-1/carbon monoxide: Novel therapeutic strategies in critical care medicine. *Curr Drug Targets* 2010;11:1485–94.
24. Wegiel B, Hanto DW, Otterbein LE. The social network of carbon monoxide in medicine. *Trends Mol Med* 2013;19:3–11.
25. Mitchell LA, Channel MM, Royer CM, et al. Evaluation of inhaled carbon monoxide as an anti-inflammatory therapy in a nonhuman primate model of lung inflammation. *Am J Physiol* 2010;299:L891–97.
26. Mayr FB, Spiel A, Leitner J, et al. Effects of carbon monoxide inhalation during experimental endotoxemia in humans. *Am J Respir Crit Care Med* 2005;171:354–60.
27. Bathoord E, Slebos DJ, Postma DS, et al. Anti-inflammatory effects of inhaled carbon monoxide in patients with COPD: A pilot study. *Eur Respir J* 2007;30:1131–1137.
28. Johnson JD, Fleshner M. Releasing signals, secretory pathways, and immune function of endogenous extracellular heat shock protein 72. *J Leukoc Biol* 2006;79(3):425–34.
29. Asea A, Kraeft SK, Kurt-Jones EA, et al. HSP70 stimulates cytokine production through a CD14-dependant pathway, demonstrating its dual role as a chaperone and cytokine. *Nat Med* 2000;6(4):435–42.
30. Asea A, Rehli M, Kabingu E, et al. Novel signal transduction pathway utilized by extracellular HSP70: Role of toll-like receptor (TLR) 2 and TLR4. *J Biol Chem* 2002;277(17):15028–34.
31. Wheeler DS, Dunsmore KE, Denenberg AG, et al. Biological activity of truncated C-terminus human heat shock protein 72. *Immunol Lett* 2011;135(1–2):173–9.
32. Zheng H, Nagaraja GM, Kaur P, et al. Chaperokine function of recombinant Hsp72 produced in insect cells using a baculovirus expression system is retained. *J Biol Chem* 2919;285:349–56.
33. Wong HR, Salisbury S, Xiao Q, et al. The pediatric sepsis biomarker risk model. *Crit Care* 2012;16(5):R174.
34. Ganter MT, Ware LB, Howard M, et al. Extracellular heat shock protein 72 is a marker of the stress protein response in acute lung injury. *Am J Physiol Lung Cell Mol Physiol* 2006;291:L354–61.
35. Madach K, Molvarec A, Rigo JJ, et al. Elevated serum 70 kDa heat shock protein level reflects tissue damage and disease severity in the syndrome of hemolysis, elevated liver enzymes, and low platelet count. *Eur J Obset Gyncecol Reprod Biol* 2008;139:133–8.

36. Molvarec A, Tamasi L, Losonczy G, et al. Circulating heat shock protein 70 (HSPA1A) in normal and pathologic pregnancies. *Cell Stress Chaperones* 2010;15:237–47.

37. Zhang Z, Tanquay RM, He M, et al. Variants of HSPA1A in combination with plasma Hsp70 and anti-Hsp70 antibiody levels associated with higher risk of acute coronary syndrome. *Cardiology* 2011;119:57–64.

38. Jenei ZM, Szeplaki G, Merkely B, et al. Persistently elevated extracellular HSP70 (HSPA1A) level as an independent prognostic marker in post-cardiac arrest patients. *Cell Stress Chaperones* 2013;18:447–54.

39. Ryan M, Levy MM. Clinical review: Fever in intensive care unit patients. *Crit Care* 2003;7(3):221–25.

40. Launey Y, Nesseler N, Malledant Y, et al. Clinical review: Fever in septic ICU patients—Friend or foe? *Crit Care* 2011;15(3):222.

41. Ziegler TR, Ogden LG, Singleton KD, et al. Parenteral glutamine increases serum heat shock protein 70 in critically ill patients. *Intensive Care Med* 2005;31:1079–86.

42. Wischmeyer PE. The glutamine story: Where are we now? *Curr Opin Crit Care* 2006;12(2):142–8.

43. Murry CE, Jennings RB, Reimer KA. Preconditioning with ischemia: A delay of lethal cell injury in ischemic myocardium. *Circulation* 1986;74:1124–36.

44. Sanada S, Kitakaze M. Ischemic preconditioning: Emerging evidence, controversy, and translational trials. *Int J Cardiol* 2004;97:263–76.

45. Das DK, Maulik N. Cardiac genomic response following preconditioning stimulus. *Cardiovasc Res* 2006;70:254–63.

46. Sharp FR, Ran R, Lu A, et al. Hypoxic preconditioning protects against ischemic brain injury. *J Am Soc Exp Neuro Therap* 2004;1:26–35.

47. Hausenloy DJ, Yellon DM. Survival kinases in ischemic preconditioning and postconditioning. *Cardiovasc Res* 2006;70:240–53.

48. Wang Z, Hernandez F, Pederiva F, et al. Ischemic preconditioning of the graft for intestinal transplantation in rats. *Pediatr Transplant* 2011;15:65–9.

49. Sitzer M, Foerch C, Neumann-Haefelin T, et al. Transient ischaemic attack preceding anterior circulation infarction is independently associated with favourable outcome. *J Neurol Neurosurg Psychiatr* 2004;75:659–60.

50. Alreja G, Bugano D, Lotfi A. Effect of remote ischemic preconditioning on myocardial and renal injury: Meta-analysis of randomized controlled trials. *J Invasive Cardiol* 2012;24:42–8.

51. Cheung MM, Kharbanda RK, Konstantinov IE, et al. Randomized controlled trial of the effects of remote ischemic preconditioning on children undergoing cardiac surgery: First clinical application in humans. *J Am Coll Cardiol* 2006;47:2277–82.

52. Luo W, Zhu M, Huang R, et al. A comparison of cardiac postconditioning and remote pre-conditioning in paediatric cardiac surgery. *Cardiol Young* 2011;21:266–70.

53. Pedersen KR, Ravn HB, Povlsen JV, et al. Failure of remote ischemic preconditioning to reduce the risk of postoperative acute kidney injury in children undergoing operation for complex congenital heart disease: A randomized single-center study. *J Thorac Cardiovasc Surg* 2012;143:576–83.

54. Pavione MA, Carmona F, de Castro M, et al. Late remote ischemic preconditioning in children undergoing cardiopulmonary bypass: A randomzied controlled trial. *J Thorac Cardiovasc Surg* 2012;144:178–83.

55. Semenza GL. Surviving ischemia: Adaptive responses mediated by hypoxia-inducible factor 1. *J Clin Invest* 2000;106(7):809–12.

56. Semenza GL. HIF-1: Mediator of physiological and pathophysiological responses to hypoxia. *J Appl Physiol* 2000;88:1474–80.

57. Lisy K, Peet DJ. Turn me on: Regulating HIF transcriptional activity. *Cell Death Differ* 2008;15:642–49.

58. Mole DR, Maxwell PH, Pugh CW, et al. Regulation of HIF by the von Hippel–Lindau tumour suppressor: Implications for cellular oxygen sensing. *IUBMB Life* 2001;52(1–2):43–7.

59. Hashmi S, Al-Salam S. Hypoxia-inducible factor-1 alpha in the heart: A double agent? *Cardiol Rev* 2012;20:268–73.

60. Prabhakar NR, Semenza GL. Adaptive and maladaptive cardiorespiratory responses to continuous and intermittent hypoxia mediated by hypoxia inducible factors 1 and 2. *Physiol Rev* 2012;92:967–1003.

61. Luo W, Zhong J, Chang R, et al. Hsp70 and CHIP selectively mediate ubiquitination and degradation of hypoxia-inducible (HIF)-1alpha but not HIF-2alpha. *J Biol Chem* 2010;285:3651–63.

62. Holmquist-Mengelbier L, Fredlund E, Lofstedt T, et al. Recruitment of HIF-1alpha and HIF-2alpha to common target genes is differentially regulated in neuroblastoma: HIF-2alpha promotes an aggressive phenotype. *Cancer Cell* 2006;10:413–23.

63. Koh MY, Lemos RJ, Liu X, et al. The hypoxia-associated factor switches cells from HIF-1alpha to HIF-2alpha-dependent signaling promoting stem cell characteristics, aggressive tumor growth and invasion. *Cancer Res* 2011;71:4015–27.

64. Koh MY, Powis G. Passing the baton: The HIF switch. *Trends Biochem Sci* 2012;37:364–72.

65. Fan H, Cook JA. Molecular mechanisms of endotoxin tolerance. *J Endotoxin Res* 2004;10:71–84.

66. Cavaillon J-M, Adrie C, Fitting C, et al. Endotoxin tolerance: Is there a clinical relevance? *J Endotoxin Res* 2003;9:101–7.

67. Cavaillon JM, Adib-Conquy M. Bench-to-bedside reivew: Endotoxin tolerance as a model of leukocyte reprogramming in sepsis. *Crit Care* 2006;10:233.

68. Biswas SK, Lopez-Collazo E. Endotoxin tolerance: New mechanisms, molecules and clinical significance. *Trends Immunol* 2009;30:475–87.

69. Chan C, Li L, McCall CE, et al. Endotoxin tolerance disrupts chromatin remodeling and NF-kappaB transactivation at the IL-1beta promoter. *J Immunol* 2005;175:461–68.

70. El Gazzar M, Yoza BK, Chen X, et al. Chromatin-specific remodeling by HMGB1 and linker histone H1 silences proinflammatory genes during endotoxin tolerance. *Mol Cell Biol* 2009;29(7):1959–71.

71. El Gazzar M, Yoza BK, Chen X, et al. G9a and HP1 couple histone and DNA methylation to TNFalpha transcription silencing during endotoxin tolerance. *J Biol Chem* 2008;283(47):32198–208.

72. El Gazzar M, Yoza BK, Hu JY, et al. Epigenetic silencing of tumor necrosis factor alpha during endotoxin tolerance. *J Biol Chem* 2007;282:26857–64.

73. El Gazzar M, McCall CE. MicroRNAs distinguish translational from transcriptional silencing during endotoxin tolerance. *J Biol Chem* 2010;285:20940–51.

74. Nahid MA, Satoh M, Chan EK. MicroRNA in TLR signaling and endotoxin tolerance. *Cell Mol Immunol* 2011;8:388–403.

75. Murphey ED, Fang G, Varma TK, et al. Improved bacterial clearance and decreased mortality can be induced by LPS tolerance and is not dependent upon IFN-gamma. *Shock* 2007;27:289–95.

76. Wheeler DS, Lahni PM, Denenberg AG, et al. Induction of endotoxin tolerance enhances bacterial clearance and survival in murine polymicrobial sepsis. *Shock* 2008;30:267–73.

77. Natarajan S, Kim J, Remick DG. Acute pulmonary lipopolysaccharide tolerance decreases TNF-alpha without reducing neutrophil recruitment. *J Immunol* 2008;181:8402–8.

78. Murphey ED, Fang G, Sherwood ER. Endotoxin pretreatment improves bacterial clearance and decreases mortality in moce challenged with Staphylococcus aureus. *Shock* 2008;29:512–18.

79. Shi DW, Zhang J, Jiang HN, et al. LPS pretreatment ameliorates multiple organ injuries and improves survival in a murine model of polymicrobial sepsis. *Inflamm Res* 2011;60:841–49.

80. Landoni VI, Chiarella P, Martire-Greco D, et al. Tolerance to lipopolysacchardie promotes an enhanced neutrophil extracellular traps formation leading to a more efficient bacterial clearance in mice. *Clin Exp Immunol* 2012;168:153–63.

81. Mathers J, Fraser JA, McMahon M, et al. Antioxidant and cytoprotective responses to redox stress. *Biochem Soc Symp* 2004;(71):157–76.

82. McCord JM. Superoxide dismutase in aging and disease: An overview. *Methods Enzymol* 2002;349:331–41.

83. Burke-Gaffney A, Callister ME, Nakamura H. Thioredoxin: Friend or foe in human disease? *Trends Pharmacol Sci* 2005;26(8):398–404.

84. Callister ME, Burke-Gaffney A, Quinlan GJ, et al. Persistently low plasma thioredoxin is associated with meningococcal septic shock in children. *Intensive Care Med* 2007;33(2):364–7.

85. Delcuve GP, Rastegar M, Davie JR. Epigenetic control. *J Cell Physiol* 2009;219(2):243–50.

86. Carson WF, Cavassani KA, Dou Y, et al. Epigenetic regulation of immune cell functions during post-septic immunosuppression. *Epigenetics* 2011;6(3):273–83.

87. Chan C, Li L, McCall CE, et al. Endotoxin tolerance disrupts chromatin remodeling and NF-kappaB transactivation at the IL-1beta promoter. *J Immunol* 2005;175(1):461–8.

88. Foster SL, Hargreaves DC, Medzhitov R. Gene-specific control of inflammation by TLR-induced chromatin modifications. *Nature* 2007;447(7147):972–8.

89. Brogdon JL, Xu Y, Szabo SJ, et al. Histone deacetylase activities are required for innate immune cell control of Th1 but not Th2 effector cell function. *Blood* 2007;109(3):1123–30.

90. Tsaprouni LG, Ito K, Adcock IM, et al. Suppression of lipopolysaccharide- and tumour necrosis factor-alpha-induced interleukin (IL)-8 expression by glucocorticoids involves changes in IL-8 promoter acetylation. *Clin Exp Immunol* 2007;150(1):151–7.

91. Nicodeme E, Jeffrey KL, Schaefer U, et al. Suppression of inflammation by a synthetic histone mimic. *Nature* 2010;468(7327):1119–23.

92. Skrupky LP, Kerby PW, Hotchkiss RS. Advances in the management of sepsis and the understanding of key immunologic defects. *Anesthesiology* 2011;115(6):1349–62.

93. Czaja AS, Zimmerman JJ, Nathens AB. Readmission and late mortality after pediatric severe sepsis. *Pediatrics* 2009;123(3):849–57.

94. Quartin AA, Schein RM, Kett DH, et al. Magnitude and duration of the effect of sepsis on survival. Department of Veterans Affairs Systemic Sepsis Cooperative Studies Group. *JAMA* 1997;277(13):1058–63.

95. Winters BD, Eberlein M, Leung J, et al. Long-term mortality and quality of life in sepsis: A systematic review. *Crit Care Med* 2010;38(5):1276–83.

96. Ishii M, Wen H, Corsa CA, Liu T, et al. Epigenetic regulation of the alternatively activated macrophage phenotype. *Blood* 2009;114(15):3244–54.

97. Wen H, Dou Y, Hogaboam CM, et al. Epigenetic regulation of dendritic cell-derived interleukin-12 facilitates immunosuppression after a severe innate immune response. *Blood* 2008;111(4):1797–804.

98. Wen H, Schaller MA, Dou Y, et al. Dendritic cells at the interface of innate and acquired immunity: The role for epigenetic changes. *J Leukoc Biol* 2008;83(3):439–46.

99. Wong HR, Freishtat RJ, Monaco M, et al. Leukocyte subset-derived genomewide expression profiles in pediatric septic shock. *Pediatr Crit Care Med* 2010;11(3):349–55.

CHAPTER 21 ■ SHOCK, ISCHEMIA, AND REPERFUSION INJURY

BASILIA ZINGARELLI

KEY POINTS

Ischemia and Reperfusion

1. Ischemia results from a dramatic reduction of oxygen supply to tissues and/or organs and rapidly results in cell metabolic derangement, molecular alterations, and dysfunction sequelae.

2. Timely reperfusion of the ischemic tissue is the mandatory treatment of patients with clinical conditions of ischemia. However, reperfusion initiates a cascade of events that causes additional cell injury, a phenomenon called *reperfusion injury*.

Oxidative and Nitrosative Stress

3. The production of excessive quantities of reactive oxygen species (ROS) and reactive nitrogen species (RNS) is an important mechanism of reperfusion injury. These reactive species mediate tissue injury by two main mechanisms: directly, by inducing damage of important cellular macromolecules, and indirectly, by activating signal transduction pathways.

4. As highly reactive species, ROS and RNS induce the alteration of the structure and function of many enzymes, proteins, lipids, and DNA.

Activation of Signaling Pathways

5. Pathogen-associated molecular patterns (PAMPs) and damage-associated molecular patterns (DAMPs) contribute to activation of inflammatory signaling pathway by recruiting toll-like receptors (TLRs) in the host cells.

6. ROS and RNS initiate signaling cascades that result in a prompt production of inflammatory mediators, such as cytokines, adhesion molecules, chemokines, and metabolic enzymes, thus determining the functional outcome of the cell in response to ischemia.

7. The complement system is activated in an attempt to induce lysis of foreign organisms and to promote phagocytic clearance of immune complexes and the recruitment of inflammatory cells at the site of injury. However, this system can amplify endothelial dysfunction and the parenchymal damage during reperfusion.

Endothelial Dysfunction and Organ Injury

8. Endothelial dysfunction is triggered by the endothelial generation of ROS and RNS and is characterized by the development of a procoagulant phenotype, loss of vascular responsiveness to vasodilator and vasoconstrictor agents, increased vascular permeability, and adhesiveness to platelets and leukocytes.

9. In the early phase of shock and reperfusion, leukocytes are present mainly in the intravascular space (attached to the endothelium), and they play an important role in endothelial injury. At later stages, leukocytes migrate into the tissues and exacerbate parenchymal damage.

10. The production of ROS and RNS, endothelial injury, activation of the complement system, release of neutrophil-attractive factors, and leukocyte infiltration (leading to further production of reactive species and proteolytic enzymes) constitute a vicious cycle, which is ultimately responsible for organ injury.

Future Prospects

11. Current experimental research has raised the exciting prospect that pharmacologic intervention aimed at interrupting the various levels of the ischemia–reperfusion injury cycle may ameliorate cell dysfunction and prevent death. However, large clinical trials are necessary to determine whether these novel therapeutic interventions may be beneficial to the patient.

Ischemia and reperfusion injury is a critical pathophysiologic sequence common to several clinical conditions, including myocardial infarction, intestinal ischemia, stroke, cardiopulmonary bypass, solid-organ transplantation, soft-tissue flaps, and extremity reimplantation. It also occurs as a consequence of collapse of systemic circulation, as in shock with low cardiac output, which results in inadequate tissue perfusion (ischemia) and typically requires cardiovascular resuscitation (reperfusion).

Ischemia can result from a dramatic reduction of oxygen supply in the whole organism or in defined tissue regions and rapidly results in cellular metabolic derangements, molecular alterations, and dysfunction sequelae. Occasionally, ischemia may occur (despite adequate oxygen delivery) from either increased metabolic requirements or impaired oxygen utilization at the cellular level. If not reversed within a short period, the altered cellular metabolism progresses to complete depletion of the energetic pools, accumulation of waste and toxic products, and eventually, to cell death.

The main therapeutic intervention in clinical conditions of ischemia requires the restoration of blood flow (reperfusion) and/or recovery of the normal oxygen levels (reoxygenation) by providing circulatory and respiratory support. Once perfusion is reestablished, tissue ischemia is generally reversed. However, restoration of blood flow initiates a paradoxical injury process known as *reperfusion injury*, which is characterized by dysregulation of the inflammatory and innate immune responses and may lead to cellular death and further organ dysfunction. The intense inflammation triggered by ischemia and reperfusion injury may also precipitate inflammatory damage in organs not involved in the initial ischemic insult. This condition is termed *multiple organ dysfunction syndrome* (MODS) (see Chapter 23) and is the leading cause of death in ICUs.

The biochemical and molecular changes of ischemia and reperfusion are complex; these include (a) the formation of toxic inflammatory mediators, reactive oxygen species (ROS) and reactive nitrogen species (RNS) by inflammatory and parenchymal cells, (b) the disturbances of the microcirculation and endothelium barrier, and (c) the alteration of the coagulation and complement cascades. To counteract this deleterious inflammatory response, the tissues also attempt to adapt within the altered metabolic environment by deploying cellular mechanisms of defense (see Chapter 20).

OXYGEN DELIVERY AND ACUTE CELLULAR OXYGEN DEFICIENCY

According to the Fick equation, oxygen delivery (Do_2) depends on both the arterial oxygen content (Cao_2) and the cardiac output (CO). The CO depends on the heart rate and the stroke volume and the stroke volume is determined by myocardial contractility and ventricular preload and afterload. In infants and children, CO depends more on heart rate than on stroke volume because of an incomplete development of myocardial contractile mass. Compensatory changes in the local vasomotor tone modify the systemic vascular resistance and adjust CO to maintain tissue perfusion and meet metabolic demands (Fig. 21.1).

Therefore, *acute cellular oxygen deficiency* may result from a reduction of Do_2 due to local tissue ischemia within the perfusion territory of an occluded artery (myocardial or splanchnic infarction, cerebral ischemia, solid-organ transplantation, soft-tissue and limb reimplantation). Conversely, decreased CO may cause global tissue ischemia observed in conditions of cardiogenic shock. However, in some clinical conditions, inadequate tissue energetic metabolism may derive from an increase of total body oxygen consumption ($\dot{V}o_2$), despite a normal Do_2. For example, during septic shock tissue oxygenation may be inadequate even in the presence of even increased blood flow due to a major increase in metabolic demand and impaired oxygen extraction.

DEFINITION AND CLASSIFICATION OF SHOCK

Shock is defined as a state of acute circulatory dysfunction that results in a failure to deliver sufficient oxygen and other nutrients to meet the metabolic demands of the tissues (1). Shock is a progressive process whose three stages are characterized by the causative factors, the cellular compensatory responses, and the ischemia and reperfusion injury. In the early or *compensated stage*, a number of neurohormonal compensatory physiologic mechanisms act to maintain blood pressure and preserve adequate tissue perfusion. At this stage, shock may be reversible,

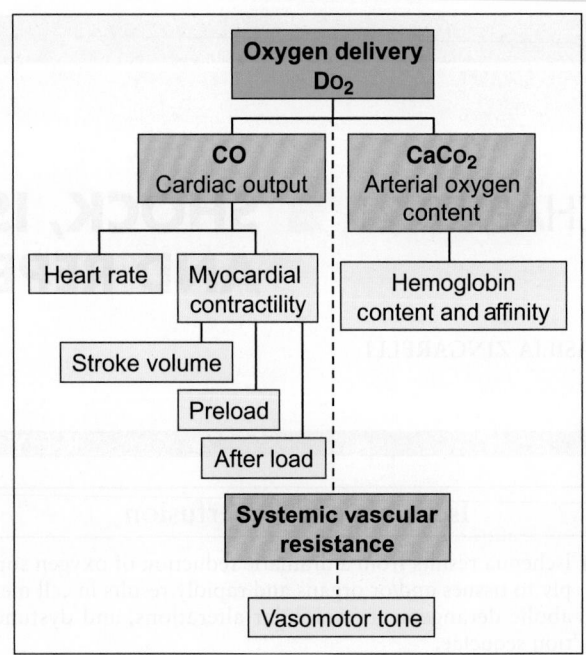

FIGURE 21.1. Variables of oxygen delivery. Oxygen delivery (Do_2) depends on cardiac output (CO) and arterial oxygen content (Cao_2). CO depends on heart rate and stroke volume, which is determined by myocardial contractility and the ventricular preload and afterload. Cao_2 depends on hemoglobin content, affinity, and saturation. Modification of the systemic vascular resistance contributes to maintenance of tissue perfusion through changes in the local vasomotor tone and affects CO by altering afterload.

even without therapeutic intervention. When the compensatory mechanisms fail, shock progresses to an *uncompensated stage* that requires, and still responds to, therapeutic interventions. In the *irreversible stage*, shock progresses to a remarkable degree of organ and tissue injury, which is unresponsive to conventional therapy and leads to the death of the patient.

Five main types of shock are described (Table 21.1). (a) *Hypovolemic shock* is the most common type of shock in children and is caused by a reduction in the volume of blood by hemorrhage or dehydration (especially in young children). (b) *Cardiogenic shock* is caused by a decline in CO secondary to myocardial damage and/or dysfunction. This type of shock is less frequent in children but may be seen in neonates with congenital heart disease, in older patients immediately after repair of congenital heart defects, and in patients with myocarditis, thyrotoxicosis, and pheochromocytoma. Septic shock may be included in cardiogenic shock because of the occurrence of myocardial depression induced by inflammatory mediators. (c) *Distributive shock* results from abnormalities in flow distribution secondary to impaired vasomotor tone, despite a normal or high CO. The most common cause of distributive shock in children is sepsis, especially in the early stage. Other types of distributive shock are *anaphylactic shock* from systemic allergic reactions and *neurologic shock* from spinal cord injuries. Drug intoxication by barbiturates, phenothiazines, and antihypertensives may also cause maldistribution of blood flow. (d) *Obstructive shock* is uncommon in children and is caused by a mechanical obstruction that impairs CO. The common causes include pericardial tamponade, congenital heart lesions characterized by left ventricular outflow obstruction (e.g., critical aortic stenosis, hypertrophic cardiomyopathy), tension pneumothorax and, less frequently, pulmonary embolism. (e) *Dissociative shock* is also uncommon

TABLE 21.1

CLASSIFICATION OF SHOCK

■ TYPE	■ CLINICAL SYNDROME
Hypovolemic	Hemorrhage
	Nonhemorrhagic fluid depletion
	Vomiting
	Diarrhea
	Severe burn
	Internal sequestration
	Diabetes (mellitus or insipidus)
	Nephrotic syndrome
	Other form of dehydration
Cardiogenic	Myocardial infarction
	Severe congestive failure
	Cardiac surgery
	Dysrhythmias
	Myocarditis
	Cardiopulmonary bypass
	Septic shock
	Drug intoxication
Distributive	Septic shock
	Toxic shock syndrome
	Anaphylaxis
	Neurogenic shock
	Endocrinologic shock
	Drug intoxication
Obstructive	Cardiac tamponade
	Pneumothorax
	Massive pulmonary embolus
Dissociative	Methemoglobinemia
	Carbon monoxide poisoning

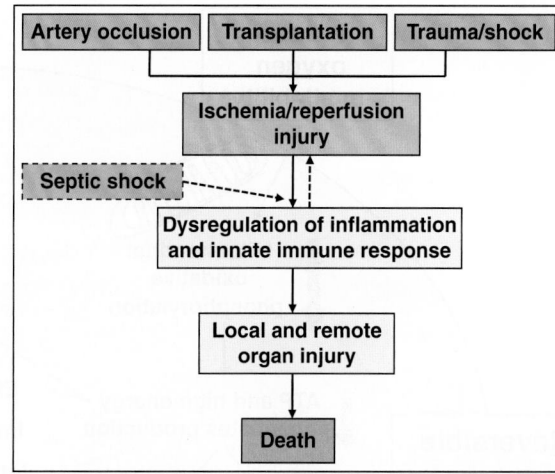

FIGURE 21.2. Kinetics of pathophysiologic events of shock and reperfusion. The pathophysiologic effects of acute local ischemia (after artery occlusion or organ transplantation) or acute global ischemia (after trauma and severe hemorrhage) are related predominantly to the acute deficiency of oxygen delivery and the subsequent reperfusion injury at the time of reoxygenation. In septic shock, an overwhelming inflammatory response is first activated by bacterial products and precedes the hemodynamic compromise and widespread tissue ischemia and reperfusion injury.

in children and results from clinical conditions associated with inadequate tissue oxygenation secondary to abnormal affinity of hemoglobin for oxygen, such as methemoglobinemia and carbon monoxide poisoning.

The specific pattern of response and related pathophysiology, clinical manifestations, and treatments vary with the etiology of shock (see Chapter 28).

CELLULAR AND MOLECULAR MECHANISMS OF INJURY

Metabolic Derangement and Energy Failure during Ischemia

The cells of all tissues undergo metabolic changes when deprived of oxygen and other nutrients. The quantitative and kinetic features of these metabolic responses are different for each specialized cell type and depend on the function and structure of the cell. Brain and myocardium are the most vulnerable tissues to acute oxygen deficiency, and even a short period of ischemia can lead to deleterious and irreversible effects.

The cause of shock or ischemia also has profound effects on many fundamental aspects of cell metabolism and function. The pathophysiologic effects of cardiogenic and hypovolemic shock are related predominantly to the acute decline in Do_2, whereas the pathophysiologic effects of sepsis result largely from the overwhelming production of inflammatory mediators. In shock associated with sepsis, in fact, bacterial products interact directly with several cell types, including macrophages, neutrophils, monocytes, endothelial cells,

and myocytes to activate the innate immune response and to stimulate the production of numerous inflammatory toxic mediators. The excessive inflammatory response is then responsible for hemodynamic compromise, widespread tissue ischemia, and reperfusion injury (Fig. 21.2).

Independent of the cause of ischemia or cell specificity, a time-dependent cascade of metabolic responses is shared among all cell types during ischemia (Fig. 21.3). Under normal conditions, glucose is converted into pyruvate via the glycolytic pathway. Pyruvate in turn is taken up by mitochondria and enters the Krebs cycle, where it is used in the production of adenosine triphosphate (ATP) via the electron transport chain (a process referred to as aerobic metabolism). After only a few seconds of ischemia, oxidative phosphorylation and mitochondrial ATP production are seriously compromised. The cell shifts from oxidative metabolism to an inefficient anaerobic glycolysis, where pyruvate remains in the cytoplasm and is converted into lactate, a process that produces only 2 moles of ATP per 1 mole of glucose, instead of the 38 moles of ATP normally produced during aerobic metabolism. Therefore, levels of ATP and other high-energy phosphates—mainly creatine phosphate—decline rapidly, and the breakdown products of adenine nucleotides, such as inorganic phosphate and adenosine, accumulate. This collapse of high-energy phosphate compounds impairs the energy-dependent cell processes, especially membrane ion pumps (Na^+/H^+ exchanger). DNA and protein synthesis are also suppressed, although some specific proteins, for example, heat shock protein 70 (Hsp70) and protein kinase C (PKC), may be induced in an attempt by the cell to adapt to the hypoxic environment (see Chapter 20).

Increased anaerobic glycolysis also leads to the accumulation of hydrogen ions, lactate, and intracellular acidosis. The elevated lactate levels can be measured in the serum and used as a biomarker of the ensuing shock state. Membrane depolarization and failure of ATP-dependent ion pumps lead to an efflux of potassium and influx of sodium and calcium. The increase of intracellular sodium concentration is accompanied by water influx into the cell, leading to swelling of the

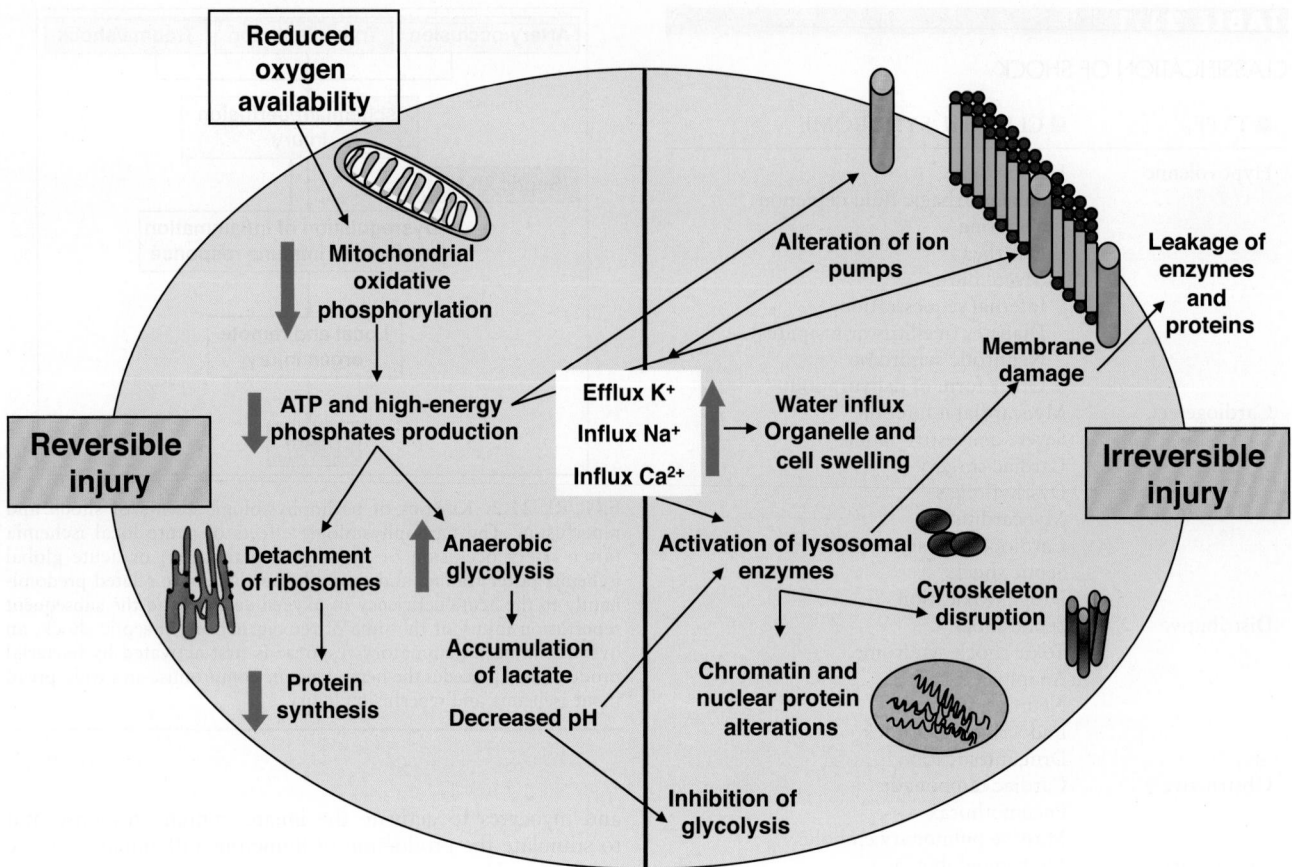

FIGURE 21.3. Metabolic and cellular derangement during ischemia. Reduction in oxygen availability compromises mitochondrial oxidative phosphorylation. Levels of ATP and other high-energy phosphates rapidly decline. The cell shifts from oxidative metabolism to an inefficient anaerobic glycolysis, producing less ATP. This energy failure slows the rate of protein synthesis and impairs the energy-dependent ion pumps, leading to an increase of intracellular levels of sodium (Na^+) and calcium (Ca^{2+}), an influx of water, and a decrease of intracellular levels of potassium (K^+). Water influx into the cell leads to swelling of the cytoplasm and organelles, such as mitochondria and endoplasmic reticulum, further impairing mitochondrial oxidative phosphorylation and protein synthesis. Accumulation of hydrogen ions and lactate results in intracellular acidosis and inhibition of glycolysis. At this time, if oxygen supply is not restored, cell injury becomes irreversible. Increase of intracellular Ca^{2+} causes activation of lysosomal enzymes and disrupts mitochondria, further uncoupling oxidative phosphorylation. Activated proteases also cleave cytoskeletal filaments and impair membrane permeability. Finally, physical disruption of the cell membrane occurs and is associated with leakage of cellular enzymes and proteins into the plasma.

cytoplasm and organelles such as mitochondria and endoplasmic reticulum. These abnormalities become rapidly severe and may reduce cellular functions within minutes. In the heart, this metabolic derangement causes a reduction of the contractile force generated by actin–myosin cross-bridging interactions. In the gut, the result is an altered intestinal absorptive function that is associated with translocation of bacteria from the intestine to the lymphatic vessels and blood stream. At this point, cell injury is reversible if oxygen supply is restored.

However, if ischemia persists, cell injury may become irreversible. The calcium concentration in the cytosol and mitochondria also increases due to changes in the cell ATPase-dependent ion transport systems. Mitochondria show amorphous matrix densities and granular dense bodies of calcium phosphate, which are considered the earliest sign of irreversible ischemic cell injury. The excessive energy demand and the resulting decrease in adenine nucleotide concentration represent crucial factors in the ensuing irreversible damage of cells.

This altered metabolic milieu, with a sustained increase in cytosolic and mitochondrial calcium and low internal pH (pHi), causes the activation of a number of enzymes (proteases, phospholipases, ATPases), which disrupt mitochondrial

and lysosomal membranes, further uncoupling mitochondrial oxidative phosphorylation and promoting the release of other acid hydrolases. Activated proteases also cleave cytoskeletal filaments and impair their anchoring and stabilizing function. These changes collectively lead to a progressive increase in membrane permeability, severe derangements of intracellular electrolytes, and ATP exhaustion (2).

The terminal event after prolonged ischemia is cell death, which occurs mainly by necrosis and is associated with physical disruption of the cell membrane and leakage of cellular enzymes and proteins across the cell membrane and into the plasma. This latter phenomenon may provide important diagnostic tools of cell damage, such as the serum increase of creatine kinase and troponin levels for the diagnosis of myocardial infarction.

Reperfusion Injury

Rapid and sustained restoration of oxygen and nutrient supply to the ischemic tissue is the major goal in the treatment of patients with clinical conditions of global or local ischemia. This therapeutic intervention has the potential to relieve ischemia and can result in the recovery of cell function and prevention of cell death. Upon reperfusion, if the cell injury is still reversible, electron transfer and ATP synthesis restart, the pHi is restored, and other metabolic processes are reestablished. The intensity and duration of ischemia are the main factors that influence recovery: earlier reperfusion and reoxygenation are associated with a more favorable clinical outcome.

Paradoxically, reoxygenation or restoration of blood flow initiates a cascade of events that results in even further cell injury, known as *reperfusion injury*. The underlying pathophysiologic mechanisms of this phenomenon are complex and involve inflammatory reactions as well as activation of the innate immune system. Major contributing events to reperfusion injury are oxidative and nitrosative stress, endothelial dysfunction, microvascular injury, neutrophil activation, and complement system activation.

Oxidative and Nitrosative Stress

The production of excessive quantities of ROS and RNS is an important mechanism of reperfusion injury. These reactive species include highly unstable oxygen and nitrogen molecules, such as superoxide (O_2^-), hydrogen peroxide (H_2O_2), oxidized lipoproteins, lipid peroxides, nitric oxide (NO), and peroxynitrite (ONOO) (3). ROS and RNS can be formed by several mechanisms; they can be produced by a reduction of molecular oxygen in altered mitochondria; by enzymes such as xanthine oxidase (XO), nicotinamide adenine dinucleotide phosphate (NADPH) oxidase (also called Nox), cytochrome P450, nitric oxide synthase (NOS), and cyclooxygenase (COX); and by auto-oxidation of catecholamines. The source of reactive species varies from cell to cell and from stage to stage during the ischemia and reperfusion event. For example, in myocytes, but to a much lesser extent than in other cell types, the production of oxyradicals starts early in the ischemic period in altered mitochondria and is further enhanced during reperfusion. At reperfusion, a massive activation of XO is a major source of ROS in endothelial cells, and COX may contribute to this oxidative stress. Cytochrome P450 accounts for the production of ROS in lung epithelial cells, and NADPH oxidase accounts for ROS production in neutrophils that have infiltrated the affected tissues. The production of potent RNS appears to be more ubiquitous because a number of inflammatory mediators may lead to the induction of NOS in several cell types. In addition, the antioxidant mechanisms of the cell may be compromised and may further favor the accumulation of reactive species.

These reactive species mediate tissue injury by two main mechanisms: (a) directly, by inducing the damage of important cellular macromolecules, and (b) indirectly, by activating signal transduction pathways that regulate the inflammatory and innate immune responses, and programmed cell death by apoptosis.

Sources of Reactive Oxygen and Nitrogen Species

Mitochondria

The generation of ROS starts during ischemia in the mitochondria. Although it might be expected that ischemia, leading to a low intracellular partial pressure of oxygen, would decrease oxyradical production, the paradoxic increase in ROS is secondary to the altered redox balance of the mitochondria. With ischemia, the metabolic reduction of the adenine nucleotide pool leaves the respiratory chain cytochromes in a more fully reduced state, allowing them to directly transfer (i.e., "leak") electrons to the residual molecular oxygen entrapped within the inner mitochondrial membrane. This electron leakage appears capable of producing large amounts of superoxide radical. While reintroduction of oxygen with reperfusion re-energizes the mitochondria, the low ADP content also allows further electron leakage, thus enabling more reactions with molecular oxygen and yielding the excessive "burst" of ROS.

Within a few minutes of reperfusion, the pHi returns to normal values. However, in this altered milieu of calcium overload, high phosphate concentrations, and depletion of adenine nucleotides, the pH normalization favors the opening of the *mitochondrial permeability transition pore*, a high-conductance channel whose opening leads to an increase of mitochondrial inner membrane permeability to solutes with molecular masses up to 1500 Da. This event plays a major role in the progression toward cell death. The opening of these pores releases stored calcium into the cytosol, and dissipation of the mitochondrial inner transmembrane potential uncouples the electron transport system from ATP hydrolysis. These events further abolish mitochondrial ATP production, leading to energy failure, enhanced production of ROS, and the release of apoptotic factors, thus contributing to cell death by apoptosis (4,5).

Xanthine Oxidoreductase System and NADPH Oxidase Systems

The xanthine oxidoreductase (XOR) enzyme system is an important enzymatic complex for the catabolism of purines, catalyzing the oxidation of hypoxanthine to xanthine and the oxidation of xanthine to uric acid. The system consists of two interconvertible forms, XO and xanthine dehydrogenase (XDH) (6). During ischemia, XDH is converted to the oxidase form by a protease activated by the intracellular overload of calcium. At the same time, degradation of ATP leads to an accumulation of hypoxanthine in the ischemic tissue. During reperfusion, with the presence of large quantities of molecular oxygen and high concentrations of hypoxanthine, XO yields a burst of superoxide (**Fig. 21.4**). During ischemia, the intracellular acidic conditions also allow the XOR enzyme system to catalyze the reduction of nitrates and nitrites to nitrites and NO, respectively, thus contributing to nitrosative stress.

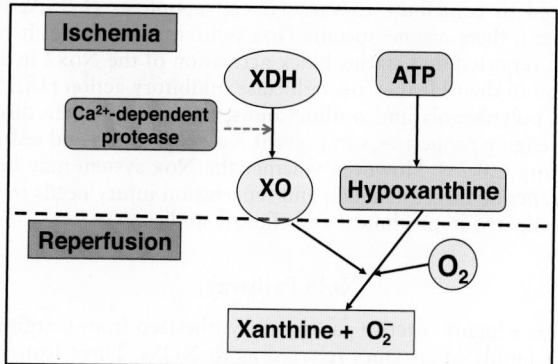

FIGURE 21.4. Superoxide production by xanthine oxidase. During ischemia, xanthine dehydrogenase (XDH) is converted to xanthine oxidase (XO) by a protease activated by the intracellular overload of calcium. At the same time, degradation of ATP leads to accumulation of hypoxanthine in the ischemic tissue. At reperfusion, large quantities of molecular oxygen are reintroduced into the cell. Both molecular oxygen and hypoxanthine then serve as substrates for XO to produce superoxide.

Furthermore, ischemia and reperfusion in any tissue leads to the release of XOR into the circulation. Elevated plasma levels of XOR have been reported in adults subjected to limb ischemia–reperfusion (7) or liver transplantation (8). In critically ill infants and children with shock subsequent to severe sepsis, trauma, or major surgery, high XO activity has been detected in urine. This elevation in the XO activity index appears to correlate with high blood levels of oxidized glutathione (a marker of oxidative stress) and with the clinical symptoms of an excessive proinflammatory response (9). It has been suggested that, once in the circulation, XOR may contribute to the development of MODS. These circulating levels may, in fact, bind to the endothelial cells of distant sites and contribute to the initiation of oxidative damage in organs remote from the original ischemic tissue (6).

The hypothesis that generation of superoxide by XO may play an important pathogenetic role in reperfusion injury has been supported by experimental studies in animals demonstrating that the inactivation of XO with allopurinol ameliorates reperfusion-induced tissue damage (10,11). A recent clinical study reported that allopurinol treatment might afford neuroprotective effects in moderately asphyxiated infants (12). Despite this human study and the beneficial effects reported in animal models, there is no other evidence of favorable effects of XOR inhibition in human conditions of reperfusion injury (10,11,13).

The NADPH oxidase family consists of seven Nox proteins: Nox1 to Nox5, Duox1 and Duox2. These proteins differ in their cell type expression, subunit composition, and function. In addition to phagocytic cells and neutrophils, where they mediate bacterial killing by producing a burst of superoxide anion, Nox enzymes are highly expressed in endothelial cells, vascular smooth muscle cells, cardiomyocytes, and renal tubular cells (14). A considerable number of experimental studies on mice genetically deficient of Nox proteins or their complex subunits suggest that this class of enzymes contribute to ischemia and reperfusion injury. Nox2 appears to contribute to lung, and brain reperfusion injury, as well as the remodeling process in the heart after infarction (14). Contribution of Nox enzymes in ischemia and reperfusion injury is suggested by clinical data demonstrating an upregulation of Nox2 and Nox5 in cardiomyocytes and intramyocardial blood vessels of patients who had died after myocardial infarction (15,16). Other clinical studies have reported that platelet-derived microparticles or exosomes, which were obtained from patients with septic shock, contained several Nox subunits and appeared to contribute to vascular cell apoptosis (17). At the present, there are no specific Nox inhibitors available. It has been reported that statins block activation of the Nox2 in addition to their HMG-CoA reductase inhibitory action (18,19); and polyphenols and anthocyanins, apart from their direct scavenging properties, can prevent Nox expression and reduce activity (20,21). However, whether the Nox system may be a therapeutic target in shock and reperfusion injury needs to be investigated in preclinical and clinical studies.

NOS Pathway

NO is a highly reactive gas that is synthesized from L-arginine by a family of enzymes referred as to NOSs. Three isoforms of NOS have been characterized: neuronal (nNOS, or type 1), inducible (iNOS, or type 2), and endothelial (eNOS, or type 3) (22). The eNOS and nNOS isoforms are constitutively expressed, are calcium/calmodulin dependent, and produce low amounts of NO. The designation of these constitutive isoforms does not strictly reflect their tissue expression because eNOS and nNOS are not only found in endothelial and neuronal cells but also in other cell types, including cardiomyocytes and muscle cells. The iNOS isoform is a calcium/calmodulin-independent enzyme that is responsible for the production of large amounts of NO. Although not detected under normal conditions, the expression of the iNOS isoform is induced in response to microbial products, inflammatory cytokines, and growth factors in almost every cell type during diverse pathologic conditions, including sepsis, hemorrhagic shock, trauma, and ischemia (22).

Under normal conditions, the constitutive forms of NOS release low concentrations of NO, which are critical to normal physiology. For example, the nNOS-derived NO acts as a neurotransmitter and a second messenger. The eNOS-derived NO is the physiologic mediator of normal vascular tone. Once formed by vascular endothelial cells, NO diffuses to adjacent smooth muscle cells, activates soluble guanylate cyclase, produces cyclic guanosine monophosphate (cGMP), and reduces intracellular calcium concentration, thus resulting in vasodilatation. Apart from its direct vasodilatory effect, the endothelium-derived NO also maintains normal tissue perfusion and vascular permeability by inhibiting platelet aggregation, leukocyte adherence, and smooth muscle proliferation in the vascular system. In cardiomyocytes, under physiologic conditions, both constitutive forms of NOS (types 1 and 3) have been described to release NO, which regulates cardiac function through their direct effects on several aspects of cardiomyocyte contractility, from the fine regulation of excitation–contraction coupling (with positive inotropic and lusitropic effects) to modulation of autonomic signaling and mitochondrial respiration (22,23).

The activation of the NOS enzymes and the production of NO change during ischemia and reperfusion injury. The best characterized events are the impairment of eNOS activity, induction of iNOS, and uncoupling of their enzymatic activity (Fig. 21.5). During sepsis (or at the onset of reperfusion after prolonged ischemia), oxidants scavenge NO, reducing its availability in the endothelium (24), and proinflammatory cytokines reduce NO production from the constitutive eNOS by reducing eNOS mRNA stability and expression (25). During ischemia and reperfusion, especially under conditions that induce oxidation of the enzyme cofactor tetrahydrobiopterin, NOS isoforms may become uncoupled and lose their ability to produce NO while producing superoxide anion, further contributing to oxidative stress (26). This reduced availability of NO is a major contributing factor in the development of endothelial dysfunction after ischemia and reperfusion in the heart and other vascular beds. In fact, the reduction of NO release from the endothelium impairs vascular relaxation to endothelium-dependent vasodilators and predisposes the vascular endothelium to platelet aggregation and leukocyte adhesion. Because of the very important effects of NO on vascular tone and thrombogenicity, drugs that can modulate NO levels (e.g., nitroglycerin) have long been used as therapeutic agents for the various angina syndromes, and they are used in congestive heart failure and in patients with left ventricular dysfunction. Because the local vasodilatory effects of NO in the lung vascular bed appear to improve oxygenation, inhaled NO gas has been used in sepsis-associated pulmonary hypertension (27).

In severe shock, high levels of NO are produced by iNOS and may be responsible for noxious effects. Vasodilation, caused by elevated levels of NO, contributes to circulatory failure in sepsis. Furthermore, NO can have damaging effects on proteins and DNA either directly or by formation of reactive NO-derived by-products. As a highly unstable gas with an unpaired electron, NO causes direct oxidation or S-nitrosylation of biomolecules. Moreover, the inherent radical nature of NO allows reactions with other free radicals or oxygen to yield other reactive intermediates, which then contribute to cell dysfunction and death. One of the most potent reactive intermediates is peroxynitrite (ONOO), which is formed from the reaction of NO with superoxide anion. Peroxynitrite causes

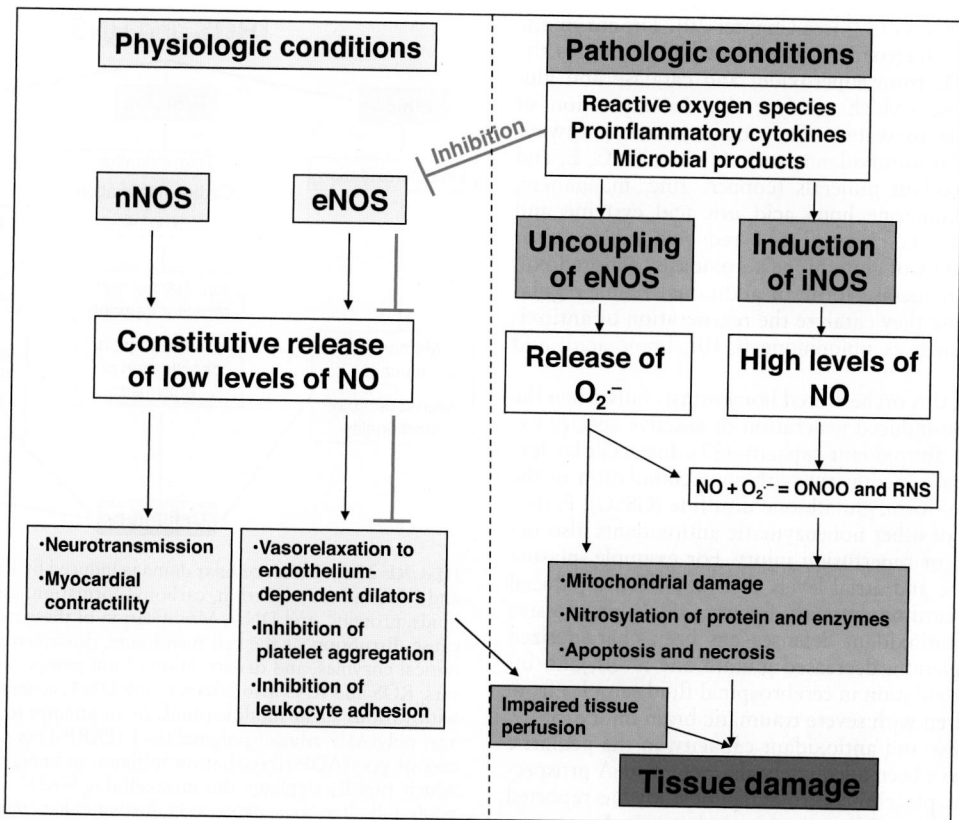

FIGURE 21.5. Activation of nitric oxide synthase (NOS) enzymes during physiologic conditions and during pathologic conditions after shock and reperfusion injury. Under normal conditions, the constitutive forms of NOS (nNOS and eNOS) release low concentrations of NO, which acts as a neurotransmitter, modulator of myocardial contractility, or modulator of vascular tone. The endothelium-derived NO also maintains normal tissue perfusion and vascular permeability by inhibiting platelet aggregation and leukocyte adherence. After prolonged ischemia and immediately at the onset of reperfusion, reactive oxygen species, several inflammatory mediators, and bacterial products may reduce NO production from the constitutive eNOS, impairing vascular relaxation to endothelium-dependent vasodilators and predisposing the endothelium to platelet aggregation and leukocyte adhesion. The eNOS also becomes uncoupled and converts oxygen to superoxide anion. In prolonged shock and severe ischemia and reperfusion, an inducible form of NOS (iNOS) is activated and produces large amounts of NO. Cytotoxic effects may be mediated directly by high levels of NO and/or indirectly by other reactive nitrogen species (RNS) and peroxynitrite, which is formed from the reaction of NO with superoxide. NO and RNS may inhibit the mitochondrial respiratory chain, induce nitrosylation of proteins and enzymes, and cause cell apoptosis and necrosis.

the oxidation of sulfhydryls, lipid peroxidation, and RNA and DNA breakage (28–30); it reacts with thiols and induces the nitration of tyrosine residues in proteins to form nitrotyrosine, thus altering protein structure and function. In the highly oxidative milieu of reperfused tissue, nitrite, hypochlorous acid, and peroxidases are involved in chemical reactions that induce tyrosine nitration and contribute to tissue damage (29). The deleterious effects of RNS are mainly related to mitochondrial damage, collapse of the energetic capacity, the induction of apoptosis by the release of proteins from the mitochondria, and the induction of necrosis by lysis of plasma membrane (29,31).

Nitrates and nitrites are stable end-products of NO and can be measured in plasma, serum, urine, and other biologic fluids. Although the concentration of these metabolites may be influenced by liver and kidney function, dietary intake of nitrates, or pharmacologic intake of NO donors, increased levels of nitrite/nitrate in biologic samples indicate increased activation of NOS in septic patients and correlate with severity of illness and mortality scores (32). High levels of nitrites and nitrates can be also found in shock without sepsis or after organ transplantation, and they are suggestive of an exaggerated proinflammatory response with poor outcome (33).

Despite the deleterious effect of nitrosative stress on biomolecules, the use of inhibitors of NO synthesis does not appear to have any clinical utility in shock (34). In an effort to reverse the severe hypotension in septic patients, nonselective pharmacologic NOS inhibitors, which can repress NO production from both the constitutive and the inducible isoforms, have been tested in clinical trials in adults. Although treatment with these NOS inhibitors is able to increase mean arterial blood pressure, mortality is increased as well (35,36). Use of iNOS inhibitors has not been tested in the pediatric population.

Therefore, it appears that NO possesses complex functions serving either as a cytoprotective or cytotoxic agent. The functions depend on the amount of gas produced, the intracellular redox state, and the presence of other inflammatory mediators and free radicals. The complexity of these interactions adds to the difficulty of developing therapies that target this gas.

Decreased Activity of Antioxidant Mechanisms

Under physiologic conditions, cells have a substantial ability to tolerate reactive species by safely metabolizing them to water and other stable molecules through enzymatic and nonenzymatic pathways (37) (see Chapter 20). The enzymatic pathways involve superoxide dismutase (which catalyzes the formation of H_2O_2 from superoxide) and catalase and glutathione peroxidase (which catalyze the decomposition of hydrogen peroxide to water). The nonenzymatic pathways include intracellular antioxidants, such as vitamins C, E, and β-carotene, antioxidant minerals (copper, zinc, manganese, and selenium), ubiquinone, lipoic acid, uric acid, cysteine, and glutathione (GSH). (GSH serves as a reducing substrate for the enzymatic activity of glutathione peroxidase.) Thioredoxin and thioredoxin reductase form an additional redox regulatory system because they catalyze the regeneration of antioxidant molecules, such as ubiquinone (Q10), lipoic acid, and ascorbic acid.

Unfortunately, this orchestrated homeostasis fails when the robust reperfusion-induced generation of reactive species exceeds the cellular antioxidant capacity (37). Intracellular levels of GSH decline concomitant with an accumulation of the oxidized (inactive) form, glutathione disulfide (GSSG). Pathological decreases of other nonenzymatic antioxidants also occur during shock or reperfusion injury. For example, plasma levels of ascorbate and atrial levels of vitamin E are reduced in patients after cardiopulmonary bypass (38). A progressive compromise of antioxidant defenses has been characterized by ascorbate depletion, decreased glutathione levels, and increased lipid peroxidation in cerebrospinal fluid samples from infants and children with severe traumatic brain injury (39).

Oxidative stress and antioxidant capacity, in the pediatric age group, have not been adequately characterized. A prospective, double-blind, placebo-controlled, pilot study has reported that supplementation with antioxidants (vitamin E, vitamin C, and zinc) protected against oxidative stress and improved wound healing in burned children (40). Despite promising data from models of reperfusion injury and the availability of a wide array of antioxidant agents, it is still undetermined whether antioxidant supplementation has any clinical application in ischemia and reperfusion (41,42).

Direct Cytotoxic Effects of ROS and RNS

Damage of Macromolecules

ROS and RNS are extremely reactive and cause direct structural damage to many enzymes, proteins, lipids, and DNA. The most common chemical reactions include the oxidation of sulfhydryl groups and thioethers, as well as the nitration and hydroxylation of aromatic compounds. Modification of these macromolecules can cause the inactivation of critical enzymes and can induce denaturation that renders proteins nonfunctional. For example, tyrosine nitration induced by peroxynitrite or nitrogen derivatives can lead to the dysfunction of superoxide dismutase and cytoskeletal actin (31,37). Lipid peroxidation results in the disruption of the cell membrane and the membranes of cellular organelles, it also causes the release of highly cytotoxic products such as malondialdehyde. Oxidation of sulfhydryl groups is responsible for the inhibition of critical mitochondrial enzymes of the respiratory chain (28) (Fig. 21.6).

DNA Damage and Activation of Poly(ADP-Ribose) Polymerase-1

Another important interaction of ROS and RNS occurs with nucleic acids. Oxidative attack on the deoxyribose moiety will lead to the release of free bases from DNA, generating strand breaks with various sugar modifications and simple abasic sites (neither a purine nor pyrimidine base). Nitrosative attack will lead to nitrated guanine nucleosides and nucleotides,

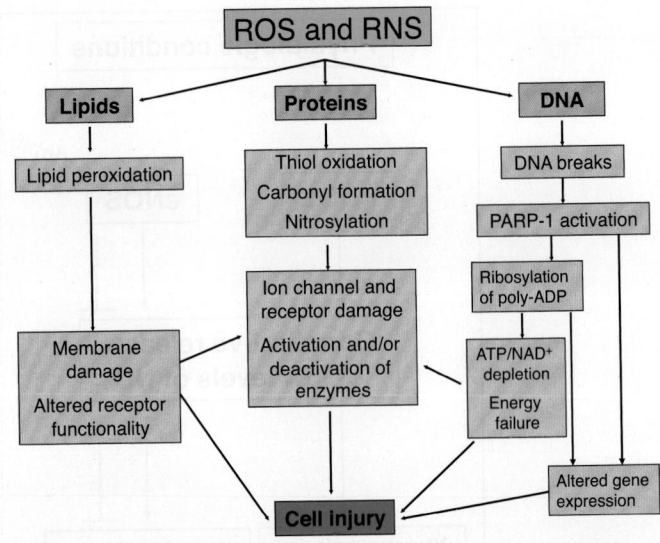

FIGURE 21.6. Direct cellular damage induced by ROS and RNS. ROS and RNS induce oxidation, carbonyl formation, and nitrosylation of lipids, proteins, and DNA. Modification of these macromolecules can cause disruption of the cell membrane, deactivation or activation of critical enzymes, and denaturation of ion pumps or membrane receptors. ROS and RNS also interact with DNA, generating strand breaks with various sugar modifications. In an attempt to repair DNA damage, poly(ADP-ribose) polymerase-1 (PARP-1) is activated. The process of poly(ADP-ribosyl)ation initiates an energy-consuming cycle, which rapidly depletes the intracellular NAD^+ and ATP energetic pools and alters gene expression, further enhancing cell injury.

which may further contribute to oxidative stress via the production of superoxide (mediated by various reductases) and may disturb or directly modulate various important enzymes, such as guanosine triphosphate (GTP)-binding proteins and cGMP-dependent enzymes. Alteration of the genetic material contributes then to the general decline in cellular functions and, ultimately, to cell death (29).

To maintain genomic stability, the cell employs many different repair pathways to remove DNA damage. Poly(ADP-ribose) polymerase (PARP)-1 is a chromatin-associated nuclear enzyme that recognizes DNA nicks and breaks and possesses DNA repair function. Once activated, PARP-1 cleaves NAD^+ into ADP-ribose and nicotinamide and attaches ADP-ribose polymers to various nuclear proteins. Although poly(ADP-ribosyl)ation is an attempt by the cell to repair DNA, this process is a *suicide phenomenon* that further amplifies tissue damage. PARP-1, in fact, initiates an energy-consuming cycle that rapidly depletes intracellular NAD^+ and ATP energetic pools, slows the rate of glycolysis and mitochondrial respiration, and progresses to a loss of cellular viability (43). Several experimental reports in rodents have demonstrated that the activation of PARP-1 is a major cytotoxic pathway of tissue injury in different pathologies associated with shock and reperfusion injury, including hemorrhagic shock, cardiopulmonary bypass, sepsis, and myocardial, cerebral, or splanchnic infarction (30,43–46). In addition to the energetic failure, PARP-1 activation and poly(ADP-ribosyl)ation also causes tissue damage by playing a role in gene expression. Experimental reports have suggested that PARP-1 alters the function of a variety of transcription factors, including the proinflammatory factor nuclear factor (NF)-κB and the cytoprotective heat shock factor-1 (HSF-1), thus modulating the gene expression of several inflammatory mediators (45,46). With respect to clinical studies, elevated plasma levels of oxidative DNA adducts were found in patients with myocardial infarction and were associated with increased activity of PARP-1 in circulating leukocytes (47). Activation of PARP-1 was also found in human skeletal muscle biopsies of children with severe burn injury (48). No study has evaluated the beneficial effect of PARP-1 inhibitors in critically ill patients.

Cytotoxic Effects by Activation of Molecular Signaling Pathways

Recruitment of Toll-Like Receptors by Pathogen and Damage-Associated Molecular Patterns

Pathophysiologic molecular mechanisms are triggered during shock and reperfusion, and they represent the first line of defense of the innate immune response to injury. Among these events, activation of toll-like receptors (TLRs) is a well-characterized phenomenon. TLRs are widely expressed on immune cells and on a variety of other cells, including vascular endothelial cells, adipocytes, cardiac myocytes, epithelial cells, and other parenchymal and nonparenchymal cells of tissues and organs (49). These receptors recognize exogenous PAMPs, such as lipopolysaccharides, lipoproteins, glycolipids and the DNA from bacteria, mycoplasma, and viruses during infection. TLRs also recognize DAMPs, which are endogenously released from dying host cells during ischemia and reperfusion even in the absence of infection (50). DAMPs include heat shock proteins, hyaluronic acid, heme, fibrinogen, surfactant protein A, heparin sulfate, and the nuclear high-mobility group box-1 protein. The specificity for ligand recognition depends on the recruitment of other co-receptors and adaptor proteins. Once activated, TLR-signaling cascades involve the activation of certain mitogen-activated protein kinases (MAPKs) and ultimately lead to the nuclear translocation of the transcription factor NF-κB with subsequent inflammatory mediator production. Genetic variability in these receptors has been proposed to result in differences in susceptibility to infectious diseases in adults and in children (51). Similarly, genetic polymorphisms or mutations of these receptors have been associated with genetic variability in outcomes after transplantation (52). For example, TLR4 and TLR2 gene polymorphisms have been associated with chronic allograft nephropathy among pediatric renal transplantation patients (53) and the mutation of TLR3 has been associated with a lower rate of acute rejection in adult liver transplanted patients (54). Because of the essential role of TLRs in shock and reperfusion, recent trials have tested the use of TLR antagonists to prevent the induction of the inflammatory cascade. Eritoran, a TLR4 antagonist, has been tested in sepsis (55,56). Initially found to be beneficial with a trend toward decreased mortality in a phase II randomized controlled trial (57), treatment with Eritoran failed to demonstrate an improvement in mortality in a phase III randomized trial in patients with severe sepsis (58). Eritoran has also been evaluated in renal and myocardial ischemia and reperfusion injury; in rodents, Eritoran reduced the inflammatory response and improved the course of organ injury (59,60). The therapeutic potentials of TLR antagonists in clinical settings of reperfusion injury are yet to be proven.

Activation of MAPKs and Transcription Factors

In addition to directly injuring cells, ROS and RNS have the potential to induce tissue damage through the regulation of signal transduction pathways that modulate the proinflammatory phenotype of the cell. Because of their reactivity, ROS and RNS induce structural and functional changes within the critical thiol groups or amino acid residues of MAPKs, which are important components of an extensive network of signal transduction pathways (61). MAPKs also mediate the transduction of extracellular signals from the receptor levels, for example, from TLRs to the nuclear transcription factors (see Chapter 19). These kinases activate each other by sequential steps of phosphorylation, whereas their inactivation is mediated through dephosphorylation by phosphatases. Important oxidant-sensitive kinases in shock and reperfusion injury include the extracellular signal-regulated kinase 1 and 2 (ERK 1/2), c-Jun amino-terminal kinase (JNK), p38 MAPK, and inhibitor κB kinase (IκK). Phosphorylation of ERK, JNK, p38, and IκK activates nuclear proteins and transcription factors and ultimately regulates the transcription of several genes of inflammatory mediators and immune modulators (61).

At the nuclear level, NF-κB is important in the expression of many genes, the proteins of which are involved in the inflammatory response (see Chapter 19). NF-κB is ubiquitously found in all mammalian cells and is usually present in the cytoplasm of the cell in an inactive state bound to an inhibitory protein known as inhibitor κBα (IκBα). A common pathway for the activation of NF-κB occurs when its inhibitor protein, IκBα, is phosphorylated by the upstream kinase IκK. After IκBα is phosphorylated, a process of proteolytic digestion of this protein is activated. Degradation of IκBα allows NF-κB to migrate to the nucleus, where it activates the transcription of target genes (62).

Specific MAPKs, such as JNK, control the activation of *fos* and *jun* family protooncogenes and their protein products (c-Fos, c-Jun, and others). These "early response protooncogene" products dimerize to form the activator protein (AP)-1, another nuclear transcription factor that is also purportedly regulated by ROS and RNS and involved in the expression of genes of inflammatory mediators (61). The final event of these signaling cascades is the rapid production of inflammatory mediators, which determine the functional outcome in response to stress. Downstream products of NF-κB and AP-1 activation include cell adhesion molecules and inflammatory cytokines (messenger molecules) that are important for leukocyte activation and leukocyte recruitment, for example, tumor necrosis factor (TNF)-α and NOS (regulator of vascular tone). It is important to note that several of the inflammatory mediators that are regulated by NF-κB and/or AP-1 (e.g., TNF-α and interleukin [IL]-1) can, in turn, further activate these transcription factors, thus creating a self-maintaining inflammatory cycle that increases the severity and duration of the inflammatory response (61,62) (**Fig. 21.7**).

Clinical data suggest a pathologic role for NF-κB in reperfusion injury, sepsis, and multiple organ failure. NF-κB binding has been shown in peripheral leukocytes of septic patients. Increased NF-κB-binding activity positively correlated with severity of illness, and it was significantly increased in nonsurvivors, compared with survivors, of septic shock (63,64). On the contrary, resolution of inflammation is associated with low DNA binding of the transcription factor. In patients with acute appendicitis, NF-κB DNA binding was elevated and correlated with the severity of symptoms. This increased activity returned to baseline values within 18 hours after appendectomy (65). In patients who underwent major vascular surgery, activation of NF-κB in neutrophils was significantly elevated and correlated with a higher incidence of postoperative organ dysfunction in comparison with patients who did not exhibit a marked elevation of NF-κB activation (66). In children who underwent congenital heart surgery on cardiopulmonary bypass, NF-κB nuclear translocation was examined in myocardial tissue samples, and it was found that the myocardial activation of NF-κB and the subsequent inflammatory cascade might contribute to the postoperative pathophysiology of congenital heart disease in infants and children (67).

These clinical findings suggest that NF-κB may represent a therapeutic target during shock and reperfusion injury. Numerous reports have demonstrated that pharmacologic

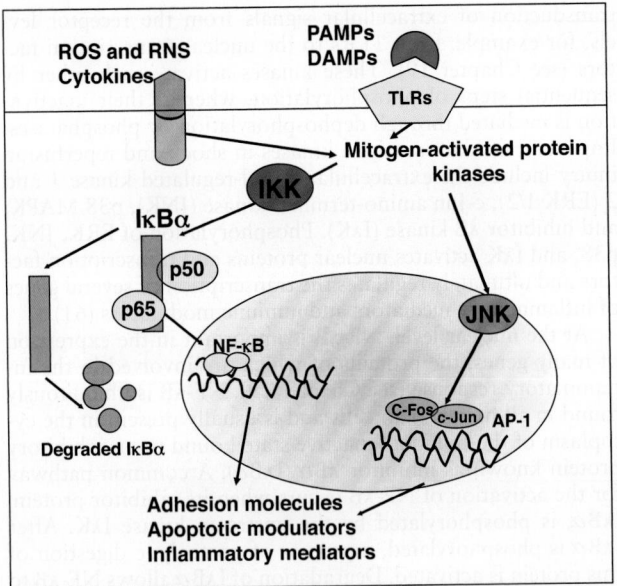

FIGURE 21.7. Activation of signal inflammatory pathways. ROS, RNS, cytokines, pathogen-associated molecular patterns (PAMPs) and damage-associated molecular patterns (DAMPs) are potent stimuli for the activation of a cascade of mitogen-activated protein kinases through various surface receptors, including toll-like receptors (TLRs). At the downstream of this cascade, the inhibitor κB kinase (IκK) phosphorylates inhibitor κBα (IκBα), allowing its proteolytic degradation. This event unmasks the nuclear factor-κB (NF-κB), which is free to translocate into the nucleus to initiate gene transcription. Similarly, c-Jun amino-terminal kinase (JNK) phosphorylates c-Jun, allowing its dimerization with c-Fos, thus forming the transcription factor activator protein (AP)-1. Activation of both NF-κB and AP-1 induces production of adhesion molecules, apoptotic modulators, and inflammatory mediators, such as cytokines and enzymes.

inhibitors of NF-κB exert beneficial effects in models of myocardial ischemia and reperfusion injury, hemorrhagic shock, and sepsis (62). This potential therapeutic approach has yet to be investigated in human studies.

Complement System Activation

The complement system is another important pathway of reperfusion injury. The principal biologic functions include cell lysis of foreign organisms, phagocytic clearance of immune complexes, antigen presentation to lymphocytes, and recruitment of inflammatory cells to the site of injury. The complement system consists of more than thirty plasma proteins, glycoproteins, and soluble or membrane-bound receptors. Most complement system proteins exist in plasma as inactive precursors that cleave and activate each other in a proteolytic cascade in response to different mechanisms. Three different pathways of activation have been described: *classical*, *alternative*, and *lectin-binding* (Fig. 21.8). The classical pathway is initiated by antigen–antibody complexes and/or inflammatory proteins, such as C-reactive protein and serum amyloid protein. The alternative pathway is initiated by surface molecules that contain carbohydrates and lipids, such as bacteria, fungal yeast cells, and some parasite surface molecules. The lectin-binding pathway is initiated by the binding of mannose-binding lectin protein (MBL) with carbohydrate ligands, resulting in the activation of MBL-associated serine-proteases (MASPs). Complement system components are numbered in the order in which they were discovered, which

is almost the same as the order in which they function in the activation cascade. Although the stimulating factors for each pathway are distinct, each one has a similar terminal sequence that creates the active factors C5a and the complex C5b–C59, also known as the *membrane attack complex* (MAC), which is believed to mediate tissue injury. C5a is one of the most proinflammatory peptides with pleiotropic functions. Upon binding to high-affinity receptors, such as the C5aR receptor on neutrophils, monocytes, and macrophages, C5a serves as a powerful *chemoattractant* for these cells and promotes their activation, leading to the oxidative burst and release of lysosomal enzymes and proinflammatory cytokines (68). C5a can also bind to specific C5aR receptor in epithelial cells and activate the release of inflammatory mediators, such as cytokines. MAC is the *killer* molecule of the complement system. Its main function is to disrupt the phospholipid bilayer of target cells, leading to cell lysis and death by the formation of transmembrane channels. MAC also has other important functions, which it shares with C5a. They activate the coagulation pathway, induce expression of adhesion molecules on endothelial cells and decrease the release of NO (causing vasoconstriction), thus amplifying the loss of vascular homeostasis and endothelial dysfunction (68,69). In addition, the classical, alternative, and lectin-binding pathways have as their by-products a number of *anaphylatoxins* and *opsonins*. Anaphylatoxins cause increased vascular permeability, smooth muscle contraction, and mast cell degranulation. Complement system fragments called *opsonins* adhere to microorganisms and promote leukocyte chemoattraction, antigen binding, phagocytosis, and the activation of macrophage and neutrophil-killing mechanisms. Under physiologic conditions, numerous inhibitory molecules are present in the plasma (serum proteases and complement system inhibitors) and on the endothelial surface (decay-accelerating factor and membrane cofactor protein), which protect the host against complement system injury (68,69).

Animal studies of ischemia and reperfusion injury in various organ systems, as well as clinical studies, support the concept that activation of the complement system is a crucial pathogenetic event of tissue injury (68,70). All three pathways are activated in ischemia and reperfusion injury and seem to be involved in an organ-dependent manner (69). Complement system activation has been demonstrated in myocardial infarction, in ischemia of the intestine, hind limb, kidney and liver, hemorrhagic shock, and sepsis. During cardiopulmonary bypass, the contact of blood with the artificial surfaces of the bypass equipment can also activate complement system proteins (69). In addition, endothelial dysfunction during reperfusion may alter the protective mechanism mediated by the complement system inhibitors, thus contributing to its exaggerated activation.

Numerous experimental studies have demonstrated beneficial effects of complement system inhibition in ischemia and reperfusion–induced injury (71). However, only a few clinical trials have been conducted. An evaluation of a C5 complement system monoclonal antibody, pexelizumab, in patients with myocardial infarction undergoing primary percutaneous coronary intervention, revealed no clinical benefit of treatment (72). Meta-analyses, regrouping data from trials in adults with coronary artery bypass graft surgery, suggested a selective reduction of mortality in high-risk patients (73,74). A recombinant soluble complement receptor type 1 (TP-10) has been developed for the potential treatment of reperfusion injury (following surgery, ischemic disease, and organ transplantation), organ rejection, acute inflammatory injury to the lungs, and autoimmune diseases (75). A phase I/II trial of TP-10 conducted in 15 children below 12 months of age who were undergoing cardiac surgery for congenital heart defects showed that TP10 administration was safe and appeared to decrease the complement system activation induced

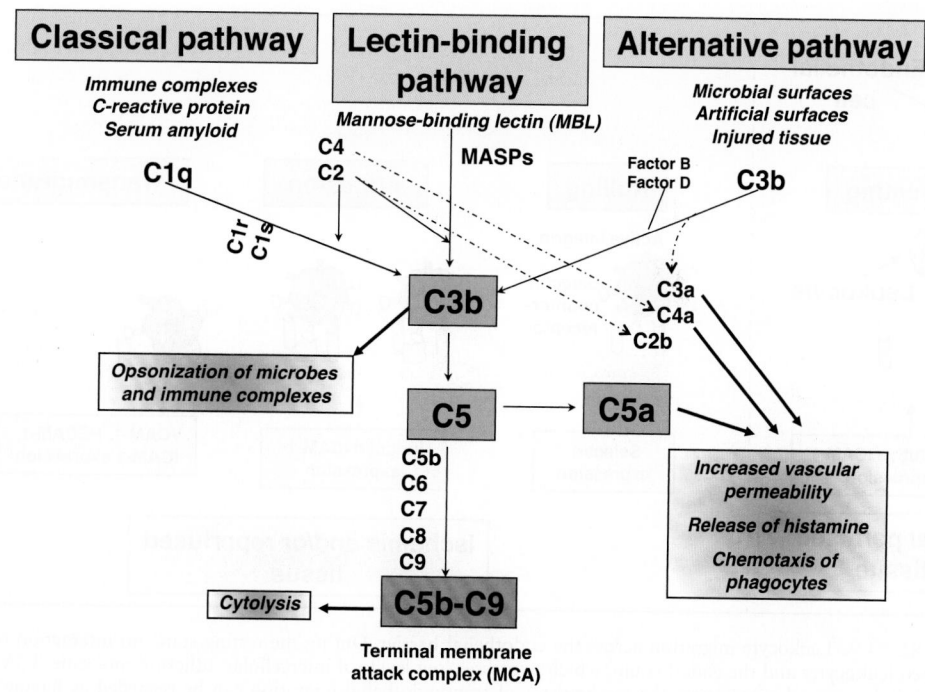

FIGURE 21.8. Activation of complement system. Three different pathways activate the complement system during shock and reperfusion: classical, lectin, and alternative pathway. The classical pathway is initiated by antigen–antibody complexes or inflammatory proteins, such as C-reactive protein and serum amyloid protein. The lectin pathway is initiated by the binding of mannose-binding lectin protein (MBL), resulting in activation of MBL-associated serine-proteases (MASPs). The alternative pathway is initiated by surface molecules that contain carbohydrates and lipids, such as bacterial, fungal yeast cell, and some parasite surface molecules. The terminal common step of these pathways is the activation of C5a and the complex C5b–C59, also known as the *membrane attack complex* (MAC), which mediates tissue injury. Other by-products of the complement cascade, *anaphylatoxins* and *opsonins*, contribute to tissue injury by facilitating phagocytosis and by increasing vascular permeability, smooth muscle contraction, and mast cell degranulation.

by cardiopulmonary bypass and to protect vascular function (76). Although unconfirmed, these clinical reports suggest that strategies to inhibit the complement system pathway may offer new therapeutic approaches to manage critically ill patients at risk for ischemia-reperfusion injury.

Endothelial Dysfunction

As a continuous monolayer on the luminal surfaces of both arteries and veins, the endothelium plays an essential role in the homeostasis of coagulation, fibrinolysis, angiogenesis, and vascular tone. In ischemia and reperfusion injury, the endothelium is one of the first organs to demonstrate signs of dysfunction and modification. As a result of oxidative stress and reduced bioavailability of the constitutive production of NO, vasodilation is impaired and vascular permeability increases, leading to edema formation and enhancement of interstitial pressure. When these detrimental changes occur in capillaries and arterioles, the local circulation of blood may be impaired, a phenomenon known as *no reflow*. Changes in endothelial adhesiveness occur that allow the recruitment of circulating leukocytes from the bloodstream into the ischemic tissue. This event plays an important physiologic role in the resolution of the damage, as leukocytes participate in the destruction of foreign antigens and in the remodeling of injured tissue. However, the recruitment and transmigration of leukocytes may further compromise the integrity of the endothelial barrier and augment damage to parenchymal cells. Activated leukocytes, indeed, release proteolytic enzymes (e.g., elastase, collagenase,

cathepsin, hyaluronidase), proinflammatory mediators and augment the oxidative burden by producing ROS and RNS. Furthermore, physical plugging of postcapillary venules and small arterioles by leukocytes contributes to the no-reflow phenomenon and exacerbates ischemic damage. Additionally, alteration of the endothelial surface and the aggregation and activation of platelets trigger dysregulation of the coagulation and fibrinolytic systems (77).

Recruitment and Transmigration of Leukocytes

The emigration of circulating leukocytes from the blood into the inflamed tissue involves a sequence of three complex steps: rolling, firm adhesion, and transmigration of leukocytes. This multistep process is coordinated by endothelial adhesion molecules, which are expressed on the endothelial surface and recognized by specific receptors on the leukocyte membrane (**Fig. 21.9**). Three families of adhesion molecules have been identified: the selectins, the immunoglobulin gene superfamily, and the integrins (78).

The selectin family mediates the initial interaction between leukocytes and endothelium, which results in the *rolling* of leukocytes along the wall of postcapillary venules at a very slow velocity, distinctly below that of flowing blood. Three members of the selectin family are named according to the cells in which they were originally discovered: P-selectin (platelets and endothelial cells), E-selectin (endothelial cells), and L-selectin

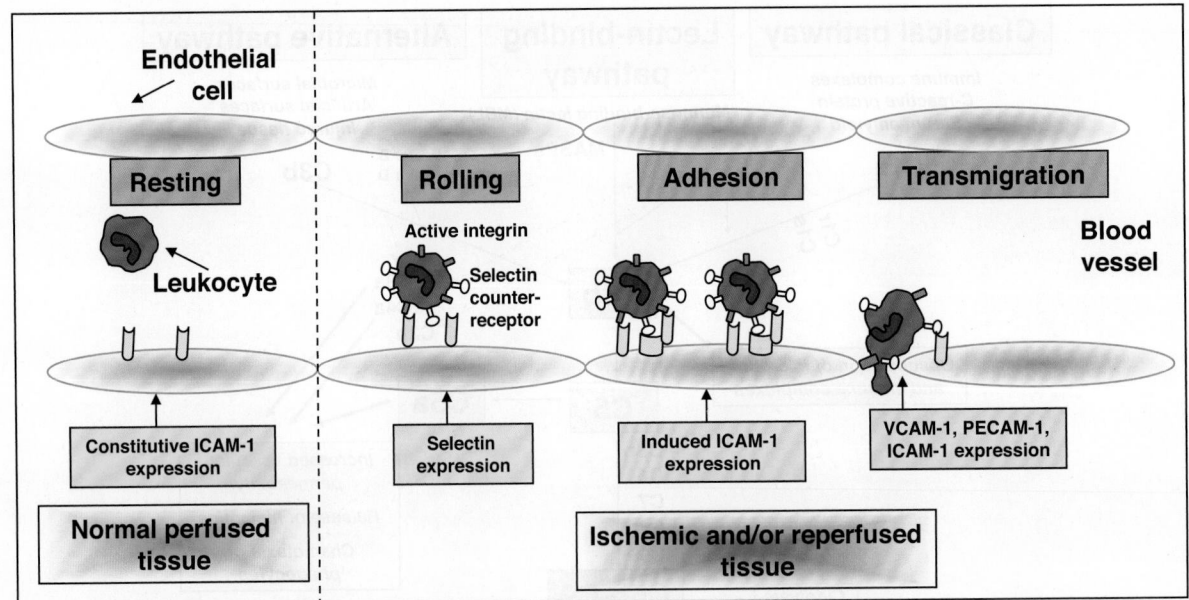

FIGURE 21.9. Leukocyte migration across the endothelial barrier. During the resting state, no interaction occurs between leukocytes and the endothelium, which expresses low levels of intercellular adhesion molecule (ICAM)-1. During ischemia and reperfusion, the mechanisms of transendothelial migration can be regarded as having three steps: rolling, adhesion, and transmigration. During the *rolling* phase, selectins are expressed on the surface of endothelial cells and corresponding ligands for selectins are expressed on leukocytes, leading to a slowing and attachment of circulating leukocytes to the vessel wall. During the *adhesion* and *transmigration phases, the interaction of* β_2 and β_1 integrins on the surface of leukocytes with immunoglobulin gene superfamily members, such as ICAM-1, VCAM-1, and PECAM-1, allows firm adhesion of leukocytes and their transmigration into the parenchyma.

(leukocytes). P-selectin is preformed and stored in α-granules of platelets and Weibel-Palade bodies of endothelial cells. It is rapidly translocated to the cell surface upon exposure to ROS and RNS, thrombin, histamine, or complement. E-selectin is expressed on the endothelial cells after stimulation with proinflammatory cytokines (TNF-α and IL-1) several hours following ischemia and reperfusion injury. The corresponding ligands for selectins on the surface of the leukocyte are sialylated Lewis^x and A blood-group antigens. The L-selectin of leukocytes also binds to a specific sulfated Lewisx ligand on endothelial cells and contributes to the rolling phase (78).

The rolling leukocytes require firm adhesion interactions to the vessel wall to migrate across the vascular endothelium into the tissues (78). *Firm adhesion* and *transmigration* are mediated by the interaction of β_2 integrins (also known as CD11/CD18) and β_1 integrins on the surface of leukocytes, with immunoglobulin gene superfamily members expressed by endothelium (78). Leukocyte integrins are activated by cytokines (IL-18), chemoattractants (e.g., leukotriene B4, C5a, platelet-activating factor), and chemoattractive chemokines during reperfusion injury. A detailed discussion of the mechanisms and the role of other chemokines is presented in Chapter 19.

The intercellular adhesion molecules (ICAMs), ICAM-1, ICAM-2, and ICAM-3; vascular cellular adhesion molecule (VCAM-1); and platelet–endothelial cell adhesion molecule (PECAM) are members of the immunoglobulin superfamily. ICAM-1 is the most characterized molecule for firm adhesion. It is constitutively expressed at low levels on the endothelium and further enhanced during inflammation on endothelial cells after exposure to oxidants or cytokines (78). In addition to endothelial cells, ICAM-1 is also present on leukocytes, epithelial cells, cardiomyocytes, and fibroblasts, thus allowing ICAM-1 to contribute to the tissue margination of leukocytes (79).

As a consequence of the modification of endothelial adhesiveness, platelets also accumulate in the vessels, resulting in further impairment of microcirculation and contributing to the prothrombotic phenotype of the endothelium. Circulating platelets roll, adhere to the endothelium or subendothelial matrix (using similar adhesion molecules), and release substances that cause further chemotaxis and migration of circulating leukocytes. This process is particularly relevant in the brain microvasculature, where shear forces are high, adhesion molecule expression is low, and platelets may play an important role as a bridge between the leukocytes and endothelium (80).

After expressed on the cell surface, adhesion molecules are rapidly shed into the bloodstream. The detection of these circulating adhesion molecules has been employed as a sensitive marker of endothelium dysfunction and has been widely reported in patients with sepsis or ischemic conditions. For example, increased blood levels of ICAM-1 in septic adults correlate well with the severity of inflammation and the course of sepsis (i.e., MODS and death) (81,82). In pediatric heart transplant recipients, systemic expression of adhesion molecules and plasma coagulation markers correlates with the occurrence of transplant coronary artery disease and/or rejection (83). Similarly, the upregulation and expression of soluble P-selectin indicates neutrophil activation in children who undergo cardiopulmonary bypass and correlates with length of surgery, aortic cross-clamping duration, inotropic support, postoperative Pediatric Risk of Mortality score, hypotension, and tachycardia (84).

Leukocyte transmigration into parenchyma is also dependent on focal matrix degradation mechanisms by the matrix metalloproteinases (MMPs) (85). MMPs are a family of specialized zinc-dependent proteases that play key roles in the physiological processes of remodeling and tissue repair. However, inappropriate or prolonged activation of MMPs may have harmful consequences in shock or reperfusion. In human orthotopic liver transplantation, the plasma concentration of MMP-9 after surgery correlated with elevation of aspartate aminotransferase levels and liver damage (86). Upregulation of MMP-9 expression, in the proximal tubule in renal allograft biopsies of children and adults, was associated with an increased risk for acute cellular rejection (87). Early increase of plasma MMP-2 was predictive of infarct size and ventricular dysfunction in patients with myocardial infarction (88). The exacerbation of MMP activity is also consequent to impairment of the regulatory tissue inhibitors of metalloproteinases (TIMP 1-4) during oxidative stress (89,90). Elevated plasma MMPs and TIMPs have also been detected in clinical studies of patients with severe sepsis. Only MMP-7 and MMP-9 appear to negatively correlate with disease severity (multiple organ dysfunctions) in adults (91). Increased MMP-8 mRNA expression and activity correlates with decreased survival and increased organ failure in children with septic shock (92).

Because the abnormal sequestration of leukocytes is a central component in the development of reperfusion injury, therapeutic strategies that employ the use of antibodies raised against adhesion molecules have been attempted to inhibit the inflammatory response. Experimental studies in a number of animal models of myocardial, splanchnic, cerebral, and hepatic ischemia and reperfusion injury have been promising (93). Experimental studies in rodents have further confirmed the pathogenetic role of MMPs in shock, and reperfusion as genetic or pharmacological inhibition of MMPs confers resistance to ischemia and reperfusion injury (94) and sepsis (92). In the clinical setting, however, antibodies raised against adhesion molecules have not been efficacious in organ transplantation, hemorrhagic shock, or myocardial infarction (79,93,95–97). More promising results have been reported with the use of MMP inhibitors, such as the tetracycline class of antibiotics, in patients undergoing endovascular aneurysm repair (98).

LABORATORY TESTS AND BIOMARKERS

Although there are no specific or gold standard biomarkers for shock, current laboratory tests have focused on markers associated with the different components of the ischemic cascade and the reperfusion injury, including the oxygenation state, oxidative and inflammatory processes, endothelial dysfunction, and tissue necrosis. When interpreted in the clinical context, these biomarkers provide information on the progression of shock and are valid complementary tools to monitor and titrate therapy.

Oxygen delivery, oxygen consumption, and tissue acidosis are the main variables that are evaluated for determining tissue perfusion and oxygenation. The mixed venous O_2 saturation ($S\bar{v}O_2$) or the central venous O_2 saturation ($ScvO_2$), serum lactate, and base deficit are the most commonly used parameters to provide information about the degree of oxygenation and anaerobic metabolism (99).

In critically ill patients, sustained $ScvO_2$ levels below 65% indicate ineffective Do_2 (see also **Fig. 21.1**). However, these biomarkers must be interpreted in the clinical context of the specific disease or type of shock. For example, normal $ScvO_2$ levels or above 75% can also be indicative of ineffective oxygen consumption when there is impaired cellular or mitochondrial oxygen extraction capability in patients with distributive septic shock or cyanide poisoning (100).

The onset of anaerobic metabolism is characterized by an increase in *serum lactate* levels (101). With the ongoing tissue hypoxia, other mechanisms can cause or contribute to hyperlactemia. Such mechanisms include excessive, or prolonged, catecholamine release, which stimulates glycolysis, and hepatic failure causing decreased lactic acid clearance. Several clinical studies have demonstrated a correlation between serum

lactate and outcome; both the duration and degree of hyperlactemia are important predictors of morbidity and mortality (102–104). Similarly, the resolution of hyperlactemia is associated with survival in critically ill patients (105,106).

Serial *C-reactive protein (CRP)* measurements may reflect the progression of the inflammatory process. It is an acute phase reactant, which is synthesized by hepatocytes in response to cytokine stimulation. Normal plasma levels of CRP are usually <10 mg/L. Plasma levels increase within 4–6 hours after initial tissue injury and continue to increase several hundred fold within 24–48 hours. CRP remains elevated during the acute phase response and returns to normal with resolution of tissue damage.

Procalcitonin (PCT) is considered a sensitive biomarker for sepsis. PCT in healthy individuals is secreted only in neuroendocrine cells of the thyroid. However, during a state of infection, especially in sepsis, PCT is released from nearly all tissues and cell types in the body in response to cytokines and bacterial products (107). Serial PCT levels have been correlated to severity of disease, multiple organ failure, and mortality, indicating that PCT appears to be a useful indicator of outcome (108).

With the onset of inflammation and endothelial dysfunction, a number of other markers such as inflammatory cytokines (IL-1β, IL-6, IL-8, TNF-α), metabolites of iNOS, and soluble adhesion molecules are also elevated in the serum of critically ill patients (81,108). These markers have been evaluated for their predictive value of the development of multiple organ failure and subsequent mortality in several clinical trials. Unfortunately, they do not appear to have a reliable prognostic value and, therefore, are not used in the routine diagnostic assessment of the patients.

In the presence of cell dysfunction and necrosis, many biomarkers are able to detect whether tissue or organ is damaged. For example, functional biomarkers such as serum creatinine measurement add diagnostic and prognostic utility in kidney injury. Recently, neutrophil gelatinase-associated lipocalin has been proposed as a plasma or urine biomarker for the early diagnosis of acute kidney injury and for the prediction of clinical outcomes such as dialysis requirement and mortality in several critical care scenarios (109). Similarly, increases above reference values in serum activities of cardiac, hepatic, or pancreatic enzymes, which are leaking from dying cells, are indicative of disease in that organ.

Because of the complexity of the molecular mechanisms of shock and reperfusion injury, it must be considered that no single marker can accurately predict clinical course and outcome. Laboratory parameters may have to be combined and, of course, complemented with other diagnostic tools. With the completion of the human genome project, recent studies are proposing novel and exciting approaches using genome-wide expression profiling in pediatric septic shock (108). These studies are allowing the identification of pools of new candidate genes as biomarkers, which can be used as new diagnostic tests to stratify patients and guide therapy.

CONCLUSIONS AND FUTURE DIRECTIONS

Several mechanisms cooperate in a complementary and synergistic manner in the pathophysiology of ischemia and reperfusion injury. The knowledge of the precise sequence of these biochemical and molecular events has enormous clinical relevance because it would imply the possibility of improving recovery using specific interventions that would target these cellular pathways. As described throughout the chapter, most basic science studies, which have been conducted in experimental animals, have reported that the use of antioxidants, antibodies against adhesion molecules, or the inhibition of complement factors, MMPs, PARP-1, and/or NF-κB, may prevent, or delay, cell death. Despite many studies, no definitive clinical indications have been revealed for the clinical application of these novel agents in shock and reperfusion injury. Multiple clinical trials have attempted to alter the progression of the inflammatory response in adults. Although successful progress in some clinical trials has been reported, other novel strategies have failed. Reasons for these equivocal results may include individual injury patterns, inappropriate timing of drug administration, suboptimal drug levels at the target site, and inadequate stratification or selection of patients. In addition, study protocols have focused on single mechanisms, whereas the inflammatory network of reperfusion is complex, including several concomitant and interconnected pathways. In the PICU, novel therapeutic drug protocols are limited by the paucity of information related to these agents in children. In the future, a better understanding of the pathologic mechanisms at the site of injury will identify exact primary targets for drug interventions. In addition, progress in diagnostic tools for the monitoring of inflammatory status may provide valuable information for the appropriate timing and management of critically ill patients.

References

1. American Heart Association. 2005 American Heart Association guidelines for cardiopulmonary resuscitation and emergency cardiovascular care of pediatric and neonatal patients: Pediatric advanced life support. *Pediatrics* 2006;117:E1005–28.
2. Taegtmeyer H, King LM, Jones BE. Energy substrate metabolism, myocardial ischemia, and targets for pharmacotherapy. *Am J Cardiol* 1998;82:K54–60.
3. Ferdinandy P, Schulz R. Nitric oxide, superoxide, and peroxynitrite in myocardial ischaemia-reperfusion injury and preconditioning. *Br J Pharmacol* 2003;138:532–43.
4. Bernardi P, Krauskopf A, Basso E, et al. The mitochondrial permeability transition from in vitro artifact to disease target. *FEBS J* 2006;273:2077–99.
5. Halestrap AP. A pore way to die: The role of mitochondria in reperfusion injury and cardioprotection. *Biochem Soc Trans* 2010;38:841–60.
6. Meneshian A, Bulkley GB. The physiology of endothelial xanthine oxidase: From urate catabolism to reperfusion injury to inflammatory signal transduction. *Microcirculation* 2002;9:161–75.
7. Friedl HP, Smith DJ, Till GO, et al. Ischemia-reperfusion in humans: Appearance of xanthine oxidase activity. *Am J Pathol* 1990;136:491–5.
8. Pesonen EJ, Linder N, Raivio KO, et al. Circulating xanthine oxidase and neutrophil activation during human liver transplantation. *Gastroenterology* 1998;114:1009–15.
9. Nemeth I, Boda D. Xanthine oxidase activity and blood glutathione redox ratio in infants and children with septic shock syndrome. *Intensive Care Med* 2001;27:216–21.
10. Lee BE, Toledo AH, Anaya-Prado R, et al. Allopurinol, xanthine oxidase, and cardiac ischemia. *J Investig Med* 2009;57:902–9.
11. Pacher P, Nivorozhkin A, Szabó C. Therapeutic effects of xanthine oxidase inhibitors: Renaissance half a century after the discovery of allopurinol. *Pharmacol Rev* 2006;58:87–114.
12. Kaandorp JJ, Van Bel F, Veen S, et al. Long-term neuroprotective effects of allopurinol after moderate perinatal asphyxia: Follow-up of two randomised controlled trials. *Arch Dis Child Fetal Neonatal Ed* 2012;97:F162–6. Randomized Clinical Trial.
13. Chaudhari T, McGuire W. Allopurinol for preventing mortality and morbidity in newborn infants with suspected hypoxic-ischaemic encephalopathy. *Cochrane Database Syst Rev* 2008;CD006817. Meta-analysis.
14. Brandes RP, Weissmann N, Schröder K. NADPH oxidases in cardiovascular disease. *Free Radic Biol Med* 2010;49(5):687–706.
15. Hahn NE, Meischl C, Kawahara T, et al. NOX5 expression is increased in intramyocardial blood vessels and cardiomyocytes after acute myocardial infarction in humans. *Am J Pathol* 2012;180:2222–9.
16. Krijnen PA, Meischl C, Hack CE, et al. Increased Nox2 expression in human cardiomyocytes after acute myocardial infarction. *J Clin Pathol* 2003;56:194–9.
17. Janiszewski M, Do Carmo AO, Pedro MA, et al. Platelet-derived exosomes of septic individuals possess proapoptotic NAD(P)H oxidase activity: A novel vascular redox pathway. *Crit Care Med* 2004;32:818–25.
18. Ago T, Kuroda J, Kamouchi M, et al. Pathophysiological roles of NADPH oxidase/nox family proteins in the vascular system. Review and perspective. *Circ J* 2011;75:1791–800.
19. Wagner AH, Köhler T, Rückschloss U, et al. Improvement of nitric oxide-dependent vasodilatation by HMG-CoA reductase inhibitors through attenuation of endothelial superoxide anion formation. *Arterioscler Thromb Vasc Biol* 2000;20:61–9.
20. Al-Awwadi NA, Araiz C, Bornet A, et al. Extracts enriched in different polyphenolic families normalize increased cardiac NADPH oxidase expression while having differential effects on insulin resistance, hypertension, and cardiac hypertrophy in high-fructose-fed rats. *J Agric Food Chem* 2005;53:151–7.
21. Lambeth JD, Krause KH, Clark RA. NOX enzymes as novel targets for drug development. *Semin Immunopathol* 2008;30:339–63.
22. Bian K, Murad F. Nitric oxide: Biogeneration, regulation, and relevance to human diseases. *Front Biosci* 2003;8:D264–78.
23. Massion PB, Feron O, Dessy C, et al. Nitric oxide and cardiac function: Ten years after, and continuing. *Circ Res* 2003;93:388–98.
24. Ma XL, Weyrich AS, Lefer DJ, et al. Diminished basal nitric oxide release after myocardial ischemia and reperfusion promotes neutrophil adherence to coronary endothelium. *Circ Res* 1993;72:403–12.
25. Schulz R, Kelm M, Heusch G. Nitric oxide in myocardial ischemia/reperfusion injury. *Cardiovasc Res* 2004;61:402–13.
26. Kietadisorn R, Juni RP, Moens AL. Tackling endothelial dysfunction by modulating NOS uncoupling: New insights into its pathogenesis and therapeutic possibilities. *Am J Physiol Endocrinol Metab* 2012;302:E481–95.
27. Kinsella JP, Abman SH. Inhaled nitric oxide therapy in children. *Paediatr Respir Rev* 2005;6:190–8.
28. Alvarez B, Radi R. Peroxynitrite reactivity with amino acids and proteins. *Amino Acids* 2003;25:295–311.
29. Halliwell B. Free radicals, proteins, and DNA: Oxidative damage versus redox regulation. *Biochem Soc Trans* 1996;24:1023–7.
30. Zingarelli B, O'Connor M, Wong H, et al. Peroxynitrite-mediated DNA strand breakage activates poly-adenosine diphosphate ribosyl synthetase and causes cellular energy depletion in macrophages stimulated with bacterial lipopolysaccharide. *J Immunol* 1996;156:350–8.
31. Ischiropoulos H. Biological selectivity and functional aspects of protein tyrosine nitration. *Biochem Biophys Res Commun* 2003;305:776–83.
32. Carcillo JA, Fields AI, American College of Critical Care Medicine Task Force Committee Members. Clinical practice parameters for hemodynamic support of pediatric and neonatal patients in septic shock. *Crit Care Med* 2002;30:1365–78.
33. Wong HR, Carcillo JA, Burckart G, et al. Nitric oxide production in critically ill patients. *Arch Dis Child* 1996;74:482–9.
34. De Cruz SJ, Kenyon NJ, Sandrock CE. Bench-to-bedside review: The role of nitric oxide in sepsis. *Expert Rev Respir Med* 2009;3:511–21.
35. Lopez A, Lorente JA, Steingrub J, et al. Multiple-center, randomized, placebo-controlled, double-blind study of the nitric oxide synthase inhibitor 546C88: Effect on survival in patients with septic shock. *Crit Care Med* 2004;32:21–30. Randomized Clinical Trial.

36. Watson D, Grover R, Anzueto A, et al. Cardiovascular effects of the nitric oxide synthase inhibitor NG-methyl-L-arginine hydrochloride (546C88) in patients with septic shock: Results of a randomized, double-blind, placebo-controlled multicenter study (study no. 144–002). *Crit Care Med* 2004;32:13–20. Randomized Clinical Trial.

37. Nordberg J, Arner ES. Reactive oxygen species, antioxidants, and the mammalian thioredoxin system. *Free Radic Biol Med* 2001;31:1287–312.

38. Ballmer PE, Reinhart WH, Jordan P, et al. Depletion of plasma vitamin C but not of vitamin E in response to cardiac operations. *J Thorac Cardiovasc Surg* 1994;108:311–20. Randomized Clinical Trial.

39. Bayir H, Kagan VE, Tyurina YY, et al. Assessment of antioxidant reserves and oxidative stress in cerebrospinal fluid after severe traumatic brain injury in infants and children. *Pediatr Res* 2002;51:571–8.

40. Barbosa E, Faintuch J, Machado Moreira EA, et al. Supplementation of vitamin E, vitamin C, and zinc attenuates oxidative stress in burned children: A randomized, double-blind, placebo-controlled pilot study. *J Burn Care Res* 2009;30:859–66. Randomized Clinical Trial.

41. Granot E, Kohen R. Oxidative stress in childhood—In health and disease states. *Clin Nutr* 2004;23:3–11.

42. Mishra V. Oxidative stress and role of antioxidant supplementation in critical illness. *Clin Lab* 2007;53:199–209.

43. Chiarugi A. Poly(ADP-ribose) polymerase: Killer or conspirator? The "suicide hypothesis" revisited. *Trends Pharmacol Sci* 2002;23:122–9.

44. Zingarelli B. Importance of poly (ADP-ribose) polymerase activation in myocardial reperfusion injury. In: Szabó C, ed. *Cell Death: The Role of Poly(ADP-ribose) Polymerase*. Boca Raton, FL: CRC Press LLC, 2000:41–60.

45. Zingarelli B, Hake PW, O'Connor M, et al. Absence of poly(ADP-ribose) polymerase-1 alters nuclear factor-κB activation and gene expression of apoptosis regulators after reperfusion injury. *Mol Med* 2003;9:143–53.

46. Zingarelli B, Hake PW, O'Connor M, et al. Differential regulation of activator protein-1 and heat shock factor-1 in myocardial ischemia and reperfusion injury: Role of poly(ADP-ribose) polymerase-1. *Am J Physiol Heart Circ Physiol* 2004;286:H1408–15.

47. Tóth-Zsámboki E, Horváth E, Vargova K, et al. Activation of poly(ADP-ribose) polymerase by myocardial ischemia and coronary reperfusion in human circulating leukocytes. *Mol Med* 2006;12:221–8.

48. Oláh G, Finnerty CC, Sbrana E, et al. Increased poly(ADP-ribosyl)ation in skeletal muscle tissue of pediatric patients with severe burn injury: Prevention by propranolol treatment. *Shock* 2011;36:18–23.

49. Akira S, Takeda K, Kaisho T. Toll-like receptors: Critical proteins linking innate and acquired immunity. *Nat Immunol* 2001;2:675–80.

50. Lorne E, Dupont H, Abraham E. Toll-like receptors 2 and 4: Initiators of non-septic inflammation in critical care medicine? *Intensive Care Med* 2010;36:1826–35.

51. Netea MG, Wijmenga C, O'Neill LA. Genetic variation in toll-like receptors and disease susceptibility. *Nat Immunol* 2012;13:535–42.

52. Krüger B, Schröppel B, Murphy BT. Genetic polymorphisms and the fate of the transplanted organ. *Transplant Rev (Orlando)* 2008;22:131–40.

53. Mutlubas F, Mir S, Berdeli A, et al. Association between toll-like receptors 4 and 2 gene polymorphisms with chronic allograft nephropathy in Turkish children. *Transplant Proc* 2009;41:1589–93.

54. Citores MJ, Baños I, Noblejas A, et al. Toll-like receptor 3 L412F polymorphism may protect against acute graft rejection in adult patients undergoing liver transplantation for hepatitis C-related cirrhosis. *Transplant Proc* 2011;43:2224–6.

55. Makkouk A, Abdelnoor AM. The potential use of toll-like receptor (TLR) agonists and antagonists as prophylactic and/or therapeutic agents. *Immunopharmacol Immunotoxicol* 2009;31:331–8.

56. Wittebole X, Castanares-Zapatero D, Laterre PF. Toll-like receptor 4 modulation as a strategy to treat sepsis. *Mediators Inflamm* 2010;2010:568396.

57. Tidswell M, Tillis W, Larosa SP, et al. Phase 2 trial of eritoran tetrasodium (E5564), a toll-like receptor 4 antagonist, in patients with severe sepsis. *Crit Care Med* 2010;38:72–83.

58. Matsuyama K. Eisai's sepsis drug eritoran fails to save more lives in final-stage study. Bloomberg Web site 2011. http://www.bloomberg.com/news/2011-01-25/eisai-s-sepsis-drug-eritoran-fails-to-save-more-lives-in-final-stage.html

59. Liu M, Gu M, Xu D, et al. Protective effects of toll-like receptor 4 inhibitor eritoran on renal ischemia-reperfusion injury. *Transplant Proc* 2010;42:1539–44.

60. Shimamoto A, Chong AJ, Yada M, et al. Inhibition of toll-like receptor 4 with eritoran attenuates myocardial ischemia-reperfusion injury. *Circulation* 2006;114(suppl 1):I270–4.

61. Yoshizumi M, Tsuchiya K, Tamaki T. Signal transduction of reactive oxygen species and mitogen-activated protein kinases in cardiovascular disease. *J Med Invest* 2001;48:11–24.

62. Zingarelli B, Sheehan M, Wong HR. Nuclear factor-κB as a therapeutic target in critical care medicine. *Crit Care Med* 2003;31:S105–11.

63. Bohrer H, Qiu F, Zimmermann T, et al. Role of NF-κB in the mortality of sepsis. *J Clin Invest* 1997;100:972–85.

64. Paterson RL, Galley HF, Dhillon JK, et al. Increased nuclear factor κB activation in critically ill patients who die. *Crit Care Med* 2000;28:1047–51.

65. Pennington C, Dunn J, Li C, et al. Nuclear factor-κB activation in acute appendicitis: A molecular marker for extent of disease? *Am Surg* 2000;66:914–8.

66. Foulds S, Galustian C, Mansfield AO, et al. Transcription factor NF-κB expression and postsurgical organ dysfunction. *Ann Surg* 2001;233:70–8.

67. Mou SS, Haudek SB, Lequier L, et al. Myocardial inflammatory activation in children with congenital heart disease. *Crit Care Med* 2002;30:827–32.

68. Guo RF, Ward PA. Role of C5a in inflammatory responses. *Annu Rev Immunol* 2005;23:821–52.

69. Hart ML, Walsh MC, Stahl GL. Initiation of complement activation following oxidative stress: *In vitro* and *in vivo* observations. *Mol Immunol* 2004;41:165–71.

70. Arumugam TV, Shiels IA, Woodruff TM, et al. The role of the complement system in ischemia-reperfusion injury. *Shock* 2004;21:401–9.

71. Bhole D, Stahl GL. Therapeutic potential of targeting the complement cascade in critical care medicine. *Crit Care Med* 2003;31(suppl 1):S97–104.

72. Martel C, Granger CB, Ghitescu M, et al. Pexelizumab fails to inhibit assembly of the terminal complement complex in patients with ST-elevation myocardial infarction undergoing primary percutaneous coronary intervention. Insight from a substudy of the assessment of pexelizumab in acute myocardial infarction (APEX-AMI) trial. *Am Heart J* 2012;164:43–51. Randomized Clinical Trial.

73. Smith PK, Shernan SK, Chen JC, et al. Effects of C5 complement inhibitor pexelizumab on outcome in high-risk coronary artery bypass grafting: Combined results from the PRIMO-CABG I and II trials. *J Thorac Cardiovasc Surg* 2011;142:89–98. Randomized Clinical Trial.

74. Testa L, Van Gaal WJ, Bhindi R, et al. Pexelizumab in ischemic heart disease: A systematic review and meta-analysis on 15,196 patients. *J Thorac Cardiovasc Surg* 2008;136:884–93. Meta-analysis.

75. Rioux P. TP-10 (AVANT immunotherapeutics). *Curr Opin Investig Drugs* 2001;2:364–71.

76. Li JS, Sanders SP, Perry AE, et al. Pharmacokinetics and safety of TP10, soluble complement receptor 1, in infants undergoing cardiopulmonary bypass. *Am Heart J* 2004;147:173–80.

77. Seal JB, Gewertz BL. Vascular dysfunction in ischemia-reperfusion injury. *Ann Vasc Surg* 2005;19:572–84.

78. Malik AB, Lo SK. Vascular endothelial adhesion molecules and tissue inflammation. *Pharmacol Rev* 1996;48:213–29.

79. Yonekawa K, Harlan JM. Targeting leukocyte integrins in human diseases. *J Leukoc Biol* 2005;77:129–40.

80. Liu L, Kubes P. Molecular mechanisms of leukocyte recruitment: Organ-specific mechanisms of action. *Thromb Haemost* 2003;89:213–20.

81. Reinhart K, Bayer O, Brunkhorst F, et al. Markers of endothelial damage in organ dysfunction and sepsis. *Crit Care Med* 2002;30:S302–12.

82. Sessler C, Windsor A, Schwartz M. Circulating ICAM-1 is increased in septic shock. *Am J Respir Crit Care Med* 1995;151:1420–7.

83. Hilgendorff A, Kraemer U, Afsharian M, et al. Value of soluble adhesion molecules and plasma coagulation markers in assessing transplant coronary artery disease in pediatric heart transplant recipients. *Pediatr Transplant* 2006;10:434–40.

84. Lotan D, Prince T, Dagan O, et al. Soluble P-selectin and the postoperative course following cardiopulmonary bypass in children. *Paediatr Anaesth* 2001;11:303–8.

85. Sternlicht MD, Werb Z. How matrix metalloproteinases regulate cell behavior. *Annu Rev Cell Dev Biol* 2001;17:463–516.

86. Kuyvenhoven JP, Ringers J, Verspaget HW, et al. Serum matrix metalloproteinase MMP-2 and MMP-9 in the late phase of ischemia and reperfusion injury in human orthotopic liver transplantation. *Transplant Proc* 2003;35:2967–9.

87. Kitajima K, Koike J, Nozawa S, et al. Irreversible immunoexpression of matrix metalloproteinase-9 in proximal tubular epithelium of renal allografts with acute rejection. *Clin Transplant* 2011;25:E336–44.

88. Nilsson L, Hallén J, Atar D, et al. Early measurements of plasma matrix metalloproteinase-2 predict infarct size and ventricular dysfunction in ST-elevation myocardial infarction. *Heart* 2012;98:31–6. Randomized Clinical Trial.

89. Baker AH, Edwards DR, Murphy G. Metalloproteinase inhibitors: Biological actions and therapeutic opportunities. *J Cell Sci* 2002;115:3719–27.

90. Donnini S, Monti M, Roncone R, et al. Peroxynitrite inactivates human-tissue inhibitor of metalloproteinase-4. *FEBS Lett* 2008;582:1135–40.

91. Yazdan-Ashoori P, Liaw P, Toltl L, et al. Elevated plasma matrix metalloproteinases and their tissue inhibitors in patients with severe sepsis. *J Crit Care* 2011;26:556–65.

92. Solan PD, Dunsmore KE, Denenberg AG, et al. A novel role for matrix metalloproteinase-8 in sepsis. *Crit Care Med* 2012;40:379–87.

93. Anaya-Prado R, Toledo-Pereyra LH, Lentsch AB, et al. Ischemia/reperfusion injury. *J Surg Res* 2002;105:248–58.

94. Coito AJ. Leukocyte transmigration across endothelial and extracellular matrix protein barriers in liver ischemia/reperfusion injury. *Curr Opin Organ Transplant* 2011;16(1):34–40.

95. Baran KW, Nguyen M, McKendall GR, et al. Double-blind, randomized trial of an anti-CD18 antibody in conjunction with recombinant tissue plasminogen activator for acute myocardial infarction: Limitation of myocardial infarction following thrombolysis in acute myocardial infarction (LIMIT AMI) study. *Circulation* 2001;104:2778–83. Randomized Clinical Trial.

96. Faxon DP, Gibbons RJ, Chronos NA, et al. The effect of blockade of the CD11/CD18 integrin receptor on infarct size in patients with acute myocardial infarction treated with direct angioplasty: The results of the HALT-MI study. *J Am Coll Cardiol* 2002;40:1199–204. Randomized Clinical Trial.

97. Rhee P, Morris J, Durham R, et al. Recombinant humanized monoclonal antibody against CD18 (rhuMAb CD18) in traumatic hemorrhagic shock: Results of a phase II clinical trial. Traumatic Shock Group. *J Trauma* 2000;49:611–20.

98. Hackmann AE, Rubin BG, Sanchez LA, et al. A randomized, placebo-controlled trial of doxycycline after endoluminal aneurysm repair. *J Vasc Surg* 2008;48:519–26. Randomized Clinical Trial.

99. Wilson M, Davis DP, Coimbra R. Diagnosis and monitoring of hemorrhagic shock during the initial resuscitation of multiple trauma patients: A review. *J Emerg Med* 2003;24:413–22.

100. Walley KR. Use of central venous oxygen saturation to guide therapy. *Am J Respir Crit Care Med* 2011;184:514–20.

101. Kjelland CB, Djogovic D. The role of serum lactate in the acute care setting. *J Intensive Care Med* 2010;25:286–300.

102. Manikis P, Jankowski S, Zhang H, et al. Correlation of serial blood lactate levels to organ failure and mortality after trauma. *Am J Emerg Med* 1995;13:619–22. Prospective observational study.

103. Trzeciak S, Dellinger RP, Chansky ME, et al. Serum lactate as a predictor of mortality in patients with infection. *Intensive Care Med* 2007;33:970–7. Post-hoc Analysis of a Prospectively Compiled Registry.

104. Khosravani H, Khosravani H, Shahpori R, et al. Occurrence and adverse effect on outcome of hyperlactatemia in the critically ill. *Crit Care* 2009;13:R90. Multicenter Retrospective Clinical Study.

105. Jansen TC, van Bommel J, Schoonderbeek FJ, et al. Early lactate-guided therapy in intensive care unit patients: A multicenter, open-label, randomized controlled trial. *Am J Respir Crit Care Med* 2010;182:752–61. Randomized Clinical Trial.

106. Nguyen HB, Rivers EP, Knoblich BP, et al. Early lactate clearance is associated with improved outcome in severe sepsis and septic shock. *Crit Care Med* 2004;32:1637–42. Prospective Observational Study.

107. Riedel S. Procalcitonin and the role of biomarkers in the diagnosis and management of sepsis. *Diagn Microbiol Infect Dis* 2012;73:221–7.

108. Standage SW, Wong HR. Biomarkers for pediatric sepsis and septic shock. *Expert Rev Anti Infect Ther* 2011;9:71–9.

109. Devarajan P. Neutrophil gelatinase-associated lipocalin: A troponin-like biomarker for human acute kidney injury. *Nephrology* 2010;15:419–28.

CHAPTER 22 ■ PHARMACOLOGY

ATHENA F. ZUPPA

KEY POINTS

Scientific Foundations

1 An understanding of pharmacokinetics and pharmacodynamics can allow for a rational approach toward prescribing medications for critically ill children.

2 Drug absorption, distribution, metabolism, elimination, and the response to medications are impacted by age and disease state.

Application to Pediatric Intensive Care

3 Many medications are prescribed for children based on dosing guidance from adult studies.

4 Care providers must be cautious of the high risk of drug interactions and adverse reactions in the intensive care setting.

The word *pharmacology* is derived from the Greek "pharmacon," or drug, and "logos," or science. It is more formally defined as the study of how chemical substances interact with living systems. If these substances have medicinal properties, they are typically referred to as *pharmaceuticals*. Pharmacology, then, encompasses drug composition, drug properties, interactions, toxicology, and desirable effects that can be used in therapy of diseases. Underlying the discipline of pharmacology are the fields of *pharmacokinetics* (PK) and *pharmacodynamics* (PD), which focus on the movement of the various molecular entities contained within a pharmaceutical as it traverses bodily space and the actions of the active moieties once they arrive at the intended physiologic site within the body. Each of these disciplines can be further defined by the underlying processes that dictate specific pathways (e.g., absorption, distribution, metabolism, elimination). Hence, pharmacology is essential to our understanding of how drugs work and how to guide their administration.

Pediatric pharmacotherapy can be challenging due to developmental changes that may alter drug kinetics, pathophysiologic differences that may alter pharmacodynamics, disease etiologies that may differ from those of adults, and other factors that may result in great variation in safety and efficacy outcomes. The situation becomes more convoluted when one considers critically ill children and the paucity of well-controlled pediatric clinical trials in this vulnerable population. Caregivers who prescribe medications to critically ill children must have some understanding of the basic processes that govern the current dosing recommendations for their patients. In many situations, understanding the source and nature of the data used to support such guidance is helpful from the standpoint of managing expectations of patient response to pharmacotherapy and considering whether dosing modifications should be made. Our comfort in using drugs in critically ill children is often based on the populations previously studied (adults, healthy pediatric patients, etc.) and the knowledge gained from previous experience.

A review of the pharmacologic principles that generally guide pharmacotherapy is provided in this chapter, with a focus on specific topics relevant to the research and development of pharmaceuticals in critically ill children. In addition, the current knowledge on dosing medications commonly prescribed for critically ill children is reviewed.

SCIENTIFIC FOUNDATIONS

Pharmacokinetics

Absorption

Absorption is the process of drug transfer from its site of administration to the bloodstream. The rate and efficiency of absorption depend on the route of administration (including but not limited to oral, inhaled, topical). For intravenous (IV) administration, absorption is complete; the total dose reaches the systemic circulation. Drugs administered enterally may be absorbed by either passive diffusion or active transport.

Bioavailability

The *bioavailability* (F) of a drug is defined by the fraction of the administered dose that reaches the systemic circulation. If a drug is administered intravenously, the bioavailability is 100% and F = 1.0. When drugs are administered by routes other than IV, the bioavailability is usually <100%. Bioavailability is reduced by incomplete absorption, first-pass metabolism, and distribution into other tissues.

Distribution

The volume of distribution (V_d) is a hypothetical volume of fluid through which a drug is dispersed. A drug rarely disperses solely into the water compartments of the body. Instead, most drugs disperse to several compartments (including adipose tissue) and bind to plasma proteins. The total volume into which a drug disperses is called the *apparent volume of distribution*. This volume is not a physiologic space, but rather a conceptual parameter. It relates the total amount of drug (Drug) in the body to the concentration of drug (C_p) in the blood or plasma:

$$V_d = Drug/C_p \qquad [22.1]$$

Figure 22.1 represents the fate of a hypothetical drug after IV administration. After administration, a maximal plasma concentration is achieved, and the drug is immediately distributed. The plasma concentration then decreases over time. This initial phase is called the *α-phase* of drug distribution, in

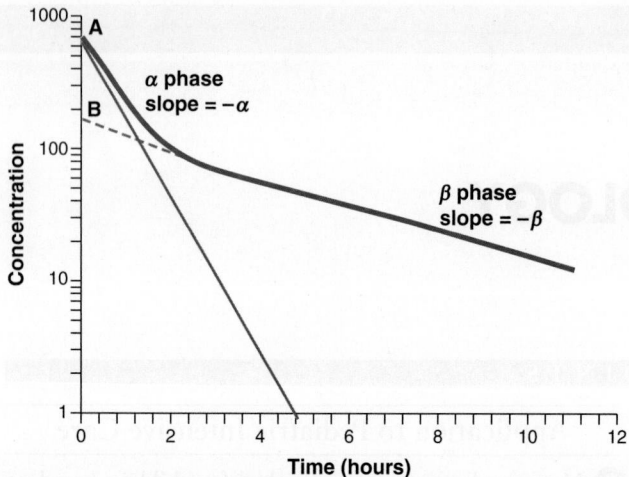

FIGURE 22.1. Semilogarithmic plot of concentration versus time after an IV administration of a drug that follows two-compartment pharmacokinetics.

which the decline in plasma concentration reflects the distribution of the drug. Once a drug is distributed, it undergoes metabolism and elimination. The second phase is called the *β-phase*, in which the decline in plasma concentration reflects drug metabolism and clearance. In equations, the terms *A* and *B* are intercepts with the *Y*-axis. The extrapolation of the *β*-phase defines *B*. The dotted line is generated by subtracting the extrapolated line from the original concentration line. This second line defines *α* and *A*. The serum concentration (*C*) can be determined using the formula:

$$C = Ae^{-\alpha t} + Be^{-\beta t} \qquad [22.2]$$

The distribution and elimination half-lives can be determined by Equations 22.3 and 22.4, respectively (1,2):

$$t_{1/2\alpha} = 0.693/\alpha \qquad [22.3]$$

and

$$t_{1/2\beta} = 0.693/\beta \qquad [22.4]$$

For drugs in which distribution is homogenous along the varied physiologic spaces, the distinction between the *α* and *β* phases may be subtle and, essentially, a single phase best describes the decline in drug concentration.

Metabolism

The metabolic transformation of drugs is catalyzed by enzymes, and most reactions follow Michaelis–Menten kinetics:

$$V = [(V_{max}) (C)/(K_m + C)] \qquad [22.5]$$

where

V is the rate of drug metabolism
C is the drug concentration
K_m is the Michaelis–Menten constant.

In most situations, the drug concentration is much less than K_m, and Equation 22.5 simplifies to

$$V = (V_{max}) (C)/K_m \qquad [22.6]$$

In this case, the rate of drug metabolism is directly proportional to the concentration of free drug, and follows first-order kinetics. A constant percentage of the drug is metabolized over time, and the rate of elimination is proportional to the amount of drug in the body. Most drugs used in the clinical setting are eliminated in this manner. The concentration–time curve of drug that follows first-order elimination is represented in **Figure 22.2**. A semilogarithmic plot results in a straight line (**Fig. 22.3**).

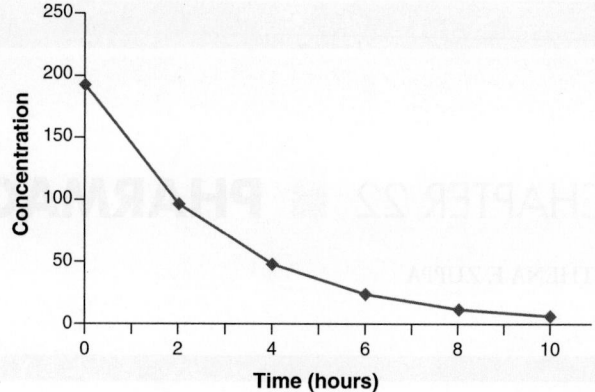

FIGURE 22.2. Concentration versus time profile of a drug demonstrating first-order elimination.

A few drugs, such as aspirin, ethanol, and phenytoin, are used at higher doses in certain clinical scenarios, resulting in higher plasma concentrations than would be seen at standard doses. In these situations, *C* is much greater than K_m, and Equation 22.5 reduces to:

$$V = (V_{max}) (C)/(C) = V_{max} \qquad [22.7]$$

The enzyme system becomes saturated by a high free-drug concentration, and the rate of metabolism is constant over time. This condition is called *zero-order kinetics*, and a constant amount of drug is metabolized per unit of time. A large increase in serum concentration can result from a small increase in dose for drugs that follow zero-order elimination. A plot of concentration versus time will result in a straight line (**Fig. 22.4**). A semilogarithmic plot of concentration versus time demonstrates a convex line (**Fig. 22.5**).

Phase I and Phase II Biotransformation. The liver is the principal organ of drug metabolism. Other tissues that display considerable drug metabolic activity include the gastrointestinal tract, lungs, skin, and kidneys. Following oral administration, many drugs are absorbed intact from the small intestine and transported via the portal system to the liver, where they are metabolized. This process is called *first-pass metabolism* and may greatly limit the bioavailability of orally administered drugs.

In general, the metabolic reactions involved in drug metabolism can be classified as either phase I or phase II biotransformation reactions. Biotransformation is the process in which a modification is made on a chemical by an organism. Phase I reactions usually convert a parent drug to a polar

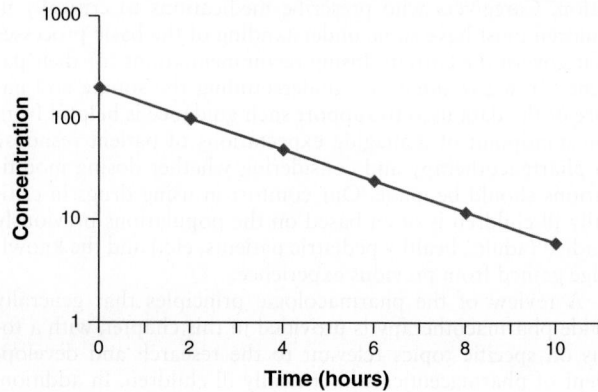

FIGURE 22.3. Semilogarithmic plot of concentration versus time of a drug demonstrating first-order elimination.

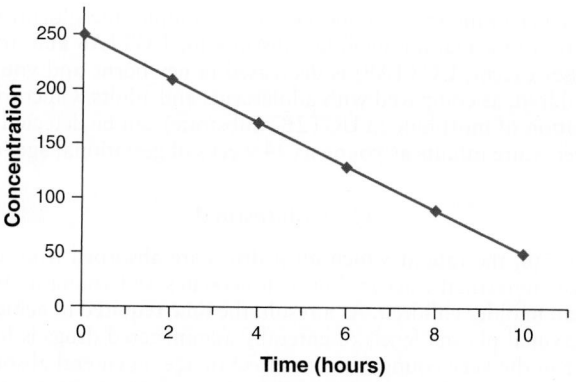

FIGURE 22.4. Concentration versus time of a drug demonstrating zero-order elimination.

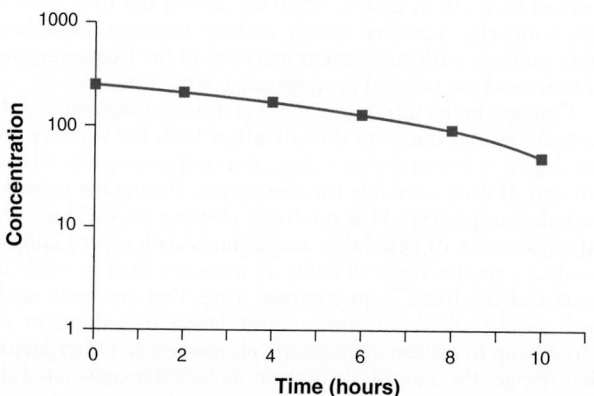

FIGURE 22.5. Semilogarithmic plot of concentration versus time of a drug demonstrating zero-order elimination.

metabolite by introducing or unmasking a more polar site (e.g., –OH, –NH$_2$). Phase I metabolites are generally less active, and because they are more polar, they are more readily excreted. However, many phase I metabolites undergo a subsequent, phase II, reaction in which endogenous substances, such as glucuronic acid, sulfuric acid, or an amino acid, combine with the metabolite to form a highly polar conjugate (conjugation reaction). Many drugs undergo these sequential reactions. However, phase II reactions may precede phase I reactions, as in the case of isoniazid.

Phase I reactions are usually catalyzed by enzymes of the cytochrome P450 system. These drug-metabolizing enzymes are located in the lipophilic membranes of the endoplasmic reticulum of the liver and other tissues. Three families, CYP1, CYP2, and CYP3, are responsible for most drug biotransformations. The CYP3A subfamily accounts for >50% of phase I drug metabolism, predominantly by the CYP3A4 subtype. CYP3A4 is responsible for the metabolism of drugs commonly used in the intensive care setting, including acetaminophen, cyclosporine, diazepam, methadone, midazolam, spironolactone, and tacrolimus. Most other drug biotransformations are performed by CYP2D6 (e.g., clozapine, codeine, flecainide, haloperidol, oxycodone), CYP2C9 (e.g., phenytoin, S-warfarin), CYP2C19 (e.g., diazepam, omeprazole, propranolol), CYP2E1 (e.g., acetaminophen, enflurane, halothane), and CYP1A2 (e.g., acetaminophen, caffeine, theophylline, warfarin). Drug biotransformation reactions may be enhanced or impaired by multiple factors, including age, enzyme induction or inhibition, pharmacogenetics, and the effects of other disease states (3,4).

Elimination

Elimination is the process by which a drug is removed or "cleared" from the body. *Clearance* (CL) is usually considered to be the amount of blood from which all drug is removed per unit of time (volume/time). The kidneys and liver are the main organs responsible for drug clearance. The total body clearance of a drug is equal to the sum of the clearances from all mechanisms, typically partitioned into renal and nonrenal clearance. Most elimination by the kidneys is accomplished through glomerular filtration. Glomerular integrity, the size and charge of the drug, water solubility, and the extent of protein binding determine the amount of drug filtered at the glomerulus. Highly protein-bound drugs are not readily filtered. Glomerular filtration rate has traditionally served as an approximation of renal function.

In addition to glomerular filtration, drugs may be eliminated from the kidneys via active secretion. Secretion occurs predominantly at the proximal tubule, where active transport systems secrete primarily organic acids and bases. Organic acids include most cephalosporins, loop diuretics, methotrexate, nonsteroidal anti-inflammatories, penicillins, and thiazide diuretics. Organic bases include ranitidine and morphine.

As drugs move toward the distal convoluting tubule, the concentration increases. High urine flow rates decrease the concentration of drug in the distal tubule, decreasing the likelihood that a drug will diffuse from the lumen. For both weak acids and bases, the nonionized form of the drug is reabsorbed more readily. Altering the pH (ion trapping) can minimize reabsorption by placing a charge on the drug and preventing its diffusion. For example, salicylate is a weak acid. In case of salicylate toxicity, urine alkalinization places a charge on the molecule and increases its elimination by reducing tubular reabsorption.

The liver also contributes to elimination through metabolism or excretion into the bile. After a drug is secreted in the bile, it may be either excreted into the feces or reabsorbed via enterohepatic recirculation (1,3,4).

The half-life of elimination is the time it takes to clear half of the drug from plasma. It is directly proportional to the V_d and inversely proportional to CL (1):

$$t_{1/2\beta} = (0.693)(V_d)/CL \qquad [22.8]$$

Organ Dysfunction

Renal Dysfunction

Renal failure can impact drug pharmacokinetics through several mechanisms. The binding of acidic drugs to albumin is reduced because accumulated organic acids compete with albumin-binding sites and because uremia changes the structure of albumin. Altered albumin binding leads to altered V_d and, consequently, to altered elimination half-life (4). Renal insufficiency is likely to decrease the clearance of drugs that are normally >30% eliminated unchanged in the urine, which results in a prolonged $t_{1/2\beta}$ of drugs such as milrinone, digoxin, aminoglycosides, insulin, and others (4).

Hepatic Dysfunction

Drugs that undergo extensive first-pass metabolism may have a significantly higher oral bioavailability in patients with liver failure than in normal subjects. Gut hypomotility may delay the peak response to enterally administered drugs in these patients. Hypoalbuminemia or altered glycoprotein levels may affect the fractional protein binding of acidic or basic drugs, respectively. Altered plasma protein concentrations may affect the extent of tissue distribution of drugs that are normally highly protein bound. The presence of significant edema and ascites may alter the V_d of highly water-soluble agents, such as aminoglycoside antibiotics. The capacity of the liver to metabolize drugs depends on hepatic blood flow and liver enzyme activity, both of which can be affected by liver disease. In addition, liver disease affects P450 isoforms in a variable manner; some P450 isoforms are more dysfunctional in the context of liver disease than others. This variability in susceptibility leads to the heterogeneous effects of liver disease on P450-dependent drug metabolism (4,5).

Cardiac Dysfunction

Circulatory failure, or shock, can alter the pharmacokinetics of drugs frequently used in the intensive care setting. Drug absorption may be impaired because of bowel wall edema. Passive hepatic congestion may impede first-pass metabolism, resulting in higher plasma concentrations. Peripheral edema inhibits absorption by intramuscular parenteral route. The balance of tissue hypoperfusion versus increased total body water with edema may unpredictably alter V_d. In addition, liver hypoperfusion may alter drug-metabolizing enzyme function, especially flow-dependent drugs such as lidocaine (4).

❷   Physiologic Differences in Children That Affect Drug Disposition

As children develop and grow, changes in body composition, development of metabolizing enzymes, and maturation of renal and liver function all have an impact on drug disposition (1,2).

Renal

Glomerular filtration and tubular secretion are significantly reduced in the premature and full-term neonate, as compared with older children. Maturation of renal function is a dynamic process that begins during fetal life and is complete by early childhood. Maturation of tubular function is slower than that of glomerular filtration. The glomerular filtration rate is ~2–4 mL/min/1.73 m^2 in term neonates, but it may be as low as 0.6–0.8 mL/min/1.73 m^2 in preterm neonates. The glomerular filtration rate increases rapidly during the first 2 weeks of life and continues to rise until adult values are reached at 8–12 months of age. For drugs that are dependent on renal elimination, impaired renal function decreases clearance and increases the half-life. Therefore, for drugs that are primarily eliminated by the kidney, dosing should be performed in an age-appropriate fashion that takes into account maturational changes in kidney function (1,2,6).

Hepatic

Hepatic biotransformation reactions are substantially reduced in the neonatal period. At birth, the cytochrome P450 system is 28% that of the adult (1,2). The expression of phase I enzymes (such as the P450 cytochromes) changes markedly during development. CYP3A7, the predominant CYP isoform expressed in fetal liver, peaks shortly after birth and then declines rapidly to levels that are undetectable in most adults. Within hours after birth, CYP2E1 activity surges, and CYP2D6 becomes detectable soon thereafter. CYP3A4 and CYP2C (CYP2C9 and CYP2C19) appear during the first week of life, whereas CYP1A2 is the last hepatic CYP to appear, at 1–3 months of life (6). The ontogeny of phase II enzymes is less well established than the ontogeny of reactions that involve phase I enzymes. Available data indicate that the individual isoforms of *uridine diphosphate glucuronosyltransferase* (UGT) have unique maturational profiles with

pharmacokinetic consequences. For example, the glucuronidation of acetaminophen (a substrate for UGT1A6 and, to a lesser extent, UGT1A9) is decreased in newborns and young children, as compared with adolescents and adults. Glucuronidation of morphine (a UGT2B7 substrate) can be detected in premature infants as young as 24 weeks of gestational age (6).

Gastrointestinal

Overall, the rate at which most drugs are absorbed from the gastrointestinal tract is slower in neonates and young infants than in older children. As a result, the time required to achieve maximal plasma levels of enterally administered drugs is longer in the very young (6). The effect of age on enteral absorption is not uniform, and it is difficult to predict (1,2). Gastric emptying and intestinal motility are the primary determinants of the rate at which drugs are presented to, and dispersed along, the mucosal surface of the small intestine. At birth, the coordination of antral contractions improves, resulting in a marked increase in gastric emptying during the first week of life. Similarly, intestinal motor activity matures throughout early infancy, with consequent increases in the frequency, amplitude, and duration of propagating contractions (6).

Changes in the intraluminal pH in different segments of the gastrointestinal tract can directly affect both the stability and the degree of ionization of a drug, thus influencing the relative amount of drug available for absorption. During the neonatal period, intragastric pH is relatively elevated (>4). Thus, oral administration of acid-labile compounds such as penicillin G produces greater bioavailability in neonates than in older infants and children (7). In contrast, drugs that are weak acids, such as phenobarbital, may require larger oral doses in the very young to achieve therapeutic plasma levels. Other factors that impact the rate of absorption include age-associated development of villi, splanchnic blood flow, changes in intestinal microflora, and intestinal surface area (6).

Body Composition

Age-dependent changes in body composition alter the physiologic spaces into which a drug may be distributed (6). The percentage of total body water drops from ~85% in premature infants to 75% in full-term infants to 60% in the adult. Extracellular water decreases from 45% in the infant to 25% in the adult. Total body fat in the premature infant can be as low as 1%, as compared to 15% in the normal term infant. Many drugs are less bound to plasma proteins in the neonate and infant than in the older child (1,2).

Much of drug distribution is a result of simple passive diffusion along concentration gradients and subsequent binding of the drug to tissue components. However, tissue transporters capable of producing a biologic barrier also contribute to drug distribution. An example is P-glycoprotein, a member of the ATP-binding cassette family of transporters that functions as an efflux transporter capable of extruding selected substances from cells. The expression and localization of P-glycoprotein in specific tissues facilitates its ability to limit the cellular uptake of selected substrates to these sites (e.g., the blood–brain barrier, hepatocytes, renal tubular cells, and enterocytes). Limited data are available regarding the ontogeny of P-glycoprotein expression in humans. A single study of the expression of P-glycoprotein in the central nervous system (CNS) using tissue obtained postmortem from neonates born at 23–42 weeks of gestational age suggests a pattern of localization similar to that in adult mice late in gestation and at term. However, the level of P-glycoprotein expression appeared to be lower than that in adults (8). Limited data in neonates suggest that the passive diffusion of drugs into the CNS is age dependent, as reflected by the progressive increase in the ratios of brain phenobarbital to plasma phenobarbital from 28 to 39 weeks of gestational age, demonstrating the increased transport of phenobarbital into the brain (9).

Pharmacodynamics

Pharmacodynamics, in general terms, seeks to define what the drug does to the body (i.e., the effects or response to drug therapy). Pharmacodynamics modeling attempts to characterize measured, physiologic parameters before and after drug administration, with the effect defined as the change in a physiologic parameter relative to its predose or baseline value. *Baseline* is defined as the physiologic parameter without drug administration and may be complicated in certain situations due to diurnal variations. Efficacy can be defined numerically as the expected sum of all beneficial effects following treatment. Similarly, toxicity can be characterized by either the time course of a specific toxic event or the composite of detrimental responses attributed to a common toxicity.

Overview

Pharmacodynamic response to drug therapy evolves only after active drug molecules reach their intended site(s) of action. Hence, the link between pharmacokinetic and pharmacodynamic processes is implicit. Differences in pharmacodynamic time course among drug entities can be broadly associated with the nature of the concentration–effect relationship as being *direct* (effect is directly proportional to concentration at the site of measurement, usually the plasma) or *indirect* (effect exhibits some type of temporal delay with respect to drug concentration either because of differences between the drug's site of action and measurement of effect or because the effect of interest results after other physiologic or pharmacologic conditions are satisfied).

Direct effect relationships are easily observed with cardiovascular agents. Pharmacologic effects such as blood pressure, ACE (angiotensin-converting-enzyme) inhibition, and inhibition of platelet aggregation can be characterized by direct response relationships. Such relationships can usually be defined by three typical patterns: linear, hyperbolic maximum effect observed (E_{max}), and sigmoid E_{max} functions (**Fig. 22.6**). In each case, the plasma concentration and drug concentration at the effect site are proportional. Likewise, the concentration–effect relationship is assumed to be independent of time.

Other drugs exhibit an indirect relationship between concentration and response. In this case, the concentration–effect relationship is time dependent. One explanation for such effects is hysteresis. *Hysteresis* refers to the phenomenon in which a time lapse exists between the cause and its effect. With respect to pharmacodynamics, this time lapse most often indicates a situation in which a delay exists in equilibrium between plasma drug concentration and the concentration of active substance at the effect site. Three broad conditions can account for this phenomenon: the active drug response site is not in the central compartment, the mechanism of drug action involves new protein synthesis, or the particular drug has active metabolites.

More complicated models (indirect response models) have been used to express the same observations but typically necessitate a greater understanding of the underlying physiologic process (e.g., cell trafficking, enzyme recruitment, etc.). The salient point is that pharmacodynamic characterization and dosing guidance derived from such characterization tend to be more informative than drug concentrations alone.

Pharmacogenomics

Pharmacogenomics is the study of how an individual's genetic inheritance affects his or her response to drugs. Pharmacogenomics holds the promise that drugs might one day be tailored to individuals and adapted to each person's own genetic makeup. Environment, diet, age, lifestyle, and state of health all can influence a person's response to medicines, but understanding an individual's genetic composition is thought to be a key to creating personalized drugs with greater efficacy and safety. Pharmacogenomics combines traditional pharmaceutical sciences, such as biochemistry, with annotated knowledge of genes, proteins, and single nucleotide polymorphisms (see Chapter 18).

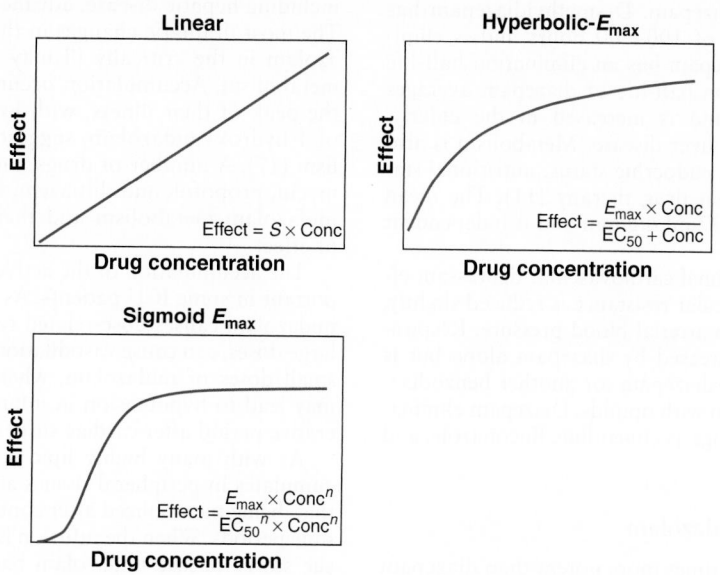

FIGURE 22.6. Representative pharmacodynamic relationships for drugs that exhibit direct responses: linear, hyperbolic, and sigmoid E_{max} relationships shown. S is the slope of the linear response; E_{max} refers to the maximum effect observed; EC_{50} refers to the concentration at which 50% of the maximal response is achieved, and n is the degree of sigmoidicity or shape factor (sometimes referred to as the Hill coefficient).

❸ APPLICATION TO PEDIATRIC INTENSIVE CARE

Benzodiazepines

Benzodiazepines are often used to provide sedation and amnesia. Benzodiazepines exert their anxiolytic, amnestic, anticonvulsant, and muscle-relaxing effects through interaction at specific binding sites on neuronal γ-aminobutyric acid (GABA) receptors (10). Benzodiazepines facilitate the inhibitory action of GABA on neuronal impulse transmission. The potency of individual medications is determined by their receptor affinity. Benzodiazepines enhance inhibitory synaptic transmission by mimicking and increasing the actions of GABA-mediated chloride influx at the GABA receptor.

Chronic administration of benzodiazepines can lead to decreased receptor activity and drug tolerance. Tolerance is a common finding in ICU patients who receive benzodiazepines or other sedative agents for periods >24 hours. Withdrawal syndromes have been reported with the cessation of midazolam and other benzodiazepine infusions. Risk factors for acute withdrawal include high infusion rates, prolonged duration, and abrupt cessation. For these reasons, gradual tapering of sedative infusions and substitution with longer-acting agents (e.g., diazepam) are suggested to reduce the chance of withdrawal reactions. Benzodiazepines also are noted for occasionally producing paradoxical reactions, including increased agitation and delirium (11).

Diazepam

Diazepam is highly lipid soluble and protein bound, and distributes quickly into the brain. It is available in IV and oral preparations. Diazepam administration results in antegrade but not retrograde amnesia. It reduces the cerebral metabolic rate for oxygen consumption and thus decreases cerebral blood flow in a dose-dependent manner. Diazepam, like the other benzodiazepines, raises the seizure threshold (11). After enteral dosing, diazepam demonstrates a bioavailability of 100%. It has a V_d of 1.1–2.9 L/kg (11,12) and is 98% protein bound (12). Diazepam is metabolized by hepatic microsomal enzymes (CYP2C19) to active compounds such as desmethyldiazepam and oxazepam. Desmethyldiazepam has a long elimination half-life of 100–200 hours and is eliminated by the kidneys. Oxazepam has an elimination half-life of 10 hours. The elimination half-life of diazepam averages 72 hours, varies widely, and is increased in the elderly, neonates, and patients with liver disease. Metabolism is also affected by genetics, gender, endocrine status, nutritional status, smoking, and concurrent drug therapy (11). The mean plasma clearance is 0.27–0.37 mL/kg/min and is independent of liver blood flow (13).

Diazepam alone has minimal cardiovascular depressant effects, although systemic vascular resistance is reduced slightly, producing a small decline in arterial blood pressure. Respiratory drive is minimally decreased by diazepam alone but is profoundly depressed when diazepam (or another benzodiazepine) is used in combination with opioids. Diazepam elimination is decreased by such drugs as cimetidine, fluconazole, and valproic acid (11).

Midazolam

Midazolam is three to four times more potent than diazepam (11). It is rapidly absorbed after administration of the oral syrup formulation, with adolescents absorbing the drug at approximately half the rate observed in younger children (ages 2 to <12 years). In children 6 months to 16 years, the absolute bioavailability of oral midazolam averaged 36%, with a very broad range (9%–71%). No relationship between midazolam bioavailability and age was observed (14). The pKa of midazolam (6.1) is especially important because it permits a conformational change in midazolam's structure, depending on pH. As currently marketed, midazolam is buffered to a pH of 3.5, opening its imidazole ring and increasing its water solubility. At physiologic pH, however, the diazepine ring closes rapidly and midazolam becomes lipid soluble. As a consequence, the effects of midazolam are rapid.

Midazolam is 95% protein bound, with a V_d of 1.9 L/kg (11). Midazolam undergoes extensive metabolism by the cytochrome P4503A subfamily (e.g., CYP3A4 and CYP3A5) to major (1-OH-midazolam) and minor (4-OH-midazolam) hydroxylated metabolites. 1-OH-midazolam is equipotent to midazolam. Both hydroxylated metabolites are subsequently glucuronidated by uridine diphosphate glucuronosyltransferases (UGTs). 1-OH-midazolam-glucuronide also appears to have sedative properties when concentrations are high, as has been observed in adult patients with renal failure (15).

In healthy children 6 months to <2 years, 2 years to <12 years, and 12 years to <16 years, midazolam clearance was 11.3, 10, and 9.3 mL/kg/min, respectively (14). Adult clearance is estimated at 6.6 mL/kg/min (12). CYP3A4/5 activity reaches adult levels at between 3 and 12 months of postnatal age (16). Developmental differences in CYP3A activity may therefore alter the pharmacokinetics of midazolam in pediatric intensive care patients of different ages. Similarly, the UGTs exhibit developmental changes in activity. However, because the specific UGTs involved in the conjugation of 1-OH-midazolam are not yet known, the impact of ontogeny on this reaction remains to be determined (15).

Less than 1% of midazolam is excreted unchanged in the urine. The elimination half-life of midazolam is 2 hours in young, healthy adults but increases rapidly in the elderly and following major surgery (11). 1-OH-midazolam-glucuronide is renally excreted, with an elimination half-life of 1 hour with normal renal function (15). This results in high concentrations in the presence of renal failure and is responsible for prolonged sedation (13).

Midazolam is metabolized by hepatic microsomal oxidation. The oxidative pathway is susceptible to many factors, including hepatic disease, advanced age, and drug inhibition. The most dramatic changes in the pharmacokinetics of midazolam in the critically ill may result from altered hepatic metabolism. Accumulation occurs in critically ill patients at the peak of their illness, with low or absent concentrations of 1-hydroxymidazolam, suggesting failure of liver metabolism (17). A number of drugs, including cimetidine, erythromycin, propofol, and diltiazem, have been reported to delay midazolam metabolism and therefore increase its duration of effect.

The accumulation of the active metabolite also may be important in some ICU patients. As with other benzodiazepines, midazolam causes dose-related respiratory depression and, in large doses, can cause vasodilation and hypotension (11). Even small doses of midazolam, when combined with an opioid, may lead to hypotension in infants in the immediate postoperative period after cardiac surgery.

As with many highly lipid soluble drugs, midazolam accumulates in peripheral tissues and in the bloodstream rather than being metabolized after continuous infusion for extended time periods. When the infusion is discontinued, peripheral tissue stores release midazolam back into the plasma, and the duration of clinical effect can be prolonged. Obese patients with larger volumes of distribution and elderly patients with decreased hepatic and renal function may be at higher risk for prolonged sedation from midazolam (18).

Lorazepam

Lorazepam is the least lipid soluble of the three benzodiazepines and traverses the blood–brain barrier most slowly, resulting in delayed onset and prolonged duration of effect (11). Lorazepam is well absorbed orally and demonstrates a bioavailability of 93% after oral administration (12). It is absorbed rapidly after intramuscular injection, and plasma concentrations peak within 60 minutes. It is ~90% protein bound and has a V_d of 2 L/kg. Lorazepam is metabolized to inactive products by hepatic glucuronidation. The pharmacokinetics of lorazepam does not change significantly in the elderly or in critically ill populations. The elimination half-life ranges from 10 to 20 hours but is prolonged by liver and end-stage kidney disease (11). CL is estimated at 1.1 mL/kg/min (12). Because lorazepam is insoluble in water, it is manufactured with a vehicle that contains polyethylene glycol, benzyl alcohol, and propylene glycol. This drug vehicle may be associated with lactic acidosis, hyperosmolar coma, and a reversible nephrotoxicity after high doses or prolonged infusions and a "gasping syndrome" in neonates (11).

Flumazenil

Flumazenil acts at the benzodiazepine binding site on the GABA receptor to antagonize the effects of benzodiazepine agonists. Flumazenil is chemically and structurally similar to other benzodiazepine receptor agonists. Flumazenil produces a reversal of benzodiazepine-induced sedative and amnestic effects. Clinical effects are seen immediately after IV administration. Flumazenil does not reverse the effects of opioids, barbiturates, alcohol, or other GABA-mimetic agents (11). Flumazenil is short acting, and careful clinical observation is crucial if the therapeutic intent is to avoid the recurrence of benzodiazepine-induced sedation. Repeated administrations may be necessary to maintain its antagonistic action (19).

Flumazenil is 40%–50% plasma protein bound, with a V_d of 0.6–1.6 L/kg (12,19). It is cleared rapidly from the plasma by hepatic metabolism. Less than 0.2% of an IV dose is recovered unchanged in the urine, and three metabolites of flumazenil have been identified (19). The elimination half-life of flumazenil is ~1 hour, which is significantly shorter than that of many of the benzodiazepine compounds used clinically. The CL is estimated at 17 mL/kg/min (12). Flumazenil can precipitate withdrawal and/or seizures in patients with benzodiazepine dependence caused by chronic exposure (11).

Barbiturates

Barbiturates are weak acids that are absorbed and rapidly distributed to all tissues and fluids, with high concentrations in the brain, liver, and kidneys. High lipid solubility is the dominant factor in the distribution of barbiturates within the body. The more lipid soluble the barbiturate, the more rapidly it penetrates all tissues of the body. Barbiturates are bound to plasma and tissue proteins to varying degrees, with the degree of binding increasing directly as a function of lipid solubility. Barbiturates are absorbed in varying degrees following oral, rectal, or parenteral administration.

Pentobarbital

Pentobarbital is a commonly used barbiturate for sedation, hypnosis, and intracranial pressure (ICP) management. Pentobarbital has two enantiomeric forms: R- and S-pentobarbital. The S-enantiomer causes a longer duration of sedation than does the R-enantiomer in humans. High-dose pentobarbital infusions have been advocated as an effective adjunct in controlling persistent intracranial hypertension after severe head

trauma in patients who are refractory to conventional therapy. Pentobarbital's beneficial effects in patients with increased ICP include both a direct vasoconstriction of cerebral blood vessels and a reduction of blood flow through reduction in cerebral metabolic rate. Pentobarbital has a potent effect on GABA-sensitive chloride channels and is a potent CNS depressant. Following IV administration, the onset of action is almost immediate for pentobarbital. Pentobarbital enters the brain more rapidly than do phenobarbital or diazepam and is a very potent antiepileptic drug. Pentobarbital has also been recommended as a sedative agent for diagnostic imaging studies (20,21). Pentobarbital administration has potential respiratory-depressant and hypotensive side effects. Myocardial depression contributes to the hypotension and may require epinephrine infusion in patients with high ICP to maintain cerebral perfusion pressure. Phenylephrine administration alone for pentobarbital-induced hypotension may not overcome the myocardial depression nor improve the cerebral perfusion pressure. Tolerance may develop with prolonged use.

Pentobarbital is metabolized primarily by the hepatic microsomal enzyme system, and the metabolic products are excreted in the urine and, less commonly, in the feces (22). The CL of the S-enantiomer is less than that of the R-enantiomer (43 vs. 32 mL/min), and the V_d of the S-enantiomer is slightly less than the R-enantiomer (1.1 vs. 1.2 L/kg). The S-enantiomer is also more strongly protein bound in plasma (73.5% vs. 63.4% for the R-enantiomer) (23). In a study of seven healthy adult men and women, 100 mg of pentobarbital was administered as an IV bolus. A two-compartment model determined the central V_d to be 0.44 L/kg, with a peripheral V_d of 0.56 L/kg (V_d = 1 L/kg). The elimination half-life was 22.3 hours (24). Pentobarbital pharmacokinetics was assessed in 10 adults with severe nonpenetrating head injury. An IV loading dose (10 mg/kg) was infused over 1 hour, followed by a continuous infusion at 0.5–3.0 mg/kg/h. The mean $t_{1/2}$ and V_d were significantly less than the values reported for the healthy control subjects (25). In another study of six adult patients with severe head injury, the mean CL was 0.7 mL/kg/min, with a V_d of 1 L/kg and an elimination half-life of 19.1 hours. Considerable variation in individual patient parameters was observed (26).

The pharmacokinetics of pentobarbital in neonates, infants, and young children with congenital heart disease after open-heart surgery were determined in 35 subjects (3.0 days to 4.4 years) after open-heart surgery who received pentobarbital as standard of care. A population-based, nonlinear mixed-effects modeling approach was used to characterize pentobarbital pharmacokinetics. A two-compartment model with weight as a covariate allometrically expressed on all parameters, bypass time as a covariate on CL and central volume of distribution, and age and ventricular physiology as covariates on CL described the pharmacokinetics. A typical infant (two-ventricle physiology, 6.9 kg, 5.2 months, and bypass time of 60 minutes) had a CL of 0.12 L/kg/h (2 mL/kg/min), central volume of distribution of 0.45 L/kg, and peripheral volume of distribution of 0.98 L/kg. The bypass effect was poorly estimated. For subjects <12 months age, an age effect on CL remained after accounting for weight and was precisely estimated. Subjects with single-ventricle physiology demonstrated a 15% decrease in CL when compared with subjects with two-ventricle physiology (27). An older study reported pharmacokinetics of pentobarbital in 11 children with Reye syndrome, hypoxic encephalopathy, or acute head injury. Nine of these patients were hypothermic (<32°C). The total CL and V_d were, respectively, 0.4 mL/kg/min and 0.8 L/kg—less than that reported in the normothermic pediatric population after open-heart surgery, suggesting that hypothermia may be associated with a reduction in pentobarbital CL. The elimination half-life of 25.5 hours was not significantly different from previously reported values (28).

Opioids

Opioids are endogenous or exogenous substances that bind to receptors found in the CNS and peripheral tissue. Three classes of opiate receptors have been characterized: $\mu 1$ and 2, $\kappa 1$–3, and $\delta 1$ and 2. The $\mu 1$ (spinal) and $\mu 2$ (supraspinal) subtypes are present in the CNS. Stimulation of these receptors produces analgesia, respiratory depression, and miosis. The primary opioids stimulating the μ receptors include fentanyl, methadone, morphine, and sufentanil. The $\kappa 1$ receptors elicit spinal analgesia when stimulated. The pharmacologic properties of $\kappa 2$ receptors remain unknown. The analgesic effects of $\kappa 3$ receptors are exerted through supraspinal mechanisms. Drugs with higher affinity for κ receptors include butorphanol, levorphanol, naloxone, and nalbuphine.

The primary activity of enkephalins, endogenous analgesic ligands in the brain and adrenal glands, is to trigger the activation of δ receptors. The stimulation of δ receptors induces spinal and supraspinal analgesia. Two subtypes of δ receptors are present: $\delta 1$ and $\delta 2$. Sufentanil is the only analgesic with known agonism for the δ receptor, although it has less affinity for δ and κ receptors than for μ receptors (29).

Opioids lead to a dose-dependent, centrally-mediated respiratory depression, mediated by the $\mu 2$ receptors in the medulla. The carbon dioxide response curve is shifted to the right, and the ventilatory response to hypoxia is obliterated. Opioids have little hemodynamic effect on euvolemic patients whose blood pressure is not sustained by ongoing sympathetic nervous system stimulation, but may cause hypotension in the hypovolemic patient or those who are normotensive despite sympathetic stimulation (pain, early sepsis). Opioid side effects include nausea, vomiting, decreased gastrointestinal motility (constipation), urinary retention, and pruritus (18). A withdrawal syndrome characterized by irritability, agitation, hypertension, nausea, vomiting, diarrhea, or sweating will occur if opioid administration is weaned abruptly after prolonged usage.

Morphine

Morphine is a potent μ-receptor agonist with additional κ-receptor activity (29). Morphine's onset of action is relatively slow (5–10 minutes after IV administration) because of low lipid solubility (peak respiratory depression is ~30 minutes after IV administration). The duration of action is dose dependent, but is ~4 hours after a single dose (18). Morphine has a bioavailability of 24%. It is 35% protein bound, with a V_d estimated at 3.3 L/kg (12). The elimination half-life is 1.9 hours, and CL is estimated at 24 mL/kg/min (12). Metabolism primarily occurs through the liver by glucuronide conjugation, and excretion occurs through the kidney. Morphine's predominant metabolite, *morphine-6-glucuronide*, is an active analgesic and may accumulate in patients with renal failure. This active metabolite is several times more potent than morphine itself. Morphine-3-glucuronide is the second metabolite of morphine. It is not active as an opioid agonist, but does have some action as a convulsant, which does not appear to be mediated through opioid receptors but instead by the GABA/glycinergic system. Renal failure may lead to its accumulation and result in seizures (29). The pharmacologic effects of morphine include analgesia, respiratory depression, gastrointestinal effects (nausea and vomiting), orthostatic hypotension, sedation, and altered mentation (29). Morphine administration may cause histamine release which may contribute to vasodilation or bronchoconstriction (18).

Hydromorphone

Hydromorphone (aka dilaudid) is a morphine-like agonist and a semisynthetic opioid analgesic with roughly three- to fourfold greater potency than morphine. Hydromorphone, like morphine, provides analgesic effects within 15–30 minutes of IV administration (29). It is metabolized primarily by the liver to hydromorphone-3-glucuronide. Although it has been recommended as an alternative to morphine for patients in renal failure (30), hydromorphone's metabolite may accumulate in renal failure, resulting in neuroexcitability and cognitive impairment (29).

Meperidine

Meperidine (aka demerol) is primarily a μ-receptor agonist and has approximately one-tenth the potency of morphine. The analgesic effects of meperidine are detectable within 5 minutes of IV administration and 10 minutes after intramuscular or subcutaneous administration (29). Meperidine is useful for drug-induced rigors and pain symptoms, such as those that accompany administration of amphotericin B. Meperidine has a bioavailability of 52%. It is 58% protein bound, with a V_d of 4.4 L/kg (12). It is metabolized through the liver to an active metabolite, normeperidine, which has a half-life of 15–30 hours (29). Meperidine has an elimination half-life of 3.2 hours, with a CL of 17 mL/kg/min (12). Normeperidine accumulation produces neurotoxicity, which may result in tremors, myoclonic jerks, and seizures. Case reports of seizures with meperidine have been noted with administration by patient-controlled analgesia pumps (31). Risk for seizures secondary to normeperidine toxicity is reported in patients with renal insufficiency, with sickle cell anemia, and in those receiving high-dose meperidine (29). Hence, meperidine is now used only rarely.

Fentanyl

Fentanyl is a synthetic opioid commonly used in anesthesia and in the ICU for pain management and sedation. Fentanyl is 50–100 times more potent than morphine and has a relatively quick (almost immediate) onset of action and short duration of action (~0.5–1 hour). Fentanyl is more lipid soluble than morphine and has a more rapid onset of action due to quicker penetration of the CNS. Fentanyl may be administered by the IV, IM, epidural, transdermal, intranasal, and intrathecal routes (29,32). Fentanyl has a very low bioavailability due to a high first-pass effect and, consequently, is not administered by the oral route. It is 84% protein bound, with a V_d of 4 L/kg (12).

Fentanyl is metabolized by the liver to inactive metabolites that are eliminated by the kidney. It has an elimination half-life of 3.7 hours and a CL of 13 mL/kg/min. Metabolism is determined primarily by liver perfusion, and diseases that decrease liver blood flow, such as cardiac failure, may decrease the CL of fentanyl. Although renal failure does not significantly alter the pharmacokinetics and pharmacodynamics of fentanyl in most patients, a few studies have demonstrated increases in the V_d and $t_{1/2}$ in critically ill patients with renal failure who are receiving continuous fentanyl infusions (12,32). Long-term, continuous infusions of fentanyl may result in a prolonged elimination half-life and duration of action as a result of drug accumulation in peripheral tissues. Unlike morphine, fentanyl is not associated with mast cell histamine release and may be preferred in patients who are susceptible to the cardiovascular effects of morphine (32). Rapid administration has been associated with rigidity of the chest wall, which produces apnea and inability to apply assisted ventilation until the patient receives neuromuscular blockade.

Remifentanil

Remifentanil is a potent ultrashort-acting synthetic opioid. Remifentanil is used for analgesia and sedation and, when combined with other medications, in general anesthesia. Unlike other synthetic opioids which are hepatically metabolized, remifentanil has an ester linkage which undergoes rapid hydrolysis by nonspecific tissue and plasma esterases. Therefore, drug accumulation does not occur. Remifentanil will be rapidly eliminated from the body once an infusion is discontinued, and the effects of the drug will diminish quickly, even after prolonged infusions. Remifentanil is a specific μ-receptor agonist resulting in a reduction in sympathetic nervous system tone, respiratory depression, and analgesia. The drug's effects include a dose-dependent decrease in heart rate and arterial pressure and respiratory rate and tidal volume. Muscle rigidity is sometimes noted. Nausea can occur as a side effect of remifentanil; however, it is usually transient in nature due to the drug's short half-life (33).

Naloxone

Naloxone is an opioid antagonist. Small doses can result in the prompt reversal of opioid-induced respiratory depression, sedation, analgesia, and hypotension. Naloxone can be administered IV or endotracheally. The duration of action is 1–4 hours, and the V_d is 2.1 L/kg. Naloxone undergoes significant first-pass metabolism and is metabolized in the liver by conjugation with glucuronic acid. CL is estimated at 22 mL/kg/min, with an elimination half-life of 1.1 hours (12). Caution must be used when treating opioid overdose in a patient with pain. Doses of 0.001–0.010 mg/kg should be titrated to achieve the desired clinical effect.

Ketamine

Ketamine is an N-methyl-D-aspartate (NMDA) receptor antagonist, and inhibits glutamate activation of the channel in a noncompetitive manner (18,34). It is a racemic mixture consisting of two optical enantiomers, R(–) and S(+). Administration produces a dose-dependent CNS depression that leads to a dissociative state, characterized by profound analgesia and amnesia but not necessarily loss of consciousness. Ketamine is a bronchodilator that causes minimal respiratory depression, and protective airway reflexes are more likely to be preserved than with other anesthetics. However, increased oral secretions can occur with its use. It is used clinically for indications such as induction of anesthesia in hemodynamically compromised patients or active asthmatic disease; intramuscular sedation of uncooperative patients, particularly children; supplementation of incomplete regional or local anesthesia; sedation in the intensive care setting; and for short, painful procedures, such as dressing changes in burn patients.

Ketamine is minimally protein bound and has a V_d of 1.8 L/kg. The $t_{1/2}$ is 2.3 hours, and CL is 15 mL/kg/min. The compound is metabolized extensively by the hepatic cytochrome P450 system. The primary metabolite, norketamine, is only one-third to one-fifth as potent as the original compound but may be involved in the prolonged analgesic actions of ketamine. The metabolites of norketamine are excreted by the kidneys (12,34). Common side effects include emergence delirium and severe hallucinations. These effects can be reduced with concomitant administration of a benzodiazepine, such as midazolam. Although ketamine administration is generally associated with increases in heart rate, cardiac output, and blood pressure, hypotension from direct myocardial depression can occur in patients with minimal physiologic reserves (catecholamine depletion) (18).

Propofol

Propofol is an alkylphenol IV anesthetic. Its exact mechanism of action is unclear, but it is thought to act at the GABA receptor. It is an oil at room temperature and is prepared as a lipid emulsion. Propofol is highly lipid soluble and rapidly crosses the blood–brain barrier. Onset of sedation is rapid (1–5 minutes), and duration of action is dose dependent but usually very short (2–8 minutes) because of rapid redistribution to peripheral tissues. When continuous infusions are used, the duration of action may be increased, but it is rare for the effect to last longer than 60 minutes after the infusion is stopped (18). Propofol is a hypnotic agent that, like benzodiazepines, provides a dose-dependent suppression of awareness from mild depression of responsiveness to obtundation. It is a potent anxiolytic, an amnestic agent (only at high doses), but does not possess analgesic properties (18).

The pharmacokinetics of propofol in healthy individuals who are undergoing surgery is characterized by a rapid distribution phase of 1.3 minutes and a rapid redistribution phase of 30 minutes (13). Propofol is metabolized primarily by conjugation in the liver to inactive glucuronide and sulfate metabolites, which are then cleared by the kidney. The elimination half-life is 4–7 hours. Metabolism of propofol does not appear to be significantly altered by hepatic or renal disease. However, in critical care populations, CL is generally slower than that in the general population, probably secondary to decrease in hepatic blood flow (13).

Propofol pharmacokinetics is distinct and can be contrasted with the pharmacokinetics of other commonly used IV-administered sedatives. Propofol pharmacokinetics is best described by a three-compartment model: a central compartment (essentially blood volume), a rapidly equilibrating compartment, and a slowly equilibrating, or deep tissue, compartment (35). Following an IV bolus dose, rapid equilibration occurs between blood and the highly perfused tissue of the brain, thus accounting for the rapid onset of anesthesia. Plasma levels initially decline rapidly as a result of both rapid distribution and metabolism. Distribution, however, is not complete, and a true steady state is not rapidly achieved. Initiation of a continuous IV infusion (CIVI) can maintain a pseudo–steady-state plasma drug concentration. The deep tissue compartment eventually is saturated, which results in an increase in plasma drug concentrations if infusions are maintained at a constant rate. The rate at which equilibration occurs is a function of the rate and duration of the infusion. Another important aspect of propofol pharmacokinetics is that the drug can limit its own CL. Propofol is eliminated by hepatic conjugation to inactive metabolites, which are excreted by the kidney. Studies have indicated that after a 2-mg/kg bolus dose of propofol for induction of cardiac anesthesia, blood flow in the liver is reduced by 14%. Bolus doses of propofol may cause a small but persistent change in blood flow to the liver, which results in decreased CL that leads to plasma concentrations that are higher than those predicted by an infusion. In addition to hepatic blood flow, other factors, such as age, lean body mass, and central blood volume, have been found to affect the induction dose of anesthesia. Younger children require larger doses for induction (36), and critically ill patients with low cardiac output usually require smaller doses (9). In addition, the presence of opioids (fentanyl) decreases the amount of propofol needed by 50%–55% (37).

Apnea may occur after a loading dose. Administration can cause significant decreases in blood pressure, especially in hypovolemic patients, mainly as a result of preload reduction from the dilation of venous capacitance vessels. A lesser effect is mild myocardial depression. Because it is delivered in a lipid carrier, hypertriglyceridemia is a possible side effect of propofol (18). Lactic acidosis has been associated with its use in the pediatric population (propofol-related infusion syndrome [PRIS]) (38). Recent reports of dysrhythmia, heart failure, metabolic acidosis, hyperkalemia, and rhabdomyolysis have been described in adults treated with high doses of propofol (>80 mcg/kg/min) (39). Although propofol is highly effective for procedural sedation in the PICU, it is not approved for long-term continuous sedation because of the risk of rhabdomyolysis, acidosis, infection, and death after prolonged administration in children.

Etomidate

Etomidate is an ultrashort-acting, nonbarbiturate, sedative/hypnotic agent without analgesic effects. IV administration of 0.3 mg/kg will induce sleep for ~5 minutes. Cardiovascular and respiratory adverse events are minimal (12). Etomidate administration is associated with a transient 20%–30% decrease in cerebral blood flow. Etomidate is rapidly metabolized in the liver to inactive metabolites, and ~75% of the administered dose is excreted in the urine during the first day after injection (3). Involuntary muscle movements are a frequent occurrence. Etomidate may inhibit adrenal steroidogenesis, causing a decrease in plasma cortisol concentrations (12). The effect of etomidate on steroidogenesis has recently led to controversy regarding its use in the care of critically ill patients (40). Although a single administration can be highly effective, we recommend avoiding repeated administration of etomidate in a critically ill patient because of its effect on steroidogenesis. There is controversy surrounding the safety of *single* dose etomidate for rapid sequence induction in patients with sepsis. Pending a large randomized controlled trial in children, we advise caution in using etomidate in septic patients (unless there are no other options considered hemodynamically safe) because of the incompletely defined risks of adrenal suppression and increased mortality (41).

Dexmedetomidine

Dexmedetomidine is a highly selective α_2 agonist, with sedative/hypnotic and anxiolytic properties attributed to the α_{2A} adrenoreceptors in the locus ceruleus. Analgesic properties are a result of the stimulation of α_2 adrenoreceptors in the brain, spinal cord, and peripheral sites (42). Dexmedetomidine is being increasingly used in the adult ICU setting because it allows postoperative patients to remain sedated but to be aroused easily with gentle stimulation (43). Furthermore, it produces sedation with less respiratory depression or risk of a withdrawal syndrome after prolonged infusion than usual sedatives. Only limited pharmacokinetic data are currently available to help guide dosing in children.

Dexmedetomidine demonstrates a rapid distribution phase, with a distribution half-life of ~6 minutes. The steady-state V_d of dexmedetomidine is 1.6 L/kg. Protein binding in healthy adult male and female volunteers was 94%. Dexmedetomidine undergoes almost complete biotransformation, with very little unchanged dexmedetomidine excreted in urine or feces. Biotransformation involves both direct glucuronidation and cytochrome P450-mediated metabolism. The major metabolic pathways of dexmedetomidine are: (a) direct N-glucuronidation to inactive metabolites; (b) aliphatic hydroxylation (mediated primarily by CYP2A6) of dexmedetomidine to generate 3-hydroxy dexmedetomidine, the glucuronide of 3-hydroxy dexmedetomidine, and 3-carboxy dexmedetomidine; and (c) N-methylation of dexmedetomidine to generate 3-hydroxy N-methyl dexmedetomidine, 3-carboxy N-methyl dexmedetomidine, and N-methyl O-glucuronide dexmedetomidine. The elimination half-life of dexmedetomidine is ~2 hours, and CL is estimated to be 9 mL/kg/min in adults. Approximately 95% of the administered dose is recovered as metabolites in the urine, and 4% in the feces. In clinical studies, hypotension and bradycardia were the significant treatment-emergent adverse events reported in dexmedetomidine patients compared with placebo patients (44). The pharmacokinetics and safety were reported for 36 infants, aged 1–24 months, after open-heart surgery. Cohorts of 12 infants requiring mechanical ventilation after open-heart surgery were enrolled sequentially to one of the three initial loading dose-continuous IV infusion regimens: 0.35–0.25, 0.7–0.5, or 1–0.75 mcg/kg/h. Pharmacokinetic parameters of dexmedetomidine were estimated using a two-compartment disposition model with weight allometrically expressed as a covariate on all parameters, total bypass time as a covariate on CL and central volume of distribution, and age and ventricular physiology as covariates on CL. A typical 7-kg infant demonstrated a CL of 17.3 mL/min/kg, central volume of distribution of 1.2 L/kg, and peripheral volume of distribution of 1.5 L/kg. Initial loading doses in the range of 0.35–1 mcg/kg over 10 minutes and infusions of 0.25–0.75 mcg/kg/h were well tolerated in this infant population (45).

Neuromuscular Blockers

During neurotransmission, the neurotransmitter acetylcholine is synthesized, stored in vesicles at the neuromuscular junction, released into the synapse, bound to nicotinic receptors in the muscle endplate, and acts as an agonist at the neuromuscular junction. Muscle contraction occurs when the impulse generated in a neuron creates an action potential that is chemically transmitted across the synapse. The postsynaptic nicotinic receptor at the neuromuscular junction is the major site of action of depolarizing and nondepolarizing neuromuscular blockers. Nondepolarizing neuromuscular blockers act as antagonists, combine with the nicotinic receptors, and block the action of acetylcholine. They also antagonize presynaptic nicotinic acetylcholine release, possibly contributing to blockade. Succinylcholine and depolarizing agents act by a different mechanism that is less well understood.

Succinylcholine

Succinylcholine is a depolarizing neuromuscular blocking agent and is structurally similar to acetylcholine. Like acetylcholine, succinylcholine depolarizes the membrane and opens sodium channels. Because succinylcholine is fairly resistant to acetylcholinesterase and not metabolized locally at the neuromuscular junction, it persists longer than acetylcholine and results in longer depolarization and a brief initial period of fasciculation. This is followed by a block in neurotransmission and the onset of flaccid paralysis, both of which are secondary to the inability of acetylcholine to initiate a propagating action potential at an already depolarized endplate. Succinylcholine is used because of its favorable pharmacokinetic profile, with quick onset and short duration (46). Administration is followed by muscle fasciculations and subsequent neuromuscular blockade 30–60 seconds after IV dosing. The blockade remains for ~5–10 minutes (2). Succinylcholine is eliminated by plasma cholinesterase, has a very short duration of action, and can be used independent of a patient's renal and hepatic status. Prolongation of blockade occurs in patients with conditions associated with plasma cholinesterase deficiency and with high doses (46). The elimination half-life is 3 hours (2). Succinylcholine can cause severe, although uncommon, adverse drug reactions, such as malignant hyperthermia (MH), increased intraocular pressure, masseter muscle rigidity, rhabdomyolysis, bradycardia, and hyperkalemia (2,46). It is contraindicated in patients with risk for MH, spinal cord injury (>24 hours old), severe burns, severe crush injuries, neuromuscular disorders, dysrhythmia, or preexisting hyperkalemia.

Pancuronium

Pancuronium is a nondepolarizing neuromuscular blocking agent. Onset of action occurs 4–6 minutes after administration and remains for 120–180 minutes (12). Pancuronium is

7% protein bound, with a V_d of 0.26 L/kg. The CL is estimated at 1.8 mL/kg/min (12). Approximately 60%–80% of pancuronium is eliminated by the kidney (2). In patients with renal failure, pancuronium CL is decreased significantly (46). Pancuronium is largely excreted unchanged in the urine, but a small percentage is metabolized to 3-desacetylpancuronium, which may accumulate after prolonged infusion. Although only 10% is eliminated by the liver, pancuronium also accumulates in fulminant hepatic failure (2,13). Its administration causes tachycardia, largely because of the blocking of cardiac muscarinic cholinergic receptors (2).

Vecuronium

Vecuronium, a steroid-based compound derived from pancuronium, is also a nondepolarizing neuromuscular blocker (13). The onset of action occurs 2–4 minutes after administration and remains for 30–40 minutes. The V_d is 0.2 L/kg (12). Vecuronium, like pancuronium, is deacetylated in the liver to produce 3-desacetyl, 17-desacetyl, and 3,17-desacetyl derivatives, which are, respectively, 2 times, 17 times, and 35 times less potent than the parent vecuronium compound (13). Even though it is primarily metabolized, cumulative effects of vecuronium are evident in renal transplant recipients and patients with severe renal failure. This effect is attributable to its metabolite, 3-desacetyl vecuronium, which has 80% of the activity of the parent drug and reportedly accumulates to a greater degree in patients with renal failure. Vecuronium may also accumulate in patients with hepatic failure because of decreased biliary uptake (2). In the presence of normal hepatic and renal function, the elimination half-life of vecuronium is 1.33–1.8 hours (13). Vecuronium's active metabolites are associated with prolonged effects lasting hours to days, which may be seen in patients with end-stage renal disease (46).

Atracurium and Cisatracurium

Atracurium is a nondepolarizing neuromuscular blocker of intermediate duration (13). The onset of action occurs 2–4 minutes after administration and remains for 30–40 minutes. Atracurium has a V_d of 0.16 L/kg, an elimination half-life of 0.3 hours, and a CL of 6.2 mL/kg/min (12). Atracurium and cisatracurium are eliminated by Hofmann elimination, which is a spontaneous nonenzymatic degradation at physiologic pH and temperature. Because of these pharmacokinetic properties, they are commonly regarded as appropriate agents when neuromuscular blockade is necessary in patients with multiorgan dysfunction. In contrast to atracurium, cisatracurium is associated with less risk of dose-dependent histamine release and hence less risk of urticaria, bronchospasm, or hypotension.

Atracurium is metabolized to the inactive metabolites laudanosine and a monoquaternary acrylate, both of which may be toxic. Laudanosine may accumulate in patients with renal insufficiency and in those receiving long-term infusions. Rare instances have been reported of patients developing seizures while receiving prolonged infusions of atracurium, presumably because of laudanosine accumulation. However, at therapeutic doses of atracurium, laudanosine concentrations may not reach adequate levels to produce a neurotoxic effect. Laudanosine and the monoacrylate are further metabolized, conjugated, and excreted in the urine. The activity of these final metabolites is unknown. Hypothermia and acidosis decrease the CL of atracurium, because Hofmann elimination is pH- and temperature dependent (46).

Mivacurium

Mivacurium is a nondepolarizing neuromuscular blocker (13). Onset of action occurs 2–4 minutes after administration and remains for 12–18 minutes (12). Mivacurium is eliminated by plasma cholinesterase, has a very short duration of action, and can be used independent of a patient's renal and hepatic status (46). As with succinylcholine, plasma cholinesterase deficiency prolongs the action of mivacurium. Higher doses are associated with histamine release (12). In the United States, mivacurium has largely been replaced by another nondepolarizing neuromuscular blocker with a safer cardiovascular profile.

Rocuronium

Rocuronium is a nondepolarizing neuromuscular blocker. Both the onset and duration of action are dose dependent. A dose of 0.6 mg/kg produces muscle relaxation in 1 minute, which lasts for 27 minutes (1–12-year-olds) to 41 minutes (3–12-month-olds). However, the 0.6-mg/kg dose may not result in optimal intubating conditions. Several trials have suggested that a higher dose of 1–1.2 mg/kg results in optimal intubating conditions in <1 minute, making rocuronium a useful alternative to succinylcholine for rapid sequence intubation (47). The higher dose is associated with a longer duration of action such that the clinician must weigh the risks and benefits of longer paralysis versus the risks and benefits of succinylcholine-associated complications. Rocuronium is metabolized in the liver and excreted in bile and urine.

Sympathomimetics

Dopamine

Dopamine is the metabolic precursor of norepinephrine and epinephrine. It is a central neurotransmitter, also found in the sympathetic nervous system and in the adrenal medulla. Dopamine stimulates dopamine (D_1 and D_2) receptors in the brain and in the vascular beds of the kidneys, mesentery, and coronary arteries. By activating cyclic AMP, D_1-receptor activation leads to vasodilation. It also stimulates α and β receptors, although its affinity for these receptors is lower (48). Low infusion rates (1–5 mcg/kg/min) augment renal sodium excretion through dopamine receptor agonism. Intermediate dosing (5–10 mcg/kg/min) results in chronotropic and inotropic effects through β-receptor agonism. Administration of these doses usually results in an increase in systolic blood pressure, minimal change in diastolic pressure, and a subsequent increase in pulse pressure. Systemic vascular resistance is unchanged secondary to the balance of dopamine's ability to reduce regional arteriolar resistance in the mesentery and kidneys, with only a minor increase in other vasculature. Higher doses (10–20 mcg/kg/min) result in increased vascular resistance secondary to a predominant α effect (12).

Dopamine hydrochloride is only used intravenously (12). As for all sympathomimetics, the central venous route is preferred over a peripheral vein. In hemodynamically stable adult patients, the steady-state V_d and the elimination half-life increased with the dose. At a dose of 3 mcg/kg/min, the V_d was 0.78 L/kg and the elimination half-life was 22 minutes, increasing to 1.58 L/kg and 38 minutes, respectively, with a dose of 6 mcg/kg/min (49). Similar values (elimination half-life of 26 minutes) were reported in hemodynamically stable children, aged 3 months to 13 years, who were recovering from cardiac surgery or shock (50). In critically ill newborn infants with sepsis and hypotensive shock, the V_d averaged 1.8 L/kg, and total body CL averaged 115 mL/kg/min (51). Dopamine is a substrate for monoamine oxidase (MAO) and catechol-O-methyltransferase (COMT) (12). In hemodynamically stable adult patients, dopamine CL ranged between 50 and 56 mL/kg/min and was independent of the dose (49). Plasma dopamine CL ranges from 60 to 80 mL/kg/min in adults and is lower in patients with renal or hepatic disease. CL in children

<2 years of age is approximately twice that in older children (82 vs. 46 mL/kg/min) (48).

A marked variation in CL was thought to explain the variation in dose amount required to achieve a desired clinical response in critically ill newborn infants (51). A study that evaluated the impact of hemodialysis on dopamine pharmacokinetics in seven adult patients reported that the fraction removed by dialysis was only 2.5% (52). Dopamine toxicity includes tachycardia, hypertension, dysrhythmias, and an increase in myocardial oxygen consumption. Dopamine depresses the ventilatory response to hypoxemia by as much as 60%. It can decrease arterial Po_2 by interfering with hypoxic pulmonary vasoconstriction. Dopamine administration may also suppress the release of thyrotropin (53).

Dobutamine

Dobutamine resembles dopamine structurally and is delivered as a racemate. The (+) isomer is a strong β agonist and α_1 antagonist, whereas the (−) dobutamine isomer is a weak β antagonist and a potent α_1 agonist. Dobutamine has somewhat greater selectivity for β_1 than β_2 receptors. As a result of opposing α_1 activities, dobutamine produces significant inotropic support, with less chronotropic and vasopressor activity (12). Doses of 5–20 mcg/kg/min are employed for inotropic support.

Dobutamine hydrochloride is used only intravenously. Dobutamine's V_d is 0.2 L/kg, with steady-state concentrations achieved within 10 minutes of the initiation of the infusion (12). In 10 children who were post–cardiac surgery and in 17 with shock, who ranged in age from 0.13 to 16.6 years, the elimination half-life was 25.8 minutes (54). Dobutamine's major metabolites are conjugates of dobutamine and 3-O-methyl dobutamine (12). Typical CL values in sick children are 70–100 mL/kg/min (55). In a study of 12 critically ill children aged 1 month to 17 years, dobutamine plasma CL rates ranged from 40 to 130 mL/kg/min, and dobutamine pharmacokinetics followed a first-order kinetic model (54,55). Dobutamine increases myocardial oxygen demand and may predispose to arrhythmias (12). Acute high-dose dobutamine lowers thyroid-stimulating hormone by an unknown mechanism (56).

Epinephrine

Epinephrine is useful in treating shock associated with myocardial dysfunction and hypotension. Epinephrine activates α_1, β_1, and β_2 receptors. It is a principal hormone of stress, and produces widespread metabolic and hemodynamic effects. β_1 receptors are affected by very low plasma concentrations of epinephrine, seen at doses of 0.05–0.1 mcg/kg/min. The earliest effects of epinephrine are an increase in heart rate and inotropy. Myocardial oxygen utilization may increase out of proportion to the increase in force of contraction. At these doses, stimulation of β_2 receptors promotes relaxation of resistance arterioles, promoting a decrease in systemic vascular resistance and diastolic blood pressure. Higher plasma concentrations result in activation of α_1 receptors, with a subsequent increase in systemic vascular resistance. At moderate doses (0.1–1 mcg/kg/min), the α stimulation is often balanced by the improved cardiac output and relaxation of the arteriolar beds. High-dose infusions (1–2 mcg/kg/min) are associated with significant vasoconstriction and possible compromise of blood flow to individual organs. The most predominant vascular effects are seen in the smaller arterioles, although veins and large arteries also have a response. The effect of epinephrine infusions on blood flow to hepatic, splanchnic, and renal vascular beds is variable and depends on baseline hemodynamics, disease state, and epinephrine dose. Even when epinephrine infusion leads to improved blood pressure and cardiac output, blood flow to abdominal viscera may decrease as flow is diverted to heart, brain, and skeletal muscle.

Epinephrine has many uses. It is commonly used in the treatment of respiratory diseases with elements of bronchospasm. It can also be used to treat the symptoms of hypersensitivity reactions to drugs and other allergens (12). In the pediatric critical care environment, the most frequent indications for IV epinephrine are cardiogenic shock and septic shock with reduced stroke volume. Patients with septic shock who do not improve after aggressive volume repletion and treatment with dopamine and/or dobutamine may benefit from epinephrine. Epinephrine is the principal drug used in CPR (cardiopulmonary resuscitation) after cardiac arrest (see Chapter 25).

Epinephrine is not effective after oral administration because it is rapidly oxidized and conjugated in the gastrointestinal mucosa and liver. Absorption from subcutaneous tissues is slow because of vasoconstriction. When inhaled, the actions of the drug are largely restricted to the respiratory system; however, systemic tachycardia can occur (12). Enhanced automaticity and increased oxygen consumption are the major toxicities. A severe imbalance of myocardial oxygen delivery and consumption may produce electrocardiographic changes consistent with ischemia. Hypokalemia secondary to β_2-adrenergic stimulation and hyperglycemia secondary to α-adrenergic–mediated insulin suppression are associated with epinephrine administration.

Norepinephrine

Dopamine is carboxylated at the β carbon to produce norepinephrine. Norepinephrine differs from epinephrine in that it lacks the methyl substitution on the amino group. Norepinephrine has little β_2 activity but is a potent α_1 and β_1 agonist. Infusions in normal subjects result in elevations of systemic vascular resistance because the α_1 effects are not opposed by β_2 stimulation. Reflex vagal activity reduces the heart rate, blunting the expected chronotropic effect of β_1 stimulation. Stoke volume increases, but cardiac output changes minimally. Peripheral vascular resistance increases in most vascular beds, including the kidney, liver, and skeletal muscle. Glomerular filtration is maintained, unless the decrease in renal blood flow is very substantial. Mesenteric vessels are also constricted, decreasing splanchnic and hepatic blood flow. Coronary blood flow increases because of direct coronary dilation and increase in blood pressure (12).

Norepinephrine is administered intravenously (12). The elimination half-life of IV norepinephrine is 2–2.5 minutes. Norepinephrine is metabolized by enzymatic degradation by either COMT or MAO. It is also cleared from the plasma by neuronal and tissue uptake. The CL of norepinephrine in healthy adults is 24–40 mL/kg/min. Limited pediatric pharmacokinetic data are available (57). Norepinephrine administration may result in compromised organ blood flow. It may improve blood pressure without improving perfusion, most commonly seen with a low cardiac index and elevated capillary wedge pressure (58,59).

Isoproterenol

Isoproterenol, the synthetic N-isopropyl derivative of norepinephrine, is a potent, nonselective β-adrenergic agonist with very low affinity for α-adrenergic receptors. The principal cardiovascular effects relate to its inotropic, chronotropic, and peripheral vasodilator effects. Isoproterenol increases heart rate and enhances contractility. Peripheral vasodilatation produces a decrease in systemic vascular resistance. The increase in inotropy and chronotropy in the face of decreased systemic vascular resistance results in an increase of cardiac output. Isoproterenol relaxes almost all smooth muscle but has a significant impact on bronchial and gastrointestinal smooth muscle. Pulmonary bronchial and vascular bed β_2-adrenergic receptor agonism results in bronchodilation and pulmonary vasodilation. If normal prior to the isoproterenol infusion, mesenteric and renal perfusion decrease. However, if isoproterenol is administered in a shock state, the increase in cardiac output may result in increase in blood flow to these tissues (12).

Isoproterenol can be given parenterally or as an aerosol. Isoproterenol is metabolized predominantly by COMT (12). The pharmacokinetics of isoproterenol in infants and children was studied in pediatric patients who were either postoperative from cardiac surgery or being treated for reactive airway disease. The volume of distribution was 0.2 L/kg. The average CL was 42.5 mL/kg/min, and the average plasma half-life was 4.2 minutes (30). Isoproterenol increases myocardial demand for oxygen and decreases supply by decreasing coronary filling. If the patient is intravascularly fluid depleted and not provided with fluid resuscitation, hypotension may occur with the institution of the drug (12).

Phenylephrine

Phenylephrine demonstrates predominantly α_1-adrenergic agonism. It causes marked vasoconstriction of the arterial and venous capacitance vessels, resulting in a rise in blood pressure and a sinus bradycardia owing to vagal reflexes (60).

Vasodilators

Sodium Nitroprusside

Despite its widespread use, quality pharmacokinetic and pharmacodynamic data regarding the use of sodium nitroprusside (SNP) in children are limited. Experiences with SNP used to induce deliberate hypotension in small cohorts of children have been described (61,62). Investigators observed that younger subjects required more SNP than did older subjects to achieve comparable degrees of blood pressure control. In their small retrospective cohort, doses of 10 mcg/kg/min were necessary to achieve satisfactory blood pressure response. Three possible responses to nitroprusside administration in children were described: (a) a constant response to "conventional" doses <3 mcg/kg/min, (b) a tachyphylactic response characterized by continuously escalating dose requirement (>3 mcg/kg/min) to achieve a satisfactory blood pressure, and (c) resistance to the blood pressure–lowering effects of the drug. They cautioned against using total doses that exceeded 3 mcg/kg/min or continuing administration of nitroprusside in the latter two scenarios. Another group compared SNP to nitroglycerin for inducing hypotension in a group of 14 adolescents; they found that doses of SNP between 6 and 8 mcg/kg/min were superior to nitroglycerin at any dose in the reliable induction of hypotension for children and adolescents undergoing scoliosis, craniofacial, or hepatic surgery (63). In a randomized trial comparing nitroprusside to nicardipine in 20 healthy adolescents with idiopathic scoliosis undergoing spinal fusion, target blood pressures were easily obtainable in both groups, and operating conditions were comparable (64). The time to restoration of baseline blood pressure after termination of the infusion was significantly longer in the nicardipine group. Interestingly, blood loss was significantly greater in the SNP group. Details on nitroprusside dose requirements were not provided.

A well-described potential side effect of nitroprusside is cyanide and/or thiocyanate toxicity. IV SNP degradation results in the release of free cyanide. Cyanide accumulation can cause a metabolic acidosis (with an elevated venous oxygen saturation), arrhythmia, excessive hypotension, and death. Cyanide can subsequently be converted to serum thiocyanate using thiosulfate. Thiocyanate is ultimately renally eliminated (3). SNP metabolism was described in 10 children who received SNP at doses up to 10 mcg/kg/min (mean infusion rate, 6 mcg/kg/min) while undergoing cardiopulmonary bypass for repair of complex congenital cardiac defects (65). Cyanide levels rose as a function of time while SNP was infused, and they rapidly fell when SNP was discontinued. Despite the fact that some children demonstrated plasma cyanide levels above the generally accepted threshold of 0.5 mcg/mL, no patients developed clinically apparent toxicity. Adverse effects include nausea, vomiting, agitation, and muscular twitching. Acute psychosis from thiocyanate intoxication can result from prolonged therapy, especially in patients with renal failure.

Hydralazine

Hydralazine causes the direct relaxation of arteriolar smooth muscle. Venous capacitance vessels are not dilated, and postural hypotension is uncommon. IV hydralazine may be used for hypertensive emergencies but is rarely the sole agent with which to treat hypertension (12). It is well absorbed but undergoes significant first-pass metabolism, making the systemic bioavailability low. It is 87% protein bound, and has a V_d of 1.5 L/kg. The rate of acetylation is genetically determined, with ~50% of the US population being fast acetylators and the other 50%, slow. The elimination half-life is 1 hour, although the systemic effect may remain for up to 12 hours. The CL is 50 mL/kg/min (12). Sympathetic stimulation can result in an increased heart rate, increased renin activity, and subsequent fluid retention. Side effects include headache, nausea, flushing, and palpitations. Administration can result in a syndrome that resembles systemic lupus and is characterized by serum sickness, hemolytic anemia, vasculitis, and glomerulonephritis (12).

Nicardipine

Nicardipine is a calcium entry blocker (slow-channel blocker or calcium ion antagonist) that inhibits the transmembrane influx of calcium ions into cardiac muscle and smooth muscle without changing serum calcium concentrations. The effects of nicardipine are more selective to vascular smooth muscle than to cardiac muscle. In animal models, nicardipine produces a relaxation of coronary vascular smooth muscle at drug levels that cause little or no negative inotropic effect. In humans, nicardipine produces a significant decrease in systemic vascular resistance. The degree of vasodilation and the resultant hypotensive effects are more prominent in hypertensive patients. In hypertensive patients, nicardipine reduces the blood pressure at rest and during exercise. In normotensive patients, a small decrease in systolic and diastolic blood pressure may occur.

Rapid dose-related increases in nicardipine plasma concentrations are seen during the first 2 hours after initiation of an infusion, and concentrations reach a steady state at ~24–48 hours. On termination of the infusion, plasma concentrations rapidly decline, with at least a 50% decrease during the first 2 hours. The V_d is ~8.3 L/kg, and the elimination half-life in adults is 8.6 hours (66).

Nicardipine undergoes extensive hepatic metabolism via the P450 pathway. Transformation of the N-benzyl side-chain position 3 is the primary site of breakdown. Oxidation to the pyridine analog is another source of metabolism (67). Virtually no unchanged drug is found in the urine. Although nicardipine is principally metabolized by the liver, lower CL has been reported in patients with renal impairment (66). Cimetidine increases plasma levels. Patients receiving the two drugs concomitantly should be carefully monitored. Concomitant administration of nicardipine and cyclosporine results in elevated plasma cyclosporine levels. Plasma concentrations of cyclosporine should therefore be closely monitored, and its dosage reduced accordingly, in patients treated with nicardipine (66).

Steroids

Glucocorticoids play a role in appetite regulation, fuel mobilization, immunosuppression, and blood pressure regulation. Mineralocorticoids are predominantly responsible for the regulation of electrolyte balance.

Glucocorticoids

Cortisol is synthesized in the zona fasciculata of the adrenal gland. It is released in response to adrenocorticotropic hormone (ACTH), produced in the pituitary. ACTH release is mediated through hypothalamic release of corticotropin-releasing hormone (CRH) from the hypothalamus. Glucocorticoids are lipid-soluble cholesterol derivatives that diffuse across the plasma membrane where they bind to intracellular receptors. Natural and synthetic glucocorticoids display wide ranging receptor-binding affinities. The relative potency of glucocorticoids has been historically defined on the basis of pituitary ACTH suppression on the morning following a single dose (1,68).

Adrenal insufficiency is a glucocorticoid deficient state that may or may not be associated with mineralocorticoid deficiency. Primary adrenal insufficiency is due to adrenal disease and is characterized by an elevated ACTH level. Secondary adrenal insufficiency is a glucocorticoid deficient state that is due to hypothalamic and/or pituitary dysfunction. Commonly administered glucocorticoids included prednisone, methylprednisone, hydrocortisone, and dexamethasone. Each of these drugs varies in their pharmacokinetic half-life, pharmacodynamic (relative effect) half-life, glucocorticoid-receptor affinity, and mineralocorticoid-receptor affinity (1) (**Table 22.1**). A recent systematic review of corticosteroid use in the setting of sepsis concluded that various doses of corticosteroids have been used for >50 years, with no clear benefit on mortality. This question remains unresolved; current pediatric sepsis guidelines recommend corticosteroid administration for catecholamine-resistant and fluid-resistant septic shock (69).

Mineralocorticoids

Aldosterone is synthesized in the zona glomerulosa of the adrenal gland under the influence of angiotensin II and ACTH. Aldosterone synthesis is increased when the renal juxtaglomerular apparatus senses insufficient circulatory volume, stimulating renin release, and formation of angiotensin II. Primary mineralocorticoid deficiency occurs in Addison disease and other adrenal diseases. This characterized by hyperkalemia, hyponatremia, postural hypotension, and low plasma aldosterone. Fludrocortisone is the mainstay of therapy for primary mineralocorticoid deficiency. Fludrocortisone has a high affinity for glucocorticoid

receptors, but a much higher affinity for the mineralocorticoid receptor. Therefore, the doses used in the replacement of mineralocorticoid deficiency have minimal glucocorticoid effect (1).

Miscellaneous

Nitric Oxide

Nitric oxide (NO) is produced by many cells of the body. It relaxes vascular smooth muscle by binding to the heme moiety of cytosolic guanylate cyclase, activating guanylate cyclase, and increasing intracellular levels of cyclic guanosine $3',5'$-monophosphate, which then leads to vasodilation. NO has a half-life of only a few seconds in vivo. However, because it is soluble in both aqueous and lipid media, it readily diffuses through the cytoplasm and plasma membranes. NO has effects on neuronal transmission and on synaptic plasticity in the CNS. When inhaled, NO produces pulmonary vasodilation and thus finds its principal use in the treatment of pulmonary hypertension.

Inhaled NO appears to increase the PaO_2 by dilating pulmonary vessels in better-ventilated areas of the lung, redistributing pulmonary blood flow away from lung regions with low ventilation-to-perfusion ratios toward regions with normal ratios. Although this therapy transiently improves oxygenation in patients with acute respiratory failure, it has not improved long-term outcomes.

In addition to its hemodynamic effects, inhaled NO may inhibit platelet aggregation. These effects are dose dependent, in that both excesses and deficiencies of the gas have been implicated in the genesis and/or evolution of many significant diseases. At high concentrations (>80–100 ppm), inhaled NO has proinflammatory and pro-oxidant effects, increasing macrophage production of tumor necrosis factor (TNF)-α, interleukin (IL)-1, and reactive oxygen species (70,71). Concentrations up to 80 ppm appear to reduce the number and activity of pulmonary neutrophils. The dose of 50 ppm appears to reduce the migration of neutrophils from the vascular compartment to the airways and inhibits chemotaxis (72).

The pharmacokinetics of NO has been studied only in adults. NO is absorbed systemically after inhalation. Most of it traverses the pulmonary capillary bed, where it combines with hemoglobin that is 60%–100% oxygen saturated. At this level of oxygen saturation, NO combines predominantly with oxyhemoglobin to produce methemoglobin and nitrate. At low oxygen saturation, NO can combine with deoxyhemoglobin to transiently form nitrosylhemoglobin, which is converted to nitrogen oxides and methemoglobin on exposure to oxygen. Within the pulmonary system, NO can combine with oxygen and water to produce nitrogen dioxide (NO_2) and nitrite, respectively, which interact with oxyhemoglobin to produce methemoglobin and nitrate. Thus, the end products of NO that enter the systemic circulation are predominantly methemoglobin and nitrate. Nitrate has been identified as the predominant

TABLE 22.1

COMPARISON OF GLUCOCORTICOID POTENCY AND HALF-LIFE

	■ GLUCOCORTICOID POTENCY	■ MINERALOCORTICOID POTENCY	■ EQUIVALENT DOSE (mg)	■ PK HALF-LIFE (min)	■ PD HALF-LIFE (h)
Dexamethasone	25–30	0	0.75	200	36–54
Methylprednisone	5	0	4	214	18–36
Prednisone	4	+	5	200	18–36
Hydrocortisone	1	++	20	80–110	8–12

From Carruthers SG, Hoffman BB, Melmon KL, eds. *Melmon and Morrelli's Clinical Pharmacology.* New York, NY: McGraw-Hill, 2000.

NO metabolite excreted in the urine, accounting for >70% of the NO dose inhaled. Nitrate is cleared from the plasma by the kidney at rates approaching the rate of glomerular filtration. No studies have been conducted to assess the interaction of inhaled NO with other drugs. Hence, clinical interactions with other medications used in the treatment of respiratory failure cannot be ruled out. Inhaled NO has been administered in combination with dopamine, dobutamine, corticosteroids, and surfactant without interactions being detected (73).

Both relative and absolute contraindications have been described for the use of NO. An absolute contraindication is warranted in the rare condition of methemoglobin reductase deficiency. The primary concerns related to the administration of inhaled NO are the formation of NO_2, methemoglobinemia, and the "rebound effect." The latter describes a phenomenon in which significant increases in pulmonary vascular resistance (rebound pulmonary hypertension) occur following termination of inhaled NO. NO_2 production is another potential concern with the use of inhaled NO. NO_2 is produced from NO and oxygen and can cause oxidative pulmonary damage, resulting in the generation of free radicals, which can oxidize amino acids and begin lipid peroxidation of the cellular membrane (73,74).

Milrinone

Milrinone has combined inotropic and vasodilating effects ("inodilator"), as well as lusitropic effects (75). It is a bipyridine derivative of amrinone, primarily used for the treatment of congestive heart failure and commonly used to support cardiac output after congenital heart surgery in neonates, infants, and children. The drug is primarily cleared through renal secretion (85%), with 15% undergoing glucuronidation, and is 70% protein bound (76). Pharmacokinetic studies suggest that the CL of milrinone is greater and its V_d is larger in children than in adults (77,78), but infants appear to have lower milrinone CL than do children (78).

A recent study of pediatric patients <6 years of age who received milrinone as a slow-loading dose followed by a constant-rate infusion after cardiac surgery used population modeling to describe milrinone pharmacokinetics (79). The pharmacokinetics was best described by a weight-normalized, one-compartment model. The V_d of 482 mL/kg was independent of age, whereas CL increased linearly with age. A comparable two-compartment model had a central V_d of 66 mL/kg, peripheral V_d of 269 mL/kg, CL of 6.29 mL/kg/min, and an intercompartmental CL of 4.75 mL/kg/min. In pediatric patients who underwent biventricular cardiac surgery, the V_d and CL of milrinone were reported as 900 mL/kg and 3.8 mL/kg/min for infants and 700 mL/kg and 5.9 mL/kg/min for children, respectively (78). In a population of neonates who underwent Norwood Stage I single-ventricle palliation, a loading dose of 100 mcg/kg during cardiopulmonary bypass resulted in plasma peak and trough milrinone concentrations similar to those achieved with 50-mcg/kg loading doses in other clinical settings (80).

Because of impaired renal CL during the immediate postoperative period, a standard infusion of 0.5 mcg/kg/min resulted in drug accumulation during the initial 12 hours of drug administration. Immediately postoperatively, milrinone CL was significantly impaired (0.4 mL/kg/min), improved by the 12th postoperative hour, and approached steady-state CL by postoperative day 4. The weight-normalized population estimate for steady-state CL in this population was 2.6 mL/kg/min, which is less than that reported for older infants postoperative from cardiac surgery (81).

Vasopressin

Vasopressin is an exogenous, parenteral form of antidiuretic hormone. Antidiuretic hormone is produced in the parvocellular and magnocellular neurons within the supraoptic and paraventricular nuclei of the hypothalamus. It is stored and released by the posterior pituitary gland in response to increases in plasma osmolality or as a baroreflex response to decreases in blood pressure and/or blood volume.

The cellular effects of vasopressin are mediated by two major receptors: V_1 and V_2. V_1 receptors have been further subdivided as V_{1a} and V_{1b}. The V_{1a} receptor is the most widespread and is found in vascular smooth muscle, myometrium, the bladder, adipocytes, hepatocytes, platelets, renal medullary interstitial cells, vasa recta in the renal circulation, epithelial cells in the renal cortical collecting duct, spleen, testis, and many CNS structures. Only the adenohypophysis is known to contain V_{1b} receptors. V_2 receptors are predominantly found in the principal cells of the renal collecting duct system. V_2 receptors mediate the most predominant renal response to vasopressin, resulting in increased water permeability in the collecting duct. These V_2-mediated effects occur at much lower concentrations than are required to engage V_1-receptor–mediated actions. Other renal activities mediated by V_2 include increased urea and sodium (Na^+) transport, increasing the urine concentrating ability of the kidneys.

The cardiovascular effects of vasopressin are complex. Vasopressin administration results in significant vasoconstriction, mediated by V_1 receptors. Vascular smooth muscle in the skin, skeletal muscle, fat, pancreas, and thyroid gland appear to be most sensitive, with vasoconstriction also occurring in gastrointestinal tract, coronary vessels, and brain. Activation of V_2 receptors increases circulating concentrations of procoagulant factor VIII and von Willebrand factor, and vasopressin is presumed to stimulate the secretion of these factors from storage sites in the vascular endothelium (12).

Diabetes insipidus is a disease of impaired renal conservation of water, either secondary to an inadequate secretion of vasopressin (central diabetes insipidus), as seen with many patients who have sustained traumatic brain injury, or an insufficient renal response to vasopressin (nephrogenic diabetes insipidus). Vasopressin is most commonly indicated in the treatment of patients with high urine flow owing to central diabetes insipidus (82).

Because of its vasoactive effects, vasopressin therapy has been evaluated in the specific setting of cardiac arrest and refractory hypotension in septic shock (83). It was recently recommended by the American Heart Association as an alternative to epinephrine for adult patients in ventricular fibrillation, and it is used to control upper gastrointestinal hemorrhage given its ability to cause vasoconstriction of the mesenteric vasculature.

Vasopressin must be administered parenterally because it is degraded by trypsin in the gastrointestinal tract. The duration of antidiuretic effect following intramuscular or subcutaneous administration is ~2–8 hours. The hormone distributes throughout the extracellular fluid but does not bind to plasma proteins. Vasopressin is degraded primarily in the liver and kidneys, and has a plasma half-life of 10–35 minutes. Approximately 5% of a subcutaneously administered dose is excreted unchanged in the urine within 4 hours (84). Large doses can result in cardiac complications, such as arrhythmias and decreased cardiac output.

CURRENT ISSUES SURROUNDING PHARMACOTHERAPY

Based on the Food and Drug Administration's (FDA) Web site (http://www.fda.gov/Drugs/DrugSafety/DrugShortages/default.htm), in 2010, there were 178 drug shortages reported to the U.S. FDA. In 2011, there were 251 drug shortages reported, 183 of which involved sterile injectable drugs. These shortages have involved cancer drugs, anesthetics, drugs needed for emergency medicine, and electrolytes needed for patients on IV feeding. The major reasons for these shortages have been quality/manufacturing issues, production delays at the manufacturer, and delays receiving raw materials and components from suppliers. The discontinuations of older drugs by companies in favor of newer, more profitable drugs also contribute to these shortages. In 2012, the FDA averted >100 drug shortages by working with manufacturers to find alternatives and by expediting drug reviews and approvals. The FDA and the American Hospital Association say that the shortages have already caused thousands of cancer patients to delay treatment and nearly every hospital to ration supplies, and hundreds of clinical trials have had to be halted or delayed for lack of drugs. It is estimated that 1 in 10 anesthesiologists has postponed or canceled procedures because of a lack of appropriate drugs. Hospitals are faced with the growing need to educate medical staff about replacement products, impacting patient safety. These current drug shortages have resulted in suboptimal treatment of many patients. It is the responsibility of the drug prescriber to identify safe and effective alternates to drugs that have been subject to these shortages (85).

SUMMARY

Pharmacology is an important discipline that underlies the management of pharmacotherapy, or the safe and effective administration of pharmaceuticals. Understanding pharmacologic principles is essential for the proper application of pharmacotherapeutic modalities in critically ill children. Although much of the pharmacologic knowledge used to derive dosing guidance for critically ill children is obtained from adult and other pediatric populations, research into understanding the dose requirements for critically ill children is more active than ever before.

Because children are typically not subject to dose-escalation studies similar to those conducted in the adult population, initial estimation of dose requirements in pediatrics is often based on various arbitrary descriptors of body size; the lack of well-conducted pharmacodynamic and pharmacokinetic studies is often replaced by extrapolation from adult or animal data. Likewise, the pediatric susceptibility to adverse drug reactions is often difficult to predict. Past therapeutic mishaps have clearly shown that dosing derived from adult studies cannot easily be extrapolated to infants and children. In addition, many adult dosage forms, such as tablets and capsules, are inappropriate for neonates, infants, and preschool children. Likewise, targeted investigations in critically ill pediatric populations are now occurring with greater frequency, as the scientific community has a greater appreciation of the risk of ignorance and the incredible burden placed on the caregivers of this population. As these data become available, it is likewise incumbent on caregivers to educate themselves to this guidance and be able to apply such knowledge to their own practice.

References

1. Carruthers SG, Hoffman BB, Melmon KL, David Nierenberg eds. *Melmon and Morrelli's Clinical Pharmacology*. New York, NY: McGraw-Hill, 2000.
2. Chernow B, ed. *The Pharmacologic Approach to the Critically Ill Patient*. Baltimore, MD: Williams & Wilkins, 1994.
3. Katzung B, ed. *Basic and Clinical Pharmacology*. New York, NY: McGraw Hill, 2001.
4. Krishnan V, Murray P. Pharmacologic issues in the critically ill. *Clin Chest Med* 2003;24(4):671–88.
5. Rodighiero V. Effects of liver disease on pharmacokinetics. An update. *Clin Pharmacokinet* 1999;37(5):399–431.
6. Kearns GL, et al. Developmental pharmacology—Drug disposition, action, and therapy in infants and children. *N Engl J Med* 2003;349(12):1157–67.
7. Huang NN, High RH. Comparison of serum levels following the administration of oral and parenteral preparations of penicillin to infants and children of various age groups. *J Pediatr* 1953;42(6):657–8.
8. Tsai CE, et al. P-glycoprotein expression in mouse brain increases with maturation. *Biol Neonate* 2002;81(1):58–64.
9. Painter MJ, et al. Phenobarbital and phenytoin in neonatal seizures: Metabolism and tissue distribution. *Neurology* 1981;31(9):1107–12.
10. Mendelson WB. Neuropharmacology of sleep induction by benzodiazepines. *Crit Rev Neurobiol* 1992;6(4):221–32.
11. Young CC, Prielipp RC. Benzodiazepines in the intensive care unit. *Crit Care Clin* 2001;17(4):843–62.
12. Hardman JG, et al., eds. *Goodman and Gilman's The Pharmacologic Basis of Therapeutics*. New York, NY: McGraw-Hill, 1996.
13. Power BM, et al. Pharmacokinetics of drugs used in critically ill adults. *Clin Pharmacokinet* 1998;34(1):25–56.
14. Reed MD, et al. The single-dose pharmacokinetics of midazolam and its primary metabolite in pediatric patients after oral and intravenous administration. *J Clin Pharmacol* 2001;41(12):1359–69.
15. de Wildt SN, et al. Population pharmacokinetics and metabolism of midazolam in pediatric intensive care patients. *Crit Care Med* 2003;31(7):1952–8.
16. Lacroix D, et al. Expression of CYP3A in the human liver—Evidence that the shift between CYP3A7 and CYP3A4 occurs immediately after birth. *Eur J Biochem* 1997;247(2):625–34.
17. Shelly MP, Mendel L, Park GR. Failure of critically ill patients to metabolise midazolam. *Anaesthesia* 1987;42(6):619–26.
18. Gehlbach BK, Kress JP. Sedation in the intensive care unit. *Curr Opin Crit Care* 2002;8(4):290–8.
19. Klotz U, Kanto J. Pharmacokinetics and clinical use of flumazenil (Ro 15-1788). *Clin Pharmacokinet* 1988;14(1):1–12.
20. Greenberg SB, Adams RC, Aspinall CL. Initial experience with intravenous pentobarbital sedation for children undergoing MRI at a tertiary care pediatric hospital: The learning curve. *Pediatr Radiol* 2000;30(10):689–91.
21. Hubbard AM, et al. Sedation for pediatric patients undergoing CT and MRI. *J Comput Assist Tomogr* 1992;16(1):3–6.
22. Physicians' Desk Reference. Montvale, NJ: Thomson Healthcare, 2006.
23. Cook CE, et al. Pharmacokinetics of pentobarbital enantiomers as determined by enantioselective radioimmunoassay after administration of racemate to humans and rabbits. *J Pharmacol Exp Ther* 1987;241(3):779–85.
24. Ehrnebo M. Pharmacokinetics and distribution properties of pentobarbital in humans following oral and intravenous administration. *J Pharm Sci* 1974;63(7):1114–8.
25. Bayliff CD, Schwartz ML, Hardy BG. Pharmacokinetics of high-dose pentobarbital in severe head trauma. *Clin Pharmacol Ther* 1985;38(4):457–61.
26. Wermeling DP, et al. Pentobarbital pharmacokinetics in patients with severe head injury. *Drug Intell Clin Pharm* 1987;21(5):459–63.
27. Zuppa AF, et al. Population pharmacokinetics of pentobarbital in neonates, infants, and children after open heart surgery. *J Pediatr* 2011;159(3):414–9 e1–3.
28. Schaible DH, et al. High-dose pentobarbital pharmacokinetics in hypothermic brain-injured children. *J Pediatr* 1982;100(4):655–60.
29. Hall LG, Oyen LJ, Murray MJ. Analgesic agents. Pharmacology and application in critical care. *Crit Care Clin* 2001;17(4):899–923.
30. Reyes G, et al. The pharmacokinetics of isoproterenol in critically ill pediatric patients. *J Clin Pharmacol* 1993;33(1):29–34.
31. Hagmeyer KO, Mauro LS, Mauro VF. Meperidine-related seizures associated with patient-controlled analgesia pumps. *Ann Pharmacother* 1993;27(1):29–32.
32. Volles DF, McGory R. Pharmacokinetic considerations. *Crit Care Clin* 1999;15(1):55–75.
33. Patel SS, Spencer CM. Remifentanil. *Drugs* 1996;52(3):417–27; discussion 428.
34. Kohrs R, Durieux ME. Ketamine: Teaching an old drug new tricks. *Anesth Analg* 1998;87(5):1186–93.

35. Schuttler J, Ihmsen H. Population pharmacokinetics of propofol: A multicenter study. *Anesthesiology* 2000;92(3):727–38.

36. Kazama T, et al. Relation between initial blood distribution volume and propofol induction dose requirement. *Anesthesiology* 2001;94(2):205–10.

37. Kazama T, Ikeda K, Morita K. Reduction by fentanyl of the Cp50 values of propofol and hemodynamic responses to various noxious stimuli. *Anesthesiology* 1997;87(2):213–27.

38. Cray SH, Robinson BH, Cox PN. Lactic acidemia and bradyarrhythmia in a child sedated with propofol. *Crit Care Med* 1998; 26(12):2087–92.

39. Cremer OL, et al. Long-term propofol infusion and cardiac failure in adult head-injured patients. *Lancet* 2001;357(9250):117–8.

40. Annane D. ICU physicians should abandon the use of etomidate! *Intensive Care Med* 2005;31(3):325–6.

41. Chan CM, Mitchell AL, Shorr AF. Etomidate is associated with mortality and adrenal insufficiency in sepsis: A meta-analysis. *Crit Care Med* 2012;40:2945–53.

42. Bhana N, Goa KL, McClellan KJ. Dexmedetomidine. *Drugs* 2000;59(2):263–8; discussion 269–70.

43. Venn RM, Grounds RM. Comparison between dexmedetomidine and propofol for sedation in the intensive care unit: Patient and clinician perceptions. *Br J Anaesth* 2001;87(5):684–90.

44. Abbot, Precedex Product Label.

45. Su F, et al. Population pharmacokinetics of dexmedetomidine in infants after open heart surgery. *Anesth Analg* 2010;110(5): 1383–92.

46. McManus MC. Neuromuscular blockers in surgery and intensive care, Part 1. *Am J Health Syst Pharm* 2001;58(23):2287–99.

47. Perry JJ, Lee JS, Sillberg VAH, et al. Rocuronium versus succinylcholine for rapid sequence induction intubation. *Cochrane Database Syst Rev* 2008;2(CD002788).

48. Notterman DA, et al. Dopamine clearance in critically ill infants and children: Effect of age and organ system dysfunction. *Clin Pharmacol Ther* 1990;48(2):138–47.

49. Le Corre P, et al. Steady-state pharmacokinetics of dopamine in adult patients. *Crit Care Med* 1993;21(11):1652–7.

50. Eldadah MK, et al. Pharmacokinetics of dopamine in infants and children. *Crit Care Med* 1991;19(8):1008–11.

51. Bhatt-Mehta V, et al. Dopamine pharmacokinetics in critically ill newborn infants. *Eur J Clin Pharmacol* 1991;40(6):593–7.

52. Allen E, et al. Alterations in dopamine clearance and catechol-O-methyltransferase activity by dopamine infusions in children. *Crit Care Med* 1997;25(1):181–9.

53. Van den Berghe G, de Zegher F, Lauwers P. Dopamine suppresses pituitary function in infants and children. *Crit Care Med* 1994;22(11):1747–53.

54. Schwartz PH, Eldadah MK, Newth CJ. The pharmacokinetics of dobutamine in pediatric intensive care unit patients. *Drug Metab Dispos* 1991;19(3):614–9.

55. Habib DM, et al. Dobutamine pharmacokinetics and pharmacodynamics in pediatric intensive care patients. *Crit Care Med* 1992;20(5):601–8.

56. Lee CY, et al. Non-exercise stress transthoracic echocardiography: Transesophageal atrial pacing versus dobutamine stress. *J Am Coll Cardiol* 1999;33(2):506–11.

57. Steinberg C, Notterman DA. Pharmacokinetics of cardiovascular drugs in children. Inotropes and vasopressors. *Clin Pharmacokinet* 1994;27(5):345–67.

58. Desjars P, et al. Norepinephrine therapy has no deleterious renal effects in human septic shock. *Crit Care Med* 1989;17(5): 426–9.

59. Fukuoka T, et al. Effects of norepinephrine on renal function in septic patients with normal and elevated serum lactate levels. *Crit Care Med* 1989;17(11):1104–7.

60. Cooper DW, et al. Fetal and maternal effects of phenylephrine and ephedrine during spinal anesthesia for cesarean delivery. *Anesthesiology* 2002;97(6):1582–90.

61. Bennett NR, Abbott TR. The use of sodium nitroprusside in children. *Anaesthesia* 1977;32(5):456–63.

62. Davies DW, et al. Sodium nitroprusside in children: Observations on metabolism during normal and abnormal responses. *Can Anaesth Soc J* 1975;22(5):553–60.

63. Yaster M, et al. A comparison of nitroglycerin and nitroprusside for inducing hypotension in children: A double-blind study. *Anesthesiology* 1986;65(2):175–9.

64. Hersey SL, et al. Nicardipine versus nitroprusside for controlled hypotension during spinal surgery in adolescents. *Anesth Analg* 1997;84(6):1239–44.

65. Przybylo HJ, et al. Sodium nitroprusside metabolism in children during hypothermic cardiopulmonary bypass. *Anesth Analg* 1995;81(5):952–6.

66. Wyeth Laboratories. Product Information: Cardene IV, n. Philadelphia, 1999.

67. Urien S, et al. Plasma protein binding and erythrocyte partitioning of nicardipine in vitro. *J Cardiovasc Pharmacol* 1985;7(5):891–8.

68. Meikle AW, Tyler FH. Potency and duration of action of glucocorticoids. Effects of hydrocortisone, prednisone and dexamethasone on human pituitary-adrenal function. *Am J Med* 1977;63(2):200–7.

69. Brierley J, et al. Clinical practice parameters for hemodynamic support of pediatric and neonatal septic shock: 2007 update from the American College of Critical Care Medicine. *Crit Care Med* 2009; 37:666–88.

70. Wang YG, Rechenmacher CE, Lipsius SL. Nitric oxide signaling mediates stimulation of L-type Ca^{2+} current elicited by withdrawal of acetylcholine in cat atrial myocytes. *J Gen Physiol* 1998;111(1):113–25.

71. Weinberger B, et al. Inhaled nitric oxide primes lung macrophages to produce reactive oxygen and nitrogen intermediates. *Am J Respir Crit Care Med* 1998;158(3):931–8.

72. Sato Y, et al. Nitric oxide reduces the sequestration of polymorphonuclear leukocytes in lung by changing deformability and CD18 expression. *Am J Respir Crit Care Med* 1999;159(5 pt 1):1469–76.

73. Gianetti J, Bevilacqua S, De Caterina R. Inhaled nitric oxide: More than a selective pulmonary vasodilator. *Eur J Clin Invest* 2002;32(8):628–35.

74. Troncy E, et al. Inhaled nitric oxide in acute respiratory distress syndrome: A pilot randomized controlled study. *Am J Respir Crit Care Med* 1998;157(5 pt 1):1483–8.

75. Shipley JB, et al. Milrinone: Basic and clinical pharmacology and acute and chronic management. *Am J Med Sci* 1996; 311(6):286–91.

76. Young RA, Ward A. Milrinone. A preliminary review of its pharmacological properties and therapeutic use. *Drugs* 1988; 36(2):158–92.

77. Hoffman TM, et al. Efficacy and safety of milrinone in preventing low cardiac output syndrome in infants and children after corrective surgery for congenital heart disease. *Circulation* 2003;107(7):996–1002.

78. Ramamoorthy C, et al. Pharmacokinetics and side effects of milrinone in infants and children after open heart surgery. *Anesth Analg* 1998;86(2):283–9.

79. Bailey JM, et al. A population pharmacokinetic analysis of milrinone in pediatric patients after cardiac surgery. *J Pharmacokinet Pharmacodyn* 2004;31(1):43–59.

80. Bailey JM, et al. Pharmacokinetics of intravenous milrinone in patients undergoing cardiac surgery. *Anesthesiology* 1994; 81(3):616–22.

81. Zuppa AF, et al. Population pharmacokinetics of milrinone in neonates with hypoplastic left heart syndrome undergoing stage I reconstruction. *Anesth Analg* 2006;102(4):1062–9.

82. David JL. Desmopressin and hemostasis. *Regul Pept* 1993; 45(1–2):311–7.

83. Rosenzweig EB, et al. Intravenous arginine-vasopressin in children with vasodilatory shock after cardiac surgery. *Circulation* 1999;100(suppl 19):II182–6.

84. Holmes CL, et al. Physiology of vasopressin relevant to management of septic shock. *Chest* 2001;120(3):989–1002.

85. Wilson D. Deepening drug shortages. *Health Aff (Millwood)* 2012;31(2):263–6.

CHAPTER 23 ■ MULTIPLE ORGAN DYSFUNCTION SYNDROME

SCOTT L. WEISS, YONG Y. HAN, THOMAS P. SHANLEY, AND JOSEPH A. CARCILLO

KEY POINTS

1 Multiple organ dysfunction syndrome (MODS) can be triggered by a number of pathologic insults (e.g., sepsis, multiple trauma, hypoxia-ischemia) and is among the most common causes of death of children in intensive care units.

2 Consensus definitions for pediatric-specific, physiologic criteria for MODS have recently been proposed so that clinicians and investigators can achieve greater uniformity in determining the epidemiology of and outcomes from pediatric MODS.

3 Living organisms achieve survival by maintaining precise physiologic homeostasis. Evolution to a multiorgan species creates an increasingly complex interplay among the systems (e.g., transport, [energy] metabolism, and communication/regulation) needed for survival. Within this paradigm, perturbations leading to a failure to main-

tain normal function within these systems can result in physiologic derangement and organ dysfunction.

4 A number of theories are attributed to the development of MODS including (a) dysregulated immunoinflammation, (b) intestinal barrier failure resulting in bacterial translocation, (c) hypercoagulability with microvascular thrombosis, and (d) bioenergetic failure/apoptosis.

5 In pediatric critical care medicine, the mainstay of therapy for MODS remains general supportive care through careful orchestration and balancing of multiple therapeutic modalities.

6 Future studies will need to determine the impact of tight glucose control, lung-protective strategies of mechanical ventilation, anticoagulation therapy, and renal replacement therapy/plasmapheresis on the progression of and outcome from MODS.

INTRODUCTION

There is perhaps no clinical entity that best epitomizes the discipline of critical care medicine as multiple organ dysfunction syndrome (MODS). The numerous pharmacologic and technologic advances reviewed in accompanying chapters have led to substantial improvements in the stabilization and support of the acutely presenting, critically ill patient such that the past decades have witnessed dramatic decreases in mortality rates from once almost universally lethal diseases. However, concomitant with the ability to alter the natural course of acute illness arose a new clinical dilemma characterized by the evolution of averted acute fatalities into protracted deaths marked by progressive dysfunction of multiple organs. Irrespective of the myriad of initial, life-threatening primary insults, the consequent progression through sequential organ dysfunction that has come to be called *MODS* has emerged as a final common pathogenic pathway that threatens the survival of critically ill children and challenges the clinical acumen of critical

1 care teams. Despite readily recognizing the clinical manifestations of MODS and its associated epidemiologic causes and prognostic implications, our understanding of underlying pathophysiologic mechanisms remains incomplete and specific and targeted therapies remain limited. Numerous theories supported by both experimental and observational data have been espoused in an attempt to elucidate the mechanisms of MODS as well as to identify novel means for treating this too-often-fatal syndrome. Herein, we provide a review of the definition and epidemiology of pediatric MODS, a discussion of some of the prevailing mechanistic theories regarding the pathogenesis and pathophysiology of MODS, and a brief description

of therapeutic interventions that may impact on the clinical course of MODS.

RECOGNIZING AND DEFINING MODS

The emergence of MODS as a clinical entity is one of the hallmark challenges of the modern era of critical care medicine. Establishment of modern intensive care units in the mid-1950s and the successful developments of contemporary life-support technologies have enabled patients afflicted with acute, life-threatening critical illness to increasingly survive their primary injury. As further advances in surgery, anesthesiology, and medicine empowered physicians with life-saving interventions, intensivists recognized that their initial resuscitative efforts were later thwarted by the onset of numerous, secondary physiologic derangements in organs previously spared by the primary insult. Initial reports of this phenomenon often focused on single organ dysfunction, such as respiratory failure, as a complicating feature of the primary disease process or of the resuscitation itself. As early as 1950, Jenkins et al. (1) provided one of the earliest pathologic descriptions of what would later be recognized as acute respiratory distress syndrome (ARDS), which the authors identified as a complication of fluid resuscitation for shock. The notion that this clinical entity could involve *multiple systems* was suggested as early as 1963 by Burke et al. (2) who described "high output respiratory failure" as an important cause of death from peritonitis or ileus. While this study also focused primarily on respiratory derangements, the authors acknowledged the contributions of hematologic, renal, and cardiovascular system dysfunction leading to patient demise.

That overwhelming infections could lead to MODS dates back to reports from the late 1960s. MacLean et al. (3) described the progression of septic shock in a large case series and detailed the sequential evolution of organ failure in this cohort. Shortly thereafter, Skillman et al. (4) described the clinical syndrome of serial respiratory, cardiovascular, and hepatic failure following hemorrhage from acute gastric stress ulcers complicated by gram-negative sepsis. Eventually, noninfectious triggers of MODS were observed, and in a related manner, Tilney et al. (5) described sequential failure of multiple organs in their seminal series of patients undergoing repair of ruptured aortic aneurysms. Shortly after these reports, Baue wrote what remains a landmark editorial in 1975 proposing that this observed "multiple, progressive, or sequential systems failure" represented a distinct clinical entity that was indeed more often difficult to combat and refractory to medical therapy than the triggering insult itself (6). Over the ensuing years, additional terms have been utilized to describe this clinical entity including "multiple organ failure" (MOF), "remote organ failure," and "multiple organ system failure" (MOSF). Relevant to pediatric critical care medicine, Wilkinson et al. (7) provided the first description of MOSF in children after having derived age-adjusted criteria for organ failure.

Because of varying terminology, an *American College of Chest Physicians (ACCP)/Society of Critical Care Medicine (SCCM)* Consensus Conference was convened "to provide a conceptual and a practical framework to define the systemic inflammatory response to infection, which is a progressive injurious process that falls under the generalized term 'sepsis' and includes sepsis-associated organ dysfunction" (8). The participants emphasized that MODS reflected a *continuum of dysfunction* rather than a *dichotomous state* of normal function versus failure, that this condition was potentially *reversible*, and that the degree of organ dysfunction could change over time. The consensus group acknowledged that numerous host, pathogen, and treatment factors could impact the occurrence and course of MODS (8). Finally, conference delegates proposed the use of "multiple organ dysfunction syndrome" as the preferred term to describe this common clinical entity.

Moreover, to reflect differences in pathophysiologic triggers leading to MODS, the concepts of *primary* versus *secondary* MODS were introduced. Primary MODS referred to its occurrence resulting from a well-defined insult in which organ failure occurred early and could be directly attributed to the insult itself (e.g., meningococcemia). In contrast, the concept of secondary MODS referred to its emergence after a latent period from the initial insult and likely as a consequence of a maladaptive host response to the injury, most commonly an infectious complication.

In differentiating between primary versus secondary MODS in children, Proulx et al. (9) presented alternative, time-based definitions. These authors defined primary MODS as occurring within the first week of PICU admission without evidence of sequential organ dysfunction; whereas secondary MODS was defined as the onset of MODS more than 7 days after PICU admission or sequential organ dysfunction to maximal number of organs failing occurring more than 72 hours after the initial diagnosis of MODS (10). At this time, it remains uncertain whether the etiology-based or time-based definition of primary versus secondary MODS will be adopted for pediatric MODS, and appropriate clarification should be noted when discussing these concepts particularly in the setting of clinical research efforts.

While intensivists caring for adults reached consensus in concept, definition, and specific physiologic criteria for MODS, it was not until 2002 that a similar consensus expert panel in pediatric critical care medicine met to address *pediatric-specific* definitions and criteria for sepsis and organ dysfunction (11,16). In a similar time frame, and nearly a decade after the 1991 *ACCP/SCCM* Conference, these definitions were revisited during a joint consensus conference sponsored by the *SCCM*, the *European Society of Intensive Care Medicine*, the *ACCP*, the *American Thoracic Society*, and the *Surgical Infection Society* (12). Conference participants concluded that although the definitions from 1991 were generally robust enough for continued clinical application, they did not allow for a precise "staging" of the host response to an inflammatory trigger. To address this, a suggestion to employ a "staging system," similar to that used for cancer biology, based on a so-called **PIRO** System was proposed (**Table 23.1**): the Predisposition of the host to be affected, the Insult/Infection triggering

TABLE 23.1

THE PIRO SYSTEM

■ DOMAIN	■ PRESENT	■ FUTURE	■ RATIONALE
Predisposition	Premorbid illness, age, sex, cultural beliefs	Genetic polymorphisms in components of the inflammatory response; better understanding of host–pathogen interaction	Premorbid factors impact on the morbidity and mortality of an acute trigger; consequences of insult are genetically influenced
Insult/infection	Culture and sensitivity of pathogens, detection of diseases amenable to source control	Assay of microbial products (e.g., LPS, PCR for DNA); gene transcript profiles	Characterizing insult in order to target specific therapies against triggering insult/pathogen
Response	SIRS; other signs of sepsis (e.g., CRP)	Markers of inflammation (IL-6, PCT); impaired host response, detection of specific therapeutic targets (LPS, TNF)	Mortality and response to therapy vary with measures of disease severity; mediator-targeted therapy
Organ dysfunction	Measured as number of failing organs or score (MODS, SOFA, LODS, PEMOD, PELOD)	Dynamic measures of cellular response to insult: apoptosis, cell stress	Response to therapy not possible if damage present; identifying cellular injury in order to utilize therapies

PIRO, Predisposition of the host to be affected, the Insult/Infection triggering the response, the Response of the host, and the degree of Organ dysfunction; LPS, lipopolysaccharide; PCR, polymerase chain reaction; CRP, c-reactive protein; PCT, procalcitonin; TNF, tumor necrosis factor; MODS, Multiple Organ Dysfunction Score; SOFA, Sequential Organ Failure Assessment; LODS, Logistic Organ Dysfunction Score; PEMOD, Pediatric Multiple Organ Dysfunction; PELOD, Pediatric Logistic Organ Dysfunction.
From Levy MM, Fink MP, Marshall JC, et al. 2001 SCCM/ESICM/ACCP/ATS/SIS International Sepsis Definitions Conference. *Crit Care Med* 2003;31:1250–6, with permission.

the response, the Response of the host (e.g., presence of the systemic inflammatory response syndrome [SIRS], biomarkers), and the degree of Organ dysfunction (12). Quantification of organ dysfunction and improved mechanistic understanding of the pathophysiology of MODS remain essential goals of ongoing critical care research.

SCORING SYSTEMS

A number of proposed scoring systems have been developed, variably validated, and applied to multiple clinical series with the goal of "quantifying" the severity of MODS. Unfortunately, the heterogeneity of these numerous scoring systems has complicated the consistency of objectively recording MODS severity for the purposes of study comparison, as well as for mortality prediction. In adults, the main scoring systems include MODS, the Logistic Organ Dysfunction Score (LODS), and Sequential Organ Failure Assessment (SOFA) score, each of which has aimed to quantify the severity of

MODS as a single score and correlate this score to outcome in adult patients.

During the early evolution of pediatric MODS quantification (that pre-dated the 1991 ACCP/SCCM Consensus Conference), organ dysfunction was viewed dichotomously rather than in a continuum, and the total number of organs with dysfunction (0 to 5, 6, or 7 depending on the inclusion(s) of the hepatic and gastrointestinal systems) was used to score the severity of MODS in children. As would have been predicted, this score (sometimes referred to as the Organ Failure Index score) correlated to mortality. As mentioned in the preceding section, Wilkinson et al. (7) presented the first series of age-specific criteria to reflect organ dysfunction in children, which were modestly refined to include criteria for hepatic and gastrointestinal failures (10,13). The adult-based criteria that the diagnosis of MODS required the simultaneous involvement of two or more organ systems was also adopted for pediatric MODS.

Although the age-adjusted criteria for organ *failure* defined by Wilkinson and Proulx provided a set of diagnostic criteria by which clinicians could identify MODS (Table 23.2), it was

TABLE 23.2

CRITERIA FOR PEDIATRIC ORGAN SYSTEM FAILURE IN INFANTS AND CHILDREN

Cardiovascular System
1. Systolic blood pressure <40 mm Hg for patients <1 y of age, or <50 mm Hg for patients >1 y of age
2. Heart rate <50 beats/min or >220 beats/min for patients <1 y of age, or <40 beats/min or >200 beats/min for patients >1 y of age
3. Cardiac arrest
4. Serum pH <7.2 with a normal $Paco_2$
5. Continuous intravenous infusion of inotropic or vasopressor agents to maintain blood pressure and/or cardiac output (excluding dopamine ≤5 μg/kg/min)

Respiratory System
1. Respiratory rate >90 breaths/min for patients <1 y of age, or >70 breaths/min for patients >1 y of age
2. $Paco_2$ >65 Torr
3. Pao_2 <40 Torr in the absence of cyanotic congenital heart disease
4. Mechanical ventilation (>24 h in the postoperative period)
5. Pao_2/Fio_2 ratio <200 in the absence of cyanotic congenital heart disease

Central Nervous System
1. Glasgow Coma Score <5
2. Fixed and dilated pupils in the absence of mydriatic medications

Hematologic System
1. Hemoglobin level <5 g/dL
2. White blood cell count <3000 cells/mm^3
3. Platelet count <20,000 cells/mm^3
4. D-dimer >0.5 μg/mL with prothrombin time >20 s and partial thromboplastin time >60 s in the absence of antithrombotic medications and/or primary liver disease

Renal System
1. Serum urea nitrogen level >100 mg/dL
2. Serum creatinine level >2 mg/dL in the absence of preexisting renal disease
3. Need for acute dialysis

Hepatic System
Total serum bilirubin >3 mg/dL in the absence of hemolysis, hyperbilirubinemia of the newborn, breast feeding–related hyperbilirubinemia, or primary liver disease

Gastrointestinal System
Gastroduodenal bleeding plus one of the following thought to be directly the result of gastroduodenal bleeding:
1. Decrease of hemoglobin of >2 g/dL
2. Requirement for blood transfusion
3. Hypotension
4. Need for gastric or duodenal surgery
5. Death

MODS is defined as the simultaneous occurrence of at least two organ dysfunctions.
Information in table is as derived by Wilkinson JD, Pollack MM, Glass NL, et al. Mortality associated with multiple organ system failure and sepsis in pediatric intensive care unit. *J Pediatr* 1987;111:324–8, and later modestly modified by Proulx F, Fayon M, Farrell CA, et al. Epidemiology of sepsis and MODS in children. *Chest* 1996;109:1033–7.

not until 1999 that a formal attempt to develop and validate a pediatric organ *dysfunction* score was reported. Leteurtre et al. (14) used two developmental methods: the PEdiatric Multiple Organ Dysfunction (PEMOD) system and the PEdiatric Logistic Organ Dysfunction (PELOD) score. The intended purpose for adapting a scoring system was not necessarily to predict mortality, which was substantially lower as compared with adults, but rather to more accurately quantify clinical complications among PICU patients by using changes in the organ dysfunction score as a surrogate outcome measure.

The creation of the PEMOD and PELOD scoring systems was carefully described in the initial report. In contrast to adults, age-dependent physiologic variables (e.g., HR) were stratified into four groups: neonates (<1 month), infants (1–12 months), children (1–12 years), and adolescents (>12 years). The weight of each variable in predicting mortality was independently determined and four levels of increasing severity were defined to which weighted "values" were assigned. In the final derivation, the weight of each organ dysfunction and severity were integrated into a score with 12 variables retained (**Table 23.3**). Following its description, the PELOD score was subjected to a further validation study that included more than 1,800 children in seven PICUs across Europe and North America (15). The predictive value of PELOD score for mortality end point was fairly accurate during the first 5 days of admission to the PICU (ROC curve area, 0.79–0.85). However, it is important to acknowledge the difference in a scoring system such as PELOD, which was designed to serve as a surrogate measure of outcome, with that of actual prognosticating scoring systems such as PRISM or PIM designed specifically to maximize mortality prediction.

As mentioned, first in 2002 (16) and then in 2004 (17), a consensus PCCM expert panel reviewed available scoring systems for pediatric MODS. The primary goal was to generate a reproducible assessment of organ dysfunction that would enable tracking of either improvement or decline in function, which could then serve as a meaningful end point for clinical trials. While no one scoring system was favored, the panel did develop specific criteria for defining organ dysfunction based on these summary scoring systems (**Table 23.4**) (16). They advised that for MODS study enrollment purposes, cardiovascular and respiratory organ dysfunction should be present with subsequent monitoring of other organ system function. They also proposed using *organ dysfunction-free days* as a study end point as was designed into the Resolution of Organ Failure in Pediatric Patients with Severe Sepsis (RESOLVE) Trial that examined the efficacy of drotrecogin alpha (i.e., recombinant activated protein C) to hasten resolution of organ failure in pediatric severe sepsis (see Treatment of MODS section below) (18). It remains uncertain how well this metric

TABLE 23.3

PEDIATRIC LOGISTIC ORGAN DYSFUNCTION (PELOD) SCORE

ORGAN SYSTEM AND VARIABLES	Points by Level of Severity for Each System			
	0	1	10	20
Respiratory System				
Pao₂/Fio₂	>70 and		≤70 or	
Paco₂	≤90 and		>90	
Mechanical ventilation	No ventilation	Ventilation		
Cardiovascular System				
HR (beats/min)				
<12 y	≤195		>195	
≥12 y	≤150		>150	
Systolic BR	and		or	
<1 mo	>65		35–65	<35
1 mo–1 y	>75		35–75	<35
1–12 y	>85		45–85	<45
>12 y	>95		55–95	<55
Neurologic System				
GCS	12–15 and	7–11	4–6 or	3
Pupillary reaction	Both reactive		Both fixed	
Hepatic System				
ALT	<950 and	≥950 and		
PT/INR	>60 or <1.4	≤60 or ≤1.4		
Renal System: Creatinine				
<7 d	<1.59		≥1.59	
7 d–1 y	<0.62		≥0.62	
1–12 y	<1.13		≥1.13	
>12 y	<1.59		≥1.59	
Hematologic System				
White blood cell count	>4.5 and	1.5–4.4 or	<1.5	
Platelet count	≥35,000	<35,000		

GCS, Glasgow Coma Score; ALT, alanine aminotransferase; PT, prothrombin time; INR, International Normalized Ratio.
From Leteurtre S, Martinot A, Duhamel A, et al. Development of a pediatric multiple organ dysfunction score: Use of two strategies. *Med Decis Making* 1999;19:399–410, and Leteurtre S, Martinot A, Duhamel A, et al. Validation of the paediatric logistic organ dysfunction (PELOD) score: Prospective, observational, multicentre study. *Lancet* 2003;362:192–7.

TABLE 23.4

PEDIATRIC ORGAN DYSFUNCTION CRITERIA: THE DIAGNOSTIC CRITERIA FOR PEDIATRIC MODS BASED ON 2002 INTERNATIONAL PEDIATRIC SEPSIS CONSENSUS CONFERENCE

Cardiovascular Dysfunction: Despite administration of isotonic intravenous fluid bolus ≥40 mL/kg in 1 h:
- Decrease in BP (hypotension) <5 percentile for age or systolic BP <2 SD below normal for age
  OR
- Need for vasoactive drug to maintain BP in normal range (dopamine ≥5 µg/kg/min or dobutamine, epi or norepi at any dose)
  OR
- Two of the following
- Unexplained metabolic acidosis: base deficit >5.0 mEq/L
- Increased arterial lactate >2 times upper limit of normal
- Oliguria: urine output <0.5 mL/kg/h
- Prolonged capillary refill: >5 s
- Core to peripheral temperature gap >3°C

Respiratory System
- Pao_2/Fio_2 ratio <300 in the absence of cyanotic congenital heart disease or preexisting lung disease
  OR
- $Paco_2$ >65 Torr or 20 mm Hg above baseline $Paco_2$
  OR
- Proven need or >50% Fio_2 to maintain saturation ≥92%
  OR
- Need for nonelective invasive or noninvasive mechanical ventilation

Central Nervous System
- Glasgow Coma Score ≤11
  OR
- Acute change in mental status with a decrease in GCS ≥3 points from abnormal baseline

Hematologic System
- Platelet count <80,000/mm³ or a decline of 50% in platelet count from highest valued recorded over the past 3 d (for chronic heme-onc patients)
  OR
- INR >2

Renal System
- Serum creatinine level >2 times upper limit for age or twofold increase in baseline creatinine

Hepatic System
- Total serum bilirubin ≥4 mg/dL (in the absence of hemolysis, hyperbilirubinemia of the newborn, or primary liver disease)
  OR
- ALT 2 times upper limit of normal for age

BP, blood pressure; SD, standard deviations; GCS, Glasgow Coma Score; INR, International Normalized Ratio; ALT, alanine aminotransferase.
From Goldstein B, Giroir B, Randolph A. International pediatric sepsis consensus conference: Definitions for sepsis and organ dysfunction in pediatrics. *Pediatr Crit Care Med* 2005;6:2–8, with permission.

will perform over time. The ultimate goal is to assimilate scoring systems such as the PELOD score, with additional biologic information (e.g., biomarkers, genetic predisposition, and pharmacogenomics) in order to more accurately determine the beneficial effects of newly developed therapeutic strategies for sepsis and MODS subjected to interventional trials.

EPIDEMIOLOGY OF MODS

Incidence

Established consensus agreement on MODS definitions and scoring systems facilitates the determination of the incidence of MODS in adults and children. The incidence of MODS in adult cohorts has ranged broadly from 14% to 54% depending on the specific patient population admitted to various ICUs (19), though the highest rates are consistently observed in adults with sepsis and/or postsurgical status (19,20).

In pediatric studies, the incidence of MODS among general PICU populations has ranged from 11% to 57% (**Table 23.5**) (7,9,10,13,15,21–23). Clearly, the incidence of MODS depends on a number of factors including surgical/postoperative status (e.g., trauma vs. transplantation vs. congenital heart repair), premorbid conditions (e.g., cancer, immunodeficiency, stem cell transplant [up to 50% with MODS]), and the triggering insult (e.g., 95% of infants presenting with postasphyxial injury had MODS) (24).

The most comprehensive evaluation of the incidence of MODS in hospitalized children was reported by Johnston et al. (25). These investigators utilized the Healthcare Cost and Utilization Project Kids' Inpatient Database (KID), which included administrative data on over 1.1 million pediatric patients from 22 states to estimate the overall incidence of MODS in children. More than 50,000 (4.5%) were admitted with at least one organ system dysfunction, and depending on how MODS was defined from the coding system, the incidence of MODS was estimated between 0.5% and 3.3% (25). While this relatively low incidence of MODS among all hospitalized children might deceptively suggest that the overall burden of pediatric MODS is minor, this study highlighted the substantial and disproportionate impact that MODS carried on the length of stay, resource utilization, and mortality for this minority of infants and children unfortunate to suffer organ dysfunction.

Specific Etiologies

As a result of only limited studies describing MODS in children, there is an incomplete description of the various factors that contribute to both the initiation of, and outcome from, pediatric MODS including age, triggering pathology, and premorbid conditions (i.e., chronic illness, immunosuppression, etc.). Despite this limitation, there are some clear patterns that emerge from the reports to date. It is clear that sepsis is a principle trigger of MODS not only among adult ICU patients, but also in the pediatric ICU population where the incidence of MODS in children with sepsis ranges from 24% to 73% (Table 23.5) (26–28). Other inciting triggers associated with pediatric MODS include asphyxial insults, inborn errors of metabolism, hypoxemic respiratory failure, acute renal failure, pancreatitis, intracranial hemorrhage, and neurodegenerative diseases (9). MODS also presents in pediatric surgical patients with the incidence varying by study cohorts that include postcardiac surgery, multiple trauma, liver transplantation, and bowel obstruction (9). Less is known regarding the influence of chronic diseases and premorbid conditions on the incidence of MODS. However, information on specific patient populations exists such as for allogeneic bone marrow transplantation (relative risk of MODS estimated to be 38.67 [CI 5.47–273.2]) (29) or oncologic patients admitted to the PICU for complications arising in the course of chemotherapy (MODS incidence on the order of 50%).

Outcome

Again, due to variations in criteria defining organ dysfunction and other factors, the mortality rate for children meeting MODS criteria has ranged widely from 12% to 57% in the general PICU population (Table 23.5). Additionally, the mortality rate for specific subpopulations as defined by their underlying disease, premorbidities, and surgical status varies with the subpopulation of patients with sepsis being most closely examined. While adult studies suggest that patients with sepsis-related MODS carry a higher mortality risk than other etiologies, early pediatric studies did not corroborate this observation (10,13). However, more recent pediatric studies have corroborated the observation in adults that sepsis portends a negative survival impact for patients with MODS (22,23).

Regardless of the triggering insult, every epidemiologic report has substantiated the observation that mortality correlates to the number of organs failing. In pediatrics, it is revealing that more than 90% (in some cases 100%) of all deaths occurring in PICUs have been associated with MODS (Table 23.5). Given this substantial impact on outcome, these data drive the imperative of gaining an improved mechanistic understanding of the pathophysiology of MODS to either attenuate the degree of organ dysfunction upon initiation and/or reverse the process once established. The following section will address mechanistic theories ascribed to explain the development of MODS.

PATHOPHYSIOLOGY OF MODS

Although the definition proposed by the *ACCP/SCCM* Consensus Conference broadly describes MODS as the "presence of altered organ function in an acutely ill patient such that homeostasis cannot be maintained without intervention" (8), the dominant conceptual framework upon which the pathogenesis of MODS has traditionally been viewed has been in the context of dysregulated inflammation. Early theories asserted that widespread organ dysfunction was a manifestation of unintended collateral organ damage stemming from an exaggerated or uncontrolled SIRS secondary to a severe inciting injury. However, continued failure of anti-inflammatory strategies to improve patient outcomes strongly suggests that this hyperinflammation model was incomplete. Additionally, the growing realization that an endogenous compensatory anti-inflammatory response syndrome (CARS) existed (30) and that an equally dysregulated anti-inflammatory response could also deleteriously modulate the host response to injury have led to more recent theories promoting the notion that MODS reflects an imbalance or *dissonance* between these pro- and anti-inflammatory processes. While there are extensive experimental and clinical data to support a dysregulated inflammation hypothesis as an important contributor to the pathogenesis of MODS, it is likely that explaining MODS only through this "inflammatory lens" represents an incomplete picture of a larger network of interdependent processes that go awry in MODS. For example, emerging data identify bioenergetic and metabolic derangements as integral to the development MODS. In this regard, it is informative to briefly review physiologic organ homeostasis in order to have a more comprehensive picture of how this homeostasis can be altered leading to dysfunction.

What Constitutes Normal Physiologic Homeostasis?

As the concept of MODS is inherently tied to that of *homeostasis* (or more precisely, the *loss* of homeostasis), what constitutes normal physiologic homeostasis should be understood. Fundamentally, homeostasis can be viewed as a state of dynamic equilibrium in which the internal environment of a living entity is maintained in a relatively narrow physiologic range while resisting perturbations caused by variations in its external environment. When applied to a single cell or simple organism, this concept is relatively easy to comprehend since the internal and external environments are clearly demarcated by a cell wall or membrane. However, also inherent to its very definition, MODS is a clinical syndrome that can arise only in sophisticated, multiorgan, higher-order species; and in this context the concept of homeostasis encompasses additional complexity as it must address spatial and hierarchical considerations related to the sheer increase in size and specialization of physiologic functions that characterize the higher-order organism. In other words, the concept of homeostasis relevant to MODS carries both micro- and macro-environmental meanings as multiple dynamic equilibriums simultaneously maintained at the local (i.e., cellular) and regional (i.e., tissue or organ) levels collectively integrate in a highly organized, well-orchestrated, and hierarchical manner to support the global dynamic equilibrium of the whole organism. Although at first glance this latter, multidimensional notion of homeostasis might be viewed as overly complex, it is possible to systematically deconstruct and reconstruct its multiple layers to provide some clarity to this intricate picture.

All complex, higher-order species start life as a single-cell entity, and subsequent embryological development proceeds through a well-ordered sequence of steps that demonstrates remarkable similarities to the march of evolution from primordial single-cell organism to modern complex, multiorgan life forms. Drawing parallels to this evolutionary and embryonic development, the same types of physical, spatial, physiologic, and logistical obstacles to evolutionary progress can be

TABLE 23.5

SUMMARY OF EPIDEMIOLOGIC STUDIES EXAMINING PEDIATRIC MODS AND SEPSIS-RELATED MODS[a]

	MODS – PICU								MODS – Hospital	Sepsis – PICU		
	WILKINSON 1986 (56)	WILKINSON 1987 (55)	PROULX 1994 (39)	PROULX 1996 (38)	GOH 1999 (16)	LETEURTE 2003 (30)	TANTALEAN 2003 (47)	LECLERC 2005 (28)	JOHNSTON 2004 (41)	SAEZ-LLORENS 1995 (43)	DUKE 1997 (13)	KUTKO 2003 (27)
Setting	1 PICU – USA	5 PICUs – USA	1 PICU – France	1 PICU – France	1 PICU – Malaysia	7 PICUs – France/Canada/Switzerland	1 PICU – Peru	3 PICUs – France/Canada	22 state database – USA	1 PICU – Panama	1 PICU – Australia	1 PICU – USA
Study Design	prospective	prospective	prospective	prospective	partly prospective	prospective	prospective	prospective	retrospective	retrospective	prospective	retrospective
Study Dates	1980–1982	1984–1985	1990–1991	1991–1992	1995–1996	1998–2000	1996–1997	1997	1997	1981–1992	?	1998–1999
Study Duration	13.5 mo	7 mo	9 mo	13 mo	19 mo	18 mo	6 mo	5 mo	12 mo	12 y	?	2 y
Number of Admissions	831	726	777	1,058	495	1,806	276	593	1,152,854	4,529	?	2,346
MODS Definition/Criteria	modified Wilkinson 1986 (56) study [b]	modified Wilkinson 1986 (56) study	modified Wilkinson 1986 (56)	modified Wilkinson 1987 (55)	Wilkinson 1987 (55)	Leteurtre 1999 [PELOD] (29)	study	Leteurtre 1999 [PELOD] (29)	ICD-9-CM coding	study	modified Wilkinson 1987 (55)	modified Wilkinson 1987 (55)
Maximum MODS (i.e. OFI)	5	7	5	7	7	6	7	6	6	5	6	7
MODS Incidence	226/831 (27.2%)	177/726 (24.4%)	85/777 (10.9%)	191/1058 (18.1%)	84/495 (17.0%)	965/1806 (53.4%)	156/276 (56.5%)	269/593 (45.4%)	6112/1152854 (0.5%) [d]; 37682/1152854 (3.3%) [e]			
Overall MODS Mortality	60/226 (26.5%)	83/177 (46.9%)	43/85 (50.6%)	68/191 (35.6%)	48/84 (57.1%)	111/965 (11.5%)	65/156 (41.7%)	51/269 (19.0%)	1633/6112 (26.7%) [d]; 3684/37682 (9.8%) [e]			
1 OD Mortality	2/241 (0.8%)					3/471 (0.6%)	6/85 (7.1%)	0/150 (0%)	1856/45274 (4.1%)			
2 OD Mortality	15/142 (10.6%)	25/97 (25.8%)	2/34 (5.9%)	?/86	20/45 (44.4%)	14/457 (3.1%)	23/78 (29.5%)	7/156 (4.5%)	1048/4854 (21.6%)			
3 OD Mortality	36/62 (58.1%)	30/48 (62.5%)	29/36 (80.6%)	?/59	16/26 (61.5%)	29/285 (10.2%)	21/54 (38.9%)	16/75 (21.3%)	441/1007 (43.8%)			
4 OD Mortality	9/12 (75.0%)	28/32 (87.5%)	7/9 (77.8%)	?/24	12/13 (92.3%)	24/125 (19.2%)	16/19 (84.2%)	19/27 (70.4%)	144/251 (57.4%)			
5 OD Mortality	no patients	included in 4 OD	5/6 (83.3%)	?/13	included in 4 OD	30/70 (42.9%)	4/4 (100%)	7/9 (77.8%)	included in 4 OD			

6 OD Mortality	xxxxx	included in 4 OD	xxxxx	?/6	14/28 (50%)	included in 4 OD	1/1 (100%)	2/2 (100%)	included in 4 OD			
7 OD Mortality	xxxxx	included in 4 OD	xxxxx	?/3	xxxxx	included in 4 OD	no patients	xxxxx	xxxxx			
Sepsis Definition	N/A	study	N/A	modified 1991 ACCP/SCCM (2)	N/A	modified 1991 ACCP/SCCM (2)	modified 1991 ACCP/SCCM (2)	modified 1991 ACCP/SCCM (2)	ICD-9-CM coding	study	modified 1991 ACCP/SCCM (2)	2002 ACCM Guidelines (9)
Sepsis Incidence		21%, 21%, 24% [c]		316/1058 (29.9%)			127/276 (46.0%)	138/593 (23.3%)		815/4529 (18.0%)		147/2346 (6.3%)
Sepsis Mortality				?/316		27/44 (61.4%)	47/127 (37.0%)	27/138 (19.6%)		319/815 (39.1%)	10/31 (32.2%)	18/143 (12.6%)
Sepsis Category Mortality												
Sepsis				?/245			16/76 (21.1%)	9/103 (8.7%)		27/171 (15.8%)		N/A
Severe Sepsis				?/46			17/30 (56.7%)	6/17 (35.3%)		201/497 (40.4%)		N/A
Septic Shock				?/25			14/21 (66.7%)	12/18 (66.7%)		91/147 (61.9%)		13/96 (13.5%)
Among MODS Patients												
Sepsis Incidence		84/177 (47.5%)	19/85 (22.4%)	72/191 (37.7%)		44/84 (52.4%)	87/156 (55.8%)	98/269 (36.4%)				
No Sepsis Mortality		44/93 (47.3%)		45/119 (37.8%)		21/40 (52.5%)	20/69 (29.0%)	24/171 (14.0%)				
Sepsis Mortality		39/84 (46.4%)		23/72 (31.9%)		27/44 (61.4%)	45/87 (51.7%)	27/98 (27.6%)				
Sepsis Category Mortality												
Sepsis				9/41 (22.0%)		2/9 (22.2%)		9/68 (13.2%)				
Severe Sepsis				2/8 (25.0%)		13/20 (65.0%)		6/13 (46.2%)				
Septic Shock				12/23 (52.2%)		12/15 (80.0%)		12/17 (70.6%)				
Among Sepsis Patients												
MODS Incidence								98/138 (71.0%)		197/815 (24.2%)	11/29 (37.9%)	70/96 (72.9%)
No MODS Mortality								0/40 (0%)		175/618 (28.3%)	3/20 (15.0%)	0/26 (0%)

(continued)

TABLE 23.5 *(continued)*

SUMMARY OF EPIDEMIOLOGIC STUDIES EXAMINING PEDIATRIC MODS AND SEPSIS-RELATED MODS

	MODS – PICU									MODS – Hospital		Sepsis – PICU		
	■ WILKINSON 1986 (56)	■ WILKINSON 1987 (55)	■ PROULX 1994 (39)	■ PROULX 1996 (38)	■ GOH 1999 (16)	■ LETEURTE 2003 (30)	■ TANTALEAN 2003 (47)	■ LECLERC 2005 (28)	■ JOHNSTON 2004 (41)	■ SAEZ–LLORENS 1995 (43)	■ DUKE 1997 (13)	■ KUTKO 2003 (27)
MODS Mortality								27/98 (27.6%)		144/197 (73.1%)	7/11 (63.6%)	13/70 (18.6%)
Overall Mortality	62/831 (7.5%)	83/726 (11.4%)	43/777 (5.5%)	68/1058 (6.4%)	50/495 (10.1%)	115/1806 (6.4%)	71/276 (25.7%)	51/593 (8.6%)	4635/1152854 (0.4%)			
Mortality without MODS	2/62 (3.2%)	0/83 (0%)	0/43 (0%)	0/68 (0%)	2/50 (4%)	4/115 (3.5%)	6/71 (8.5%)	0/51 (0%)				
Mortality with MODS	60/62 (96.8%)	83/83 (100%)	43/43 (100%)	68/68 (100%)	48/50 (96%)	111/115 (96.5%)	65/71 (91.5%)	51/51 (100%)				

[a]Many of these data were not explicitly reported in the original studies and have been extracted from the text through interpolation and reverse calculations.
[b]The mortality rate was reported as 54% in the original paper.
[c]Incidence of sepsis reported from three of the five PICUs in the study.
[d]MODS defined by dysfunction of two or more organs.
[e]MODS defined by study.
MODS, multiple organ dysfunction syndrome; OD, organ dysfunction; OFI, organ failure index; PELOD, pediatric logistic organ dysfunction.

applied to the development from a single-cell organism into a complex, mature life form. Certain vital physiologic functions must be sequentially gained at each step of development, and disruption of any of these basic functions at earlier stages prohibits the progression to later stages. Therefore, examining these obligatory gains in homeostatic function through the progression of evolution can provide insight into human biologic development and thus reveal potential areas of vulnerability with respect to the development of MODS.

Taking this approach, one can identify the necessary elements for a unicellular organism to maintain homeostasis and sustain life: transport, (energy) metabolism, and communication/regulation. At the most fundamental level, all living organisms are organic, water-filled biologic systems composed of proteins, carbohydrates, lipids, and nucleic acids enclosed by physical barriers that demarcate an internal milieu distinct from its external environment. The presence of this physical barrier necessitates that cells must adapt *transport* mechanisms to import essential biomolecules and substrates needed to build and maintain its internal biological system (and conversely, export undesired biological "waste"). However, simply combining these bio-elements does not itself constitute a living entity but in addition the organism ultimately requires this transport system facilitate active use of substrates via cellular *metabolism*. Metabolism entails both anabolic and catabolic activities and encompasses DNA replication, protein synthesis, maintenance of cell membrane integrity as well as a host of other vital cellular functions. The most critical facet of cellular metabolism involves the generation of adequate *energy* or fuel to drive this cellular machinery. Finally, it is imperative to recognize that while cellular transport assembles the components of the life machine and energy metabolism sets this machine into motion, precise regulatory control of cellular activity is needed to maintain the ongoing operation of the life machine. This regulatory control implies the presence of a sophisticated "communication network" that senses changes in both internal and external conditions to signal appropriate responses to regain equilibrium from any perturbation. This "network" must simultaneously adjust the flux of biomaterials and rate of energy production to meet specific demands imposed on the cell at any particular moment. For example, the highly conserved heat shock response can be viewed as series of regulatory communication switches that are triggered in response to high ambient temperature (as well as other stressors) which mobilize factors to assist in proper protein folding to protect against protein degradation (31) (see Chapter 20). As another example, a cell preparing for mitosis actively imports nucleic acids for DNA replication and escalates energy production (i.e., imports and consumes more glucose or lipid) in order to meet increased metabolic demands (32). Alternatively, it may sense that insufficient biomaterials are available and instead signal to abort mitosis altogether. Thus, at the cellular level, a series of regulatory controls and feedbacks that are closely tied to continuous environmental sensing are necessary to maintain homeostasis. Before proceeding to discuss how these concepts of transport, energy metabolism, and communication/regulation become modified as organisms evolve from a unicellular to multicellular entities, a specific aspect of cellular energy metabolism deserves special attention.

Many proto-eukaryotic cells and plant life are able to harness light energy directly from their environment; however, most other cell types extract their energy from the controlled breakage of high-energy carbon–carbon bonds in organic material (e.g., glucose) that is ultimately converted into the universal energy currency of adenosine triphosphate (ATP). In the absence of oxygen, cellular capacity to generate ATP is restricted to 2 ATPs per glucose molecule consumed, and although primitive life forms can still exist with this rudimentary metabolic machinery, advanced evolutionary progress

through anaerobic energy metabolism is impossible. Hence, biologic transformation from anaerobic to aerobic metabolism, characterized by the emergence of mitochondria as subcellular organelles that utilize *oxygen* to perform oxidative phosphorylation (also known as *cellular respiration*), marked a critical leap in evolutionary development. This exponential increase in ATP-generating capacity per organic substrate consumed (theoretically up to 36–38 ATPs per glucose molecule) provided the fuel to support a vast array of cellular activities. Importantly, this functional transformation came with a risk, as strict aerobic entities like mammalian cells became critically vulnerable to periods of anoxia or hypoxia or to any impairment of mitochondrial function. Additionally, inadvertent release of toxic oxygen moieties (i.e., reactive oxygen species [ROS]) from occasional basal errors in oxidative phosphorylation can occur. Thus, the same oxidative properties of oxygen that afford more efficient ATP production can also inflict "self-injury" by damaging sensitive parts of the cellular machinery. In fact, the very mitochondria that unintentionally produce these toxic oxygen moieties are probably most at risk for self-injury (33). A self-amplifying cycle can be set into motion by which mitochondrial oxidant injury can lead to increased errors in oxidative phosphorylation leading to further increased production of ROS, and consequently more self-injury. This damaging cycle, left unchecked, ultimately leads to a functional anaerobic state and bioenergetic failure even despite adequate oxygen availability. Hence, an indispensable function that cells must perform in tandem with the transition from anaerobic to aerobic energy metabolism is the establishment of a powerful antioxidant defense system to prevent rampant proliferation of this autodestructive cycle (see Chapter 20). Of note, one theory of aging (which can be viewed in some respects as the development of MODS over a much more prolonged time frame) hypothesizes that incremental oxidative damage to mitochondrial DNA encoding components of the electron transport chain increase over time and lead to progressive decline in cellular energy-production capacity, limited compensatory reserves to tolerate stress, and ultimately to cellular demise (34).

In observing that cellular energy metabolism in higher-order organisms is dependent on a constant oxygen (and nutrient) supply, mitochondrial integrity, and robust antioxidant defense mechanisms, one can begin to appreciate how critical perturbations to the delicate balance of these elements can set the stage for the development of bioenergetic derangements observed in organ failure present in MODS.

Transport and Energy Metabolism

As described earlier, cellular transport at the single-cell level principally involves the import of biomaterial into the cell, most notably vital nutrients like carbohydrates or lipids needed for energy metabolism. While gases like oxygen and small lipophilic molecules can diffuse across cell membranes along a concentration gradient, cellular transport is often facilitated by specialized channels or transport proteins that selectively recognize specific substrates. Although it is not typically considered in the single-cell setting, the most basic concept of *shock*, which is the state when cellular metabolic demand cannot be met due to insufficient nutrient supply or mitochondrial dysfunction, can be applied to describe conditions of oxygen depletion (hypoxic shock) and glucose depletion (hypoglycemic shock). In the absence of limited exogenous nutrient supply, the flux of biomaterials is regulated by internal signals that control the activity of these channels or transport proteins.

Evolution from a single cell into a simple, multicellular organism requires little change in transport function since each individual cell is within proximity to the outside environment and can obtain sufficient nutrients for survival from diffusion. However, as the multicellular entity gains additional complexity and increases in size, its metabolic needs exceed that which can be supported by diffusion alone. Thus, it must adapt a means to transport vital biomaterials across large spatial domains so that every cell receives a continuous nutrient supply irrespective of its location within the organism. This critical adaptation of transport function in the higher-order organism is fundamentally fulfilled by a *circulatory system*—the intimate link between transport and energy metabolism. As a result, derangements in the physiologic components of this functional "pump" mechanism—preload, contractility, afterload—give rise to the more familiar classifications of shock states—hypovolemic, cardiogenic, and distributive—that are associated with global circulatory collapse. It is important to note that although circulatory compromise results in a state of energy deficit caused by an imbalance between energy production and energy expenditure that we call "shock," it is a state not contingent on hypotension as cellular energy deficits may continue to mount despite preservation of normal blood pressures. Furthermore, with improved monitoring, it is increasingly appreciated that despite restoration of global circulation, microcirculatory perfusion defects from evolving microvascular derangements may still continue and lead to persistent *regional* shock that may herald progressive organ dysfunction (34a).

Communication/Regulation

As described earlier, cell communication at the unicellular level is primarily *intra*cellular and directed solely for self-regulation of biologic activity in response to changes in internal and external signals. A host of both negative and positive feedback loops keep the internal conditions of the cell within the narrow and optimal physiologic range necessary to maintain general cellular metabolism. External stimuli are sensed through specialized receptor complexes, typically located on the cell surface but may also be present in the cell nucleus, that upon binding by specific chemical signals (i.e., ligands) activate a conditioned response from the cell. For example, ligand binding of the tyrosine–kinase family of receptors may, after signal transduction and a series of signal amplification and regulatory sequences, initiate important steps for cellular growth and differentiation (35).

As the organism becomes multicellular, communication by necessity expands to encompass *inter*cellular dimensions in order to regulate cell–cell interactions and coordinate cellular functions so that the composite organism functions optimally as a single unit. Even in less complex organism, the simple task of initiating cell–cell contact still requires that the cells of the organism gain the ability to distinguish "self" from "nonself" which is facilitated through mutual cell surface ligand–receptor bindings via expression of specific adhesion molecules. This important capacity to discriminate "friend" from "foe" becomes especially relevant as an array of Toll-like receptors evolved to identify foreign pathogens (36). These and other components of the *innate immune system* in primitive organisms (and conserved in later, higher-order life forms) play a critical role in defending against pathogens as well as endogenous molecules signaling injury to the host (so-called "alarmins") (37) (see Chapter 19).

As organisms grew more complex, there arose the need for specialized cellular functions and consequently differentiation into specific tissues and organs, but with obligate interdependence. Therefore, a vast hierarchical intercellular communication network had to evolve simultaneously. Despite the profound intricacies of this network, the mode of intercellular communication remains remarkably similar to the single-cell paradigm as "effector" cells release signals that bind to specific receptors on recipient cells to elicit a desired response.

Cells that are in direct contact through specialized adhesion molecules or in close proximity to each other communicate via *paracrine* signals, whereas far-reaching communication (made feasible by the emergence of the circulatory system) is afforded by *endocrine* signals. Regulatory control for entire organisms required the evolution of specialized neuroendocrine cells that further differentiate into neuronal cells that form the critical central and peripheral nervous systems and a variety of discrete endocrine cells that collectively form the endocrine system. Through mutual coordination—still incompletely understood in the human—they serve to regulate global physiologic functions via neurotransmitter/electrical signals and specific hormonal signals. In this context, it is remarkable how a single cell can manage to integrate hundreds and perhaps thousands of different signals being transmitted at any given moment into an appropriate functional response. This remarkable physiologic task is even more noteworthy when considering how a group of cells can coordinate their activities to collectively function in unison as a single entity (i.e., an organ). On the other hand, given this complexity, it is easy to see how aberrant or imbalance of signals, disruption of signal processing, or inadequate or improper response to regulatory signals can have far-reaching consequences that may jeopardize the delicate homeostatic physiologic balance of the organism.

Linking Transport and Communication Functions with the Immune and Coagulation Systems

The development of the circulatory system stemmed from the evolutionary need to overcome diffusion limitation as organisms grew larger, more complex, and more metabolically active. These same evolutionary pressures lead to the development of specialized cells (e.g., erythrocytes) to enhance oxygen transport in the circulation to overcome the limited solubility of oxygen in liquid phase. The organism's dependence on these circulatory components has led to the concepts of hemorrhagic and anemic shock resulting from inadequate oxygen transport.

Circulatory systems have been classified into two distinct types, open (seen in more primitive life forms, e.g., insects) and closed (seen in higher-order mammals including human beings). In an open circulatory system there is no real distinction between intravascular and interstitial space. As such a simple breech of the outer body would allow loss of all extracellular fluid (hemolymph) (38) as well as provide an opening for bacterial invasion and infection. Pathogen invasion quickly becomes systemic as bacteria use the convective flow of hemolymph to spread throughout the organism. Adaptive mechanisms developed to seal the tear in the body wall to prevent further loss of bodily fluid and to kill and eliminate the foreign invaders. This evolutionary adaptation involved the development of a specialized cell known as a hemocyte, which is believed to be the precursor to the pluripotent hematopoetic cell before it diverged into the three lines (leukocytes, megakaryocytes, and erythrocytes) associated with closed circulatory systems (39). In addition to its erythrocyte-like oxygen-carrying function, the primitive hemocyte bears the earliest semblance of the cellular component of the innate immune system, possessing the ability to distinguish "self" from "nonself." Through specialized receptors on its surface, homologous to Toll-like receptors, the hemocyte recognizes unique bacterial components and becomes activated to mobilize cellular defenses. It releases chemokine-like signals to recruit other hemocytes to the site of injury and also releases fibrin-like substances that can form a "clot" that seals the breech in the body wall and immobilizes bacteria to facilitate phagocytosis and pathogen killing (40). Thus, in the open circulatory system, combined *coagulation* and *inflammatory* responses serve to achieve the common goals of gaining *hemostasis* and *pathogen eradication*.

In identifying the components of an open circulatory system, it is clear how cells that are key to the modulation of inflammation in an open circulatory system are related to those fulfilling the functions of energy metabolism as well as hemostatic function.

Systemic Inflammatory Response and Immune Dysregulation

Because sepsis-induced inflammation is a principal trigger for the development of MODS, it is important to have a thorough understanding of the physiologic function of this inflammatory response. Inflammation occurring in the setting of a closed circulatory system entails a series of communication cascades triggered by cellular or tissue injury that orchestrate the mobilization of reparative mechanisms in order to restore function at the affected site of injury. For example, localized trauma, involving crush or sheer injury to soft tissue, releases chemical substances, such as tumor necrosis factor (TNF)-α and interleukin (IL)-1β, into the circulation. These cytokines cause local vasodilation through relaxation of vascular smooth muscle cells, activate endothelial cells to increase capillary permeability, and attract circulating leukocytes to the site of injury. These events culminate in exudation of fluid and plasma proteins, leukocyte transmigration, and the classic findings of *rubor* (redness), *calor* (heat), *tumor* (swelling), and *dolor* (pain). Several plasma protein cascades (complement, coagulation/fibrinolysis, and bradykinin) are activated as part of this evolutionarily imprinted response to injury.

During this response, the first wave of leukocytes recruited to the site of injury are primarily circulating neutrophils, which are "caught" at the affected vascular site by a complex leukocyte–endothelial adhesion cascade involving "rolling," cell adhesion, and consequent transmigration from the circulation to a site of injury (41). The initial phase of rolling is mediated by members of the selectin family of adhesion molecules (e.g., E-selectin) that are upregulated on the endothelium and mediate an interaction with sialylated oligosaccharides that are constitutively expressed on neutrophils. Next, other adhesion molecules (e.g., ICAM-1) bind to neutrophil adhesion molecules (e.g., β2-integrins), both of which are upregulated in response to early cytokine (TNF-α and IL-1β) release. Finally, adherent neutrophils on the endothelial surface are recruited by chemotactic molecules including chemokines (e.g., IL-8/CXCL8), complement products (e.g., C5a), and leukotrienes (e.g., LTB4) to an extravascular site of injury (41). Neutrophil recruitment is critical to combating pathogens through phagocytosis and release of lysosomal enzymes (e.g., proteases and myeloperoxidases) that kill organisms as well as scavenge cellular debris and breakdown damaged scaffolding proteins to facilitate the reparative process.

A subsequent wave of cells recruited to a site of "injury" involves those from the monocyte/macrophage and fibroblast lineages drawn in by a different group of cytokines and chemokines. These cells are enlisted to repopulate the site, lay down scaffolding proteins, and reestablish intercommunication pathways. Even as this local activity reaches a maximal level, additional signals from immune cells modulate the downregulation of this proinflammatory cascade. A well-defined CARS (42,30) results from a coordinated action by a series of mediators (e.g., IL-10, TGF-β, IL-1 receptor antagonist protein [IL1Ra], among other cytokines) to reduce proinflammatory gene expression, stop further leukocyte trafficking, assist in reabsorbing extravascular fluid, and begin reparative processes to reestablish normal cellular function.

Most commonly, the degree to which this inflammatory response is activated and consequently regulated parallels the degree of tissue injury such that small injuries remain completely localized. Thus, the vast majority of the time this coordinated cascade effectively serves the human host to contain and eradicate pathogens and repair injured tissue without any harmful consequences. However, for reasons that remain incompletely understood, either inadequate "containment" or overexuberance of the inflammatory signals for this normally beneficial response result in physiologic perturbations that lead to MODS. In these instances, what was intended to be a beneficial local host response becomes an overwhelming perturbation of systemic homeostasis characterized by significant elevations in cytokines (TNF-α and IL-1β) and upregulation of the inducible form of nitric oxide synthase (iNOS). These mediators, in concert with others, cause loss of vasomotor tone, capillary leak, and myocardial depression culminating in inadequate cardiac output and shock. Without aggressive fluid and inotropic/vasopressor resuscitation, persistent global shock leads to ongoing hypoxic-ischemic injury, eliciting even more inflammatory signals and creating a self-amplifying cycle that can be exacerbated by cell-injury-derived alarmins. This physiologic paradigm also supports an additional theory regarding the cause of MODS: the so-called "gut hypothesis." This hypothesis states that during a period of hypotension or shock, hypoperfusion of the intestines compromises the integrity of immunological barriers allowing for *translocation* of endogenous gut flora or their bacterial products (e.g., endotoxin) into the systemic circulation thereby triggering, or perhaps amplifying, the systemic inflammatory response (43). This "gut hypothesis" would explain the high prevalence of bacteremia in the absence of an identifiable septic focus in patients with MODS and the fact that enteric bacteria are the most commonly isolated organisms.

This pathobiology explains the early traditional paradigm in which massive activation and dysregulation of pro-inflammation was believed to be the culprit for MODS development. As a result, it was believed that attenuating the magnitude of this hyperinflammatory response might enhance the restoration of homeostasis. Unfortunately, numerous anti-inflammatory strategies have failed to translate into clinical improvements in combating the development of and outcomes from MODS. This realization occurred around the same time that clinicians began to recognize that many people dying from MODS had either persistent infection, often with atypical pathogens, or were prone to acquiring new (often nosocomial) infections. Additionally, translational investigators were providing a better understanding of the natural communication sequence of inflammation and the important contribution of endogenous counter-regulatory signals comprising CARS and hypothesized that this, too, might become dysregulated (42). In pursuing this hypothesis, a population of patients was identified that demonstrated an inability to mount an appropriate inflammatory response to typical triggers. Such patients were characterized as functionally immunodeficient or immunocompromised; some clinician-investigators referred to this cohort as "immunoparalyzed" (44), a state of immune *dissonance* that placed them at risk of being unable to clear invading pathogens. This speculation has led to an alternative theory that a "second hit" (infectious or otherwise) causes the clinical progression to MODS.

With such reasoning, it has been suggested that "boosting" the immune response (using, e.g., GM-CSF or interferon-γ) may benefit patients with MODS by helping clear persistent infections or augment their ability to avoid secondary infectious challenges (e.g., ventilator-associated pneumonia) (45). Whether this approach will be successful remains to be determined and success is dependent on clinicians being able to readily identify which patients are actively demonstrating this *immune phenotype*.

In summary, viewing this physiology within the framework of normal immune responses, dysregulation of these evolutionary beneficial processes provides the underpinnings for a number of theories used to explain the pathophysiology of MODS.

Coagulation/Thrombosis and Microcirculatory Impairment

Given the early combined phylogenetic functions of the coagulation and innate immune systems, it should come as no surprise that both systems become activated when infection and/or tissue injury occurs. Perhaps nothing exemplifies activation of both systems better than the thrombotic complications of *purpura fulminans* resulting from disseminated bacteremia with meningococcus. Historically, concerns about coagulation abnormalities focused on excessive bleeding risks from impaired hemostatic function, including disseminated intravascular coagulation (DIC), and less so on thromboembolic pathology and particularly microangiopathic pathology. However, we now know that the same destructive injuries that incite the "cytokine storm" of inflammation and precipitate shock concomitantly activate the coagulation cascade and impair fibrinolysis, resulting in a functional hypercoagulable state that can lead to disseminated microvascular thrombosis (46). The intrinsic link between coagulation and inflammation and their combined roles in the development of MODS is further supported by autopsy findings demonstrating neutrophils in addition to platelets and fibrin as comprising clots in the microcirculation (47). Clearly, the development of microthrombi throughout multiple organs contributes to local ischemia and inadequate substrate delivery and further organ injury and dysfunction. Even with reestablishment of global circulation with early resuscitation, ongoing microvascular thrombosis (often manifest clinically as new-onset thrombocytopenia) can cause persistent microcirculatory ischemia and tissue injury that continue to fuel the vicious cycle of ischemia/shock–(re)injury–inflammation described earlier. In this regard, the idea that persistent *regional* shock contributes to the development of MODS has gained broader appeal.

As a result of this pathology an additional cause of MODS has emerged, described as thrombocytopenia-associated multiple organ failure (TAMOF) (48). TAMOF is described as a thrombotic microangiopathic process akin to thrombotic thrombocytopenic purpura (TTP) and characterized by decreased ADAMTS13 protease activity resulting in accumulation of large, multimeric von Willebrand Factor (vWF) leading to MODS development (49). vWF is a pro-thrombogenic protein, produced by the vascular endothelium and platelets, whose function is to assist in hemostatic function at a site of vascular/endothelial injury. vWF is normally released into the circulation as large multimeric complexes whose size correlates to platelet thrombogenicity (50). However, the propensity to form spontaneous clot is minimized in part by circulating in a compact, less thrombogenic form and also by the presence of circulating proteases, notably ADAMTS13, that degrade vWF into smaller multimers. After localized vascular injury, the activation of the endothelium, or increased shear stress at the site, causes the large vWF multimers to unfold, which uncovers their full thrombogenic potential. This causes the trapping of platelets and the formation of platelet-vWF clot that serves to create a platelet plug. Once hemostasis has been achieved, the balance between thrombosis/fibrinolysis shifts in favor of increased fibrinolytic activity and eventual restoration of normal microcirculatory flow and function. This homeostatic function may go awry in the setting of severe injury that triggers massive systemic endothelial (and platelet) activation. Alternatively, the systemic release of proinflammatory mediators (e.g., TNF-α) can activate formation of large vWF multimers while reducing ADAMTS13 amount and/or activity resulting in disseminated microvascular thrombosis and organ failure (50).

The presence of this pathology raise the possibility that plasma exchange, by clearing large vWF multimers and replacing ADAMTS13 with fresh plasma, may improve MODS by diminishing circulating vWF multimers.

This "microcirculatory hypothesis" of MODS becomes even more complicated when the additional biologic complexity introduced by the reestablishment of adequate blood flow to organs is considered. The phenomenon of *reperfusion injury* that follows a period of thrombosis-mediated ischemia can result in substantial cellular and tissue injury as a result of oxygen radical generation as described above and reviewed elsewhere (51) (see Chapter 21). Thus, even when the primary insult of hypoperfusion is addressed with the reestablishment of flow of oxygenated blood, a second wave of injurious mediators in the form of oxidant stresses may be generated. Provision of antioxidant therapies has shown some clinical benefits in specific situations of reperfusion injury (52), though whether this effect can be achieved globally in the setting of resuscitation from hypoxic-ischemic insult to prevent MODS remains to be determined.

Mitochondrial Dysfunction, Bioenergetic Failure, and Apoptosis

Given the requirement of higher-order organisms to maintain aerobic energy metabolism for their survival, the accumulation of cellular energy deficits arising from global and/or regional shock states may also result in the development of MODS. In this regard, rapid reversal of shock through aggressive restoration of adequate delivery of oxygen and nutrients is paramount for the prevention of complete bioenergetic failure and necrotic cell death. Occasionally, despite restoration of oxygen delivery, a condition develops in which cells appear unable to effectively utilize delivered oxygen. The clinical scenario involves an increasing lactic acidosis in the face of diminished oxygen extraction and abnormally elevated mixed venous oxygen saturations and is referred to as "cytopathic hypoxia" (53). The purported mechanism for this impaired oxygen utilization stems from an acquired state of mitochondrial dysfunction related to mitochondrial oxidant self-injury from the inadvertent release of free radicals from oxidative phosphorylation. In addition to mitochondria serving as an important source for ROS production, ROS can also be generated elsewhere under pathologic conditions. Other possible sources include the production of superoxide for bacterial killing by neutrophils, the reversible inhibition of complex IV of the mitochondrial electron transport chain (ETC) (54) by nitric oxide overproduction secondary to upregulation of iNOS in endothelial cells during acute inflammation, and the combination of nitric oxide with superoxide to form peroxynitrite, a considerably stronger free radical, capable of damaging a wide range of cellular components including DNA, proteins, lipid membranes, and mitochondria. Regardless of source, the onslaught of reactive oxygen and nitrogen species (RONS) ultimately overwhelms cellular antioxidant defenses that typically attenuate RONS-mediated damage. Resultant mitochondrial damage further precipitates a self-destructive cycle and impairs the energy-production capacity needed to escape energy debt. Furthermore, RONS (and potentially other inflammatory mediators) can directly inhibit the mitochondrial ETC and impair or downregulate certain mitochondrial enzymes involved in energy metabolism (e.g., pyruvate dehydrogenase, cis-aconitase) upstream to the ETC (55). This impairment contributes to further loss of the mitochondrial membrane potential ($\Delta\Psi$), the proton gradient across the inner mitochondrial membrane that drives oxidative phosphorylation, to ultimately result in cellular bioenergetic failure and classic apoptotic cell death. Interestingly, it has been hypothesized that early perturbations in mitochondrial activity may actually be protective, allowing for cellular "hibernation" in the face of limited oxygen and nutrient supply as an alternative to cell death (56). Although cell, and ultimately organ, dysfunction may become manifest, recovery of mitochondrial function and enhanced mitochondrial biogenesis concurrent with restoration of oxygen and/or nutrient delivery lead to resolution of this transient organ dysfunction. However, failure to restore mitochondrial function and deficient mitochondrial biogenesis results in a state of persistent cellular bioenergetic failure, cell death, and progressive MODS (56).

Necrotic cell death and "programmed cell death" or apoptosis are the two characterized pathways by which cells die as organ dysfunction/failure occurs. The role apoptosis plays in the setting of critical illness remains unclear. However, mitochondria are involved in the trigger by key inflammatory signals (e.g., TNF-α, Fas) or other endogenous signals (e.g., DNA damage, p53) toward apoptosis (57). That mitochondria would play such a role is logical given that these organelles gauge the energy costs associated with restoration of cellular homeostasis that may be too excessive in the setting of limited "resources" (i.e., shock), leaving apoptosis as a better option for the whole organism. While a comprehensive review is beyond the scope of this chapter (reviewed in (58)), a brief overview of the important mechanisms of mitochondrial-mediated apoptosis is warranted.

A number of cellular stressors, such as oxidant stress or low ATP states, are thought to trigger conformational alignment of various mitochondrial proteins integral to its outer and inner membranes such that physical "pores" are formed, allowing free passage of molecules <1.5 kDa (59). Creation of these pores effectively "short circuits" the mitochondrion thereby collapsing $\Delta\Psi$ that drives oxidative phosphorylation and ATP production. In addition, the osmotic influx of water into the mitochondrial matrix leads to significant swelling and rupture of the outer membrane that allows the release of cytochrome c, a non–membrane-bound component of the mitochondrial ETC, along with other pro-apoptotic proteins into the cytosol. In the cytosol, cytochrome c binds with apoptotic protease activating factor 1 (Apaf-1) to form a multimeric structure called the apoptosome. This apoptosome recruits procaspase-9, which then becomes activated to caspase-9, and in turn cleaves and activates procaspase-3 to caspase-3, the key executioner of apoptosis (reviewed in (60)).

Unfortunately for the intensivist, understanding the mechanisms of apoptosis is irrelevant unless these processes can be therapeutically manipulated for patient benefit. In this regard, the development of target "therapies" to alter apoptotic signaling has been especially challenging because the tightly regulated process of apoptosis serves an important functional role in maintaining the homeostasis of the organism. Although cell death is often viewed as a negative consequence, the careful, controlled elimination of cells benefits the organism by creating room for new, more robust cells—a crucial mechanism of development. Clearly, any potential intervention will need to selectively target *pathologic* apoptosis while sparing *physiologic* apoptosis to have any clinical therapeutic relevance.

TREATMENT OF MULTIPLE ORGAN DYSFUNCTION SYSTEM

One of the more disappointing realizations for intensive care physicians has been the inability to consistently alter the outcome of MODS after it has developed. Thus, *prevention* has been embraced as an important approach when dealing with patients at risk for developing MODS. From the perspective that MODS reflects a loss of homeostasis due to a number of derangements in normal cellular function, the logical goal in approaching MODS avoidance is to prevent this loss of homeostasis. To maintain biologic homeostasis, clinicians must provide "supportive care" by utilizing effective, early resuscitation in the form of restoration of ventilation, oxygenation, intravascular volume, adequate hemoglobin levels, and the maintenance of adequate organ perfusion (61). While these are intuitively obvious goals, how they are achieved may have impact on the severity and outcome of MODS.

The application of mechanical ventilation can be a lifesaving therapy and can also have detrimental consequences. The use of high inspiratory pressures (*barotrauma*), excessive tidal volumes (*volutrauma*), and inadequate PEEP (*atelectatrauma*) has the potential to produce ventilator-induced lung injury (VILI) and result in the systemic release of inflammatory mediators from the lung—a pathophysiologic principle collectively termed *biotrauma* (62). Evidence supporting this notion of VILI include inflammatory gene expression in lungs caused by injurious ventilation (63), the spread of this reaction outside the lung (64), and a decrease in systemic cytokine expression and MODS associated with protective ventilatory strategy (65). Other associations that include VILI involve the promotion of bacterial translocation (66), the release of pro-apoptotic factors from the lung, and the suppression of peripheral immune responses related to counter-regulation of lung inflammation (67). Regardless of the precise causes, these observations have led to the therapeutic principle of a protective lung strategy achieved by limiting tidal volumes and/or plateau pressures and avoiding excessive lung collapse by utilizing sufficient PEEP.

Instituting the common principles of hemodynamic support, though not always assuring a favorable outcome, has been shown to influence MODS progression. Perhaps the best example of the effectiveness of this approach is the observation that successful, goal-directed therapy in adults with sepsis often attenuates the severity of organ dysfunction (as estimated by surrogate APACHE scores) (68). Whether achieving early, goal-directed targets such as superior vena cava oxygen saturation levels >70% is as effective at reducing organ failure and mortality in pediatric patients as has been shown in adults remains an incompletely answered question. Nevertheless, despite what otherwise appears to be adequate delivery of oxygen as reflected by normal cardiac output and oxygen saturation levels, it is clear that in many circumstances this is insufficient to meet the patient's metabolic demands. This relative failure or inadequacy of typically "normal" oxygen delivery has been termed *pathologic supply-dependent oxygen consumption* by some and implies that a critical imbalance between oxygen delivery and consumption has been reached (53). Unfortunately, *supranormal* delivery of oxygen achieved by augmenting cardiac output, hemoglobin concentration and/or hemoglobin oxygen saturation does not consistently reverse this physiologic state. Certain theories, backed by scant experimental evidence, have been put forward to explain this phenomenon including maldistribution of perfusion at the microcirculatory level (69), initiation of a futile energy cycle of the cell mediated by inflammatory cytokines (70), or molecular alterations in cellular respiration affecting oxygen uptake by the cell (71). Regardless of the ultimate pathologic cause, it is humbling that strict adherence to long-practiced principles of hemodynamic support will not always prevent the progression of MODS in our patients and keeps pursuit of the "insulin for oxygen" one of the most important targets in MODS research.

Other mainstays of therapy aimed at preventing and/or reversing MODS include "source" control of the injury, early institution of enteral feeding, and avoiding excessive fluid overload. Whether the trigger is traumatic in nature or related to an identifiable nidus of infection, "source control" achieved by institution of timely (goal of within 60 minutes of suspected infection) and accurate (i.e., targeting causative pathogen) antibiotic coverage remains of one of the most important predictors of outcome in critically ill patients (71a). Early initiation of enteral nutrition has been consistently demonstrated to improve ICU outcomes, including the degree of MODS in some studies of critically ill adults. However, some studies have questioned whether the enteral route is indeed superior to parenteral nutrition and capable of preventing MODS if a positive nitrogen balance is maintained and adequate caloric delivery achieved. Also, whether adding enteral bacterial decontamination or immunoactive nutritional supplements (e.g., glutamine) to the nutritional approach ultimately affects the incidence and outcome of MODS remains incompletely studied. The role for antioxidant or other mitochondrial-targeted therapies to either prevent or reverse MODS is also unproven. Finally, there is an association between fluid overload and MODS in critically ill pediatric patients (11). It has been suggested that using continuous renal replacement therapy early in the course of illness to avoid excessive fluid overload (>15% above dry weight) may improve mortality in patients with established MODS (11). However, whether this approach translates broadly to the pediatric ICU population remains to be determined.

Finally, two recent therapeutic approaches in the critically ill children at risk for MODS deserve comment: targeting the coagulation cascade and tight glucose control. In light of the link between inflammation and coagulation with MODS, it was hypothesized that pharmacologically targeting both systems may prove beneficial in patients with severe sepsis who were at substantial risk for developing MODS. Activated protein C (APC), or drotrecogin alpha, has been shown to possess both anticoagulant and anti-inflammatory activity (72). While initial studies proved promising with an observed absolute reduction in mortality of 6.1% in adults with severe sepsis (73), later results have not continued to demonstrate the same degree of efficacy. In light of this lack of efficacy combined with an increased risk of bleeding associated with drotrecogin alpha use (74), the drug was removed from the market. This ultimate result paralleled the findings in pediatrics. One of the largest multicenter trials in pediatric critical care, the RESOLVE Trial (RESolution of Organ faiLure in pediatric patients with seVEre sepsis), tested the efficacy of drotrecogin alpha to decrease the number organ-failure-free days was terminated early for lack of efficacy (75). Whether this reflects a misdirected therapeutic approach in the setting of MODS remains unclear, as there are ample data supporting the pathophysiologic role of inflammation and microvascular thrombosis in *some* patients with MODS. Instead, it may be that better stratification of the cohort of patients at risk for or with existing MODS may assist in identifying the subset of patients that might derive benefit from a compound targeting these pathways.

Over the past decade, intensivists have become familiar with the concept of striving to achieve tight glycemic control (TGC) in patients with hyperglycemia. In one of the earliest studies of tight glycemic control, van den Berghe et al. (76,77) demonstrated that maintaining blood glucose at a level between 80 and 110 mg/dl reduced mortality in an adult surgical ICU from 8.0% to 4.6% ($p < 0.04$) with the greatest reduction in mortality involving deaths due to MODS with a proven septic focus. Since this report, a number of studies have attempted to corroborate the finding in broader patient populations with inconsistent results (78). With regard to children, it appears that hyperglycemia may also be associated with increased mortality and organ failure in children (79), although when adjusted for severity of illness, the risk related to hyperglycemia is insignificant. Instead, consequent hypoglycemia resulting from overly aggressive correction of hyperglycemia may be equally as bad in the developing child (80). In fact, consistent with the hypothesis of dysregulated homeostasis presented above, the worst outcomes have been observed in those children demonstrating the greatest degree of variability in serum glucose (i.e., from lowest to highest value) suggesting that the normal physiologic regulation of this system has been lost (80). Whether the clinical benefits observed with tight glycemic control derive from attenuating the effects of high glucose on impairing physiologic function, i.e., *glucose toxicity*, or are a result of insulin being a beneficial, therapeutic modulator of critical illness remains incompletely known (reviewed in (81)). In the largest pediatric study to date, a total of 1369 children ≤ 16 years of age admitted to a pediatric intensive care unit at 13 centers in England were randomized to either tight (glucose 72–126 mg/dL) or conventional (glucose <216 mg/dL) control in the CHIP study (82,83). There was no difference in primary outcome of number of days alive and free from mechanical ventilation at 30 days or other secondary outcomes, except for a slight decrease in 12-month costs in the tight glycemic control group. However, 60% of the children in this study had undergone cardiac surgery. Whether the same approach of tight glucose control in a general cohort of critically ill children with MODS has a favorable outcome remains to be studied in the context of the planned Heart And Lung Failure—Pediatric INsulin Titration Trial (HALF-PINT) Study (http://clinicaltrials.gov/ct2/show/NCT01565941). In summary, it remains to be seen as to whether tight glucose control ultimately confers any benefit to critically ill children with MODS. Clearly, an improved mechanistic understanding of the biologic processes mediating the initiation, propagation, and resolution of organ dysfunction in critically ill children is needed before similar improvements in our therapeutic armamentarium are gained.

CONCLUSIONS AND FUTURE DIRECTIONS

Our clinical and epidemiologic understanding of pediatric MODS has expanded substantially since its initial recognition as a distinct clinical entity, though the interpretation of the cumulative data has been complicated by the methodological heterogeneity between studies. With recent consensus agreements reached for *pediatric-specific* definitions and criteria for MODS, greater epidemiologic and mechanistic understanding should emerge through more uniformity in future investigations. Yet, despite our increasing ability to recognize the clinical manifestations of MODS and its associated epidemiologic and prognostic implications, ICU physicians remain frustrated by the current limitations to our therapeutic armamentarium. As a result, as with every challenging clinical syndrome that prematurely robs the precious lives of the children whom we care for, our discipline must remain committed to advancing our biologic and mechanistic understanding of this fatal syndrome so that future development of novel, viable therapies for MODS can be realized.

To assist with this, we have presented a conceptual paradigm to support the view that MODS reflects the ultimate loss of homeostasis at the cellular, tissue/organ, and whole body levels. From this perspective, it is possible to make connections between many of the prevailing theories that have attempted to explain the pathogenesis of MODS. Despite the promise of our expanding knowledge base and increasingly advanced life-sustaining technologies for improving patient outcomes, the looming presence of potential death from MODS remains. In the near future, the impact of intensive glucose control, early goal-directed therapy (perhaps with novel, noninvasive measures of oxygen delivery), and the influence of lung-protective ventilatory strategy on organ failure and outcomes in children will become clearer. Meanwhile, amid the struggle to achieve physiologic balance at the patient's bedside perhaps there is no better virtue to exhibit than patience. It may be as important to know what *not to do* as it is to know what to do, particularly as evidence of therapeutic advances realized in adults are either not replicated or even studied in children. As stated in the introduction of this chapter, MODS epitomizes our discipline of critical care medicine. As such, we must continue to "balance" the concerns of each of our subspecialty colleagues regarding their particular organ system of interest as it is our responsibility to orchestrate the multiple therapeutic modalities aimed to restore global homeostasis. Finally, it is important not to lose sight of the humanistic side of our profession as family members of those children whom we care often place their faith in spiritual and religious "forces" even as they place their faith and trust in our clinical judgment.

References

1. Jenkins MT, Jones RF, Wilson B, et al. Congestive atelectasia complication of the intravenous infusion of fluids. *Ann Surg* 1950;132(3):327–47.
2. Burke JF, Pontoppidan H, Welch CE. High output respiratory failure: An important cause of death ascribed to peritonitis or ileus. *Ann Surg* 1963;158:581–95.
3. MacLean LD, Mulligan WG, McLean AP, et al. Patterns of septic shock in man—a detailed study of 56 patients. *Ann Surg* 1967;166(4):543–62.
4. Skillman JJ, Bushnell LS, Goldman H, et al. Respiratory failure, hypotension, sepsis, and jaundice. A clinical syndrome associated with lethal hemorrhage from acute stress ulceration of the stomach. *Am J Surg* 1969;117(4):523–30.
5. Tilney NL, Bailey GL, Morgan AP. Sequential system failure after rupture of abdominal aortic aneurysms: An unsolved problem in postoperative care. *Ann Surg* 1973;178(2):117–22.
6. Baue AE. Multiple, progressive, or sequential systems failure. A syndrome of the 1970s. *Arch Surg* 1975;110(7):779–81.
7. Wilkinson JD, Pollack MM, Ruttimann UE, et al. Outcome of pediatric patients with multiple organ system failure. *Crit Care Med* 1986;14(4):271–4.
8. American College of Chest Physicians/Society of Critical Care Medicine Consensus Conference. Definitions for sepsis and organ failure and guidelines for the use of innovative therapies in sepsis. *Crit Care Med* 1992;20(6):864–74.
9. Proulx F, Gauthier M, Nadeau D, et al. Timing and predictors of death in pediatric patients with multiple organ system failure. *Crit Care Med* 1994;22(6):1025–31.
10. Proulx F, Fayon M, Farrell CA, et al. Epidemiology of sepsis and multiple organ dysfunction syndrome in children. *Chest* 1996;109(4):1033–7.
11. Goldstein SL, Somers MJ, Baum MA, et al. Pediatric patients with multi-organ dysfunction syndrome receiving continuous renal replacement therapy. *Kidney Int* 2005;67(2):653–8.
12. Levy MM, Fink MP, Marshall JC, et al. 2001 SCCM/ESICM/ACCP/ATS/SIS International Sepsis Definitions Conference. *Crit Care Med* 2003;31(4):1250–6.
13. Wilkinson JD, Pollack MM, Glass NL, et al. Mortality associated with multiple organ system failure and sepsis in pediatric intensive care unit. *J Pediatr* 1987; 111(3):324–8.
14. Leteurtre S, Martinot A, Duhamel A, et al. Development of a pediatric multiple organ dysfunction score: Use of two strategies. *Med Decis Making* 1999;19(4):399–410.
15. Leteurtre S, Martinot A, Duhamel A, et al. Validation of the paediatric logistic organ dysfunction (PELOD) score: Prospective, observational, multicentre study. *Lancet* 2003;362(9379):192–7.
16. Goldstein B, Giroir B, Randolph A. International pediatric sepsis consensus conference: Definitions for sepsis and organ dysfunction in pediatrics. *Pediatr Crit Care Med* 2005;6(1):2–8.
17. Brilli RJ, Goldstein B. Pediatric sepsis definitions: Past, present, and future. *Pediatr Crit Care Med* 2005;6(suppl 3):S6–8.
18. Nadel S, Goldstein B, Williams MD, et al. Drotrecogin alfa (activated) in children with severe sepsis: A multicentre phase III randomised controlled trial. *Lancet* 2007;369(9564):836–43.
19. Moreno R, Vincent JL, Matos R, et al. The use of maximum SOFA score to quantify organ dysfunction/failure in intensive care. Results of a prospective, multicentre study. Working Group on Sepsis related Problems of the ESICM. *Intensive Care Med* 1999;25(7):686–96.
20. Guidet B, Aegerter P, Gauzit R, et al. Incidence and impact of organ dysfunctions associated with sepsis. *Chest* 2005;127(3):942–51.
21. Goh A, Lum L. Sepsis, severe sepsis and septic shock in paediatric multiple organ dysfunction syndrome. *J Paediatr Child Health* 1999;35(5):488–92.
22. Leclerc F, Leteurtre S, Duhamel A, et al. Cumulative influence of organ dysfunctions and septic state on mortality of critically ill children. *Am J Respir Crit Care Med* 2005;171(4):348–53.
23. Tantalean JA, Leon RJ, Santos AA, et al. Multiple organ dysfunction syndrome in children. *Pediatr Crit Care Med* 2003;4(2):181–5.
24. Shah P, Riphagen S, Beyene J, et al. Multiorgan dysfunction in infants with post-asphyxial hypoxic-ischaemic encephalopathy. *Arch Dis Child Fetal Neonatal Ed* 2004;89(2):F152–5.
25. Johnston JA, Yi MS, Britto MT, et al. Importance of organ dysfunction in determining hospital outcomes in children. *J Pediatr* 2004;144(5):595–601.
26. Duke TD, Butt W, South M. Predictors of mortality and multiple organ failure in children with sepsis. *Intensive Care Med* 1997;23(6):684–92.
27. Kutko MC, Calarco MP, Flaherty MB, et al. Mortality rates in pediatric septic shock with and without multiple organ system failure. *Pediatr Crit Care Med* 2003;4(3):333–7.
28. Saez-Llorens X, Vargas S, Guerra F, et al. Application of new sepsis definitions to evaluate outcome of pediatric patients with severe systemic infections. *Pediatr Infect Dis J* 1995;14(7):557–61.
29. Diaz MA, Vicent MG, Prudencio M, et al. Predicting factors for admission to an intensive care unit and clinical outcome in pediatric patients receiving hematopoietic stem cell transplantation. *Haematologica* 2002;87(3):292–8.
30. Bone RC. Sir Isaac Newton, sepsis, SIRS, and CARS. *Crit Care Med* 1996;24(7):1125–8.
31. Hendrick JP, Hartl FU. Molecular chaperone functions of heat-shock proteins. *Annu Rev Biochem* 1993;62:349–84.
32. Gelfant S. The energy requirements for mitosis. *Ann N Y Acad Sci* 1960;90:536–49.
33. Kirby DM, Thorburn DR. Approaches to finding the molecular basis of mitochondrial oxidative phosphorylation disorders. *Twin Res Hum Genet* 2008;11(4):395–411.
34. Scialo F, Mallikarjun V, Stefanatos R, et al. Regulation of lifespan by the mitochondrial electron transport chain: Reactive oxygen species-dependent and reactive oxygen species-independent mechanisms. *Antioxid Redox Signal* 2012;19(16):1953–69.
34a. Vincent JL, De Backer D. Microvascular dysfunction as a cause of organ dysfunction in severe sepsis. *Crit Care.* 2005;9(Suppl 4):S9–12.
35. Cornell TT, Shanley TP. Signal transduction overview. *Crit Care Med* 2005;33(suppl 12):S410–3.
36. Medzhitov R, Shevach EM, Trinchieri G, et al. Highlights of 10 years of immunology in nature reviews immunology. *Nat Rev Immunol* 2011;11(10):693–702.
37. Chan JK, Roth J, Oppenheim JJ, et al. Alarmins: Awaiting a clinical response. *J Clin Invest* 2012;122(8):2711–9.
38. Dushay MS. Insect hemolymph clotting. *Cell Mol Life Sci* 2009;66(16):2643–50.
39. Grigorian M, Hartenstein V. Hematopoiesis and hematopoietic organs in arthropods. *Dev Genes Evol* 2013;223(1–2):103–15.
40. Cerenius L, Jiravanichpaisal P, Liu HP, et al. Crustacean immunity. *Adv Exp Med Biol* 2010;708:239–59.

41. Shanley TP, Warner RL, Ward PA. The role of cytokines and adhesion molecules in the development of inflammatory injury. *Mol Med Today* 1995;1(1):40–5.

42. Bone RC. Immunologic dissonance: A continuing evolution in our understanding of the systemic inflammatory response syndrome (SIRS) and the multiple organ dysfunction syndrome (MODS). *Ann Intern Med* 1996;125(8):680–7.

43. Deitch EA, Morrison J, Berg R, et al. Effect of hemorrhagic shock on bacterial translocation, intestinal morphology, and intestinal permeability in conventional and antibiotic-decontaminated rats. *Crit Care Med* 1990;18(5):529–36.

44. Volk HD, Reinke P, Docke WD. Clinical aspects: From systemic inflammation to 'immunoparalysis'. *Chem Immunol* 2000;74:162–77.

45. Hall MW, Knatz NL, Vetterly C, et al. Immunoparalysis and nosocomial infection in children with multiple organ dysfunction syndrome. *Intensive Care Med* 2011;37(3):525–32.

46. Gando S. Microvascular thrombosis and multiple organ dysfunction syndrome. *Crit Care Med* 2010;38(suppl 2):S35–42.

47. Hook KM, Abrams CS. The loss of homeostasis in hemostasis: New approaches in treating and understanding acute disseminated intravascular coagulation in critically ill patients. *Clin Transl Sci* 2012;5(1):85–92.

48. Nguyen TC, Carcillo JA. Bench-to-bedside review: Thrombocytopenia-associated multiple organ failure—a newly appreciated syndrome in the critically ill. *Crit Care* 2006;10(6):235.

49. Nguyen T, Hall M, Han Y, et al. Microvascular thrombosis in pediatric multiple organ failure: Is it a therapeutic target? *Pediatr Crit Care Med* 2001;2(3):187–96.

50. Claus RA, Bockmeyer CL, Sossdorf M, et al. The balance between von-Willebrand factor and its cleaving protease ADAMTS13: Biomarker in systemic inflammation and development of organ failure? *Curr Mol Med* 2010;10(2):236–48.

51. Granger DN. Role of xanthine oxidase and granulocytes in ischemia-reperfusion injury. *Am J Physiol* 1988;255(6 ptt 2):H1269–75.

52. Rayner BS, Duong TT, Myers SJ, et al. Protective effect of a synthetic anti-oxidant on neuronal cell apoptosis resulting from experimental hypoxia re-oxygenation injury. *J Neurochem* 2006;97(1):211–21.

53. Fink MP. Bench-to-bedside review: Cytopathic hypoxia. *Crit Care* 2002;6(6):491–9.

54. Brown GC. Nitric oxide inhibition of cytochrome oxidase and mitochondrial respiration: Implications for inflammatory, neurodegenerative and ischaemic pathologies. *Mol Cell Biochem* 1997;174(1–2):189–92.

55. Haynes V, Elfering SL, Squires RJ, et al. Mitochondrial nitric-oxide synthase: Role in pathophysiology. *IUBMB Life* 2003;55(10–11):599–603.

56. Singer M. Mitochondrial function in sepsis: Acute phase versus multiple organ failure. *Crit Care Med* 2007;35(suppl 9):S441–8.

57. Liu X, Kim CN, Yang J, et al. Induction of apoptotic program in cell-free extracts: Requirement for dATP and cytochrome c. *Cell* 1996;86(1):147–57.

58. Exline MC, Crouser ED. Mitochondrial mechanisms of sepsis-induced organ failure. *Front Biosci* 2008;13:5030–41.

59. Zoratti M, Szabo I. The mitochondrial permeability transition. *Biochim Biophys Acta* 1995;1241(2):139–76.

60. Jin Z, El-Deiry WS. Overview of cell death signaling pathways. *Cancer Biol Ther* 2005;4(2):139–63.

61. Carcillo JA, Fields AI. Clinical practice parameters for hemodynamic support of pediatric and neonatal patients in septic shock. *Crit Care Med* 2002;30(6):1365–78.

62. Plotz FB, Slutsky AS, van Vught AJ, et al. Ventilator-induced lung injury and multiple system organ failure: A critical review of facts and hypotheses. *Intensive Care Med* 2004;30(10):1865–72.

63. Wilson MR, Choudhury S, Goddard ME, et al. High tidal volume upregulates intrapulmonary cytokines in an in vivo mouse model of ventilator-induced lung injury. *J Appl Physiol* 2003;95(4):1385–93.

64. Ranieri VM, Suter PM, Tortorella C, et al. Effect of mechanical ventilation on inflammatory mediators in patients with acute respiratory distress syndrome: A randomized controlled trial. *JAMA* 1999;282(1):54–61.

65. Ventilation with lower tidal volumes as compared with traditional tidal volumes for acute lung injury and the acute respiratory distress syndrome. The Acute Respiratory Distress Syndrome Network. *N Engl J Med* 2000;342(18):1301–8.

66. Lin CY, Zhang H, Cheng KC, et al. Mechanical ventilation may increase susceptibility to the development of bacteremia. *Crit Care Med* 2003;31(5):1429–34.

67. Vreugdenhil HA, Heijnen CJ, Plotz FB, et al. Mechanical ventilation of healthy rats suppresses peripheral immune function. *Eur Respir J* 2004;23(1):122–8.

68. Rivers E, Nguyen B, Havstad S, et al. Early goal-directed therapy in the treatment of severe sepsis and septic shock. *N Engl J Med* 2001;345(19):1368–77.

69. De Blasi RA, Palmisani S, Alampi D, et al. Microvascular dysfunction and skeletal muscle oxygenation assessed by phase-modulation near-infrared spectroscopy in patients with septic shock. *Intensive Care Med* 2005;31(12):1661–8.

70. Soriano FG, Liaudet L, Szabo E, et al. Resistance to acute septic peritonitis in poly(ADP-ribose) polymerase-1-deficient mice. *Shock* 2002;17(4):286–92.

71. Kozlov AV, Staniek K, Haindl S, et al. Different effects of endotoxic shock on the respiratory function of liver and heart mitochondria in rats. *Am J Physiol Gastrointest Liver Physiol* 2006;290(3):G543–9.

71a. Kumar, et al. Duration of hypotension before initiation of effective antimicrobial therapy is the critical determinant of survival in human septic shock. *Crit Care Med* 2006;34(6): 1589–96.

72. Joyce DE, Nelson DR, Grinnell BW. Leukocyte and endothelial cell interactions in sepsis: Relevance of the protein C pathway. *Crit Care Med* 2004;32(suppl 5):S280–6.

73. Bernard GR, Ely EW, Wright TJ, et al. Safety and dose relationship of recombinant human activated protein C for coagulopathy in severe sepsis. *Crit Care Med* 2001;29(11):2051–9.

74. Fumagalli R, Mignini MA. The safety profile of drotrecogin alfa (activated). *Crit Care* 2007;11(suppl 5):S6.

75. Goldstein B, Nadel S, Peters M, et al. ENHANCE: Results of a global open-label trial of drotrecogin alfa (activated) in children with severe sepsis. *Pediatr Crit Care Med* 2006;7(3):200–11.

76. van den Berghe G, Wouters P, Weekers F, et al. Intensive insulin therapy in the critically ill patients. *N Engl J Med* 2001;345(19):1359–67.

77. Van den Berghe G, Wilmer A, Hermans G, et al. Intensive insulin therapy in the medical ICU. *N Engl J Med* 2006;354(5):449–61.

78. Van den Berghe G, Mesotten D, Vanhorebeek I. Intensive insulin therapy in the intensive care unit. *CMAJ* 2009;180(8):799–800.

79. Faustino EV, Apkon M. Persistent hyperglycemia in critically ill children. *J Pediatr* 2005;146(1):30–4.

80. Wintergerst KA, Buckingham B, Gandrud L, et al. Association of hypoglycemia, hyperglycemia, and glucose variability with morbidity and death in the pediatric intensive care unit. *Pediatrics* 2006;118(1):173–9.

81. Van den Berghe G. How does blood glucose control with insulin save lives in intensive care? *J Clin Invest* 2004;114(9):1187–95.

82. Agus MS, Steil GM, Wypij D, et al. Tight glycemic control versus standard care after pediatric cardiac surgery. *N Engl J Med* 2012;367(13):1208–19.

83. Macrae, et al. A randomized trial of hyperglycemic control in pediatric intensive care. *NEJM* 2014;370(2):107–118

PART TWO ■ EMERGENCY CARE AND ACUTE MANAGEMENT

CHAPTER 24 ■ AIRWAY MANAGEMENT

DOMINIC CAVE, JONATHAN P. DUFF, ALLAN DE CAEN, AND MARY FRAN HAZINSKI

KEY POINTS

❶ To provide successful and safe airway management, providers must have an appreciation of the unique developmental anatomy and physiology of the child's airway.

❷ Successful acute airway management requires that providers anticipate the development of a difficult airway and have a primary and secondary plan for management.

❸ The difficult pediatric airway is best managed not by heroic intervention and uncommonly used techniques but, rather, by anticipation and planning, careful patient posi-

tioning, effective bag-mask ventilation, and advanced airway insertion, as needed.

❹ Successful airway support requires careful choice of equipment (type and size), appreciation of the pathology requiring intubation, and presence of personnel with the requisite skills.

❺ Children rapidly develop hypoxemia; hence, time for deliberation is limited when airway support is needed. Modification of the standard rapid sequence intubation technique may therefore be necessary.

The accurate assessment and safe management of the airway is fundamental to the care of critically ill or injured children. The anatomy, development, and evaluation of the pediatric airway, basic airway management, and management of the difficult airway are reviewed in this chapter, with emphasis on techniques for securing the airway.

ANATOMY AND AIRWAY DEVELOPMENT

The Anatomy of the Airway

The normal pediatric airway can be divided into supraglottic, glottic, and subglottic structures. Dividing the airway in this way allows us to consider the impact of pediatric airway development in a way that aligns with interventions and management.

The *supraglottic* structures include the elements of the upper airway: the tongue, palate, posterior pharyngeal space, and epiglottis. Supraglottic sensation is mediated by the superior laryngeal nerve.

The *glottis* is made up of the cartilages and muscular structures of the larynx. The larynx consists of nine cartilages, including the thyroid, cricoid, and epiglottis, and the corniculate, cuneiform, and arytenoid cartilages. These cartilages are covered by folds of mucosa, connective tissue, and muscle; laryngeal tissue folds define the glottis. The superior, inferior, and recurrent laryngeal nerves innervate the larynx. The recurrent laryngeal nerve provides most laryngeal motor innervation. Only the cricothyroid muscle is innervated by the superior laryngeal nerve.

The *subglottis* or *infraglottis* consists of the cricoid cartilage and the tracheal rings and mucosal surfaces of the upper trachea. This region also includes the trachea itself and the initial branches of the bronchial tree. Infraglottic sensation is mediated by the inferior laryngeal nerve. The airway is lined with ciliated and squamous epithelium that is highly vascular and overlies a rich network of lymphatic vessels.

❶ ### Developmental Airway Considerations

The anatomy of the pediatric airway differs from the adult airway until it reaches mature position at ~8–14 years of age. The major differences between pediatric and adult airway structures are size, shape, and position in the neck (**Fig. 24.1**).

The infant's tongue is large in proportion to the rest of the oral cavity and is closer to the palate; therefore, it can easily obstruct the airway. Laryngoscopic stabilization of the tongue may be more difficult in the infant and child than in the adult. The epiglottis is proportionally larger in the child than in the adult, and the ligamentous connection between the base of the tongue and the epiglottis (the hyoepiglottic ligament) is not as strong in the young child as in the adult. These differences can influence the selection of laryngoscope blade (straight vs. curved) for the intubation of young children (see discussion in the section *Endotracheal Intubation— Intubation Procedure*, later).

Tracheal diameter and length increase with age. Tracheal dimensions reported from postmortem examinations have been verified using magnetic resonance imaging (MRI) (1) (**Table 24.1**). Because the diameter of the pediatric trachea is small, relatively minor compromise in tracheal radius can significantly increase resistance to airflow and work of breathing. Resistance to airflow is inversely related to the *fourth* power of the radius during quiet breathing, when airflow is laminar, but is inversely related to the *fifth* power of the radius when airflow is turbulent. When respiratory distress is present, providers should attempt to keep the child as quiet as possible to minimize agitation and to reduce turbulent flow, airway resistance, and work of breathing.

The glottic opening lies at approximately the level of cervical vertebrae C2 or C3 in the infant or child and at the level of C3 or C4 in the adolescent or adult. This position places the glottic opening of the infant or child at the base of the proportionally larger and predominantly intraoral tongue (**Fig. 24.1**). This position of the pediatric glottis has been described as *anterior* when compared to the mature laryngeal structures, because the airway may become hidden

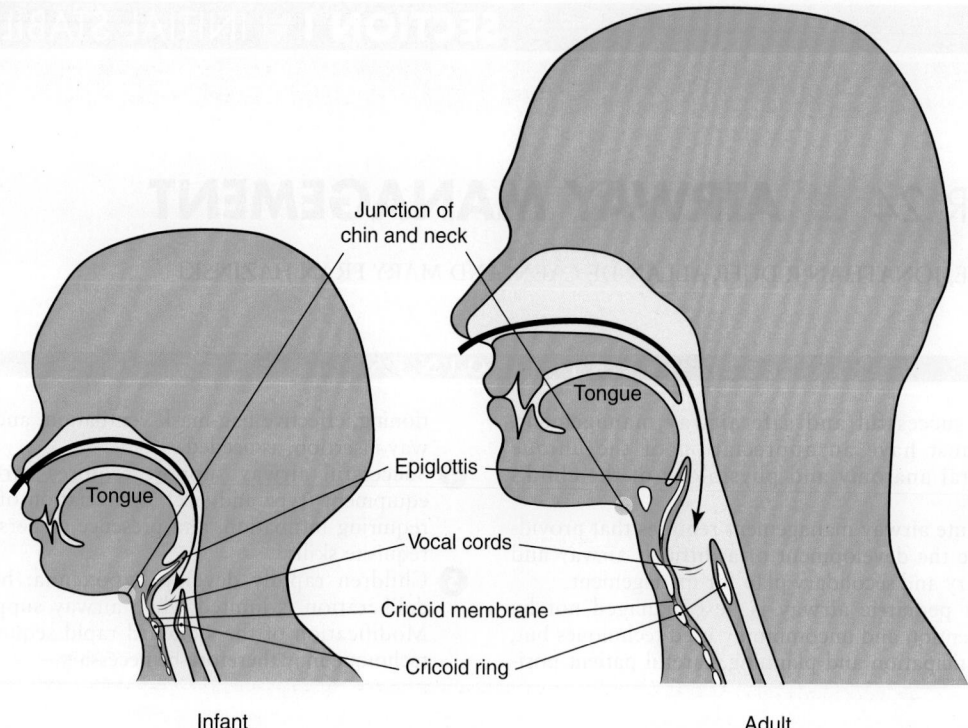

Junction of
chin and neck

Tongue

Epiglottis

Vocal cords

Cricoid membrane

Cricoid ring

Tongue

Infant   Adult

FIGURE 24.1. The anatomic differences particular to children are these: (1) higher, more anterior position of the glottic opening (note the relationship of the vocal cords to the chin/neck junction); (2) relatively larger tongue in the infant, which lies between the mouth and glottic opening; (3) relatively larger and more floppy epiglottis in the child; (4) the cricoid ring is the narrowest portion of the pediatric airway versus the vocal cords in the adult; (5) position and size of the cricothyroid membrane in the infant; (6) sharper, more difficult angle for blind nasotracheal intubation; and (7) larger relative size of the occiput in the infant. (From Luten RC, Kissoon NJ. In: Walls R, Murphy MF, Luten LC, et al., eds. *Manual of Emergency Airway Management.* 2nd ed. Philadelphia, PA: Lippincott Williams & Wilkins, 2004:217, with permission.)

by the tongue during laryngoscopy. The pediatric glottis is actually more *superior* (i.e., higher or more cephalad) and more *anterior* than in the adult airway. The larynx itself has an angulation, with the superior portion angled toward the provider. This can make it difficult to pass an endotracheal tube (ETT), particularly during nasal intubation. MRI

studies in children document anterior angulation (nearly 10 degrees from the vertical) at approximately the level of the sternal notch (1).

On the basis of cadaver studies, it has long been accepted that the child's larynx is cylindrical from side to side but conical in the transverse or anterior–posterior dimension, with the

TABLE 24.1

TRACHEAL DIMENSIONS

■ AGE (YEARS)	■ TRACHEAL DIAMETER (MM)	■ COMBINED TRACHEAL LENGTH (MM)	■ APPROXIMATE ENDOTRACHEAL TUBE (MM INTERNAL DIAMETER) SIZE	■ LENGTH/DEPTH OF TRACHEAL TUBE FROM TIP TO LIPS WITH ORAL INSERTION (APPROXIMATE MM WITH CM IN PARENTHESES)
0–1	4.91 ± 0.88	44.68	3.0–3.5	85–120 (8.5–12.0)
1–2	6.68 ± 3.37	50.65	3.5–5.5	120–140 (12.0–14.0)
2–4	6.38 ± 1.86	58.23	4.5–6.0	135–150 (14.5–15.0)
4–6	8.4 ± 0.98	63.72	5.5–6.5	150–160 (15.0–16.0)
6–8	8.88 ± 1.51	64.88	5.5–6.5	160–180 (16.0–18.0)
8–10	9.35 ± 1.70	75.00	6.0–7.0	170–195 (17.0–19.5)
10–12	9.55 ± 1.14	72.56	6.5–7.5	200–210 (20.0–21.0)
12–14	10.46 ± 2.32	82.00	7.0–8.0	210 (21.0)
≥14	12.99 ± 1.35	91.51	7.0–8.0	210 (21.0)

Measurements are listed ± sample SD. From Reed JM, O'Conner DM, Myer CM III. Magnetic resonance imaging determination of tracheal orientation in normal children: Practical implications. *Arch Otolaryngol Head Neck Surg* 1996;122(6):605–8, with permission.

tip of the cone at the level of the cricoid cartilage. Pediatric studies using MRI have confirmed this conical shape. In these studies of anesthetized, spontaneously breathing children, the smallest transverse diameter of the larynx was at and immediately below the level of the vocal cords, rather than at the cricoid cartilage (2). However, because the vocal cords and subglottic tissues can be distended, the rigid cricoid ring is still the smallest functional part of the infant airway (2). As the child grows to adulthood, the larynx becomes more cylindrical in shape, with the narrowest segment at the level of the vocal cords (see **Fig. 24.1, Table 24.2**).

The child's subglottic airway is smaller and more compliant, and the supporting cartilage is less well developed than in the adult. As a result, upper airway obstruction (e.g., caused by croup, epiglottitis, or extrathoracic foreign body) can produce tracheal collapse and stridor. Although most of the child's laryngeal mucosa is loosely connected to the underlying tissues, it is tightly connected in the area of the vocal cords and at the laryngeal surface of the epiglottis. Subglottic inflammation is typically contained below this level; however, with little room to accommodate even modest inflammation at the level of the vocal cords or epiglottis, such inflammation can lead to a gross distortion of tissue planes and anatomy and to airway obstruction.

These anatomic variations have long been thought to cause difficulty in intubating the child, requiring more expertise than intubating the adult. More recent evidence suggests that the general incidence of difficult laryngoscopy in children (0.58%–3%) is lower than that reported in adults (9%–13%). In a recent report of 8434 children intubated for 11,219 procedures, Heinrich et al. (3) found an overall incidence of difficult intubation in 1.35% of all children, with the risk highest in neonates (3.2%) and infants (5%). They also found a correlation with severity of presenting illness, with difficult intubation reported in 3.8% of the sickest children (compared with 0.8% of the children who were less ill). Although the incidence of difficulty intubating children in general may be low, children with significant illness, such as those presenting in an ICU are more likely to be difficult to intubate. It should also be noted that the above study looked at experienced practitioners in pediatric anesthetic practice. Other work has shown a high (50%) failure rate on first intubation attempt among pediatric residents (4) and fellows intubating neonates (5).

Selection of ETT size can be challenging, and precise selection is extremely important. If the ETT is too large, it can cause subglottic pressure ischemia and necrosis, leading to subglottic stenosis. If the ETT is too small, it provides significant resistance to air flow and typically is associated with a large air leak that may complicate support of ventilation.

Oral intubation with direct laryngoscopy requires the establishment of a line of vision from the mouth and teeth to the vocal cords (i.e., the glottic opening). This line of vision requires the alignment of three axes: the oral, pharyngeal, and laryngeal. Normally, the laryngeal axis is perpendicular to the oral axis and forms a 45-degree angle with the pharyngeal axis. The provider must position the patient to align these axes for optimal airway patency and for successful intubation.

The provider aligns the three axes in an older child or adult by placing a towel or other support beneath the occiput to tilt the neck forward (from the shoulders) and by lifting the chin to extend the neck (i.e., the *sniffing position*) (**Fig. 24.2**). Because

TABLE 24.2

ANATOMIC DIFFERENCES BETWEEN ADULT AND PEDIATRIC AIRWAYS

■ ANATOMY	■ CLINICAL SIGNIFICANCE
Tongue occupies relatively large portion of the oral cavity	The tongue may obstruct the upper airway in the supine, unconscious child
Epiglottis relatively larger and less tethered by the hyoepiglottic ligament in children than in adults	Straight blade preferred over curved blade to push distensible anatomy (specifically the epiglottis) out of the way to visualize the larynx
High tracheal opening (relative to cervical vertebrae): C1 in infancy C3 to C4 at 7 y of age C4 to C5 in the adult	High anterior view of the glottic opening compared with that in adults may contribute to difficulty intubating the child
Large occiput may cause flexion of the airway, and large tongue can fall against the posterior pharynx when child is supine	Sniffing position opens the airway. The larger occiput actually elevates the head toward the sniffing position in most infants and children (neck must be extended). A towel may be required under shoulders to elevate torso relative to head in small infants
Cricoid ring is the narrowest portion of the child's trachea (vocal cords are the narrowest portion in the adult)	Uncuffed tubes may provide adequate seal, as they can fit snugly at the level of the cricoid ring Selection of correct tube size is essential because use of excessively large tube may cause mucosal injury
Consistent anatomic variations with age, with fewer anatomic abnormal variations related to body habitus, arthritis, and chronic disease	Age-related variations: <2 y: high anterior airway 2–8 y: transition >8 y: small adult
Large tonsils and adenoids may bleed. More acute angle between epiglottis and laryngeal opening makes endotracheal intubation difficult	Blind nasotracheal intubation not indicated in children May cause failure of attempted nasotracheal intubation
Small cricothyroid membrane	Needle cricothyrotomy difficult; surgical cricothyrotomy is extremely difficult in infants and small children

Adapted from Luten RC, Kissoon NJ. Approach to the pediatric airway. In: Walls R, Murphy MF, Luten LC, et al., eds. *Manual of Emergency Airway Management*. 2nd ed. Philadelphia, PA: Lippincott Williams & Wilkins, 2004.

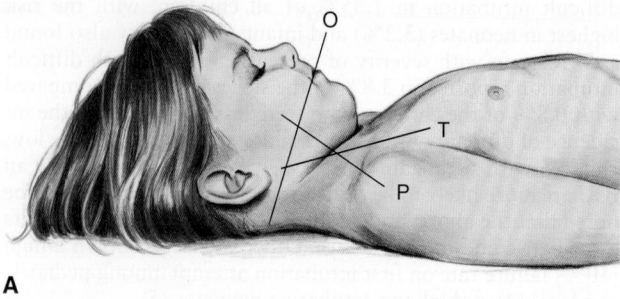

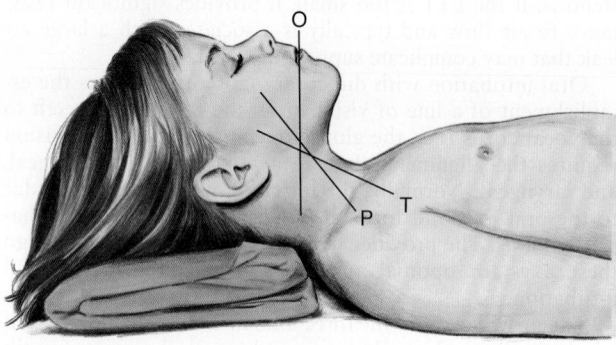

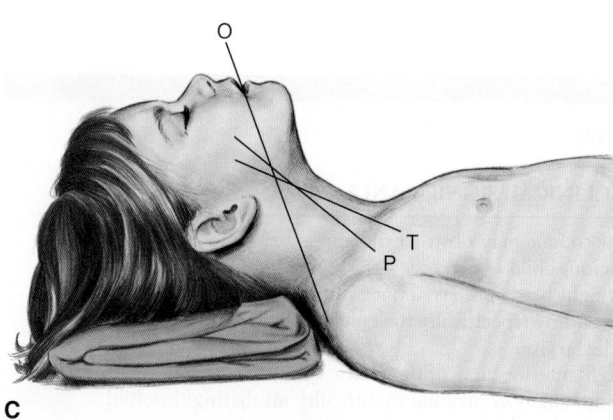

FIGURE 24.2. Correct positioning of the child over 2 years of age for ventilation and tracheal intubation. The oral (*O*), pharyngeal (*P*), and laryngeal/tracheal (*T*) axes are optimally aligned for intubation when the child is placed in the "sniffing" position. For infants and children <2 years of age, the prominent occiput often provides the needed movement of the head forward of the shoulders. In the child >2 years of age (shown here), a small towel is placed under the head (to lift the head forward) and the neck is slightly extended. The opening of the ear canal should be above or just anterior to the front of the child's shoulder. **A:** Resting position. **B:** Proper forward movement of head relative to shoulders. **C:** Proper positioning with both head position and neck extension for intubation. The oral, pharyngeal, and laryngeal/tracheal axes are aligned. (From Pediatric Advanced Life Support. American Heart Association, Inc., 2002, with permission.)

children younger than ~2 years have a relatively large occiput, it is unnecessary to place a towel or other support under the occiput to tilt the neck. Such tilting naturally occurs when the child lies supine on a flat surface. The provider may only need to lift the chin to produce slight extension of the neck and align

the axes. Providers should avoid hyperextension of the infant's neck because it can cause airway obstruction. In fact, for small infants, it may be necessary to balance the disproportionate occipital size by placing a small support under the shoulders. In all ages, the axes are correctly aligned for laryngoscopy if the external auditory canal is anterior to the front edge of the shoulders of the supine infant or child (see **Fig. 24.2**).

INITIAL AIRWAY ASSESSMENT

Before performing any invasive airway procedure, the provider must assess the child to identify the potentially difficult airway. The three basic components of this assessment are as follows:

- The oropharyngeal examination—assessing tongue protrusion, mouth opening, and *Mallampati score*
- Evaluation of atlantooccipital joint extension—extension and flexion with hands on shoulders
- Measurement of the potential mandibular displacement area—the *thyromental distance*

Although the combination of these three assessments predicts the difficult adult airway, no comparative pediatric data exist.

The Oropharyngeal Examination

The degree of mouth opening enables assessment of the palate, the range of motion of the temporomandibular joint, and the size of the tongue relative to the oral cavity. The *Mallampati assessment* (6) (**Fig. 24.3**) classifies the degree of airway difficulty based on the ability to visualize the tonsillar (also called faucial) pillars, soft palate, and uvula with exposure of the glottis. With a Class 1 airway, all three pharyngeal structures can be visualized, and laryngoscopy yields adequate laryngeal exposure in >99% of adult patients. With a Class 3 airway, the glottis cannot be exposed, and laryngoscopy yields adequate laryngeal exposure in only 7% of adult patients (6). Limited pediatric data suggest that this technique has a high (50%) false-positive rate for identifying difficult pediatric airways (7).

Evaluation of Atlantooccipital Joint Extension

Reduced range of neck motion (reduced *atlantooccipital joint extension*) will preclude successful alignment of the airway axes, making it difficult to visualize the glottic opening. An atlantooccipital extension of 35 degrees is normal for adults, with no comparable pediatric data.

Evaluation of Potential Mandibular Displacement Area

To perform successful laryngoscopy, the intubator must be able to deflect supraglottic soft-tissue structures, such as the tongue into the pharyngeal space. This potential space is defined by the space from the lateral and anterior aspects of the mandible to the hyoid bone. Reduction in the volume of this potential space (e.g., mandibular hypoplasia or an increase in the volume of submandibular soft tissue) or an increase in the volume of soft tissue (e.g., enlarged tongue) that must be displaced will make it difficult to visualize the larynx.

The size of the potential pharyngeal space can be estimated with the neck extended by evaluating the *thyromental*

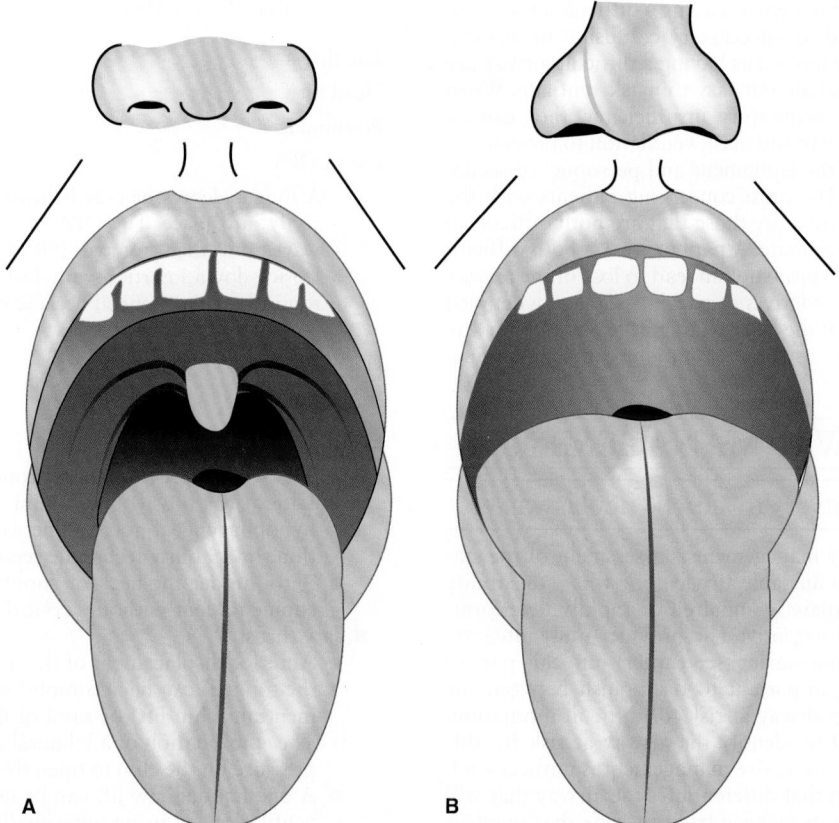

FIGURE 24.3. A: Tonsillar (also called faucial) pillars, soft palate, and uvula are clearly visualized—a Class 1 airway. **B:** None of the pharyngeal structures are visualized—a Class IV airway. (From Mallampati SR, Gatt SP, Gugino LD, et al. A clinical sign to predict difficult tracheal intubation: A prospective study. *Can Anaesth Soc J* 1985;32:429–34, with permission.)

distance, the distance between the upper aspect of the thyroid cartilage/hyoid bone and the lower aspect of the mandible. When this distance is small, the angle between the pharyngeal and laryngeal axes will be more acute, making it difficult to align these axes to visualize the larynx. The potential mandibular displacement area is considered adequate for the adult and child if, with the head in neutral position, two fingers (3 cm) can be placed between the hyoid bone and the anterior ramus of the mandible. The minimum threshold for the hyoid-to-mandible distance for an infant is 1.5 cm (8).

IDENTIFYING THE DIFFICULT AIRWAY

Definition and Priorities

A difficult airway is present if the provider has trouble delivering effective bag-mask ventilation or intubating the trachea. Identifying the difficult airway is a crucial part of patient assessment. The risk of failure of airway management is significantly increased in the difficult airway. This risks a situation where it is not possible to secure the airway or to provide adequate oxygenation or ventilation (i.e., the "can't intubate, can't oxygenate" or "can't intubate, can't ventilate" scenario, or both). Although it may not be possible to anticipate all difficult airways, those that we can identify prospectively will allow us to prepare an appropriate airway management strategy to reduce the risk to the patient as much as possible.

The difficult pediatric airway is best managed not by heroic intervention and uncommonly used techniques but, instead, by anticipation and careful planning. Much of the information that will guide risk assessment and management decisions can be obtained from a careful patient history and a focused physical examination.

Clues to Identification

Caregivers should be questioned and old records obtained to determine if previous intubations have been difficult. A history of previous acute or chronic upper airway obstruction, including symptoms of stridor, snoring, or sleep apnea, suggests a potentially difficult airway. A history of obesity, limited jaw or neck movement, facial trauma, or laryngeal abnormalities may also create problems during intubation. Craniofacial anomalies can be associated with difficult airways; they may be isolated or they may be associated with syndromes or other organ system dysfunction that could complicate intubation. As noted earlier (see earlier section, *Developmental Airway Considerations*), any condition that interferes with alignment of the oral, pharyngeal, and laryngeal axes will complicate and may prevent intubation.

The child is positioned appropriately for intubation/laryngoscopy if the external auditory canal is anterior to the front edge of the supine patient's shoulders. While assessment of the visibility of the uvula, tonsils, and posterior pharyngeal wall can help predict a difficult airway, these techniques have not been validated in children and may be difficult to perform in an uncooperative, critically ill child.

The designation of a patient as having a difficult airway can be insufficient and lead to unnecessary confusion or anxiety. Many patients who are labeled as having a difficult airway are actually difficult to intubate but easy to mask ventilate. When these patients develop respiratory insufficiency, they can be safely maintained with bag and mask ventilation to provide the time needed to obtain the equipment and personnel to secure a difficult intubation. The most concerning patients with the difficult airway designation are those that are both difficult to mask ventilate and to intubate. A patient who is both difficult to mask ventilate and to intubate can lead to loss of the airway with administration of sedatives or paralytics. Having detailed information displayed at the bedside about the patient's airway concerns and previously useful interventions can be lifesaving.

BASIC AIRWAY MANAGEMENT

Initial Maneuvers to Open the Airway

The first step in airway management is assessment of the stability of the airway. An unstable airway (one where the ability to oxygenate and ventilate is impaired or rapidly deteriorating) must be managed urgently. The provider must integrate the anatomic airway assessment (see earlier) into this part of the management. It is important to distinguish between the normal airway and the airway at risk for difficult intubation. It is even more critical to identify the airway at risk for difficult mask ventilation if invasive management is unsuccessful. It is this last distinction that differentiates the airway that will simply be troublesome to manage from the one that involves a significant risk to life. Any airway that is assessed as having increased risk requires the presence of the most skilled airway practitioner available where time allows. This may include an anesthesiologist or otolaryngologist.

Whenever there are concerns regarding patient stability and when airway management is anticipated, providers must initiate appropriate monitoring and provide supplementary inspired oxygen. Equipment should be immediately available for the level of airway intervention anticipated at the difficulty level anticipated, as well as for the next level above that.

The target of airway management is to achieve adequate oxygenation and ventilation in a safe manner. Often the minimum level of intervention that achieves this aim is the appropriate one, as all increases in intervention bring with them new risks. If the child is awake, with mild-to-moderate airway obstruction and no suspected cervical spine injury, the child should be allowed to assume a position of comfort. The provider suctions the airway as needed and administers oxygen. If the child is obtunded, the airway can become obstructed by a combination of neck flexion, jaw relaxation, displacement of the tongue against the posterior pharyngeal wall, and collapse of the hypopharynx. A simple jaw-thrust maneuver is the most effective method of opening the airway, although a head-tilt–chin-lift may also be successful (see **Box 24.1**). Providers should perform the jaw thrust to open the airway during bag-mask ventilation. It is the preferable technique to open the airway if cervical spine injury is suspected. If no cervical spine injury is suspected. If no cervical spine injury is suspected, or if the airway cannot be opened using the jaw thrust, the provider should open the airway using a head-tilt–chin-lift maneuver. Both of these maneuvers are intended to create a patent airway for spontaneous ventilation and oxygenation without more invasive intubation. The initial steps for airway management depend on patient condition and neck stability but can include the following:

- Positioning
  - Prone positioning may be effective in children with glossoptosis (Pierre Robin anomalad, Trisomy 21,

BOX 24-1: Basic Airway Management

Jaw thrust

Head tilt

Positioning

Use of OPA

> A tongue depressor may be used to insert the OPA directly into place. The OPA may also be inserted sideways and then rotated (90 degrees) into position. Upside-down insertion with 180-degree rotation is not routinely recommended because it may injure tissues or push the tongue posteriorly

Use of NPA

Beckwith–Wiedemann syndrome).
  - Lateral (or tonsil) positioning may be effective with hypopharyngeal and tongue weakness (residual sedation) or inability to handle secretions.
  - A roll under the neck or shoulders may be helpful in supine patient without cervical spine instability.
- Jaw thrust
  - Anterior displacement of the mandible (and indirectly the tongue) can be accomplished with pressure on the mentum (chin lift) or rami of the mandible (jaw lift). The combination of a bilateral jaw lift and downward pressure on the chin to open the mouth is a jaw thrust.
  - A one-handed jaw lift can be used initially with mask ventilation by using anterior (lifting) pressure on the mandibular ramus with the fifth finger.
  - If a one-handed jaw lift and oral airway are unsuccessful during mask ventilation, the ultimate maneuver to overcome tongue obstruction during mask ventilation is a two-handed jaw lift with the oral airway still in place. This requires a helper to provide mask ventilation.
- Head tilt
  - Extension of the cranium at the junction with the cervical spine is a head tilt.
  - The combination of head tilt with flexion at the junction of the cervical and thoracic spine produces the sniffing position. The sniffing position is optimal for intubation conditions but can also improve airway obstruction.
- Oropharyngeal airway (OPA)
  - A tongue depressor may be used to insert the OPA directly into place. The OPA may also be inserted sideways and then rotated (90 degrees) into position. Upside-down insertion with 180-degree rotation is not routinely recommended because it may injure tissues or push the tongue posteriorly.
- Nasopharyngeal airway (NPA)
  - The NPA may be better tolerated by a patient who is responsive to stimuli. Insertion of the NPA should be done carefully as hemorrhage is a potential complication that can complicate airway management.

If spontaneous respiratory effort is absent or insufficient to adequately ventilate or oxygenate the patient, bag-mask ventilation is required. If the airway is not patent following the jaw-thrust and chin-lift maneuvers, either these maneuvers have been insufficient to relieve the obstruction or the obstruction is at or below the level of the glottis. If the obstruction is above the level of the glottis, a supraglottic airway (OPA or NPA) will bypass supraglottic obstruction. However, if the obstruction is at or below the glottis, more invasive airway management is indicated.

Oral and Nasal Airways

Oropharyngeal Airways

The *oropharyngeal airway* consists of a flange, a short bite-block segment, and a curved plastic body that provides an airway and suction channel through the mouth to the pharynx. It is designed to relieve airway obstruction by fitting over the tongue to hold it and the soft hypopharyngeal structures away from the posterior wall of the pharynx. An OPA may be used in the *unconscious* child if manual attempts to open the airway (e.g., head-tilt–chin-lift or jaw thrust) fail to provide and maintain a clear, unobstructed airway. Use of an OPA is not recommended in patients with intact cough or gag reflexes, because it may stimulate gagging and vomiting.

A correctly sized OPA will extend from the corner of the mouth to the angle of the jaw. If the OPA is too large, it may obstruct the pharynx; if it is too small, it may push the base of the tongue back against the posterior pharynx (9).

Nasopharyngeal Airways

A *nasopharyngeal airway* is a soft rubber or plastic tube (a shortened ETT can be used) that provides an airway and channel for suctioning between the nares and the pharynx. NPAs may be used in patients with or without an intact cough and gag reflex.

NPAs are available in sizes 12–36 French. A 12-French NPA (approximately the size of a 3-mm ETT) will generally fit the nasopharynx of a full-term infant. The NPA should be smaller than the inner aperture of the nares, and its proper length is approximately equal to the distance from the tip of the nose to the tragus of the ear. If the NPA is too long, it may cause vagal stimulation and bradycardia, or it may injure the epiglottis or vocal cords.

After the airway is inserted, the provider must frequently reevaluate the airway and the surrounding tissues. If the airway is too large, it will cause sustained blanching of the alae nasi (nostrils) after insertion. The airway can irritate the mucosa or lacerate adenoidal tissue and cause bleeding. These complications may aggravate airway obstruction and complicate airway management. Physical irritation of the larynx may stimulate coughing, vomiting, or laryngospasm.

Bag-Mask Ventilation

Bag-mask ventilation is an essential skill that requires adequate training and frequent use or periodic retraining. The ability to provide effective bag-mask ventilation is the single difference between the "can't intubate, but can ventilate" patient challenge and the "can't intubate and can't ventilate" life-threatening event. It is the single most important aspect of airway management; unfortunately, it is infrequently practiced.

The most common technique for single-rescuer bag-mask ventilation involves the "E-C clamp" technique. The rescuer tilts the child's head and uses the last three fingers of one hand (forming a capital letter "E") to lift the jaw while pressing the mask against the face with the thumb and forefinger of the same hand (creating a "C"). The second hand squeezes the bag to deliver each breath over 1 second to produce visible chest rise. It is important that the jaw is lifted to open the airway and the mask is simultaneously held tightly against the face. The rescuer should not simply press the mask down on the face, because this can close the airway and prevent effective ventilation, rather the mandible should be pulled up into the mask to create an effective seal.

For larger patients, those with a difficult airway, or those with reduced lung compliance, a two-person bag-mask technique may be necessary. The first rescuer uses both hands to lift the jaw and open the airway while holding the mask to the face; the second rescuer squeezes the bag. Both rescuers should ensure that each breath produces visible chest rise.

It is essential that a provider acquire and maintain a patent airway during bag-mask ventilation to avoid hypoventilation, inadequate oxygenation, and preferential inflation of the stomach. Gastric inflation can produce complications, including distension, regurgitation, and increased airway pressures. Providers must be proficient in selecting the correct mask size, opening the airway, making a tight seal between the mask and face, delivering effective ventilation, and monitoring the patient. In the out-of-hospital setting, bag-mask ventilation can be as effective as endotracheal intubation (ETI) when the transport interval is short, particularly when providers have limited training or experience in pediatric intubation (10,11).

It is critical to use the maneuvers described earlier to overcome tongue obstruction of the airway rather than use high ventilation pressure in the unintubated airway. The lower esophagus provides a functional sphincter that produces resistance to gas entry into the stomach up to ~20 cm H_2O. With cardiac arrest, the competency of this functional sphincter falls to 0 cm H_2O and stomach overdistension more easily occurs. Gastric overdistension reduces lung functional residual capacity (FRC), which can increase hypoxemia or the rapidity of desaturation when bag-mask ventilation is stopped for intubation attempts. The effect of gastric overdistension is more significant in neonates and infants who consume the oxygen in the FRC at a much higher rate than older children.

When, despite manipulation of the upper airway, it is not possible to maintain a patent airway, or if the airway is not expected to remain patent for the length of time assistance is likely to be required, it is time to consider the merits of an advanced airway.

ADVANCED AIRWAY MANAGEMENT

Advanced airways should be placed within a healthcare system that has established processes for continuous quality improvement, including protocols (e.g., indications for intubation, device selection, medications, and technique for confirmation of tube placement), verification of healthcare provider training and experience, monitoring of complication rates, and a system for remedial training.

General Indications for an Advanced Airway

The general indications for advanced airway placement include actual or anticipated compromise in airway patency, ventilation, or oxygenation. An unstable airway may result from an altered level of consciousness or compromised airway reflexes, from intrinsic airway or lung parenchymal disease, or from hemodynamic compromise. Specific examples include loss of airway protection from impaired central nervous system function or from inflammation or edema of the airway, inadequate ventilation or ventilatory drive, or hypoxemia despite oxygen administration. Advanced airway placement may be appropriate if deterioration of the patient's respiratory status is anticipated or if a borderline patient must be moved into a poorly monitored or poorly controlled environment (e.g., sedation of a patient in the CT scanner or the interhospital transport of a child).

Choice of Advanced Airway

Advanced airway choices can be divided into the supraglottic airways and the transglottic airways. Recently, supraglottic airways or variations of the laryngeal mask airway (LMA) have established themselves as alternatives to both bag-mask ventilation and tracheal (i.e., transglottic) intubation, and also as bridges to a transglottic airway, whether by blind advancement of an ETT through the airway or by fiber-optic placement of an ETT through the device (12). In addition, hybrid airways, such as the Combitube, have demonstrated ease of use in some patient populations.

The ETT has long been considered the optimal advanced airway. However, evidence in a prehospital setting documented that ETI may offer no survival benefit over bag-mask ventilation when the transport interval is short (10). In addition, when personnel assigned to intubate the patient lack adequate training and experience, the incidence of complications, such as unrecognized esophageal intubation, is unacceptably high (10,11). The final common pathway for all difficult airway algorithms remains the subglottic surgical airway, specifically the percutaneous cricothyrotomy or surgical tracheostomy.

Data are inadequate to support the routine use of any single approach to advanced airway management in pediatric critical care. The optimal technique and device is affected by the clinical situation (patient condition and available resources) and the competence of the provider. The provider must weigh potential benefits of the advanced airway against potential risks of the procedure, and should verify correct advanced airway placement immediately after insertion, when the patient is moved (e.g., from patient bed to a gurney), and with any clinical deterioration (13).

Placement of an advanced airway during cardiopulmonary resuscitation (CPR) also requires the weighing of potential risks and benefits. During CPR, intubation may lead to interruption of lifesaving interventions, such as cardiac compressions, and it may cause hypoxemia, reflux, and aspiration. Unrecognized tube misplacement is likely to be fatal. The rescuer must weigh these risks against the potential benefit of establishing an advanced airway in a timely fashion. An advantage of advanced airway placement during CPR is that, after placement, compressions can be provided continuously, without pauses for ventilation. The presence of an expert in ETT placement and the use of end-tidal CO_2 confirmation of tracheal intubation can minimize potential delays and incorrect placement. The provider should always have a second strategy to provide oxygenation and ventilation if the initial airway approach fails. Bag-mask ventilation may provide this second strategy.

Endotracheal Intubation

ETI requires the preparation of equipment and personnel, patient assessment and positioning, and provision of adequate monitoring, oxygenation, and ventilation. Orotracheal intubation is usually performed initially because it is typically a faster route of insertion with fewer complications.

Preparation

Preparation for laryngoscopy and intubation is essential; many airways assessed as difficult are simply airways that are inadequately supported. While providing effective oxygenation and ventilation using a bag and mask, the provider should quickly perform a basic airway assessment (see earlier section, *Basic Airway Management*) before attempting intubation. While establishing that the airway can be intubated, the provider should request immediate assistance to assemble the necessary equipment and personnel and establish monitoring (**Table 24.3**).

Because infants and children vary widely in size, the use of a reference device, such as a length-based resuscitation tape, is helpful in guiding the selection of intubation equipment. Although the use of age-based formulas (**Table 24.4**) to estimate the initial choice of cuffed and uncuffed ETTs is more reliable than estimates based on the size of the fifth finger, these formulas are not as accurate as length-based tapes in predicting appropriate ETT size (9,13,14).

It may be necessary to modify equipment selection based on the patient's condition. For example, providers generally use smaller-than-predicted ETTs in the setting of upper airway obstruction. As noted earlier, the provider must always have an alternate approach in mind to manage the airway in the event that the initial approach fails.

Appropriate positioning of the patient prior to intubation is critical. To directly visualize the glottis, the provider must position the child to align the axes of the mouth, pharynx, and trachea ("the sniffing position"; see discussion in the previous section, *Developmental Airway Considerations*). Incomplete extension or hyperextension of the neck or failure to use appropriate age-related head positioning can convert a normal airway into a difficult one. The provider should avoid manipulation of the neck if a risk exists of cervical spinal instability.

Intubation Procedure

Procedural monitoring is essential during ETI, including the monitoring of heart rate, blood pressure, oxygen saturation, and end-tidal capnometry/capnography prior to and immediately following ETI. Children have higher oxygen consumption (per kilogram body weight) than do adults and may rapidly become hypoxemic during the procedure, so the provider must ensure adequate oxygenation before the intubation attempt. It is important to terminate ETI efforts and initiate bag-mask ventilation if the patient's heart rate, oxygenation, or clinical appearance deteriorates.

A curved blade is often more effective for intubation of the older child (>2 years), whereas a straight blade is typically reserved for younger children and those with a difficult airway. However, no rule has been established to determine the ideal blade to be used. Both curved and straight blades should be available.

After pharmacologic preparation of the patient (if appropriate), bag-mask ventilation should be interrupted to insert the ETT under direct visualization. The laryngoscope blade is used to deflect the tongue and lift the supraglottic structures (or tent the epiglottis) to visualize the glottis. The ETT is inserted through the vocal cords.

If, despite appropriate head positioning, the intubator cannot see the glottis during the attempt, an assistant should perform external laryngeal manipulation (*b*ackward—posterior, *u*pward—cephalad, and *r*ightward *p*ush [BURP]) to attempt to bring the glottis into view. If the glottis is still difficult to visualize, bag-mask ventilation should be provided and the patient's head repositioned, with verification that the external auditory canal is anterior to the front edge of the patient's shoulder. It may be helpful to ask an assistant to place a finger in the right side of the patient's mouth and pull to the right, which may create more room to successfully visualize the glottis. If the provider can only visualize the posterior aspects of the glottis, successful intubation may be possible by using a stylet to create a bend ("hockey stick") in the end of the tracheal tube. Providers must ensure that the tip of the stylet does not protrude beyond the end of the tracheal tube.

Many uncuffed ETTs have depth indicators (varies by manufacturer) that should be positioned at or slightly distal to the vocal cords. Using the depth indicator helps ensure

TABLE 24.3

EQUIPMENT FOR ENDOTRACHEAL INTUBATION

Monitoring equipment (apply before intubation if at all possible)
Cardiorespiratory monitor (including monitoring of blood pressure, if possible)
Pulse oximeter
Length-based tape to estimate tube and equipment sizes

Confirmation devices
Continuous waveform capnography preferred. In absence of continuous waveform capnography, the following may be used:
- Exhaled CO_2 colorimetric detector (pediatric size for patients <15 kg, adult size for patients >15 kg)
- Esophageal detector device (for children >20 kg with a perfusing rhythm) may be used

Suction equipment
Tonsil-tipped suction device or large-bore suction (to suction pharynx)
Suction catheter of appropriate size (to suction endotracheal tube)
Suction canister and device capable of generating suction of −80 to −120 mm Hg (a wall-suction device capable of generating −300 mm Hg is preferred)

Bag and mask
Check size and oxygen connections
Connected to high-flow oxygen source with reservoir (capable of providing ~100% oxygen)

Medications
Anticholinergics (atropine)
Sedatives
Paralytics
Appropriate IV equipment and syringes for administration of medications

Intubation equipment
Stylet
Cuffed and uncuffed tubes of estimated size and cuffed and uncuffed tubes that are 0.5 mm larger and smaller than estimated sizes
Laryngoscope blades (curved and straight) and handle with working light (keep extra batteries and bulb ready)
Water-soluble lubricant
Syringe to inflate tube cuff (if appropriate)
Towel or pad to place under patient (if appropriate)

Tape/device to secure tube
Tape and tincture of benzoin or commercial device

---

adequate depth while minimizing the risk of mainstem bronchus intubation. Cuffed tubes should be placed so that the cuff is positioned immediately below the level of the cords. Correct depth of insertion can be estimated from formulas using the child's age or the ETT size (see **Tables 24.1 and 24.4**).

Nasotracheal Intubation

Nasotracheal intubation is rarely performed as a primary intubation technique in the emergently ill or injured child. It is more commonly performed electively after primary oral

TABLE 24.4

FORMULAS FOR ESTIMATION OF ENDOTRACHEAL TUBE SIZE AND DEPTH OF INSERTION

■ SIZE

Uncuffed tube for infant: 3.0–3.5 mm ID
Uncuffed tube for child 1–2 y: 3.5–4.5 mm ID
Uncuffed tubes for children >2 y, size can be estimated with the following formula[a]:

$$\text{Endotracheal tube (internal diameter (ID) in mm)} = \frac{\text{Age (y)}}{4} + 4$$

Cuffed tube for infant ≥3.5 kg and <1 y: 3.0 mm ID
Cuffed tube for child 1–2 y: 3.5 mm ID
Cuffed tubes for children >2 y, size can be estimated with the following formula[a]:

$$\text{Endotracheal tube (ID in mm)} = \frac{\text{Age (y)}}{4} + 3$$

■ DEPTH OF INSERTION

Depth of insertion (cm) = (age in years/2) + 12
Depth of insertion = (ETT internal diameter) × 3

[a]Note: See, also, Table 24.1 for approximate tracheal tube size and depth of insertion.
ID: Internal Diameter.

intubation, with the hopes of improving patient comfort (e.g., reducing gagging) or increasing ease of tube stabilization (with reduced kinking or biting, when compared to oral tracheal tubes, and reduced secretion-induced tube slippage) (15). Relative contraindications to nasotracheal intubation include coagulopathy, maxillofacial injury, or basilar skull fracture.

To perform nasotracheal intubation, the lubricated ETT is passed through one of the nares and guided through the larynx with McGill forceps during oral laryngoscopy. If an orotracheal tube is in place, request an assistant to remove it when the nasotracheal tube is in position and the glottis is well visualized. Care is taken to avoid lacerating or rupturing the ETT cuff during manipulation with the McGill forceps.

Blind nasotracheal intubation, as taught for awake intubation of adults, is generally difficult to perform in children. Several anatomic characteristics of the pediatric airway and the need for a cooperative patient limit the feasibility of this procedure in children <8–10 years of age.

Complications of nasotracheal intubation include nosebleed (especially problematic if no other airway is in place), pressure-induced ischemic tissue injury to the rim of the nares, and nasal deformity due to nasal septal pressure necrosis (more likely when a tube is in place for long periods in premature infants). In older children, nasal intubation may be associated with a greater risk of sinusitis or otitis media than is oral intubation.

❺   Rapid Sequence Intubation

General Principles

Rapid sequence intubation (RSI) is a technique used to secure the airway in the patient who presents with a full (or presumed full) stomach, where even moderate preintubation gastric insufflation with bag-mask ventilation may cause gastric regurgitation and risk of pulmonary aspiration. Medications are preselected and doses prepared to facilitate intubation. The medications, including premedications (e.g., atropine, lidocaine or a defasciculating dose of a paralytic), a sedative, and a neuromuscular blocker are administered in rapid sequence (immediately following one other), without awaiting the full effect of the preceding drug(s) (16). Intubation occurs after a timed delay that is based on the expected onset of action of the paralytic agent used. During a true RSI, in an effort to avoid gastric distension and regurgitation, no assistance to ventilation is provided between cessation of spontaneous respiration and intubation. As a result, this time must be minimized to avoid development of severe hypoxia.

The steps of the classic RSI include the following (16):

- A basic airway assessment, including relevant patient history using the *SAMPLE* mnemonic (*s*igns and symptoms, *a*llergies, *m*edications, *p*ast history, *l*ast meal, *e*vents leading to intubation) to assess the risk/suitability for the use of anesthetics or paralytics
- Preparation of personnel and equipment and establishment of monitoring
- Preoxygenation with 100% O_2 for a period adequate to replace the majority of the 79% nitrogen in the patient's FRC (six deep breaths in a cooperative patient) helps to maintain oxygenation during the period of apnea that follows
- Administration of an IV amnestic/sedative/analgesic and almost simultaneous delivery of a muscle relaxant
- Application of cricoid pressure (once patient is deeply sedated) (see section, *Cricoid Pressure* for important caveats)

- A brief period of apnea until the patient has adequate muscle relaxation
- Tracheal intubation
- Removal of cricoid pressure only after tube position is confirmed and the tube cuff (if present) is inflated

RSI in children is particularly challenging for several reasons. As discussed earlier, the normal child can rapidly develop arterial oxygen desaturation (hypoxemia) after relatively short periods of apnea. The desaturation will be more rapid and more significant if the child is hypoxemic prior to the procedure.

Some patients who require emergent intubation (e.g., those with intracranial or pulmonary hypertension) will be intolerant of even brief periods of hypercapnia associated with apnea. For these reasons, a modified RSI technique is often used in the intubation of critically ill children. After establishment of monitoring, some degree of bag-mask ventilation is provided and cricoid pressure is often applied in an attempt to minimize gastric distention. This technique should prevent or delay the onset of hypoxemia and hypercarbia and their sequelae. A modified RSI is also sometimes used in patients whose risk of being difficult to intubate or ventilate is greater than their risk of aspiration, and ventilation is tested with cricoid pressure before the paralytic is administered.

Before initiating RSI, the provider must determine if the patient will tolerate the procedure. Some patients have tenuous airways that allow for some oxygenation during spontaneous ventilation. Administration of sedatives will decrease and neuromuscular blockers will eliminate spontaneous respiratory effort. If the provider is unable to maintain the patient's airway (with or without intubation), hypoxemia and hypercarbia can develop rapidly. Examples of scenarios in which RSI may lead to "losing the airway" (i.e., "can't intubate and can't ventilate") include patients with significant airway obstruction, facial trauma, or congenital craniofacial anomalies.

Medications

No perfect combination of drugs exists for RSI of all patients, so providers must select drugs based on the patient's condition and the provider's expertise. Not every patient needs general anesthesia for intubation, but appropriate sedation will facilitate intubation, minimize physiologic response, and reduce awareness of paralysis and intubation.

Bradycardia with intubation, whether due to airway manipulation or specific medications, can significantly reduce oxygen delivery, especially in patients with limited cardiac output. The American Heart Association Pediatric Advanced Life Support guidelines (9,13) and the American College of Emergency Physicians (17) recommend the use of atropine for RSI for infants <1 year of age, for children 1–5 years of age who are receiving succinylcholine, and for adolescents who are receiving a second dose of succinylcholine. However, atropine may not always be effective in preventing bradycardia (18–20). Controversy still exists as to the necessity/propriety of universal prophylactic atropine administration (i.e., before bradycardia occurs) with intubation, as opposed to administration only in the setting of vasodilatory states or with the concurrent use of succinylcholine (20). Although atropine can reduce oral secretions (facilitating airway visualization), the time to the onset of this effect is longer (15–30 minutes) than most practitioners are prepared to wait before instrumenting the airway.

The choice of sedative or anesthetic for intubation (see **Table 24.5**) must be tailored to the individual patient and the clinical scenario. The potentially difficult airway may best be approached by calling for backup (e.g., an anesthesia or ear, nose, and throat specialist) while allowing the patient to breath spontaneously, and using a sedative agent to facilitate laryngoscopy, thereby avoiding induction of full anesthesia. Hemodynamically unstable children that require intubation are likely to develop hypotension with the use of anesthetics that have significant vasodilatory properties (e.g., propofol or thiopental), but might well tolerate other anesthetic agents, such as ketamine or etomidate. Ketamine's bronchodilator properties are helpful when intubating children with asthma or other reactive airways disease.

Neuromuscular blocking (NMB) agents are used to facilitate the visualization and intubation of the airway. The use of these agents during RSI has been shown to increase the likelihood of successful intubation (21). Clinical indicators of adequate neuromuscular blockade include lack of spontaneous movements, respiratory effort, and blink reflex, as well as jaw relaxation, manifested by the ability to fully open the patient's mouth without resistance.

The two broad groups of NMB agents are the depolarizing and nondepolarizing agents, distinguished by their action on receptors at the neuromuscular junction. *Depolarizing neuromuscular blockers* bind the postsynaptic receptor of the neuromuscular junction, leading to unsynchronized depolarization of the postsynaptic membrane, which causes transient muscular fasciculation (seen less commonly in smaller infants) and then paralysis as the receptors remain occupied. Succinylcholine is the most commonly used agent in this group. The advantages of this drug include rapid onset and relatively short duration of action. Pharmacokinetics and dosing characteristics vary with patient age (see **Table 24.5**). Complications occur in 0.3%–1% of children (22), including malignant hyperthermia and masseter spasm with subsequent airway obstruction. This drug normally causes a modest rise in serum potassium (typically 0.5–1 mEq/L), but may produce significant hyperkalemia in specific at-risk patients (23); these include patients with burns (the response is proportional to the extent of the burn), peripheral nerve injury, renal failure, neuromuscular disease, or major trauma with rhabdomyolysis. The risk of acute hyperkalemia in the child with previously undiagnosed neuromuscular disease triggered a U.S. Food and Drug Administration warning that succinylcholine is contraindicated in pediatric intubation ". . . except when used for emergency tracheal intubation or in instances where immediate securing of the airway is necessary" (24). Although the risk of hyperkalemia may be reduced by the simultaneous use of defasciculating, nondepolarizing agents (25), such drugs will substantially increase succinylcholine dose requirements. Because nondepolarizing neuromuscular blockers are available with rapid onset of action, succinylcholine's role in pediatric neuromuscular blockade may be extremely limited. Despite the theoretical contraindications to succinylcholine in the setting of ocular trauma and increased intracranial pressure (ICP), limited clinical literature documents these concerns (26).

Nondepolarizing neuromuscular blockers (e.g., rocuronium and atracurium) bind the postsynaptic receptors of the neuromuscular junction, without causing postsynaptic depolarization and neuromuscular transmission. The literature shows that high doses of these agents can create adequate conditions for intubation in times similar to those of succinylcholine. The onset of action is shortened if a priming dose is given 3–5 minutes prior to the intubation, but this will prolong the period of muscle relaxation (27). The provider must be ready to assume control of the airway and ventilation when a priming dose is used in children, because some will develop profound muscle weakness with a priming dose. These nondepolarizing agents have a duration that is significantly longer than succinylcholine, and they are not reversible in a clinically acceptable time to allow spontaneous ventilation if the patient cannot be intubated or ventilated. Their use must be considered carefully in a patient with a potential difficult airway.

Cricoid Pressure

Cricoid pressure, also known as the "Sellick maneuver," puts direct pressure on the cricoid cartilage, compressing the upper esophageal sphincter, in order to prevent reflux of gastric contents from the esophagus into the airway (aspiration) and gastric distension from the insufflation of air into the stomach during positive-pressure ventilation (PPV). While cricoid pressure may be used in some settings, there is little evidence to support its consistent use, and consequently the practitioner should individualize its application. Cricoid pressure can distort the upper airway, preventing effective visualization of the airway and effective bag-mask ventilation. The application of cricoid pressure commonly (in as many as 91% of patients) displaces the esophagus laterally, leaving the compression of the upper esophagus incomplete (28). Consequently, the maneuver may be ineffective in protecting the upper airway from gastric regurgitation. The use of cricoid pressure in patients with laryngeal or cervical spine pathology is controversial because it may cause cervical spine movement. It is contraindicated in patients with a cough or gag reflex.

Adjuncts to Direct Laryngoscopy

Gum Elastic Bougie

The *gum elastic bougie* can be inserted blindly into the airway and then used as a guide for insertion of an ETT (29). "Clicks" may be felt as the bougie is inserted through the tracheal rings. The bougie can also be used to guide LMA placement (see section, *Laryngeal Mask Airway*).

Airway Exchange Catheter

The *airway exchange catheter* was designed to be placed through an ETT already in place to allow exchange of the existing ETT with a new one. It can also be used to intubate the larynx directly if an ETT would not pass through the larynx. The exchange catheter is inserted into the larynx, and an ETT is then threaded over the exchange catheter into the airway. The airway exchange catheter has a central lumen allowing oxygenation, or it can be threaded over a guidewire (i.e., during retrograde intubation).

Lighted Intubation Stylet

The *lighted intubation stylet*, also known as the light wand, is essentially a rigid stylet with a fiber-optic light at the end. Pediatric versions are available and can accommodate tracheal tubes as small as 2 mm (30). The lighted stylet is portable, produces less irritation than laryngoscopy, and is relatively inexpensive. It can be used as a traditional stylet with direct laryngoscopy or blindly if direct laryngoscopy is impossible. The lighted stylet takes time to insert and may not be tolerated in the already hypoxemic patient. It is therefore relatively contraindicated in the "can't intubate, can't oxygenate" scenario. It requires that the airway be midline, so it is contraindicated in conditions where the glottis is deviated laterally or when there is laryngeal pathology. Any condition limiting transmission of light through the anterior neck, such as mass lesions, scarring or massive edema, or obesity, will also interfere with its use. Airway injury is uncommon (30).

Flexible Bronchoscopy

ETI over a flexible fiber-optic bronchoscope has become an important technique, particularly when direct ETI is impossible.

TABLE 24.5

RAPID SEQUENCE INTUBATION DRUGS AND DOSES

■ DRUG	■ DOSE/ROUTE	■ DURATION	■ COMMENTS
Cardiovascular adjuncts			
Atropine	IV: 0.01–0.02 mg/kg (max: 1 mg)	>30 min	■ Inhibits bradycardic response to hypoxia; may cause tachycardia ■ May cause pupil dilation
Glycopyrrolate	IV: 0.005–0.01 mg/kg (max: 0.2 mg)	>30 min	■ Inhibits bradycardic response to hypoxia; may cause tachycardia
Sedative hypnotic agents/analgesics			
Diazepam	IV: 0.1–0.2 mg/kg (max: 4 mg)	30–90 min	■ May cause respiratory depression or potentiate depressant effects of narcotics and barbiturates
Lorazepam	IV: 0.05–0.1 mg/kg (max: 4 mg)	4–6 h	■ May cause hypotension ■ Minimal cardiac depression
Midazolam	IV: 0.1–0.3 mg/kg (max: 4 mg)	1–2 h	■ Occasional respiratory depression ■ No analgesic properties
Fentanyl citrate	IV, IM: 2–5 μg/kg	IV: 30–60 min IM: 1–2 h	■ May cause respiratory depression, hypotension, chest wall rigidity with high-dose (>5 mg/kg) infusions ■ May elevate ICP
Anesthetic agents (in doses indicated)			
Thiopental	IV: 2–5 mg/kg	5–10 min	■ Negative inotropic effects and often causes hypotension ■ Decreases cerebral metabolic rate and ICP ■ Potentiates respiratory depressive effects of narcotics and benzodiazepines ■ No analgesic properties
Etomidate	IV: 0.2–0.4 mg/kg	5–15 min	■ Decreases cerebral metabolic rate and ICP ■ May cause respiratory depression ■ Minimal cardiovascular effects ■ Causes myoclonic activity; may lower seizure threshold ■ Causes cortisol suppression; contraindicated in patients dependent on endogenous cortisol response ■ No analgesic properties
Lidocaine	IV: 1–2 mg/kg	~30 min	■ Causes myocardial and CNS depression with high doses ■ May decrease ICP during RSI ■ Hypotension occurs infrequently
Ketamine	IV: 1–2 mg/kg IM: 3–5 mg/kg	30–60 min	■ May increase blood pressure, heart rate, cardiac output ■ May cause increased secretions, laryngospasm ■ Causes limited respiratory depression ■ Bronchodilator ■ May cause hallucinations, emergence reactions
Propofol	IV: 2 mg/kg (up to 3 mg/kg in young children)	3–5 min	■ May cause hypotension, especially in hypovolemic patients ■ May cause pain on injection ■ Highly lipid soluble ■ Causes less airway reactivity than barbiturates
Neuromuscular blocking agents			
Succinylcholine	Infant IV: 2 mg/kg Child IV: 1–1.5 mg/kg IM: Double the IV dose	3–5 min	■ Depolarizing muscle relaxant; causes muscle fasciculation ■ May cause rise in ICP and intraocular and intragastric pressures ■ May cause rise in serum potassium ■ May cause hypertension ■ Avoid in renal failure, burns, crush injuries, or hyperkalemia
Atracurium	IV: 0.5 mg/kg	30–40 min	■ Metabolized by plasma hydrolysis ■ May cause mild histamine release
cis-Atracurium	IV: 0.1 mg/kg, then 1–5 mg/kg/min	20–35 min	■ Metabolized by plasma hydrolysis ■ May cause mild histamine release
Rocuronium	IV: 0.6–1.2 mg/kg	30–60 min	■ Few cardiovascular effects
Vecuronium	IV: 0.1–0.2 mg/kg	30–60 min	■ Few cardiovascular effects

Adapted from Hazinski M, Zaritsky A, Nadkarni V, et al. Rapid sequence intubation. In: *PALS Provider Manual*. Dallas, TX: American Heart Association, 2002; Venkataraman ST, Khan N, Brown A. Validation of predictors of extubation success and failure in mechanically ventilated infants and children. *Crit Care Med* 2000;28(8):2991–6.

The fiber-optic scope can also be passed through an LMA to aid passage through the oropharynx.

The bronchoscope has an operator-guided flexible port and a port that can be used for administering medications, providing suction, or passing a guidewire. Once the fiber-optic bronchoscope is inserted into the trachea, a guidewire can be passed through the suction port or preferably a preloaded ETT can be passed over the scope into the trachea. The fiber-optic scope also allows direct visualization of the larynx to identify trauma or congenital anomalies, and to evaluate the dynamic function of the larynx to rule out conditions, such as laryngomalacia. It also can be used in intubated patients to assess persistent atelectasis, airway injury, or pulmonary hemorrhage, and to perform bronchial alveolar lavage.

Very small, ultrathin bronchoscopes are available for tube sizes as small as 3 mm, although most of these scopes do not have a suction port, are very delicate, and are difficult to control. Cooperative older children may tolerate flexible laryngoscopy awake, but most patients will require sedation to minimize gagging and laryngospasm. Topical anesthesia can be given through the scope to attenuate airway-protective reflexes.

Videolaryngoscopy

Videolaryngoscopes are intubation devices with a camera on the distal end of the blade. It can provide a more anterior laryngeal view and improve the view of the glottis when compared to direct laryngoscopy alone. They also often require less extension of the head to provide a view of the glottis and so may minimize the need to move the neck of a patient with cervical instability.

In elective intubations of pediatric patients with normal airways in the operating suite the videolaryngoscope (GlideScope) improved time to view of the glottis, although this was not always associated with an improved time to insertion of the ETT (31–33). Using the GlideScope with a blade size smaller than would be predicated by the patient's weight may provide a better view (34). Care must be taken when inserting a styleted ETT into the mouth with attention focused on the video screen and not the introduction of the ETT, as perforation of the soft palate has occurred in this situation.

Bullard Laryngoscope

The Bullard laryngoscope is another rigid fiber-optic laryngoscope that can aid with visualization of the glottis. More pediatric experience is needed but in simulation studies, inexperienced providers have a high rate of success using this device (35).

Supraglottic Airways

Laryngeal Mask Airway

The LMA consists of a small mask with an inflatable cuff that is connected to a plastic tube with a universal adaptor. It is placed in the oropharynx with its tip in the hypopharynx and the base of the mask at the epiglottis. When the cuff of the mask is inflated, it creates a seal with the supraglottic area, allowing air flow between the tube and the trachea.

The LMA can be used to allow spontaneous ventilation, to deliver PPV, or as a guide for insertion of another airway device, such as an ETT, airway exchange catheter, lighted stylet, or flexible fiber-optic bronchoscope. The maximum seal pressure possible is ~25 cm H_2O, which may limit effective PPV in critically ill children. Use in conscious patients requires sedation to minimize airway-protective reflexes, including laryngospasm and bronchospasm.

The ease of insertion and relatively low complication rate have made the LMA an important component of the management of patients with difficult airways (12). However, because it is a supraglottic device, it is less effective in patients with glottic or subglottic pathology. It also does not protect the airway against the risk of aspiration. Complications due to malpositioning of the device (resulting in airway obstruction) or increased difficulty of insertion are more common in younger children (36), but the complication rate decreases with increased operator experience (37).

As of 2014, no clinical reports of LMA use during pediatric cardiac arrest were available, although in a simulation study of cardiac arrest, use of a LMA resulted in faster and more effective ventilations with fewer complications when compared to ETI (38). However, LMAs have successfully been used clinically in neonatal resuscitation (39,40).

The original LMA, the LMA Classic, is a multiuse device with sizes for neonates through adults (**Table 24.6**). It is important to choose the correct size; if the LMA is too large, it will be difficult to place, and if it is too small, it will not maintain an adequate seal to deliver effective PPV. The combined widths of the patient's index, middle, and ring fingers can be used to estimate the size of the LMA (41).

Several techniques have been described for inserting LMAs in children. Classically, the LMA is inserted with the patient positioned as for ETI. The LMA can be inserted with the cuff fully deflated and lubricated; it is advanced with the aperture of the mask facing toward the tongue until the rescuer feels resistance, and the cuff then is inflated. Cuff inflation may push the LMA slightly out of the mouth, which may indicate that

TABLE 24.6

LMA AIRWAY SELECTION AND CUFF INFLATION VOLUMES

■ LMA MASK SIZE (CLASSIC, CLASSIC EXCEL, AND PROSEAL)	■ PATIENT SIZE	■ MAXIMUM CUFF INFLATION VOLUMES (ML)[a]
1	Neonates/infants up to 5 kg	4
1½	Infants 5–10 kg	7
2	Infants/children 10–20 kg	10
2½	Children 20–30 kg	14
3	Children 30–50 kg	20
4	Adults 50–70 kg	30
5	Adults 70–100 kg	40
6 (LMA Classic Only)	Adults >100 kg	50

[a]These are maximum clinical volumes that should never be exceeded. It is recommended that the cuff be inflated to 60 cm H_2O intracuff pressures.
From LMA. http://www.lmana.com/files/flexiblequick-reference-card.pdf. Accessed January 14, 2014.

it is fully seated. The LMA may also be inserted with the cuff partially inflated (i.e., with half of the recommended volume) and the LMA mask inverted or turned to the side. Once the LMA is fully inserted, it is rotated to normal position and the cuff is fully inflated (42,43).

Newer models have been designed that have some benefits over the classic LMA, including better seals, delivery of higher tidal volumes, and with no increase in adverse events (44). Other LMA devices, such as the AirQ, allow for direct passage of an ETT down through the LMA to facilitate ETI. LMA insertion causes less airway trauma and hemodynamic changes than laryngoscopy.

The Combitube

The *Combitube* is a dual-lumen, dual-cuff airway device. The smallest size is designed for patients over 4 ft in height, so its use in pediatrics is limited.

The tube is blindly placed in the esophagus and the two cuffs are inflated, one distal in the esophagus and the second in the oropharynx. The inflation of the cuffs traps the larynx between the two cuffs, and ventilation can be provided through the pharyngeal lumen. If the tip of the tube is placed in the trachea (<5% of insertions), then the second lumen is used for ventilation.

Techniques Used to Verify Placement of Advanced Airway

Both clinical assessment (of chest rise, auscultation, and vapor in the tube) and a device should be used to confirm advanced airway placement immediately after insertion, when the patient is moved from one location to another (e.g., from a gurney to a bed), and whenever the intubated patient deteriorates (13).

Once the tube has been placed, it should be held firmly while correct placement is verified with clinical examination and a confirmation device. No single method for confirmation of tube placement is completely accurate and reliable; therefore, both clinical assessment and a confirmation device are necessary. To perform clinical confirmation, bag-tube ventilation is delivered while the provider observes for chest rise, auscultating over the stomach (breath sounds should not be heard over the stomach), and bilaterally over the anterior chest and both axillae. The provider also observes for water vapor in the tracheal tube on exhalation. In addition to the clinical findings, demonstration of end-tidal CO_2 after the insertion of an ETT or LMA is a monitoring standard among anesthesiologists and is recommended.

After confirmation of correct tube position, the tube should be taped in place and the depth of insertion should be recorded (in centimeters) at the lip. Hand ventilation is provided using a bag with attached manometer to assess for the presence of leak around the tracheal tube. Correct tube selection should permit an audible air leak around the tube when the inflation pressure exceeds 15–25 cm H_2O. Absence of a leak with this pressure suggests that the tube is too large or that the cuff inflation pressure is too high; either condition can cause tracheal mucosal injury. If a cuffed tube is used, the cuff should be deflated until an air leak is detectable at the appropriate pressures, and cuff pressure should be maintained at a pressure consistent with that recommended by the manufacturer, generally <20–25 cm H_2O. If an uncuffed tube is in place, and no air leak is detected with the application of 15–25 cm H_2O pressure, it may be necessary to replace the tube with a smaller size when the patient is stable.

If a leak is present at inspiratory pressures of <10–15 cm H_2O, the tube may be too small or the cuff may be incompletely inflated. Such an air leak can prevent the creation of any positive end-expiratory pressure (PEEP) and may complicate mechanical ventilation. Although most ventilators can compensate for some air leak, excessive air leak is undesirable. Further inflation of the cuff may help, provided the cuff inflation pressure remains at <20–25 cm H_2O. If an uncuffed tube is used, and it is impossible to provide adequate ventilation, replacement of the tube with a larger or cuffed tube should be considered.

Exhaled Carbon Dioxide Detector

Accuracy of exhaled CO_2 monitors and esophageal detector devices to confirm tracheal tube placement in children has been reported, but accuracy of these devices has not been reported with pediatric use of other advanced airways, such as LMAs. An important caveat of exhaled CO_2 monitoring is that CO_2 may be detected with placement of a supraglottic airway, such as an LMA. While this confirms that the supraglottic airway is capturing exhaled gas from the trachea and that ventilation is occurring, it does not necessarily confirm *tracheal* placement of the tube (45).

Following placement of a transglottic airway, such as an ETT, with a perfusing rhythm the detection of exhaled CO_2 after six initial breaths (to wash out any CO_2 that entered the stomach during bag-mask ventilation) reliably indicates placement of the ETT in the trachea. In a child with a perfusing rhythm, the detection of exhaled CO_2 using a colorimetric detector or capnometer is both sensitive and specific for ETT placement (9,13).

In cardiac arrest, or with a large pulmonary embolus, pulmonary blood flow may be extremely low; therefore, inadequate CO_2 may be detected despite correct tracheal tube placement. Bolus IV epinephrine administration during resuscitation may transiently reduce pulmonary blood flow, reducing the exhaled CO_2 below the limits of detection (46,47). In experimental pediatric cardiac arrest, the sensitivity of CO_2 detection was 85% and the specificity was 100% for tracheal tube placement (48). If tube position is in doubt during CPR, the rescuer should confirm tube position with direct laryngoscopy.

Two sizes of colorimetric exhaled CO_2 devices are available: one for children who weigh <15 kg and the other for patients who weigh >15 kg. Use of the larger detector with a small child could result in failure to detect exhaled CO_2 despite correct tracheal tube placement. In addition, use of even the smaller detector in infants who weigh <2 kg will add substantial dead space to the ventilator circuit (9).

Severe airway obstruction (e.g., status asthmaticus) and pulmonary edema may impair CO_2 elimination sufficiently to cause failure to detect exhaled CO_2 in adults, but this problem has not been reported in children. If the detector is contaminated with acidic gastric contents or acidic drugs, such as tracheally administered epinephrine, the colorimetric detector may not reliably reflect the presence of exhaled CO_2 (44,45). Despite these potential limitations, monitoring exhaled CO_2 is an important tool for confirming the initial placement and position of a tracheal tube. An abrupt fall in exhaled CO_2 indicates tube displacement more rapidly and reliably than pulse oximetry (49).

When time permits, a chest radiograph should be obtained to confirm the proper depth of tube insertion. The tip of the tube should be in midtrachea, at approximately the level of the third or fourth thoracic vertebra. Most commercially available ETTs have marks that indicate depth of insertion; the depth marker at the child's teeth or lips should be noted before the tube is secured and throughout intubation. Position of the tip of the ETT will move with changes in head position; the tube will move further into the trachea when the neck is flexed and will move out of the trachea when the neck is extended (50).

Esophageal Detector Device

The esophageal detector device is accurate when used to confirm ETT placement in children >20 kg in weight who have a perfusing rhythm (51). As of 2014, no published evidence was available regarding the sensitivity or reliability of the device in children in cardiac arrest.

Support of a Patient with an Advanced Airway

The patient with an advanced airway requires specialized medical and nursing care and constant assessment. These patients should be monitored in a high-acuity environment with sufficient staff to ensure that the patient and the airway are protected. Constant monitoring is particularly important if the child is sedated, because sedation may mask overt signs of hypoxia or inadequate ventilation.

The advanced airway bypasses the humidification and warming functions of the upper airway; therefore, warmed and humidified inspired gas (with supplementary oxygen as needed) must be provided. Sedation should be titrated to maintain patient comfort. Periodic suctioning of the airway is required because secretion clearance is impaired. Providers must frequently verify tube patency and proper tube position. Continuous monitoring of exhaled CO_2 is recommended.

Complications of Endotracheal Intubation

Complications of ETI can be divided into immediate, or procedure, complications (associated with the placement of the artificial airway) and later complications. Later complications include those that occur while the artificial airway is in place and those that develop during and following extubation.

Procedure Complications

Any airway intervention may convert a *potentially* compromised airway to an *actually* compromised airway and may create hypoxemia and hypercarbia. In addition, placement of an advanced airway often requires interruption or postponement of other interventions (e.g., chest compressions during CPR) that may have a greater impact on patient survival. In some settings (e.g., in the prehospital setting with short transport intervals (10) or healthcare settings in which providers have limited opportunities for intubation), more emphasis should be placed on good basic airway management than on advanced airway placement.

Immediate complications of intubation can result from the medications required for intubation, trauma to (e.g., laceration of) airway structures, injury to the cervical spine, and from the physiologic effects of laryngoscopy and PPV. Laryngoscopy can cause increased intracranial and intraocular pressures, coughing, regurgitation, aspiration, and laryngospasm, especially in the patient with inadequate sedation. The potential for airway injury increases with a difficult airway and with multiple intubation attempts. Dental injury is common in school-aged children with loose deciduous teeth. The risk of injury can be minimized by careful laryngoscopy (with appropriate patient sedation) and selection of appropriate tube size.

Accurate initial and ongoing assessment of ETT placement is essential. Esophageal intubation and gastric distension will quickly result in hypoxemia and increase the risk of aspiration. A misplaced tube should be detected immediately with careful clinical assessment and evaluation of exhaled CO_2. Mainstem bronchus intubation (more commonly to the right side) can result in atelectasis, hypoxemia, and pneumothorax.

Late Complications

While the tube is in place, providers should assess the nares (when a nasotracheal tube is in place) or the lip, gum, and tongue (when an orotracheal tube is in place) for signs of pressure injury. Ulcers may develop on the arytenoids, posterior vocal cords, subglottic area, anterior tracheal wall, and epiglottis. Oropharyngeal aspiration has been documented in 28% of intubated pediatric patients, and it is more likely to occur with oral intubation and in patients with lower sedation scores (52). The use of cuffed ETTs may decrease this risk. Ventilator-associated pneumonia and sinusitis can also be sources of morbidity in intubated patients.

Intubation results in hyperemia, edema, and mucosal hemorrhage, which can progress to ulceration, erosion, and eventual chronic fibrosis. Fibrosis typically develops in the subglottic region; it is circumferential but may be asymmetric and may result in granuloma formation, especially posteriorly.

Late complications can develop up to 6 weeks after extubation and include laryngeal and tracheal granulomas and vocal cord paralysis. Subglottic stenosis following extubation has been reported in <8% of intubated neonates in retrospective studies (53). In a recent prospective study following extubation, 11% of children had subglottic stenosis on routine follow-up; of those affected, 86% required surgical repair (54). There was no association with age, number of intubations, or use of a cuffed ETT. Duration of intubation was associated with an increased risk of subglottic stenosis, although injuries have been reported even after relatively short-term intubations. In that no apparent "safe" duration of intubation has been defined, the decision to switch from an ETT to a tracheostomy should be patient specific and not related to an arbitrary time limit.

Planned Extubation and Postextubation Care

Weaning from mechanical ventilation and extubation may be attempted after resolution of the conditions that necessitated intubation. To be ready for extubation, the patient should have adequate airway-protective reflexes, as demonstrated by an intact cough, gag, and swallow. Sedation should be weaned so that the patient has adequate airway reflexes and ventilatory drive. Neuromuscular blockade should be completely reversed and confirmed by train-of-four testing or documentation of spontaneous movement and adequate strength.

Oxygenation and ventilation should be adequate with minimal ventilatory support (e.g., ≤4–6 cm H_2O positive end-expiratory pressure, and minimal FIO_2). Weaning of ventilation can be accomplished either by gradual reduction in ventilator support or by performing a daily extubation readiness trial in eligible patients (55). Aggressive use of extubation readiness trials may identify children ready for extubation faster than typical practice (56), although this is not clear across all trials (57). These trials are typically performed by placing the patient on a spontaneous breathing mode (pressure or volume support) with a small amount of continuous positive airway pressure (CPAP) or with a T-piece. Some authors have suggested that there is a requirement to maintain a high level of pressure support to overcome ETT resistance, especially in small children, although evidence for this is lacking (58) and may overestimate extubation readiness (59). Successful completion of a trial may reliably predict extubation readiness in children ventilated for >48 hours (59). Other indices, such as tension-time index, have been evaluated as a method of predicting extubation failure with mixed results (60–62).

Ideally, the patient should have an air leak around the ETT with inflation pressures of <15–25 cm H_2O, although this test has poor sensitivity for predicting postextubation stridor or extubation failure, especially in younger children (63). Finally, cardiac function should be adequate to tolerate the increase in left ventricular afterload that develops with the withdrawal of PPV.

Once criteria for extubation are met, the ETT and oropharynx are suctioned to help prevent aspiration and laryngospasm. Oral or gastric feeding is suspended for 4–6 hours prior to extubation in case reintubation is required. If a cuffed tube is in place, the cuff is deflated prior to extubation. Oxygen (100%) is provided (a buffer for possible laryngospasm), and the lungs are fully inflated (to promote an exhalation or cough if secretions have accumulated in the supraglottic) as the tube is withdrawn. For children with airway anomalies, extubation in the operating suite may be appropriate.

After extubation, humidified inspired oxygen is provided, and the patient is monitored for signs of extubation failure. Extubation failure occurs in 4.1%–29% of patients (depending on the definition of failure and the study population) and results in increased PICU and hospital lengths of stay and possibly in mortality (64). Upper airway obstruction, pulmonary dysfunction, and respiratory muscle weakness are the most common causes of failure (64). Patients who fail extubation tend to be younger and have chronic medical problems (55,64,65).

Noninvasive ventilation has been touted as a treatment for patients who develop postextubation respiratory failure. In a recent study, it was more likely to be successful in patients with chronic respiratory conditions (66).

The complications of extubation include aspiration, laryngospasm, bronchospasm, and upper airway edema, causing stridor. Risk of aspiration can be reduced by ensuring that the stomach is empty, the patient is awake, and the oropharynx is clear of secretions before extubation. Laryngospasm results from stimulation of the larynx by secretions or by the ETT, especially in a patient who is not fully awake. Under most circumstances, it can be treated by the application of continuous positive airway pressure until the spasm resolves, although some patients require sedation, neuromuscular blockade, and reintubation. Some experts recommend application of firm pressure just posterior to the mandibular ramus (medial to the earlobe) to break laryngospasm (67). Bronchospasm is common in asthmatic patients after extubation and can be treated with inhaled β-adrenergic agonists.

Postextubation stridor is more common in patients who are 1–4 years of age, those who have traumatic or multiple intubations, and those with airway abnormalities (68). Postextubation stridor has also been associated with excessive tube movement and use of a relatively large ETT (68). Hoarseness and croupy cough, with or without respiratory insufficiency, develop within the first 3 hours after extubation, peak within 8 hours, and usually resolve by 24 hours, although residual hoarseness can persist for up to 72 hours (61,68). The stridor is often caused by subglottic edema but may result from neurologic impairment, laryngomalacia, subglottic stenosis, or vocal cord paralysis. In an endoscopic survey of children with persistent postextubation stridor (69), most had laryngotracheitis with or without neurologic dysfunction. Only 20% of children had structural airway problems, such as stenosis or vocal cord paralysis.

The treatment of postextubation stridor includes administration of humidified air or oxygen, racemic epinephrine, and possible corticosteroids. Nebulized epinephrine has been used to produce vasoconstriction and reduce edema, although its efficacy is not clearly established (9,70). The use of dexamethasone for the prevention and treatment of postextubation stridor remains controversial. A meta-analysis of trials of dexamethasone (0.25–0.5 mg/kg/dose) found that it reduced the incidence of postextubation stridor but did not significantly reduce the reintubation rate (71). However, other than hyperglycemia, this regimen of dexamethasone produces no significant side effects. Oxygen in helium may be administered because this mixture is less dense than pure oxygen, allows higher inspiratory flow at lower resistance, and can improve comfort. However, patients who require >40% inspired O_2 concentration may not receive sufficient helium to experience benefit. Extubation failure may require reintubation until the reason for the failure can be treated or resolved. Persistent postextubation stridor is an indication for diagnostic bronchoscopy.

Unplanned extubation increases hospital and PICU lengths of stay and occurs in 0.11–2.7 per 100 intubation days (72). Risk factors for unplanned extubation include younger age, oral intubation, delirium or agitation, increased secretions, inadequate tube fixation, and a less than 1-to-1 patient-to-nurse ratio (72,73). In a recent study (72), only half of patients reported to have unplanned extubation required reintubation, suggesting the need for more aggressive identification of patients who are ready for extubation. A number of different quality improvement initiatives have been shown to be effective in reducing the rate of unplanned extubation in the PICU (74–76).

MANAGEMENT OF THE DIFFICULT AIRWAY

General Principles of Difficult Airway Management

The most critical aspects of management of the difficult airway are the anticipation of difficulties and the development of a suitable backup plan or plans. Obtaining a thorough history to identify previous airway problems and their management and performing careful physical examination are keys to predicting difficulty in securing an airway. These are required with each intubation, whether the provider anticipates a difficult airway or not.

The American Society of Anesthesiologists has developed an algorithm for the approach to and management of the difficult airway (77,78). Often, the most difficult decision is whether to attempt conventional intubation or to proceed directly to more advanced techniques. If the patient can be ventilated with a bag-mask device, the provider has some time for decision making and preparation for additional interventions, avoiding the "can't intubate, can't ventilate" scenario.

If a difficult airway is suspected, the provider must consider a number of factors. A portable kit with the necessary equipment to deal with the difficult airway must be readily available and include different types and sizes of laryngoscope blades, ETTs and LMAs, forceps, stylets, a needle cricothyrotomy/tracheostomy kit, and a fiber-optic device, such as an intubating bronchoscope or videolaryngoscope. Providers should practice often with advanced airway equipment and techniques to become comfortable with them. The appropriate personnel should be notified in case more advanced techniques, such as bronchoscopy or a surgical airway, are necessary. If time permits, consideration should be given to moving the child to an appropriate environment (such as the operating suite) where more specialized equipment and personnel are available.

When intervention is needed, short-acting and/or reversible sedative agents are preferred, but the safety of the airway is the priority over patient comfort. Having an extra set of hands to manage sedation is helpful to allow one provider to focus on the airway. Adequate preoxygenation with 100% oxygen can also delay the development of hypoxemia and bradycardia if intubation requires more time than anticipated.

If initial tracheal intubation fails, it is important to make some change in technique or personnel before another attempt. Calling for help or using an alternative airway strategy early is preferable to repeated unsuccessful intubation attempts, which can lead to patient instability and airway trauma. If visualization of the glottis is poor, the provider should reassess the patient's position to improve alignment of the oral–pharyngeal–laryngeal axes. External laryngeal manipulation (BURP) can be used to bring the larynx into view. A different laryngoscope blade may provide a better view of the larynx. If these techniques are not successful when performed by an experienced provider, the provider should consider use of a supraglottic airway (such as an LMA) or a fiber-optic device.

The same careful preparations are required for extubation as for intubation because reintubation may be required and edema may make the reintubation even more difficult than the initial intubation. Providers must assemble the appropriate equipment and personnel (see earlier sections, *Endotracheal Intubation—Preparation* and *Adjuncts to Direct Laryngoscopy*).

Surgical Airways: Percutaneous Needle Cricothyrotomy/Tracheostomy

Needle cricothyrotomy or tracheostomy are indicated as life-saving procedures in patients who present with, or progress to, the "can't intubate, can't oxygenate" scenario. Although there is limited literature and clinical experience to support this technique, clinicians who manage pediatric emergencies must be familiar with the procedure and its equipment and indications. It can be used in patients with obstruction proximal to the glottic opening, or in patients with abnormal anatomy that precludes laryngoscopic visualization of the glottic opening. Other clinical indications include facial trauma and angioedema. The procedure is rarely helpful in foreign-body aspiration if the object cannot be visualized by direct laryngoscopy, because it is unlikely that the obstruction is located proximal to the level of the cricothyroid membrane. It also will be of questionable value in the patient with croup because a small ETT can usually bypass the subglottic obstruction.

Equipment

If the procedure is necessary, the use of familiar equipment, such as an IV catheter with ventilation bag, is recommended. Bag-catheter ventilation can provide effective oxygenation but not effective ventilation (i.e., hypercarbia will persist). It is a good practice to preassemble a needle cricothyrotomy/tracheostomy kit (premade kits are available), seal it in a transparent bag, and tape it in an accessible place in the resuscitation area. Providers should practice with the equipment (especially manual ventilation through the catheter) prior to use. The simplest equipment, appropriate for use in infants consists of a 14-gauge over-the-needle catheter, a 3-mm ETT adapter, and a 5-mL syringe.

A number of commercial devices are available, some using a Seldinger technique to facilitate placement of the airway. However, there are little published data to justify the use of one over another. A new device (the Quicktrach baby; Rusch, CCR Medical, St Petersburg, FL) has been shown to be effective in an infant animal model (79).

Procedure

The child is placed in the supine position with a towel under the shoulders to produce exaggerated neck extension. This position forces the trachea anteriorly so that it is easily palpable and can be stabilized with two fingers of one hand.

The upper trachea should be considered functionally as a large palpable vein that the provider must isolate and cannulate, with the catheter directed at the shallowest angle practical. Although it is ideal to puncture the cricothyroid membrane (the cricoid ring is less likely to narrow during healing), this membrane may be difficult to palpate in infants, and insertion of the catheter through adjacent tracheal structures is unlikely to cause life-threatening complications. For this reason, the procedure is probably better called *percutaneous needle tracheostomy*; the priority is to quickly establish adequate airway and oxygenation through a needle or catheter placed in the trachea.

Once the catheter is in place, the 3-mm ETT adapter and a ventilation bag with oxygen are attached to the catheter or airway hub, and bag-catheter ventilation is provided. Placement is confirmed by clinical examination (chest rise and breath sounds may be difficult to appreciate) and detection of exhaled CO_2. The small catheter radius will normally provide high resistance to ventilation that should not be mistaken for signs of a misplaced catheter, poor lung compliance, or a pneumothorax. The inspiratory pressures required to produce flow through the catheter are well above the limits of the pop-off valve for any ventilation bag; therefore, the valve must be occluded to deliver gas flow through the catheter.

The catheter can be exchanged for a more secure device using a modified Seldinger technique, although there is a risk of catheter displacement and complete loss of airway with these techniques. If adequate oxygenation is obtained using the catheter, it should be maintained until additional personal are available to establish a more secure airway. If bag-catheter ventilation does not provide adequate oxygenation, jet ventilation can be provided, although preferably only in older children. Begin ventilation with low psi (20 mm Hg) and titrate to adequate chest excursion and oxygen saturation. Extreme caution is required to avoid the complications of excessive flow and resultant barotrauma.

MANAGEMENT OF SPECIFIC PROBLEMS

Full Stomach

One of the risks associated with instrumenting the pediatric airway is the potential for reflux and aspiration of gastric contents. Airway reflexes that usually protect against aspiration may be suppressed by sedatives and anesthetics, neuromuscular blockers, or underlying disease or injury. Aspiration of as little as 0.4 mL/kg of gastric contents can cause significant acute lung injury (80). Acidic gastric fluid (especially when the pH is <2.5) is particularly injurious. Other factors that influence the severity of aspiration include the size of the particles involved, the bacterial content, and the patient's underlying cardiopulmonary status. Immediate sequelae of aspiration can include bronchospasm, acute pneumonitis, and acute respiratory distress syndrome (ARDS).

Providers should attempt to minimize the risk of aspiration by withholding oral intake (i.e., making the patient nil per os [NPO]) as soon as the possibility of intubation arises. However, it may be impossible to delay intubation to allow time for gastric emptying. Because time to gastric emptying can be prolonged by acute illness and some medications, even patients who have had nothing by mouth for ≥6 hours may still be at risk. Altered bowel motility and processes that increase intra-abdominal pressure (e.g., obesity, ascites, or abdominal masses) can also increase risk of gastric reflux and aspiration.

Therapy to modify the pH (e.g., antacids or H_2 blockers) prior to intubation is thought to reduce lung injury from the aspiration of gastric contents, but little data support this claim. Although some drugs given 60–90 minutes prior to intubation may reduce the volume and acidity of pediatric gastric secretions (81), this option is not practical if the airway must be secured emergently.

If the child requiring intubation may have a full stomach, RSI (see earlier) is the technique of choice unless contraindications exist. Preferentially intubation should be performed before any PPV is applied; however, if the patient will not tolerate the delay for intubating conditions to be achieved, then the use of cricoid pressure during ventilation may reduce the risk of aspiration. Placing a nasogastric tube before intubation may not reliably empty the stomach and may increase the risk of aspiration by reducing the lower esophageal sphincter opening pressure.

Awake Intubation

Although awake intubation (i.e., intubation without sedation) is an important strategy for use in an adult patient with a difficult airway, it can be very difficult to perform in an uncooperative child. The risks of intubating an awake, struggling, frightened child must be weighed against the need for maintaining spontaneous breaths if intubation fails. Intubation without sedation is appropriate in cardiopulmonary arrest and may be appropriate for the child in severe shock.

Sedation may be titrated to minimize discomfort but avoid deep sedation. This approach allows intubation without severely compromising airway reflexes, respiratory drive, or hemodynamics. However, intubation of the sedated, spontaneously breathing child should only be attempted by individuals experienced with the technique, who can judge the relative risks of a full stomach or laryngospasm versus the risk of general anesthesia and paralysis in a patient with a difficult airway.

If available, a relatively short-acting inhalation anesthetic, such as sevoflurane, can create appropriate conditions for intubation and maintains respiratory drive. Short-acting medications, such as propofol, ketamine, or benzodiazepines, may be titrated to balance patient cooperation and cardiopulmonary stability. However, this balance can be difficult to maintain, especially in younger children. Lidocaine spray may minimize gagging and laryngospasm.

Cervical Spine Abnormalities and Injuries

Cervical spine anomalies, trauma, and conditions that limit neck movement interfere with visualization of the larynx. Cervical spine abnormalities may be associated with conditions, such as Goldenhar and Klippel–Fiel syndromes, juvenile idiopathic arthritis, spondyloarthropathies, and neuromuscular scoliosis. Airway management in these patients is further complicated if the disease process affects the temporomandibular joint, limiting mouth opening.

In patients with an unstable cervical spine, movement of the neck required for direct laryngoscopy could result in subluxation of the spine and spinal cord injury. Atlantoaxial instability occurs in 10%–30% of patients with Down syndrome (82). Evaluation of the child's history of neurologic symptoms and of any flexion/extension cervical spine radiographs can help to screen for these patients but may not be reliable. In cases of uncertainty, it is prudent to treat all children with Trisomy 21 as if they have unstable cervical spines. In trauma patients, cervical spine instability is assumed to be present in all patients with a head or neck injury or a mechanism of injury consistent with application of force to the head or neck.

In patients with presumed or diagnosed cervical spine instability, one healthcare provider must be responsible for stabilizing the neck during airway manipulation until the airway is secured and immobilization devices can be applied. In these cases, a straight blade may provide a better view of the glottic structures, although more advanced airway techniques, such as fiber-optic intubation, are sometimes required. In studies of simulated cervical spine instability, the use of a GlideScope actually worsened views of the glottic structures (83) although the use of a Bullard laryngoscope dramatically improved them (84). Although it is important to minimize movement of the neck in these patients, establishment of an adequate airway is a priority.

Intracranial Hypertension

Successful airway management for a patient with increased ICP includes both advanced airway placement and prevention of secondary neurologic injury. Laryngoscopy and intubation will trigger spikes in ICP just as airway suction does in already intubated patients being monitored for increased ICP in the PICU. In addition, intubation may be complicated by the presence of facial trauma or a potentially unstable cervical spine.

For intubation of patients with isolated intracranial hypertension, anesthetic agents, such as thiopental (not available in the United States) and propofol, may be beneficial. Although fentanyl has been shown to raise ICP (85), an increasing volume of literature (86,87) suggests that ketamine might actually lower ICP. While lidocaine treatment prior to intubation in the patient at risk for increased ICP may help prevent an ICP spike, the only evidence to support this practice is extrapolated from reports of the use of lidocaine to prevent increased ICP associated with suctioning or similar scenarios (88).

Sedation with neuromuscular blockade is thought to allow for a safer intubation with smaller rises in ICP, but these effects probably result from the simultaneous use of anesthetic agents. Controversy still exists as to whether succinylcholine's rapid action offsets its potential side effects, including drug-induced fasciculation and consequent increases in ICP. Because patients with increased ICP do not tolerate the mild hypoxemia and hypercapnia that can develop with a traditional RSI protocol, a modified RSI technique is typically used. Hyperventilation that may reduce cerebral blood flow is avoided unless the patient is herniating or already hyperventilating themselves.

When intubating the trachea of a patient with intracranial hypertension associated with multisystem disease, providers should remember that what is theoretically good for the brain might not benefit the rest of the body. Many anesthetic agents produce vasodilation that may compound the abnormal hemodynamics seen with trauma and septic shock.

Shock

When intubating the trachea of a child in shock, the provider must be aware of normal cardiopulmonary interactions. The reduced left ventricular afterload that results from PPV may be beneficial when myocardial contractility is poor. However, securing the airway of these patients carries risk. PPV reduces preload, potentially reducing cardiac output (89,90). Small infants can have an augmented vagal response to PPV, leading to bradycardia and further reduction in cardiac output. These changes with PPV can be exacerbated by hypovolemia or reduced cardiac contractility.

The provider should assume that the child in shock has a full stomach and should use an RSI technique for placement of an advanced airway. It may be necessary to optimize hemodynamics by administering bolus intravenous fluids or inotropes before attempting the intubation. Potential bradycardia (resulting from vagal or drug-related effects) should be anticipated, and prophylactic use of atropine may be appropriate.

Intubation sedatives/anesthetics should be selected with careful consideration of their associated hemodynamic effects; no anesthetic agent is risk free. Drugs with potent vasodilatory effects, such as propofol and thiopental, should be used with extreme caution. Ketamine is a useful drug in the hemodynamically unstable patient, but even it has negative inotropic effects. Fentanyl at low doses is commonly used but also has some vasodilatory effects. Etomidate maintains blood pressure during intubation but has potential adrenal suppressive effects, especially in septic patients; these effects can worsen hemodynamic instability.

Facial or Laryngotracheal Injury

Although trauma to the airway structures is relatively uncommon, it can significantly complicate airway management. Facial injuries may be associated with profuse bleeding, fractures, and aspiration of blood, gastric contents, or teeth. Concurrent orbital and intracranial injuries are common and can affect management (see the next section, *Open Globe*). A free-floating (fractured) maxilla can cause compression of the nasopharynx and airway obstruction.

If the patient is breathing spontaneously with no signs of obstruction, oxygen administration by mask may be adequate. However, ongoing hemorrhage and edema may create the need for an advanced airway. Orotracheal intubation with BURP (external laryngeal manipulation with BURP) and aggressive suctioning is often all that is required. If injury or uncontrolled bleeding obstructs the view of the larynx, fiber-optic or surgical techniques may be needed. Nasotracheal intubation is contraindicated until basilar skull fracture can be ruled out because the tube can migrate intracranially when a basilar skull fracture and dural tear are present.

Neck injuries can result in direct trauma to the larynx. Soft-tissue injury, including edema, hematoma, arytenoid dislocation, laryngotracheal separation, and vocal cord paralysis, can occur. Fractures are rare. Laryngeal injuries should be suspected in any patient with anterior neck trauma and hoarseness, stridor, subcutaneous emphysema, or pneumomediastinum/pneumothorax. Injuries to other structures in the neck, such as the great vessels, esophagus, and cervical spine, must be ruled out. When laryngeal injury is present, it is helpful to evaluate it endoscopically before intubation to exclude laryngotracheal separation that will increase the risk of soft-tissue intubation.

Many injuries and problems can cause progressive and potentially life-threatening laryngeal swelling. For these problems, early airway intervention is crucial before increasing edema makes intubation impossible. Inhalation injury should be anticipated in any burn patient with facial burns, singed nasal hairs, carbonaceous debris in the airway, or a history of closed-space exposure (91). Caustic ingestion can have a similar effect on airway structures. Anaphylaxis and hereditary angioedema are abrupt reactions that can result in severe airway edema, obstruction, and cardiovascular collapse. In these conditions, epinephrine and early airway management are keys to therapy.

Iatrogenic injuries can cause airway obstruction. Vocal cord paralysis results from damage to the recurrent laryngeal nerve and can result from central causes (head injury, hydrocephalus) or direct injury (e.g., difficult birth or mediastinal or neck surgery, such as coarctation repair). Stridor, aspiration, and a weak cry are common symptoms. Subglottic stenosis, congenital or secondary to intubation, may necessitate use of a smaller-than-predicted ETT.

Open Globe

When a child has a penetrating eye injury, extrusion of vitreous contents can occur during intubation. Rises in ocular pressure, produced by any Valsalva maneuver (such as crying, coughing, gagging, or straining), will exacerbate this risk. The best approach to intubate such patients is RSI with adequate amounts of analgesia and sedation. Intravenous lidocaine may be helpful in preventing the rise in intraocular pressure. Succinylcholine and ketamine have historically been associated with vitreous extrusion in this setting (92), although adult data challenge this dogma (93). Once intubated, the patient requires ongoing sedation/analgesia to prevent straining against the tracheal tube or gagging, which could result in increased ocular pressure.

Mediastinal Mass

The anterior mediastinal space can occasionally be occupied by masses, most commonly neoplasms. Malignant lesions, such as lymphoma (Hodgkins or non-Hodgkins), are common, but nonmalignant lesions can occur as well. The diagnosis may be made during preanesthesia respiratory function testing, with a finding of partial intrathoracic airway obstruction. The diagnosis may also be made through the use of chest radiographs, CT scans, echocardiography, or MRI.

High-risk patients often present with positional symptoms. The patient with a mediastinal mass compressing the airway or cardiovascular structures can be relatively asymptomatic until the patient lies supine, when dyspnea develops. Patients who sleep sitting up often do so to prevent airway collapse. Such children can develop severe airway compromise when anesthesia is initiated, so extreme caution is needed.

The presence of at least three respiratory signs or symptoms (including cough, shortness of breath, orthopnea, pleural effusion, the use of accessory muscles, stridor) during preanesthetic assessment of children with anterior mediastinal masses has been associated with an increased risk of cardiorespiratory complications during anesthesia (94). Changes in airway tone or chest wall compliance that result from anesthesia or neuromuscular blockade can lead to collapse or compression of the airway and nearby vascular structures, with consequent cardiorespiratory collapse. Although it may be possible to insert an ETT, the mass may compress the trachea distal to the end of the tube, precluding effective oxygenation and ventilation even after intubation. Respiratory distress may also result from a malignant pleural effusion or from partial intrathoracic airway obstruction. Compression of mediastinal vascular structures can lead to superior vena cava syndrome.

The basic principle of management of the patient with a mediastinal mass is to keep the patient breathing spontaneously. The anesthetic agent should be chosen with this goal in mind. Choices include ketamine, dexmedetomidine, and inhalational agents, although careful titration of other agents (e.g., narcotics) can be effective (95). The hemodynamic effects of these agents may need to be balanced by hemodynamic intervention (e.g., administration of fluids or vasoactive drugs). It may be necessary to stop the anesthetic and awaken the patient if hemodynamic compromise develops (95).

The supine position may worsen airway and cardiovascular compromise, and the lateral or even prone position may minimize airway compression. While preparations are made for intubation, elevating the head of the bed can help to maintain lung volumes.

Because the transition from spontaneous breathing to PPV is a high-risk moment for the child with mediastinal mass, it is prudent to briefly (and gently) assist spontaneous respiratory efforts with PPV. This enables assessment of the child's tolerance of PPV. If the child does not tolerate PPV, the child can resume spontaneous breathing and the provider will then plan additional support and alternative approaches.

Before anesthesia is administered, preload is optimized with IV fluids to counteract the mass compression of vascular structures, and providers must support an adequate heart rate. Acute airway obstruction may be successfully managed with the use of rigid bronchoscopy or extracorporeal life support (transthoracic or femoral–femoral). These solutions will only be possible if airway obstruction is anticipated and equipment and personnel are prepared in advance.

Craniofacial Abnormalities

Craniofacial anomalies, such as Pierre Robin, Treacher Collins, and Goldenhar syndromes, can create a difficult airway. Visualization of the glottis by direct laryngoscopy can be difficult—if not, impossible—in these conditions.

Micrognathia is common in these conditions and causes a cephalad positioning of the larynx, thus resulting in a more "anterior" airway with a smaller anterior mandibular space for displacement of the tongue during laryngoscopy. Glossoptosis, the downward and backward displacement of the tongue, will also interfere with visualization of the larynx. Other craniofacial anomalies that can complicate airway management include gross macrocephaly, midface hypoplasia, maxillary protrusion, facial asymmetry and a high arched palate, a small mouth, a short muscular or immobile neck, and facial clefts. Patients with cleft palate can develop obstruction of the oropharynx during sedation if the tongue falls into the cleft, although this can be prevented with the use of an OPA. The LMA can provide an effective airway for children with craniofacial anomalies (96).

Infiltration of Soft Tissues

Infiltration of the soft tissues will result in a decreased area for displacement of upper airway structures during laryngoscopy, making it more difficult to view the glottis. In addition, the infiltration can distort the glottis.

Hemangiomas grow rapidly during infancy and can cause airway compromise either from mass effect or acute airway hemorrhage. Subglottic hemangiomas can cause complete airway obstruction in infants. Venous lymphatic malformations (cystic hygromas) can continue to grow through childhood; they may grow rapidly as the result of infection or hemorrhage and produce airway obstruction.

Macroglossia (enlargement of the tongue), present in patients with Beckwith–Wiedemann syndrome and Trisomy 21, can also make laryngoscopy difficult. These conditions are also associated with hypotonia that can make bag-mask ventilation difficult. Management of these problems requires early detection and possible insertion of an advanced airway. A curved blade may be preferable for visualization of the vocal cords in these patients (97).

The deposition of mucopolysaccharides in the airways (mucopolysaccharidosis) leads to macroglossia, tonsillar hypertrophy, thickening of the oral mucosa, and obstruction of nasal passages. A short neck is common. The temporomandibular joints and cervical spine may be involved, limiting jaw and neck mobility. Patients with Morquio syndrome are at risk for atlantoaxial subluxation. The airway infiltration worsens with age; therefore, intubation becomes more difficult (and sometimes impossible) as the child ages. These problems can develop in patients with Hurler syndrome as early as 2 years of age. The LMA or videolaryngoscope are useful airway adjuncts in this population but some patients can only be intubated with a fiber-optic bronchoscope (98,99). The airway infiltration in the mucopolysaccharidosis can also increase the difficulty of emergency surgical tracheostomy.

Obesity

The obese child can present challenges during basic (noninvasive) and advanced airway and ventilation support. Children with obesity have limited oxygen reserve. Increased chest wall and abdominal tissue and reduced chest compliance all compromise diaphragm excursion and reduce FRC during both spontaneous and assisted ventilation. Oxygenation is often further compromised by ventilation–perfusion mismatch. Chronic airway obstruction and hypoventilation can produce alveolar hypoxia and pulmonary hypertension that may be detected during preanesthetic clinical exam, augmented by electrocardiogram and echocardiogram (revealing right ventricular strain).

Obese children often have relatively short necks with fatty infiltration of the upper airway structures, creating a relative macroglossia. Fatty infiltration may also distort the airway. When combined with commonly associated airway anomalies (e.g., tongue size and position in the child with Down syndrome), airway obstruction is likely. Superimposed infection, even from "benign" upper respiratory viral illnesses, or altered airway tone with sleep, anesthesia, or muscle relaxation, can further compromise the airway.

It can be difficult for one person to hold the airway open and provide bag-mask ventilation for the very obese child because the child's jaw, head, and neck are very heavy. Two rescuers or the insertion of a nasal/oral airway may be required. The supine position may be associated with reduction in FRC, so induction of anesthesia may occur with the head of the bed elevated. Elevation of the head of the bed during intubation will help prevent the reduction in FRC that is likely to occur when the child is placed supine. Positioning of the obese child's airway may be complicated by the presence of fatty infiltration of the posterior thorax. Only limited additional padding under the torso may be necessary to place the child in the sniffing position; in fact, doing so may hyperextend the neck, partially obstructing the airway and compromising visualization during laryngoscopy.

Medication doses should generally be based on ideal body weight. However, a greater volume of adipose tissue will increase the volume of distribution of some medications used in RSI (such as fentanyl, succinylcholine, and rocuronium), and these must be dosed based on actual body weight (100).

Although advanced airway size is based on ideal body weight, the use of large laryngoscope blades and short laryngoscope handles may be necessary to adequately visualize the obese child's larynx. When intubation is planned, preparations should be made for management of a difficult airway before intubation is attempted. If intubation attempts fail, alternative airway devices, such as LMAs, can be used.

As a final option, cricothyrotomy can be performed. If it is difficult to identify the traditional landmarks, the incision is made halfway between the hyoid bone and the sternal notch, because this approximates the position of the cricothyroid membrane (101).

Acute Infectious Airway Obstruction

Infections of the deep neck space, including parapharyngeal, retropharyngeal, and peritonsillar infections, can lead to airway compromise. A high index of suspicion is required for diagnosis, because these infections are relatively rare. Symptoms include fever, neck swelling, pain, torticollis, limited neck movement, drooling, and trismus (102). A protruding tongue can suggest infection in the submandibular or sublingual space (Ludwig angina). These conditions can rapidly progress to airway compromise. Therapy includes early antibiotics and surgical evaluation.

Laryngotracheobronchitis (croup) presents with hoarseness, barky cough, and stridor and is almost always viral in origin. Only the most severe cases that are not responsive to steroids and nebulized racemic epinephrine require intubation. Subglottic narrowing may necessitate use of a much smaller ETT than predicted.

Bacterial laryngotracheobronchitis (bacterial tracheitis) is most commonly caused by *Staphylococcus aureus*. It often begins with a viral prodrome similar to croup but progresses rapidly with high fever, severe stridor, and respiratory distress.

Acute epiglottitis is an airway emergency characterized by acute inflammation of the supraglottic region. Fortunately, this problem has almost vanished with the introduction of the *Haemophilus influenzae* type B vaccine. Epiglottitis is marked by sudden onset of fever, dysphagia, drooling, a "hot-potato voice," and toxemia. Unlike croup and bacterial tracheitis, cough is rarely present. Older patients often present in the "tripod" position to maximize air entry (i.e., sitting and leaning forward braced on both arms). Antibiotic therapy is a priority in management.

Patients with impending airway obstruction from upper airway infection or any other rapidly progressive process should be taken immediately to the operating suite or ICU for assessment. Urgent consultation with pediatric anesthesia and ear, nose, and throat specialists is required. Control of the airway is the priority. It is imperative to keep the child calm and allow the child to remain in the position of comfort; placing the child supine or performing unnecessary procedures, such as blood sampling, can trigger laryngospasm and irreversible airway obstruction. Examinations should be limited until all necessary equipment and personnel are available to treat airway collapse. Patients should always be accompanied by a physician skilled in airway procedures. The utility of a lateral neck radiograph in these patients is controversial and can cause agitation and result in further airway compromise.

Intubation in the operating suite using an inhalational anesthetic is preferred. Swelling and distortion of upper airway structures can be so extreme that intubation is impossible and a surgical airway is required. In the spontaneously breathing child, the visualization of air bubbles during exhalation can help to locate the glottic opening, and the ETT can be blindly placed in that area. The appropriate tube size will allow a small amount of air leak and is usually 0.5–1.0 mm smaller in diameter than the predicted ETT size. It is important to remember that normal smaller-diameter tubes may not be sufficiently long for larger patients and special microlaryngeal tracheal (MLT) tubes may be required (longer lengths for same external diameter) from the operating suite. Neuromuscular blockers are contraindicated until the airway is secure. If the child collapses acutely and experienced personnel are not yet available, bag-mask ventilation should be attempted while personnel and equipment are assembled.

The resolution of acute airway obstruction can result in *postobstructive pulmonary edema (POPE)*. It has been reported in 2%–10% of all patients with upper airway obstruction and in a higher percentage of those patients who require intubation (103). Various etiologies of airway obstruction have been associated with the development of pulmonary edema, including foreign bodies, laryngospasm, obstructed ETT, and croup. POPE usually develops within a few minutes to a few hours following the onset of airway obstruction, and usually resolves within 72 hours. Proposed mechanisms include negative intrapleural pressure transmitted to the alveoli, creating a hydrostatic gradient that favors extravascular fluid movement. Negative intrapleural pressure can increase venous return to the right heart with bowing of the interventricular septum (increasing left ventricular end-diastolic pressure and thus pulmonary venous pressure) and increased right ventricular output and pulmonary blood flow (103). The edema is often asymptomatic, and treatment is supportive. PPV with positive end-expiratory pressure is occasionally required.

Foreign-Body Aspiration

Foreign-body aspiration is a common cause of airway obstruction in children <2 years of age. Food, especially nuts and seeds, are the most commonly aspirated foreign objects. They can lodge in any part of the airway from the nasal passage to the lung parenchyma. The trachea and the mainstem bronchi are common sites of foreign-body deposition. Because the left bronchus angles more acutely from the trachea in older children and adults, more right-bronchus foreign-body aspiration is observed in these older patients. Because the angle of the left bronchus is not as acute, left-bronchus foreign-body aspiration is more common in smaller children than in adults.

A high index of suspicion is necessary to diagnose foreign-body aspiration because many choking episodes are not witnessed, and findings in physical and radiographic examinations are nonspecific. Cervical and chest films should be obtained, especially in the case of a radiopaque foreign body. If the inspiratory chest film is normal, an expiratory chest film can demonstrate air trapping due to endobronchial foreign bodies causing partial bronchial obstruction. If foreign-body aspiration is at all suspected, endoscopy is indicated. Any sharp object or any object causing acute upper airway obstruction with respiratory failure should be removed on an urgent basis. Back slaps/chest thrusts in responsive infants and abdominal thrusts in responsive older children can be attempted if endoscopy is not immediately available. Flexible bronchoscopy can be used for diagnosis, but a rigid scope is almost always required for removal.

CONCLUSIONS AND FUTURE DIRECTIONS

Successful acute airway management requires adequate training, frequent experience, and a process of continuous quality improvement. However, the need for provider experience must be weighed against the need of the child for an experienced provider to establish an airway under urgent conditions.

High-resolution visual imaging using cameras on the distal end of the tracheal tube, light wand stylets, and laryngoscopes are rapidly being developed. Realistic simulation manikins can facilitate training and experience before a clinical need for airway intervention arises. In addition, the use of simulation programs can enhance the development of teamwork, improve skill performance, enhance the quality of the practice, and enable evaluation of preparation and protocols before clinical use.

The use of quality assurance bundles (with elements such as protocols for weaning and extubation) has been shown to reduce intubation complications in adults (104). Simulation allows "just-in-time" training where healthcare professionals can practice managing an airway prior to performing it with a patient (105).

Intensive and continuous quality improvement using such tools as the National Emergency Airway Registry can provide feedback and data on the impact of these technologies on airway management (21). More information is necessary, however, on the effectiveness of simulator mannequin training and the necessary intervals for retraining in airway techniques.

ACKNOWLEDGMENT

The authors gratefully acknowledge the insights and expertise of Ashraf Coovadia, Robert Luten, and Ann E. Thompson, who contributed to the previous edition of this chapter. That version of the chapter provided the foundation for this revised chapter.

References

1. Reed JM, O'Conner DM, Myer CM III. Magnetic resonance imaging determination of tracheal orientation in normal children: Practical implications. *Arch Otolaryngol Head Neck Surg* 1996;122(6):605–8.
2. Litman RS, Weissend EE, Shibata D, et al. Developmental changes of laryngeal dimensions in unparalyzed, sedated children. *Anesthesiology* 2003;98:41–5.
3. Heinrich S, Birkholz T, Ihmsen H, et al. Incidence and predictors of difficult laryngoscopy in 11,219 pediatric anesthesia procedures. *Paediatr Anaesth* 2012;22(8):729–36.
4. Sanders RC Jr, Giuliano JS Jr, Sullivan JE, et al.; National Emergency Airway Registry for Children Investigators and Pediatric Acute Lung Injury and Sepsis Investigators Network. Level of trainee and tracheal intubation outcomes. *Pediatrics* 2013;131(3):e821–8.
5. Haubner LY, Barry JS, Johnston LC, et al. Neonatal intubation performance: Room for improvement in tertiary neonatal intensive care units. *Resuscitation* 2013;10(84):1359–64.
6. Mallampati SR, Gatt SP, Gugino LD, et al. A clinical sign to predict difficult tracheal intubation: A prospective study. *Can Anaesth Soc J* 1985;32:429–34.
7. George E, Haspel KL. The difficult airway. *Int Anesthesiol Clin* 2000;38:47–63.
8. Berry F. Anesthesia for the child with a difficult airway. In: Berry F, ed. *Anesthetic Management of Difficult and Routine Pediatric Patients*. New York, NY: Churchill Livingstone, 1990:167–98.
9. Chameides L, Samson RA, Schexnayder SM, et al. *Pediatric Advanced Life Support Provider Manual*. Dallas, TX: American Heart Association, 2011.
10. Gausche M, Lewis RJ. Out-of-hospital endotracheal intubation of children. *JAMA* 2000;283:2790–2.
11. Stockinger ZT, McSwain NE Jr. Prehospital endotracheal intubation for trauma does not improve survival over bag-valve-mask ventilation. *J Trauma* 2004;56:531–6.
12. Hubble MW, Wilfong DA, Brown LH, et al. A meta-analysis of prehospital airway control techniques part II: Alternative airway devices and cricothyrotomy success rates. *Prehosp Emerg Care* 2010;4(14):515–30.
13. Kleinman ME, de Caen AR, Chameides L, et al.; Pediatric Basic and Advanced Life Support Chapter Collaborators. Part 10: Pediatric basic and advanced life support: 2010 International Consensus on Cardiopulmonary Resuscitation and Emergency Cardiovascular Care Science with Treatment Recommendations. *Circulation* 2010;122(16, suppl 2):S466–515.
14. Daugherty RJ, Nadkarni V, Brenn BR. Endotracheal tube size estimation for children with pathological short stature. *Pediatr Emerg Care* 2006;22:710–7.
15. Kim HJ, Kim JT, Kim HS, et al. A comparison of GlideScope videolaryngoscopy with direct laryngoscopy for nasotracheal intubation in children. *Paediatr Anaesth* 2011;21(11):1165–6.
16. Hazinski M, Zaritsky A, Nadkarni V, et al. Rapid sequence intubation. In: *PALS Provider Manual*. Dallas, TX: American Heart Association, 2002.
17. Thompson A. Pediatric airway management. In: Fuhrman B, Zimmerman J, eds. *Pediatric Critical Care*. 3rd ed. Philadelphia, PA: Mosby, 2005.
18. Fastle RK, Roback MG. Pediatric rapid sequence intubation: Incidence of reflex bradycardia and effects of pretreatment with atropine. *Pediatr Emerg Care* 2004;20:651–5.
19. McAuliffe G, Bissonnette B, Boutin C. Should the routine use of atropine before succinylcholine in children be reconsidered? *Can J Anaesth* 1995;42:724–9.
20. Jones P, Dauger S, Denjoy I, et al. The effect of atropine on rhythm and conduction disturbances during 322 critical care intubations. *Pediatr Crit Care Med* 2013;14(6):e289–97.
21. Sagarin MJ, Chiang V, Sakles JC, et al. Rapid-sequence intubation for pediatric emergency airway management. *Pediatr Emerg Care* 2002;18:417–23.
22. McAllister JD, Gnauck KA. Rapid sequence intubation of the pediatric patient. Fundamentals of practice. *Pediatr Clin North Am* 1999;46:1249–84.
23. Zelicof-Paul A, Smith-Lockridge A, Schnadower D, et al. Controversies in rapid sequence intubation in children. *Curr Opin Pediatr* 2005;17:355–62.
24. Food and Drug Administration; Pediatric Advisory Committee; Rosenthal A (Chair). Transcript of June 21, 2010 meeting of the FDA Pediatric Advisory Committee. Bethesda, MD. http://www.accessdata.fda.gov/drugsatfda_docs/label/2010/008453s027lbl.pdf. Accessed October 1, 2014.
25. Theroux MC, Rose JB, Iyengar S, et al. Succinylcholine pretreatment using gallamine or mivacurium during rapid sequence induction in children: A randomized, controlled study. *J Clin Anesth* 2001;13:287–92.
26. Vachon CA, Warner DO, Bacon DR. Succinylcholine and the open globe. Tracing the teaching. *Anesthesiology* 2003;99:220–3.
27. Cheng CA, Aun CS, Gin T. Comparison of rocuronium and suxamethonium for rapid tracheal intubation in children. *Paediatr Anaesth* 2002;12:140–5.
28. Smith KJ, Dobranowski J, Yip G, et al. Cricoid pressure displaces the esophagus: An observational study using magnetic resonance imaging. *Anesthesiology* 2003;99(1):60–4.
29. Arora MK, Karamchandani K, Trikha A. Use of a gum elastic bougie to facilitate blind nasotracheal intubation in children: A series of three cases. *Anaesthesia* 2006;61:291–4.
30. Fisher QA, Tunkel DE. Lightwand intubation of infants and children. *J Clin Anesth* 1997;9:275–9.
31. Fiadjoe JE, Gurnaney H, Dalesio N, et al. A prospective randomized equivalence trial of the GlideScope Cobalt(R) video laryngoscope to traditional direct laryngoscopy in neonates and infants. *Anesthesiology* 2012;116:622–8.
32. Kim JT, Na HS, Bae JY, et al. GlideScope video laryngoscope: A randomized clinical trial in 203 paediatric patients. *Br J Anaesth* 2008;101:531–4.
33. Armstrong J, John J, Karsli C. A comparison between the GlideScope video laryngoscope and direct laryngoscope in paediatric patients with difficult airways—A pilot study. *Anaesthesia* 2010;65:353–7.
34. Lee JH, Park YH, Byon HJ, et al. A comparative trial of the GlideScope(R) video laryngoscope to direct laryngoscope in children with difficult direct laryngoscopy and an evaluation of the effect of blade size. *Anesth Analg* 2013;117:176–81.
35. Kalbhenn J, Boelke AK, Steinmann D. Prospective model-based comparison of different laryngoscopes for difficult intubation in infants. *Paediatr Anaesth* 2012;22:776–80.
36. Park C, Bahk JH, Ahn WS, et al. The laryngeal mask airway in infants and children. *Can J Anaesth* 2001;48:413–7.
37. Mathis MR, Haydar B, Taylor EL, et al. Failure of the laryngeal mask airway unique™ and classic™ in the pediatric surgical patient: A study of clinical predictors and outcomes. *Anesthesiology* 2013;119(6):1284–95.

38. Chen L, Hsiao AL. Randomized trial of endotracheal tube versus laryngeal mask airway in simulated prehospital pediatric arrest. *Pediatrics* 2008;122(2):e294–7.

39. Zanardo V, Weiner G, Micaglio M, et al. Delivery room resuscitation of near-term infants: Role of the laryngeal mask airway. *Resuscitation* 2010;81(3):327–30.

40. Zhu XY, Lin BC, Zhang QS, et al. A prospective evaluation of the efficacy of the laryngeal mask airway during neonatal resuscitation. *Resuscitation* 2011;82(11):1405–9.

41. Gallart L, Mases A, Martinez J, et al. Simple method to determine the size of the laryngeal mask airway in children. *Eur J Anaesthesiol* 2003;20:570–4.

42. Kundra P, Deepak R, Ravishankar M. Laryngeal mask insertion in children: A rational approach. *Paediatr Anaesth* 2003;13:685–90.

43. Nakayama S, Osaka Y, Yamashita M. The rotational technique with a partially inflated laryngeal mask airway improves the ease of insertion in children. *Paediatr Anaesth* 2002;12:416–9.

44. Zhang X, Chen M, Li Q. The ProSeal Laryngeal Mask Airway is more effective than the LMA-Classic in pediatric anesthesia: A meta-analysis. *J Clin Anesth* 2012;24(8):639–46.

45. Chhibber AK, Kolano JW, Roberts WA. Relationship between end-tidal and arterial carbon dioxide with laryngeal mask airways and endotracheal tubes in children. *Anesth Analg* 1996;82(2):247–50.

46. Cantineau JP, Merckx P, Lambert Y, et al. Effect of epinephrine on end-tidal carbon dioxide pressure during prehospital cardiopulmonary resuscitation. *Am J Emerg Med* 1994;3(12):267–70.

47. Lindberg L, Liao Q, Steen S. The effects of epinephrine/norepinephrine on end-tidal carbon dioxide concentration, coronary perfusion pressure and pulmonary arterial blood flow during cardiopulmonary resuscitation. *Resuscitation* 2000;43(2):129–40.

48. Bhende MS, Karasic DG, Karasic RB. End-tidal carbon dioxide changes during cardiopulmonary resuscitation after experimental asphyxial cardiac arrest. *Am J Emerg Med* 1996;14:349–50.

49. Poirier MP, Gonzalez Del-Rey JA, McAneney CM, et al. Utility of monitoring capnography, pulse oximetry, and vital signs in the detection of airway mishaps: A hyperoxemic animal model. *Am J Emerg Med* 1998;16(4):350–2.

50. Kuhns LR, Poznanski AK. Endotracheal tube position in the infant. *J Pediatr* 1971;78:991–6.

51. Sharieff GQ, Rodarte A, Wilton N, et al. The self-inflating bulb as an airway adjunct: Is it reliable in children weighing less than 20 kilograms? *Acad Emerg Med* 2003;10:303–8.

52. Amantea SL, Piva JP, Sanches PR, et al. Oropharyngeal aspiration in pediatric patients with endotracheal intubation. *Pediatr Crit Care Med* 2004;5:152–6.

53. Walner DL, Loewen MS, Kimura RE. Neonatal subglottic stenosis—Incidence and trends. *Laryngoscope* 2001;111:48–51.

54. Manica D, Schweiger C, Maróstica PJ, et al. Association between length of intubation and subglottic stenosis in children. *Laryngoscope* 2013;123(4):1049–54.

55. Newth CJ, Venkataraman S, Willson DF, et al. Weaning and extubation readiness in pediatric patients. *Pediatr Crit Care Med* 2009;10(1):1–11.

56. Foronda FK, Troster EJ, Farias JA, et al. The impact of daily evaluation and spontaneous breathing test on the duration of pediatric mechanical ventilation: A randomized controlled trial. *Crit Care Med* 2011;39(11):2526–33.

57. Randolph AG, Wypij D, Venkataraman ST, et al. Effect of mechanical ventilator weaning protocols on respiratory outcomes in infants and children: A randomized controlled trial. *JAMA* 2002;288(20):2561–8.

58. Keidan I, Fine GF, Kagawa T, et al. Work of breathing during spontaneous ventilation in anesthetized children: A comparative study among the face mask, laryngeal mask airway and endotracheal tube. *Anesth Analg* 2000;91(6):1381–8.

59. Ferguson LP, Walsh BK, Munhall D, et al. A spontaneous breathing trial with pressure support overestimates readiness for extubation in children. *Pediatr Crit Care Med* 2011;12(6):e330–5.

60. Venkataraman ST, Khan N, Brown A. Validation of predictors of extubation success and failure in mechanically ventilated infants and children. *Crit Care Med* 2000;28(8):2991–6.

61. Kline-Tilford AM, Sorce LR, Levin DL, et al. Pulmonary disorders: Weaning from mechanical ventilatory support. In: Hazinski MF, ed. *Nursing Care of the Critically Ill Child.* 3rd ed. St Louis, MO: Elsevier Mosby, 2013.

62. Harikumar G, Egberongbe Y, Nadel S, et al. Tension-time index as a predictor of extubation outcome in ventilated children. *Am J Respir Crit Care Med* 2009;180(10):982–8.

63. Mhanna MJ, Zamel YB, Tichy CM, et al. The "air leak" test around the endotracheal tube, as a predictor of postextubation stridor, is age dependent in children. *Crit Care Med* 2002;30:2639–43.

64. Kurachek SC, Newth CJ, Quasney MW, et al. Extubation failure in pediatric intensive care: A multiple-center study of risk factors and outcomes. *Crit Care Med* 2003;31:2657–64.

65. Edmunds S, Weiss I, Harrison R. Extubation failure in a large pediatric ICU population. *Chest* 2001;119:897–900.

66. James CS, Hallewell CP, James DP, et al. Predicting the success of non-invasive ventilation in preventing intubation and reintubation in the paediatric intensive care unit. *Intensive Care Med* 2011;37(12):1994–2001.

67. Membership of the Difficult Airway Society Extubation Guidelines Group; Popat M, Mitchell V, Dravid R, et al. Difficult Airway Society Guidelines for the management of tracheal extubation. *Anaesthesia* 2012;67:318–40.

68. Koka BV, Jeon IS, Andre JM, et al. Postintubation croup in children. *Anesth Analg.* 1977;56(4):501–5.

69. Lin CD, Cheng YK, Chang JS, et al. Endoscopic survey of post-extubation stridor in children. *Acta Paediatr Taiwan* 2002;43:91–5.

70. da Silva PS, Fonseca MC, Iglesias SB, et al. Nebulized 0.5, 2.5 and 5 ml L-epinephrine for post-extubation stridor in children: A prospective, randomized, double-blind clinical trial. *Intensive Care Med* 2012;38(2):286–93.

71. Markovitz BP, Randolph AG. Corticosteroids for the prevention of reintubation and postextubation stridor in pediatric patients: A meta-analysis. *Pediatr Crit Care Med* 2002;3:223–6.

72. da Silva PS, de Carvalho WB. Unplanned extubation in pediatric critically ill patients: A systematic review and best practice recommendations. *Pediatr Crit Care Med* 2010;11(2):287–94.

73. Marcin JP, Rutan E, Rapetti PM, et al. Nurse staffing and unplanned extubation in the pediatric intensive care unit. *Pediatr Crit Care Med* 2005;6(3):254–7.

74. Sadowski R, Dechert RE, Bandy KP, et al. Continuous quality improvement: Reducing unplanned extubations in a pediatric intensive care unit. *Pediatrics* 2004;114(3):628–32.

75. da Silva PS, de Aguiar VE, Neto HM, et al. Unplanned extubation in a paediatric intensive care unit: Impact of a quality improvement programme. *Anaesthesia* 2008;63(11):1209–16.

76. Rachman BR, Mink RB. A prospective observational quality improvement study of the sustained effects of a program to reduce unplanned extubations in a pediatric intensive care unit. *Paediatr Anaesth* 2013;23(7):614–20.

77. Henderson JJ, Popat MT, Latto IP, et al. Difficult Airway Society guidelines for management of the unanticipated difficult intubation. *Anesthesia* 2004;59:675–94.

78. Apfelbaum JL, Hagberg CA, Caplan RA, et al.; American Society of Anesthesiologists Task Force on Management of the Difficult Airway. Practice guidelines for management of the difficult airway: An updated report by the American Society of Anesthesiologists Task Force on Management of the Difficult Airway. *Anesthesiology* 2013;118(2):251–70.

79. Metterlein T, Frommer M, Kwok P, et al. Emergency cricothyrotomy in infants—Evaluation of a novel device in an animal model. *Paediatr Anaesth* 2011;21(2):104–9.

80. Raidoo DM, Rocke DA, Brock-Utne JG, et al. Critical volume for pulmonary acid aspiration: Reappraisal in a primate model. *Br J Anaesth* 1990;65:248–50.

81. Maekawa N, Nishina K, Mikawa K, et al. Comparison of pirenzepine, ranitidine, and pirenzepine-ranitidine combination for reducing preoperative gastric fluid acidity and volume in children. *Br J Anaesth* 1998;80:53–7.

82. McKay SD, Al-Omari A, Tomlinson LA, et al. Review of cervical spine anomalies in genetic syndromes. *Spine* 2012;37(5): E269–77.

83. Vlatten A, Litz S, MacManus B, et al. A comparison of the GlideScope video laryngoscope and standard direct laryngoscopy in children with immobilized cervical spine. *Pediatr Emerg Care* 2012;28(12):1317–20.

84. Nileshwar A, Garg V. Comparison of Bullard laryngoscope and short-handled Macintosh laryngoscope for orotracheal intubation in pediatric patients with simulated restriction of cervical spine movements. *Paediatr Anaesth* 2010;20(12):1092–7.

85. de Nadal M, Ausina A, Sahuquillo J, et al. Effects on intracranial pressure of fentanyl in severe head injured patients. *Acta Neurochir Suppl* 1998;71:10–2.

86. Albanese J, Arnaud S, Rey M, et al. Ketamine decreases intracranial pressure and electroencephalographic activity in traumatic brain injury patients during propofol sedation. *Anesthesiology* 1997;87:1328–34.

87. Bar-Joseph G, Guilburd Y, Tamir A, et al. Effectiveness of ketamine in decreasing intracranial pressure in children with intracranial hypertension. *J Neurosurg Pediatr* 2009;4(1):40–6.

88. Mathieu A, Guillon A, Leyre S, et al. Aerosolized lidocaine during invasive mechanical ventilation: In vitro characterization and clinical efficiency to prevent systemic and cerebral hemodynamic changes induced by endotracheal suctioning in head-injured patients. *J Neurosurg Anesthesiol* 2013;25(1):8–15.

89. Pepe PE, Raedler C, Lurie KG, et al. Emergency ventilatory management in hemorrhagic states: Elemental or detrimental? *J Trauma* 2003;54:1048–55; discussion 1055–57.

90. Kline-Tilford AM, Sorce LR, Levin DL, et al. Pulmonary disorders: Cardiopulmonary interactions. In: Hazinski MF, ed. *Nursing Care of the Critically Ill Child*. 3rd ed. St Louis, MO: Elsevier Mosby, 2013.

91. Caruso TJ, Janik LS, Fuzaylov G. Airway management of recovered pediatric patients with severe head and neck burns: A review. *Paediatr Anaesth* 2012;22(5):462–8.

92. Halstead SM, Deakyne SJ, Bajaj L, et al. The effect of ketamine on intraocular pressure in pediatric patients during procedural sedation. *Acad Emerg Med* 2012;19(10):1145–50.

93. Moeini HA, Soltani HA, Gholami AR, et al. The effect of lidocaine and sufentanil in preventing intraocular pressure increase due to succinylcholine and endotracheal intubation. *Eur J Anaesthesiol* 2006;23(9):739–42.

94. Ng A, Bennett J, Bromley P, et al. Anaesthetic outcome and predictive risk factors in children with mediastinal tumours. *Pediatr Blood Cancer* 2007;48(2):160–4.

95. Marks R, Tanner L, Wenleder B. Management of a tumor in the distal trachea while maintaining spontaneous ventilation. *J Anesth* 2010;24(6):932–4.

96. Brambrink AM, Braun U. Airway management in infants and children. *Best Pract Res Clin Anaesthesiol* 2005;19:675–97.

97. Infosino A. Pediatric upper airway and congenital anomalies. *Anesthesiol Clin North America* 2002;20:747–66.

98. Osthaus WA, Harendza T, Witt LH, et al. Paediatric airway management in mucopolysaccharidosis 1: A retrospective case review. *Eur J Anaesthesiol* 2012;29(4):204–7.

99. Khan FA, Khan FH. Use of the laryngeal mask airway in mucopolysaccharidoses. *Paediatr Anaesth* 2002;12:468.

100. Brunette DD. Resuscitation of the morbidly obese patient. *Am J Emerg Med* 2004;22:40–7.

101. Ray RM, Senders CW. Airway management in the obese child. *Pediatr Clin North Am* 2001;48:1055–63.

102. Rafei K, Lichenstein R. Airway infectious disease emergencies. *Pediatr Clin North Am* 2006;53:215–42.

103. Ringold S, Klein EJ, Del Beccaro MA. Postobstructive pulmonary edema in children. *Pediatr Emerg Care* 2004;20:391–5.

104. Jaber S, Jung B, Corne P, et al. An intervention to decrease complications related to endotracheal intubation in the intensive care unit: A prospective, multiple-center study. *Intensive Care Med* 2010;36(2):248–55.

105. Nishisaki A, Donoghue AJ, Colborn S, et al. Effect of just-in-time simulation training on tracheal intubation procedure safety in the pediatric intensive care unit. *Anesthesiology* 2010;113(1):214–23.

CHAPTER 25 ■ CARDIOPULMONARY RESUSCITATION

ROBERT A. BERG, KATSUYUKI MIYASAKA, ANTONIO RODRÍGUEZ-NÚÑEZ, MARY FRAN HAZINSKI, DAVID ANTHONY ZIDEMAN, AND VINAY M. NADKARNI

KEY POINTS

1 Effective cardiopulmonary resuscitation (CPR) and advanced life support (ALS) targeted to the etiology, timing, intensity, and duration of the cardiac arrest can optimize the potential to restore an apparently dead child back to life.

2 Sudden arrhythmogenic ("electrical") cardiac arrests are typically due to ventricular fibrillation (VF) or rapid ventricular tachycardia (VT) and respond to rapid electrical defibrillation.

3 Mechanical ("pump") cardiomyopathic arrests are typically due to inadequate myocardial oxygen delivery from asphyxial, ischemic, metabolic, or pharmacologic problems, and usually require mechanical support (CPR) to restore perfusion.

4 Cardiac arrest has at least four phases: prearrest, no-flow (untreated cardiac arrest), low-flow (during CPR efforts), and postresuscitation. The interventions needed in each phase are specific to the phase of resuscitation.

5 Animal and human data indicate that well-performed CPR for children is quite effective and that high-quality basic life support (BLS) early is more important than ALS late.

6 Outcomes following pediatric out-of-hospital arrests appear to be worse than those following in-hospital arrests. Two common types of out-of-hospital cardiac arrests have especially poor outcomes: traumatic arrests and those associated with sudden infant death syndrome (SIDS).

7 The incidence of VF varies by setting and age. In special circumstances, such as tricyclic antidepressant overdose, hyperkalemia, cardiomyopathy, postcardiac surgery, and prolonged QT syndromes, VF is a more likely rhythm during cardiac arrest.

8 Defibrillation (termination of VF) is necessary for successful resuscitation from VF cardiac arrest. Defibrillation can result in asystole, pulseless electrical activity (PEA), or a perfusing rhythm. Successful defibrillation is achieved by attaining current flow adequate to depolarize a critical mass of myocardium.

9 One of the most common precipitating events for cardiac arrest in children is respiratory insufficiency. Adequate oxygen delivery to meet metabolic demands and removal of carbon dioxide are the goals of initial assisted ventilation.

10 Providing BLS with continuous effective chest compressions and minimal pauses and interruptions is generally the best way to provide circulation during cardiac arrest. In selected settings, particularly in the pediatric intensive care unit (PICU), goal-directed therapies targeted to hemodynamics are possible.

11 Targeted temperature management with close attention to avoid hypotension and hyperoxia is a promising goal-directed, postresuscitation therapy. However, benefits from these treatments deserve further rigorous study in infants, children, and adults.

12 Optimal treatment of postarrest myocardial dysfunction has not been rigorously established; it has been treated with various continuous inotropic/vasoactive agents in both children and adults.

13 Extracorporeal membrane oxygenation (ECMO) may provide optimized control of postresuscitation temperature and vital organ perfusion, and has been demonstrated to facilitate good outcomes in selected resuscitation circumstances. The concomitant administration of anticoagulants may optimize microcirculatory flow.

14 Despite evidence-based guidelines, extensive provider training, and provider credentialing in resuscitation medicine, the quality of CPR is typically poor. Slow compression rates, inadequate depth of compression, and substantial pauses are the norm. A focus on "push hard, push fast, minimize interruptions, allow full-chest recoil, and don't overventilate" can markedly improve myocardial, cerebral, and systemic perfusion and improve outcomes.

Cardiopulmonary resuscitation (CPR), sometimes termed "cardiocerebral resuscitation," delivers oxygen and blood to the vital organs (heart and brain). Life-sustaining CPR can temporarily support myocardial and cerebral blood flow and oxygen delivery during cardiac arrest or "near cardiac arrest," such as very low-flow conditions associated with severe hypotension or hemodynamically compromising bradycardia. Most commonly, CPR is delivered very simply, by pushing hard and fast in the center of the chest. Chest compression, "closed-chest" or "open-chest," can be delivered with or without assisted ventilation and/or supplemental oxygen. High-quality CPR can provide sufficient myocardial and cerebral blood flow to attain return of spontaneous circulation (ROSC) (e.g., defibrillation of VF) or can be a bridge to extracorporeal life support (ECLS) and more definitive therapy (e.g., ECLS to allow time for a reversible cardiomyopathy to improve postcardiopulmonary bypass or myocarditis, or to receive a transplant).

DEFINITION OF CARDIAC ARREST

Pulseless cardiac arrest is typically defined as the cessation of cardiac mechanical activity, determined by unresponsiveness, apnea, and lack of evidence of an effective circulation (e.g., nonpalpable central pulse). Separating severe hypoxic-ischemic shock with poor perfusion from the nonpulsatile state of cardiac arrest (e.g., pulseless electrical activity) can be challenging at any age, especially when invasive arterial blood pressure monitoring is not present. In adults, a rescuer's ability to determine pulselessness by palpation is neither sensitive nor specific (1,2), with rescuer threshold for detection of pulses usually around a systolic blood pressure >50 mm Hg. Assessment of pulselessness by palpation is especially challenging in infants and children because of their anatomic and physiologic characteristics. Normal systolic blood pressure in neonates is ~60 mm Hg, and during hypotension, the systolic pressure is below the threshold that most rescuers can detect by palpation (3). While the carotid is the strongest accessible central arterial pulse to palpate in an adult, the short, fleshy neck of a baby (as well as the potential to compress the airway and impede respiration) limits the appropriateness of using the carotid location to assess central pulse presence in infants. Early detection of impending cardiac arrest is important because lack of prompt recognition and effective early intervention often results in death or profound hypoxic-ischemic neurologic injury. Effective CPR and ALS targeted to the etiology, timing, intensity, and duration of the cardiac arrest can optimize the potential to restore an apparently dead child back to life.

MECHANISM OF DISEASE

Cardiac arrest is the end result of diverse etiologies and pathophysiologic mechanisms, ultimately leading to an electrical or mechanical cardiac arrest due to progressive hypoxic-ischemic events or metabolic disturbances.

Arrhythmogenic ("electrical") cardiac arrests are typically associated with ventricular fibrillation (VF) or rapid ventricular tachycardia (VT). These arrhythmias can result from (a) *congenital cardiac abnormalities* associated with myocardial ischemia (e.g., coronary artery anomalies), genetic channelopathies associated with prolonged QT syndrome, familial cardiomyopathies (e.g., Duchenne muscular dystrophy, hypertrophic cardiomyopathy, dilated cardiomyopathies, arrhythmogenic right ventricular dysplasia), or mitochondrial diseases, or from (b) *acquired cardiomyopathies* associated with drugs/toxins (e.g., doxorubicin cardiomyopathy, drug-induced prolonged QT syndrome), a hypoxic-ischemic event with inadequate myocardial oxygen delivery, cardiac surgical injury, commotio cordis, mechanically induced VF, ischemia during CPR, and inappropriate unsynchronized cardioversion shock.

Mechanical ("pump") cardiomyopathic arrests are typically due to inadequate myocardial oxygen delivery from asphyxia, ischemia, metabolic disturbances (e.g., hypocalcemia, hypomagnesemia, severe acidosis), or pharmacologic (e.g., β-blocker, calcium channel blocker, barbiturate) toxicity. A myriad of events that lead to asphyxia, severe hypoxia, severe ischemia, or a combination of all three, ultimately result in myocardial pump failure and cardiac arrest. These problems typically manifest as hypoxic-ischemic cardiac dysfunction and circulatory shock with a cardiogenic component before progressing to cardiac arrest. Therefore, the best outcomes from these processes occur with early recognition, monitoring, and aggressive intervention to treat the prearrest condition, thereby preventing progression to pulseless cardiac arrest.

PHASES OF CARDIAC ARREST AND CARDIOPULMONARY RESUSCITATION

Interventions to improve outcome from pediatric cardiac arrest should be targeted to optimize therapies according to the

etiology, timing, duration, intensity, and "phase" of resuscitation, as suggested in **Table 25.1**. Cardiac arrest has at least four phases: prearrest, no-flow (untreated cardiac arrest), low-flow (CPR), and postresuscitation. The prearrest phase represents the greatest opportunity to impact patient survival by preventing pulseless cardiopulmonary arrest.

Interventions during the no-flow phase of untreated, pulseless cardiac arrest focus on early recognition of cardiac arrest and initiation of high-quality BLS with rapid recognition and treatment of shockable ECG rhythms, if present. When blood flow and oxygen delivery to the brain or heart is insufficient, CPR should be started. The goal of effective CPR is to optimize cerebral and coronary perfusion. BLS using minimally interrupted, effective chest compressions (i.e., push hard, push fast, allow full-chest recoil, minimize interruptions, and do not overventilate) is the emphasis in this phase. While the concepts are simple, effective implementation is a challenge (4–8).

The postresuscitation phase is a high-risk period for hypotension, hyperoxia, ventricular arrhythmias, hyperglycemia, seizures, hyperthermia, brain injury, and reperfusion injuries to multiple organs (9,10). Injured cells can follow many pathways: they can die rapidly, die slowly, undergo apoptosis, hibernate, or partially or fully recover function. Overventilation (hyperventilation or overdistension) is common, and can have adverse effects during and following CPR (see below for details). Hyperoxia is common after ROSC and potentially associated with harm. Interventions such as induction of systemic hypothermia during and immediately following ROSC may minimize reperfusion injury and support cellular recovery in selected settings. The postarrest phase may have the most potential for innovative advances in the understanding of cell injury and death, inflammation, apoptosis, and hibernation and to ultimately lead to novel interventions. Thoughtful attention to goal-directed therapies including targeted temperature management, glycemic control, titration of vasoactive medications, seizure detection and treatment, targeted ventilation, and rehabilitative therapies may be particularly important to avoid secondary organ injury and enhance recovery. The rehabilitation stage of postresuscitation concentrates on the salvage of injured cells, recruitment of hibernating cells, and reengineering of the reflex and voluntary communications of these cell and organ systems to improve functional outcome.

The specific phase of resuscitation should dictate the timing, intensity, duration, and focus of interventions. Emerging data suggest that interventions that can improve short-term outcome during one phase may be deleterious during another. For example, intense vasoconstriction (induced by epinephrine or vasopressin) during the low-flow phase of cardiac arrest may improve coronary perfusion pressure and the probability of ROSC but during the postresuscitation phase may increase left ventricular afterload and worsen myocardial strain and dysfunction. Our current management of the physiology of cardiac arrest and recovery consists of the crude titration of blood pressure, global oxygen delivery and consumption, body temperature, inflammation, coagulation, and other physiologic parameters to attempt to optimize outcome. Future strategies will likely take advantage of emerging discoveries in cellular inflammation modulation, thrombosis, reperfusion, mediator cascades, mitochondrial function, cellular markers of injury and recovery, and transplantation technology.

IS CARDIOPULMONARY RESUSCITATION EFFECTIVE FOR CHILDREN?

In the original 1960 report of successful resuscitation using closed-chest cardiac compression, asphyxiated children

TABLE 25.1

PHASES OF CARDIAC ARREST AND RESUSCITATION

■ PHASE	■ INTERVENTIONS
Prearrest phase (protect)	Optimize community education regarding child safety
	Optimize patient monitoring and rapid emergency response
	Recognize and treat respiratory failure and/or shock to prevent cardiac arrest
Arrest (no-flow) phase (preserve)	Minimize interval to BLS and ALS (organized response)
	Minimize interval to defibrillation, when indicated
Low-flow (CPR) phase (resuscitate)	"Push hard, push fast"
	Allow full-chest recoil
	Minimize interruptions in compressions
	Avoid overventilation
	Titrate CPR to optimize myocardial blood flow (coronary perfusion pressures and exhaled CO_2)
	Consider adjuncts to improve vital organ perfusion during CPR
	Consider ECMO if standard CPR/ALS not promptly successful
Postresuscitation phase: Short-term rehabilitation	Optimize cardiac output and cerebral perfusion
	Treat arrhythmias, if indicated
	Avoid hyperglycemia, hyperthermia, hyperventilation
	Consider mild postresuscitation systemic hypothermia
	Debrief to improve future responses to emergencies
Postresuscitation phase: Longer-term rehabilitation (regenerate)	Early intervention with occupational and physical therapy
	Bioengineering and technology interface
	Possible future role for stem cell transplantation

BLS, basic life support; ALS, advanced life support; ECMO extracorporeal membrane oxygenation; CPR, cardiopulmonary resuscitation.

and adults who received immediate, effective resuscitation attained remarkably good outcomes (11). When cardiac arrest is witnessed and is of short duration, excellent outcomes *can* occur after various types of bystander CPR, including mouth-to-mouth rescue breathing alone, chest compressions alone, or standard chest compressions and mouth-to-mouth rescue breathing. Nevertheless, some reports in the 1980s and 1990s questioned the effectiveness and advisability of out-of-hospital pediatric CPR, and also indicated that survival rates from in-hospital CPR were <10%. Studies from that era, which included infants with sudden infant death syndrome (SIDS), demonstrated that <5% of children receiving out-of-hospital CPR survived to hospital discharge and that many of the survivors were neurologically devastated. These findings led to suggestions that out-of-hospital CPR for children was futile. More contemporary large epidemiologic studies from North America, the Netherlands, Sweden, and Japan show that children are more likely to survive out-of-hospital CPR than adults, and that ~10% of children older than one year survive to hospital discharge. Many of the children in these studies survived with favorable neurologic outcomes (12–17).

In-hospital CPR studies in the 1980s revealed that <10% of these children survived to hospital discharge. The American Heart Association (AHA) developed the Pediatric Advanced Life Support (PALS) course to focus on prevention of cardiac arrests by prompt recognition and treatment of respiratory failure and shock, in addition to treatment of pulseless cardiac arrest. More recent studies have established that 25%–60% of children treated with in-hospital CPR and aggressive postresuscitative care survive to hospital discharge, and 70%–90% of survivors have favorable neurologic outcomes (18–22). The message is increasingly clear: CPR is "a chance to save a life."

EPIDEMIOLOGY

Pediatric In-Hospital Arrests

The true incidence of pediatric pulseless arrest is difficult to estimate due to inconsistent definitions and challenges for assessment of pulselessness in children. Based on registry and administrative data, more than 6000 children in the United States receive in-hospital CPR each year, mostly in pediatric intensive care units (PICUs) (22,23). Cardiac arrest rates of children admitted to the PICU in the 1990s were 1.8% in the United States (24) and 6% in Finland (25). More recent data from three single-center pediatric *cardiac* PICU studies demonstrate cardiac arrests in 3%–6% of children admitted (18,26–28). Despite increasing numbers of PICU admissions in the United States in the last two decades, the incidence of CPR events among PICU patients has remained relatively constant. Among 10,040 children prospectively evaluated in the eight academic PICUs from 2010–2013, 139 (1.4%) of the children were treated with CPR (Berg, personal communication). In addition, a population-based study from a nationwide administrative database in the United States reported that 5807 children received in-hospital CPR (95% CI, 5259–6355) in 2006, ~0.77 children received CPR per 1000 hospital admissions (23). With the intense interest in preventing cardiac arrests on hospital wards by using rapid response or medical emergency teams, it is not surprising that >95% of CPR events in the United States are now occurring in PICUs (22).

Many in-hospital pediatric CPR investigations with longer-term follow-up have established that pediatric CPR and ALS can be remarkably effective (19,20,29,30). Although most of these arrests/events occurred in PICUs and were due to progressive life-threatening illnesses that had not responded to treatment despite critical care, more than 67% attained ROSC following CPR. Among hospitals in the AHA Get With The Guidelines-Resuscitation (GWTG-R) registry, survival to discharge rates improved from ~25% (2000–2005) to >40% (since 2006) with 70%–90% having favorable neurologic outcomes (22,31).

The improvement in survival with favorable neurological outcome following in-hospital CPR has been associated with the increased shift of CPR events from ward to ICU settings, where staff-to-patient ratios, resuscitation experience and expertise are better. In addition, published approaches to improve PICU CPR education and implementation may have affected the quality of PICU resuscitation efforts (19,32,33). Over the last two decades, studies have increasingly used the more rigorous Utstein-style reporting (34–36) for in-hospital pediatric cardiac arrests and CPR, many of which are derived from the multicentered AHA GWTG-R registry (21). The large size, scope, and quality of the National registry distinguish these North American data, which characterize the process and outcome of pediatric in-hospital CPR events.

In the GWTG-R reports, a cardiac arrest is explicitly defined as cessation of cardiac mechanical activity, determined by the absence of a palpable central pulse, unresponsiveness, and apnea. Events are excluded if the cardiac arrest began out-of-hospital, involved a newborn in a delivery room or NICU, or was limited to a shock by an implanted cardioverter-defibrillator. Most of these arrests occurred in children with progressive respiratory insufficiency and/or progressive circulatory shock. These children often had progressive underlying critical illnesses despite aggressive critical care monitoring and therapy. Therefore, >95% of these arrests were witnessed and/or monitored, and less than 5% occurred on a general pediatric ward. Before the arrest, approximately three-quarters of these children were mechanically ventilated, 50% had continuous vasopressor infusions, and one-third had continuous direct arterial blood pressure monitoring (20–22,31). In a different research network, 60% of the PICU cardiac arrests had direct arterial pressure monitoring at the time of the event (Berg, personal communication).

Of importance, almost one-half of children have severe bradycardia and poor perfusion rather than a pulseless cardiac arrest (30,37) at the time that chest compressions are initiated in hospitals. As expected, children who received chest compressions initiated for bradycardia with pulses present have a much higher survival-to-hospital discharge rate (41%) than those whose chest compressions are initiated for nonshockable *pulseless* cardiac arrest (25%, $p < 0.001$). Notably, the 59% mortality rate in the group receiving CPR for bradycardia and poor perfusion, and the similarity of this cohort to the children with CPR for asystole and pulseless electrical activity (PEA), suggest that the CPR was provided during severe asphyxial or ischemic insults likely to otherwise progress to pulseless cardiac arrests and death without CPR. These data provide support for the PALS approach to initiate chest compressions for the pediatric patient when bradycardia and poor perfusion persist despite adequate oxygenation and ventilation, before progression to a pulseless cardiac arrest.

Pediatric Out-of-Hospital Arrests

Outcomes following pediatric out-of-hospital cardiac arrests (OHCAs) are worse than those following in-hospital arrests. These poor outcomes are in part due to prolonged periods of "no-flow" and disease processes with especially poor outcomes. Many pediatric out-of-hospital cardiac arrests are not witnessed, and many children with an out-of-hospital cardiac arrest are not provided with bystander CPR. Therefore, the no-flow period is often quite prolonged before EMS personnel provide CPR, and neurologic outcomes are generally worse among children who are survivors of out-of-hospital arrest compared with those with in-hospital arrests.

Large-scale population-based studies from North America, Japan, The Netherlands, and Finland demonstrate an incidence of 8–10 pediatric out-of-hospital cardiac arrests/100,000 person-years (15,38–41). Accordingly, more than 5000 children experience a nontraumatic pediatric out-of-hospital cardiac arrest each year in the United States (38). Infants have a tenfold higher incidence than older children, and a much higher mortality rate. The most common diagnosis is SIDS. Factors that influence survival include the environment in which the arrest occurs, the child's preexisting condition, the duration of no-flow before resuscitation, provision of bystander CPR, shockable versus nonshockable rhythms, and the quality of the basic and advanced life support interventions. Many infants treated with CPR in the prehospital setting are found pulseless in the morning by a parent long after the apparent SIDS event. Not surprisingly, their outcomes are dismal. In addition, for children who have prehospital cardiac arrests from traumatic hemorrhagic shock, CPR is challenged by inadequate intravascular volume, so, not surprisingly, outcomes are again dismal.

Although many adult OHCAs are caused by primary cardiac disease, pediatric OHCAs are more than twice as likely to be attributable to noncardiac causes as to primary cardiac disease. Nevertheless, outcomes after OHCAs are better among children than adults (16,38,40)

Bystander CPR

The AHA's Chain of Survival for pediatric cardiac arrest highlights five elements: Prevention, Early CPR, Call for Help, Rapid Implementation of Advanced Life Support, and Aggressive Postresuscitation Care. Bystander CPR is one of the key elements in increasing survival from OHCA, yet only one-third to one-half of children are provided with bystander CPR (similar to the rates for adults) (38–40). Not surprisingly, outcomes are worse without bystander CPR because of the prolonged no-flow period during the typical 6–15 minutes before emergency medical services personnel arrive.

What is the role for hands-only bystander CPR in children? For children with sudden collapse cardiac arrests of presumed cardiac etiology, hands-only bystander CPR is as effective as chest compression plus rescue breathing because: (a) the reservoir of oxygen in the lungs is adequate to oxygenate blood perfusing through the lungs during the low-flow state of CPR for 5–15 minutes, (b) gas exchange occurs with gasping during CPR, and (c) gas enters the lungs during the relaxation phase of chest compressions because of negative pressure generated with chest recoil. In a nationwide, prospective, population-based, observational study that enrolled 5170 children aged 17 years and younger who had an OHCA from January 1, 2005, to December 31, 2007, 3675 (71%) children had arrests of noncardiac causes and 1495 (29%) presumed cardiac causes. 1551 (30%) received conventional CPR and 888 (17%) compression-only CPR. Children who were given CPR by a bystander had a significantly higher rate of favorable neurological outcome than did those not given bystander CPR (4.5% vs. 1.9%; adjusted odds ratio [OR] 2.59, 95% CI, 1.81–3.71). In children with *noncardiac causes*, conventional CPR (with rescue breathing) produced more favorable neurological outcome than did compression-only CPR (7.2% vs. 1.6%; OR 5.54, 2.52–16.99). However, in children aged 1–17 years who had arrests of cardiac causes, favorable neurological outcome did not differ between conventional and compression-only CPR (9.9% vs. 8.9%; OR 1.20, 0.55–2.66). Thus, for children who have out-of-hospital cardiac arrests from noncardiac causes, conventional CPR (with rescue breathing) by bystander is the preferable approach to resuscitation. For arrests of cardiac causes, either conventional or compression-only CPR is similarly effective (12,39).

Outcomes following sudden collapse with shockable rhythms of presumed cardiac etiology in children are substantially better than pulseless cardiac arrest due to presumed asphyxia etiology. Most pediatric OHCAs result from an asphyxial event, so the lungs are depleted of oxygen by the time cardiac arrest occurs, and gasping during CPR may be less frequent when the brain is perfused with profoundly hypoxemic blood. Therefore, providing some oxygen to the lungs with rescue breathing substantially improves outcome from asphyxia cardiac arrests. Because appreciating the difference between a sudden collapse cardiac arrest and an acute asphyxial event is a complex task for a bystander, and because most pediatric OHCAs are secondary to acute asphyxia, chest compression plus rescue breathing is the recommended approach for pediatric OHCAs. The AHA recommends a C-A-B (compressions-airway-breathing) rather than the A-B-C (airway-breathing-compressions) approach because: (a) there is no flow until chest compressions are initiated and (b) providing rescue breathing is complex and time-consuming, thereby delaying time to restarting circulation to vital organs.

Outcomes

Although rates of survival to discharge following OHCA in children vary from 3% to 24% (15,38–41), the largest population-based studies suggest: (a) overall 3%–10% survive to hospital discharge, (b) infant survival rate is only 3%–5%, and most surviving infants are severely neurologically impaired, (c) beyond infancy survival rate is ~10%, and (d) survival rate with a shockable rhythm (pulseless VT or VF) is ~20% (38–40), with >70% favorable neurologic outcome. Two common types of OHCAs consistently have especially poor outcomes: traumatic arrests and those associated with SIDS. The large OHCA registries in North America and Japan have both shown that survival rates are higher among children compared with adults (38–40).

PEDIATRIC VF

VF is an uncommon but not rare electrocardiographic rhythm during pediatric OHCA. Several studies reported VF as the initial rhythm in 19%–24% of pediatric OHCA. Unlike other investigations with VF prevalence in the range of 6%–10% (38,41–50), these studies excluded SIDS deaths because nearly all SIDS victims had been dead and nonresuscitable at the time of discovery. Perhaps VF is even more common, but electrocardiographic rhythms are often not attained as promptly in children as in adults, and VF eventually converts into asystole over time. Therefore, the reported prevalence of VF depends on the aggressiveness and timing of monitoring and the inclusion criteria for the report.

7 The incidence of VF varies by setting and age. In special circumstances, such as tricyclic antidepressant overdose, cardiomyopathy, renal failure with hyperkalemia, post–cardiac surgery, and prolonged QT syndromes, VF is a more likely rhythm during cardiac arrest. Commotio cordis, or mechanically initiated VF due to relatively low-energy chest-wall impact during a narrow window of repolarization (10–30 ms before the T wave peak in swine models), is reported predominantly in children 4–16 years old. Out-of-hospital VF cardiac arrest, uncommon in infants, occurs more frequently in children and adolescents. The variance of VF prevalence by age was highlighted in a study that documented VF/VT in only 3% of children in cardiac arrest who were 0–8 years old versus 17% of children who were 8–19 years old (51). This has been corroborated in large North American and Japanese registry studies with first documented rhythm of VF in 15%–18% of adolescents (38,40). Although VF is often associated with underlying heart disease and generally considered the "immediate cause" of cardiac arrest, "subsequent" VF can also occur during resuscitation efforts. In studies of VF among asphyxiated piglets, the incidence of VF was 28%–33% during resuscitation. Asphyxia-associated VF is also well documented among pediatric near-drowning patients (13,52,53).

The shockable rhythms of VF and pulseless VT occurred in 27% of in-hospital pediatric cardiac arrests at some time during the arrest and resuscitation (54), although the first documented rhythms during most in-hospital cardiac arrests (both in children and in adults) are asystole and PEA. Among the first 1005 pediatric in-hospital cardiac arrests in the GWTG-R registry (54), 10% had an initial rhythm of VF/VT, and an additional 15% had subsequent VF/VT (i.e., later during the resuscitation efforts).

Traditionally, VF and VT have been considered "good" cardiac arrest rhythms, resulting in better outcomes than asystole and PEA. Of note, survival to discharge was much more common among children with an initial shockable rhythm than among children with shockable rhythms that occurred later during the resuscitation. Even in the setting of progressive respiratory failure and shock with an initial electrocardiogram of asystole or PEA, a substantial number of these children developed subsequent shockable VF/VT during CPR. Surprisingly, the subsequent VF/VT group had worse outcomes than children with asystole/PEA who never developed VF/VT during the resuscitation: 11% survival to hospital discharge with subsequent VF/VT during resuscitation from asystole/PEA versus 27% with asystole/PEA alone. These data suggest that outcomes after *initial* VF/VT are "good," but outcomes after *subsequent* VF/VT are substantially worse, even compared with asystole/PEA rhythms. These observations have been corroborated in other pediatric and adult investigations (47,55).

Why was the outcome so poor in the subsequent VF/VT group? Plausible explanations include: (a) a delay in the diagnosis of subsequent VF/VT during the resuscitative efforts, (b) adverse effects of resuscitative interventions (e.g., too much epinephrine), and (c) subsequent VF/VT is a marker of severe underlying myocardial pathology, refractory hypoxemia, or tissue hypoxia.

Termination of VF: Defibrillation

8 Defibrillation (defined as termination of VF) is necessary for the successful resuscitation from VF cardiac arrest. Note that termination of fibrillation can result in asystole, PEA, or a perfusing rhythm. The goal of defibrillation is the return of an organized electrical rhythm with pulse. When prompt defibrillation is provided soon after the induction of VF in a cardiac catheterization laboratory, the rates of successful defibrillation and survival approach 100%. When automated external defibrillators are used within 3 minutes of adult-witnessed VF, long-term survival can occur in >70% (56,57). In general, the mortality increases by 7% to 10% per minute of delay to defibrillation. Early and effective, near-continuous chest compressions can attenuate the incremental increase in mortality with delayed defibrillation. The provision of high-quality CPR can improve outcome and save lives. Because pediatric cardiac arrests are commonly due to progressive asphyxia and/or shock, the initial treatment of choice is prompt CPR. Therefore, rhythm recognition is relatively less emphasized compared with adult cardiac arrests. However, successful resuscitation from VF does require defibrillation. The earlier VF can be diagnosed, the more successfully it can be treated.

Determinants of Defibrillation (Termination of VF)

Successful termination of VF (defibrillation) is achieved by attaining current flow adequate to depolarize a critical mass of myocardium. Current flow (amperes) is primarily determined by the shock energy (joules), which is selected by the operator, and the patient's transthoracic impedance (ohms).

During the 1970s, animal studies using monophasic shock waveforms established that adequate electrical current flow through the myocardium led to successful defibrillation, and too much current flow resulted in postresuscitation myocardial damage and necrosis. In addition, factors that affected transthoracic impedance were identified as paddle size, thoracic gas volume, electrode/paddle contact, and conducting paste. Small paddle size increases resistance and thereby decreases current through the myocardium. On the other hand, paddles/pads larger than the heart result in current flow through extramyocardial pathways and less current through the heart (consequently, less flow for effective defibrillation). Poor electrode paddle contact and larger lung volumes (gas) result in greater impedance, whereas conducting paste and increased pressure at the paddle-skin contact decrease impedance. Transthoracic impedance could be decreased with multiple "stacked" shocks, partly due to increased skin blood flow after electrical shocks. However, pediatric and adult observational studies (58,59) with biphasic defibrillators suggest that the time to defibrillation attempt is much more important than the impedance, and thus enthusiasm for stacking of shocks with longer interruptions of chest compressions has waned. Current density (current flow through the myocardium) is the primary determinant of both the effectiveness of the shock and myocardial damage.

Pediatric Defibrillation Dose

Early recommendations (from the 1970s) for initial defibrillation doses as high as 200 J for all children were extrapolated from adult data. Despite clinical experience indicating that such doses were effective, providing these large energies to infants and children seemed potentially dangerous, with animal data (60) demonstrating histopathologic myocardial damage at doses >10 J/kg. Other animal data indicated that 0.5–10 J/kg was adequate for defibrillation in a variety of species.

In a retrospective study of the efficacy of the 2-J/kg pediatric defibrillation strategy, 71 transthoracic defibrillation attempts on 27 children were evaluated (61). These children were 3 days to 15 years old and weighed 2.1–50 kg. Fifty-seven of 71 shocks were within 10 J of the 2-J/kg pediatric doses, and 91% (52/57) of these shocks were effective at terminating VF. The authors did not report any other outcome measures (e.g., successful termination of fibrillation to a perfusing rhythm, 24-hour survival, survival to discharge). Subsequent clinical usage suggests that the 2-J/kg dose is effective for short-duration, in-hospital defibrillation, although this conclusion has not been rigorously evaluated.

As noted earlier, current density determines the effectiveness and harm of the shock. Moreover, differences in paddle size, defibrillation energy dose, and the individual's transthoracic impedance are the main determinants of current density. Therefore, investigators explored the effects of paddle size, age, and weight on transthoracic impedance in children (62) (**Fig. 25.1**). As expected, transthoracic impedance increased substantially with pediatric paddles. Based on those data, the AHA recommends that "pediatric" or "small" paddles only be used in infants (63). More importantly, the authors of this study established that the relationship between transthoracic impedance and weight is not linear. The mean transthoracic impedance in their children was ~50 Ω with adult (83 cm²) paddles and varied threefold among children. With pediatric or small (44 cm²) paddles, the mean impedance was ~70 Ω in 3.8 to 36-kg children. The impedances of their infants were

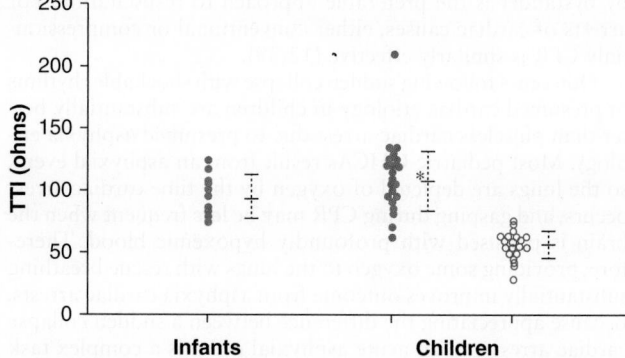

FIGURE 25.1. Effect of paddle size and age on transthoracic impedance (TTI). •, pediatric paddles; ○, adult paddles; *, $p < 0.001$ versus adult paddles; bar indicates standard deviation. (From Atkins DL, Sirna S, Kieso R, et al. Pediatric defibrillation: Importance of paddle size in determining transthoracic impedance. *Pediatrics* 1988;82:914–8, with permission.)

slightly lower than those of their older children, but the range of each was wide, and the overlap substantial (62). Note that the mean transthoracic impedance in adults is ~60–80 Ω and that it also varies by more than threefold. These data suggest that the adjustment of pediatric energy dose to weight (2–4 J/kg) requires further study.

Pediatric Defibrillation Doses for Prolonged VF

Of the >11,000 children with cardiac arrest each year in North America, only 5%–20% present with VF as the initial rhythm. Very little data have been published regarding pediatric defibrillation doses for refractory or prolonged VF. Therefore, the approach to pediatric refractory VF is extrapolated from adult recommendations. For adults, the same defibrillation dose is recommended after brief-duration or prolonged-duration VF. The previously used monophasic 200-J dose was often less effective at terminating prolonged VF (~60% termination of prolonged VF compared with >90% for short-duration VF). Defibrillation using biphasic defibrillators or the 150-J or 200-J biphasic adult automated external defibrillator (AED) dosage is nearly 90% successful at terminating prolonged VF (much better than the ~60% effectiveness with 200-J monophasic defibrillation). The presently recommended pediatric VF dose of 2 J/kg by monophasic waveform is safe, but data are limited regarding effectiveness for prolonged VF. An animal study (60) regarding monophasic defibrillation after 7 minutes of untreated VF in 4- to 24-kg piglets suggests that 2 J/kg may not be adequate. Twenty-four piglets were shocked with 2 J/kg, followed by 4 J/kg. The pediatric dose of 2 J/kg monophasic shocks was uniformly unsuccessful at terminating fibrillation in all 24 piglets. This should not be overinterpreted; interspecies differences could exist in defibrillation thresholds.

However, a small clinical study of pediatric defibrillation (50) attempts also confirms that a 2-J/kg monophasic defibrillation dose is often unsuccessful. Eleven children received 14 pediatric-dose shocks for VF in the Tucson EMS over a 5-year period, using the same definition as the earlier-mentioned pediatric in-hospital (i.e., brief duration) defibrillation study (2 J/kg ±10 J) (61). Only 7 of 14 shocks (50%) terminated out-of-hospital (prolonged) VF, versus 52 of 57 shocks (91%) in their 27 in-hospital patients ($p < 0.01$). This small series suggests that further evaluation of shock dose for refractory or prolonged VF is important.

Additional concerns emanate from a retrospective evaluation of pediatric defibrillation dosage from the GWGT-R database (64). Of 266 children with 285 VF/VT events, 173 of 285 (61%) survived the event, and 61 of 266 (23%) survived to discharge. Termination of fibrillation after the initial shock was achieved for 152 of 285 (53%) events. Termination of fibrillation with 2–10 J/kg was much less frequent than that seen among historic control subjects (56% vs. 91%; $p = 0.001$), but not different than 4 J/kg. Compared with 2 J/kg, an initial shock dose of 4 J/kg was associated with lower rates of return of spontaneous circulation (odds ratio: 0.41 [95% CI, 0.21–0.81]) and event survival (odds ratio: 0.42 [95% CI, 0.18–0.98]). The authors concluded that: (a) the currently recommended 2 J/kg initial shock dose for in-hospital cardiac arrest was substantially less effective than previously published; (b) a higher initial shock dose (4 J/kg) was not associated with superior termination of VF or pulseless VT or improved survival rates; and (c) the optimal pediatric defibrillation dose remains unknown. Similar findings in smaller Australian and Spanish observational studies led those authors to recommend a higher dose simply because 2 J/kg was so often ineffective, although data to support the higher-dose recommendation as safe and effective are not confirmed (47,65,66). In the absence of clear superiority of a specific defibrillation protocol, we recommend 2 J/kg on the first attempt and then 4 J/kg or more on subsequent attempts (maximum 10 J/kg). Clearly, more research is needed in this area.

Pediatric Automated External Defibrillators

VF is prolonged in nearly all children with out-of-hospital VF by the time EMS personnel and defibrillators arrive. AEDs have been recommended for children <8 years old (63,67). Before such recommendations could be made, two issues were considered: (a) the safety and efficacy of the AED diagnostic rhythm-analysis program in children and (b) the safety and efficacy of the AED shock dosage.

An important concern was that babies and small children with sinus tachycardia or supraventricular tachycardia can have very high heart rates that might be misinterpreted as "shockable" by AEDs with diagnostic programs developed for adult arrhythmias. Fortunately, published studies regarding the rhythm-analysis programs from modern AEDs have established that they are quite sensitive and specific in detecting the shockable rhythm of VF (68,69). Algorithms were less sensitive at detecting the very uncommon shockable rhythm of VT, but were quite specific (i.e., the algorithm did not misinterpret other rhythms as VT and therefore did not recommend shocking a "nonshockable" rhythm). Ideally, the device should demonstrate high specificity for pediatric shockable rhythms.

Standard weight-based dosing strategy for pediatric defibrillation is not easily implemented in AEDs. Manufacturers have developed alternatives that attenuate the pediatric dose to 50–86 J biphasic. This dose is safe and effective in piglets after either brief or prolonged VF. In addition, 50-J/75-J/86-J shocks were more effective than a weight-based 2-J/kg dose at initial termination of fibrillation after prolonged VF. In addition, in piglet studies that modeled prolonged out-of-hospital pediatric VF (7 minutes of untreated VF), adult biphasic shocks of 200-J/300-J/360-J were compared with a "pediatric" biphasic AED dose of 50-J/75-J/86-J. Pediatric dosing resulted in fewer elevations of cardiac troponin T levels (70), less postresuscitation myocardial dysfunction (i.e., lesser decreases of left ventricular ejection fraction 1–4 hours postresuscitation), and superior 24-hour survival with good neurologic outcome. These data support the use of attenuating electrodes with adult AEDs for pediatric defibrillation.

It is important to remember that the lack of shock delivery for pediatric VF is 100% lethal. Therefore, adult defibrillation doses are preferable to no defibrillation dose. Elevations of cardiac troponin are not uncommon following pediatric defibrillation (71). A case report suggested that an adult AED dose could save the life of a 3-year-old child in VF. That child was defibrillated with a biphasic shock of 150 J (9 J/kg) (72). He survived without any apparent adverse effects. In particular, he had no elevations of serum creatine kinase or cardiac troponin I and had normal postresuscitation ventricular function on echocardiogram.

INTERVENTIONS DURING THE PREARREST PHASE

Interventions during the prearrest phase focus on recognition and prevention. For example, infant safety seats and safe driving to prevent traumatic arrests, water safety programs to prevent drowning arrests, and medication safety caps to prevent drug poisoning arrests are all well-known, highly effective efforts to prevent cardiac arrests. Because early recognition, prevention, and anticipation of cardiac arrest are better than treatment, early warning scores and medical emergency teams (rapid response teams) are being implemented to recognize and intervene when cardiac arrest is impending. Because many pediatric cardiac arrests are due to progressive respiratory failure and shock, the main focus of various early warning systems and medical emergency teams (METs) is the early recognition and treatment of respiratory failure and shock in children (i.e., prevention of cardiac arrest during the prearrest phase). Although it is difficult to document a statistically significant impact of these METs on outcome, their implementation has decreased the incidence of CPR on wards and is associated with improving survival rates (28,73–79).

INTERVENTIONS DURING THE CARDIAC ARREST (NO-FLOW) PHASE AND CARDIOPULMONARY (LOW-FLOW) PHASE: CARDIOPULMONARY RESUSCITATION

Circulation

Providing BLS with continuous effective chest compressions is generally the best way to provide circulation during cardiac arrest. BLS is often provided poorly or not provided at all. The most critical elements are to *push hard* and *push fast*. Because no blood flow occurs without chest compressions, it is important to minimize interruptions in chest compressions. To allow adequate venous return in the decompression phase of closed-chest compressions, it is important to allow full-chest recoil and to avoid overventilation. The latter can prevent venous return because of increased intrathoracic pressure.

The use of closed-chest cardiac compression to provide adequate circulation during cardiac arrest was initially demonstrated in small dogs with compliant chest walls. On the basis of reasonable extrapolation, these investigators felt that closed-chest cardiac massage would be effective with children but might not be effective with adults. Therefore, the first patients successfully treated with closed-chest cardiac massage were children. The presumed mechanism of blood flow involved compression of the heart between the sternum and the spine (cardiac pump mechanism) that was facilitated by the compliant chest wall of children. Later investigations indicated that blood could also be circulated during CPR by the thoracic pump mechanism in which intrathoracic pressure generates a gradient for blood to flow from the pulmonary vasculature, through the heart, and into the peripheral circulation without the need for compression of the heart. Regardless of mechanism, cardiac output during CPR seems to be greater in children (and immature animals) with compliant chest walls than in adults with less-compliant chest walls. Interestingly, recent GWTG-R data indicate that outcomes from in-hospital cardiac arrest are substantially better in infants than in older children (80), perhaps because of superior perfusion during CPR.

Why C-A-B Instead of A-B-C?

Although most pediatric cardiac arrests are precipitated by respiratory compromise (i.e., asphyxia), chest compressions are necessary to provide circulatory support. Nearly all in-hospital cardiac arrests are witnessed and/or monitored, so a rapid response should be the norm, and the first rescuer should be able to start chest compressions almost immediately. In contrast, positioning the head and attaining a seal for mouth-to-mouth or a bag-mask apparatus for rescue breathing take time and delay the initiation of chest compressions. Therefore, since 2010, the AHA has recommended that the first responders call for help and immediately start chest compressions while the second and subsequent responders address the airway/breathing and rhythm issues. If the cause of the arrest is a shockable rhythm (VF/VT), chest compressions and defibrillation are the mainstays of treatment. When the cause is more commonly asphyxia or hypotension, prompt chest compressions can reestablish the circulation while personnel and respiratory equipment become rapidly available. For OHCA, the concepts are similar, but the initial responder may be a single lay rescuer. Because it is easier to provide good chest compressions than chest compressions plus rescue breathing, and because the combination of chest compressions plus rescue breathing is difficult to perform, it is reasonable to start with chest compressions. Observational data suggest that outcomes are comparable with chest compression–only bystander CPR versus chest compression plus rescue breathing for children whose cardiac arrest is from a cardiac cause (39), but animal studies and a large observational study have established that chest compressions alone are simply inadequate for children with OHCA due to noncardiac etiologies (i.e., primarily respiratory cause) (40). For these children, C-A-B is fine, but chest compressions alone are not.

What Should Be the Immediate Goal of Chest Compressions?

10

Animal studies have shown that CPR results in successful resuscitation only if it maintains adequate coronary perfusion pressure, the primary determinant of myocardial blood flow (5,81–85). The coronary perfusion pressure is the arterial pressure minus the right atrial pressure during the relaxation phase of CPR. The experimental data indicate that a coronary perfusion pressure >20 mm Hg or arterial "diastolic/relaxation" pressure >30 mm Hg is associated with successful resuscitation (5,81–85). Limited data from adult out-of-hospital cardiac arrests are consistent with the animal data (86). Recent swine studies suggest that focusing on efforts to target a coronary perfusion pressure >20 mm Hg is more effective than following anatomic targets of depth and frequency of epinephrine administration (5,85). Importantly, most in-hospital cardiac arrests occur in ICUs, and more than 60% of these patients have arterial catheters at the time of CPR. Therefore, titration of CPR efforts to adequate arterial pressures during the relaxation phase is often feasible.

When an arterial catheter is not available, end-tidal carbon dioxide ($ETCO_2$) measurements are often available. Animal studies suggest that $ETCO_2$ during CPR correlates with cardiac output and survival (87,88). Also, adult studies have confirmed that attaining $ETCO_2 > 15$ mm Hg is associated with survival (89,90). Although published pediatric data associating $ETCO_2$ during CPR with hemodynamics and survival outcomes are limited (91), the American Heart Association (AHA) extrapolates from adult data to recommend monitoring of $ETCO_2$ during pediatric CPR (92).

Circumferential Versus Focal Sternal Compressions

In adults and animal models of cardiac arrest, circumferential (e.g., Vest) CPR provides better CPR hemodynamics than point compressions. In smaller infants, it is often possible to encircle the chest with both hands and depress the sternum with the thumbs, while compressing the thorax circumferentially. In an infant model of CPR (93,94), this "two-thumb" method of compression resulted in higher systolic and diastolic blood pressures and a higher pulse pressure than did traditional two-finger compression of the sternum. Load distributing band circumferential chest compressions in larger animals and adults also results in better hemodynamics, but has not consistently been associated with superior outcomes in OHCA (95).

Duty Cycle

Duty cycle is the ratio of the duration of the compression phase to the entire compression–relaxation cycle. In a model of human adult cardiac arrest (96,97), cardiac output and coronary blood flow are optimized when chest compressions last for 30% of the total cycle time. As the duration of CPR increases, the optimal duty cycle may change from 30% to 50%. In a juvenile swine model, a relaxation period of 250–300 ms (a duty cycle of 40%–50% if 120 compressions are delivered per minute) correlated with improved cerebral perfusion pressure when compared with shorter duty cycles of 30% (98).

Open-Chest Compressions

Excellent closed-chest compressions during CPR generates ~10%–25% of baseline myocardial blood flow and a cerebral blood flow that is ~50% of normal. By contrast, open-chest compressions can generate a cerebral blood flow that approaches normal. Although open-chest massage improves coronary perfusion pressure and increases the chance of successful defibrillation in animals and humans, surgical thoracotomy is not practical or desirable in many situations. A retrospective review of 27 cases of CPR following pediatric blunt trauma (15 with open-chest CPR and 12 with closed-chest CPR) demonstrated that open-chest CPR increased hospital costs without altering ROSC or survival to discharge rates (99). However, survival in both groups was 0%, indicating that the population may have been too severely injured or too late in the process to benefit from this aggressive therapy. Open-chest CPR is often provided to children after cardiac surgery and sternotomy. The earlier institution of open-chest CPR may warrant study in selected special resuscitation circumstances.

Airway and Breathing

The most common precipitating event for cardiac arrest in children is respiratory insufficiency. Adequate oxygen delivery to meet metabolic demands and the removal of carbon dioxide are the goals of initial assisted ventilation. High-quality bag-mask ventilation remains the cornerstone of providing effective emergency ventilation. Effective ventilation during CPR does not necessarily require a tracheal tube. In one randomized, controlled study of children with out-of-hospital respiratory arrest (100), children who were treated with bag-mask ventilation did as well as children treated with prehospital endotracheal intubation. Emergency airway techniques such as transtracheal jet ventilation and emergency cricothyroidotomy are rarely, if ever, required during CPR. During CPR, cardiac output and pulmonary blood flow are ~10%–25% of that during normal sinus rhythm. Consequently, much less ventilation is necessary for adequate gas exchange from the blood traversing the pulmonary circulation during CPR. *Overventilation during CPR* is an important concern based on both preclinical and adult data that indicate that it is common (6) and can substantially compromise venous return and cardiac output (101). Overventilation can be due to too frequent breaths (hyperventilation), which can increase the interference with the generation of negative intrathoracic pressure during the relaxation phase of chest compression. Overventilation can also be due to too large breaths (overdistension) that may cause excessively increased intrathoracic pressure (and vascular resistance) and further compromise venous return. A third concern is that, in nonintubated patients, interposing ventilations and compressions during rescue breathing increases the number of pauses in chest compression delivery (decreasing the chest compression ratio and increasing the no-flow fraction) and can contribute to worse survival outcomes. The final concern is that continued overventilation during ROSC and postresuscitation care may cause alkalosis, cerebral vasoconstriction, and limit cerebral blood flow.

Although airway and breathing are prioritized in the ABC (airway, breathing, circulation) assessment approach, special circumstances may impact that priority order. In animal models of sudden VF cardiac arrest, acceptable Pao_2 and $Paco_2$ persist for 4–8 minutes during chest compressions without rescue breathing. Moreover, many animal studies indicate that outcomes from sudden, short-duration VF cardiac arrests are at least as good with chest compressions alone as with chest compressions plus rescue breathing. In addition, several retrospective studies of witnessed VF cardiac arrest in adults also suggest that outcomes are similar after bystander-initiated CPR with either chest compressions alone or chest compressions plus rescue breathing. A randomized, controlled study of dispatcher-assisted, bystander CPR in adults found a trend toward improved survival in those patients who received chest compressions alone compared with those who received dispatcher-instructed ventilation and chest compressions (102). In contrast, animal studies of asphyxia-precipitated cardiac arrests have established that rescue breathing is a critical component of successful CPR under those circumstances (103).

If adequate oxygenation and ventilation are important for survival from any cardiac arrest, why is rescue breathing not initially necessary for VF, yet quite important in asphyxia? Immediately after an acute fibrillatory cardiac arrest, aortic oxygen and carbon dioxide concentrations do not vary from the prearrest state because there is no blood flow, and aortic oxygen consumption is minimal. Therefore, when chest compressions are initiated, the blood flowing from the aorta to the coronary and cerebral circulations provides adequate oxygenation at an acceptable pH. At that time, myocardial oxygen delivery is limited more by blood flow than by oxygen content. Adequate oxygenation and ventilation can continue without rescue breathing because the lungs serve as a reservoir for oxygen during the low-flow state of CPR. In addition, ventilation can occur due to chest compression–induced gas exchange and spontaneous gasping during CPR in victims of sudden cardiac arrest. Therefore, arterial oxygenation and pH can often be adequate using chest compressions alone for VF arrests.

For the infant or child, forgoing ventilation may not be appropriate because respiratory arrest and asphyxia generally precede pediatric cardiac arrest. During asphyxia, blood continues to flow to tissues; therefore, arterial and venous oxygen saturations decrease while carbon dioxide and lactate

increase. In addition, continued pulmonary blood flow before the cardiac arrest depletes the pulmonary oxygen reservoir. Therefore, asphyxia results in significant arterial hypoxemia and acidemia prior to resuscitation, in contrast to VF. In this circumstance, rescue breathing can be lifesaving.

Ratio of Compressions to Ventilation

Compression:ventilation (C:V) ratios and tidal volumes recommended during CPR are based on rational conjecture and educational retention theory. Ideal C:V ratios for pediatric patients are unknown. Recent physiologic estimates suggest the amount of ventilation needed during CPR is much less than the amount needed during a normal perfusing rhythm because the cardiac output during CPR is only 10%–25% of that during normal sinus rhythm (104). The benefits of positive-pressure ventilation (increased arterial content of oxygen and carbon dioxide elimination) must be balanced against the adverse consequence of impeding circulation.

Maximizing systemic oxygen delivery during single-rescuer CPR requires a tradeoff between time spent doing chest compressions and the time spent doing mouth-to-mouth ventilations. Theoretically, neither compression-only nor ventilation-only CPR can sustain systemic oxygen delivery. The best ratio depends on many factors, including the compression rate, tidal volume, blood flow generated by compressions, and the time that compressions are interrupted to perform ventilations. A C:V ratio of 15:2 delivered the same minute ventilation as CPR with a chest C:V ratio of 5:1 in a mannequin model of pediatric CPR, but the number of chest compressions delivered was 48% higher with the 15:2 ratio (105,106).

In adults, mathematical models (107) of oxygen delivery during CPR performed with variable ratios of healthcare-provider chest compressions to ventilations suggest that the optimal C:V ratio is ~30:2 and, for lay rescuers, closer to 50:2. Mathematical models of C:V ratios suggest that matching the amount of ventilation to the amount of reduced pulmonary blood flow during closed-chest cardiac compressions should favor very high compression-to-ventilation ratios. The effect of C:V ratio on oxygen delivery to peripheral tissues has been demonstrated (107). Ignoring the amount of ventilation provided by chest compressions alone, neither compression-only nor ventilation-only CPR can sustain oxygen delivery to the periphery for prolonged periods of CPR. As mentioned earlier, the best ratio depends on many factors (i.e., compression rate, tidal volume, blood flow generated by compressions, and time that compressions are interrupted to perform ventilations). These factors can be related in a mathematical formula based on physiology, because they change as a function of the size of the patient. Such considerations may help refine the amount of ventilation recommended for both adults and children. The ratio of chest compressions to ventilations during no-flow and low-flow phases of cardiopulmonary-cerebral resuscitation remains an area of interest, controversy, and future research. These formulas, adjusted to the known physiologic variables in children, have suggested the potential to simplify the C:V ratio of 15 chest compressions to two ventilations in children prior to intubation (106, 108). Once the trachea is intubated, pauses in chest compressions during ventilations are no longer recommended and so ventilations are provided with near continuous chest compressions (63, 109).

Intraosseous Vascular Access

Intraosseous (IO) vascular access provides access to a noncollapsible marrow venous plexus, which serves as a rapid, safe, and reliable route for the administration of drugs, crystalloids, colloids, and blood during resuscitation. Intraosseous vascular access can often be achieved in 30–60 seconds. A specially designed IO bone marrow needle with a stylet is preferred to prevent obstruction of the needle with cortical bone. The IO needle is typically inserted into the anterior proximal tibial bone marrow; alternative sites include the distal femur, medial malleolus, anterior superior iliac spine, and the distal tibia. In adults and older children, the medial malleolus, distal radius, and distal ulna are optional locations. Mechanical drills to insert IO needles are now widely available in resourced settings.

Resuscitation drugs, fluids, continuous catecholamine infusions, and blood products can be safely administered through the IO route. The onset of action and drug levels following IO infusion during CPR are comparable to those achieved following central vascular administration. Intraosseous vascular access may also be used to obtain blood specimens for chemistry, blood gas analysis, and blood typing and cross-matching (110).

Complications have been reported in <1% of patients following IO infusion; these include tibial fracture, lower extremity compartment syndrome, severe extravasation of drugs, and osteomyelitis. Most of these complications may be avoided by careful technique. Although microscopic pulmonary fat and bone marrow emboli have been demonstrated in animal models (111), they have never been reported clinically and appear to occur just as frequently during cardiac arrest without IO drug administration. Animal data and one human follow-up study indicate that the local effects of IO infusion on the bone marrow and bone growth are minimal.

Endotracheal Drug Administration

Intraosseous vascular access has largely replaced the need for endotracheal drug administration (in the past, important drugs were commonly administered via the endotracheal tube before vascular access was achieved). In particular, epinephrine, atropine, naloxone, and lidocaine were commonly administered via the endotracheal route. Sodium bicarbonate and calcium may be very irritating to the airways and lung parenchyma and are not recommended for endotracheal administration.

Absorption of drugs into the circulation after endotracheal administration depends on dispersion over the respiratory mucosa, pulmonary blood flow, and the matching of the ventilation (drug dispersal) to perfusion. The small volumes of drug that remain as droplets in the tracheal tube are obviously not effective. Inadequate chest compressions that result in poor pulmonary blood flow will also limit absorption of the drug and prevent its delivery to the heart and systemic circulation. Preexisting pathophysiologic conditions such as pulmonary edema, pneumonitis, and airway disease also affect the pharmacokinetics of endotracheally administered drugs. Another confounding factor is that the vasoconstrictive effects of epinephrine may limit local pulmonary blood flow, thereby diminishing drug uptake and delivery. It is therefore not surprising that drug absorption varies greatly and that optimal drug doses have not been determined. Animal studies reveal a wide variability in plasma epinephrine levels and physiologic effects after endotracheal administration. On average, 10 times as much endotracheal epinephrine is required to attain peak plasma levels comparable to those of IV administration (112). Moreover, a prolonged depot effect typically occurs after endotracheal epinephrine administration, which can lead to postresuscitation hypertension, tachycardia, and ventricular arrhythmias.

Medication Use During Cardiac Arrest

Although animal studies indicate that epinephrine can improve initial ROSC after both asphyxial and VF cardiac arrests, no single medication has been shown to improve survival outcome from pediatric cardiac arrest.

Vasopressors

During CPR, epinephrine's α-adrenergic effect on vascular tone increases systemic vascular resistance, thereby increasing diastolic blood pressure, which, in turn, increases coronary perfusion pressure and blood flow and increases the likelihood of ROSC. Epinephrine also increases cerebral blood flow during CPR because peripheral vasoconstriction directs a greater proportion of flow to the cerebral circulation. However, the β-adrenergic effect increases myocardial oxygen consumption, perhaps worsening the already tenuous relationship of oxygen supply and demand during CPR. Perhaps this effect is one of the reasons for demonstrable worsening of post–cardiac arrest myocardial function with epinephrine administration in animal models. Importantly, animal studies indicate that epinephrine administration during CPR can diminish microcirculatory flow in the brain and other tissues presumably through its α-adrenergic-mediated vasoconstriction. Epinephrine also increases the vigor and intensity of VF, increasing the likelihood of successful defibrillation, presumably because of increased coronary perfusion.

High-dose epinephrine (0.05–0.2 mg/kg) improves myocardial and cerebral blood flow during CPR more than standard-dose epinephrine (0.01–0.02 mg/kg) and may increase the incidence of initial ROSC (113–115). The administration of high-dose epinephrine, however, can worsen a patient's postresuscitation hemodynamic condition by causing increased myocardial oxygen demand, ventricular ectopy, hypertension, and myocardial necrosis (116). Prospective and retrospective studies indicate that the use of higher doses of epinephrine in adults or children does not improve survival and may be associated with a worse neurologic outcome (115–119).

A randomized, controlled trial of rescue high-dose epinephrine versus standard-dose epinephrine following failed initial standard-dose epinephrine for pediatric in-hospital cardiac arrest demonstrated a worse 24-hour survival in the high-dose epinephrine group (1/27 vs. 6/23, $p < 0.05$) (120). In particular, high-dose epinephrine seemed to worsen the outcome of patients with asphyxia-precipitated cardiac arrest. High-dose epinephrine cannot be recommended routinely for initial therapy or rescue therapy.

Wide variability in catecholamine pharmacokinetics and pharmacodynamics dictates individual titration. A lifesaving dose during CPR for one patient may be life-threatening to another. High-dose epinephrine should be considered as an alternative to standard-dose epinephrine in special circumstances of refractory pediatric cardiac arrest (e.g., patient on high-dose epinephrine infusion prior to cardiac arrest) and/or when continuous direct arterial blood pressure monitoring allows titration of the epinephrine dosage to diastolic (decompression phase) arterial pressure during CPR. Nevertheless, high-dose epinephrine has not been demonstrated to improve outcome and should only be used with caution.

Data from adult OHCA raise the possibility that any dose of epinephrine during CPR might be harmful. Consistent with animal studies, several observational studies indicate that epinephrine improves initial success of resuscitation (121–123). However, none of the observational studies showed benefit for survival to discharge or survival with favorable neurological outcomes (121–124), and some studies showed an association of epinephrine during CPR and lower rates of survival to discharge and/or survival with favorable neurological outcomes (121–123). In the only RCT with 262 adults receiving epinephrine and 262 receiving placebo, epinephrine improved ROSC (23.5% vs. 8.4%; OR 3.4; 95% CI, 2.0–5.6). (115), and the survival rate was not demonstrably different (4% vs. 1.9%; OR 2.2; 95% CI, 0.7–6.3). Importantly, most adults with OHCA have coronary artery disease, and the cause of the arrest in many of these patients is an acute coronary syndrome.

How do these data relate to the use of epinephrine for children in cardiac arrest? First, the animal data are quite clear that adequate coronary perfusion is necessary to attain ROSC. If a child does not have adequate coronary perfusion during CPR by invasive hemodynamic monitoring despite excellent chest compressions, the risk of not increasing the coronary perfusion pressure with a vasoactive agent presumably exceeds the potential secondary risks of epinephrine vasoconstriction. Second, the only RCT in adults shows higher rates of ROSC with epinephrine and a presumably underpowered tendency for higher survival to discharge rates as well. Third, the adverse effects of epinephrine may be more problematic for adults with acute coronary syndromes than for children in cardiac arrest. Nevertheless, the concerns about potential adverse effects of epinephrine during CPR should not be dismissed.

Vasopressin is a long-acting endogenous hormone that acts at specific receptors to mediate systemic vasoconstriction (V_1 receptor) and reabsorption of water in the renal tubule (V_2 receptor). In experimental models of cardiac arrest (125,126), vasopressin increases blood flow to the heart and brain, and improves long-term survival when compared with epinephrine. Vasopressin may decrease splanchnic blood flow during and following CPR, and the increased afterload with this long-acting agent may exacerbate post–cardiac arrest myocardial dysfunction. In randomized, controlled trials of in-hospital and out-of-hospital arrest in adults (127,128), vasopressin had comparable efficacy to epinephrine. Vasopressin did not improve outcome compared with epinephrine.

In a piglet model of prolonged VF, the use of vasopressin and epinephrine in combination resulted in higher left ventricular blood flow than either pressor alone, and both vasopressin alone, and vasopressin plus epinephrine resulted in superior cerebral blood flow than did epinephrine alone (126,129). By contrast, in a piglet model of *asphyxial* cardiac arrest, return of spontaneous circulation was more likely in piglets treated with epinephrine than in those treated with vasopressin. A case series of four children who received vasopressin during six prolonged cardiac arrest events suggests that the use of bolus vasopressin may result in ROSC when standard medications have failed (130). Vasopressin has also been reported to be useful in low-cardiac-output states associated with sepsis syndrome and organ recovery in children. Although vasopressin will not likely replace epinephrine as a first-line agent in pediatric cardiac arrest, preliminary data suggest that its use in conjunction with epinephrine deserves further investigation.

Calcium

For in-hospital pediatric cardiac arrests, hypocalcemia is not uncommon. Although calcium administration is recommended only during cardiac arrest for documented hypocalcemia, hyperkalemia, hypermagnesemia, and calcium-channel-blocker overdose, it is commonly used for in-hospital pediatric cardiac arrests, especially those that occur post–cardiac surgery. The administration of calcium has not been demonstrated to improve outcome in cardiac arrest (131). Animal studies suggest that calcium administration may worsen reperfusion injury (132). Observational studies of in-hospital pediatric cardiac arrests consistently show that calcium administration during CPR is associated with worse outcomes (133–135). Although epidemiologic associations cannot establish causality, it is concerning that there are no available data to demonstrate the effectiveness of calcium administration during CPR.

Buffer Solutions

Cardiac arrest results in lactic acidosis from inadequate organ blood flow and poor oxygen delivery. Acidosis depresses myocardial function, reduces systemic vascular resistance, and inhibits defibrillation. Nevertheless, the routine use of sodium bicarbonate for a child in cardiac arrest is not recommended. Like calcium, bicarbonate administration during in-hospital pediatric CPR is associated with worse outcomes (133). Clinical trials that involved critically ill adults with severe metabolic acidosis did not demonstrate a beneficial effect of sodium bicarbonate. However, because the presence of acidosis may depress the action of catecholamines, some pediatric intensivists have used sodium bicarbonate in an acidemic child who is refractory to catecholamine administration despite the lack of data showing a benefit to this approach. The administration of sodium bicarbonate is more clearly indicated in the patient with hyperkalemia, a tricyclic antidepressant overdose, or sodium-channel-blocker poisoning.

The buffering action of bicarbonate occurs when a hydrogen cation and a bicarbonate anion combine to form carbon dioxide and water. If carbon dioxide is not effectively cleared through ventilation, its buildup will counterbalance the buffering effect of bicarbonate. Other side effects with sodium bicarbonate include hypernatremia, hyperosmolarity, and metabolic alkalosis. THAM is a non–carbon-dioxide-generating buffer that can be used during cardiac arrest. Note that excessive alkalosis decreases calcium and potassium concentration and shifts the oxyhemoglobin dissociation curve to the left and may cause cerebral vasoconstriction.

Antiarrhythmic Medications: Lidocaine and Amiodarone

The administration of antiarrhythmic medications should not delay the use of defibrillation for a patient with VF. However, after unsuccessful attempts at electrical defibrillation, medications to increase the effectiveness of defibrillation should be considered. In both pediatric and adult patients, after an unsuccessful defibrillation attempt, the first administered medication is epinephrine (with or without vasopressin) and a subsequent repeat attempt to defibrillate. If this attempt is unsuccessful, the antiarrhythmic agents amiodarone or lidocaine should be considered.

Lidocaine has been recommended traditionally for shock-resistant VF in adults and children. However, amiodarone is the only antiarrhythmic agent that has been prospectively determined to improve survival to hospital admission in the setting of shock-resistant VF when compared with placebo (136,137). Furthermore, patients who received amiodarone for shock-resistant out-of-hospital VF had a higher rate of survival to hospital admission than did patients who received lidocaine alone. Neither of these (136,137) randomized, controlled trials included children. Although no comparisons of antiarrhythmic medications for pediatric refractory VF have been published, extrapolation of the adult studies has led to the recommendation of amiodarone as the preferred antiarrhythmic agent for children.

POSTRESUSCITATION INTERVENTIONS

Targeted Temperature Management

Mild, induced hypothermia is a promising goal-directed, postresuscitation therapy. Two seminal articles suggested that induced hypothermia (32°–34°C) could improve outcome for comatose adults after resuscitation from witnessed out-of-hospital VF cardiac arrest (138,139). In both of these randomized, controlled trials, the inclusion criteria were patients >18 years who were persistently comatose after successful resuscitation from nontraumatic VF. The multicentered European study had a goal of 32°–34°C for the first 24 hours postarrest

(139). The mean time until attainment of this temperature goal was 8 hours. Six-month survival with good neurologic outcome was superior in 75/136 (55%) in the hypothermic group versus 54/137 (39%) in the normothermic group (RR, 1.40; CI, 1.08–1.81). Similarly, death at 6 months postevent occurred less often in the hypothermic group (56/137; 41%) versus (76/138; 55%) in the normothermic group (RR, 0.74; CI, 0.58–0.95). The second study from Australia reported good outcomes in 21/43 (49%) of the hypothermic group versus 9/34 (26%) of the control group (*p* = 0.046, OR 5.25; CI, 1.47–18.76) (138). Importantly, hypotension occurred among over half of the patients in both groups and was aggressively treated with vasoactive infusion in the European study. Similarly, more than half of the Australian patients received epinephrine infusions during the first 24 hours postresuscitation. More recent adult studies suggest that a targeted temperature management with close attention to postresuscitation supportive care is equally effective at 32°C as at 36.5°C (140,141).

Interpretation and extrapolation of these studies to children is difficult. Fever following cardiac arrest, brain trauma, stroke, and ischemia is associated with poor neurologic outcome. Hyperthermia following cardiac arrest is common in children (142). It is reasonable to believe that mild, induced, systemic hypothermia may benefit children who are resuscitated from cardiac arrest. However, a retrospective observational pediatric study showed no difference in outcome with hypothermia (143). Further randomized controlled trials of Therapeutic Hypothermia after Pediatric Cardiac Arrest (THAPCA), out-of-hospital and in-hospital cohorts, should provide greater clarity about these issues. At this time, avoiding, and actively treating, hyperthermia following CPR is indicated.

Postresuscitation Myocardial Support

Postarrest myocardial stunning occurs commonly after successful resuscitation in animals, adults, and children. In addition, most adults who survive to hospital admission after OHCA die early in the postresuscitation phase, many due to progressive myocardial dysfunction. Animal studies demonstrate that postarrest myocardial stunning is characterized by a global biventricular systolic and diastolic dysfunction and typically resolves after 1 or 2 days (144,145). Postarrest myocardial stunning is pathophysiologically similar to sepsis-related myocardial dysfunction and postcardiopulmonary bypass myocardial dysfunction, including increases in inflammatory mediator and nitric oxide production. Postarrest myocardial stunning is worse after a more prolonged untreated cardiac arrest, after more prolonged CPR, after defibrillation with higher energy shocks, and after a greater number of shocks.

Optimal treatment of postarrest myocardial dysfunction has not been rigorously established. As noted earlier, this myocardial dysfunction has been treated with various continuous inotropic/vasoactive agents (including dopamine, dobutamine, and epinephrine) in both children and adults. The inodilator milrinone improves the hemodynamic status of children with post–cardiopulmonary bypass myocardial dysfunction and septic shock. A new inotropic agent levosimendan has been effective in the treatment of animal models of postresuscitation myocardial dysfunction (146), treatment of myocardial stunning in adults (147), and pediatric low-cardiac output (148).

Although prospective, controlled trials in animals have demonstrated that the myocardial dysfunction can be effectively treated with vasoactive agents, no data demonstrate improvements in outcome. Nevertheless, because myocardial dysfunction is common (149) and can lead to secondary ischemic injuries to other organ systems or even cardiovascular collapse, treatment with vasoactive medications is a rational therapeutic choice that may improve outcome. The hemodynamic benefits in animal studies of postarrest myocardial dysfunction, pediatric studies of post–cardiopulmonary bypass myocardial dysfunction, and pediatric sepsis-related myocardial dysfunction support the use of inotropic/vasoactive agents in this setting (150–155). In addition, adult studies document the common occurrence of postarrest hypotension and/or poor myocardial function "requiring" inotropic/vasoactive agents. In summary, because treatment of postarrest myocardial dysfunction with inotropic/vasoactive infusions can improve the patient's hemodynamic status, such treatment should be routinely considered and titrated to effect. Unfortunately, evidence-based therapeutic targets for goal-directed therapy are ill defined.

Blood Pressure Management

It has been demonstrated that 55% of adults who survived OHCA required in-hospital vasoactive infusions for hypotension unresponsive to volume boluses (156). Among 138 children who survived to PICU admission following OHCA, 70% were treated with vasoactive infusions for hypotension or myocardial dysfunction (157). Post-ROSC hypotension in adults is a predictor of in-hospital death and is associated with diminished functional status among the survivors (158). Among 383 children, 56% had at least one hypotensive episode in the first 6 hours post–ROSC, and those with hypotension were much more likely to die during that hospitalization (adjusted OR = 1.71; 95% CI, 1.02–2.89) and to have an unfavorable neurological outcome if they survived to hospital discharge (adjusted OR = 1.83; 95% CI, 1.06–3.19). Aggressive PICU monitoring and supportive care to prevent hypotension should be a mainstay of post–cardiac arrest care.

Glucose Control

Hyperglycemia following adult cardiac arrest is associated with worse neurologic outcome after controlling for duration of arrest and presence of cardiogenic shock (159). In animal models of asphyxial and ischemic cardiac arrest, the administration of insulin and glucose, but not the administration of glucose alone, improved neurologic outcome compared with administration of normal saline (160). Data for evidence-based titration of specific end points is not available.

Post–Cardiac Arrest Seizures

Seizures after pediatric cardiac arrest are common. In one study, 42% of children treated with hypothermia after cardiac arrest had seizures, and 32% had status epilepticus (161). It is very important to note that two-thirds of these children had nonconvulsive seizures that would have been undetected without continuous EEG. This is especially important because electrographic status epilepticus is associated with mortality and worse short-term neurologic outcome in critically ill children (162). Furthermore, continuous and reactive background patterns on EEG are associated with good outcome, whereas burst-suppression and discontinuous backgrounds are associated with poor outcome (163). Continuous EEG monitoring can provide useful information to help minimize brain injury and enhance prognostication.

Postresuscitation Hyperoxia

The administration of 100% oxygen after ROSC following cardiac arrest is associated with worse neurological outcomes than lower oxygen concentrations in animal models (thought to be associated with free radical injury and oxidative stress) (164).

Consistent with these findings, a study of 6326 ICU adults admitted to an ICU post–ROSC showed that hyperoxia on the first blood gas was associated with increased in-hospital mortality (165). A larger study of 12,108 adults in an ICU post–ROSC was unable to confirm any adverse effect of post-ROSC hyperoxia (166). Among 1875 children in the Pediatric Intensive Care Audit Network of 33 PICUs in the United Kingdom and Ireland, post-ROSC hypoxemia was strongly associated with increased mortality and, to a lesser extent, post-ROSC hyperoxia was also associated with increased mortality (164–166). In contrast, a smaller single-center study of 74 children did not show any relationship of hyperoxia with mortality (167). Until more is known, it is prudent to wean children from 100% oxygen post–ROSC while titrating oxygen therapy to maintain adequate oxygen saturations in vital organs.

Extracorporeal Membrane Oxygenation—Cardiopulmonary Resuscitation

Extracorporeal membrane oxygenation (ECMO) is a technology that can be used to control postresuscitation temperature and hemodynamic parameters. The concomitant administration of heparin may facilitate microcirculatory flow. The use of venoarterial ECMO to reestablish circulation and provide controlled reperfusion following cardiac arrest has been published, but prospective, controlled studies are lacking. Nevertheless, these series have reported extraordinary results with the use of ECMO as a rescue therapy for pediatric cardiac arrests, especially from potentially reversible acute postoperative myocardial dysfunction or arrhythmias. In one study, 11 children in the PICU who suffered cardiac arrest after cardiac surgery were placed on ECMO during CPR (E-CPR) (168). Prolonged CPR (20–110 minutes) was continued until ECMO cannulae, circuits, and personnel were available. Six of these 11 children were long-term survivors without apparent neurologic sequelae. More recently, two centers have reported an additional eight remarkable pediatric cardiac patients who were provided with mechanical cardiopulmonary support during CPR within 20 minutes of the initiation of CPR. All eight survived to hospital discharge (169). CPR and ECMO are not curative treatments. They are cardiopulmonary supportive measures that provide tissue perfusion and viability until recovery from the precipitating disease process. As such, they can be powerful tools. Most remarkably, in 66 children placed on E-CPR over a 7-year period, the median duration of CPR prior to ECMO was 50 minutes, and 23 (35%) survived to hospital discharge (169). Additional centers have corroborated this finding (135). It is important to emphasize that these children had brief no-flow periods, excellent CPR during the low-flow period, and a well-controlled postresuscitation phase.

The potential advantages of E-CPR come from its ability to maintain a tight control of physiologic parameters after resuscitation: blood flow rates, oxygenation, ventilation, anticoagulation, and body temperature can be precisely manipulated using ECMO support. As we learn more about the processes of secondary injury following cardiac arrest, ECMO might enable controlled perfusion and temperature management to minimize reperfusion injury and maximize cell recovery.

DURATION OF CARDIOPULMONARY RESUSCITATION: WHAT IS REASONABLE?

Two sets of studies have created confusion and hope for pediatric intensivists regarding the appropriate duration of CPR.

As noted above, E-CPR can be successfully instituted after >50 minutes of CPR with survival and favorable neurological outcomes in some patients. In addition, two GWTG-R studies, one adult and one pediatric, establish that prolonged CPR can result in survival with favorable neurological outcomes without E-CPR (20,170). In a GWTG-R study, 994 of 3419 children with in-hospital CPR (29%) had CPR for >35 minutes, and of those, 158 (15.9%) survived to hospital discharge (20). Notably, >84% did not survive after CPR for >35 minutes. The survival rate with CPR >35 minutes was much lower among trauma patients than among medical or surgical noncardiac patients, and highest among the cardiac surgical patients. Among survivors, favorable neurological outcome occurred in 70% undergoing <15 minutes of CPR and 60% undergoing CPR >35 minutes.

The observational GWTG-R data do not provide sufficient information to elucidate why providers continued CPR so long in a subset of these children. Presumably, some of these providers felt that continued CPR was a potential bridge to survival for some children, and the surprisingly good outcomes emanate from this thoughtful clinical judgment. Importantly, these findings should help dispel common perceptions that CPR is futile beyond 20 minutes. On the other hand, providers may realize that CPR is not a viable bridge for some patients and should therefore not be continued so long. This study was not designed to offer decision rules about when to discontinue CPR in individual patients.

POSTRESUSCITATION OUTCOMES

The most important postresuscitation outcomes are survival with favorable neurologic outcome and acceptable quality of life. Many studies report end points of ROSC or survival to hospital discharge. Information is limited about neurologic outcomes and predictors of neurologic outcome after both adult and pediatric cardiac arrests. Barriers to the assessment of neurologic outcomes of children after cardiac arrests include the constantly changing developmental context that occurs with brain maturation. Prediction or prognosis for future neuropsychologic status is a complex task, particularly after an acute neurologic insult. Little information is available regarding the predictive value of clinical neurologic examinations, neurophysiologic diagnostic studies (e.g., electroencephalogram or somatosensory-evoked potentials), biomarkers, or imaging (CT, MRI, or positron-emission tomography) on eventual outcomes following cardiac arrest or other global hypoxic-ischemic insults in children. CT scans are not sensitive in detecting early neurologic injury. The value of MRI studies following pediatric cardiac arrest is not yet clear. However, MRI with diffusion weighting should provide valuable information about hypoxic-ischemic injury in the subacute and recovery phases. For example, a small single-center study of 28 children, showed that increased T-2 intensity in the basal ganglia and restricted diffusion in brain lobes were associated with unfavorable neurologic outcomes. Emerging data suggest that burst-suppression pattern on postarrest electroencephalogram is sensitive and specific for poor neurologic outcome (163,171). One study showed somatosensory-evoked potential was highly sensitive and specific in pediatric patients after cardiac arrest (172). However, somatosensory-evoked potentials are not standardized in the pediatric population, and they are difficult to interpret. Many children who suffer a cardiac arrest have substantial preexisting neurologic problems. For example, 17% of the children with in-hospital cardiac arrests from the GWTG national registry of CPR were neurologically abnormal before the arrest (21). Thus, comparison to prearrest neurologic function of a child is difficult and adds another barrier to the assessment and prediction of postarrest neurologic status. Rather than reporting neurologic deficits or neurologic outcome post–resuscitation, reporting new neurologic deficits or change in neurologic status would be useful.

Biomarkers are emerging tools with which to predict neurologic outcome. In an adult study, the serum level of neuron-specific enolase and S100b protein showed prognostic value. Neuron-specific enolase of $>33\ \mu g/L$ and S100b of $>0.7\ \mu cg/L$ were highly sensitive and specific for poor neurologic outcome (death or persisting unconsciousness) (173). Similarly, serum neuron-specific enolases levels were associated with outcomes in pediatric postarrest patients, but thresholds for prediction were demonstrable in contrast to the adult data (174). The S100b levels in children post–arrest were associated with survival, but not neurological outcome among survivors.

Most pediatric cardiac arrest outcome studies have not included formal neurologic assessments and long-term follow-up of important quality of life assessments. Investigations that include neurologic outcomes have generally used the Pediatric Cerebral Performance Category, a gross outcome scale. Many neuropsychologic tests can detect more subtle, clinically important neuropsychologic sequelae from neurologic insults. Neuropsychologic outcomes are important issues for future pediatric cardiac arrest outcome studies.

QUALITY OF CARDIOPULMONARY RESUSCITATION AND RESUSCITATION INTERVENTIONS

Despite evidence-based guidelines, extensive provider training, and provider credentialing in resuscitation medicine, the quality of CPR is typically poor. Slow compression rates, inadequate depth of compression, and substantial pauses are the norm. The mantra of "push hard, push fast, minimize interruptions, allow full-chest recoil, and don't overventilate" can markedly improve myocardial, cerebral, and systemic perfusion and improve outcomes (175). The quality of postresuscitative management has also been demonstrated to be critically important to improve resuscitation survival outcomes (176).

Post–Cardiac Arrest Evaluation of Sudden Death

Channelopathies

Genetic mutations that lead to channelopathies are relatively common among infants and children with OHCAs. The evaluation of these patients and their families for channelopathies is especially important because 25%–53% of first- and second-degree relatives have these inherited arrhythmogenic diseases. Therefore, when a child or young adult has an unexplained sudden death, a full past medical history and family history should be obtained, and family members should be referred for evaluation regarding potential channelopathies (109). An autopsy is recommended and, if possible, genetic tissue evaluation.

Hypertrophic Cardiomyopathy

Hypertrophic cardiomyopathy occurs among 1 in 500 in the general population (177). The annual risk of death is 1% for affected patients, and such deaths are often caused by ventricular arrhythmias. Because hypertrophic cardiomyopathy is the most common cause of sudden cardiac death among young athletes and often has no preceding symptoms, evaluation for hypertrophic cardiomyopathy is appropriate for young athletes with sudden cardiac arrests either by echocardiography or postmortem examination (177).

Coronary Artery Abnormalities

Coronary artery abnormalities (generally aberrant coronary arteries with extrinsic obstruction) are the second leading cause of sudden death in athletes. Up to 17% of sudden deaths among young athletes have been attributed to anomalous coronary arteries (178). Diagnoses of these anomalies may require postmortem examination by pathologists with special expertise.

CONCLUSIONS AND FUTURE DIRECTIONS

Outcomes from pediatric cardiac arrest and CPR are improving. An evolving understanding of the pathophysiology of events and titration of the interventions to the timing, etiology, duration, and intensity of the cardiac arrest event can improve resuscitation outcomes. Exciting discoveries in basic and applied science are on the immediate horizon for study in specific populations of cardiac arrest victims. By strategically focusing therapies to the specific phases of cardiac arrest and resuscitation and to evolving pathophysiology, critical care interventions can lead the way to more successful cardiopulmonary and cerebral resuscitation in children. In the future, the treatment of sudden death in children should involve interventions that are more evidence-based and less anecdotal. Timing of therapeutic interventions to prevent arrest and to protect, preserve, and promote the restoration of intact neurologic function and survival is of the highest priority. Emerging technology interfaced with evolving teams and systems of postresuscitative care will likely facilitate high-quality interventions and ensure optimal odds for survival.

Exciting new epidemiologic studies, such as GWTG-R for in-hospital cardiac arrests and the large-scale, multicentered Resuscitation Outcome Consortium, are providing new data to guide our resuscitation practices and generate hypotheses for new approaches to improve outcomes. It is increasingly clear that excellent quality BLS is often not provided. Innovative technical advances, such as directive and corrective real-time feedback with after-event debriefing, can increase the likelihood of effective BLS. In addition, team dynamic training and debriefing can substantially improve self-efficacy and operational performance, leading to improved survival outcomes (19).

Targeted temperature management, chemical hibernation, controlled reanimation, and emergency preservation and resuscitation techniques are being considered. Mechanical interventions such as ECMO or other cardiopulmonary bypass systems are already commonplace interventions during prolonged or refractory in-hospital cardiac arrests. Technical advances are likely to further improve our ability to provide such mechanical support.

In the past, the concept of evidence-based pediatric cardiac arrest resuscitation recommendations seemed remote. Pediatric recommendations were based on extrapolated animal and adult data and expert consensus. Informative and evidence-based pediatric cardiac arrest clinical trials have started with the randomized controlled trial of high-dose epinephrine versus standard-dose epinephrine as rescue therapy for in-hospital pediatric cardiac arrests, and therapeutic hypothermia after pediatric cardiac arrest trials. It is likely that the evolution of systems such as "cardiac arrest centers," similar to trauma, stroke, and myocardial infarction centers, will be established and will facilitate the appropriate intensive care for patients who require specialized postresuscitation care.

References

1. Eberle B, Dick WF, Schneider T, et al. Checking the carotid pulse check: Diagnostic accuracy of first responders in patients with and without a pulse. *Resuscitation* 1996;33:107–16.

2. Moule P. Checking the carotid pulse: Diagnostic accuracy in students of the healthcare professions. *Resuscitation* 2000;44:195–201.

3. Tibballs J, Russell P. Reliability of pulse palpation by healthcare personnel to diagnose paediatric cardiac arrest. *Resuscitation* 2009;80:61–4.

4. Sutton RM, Niles D, French B, et al. First quantitative analysis of cardiopulmonary resuscitation quality during in-hospital cardiac arrests of young children. *Resuscitation* 2014;85(1):70–4.

5. Sutton RM, Wolfe H, Nishisaki A, et al. Pushing harder, pushing faster, minimizing interruptions, but falling short of 2010 cardiopulmonary resuscitation targets during in-hospital pediatric and adolescent resuscitation. *Resuscitation* 2013;84(12):1680–4.

6. McInnes AD, Sutton RM, Orioles A, et al. The first quantitative report of ventilation rate during in-hospital resuscitation of older children and adolescents. *Resuscitation* 2011;82(8):1025–9.

7. Sutton RM, Maltese MR, Niles D, et al. Quantitative analysis of chest compression interruptions during in-hospital resuscitation of older children and adolescents. *Resuscitation* 2009;80(11):1259–63.

8. Sutton RM, Niles D, Nysaether J, et al. Quantitative analysis of CPR quality during in-hospital resuscitation of older children and adolescents. *Pediatrics* 2009;124(2):494–9.

9. Neumar RW, Nolan JP, Adrie C, et al. Post-cardiac arrest syndrome: Epidemiology, pathophysiology, treatment, and prognostication. A consensus statement from the International Liaison Committee on Resuscitation (American Heart Association, Australian and New Zealand Council on Resuscitation, European Resuscitation Council, Heart and Stroke Foundation of Canada, InterAmerican Heart Foundation, Resuscitation Council of Asia, and the Resuscitation Council of Southern Africa); the American Heart Association Emergency Cardiovascular Care Committee; the Council on Cardiovascular Surgery and Anesthesia; the Council on Cardiopulmonary, Perioperative, and Critical Care; the Council on Clinical Cardiology; and the Stroke Council. *Circulation* 2008;118(23):2452–83.

10. Morrison LJ, Neumar RW, Zimmerman JL, et al. Strategies for improving survival after in-hospital cardiac arrest in the United States: 2013 consensus recommendations: A consensus statement from the American Heart Association. *Circulation* 2013;127(14):1538–63.

11. Kouwenhoven WB, Jude JR, Knickerbocker GG. Closed-chest cardiac massage. *JAMA* 1960;173:1064–7.

12. Kitamura T, Kiyohara K, Nitta M, et al. Survival following witnessed pediatric out-of-hospital cardiac arrests during nights and weekends. *Resuscitation* 2014;85(12):1692–8.

13. Nitta M, Kitamura T, Iwami T, et al. Out-of-hospital cardiac arrest due to drowning among children and adults from the Utstein Osaka Project. *Resuscitation* 2013;84(11):1568–73.

14. Okamoto Y, Iwami T, Kitamura T, et al. Regional variation in survival following pediatric out-of-hospital cardiac arrest. *Circ J* 2013;77(10):2596–603.

15. Donoghue AJ, Nadkarni V, Berg RA, et al; CanAm Pediatric Cardiac Arrest Investigators. Out-of-hospital pediatric cardiac arrest: An epidemiologic review and assessment of current knowledge. *Ann Emerg Med* 2005;46(6):512–22.

16. Michiels EA, Dumas F, Quan L, et al. Long-term outcomes following pediatric out-of-hospital cardiac arrest. *Pediatr Crit Care Med* 2013;14(8):755–60.

17. Kuisma M, Suominen P, Korpela R. Paediatric out-of-hospital cardiac arrests—Epidemiology and outcome. *Resuscitation* 1995;30(2):141–50.

18. Gupta P, Jacobs JP, Pasquali SK, et al. Epidemiology and outcomes after in-hospital cardiac arrest after pediatric cardiac surgery. *Ann Thorac Surg* 2014;98(6):2138–44.

19. Wolfe H, Zebuhr C, Topjian AA, et al. Interdisciplinary ICU cardiac arrest debriefing improves survival outcomes. *Crit Care Med* 2014;42(7):1688–95.

20. Matos MR, Watson RS, Nadkarni VM, et al. Duration of cardiopulmonary resuscitation and illness category impact survival and neurologic outcomes for in-hospital pediatric cardiac arrests. *Circulation* 2013;128(7):e102–e103.

21. Nadkarni VM, Larkin GL, Peberdy MA, et al; National Registry of Cardiopulmonary Resuscitation Investigators. First documented rhythm and clinical outcome from in-hospital cardiac arrest among children and adults. *JAMA* 2006;295(1):50–7.

22. Berg RA, Sutton RM, Holubkov R, et al. Ratio of PICU versus ward cardiopulmonary resuscitation events is increasing. *Crit Care Med* 2013;41:2292–7.

23. Knudson JD, Neish SR, Cabrera AG, et al. Prevalence and outcomes of pediatric in-hospital cardiopulmonary resuscitation in the United States: An analysis of the Kids' Inpatient Database. *Crit Care Med* 2012;40:2940.

24. Slonim AD, Patel KM, Ruttimann UE, et al. Cardiopulmonary resuscitation in pediatric intensive care units. *Crit Care Med* 1997;25:1951–5.

25. Suominen P, Olkkola KT, Voipio V, et al. Utstein style reporting of in-hospital paediatric cardiopulmonary resuscitation. *Resuscitation* 2000;45:17–25.

26. Peddy SB, Hazinski MF, Laussen PC, et al. Cardiopulmonary resuscitation special considerations for infants and children with cardiac disease. *Cardiol Young* 2007;17:116–26.

27. Parra DA, Totapally BR, Zahn E, et al. Outcome of cardiopulmonary resuscitation in a pediatric cardiac intensive care unit. *Crit Care Med* 2000;28:3296–300.

28. Rhodes JF, Blaufox AD, Seiden HS, et al. Cardiac arrest in infants after congenital heart surgery. *Circulation* 1999;100(suppl 2):II194–II199.

29. Del Castillo J, López-Herce J, Canadas S, et al; Iberoamerican Pediatric Cardiac Arrest Study Network RIBEPCI. Cardiac arrest and resuscitation in the pediatric intensive care unit: A prospective multicenter multinational study. *Resuscitation* 2014;85(10):1380–6.

30. López-Herce J, Del Castillo J, Matamoros M, et al; Iberoamerican Pediatric Cardiac Arrest Study Network RIBEPCI. Factors associated with mortality in pediatric in-hospital cardiac arrest: A prospective multicenter multinational observational study. *Intensive Care Med* 2013;39(2):309–18.

31. Girotra S, Spertus JA, Li Y, et al; American Heart Association Get With the Guidelines-Resuscitation Investigators. Survival trends in pediatric in-hospital cardiac arrests: An analysis from Get With the Guidelines-Resuscitation. *Circ Cardiovasc Qual Outcomes* 2013;6(1):42–9.

32. Zebuhr C, Sutton RM, Morrison W, et al. Evaluation of quantitative debriefing after pediatric cardiac arrest. *Resuscitation* 2012;83(9):1124–8.

33. Sutton RM, Niles D, Meaney PA, et al. Low-dose, high-frequency CPR training improves skill retention of in-hospital pediatric providers. *Pediatrics* 2011;128(1):e145–e151.

34. Jacobs I, Nadkarni V, Bahr J, et al. Cardiac arrest and cardiopulmonary resuscitation outcome reports: update and simplification of the Utstein templates for resuscitation registries: A statement for healthcare professionals from a task force of the International Liaison Committee on Resuscitation (American Heart Association, European Resuscitation Council, Australian Resuscitation Council, New Zealand Resuscitation Council, Heart and Stroke Foundation of Canada, InterAmerican Heart Foundation, Resuscitation Councils of Southern Africa). *Circulation* 2004 Nov 23;110(21):3385-97.

35. Jacobs I, Nadkarni V, Bahr J, et al; International Liaison Committee on Resuscitation. Cardiac arrest and cardiopulmonary resuscitation outcome reports: Update and simplification of the Utstein templates for resuscitation registries. A statement for healthcare professionals from a task force of the international liaison committee on resuscitation (American Heart Association, European Resuscitation Council, Australian Resuscitation Council, New Zealand Resuscitation Council, Heart and Stroke Foundation of Canada, InterAmerican Heart Foundation, Resuscitation Council of Southern Africa). *Resuscitation* 2004;63(3):233–49.

36. Perkins GD, Jacobs IG, Nadkarni VM, et al. Cardiac arrest and cardiopulmonary resuscitation outcome reports: Update of the

Utstein resuscitation registry templates for out-of-hospital cardiac arrest [published online ahead of print on November 25, 2014]. *Resuscitation*. doi:10.1016/j.resuscitation.2014.11.002

37. Donoghue A, Berg RA, Hazinski MF, et al; American Heart Association National Registry of CPR Investigators. Cardiopulmonary resuscitation for bradycardia with poor perfusion versus pulseless cardiac arrest. *Pediatrics* 2009;124(6):1541–8.

38. Atkins DL, Everson-Stewart S, Sears GK, et al; Resuscitation Outcomes Consortium Investigators. Epidemiology and outcomes from out-of-hospital cardiac arrest in children: The Resuscitation Outcomes Consortium Epistry-Cardiac Arrest. *Circulation* 2009;119(11):1484–91.

39. Kitamura T, Iwami T, Kawamura T, et al; Implementation working group for All-Japan Utstein Registry of the Fire and Disaster Management Agency. Conventional and chest-compression-only cardiopulmonary resuscitation by bystanders for children who have out-of-hospital cardiac arrests: A prospective, nationwide, population-based cohort study. *Lancet* 2010;375(9723):1347–54.

40. Nitta M, Iwami T, Kitamura T, et al. Age-specific differences in outcomes after out-of-hospital cardiac arrests. *Pediatrics* 2011;128(4):e812–e820.

41. Bardai A, Berdowski J, van der Werf C, et al. Incidence, causes, and outcomes of out-of-hospital cardiac arrest in children. A comprehensive, population-based study in the Netherlands. *J Am Coll Cardiol* 2011;57(18):1822–8.

42. Nishiuchi T, Hayashino Y, Iwami T, et al; Utstein Osaka Project Investigators. Epidemiological characteristics of sudden cardiac arrest in schools. *Resuscitation* 2014;85(8):1001–6.

43. Mitani Y, Ohta K, Ichida F, et al. Circumstances and outcomes of out-of-hospital cardiac arrest in elementary and middle school students in the era of public-access defibrillation. *Circ J* 2014;78(3):701–7.

44. Foltin GL, Richmond N, Treiber M, et al. Pediatric prehospital evaluation of NYC cardiac arrest survival (PHENYCS). *Pediatr Emerg Care* 2012;28(9):864–8.

45. De Maio VJ, Osmond MH, Stiell IG, et al; CanAm Pediatric Study Group. Epidemiology of out-of-hospital pediatric cardiac arrest due to trauma. *Prehosp Emerg Care* 2012;16(2):230–6.

46. Moler FW, Donaldson AE, Meert K, et al; Pediatric Emergency Care Applied Research Network. Multicenter cohort study of out-of-hospital pediatric cardiac arrest. *Crit Care Med* 2011;39(1):141–9.

47. Rodríguez-Núñez A, López-Herce J, García C, et al; Spanish Study Group of Cardipulmonary Arrest in Children. Pediatric defibrillation after cardiac arrest: Initial response and outcome. *Crit Care* 2006;10(4):R113.

48. Smith BT, Rea TD, Eisenberg MS. Ventricular fibrillation in pediatric cardiac arrest. *Acad Emerg Med* 2006;13(5):525–9.

49. López-Herce J, García C, Domínguez P, et al; Spanish Study Group of Cardiopulmonary Arrest in Children. Outcome of out-of-hospital cardiorespiratory arrest in children. *Pediatr Emerg Care* 2005;21(12):807–15.

50. Berg MD, Samson RA, Meyer RJ, et al. Pediatric defibrillation doses often fail to terminate prolonged out-of-hospital ventricular fibrillation in children. *Resuscitation* 2005;67(1):63–7.

51. Appleton GO, Cummins RO, Larson MP, et al. CPR and the single rescuer: At what age should you "call first" rather than "call fast?" *Ann Emerg Med* 1995;25(4):492–4.

52. Graf WD, Cummings P, Quan L, et al. Predicting outcome in pediatric submersion victims. *Ann Emerg Med* 1995;26:312–9.

53. Quan L, Mack CD, Schiff MA. Association of water temperature and submersion duration and drowning outcome. *Resuscitation* 2014;85(6):790–4.

54. Samson RA, Nadkarni VM, Meaney PA, et al. Outcomes of in-hospital ventricular fibrillation in children. *N Engl J Med* 2006;354:2328–39.

55. Meaney PA, Nadkarni VM, Kern KB, et al. Rhythms and outcomes of adult in-hospital cardiac arrest. *Crit Care Med* 2010;38(1):101–8.

56. Caffrey SL, Willoughby PJ, Pepe PE, et al. Public use of automated external defibrillators. *N Engl J Med* 2002;347:1242–7.

57. Valenzuela TD, Roe DJ, Nichol G, et al. Outcomes of rapid defibrillation by security officers after cardiac arrest in casinos. *N Engl J Med* 2000;343:1206–9.

58. Niles DE, Nishisaki A, Sutton RM, et al. Analysis of transthoracic impedance during real cardiac arrest defibrillation attempts in older children and adolescents: Are stacked shocks appropriate? *Resuscitation* 2010;81(11):1540–3.

59. White RD, Blackwell TH, Russell JK, et al. Transthoracic impedance does not affect defibrillation, resuscitation or survival in patients with out-of-hospital cardiac arrest treated with non-escalating biphasic waveform defibrillator. *Resuscitation* 2005;64(1):63–9.

60. Berg RA, Chapman FW, Berg MD, et al. Attenuated adult biphasic shocks compared with weight-based monophasic shocks in a swine model of prolonged pediatric ventricular fibrillation. *Resuscitation* 2004;61:189–97.

61. Gutgesell HP, Tacker WA, Geddes LA, et al. Energy dose for ventricular defibrillation of children. *Pediatrics* 1976;58:898–901.

62. Atkins DL, Sirna S, Kieso R, et al. Pediatric defibrillation: Importance of paddle size in determining transthoracic impedance. *Pediatrics* 1988;82:914–8.

63. Field JM, Hazinski MF, Sayre MR, et al. Part 1: Executive Summary: 2010 American Heart Association Guidelines for Cardiopulmonary Resuscitation and Emergency Cardiovascular Care. *Circulation* 2010;122:S640–S656.

64. Meaney PA, Nadkarni VM, Atkins DL, et al; American Heart Association National Registry of Cardiopulmonary Resuscitation Investigators. Effect of defibrillation energy dose during in-hospital pediatric cardiac arrest. *Pediatrics* 2011;127(1):e16–e23.

65. Tibballs J, Carter B, Kiraly NJ, et al. External and internal biphasic direct current shock doses for pediatric ventricular fibrillation and pulseless ventricular tachycardia. *Pediatr Crit Care Med* 2011;12(1):14–20.

66. Rodríguez-Núñez A, López-Herce J, del Castillo J, et al; Iberian-American Paediatric Cardiac Arrest Study Network RIBEPCI. Shockable rhythms and defibrillation during in-hospital pediatric cardiac arrest. *Resuscitation* 2014;85(3):387–91.

67. Samson RA, Berg RA, Bingham R, et al. Use of automated external defibrillators for children: An update: An advisory statement from the Pediatric Advanced Life Support Task Force, International Liaison Committee on Resuscitation. *Circulation* 2003;107:3250–5.

68. Atkinson E, Mikysa B, Conway JA, et al. Specificity and sensitivity of automated external defibrillator rhythm analysis in infants and children. *Ann Emerg Med* 2003;42:185–96.

69. Cecchin F, Jorgenson DB, Berul CI, et al. Is arrhythmia detection by automatic external defibrillator accurate for children? Sensitivity and specificity of an automatic external defibrillator algorithm in 696 pediatric arrhythmias. *Circulation* 2001;103:2483–8.

70. Berg RA, Samson RA, Berg MD, et al. Better outcome after pediatric defibrillation dosage than adult dosage in a swine model of pediatric ventricular fibrillation. *J Am Coll Cardiol* 2005;45:786–9.

71. Checchia PA, Sehra R, Moynihan J, et al. Myocardial injury in children following resuscitation after cardiac arrest. *Resuscitation* 2003;57(2):131–7.

72. Gurnett CA, Atkins DL. Successful use of a biphasic waveform automated external defibrillator in a high-risk child. *Am J Cardiol* 2000;86:1051–3.

73. Sharek PJ, Parast LM, Leong K, et al. Effect of a rapid response team on hospital-wide mortality and code rates outside the ICU in a Children's Hospital. *JAMA* 2007;298(19):2267–74.

74. Brilli RJ, Gibson R, Luria JW, et al. Implementation of a medical emergency team in a large pediatric teaching hospital prevents respiratory and cardiopulmonary arrests outside the intensive care unit. *Pediatr Crit Care Med* 2007;8(3):236–46; quiz 247.

75. Hunt EA, Zimmer KP, Rinke ML, et al. Transition from a traditional code team to a medical emergency team and categorization of cardiopulmonary arrests in a children's center. *Arch Pediatr Adolesc Med* 2008;162(2):117–22.

76. Joffe AR, Anton NR, Burkholder SC. Reduction in hospital mortality over time in a hospital without a pediatric medical emergency team: Limitations of before-and-after study designs. *Arch Pediatr Adolesc Med* 2011;165(5):419–23.

77. Tibballs J, Kinney S. Reduction of hospital mortality and of preventable cardiac arrest and death on introduction of a pediatric medical emergency team. *Pediatr Crit Care Med* 2009;10(3):306–12.

78. Brady PW, Muething S, Kotagal U, et al. Improving situation awareness to reduce unrecognized clinical deterioration and serious safety events. *Pediatrics* 2013;131(1):e298–e308.

79. Bonafide CP, Localio AR, Song L, et al. Cost-benefit analysis of a medical emergency team in a children's hospital. *Pediatrics* 2014;134(2):235–41.

80. Meaney PA, Nadkarni VM, Cook EF, et al. Higher survival rates among younger patients after pediatric intensive care unit cardiac arrests. *Pediatrics* 2006;118:2424–33.

81. Berg RA, Kern KB, Hilwig RW, et al. Assisted ventilation during "bystander" CPR in a swine acute myocardial infarction model does not improve outcome. *Circulation* 1997;96:4364–71.

82. Michael JR, Guerci AD, Koehler RC, et al. Mechanisms by which epinephrine augments cerebral and myocardial perfusion during cardiopulmonary resuscitation in dogs. *Circulation* 1984;69:822–35.

83. Kern KB, Ewy GA, Voorhees WD, et al. Myocardial perfusion pressure: A predictor of 24-hour survival during prolonged cardiac arrest in dogs. *Resuscitation* 1988;16:241–50.

84. Sanders AB, Ewy GA, Taft TV. Prognostic and therapeutic importance of the aortic diastolic pressure in resuscitation from cardiac arrest. *Crit Care Med* 1984;12:871–3.

85. Friess SH, Sutton RM, Bhalala U, et al. Hemodynamic directed cardiopulmonary resuscitation improves short-term survival from ventricular fibrillation cardiac arrest. *Crit Care Med* 2013;41(12):2698–704.

86. Paradis NA, Martin GB, Rivers EP, et al. Coronary perfusion pressure and the return of spontaneous circulation in human cardiopulmonary resuscitation. *JAMA* 1990;263(8):1106–13.

87. Kern KB, Sanders AB, Voorhees WD, et al. Changes in expired end-tidal carbon dioxide during cardiopulmonary resuscitation in dogs: A prognostic guide for resuscitation efforts. *J Am Coll Cardiol* 1989;13(5):1184–9.

88. Ornato JP, Garnett AR, Glauser FL. Relationship between cardiac output and the end-tidal carbon dioxide tension. *Ann Emerg Med* 1990;19(10):1104–6.

89. Sanders AB, Kern KB, Otto CW, et al. End-tidal carbon dioxide monitoring during cardiopulmonary resuscitation. A prognostic indicator for survival. *JAMA* 1989;262(10):1347–51.

90. Levine RL, Wayne MA, Miller CC. End-tidal carbon dioxide and outcome of out-of-hospital cardiac arrest. *N Engl J Med* 1997;337(5):301–6.

91. Hamrick JL, Hamrick JT, Lee JK, et al. Efficacy of chest compressions directed by end-tidal CO_2 feedback in a pediatric resuscitation model of basic life support. *J Am Heart Assoc* 2014;3(2):e000450.

92. Berg MD, Schexnayder SM, Chameides L, et al. Part 13: Pediatric basic life support: 2010 American Heart Association Guidelines for Cardiopulmonary Resuscitation and Emergency Cardiovascular Care. *Circulation* 2010;122(18, suppl 3):S862–S875.

93. Houri PK, Frank LR, Menegazzi JJ, et al. A randomized, controlled trial of two-thumb vs. two-finger chest compression in a swine infant model of cardiac arrest. *Prehosp Emerg Care* 1997;1:65–7.

94. Menegazzi JJ, Auble TE, Nicklas KA, et al. Two-thumb versus two-finger chest compression during CRP in a swine infant model of cardiac arrest. *Ann Emerg Med* 1993;22:240–3.

95. Dorfsman ML, Menegazzi JJ, Wadas RJ, et al. Two-thumb vs. two-finger chest compression in an infant model of prolonged cardiopulmonary resuscitation. *Acad Emerg Med* 2000;7(10):1077–82.

96. Feneley MP, Maier GW, Kern KB, et al. Influence of compression rate on initial success of resuscitation and 24-hour survival after prolonged manual cardiopulmonary resuscitation in dogs. *Circulation* 1988;77:240–50.

97. Halperin HR, Tsitlik JE, Guerci AD, et al. Determinants of blood flow to vital organs during cardiopulmonary resuscitation in dogs. *Circulation* 1986;73:539–50.

98. Dean JM, Koehler RC, Schleien CL, et al. Age-related changes in chest geometry during cardiopulmonary resuscitation. *J Appl Physiol* 1987;62:2212–9.

99. Sheikh A, Brogan T. Outcome and cost of open- and closed-chest cardiopulmonary resuscitation in pediatric cardiac arrests. *Pediatrics* 1994;93:392–8.

100. Gausche M, Lewis RJ. Out-of-hospital endotracheal intubation of children. *JAMA* 2000;283:2790–2.

101. Aufderheide TP, Lurie KG. Death by hyperventilation: A common and life-threatening problem during cardiopulmonary resuscitation. *Crit Care Med* 2004;32(9, suppl):S345–S351.

102. Hallstrom AP, Cobb LA, Johnson E, et al. Dispatcher-assisted CPR: Implementation and potential benefit. A 12-year study. *Resuscitation* 2003;57:123–9.

103. Berg RA, Hilwig RW, Kern KB, et al. "Bystander" chest compressions and assisted ventilation independently improve outcome from piglet asphyxial pulseless "cardiac arrest." *Circulation* 2000;101:1743–8.

104. Idris AH, Staples ED, O'Brien DJ, et al. Effect of ventilation on acid-base balance and oxygenation in low blood-flow states. *Crit Care Med* 1994;22:1827–34.

105. Kinney SB, Tibballs J. An analysis of the efficacy of bag-valve-mask ventilation and chest compression during different compression-ventilation ratios in manikin-simulated paediatric resuscitation. *Resuscitation* 2000;43:115–20.

106. Srikantan SK, Berg RA, Cox T, et al. Effect of one-rescuer compression/ventilation ratios on cardiopulmonary resuscitation in infant, pediatric, and adult manikins. *Pediatr Crit Care Med* 2005;6:293–7.

107. Babbs CF, Kern KB. Optimum compression to ventilation ratios in CPR under realistic, practical conditions: A physiological and mathematical analysis. *Resuscitation* 2002;54:147–57.

108. Babbs CF, Nadkarni V. Optimizing chest compression to rescue ventilation ratios during one-rescuer CPR by professionals and lay persons: Children are not just little adults. *Resuscitation* 2004;61:173–81.

109. Kleinman ME, de Caen AR, Chameides L, et al; Pediatric Basic and Advanced Life Support Chapter Collaborators. Part 10: Pediatric basic and advanced life support: 2010 International Consensus on Cardiopulmonary Resuscitation and Emergency Cardiovascular Care Science with Treatment Recommendations. *Circulation* 2010;122(16, suppl 2):S466–S515.

110. Johnson L, Kissoon N, Fiallos M, et al. Use of intraosseous blood to assess blood chemistries and hemoglobin during cardiopulmonary resuscitation with drug infusions. *Crit Care Med* 1999;27:1147–52.

111. Orlowski JP, Julius CJ, Petras RE, et al. The safety of intraosseous infusions: Risks of fat and bone marrow emboli to the lungs. *Ann Emerg Med* 1989;18:1062–7.

112. Hornchen U, Schuttler J, Stoeckel H, et al. Endobronchial instillation of epinephrine during cardiopulmonary resuscitation. *Crit Care Med* 1987;15:1037–9.

113. Brown CG, Martin DR, Pepe PE, et al. A comparison of standard-dose and high-dose epinephrine in cardiac arrest outside the hospital. The Multicenter High-Dose Epinephrine Study Group. *N Engl J Med* 1992;327:1051–5.

114. Lindner KH, Ahnefeld FW, Bowdler IM. Comparison of different doses of epinephrine on myocardial perfusion and resuscitation success during cardiopulmonary resuscitation in a pig model. *Am J Emerg Med* 1991;9:27–31.

115. Jacobs IG, Finn JC, Jelinek GA, et al. Effect of adrenaline on survival in out-of-hospital cardiac arrest: A randomized double-blind placebo controlled trial. *Resuscitation* 2011;82(9):1138–43.

116. Berg RA, Otto CW, Kern KB, et al. High-dose epinephrine results in greater early mortality after resuscitation from prolonged cardiac arrest in pigs: A prospective, randomized study. *Crit Care Med* 1994;22:282–90.

117. Behringer W, Kittler H, Sterz F, et al. Cumulative epinephrine dose during cardiopulmonary resuscitation and neurologic outcome. *Ann Intern Med* 1998;129:450–6.

118. Callaham M, Madsen C, Barton C, et al. A randomized clinical trial of high-dose epinephrine and norepinephrine versus standard-dose epinephrine in prehospital cardiac arrest. *JAMA* 1992;268:2667–72.

119. Arrich J, Sterz F, Herkner H, et al. Total epinephrine dose during asystole and pulseless electrical activity cardiac arrests is associated with unfavourable functional outcome and increased in-hospital mortality. *Resuscitation* 2012;83(3):333–7.

120. Perondi MB, Reis AG, Paiva EF, et al. A comparison of high-dose and standard-dose epinephrine in children with cardiac arrest. *N Engl J Med* 2004;350:1722–30.

121. Hagihara A, Hasegawa M, Abe T, et al. Prehospital epinephrine use and survival among patients with out-of-hospital cardiac arrest. *JAMA* 2012;307(11):1161–8.

122. Olasveengen TM, Wik L, Sunde K, et al. Outcome when adrenaline (epinephrine) was actually given vs. not given—Post hoc analysis of a randomized clinical trial. *Resuscitation* 2012;83(3):327–32.

123. Herlitz J, Ekstrom L, Wennerblom B, et al. Adrenaline in out-of-hospital ventricular fibrillation. Does it make any difference? *Resuscitation* 1995;29(3):195–201.

124. Ong ME, Tan EH, Ng FS, et al; Cardiac Arrest and Resuscitation Epidemiology Study Group. Survival outcomes with the introduction of intravenous epinephrine in the management of out-of-hospital cardiac arrest. *Ann Emerg Med* 2007;50(6):635–42.

125. Voelckel WG, Lindner KH, Wenzel V, et al. Effects of vasopressin and epinephrine on splanchnic blood flow and renal function during and after cardiopulmonary resuscitation in pigs. *Crit Care Med* 2000;28:1083–8.

126. Voelckel WG, Lurie KG, Lindner KH, et al. Comparison of epinephrine and vasopressin in a pediatric porcine model of asphyxial cardiac arrest. *Circulation* 1999;36:1115–8.

127. Stiell IG, Hebert PC, Wells GA, et al. Vasopressin versus epinephrine for inhospital cardiac arrest: A randomised controlled trial. *Lancet* 2001;358:105–9.

128. Wenzel V, Krismer AC, Arntz HR, et al. A comparison of vasopressin and epinephrine for out-of-hospital cardiopulmonary resuscitation. *N Engl J Med* 2004;350:105–13.

129. Lurie K, Voelckel W, Plaisance P, et al. Use of an inspiratory impedance threshold valve during cardiopulmonary resuscitation: A progress report. *Resuscitation* 2000;44:219–30.

130. Mann K, Berg RA, Nadkarni V. Beneficial effects of vasopressin in prolonged pediatric cardiac arrest: A case series. *Resuscitation* 2002;52:149–56.

131. Stueven HA, Thompson B, Aprahamian C, et al. The effectiveness of calcium chloride in refractory electromechanical dissociation. *Ann Emerg Med* 1985;14:626–39.

132. Katz AM, Reuter H. Cellular calcium and cardiac cell death. *Am J Cardiol* 1979;44:188–90.

133. Meert KL, Donaldson A, Nadkarni V, et al. Multicenter cohort study of in-hospital pediatric cardiac arrest. *Pediatr Crit Care Med* 2009;10(5):544–53.

134. Srinivasan V, Morris MC, Helfaer MA, et al; American Heart Association National Registry of CPR Investigators. Calcium use during in-hospital pediatric cardiopulmonary resuscitation: a report from the National Registry of Cardiopulmonary Resuscitation. *Pediatrics* 2008;121(5):e1144–e1151.

135. de Mos N, van Litsenburg RR, McCrindle B, et al. Pediatric in-intensive-care-unit cardiac arrest: Incidence, survival, and predictive factors. *Crit Care Med* 2006;34:1209–15.

136. Dorian P, Cass D, Schwartz B, et al. Amiodarone as compared with lidocaine for shock-resistant ventricular fibrillation. *N Engl J Med* 2002;346:884–90.

137. Kudenchuk PJ, Cobb LA, Copass MK, et al. Amiodarone for resuscitation after out-of-hospital cardiac arrest due to ventricular fibrillation. *N Engl J Med* 1999;341:871–8.

138. Bernard SA, Gray TW, Buist MD, et al. Treatment of comatose survivors of out-of-hospital cardiac arrest with induced hypothermia. *N Engl J Med* 2002;346:557–63.

139. Hypothermia after Cardiac Arrest Study Group. Mild therapeutic hypothermia to improve the neurologic outcome after cardiac arrest. *N Engl J Med* 2002;346:549–56.

140. Nielsen N, Wettersley J, Cronberg T, et al; TTM Trial Investigators. Targeted temperatures management at 33°C versus 36°C after cardiac arrest. *N Engl J Med* 2013;369(23):2197–206.

141. Rittenberger JC, Callaway CW. Targeted temperature management after cardiac arrest. *N Engl J Med* 2014;370(14):1360–1.

142. Hickey RW, Kochanek PM, Ferimer H, et al. Hypothermia and hyperthermia in children after resuscitation from cardiac arrest. *Pediatrics* 2000;106:118–22.

143. Doherty DR, Parshuram CS, Gaboury I, et al; Canadian Critical Care Trials Group. Hypothermia therapy after pediatric cardiac arrest. *Circulation* 2009;119(11):1492–500.

144. Gazmuri RJ, Weil MH, Bisera J, et al. Myocardial dysfunction after successful resuscitation from cardiac arrest. *Crit Care Med* 1996;24:992–1000.

145. Kamohara T, Weil MH, Tang W, et al. A comparison of myocardial function after primary cardiac and primary asphyxial cardiac arrest. *Am J Respir Crit Care Med* 2001;164:1221–4.

146. Huang L, Weil MH, Sun S, et al. Levosimendan improves postresuscitation outcomes in a rat model of CPR. *J Lab Clin Med* 2005;146:256–61.

147. García González MJ, Domínguez Rodríguez A. Pharmacologic treatment of heart failure due to ventricular dysfunction by myocardial stunning: Potential role of levosimendan. *Am J Cardiovasc Drugs* 2006;6:69–75.

148. Egan JR, Clarke AJ, Williams S, et al. Levosimendan for low cardiac output: A pediatric experience. *J Intensive Care Med* 2006;21:183–7.

149. Conlon TW, Falkensammer CB, Hammond RS, et al. Association of left ventricular systolic function and vasopressor support with survival following pediatric out-of-hospital cardiac arrest. *Pediatr Crit Care Med* 2015;16(2):146-54. doi: 10.1097/PCC.0000000000000305.

150. Abdallah I, Shawky H. A randomised controlled trial comparing milrinone and epinephrine as inotropes in paediatric patients undergoing total correction of Tetralogy of Fallot. *Egypt J Anaesth* 2003;19:323–9.

151. Ceneviva G, Paschall JA, Maffei F, et al. Hemodynamic support in fluid-refractory pediatric septic shock. *Pediatrics* 1998;102:e19.

152. Hoffman TM, Wernovsky G, Atz AM, et al. Efficacy and safety of milrinone in preventing low cardiac output syndrome in infants and children after corrective surgery for congenital heart disease. *Circulation* 2003;107:996–1002.

153. Innes PA, Frazer RS, Booker PD, et al. Comparison of the haemodynamic effects of dobutamine with enoximone after open heart surgery in small children. *Br J Anaesth* 1994;72:77–81.

154. Laitinen P, Happonen JM, Sairanen H, et al. Amrinone versus dopamine-nitroglycerin after reconstructive surgery for complete atrioventricular septal defect. *J Cardiothorac Vasc Anesth* 1997;11:870–4.

155. Laitinen P, Happonen JM, Sairanen H, et al. Amrinone versus dopamine and nitroglycerin in neonates after arterial switch operation for transposition of the great arteries. *J Cardiothorac Vasc Anesth* 1999;13:186–90.

156. Laurent I, Monchi M, Chiche JD, et al. Reversible myocardial dysfunction in survivors of out-of-hospital cardiac arrest. *J Am Coll Cardiol* 2002;40:2110–16.

157. Moler FW, Meert K, Donaldson AE, et al; Pediatric Emergency Care Applied Research Network. In-hospital versus out-of-hospital pediatric cardiac arrest: A multicenter cohort study. *Crit Care Med* 2009;37(7):2259–67.

158. Trzeciak S, Jones AE, Kilgannon JH, et al. Significance of arterial hypotension after resuscitation from cardiac arrest. *Crit Care Med* 2009;37(11):2895–903.

159. Langhelle A, Tyvold SS, Lexow K, et al. In-hospital factors associated with improved outcome after out-of-hospital cardiac arrest.

A comparison between four regions in Norway. *Resuscitation* 2003;56:247–63.

160. Berger PB. A glucose-insulin-potassium infusion did not reduce mortality, cardiac arrest, or cardiogenic shock after acute MI. *ACP J Club* 2005;143:4–5.

161. Abend NS, Topjian A, Ichord R, et al. Electroencephalographic monitoring during hypothermia after pediatric cardiac arrest. *Neurology* 2009;72(22):1931–40.

162. Topjian AA, Gutierrez-Colina AM, Sanchez SM, et al. Electrographic status epilepticus is associated with mortality and worse short-term outcome in critically ill children. *Crit Care Med* 2013;41(1):215–23.

163. Kessler SK, Topjian AA, Gutierrez-Colina AM, et al. Short-term outcome prediction by electroencephalographic features in children treated with therapeutic hypothermia after cardiac arrest. *Neurocrit Care* 2011;14(1):37–43.

164. Pilcher J, Weatherall M, Shirtcliffe P, et al. The effect of hyperoxia following cardiac arrest—A systematic review of meta-analysis of animal trials. *Resuscitation* 2012;83(4):417–22.

165. Kilgannon JH, Jones AE, Shapiro NI, et al; Emergency Medicine Shock Research Network (EMShockNet) Investigators. Association between arterial hyperoxia following resuscitation from cardiac arrest and in-hospital mortality. *JAMA* 2010;303(21):2165–71.

166. Bellomo R, Bailey M, Eastwood GM, et al. Arterial hyperoxia and in-hospital mortality after resuscitation from cardiac arrest. *Crit Care* 2011;15(2):R90.

167. Guerra-Wallace MM, Casey FL III, Bell MJ, et al. Hyperoxia and hypoxia in children resuscitated from cardiac arrest. *Pediatr Crit Care Med* 2013;14(3):e143–e148.

168. Duncan BW, Ibrahim AE, Hraska V, et al. Use of rapid-deployment extracorporeal membrane oxygenation for the resuscitation of pediatric patients with heart disease after cardiac arrest. *J Thorac Cardiovasc Surg* 1998;116:305–11.

169. Morris MC, Wernovsky G, Nadkarni VM. Survival outcomes after extracorporeal cardiopulmonary resuscitation instituted during active chest compressions following refractory in-hospital pediatric cardiac arrest. *Pediatr Crit Care Med* 2004;5:440–6.

170. Goldberger ZD, Chan PS, Berg RA, et al. Duration of resuscitation efforts and survival after in-hospital cardiac arrest: an observational study. American Heart Association Get With The Guidelines—Resuscitation (formerly National Registry of Cardiopulmonary Resuscitation) Investigators. *Lancet* 2012;380(9852):1473–81. doi: 10.1016/S0140-6736(12)60862-9.

171. Nishisaki A, Sullivan J III, Steger B, et al. Retrospective analysis of the prognostic value of electroencephalography patterns obtained in pediatric in-hospital cardiac arrest survivors during three years. *Pediatr Crit Care Med* 2007;8:10–7.

172. Schellhammer F, Heindel W, Haupt WF, et al. Somatosensory evoked potentials: A simple neurophysiological monitoring technique in supra-aortal balloon test occlusions. *Eur Radiol* 1998;8:1586–9.

173. Piazza O, Cotena S, Esposito G, et al. S100B is a sensitive but not specific prognostic index in comatose patients after cardiac arrest. *Minerva Chir* 2005;60:477–80.

174. Topjian AA, Lin R, Morris MC, et al. Neuron-specific enolase and S-100B are associated with neurologic outcome after pediatric cardiac arrest. *Pediatr Crit Care Med* 2009;10(4):479–90. doi: 10.1097/PCC.0b013e318198bdb5.

175. Edelson DP, Abella BS, Kramer-Johansen J, et al. Effects of compression depth and pre-shock pauses predict defibrillation failure during cardiac arrest. *Resuscitation* 2006;71:137–45.

176. Sunde K, Pytte M, Jacobsen D, et al. Implementation of a standardised treatment protocol for post resuscitation care after out-of-hospital cardiac arrest. *Resuscitation* 2007;73:29–39.

177. Berger S, Dhala A, Dearani JA. State-of-the-art management of hypertrophic cardiomyopathy in children. *Cardiol Young* 2009;19(suppl 2):66–73.

178. Maron BJ, Shirani J, Poliac LC, et al. Sudden death in young competitive athletes. Clinical, demographic, and pathological profiles. *JAMA* 1996;276(3):199–204.

CHAPTER 26 ■ STABILIZATION AND TRANSPORT

MONICA E. KLEINMAN, AARON J. DONOGHUE, RICHARD A. ORR, AND NIRANJAN "TEX" KISSOON

KEY POINTS

1 Pediatric critical care transport programs are designed to improve the safety and outcome for critically ill or injured children who require interfacility transfer for specialized care. Resuscitation and stabilization prior to transport are important principles to prevent patient deterioration en route between hospitals.

2 Providing intensive care in a mobile environment is associated with unique challenges and risks in comparison to the inpatient setting. Aeromedical transport is associated with additional physiologic stresses that should be considered when preparing a patient for interfacility transport.

3 Most critical care therapies can be provided during transport, although little evidence exists for specific treatments that improve patient outcome.

4 Specialized pediatric transport teams appear to have advantages over general critical care teams in terms of appropriateness of therapy and adverse events and, in retrospective studies, reduced mortality. In most cases, children are more likely to benefit from the expertise of the transport team members than from the speed of travel.

5 Healthcare providers involved in interfacility transports should be familiar with the resources of receiving hospitals with regard to pediatric emergency, intensive care, and trauma services, as well as the responsibilities of referring physicians specified by federal regulations.

In developed countries, pediatric critical care is delivered in dedicated specialty units in which trained personnel and advanced resources are concentrated, usually within tertiary care centers. Critically ill or injured children who are admitted to a PICU have an improved outcome compared with children who are admitted to an adult ICU (1). Therefore, it is often necessary to transfer critically ill or injured children to another facility to obtain the appropriate level of pediatric critical care services. Transport is a particularly high-risk phase of a child's care due to the limitations of a mobile environment with restricted space and resources. Through access to critical care services that traditionally are not available until arrival at the tertiary care center, the use of a specialty transport team may improve patient safety and outcome either by the prevention of deterioration or by the initiation of specific therapies. Pediatric transport programs permit hospitals to extend critical care services into the community so that patients can benefit from specialty care prior to and during interfacility transfer.

HISTORIC DEVELOPMENT OF PEDIATRIC TRANSPORT PROGRAMS

The history of pediatric transport medicine is relatively short compared with other aspects of emergency and critical care. The first formal guidelines for air and ground transports of children were issued by the American Academy of Pediatrics (AAP) in 1986 (2). Shortly thereafter, the AAP granted task force status to Interhospital Transport, and the Section on Transport Medicine was officially established in 1995. More comprehensive guidelines were published in 1993 (3), with subsequent revisions in 1999 and 2006 (4,5).

TRANSPORT IN DEVELOPING COUNTRIES

Most of this chapter focuses on the development and attributes of highly sophisticated tertiary care transport systems in developed countries; however, many alternatives and ingenious systems have evolved in resource-limited settings or less-developed emergency medical and tertiary care networks. Transport is a neglected aspect of care in many areas of the world due to lack of resources (trained personnel, vehicles, resources to pay personnel, lack of roads, and attacks on transport vehicles during conflicts) (6). Under these circumstances, adverse events are high, and improvement in outcomes is not demonstrated. Deciding whether developing and transitional countries should have PICU transport involves a balance of the overall health priorities of that community, and decisions can only be made locally with full knowledge of continuous quality improvement (QI) data. Sophisticated transport systems are unlikely to decrease overall mortality if resources are simply diverted from one entity to another. Sophisticated transport efforts may be of little benefit and may not lead to improved outcomes if pre-PICU practice (IV fluids, supplemental oxygen, bag-valve-mask ventilation and intubation equipment, proper monitoring and resuscitation protocols, etc.) and tertiary PICU facilities are not improved first (7). In resource-limited settings, the cost benefit of a retrieval team must be balanced against compelling and competing primary healthcare priorities such as nutrition, primary care, and immunizations (8). These competing interests and limitations aside, home-grown solutions include bicycles with trailers, tricycles with platforms, motor boats, ox carts in Tanzania, and taxis and buses driven by drivers with training in prehospital emergency management in Ghana. In many other areas of the world, no transport options are available. Despite severely limited resources for such communities, from a patient perspective, the principles and considerations for sound transport medicine are the same in resource-rich and resource-poor settings.

ORGANIZATION OF PEDIATRIC TRANSPORT SYSTEMS

Pediatric critical care transport programs are part of the continuum of care of emergency medical services (EMS) for children and are intended to provide a safe environment during transfer between healthcare institutions. In designing a pediatric transport program to meet the specific needs of the region served, considerations should include the resources of the referring and receiving hospitals, the characteristics of the patient population, and the area's geography and accessibility.

Most specialty pediatric transport services are hospital based. Several models exist, including the use of on-duty staff who are relieved of other duties to perform patient transport, "on-call" staff who respond from home, and dedicated pediatric transport team members who are on-site and do not have other patient care responsibilities. Each program design has obvious advantages and disadvantages in terms of mobilization time, personnel utilization, and cost. No consensus exists concerning the volume of patient transfers required to justify a dedicated pediatric transport team, and each institution must consider the economic and staffing implications of the various program structures.

Established transport services have certain organizational features in common. In addition to trained and qualified staff, essential components include (a) online medical control by qualified physicians, (b) ground and air ambulance capabilities, (c) a coordinated communications system, (d) written clinical and operational guidelines, (e) a comprehensive program for quality and performance improvement, (f) a database to track activity and permit patient follow-up, (g) medical and nursing leadership, (h) administrative resources, and (i) institutional endorsement and financial support (5).

Administrative Issues

While the pediatric transport team's primary objective is to provide high-quality critical care services, there are myriad administrative considerations that distinguish operation of a transport program from other hospital-based activities. Among other things, the transport program leadership has responsibility for treatment protocols, ambulance licensure, emergency vehicle operation and maintenance, and transfer agreements. Clinicians, medical directors, and administrative leaders must closely collaborate to ensure the safety and quality of all aspects of the transport system. A full discussion of the administrative issues is beyond the scope of this chapter, but there are several excellent resources in print and online (5) (http://www.emscnrc.org/EMSC_Resources/Publications.aspx).

Training, Certification, and Licensure

Most transport teams are multidisciplinary and include members with expertise in communications and out-of-hospital care and highly trained hospital-based providers. At present, no uniform national curriculum exists for critical care transport clinicians, either adult or pediatric. Several organizations have nationally recognized certification programs for certain types of transport team members, such as flight nurses and critical care paramedics. Although board certification or a certificate

of special competency in transport medicine has not yet been established, most physicians who provide medical direction or participate in patient care during transport are trained in emergency medicine, critical care, or neonatology. Attending physicians who provide medical control to the team must be licensed to practice medicine in the state in which the base hospital is located. If physicians in training (fellows or residents) are part of the transport team, requirements for participation, supervision, and evaluation must be developed. Orientation to the specialized transport equipment and safety considerations in the mobile environment are essential, as many physicians have never practiced acute care outside a hospital setting.

Multiple standardized life support courses provide certification in specialty areas such as neonatal resuscitation, pediatric resuscitation, advanced trauma care, and disaster management. While these programs provide an opportunity for skills review and to practice a consistent approach to common acute situations, they are not adequate to establish competency in a specific area of clinical care. While there are no evidence-based guidelines for initial training requirements for nonphysician transport providers, recommendations have been published for procedural training for pediatric and neonatal transport nurses, as well as guidelines for skill assessment and retention (9,10).

The term "scope of practice" describes the clinical abilities and skill set for each team member, and may vary depending on an individual's educational background or experience, even among staff with the same professional degree. Scope of practice is also used to refer to the specific clinical activities permitted by a healthcare facility or state regulatory agency such as the Department of Health. As healthcare providers, transport team members must be licensed for their professional practice according to the regulations of the state in which their service is based.

Standard operating procedures, protocols, and guidelines should be established for transport team members by the team's administrative and medical leadership. Patient care protocols define a team's usual approach to specific patient problems and, for nonphysician teams, provide standing orders for therapies that can be provided without contact with medical control. Protocols also allow the team to function in the event that a patient's condition changes and the medical control physician cannot be immediately contacted.

Many transport teams provide services in multiple states or even in multiple countries. It is not necessary for each transport team professional to be licensed in every jurisdiction in which the team may provide patient care; instead, transport personnel are considered to be practicing within their home state for purposes of licensure, regardless of the patient's location. Transport team members are typically credentialed by the institution where they are based or with which they are primarily affiliated. However, by the nature of their work, they regularly provide patient care in facilities in which they do not have clinical privileges. This situation is best addressed by the creation of preapproved interfacility transfer agreements between the referring and receiving institutions.

Finances and Reimbursement

Just as emergency medical care for critically ill or injured children should be provided regardless of the patient's insurance status or ability to pay, a transport team's response to a request for emergent interfacility transfer should not depend on financial factors. Regardless, it is important to recognize that transport services are resource intensive and, when considered in isolation, typically represent a source of revenue loss for an individual patient. Administrators must understand that transport teams facilitate patient entry into the hospital's system and cannot be expected to be independently profitable.

On a less-measurable basis, the availability of high-quality interfacility transport services is expected to promote satisfaction and appreciation among referring physicians and families.

Reimbursement for critical care transport services varies widely among states and between insurance providers. As in other areas of healthcare, reimbursement for transport services has consistently declined while costs have increased. If the transport team composition includes an attending physician, CPT codes exist for face-to-face care of a child during transport. Additional codes include those for telephone consultation with the referring physician prior to the transport team's arrival, and non–face-to-face medical direction provided by the medical control physician.

Most costs (e.g., equipment and salaries) associated with operating a critical care transport service are fixed. Significant expenses include vehicle maintenance, repairs, and insurance; durable medical equipment; and disposable supplies. As in other areas of healthcare, personnel salaries and benefits constitute most of a transport team's budget, and as team members are often more senior and experienced, their salaries may be accordingly higher.

Legal Considerations

In the United States, the practice of interfacility patient transfer is regulated by federal laws that serve to protect patients who present to Medicare-participating hospitals with an emergency condition. The Consolidated Omnibus Budget Reconciliation Act (COBRA) was first passed in 1986; one component of this legislation was the Emergency Medical Transportation and Labor Act (EMTALA). EMTALA was created to prevent "patient dumping"; that is, the transfer to another facility of an individual presenting for emergency care without assessment or stabilizing treatment (Table 26.1). EMTALA was last revised in 2010, and regular revisions can be expected in the future (http://www.cms.hhs.gov/EMTALA) (11). Physicians who transfer patients under emergency circumstances should be aware of the regulations in their practice locale and be familiar with the requirements for communication and documentation (12).

Risk Management and Insurance

Unlike personnel who function solely within a hospital setting, transport team members provide care in hazardous environments during ground and air transports. Because they are exposed to an increased risk of injury and death, programs

TABLE 26.1

REQUIREMENTS OF THE EMERGENCY MEDICAL TRANSPORTATION AND LABOR ACT

1. The transferring hospital provides medical treatment to the best of its ability, based on available resources.
2. The transferring physician contacts the receiving facility to determine that qualified personnel and space are available for treatment and to identify a receiving physician who will accept the patient.
3. The transferring hospital sends copies of all available medical records related to the patient's emergency medical condition.
4. The transfer is affected through qualified personnel and transportation equipment, including the use of advanced life support, if appropriate.

should consider requesting additional insurance coverage for staff participating in critical care transport. Collisions and crashes involving pediatric and neonatal teams are uncommon, with surveillance data suggesting that one collision or crash occurs for every 1000 patient transports. Collisions or crashes resulting in serious injuries or death are even less common and occur at a rate of 0.55 injuries or deaths per 1000 transports (13). Although most fatal events are the result of aircraft crashes, ground collisions account for most transport-related injuries and are often moderate or severe in nature. Because transport team members tend to be young, with many productive years ahead of them, disability coverage is important to provide financial security following an accident or work-related injury.

Transfer Agreements

It is important to cultivate relationships with transferring facilities to promote patient referrals and to improve the coordination of patient care. In the current financial climate, many smaller hospitals are reducing pediatric subspecialty services and referring sicker children to tertiary facilities. Transfer agreements establish policies that clearly define administrative procedures and the roles and responsibilities of the referring and receiving facilities. These agreements may include language that indicates acceptance of acutely ill patients by the receiving hospital, as well as an understanding that recuperating patients will be returned to the referring facility. Transfer agreements must comply with local, state, and federal mandates. The EMS for Children (EMSC) program has published sample pediatric transfer guidelines for adoption by different states or programs (http://www.emscnrc.org).

Quality Improvement and Accreditation

The construction of a well-functioning transport program begins with a strong foundation of personnel, training, equipment, communication system, and vehicles (ambulance, helicopter, and/or fixed-wing aircraft). Continued monitoring and evaluation of the transport program are critical to ensuring quality patient care and promoting the program's success. A written QI plan is essential and should begin with an explanation of the mission of the transport service and the goals for the QI program. It should delineate the lines of authority for performing quality measurement activities and should demonstrate how that authority interfaces with the governing body for the transport service. A QI program should establish criteria to ensure that the standards of care are practiced by individuals and groups, linking the transport team with the medical director, administrative team, risk management, and other pertinent disciplines to identify opportunities to improve care. Transport programs should analyze every component of the services that they provide to ensure effective, consistent, safe, and state-of-the-art care.

The medical director must actively participate in the QI process if it is to be a viable component of the transport program. The medical director serves in various capacities as a resource, supervisor, moderator, evaluator, and educator. Activities for the medical director related to QI include interviewing, hiring, educating personnel, developing treatment protocols, and reviewing and critiquing clinical care. Supervision of patient care during transport (i.e., online medical control) via direct communication is another important component of ensuring quality of care. The medical director should oversee the posttransport case review process, including audits of charts, recorded audiotapes, and morbidity and mortality conferences.

The Commission on Accreditation of Medical Transport Systems (CAMTS) is an organization that aims to improve the quality of patient care and safety of the transport environment through its voluntary accreditation process. Although originally focused on air transport services, CAMTS now surveys ground, rotor-wing, and fixed-wing programs. Accreditation consists of an application process, site survey, and program review to evaluate the transport service using measurable standards and objective criteria. Accreditation standards are revised every 2–3 years with input from representatives of the medical profession to reflect the dynamic nature of the critical care transport field. As of October 2012, 149 services in North America were accredited by CAMTS. The most recent CAMTS standards for accreditation (9th edition) were released in August 2012 and updated in November 2012 (http://www.camts.org).

THE TRANSPORT ENVIRONMENT

Prehospital Care versus Critical Care Transport

EMS include all aspects of basic life support, advanced life support, and critical care transport in which emergency care is provided at a scene and/or in a vehicle. EMS encompass the prehospital and interfacility components of transport and include hospital-based specialty teams. Most pediatric critical care transport programs provide interfacility transport but do not routinely respond to the scene of an accident or emergency, except if a crash is encountered during travel or if a multicasualty incident or disaster occurs.

Prehospital care providers have variable educational backgrounds and experience in the care of critically ill or injured children. Less than 10% of all ambulance calls nationwide are for infants and children; only a few involve advanced life support, and even less can be classified as critical care. Overall, this frequency translates into three pediatric patient encounters per month for ~60% of the nation's paramedics, with <3% of the nation's paramedics providing emergency care for ≥15 children per month (14).

Limited provider exposure to critically ill children presents a challenge to maintaining pediatric assessment and treatment skills. For example, in a moderately-sized EMS system with 50 active advanced life support providers, each provider would be expected to have one pediatric bag-valve-mask case every 1.7 years, one pediatric intubation case every 3.3 years, and one intraosseous cannulation case every 6.7 years (15). It has also been demonstrated that the ability of a prehospital provider to intubate or provide bag-valve-mask ventilation for a child deteriorates significantly in the 6 months following initial training (16). These data should be considered when selecting the appropriate mode of interfacility transport for an ill or injured child.

Currently, no federal regulations specifically address the interfacility transfer of children, other than EMTALA which pertains to all age groups. The federally funded EMSC program (http://www.emscnrc.org), founded in 1984, has as its mission to ensure that all children and adolescents receive state-of-the-art emergency care throughout the EMS system, from prevention through rehabilitation. The EMSC program provides grants to states to improve existing EMS systems and to develop and evaluate protocols and procedures for treating children.

Mobile Intensive Care

The care of critically ill or injured children during interfacility transport presents unique challenges for assessment, monitoring, diagnosis, and treatment. Thorough preparation and appropriate equipment are required to permit safe and effective management during transport. The clinical assessment of patients, both by physical examination and through the use of monitoring equipment, is more difficult in a mobile environment as compared to within the ICU. Both ground and air transports result in noise levels that can prohibit auscultation of lung and heart sounds. Vehicular motion and vibration can result in artifacts in pulse oximetry, electrocardiography, and oscillometric blood pressure monitoring. Despite these limitations, it is possible to perform advanced procedures in a mobile environment. Published reports have described successful endotracheal intubation, pleural decompression, and intraosseous access during both air and ground transports. In general, however, the risk of performing a procedure during transport is considered higher than that in a stationary setting. As a result, the threshold for establishing a secure airway, for example, is lower when interfacility transport is required.

The capacity for laboratory analysis during transport has traditionally been limited, other than the use of reagent strips or glucometers for blood glucose measurement. Recent technologic advances have produced handheld and portable devices that enable point-of-care (POC) testing through the use of rapid assays, thus permitting the analysis of whole-blood chemistries and blood gases. A retrospective review, over 5 years, by a single institution's critical care transport team showed that POC testing led to significant management changes in 30% of patients, with bedside blood gas analysis having the highest impact on therapy (17). A similar prospective study was performed in which the transport team sampled arterial blood at the referring hospital and during transport; the results influenced management in 86.2% of the patients, with adjustment in mechanical ventilation being most common (18).

With advances in technology, most therapies available in the ICU can be employed during critical care transport; examples include mechanical ventilation (invasive and noninvasive), continuous infusions, administration of inhaled nitric oxide (iNO), and cardiac pacing. Limitations to the performance of specific therapies are largely due to the inability to safely secure equipment for travel. Despite this, several programs have invested in the necessary vehicle modifications to permit such advanced therapies as extracorporeal membrane oxygenation (ECMO) and high-frequency oscillatory ventilation (HFOV) during interfacility transport (19–21).

Ground Transport Considerations

Transport by ground is the most common modality of interfacility and prehospital transport. The advantages of ground transport include virtually ubiquitous access, low cost, and ability to respond in most weather conditions. Ambulances are more spacious than most aeromedical transport vehicles and provide the option to perform procedures or clinical interventions in a stationary setting when necessary. Specially equipped ambulances for children have the capability to transport newborns and small infants in isolettes and can be modified to provide adequate infant and child restraint devices, even for critically ill patients.

The disadvantages of ground transport include the impact of severe winter weather, traffic congestion, and road and highway conditions. The use of sirens to facilitate navigation through traffic, although helpful in expediting transport in urban areas, can impair the ability of the team to perform clinical tasks dependent on auscultation. Teams that perform only ground transports should develop a strong working relationship with teams that provide rotor- and fixed-wing transports to allow for optimal coordination of efforts for transports of critically ill children that are time sensitive or involve travel over long distances.

Aeromedical Transport

Aeromedical transport is widely available in the United States and other developed countries. Both rotor-wing (helicopter) and fixed-wing (airplane) aircraft can be adapted for use as critical care transport vehicles. The use of aeromedical services requires an understanding of the unique physiologic stresses and logistic issues associated with rotor- and fixed-wing transports.

Barometric pressure is defined as the sum of the partial pressures of each of the component gases in the atmosphere; it represents the force or weight exerted by the atmosphere at any given altitude. Barometric pressure at sea level is 760 mm Hg and decreases as altitude increases. The component gases exist in constant proportions: nitrogen (78%), oxygen (21%), and very small percentages of other gases, such as carbon dioxide, helium, and hydrogen.

Dalton's law states that the total pressure of a gas represents the sum of the partial pressures of the different gas components:

$$P_T = P_1 + P_2 + P_3. \qquad [26.1]$$

As total barometric pressure decreases with increasing altitude, the partial pressure of each gas is reduced. Likewise, the addition of another gas to the mixture decreases the partial pressure of all other gases.

The partial pressure of any inspired gas is determined by the barometric pressure (P_B) and the fraction of the atmospheric gas it represents. In the case of oxygen, for example, P_{IO_2} at sea level can be calculated as follows:

$$P_{IO_2} = P_B \times F_{IO_2}$$

$$= 760 \text{ mm Hg} \times 0.21$$

$$= 159 \text{ mm Hg} \qquad [26.2]$$

At an altitude of 8000 feet, the partial pressure of inspired oxygen is reduced as follows:

$$P_{IO_2} = P_B \times F_{IO_2}$$

$$= 565 \text{ mm Hg} \times 0.21$$

$$= 118 \text{ mm Hg} \qquad [26.3]$$

Whereas P_{IO_2} represents the partial pressure of inspired oxygen, the actual partial pressure of oxygen at the alveolar level is affected by the presence of water vapor and carbon dioxide, both of which reduce the partial pressure of oxygen in accordance with Dalton's law. The amount of carbon dioxide in the alveolar space is, in part, determined by the patient's metabolism—that is, *the respiratory quotient*.

The *alveolar gas equation* defines the relationship between the alveolar partial pressure of oxygen (P_{aO_2}), P_B, fraction of oxygen in inspired gas (F_{IO_2}), alveolar partial pressure of carbon dioxide (P_{aCO_2}), and respiratory quotient (R), as follows:

$$P_{aO_2} = (P_B - P_{H_2O}) \times F_{IO_2} - (P_{aCO_2}/R) \qquad [26.4]$$

Assuming that R is 0.8, P_{aCO_2} is normal (i.e., ~40 mm Hg), and the partial pressure of water vapor at body temperature (37°C) is 47 mm Hg, the P_{aO_2} while breathing room air at sea level is calculated as follows:

$$P_{aO_2} = (760 \text{ mm Hg} - 47 \text{ mm Hg}) \times 0.21 - (40/0.8)$$

$$= 99 \text{ mm Hg} \qquad [26.5]$$

Thus, with increasing altitude and decreasing P_B, the resultant P_{aO_2} will decrease. P_{aO_2} can be restored to baseline values by increasing the F_{IO_2}. If other factors remain constant, the F_{IO_2} required to maintain the same P_{aO_2} at a lower barometric pressure can be calculated as follows:

$$F_{IO_{2(1)}} \times P_{B_{(1)}} = F_{IO_{2(2)}} \times P_{B_{(2)}} \qquad [26.6]$$

The maintenance of a specific barometric pressure in the cabin of an aircraft (i.e., cabin pressurization) ameliorates this effect to some extent, but this is possible only in fixed-wing aircraft and not in helicopters.

For the patient with severe cardiac or pulmonary disease who is already requiring a F_{IO_2} of 1.0 at ground level, the effects of altitude can worsen the degree of hypoxemia. For example, a child with ARDS (Acute Respiratory Distress Syndrome) and P_{aO_2} of 50 mm Hg on a F_{IO_2} of 1.0 will be exposed to the equivalent of a F_{IO_2} of 0.8 at an altitude of 5000 feet. An infant with cyanotic heart disease is similarly vulnerable to developing a critical level of tissue hypoxia.

A decrease in the ambient barometric pressure has the potential to affect any gas-filled compartment in the body. *Boyle's law* states that an inverse relationship exists between volume and pressure of a gas; therefore, a decrease in pressure results in an increase in volume. The formula for Boyle's law is:

$$P_1V_1 = P_2V_2 \qquad [26.7]$$

where P_1 = pressure at altitude 1, V_1 = volume at altitude 1, P_2 = pressure at altitude 2, and V_2 = volume at altitude 2.

The significance of decreased barometric pressure is dependent on the altitude at which an unpressurized aircraft operates or to which the cabin of a fixed-wing aircraft is pressurized. Most medical helicopters travel at between 1500 and 5000 feet above ground level. If ground level represents sea level, then barometric pressure will decrease by 20% at 5000 feet, with a consequent 20% increase in gas volume. Most commercial aircraft will maintain a cabin pressure that is equivalent to ~8000 feet above sea level, corresponding to a 30% decrease in barometric pressure and a 30% increase in the volume of air-filled spaces.

Gas in normal anatomic compartments (e.g., bowel, middle ears) or in abnormal locations (e.g., pneumothorax) has the potential to undergo physical changes as a result of increased altitude, as does air in devices with gas-inflated medical components (e.g., sequential compression devices, endotracheal tube cuffs, etc.). In a study of intubated adults undergoing aeromedical transport, the tracheal cuff pressures increased by an average of 23 cm H_2O at an altitude of 3000 feet (22). It is essential to anticipate and address the potential for gas expansion by such interventions as gastric drainage, pleural decompression, and replacement of air in an endotracheal tube cuff (using saline) prior to transport.

Rotor-Wing (Helicopter) Transport

Rotor-wing transport is much more common than fixed-wing transport and has a long history of use in prehospital and interfacility patient transport. The greatest advantage of helicopter transport is the speed with which a helicopter can be deployed and can complete a trip. This advantage may be important in densely populated urban areas, where traffic can impede expeditious ground-based transport, but it is particularly significant for rural areas, where greater distances must be covered. Delays in helicopter response due to need for refueling, reconfiguration, or pilot duty time may reduce the impact of air transport on mobilization and transport times. Although significant variability is involved due to geography, staffing, helipad accessibility, and the need for refueling or reconfiguration, helicopter transport is generally faster than ground transport if the patient is >45 miles from the receiving facility (23).

The disadvantages of helicopter transport include a high level of noise, which impairs or sometimes totally eliminates the ability to use a stethoscope, and vibration, which can interfere with patient evaluation. Esophageal stethoscopes designed to fit under flight headphones may ameliorate the difficulty with auscultation, but they are in limited use. Hypothermia is a major risk for infants during helicopter transport if an isolette is not used. In the unpressurized cabin of a helicopter, ambient air has less moisture, which leads to increased risk of airway plugging from secretions. Humidified gases should be used as early as possible.

The use of transport helicopters also requires the presence of a helipad or a suitable landing zone; in the case of interfacility transport, it may be necessary for a helicopter to land at a local airport if the referring hospital has no on-site helipad. Time saved by air transport can be diminished by the need for ground ambulance transfer between the helicopter and the referring and/or receiving hospital. Weather has a more profound effect on helicopter transport than other vehicular modalities, and helicopter flights can be unavailable due to weather as frequently as 20% of the time, depending on the region.

Cost is another significant disadvantage of helicopter transport. The cost-effectiveness of scene flights by prehospital aeromedical teams, primarily for trauma patients, has been called into question for both adults and children (24). Investigations into whether air transport has a significant impact on patient outcomes have yielded mixed results (see Outcomes section). Several studies have demonstrated that air transport is an overutilized resource for children, most likely reflecting the discomfort of community providers with the management of children (25). In one retrospective review, 33% of pediatric trauma patients transported by helicopter were discharged home from the emergency department (ED); among the same population, only 4% were taken directly to the operating room (26).

Fixed-Wing (Airplane) Transport

Fixed-wing transport is typically reserved for travel over long distances or over open water. It has the advantage of the fastest speed of the three commonly used transport modalities. Additional advantages include cabin pressurization, which minimizes the adverse physiologic effects of altitude, and the ability to fly in weather conditions that may not be favorable for helicopter transport. The disadvantages of fixed-wing transport include the same considerations with regard to noise and movement as encountered in a helicopter. Additionally, the available workspace in a fixed-wing vehicle is usually less than that in either helicopters or ambulances. Use of fixed-wing transport also requires the presence of airports close to both referring and receiving hospitals, and such a transport necessarily entails ground transportation to and from the airports, with multiple patient transfers from ambulance to aircraft. Fixed-wing transport requires additional time to mobilize due to the need to file a flight plan. Finally, very high cost remains a disadvantage.

Intrahospital Transport

The transport of a critically ill child outside the PICU occurs commonly due to the need for diagnostic evaluation and procedures in areas such as the radiology suite and operating room. Intrahospital transport presents challenges that are similar to interfacility transport, namely, the need to provide critical care in a nonoptimal environment with limited resources.

For any given procedure or test that requires travel outside the ICU, the clinician must weigh the risks and benefits to the patient. A patient whose condition has not been stabilized or who may deteriorate if specific therapies are interrupted should only be transported if the proposed study or intervention is essential to direct therapy or definitively manage a critical problem. The requirements for such a transport include adequate personnel, equipment, monitoring, and medications such that the level of care and monitoring provided during the time spent outside the ICU is similar to that in the ICU. Monitoring, at a minimum, must include electrocardiography, pulse oximetry, and noninvasive blood pressure. Most portable monitors are also equipped with the capability to measure arterial blood pressure, intracardiac or pulmonary artery pressure, central venous pressure, and intracranial pressure. Capnography during transport is essential for the intubated patient, both to provide a noninvasive measure of ventilation and to ensure early recognition of a displaced or obstructed endotracheal tube. Equipment and medications for emergent airway management should be available for all patients who have an artificial airway or who may require assisted ventilation. All monitors and equipment must be portable and capable of operation by battery power, with verification of a fully charged state prior to leaving the ICU. It is important not to rely on the presence or availability of such equipment in the other hospital areas to which the patient is being transported.

Respiratory support during intrahospital transport is commonly indicated; a respiratory therapist or other provider familiar with the devices being used for the patient in the ICU should be present on all such transports. A patient may be ventilated using either a manual resuscitation bag or a portable transport ventilator. In general, manual ventilation results in significantly increased variability in end-tidal carbon dioxide concentration as compared to transport ventilators (27). In a cohort of 12 children undergoing repeated $Paco_2$ measurements during intrahospital transport, unintentional hyperventilation was very common, with resultant $Paco_2$ levels of <25 mm Hg occurring in 62% of measurements taken (28). It is also essential to have access to an adequate supply of oxygen and/or compressed air during the anticipated travel time. Most patients can be safely ventilated with 100% oxygen during brief intrahospital transports.

The largest study of adverse occurrences during pediatric intrahospital transport found that, during 269 events, significant physiologic derangements, as evidenced by vital sign changes, occurred 72% of the time and that equipment-related problems occurred during 10% of the transports (29). A significant therapeutic intervention was necessary in 14% of patients. Adverse occurrences were more common in patients who received mechanical ventilation, and interventions were also more commonly necessary in this group (34%, as compared to 9% of nonventilated patients). Multivariate analysis demonstrated an association between length of transport and the likelihood of an adverse event, whereas no association was found with age of patient or number of team members accompanying the patient.

Safety Considerations

By its nature, interfacility transport carries additional potential risks for healthcare providers, patients, and other individuals (parents). Collisions during air and ground interfacility transports are uncommon but can result in death or injury for patients, clinicians, and vehicle operators or disruption of care delivery systems due to lost work days and damage to vehicles and equipment. A survey of transport teams composed of National Association of Children's Hospitals and Related Institutions (NACHRI) members found that a total of 66 collisions were reported over 5 years (13). No association between number of collisions and total number of transports by the team was apparent, and all fatalities occurred secondary to air transport crashes.

Despite the known advantages of appropriate child restraint devices, their use in ground ambulances is uncommon because of the perception that children cannot be adequately monitored and treated while restrained. In a recent survey of prehospital EMS providers, only half reported that they had adequate knowledge about securing a critically ill child for transport, and 23% indicated that they permitted children to travel while sitting on an adult's lap at least some of the time (30). In comparison, none of the specialty pediatric transport personnel surveyed permitted this practice. Ground transport providers should be familiar with state and local regulations regarding child restraint, which often do not exempt emergency vehicles.

PATIENT CARE DURING TRANSPORT

Optimal pediatric critical care transport achieves a seamless transition from the referring hospital to the receiving institution, with no decrement in the level of care or monitoring during travel. The initiation of specific critical care therapies prior to transport is indicated if they will improve the safety and outcome of the transport. Transferring a child prior to stabilization is associated with significant risk of deterioration en route and a delay in receiving appropriate care. For the few situations in which a time-sensitive, lifesaving intervention is needed that cannot be provided at the referring hospital, such as a craniotomy for an expanding epidural hematoma, one-way transfer using the referring hospital staff may be preferable.

Resuscitation and Stabilization

The referring physician is responsible for determining whether the benefit of transferring a child to another center outweighs the risk of the transport itself, and should use his/her best available resources to stabilize a child prior to transport. Further interventions by the transport team may be necessary; the goals of such additional measures are to optimize patient care and safety during travel while minimizing additional time at the referring facility. These include ensuring the security and proper function of vascular lines, assessing endotracheal tube patency and position, evaluating oxygenation and ventilation, and administering additional medications such as sedatives or analgesics. POC laboratory testing may be utilized when appropriate.

Not surprisingly, time spent by transport teams at referring institutions has been shown to be significantly increased when patients require advanced procedural interventions, such as endotracheal intubation, central venous or arterial access, or thoracostomy tube placement; by contrast, simpler procedures, such as IV placement, blood gas analysis, and nasogastric tube placement have not been associated with such delays (31). Obtaining a postintubation chest radiograph at the referring facility prior to transport resulted in repositioning the endotracheal tube in 50% of neonatal and 42% of pediatric patients (32). A study of pediatric endotracheal tube cuff pressures in children intubated prior to transport team arrival showed that 41% had cuff pressures above the 30 cm H_2O cutoff and 30% of those elevated cuff pressures were >60 cm H_2O (33). Length of stabilization time prior to transport does not appear to have an impact on early ICU mortality for critically ill children transported to receive intensive care (34). The transport team and medical control physician must weigh the benefits of remaining at the referring hospital to perform procedures or to place catheters for invasive monitoring against the risk of further delays in patient transfer to the tertiary center.

Preparation for Transport

For the referring facility, preparation for the transport of children begins with a baseline level of readiness for pediatric assessment, resuscitation, and treatment. Unfortunately, multiple studies have documented that many facilities have considerable deficiencies in the availability of specialized equipment and medications and inadequate training for hospital personnel in the care of the critically ill child (35). No uniform requirements exist for specific credentials or certifications for hospital ED personnel; these are determined by individual institutions. Facilities staffed by board-certified emergency medicine physicians may provide a higher level of pediatric emergency care; however, medical command physicians and transport teams from receiving hospitals should not make assumptions about any given level of knowledge or skill.

Community hospitals should maintain a current list of receiving hospitals and their contact numbers. Once the process of transporting a child is initiated, the referring hospital should be requested to prepare the appropriate documentation, which often includes chart duplication and copies or digital images of radiographs. When possible, it is preferable for the parent(s) or caretaker(s) to remain with the patient until the transport team arrives, to provide informed consent for the transport. All communications should be well documented, ideally through the use of continuously recorded telephone lines that can be used for all transport-related conversations.

Prior to their arrival, the transport team members should discuss and anticipate the patient's needs to ensure an appropriate level of continued care while in transit. Devices for respiratory support and vascular access should be carried by the team, and their function should be checked prior to departure. Medications in weight-appropriate doses and infusions (either in use at the time of transport or anticipated to become necessary) should be prepared in advance. Portable monitors should include the capability for invasive monitoring (arterial, intracranial, capnography) when such monitors are known to be in use or believed to be necessary for the patient's management during transport. The team should know the patient's ongoing medical issues to be able to devise a plan in case of deterioration or complications; in some instances, this may involve consultation with the medical command physician and/or relevant specialists by telephone during stabilization and transport. Additional assessment and stabilization should be thorough but efficient; the adequacy of the resuscitation and stabilization is more important than the amount of time spent on scene at the referring institution.

Communication

Initial communication should include a direct conversation between the referring physician and the receiving physician. Information provided by the referring facility should include the patient's history; the clinical status, including a complete set of vital signs; and an assessment of respiratory, cardiovascular, and neurologic functions. The patient's management through the time of the call should be described completely.

The receiving physician may be asked for medical advice pertaining to the ongoing treatment of the patient. Such advice should be clearly documented. Giving medical advice to a referring facility, depending on the level of comfort and capability of the referring facility with respect to critically ill or injured children, can be fraught with potential difficulty. It is essential to provide such advice in a constructive and diplomatic way and not to convey any sense of criticism. Training for physicians who act as medical control for transported patients should include attention to the importance of effective communication.

Communication with family members prior to transport may be challenging. Time constraints and the need for rapid interventions and evacuation very frequently result in conversations that are brief and hurried, despite an often increased level of concern and anxiety in family members. At a minimum, the risks and benefits of interfacility transfer must be explained and consent obtained, either in person or by phone. Studies have demonstrated that these brief encounters, while difficult, can be very effective at achieving levels of communication that parents view as satisfactory and that the cost incurred by delays on the order of minutes by longer family encounters is small (36). Training program educators should be mindful of these concerns and should include specific training directed toward optimizing such communication skills.

Family and Ethical Considerations

Do-Not-Attempt-Resuscitation Orders

The improved ability to treat disorders that were previously fatal in childhood has resulted in many patients surviving with chronic conditions for longer periods of time. With this trend, advanced directives and do-not-attempt-resuscitation (DNAR) orders have become more prevalent for children. The expressed wishes of a patient and/or the family can vary considerably with respect to interventions and measures that are included in the advanced directives.

The existence of a DNAR order or advanced directive does not imply that the child should not receive any treatment; in general, these orders address specific interventions at the time of a respiratory or cardiorespiratory arrest. Children for whom a DNAR order has been written may still present for emergency care due to issues with pain management, fear or uncertainty about the trajectory of deterioration, or unanticipated changes in condition. Existing data from pediatric EDs have demonstrated that patients with DNAR orders frequently present to these settings when acutely ill. Therefore, pediatric transport teams may be requested to transport a child with an existing DNAR order to a tertiary facility. The consent by a patient or parent to be transported is generally regarded as a request for a higher level of care when, in fact, many factors may lead to a request for transfer: desire for end-of-life care by familiar caretakers, uncertainty as to whether the patient is actually at end of life, or inability to control symptoms such as pain or anxiety. Nonetheless, the possibility still exists that patients or their caretakers may have preexisting preferences with respect to interventions or procedures that they would not want performed regardless of circumstances. A complete exploration of these preferences in the face of such an ambiguous situation, coupled with ongoing acute illness and the need for expedient care, can be extremely challenging. Although attempts to generate systems to track advanced directives in children in EDs are made, they are limited by design to individual hospitals and their referral areas.

Transport team members should inquire about the presence of advanced directives for patients in their care, and they should not assume that such inquiries would have been made by the providers at the referring facility. Transport team members should also obtain specific details about the terms of an advanced directive. When the patient's deterioration appears rapid, it is important to discuss the potential events during transport with family members who have decision-making capacity. When ambiguity exists or family members appear uncertain about their decisions, it is highly preferable for them to accompany the patient on the transport if possible (see Family Presence section). If family members are unavailable or unable to reach consensus, it may be appropriate to offer limited resuscitation measures in an effort to reach the receiving hospital, at which point life-sustaining care can be withdrawn if appropriate.

Death on Transport

It is unusual for children to die during interfacility transport. By policy, most critical care transport programs will not depart from the referring facility with active cardiopulmonary resuscitation (CPR) in progress. Exceptions to this rule include situations such as accidental hypothermia, in which a prolonged period of cardiac arrest may be tolerated without severe neurologic injury. Pediatric transport services may respond to a referring facility to find that a patient has failed to respond to resuscitative measures but the resuscitation team chose to continue efforts until arrival of the team. Transport team members should review the patient's status for any potentially reversible causes of refractory arrest and, in consultation with the medical control physician, use usual and customary criteria to discontinue resuscitation. They may be called on to provide emotional support for the family as well as the referring hospital staff.

Transport team members should be familiar with state regulations regarding notification of the regional organ procurement organization and medical examiner's office following the death of a child. In most states in the United States, it is illegal for anyone other than authorized funeral homes and the medical examiner's office staff to transport a patient who has been pronounced dead. Transporting a child's body from the referring facility for autopsy at a tertiary care center, for example, requires that the child be sent to the referring hospital's morgue and then transported by an authorized party. In general, if cardiac arrest occurs after the team departs from the referring facility, the team should continue resuscitative efforts until arrival at the receiving facility. Under certain circumstances and in consultation with the medical control physician, it may be appropriate to divert to a closer facility.

Family Presence

Permitting family members to remain physically present during acute medical care for their children is an issue that has been systematically evaluated with respect to CPR and invasive procedures (37,38). Policy statements that encourage family presence in these situations now exist, but to date, no such formal recommendations have been formulated with respect to family presence during critical care transport.

Special considerations related to the presence of a family member or caretaker during interfacility transport include the effect on care delivery, safety, and the emotional milieu for patients, parents, and staff. Additional seats for passengers are present in most ambulances and approximately one-half of helicopters used for transport in the United States, but opinions and policies regarding the presence of parents during critical care transport vary greatly. Possible advantages associated with parental presence include emotional benefit to the patient, decreased parental anxiety, caretaker availability for procedural consent when necessary, and improved public relations. Disadvantages include limitations of space, distraction or increased anxiety for the crew, and increased parental or patient anxiety.

Data on the effect of parental presence during transport is limited but, for the most part, report its safety without impedance of care. A national survey of pediatric transport programs showed that 63% of 103 responding programs permitted parents to travel with their children in the ambulance, but parents actually accompanied the team during only 28% of transports (39). Parents who accompanied their children during transport reported less anxiety in themselves and their children, compared with parents whose children were transported without parental accompaniment (40). Physicians and nurses experienced very little additional stress or difficulty performing interventions when necessary, and the majority of practitioners described the experience as beneficial (41). Adverse events occurred in only 11 of 279 (3%) transports, and most of the recorded adverse events were parent related as opposed to patient related. This study resulted in the adoption of parental presence as standard practice for the South Thames Retrieval Service, one of the largest pediatric transport services in the United Kingdom.

TRANSPORT CONSIDERATIONS FOR SPECIFIC POPULATIONS

Pediatric critical care transport team members must have a diverse set of skills and the flexibility to adapt to changing environments and situations—all perhaps within a single shift or day of the week. Familiarity with the special considerations for unique populations will contribute to the transport service's effectiveness and quality of care.

Pediatric Emergency Department Considerations

It is estimated that <10% of hospitals in the United States have dedicated pediatric EDs. The majority of pediatric emergency care, therefore, is provided in EDs that serve both adults and children, and whose resources for pediatric emergency care are variable. The AAP and American College of Emergency Physicians have jointly published guidelines for the care of children in the ED, addressing leadership, personnel, equipment, and policies and procedures (42). At present, no method is uniformly accepted for categorizing EDs based on their capabilities with regard to pediatric emergency care. The AAP has endorsed a statement by the Society for Academic Emergency Medicine that, whereas physically separate care areas for children are ideal, they are not mandatory for the provision of quality pediatric emergency care (43). Despite the existence of recommendations from national organizations, many EDs are underequipped for the treatment of critically ill or injured children.

Trauma Centers

Trauma is the leading cause of death for children between the ages of 6 months and 14 years; consequently, the interfacility transport of critically injured children is a frequent occurrence. It is essential that pediatric transport team members be familiar with the trauma capabilities of receiving institutions. The American College of Surgeons Committee on Trauma offers site visits to review trauma programs based on predefined criteria for staffing, facilities, and other resources. While the designation as a trauma center is based on individual state regulations, the ACS (American College of Surgeons) uses a process known as *verification* to indicate that the facility meets criteria for a specific trauma center level (http://www.facs.org/trauma/vcprogram.html). Level 1 trauma centers may be classified as level 1 pediatric and/or adult trauma centers. As expected, to be so designated, these facilities must meet additional requirements for specially trained pediatric medical and surgical specialists. Guidelines for prehospital transport destination based on trauma center level are typically determined by state or regional EMS protocols. Pediatric trauma patients may or may not be given special consideration within a state's trauma system, depending on the availability and accessibility of pediatric trauma centers in the region.

Most pediatric trauma patients suffer blunt injuries that are typically managed nonoperatively. Pediatric trauma resuscitation focuses on airway management, ventilatory support, and restoration of intravascular volume. Approximately 30% of pediatric trauma patients will require an operation at some point during their hospitalization. A retrospective review was performed of over 68,000 trauma patients under the age of 18 whose information was available through the National Trauma Data Bank (44). Excluding patients with isolated orthopedic injuries, 7.8% of patients with blunt trauma underwent emergent surgical procedures defined as surgery within 4 hours following admission. The indications for surgery were general surgical (4.5%), neurosurgical (2.1%), or other (1.2%). When the patient population was limited to children ≤13 years of age, only 5.5% of patients underwent emergency operative procedures other than orthopedic surgery.

A small percentage of injured children (e.g., patients with expanding epidural hematomas) will require immediate surgery on arrival to the trauma center. In these cases, it is important that transport programs work with receiving hospitals to develop procedures for direct admission of selected patients to the operating room or other appropriate location. Components of a "direct-to-the-OR" protocol include a communication system to notify the appropriate surgical service(s) and other essential personnel (e.g., anesthesia, operating room nursing, blood bank, radiology). In most cases, eligible patients should already have a secure airway and any imaging that would be considered essential (e.g., CT scan) prior to surgery.

For most pediatric trauma patients, the most common complication during interfacility transport is airway compromise. As discussed earlier, despite the importance of pretransport stabilization, it is common for injured children to be rapidly transferred from community facilities because of their lack of comfort with pediatric patients. Children who were transported by helicopter were likely to be transferred significantly more quickly from referring hospitals than were adults with equal severity of injury (45).

Given the nonoperative nature of most pediatric trauma cases, trauma specialists and transport providers continue to debate whether direct transfer from the scene of the injury to a trauma center is preferable to secondary transfer after stabilization at a nontertiary hospital. Proponents of the former method cite rapid access to diagnostic and surgical services, whereas proponents of the latter emphasize the importance of early airway and shock management. Several studies have supported the position that early and ongoing resuscitation of the pediatric trauma patient improves outcome and should not be compromised in the interest of rapid transfer. The outcomes of injured children transported from the scene directly to a trauma center were compared with those of children who were first stabilized in a community hospital and later transferred by air (46). The patients were stratified by injury severity (minor = index injury severity score <15, major = index injury severity score >15). The overall mortality rate was lower for the group that underwent secondary interfacility transport (5.5% vs. 8.7%, $p < 0.05$). The most severely injured patients were the most likely to benefit, with a mortality of 15.5% versus 26.7%. The authors concluded that stabilization at a community hospital prior to transfer to a trauma center might improve survival for injured children.

PICU Considerations

As with trauma centers and NICUs, PICUs may be classified by level based on their resources and capabilities. Guidelines for PICUs have been updated by the AAP and the Society of Critical Care Medicine (47). Level I facilities are those that provide a full range of pediatric subspecialty services and meet specific requirements for availability of personnel, equipment, and support services on a 24-hour basis. For level II facilities, some of these resources are considered optional, with continued minimum requirements for staffing and other services. In most states, the classification of PICUs is an informal practice that has no bearing on patient triage or transfer or the type or complexity of care that is permitted at a particular institution. The availability of certain services, however, may be regulated by a state agency such as the Department of Public Health, which often has the authority to license ICU beds, approve expansion of services and physical facilities, and control expenditures for capital resources. Such regulations may impact hospital-based transport programs, which may be required to demonstrate sufficient need in the region or state to expand physical facilities or enact major purchases, such as aircraft.

Despite evidence that supports improved outcomes with admission to PICUs, a significant number of critically ill infants and children continue to be admitted to hospitals that lack pediatric specialty facilities or expertise (48). Nearly 10% of all US hospitals without PICU facilities admit critically ill and injured children, and 7% of these hospitals routinely admit these children to adult ICUs rather than transferring them to a pediatric facility. Of the hospitals that keep children, few have protocols for obtaining pediatric consultation for emergencies, and many do not have appropriately sized equipment for children (48).

Burn Centers

The management of the pediatric burn patient may require specific resources because serious burns are both uncommon and highly complex. Although adult burn units are commonly found at major medical centers, specialized care for pediatric burn patients is concentrated among a small number of facilities, such as the Shriners Hospital system. Transfer to a pediatric burn center is often a secondary or even tertiary transport following resuscitation and/or stabilization at a community hospital or trauma center without a burn unit.

Critical care transport programs should work with the closest regional pediatric burn center to develop procedures for the triage of seriously burned children either directly to the burn center or in secondary transfer following resuscitation and stabilization at another facility. The American Burn Association (http://www.ameriburn.org) has developed guidelines for the transfer of children to a pediatric burn center (49) (Table 26.2). Burn patients are often transported by helicopter, but in many instances, air transport may be unnecessary due to an observed practice of "overtriage." Studies have shown that referring physicians regularly overestimate burn size, favoring the use of air transport and thus increasing the costs of acute burn care (50,51).

NICU Considerations

Unlike trauma centers or PICUs, NICUs are typically licensed by the individual state to provide a specific level of services for neonatal patients. The level of NICU care is usually designated by the state's hospital regulatory agency, such as the

TABLE 26.2

AMERICAN BURN ASSOCIATION BURN UNIT REFERRAL CRITERIA

1. Partial thickness burns >10% total body surface area
2. Burns that involve the face, hands, feet, genitalia, perineum, or major joints
3. Third-degree burns in any age group
4. Electrical burns, including lightning injuries
5. Chemical burns
6. Inhalation injury
7. Burn injury in patients with preexisting medical disorders that could complicate management, prolong recovery, or affect mortality
8. Any patients with burns and concomitant trauma (e.g., fractures) in which the burn injury poses the greatest risk of morbidity or mortality. In such cases, the patient may be initially stabilized in a trauma center before being transferred to a burn unit. Physician judgment will be necessary in such situations and should be in concert with the regional medical control plan and triage protocols.
9. Burned children in hospitals without qualified personnel or equipment for the care of children
10. Burn injury in patients who will require special social, emotional, or long-term rehabilitative intervention

Department of Public Health, whose definitions may vary from state to state. The AAP recommends a uniform classification and subclassification of NICUs based on their capabilities (52) (Table 26.3).

Extracorporeal Membrane Oxygenation and Inhaled Nitric Oxide

ECMO, a form of extracorporeal life support, is provided at ~120 centers in the United States, a number that has remained stable over the past 5 years (http://www.elsonet.org), reflecting the decreased demand for ECMO due to the use of therapies such as HFOV, iNO, and surfactant replacement.

In 1999, the Food and Drug Administration approved the use of iNO for the treatment of hypoxic respiratory failure in term and near-term neonates with clinical or echocardiographic evidence of pulmonary hypertension. As a result, many newborn ICUs, including facilities that do not have ECMO capabilities, began to provide iNO therapy. The initiation of iNO therapy in a non-ECMO center is controversial, because it may delay transfer to a facility with ECMO capability. This practice has major implications for critical care transport teams, who may be called on to urgently transfer a critically ill newborn who is already receiving maximal medical therapy, including iNO, in a non-ECMO facility. Therefore, it is essential that non-ECMO centers that provide iNO therapy for neonatal respiratory failure work closely with an ECMO center to develop criteria for the transfer of these infants, with a goal of ensuring a "window of opportunity" during which the transport can be safely accomplished. These guidelines should be evaluated regularly by reviewing the outcome of infants transported for ECMO. A certain incidence of "unnecessary" transports (i.e., infants who are referred for, but ultimately do not require, ECMO) may be necessary if the transfer criteria are adequately conservative. Furthermore, any transport team that may be called on to transport a newborn who is already receiving iNO therapy must have the capability of providing iNO during transport, because abrupt discontinuation may result in serious deleterious effects (53,54).

TABLE 26.3

LEVELS OF NEONATAL INTENSIVE CARE UNITS

Level I (Basic)
Neonatal resuscitation
Postnatal care of healthy newborns
Care of infants born at 35–37 wk of gestation who are
  physiologically stable
Stabilization of sick newborns or those who are <35 wk of
  gestational age prior to transfer to a higher-level facility

Level II (Specialty)
Neonatal resuscitation
Postnatal care of infants born at >32 wk of gestation and
  birth weight >1500 g, and care of newborns who are moderately ill and do not require urgent subspecialty services
Care of premature infants who are convalescing after a
  course in a level III nursery

Level III (Subspecialty)
Neonatal resuscitation
Postnatal care that includes advanced life support and/or
  comprehensive care for high-risk or critically ill newborns

The decision to initiate iNO on transport should reflect a consideration of the potential risks and benefits of its use outside the ICU, including the severity of illness and distance or time to the receiving facility. The practice of empirically initiating iNO on transport to facilitate the transition from HFOV to conventional mechanical ventilation has been reported, but no evidence suggests that it improves patient safety or outcome (55).

Ideally, a newborn with hypoxic respiratory failure whose trajectory predicts the need for ECMO will be transferred to an ECMO center prior to meeting criteria for cannulation or becoming too unstable to transport. When this is not possible, a few select programs have the capability to respond to requests for transport by mobilizing an ECMO team that is capable of cannulating the patient at the referring facility, then transporting while on ECMO to the base institution (19–21). Although labor intensive, expensive, and associated with high risk, this practice has been carried out safely and successfully in both civilian and military programs.

In general, the Extracorporeal Life Support Organization recommends that a neonate whose condition is deteriorating be transferred at a time when the conversion to conventional ventilation can still be tolerated and suggests that an infant who has not improved after 6 hours of HFOV be considered a candidate for expedient transfer (56). Individual institutions may use the alveolar–arterial oxygen difference, the oxygenation index, or the persistence of a Pao_2 of <50 torr as predictors of the need for ECMO. Unfortunately, published experience indicates that the transfer of newborns for ECMO often occurs after the patient has reached commonly-agreed-upon criteria for cannulation (57).

The staff at the ECMO center that accepts a newborn in transfer should clearly indicate to the referring physician that the patient is being transported as an ECMO candidate, without a guarantee that ECMO will be provided. This approach minimizes the possibility that the referring hospital or the family will question the decision to transport in the event that ECMO is not required. Furthermore, it communicates the fact that the ECMO center will be evaluating the patient and determining if the infant is an appropriate candidate for ECMO after arrival.

The decision to cannulate for ECMO may be facilitated by requesting that the referring facility perform certain diagnostic studies while the transport team is mobilizing and responding.

These studies include an echocardiogram to evaluate for non-correctable conditions or cyanotic heart disease that might have been misdiagnosed as pulmonary hypertension. In addition, a cranial ultrasound to assess for the presence of intracranial hemorrhage may be helpful. Because the receiving facility will need to type and crossmatch the patient's blood, it is unnecessary to perform this at the referring hospital, unless a need for the transfusion of blood products during transport is anticipated.

Resident Education in Transport Medicine

Transport represents an excellent educational opportunity for residents in training but may conflict with the efficiency and effectiveness of a dedicated transport team. Interfacility transport requires a unique set of skills, distinct from the traditional hospital-based training of most residency programs. It is essential that personnel utilized to provide care during interfacility transport be properly trained, familiar with the unique demands of providing care in a mobile environment, and prepared to handle the variety of patient contingencies that may arise during ground and air transports. The addition of a trainee to the transport team composition should only occur with adequate preparation and education so that patient and team safety are not jeopardized. Practically, space or weight considerations may be an issue, because vehicles used by transport teams have limited room and capacity. Further studies are warranted to determine if pediatric resident involvement in a transport medicine rotation improves the resident's level of skill and confidence or adds value to the service.

The Residency Review Committee of the Accreditation Council for Graduate Medical Education refers to pediatric resident involvement in critical care transport in its program requirements for residency education in pediatrics as follows: (a) participation in decision making in admitting, discharging, and transferring of patients to the ICU; and (b) resuscitation, stabilization, and transportation of patients to the ICU and within the hospital (http://www.acgme.org). In a recent survey of 138 pediatric residency programs, 80% of base hospitals operated a pediatric critical care transport team (25). Team leadership was provided by nurses in 44% of pediatric transports. Of the remaining programs, 70% used residents as team leaders. The prerequisites for resident participation were variable, but most often included completion of a NICU or PICU rotation (85%) or certification in the Neonatal Resuscitation Program or Pediatric Advanced Life Support (94%). If a residency program elects to include transport medicine as a clinical rotation, a specific curriculum should be developed for resident physicians in training.

OUTCOMES

It is difficult to measure the impact of interfacility transport care or events on the ultimate outcome of a critically ill patient. Most studies have used surrogate end points rather than long-term clinical outcomes or mortality. In a systematic review of outcomes of interfacility transport for adult patients who were intubated and mechanically ventilated, data were insufficient to conclude risk factors for morbidity and mortality (58). Evidence for or against a particular practice or specific therapy is limited by the absence of randomized, controlled trials, especially in pediatric critical care transport. Two national leadership conferences have identified key questions in the field, most of which would require multicentered studies for answers (59,60).

Transport Scoring Systems

In contrast to transported neonates, the ability to predict which children are at high risk for deterioration during interfacility transport has been elusive (61). Several scoring systems have been developed based on pretransport data, but their utility is limited by the subjective nature and variable accuracy of referring physicians' assessments. The association between pretransport variables and inhospital mortality was studied, and factors identified at the time of referral for transport that were predictive of mortality were systolic blood pressure, respiratory rate, oxygen requirement, and altered mental status, similar to those variables that are used to evaluate risk of mortality at the time of admission to the ICU (62). Importantly, the risk of mortality correlated with the likelihood of deterioration and the need for major interventions or procedures during transport. The Transport Risk Assessment in Pediatrics (TRAP) score uses physiologic variables to predict need for PICU admission and may support triage decision making (63).

Team Composition

Pediatric critical care transport teams may be staffed with a variety of personnel combinations including registered nurses or nurse practitioners, physicians, respiratory therapists, and paramedics. A consensus does not exist among transport experts as to the ideal team composition, and optimal staffing may depend on the patient's condition, anticipated clinical needs, and available resources at the referring facility. In many European countries and Australia, it is commonplace for physicians to serve as team members for both prehospital and interhospital transports. Several adult studies have demonstrated improved survival for trauma patients when physicians are included in the team composition (64), whereas others have shown no benefit. To date, no studies have been conducted to evaluate the effect of physician-versus-nonphysician team composition on the outcome of transported children.

With adequate pretransport stabilization, most pediatric transports occur without the need for advanced procedures (65). With regard to specific skills, nonphysician teams compare favorably with physician-staffed teams. A 95.1% success rate has been reported for endotracheal intubation in children <13 years of age by a single, nonspecialty, nurse–paramedic, critical care transport team (66). In contrast, other aeromedical transport programs have reported worse performance when comparing adult with pediatric intubations. It was concluded in all of these studies that additional training in airway management in children and the use of medications (e.g., neuromuscular blockade) to facilitate intubation would likely result in a greater success rate.

As might be expected, when cognitive skills are considered, a greater difference is observed between physicians and nonphysicians. The training and performance of pediatric transport nurses were compared with those of third-year pediatric residents with regard to radiographic interpretation (67). The transport nurses had <10 hours of instruction, whereas the residents had an average of 133 hours of formal training in radiology. The correlation with a radiologist's interpretation was ~66% for the house staff and ~34% for the transport nurses. The transport nurses' training was apparently more focused, and they had higher scores on the assessment of radiographs with pneumothoraces.

④ Specialty Pediatric Teams versus General Teams

Pediatric critical care transport exposes patients to risks that may be mitigated by the use of specially trained and equipped personnel. In a prospective study to evaluate the morbidity associated with interhospital transport by a nonspecialty team, the risk of adverse events was compared between patients who underwent interfacility transport and a control group of patients admitted to the PICU from within the receiving institution (68). Of 177 transported patients, significant adverse events occurred in 15.3%, whereas the incidence of adverse events was 3.6% in the 195 control patients. Although the severity of illness was slightly greater in the group of patients who required transport, the difference in adverse events persisted among the most severely ill patients when controlling for risk of mortality.

Inadequate stabilization and adverse events were reduced when transport team members received specialized pediatric training (69). In this study, 72% of all preventable insults on transport occurred with emergency medical attendants who had no formalized pediatric training; 20% occurred with emergency medical attendants who had received an intensive 18-month pediatric training module; and only 8% occurred when the patients were transported by a pediatric intensive care team. Similarly, it was demonstrated that children who were transported by nonspecialized teams had a 10-fold increase in transport-related adverse events (e.g., inadvertent extubation) compared with patients who were transported by pediatric specialty teams, after adjusting for severity of illness and number of interventions (70).

A study from the Netherlands prospectively compared patient care during interhospital transport when children were accompanied either by the referring physicians or by the specialty transport (retrieval) teams (71). Patients transported by referring physicians had a higher incidence of respiratory insufficiency (56.9% vs. 41.1%) and a lower incidence of circulatory insufficiency (27.0% vs. 41.1%) as their primary diagnosis. Despite this, fewer of the children transported by the referring physician received ventilatory support (47.4% vs. 72.3%). Notably, they also had a higher rate of significant complications and need for acute interventions immediately on arrival at the receiving hospital's PICU.

In a prospective risk assessment of 1085 children transported to a children's hospital, patients who were transported by nonspecialized transport teams were more likely to suffer from an unplanned event (odds ratio, 22.2) and inhospital mortality (odds ratio, 2.4) when compared with children who were transported by specialized teams, after adjusting for severity of illness, age, and diagnosis (72). Mobilization time, scene time, and total transport time did not predict unplanned events or death.

A systematic review of the literature to evaluate the evidence that supported the use of specialist transport personnel for critically ill adults and children included a total of 4534 patients from six cohort studies (73). When adjusted for severity of illness, only one study demonstrated a clinically relevant improvement in outcome—survival to 6 hours—when specialty personnel accompanied the patient. However, in the largest study to date involving 17,649 patients transferred from other hospitals, patients admitted to the PICU from within the same hospital had a lower risk-adjusted mortality rate. Multivariate analysis showed that use of a pediatric specialty transport team was associated with improved survival (74). A study of 1085 infants and children in Pittsburgh transported by a nonspecialized team versus a specialized team showed (with adjustment for severity) greater unplanned events (61% vs. 1.5%) and greater death (23% vs. 9%) with the nonspecialized team (75).

In addition to outcome, transport by specialty teams has also been shown to impact costs. A case-controlled study of head-injured children was conducted, and costs associated with secondary adverse events during transport were calculated, with the Glasgow Coma Scale score used for case severity adjustment (76). Investigators found more preventable insults among those patients transported by untrained escorts than among those transported by trained escorts, with the majority of insults in the untrained escort group occurring due to hypoxia. It was determined that the additional cost of care resulting from secondary adverse events that occurred during transport by untrained escorts was $135,952.

Air versus Ground Transport

The primary difference between transport by air and transport by ground is the reduction in time to arrival at the tertiary facility; the patients most likely to benefit are those with emergent conditions that require an intervention that is not available at the referring hospital or during transport. Examples include patients with neurosurgical conditions (shunt malfunction, intracranial hemorrhage) or those with airway obstruction that requires specialized management (e.g., foreign body aspiration, congenital anomalies). In a retrospective analysis of children transported to an urban trauma center, it was found that patients transported by air had higher injury severity scores and were more likely to require ICU admission and rehabilitation services. After adjusting for injury severity, patients transported by air were found to have improved survival rates (77). It was estimated that approximately one patient was saved (i.e., an unexpected survivor) for every 100 helicopter transports.

The adult literature contains multiple studies that show improvement in mortality for severely injured patients transported by helicopter, while at the same time acknowledging that the majority of trauma patients have non–life-threatening injuries. A meta-analysis of adult trauma patients transported from the scene of injury to a trauma center analyzed 22 studies and 37,350 patients (78). A non–life-threatening injury was defined as one with a >90% survival based on trauma score–injury severity score methodology. Approximately 60% of patients had minor injuries based on their scores. A total of 25.8% of patients were discharged within 24 hours after arrival at the trauma center. The challenge for aeromedical transport teams, therefore, is to more accurately predict which patients are likely to benefit from scene transport by helicopter.

No studies have directly compared interfacility ground and air transports for children. The decision to use a particular mode of transport must balance the anticipated benefits to the individual patient with the potential threats to patient and team safety.

Telemedicine

One obvious justification for the use of critical care transport services is the need for evaluation by experts who are located in another facility. New technology makes it possible for patient assessment or test interpretation to be performed remotely, potentially improving pretransport care or, at the other extreme, obviating the need for patient transfer. The feasibility of telemedicine use during pediatric critical care transport was demonstrated in a cohort of 15 patients between the ages of 3 months and 14 years (79). Patients who presented to the ED were simultaneously evaluated directly by a pediatric emergency medicine physician and remotely by a pediatric critical care physician via a broadband audiovisual link. With regard to important clinical findings, the telemedicine physician performed with a sensitivity of 87.5% for abnormal findings and a specificity of 93% for normal findings.

A specific area in which the benefits of telemedicine have been demonstrated is the use of remote echocardiography interpretation. *Tele-echocardiography* has been used successfully to evaluate newborns with suspected congenital heart

disease, preventing unnecessary transport for diagnostic testing for those infants who are clinically well. The use of remote interpretation of neonatal echocardiograms was reported at two community hospitals in South Dakota. Of 72 patients, transport was deemed necessary for only 8 (11%) newborns with cardiac disease or persistent pulmonary hypertension (80). A study of a larger series of patients described the use of real-time echocardiogram interpretation by pediatric cardiologists using videoconferencing technology (81). Of the 500 studies performed, 266 revealed significant findings, including complex congenital heart disease and decreased cardiac function. The tele-echocardiography results had an immediate impact on patient management in 151 cases. Importantly, only 19 patients required emergency transport to the tertiary care center, and the average time interval between request for echocardiogram and the availability of results was reduced from over 12 hours to 28 minutes.

CONCLUSIONS AND FUTURE DIRECTIONS

Historically, the incorporation of new therapies and strategies into the transport environment has lagged behind their implementation in the ICU, largely due to cost and logistical issues (e.g., portability). Importantly, this delay provides the opportunity to evaluate whether the potential benefit of a specific treatment or technique merits its adaptation for use in a mobile setting. It is essential to remember that the most valuable resource is the trained and prepared transport team member who can anticipate the patient's trajectory of illness and respond to changes in the patient's condition. Ultimately, the safety of the journey and the outcome for the patient depend most on the expertise and skill of the healthcare providers and the strength of the system within which they practice.

References

1. Pollack MM, Alexander SR, Clarke N, et al. Improved outcomes from tertiary center pediatric intensive care: A statewide comparison of tertiary and nontertiary intensive care facilities. *Crit Care Med* 1991;19:150–9.
2. American Academy of Pediatrics, Committee on Hospital Care. Guidelines for air and ground transportation of pediatric patients. *Pediatrics* 1986;78:943–50.
3. *Guidelines for Air and Ground Transportation of Neonatal and Pediatric Patients.* Elk Grove Village, IL: American Academy of Pediatrics, 1993.
4. MacDonald MG, Ginzburg HM, eds. *Guidelines for Air and Ground Transport of Neonatal and Pediatric Patients.* 2nd ed. Elk Grove Village, IL: American Academy of Pediatrics, 1999.
5. Woodward GA, Insoft RM, Kleinman ME, eds. *Guidelines for Air and Ground Transport of Neonatal and Pediatric Patients.* 3rd ed. Elk Grove Village, IL: American Academy of Pediatrics, 2006.
6. Duke T. Transport of seriously ill children: A neglected global issue. *Intensive Care Med* 2003;29:1414–6.
7. Hatherill M, Waggie Z, Reynolds L. Transport of critically ill children in a resource-limited setting. *Intensive Care Med* 2003;29(9):1547–54.
8. Goh AY, Abdel-Latif M, Lum LC. Outcome of children with different accessibility to tertiary pediatric intensive care in a developing country—A prospective cohort study. *Intensive Care Med* 2003;29(1):97–102.
9. King BR, Woodward GA. Procedural training for pediatric and neonatal transport nurses: Part I—Training methods and airway training. *Pediatr Emerg Care* 2001;17:461–4.

10. King BR, Woodward GA. Procedural training for pediatric and neonatal transport nurses: Part 2—Procedures, skills assessment, and retention. *Pediatr Emerg Care* 2002;18:438–41.

11. Centers for Medicare and Medicaid Services (CMS), HHS. Medicare program: Clarifying policies related to the responsibilities of Medicare-participating hospitals in treating individuals with emergency medical conditions. Final rule. *Fed Reg* 2003;68:53222–64.

12. McDonnell WM, Roosevelt GE, Bothner JP. Deficits in EMTALA knowledge among pediatric physicians. *Pediatr Emerg Care* 2006;22:555–61.

13. King BR, Woodward GA. Pediatric critical care transport—The safety of the journey: A five-year review of vehicular collisions involving pediatric and neonatal transport teams. *Prehosp Emerg Care* 2002;6:449–54.

14. Scribano PV, Baker MD, Holmes J, et al. Use of out-of-hospital interventions for the pediatric patient in an urban emergency medical services system. *Acad Emerg Med* 2000;7:745–50.

15. Babl FE, Vinci RJ, Bauchner H, et al. Pediatric prehospital advanced life support care in an urban setting. *Pediatr Emerg Care* 2001;17:36–7.

16. Henderson DP. Education of paramedics in pediatric airway management effects of different retaining methods on self-efficacy and skill retention. *Acad Emerg Med* 1998;171:429 (abstract).

17. Gruszecki AC, Hortin G, Lam J, et al. Utilization, reliability, and clinical impact of point-of-care testing during critical care transport: Six years of experience. *Clin Chem* 2003;1017–9.

18. Vos G, Engel M, Ramsay G, et al. Point-of-care blood analyzer during the interhospital transport of critically ill children. *Eur J Emerg Med* 2006;13:304–7.

19. Foley DS, Pranikoff T, Younger JG, et al. A review of 100 patients transported on extracorporeal life support. *ASAIO J* 2002;48:612–9.

20. Linden V, Palmer K, Reinhard A, et al. Inter-hospital transportation of patients with severe acute respiratory failure on extracorporeal membrane oxygenation—National and international experience. *Intensive Care Med* 2001;27:1643–8.

21. Wilson BJ Jr, Heiman HS, Butler TJ, et al. A 16-year neonatal/pediatric extracorporeal membrane oxygenation transport experience. *Pediatrics* 2002;189–93.

22. Henning J, Sharley P, Young R. Pressures within air-filled tracheal cuffs at altitude—An in vivo study. *Anaesthesia* 2004;59:252–4.

23. Diaz MA, Hendy GW, Bivins HG. When is the helicopter faster? A comparison of helicopter and ground ambulance transport times. *J Trauma* 2005;58:148–53.

24. Brathwaite CE, Rosko M, McDowell R, et al. A critical analysis of on-scene helicopter transport on survival in a statewide trauma system. *J Trauma* 1998;45:140–4.

25. Fazio RF, Wheeler DS, Poss WB. Resident training in pediatric critical care transport medicine: A survey of pediatric residency programs. *Pediatr Emerg Care* 2002;16:166–9.

26. Eckstein M, Jantos T, Kelly N, et al. Helicopter transport of pediatric trauma patients in an urban emergency medical services system: A critical analysis. *J Trauma* 2002;53:340–4.

27. Dockery WK, Futterman C, Keller SR, et al. A comparison of manual and mechanical ventilation during pediatric transport. *Crit Care Med* 1999;27:802–6.

28. Tobias JD, Lynch A, Garrett J. Alterations of end-tidal carbon dioxide during the intrahospital transport of children. *Pediatr Emerg Care* 1996;12:249–51.

29. Wallen E, Venkataraman ST, Grosso MJ, et al. Intrahospital transport of critically ill pediatric patients. *Crit Care Med* 1996;23:1588–95.

30. Johnson TD, Lindholm D, Dowd D. Child and provider restraints in ambulances: Knowledge, opinions, and behaviors of emergency medical services providers. *Acad Emerg Med* 2006;13:886–92.

31. Chen P, Macnab AJ, Sun C. Effect of transport team interventions on stabilization time in neonatal and pediatric interfacility transports. *Air Med J* 2005;24:244–7.

32. Sanchez-Pinto N, Giuliano JS, Schwartz HP, et al. The impact of postintubation chest radiograph during pediatric and neonatal critical care transport. *Pediatr Crit Care Med* 2013;14:e213–7.

33. Tollefson WW, Chapman J, Frakes M, et al. Endotracheal tube cuff pressures in pediatric patients intubated before aeromedical transport. *Pediatr Emerg Care* 2010;26:361–3.

34. Borrows EL, Lutman DH, Montgomery MA, et al. Effect of patient- and team-related factors on stabilization time during pediatric intensive care transport. *Pediatr Crit Care Med* 2010;11:451–6.

35. McGillivray D, Nijssen-Jordan C, Kramer MS, et al. Critical pediatric equipment availability in Canadian hospital emergency departments. *Ann Emerg Med* 2001;37:371–6.

36. Macnab AJ, Gagnon F, George S, et al. The cost of family-oriented communication before air medical interfacility transport. *Air Med J* 2001;20:20–2.

37. American Heart Association. Guidelines for cardiopulmonary resuscitation and emergency cardiovascular care, Part 2: Ethical issues. *Circulation* 2005;112:IV-6–11.

38. Henderson DP, Knapp JF. Report of the national consensus conference on family presence during pediatric cardiopulmonary resuscitation and procedures. *J Emerg Nurs* 2006;32:23–9.

39. Woodward GA, Fleegler EW. Should parents accompany pediatric interfacility ground ambulance transports? The parent's perspective. *Pediatr Emerg Care* 2000;16:383–90.

40. Woodward GA, Insoft RM, Shaver AL, et al. The state of pediatric interfacility transport: consensus of the second national Pediatric and Neonatal Interfacility Transport Medicine Leadership Conference. *Pediatr Emerg Care* 2002;18:38–43.

41. Davies J, Tibby SM, Murdoch IA. Should parents accompany critically ill children during inter-hospital transport? *Arch Dis Child* 2005;90:1270–3.

42. American Academy of Pediatrics, Committee on Pediatric Emergency Medicine, American College of Emergency Physicians. Care of children in the emergency department: Guidelines for preparation. *Pediatrics* 2001;107:777–81.

43. American Academy of Pediatrics, Statement of Endorsement. Pediatric care in the emergency department. *Pediatrics* 2004; 113:420.

44. Acierno SP, Jurkovich GJ, Nathens AB. Is pediatric trauma still a surgical disease? Patterns of emergent operative intervention in the injured child. *J Trauma* 2004;56:960–4.

45. Harrison T, Thomas SH, Wedel SK. Interhospital aeromedical transports: Air medical activation intervals in adult and pediatric trauma patients. *Am J Emerg Med* 1997;15:122–4.

46. Larson JT, Dietrich AM, Abdessalam SF, et al. Effective use of the air ambulance for pediatric trauma. *J Trauma* 2004;56:89–93.

47. American Academy of Pediatrics, Section on Critical Care and Committee on Hospital Care. Guidelines and levels of care for pediatric intensive care units. *Pediatrics* 2004;114:1114–25.

48. Athey J, Dean JM, Ball J, et al. Ability of hospitals to care for pediatric emergency patients. *Pediatr Emerg Care* 2001;17:170–4.

49. American College of Surgeons, Committee on Trauma. *Resources for the Optimal Care of the Injured Patient: Guidelines for the Operations of Burn Units*, 1999; Chicago, IL.

50. Saffle JR, Edelman L, Morris SE. Regional air transport of burn patients: A case for telemedicine? *J Trauma* 2004;57:57–64.

51. Slater H, O'Mara MS, Goldfarb IW. Helicopter transport of burn patients. *Burns* 2002;28:70–2.

52. American Academy of Pediatrics, Committee on Fetus and Newborn. Levels of neonatal care. *Pediatrics* 2004;114:1341–7.

53. American Academy of Pediatrics, Committee on Fetus and Newborn. Use of inhaled nitric oxide. *Pediatrics* 2000;106:344–5.

54. Westrope C, Roberts N, Nichani S, et al. Experience with mobile inhaled nitric oxide during transport of neonates and children with respiratory insufficiency to an extracorporeal membrane oxygenation center. *Pediatr Crit Care Med* 2004:5;542–6.

55. Kinsella JP, Griebel J, Schmidt JM, et al. Use of inhaled nitric oxide during interhospital transport of newborns with hypoxemic respiratory failure. *Pediatrics* 2002;109:158–61.

56. Van Meurs K, Lally KP, Peek G, et al., eds. *ECMO: Extracorporeal Cardiopulmonary Support in Critical Care.* 3rd ed. Ann Arbor, MI: Extracorporeal Life Support Organization, 2002.

57. The Neonatal Inhaled Nitric Oxide Study Group. Inhaled nitric oxide in full-term and nearly full-term infants with hypoxic respiratory failure. *N Engl J Med* 1997;336:597–604.

58. Fan E, MacDonald RD, Adhikari NK, et al. Outcomes of interfacility critical care adult patient transport: A systematic review. *Crit Care* 2005;10(1):R6.

59. Day S, McCloskey K, Orr R, et al. Pediatric interhospital critical care transport: Consensus of a national leadership conference. *Pediatrics* 1991;88:696–704.

60. Woodward GA, Fleegler EW. Should parents accompany pediatric interfacility ground ambulance transports? Results of a national survey of pediatric transport team managers. *Pediatr Emerg Care* 2001;17:22–7.

61. Broughton SJ, Berry A, Jacobe S, et al.; The Neonatal Intensive Care Unit Study Group. The mortality index for neonatal transportation score: A new mortality prediction model for retrieved neonates. *Pediatrics* 2004;114:e424–8.

62. Orr RA, Venkataraman ST, McCloskey KA, et al. Measurement of pediatric illness severity using simple pretransport variables. *Prehosp Emerg Care* 2001;5;127–33.

63. Kandil SB, Sanford HA, Northrup V, et al. Transport disposition using the Transport Risk Assessment in Pediatrics (TRAP) score. *Prehosp Emerg Care* 2012;16:366–73.

64. Garner A, Rashford S, Lee A, et al. Addition of physicians to paramedic helicopter services decreases blunt trauma mortality. *ANZ J Surg* 1999;69:697–701.

65. King BR, Foster RL, Woodward GA, et al. Procedures performed by pediatric transport nurses: How "advanced" is the practice? *Pediatr Emerg Care* 2001;17:410–3.

66. Harrison TH, Thomas SH, Wedel SK. Success rates of pediatric intubation by a non-physician staffed critical care transport service. *Pediatr Emerg Care* 2004;20(2):101–7.

67. King BR, Wolfson BJ, Geller E. A comparison of the radiographic interpretation skills of pediatric transport nurses and pediatric residents. *Pediatr Emerg Care* 1999;15:373–5.

68. Kanter RK, Boeing NM, Hannan WP, et al. Excess morbidity associated with interhospital transport. *Pediatrics* 1992;90:893–8.

69. Macnab AJ. Optimal escort for interhospital transport of pediatric emergencies. *J Trauma* 1991;31:205–9.

70. Edge WE, Kanter RK, Weigle CG, et al. Reduction of morbidity in interhospital transport by specialized pediatric staff. *Crit Care Med* 1994;22:1186–91.

71. Vos GD, Nissen AC, Nieman FH, et al. Comparison of interhospital pediatric intensive care transport accompanied by a referring specialist or a specialist retrieval team. *Intensive Care Med* 2004;30:302–8.

72. Orr R, Venkataraman S, Seidberg N. Pediatric specialty care teams are associated with reduced morbidity during pediatric interfacility transport. *Crit Care Med* 1999;27:A30.

73. Belway D, Henderson W, Keenan SP, et al. Do specialist transport personnel improve hospital outcome in critically ill patients transferred to higher centers? A systematic review. *J Crit Care* 2006;21:8–17.

74. Ramnarayan P, Thiru K, Parslow RC, et al. Effect of specialist retrieval teams on outcomes in children admitted to paediatric intensive care units in England and Wales: A retrospective cohort study. *Lancet* 2010;76:698–704.

75. Orr RA, Felmet KA, Han Y, et al. Pediatric specialized transport teams are associated with improved outcomes. *Pediatrics* 2009;124:40–8.

76. Macnab AJ, Wensley DF, Sun C. Cost-benefit of trained transport teams: Estimates for head-injured children. *Prehosp Emerg Care* 2001;5:1–5.

77. Moront ML, Gotschall CS, Eichelberger MR. Helicopter transport of injured children: System effectiveness and triage criteria. *J Pediatr Surg* 1996;31:1183–6.

78. Bledsoe BE, Wesley AK, Eckstein M, et al. Helicopter scene transport of trauma patients with nonlife-threatening injuries: A meta-analysis. *J Trauma* 2006;60:1257–65.

79. Kofos D, Pitetti R, Orr R, et al. Telemedicine in pediatric transport: A feasibility study. *Pediatrics* 1998;102:e58.

80. Awadallah S, Halaweish I, Kutayli F. Tele-echocardiography in neonates: Utility and benefits in South Dakota primary care hospitals. *S D Med* 2006;59:97–100.

81. Sable CA, Cummings SD, Pearson GD, et al. Impact of telemedicine on the practice of pediatric cardiology in community hospitals. *Pediatrics* 2002;109:e3.

CHAPTER 27 ■ INVASIVE PROCEDURES

STEPHEN M. SCHEXNAYDER, PRAVEEN KHILNANI, AND NAOKI SHIMIZU

KEY POINTS

1 Central venous catheterization is frequently required in the PICU. Femoral, subclavian, and internal jugular site choices in children are largely a function of operator experience and local practice.

2 Intraosseous infusion is an emergency vascular access technique appropriate for children and adolescents of all ages.

3 Thoracostomy is frequently required in critical care, and newer wire-guided techniques are increasingly used.

4 Arterial catheterization remains the gold standard for arterial pressure monitoring and is necessary in many critically ill patients.

5 Pericardiocentesis may be required emergently for pericardial tamponade, but imaging modalities (ultrasound or fluoroscopy) may improve safety when time permits.

6 Transpyloric feeding tube placement may be performed blindly at the bedside with good success rates; magnet-tipped and pH-guided tubes may be useful in experienced hands.

7 Abdominal paracentesis is useful for both diagnostic and therapeutic purposes in the PICU.

8 Bladder pressure monitoring via a transurethral bladder catheter can allow monitoring of bladder pressure as a surrogate marker for intra-abdominal pressure. Pressures >12 mm Hg are considered high, and >25 mm Hg may require surgical intervention.

9 Infectious complications, one of the most frequent adverse events of invasive procedures, can be reduced by strict attention to full surgical barrier precautions, skin disinfection with chlorhexidine, and by removing invasive devices as quickly as possible. Antibiotic catheters may also reduce infectious complications as well.

10 Ultrasound is a promising bedside technology for the reduction of risks in many procedures. As clinicians gain experience with this technology, success rates and safety of the procedures will likely improve.

Invasive procedures are necessary for the routine care of many critically ill children. Complications from these procedures can be life-threatening, necessitating careful assessment and informed consent of the risk versus benefit. Anatomically realistic task trainers (e.g., mannequins) are not available for many procedures; therefore, procedures are frequently learned on real patients under the guidance of experienced clinicians. Invasive procedural competence must first be attained, and then retained. Ongoing performance of procedures is important to assess and maintain competence and reduce the risk of complications.

CENTRAL VENOUS CATHETERIZATION

Central venous catheter (CVC) placement is frequently required in the care of critically ill and injured children. Common indications for placement include reliable venous access for medication administration, monitoring of central venous pressure and central venous oxygen saturation, parenteral nutrition, and frequent blood sampling. The decrease in use of pulmonary artery catheters has resulted in an increased use of CVCs for goal-directed therapies in the ICU. CVCs are also placed for hemodialysis, hemofiltration, and apheresis in the PICU.

Contraindications for the procedure are based on balancing the benefits and risks: bleeding, infection, thrombosis, air or clot embolus, vessel puncture or injury, nerve or lymphatic injury, catheter malfunction, wire-induced arrhythmia, or catheter displacement. Bleeding complications may be the most common immediate adverse associated events, and subclavian catheters are frequently avoided in very young and coagulopathic patients because of inability to effectively compress the subclavian vessels. With appropriate training, vessel cannulation complications can be reduced using bedside ultrasound. Recent advances demonstrate that catheter-related bloodstream infection (CRBSI), a common complication of CVC, can be substantially reduced by using a "bundle" of practices during insertion and ongoing care of CVCs (1). Collaborative efforts among PICUs have reduced catheter-related infection rates dramatically over the past decade (2).

Three sites are commonly used for pediatric CVC placement: femoral, internal jugular, and subclavian. Increasingly, peripherally inserted central catheters (PICCs) are used from both upper and lower extremity sites, often by interventional radiologists in infants and children, but these techniques will not be described here. Although data from adults indicate a lower risk of infection from subclavian sites, conclusive data in children are lacking. Regardless of site, attention to detail in CVC placement can reduce CVC infections. Recommended insertion techniques for all sites include strict hand scrubbing prior to placement, skin antisepsis with chlorhexidine, and full barrier precautions (operator wearing hair covering, mask, sterile gown, and gloves, and use of a large sterile-field drape), with attention to visibility of the tracheal tube/ventilator tubing and peripheral vascular access site where medications are being administered. Sedation and analgesia plus local anesthesia should be routinely used for pediatric CVC placement, both for patient comfort and to facilitate placement and reduce complications related to patient movement. If possible, an additional provider should be monitoring the administration of sedation and analgesia while the operator is concentrating on the vascular access procedure itself.

Most CVCs are placed using the wire-guided (Seldinger) technique, in which a needle or catheter-over-needle unit is introduced into the desired vein, blood is aspirated, and a guidewire is placed through the needle or catheter. Advancing the guidewire through the veins into the chambers of the heart, particularly into the ventricle, may cause cardiac arrhythmias. With soft or larger catheters, a dilation step is frequently required and is performed by passing the dilator over the guidewire after the needle has been removed. Care must be taken to insert the dilator only to the estimated depth of the vessel, as the stiffness of the dilator may penetrate the posterior wall of the vessel. Catheters should first be flushed and then filled with saline or diluted heparin flush solution prior to insertion, and then occluded to reduce the chance of air embolism. In hypovolemic patients, volume resuscitation through a peripheral or intraosseous site prior to attempted CVC placement may increase vein size and facilitate successful cannulation.

In children with severe hypoxemia or cyanotic congenital heart disease, recognition of inadvertent arterial puncture or placement can be difficult owing to poorly saturated arterial blood. In general, it is a good idea to check that the catheter is not inserted into an adjacent artery. This is often accomplished with some combination of a fluid-column drop test, the use of a pressure transducer in line, or analyzing a blood sample from the line for blood gas results. A sterile, saline-filled, extension tubing set may be attached to the needle or short catheter prior to dilation of the vessel. The distal end of the IV tubing should be opened, and the tubing should be raised to ~10 cm above the body surface (e.g., above the level of the presumed central venous pressure of the patient). Arterial placement should result in pulsatile blood that pushes saline from the tubing at this level, while venous placement frequently results in oscillations of the fluid column with respiration. In patients with low venous pressures, the fluid will frequently flow toward the patient at the 10-cm height, and care should be taken to avoid air embolism. In equivocal cases, a sterile pressure transducer set can be attached to the tubing to verify pressures and differentiate arterial and venous waveforms. The preferred location for the tip of the catheter is controversial. Most authorities recommend placement at or just above the junction of the superior vena cava and right atrium for upper body catheters (3), to minimize risk of atrial perforation or ventricular arrhythmia. The catheter should be secured with suture or a sutureless catheter securement device, as per the hospital policy and procedure, with attention not to kink the catheter at the site of skin entry. Confirmation and documentation of catheter tip location with ultrasound and/or x-ray according to hospital policy and procedure is recommended.

Femoral Venous Catheterization

For femoral venous cannulation, the lower extremity should be positioned with slight external rotation at the hip and flexion at the knee (frog-leg appearance). A rolled towel under the buttock may facilitate successful venous access, particularly in smaller children. Restraining the leg in the desired position will help to maintain optimal conditions. The femoral artery should be located by palpation and/or ultrasound or, in the pulseless patient, assumed to be at the midpoint between the pubic symphysis and anterior superior iliac spine. Local anesthesia to the area over the intended puncture site should be considered and can reduce the need for sedation and analgesia. During cardiopulmonary resuscitation, pulsations may be felt in the femoral vein or artery; therefore, if cannulation is not successful medial to the pulsations, one should aim for the pulsation during cardiopulmonary resuscitation. The needle should be inserted 1–2 cm below the inguinal ligament, just medial to the femoral artery, and slowly advanced while negative pressure is applied to a syringe attached to the introducer needle (**Fig. 27.1**). The needle should be directed at a 15–60-degree angle toward the

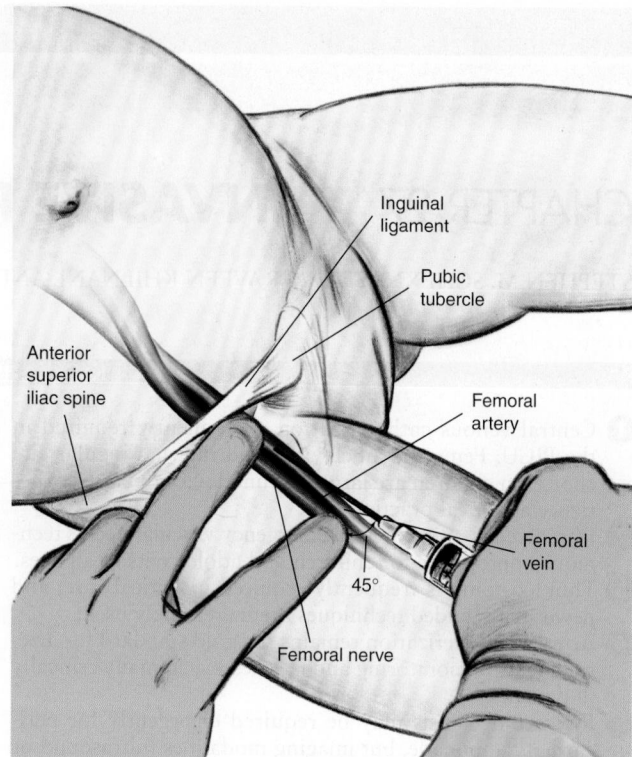

FIGURE 27.1. Femoral vein cannulation technique.

umbilicus, depending on the size of the child, with a flatter approach used in infants than in older children. Once the free flow of venous blood is observed, the syringe should be removed while the needle is carefully stabilized and the guidewire is introduced gently. Some manufacturers include a specially designed syringe (Raulerson) that allows the guidewire to pass through the syringe without removing the needle when placing larger catheters. The guidewire should pass easily with minimal resistance; *force should not be applied* to overcome a great deal of resistance. Once the guidewire is in place, the Seldinger technique (as described earlier) should be employed. Checking for venous and not arterial placement should be done as described earlier. Some experts recommend confirmation with ultrasound or a lateral abdominal x-ray when femoral venous catheters are placed to document that the catheter has not been placed in the lumbar venous plexus (4). The catheter should be secured with suture or sutureless catheter securement device, as per the hospital policy and procedure, with attention not to kink the catheter at the site of skin entry.

Subclavian Venous Catheterization

For cannulation of the subclavian vein, positioning of the patient in a head-down position (Trendelenburg) of ~30 degrees increases upper body venous pressures, which causes distention of the central veins. This positioning also minimizes the risk of introduced air embolism traveling to the brain. Positioning of the patient to optimize cannulation is important, but controversial. The most common positioning technique is to extend the patient's neck, turn the patients head away from the site of cannulation, and place a rolled towel beneath the patient's shoulder blades, along the axis of the thoracic spine. However, some authorities recommend keeping the head in a neutral (midline) position in children to optimize the diameter of the vein (5) or slightly flexing the neck and turning the head toward the puncture site when using the right side approach in infants (6). The shoulders should be maintained in neutral position with the arms at the patient's side (7).

In the smaller intubated patient, sedation, analgesia, and temporary neuromuscular blockade will facilitate proper patient positioning and reduce complications related to patient movement. In intubated patients, care should be taken to avoid kinking, disconnecting, or dislodging the tracheal tube. Bilateral breath sounds should be verified after proper patient positioning. The infraclavicular approach is most commonly used and will be described here. Alternative approaches include the supraclavicular approach using ultrasound guidance (8). The junction of the middle and proximal thirds of the clavicle should be located, and a small (25 gauge) needle should be used to infiltrate local anesthesia when the patient is not anesthetized. The needle should be introduced just under the clavicle at the junction of the middle and medial thirds and slowly advanced while negative pressure is applied with an attached syringe (**Fig. 27.2**). The needle should be inserted parallel with the frontal plane and directed medially and slightly cephalad, under the clavicle toward the lower end of the fingertip in the sternal notch. When patients are mechanically ventilated, the needle is advanced while someone holds the ventilator in an expiratory hold position to minimize the risk of pneumothorax. When free flow of venous blood is obtained, the needle should be stabilized and the syringe removed while a fingertip is placed over the needle hub to prevent air entrainment. The guidewire should be introduced during inspiration in a patient on positive-pressure ventilation or during exhalation in a spontaneously breathing patient (to avoid air embolus). The Seldinger technique as described earlier should then be followed. Once the CVC is placed, nonarterial cannulation should be determined, the catheter should be secured with suture or with a sutureless securement device, and a chest x-ray should be obtained to verify catheter location prior to using the catheter and to rule out complications, such as pneumothorax or hemothorax.

Internal Jugular Catheterization

Internal jugular catheterization can be achieved via multiple approaches. When available, ultrasound guidance is preferable. Right-sided approaches are preferred owing to potential injury to the thoracic duct on the left side. The carotid artery should be palpated, as it lies medial to the internal jugular vein within the carotid sheath. For all approaches, the patient should be positioned supine and in a slight (15–30 degree) Trendelenburg position, with a roll under the shoulders and with the head turned away from the puncture site. Consider performing beside ultrasound before positioning and draping, and using ultrasound dynamically during needle insertion.

There are three basic approaches to catheterization of the internal jugular vein: anterior, middle, and posterior approaches. In the anterior approach, the needle is introduced along the anterior margin of the sternocleidomastoid muscle, halfway between the mastoid process and sternum and directed toward the ipsilateral nipple (**Fig. 27.3A**). In the middle approach, the needle enters the apex of a triangle formed by the clavicle and the heads of the sternocleidomastoid muscle (**Fig. 27.3B**). The skin should be punctured with the needle at a 30–60-degree angle while the needle is directed toward the ipsilateral nipple. For the posterior approach, the needle should be introduced along the posterior border of the sternocleidomastoid cephalad to its bifurcation into the sternal and clavicular heads (**Fig. 27.3C**). The needle should be aimed toward the suprasternal notch. In all approaches, the needle should be advanced during exhalation to minimize the chance of pneumothorax, and the syringe should be aspirated as the needle is advanced. When the vein is entered and free flow of venous blood is established, the needle should be stabilized and the syringe removed while the hub of the needle is covered to prevent air entrainment. The guidewire should then be introduced and advanced a distance that approximates the distance to the junction of the superior vena cava and right atrium. During guidewire introduction it is helpful to have an assistant watching the patient's electrocardiogram (ECG) and announcing the provocation of dysrhythmias by the guidewire. Nonarterial placement confirmation, securing, and chest x-ray should be obtained as mentioned before.

Complications

Early complications include perforations (vessels and other structures) that may be related to the needle, guidewire, dilator, or catheter, or later perforations related to catheter-induced erosion. Hemothorax, hydrothorax, and pericardial tamponade may occur with upper body CVCs or long femoral

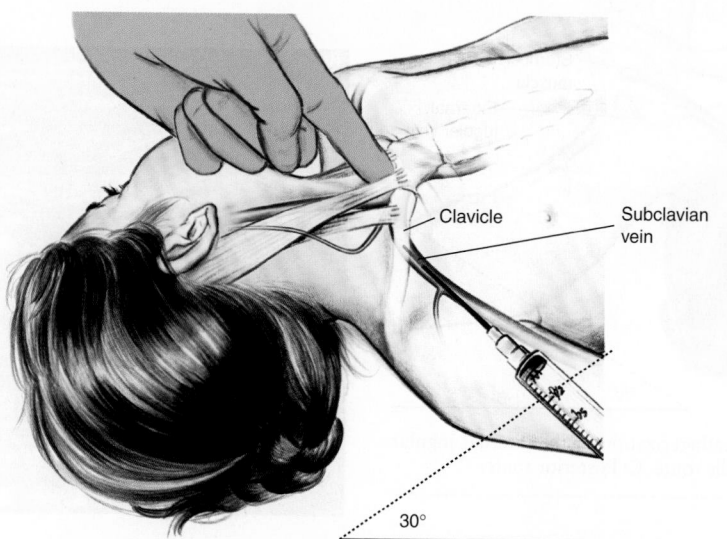

FIGURE 27.2. Cannulation of the subclavian vein.

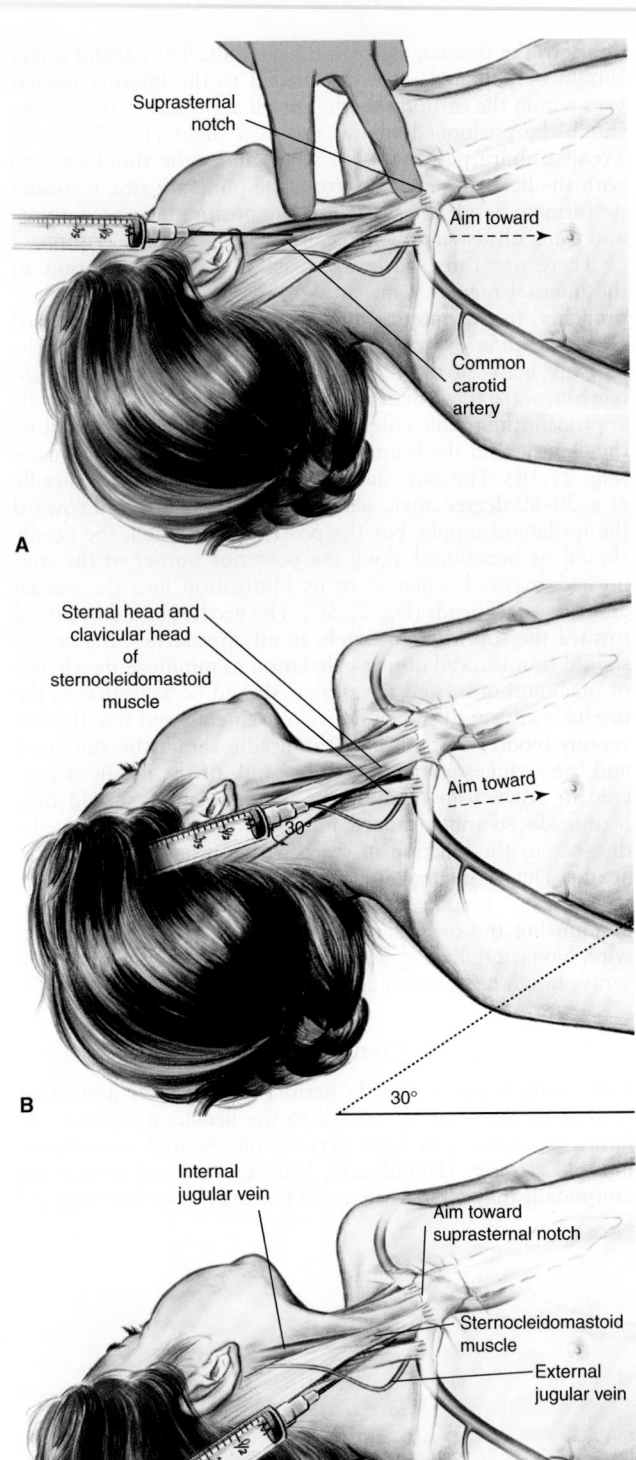

A

Suprasternal notch

Aim toward

Common carotid artery

B

Sternal head and clavicular head of sternocleidomastoid muscle

Aim toward

30°

30°

C

Internal jugular vein

Aim toward suprasternal notch

Sternocleidomastoid muscle

External jugular vein

30°

FIGURE 27.3. Technique for catheterization of the internal jugular vein. **A:** Anterior route. **B:** Middle route. **C:** Posterior route.

CVCs. The risk of catheter-induced erosion increases with stiffer catheters, when the catheter tip rubs against a vessel bifurcation or the thin right atrium, or remains in place for a long time. Pneumothoraces may occur using the subclavian and internal jugular approaches, whereas retroperitoneal hemorrhage may occur using femoral approaches. Hemorrhagic complications may be reduced through the correction of coagulopathies prior to CVC attempts and the use of imaging (e.g., ultrasound or fluoroscopy) during insertion. Catheter or wire fracture may occur at any point and may require retrieval under fluoroscopy. Looping of the guidewire and/or catheter may occur within the vessel and may require interventional radiology assistance for removal (9).

CRBSI is a common complication of CVC and can be reduced by employing strict attention to the insertion technique and ongoing maintenance for the duration of its placement. In addition to insertion technique, minimizing entry into the catheter, daily assessment of the continued need for the catheter, and employing chlorhexidine skin prep during dressing changes are recommended (2). For longer-term catheters, a vancomycin–heparin lock solution reduces CRBSI when the catheters are not being used (10,11), although daily evaluation for the continued need for the catheter is considered an important part of CRBSI-reduction strategies. Both antibiotic- and antiseptic-impregnated catheters have been shown to reduce CRBSI; comparisons between the two products have demonstrated lower CRBSI rates, with rifampin/minocycline catheters compared to chlorhexidine/silver sulfadiazine–treated products (12). Deep venous thrombosis is found with all catheters sites and is associated with diabetic ketoacidosis, as well as oncologic conditions (13,14).

Ultrasound Assistance in Central Venous Catheter Placement

Ultrasonography is used increasingly at the bedside to assist in the placement of CVCs. Ultrasound is recommended for routine use in CVC placement; reports demonstrate that its use reduces complications in infants and children (15–18). A number of commercial systems are available with high-frequency transducers for use in pediatrics, as a higher-frequency probe is necessary for good anatomic detail in children. The anatomy seen for internal jugular catheter placement is demonstrated in **Figure 27.4**.

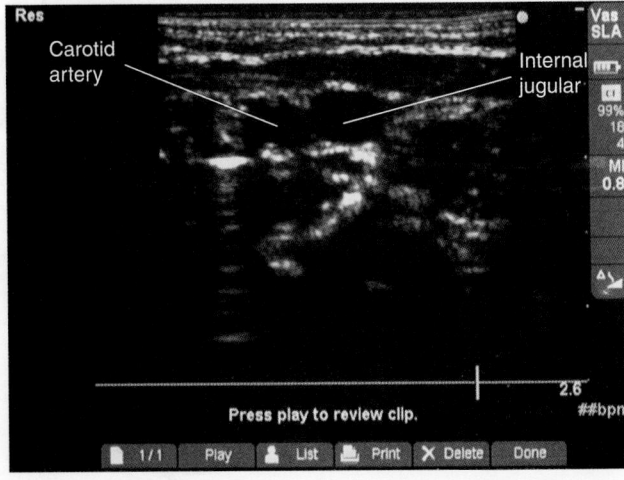

Res

Carotid artery

Internal jugular

Press play to review clip.

1/1   Play   List   Print   Delete   Done

FIGURE 27.4. Anatomy seen during an ultrasound-assisted placement of a central venous line.

A meta-analysis of published pediatric trials demonstrated an overall risk reduction of 85% for failed placement and a 73% risk reduction in complications when using ultrasound for internal jugular approaches (19). As the use of ultrasound technology has grown, its use has spread to all sites for central venous access, including subclavian (20).

Some operators use the technology to mark the vein prior to attempted puncture (static technique), while others use real-time imaging to guide the needle puncture and CVC placement (dynamic technique). Higher success rates are generally found when real-time images are obtained and used to guide needle and catheter insertion during the procedure. In children, an assistant can be very helpful to keep the transducer in the correct position. To maintain strict antisepsis, the assistant must utilize full barrier precautions and use a long, sterile sheath to maintain the integrity of the sterile field. Ultrasonic gel is also required inside the sterile sheath.

To train providers on CVC placement, anatomic models can be used to simulate ultrasound-guided CVC placement. Other nonanatomically correct models allow practicing the use of ultrasound for the puncture of smaller vessels, and some centers use turkey thighs for practicing vessel cannulation using ultrasound guidance.

INTRAOSSEOUS INFUSION

Intraosseous (IO) needle placement and infusion are essential techniques for pediatric resuscitation. American Heart Association guidelines recommend IO access for all ages during cardiopulmonary arrest when no vascular access is present (21). IO infusions (IOIs) have drug delivery-times equivalent to peripheral and central IVs and can be used to administer all medications that can be given IV. Blood can be drawn for laboratory analyses and culture, and this route can deliver continuous medication infusions. The IO route is preferred over endotracheal administration for drug delivery during cardiopulmonary resuscitation.

The most common site for IO placement is the proximal tibia. The distal tibia, distal femur, calcaneus, and anterior superior iliac spine are alternate lower body sites (**Fig. 27.5**). For the upper body, use of the humerus and radius has been

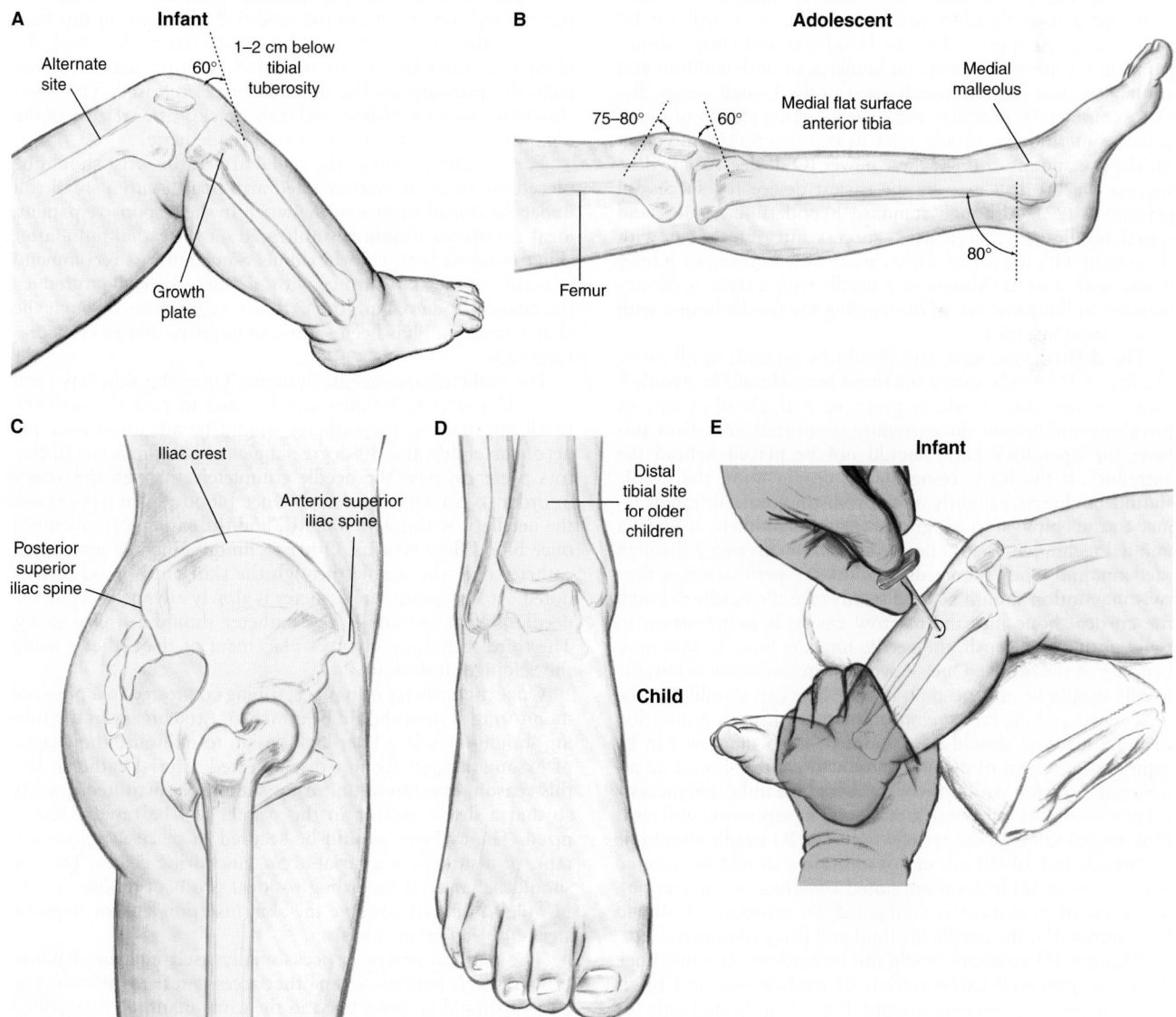

FIGURE 27.5. A: Locations for IOI in an infant. **B:** Locations for IOI in the distal tibia and the femur in older children. **C:** Location for IOI in the iliac crest. **D:** Location for IOI in the distal tibia. **E:** Technique for IOI needle insertion.

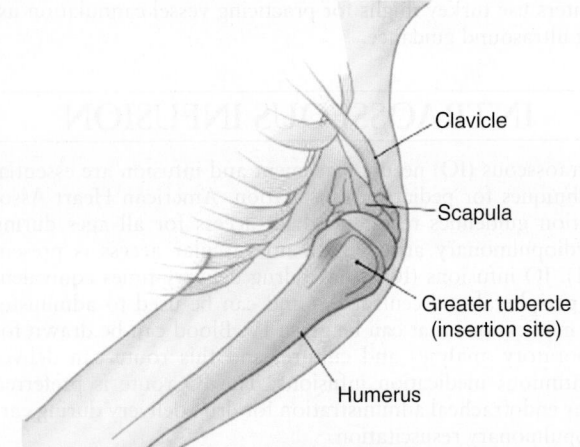

Clavicle

Scapula

Greater tubercle
(insertion site)

Humerus

FIGURE 27.6. Placement of intraosseous needle in the humerus.

described (**Fig. 27.6**). A sternal IO catheter placement system
is available in both adult and pediatric sizes. A drill for IO
access has been approved by the U.S. Food and Drug Administration for use in the tibia and humerus of both children and
adults, and has become widely used in the United States. Because commercial products and their insertion techniques vary
widely, practitioners should refer to manufacturers' direction
for the use and insertion of these newer IO devices. Some data
suggest the IO drill may be the easiest device for successful
placement (22). Although standard hypodermic needles and
spinal needles have been used, success rates are lower with
these than with the use of a bone marrow aspiration or biopsy
needle with a stylet. Moreover, a needle with a stylet is recommended to limit the risk of obstructing the needle lumen with
bone during insertion.

The desired placement site should be located; in all cases,
placing an IO needle into a fractured bone should be avoided.
The overlying skin should be prepared with chlorhexidine or
povidone–iodine and the extremity supported on a firm surface; the operator's hand should not be placed behind the
extremity. If the IO is being placed near a joint, the needle
should be directed slightly away from the joint, although injury to the epiphysis (e.g., growth plate) is unlikely. If using a
manual technique, the IO needle should be advanced through
the skin, and when the needle reaches the periosteum, a firm
twisting motion should be used to advance the needle through
the cortical bone into the marrow cavity. It is important to
twist, rather than push, the needle into the bone to minimize
bending of the needle. Once a decrease in resistance is felt, the
needle should be advanced no further. The cap should then be
unscrewed and the stylet removed from the needle. Aspiration
of bone marrow should be attempted; if no marrow can be
aspirated, infusion of a small amount of saline should be attempted. Infusion with little or no resistance indicates successful placement. At this point, a reattempt at aspiration will yield
pink-tinged saline in the syringe hub. The IO needle should be
stabilized, and 10–20 mL of normal saline should be injected
while signs of infiltration are noted (swelling or induration).
If successful placement is confirmed, an infusion set should
be connected to the needle for fluid and drug administration.

Multiple IO attempts should not be made in the same bone
owing to potential extravasation of medications and fluids
from the site of a previous attempt. IOIs are indicated only for
short-term use (hours) until more reliable vascular access can
be obtained. Complications of IOI are rare, and include fluid
or drug extravasation, infection, compartment syndrome, and,
potentially, growth failure if the IO is placed in the epiphysis.

The area should be frequently observed during fluid administration in order to detect infiltration as early as possible. While
fat emboli have been documented in the pulmonary circulation
of animals that have an IO placed, no effects on gas exchange
or pulmonary shunt were observed (23). The IO should be removed as soon as sufficient IV access has been established.

ARTERIAL CATHETERIZATION

Arterial access is frequently used in the care of critically ill
infants and children for arterial blood gas and other blood
sampling, as well as continuous blood pressure monitoring.
Like central venous catheterization, sedation and analgesia
plus local anesthesia facilitate the successful placement of
arterial lines. To minimize infection risks, sterile technique
should be employed in the placement of arterial catheters.
Clinicians increasingly use real-time ultrasound for arterial
catheter placement (24).

Radial artery catheterization is frequently performed in
the PICU, although radial artery catheter placement can be
difficult in patients with shock. Some authorities recommend
verifying and documenting collateral circulation through the
palmar arch via the use of the modified Allen test. In this bedside test, the blood is displaced from the hand while both the
ulnar and radial arteries are occluded. After the hand becomes
pale, the pressure on the ulnar artery is released. The hand
should regain its well-perfused state quickly after release of the
ulnar artery if collateral circulation is adequate.

For catheterization of the radial artery, the wrist should be
placed on an appropriately sized arm board with a small roll
under the dorsal surface of the wrist. In the responsive patient,
local anesthesia should be infiltrated on the radial pulse after
skin antisepsis with chlorhexidine. Some authors recommend
puncture of the skin surface with a 20-gauge needle to reduce
the chance of damaging the catheter as it passes through the
skin. Ultrasound has been shown to improve first-pass success
rates (25).

For catheter-over-needle systems: Once the skin has been
entered, several techniques can be used to pass the catheter. In
all approaches, the catheter should be advanced over the
needle assembly at a 30-degree angle to the skin. Some operators prefer to pass the needle completely through the artery
in order to transfix the vessel. Once blood return has ceased,
the needle is withdrawn slightly, and the catheter is advanced
once blood flow returns. Other techniques include inserting a
catheter over the needle through the skin until blood flow is
noted. At that point, the catheter is slowly advanced while the
needle is kept immobile. The catheter should advance easily.
The third technique involves placement of the catheter using
the Seldinger technique.

Once the catheter is in place, tubing connected to a pressure
monitoring system should be attached. Attachment of the tubing should include a Luer-lock design to minimize the chance
of exsanguination from a disconnected arterial catheter. For
this reason, pressure monitoring should be instituted quickly
so that a disconnection in the system will be rapidly recognized. The catheter should be secured in place using suture,
tape, or a sutureless arterial access anchoring device. The site
should be covered according to local protocol taking care to
be able to directly observe the skin insertion site for ongoing
signs of bleeding or infection.

The femoral artery is occasionally used in hemodynamically unstable patients when other access sites are difficult. The
patient should be positioned in the same manner as described
for femoral venous catheterization. The site of puncture
should be directly over the point of maximal pulsation in the
femoral triangle, or with ultrasound guidance. Because of the
relatively deeper location of the femoral artery, the Seldinger

technique is recommended for this site. Complications include hematoma formation, limb ischemia, and thrombosis of the artery. Emboli from the femoral artery may travel distally and cause foot or toe ischemia.

Both the dorsalis pedis and posterior tibial arteries can be cannulated in the foot. The posterior tibial artery is best approached with the foot dorsiflexed, while the dorsalis pedis artery is cannulated with the foot in midplantar flexion.

The axillary artery is rarely used in children but can occasionally be a useful location when other sites have been exhausted or the condition of overlying skin prohibits their use (26). The Seldinger technique is preferred for this site. When the axillary artery is used, great care should be taken to eliminate all bubbles from the tubing circuit, as flushing can introduce air bubbles in a retrograde fashion into the subclavian artery, and they potentially can move into the carotid and cerebral circulation. Owing to the absence of collateral circulation, the brachial artery is not recommended for arterial access.

For radial (and presumably other peripheral) catheters, use of a papaverine-containing heparin saline solution has been demonstrated to prolong arterial catheter life (27).

THORACENTESIS/TUBE THORACOSTOMY

Tube thoracostomy or thoracentesis is sometimes required in the management of critically ill and injured infants and children. Both procedures may be rapidly required for patients in extremis, or they may be performed in a purely elective manner. Both procedures may be required to drain abnormal accumulations within the chest, which may include air (pneumothorax), blood (hemothorax), fluids (hydrothorax), or pus (empyema). Any abnormal collection in the pleural space may interfere with respiratory function and, in severe cases, will impair cardiovascular function.

Not all pneumothoraces require drainage. In small pneumothoraces in spontaneously breathing patients, observation alone may be sufficient, although data in children are lacking.

Needle Thoracostomy

Emergent decompression is indicated when a tension pneumothorax is suspected in a deteriorating patient. In these circumstances, awaiting a confirmatory chest x-ray is unnecessary. A needle or catheter-over-needle unit (IV catheter) is inserted perpendicular to the chest wall and advanced along the superior border of the third rib (second intercostal space) in the midclavicular line until a rush of air is heard. A syringe with three-way stopcock may also be attached to the end of the needle–catheter unit and air aspirated as the procedure is completed. When a catheter-over-needle unit is used, the needle is removed and the catheter is left in place. When spontaneous respirations are present, a one-way valve or stopcock should be attached to prevent air entry into the chest during negative pressure spontaneous breathing. Repeated aspiration of air through a syringe attached to the stopcock may be required until a tube thoracostomy can be performed.

Thoracentesis

Thoracentesis may be used to symptomatically relieve respiratory distress in patients with large effusions (e.g., postoperative cardiac surgery patients) and capillary leak syndromes (e.g., sepsis) and to obtain pleural fluid for diagnostic studies.

Contraindications to thoracentesis are relative and must be weighed against the risks and benefits. If a small volume of fluid is present, the risks are substantially higher, as they are in patients who are coagulopathic or uncooperative or in patients who are being ventilated with positive pressure. Local anesthetic, sedation, and analgesia are generally required in pediatric patients and are discussed in Chapter 14. Topical anesthetics, such as lidocaine–prilocaine or liposomal lidocaine, applied at least 1 hour prior to the procedure may reduce the discomfort of the infiltration of local anesthetics.

When possible, larger patients may be positioned in a seated, upright position to obtain pleural fluid. A young child may be held in an upright position by an assistant, or an older child may be positioned leaning over a padded tray table. In mechanically ventilated or deeply sedated patients, using a partial lateral decubitus position, with the side containing the fluid in the dependent position (generally with the patient at a 30–45-degree angle to the bed), may facilitate obtaining fluid. For simple aspiration of air, the supine position can be used with the technique described under needle decompression.

The usual site for a thoracentesis to obtain fluid is the posterior axillary line near the tip of the scapula, which represents the seventh intercostal space during full inspiration. Bedside ultrasound may be very helpful in localizing the best location for aspiration or tube placement. The area is cleaned with an antiseptic, such as chlorhexidine or povidone–iodine, and the area is infiltrated with local anesthetic using a fine (27–30 gauge) needle. A longer, 22–25-gauge needle is then used to infiltrate local anesthetic into the deeper soft tissue and to locate the superior border of the rib, to avoid the neurovascular bundle that runs under the inferior surface of the rib. The periosteum is infiltrated, and the needle is advanced into the pleural space until fluid is aspirated. The depth at which the fluid is obtained should be noted and can be marked by clamping a sterile hemostat to the needle at the skin when the proper insertion depth is noted. If a catheter-over-needle unit is used, the unit is advanced just past the point at which fluid is obtained; the plastic catheter is then advanced into the chest cavity. The needle is then removed, and a stopcock or extension tubing is attached. If the fluid is very viscous, a larger (14–16 gauge) needle or catheter will facilitate successful removal of the fluid, while a smaller gauge (20–22 gauge) may be sufficient for thin fluid. Aspiration should be continued until the desired volume for diagnostic studies is aspirated or until respiratory distress is relieved if the procedure is for symptom control.

Pneumothorax may occur after thoracentesis, and a chest x-ray is frequently obtained after the procedure. Pneumothorax is more common when patients are undergoing positive-pressure ventilation. Hemothorax may also occur. Pulmonary edema from a large volume of fluid removal has not been described in children, although it has been noted in adults when >1 L of fluid is removed. Ultrasound is increasingly used to isolate fluid location during the procedure although published data that demonstrated a benefit are lacking.

Tube Thoracostomy

Tube thoracostomy is performed in the PICU setting for the ongoing drainage of air or pleural fluid. Tube thoracostomy may also be required in the care of postoperative cardiac patients for the management of pleural effusions and chylothoraces. As with thoracentesis, no definite contraindications are associated with tube thoracostomy, but coagulopathies should be corrected when feasible in non–life-threatening situations. In patients with hemothorax, the hemothorax may tamponade ongoing bleeding; therefore, adequate vascular access and volume resuscitation should precede drainage, and blood should be readily available to anticipate the need for rapid blood transfusion.

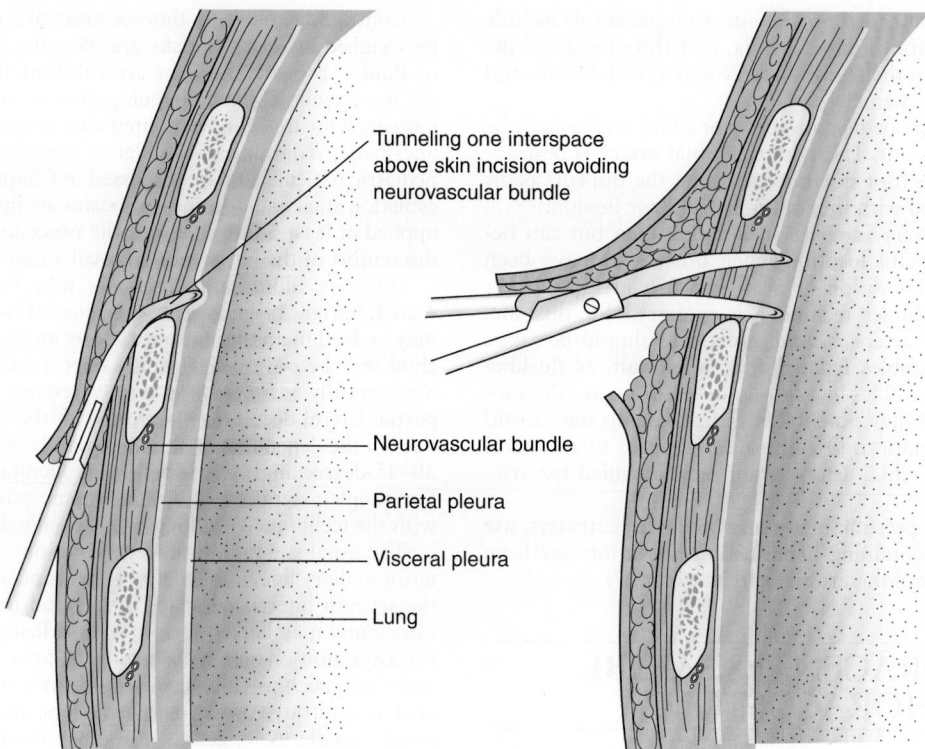

Tunneling one interspace
above skin incision avoiding
neurovascular bundle

Neurovascular bundle

Parietal pleura

Visceral pleura

Lung

FIGURE 27.7. Chest tube thoracostomy.

Sedation and analgesia are generally required in pediatric patients, as this procedure is painful. Generous local anesthesia will decrease sedation and analgesia requirements, although care must be taken with small children to avoid inadvertent administration of a toxic dose of local anesthesia (maximum dose of lidocaine without epinephrine, 5 mg/kg or 1 mL/kg of a 0.5% solution; lidocaine with epinephrine, 7 mg/kg or 1.4 mL/kg of a 0.5% solution). The usual site of entry is into the fourth or fifth intercostal space in the anterior or midaxillary line. As with thoracentesis, ultrasound can be helpful in advance to characterize the amount and character of the fluid, and can be used dynamically to facilitate localization. In the prepubertal child, the nipple usually overlies the fourth intercostal space. After puberty, the fourth intercostal space is usually located at the inferior border of the breast. The skin entry site should be infiltrated one intercostal space inferior to the anticipated entry to the chest wall, continuing along the anticipated track of the catheter and between the intercostal spaces, as noted previously.

The skin should be prepared with an antiseptic solution, such as chlorhexidine or povidone–iodine. For classical chest tube placement, a skin incision in an axis parallel to the rib is made through the area and blunt dissection is performed using a curved hemostat or Kelly clamp through the incision site and directed up to the superior intercostal space that has been chosen for chest wall entry (**Fig. 27.7**). The clamp should be inserted with the tip closed; the tip is then spread to dissect the tissues. When the dissection has reached the area chosen for pleural penetration, the clamp should be pushed firmly through the pleura while control is maintained so that the chest wall is not penetrated too deeply. In larger children, a finger can be inserted through the tract to manually break up any adhesions that can be felt. The clamp can be placed through the most distal side hole of the tube and clamped at the end of the tube to facilitate guiding the tube. A second clamp placed near the distal end of the tube prevents the free flow of pleural fluid or blood once the tube is in place.

Once the tube tip is within the thorax, the clamp should be opened and the tube advanced sufficiently so that the most proximal hole of the tube is within the thoracic cavity. While the tube is held securely, the drainage system should be connected, and the distal clamp on the tube released to allow drainage. Several techniques for securing the tube have been described, including a purse-string suture and sutures on each side of the skin incision. Commercial devices for securing tubes without sutures are available. Tapes may also be applied to reinforce the stability of the tube.

A number of percutaneous chest-drainage systems are available, including pigtail catheters and tube-over-obturator systems (ThalQuik, Cook Critical Care, Bloomington, IN). Most of these systems involve needle puncture into the thorax, followed by placement of a reinforced wire through the needle, dilation of the track, and finally, tube placement using an obturator introducer over the wire (**Fig. 27.8**). Care should be taken with these systems to avoid deeply inserting stiff dilators into the chest, with the subsequent risk of injury. The dilator should only be inserted to the depth needed to penetrate the chest wall and facilitate passage of the tube into the thorax.

Once the tube is in place, it should be observed for air leaks. If an air leak persists for more than a few minutes, all connections should be checked to ensure that air is not being entrained through a loose connection. Once the tube is secured, an x-ray should be taken to verify the tube position and observe resolution of the pneumothorax or effusion. If pneumothorax is ongoing despite a working thoracostomy tube, an airway injury or bronchopleural fistula may be present.

In general, when tube drainage has fallen to <2–3 mL/kg over 24 hours, the tube may be considered for removal. If the tube was placed for a pneumothorax and no active air leak is present, a several-hour trial of observation without suction (water seal) is recommended, obtaining another x-ray to assess reaccumulation of the pneumothorax prior to removing

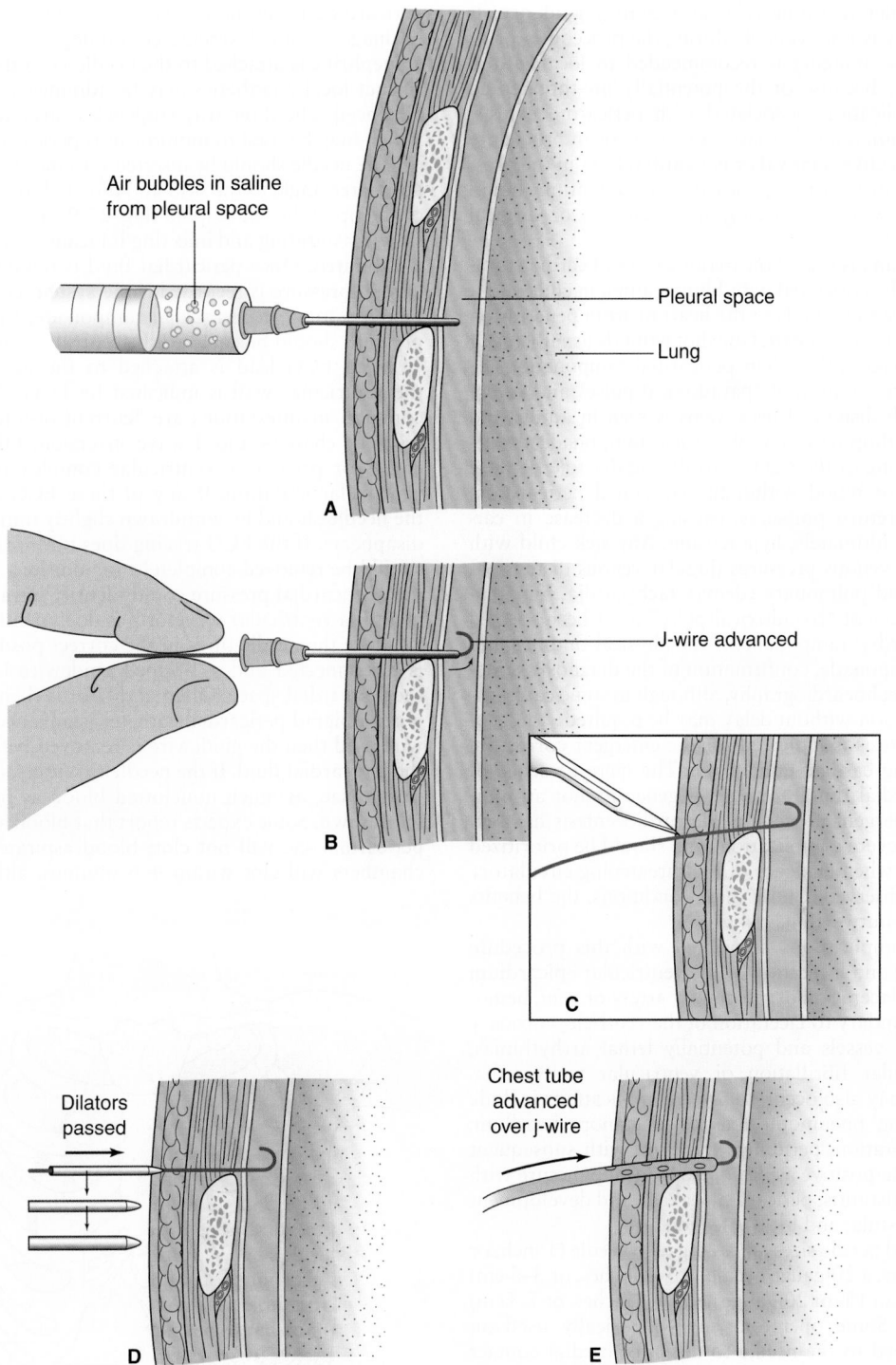

Air bubbles in saline
from pleural space

Pleural space

Lung

A

J-wire advanced

B

C

Dilators
passed

D

Chest tube
advanced
over j-wire

E

FIGURE 27.8. Wire-guided placement of chest-drainage system.

the tube. Water seal is a preferable method since it prevents
the development of tension pneumothorax if a small ongoing air leak persists. Most significant reaccumulations have
been shown to be clinically evident using this method (28,29).
When the decision is made to remove the tube, treatment with
analgesics will reduce discomfort. Topically applied anesthetic
creams have been shown to reduce pain and to be superior to
IV morphine when left in place for 3 hours (30). Intrapleural
bupivacaine has also been used but has not been demonstrated
to be effective in adult trials (31).

PERICARDIOCENTESIS

Pericardiocentesis is required for life-threatening cardiac tamponade or for elective removal of fluid for diagnostic purposes.
This procedure may be required after pediatric cardiovascular
surgery or during the initial stabilization of pediatric trauma.
When practical, pericardiocentesis may be performed in the
cardiac catheterization laboratory with electrocardiographic
and hemodynamic monitoring and fluoroscopic imaging or,

alternatively, under real-time echocardiography guidance. If echocardiography is not available during the procedure, prior echocardiographic imaging is recommended to localize and size the effusion. Because of the potentially life-threatening immediate complications associated with pericardiocentesis, surgical exploration is an alternative to an emergent procedure if time allows. Elective removal of pericardial fluid in the presence of a chronic or recurrent pericardial accumulation should be accomplished with echocardiography guidance or surgical exploration to enhance safety.

Although trauma is one of the major causes of cardiac tamponade, it is rarely associated with blunt trauma in children. It may result from stab wounds to the heart or from penetration of a fractured rib into the heart. Gunshot wounds usually result in fatal hemorrhage rather than pericardial tamponade. The classic clinical presentation of "paradoxical pulse" and severe hypotension with distended neck veins is seen in adults and children. The pathophysiology of cardiac tamponade results from reduced filling of the right heart during diastole because of the pressure of blood within the contained pericardium exceeds venous return pressures, causing a decrease in cardiac output and, ultimately, hypotension. Any sick child with signs of elevated venous pressures (jugular venous distension, hepatomegaly, and pulmonary edema), tachycardia, hypotension, and a prominent "paradoxical pulse" must be suspected of having pericardial tamponade. If the physical findings and signs suggest tamponade, confirmation of the diagnosis is ideally obtained by echocardiography, although in some cases immediate intervention without delay may be required.

Pericardiocentesis is indicated for the emergent correction of life-threatening cardiac tamponade. The mere presence of excessive pericardial fluid, however, is generally not an indication for an emergent procedure. Pericardiocentesis has several potentially severe complications and should be prioritized for emergencies, when evidence of life-threatening circulatory compromise is observed. Under these conditions, the benefits of the procedure outweigh its risks.

Immediate complications associated with this procedure include puncture and laceration of the ventricular epicardium or myocardium, laceration of a coronary artery or vein, hemopericardium secondary to laceration of the ventricle, coronary vessels, or great vessels and potentially lethal arrhythmias, such as ventricular fibrillation or ventricular tachycardia. Pneumothorax may also occur. Delayed complications include slowly developing pneumothorax and pneumopericardium, diaphragm perforation, peritoneal puncture with subsequent peritonitis or false-positive aspirate, esophageal puncture with subsequent mediastinitis, pericardial leakage and development of a cutaneous fistula, and local infection.

Recommended needle sizes are a 20-gauge needle (1 inch, or 2.5 cm) for infants, a 20-gauge needle (1.5–2 inches, or 3–5 cm) for children, and an 18- or 20-gauge needle (3 inches, or 7.5 cm) for adolescents. Some operators have historically used an ECG lead attached to the needle to detect epicardial contact of the needle. Over-the-needle IV catheters may also be used in smaller children, but most do not allow attachment of an ECG lead.

The child's vital signs should be monitored during and after the procedure. If the patient is not intubated, airway management and resuscitation equipment, including a defibrillator, should be immediately available. The xiphoid and subxiphoid areas and thorax should be disinfected. The child should be placed in a head-up position, if possible, to promote anterior pooling of the effusion.

The overlying skin should be infiltrated with lidocaine, and a small stab incision should be made with a blade just below and to the left of tip of the xiphoid process to facilitate easier passage of the needle. Some experts prefer to enter the chest just to the right of the xiphoid tip. An 18- or 20-gauge

pericardiocentesis needle is recommended for percutaneous drainage. A small syringe containing 1% lidocaine without epinephrine is attached to the needle via a three-way stopcock so that local anesthetics may be administered as the needle is advanced. The three-way stopcock is also attached to tubing, which may be used to monitor intrapericardial pressure.

The needle should be inserted into the skin incision site at a 45-degree angle to the skin and directed toward the left nipple or the tip of the left scapula (**Fig. 27.9**). The needle is advanced slowly, aspirating and injecting lidocaine until pericardial fluid is aspirated. Once pericardial fluid is obtained, the intrapericardial pressure is recorded if the system is being transduced. In the setting of pericardial tamponade, the intrapericardial pressure should be equal to the central venous pressure.

If an ECG lead is attached to the needle, contact with the ventricular wall is indicated by ECG changes. The most common manifestations are "current-of-injury" patterns (ST segment changes and T-wave inversion, QRS complex widening) or premature ventricular complex (PVCs) caused by ventricular irritation. If any of these ECG changes are seen, the needle should be withdrawn slightly until the ECG change disappears. If the ECG tracing does not normalize, the needle should be removed completely. In addition, a recording of the intrapericardial pressure could identify intraventricular placement if a ventricular waveform is documented.

Once the needle tip is in the correct position, the stopcock is disconnected and a J-tipped guidewire is introduced into the pericardial space. Often, a dilator is then inserted over the wire, a pigtail pericardial catheter is advanced over the guidewire, and then the guidewire is removed before evacuation of the pericardial fluid. If the needle tip enters a blood-filled pericardial sac, as much nonclotted blood as possible should be withdrawn. Some experts report that blood aspirated from the pericardial sac will not clot; blood aspirated from the heart chambers will clot within 4–6 minutes, although this is not

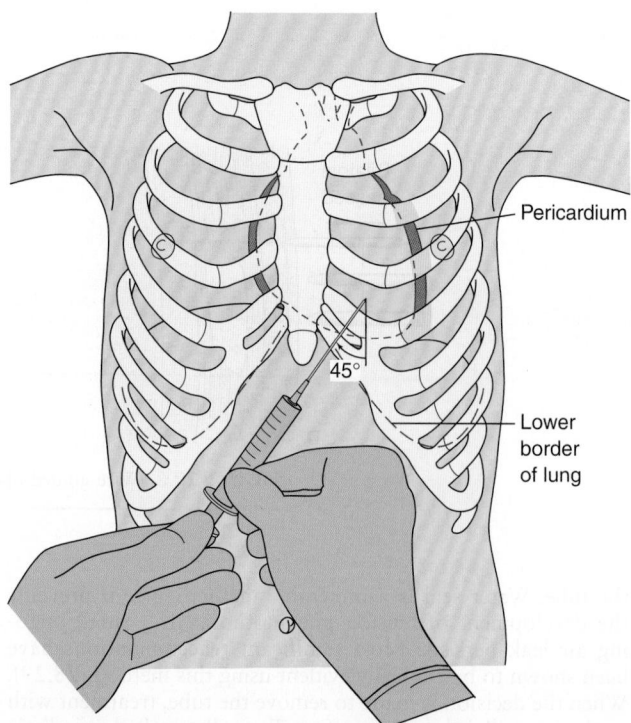

FIGURE 27.9. Needle placement for pericardiocentesis. The needle should be inserted into the skin incision site at a 45-degree angle to the skin and directed toward the left nipple or the tip of the left scapula.

universally accepted. Whether the blood clots or not depends on its source of origin. For instance, if the cause of the pericardial tamponade is catheter perforation of a heart chamber, the pericardial blood will often clot even though it is not drawn directly from the heart chamber. Fluid aspirated at the time of pericardiocentesis should be sent for the laboratory examinations.

Even in an emergency setting, it is preferable to use a pericardiocentesis needle, guidewire, and catheter rather than a needle alone, although an 18- or 20-gauge catheter-over-needle system may be substituted if necessary. It is quite hazardous to attempt to drain a pericardial effusion with a needle alone because of the possibility of laceration of the myocardium or coronary vessels. As much fluid as possible should be aspirated, and the intrapericardial pressure following the procedure should be <3 mm Hg, with negative deflections during spontaneous inspiration.

The catheter may be withdrawn immediately after the procedure or left in place for up to 24–48 hours if reaccumulation of fluid is of concern. Echocardiography should be performed following the procedure to document evacuation of the fluid and to determine catheter position. If echocardiography is immediately available, it can be used during the procedure to verify correct catheter placement and ensure adequate drainage during the procedure.

TRANSPYLORIC FEEDING TUBE PLACEMENT

Nutrition is an integral part of the management of critically ill and injured children. Either parenteral or enteral routes can provide nutritional support. Whenever possible, enteral nutrition is the method of choice, as it reduces complication rates and maintains gut integrity.

Nasogastric tube feeding is the first choice of enteral nutrition, but it may be poorly tolerated in critically ill children as a result of gastroparesis. In this setting, transpyloric placement of a feeding tube into the duodenum or jejunum is often recommended to support early feeding, improve tolerance of enteral nutrition, and decrease the risk of aspiration pneumonia. However, achieving small-bowel feeding tube placement can be difficult, time consuming, costly, and it may delay the initiation of enteral nutrition. Transpyloric tube feeding is commonly indicated when children are unable to tolerate oral or gastric feeding but have adequate gastrointestinal function.

Blind insertion of a transpyloric tube is usually performed at bedside using a weighted or unweighted tube. Right lateral decubitus positioning and motility (prokinetic) agents, such as metoclopramide or erythromycin, are occasionally used. Even if postpyloric position is not achieved soon after the insertion, the tube may migrate through the pylorus over time.

An immediate x-ray to confirm transpyloric placement may not always be necessary. Ultrasonography can also be used for placement confirmation (32). If a child is stable and requires early establishment of feeding, fluoroscopic-guided insertion may be considered, although if bedside fluoroscopy is not available, the risks of moving critically ill children to the radiology suite should be considered. Various alternative bedside techniques, including pH assisted, magnet/endoscope guided, and spontaneous passage with or without motility (prokinetic) agents, have been suggested as alternative techniques to facilitate tube passage through the pylorus.

Complications during insertion include gastrointestinal tract perforation and tube misplacement. Similar to malplacement of a nasogastric tube, tracheal or bronchial intubation may occur during feeding tube placement, particularly in patients who are receiving sedation and neuromuscular blockade.

Perforations of the gastrointestinal tract and formation of an enterocutaneous fistula are reported, particularly in infants. Development of pyloric stenosis during transpyloric tube feeding has also been reported in infants (33). Obstruction of a long, narrow transpyloric tube is one of the more common problems.

Gastric air insufflation may allow rapid placement of feeding tubes into the small bowel with fewer attempts, compared with a standard insertion technique in children (34,35). For this technique, an unweighted nasoenteric feeding tube attached to a three-way stopcock and a 60-mL syringe is inserted through the nares into the stomach. After 10 mL/kg of air is injected, the tube is advanced a distance estimated to position the tip of the tube proximal to the pylorus. An additional 10 mL/kg of air is then injected, and the tube is advanced the distance necessary to place the tube in the fourth part of the duodenum. The success rate using this technique was reported in multiple pediatric studies as 86%–92%, compared to <50% in the control group (34).

Another placement technique uses a feeding tube with a pH sensor at the distal tip. pH-assisted transpyloric tube placement was reported as a safe, easy bedside alternative to other techniques in critically ill infants and small children. The success rate using this technique was reported in a pediatric study as 97%, compared with 53% in the control group (36).

Recently, the use of a magnet-tipped feeding tube, dragged into proper position with an external magnet, has been described (37). The feeding tube is manufactured to include a magnet and a magnet field sensor in the distal tip, connected by a thin insulated wire to a small light at the proximal end. A larger handheld magnet is held over the epigastrium to magnetically capture the tube tip, indicated by the illumination of the proximal light. The tube tip is then maneuvered by the handheld magnet along the lesser curvature of the stomach, through the pylorus, and into the duodenum. The success rate has been reported between 60% and 95% inconsistently (38).

Endoscopic tube placement provides additional anatomic information and may allow for earlier initiation of enteral feedings. However, the efficacy and success rate is not uniform, and it requires the availability of an experienced pediatric endoscopist. Some studies demonstrate a failure to improve transpyloric intubation rates and tube dislodgement during endoscope removal.

The use of metoclopramide, a prokinetic agent, has been recommended to achieve transpyloric placement, but its efficacy is controversial. A *Cochrane Database Systematic Review* of four clinical studies reported no statistically significant difference between IV and intramuscular metoclopramide administered to promote tube migration (39). IV administration of 10 and 20 mg of metoclopramide was equally ineffective in facilitating transpyloric intubation in adults.

Some studies reported that gastric feeding using erythromycin as a prokinetic is equivalent to transpyloric feeding in meeting the nutritional goals of the critically ill (40). Erythromycin has been tried as a prokinetic agent instead of metoclopramide, to enhance gastric motor activity and emptying; however, its efficacy is inconsistent. Some reports described that erythromycin infusion (3 mg/kg) and electromyogram signal guidance can facilitate rapid transpyloric feeding tube placement with an initial success rate of 80%.

ABDOMINAL PARACENTESIS

Abdominal paracentesis is a percutaneously performed procedure for sampling and drainage of the peritoneal cavity in patients with ascites, peritonitis, or blunt abdominal trauma. Therapeutic indications for this procedure include an increase in intra-abdominal pressure (IAP) that causes some combination of significant respiratory distress, cardiovascular compromise, oliguria, acidosis, or raised intracranial pressure. In the PICU, common etiologies of massive ascites include fluid resuscitation for treatment of shock (e.g., in meningococcemia), viral hemorrhagic shock (e.g., Dengue shock syndrome), trauma, severe burns, and multiorgan dysfunction with fluid overload from capillary leak syndromes.

Diagnostic indications include new onset ascites, chronic ascites with clinical deterioration and suspected peritonitis, pancreatitis, and intraperitoneal bleeding. Diagnostic peritoneal lavage is not routinely recommended in the evaluation of patients with blunt trauma because of high false-negative rates (41) and the widespread and rapid availability of CT scanning, which is noninvasive and provides more organ-specific information to guide potential surgical intervention. Various causes of ascites include portal hypertension, inferior vena cava obstruction, heart failure, nephrotic syndrome, lymphomas, leukemias or neoplasms that involve liver or mediastinum, chronic pancreatitis, or cirrhosis of the liver. The differential diagnosis of clinical symptomatology related to ascites is shown in Table 27.1 (42).

No absolute contraindications are associated with abdominal paracentesis. It should be avoided in a patient with an acute abdomen who requires immediate surgery. Coagulopathies and thrombocytopenia in patients with chronic liver disease are associated with a very low risk of bleeding (<1%); therefore, prophylactic platelets or fresh frozen plasma is not recommended before this procedure. Disseminated intravascular coagulopathy (DIC) is an exception to the rule and DIC patients should receive platelets and rarely fresh frozen plasma before paracentesis.

Special caution is necessary in patients with severe bowel distension, history of previous abdominal or pelvic surgery, or distended bladder not adequately drained by a Foley catheter. Insertion sites where abdominal scar or cellulitis is apparent should be avoided owing to the possibility of adherent bowel

with scars and introduction of infection with cellulitis. While abdominal paracentesis is a relatively safe procedure (43), perforation of bowel and bladder, persistent leakage of fluid, intra-abdominal bleeding, infection, and hypovolemic shock may occur.

Paracentesis kits are usually available. When they are not, the following supplies should be assembled: skin disinfectant, sterile gloves and mask, sterile drape, local anesthetic, 3–10-mL syringe with small (25 gauge) needle for anesthesia, 20–22-gauge over-the-needle catheter for smaller children, and a 16–20-gauge catheter for larger children. Large syringes and a three-way stopcock should be available. When ongoing drainage is planned, a pigtail catheter kit should be available, along with a collection bag to drain the removed fluid.

The diagnosis of ascites should be clinically confirmed by shifting dullness, flank dullness, and fluid waves on abdominal examination (44). Clinical examination will usually identify patients with moderate-to-severe ascites, but some patients with mild-to-moderate ascites may be missed (45). Abdominal ultrasound can detect even small quantities of fluid (as low as 150 mL) and should be used to aid in diagnosis and to perform ultrasound-guided aspiration. Sedation is usually required and is discussed in Chapter 14.

In ascites, the bowel tends to float in the nondependent midline area. Therefore, the area of needle insertion should be dependent and lateral in children (46), although some authorities prefer the midline 2 cm below the umbilicus (47). The patient should be placed in a supine position, with head elevated and the bladder empty. Using sterile technique, the insertion site is prepared with chlorhexidine or povidone–iodine. The skin and subcutaneous tissue are infiltrated with a local anesthetic. Alternatively, lateral insertion can be accomplished, preferably in the left lower quadrant, a few centimeters above the inguinal ligament, lateral to the rectus abdominis muscle (43,48). A Z-track method minimizes the risk of fluid leak, compared with a direct linear-track insertion. The Z-track

TABLE 27.1

DIFFERENTIAL DIAGNOSES OF FLUID IN ABDOMEN

Ascites associated with abdominal tenderness
Peritonitis
Pancreatitis
Congestive heart failure
Constrictive pericarditis
Biliary peritonitis
Hepatitis
Hepatic venous obstruction (Budd–Chiari syndrome)
Intraperitoneal bleeding (trauma, ectopic pregnancy)
Hepatic abscess

Ascites associated with no abdominal tenderness and low serum albumin
Protein-losing enteropathy
Nephrotic syndrome
Malnutrition
Portal hypertension
Congenital syphilis
Cirrhosis

Ascites associated with no abdominal tenderness and normal serum albumin
Portal hypertension
Tuberculous peritonitis
Chylous ascites
Renal disease
Malignancy
Obstructive uropathy
Wilson disease
Hematocolpos

can be applied by placing caudal traction on the skin after the needle has been inserted perpendicular to the abdominal wall.

Once the initial needle insertion is made through the skin and subcutaneous tissues, negative pressure is maintained with the syringe, while the needle is advanced further until a pop is felt as the needle enters the peritoneal cavity and free fluid is aspirated. If a catheter-over-needle system is used, the catheter is advanced over the needle into the peritoneal cavity and the needle is removed. Approximately 20–30 mL of fluid is usually enough for diagnostic studies, but for therapeutic drainage, more fluid may be required until the abdomen is visibly lax and the patient's respiratory distress improves. Ascitic fluid may be sent for cell count with differential count, specific gravity, glucose, total protein, alkaline phosphatase, albumin, amylase, LDH, ammonia, creatinine, potassium, bilirubin, triglycerides, cellular morphology, aerobic and anaerobic cultures, viral and fungal cultures, acid-fast bacilli stain and culture, and Gram stain, as clinically indicated. Corresponding serum chemistries should also be sent. A large volume drained quickly can result in shock and hypotension; therefore, no more than 15–20 mL/ kg should be drained at one time (49). Positional change may be necessary to facilitate drainage of the ascitic fluid. A pigtail catheter may be used if drainage is required over the following 24–48 hours, leaving the catheter in place. After the removal of the needle or the catheter, a sterile pressure dressing should be applied.

The rate of complications is reported as 1%–3% (44). Complications include bowel or bladder perforation, bleeding, subcutaneous hematoma, infection, persistent leak, scrotal edema, and hypotension. Perforation of the bladder can be prevented if care is taken to empty the bladder prior to the procedure (48). As the risk of bowel perforation is high in patients with a history of previous surgery and adhesions, it can be prevented by avoiding old scars at the insertion site, to prevent injury to an adherent bowel loop (50). Ultrasound-guided paracentesis will also reduce risk in this setting.

Bowel perforation will usually close quickly without leak unless intraluminal pressure is high. Blood vessel perforation may result in bleeding, which usually stops quickly unless portal hypertension or severe coagulopathy is present. Perforation of solid organs can occur, but usually bleeding will stop spontaneously. Introduction of infection into the peritoneal cavity is possible; therefore, strict aseptic technique should be used. Scrotal edema (or labial edema in females) has been reported in patients with massive ascites (presumably from the tracking of fluid along tissue planes), and the use of small needles may prevent this complication. The persistent leak of ascitic fluid is rare but usually responds to pressure and potentially may be prevented by use of the Z-track method. Hypotension from hypovolemia can occur if >20 mL/kg of fluid is aspirated from the peritoneal cavity.

The fluid is initially evaluated by visual inspection. The fluid is normally straw-colored but may be turbid in chemical or infectious peritonitis. Chylous ascites will yield milky or yellowish fluid (51). Bile-stained fluid may be associated with pancreatitis or gall bladder or common bile duct perforation (52). Blood-tinged fluid is seen with visceral disruption or traumatic paracentesis (44).

In peritonitis, >50% polymorphonuclear leukocytes will be seen. Lymphocytes will predominate with chylous ascites (usually >90% lymphocytes) or tuberculous peritonitis (44). If paracentesis is used to diagnose the need for surgery in necrotizing enterocolitis, brownish fluid indicates perforation or necrotic bowel. If Gram stain reveals bacteria, surgery or drainage procedures may be considered for necrotizing enterocolitis (53).

Low glucose is seen with bacterial or tuberculous peritonitis. An absolute glucose of <60 mg/dL is considered low, or if the ascitic fluid glucose is less than two-thirds of the serum glucose level. Total protein of <2.5 g/dL, a fibrinogen level of 0.3%–4% of total protein, a fluid-to-serum protein ratio of <0.5, and specific gravity of <1.015 are consistent with a transudate. Alkaline phosphatase is greater than twice the serum level in patients with perforated or necrotic viscus. The ammonia level is twice as high as serum ammonia in patients with strangulated bowel and duodenal perforation. Ascitic fluid amylase is greater than serum amylase in patients with pancreatitis, pancreatic pseudocyst, intestinal perforation, or strangulation. In urinary ascites, ammonia, creatinine, and potassium concentrations will be elevated (12). Serum-ascitic albumin gradient is defined as the difference between serum and ascitic fluid albumin concentrations. A gradient of ≥1.1 g correlates with portal hypertension (54). A comparison of ascitic fluid composition in different types of ascites is shown in **Table 27.2.**

TRANSURETHRAL BLADDER CATHETER PLACEMENT AND BLADDER PRESSURE MONITORING

Transurethral bladder catheter placement is commonly performed in the PICU as an integral part of strict intake and output monitoring of fluid balance, and it has recently been used in certain specific situations for monitoring IAP. Contraindications to transurethral catheter placement include urethral trauma or blood at the tip of the meatus, prostatic displacement on rectal examination in males, obvious pelvic fracture, or perineal hematoma. Complications include trauma to the urethra and bladder, vaginal catheterization, urinary tract infection, intravesical knotting of the catheter, paraphimosis, and hematuria.

The measurement of bladder pressure as a surrogate for IAP is used to detect intra-abdominal hypertension (IAH), leading to abdominal compartment syndrome (ACS). A number of physiologic derangements have been described with IAH, including cardiovascular, pulmonary, and renal effects (13). Many pediatric reports suggest the importance of monitoring IAP in an attempt to detect IAH early, allowing early intervention and potentially preventing associated complications (55–58).

Among the common clinical situations in which IAP can increase is trauma that leads to accumulation of blood, fluid, or edema; nontraumatic bowel ischemia, infarction, and gastrointestinal hemorrhage can also lead to increased IAP owing to edema or fluid collection. IAP increases in the PICU are commonly seen in (a) children with septic shock with capillary leak, (b) children with multiorgan dysfunction syndrome (MODS), (c) severely burned or trauma patients with ischemia–reperfusion injury following fluid resuscitation, and (d) those who are post–liver transplantation or post–surgical closure of an abdominal wall defect. Although specific pediatric indications for IAP monitoring have not been established, patients at risk for significant increases in IAP include (a) those with blunt abdominal injury; (b) those with MODS, meningococcemia, dengue shock syndrome, severe burns, or high cumulative fluid balance who are mechanically ventilated; and (c) those who are postoperative with abdominal packing.

Increased IAP can lead to inferior vena cava compression with a reduction of venous return, which causes a low cardiac output with impaired renal perfusion and oliguria. In severe cases, raised IAP can lead to intra-abdominal arterial occlusion. It can also lead to respiratory compromise because of impaired diaphragmatic excursion, raised airway pressures, and reduction of pulmonary blood flow, with consequent hypoxemia and hypercarbia. Abdominal tamponade also leads to increased

TABLE 27.2

COMPARISON OF ASCITIC FLUID OF DIFFERENT ETIOLOGIES

Spontaneous bacterial peritonitis	>250 cells/mL
	Total protein is >1 g/dL
	LDH and glucose may be normal
	pH may be low or normal
	Culture and Gram stain may be negative
	Serum/ascites albumin gradient is usually >1.1 g
Secondary bacterial peritonitis	>500 cells/mL with polymorphonuclear predominance
	Total protein is <3 g/dL
	LDH > serum LDH
	Glucose is <50 mg/dL
	pH is not a reliable correlate of bacterial peritonitis
	Gram stain is positive
	Serum/ascites albumin gradient is <1.1 g/dL
Chylous ascites	Milky or yellow fluid, but may be clear
	WBC = 1000–5000, with lymphocytic predominance (usually >90%)
	Triglyceride level >> serum triglycerides (>1500 g/dL)
	Total protein is <3 g/dL
Pancreatic ascites	Turbid, tea-colored, or bloody fluid
	Elevated total WBC count and protein
	Amylase and lipase > serum levels; in patients <4–6 months of age, amylase may be low, but lipase is always higher
Tuberculous ascites	Bloody or yellow fluid, firm clots
	Total protein is >2.5 g/dL
	WBC is >1000 with predominant lymphocytes
	Glucose is <30 mg/dL
Urine ascites	Protein is <1 g/dL
	Potassium and creatinine > serum
	Malignant ascites
	Bloody fluid
	⇑ Protein and LDH
	⇓ Glucose
	Serum-ascitic albumen gradient is <1.1 g/dL
Nephrotic syndrome	Total protein is <2.5 g/dL
Biliary ascites	Bile-stained fluid
	Bilirubin >> serum bilirubin (100–400 mg/dL)

LDH, lactate dehydrogenase; WBC, white blood count.

intracranial pressure and reduction in cerebral perfusion pressure. In summary, signs of ACS include abdominal distension, oliguria, hypoxia, hypotension, and acidosis. Early monitoring of IAP should be considered in situations in which the patient is already exhibiting signs of ACS or is at high risk of developing it.

Although various techniques of IAP monitoring (intragastric or intravesical pressure) have been described, measurement of intravesical pressure is considered a gold standard for IAP measurement. The technique for intravesical pressure measurement was first described by Kron et al. (59) and later modified by Cheatham and Safcsak (60). Recent reports suggest the inaccuracy of clinical examination in detecting IAH (61). Although measurement of IAP has been recommended in pediatric patients with abdominal wall defects (49) and in children with major burns, routine measurement of intra-abdominal bladder pressure is not yet a common practice in the PICU. In pediatric patients, various indirect methods of measuring intravesical pressure have been compared recently (62). The setup is schematically shown in **Figure 27.10**.

To monitor intravesical pressure, the urinary catheter must have a closed drainage system, and the patient must be in the supine position. The transducer system should be connected to the monitor, with connection to a bag of saline. A 30-mm or 60-mm pressure scale on the monitor is selected, a 60-mL syringe is attached to the distal stopcock, and the symphysis pubis is taken as the zero reference point. The bladder drainage system is clamped distal to the catheter and drainage bag connection. The sampling port of the catheter is cleaned with an antiseptic swab, and a large (18 gauge) needle is inserted into the sampling port. The stopcock attached to the syringe is turned off to the patient. The saline bag is then opened toward the syringe, and the syringe is filled with saline flush. The stopcock is turned off to the pressure bag, and 1 mL/kg of saline from the syringe is injected into the bladder. Any air seen between the clamp and the urinary catheter should be expelled by opening the clamp and allowing the saline to flow back past the clamp before reapplying the clamp. The pressure waveform typically shows a small variation between inspiration and expiration, with the end-expiratory pressure taken as the IAP. A printed strip facilitates measurement of the IAP. Once the pressure measurement is made, the needle is removed from the sampling port and catheter drainage tubing is

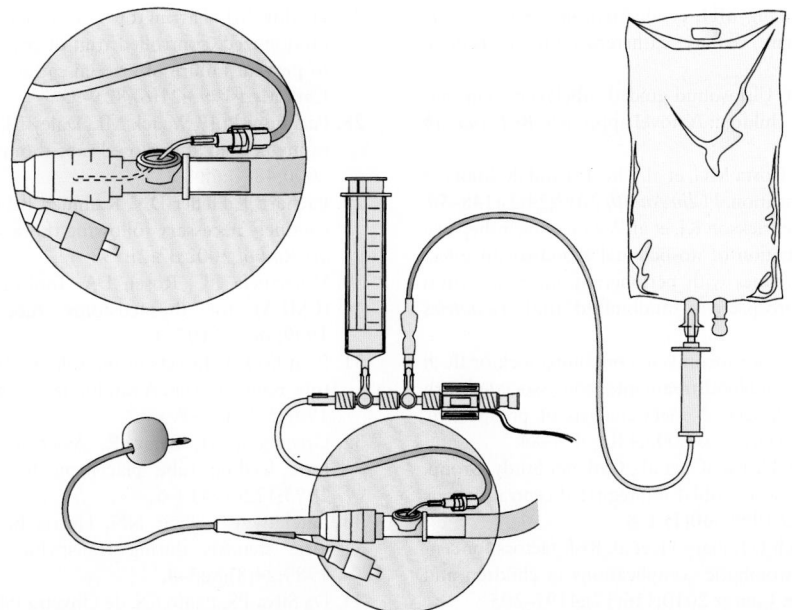

FIGURE 27.10. A closed, needle-free system for measurement of intravesicular pressure. Normal saline (1000 mL), a 60-mL Luer-lock syringe, and a segment of pressure tubing are attached to a disposable pressure transducer connected to two stopcocks. An 18-gauge angiocatheter is inserted into the culture aspiration port of the urinary drainage tubing, and the needle is removed, with the plastic infusion catheter left in place. The infusion catheter is connected to the pressure tubing, and the system is flushed with normal saline. The infusion catheter may be taped to the urinary drainage tubing for added security.

unclamped. The amount of saline injected should be accounted for in the output charting.

When a transducer is not available, the catheter tubing is simply raised vertically above the symphysis pubis at a 90-degree angle to the patient's pelvis, and the tubing is unclamped. The distance in centimeters between the symphysis pubis zero point and the maximal height of the fluid column is recorded (60). This minimally invasive technique is popular in some institutions because it is quick and can be easily performed by the staff, without the need for a transducer setup. A closed commercial monitoring and drainage system that utilizes an inline valve allows monitoring without the need to use a needle to connect to the sampling port of the catheter (AbViser, ConvaTec Inc., Skillman, NJ).

Normal pediatric values are not established for IAP. Based on adult data (16), normal range of IAP is considered to be 0–12 mm Hg. IAH is defined as an IAP of >12 mm Hg. ACS may occur with an IAP of >20 mm Hg. The severity of IAH has also been described as mild (10–20 mm Hg), moderate (>20–40 mm Hg), and severe (>40 mm Hg). The incidence of ACS is 15% in adult studies, much higher than the reported pediatric incidence of 0.7% (63), which may reflect a failure to recognize this condition in the pediatric population. In patients who are at a high risk of developing ACS, a high index of suspicion and early measurement of IAP are required to recognize this condition.

Various interventions to reduce IAP include gastric suction, enemas, diuretics, muscle relaxants, paracentesis, and surgical decompression as clinically indicated. Because the level of IAP at which ACS occurs in children is unknown, some have suggested that a distended abdomen, oliguria, and/or hypoxia and hypercarbia plus increased airway pressure justify abdominal decompression (57). Some authors recommend decompression at >25 mm Hg in patients who are treated by silo decompression (55). Paracentesis may provide an alternative to operative intervention in pediatric patients.

CONCLUSIONS AND FUTURE DIRECTIONS

Invasive procedures are a routine part of pediatric critical care. Complications can range from trivial to life-threatening, requiring an assessment of the risk and benefit for each procedure. Informed consent is appropriate in less-urgent circumstances. Operator training, practice, experience, and real-time ultrasound can reduce risks. Future improvements in device technology may also reduce infectious and mechanical complications. Sedation and analgesia are often required when performing invasive procedures in children.

References

1. O'Grady N, Alexander M, Burns LA, et al. 2011 guidelines for the prevention of intravascular catheter-related infections. http://www.cdc.gov/hicpac/BSI/01-BSI-guidelines-2011.html. Updated April 1, 2011. Accessed December 2, 2013.
2. Miller MR, Niedner MF, Huskins WC, et al. Reducing PICU central line-associated bloodstream infections: 3-year results. *Pediatrics* 2011;128(5):e1077–83.
3. Polderman KH, Girbes AJ. Central venous catheter use. Part 1: Mechanical complications. *Intensive Care Med* 2002;28(1):1–17.
4. Chen CC, Tsao PN, Yau KI. Paraplegia: Complication of percutaneous central venous line malposition. *Pediatr Neurol* 2001;24(1):65–8.
5. Lukish J, Valladares E, Rodriguez C, et al. Classical positioning decreases subclavian vein cross-sectional area in children. *J Trauma* 2002;53(2):272–5.
6. Jung CW, Bahk JH, Kim MW, et al. Head position for facilitating the superior vena caval placement of catheters during right subclavian approach in children. *Crit Care Med* 2002;30(2):297–9.

7. Tan BK, Hong SW, Huang MH, et al. Anatomic basis of safe percutaneous subclavian venous catheterization. *J Trauma* 2000;48(1):82–6.

8. Pirotte T, Veyckemans F. Ultrasound-guided subclavian vein cannulation in infants and children: A novel approach. *Br J Anaesth* 2007;98(4):509–14.

9. Vertrugno L, Piccoli G, Costa MG, et al. The dos and do knots of central venous catheterization. *J Clin Anesth* 2012;24(2):148–50.

10. Garland JS, Alex CP, Henrickson KJ, et al. A vancomycin-heparin lock solution for prevention of nosocomial bloodstream infection in critically ill neonates with peripherally inserted central venous catheters: A prospective, randomized trial. *Pediatrics* 2005;116(2):e198–205.

11. Safdar N, Maki DG. Use of vancomycin-containing lock or flush solutions for prevention of bloodstream infection associated with central venous access devices: A meta-analysis of prospective, randomized trials. *Clin Infect Dis* 2006;43(4):474–84.

12. Darouiche RO, Raad II, Heard SO, et al.; Catheter Study Group. A comparison of two antimicrobial-impregnated central venous catheters. *N Engl J Med* 1999;340(1):1–8.

13. Revel-Vilk S, Yacobovich J, Tamary H, et al. Risk factors for central venous catheter thrombotic complications in children and adolescents with cancer. *Cancer* 2010;116(17):4197–205.

14. Worly JM, Fortenberry JD, Hansen I, et al. Deep venous thrombosis in children with diabetic ketoacidosis and femoral central venous catheters. *Pediatrics* 2004;113(1, pt 1):e57–60.

15. Verghese ST, McGill WA, Patel RI, et al. Ultrasound-guided internal jugular venous cannulation in infants: A prospective comparison with the traditional palpation method. *Anesthesiology* 1999;91(1):71–7.

16. Chuan WX, Wei W, Yu L. A randomized-controlled study of ultrasound prelocation vs anatomical landmark-guided cannulation of the internal jugular vein in infants and children. *Paediatr Anaesth* 2005;15(9):733–8.

17. Froehlich CD, Rigby MR, Rosenberg ES, et al. Ultrasound-guided central venous catheter placement decreases complications and decreases placement attempts compared with the landmark technique in patients in a pediatric intensive care unit. *Crit Care Med* 2009;37(3):1090–6.

18. Keenan SP. Use of ultrasound to place central lines. *J Crit Care* 2002;17(2):126–37.

19. Hind D, Calvert N, McWilliams R, et al. Ultrasonic locating devices for central venous cannulation: Meta-analysis. *BMJ* 2003;327(7411):361.

20. Rhondali O, Attof R, Combet S, et al. Ultrasound-guided subclavian vein cannulation in infants: Supraclavicular approach. *Paediatr Anaesth* 2011;21(11):1136–41.

21. Kleinman ME, Chameides L, Schexnayder SM, et al. Part 14: Pediatric advanced life support: 2010 American Heart Association Guidelines for Cardiopulmonary Resuscitation and Emergency Cardiovascular Care. *Circulation* 2010;122(18, suppl 3): S876–908.

22. Weiser G, Hoffmann Y, Galbraith R, et al. Current advances in intraosseous infusion—A systematic review. *Resuscitation* 2012;83(1):20–6.

23. Orlowski JP, Julius CJ, Petras RE, et al. The safety of intraosseous infusions: Risks of fat and bone marrow emboli to the lungs. *Ann Emerg Med* 1989;18(10):1062–7.

24. Gu WJ, Tie HT, Liu JC, et al. Efficacy of ultrasound-guided radial artery catheterization: A systematic review and meta-analysis of randomized controlled trials. *Crit Care* 2014;18(3):R93.

25. Ueda K, Puangsuvan S, Hove MA, et al. Ultrasound visual image-guided vs Doppler auditory-assisted radial artery cannulation in infants and small children by non-expert anaesthesiologists: A randomized prospective study. *Br J Anaesth* 2013; 110(2):281–6.

26. Greenwald BM, Notterman DA, DeBruin WJ, et al. Percutaneous axillary artery catheterization in critically ill infants and children. *J Pediatr* 1990;117(3):442–4.

27. Heulitt MJ, Farrington EA, O'Shea TM, et al. Double-blind, randomized, controlled trial of papaverine-containing infusions to prevent failure of arterial catheters in pediatric patients. *Crit Care Med* 1993;21(6):825–9.

28. Pacanowski JP, Waack ML, Daley BJ, et al. Is routine roentgenography needed after closed tube thoracostomy removal? *J Trauma* 2000;48(4):684–8.

29. Pacharn P, Heller DN, Kammen BF, et al. Are chest radiographs routinely necessary following thoracostomy tube removal? *Pediatr Radiol* 2002;32(2):138–42.

30. Valenzuela RC, Rosen DA. Topical lidocaine-prilocaine cream (EMLA) for thoracostomy tube removal. *Anesth Analg* 1999;88(5):1107–8.

31. Puntillo KA. Effects of interpleural bupivacaine on pleural chest tube removal pain: A randomized controlled trial. *Am J Crit Care* 1996;5(2):102–8.

32. Greenberg M, Bejar R, Asser S. Confirmation of transpyloric feeding tube placement by ultrasonography. *J Pediatr* 1993;122(3):413–5.

33. Latchaw LA, Jacir NN, Harris BH. The development of pyloric stenosis during transpyloric feedings. *J Pediatr Surg* 1989;24(8):823–4.

34. Da Silva PS, Paulo CS, de Oliveira ISB, et al. Bedside transpyloric tube placement in the pediatric intensive care unit: A modified insufflation air technique. *Intensive Care Med* 2002;28(7):943–6.

35. Spalding HK, Sullivan KJ, Soremi O, et al. Bedside placement of transpyloric feeding tubes in the pediatric intensive care unit using gastric insufflation. *Critical Care Med* 2000;28(6):2041–4.

36. Dimand RJ, Veereman-Wauters G, Braner DA. Bedside placement of pH-guided transpyloric small bowel feeding tubes in critically ill infants and small children. *JPEN J Parenter Enteral Nutr* 1997;21(2):112–4.

37. Gabriel SA, Ackermann RJ. Placement of nasoenteral feeding tubes using external magnetic guidance. *JPEN J Parenter Enteral Nutr* 2004;28(2):119–22.

38. Boivin M, Levy H, Hayes J; Magnet-Guided Enteral Feeding Tube Study Group. A multicenter, prospective study of the placement of transpyloric feeding tubes with assistance of a magnetic device. *JPEN J Parenter Enteral Nutr* 2000;24(5):304–7.

39. Silva CC, Saconato H, Atallah AN. Metoclopramide for migration of naso-enteral tube [review]. *Cochrane Database Syst Rev* 2002;(4):CD003353.

40. Gharpure V, Meert KL, Sarnaik AP. Efficacy of erythromycin for postpyloric placement of feeding tubes in critically ill children: A randomized, double-blind, placebo controlled study. *JPEN J Parenter Enteral Nutr* 2001;25(3):160–5.

41. Heller M, Jehle D. *Ultrasound in Emergency Medicine.* Philadelphia, PA: WB Saunders, 1995.

42. Simon JE. Abdominal distension. In: Fleisher GR, Ludwig S, Henretig FM, et al., eds. *Textbook of Pediatric Emergency Medicine.* 4th ed. Baltimore, MD: William & Wilkins, 2000.

43. Runyon BA. Paracentesis of ascitic fluid: A safe procedure. *Arch Intern Med* 1986;146:2259–61.

44. Cochran WJ. Ascites. In: McMillan JA, De Angelis CD, Feigin RD, eds. *Oski's Pediatrics: Principles and Practice.* Philadelphia, PA: Lippincott, 1994.

45. Glauser JM. Paracentesis. In: Roberts JR, Hedges JR, eds. *Clinical Procedures in Emergency Medicine.* Philadelphia, PA: WB Saunders, 1991.

46. Tuggle DW. Abdominal paracentesis. In: Blumer JL, ed. *A Practical Guide to Pediatric Intensive Care.* St Louis, MO: Mosby Year Book, 1990.

47. Ruddy RM. Section VII procedures: Peritoneal tap. In: Fleisher GR, Ludwig S, Henretig FM, et al., eds. *Textbook of Pediatric Emergency Medicine.* Baltimore, MD: William & Wilkins, 2000.

48. Mallory A, Schaefer JW. Complication of diagnostic paracentesis in patients with liver disease. *JAMA* 1978;239:628–30.

49. Lacey SR, Bruce J, Brooks SP, et al. The relative merits of various methods of indirect measurement of intraabdominal pressure

as a guide to closure of abdominal wall defects. *J Pediatr Surg* 1987;22(12):1207–11.

50. Smith SD, Vasquez WD. Ascites. In: O'Neill JA, Rower MI, Grossfield JL, et al., eds. *Pediatric Surgery*. Baltimore, MD: Mosby Year Book, 1998.

51. Unger SW, Chandler JG. Chylous ascites in infants and children. *Surgery* 1983;93:455–61.

52. Athow AC, Wilkins ML, Saunders AJ. Pancreatic ascitis presenting in infancy, with review of literature. *Dig Dis Sci* 1991;36:245–7.

53. Kosloske AM, Papile L, Burstein J. Indication for operation in acute necrotizing enterocolitis. *Surgery* 1980;87:502–6.

54. Kandel G, Diamant NE. A clinical view of recent advances in ascites. *J Clin Gastroenterol* 1986;8:85–99.

55. DeCou JM, Abrams RS, Miller RS, et al. Abdominal compartment syndrome in children: Experience with three cases. *J Pediatr Surg* 2000;35:840–2.

56. Aman MG, Arnold LE, McDougle CJ, et al. Acute and long-term safety and tolerability of risperidone in children with autism. *J Child Adolesc Psychopharmacol* 2005;15(6):869–84.

57. Kawar B, Siplovich L. Abdominal compartment syndrome in children: The dilemma of treatment. *Eur J Pediatr Surg* 2003;13(5):330–3.

58. Neville HL, Lally KP, Cox CS Jr. Emergent abdominal decompression with patch abdominoplasty in the pediatric patient. *J Pediatr Surg* 2000;35(5):705–8.

59. Kron IL, Harman PK, Nolan SP. The measurement of intra-abdominal pressure as a criterion for abdominal re-exploration. *Ann Surg* 1984;199(1):28–30.

60. Cheatham ML, Safcsak K. Intraabdominal pressure: A revised method for measurement. *J Am Coll Surg* 1998;186(5):594–5.

61. Kirkpatrick AW, Brenneman FD, McLean RF, et al. Is clinical examination an accurate indicator of raised intra-abdominal pressure in critically injured patients? *Can J Surg* 2000;43(3):207–11.

62. Davis PJ, Koottayi S, Taylor A, et al. Comparison of indirect methods of measuring intra-abdominal pressure in children. *Intens Care Med* 2005;31(3):471–5.

63. Beck R, Halberthal M, Zonis Z, et al. Abdominal compartment syndrome in children. *Pediatr Crit Care Med* 2001;2:51–6.

CHAPTER 28 ■ RECOGNITION AND INITIAL MANAGEMENT OF SHOCK

RUCHI SINHA, SIMON NADEL, NIRANJAN "TEX" KISSOON, AND SUCHITRA RANJIT

KEY POINTS

1 Clinical evaluation must include full assessment of respiratory and cardiovascular status, including oxygenation, respiratory rate, work of breathing, heart rate, blood pressure, peripheral perfusion, urine output, as well as level of consciousness.

2 Laboratory evaluation should include markers of global oxygenation, particularly arterial blood gas, lactate measurement, and mixed (or central) venous oxygen saturation.

3 Cardiac output monitoring, including noninvasive methods, should be considered for assessing trends and guiding fluid administration and use of vasoactive drugs.

4 Many methods of evaluation of regional tissue oxygenation and microvascular blood flow are being developed;

the most useful include near-infrared spectroscopy and orthogonal polarization spectral imaging.

5 The "Holy Grail" of shock management would be a rapid, noninvasive, reliable method of assessing deficits in both regional and local oxygenation.

6 Management is dependent on understanding the causes of shock and giving both cause-directed and early goal-directed therapies.

7 Well-controlled, randomized trials for children with shock states are urgently required to evaluate the most appropriate and effective aspects of therapy.

Shock is a complex clinical syndrome characterized by acute failure of the cardiovascular system to deliver adequate substrate to, and remove metabolic waste from, tissues resulting in anaerobic metabolism and tissue acidosis. This impaired utilization of essential cellular substrates eventually leads to loss of normal cellular function.

Shock may occur suddenly (as seen in major trauma) or can develop insidiously (as in sepsis). From the clinician's viewpoint shock often progresses through three stages. Initially, neurohumoral mechanisms maintain blood pressure (BP) and preserve tissue perfusion producing a *compensated* stage, during which shock reversal is possible with appropriate therapy. When these compensatory mechanisms are exhausted, the pathophysiologic derangements become more pronounced and the *progressive* stage begins. Without aggressive support the patient develops severe organ and tissue injury that lead to a *refractory stage*, which culminate in multiple organ failure and death.

Shock is a clinical diagnosis, but its recognition remains problematic in children. Symptoms and signs of shock include tachypnea, tachycardia, decreased peripheral perfusion (reduced pulse volume, prolonged capillary refill time (CRT), peripheral vasodilation [warm shock], or cool extremities [cold shock]), altered mental status, hypothermia or hyperthermia, and reduction of urine output (1). The presence of systemic hypotension is not required to make the diagnosis of shock in children, because children will often maintain their BP until the late stages of shock. Laboratory evidence includes the finding of metabolic acidosis, decreased mixed venous oxygen saturation, and increased blood lactate levels.

CLASSIFICATION OF SHOCK

Shock is often classified based on five mechanisms that have important therapeutic implications:

- *Hypovolemic shock* includes hemorrhagic and nonhemorrhagic causes of fluid depletion.
- *Cardiogenic shock* occurs when cardiac compensatory mechanisms fail and may occur in children and infants with preexisting myocardial disease or injury.
- *Obstructive shock* is due to increased afterload of the right or left ventricle; examples include cardiac tamponade, pulmonary embolism, and tension pneumothorax.
- *Distributive shock*, such as septic and anaphylactic shock, is often associated with peripheral vasodilatation, pooling of venous blood, and decreased venous return to the heart.
- *Dissociative shock* occurs as a result of inadequate oxygen releasing capacity; examples include profound anemia, carbon monoxide poisoning, and methemoglobinemia.

This distinct categorization of shock may be beneficial when present in pure form; however, in many cases several mechanisms often contribute in the same patient and the relative contribution of each mechanism may change over time. Thus, the clinician is well advised to repeatedly examine the patient, especially after administering any therapeutic intervention.

PATHOPHYSIOLOGY

The pathophysiology of shock can be explained in terms of derangements in oxygen delivery and consumption.

Oxygen Delivery

Circulatory failure results in a decrease in oxygen delivery (DO_2) to the tissues and is associated with a decrease in cellular partial pressure of oxygen (PO_2). When a critical PO_2 is reached, oxidative phosphorylation is limited by the lack of oxygen, leading to a shift from aerobic to anaerobic metabolism. This shift results in a rise in cellular and blood lactate concentration and a concomitant decrease in ATP synthesis. Because ATP is the source of energy for cellular function, insufficient ATP becomes the final common pathway to cellular insult in all forms of shock. Insufficient ATP leads to accumulation of ADP and hydrogen ion, which together with an increase in serum lactate results in metabolic and lactic acidosis.

DO_2 depends on two variables: the arterial oxygen content (CaO_2) and the cardiac output (CO). CaO_2 is the product of Hb content, arterial saturation, and hemoglobin (Hb) carrying capacity. CO depends on HR (heart rate) and SV (stroke volume), the latter of which is determined by myocardial contractility, ventricular preload, and ventricular afterload. In children, CO depends more on the HR than on SV because of myocardial immaturity.

Adequate tissue oxygenation is not an absolute number, but relies on a DO_2 sufficient to meet tissue oxygen demand (2). Oxygen demand varies according to tissue type and time. Although oxygen demand cannot be measured or calculated, oxygen uptake or consumption ($\dot{V}O_2$) and DO_2 can both be quantified and are linked by the relationship:

$$\dot{V}O_2 = DO_2 \times O_2ER$$

where O_2ER = oxygen extraction ratio (O_2ER in %, $\dot{V}O_2$ and DO_2 in mL O_2/kg/min) and DO_2 = total flow of oxygen in arterial blood, which is related to CO and arterial oxygen content (CaO_2): $DO_2 = CO \times CaO_2$. CaO_2 is the product of Hb (g/100 mL), arterial oxygen saturation (SaO_2%), and Hb's oxygen-carrying capacity (1.39 mL O_2/g Hb):

$$CaO_2 = Hb \times SaO_2 \times 1.39$$

Under normal conditions, oxygen demand equals $\dot{V}O_2$ (roughly equivalent to 2.4 mL O_2/kg/min for a DO_2 of 12 mL O_2/kg/min, which corresponds to an O_2ER of 20%). The rate of oxygen delivery must remain greater than the rate of uptake or consumption; that is, DO_2 adjusts to oxygen demand. When demand increases (e.g., during exercise), DO_2 must adapt and increase.

During circulatory shock or hypoxemia, as DO_2 declines, $\dot{V}O_2$ is maintained by a compensatory increase in O_2ER; $\dot{V}O_2$ and DO_2 therefore remain independent. However, if DO_2 falls further, a critical point is reached (DO_2crit) when O_2ER can no longer increase to compensate for the fall in DO_2. At this point, $\dot{V}O_2$ becomes dependent on DO_2. If $\dot{V}O_2$ increases, then DO_2crit also increases (**Fig. 28.1**).

O_2ER increases because of redistribution of blood flow and capillary recruitment. Redistribution of blood flow occurs via an increase in sympathetic adrenergic tone and central vascular contraction in organs (e.g., the skin and gut), which have a low O_2ER. Blood is often preferentially redirected to maintain perfusion of critical organs (e.g., the brain and heart) that have a high O_2ER. Capillary recruitment is responsible for peripheral vasodilatation.

Mixed Venous Oxygen Saturation

Measurements of global oxygen consumption ($\dot{V}O_2$) are sometimes used to assess the adequacy of DO_2, on the assumption that if DO_2 is inadequate, $\dot{V}O_2$ becomes supply dependent as mentioned above. $\dot{V}O_2$ can be measured directly by gas analysis techniques, which require specialized equipment, or, more easily can be calculated from CO and arterial and mixed venous

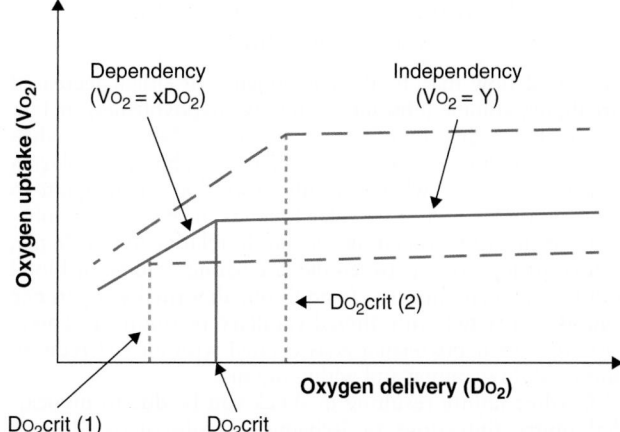

FIGURE 28.1. Relationship of oxygen uptake (VO_2) to oxygen delivery (DO_2) (*solid line*): When $\dot{V}O_2$ is supply independent (independency), whole-body O_2 needs are met. When $\dot{V}O_2$ becomes dependent on DO_2 (dependency), $\dot{V}O_2$ becomes linearly dependent on DO_2 at the critical DO_2 (DO_2crit), which corresponds to the definition of "dysoxia." DO_2crit is influenced by global oxygen requirements: When $\dot{V}O_2$ is decreased (i.e., during sedation and hypothermia—*lower dotted line*), the DO_2crit is also decreased [DO_2crit (1)]. When $\dot{V}O_2$ is increased (i.e., agitation, hyperthermia, sepsis—*upper dotted line*), DO_2crit is increased [DO_2crit (2)].

oxygen content using the inverse Fick principle. According to the Fick equation, tissue $\dot{V}O_2$ is proportional to CO:

$$\dot{V}O_2 = CO \times (CaO_2 - CvO_2)$$

where CvO_2 = mixed venous blood oxygen content. To some extent, CaO_2 and CvO_2 are proportional to SaO_2 and SvO_2, respectively, by the relationship:

$$\dot{V}O_2 \text{ is proportional to } CO \times (SaO_2 - SvO_2) \times Hb \times 1.39$$

Therefore, it becomes apparent that:

$$SvO_2 \text{ is proportional to } SaO_2 - \dot{V}O_2/(CO \times Hb \times 1.39)$$

An examination of this relationship reveals that four conditions may cause SvO_2 to decrease: hypoxemia (decrease in SaO_2), increase in $\dot{V}O_2$, reduction in CO, and decrease in Hb concentration.

At DO_2crit, SvO_2 is approximately 40% (SvO_2crit), with an O_2ER of 60% and a SaO_2 of 100%. For the same decrease in CaO_2 (induced by a decrease in either Hb or SaO_2), the decrease in SvO_2 will be more pronounced if CO cannot increase proportionately (9). Hence, SvO_2 represents adequacy of the response of global CO to CaO_2 decrease.

A 40% SvO_2 can be taken as an imbalance between arterial blood O_2 supply and tissue O_2 demand, with evident risk of dysoxia. In the clinical setting, a decrease in SvO_2 of 5% from its normal value (65%–77%) represents a significant fall in DO_2 and/or an increase in O_2 demand. If treatment is instituted to restore SvO_2 to the normal range (such as fluid resuscitation, inotropic therapy, or red cell transfusion), the measurement of CO, as well as SaO_2 and Hb, should be instituted to choose (and monitor response to) therapy.

Decreased Oxygen Delivery (Quantitative Shock)

Oxygen delivery is dependent on both blood flow and oxygen content, and each can be considered independently in the pathophysiology of shock.

Decreased Flow (e.g., Hypovolemic, Cardiogenic Shock)

Decreased flow may be the consequence of either decreased circulating volume (absolute or relative hypovolemia) or failure of the cardiac pump. Hypovolemia is "absolute" when there is dehydration from extracellular fluid, blood, or plasma loss; and "relative" when fluid administration is inadequate to compensate for loss of vascular tone (as in sepsis or anaphylaxis, or due to vasodilating agents). In relative hypovolemia, a discrepancy exists between the circulating volume of blood and the vascular capacity. In addition, abnormal sympathetic tone is associated with altered capillary recruitment. Therefore, relative hypovolemia is associated with altered redistribution of flow among and within organs.

Cardiac failure resulting in shock can be due to myocardial injury (infectious or ischemic) or obstructive lesions (increased right ventricular afterload, increased pulmonary vascular resistance, increased left ventricular afterload, increased systemic vascular resistance [SVR]), or lack of ventricular filling (decreased right ventricular or left ventricular preload, valvular lesions, decrease in filling time due to tachycardia).

Decreased Oxygen Content (e.g., Hemorrhagic Shock, Acute Hypoxemic Respiratory Failure, Poisoning)

Hemorrhagic shock is usually a result of hypovolemia and anemia. However, anemia is not necessarily associated with hypovolemia (e.g., in hemolysis). When anemia is associated with hemorrhage (hypovolemia), the decrease in oxygen delivery (Do_2) is substantially greater than either insult alone. Decreased oxygen-carrying capacity of Hb, and therefore inadequate Do_2, may also result in shock. For instance, with carbon monoxide poisoning, a decrease in Do_2 results from competitive binding of carbon monoxide in preference to O_2. This process is exacerbated by abnormal O_2 utilization, as carbon monoxide interferes with oxidative phosphorylation, resulting in a decreased O_2ER. In this case, shock is both distributive and quantitative. In any respiratory cause of acute hypoxia, decreased Sao_2 leads to a decrease in Do_2 as soon as CO is unable to compensate for metabolic needs.

Decreased Oxygen Extraction (Distributive Shock)

Distributive shock often coexists with hypovolemic and/or cardiogenic shock. Distributive shock occurs when blood is redistributed among organs, as in sepsis, anaphylaxis, or with the use of vasodilating agents. In addition, especially in sepsis, a decrease in capillary recruitment secondary to altered vascular reactivity, disseminated intravascular coagulation, endothelial cell dysfunction, increased blood cell adhesiveness, and/or abnormal mitochondrial function (mitochondrial injury or dysfunction) may be present. These changes contribute to the inability to fully utilize oxygen that is delivered.

Spinal cord injury is a specific form of distributive shock that leads to profound hemodynamic derangement. The loss of sympathetic outflow from the spinal cord leads to a sudden decrease in SVR and CO, while central venous pressure (CVP) remains unchanged. The hypotension improves within days due to reasons that are not totally understood but may include synaptic reorganization or hyperresponsiveness of α receptors.

ASSESSMENT

History

In many cases, the cause of shock is obvious. However, a detailed history in less obvious situations is vital to decisions regarding appropriate management. The early diagnosis of shock requires knowledge of the conditions that predispose children of different ages and comorbidities to shock. For instance, a history of congenital heart disease, immunodeficiency, trauma, surgery, toxin ingestion, or allergies is important.

Children who are febrile, who have an identifiable source of infection, or who are hypovolemic are at increased risk of developing shock. In neonates, the maternal and birth history with regard to timing and duration of rupture of membranes, maternal fever, blood loss, fetal distress, and other obstetric information are important. In the case of trauma, history regarding the mechanism and timing of injury, whether excessive blood loss has occurred, and the level of consciousness before hospital arrival is vital. A history of immunodeficiency, use of immunosuppressive agents, duration and height of fever, and associated features, such as lethargy, vomiting, diarrhea, decreased oral intake, and decreased level of consciousness or awareness, may suggest infection and the possibility of septic shock or dehydration. Other details, such as environmental exposure, drug ingestion, previous medical history, and allergies, are also important.

Physical Examination

As children will maintain BP until they are severely ill (5), the presence of systemic hypotension is not required to make the diagnosis of shock. In guidelines published by the American College of Critical Care Medicine (ACCM), shock in children is characterized by tachycardia (which may be absent in the hypothermic patient), with signs of decreased organ or peripheral perfusion, including decreased peripheral pulses compared with central pulses, altered alertness, flash capillary refill or capillary refill >2 seconds, mottled or cool extremities, or decreased urine output (1). Hypotension is a late sign of shock and should not be relied on to make the diagnosis. Moreover, the classifications of shock in children (e.g., warm and cold shock, fluid-refractory shock, or catecholamine-resistant shock) are not helpful for diagnosis, but may dictate therapy. Shock in children can be recognized before hypotension occurs by clinical as well as laboratory signs that include metabolic acidosis, or increased blood lactate.

In the early, compensated stage, homeostatic mechanisms attempt to maintain vital organ perfusion. BP, urine output, and cardiac function may all appear normal; however, early cellular metabolic alterations are already underway. In decompensated shock, circulatory compensation fails because of dysoxia, ischemia, endothelial cell injury and dysfunction, the upregulation and elaboration of inducible gene products, and the release of toxic materials from host cells and microorganisms (either invasive or from the patient's gut). Eventually, cellular function deteriorates, and widespread abnormalities occur in all organ systems, which lead to multiorgan failure. When this process has caused such widespread organ dysfunction, shock is irreversible and death is inevitable despite temporary support. The point at which irreversibility is reached is becoming more extended as technology and supportive care improves.

The physical examination may reveal a decrease in tissue perfusion, which is identified by changes in body surface temperature, prolonged CRT, and impaired organ function. Decreased skin perfusion and temperature reflect the sympathetic neurohumoral response to hypovolemia (6). Skin temperature is measured using the dorsal surface of the examiner's hands or fingers because these areas are most sensitive to temperature perception. Patients are considered to have cool extremities if all extremities are cool to the examiner or if only the lower extremities are cool, in the absence of peripheral vascular disease. Clinical signs of poor peripheral perfusion consist of cold, pale, clammy, and mottled skin, associated with an increase in CRT. In particular, skin temperature and CRT have been advocated as an indicator of the adequacy of peripheral perfusion (3,7,8,10). Cool peripheries as a marker of peripheral perfusion is associated with higher blood lactate levels and lower CO in adult patients in the ICU, indicating more severe tissue hypoxia (7).

CRT has become widely accepted as a reflection of intravascular volume, especially in children and in the assessment of trauma. A value ≤2 seconds at normal ambient temperature is considered adequate. CRT has been validated as a measure of peripheral perfusion, with significant variation in children and adults. A study on a normal population reported that CRT varied with age and sex (9). It was found that a CRT of <2 seconds was a normal value for most young children and young adults (most ≤1 second), but that CRT varied with age, being substantially higher in healthy women (2.9 seconds) and in the elderly (4.5 seconds). A poor correlation may exist between CRT, HR, BP, and CO (9,10); however, prolonged CRT in pediatric patients has been found to be a good predictor of dehydration, reduced SV, and increased blood lactate levels (3,8). The findings of these studies show that monitoring of skin temperature and CRT are valuable in hemodynamic monitoring during circulatory shock and should be the first approach to assess any critically ill patient. A few data are available regarding the clinical utility of these measures once the patient has been admitted to the ICU.

Laboratory Markers of Shock

Serial blood gas and arterial lactate evaluations are widely used to complement the clinical assessment of systemic perfusion. They help quantify the extent of tissue hypoperfusion and provide trends with which to titrate therapy. Normalization of BP may not indicate reversal of the shock state in a patient who has ongoing metabolic acidosis and/or elevated arterial lactate. Similarly, tissue hypoxia may be present before derangements in lactate, acid levels, or hemodynamic stability. In such instances, decreased mixed venous oxygen saturation can detect imbalances in Do_2 and $\dot{V}o_2$.

Mixed venous O_2 saturation (SvO_2) can be useful in assessing whole-body $\dot{V}o_2$–Do_2 relationships. Recent studies have used central venous oxygen saturation ($ScvO_2$) to detect global O_2 deficiency (11). It has been shown that although $ScvO_2$ tracks SvO_2, the former tends to be up to 7% higher. Furthermore, changes in $ScvO_2$ paralleled SvO_2 changes 90% of the time when SvO_2 changed by 5% or more. So if threshold values of $ScvO_2$ are to be used to guide therapy, then higher thresholds may be needed to detect potential tissue hypoperfusion (12).

Early identification of patients with severe sepsis and shock and rapid initiation of goal-directed therapy to achieve adequate tissue oxygenation by improving Do_2 ($ScvO_2$ monitoring) has been shown to significantly improve mortality (11). Continuous monitoring of $ScvO_2$ with fiber-optic probes offers the advantage of real-time assessments in patients.

A decrease in SvO_2 of 5% from its normal value (65%–77%) represents a significant fall in Do_2 and/or an increase in O_2 demand. In order to determine the appropriate therapy to restore SvO_2, measurements of CO, as well as SaO_2 and Hb, are necessary. The strategy for managing shock relies on early and rapid estimation of O_2 deficit, rapidly followed by

corrective therapy and ongoing monitoring, dependent on the most likely cause of dysoxia (11).

While lactate and base deficit estimations together with $ScvO_2$ measurement are invaluable for detection and monitoring of global O_2 deficiency, regional and tissue perfusion may not be accurately assessed using these indices.

Assessment of Global Blood Flow

Global blood flow is dependent on preload, myocardial function, afterload, and HR. Regional flow distribution is not homogeneous and is dependent on central and peripheral vascular tone, which determine SVR. As a gross simplification, mean arterial pressure (MAP) can be estimated as the product of flow and SVR. If flow decreases, MAP remains stable when SVR increases (an increase in sympathetic adrenergic tone, central volume contraction in low-O_2ER organs, and preserved vasodilatation in high-O_2ER organs). Under these circumstances, overall O_2ER increases and SvO_2 decreases.

In children, good data are not available to determine threshold BPs that should be maintained in these situations. Arbitrary values of systolic pressure of 90 mm Hg or MAP of 60 mm Hg in adults have been chosen, with population standards for age in children (13). During circulatory shock, when Do_2crit is breached, $\dot{V}o_2$–Do_2 dependency is associated with a rise in blood lactate level and implies oxygen debt. In adults and children, hyperlactemia (and thus oxygen debt) is related to the likelihood of multiorgan failure and mortality (14,15).

The hemodynamic variables important in shock also relate to flow to vital organs. Flow (Q) varies directly with perfusion pressure (dP) and inversely with resistance (R), mathematically represented by:

$$Q = dP/R$$

For the whole body, this relationship is represented by:

$$CO = MAP - CVP/SVR$$

This relationship also holds for organ perfusion. In the kidney, for example:

Renal blood flow = mean renal arterial pressure − mean renal venous pressure/renal vascular resistance

Some organs, including the kidney and brain, have vasomotor autoregulation that maintains flow in low-pressure states. However, even in organs with autoregulation capabilities, at some critical point (lower limit of pressure autoregulation), perfusion pressure is reduced below the ability to maintain blood flow. The purpose of the treatment of shock is to maintain perfusion pressure above the critical point for blood flow in individual organs.

Because the kidney receives the second highest blood flow of any organ in the body, measurement of urine output can be used as an indicator of adequate perfusion pressure (except in hyperosmolar states leading to osmotic diuresis). In this regard, maintenance of MAP with norepinephrine has been shown to improve urine output and creatinine clearance in hyperdynamic sepsis. However, maintenance of supranormal MAP above this point is likely of no benefit (16).

Cardiac index (CI) × (arterial oxygen content − mixed venous oxygen) has been proposed as a useful measure of CO and oxygen consumption in patients with persistent shock, because a CI between 3.3 and 6.0 L/min/m² and oxygen consumption of >200 mL/min/m² are associated with improved survival (17). Assuming a Hb concentration of 10 g/dL and 100% SaO_2, a CI of >3.3 L/min/m² would correlate to a mixed venous oxygen saturation of 70% in a patient with a normal oxygen consumption of 150 mL/min/m².

Pulmonary Artery Catheter Thermodilution

The Society of Critical Care Medicine Pulmonary Artery Catheter Consensus conference document (18) suggests that the use of pulmonary artery catheter (PAC) clarifies cardiopulmonary physiology in pediatric patients with refractory shock. However, randomized controlled studies to support the use of PAC in children are not available. Also, catheter placement and interpretation of the hemodynamic data derived from it require experienced healthcare providers to avoid complications and misguided decision making.

In the absence of definitive studies, various professional groups have developed guidelines for PAC use. However, their role has been increasingly challenged because several large trials have questioned a positive effect of their use on outcome in critically ill patients, and because alternative, less invasive methods have become available.

Doppler Ultrasound

③ Doppler ultrasound cardiac monitors provide a rapid, noninvasive measure of cardiac function. It can be measured via the transthoracic route or continuously via the esophageal route. Validation studies against thermodilution show these devices to be inaccurate, particularly when used in children (19). However, if the probe is well positioned in the esophagus, these devices can be used as trend monitors and rapidly detect changes in CO, making them useful for monitoring therapeutic interventions, such as fluid administration in critically ill patients.

The recent ACCM guidelines recommend the use of pulmonary artery thermodilution (PATD), pulse contour analysis or Doppler ultrasound for monitoring CO in patients with septic shock. Of all three methods, Doppler ultrasound is the least invasive, and being used in emergency departments where the equipment and expertise to perform PATD or pulse contour analysis is not usually available.

Pulse Contour Analysis

One of the less invasive methods for measuring CO is pulse contour analysis. Pulse contour analysis estimates global End-diastolic Volume (EDV) and can be used to assess whether preload is adequate. Stroke volume variability (SVV), a functional parameter of preload, has been suggested as a better determinant of preload compared with other measurements, such as cardiac filling pressures (CVPs) (pulmonary capillary wedge pressure), volumetric parameters (right ventricular end diastolic volume, PATD), and left ventricular end diastolic area (measured by echocardiography).

SVV is derived from pulse contour analysis, which uses the area under the systolic portion of the arterial pressure curve for beat-to-beat determination of SV and its variability over the respiratory cycle. Several studies have shown that as CO increased after volume loading, intrathoracic blood volume increased and SVV during positive pressure ventilation decreased. There is reportedly a good agreement between CO assessed by PATD and that assessed via pulse contour analysis in stable patients (18). Pulse contour–derived SVV has been described as a valuable estimate of fluid responsiveness in mechanically ventilated, stable patients.

Plethysmography

Pulse oximetry is a noninvasive monitoring tool routinely used to assess oxygenation. The oximeters use photoelectric plethysmography to detect changes in blood volume at the site of measurement. This waveform measures volume changes and pulse plethysmographic variation and has shown significant correlation with pulse pressure variation associated with

fluid responsiveness (20,21). The waveform is generated by blood volume changes in both arterial and venous vessels. Its amplitude depends on intravascular pulse pressure as well as distensibility of the vascular wall. It has, however, been shown that pulse pressure variation is a reliable indicator of fluid responsiveness only when tidal volume is at least 8–12 mL/kg (22). Studies have confirmed that prediction of fluid responsiveness by pulse pressure variation should be performed with caution in critically ill patients with low-to-normal tidal volume (23).

Echocardiography

Echocardiography is an appropriate noninvasive tool to rule out the presence of pericardial effusion, evaluate contractility, and depending on the skills of the operator, check ventricular filling. Doppler echocardiography can be used to measure CO and Superior vena cava (SVC) flow.

In summary, CO monitoring in children may help guide therapy; however, there is no conclusive evidence linking their use to improved outcomes in critically ill patients.

Assessment of Regional Blood Flow

Skin Temperature Gradient

Body temperature gradients have long been used as a parameter of peripheral perfusion. In the presence of a constant environmental temperature, changes in skin temperature are the result of changes in skin blood flow (13). The temperature gradients, peripheral-to-ambient (dTp-a) and central-to-peripheral (dTc-p), can better reflect cutaneous blood flow than skin **④** temperature itself. In the presence of constant environmental conditions, dTp-a decreases and dTc-p increases during vasoconstriction. A gradient of 3°C–7°C occurs in patients who are hemodynamically stable (24). Moreover, an increase in dTp-a of >4°C–6°C over 12 hours was observed in survivors of hypovolemia and low CO (25).

Optical Monitoring

Optical methods apply light with different wavelengths directly to tissue components, using the scattering characteristics of tissue to assess various states of these tissues. At physiologic concentrations, the molecules that absorb most light are Hb, myoglobin, cytochrome, melanins, carotenes, and bilirubin. These substances can be quantified and measured in tissues using simple optical methods. The assessment of tissue oxygenation is based on the specific absorption spectrum of oxygenated Hb (HbO_2), deoxygenated Hb, and cytochrome aa3 (Cytaa3). Commonly used optical methods for peripheral monitoring are perfusion index, near-infrared spectroscopy (NIRS), laser-Doppler flowmetry, and orthogonal polarization spectral (OPS) imaging.

Peripheral Perfusion Index

The peripheral perfusion (flow) index (PFI) is derived from the photoelectric plethysmographic signal of pulse oximetry and has been used as a noninvasive measure of peripheral perfusion in critically ill patients (26). The principle of pulse oximetry is based on two light sources with different wavelengths (660 and 940 nm) transmitted through the cutaneous vascular bed of a finger or earlobe. Deoxygenated Hb absorbs more light at 660 nm, and HbO_2 absorbs more light at 940 nm. A detector measures the intensity of the transmitted light at each wavelength, and the oxygen saturation is derived by the ratio between the red light (660 nm) and the infrared light (940 nm) absorbed. As other tissues, such as connective tissue, bone, and venous blood, also absorb light, pulse oximetry distinguishes the pulsatile component of arterial blood from the nonpulsatile component of other tissues. Using a two-wavelength system, the nonpulsatile component is then discarded, and the pulsatile component is used to calculate the SaO_2. The overall Hb concentration can be determined by a third wavelength at 800 nm, with a spectrum that resembles that of both Hb and HbO_2. The resulting variation in intensity of this light can be used to determine the variation in arterial blood volume (pulsatile component). The PFI is calculated as the ratio of the light that reaches the detector of the oximeter between the pulsatile component (arterial compartment) and the nonpulsatile component (other tissues) and is calculated independently of the patient's oxygen saturation. Alteration in peripheral perfusion is accompanied by variation in the pulsatile component, and because the nonpulsatile component does not change, the ratio changes. As a result, the value displayed on the monitor reflects changes in peripheral perfusion.

Near-Infrared Spectroscopy

NIRS offers a technique for continuous, noninvasive, bedside monitoring of tissue oxygenation. As with pulse oximetry, NIRS uses the principles of light transmission and absorption to measure the concentrations of Hb, tissue oxygen saturation (StO_2), and Cytaa3 in tissues. NIRS has a greater tissue penetration than pulse oximetry and provides a global assessment of oxygenation in all vascular compartments (arterial, venous, and capillary). In addition to blood flow, evaluation of HbO_2 and Hb, NIRS can assess the Cytaa3 redox state. Cytaa3 is the end receptor in the oxygen transport chain that reacts with oxygen to form water, and most cellular energy is derived from this reaction. Cytaa3 remains in a reduced state during hypoxemia. The absorption spectrum of Cytaa3 in its reduced state shows a weak peak at 70 nm, whereas the oxygenated form does not. Therefore, monitoring changes in the Cytaa3 redox state can provide a measure of the adequacy of oxidative metabolism.

The use of NIRS in deltoid muscle during resuscitation from trauma has shown a strong association between elevated serum lactate levels and elevated Cytaa3 redox state during 12 hours of shock resuscitation and the development of multiorgan failure (27). A good relationship was also shown between tissue O_2 (StO_2), systemic oxygen delivery, and lactate during and after resuscitation in severely injured patients over a period of 24 hours (28). A study in septic and nonseptic adults used NIRS to measure both regional blood flow and oxygen consumption after venous occlusion (29). The potential to monitor regional perfusion and oxygenation noninvasively at the bedside makes clinical application of both PFI and NIRS technology of particular interest in intensive care.

Orthogonal Polarization Spectral Imaging

OPS imaging is a noninvasive technique that uses reflected light to produce real-time images of the microcirculation. Light from a source passes through the first polarizer and is directed toward the tissue by a set of lenses. As the light reaches the tissue, the depolarized light is reflected back through the lenses to a second polarizer or analyzer and forms an image of the microcirculation, which can be recorded. The technology has been incorporated into a small handheld video-microscope, which can be used in both research and clinical settings.

OPS imaging can assess tissue perfusion using functional capillary density, that is, the length of perfused capillaries per observation area (measured as cm/cm^2). Functional capillary density is a very sensitive parameter for determining the status of perfusion to the tissue, and it is an indirect measure of oxygen delivery.

One of the most easily accessible sites in humans for perfusion monitoring is the mouth. OPS imaging produces clearly defined images of the sublingual microcirculation by placement of the probe under the tongue. The use of OPS imaging to assess the sublingual tissues provides information about the dynamics of microcirculatory blood flow and, therefore, has been used to monitor the perfusion during clinical treatment of circulatory shock. It has shown the effects of improvements in microcirculatory blood flow with dobutamine and nitroglycerin in volume-resuscitated septic patients (30,31). Limitations of the technique include movement artifacts, semiquantitative measures of perfusion, the presence saliva or blood, observer-related bias, and inadequacy of sedation to prevent patients from moving or damaging the device. In septic patients, OPS imaging has shown that microvascular alterations are more severe in patients with a worse outcome and that these microvascular alterations can be reversed using vasodilators (32).

In patients with cardiac failure and cardiogenic shock, the number of small vessels and the density of perfused vessels are lower than those in controls, and the proportion of perfused vessels is higher in survivors than that in nonsurvivors (33). Although alterations in the sublingual microcirculation may not be representative of other microvascular beds, changes in the sublingual circulation evaluated by capnometry during hemorrhagic shock have reflected changes in perfusion of splanchnic organs (34).

Transcutaneous Oxygen and Carbon Dioxide Measurements

Oxygen sensors for transcutaneous electrochemical measurements are based on polarography: an amperometric transducer is used in which the rate of a chemical reaction is detected by the current drained through an electrode. The sensor heats the skin to 43°C–45°C, which causes dermal capillary hyperemia and increases local oxygen tension by shifting the oxygen dissociation curve in the heated dermal capillary blood. Transcutaneous sensors enable the estimation of arterial oxygen pressure (PaO_2) and arterial carbon dioxide pressure ($PaCO_2$) and have been successfully used for monitoring these values in both neonates and in adults.

This technique is well suited for the newborn infant because of its thin epidermal layer. However, in older children and adults, the skin is thicker, causing the transcutaneous oxygen partial pressure ($PtcO_2$) to be lower than PaO_2. The correlation between $PtcO_2$ and PaO_2 also depends on the adequacy of blood flow. Low blood flow caused by vasoconstriction during shock overcomes the vasodilatory effect of the $PtcO_2$ sensor, resulting in tissue hypoxia beneath the $PtcO_2$ sensor. The fact that the $PtcO_2$ sensor does not accurately reflect the PaO_2 in low-flow states, such as shock, enables the estimation of cutaneous blood flow through the relationship between the two variables. Some have suggested the use of a transcutaneous oxygen index (tc-index), that is, the changes in $PtcO_2$ relative to changes in PaO_2 (35).

When blood flow is adequate, $PtcO_2$ and PaO_2 values are almost equal and the tc-index is close to 1. During low-flow states, such as shock, the $PtcO_2$ drops and becomes dependent on the PaO_2 value, and the tc-index decreases. A tc-index below 0.7 has been associated with hemodynamic instability. One group found a good correlation ($r = 0.86$) between tc-index and CI in patients with shock (35). However, the relationship between tc-index and CI appeared less reliable in hyperdynamic shock.

Transcutaneous carbon dioxide partial pressure ($PtcCO_2$) has been also used as an index of cutaneous blood flow. Differences between $PaCO_2$ and $PtcCO_2$ have been explained by local accumulation of CO_2 in the skin because of hypoperfusion. Because the diffusion constant of CO_2 through skin is approximately 20 times greater than O_2, $PtcCO_2$ is less sensitive to changes in hemodynamics than $Ptco_2$.

$Ptco_2$ and $PtcCO_2$ have also been used as early indicators of tissue hypoxia and subclinical hypovolemia in acutely ill patients in the emergency department (36) and operating room (37). Nonsurvivors had lower $Ptco_2$ values and higher $PtcCO_2$ values than did survivors. These differences were evident even shortly after the patient's arrival. The authors reported critical tissue perfusion threshold values of a $Ptco_2$ of 50 mm Hg for more than 60 minutes and a $PtcCO_2$ of 60 mm Hg for more than 30 minutes. Patients with these critical thresholds had 89%–100% mortality.

One of the main limitations of this technique is the necessity of blood gas analysis to obtain the tc-index and $PaCO_2$. In addition, the sensor position must be changed every 1–2 hours to avoid burns. After each repositioning, a period of 15–20 minutes is required for stability, which limits its use in emergency situations. Also, the time required for calibration limits its early use in the emergency department, and critical $Ptco_2$ and $PtcCO_2$ values have not yet been established. Therefore, this technology has not gained widespread acceptance in clinical practice.

Tissue Capnometry

Measurement of the tissue-arterial CO_2 tension gradient has been used to reflect the adequacy of tissue perfusion. Gastric and ileal mucosal CO_2 clearance has been the primary reference for measurements of regional PCO_2 gradient during circulatory shock (38). The regional PCO_2 gradient represents the balance between regional CO_2 production and clearance. In low-flow states, tissue CO_2 increases as a result of a stagnation phenomenon (39). Comparable decreases in tissue blood flow during circulatory shock have also been demonstrated by measuring the sublingual tissue PCO_2 ($PslCO_2$) (40).

The currently available system for measuring $PslCO_2$ consists of a disposable PCO_2 sensor and a battery-powered, handheld instrument. Clinical studies have suggested that $PslCO_2$ is a reliable marker of tissue hypoperfusion. In one study of emergency department patients, patients with physical signs of circulatory shock and high blood lactate levels had higher $PslCO_2$ values, and a $PslCO_2$ threshold value of 70 mm Hg was predictive for the severity of circulatory failure (41).

As with PCO_2 in the gut mucosa, $PslCO_2$ is also influenced by $PaCO_2$. Hence, the gradient between $PslCO_2$ and $PaCO_2$ (Psl-aCO_2) may be more specific for tissue hypoperfusion. In one study, the Psl-aCO_2 gradient was a sensitive marker for tissue perfusion and a useful endpoint for the titration of goal-directed therapy (42). Psl-aCO_2 differentiated better than $PslCO_2$ alone between survivors and nonsurvivors, and a difference of >25 mm Hg indicated a poor prognosis. Limitations of this technique include the necessity of blood gas analysis to obtain $PaCO_2$. In addition, normal and pathologic Psl-aCO_2 values are not well defined.

Monitoring Dilemmas and Pitfalls

Clinical indicators of end-organ perfusion and biochemical parameters of global perfusion, such as central venous oxygen saturation ($Scvo_2$), blood lactate and base deficit, as well as invasive central venous and arterial pressure monitoring, are often poorly correlated with CO (43). Indeed, several studies have shown that clinical monitoring is not reliable in predicting volume status or CO in critically ill patients (44,45). The recent update of the ACCM guidelines for the management of pediatric septic shock encourages the use of CO monitoring to direct therapy. Some of these techniques aim to measure CI and SVR index. Others seek to measure fluid responsiveness

by monitoring increases in CO through a rise in preload, such as by the observation of an improvement (reduction) in SVV. The effect of fluid therapy can be determined by measuring CO before and after fluid bolus. If SV increases by 10%–15%, the patient is considered fluid responsive. Results from adult and pediatric studies have shown that only a proportion of patients in shock who receive a fluid challenge demonstrate an increased SV (46–48). To avoid fluid overload, therefore, it would be useful to predict fluid responsiveness. This can be done through static variables, such as CVP, HR, and global end diastolic volume index; or by dynamic variables, such as arterial pressure variations that result from mechanical ventilation. CVP alone does not predict fluid responsiveness and only poorly reflects preload in adults and children. In general, dilution techniques deliver a reliable CO measurement in children >3.5 kg, but require invasive monitoring. Less invasive methods are often less reliable. The method of transpulmonary thermodilution also offers measurement of extravascular lung water (EVLW), which may reflect pulmonary edema. In adults, EVLW measurement has been validated in many studies, but this is not well validated in children. In addition, it cannot be reliably measured in patients with significant left-to-right or right-to-left shunts.

Classically, CO monitoring had been performed via PAC thermodilution, which is not only technically difficult in children, but also has significant complication risks. Because of this, over the last decade, there has been increasing use of noninvasive and partially invasive CO monitoring modalities. The ideal CO monitor should be noninvasive, valid, and reliable under various hemodynamic conditions, operator independent, easy to use, and cost-effective. Noninvasive assessment of CO using conventional echocardiography is well described, but requires sequential measurements, a skilled technician, and a cardiac grade ultrasound machine, all of which are not often readily available at all times. Other means of continuously assessing CO include Doppler ultrasound and arterial pulse contour analysis, which is derived from the arterial pulse wave. Doppler ultrasound is a well-accepted, noninvasive method for CO monitoring. The advantage is that it can be used early to direct therapy. However, agreement between Doppler ultrasound and echocardiography has shown to be poor, and there is high interuser variability in newborns (49). Pulse contour analysis is less reliable as a trend marker as it often fails to compensate for circulatory changes, such as peripheral vascular resistance. Other CO monitoring techniques include thoracic bioimpedance and pulse oximetry plethysmographic waveform analysis. Both of these methods have several limitations in critically ill patients. It is important to note, however, that there is no evidence that these hemodynamic monitoring techniques improve mortality or morbidity in critically ill patients.

MANAGEMENT

Monitoring

In addition to repeated clinical examinations, monitoring for patients who are in either incipient or actual shock includes continuous electrocardiography, pulse oximetry, measurement of urine output, and either continuous invasive or rapid and regular noninvasive measurements of BP. A central venous catheter allows CVP monitoring, which may help determine the need for fluid administration. In addition, the catheter allows rapid infusion of drugs and fluids and monitoring of $Scvo_2$ (if placed in the SVC distribution). However, a central venous catheter insertion for CVP monitoring is not essential in the early stages of management of a child in shock.

In the sedated, ventilated patient, recordings of systolic pressure variation and/or pulse pressure variation may be helpful. The heart remains preload dependent until systolic pressure variation is <10 mm Hg, and/or pulse pressure variation is <10% (50). Blood gas analysis, which examines metabolic acidosis and lactate concentration, gives an indication of global oxygenation, which reflects the adequacy of CO and oxygen delivery.

As outlined earlier, hemodynamic monitoring techniques, such as a PAC (ideally with continuous CO monitoring and with a fiber-optic SvO2 device) and/or noninvasive flow assessment (pulse contour analysis, transesophageal Doppler or echocardiography), may be considered when CO is difficult to assess. In this context, the effect of fluid administration on CO and oxygen delivery/consumption can be assessed and titrated.

General Supportive Measures

The appropriate recognition and management of shock is essential as evidence shows that early normalization of hemodynamic status can improve outcome (51,52). Initial management should focus on interpreting and treating hemodynamic derangements, with targeted therapeutic interventions aimed at improving tissue perfusion and restoring balance between Do_2 and demand. This therapeutic approach has been labeled "early goal-directed therapy" and includes prompt fluid resuscitation, targeted vasoactive therapy, early empiric antimicrobial therapy, and continuous monitoring of hemodynamic status. Rivers et al. (11) demonstrated a lower mortality in adults with sepsis when they achieved hemodynamic and oxygenation goals using aggressive treatment with fluid administration, early red cell transfusions, and early vasoactive therapy. The ACCM has made a series of recommendations emphasizing first-hour fluid resuscitation and vasoactive drug therapy directed to targeted goals of threshold HRs, BP, and CRT. They have also made recommendations for subsequent intensive care hemodynamic support directed to goals achieving Scvo2 >70% and CI of 3.3–6.0 L/min/m². The recent update of this guideline advocated the use of peripheral inotropes until central venous access is established and also encourages the use of noninvasive CO monitoring to direct therapies to achieve a CI of 3.3–6.0 L/min/m² (53).

Emergency therapy should be given to all patients while the specific diagnosis is being established. Support of the airway and breathing is essential to maximize Do_2. Supplemental oxygen should be delivered to all patients with signs of shock and early tracheal intubation may be necessary. Supplemental O_2 and respiratory support should be titrated in response to acute respiratory failure whether primary (acute lung injury) or secondary (result of shock). Acute circulatory failure should be initially treated by fluid challenge. If intravascular volume is optimized and myocardial contractility remains reduced, support with vasoactive agents will be necessary. In the case of distributive shock (e.g., anaphylaxis or acute vasodilation), adrenaline or vasoconstrictors should be considered early. Suggested protocols for management in the emergency department and shortly after transition to the ICU are outlined in **Figures 28.2** and **28.3**.

Fluid Resuscitation

The goal of fluid administration is to optimize left ventricular preload to improve Do_2 by increasing CO via the Frank–Starling mechanism. However, overaggressive fluid administration increases the risk of pulmonary interstitial edema. Up to 60 mL/kg fluid may be given in the first hour of therapy to children with septic shock, without increasing the risk of pulmonary edema, while resulting in a consequent improvement in outcome (51). The "surviving sepsis" and ACCM guidelines suggest initial resuscitation with infusion of crystalloid, with boluses of 20 mL/kg, over 5–10 minutes, titrated to clinical estimation of CO (53–55).

Early, aggressive, goal-directed fluid administration has been the cornerstone of the management of children in septic shock. Failure to adhere to the ACCM guidelines was associated with a significantly increased risk of mortality (52,56). Recently, the Fluid Expansion as Supportive Therapy (FEAST) study (57), a randomized trial of fluid bolus therapy versus maintenance fluid only therapy in 3144 African children with severe febrile illness and signs of poor perfusion, compared outcomes in those that received fluid boluses. This study found significantly higher mortality rates in the fluid bolus group. There were several limitations to the FEAST study. Firstly, the inclusion criteria were broader than most shock classification systems, focusing mainly on poor perfusion rather than shock. Secondly, many of the children had severe anemia. Fluid boluses in this population can further dilute Hb and so effectively reduce tissue oxygen delivery and exacerbate cardiac failure. However, the study highlighted the need for further investigation of fluid therapy in septic shock, especially in resource limited environments. Indeed, it has been shown that adult patients treated for shock in the ICU with raised CVP and positive fluid balance have an increased risk of mortality (58). However, the results of the FEAST study cannot be readily extrapolated to patients in developed countries with a different pediatric population and the availability of intensive care facilities to deal with the consequences of aggressive fluid therapy. Because of concerns regarding the risks of fluid overload, the ACCM guidelines recommend that fluid removal using diuretics, peritoneal dialysis, or continuous renal replacement therapy (CRRT) is indicated in patients who have been adequately fluid resuscitated, but cannot subsequently maintain an even fluid balance via their native urine output in the ICU (53).

Emergent fluid requirement is usually determined by a combination of clinical parameters, including HR, BP, peripheral perfusion, and urine output. These can be supplemented by monitoring of CVP, arterial pressure, central venous oxygen saturation, serum lactate, and base deficit. However, as outlined earlier, these clinical indicators of end-organ perfusion are often poor correlates of CO.

Fluid-refractory shock is defined as the persistence of shock after the administration of sufficient fluids to achieve a CVP of 8–12 mm Hg and/or signs of fluid overload (hepatic congestion, pulmonary edema). Additional therapy, such as vasopressors/inotropes, should be administered.

Choice of Fluids

The choice of fluid for resuscitation is also a subject of intense debate. Several studies have cast doubt on previously accepted theories that colloid solutions are better for fluid replacement in critical illness, as colloids were thought to be more likely to be retained intravascularly and thus less likely to exacerbate capillary leakage, especially in the lung. A meta-analysis by the Cochrane Albumin Reviewers suggested that 4.5% human albumin solution (HAS) may be associated with excess mortality when compared with saline for various indications, including hypovolemia (59). However, other investigators have suggested that the use of 4.5% HAS may be associated with improvements in morbidity (60). These meta-analyses prompted a large, randomized, controlled study in nearly 7000 critically ill adults that showed that use of either 4% HAS or normal saline for fluid resuscitation in patients in ICUs resulted in similar outcomes at 28 days (61). However, in subgroup analyses of patients included in this study, HAS seemed to have a protective effect in patients with septic shock, and normal saline

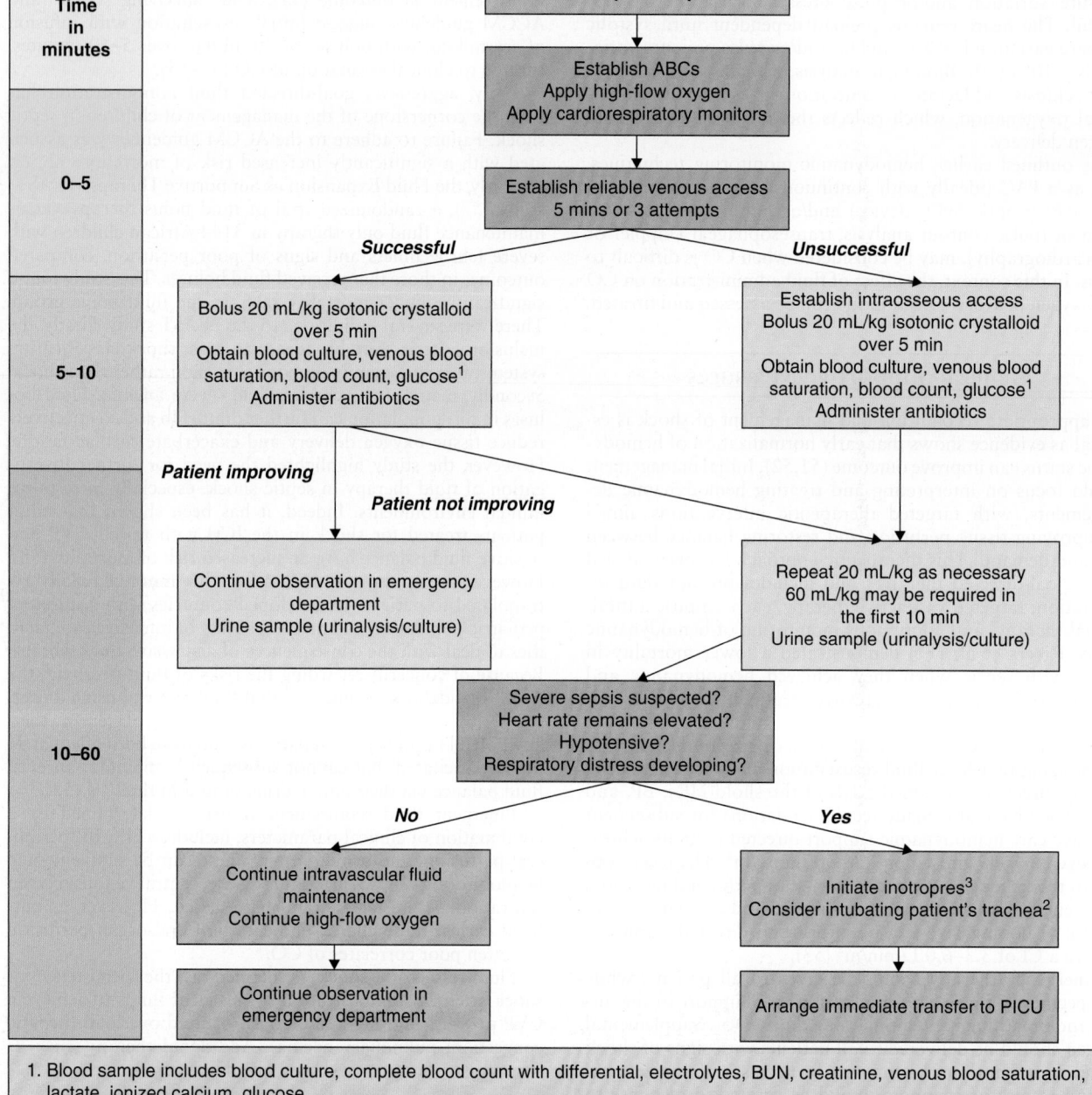

Time in minutes	

Severe sepsis suspected

Establish ABCs
Apply high-flow oxygen
Apply cardiorespiratory monitors

0–5

Establish reliable venous access
5 mins or 3 attempts

Successful ← → *Unsuccessful*

Bolus 20 mL/kg isotonic crystalloid over 5 min
Obtain blood culture, venous blood saturation, blood count, glucose[1]
Administer antibiotics

Establish intraosseous access
Bolus 20 mL/kg isotonic crystalloid over 5 min
Obtain blood culture, venous blood saturation, blood count, glucose[1]
Administer antibiotics

5–10

Patient improving

Patient not improving

Continue observation in emergency department
Urine sample (urinalysis/culture)

Repeat 20 mL/kg as necessary
60 mL/kg may be required in the first 10 min
Urine sample (urinalysis/culture)

Severe sepsis suspected?
Heart rate remains elevated?
Hypotensive?
Respiratory distress developing?

10–60

No ← → *Yes*

Continue intravascular fluid maintenance
Continue high-flow oxygen

Initiate inotropres[3]
Consider intubating patient's trachea[2]

Continue observation in emergency department

Arrange immediate transfer to PICU

1. Blood sample includes blood culture, complete blood count with differential, electrolytes, BUN, creatinine, venous blood saturation, lactate, ionized calcium, glucose.

2. Consider: Vagolytic (atropine 20 μg/kg); Induction agent with minimal hypotensive effect (ketamine 1 mg/kg); Paralytic (rocuronium 1 mg/kg or succinylcholine 2 mg/kg).

3. Recommended inotropes if peripheral access only: dopamine 10 μg/kg/min, epinephrine 0.1–0.2 μg/kg/min.
Recommended inotropes if central access: dopamine 10 μg/kg/min, epinephrine 0.05–2 μg/kg/min, norepinephrine 0.05–2 μg/kg/min.

FIGURE 28.2. Suggested emergency department sepsis protocol.

seemed to have a protective effect in patients with traumatic brain injury. The reasons for these subgroup findings are unclear. These results have led to the recommendation for use of either crystalloid or colloid for early resuscitation of patients with sepsis [see the Surviving Sepsis Campaign Guidelines—(54,55)]. However, there is emerging evidence that choice of fluid may influence outcome in different populations of patients. For example, colloids should not be used in trauma and

hydroxyethyl starch has been shown to increase the risk of death and the need for CRRT in septic patients (62).

A few large, properly controlled studies of the differences between various fluids for resuscitation of pediatric shock have been conducted. In one analysis of children with dengue shock syndrome, no difference was seen between patients resuscitated with crystalloid or colloid solutions (63). However, this is a very specific form of septic shock in which, despite

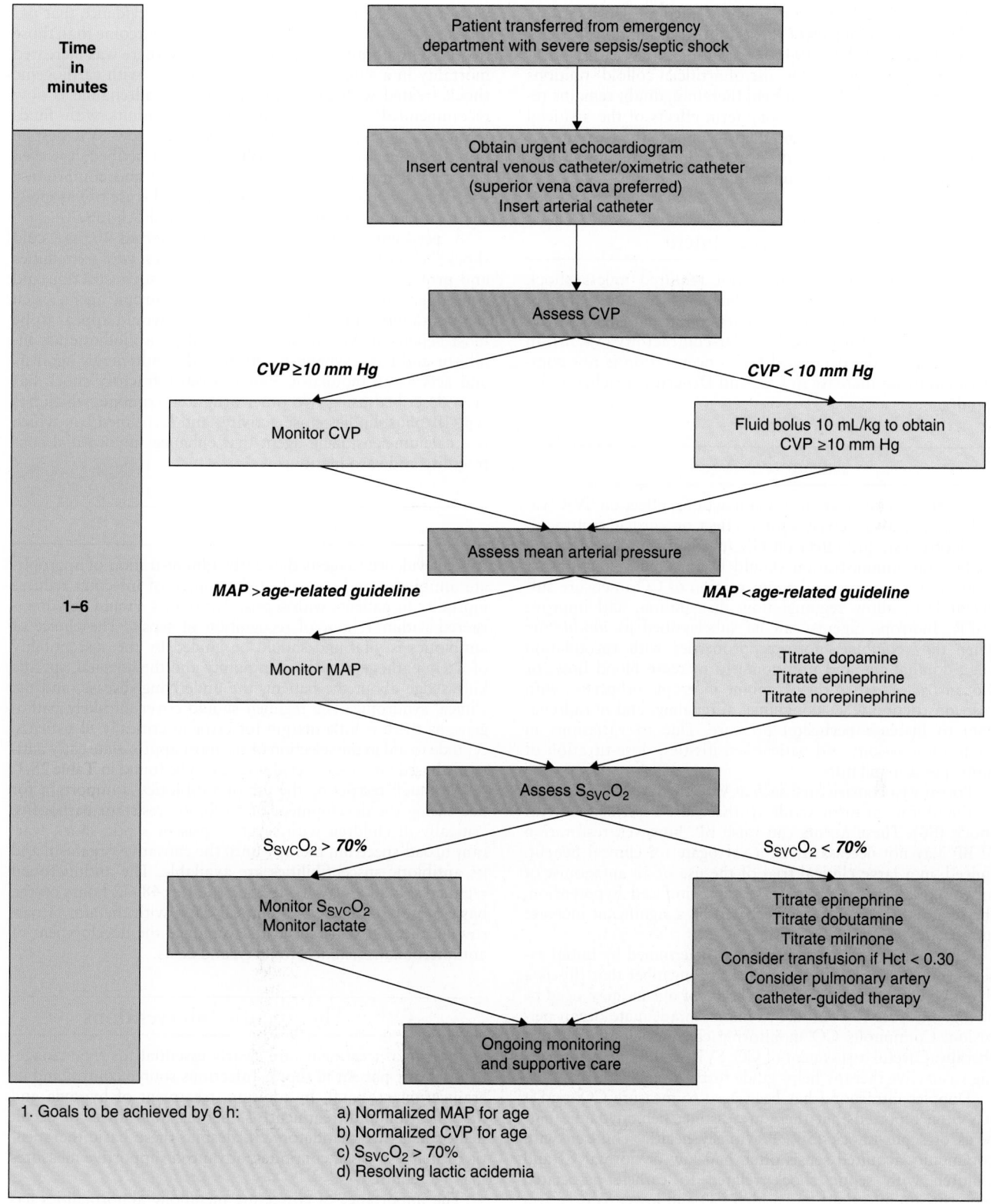

FIGURE 28.3. Suggested PICU sepsis protocol.

increased capillary permeability, patients become hemoconcentrated, a condition not seen in other forms of septic shock. A systematic review in pediatric shock and severe infection also showed insufficient evidence to support the preferred use of colloids or crystalloids in sepsis (64). More recently, however, a meta-analysis examining the role of albumin as a resuscitation fluid for patients with sepsis showed an association between albumin administration and a reduction in mortality (65). This included both adult and pediatric studies. The results of the following randomized trials examining this are awaited: ALBIOS (Albumin Italian Outcome Sepsis Study) (NCT00707122) and PRECISE (Fluid Resuscitation in Early Septic Shock) (NCT00819416). In addition, few large, properly conducted studies of the use of artificial colloid solutions have been performed in children; therefore, doubt remains regarding the short-term and long-term effects of the artificial colloid solutions. There is no data to oppose the current recommendation for the use of normal saline as the initial fluid for shock resuscitation in children (4).

Blood Replacement

Usually, blood replacement is not required unless shock is due to acute hemorrhage or anemia. However, a Hb of >8–10 g/dL is thought to be beneficial in patients with severe sepsis and/or decreased cardiac contractility (54,55). In these patients, the decreased Hb concentration is not compensated by an increase in CO, and Do_2crit is reached more rapidly.

Vasoactive Agents

Vasoactive agents have three main actions: effect on SVR (vasodilators and vasoconstrictors), effect on cardiac contractility (inotropes), and effect on HR (chronotropes). Vasoactive medication administration should be directed at restoration of perfusion pressure and augmentation of CO to ensure sufficient Do_2, allow regional flow distribution, and improve O_2ER. Inotropic agents can be subclassified as *inodilators* when they combine inotropic properties with vasodilation (e.g., dobutamine and milrinone) to increase blood flow, or *inoconstrictors* when they combine inotropic properties with vasoconstriction (e.g., dopamine, adrenaline, and noradrenaline) to increase perfusion pressure. Due to variations in medication actions and patient sensitivities, dose titration of inotropes is mandatory.

Potent vasoconstrictors, such as vasopressin, its derivatives, and inhibitors of nitric oxide synthase, are described to treat shock (66). These agents can raise BP; however, restoration of BP may not necessarily be a surrogate for clinical benefit. Indeed, in a large clinical trial of the use of an antagonist of nitric oxide synthase to reverse sepsis-induced hypotension, the required rise in BP was mirrored by a significant increase in mortality (67).

The choice of vasoactive agent is determined by initial assessment; however, it is important to remember that this is a dynamic condition so that the choice of agents may need to change in order to continue to maintain adequate organ perfusion. Continuous CO monitoring can be helpful to direct therapy. Careful assessment of CO, SVR, and BP after instituting vasoactive therapy helps guide further management.

Doppler ultrasound has been used to measure CO, and it has been reported that there are distinct hemodynamic patterns of septic shock (56). Previously healthy children with community-acquired sepsis often had low or normal CI and children with septic shock related to catheter-associated bloodstream infections had a high CO and lower SVR (warm shock) pattern. Unlike adults, low CO, not low SVR, is associated with mortality in pediatric septic shock; achieving a therapeutic goal of CI 3.3–6.0 L/min/m^2 may result in improved survival (53).

In vasodilated ("warm") shock (bounding pulses, warm extremities, normal CRT), the use of vasoconstrictor agents (e.g., noradrenaline) appears beneficial. Dopamine remains the first-line vasopressor for fluid-refractory hypotensive shock

with low SVR. However, there is emerging evidence that patients treated with dopamine have a worse outcome than those treated with noradrenaline (68). Certainly, there was increased mortality in a subgroup analysis of patients with cardiogenic shock treated with dopamine. Indeed, noradrenaline is now recommended as the first-line agent in adults with fluid-refractory shock. In cases with persistently low SVR despite noradrenaline, use of vasopressin has been described; however, this may significantly elevate the afterload and compromise CO. There is no clear evidence to support the use of vasopressin in children or adults with severe septic shock (69,70).

A predominantly poor CO state referred to as "cold shock," clinically manifested by weak pulses, cool extremities and prolonged CRT, is associated with vasoconstriction and consequent increase in afterload. Using inotropic agents, such as dobutamine, adrenaline, or milrinone, would appear to be most beneficial. Milrinone is a type III phosphodiesterase inhibitor and has a synergistic effect with β-adrenergic agonists and acts as an inodilator. Rescue from refractory shock has been described using two other drugs: enoximone, which has type III phosphodiesterase activity; and levosimendan, which is a calcium-sensitizing agent that enhances myocardial contractility and vasodilation.

Antibiotic Therapy

Ample evidence suggests that early administration of appropriate antibiotics and control of the source of infection reduces mortality in patients with sepsis. Antibiotics should be administered within 1 hour of recognition of sepsis. The choice of antibiotics is vital and should be guided by the susceptibility of likely pathogens in the community and the hospital, specific knowledge about the patient, the underlying disease, and the clinical syndrome. The regimen should cover all likely pathogens, as there is little margin for error in critically ill patients. A guide to aid in the selection of the most appropriate early antibiotic based on the suspected source can be found in **Table 28.1**.

Although restricting the use of antibiotics is important for decreasing the development of antibiotic-resistant pathogens, critically ill children with severe sepsis or septic shock warrant broad-spectrum therapy until the causative organism and its antibiotic susceptibilities are available. The antimicrobial regimen should always be reassessed after 48–72 hours on the basis of microbiologic and clinical data, with the aim of narrowing the antibiotic spectrum to reduce the development of antimicrobial resistance, toxicity, and costs.

Other Therapeutic Interventions

A number of treatments are clearly essential for the management of any patient in shock. Infectious source control and its eradication are vital. In addition, treatment of hypoxia and identification and treatment of ongoing fluid losses or occult hemorrhage are mandatory. If, despite these basic therapeutic principles, shock continues, advanced supportive measures may be required.

The importance of correcting metabolic abnormalities has been emphasized in treatment guidelines for children with meningococcal shock (71). However, clinical studies of the use of bicarbonate therapy to correct shock-induced metabolic acidosis failed to show any improvement in CO or reduction in inotrope requirement, regardless of the degree of acidemia (72).

Replacement low-dose steroid therapy has been shown to be beneficial in patients with septic shock and evidence of adrenal hyporesponsiveness, especially in those with high or

TABLE 28.1

PEDIATRIC ANTIMICROBRIAL TREATMENT GUIDE

	■ NEONATE (<1 mo)	■ INFANT (1–3 mo)	■ PEDIATRIC (>3 mo)

Sepsis Unknown Source	Ampicillin + [gentamicin or cefotaxime]
	    Ampicillin 50 mg/kg/dose IV q6h (q8h if <1 wk old) **plus**
	    Gentamicin 2.5 mg/kg/dose IV q8h (q12h if <1 wk old) and Acyclovir 20 mg/kg/dose IV q8h
	 OR
	    Ampicillin 50 mg/kg/dose IV q6h (q8h if <1 wk old) **plus**
	    Cefotaxime 50 mg/kg/dose IV q8h (q12h if <1 wk old)
		Ampicillin + cefotaxime
		    Ampicillin 50 mg/kg/dose IV q6h **plus**
		    Cefotaxime 50 mg/kg/dose IV q6h
			Cloxacillin + cefotaxime
			    Cloxacillin 50 mg/kg/dose IV q6h (max 2 g/dose) **plus**
			    Cefotaxime 50 mg/kg/dose IV q6h (max 2 g/dose)

CNS Suspected Source			Cefotaxime ± vancomycin
			    Cefotaxime 75 mg/kg/dose IV q6h (max 2 g/dose) **plus**
			    Vancomycin 20 mg/kg IV × 1 dose, then 15 mg/kg/dose IV q6h
			
			 Shunt/EVD
			    Meropenem 40 mg/kg dose IV q8h (max 2 g/dose) **plus**
			    Vancomycin 20 mg/kg IV × 1 dose, then 15 mg/kg/dose IV q6h

Pneumonia Suspected Source		Cloxacillin + cefotaxime
		    Cloxacillin 50 mg/kg/dose IV q6h (max 2 g/dose) **plus**
		    Cefotaxime 50 mg/kg/dose IV q6h (max 2 g/dose)
			Cloxacillin + cefotaxime +/− azithromycin
			    Cloxacillin 50 mg/kg/dose IV q6h (max 2 g/dose) **plus**
			    Cefotaxime 50 mg/kg/dose IV q6h (max 2 g/dose) **plus**
			    Azithromycin 10 mg/kg/dose PO/IV × 1 dose (max 500 mg), then 5 mg/kg/dose PO/IV q24h (max 250 mg/dose) × 5 d

GU Suspected Source	No known anatomic abnormalities or first presentation:
	 Ampicillin + gentamicin
	    Ampicillin 50 mg/kg/dose IV q6h (q8h if <1 wk old) **plus**
	    Gentamicin 2.5 mg/kg/dose IV q8h (q12h if <1 wk old)
		>1 mo old:
		 No known anatomic abnormalities or first presentation:
		 Ampicillin + gentamicin
		    Ampicillin 50 mg/kg/dose IV q6h (max 3 g/dose) **plus**
		    Gentamicin 7 mg/kg/dose IV q24h	

	Known abnormality of GU tract:
	 Piperacillin + gentamicin
	    Piperacillin 75 mg/kg/dose IV q6h (q8h if <1 wk old) **plus**
	    Gentamicin 2.5 mg/kg/dose IV q8h (q12h if <1 wk old)
		Known abnormality of GU tract:
		 Piperacillin/tazobactam + gentamicin
		    Piperacillin/tazobactam 75 mg/kg/dose piperacillin component IV q6h (max 4 g/dose) **plus**
		    Gentamicin 7 mg/kg/dose IV q24h	

Skin/Soft Tissue Suspected Source	Clindamycin + penicillin + gentamicin
	 OR
	 Clindamycin + cefotaxime
	    Clindamycin 5 mg/kg/dose IV q6h (q8h if <1 wk old) **plus**
	    Penicillin 50,000 units/kg/dose IV q6h (q8h if <1wk old) **plus**
	    Gentamicin 2.5 mg/kg/dose IV q8h (q12h if <1wk old)
	 OR
	    Clindamycin 5 mg/kg/dose IV q6h (q8h if <1wk old) **plus**
	    Cefotaxime 50 mg/kg/dose IV q8h (q12h if <1 wk old)
		>1 mo old:
		 Clindamycin + penicillin + gentamicin
		 OR
		 Clindamycin + cefotaxime
		    Clindamycin 13 mg/kg/dose IV q8h (max 900 mg/dose) **plus**
		    Penicillin 65,000 units/kg/dose IV q4h (max 4 million units/dose) **plus**
		    Gentamicin 7 mg/kg/dose IV q24h
		 OR
		    Clindamycin 13 mg/kg/dose IV q8h (max 900 mg/dose) **plus**
		    Cefotaxime 50 mg/kg/dose IV q6h (max 2 g/dose)
		
		 if Group A Strep suspected
		 Add IV immunoglobulin (IVIG) 1 g/kg/dose IV q24h × 2 doses
		 Ordered from blood bank	

Immunocompromised/Febrile Neutropenic Patient		>1 mo old:
		 Piperacillin/tazobactam + gentamicin
		    Piperacillin/tazobactam 75 mg/kg/dose piperacillin component IV q6h (max 4 g/dose) **plus**
		    Gentamicin 7 mg/kg/dose IV q24h	

increasing requirements for inotropes (73). This benefit has not yet been demonstrated in pediatric patients. However, similar adrenal hyporesponsiveness has been shown in children (74), and stress doses of steroids are now commonly used in children with fluid-refractory, catecholamine-resistant shock.

CONCLUSIONS AND FUTURE DIRECTIONS

Shock is a clinical diagnosis. The mainstay of therapy is to recognize the seriously ill child before shock progresses to irreversibility. Once shock is present, attempts must be made to prevent its progression. Without a specific marker to determine the irreversible point in shock, heroic efforts to reverse shock, such as the use of extracorporeal devices for cardiac support, may be reasonable. However, regardless of the initial type of shock, by the time shock advances to gross abnormalities in volume status, vascular tone, cardiac function, cellular energetics, and multiorgan function, it is very likely that purely mechanical devices will not correct all of these existent abnormalities (75). Further definition of specific goal-directed therapies, with evidence-based targets for prevention or nonprogression of shock, is on the horizon.

References

1. Carcillo JA, Fields AI; American College of Critical Care Medicine Task Force Committee Members. Clinical practice parameters for hemodynamic support of pediatric and neonatal patients in septic shock. *Crit Care Med* 2002;30:1365–78.
2. Vallet B, Tavernier B, Lund N. Assessment of tissue oxygenation in the critically ill. *Eur J Anaesthesiol* 2000;17:221–9.
3. Steiner MJ, DeWalt DA, Byerley JS. Is this child dehydrated? *JAMA* 2004;291:2746–54.
4. Boluyt N, Bollen CW, Bos AP, et al. Fluid resuscitation in neonatal and pediatric hypovolemic shock: A Dutch Pediatric Society evidence-based clinical practice guideline. *Intensive Care Med* 2006;32(7):995–1003.
5. Zaritsky AL, Nadkarni VM, Hickey RW, et al., eds. *Pediatric Advanced Life Support Provider Manual.* Dallas, TX: American Heart Association, 2002.
6. Lima AP, Beelen P, Bakker J. Use of a peripheral perfusion index derived from the pulse oximetry signal as a noninvasive indicator of perfusion. *Crit Care Med* 2002;30:1210–3.
7. Kaplan LJ, McPartland K, Santora TA, et al. Start with a subjective assessment of skin temperature to identify hypoperfusion in intensive care unit patients. *J Trauma* 2001;50:620–7.
8. McGee S, Abernethy WB III, Simel DL. Is this patient hypovolemic? *JAMA* 1999;281:1022–9.
9. Schriger DL, Baraff L. Defining normal capillary refill: Variation with age, sex, and temperature. *Ann Emerg Med* 1988;17:932–5.
10. Tibby SM, Hatherill M, Murdoch IA. Capillary refill and core-peripheral temperature gap as indicators of haemodynamic status in paediatric intensive care patients. *Arch Dis Child* 1999;80:163–6.
11. Rivers E, Nguyen B, Havstad S, et al. Early goal-directed therapy in the treatment of severe sepsis and septic shock. *N Engl J Med* 2001;345:1368–77.
12. Reinhart K, Kuhn HJ, Hartog C, et al. Continuous central venous and pulmonary artery oxygen saturation monitoring in the crtitically ill. *Intensive Care Med* 2004;30:1572–8.
13. Guyton AC. Body temperature, temperature regulation, and fever. In: Guyton AC, Hall JE, eds. *Textbook of Medical Physiology.* Philadelphia, PA: Saunders, 1996:911–22.
14. Hatherill M, Waggie Z, Purves L, et al. Mortality and the nature of metabolic acidosis in children with shock. *Intensive Care Med* 2003;29:286–91.
15. Husain FA, Martin MJ, Mullenix PS, et al. Serum lactate and base deficit as predictors of mortality and morbidity. *Am J Surg* 2003;185:485–91.
16. LeDoux D, Astiz ME, Carpati CM, et al. Effects of perfusion pressure on tissue perfusion in septic shock. *Crit Care Med* 2000;28:2729–32.
17. Hamzaoui O, Monnet X, Richard C, et al. Effects of changes in vascular tone on the agreement between pulse contour and transpulmonary thermodilution cardiac output measurements within an up to 6 hour calibration-free period. *Crit Care Med* 2008;36:434–40.
18. Pulmonary artery catheter consensus conference. *Crit Care Med* 1997;25:910–25.
19. Critchley LA, Lee A, Ho AMH. A critical review of the ability of continuous cardiac output monitors to measure trends in cardiac output. *Anesth Analg* 2010;111:1180–92.
20. Cannesson M, Besnard C, Durand PG, et al. Relation between respiratory variations in pulse oximetry plethysmographic waveform amplititude and arterial pulse pressure in ventilated patients. *Crit Care* 2005;9:R562–8.
21. Natalini G, Rosano A, Franceschetti ME, et al. Variation in arterial blood pressure and photoplethysmography during mechanical ventilation. *Anesth Analg* 2006;103:1182–8.
22. De Backer D, Henenan S, Oiagnarelli M, et al. Pulse pressure variations to predict fluid responsiveness: Influence of tidal volume. *Intensive Care Med* 2005;31:517–23.
23. Natalini G, Rosano A, Taranto M, et al. Arterial versus plethysmographic dynamic indices to test responsiveness for testing fluid administration in hypotensive patients. *Anesth Analg* 2006;103:1478–84.
24. Curley FJ, Smyrnios NA. Routine monitoring of critically ill patients. In: Irwin RS, Cerra FB, Rippe JM, eds. *Intensive Care Medicine.* New York, NY: Lippincott Williams & Wilkins, 2003:250–70.
25. Henning RJ, Wiener F, Valdes S, et al. Measurement of toe temperature for assessing the severity of acute circulatory failure. *Surg Gynecol Obstet* 1979;149:1–7.
26. Lima A, Bakker J. Noninvasive monitoring of peripheral perfusion. *Intensive Care Med* 2005;31:1316–26.
27. Cairns CB, Moore FA, Haenel JB, et al. Evidence for early supply independent mitochondrial dysfunction in patients developing multiple organ failure after trauma. *J Trauma* 1997;42:532–6.
28. McKinley BA, Marvin RG, Cocanour CS, et al. Tissue hemoglobin O_2 saturation during resuscitation of traumatic shock monitored using near infrared spectrometry. *J Trauma* 2000;48:637–42.
29. Girardis M, Rinaldi L, Busani S, et al. Muscle perfusion and oxygen consumption by near-infrared spectroscopy in septic shock and non-septic-shock patients. *Intensive Care Med* 2003;29:1173–6.
30. De Backer D, Creteur J, Dubois MJ, et al. The effects of dobutamine on microcirculatory alterations in patients with septic shock are independent of its systemic effects. *Crit Care Med* 2006;34:403–8.
31. Spronk PE, Ince C, Gardien MJ, et al. Nitroglycerin in septic shock after intravascular volume resuscitation. *Lancet* 2002;360:1395–6.
32. De Backer D, Creteur J. Regional hypoxia and partial pressure of carbon dioxide gradients: What is the link? *Intensive Care Med* 2003;29:2116–8.
33. De Backer D, Creteur J, Dubois MJ, et al. Microvascular alterations in patients with acute severe heart failure and cardiogenic shock. *Am Heart J* 2004;147:91–9.
34. Jin X, Weil MH, Sun S, et al. Decreases in organ blood flows associated with increases in sublingual PCO_2 during hemorrhagic shock. *J Appl Physiol* 1998;85:2360–4.
35. Tremper KK, Shoemaker WC. Transcutaneous oxygen monitoring of critically ill adults, with and without low flow shock. *Crit Care Med* 1981;9:706–9.
36. Waxman K, Sadler R, Eisner ME, et al. Transcutaneous oxygen monitoring of emergency department patients. *Am J Surg* 1983;146:35–8.

37. Tatevossian RG, Wo CC, Velmahos GC, et al. Transcutaneous oxygen and CO_2 as early warning of tissue hypoxia and hemodynamic shock in critically ill emergency patients. *Crit Care Med* 2000;28:2248–53.

38. Fiddian-Green RG, Baker S. Predictive value of the stomach wall pH for complications after cardiac operations: Comparison with other monitoring. *Crit Care Med* 1987;15:153–6.

39. De Backer D, Creteur J, Preiser JC, et al. Microvascular blood flow is altered in patients with sepsis. *Am J Respir Crit Care Med* 2002;166:98–104.

40. Povoas HP, Weil MH, Tang W, et al. Comparisons between sublingual and gastric tonometry during hemorrhagic shock. *Chest* 2000;118:1127–32.

41. Weil MH, Nakagawa Y, Tang W, et al. Sublingual capnometry: A new noninvasive measurement for diagnosis and quantitation of severity of circulatory shock. *Crit Care Med* 1999;27:1225–9.

42. Marik PE, Bankov A. Sublingual capnometry versus traditional markers of tissue oxygenation in critically ill patients. *Crit Care Med* 2003;31:818–22.

43. Tibby SM, Hatherill M, Marsh MJ. Clinicians' abilities to estimate cardiac index in ventilated children and infants. *Arch Dis Child* 1997;77:516–8.

44. Cooper ES, Muir WW. Continuous cardiac output monitoring via arterial pressure waveform analysis following severe haemorrhagic shock in dogs. *Crit Care Med* 2007;35:1724–9.

45. Michard M. Pulse contour analysis: Fairy tale or new reality? *Crit Care Med* 2007;35(7):1791–2.

46. Marik PE, Cavallazi R, Vasu T, et al. Dynamic changes in arterial waveform derived variables and fluid responsiveness in mechanically ventilated patients: A systematic review of the literature. *Crit Care Med* 2009;37:2642–7.

47. Choi DY, Kwak HJ, Park HY, et al. Respiratory variation in aortic blood flow velocity as a predictor of fluid responsiveness in children after repair of ventricular septal defect. *Pediatr Cardiol* 2010;31(8):1166–70.

48. Durand P, Chevret L, Essouri S, et al. Respiratory variations in aortic blood flow predict fluid responsiveness in ventilated children. *Intensive Care Med* 2008;34(5):888–94.

49. Patel N, Dodsworth M, Mills JF. Cardiac output measurement in newborn infants using the ultrasonic cardiac output monitor: An assessment of agreement with conventional echocardiography, repeatability and new user experience. *Arch Dis Child Fetal Neonatal Ed* 2011;96:F206–11.

50. Michard F, Boussat S, Chemla D, et al. Relation between respiratory changes in arterial pulse pressure and fluid responsiveness in septic patients with acute circulatory failure. *Am J Respir Crit Care Med* 2000;162:134–8.

51. Han YY, Carcillo JA, Dragotta MA, et al. Early reversal of pediatric-neonatal septic shock by community physicians is associated with improved outcome. *Pediatrics* 2003;112:793–9.

52. Inwald DP, Tasker RC, Peters MJ, et al. Emergency management of children severe sepsis in the United Kingdom: The results of the Paediatric Intensive Care Society Sepsis Audit. *Arch Dis Child* 2009;94:348–53.

53. Brierley, J, Carcillo JA, Choong K, et al; American College of Critical Care Medicine Task Force Committee Members. Clinical practice variables for hemodynamic support of pediatric and neonatal patients in septic shock. *Crit Care Med* 2009;37:666–88.

54. Dellinger RP, Carlet JM, Masur H, et al. Surviving Sepsis Campaign guidelines for management of severe sepsis and septic shock. *Crit Care Med* 2004;32:858–73.

55. Dellinger RP, Levy MM, Carlet JM, et al. Surviving Sepsis Campaign: International guidelines for management of severe sepsis and septic shock: 2008. *Crit Care Med* 2008;36:296–327.

56. Brierley J, Peters M. Distinct hemodynamic patterns of septic shock at presentation to pediatric intensive care. *Pediatrics* 2008;122:752–9.

57. Maitland K, Kiguli S, Opoka RO, et al. Mortality after fluid bolus in African children with severe infection. *N Eng J Med* 2011;364:2483–96.

58. Boyd JH, Forbes J, Nakada TA, et al. Fluid Resuscitation in septic shock: A positive fluid balance and elevated central venous pressure is associated with increased mortality. *Crit Care Med* 2011;39:259–65.

59. Alderson P, Bunn F, Lefebvre C, et al. Human albumin solution for resuscitation and volume expansion in critically ill patients. *Cochrane Database Syst Rev* 2004;4:CD001208.

60. Vincent JL, Navickis RJ, Wilkes MM. Morbidity in hospitalized patients receiving human albumin: A meta-analysis of randomized, controlled trials. *Crit Care Med* 2004;32:2029–38.

61. Finfer S, Bellomo R, Boyce N, et al. A comparison of albumin and saline for fluid resuscitation in the intensive care unit. *N Engl J Med* 2004;350:2247–56.

62. Perner A, Haase N, Guttormsen AB, et al. Hydroxyethyl starch 130/0.42 versus Ringer's acetate in severe sepsis. *N Eng J Med* 2012;367:124–34.

63. Wills BA, Nguyen MD, Ha TL, et al. Comparison of three fluid solutions for resuscitation in dengue shock syndrome. *N Engl J Med* 2005;353:877–89.

64. Akech S, Ledermann H, Maitland K. Choice of fluids for resuscitation in children with severe infection and shock: A systematic review. *BMJ* 2010;341:c4416.

65. Delaney AP, Dan A, McCaffrey J, et al. The role of albumin as a resuscitation fluid for patients with sepsis: A systematic review and meta-analysis. *Crit Care Med* 2011;39:386–91.

66. Matok I, Vard A, Efrati O, et al. Terlipressin as rescue therapy for intractable hypotension due to septic shock in children. *Shock* 2005;23:305–10.

67. Lopez A, Lorente JA, Steingrub J, et al. Multiple-center, randomized, placebo-controlled, double-blind study of the nitric oxide synthase inhibitor 546C88: Effect on survival in patients with septic shock. *Crit Care Med* 2004;32:21–30.

68. De Backer D, Biston P, Devriendt J, et al. Comparison of dopamine and norepinephrine in the treatment of shock. *N Engl J Med* 2010;362:779–89.

69. Choong K, Bohn D, Ward RE, et al. Vasopressin in pediatric vasodilatory shock: A multicenter randomized controlled trial. *Am J Respir Crit Care Med* 2009;180:632–9.

70. Russell JA, Walley KR, Ayers D, et al. Vasopressin versus norepinephrine infusion in patients with septic shock. *N Engl J Med* 2008;358:877–87.

71. Pollard AJ, Britto J, Nadel S, et al. Emergency management of meningococcal disease. *Arch Dis Child* 1999;80:290–6.

72. Forsythe SM, Schmidt GA. Sodium bicarbonate for the treatment of lactic acidosis. *Chest* 2000;117:260–7.

73. Annane D, Sebille V, Charpentier C, et al. Effect of treatment with low doses of hydrocortisone and fludrocortisone on mortality in patients with septic shock. *JAMA* 2002;288:862–71.

74. Pizarro CF, Troster EJ, Damiani D, et al. Absolute and relative adrenal insufficiency in children with septic shock. *Crit Care Med* 2005;33:855–9.

75. Werns SW. Percutaneous extracorporeal life support: Reserve for patients with reversible causes of shock and cardiac arrest. *Crit Care Med* 2003;31:978–80.

CHAPTER 29 ■ RAPID RESPONSE SYSTEMS

CHRISTOPHER P. BONAFIDE, RICHARD J. BRILLI, JAMES TIBBALLS, CHRISTOPHER S. PARSHURAM, PATRICK W. BRADY, AND DEREK WHEELER

KEY POINTS

1 Rapid response systems (RRSs) aim to identify hospitalized general ward children who exhibit early signs of clinical deterioration and to intervene before respiratory or cardiac arrest occurs.

2 RRSs operate on the assumptions that early, reversible clinical deterioration can be identified and that assistance from a team of critical care experts can improve patients' outcomes.

3 RRSs include two clinical components (afferent and efferent limbs) and two organizational components (process improvement and administrative limbs).

4 The role of the afferent limb of RRSs is to identify patients at risk of deterioration and trigger an appropriate response based on the level of risk.

5 The role of the efferent limb of RRSs is to deploy specialized teams of skilled personnel to hospital wards to address urgent care needs.

6 The effectiveness of medical emergency teams in reducing hospital arrest rates and mortality is controversial; no cluster-randomized trial shows benefit, but several pediatric before-and-after studies show improvements in outcomes.

7 The role of the process improvement limb of RRSs is to assess the overall success, assess opportunities to optimize the system, and design tailored improvement interventions.

8 The role of the administrative limb of RRSs is to manage each of the RRS components, focus on implementing the system, and support its ongoing operation.

The rate of urgent requests to the pediatric critical care team to provide expert advice and management for patients on the wards exhibiting early signs of clinical deterioration continues to increase. The systems that focus on the prediction, detection, and management of clinical deterioration in non–intensive care areas are known as rapid response systems (RRSs) (1). The hallmark of RRSs is their focus on identifying and mitigating reversible early signs of clinical deterioration in ward

1 settings to prevent respiratory and cardiac arrest. They operate on the assumptions that, in at least a subset of patients, (a) early, reversible clinical deterioration can be identified using tools that facilitate detection and standardize escalation of care on the wards, and (b) consulting a multidisciplinary team of critical care experts with the capability to rapidly intervene

2 at the bedside can improve patients' outcomes. The organizational structure of RRSs includes two clinical components (afferent and efferent limbs) and two organizational components

3 (process improvement and administrative limbs).

The objectives of this chapter are (a) to provide the pediatric intensivist with an overview of RRSs and their components, (b) to review early warning scores (EWSs) and the *calling criteria* that comprise the afferent limb, (c) to summarize the response mechanisms that comprise the efferent limb, (d) to provide a set of process improvement measures that can be used to evaluate RRS effectiveness, and (e) to discuss the administrative issues associated with implementing and managing an RRS.

ORIGINS, DISSEMINATION, AND PREVALENCE OF PEDIATRIC RAPID RESPONSE SYSTEMS

Origins

Over the past two decades, RRSs that are focused on identifying and managing pre-arrest status have been implemented in thousands of hospitals throughout the world. The medical emergency team (MET) concept was first reported in an adult hospital in Australia in 1995 (2). The team was developed to rapidly detect and correct vital sign abnormalities that represent early disturbances in cardiorespiratory function that precede arrest in patients with severe trauma. Team members included medical and nursing staff with training in resuscitation. The team could be activated when urgent help was required or when calling criteria based on specified vital sign parameters or conditions were attained (2). Definitions for MET, rapid response team, and critical care outreach team are provided in the section on The Efferent Limb.

Ten years later, Tibballs, Kinney, and colleagues reported the first pediatric RRS implementation at Royal Children's Hospital in Australia (3). The team was composed of physicians and nurses from the ICU and emergency department, as well as a medical registrar (analogous to a physician fellow in the US system). Like the adult system, the team could be activated at any time by a concerned nurse or physician or when calling criteria were attained. An important innovation from this pediatric implementation was the inclusion criteria based on age-specific parameters for heart rate, blood pressure, and respiratory rate.

Dissemination

In the years that followed, hospitals around the world began describing their results after implementing RRSs, and patient safety organizations took notice. In 2005, the Institute for Healthcare Improvement launched the 100,000 Lives Campaign, a nationwide initiative to reduce morbidity and mortality in the American healthcare system (4). The campaign expanded in 2006 as the 5 Million Lives Campaign and included over 4000 participating hospitals (5). One of the key components of these campaigns was the implementation of RRSs as a means of rapidly responding to early signs of patient deterioration.

In 2008, the Joint Commission, an organization that accredits and certifies more than 19,000 healthcare organizations and programs in the United States, set a National Patient Safety Goal requiring that hospitals seeking accreditation "empower staff, patients, and/or families to request additional assistance when they have a concern about the patient's condition" (6). While compliance with this safety goal did not require implementation of a formal RRS, the issuance of this goal likely contributed to further uptake of RRSs.

Organizational bodies outside the United States (in Canada, the United Kingdom, and Australia) supported RRS implementation to varying degrees and with differing models (7–9).

Prevalence

Estimates of the prevalence of pediatric RRSs began to emerge in the mid-2000s. A 2005 survey of 181 children's hospitals in the United States and Canada showed that 100% had an immediate-response code blue team that responded for cardiopulmonary arrest, and that 17% had an MET that responded to children clinically deteriorating but not at risk of imminent cardiopulmonary arrest. In 21% of the hospitals with METs, discrete calling criteria were used to determine when to activate the team (10). A 2010 survey to estimate the prevalence and characteristics of pediatric RRSs among 130 US children's hospitals with PICUs found that 79% had an MET that "quickly responds to patients on the general wards at early stages of instability" (11). They also found that 34% used automatic triggers, defined as predetermined changes in the patient's vital signs or overall clinical status, to activate the MET.

THE AFFERENT LIMB

The role of the afferent limb of RRSs is to identify, or track, patients at risk of deterioration and trigger an appropriate response based on the level of risk. In a consensus statement on the afferent limb of RRSs, systems for prediction of deterioration were distinguished from systems for detection of deterioration (12). Predictive tools focus on "traits" (such as a diagnosis of epilepsy) rather than "states" (such as a heart rate of 200) and do not require continuous data collection. Detective tools, in contrast, focus on identifying states consistent with critical illness by recognizing signs of deterioration using highly time-varying data like vital signs. Detective systems require frequent intermittent measurements or continuous data collection to provide early identification of departures from clinical stability and prevent progressive deterioration.

Predicting Deterioration

In comparison to detective tools, little work has been performed in the area of developing tools to predict clinical deterioration in hospitalized children using patient characteristics. The first detailed case series of hospitalized children provided with urgent assistance from an MET described the clinical characteristics of the patients: 44% had surgery during the hospital admission, 36% had an ICU admission, and 20% had a diagnosis of chronic encephalopathy (13). Additional chronic conditions that occurred frequently included congenital syndromes, chronic lung disease, and abnormal upper airways. This case series provided a snapshot of the populations at risk of deterioration; however, estimates of association between these conditions and pediatric deterioration could not be determined.

More recently, a predictive model for clinical deterioration using non–vital sign patient characteristics was developed using a case-control design (14). The predictive model resulted in a 7-item weighted score that included age under 1 year, epilepsy, congenital/genetic conditions, history of transplant, presence of an enteral tube, hemoglobin less than 10 g/dL, and blood culture drawn in the preceding 72 hours. Patients were grouped into risk strata based on their scores. The very low-risk group's probability of deterioration was less than half of baseline risk. The high-risk group's probability of deterioration was more than 80-fold higher than the baseline risk. Predictive tools like this have the potential to assist in identifying and triaging a subset of high-risk children who should be intensively monitored for early signs of deterioration at the time of admission. The converse may also be helpful; the predictive tool may help identify very low-risk children who, in the absence of other clinical concerns, can be monitored less intensively.

Detecting Deterioration

Single-Parameter Calling Criteria

The simplest and most widely used form of a detective tool is a set of single-parameter calling criteria. They are easy for bedside clinicians to use; if any one of the criteria is met, the efferent limb should be activated. While the parameters are commonly objective clinical findings such as vital signs, they can also include diagnoses (such as suspected shock), events (such as seizures), subjective observations (such as increased work of breathing), and intuitive concerns (such as worried about the patient). Parameters for heart rate, respiratory rate, and blood pressure are usually presented within distinct groups to account for variability by age. The differences in parameter cut points across studies reflect that evidence supporting age-based vital sign parameters is very limited. A list of single-parameter calling criteria is given in **Table 29.1**.

Multiparameter Early Warning Scores

Multiparameter tools combine several of the core components of single-parameter calling criteria into EWSs. The first EWS was developed to detect deterioration among hospitalized adults in 1997 (15). These scores trade increased complexity for potentially better accuracy in identifying deterioration. The scores may be either weighted or unweighted; weighted scores allocate a variable number of points based on the degree to which patients' vital signs deviate from a (usually arbitrarily developed) "normal" or "expected" range. The scores are periodically calculated either by hand or within the electronic health record, and the sum total score is used to trigger the efferent limb.

TABLE 29.1

PRE-ARREST SINGLE-PARAMETER CALLING CRITERIA USED IN RECENT MET STUDIES

	BRILLI ET AL. (51)	HANSON ET AL. (48)	HUNT ET AL. (52)	KOTSAKIS ET AL. (7)	SHAREK ET AL. (47)	TIBBALLS ET AL. (50)	ZENKER ET AL. (49)
Heart rate		•		•	•	•	•
Respiratory rate		•		•	•	•	•
Blood pressure		•		•	•	•	•
Oxygen saturation	•	•	•	•	•	•	•
Respiratory distress	•	•	•	•			•
Airway threat		•		•		•	
Circulatory compromise/shock				•			•
Cardiac dysrhythmias				•			
Mental/neurologic status	•	•	•	•	•	•	•
Seizures		•	•			•	
Staff concern	•	•	•	•	•	•	•
Family concern	•	•	•			•	•

An ideal score would balance high sensitivity (minimizing the number of children who deteriorate without being identified by the score) with high specificity (minimizing the number of children who trigger the MET but are not deteriorating, unnecessarily consuming pediatric intensive care resources). The achievement of high sensitivity and specificity when identifying a broadly defined condition such as clinical deterioration is challenging.

Two scores: The Paediatric Early Warning Score (PEWS) developed in England and the Bedside Paediatric Early Warning System Score (Bedside PEWS) developed in Canada are the most rigorously evaluated.

Pediatric Early Warning Score. The PEWS, first described in 2005, was developed using concepts from adult systems and is composed of three components: behavior, cardiovascular, and respiratory (**Table 29.2**) (16). The total PEWS corresponded with a color, which was then used to indicate a suggested staff response, including, at the highest scores, calling the critical care outreach team.

Being the first EWS for children, the PEWS was widely disseminated and evaluated. In a 1-year study in which the PEWS was part of clinical care and evaluated in an observational design, the score performed well in an analysis that used transfer to the ICU as the outcome and the highest score a patient had during hospitalization as the exposure (17). At a score of 7 or higher (their recommended "automatic" MET activation cut point), the sensitivity was 33%, specificity 99%, positive predictive value 49%, and negative predictive value 99%. However, use of transfer alone as an outcome in a study in which the score was calculated as part of clinical care and as such may have directly influenced decision making about transfer introduces substantial limitations, as does using the highest score occurring during a hospitalization without regard to the timing of that score in relationship to the transfer.

In a subsequent case series of patients, who required assistance from an MET or code blue team, the PEWS was applied retrospectively to the 24 hours preceding the event (18). Using a lower score cut point of 4, the researchers found that the score had a sensitivity of 86%. They did not report the specificity or any other test characteristics. In summary, PEWS has undergone some formal evaluation, but its test characteristics

TABLE 29.2

THE PEWS TOOL

	Component Subscore			
COMPONENT	**0**	**1**	**2**	**3**
Behavior	Playing/appropriate	Sleeping	Irritable	Lethargic/confused. Reduced response to pain
Cardiovascular	Pink or capillary refill 1–2 s	Pale or capillary refill 3 s	Gray or capillary refill 4 s. Tachycardia of 20 above normal rate	Gray and mottled or capillary refill $\geq$ 5 s. Tachycardia of 30 above normal rate or bradycardia
Respiratory	Within normal parameters, no recession or tracheal tug	>10 above normal parameters, using accessory muscles $F_{IO_2} \geq 30\%$ or 4 L/min	>20 above normal parameters, recessing, tracheal tug $F_{IO_2} \geq 40\%$ or 6 L/min	5 below parameters with sternal recession, tracheal tug, or grunting $F_{IO_2} \geq 50\%$ or 8 L/min

Score 2 extra points for ¼ hourly nebulizers or persistent vomiting following surgery.
The total score is calculated as the sum of the subscores from each of the three components.
Adapted from Monaghan A. Detecting and managing deterioration in children. *Paediatr Nurs* 2005;17(1):32–5.

to predict a meaningful clinical deterioration outcome are still not clear. Nevertheless, the score is widely used on pediatric wards.

Bedside PEWS. The Bedside PEWS was first described by Duncan, Hutchison, and Parshuram in 2006 and has been iteratively refined in subsequent studies (19–21). The initial score was developed using expert opinion and consensus methods, and refined using statistical methods. The 7-item score includes heart rate, systolic blood pressure, capillary refill time, respiratory rate, respiratory effort, oxygen therapy, and oxygen saturation (**Table 29.3**). Bedside PEWS has performed well in multiple retrospective evaluations, including, most recently, a multicenter validation study (21). That study used an outcome of a clinical deterioration event resulting in either an immediate call to the resuscitation team or an urgent ICU admission and an exposure of the maximum Bedside PEWS for the 12 hours ending 1 hour before the deterioration event. Among case patients, the Bedside PEWS significantly increased over the 24 hours leading to the event. At a score of 7 or higher, the sensitivity was 64% and the specificity was 91%. Positive and negative predictive values were appropriately not reported since this was a case-control design, but the positive predictive value was estimated at 9%, assuming a baseline clinical deterioration rate of 10 per 1000 patient-days.

Most importantly, the Bedside PEWS is currently being evaluated in the Evaluating Processes of Care & the Outcomes of Children in Hospital (EPOCH) study. EPOCH is a prospective, cluster-randomized trial that will determine the effect of its implementation on mortality, cardiac arrest rates, and processes of care among children hospitalized outside ICUs (22).

Other Pediatric Early Warning Score Systems. Other scoring systems similar to PEWS and Bedside PEWS have been developed, including the Cardiff and Vale Paediatric Early Warning System (23) and the Bristol Paediatric Early Warning Tool (24). Since neither of these has been prospectively validated, they may be less well-suited for clinical implementation than the two scores described earlier.

Family Concern as an Afferent Trigger

In 2001, an 18-month-old girl named Josie King died on an inpatient ward at Johns Hopkins Children's Center. The death was highly publicized and was attributed in part to critical delays in escalation of Josie's care despite her family's persistently verbalized concern (25). As a result, Children's Hospital of Pittsburgh launched a program called Condition HELP, a program that enables families who detect concerning changes in their children's conditions to directly activate a multidisciplinary immediate-response team to the patient's bedside. Other hospitals have followed suit, implementing family activation in both pediatric (26–28) and adult (29–33) hospital settings. A recent survey of US hospitals revealed that 79% have an MET, of which 69% have mechanisms for families to activate the team (11).

Data are scant regarding the effectiveness and unintended consequences of including family concern as an afferent trigger for METs. Existing reports suggest that families infrequently activate these systems and that, when activated, the calls for assistance rarely represent urgent critical care needs. When calls occur, they are most often requests to address communication and coordination issues between patients and providers (26,29,32,33) and perceived delays in care (30). In 6.25 hospital-years described across seven published reports that provided call outcomes, 6 of 117 (5%) family activations

TABLE 29.3

THE BEDSIDE PEWS TOOL

		Item Subscore			
■ ITEM	■ AGE GROUP	■ 0	■ 1	■ 2	■ 4
Heart rate	0 to <3 mo	>110 and <150	≥150 or ≤110	≥180 or ≤90	≥190 or ≤80
	3 to <12 mo	>100 and <150	≥150 or ≤100	≥170 or ≤80	≥180 or ≤70
	1 to <4 y	>90 and <120	≥120 or ≤90	≥150 or ≤70	≥170 or ≤60
	4 to 12 y	>70 and <110	≥110 or ≤70	≥130 or ≤60	≥150 or ≤50
	>12 y	>60 and <100	≥100 or ≤60	≥120 or ≤50	≥140 or ≤40
Systolic blood pressure	0 to <3 mo	>60 and <80	≥80 or ≤60	≥100 or ≤50	≥130 or ≤45
	3 to <12 mo	>80 and <100	≥100 or ≤80	≥120 or ≤70	≥150 or ≤60
	1 to <4 y	>90 and <110	≥110 or ≤90	≥125 or ≤75	≥160 or ≤65
	4 to 12 y	>90 and <120	≥120 or ≤90	≥140 or ≤80	≥170 or ≤70
	>12 y	>100 and <130	≥130 or ≤100	≥150 or ≤85	≥190 or ≤75
Capillary refill time		<3 s			≥3 s
Respiratory rate	0 to <3 mo	>29 and <61	≥61 or ≤29	≥81 or ≤19	≥91 or ≤15
	3 to <12 mo	>24 or <51	≥51 or ≤24	≥71 or ≤19	≥81 or ≤15
	1 to <4 y	>19 or <41	≥41 or ≤19	≥61 or ≤15	≥71 or ≤12
	4 to 12 y	>19 or <31	≥31 or ≤19	≥41 or ≤14	≥51 or ≤10
	>12 y	>11 or <17	≥17 or ≤11	≥23 or ≤10	≥30 or ≤9
Respiratory effort		Normal	Mild increase	Moderate increase	Severe increase/ any apnea
Saturation (%)		>94	91–94	≤90	
Oxygen therapy		Room air		Any to <4 L/min or <50%	≥4 L/min or ≥50%

The total score is calculated as the sum of the subscores from each of the items.
Reprinted from Parshuram CS, Duncan HP, Joffe AR, et al. Multi-centre validation of the Bedside Paediatric Early Warning System score: A severity of illness score to detect evolving critical illness in hospitalized children. *Crit Care* 2011;15(4):R184, an open access article distributed under the terms of the Creative Commons Attribution License (http://creativecommons.org/licenses/by/2.0), which permits unrestricted use, distribution, and reproduction in any medium, provided the original work is properly cited.

required critical interventions and/or transfer to a higher level of care (26–30,32,33). Enabling families to directly activate a team may not represent the optimal method for families to participate in monitoring their children. There may be complex unintended consequences from the use of family concern as an afferent trigger; these include the misuse of the MET, expectations placed on parents to make assessments without clinical training, undermining of therapeutic relationships, and burden placed on families (34). It is interesting that in one adult study, the implementation of family activation resulted in very few family activations, but increased staff activations of the MET by fourfold (31). Future research in this area should focus on the development of methods to optimize shared decision making between families and clinicians to capitalize on the strengths of families in recognizing changes from their children's baseline and the expertise of clinicians in identifying the need for intensive care.

Technologic Advancements

Intermittently Assessed Deterioration Surveillance

EWSs have been integrated into the electronic health records of major children's hospitals, including The Children's Hospital of Philadelphia, Children's Hospital Boston, and Cincinnati Children's Hospital Medical Center (35). These tools leverage the benefits of discrete vital sign data and subjective observations manually entered into electronic flow sheets with the ability to perform calculations and provide immediate clinical decision support to frontline staff. This includes sending alerts when scores exceed a predetermined threshold to warn clinicians of possible signs of deterioration and prompt staff to activate the MET.

In addition, systems that detect signs of deterioration using afferent tools integrated into physiologic monitoring devices have been developed for adult settings. For example, a bedside electronic advisory vital signs monitor that assists in the intermittent acquisition of vital signs and calculation of EWSs has been described (36). For patients with elevated scores, the device displays the total score in red as well as an advisory message that guides the nurse toward an appropriate response, including informing the charge nurse, escalating physiologic monitoring, and activating the MET. Implementation of the device into clinical practice across 10 hospitals led to an improvement in survival among patients evaluated by the MET, although this may have been due to an increase in calls for less critically ill patients (36).

Continuous Deterioration Surveillance

While intermittently measured EWSs have had some success in detecting deterioration using data with low temporal resolution, the nature of their intermittent measurement makes them unlikely to detect fast-developing deterioration events (37). In theory, continuous multiparameter monitoring for early signs of deterioration offers the potential benefit of detecting critical illness earlier, without requiring manual measurement of vital signs or frequent calculation of complex scores. These integrated monitoring systems gather data continuously, synthesize them, and alert staff to potential instability. While there have been no reports of integrated systems for children hospitalized on wards, there have been reports of integrated systems developed for adult patients. Visensia, previously known as BioSign, integrates four continuously measured physiologic parameters (heart rate, respiration rate, oxygen saturation, and skin temperature) with one intermittently measured parameter (blood pressure) to generate a numerical patient status index (38). The index represents the amount of deviation of

the patient's combined vital signs from a model of physiologic normality derived from a training data set of hospitalized adult patients. In a study of 326 adult step-down unit patients who had their monitor signals evaluated by this device in a blinded fashion, the device detected all seven MET activations for cardiorespiratory events during the study period, reflecting the high sensitivity of the integrated system (39). The false alarm rate and the impact of implementing such a system on patient outcomes have not yet been thoroughly evaluated. Despite their promise, the feasibility of managing these systems and responding to their alarms across a large number of general wards with low nurse-to-patient ratios is unknown.

THE EFFERENT LIMB

The role of the efferent limb of RRSs is to provide a means of quickly dispatching teams of skilled personnel to address urgent care needs in patients on general medical and surgical wards. Teams may be reactive or proactive. Conventional "code blue" teams are an example of reactive teams; they are widely available to immediately respond to patients with existing respiratory or cardiac arrest. The introduction of formal RRSs over the past 20 years brought a focus on responding to patients at earlier stages of clinical deterioration with the aim of preventing progression to respiratory or cardiac arrest. The composition of these teams varies, but typically includes at least one critical care attending physician or fellow, at least one nurse, and often a respiratory therapist (40). While the terms MET, rapid response team, and critical care outreach team are often used interchangeably, they have subtle differences according to terminology from a 2006 consensus statement (41). The terms were defined as follows: MET refers to a physician-led team with full critical care capabilities, including (a) the ability to prescribe therapy, (b) advanced airway skills, (c) central venous access skills, and (d) the ability to initiate intensive care at the bedside (41). Rapid response team refers to a team that does not necessarily have all of these capabilities, and may include only nonphysician responders with rapid access to physician assistance if needed (40,41). Rover team or critical care outreach team refers to a team structured like a rapid response team, with the addition of providing proactive outreach for patients at high risk of deterioration, such as those recently discharged from an ICU (42,43). Finally, some teams exist with the primary goal of responding to the concerns of families. Each of these teams may function independently with distinct members, or they may comprise overlapping members who respond to different needs throughout the hospital.

Medical Emergency Teams

The most widely researched aspect of RRSs has been METs. A meta-analysis of MET implementation studies showed a 34% reduction in cardiopulmonary arrest outside the ICU but no reduction in hospital mortality in adults, and a 38% reduction in cardiopulmonary arrest outside the ICU and a 21% reduction in hospital mortality in children (44). Most studies included in these analyses were quasi-experimental before-and-after designs, with varying degrees of statistical rigor. These study designs do not account for secular trends or the influences of other quality improvement interventions implemented during the same time periods. One multicenter cluster-randomized study, the Medical Emergency Response and Intervention Trial (MERIT), showed reductions in cardiac arrest and unexpected death rates from baseline to the study period in both intervention (MET team) and control (usual functioning) hospitals combined, but no significant difference between control and intervention hospitals (45). The improved outcomes seen in the control group of MERIT were similar in magnitude to the improvements demonstrated in before-and-after studies of MET implementation. This implies that interventions other than the MET may have been responsible for reductions in morbidity and mortality in this study as well as in other before-and-after studies that showed significant differences pre- and post-MET implementation (46).

A summary of key pediatric MET studies is shown in **Table 29.4**. The studies are all single-center before-and-after designs without adjustment for other key variables, with the exception of the Sharek et al. study (47) that used sophisticated time series modeling and adjustment for season and case mix index and the multicenter Kotsakis et al. study (7) that included adjustment by hospital. Two of the seven studies showed no impact on arrest or mortality rates (48,49). One showed an impact on mortality only in a group of patients readmitted to the PICU (7). Two demonstrated reductions in hospital-wide mortality (47,50), two demonstrated reductions in combined respiratory and cardiac arrests outside the ICU (47,51), and one demonstrated a reduction only in respiratory arrests outside the ICU (52). While these findings generally support implementation, the variability in findings and the limitations of design lead some experts to argue that it is unclear if MET implementation has a direct effect on mortality and arrest rates in children's hospitals, or if the improvements are due to other patient safety initiatives (46).

Proactive Rover and Outreach Teams

Rover and critical care outreach teams are structured like an MET, with the addition of providing proactive outreach for patients at high risk of deterioration. Within 3 months of the implementation of an MET at Duke University's Children's Center, it was noticed that their team would frequently be used as a resource in the care of other patients who were not the focus of the original call for urgent assistance. In response, they launched a proactive rover team (42). The rover team, separate in name but comprising the same members as the hospital's MET, includes a pediatric critical care nurse practitioner or fellow, the PICU charge nurse, and a PICU respiratory therapist. The team makes scheduled rounds to each of the inpatient care areas and discusses any at-risk patients identified by each ward's charge nurse and on-call senior resident. The team also evaluates all children who were discharged from the PICU in the preceding 12 hours and all new admissions to the progressive care unit. Because the rover team was implemented and evaluated concurrently with MET implementation, it is not possible to evaluate the effect of rover team implementation on outcomes in that study.

Family Concern Teams

Teams also exist to respond to the concerns of families related to their children's conditions. The most well-known is Condition HELP, implemented at Children's Hospital of Pittsburgh (26). The team comprises a physician, a nursing supervisor, and a patient advocate and is capable of identifying, triaging, and escalating medical, social, and care coordination issues as necessary. On admission, families receive a verbal explanation of the program from their nurse, receive a brochure, and view a video presentation. Families are asked to voice concerns to their ward team first, and, if not addressed, to activate Condition HELP. Examples of situations that might necessitate a Condition HELP call include medical changes in a patient not addressed by the healthcare team, breakdowns in communication, or a patient receiving a medication that the family feels will have an adverse effect on the child (26). In the first 2 years

of activity, the team received 42 calls, 15 related to management/coordination of care, 9 related to medications or pain control, 6 related to discharge, 6 related to dietary status, and 6 related to delays in service or amenities (26).

Other children's hospitals have given families direct access to the MET (27,28). North Carolina Children's Hospital, in the absence of a specialized family concern team like Condition HELP, implemented a system in which families were given the same telephone number that staff members use to directly activate the MET. Over the 1-year period after implementation, only two calls were made by families but the number of calls initiated by staff increased (28). A similar implementation at Duke University Children's Hospital and Health Center yielded two calls over a 12-week pilot period (27).

PROCESS IMPROVEMENT LIMB

The role of the process improvement limb of RRSs is to take a data-driven approach to evaluating system success, avoid potential threats to success, seize opportunities to optimize the system, and design tailored improvement interventions. This limb works with the administrative limb and should include membership/oversight from clinicians (including each discipline on team and members of activating and responding teams) as well as improvement science experts with experience in time series data analysis and improvement interventions. This limb addresses three categories of measures through the following three questions:

1. Do we see signs of improvement in patient outcomes? (outcome measures)
2. Is the RRS working as planned? (process measures)
3. What are the unintended consequences? (balancing measures).

Outcome Measures

Several outcome measures have been reported in the context of RRS intervention effectiveness studies and quality improvement work. The most frequent outcome measures have been rates of hospital-wide mortality, cardiac arrests, and respiratory arrests outside the ICU. The hospital-wide mortality rate is relatively easy to acquire using administrative data. However, its analysis and interpretation present challenges when using the data for improvement purposes. Identifying deaths that were potentially preventable by an RRS versus those that occurred following a complex ICU course can be difficult and requires expertise. The rate of cardiopulmonary arrests occurring outside the ICU may be a better outcome measure for improvement work, in that the events are discrete and measurable, and research describing clinical antecedents to arrests suggests that many of these events are preventable by METs (53). Whether all of these are preventable is a subject of some debate and has led to measures like the MET-preventable code (51). MET-preventable metrics offer the advantage in improvement efforts of targeting zero events as the goal; however, the subjectivity of such distinctions may be problematic.

The relative rarity of cardiac and respiratory arrests outside the ICU is an additional challenge when analyzing and drawing conclusions using data from a single hospital. The rate of cardiopulmonary arrests in the after phase of RRS implementation at five studies in a recent systematic review is 5.9 arrests per 10,000 patients (44). These challenges have led to a focus on proximal outcome measures that capture clinically important deterioration at a stage pre-arrest and that occurs more commonly and hence a more responsive measure at a single-center level. The Children's Resuscitation Intensity Scale defines

TABLE 29.4

PEDIATRIC MEDICAL EMERGENCY TEAM IMPLEMENTATION STUDIES

■ SOURCE/ COUNTRY	■ STUDY DESIGN	■ CENTERS	■ TEAM COMPOSITION	■ YEARS OF STUDY	■ VARIABLES ADJUSTED FOR	■ STATISTICALLY SIGNIFICANT CHANGE IN ARREST OR MORTALITY RATES?
Brilli et al. (51), United States	Before and after	1	■ PICU fellow ■ Resident ■ PICU nurse ■ Respiratory therapist ■ Nursing supervisor	2003–2006	None	Reduction in combined respiratory and cardiac arrests outside ICU
Hanson et al. (48), United States	Before and after	1	■ PICU fellow ■ Resident ■ PICU nurse ■ Respiratory therapist	2003–2007	None	No[a]
Hunt et al. (52), United States	Before and after	1	■ PICU fellow ■ 3 Residents ■ PICU nurse ■ Respiratory therapist ■ Nursing supervisor	2003–2005	None	Reduction in respiratory arrests outside ICU
Kotsakis et al. (7), Canada	Before and after	4	■ PICU attending and/or fellow and/or resident ■ PICU nurse ■ Respiratory therapist	2004–2009	Center	Reduction in mortality rate among patients readmitted to PICU within 48 h of being discharged
Sharek et al. (47), United States	Before and after with ARIMA time series modeling	1	■ PICU attending or fellow ■ PICU nurse ■ Respiratory therapist ■ Nursing supervisor	2001–2007	Season and case mix	Reduction in combined respiratory and cardiac arrests outside ICU and hospital-wide mortality
Tibballs et al. (50), Australia	Before and after	1	■ PICU consultant or registrar ■ PICU nurse ■ Emergency department physician ■ Emergency department registrar	1999–2006	None	Reductions in hospital-wide mortality, hospital ward unexpected deaths, hospital ward preventable cardiac arrests, mortality from preventable hospital ward cardiac arrests
Zenker et al. (49), United States	Before and after	1	■ PICU nurse ■ Respiratory therapist	2004–2006	None	No

[a]Changes in arrest and mortality rates were not significant. There was a significant increase in the mean number of patient-days between ward cardiac arrests; however, this metric ignores the patient-time at risk of the event and is thus a poor measure of improvement.[55]
ARIMA, autoregressive integrated moving average.

intermediate and late transfers based on aggressive respiratory and circulatory interventions occurring in the 12 hours before transfer to the ICU; the rate of late transfers has been shown to decrease in association with the use of an EWS (54). Bonafide and colleagues (55,55a) have demonstrated the validity of a "critical deterioration" metric defined as events resulting in ICU transfer and noninvasive ventilation, intubation, or vasopressor infusion in the 12 hours following arrival in the ICU. Critical deterioration was associated with a >13-fold risk of mortality and occurred more than 8 times more commonly than arrests outside the ICU. Unrecognized situation awareness failure events (UNSAFE transfers) are another proximate outcome measure for RRS effectiveness. These are defined as ward-to-ICU transfers where patients are intubated, placed on vasopressors, or receive three or more fluid boluses within the first 1 hour after transfer. An intervention to improve the afferent arm of the RRS has been associated with a significant and sustained reduction in UNSAFE transfers (56).

Process Measures

Process measures are needed to assess both underuse (e.g., missed MET calls) and overuse (e.g., unnecessary MET workload) of RRSs. The most commonly used measure is the number of MET calls, expressed as a rate per admission, patient-day, or non-ICU patient-day. This rate differs by more than fourfold in the literature, causing uncertainty about what the optimal rate is (44). A complementary measure to this is the percentage of MET calls that result in transfer to the ICU. Although the optimal percentage is not known, 100% of MET calls resulting in ICU transfer likely reflects underuse. The time between initial physiologic abnormality and admission to ICU, or "score to door time" (57), is a measure reflecting RRS efficiency, and may be helpful in setting expectations among activating teams and determining when more responding team resources may be needed. Similarly the timing of calls (e.g., during the day vs. night or weekday vs. weekend) may help with allocation of resources as well as reveal potential vulnerabilities in the usual care provided to hospitalized patients. Reasons for MET calls can be potentially rich sources for learning and improvement, particularly those that relate to quantitative triggers like EWSs or to family activations where tailored education may be needed. Evaluation of EWSs should include their sensitivity, specificity, positive predictive value, and negative predictive value at various cut points for outcomes such as MET activation, ICU transfer, and proximate outcome measures.

Balancing Measures

Balancing measures are particularly important for a complex intervention like RRSs; however, work to date on measures is limited. Qualitative data from the responding and activating teams are needed to measure team function as well as unintended consequences. Qualitative data on RRSs are generally lacking in pediatrics, but several adult studies have identified reasons for failure to activate the MET, including primary team belief that the situation was "under control," poor communication, leadership challenges, and organizational culture (58–60). In an institution where calling the MET was not required (discretionary) (50), staff experienced multiple barriers to activating the system. In a pediatric study of 280 nurses and 127 doctors, 41% of nurses and 12% of doctors reported they received active discouragement by colleagues to activate the RRS (61). Many reported that they feared criticism by colleagues. There also appeared an inability to recognize serious illness as evidenced by unwillingness to

activate the system when calling criteria had been attained and an admission that in retrospect they should have called MET when they had not. Overcoming such barriers is a complex challenge. Potential solutions include making reeducation by means of simulation exercises a requirement (62) or mandating the activation of an MET when calling criteria are attained. For improvement purposes, data like these can be invaluable for identifying and addressing barriers to effective RRS functioning. This is particularly important in the initial stages of MET implementation. Less resource-intensive methods such as survey tools exist in the literature (51). The Agency for Healthcare Research and Quality (AHRQ) Hospital Survey on Patient Safety Culture is one that may be useful in measuring expected improvements as well as unintended consequences, although supplemental tailored questions may be needed. One center saw an unexplained initial worsening in AHRQ Patient Safety Culture survey results in association with the beginning of a broad patient safety program that included an RRS before realizing a subsequent sustained improvement in reduced serious safety events in the years that followed (63).

ADMINISTRATIVE LIMB

The role of the administrative limb of RRSs is to implement the system, manage each of its components, and support its ongoing operation. This includes managing personnel and associated costs, determining equipment requirements, and ensuring that the needs for ongoing clinician and patient/family education are satisfied (41). This requires a formal committee structure, which may be combined with the hospital's resuscitation/code blue committee. Membership should include nurses, physicians, and respiratory therapists in frontline clinical roles as well as leadership roles in ICU and ward settings. In addition, at least one participant should be experienced in patient safety and quality improvement methodology in order to guide the group's decision making with regard to incrementally evaluating and optimizing the RRS.

Implementing a Rapid Response System

Successfully implementing and operating an RRS requires commitment and support from hospital leaders, as well as buy-in from the frontline staff that comprise the response teams and from those who will be calling for help from the wards. The Ontario Pediatric Critical Care Response Team Collaborative recently published a detailed RRS implementation strategy, which is broadly generalizable (64). Their guide included gathering baseline data, developing project plans, recruiting and training champions and MET providers, developing a strategy for promoting the RRS across the hospitals, a limited rollout to obtain feedback and refine the system, and finally a full-time rollout that included ongoing education and quality improvement data collection (64).

RRS Operating Costs

While their potential to reduce costs is often mentioned in the discussion sections of RRS manuscripts, formal cost-effectiveness analysis of RRS implementation has not been performed. Hospital administration must make the decision of whether to staff METs with clinicians who have concurrent responsibilities in the PICU or to identify additional staff without other patient care responsibilities to serve as responding team members. Most pediatric centers will not have sufficient MET call volume to justify a completely stand-alone MET.

Therefore, most members of the MET will have other clinical responsibilities that will need to be balanced. If members of the responding team are pulled away from a critically ill ICU patient to attend to a less ill patient on a hospital ward, the MET call may be a net negative in improving quality of care for the two patients. Further work is needed to better define this issue and develop workload measures for METs.

SUMMARY AND FUTURE DIRECTIONS

RRSs have emerged at hospitals throughout the world despite what some experts believe is a lack of definitive evidence. Several before-and-after studies of MET implementation have demonstrated reductions in cardiac arrests, respiratory arrests, and mortality following MET implementation; however, other concomitantly implemented patient safety interventions make it difficult to ascribe the aforementioned outcomes to MET implementation alone. Given their wide dissemination, identifying sites for a cluster-randomized trial of MET implementation is not likely. Therefore, we must rely on meta-analyses of quasi-experimental studies to ultimately determine their value in improving patient outcomes.

A number of additional questions about RRSs remain, and should be addressed in the coming years. Comparative effectiveness studies are needed in order to determine the best afferent tools and efferent mechanisms to reduce morbidity and mortality among patients at risk of deterioration on the wards. With regard to the afferent limb, it is important to identify which calling criteria and EWSs are most effective. It is also important to identify how the volumes of physiologic data collected every day on bedside monitors can be harnessed to accurately detect early deterioration in children and alert clinicians to rapidly intervene. The ability to analyze and apply predictive models to continuous streams of multiparameter physiologic data combined with data from electronic health records in real time will likely emerge as an area of active research and innovation in the coming years. With regard to the process improvement limb, it is necessary to determine the optimal ratio of MET calls to ICU admissions in order to help administrators make decisions about resource allocation. Finally, efforts should be undertaken to develop better systems to involve families in their children's ongoing assessment in order to take advantage of their ability to recognize subtle changes and share those findings with clinicians in a meaningful, ongoing way.

References

1. Tibballs J, Brilli RJ. Pediatric RRSs. In: DeVita MA, Hillman K, Bellomo R, eds. *Textbook of Rapid Response Systems: Concept and Implementation.* New York, NY: Springer Science + Business Media, 2011:231–43.

2. Lee A, Bishop G, Hillman KM, et al. The medical emergency team. *Anaesth Intensive Care* 1995;23(2):183–6.

3. Tibballs J, Kinney S, Duke T, et al. Reduction of paediatric inpatient cardiac arrest and death with a medical emergency team: Preliminary results. *Arch Dis Child* 2005;90(11):1148–52.

4. Institute for Healthcare Improvement. *Overview of the 100,000 Lives Campaign.* http://www.ihi.org/offerings/Initiatives/PastStrategicInitiatives/5MillionLivesCampaign/Documents/Overview%20of%20the%20100K%20Campaign.pdf. Accessed April 28, 2014

5. Institute for Healthcare Improvement. *Overview of the Institute for Healthcare Improvement Five Million Lives Campaign.* http://www.ihi.org/offerings/Initiatives/PastStrategicInitiatives/5MillionLivesCampaign/Pages/default.aspx. Accessed April 28, 2014

6. The Joint Commission. *The Joint Commission 2008 National Patient Safety Goals.* http://www.jointcommission.org/ PatientSafety/NationalPatientSafetyGoals/08_hap_npsgs.htm. Accessed April 6, 2008.

7. Kotsakis A, Lobos A-T, Parshuram C, et al. Implementation of a multicenter rapid response system in pediatric academic hospitals is effective. *Pediatrics* 2011;128(1):72–8.

8. UK National Institute for Health and Clinical Excellence (NICE). *Acutely Ill Patients in Hospital: Recognition of and Response to Acute Illness in Adults in Hospital, 2007.* http://publications.nice. org.uk/acutely-ill-patients-in-hospital-cg50. Accessed April 28, 2014

9. Australian Commission on Safety and Quality in Health Care. *National Safety and Quality Health Service Standards, 2011.* http://www.safetyandquality.gov.au/wp-content/uploads/2011/09/ NSQHS-Standards-Sept-2012.pdf. Accessed April 28, 2014

10. VandenBerg SD, Hutchison JS, Parshuram CS. A cross-sectional survey of levels of care and response mechanisms for evolving critical illness in hospitalized children. *Pediatrics* 2007;119(4): e940–6.

11. Chen JG, Kemper AR, Odetola F, et al. Prevalence, characteristics, and opinions of pediatric rapid response teams in the United States. *Hosp Pediatr* 2012;2(3):133–40.

12. DeVita MA, Smith GB, Adam SK, et al. "Identifying the hospitalised patient in crisis"—A consensus conference on the afferent limb of rapid response systems. *Resuscitation* 2010;81(4):375–82.

13. Kinney S, Tibballs J, Johnston L, et al. Clinical profile of hospitalized children provided with urgent assistance from a medical emergency team. *Pediatrics* 2008;121(6):e1577–84.

14. Bonafide CP, Holmes JH, Nadkarni VM, et al. Development of a score to predict clinical deterioration in hospitalized children. *J Hosp Med* 2012;7(4):345–49.

15. Morgan R, Williams F, Wright M. An early warning scoring system for detecting developing critical illness. *Clin Intensive Care* 1997;8:100.

16. Monaghan A. Detecting and managing deterioration in children. *Paediatr Nurs* 2005;17(1):32–5.

17. Tucker KM, Brewer TL, Baker RB, et al. Prospective evaluation of a pediatric inpatient early warning scoring system. *J Spec Pediatr Nurs* 2009;14(2):79–85.

18. Akre M, Finkelstein M, Erickson M, et al. Sensitivity of the Pediatric Early Warning score to identify patient deterioration. *Pediatrics* 2010;125(4):e763–69.

19. Duncan H, Hutchison J, Parshuram CS. The Pediatric Early Warning System score: A severity of illness score to predict urgent medical need in hospitalized children. *J Crit Care* 2006;21(3):271–8.

20. Parshuram CS, Hutchison J, Middaugh K. Development and initial validation of the Bedside Paediatric Early Warning System score. *Crit Care* 2009;13(4):R135.

21. Parshuram CS, Duncan HP, Joffe AR, et al. Multi-centre validation of the Bedside Paediatric Early Warning System score: A severity of illness score to detect evolving critical illness in hospitalized children. *Crit Care* 2011;15(4):R184.

22. The Hospital for Sick Children. *Evaluating Processes of Care & the Outcomes of Children in Hospital (EPOCH).* http://clinicaltrials .gov/show/NCT01260831. Accessed April 28, 2014

23. Edwards ED, Powell CVE, Mason BW, et al. Prospective cohort study to test the predictability of the Cardiff and Vale Paediatric Early Warning System. *Arch Dis Child* 2009;94(8):602–6.

24. Haines C, Perrott M, Weir P. Promoting care for acutely ill children—development and evaluation of a paediatric early warning tool. *Intensive Crit Care Nurs* 2006;22(2):73–81.

25. King S. Our story. *Pediatr Radiol* 2006;36(4):284–6.

26. Dean BS, Decker MJ, Hupp D, et al. Condition HELP: A pediatric rapid response team triggered by patients and parents. *J Health Qual* 2008;30(3):28–31.

27. Hueckel RM, Mericle JM, Frush K, et al. Implementation of condition help: Family teaching and evaluation of family understanding. *J Nurs Care Qual* 2012;27(2):176–81.

28. Ray EM, Smith R, Massie S, et al. Family alert: Implementing direct family activation of a pediatric rapid response team. *Jt Comm J Qual Patient Saf* 2009;35:575–80.

29. Bogert S, Ferrell C, Rutledge DN. Experience with family activation of rapid response teams. *Medsurg Nurs* 2010;19(4):215–23.

30. Dunning E, Brzozowicz K, Noel E, et al. FAST track beyond RRTs. *Nurs Manage* 2010;41(5):38–41.

31. Gerdik C, Vallish RO, Miles K, et al. Successful implementation of a family and patient activated rapid response team in an adult level 1 trauma center. *Resuscitation* 2010;81(12):1676–81.

32. Greenhouse PK, Kuzminsky B, Martin SC, et al. Calling a condition H(elp). *Am J Nurs* 2006;106(11):63–6.

33. Odell M, Gerber K, Gager M. Call 4 Concern: Patient and relative activated critical care outreach. *Br J Nurs* 2010;19(22):1390–95.

34. Paciotti B, Roberts KE, Tibbetts KM, et al. Physician Attitudes Toward Family-Activated Medical Emergency Teams for Hospitalized Children. Joint Commission Journal on Quality and Patient Safety. 2014;40(4):187-192.

35. Bonafide CP, Keren R, Nadkarni VM, et al. Improving recognition of children at risk of cardiopulmonary arrest through EHR-integrated pediatric rapid response team activation criteria. *Paper presented at: American Medical Informatics Association Annual Symposium.*

36. Bellomo R, Ackerman M, Bailey M, et al. A controlled trial of electronic automated advisory vital signs monitoring in general hospital wards. *Crit Care Med* 2012;40(8):2349–61.

37. Taenzer AH, Pyke JB, McGrath SP. A review of current and emerging approaches to address failure-to-rescue. *Anesthesiology* 2011;115(2):421–31.

38. Tarassenko L, Hann A, Young D. Integrated monitoring and analysis for early warning of patient deterioration. *Br J Anaesth* 2006;97(1):64–8.

39. Hravnak M, Edwards L, Clontz A, et al. Defining the incidence of cardiorespiratory instability in patients in step-down units using an electronic integrated monitoring system. *Arch Intern Med* 2008;168(12):1300–8.

40. Jones DA, DeVita MA, Bellomo R. Rapid-response teams. *N Engl J Med* 2011;365(2):139–46.

41. DeVita MA, Bellomo R, Hillman K, et al. Findings of the first consensus conference on medical emergency teams. *Crit Care Med* 2006;34(9):2463–78.

42. Hueckel RM, Turi JL, Cheifetz IM, et al. Beyond rapid response teams: Instituting a "rover team" improves the management of at-risk patients, facilitates proactive interventions, and improves outcomes. In: Henriksen K, Battles JB, Keyes MA, et al, eds. *Advances in Patient Safety: New Directions and Alternative Approaches. Vol 3. Performance and Tools.* Rockville, MD: Agency for Healthcare Research and Quality, 2008. AHRQ Publication No 08-0034-3.

43. Ball C, Kirkby M, Williams S. Effect of the critical care outreach team on patient survival to discharge from hospital and readmission to critical care: Non-randomised population based study. *BMJ* 2003;327(7422):1014.

44. Chan PS, Jain R, Nallmothu BK, et al. Rapid response teams: A systematic review and meta-analysis. *Arch Intern Med* 2010;170(1):18–26.

45. Hillman K, Chen J, Cretikos M, et al. Introduction of the medical emergency team (MET) system: A cluster-randomised controlled trial. *Lancet* 2005;365(9477):2091–7.

46. Joffe AR, Anton NR, Burkholder SC. Reduction in hospital mortality over time in a hospital without a pediatric medical emergency team: Limitations of before-and-after study designs. *Arch Pediatr Adolesc Med* 2011;165(5):419–23.

47. Sharek PJ, Parast LM, Leong K, et al. Effect of a rapid response team on hospital-wide mortality and code rates outside the ICU in a children's hospital. *JAMA* 2007;298(19):2267–74.

48. Hanson CC, Randolph GD, Erickson JA, et al. A reduction in cardiac arrests and duration of clinical instability after implementation of a paediatric rapid response system. *Postgrad Med J* 2010;86(1015):314–8.

49. Zenker P, Schlesinger A, Hauck M, et al. Implementation and impact of a rapid response team in a children's hospital. *Jt Comm J Qual Patient Saf* 2007;33(7):418–25.

50. Tibballs J, Kinney S. Reduction of hospital mortality and of preventable cardiac arrest and death on introduction of a pediatric medical emergency team. *Pediatr Crit Care Med* 2009;10(3):306–12.

51. Brilli RJ, Gibson R, Luria JW, et al. Implementation of a medical emergency team in a large pediatric teaching hospital prevents respiratory and cardiopulmonary arrests outside the intensive care unit. *Pediatr Crit Care Med* 2007;8(3):236–46.

52. Hunt EA, Zimmer KP, Rinke ML, et al. Transition from a traditional code team to a medical emergency team and categorization of cardiopulmonary arrests in a children's center. *Arch Pediatr Adolesc Med* 2008;162(2):117–22.

53. Schein RM, Hazday N, Pena M, et al. Clinical antecedents to in-hospital cardiopulmonary arrest. *Chest* 1990;98(6):1388–92.

54. Parshuram CS, Bayliss A, Reimer J, et al. Implementing the Bedside Paediatric Early Warning System in a community hospital: A prospective observational study. *Paediatr Child Health* 2011;16(3):e18–22.

55. Bonafide CP, Roberts KE, Priestley MA, et al. Development of a pragmatic measure for evaluating and optimizing rapid response systems. *Pediatrics* 2012;129(4):e874–81.

55a. Bonafide CP, Localio AR, Roberts KE, Nadkarni VM, Weirich CM, Keren R: Impact of rapid response system implementation on critical deterioration events in children. *JAMA Pediatrics* 2014;168(1):25–33.

56. Brady PW, Muething SE, Kotagal UR, et al. Improving situation awareness to reduce unrecognized clinical deterioration and serious safety events. *Pediatrics* 2013;131(1):e298–308.

57. Oglesby KJ, Durham L, Welch J, et al. 'Score to Door Time', a benchmarking tool for rapid response systems: A pilot multi-centre service evaluation. *Crit Care* 2011;15(4):R180.

58. Nembhard IM, Edmondson AC. Making it safe: The effects of leader inclusiveness and professional status on psychological safety and improvement efforts in health care teams. *J Organ Behav* 2006;27(7):941–66.

59. Mackintosh N, Rainey H, Sandall J. Understanding how rapid response systems may improve safety for the acutely ill patient: Learning from the frontline. *BMJ Qual Saf* 2012;21(2):135–44.

60. Shearer B, Marshall S, Buist MD, et al. What stops hospital clinical staff from following protocols? An analysis of the incidence and factors behind the failure of bedside clinical staff to activate the rapid response system in a multi-campus Australian metropolitan healthcare service. *BMJ Qual Saf* 2012;21(7):569–75.

61. Azzopardi P, Kinney S, Moulden A, et al. Attitudes and barriers to a medical emergency team system at a tertiary paediatric hospital. *Resuscitation* 2011;82(2):167–74.

62. Theilen U, Leonard P, Jones P, et al. Regular in situ simulation training of paediatric medical emergency team improves hospital response to deteriorating patients. *Resuscitation* 2013;84(2):218-222.

63. Muething SE, Goudie A, Schoettker PJ, et al. Quality improvement initiative to reduce serious safety events and improve patient safety culture. *Pediatrics* 2012;130(2):e423–31.

64. Lobos AT, Costello J, Gilleland J, et al. An implementation strategy for a multicenter pediatric rapid response system in Ontario. *Jt Comm J Qual Patient Saf* 2010;36(6):271–80; 241.

CHAPTER 30 ■ **MULTIPLE TRAUMA**

JOHN SCOTT BAIRD AND ARTHUR COOPER

KEY POINTS

Epidemiology of Pediatric Trauma

❶ Trauma is the leading cause of pediatric deaths in developed countries; most children suffer significant morbidity following major trauma.

❷ Further reductions in morbidity and mortality related to pediatric trauma are possible but will require a multidisciplinary approach.

Pediatric Injury: Mechanisms and Patterns

❸ Blunt trauma is more frequent than penetrating trauma, although the latter is associated with a higher mortality rate.

❹ The mechanism of injury often predicts the pattern of injuries and suggests a management strategy.

Pathophysiology

❺ Genotypic innate response to injury, involving a multitude of molecular products, may be an important determinant of outcome following trauma.

Initial Assessment

❻ The ABCDs (airway, breathing, circulation, and disability) are the focus of the primary survey and mandate appropriate interventions and continued reassessment during the "golden hour" (or "platinum half hour") following injury.

❼ Respiratory failure is a frequent complication of major pediatric trauma, whereas hypotension is less common and a late finding (compared with adults).

❽ The goal of the secondary survey is to definitively evaluate the injured child, and it should proceed concurrently with ongoing resuscitation efforts by a multidisciplinary team; laboratory examinations are an important component.

❾ Common visceral injuries in children include contusions, hematomas, and lacerations of the lungs, liver, spleen, or kidneys, as well as pneumothorax, hemothorax, rib fractures, and gastrointestinal tract injury.

❿ Important aspects of these injuries in children include the role of nonoperative management and the provision of meticulous intensive care.

Child Abuse

⓫ When the extent of pediatric injury is inconsistent with the history of injury, the possibility of child abuse must be considered.

Complications

⓬ Common complications of major pediatric trauma include functional limitations, troublesome anxiety and stress, and infection (often related to treatment). The optimal recognition and management of each of these problems remains to be determined.

EPIDEMIOLOGY OF PEDIATRIC TRAUMA

Trauma is the forceful disruption of bodily homeostasis and is the leading cause of death in children and young adults in developed countries (**Fig. 30.1**). It comprises unintentional as well as intentional injuries, including child abuse. Approximately half of all injuries to children involve multiple organs or body regions, and these injuries are associated with a higher case-based fatality rate. Blunt injury is far more common than penetrating injury in children, although the latter is more deadly ❶ (**Table 30.1**). During the last three decades in the United States, the population-based mortality rate for unintentional pediatric injury has fallen by more than 50%, although it remains the most common cause of death for all pediatric patients in the most recent year for which statistics are available (2009) (1), followed in older adolescents by homicide and suicide. Indeed, although mortality rates for the leading causes of pediatric

death have declined in developed countries, the decline is least for trauma (**Fig. 30.2**). Most pediatric deaths from trauma are associated with motor vehicles and occur prior to hospital admission. The morbidity of pediatric trauma increases with increasing severity of injury and is manifested frequently by functional limitations following major injury; the overall cost is difficult to estimate, although it is likely enormous.

Trauma remains the "neglected disease of modern society," as it was originally described in a monograph by the National Academy of Sciences over 40 years ago (2). Organizing a community for pediatric trauma care requires not only specialized knowledge of the evaluation and management of childhood injury, but also the ability to ensure that the special needs of children are met throughout the entire continuum of trauma care—from prevention, through prehospital care, transport, emergency care, operative and intensive care, recovery, and re- ❷ habilitation. Reductions in the rates of pediatric trauma morbidity and mortality are the result of concerted efforts during the last few decades, which have involved research, education,

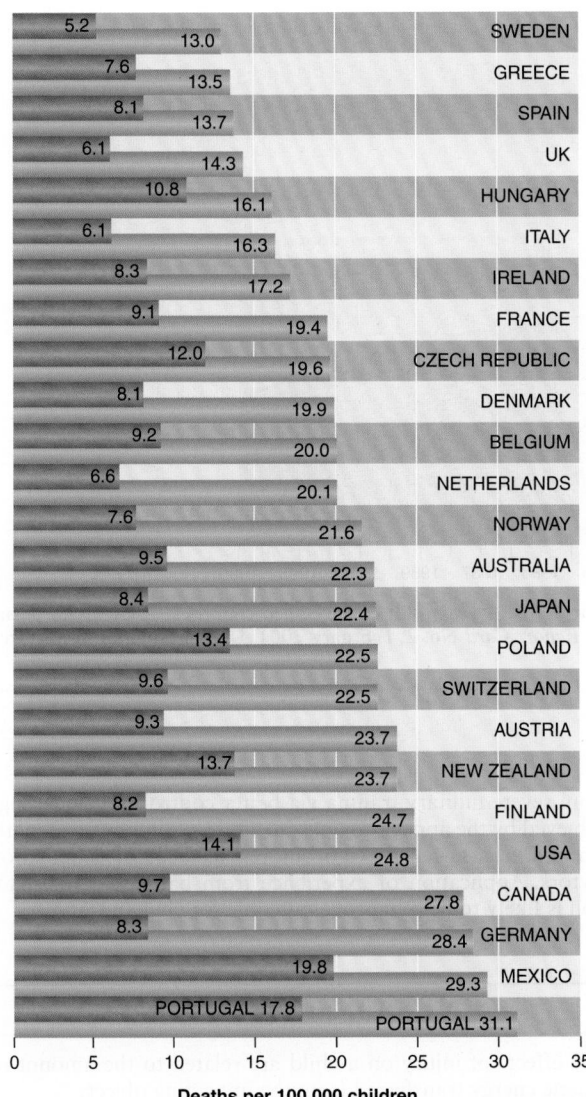

FIGURE 30.1. Annual deaths due to injury in children during the 1970s (*long bars*) and 1990s (*short bars*). (From UNICEF. A league table of child deaths by injury in rich nations. *Innocenti Report Card* No. 2, February 2001. UNICEF Innocenti Research Centre, Florence. © The United Nations Children's Fund, 2001.)

TABLE 30.1

INCIDENCE AND MORTALITY OF PEDIATRIC TRAUMA

■ INJURY MECHANISM	■ INCIDENCE (%)	■ MORTALITY (%)
Blunt	92	3
Fall	27	<1
Motor vehicle injury—occupant	21	4
Motor vehicle injury—pedestrian	12	5
Bicycle	9	2
Penetrating	8	5
Gunshot wound	2	10
Stabbing	3	3
Crush	<1	3

Adapted from Cooper A. Early assessment and management of trauma. In: Ashcroft KW, Holcomb GW, Murphy JP, eds. *Pediatric Surgery*. Philadelphia, PA: Elsevier, 2005:168–84.

PEDIATRIC INJURY: MECHANISMS AND PATTERNS

Intracranial injuries are the cause of most pediatric trauma deaths (due at least in part to the untoward effects of traumatic coma on airway patency, breathing control, cerebral perfusion, and to the pediatric anatomy). The evaluation and management of neurologic injuries is reviewed elsewhere in Chapter 61. Most blunt trauma in childhood is unintentional, but 7% of serious injuries are due to intentional physical assault (of which nearly half, or 3%, are due to child abuse) (4). Blunt injuries outnumber penetrating injuries in children by a ratio of 12:1, a ratio that has decreased in recent years. While blunt injuries are more common, penetrating injuries are more lethal.

Injury mechanism is the main predictor of injury pattern (**Table 30.2**). Pedestrian motor vehicle trauma may result in the *Waddell triad* of injuries to the head, torso, and lower extremities, while occupant injuries include head, face, and neck trauma in unrestrained passengers, and cervical spine injuries, bowel disruption or hematoma, and Chance fractures of the spine in restrained passengers. Bicycle trauma results in head injury in unhelmeted riders and upper extremity and upper abdominal injuries (results from contact with the handlebar). Low falls, the most common cause of childhood injury, rarely produce significant trauma, but high falls (from the second story or higher) are associated with serious head injuries, with the addition of long-bone fractures (at the third story), and intrathoracic and intra-abdominal injuries (at the fifth story, the height from which 50% of children can be expected to die) (5). With the growing popularity of extreme sports (including extreme skiing and surfing, inline skating, mountain bicycling, rock climbing, skateboarding, snowboarding, and ultraendurance racing) in which risk is very high and often underappreciated, patterns of adolescent traumatic injury are likely to change.

While it is important to realize that the involvement of multiple organ systems is typical following major trauma in children (due chiefly to their small size, the proportionately larger size of the head, and the proportionately smaller size of the torso), major pediatric blunt trauma is more a disease of airway and breathing than of bleeding and shock.

Though uncommon in most pediatric trauma, hemorrhagic shock remains an important problem in major trauma, and advances have come from recent experience in the battlefield. We will review research, which suggests improved outcome

legislation, and an investment in medical services at all levels. Further declines in pediatric trauma morbidity and mortality in the United States will require an even broader and more vigorous public health approach, probably modeled after some of the more successful systems in European countries such as Sweden, Italy, the UK, and the Netherlands.

Injuries are, for the most part, not true "accidents," but predictable events rooted in a complex web of social, cultural, and economic factors that impact upon the host, agent, and environment. Injury rates have been shown to respond to established harm-reduction strategies based within the community. The National Safe Kids Campaign (www.safekids.org) and the Injury Free Coalition for Kids (www.injuryfree.org) have both proven effective in reducing the burden of childhood injury (3). Comorbidities common to many injured children and adolescents include limited access to health care, altered family dynamics (including child abuse), increased risk-taking behavior (including substance abuse and intoxications), and suicidal intent, among others. Strategies to limit such comorbidities are likely to prove useful in reducing childhood injuries.

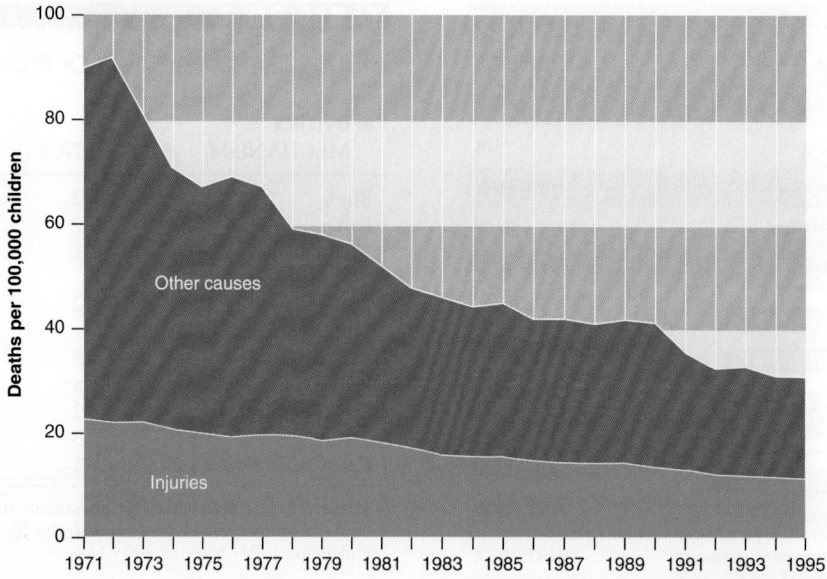

FIGURE 30.2. Death rates from injuries versus all other causes in children (up to 14 years old) of developed countries, 1971–1995. (From UNICEF. A league table of child deaths by injury in rich nations. *Innocenti Report Card* No. 2, February 2001. UNICEF Innocenti Research Centre, Florence. © The United Nations Children's Fund, 2001.)

TABLE 30.2

COMMON INJURY MECHANISMS AND CORRESPONDING INJURY PATTERNS IN CHILDHOOD TRAUMA

■ INJURY MECHANISM	■ DETAILS	■ INJURY PATTERN
Motor vehicle injury—occupant	Unrestrained	Head/neck injuries
		Scalp/facial lacerations
	Restrained	Abdomen injuries
		Lower spine fractures
Motor vehicle injury—pedestrian	Single injury	Lower extremity fractures
	Multiple injuries	Head/neck injuries
		Chest/abdomen injuries
		Lower extremity fractures
Fall from height	Low	Upper extremity fractures
	Medium	Head/neck injuries
		Scalp/facial lacerations
		Upper extremity fractures
	High	Head/neck injuries
		Scalp/facial lacerations
		Chest/abdomen injuries
		Extremity fractures
Fall from bicycle	Unhelmeted	Head/neck injuries
		Scalp/facial lacerations
		Upper extremity fractures
	Helmeted	Upper extremity fractures
	Handlebar impact	Abdomen injuries

Adapted from Cooper A. Early assessment and management of trauma. In: Ashcroft KW, Holcomb GW, Murphy JP, eds. *Pediatric Surgery*. Philadelphia, PA: Elsevier, 2005:168–84.

from severe military trauma via better control of hemorrhage achieved by the application of tourniquets following traumatic amputation as well as vigorous replacement of coagulation factors. Application of experience from battlefield resuscitation is likely to help improve outcome for civilian trauma.

PATHOPHYSIOLOGY

The effects of injury on a child are related to the amount of kinetic energy transferred from the impacting object:

$$\text{Kinetic energy (J)} = 0.5 \times \text{Mass (kg)} \times \text{Velocity}^2 \text{ (m/sec}^2).$$

Because the child's body is smaller, this energy is compacted into a smaller space. As a result, involvement of many organ systems is common after significant pediatric trauma. In addition, the increased elasticity of immature bone results in increased soft-tissue injury when the impact is confined to a smaller space. In blunt trauma, the forces of impact are dependent upon such factors as the size and speed of the vehicle or the vertical displacement following a fall. In penetrating trauma, the forces of violation are dependent upon the weapon used (e.g., the size of the missile it discharges and the velocity with which it is delivered).

Irrespective of the exact mechanism of injury, the body's physiologic responses to trauma and hemorrhage tend to be similar and essential for survival: reflexive, catecholamine-mediated, increases in vasomotor tone and cardiac output help to maintain effective circulating blood volume and vital organ perfusion. Organs involved in these and related reflex arcs following acute traumatic injury include the central and peripheral nervous systems, the cardiovascular system, the adrenal glands, the kidneys, and the liver. The resultant collection of reflex responses mediated by these organ systems helps to define the stress response following injury. Without these responses, changes in intravascular volume and systemic vascular resistance following major trauma could compromise oxygen delivery.

Baroreceptors located in the walls of large arteries in the thorax and neck respond to changes in blood pressure by exciting or inhibiting the medullary vasoconstrictor and vagal parasympathetic centers, with resultant changes in vasomotor tone, chronotropy, and inotropy. Maximum sympathetic vasoconstriction may occur, at least for the first few minutes following trauma that results in global brain ischemia. Other responses to the stress of trauma include the release of angiotensin by the kidneys, cortisol, and aldosterone by the adrenal glands, vasopressin by the posterior pituitary gland, and various local compensatory mechanisms, which help to contract circulation or shift fluid into the intravascular compartment in the presence of diminished blood volume. Tissue injury may also activate cascades that contribute to the stress response and that include complement, cytokines, eicosanoids, histamine, kinins, nitric oxide, serotonin, and a variety of hormonal mediators.

The stress response is usually self-limited and adaptive, but when severe injury occurs, the response may be profound and result in a hypermetabolic state, which increases substrate consumption and may become pathologic when persistent. A persistent and unopposed hypermetabolic state may occur in severely injured children, is characterized by prolonged catabolism, and results in impaired healing and immunodeficiency. A shift in protein production to acute-phase proteins (α1-antitrypsin, C-reactive protein, complement components, fibrinogen, and haptoglobin, etc.) is common and appears to be mediated by cytokines, such as interleukin (IL)-1, IL-6, and IL-8 (6). Inflammation remote to the site of injury may occur and manifest as systemic inflammatory response syndrome and/or multiple organ dysfunction syndrome, although the incidence of these entities following trauma appears to be lower in children compared with adults (7).

Recently, attention has been focused on the contribution of genotype to trauma outcome. Many different genes are likely to modulate the stress response, improve healing, and reduce morbidity. This genetic contribution to post-traumatic inflammation is complex and difficult to study in the laboratory. The defense mechanisms utilized by cells in animal models include innate (as opposed to adaptive) immune components that appear to exert a powerful effect on outcome following inflammation and/or injury. Innate responses to inflammation and injury include many of the mediators and/or cascades noted previously, as well as toll-like receptors and the transcription factor known as nuclear factor (NF)-κB. Activation of both has been described in animal models following trauma, and evidence of NFκB activation in adults with severe trauma has been observed (8). Activation of NFκB results in the expression of hundreds of genes, including those responsible for the production of adhesion molecules, cytokines, immune recognition receptors, neutrophil adhesion receptors, and proteins involved in antigen presentation. These mediators (cytokines in particular) appear to be responsible for remote inflammation in the setting of major trauma and sepsis.

The production of various acute-phase proteins in the liver appears to be mediated by specific cytokines after activation and translocation of NFκB to the nucleus (**Fig. 30.3**): IL-1–like cytokines [IL-1α, IL-1β, tumor necrosis factor (TNF)-α, and TNF-β] are associated with the production of C-reactive protein and complement C3, whereas IL-6–like cytokines (IL-6, leukemia inhibitory factor, IL-11, and others) are associated with the production of fibrinogen, haptoglobin, α1-antitrypsin, etc. The various functions of these acute-phase proteins include bacterial killing and phagocytosis, thrombosis, and fibrinolysis, control of proteolysis, and various repair processes. These proteins work to restore homeostasis following inflammation or injury and are part of a carefully orchestrated response.

It is probable that trauma is, in large part, an inflammatory critical illness much like sepsis, and that both may be characterized by a vigorous cytokine response (9). As trauma victims often have diminished cellular and humoral immunity,

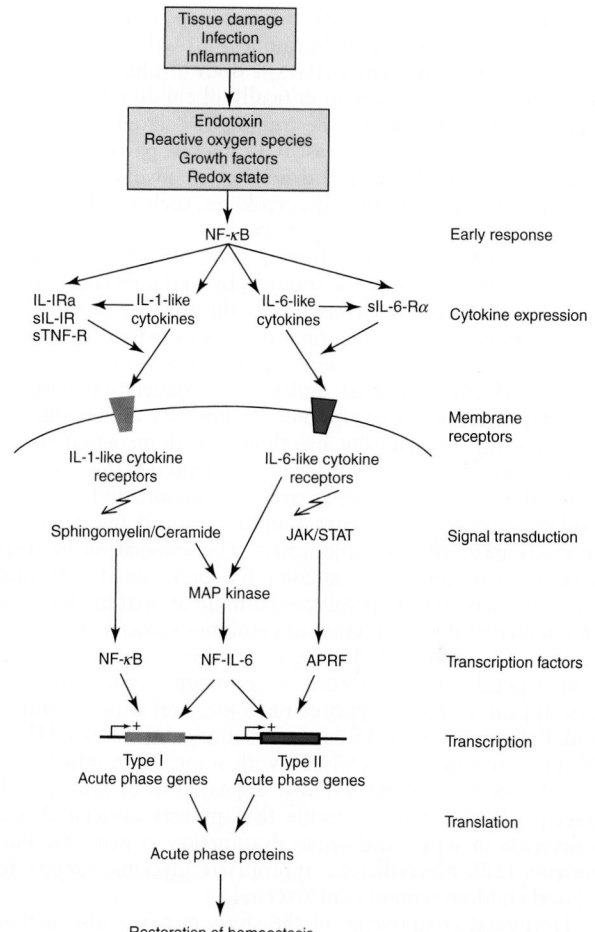

FIGURE 30.3. Main events leading to the acute-phase response in trauma, infection, or inflammation, including the role of NFκB and cytokines in the induction of protein translation. (From Moshage H. Cytokines and the hepatic acute phase response. *J Pathol* 1997;181:257–66.)

an increased risk of multiple organ dysfunction (even in organ systems remote from the site of injury), and other evidence of systemic inflammation, investigators have searched for a common cause. Cytokines participate in immunity, multiple organ dysfunction, and systemic inflammation: These low-molecular-weight proteins are extraordinarily potent and influence a broad range of cellular functions. The increase in cytokines following major trauma occurs locally at the site of injury (and perhaps in sites remote from injury) and often extends systemically to produce systemic inflammation. Recent evidence suggests that severity of injury (10–13), progression to multiorgan system failure (14), and mortality (13) are associated with plasma concentrations of IL-2, IL-6, and/or IL-8 that increase within hours of multiple trauma. Marked elevations in IL-6 have been noted in hemorrhage associated with trauma (15). As similar traumatic insults produce varied outcomes, it is likely that genetic polymorphisms at multiple alleles (particularly those involved in cytokine production) contribute to the variability in outcome. The developmental aspects that involve differences in these responses have not yet been explored. In addition, the hypothesis that excessive cytokine release following trauma may be maladaptive and contribute to worsening injury requires further investigation.

The trauma-associated hypermetabolic state in children involves a shift in the hormonal milieu from anabolic to catabolic mediators that include increases in cortisol, epinephrine, and glucagon concurrent with a decrease in activity of insulin and the somatotropic axis hormones (growth hormone and insulin-like growth factors [IGFs]). Both insulin and growth hormone resistance occur in critically ill children with major trauma and contribute to the trauma-associated hypermetabolic state. Antagonism against IGFs may be partially responsible for decreased levels and activity of insulin and cause insulin resistance. Additionally, cytokines, such as TNF-α, may further inhibit the somatotropic axis.

Stress hyperglycemia (serum glucose of >200 mg/dL) is common following pediatric trauma (16) and is related to insulin and growth hormone resistance in the presence of enhanced gluconeogenesis. An association appears to exist between hyperglycemia and poor outcome in adults with traumatic injury (17,18). Mechanisms that underlie the association between hyperglycemia and poor outcome are not fully understood, although a shift to anaerobic metabolism with increased lactate production and brain tissue acidosis, impaired neutrophil activation due to impaired superoxide production, and increased oxidant stress from the generation of advanced glycation end-products have all been implicated. The association between hyperglycemia and poor outcome has been noted with both early and persistent hyperglycemia. In an animal model, insulin attenuated the production of cytokines associated with the acute stress response following thermal injury (19). Children with hyperglycemia and burn or traumatic brain injury (20) also appear to have a poorer outcome, and insulin reduced both IL-1β and TNF-α 15 days after injury and increased IL-10 30 days after injury in children with severe burn injury (21). The change in cytokine response appeared to be unrelated to glycemic level. Intensive insulin therapy was associated with a decrease in sepsis and organ dysfunction in pediatric burn patients (22). Nevertheless, appropriate glycemic targets for injured children remain controversial.

Hormonal components of the stress response also include arginine vasopressin (AVP). The release of AVP from the posterior pituitary is stimulated by increasing plasma osmolality or declining extracellular fluid volume, the latter mediated via stretch receptors in the atria and the baroreceptor reflex arc. AVP release is more sensitive to small increases in plasma osmolality, but large declines in extracellular fluid volume produce rapid increases in AVP regardless of plasma osmolality. AVP release is also stimulated by factors associated with the stress response (dopamine, hypoxemia, and hypocapnia) as well as certain cytokines. Once released, AVP activates specific renal tubular receptors that are responsible for free water control, as well as vessel wall receptors responsible for the regulation of vasomotor tone. AVP release may result in the syndrome of inappropriate antidiuretic hormone following pediatric trauma, particularly head trauma (23) and result in water retention with hyponatremia in the absence of hypovolemia. Alternatively, AVP release may be deficient following pediatric head trauma, resulting in a dilute diuresis with hypernatremia-associated diabetes insipidus.

INITIAL ASSESSMENT AND STABILIZATION

Emergency Medical Services

Pediatric trauma resuscitation should begin as soon as possible after the injury, ideally through pediatric-capable emergency medical dispatchers who provide instructions to lay rescuers at the scene. It continues upon the arrival of prehospital professionals, including first responders, emergency medical technicians, and paramedics. During prehospital pediatric trauma care, the emphasis is on aggressive support of vital functions and is referred to as *the platinum half hour*.

The transport of critically injured children requires special expertise: paramedics who routinely perform these tasks receive extra pediatric training, as well as support from experienced physicians, nurses, and other health-care professionals. Additional support, which is essential for this type of service, includes an ongoing review of adverse events, equipment, personnel, policies, and procedures. Prehospital transport of critically injured children frequently presents a difficult decision for emergency medical personnel between "scoop and run" or "stay and play." Although a universal answer to this dilemma is not possible, it is clear that as time is spent at the trauma site, the "platinum half hour" ticks away and that delay should be avoided whenever possible. Transport between health-care facilities is often appropriate for injured children who require special medical expertise available at another hospital or as a component of regionalization of pediatric critical care. Some pediatric hospitals have established specialized teams for this type of interhospital transport of critically ill and injured patients. Private ambulance services with pediatric expertise in the prehospital or interhospital setting is an alternative in many communities. Yet, transport of critically injured children is not risk-free, because adverse events (obstruction of endotracheal tubes or loss of vascular access) occur (twice the rate during interhospital transport as in the pediatric intensive care unit (PICU) and 10 times more frequently with nonspecialized teams than with specialized teams). At a minimum, transport providers must be capable of critical pediatric assessment and monitoring, and they must be highly skilled in the techniques of pediatric endotracheal intubation, vascular access, as well as in fluid and drug administration in critically ill and injured children. Whenever possible, interhospital transport of such patients should be conducted by specialized pediatric transport teams staffed by physicians and nurses with special training.

Trauma Centers and Field Triage Recommendations

Trauma centers are hospitals with special expertise in trauma care, and *classification of trauma centers* is provided for centers verified by the American College of Surgeons. Trauma centers are classified as Level One (with the most comprehensive array of specialists and services, often located in large academic medical centers), Level Two (with most but not all of the specialists and services available in Level One), and Level Three (only core specialists and services are available; usually located in smaller community hospitals). In some states, pediatric trauma centers have also been designated and are similarly classified. Hospitals and clinics without trauma center designation (nontrauma centers) are still part of the regional trauma system and should be capable of routine resuscitation and stabilization of injured patients.

Severely injured children in the United States who are cared for in hospitals with a PICU or in pediatric trauma centers have an improved outcome (24,25). The common denominator for these sites is accumulated expertise caring for critically ill children, and this expertise is both essential and difficult to quantify. However, as few institutions possess the resources to provide such a level of care, the number of qualified centers is limited, even in larger metropolitan areas, where a full range of pediatric specialty services may be available at more than one institution. Referral of critically ill and injured children to qualified centers (i.e., regionalization) is a well-established practice, and critically injured children should undergo primary transport to these institutions wherever possible. However, not all injured children require the highest level of care: triage of less-severely injured children to local centers may help avoid overloading higher-level trauma centers and increase cost effectiveness. Recently revised triage guidelines (26) suggest abnormal vital signs and Glasgow Coma Scale (GCS) scores as early triage criteria sufficient for trauma center referral of injured children, though "when in doubt, transfer to a trauma center (26)." Regardless, every receiving hospital must be capable of initiating resuscitation and stabilizing critically injured children, and have transfer agreements in place with hospitals that have full pediatric capabilities. See Chapter 34 for a full discussion of mass casualty events.

Scoring

A global assessment that is represented by a single number and is capable of stratifying risk and survival following traumatic injury has long been a goal among trauma researchers. Current scoring systems include the Injury Severity Score and the Revised Trauma Score, although neither specifically addresses children. The GCS is used to assess gross neurologic status following injury (can be modified for infants and small children; see Chapter 61), while the Pediatric Risk of Mortality III and Pediatric Index of Mortality II are focused on the outcome of all patients admitted to a PICU.

The Pediatric Trauma Score (**Table 30.3**) is acceptable for field use to assess and predict outcome in critically injured children and is recognized by the American College of Surgeons Committee on Trauma and the American Pediatric Surgical Association Trauma Committee. A Pediatric Trauma Score of <9 is consistent with significant risk of mortality, and identifies patients with an Injury Severity Score of >9. However, the Pediatric Trauma Score has not consistently proven superior to other scores, particularly the Revised Trauma Score (**Table 30.4**). At present, reliance on anatomic, physiologic, and mechanistic criteria for primary transport to a trauma center with pediatric expertise is the currently preferred method for field triage of injured adults and children by the American College of Surgeons Committee on Trauma.

Primary Survey

The body regions most frequently injured in major childhood trauma are the head and neck, abdomen, and lower extremities, while in minor childhood injury, soft tissue and upper extremity injuries predominate. Because most pediatric trauma is blunt trauma that involves the head, it is primarily a disease of airway and breathing, rather than circulation, bleeding, or shock. While neuroventilatory derangements (abnormalities in

GCS and respiratory rate) are five times more common than hemodynamic derangements (abnormalities in blood pressure) in the children with significant mortality risk in the National Pediatric Trauma Registry, children with hemodynamic problems have double the mortality compared with those with neuroventilatory derangements. The primary survey (the ABCs: airway, breathing, and circulation with D added for disability/gross neurologic impairment and E for exposure/environment, see below) is vitally important in the evaluation and treatment of pediatric victims of multiple or severe trauma, and repeated evaluation is necessary. Resuscitation of the pediatric trauma victim and the primary survey are conducted concurrently using a continuous cycle of assessment, intervention, and reassessment.

The primary survey requires full exposure (i.e., undressing the injured child) to fully assess injury. In an environment at room temperature, children rapidly lose heat due to their large body surface area (relative to their body mass), their increased minute ventilation (heat effect of vaporization), and decreased subcutaneous tissue (for heat insulation) in young children. It is incumbent on the clinical team to prevent hypothermia in this setting, as it may further compromise control of hemorrhage and cardiorespiratory function.

Airway (and Cervical Spine Stabilization)

All else will be futile if the first step of trauma management, airway control, is ineffective. As a corollary, consideration of cervical spine stabilization is mandatory with this first step, and the best approach is a plan formulated well in advance. When tracheal intubation is required (for respiratory failure, airway protection, or hyperventilation), rapid-sequence oral–tracheal intubation using cervical spine protection is recommended (assume that patient has a full stomach). Tracheal intubation may also be necessary for the child in decompensated shock. Exceptions to this approach will be reviewed.

All patients undergoing a primary survey should receive supplemental oxygen with an FIO_2 of 1. An airway obstructed by soft tissues and secretions is opened (utilizing the modified jaw thrust maneuver with or without an oropharyngeal airway to displace the mandible) while proper cervical spine precautions are taken (maintaining the cervical spine in a neutral position with bimanual cervical spine stabilization, followed by application of a semirigid cervical extrication collar and long backboard). The airway is then cleared utilizing a

TABLE 30.3

TRAUMA SCORES COMMONLY USED IN CHILDREN: PEDIATRIC TRAUMA SCORE

■ POINTS	■ +2	■ +1	■ −1
Size (kg)	>20	10–20	<10
Airway	Normal	Maintained	Unmaintained
Systolic blood pressure (mm Hg)	>90	50–90	<50
Central nervous system (CNS)	Awake	Obtunded	Coma
Open wound	None	Minor	Major
Skeletal trauma	None	Closed	Open-Multiple

TABLE 30.4

TRAUMA SCORES COMMONLY USED IN CHILDREN: REVISED TRAUMA SCORE

■ POINTS	■ 4	■ 3	■ 2	■ 1	■ 0
Glasgow Coma Scale (GCS)	13–15	9–12	6–8	4–5	3
Systolic blood pressure (mm Hg)	>89	76–89	50–75	1–49	0
Respiratory rate (breaths/min)	10–29	>29	6–9	1–5	0

large-bore, Yankauer-type suction device, and assessment can proceed to the next step. A head tilt is avoided in patients with possible cervical spine injury. The larynx is more superior and anterior in children (see Chapter 24), and oral intubation can be difficult for those without pediatric experience.

Important considerations regarding pediatric endotracheal intubation include the following: (a) nasal intubation is contraindicated in patients with severe facial or head trauma (in particular those with cerebrospinal fluid leak) and blind tracheal intubation is discouraged; (b) trauma patients should be considered to have a full stomach, independent of their last documented meal, as gastric emptying time may be delayed in this setting; (c) children are more likely to develop respiratory failure than are adults with equivalent injury; (d) the patient's hemodynamic status will help to determine the most appropriate therapeutic approach; and (e) while uncuffed endotracheal tubes may be utilized, a cuffed endotracheal tube may reduce the need for tube changes due to size issues and may be indicated if respiratory compliance appears to be significantly diminished during bag valve mask ventilation. Noninvasive ventilation may be contraindicated in injured children with head, face, or neck injury. Finally, children are less tolerant of prolonged hypoxia; with full denitrogenation, an adult can sustain 4 minutes of apnea without hypoxia while infants may only tolerate 30 seconds of apnea because the infant's functional residual capacity is relatively smaller while oxygen consumption is greatly increased. Denitrogenation is thus essential in children and accomplished by prior administration of an F_{IO_2} of 1.

The details of pediatric rapid-sequence intubation, including appropriate medications and algorithms, are reviewed in Chapter 24. In most pediatric victims of multiple trauma, the indications, practice, and complications of endotracheal intubation are clear and easily understood. When endotracheal intubation is unsuccessful, or in patients with significant facial, head, neck, and/or airway injury, the laryngeal mask airway can be inserted blindly but has the limitation of not completely sealing the airway and is not as protective against aspiration. It can provide a temporary rescue until an alternative method of tracheal intubation is accomplished (videolaryngoscopic, fiber-optic, or surgical placement). Fiber-optic–assisted intubation may be helpful in patients with injury to the upper airway particularly as endoscopy is required for evaluation of suspected injury to the larynx, trachea, or bronchi.

Surgical approaches to establish an airway for trauma patients include needle and surgical cricothyroidotomy. A needle cricothyroidotomy is appropriate for trauma patients with upper airway obstruction (above the larynx) after failed orotracheal intubation or because significant upper airway injury renders an attempt at intubation futile, but it is contraindicated in the presence of laryngotracheal injury as it may exacerbate the injury. A needle cricothyroidotomy is merely a temporary expedient, and plans for the next step should be made concurrently. An emergent surgical cricothyroidotomy is indicated for trauma patients with significant laryngeal injury or following failed procedures to secure an airway; some practitioners also perform an urgent tracheostomy for acute, posttraumatic asphyxia. Adequate support for both procedures in a setting outside the operating room is essential, as it is very easy to lose the airway due to hemorrhage, edema, subcutaneous air, or relaxation of muscle tone following anesthesia.

Breathing

As soon as a patent airway is assured, the patient should continue to receive an F_{IO_2} of 1. If ventilation is inadequate, positive-pressure ventilation (PPV) assistance should be offered. Inadequate ventilation is characterized by decreased breath sounds, an abnormal respiratory pattern, and clinical evidence of hypercarbia (including an increase in sympathetic tone, which may be unappreciated in the setting of major trauma). Hypercarbia may rise rapidly without obvious signs, although decreased

responsiveness is the rule. Hypoxia prevention can include titration of the F_{IO_2} to maintain an oxygen saturation of ~95%.

Laboratory examinations, often helpful in this setting, should not be relied upon to determine therapy; a chest radiograph or even an arterial blood gas level generally confirms what is clinically obvious. Waiting for the chest radiograph to drain a tension pneumothorax (indicated by decreased breath sounds, deviated trachea, progressive respiratory distress, and hemodynamic compromise) in a patient with multiple trauma is not helpful. Nor is it helpful to rely on the arterial blood gas level to decide whether to intubate a patient; that decision is based on the clinical appearance of the patient's ability to adequately exchange gas and on the need to maintain and protect the airway.

Ensuring adequate minute ventilation and oxygenation during PPV for children of various ages involves making appropriate decisions during stressful situations about technology that changes often. It is essential that pediatric intensivists be involved in the prescription for mechanical ventilation early in the course. Age-appropriate initial settings are reviewed in Chapter 38.

Circulation

Attention devoted to the maintenance of adequate circulation will help attenuate the stress response and may prevent delayed inflammatory complications of major trauma. The basic steps in the management of hemorrhagic shock are control of active hemorrhage, placement of intravascular access, and appropriate volume replacement or resuscitation.

Control of Active Hemorrhage. Most children in hypotensive shock following traumatic injury are victims of uncontrolled hemorrhage, which can be reversed only if promptly recognized and appropriately treated. Potential sites of unrecognized hemorrhage include those body cavities large enough to sequester significant volumes of blood (hemithorax, retroperitoneum, pelvis, thigh compartments). Control of active hemorrhage involves the principles of hemostasis, which have not changed in several decades and include as the first and most important step direct pressure over all actively bleeding wounds.

Tourniquets and Traumatic Amputation. Current military experience suggests a role for tourniquets in control of exsanguinating hemorrhage from a traumatic amputation (27). The use of tourniquets on the battlefield is associated with decreased mortality and no increase in limb amputations. Their use after the onset of shock was less helpful and as a result, prehospital use is recommended (27). A recent review of a military trauma registry, which included pediatric trauma victims, suggested a similar role in severely injured children (28). Military antishock trousers are unlikely to be useful.

Trauma-Associated Coagulopathy. Coagulopathies in injured children are typically related to dilution of platelet and plasma coagulation factors during extensive resuscitation and massive transfusion, although hypothermia and acidosis may also contribute. Massive transfusion is generally defined in adults as transfusion of >10 units of packed red blood cells (PRBC) over a 24 hours *or* transfusion of >4 units of PBRC over 1 hour with ongoing uncontrolled bleeding (see also Chapter 42). The definition of massive transfusion in children is more complex, because the estimated blood volume (EBV) varies with size such that:

- Term infant EBV: 80–90 mL/kg
- Child >3 months EBV: 70 mL/kg
- Adult EBV: 60–65 mL/kg

Hence, Diab et al. (29) define massive transfusion in children as:

- Transfusion of >50% EBV over 3 hours, or
- Transfusion 100% EBV of 24 hours, or
- Transfusion to replace ongoing blood loss at >10% EBV per minute.

The following developments frame the current approach to trauma-associated coagulopathy:

1. The military experience with massive transfusion after multiple trauma has suggested early administration of fresh frozen plasma (FFP) and platelets in ratios of ~1:1:1 for packed red cells:FFP:platelets. This is part of an approach known as damage-control resuscitation (DCR) that relies on a formal massive transfusion protocol (MTP) (30).
2. Most trauma centers have adopted MTPs to organize the responses of the trauma team and the blood bank with the goal of preventing significant coagulopathy following massive transfusion.
3. It is unknown whether MTP with early FFP and platelet administration improves outcomes in children. Two small pediatric series showed no effect of MTP on outcome (31,32).

The DCR/MTP approach grew out of experience with combat casualties who required massive transfusions and suggested that a 1.4:1 ratio of PRBC:FFP was associated with a lower mortality rate compared to less vigorous use of FFP (33). Other studies suggested that the outcome of trauma patients requiring massive transfusion may be improved utilizing protocols that emphasize empiric replacement of FFP and platelets with a ratio of 1:1:1 (PRBC:FFP:platelets) (34). This approach in injured children with massive, exsanguinating hemorrhage is reasonable, although appropriately powered studies are still needed to assess the impact of the DCR/MTP approach on survival in children. MTPs have varied widely among institutions. **Figure 30.4** shows an example of one institution's MTP for children (35).

The threshold platelet count that should mandate platelet transfusion in a bleeding child remains controversial. Nevertheless, it is appropriate to begin a platelet transfusion, when the

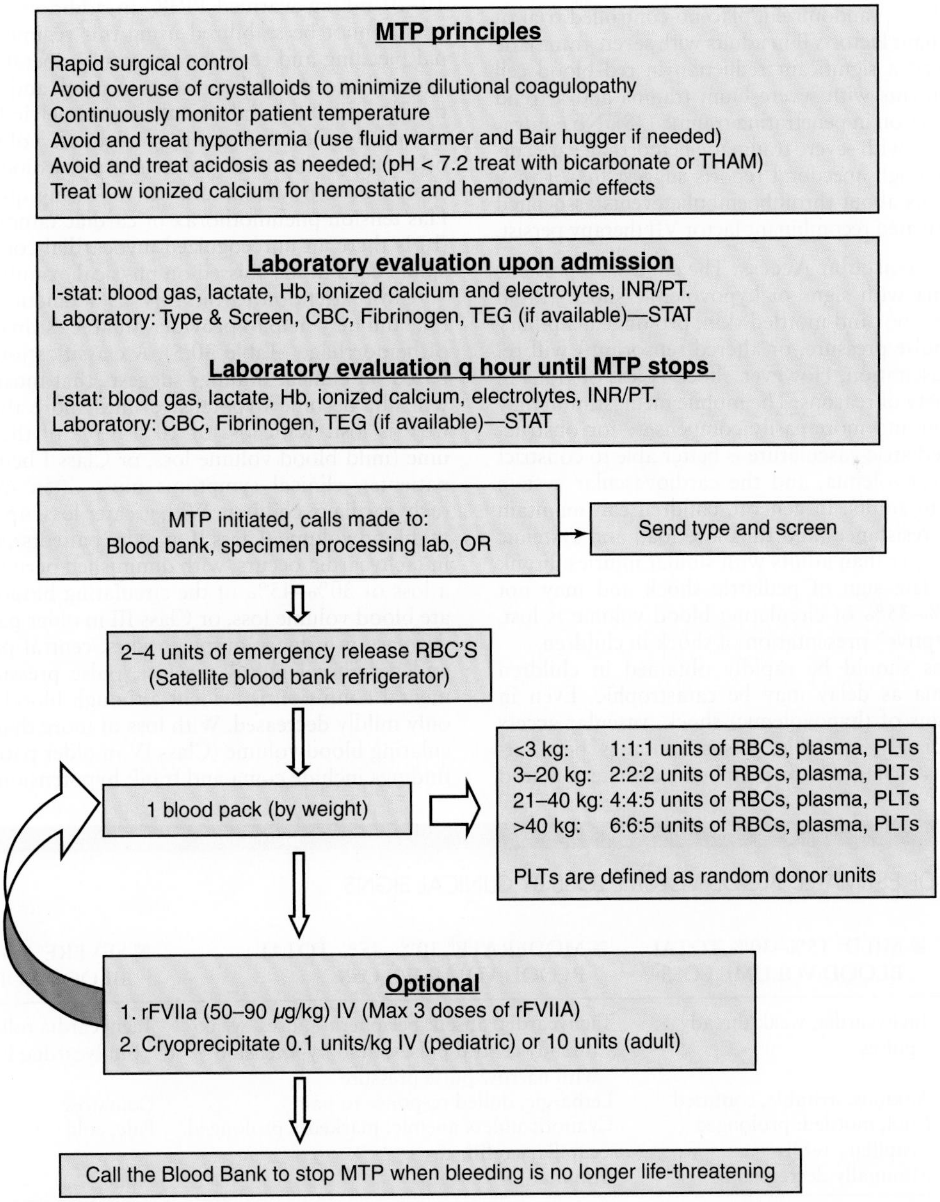

MTP principles

Rapid surgical control
Avoid overuse of crystalloids to minimize dilutional coagulopathy
Continuously monitor patient temperature
Avoid and treat hypothermia (use fluid warmer and Bair hugger if needed)
Avoid and treat acidosis as needed; (pH < 7.2 treat with bicarbonate or THAM)
Treat low ionized calcium for hemostatic and hemodynamic effects

Laboratory evaluation upon admission

I-stat: blood gas, lactate, Hb, ionized calcium and electrolytes, INR/PT.
Laboratory: Type & Screen, CBC, Fibrinogen, TEG (if available)—STAT

Laboratory evaluation q hour until MTP stops

I-stat: blood gas, lactate, Hb, ionized calcium, electrolytes, INR/PT.
Laboratory: CBC, Fibrinogen, TEG (if available)—STAT

MTP initiated, calls made to:
Blood bank, specimen processing lab, OR → Send type and screen

2–4 units of emergency release RBC'S
(Satellite blood bank refrigerator)

1 blood pack (by weight)

<3 kg: 1:1:1 units of RBCs, plasma, PLTs
3–20 kg: 2:2:2 units of RBCs, plasma, PLTs
21–40 kg: 4:4:5 units of RBCs, plasma, PLTs
>40 kg: 6:6:5 units of RBCs, plasma, PLTs

PLTs are defined as random donor units

Optional
1. rFVIIa (50–90 μg/kg) IV (Max 3 doses of rFVIIA)
2. Cryoprecipitate 0.1 units/kg IV (pediatric) or 10 units (adult)

Call the Blood Bank to stop MTP when bleeding is no longer life-threatening

FIGURE 30.4. Massive Transfusion Protocol for Children. The protocol calls for the sequential administration of "packages" of blood products that contain packed red cells, fresh frozen plasma, and platelets in approximately 1:1:1 ratios. THAM, tris-hydroxymethyl aminomethane; MTP, massive transfusion protocol; CBC, complete blood count; TEG, thromboelastogram; RBCs, red blood cells. (From Dressler AM, Finck CM, Carroll CL, et al. Use of a massive transfusion protocol with hemostatic resuscitation for severe intraoperative bleeding in a child. *J Pediatr Surg* 2010;45:1530–3. With permission.)

platelet count falls below 50,000–100,000/mm^3 in a trauma patient with massive bleeding. A general guideline is to administer 6 whole blood-derived platelet units to an adult or 0.1–0.2 units/kg to a child. Empiric platelet and FFP transfusions should be considered when massive transfusion is diagnosed and the MTP is activated. Laboratory tests of the coagulation system (the prothrombin time, partial thromboplastin time, and platelet count) are used to guide replacement therapy but blood product administration should not be delayed in the massively bleeding, unstable patient. The thromboelastogram or rotational thromboelastometry are point-of-care assays that graphically represent the entire hemostatic system and may allow timely, goal-directed treatment of trauma-associated coagulopathy (29).

In addition to the replacement of coagulation components and avoiding the inhibition of coagulation factors, both aminocaproic acid and activated factor VII are useful in selected patients. Aminocaproic acid has been used successfully in injured children to control hemorrhage associated with severe head injury (36) or extracorporeal membrane oxygenation (ECMO) (37). A large, randomized, placebo-controlled trial of activated recombinant factor VII in adults with severe traumatic hemorrhage showed a significant reduction in red blood cell transfusions in patients with severe blunt trauma and a trend to transfusion reduction in penetrating trauma (38). No equivalent trials in children with severe traumatic hemorrhage are currently available, though anecdotal reports suggest that it may be helpful. Concerns about thromboembolic events associated with the use of activated recombinant factor VII therapy persist.

Placement of Intravascular Access. The child who presents with major trauma with signs of hypovolemic shock (rapid and thready pulse, cool and mottled skin, prolonged capillary refill, decreased pulse pressure, or altered sensorium) will require volume resuscitation. However, shock is less obvious in children for a variety of reasons: The mobile mediastinum may shift under tension and more easily compensate for obstructive lesions, the pediatric vasculature is better able to constrict in response to hypovolemia, and the cardiovascular system is healthier than in adults. In general, children can maintain systemic vascular resistance (and thus afterload and systemic blood pressure) longer than adults with similar injuries. Frank hypotension is a late sign of pediatric shock and may not develop until 30%–35% of circulating blood volume is lost, leading to a "deceptive" presentation of shock in children.

Vascular access should be rapidly obtained in children with major trauma as delay may be catastrophic. Even in the absence of signs of (hypovolemic) shock, vascular access should be immediately available. Resuscitation is best carried out by means of large-bore peripheral catheters placed percutaneously in median antecubital veins at the elbow or saphenous veins at the ankle. In the event that access cannot be established rapidly in younger children, intraosseous access may be utilized. Access by central venous catheter in the femoral, internal jugular, or subclavian veins or by cutdown in the ankle or groin is helpful during resuscitation if experienced operators are immediately available and other means of vascular access are inadequate. Femoral or saphenous vein (lower extremity) intravenous catheters may not be helpful in children with abdominal trauma (due to vascular disruption or abdominal compartment syndrome), and upper body sites are preferred in those cases. Following acute resuscitation, arterial and central venous catheterization is indicated for children with ongoing cardiorespiratory compromise.

Volume Replacement. Simple hypovolemia usually responds to 20–40 mL/kg of warmed isotonic solution, but frank hypotension (clinically diagnosed by a systolic blood pressure <70 mm Hg plus twice the age in years) typically requires 10–20 mL/kg warmed PRBC in addition. Any injured child who cannot be stabilized using this regimen likely has internal bleeding and requires emergency operation for control of hemorrhage. If a child presents in shock and has no signs of intrathoracic, intra-abdominal, or intrapelvic bleeding, but fails to improve despite seemingly adequate volume resuscitation, other forms of shock (obstructive, cardiogenic, neurogenic) should be considered, and the following questions asked: (a) Has tension pneumothorax or cardiac tamponade developed? (b) Is there an unrecognized myocardial contusion? (c) Was a spinal cord injury missed on physical examination?

Close attention to the EBV as a function of size is essential, and may help to provide valuable estimates of the severity of hemorrhage (Table 30.5). A classification of hypovolemia based on clinical findings suggests that most injured children will not become hypotensive until more than 30% of their EBV is lost. With loss of 10%–15% of the total blood volume (mild blood volume loss, or Class I hemorrhage in older patients), clinical symptoms most often include only mild tachycardia in children. With greater loss, up to 30% of the total blood volume (Class II in older patients), a further increase in tachycardia occurs, with diminished peripheral pulses. With a loss of 30%–45% of the circulating blood volume (moderate blood volume loss, or Class III in older patients), a marked decrease in urinary output occurs, central pulses are thready and peripheral pulses are lost, pulse pressure narrows, and mental confusion is evident although blood pressure may be only mildly decreased. With loss of more than 45% of the circulating blood volume (Class IV in older patients), the clinical findings include coma and frank hypotension.

TABLE 30.5

CLASSIFICATION OF ESTIMATED BLOOD VOLUME LOSS BY CLINICAL SIGNS

■ SYSTEM	■ MILD^a 15%–30% TOTAL BLOOD VOLUME LOSS	■ MODERATE^b 30%–45% TOTAL BLOOD VOLUME LOSS	■ SEVERE^c >45% TOTAL BLOOD VOLUME LOSS
Cardiovascular	Tachycardia, weak/thready pulses	Tachycardia, absent peripheral pulses, weak/thready central pulses; mild hypotension with narrow pulse pressure	Tachycardia followed by bradycardia; hypotension
Neurologic	Anxious, irritable, confused	Lethargic, dulled response to pain	Comatose
Skin	Cool, mottled; prolonged capillary refill	Cyanotic unless anemic; markedly prolonged capillary refill	Pale, cold
Urine output	Minimally decreased	Minimal	None

^{a}Corresponds to Class I/II blood loss in adults.
^{b}Corresponds approximately to Class III blood loss in adults.
^{c}Corresponds approximately to Class IV blood loss in adults.
Adapted from American College of Surgeons Committee on Trauma. *Advanced Trauma Life Support Program for Doctors.* 7th ed. Chicago: American College of Surgeons Committee on Trauma, 2004.

The ongoing controversy regarding colloid versus crystalloid resuscitation fluids has abated somewhat in the last few years. Meta-analyses of trials in critically ill (mostly adult) patients (39,40) suggest that outcome following resuscitation with albumin or other colloid solutions is no different when compared to crystalloid solutions. In addition, studies in young trauma patients treated with colloids or crystalloids showed no differences in the development of pulmonary edema or in pulmonary dysfunction. Crystalloid solutions are generally cheaper than colloids and immediately available are popular for the initial resuscitation of injured children. However, an animal model of hemorrhagic shock suggests that resuscitation with albumin is associated with lower levels of inflammatory cytokines in the lungs and the circulation (41), as well as a decrease in lung apoptosis (42), compared to resuscitation with lactated Ringer's solution. In addition, the possibility that infusion of a colloid solution could more rapidly restore the adequacy of circulation (perhaps in specific subgroups with shock) remains a tantalizing prospect, and the use of colloid solutions in trauma resuscitation is not likely to disappear soon. In any case, severe exsanguinating hemorrhage mandates blood product replacement, and volume replacement with crystalloid in these patients may contribute to trauma-associated coagulopathy.

Resuscitation with hypotonic solution is contraindicated for several reasons: (a) excess free water will exacerbate edema formation, particularly in the central nervous system (CNS); (b) subsequent changes in osmolality are poorly tolerated in critically ill patients; and (c) blood products and other parenteral medications may not be compatible with these solutions.

Isotonic crystalloid solutions commonly utilized for resuscitations (often while blood products are being prepared) include normal saline and lactated Ringer's solution. The excessive use of normal saline may lead to a hyperchloremic metabolic acidosis, which can obscure underlying metabolic acidosis secondary to hypoperfusion. The lactate in lactated Ringer's solution is metabolized by the liver to bicarbonate; therefore, this solution provides a buffer, so long as hepatic function remains intact. In patients with severe hepatic injury, it may be reasonable to limit lactate intake. Plasmalyte is another isotonic solution that provides buffer as acetate and gluconate, although it may not be available at some sites.

Hypertonic saline may offer some benefits in hemorrhagic shock, including a redistribution of extracellular water due to tonicity changes; as hypertonic saline increases extracellular fluid osmolality, a tonicity gradient helps to pull water from the intracellular compartment. In animal models, hemodynamic effects include an improvement in inotropy (43,44), as well as less neutrophil activation and less gut and lung injury compared to that with lactated Ringer's solution (45,46). Even small volumes of hypertonic saline may be helpful in this regard, and the concept of small-volume hyperosmolar resuscitation may have utility in pediatric trauma. In some patients with multiple trauma, including neurologic injury, the judicious use of hypertonic (3%) saline may therefore be appropriate, although data from large clinical trials are not yet available, nor are extensive clinical data in children without neurologic injury, and appropriate limits for extracellular osmolality are still controversial. It is also likely that an equivalent amount of chloride from 3% saline contributes equally to the development of hyperchloremic metabolic acidosis, similar to that occurring with normal saline. Reliance on hypertonic saline to the exclusion of isotonic resuscitation fluids is not supported at this time.

Albumin (molecular weight: 69 kDa) is a naturally occurring plasma protein that provides ~80% of the intravascular colloid oncotic pressure. It is a human blood product, although heat treated; therefore, it is not associated with infectious disease risks. Both 5% and 25% (or "salt-poor") albumin have been used in the resuscitation of pediatric trauma patients;

5% albumin is preferred for acute resuscitation. Other colloid solutions include 6% hydroxyethyl starch and low-molecular-weight dextran (the latter agent is seldom used in the trauma setting, because it induces platelet dysfunction, interferes with cross-matching of blood, and may be filtered by the renal tubules, leading to renal failure). Hydroxyethyl starch is a synthetic colloid that consists of a hydroxyethyl-substituted, branched-chain amylopectin with a molecular weight of 69 kDa. Although its elimination half-life is 17 days, in clinical practice, it expands the plasma volume for only 24–36 hours. Adverse effects include an inhibition of platelet aggregation following the administration of more than 15–20 mL/kg.

The treatment of hemorrhagic shock must include transfusion of blood products, particularly in patients with moderate to severe blood volume loss (i.e., Class III and Class IV in older patients). The hematocrit of a unit of PRBC will depend on the anticoagulant used. With citrate phosphate dextrose, the average hematocrit is 65%–75%, whereas the more commonly used adenine anticoagulants are associated with hematocrits of 50%–60%. In the emergent resuscitative phase of therapy in Class III and Class IV patients, time may not allow a full type and cross-match to be accomplished before transfusion. When using uncross-matched blood, it is best to obtain at least an ABO and Rh type and partial cross-match. If time does not permit even a preliminary screen, ABO and Rh type-specific, uncross-matched blood is still preferable (and more abundant) to type O-negative, Rh-negative, uncross-matched blood. In the absence of type-specific blood, the latter can be used, although cross-matching may still be helpful to ensure the absence of A and/or B antibodies. Blood warmers should be used whenever possible, especially if the delivered fluid volume is great or if the patient is small. Several types of fluid warmers are available, and they are often found in the operating room. The use of blood replacement products, such as stroma-free hemoglobin and human polymerized hemoglobin, holds great promise and possible benefit in adult hemorrhagic shock; however, their use in children is still investigational.

Although the majority of patients will respond to timely intravascular repletion of volume and hemoglobin, some severely injured patients in Class III and/or Class IV have persistent perfusion defects that will not correct without immediate surgical intervention.

Disability (Abbreviated Neurologic Exam)

Assessment of disability and the neurologic status completes the primary survey ("ABCD") and includes ascertainment of the GCS (to assess level of consciousness), the pupillary responses (to exclude mass lesions), and evidence of an altered mental status. Traumatic coma (GCS ≤8) and pupillary asymmetry mandate immediate involvement of neurosurgical consultants. It is important to make at least a preliminary assessment of the neurologic status while the severely injured patient is being prepared for endotracheal intubation, although this exercise should not divert the clinician; rather, a few seconds should be sufficient to make a mental note of the pupillary responses and GCS. Documentation can wait, but cannot be ignored, since serial measurements of GCS are no less valuable than the initial measurement.

Monitoring Resuscitation

Resuscitation proceeds concurrently with continuous reevaluation at this stage, and the most sensitive monitors of adequate circulation in children include the vital signs, perfusion, filling pressures, and urinary output. Although noninvasive monitoring (e.g., SpO$_2$, ETCO$_2$) will suffice for many patients, the use of invasive monitoring may be warranted in selected patients. However, continuous reassessment by a knowledgeable and observant bedside physician will still be needed to guide resuscitation.

The most sensitive monitor of cardiac output and volume status in a child is the heart rate. The adequacy of circulation is assessed by noting the quality, rate, and regularity of the pulse and secondarily by obtaining the blood pressure. Progressively weakening central pulses, particularly with other signs of poor perfusion, suggest an impending cardiac arrest. On the other hand, bounding peripheral pulses with an active precordium do not guarantee that all is well in patients with a stress response following severe trauma. Respiratory rates in children generally require careful assessment, as a cursory examination over a few seconds is likely to miss periods of apnea, intermittent distress, or progressive deterioration. A respiratory rate of 25 per minute is inappropriately low in the injured infant, while a respiratory rate of 50 per minute is inappropriately high in the injured adolescent. Blood pressure may be normal despite a 25%–30% loss of total blood volume. Nevertheless, beat-to-beat monitoring of blood pressure via an intra-arterial catheter is an important component of pediatric intensive care, and such catheters provide ready access for blood sampling.

The perfusion of distal extremities is monitored by assessing capillary refill and skin turgor and by looking for cyanosis or other signs of circulatory embarrassment. A capillary refill greater than 2 seconds suggests poor distal perfusion. Adequate lighting is essential to detect such findings, as is maintenance of normal body temperature.

The central venous pressure may be a helpful marker of intravascular volume, particularly in patients with extensive fluid resuscitation. It is measured from a catheter within the vena cava, as near to the right atrium as possible and, when measured at end-expiration/end-diastole, offers a good estimate of right atrial and right ventricular pressure (in the absence of pericardial or other cardiovascular disease). Although a single determination of central venous pressure may not accurately reflect effective circulating blood volume, repeated determinations, particularly following carefully monitored fluid boluses, may more accurately reflect filling pressure and blood volume. The *Weil criteria* for central venous pressure change with hypovolemia following intravascular fluid bolus therapy, also known as the "2–5 rule," may be helpful in deciding when to offer further volume resuscitation: If the response to a fluid bolus within 10 minutes of starting the bolus is an increase in central venous pressure of <2 mm Hg or >5 mm Hg, it is continued or discontinued, respectively (47). A flow-directed, balloon-tipped pulmonary artery catheter to measure pulmonary capillary wedge pressure (potentially a good estimate of left atrial pressure) may offer a survival benefit in the most severely injured adult trauma patients (48).

Urinary output should be measured in all seriously injured children as an indicator of renal perfusion, because this may be a surrogate for tissue perfusion of other vital organs. As such, urinary output provides a valuable marker for the adequacy of fluid resuscitation. Hourly trends are more important and clinically relevant than average daily results and should be at least 1–2 mL/kg/h in infants and younger children and at least 0.5–1 mL/kg/h in older children and adolescents. Hourly output may vary due to technologic issues, and attention must be paid to ensure accuracy. Leaking around catheters is common, and measurement of fluid losses in wet clothing and sheets improves accuracy. Occasionally, sediment occludes the small catheters utilized in infants and children, and catheter flushes with small amounts of sterile saline may be helpful. Placement of a urinary catheter via the transurethral route should be deferred in patients with urethral injury, including those with pelvic fractures and/or gross hematuria.

Urinary output and other clinical markers, including the vital signs, may not always permit discrimination between those with compensated and uncompensated shock, or allow recognition of adequate volume resuscitation. Additional helpful markers of adequate resuscitation include mixed venous oxygen saturation, arterial lactate concentration, and the base deficit. These should be measured serially and trended to provide the most information. Lack of improvement in arterial lactate concentration and/or base deficit despite appropriate volume resuscitation may indicate ongoing hemorrhage and increased risk of mortality.

SECONDARY SURVEY

Complete History and Physical Examination

Once the primary survey is complete, resuscitation is ongoing, and shock is being effectively treated, a secondary survey is undertaken for the definitive evaluation of the injured child. The primary survey and associated resuscitation efforts should be well advanced within 15 minutes of arrival in the trauma resuscitation area. The secondary survey consists of a "SAMPLE" history (*symptoms, allergies, medications, past illnesses, last meal, events,* and *environment*) and a complete head-to-toe examination that addresses all body regions and organ systems, along with a complete history of the injury. Continued reassessment and resuscitation must proceed concurrent to the secondary survey. The examination should be targeted to the head and neck (for any history of blunt injury above the clavicles, alteration in level of consciousness, or neck pain or swelling), to the chest (for any history of chest pain, noisy or rapid breathing, respiratory insufficiency, or hemoptysis), and to the abdomen (for any history of abdominal pain, bruising or tenderness, distention, pelvic instability, or vomiting, especially if the emesis is stained with blood or bile). In examining the child, the physician's first responsibility is to identify life-threatening injuries that may have been overlooked during the primary survey, such as tension pneumothorax, massive hemothorax (unilaterally decreased breath sounds with dullness to percussion and a displaced trachea), and gastric dilatation (upper abdominal distention with hyperresonance to percussion).

Any drainage from the nose or ears or any evidence of midface instability suggests the presence of a basilar skull fracture (which precludes the passage of a nasogastric tube) or an oromaxillofacial fracture (which may compromise the airway). *Hemotympanum* or *Battle sign* (post-auricular ecchymosis) points toward a basilar skull fracture. A neurologic examination as complete as circumstances allow should be performed. Following the lateral cervical spine radiograph (omitted acutely if it distracts from ongoing resuscitation, so long as the cervical spine is protected), the neck is examined for tenderness, swelling, torticollis, or spasm, suggesting the presence of a cervical spine fracture (which may not be detected on lateral cervical spine films, i.e., *spinal cord injury without radiologic abnormality,* or *SCIWORA*). The trachea should be midline, and the large vessels of the neck examined. A chest that discloses (a) point tenderness, palpable bony deformity, crepitus, or subcutaneous emphysema (on inspection or palpation); (b) inadequate chest rise or air entry (on auscultation or percussion); or (c) asymmetry in excursion suggests the presence of a rib fracture or air or blood in the thorax (mandating a search for a pneumothorax or hemothorax). Muffled or distant heart sounds with jugular venous distention may suggest cardiac tamponade (although jugular venous distention may be difficult to detect if the child has a short, fat neck; it may also be absent with concurrent hypovolemia). An abdomen that remains distended following gastric decompression suggests the presence of intra-abdominal bleeding (most often from the spleen or liver) or a disrupted hollow viscus (especially if fever, tenderness, or guarding is found together with abdominal distention or nasogastric aspirate stained with blood or bile).

All skeletal components should be palpated for evidence of instability or discontinuity, especially bony prominences (such as the anterior superior iliac spines), which are commonly injured in major blunt trauma. In the absence of obvious deformities, fractures should be suspected if bony point tenderness (or hematoma or spasm of overlying muscles), an unstable pelvic girdle, or perineal swelling or discoloration is appreciated. Most long-bone fractures will be self-evident, but such injuries are occasionally missed during the secondary survey, emphasizing the need to assume that a fracture is present on the basis of history alone (even if no deformity is obvious) until proven otherwise; in addition, frequent reexamination of all injured extremities for evidence of pain, pallor, pulselessness, paresthesias, and paralysis (the classic signs of associated vascular trauma, or, when advanced, compartmental hypertension) is necessary. The back should be completely examined. Appropriate components of the secondary survey should be repeated at intervals.

Laboratory Examinations

Although screening laboratory examinations may be of limited value in injured children, they are an integral part of the secondary survey, and their utility increases with severity of injury. Selected laboratory examinations may serve to provide early warning to the treating physician of impending deterioration, especially when physical findings are minor or questionable. Arterial blood gases are of paramount importance in determining the adequacy of ventilation ($PaCO_2$), oxygenation (PaO_2), and perfusion (base deficit), although the critically important determinant of blood oxygen content and, hence, tissue oxygen delivery (assuming the PaO_2 exceeds 60 mm Hg) is the blood hemoglobin concentration. Serial hematocrits (obtained at regular intervals until the patient is stable) are essential to the management of severely injured children, as is a type and cross-match sent as early as possible from the emergency department. In the presence of abdominal injury or occult hemorrhage, elevation in serum transaminases, amylase, and lipase suggests injury to the liver or pancreas; the infrequency of pancreatic injury makes the latter far less cost effective than the former. Coagulopathy is common in children with extensive resuscitation or traumatic brain injury, and a screen that includes the prothrombin time and partial thromboplastin time should be performed in these patients. Urinalysis should be performed on children with suspected abdominal injury; urine that is grossly bloody or is positive for blood by dipstick (myoglobin may yield false-positive results) or microscopy (20 or more red blood cells per high-power field) suggests renal trauma and possible damage to adjacent organs (high incidence of associated injuries). A pregnancy test is advisable for injured adolescent females. Point-of-care laboratory examinations may be particularly helpful, because results are immediately available and, when appropriately chosen, likely to be clinically relevant.

Radiologic examinations are an integral part of the secondary survey. Arrangements should be made, before plain films are ordered, to obtain CT scans, as indicated. Once the CT scans are completed, the required plain films are obtained. However, at no time should imaging studies take precedence over resuscitation from life-threatening injuries, an unstable patient be taken to the radiology department, or the physician and nurse fail to accompany and continuously monitor a critically injured child. CT scans of the head should be obtained whenever the patient has suffered a loss of consciousness or neurologic injury is suspected. To the extent that hemodynamic stability permits, CT scans of the abdomen should be obtained in the presence of signs of internal bleeding (abdominal tenderness, distention, bruising, or gross hematuria), a

history of hypotensive shock (which has responded to volume resuscitation), penetrating injury, or major trauma. Children with severe, multiple trauma that prevents a complete physical examination will benefit from routine CT of the head, thorax, abdomen, and pelvis (normal results do not exclude injury); spiral or helical CT scanners in this setting may allow for optimal use of IV contrast, given the increased rapidity and resolution of such scans.

Angiography, often following preliminary identification of such injury by CT, is appropriate for further study of injuries to large vessels in selected patients. Interventional radiologists may then be able to offer an alternative to surgical intervention, including embolization or stenting. When interventional radiology procedures are not advisable, such information obtained by angiography may still prove helpful for vascular surgical intervention.

Although the incidence of SCIWORA (almost exclusively a pediatric diagnosis and uncommon even when originally described several decades ago) is low, it is a frequent cause of spinal cord injury in children. SCIWORA is a result of high-energy injuries, usually associated with automobile accidents, and is characterized by normal radiographic studies (either plain films or CT scans) with demonstrable defects on MRI. In some children with SCIWORA, a delayed clinical presentation of neurologic injury occurs, and the optimal time for MRI following such injury is still unknown.

Focused assessment by sonography in trauma (FAST) may be useful in detecting intra-abdominal blood, with the additional advantage that assessments can be performed serially at the patient's bedside. The role of FAST in the diagnosis of abdominal injury is likely to increase, while the role of diagnostic peritoneal lavage decreases. However, FAST is not yet sufficiently reliable to exclude abdominal injury. A detailed sonographic examination may be useful for those cases in which intra-abdominal injury is suspected and CT cannot be obtained, either due to lack of equipment, a history of allergy to iodinated contrast agents, or pregnancy. Echocardiography is often helpful in the evaluation of thoracic injury, because it may reveal anatomic or functional cardiovascular injury or injury adjacent to cardiovascular structures.

MANAGEMENT

The management of pediatric trauma is the responsibility not of a single individual or specialty, but of a multidisciplinary team of pediatric-capable health professionals. It continues with the secondary survey and frequent reevaluation of vital functions and concludes with rehabilitation. It encompasses the operative, critical, acute, and convalescent phases of care. Avoidance of secondary injury (injury due to persistent or recurrent hypoxia or hypoperfusion) is a major goal and mandates reliance on continuous monitoring.

Any child who requires resuscitation should initially receive no oral intake because of the temporary paralytic ileus that often accompanies major blunt abdominal trauma, and because general anesthesia may later be required. However, isotonic IV fluid should be administered at a maintenance rate, presuming both normal hydration at the time of the injury and normalization of both vital signs and perfusion status following resuscitation. Gastric tube decompression and a urinary catheter should be placed unless proscribed by signs of a craniofacial or pelvic fracture, respectively.

With few exceptions, hypotensive pediatric trauma patients require immediate operation, while nonoperative management of blunt visceral trauma is most often successful. Penetrating injuries of the head, neck, and abdomen also require surgical intervention, but most intrathoracic injuries, whether blunt or penetrating, require only tube thoracostomy. Resuscitative emergency department thoracotomy has a dismal outcome in children, and is no longer routinely performed. Survival approaches zero for blunt trauma with cardiac arrest at any point during resuscitation, and for penetrating trauma with cardiac arrest and absent signs of life in the field or in the emergency department. Emergency thoracotomy in the operating room is also rarely performed in children, except for massive hemothorax (20 mL/kg), ongoing hemorrhage (2–4 mL/kg/h) from the chest tube, and persistent massive air leak or food or salivary drainage from the chest tube. Laparotomy is always required for gunshot wounds to the abdomen, as well as for penetrating abdominal injury associated with hemorrhagic shock, peritonitis, or evisceration. Thoracoabdominal injury should be suspected (a) whenever the torso is penetrated between the nipple line and the umbilicus (anteriorly) or the costal margin (posteriorly), (b) if peritoneal irritation develops following thoracic penetration, (c) if food or chyme is recovered from the chest tube, or (d) if injury trajectory imaging studies suggest the possibility of diaphragmatic penetration. If one or more of these signs is present, tube thoracostomy should be performed expeditiously, followed by laparotomy or laparoscopy for repair of the diaphragm and damaged organs. Skeletal injuries constitute the majority of cases in which surgical intervention is necessary. All penetrating wounds are contaminated and must be treated as infected, while accessible missile fragments should be removed (once swelling has subsided) to prevent the development of lead poisoning (especially those in contact with bone or joint fluid).

Analgesia appropriate for the injury is essential and may require frequent titration by experienced nursing staff. Most children with multiple trauma benefit from parenteral opiate therapy. Age-appropriate rating devices to assess for pain are available and should be monitored frequently during the first few days following injury. Physician staff should be notified when increasing needs for analgesia are noted. Patient-controlled analgesia (also with parenteral opiate) is indicated for children with significant injury-associated pain. Alternative methods of analgesia that may be valuable for some patients include local anesthesia, regional and epidural analgesia, and nonopioid analgesia; adjunctive use of sedative-hypnotic agents may also be helpful in some injured children.

Glucose supplementation is unnecessary in most noninfant trauma victims, at least during the first day of therapy following major trauma, unless hypoglycemia or underlying disease is noted. Patients who receive supplemental glucose and those with an increased risk for hyperglycemia (i.e., a history of diabetes) should be closely monitored. Although the appropriate threshold for intervention in hyperglycemia associated with pediatric trauma is unknown, it is common practice to treat patients with glycosuria. When an insulin infusion is used to treat hyperglycemia, close attention to avoid hypoglycemia is essential. Following the acute injury and recovery, euglycemia is a reasonable goal, with maximized caloric intake.

Early involvement of social services, psychiatric support, pastoral care, and the appropriate law enforcement and child protective agencies is mandatory (especially in cases of intentional injury). Efforts must be made to attend to the emotional needs of the child and family, especially for those families who suffer the death of a child. In addition to loss of control over their child's destiny, parents of seriously injured children may also feel enormous guilt, whether or not these feelings are warranted. The responsible physician should attempt to create as normal an environment as possible for the child and to allow parents to participate meaningfully in postinjury care. In so doing, treatment interventions will be facilitated, as the child perceives that parents and staff are working together to ensure an optimal recovery.

The care of children with major traumatic injury also involves nutritional support with protein (even more than

calories) and, in patients who are not eating, prophylactic therapy to prevent gastric stress ulcer bleeding. Tetanus-prone wounds require tetanus toxoid, with or without tetanus-immune globulin, depending on immunization status and degree of contamination.

A critical result of the secondary survey in severe pediatric trauma is the decision about ensuing disposition: the radiology department, the operating room, or the PICU. The subsequent intrahospital transport of severely injured children requires planning, equipment, and professional support. Both the nurse responsible for the patient and the primary resuscitating physician should accompany a critically injured child, allowing for the transfer of important data and a plan of management. The design of an emergency department with on-site radiology and operating room and a co-located PICU may facilitate trauma care.

Definitive Management of Non-Neurologic Injuries

The definitive management of childhood trauma begins once sustentative care (the primary survey and resuscitation phases) has concluded. Definitive management of childhood trauma depends on the type, extent, and severity of the injuries sustained. Injuries to the torso (chest and abdomen) and skeleton are reviewed in this section. In patients treated with or without acute surgical intervention, it is important to note that later surgical interventions may be required, particularly in patients with persistent or worsening organ dysfunction.

Chest Trauma

Intrathoracic injuries occur in 6% of pediatric trauma victims (49), with the majority (86%) due to blunt injury, mostly (74%) automobile related. Most of these injuries will be manifest during the primary survey, although occasionally (with pulmonary contusions or lacerations, tracheobronchial injuries, etc.), identification will be delayed for several hours following injury. About 50% of children with thoracic injury require a thoracostomy. The thoracic injury pattern includes lung contusion and laceration (48%), pneumothorax and hemothorax (41%), and rib and sternal fractures (32%). Thus, a routine portable chest radiograph (anterior–posterior) will be helpful in most patients. Injuries to the heart, diaphragm, great vessels, bronchi, and esophagus occur less frequently. A chest CT scan is often helpful in patients with severe thoracic injuries, and may help to grade the severity of lung injury, including contusion. Because blunt trauma is nearly 10 times more deadly when associated with major intrathoracic injury, intrathoracic injury serves as a marker of severity, even though it is the proximate cause of death in <1% of all pediatric blunt trauma.

The child compensates poorly for respiratory derangements associated with serious thoracic injury, due to (a) larger oxygen consumption (as noted previously); (b) a smaller functional residual capacity compared to closing capacity, with a resultant tendency to atelectasis; (c) lesser pulmonary compliance, yet greater chest wall compliance (which dictate chiefly a tachypneic response to hypoxia); and (d) horizontally aligned ribs and rudimentary intercostal musculature (which make the infant or small child a diaphragmatic breather). The chest wall of the child often escapes major harm because the pliable nature of the cartilaginous ribs permits compression without radiographic fracturing. Pulmonary contusions are the typical result, and they are seldom life threatening. Pneumothorax and hemothorax, due to lacerations of the lung parenchyma and intercostal vessels, are less common results but place the child in grave danger of sudden, marked ventilatory and circulatory compromise as the mediastinum shifts. A flail chest is unlikely until ribs are more completely ossified. Traumatic asphyxia secondary to blunt thoracic trauma with a closed glottis results in petechial hemorrhages in the upper portion of the body but may require only a few days of mechanical ventilatory support.

Critical care of the respiratory insufficiency that accompanies severe thoracic injury emphasizes the avoidance of further injury related to atelectrauma, barotrauma, biotrauma, and volutrauma, using the least amount of oxygen and respiratory support necessary to maintain the PaO_2 at 70–80 mm Hg (hence, an SpO_2 of 90%–100%). In the absence of acute lung injury (ALI, $PaO_2/FIO_2 = 200$–300), normocarbia is recommended. If ALI is present or likely to develop, volutrauma should be avoided by using tidal volumes of 6–8 mL/kg and permissive hypercapnia, so long as head injury is not present, to attenuate further lung injury and lessen progression to acute respiratory distress syndrome (ARDS, $PaO_2/FIO_2 < 200$). Positive end-expiratory pressure sufficient to prevent end-expiratory collapse of small airways should be used to minimize atelectrauma. If peak inspiratory pressure cannot be maintained below 30 cm H_2O with minimal attendant barotraumas (less in the presence of air leak syndromes or fresh bronchial or pulmonary suture lines), alternative strategies should be considered, including high-frequency oscillatory ventilation, pronation, and lung surfactant. The role of ECMO for trauma patients remains uncertain due to the possibility of further hemorrhage during mandatory anticoagulation, although a recent case series included five children with respiratory failure and abdominal and/or thoracic injury treated successfully with veno-venous ECMO. Median mechanical ventilation prior to ECMO was 6 days. Hemorrhage occurred frequently during ECMO, but it was manageable (50).

Pulmonary Contusion, Laceration, and Hematoma.
Pulmonary parenchymal injury due to blunt trauma is characterized by alveolar hemorrhage, consolidation, and edema, leading to decreased gas exchange and pulmonary compliance. It may manifest as hemoptysis, subcutaneous emphysema, and respiratory distress, and occurs commonly in children with thoracic injury. Laboratory examinations may reveal hypoxemia on an arterial blood gas and a density in the lung fields on chest radiograph. A laceration in the pulmonary parenchyma may result from blunt or penetrating thoracic trauma and manifest as hemoptysis or hemothorax, often with an associated pneumothorax. Most pulmonary lacerations are minor and do not require specific therapy. Persistent hemorrhage from a laceration or contusion may result in a pulmonary hematoma; distinction of this entity from a simple contusion is not clearly defined.

Secondary complications of pulmonary contusion are not uncommon and include aspiration and infection; ARDS develops in up to one-fifth of children with pulmonary contusion (51). Careful attention to fluid intake is essential in patients with pulmonary contusion. The management of respiratory insufficiency in patients with these complex injuries was reviewed earlier. Pulmonary contusions uncomplicated by aspiration, overhydration, or infection can be expected to resolve in 7–10 days, mandating the judicious use of pulmonary toilet, crystalloid fluid (i.e., avoiding overhydration), loop diuretics, and selective antibiotic therapy to preclude the development of ARDS. Fluid and blood in lung parenchyma provide an excellent "culture medium" for bacterial infection, and care must be taken to recognize early signs of superinfection of a pulmonary contusion.

Hemopneumothorax.
Blunt or penetrating trauma that leads to a communication between the pleural space and the atmosphere results in an immediate accumulation of air (and possibly blood) into the pleural space, with contralateral mediastinal shift. Often, these injuries are associated with rib fractures. Penetrating trauma is associated with a higher incidence of hemopneumothorax than is blunt trauma. Air passes freely in and out of a large chest wall defect, but if the opening is small, ingress may occur during inspiration and obstruction may occur during expiration, filling the pleural space and causing shift of the mediastinum (i.e., tension pneumothorax). As more air and/or blood collects in the thorax with worsening mediastinal shift, obstruction to venous return and cardiac output lead to shock. However, some patients may be minimally symptomatic, and a screening chest radiograph is appropriate in children with thoracic trauma. In any case, collections of blood and/or air in the pleural space of an injured child should be expeditiously drained.

Initial therapy of hemopneumothorax in this setting includes a sterile, occlusive dressing to convert the open chest wall injury to a closed injury. A tube thoracostomy inserted via the fifth intercostal space in the mid-axillary line via open or Seldinger technique is then connected to a collection chamber with an applied pressure of –20 cm H_2O; a water-seal chamber connected in series will facilitate the identification of air leaks in the system. In young children with thin chest walls, a short subcutaneous tunnel created between the skin incision and the entry point into the pleural space helps prevent air leaks around the tube. The management of a tube thoracostomy requires significant nursing skills, including knowledge of appropriate dressings, the ability to troubleshoot the system (including both air leak and obstruction scenarios), and an understanding of the patient's tolerance and analgesia requirements. The water-seal chamber should be frequently checked to assess for air leaks, while the collection chamber may reveal blood, serosanguineous, or other exudative fluid. Video-assisted thoracoscopy may be helpful when residual collections of blood persist. Definitive management of an open chest wound requires surgical intervention in the controlled environment of the operating room following stabilization.

Rib Fractures and Flail Chest.
Rib fractures occur in approximately one-third of children with blunt thoracic trauma (49), and their occurrence suggests a mechanism of injury characterized by significant energy transfer. The presence of rib fractures in an injured child appears to be a marker of more severe injury and increased risk of mortality. Rib fractures in infants and young children are frequently associated with child abuse, particularly in the absence of a history of major blunt trauma. Cardiopulmonary resuscitation is rarely associated with anterior rib fractures. Fracture of a first rib may be a marker of major vascular injury in children. Treatment of isolated rib fractures includes adequate analgesia and chest physiotherapy to prevent atelectasis and pneumonia. Older children may be able to use incentive spirometry and deep-breathing exercises.

A flail chest is rare in children and is characterized by a chest wall segment that has lost continuity with the thorax and moves paradoxically with changes in intrathoracic pressure: *in* with inspiration and *out* with expiration. This injury is the result of major thoracic blunt trauma and is usually associated with multiple rib fractures (contiguous ribs have two or more fractures) as well as a pulmonary contusion. Diagnosis is made by the visual inspection of paradoxical movement of the chest wall, although it may be less obvious or absent in young children with small flail segments. Definitive management includes controlled mechanical ventilation; the inflated lung acts as a splint, stabilizes the rib fractures, and decreases pain associated with the chest wall injury. Continued therapy is mainly directed at the underlying pulmonary contusion. Intercostal or epidural analgesia may be helpful. Prolonged mechanical ventilatory support and surgical fixation may be necessary in rare cases.

Myocardial Contusion.
Although myocardial contusion may occur in adults with significant thoracic trauma (mainly automobile drivers whose chests are crushed against the

steering column), similar injuries are rare in children. Symptoms include chest pain, dysrhythmias, and myocardial dysfunction. Signs on physical examination include tachycardia or dysrhythmia, a gallop rhythm, and findings consistent with cardiogenic pulmonary edema. Laboratory examinations may reveal the presence of cardiomegaly, as well as myocardial dysfunction on electrocardiography and/or echocardiography, and elevated myocardial enzymes. Treatment is primarily supportive. Because children with myocardial contusion are at risk for sudden and lethal dysrhythmias, even if the initial electrocardiogram is unremarkable, they require admission to a PICU and continuous cardiac monitoring.

Sudden death that occurs with a relatively minor blunt injury to the chest is known as *commotio cordis* and is seen principally in male adolescents in association with athletic events (e.g., baseball struck by a bat to the chest). The mechanism of injury appears to be ventricular dysrhythmia, and because the energy of impact is often low, associated injury is not generally present. Survival is low but would likely improve with more widespread community access to defibrillation.

Cardiac Tamponade. Pericardial contusions and lacerations may lead to hemopericardium and subsequent cardiac tamponade, although this appears to be an uncommon complication in children. Rising pericardial pressure obstructs both venous return and cardiac output, leading to *Beck's triad* (pulsus paradoxus, a quiet precordium, and distended neck veins) in some affected adolescents and adults; shock is the result. In younger victims of major thoracic trauma, unexplained tachycardia may be an early sign of tamponade, and examination of neck veins may be less revealing. Additional data that may be helpful include a jugular venous pressure tracing with absent Y descent (in older patients with a central venous catheter) and, occasionally, the presence of *pulsus alternans*. Treatment in severely injured patients with a suggestive history and physical examination should not be delayed. FAST examination in selected patients may be quite helpful, while a CT scan may be useful for patients at increased risk and in whom the clinical suspicion is lower. Other helpful laboratory tests include a chest radiograph, electrocardiography, and echocardiography (in particular, the presence of right atrial diastolic collapse in patients with a pericardial effusion). Expansion of intravascular volume is a helpful temporizing measure as the patient is prepared for a pericardiocentesis or operative placement of a pericardial window. Because most anesthetic agents are associated with a decrease in systemic vascular resistance and a subsequent fall in preload, local anesthesia may be a good choice for emergency pericardiocentesis. Positive-pressure ventilation, with or without intubation, is not well tolerated in these patients either, until at least partial decompression has occurred. When either general sedation or tracheal intubation is used, preparation at the bedside with resuscitation agents and defibrillator is requisite. Sedation with agents that permit spontaneous ventilation without significant decreases in myocardial contractility and systemic vascular resistance is helpful in patients who are unable to tolerate the procedure; ketamine and etomidate have been used. Bedside pericardiocentesis with contemporaneous placement of a drainage catheter via Seldinger technique may help temporize unstable patients until definitive repair in the operating room can be undertaken.

Rupture of the Diaphragm. Traumatic rupture of the diaphragm results from severe compression forces over the lower chest and upper abdomen, and patients generally have severe associated injuries. This injury has been recognized with increased frequency in the pediatric trauma patient following blunt trauma or with lap-belt injuries. Rupture is far more common on the left side, almost certainly because the right diaphragm is buttressed, and partially occluded, by the liver. A small tear in the diaphragm may not cause immediate symptoms, but eventually results in progressive herniation of abdominal contents through the diaphragmatic defect, as negative intrathoracic pressure gradually sucks abdominal viscera through the defect. The diagnosis should be suspected when the left diaphragm is not clearly visualized or is abnormally elevated or shaped, when abdominal visceral shadows are abnormally located on the initial chest radiograph, or when a nasogastric tube terminates in the hemithorax. Radiographic evaluation may be unreliable in the setting of penetrating injury. Treatment is operative repair. Unfortunately, significant delays in diagnosis are not uncommon.

Aortic Disruption. Although injury to the aorta is uncommon in children, it may occur following severe deceleration injuries and/or a fall from extreme heights. It is associated with a high mortality rate and other significant thoracic injuries, and most children with this injury die at the scene. Among the rare survivors, clinical symptoms and signs include back pain, a machinery-type heart murmur that classically radiates to the back, and hemorrhagic shock. A widened mediastinum, loss of the aortic knob, deviation of the trachea to the right, fracture of the first or second ribs, and apical capping may also suggest its presence in this setting. Arch aortography, a chest CT or MRI, and transesophageal echocardiography are frequently needed to adequately delineate the injury. Preoperative β-blockade may be appropriate in selected patients. Treatment is emergent thoracotomy and surgical repair, most often under cardiopulmonary bypass.

Tracheobronchial Tears. Rupture of the tracheobronchial tree due to blunt or penetrating thoracic trauma is often difficult to diagnose; most patients with major tracheobronchial tears die at the scene. Survivors may include some children suffering "clothesline" injuries to the neck, in whom an airway can be established distal to the injury. Affected patients often have symptoms and signs of airway obstruction (dyspnea and stridor), as well as pneumothorax, pneumomediastinum, and subcutaneous emphysema. A persistent, and often large, air leak following tube thoracostomy also suggests the possibility of a tracheobronchial tear, usually located near the carina in children with severe thoracic trauma. Blind airway suctioning is contraindicated when tracheobronchial tears are suspected, and bronchoscopy may be diagnostic. Because PPV may exacerbate the leak, careful management of airway pressures and fluid intake is essential. High-frequency oscillatory ventilation and other therapeutic modalities may be helpful and should be considered early in the course of injury. Some patients require multiple tube thoracostomies or emergent operative intervention to repair the leak. Isolation of the affected airway with one-lung ventilation or even ECMO may be life saving.

Abdominal Trauma

The abdomen of the child is vulnerable to injury for several reasons. Flexible ribs cover only the uppermost portion of the abdomen; thin layers of muscle, fat, and fascia provide little protection to the large solid viscera; the pelvis is shallow, lifting the bladder into the abdomen. Moreover, the overall small size of the abdomen predisposes the child to multiple rather than single injuries. Finally, gastric dilatation due to air (which often confounds abdominal examination by simulating peritonitis) leads to ventilatory and circulatory compromise by limiting diaphragmatic motion, increasing risk of aspiration, and causing vagally mediated dampening of the normal tachycardic response to hypovolemia.

Serious intra-abdominal injuries occur in 8% of pediatric trauma victims (49) and include injuries to the liver (27%), spleen (27%), kidneys (25%), and gastrointestinal tract (21%). Injuries to the genitourinary tract, pancreas, abdominal blood vessels, and pelvis are infrequent (5% or less) and, with the exception of injuries to abdominal blood vessels, account for few of the deaths that result from intra-abdominal injury. Penetrating abdominal injury is much less common than blunt trauma in children, and most of these patients will need surgical exploration following resuscitation and stabilization.

Physical signs of significant abdominal injury in children include diminished bowel sounds, tenderness to palpation, guarding, rebound tenderness, and other signs of peritoneal irritation. Depending on the mechanism of injury, some children may develop an abdominal wall hematoma (i.e., the "seatbelt sign" due to a restraint). Although the physical examination is usually abnormal in children with significant intra-abdominal injury, the findings may not be specific. Frequent reexamination is essential, because the possible need for intervention does not abate immediately following the injury.

Laboratory examinations that should be reviewed in the child with abdominal injury (as noted previously) include serial hematocrits, a type and cross-match, a complete blood count, serum transaminases, a coagulation screen (prothrombin time and partial thromboplastin time), urinalysis, and amylase and lipase in patients at increased risk. Abdominal radiographs should be assessed for evidence of free air. Following plain abdominal radiographs in children with suspected abdominal injury, CT scanning is the imaging study of choice; it is readily available, noninvasive, and has helped reduce the need for acute surgical interventions. It is recommended for both blunt and penetrating injury. Because the extent of abdominal injury may be more difficult to appreciate from the pediatric physical examination than is the extent of thoracic injury, imaging results often help guide resuscitation.

Although intravenous contrast is essential (in the absence of renal failure or allergy) to optimize the information from an abdominal CT scan, some controversy exists about the role of intraluminal contrast. Time spent preparing the patient for the scan is increased, there may be an increased risk of aspiration, and the contrast may traverse the alimentary canal slowly in patients with major trauma; in addition, common abdominal injury patterns in children typically involve solid rather than hollow viscera, potentially limiting the utility of intraluminal contrast. Nevertheless, double (intraluminal and intravenous) contrast CT scans of the abdomen are quite helpful in many injured children, and are preferred in many trauma centers.

Key findings on abdominal CT scans include vascular blush and other signs of contrast extravasation, although evidence of extravasation does not mandate emergency laparotomy, as is true for adults. A FAST examination may be useful to confirm abnormalities in children but is less helpful when negative. Subsequent imaging procedures that may prove useful include radionuclide scans and an intravenous urogram for renal trauma in selected patients.

Most solid visceral injuries are successfully treated nonoperatively, especially those involving kidneys (98%), spleen (95%), and liver (90%) (52). Acute management should follow consensus guidelines. The extent of intra-abdominal injury in a child may be difficult to determine because of an inadequate history, a presumed inconsequential injury, or the frequent absence of external clinical signs of internal injury. Bleeding from renal, splenic, and hepatic injuries is mostly self-limited and resolves spontaneously in nearly 100%, 95%, and 90% of such cases, respectively, unless the patient presents in hypotensive shock or the transfusion requirement exceeds 40 mL/kg of body weight (half of the circulating blood volume) within 24 hours of injury. Although uncommon, vascular injury (excluding solid-organ injuries) in children, whether in the thorax or abdomen, is associated with high mortality. The role of peritoneal lavage to diagnose intra-abdominal hemorrhage in children has markedly declined, with an increased reliance on imaging and nonoperative management. The indications

for immediate abdominal surgery in pediatric trauma patients include evidence of ongoing intra-abdominal hemorrhage (shock), evidence of hollow viscus perforation (peritonitis), and evisceration. Some experts would add major renal and collecting system disruption as well as major pancreatic ductal disruption to this list, although nonoperative management has also been advocated for these injuries. When hemorrhage is ongoing, the transfusion of blood products requires careful attention; rapid transfusions may be best accomplished using specific devices and catheters, warming of blood products is essential, and close monitoring of blood chemistry will help to prevent or treat resultant electrolyte problems (hyperkalemia and hypocalcemia) and metabolic acidosis. Laparotomy for the management of renal, pancreatic, gastrointestinal, and genitourinary injuries is performed utilizing damage-control methods for patients in extremis and staged closure for patients with abdominal compartment syndrome. Resuscitation in the PICU of patients treated with a damage-control approach may permit a more controlled reoperation, with an improved outcome as observed in adult patients (data in children are lacking). In any case, an open abdomen following either damage control or decompressive laparotomy mandates adequate protection of the viscera from microbial contamination, evaporative water and heat loss, and desiccation.

Appreciation of the likelihood of multiple injuries in children mandates prioritization; for example, "uncontrolled intra-abdominal hemorrhage takes precedence over a stable thoracic aorta tear" (53). Angiographic interventional radiology may be useful in selected cases, particularly where bleeding is severe and easily accessible.

Liver and Spleen. The spleen and liver are the most commonly injured organs in blunt abdominal trauma, and each accounts for approximately one-fourth of all intra-abdominal injuries. Diagnosis is made by abdominal CT in hemodynamically stable patients. A grading system for anatomic findings in splenic and hepatic injury has been developed by the American Association for the Surgery of Trauma (54) (**Table 30.6**); this system may also prove helpful in predicting outcome. In hemodynamically unstable patients, diagnosis is based on operative findings. However, conservative management is the rule, because the majority of patients are not hemodynamically unstable and most do not progress to frank, uncontrolled intra-abdominal hemorrhage. Nevertheless, operative intervention must be readily available if nonoperative management is contemplated. Complications specific to conservative management have not yet been completely characterized.

Of particular importance in the evaluation of patients for potential surgical intervention is hemodynamic stability: Is the hematocrit stable, even if low? If so, hemorrhage may have stopped; continuing hemorrhage is indicated by a falling hematocrit. An ongoing requirement for transfusion in the first few hours of resuscitation may also indicate an increased risk for vascular injury that requires surgery. Is there evidence of continued intra-abdominal hemorrhage on imaging procedures or are the base deficit and serum lactate concentrations continuing to worsen? If so, a laparotomy may be indicated.

An evidence-based guideline utilizing CT scan findings for the treatment of children with liver and spleen injuries below grade V has been proposed and includes ICU admission for patients with grade IV injury, several weeks of activity restriction depending on grade of injury, and no need for routine follow-up imaging (52). However, the relatively small study size, given the infrequency of late solid-organ hemorrhage, suggests that continued outcomes research is needed.

Kidneys and Urinary Tract. Children are more susceptible to renal trauma than adults are due to the reasons cited earlier; in addition, the child's kidney occupies a proportionally larger retroperitoneal space. Blunt trauma is more frequent than

TABLE 30.6

GRADING SYSTEM[a] FOR HEPATIC AND SPLENIC INJURIES

INJURY	GRADE I	GRADE II	GRADE III	GRADE IV	GRADE V	GRADE VI
Hematoma: liver, spleen	Subcapsular, <10% surface area	Subcapsular, 10%–50% surface area; intraparenchymal diameter <10 cm (liver) vs. <5 cm (spleen)	Subcapsular, >50% surface area or expanding; ruptured subcapsular or parenchymal hematoma; intraparenchymal hematoma >10 cm (liver) vs. >5 cm (spleen) or expanding			
Laceration: liver	Capsular tear <1 cm parenchymal depth	1–3 cm parenchymal depth, <10 cm in length (liver) vs. not involving a trabecular vessel (spleen)	>3 cm parenchymal depth or involving trabecular vessels (spleen)	Parenchymal disruption of 25%–75% of hepatic lobe, or 1–3 segments within a lobe	Parenchymal disruption >75% of hepatic lobe, or >3 segments within a lobe	
Laceration: spleen				Shattered spleen		
Vascular injury: liver			Involvement of hilar vessels with >25% devascularization		Juxtahepatic venous injuries Hilar injury with devascularization	Hepatic avulsion
Vascular injury: spleen						

[a]Advance one grade for multiple injuries, up to grade III.
Adapted from Moore EE, Cogbill TH, Jurkovich GJ, et al. Organ injury scaling: Spleen and liver (1994 revision). J Trauma 1995;38:323–4.

TABLE 30.7

GRADING SYSTEM[a] FOR RENAL INJURY

■ INJURY	■ GRADE I	■ GRADE II	■ GRADE III	■ GRADE IV	■ GRADE V
Contusion	Microscopic or gross hematuria, normal urologic studies				
Hematoma	Subcapsular, nonexpanding	Nonexpanding perirenal hematoma confined to renal retroperitoneum			
Laceration		<1 cm parenchymal depth (renal cortex) without urinary extravasation	>1 cm parenchymal depth (renal cortex) without urinary extravasation	Extending through renal cortex, medulla, and collecting system	Shattered kidney
Vascular injury				Main renal artery or vein injury with contained hemorrhage	Avulsion of renal hilum

[a]Advance one grade for multiple injuries to the same organ.
Adapted from Moore EE, Shackford SR, Pachter HL, et al. Organ injury scaling: Spleen, liver, and kidney. *J Trauma* 1989;29:1664–6.

penetrating trauma, usually leading to a hematoma. However, lacerations of the kidney are not uncommon and result mostly from crush injuries against the ribs or spine.

Gross hematuria remains the most reliable indicator of serious urologic injury and mandates radiographic examination. Microscopic hematuria is less sensitive in this regard, although the degree of hematuria does not necessarily correlate with severity of urologic injury. Because insertion of a urethral catheter itself can cause hematuria, the urine that is examined should ideally be a spontaneously voided specimen. Because rhabdomyolysis following crush injury may present with pigmented urine and a urinalysis positive for heme, it is important to distinguish this entity. Red blood cells on microscopic analysis of urine suggest urologic hemorrhage rather than myoglobinuria. An abdominal CT scan with intravenous contrast is the most appropriate initial test for hemodynamically stable children with suspected renal trauma. The American Association for the Surgery of Trauma developed a grading system (Table 30.7) for renal injury utilizing CT scan results, which has been used in management (55). A "one-shot" trauma intravenous urogram, which may be performed in the operating room for patients who require emergent surgical exploration, provides some gross information about renal function.

The conservative management of renal injury in grades I to III is routine. In children with grades IV and V renal injury, indications for surgical exploration include persistent hemorrhage, expanding or uncontained retroperitoneal hematoma, or suspected renal pedicle avulsion. In addition, those with substantial devitalized renal parenchyma and/or urinary extravasation may also be candidates. Occasionally angiographic control of renal hemorrhage is feasible.

The ureters are protected by muscle and soft tissue and are rarely injured, although ureteropelvic junction disruption may occur following severe abdominal trauma; delayed radiographic imaging may be helpful in this setting. Surgical repair of these injuries may include multiple reconstruction procedures following acute recovery. The bladder is less protected in children due to its position. Rupture of the bladder dome (the weakest area) leads to an intraperitoneal leak, whereas pelvic fractures associated with rupture of the bladder wall or base give rise to an extraperitoneal leak. If the bladder is not filled with contrast for a CT scan, diagnosis may be delayed. The approach for surgical repair of a ruptured bladder depends on the site of the leak; a cystostomy is often helpful.

Pelvic fractures are also associated with urethral injury, particularly in males, and blood is generally present at the urethral meatus of affected patients. Diagnosis mandates retrograde urethrography. Management depends on the severity and site of urethral injury and may include multiple reconstruction procedures and cystostomy.

Rhabdomyolysis secondary to crush injuries may be associated with renal dysfunction and failure; serum muscle enzymes are dramatically elevated, and early treatment with hydration (and possibly urinary alkalinization) is helpful. Renal replacement therapy is appropriate for patients with trauma-associated renal failure, whether or not rhabdomyolysis is present. This therapy may permit optimization of nutritional support, especially when meticulous fluid balance is essential. The threshold for initiation of renal replacement therapy in trauma-associated renal insufficiency, particularly in children, remains controversial.

Gastrointestinal Tract. The esophagus is a thoracic organ, although rarely injured by blunt thoracic trauma. Blunt injuries to the remainder of the gastrointestinal tract may follow several patterns, including crush injury (the organ is compressed against the spine), burst injury (the filled, distended viscus is compressed rapidly), and shear injury (tethers, including neurovascular structures, of an organ are damaged by rapid acceleration/deceleration). Subsequent damage may include hematoma, laceration, perforation, or transection of the gastrointestinal tract, and symptomatology may change over hours or days. Blunt stomach injury is more frequent in children than in adults and usually results in a perforation or "blowout" injury along the greater curvature. Nasogastric drainage may be bloody, and radiographic studies are generally positive for free air. Duodenal injuries are less frequent than other injuries of the gastrointestinal tract due in part to a retroperitoneal—and somewhat protected—location. Because this location may also serve to hide clinical signs of injury, it is reassuring to note that CT scans (preferably with double contrast) appear to differentiate well between duodenal hematoma and perforation in children. Hematomas and/or perforations that involve the remainder of the small bowel may be difficult to diagnose early, because peritoneal signs may take several hours to develop fully. Significant blunt injuries to the large bowel generally lead to the rapid development of symptoms and an abnormal physical examination. Diagnosis of gastrointestinal tract perforation following trauma in children is mostly the result of careful, repeated physical examination, although CT scans and other laboratory examinations are helpful, particularly in patients who are unable to respond appropriately or comply with the examination.

The management of gastrointestinal tract perforation in children is surgical; nonoperative management of duodenal hematomas has also been used successfully and is indicated as initial treatment. Because adults with a hematoma in the colonic wall may develop delayed perforation, the appropriate management strategy for this entity in children is debated. A colostomy may also be necessary for extensive large bowel injury with perforation and significant fecal contamination, although in its absence, primary repair is often feasible in an otherwise healthy child without shock or the need for multiple blood transfusions.

Pancreas. Although infrequently injured in children due in part to its retroperitoneal location, the pancreas may be injured with severe blunt abdominal trauma; a delay in diagnosis may occur, and affected children generally have multiple associated injuries. Diagnosis depends mainly on CT scan results, although clinical and laboratory data may also be useful. Endoscopic retrograde cholangiopancreatography with possible stenting may be helpful for selected patients with duct disruption. Routine surgical intervention is not recommended, but distal pancreatectomy may have a role in selected patients. Pseudocyst formation related to duct disruption has been reported in approximately one-third of children with pancreatic injuries (56); nonoperative management with parenteral nutrition, gut rest, and drainage procedures, when appropriate, are recommended.

Abdominal Compartment Syndrome. Trauma-associated abdominal compartment syndrome is not common in children but may occur following blunt trauma or burn injury. Massive fluid resuscitation may be associated with the development of this syndrome. The syndrome is recognized by increasing intra-abdominal pressure, and the pathophysiology involves decreased abdominal organ perfusion with decreased venous return from the lower half of the body. Hypoperfusion injury leads to further tissue edema and progressive hypoperfusion, and abdominal distention with organ dysfunction occurs. Oliguria and respiratory insufficiency are common clinical findings in children.

Diagnosis involves instilling 1 mL/kg of sterile saline via the bladder catheter and measuring the intravesical pressure; pressure greater than 25 mm Hg (or ~18 cm H_2O) is diagnostic (the reference point is the symphysis pubis). A lower pressure threshold (16 mm Hg, or ~12 cm H_2O) for the diagnosis of abdominal compartment syndrome in children with organ dysfunction has been suggested (57) and may prove more clinically relevant. The mortality rate associated with this complication is high, but the condition itself is easily treated by decompressive laparotomy, often with temporary patch abdominoplasty.

Skeletal Trauma

The porous nature of immature cortical bone may lead to an increased incidence of fractures in children compared to adults. As immature bone is also more elastic, fractures in children are often incomplete or nondisplaced. Fractures in childhood are also unique as a result of the presence of growth plates, the rapid rate of healing, a tendency to remodel in the plane of the fracture, and a high incidence of ischemic vascular injuries. In addition, long-term growth disturbances may complicate childhood fractures. Diaphyseal fractures of the long bones cause significant overgrowth, while physeal (growth

plate) fractures, particularly if severe (Salter-Harris types 3 and 4), cause significant undergrowth. Joint dislocations and ligamentous injury are less common in children. The periosteum is also thicker in children and may assist in stabilization of underlying fractures.

Fractures are rarely an immediate cause of death in blunt trauma, although they are the leading cause of disability; they are present in 26% of serious blunt injury cases and constitute the principal anatomic diagnosis in 22%. Upper extremity fractures outnumber lower extremity fractures by 7:1, although in serious blunt trauma, this ratio is 2:3. The most common long-bone fractures sustained during childhood pedestrian motor vehicle crashes are fractures of the femur and tibia, whereas falls are typically associated with both upper and lower extremity fractures if fall height is significant (from the top of a bunk bed or the window of a high-rise dwelling, not from falls from standard-height beds or down the stairs). The delayed diagnosis of fractures in multiply injured children occurs and the frequency of this depends on the child's age and the diagnostic method.

Because isolated long-bone and pelvic fractures are rarely associated with significant hemorrhage, a diligent search must be made for another source of bleeding if signs of hypotensive shock are observed. This search frequently leads to the abdomen, although infants and children may also lose substantial amounts of blood in the thorax or head. For a more detailed discussion of open fractures, amputations, and other forms of severe skeletal trauma, the reader is referred to orthopedic texts.

Fractures. Because long-bone fractures are rarely life threatening unless associated with major bleeding (bilateral femur fractures or unstable pelvic fractures), the general care of the injured patient takes precedence over orthopedic care, but early stabilization will serve both to decrease patient discomfort and to limit the amount of blood loss. Closed treatment predominates for fractures of the clavicle, upper extremity, and tibia, while fractures of the femur increasingly involve the use of internal fixation. Careful inspection of all wounds is necessary, as an open fracture may be associated with an innocuous-appearing puncture wound. If an open fracture is suspected, do not reexamine it repeatedly; a simple dressing with immobilization of the extremity is appropriate. It is worth noting that open fractures significantly increase the risk of developing a compartment syndrome. Operative treatment is required for complex open fractures (for debridement and irrigation), displaced supracondylar fractures (due to their association with ischemic vascular injury), and major or displaced physeal fractures (which must be reduced anatomically). Owing to the ability of most long-bone fractures to remodel, reductions need not be perfectly anatomic, but remodeling is limited in torus and greenstick fractures, as the hyperemia typical of complete fractures is unlikely to occur.

The critical care of skeletal injuries consists of careful immobilization as appropriate, with emphasis on the prevention of immobilization-related complications (such as friction burns and decubitus ulcers) through the use of supportive and assistive devices (such as egg-crate or similar mattresses and a trapeze to permit limited freedom of movement). Prolonged skeletal traction in children with fractures may be associated with hypertension and hypercalcemia, although a direct relationship appears unlikely; both respond to mobilization. Frequent neurovascular checks are essential to assess for the development of arterial insufficiency, a hallmark of the compartment syndrome.

The care of open fractures includes antibiotics, generally a first-generation cephalosporin unless there is significant comminuted bone from a high-energy injury (in which case, addition of an aminoglycoside is reasonable). Complications, including traumatic fat embolism following long-bone fracture and rhabdomyolysis following severe crush injury, are rare, but require aggressive care when present. The former may be associated with ARDS and/or emboli to other organs, and early stabilization of long-bone fractures is helpful, while the latter is treated as previously noted. Early rehabilitation is vital to optimal recovery and mandates routine physiatric consultation on admission to the PICU.

Compartment Syndrome. Fracture-associated arterial insufficiency is recognized by the presence of a pulse deficit on serial examination, but detection of the compartment syndrome usually requires the measurement of compartment pressures. Elevated compartment pressures impair capillary perfusion, and ischemia develops rapidly. This syndrome can develop occasionally, even in the absence of trauma, with extravasation of IV fluid. Symptoms include the 5 Ps: pallor, pulselessness, paresthesia, paralysis, and pain. The last, pain, is the earliest sign of the syndrome, is often out of proportion to the injury, and may be difficult to treat, even with opiates. Frequent, repeated neurovascular checks of multiply traumatized children are essential to detect this devastating complication early.

Fasciotomy is indicated when the compartment pressure is greater than 40 cm H_2O, although lower pressures may mandate treatment if the child is symptomatic or if the capillary perfusion pressure is reduced. The utility of an absolute pressure limit for children of different ages is controversial, and the diagnosis remains, in part, a clinical one. Fasciotomy in the lower extremities is often performed simultaneously for all adjacent compartments and, following fasciotomy, the skin wounds are left open to heal by delayed primary closure or skin grafting.

CHILD ABUSE

(11) When the history of injury in a child is inconsistent with the severity of injury, child abuse must be considered. Child abuse is the presumed underlying cause of 3% of major traumatic injuries in children, although the actual incidence is difficult to determine. A detailed review of the mechanisms, patterns, presentation, and findings of physical abuse is beyond the scope of this chapter, but child abuse should be suspected whenever a delay in obtaining treatment is unexplained; when the history is vague or otherwise incompatible with the observed physical findings; when the caretaker blames siblings, playmates, or other third parties; or when the caretaker protects other adults rather than the child. Although the recognition and sociomedicolegal management of suspected cases of child abuse require a team approach, assessment and medical treatment of physical injuries is no different than for any other mechanism of injury. Confrontation and accusation hinder treatment and rehabilitation and have no place in the management of any injured child, regardless of the nature of the injury (although reports of suspected child abuse must be filed with local child protective services in every state and territory in the United States).

Victims of child abuse are younger, more severely injured, and more likely to die from their injuries than are other pediatric trauma patients. More importantly, morbidity in this group is worse. These patients are more likely to require custodial care and have more significant functional limitations (58). The "shaken baby syndrome" comprises a unique set of symptoms and signs peculiar to nonaccidental trauma; this entity is also known as the "whiplash shaken infant syndrome" (59). These patients have intracranial and intraocular hemorrhages in the absence of external trauma to the head or fracture of the calvaria, and the "shaking" injuries are the result of bleeding from the easily torn bridging veins of the infant's meninges during rapidly applied forces of acceleration–deceleration,

forces which are dramatically increased if concomitant impact is also present. Ophthalmologic examination often reveals retinal hemorrhages of varying severity, occasionally with retinal detachment. The prognosis is poor for many affected infants. Additional patterns of injury secondary to physical abuse include burns (particularly shapes suggesting a mechanism such as a cigarette or hot iron) and contusions (e.g., fingerprint contusions) as well as asphyxiation, blunt abdominal injury, multiple fractures of various ages, and sexual abuse.

The physical examination is often normal in abused infants and children; it may also be normal initially and change over several hours, mandating frequent reexamination. Findings on physical examination may include signs of general neglect, such as poor skin hygiene, malnutrition, failure to thrive, hematomas, and petechiae of various ages and distribution (although the color of cutaneous contusions is not generally a sensitive and specific indicator of contusion age), bite marks, burn injuries, abrasions, strap or belt injuries, and soft-tissue swelling (Fig. 30.5). An ophthalmologic examination is mandatory in infants who are possible abuse victims; pupillary dilatation should be performed sequentially, using shorter-acting agents to avoid prolonged, bilateral mydriasis. Particular attention should also be directed at evidence of sexual abuse, such as condylomata, perianal and genital hematoma, other venereal disease (oral and genital), and pain in the anogenital area.

In addition to routine laboratory examinations for childhood trauma, infant victims of abuse require an examination for skeletal injury; either a skeletal survey with chest radiograph (possibly including oblique rib films) or a bone scan is commonly used. Further testing, including radiographic imaging, will depend on the presentation and differential diagnosis. Radiographic manifestations of child abuse include new and old injuries, subperiosteal hemorrhages, epiphyseal separations, periosteal shearing, metaphyseal fragmentations, previously healed periosteal calcifications, and shearing of the metaphysis.

The diagnosis of child abuse is uncomfortable, even for experienced physicians; it is frequently a diagnosis of exclusion, considered only after more "acceptable" diagnoses are ruled out. However, the diagnosis of child abuse is rarely made with absolute certainty on the initial presentation, and the physician's role is to serve as an advocate for children. The possibility of abuse should therefore be investigated expeditiously, because it is equally important to protect siblings still in the home. The prompt involvement of social services and responsible child protective services allows the intensive care unit staff to attend to the child's medical problems.

COMPLICATIONS

(12) The case fatality rate following pediatric trauma is ~2.5% overall, but the morbidity associated with pediatric trauma is much greater and increases with increasing severity of injury. Mild-to-moderate functional limitations are present at discharge in one-fourth of injured children without traumatic neurologic injury (60). The incidence is much higher in children with traumatic neurologic injury, and severe functional limitations, including cognitive impairment, behavioral disturbances, and a decline in academic performance, are all generally associated with traumatic brain injuries. Severe functional limitations are present in most children following major trauma and may persist for months or longer. The direct cost of pediatric trauma care in the United States is enormous, but the burden, including direct and indirect costs, related to pediatric trauma morbidity is unknown, although likely just as significant. Rehabilitation and physical therapy appear to be underutilized in some injured children, and more appropriate

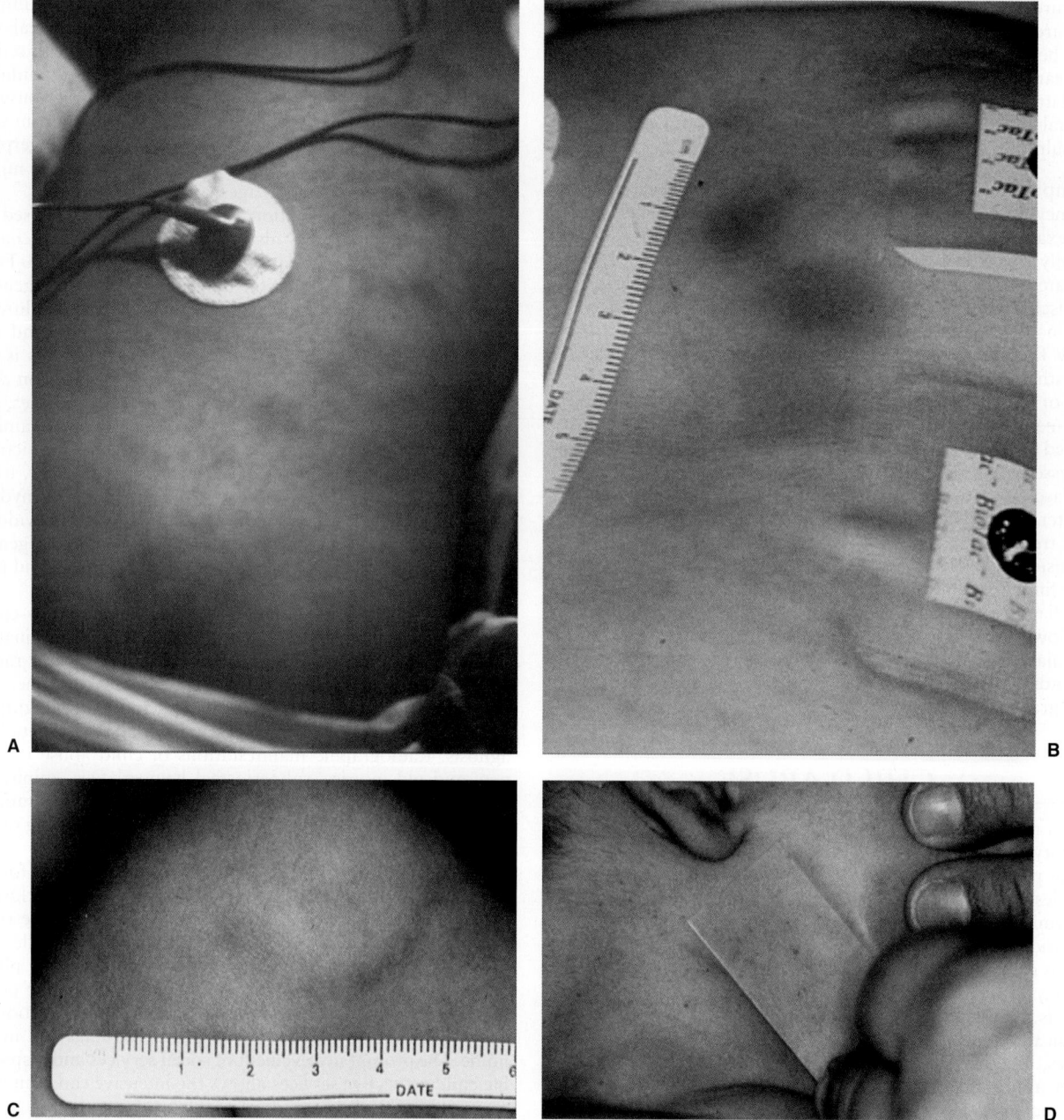

FIGURE 30.5. Cutaneous findings in child abuse. **A** and **B:** Fingerprint contusions of various ages on back of one baby and chest wall of another. **C:** Bite mark on knee. **D:** Petechiae on neck of asphyxiated baby.

use of these services could help reduce this burden. Referrals for these services should be made early in the hospital course. Of note, socially disadvantaged families may experience barriers to long-term follow-up services for their injured children (61). Vigilance to ensure appropriate follow-up in all injured children should be the goal.

Primary and secondary injuries, including its complications, contribute to morbidity and mortality; of note, injury-related complications appear to be more frequent than treatment-related complications. Functional limitations, troublesome episodes of anxiety and stress, and infection (often treatment related) are all common complications of pediatric trauma. Thromboembolic events and ventilator-associated pneumonia occur less frequently than in injured adults.

Acute Stress and Post-Traumatic Stress Disorder

The anxiety and stress associated with pediatric traumatic injury impact the patient, the family, and, often, the community. It would not be surprising if these symptoms persisted for some time, although the time course and incidence are not yet well described. Symptoms of stress immediately following childhood injuries involving automobiles were reported in 88% of pediatric patients and 83% of their parents (62). In addition, 40% of these families (patients and/or parents) experienced "broad distress" (significant symptoms across multiple symptom categories). These families benefit from referral to behavioral health specialists with expertise in treating families after traumatic events.

When symptoms are present more than a month following a traumatic event, post-traumatic stress disorder (PTSD) may be diagnosed; this diagnosis is suggested by avoidance of reminders of the event, persistent hyperarousal symptoms, and unwanted recollections of the event. The occurrence of PTSD in children appears to be high, irrespective of the severity of injury. Between one-fourth and one-third of all children are affected up to 18 months following injury (63–65). Not surprisingly, it is also high in the parents and family members of victims. Although research on treatment methods is scant, referral for psychologic care should be considered for all patients and families with suggestive symptoms. Therapeutic options include pharmacotherapy, behavioral therapy, and various educational initiatives, among others.

Infection

Because fever, leukocytosis, and other signs of inflammation are commonly observed in injured children during the acute-phase response, they are neither sensitive nor specific to infection. Resorption of large hematomas, atelectasis, long-bone fractures, and retained necrotic tissue all may contribute to or suggest an inflammatory response. Continued vigilance is necessary to ensure that occult infection does not complicate the care of injured children.

Approximately 10% of severely injured children develop infection, and the majority of these are nosocomial (66), including catheter-related sepsis, urinary tract infection in patients with indwelling urinary catheters, and ventilator-associated pneumonia. Trauma-related infections are much less common and typically involve the wound, abdomen, or CNS. Broad-spectrum IV antibiotics are often prescribed following significant penetrating trauma and/or open fractures, but not following blunt trauma. Routine antibiotic therapy following trauma, including burn injury, is not indicated, because it may lead to the selection of resistant organisms and does not seem to prevent infection.

Injured children who develop an infection have a longer hospital stay, but mortality is generally unaffected (66), in part because significant clinical deterioration during hospitalization usually mandates empiric, broad-spectrum antibiotic therapy. Antibiotic therapy is also begun for severely injured children with wound infection, cellulitis, or thoracostomy tube. A urinary tract infection in a child with an indwelling catheter usually mandates catheter removal or at least catheter exchange, whereas venous catheter–related sepsis mandates a new venous catheter and empiric antibiotic therapy.

Thromboembolic Events

The incidence of thromboembolic events appears to be very low in injured children compared with adults, although epidemiologic data are lacking. Significant deep venous thromboses and/or pulmonary emboli have been noted in less than 0.1% of children who are hospitalized for traumatic injury (67,68). As a result, routine prophylaxis is not indicated for infants and children who are hospitalized with traumatic injury. While it is possible that adolescents have a gradually increasing risk of thrombotic events after acute traumatic injury, to date, little evidence supports this. Compression stockings and pneumatic sequential decompression devices may be appropriate for older adolescents who are likely to require prolonged bed rest or in the presence of other risk factors. Assuming that hemorrhage has been controlled, further therapy to prevent thrombotic complications should be considered for those adolescents with a history of venous stasis and/or injury or prothrombotic conditions. Individualized therapy that involves the trauma surgeon and a pediatric hematologist is most helpful in this setting, at least until the promulgation of well-supported clinical guidelines.

In the presence of deep venous thrombosis and/or pulmonary embolism in injured children, the decision to employ therapeutic anticoagulation must be carefully evaluated by the entire trauma team. Both therapeutic anticoagulation and vena cava filters have been used successfully in injured pediatric patients (69) although the evidence is limited. Even less evidence supports the role for thrombolysis, surgical thrombectomy, or other vascular procedures (i.e., stenting) in injured children with thrombotic complications that involve large veins. The management of arterial injuries, including surgical (for threatened limbs) and conservative approaches ("watch and wait" with anticoagulation for nonthreatened but mildly ischemic limbs), has been successful in children.

CONCLUSIONS AND FUTURE DIRECTIONS

Among the areas of basic science research, the effect of genotype—in particular the contribution of factors such as NFκB—is a target of vigorous current research. Improvements in clinical care, including analgesia, particularly of younger patients, optimal control of glucose in critically injured children, the early institution of rehabilitative services, and improvement in our ability to address the emotional needs of injured children and their parents also deserve further investigation. Continued improvements in monitoring equipment may offer early evidence of clinically significant physiologic derangements without the problems associated with invasive devices. Epidemiologic investigations in risk, and the prevention, of injury are likely to identify important targets for intervention. However, it is worth reemphasizing that further declines in morbidity and mortality associated with pediatric trauma are most likely to come from a concerted social, cultural, and economic approach involving prevention and including education, legislation, and the expansion of pediatric emergency medical services at every level. Pediatric critical care practitioners should play an important role in this effort.

References

1. Kochanek KD, Kirmeyer SE, Martin JA, et al. Annual summary of vital statistics: 2009. *Pediatrics* 2012;129:338–48.
2. Committee on Trauma and Committee on Shock, Division of Medical Sciences. National Research Council, National Academy of Sciences, ed. *Accidental Death and Disability: The Neglected Disease of Modern Society*. Washington, DC: National Academy of Sciences, 1966.
3. Davidson LL, Durkin MS, Kuhn L, et al. The impact of the Safe Kids/Healthy Neighborhoods Injury Prevention Program in Harlem, 1988 through 1991. *Am J Public Health* 1994;84:580–6.
4. DiScala C. *National Pediatric Trauma Registry Annual Report*. Boston, MA: Tufts University Rehabilitation and Childhood Trauma Research and Training Center, 2002.
5. Barlow B, Niemirska M, Gandhi RP, et al. Ten years of experience with falls from a height in children. *J Pediatr Surg* 1983;18:509–11.
6. Moshage H. Cytokines and the hepatic acute phase response. *J Pathol* 1997;181:257–66.
7. Dilley A, Wesson DE. Pediatric organ failure. In: Wesson DE, ed. *Pediatric Trauma*. New York, NY: Taylor & Francis Group, 2006;197–209.
8. Nakamori Y, Ogura H, Koh T, et al. The balance between expression of intranuclear NF-κB and glucocorticoid receptor

in polymorphonuclear leukocytes in SIRS patients. *J Trauma* 2005;59:308–14; discussion 14–5.

9. Bone RC. Toward a theory regarding the pathogenesis of the systemic inflammatory response syndrome: What we do and do not know about cytokine regulation. *Crit Care Med* 1996;24:163–72.

10. Hoch RC, Rodriguez R, Manning T, et al. Effects of accidental trauma on cytokine and endotoxin production. *Crit Care Med* 1993;21:839–45.

11. Roumen RM, Hendriks T, van der Ven-Jongekrijg J, et al. Cytokine patterns in patients after major vascular surgery, hemorrhagic shock, and severe blunt trauma. Relation with subsequent adult respiratory distress syndrome and multiple organ failure. *Ann Surg* 1993;218:769–76.

12. Svoboda P, Kantorova I, Ochmann J. Dynamics of interleukin 1, 2, and 6 and tumor necrosis factor alpha in multiple trauma patients. *J Trauma* 1994;36:336–40.

13. Yagmur Y, Ozturk H, Unaldi M, et al. Relation between severity of injury and the early activation of interleukins in multiple-injured patients. *Eur Surg Res* 2005;37:360–4.

14. Partrick DA, Moore FA, Moore EE, et al. Jack A. Barney Resident Research Award winner. The inflammatory profile of interleukin-6, interleukin-8, and soluble intercellular adhesion molecule-1 in postinjury multiple organ failure. *Am J Surg* 1996;172:425–9; discussion 429–31.

15. Murata A, Ogawa M, Yasuda T, et al. Serum interleukin 6, C-reactive protein and pancreatic secretory trypsin inhibitor (PSTI) as acute phase reactants after major thoraco-abdominal surgery. *Immunol Invest* 1990;19:271–8.

16. Valerio G, Franzese A, Carlin E, et al. High prevalence of stress hyperglycaemia in children with febrile seizures and traumatic injuries. *Acta Paediatr* 2001;90:618–22.

17. Laird AM, Miller PR, Kilgo PD, et al. Relationship of early hyperglycemia to mortality in trauma patients. *J Trauma* 2004;56:1058–62.

18. Yendamuri S, Fulda GJ, Tinkoff GH. Admission hyperglycemia as a prognostic indicator in trauma. *J Trauma* 2003;55:33–8.

19. Jeschke MG, Einspanier R, Klein D, et al. Insulin attenuates the systemic inflammatory response to thermal trauma. *Mol Med* 2002;8:443–50.

20. Gore DC, Chinkes D, Heggers J, et al. Association of hyperglycemia with increased mortality after severe burn injury. *J Trauma* 2001;51:540–4.

21. Jeschke MG, Klein D, Herndon DN. Insulin treatment improves the systemic inflammatory reaction to severe trauma. *Ann Surg* 2004;239:553–60.

22. Jeschke MG, Kulp GA, Kraft R, et al. Intensive insulin therapy in severely burned pediatric patients: A prospective randomized trial. *Am J Respir Crit Care Med* 2010;182:351–9.

23. Gionis D, Ilias I, Moustaki M, et al. Hypothalamic-pituitary-adrenal axis and interleukin-6 activity in children with head trauma and syndrome of inappropriate secretion of antidiuretic hormone. *J Pediatr Endocrinol Metab* 2003;16:49–54.

24. Farrell LS, Hannan EL, Cooper A. Severity of injury and mortality associated with pediatric blunt injuries: Hospitals with pediatric intensive care units versus other hospitals. *Pediatr Crit Care Med* 2004;5:5–9.

25. Potoka DA, Schall LC, Gardner MJ, et al. Impact of pediatric trauma centers on mortality in a statewide system. *J Trauma* 2000;49:237–45.

26. Sasser SM, Hunt RC, Sullivent EE, et al. Guidelines for field triage of injured patients. Recommendations of the National Expert Panel on Field Triage. *MMWR Recomm Rep* 2009;58:1–35.

27. Kragh JF Jr, Walters TJ, Baer DG, et al. Survival with emergency tourniquet use to stop bleeding in major limb trauma. *Ann Surg* 2009;249:1–7.

28. Kragh JF Jr, Cooper A, Aden JK, et al. Survey of trauma registry data on tourniquet use in pediatric war casualties. *Pediatr Emerg Care* 2012;28:1361–5.

29. Diab YA, Wong ECC, Luban NLC. Massive transfusion in children and neonates. *Br J Haematol* 2013;161:15–26.

30. Spinella PC, Holcomb JB. Resuscitation and transfusion principles for traumatic hemorrhagic shock. *Blood Rev* 2009;23(6):231–40.

31. Chidester SJ, Williams N, Wang W, et al. A pediatric massive transfusion protocol. *J Trauma Acute Care Surg* 2012;73:1273–7.

32. Hendrickson JE, Shaz BH, Pereira G, et al. Implementation of a pediatric trauma massive transfusion protocol: One institutions experience. *Transfusion* 2012;52:1228–36.

33. Borgman MA, Spinella PC, Perkins JG, et al. The ratio of blood products transfused affects mortality in patients receiving massive transfusions at a combat support hospital. *J Trauma* 2007;63:805–13.

34. Malone DL, Hess JR, Fingerhut A. Massive transfusion practices around the globe and a suggestion for a common massive transfusion protocol. *J Trauma* 2006;60:S91–S96.

35. Dressler AM, Finck CM, Carroll CL, et al. Use of a massive transfusion protocol with hemostatic resuscitation for severe intraoperative bleeding in a child. *J Pediatr Surg* 2010;45:1530–3.

36. Morenski JD, Tobias JD, Jimenez DF. Recombinant activated factor VII for cerebral injury-induced coagulopathy in pediatric patients. Report of three cases and review of the literature. *J Neurosurg* 2003;98:611–6.

37. Fortenberry JD, Meier AH, Pettignano R, et al. Extracorporeal life support for posttraumatic acute respiratory distress syndrome at a children's medical center. *J Pediatr Surg* 2003;38:1221–6.

38. Boffard KD, Riou B, Warren B, et al. Recombinant factor VIIa as adjunctive therapy for bleeding control in severely injured trauma patients: Two parallel randomized, placebo-controlled, double-blind clinical trials. *J Trauma* 2005;59:8–15; discussion 15–8.

39. Alderson P, Bunn F, Lefebvre C, et al. Human albumin solution for resuscitation and volume expansion in critically ill patients. *Cochrane Database Syst Rev* 2004:CD001208.

40. Roberts I, Alderson P, Bunn F, et al. Colloids versus crystalloids for fluid resuscitation in critically ill patients. *Cochrane Database Syst Rev* 2004:CD000567.

41. Zhang H, Voglis S, Kim CH, et al. Effects of albumin and Ringer's lactate on production of lung cytokines and hydrogen peroxide after resuscitated hemorrhage and endotoxemia in rats. *Crit Care Med* 2003;31:1515–22.

42. Deb S, Sun L, Martin B, et al. Lactated Ringer's solution and hetastarch but not plasma resuscitation after rat hemorrhagic shock is associated with immediate lung apoptosis by the up-regulation of the Bax protein. *J Trauma* 2000;49:47–53; discussion 53–5.

43. Rowe GG, McKenna DH, Corliss RJ, et al. Hemodynamic effects of hypertonic sodium chloride. *J Appl Physiol* 1972;32:182–4.

44. Wildenthal K, Mierzwiak DS, Mitchell JH. Acute effects of increased serum osmolality on left ventricular performance. *Am J Physiol* 1969;216:898–904.

45. Deitch EA, Shi HP, Feketeova E, et al. Hypertonic saline resuscitation limits neutrophil activation after trauma-hemorrhagic shock. *Shock* 2003;19:328–33.

46. Shi HP, Deitch EA, Da Xu Z, et al. Hypertonic saline improves intestinal mucosa barrier function and lung injury after trauma-hemorrhagic shock. *Shock* 2002;17:496–501.

47. Weil MH, Henning RJ. New concepts in the diagnosis and fluid treatment of circulatory shock. Thirteenth annual Becton, Dickinson and Company Oscar Schwidetsky Memorial Lecture. *Anesth Analg* 1979;58:124–32.

48. Friese RS, Shafi S, Gentilello LM. Pulmonary artery catheter use is associated with reduced mortality in severely injured patients: A National Trauma Data Bank analysis of 53,312 patients. *Crit Care Med* 2006;34:1597–601.

49. Cooper A, Barlow B, DiScala C, et al. Mortality and truncal injury: The pediatric perspective. *J Pediatr Surg* 1994;29:33–8.

50. Fortenberry JD, Meier AH, Pettignano R, et al. Extracorporeal life support for posttraumatic acute respiratory distress syndrome at a children's medical center. *J Pediatr Surg* 2003;38:1221–6.

51. Allen GS, Cox CS Jr. Pulmonary contusion in children: Diagnosis and management. *South Med J* 1998;91:1099–106.

52. Stylianos S. Evidence-based guidelines for resource utilization in children with isolated spleen or liver injury. The APSA Trauma Committee. *J Pediatr Surg* 2000;35:164–7; discussion 7–9.

53. Bliss D, Silen M. Pediatric thoracic trauma. *Crit Care Med* 2002;30:S409–S415.

54. Moore EE, Cogbill TH, Jurkovich GJ, et al. Organ injury scaling: Spleen and liver (1994 revision). *J Trauma* 1995;38:323–4.

55. Moore EE, Shackford SR, Pachter HL, et al. Organ injury scaling: Spleen, liver, and kidney. *J Trauma* 1989;29:1664–6.

56. Shilyansky J, Sena LM, Kreller M, et al. Nonoperative management of pancreatic injuries in children. *J Pediatr Surg* 1998;33:343–9.

57. Beck R, Halberthal M, Zonis Z, et al. Abdominal compartment syndrome in children. *Pediatr Crit Care Med* 2001;2:51–6.

58. DiScala C, Sege R, Li G, et al. Child abuse and unintentional injuries: A 10-year retrospective. *Arch Pediatr Adolesc Med* 2000;154:16–22.

59. Caffey J. The whiplash shaken infant syndrome: Manual shaking by the extremities with whiplash-induced intracranial and intra-ocular bleedings, linked with residual permanent brain damage and mental retardation. *Pediatrics* 1974;54:396–403.

60. Aitken ME, Jaffe KM, DiScala C, et al. Functional outcome in children with multiple trauma without significant head injury. *Arch Phys Med Rehabil* 1999;80:889–95.

61. Keenan HT, Runyan DK, Nocera M. Child outcomes and family characteristics 1 year after severe inflicted or noninflicted traumatic brain injury. *Pediatrics* 2006;117:317–24.

62. Winston FK, Kassam-Adams N, Vivarelli-O'Neill C, et al. Acute stress disorder symptoms in children and their parents after pediatric traffic injury. *Pediatrics* 2002;109:E90.

63. de Vries AP, Kassam-Adams N, Cnaan A, et al. Looking beyond the physical injury: Posttraumatic stress disorder in children and parents after pediatric traffic injury. *Pediatrics* 1999;104:1293–9.

64. Landolt MA, Vollrath M, Ribi K, et al. Incidence and associations of parental and child posttraumatic stress symptoms in pediatric patients. *J Child Psychol Psychiatry* 2003;44:1199–207.

65. Schreier H, Ladakakos C, Morabito D, et al. Posttraumatic stress symptoms in children after mild to moderate pediatric trauma: A longitudinal examination of symptom prevalence, correlates, and parent-child symptom reporting. *J Trauma* 2005;58:353–63.

66. Patel JC, Mollitt DL, Tepas JJ III. Infectious complications in critically injured children. *J Pediatr Surg* 2000;35:1174–8.

67. Azu MC, McCormack JE, Scriven RJ, et al. Venous thromboembolic events in pediatric trauma patients: Is prophylaxis necessary? *J Trauma* 2005;59:1345–9.

68. Truitt AK, Sorrells DL, Halvorson E, et al. Pulmonary embolism: Which pediatric trauma patients are at risk? *J Pediatr Surg* 2005;40:124–7.

69. Grandas OH, Klar M, Goldman MH, et al. Deep venous thrombosis in the pediatric trauma population: An unusual event: Report of three cases. *Am Surg* 2000;66:273–6.

CHAPTER 31 ■ DROWNING

KATHERINE V. BIAGAS AND LINDA APONTE-PATEL

KEY POINTS

1 Drowning injury is a leading cause of accident-related childhood death and disability.
   a. Two age groups are primarily affected (infant/toddler and adolescent).
   b. Epidemiology is related to developmental risks and behaviors at these ages.

2 Therapy at the scene focuses on initial restoration of respiration and circulation.
   a. Rapid transportation to a hospital is essential for those who remain "lifeless" with consideration of appropriate transfer to a specialty center for definitive care (cerebral resuscitation).

3 Drowning events are distinct from more usual forms of cardiac arrest in that drowning is an asphyxia event with subsequent cessation of cardiac function.
   a. Rescue breathing and chest compressions, rather than chest compressions alone, are indicated for those who remain "lifeless."

4 Cerebral resuscitation is primary. Evidence extrapolated from clinical events and laboratory experiments supports the consideration of mild hypothermia as a cerebral resuscitation method.
   a. Temperature monitoring to maintain body cooling in the emergency department and pediatric intensive care unit is indicated.
   b. Rewarming should be reserved for those with persistent nonperfusing rhythms.

5 Treatment of injury to the lungs and cardiovascular system contributes to the potential for brain resuscitation.
   a. A "protective lung strategy" should be adopted as long as it does not contribute to increased intracranial pressure.

6 Prognosis is difficult to determine in the early phases of care.
   a. A picture of likely outcome develops over time with repeated neurological examinations and adjunctive studies such as magnetic resonance imaging (MRI) scans.

7 The pediatric intensivist can be an important advocate for responsible community action focusing on drowning prevention.

In 2005, the World Health Organization (WHO) defined drowning as "... the process of experiencing respiratory impairment from submersion/immersion in liquid" (1). The WHO estimates that nearly 400,000 persons die from drowning annually. In many countries, drowning is the second or third most frequent cause of childhood death (2). In the United States, drowning events account for ~1000 deaths and more than 3000 emergency department (ED) visits annually for children less than 19 years of age (3). In some states, drowning is the leading cause of death for children under the age of five (4). Despite recent efforts to prevent such events and advances in medical care, outcomes for many drowning injuries remain quite poor.

The previous terminology describing drowning events was confusing and much of it is no longer used. Terms such as "wet drowning," "dry drowning," "near-drowning," and "drowning injury" did not offer clinically important distinctions and have been abandoned in favor of using the definition mentioned above and the general term "drowning" for all (1). Similarly, the terms used for the outcomes from drowning have been simplified to death, morbidity, and no morbidity.

EPIDEMIOLOGY

Sociodemographic considerations have significant effects on the epidemiology of drowning events (**Table 31.1**). The majority of drowning events occur in freshwater with a large proportion of these occurring in natural bodies of water—rivers, creeks, lakes, and ponds. Drowning also occurs frequently in domestic sites—home pools, spas, or bathtubs—and recreational community pools, water parks, schools, etc. As few as 4% of events occur in salt water, although this incidence is higher in coastal communities (5). The three groups of children at particular risk for drowning include the very young, male adolescents, and African-American children. Drowning events that involve infants and toddlers commonly occur in sources of water in the home (5,6). Infants 6–11 months of age drown in bathtubs and these are not prevented by the use of bathtub seats (5,7). Older infants and toddlers drown as the result of a fall into a shallow body of water (i.e., a wading pool) as well as in bathtubs (5,7). Outcomes in these children are usually poor. Infants and toddlers are the group least likely to have a witnessed drowning event, which is associated with longer drowning time. In this age group, males and females drown with equal frequency; in all other age groups the prevalence of drowning is higher in males (5,7).

Boys 15–19 years of age have the second highest drowning rate. Events in this age group are generally related to recreational water activities. These male adolescents have the highest rate of drowning while swimming, boating, or driving a car even when compared with adults who over a lifetime engage in such activities to a greater extent (7). African-American children have higher drowning rates and the highest drowning mortality rates are seen in 15 to 19-year-old African-American males as compared with Caucasian and Hispanic counterparts (8).

Certain medical conditions may predispose children to drowning. Drowning risk is elevated in children with epilepsy and certain neurologic conditions with the most events occurring in bathtubs and pools. Epilepsy, excluding other

TABLE 31.1

EPIDEMIOLOGIC, SOCIODEMOGRAPHIC, AND PREVENTION CONSIDERATIONS IN DROWNING ACCIDENTS

■ AGE GROUP	■ MORTALITY	■ GENDER	■ COMMON MECHANISMS	■ SOCIODEMOGRAPHIC FACTORS	■ PREVENTION MEASURES
0–4 y	2.5/100,000 (overall), 4/100,000 (1–3 y)	M = F	■ Infants: bathtubs, water containers ■ Toddlers: domestic and community water sources (inflatable pools, ponds)	■ "Inattention" events: ■ Times of inattentive adult supervision (dinner preparation) ■ Unsupervised "bath time" or use of unreliable aids such as "bathtub rings"	■ Anticipatory guidance: usual hazards ■ Attentive adult supervision ■ Early swimming training has limited but possible utility
4–12 y	0.85–1/100,000	M > F (2:1)	Community or domestic water sources such as ponds, swimming pools, open water sources	■ Gender difference in incidence related to the initiation of greater engagement in risk-taking behaviors by males	■ Swimming lessons (drowning prevention skills) for >4 year-olds is endorsed by AAP ■ Latched, 4-sided pool fencing
Adolescents	2.6/100,000	M > F (nearly 10:1)	Open water sources, boating accidents	■ Highest death rate of all groups for African-American adolescents (4.5/100,000) ■ Death attributable to alcohol intoxication in 10%–30%	■ Swimming instruction and water survival training ■ Education about drug and alcohol abuse

Data drawn from recent American Academy of Pediatrics sources. American Academy of Pediatrics Committee on Injury, Violence, and Poison Prevention. Prevention of drowning. *Pediatrics* 2010;126:178–85; Meyer RJ, Theodorou AA, Berg RA. Childhood drowning. *Pediatr Rev* 2006; 27:163–8; quiz 9.

neurologic disabilities, results in a 10-fold increased risk of drowning (9). In one report, 7% of pediatric drowning victims had a prior history of seizure (7). Hyperventilation with swimming exertion may predispose a child with epilepsy to have a seizure, precipitating the drowning event. The risk of drowning is also greater in children with autism (10) or mental retardation.

Patients with long QT syndrome (LQTS) or other cardiac "channelopathies" are also at increased risk of drowning (11,12). In these patients, ventricular tachyarrhythmias may be exacerbated by swimming. In one report, 91% of patients presenting for cardiac evaluation who also had a personal or family history of swimming-related syncope had mutations in the LQTS1 gene (11). Similar results have been found with other genes associated with LQTS (13). Swimming is an arrhythmogenic trigger with activation of the "diving reflex," which alters autonomic stability (14). The "diving reflex" is elicited in mammals by contact of the face with cold water and consists of breath-holding, bradycardia, and intense peripheral vasoconstriction. Swimming also involves physical exertion, which may be a syncopal trigger in some. Screening of relatives is recommended for anyone suspected of having a swimming-related arrhythmia syndrome. Counseling regarding safe water-related activities and β-blockade therapy are recommended for affected individuals.

The use of alcohol or other intoxicating substances is associated with drowning in adolescents and adults. Thirty to seventy percent of boating and swimming fatalities in these age groups have measurable blood alcohol levels (15). Moreover, the intoxicated victim may vomit and aspirate gastric contents. Other medical conditions that less frequently predispose to drowning include depression, coronary artery disease, cardiomyopathy, hypoglycemia, and hypothermia.

Drowning injuries in older children and adolescents may be associated with cervical spine injury. The incidence of such injury is low, estimated at 0.5%–5.0% of drowning events (4). The mechanism of injury is diving or falling into a body of water with a blow that hyperextends the cervical spine. A history of diving is usually elicited. When evaluating victims of unwitnessed events, the possibility of associated cervical spine injury should be considered. Immobilization of the cervical spine at the scene is important. As with other injuries of the spine, the diagnosis is a clinical one and is based on suspicion about the mechanism of injury and the patient's neurologic condition. Radiographs of the cervical spine may be normal despite debilitating cord injury and MRI is usually necessary to confirm the clinical suspicion.

PATHOPHYSIOLOGY

The initial sequence of events in drowning was studied in the 1930s in animals and consists of the following: an initial struggle sometimes with a surprise inhalation, suspension of movement and exhalation of a little air frequently followed by swallowing, violent struggle, convulsions with spasmodic respiratory efforts through an open mouth, loss of reflexes, and death. This sequence has been confirmed in many cases by bystanders who witness this progression. During the initial seconds of drowning, small amounts of aspirated fluid often cause laryngospasm. Victims who are resuscitated at this phase will have little water aspiration, but ventilation by rescue breathing may be difficult because of glottic closure. If the victim loses muscle tone while submerged, larger quantities of fluid may be aspirated. In addition, a victim may swallow a large amount of fluid, vomit, and aspirate gastric contents.

The development of hypothermia is common with drowning and the presence of hypothermia should not be interpreted as a *cold water drowning* (discussed later). Hypothermia during drowning is usually secondary to rapid radiant heat losses in tepid water. As core temperature drops below 32°–35°C, unconsciousness and muscular weakness develop and the risk of aspiration is increased. Atrial fibrillation occurs with core temperatures in the low 30°C and ventricular fibrillation or asystole with severe hypothermia at a core temperature less than 28°C.

Cardiorespiratory Arrest

Drowning is an asphyxial cardiac arrest (ACA), which is distinct from more usual forms of primary cardiac arrest (CA) such as ventricular fibrillation. This distinction has implication for brain resuscitation therapies (discussed below). In ACA, victims have cessation of gas exchange first with resultant hypoxic deterioration and eventual CA. For the ACA victim, hypoxemia precedes ischemia and may augment injury.

Respiratory and Cardiovascular Dysfunction

In drowning victims with brief episodes of hypoxia, hypoxemia is limited to the duration of hypopnea or apnea and resolves with rescue or initial resuscitation efforts. However, in patients with longer hypoxic episodes and alveolar aspiration, these processes are more aggressive with surfactant washout, resultant lung collapse, alveolar derecruitment, intrapulmonary shunting, raised pulmonary vascular resistance, and ventilation–perfusion mismatching. In combination, these processes create the clinical syndromes of acute lung injury (ALI) and acute respiratory distress syndrome (ARDS). Aspiration of gastric contents may add caustic injury to airways and alveoli, worsening ALI. Lastly, neurogenic pulmonary edema may contribute to deficits in gas exchange and lung function.

The hallmark of cardiovascular dysfunction associated with drowning is decreased myocardial contractility with hypoxemia. Ventricular end-diastolic pressures are raised, as are atrial pressures, with resultant congestion of central and pulmonary veins. Poor myocardial contractility, in combination with raised systemic vascular resistance, results in lower cardiac output. Cessation of cardiac function occurs as body temperature or oxygenation decreases as previously discussed.

Brain Injury

The important sequela of ACA is hypoxic–ischemic brain injury. Metabolically active areas, such as subcortical tissues, and regions with so-called "watershed" perfusion are the most vulnerable. Global brain involvement is seen in the most severe cases. The combination of hypoxemia and low-flow states results in a host of pathologic processes including energy failure, lipid peroxidation, production of free radicals, inflammatory responses, and release of excitotoxic neurotransmitters. There is disruption of neuronal and glial functions. Neuronal losses occur in selectively vulnerable zones with "delayed neuronal drop out." ACA may differ importantly from CA in the development of microinfarctions in addition to selective neuronal injury (16). The reader is referred to the thorough review of brain injury and resuscitation after ACA by Topjian et al. (17) for a more complete discussion of research on the unique mechanisms of ACA and putative therapeutic targets.

Drowning in Ice-Cold Water

The terms "cold water" or "ice water" drowning are worth retaining when used correctly. Brain function may be preserved in "ice-cold water drowning" with good and even normal neurologic outcomes observed despite extensive submersion times. Numerous reports have documented dramatic cases of intact neurological functioning in children who drowned in ice-cold water (6,18,19). The term "cold water drowning" is a misnomer in that the drowning must occur in ice-cold water and, with very rare exceptions, is a phenomenon restricted to cold weather climates (18). Patients who have drowned in more temperate water but who have become hypothermic should be considered to have hypothermia from prolonged submersion. Such secondary hypothermia is often a poor prognostic sign associated with prolonged submersion before rescue.

Young children are particularly susceptible to rapid cooling of the brain in ice-cold water because of little subcutaneous fat and large head-to-body ratio. Moreover, brain preservation may be augmented by activation of the "diving reflex," which slows metabolism and may preserve some perfusion to the heart and brain. Additionally, neurologic preservation can be seen when the lower body is submersed in ice water and the head remains above water allowing the victim to continue to breathe. The result is rapid brain cooling in the face of residual perfusion and provision of brain substrates.

It should be noted that ice-cold water drowning is associated with a rather high incidence of arrhythmias. Shattock and Tipton (20) studied this phenomenon by investigating the parasympathetic and sympathetic responses in healthy volunteers to ice water immersion of the face. Simultaneous activation of the diving response and the breath-holding response was noted inducing responses of bradycardia and tachycardia, respectively. They refer to this phenomenon as "autonomic conflict" and point to it as a cause of arrhythmias (20).

MANAGEMENT

Prehospital Management

The clinical management of drowning begins at the scene and continues during transport, at the ED, and when necessary into the pediatric intensive care unit (PICU) followed by a rehabilitation center. **Table 31.2** outlines the three most active areas of acute management. Management at the scene should focus on rapid restoration of oxygenation and spontaneous circulation with basic cardiopulmonary resuscitation. Emergency services should be summoned as quickly as possible. In contradistinction to the recommendations of chest compressions only for victims of CA, the victims of drowning have suffered ACA and rescue breathing as well as chest compressions should be administered by bystanders (17). Of these, early initiation of rescue breathing is paramount. In patients who have suffered respiratory arrest and continue to have some spontaneous circulation, reestablishing ventilation usually results in recovery with no serious morbidity (14). Time should not be wasted by attempting to drain water from the lungs before rescue breathing commences. If possible, bystanders should perform mouth-to-mouth breathing before the patient is removed from the water. Trained rescuers, equipped with buoyant rescue aids, should attempt in-water rescue breathing of the victim found in deep water (21). Once on solid ground, chest compressions should be initiated unless signs of life are present. Cervical spine immobilization should be performed in cases with a history of diving, or when the cause of drowning is not known. Spinal immobilization is otherwise unnecessary and should not interfere with resuscitative efforts.

TABLE 31.2

IMPORTANT PRINCIPLES IN THE MANAGEMENT OF CHILDREN WITH DROWNING EVENTS ARRANGED BY PHASE OF CARE

■ PHASE OF CARE	■ FOCUS OF THERAPY	■ SPECIFIC MEASURES
Prehospital	Initial rescue	■ Removal from water
		■ Activate EMS system
	Resuscitation	■ Rescue breathing
		■ Rescue breathing + chest compressions if "lifeless" appearing
		■ Consider cervical collar for diving accidents
Emergency department	Oxygenation and ventilation	■ Supply supplemental oxygen
		■ Intubation if unable to protect airway
		■ Ventilation to provide normocarbia
	Brain resuscitation	■ Temperature monitoring to maintain body cooling
		■ Rewarming for persistent nonperfusing rhythms
	Circulation	■ Vasoactive agents for hypotension
	Disposition	■ Transfer victims not fully alert for definitive care
PICU	Brain resuscitation	■ Consider therapeutic hypothermia (32°C–34°C for 12–72h)
		■ Control of fevers and seizures
	Respiratory management	■ "Lung protective" strategy ventilation for ALI/ARDS unless contributes to increased ICP
	Treatment of hypotension/shock	■ Vasoactive infusions
	Restore homeostatic systems	■ Control of dysglycemia
		■ Measurement and monitoring of electrolyte and fluid abnormalities
	Assessment of prognosis	■ Repeated neurologic exams
		■ CT if concern for trauma
		■ MRI/MRS
		■ Electrophysiologic studies
		■ Measurement of biomarkers—future measure

EMS, emergency medical services; ALI, acute lung injury; ARDS, acute respiratory distress syndrome; ICP, intracranial pressure; CT, computerized tomography; MRI, magnetic resonance imaging; MRS, magnetic resonance spectroscopy.

Advanced life support should be initiated by paramedics for victims who do not regain spontaneous breathing and consciousness with rescue breaths. Bag valve mask ventilation with supplemental oxygen is sufficient to restore circulation in some. Endotracheal intubation with manual ventilation, administration of fluid boluses, defibrillation, and administration of bolus vasoactive medications may be required in others. However, these efforts should not be pursued to the extent that transportation of the victim to a hospital is delayed. Many hospitals are not prepared to handle the critical care needs of children requiring brain resuscitation after ACA. Prehospital providers should weigh the advantages and disadvantages of transport of such children to the nearest hospital versus one with more specialized capabilities. Expedient, initial stabilization may be preferred but if the initial hospital is not prepared to provide pediatric critical care services, then later transport to a specialty center is indicated.

Management in the Emergency Department

Definitive care begins in the ED. Advanced life support should focus on establishment of adequate of oxygenation and ventilation, adequate circulation, and determination of neurologic functioning. Intubation and positive pressure ventilation is required for patients who cannot protect their airway or remain unconscious. Continuous positive pressure or noninvasive, bi-level ventilation may be sufficient support for those who are partially or fully conscious but who have alterations in gas exchange. With any method of respiratory support the goals are to avoid or treat hypoxemia and to minimize hyperoxemia. Support of circulatory function may be required for hypotension associated with passive rewarming of the victim in the ambient environment of the ED. Continuous infusions of vasopressor or inotropic agents should be administered to maintain a normal blood pressure range. Initial neurologic status is approximated using the Glasgow Coma Score (GCS) with a more thorough neurological examination performed later. Repeated GCS determinations during the first 12 hours of treatment and repeated neurological examinations throughout hospitalization are necessary to document improvement or deterioration in function.

Temperature management of patients is a key component of brain resuscitation. Core temperature should be measured continuously or frequently. In the ED, core temperature measurement with an esophageal or rectal probe is easiest. In the PICU, continuous temperature monitoring can be accomplished by the use of these or an intravenous catheter with thermistor. A recent literature review advocates for abandoning aggressive rewarming (17). Studies of hypothermic treatment in adults with CA suggest that brain cooling may be neuroprotective and that better-than-expected neurologic outcomes are possible (22,23). Given these encouraging data, consideration should be given to maintaining mild hypothermia (core temperature of 32°C–34°C) for 12–72 hours in children who remain comatose after drowning (17). However, for victims with sustained ventricular fibrillation, rewarming may be necessary to establish a perfusing rhythm. For these, the simplest warming techniques include the use of warmed intravenous fluids, external radiant heat, and ventilation with heated gas. More aggressive efforts are sometimes needed and include warmed peritoneal lavage or dialysis fluids and bladder washes with warm fluids. With severe hypothermia and in the absence of a perfusing rhythm, rewarming on cardiopulmonary bypass or extracorporeal cardiopulmonary resuscitation has been described and remains option for consideration. A note of caution, rewarming can induce "rewarming shock," with peripheral vasodilatation and impaired cardiac output. This is especially seen in severely hypothermic patients. If rewarming efforts are used, they should be employed solely to reestablish a perfusing rhythm and stopped as early as possible to prevent overshoot and hyperthermia. In cases in which continued hypothermia is employed, rewarming to keep patient ≤34°C for the first 48–72 hours may be indicated.

Management in the PICU

Children who do not regain full consciousness in the ED, or those with concerns for severe injuries and life-threatening complications should be transferred to a pediatric intensive care facility. Ongoing efforts should be directed to aggressively treat any organ dysfunction. The main focus of PICU care should be on restoration of cerebral function. There is no definitive treatment that reverses neuronal injury or microinfarction and the neurologic critical care is largely supportive. Hypermetabolic states of the brain, such as seizures and fevers, should be aggressively treated. Seizures are common sequelae of hypoxic–ischemic brain injury and their clinical detection is sometimes difficult. Accordingly, routine electroencephalography (EEG) may be needed to detect subclinical events and to titrate antiepileptic therapy.

The use of therapeutic hypothermia as a neuroprotective treatment strategy for drowning injuries has largely been extrapolated from the findings in other types of brain injuries. That said, hypothermia represents the sole brain resuscitation option in current practice. In the late 1970s, therapy included moderate dehydration, controlled hyperventilation, deep hypothermia (30°C), barbiturate coma, corticosteroids, and continuous muscular paralysis over 48–72 hours (24). Subsequent retrospective studies in children showed that deep hypothermia for pulseless victims resulted in more survivors who suffered a persistent vegetative state (18,25) and increased infectious complications (25). The promising results of moderate hypothermia in treating adults following witnessed out-of-hospital CA (23,26) and in multiple studies of asphyxiated newborns (see reviews in References 27 and 28), as well as data from animal models of ACA (17) suggest possible usefulness of this therapy. In their systematic review of the subject, Topjian et al. (17) recommend maintaining a target core temperature of 32°–34°C for 12–72 hours. Use of moderate hypothermia comes with a caveat: To maintain hypothermia, patients may require the use of neuromuscular blocking agents that interfere with the neurologic examination. Much of the remainder of discussion in this section will focus on the major therapeutic considerations for extracranial organ systems. There will be particular emphasis on the effects of these therapies on brain resuscitation.

For patients with ALI or ARDS, an "open-lung strategy" should be employed. Usual ventilator management includes limiting peak pressures to 25 torr, tidal volumes to 6–8 mL/kg, fraction of inspired oxygen to <0.60, and increasing positive end-expiratory pressure (PEEP) (to improve oxygenation). Ventilator management may need to be altered if significant brain injury is detected. Permissive hypercapnia, a commonly used lung protective strategy, may adversely affect intracranial pressure (ICP) as elevations in Pco_2 may further increase ICP. Moreover, the increase in intrathoracic pressure associated with high levels of PEEP be transmitted to the intracranial space and further increase ICP as well as diminish cerebral venous return.

Lung injury following drowning is at least partly related to surfactant washout; however, efficacy of surfactant administration has only been shown in case reports (29,30). Routine administration of exogenous surfactant is not supported by present evidence. Its use should be limited to those with severe hypoxemic respiratory failure. Other extraordinary methods of lung support, including extracorporeal membrane oxygenation (31,32), inhaled nitric oxide, and prone positioning (33), have been suggested and are considered for cases with severe ALI/ARDS.

The brain is greatly aided when normal cardiovascular functions are maintained. Continuous vasoactive infusions may be required to treat myocardial dysfunction and to correct abnormal peripheral vascular resistance; although, the need for sustained cardiovascular support is rare. Treatment should concentrate on normalizing blood pressure, organ perfusion, and gas exchange for as long as needed.

Both hypo- and hyperglycemia are associated with critical illness and both conditions are associated with increased mortality and morbidity (34). In addition, hyper- or hypoglycemia in children with brain injury may worsen neurologic outcome. The injured brain may be particularly susceptible to alterations in serum glucose as glucose is the primary metabolic substrate for brain and its supply across the blood–brain barrier may be limited by injury. Accordingly, normoglycemia should be maintained in patients after drowning (recommendations for therapeutic ranges of glucose in brain injury are under investigation). Frequent assessments of serum or whole blood glucose are indicated and periodic adjustments in glucose infusion rates may be necessary.

Much has been made of possible fluid shifts and electrolyte disturbances in drowning. Postmortem examinations demonstrate mild to moderate hyponatremia and hypotonic hemolysis in victims who drowned in freshwater and moderate hypernatremia and hyperchloremia after salt water drowning. However, clinically important abnormalities in serum electrolyte concentrations are not usually found in patients who survive the event. Exceptions to this generality are found in drowning that occurs in high-salinity water, such as the Dead Sea. Important disorders of vascular volume are not often seen after drowning. Hemodilution and hypervolemia may be found with fresh-water-associated drowning but these are generally mild as the absorbed fluid is readily excreted in survivors. These findings do not require therapy and are not considered to contribute greatly to brain injury. Volume contraction after salt water drowning may be seen in cases of severe ingestion, but such victims do not usually survive. The critical care practitioner should measure electrolytes and assess the volume status of drowning victims but corrective therapy is rarely required.

Neuromonitoring is another important consideration. Evaluation of change is accomplished by frequent neurologic examinations. Evidence of higher cortical function is usually associated with a potential for a good neurologic outcome while deterioration in brainstem functions suggests poor prognosis. Continuous EEG monitoring may be helpful to detect presence of subclinical seizures or response to antiepileptic therapy in the presence of neuromuscular blockade during hypothermia. Intracranial hypertension is a consideration in those with severe ACA and is a marker of poor prognosis but there is no evidence that ICP management in drowning affects outcome. The clinical practice of ICP-directed therapy is not generally supported. An exception may include the use of ICP monitoring in those with severe ARDS to help determine the impact of permissive hypercarbia, low oxygen saturation, and intrathoracic pressure levels (due to PEEP) on ICP. Another consideration for the use of ICP monitoring is to determine if neurologic deterioration during rewarming is due to an exacerbation of intracranial hypertension in the patient who was therapeutically cooled.

PREVENTION

The usual role of the pediatric intensivist is to care for a victim after the fact. Yet, the pediatric intensivist can be an effective advocate for injury prevention. Community efforts focused on responsible water safety tend to get their start after the tragic death or injury of a drowned child. Pediatric intensivists can greatly aid these efforts by relating their unique personal observations about the toll of such injuries. Community activism combined with effective physician advocacy can create powerful responses to unsafe water hazards and support effective child-care practices. Interested pediatric intensivists are encouraged to get involved in local and state advocacy efforts.

Prevention strategies should focus on the supervision of young children around any water, the risks of recreation-related incidents, the need for CPR training of parents and caretakers, and the use of effective pool and water hazard barriers (15). Supervision of young children around water sources is paramount. Slogans such as "Don't Turn Your Back On Me" alert parents to the proper supervision of infants and toddlers. Parents and caretakers need to be knowledgeable about the risks of all water hazards, including wading pools, spas, drainage ditches, toilets, buckets, and moderate-sized containers. A water-filled 5-gallon bucket has sufficient depth to cause a toddler to drown. Other alerts focus on specific events, for example the installation of a home pool. Most pool-related drowning occurs within the first six months of pool exposure (35). The absence of proper pool fencing may increase the odds of pool-related drowning by as much as three- to fivefold (35)

Additional prevention campaigns focus on the family pediatrician. The American Academy of Pediatrics (AAP) updated its policy statement in 2010 to guide pediatricians in incorporating regular, age-appropriate teaching about water safety in their anticipatory guidance, as well as highlighting other topics such as drain-entrapment hazards, the dangers of inflatable pools, and possible benefit of swimming lessons for young children (15). Their recommendations can be found on the AAP website at http://www.aap.org/en-us/about-the-aap/aap-press-room/Pages/AAP-Gives-Updated-Advice-on-Drowning-Prevention.aspx. Additional prevention tips and information on safety barriers can be found on the Consumer Product Safety Commission website http://www.cpsc.gov/en/Safety-Education/Neighborhood-Safety-Network/Toolkits/Drowning-Prevention/. Such educational strategies have been met with demonstrable success. Reduction in some types of drowning events was noted in 2002 in the United Kingdom (36), and the AAP reports a 20-year reduction in drowning rates (37).

OUTCOMES

Outcome from drowning is often related to the extent of neurologic injury, which is often difficult to initially predict. Poor prognostic signs include an unwitnessed event, prolonged time to resuscitation, the need for CPR at the scene, the need for continued CPR in the ED, (38), and prolonged coma. The best independent predictor of survival is drowning time (14,39); however, these data are not known for many patients. In Toronto, investigators found the presence of a detectable heartbeat and hypothermia on initial examination in the ED to be discriminate predictors of good outcome from death or persistent vegetative state (25). These findings may not be generalizable; rather they may reflect the somewhat unique occurrence

in Ontario of drowning in ice water. In the ED, a physical examination remarkable for nonreactive pupils or a Glasgow Coma Scale score of ≤5 predicts poor neurologic outcome (40) but is not absolute. Predictors of outcomes at the time of PICU admission are also of mixed certainty (41). Drowning victims who are awake on admission have generally good outcomes. The opposite statement cannot be made. Those who remain nonresponsive at 24 hours after admission do not necessarily have poor outcome (42). Moreover, gross neurological examination of drowned children at the time of discharge may not reveal all sequelae (41). Follow-up neuropsychological and behavioral evaluation is indicated for many.

Specific prognostic scales are similarly less satisfactory in discriminatory function. The Pediatric Risk of Mortality Score, a predictor of mortality in critical illness, discriminates between death and the presence or absence of poor outcome, but is unable to distinguish between different degrees of neurologic dysfunction (43). Other clinical classification systems developed specifically for drowning events have been similarly inadequate (1,44). A reasonable approach, therefore, is to avoid using prognostic factors and instead use a "treat them all approach" with aggressive efforts despite initial lack of heartbeat (40). Prognosis is deferred until circulation is restored and perfusion optimized. At that time, the patient can be more completely examined.

Adjunct radiographic studies can aid in the determination of the extent of the initial injury and contribute to the understanding of ongoing disease. Brain CT is often used in the initial assessment of patients, especially in patients with a history of a possible associated traumatic injury. Repeated brain CT scans add little information unless the neurological examination is particularly grim, such as a CT scan done when the clinical findings suggest the loss of all brainstem reflexes. With extensive insults, CT scan may show a "reversal sign" or global "ground glass" appearance with attenuation of signal in the supratentorial intracranial contents or the entire brain, respectively.

MRI and MR spectroscopy (MRS) scans detect more subtle injury (45,46). Diffusion-weighted imaging detects early (minutes to hours) injury after CA and may provide information about poor prognosis (47). Repeat MR scans obtained 4–7 days after injury may be the most predictive (48) and MRS may aid in this determination (45).

Electrophysiologic studies may provide additional information. Brain stem auditory-evoked responses (BSAER) have been used to evaluate prolonged functional outcome with some success (49). Absence of bilateral N20 somatosensory evoked potentials (SSEP) suggest poor outcome in adults after CA (42). A series of electrophysiological modalities, including sleep recordings, BSAER, SSEP, and polysomnography, was used to generate a more complete picture of functioning in five children who remained comatose after drowning (50). Better prediction may be attained using all of these modalities over the use of EEG alone (50); however, cost issues and availability of resources may make this an impractical approach.

One might expect that biomarkers would be ideal predictors of outcome. Biomarkers are proteins or protein conjugates that are breakdown products from organ injury. Biomarkers that discriminate between good, functional, and poor outcomes in drowning victims are not known. Some use can be extrapolated from data on biomarkers in stress or CA. Using this approach, putative biomarkers fall into two categories, those associated with severe critical illness or with brain injuries. Blood glucose, serum lactate, and pro-calcitonin levels are nonspecific stress biomarkers. High blood glucose on presentation has been associated with death or persistent vegetative state in children who drowned (51). Neuron-specific enolase (NSE) is a brain biomarker that has undergone very limited study in drowning victims. A single case report exists of a patient with good outcome who had a peak serum NSE level below the cutoff value of 33 μg/L—a value established in guidelines associated with extensive brain injury after CA (52,53). However, the usefulness of NSE may be limited in the presence of trauma as NSE is also an erythrocytic protein and bleeding or hemolysis may cause elevation unrelated to brain injury. The brain-specific biomarkers S-100B and glial fibrillary protein are being investigated in brain injury and CA and their usefulness remains to be established.

In summary, no prognostic test or assessment reliably predicts functional neurologic outcomes after drowning; moreover, no indicator is sufficiently reliable to be the determinant of a decision to withdraw or withhold therapy in drowning victims. It is recommended that care be continued until the likely prognosis can be discerned from multiple sources of information. And the best source of information remains changes over time in the neurological examination (41).

CONCLUSIONS AND FUTURE DIRECTIONS

Drowning injury is one of the leading causes of accident-related mortality and morbidity in childhood. The pathophysiologic processes of such injury are those of ACA. At present, therapy is focused on restoration of oxygenation, ventilation, and circulation at the scene with rapid transfer to an ED and pediatric intensive care facility when the patient does not experience rapid, full recovery. At present, therapy for brain injury is largely limited to good supportive care and avoidance of secondary insults. Hypothermia is the only current therapy with putative benefit in ACA. On the basis of very limited data for this specific condition, its use can be supported. Advancements in general critical care such as treating ALI/ARDS, managing transient cardiac dysfunction and arrhythmias, and supporting end-organ function remain the mainstays of extracerebral care. Prognostic indicators of outcome can be detected, although there is no one such indicator or time point of measurement. Thorough and repeated neurologic examinations and adjunct studies such as brain MRIs remain the best guides about prognosis. In the near term the greatest benefit may be realized by prevention and community activism about this public health problem.

References

1. van Beeck EF, Branche CM, Szpilman D, et al. A new definition of drowning: Towards documentation and prevention of a global public health problem. *Bull World Health Organ* 2005;83:853–6.
2. Peden M. World report on child injury prevention appeals to "Keep Kids Safe". *Inj Prev* 2008;14:413–4.
3. Moon RE, Long RJ. Drowning and near-drowning. *Emerg Med (Fremantle)* 2002;14:377–86.
4. Wintemute GJ. Childhood drowning and near-drowning in the United States. *Am J Dis Child* 1990;144:663–9.
5. Ibsen LM, Koch T. Submersion and asphyxial injury. *Crit Care Med* 2002;30:S402–S408.
6. Agran PF, Anderson C, Winn D, et al. Rates of pediatric injuries by 3-month intervals for children 0 to 3 years of age. *Pediatrics* 2003;111:e683–e692.
7. Lienhart HG, John W, Wenzel V. Cardiopulmonary resuscitation of a near-drowned child with a combination of epinephrine and vasopressin. *Pediatr Crit Care Med* 2005;6:486–8.
8. Weiss J; American Academy of Pediatrics Committee on Injury, Violence, and Poison Prevention. Prevention of drowning. *Pediatrics* 2010;126:e253–e262.
9. Pearn J, Bart R, Yamaoka R. Drowning risks to epileptic children: A study from Hawaii. *Br Med J* 1978;2:1284–5.
10. Shavelle RM, Strauss DJ, Pickett J. Causes of death in autism. *J Autism Dev Disord* 2001;31:569–76.
11. Choi G, Kopplin LJ, Tester DJ, et al. Spectrum and frequency of cardiac channel defects in swimming-triggered arrhythmia syndromes. *Circulation* 2004;110:2119–24.
12. Quan L, Cummings P. Characteristics of drowning by different age groups. *Inj Prev* 2003;9:163–8.
13. Ackerman MJ, Tester DJ, Porter CJ, et al. Molecular diagnosis of the inherited long-QT syndrome in a woman who died after near-drowning. *N Engl J Med* 1999;341:1121–5.
14. Quan L, Wentz KR, Gore EJ, et al. Outcome and predictors of outcome in pediatric submersion victims receiving prehospital care in King County, Washington. *Pediatrics* 1990;86:586–93.
15. American Academy of Pediatrics Committee on Injury, Violence, and Poison Prevention. Prevention of drowning. *Pediatrics* 2010;126:178–85.
16. Vaagenes P, Safar P, Moossy J, et al. Asphyxiation versus ventricular fibrillation cardiac arrest in dogs. Differences in cerebral resuscitation effects—a preliminary study. *Resuscitation* 1997;35:41–52.
17. Topjian AA, Berg RA, Bierens JJ, et al. Brain resuscitation in the drowning victim. *Neurocrit Care* 2012;17:441–67.
18. Bohn DJ, Biggar WD, Smith CR, et al. Influence of hypothermia, barbiturate therapy, and intracranial pressure monitoring on morbidity and mortality after near-drowning. *Crit Care Med* 1986;14:529–34.
19. Gilbert M, Busund R, Skagseth A, et al. Resuscitation from accidental hypothermia of 13.7 degrees C with circulatory arrest. *Lancet* 2000;355:375–6.
20. Shattock MJ, Tipton MJ. 'Autonomic conflict': A different way to die during cold water immersion? *J Physiol* 2012;590:3219–30.
21. Perkins GD. In-water resuscitation: A pilot evaluation. *Resuscitation* 2005;65:321–4.
22. Arrich J, Holzer M, Havel C, et al. Hypothermia for neuroprotection in adults after cardiopulmonary resuscitation. *Cochrane Database Syst Rev* 2012;9:CD004128.
23. Bernard SA, Gray TW, Buist MD, et al. Treatment of comatose survivors of out-of-hospital cardiac arrest with induced hypothermia. *N Engl J Med* 2002;346:557–63.
24. Conn AW, Edmonds JF, Barker GA. Cerebral resuscitation in near-drowning. *Pediatr Clin North Am* 1979;26:691–701.
25. Biggart MJ, Bohn DJ. Effect of hypothermia and cardiac arrest on outcome of near-drowning accidents in children. *J Pediatr* 1990;117:179–83.
26. Hypothermia after Cardiac Arrest Study Group. Mild therapeutic hypothermia to improve the neurologic outcome after cardiac arrest. *N Engl J Med* 2002;346:549–56.
27. Higgins RD, Raju TN, Perlman J, et al. Hypothermia and perinatal asphyxia: Executive summary of the National Institute of Child Health and Human Development workshop. *J Pediatr* 2006;148:170–5.
28. Shah PS. Hypothermia: A systematic review and meta-analysis of clinical trials. *Semin Fetal Neonatal Med* 2010;15:238–46.
29. Onarheim H, Vik V. Porcine surfactant (Curosurf) for acute respiratory failure after near-drowning in 12 year old. *Acta Anaesthesiol Scand* 2004;48:778–81.
30. Varisco BM, Palmatier CM, Alten JA. Reversal of intractable hypoxemia with exogenous surfactant (calfactant) facilitating complete neurological recovery in a pediatric drowning victim. *Pediatr Emerg Care* 2010;26:571–3.
31. Eich C, Brauer A, Kettler D. Recovery of a hypothermic drowned child after resuscitation with cardiopulmonary bypass followed by prolonged extracorporeal membrane oxygenation. *Resuscitation* 2005;67:145–8.
32. Guenther U, Varelmann D, Putensen C, et al. Extended therapeutic hypothermia for several days during extracorporeal membrane-oxygenation after drowning and cardiac arrest. Two cases of survival with no neurological sequelae. *Resuscitation* 2009;80:379–81.

33. Tulleken JE, van der Werf TS, Ligtenberg JJ, et al. Prone position in a spontaneously breathing near-drowning patient. *Intensive Care Med* 1999;25:1469–70.

34. Hirshberg E, Larsen G, Van Duker H. Alterations in glucose homeostasis in the pediatric intensive care unit: Hyperglycemia and glucose variability are associated with increased mortality and morbidity. *Pediatr Crit Care Med* 2008;9:361–6.

35. Thompson DC, Rivara FP. Pool fencing for preventing drowning in children. *Cochrane Database Syst Rev* 2005:CD001047.

36. Sibert JR, Lyons RA, Smith BA, et al. Preventing deaths by drowning in children in the United Kingdom: Have we made progress in 10 years? Population based incidence study. *BMJ* 2002;324:1070–1.

37. Meyer RJ, Theodorou AA, Berg RA. Childhood drowning. *Pediatr Rev* 2006;27:163–8; quiz 9.

38. Horisberger T, Fischer E, Fanconi S. One-year survival and neurological outcome after pediatric cardiopulmonary resuscitation. *Intensive Care Med* 2002;28:365–8.

39. Suominen P, Baillie C, Korpela R, et al. Impact of age, submersion time and water temperature on outcome in near-drowning. *Resuscitation* 2002;52:247–54.

40. Lavelle JM, Shaw KN. Near drowning: Is emergency department cardiopulmonary resuscitation or intensive care unit cerebral resuscitation indicated? *Crit Care Med* 1993;21:368–73.

41. Suominen PK, Vahatalo R. Neurologic long term outcome after drowning in children. *Scand J Trauma Resusc Emerg Med* 2012;20:55.

42. Zandbergen EG, Hijdra A, Koelman JH, et al. Prediction of poor outcome within the first 3 days of postanoxic coma. *Neurology* 2006;66:62–8.

43. Gonzalez-Luis G, Pons M, Cambra FJ, et al. Use of the Pediatric Risk of Mortality Score as predictor of death and serious neurologic damage in children after submersion. *Pediatr Emerg Care* 2001;17:405–9.

44. Christensen DW, Jansen P, Perkin RM. Outcome and acute care hospital costs after warm water near drowning in children. *Pediatrics* 1997;99:715–21.

45. Dubowitz DJ, Bluml S, Arcinue E, et al. MR of hypoxic encephalopathy in children after near drowning: Correlation with quantitative proton MR spectroscopy and clinical outcome. *AJNR Am J Neuroradiol* 1998;19:1617–27.

46. Kreis R, Arcinue E, Ernst T, et al. Hypoxic encephalopathy after near-drowning studied by quantitative 1H-magnetic resonance spectroscopy. *J Clin Invest* 1996;97:1142–54.

47. Wijman CA, Mlynash M, Caulfield AF, et al. Prognostic value of brain diffusion-weighted imaging after cardiac arrest. *Ann Neurol* 2009;65:394–402.

48. Christophe C, Fonteyne C, Ziereisen F, et al. Value of MR imaging of the brain in children with hypoxic coma. *AJNR Am J Neuroradiol* 2002;23:716–23.

49. Fisher B, Peterson B, Hicks G. Use of brainstem auditory-evoked response testing to assess neurologic outcome following near drowning in children. *Crit Care Med* 1992;20:578–85.

50. Cheliout-Heraut F, Rubinsztajn R, Ioos C, et al. Prognostic value of evoked potentials and sleep recordings in the prolonged comatose state of children. Preliminary data. *Neurophysiol Clin* 2001;31:283–92.

51. Ashwal S, Schneider S, Tomasi L, et al. Prognostic implications of hyperglycemia and reduced cerebral blood flow in childhood near-drowning. *Neurology* 1990;40:820–3.

52. Friberg H, Rundgren M. Submersion, accidental hypothermia and cardiac arrest, mechanical chest compressions as a bridge to final treatment: a case report. *Scand J Trauma Resusc Emerg Med* 2009;17:7.

53. Wijdicks EF, Hijdra A, Young GB, et al; Quality Standards Subcommittee of the American Academy of Neurology. Practice parameter: Prediction of outcome in comatose survivors after cardiopulmonary resuscitation (an evidence-based review): Report of the Quality Standards Subcommittee of the American Academy of Neurology. *Neurology* 2006;67:203–10.

CHAPTER 32 ■ BURNS AND SMOKE INHALATION

ROGER W. YURT, JAMES J. GALLAGHER, JOY D. HOWELL, AND BRUCE M. GREENWALD

KEY POINTS

1 Initial evaluation of the patient includes determination of depth of injury and extent of surface area involved. These are trauma patients and may have other injuries in addition to the burn.

2 Fluid resuscitation in the first 24 hours is based on a formula to calculate the amount of lactated Ringer solution to infuse. The formula is only a guide; adjustments are made on the basis of vital signs and urine output.

3 Silver sulfadiazine is the topical agent most commonly used for burn wounds. Early excision of the wound is now standard of care in the burn-injured patient.

4 Hypermetabolism is very prominent in the burn-injured child. Proteins and calories must be provided to address these needs, beginning on the day of injury. Hypermetabolism persists for 9–12 months postinjury.

5 Outcomes have improved to the extent that all children should be resuscitated regardless of extent of injury.

The derangements of physiology that occur after major burn injury in a child are among the most challenging problems in modern medical care. The loss of skin integrity exposes the child to the exterior environment of bacterial, fungal, and viral pathogens. At the same time, the wounds provide a portal for loss of fluid and body heat. Beyond these local changes are the systemic responses that further stress the homeostatic mechanisms that usually maintain a stable internal environment for the patient. This chapter addresses the evaluation and care of the child with a major burn, electrical injury, and/or smoke inhalation injury. Information will also be provided regarding lesser wounds, as it is not uncommon for patients to present with multisystem injury in addition to their burns.

EVALUATION OF THE PATIENT

The distraction created by the appearance of large areas of blistering, tissue loss, and disfigurement associated with a burn injury can lead to a fixation on that injury and a lack of recognition that burn-injured patients are trauma patients. In that regard, initial evaluation should be the same as for any patient who has sustained injury. Thus, the ABCs of ensuring adequacy of an airway, that the patient is ventilating, and that circulation is intact must be addressed. A rapid overall evaluation of the patient is performed as resuscitation is initiated. The specific details of evaluating a child with burn injury will be addressed here. The aspects of evaluation of additional traumatic injury are addressed in Chapter 30.

Extent of Burn Injury

The extent of tissue injury caused by a burn is quantified by the surface area (SA) and the depth of injury. Determination of the extent of injury provides a basis for estimation of fluid requirements for resuscitation and for determining an overall care plan. In addition, in that a positive correlation exists between extent of injury and mortality, this determination

provides information on prognosis. For estimation of the extent of SA involved, a Lund & Browder chart or Berkow's formula should be used. The "rule of nines" cannot be used in children <15 years of age. The distribution of SA by age is shown in the chart in **Table 32.1**.

Evaluation of depth of injury is readily determined at the extremes of depth, such that partial-thickness injury is easy to differentiate from full-thickness injury. A first-degree burn is characterized as erythematous, painful, and dry, while a third-degree burn, also known as a full-thickness burn, is leathery, dry, and insensate. Burn injuries at an intermediate depth of partial thickness are more difficult to assess. They are divided into superficial and deep partial-thickness wounds. Whether superficial or deep, these wounds appear very similar on physical examination. They are erythematous, moist, and sensate. Evaluation of these wounds is complicated by the fact that

TABLE 32.1

DISTRIBUTION OF BODY SURFACE AREA BY AGE AS PERCENTAGE OF TOTAL BODY SURFACE AREA

■ AREA	■ 0–1	■ 1–4	■ 5–9	■ 10–14	■ 15
			AGE IN YEARS		
Head	19	17	13	11	9
Neck	2	2	2	2	2
Anterior trunk	13	13	13	13	13
Posterior trunk	13	13	13	13	13
Each buttock	2.5	2.5	2.5	2.5	2.5
Genitalia	1	1	1	1	1
Each upper arm	4	4	4	4	4
Each lower arm	3	3	3	3	3
Each hand	2.5	2.5	2.5	2.5	2.5
Each thigh	5.5	6.5	8	8.5	9
Each leg	5	5	5.5	6	6.5
Each foot	3.5	3.5	3.5	3.5	3.5

they evolve over time, are frequently not homogeneous with regard to depth, and dynamically change over the first days after injury. Previous attempts to use advanced instrumentation, such as laser Doppler and infrared sensing devices, did not demonstrate proven value in routine evaluation of this depth of injury. However, a more recent report suggests that laser Doppler imaging may be useful in estimating depth of injury in children (1). The importance of differentiating depth of injury relates to the fact that a superficial partial-thickness burn will reepithelialize in 2 weeks, whereas a deep partial-thickness wound heals by epithelialization and contraction. To avoid scarring, the deeper wound must be treated by skin grafting. Except for small-SA wounds, full-thickness wounds should either should be excised and closed primarily or grafted with the patient's skin. A cross section of skin with indication of the various depths of injury is depicted in **Figure 32.1.**

Types of Injury

The depth of the injury in burns that are caused by scalding, flame, or contact with a hot object is directly related to the temperature, duration of exposure, and thickness of the tissue. Three zones of injury have been identified in burn-injured skin. The outer *zone of coagulative necrosis* includes necrotic tissue that is irreversibly damaged by heat or chemical. Below that is the *zone of stasis* in which some viable tissue remains. This dynamic region is subject to further necrosis if it is not protected from further physical damage. Care must be taken to avoid aggressive methods of debridement and harsh cleansing agents. In addition, delivery of nutrient blood flow and oxygen is important in this region, and compromised cardiac output due to inadequate resuscitation can increase the depth of injury. The zone adjacent to the zone of stasis is the *zone of hyperemia*, and is characterized by increased blood flow and local inflammatory response to the injury.

Chemical burns cause denaturation of protein and disruption of cellular integrity. The degree of injury is dependent on the time of exposure, the strength of the agent, and the solubility of the agent in tissue. Alkaline agents tend to penetrate deeper into tissues than do acids, with an exception being hydrofluoric acid, which penetrates lipid membranes readily.

Electrical injury accounts for 2%–3% of the burns in children that require evaluation in an emergency department (2). Electricity is the flow of electrons, the force (or gradient) behind the flow is the voltage, the volume of the flow is the current measured in amperes, and the resistance to that flow is measured in ohms. Electrical injury can occur from direct contact or by an arc such as a lightning strike. Direct contact often causes damage at the entry and exit sites and along the path of the current. Arcs associated with high voltage can be

extremely hot and cause deep thermal burns at the entrance site as well as current injury along the path. Domestic electricity in North America ranges 120/240 V. Low voltage is defined as <500–1000 V and is usually associated with less morbidity (less tissue injury from burns or blunt trauma) if there is no cardiac or respiratory arrest. Electricity occurs in two forms, alternating current (AC) where the current flows back and forth, and direct current (DC) where flow is in one direction. AC is in common use in North America and standardly runs at 60 cycles per second or 60 Hz (3). Battery power and lightning are examples of DC current. AC is more dangerous at a given voltage because of its ability to produce a tetanic muscular contraction that can prevent the victim from letting go and prolong the contact with electricity.

Electrical injury has both direct and indirect mechanisms for injury; direct damage comes from current passing through living tissues causing arrhythmias and tissue necrosis by conversion of electrical into thermal energy. Indirect injury is commonly from muscle contractions that can cause falls or even asphyxia from tetanic contraction of the respiratory muscles. Spinal cord injuries can occur from direct passage of current but more commonly are the result of a fall from loss of consciousness and/or muscle contraction (2). The extent of an electrical injury is normally proportional to the current that passed through the victim. By Ohm's law, current is equal to voltage/resistance. When resistance is high, conversion of electrical to thermal energy is high, causing greater tissue damage. The resistance of wet skin is almost zero. In this situation, more damage can occur to internal organs, and the skin appears minimally damaged. This general point of normal tissue overlying extensive deeper injury is important when evaluating a victim of electrical injury. Additionally, when considering the possible damage caused by electrical injury, care must be taken to consider the course the electricity took through the body. Current passing in the region of the heart, even at low voltage, can cause arrhythmia and death. Severity of cutaneous burn injury from electricity is dependent on the SA of contact, current flow, and duration of contact. Tissues with higher resistance like bone and tendon convert more electrical energy to thermal and can lead to increased damage where these tissues predominate, such as the elbow or shoulder versus the mid arm and forearm, where muscle predominates. In high-voltage injury, muscle necrosis and compartment syndromes need aggressive evaluation to avoid more tissue loss and possible renal failure from rhabdomyolysis. Surgical decompression and early excision of dead muscle may be needed to prevent these complications.

Lightning injury is unique with its extremely high DC current of more than 1 million volts. This energy is transformed into an arc of current releasing light and extreme heat. Despite this massive energy release, flash over effect without conduction of the current through the victim results in fewer than 5% having deep cutaneous burns (2). Eyes and ears may be points of entry or damaged by blast effect. Up to 50% of patients from a lightning strike will have ruptured tympanic membranes. Transient autonomic disturbances may cause fixed and dilated pupils coupled with unconsciousness simulating death. Asystole may respond to CPR (Cardiopulmonary Resuscitation), or the heart may restart from asystole spontaneously. Cataracts can form late with any electrical injury where the current passes through the eyes. Lightning strike, in particular, is known for this late complication (2).

The major concern in evaluating patients who sustain electrical injuries is that the surface injury, which may appear similar to other burn injuries, is often not indicative of the extent of injury to subcutaneous tissues, muscle, and bone. Electrical current follows the path of least resistance and passes through nerve and blood vessels preferentially, causing injury to these tissues. If the current passes through the torso, visceral organ

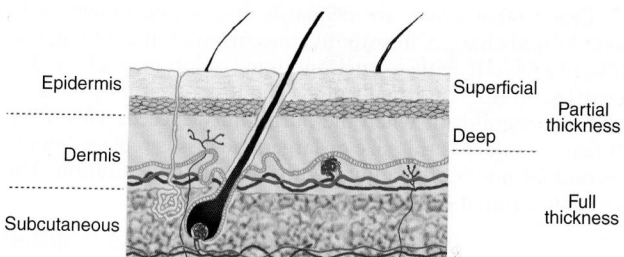

FIGURE 32.1. Schematic depiction of a cross section through skin. The epidermis, dermis, and subcutaneous layers are shown. The levels of burn injury are divided into partial thickness, which may be superficial or deep, and full thickness.

injury may result, including injuries of the pancreas and gastrointestinal tract. Injury of the heart is primarily associated with dysrhythmia. Practice guidelines for the management of electrical injury suggest that a patient who contacts a low-voltage (<1000 V) source can be cared for as an outpatient if they have no electrocardiographic abnormalities, no history of loss of consciousness, and no other reason for admission (4). Patients who contact high-voltage sources should be admitted and placed on cardiac monitoring. Creatine kinase levels, including the MB subunit, do not reliably indicate the extent of myocardial injury, and the published guidelines indicate that data are insufficient to determine whether troponin levels give an accurate index of the extent of injury. Care providers should have a high index of suspicion that deep injury has occurred and that exploration of extremities is necessary if compartment pressures rise, perfusion is compromised, or neurologic changes occur. Late sequelae of electrical injury, which may occur months or even years after injury, include the development of cataracts and transverse myelitis of the spinal cord.

Injury caused by exposure to ionizing radiation may be limited to the skin, but is often deeper. Because these wounds do not heal well, care must be taken to avoid additional damage of the tissue. The vasculitis that is associated with these injuries is usually a life-long problem.

RESUSCITATION

General Principles

Peripheral venous cannulation is preferred over central venous access and may be performed through burn-injured tissue if access through noninjured sites is not available. Children with more than 10% total body surface area (TBSA) injury require IV fluid resuscitation and should have a urinary catheter. In addition, patients who have sustained a major injury should have a nasogastric tube placed to decompress the stomach. During transport and resuscitation, every effort should be made to maintain body temperature. Patients should be wrapped in clean sheets or blankets and, in the initial phase in the emergency care area, both the room and resuscitation fluids should be warmed.

Fluid Resuscitation

Burn injury leads to intravascular volume depletion because fluid is lost into burn-injured tissue, through the wound, and into noninjured tissue. The major losses occur during the first 24 hours following the injury, and it is generally agreed that during this period, crystalloid solutions should be used. As fluid shifts from the vascular space are massive in major injuries, formulas have been developed to provide an estimate of fluid requirement. In addition to intravascular volume loss, myocardial depression occurs in the first 24–36 hours after injury. Every guideline that has been developed carries with it the mandate that the patient's response to resuscitation—not the formula—be used as the actual determinant of fluid administration. The goal of resuscitation is to maintain adequate intravascular volume to support tissue perfusion and thereby preserve organ function. The adequacy of resuscitation in burn injury is based on observation of urine output as the primary end point of resuscitation. Clinical causes of false elevation in urine output should be considered when using renal perfusion as a marker of overall tissue perfusion. Vital signs in burn injury are deranged by shock and the therapy associated with care from narcotics, sedatives, and mechanical ventilation. Fluid resuscitation of major burn injury requires

at least hourly reassessment of a variety of parameters. Fluids are titrated to maintain hourly urine output of 1 mL/kg/hour in the infant and young child and 0.5 mL/kg/hour in the child >12 years of age or >50 kg in weight. Importantly, urine output above these goals should motivate the clinician to decrease resuscitation fluid volumes. The Parkland formula is a crystalloid-based formula that provides the foundation for current methods of resuscitation (5). This formula calls for the initiation of resuscitation with lactated Ringer solution at a rate based on the BSA of burn injury and the patient's body weight. The calculated resuscitation volume for the first 24 hours is:

$$(4 \text{ mL/Kg} \times \%\text{BSA burn}) + \text{Maintenance fluids} \quad [32.1]$$

Maintenance fluids (5% dextrose in lactated Ringer solution) should be estimated (100 mL/kg for the first 10 kg, 50 mL/kg for the second 10 kg, and 20 mL/kg above 20-kg body weight) for children who weigh <40 kg. For adults and children who weigh >40 kg, maintenance fluids are not included in the estimate of fluid requirements. Half of the resuscitation volume is given in the first 8 hours after injury, and the other half is given in the following 16 hours. To minimize the volume of fluid used during resuscitation, hypertonic fluids have been tried for resuscitation; however, they result in higher complication and mortality rates compared with historic use of lactated Ringer solution (6).

At the Shriners Burn Center in Galveston, Texas, an alternative formula used for calculating resuscitation fluid for the first 24 hours after injury calls for lactated Ringer solution based upon SA of injury in square meters with maintenance fluid (5% dextrose in lactated Ringer solution) based on total BSA in square meters:

$$(5000 \text{ mL} \times \text{SA burn}) + (2000 \text{ mL} \times \text{Total BSA}) \quad [32.2]$$

The current evidence continues to support a crystalloid-based regimen in the range of 2–4 mL/kg/% BSA burn in the first 24 hours. However, more recent data indicate that patients who have sustained inhalation injury—and all patients in general—are receiving more than estimated needs. This change, which Pruitt reviewed and called "fluid creep" (7), may be due in part to a much more aggressive use of analgesics in recent years, which appears to cause vasodilatation and exacerbation of the discrepancy between intravascular volume and the capacity of the intravascular space (8). Of concern are the complications associated with excessive volume resuscitation, which include pulmonary edema and increased subeschar pressures in the extremities and the abdomen, leading to compartment syndrome.

After the first 24 hours, fluids are given to meet maintenance requirements and to replace ongoing losses. The hourly evaporative fluid loss from the patient's wounds can be estimated as:

$$(25 + \%\text{BSA burn}) \times \text{Total BSA} \quad [32.3]$$

Evaporative losses are primarily free water. However, to avoid rapid changes in sodium concentration in children, this loss is replaced with a salt-containing solution, such as 5% dextrose in 0.2% normal saline. The loss of serum protein is clinically significant when the burn injury exceeds 40% BSA. When the injury is this size or larger, the loss is replaced in the second 24 hours after injury with 5% albumin solution. The volume required can be estimated as:

$$0.3-4 \text{ mL/kg} \times \%\text{BSA burn} \quad [32.4]$$

The ultimate goal in the postresuscitation period is to maintain normal blood pressure, heart rate, urine output, and serum sodium. Calculation of expected resuscitation volume is critical when caring for patients in burn shock. The volume each patient receives should be driven by the clinical parameters outlined above; however, knowledge of expected volumes can help identify patients who fail to adequately resuscitate. These patients may have a missed injury, unreported delay in care, or previously unknown cardiac dysfunction. The expected course of burn shock must be known if outliers are to be identified and care modified. The risks in children are magnified given the possibility of burn injury being used to cover other forms of child abuse.

Inhalation Injury

Although it is commonly thought that inhalation injury to the upper airway and parenchyma of the lung is due to thermal injury to the airway, this is almost never the case. The upper airway can dissipate heat effectively, and only occasionally has direct inhalation of superheated steam been found to cause inhalation injury. Inhalation injury is most clearly understood when considered in three components: upper airway direct thermal burn, chemical pneumonitis from products of combustion, and systemic poisoning from inhalation of cyanide and carbon monoxide.

The morbidity from unnecessary tracheal intubation should be appreciated. The decision to intubate a burn victim is straightforward if the victim is unconscious and not able to protect his airway or has stridor. More commonly, a stable patient presents with soot on the face and in the mouth. In this case, a careful history and physical examination looking for evidence of the child having been trapped in a space with smoke, and physical findings of a change in voice, hoarseness, or increased work of breathing suggest that the airway may become compromised. In some situations laryngoscopy is performed to rule out upper airway injury, but this can be difficult depending on the age of the child. If there is no sign of upper airway compromise, inhalation injury may be present, but without upper airway burn or immediate need for intubation. Other components of inhalation injury, including pneumonitis, are usually best managed without intubation and mechanical ventilation. Decisions surrounding airway management are some of the most challenging, and early involvement of the burn team along with pediatric critical care or anesthesia is recommended. In children with scald burns, upper airway injury and edema associated with aspiration of hot liquids at the time of injury is rare, requiring a child to be positioned with the face upward and the mouth open allowing the hot liquid to directly burn the pharynx.

Pulmonary parenchymal pathology following inhalation injury evolves and peaks 3–5 days following the fire. This timing is dependent upon the combustibles present in the fire. Common plastics when burned produce cyanide gas and carbon monoxide, which cause the systemic poisoning seen in inhalation injury. The pneumonitis associated with inhalation injury is produced from chemicals that are inhaled and deposited in the airways. These toxins cause erythema and edema of the airway and lead to the blistering, ulceration, erosions, and sloughing of the mucosa, seen on bronchoscopy. The local edema, infiltration of the tissue with polymorphonuclear leukocytes (PMNs), and sloughing of bronchial mucosa can lead to the formation of an endobronchial cast and obstruction of terminal bronchioles. Pulmonary edema occurs from increases in pulmonary lymph flow and microvascular permeability. The debris in the airway cannot be cleared because of the mucosal injury and disruption of the mucociliary transport mechanism. Patients who are initially managed without intubation can deteriorate in the days after the injury and require intubation and mechanical ventilation. The obstruction of the small airways and the accumulation of carbonaceous material and necrotic debris provide a fertile environment for the development of infection. The incidence of pneumonia in patients with inhalation injury may be as high as 70% within a week of injury (9).

In the management of patients with burns and trauma, airway evaluation and management are of paramount importance and begin with an assessment of airway patency and quality of respirations. Chest radiograph, arterial blood gas determination, and pulmonary function testing are usually normal during the first 3 days following injury. Patients, who sustain injury in a closed space, have burns above the clavicle, singeing of facial hair, hoarseness, or carbonaceous sputum, should be assumed to have an inhalation injury. Diagnostic bronchoscopy is performed on all patients who require intubation for confirmation of inhalation injury and evaluation of severity. Therapeutic bronchoscopy may also be necessary to aid in the removal of bronchial casts that form, often on a daily basis. Elevated carboxyhemoglobin levels confirm exposure to carbon monoxide but are not diagnostic for injury to the lung. Because the primary concern early after inhalation injury is obstruction of the airway, the upper airway should be evaluated immediately by flexible bronchoscopy, usually in the emergency department. Xenon ventilation/perfusion scan shows air trapping when parenchymal injury is present; however, this test does not provide quantitative information on the extent of injury and should not be performed routinely.

Management of Inhalation Injury

Therapy for inhalation injury consists of aggressive pulmonary toilet, use of mucolytics, and early identification and treatment of infection and supportive care. Administration of *nebulized heparin* is associated with reduced atelectasis and improved pulmonary function, compared with historic controls (10). The combination of *N*-acetylcysteine and nebulized heparin has been used for smoke inhalation treatment in adults and was associated with improved survival (11). Prophylaxis with antibiotics is not used; corticosteroids are of no benefit and are potentially harmful (12).

The level of support that is required may range from supplemental oxygen to advanced modes of assisted ventilation and hyperbaric oxygen (HBO) therapy. For patients with evidence of inhalation injury, supplemental oxygen should be provided via nasal cannula or simple facemask, both of which will add additional humidification. If stridor due to upper airway inflammation and edema is present, racemic epinephrine may be employed to transiently relieve the obstruction to airflow. Helium/oxygen admixtures (Heliox) reduce resistance to turbulent airflow, increase laminar flow, and, in turn, improve the work of breathing in the presence of upper airway obstruction. Heliox, most frequently, is used to treat upper airway obstruction that follows extubation in patients with subglottic edema. Patients in whom the airway is compromised should be intubated to permit definitive assessment and airway control. Based on a recent survey of pediatric burn centers, approximately 12% of pediatric burn victims require intubation, with approximately 70% of those intubated having sustained inhalation injury (13). Intubation is recommended if the burn exceeds 50% of the BSA, in anticipation of a large volume resuscitation and associated edema.

Evidence suggests that cuffed endotracheal tubes can be safely and effectively used in critically ill and burned pediatric patients. When using a cuffed tube the size of the endotracheal tube should be 0.5–1.0 cm smaller than an uncuffed tube. The current Pediatric Advanced Life Support guidelines recommend use of the formulas: (age/4) + 3 for cuffed endotracheal tubes and (age/4) + 4 for uncuffed tubes (14).

The prevalence of acute respiratory distress syndrome (ARDS) in mechanically ventilated adults with major burns has been estimated to be as high as 54% (15). Although the prevalence in pediatric burn patients is likely lower, acute lung injury and ARDS represent significant clinical challenges, especially in very young patients. Ventilator modes for children with respiratory failure vary among burn centers. The mode of mechanical ventilation employed in the care of the pediatric burn patient should be governed by the level of pulmonary dysfunction. Synchronized intermittent mandatory ventilation plus pressure support is a reasonable choice when there is little-to-no lung disease. Pressure-control ventilation and pressure-regulated volume control are alternatives, especially in patients who demonstrate high peak pressures. Cuffed endotracheal tubes and lung-protective ventilator strategies should be employed in patients at risk for acute lung injury. Low tidal volume/high positive end-expiratory pressure (PEEP) is used initially and progresses to airway pressure release ventilation or high-frequency oscillatory ventilation (HFOV) in patients who require PEEP in excess of 10 cm of H_2O (16). It should be noted that the practice guidelines for burn care, developed by the American Burn Association, indicate that insufficient data exist to support a standard treatment guideline (17). Early excision and closure of the burn wound, as well as lung-protective ventilation strategies, are the two major priorities in the management of burn patients with ARDS.

HFOV has been used as a rescue therapy in burn patients with ARDS who fail conventional mechanical ventilation. One center has reported the use of HFOV not only as rescue therapy, but also as a modality employed in the operating room for treating patients who require surgical intervention. As the timing of burn excision has a significant impact on survival, the ability to use HFOV in the operating room may be important in maximizing survival. Also, inhalation injury worsens outcome in burn patients who require HFOV (15). The use of high-frequency percussive ventilation has been reported in adult burn patients with ARDS but not pediatric burn victims.

A major concern in the management of inhalation injury is the possibility of carbon monoxide (CO) poisoning. Blood sampling for the presence of CO should be performed on admission. When interpreting COHb levels it is important to note that earlier administration of hydroxycobalamin (see next paragraph) may falsely lower COHb levels and result in an underestimation of the severity of CO poisoning (18). Treatment for CO poisoning begins with the administration of 100% oxygen. There is a lack of clarity regarding the treatment of inhalation injury–associated carbon monoxide (CO) poisoning with HBO therapy. The existing evidence is insufficient to mandate the use of HBO for CO as there are not clear groups that HBO will benefit or harm; a large study is needed to answer the question of a benefit from HBO for CO poisoning (19–21). The suggested indications for HBO treatment include loss of consciousness, ischemic cardiac changes, neurologic deficits, significant metabolic acidosis, or COHb level >25% (20). If used, HBO treatment should be initiated within 6 hours (no benefit is likely after 12 hours) and for at least one session at 2.5–3 atm (there is a lack of data about the need for additional sessions). In situations when the patient must be transferred to receive HBO therapy, the lack of proof of benefit and the risk to an unstable patient need to be considered. Hyperbaric treatment is not directed at the serum CO level, which rapidly decreases on 100% oxygen, but rather the effects of CO on the nervous system. The long-term central nervous system effects of CO poisoning appear to be related to the production of reactive oxygen species, lipid peroxidation, activation of inflammation, and the induction of apoptosis. Evidence is also lacking to direct the use of acute (or delayed) HBO therapy in the prevention (or treatment) of long-term neurologic changes caused by the *delayed neuropsychiatric syndrome* or *posthypoxic leukoencephalopathy* that

are associated with CO poisoning. The clinical goal of treatment is to minimize sequelae of CO poisoning and to optimize long-term neurologic outcome.

Cyanide poisoning can occur with inhalation injury when significant quantities of plastics are burned. Cyanide gas poisoning can be rapidly fatal; therefore, in recent years, cyanide antidote kits have been provided and used by first responders. Cyanide poisoning should be considered in patients with unexplained metabolic acidosis (especially if they also have elevated venous oxygen saturation) and treated when suspected, even before diagnosis is confirmed. The antidote, hydroxycobalamin (a precursor to vitamin B_{12} and FDA approved), is administered by the IV route as 70 mg/kg (max dose 5 g). Cyanide has a greater affinity for cobalamin than cytochrome oxidase and forms cyanocobalamin, which is stable and eliminated in the urine. Notably the urine becomes dark purple or red color for several days following administration. It is important to note that the use of antidotes that induce the formation of methemoglobin (amyl nitrite and sodium nitrite found in some cyanide antidote kits) will worsen the toxicity from carbon monoxide. Treatment that produces methemoglobin should be avoided until it is determined that CO is not present in the blood (use carboxyhemoglobin level).

Timing of Tracheostomy in Pediatric Burn Victims

Tracheostomy is classically utilized in patients following a prolonged course of endotracheal intubation. However, early tracheostomy has also been used safely in a cohort of pediatric burn patients. A retrospective review of 38 children with burn injury who underwent early tracheostomy over a 2 1/2-year period reported no cases of tracheal stenosis, tracheomalacia, or acute airway emergencies in 38 children with burn injury in whom early tracheostomy was performed 2–4 days after the initiation of assisted ventilation (22). The patient population consisted mainly of children with burns of the face and head, and approximately 67% had inhalation injury. Thirteen percent had ARDS, and the mean $Pao_2:Fio_2$ ratio prior to tracheostomy was 300. The average time to decannulation was 6 weeks. The authors concluded, lack of complications and modest (15%) improvement in the $Pao_2:Fio_2$ ratio (300.6–348.6, $p < 0.05$), that tracheostomy should be considered in all children with severe burns in whom a prolonged course of mechanical ventilation is anticipated (22). Further study is warranted to define precisely both the appropriate patient population and timing of tracheostomy placement in pediatric burn victims. Currently, tracheostomy is generally reserved for patients who have failed extubation or for those projected to require chronic mechanical ventilation, that is neurologically devastated patients.

Decision to Transfer to Specialized Care

The resources required to care for patients with significant burn injury are not available at many medical centers. For this reason, a regionalized system for care of the burn-injured patient has been developed. Although travel time and distance to a burn center are of concern, transfer of burn-injured patients after initial evaluation has been shown to be safe, especially if initiated early after injury. Patients with burns >30% of their BSA, children with injury of critical body parts, such as genitalia, and those with significant preexisting disease should be cared for in a burn center. Specific guidelines have been published by the American Burn Association (23) (**Table 32.2**).

TABLE 32.2

CRITERIA FOR REFERRAL FOR CARE OF A PATIENT WITH A BURN INJURY TO A REGIONAL BURN CENTER

For adults and children with second- and third-degree cutaneous burns, burn center candidates are identified according to the following:

1. Partial-thickness burns >10% total body surface area
2. Burns that involve the face, hands, feet, genitalia, perineum, or major joints
3. Third-degree burns in any age group
4. Electrical burns, including lightning injury
5. Chemical burns
6. Inhalation injury
7. Burn injury in patients with preexisting medical disorders that could complicate management, prolong recovery, or affect mortality
8. Any patients with burns and concomitant trauma (such as fractures) in which the burn injury poses the greatest risk of morbidity or mortality. In such cases, if the trauma poses the greater immediate risk, the patient may be initially stabilized in a trauma center before being transferred to a burn unit. Physician judgment will be necessary in such situations, and should be in concert with the regional medical control plan and triage protocols
9. Burned children in hospitals without qualified personnel or equipment for the care of children
10. Burn injury in patients who will require special social, emotional, or long-term rehabilitative intervention

From *Guidelines for the Operations of Burn Units* (pp. 55–62), Resources for Optimal Care of the Injured Patient: 1999, Committee on Trauma, American College of Surgeons.

Collaborative Practice

The management of severe burn injury in infants and young children, especially those with inhalation injury and/or multiple organ dysfunction syndrome, has been particularly challenging for many burn centers. We have developed a collaborative comanagement model of care that utilizes the strengths and personnel from both the Burn Center and the Pediatric Intensive Care Unit (PICU). The location of care is based upon a standardized algorithm (Table 32.3), and includes physicians, nurses, and respiratory, physical, and occupational therapists from both services, as well as social workers and child life specialists. Children under 6 years of age with critical burn injury are admitted to the PICU on the basis of standardized criteria. Upon stabilization and recovery, they are transferred to the burn unit for ongoing management of the burn injury.

TABLE 32.3

BURN PATIENTS ADMITTED/TRANSFERRED TO THE PEDIATRIC INTENSIVE CARE UNIT

1. All endotracheally intubated patients under 1 year of age
2. Endotracheally intubated patients 1–5 years of age with:
   A. Acute lung injury ($PaO_2/FiO_2 < 300$) and/or
   B. 50% or greater body surface area burns
3. Patients 12 years of age or under with complex multisystem disease (by agreement between Pediatric Critical Care and Burn Service)

Inherent to the success of comanagement is the recognition that the expertise required to accurately assess and manage burned tissue, particularly as it pertains to transitional areas of injury (i.e., between zones of coagulation and stasis), is typically found only in burn centers. Yet resuscitation of the critically ill and injured pediatric patients, especially those with respiratory failure and shock, calls upon expertise routinely housed within the PICU. The processes developed in this combined approach allow children of all ages to fully benefit from the strengths and experience of both the PICU and the burn teams. Regardless of the location of care (burn unit or PICU), bedside rounds and the determination of physiologic goals of therapy are collaborative. For patients in the PICU, specific management of the airway, respiratory failure, shock, organ system dysfunction, attainment of vascular access, and monitoring of physiologic parameters are supervised by pediatric intensivists. Detailed assessment of extent of injury, cleaning and excision of nonviable tissue, prescription of topical medications and dressings, timing of grafting, and other surgical procedures are performed by the burn unit team. Coordination of care is optimized when the burn team performs dressing changes, debridement, and cleaning of wounds, while the PICU team facilitates patient readiness and administers appropriate analgesia and sedation for these procedures.

A great strength of specialized burn centers is the significant nursing expertise developed in the area of wound care. Experience and familiarity with a variety of dressings, application and removal of topical agents, and debridement techniques that are minimally traumatic yet effective are among the skills required. Scheduled dressing changes may be extensive and encompass substantial percentages of TBSA. Deep sedation or general anesthesia is often required, particularly in the pediatric population, to safely and effectively perform wound care. With appropriate training, some dressing changes can be conducted by the PICU nursing staff, but ideally dressing changes, especially when extensive, are performed in a coordinated fashion between PICU and burn unit nursing.

In addition to physicians and nurses, care of the critically ill child with burn injury requires a team of professionals with special expertise in pediatric burns. Questions of adequacy of parental supervision, possibility of intentional trauma, and appropriateness of parental or caregiver support require the skills of a pediatric social worker. Rehabilitation, including both physical and occupational therapy, begins at the time of admission and requires specialized training and experience with pediatric burns. Burn injuries are associated with physical as well as emotional trauma that can be compounded by secondary trauma associated with wound care. Active participation by child life therapists as well as child psychiatrists often helps patients cope with their injuries and treatments and should yield the best psychological outcome.

At our center, adoption of the multiprofessional collaborative model described above has resulted in significant improvement in care for infants and toddlers with significant burn injury. This improvement has been particularly important in patients under 6 years of age with >50% total body surface and those with severe inhalation injury.

Neglect and Abuse

The incidence of child abuse has been reported as high as 16% of children admitted to burn centers (24) so that an appropriate level of suspicion should be maintained. Most nonaccidental injuries occur in children between 2 and 4 years of age. The determination of whether abuse or neglect has occurred is based on the characteristics of the wounds and the history provided. A history that is inconsistent with the findings on physical exam is sufficient reason to launch a deeper investigation into the injury. Conflicting histories should also lead to a search for additional information about the incident.

Well-defined lines of demarcation between burned and unburned skin in a scald burn and the absence of splash burns are suggestive of intentional injury. However, splash burns can also be seen in intentional scald-burning cases. In addition, sparing of areas of skin may be suggestive of an intentional injury, particularly when the extremity is held in flexion and the area around the joint is protected and spared. Contact burns also present with well-defined margins; the object that caused the injury can often be determined by the outline of the wound.

A recent study reported that 70% of children admitted to the burn center were victims of neglect, and that the incidence was highest in 3–6-year-olds, those with low socioeconomic status, and those with a family size of six or more (25). All states in the United States require the reporting of suspected neglect and/or abuse of children.

WOUND CARE
General Principles

The objective of wound care is to avoid infection and protect the wound from further injury. Small (<2 cm) blisters are often left intact, whereas larger blisters and full-thickness wounds should be debrided and covered with a topical agent. Debridement is often painful and is therefore carried out under deep sedation or general anesthesia. Ketamine may be useful because of its profound cutaneous analgesia and the ability to administer by the IM route. Propofol is an alternative, although associated with a greater risk of hypotension and the need for supplementation with an opioid for painful procedures. Even in the absence of debridement, burns are painful, and patients usually require opioid analgesia. Pain management is discussed in detail in Chapter 14.

Inpatient wound care is provided in a warm environment in an area reserved for wound care. Agents that may cause additional tissue damage are avoided, and the circulation of the wound is protected by avoiding hypotension, hypoxemia, hypothermia, and the use of α-adrenergic agents. Sterile gloves should be worn at all times when the wound is manipulated. Chemical injury of tissue is treated with irrigation with copious amounts of either normal saline or tap water for as long

as 6 hours. Neutralizing agents are not used because they can lead to additional tissue damage resulting from heat generated in an exothermic reaction between the chemicals. Hydrofluoric acid injuries can lead to systemic hypocalcemia and be rapidly fatal; therefore, brief irrigation should be followed by topical application of calcium gluconate gel. If pain persists, clysis of the wound with calcium gluconate can be considered except in digits.

Prophylaxis against Wound Infection

Systemic antimicrobial prophylaxis is not used in patients who are admitted to the hospital. The wounds are closely observed for infection, and treatment is initiated if infection occurs. Opinions vary regarding the use of antibiotics in the outpatient setting. If it is anticipated that compliance with a topical therapy regimen will be poor, systemic prophylaxis may be provided.

The advent of effective topical antimicrobial agents has substantially reduced the mortality associated with burn-wound infection. The commonly used agents and their advantages and disadvantages are listed in **Table 32.4**. The ideal topical regimen rests on the use of an agent with good prophylactic antimicrobial activity that also provides an opportunity to easily evaluate the wound and to perform regular physical therapy. According to a recent international survey (26), silver sulfadiazine is the topical agent most commonly used for partial-thickness (32% of centers), mixed partial- and full-thickness (34% of centers), and full-thickness (30% of centers) burn wounds. An aqueous solution of silver nitrate (0.5%) has been used for years for its topical antimicrobial activity; however, only 4% of centers currently use this agent as a primary topical. Because these agents do not penetrate burn wounds well, they are indicated for prophylaxis against infection, but not for therapy. Mafenide acetate does penetrate the wound and is the agent used for therapy of burn-wound infection. More recent approaches include the use of silver as an antimicrobial in multiday dressings. The advantages of silver-containing dressings are that the dressing does not have to be changed, and antimicrobial activity is equivalent to silver sulfadiazine. Ease of movement and flexibility were decreased with this product, compared with silver sulfadiazine. Silver sulfadiazine is not used in infants <2 months of age or in patients with a near-term pregnancy, given the association

TABLE 32.4

TOPICAL ANTIMICROBIAL AGENTS FOR TREATMENT OF BURN INJURY BY TYPE

	■ APPLICATION	■ ADVANTAGES	■ DISADVANTAGES
Ointment			
Bacitracin	Second-degree burns, small areas	Not water soluble, good on face	Not indicated for large surface area
Cream			
Silver sulfadiazine	Second- and third-degree burns	Soothing, good for range of motion	Possible neutropenia; little penetration
Mafenide acetate	Second- and third-degree burns	Penetrates eschar	Painful, metabolic acidosis
Solution			
Aqueous silver nitrate (0.5%)	Second- and third-degree burns	Good antimicrobial	Hyponatremia, stains wound, little penetration
Mafenide acetate (5%)	Graft dressing, open wound soak	Broad activity, moist dressing	Not used for unexcised wound
Impregnated Dressings			
Acticoat	Second-degree burns	Dressing change every 3 days	Only second degree
Aquacel Ag	Second-degree burns	Leave on for 21 days	Less flexibility and ease of motion; only second-degree burns

between kernicterus and exposure to sulfonamides. An algorithm for wound care is shown in **Figure 32.2**.

Surgical Care

Commonly, the burn surgeon evaluates the burn wound and determines the care it will receive. First-degree burns require no specific treatment and will heal without a scar. Third-degree burns require surgery for wound closure unless they are very small. Second-degree burns include deep and superficial burns with varying degrees of healing potential. The three goals in burn surgery (closure of the wound, normal function, and cosmetic excellence of the result) are considered in the decision to treat the wound. Scar development and contracture formation are minimized by the experienced burn surgeon exercising judgment in the surgical care of the burn wounds. With small burns, cosmetic and functional results are often the primary concern. However, as the burn size increases, wound closure is of paramount importance for survival. Excision and closure of wounds have the advantage of reducing the extent of injury and eliminating the risk of wound infection.

One of the major advances in burn care has been the recognition that patients in whom the wounds are excised early after injury have fewer complications. The usual approach is to begin excision within the first 3–4 days after injury (27). Although no randomized, prospective study has indicated that outcome is affected by early intervention, it is widely held that the overall improved outcome in burn-injured patients over the past 20 years is in large part due to this approach. Excision has been initiated by some within the first 24 hours after injury (28). However, most authors suggest that 24 hours is too early, and excision is better performed when the patient with a large burn has been stabilized. In addition to the stability of the patient, other factors (coexistent injuries, inhalation injury) affect the timing of operative intervention. In the patient with extensive wounds that require grafting (i.e., deep partial and full thickness over >40% of the BSA), a strategy for surgical intervention must take into account the availability of donor sites, while maintaining a goal of reducing the amount of open wound as quickly as possible. In such cases, closure of the wound takes precedence over cosmetic and functional considerations.

At the present time, the ultimate closure of the excised wound requires the use of autograft. If sufficient donor sites are available, the preferred skin graft in children is a split-thickness autograft (0.15–0.20 mm in thickness). A thicker, full-thickness graft is preferred for cosmetic reconstruction and in areas where scarring would lead to functional compromise.

However, this thickness of donor skin requires that the donor site be grafted. When donor sites are limited, autograft can be expanded by passing it through a mechanical meshing device that allows it to be enlarged up to six times the SA of the original donor skin. For practical purposes, the skin is not usually meshed to a size greater than four times the initial area.

Closure of the excised wound may be staged by temporarily covering it with biologic or manufactured dressings. Allograft provides for closure of the wound and may also be used as a test graft in areas where infection is of concern or when the adequacy of the excised wound bed is suspect. If an allograft is left in place for longer than 10–14 days, it becomes incorporated into the wound, and the wound must be excised to remove it. In recent years, a number of skin substitutes have been developed that replace the function of some or all layers of the skin.

Integra Life Sciences Corporation provides a temporary epidermis as an outer layer of silastic and an inner layer matrix for the growth of a neodermis. Success with use of this product has been reported, noting improvement in cosmesis and function, but increased rate of infection when the wound bed was contaminated. A thin layer of epidermis must ultimately be grafted onto the neodermis. *AlloDerm* is an acellular, human dermis, tissue matrix that has been processed to extract cells and their components. The remaining nonantigenic matrix provides a scaffold for a new dermis upon which a thin epidermal graft may be placed. This product allows the placement of a thin epidermal graft and improves cosmetic outcome. The advantage that these products offer, for patients with a large SA of injury, is that donor sites are available in shorter time frames for recropping of epidermis for further grafting.

Immediate application of other products (pigskin or a commercially available synthetic membrane composed of silastic covered with a chondroitin sulfate–coated surface) on a partial-thickness wound moderates pain and eliminates the need to change dressings, but these slough off when applied to deep partial-thickness wounds.

Circumferential Burns

Circumferential burn wounds present unique problems associated with the compromise of tissue beneath the wound. In the extremities, the combination of increased extravascular fluid in the wound and underlying tissues and the lack of elasticity of the burn wound can lead to subeschar pressures that compromise blood flow to viable tissue. All extremities with circumferential full-thickness burns should be

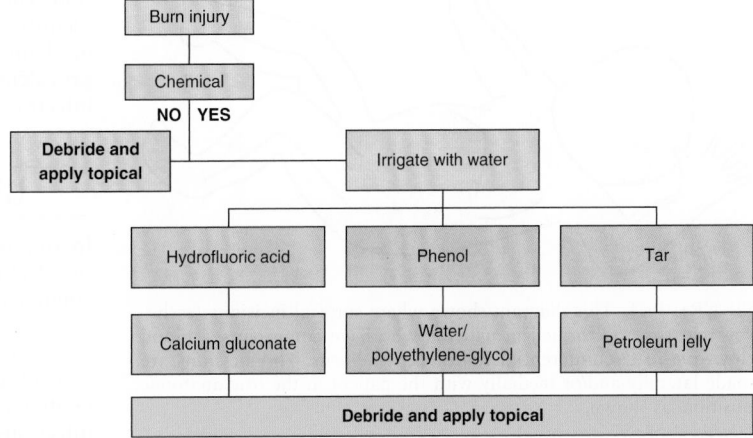

FIGURE 32.2. An algorithm for burn-wound care. Chemical injuries require irrigation and, in some cases, additional treatment prior to debridement and application of topical antimicrobials.

elevated to minimize edema formation and should be evaluated hourly for the classic signs of vascular compromise: pallor, pain, paresthesia, paralysis, and poikilothermia. Because these signs are often difficult to evaluate in a burn-injured extremity, additional assessment of Doppler-measured blood flow in the distal extremity should also be performed. Loss of a Doppler signal may not be seen until after damage has occurred; therefore, the threshold for performing an escharotomy to release subeschar pressure should be low. An escharotomy is performed by making an incision through the eschar on the lateral surface of the extremity. An additional escharotomy may be required on the medial surface as well. The preferred sites for escharotomy are indicated in **Figure 32.3.** A multicentered study has suggested that delay in decompression of extremities may be associated with occult intracompartmental infection (29). Decompression of the hand should be performed when full-thickness burn injury leads to compromise of blood flow and function. Escharotomies are performed in fingers (2–5) in the midaxial line, on the ulnar side, and on the radial side of the thumb, so as to preserve tactile sensation of the surfaces of opposition of the fingers and thumb.

In a similar way, a "compartment syndrome" can occur in the chest or abdomen in patients with circumferential full-thickness burn injury in these areas. A decrease in pulmonary system compliance in these patients may indicate that decompression is necessary. Escharotomy of the chest in the anterior axillary line will often decrease the inspiratory pressures required to maintain tidal volume. If circumferential full-thickness burns of the abdomen and back are present, an escharotomy following the costal margin may be necessary. Incision of the eschar may be performed with a scalpel, but is often done with electrocautery so that minor bleeding can be controlled. Because full-thickness wounds are insensate and avascular, anesthesia is not necessary, and these procedures may be performed under sterile conditions at the bedside. Circumferential full-thickness burns on the abdominal wall can contribute to the development of increased intra-abdominal pressure during resuscitation. If an abdominal compartment syndrome develops, it may be relieved by escharotomy, drainage of peritoneal fluid, or decompressive laparotomy. Monitoring of intra-abdominal pressure may be accomplished by measurement of bladder pressure.

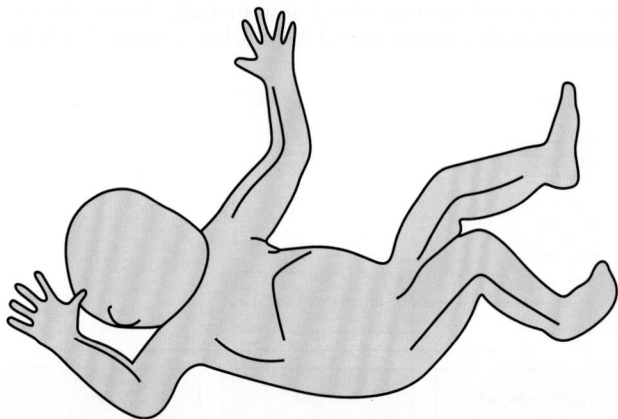

FIGURE 32.3. This diagram shows where surgical incisions (escharotomies) are performed in patients who have compromised blood flow due to circumferential full-thickness burns. The incisions are made laterally and/or medially with the patient in the true anatomic position, as shown.

INFECTION
General Aspects in Burn Injury

The systemic inflammatory response that is associated with a major burn ignites a cascade of events that presents as a clinical syndrome that is difficult to distinguish from infection. Most children that sustain burn injury have fever; severely burn-injured patients often have core body temperatures of 39°C–39.5°C, develop intestinal ileus, become disoriented, develop hyperglycemia, and sustain changes in fluid balance. The burn wound has been described as a "black box" in which a local inflammatory process occurs that leads to introduction of mediators of inflammation into the systemic circulation and causes activation of cells as they pass through the milieu of the wound. These events compound the responses to injury and distinguish the burn-injured patient from patients with other injuries. It appears that the incidence of infection is higher in burn-injured children compared to other critically ill children. Reported nosocomial infection rates in burn-injured children are high in all cases, with a central catheter infection rate of 4.9/1000 catheter days, a burn-wound infection rate of 5.6/1000 burn unit days, a ventilator-associated pneumonia rate of 11.4/1000 ventilator days, and a urinary catheter-related urinary tract infection rate of 13.2/1000 urinary catheter days (30).

An increased susceptibility to infection related to the extent of burn injury has also been suggested experimentally in animal models that demonstrate the activation of PMNs. Serum cytokine levels following a burn injury in children are elevated within the first week. Both proinflammatory (IL-6, IL-8, IL-1β, monocyte chemoattractant protein 1, macrophage inflammatory protein 1β, IL-13, IL-5, and IL-7) and anti-inflammatory (IL-10, granulocyte colony-stimulation factor, IL-17, interferon [IFN]-γ, IL-12, p70, and IL-4) serum cytokine levels have been found in significantly higher amounts in burn-injured children compared to normal controls (31). The net result of the activation of these cells and mediators appears to be the indiscriminant recruitment of the pathways that normally maintain homeostasis, leading to susceptibility to infection, further local tissue injury, and distant organ dysfunction.

Recently, published consensus definitions for infection in burn patients aim to serve as a necessary step in the burn community to compare and study outcomes. The recognition of the marked derangements in physiology outlined above is addressed in these guidelines. Identification of baseline changes in temperature, heart rate, blood pressure, and other vital signs used in other definitions of infection are considered and modified for the burn patient. In particular, patients with large burns are in a state of chronic systemic inflammatory stimulation. Therefore, the standard SIRS criteria are of little value in identifying infection in burn victims, and should not be utilized for that purpose (32). In our center, elevated levels of procalcitonin appear to show promise in identifying bacterial infection in febrile burn patients.

BURN-WOUND INFECTION

In an attempt to standardize the evaluation and classification of infection in the wounds of the burn-injured patient, a subcommittee of the American Burn Association has provided a proposal for categorization of these infections (33). Although these guidelines are open for comment at this time, they provide a foundation for describing the four categories of wound-related infection and are used here as a basis for describing the infections that occur in the patient with burn injury.

Impetigo

Impetigo is an infection that "involves the loss of epithelium from a previously reepithelialized surface such as a grafted burn, a partial-thickness burn allowed to heal by secondary intention, or a healed donor site" (34). This condition assumes that no other cause for epithelial loss is present such as mechanical damage, hematoma formation, or tissue ischemia. This infection, also termed "melting graft syndrome," is not necessarily associated with systemic signs of infection, fever, or an elevated white blood cell count. Although it is often caused by streptococcal or staphylococcal species, it may be caused by other organisms as well. Burn-wound surface cultures, which give no insight into what is occurring within the wound, are helpful in determining the inciting organism in these infections. Treatment consists of local care of the wound and systemic antibiotics.

Open Surgical Wound Infection

Open surgical wound infections are associated with a surgical intervention that has not healed. As defined by the subcommittee, they may occur in an ungrafted, excised burn or at unhealed donor sites and are associated with culture-positive purulent exudates. In addition, at least one of the following is present: (a) loss of synthetic or biologic covering of the wound; (b) changes in wound appearance, such as hyperemia; (c) erythema in the uninjured skin surrounding the wound; or (d) systemic signs, such as fever or leukocytosis.

These infections require a change in local wound care, usually the addition of a topical antimicrobial agent, more frequent dressing changes, and the administration of systemic antibiotics.

Cellulitis

Burn-associated *cellulitis* presents as erythema and edema. It must be differentiated from the normal local inflammatory response to a burn injury that is manifest as erythema localized <1–2 cm from the margin of the wound and by the lack of extension beyond that zone. The definition of cellulitis also requires at least one of the following: (a) localized pain, tenderness, swelling, or warmth at the affected site; (b) systemic signs of infection, such as hyperemia, leukocytosis, or septicemia; (c) progression of erythema and swelling; or (d) signs of lymphangitis, lymphadenitis, or both. The presence of cellulitis necessitates antibiotic treatment.

Invasive Infection

The diagnosis of *invasive infection* of a burn wound rests on the recognition of changes in the wound (black, purple, or reddish discoloration; maceration; or early separation of eschar) and systemic manifestations of infection. In addition to the clinical assessment of the wound, biopsy may be performed for quantitative culture or histologic evaluation. A tissue culture with >100,000 organisms cultured from a gram of tissue is considered positive. However, considerable variability in results with this technique and the lack of correlation with histologic findings have limited utility for identification of organisms in wounds. Histologic evaluation, although not readily available at most institutions, is diagnostic for invasive infection when organisms are identified in viable tissue. Invasive wound infection requires surgical excision of the wound to the level of viable tissue and administration of systemic

antibiotics. The topical antimicrobials, with the exception of mafenide acetate, which may be used in preparation for excision, are not used for therapy for invasive burn-wound infection because they do not penetrate eschar.

The criteria for diagnosis of invasive infection, as outlined in the American Burn Association guidelines, include the following:

- Inflammation of the surrounding uninjured skin
- Histologic examination that shows invasion by the infectious organism into adjacent viable tissue
- Isolation of an organism from the blood in the absence of other infection
- Signs of the systemic inflammatory response syndrome (such as hyperthermia, hypothermia, leukocytosis, tachypnea, hypotension, oliguria, or hyperglycemia at a previously tolerated level of carbohydrate intake) and mental status changes.

Pneumonia

The use of effective topical antimicrobials for prevention and therapy of wound infection, along with earlier surgical intervention in wound care, has led to a decrease in the incidence of wound infection. Because of the decrease in the rate of wound infections, respiratory failure is now the leading cause of death in the patient with thermal injury. Although inhalation injury is a prominent cause of respiratory complications in these patients, the incidence of pneumonia and ARDS is high, even when direct lung injury is not present. A review of autopsies on burn-injured children revealed that 44% had pneumonia at the time of death (35). Standard care includes early detection of pulmonary infection by Gram stain of sputum, culture of endotracheal secretions, assisted ventilation if respiratory failure develops, and appropriate antimicrobial therapy. The issue of how to make the diagnosis of pneumonia in a burn-injured patient remains unresolved. Pneumonia was diagnosed clinically in only 28% of children who had findings of pneumonia present at autopsy (35). This same study showed a poor correlation with bronchoalveolar lavage (BAL) and protected bronchial brush (PBB) results. Additional studies suggest that BAL, with a positive result defined as >1000 colony-forming units (CFU) per milliliter, and PBB are not sensitive enough in children to make the diagnosis of pneumonia but are helpful in detecting tracheobronchitis after inhalation injury (33). BAL has been reported to be useful in diagnosis and directing therapy in adult burn-injured patients with ventilator-associated pneumonia (36). In those studies, a positive BAL was considered to be at least 10,000 CFU/mL. The presence of white blood cells and bacteria in the sputum associated with other signs of infection should prompt the initiation of systemic antimicrobials that target the organisms that predominate in the flora of the unit at the time. Specific antimicrobials are then selected when culture results are available.

Suppurative Thrombophlebitis

Bacterial colonization of central venous catheters in burn-injured patients in the ICU has been reported to be as high as 25%. No general consensus exists regarding how to minimize catheter-related infections. Some centers require that all peripheral, central venous, and arterial catheters be changed over a guidewire on day 3 and that a new site be used on day 6. Others have suggested that once-a-week catheter replacement is sufficient to maintain an acceptable rate of catheter-related bloodstream infection in children (37). The reason for concern, especially in burn-injured individuals, is that suppurative thrombophlebitis can be an insidious and life-threatening infection. The only findings may be persistent fever and a bacteremia that continues despite appropriate antibiotic treatment. The classic findings of edema, erythema, pain, and a palpable cord at an IV site, associated with phlebitis, may not be identifiable. Diagnosis is confirmed by aspiration of purulent material from the affected vein. Treatment consists of excision of the involved vein to the point at which bleeding is encountered and the remaining vessel is normal.

Suppurative Chondritis

The cartilage of the ear has minimal protection with low blood supply and is highly susceptible to infection when the overlying tissue is damaged. Dressings should not be applied to the ear, and pillows should not be used. Auricular burns should be treated with twice-daily open wound care and gentle debridement. The topical agent of choice is mafenide acetate because it penetrates eschar and avascular cartilage. When suppurative chondritis occurs, systemic antibiotics are of little value due to the avascular nature of the tissue, and the ear must be surgically drained under anesthesia by bivalving of the ear, with excision of infected and necrotic tissue.

Bacteremia Associated with Wound Manipulation

It is anticipated that debridement and surgical excision of burn wounds lead to bacteremia; however, the data to support this assertion are variable. Sasaki et al. (38) observed transient bacteremia in 21% of patients after burn-care procedures, while others have reported that more than 40% of burn patients had positive blood cultures following burn excision (39). It appears that the incidence of bacteremia following wound manipulation is related to the extent of injury. This finding is supported by the 8% incidence of bacteremia in patients with 31%–60% TBSA burns, compared to a 75% incidence in those with >60% TBSA burns. More recent studies have suggested that the incidence of bacteremia associated with wound manipulation is low in the early period after injury. Nevertheless, bacteria may seed distant sites such as cardiac valves or the brain, and it is likely that in this population of patients, perioperative administration of antibiotics that are active against the flora of the wound is of benefit.

Other Infections

As in any seriously injured patient, immunocompromise may set the stage for infection at any site. Burn-injured patients have a high incidence of urinary tract infections and pneumonia. They may also develop other infections, such as appendicitis, but often do not present with classic features due to a suppressed inflammatory response. A high index of suspicion is necessary to detect these infections. Additional infections of concern in the burn-injured patient are listed below.

Sinusitis

One source of sepsis that is frequently overlooked in the burn patient is nosocomial sinusitis. Factors that predispose to sinusitis include nasogastric, nasoduodenal, and nasotracheal intubation, especially in patients with inhalation injury. The clinical diagnosis of nosocomial sinusitis is difficult because a purulent nasal discharge is absent in 73%, a majority of cases. The diagnosis is made by culture of drainage fluid and by CT

scan of the sinuses. Once the diagnosis is made, treatment consists of removal of all tubes, initiation of appropriate antibiotic therapy, and drainage. If a nasotracheal tube is present, it should be changed to the orotracheal route. In some cases, it may be necessary to perform a tracheostomy to adequately control the infectious process.

Bacterial Endocarditis

Immune compromise, recurrent bacteremia, and the frequent use of central venous catheters in the patient with burn injury are risk factors for the development of endocarditis. The association of central venous and pulmonary artery catheters with the development of bacterial endocarditis in burn-injured patients is well documented. Similar to suppurative thrombophlebitis, bacterial endocarditis is insidious and should be suspected when blood cultures are positive without an obvious source and with a fever of unknown origin—particularly in burn-injured patients, as the incidence of bacterial endocarditis has been reported to be as much as 14–70 times higher than in other ICU patients. The presence of a new cardiac murmur supports the diagnosis, which should be confirmed by echocardiography. In the past, bacterial endocarditis was associated with nearly 100% mortality in the patient with burn injury. Early diagnosis with surgical intervention has led to improved survival in recent years. Antibiotic therapy is based upon blood culture results and should continue for 4–6 weeks.

HYPERMETABOLISM AND NUTRITION

The classic description of the metabolic response to injury includes an early ebb phase that is characterized by low cardiac output and a decreased metabolic rate followed by a hypermetabolic phase that begins 24–36 hours after injury. An approximate 50% increase in protein metabolism and energy expenditure occurs due to hypermetabolism, fluid losses, sepsis, and inflammation in children following a large burn injury. This increased catabolic state can persist for 9–12 months. The stress hormones (cortisol, epinephrine, and glucagon) all increase, mediating increased gluconeogenesis, glycogenolysis, muscle breakdown, and bone loss. Furthermore, the anabolic effects of insulin and growth hormone are antagonized in patients with burns. Early and aggressive nutritional support has been shown to reduce the elevated resting energy expenditure (REE) in burn victims. Most investigations have led to the conclusion that measurement of REE by indirect calorimetry is the best way to estimate caloric needs in children during the hypermetabolic phase. The use of the Harris–Benedict formula, the World Health Organization formula, or the Schofield-HW equation showed poor correlation with REE in children after major burn injury (40). It has been shown that male children have a higher metabolic rate than females after injury and that children who are <3 years of age have only a slight increase in metabolic rate (41). Furthermore, studies confirm that hypermetabolism persists for over 12 months following injury. Nutritional support in the burn patient is usually guided by a formula, such as that used at the Shriners Burn Center, especially when indirect calorimetry is not available (Table 32.5).

The enteral route is the preferred route for administration of nutrition. A nasogastric or nasoduodenal tube should be placed as soon as initial evaluation and burn resuscitation are complete. In the absence of contraindications, enteral feeds should be initiated within 24 hours of injury. There is insufficient data to make recommendations regarding the optimal route for enteral feeding (gastric vs. transpyloric);

TABLE 32.5

FORMULA FOR NUTRITIONAL SUPPORT IN THE
BURN PATIENT

Infants (0–12 months)	$2100 \text{ kcal/m}^2 + 1000 \text{ kcal/m}^2$ burn
Children 1–11 years	$1800 \text{ kcal/m}^2 + 1300 \text{ kcal/m}^2$ burn
Children 12 years and older	$1500 \text{ kcal/m}^2 + 1500 \text{ kcal/m}^2$ burn

there is no difference in the incidence of microaspiration, tube feed displacement, and feeding intolerance based on route of delivery (42).

Feeding intolerance, as evidenced by significant gastric residual volume and diarrhea, may limit use of the gastrointestinal tract for caloric delivery. Diarrhea is a commonly encountered problem in the burn population. The etiology is likely multifactorial, and the commonly proposed reasons include antibiotic use, nosocomial infection, bowel wall edema, hyperosmolarity, insufficient fiber content of enteral formulas, and compromised mucosal integrity. However, diarrhea is usually noninfectious and, despite physiologic plausibility, is not worsened by hypoalbuminemia. Factors associated with a decreased incidence of diarrhea in burn victims include fat intake <20% of overall caloric intake, vitamin A intake >10,000 IU/day in adults, and early implementation of enteral feeds (<48 hours post-burn) (43).

In addition to vitamin A, other vitamins, minerals, and trace elements may be required in excess of recommended daily allowances, including calcium, magnesium, vitamin D, zinc, copper, and other micronutrients. It is believed that upregulation of the parathyroid gland calcium-sensing receptor contributes to hypocalcemia and hypomagnesemia. The current standard is to supplement calcium and magnesium until serum levels are within the normal range. Zinc and copper levels are also diminished following thermal injury. These micronutrients have important roles in bone matrix formation, linear growth, wound healing, and immunity (44). Levels are thought to be low because of wound losses, increased urinary excretion, and the activity of IL-1 and other cytokines produced during the acute-phase response. Calcium supplementation can impair zinc absorption and decrease copper retention. No clear consensus exists regarding appropriate zinc and copper supplementation in burn-injured patients.

In addition to early and aggressive nutritional support, attempts have been made to pharmacologically mitigate the persistent hypermetabolic state that follows burn injury. The hypermetabolism, which can be blunted to some extent by β-blockade, has led some to recommend the use of propranolol in children. A 2006, randomized, prospective, placebo-controlled study showed that propranolol given via nasogastric tube in doses of 0.3–1.0 mg/kg body weight every 4–6 hours decreases heart rate by 11% (45). This study also showed a reduction in the hepatomegaly that routinely occurs in severely burn-injured. In a long-term study of propranolol use, the significant improvement in preservation of lean body mass that was seen at 3 and 6 months post-burn in the propranolol group was matched by the control group at 9 and 12 months. Propranolol may also improve outcome by reducing the development of post-traumatic stress and anxiety (32).

Muscle wasting, decreased bone mineralization, and retarded linear growth can be profound. In the early 1990s, recombinant human growth hormone was evaluated, initially in adults and later in children. Safety concerns surrounding its use were noted in several European studies. Although children did not appear to have the same issues, daily subcutaneous injections limited patient compliance. In the mid-1990s,

testosterone was shown to improve protein synthesis; however, hepatotoxicity, acne, hirsutism, and virilization in females limited its utility. In the late 1990s, a synthetic testosterone analog, oxandrolone, was studied in adult and pediatric burn patients. In a 12-month randomized, placebo-controlled, double-blinded study in pediatric patients with burns of 40% BSA or greater, it was found to produce an earlier normalization of serum albumin, prealbumin, and retinol-binding protein and to improve lean body mass and bone mineral content. In treated patients, as compared to controls, this study reported no acne, facial hair, hirsutism, or hepatotoxicity (46). Despite these results, oxandrolone is not yet considered to be standard care following burn injury in children.

Hypoalbuminemia

In burn patients, hypoalbuminemia is a frequent finding, and the etiology is multifactorial. Increased losses of albumin occur directly via drainage from burn wounds, as well as diffusely, as a consequence of profound capillary leakage ignited by the cascade of inflammatory mediators triggered by the burn injury. Albumin production is also reduced in critical illness, likely due to an increase in the production of acute-phase proteins. Additionally, in the immediate postresuscitation phase, a dilutional contribution to hypoalbuminemia may occur if intravascular volume is increased. Chronic illness and malnutrition are other potential causes of nonacute hypoalbuminemia.

Albumin contributes 80% of the normal colloid oncotic pressure (47); therefore, hypoalbuminemia is associated with edema, particularly of the pulmonary interstitium and bowel wall. Albumin is often administered in an effort to avoid exacerbating acute lung injury, diarrhea, feeding intolerance, and impaired wound healing.

The therapeutic use of albumin in burn patients and in those with critical illness has been extensively studied, with great variability in results. Although some studies have suggested an increased risk of mortality associated with hypoalbuminemia, when the data from these studies are carefully analyzed, increased mortality is primarily seen in patients whose serum albumin was low at the time of presentation and in patients with extensive burns, infectious complications, chronic illness, and malnutrition (47). The extent of burn injury and incidence of sepsis appear to be the true risk factors for mortality. Studies that suggest an increased mortality associated with the administration of albumin have been refuted by a recent multi-institutional, randomized, double-blinded study that showed no difference in mortality in adult ICU patients resuscitated with saline versus albumin (48).

When considering albumin replacement in burn patients, it is best to separate the administration into three distinct scenarios (17). Albumin supplementation during the resuscitation of major burns in the first 48 hours: This practice, although well studied, remains controversial in the burn community with most specialists using albumin supplementation in larger burns. Recently, albumin (5% solution) has been recommended as a rescue fluid in an effort to prevent large volume over resuscitation (4,49). The use of albumin during acute sepsis: There is little literature specifically addressing the use of albumin in the septic burn patient. Its use should be based on the available evidence in non-burn critically ill patients at this time. An article from 2004 with nearly 7000 patients prospectively randomized evaluating crystalloid versus colloid in a mixed ICU population showed no difference in mortality with respect to the resuscitation fluid used (35,50). Albumin in the chronic ICU setting: Should a goal for albumin level be maintained throughout the ICU stay by periodic repletion? The answer to this question is unknown in the burn population. Albumin replacement for this indication remains commonplace despite the lack of evidence. The precise threshold at which hypoalbuminemia actually becomes clinically significant has only been investigated in animal studies. In humans, the preponderance of evidence from randomized, controlled trials that evaluate feeding intolerance, diarrhea, pulmonary dysfunction, and mortality as end points demonstrated that mild-to-moderate hypoalbuminemia is well tolerated in previously healthy patients (51). Among burn patients with hypoalbuminemia, serum albumin gradually normalizes, especially in the context of aggressive nutritional support, and higher serum albumin concentration is seen in patients who receive enteral, as compared with parenteral, nutrition. Therefore, routine albumin repletion may not be warranted, but more rigorously conducted studies are necessary to clarify the issue. The present practice at our center is to ensure appropriate caloric delivery preferably by the enteral route, as quickly as possible. In critically ill children, 25% albumin is administered if the serum level is below 2 mg/dL and the patient is symptomatic.

Glycemic Control

As noted previously, protein metabolism and energy expenditure increase by approximately 50% in children following a large burn injury. The etiology of this catabolic state is multifactorial but favorably impacted by insulin administration. Hyperglycemia in burn patients is associated with increased morbidity and mortality. Additionally, maintenance of normoglycemia has been shown to be associated with improved outcomes in single-center studies involving critically ill adults or children with severe burn injury (52–54). Administration of exogenous insulin can overcome insulin resistance, retard protein catabolism, and promote normoglycemia. In children, modest glycemic control has been favored over tight control in view of the risk of significant hypoglycemia. The combined benefits of glycemic control in the critically ill patient and the favorable effects of insulin in promoting protein synthesis and preventing protein catabolism support the use of insulin administration to prevent significant hyperglycemia in the burn patient. No blood glucose goal has been established for the critically ill pediatric burn patient; however, a reasonable target for blood glucose should be levels that range between 120 and 180 mg/dL (54,55). Members of the healthcare team participating in the care of pediatric burn patients should be sensitized to the importance of glucose monitoring and the recognition of both hyperglycemia and hypoglycemia, especially in very young or nonverbal children. Standing insulin orders should be limited to patients who demonstrate persistent hyperglycemia during a constant glucose delivery (enteral tube feedings or parenteral nutrition) and are regularly monitored for hypoglycemia.

OUTCOME

Survival after burn injury has improved significantly during the past 20 years and appears to have reached a plateau over the past 10 years (56). Because mortality rates have changed, the suggestion of two decades ago that mortality could be estimated as the sum of age and percentage of the BSA that sustained thermal injury no longer holds true. However, multiple studies have confirmed that patient age and extent of injury are still the two most powerful predictors of outcome. Review of the records of more than 187,000 victims of burn injury indicates that mortality has decreased from 6.2% in 1995 to 4.7% in 2005 (57). These data also demonstrate the significant contribution of age to mortality risk in children. The mortality for a burn injury of 60%–69.9% TBSA was 50% in

the newborn to 1.9-year-old group, 22.6% in those between 2 and 4.9 years of age, and 18.3% in those between 5 and 19.9 years of age. Although it has been suggested that the rate of survival in girls is greater than in boys, this was unconfirmed by a 2005 study (58).

It is well recognized that mortality rate is increased as much as 20% when inhalation injury accompanies thermal injury. A comparative study of patients matched for burn size and age reported a mortality rate of 9.6% in patients without inhalation injury, compared to 46.6% in those with inhalation injury (9). Multivariate statistical techniques (probit or regression analysis) have been suggested for improving accuracy in outcome prediction for burn patients.

REHABILITATION

Advances in medical care leading to increased survival from thermal injury have led to a renewed emphasis on quality of life after these injuries. Rehabilitation of the patient with a burn injury should begin with the initial medical care, be intensely administered in the first year after injury, and, often continued for life. Splinting of injured extremities begins as soon as the patient is stabilized, and range-of-motion exercises begin within the first 24 hours. The team approach is important to coordinate therapy, surgical intervention, and medical care. As soon as wounds have a stable epidermal closure, usually within 2 weeks after grafting or primary healing has occurred, attention is turned to wound and scar management. Garments that apply pressure to the wounds are tailor-made for the patient and worn 24 hours per day. The opportunity to modulate the development of cicatrix is restricted to the time when the wound is immature and actively remodeling. This period may extend up to a year postinjury, but mechanical intervention is of little benefit beyond that time. Surgical intervention for cosmetic deformity is usually delayed until the wound is mature, as is intervention for functional restriction, unless a surgical procedure is necessary to allow for physical therapy.

CONCLUSIONS AND FUTURE DIRECTIONS

Advances in the care of the burn-injured child have paralleled progress in critical care, with additional improvements in resuscitation and wound care leading to a decrease in mortality from burn injury. The current challenge is to improve the quality of life after major injury, and future directions include advances to improve texture, color, and elasticity of grafted areas. Microvascular techniques for reconstruction will become increasingly important to replace major tissue loss and improve cosmetic outcomes.

References

1. La Hei ER, Holland AJA, Martin HCO. Laser Doppler imaging of pediatric burns: Burn wound outcome can be predicted independent of clinical examination. *Burns* 2006;32:550–3.
2. Koumbourlis AC. Electrical injuries. *Crit Care Med* 2002;30(11)(suppl):S424–30.
3. Jain S, Bandi V. Electrical and lightning injuries. *Crit Care Clin* 1999;15:319–31.
4. Arnoldo B, Klein M, Gibran NS. Practice guidelines for the management of electrical injuries. *J Burn Care Res* 2006;27:439–47.
5. Baxter CR, Shires T. Physiologic response to crystalloid resuscitation of severe burns. *Ann N Y Acad Sci* 1968;150:874–94.

6. Huang PP, Stucky FS, Dimick AR. Hypertonic sodium resuscitation is associated with renal failure and death. *Ann Surg* 1995;221:543–57.

7. Pruitt BA Jr. Protection from excessive resuscitation "pushing the pendulum back." *J Trauma* 2000;49:567–8.

8. Sullivan SR, Friedrich JB, Engrav LH, et al. "Opioid creep" is real and may be the cause of "fluid creep." *Burns* 2004;30:583–90.

9. Shirani KZ, Pruitt BA Jr, Mason AD. The influence of inhalation injury and pneumonia on burn mortality. *Ann Surg* 1986;205:82–7.

10. Desai MH, Mlcak R, Richardson J, et al. Reduction in mortality in pediatric patients with inhalation injury with aerosolized heparin/N-acetylcystine therapy. *J Burn Care Rehabil* 1998;19:210–2.

11. Miller AC, Rivero A, Ziad S, et al. Influence of nebulized unfractionated heparin and N-acetylcysteine in acute lung injury after smoke inhalation injury. *J Burn Care Res* 2009;30:249–56.

12. Levine BA, Petroff PA, Slade CL, et al. Prospective trials of dexamethasone and aerosolized gentamicin in the treatment of inhalation injury in the burned patient. *J Trauma* 1978;18:188–93.

13. Silver GM, Freiburg C, Halerz M, et al. A survey of airway and ventilator management strategies in North American pediatric burn units. *J Burn Care Rehabil* 2004;25:435–40.

14. 2005 American Heart Association guidelines for cardiopulmonary resuscitation and emergency cardiovascular care, part 12: Pediatric advanced life support. *Circulation* 2005;112(suppl I):IV-167–187.

15. Cartotto R, Ellis S, Smith T. Use of high-frequency oscillating ventilation in burn patients. *Crit Care Med* 2005;33(3):S175–81.

16. Habashi NM. Other approaches to open-lung ventilation: Airway pressure release ventilation. *Crit Care Med* 2005;33(3)(suppl):228–40.

17. Ahrenholz DH, Cope N, Dimick AR, et al. Inhalation injury: Initial management in practice guidelines for burn care. *J Burn Care Rehabil* 2001;(suppl):23S–6S.

18. Livshits Z, Lugassy DM, Shawn LK, et al. Falsely low carboxyhemoglobin level after hydroxocobalamin therapy. *N Engl J Med* 2012;367:1270–1.

19. Wolf FJ, Lavonas EJ, Sloan EP, et al. Clinical policy: Critical issues in the management of adult patients presenting to the emergency department with acute carbon monoxide poisoning. *Ann Emerg Med* 2008;51:138–52.

20. Hampson NB, Piantadosi CA, Thom SR, et al. Practice recommendations in the diagnosis, management, and prevention of carbon monoxide poisoning. *Am J Respir Crit Care Med* 2012;186:1095–101.

21. Buckley NA, Juurlink DN, Isbister G, et al. Hyperbaric oxygen for carbon monoxide poisoning. *Cochrane Database Syst Rev* 2011;13(4):CD002041.

22. Palmieri TL, Jackson W, Greenhalgh DG. The benefits of early tracheostomy in severely burned children. *Crit Care Med* 2002;30(4):922–4.

23. Committee on Trauma. Guidelines for the operations of burn units in resources for optimal care of the injured patient. *Bull Am Coll Surg* 1999; vol 84;55–62.

24. Hight DW, Bakalar HR, Lloyd JR. Inflicted burns in children. *JAMA* 1979;242:517–20.

25. Yasti AC, Tumer AR, Atli M, et al. A clinical forensic scientist in the burns unit: Necessity or not? A prospective clinical trial. *Burns* 2006;32:77–82.

26. Hermans MHE. Results of a survey on the use of different treatment options for partial and full-thickness burns. *Burns* 1998;24:539–51.

27. Tompkins RG, Remensnyder JP, Burke JF, et al. Significant reductions in mortality for children with burn injuries through the use of prompt eschar excision. *Ann Surg* 1988;208:577–85.

28. Still JM, Law EJ, Craft-Coffman B. An evaluation of excision with application of autografts or porcine xenografts within 24 hours of injury. *Ann Plast Surg* 1996;36:176–9.

29. Sheridan RL, Tompkins RG, McManus WF, et al. Intercompartmental sepsis in burn patients. *J Trauma* 1994;36:301–5.

30. Weber JM, Sheridan RL, Pasternak MS, et al. Nosocomial infections in pediatric patients. *Am J Infect Control* 1997;25:195–201.

31. Finnerty CC, Herndon DN, Przkora R, et al. Cytokine expression profile over time in severely burned pediatric patients. *Shock* 2006;26:13–9.

32. Greenhalgh DG, Saffle JR, Holmes JH IV, et al. American burn association consensus conference to define sepsis and infection in burns. *J Burn Care Res* 2007;28:776–90.

33. Peck MD, Weber J, McManus A, et al. Surveillance of burn wound infections: A proposal for definitions. *J Burn Care Rehabil* 1998;19:386–9.

34. Ramzy PI, Jeschke MG, Wolf SE. Correlation of bronchoalveolar lavage with radiographic evidence of pneumonia in thermally injured children. *J Burn Care Rehabil* 2003;24:382–5.

35. Barret JP, Ramzy PI, Wolf SE, et al. Sensitivity and specificity of bronchoalveolar lavage and protected bronchial brush in the diagnosis of pneumonia in pediatric burn patients. *Arch Surg* 1999;134:1243–6.

36. Wahl WL, Ahrns KS, Brandt MM, et al. Bronchoalveolar lavage in diagnosis of ventilator-associated pneumonia in patients with burns. *J Burn Care Rehabil* 2005;26:57–61.

37. Sheridan RL, Weber JM. Mechanical and infectious complications of central venous cannulation in children: Lessons learned from a 10-year experience placing more than 1000 catheters. *J Burn Care Res* 2006;27:713–8.

38. Sasaki TM, Welch GW, Herndon DN, et al. Burn wound manipulation-induced bacteremia. *J Trauma* 1979;19(1):46–8.

39. Beard CH, Ribeiro CD, Jones DM. The bacteraemia associated with burns surgery. *Br J Surg* 1975;62:638–41.

40. Suman OE, Mlcak RP, Chinkes DL, et al. Resting energy expenditure in severely burned children: Analysis of agreement between indirect calorimetry and prediction equations using the Bland-Altman method. *Burns* 2006;32:335–42.

41. Mlcak RP, Jeschke MG, Barrow RE, et al. The influence of age and gender on resting energy expenditure in severely burned children. *Ann Surg* 2006;244:121–30.

42. Mehta NM. Approach to enteral feeding in the PICU. *Nutr Clin Pract* 2009;24:377.

43. Gottschlich MM, Warden GD, Havens MM, et al. Diarrhea in tube-fed burn patients: Incidence, etiology, nutritional impact, and prevention. *JPEN J Parenter Enteral Nutr* 1988;12(4):338–45.

44. Voruganti VS, Klein GL, Lu H, et al. Impaired zinc and copper status in children with burn injuries: Need to reassess nutritional requirements. *Burns* 2005;31:711–6.

45. Barrow RE, Wolfe RR, Dasu MR, et al. The use of beta-adrenergic blockade in preventing trauma-induced hepatomegaly. *Ann Surg* 2006;243:115–20.

46. Hart DW, Wolf SE, Ramzy PI, et al. Anabolic effects of oxandrolone after severe burn. *Ann Surg* 2001;233(4):556–64.

47. Greenhalgh DG, Housinger TA, Kagan RJ, et al. Maintenance of serum albumin levels in pediatric burn patients: A prospective, randomized trial. *J Trauma* 1995;39(1):67–74.

48. Finfer S, Norton R, Bellomo R, et al. The SAFE study: Saline vs. albumin for fluid resuscitation in the critically ill. *Vox Sang* 2004;87(suppl 2):S123–31.

49. Park SH, Hemmila MR, Wahl WL. Early albumin use improves mortality in difficult to resuscitate burn patients. *J Trauma Acute Care Surg* 2012;73:1294–7.

50. Finfer S, Bellomo R, Boyce N, et al; SAFE Study Investigators. A comparison of albumin and saline for fluid resuscitation in the intensive care unit. *N Engl J Med* 2004;350:2247–56.

51. Sheridan RL, Prelack K, Cunningham JJ. Physiologic hypoalbuminemia is well tolerated by severely burned children. *J Trauma* 1997;43(3):448–52.

52. Van den Berghe G, Wouters PJ, Bouillon R, et al. Outcome benefit of intensive insulin therapy in the critically ill: Insulin dose versus glycemic control. *Crit Care Med* 2003;31(2):359–66.

53. Vlasselaers D, Milants I, Desmet L, et al. Intensive insulin therapy for patients in paediatric intensive care: A prospective, randomized controlled study. *Lancet* 2009;373:547–56.

54. Jeschke MG, Kulp GA, Kraft R, et al. Intensive insulin therapy in severely burned pediatric patients: A prospective randomized trial. *Am J Respir Crit Care Med* 2010;182:351–9.

55. Dellinger RP, Levy MM, Rhodes A, et al; Surviving Sepsis Campaign Guidelines Committee including the Pediatric Subgroup. Surviving sepsis campaign: international guidelines for management of severe sepsis and septic shock: 2012. *Crit Care Med* 2013;41(2):580–637.

56. Ryan CM, Schoenfeld DA, Thorpe WP, et al. Objective estimates of the probability of death from burn injuries. *N Engl J Med* 1998;338:362–6.

57. Miller SF, Bessey PQ, Schurr MJ, et al. National burn repository 2005: A ten-year review. *J Burn Care Res* 2006;27:411–3.

58. Barrow RE, Przkora R, Hawkins HK, et al. Mortality related to gender, age, sepsis, and ethnicity in severely burned children. *Shock* 2005;23:485–7.

CHAPTER 33 ■ INJURY FROM CHEMICAL, BIOLOGIC, RADIOLOGIC, AND NUCLEAR AGENTS

PETER SILVER, F. MERIDITH SONNETT, AND GEORGE L. FOLTIN

KEY POINTS

1 Because of their unique physiology, chemical, biologic, radiologic, and nuclear (CBRN) events will affect a disproportionate number of children.

2 The most important first step in responding to a chemical, biologic, or radiologic event is rapid and thorough decontamination of victims by healthcare workers requiring adequate personal protective equipment.

3 Nerve agent inhalation presents with signs of muscarinic and nicotinic excess, and should be treated with atropine and pralidoxime until symptoms abate.

4 Cyanide exposure causes cellular anoxia by inhibiting cytochrome oxidase. If symptomatic, patients should be treated with sodium nitrate and sodium thiosulfate.

5 Supportive measures are the mainstay of treatment for survivors of CBRN attacks; however, certain exposures require specific pharmacologic and medical interventions.

6 All physicians should recognize the patterns of clinical illness that could indicate the first manifestations of a bioterrorist attack.

7 Bacterial biologic agents (anthrax, plague, and tularemia) require prompt administration of appropriate antibiotics.

8 All critical care physicians should be cognizant of the status of surge equipment, supplies, and availability of personnel at their institutions.

9 Coordination should occur between hospitals and regional, municipal, state, and federal entities, both in the planning stages and in the event of a true CBRN emergency.

10 Historically, the needs of pediatric victims of CBRN attacks had not been sufficiently addressed in formal disaster preparedness strategies. However, over the past 5 years, progress has been made in terms of formally incorporating pediatric-specific treatment and management guidelines for CBRN exposures in this vulnerable population.

11 Facilities that have PICUs have a role to support facilities that do not have PICU resources. Strategies for coordination should be established and regularly practiced.

The deliberate use of toxic materials to inflict injury or death is not a new phenomenon. For centuries, poisons have been used as weapons against individual victims. However, a major development occurred in World War I, when the industrial capabilities of the main combatants led to the use of chemical weapons on an immense scale. Subsequently, a series of international agreements to ban the use of such means of warfare were made, albeit with varying degrees of success. A significant, unfortunate development in recent times has been an increase in the use of chemical, biologic, radiologic, or nuclear (CBRN) agents in order to cause deliberate harm to unprotected civilians (1). Today, the potential of CBRN weapons in the hands of a terrorist or rogue state is one of the greatest threats to the security of the United States and other nations. These weapons challenge the healthcare system of the United States and other **1** nations beyond their capacity to provide treatment (2).

Children comprise a specifically vulnerable population, and are at disproportionally higher risk for morbidity and mortality from these types of attacks. Some important factors associated with this increased risk to children compared with adults are their smaller size, thinner skin (greater dermal absorption), smaller pulmonary reserve (increased minute volume), increased central nervous system permeability, underdeveloped communication skills, and unsophisticated coping strategies (3).

This chapter reviews those CBRN agents which pose the greatest threat.

CHEMICAL AGENTS

Chemical agents include nerve agents, asphyxiants, choking/pulmonary agents, and blistering/vesicant agents. These agents of chemical terrorism may originate from military, industrial, medical, or other sources.

Initial Approach to Chemical Attack

The single most important first step for treating all chemical exposures is the initial decontamination strategy. Removal **2** of patient clothing can eliminate ~90% of contaminants; this should be done as early as possible after the exposure, as the effectiveness of decontamination rapidly decreases with time (4). After the clothing is removed and put in sealed bags, the patient's skin and eyes may require decontamination. In most cases, decontamination of skin can be accomplished by gentle and thorough washing with water and soap. Decontamination should ideally be done at the scene of the incident by prehospital personnel, but many victims will bypass decontamination at the scene and self-present to hospitals; therefore, hospitals must be prepared for decontamination of potential victims (5). Special challenges are encountered in decontaminating pediatric patients, including susceptibility to hypothermia, particularly in cold weather, behavioral regression, and the need to decontaminate caretakers.

Nerve Agents

Pathophysiology

Nerve agents, including Sarin, Soman, Tabun, and Venom X (VX), are organophosphate compounds that inhibit acetylcholinesterase, resulting in accumulation of acetylcholine at the neural junctions, resulting in a syndrome of cholinergic crisis. These agents are generally colorless, odorless, tasteless, and nonirritating to the skin. Nerve agent vapors are denser than air and tend to accumulate in low-lying areas, putting children (with their shorter stature) at risk for higher exposure. Exposure can result from inhalational, dermal, or gastrointestinal absorption (6).

Clinical Signs and Symptoms

Symptoms of cholinergic crisis include both muscarinic and nicotinic effects. Muscarinic effects involve multiple organ systems, including the respiratory (shortness of breath, rhinorrhea, bronchorrhea, bronchospasm), cardiovascular (bradycardia, arrhythmias), gastrointestinal (salivation, nausea, vomiting, diarrhea, abdominal cramping), ophthalmologic (miosis, lacrimation), and genitourinary (incontinence)

systems. Nicotinic effects include muscle fasciculations that progress to weakness and flaccid paralysis, as well as sympathetic effects such as tachycardia and hypertension. Central nervous system symptoms include altered levels of consciousness ranging from agitation or lethargy to coma, and seizures (3,6). Patients with severe exposure may present with unconsciousness, convulsions, apnea, and flaccid paralysis (7).

Management

Emergent treatment of nerve agent toxicity is described in **Tables 33.1–33.3**. In addition to securing the airway, initial treatment includes administration of atropine followed by pralidoxime (2-PAM, 2-pyridine aldoxime methyl chloride), and the liberal use of benzodiazepines. Autoinjector kits ("Mark 1") containing a 2-mg dose of atropine and 600-mg dose of pralidoxime are now available in the prehospital setting. Although pediatric-sized atropine autoinjectors ("Atropen," containing 0.25, 0.5, or 2 mg of atropine) and larger 2-PAM autoinjectors (600 mg) are commercially available (8), corresponding pralidoxime autoinjectors for smaller pediatric patients are not available. Administration of intravenous atropine has resulted in ventricular fibrillation in hypoxic animals with nerve agent poisoning. Therefore, it is recommended that hypoxia be corrected prior to atropine administration, or that the atropine be given intramuscularly via autoinjector (to slow time to peak blood level) for the first dose in a hypoxic patient suffering from nerve agent exposure (**Table 33.2**). However, atropine should not be withheld due to fears of ventricular fibrillation (7). Adult survivors of nerve gas exposure have required as much as 20 mg of atropine over the first 24 hours, along with frequent pralidoxime doses or a continuous

TABLE 33.1

FINDINGS AND MANAGEMENT OF SPECIFIC CHEMICAL AGENTS

■ AGENT	■ FINDINGS	■ TREATMENT
Nerve agents Sarin Soman Tabun VX	Rhinorrhea Bronchorrhea Eye pain Bronchospasm Apnea Respiratory muscle paralysis Unconsciousness Convulsions	Airway, breathing, circulation support, 100% oxygen Atropine IM (autoinjector) or IV, at 2–5 min for secretions and respiratory symptoms—see **Table 33.2** for dosing *THEN* Pralidoxime (2-PAM) IM (autoinjector) or IV—see **Table 33.2** for dosing Diazepam or midazolam for seizures or if seriously ill[a]—see **Table 33.3** for dosing

Asphyxiant
Cyanide
	Cherry-red skin
	Tachypnea
	Seizures
		Airway, breathing, circulation support, 100% oxygen
		If conscious
		  No antidote
		If unconscious
		  Sodium nitrate 3%: 0.12–0.33 mL/kg (max 10 mL) slow IV (minimum 5 min); causes orthostatic hypotension
		  Sodium thiosulfate 25%: 1.65 mL/kg (max 50 mL) IV over 10–20 min
		  Sodium bicarbonate for acidosis after above if unresponsive

Choking agents Chlorine Phosgene	Ear, nose, throat irritation Stridor Bronchospasm Pulmonary edema (esp. phosgene)	Symptomatic care Possible bronchoscopy Aggressive management of pulmonary edema
Blistering/vesicants Sulfur mustard Lewisite	Skin erythema Bullae, ulcers Skin sloughing Ocular inflammation Respiratory tract inflammation Hyperexcitability, seizures	Symptomatic care Burn care Cycloplegics for eyes Possible use of hematopoietic growth factors BAL (dimercaprol, if available) 3 mg/kg IM q4–6h for systemic effects in severe cases

[a]Some authorities recommend seizure prophylaxis with benzodiazepines, others suggest use be reserved for treatment of seizures.
IM, intramuscular; IV, intravenous; BAL, British anti-Lewisite.

TABLE 33.2

DOSING OF ATROPINE AND PRALIDOXIME (2-PAM) FOR SEVERE NERVE AGENT EXPOSURE

	■ ATROPINE[a,b]	■ 2-PAM[c]
Infant (0–2 y)	0.1 mg/kg given IM or via autoinjector (0.25 or 0.50 mg available) or 0.1 mg/kg IV	45 mg/kg IM or 50 mg/kg IV over 20–30 min
Small child (3–7 y) 13–25 kg	0.1 mg/kg IM/IV or 1 (2 mg) autoinjector/IM	45 mg/kg IM; use 1 autoinjector (600 mg)[d] or 50 mg/kg IV over 20–30 min
Larger child (8–14 y) 26–50 kg	4 mg IM/IV or 2 (2 mg) autoinjectors/IM	45 mg/kg IM; use 2 autoinjectors (1200 mg)[d] or 50 mg/kg over 20–30 min (max 2 g)
Adolescent (>14 y) or adult	6 mg IM/5 mg IV or 3 (2 mg) autoinjectors	Use 3 autoinjectors (1800 mg) or 50 mg/kg over 20–30 min (max 2 g)

[a]Intramuscular dosing preferred, especially in hypoxic patients (see text).
[b]Repeat atropine at 2- to 5-minute intervals until secretions have diminished, breathing is comfortable, and airway resistance has returned to normal. Recommendations for repeat doses: for infants 0–3 years, 0.05 mg/kg (0.25–0.50 mg); for children 3–7 years, 1 mg; and for patients ≥8 years, 2 mg.
[c]Repeat 2-PAM dose hourly for two doses, and then every 10–12 hours as needed; if clinically possible, instead start continuous infusion 10–20 mg/kg/h (max 500 mg/h).
[d]Use of 2-PAM autoinjectors in pediatric patients is off-label (not FDA-approved).
Adapted from U.S. Department of Health & Human Services, Chemical Hazard Emergency Medical Management; U.S. Food and Drug Administration.

TABLE 33.3

TREATMENT FOR NERVE AGENT–INDUCED SEIZURES

	■ DIAZEPAM	■ MIDAZOLAM
Infant (0–2 y)	IM: Initial dose 0.2–0.5 mg/kg, repeat PRN every 2–5 min IV: Initial dose 0.2–0.5 mg/kg, repeat PRN every 15–30 min Total max dose: 5 mg	0.15 mg/kg IM, repeat PRN every 10 min Total max dose: 0.3 mg/kg
Child <5 y	IM: Initial dose 0.2–0.5 mg/kg, repeat PRN every 2–5 min IV: Initial dose 0.2–0.5 mg/kg, repeat PRN very 15–30 min Total max dose: 5 mg	0.15 mg/kg IM not to exceed 5 mg, repeat PRN every 10 min Total max dose: 0.3 mg/kg
Child 5–12 y	IM: Initial dose 0.2–0.5 mg/kg, repeat PRN every 2–5 min IV: Initial dose 0.2–0.5 mg/kg, repeat PRN every 15–30 min Total max dose: 10 mg May use 1 CANA autoinjector[a]	0.15 mg/kg IM not to exceed 10 mg, repeat PRN every 10 min Total max dose: 0.3 mg/kg
Adolescent/Adult	IM: 2–3 CANA autoinjectors[a] IV: 5–10 mg, repeat PRN every 15 min Total max dose: 30 mg	10 mg IM, repeat PRN every 10 min Total max dose: 20 mg

[a]Convulsant antidote for nerve agent (CANA); one CANA autoinjector contains 10 mg diazepam.
Adapted from U.S. Department of Health & Human Services, Chemical Hazard Emergency Medical Management.

infusion of 500 mg/h; patients surviving nerve gas attacks will likely need atropine for several days.

Benzodiazepines are the most effective medication for nerve agent–induced seizure activity (**Table 33.3**). Diazepam or midazolam should be given to all patients having seizure activity, unconsciousness, diffuse muscle twitching, or if more than one organ system is involved. Consideration should be given for including diazepam as part of the initial therapy for any seriously ill patient exposed to nerve agents. Early doses of atropine will also have an anticonvulsant effect (7). Topical cycloplegics may reduce nerve agent–induced ocular pain (9,10).

Asphyxiants

Pathophysiology

Asphyxiants are toxic compounds that inhibit cytochrome oxidase, thereby interfering with normal mitochondrial oxidative metabolism, causing cellular anoxia and lactic acidosis (high anion gap). Hydrogen cyanide, the most commonly known toxicant in this class, is a colorless liquid or gas that smells like bitter almonds, and has a strong chemical affinity for the heme ring. In addition, cyanide is believed to be a direct neurotoxin contributing to an excitatory injury in the brain,

likely mediated by glutamate stimulation of N-methyl-D-aspartate (NMDA) receptors. Cyanide's efficacy as a weapon of chemical terrorism is considered somewhat limited by its volatility in open air and relatively low lethality compared with nerve agents. However, if it were to be released in closed, crowded quarters, the effects would be severe (11).

Clinical Signs and Symptoms

Clinical manifestations of cyanide toxicity depend on the acuity of the exposure, but reflect the effects of cellular anoxia on different organ systems. With exposure to low concentrations of vapor, early findings include tachypnea and hyperpnea, tachycardia, flushing, dizziness, headache, and diaphoresis. As exposure continues, symptoms may progress to those associated with exposures to high concentration of vapor. These symptoms include rapid onset of tachypnea and hyperpnea (15 seconds), followed by seizures (30 seconds), coma and apnea (2–4 minutes), and cardiac arrest (4–8 minutes). Classical signs of cyanide poisoning include severe dyspnea without cyanosis, cherry-red skin (due to a lack of peripheral oxygen use), and a bitter almond odor to the breath and body fluids, although these signs are not always present. Laboratory abnormalities include metabolic acidosis with a large anion gap, increased serum lactate, and an abnormally high mixed venous oxygen saturation (again, due to decreased use of peripheral oxygen). Blood cyanide levels can be determined but usually not on an emergent basis. Although the symptoms of cyanide and nerve agent toxicity may be hard to distinguish, it should be remembered that in the presence of a high concentration of cyanide, seizures occur within seconds and death within minutes. This is in contrast to the course following nerve agent inhalation, which is typically longer and accompanied by copious secretions, muscle fasciculations, and cyanosis prior to death (11).

Management

Initial management of cyanide poisoning includes removal of the victim from the contaminated environment into fresh air, early administration of 100% oxygen, correction of acidosis with sodium bicarbonate, and seizure control with benzodiazepines. Specific antidotal therapy is a multiple-step process (**Table 33.1**). First, inhaled amyl nitrite and intravenous sodium nitrite are given, as methemoglobin-forming agents. Methemoglobin has a higher affinity for cyanide and thus dissociates it from cytochrome oxidase to form cyanomethemoglobin, which helps to restore normal cellular respiration. The second step is to administer intravenous sodium thiosulfate, as a sulfur donor, which provides substrate for conversion of cyanide to thiocyanate, which can then be eliminated in the urine. Nitrite administration should be done with caution, as it may cause hypotension, or lead to the production of excess amounts of methemoglobin, which may compromise oxygen-carrying capacity. Intravenous hydroxocobalamin is an alternative antidote for cyanide poisoning and while it may be synergistic, it should not be given in the same intravenous line as thiosulfate. Patients who survive the initial exposure and receive specific treatment will likely require intensive care to manage the effects of cellular anoxia, including acidosis, respiratory failure, acute respiratory distress syndrome, shock, and seizures.

Choking/Pulmonary Agents

Pathophysiology

Choking agents include chlorine and phosgene, which are in the gaseous form at room temperature. Unlike other chemical agents described in this chapter, millions of tons of these chemicals are produced in the United States each year for manufacturing purposes, including for the textile, paint, and dye industries. Because these agents are easy both to acquire and to handle, their use in terrorist acts remains a threat. They may also be released as a consequence of an industrial accident. When inhaled, the pulmonary agents produce massive mucosal irritation and edema, and damage to lung parenchyma. Chlorine has a strong, characteristic odor. It acts primarily on the tracheobronchial tree at the level of the respiratory epithelium of the bronchi and larger bronchioles. The result includes necrosis and denudation, often with the formation of pseudomembranes. Phosgene also has a characteristic odor of "freshly mown hay." Unlike the large airway effects of chlorine, phosgene tends to harm the gas-exchange regions of the respiratory system (bronchioles, alveolar ducts, and alveoli), which results in pulmonary edema. Both chlorine and phosgene are heavier than air and settle closer to the ground, which may have added significance for small children.

Clinical Signs and Symptoms

Chlorine and phosgene gasses have both immediate and delayed effects depending on the level of exposure. Initial symptoms of chlorine poisoning include a sensation of choking and mucosal irritation of the eyes, nose, and upper airways. Greater exposure leads to respiratory symptoms that progress from coughing and choking to hoarseness, aphonia, stridor, and bronchospasm. Dyspnea indicates the presence of pulmonary edema. Phosgene toxicity typically presents with coughing and sneezing. Dyspnea is often not present initially but after a several hour period of latency, progressive respiratory distress due to pulmonary edema typically occurs (12).

Management

After decontamination, which may require copious water irrigation of the eyes and mucosal membranes, management is largely supportive and follows standard recommendations for acute lung injury (administration of oxygen, bronchodilators, racemic epinephrine for stridor, and mechanical ventilation with appropriate levels of positive end-expiratory pressure for pulmonary edema, see **Table 33.1**). The value of corticosteroids is less clear but may be beneficial in patients with bronchospasm or history of asthma. Pseudomembrane formation may lead to airway obstruction, and bronchoscopy is often necessary to remove pseudomembranous debris. Secondary bacterial infection often occurs 3–5 days after exposure, and early, aggressive antibiotic coverage directed against culture-documented organisms is imperative. Prophylactic antibiotic administration is of no value (13).

Blistering/Vesicant Agents

Pathophysiology

The term "vesicant" refers to chemical agents that cause blistering of the skin, and include sulfur mustard and Lewisite. Sulfur mustard is stockpiled in several countries (including the United States) and has been used in military actions. Although these agents are associated with a lower mortality than that caused by other chemical agents, vesicant exposure on a large scale would be associated with significant and prolonged morbidity that could overwhelm a nation's health resources. Sulfur mustard is an alkylating agent that is highly toxic to rapidly reproducing and poorly differentiated cells (e.g., skin, pulmonary parenchyma, and bone marrow). It has an odor similar to garlic or mustard, has low volatility, and as both a liquid and vapor can penetrate most clothes. It is rapidly absorbed by tissue surfaces, and exerts cellular damage within minutes. Lewisite is an arsenical compound that affects skin and eyes immediately upon exposure (11).

Clinical Signs and Symptoms

The first skin findings occur within 2–48 hours after exposure to sulfur mustard, and progress from erythema resembling sunburn to yellow blisters, which coalesce into bullae and then ulcers, which may take months to heal (**Table 33.1**). If the exposure is severe, the victim may present instead with full-thickness skin sloughing. Ocular symptoms include conjunctivitis, corneal ulceration, and globe perforation (in severe exposures). Both the proximal and distal parts of the respiratory tract are affected, with symptoms ranging from hoarseness and cough to respiratory failure due to epithelial necrosis and the development of pseudomembranes which obstruct the airway. Secondary bacterial pneumonia may occur. All cellular elements of the bone marrow can be affected; megakaryocyte and granulocyte precursors are more susceptible than erythrocyte precursors. Gastrointestinal symptoms result both from general cholinergic activity of sulfur mustard and from direct mucosal injury, which leads to severe abdominal pain, vomiting, and diarrhea. Central nervous manifestations include hyperexcitability, convulsions, and coma.

Management

The most effective treatment for mustard exposure is prompt decontamination, because of the rapid absorption (3–10 minutes) and irreversible effects on tissues. Self-decontamination is preferred; anyone assisting an exposed victim must take proper precautions. Because there is no specific antidote for mustard exposure, therapy is supportive. Skin lesions are treated similar to that of burn victims, although there is usually less fluid loss. Eye treatment includes copious irrigation to remove the agent, cycloplegics for comfort and prevention of synechiae formation, and topical antibiotics with lubricating agents to prevent adhesions and scarring. Although mild respiratory symptoms can be treated noninvasively, more significant lung involvement will often require positive pressure ventilation and frequent bronchoscopy to remove necrotic tissue and pseudomembranes. Culture-proven secondary pulmonary infection should be treated with intravenous antibiotics. The use of hematopoietic growth factors, such as granulocyte colony-stimulating factor and granulocyte–macrophage colony-stimulating factor, may shorten the duration of sulfur mustard–induced bone marrow suppression (14–16). Treatment for Lewisite is also supportive but with the additional use of the specific antidote British anti-Lewisite (BAL), also called Dimercaprol. This is a chelating agent that, if available, should be administered only to the victims of Lewisite exposure who have signs of shock or significant pulmonary injury (9).

BIOTERRORISM/BIOLOGIC AGENTS

Bioterrorism involves the intentional release of bacteria, viruses, or other infectious agents that result in morbidity, mortality, and/or physical damage to those exposed, which may include humans, livestock, and crops. The Soviet Union, the United States, and Japan all developed biological weapons programs during the 20th century. The Convention of the Prohibition of the Development, Production, and Stockpiling of Bacteriologic and Toxic Weapons was held in 1972, with >140 nations signing. Despite this treaty, some supplies of biologic agents remain, and the threat of biologic warfare continues with the rise of certain terrorist groups (3).

The Centers for Disease Control and Prevention (CDC) groups these potential biological agents into three categories, based on their relative risk to national security. Category A agents are of the highest national priority, because of the following associations:

- Ease of transmission or dissemination
- Potential for high rates of mortality
- Potential for major public health impact
- Risk of public panic and social disruption
- Need for special action plans for public health preparedness

Category A agents include the bacteria *Bacillus anthracis* (anthrax), *Yersinia pestis* (plague), and *Francisella tularensis* (tularemia); variola virus (smallpox) and viral hemorrhagic fevers (Ebola virus and Marburg hemorrhagic fever); and toxin-mediated botulism from *Clostridium botulinum* (17). Category B agents constitute the second highest priority. They are moderately easy to disseminate, but in contrast to Category A agents they result in a lower mortality. Examples of Category B agents include brucellosis, food safety threats (e.g., *Salmonella* and *Shigella* spp.), ricin toxin, and water safety threats (e.g., *Vibrio cholerae*). Category C agents are emerging infectious diseases, including those caused by Nipah virus and Hantavirus.

The ability to recognize that an attack has occurred and the ability to differentiate this from a natural outbreak can be difficult as symptoms of these agents may be delayed for days after exposure. It is crucial that physicians recognize patterns of clinical illness that could indicate the presence of a bioterrorist attack. A sudden outbreak of an unusual illness is likely to be the first indication (3).

Terror-Related Bacterial Agents

Bacillus anthracis (Anthrax)

Pathophysiology. Anthrax disease is caused by spores from *B. anthracis*, an aerobic gram-positive rod-shaped bacterium. Although anthrax can be found naturally in soil, affecting domestic and wild animals in developing countries (typically in Central and South America, central and southwestern Asia, and the Caribbean), it is very rare in the United States. However, because anthrax spores are easily found in nature, can be produced in the laboratory, are durable, and can be easily dispersed in powders, sprays, food, or water, anthrax remains a potential for a terrorist attack (18).

Following exposure to *B. anthracis*, anthrax infection can manifest differently depending on the route of exposure. *Cutaneous anthrax* occurs after a spore enters the skin through an open laceration or abrasion, and accounts for 95% of anthrax disease in the United States. *Gastrointestinal anthrax* occurs after consumption of food contaminated with *B. anthracis* bacilli or spores, often from eating the meat of an animal that died of the disease. *Inhalation anthrax* occurs as a result of breathing in airborne *B. anthracis* spores. In both cutaneous and gastrointestinal anthrax, infection typically originates at a low level, with local edema and necrosis. In inhalation anthrax, and some cases of cutaneous and gastrointestinal anthrax, *B. anthracis* spores undergo phagocytosis by macrophages and are transported to regional lymph nodes where they germinate into toxin-producing bacteria and cause regional hemorrhagic lymphadenitis and subsequent septicemia (19). The secretion of two toxins by *B. anthracis* (*edema toxin* and *lethal toxin*, which enter the cytosol of almost every cell type) has been demonstrated to subvert the host immune response and is thought to be largely responsible for the severe edema, bacteremia, and toxemia that occurs with anthrax infections (20).

Clinical Signs and Symptoms. Cutaneous lesions develop after a *B. anthracis* spore enters the skin through an open laceration or abrasion, following an incubation period of 1–12 days. The skin lesions progress from pruritic papules or vesicles into painless, depressed black eschars (necrosis) surrounded by moderate to severe edema. In addition to the cutaneous findings, cutaneous anthrax is associated with systemic findings, including fever, headache, and lymphadenopathy. The most common signs and symptoms of gastrointestinal anthrax in children are fever, abdominal pain, vomiting, diarrhea, and bloody stools (21). The incubation period of inhalation anthrax is typically 1–7 days, but may be as long as 6–8 weeks. Inhalational illness is biphasic, with an initial period of nonspecific signs such as fever, fatigue, cough, and myalgia. There may be a brief improvement, followed by a more fulminant phase with high fever, respiratory failure (pleural effusions, pulmonary hemorrhage), and spread of bacteria through the blood resulting in severe edema and shock (19). Chest radiographs may be notable for pleural effusion (69%) and widened mediastinum (52%). In adults, meningoencephalitis occurs in ~50% of cases of inhalation anthrax; the incidence is unknown in children (22). The incidence of mortality associated with inhalation anthrax is 40% with treatment and nearly 100% without treatment (23).

TABLE 33.4

CENTERS FOR DISEASE CONTROL'S CATEGORY A BIOLOGIC AGENTS

■ AGENT	■ FINDINGS	■ TREATMENT
Inhalational anthrax	Fever, respiratory failure, effusions, widened mediastinum, sepsis	Ciprofloxacin (10 mg/kg/dose) IV (max 400 mg) q12h OR doxycycline 2.2 mg/kg/dose IV (max 100 mg) q12h AND 1–2 other drugs[a]
Plague	Fever, hemoptysis, pneumonia, sepsis	Streptomycin OR gentamicin 2.5 mg/kg/dose IV q8h OR doxycycline 2.2 mg/kg/dose IV (max 100 mg) q12h OR ciprofloxacin (10 mg/kg/dose) IV (max 400 mg) q12h OR chloramphenicol 25 mg/kg q6h IV (max 4 g/d)[b]
Tularemia	Necrotizing pneumonia, hilar adenopathy, effusions	Streptomycin OR gentamicin 2.5 mg/kg/dose IV q8h OR doxycycline 2.2 mg/kg/dose IV (max 100 mg) q12h OR ciprofloxacin (10 mg/kg/dose) IV (max 400 mg) q12h
Smallpox	Fever, multiple firm pustules all in the same stages of evolution	Vaccination for exposure within 72–96 h Potential use of ribavirin and cidofovir
Viral hemorrhagic fevers	Fever, gastrointestinal losses, hemorrhage, shock	Supportive care Aggressive rehydration and maintenance of electrolytes Potential use of monoclonal antibody Strict adherence to isolation precautions
Botulism	Afebrile, descending paralysis, autonomic instability	Supportive care Antitoxin

[a]Penicillin, amoxicillin, and clindamycin. Most authorities would treat with three to four drugs for 2 weeks, and then change to monotherapy or dual therapy once sensitivities are known, to complete a 60-day course. Anthrax may have either natural or engineered resistance elements.
[b]Recommended for plague meningitis. Serum levels and hematologic adverse events must be monitored.

Management. Specific multiagent antimicrobial therapy is required, as well as aggressive ventilatory and circulatory support for the multiorgan failure that occurs in severely affected patients. Antimicrobial treatment is detailed in **Table 33.4.** Drainage of pleural effusions and ascites, which may have high concentrations of toxin, is often indicated. Although there are only limited studies about the use of corticosteroids in the treatment of anthrax, adjunctive corticosteroids are indicated in the event of suspected or confirmed adrenal failure, and may have a role in the management of anthrax meningoencephalitis (24). Two antitoxin products for the treatment of anthrax are in the U.S. Strategic National Stockpile: raxibacumab (a humanized monoclonal antibody) and anthrax immune globulin (AIG, a polyclonal human immunoglobulin). The use of antitoxin in addition to systemic antimicrobial agents with highly suspected or confirmed systemic anthrax is recommended by the CDC (22).

Yersinia pestis (Plague)

Pathophysiology. Plague is a disease caused by the bacterium *Yersinia pestis*, and occurs most commonly in three forms: bubonic, septicemic, and pneumonic. *Bubonic plague* occurs in humans following a bite from a rodent flea or by handling an infected animal with plague. *Septicemic plague* occurs either as the spread of bubonic plague or as the first symptom of plague. *Pneumonic plague* is the most serious form of the disease, and although it can be the result of hematogenous spread of other forms of plague, it can also be caused by inhalation of aerosolized *Y. pestis*, delivered for the purpose of bioterrorism. The bacillus causes a multilobar hemorrhagic and necrotizing bronchopneumonia (25).

Clinical Signs and Symptoms. Signs and symptoms appear after an incubation period of 2–8 days (less for aerosolized exposure). In bubonic plague, patients develop fever, headache, weakness, and one or more swollen and tender lymph nodes, usually in the area of a bite from an infected flea. Symptoms of septicemic plague include fever, chills, extreme weakness, hemorrhage (including into the skin), and shock. Pneumonic plague presents with fever, cough with purulent sputum (gram-negative rods may be present), hemoptysis, and desaturation. Pneumonia, evident on chest radiograph, rapidly progresses and leads to respiratory failure and shock.

Management. *Y. pestis* can be isolated from multiple sources, including lymph node aspiration, blood culture, and sputum culture or bronchial washing. It can also be rapidly confirmed by polymerase chain reaction (PCR) testing (26). However, because of the potential for rapid progression, particularly in the case of pneumonic plague, prompt treatment is essential and should not be delayed for diagnostic testing. Gentamicin or streptomycin administered intramuscularly or intravenously are equally effective and are the antibiotics of choice (**Table 33.4**). Tetracycline, doxycycline (for children ≥8 years of age), chloramphenicol, and ciprofloxacin are alternative agents. Fluoroquinolone or chloramphenicol is an appropriate treatment for plague meningitis (27). Patients with pneumonic plague should be placed in isolation, and droplet precautions should be utilized until they have received 72 hours of antibiotic therapy (28).

Francisella tularensis (Tularemia)

Pathophysiology. *F. tularensis* is a highly virulent, small, nonmotile, aerobic, gram-negative bacillus that causes tularemia. It multiplies within macrophages, allowing it to invade the lymph nodes, lungs, pleura, spleen, and liver. Humans can become infected via several routes, including tick or deer fly bites, skin contact with infected animals (rodents, rabbits), or inhalation of contaminated dusts or aerosols. Multiple forms of tularemia include ulceroglandular (most common), glandular, oculoglandular, oropharyngeal, and pneumonic. *Pneumonic tularemia* is the most severe type, and results either from direct inhalation or from hematogenous spread from other sites. As many as 203 cases of tularemia occurred naturally as non-terror acts in the United States from 2004 to 2013, but because of its virulence, and the severity of pulmonary disease, the airborne spread of *F. tularensis* as an act of bioterrorism is a risk (29–31).

Clinical Signs and Symptoms. From 1 to 14 days postexposure, patients initially develop a viral-like illness, with fever, chills, headache, and often an atypical pneumonia, with hilar adenopathy on chest radiograph. In *ulceroglandular tularemia*, there is a skin ulcer at the point of contact, with swelling of regional lymph nodes. After inhalational exposure, hemorrhagic inflammation of the airways develops and progresses to necrotizing pneumonia. Pleural disease is common. Bacteremia may also be common, particularly in the early stages.

Management. Streptomycin or gentamicin is recommended for treatment of tularemia (**Table 33.4**), and doxycycline (for children >8 years of age) is recommended for an alternative treatment (27). Given the lack of person-to-person spread, standard precautions are the only infection control measures required (32,33).

Terror-Related Viral Agents

Variola Virus (Smallpox)

Pathophysiology. Smallpox is caused by Variola virus, which emerged in humans thousands of years ago (34). The last naturally occurring case in the world occurred in Somalia in 1977. As a result of smallpox eradication, routine vaccination against smallpox is no longer necessary for prevention and is no longer done. Despite elimination of smallpox as a disease entity, smallpox still exists in laboratory stockpiles, and could potentially be used as a bioterrorism agent. A single case of smallpox anywhere in the world should therefore be evidence that a bioterror attack has occurred. Smallpox is spread either by direct contact with infected body fluids, respiratory secretions, or contaminated objects, or by prolonged face-to-face contact with an infected individual. Variola infection follows the transmission of infected droplets to the oropharyngeal or respiratory mucosa. The infective dose is thought to be only a few virions. Macrophages are the first cells infected; the virus then migrates along the lymphatics and multiplies in regional lymph nodes. Infected macrophages migrate from these vessels into the epidermis, with subsequent edema and necrosis. Polymorphonuclear leukocytes then migrate into these areas, forming pustules (33).

Clinical Signs and Symptoms. The clinical illness for each stage of smallpox is depicted in **Table 33.5**. Historically, mortality rates in unimmunized patients were as high as 30%, and occurred from multiorgan failure secondary to overwhelming viremia.

Management. There are no proven treatments for smallpox; medical care is generally supportive. Dehydration and electrolyte abnormalities may occur during the vesicular and pustular stages of rash, and should be treated specifically. Bacterial superinfections can also occur, and should be treated with appropriate antibiotics (34). Several antiviral agents, including ribavirin and cidofovir, have been shown experimentally to inhibit replication of variola, but their effect in potential human patients with smallpox is not known (35–37). If smallpox occurs, mass vaccination campaigns must take place; vaccination within 72–96 hours of exposure provides good protection against disease and excellent protection against fatal disease (38). The CDC reports that vaccine stockpiles are large enough to vaccinate everyone in the United States in the event of a smallpox emergency. Patients hospitalized with smallpox should be cared for in a negative-pressure environment, utilizing both airborne and contact precautions. Ideally, only staff previously vaccinated for smallpox should care for victims.

Viral Hemorrhagic Fevers

Pathophysiology. The viral hemorrhagic fevers are a group of infections caused by a variety of viral agents, most notably Ebola and Marburg viruses, both members of the filovirus family. There continues to be sporadic outbreaks throughout Africa, most recently with Ebola virus in West Africa (Sierra Leone, Liberia, Guinea, and Mali), in 2014. Spread of viral hemorrhagic fevers occurs rapidly, through direct contact with blood, body fluids, and contaminated objects.

Clinical Signs and Symptoms. After an incubation period of 2–21 days (shorter for Marburg virus), patients develop fever, severe headache, and muscle ache. Gastrointestinal symptoms include abdominal pain, vomiting, and voluminous diarrhea

---

TABLE 33.5

CLINICAL STAGES OF VARIOLA VIRUS (SMALLPOX)

■ PERIOD	■ DURATION (d)	■ TRANSMISSION	■ CLINICAL ILLNESS
Incubation	7–17	Not contagious	Asymptomatic
Prodrome	2–4	Sometimes contagious	High fever, malaise, vomiting, head and body aches
Early rash	4	Most contagious	Small red spots on tongue and mouth, which develop into sores that break open
			Macular rash then spreads from face to arms and legs, and then to hands and feet
			Macular rash progresses through papular and vesicular stages, with depression in center and filled with opaque fluid
Pustular rash	5	Contagious	Lesions become sharply raised, firm pustules
Pustules and scabs	5	Contagious	Pustules form a crust and then scab
Resolving scabs	6	Contagious	Scabs fall off
Scabs resolved		Not contagious	

Adapted from Centers for Disease Control and Prevention. ANNEX I: Overview of smallpox, clinical presentations, and medical care of smallpox patients. www.emergency.cdc.gov/agent/smallpox/response-plan/files/annex-1-part1of3.pdf. Accessed October 29, 2014.

(as much as 3–5 L/d in adults). The clinical course can progress to massive hemorrhage, shock, and multiorgan dysfunction. Diagnosis can be made by antigen-capture enzyme-linked immunosorbent assay (ELISA) testing, PCR, or IgM-capture ELISA.

Management. Treatment is supportive, including aggressive intravenous rehydration, replacement of potassium and calcium from gastrointestinal loss, and administration of blood products as needed. An experimental monoclonal antibody (ZMapp, Mapp Pharmaceutical, San Diego, CA) has been used in the 2014 Ebola outbreak, but its effect is not clearly known (39). During outbreaks, disease can spread quickly within a healthcare setting. Healthcare providers and family in close contact with victims are at risk because of the risk of contact with infected blood or body fluids from sick patients. As a result, the care for these patients should include the use of dedicated medical equipment (disposable if possible), proper sterilization of nondisposable equipment, the use of appropriate personal protective equipment, including masks, gloves, gowns, and eye protection, and isolation from other patients. Mortality from viral hemorrhagic fevers has historically ranged from 40% to 90%. However, a case series reporting the successful care of persons who contracted Ebola virus in West Africa but were treated aggressively in the United States with aggressive fluid and electrolyte replacement suggests that the provision of early care is likely associated with a better outcome (17,39).

Terror-Related Toxin-Mediated Disease

Pathophysiology

Botulism is a neuroparalytic illness caused by a toxin produced by the *Clostridium botulinum* bacterium that is found ubiquitously in soil and water. In addition to foodborne botulism, other forms of naturally occurring botulism include infantile botulism and wound botulism. *Inhalational botulism* does not occur naturally, and occurs after botulinum toxin has been intentionally released via aerosolization. Botulinum toxin exerts its effect by inhibiting acetylcholine release, thereby decoupling the nervous system from skeletal muscle, leading to weakness, which results in aspiration, respiratory failure, and death. Recovery from botulism occurs in part by recovery of function in poisoned presynaptic terminals. Axonal sprouting, with creation of new presynaptic terminals, is of equal or greater importance in recovery (40,41).

Clinical Signs and Symptoms

The epidemiology of a botulism terror attack would likely include multiple victims presenting for care between hours to 3 days of exposure. Lack of acetylcholine release at the neuromuscular junction leads to symmetrical cranial neuropathy, progressing to symmetric descending weakness, respiratory failure, and flaccid paralysis. Inhibition of acetylcholine release also occurs at the parasympathetic terminals, leading to autonomic signs and symptoms. Mental status and sensation remain intact.

Management

The mainstays of therapy are supportive care, including bedside pulmonary function testing to assess for the need for mechanical ventilation, and timely treatment with botulinum antitoxin, the only specific treatment for botulism. Antitoxin can arrest the progression of paralysis, but it is best used when given early in the course of illness, because it neutralizes only toxin molecules that are still unbound to nerve endings.

Antitoxin is an equine product and therefore has a risk of serum sickness; skin testing and possible desensitization are necessary. National stockpiles of a heptavalent botulism antitoxin have been purchased by the CDC. Botulism is not transmitted between people, and patients do not need to be isolated once the diagnosis is confirmed; only standard precautions need to be exercised. Complete recovery of muscle function may take as long as 3–6 months. Given the protracted course of the illness, even a small bioterror attack with botulism can consume considerable resources, including the use of mechanical ventilators (42,43).

RADIOLOGIC/NUCLEAR AGENTS

Unfortunately, even many decades after the world witnessed the devastating effects of nuclear attack (Japan, 1945) and those of radiation exposure (Chernobyl, Russia, 1986), the world remains under threat of nuclear and radiologic terrorism. Increased reliance on nuclear energy to decrease dependence on fossil fuels; deterioration of the 20th century's nuclear nonproliferation principles; and the possibility of misuse of a nuclear weapon nation's enriched uranium, weapon-grade plutonium, or nuclear devices by terrorist group, all increase the potential for radiologic/nuclear terrorism. In May of 2010, President Barack Obama of the United States, in a report on security strategy, said "the American people face no greater or more urgent danger than a terrorist attack with a nuclear weapon" (44,45). Radiological terrorism could include detonation of one or more nuclear weapons, deployment of a conventional explosive to deploy radioactive materials (e.g., "dirty bomb"), or, more simply, placement of a radioactive source (e.g., nuclear waste material) in a public location (11). Radiologic and nuclear terrorism have a wide spectrum of possible effects. In addition to damage and contamination in the geographic area involved, widespread panic will occur within the affected areas, which will undoubtedly lead to further injuries, and civic disruption.

A nuclear attack involves fission and immediate morbidity and mortality result from the explosive force of the detonation. Acute radiation syndrome, or "radiation sickness," can occur in the survivors of a nuclear attack. Despite concerns over potential attacks on nuclear power plants, designs of nuclear power reactors in the United States include a layered system of physical safety shields and walls. The primary hazard of such an attack would likely be downwind exposure of radioactive iodine gas, as opposed to a full-blown nuclear event. Nuclear power reactors cannot detonate like a nuclear bomb, because reactor fuel does not contain the highly enriched uranium needed for detonation (11,46).

Decontamination

Unlike some of the chemical and biological scenarios described previously, decontamination of radiologic victims is less time sensitive. Critical and life-threatening conditions should be treated before decontamination occurs. As with chemical exposures, removal of clothing eliminates 90% of contamination. If a patient is exposed to radioactive material and is alive upon arrival to the hospital, it is unlikely that he/she would be sufficiently contaminated to cause harm to healthcare workers. After stabilization of conventional injuries, the patient can be disrobed and washed with soap and water; runoff should be contained, and the discarded clothes should be placed in a double-bag, following hazardous waste guidelines. The eyes may then be flushed. Care should be taken not to irritate or abrade the skin. The patient should be monitored with a radiation meter, and the washings should continue until the radiation survey indicates that the patient's radiation level is no more than twice the background level, or the level remains unchanged. Standard precautions are the only measures required for healthcare workers who do not come into direct contact with radioactive dust or debris (11,47).

Pathophysiology

For both radiological and nuclear victims, a dose- and time-dependent illness occurs at predictable intervals after exposure. Acute radiation syndrome is most likely to occur in those who were exposed to a nuclear detonation but were far enough away not to die from the blast effects. A radiological dispersal device is much less likely to cause acute radiation syndrome. Military, industrial, and medical exposures can also lead to acute radiation syndrome.

On a cellular level, sensitivity to radiation varies according to cell cycle length (i.e., the rate at which a cell replicates and divides). Cells are most vulnerable to radiation during mitosis, when genetic material is most exposed. Cells with active mitoses including spermatogonia, lymphocytes, erythroblasts, other hematopoietic cells, and cells of the gastrointestinal tract are very radiosensitive. Muscle, bone, and collagen-producing cells being less mitotically active are therefore less sensitive to the effects of radiation (48).

Clinical Signs and Symptoms

Victims of radiation exposure with acute radiation syndrome follow a course that is divided into four clinical stages: the prodromal, latent, manifest illness, and recovery stages. In the *prodromal stage of radiation syndrome*, nausea and vomiting predominate, with other nonspecific signs and symptoms, including fever, headache, abdominal cramping, and skin erythema. This stage typically lasts up to 48 hours. In the *latent stage*, the patient experiences apparent clinical improvement, for a period of a few hours or even up to a few weeks. During this stage, the patient's reservoir of pluripotent stem cells is critically depleted. The next stage is the *manifest illness stage*, during which the effects of the loss of stem cells are fully manifested. Patients suffer total loss of their hematopoietic system and so hemorrhage and sepsis are common. Effects on the gastrointestinal system include mucosal sloughing, hemorrhage, obstruction, and sepsis. Radiation pneumonitis can occur and requires aggressive ventilatory support. High doses of radiation can cause microvascular injury of the central nervous system, leading to cerebral edema, increased intracranial pressure, and intractable seizures. The fourth stage is the *recovery stage*, which can last for several weeks to years (48).

Treatment

Removal of external contamination, dose estimation, supportive care (including psychological support of the patient and family), symptomatic treatment, and replacement of fluid and electrolytes should be the goals of early medical management. As patients become neutropenic, the risk of infection increases, and hematopoietic growth factors (granulocyte colony-stimulating factor and granulocyte–macrophage colony-stimulating factor) should be administered (16). The full spectrum of radiation sickness is beyond the scope of this text, but important points to consider include the following:

- Health physicists and/or nuclear medicine physicians will help to determine the specific exposure and prognosis.

- Life-threatening injuries should be treated before decontamination occurs.
- Specific antidotes are unlikely to be helpful in the critical care environment (it is possible that some victims will have been given potassium iodide in an attempt to avoid the carcinogenic effects of radioactive iodine, which could be released in a nuclear power plant incident), but some chelating agents may have efficacy.

While all PICUs should have the ability to treat one or more victims of severe radiation exposure, these patients will require a huge amount of resource, and so surge capacity may be quickly overwhelmed. Expert nuclear medicine and health physicist advice and guidance will be critical in determining which victims are most likely to benefit from critical care interventions and if exposure-specific treatments are available.

CONCLUSIONS AND FUTURE DIRECTIONS

Emergency preparedness remains a high-priority endeavor and a critical necessity for healthcare and governmental institutions. Successful emergency and critical care of CBRN attack victims will require ongoing coordination with federal, state, regional, and municipal agencies. For decades, plans that appropriately and adequately provided for the treatment and management of children lagged behind the developed strategies that addressed adult mass casualty victims. The National Center for Disaster Preparedness, in consensus reports in 2003, 2007, and 2009, highlighted deficiencies in the structure of a response to a CBRN attack that involved children. They identified multiple items that needed immediate attention, including the development of an expert advisory group to maintain and update recommendations on medical countermeasures for pediatric patients to all known and emerging CBRN threats; improved funding of local, regional, and state agencies; and improved coordination between these agencies and the federal government before and after a disaster (49).

On a positive note, since 2009 there have been a number of efforts, including the creation of working groups, task forces, and federal funding initiatives, dedicated to disaster preparedness for children who have addressed many of these issues. Specifically, these efforts have included:

- Establishment of the Children's Health and Human Resources Interagency Leadership on Disasters (CHILD) Working Group (2012), to facilitate identification and comprehensive integration of activities related to the needs of children across all disaster activities and operations (50).
- Creation of the Department of Homeland Security Grant Program for Children in Disasters Guidance (2012), which provides grants to enhance existing or creation of new pediatric-specific planning and preparedness initiatives, including the planning and purchasing of pediatric-specific supplies and the provision of training to a broad range of child-specific provider agencies, including for activities such as evacuation, sheltering, and emergency medical care of children (51).
- Passage of the Pandemic and All-Hazards Preparedness Reauthorization Act (2013), which established the National Advisory Committee on Children and Disasters. The purpose of this committee is to provide expert advice and consultation to the federal government on the comprehensive planning and creation of policies to meet the needs of children before, during, and after a disaster or other public health emergencies (52,53).

References

1. Chilcott RP. CPRN contamination. In: *Textbook of Environmental Medicine*. London, United Kingdom: Hodder Arnold, 2010:475–86.

2. Stone FP. The "worried well" response to CBRN events: Analysis and solutions. Montgomery, AL: USAF Counterproliferation Center, Maxwell Air Force Base, Air University, 2007.

3. Hamele M, Poss WB, Sweeney J. Disaster preparedness: Pediatric considerations in primary, blast injury, chemical, and biological terrorism. *World J Crit Care Med* 2014;3:15–23.

4. U.S. Department of Health & Human Services, Chemical Hazard Emergency Medical Management. Information for hospital providers. chemm.nlm.nih.gov/hospitalproviders.htm. Accessed December 26, 2014.

5. Heon D, Foltin GL. Principles of pediatric decontamination. *Clin Pediatr Emerg Med* 2009;10:186–91.

6. Foltin G, Tunik M, Curran J, et al. Pediatric nerve agent poisoning: Medical and operational considerations for Emergency Medical Services in a large American city. *Pediatr Emerg Care* 2006;22:239–44.

7. U.S. Department of Health & Human Services, Chemical Hazard Emergency Medical Management. Nerve agents—Emergency department/hospital management. chemm.nlm.nih.gov/na_hospital_mmg.htm#top. Accessed January 2, 2015.

8. U.S. Food and Drug Administration. PROTOPAM Chloride (pralidoxime chloride) for injection; September 8, 2010. www.accessdata.fda.gov/drugsatfda_docs/label/2010/014134s022lbl.pdf. Accessed December 29, 2014.

9. Agency for Toxic Substances and Disease Registry. Toxic substances portal: Blister agents: Lewisite and mustard-Lewisite mixture. www.atsdr.cdc.gov/mhmi/mmg163.pdf. Accessed December 28, 2014.

10. Quail MT, Shannon MW. Pralidoxime safety and toxicity in children. *Prehosp Emerg Care* 2007;11:341.

11. Foltin GL, Schonfeld DJ, Shannon MW. *Pediatric Terrorism and Disaster Preparedness: A Resource for Pediatricians*. Elk Grove, IL: American Academy of Pediatrics, 2006. Agency for Healthcare Research and Quality publication no. 06(07)-0056.

12. Agency for Toxic Substances and Disease Registry. Toxic substances portal: Chlorine. www.atsdr.cdc.gov/mhmi/mmg172.pdf. Accessed December 27, 2014.

13. Russell D, Blain PG, Rice P. Clinical management of casualties exposed to lung damaging agents: A critical review. *Emerg Med J* 2006;23:421–4.

14. Anderson DR, Holmes WW, Lee RB. Sulfur mustard-induced neutropenia: Treatment with granulocyte colony-stimulating factor. *Mil Med* 2006;171:448–53.

15. Rice P. Sulphur mustard. *Medicine* 2007;35:578–9.

16. Treleaven JG. The normal bone marrow and management of toxin-induced stem cell failure. In: Marrs TC, Maynard RL, Sidell FR, eds. *Chemical Warfare Agents: Toxicology and Treatment*. 2nd ed. Chichester, United Kingdom: Wiley, 2007:443–66.

17. Centers for Disease Control and Prevention. Bioterrorism agents/diseases. CDC Emergency Preparedness and Response. emergency.cdc.gov/agent/agentlist-category.asp. Accessed October 19, 2014.

18. Centers for Disease Control and Prevention. Anthrax. cdc.gov/anthrax/bioterrorism/threat.html. Accessed October 6, 2014.

19. Bradley J, Peacock G, Krug G, et al. Pediatric anthrax clinical management. *Pediatrics* 2014;133:e1411–e1436.

20. Baldari CT, Tonello F, Paccani SR, et al. Anthrax toxins: A paradigm of bacterial immune suppression. *Trends Immunol* 2006;27:434–40.

21. Bravata DM, Holty JE, Wange E, et al. Inhalational, gastrointestinal, and cutaneous anthrax in children: A systematic review of cases 1900-2005. *Arch Pediatr Adolesc Med* 2007;161:896–905.

22. Holty JE, Bravata DM, Liu H, et al. Systemic review: A century of inhalational anthrax cases from 1900 to 2005. *Ann Intern Med* 2006;144:270–80.

23. Beatty ME, Ashford DA, Griffin PM, et al. Gastrointestinal anthrax: Review of the literature. *Arch Intern Med* 2003;163:2527–31.

24. Sejvar JJ, Tenover FC, Stephens DS. Management of anthrax meningitis. *Lancet Infect Dis* 2005;5:287–95.

25. Centers for Disease Control and Prevention. Plague. cdc.gov/plague. Accessed September 6, 2014.

26. Zasada AA, Formińska K, Zocharczuk K. Fast identification of *Yersinia pestis*, *Bacillus anthracis* and *Francisella tularemis* based on conventional PCR. *Pol J Microbiol* 2013;62:453–5.

27. Committee on Infectious Diseases, American Academy of Pediatrics. In: Pickering LP, ed. *Red Book*. 29th ed. Elk Grove Village, IL: American Academy of Pediatrics, 2012.

28. Pohanka M, Skladal P. *Bacillus anthracis*, *Francisella tularensis* and *Yersinia pestis*: The most important bacterial warfare agents—Review. *Folia Microbiol* 2009;54:263–72.

29. Centers for Disease Control and Prevention. Tularemia. cdc.gov/tularemia. Accessed September 15, 2014.

30. Patt HA, Feigin RD. Diagnosis and management of suspected cases of bioterrorism: A pediatric perspective. *Pediatrics* 2002;109:685–92.

31. Scarfone RJ, Henretig FM, Cieslak TJ, et al. Emergency department recognition and management of victims of biological and chemical terrorism. In: Fleisher G, Ludwig S, eds. *Textbook of Pediatric Emergency Medicine*. 6th ed. Philadelphia, PA: Lippincott Williams & Wilkins, 2010:125–52.

32. Dennis DT, Inglesby TV, Henderson DA, et al. Consensus statement: Tularemia as a biological weapon: Medical and public health management. *JAMA* 2001;285:2763–73.

33. Leggiadro RJ. The threat of biological terrorism: A public health and infection control reality. *Infect Control Hosp Epidemiol* 2000;21:53–6.

34. Centers for Disease Control and Prevention. ANNEX I: Overview of smallpox, clinical presentations, and medical care of smallpox patients. www.emergency.cdc.gov/agent/smallpox/response-plan/files/annex-1-part1of3.pdf. Accessed October 29, 2014.

35. Baker RO, Bray M, Huggins JW. Potential antiviral therapies for smallpox, monkeypox, and other orthopoxvirus infections. *Antiviral Res* 2003;57(1–2):13–23.

36. Buller RM, Owens G, Schriewer J, et al. Efficacy of oral active ether lipid analogs of cidofivir in a lethal mousepox model. *Virology* 2004;318:474–81.

37. Henderson DA, Inglesby TV, Bartlett JG, et al. Smallpox as a biological weapon: Medical and public health management. *JAMA* 1999;281:2127–37.

38. Brennan JG, Henderson DA. Diagnosis and management of smallpox. *N Engl J Med* 2002;346:1300–8.

39. Lyon GM, Mehta AK, Varkey JB, et al. Clinical care of two patients with Ebola virus disease in the United States. *N Engl J Med* 2014;371:2402–9.

40. Erbguth FJ. From poison to remedy: The chequered history of botulinum toxin. *J Neural Transm* 2008;115:559–65.

41. Thompson JA, Glasgow LA, Warpinski JR, et al. Infant botulism: Clinical spectrum and epidemiology. *Pediatrics* 1980;66:936–42.

42. Chang GY, Ganguly G. Early antitoxin treatment in wound botulism results in better outcome. *Eur Neurol* 2003;49:151–3.

43. Sobel J. Botulism. *Clin Infect Dis* 2005;41:1167–73.

44. Jaspal ZN. Nuclear/radiological terrorism: Myth or reality. *J Pol Stud* 2012;19:91–111.

45. Obama B. National security strategy, May 2010. www.whitehouse.gov/sites/default/files/rss_viewer/national_security_strategy.pdf. Accessed December 20, 2014.

46. Behrens C, Holt M. Nuclear power plants: Vulnerability to terrorist attack. Library of Congress, DC: Congressional Research Service, 2005.

47. Centers for Disease Control and Prevention. Radiological terrorism: Emergency pocket guide for clinicians, 2005. emergency.cdc.gov/radiation/pdf/clinicianpocketguide.pdf. Accessed December 1, 2014.

48. Donnelly EH, Nemhauser JB, Smith JM, et al. Acute radiation syndrome: Assessment and management. *South Med J* 2010;103:541–4.

49. Garrett AC, Redlener IE. Pediatric emergency preparedness for natural disasters, terrorism, and public health emergencies: A national consensus conference, 2009 update. http://academiccommons.columbia.edu/catalog/ac:126143. Accessed December 22, 2014.

50. U.S. Department of Health & Human Services. 2011 update on children and diseases: Summary of recommendations and implementation (April 2012). www.phe.gov/Preparedness/planning/abc/Documents/2011-children-disasters.pdf. Accessed December 28, 2014.

51. U.S. Department of Homeland Security. Homeland Severity Grant Program: Children in Disasters Guidance (2012). www.fema.gov/pdf/government/grant/2012/fy_12_hsgp_children.pdf. Accessed December 30, 2014.

52. U.S. Department of Health & Human Services. New committee to advise HHS on needs of children in disasters. January 22, 2014. www.hhs.gov/news/press/2014pres/01/20140122a.html. Accessed January 1, 2015.

53. U.S. Department of Health & Human Services, Office of the Assistant Secretary for Preparedness and Response. Public health emergency: Pandemic and All-Hands Preparedness Reauthorization Act. www.phe.gov/Preparedness/legal/pahpa/Pages/pahpra.aspx. Accessed December 29, 2014.

CHAPTER 34 ■ MASS CASUALTY EVENTS

MARIA CRISTINA ESPERANZA

KEY POINTS

1. Mass casualty events (MCEs) from natural or terrorist-related events affect a significant number of children.
2. Children have unique anatomic, physiologic, developmental, and psychological needs compared with adult victims of MCEs.
3. Pediatric disaster response requires multiagency cooperation.
4. A universal pediatric disaster triage tool needs to be developed, applied, and studied.
5. A significant portion of the healthcare and private community sectors still lack pediatric disaster readiness.
6. All hospitals and physicians, regardless of training, should be prepared to treat pediatric victims of MCEs.
7. Secondary transfer of patients for definitive care is part of the pediatric response. Facilities with PICUs should support neighboring facilities that do not have PICU resources.
8. Awareness of surge plans, equipment, supply availability, and staffing patterns during an MCE is required of all healthcare workers.
9. Pediatric victims of terror-related events utilize more healthcare resources than the general trauma population.
10. Rapid and thorough decontamination of victims exposed to a chemical or radiological event is the single most important facet of treatment.
11. Pediatric victims of MCEs have increased mental health needs after the event.

With the effects of climate change and the presence of political unrest in many areas of the world, there is an increasing number of events with multiple casualties. There were 211 million people affected by natural disasters (1) and 54,000 terrorist-related casualties (2) in 2008. With 74 million children in the United States in 2011 (3,4), the odds of having significant pediatric casualties are high.

The healthcare community has been developing an increasing awareness of the need for disaster preparedness. Mass casualty events (MCEs) are nondiscriminatory. They are not limited by geographic boundaries nor do they target a specific population demographic. During MCEs, the local health systems may be easily overwhelmed, requiring redistribution of casualties and request for external assistance. Collaboration and resource sharing among regional hospitals will provide the most optimal response. Every hospital and healthcare provider should be familiar with the management of victims of MCEs.

Pediatric emergency care expertise and resources are not uniformly accessible even in the United States (5,6). With children accounting for one-third of the victims of MCEs, provisions for children in community, hospital, state, and federal disaster planning should be made. Pediatric intensive care physicians are looked to as a valuable resource in the planning and management of MCEs. An understanding of the status of pediatric emergency preparedness, general principles of disaster medicine and epidemiology, and management of disaster-related injuries is essential. It is impossible to exhaustively cover the breadth of literature on disaster preparedness and terrorism. This chapter will provide the clinician with a framework to understand the public health and clinical management issues surrounding terrorism and disaster preparedness. At the end of this chapter, one will be able to:

- Describe the status of pediatric emergency preparedness
- Discuss the principles of mass casualty medicine as it pertains to planning, triage, and surge capacity
- Describe unique aspects of children with regard to patterns of injury and management
- Describe the presentation, characteristics, and management of different agents of terrorism.

BACKGROUND

An MCE is an incident that results in multiple injuries or deaths and that can have an impact on health care and access to vital services. It affects at least 10 patients, with 3–4 severely wounded patients arriving to the same hospital (7). MCEs can be due to natural or man-made disasters (Table 34.1).

While infrequent, MCEs have the capacity to overwhelm and paralyze healthcare delivery systems. Therapeutic capacities of local healthcare services are exceeded, and external assistance is required. Access may be prevented because the local infrastructure such as roads or hospital buildings may be destroyed. Sustained effects on the community may lead to changes in environmental hazards such as an increased susceptibility to infections or to respiratory diseases (e.g., after the 2001 attack on the World Trade Center [WTC]) (8,9). Events may also cause large population movements (e.g., after Hurricane Katrina). The geographic areas with population surge may not have the resources to handle the healthcare needs of

TABLE 34.1

CAUSES AND EXAMPLES OF DISASTERS AND MASS CASUALTY EVENTS

Nature and weather-related disasters	Earthquakes
	Tornadoes
	Hurricanes
	Flooding
	Tsunamis
Transportation accidents	Airplane crash
	Train derailments/collision
	Multiple car collisions
Civilian disasters	Bridge collapse
	Building collapse
	Fires
Terrorist-related	Bombings
	Chemical disaster
	Radioactive/nuclear disaster
Pandemics	SARS
	Small pox
	Influenza
	Anthrax

SARS, severe acute respiratory syndrome.

the displaced segment of the population and perpetuate the MCE (10).

The nature of the event dictates the scope, type, and severity of injuries. Much of the emergency response to MCEs is directed toward the management of trauma-related injuries. Emergency and critical care providers must also be ready to deal with environmental effects such as hypothermia, heat stroke, electrolyte imbalance, dehydration, infections, and psychological stress. An increase in mental health services is particularly necessary due to the prevalence of psychological stresses on the population (4,10–13). A multidisciplinary team is best equipped to deal with victims of MCEs.

The National Commission on Children and Disasters in its 2010 report to the US President and Congress called for the development of a National Strategy for Children and Disasters. A unified platform for the development of short- and long-term goals, objectives, and capabilities to cohesively address gaps in disaster preparedness, response, and recovery for children is needed. The "at-risk" population designation for pediatrics has not drawn sufficient attention and resources to its needs. Pediatrics has not always been viewed as a separate and distinct stage in growth and requires separate study and planning (14). Modifications to existing plans formulated for the adult population are not enough given the unique needs and vulnerabilities of children. These needs could be predicted and planned for. All disaster management agencies should be required to have distinct and separate plans for pediatrics in their daily and disaster response activities (15) (Table 34.2).

THE STATE OF PEDIATRIC EMERGENCY PREPAREDNESS

MCEs usually consist of 8%–30% of the victims under the age of 17 (16–18). Emergency department (ED) utilization rates are high, ranging from 61% to 97% of victims, and admission rates are also higher than normal at 13%–58% (19).

It is well recognized that pediatric healthcare delivery is uneven. Knowledge, logistical, and infrastructure support is highly variable. This problem extends to the state of pediatric emergency preparedness. MCEs require a high level of coordination among prehospital and hospital personnel, and local, regional, state, and federal agencies. Any weakness in planning and execution at any level severely affects the disaster response. The National Commission on Children and Disasters

TABLE 34.2

PEDIATRIC-SPECIFIC VULNERABILITIES DURING MASS CASUALTY EVENTS

Increased susceptibility to effects of exposure to terrorism-related agents	Increased respiratory exposure	■ Higher minute ventilation ■ Located closer to the ground
	Increased dermal exposure	■ Thinner, more permeable skin, less fat ■ Larger BSA/mass ratio
	More virulent disease manifestations from infectious agents	■ Immature immune system
	Less capable of escaping attack and taking appropriate protective actions	■ Motor and cognitive immaturity ■ Dependence on caregivers
More susceptible to development of secondary medical problems	Increased risk of dehydration due to toxin-induced vomiting and diarrhea	■ Decreased intravascular volume, larger BSA/mass ratio ■ May be dependent on caregivers for access to fluids
	Increased risk of hypothermia	■ Larger BSA/mass ratio ■ Immature temperature regulation in infants
	Increased incidence of multiple organ injury	■ Thoracic cage less developed ■ Small size with more force applied per unit body area ■ Less fat protecting internal organs
	Increased incidence of head injury	■ Larger head-to-body ratio ■ Thinner calvarium
	Increased fractures	■ Incomplete ossification of skeletal system ■ Smaller body mass
	Increased mental health needs	■ Separation from primary caregiver, need for reunification ■ Developmental immaturity

Adapted from Henretig FM, Ciesiak TJ, Eitzen EM Jr. Biologic and chemical terrorism. *J Pediatr* 2002;141:311–26.

recognizes the gaps in knowledge, training, and access to health care in their 2010 report (15).

5 State and regional emergency preparedness plans are crucial in MCE events because local conditions will delay federal and neighboring state responses to the event. In 1997, the Federal Emergency Management Agency (FEMA) showed that no state had pediatric-specific plans for disaster response (20). In 2002, most states (94%) reported the presence of a statewide disaster plan, but only half were tested by activation and only one-third of the plans contained a bioterrorism component. A minority of states, 10%, required disaster training of medical professionals (21). A decade later, only 17 states have plans for four key components of the pediatric disaster response: evacuation/relocation, family and child reunification, children with special needs, and a K-12 multiple disaster plan. Five states have not met any of the standards (22).

Prehospital provider preparedness in pediatric MCEs is still uncertain. Prehospital providers receive limited disaster, MCE (23), and pediatric training (24). As children make up very few ambulance calls, prehospital providers have very little practical experience in general pediatrics let alone pediatric MCE events. Participation in disaster drills can fill this gap; however, only half of the drills included pediatric victims (25). While most (72%) prehospital EMS agencies have a written disaster plan, only 13% had a pediatric-specific plan. Only 19% utilize pediatric triage protocols, and the majority do not address MCEs at schools, or have accommodations for people with special healthcare needs (25). Availability of pediatric equipment on ambulances is also poor as shown by several studies (24,26).

There is marked variability in hospitals' pediatric capabilities. Outcomes for pediatrics are tied to availability of pediatric trained personnel, dedicated pediatric services and presence of pediatric-specific equipment (27). Most hospitals have low pediatric volumes, with about 50% having less than 4000 ED visits per year. While 60% of EDs have pediatric attending coverage, only 23% utilize pediatric emergency medicine physicians. Less than 15% of hospitals have a PICU or pediatric trauma service, opting instead to transfer patients requiring specialized care. Availability of equipment is also a concern, with only 5% of EDs having all recommended pediatric supplies, and most have 80% of the list (28). The availability of interfacility transport to tertiary children's hospitals allows most children relatively easy access to specialized pediatric **6** services. However, in an MCE, all hospitals must prepare to **7** receive and stabilize critically injured children before a secondary interfacility transport for definitive care. Less critically ill children may need to be admitted and treated at a non-children's hospital. Those hospitals will need to provide a level of care beyond what they would normally provide (27). To highlight these shortcomings, only 13% of hospitals have a pediatric mass casualty protocol, and only 64% participate in disaster drills with pediatric patients (29).

PEDIATRIC DISASTER TRIAGE

Triage is a system by which treatment is rendered by prioritization according to clinical need as patient volume outstrips the available resources (30). The finite amount of resources dictates that care is provided to patients with survivable injuries. Casualties with very severe injuries should be provided expectant management and not be transferred for definitive care.

8 As many individuals perform triage, variability can negatively impact patient outcomes and resource utilization. A high rate of undertriage (underestimation of the severity of injuries) will lead to missed injuries and avoidable deaths. Hence, MCE response favors the overtriage (overestimation of the severity of injuries) of patients in order not to miss potentially salvageable patients. However, the rate of overtriage positively

correlates with worse outcomes (31). When overtriage rates are high, hospitals will be flooded with patients that could have received delayed care. The high influx of patients lowers the hospital's surge capacity (32). Acceptable undertriage and overtriage rates by the American College of Surgeons are 5%–10% and 30%–50%, respectively (33).

An attempt at standardization has been made through the introduction and use of triage tools and algorithms. A triage tool must be quick and simple to use. Different prehospital providers use different triage algorithms in their protocols. The Simple Treatment and Rapid Transport (START) protocol is most commonly used in the United States, and includes an assessment of mobility, the frequency of respirations, the presence of a palpable pulse, and the ability to follow commands. Patients are classified into four categories on the basis of their needs for advanced care: deceased or expected to die from incident (black); immediate (red); delayed (yellow); or ambulatory (green).

There is no evidence to support the use of one triage tool over another (30,34). Existing triage algorithms have not been validated and have unknown rates of interobserver and intraobserver reliability. Applicability in events with biological, chemical, or radiological toxins is also questionable. Most of the tools are static and assess patient status without regard for available resources. As the MCE event unfolds, patients who earlier may have been eligible for certain interventions, may not be able to receive them due to exhaustion of resources. The Sacco triage method (a computer mathematical model) orders patients on the basis of their probability of survival, potential for deterioration, and available resources (35). When applied to pediatric data in the National Trauma Database, it showed high reliability in predicting mortality (36). Shortcomings, however, include that the method has not been field-tested and requires software support, data entry, communication lines to an incident command center, and data on resource availability.

Clinical reevaluation of patients for improvement or deterioration is not built into most triage tools. The performance of secondary triage in the field through the Secondary Assessment of Victim Endpoint (SAVE) methodology establishes the order with which patients receive care at the hospital, or in the setting of delayed transport, at the scene. It is most effective in MCEs where transport to definitive care cannot be carried out and **4** treatment continues under less than ideal conditions (35,37).

Modifications to triage tools were necessary to account for acceptable vital sign ranges in pediatrics. If used in an unmodified form, the age-dependent normal physiologic variables in children will result in an artificially high triage priority leading to overtriage. Pediatric-specific triage tools such as Jump-START (for 1–8 years of age) and Pediatric Triage Tape (PTT) are modifications to adult triage tools. The Care Flight triage tool uses qualitative observations and requires no vital sign measurements rendering it amenable to pediatric use (38). None of the tools mentioned have been field-tested. Comparing all three tools, Wallis and Carley (34) showed similarly poor sensitivity rates at detecting critically ill children. Further study is needed to arrive at a universally accepted, validated pediatric triage tool.

HOSPITAL RESPONSE TO MASS CASUALTY EVENTS

8 Each MCE is unique due to the interplay of factors, which include the nature of the precipitating event; location, date, and time of event; weather patterns; and population density. The type and magnitude of response are equally affected by these variables. It is impossible to make disaster plans tailored to every MCE. Disaster response must be made with an all-hazards approach. This will address the aspects of response that is common to all types of MCEs (e.g., evacuation plans, allocation of supplies and personnel, etc.).

Surge Response

MCEs can be thought of as either "big bang" events that occur suddenly (e.g., earthquakes, transport accidents, or terrorist bombing) or "rising tide" events that develop slowly (e.g., pandemics or flooding). In the latter, the precipitating event may not be apparent, but with monitoring for unusual clusters of symptoms or syndromic surveillance, a pattern of disease emerges (30). In "big bang" MCEs, almost all casualties are created at the time of the event and the number remains relatively constant. In rising tide events, the number of patients gradually increases at an unknown rate, the duration of the MCE is unknown, and resources may exhaust due to the protracted course of the disease. Big bang events have greater capacity to immediately paralyze health systems. As such, disaster planning is made with this type of scenario in mind.

After the MCE, patients arrive at emergency facilities in three phases. A sudden influx of patients (50% within the first hour) is seen, many of whom self-triage and have minor injuries (39). They usually need little intervention but may require observation for the development of complications. The second wave consists of more critically injured patients. They may arrive as early as 15 minutes after the beginning of the event (19,40). Eighty percent of all casualties arrive within 90 minutes of the event. The final phase, which may last for days, consists of patients with minor injuries and emotional stress (**Fig. 34.1**).

After arrival and treatment in the ED, one-way flow of patients must occur during the MCE response. Patient should move forward through the system and not have any opportunity to backtrack. Once patients are evaluated and stabilized in the ED, they must move toward the operating room (OR) or the ICU. Patients that go to radiology must also move to the OR or the ICU on the basis of the study findings. A seamless flow of patient movement can help optimize outcomes as indicated by a low critical mortality rate (40).

Pediatric victims from MCEs have a high overtriage rate, with 4% requiring ICU admission (41). Children presenting with multiple injuries require more surgical interventions and have longer hospital stays (42). The majority (75%) receive mechanical ventilation. The high acuity of admitted survivors makes PICU surge capacity an integral part of any MCE response.

Soon after receiving ED notification of the event, the PICU should plan for an anticipated 300% increase in critical care bed capacity (43). Satellite critical care units may be established in the following areas in descending order of preference: postanesthesia care units, intermediate care units, large procedure suites, telemetry units, and hospital floors (44). While the use of the ED may be considered as a satellite critical care area, the incident command center should consider the likelihood of continued influx into the ED of MCE casualties. Hospitals in certain geographic regions may be required to increase critical care surge capacity above the suggested 300%. These areas will be at high risk for mass critical care events, may have inadequate ICU beds for their catchment area at baseline, or are too remote from any ICU. Interfacility transfers and sharing of healthcare systems resource are necessary to surge pediatric care regionally (17,27,45,46).

The amount of supplies and equipment must last for at least 10 days at the 300% capacity (47). Emphasis is on procuring the following resources: all supplies for mechanical ventilation, intravenous fluids, vasopressors, antidotes and antimicrobials, and sedatives and analgesics (45).

Maintenance of normal staffing patterns will be difficult. Hospital personnel and their families may be affected by the event. Staff may be reluctant to report to work during a radiologic, infectious, or chemical-related event (48). Recent protocols have considered increasing stockpiles of antidotes and antimicrobials to cover hospital personnel and their family members to address this concern (49). In the event of limited personnel, altered staffing patterns may have to be adopted. The most experienced clinicians should take patient assignments, and these should be based on experience and staff abilities. Certain staff responsibilities may have to be delegated to other healthcare providers. To minimize risk to patients, existing policies and procedure should be followed to minimize variability and iatrogenic complications (44).

Alternate Levels of Care and Allocation of Scarce Resources

Every attempt should be made to maintain existing standards of care in the face of an MCE. Acquisition of supply of scarce resources is recommended. Transfer of patients to other healthcare facilities to decrease the caseload must also be undertaken. However, when these attempts are exhausted, alternative allocation of resources and standards of care may be performed (44). With alteration of standards of care to quadruple ICU and non-ICU capacity, mortality may drop by 24% (50). Stepwise changes in resource utilization are recommended until reallocation is the only feasible option (**Fig. 34.2**). Explicit policies and procedures should detail how hospitals will proceed in changing standards of care (45). These modifications should be appropriate for different surge requirements. The authority to alter standards for health care during mass critical care should be made by local or state emergency management systems (27,45).

Children with Special Needs and the Technology-Dependent Child

As disaster risk is distributed to reflect preexisting inequalities, children with disabilities have an increased risk of poor outcome (51). They lack access to economic and social resources,

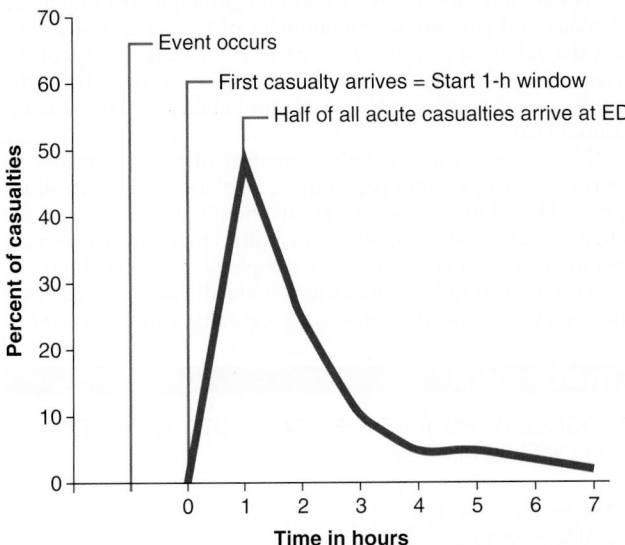

FIGURE 34.1. Timeline for arrival of victims of an MCE at emergency facilities. (From Centers for Disease Control and Prevention. *Mass Casualties Predictor*. Department of Health and Human Services, Centers for Disease Control and Prevention, 2003.)

Little clinical impact   Major clinical impact

Minimal patient need/   Overwhelming patient need/
resource balance   resource balance

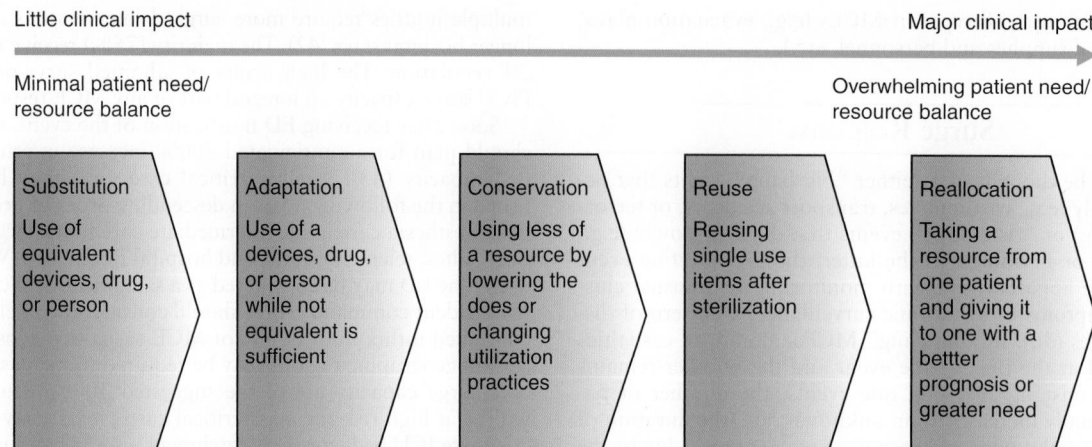

Substitution

Use of equivalent devices, drug, or person

Adaptation

Use of a devices, drug, or person while not equivalent is sufficient

Conservation

Using less of a resource by lowering the does or changing utilization practices

Reuse

Reusing single use items after sterilization

Reallocation

Taking a resource from one patient and giving it to one with a bettter prognosis or greater need

FIGURE 34.2. Stepwise approach to altered resource utilization and standard of care. (Adapted from Christian MD, Deveraux AV, Dichter JR, et al. Definitive care for the critically ill during a disaster: Current capabilities and limitations from a Task Force for Mass Critical Care Summit meeting, January 26–27, 2007, Chicago, IL. *Chest* 2008;133(5 suppl):8S–17S.)

have limited autonomy, and restricted social capital (52). There are 2.8 million children (5.2% of all school-aged children) in the United States and 200 million worldwide that have disabilities (US census bureau) (52), and represent a significant at-risk population. The majority of children with disabilities have cognitive difficulties. A medical needs approach to emergency preparedness is insufficient; a functional-needs approach helps define the extent of support these individuals require in the areas of medical health, communication, functional independence, supervision, and transportation (53) (**Table 34.3**).

The FEMA has worked on addressing the deficiencies in planning for this population. In seven of its recent emergency preparedness plans issues of integration, inclusion and accessibility were addressed. FEMA also provides support to the individual state's efforts to increase preparedness for individuals with disabilities (54).

Children with disabilities will often present to the hospital due to a failure in medical planning. Loss of electricity and consumption of resources such as medications, formula, or oxygen will require these patients to present to a hospital.

TABLE 34.3

⑪ VULNERABILITIES OF CHILDREN WITH SPECIAL NEEDS

Medical	Exacerbation of preexisting diseases
	Supplies, equipment, special formula, and medication lost or consumed and not replenished
	Lack of access to healthcare services
Infrastructure	Less likely to evacuate
	Power outage affects patients on medical equipment
	Access to shelters more difficult for patients with disabilities
	Shelter setup not conducive to needs of patients
Psychological	Dependence on parents and primary caregivers
	May exhibit an increase in separation anxiety, aggressive and oppositional behavior
	At higher risk for PTSD

Hospitals should consider creation and staffing of an area where these patients may be cared for until their home healthcare supplies are replenished.

BOMBINGS AND BLAST INJURIES

Background

Even with increasing concern for the use of guns and biological, chemical, or radioactive weapons of mass destruction, the use of explosives remains the most common cause of mass casualty incidents. Urban explosions have the potential to have far reaching effects. In addition to casualties from the immediate area, first responders and onlookers may be wiped out by a subsequent blast, fire, or building collapse. This was illustrated by the WTC bombings in 2001, the US Marine barracks bombings in Beirut in 1982, and the maritime explosions in Texas City, Texas (1947) and Halifax, Nova Scotia (1917). Terrorists have used this "second-hit principle" to maximize damage and casualties. Containment of the scene and ensuring the safety of responders is part of on-scene management. Protection of medical assets by keeping them away from the explosion and areas with a high probability of attack is essential (55).

Blast injuries can present in a number of patterns, including burns, as well as blunt, penetrating, inhalational, and crush injuries. The relationships between the bomb, the victim, and the environment produce multisystem injuries that render pre-event planning and management more complex (55) (**Table 34.4**).

Different bombing incidents showed common patterns of injury and death (immediate casualty rates 5%–68%).

TABLE 34.4

PROGNOSTIC FACTORS AFFECTING OUTCOME AFTER TERRORIST BOMBINGS

Magnitude of explosion
Building collapse
Triage accuracy
Time interval to treatment
Urban vs. isolated setting
Indoor vs. open-air location

Incidents with structural collapse, such as the WTC, Oklahoma City Murrah Federal Building, and Argentine Israeli Mutual Association building, are associated with higher immediate mortality rates (87% to >99%) (31,55).

Most survivors have noncritical injuries (31,55). Soft tissue and bone injuries predominate, and these may receive delayed care. Critically injured patients, those with an injury severity score (ISS) >16, comprise 8%–34% of survivors. Critical mortality rate (number of mortalities per number of critically injured survivors) is 12%–37% (55).

Multisystem injury is common in the immediate period. Head injuries are most common followed by pulmonary, abdominal, and chest injuries. The mortality rate associated with head injury is low as most are noncritical. In contrast, a greater proportion of casualties with chest and abdominal injuries or traumatic amputations die. These injuries can be a marker of severity of injury, and their presence should prompt aggressive care (55).

Two studies from Israel and from the Oklahoma City bombing described patterns of injury in children associated with these bombing incidents. Pediatric MCE trauma victims are more severely injured than the typical pediatric trauma population as evidenced by more torso, head, extremity, and penetrating injuries and a higher proportion with ISSs >25 (17). They also require more operative interventions, ICU admissions, and longer hospital stays. Pediatric organ-specific mortality rates for chest and abdominal injuries are similar to those described for adults (56). However, the organ-specific mortality rate for head injuries is higher. Head injuries are more prevalent in children 1–3 years of age. The practice of suicide bombers to wear torso-level explosive belts may explain this observation (56,57).

Pediatric survivors appear to be less debilitated than adults, with fewer discharges to rehabilitation centers. Compared with non-MCE pediatric trauma victims, children from MCEs are more debilitated at discharge, with higher rehabilitation center admission rates (17% vs. 1%).

Mechanisms, Manifestations, and Management of Blast Injuries

Bomb blasts involve the rapid transformation of a combustible liquid or solid into a gas. The explosion generates a blast wave, a shock wave of high pressure, which travels at the speed of sound away from the detonation center. As the wave travels, it rapidly loses pressure and velocity. It may be reflected off solid surfaces (multiplying 8–9 times) and lead to greater injury. The magnitude and duration of the blast wave is dependent on the type of explosive and the medium, air or water, through which it travels. As the blast wave displaces surrounding air, it generates wind of significant velocity, blast wind, which propels individuals and bomb fragments, causing additional injury. The effect is also worsened by the low pressure (negative pressure phase) that moves through a space caused by void of the displaced air (58–61) (Fig. 34.3).

The interaction between the bomb, the victim, and the surrounding environment will produce different mechanisms and patterns of injury. Explosion-related injuries are classified into four categories according to the mechanism: primary, secondary, tertiary, or quaternary. *Primary blast injuries* are due to barotrauma from the blast wave, and are most severe when they occur in confined space bombings. As the blast wave enters the body, it creates stress, shock, and shear waves. Stress waves are longitudinal pressure forces that create a spalling effect (breaking into small pieces) at air–fluid interfaces causing microvascular damage and tissue disruption. Gas-filled organs such as the middle ear, lung, and gastrointestinal tract are most commonly affected. Shear waves are transverse waves

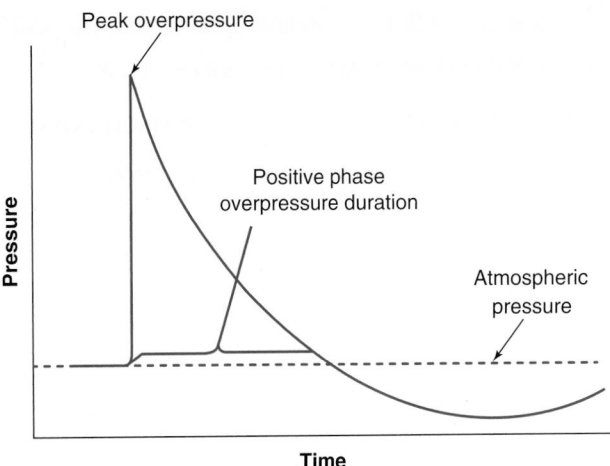

FIGURE 34.3. Idealized blast overpressure waveform. (From Ritenour AE, Baskin TW. Primary blast injury: Update on diagnosis and treatment. *Crit Care Med* 2008;36(7):S311–S317.)

that cause asynchronous movement of tissue and possible tissue disruption and traumatic amputation (58,59).

Secondary blast injuries are caused by projectile particles from the explosive device and from the effect of the explosion on surrounding materials. Highest rates of secondary blast injuries occur in open-air bombings. Victims typically present with penetrating soft tissue injuries. These injuries are the leading cause of death and injury in terrorist attacks (19).

Tertiary blast injuries are caused by the blast wind. Victims may be thrown against fixed objects, resulting in fractures, intracranial injuries, and other solid organ injuries. Different body parts may also undergo acceleration causing amputation.

The effect of the explosion on surrounding building structures and vehicles can cause building collapse and fires, resulting in *quaternary blast injuries*. Few victims survive such incidents. Timely extraction and initiation of therapy is not always possible when dealing with a building collapse or fire. Fatality rates can double when victims are trapped for more than 24 hours even if they reach the hospital alive (62). Survivors may present with burns, fractures, compartment syndrome, inhalational, head, and crush injuries. Late complications such as acute respiratory distress syndrome (ARDS), acute kidney injury, effects of chemical and radiation exposure, and exacerbation of preexisting conditions may be present (**Table 34.5**).

Aural Injuries

Of the primary blast injuries, rupture or perforation of the tympanic membrane (TM) is most common. Patients may present with deafness, tinnitus, or vertigo. Under sufficiently high pressures, the ossicles of the middle ear can be dislocated. The traumatic disruption of the oval or round window may lead to permanent hearing loss. Evaluation for ruptured TM was previously used as a screening tool to identify patients at risk for the development of other primary blast injuries. In the absence of middle ear injury, other primary blast injuries are less likely although not entirely impossible (61). Different case series have reported anywhere from 10% to 50% of patients with primary blast injuries with no middle ear findings (63–65). Leibovici et al. (66) found that patients with isolated TM rupture did not develop symptoms of late onset blast injury. Hence, in the absence of other symptoms of organ dysfunction, the finding of a ruptured TM is a poor biomarker for severity of blast injury, and clinicians are discouraged from using otoscopic examination as a screening tool.

TABLE 34.5

INJURY DETERMINANTS AND EFFECTS IN EXPLOSION

■ DETERMINANT		■ MECHANISM	■ EFFECT	■ CATEGORY
Bomb	Magnitude and type of blast	Barotrauma	■ Pulmonary blast injury—pulmonary contusion, pneumothorax, pneumomediastinum, subcutaneous emphysema, blast lung syndrome, air embolism ■ Auditory blast injury—hearing loss, ruptured TM, ossicle injury, vertigo ■ Abdominal blast injury—ruptured viscus, solid organ injury, subserosal hemorrhage ■ CNS blast injury—brain and SCI ■ Traumatic amputations	Primary
		Primary shrapnel from bomb contents or casing	Penetrating injuries	Secondary
		Blast wind accelerates victims against fixed objects	Blunt deceleration injuries	Tertiary
		Blast wind differentially accelerates exposed body parts	Traumatic amputations	Primary Tertiary
		Blast heat	Flash burns on exposed skin	Quaternary
Environment	Space in which blast wave occurs	Amplitude of reflected blast waves increases in smaller confined spaces	Primary blast injuries increase in confined space	Primary
		Duration of exposure to blast overpressure increases in smaller confined spaces	Pulmonary blast injury increases disproportionately in smaller confined space	Primary
		Duration of exposure to blast heat increases in smaller confined space	Percentage of BSA affected by flash burns increases	Quaternary
	Material upon which blast wave acts	Secondary shrapnel from environmental destruction	Penetrating injuries from glass, wood, structural material	Secondary
	Environmental effects of the blast	Structural collapse	Blunt injuries, compartment syndrome, inhalation injury, hypothermia	Quaternary
		Fire	Thermal burns, inhalational injury	Quaternary
Victim	Distance from detonation point	Blast wave and heat exponentially decays with distance	■ Primary blast injuries, traumatic amputations, blast burns occur near detonation point ■ Penetrating injuries occur farthest away from detonation point ■ Injury severity decreases with distance from detonation point	
	Protective barriers	Clothing, shoes, protect from minor blast effects	■ Minor penetrating injuries and flash burns affect exposed body areas	

Arnold JL, Tsai M, Halpern P, et al. Mass-casualty, terrorist bombings: Epidemiological outcomes, resource utilization, and time course of emergency needs (Part I). *Prehosp Disaster Med* 2003;18(3):220.

Treatment is expectant as small perforations heal in several weeks. Ototopical antibiotics may be used, and avoidance of probing or irrigation of the auditory canal is recommended. Tympanoplasty may be required if healing does not occur and survivors should receive audiologic screening.

Blast Lung Injury

Pulmonary injuries typically are life threatening and are the most common critical injury. The pressure differential across the alveolar–capillary barrier causes disruption of alveolar septa and capillaries, leading to acute pulmonary hemorrhage, pulmonary edema, and hypoxic respiratory failure. Pneumothorax, hemothorax, pneumomediastinum, and subcutaneous emphysema have also been described. Acute gas embolism from pulmonary disruption can cause sudden death (58,61).

Cellular changes include activation of endothelial cells and macrophages with the recruitment of neutrophils and other immune responses. Reactive oxygen species, superoxide (O_2^-), peroxide (H_2O_2), and hydroxyl (OH) radicals, and reactive nitrogen species, nitric oxide (NO) and peroxynitrite (ONOO⁻), alter biological membrane function and lead to the development of acute lung injury (ALI) or ARDS (67). Animal models of blast overpressure have shown an increase in markers of inflammatory cell activation and formation of reactive oxygen and nitrogen species during the first 24–48 hours. Levels subside 5 days after the injury and may be secondary to effects of antioxidant enzymes such as manganese-containing superoxide dismutase and heme-oxygenase-1 (67).

Diagnosis of blast lung injury should be suspected in patients presenting with apnea, bradycardia, or hypotension. Patients may also be dyspneic or hypoxemic. Chest x-ray shows the characteristic butterfly or batwing infiltrates (**Fig. 34.4**) caused by reflection of the blast wave off the mediastinal structures. X-ray findings may appear as early as 90 minutes or as late as 48 hours after the blast (61). Physical examination may reveal diminished breath sounds and crepitus.

Patients require ICU admission and close monitoring. FiO₂ of 1.0 should be administered and avoidance of positive-pressure ventilation if possible is recommended. In the setting of severe pulmonary hemorrhage and hypoxemia, endotracheal intubation and mechanical ventilation are necessary. The use of lung protective strategies such as pressure-limited, volume-controlled ventilation with permissive hypercapnia is recommended. The use of high-frequency oscillatory ventilation, high-frequency jet ventilation, nitric oxide, and extracorporeal membrane oxygenation may also be considered (68). Patients are at high risk for developing pneumothoraces and the index of suspicion should remain high. Early detection and prompt tube thoracostomy is necessary. Prophylactic tube thoracostomy may be considered prior to aeromedical transport. Providers must be cautious with intravenous fluid administration and avoid worsening pulmonary edema by causing a fluid overload state. There is no evidence suggesting the routine use of corticosteroids or antibiotics for blast lung injury (58). With meticulous critical care, survival rates of 88% have been reported (69).

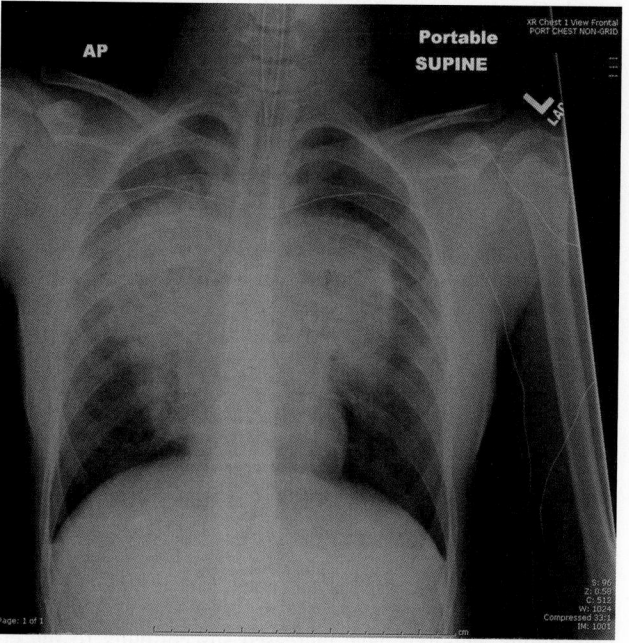

FIGURE 34.4. Pediatric blast lung injury with typical butterfly pattern. (From Ratto J, Johnson BK, Condra CS, et al. Pediatric blast lung injury from a fireworks-related explosion. *Pediatr Emerg Care* 2012;28(6):573–6.)

Gastrointestinal Blast Injury

Gastrointestinal (GI) blast injuries are rare with an incidence of 0.3%–0.6% among survivors. The rapid compression and expansion of air in gas-filled organs result in contusions, intramural hemorrhage, and perforation. Tearing of mesenteric vessels leading to mesenteric ischemia or infarction presents later. Given sufficient force from tertiary blast injury, rupture of solid organs (liver, spleen, or kidney) with resulting hemorrhage can occur (59). Pancreatic rupture is uncommon.

Manifestations of GI injuries are usually delayed, presenting 8–36 hours postevent. Signs and symptoms include abdominal pain, nausea, vomiting, hematemesis, melena and rebound tenderness or abdominal rigidity. Hemodynamic instability may be seen with mesenteric vessel and solid organ injury. Pneumoperitoneum, free fluid, and a sentinel clot adjacent to bowel wall or mesentery may be seen on abdominal CT scan. Pneumoperitoneum is a nonspecific sign and is associated with bowel perforation in only 44% of patients (70).

Treatment is supportive. Hemodynamically stable patients should receive bowel rest with nasogastric tube decompression. Patient deterioration requires an exploratory laparotomy to control possible hemorrhage and GI contamination of the peritoneal cavity (59).

Cardiovascular Effects of Blast injury

Cardiac contusion and air embolization to the coronary arteries may occur from blast wave and blast wind. Animal studies have demonstrated a triad of bradycardia, apnea, and hypotension thought to be mediated by vagal stimulation (71,72). Hemodynamic measurements reveal a low cardiac index and stroke volume with normal systemic vascular resistance (72). Apnea occurs immediately, is short-lived, and is followed by tachypnea with a gradual return to baseline. Bradycardia has a rapid onset, is severe, and is typically protracted in humans (71). Blast survivors may lose the ability to mount a tachycardic response to hemorrhage. Knowledge of these patterns of physiologic response may be useful when victims are not responding to standard resuscitation efforts. The use of atropine may be considered for blast-induced bradycardia (59).

Traumatic Amputations

The presence of a traumatic amputation is an indicator of the severity of the blast wave (31). A search for occult injuries should be carefully made, given the high correlation of a traumatic amputation with coexisting central nervous system (CNS), chest, or abdominal injury. The transmission of energy through the extremities causes fracture through the shaft rather than the joint. Flailing of the extremity from blast wind completes the amputation (61). Soft tissue damage from the primary blast is minimal and confined to the area of amputation. Secondary and tertiary soft tissue injury results from shrapnel and debris from structural collapse. Open wounds, lacerations, and crush injuries should be managed using general trauma principles. Wounds should be irrigated, debrided, and left for delayed primary closure. Serial assessment of vascular integrity should be performed as victims are at high risk for the development of delayed vascular occlusion (59,73).

Neurologic Injuries

Previously thought to be due to secondary and tertiary blast injuries, there is now evidence that primary blast injury from the blast wave can lead to neurologic injury. Fractures around sinuses, air embolism in cerebral vessels, cerebral contusion, and intracranial hemorrhage have all been described. Shearing and diffuse axonal injury with activation of inflammatory mechanisms produce immediate and delayed symptoms including posttraumatic stress disorder (PTSD) and memory impairment (59). EEG testing has shown a variety of disorders, including hypersynchronous, discontinuous, or irregular activity with theta activity consistent with cortical dysfunction (61).

Immediate management should center on identification of life-threatening conditions such as intracranial hemorrhage, the presence of a foreign body in the brain or a spinal cord injury (SCI). Neurosurgical intervention is almost always necessary and general principles of traumatic brain injury (TBI) and SCI management should be followed.

As seen in adult patients, pediatric survivors with head injury are at increased risk for CNS dysfunction. Children are more likely to demonstrate persistent functional deficits in neuropsychological, behavioral, adaptive, and academic outcomes (74,75). These may present as a mood disorder, impaired memory and poor concentration, and academic performance. However, improvements over time in neuropsychological, adaptive, and academic outcomes have been demonstrated (74). All patients should be referred for psychologic evaluation and cognitive testing. Families should be forewarned that symptoms may develop over time and that counseling and treatment will be necessary (**Table 34.6**).

Patient Risk Stratification

Whenever possible, gathering a focused history is a helpful tool to assess patient risk for severe injury. Key components include (a) the type of explosive device; (b) geography of the detonation site; (c) victim details such as distance from the detonation center, surrounding structures, and personal protective equipment (PPE); and (d) status of other casualties. If no history is

TABLE 34.6

OVERVIEW OF EXPLOSIVE-RELATED INJURIES

■ SYSTEM	■ INJURY OR CONDITION
Auditory	TM rupture, ossicular disruption, cochlear damage, foreign body
Eye, orbit, face	Perforated globe, hyphema, foreign body, air embolism, fractures
Respiratory	Blast lung, hemothorax, pneumothorax, pulmonary contusion and/or hemorrhage, AV fistulas, airway epithelial damage, aspiration, pneumonitis, sepsis
Gastrointestinal	Bowel perforation, hemorrhage, liver/spleen/kidney rupture, mesenteric ischemia from air embolism
Cardiovascular	Cardiac contusion, coronary air embolism with myocardial infarction, shock, vasovagal hypotension, peripheral vascular injury
Neurological	Concussion, open and closed brain injury, stroke, SCI, air embolism–induced injury
Renal injury	Renal contusion, laceration acute renal failure from rhabdomyolysis, hypotension, hypovolemia
Extremity injury	Traumatic amputation, fractures, crush injuries, compartment syndrome, burns, lacerations, vascular injury, air embolism–induced injury

AV, arteriovenous.
From National Center for Injury Prevention and Control. http://www.bt.cdc.gov/masscasualties/explosions.asp. Accessed June 28, 2013.

obtained, assessment for injuries that have a high correlation with increased rates of blast injuries such as burns or traumatic amputations can assist in patient risk stratification.

SCHOOL MASS SHOOTINGS

The public and healthcare communities have a heightened awareness of schools shootings as a source of pediatric MCE victims. The scope of the problem is difficult to establish because of a lack of a universal definition and of a central repository for information. The Congressional Research Service (CRS) has defined public mass shooting as an incident occurring in a public place involving four or more deaths (excluding the gunman) with indiscriminate victim selection (76). The violence in these cases is not a means to an end such as robbery or terrorism.

The CRS has identified 78 public mass shootings in the United States since 1983. There have been 547 deaths and 476 injured victims. Since the 9/11 attacks, the CRS estimates that 281 people have died from 38 public mass shootings (76). High-profile cases including the Columbine, Virginia Tech, and Sandy Hook shootings have drawn attention to public mass shootings at academic institutions. It is estimated that 15% of public mass shootings occur in academic institutions (67% occur at primary or secondary schools) (**Table 34.7**).

Emergency preparedness by schools and other childcare facilities is a priority as recognized by the National Commission on Children and Disasters (15). Schools and other childcare facilities receive federal support on funding, training and operations for emergency preparedness, and pediatric disaster mental and behavioral health. While many schools have disaster plans, a significant number do not address children with special healthcare needs or postdisaster counseling (77,78).

Little information is available on the nature of injuries and patient outcomes from school mass shootings or gun-related MCEs. In a review of terror-related mortalities in Israel, Shapira et al. (79) showed high immediate mortality rates (77%) for shooting events. Of the survivors, 17% die within 24 hours of the event, three times higher than for bombing casualties with similar severity of injury and thought to be due to delayed evacuation. While 60% of bombing victims are at the hospital within 30 minutes, only 22% of shooting victims arrive during that time frame. At the end of the first hour, 87% versus 78% have arrived, respectively.

MCE-related shooting patients had higher mortality (2.75 times) than for non-MCE shooting casualties (80). Operative mortality was higher in MCE patients implying a difference in the standard of care between the two events. Both of these studies highlight the fact that outcomes in MCEs may be more affected by patterns of healthcare delivery rather than by the mechanism of injury.

CHEMICAL AND RADIOLOGIC MASS CASUALTY EVENTS

Children may be exposed to chemical and radiologic agents through industrial accidents or acts of terrorism. Compared with adults, children have increased susceptibility to the effects of these agents. In contrast with MCEs from bombing events or from natural causes that present with trauma injuries, victims of chemical and radiologic MCEs present with symptoms from organ dysfunction (e.g., respiratory distress, weakness, or encephalopathy).

TABLE 34.7

UNITED STATES SCHOOL-ASSOCIATED PUBLIC MASS SHOOTINGS, 1996–2012

■ YEAR	■ INSTITUTION	■ NUMBER OF WOUNDED	■ KILLED
1996	Frontier Junior High School, Moses Lake, WA		3
1997	Health High School, Paducah, KY	5	3
1998	West Side Middle School, Jonesboro, AK	10	5
1999	Columbine High School, Littleton, CO	26	13
2005	Red Lake Senior High School, Red Lake, MN	5	7
2006	Nickel Mines, PA		5
2007	Virginia Tech, Blacksburg, VA		32
2012	Chardon High School, Chardon, OH	2	3
2012	Sandy Hook Elementary School, Newton, CT		26

USA Today. From Sandy Hook to Dunblane, shootings leave unforgettable legacies. December 14, 2012.

Chemical Mass Casualty Events

Chemical agents are more prevalent than radiologic due to their application in nearly all sectors of society. They are ideal for use in terrorism as they are easy to manufacture, transport, and cause instantaneous confusion and illness (49). Most enter the body through inhalation, ingestion, absorption, or inoculation. With their rapid minute ventilation and large body surface area (BSA), children are at increased risk for serious toxicity. The chemical agents are often classified as (a) nerve agents, (b) vesicants, (c) choking agents, or (d) asphyxiants.

10   Duration of contact with the agent increases the likelihood of severe illness. Rapid decontamination of the victim is the first step in management. Patient stabilization may need to be delayed until decontamination is performed. This delay should not put the patient at additional risk. Field triage should determine the priority of treatment and decontamination. Decontamination procedures need to be flexible owing to the range of severity of illness, the physical nature of the agent, as well as the season and weather conditions (81).

These principles of decontamination should be followed (82):

- Decontaminate as soon as possible
- Decontaminate by priority of patients needing stabilization
- Decontaminate only what is necessary
- Decontaminate as far forward (away from the hot zone) as possible

Effective decontamination of the victim reduces the risk of secondary contamination of healthcare workers.

Decontamination of children requires careful planning due to developmental and physiological differences from adults. Children are more prone to developing hypothermia. The use of a heated room, water warmed to 37.8°C, and the availability of new clothing should minimize this risk. Children may be nonambulatory due to their developmental stage or injuries, and health providers should be ready to provide assistance. At least one decontamination bay should be set up to accommodate a wheelchair or gurney. Attempts should be made to keep family units together even during decontamination. Family presence may minimize the child's fear and decrease the chances of psychological trauma. In the event the patient is alone, hospital staff should be sensitive, and a child life specialist should be utilized if available (49,83).

Nerve Agents

Nerve agents, such as tabun, sarin, and VX, act as acetylcholine (ACh) receptor agonists on the postsynaptic receptor of the cholinergic synapses. They prevent the degradation of ACh by binding to and inhibiting acetylcholinesterase (AChE). These AChE inhibitors produce signs and symptoms of a cholinergic toxidrome characterized by muscarinic excess (excess secretions and smooth muscle contractions) and nicotinic excess (muscle fasciculation and weakness). Respiratory distress can be secondary to bronchorrhea and bronchospasm mimicking status asthmaticus. Respiratory muscle weakness or paralysis may also be present. Cardiovascular effects include tachycardia or bradycardia. CNS toxicity includes encephalopathy, agitation, headache, and seizures (84).

Management consists of administration of atropine and pralidoxime and supportive care for seizures and respiratory failure. With "aging" (a chemical change in the nerve agent–AChE complex that occurs over time varies by nerve agent and renders AChE irreversibly inactive), the bonding of the two compounds becomes irreversible and limits the effectiveness of pralidoxime to overcome the nerve agent–AChE bond. Because nerve agents have different rates of aging, pralidoxime administration may still be able to remove the nerve agent from AChE and some therapeutic benefit may occur. Atropine, as a competitive antagonist of the ACh muscarinic receptor, reduces the ACh overload and is the primary antidote for nerve agent exposure. Autoinjector kits ("Mark 1" kits) containing pralidoxime and atropine are available for prehospital use. Repeated dosing may be necessary.

Vesicants

Vesicants such as mustard gas and nitrogen mustard produce blisters upon contact. These are alkylating agents that exist in solid, liquid, or gaseous form. They enter the body following inhalational, dermal, or oral exposure. Patients usually present within 12–24 hours of exposure with complaints that include burning, itching, and erythema followed by vesicle formation. Airway manifestations include rhinorrhea, hoarseness, and cough. GI symptoms include vomiting, diarrhea, and abdominal pain. Electrolyte imbalance and dehydration can occur if the affected BSA is large. Bone marrow suppression is also possible with depletion of all cell lines. Decontamination with a 0.5% hypochlorite solution (dilute bleach) may be considered instead of decontamination with water but should not be used in contact with eyes, nervous tissue, or open chest or abdominal wounds. No antidote exists and general supportive care should be provided.

Choking Agents

Choking agents produce respiratory symptoms. They induce the sense of choking and can cause upper airway damage and

TABLE 34.8

CHEMICAL AGENTSAND THEIR PROPERTIES

■ AGENT TYPE	■ NERVE	■ VESICANT	■ CHOKING	■ ASPHYXIANT
Example	Tabun, Sanrin, VX	Mustard gas Nitrogen mustard	Chlorine Phosgene	Cyanide
Symptoms	Bronchospasm Bronchorrhea Muscle weakness Seizures Encephalopathy Increased secretions	*Eyes*: tearing, itching, burning *Skin*: erythema and blisters *Airways*: rhinorrhea, cough, dyspnea	Cough Dyspnea Pulmonary edema	Dyspnea without hypoxia "Cherry red skin" Encephalopathy
Antidotes	Atropine 0.05–0.1 mg/kg IV/IM (max 5 mg) Pralidoxime >15 kg 600 mg autoinjector <15 kg 25–50 mg/kg IV/ IM (max 1 g IV, 2 g IM)	None	None	Amyl nitrate 1–2 amps crushed, inhaled; Sodium nitrite 4–10 mg/kg (max 300 mg) Sodium thiosulfate 250 mg/kg (max 12.5 g)
Provider precautions	Removal of clothes Decontamination PPE			

IV, intravenous; IM, intramuscular.
Adapted from Chung S, Shannon M. Hospital planning for acts of terrorism and other public health emergencies involving children. *Arch Dis Child* 2005;90(12):1300–7.

pulmonary edema. Chlorine and phosgene are easily acquired because of their industrial applications. Symptoms depend on the duration of exposure. Children may be more severely affected because of their high minute ventilation rate. Patients present with varying degrees of airway edema as well as pulmonary congestion, edema, and hemorrhage. There is no antidote for these agents. Removal of the individual from the environment is the primary goal. First responders should be aware of possible exposure and take precautions. Management consists of supportive care with oxygen, bronchodilators, and tracheal intubation with mechanical ventilation when indicated.

Asphyxiants

The asphyxiants are toxic compounds that act on cytochrome oxidase and inhibit oxidative phosphorylation which leads to cellular hypoxia and death. Cyanide salts are commonly used in metal cleaning, photographic processes, jewelry cleaning, and laboratory assays. Combustion of plastic-containing compounds liberates cyanide gas. Toxicity presents with dyspnea (without hypoxemia), tachycardia, confusion, weakness, seizures, and death. Progression of symptoms may be quick, and death may occur as early as 8 minutes after exposure. To make the diagnosis, one needs a high index of suspicion. Initial management concentrates on decontamination and the ABCs. Patients should receive 100% oxygen. Antiarrhythmics, vasoactive agents, and benzodiazepines may be needed to treat arrhythmias, shock, and seizures. Inhaled amyl nitrite and intravenous sodium nitrite are administered to produce methemoglobinemia. Methemoglobin binds cyanide and liberates cytochrome oxidase. Thiosulfate is a substrate for the mitochondrial enzyme rhodanese, which converts cyanide to thiocyanate. This reaction occurs too slowly in the body to be effective during acute toxicity. Thiosulfate must therefore be used alongside the nitrites. In 2006, the FDA approved hydroxocobalamin for the treatment of cyanide intoxication. It binds to cyanide to form cyanocobalamin, which is then excreted by the kidneys. Either protocol may be used but not both. Patients who survive the initial exposure will need

intensive care to manage respiratory failure, ARDS, shock, and seizures (**Table 34.8**).

Radiological/Nuclear Mass Casualty Events

Radiation exposure can result from a nuclear power plant event, detonation of a nuclear weapon, or the release of a radioactive dispersal device (RDD, also called a dirty bomb). Blast injuries may coexist with the effects of radiation exposure. In these scenarios, stabilization and treatment of life-threatening conditions should occur before decontamination. Regular decontamination procedures should be followed.

Effects of a nuclear MCE will not be immediately evident. Acute radiation syndrome (toxicity may occur within minutes and usually in <24 hours) will develop in individuals exposed to a nuclear detonation and are close enough to sustain blast injuries. Rapidly dividing cells of the reproductive, hematopoietic, and gastrointestinal systems will be most affected. Nonspecific symptoms such as malaise and fatigue are first to appear. This is followed by bone marrow depression affecting all cell lines. Hemorrhage and sepsis may develop. Radiation pneumonitis may occur, requiring ventilatory support. CNS injury may present as seizures and increased intracranial pressure.

Treatment is supportive. Fluids, antibiotics, hematopoietic growth factors, nutrition, and skin care are provided when indicated. Administration of potassium iodide within 8 hours after exposure is recommended. This agent is taken up by the thyroid and prevents the incorporation of inhaled or ingested radioiodines with the hope of reducing the possibility of thyroid cancer. Other antidotes include Prussian blue for exposure to cesium-137 and thallium. It enhances excretion but does not treat complications of radiation. For plutonium, curium, and americium exposures, treatment is through chelation with pentetate calcium trisodium, pentetate zinc trisodium, or 2,3-dimercaptopropane-1-sulfonic acid, which bind radioactive elements/heavy metals and remove them through the urine.

CONCLUSIONS AND FUTURE DIRECTIONS

Pediatric emergency preparedness is a high-priority endeavor for governmental and healthcare institutions. The changing climate and increasingly tense political environment lend an increased urgency for enhanced preparedness. Plans and resources, as well as the current knowledge base, used in the treatment and management of children are lagging behind the developed strategies that address adult mass casualty victims. Further study and research is required to formulate evidence-based standards and performance measures for children. Education, training, and community emergency preparedness are key components to the disaster response. Equally important are the efforts to address mental health, education, and child care needs after the event. Government, healthcare, and community agencies need to continue to advocate for the needs of the children.

References

1. World Health Organization. *Health Action in Crises: Annual Report 2008*. Geneva, Switzerland: World Health Organization, 2009:1–44.
2. National Counterterrorism Center. *2008 Report on Terrorism*. Washington, DC: Office of the Director of National Intelligence, National Counterterrorism Center, 2009:1–68.
3. Federal Interagency Forum on Child and Family Statistics. Child population: number of children ages 0–17 in the United States by age, 1950–2011 and projected 2012–2050. http://www.childstats.gov/americaschildren/tables/pop1.asp?popup=true. Accessed June 25, 2013.
4. Federal Interagency Forum on Child and Family Statistics. Children as a percentage of the population: persons in selected age groups as a percentage of the total U.S. population, and children ages 0–17 as a percentage of the dependent population, 1950–2011 and projected 2012–2050. http://www.childstats.gov/americaschildren/tables/pop2.asp?popup=true. Accessed June 25, 2013.
5. Odetola FO, Miller WC, Davis MM, et al. The relationship between the location of pediatric intensive care unit facilities and child death from trauma: A county-level ecologic study. *J Pediatr* 2005;147(1):74–7.
6. Institute of Medicine Committee of the Future of Emergency Care in the U.S. Health System. Emergency care for children: Growing pains. https://www.iom.edu/Reports/2006/Emergency-Care-for-Children-Growing-Pains.aspx. Published on June 13, 2006.
7. Einav S, Aharonson-Daniel L, Weissman C, et al. In-hospital resource utilization during multiple casualty incidents. *Ann Surg* 2006;243(4):533.
8. Prezant DJ, Weiden M, Banauch GI, et al. Cough and bronchial responsiveness in firefighters at the World Trade Center site. *N Engl J Med* 2002;347(11):806–15.
9. Herbstman JB, Frank R, Schwab M, et al. Respiratory effects of inhalation exposure among workers during the cleanup effort at the World Trade Center disaster site. *Environ Res* 2005;99(1):85–92.
10. Noji EK. Disaster epidemiology. *Emerg Med Clin North Am* 1996;14(2):289–300.
11. Stellman JM, Smith RP, Katz CL, et al. Enduring mental health morbidity and social function impairment in World Trade Center rescue, recovery, and cleanup workers: The psychological dimension of an environmental health disaster. *Environ Health Perspect* 2008;116(9):1248.
12. Boscarino JA, Adams RE, Figley CR. Mental health service use 1-year after the World Trade Center disaster: Implications for mental health care. *Gen Hosp Psychiatry* 2004;26(5):346–58.
13. Mandell DJ. Children's mental health after disasters: The impact of the World Trade Center attack. *Curr Psychiatry Rep* 2003;5(2):101–7.
14. Ginter PM, Wingate MS, Rucks AC, et al. Creating a regional pediatric medical disaster preparedness network: Imperative and issues. *Matern Child Health J* 2006;10(4):391–6.
15. National Commission on Children and Disasters. *2010 Report to the President and Congress*. AHRQ Publication No. 10-M037. Rockville, MD: Agency for Healthcare Research and Quality. October, 2010.
16. Gnauck KA, Nufer KE, LaValley JM, et al. Do pediatric and adult disaster victims differ? A descriptive analysis of clinical encounters from four natural disaster DMAT deployments. *Prehosp Disaster Med* 2007;22(1):67–73.
17. Aharonson-Daniel L, Waisman Y, Dannon YL, et al; Members of the Israel Trauma Group. Epidemiology of terror-related versus non-terror-related traumatic injury in children. *Pediatrics* 2003;112(4):e280.
18. Peleg K, Aharonson-Daniel L, Michael M, et al; Israel Trauma Group. Patterns of injury in hospitalized terrorist victims. *Am J Emerg Med* 2003;21(4):258–62.
19. Arnold JL, Tsai M, Halpern P, et al. Mass-casualty, terrorist bombings: Epidemiological outcomes, resource utilization, and time course of emergency needs (Part I). *Prehosp Disaster Med* 2003;18(3):220.
20. Federal Emergency Management Agency. *Report on State Emergency Preparedness*. Washington, DC: Federal Emergency Management Agency, U.S. Department of Homeland Security, 1999.
21. Mann NC, MacKenzie E, Anderson C. Public health preparedness for mass-casualty events: A 2002 state-by-state assessment. *Prehosp Disaster Med* 2004;19(03):245–55.
22. Save The Children. *A National Report Card on Protecting Children During Disasters: 2012*. U.S. Center for Child Development and Resiliency, 2012.
23. Chaput CJ, Deluhery MR, Stake CE, et al. Disaster training for prehospital providers. *Prehosp Emerg Care* 2007;11(4):458–65.
24. Graham CJ, Stuemky J, Lera TA. Emergency medical services preparedness for pediatric emergencies. *Pediatr Emerg Care* 1993;9(6):329–31.
25. Shirm S, Liggin R, Dick R, et al. Prehospital preparedness for pediatric mass-casualty events. *Pediatrics* 2007;120(4):e756–e761.
26. Seidel JS, Hornbein M, Yoshiyama K, et al. Emergency medical services and the pediatric patient: Are the needs being met? *Pediatrics* 1984;73(6):769–72.
27. Barfield WD, Krug SE, Kanter RK, et al. Neonatal and pediatric regionalized systems in pediatric emergency mass critical care. *Pediatr Crit Care Med* 2011;12(6):S128–S134.
28. Middleton KR, Burt CW. *Availability of Pediatric Services and Equipment in Emergency Departments, United States, 2002-03*. US Department of Health and Human Services, Centers for Disease Control and Prevention, National Center for Health Statistics, 2006.
29. Thompson T, Lyle K, Mullins SH, et al. A state survey of emergency department preparedness for the care of children in a mass casualty event. *Am J Disaster Med* 2009;4(4):227–32.
30. Kilner T, Brace SJ, Cooke M, et al. In 'big bang' major incidents do triage tools accurately predict clinical priority? A systematic review of the literature. *Injury* 2011;42(5):460–8.
31. Frykberg ER, Tepas JJ. Terrorist bombings. Lessons learned from Belfast to Beirut. *Ann Surg* 1988;208(5):569.
32. Hirshberg A, Scott BG, Granchi T et al. How does casualty load affect trauma care in urban bombing incidents? A quantitative analysis. *J Trauma* 2005;58(4):686–95.
33. American College of Surgeons - Committee on Trauma. *Resources for Optimal Care of the Injured Patient: 1999*. Chicago, IL: American College of Surgeons, 1998.
34. Wallis L, Carley S. Comparison of paediatric major incident primary triage tools. *Emerg Med J* 2006;23(6):475–8.

35. Jenkins JL, McCarthy ML, Sauer LM, et al. Mass-casualty triage: Time for an evidence-based approach. *Prehosp Disaster Med* 2008;23(1):3–8.

36. Cross KP, Cicero MX. Independent application of the Sacco Disaster Triage Method to pediatric trauma patients. *Prehosp Disaster Med* 2012;27(4):306–11.

37. Benson M, Koenig KL, Schultz CH. Disaster triage: START, then SAVE—a new method of dynamic triage for victims of a catastrophic earthquake. *Prehosp Disaster Med* 1996;11(02):117–24.

38. Garner A, Lee A, Harrison K, et al. Comparative analysis of multiple-casualty incident triage algorithms. *Ann Emerg Med* 2001;38(5):541–8.

39. Centers for Disease Control and Prevention. *Mass Casualties Predictor*. Department of Health and Human Services, Centers for Disease Control and Prevention, 2003.

40. Aylwin CJ, König TC, Brennan NW, et al. Reduction in critical mortality in urban mass casualty incidents: Analysis of triage, surge, and resource use after the London bombings on July 7, 2005. *Lancet* 2007;368(9554):2219–25.

41. Peleg K, Rozenfeld M, Dolev E. Children and terror casualties receive preference in ICU admissions. *Disaster Med Public Health Prep* 2012;6(1):14.

42. Waisman Y, Aharonson-Daniel L, Mor M, et al. The impact of terrorism on children: A two-year experience. *Prehosp Disaster Med* 2003;18(3):242–8.

43. Kissoon N. Deliberations and recommendations of the Pediatric Emergency Mass Critical Care Task Force: Executive summary. *Pediatr Crit Care Med* 2011;12(6):S103–S108.

44. Devereaux A, Christian MD, Dichter JR, et al. Summary of suggestions from the task force for mass critical care summit, January 26–27, 2007. *Chest* 2008;133(5 suppl):1S–7S.

45. Christian MD, Devereaux AV, Dichter JR, et al. Definitive care for the critically ill during a disaster: Current capabilities and limitations from a Task Force for Mass Critical Care summit meeting, January 26–27, 2007, Chicago, IL. *Chest* 2008;133(5 suppl):8S–17S.

46. Devereaux AV, Dichter JR, Christian MD, et al; Task Force for Mass Critical Care. Definitive care for the critically ill during a disaster: A framework for allocation of scarce resources in mass critical care: From a Task Force for Mass Critical Care summit meeting, January 26–27, 2007, Chicago, IL. *Chest* 2008;133(5 suppl):51S–66S.

47. Bohn D, Kanter RK, Burns J, et al. Supplies and equipment for pediatric emergency mass critical care. *Pediatr Crit Care Med* 2011;12(6):S120–S127.

48. Qureshi K, Gershon MR, Sherman MM, et al. Health care workers' ability and willingness to report to duty during catastrophic disasters. *J Urban Health* 2005;82(3):378–88.

49. Chung S, Shannon M. Hospital planning for acts of terrorism and other public health emergencies involving children. *Arch Dis Child* 2005;90(12):1300–7.

50. Kanter RK. Strategies to improve pediatric disaster surge response: Potential mortality reduction and tradeoffs. *Crit Care Med* 2007;35(12):2837–42.

51. Peek L, Stough LM. Children with disabilities in the context of disaster: A social vulnerability perspective. *Child Dev* 2010;81(4):1260–70.

52. Morrow BH. Identifying and mapping community vulnerability. *Disasters* 1999;23(1):1–18.

53. Kailes JI, Enders A. Moving beyond "special needs" a function-based framework for emergency management and planning. *J Disabil Pol Stud* 2007;17(4):230–7.

54. Federal Emergency Management Agency. *2013 National Preparedness Report*. Washington, DC: Federal Emergency Management Agency, U.S. Department of Homeland Security, 2013.

55. Frykberg ER. Medical management of disasters and mass casualties from terrorist bombings: How can we cope? *J Trauma* 2002;53(2):201–12.

56. Amir LD, Aharonson-Daniel L, Peleg K, et al. The severity of injury in children resulting from acts against civilian populations. *Ann Surg* 2005;241(4):666.

57. Jaffe DH, Peleg K. Terror explosive injuries: A comparison of children, adolescents, and adults. *Ann Surg* 2010;251(1):138–43.

58. DePalma RG, Burris DG, Champion HR, et al. Blast injuries. *N Engl J Med* 2005;352(13):1335–42.

59. Ritenour AE, Baskin TW. Primary blast injury: Update on diagnosis and treatment. *Crit Care Med* 2008;36(7):S311–S317.

60. Wolf SJ, Bebarta VS, Bonnett CJ, et al. Blast injuries. *Lancet* 2009;374(9687):405–15.

61. Born C. Blast trauma: The fourth weapon of mass destruction. *Scand J Surg* 2005;94(4):279.

62. Oda J, Tanaka H, Yoshioka T, et al. Analysis of 372 patients with crush syndrome caused by the Hanshin-Awaji earthquake. *J Trauma Acute Care Surg* 1997;42(3):470–6.

63. Harrison CD, Bebarta VS, Grant GA. Tympanic membrane perforation after combat blast exposure in Iraq: A poor biomarker of primary blast injury. *J Trauma Acute Care Surg* 2009;67(1):210–1.

64. Katz E, Ofek B, Adler J, et al. Primary blast injury after a bomb explosion in a civilian bus. *Ann Surg* 1989;209(4):484.

65. Xydakis MS, Bebarta VS, Harrison CD, et al. Tympanic-membrane perforation as a marker of concussive brain injury in Iraq. *N Engl J Med* 2007;357(8):830–1.

66. Leibovici D, Gofrit ON, Shapira SC. Eardrum perforation in explosion survivors: Is it a marker of pulmonary blast injury? *Ann Emerg Med* 1999;34(2):168–72.

67. Chavko M, Prusaczyk WK, McCarron RM. Lung injury and recovery after exposure to blast overpressure. *J Trauma Acute Care Surg* 2006;61(4):933–42.

68. Avidan V, Hersch M, Armon Y, et al. Blast lung injury: Clinical manifestations, treatment, and outcome. *Am J Surg* 2005;190(6):945–50.

69. Sorkine P, Szold O, Kluger Y, et al. Permissive hypercapnia ventilation in patients with severe pulmonary blast injury. *J Trauma Acute Care Surg* 1998;45(1):35–8.

70. Cripps NP, Glover MA, Guy RJ. The pathophysiology of primary blast injury and its implications for treatment. Part II: The auditory structures and abdomen. *J R Nav Med Serv* 1999;85(1):13–24.

71. Guy RJ, Kirkman E, Watkins PE, et al. Physiologic responses to primary blast. *J Trauma Acute Care Surg* 1998;45(6):983–7.

72. Irwin RJ, Lerner MR, Bealer JF, et al. Cardiopulmonary physiology of primary blast injury. *J Trauma Acute Care Surg* 1997;43(4):650–5.

73. Halpern P, Tsai M, Arnold J, et al. Mass casualty, terrorist bombings: Implications for emergency department and hospital emergency response (Part II). *Prehosp Disaster Med* 2003;18(3):235, 236–241.

74. Fay TB, Yeates KO, Wade SL, et al. Predicting longitudinal patterns of functional deficits in children with traumatic brain injury. *Neuropsychology* 2009;23(3):271.

75. Ewing-Cobbs L, Prasad MR, Kramer L, et al. Late intellectual and academic outcomes following traumatic brain injury sustained during early childhood. *J Neurosurg* 2006;105(4 suppl):287.

76. Bjelopera J, Bagalman E, Caldwell S, et al. Public Mass Shootings in the United States: Selected Implications for Federal Public Health and Safety Policy. March 18, 2013. Congressional Research Service.

77. Graham J, Shirm S, Liggin R, et al. Mass-casualty events at schools: A national preparedness survey. *Pediatrics* 2006;117(1):e8–e15.

78. Wisniewski R, Dennik-Champion G, Peltier JW. Emergency preparedness competencies: Assessing nurses' educational needs. *J Nurs Adm* 2004;34(10):475–80.

79. Shapira SC, Adatto-Levi R, Avitzour M, et al. Mortality in terrorist attacks: A unique modal of temporal death distribution. *World J Surg* 2006;30(11):2071–7.

80. Peleg K, Rozenfeld M, Stein M. Poorer outcomes for mass casualty events victims: Is it evidence based? *J Trauma Acute Care Surg* 2010;69(3):653–9.

81. Okumura T, Kondo H, Nagayama H, et al. Simple triage and rapid decontamination of mass casualties with colored clothes pegs (STARDOM-CCP) system against chemical releases. *Prehosp Disaster Med* 2007;22(3):233.

82. Ramesh AC, Kumar S. Triage, monitoring, and treatment of mass casualty events involving chemical, biological, radiological, or nuclear agents. *J Pharm Bioallied Sci* 2010;2(3):239.

83. Timm N, Reeves S. A mass casualty incident involving children and chemical decontamination. *Disaster Manage Resp* 2007;5(2):49–55.

84. Rotenberg JS, Newmark J. Nerve agent attacks on children: Diagnosis and management. *Pediatrics* 2003;112(3):648–58.

CHAPTER 35 ■ POISONING

MICHAEL A. NARES, G. PATRICIA CANTWELL, AND RICHARD S. WEISMAN

KEY POINTS

1. Childhood poisoning requires a continuum of care from the prehospital environment to the emergency department and the ICU that can quickly distinguish ingestions that pose significant risk from those that are inconsequential.

2. A comprehensive history, focused physical examination, and thoughtful laboratory evaluation provide an excellent template for assessing risk of toxicity and enabling the practitioner to avail of the use of a multitude of poisoning resources.

3. Identification of toxidromes (sympathomimetic/adrenergic, cholinergic, anticholinergic, and opioid) requires meticulous attention to clinical signs and symptoms.

4. The laboratory evaluation generally serves to confirm a toxicologic diagnosis, but a negative screen does not exclude the possibility of toxic exposure. Targeted determination of electrolytes, osmolality, glucose, electrocardiogram, urinalysis, and radiographic imaging may be particularly helpful in eliciting the etiology of a suspected toxin.

5. Familiarity with specific toxins and their antidotes enables immediate initiation of therapy, as well as the ability to definitively identify certain toxins.

6. Toxicokinetic principles focus on the processes of absorption, distribution, metabolism, and elimination of drugs or toxins and provide the mainstay of specific management of the poisoned child.

7. Supportive care remains the crux of therapy and requires aggressive airway management with attention to airway reflexes, careful evaluation and maintenance of ventilation, recognition and correction of hemodynamic compromise, and anticipation of aberrations in the cardiopulmonary and neurologic systems.

8. Prevention strategies are key in decreasing morbidity and mortality. All healthcare providers in the United States must be familiar with the Universal Poison Control number: 1-800-222-1222.

Childhood poisoning remains a common occurrence despite widespread educational efforts by healthcare providers and the utilization of childproof medication dispensers. The challenge to the pediatric intensivist can be daunting in determining which ingestions are potentially high risk and which are inconsequential. Yearly data collection reveals that more than 2 million exposures to toxic substances are reported to poison centers throughout the United States. The overwhelming majority of toxic exposures cause minimal to no effect; morbidity and mortality associated with these exposures are extremely uncommon (1). Poisoning that occurs in children less than 5 years of age is generally accidental and accounts for ~85%–90% of pediatric poisoning. Poisoning in a child older than 5 years is generally considered intentional and comprises the remaining 10%–15% of childhood poisonings (2). Unintentional overdoses may occasionally occur in teenagers who take alcohol and street drugs. Teenagers are also subject to hospitalization following suicide attempts or suicide gestures. The Toxic Exposure Surveillance System of the American Association of Poison Control Centers reports ingestion to be the primary route of exposure to toxic substances (1). Risk factors for childhood exposure include exploratory behavior, child abuse, the possibility of environmental exposures, suicide attempts in children, and neonates exposed to toxins in utero.

EPIDEMIOLOGY

Poisoning may occur with differing modes of exposure. Exposures may occur via ingestion, ocular exposure, topical exposure, envenomation, inhalation, and transplacental exposure.

The ingestion of poisonous plants is common in children and may account for ~5%–10% of calls to poison control centers. It is difficult to establish a clear-cut list of problem plants, as many plants have both edible and toxic parts, are difficult for nonbotanists to identify accurately, and have variable plant names, and for many plants, the quantity necessary to produce toxicity is unclear.

Management of childhood poisoning is challenging owing to the large variety of prescription medications, household chemicals, stings, envenomations, illicit drugs and designer drugs, as well as an increase in the use of nonprescription and herbal medications. Pediatric fatalities are most often associated with the following agents: analgesics, hydrocarbons, antidepressants, gases and fumes, stimulants, street drugs, cardiovascular drugs, anticonvulsants, sedative/hypnotics, antipsychotics, and chemicals. The agents that most frequently prompt calls to poison control centers are cosmetics and personal care products, cleaning substances, analgesics, foreign bodies, topical agents, and plants.

CLINICAL APPROACH TO THE POISONED CHILD

The acute management of the poisoned child generally begins in the emergency department. Recommendations for the management of the poisoned child have been challenging owing to limited research based upon small-case series, animal studies, and case reports. Initial evaluation involves the process of triage and the determination of appropriate decontamination and treatment regimens. The intensivist may be immediately involved, as aggressive interventions are often required before it is possible to determine a comprehensive history, physical examination, and diagnostic testing. Urgent priorities include the focus on a primary survey that involves attention to the patient's airway, breathing, and circulation (ABC). Following the establishment of life-saving supportive care, a detailed evaluation can be meticulously performed. Toxins may cause respiratory failure by depression of the respiratory drive, hypoperfusion of the central nervous system (CNS), coma with impaired/absent protective airway reflexes, or direct toxic effects on the pulmonary system. Airway management mandates a low threshold for rapid-sequence intubation in view of the potential for loss of protective airway reflexes and expectation of a full stomach, with risk of aspiration. Many toxins may cause extreme hemodynamic instability due to dysrhythmias and/or hypotension. Comprehensive stabilization involves attention to respiratory, cardiovascular, neurologic, and metabolic aberrancies. It is critical for healthcare providers to ensure safety of personnel in initiating treatment; decontamination and proper personal protective equipment may be required prior to proceeding with management. Optimal clinical management of the critically ill, poisoned patient mandates a seamless transfer of information and patient care from the emergency department to the ICU. The mainstay of intensive care management is meticulous supportive care with attention to emergent airway management (Chapter 24), respiratory failure (Chapters 49 and 50), hemodynamic collapse (Chapter 28), and management of the comatose patient (Chapter 57). These entities are discussed in detail in respective chapters, while specifics related to particular poisons are highlighted below.

Patient History

A comprehensive history for the potential of toxic exposure may be obtained from witnesses, family members, friends, and emergency medical services personnel. It is important to obtain a list of all available toxins within the household, including over-the-counter medications and nonpharmaceutical agents (e.g., plants, cleaning agents). A comprehensive history must also include focused information about the environment, circumstances preceding and surrounding a toxic exposure, smells or unusual items, the occupation of those in the home, and queries regarding the presence of a suicide note. Obtaining an accurate history in adolescent poisonings is especially challenging owing to the potential use of multiple substances, possible drugs of abuse, prolonged time between ingestion and presentation, and attempts at concealing accurate information. Additional information includes the maximum amount of toxin available and the minimum amount per kilogram that produces symptoms. It is helpful to estimate the quantity of liquid toxins by quantifying a swallow: 5–10 mL in a young child and 10–15 mL in an adolescent. A useful mnemonic is the "over-the-counter" or "OTC" designation for medications, which can also mean "oblivious to toxic contents" (3). The history must include potential illnesses of family members, which can serve to identify other medications in the home. It is vital to obtain product containers or medication labels to identify specific toxic contents. Extremely dangerous single agents are camphor, chloroquine, hydroxychloroquine, imipramine, desipramine, quinine, methyl salicylate, theophylline, thioridazine, and chlorpromazine. A number of medications have been determined to be potentially lethal to a child who weighs 10 kg and ingests just one tablet, capsule, or teaspoonful (4) (Table 35.1).

A comprehensive history must include evaluation for indoor air pollutants, which may include carbon monoxide, cyanide, ozone, smoke, volatile hydrocarbons, and mercury vapor.

After obtaining the history, early contact with the *regional poison control center (1-800-222-1222)* provides rapid access to a toxicology consult. Specific signs and symptoms can serve to focus a differential diagnosis. Prompt assimilation of metabolic and kinetic information allows the determination of a potential clinical course. The clinician may be caught off-guard in cases of delays between the onset of ingestion and development of symptoms. It is especially helpful to obtain assistance in identifying and managing drugs and chemicals unfamiliar to the practitioner. Centralized databases provide information about possible public health threats in the event of multiple poisonings.

Physical Examination

General

A comprehensive physical examination can be crucial in determining which agents are involved in causing toxic symptoms. Careful assessment of vital signs combined with a thorough physical examination serves to narrow a broad array of differential diagnoses and allows for specific initial treatment interventions. The intent of this chapter is not to review every possible poisoning, but rather to provide a methodical

TABLE 35.1

TOXICITY LEVELS OF SELECTED MEDICATIONS AND MEDICATION CLASSES

■ AGENTS	■ MINIMUM POTENTIAL LETHAL DOSE	■ MAXIMUM DOSE AVAILABLE	■ POTENTIALLY FATAL UNITS IN A 10-kg CHILD
Antimalarials			
Chloroquine	20 mg/kg	500 mg	1
Hydroxychloroquine	20 mg/kg	200 mg	1
Camphor	100 mg/kg	200 mg/mL	5 mL
Imidazolines			
Clonidine	0.01 mg/kg	0.3 mg; 7.5 mg/patch	1
Tetrahydrozoline	2.5–5 mL	0.1%	2.5–5 mL
Methyl salicylates	150–200 mg/kg	1400 mg/mL	1.1–1.4 mL
Sulfonylureas			
Glipizide	0.1 mg/kg	5 mg	1
Glyburide	0.1 mg/kg	10 mg	1

From Matteucci MJ. One pill can kill: Assessing the potential for fatal poisonings in children. *Pediatr Ann* 2005;34:964–968, with permission.

approach to organizing physical findings that can focus therapy and guide specific diagnostic evaluations. The signs and symptoms that suggest specific classes of poisoning are generally grouped into syndromes and referred to as toxidromes. These groupings are essential for the successful recognition of poisoning patterns. Herbal poisoning and dietary supplements have also been implicated with a host of typical symptomatologies (5) (**Tables 35.2 and 35.3**). An approach to the classic toxidromes can be misleading, depending on the amount of toxic exposure, competing toxins or medications, and patient comorbidities. The classic toxidromes may be grouped into four categories: sympathomimetic/adrenergic, cholinergic, anticholinergic, and opiate–sedative–ethanol syndromes.

Many nonspecific findings are related to the gastrointestinal (GI) system and include nausea, vomiting, abdominal pain, and loose stools. Elevated body temperature serves to identify specific toxic agents. Careful physical examination elucidates findings of significant concern that can serve to identify the heralding features of a particular toxidrome.

Cardiopulmonary

As noted in the primary survey, the priority is to recognize life-threatening compromise of ABC. Toxins may cause an array of aberrations of the cardiovascular system, including hypertension/hypotension due to direct action of the toxin on vascular smooth muscle, neurogenic effects on autonomic nervous centers, and direct cardiogenic or renal effects. These specific physical findings are best expressed in **Table 35.4** (6).

Neurologic

The neurologic examination is especially important, as many toxins can be expected to depress the level of consciousness by directly interfering with respiratory drive or hypoxia from loss of protective airway reflexes. Neurologic deterioration can be catastrophic; therefore, the patient should be examined frequently. One must anticipate the potential for seizures. The pupillary exam is an extremely useful neurologic finding. Various toxins interfere with the autonomic innervation of the pupil and may manifest as miosis or mydriasis. Symmetrical pupillary changes are typical of toxic exposures, with asymmetry pointing to a structural or focal neurologic abnormality. It is essential to recognize that polydrug toxicity may involve agents with competing actions on the pupillary response. Management based on the isolated evaluation of pupil size may lead to misdiagnosis. Further confounding the exam may be the possibility of traumatic brain injury or intracranial hemorrhage that stems from the toxic exposure. An extensive list of toxins that includes over-the-counter medications, common household products, and drugs of abuse is associated with an altered sensorium. Additionally, one must be cognizant of potential abstinence syndromes in patients suffering from chronic substance abuse. Drug withdrawal may be heralded by agitation, abnormal vital signs, irritability, and an altered sensorium. Nystagmus, tinnitus, and visual disturbances are commonly observed neurologic findings in selected intoxications.

Dermatologic Manifestations and Telltale Odors

Dermatologic examination may yield the identification of varied toxins. Inhalant abuse may lead to skin rashes around the nose and the mouth. Needle tracks or characteristic tattooing are suggestive of IV drug use. Meticulous skin examination must focus on commonly employed intravascular access sites, including the groin, neck, supraclavicular areas, dorsum of the feet, and tongue. Adverse drug reactions and allergic dermatitis may occur from exposure to drugs, plants, or chemicals. Alopecia can lead to the identification of long-term exposure to a variety of toxic chemicals. Jaundice is another dermatologic finding of significance that should suggest consideration of specific toxic exposures in the differential diagnosis. Telltale odors are another means of compartmentalizing a variety of toxins (**Table 35.5**). Agents may have saturated the clothing or skin, or may be emanated via the breath.

TABLE 35.2

EXAMPLES OF KNOWN HERBAL PRODUCTS AND THEIR ASSOCIATED TOXIC EFFECTS

■ HERBAL PRODUCT	■ TOXIC CHEMICALS	■ EFFECT OR TARGET ORGAN
Monkshood (*Aconitum* sp.)	Aconite	Cardiac arrhythmias, shock, weakness, seizures, coma, paresthesias, nausea, emesis
Wormwood (*Artemisia absinthium*)	Thujone	Seizures, dementia, tremors, headache, ataxia
Chaparral (*Larrea divericata*)	Nordihydroguaiaretic acid	Nausea, emesis, hepatitis
Cinnamon oil (*Cinnamomum* sp.)	Cinnamaldehyde	Dermatitis, abuse syndrome
Comfrey (*Symphytum officinale*)	Pyrrolizidines	Hepatic veno-occlusive disease
Crotalaria sp.	Pyrrolizidines	Hepatic veno-occlusive disease
Eucalyptus (*Eucalyptus globulus*)	1,8-Cineol	Drowsiness, ataxia, seizures, nausea, vomiting, coma
Garlic (*Allium sativum*)	Allicin	Nausea, emesis, anorexia, weight loss, bleeding, platelet dysfunction
Heliotropium sp.	Pyrrolizidines	Hepatic veno-occlusive disease
Jin bu huan	Tetrahydropalmatine	Hepatitis
Kava (*Piper methysticum*)	Kavapyrones	Hepatitis, cirrhosis
Laetrile	Cyanide	Coma, seizures, death, respiratory failure
Licorice (*Glycyrrhiza glabra*)	Glycyrrhetic acid	Hypertension, hypokalemia, dysrhythmias
Ma Huang (*Ephedra sinica*)	Ephedrine	Hypertension, dysrhythmias, stroke, seizures
Nutmeg (*Myristica fragrans*)	Myristicin, eugenol	Hallucinations, emesis, headache
Strychnos nux-vomica	Strychnine	Seizures, abdominal pain, respiratory failure
Pennyroyal (*Mentha pulegium*; *Hedeoma* sp.)	Pulegone	Centrilobular liver necrosis, fetotoxicity, abortion
Senecio sp.	Pyrrolizidines	Hepatic veno-occlusive disease

From Woolf AD. Herbal remedies and children: Do they work? Are they harmful? *Pediatrics* 2003;112:240–246, with permission.

TABLE 35.3

TWELVE MOST DANGEROUS DIETARY SUPPLEMENTS

■ NAME (ALSO KNOWN AS)	■ DANGERS
DEFINITELY HAZARDOUS *Documented organ failure and known carcinogenic properties* ***ARISTOLOCHIC ACID*** *Aristolochia* sp. (birthwort, snakeroot, snakeweed, sangree root, sangrel, serpentary, serpentaria); *Asarun canadens* (wild ginger)	Potent human carcinogen; can cause kidney failure and death
(a) VERY LIKELY HAZARDOUS *Banned in some countries, FDA warning, or adverse effects in studies*	
COMFREY *Symphytun officinale* (ass ear, black root, blackwort, bruisewort, consolidate radix, consound, gum plant, healing herb, knitback, knitbone, salsify, slippery root, symphytum radix, wallwort)	Abnormal liver function or irreversible damage; deaths reported
ANDROSTENEDIONE *4-Androstene-3* (17-dione, andro, androstene)	Increased cancer risk; decrease in HDL cholesterol
CHAPARRAL *Larrea divaricate* (creosote bush, greasewood, hediondilla, jarilla, larreastat)	Abnormal liver function or irreversible damage; deaths reported
GERMANDER *Teucrium chamaedrys* (wall germander, wild germander)	Abnormal liver function or irreversible damage; deaths reported
KAVA *Piper methysticum* (ava, awa, gea, gi, intoxicating pepper, kao, kavain, kawa-pfeffer, kew, long pepper, malohu, maluk, meruk, milik, rauschpfeffer, sakau, tonga, wurzelstock, yagona, yangona)	Abnormal liver function or irreversible damage; deaths reported
(b) LIKELY HAZARDOUS *Adverse events reported, theoretical risks*	
BITTER ORANGE *Citrus aurantium* (green orange, kijitsu, neroli oil, Seville orange, and shangzhou zhiqiao, sour orange, zhi oiao, zhi xhi)	High blood pressure; risk of arrhythmias, heart attack, and stroke
LOBELIA *Lobelia inflata* (asthma weed, bladderpod, emetic herb, gagroot, lobelie, Indian tobacco, pukeweed, vomit wort, wild tobacco)	Breathing difficulty, rapid heartbeat, low blood pressure, diarrhea, dizziness; possible related deaths reported
ORGAN/GLANDULAR EXTRACTS Brain, adrenal, pituitary, placenta, other gland "substance" or "concentrate"	Theoretical risk of mad cow disease, especially from brain extracts
PENNYROYAL OIL *Hedeoma pulegioides* (lurk-in-the-ditch, mosquito plant, piliolerial, pudding grass, pulegium, run-by-the-ground, squaw balm, squawmint, stinking balm, tickweed)	Liver and kidney failure, nerve damage, convulsions, abdominal tenderness, burning of the throat; deaths reported
SCULLCAP *Scutellaria lateriflora* (blue pimpernel, helmet flower, hoodwort, mad weed, mad-dog herb, mad-dog weed, quaker bonnet, scutelluria, skullcap)	Abnormal liver function or damage
YOHIMBE *Pausinystalia yobimbe* (johimbi, yohimbehe, yohimbine)	Changes in blood pressure, arrhythmias, respiratory depression, myocardial infarction; deaths reported

From Natural Medicines Comprehensive Database 2004 and Consumers Union's medical and research consultants. Data extracted from *Consumer Reports*, May 2004.

TABLE 35.4

CLINICAL MANIFESTATIONS OF POISONING

SKIN

Cyanosis (unresponsive to oxygen-methemoglobinemia)	Nitrates, nitrites, phenacetin, benzocaine
Red flush	Carbon monoxide, cyanide, boric acid, anticholinergics
Sweating	Amphetamines, LSD, organophosphates, cocaine, barbiturates
Dry	Anticholinergics
Bullae	Barbiturates, carbon monoxide
Jaundice	Acetaminophen, mushrooms, carbon tetrachloride, iron, phosphorus
Purpura	Aspirin, warfarin, snakebite

TEMPERATURE

Hypothermia	Sedative hypnotics, ethanol, carbon monoxide, phenothiazines, TCAs, clonidine
Hyperthermia	Anticholinergics, salicylates, phenothiazines, TCAs, cocaine, amphetamines, theophylline

BLOOD PRESSURE

Hypertension	Sympathomimetics (especially phenylpropanolamine in over-the-counter cold remedies) organophosphates, amphetamines, PCP
Hypotension	Narcotics, sedative hypnotics, TCAs, phenothiazines, clonidine, β-blockers, calcium channel blockers

PULSE RATE

Bradycardia	Digitalis, sedative hypnotics, β-blockers, ethchlorvynol, calcium channel blockers
Tachycardia	Anticholinergics, sympathomimetics, amphetamines, alcohol, aspirin, theophylline, cocaine, TCAs
Arrhythmias	Anticholinergics, TCAs, organophosphates, phenothiazines, digoxin, β-blockers, carbon monoxide, cyanide, theophylline

MUCOUS MEMBRANES

Dry	Anticholinergics
Salivation	Organophosphates, carbamates
Oral lesions	Corrosives, paraquat
Lacrimation	Caustics, organophosphates, irritant gases

RESPIRATION

Depressed	Alcohol, narcotics, barbiturates, sedative/hypnotics
Tachypnea	Salicylates, amphetamines, carbon monoxide
Kussmaul	Methanol, ethylene glycol, salicylates
Wheezing	Organophosphates
Pneumonia	Hydrocarbons
Pulmonary edema	Aspiration, salicylates, narcotics, sympathomimetics

CNS

Seizures	TCAs, cocaine, phenothiazines, amphetamines, camphor, lead, salicylates, isoniazid, organophosphates, antihistamines, propoxyphene, strychnine
Pupils, miosis	Narcotics (except Demerol and Lomotil), phenothiazines, organophosphates, diazepam, barbiturates, mushrooms (muscarine types)
Mydriasis	Anticholinergics, sympathomimetics, cocaine, TCAs, methanol, glutethimide, LSD
Blindness, optic atrophy	Methanol
Fasciculation	Organophosphates
Nystagmus	Diphenylhydantoin, barbiturates, carbamazepine, PCP, carbon monoxide, glutethimide, ethanol
Hypertonus	Anticholinergics, strychnine, phenothiazines
Myoclonus, rigidity	Anticholinergics, phenothiazines, haloperidol
Delirium/psychosis	Anticholinergics, sympathomimetics, alcohol, phenothiazines, PCP, LSD, marijuana, cocaine, heroin, methaqualone, heavy metals
Coma	Alcohols, anticholinergics, sedative hypnotics, narcotics, carbon monoxide, TCAs, salicylates, organophosphates, barbiturates
Weakness, paralysis	Organophosphates, carbamates, heavy metals

GASTROINTESTINAL SYSTEM

Vomiting, diarrhea, abdominal pain	Iron, phosphorus, heavy metals, lithium, mushrooms, fluoride, organophosphates, arsenic

LSD, lysergic acid diethylamide. Adapted from Guzzardi L, Bayer MJ. Emergency management of the poisoned patient. In: Bayer M, Rumack BH, Wanke LA, eds. *Toxicologic Emergencies*. Bowie, MD: Robert J. Brady, 1984.

TABLE 35.5

TOXINS ASSOCIATED WITH CHARACTERISTIC BREATH ODORS

■ TOXIN	■ CHARACTERISTIC ODOR
Acetone	Acetone
Arsenic	Garlic
Camphor	Mothballs
Chloroform	Sweet
Cyanide	Bitter almond
Ethanol	Ethanol
Hydrogen sulfide	Rotten eggs
Isopropanol	Acetone
Methyl salicylate	Wintergreen
Nicotine	Stale tobacco
Organophosphates	Garlic
N-Pyridylmethylnitrophenylurea (Vacor rat poison)	Peanuts
Paraldehyde, chloral hydrate	Pears (urine)
Phenol, cresol	Phenolic
Phosphorus	Garlic
Salicylates	Acetone
Thallium	Garlic
Turpentine	Violets

From Woolf AD. Principles of toxin assessment and screening. In: Fuhrman BP, Zimmerman J, eds. *Pediatric Critical Care*, 3rd ed. Philadelphia, PA: Mosby, Elsevier, 2006:1511–31, with permission.

Laboratory Evaluation

Basic Principles

The laboratory evaluation generally confirms a diagnosis that has already been established on the basis of the history and physical examination. In some circumstances, important decisions about therapy will be made on the basis of quantitative drug or toxin levels in blood specimens. These include acetaminophen, ethanol, methanol, ethylene glycol, lithium, salicylates, iron, lead, mercury, arsenic, phenobarbital, carbon monoxide, methemoglobin, and theophylline. It is extremely important to be aware of the spectrum of toxins screened by individual hospital laboratories. Most laboratories routinely screen for acetaminophen, ethanol, barbiturates, opiates, anticonvulsants, benzodiazepines, phenothiazines, and salicylates. A number of drugs of abuse may be included, specifically, amphetamines, cocaine, and tetrahydrocannabinol. A "negative" toxicology screen does not exclude the possibility of a toxic exposure. Opioids, such as hydrocodone, oxycodone, methadone, fentanyl, meperidine, and propoxyphene, may not be detected by some opiate screening methodology, such as the immunoassay. It is extremely helpful to be specific about identifying toxins of interest so that the laboratory personnel have input into the ideal screening evaluation. In certain instances, toxins may be better detected in urine than in blood. Analysis of gastric contents may be helpful in identifying a particular toxin if collected before absorption is likely. Although comprehensive drug screens and drug levels are often obtained, the results are generally not available in time to effect any initial interventions. Many physicians do not fully understand the limitations of toxicology screens or the implications of positive versus negative results. For example, a urine drug screen may detect the parent drug or metabolites up to a number of days following the use of a drug. It follows that a positive urine drug screen may not necessarily confirm that symptoms are due to the agent identified by the test. A number of immunoassays are poorly sensitive and specific, which

TABLE 35.6

METABOLIC ACIDOSIS [NA – (CL + HCO₃)]: MUDPILES

Methanol
Uremia
Diabetic ketoacidosis
Paraldehyde and phenformin
Isoniazid and iron
Lactic acidosis
Ethanol and ethylene glycol
Salicylates

can lead to false-positive and false-negative results. Consultation with a toxicologist at the regional poison control center (800-222-1222) is helpful in selecting and interpreting test results. The National Institute for Drug Abuse has established the commonly employed "drug of abuse screen" (NIDA-5), which utilizes immunoassay for amphetamines, marijuana, cocaine, opiates, and phencyclidine.

Prioritization of laboratory analysis is directed at the identification of immediately life-threatening situations. It is essential to obtain acetaminophen levels in virtually all poisoned patients to ensure that urgent management can be addressed, if necessary. Prompt determination of blood glucose level should be accomplished in any patient with an altered sensorium.

Anion Gap

Electrolytes and blood urea nitrogen (BUN)/creatinine levels allow for the determination of an anion gap acidosis, basic electrolytes, and the assessment of renal function. The anion gap calculation is

$$Na\ (mEq/L) - [Cl\ (mEq/L) + HCO_3\ (mEq/L)]$$

The normal anion gap is generally 3–16 mEq/L. Agents that cause an elevated anion gap metabolic acidosis are listed in **Table 35.6**.

Electrocardiogram

The 12-lead electrocardiogram is an invaluable tool in the evaluation of potential intoxication, particularly in detecting dysrhythmias and conduction abnormalities, such as widening of the QRS complex or prolongation of the QT interval. Cardiovascular toxicity is a common cause of death that results from antidepressant overdose and can manifest as myocardial depression, ventricular fibrillation, and ventricular tachycardia. The electrocardiogram is useful both in diagnosis and in management.

Urinalysis

Urine color may be helpful in the identification of a number of toxins (**Table 35.7**). It is important to obtain urine pregnancy tests on any female of child-bearing age.

TABLE 35.7

CHARACTERISTIC URINE COLOR CHANGES

Orange to red-orange
Rifampin, deferoxamine, mercury, phenazopyridine, chronic lead poisoning

Pink
Cephalosporins or ampicillin

Brown
Chloroquine or carbon tetrachloride

Green to blue
Amitriptyline

Urinalysis may reveal specific crystals (calcium oxalate crystals in ethylene glycol poisoning) or myoglobinuria. The presence of myoglobinuria is suggestive of rhabdomyolysis, which should be confirmed by determination of serum creatinine phosphokinase. A positive urine ferric chloride test (phenylpyruvic acid) is indicative of a phenothiazine or salicylate overdose.

Blood Gas Analysis

Arterial blood gas analysis is useful for the evaluation of acid–base status, and the addition of co-oximetry can diagnose carboxyhemoglobin, methemoglobinemia, and sulfhemoglobin.

Osmolality

Intoxication with methanol, ethanol, ethylene glycol, acetone, and isopropanol increases serum osmolality. Calculated serum osmolality is determined by the following:

$$2 \times Na\ (mEq/L) + BUN\ (g/L)/2.8 + glucose\ (mg/dL)/18$$

The osmolal gap is evaluated by subtracting the calculated osmolality from the measured osmolality. Normal osmolal gap range is −3 to +6 mOsm/kg H_2O. Conversion factors may be utilized to determine an estimated serum concentration of alcohols and glycols (7). Calculation of the osmolal gap may be confounded by the presence of lipemia or other osmotically active agents often used in the ICU, such as mannitol or contrast for diagnostic imaging procedures.

Ancillary Testing

Additional baseline laboratory evaluation may be particularly prudent in the evaluation of the patient. Complete blood cell count with platelets and leukocyte differential, blood clotting parameters (prothrombin time and partial thromboplastin time), liver function tests, and possible electroencephalogram may prove useful.

Radiologic Imaging

Radiographic evaluation is useful in ingestion of certain foreign bodies, as well as in the instance of a number of radiopaque drugs, metals, and chemicals. In the event of the ingestion of disc batteries, it is necessary to obtain serial chest/abdominal x-rays to document the movement of the foreign body through the GI tract. Radiographic evaluation has identified efforts at drug smuggling via body packing with cocaine-filled containers. Chest and abdominal x-rays are extremely helpful in locating a number of radiopaque pills or tablets and in determining aspiration or pulmonary edema. Pill bezoars may be identified when contrast is utilized for the study. Radiopaque compounds may be grouped by the mnemonic "COINS": chloral hydrate and cocaine packets, opiate packets, iron and heavy metals (lead, arsenic, and mercury), neuroleptics, and sustained-release or enteric-coated tablets.

MANAGEMENT

Toxicology Resources

It is essential to employ all available resources when dealing with a toxic exposure. Numerous resources enable the practitioner to have rapid access to a wealth of information regarding drug identification, pharmacokinetics, drug interactions, and precautions. It is especially important to have a link to resource information for patterns of drug toxicity and current therapies for exposure in the event of chemical terrorism. The regional poison control hotline is a mainstay for reference. Additional

helpful resources are the Poisindex computer database (Micromedex Corporation, Greenwood Village, CO) and Drug Information Centers located in most large medical centers.

Toxicokinetics

Toxicokinetics, or pharmacokinetics in the poisoned patient, can provide important conceptual information to the healthcare provider. As pharmacokinetics differ between adult and pediatric patients, it is vital to consider the differences in order to make appropriate modifications to poisoning treatment recommendations that may have been developed for adult patients. Principles of toxicokinetics focus on the dynamics of the processes of absorption, distribution, metabolism, and elimination of drugs or toxins.

Prevention or limitation of absorption is a mainstay of toxicology. Limiting the time of exposure to a toxin may dramatically reduce toxicity, for example, washing a toxin from the skin or removing a patient from an environment with a toxic gas. Preventing absorption from the GI tract is more complex, as the drug or toxin must dissolve in aqueous gastric fluids and traverse several lipophilic membranes prior to reaching the vascular compartment. Consequently, factors such as pH and pKa of the toxin and lipid solubility of the drug may alter absorption. Timely administration of activated charcoal allows adsorption of the drug or toxin within the GI lumen. Enteric-coated tablets and sustained-release formulations have been designed to delay and sustain the absorption process. Kinetically, this delayed absorption results in an increased time to achieve peak serum concentrations, which prolongs the duration of action of the drug. Whole-bowel irrigation may allow enteric-coated tablets or sustained-release formulations to transit the GI tract before absorption begins. Drugs with complex or slow dissolution or absorption are most amenable to adsorption by activated charcoal.

Distribution is the process of the drug or toxin moving from the intravascular compartment into tissue. Protein binding, pH, and lipophilicity of the drug or toxin impact this process. The volume of distribution (V_d) is equal to the amount of drug in the body divided by the peak concentration of the drug in the blood compartment.

$$V_d = \text{concentration in body/[plasma]}$$

Age-specific volume of distribution for drugs and toxins can be found in the medical literature. The larger the volume of distribution, the more likely the drug will transit from the intravascular compartment into the tissue. Toxins with a large volume of distribution include camphor, antidepressants, digoxin, opioids, phenothiazines, and phencyclidine. Drugs with a small volume of distribution include ethanol, methanol, salicylate, lithium, valproic acid, and phenobarbital. In the event that V_d is <1 L/kg, the drug or toxin can usually be removed by hemodialysis. The volume of distribution formula can also be useful in predicting peak drug or toxin levels when the amount of toxin or drug ingested is known. Some drugs with small V_d, low molecular weight, and limited protein binding that are amenable to removal by hemodialysis include

- Alcohols
- Barbiturates
- Lithium
- Procainamide
- Salicylates
- Theophylline

Protein binding plays an important role in the distribution process. Drugs and toxins that are highly bound to plasma proteins will exist in the intravascular compartment in both the bound and the unbound form. The unbound form of a drug is always the pharmacologically active component.

Albumin and α_1-acid glycoprotein are two of the most common plasma proteins that bind drugs. Drugs that are highly protein bound include carbamazepine, phenytoin, valproic acid, warfarin, and salicylate. Lower levels of plasma proteins result in a proportional increase in the unbound, active form of the drug. For example, phenytoin has a therapeutic range of 10–20 mcg/mL in a patient with a normal albumin level. A patient with a 20% reduction in albumin level may experience toxicity (nystagmus, ataxia, CNS depression) with levels in the normally reported therapeutic range. The dose should be reduced and the therapeutic goal either lowered to 8–16 mcg/mL or based on the free fraction of phenytoin to take into account the effects of protein binding on activity. A free level of 1–2 mcg/mL is generally considered therapeutic. Protein binding is also known to be pH dependent, a principle that is extremely important in the management of tricyclic antidepressant poisoning, as discussed later in this chapter.

Metabolism is an important process of inactivation and elimination that involves a complex array of enzymes that usually improve the water solubility of drugs and their by-products. Among the enzyme systems frequently involved in this process are the cytochrome P-450 monooxygenase enzymes. Many of these enzymes have specific isoenzymes that can be induced (cigarette smoke, omeprazole, rifampin) or inhibited (amiodarone, cimetidine, erythromycin, grapefruit juice, ketoconazole), resulting in toxicity or subtherapeutic levels. Patients with hepatotoxicity or poor hepatic perfusion may exhibit increased drug levels and decreased drug clearance if they are receiving a drug with a high hepatic extraction ratio.

Renal elimination is the most common route of elimination. Many drugs are metabolized in the liver to water-soluble metabolites to be cleared by the kidneys. Renal elimination and glomerular filtration rates parallel, but do not equal, the creatinine clearance. As creatinine clearance decreases and serum creatinine increases, it is likely that the drug and toxin clearance is proportionally reduced. Clearance is a valuable tool in predicting drug half-life and rates of elimination. Clearance (Cl) is equal to the volume cleared of drug/toxin per unit of time, expressed as mL/min or L/h.

$$Cl = \text{excretion rate/steady-state plasma concentration}$$

Clearance at steady state is also proportional to the dose rate, which is ratio of drug dose (mg) to dosing interval (hours).

$$Cl = \text{dose rate/steady-state plasma concentration}$$

The clearance calculation is used to determine how quickly a drug is removed from the body and whether hemodialysis with a known clearance can accelerate the elimination profile.

Decontamination

Principles

Decontamination may be individualized, depending upon the type and route of exposure and the amount of time that elapses from ingestion. The approach to the poisoned patient has evolved significantly over the years. Aggressive gastric decontamination was once the rule of thumb for the management of every child, and syrup of ipecac was routinely prescribed by the general pediatrician as a component of anticipatory guidance.

Syrup of Ipecac

Syrup of ipecac is a derivative of the ipecacuanha plant, the active components of which are emetine and cephaeline. These substances lead to vomiting by means of central chemotactic stimulation and local effects on the gastric mucosa (8). Research has shown that this agent is useful if given within

minutes of ingestion but that the benefit is extremely time limited. Most importantly, clinical evidence has not revealed that syrup of ipecac results in improved patient outcome, even with early administration. Ipecac is contraindicated in the presence of airway compromise; caustic or hydrocarbon ingestion; and symptoms of lethargy, drowsiness, and prolonged vomiting. The American Academy of Clinical Toxicology (AACT) and the European Association of Poisons Centres and Clinical Toxicologists (EAPCCT) issued a firm position statement that "syrup of ipecac should **not** be administered routinely in the management of poisoned patients... its routine administration in the emergency department should be abandoned" (9). This statement has been further supported in a more recent review of the literature relating to syrup of ipecac (10). Literature exists regarding inappropriate utilization of ipecac and lack of efficacy when administered in the home setting (11). The American Academy of Pediatrics issued a position statement that syrup of ipecac no longer be used for routine poisoning treatment at home, which is consistent with the AACT policy (12), and is outlined in current guidelines published by the American Association of Poison Control Centers (13).

Gastric Lavage

Another common method of gastric decontamination had been the utilization of gastric lavage (14). The proper technique of gastric lavage involves the insertion of a large-bore orogastric or nasogastric tube into the stomach, followed by administration and aspiration of fluid, with the intent of recovering newly ingested toxins. This technique can be particularly traumatizing to a young child and is associated with risk in a patient with impaired airway protection. Contraindications to gastric lavage include inadequate upper airway protection, ingestion of corrosive substances or hydrocarbons, and patients at risk for GI perforation or hemorrhage. Complications associated with this technique include pulmonary aspiration, respiratory compromise, mechanical injury/perforation, and electrolyte imbalances (14,15). A position statement from the AACT/EAPCCT stipulates that,

> "...gastric lavage should not be employed routinely in the management of poisoned patients...No evidence suggests that its use improves clinical outcome, and it may cause significant morbidity. [Gastric lavage] should not be considered unless a patient has ingested a potentially life-threatening amount of a poison and the procedure can be undertaken within 60 mins of ingestion. Even then, clinical benefit has not been confirmed in controlled studies (15)."

This position has been reinforced in a position paper looking at previous and newer data (16). Incorrectly performed, gastric lavage places the patient at significant risk for complications and unlikely clinical benefit. For these reasons, use of gastric lavage has progressively declined (1).

Activated Charcoal

Activated charcoal is an efficacious therapy in the management of most poisonings, as it may decrease the absorption of a broad array of toxins (**Table 35.8**). Activated charcoal adsorbs drugs and chemicals by weak Van der Waals forces to prevent GI absorption. Activated charcoal is prepared by superheating highly carbonaceous materials with activating agents (e.g., steam or carbon dioxide) to form a substance with a significant surface area, which provides the basis for its high adsorptive capacity (17). Numerous studies have shown that activated charcoal is very effective as a single agent in achieving gastric decontamination. The adsorptive utility of activated charcoal depends upon how quickly

TABLE 35.8

AGENTS NOT ADSORBED BY CHARCOAL

Common electrolytes
Iron
Mineral acids or bases
Alcohols
Cyanide
Most solvents
Most water-insoluble compounds (hydrocarbons)
Pesticides
Lithium

it can be administered after the toxic ingestion. Activated charcoal was found to reduce the mean bioavailability of drugs by 69.1% when administered within 30 minutes after ingestion. The most recent AACT/EAPCCT policy statement stipulates that,

> "activated charcoal should not be routinely administered in the management of poisoned patients.. the greatest benefit is within one hour of ingestion.. there are insufficient data to support or exclude its use after one hour of ingestion. There is no evidence that the administration of activated charcoal improves clinical outcome (18)."

A more recent review of the literature supports this previous consensus statement and offers no change (19).

Even so, widespread practice has followed the convincing indirect evidence that early administration of activated charcoal is useful in reducing enteric absorption of drugs and toxins (20). It is important to note that the inability of existing studies to show benefit after 1 hour does not exclude a potential benefit of activated charcoal administered 2–3 hours postingestion. Additional studies with larger populations, greater sensitivities, and better-defined endpoints are needed. The generally accepted dose of activated charcoal is based upon in vitro studies, which support a charcoal-to-drug ratio of 10:1. It follows that the usual dosage for unquantified ingestions is 1 g/kg. Activated charcoal is contraindicated in the event of an inadequately protected airway (absent gag reflex or extreme somnolence). If the administration of activated charcoal is indicated in a patient with inadequate airway protection, the patient should first undergo rapid-sequence intubation. Toxic agents that reduce GI motility (tricyclic antidepressants, calcium channel blockers, and opiates) may increase the risk of aspiration of stomach contents.

Activated charcoal preparations may contain sorbitol, a common cathartic. Data are conflicting regarding the administration of the combination of a charcoal-cathartic, and improvement in patient outcomes has not been documented (21). The consensus is that the isolated use of cathartics has no role in the management of the poisoned patient, and a definitive recommendation is lacking regarding the routine use of a cathartic in combination with activated charcoal (21).

Activated charcoal has additional utility when given in multiple doses for substances with prolonged half-lives and small volumes of distribution. Agents amenable to the use of multidose activated charcoal are carbamazepine, dapsone, phenytoin, phenobarbital, quinine, salicylates, and theophylline. The mechanism of action appears to be via the interruption of enterohepatic and enteroenteric recirculation of drugs by sequestration of the drug in the gut lumen due to its concentration gradient. Clinical judgment must be utilized, as the clinical benefits of this therapy have not been proven with controlled studies, and the therapy is contraindicated in the presence of decreased peristalsis or bowel obstruction.

Whole-Bowel Irrigation

The technique of whole-bowel irrigation utilizing osmotically balanced polyethylene glycol electrolyte solutions (PEG-ES) appears attractive, in that it can enhance the elimination of toxins prior to their absorption. A definite theoretical benefit can be gained in aiding elimination following ingestions of heavy metals, iron, sustained-release or enteric-coated tablets, and illegal drug packets. However, definitive clinical recommendations regarding this practice have not been established (22). Recommendations regarding dosing of PEG-ES have proposed target goals of 1500–2000 mL/h in adults, 1000 mL/h in children ages 6–12 years, and 500 mL/h in children 9 months to 6 years of age. Utilization of this technique has no role in the management of patients with an unprotected airway, hemodynamic compromise, intractable vomiting, GI hemorrhage, ileus, perforation, or obstruction (22).

Surgical Decontamination

Emergent surgical GI decontamination may prove useful in rare cases. For example, surgical intervention would be indicated in the event of mechanical bowel obstruction or bowel ischemia due to heroin or cocaine drug packets. Surgical intervention may be an option in the event of massive iron ingestion with failure to evacuate the GI tract.

Antidotes

Antidotal therapy is a vital component of management, as it may prove useful in initiating therapy and in definitively identifying a particular toxin (**Tables 35.9 and 35.10**). However, antidotes are available only for a limited number of toxins and may have potential adverse reactions. It is essential to be familiar with specific antidotes that must be readily available in both the emergency department and the ICU. The crux of management still centers on aggressive supportive care rather than administration of an antidote. Specific toxins and their antidotes as well as modes of enhancing elimination are listed in **Table 35.9**.

Flumazenil is an extremely useful benzodiazepine antagonist that can result in dramatic improvement in a depressed sensorium due to a benzodiazepine overdose. Flumazenil is a 1,4-imidazobenzodiazepine that competes with the benzodiazepines for receptor sites in the CNS that bind γ-aminobutyric acid (GABA), a primary inhibitory neurotransmitter; hence, it is classified as a benzodiazepine receptor antagonist. Flumazenil has a short duration of action; thus, the sedation and respiratory depression may recur after the reversal of long-acting benzodiazepines. The major adverse reactions reported with flumazenil use are seizures and dysrhythmias. Seizures induced by flumazenil are difficult to manage because the benzodiazepine (GABA) receptors are blocked. The association of seizures has occurred in patients who were physically dependent upon benzodiazepines, those utilizing benzodiazepines for control of seizures, those with an underlying seizure disorder, and individuals treated for a combined ingestion of benzodiazepines and tricyclic antidepressants. Flumazenil may be especially helpful in managing a pure benzodiazepine overdose, but should be avoided in unknown overdoses or in mixed ingestions.

The intensivist must be extremely familiar with the utilization of naloxone, an opiate-receptor antagonist that proves particularly useful in effecting rapid reversal of narcotic toxicity. Administration and dosing are discussed in the opioid toxidrome section of this chapter.

One of the most exciting toxicologic advances involves the use of lipid emulsion infusions (LEIs) to reverse cardiotoxicity from lipophilic drugs. First described as the use of 20% intralipid administration to treat arrhythmias secondary to local anesthetic toxicity in the operating room, LEI therapy has been used

TABLE 35.9

SELECTED ANTIDOTES AND METHODS OF ENHANCING TOXIN ELIMINATION

■ ANTIDOTE	■ TOXIN
❺ Antivenoms	
Crotalidae	
Polyvalent (ACP)	North American Pit Viper envenomation
Polyvalent immune Fab	
Micruris sp.	Eastern or Texas coral snake envenomations
Latrodectus mactans	Black widow spider envenomation
Atropine	Organophosphate (OP), carbamate poisoning, bradydysrhythmias, Centruroides envenomation
Calcium (chloride or gluconate)	Calcium channel blocker overdose, hydrofluoric acid ingestion/exposure
Cyanide antidote package	Cyanide, acetonitrile (artificial nail remover), amygdalin (peach, apricot pits),
Amyl nitrite	nitroprusside (thiosulfate only)
Sodium nitrite	
Sodium thiosulfate	
Deferoxamine	Iron
Digoxin-specific antibody fragments	Digoxin, digitoxin, natural cardiac glycosides (e.g., oleander, red squill, Bufo toad venom)
Flumazenil	Benzodiazepines
Fomepizole	Toxic alcohols (ethylene glycol, methanol)
Glucagon	Calcium channel blocker, β-blocker toxicity
Glucose (dextrose)	Sulfonylureas, insulin, hypoglycemia (multiple toxins)
Hydroxocobalamin (vitamin B_{12})[a]	Cyanide, acetonitrile, amygdalin, nitroprusside
Insulin (high dose)/euglycemia[b]	Calcium channel blocker, β-blocker toxicity
Lipid emulsion, 20%	Lipophilic drugs, local anesthetics, calcium channel blocker, β-blocker toxicity
Methylene blue	Methemoglobinemia
N-acetylcysteine	Acetaminophen, pennyroyal oil, carbon tetrachloride
Naloxone	Opioid toxicity
Octreotide	Sulfonylurea toxicity
Physostigmine	Antimuscarinic delirium (as a diagnostic tool only)
Pralidoxime	OP poisoning (insecticides, nerve agents)
Protamine sulfate	Heparins
Pyridoxine	Isoniazid, monomethylhydrazine (rocket fuel), Gyromitra mushrooms
Thiamine	Deficiency states (e.g., alcoholism, anorexia nervosa)
Sodium bicarbonate	Sodium channel blocking cardiotoxins, salicylates

■ METHOD OF REMOVAL	■ INDICATION
Dialysis	Toxic alcohols, salicylates, lithium, theophylline, valproic acid, atenolol, sotalol, others
Urinary alkalinization with sodium bicarbonate	Salicylates, phenobarbital, chlorpropamide, chlorophenoxy herbicides, methotrexate

[a]Not FDA approved for this use.
[b]Anecdotal experience.
From Barry JD. Diagnosis and management of the poisoned child. *Pediatr Ann* 2005;34:937–46, with permission.

with successful results in a wide variety of intoxications (23). The case reports of the use of LEI include intoxications with a variety of calcium channel blockers, β-blockers, and psychiatric medications. A checklist for the use of LEI therapy to treat *local anesthetic systemic toxicity* can be found on the American Society of Regional Anesthesia Web site at www.asra.com/checklist-for-local-anesthetic-toxicity-treatment-1-18-12.pdf.

Extracorporeal Elimination

Aggressive supportive therapies to enhance toxin elimination have included hemoperfusion and hemodialysis (24). Randomized, prospective, controlled studies have not established solid guidelines for the utilization of such therapies. General guidelines have been suggested for circumstances that may warrant such techniques, including progressive clinical deterioration refractory to aggressive supportive care, ingestion and/or absorption of a potentially lethal dose of toxin, blood concentrations that indicate serious intoxication, and impaired organ function that limits the normal route of toxin elimination. Hemodialysis is effective for the removal of small compounds that are concentrated in the intravascular compartment and that are loosely protein bound. Charcoal hemoperfusion is preferred in the instance of toxicity with larger, lipid-soluble compounds with greater affinity for plasma proteins.

Hemodialysis is indicated for the management of severe salicylate and lithium exposures, following toxic exposures to methanol and ethylene glycol, and occasionally when hydrophilic drugs with a low volume of distribution and low protein binding result in severe or life-threatening symptoms and other, less-invasive, therapeutic options are not available. Successful hemodialysis is dependent upon membrane permeability, correlation between the plasma drug concentration and drug toxicity, plasma levels in a potentially fatal range or the presence of a substance with a high likelihood to be metabolized to a toxic substance, and ability to significantly enhance clearance. Consultation with the poison control center and a nephrologist is often helpful in determining whether hemodialysis is indicated. Although distinct theoretical benefits support utilization of extracorporeal therapies in the management of acute intoxications, few intoxicants require these techniques.

Hemoperfusion involves the passage of blood through an extracorporeal circuit and cartridge that contains an adsorbent and return of the detoxified blood to the patient. Using hemoperfusion is advantageous to hemodialysis for selected drugs (e.g., theophylline); however, overdoses of theophylline have become extremely rare. For this reason, few institutions have experience with this technique; cartridges have become difficult to obtain and may be unavailable in many areas. Cartridges may become saturated with the toxin following 2 or more hours of use, which limits effective removal. Generous amounts of heparin are required to prevent the cartridges from clotting due to the adsorption of heparin by the charcoal. One must weigh the risk-benefit ratio of these therapies when considering their use.

Diuresis

Drug elimination may be facilitated by ensuring adequate renal flow of 2–5 mL/kg/h. This brisk diuresis will reduce drug concentration in the distal tubules, reduce the chance of reabsorption, and enhance elimination. Diuresis is occasionally combined with techniques to alter the urinary pH, a principle based upon the premise that reabsorption across the renal tubular epithelium occurs when a compound is nonionized and lipid soluble. The ionized versus nonionized portion of a drug depends upon the pKa of the drug and the pH of the urine or plasma. It is possible to alter the pH of the urine and enhance the proportion of ionized drug, which essentially traps the drug in the tubular lumen, thereby reducing reabsorption and enhancing excretion. Elimination of drugs with pKa in the range of 3.0–7.2 may be enhanced by alkalinizing the urine. Drugs and toxins with which alkalinization of the urine has shown to be effective in enhancing elimination include salicylate, phenobarbital, chlorpropamide, and the chlorophenoxy herbicides. Alkalinization of the urine may be achieved by adding sodium bicarbonate (to a concentration

of 50–75 mEq/L) to the IV fluids. It is imperative to closely follow serum potassium and sodium levels as alkalinization is accomplished. The utilization of aggressive diuresis poses a risk of fluid overload, with resultant cerebral edema, pulmonary edema, or hyponatremia. It is essential to monitor urinary pH and serum sodium, potassium, and acid–base balance during alkalinization therapy.

Several agents are particularly useful to employ as a diagnostic trial in elucidating the presence of a particular toxin (Table 35.10). Specific antibodies have been extremely efficacious in binding to a drug, reversing its toxicity, and enhancing its elimination (e.g., digoxin intoxication, discussed later). Specific antibodies are also commonly used for the treatment of viper and cobra envenomations.

TOXIDROMES

The physical examination may lend itself to the association of a constellation of signs associated with particular substances or groups of substances, most commonly referred to as toxidromes. Elucidating a toxidrome is dependent on careful review of vital signs, mental status, pupillary size and reactivity, skin characteristics (moisture, temperature, and color), bowel sounds, muscle tone, respiratory effort, and the presence of tremors. The following review of toxidromes is meant to provide a descriptive overview, with tables for rapid reference. Further in-depth discussion may be sought in medical toxicology references.

Sympathomimetic/Adrenergic Agents

Common sympathomimetic adrenergic agents are listed in Table 35.11. Signs and symptoms of sympathomimetic toxicity (Table 35.12) are dependent upon the target receptor sites. Tachycardia and hypotension due to the stimulatory and vasodilatory effects of β-agonists are common, while α-agonists are associated with severe hypertension and reflex bradycardia. Sympathetic effects may be rendered by direct adrenergic stimulation or via indirect action through release of norepinephrine. Hyperthermia, rhabdomyolysis, and myoglobinuria are attributed to increased metabolic activity. Myocardial

TABLE 35.10

USEFUL DIAGNOSTIC TRIALS

■ AGENT SUSPECTED	■ AGENT ADMINISTERED	■ DOSE	■ COMMENTS
Benzodiazepines	Flumazenil	0.01 mg/kg IV prn (maximum total dose: 1 mg)	Risk of seizures. Contraindicated for TCA overdose
Insulin reaction (hypoglycemia)	Dextrose	0.25 g/kg IV (10% Dextrose 2.5 mL/kg IV; repeat if serum glucose <60 mg/dL)	Use central venous line for 25% or 50% dextrose
Iron	Deferoxamine	40 mg/kg IM QD (maximum: 1 g/day if no transfusion)	Risk of shock with IV use
Isoniazid	Pyridoxine	70 mg/kg IV (maximum 5 g)	Seizures abate; improved consciousness
Opiates	Naloxone hydrochloride	0.03–0.1 mg/kg/dose IM/IV q 3 min (up to 4 mg)	Use 0.003–0.01 mg/kg/dose in postoperative patient to avoid sudden acute pain
Organophosphate	Atropine	0.05–0.1 mg/kg/dose IV/IM	May repeat q 10 min until muscarinic symptoms resolved
Phenothiazine (dystonia)	Diphenhydramine	1–2 mg/kg/dose IV/IM (maximum 25 mg)	Contraindicated in children <2 y.o.
Phenothiazine (neuroleptic malignant syndrome)	Dantrolene	1–3 mg/kg/dose IV (maximum 10 mg/kg/day)	Continue for 3–5 days. Use slow taper if signs of relapse.

TABLE 35.11

SYMPATHOMIMETIC AGENTS

Albuterol
Amphetamines
Caffeine
Catecholamines
Cocaine
Ephedrine
Ketamine
LSD
Methamphetamine
PCP
Phenylephrine
Phenylpropanolamine
Pseudoephedrine
Terbutaline
Theophylline

ischemia may occur, as well as ischemic or hemorrhagic stroke. This classification generally includes the amphetamines, cocaine, ephedrine, pseudoephedrine, phenylpropanolamine, and other adrenergic stimulants. The methylxanthines, caffeine and theophylline, are not sympathomimetics, but may result in similar symptomatology.

Benzodiazepines are useful in reducing CNS catecholamine release and thereby are effective in controlling severe hypertension, tachycardia, agitation, and extreme muscle activity. It is essential to recognize that use of a β-blocking agent to control tachycardia and hypertension may result in unopposed α-receptor stimulation. For this reason, β-blockers are best avoided, and a benzodiazepine alone or with nitroprusside or phentolamine should be used when control of hypertension and tachycardia becomes necessary. Hypoglycemia and hyperthermia may be present and require specific treatment. Cocaine toxicity can result in depletion of catecholamines (see below), which may cause late cardiovascular collapse. It follows that short-acting antihypertensive agents are preferred for treating these overdoses.

The sympathomimetic toxidrome is not seen with toxicity owing to such centrally acting α-agonists as clonidine. These agents result in decreased sympathetic outflow and cause reflex bradycardia, hypotension, and CNS and respiratory depression.

Cholinergic Agents

Toxins and poisons that increase the effect of the cholinergic nervous system are classified as cholinergic agonists. These substances include muscarinic agents, nicotinic agents, and cholinesterase inhibitors (**Table 35.13**). Muscarinic agents act

TABLE 35.12

SYMPATHOMIMETIC TOXIDROME

Agitation
Seizures
Mydriasis
Tachycardia
Hypertension
Diaphoresis
Pallor
Cool skin
Fever

TABLE 35.13

CHOLINERGIC TOXIDROME FEATURES

Muscarinic effects (DUMBBELLS)
  Diarrhea
  Urinary incontinence
  Miosis
  Bradycardia
  Bronchorrhea
  Emesis
  Lacrimation
  Salivation

Nicotinic effects
  Fasciculations
  Weakness
  Paralysis
  Tachycardia
  Hypertension
  Agitation

Central effects
  Lethargy
  Coma
  Agitation
  Seizures

at postganglionic, parasympathetic nerve endings and in sweat glands. The direct acting muscarinic agonists result in excessive parasympathetic activity. Nicotinic agents act at sympathetic and parasympathetic autonomic ganglia. Cholinesterase inhibitors result in an accumulation of acetylcholine at the cholinergic synapse.

This toxidrome is effectively managed with atropine. Nicotine is known to cause salivation, nausea, and vomiting. Tachycardia, hypertension, and tachypnea are generally followed by bradycardia, hypotension, and respiratory failure. Central effects include initial agitation, followed by seizures, lethargy, coma, and possible neuromuscular blockade. Management of nicotine poisoning is accomplished with aggressive supportive care.

Organophosphate pesticides and nerve agents are examples of cholinesterase inhibitors. It is possible to have a mixed toxicity, but parasympathetic toxicity is most commonly seen. The mechanism of action of organophosphate toxicity occurs by the binding and inactivation of acetylcholinesterase, with a subsequent excess of nicotinic and muscarinic activity in the peripheral system and CNS. The preponderance of acetylcholine results in depolarization of the neuromuscular junction. The enzyme is eventually phosphorylated, and cholinesterase activity resumes following synthesis of new enzyme. Carbamates, which are also used as pesticides, reversibly bind to acetylcholinesterase and ultimately undergo spontaneous hydrolysis, which results in restoration of cholinesterase activity within hours. The central manifestations of carbamate toxicity are less severe, as they do not easily penetrate the CNS. The symptoms of organophosphate toxicity depend upon the route, duration of exposure, and the absorbed dose. Dermal exposure results in local hyperhidrosis, which is followed by systemic involvement as the drug is absorbed.

Topical decontamination with utilization of personal protective equipment is essential. Inhalational exposure is marked by upper airway involvement and subsequent respiratory distress. Vomiting and drooling are most commonly seen following ingestion. Fatality is usually attributed to respiratory failure that results from bronchorrhea, bronchospasm, diminished respiratory drive, and neuromuscular blockade. Seizures and severe CNS toxicity occur following large exposures to household products or small exposures to industrial pesticides and "nerve agents."

Management of organophosphate toxicity involves expeditious administration of atropine to reverse the muscarinic effects, an oxime (Pralidoxime) to facilitate reactivation of acetylcholinesterase, which reverses the neuromuscular blockade, and benzodiazepines to control seizures. Atropine administration is guided by the effect of drying secretions rather than by heart rate or pupil size. Pralidoxime is not generally administered in the case of carbamate toxicity, because the carbamates bind to acetylcholinesterase; consequently, the effects are self-limited.

A caveat of rapid-sequence intubation in the management of organophosphate poisoning involves the potential for prolonged paralysis if succinylcholine is used, because its half-life is prolonged by the organophosphate-induced inhibition of cholinesterase production.

Anticholinergic Agents

Agents that produce antimuscarinic properties (Table 35.14) result in a constellation of symptoms and signs referred to as the anticholinergic toxidrome (Table 35.15). These agents act at muscarinic receptors of the CNS, targeting organs of the parasympathetic nervous system and the sympathetic nervous system (the sweat glands). This toxidrome is extremely similar to the sympathomimetic toxidrome, but may be distinguished by examination of the mucous membranes and skin and by auscultation for bowel sounds. Sympathomimetic toxicity results in diaphoresis and cool skin, whereas anticholinergic toxicity is notoriously marked by impaired sweating and warm, dry skin. Sympathomimetics result in hyperactive bowel sounds, whereas anticholinergics cause diminished bowel sounds and even ileus. Tachycardia, mydriasis, urinary retention, flushing, and hyperthermia are found with both sympathomimetic and anticholinergic toxicity. Hypertension also occurs with both sympathomimetic and anticholinergic exposures; however, it is generally less severe with anticholinergic toxicity than with sympathomimetic toxicity.

Management must focus on controlling agitation to minimize hyperthermia in the face of impaired sweating mechanisms. Benzodiazepines may be extremely helpful in managing symptoms. Physostigmine, a cholinesterase inhibitor, may be employed with the intent of reversing central and peripheral manifestations of the anticholinergic toxidrome; however, it is not recommended for management of tricyclic antidepressant toxicity because of reported convulsions and asystole.

TABLE 35.14

ANTICHOLINERGIC AGENTS

Antihistamines—diphenhydramine, hydroxyzine
Atropine
Benztropine mesylate
Carbamazepine
Cyclic antidepressants
Cyclobenzaprine
Hyoscyamine
Jimsonweed
Oxybutynin
Phenothiazines
Scopolamine
Trihexyphenidyl

TABLE 35.15

ANTICHOLINERGIC TOXIDROME

Agitation
Delirium
Coma
Mydriasis
Dry mouth
Warm, dry, flushed skin
Tachycardia
Hypertension
Fever
Urinary retention
Decreased bowel sounds

Associated expressions
"Mad as a Hatter"
"Blind as a Bat"
"Red as a Beet"
"Hot as a Hare"
"Dry as a Bone"

Opioid Agents

Agents that result in the opioid toxidrome are classified as opiates (substances derived from opium) and opioids (substances derived from opium and synthetically derived agents with similar properties). These terms are used interchangeably, as the pharmacologic effects are similar. Most opioids and opiates cause a triad of respiratory depression, coma, and miosis. An exception is meperidine toxicity, which manifests as respiratory depression, coma, *mydriasis*, and *seizures*. Physical findings of opioid toxicity often include bradycardia, hypotension, and decreased GI motility. Diphenoxylate and methadone present a particular hazard to toddlers owing to low-dose ingestions (25).

Management involves administration of naloxone, an opiate-receptor antagonist that results in rapid reversal of toxicity. Naloxone is generally initiated at 0.1 mg/kg/dose IV in children and 1–2 mg/dose in adolescents and adults to achieve reversal of respiratory depression. If a partial response is observed, up to 10 mg may be necessary. Alternate administration can be accomplished by a variety of routes: subcutaneous, intramuscular, and endotracheal. It is critical to note that administration of naloxone may precipitate an acute withdrawal syndrome in opiate-dependent patients. If opiate dependency is suspected, it is prudent to initiate therapy with lower doses. The duration of action of naloxone is shorter than the action of many opiates; therefore, it is essential to strongly consider subsequent dosing or administration of a continuous infusion. Naloxone has been associated with the development of pulmonary edema, although this condition may occur as a result of opiate toxicity (26). Nalmefene is a longer-acting opiate-receptor antagonist; its administration should be preceded by a test dose of naloxone to rule out the possibility of acute withdrawal (27). Nalmefene is not thought to carry significant advantages, as compared with a continuous naloxone infusion.

Clonidine is a centrally acting α-agonist that is often included in the opiate toxidrome owing to the diminished sympathetic tone, its ability to cause miosis and CNS and respiratory depression in overdose, and its occasional reversal with naloxone. Controversy exists regarding the utilization of naloxone in clonidine toxicity. In the event of respiratory failure, aggressive supportive care mandates initiation of airway management prior to the administration of naloxone.

Many opiates (e.g., codeine, hydrocodone, oxycodone, and propoxyphene) are formulated in combination with acetaminophen or aspirin. Therefore, it is extremely important to maintain a high index of suspicion for combined toxicity from such compounds. Fentanyl patches contain a high concentration of drug per patch; significant toxicity can result from ingestion or inhalation.

FOCUSED REVIEW OF COMMON TOXINS

It is beyond the scope of a textbook of pediatric critical care medicine to do justice to the field of toxicology in attempting to review specific pharmacology, pathophysiology, clinical manifestations, and management for each toxin. The earlier discussion was designed to provide a succinct, common sense approach to dealing with a poisoned child or adolescent. These tools will guide the practitioner in locating appropriate resources and adeptly stabilizing the patient. The following section will review a number of the most commonly seen toxins in the emergency department that require subsequent care in the ICU.

Acetaminophen

Acetaminophen is the most commonly ingested drug in intentional overdoses. It presents a significant concern owing to its toxicity, which can result in fulminant hepatic failure. An understanding of the pharmacokinetics of acetaminophen metabolism is essential to developing a management plan. Acetaminophen is metabolized in the liver by glucuronidation and sulfation-forming nontoxic metabolites that are renally excreted. In the event of an overdose, metabolism via the CYP2E1, CYP1A2, and CYP3A4 subfamilies of the cytochrome P-450 pathway produces N-acetyl-p-benzoquinoneimine (NAPQI), which conjugates with reduced glutathione (28). Glutathione is depleted in a significant overdose, which allows the toxic intermediate NAPQI to bind to the hepatocytes and cause cell death. This metabolite is detoxified by reduced glutathione when acetaminophen is taken in appropriate doses. Excessive doses of acetaminophen completely overwhelm the liver's ability to detoxify NAPQI, which results in hepatic necrosis (Fig. 35.1).

The clinical manifestations of acetaminophen intoxication are commonly described in four stages. The initial presentation is usually the development of nausea and vomiting within 12–24 hours of ingestion, although some patients are asymptomatic (Stage I). This is clearly a reason to screen for acetaminophen levels in all ingestions. Acidosis may be present in extreme overdoses. The liver transaminases usually elevate by 24 hours following ingestion (Stage II), at which time clinical symptoms often abate. Liver function abnormalities peak at 48–72 hours following ingestion, and symptoms return with nausea, vomiting, and anorexia (Stage III). The clinical course may result in complete recovery or fulminant hepatic failure. The recovery phase (Stage IV) generally lasts ~7–8 days. It is important to know that cases of fulminant hepatic failure with jaundice, encephalopathy, and bleeding occur infrequently. The most efficacious therapy involves the administration of N-acetylcysteine (NAC), which serves as a precursor to facilitate the synthesis of glutathione or to directly conjugate with and detoxify the reactive metabolite NAPQI (Fig. 35.1). Initiation of NAC is usually recommended within 10 hours following ingestion; however, it has been beneficial when administered up to 24 hours following ingestion. Timely utilization of NAC has been proven to reduce the incidence of hepatotoxicity.

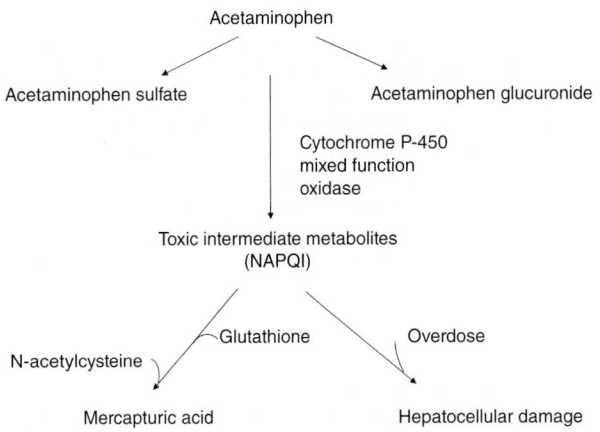

FIGURE 35.1. The intermediate metabolite NAPQI is responsible for hepatic injury associated with acetaminophen toxicity; it is ordinarily detoxified by the addition of sulfhydryl groups. Glutathione acts as a sulfhydryl group donor, but, in massive overdose, it is not present in sufficient quantity to protect the liver. N-acetylcysteine acts as a sulfhydryl group donor to detoxify NAPQI when glutathione is depleted.

A decision to employ this therapy is based upon application of the Rumack–Matthew nomogram (29) (Fig. 35.2) in plotting a serum level of acetaminophen drawn at least 4 hours following ingestion. In the event that blood levels are not immediately available, treatment decisions should be based upon a suggestive history. The therapy can be stopped if a nontoxic

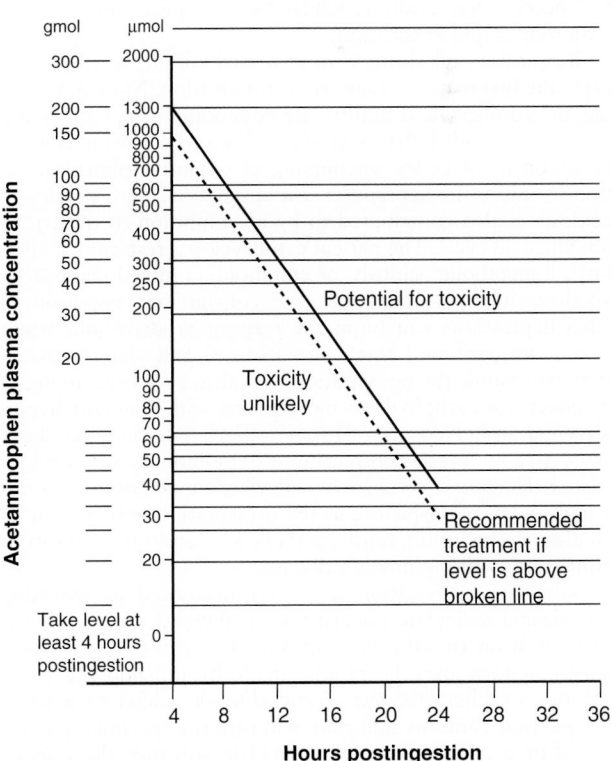

FIGURE 35.2. Use of nomogram in management of acute acetaminophen overdose. Acetaminophen level is obtained at ≥4 hours after ingestion. Level is then plotted on nomogram. Above the broken line = administer full course of acetylcysteine. Below the broken line = acetylcysteine not necessary.

level is eventually obtained. Oral dosing of NAC begins with a loading dose of 140 mg/kg, followed by maintenance therapy of 70 mg/kg every 4 hours for 17 doses. Therapy should continue until all doses are administered, even though the acetaminophen plasma level drops below the toxic range. NAC can also be administered IV in a 20-hour protocol. Initially, the patient receives a 150-mg/kg loading dose over 15 minutes, followed by 50 mg/kg over 4 hours, and then 100 mg/kg over the final 16 hours. Care must be taken to ensure that the NAC is appropriately diluted and that the patient does not become fluid overloaded.

Salicylates

It is essential that physicians in the PICU are aware of the many forms of salicylates. Acetylsalicylic acid, or aspirin, is the most commonly encountered form, but bismuth subsalicylate, sodium salicylate, and magnesium salicylate are often encountered in various drugs. Aspirin is contained in a wide variety of medications, including antihistamines, sympathomimetics, anticholinergics, opiates, and acetaminophen. Oil of wintergreen, comprised of 98% methyl salicylate, is a particularly dangerous compound. Another less commonly considered mode of intoxication occurs via exposure to topical aspirin-containing compounds that are ingested or absorbed cutaneously. In general, doses of <100 mg/kg produce minimal toxicity; however, doses that exceed 300 mg/kg can result in catastrophic clinical symptoms and often prove deadly. Aspirin with a pKa of 3.5 exists largely in the nonionized, insoluble form in the stomach. A low gastric pH causes most of the aspirin to remain in the nonionized form; hence, it dissolves inefficiently. If a patient has been taking an H_2 antagonist, a proton-pump inhibitor, or antacids, the pH of the stomach will become less acidotic, rendering the aspirin more soluble with more rapid absorption.

Respiratory alkalosis, with increased minute ventilation, is often the first feature of salicylate intoxication. Nausea, vomiting, dehydration, and tinnitus are commonly seen. CNS manifestations include lethargy, coma, and seizures. The mechanism of action involves the uncoupling of oxidative phosphorylation, resulting in hyperpyrexia and acidosis. The severity of acidosis is also contributed to by an inhibition of the tricarboxylic acid cycle. The patient can develop a respiratory alkalosis, a metabolic acidosis, or commonly a mixed respiratory alkalosis–metabolic acidosis. The concomitant ingestion of CNS depressants can blunt the respiratory drive and result in a more profound metabolic acidosis. Salicylate intoxication may mimic the presentation of diabetes mellitus owing to its effects on carbohydrate metabolism, with resultant hyperglycemia and glycosuria. Chronic salicylate toxicity has been associated with fatal complications of pulmonary and cerebral edema. Diagnosis of chronic salicylate intoxication requires a high index of suspicion, as the presentation may appear as an altered sensorium, sepsis, diabetic ketoacidosis, respiratory failure, or cardiopulmonary disease.

Salicylate intoxication is quickly diagnosed by assessing the plasma salicylate concentration, thereby measuring the concentration of salicylic acid and its metabolites. Preliminary diagnosis may be rapidly made by utilizing the ferric chloride or Phenistix test. Ferric chloride added to a urine sample that contains salicylate will turn the specimen purple. Blood or urine that contains salicylate will turn the Phenistix brown. Determination of serum salicylate levels should be made 2 and 6 hours following ingestion of immediate-release preparations. In the event of a significant overdose or ingestion of enteric-coated tablets, it is important to monitor levels every 2–4 hours to establish a peak level. Levels should be monitored for at least 24 hours in the event of an ingestion

of sustained-release or enteric-coated capsules due to erratic absorption.

Targeted therapy in salicylate ingestion includes the early use of activated charcoal to prevent absorption and the alkalinization of the urine to enhance elimination. Meticulous monitoring of urine pH is necessary to avoid significant alkalemia. Acetazolamide is not utilized to achieve an alkaline diuresis, as it results in a systemic metabolic acidosis. Hemodialysis is effective, and is recommended for extremely elevated serum salicylate levels (>100 mg/dL), presence of renal insufficiency, significant volume overload, pulmonary edema, or severe electrolyte aberrations. The benefit of hemodialysis is the ability to achieve rapid correction of fluid and electrolyte abnormalities, correct acid–base disturbances, and enhance salicylate clearance.

Alcohols

Ethanol

Not surprisingly, ethanol is the most commonly ingested alcohol and poses a hazard not only in beverage form, but also in a variety of other products in which it is contained, such as mouthwash, perfume, cologne, and topical antiseptics. Children may present with nausea, vomiting, stupor, and ataxia. Infants and toddlers may dramatically develop coma, hypothermia, and hypoglycemia when ethanol levels exceed 50–100 mg/dL. Metabolic acidosis is typically found. Adolescents tend to have more typical signs of intoxication with levels of 100–150 mg/dL. Deaths directly attributed to alcohol ingestion are usually associated with alcohol concentrations >500 mg/dL. An ingestion of ~1 g/kg of ethanol will raise the blood alcohol level to 100 mg/dL. The following estimates of toxicity may be extrapolated: beer (5% alcohol), 10–15 mL/kg; wine (14% alcohol), 4–6 mL/kg; and 80-proof liquor (40% alcohol), 1–2 mL/kg. Binge drinking has been a catastrophic activity of adolescents and college students.

Emergent assessment and management of potential respiratory compromise is a priority, as is rapid blood glucose determination. Ethanol is rapidly absorbed from the GI tract, so that GI decontamination is rarely necessary. However, in adolescents, activated charcoal is useful owing to a significant risk of a coingestion.

The metabolism of alcohol by the hepatic enzyme alcohol dehydrogenase is dose dependent. In general, the rate of reduction is reported to range from 10 to 25 mg/dL/h. Hemodialysis may increase the rate of elimination significantly, but is rarely necessary. Patients with impaired liver function or significant toxicity (levels >450–500 mg/dL) may be candidates for hemodialysis.

Isopropyl Alcohol

Isopropyl alcohol is a component of many home products, including rubbing alcohol, aftershave lotions, perfumes, skin lotions, and antifreeze compounds. Young children are at risk for accidental ingestion, whereas adolescents may utilize the products as an ethanol substitute. Ingestion is typically the most common route, but infants may be poisoned via inhalation of isopropyl vapors during sponging for a fever. The toxic dose is reported to be 1 mL/kg of 70% isopropyl alcohol; ingestion of more than a swallow is potentially toxic in children. Toxicity is manifested by vomiting, abdominal pain, and, often, hematemesis due to gastritis. Neurologic manifestations include lethargy, dizziness, ataxia, and coma. Patients who have ingested isopropyl alcohol may have the unusual findings of ketosis and ketonemia without an acidemia. Isopropyl alcohol is metabolized to acetone. Children are at extreme risk for hypoglycemia. Ethanol, fomepizole, and hemodialysis are usually not indicated in the management of isopropyl alcohol intoxication.

Methanol and Ethylene Glycol

Methanol and ethylene glycol are toxic alcohols most commonly found in antifreeze compounds, and both are known to cause CNS depression. The substances are metabolized by alcohol dehydrogenase, which results in extremely toxic metabolites. Methanol is metabolized to formic acid, which causes severe metabolic acidosis and retinal toxicity. Ethylene glycol is ultimately metabolized to oxalate, which results in severe metabolic acidosis, hypocalcemia, and renal failure.

Ingestions that exceed 0.5 mL/kg may result in significant toxicity, and ingestions >1 mL/kg may prove to be fatal. Determination of an elevated osmolal gap is helpful, as these compounds are osmotically active and may raise the measured serum osmolality. The presence of a normal osmolal gap (<10 mOsm/kg H_2O) does not exclude significant levels of toxic alcohols. Toxicity may be documented with serum levels of the parent compounds; however, in the event of a late presentation, levels may be undetectable following complete metabolism. The laboratory hallmarks of ethylene glycol and methanol poisoning are a high–anion-gap metabolic acidosis and an elevated osmolal gap.

The cornerstone of management has been aimed at blocking alcohol dehydrogenase to negate the formation of the toxic metabolites. Although ethanol has been utilized, it is fraught with difficulties in titration, as well as side effects of inebriation, CNS depression, hypoglycemia, and hypotension. Fomepizole has become the accepted drug of choice in blocking alcohol dehydrogenase. Following the administration of fomepizole, the parent alcohol compounds are renally excreted: methanol with a half-life of 54 hours and ethylene glycol with a half-life of 19.7 hours. Thiamine and pyridoxine should be administered IV every 6 hours to patients who have ingested ethylene glycol. Thiamine has been shown to stimulate the conversion of glyoxylate to α-hydroxy-β-ketoadipate, and pyridoxine stimulates the conversion of glyoxylate to nontoxic glycine. Both of these may theoretically reduce metabolism to oxalic acid and calcium oxalate; however, evidence-based benefits have not been established. Folic acid should be given to patients who have ingested methanol, as it has been shown in animals to speed the metabolism of formic acid to carbon dioxide (30). Hemodialysis is recommended in the instance of high levels of methanol or ethylene glycol, especially with concomitant metabolic acidosis, electrolyte abnormalities, and renal impairment of visual disturbance.

Caustics

The ingestion of caustic compounds requires an understanding of the differing pathophysiologic principles between alkaline and acid products. Alkaline injury results from a liquefaction necrosis caused by saponification of cellular fats and protein degradation. This process quickly results in very deep injury, mostly involving the oropharynx and proximal esophagus. Affected tissue often turns a white-gray color (saponification necrosis) and becomes friable and structurally unstable. Perforation is common with a severe exposure. Automatic dishwasher detergents possess extremely high alkalinity and are thought to be the most dangerous detergent in most households (31).

Acid ingestion results in a superficial coagulation necrosis, with marked heat production and eschar formation. Ingested acid is often absorbed, resulting in metabolic acidosis, hemolysis, and renal failure. The coagulative necrosis seen with acid

ingestions often involves the length of the esophagus, extending into the stomach. Injury potential is dependent upon the type of chemicals involved, the quantity and concentration, duration of contact, liquid versus solid, diluents present, and the vulnerability of the tissues affected.

Caustic ingestions pose risk to the GI tract and may result in respiratory damage. Significant caustic ingestions are marked by nausea, vomiting, oropharyngeal plaques, burns, tissue edema, dysphagia, drooling, and refusal to eat or drink. The clinical presentation may involve generalized systemic signs, including hyperpyrexia, respiratory distress, hemodynamic instability, hypocalcemia (with hydrofluoric acid ingestion), and metabolic acidosis (with acidic ingestion). Perforation may be marked by abdominal pain, subcutaneous emphysema, pneumothorax, pneumomediastinum, or peritonitis.

Management of the caustic toxin involves aggressive decontamination, with washing and diluting of dermal or ocular exposures, fresh air and oxygen for inhalational injury, and removal of as much substance from the mouth as possible in the ingestion of a caustic solid. The pH of the ocular fluids should be determined following irrigation to ensure neutralization of caustics; normal pH of tears is 7. Alkali eye exposures mandate an urgent ophthalmologic consult. Serial radiographs are utilized to track swallowed button batteries. Button batteries lodged in the esophagus must be expeditiously removed; those in the stomach or intestines generally pass intact.

If the patient can immediately drink a small amount of water or milk, it may help to reduce esophageal injury by washing the caustic into the stomach. Damage following the ingestion of a liquid occurs within seconds to minutes, offering little opportunity to dilute the toxin. After the immediate phase, when tissue damage is occurring, dilution of the ingested caustic is not recommended because of the limited possibility for benefit and the greater potential for harm due to perforation or even pulmonary aspiration. Tissue damage may continue for a slightly longer period when a solid caustic agent has been ingested. Additionally, with the anticipation of sedation for diagnostic endoscopy, the patient must remain with an empty stomach. Neutralization of a caustic substance is contraindicated, as the resultant exothermic reaction can yield more extensive tissue destruction. Ipecac, gastric lavage, and activated charcoal are not indicated. Endoscopy is recommended within the first 24 hours following ingestion to quantify actual tissue damage. Risk of perforation is significant if endoscopy is delayed over 48 hours owing to loss of tissue integrity. The role of steroids has been controversial in reducing inflammation, granulation, and stricture formation. Steroids may be indicated in the event of laryngeal edema and bronchospasm. Antibiotics have no role in the absence of documented bacterial involvement or an existing secondary infection. Patients must be monitored for complications of mediastinitis, pneumonitis, and peritonitis.

Iron

Iron exists in a variety of salts that contain differing proportions of elemental iron. Doses of elemental iron that exceed 20 mg/kg generally cause GI irritation. Systemic toxicity usually does not occur unless the elemental iron dose exceeds 60 mg/kg. The first phase of iron intoxication usually occurs within 30 minutes of ingestion and is marked by vomiting, diarrhea, and possible hematemesis or hematochezia. This stage may require aggressive fluid resuscitation because of profound fluid and electrolyte losses. The latent period, or second phase, is heralded by a resolution of the GI manifestations, but the patient continues to have nonspecific malaise. Tachycardia may be present following the previous fluid derangements, and metabolic acidosis may develop. The third phase occurs 12 hours following ingestion and is manifested by profound hemodynamic instability and shock. The fourth phase results in liver failure. Scarring or strictures of the GI tract may occur owing to the corrosive effect of the iron. It is highly unusual to be faced with systemic iron toxicity without the prodromal GI symptoms.

Iron toxicity warrants serious consideration of GI lavage or whole-bowel irrigation because it is not effectively adsorbed by charcoal. Whole-bowel irrigation is effective in decreasing iron absorption and is helpful in breaking up pill concretions that can result in direct mucosal injury. The coalescence of iron tablets in the stomach or duodenum has resulted in hemorrhagic infarction, with subsequent perforation, peritonitis, and death. A moderate risk of pyloric stenosis or bowel stenosis may present at 4–6 weeks following ingestion.

Serum iron levels should be determined within 6 hours of ingestion. If the patient remains asymptomatic by 6 hours following ingestion, it is highly unlikely that systemic illness will develop. Metabolic acidosis or acidemia correlates with toxicity. A white blood cell count >15,000/mm^3 with a serum glucose level >150 mg/dL may sometimes be found and may have some predictive value of elevated serum iron levels. Deferoxamine chelation (continuous infusion of 15 mg/kg/h IV) is indicated for serum iron levels >500 mcg/dL or in the event of hemodynamic collapse. Deferoxamine must be administered with caution for multiple reasons. It is derived from *Streptomyces pilosus*, and so some patients exhibit allergic reactions. If deferoxamine is administered too rapidly, it causes hypotension, and in adults, if greater than 6–8 g is administered in 24 hours, pulmonary fibrosis can occur. If symptoms appear refractory to management following 24 hours of chelation therapy, it is recommended to decrease the deferoxamine infusion in view of its association with development of acute respiratory distress syndrome. Chelation therapy is continued until the serum iron level returns to normal, the metabolic acidosis resolves, the patient clinically improves, and the urine color returns to normal. Determination of total iron-binding capacity is not useful in acute management, as the presence of free iron interferes with the assay, which results in a falsely elevated reading of total iron-binding capacity.

Critical care management must focus on the potential for cardiopulmonary failure with profound hypotension, extreme metabolic acidosis, hypo- or hyperglycemia, anemia and colloid losses due to GI hemorrhage, renal failure secondary to shock, and hepatic failure, which exacerbates the bleeding diathesis. Brisk urine output is essential for the excretion of the iron–deferoxamine complex.

Asphyxiants

Carbon Monoxide

Carbon monoxide poisoning is a major factor in deaths related to fire, but exposure may occur owing to the incomplete combustion of any carbon-containing fuel (natural gas, fuel oil, gasoline, propane, or charcoal). Such poisonings are often reported with improperly vented wood- or coal-burning stoves and from an inadequately ventilated automobile exhaust pipe. Carbon monoxide exposure results in significant tissue hypoxia owing to the extremely high binding affinity with hemoglobin (200–300 times that of oxygen) and a leftward shift and change in shape (hyperbolic configuration) of the oxyhemoglobin dissociation curve. Carbon monoxide also binds to cytochrome oxidase and interferes with electron transport and adenosine triphosphate production. Definitive diagnosis is made by co-oximetry and determination of the carboxyhemoglobin level. Frequently reported signs and symptoms are associated with a specific level of carboxyhemoglobin (**Table 35.16**); however, exact correlation between carboxyhemoglobin levels and symptomatology is often lacking. It is important to recognize that the blood carboxyhemoglobin levels will fall rapidly and may not truly reflect the degree of cellular dysfunction. Transcutaneous measurement of oxygen saturation by pulse oximetry will be falsely normal, as pulse oximetry cannot differentiate oxyhemoglobin from carboxyhemoglobin.

The mainstay of therapy is directed at removing the patient from the source of contamination and expeditious delivery of

TABLE 35.16

CARBON MONOXIDE INHALATION

CARBOXYHEMOGLOBIN LEVEL	INTOXICATION CLASSIFICATION	SYMPTOMS
5%		Impaired judgment Altered fine motor skills
20%	Mild	Headache Dyspnea Visual changes Confusion
30%	Moderate	Drowsiness, dulled sensorium Faintness Nausea/vomiting Tachycardia
40%–60%	Moderate–Severe	Weakness Poor coordination Loss of recent memory Impending cardiovascular and neurologic collapse
>60%	Severe	Coma Convulsion Death

TABLE 35.17

HALF-LIFE OF CARBOXYHEMOGLOBIN

■ OXYGEN CONCENTRATION	■ T 1/2
21%	5 h
100% (mask, ET)	90 min
Hyperbaric oxygen, 2–3 atm	30 min

ET, endotracheal.

100% oxygen. The half-life of carboxyhemoglobin is dependent upon the mode of delivery of varying oxygen concentrations (Table 35.17). Hyperbaric oxygen therapy is particularly useful in extreme cases, because it both dramatically decreases the concentration of carboxyhemoglobin and accelerates the removal of carbon monoxide from cytochrome oxidase. A caveat in consideration of hyperbaric oxygen therapy is the lack of pediatric clinical trials; it follows that utilization of hyperbaric oxygenation is controversial. However, strong consideration should be given to early consultation with a hyperbaric oxygen therapy facility for patients who have experienced loss of consciousness or syncope or who continue to exhibit neurologic symptoms while receiving oxygen therapy. Hyperbaric therapy has no role if such a transfer would compromise patient stabilization and the accessibility/capability for providing intensive care management. Complications associated with hyperbaric therapy include barotrauma (pneumomediastinum, pneumothorax, and tympanic membrane rupture), oxygen toxicity (seizures), and claustrophobic reactions in a small chamber. It is disheartening that carbon monoxide poisoning that presents with loss of consciousness or syncope, even with initially low carboxyhemoglobin levels, may ultimately result in delayed or persistent neurologic sequelae.

Cyanide

Cyanide toxicity may result from a number of differing exposures. Often used as an industrial reagent, it is also found as a component of smoke in household fires that involve plastics and other synthetic materials. Hydrogen cyanide is generated by the combustion of plastics in home and industrial fires. The seeds of a number of edible fruits (apples, cherries, peaches, and pears) contain cyanogenic glycosides that are converted to cyanide in the GI tract. Nitroprusside is metabolized to cyanide; therefore, close monitoring for toxicity is necessary when utilized in the ICU, especially with preexisting renal failure.

The ingestion of cyanide salts (sodium cyanide, potassium cyanide) results in their conversion to hydrogen cyanide by the presence of gastric acids. This compound is then absorbed. Cyanide quickly causes toxicity via the inhalational route by binding to cytochrome A3, preventing the uptake of oxygen by cytochrome oxidase and the electron transport chain. Tissue hypoxia results owing to a complete lack of oxygen utilization, with failure to produce ATP.

Management is especially challenging, as the signs and symptoms are nonspecific but reflect profound hypoxia. Death often occurs within minutes of exposure. Patients do not present with cyanosis; venous oxygen saturation is elevated, which reflects the inability of the cells to utilize oxygen. Successful treatment requires rapid diagnosis and administration of the antidote (Fig. 35.3). The antidote kit contains amyl nitrite ampules and IV sodium nitrite to produce methemoglobinemia. The amyl nitrite is administered by inhalation while IV access is obtained. Once an IV site is available, the sodium

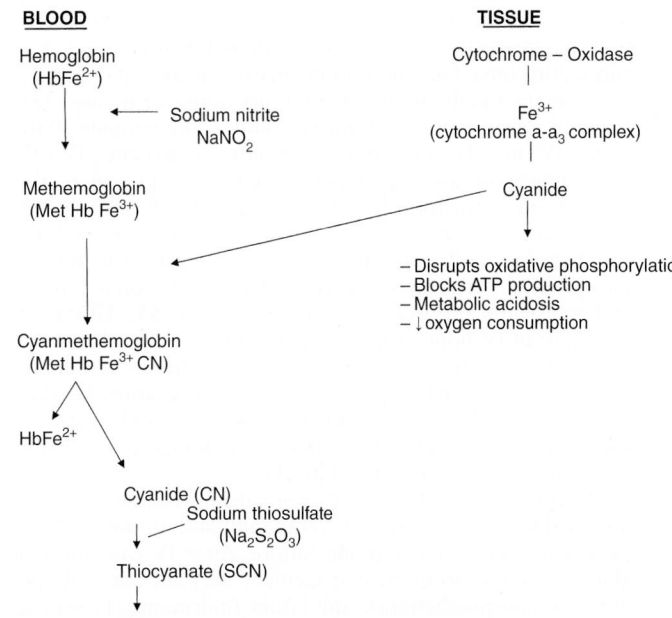

FIGURE 35.3. Sodium nitrite ($NaNO_2$) causes an oxidant stress, which results in the formation of methemoglobin. The ferric ion of methemoglobin competes with cytochrome oxidase for cyanide, dissociates cyanide from the tissue, and forms cyanmethemoglobin. Sodium thiosulfate ($Na_2S_2O_3$) facilitates the conversion of the cyanide (CN) contained in cyanmethemoglobin to thiocyanate (SCN).

nitrite is given to produce an approximate 20% methemoglobinemia. The utility of methemoglobin is that it has an even higher binding affinity for cyanide than cytochrome A3 and will remove the cyanide-forming cyanmethemoglobin. Sodium thiosulfate is then administered as a substrate for the enzyme rhodanase, which will form sodium thiocyanate and regenerate the methemoglobin to scavenge another molecule of cyanide from the cytochrome oxidase chain. The sodium thiocyanate will then be cleared by the kidneys and eliminated in the urine. It is important to judiciously administer the initial nitrites to minimize the risk of hypotension, as both are potent vasodilators. Although cyanide toxicity may be present in fire victims, nitrite administration is particularly risky because the resultant methemoglobin formation will exacerbate the already diminished oxygen-carrying capacity owing to carbon monoxide exposure.

Calcium Channel Blockers

Various calcium channel antagonists (e.g., nifedipine, amlodipine, felodipine, nicardipine, verapamil, diltiazem) are used in the management of cardiovascular and renal diseases. Calcium channel blockers are used for their action on L-type calcium channels in the heart and vascular smooth muscle. The blockade of cardiac calcium channels causes negative inotropic, chronotropic, and dromotropic effects. Vasodilation results from the blockade of calcium channels in arteriolar smooth muscle. The dihydropyridine calcium channel antagonists (nifedipine, amlodipine, felodipine, nicardipine) may result in hypotension and reflex tachycardia. The life-threatening consequences of blocked calcium channels include bradydysrhythmias (pacemaker cell inhibition and atrioventricular [AV] block) and profound hypotension (vasodilation and impaired contractility) (32). Electrocardiographic changes include prolonged PR interval, inverted P waves, AV dissociation, AV block, ST-segment changes, sinus arrest, and asystole. Cerebral hypoperfusion may present as altered mental status, seizures, and coma. GI hypomotility, ileus, and constipation may occur owing to inhibition of GI motility hormone release (33).

Fluid resuscitation with normal saline and atropine (0.02 mg/kg IV) may be successful in symptomatic patients. IV calcium, glucagon, and vasopressors may be employed in the instance of refractory hypotension and bradycardia (34). Glucagon has been considered a specific therapy for refractory hypotension because it increases cyclic adenosine monophosphate (cAMP), activates cAMP-dependent protein kinase, and transiently releases intracellular calcium (35). Glucagon dosing is an IV bolus 0.15 mg/kg, followed by an infusion of 0.05–0.1 mg/kg/h (36). Activated charcoal should be administered and repeated if the ingested calcium channel blocker was a sustained-release formulation. Whole-bowel irrigation should also be considered for patients with ingestions of sustained-release calcium channel blockers.

Because of the effects of L-type calcium channels on the myocardium, overdosage of verapamil and diltiazem may cause cardiogenic shock/pump failure. After IV calcium and glucagon administration, management may include dobutamine or phosphodiesterase inhibitors (milrinone). However, continuous invasive monitoring is required in this setting because of the risk of peripheral vasodilation and worsening hypotension.

Hyperinsulinemia/euglycemia therapy has been reported to reverse cardiogenic shock in the instance of calcium channel blocker toxicity (37). High-dose insulin (0.5–1 unit regular insulin IV bolus followed by 0.5 units/kg/h) may offset the hyperglycemia caused by impaired insulin release from the calcium channel blocker toxicity (38). Hyperglycemia should be verified before administering insulin. If the serum glucose is <150 mg/dL, administer dextrose 0.25 g/kg (10% dextrose 2.5 mL/kg) slowly followed by a continuous dextrose infusion (6–9 mg/kg/min) before administering insulin. Serum glucose should be checked q30–60 minutes. The clinician must be prepared to also administer potassium supplementation if insulin and glucose therapy is employed to treat calcium channel blocker overdose.

In severe cases that are refractory to medical management, alternative therapies may include use of transvenous pacing, a ventricular assist device, or extracorporeal life support. Lipid emulsion therapy is an exciting new treatment option for calcium channel blocker overdose (see above). Ideally, the intensivist should consult with a medical toxicologist on dosing; however, 20% lipid emulsion solution (e.g., intralipid) 1.5 mL/kg IV over 1 minute followed by an infusion of 0.25–0.5 mL/kg/min has been used successfully with resolution of hypotension as a therapeutic endpoint.

β-Blockers

β-Adrenergic antagonists are classified according to their site of receptor activity. β_1-Receptors are located in cardiac, renal, and adipose tissues. β_1-Receptor agonists result in positive inotropic and chronotropic effects, renin release, and lipolysis. β_1-Selective antagonist agents include atenolol, metoprolol, esmolol, and acebutolol. Propranolol, nadolol, and pindolol have activity at β_1- and β_2-receptors. β_2-Receptors are located in the liver and smooth muscle of blood vessels, trachea, bronchi, and GI tract. Catecholamine stimulation that targets β_2 receptors results in increased glycogenolysis or gluconeogenesis, vasodilatation, bronchial relaxation, and decreased GI motility. β-Adrenergic antagonists competitively inhibit the effects of the sympathetic neurotransmitters at the respective receptor sites. Some β-blocking agents have additional actions, such as propranolol, which causes

sodium channel blocking activity, and labetalol, which has α-receptor-blocking activity.

β-Blocker toxicity results in bradycardia, hypotension, and conduction delay. Severe toxicity may result in arrhythmias, including torsades de pointes, ventricular fibrillation, and asystole. Patients may occasionally present with bronchospasm. Hypoglycemia is frequently seen in β-blocker toxicity. Propranolol not only causes hemodynamic compromise but also, due to its lipid solubility, has the potential to cross the blood–brain barrier and result in coma and seizures. Labetalol can have conflicting actions and may cause vasodilation and β-receptor blockade. Sotalol, a β-blocker with type III antiarrhythmic activity, may cause dose-dependent prolongation of the QT interval and subsequent torsades de pointes. Acebutolol toxicity is one of the most severe toxicities, in that it predisposes to ventricular repolarization abnormalities, resulting in ventricular arrhythmias (39).

Management may merely require hemodynamic monitoring if the patient presents with asymptomatic bradycardia. Atropine is often helpful to reverse bradycardia and hypotension. It is important to consider that therapy with mixed β-agonists may result in an exacerbation of hypotension owing to β_2-receptor-mediated vasodilatation. Epinephrine infusions have been reported to be efficacious in overcoming the β-adrenergic blockade. The phosphodiesterase inhibitors amrinone and milrinone are thought to carry the benefit of blocking the breakdown of cAMP, thereby enhancing cardiac contractility. Contractility may also be enhanced by the action of glucagon, which increases intracellular cAMP. Severe toxicity may be managed with similar therapies in calcium channel blocker overdose, including transvenous pacing and extracorporeal life support. Benzodiazepines are helpful to manage seizures. Bronchospasm that is not abated with inhaled β_2-agonists might respond to anticholinergic agents.

Digoxin

Digoxin and digitalis glycosides are commonly utilized to manage cardiac failure and tachydysrhythmias. Digoxin improves cardiac contractility by increasing intracellular calcium concentration due to blockade of Na/K-ATPase. It enhances vagal tone and causes sinoatrial and AV nodal depression. Digoxin toxicity is marked by an increase in sympathetic tone and likelihood of increased automaticity.

Clinical manifestations of digoxin overdose include nausea, vomiting, altered sensorium, and cardiac dysrhythmias. The most typical dysrhythmias of digoxin toxicity are bidirectional ventricular tachycardia and atrial tachycardia with AV block. Hyperkalemia results from the blockade of Na/K-ATPase. The diagnosis of acute digoxin toxicity can be documented with a serum digoxin level.

Heart block or sinus bradycardia may be managed with atropine. In the event of serious cardiac dysrhythmias, therapy should commence with digoxin-specific Fab fragments (Digibind, DigiFab). It is absolutely essential to avoid any drugs whose action is to depress activity of the sinoatrial or AV nodes. Fab therapy restores the activity of the Na^+–K^+ pump and consequently results in resolution of hyperkalemia. Therefore, additional therapies for hyperkalemia are not indicated in digitalis intoxication. Hypokalemia exacerbates digitalis-associated dysrhythmias, and potassium administration is indicated for K^+ <3.0 mEq/L. Calcium should be avoided in view of the action of digoxin, which causes an increase in intracellular calcium.

Indications for utilization of Fab therapy in children include (a) a known ingestion of at least 0.1 mg/kg, (b) a digoxin level of >5 ng/mL and signs and symptoms of digoxin toxicity, (c) the occurrence of life-threatening arrhythmias, or (d) a serum potassium level of >6 mEq/L. The ingestion of the oleander plant, which contains cardiac glycoside, may present as digitalis toxicity. Children who have ingested oleander should receive activated charcoal and Fab therapy.

If Fab therapy is not available, the standard pediatric advanced life support algorithm with attention to ABC should be followed. Hypotension is treated with a normal saline fluid bolus. Hyperkalemia is managed with dextrose and insulin administration, but calcium administration should be avoided in digitalis intoxication. Atropine followed by cardiac pacing is used to treat heart block or other life-threatening bradydysrhythmias. Ventricular tachycardia and ventricular fibrillation are treated with cardioversion and defibrillation, respectively. Amiodarone, magnesium sulfate, and phenytoin have been used for recurrent life-threatening tachydysrhythmias associated with digitalis intoxication.

Tricyclic Antidepressants

The tricyclic antidepressants (TCAs) are utilized for a variety of disorders, such as enuresis, pain syndromes, and psychiatric disorders, consequently posing a risk of accidental and intentional ingestions. This class of medication carries the potential for serious toxicity and may result in a broad array of clinical manifestations. The tricyclic compounds have anticholinergic properties that result in the anticholinergic toxidrome. Their inhibition of α-adrenergic receptors can result in sedation and hypotension. They cause blockade of cardiac sodium channels, which results in decreased myocardial contractility and delayed conduction, manifested by widening of the QRS complex. Clinical symptoms have been related to the degree of QRS widening: seizures (QRS >100 ms) and arrhythmias (QRS >160 ms). Some investigators have reported the presence of an R wave in lead aVR ≥3 mm or an R wave:S wave ratio in lead aVR ≥0.7 to be a superior predictor of severe toxicity (40). Blockade of the potassium channel results in prolongation of the QT interval. Seizures have been attributed to effects of the tricyclics on GABA and on the reuptake of biogenic amines in the CNS. Consequently, it is possible to have a strong clinical impression of tricyclic toxicity in the presence of the anticholinergic syndrome, hypotension, widening of the QRS complex, and seizures. In general, severe toxicity is expressed very early in the course of management. Patients initially require meticulous monitoring, although in the absence of QRS widening, cardiac conduction anomalies, hypotension, altered sensorium, and seizures within the initial 6 hours, it is unlikely that the patient will deteriorate. Supportive management is indicated for the control of anticholinergic symptoms. Seizure management is generally accomplished with benzodiazepines. It is extremely important to avoid the use of flumazenil if suspicion of coingestion of benzodiazepines, as this may precipitate tricyclic-induced seizure activity. Sodium bicarbonate is utilized to achieve serum alkalinization (pH >7.4 and <7.55) when the QRS is widened or in the face of ventricular arrhythmias (41). Alkalinization significantly increases the protein binding of free drug to α_1-acid glycoprotein, resulting in rapid restoration of normal cardiac conduction. The administration of sodium bicarbonate is targeted at narrowing of the QRS and is titrated accordingly, by bolus dosing or continuous infusion. It is fairly standard practice to monitor the electrocardiogram for ~6 hours following the discontinuation of a continuous bicarbonate infusion. Patients who receive sodium bicarbonate often become hypokalemic, requiring careful monitoring and replacement therapy. TCAs block the reuptake of norepinephrine at the neuromuscular junction, leading to catecholamine depletion. For this reason, vasopressors (e.g., norepinephrine and epinephrine) may be needed to maintain adequate vascular tone

and blood pressure. Catecholamine depletion renders a poor response to dopamine, the effectiveness of which is dependent upon releasable stores of norepinephrine (42). TCA-induced hemodynamic compromise that is refractory to alkalinization therapy may benefit from lipid emulsion therapy (see above). In the case of hypotension refractory to vasopressor therapy, extracorporeal membrane oxygenation may be effective.

Certain drugs are contraindicated in the management of TCA intoxication. Flecanide (class IC antiarrhythmic agent) and procainamide (class IA antiarrhythmic agent) are contraindicated because their inhibition of rapid sodium channels is similar to the effect of TCAs on sodium channels. As a class III antiarrhythmic agent, amiodarone prolongs the cardiac action potent and is therefore hazardous in the setting of the widened QRS associated with TCA intoxication. Flumazenil may precipitate seizures in a setting of lowered seizure thresholds from TCAs. Physostigmine has been associated with cardiac arrest in TCA intoxication.

Carbamazepine toxicity may mirror the above constellation of symptoms and signs, as it is a benzodiazepine derivative structurally related to the TCAs. Toxicity has manifested following drug interactions with erythromycin, isoniazid, cimetidine, and propoxyphene. Management principles are directed at supportive care, with a high index of suspicion for respiratory failure, seizures, and hemodynamic instability. Charcoal may be utilized to prevent absorption. Vasopressors and anticonvulsant therapies may be necessary.

HERBAL TOXICITY/ NUTRITIONAL SUPPLEMENT TOXICITY

Nutritional supplements have risen to the forefront as a potential for significant toxicity. These agents have not been regularly monitored by laws or mandatory safety guidelines, and their easy availability gives the false impression of safety. The 12 most dangerous supplements with alternate names and associated clinical manifestations are listed in Table 35.3. This information can be reviewed on the Consumer Reports Web site (www.consumerreports.org). A number of herbal remedies have been reported to carry significant toxicity and are listed in Table 35.2. Management of these poisonings can be summarized by aggressive supportive care and therapies directed at control of specific symptoms.

CLUB DRUGS

The increased popularity of club drugs emerged with the rave scene—all-night, semiprivate parties characterized by techno music, dancing, visual effects with strobe lighting and lasers, and illicit use of drugs and alcohol. Substance abuse at these events most commonly includes ecstasy and amphetamines, as well as marijuana, cocaine, inhalants, ketamine, and γ-hydroxybutyrate (GHB). It is important to recognize that these agents often find themselves in the hands of adolescents. The practitioner must remain cognizant of an array of common drugs of abuse, along with their respective street names (Table 35.18).

A number of substances are abused via inhalation (Table 35.19). The inhalants are categorized by hydrocarbons (aliphatic and halogenated hydrocarbons and solvents), nitrous oxide, and nitrites. These agents are typically abused by techniques commonly referred to as sniffing, bagging, or huffing. Sniffing involves inhalation of the vapor from an open container or surface containing the volatile agent. Bagging refers to the user placing the compound into a large bag and inhaling

TABLE 35.18

COMMON DRUGS OF ABUSE AND THEIR STREET NAMES

■ CATEGORY SUBSTANCE NAME	■ STREET NAMES
Marijuana	Dope, ganja, joint, Mary Jane, pot, weed
Tobacco	Smoke, chew, beedi, snuff, cigar
Alcohol	Booze
Cocaine	Crack, candy, rock, Charlie, toot, snow
Methamphetamine	Crystal, meth, ice, speed, fire
Ritalin (methylphenidate)	MPH, Vitamin R, skippy
MDMA (methylenedioxy-methamphetamine)	Adam, Molly, clarity, ecstasy, XTC
GHB (Γ-hydroxybutyrate)	Georgia home boy, G, liquid ecstasy
Ketamine	Special K, K, Vitamin K
PCP (phencyclidine)	Angel dust
LSD (lysergic acid diethylamide)	Acid, Big D, blotters, cube
Heroin (diacetylmorphine)	Brown sugar, H, horse
OxyContin (oxycodone HCl)	Oxy, OC, killer
Vicodin (hydrocodone bitartrate with acetaminophen)	Vike, Watson-387
Benzodiazepines	Downers, sleeping pills
Rohypnol (flunitrazepam)	Roofies, roofinol, rope, R2
Anabolic steroids	Roids, juice
Inhalants	Poppers, snappers, whippets

From Nanda S, Konur N. Adolescent drug and alcohol use in the 21st century. *Pediatr Ann* 2006;35:193–9, with permission.

TABLE 35.19

COMMONLY ABUSED INHALANTS

■ SOLVENTS	■ COMMERCIAL PRODUCTS	■ MEDICAL GASES	■ ALIPHATIC NITRITES
Paint thinners	Butane lighters	Chloroform	Cyclohexyl nitrite
Gasoline	Whipping cream aerosols	Ether	Amyl nitrite
Glue	Spray paint	Halothane	Butyl nitrite
Felt-tip marker fluid	Hair and deodorant sprays	Nitrous oxide	
	Shoe polish		

Data from National Institute on Drug Abuse. *Monitoring the Future National Results on Adolescent Drug Use: Overview of Key Findings*. Bethesda, MD: National Institute on Drug Abuse, 2004. NIH Publication No. 05-5726.

directly from the bag. With huffing, the user places the inhalant into a rag or handkerchief, which is held under the nose, and inhales deeply. The rapid absorption from the lungs and the high lipid solubility of these agents result in rapid brain uptake. Clinical effects usually occur within seconds to minutes. It is essential to recognize that these compounds can cause significant organ damage (43) (**Table 35.20**). Inhalation of volatile compounds may result in chemical pneumonitis. CNS depression may result in depression of airway reflexes, which may lead to catastrophic aspiration and respiratory arrest.

Ecstasy (X, E, XTC, Adam, Molly)

Ecstasy, 3,4-methylenedioxymethylamphetamine (MDMA), is a selective serotoninergic neurotoxin that is utilized to foster a sense of enhanced empathy, relaxation, and closeness. A significant danger associated with obtaining ecstasy pills is the risk of contaminants. Contaminants such as aspirin or caffeine may exacerbate fluid losses. Other commonly found contaminants include methylenedioxyamphetamine (MDA), paramethoxyamphetamine, phencyclidine (PCP), and heroin, all of which can cause serious toxicity. Some deaths reported from ecstasy were actually felt to be secondary to high concentrations of the contaminant paramethoxyamphetamine (44). Dehydration is a frequent manifestation of ecstasy toxicity.

Mild cases may present with anxiety attacks, muscle cramping, severe trismus, or urinary retention due to spasm of the urethral sphincter. Acute intoxication with MDMA is heralded by hyperthermia, malignant hyperthermia, rhabdomyolysis, disseminated intravascular coagulation, acute renal failure, seizures, cardiac arrhythmias, intracranial hemorrhage, brain infarction, or death (45). Hyperpyrexia results from a recalibration of the central thermoregulatory center by MDMA and other amphetamine derivatives. Significant hyponatremia is commonly found and has been attributed to the consumption of large amounts of water to counteract the increased insensible fluid losses from hyperpyrexia.

γ-Hydroxybutyrate (G, Liquid Ecstasy, Liquid E)

GHB is a CNS depressant that results in a state of euphoria, disinhibition, and heightened sexuality, making it a "date-rape drug." GHB had been sold in health food stores as a sleeping aid and a stimulant of muscle growth and human growth hormone. It was declared illegal for use in the United States in 1991, followed by the illegalization of GHB precursors in 2000 (46). Dose-dependent side effects include drowsiness, dizziness, nausea, vomiting, amnesia, hallucinations, convulsions,

TABLE 35.20

EFFECTS OF INHALANTS

■ EFFECT	■ INHALANT
Hearing loss	Trichloroethylene, toluene
Peripheral neuropathies or limb spasms	Hexane, nitrous oxide
CNS or brain damage	Toluene
Bone marrow damage	Benzene
Liver and kidney damage	Toluene, chlorinated hydrocarbons
Blood oxygen depletion	Organic nitrates, methylene chloride

Data from National Institute on Drug Abuse. *Monitoring the Future National Results on Adolescent Drug Use: Overview of Key Findings*. Bethesda, MD: National Institute on Drug Abuse. 2004. NIH Publication No. 05-5726.

respiratory failure, coma, and death. Aggressive supportive care is the mainstay of management. Intubation is generally unnecessary, as patients tend to have a sudden reversal of loss of consciousness. Emergence may be marked by myoclonic jerking, confusion, or combativeness. If trismus is present, the accompanying ingestion of ecstasy or other stimulants should be suspected. Deaths reported from GHB intoxication usually result from the concomitant use of other respiratory depressants, such as alcohol or ketamine (44).

Methamphetamines (Tina, Ice, Crystal Meth, Tweak, Crank, Glass)

Methamphetamine may be taken orally, rectally, intravenously, or smoked; it is most commonly snorted intranasally. This agent is extremely physically addictive. Symptomatology follows the pattern of the sympathomimetic toxidrome. The clinical presentation may include headaches, pallor, tachycardia, hypertension, chest pain, palpitations, arrhythmias, hyperthermia, rhabdomyolysis, convulsions, and death (47). Patients will often be extremely agitated and anxious, flushed, and diaphoretic and have mydriasis. Management of these patients includes fluid and electrolyte replacement, as well as utilization of benzodiazepines that are effective in controlling agitation, hypertension, and seizures. Most patients do well with aggressive supportive care.

Cocaine

Cocaine toxicity is incorporated within the sympathomimetic toxidrome, but deserves mention with the specific club drugs. It may be used by inhalation (cocaine alkaloid, or "crack"), nasal insufflation, or the IV or GI route. It is absorbed in the hydrochloride or base form. Crack cocaine is considered the most potent and addictive form; it is also the most common form that is unintentionally ingested by small children. Infants may be exposed to cocaine in breast milk or via passive inhalation of vapors from crack cocaine (48). Cocaine results in an adrenergic storm by blocking reuptake of catecholamines at adrenergic nerve endings. Clinical manifestations include extreme CNS stimulation, along with cardiovascular and respiratory effects. Seizures, hypertension, and hyperthermia may lead to cardiac ischemia, CNS bleeding and infarction; end-organ failure may progress to hemodynamic collapse, coma, and death. An acute coronary syndrome results from the combined effects of cocaine: Stimulation of β-adrenergic myocardial receptors increases myocardial oxygen demand, whereas the α-adrenergic and 5-hydroxytryptamine agonist

effects cause coronary artery constriction. Cocaine results in a variety of dysrhythmias (wide complex tachycardia and ventricular fibrillation) owing to adrenergic stimulation and sodium channel blockade. It is difficult to accurately identify a cocaine-related myocardial infarction, because the electrocardiogram may be abnormal even in the absence of myocardial infarction. Furthermore, serum creatine kinase concentrations are typically elevated without an accompanying myocardial infarction. This elevation is attributed to rhabdomyolysis, which mandates a need for aggressive diuresis. Serum troponin levels are helpful in the evaluation for cocaine-related myocardial infarction (49).

Myocardial ischemia due to cocaine-induced vasoconstriction usually appears within 1 hour after exposure, corresponding with the time frame for peak concentration. It is important to realize that, as concentrations of cocaine's major metabolites (benzoylecgonine and ecgonine methyl ester) rise, there may be an associated delayed vasoconstriction. This pattern of metabolism explains the clinical delay often seen with myocardial ischemia or infarction.

Management commonly includes the liberal use of benzodiazepines, which control seizure activity and have also been reported to be efficacious in reducing heart rate and systemic arterial pressure (49). Hypertensive crisis must be controlled to minimize cerebrovascular or myocardial injury. Management of pediatric acute coronary syndrome may be represented by the mnemonic MONA (morphine, oxygen, nitroglycerin, aspirin). Recommended dosing of nitroglycerine in children is by IV infusion: initial dose of 0.25–0.5 mcg/kg/min, titrated by 0.5–1 mcg/kg/min every 3–5 minutes as needed; in general, the dose range is 1–3 mcg/kg/min. Cocaine-induced vasoconstriction of the coronary arteries may be reversed with phentolamine, an α-adrenergic antagonist. β-Adrenergic blockers are contraindicated in the management of cocaine-induced acute coronary syndrome.

CONCLUSIONS AND FUTURE DIRECTIONS

Management of the poisoned child is often accomplished by pediatricians and emergency medicine physicians. The intensivist becomes involved in cases of significant cardiopulmonary instability or those that require meticulous monitoring in view of the distinct potential for an ingested agent to result in clinical deterioration. Vigilant supportive care remains the hallmark of management and is important in asymptomatic poisonings and in life-threatening toxicity. Toxicology literature contains an abundance of research targeted at antidotes and decontamination strategies. The reality remains that pediatric ingestions are ideally managed by prevention, and it is essential to recognize that the only way to decrease morbidity and mortality from poisoning is to focus efforts at prevention. Parents must receive diligent anticipatory guidance about the variety of common household substances that contain often-overlooked, potentially lethal ingredients. The Universal Poison Control number should be posted in all homes, clinics, schools, and hospitals. Diligence in advancing public health education and garnering increased funding for research will ideally serve to combat morbidities associated with pediatric poisoning.

References

1. Watson WA, Litovitz TL, Lein-Schwartz W, et al. 2003 annual report of the American Association of Poison Control Centers Toxic Exposure Surveillance System. *Am J Emerg Med* 2004;22:335–404.

2. Osterhoudt KC, Shannon M, Henretig FM. Toxicologic emergencies. In: Fleisher GR, Ludwig S, eds. *Textbook of Pediatric Emergency Medicine*. 4th ed. Philadelphia, PA: Lippincott Williams & Wilkins, 2000:887–942.

3. Hochman J, Tunnessen WW Jr. Pediatric puzzler. *Contemporary Pediatr* 1995;12:121–31.

4. Matteucci MJ. One pill can kill: Assessing the potential for fatal poisonings in children. *Pediatr Ann* 2005;34:964–8.

5. Woolf AD. Herbal remedies and children: Do they work? Are they harmful? *Pediatrics* 2003;112:240–6.

6. Guzzardi L, Bayer MJ. Emergency management of the poisoned patient. In: Bayer M, Rumack BH, Wanke LA, eds. *Toxicologic Emergencies*. Bowie, MD: Brady RJ, 1984.

7. Woolf AD. Principles of toxin assessment and screening. In: Fuhrman BP, Zimmerman JJ, eds. *Pediatric Critical Care*. 3rd ed. Philadelphia, PA: Mosby, Elsevier, 2006:1511–31.

8. Chomchai CG. Ipecac syrup. In: Olson KR, ed. *Poisoning & Drug Overdose*. 4th ed. New York, NY: Lange Medical Books/McGraw-Hill, 2004:228–9.

9. Krenzelok EP, McGuigan M, Lheur P; American Academy of Clinical Toxicology; European Association of Poisons Centres and Clinical Toxicologists. Position statement: Ipecac syrup. *J Toxicol Clin Toxicol* 1997;37:699–709.

10. Hojer J, Troutman WG, Hoppu K, et al. Position paper update: Ipecac syrum for gastrointestinal decontamination. *Clin Toxicol* 2013;52(3):134–9.

11. Bond GR. Home syrup of ipecac use does not reduce emergency department use or improve outcome. *Pediatrics* 2003;112:1061–4.

12. American Academy of Pediatrics Committee on Injury, Violence, and Poison Prevention. Poison treatment in the home. American Academy of Pediatrics Committee on Injury, Violence, and Poison Prevention. *Pediatrics* 2003;112:1182–5.

13. Manoguerra AS, Cobaugh DJ; Guidelines for the Management of Poisonings Consensus Panel; American Association of Poison Control Centers. Guideline on the use of ipecac syrup in the out-of-hospital management of ingested poisons. 2004; *Clin Toxicol* 2005;1:1–10.

14. Tucker JR. Indications for, techniques of, complications of, and efficacy of gastric lavage in the treatment of the poisoned child. *Curr Opin Pediatr* 2000;12:163–5.

15. Vale JA; American Academy of Clinical Toxicology; European Association of Poisons Centres and Clinical Toxicologists. Position statement: Gastric lavage. *J Toxicol Clin Toxicol* 1997;35:711–9.

16. Benson BE, Hoppu K, Troutman WG, et al. Position paper update: Gastric lavage for gastrointestinal decontamination. *Clin Toxicol* 2013;51:140–6.

17. Howland MA. Antidotes in depth: Activated charcoal. In: Goldfrank LR, Flomenbaum NE, Lewin NA, et al, eds. *Goldfrank's Toxicologic Emergencies*. 7th ed. New York, NY: McGraw-Hill, 2002:469–74.

18. Chyka PA, Seger D; American Academy of Clinical Toxicology; European Association of Poisons Centres and Clinical Toxicologists. Position statement: Single-dose activated charcoal. *J Toxicol Clin Toxicol* 1997;35:721–41.

19. Chyka PA, Seger D, Krenzelok EP; American Academy of Clinical Toxicology; European Association of Poisons Centres and Clinical Toxicologists. Position paper: Single-dose activated charcoal. *Clin Toxicol* 2005;43:61–87.

20. Smilkstein MJ. Techniques used to prevent gastrointestinal absorption of toxic compounds. In: Goldfrank LR, Flomenbaum NE, Lewin NA, et al, eds. *Goldfrank's Toxicologic Emergencies*. 7th ed. New York, NY: McGraw-Hill, 2002:44–57.

21. Position paper: Cathartics. *J Toxicol Clin Toxicol* 2004;42:243–53.

22. Position paper: Whole bowel irrigation. *J Toxicol Clin Toxicol* 2004;42:843–54.

23. Weinberg GL. Lipid emulsion infusion: Resuscitation for local anesthetic and other drug overdose. *Anesthesiology* 2012; 117:180–7.

24. Borkan SC. Extracorporeal therapies for acute intoxications. *Crit Care Clin* 2002;18:393–420.

25. Osterhoudt KC. The toxic toddler: Drugs that can kill in small doses. *Contemp Peds* 2000;17(3):73–85.

26. Sterrent C, Brownfield J, Korn CS, et al. Patterns of presentation in heroin overdose resulting in pulmonary edema. *Am J Emerg Med* 2003;21:32–4.

27. Wang DS, Sternbach G, Varon J. Nalmefene: A long-acting opioid antagonist. Clinical applications in emergency medicine. *J Emerg Med* 1998;16(3):471–5

28. Alander SW, Dowd D, Bratton SL, et al. Pediatric acetaminophen overdose: Risk factors associated with hepatocellular injury. *Arch Pediatr Adolesc Med* 2000;154:346–50.

29. Joshi P. Toxidromes and their treatment. In: Fuhrman BP, Zimmerman JJ, eds. *Pediatric Critical Care*. 3rd ed. Philadelphia, PA: Mosby, Elsevier; 2006:1521–31.

30. Noker PE, Tephly TR. The role of folates in methanol toxicity. *Adv Exp Med Biol* 1980;132:305–15.

31. Mack RB. Dishwasher detergent toxicity—Here's looking at you, kid. *Contemp Pediatr* 1993;10:49–58.

32. Moser LR, Smythe MA, Tisdale JE. The use of calcium salts in the prevention and management of verapamil-induced hypotension. *Ann Pharmacother* 2000;34:622–29.

33. Ray JM, Squires PE, Meloche RM. L-type calcium channels regulate gastrin release from human antral G cells. *Am J Physiol* 1997;273:G281–8.

34. Belson MG, Gorman SE, Sullivan K. Calcium channel blocker ingestion in children. *Am J Emerg Med* 2000;18:581–6.

35. Papadopoulos J, O'Neil MG. Utilization of a glucagon infusion in the management of a massive nifedipine overdose. *J Emerg Med* 2000;18:453–5.

36. Bailey B. Glucagon in beta-blocker and calcium channel blocker overdoses: A systematic review. *J Toxicol Clin Toxicol* 2003;41:595–602.

37. Boyer EQ, Duic PA, Evans A. Hyperinsulinemia/euglycemia therapy for calcium channel blocker poisoning. *Pediatr Emerg Care* 2002;18:36–7.

38. Boyer EW, Shannon M. Treatment of calcium-channel-blocker intoxication with insulin infusion. *N Engl J Med* 2001;344:1721–2.

39. Love JN. Acebutolol overdose resulting in fatalities. *J Emerg Med*. 2000;18:341–344.

40. Liebelt EL, Francis PD, Woolf AD. ECG lead aVR versus QRS interval in predicting seizures and arrhythmias in acute tricyclic antidepressant toxicity. *Ann Emerg Med* 1995;26:195–201.

41. Liebelt EL. Targeted management strategies for cardiovascular toxicity from tricyclic antidepressant overdose: The pivotal role for alkalinization and sodium loading. *Pediatr Emerg Care* 1998;14:293–98.

42. Zaritsky AL. Catecholamines, inotropic medications, and vasopressor agents. In: Chernow B, ed. *The Pharmacologic Approach to the Critically Ill Patient*. 3rd ed. Baltimore, MD: Williams & Wilkins, 1994:387–404.

43. Nanda S, Konnur N. Adolescent drug and alcohol use in the 21st century. *Pediatr Ann* 2006;35:193–99.

44. Tellier PP. Club drugs: Is it all ecstasy? *Pediatr Ann* 2002;31:550–6.

45. Shannon M. Methylenedioxymethamphetamine (MDMA, "Ecstasy"). *Pediatr Emerg Care* 2000;16:377–80.

46. Shannon M, Quang LS. Gamma-hydroxy-butyrate, gamma-butylolactone, and 1,4,-butanediol: A case report and review of the literature. *Pediatr Emerg Care* 2000;6:435–40.

47. McEvoy AW, Kitchen ND, Thomas DG. Lesson of the week: Intracerebral haemorrhage in young adults: The emerging importance of drug misuse. *Br Med J* 2000;320:1322–24.

48. Winecker RE, Goldberger BA, Tebbett IR. Detection of cocaine and its metabolites in breast milk. *J Forensic Sci* 2001;46:1221–3.

49. Lange RA, Hillis LD. Cardiovascular complications of cocaine use. *N Engl J Med* 2001;345:351–8.

CHAPTER 36 ■ THERMOREGULATION

ADNAN M. BAKAR AND CHARLES L. SCHLEIEN

KEY POINTS

1 Extreme variations in environmental temperature disrupt thermoregulatory function and lead to heat-related illness.

2 Prevention is essential in avoiding the complications of heat-related illness.

3 Modulation of the systemic inflammatory response is an important determinant of compensated versus decompensated response to heat-related injury.

4 Heat stroke is a medical emergency. Prompt and aggressive cooling to below 39°C within 30 minutes of onset of illness prevents a high mortality rate.

5 The superior method of cooling has not been proven.

6 Hypothermia can occur due to exposure to cold and other etiologies when thermoregulation is overwhelmed or dysfunctional.

7 Children are at increased risk for hypothermia due to their body morphology and faster cooling rates.

8 The choice of rewarming method for hypothermia depends on the degree of hypothermia and the presence or absence of cardiac arrest.

9 Resuscitation of the hypothermic patient with cardiac arrest should be continued until the core temperature is 34°C, spontaneous circulation has occurred, or lethal injuries are identified.

10 Prevention and early recognition can limit the incidence, morbidity, and mortality of accidental hypothermia.

PHYSIOLOGY OF THERMOREGULATION

Normal body temperature is maintained constant by a balance of heat loss and heat gain with the assistance of an efficient thermoregulatory mechanism. Extreme environmental temperature variations, however, can overcome this effective **1** thermoregulatory function and lead to heat- or cold-related illnesses.

Body temperature consists of core and shell temperatures. Rectal, esophageal, bladder, and oral temperatures represent core temperature, whereas axillary and skin temperatures represent shell temperature. Core temperature determines the risk of injury to various organs in the body. Air temperature, air movement, thermal radiation, sweating, skin blood flow, and temperature of underlying tissue all influence shell temperature (1). Thermoreceptors for the shell reside in the skin. Core thermoreceptors exist in the cortex, hypothalamus, midbrain, medulla, spinal cord, and deep abdominal structures in addition to the skin (2,3). On sensing a temperature change, these receptors transmit afferent impulses via the lateral spinothalamic tract to the central thermostat located in the preoptic/anterior hypothalamus, which maintains the temperature set point (4). Thermoregulation is initiated when sensed temperature is different from the set point. The conditions associated with failed thermoregulatory mechanisms that lead to hyperthermia or hypothermia will be discussed in this chapter.

Heat Gain

Warm-blooded animals have the capacity to raise their body temperature above their environmental temperature, which occurs when endogenous or exogenous heat gain exceeds heat loss. Heat is generated in the human body from basal metabolism, physical activity, food consumption, metabolic activity, emotional change, hormonal effects, and certain medications that typically raise body metabolism. The body may also acquire heat passively when the environmental temperature exceeds body temperature.

Heat Loss

Heat is lost from the body via *conduction*, *convection*, *radiation*, and *evaporation*. In most situations, humans produce more heat than necessary and dissipate the excess heat into the environment.

Conduction is heat loss by the transfer of heat from a warmer to a cooler object when the two objects are in direct contact. The amount of heat loss depends on the contact area and the temperature difference between the body and the other surface. Typically, only 3% of body heat is lost by conduction; however, conduction may be a major source of heat loss in wet clothing or immersion incidents because of the excellent conductive properties of water.

Convection is heat loss by the movement of air or fluid that circulates around the skin. More heat is carried away from the body in windy conditions, as the movement of air rapidly removes the insulating layer of warmer air normally around the body surface. Approximately 12%–15% of body heat is lost by convection.

Radiation is heat loss due to infrared heat emission to surrounding air. Heat loss occurs primarily from the head and noninsulated areas of the body and usually occurs rapidly. Radiation can account for 55%–65% of heat loss.

Evaporation is heat loss by the change of water from a liquid (sweat) to a gas state via the skin or respiration. Evaporation normally accounts for 25% of heat loss, but depends on surface area, temperature difference, and humidity. Evaporative heat loss is highest in cold, dry, and windy conditions (5).

HYPERTHERMIA

Definitions

Hyperthermia refers to body temperature elevation beyond the hypothalamic set point because of inadequate heat loss and/or excessive heat gain. Cytokines do not mediate this temperature elevation in contrast to fever (see what follows), as the hypothalamic set point itself has not changed. Hence, antipyretics (aspirin, acetaminophen, nonsteroidal anti-inflammatories), which lower the set point, have no effect. Extreme temperature elevations (>41°C) are common in the hyperthermic patient.

Fever represents a regulated temperature elevation (>38.5°C) to a new higher set point in the hypothalamus. It is caused by the release of pyrogens from macrophages/monocytes. These include the cytokines interleukin-1 (IL-1), tumor necrosis factor (TNF), interferon (IFN)-γ, and IL-6, which are released in response to inflammatory stimuli such as infection, malignancy, autoimmune disease, and other disease states. Cytokine-induced fever rarely exceeds 41°C, with the exception of some cases of encephalitis and meningitis.

Classification of Hyperthermia Syndromes

Hyperthermia syndromes may be classified as environmental (or exertional), drug (or toxin)-induced, or of genetic/unknown origin. Considerable overlap exists among these groups, as patients with a genetic predisposition may be more susceptible to environmental/exertional or drug-induced hyperthermia.

TABLE 36.1

RISK FACTORS FOR HEAT-RELATED ILLNESS

■ FACTORS	■ DESCRIPTION
Socioeconomic factors	Lack of access to air conditioners; individuals living in upper floors of apartment buildings especially with flat roof tops; social isolation; closed doors and windows during hot weather conditions
Weather conditions	Factors that prevent heat loss from the body: reduced wind, elevated barometric pressure, high humidity, high environmental temperature at or above body temperature for prolonged periods of time
Drugs	Alcohol, anticholinergics, amphetamines, anti-Parkinson medications, β-blockers, cocaine, diuretics, ecstasy, ephedra-containing diet supplements, neuroleptics, phenothiazines, tricyclic antidepressants
Body habitus	Obesity (BMI > 85th percentile for age)
Clothing	Thick, nonabsorbable clothing
Illnesses	Mental handicap; febrile illnesses; dehydrating illnesses such as diabetes insipidus, diabetes mellitus, diarrhea, and vomiting; skin diseases such as anhidrosis; heat-producing illnesses such as thyrotoxicosis; lack of sleep, food, or water; diminished sweating as in cystic fibrosis; lack of acclimatization; previous heat stroke
Exertional heat illness	Athletes, military personnel, manual laborers, multiple same day sessions, insufficient rest/recovery between sessions, excessive physical exertion, poor acclimatization

These syndromes have similar patient presentation. However, certain aspects of the clinical presentation may be unique or exaggerated, depending on the specific entity. Hyperthermia may induce euphoria instead of discomfort, resulting in failure to seek prompt medical attention. Even in the most severe form of heat illness, early clinical signs are nonspecific. The severity of heat-related injury depends on the degree of core temperature elevation and its duration. Therefore, preventive measures, early diagnosis, and aggressive treatment are essential components of a good outcome (6).

Heat Stroke (Environmental/Exertional Heat-Related Illness)

Heat-related illnesses comprise a spectrum of diseases that ranges from heat stress—a benign condition—to heat stroke—a potentially fatal condition. The milder conditions (variously termed heat rash, heat cramps, heat edema, and heat exhaustion) generally do not require PICU management.

Between 1979 and 2002, there were 4780 heat-related deaths in the United States. Only 6% of these patients were <15 years of age, 50% were between 15 and 64 years old, and 44% were >65 years old. It is estimated that heat stroke caused more American deaths during this time period than the effects of hurricanes, lightning, earthquakes, tornadoes, and floods combined (7).

Heat stroke is characterized by an elevation of core temperature above 40°C, commonly with nervous system dysfunction manifesting in delirium, convulsions, or coma. Death associated with heat stroke has been estimated as high as 50%, and those who do survive may sustain permanent neurologic damage (8). Heat stroke is subdivided into classic (environmental) or exertional. The mechanism of classic heat stroke that follows exposure to high environmental temperature is more common in younger children who are unable to escape from the hot environment, or in those who may have an underlying condition that causes thermoregulatory dysfunction. While exertional heat stroke may occur in temperate environments, the risk is higher when the individual engages in heavy exercise in hot and humid conditions.

Exertional heat stroke often may be linked to a genetic predisposition. Individuals with a predominance of type II muscle fibers are more susceptible to exertional heat stroke. These individuals have lower exercise capacity and accumulate more lactate, which, in turn, directly activates the cell membrane sodium/potassium pump (Na/K-ATPase). Activation of Na/K-ATPase affects intracellular sodium and calcium resulting in depletion of cellular energy stores (9). The loss of mitochondrial function and disturbed calcium (Ca^{2+}) homeostasis activate phospholipase A_2, resulting in the production of free radicals, prostaglandins, leukotrienes, and calcium-dependent proteases and the eventual development of rhabdomyolysis (10). Rhabdomyolysis results from free radical–induced lipid peroxidation and overload of cellular and mitochondrial calcium, primarily resulting in muscle necrosis.

Prevention

Understanding the risk factors for heat stroke better allows for more effective preventive measures. Previously it was thought that children were more prone to heat-related illness than adults because they were less effective at regulating body temperature, incurred greater cardiovascular strain for similar amounts of work, had diminished sweating capacity, and had a lower exercise tolerance in heat (11–14). Recent studies have disproven that notion. When 9- to 12-year-old boys and girls are compared to similarly fit adults while undertaking an equivalent exercise workload under similar environmental conditions, it has been shown that children and adults have a similar cardiovascular response, exercise tolerance, and increase in rectal and skin temperatures in heat (15–17).

Multiple risk factors may increase the likelihood of heat-related illness. Current or recent illness may have residual effects on hydration status and regulation of body temperature, increasing the risk. Chronic conditions such as diabetes insipidus, diabetes mellitus, obesity, hyperthyroidism, and cystic fibrosis may also effect thermoregulation. Acclimatization can protect against heat-related illness, and typically occurs gradually over a 10- to 14-day period. Children frequently do not consume enough water to replenish fluid lost during physical activity, and should be encouraged to drink adequate quantities of fluids before and during physical activity. Generally, 3–8 oz every 20 minutes for 9- to 12-year-olds and 1–1.5 L every hour for adolescents are sufficient to minimize body water deficits. The risk factors for heat illness are listed in **Table 36.1** (6,18).

Identifying high-risk groups can prevent heat-related illness. Heat-related mortality and morbidity are reduced when safe havens are established that provide air conditioning, hydration, and medical equipment for those in need. The news media can play a key role in educating the public in the prevention of heat-related illnesses. Administration of fluid (e.g., cold tap water) to ensure hydration is recommended even when children are not thirsty (6). The addition of water flavoring with carbohydrate and salt increases fluid consumption significantly and makes heat-related illness less likely. A gradual acclimatization process should be encouraged, with the duration of intense physical activity reduced when air temperature and relative humidity are elevated.

Measurement of environmental stress can be used to prevent heat-related injuries associated with activity in hot environments. The wet-bulb globe temperature (WBGT) index is widely used to measure environmental stress as an index of heat stress. The WBGT index consists of three parameters weighted as follows:

$$\text{WBGT} = (0.7 \text{ Twb}) + (0.2 \text{ Tg}) + (0.1 \text{ Tab}) \quad [36.1]$$

The first metric, Twb, refers to wet-bulb temperature. It is obtained by covering a dry-bulb thermometer not immersed in water, with a water-saturated cloth and placing it in direct sunlight. The second metric, Tg, refers to black globe temperature and is obtained by placing, in direct sunlight, a dry bulb in a metal globe. Lastly, Tab refers to a measurement of air temperature without direct sunlight using a dry-bulb thermometer. A portable monitor is used to measure the WBGT index, with temperature values reported in Celsius or Fahrenheit. Risk category stratification is based on the result as follows: "very high risk" is associated with values over 28°C, "high risk" is in the range of 23°C–28°C, "moderate risk" falls in the range of 18°C–23°C, and temperatures below 18°C fall into the "low-risk" category. Activities should be modified according to the risk (19).

Core Pathophysiology

Compensated Response

Thermoregulation. A major portion of heat is lost from the body via the skin, and perspiration-induced evaporation is responsible for most heat loss. The skin's blood flow enhances heat loss through conduction and convection. Cutaneous vasodilation that results from increased skin blood flow brings skin temperature nearer to core temperature. The increase in cutaneous blood flow that results from an elevated core temperature is ninefold greater than the increase that results from an elevation in the skin temperature (3).

The sympathetic nervous system controls blood flow through the skin by modulating adrenergic vasoconstrictor and vasodilator fibers. During heat stress, tonic cutaneous vasoconstriction is inhibited and vasodilatation is induced, resulting in an increase in skin blood flow. An elevation in skin temperature results from convection of heat from both striated muscles and internal organs to the surface (20). Cutaneous blood flow at rest constitutes 5%–10% of total cardiac output (200–500 mL/min). Heat stress–induced vasodilatation increases cutaneous blood flow to as much as 60% of cardiac output (8 L/min).

Acclimatization. Acclimatization is an adaptation response that can take up to several weeks following exposure to a hot environment. These adaptation responses include increase in plasma volume, enhancement of cardiovascular performance, activation of renin–angiotensin–aldosterone axis, ability to increase sweating, salt retention by sweat glands and kidneys, rise of the glomerular filtration rate, and inhibition of rhabdomyolysis (21).

Systemic Inflammatory Response: Cytokine Release. Serum levels of TNF-α, IL-1, IL-6, and endotoxin are increased following body temperature elevation. The ensuing systemic inflammatory response involves epithelial and endothelial cells as well as leukocytes. Each of these cells modulates the cytokine response to heat injury, resulting in healing and repair, thereby preventing multi–organ dysfunction (22).

Cell Survival Response: Heat Shock Proteins. Heat stress induces heat shock elements, which leads to an accelerated transcription of heat shock proteins (HSPs). These proteins improve the cell's ability to survive injury. This mechanism is based on HSPs acting as molecular chaperones, that is, proteins that assist other proteins in achieving proper folding, thus preventing further protein denaturation. It has been observed that HSPs modulate baroreceptor reflex response following heat stress and blunt bradycardia and hypotension (23).

Decompensated Response

Temperature. The absolute rise in temperature and the duration of this rise determine organ injury. Body temperature in the 41°C–42°C range leads to tissue injury within 1–8 hours. A temperature that exceeds 49°C induces tissue injury within 5 minutes. Hypovolemia follows excessive dehydration, lowering preload and therefore cardiac output, with a resultant decrease in skin blood flow. Loss of heat by conduction and convection is thus limited and thermoregulation is compromised. Decreased blood volume due to hypovolemia results in less sweating, thereby reducing heat loss by evaporation. Reflexes that help to maintain central blood volume and blood pressure override thermoregulatory signals for cutaneous vasodilation, resulting in an inability to lose heat by evaporation (24).

Exaggerated Systemic Inflammatory Response. The balance between proinflammatory mediators such as TNF-α, IL-1β, IFN-γ, and anti-inflammatory mediators, such as soluble TNF-α (sTNF-α) and IL-10, determines the extent of tissue injury. The predominance of proinflammatory mediators leads to systemic inflammation with subsequent multi–organ dysfunction (25).

Gastrointestinal Ischemia. Vasodilatation-induced shift of blood flow from the core to the peripheral circulation results in reduced blood flow to the gastrointestinal tract, with subsequent intestinal ischemia. Intestinal ischemia disrupts immunologic and gut mucosal barrier function, leading to translocation of endotoxin and release of proinflammatory cytokines. Proinflammatory cytokine release promotes endothelial activation with the subsequent release of endothelin and nitric oxide. Specific to this discussion, these cytokine mediators cause thermoregulatory failure and alter hemodynamic function, resulting in the progression of heat-related illness (26–28).

Activation of Coagulation Cascade. The activation of the coagulation cascade as a result of heat injury is supported by the presence of the thrombin–antithrombin complex with decreased levels of naturally synthesized anticoagulation proteins such as protein C, protein S, and antithrombin III. The activation of fibrinolysis is indicated by the appearance of D-dimer, decreased levels of plasminogen, and the presence of the plasmin–antiplasmin complex (29). Heat injury also induces a prothrombotic state by enhancing the expression of adhesion molecules.

Inadequate Heat Shock Protein Response. Progression of heat-related illness is associated with attenuated release of HSPs. Advanced age, failure to acclimatize, and genetic factors are associated with inadequate HSP release (30).

CLINICAL FEATURES

Heat stroke affects multiple organs and results in their dysfunction. The clinical effects seen in various organs are discussed below.

Central Nervous System

Individuals who suffer from heat exposure can present with delirium, seizures, lethargy, or coma due to metabolic disturbances, cerebral edema, or ischemia. The cerebellum is particularly sensitive to high temperature (31). Neurologic complications include intracranial bleed, cerebral infarct, cerebral edema, central pontine myelinolysis, and demyelination resulting in Guillain–Barré syndrome. Intracranial bleed occurs acutely and is related to disseminated intravascular coagulation (DIC) that accompanies heat stroke. Cerebral infarct results from cerebral thrombosis secondary to hemoconcentration and the other prothrombotic effects cited earlier. Cerebral pontine myelinolysis may be related to rapid changes in serum osmolality with little alteration in serum sodium. Immune system activation by cytokines following heat stroke disrupts the blood–brain barrier and exposes peripheral nerves to antigen, resulting in the Guillain–Barré syndrome, usually seen 7–10 days after heat stroke.

Cardiovascular System

Heat elimination involves translocation of blood from the central circulation to the periphery, leading to hypotension, especially in the presence of hypovolemia. Hypotension may also be due to vasodilation secondary to the production of nitric oxide that results from heat-related illnesses (32). Patients with heat stroke may present with either a hyperdynamic or hypodynamic circulation, with elevated systemic vascular resistance, low cardiac output, and variable pulmonary vascular resistance.

Electrocardiographic Changes

Victims of heat stroke show electrocardiographic changes that include rhythm disturbances, conduction defects, and changes in the QT interval or the ST segment. Rhythm disturbances such as sinus tachycardia, supraventricular tachycardia, and atrial fibrillation may be observed. Conduction defects such as right bundle branch block and intraventricular conduction defects have been noted. Prolonged QT may be due to

hypomagnesemia, hypocalcemia, or hypokalemia (all associated with heat-related injury). The presence of ST segment changes indicates myocardial ischemia, which can lead to myocardial infarction. The predisposing factors for myocardial ischemia include tachycardia and increased oxygen demand from hyperthermia, combined with hypotension from hypovolemia.

Respiratory System

Heat stroke may result in respiratory failure secondary to acute respiratory distress syndrome (ARDS) (see Chapter 49). The exact time of onset of ARDS following heat stroke is unpredictable. DIC that accompanies heat injury may trigger the onset of ARDS.

Acid–Base, Electrolyte, and Renal Disorders

Renal System

Acute renal failure may result as a combination of hypovolemia, rhabdomyolysis, DIC, and direct effects of thermal injury. A variety of acid–base and electrolyte derangements follow from the primary heat-related illness, compounded by rhabdomyolysis and renal insufficiency.

Lactic acidosis with compensatory respiratory alkalosis occurs in exertional heat stroke. *Hyponatremia* is seen following sweat losses of >5 L/day and on rehydration especially with hypotonic solutions. It also occurs during the early stages of acclimatization to heat, during vigorous exercise (e.g., marathon or triathlon), and during prolonged and repeated exercise in the heat. *Hypokalemia* initially is seen as a consequence of respiratory alkalosis induced by hyperventilation secondary to hyperthermia, catecholamine secretion, sweat losses, and renal losses from hyperaldosteronism due to physical activity in a hot environment. Persistent high temperature, perfusion failure, and hypoxemia all lead to magnesium-dependent Na/K ATPase pump malfunction. The resultant potassium seepage from cells may cause *hyperkalemia*, which is exacerbated by renal failure. Although hyperkalemia and hypokalemia occur in heat-related injury, hypokalemia is the predominant effect observed. Acute *hypophosphatemia* occurs from the increase in glucose phosphorylation seen in alkalosis. Later in the course, sustained tissue injury leads to leakage of phosphate from the cells, which complexes with extracellular calcium, resulting in *hypocalcemia*. Hypocalcemia and hypophosphatemia are also secondary to hypomagnesemia, lack of bone responsiveness to parathyroid hormone or deficient parathyroid hormone secretion. *Hyperuricemia* occurs due to augmented release and diminished excretion of uric acid secondary to rhabdomyolysis and renal failure, respectively. The mechanisms involve release of purine from injured muscle and inhibition of uric acid excretion in the urine due to metabolic acidosis. *Hypomagnesemia* follows excessive sweating. However, a rapid decline in urinary magnesium excretion normalizes the serum magnesium level. Prolonged intense exercise can induce the uptake of magnesium by erythrocytes, mononuclear cells, and muscle, leading to clinically significant hypomagnesemia. *Hypoglycemia* occurs due to rapid depletion of glycogen, rapid utilization of glucose, and liver dysfunction from splanchnic ischemia, resulting in failure to convert lactate to glucose.

Gastrointestinal Tract

Gut ischemia results in liver dysfunction with elevated alanine transaminase, aspartate transaminase, bilirubin, γ-glutamyl transpeptidase, and lactic dehydrogenase. Peak elevation in liver enzymes occurs 72 hours following heat injury. Liver damage may be due to either direct heat injury or hypoxemia secondary to splanchnic ischemia. Fulminant liver failure is uncommon following heat injury.

Hematology and Immunology

DIC occurs and is worsened by liver dysfunction. Splanchnic ischemia leads to translocation of bacteria and resultant endotoxin production, with subsequent release of proinflammatory mediators, including TNF-α, IL-1, IL-2, IL-6, IL-8, platelet activating factor, arachidonic acid, and vasoactive amines, leading to multi–system organ dysfunction.

Musculoskeletal System

Elevated serum creatine phosphokinase (CPK) is the major sign for rhabdomyolysis, occurring in most cases of exertional heat stroke and less frequently in classical heat stroke. The consequences of rhabdomyolysis include hyperkalemia leading to cardiotoxicity, myoglobinuria resulting in renal failure, shock from sequestration of fluid into injured muscle, and muscle necrosis of the diaphragm leading to respiratory failure. Compartment syndrome can result from severe edema of the muscles of the extremities. Thus, it is important to monitor arterial pulsation, perfusion, and sensation of the swollen extremities and to measure direct tissue pressure in suspected cases of compartment syndrome.

DIFFERENTIAL DIAGNOSIS

Diagnosis of heat stroke should be suspected in anyone who presents with a core temperature of >40.6°C, hot, dry skin, and changes in mental status that include delirium, and seizures. The differential diagnosis is listed in **Table 36.2**. Septic shock closely mimics heat-related illness. A good history and physical examination can exclude many diagnostic entities such as complications related to thyroid disease, drug toxicities, and malignant hyperthermia (MH).

LABORATORY EVALUATION

Laboratory tests are performed to evaluate target organ injury and confirm the diagnosis by ruling out other disease entities.

Urine

Urine analysis may show elevated specific gravity with low urine output from dehydration and hypovolemia. Protein in the

TABLE 36.2

DIFFERENTIAL DIAGNOSES OF HEAT STROKE

■ ENTITIES	■ ETIOLOGIES
Central nervous system	Meningitis, encephalitis, and hypothalamic infarction
Thyroid	Graves disease, thyroid storm
Infection	Sepsis
Drugs	Toxicity from anticholinergic, antidepressants, amphetamines, hallucinogens, cocaine, phencyclidine, monoamine oxidase inhibitors, neuroleptics, and salicylates
Drug withdrawal	Narcotics, benzodiazepines
Metabolic	Diabetic ketoacidosis
Miscellaneous	Malignant hyperthermia

urine indicates muscle breakdown. The presence of red blood cells, myoglobin, and tubular casts denotes acute tubular necrosis as a consequence of hypovolemia and rhabdomyolysis. The finding of myoglobinuria is especially important, as it is diagnostic of rhabdomyolysis in this setting, for which specific emergency therapy is necessary (see what follows). Urine drug screen is performed when drug ingestion is suspected.

Blood Testing

Leukocytosis on a complete blood count may be due to systemic inflammation from heat-related illness or sepsis. Elevated hemoglobin and hematocrit indicate hemoconcentration due to dehydration. Thrombocytopenia, elevation in hypersegmented neutrophils, and atypical lymphocytosis are also features of heat injury. At times, spherocytes and, less commonly, schistocytes, ovalocytes, and stomatocytes are observed on the blood smear. These changes are reversed within 4–7 days following effective treatment of heat injury.

Serum chemistry typically reveals hyponatremia, hypokalemia followed by hyperkalemia, hyperphosphatemia, and hypocalcemia. Hypoglycemia is also noted in victims of heat stroke. Elevated blood urea nitrogen and creatinine levels can be observed as a consequence of dehydration and ensuing prerenal azotemia or renal failure. Increase in CPK follows rhabdomyolysis.

Elevation in aspartate aminotransferase (AST) and alanine aminotransferase (ALT) are noted due to liver dysfunction, an attribute of multi–organ failure from heat stroke.

Activation of the extrinsic pathway of coagulation following heat stroke promotes coagulopathy (DIC). Elevation in prothrombin time, partial thromboplastin time, and D-dimer and a decrease in platelets are seen as a consequence of coagulopathy.

Evaluation of arterial blood gas reveals respiratory alkalosis in cases of classic heat stroke and metabolic acidosis in cases of exertional heat stroke. Hypoxemia with low PaO_2/FIO_2 ratio occurs as a result of heat stroke complicated by ARDS.

Imaging

A chest x-ray is useful in confirming the presence of ARDS and in detecting the presence of infective or aspiration pneumonia. CT imaging of the brain is performed to diagnose central nervous system (CNS) complications of heat stroke such as cerebral infarction, hemorrhage, or edema. Patients with heat-related illnesses suffer from cardiac arrhythmias, which can be confirmed with a 12-lead electrocardiogram. An echocardiogram is indicated in patients who present with clinical suspicion of myocardial dysfunction.

Lumbar Puncture

A lumbar puncture is useful in suspected cases of meningitis or encephalitis, both of which can closely mimic the encephalopathy that accompanies heat stroke. The clinician should be cognizant of raised intracranial pressure (ICP) due to associated CNS complications, as well as DIC, which accompanies heat stroke, both of which are relative contraindications for a spinal tap.

COMPLICATIONS

Complications following heat-related illness are enumerated in **Table 36.3**.

TABLE 36.3

COMPLICATIONS OF HEAT-RELATED ILLNESS

■ ORGAN SYSTEM	■ COMPLICATIONS
Central nervous system	Encephalopathy, coma, seizures, hemiplegia, cerebellar injury
Cardiovascular	Myocardial injury
Pulmonary	Acute respiratory distress syndrome
Gastrointestinal	Ischemia or infarction
Renal	Acute renal failure
Muscular	Rhabdomyolysis
Hematology	Disseminated intravascular coagulation, thrombocytopenia
Metabolic	Lactic acidosis

TREATMENT

Heat Stroke

Heat stroke is a medical emergency that requires prompt and aggressive treatment to prevent mortality. Prompt attention to the ABCs of resuscitation is required here and in every other form of hyperthermia.

Therapy at the Scene

Emergency cooling should be undertaken without delay (8). The victim should be moved to a shaded area, tight clothing should be removed, and the victim should be sprinkled with water from any source and fanned constantly. Cooling victims to below 39°C within 30 minutes greatly improves the outcome from heat-related injury. The core temperature is measured during the application of the cooling process. Various methods of cooling are available. Currently, no prospective study recommends one method over another (33). Various methods of cooling and their advantages and disadvantages are listed in **Table 36.4**.

Supplemental oxygen should be provided to hypoxic individuals, and the airway should be secured with an endotracheal tube in comatose patients due to loss of protective airway reflexes. Shivering and consequent increase in body temperature can be prevented by the administration of diazepam. Vital signs, including core temperature via rectal or esophageal route, are monitored continuously. Vascular access is established with a wide bore catheter. Ringer's lactate or normal saline is used for hydration. Hydration status should be assessed by physical examination of skin perfusion and urine output monitoring by means of a bladder catheter. Overhydration should be avoided to minimize the development of pulmonary edema and cerebral edema that can follow heat stroke. Seizures from heat stroke can effectively be treated with a benzodiazepine. The victim should be moved to a tertiary care medical center as soon as possible.

Therapy at the Tertiary Center

Those victims who had their airway controlled are placed on positive-pressure ventilation with supplemental oxygen to correct hypoxemia. Positive end-expiratory pressure should be titrated to treat hypoxemia and to keep FiO_2 below the toxic level of 0.6. Body cooling (see **Table 36.4**) should be continued until core temperature is below 39°C with core temperature monitored every 5 minutes by one of the methods mentioned earlier. IV fluids should be given via a wide bore catheter, and a central venous line should be placed for central venous pressure measurement. Fluids are given based on perfusion status, pulse characteristics, and measurement of urine output via a bladder catheter. Overhydration must be avoided for the reasons stated earlier. Low cardiac output, elevated central venous pressure, mild right heart failure, and low systemic vascular resistance are seen in most victims of heat stroke. However, effective cooling results in vasoconstriction and increased blood pressure. Victims of heat stroke need careful titration of fluids, as they develop noncardiogenic pulmonary edema and cerebral edema. Some victims may present with low cardiac output, elevated central venous pressure,

TABLE 36.4

METHODS OF COOLING

■ COOLING METHODS	■ DESCRIPTION	■ ADVANTAGES	■ DISADVANTAGES
External Cooling			
Immersion	Immersion of body in ice water	Faster cooling, greater temperature gradient between core and periphery	Vasoconstriction; interferes with heat loss; shivering; interferes with resuscitative measures
Body-cooling unit	Spraying finely atomized water mixed with warm air to keep body temperature above 32°C–33°C	Faster cooling (mean cooling rate of 0.31°C/min or 0.56°F/min); comfortable to the patient; heat is lost by evaporation and convection	Sophisticated unit that requires maintenance and storage
Wet sheet and fan	Patients are covered with a sheet, water is sprayed over the sheet, and fans are used to blow over the wet sheet	Heat lost by evaporation; heat loss is comparable to body-cooling unit; easy maintenance	
Ice packs	Ice packs are placed over the groin, axillae, and neck	Simple and readily available; inexpensive; shorter cooling time when combined with evaporative technique	Longer cooling time compared to evaporative technique
Core Cooling			
Cold water irrigation	Gastric, bladder, peritoneal lavage, extracorporeal technique	Not well studied	Invasive, especially peritoneal and extracorporeal techniques
IV fluids	Cold IV fluid administration	Not studied	Noninvasive

and hypotension, which necessitate inotropic support. Low cardiac output, low central venous pressure, and hypotension may also be observed, necessitating liberal fluid administration. Avoidance of α-adrenergic agents to avoid vasoconstriction (which prevents heat loss from the skin) and avoidance of anticholinergic agents (which prevent sweating and increased body temperature) are important.

Blood glucose and serum electrolytes are measured frequently and corrected appropriately. Hypocalcemia is corrected cautiously due to the risk of deposition of calcium carbonate and calcium phosphate in injured skeletal muscles.

Rhabdomyolysis, identified by elevated creatine kinase and myoglobinuria, requires aggressive hydration in order to increase urine output to >3 mL/kg/h. In addition to volume expansion, mannitol 0.25 g/kg IV may be used as an osmotic diuretic to increase urine flow. The addition of sodium bicarbonate to the IV fluids prevents breakdown of myoglobin to its nephrotoxic metabolites (i.e., ferrihemate) if the urine pH is raised to >6.5. However, there are no large randomized clinical trials to demonstrate that the alkalinization of urine is better than early, aggressive hydration for treatment of rhabdomyolysis (34,35).

Once rhabdomyolysis has been diagnosed, the patient may face several additional life-threatening problems, including renal failure, pulmonary edema, worsening electrolyte derangements, and compartment syndrome. Oliguric renal failure secondary to acute tubular necrosis (see Chapter 110) may lead to pulmonary edema, unless the fluid administration rate is decreased. Hemofiltration or dialysis may be necessary to remove excess fluid volume and treat electrolyte abnormalities in the patient with heat stroke, rhabdomyolysis, and acute tubular necrosis.

Extreme hyperkalemia, hyperphosphatemia, and hyperuricemia may occur. Although standard measures to treat hyperkalemia (bicarbonate, calcium chloride, insulin, and glucose administration) apply in this setting, it is likely that the patient will already have been alkalinized. In addition, the benefits of calcium administration in preventing arrhythmias must be balanced against the risk of precipitation of calcium phosphate crystals in injured muscle. If meticulous monitoring of the ECG pattern shows signs of hyperkalemia (tall T waves, prolonged PR interval, widened QRS, any arrhythmia), then calcium administration should be undertaken. Aggressive lowering of the serum potassium level is critical with: (a) glucose 0.5 g/kg (2 mL/kg of 25% dextrose over 30 minutes) and insulin 0.1 unit/kg IV; (b) sodium polystyrene sulfonate (Kayexalate) 1 g/kg via nasogastric tube every 2–6 hours, and/or (c) dialysis. Hyperphosphatemia is managed with phosphate binders and dialysis. Hyperuricemia is managed with hydration, alkalinization, and drug therapy, including allopurinol and recombinant uricase (rasburicase).

Acute renal failure is seen in 30% of patients with exertional heat stroke and in 5% following classic heat stroke. The most important aspect in the prevention of renal failure is to maintain adequate hydration. If oliguria persists despite adequate hydration and in the presence of normal blood pressure, patients who are at high risk for pulmonary edema may need invasive monitoring (e.g., central venous pressure) to titrate fluid therapy. A trial dose of furosemide or mannitol may be given to induce diuresis. Early dialysis should be considered in those who have renal failure.

Shock can follow rhabdomyolysis from sequestration of large quantities of fluid into the injured muscles in the first 24 hours following heat injury. Intravenous fluids may contribute to edema in injured muscles leading to compartment syndrome usually occurring on the third or fourth day following injury. Compartment syndrome results in a secondary elevation of creatine kinase due to muscle necrosis from compression by trapped fluid. Documentation of compartment syndrome includes pulselessness, paresthesias, pain, or paralysis of an extremity with increased compartment pressure. Fasciotomy should be undertaken immediately with a diagnosis of compartment syndrome.

Coagulation abnormalities peak at 24–36 hours; thus, prothrombin time, partial thromboplastin time, platelet count, and fibrin split products are obtained at admission and at intervals thereafter. DIC is treated with fresh frozen plasma or cryoprecipitate if hypofibrinogenemia is also present. The use of ε-aminocaproic acid for fibrinolysis is extremely dangerous and provides no long-term benefit; it has also been shown to cause rhabdomyolysis. The other contributing factor for coagulopathy is liver dysfunction treated with supportive care. Liver transplantation is seldom needed for liver dysfunction following heat stroke.

ICP monitoring has not been reported in heat stroke victims; however, it should be individualized based on bedside clinical evaluation of elevated ICP without coagulopathy.

HYPERTHERMIA SYNDROMES

Malignant Hyperthermia

MH is a genetic syndrome that requires exposure to certain potent inhaled general anesthetics (halothane, isoflurane, sevoflurane) and/or the depolarizing muscle relaxant succinylcholine. The inheritance pattern in 50% of patients is autosomal dominant, caused by a point mutation in the gene encoding the ryanodine receptor RYR1 (the Ca^{2+} release channel of the sarcoplasmic reticulum). This mutation leads to sustained Ca^{2+} release from the sarcoplasmic reticulum on exposure to a triggering agent. Patients without a family history may have other spontaneous mutations that produce the MH phenotype. Because of the variable genotype, the diagnosis is still usually made with the halothane (or caffeine) contracture test on skeletal muscle obtained during biopsy. Patients who are suspected of having MH should undergo testing at an MH testing center, wear a "Medic Alert" bracelet, and obtain up-to-date information from the Malignant Hyperthermia Association at http://www.mhaus.org.

The incidence of MH is 1 in 4000 for mild presentations and 1 in 250,000 for the fulminant form. Patients with certain neuromuscular disorders such as muscular dystrophy, myotonia, and central core disease are at increased risk.

The cardinal features of MH include muscle rigidity (sustained contracture), which is often first detected when masseter spasm prevents opening of the mouth during tracheal intubation. The sustained muscle contracture generates heat and greatly increased muscle metabolism, which, in turn, lead to increased carbon dioxide production (increased end-tidal carbon dioxide [$ETCO_2$] concentration), acidosis, tachypnea, and tachycardia (including ventricular tachycardia). The body temperature often exceeds 41°C. In the absence of prompt medical intervention, rhabdomyolysis supervenes, with the risk of hyperkalemia, ventricular tachycardia, myoglobinuric renal failure, and cardiac arrest.

Although MH presents most commonly in the operating room, the pediatric intensivist must be thoroughly familiar with the course and management because of the possibility of recurrence of MH in the ICU. Also, the increasing use of inhaled anesthetics in the ICU to treat refractory asthma or provide sedation increases the risk of MH occurring initially in the PICU. All patients who develop intraoperative MH must be admitted to an ICU because recurrence of MH occurs in 20% of patients, especially in those with a muscular body type (36). The time between the initial onset of MH and recurrence averages 13 hours.

Therapy for MH consists of immediate discontinuation of inhaled anesthesia or other possible trigger agent. The inspired gas is converted to 100% oxygen at a high flow rate to wash out residual anesthetic as rapidly as possible. The muscle relaxant dantrolene, 2.5 mg/kg IV, is given as rapidly as possible. The dose may be repeated to control signs of hypermetabolism. Cold normal saline, 15 mL/kg, is administered rapidly if the temperature is >39°C. Emergency laboratory testing includes serum potassium, creatine kinase, arterial blood gas, and coagulation tests to evaluate hyperkalemia, rhabdomyolysis, metabolic acidosis, and DIC, respectively. Complications should be treated rapidly. Hyperkalemia is the presumed cause of any ventricular arrhythmia during MH until proven otherwise, such that glucose, insulin, bicarbonate, and calcium are added to primary antiarrhythmia therapy (e.g., amiodarone for cardioversion).

Malignant Hyperthermia-Like Syndrome

In 2003, a new syndrome resembling MH was described (37). However, in contrast to classic MH, these patients had not been exposed to anesthetics or succinylcholine; rather they presented with type II diabetic coma and a hyperglycemic, hyperosmolar nonketotic state. Hyperthermia occurred typically after administration of insulin, although exceptions have been described. The patients were usually obese African American males with acanthosis nigricans. Rhabdomyolysis, hemodynamic instability, and organ failure punctuate the course of this condition, which has been termed malignant hyperthermia-like syndrome (MHLS). The mortality rate is high (>50%).

The etiology of MHLS is unknown. The insulin preservative, m-creosol, underlying fatty acid oxidation defects (e.g., short-chain acyl-CoA dehydrogenase deficiency), and infection have all been proposed as contributing to the cause of MHLS (38). It is likely that multiple factors contribute to MHLS, and each case requires a careful workup for enzyme defects, infection, and toxins.

Therapy for MHLS should include the immediate administration of dantrolene, based on limited case reports to date (38). Because dantrolene must be diluted in sterile water, a calculated dose of hypertonic saline can be administered concurrently to prevent a rapid decline in serum osmolality, which may precipitate cerebral edema. Cooling methods outlined in Table 36.4 are indicated until the temperature is <39°C.

Meticulous use of IV fluids, glucose, and electrolytes is critical. After a sufficient volume of normal saline has been administered rapidly to restore blood pressure and perfusion, the remaining volume deficit and ongoing losses are replaced more slowly over 72 hours. Hydration alone often lowers serum glucose such that a lower dose of insulin can be used (0.05 units/kg/h) to correct hyperglycemia without precipitating rapid osmotic shifts.

Neuroleptic Malignant Syndrome

Neuroleptic malignant syndrome (NMS) is a rare clinical syndrome associated with the use of antipsychotic drugs and characterized classically by four cardinal signs: muscle rigidity, mental status changes (confusion, agitation, catatonia, bradykinesia, encephalopathy, coma), hyperthermia, and autonomic instability (tachycardia, labile hypertension, diaphoresis). Atypical presentations may occur where only two or three of the cardinal signs are present.

Every type of neuroleptic agent that antagonizes dopamine D2 receptors has been associated with NMS, including haloperidol, chlorpromazine, fluphenazine, risperidone, clozapine, and olanzapine. The antiemetic and gastric motility agents, promethazine and metoclopramide, have also been implicated in NMS. Risk factors for NMS appear to correlate with potent antipsychotics (e.g., haloperidol), rapid dose escalation, concomitant use of lithium, and comorbid diseases such as acute infection. Although no controlled trials have been reported to support specific medical therapy, dantrolene, bromocriptine, and amantadine have been tried. Most centers favor the use of dantrolene (39). All antipsychotic drugs known to trigger NMS must be discontinued emergently. Monitoring, laboratory testing, and supportive care follow the approach described for other hyperthermia syndromes. Benzodiazepines may be used to control agitation. Psychosis or catatonia may require electroconvulsive therapy. Once NMS has resolved, antipsychotic medications, preferably of lower potency and without the concomitant use of lithium, can be reintroduced gradually and titrated to effect.

Serotonin Syndrome

Serotonin syndrome (SS) is a clinical syndrome that exhibits signs of excess postsynaptic serotonergic neurotransmission, which may include hyperthermia. The classic triad of SS signs includes abnormalities of mental status (agitation, delirium, hypervigilance), neuromuscular function, (hyperreflexia, clonus, hypertonicity, tremor, hyperkinesia), and autonomic function (hyperthermia, tachycardia, hypertension, diaphoresis, vomiting, diarrhea). Clonus may be seen in multiple patterns including spontaneous, inducible, or ocular, and may be greater in the lower extremities than upper extremities (40). Given the multiplicity of potential signs and symptoms, patients usually present with variations of the classic triad, and a high index of suspicion needed in any patient who is receiving medications that increase serotonergic activity (Table 36.5).

SS is often confused with NMS, anticholinergic poisoning, or MH. Clonus is not a prominent finding in NMS, and patients with NMS usually suffer from muscle rigidity and akinesia/bradykinesia, as opposed to the hyperkinesia of SS. Furthermore, NMS develops over days to weeks, whereas SS usually develops within 24 hours, and at times within minutes of administration of the offending medication.

Patients with anticholinergic poisoning have normal reflexes and the typical toxidrome of mydriasis, delirium, dry oral mucosa, dry and hot erythematous skin, urinary retention, and an absence of bowel sounds. Anticholinergic poisoning is differentiated from SS with its absence of bowel sounds, diaphoresis with normal skin color, and neuromuscular findings.

Patients with MH often have mottled skin, muscle rigidity, and hyporeflexia. This is in contrast to the findings of normal skin color, hyperkinesia, and hyperreflexia found in SS (40).

Overall, hyperthermia occurs in 50% of patients with SS but is universal among the sickest SS patients in the PICU. The Hunter Serotonin Toxicity Criteria incorporate the most important findings (clonus, agitation, diaphoresis, tremor, hyperreflexia, hypertonicity, hyperthermia) into a decision-making rule set that is sensitive (84%) and very specific (97%) for SS (41).

The management of SS relies on supportive care, as outlined for other hyperthermia syndromes. The serotonergic drug is discontinued immediately. Agitated patients should receive benzodiazepine sedation. If the triggering agent is a monoamine oxidase inhibitor (MAOI), which has caused hypotension, then it is prudent to avoid inotropes (e.g., dopamine) that are metabolized by monoamine oxidase inhibitors. After fluid resuscitation, a direct-acting vasoconstrictor such as phenylephrine is preferred to treat hypotension. The cause of hyperthermia in SS is related to muscle activity. Therefore, severely hyperthermic patients should undergo rapid-sequence induction of anesthesia, endotracheal intubation,

TABLE 36.5

DRUGS THAT INCREASE SEROTONIN LEVELS AND MAY PRECIPITATE SEROTONIN SYNDROME

■ CLASS	■ MECHANISM	■ EXAMPLES
Dietary supplement	Increases serotonin formation	L-tryptophan
Illicit drug	Increases release of serotonin	Amphetamines, ecstasy, cocaine
Weight loss drug (amphetamine derivatives)	Increases release of serotonin	Phentermine, fenfluramine, dexfenfluramine
Herbal medication	Prevents reuptake of serotonin into the presynaptic neuron	St. John's wort
Antidepressant: selective serotonin reuptake inhibitor	Prevents reuptake of serotonin into the presynaptic neuron	Citalopram, escitalopram, fluoxetine, paroxetine, sertraline
Antidepressant: tricyclic antidepressant	Prevents reuptake of serotonin into the presynaptic neuron	Amitriptyline, amoxapine, desipramine, doxepin, imipramine, maprotiline, nortriptyline, protriptyline, trimipramine
Antidepressant: selective serotonin/norepinephrine reuptake inhibitor	Prevents reuptake of serotonin and norepinephrine into the presynaptic neuron	Bupropion, trazodone, nefazodone, venlafaxine
Antidepressant: monoamine oxidase inhibitor	Inhibits metabolism of serotonin	Phenelzine, tranylcypromine, isocarboxazid
Antibiotic: monoamine oxidase inhibitor	Inhibits metabolism of serotonin	Linezolid
Migraine drug	Activates serotonin 5-HT$_1$ receptors	Almotriptan (Axert), naratriptan (Amerge), sumatriptan (Imitrex), zolmitriptan (Zomig)
Antiemetics	Prevents reuptake of serotonin into the presynaptic neuron	Ondansetron, granisetron
Antitussive	Prevents reuptake of serotonin into the presynaptic neuron	Dextromethorphan
Analgesic	Activates serotonin 5-HT$_1$ receptors	Fentanyl

and neuromuscular blockade to eliminate motor activity until hyperthermia resolves. The antidote for SS is cyproheptadine, a histamine-1 (H$_1$) receptor antagonist with nonspecific serotonergic (5-HT$_{1A}$ and 5-HT$_{2A}$) antagonistic properties, although its efficacy has not been rigorously studied. Because cyproheptadine is only available as an oral formulation (tablet or syrup), it should be crushed and given via nasogastric tube at a total daily dose of 0.25 mg/kg divided every 6 hours. The maximum daily dose is 12 mg for children 2–6 years and 16 mg for children 7–14 years old. After discontinuation of the triggering agent and institution of supportive care plus cyproheptadine, most patients will show marked improvement within 24 hours.

Sympathomimetic and Anticholinergic-Induced Hyperthermia Syndromes

Drug-induced hyperthermia from sympathomimetic or anticholinergic poisoning is discussed in Chapter 35.

HYPOTHERMIA

Hypothermia and cold-induced injuries include a spectrum of conditions that range from frostnip and frostbite to severe hypothermia, all of which may cause minor-to-significant morbidity and mortality. Although hypothermia is most common during exposure to cold environments, it can also develop secondary to other causes, such as toxin exposures, metabolic derangements, infections, and CNS or endocrine system dysfunction. Environmental cold injury typically occurs in cold climates, but can also occur in warmer climates that have rapid temperature changes or with the use of air conditioning.

Definitions

Frostnip (also known as first-degree frostbite) is a mild form of cold injury. It is a nonfreezing injury of skin tissues, usually of the face, fingertips, or toes of patients who are exposed to cold. Ice crystals may form in superficial layers of skin, but no tissue destruction occurs. Frostnip is associated with pallor and numbness or tingling of the affected skin until warming occurs. A more significant nonfreezing injury is termed *chilblains*, which can occur as tissue temperature drops below 15°C. The walls of small vessels break and tissues swell. Treatment of frostnip and chilblains usually involves simple rewarming. Dressing warmly, covering ears, keeping hands and feet dry, and seeking a warmer environment when hands and feet feel cold usually prevent frostnip and chilblains.

Frostbite is the destruction of skin or other tissues caused by freezing. It is classified as superficial—affecting skin and subcutaneous tissues—or deep—affecting bones, joints, and tendons (42,43). During freezing, intracellular and extracellular ice crystals form causing direct cellular injury. Cells then become dehydrated through outward diffusion of water resulting in intracellular electrolyte disturbances. As tissues rewarm, tissue edema forms as the extracellular ice crystals melt.

Exposure to below-freezing temperatures leads to vasoconstriction, which reduces blood flow to extremities, exacerbates the cooling process, and causes even greater vasoconstriction. Cooling of vascular contents also increases the blood viscosity, which leads to increased microvascular damage and tissue edema. This damage also precipitates microthrombi formation and ischemia. During rewarming of frozen tissues, lysis of ice-containing cells also produces a prothrombotic environment, exacerbating tissue ischemia secondary to microthrombi formation.

Vasoconstriction may be followed by vasodilation, the so-called hunting response, which is a normal physiologic response thought to prevent the extremities from freezing. The vasodilation response is ineffective during overwhelming cold stress as the vasodilation causes a drop in core body temperature, which may lead to hypothermia (44).

Below-freezing temperatures, low windchill, high humidity, and prolonged exposure to cold are risk factors for the development of frostbite. Superficial frostbite leads to pallor, edema, blistering, and desquamation. Deep frostbite can lead to hemorrhagic blisters, anesthesia, hyperesthesia, ulceration, and gangrene. Treatment involves removal of nonadherent wet clothing, rapid rewarming, and avoidance of rubbing damaged tissue. Preparation and protection from the effects of cold weather is the best prevention for frostbite.

Hypothermia is defined as a core body temperature of <35°C (95°F). Humans adapt to their environment and maintain core temperature within a narrow range. When this adaptive thermoregulation is overwhelmed, the body cannot generate sufficient heat to continue to function naturally and hypothermia occurs. Hypothermia is classified as mild (35°C–32°C), moderate (<32°C–28°C), or severe (<28°C) based on core body temperature (45). All organ systems are affected by hypothermia, but the CNS and the cardiovascular system are the most sensitive. The degree of hypothermia dictates the expected pathophysiologic changes and appropriate therapeutic modalities.

Determining the severity of hypothermia is sometimes difficult because standard clinical thermometers measure temperature only as low as 34.4°C. Therefore, when hypothermia is suspected, it is important to record core body temperature using low-reading rectal thermometers or electronic rectal, esophageal, or bladder thermistor probes. In a tracheally intubated patient, insertion of a thermistor probe into the distal third of the esophagus is the preferred method to determine core temperature. A probe placed into the proximal esophagus may be falsely elevated due to ventilation with warmed gases. A thermistor probe placed in an insulated ear canal free of snow and cerumen, in contact with the tympanic membrane, accurately reflects brain temperature. A bladder probe may be falsely elevated during peritoneal lavage. A rectal probe may lag behind core temperature during rewarming. Measurements made with infrared thermometers are often inaccurate in patients with hypothermia (46).

Mechanisms of Disease

The pathophysiology of hypothermia is related to mechanisms of heat loss (see earlier sections), temperature homeostasis, cellular effects, and organ system response.

Temperature Homeostasis

Thermoregulation. Thermoregulatory response to cold requires input from peripheral skin receptors and core thermoreceptors along the distribution of the internal carotid arteries and the posterior hypothalamus. The cutaneous nerve-ending cold receptors are located more superficially and in greater numbers than warm receptors. Afferent impulses are transmitted via the spinothalamic tracts and relayed to the hypothalamus. Core thermoreceptors are less well understood, but the response of the peripheral vasculature to sympathetic input appears to be modulated by the temperature of circulating blood. Thermosensitive neurons are located throughout the CNS in close proximity to arteries so that blood and brain temperatures are closely coupled.

Thermogenesis. Thermogenesis, or heat production, normally occurs in obligatory ways, such as that due to basal metabolism and exercise. When cooling occurs despite this heat generation, facultative thermogenesis occurs via voluntary physical activity, shivering, or humoral response. Shivering is the production of heat by muscle tremor and produces a fivefold increase in metabolic rate. Humoral thermogenesis involves sympathetic release of norepinephrine and subsequent expression of mitochondrial uncoupling proteins, which then leads to the production of heat by uncoupling of the metabolic chain from oxidative phosphorylation in the inner membranes of mitochondria. Norepinephrine and epinephrine are also released from the adrenal medulla, inducing glycogenolysis in muscle and liver cells (47).

Heat Conservation. The conservation of heat occurs in response to cold stress. The response by the cutaneous circulation is a locally initiated and mediated vasoconstrictor response via the release of norepinephrine from sympathetic nerve endings acting on peripheral α_2-receptors and a reflex response initiated by skin cooling over the general body surface. Skin blood flow can be downregulated to nearly zero in extreme cold. Local sensory blockade can interfere with the adrenergic response, allowing for reversal to vasodilation (e.g., in the hands, during local cooling). As whole-body cooling proceeds, the prevailing vasoconstrictor mechanisms are nonadrenergic (48). Heat may be conserved with insulation secondary to subcutaneous fat and by normal behavioral responses to cold exposure, both of which may be less effective at the extremes of age.

Cellular and Tissue Effects

Cold exposure and freezing of tissue can cause direct cellular injury by the formation of extracellular ice crystals, which, in turn, produces intracellular dehydration, elevation of intracellular electrolytes, and temperature-induced protein changes. Further temperature reduction leads to intracellular crystallization and mechanical destruction of cells (43). A shift in the oxyhemoglobin dissociation curve to the left leads to further tissue hypoxia. Vasoconstriction contributes to hypoperfusion and stasis, and endothelial injury causes thromboembolism. During cooling, cyclic freezing and thawing can occur in extremities, resulting in the release of prostaglandin F2 and thromboxane A2, which potentiate vasoconstriction, platelet aggregation, and thrombosis. In mice, moderate systemic hypothermia causes accelerated microvascular arteriole and venule thrombus formation by activation of the glycoprotein (GP) IIb-IIIa fibrinogen receptor (49). Cold-induced inhibition of coagulation cascade enzymes and platelet dysfunction also occurs, which can lead to bleeding. Thawing of frozen tissue results in marked edema that is secondary to melting of ice crystals, cell damage, lack of endothelial integrity, and thrombosis.

Organ System Response to Hypothermia

All organ systems are affected by significant hypothermia. The responses at different degrees of hypothermia are summarized in **Table 36.6**. The most significant of these effects occur in the central nervous, cardiovascular, and renal systems. Even with mild systemic hypothermia, the CNS responses are slowed, and severe mental status changes and unconsciousness occur below 32°C. Myocardial irritability develops and frequently leads to initially atrial and then ventricular arrhythmias, including ventricular fibrillation below 28°C. Below 32°C, a J (Osborn) wave may be seen on electrocardiogram, represented by a hump at the QRS–ST junction in the inferior and lateral precordial leads (50).

A cold-induced diuresis occurs with mild hypothermia. Initially, increased renal blood flow occurs after peripheral vasoconstriction. However, with falling temperature, loss of distal tubular reabsorption of water and sodium and a resistance to the action of antidiuretic hormones occurs, which can result in significant intravascular volume depletion in the hypothermic patient.

TABLE 36.6

ORGAN SYSTEM RESPONSES TO HYPOTHERMIA

■ SEVERITY OF HYPOTHERMIA	■ CENTRAL NERVOUS SYSTEM	■ CARDIOVASCULAR	■ RESPIRATORY	■ METABOLIC, RENAL, ENDOCRINE	■ NEUROMUSCULAR
Mild (35°C–32°C)	Depressed cerebral metabolism; confusion; amnesia; ataxia	Vasoconstriction; tachycardia followed by bradycardia; increased cardiac output; hypertension	Tachypnea followed by progressive decrease in minute ventilation; bronchospasm; impaired mucosal function	Increased metabolism; increased oxygen consumption; cold diuresis; impairment of renal-concentrating ability; hypovolemia	Increased tone with shivering, followed by muscle fatigue
Moderate (<32°C–28°C)	Unconsciousness; pupillary dilatation; diminished gag reflex	Bradycardia; decreased contractility; slowed cardiac conduction; J waves on ECG; arrhythmias	Hypoventilation with acidosis despite decrease in CO_2 production; V/Q mismatch; decreased oxygen consumption	Decreased renal blood flow; no insulin activity	Extinction of shivering; hyporeflexia; muscle rigidity
Severe (<28°C)	Decreased or no EEG activity; nonreactive pupils; loss of ocular reflexes	Progressive decrease in BP, cardiac output, and heart rate; ventricular arrhythmias (fibrillation); asystole	Lung capillary damage; pulmonary edema; further decreased oxygen consumption; apnea	Decrease in basal metabolism; acidosis; renal failure	Areflexia; rhabdomyolysis

ECG, electrocardiogram; EEG, electroencephalogram; BP, blood pressure.

Cold Water Immersion. The organ system response to immersion in cold water versus exposure to cold air can be dramatically different at the onset of the insult. An initial "cold shock" results in uncontrolled respiratory gasping and hyperventilation, tachycardia, and hypertension. Respiratory alkalosis and cerebral vasoconstriction occur. However, the heat loss by conduction in cold water is ~20 times greater than in air, leading to very rapid cooling and decrease in organ blood flow. Conditions that involve total immersion, including the head, initiate a "diving reflex" that consists of apnea, marked bradycardia, increased peripheral vascular resistance, and increased blood supply to the brain and heart due to parasympathetic neural output in addition to the sympathetic activity from cold exposure (51). The early shunting of oxygen to essential vascular beds and the subsequent overall decrease in metabolic rate due to rapid cooling may provide an explanation for the very prolonged submersion survival times seen in children.

Etiology of Hypothermia

Common Causes

Hypothermia may occur due to a variety of causes and can be accidental or nonaccidental and environmental or nonenvironmental. Primary hypothermia occurs in an otherwise healthy individual whose ability to produce heat is overcome by the stress of excessive cold. Secondary hypothermia occurs due to an underlying condition, and death in patients with secondary hypothermia is usually due to the underlying condition (46).

The majority of cases of hypothermia are caused by environmental exposure. The diagnosis of environmental hypothermia is usually obvious in patients found in cold outdoor environments, but may be overlooked in patients found indoors. Etiologies of hypothermia include conditions that cause increased heat loss, decreased heat production, impaired thermoregulation, and other miscellaneous clinical conditions (**Table 36.7**).

Predisposing Factors

Preexisting and concomitant factors may increase the susceptibility to hypothermia. Infants and children have a high ratio of body surface area to mass and, therefore, faster cooling rates. In addition, low body fat decreases tissue insulation, and small muscle mass results in lower absolute metabolic heat production (52). Neonates and the elderly can be dysthermic at seasonal temperature extremes. Minimal differences in thermoregulation exist between eumenorrheic females and males of similar body type and fitness. However, during cold exposure, females in the luteal and follicular phase of menstruation have greater decreases in temperature than males (53).

Alcohol and sedative drugs cause cutaneous vasodilation and inhibit the shivering response to cold exposure. In addition, these substances lead to impairment in awareness of the cold and in the necessary judgment to seek shelter and warm clothing.

Clinical Presentation and Diagnosis

In that hypothermia can occur without exposure to a cold environment, the diagnosis must be considered in those patients who present with recognized clinical features and with an accurately measured core body temperature. The cardiovascular examination in patients with hypothermia is often difficult. Pulses are often difficult to palpate due to profound bradycardia and frozen extremities. Many hypothermic changes may be seen on electrocardiogram. The clinical features noted in mild, moderate, and severe hypothermia are listed in **Table 36.8**.

Laboratory Data

Hypothermia leads to acidosis, altered blood clotting, and decreased kidney and renal function. Hypokalemia and hyperkalemia occur, and hyperkalemia becomes prominent with increased severity of hypothermia. Liver function tests

TABLE 36.7

ETIOLOGIES OF HYPOTHERMIA

■ INCREASED HEAT LOSS	■ DECREASED HEAT PRODUCTION	■ IMPAIRED THERMOREGULATION	■ OTHER CLINICAL STATES
Environmental	Neuromuscular insufficiency	Central nervous system failure or abnormalities	Multisystem trauma
Immersion	Age extremes	Cerebrovascular accident	Sepsis
Nonimmersion	Impaired shivering	Trauma	Shock
Iatrogenic	Lack of adaptation	Birth asphyxia	Systemic acidoses
Exposure	Insufficient fuel	Neoplasm	Pancreatitis
Cold IV infusions	Hypoglycemia	Malformations	Uremia
Emergency childbirth	Undernutrition	Hypothalamic dysfunction	Familial dysautonomia
Heat stroke treatment	Extreme physical exertion	Metabolic failure	Water intoxication
Dermatologic	Impaired mobility	Ethanol	Major infection
Burns	Endocrinologic failure	Toxins	Episodic spontaneous hypothermia with hyperhidrosis
Exfoliative dermatitis	Hypothyroidism	Impaired shivering	
Induced vasodilation or impaired peripheral vasoconstriction	Hypopituitarism	Pharmacologic: barbiturates, narcotics, phenothiazines, lithium	
Ethanol	Hypoadrenalism	Peripheral nervous system failure	
Pharmacologic: phenothiazines, α-blockers		Neuropathies	
		Diabetes	
		Acute spinal cord transection	

are abnormal secondary to reduced cardiac output. Hyperglycemia occurs in acute hypothermia, but hypoglycemia may be seen in subacute or chronic hypothermic conditions. Previously, blood gas temperature correction was thought to be necessary for correct interpretation of acid–base and respiratory status. However, current data support the use of uncorrected blood gas values to guide therapy (54). Hypothermia results in prolongation of prothrombin and partial thromboplastin times secondary to the inhibition of the enzymatic reactions of the coagulation cascade. Thrombocytopenia can occur due to bone marrow suppression and splenic sequestration.

Clinical Management

Hypothermia is a medical emergency that requires prehospital care, and depending on the severity, may include a need for basic life support and advanced cardiac life support. All patients should be removed from the cold environment, wet clothing removed, and rewarmed. The method of rewarming is determined by the severity of hypothermia and other clinical parameters. Little evidence supports the benefit of one method of rewarming over another. However, anecdotal evidence suggests that, unless the patient has full monitoring and critical

TABLE 36.8

CLINICAL FEATURES OF HYPOTHERMIA

	■ MILD HYPOTHERMIA (35°C–32°C)	■ MODERATE HYPOTHERMIA (<32°C–28°C)	■ SEVERE HYPOTHERMIA (<28°C)
Thermoregulatory	Shivering	Extinction of shivering	No shivering
Respiratory	Tachypnea	Hypoventilation, respiratory acidosis, hypoxemia, aspiration pneumonia, atelectasis	Apnea, pulmonary edema, acute respiratory distress syndrome
Cardiovascular	Tachycardia, hypertension	Bradycardia, hypotension, prolonged QT interval, J wave, atrial arrhythmias	Pulseless electrical activity, atrial and ventricular fibrillation, asystole
Gastrointestinal	Ileus, nausea, vomiting	Pancreatitis, gastric erosions	Pancreatitis, gastric erosions
Renal/fluid/electrolyte	Cold diuresis, hypokalemia, alkalosis	Hyperkalemia, hyperglycemia, lactic acidosis	Hyperkalemia, hyperglycemia, lactic acidosis
Muscular	Hypertonia	Rigidity	Rhabdomyolysis
Hematologic		Hemoconcentration, hypercoagulability	Thrombocytopenia, disseminated intravascular coagulation, bleeding
Neurologic	Disorientation, impaired judgment, dysarthria, ataxia, hyperreflexia	Agitation, hallucination, unconsciousness, dilated pupils, diminished gag reflex, hyporeflexia	Coma, nonreactive pupils, areflexia, brain-dead-like state

care support systems, slow rewarming is safer than rapid rewarming (55).

Passive External Rewarming

Passive rewarming—the use of blankets to cover the head, neck, and body—reduces evaporative heat loss and allows rewarming at a rate of 0.5°C–4°C per hour. This method will be unsuccessful if shivering or other thermoregulatory mechanisms are absent. Passive external rewarming is usually an adequate treatment modality for patients with mild hypothermia.

Active External Rewarming

Active external warming—the application of heat directly to the skin—is only effective if the patient has an intact circulation that can return peripherally rewarmed blood to the core. Hot water bottles may cause burns to cold and vasoconstricted skin. Warm blankets and heating blankets rewarm at variable rates and may produce burns to the skin. Radiant warmers can also produce skin burns if patients are not covered with blankets. Forced-heated-air devices such as the Bair Hugger device can rewarm at a rate of 1°C–2.5°C per hour by heat transfer via convection. Warm water immersion is not recommended because the patient cannot be monitored. External methods of rewarming are usually effective for mild-to-moderate hypothermia.

Complications of active external warming include afterdrop, a decrease in core temperature secondary to the rapid return of cold peripheral blood to the heart. With use of active external and minimally invasive rewarming techniques, and with concurrent esophageal temperature measurement, afterdrop has not been reported (56). *Rescue collapse* is defined as cardiac arrest related to extrication and transport of a patient with deep hypothermia. It has been attributed to

circulatory collapse due to hypovolemia, cardiac arrhythmias triggered by interventions, and further cooling. Acidosis due to return of pooled lactic acid to the central circulation may be seen (46).

Active Internal Rewarming

The modalities for active internal rewarming have a spectrum of invasiveness and potential complications. These methods are necessary for treating patients with severe hypothermia. The rewarming method should be chosen based on available resources, monitoring, and support systems and on the presence of cardiac arrest or fibrillation.

Active internal warming methods include heated (42°C), humidified air via an endotracheal tube and heated (42°C) IV fluids via rapid infusion. Together, these methods can warm at a rate of 1°C–2°C per hour. More invasive techniques include body cavity lavage (gastric, bladder, colon, pleural, peritoneal) with warmed saline, which can warm at a rate of 1°C–4°C per hour. The most invasive methods of active internal rewarming are extracorporeal and include continuous arteriovenous or venovenous warming, hemodialysis, and cardiopulmonary bypass. The first three require the presence of a pulse and adequate blood pressure. Cardiopulmonary bypass is highly effective and can increase the core temperature by 1°C–2°C every 3–5 minutes. In addition, it provides the benefit of full circulatory support. Cardiopulmonary bypass is the method indicated for severe hypothermia associated with either the failure of less invasive, active rewarming techniques, or severe hypothermia accompanied by cardiac arrest, or a nonperfusing cardiac rhythm. In a series of young, healthy patients (including 7 children) with accidental deep hypothermia, survival with good neurologic outcome was reported in the 15 of 32 patients who received cardiopulmonary bypass (20). An algorithm for the rewarming approach to the hypothermic patient is shown in **Figure 36.1**.

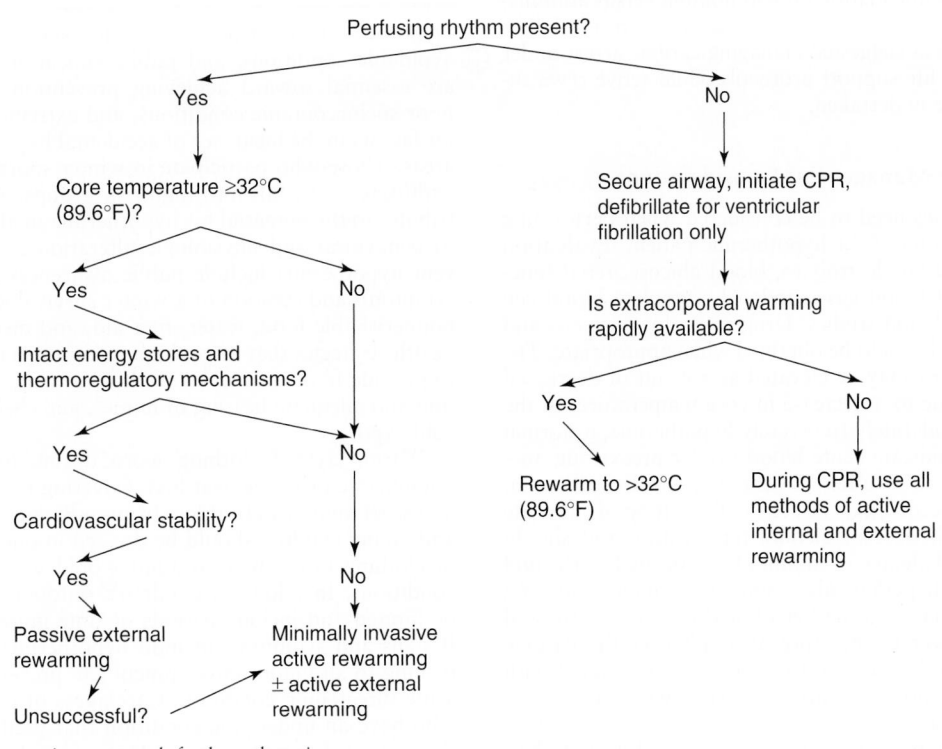

FIGURE 36.1. Rewarming approach for hypothermia.

Management of Patients with Arrhythmias and Cardiac Arrest

Patients with hypothermia develop arrhythmias. Most arrhythmias correct with rewarming alone. Initial rewarming procedures, endotracheal intubation, vascular access, and patient transport should be performed gently, as these patients are prone to develop ventricular fibrillation. When central venous access is required, it is important to ensure that the tip of the catheter or the guidewire does not enter the heart in order to minimize the risk for arrhythmia. However, these concerns should not cause a delay in performing urgent procedures.

According to the guidelines set by the American Heart Association (AHA) in 2010, CPR (cardiopulmonary resuscitation) should be administered without delay in severely hypothermic patients with cardiac arrest or nonperfusing rhythms. CPR should be initiated even if the patient appears clinically dead on initial assessment, unless there are obvious signs of death such as rigor mortis or decomposition (57). Resuscitative efforts in the severely hypothermic patient may be very prolonged, especially if extracorporeal warming is unavailable. Although a patient may appear clinically dead, resuscitative efforts should continue at least until the patient has been rewarmed to ~34°C, spontaneous circulation has been restored, or clearly lethal injuries are identified.

Previous guidelines had suggested withholding IV resuscitation medications until the core temperature was raised above 30°C. This was due to the theoretical concern that drug metabolism may be reduced and cause an accumulation to toxic levels in the severely hypothermic patient. Also, it was theorized that the hypothermic heart would be unresponsive to cardiovascular medications, pacemaker stimulation, or defibrillation. However, more recent animal studies have shown improved rates of return of spontaneous circulation and higher coronary perfusion pressure in animals treated with vasoactive medications and defibrillation than in those treated with placebo. Human trials of medication use in accidental hypothermia do not exist (57). Based on the lack of human evidence and the small number of animal studies, the AHA could not make a clear recommendation on withholding versus administering vasopressive medications during cardiac arrest in hypothermic patients, but suggested managing cardiac arrest under normal advanced life support protocols while active rewarming strategies were undertaken.

Other Management Considerations

Many abnormalities need to be considered when performing laboratory evaluation of the hypothermic patient. Evaluation should include serum electrolytes, blood glucose, renal function tests, arterial blood gases and pH, complete blood cell count, and coagulation studies. Drug toxicology screens and blood alcohol level should be obtained when appropriate. The patient's hematocrit may be elevated as a result of decreased plasma volume due to a decrease in core temperature. In the patient who is moderately to severely hypothermic, a normal hematocrit may indicate acute blood loss or preexisting anemia. Hyperglycemia is often present in acute hypothermia; however, hypoglycemia may be seen in the setting of subacute or chronic hypothermia or alcohol intoxication and should be treated. Hypokalemia is commonly associated with mild hypothermia, but hyperkalemia—common with moderate and severe hypothermia—is a marker of acidosis, cell death, and renal failure. Lower temperature also enhances the cardiac toxicity of hyperkalemia (58). Coagulopathy associated with hypothermia commonly occurs, especially when associated with major trauma.

Aggressive volume resuscitation is warranted in hypothermic patients secondary to the dehydration caused by cold diuresis and the vascular expansion associated with vasodilatation on rewarming. No evidence exists for the empiric administration of corticosteroids or antibiotics. However, stress-dose steroids should be administered in patients with a known history of adrenal insufficiency and should be considered if body temperature fails to normalize despite the use of appropriate warming techniques. Antibiotics should be administered to patients in whom it is suspected that infection is the etiology of hypothermia (59).

Outcomes

Between the years 1999 and 2004, there were a total of 3881 deaths in the United States attributed to hypothermia. The annual death rate was 0.23 per 100,000 population. The majority of deaths were in males and those older than 65 years (60).

The outcome of hypothermia depends on the cause and comorbid conditions that precipitated the hypothermia. The abnormal physiologic conditions that occur with hypothermia are generally reversible with rewarming. Reported death rates vary widely between 17% and 69% (61). The lowest initial temperatures recorded in those who survived from hypothermia were 14.2°C in a child (62) and 13.7°C in an adult (63); both had good neurologic recovery after rescue and rewarming with cardiopulmonary bypass. The presence of asphyxia or hypoxic brain damage prior to the development of hypothermia increases the risk of mortality, as does serious underlying disease. In patients with multisystem trauma, uncorrectable spontaneous hypothermia is associated with poor outcomes and death (64).

"Rewarming shock," multi–system organ dysfunction, sepsis, and tissue injury remain frequent morbidities and can contribute to mortality. Psychological and neurodevelopmental disturbances have been reported in infant and newborn survivors of accidental hypothermia (65).

Prevention

Hypothermia and frostbite are devastating and potentially avoidable conditions, and public education and preparation are essential toward achieving prevention. Urban poverty, poor socioeconomic conditions, and extremes of age are major factors in the incidence of accidental hypothermia in urban areas. Those who participate in winter sports and wilderness enthusiasts also fall into high-risk groups. Alcohol use contributes to the potential for hypothermia in all risk groups due to behavioral and physiologic alterations. Strategies to prevent hypothermia include public awareness of the signs and symptoms and creation of a winter survival kit with blankets, nonperishable food, water, first aid, and medications. Public health strategies that target high-risk groups include resources to provide frequent checks on those at risk, improved insulation and adequate heating of homes, and shelters to minimize cold exposure.

Warm, layered clothing worn during outdoor activities minimizes convective heat loss. Covering the head with a hat or a scarf minimizes heat loss from radiation. As a rule, infants and young children should be dressed in one additional layer of clothing more than an adult would wear in similar cold conditions. In addition, children's outdoor playtime should be limited and include periods of time indoors to warm up. If signs and symptoms of mild hypothermia are present, returning to an indoor environment can prevent progression to a life-threatening condition. Caretakers of children or adults who have an underlying condition that predisposes to hypothermia need anticipatory guidance on risks and prevention. Education of public safety personnel and healthcare workers to recognize hypothermia and to know effective treatment strategies can also help to prevent hypothermia-related morbidity and mortality.

CONCLUSIONS AND FUTURE DIRECTIONS

Heat-related illnesses consist of a group of disorders that range from benign heat cramps to devastating heat strokes. Early diagnosis and rapid treatment prevent the high mortality and morbidity associated with heat stroke. A preventive strategy is an important part of the overall therapeutic approach that can be effectively implemented to thwart a poor outcome.

Heat-induced inflammatory cascade cannot be interrupted once it is initiated. Corticosteroids, antiendotoxin antibodies, interleukin receptor antagonists, and nuclear factor (NF)-κB blockers have been used in experimental settings. The interruption of activated coagulation cascade by replacing deficient levels of naturally-occurring anticoagulant factors, such as activated protein C and tissue factor pathway inhibitor, may modulate the inflammatory cascade, which may ameliorate systemic inflammation and subsequent multi–organ dysfunction. Upregulation of HSPs to protect cells from heat-related illnesses is another logical therapeutic possibility aimed at preventing irreversible cell damage.

Cold-induced injuries and hypothermia are a group of disorders that range from frostnip and frostbite to devastating profound hypothermia. Early recognition of localized cold injury and rapid rewarming prevent limb-threatening conditions. Although hypothermia typically occurs after exposure to low ambient temperature, many other conditions may precipitate a fall in core body temperature. Early recognition and rapid treatment can limit the morbidity and mortality in less severe cases of hypothermia. Severe hypothermia requires the rapid initiation of complex and invasive modalities in centers that provide tertiary and quaternary care. Despite a very high expected mortality, good outcomes have been reported for patients who present clinically dead when they are treated with extracorporeal life support for rewarming and prolonged resuscitation. Preventive strategies are necessary to reduce the incidence of accidental hypothermia.

To date, no validated prognostic indicators have been identified that determine potential recovery from severe accidental hypothermia. Further study might improve treatment and rewarming algorithms. Understanding the mechanisms of circulatory dysfunction during rewarming of hypothermic patients may result in management strategies to optimize tissue oxygen delivery and vascular bed reperfusion (66). Ongoing study of organ system response to hypothermia and its treatment may also point to mechanisms by which hypothermia provides protective effects during its therapeutic use for conditions such as cardiac arrest.

References

1. Gilbert SS, van den Heuvel CJ, Ferguson SA, et al. Thermoregulation as a sleep signalling system. *Sleep Med Rev* 2004;8(2):81–93.
2. Adair ER, Black DR. Thermoregulatory responses to RF energy absorption. *Bioelectromagnetics* 2003;(suppl 6):S17–38.
3. Passlick-Deetjen J, Bedenbender-Stoll E. Why thermosensing? A primer on thermoregulation. Nephrology, dialysis, transplantation: Official publication of the European Dialysis and Transplant Association. *Eur Renal Assoc* 2005;20(9):1784–9.
4. McAllen RM. Preoptic thermoregulatory mechanisms in detail. *Am J Physiol Regul Integr Comp Physiol* 2004;287(2):R272–3.
5. Lee-Chiong TL Jr, Stitt JT. Disorders of temperature regulation. *Compr Ther* 1995;21(12):697–704.
6. Bergeron MF, Devore C, Rice SG. Policy statement-climatic heat stress and exercising children and adolescents. *Pediatrics* 2011;128(3):e741–7.
7. Heat-related mortality—Arizona, 1993–2002, and United States, 1979–2002. *MMWR Morb Mortal Wkly Rep* 2005;54(25):628–30.
8. Bouchama A, Knochel JP. Heat stroke. *N Engl J Med* 2002;346(25):1978–88.
9. Epstein Y. Predominance of type II fibres in exertional heat stroke. *Lancet* 1997;350(9071):83–4.
10. Larner AJ. Dantrolene for exertional heatstroke. *Lancet* 1992;339(8786):182.
11. Falk B, Bar-Or O, MacDougall JD. Thermoregulatory responses of pre-, mid-, and late-pubertal boys to exercise in dry heat. *Med Sci Sports Exerc* 1992;24(6):688–94.
12. Falk B. Effects of thermal stress during rest and exercise in the paediatric population. *Sports Med* 1998;25(4):221–40.
13. Wagner JA, Robinson S, Tzankoff SP, et al. Heat tolerance and acclimatization to work in the heat in relation to age. *J Appl Physiol* 1972;33(5):616–22.
14. Drinkwater BL, Kupprat IC, Denton JE, et al. Response of prepubertal girls and college women to work in the heat. *J Appl Physiol* 1977;43(6):1046–53.
15. Inbar O, Morris N, Epstein Y, et al. Comparison of thermoregulatory responses to exercise in dry heat among prepubertal boys, young adults and older males. *Exp Physiol* 2004;89(6):691–700.
16. Rivera-Brown AM, Rowland TW, Ramirez-Marrero FA, et al. Exercise tolerance in a hot and humid climate in heat-acclimatized girls and women. *Int J Sports Med* 2006;27(12):943–50.
17. Rowland T. Thermoregulation during exercise in the heat in children: Old concepts revisited. *J Appl Physiol (1985)* 2008;105(2):718–24.
18. Grogan H, Hopkins PM. Heat stroke: Implications for critical care and anaesthesia. *Br J Anaesth* 2002;88(5):700–7.
19. Armstrong LE, Epstein Y, Greenleaf JE, et al. American College of Sports Medicine position stand. Heat and cold illnesses during distance running. *Med Sci Sports Exerc* 1996;28(12):i–x.
20. Walpoth BH, Walpoth-Aslan BN, Mattle HP, et al. Outcome of survivors of accidental deep hypothermia and circulatory arrest treated with extracorporeal blood warming. *N Engl J Med* 1997;337(21):1500–5.
21. Knochel JP. Catastrophic medical events with exhaustive exercise: "White collar rhabdomyolysis". *Kidney Int* 1990;38(4):709–19.
22. Hietala J, Nurmi T, Uhari M, et al. Acute phase proteins, humoral and cell mediated immunity in environmentally-induced hyperthermia in man. *Eur J Appl Physiol Occup Physiol* 1982;49(2):271–6.
23. Li PL, Chao YM, Chan SH, et al. Potentiation of baroreceptor reflex response by heat shock protein 70 in nucleus tractus solitarii confers cardiovascular protection during heatstroke. *Circulation* 2001;103(16):2114–9.
24. Donaldson GC, Keatinge WR, Saunders RD. Cardiovascular responses to heat stress and their adverse consequences in healthy and vulnerable human populations. *Int J Hyperthermia* 2003;19(3):225–35.
25. Chang DM. The role of cytokines in heat stroke. *Immunological Invest* 1993;22(8):553–61.
26. Bosenberg AT, Brock-Utne JG, Gaffin SL, et al. Strenuous exercise causes systemic endotoxemia. *J Appl Physiol (1985)* 1988;65(1):106–8.
27. Hall DM, Baumgardner KR, Oberley TD, et al. Splanchnic tissues undergo hypoxic stress during whole body hyperthermia. *Am J Physiol* 1999;276(5 pt 1):G1195–203.
28. Hall DM, Buettner GR, Oberley LW, et al. Mechanisms of circulatory and intestinal barrier dysfunction during whole body hyperthermia. *Am J Physiol Heart Circ Physiol* 2001;280(2):H509–21.
29. Bouchama A, Bridey F, Hammami MM, et al. Activation of coagulation and fibrinolysis in heatstroke. *Thromb Haemost* 1996;76(6):909–15.
30. Moseley PL. Heat shock proteins and heat adaptation of the whole organism. *J Appl Physiol (1985)* 1997;83(5):1413–7.

31. Albukrek D, Bakon M, Moran DS, et al. Heat-stroke-induced cerebellar atrophy: Clinical course, CT and MRI findings. *Neuroradiology* 1997;39(3):195–7.

32. Alzeer AH, Al-Arifi A, Warsy AS, et al. Nitric oxide production is enhanced in patients with heat stroke. *Intens Care Med* 1999;25(1):58–62.

33. Smith JE. Cooling methods used in the treatment of exertional heat illness. *Br J Sports Med* 2005;39(8):503–7; discussion 7.

34. Bagley WH, Yang H, Shah KH. Rhabdomyolysis. *Int Emerg Med* 2007;2(3):210–8.

35. Scharman EJ, Troutman WG. Prevention of kidney injury following rhabdomyolysis: A systematic review. *Ann Pharmacother* 2013;47(1):90–105.

36. Burkman JM, Posner KL, Domino KB. Analysis of the clinical variables associated with recrudescence after malignant hyperthermia reactions. *Anesthesiology* 2007;106(5):901–6; quiz 1077–8.

37. Hollander AS, Olney RC, Blackett PR, et al. Fatal malignant hyperthermia-like syndrome with rhabdomyolysis complicating the presentation of diabetes mellitus in adolescent males. *Pediatrics* 2003;111(6 pt 1):1447–52.

38. Kilbane BJ, Mehta S, Backeljauw PF, et al. Approach to management of malignant hyperthermia-like syndrome in pediatric diabetes mellitus. *Pediatr Crit Care Med* 2006;7(2):169–73.

39. Perry PJ, Wilborn CA. Serotonin syndrome vs neuroleptic malignant syndrome: A contrast of causes, diagnoses, and management. *Ann Clin Psych* 2012;24(2):155–62.

40. Boyer EW, Shannon M. The serotonin syndrome. *N Engl J Med* 2005;352(11):1112–20.

41. Dunkley EJ, Isbister GK, Sibbritt D, et al. The Hunter Serotonin Toxicity Criteria: Simple and accurate diagnostic decision rules for serotonin toxicity. *QJM* 2003;96(9):635–42.

42. Biem J, Koehncke N, Classen D, et al. Out of the cold: Management of hypothermia and frostbite. *Can Med Assoc J* 2003;168(3):305–11.

43. Murphy JV, Banwell PE, Roberts AH, et al. Frostbite: Pathogenesis and treatment. *J Trauma* 2000;48(1):171–8.

44. Hallam MJ, Cubison T, Dheansa B, et al. Managing frostbite. *BMJ* 2010;341:c5864.

45. Ulrich AS, Rathlev NK. Hypothermia and localized cold injuries. *Emerg Med Clin N Am* 2004;22(2):281–98.

46. Brown DJ, Brugger H, Boyd J, et al. Accidental hypothermia. *N Engl J Med* 2012;367(20):1930–8.

47. Van Someren EJ, Raymann RJ, Scherder EJ, et al. Circadian and age-related modulation of thermoreception and temperature regulation: Mechanisms and functional implications. *Age Res Rev* 2002;1(4):721–78.

48. Alvarez GE, Zhao K, Kosiba WA, et al. Relative roles of local and reflex components in cutaneous vasoconstriction during skin cooling in humans. *J Appl Physiol (1985)* 2006;100(6):2083–8.

49. Lindenblatt N, Menger MD, Klar E, et al. Sustained hypothermia accelerates microvascular thrombus formation in mice. *Am J Physiol Heart Circ Physiol* 2005;289(6):H2680–7.

50. Mattu A, Brady WJ, Perron AD. Electrocardiographic manifestations of hypothermia. *Am J Emerg Med* 2002;20(4):314–26.

51. Kawakami Y, Natelson BH, DuBois AR. Cardiovascular effects of face immersion and factors affecting diving reflex in man. *J Appl Physiol* 1967;23(6):964–70.

52. Stocks JM, Taylor NA, Tipton MJ, et al. Human physiological responses to cold exposure. *Aviation Space Environ Med* 2004;75(5):444–57.

53. Kaciuba-Uscilko H, Grucza R. Gender differences in thermoregulation. *Curr Opin Clin Nutr Metabolic Care* 2001;4(6):533–6.

54. Shapiro BA. Temperature correction of blood gas values. *Respir Care Clin N Am* 1995;1(1):69–76.

55. Aslam AF, Aslam AK, Vasavada BC, et al. Hypothermia: Evaluation, electrocardiographic manifestations, and management. *Am J Med* 2006;119(4):297–301.

56. Roggla M, Frossard M, Wagner A, et al. Severe accidental hypothermia with or without hemodynamic instability: Rewarming without the use of extracorporeal circulation. *Wien Klin Wochenschr* 2002;114(8–9):315–20.

57. Vanden Hoek TL, Morrison LJ, Shuster M, et al. Part 12: Cardiac arrest in special situations: 2010 American Heart Association Guidelines for Cardiopulmonary Resuscitation and Emergency Cardiovascular Care. *Circulation* 2010;122(18 suppl 3):S829–61.

58. Mallet ML. Pathophysiology of accidental hypothermia. *QJM* 2002;95(12):775–85.

59. McCullough L, Arora S. Diagnosis and treatment of hypothermia. *Am Fam Phys* 2004;70(12):2325–32.

60. Hypothermia-related mortality—Montana, 1999–2004. *MMWR* 2007;56(15):367–8.

61. van der Ploeg GJ, Goslings JC, Walpoth BH, et al. Accidental hypothermia: Rewarming treatments, complications and outcomes from one university medical centre. *Resuscitation* 2010;81(11):1550–5.

62. Dobson JA, Burgess JJ. Resuscitation of severe hypothermia by extracorporeal rewarming in a child. *J Trauma* 1996;40(3):483–5.

63. Gilbert M, Busund R, Skagseth A, et al. Resuscitation from accidental hypothermia of 13.7 degrees C with circulatory arrest. *Lancet* 2000;355(9201):375–6.

64. Fukudome EY, Alam HB. Hypothermia in multisystem trauma. *Crit Care Med* 2009;37(suppl 7):S265–72.

65. Culic S. Cold injury syndrome and neurodevelopmental changes in survivors. *Arch Med Res* 2005;36(5):532–8.

66. Kondratiev TV, Flemming K, Myhre ES, et al. Is oxygen supply a limiting factor for survival during rewarming from profound hypothermia? *Am J Physiol Heart Circ Physiol* 2006;291(1):H441–50.

CHAPTER 37 ■ ENVENOMATION SYNDROMES

JAMES TIBBALLS AND KENNETH D. WINKEL

KEY POINTS

1 Snakebite causes most mortality attributed to envenomation, particularly in developing countries. The main snake species belong to families of Elapidae and Viperidae. Snake venoms cause neurotoxic, myotoxic, procoagulopathic and anticoagulopathic, cytotoxic, and hemolytic effects.

2 Snakebite is not always accompanied by envenomation, but its management includes first aid that consists of pressure-immobilization bandaging of the bitten limb (for neurotoxic elapid bites), resuscitation, appropriate antivenom therapy, and treatment of systemic effects of venom. Hypoxemia, hypotension, rhabdomyolysis, and disseminated intravascular coagulation may combine to cause renal failure, for which support may be needed. Antivenom administration should be preceded by the administration of subcutaneous adrenaline to prevent and ameliorate adverse reactions.

3 Bites by spiders are very common, but only a few species of spider threaten life. These include bites by Australian funnel-web spiders; they cause muscle fasciculation followed by weakness and respiratory failure, which along with bronchorrhea is due to acetylcholine release. Hypertension and coma occur secondary to catecholamine release, which later culminates in heart failure, hypotension, and pulmonary edema. An antivenom is available and pressure-immobilization bandaging of the bitten limb is an effective first-aid technique.

4 Globally, bites by comb-footed spiders, such as the Australian redback spider and the North American widow spider (genus *Latrodectus*), are the most important. They cause severe pain, inflammatory signs, and hypertension. Antivenoms are available in several countries.

5 Bites by some North and South American recluse spiders may cause dermatonecrotic lesions alone or in combination with gastrointestinal illness, coagulopathy, hemolysis, and sometimes rhabdomyolysis, with subsequent renal failure. Antivenoms are sometimes available.

6 Scorpion stings may threaten life in India, Africa, Brazil, Mexico, and the southern American States. All cause severe pain and, depending on the species, life-threatening cardiovascular effects and a wide range of neurotoxicity. The efficacy of antivenoms is debated, but judicious vasodilator and inotropic therapy, along with mechanical ventilation, may be required.

7 Bee and wasp stings worldwide and some ant stings may cause life-threatening anaphylaxis. Envenomation syndromes may occasionally be encountered with multiple stings. Prominent bee species are the common honeybee (*Apis mellifera*) and wasps of the genera *Vespa*, *Vespula*, *Provespa*, and *Polistes*. Prominent ants are the Australian *Myrmecia* species (jumping jack and bull-ants) and the American *Solenopsis* spp. (fire ants). Treatment is as for anaphylaxis and, longer term, venom immunotherapy.

8 Tick bite may cause allergy and zoonosis, especially rickettsial diseases, Lyme disease, viral encephalitis, and hemorrhagic fever. Species that cause paralysis in North America are of the genera *Dermacentor*, *Amblyomma*, and *Ixodes*; in South Africa, *Argas*; and in Australia, *Ixodes*. The onset of flaccid paralysis is slow. Mechanical ventilation may be required until spontaneous recovery after tick removal.

9 Although many species of jellyfish cause painful stings, few threaten life. Most deaths from jellyfish stings have been due to the chirodropid (jellyfish with many tentacles arising from corners of a bell) Australian box jellyfish (*Chironex fleckeri*), whose stings cause rapid cardiorespiratory failure by unknown mechanisms. An antivenom is available.

10 Similar chirodropid jellyfish inhabit the Indo-Pacific region. Of the carybdeid jellyfish (single tentacles arising from corners of a bell), the Hawaiian box jellyfish (*Carybdea alata*), Australian jimble (*Carybdea rastoni*), and irukandji (*Carukia barnesi*) cause significant pain, and stings by the latter may be accompanied by hypertension and late cardiac failure. Treatment includes pain relief, oxygen therapy, diuretics, vasodilators, inotropic support, mechanical ventilation or application of continuous positive airway pressure, and possible antihypertensive therapy.

11 Although stings by *Physalia* spp. (Portuguese man-of-war, bluebottle) are the most frequent worldwide, few deaths have been recorded.

12 Numerous fish have spines that inject venom when they are handled or trodden upon, causing very painful lesions. The most prominent are species of the genus *Synanceia* (stonefish), which inhabit the Indo-Pacific region. An antivenom is available. Occasionally, the barbs of stingrays cause severe penetrating chest trauma.

13 Several species of Australian *Hapalochlaena* (blue-ringed) octopuses inject TTX, which causes the rapid onset of flaccid paralysis, necessitating mechanical ventilation for several hours.

14 Some mollusc cone snails fire a venom-laden mini-harpoon, which bears protein toxins that cause rapid paralysis.

15 Some fish are poisonous to eat, including numerous worldwide tetrodotoxic species (order tetraodontiformes) that cause paralysis. Tropical and subtropical species cause ciguatera, an acute gastrointestinal illness that is accompanied by a polymorphic long-lasting neurologic illness for which mannitol may be effective. Scombroid poisoning is due to consumption of fish that are contaminated by bacteria that manufacture histamine, which causes flushing, tachycardia, hypotension, and bronchospasm. Consumption of some shellfish may cause toxin-related paralysis or gastrointestinal illness.

Numerous terrestrial and marine animals envenomate or poison human victims around the world causing characteristic syndromes. Children are overrepresented among the victims of envenomation. Many envenomation syndromes threaten life and cause serious illness. Treatment in some syndromes requires only mechanical ventilation and intensive cardiovascular support, but others may require specific therapies including the administration of antivenom. This chapter describes the animals, their toxins or poisons, the injuries which they cause, and outlines treatment appropriate for each. The sites of action of toxins and poisons on neuromuscular function are given in **Figure 37.1**.

SNAKEBITE

Venomous Snakes and Snakebite

The highest incidence of snakebite is in tropical developing countries. Although the true incidence of snakebite is unknown, two million bites are estimated throughout the world annually with 100,000–200,000 deaths (1) of which 46,000 occur in India (2) and 7500 in sub-Saharan Africa (3). Many more survivors have significant handicaps. The greatest burden occurs in highly populated, rural Asian regions with children being frequent victims. A worldwide massive lack of antivenoms contributes to this neglected public health problem (4).

Medically significant venomous snakes can be classified into two major families—the Elapidae and Viperidae. Elapids are front fanged terrestrial snakes, and they include most dangerous Australian snakes (taipan, brown, death adder, tiger, and black snakes), the cobras, mambas, and kraits of Asia and Africa, as well as the coral snakes of the Americas. Two coral snakes of medical importance exist in the United States—the eastern coral snake and the Texas coral snake. Elapid venoms are highly neurotoxic with an additional cytotoxicity in some species such as spitting cobras. Vipers have characteristic large front folding fangs and their venom is less likely to cause systemic toxicity than that of the elapids. The venom of vipers is notable for inducing bite site swelling and tissue destruction. These snakes include the rattlesnakes of the Americas, and the

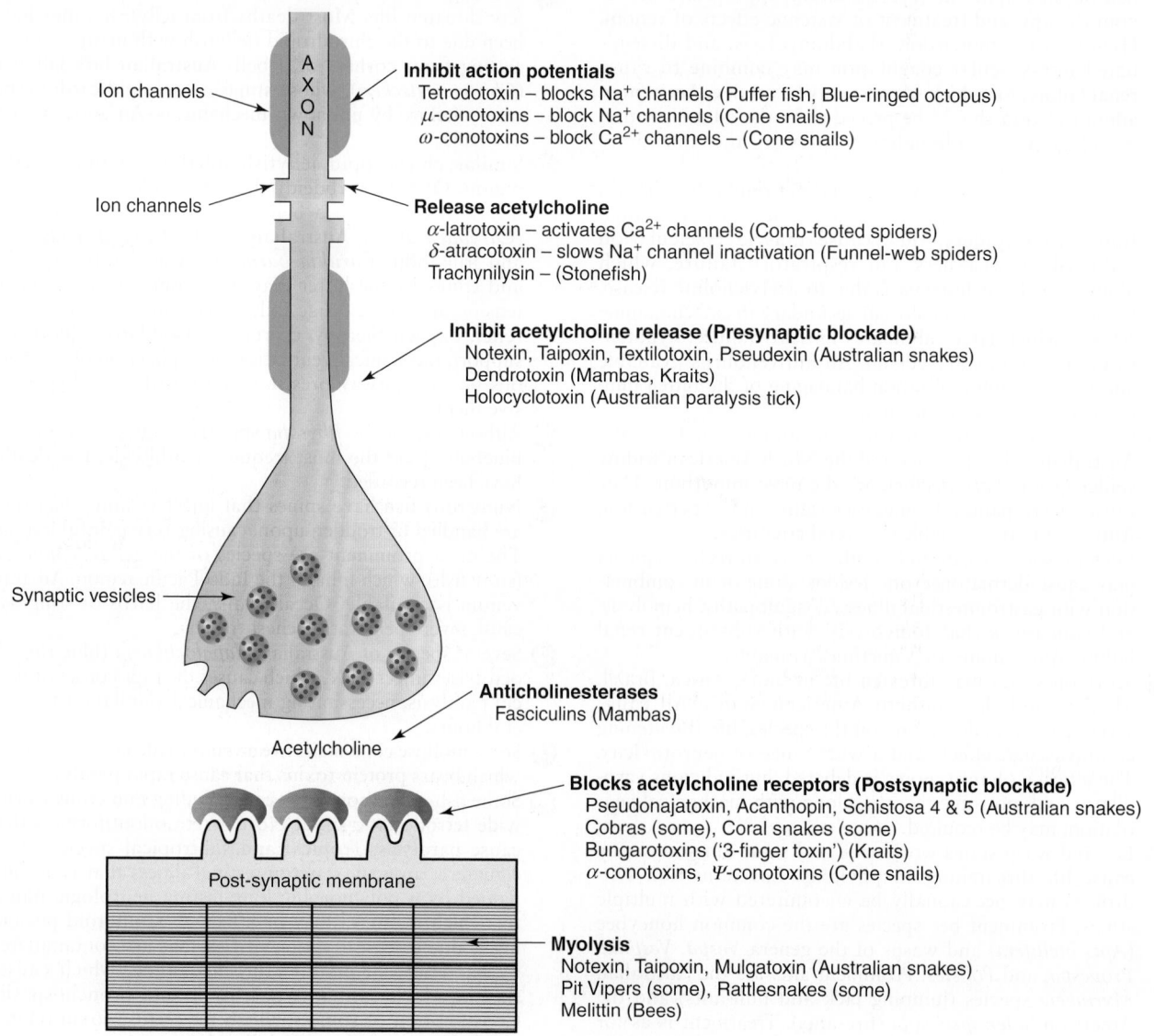

Inhibit action potentials
Tetrodotoxin – blocks Na^+ channels (Puffer fish, Blue-ringed octopus)
μ-conotoxins – block Na^+ channels (Cone snails)
ω-conotoxins – block Ca^{2+} channels – (Cone snails)

Release acetylcholine
α-latrotoxin – activates Ca^{2+} channels (Comb-footed spiders)
δ-atracotoxin – slows Na^+ channel inactivation (Funnel-web spiders)
Trachynilysin – (Stonefish)

Inhibit acetylcholine release (Presynaptic blockade)
Notexin, Taipoxin, Textilotoxin, Pseudexin (Australian snakes)
Dendrotoxin (Mambas, Kraits)
Holocyclotoxin (Australian paralysis tick)

Ion channels
Ion channels
Synaptic vesicles
Acetylcholine
Post-synaptic membrane

Anticholinesterases
Fasciculins (Mambas)

Blocks acetylcholine receptors (Postsynaptic blockade)
Pseudonajatoxin, Acanthopin, Schistosa 4 & 5 (Australian snakes)
Cobras (some), Coral snakes (some)
Bungarotoxins ('3-finger toxin') (Kraits)
α-conotoxins, Ψ-conotoxins (Cone snails)

Myolysis
Notexin, Taipoxin, Mulgatoxin (Australian snakes)
Pit Vipers (some), Rattlesnakes (some)
Melittin (Bees)

FIGURE 37.1. Sites of action of some major toxins and poisons on nerve, neuromuscular junction, and muscle.

old and new world vipers. A small number of venomous Colubridae, a family of back fanged snakes, are also medically important, such as the African Boomslang. The Hydrophiidae is a fourth family of venomous snakes and includes the sea snakes found along much of the Indo-Pacific coastline, predominantly in the tropics.

Venom

Snake venom is a complex mixture of toxic and nontoxic substances, mostly proteins that can have neurotoxic, myotoxic, procoagulant, anticoagulant, cytotoxic, and hemolytic properties. The composition of each venom influences the clinical presentation (**Table 37.1**).

Diagnosis of Envenomation

A high index of suspicion should be maintained in children who suddenly become sick while unsupervised outdoors, particularly in rural areas and in the summer months.

Signs of Snakebite (Not Necessarily Envenomation) May Include:

- Puncture marks (usually on limbs) which:
  - may be difficult to see;
  - may consist of single, double, or multiple puncture marks or scratch marks;
  - may be accompanied by bruising/bleeding/oozing/blistering;
  - may be multiple, suggesting severe envenomation (although this may occur with nonvenomous snakebites).
- Regional tender lymphadenopathy (this, also may be present after bites by nonvenomous snakes, and is thus not by itself an indication for antivenom).

Symptoms of Envenomation May Include

Local Effects
- Swelling, bruising/bleeding/oozing/blistering, pain.

Nonspecific Features
- Headache, nausea, vomiting, abdominal pain
- Collapse, unconsciousness (may be transient).

Specific Features
- Painful, tender muscles (myolysis)
- Blurred vision, diplopia, difficulty swallowing or breathing, slurred speech, weakness, paresthesia (neurotoxicity)
- Spontaneous bleeding from mucosal surfaces, continual bleeding from the bite site or venepunctures (coagulopathy).

Signs of Envenomation

- Progressive limb swelling, blistering, and discoloration
- Irritability, confusion, coma
- Bleeding from bite, venepuncture, or other sites (care should be taken with puncture of arterial or central venous sites in the presence of potential coagulopathy, and intramuscular injections should be avoided)
- Dark urine (myoglobinuria, hematuria)
- Ptosis, dysarthria, weakness/paralysis, dyspnea, respiratory failure (neurotoxicity).

Investigations

- Venom detection at bite site, in urine, or in blood using snake venom detection kit (SVDK) (available only for use in Australia and Papua New Guinea)
- Blood tests to include:
  - Coagulation studies INR/PT, APTT, ACT, D-dimer, X-FDP, and fibrinogen. If these tests are unavailable, perform a test "20-minute whole blood clotting test." A blood sample in a plain glass tube should clot within 10 minutes, if it remains unclotted at 20 minutes, coagulopathy is present.
  - Creatine kinase level to check for myolysis.
  - Renal function tests to determine if renal function is impaired secondary to myoglobinuria or hypotension.
  - Electrolytes because rhabdomyolysis may cause elevated K^+ and decreased Ca^{++} levels.
  - Complete blood count, while the white cell count is usually acutely mildly elevated, significant leucocytosis may indicate other pathology. Thrombocytopenia may occur with some snakebites in isolation, as part of disseminated intravascular coagulation (DIC), or due to microangiopathic hemolytic anemia.
- Urinalysis to check for hemoglobin, myoglobin.
- ECG and cardiac troponin in cases of suspected cardiotoxicity. This may be primary or secondary, for example in the case of hyperkalemia associated with rhabdomyolysis.

Differential Diagnosis of Venomous Snakebite

The diagnosis of snakebite may be unclear. This is more likely in young children or others unable to give a clear history (e.g., found unconscious), in patients bitten at night or in dense scrub where snakes may not be seen, or occasionally in persons engaged in catching or keeping snakes.

Differential diagnosis of venomous snakebite includes:

- nonvenomous snakebite;
- bite or sting by other venomous creature (e.g., Hymenoptera, spider, octopus, jellyfish);
- cerebrovascular accident;
- ascending neuropathy (Guillain–Barré syndrome);
- acute myocardial infarction;
- allergic reaction (allergy may also develop to snake venoms, as well as to antivenoms);
- hypoglycemia/hyperglycemia;
- drug overdose;
- closed head injury;
- sepsis.

The symptoms and signs of envenomation follow a predictable time sequence (**Table 37.2**) but may vary enormously between victims, influenced by body weight, amount of venom injected, age and state of health of the patient, time elapsed since the bite, prior bite history and allergy status, as well as the site of the bite. The amount of venom injected may vary between snake species and between snakes of the same species according to size and maturity of the snake and the time since it last injected venom.

Effects of envenomation are specific to snake genera and species. Bite site swelling and tissue necrosis may be severe after Asian cobra and pit viper bites and may lead to a compartment syndrome and even require limb amputation. Myolysis is particularly prominent in envenomations from South American pit vipers, sea snakes, and black snakes, while death adder and king cobra envenomations are specifically neurotoxic. Myolysis may lead to renal failure, a complication that

TABLE 37.1

THE CLINICAL FEATURES OF VARIOUS MEDICALLY SIGNIFICANT VENOMOUS SNAKES OF THE WORLD

■ REGION AND SPECIES	Clinical Features				
	■ NEUROTOXIC	■ COAGULOPATHIC	■ LOCAL CYTOTOXIC	■ MYOTOXIC	■ OTHER
SOUTH AMERICA					
Bothrops spp. (lance-headed vipers)	−	++	++	+	Shock, renal failure
Crotalus durrissus terrificus (pit vipers)	++	++	−	+++	Renal failure
NORTH AMERICA					
Crotalus spp. (pit vipers)	+	++	++	+	Shock, renal failure
Micrurus spp. (coral snakes)	++			++	
AUSTRALIA-PAPUA NEW GUINEA					
Oxyuranus spp. (taipan)	+++	+++		+	Renal failure
Acanthophis spp. (death adder)	+++				
Notechis spp. (tiger)	+++	+++	+	++	Renal failure
Pseudechis spp. (black)	+	++	+	+++	Renal failure
Pseudonaja spp. (brown)	++	+++			Renal failure
ASIA					
Daboia russelii (Russell's viper)	−/+	+++	++	+++	Shock, renal failure
Naja spp. (cobras)	+++		+++		Shock
Naja philippinensis (Philippines cobra)	+++	−	+	−	Shock
Ophiophagus hannah (King cobra)	+++				
Echis carinatus (saw-scaled viper)	−	++	+++	−	Shock, renal failure
Bungaris spp. (kraits)	++		−	−	
Calloselasma rhodostoma (Malayan pit viper)		+++	+++		Shock, renal failure
EUROPE					
Vipera spp. (European adders)	+/−	+	+		Shock, renal failure
AFRICA					
Cerastes cerastes (Saharan horned viper)		+++	++		Shock
Echis ocellatus (carpet viper)		+++	++		Shock, renal failure
Naja spp. (African spitting cobras)			+++		
Bitis gabonica (gaboon viper)	+	+++	+++		Cardiotoxic
Bitis arietans (puff adder)		++	+++		Cardiotoxic
Dendroaspis spp. (mambas)	+++		+/++		
INDO-PACIFIC					
Hydrophids (sea snakes)	+++			++/+++	Renal failure

The symbols represent subjective degrees of severity: −, little clinical effect; +, mild effect of envenomation; ++, moderate effect; +++, severe effect. It is only an approximate guide as the extent of the envenomation syndrome varies with the species or subspecies.

Adapted from Cheng AC, Currie BJ. Venomous snakebites worldwide with a focus on the Australia-Pacific region: Current management and controversies. *J Intensive Care Med* 2004;19:259–69; Meier J, White J. *Clinical Toxicity of Animal Venoms and Poisons*. Florida: CRC Press, 1995.

TABLE 37.2

EXPECTED SEQUENCE OF MAJOR SYSTEMIC SYMPTOMS AND SIGNS AFTER ENVENOMATION BY ELAPID SNAKE SPECIES. A MORE RAPID ILLNESS MAY DEVELOP AFTER MULTIPLE BITES OR IN SMALL CHILD

<1 hour after bite
Headache
Nausea, vomiting, abdominal pain
Transient hypotension associated with confusion or loss of consciousness
Coagulopathy (laboratory testing or whole blood clotting time)
Regional lymphadenitis
1–3 hours after bite
Paresis/paralysis of cranial nerves, e.g., ptosis, double vision, external ophthalmoplegia, dysphonia, dysphagia, and myopathic facies
Hemorrhage from mucosal surfaces and needle punctures secondary to disseminated intravascular coagulation (DIC)
Tachycardia, hypotension
Tachypnea, shallow tidal volume
>3 hours after bite
Paresis/paralysis of truncal and limb muscles
Paresis/paralysis of respiratory muscles (respiratory failure)
Peripheral circulatory failure (shock), hypoxemia, cyanosis
Rhabdomyolysis
Dark urine (due to myoglobinuria or hemoglobin)
Renal failure secondary to combinations of shock, hypoxemia, DIC, rhabdomyolysis, and hemolysis
Coma secondary to cerebral hypoxemia or ischemia, occasionally due to hemorrhage

is particularly severe in cases of Russell's viper envenomation. Some snake venoms, including many elapid species, contain both postsynaptic and presynaptic neurotoxins, the latter being difficult to reverse if the patient is not treated promptly. Coagulation disturbances, secondary to consumption procoagulopathy, fibrinolysis, or anticoagulation, are common after many elapid and viper bites, although severe hemorrhage is infrequent. Most Australian snake envenomations can be diagnosed within 12 hours of bite by disturbances of coagulation or neurological disturbances (5).

Treatment of Venomous Snakebite

First Aid

The role of first aid is important in prehospital and hospital treatment. It is prudent to treat all snakebites as potentially serious envenomations and to apply appropriate first aid even though many snakes are not venomous and a significant number of venomous snakebites, perhaps the majority, do not result in systemic envenomation because no venom or only a small amount of venom is injected. However, the severity of envenomation cannot be predicted at the time of the bite. Since at least 95% of bites occur on the limbs and ~60% involve a lower limb, they are easily treated with first aid.

There are many first-aid practices that are useless or harmful. Venom may be injected quite deeply, and consequently little venom is removed by incision or excision (cutting or sucking). These practices are not recommended, and indeed may be dangerous, particularly in the coagulopathic patient. The use of arterial tourniquets, especially for prolonged periods, may also be dangerous and not recommended for any type of venomous bite or sting. Local application of chemicals, electricity, or suction is also ineffective and may worsen local tissue damage.

Pressure-Immobilization First Aid

The pressure-immobilization first-aid technique for venomous bites and stings was developed experimentally in the 1970s by Struan Sutherland specifically for Australian elapid envenomation (6). In this technique (**Fig. 37.2**), a continuous

bandage is applied (as tightly as when binding a sprained ankle, 40–70 mm Hg) to the whole limb and then a splint applied to further prevent movement. For example for a bite on the ankle, the bandage is applied continuously from the toes upwards to include the bite site and is extended above the knee and a splint applied to prevent use and movement of the limb. The patient also needs to be kept still as even the movement of a splinted limb undermines the effectiveness of the technique. The rationale is compression of lymphatic channels and inactivation of the "muscle pump" by which lymph flows and by which venom reaches the circulation. Compression without immobilization is ineffective. By retarding the movement of venom from the bite site into the circulation, it "buys time" for the victim to reach medical care.

It is recommended for use in bites by all Australian venomous snakes and other purely neurotoxic elapids such as kraits, mambas, and coral snakes. While clinical trials are lacking, animal studies and human case reports suggest that pressure immobilization is safe and probably effective in delaying the movement of venom into the circulation (7). Its general use has been endorsed by the International Liaison Committee on Resuscitation (8). If applied correctly, pressure-immobilization first aid may be safely left in situ for several hours, unlike arterial tourniquets, which may cause ischemic or nerve damage. Additional studies support the efficacy of this technique to retard the movement of eastern diamond-back rattlesnake (9) and Indian cobra venom (10) but use in these circumstances is controversial. An elasticized bandage is preferred because it retains pressure. A variant of the technique featuring a "pressure pad" applied to Russell's viper bite sites has been trailed with modest success, in Burma (11).

The timing of removal of a pressure-immobilization bandage (PIB) is important. Once an asymptomatic patient has reached a hospital stocked with appropriate antivenom, first-aid measures may be removed. Bandages and splints should not be left in place for prolonged periods. If, on removal of first-aid measures, the patient's condition deteriorates, the bandages can be reapplied while antivenom is administered. If a patient arrives at the hospital with obvious envenomation but without pressure immobilization, it should be applied. Pressure bandages may be cut away from a bite site to allow swabs to be taken for venom detection and new bandages quickly applied.

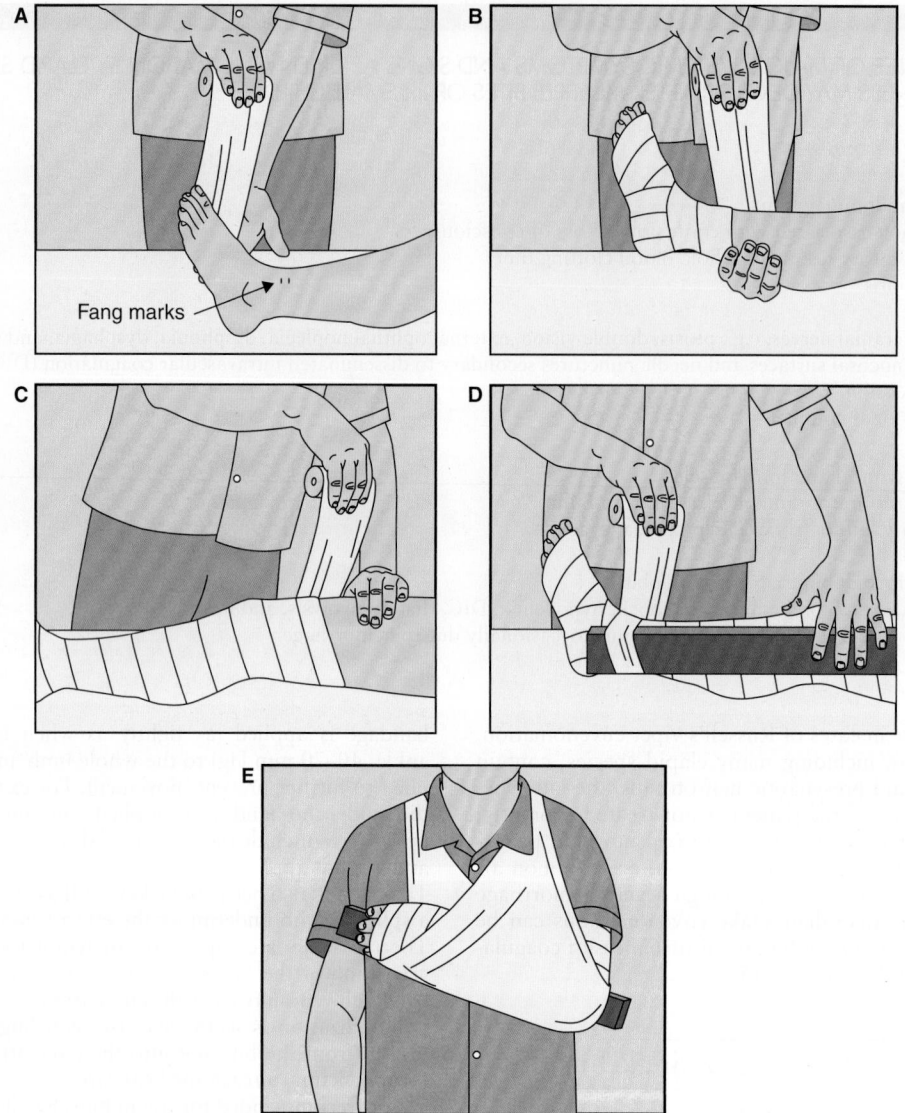

Fang marks

FIGURE 37.2. Pressure-immobilization first aid. **A–C:** Commencing distal to bite, apply bandage as tightly as binding a sprained ankle, enveloping the bite site and extending above major joint. **D** and **E:** Apply splint to prevent use of limb thereby preventing muscle use and lymph flow.

Resistance to a universal recommendation for use of pressure immobilization for snakebite has centered on concerns about potentiating local tissue damage by trapping venom locally. The rationale for this concern appears sound when the significant local toxicity of species such as North American crotalids (rattlesnakes) and Asian pit vipers is compared with the limited local effects of most Australian elapids. Therefore, immobilization without pressure remains a routine first-aid recommendation for crotalid and viper bites (12).

Medical Treatment of Envenomation

The management principles are resuscitation, antivenom administration, and treatment of specific effects of venom. A careful history and examination should be undertaken with reference to the features of envenomation described above, as well as to any previous envenomations and allergies to antivenom, to horse serum, or to other venoms, and with reference to allergic illnesses and asthma. Samples for venom detection and for investigations should be obtained, and an attempt made, if possible, to identify the genus of snake (see

below). The key question is whether or not to give antivenom, an issue that should be regularly reassessed as envenomation is a highly dynamic situation reflecting ongoing absorption of venom.

If the patient has not developed any symptoms or signs of envenomation, nor any indication of coagulopathy or myolysis within 4–6 hours after the removal of first aid (or after the bite if no first aid was used), significant envenomation has not occurred. However, the delayed onset of symptoms, particularly relating to neurotoxicity and rhabdomyolysis, for up to 24 hours after bites has been described. Particular care is required if a neurotoxic elapid bite is suspected, as few signs may be present apart from late-onset neurotoxicity. Overnight observation is highly desirable, especially if the victim is a young child or comes from a remote area. Ideally, envenomated patients should be admitted to hospital and observed for a period of at least 24 hours, depending on the clinical circumstances. Frequent neurological observations should be performed and pathology studies repeated regularly to monitor progression of the illness.

Local Effects. Vipers cause local effects such as skin blistering, limb swelling, and tissue necrosis. Although progressive limb swelling is an indication for antivenom use, its effectiveness at reducing local venom effects remains controversial. The role of fasciotomy in North American Crotaline (pit viper) envenomation causing limb swelling has been controversial but at present, fasciotomy is generally considered not useful when crotaline antivenom has been administered (13). As compartment syndrome is an infrequent complication of necrotizing snakebites, intracompartment pressures should be carefully monitored before surgical intervention (14). Local blistering may progress to full-thickness skin necrosis over 3–7 days—such sites are particularly prone to infection. Some such cases have been treated with the application of medical leeches in attempts to revitalize the affected tissue (15).

Coagulopathy. Procoagulants in Australian elapid venoms initiate the consumption of coagulation factors (16) with possible thrombotic sequelae, such as thrombotic microangiopathic renal failure. Platelets may be consumed and fibrinolysis may occur as a primary or secondary phenomenon resembling the findings in DIC caused by other conditions. After circulating venom has been neutralized, it may be 4–6 hours or longer before reconstitution of plasma clotting factors can normalize coagulation tests.

Whether to give or withhold coagulation factors, for example in the form of fresh frozen plasma (FFP), has always been a vexed question (17) in the treatment of Australian snake envenomation. While FFP would restore coagulation in the absence of free toxin, it may exacerbate the effects of coagulopathy in the presence of venom. A rational decision to give or withhold coagulation factor therapy is hampered by the lack of a rapid test for detection of exogenous enzymatically active prothrombin activator in blood. A lack of improvement in a victim's clotting times on retesting may therefore represent either insufficient antivenom or insufficient time for hepatic regeneration of clotting factors, while improvement in coagulation may represent the efficacy of antivenom or natural hepatic regeneration of clotting factors. While it is reasonable to withhold FFP unless coagulation restores itself within 6 hours after antivenom therapy, active bleeding or such risk, despite adequate quantities of antivenom, is an indication for factor replacement after antivenom. Whole blood should only be reserved for significant anemia and volume loss. In North America, extrapolation from other hematologic conditions suggests that coagulopathy with parameters exceeding critical thresholds (INR > 3, aPTT > 50 seconds, platelets < 50,000/mm^3, and fibrinogen < 75 mg/dL) is associated with a major bleeding risk of 1% over a few days and thus warrants coagulation factor replacement (18).

Neurotoxicity. Descending paralysis, starting with ptosis and external ophthalmoplegia and progressing to respiratory failure, is typical of bites by Elapidae (including sea snakes) and a few species of Viperidae (14). In severe envenomations, resulting in respiratory failure, supplemental oxygen and endotracheal intubation with mechanical ventilation are indicated. If antivenom is delayed or inadequate doses given, recovery may be prolonged (days–weeks). Additional possible neurotoxic complications of snakebite include dysgeusia and hypopituitarism (19).

Rhabdomyolysis and Renal Failure. Many factors may contribute to renal failure including shock, a direct toxic effect of venom, rhabdomyolysis, and DIC. Although various measures (such as alkalization of the urine with bicarbonate and mannitol to create a forced diuresis) have been advocated, these practices remain controversial with poor evidence of effectiveness (20). Hyperkalemia secondary to rhabdomyolysis may be treated with calcium, insulin and glucose, salbutamol, or sodium polystyrene sulfonate. Hemodialysis may occasionally be required, particularly in delayed antivenom treatment. Long-term renal morbidity may occur (21).

Shock and Cardiotoxicity. Central venous pressure monitoring may help titration of intravenous fluid in hypotensive patients not responding to volume replacement. The etiology of shock may vary with the snake species and includes fluid sequestration into necrotic tissue, altered vascular permeability, autopharmacological phenomena, acute reactions to venom or antivenom, and cardiotoxicity either direct or secondary to hypoxemia or hypotension. Shock occurs for example with *Echis* and *Bitis* species envenomation in which electrocardiographic abnormalities, such as septal T-wave inversion, sinus bradycardia, atrioventricular block, and other conduction defects are observed, but their clinical significance has not been well defined. Procoagulopathy may contribute to myocardial ischemia and pulmonary hypertension. Acute systemic hypotension after Australian brown snakebite may be lethal (22).

Other. Spitting cobras of Asia and Africa and the South African rinkhals spray venom from their fangs into a victim's eyes, potentially causing blindness (venom ophthalmia) with painful chemical conjunctivitis, corneal ulceration, anterior uveitis, and possible secondary infection (23). The eyes should be irrigated immediately with generous volumes of water followed by other treatment such as cycloplegics, topical antibiotics, and analgesia.

All victims should receive appropriate tetanus prophylaxis but antibiotic prophylaxis is only routinely warranted if the bite wound is contaminated. Rarely, the snake's fangs may break and become embedded in the wound, acting as a foreign body and a nidus for infection. Other treatments include analgesia (avoid sedating agents such as morphine if possible). Prolonged bed rest may cause contractures, which may be prevented by splinting. Rehabilitation physiotherapy should be started as early as possible (14).

Antivenom

Antivenom is the only specific treatment for bites by venomous snakes. The type of antivenom is determined by the genus or species of snake or by geographic factors if unknown.

Indications for Antivenom

Antivenom should be administered for systemic envenomation, progressive limb swelling, or limb necrosis. If pressure-immobilization first aid is in place, be aware that symptoms or signs of envenomation, including laboratory signs, may only become rapidly apparent when it is removed. Evidence of systemic envenomation includes physical symptoms or signs such as headache, nausea or vomiting, irritability, confusion, collapse, hypotension, neurologic impairment, abnormal bleeding, hematuria, or myoglobinuria. Laboratory investigations consistent with systemic envenomation include a disordered coagulation profile (or incoagulable blood in whole blood clotting test), low or undetectable levels of fibrinogen or raised levels of fibrin degradation products, elevated serum creatine kinase level, hemoglobinuria, or myoglobinuria. Puncture marks and lymphadenopathy are not indications, per se, for antivenom, as these can occur in bites from nonvenomous snakes, or in cases where little or no venom is injected. Similarly, a positive SVDK result (see below) at the bite site (or in urine or blood) is not in itself an indication for antivenom, as venom may be present on the skin or clothing, or in the circulation, but not in sufficient quantity to cause systemic envenomation.

Choice of Antivenom

The correct choice is crucial. Antivenoms only neutralize the venoms used in their production. Generally they provide little or no neutralization of other snake venoms, although some neutralization of other species, particularly within the same genus, may be expected. The correct antivenom may be selected on the basis of unequivocal morphological identification of the snake, use of a SVDK (only available in Australia and Papua New Guinea) or on geographical location, combined with a specific clinical syndrome.

Identification of the offending snake aids the choice of the appropriate antivenom and alerts clinicians to particular features characteristic of envenomation by that type of snake. In cases of snakebite involving zoo staff, herpetologists, or other experienced snake handlers, the snake's identity may be known (although this should not be relied upon, particularly in the case of amateur collectors). Identification of snakes by the general public or by hospital staff, even when the offending snake accompanies the patient to hospital, is frequently unreliable. Formal identification by a highly experienced professional herpetologist is ideal. Sometimes, the snake is not seen, or is only glimpsed in retreat, rendering species identification impossible or unreliable. In addition, especially in the case of snakebite involving small children, a history may be vague or entirely lacking. In all these circumstances a contingency plan for choice of antivenom should be based on knowledge of local species. Bites by exotic snakes, i.e., snakes from other countries or regions kept in zoos or private collections, are very problematic. Local poison information centers may be able to source appropriate antivenom. The US Antivenom Handbook is now available online for selected user groups (http://www.aza.org/antivenom-index), while the many other antivenom stockholders, stocking lists, and antivenom recommendations are available as open-access resources (http://www.who.int/bloodproducts/snake_antivenoms/en).

Australia and Papua New Guinea are the only countries that have a commercially available SVDK. This test is a rapid two-step enzyme immunoassay, which uses antibodies to the venoms of major Australian snake genera. Venom from a bite site swab and blood or urine sample reacts with specific antibodies in different reaction wells, resulting in a rapid color change indicating the snake group involved and thus helping to select the type of snake antivenom that may be required.

Bite site swabs are the most reliable sample for use in an SVDK, provided the bite site has not been washed. Blood and urine samples (or other biological sample) may also be used but are less reliable. Urine in particular may be useful when presentation is delayed, or if the bite site cannot be identified. The kit has "built-in" positive and negative controls that need to be checked to validate the test results. The test is regarded as highly reliable but, like all tests, it must have an (unknown) rate of false negatives and false positives. Initial studies suggest that the latter is likely to be very low (24).

Although a positive SVDK test of blood or urine confirms that envenomation has occurred, it is not per se an indication to give antivenom. Conversely, a negative SVDK result does not mean that envenomation has not occurred since venom may be present in concentration below the detection limit or may not yet have reached the blood or have been excreted in urine. In addition, not all snake venom is detected by the kit (25). The information should be used in conjunction with other information (such as clinical presentation, knowledge of snakes in the geographic area, identification of snakes brought to hospital with the patient) to determine which antivenom to use if the patient is significantly envenomated.

If a reliable identification of the snake cannot be made, then polyvalent antivenom or a selection of monovalent antivenoms, which covers likely species, should be used. For example,

in Australia, a combination of brown and tiger snake antivenoms is satisfactory for all snake envenomation (by indigenous species) in the state of Victoria and tiger snake antivenom alone is satisfactory for the state of Tasmania but elsewhere polyvalent antivenom containing tiger, brown, black, death adder, and taipan antivenoms is required.

Administration of Antivenom

Snake antivenoms are given intravenously. Skin testing for allergy to antivenom is not recommended, as it is unreliable and may delay urgent therapy. Antivenoms should be diluted in at least 100 mL of normal saline, 5% dextrose, Ringer's lactated solution, or Hartmann's solution immediately prior to administration. Note that some antivenoms are lyophilized for storage and must be solubilized before administration. Initial administration should be slow while the patient is observed for signs of allergic reaction. If no reaction is observed, the infusion may be run over 15–30 minutes. If the patient reacts to the antivenom, the rate may be slowed or the infusion ceased temporarily. If the reaction is severe, treatment with epinephrine, antihistamines, corticosteroids, and plasma volume expanders should be undertaken as required. The decision to recommence antivenom should be based on the clinical state of the patient. In the case of the patient with a known allergy to antivenom or to horse serum, the decision to withhold antivenom should be based on the severity of envenomation and availability of resuscitation facilities and skills. Note that prior allergy to antivenom is not an absolute contraindication to subsequent administration.

The neutralization doses of antivenoms are variable. The initial doses recommended for particular envenomations are provided by product information and are based on the *average* venom yields from the snake concerned and the severity of the presenting signs and symptoms. The amount of venom injected is quite variable. For example, 1 vial of bioCSL Ltd antivenom (10–40 mL of 17% equine Fab_2 IgG) (AAT) is comparable to 10 vials of US CroFab (26). Few rigorous clinical trials have been undertaken on the efficacy of antivenoms internationally. Further, antivenoms are often used for their "para-specific" efficacy, most notably the bioCSL Ltd sea snake antivenom (27) in that the identity of the snake is unknown and that venom from only a few, or single, species are used to manufacture polyvalent antivenoms. In Australia, there is evidence, however, that manufacturer-recommended doses may be insufficient to reverse coagulopathy associated with the bites of several Australian venomous snakes, notably the brown snake (28,29). However, some authors have also argued a contrary case (30). Larger initial doses should also be considered if there is evidence of severe envenomation (multiple bites, rapidly progressive symptoms, large snakes). The dose of antivenom for children should not be reduced according to their weight, since the amount of venom injected by the snake is independent of the victim's size.

Thus, the dose of antivenom cannot be initially specified with absolute reliability. Antivenom requirements of individual patients will vary considerably. Some patients with minimal envenomation may not require antivenom, whereas severely envenomated patients may require multiple doses. Recurrence of coagulopathy may occur, particularly with the use of newer Fab-type antivenoms, leading to the need for further doses of antivenom (18). Advice may be available from local Poisons Information (Control) Centers.

Adverse Reactions to Antivenom

As snake antivenoms are biological products manufactured by a variety of techniques from animal sources, the rate of adverse reaction varies considerably in frequency and severity. Overall, adverse reactions are common and may be divided into early hypersensitivity reactions (true anaphylactic reactions are probably less common compared with anaphylactoid reactions), pyrogenic reactions, and late allergic reactions (serum sickness). Limited data are available to estimate the incidence of each type of reaction. In general, the highest rates of acute reaction, up to 70%–80%, occur in unfractionated equine antivenoms, whereas the incidence of immediate hypersensitivity and serum sickness after ovine North American Crotaline polyvalent immune Fab antivenom is 8% and 13%, respectively (31).

Facilities and skills should be immediately at hand for dealing with complications, such as anaphylaxis, before continuing the administration of antivenoms. In particular, prior to the administration of antivenom, epinephrine (10 $\mu g/kg$) should be prepared for use in the event of hypotension or bronchospasm. Epinephrine is the treatment of choice in conjunction with bronchodilators, H_1 receptor blockers, fluid replacement, and corticosteroids.

Premedication for Antivenom

Premedication to reduce adverse antivenom reactions had been controversial but now endorsed by a systematic review and meta-analysis of studies (32). The best study is a randomized, double-blind, placebo-controlled trial of the efficacy of low-dose subcutaneous epinephrine to prevent acute adverse reactions to snake antivenom in Sri Lanka, which demonstrated a fourfold reduction in such reactions (33). In addition, no adverse reactions (such as intracranial hemorrhages) were observed in the premedicated patients, supporting the safety of this recommendation. Although this study has been criticized for lacking statistical power and its relevance to antivenoms with much lower reaction rates (20), premedication with subcutaneous epinephrine is particularly recommended for polyvalent antivenom in a low-resource setting and for higher-risk patients, such as those with equine allergy and asthma. Adults should receive 0.25 mg of epinephrine by the subcutaneous route (0.005 mg/kg for a child). Epinephrine as a premedicant should not be given intravenously because it might result in hypertension in a coagulopathic patient with the potential for bleeding. Similarly, epinephrine should not be administered intramuscularly, as this may also lead to hypertension, as well as to hematoma formation in the presence of coagulopathy. Although traditionally used, antihistamines are not recommended on the basis of ineffectiveness in a randomized, placebo-controlled trial in Brazil (34) and because they may confound the effects of venom through their sedative and hypotensive actions.

Serum Sickness

Serum sickness, due to the deposition of immune complexes, is a recognized complication of the administration of foreign protein solutions such as antivenoms. Symptoms include fever, rash, arthralgia, lymphadenopathy, and a flu-like illness. It usually occurs 7–10 days after antivenom administration. The possibility of serum sickness, and the usual symptoms and signs, should be discussed with a patient prior to discharge, so that it may be recognized and treated early. Corticosteroids should be considered if a large volume of antivenom, such as polyvalent antivenom or multiple ampules of monovalent antivenom, has been administered, or if the patient has a past history of exposure to equine protein. Both the incidence and severity of delayed serum sickness may be reduced by the administration of prednisolone, 1–2 mg/kg daily for 5 days after the administration of antivenom.

Anticholinesterase Treatment

Anticholinesterase inhibitors such as neostigmine may assist in the emergency management of predominantly postjunctional neurotoxic envenomations, such as by the Philippine cobra (35) and Papuan death adder (20), due to the curare-like actions of their neurotoxins but it is not helpful for Indian common krait (*Bungarus caerulus*) envenomation (36). It may also assist in the diagnosis of ophthalmoplegia post-snakebite (37).

SPIDERBITE

Spiders have a global distribution with thousands of species described. Consequently, spider bite is one of the commonest problems in toxicology. Fortunately, in most cases, only transient local or radiating pain, bite site redness, swelling, and itchiness occur. Since virtually nothing is known about the venom of most spiders, the most appropriate approach is symptomatic and general treatment. Spiders with the greatest potential for harm include funnel-web spiders (*Atrax* or *Hadronyche* species), comb-footed spiders (*Latrodectus* species), and the necrotizing species, the most important of which are the recluse or violin spiders (*Loxosceles* spp.). These require specific treatment.

Funnel-Web Spiders

More than 30 species of highly dangerous funnel-web spiders are found on the eastern seaboard of Australia. Funnel-web spiders are the most dangerous spiders in the world, as they can cause death within 2 hours. Fortunately, severe envenomation is uncommon and no fatalities have occurred since introduction of an antivenom in 1980 (38).

Identification and classification of funnel-webs is often difficult, and some resemble the less-dangerous trapdoor spiders. Any dark-colored or brown spider with a body size of 2–3 cm on the eastern seaboard of Australia should be regarded, from a medical perspective, as if it were a funnel-web. Capture and formal identification of the spider is helpful.

Venom

The venom of the male Sydney funnel-web spider is more toxic than that of the female (an unusual occurrence among spiders). While the venoms have many components, the key polypeptide neurotoxins of around 42 amino acids are the γ-atracotoxins, which act by slowing sodium current inactivation resulting in spontaneous repetitive generation of action potentials. This triggers the release of excessive catecholamines and eventual exhaustion of predominantly sympathetic neurotransmitters leading to a characteristic biphasic clinical syndrome. Acetylcholine is also released at neuromuscular junctions and in the autonomic nervous system.

Envenomation

The syndrome is generally characterized by two phases, the first begins within minutes of the bite, and the second when the secretions subside, typically many hours later. Historically, deaths have occurred in either phase of the envenomation. Phase 1 is characterized by the following:

Local Effects

- Bite site may be painful for days to weeks because of direct trauma and acidity of venom, but no local necrosis has been recorded.
- Local swelling and erythema.

General Effects

- Numbness around the mouth and spasms or fasciculation of the tongue
- Nausea and vomiting, abdominal pain, and acute gastric distension
- Profuse sweating, salivation, lacrimation, piloerection, and severe dyspnea
- Confusion progressing to coma
- Hypertension, tachycardia, and vasoconstriction (hypotension may occur later)
- Local and generalized muscle fasciculation and spasm, which may be prolonged and violent (facial, tongue, or intercostal muscles, and including trismus)

Phase 2 is characterized by:

- Hypotension
- Hypoventilation and apnea
- Acute noncardiogenic pulmonary edema
- Coma and finally irreversible cardiac arrest.

However, most bites by funnel-web spiders are asymptomatic.

Treatment

The key points in treatment are:

- Maintenance of airway, breathing, and circulation
- Prompt application of a PIB to affected limb, as for neurotoxic elapid snake bite. The PIB should only be removed when appropriate resuscitation can be given and antivenom is available. If the PIB is removed and the patient deteriorates, it should be reapplied. If antivenom is not available, the PIB should be kept in place, because evidence from animal experiments suggests that venom may be inactivated at the bite site
- Administration of intravenous antivenom
- Intubation and ventilation for respiratory failure and to reduce intracranial pressure. (Note: endotracheal intubation may be hindered by excessive salivary secretions and violent fasciculations)
- Supportive care (additional) may include:
  - Atropine in doses sufficient (20 μg/kg initial dose) to reduce salivation and bronchorrhea
  - Nasogastric aspiration to relieve gastric distension
  - Muscle relaxants and sedatives to facilitate mechanical ventilation
  - Sympathetic blockade for hypertension and severe tachycardia
  - Fluid resuscitation in the event of hypotension but with caution because of risk of noncardiogenic pulmonary edema.

If no symptoms or signs of envenomation occur within 4 hours after a bite or removal of the PIB, the patient may be discharged. (Most patients presenting to the hospital will not have been envenomated.) Tetanus status should be assessed and prophylaxis provided if indicated. Follow-up is needed for potential secondary infection. Although rarely required in practice, wound cultures and appropriate antibiotic therapy may be needed.

Comb-Footed (Widow) Spiders

The "comb-footed" spiders of the family Theridiidae are ubiquitous throughout the world, with more than a hundred species described within one genus alone. The *Latrodectus* genus, including the widow, button, koppie, and redback spiders, are the most medically significant. Globally this genus is probably the most important cause of spider bite, with

Latrodectus antivenom producers on every continent. In Australia, more redback spider (*L. hasselti*) antivenom is used than any other antivenom. Mortality from envenomation is extremely rare.

Venom

The exact mechanism(s) by which toxins produce the clinical effects are poorly understood, as is the precise cause of death in the rare fatalities. The key toxin, α-Latrotoxin, a high-molecular-weight protein of around 132 kDa, appears to be relatively constant among *Latrodectus* species. It forms Ca⁺⁺ permeable pores in presynaptic membranes (39) and stimulates the release of catecholamines from sympathetic nerves and acetylcholine from motor nerve endings. This action has both receptor-mediated and receptor-independent phases. In a remarkable contrast to most envenomation syndromes, widow spider envenomation may progress and persist for days to months.

Envenomation

Bites by *Lactodectus* spiders produce a recognizable syndrome "latrodectism" that may necessitate antivenom. Usually the bite is painful but it may be relatively painless and, unless the spider is seen, may initially go unnoticed. Puncture marks are uncommon and local swelling is not a common feature. The onset of symptoms and signs is highly variable, but progression of the illness is generally slow. Effects may persist for weeks after an untreated bite and have been successfully treated with black widow or redback spider antivenom weeks or even months after the bite. Signs and symptoms are summarized below:

- Local pain, radiating from the bite site involving the entire limb, which increases over the first hour and typically persists for greater than 24 hours
- Localized redness, piloerection, painful regional lymphadenopathy, and sweating (sometimes affecting only the bitten limb but can be in a distribution unrelated to the bite site)
- Systemic features including fever, hypertension, tachycardia, nausea, vomiting, abdominal pain, headache, lethargy, and insomnia
- Children generally present with irritability, local pain, erythema, and nonspecific maculopapular rashes
- Myalgia or neck spasms in children greater than 4 years of age may be a prominent feature
- Migratory arthralgia and paresthesias.

Rare complications include neurological symptoms associated with the neuromuscular blockade and possibly excessive catecholamine release (e.g., muscle weakness, twitching, myocarditis, rhabdomyolysis, paralysis, or death) (40).

Treatment

Antivenom should be administered for pain unrelieved by simple analgesia (i.e., local application of ice or oral analgesics) or with systemic symptoms or signs of envenomation such as vomiting, severe headache, abdominal pain, collapse, hypertension, arthralgia, or myalgia. When the clinical findings are atypical but the history is suggestive, a trial of antivenom may be helpful both diagnostically and therapeutically. The usual dose is a single vial but occasionally several vials may be required, especially in the setting of victims sustaining more than one bite or presenting late. Typically, antivenom is effective within the first 2 hours but symptoms can reappear necessitating a further dose. The dose should not be reduced for children, whose lower body weight renders them theoretically more susceptible to severe envenomation.

The acute reaction rate to CSL redback antivenom is low, observed in one series as 0.5%; therefore, premedication is usually not recommended, but patients with a history of horse allergy or prior exposure to equine immunoglobulin may be at higher risk of acute or delayed allergic reactions. Similarly the acute reaction rate to Merck black widow spider antivenin is very low (41) with only a few cases of anaphylaxis recorded (42) including one death (43). The incidence of delayed reaction to *Latrodectus* antivenom, serum sickness, is also low and thus corticosteroids are not routinely recommended. Several reports of redback antivenom used at different stages of pregnancy were without problems or increase in the frequency of malformation or other direct or indirect harmful effects on the fetus. Unlike most other antivenoms, administration of widow or redback spider antivenom may be effective even several weeks after a bite. A US-based randomized, placebo-controlled, double-blind clinical trial of a *Latrodectus mactans* antivenom (44) reported that although the overall reduction in pain was similar for antivenom and placebo-treated subjects, antivenom reduced pain more rapidly than placebo.

Unlike snake antivenoms, redback and widow antivenom may be administered simply by the intramuscular route. However, if envenomation is severe or if there is a poor response to IM injection, the IV route can be used. Systemic effects in envenomated patients given IV or IM redback antivenom resolved similarly (45). If given IV, the antivenom should be diluted in 100–500 mL of crystalloid solution (normal saline, Ringer's lactate, Hartmann's, or dextrose) and run over 15–30 minutes.

The redback antivenom is also effective against other widow spiders that cause "latrodectism-like" symptoms. However, more research needs to be undertaken before the full range of indications is established. For example, envenomation by the brown house, cupboard, or "false widow" spiders (*Steatoda* species), although belonging to a separate genus within the same family as redback spiders (Theridiidae), is effectively treated with redback antivenom. Like the redback-type spiders, they are found throughout the world but bites have been poorly documented. Physically they are slightly smaller in size with a similar body shape to the redback but lack the distinctive red coloration on the ventral abdominal surface. Instead they may have a yellow or cream tip or spots. With all *Steatoda* and *Latrodectus* species, the female is the larger and more dangerous (but male and juveniles may still bite and envenomate). The *Steatoda* envenomation syndrome is similar to that caused by the redback spider but less severe: bite site pain, redness, swelling, sweating, piloerection, pain radiating to involve the limb, chest pain, nausea, vomiting, shivering, lethargy, tachycardia, and hypertension have all been observed after these spider bites. It is therefore prudent to treat these bites as for *Latrodectus* envenomation.

Recluse or Violin Spiders

Loxosceles spiders are widely distributed, from equatorial to subtemperate regions. Although more than 50 species exist, only a few have been implicated in human envenomation as causing "loxoscelism" and necrotizing skin lesions (46). The important species in South America are *L. gaucho*, *L. intermedia*, and *L. laeta* while in North America are *L. deserta* and *L. reclusa*.

Venom

The venom from *Loxosceles* species has variable toxicity. For instance, *L. deserta*, *L. rufescens*, and *L. arizonica* are thought to cause relatively mild lesions. In general, the *Loxosceles* species in South America cause a higher incidence of the systemic illness. The venoms contain proteases, hydrolases, lipases, hyaluronidase, alkaline phosphatase, and collagenase, among other enzymes. Sphingomyelinase D is one of the most important components of the venom responsible for development of dermonecrosis, myolysis, and hemolysis. The mechanism of action is complex and multifactorial. The characteristic dermonecrotic lesion results from the venom's direct effect on the cellular and basal membrane components, as well as the extracellular matrix. The initial interaction between the venom and tissues causes complement activation, migration of polymorphic neutrophils (PMNs), liberation of proteolytic enzymes, cytokines, and chemokines, platelet aggregation, and blood flow alterations that result in edema and ischemia with development of necrosis.

Envenomation

The diagnosis of *Loxosceles* envenomation is usually based on the clinical findings and patient history, since the spider is seldom identified. For these reasons, the real incidence of envenomation is unknown and misdiagnosis frequent. Envenomation causes two syndromes.

Cutaneous Loxoscelism. This is characterized by a dermonecrotic lesion at the bite site taking weeks to heal. Most *Loxosceles* envenomations result in only a mild inflammatory reaction but in a small subset of victims bitten, a necrotic skin ulcer develops. This occurs within 2–6 hours after the bite with the site developing severe burning pain and accompanied by localized intradermal hemorrhage, erythema, pruritus, and swelling. It is often surrounded by a perimeter of blanched skin that results from venom-induced vasoconstriction. A larger area of erythema may also evolve in reaction to the chemical mediators that leach into the surrounding tissue. A fine, macular eruption over the entire body occurs occasionally. By the third or fourth day, the initial hemorrhagic area degrades into a central area of blue necrosis, which eventually forms an eschar that sinks below the surface of the skin. This common pattern is referred to as the "red, white and blue sign." This appearance of the wound differentiates this bite from nonnecrotic ulcers, which tend to maintain as a red lesion raised above the surrounding skin.

Eschars eventually dehisce leaving a necrotic center that heals by secondary intention, usually with scar formation. Plastic surgery is sometimes required to repair the affected area. The average time from treatment to healing of a suspected bite averages 15 days with a range from 0 to 78 days. If ulceration has not developed by 2–3 days after the bite, necrosis will not usually develop. Secondary infection at a *Loxosceles* envenomation site is rare, although a more generalized rash can simulate cellulitis. Venom-induced lymphangitis can also be confused with a secondary infection. Transient and mild constitutional signs and symptoms such as myalgia, malaise, fever, chills, nausea, vomiting, generalized rashes, and headache may accompany *Loxosceles* envenomations that are not as severe as the systemic illness, although the early stages of systemic illness may be similar.

Viscerocutaneous Loxoscelism. This severe systemic illness sometimes occurs after *Loxosceles* envenomation, in addition to the local lesion. It consists of low-grade fever, arthralgia, diarrhea, vomiting, coagulopathy, DIC, hemolysis, petechiae, thrombocytopenia, urticaria, and sometimes rhabdomyolysis. Hemolysis and rhabdomyolysis can cause acute renal failure. Although viscerocutaneous loxoscelism occurs 48–72 hours after envenomation, it has occurred as early as 24 hours (46). It has a higher incidence in children.

The prevalence of viscerocutaneous loxoscelism ranges from 0.7% to 27% and varies geographically. This difference may exist because *L. reclusa*, the predominant species in the

USA, seldom causes the systemic illness caused by *L. laeta*, the predominant South American species. Deaths, which occur, are of children, particularly those less than 7 years of age, presumably because the ratio of venom quantity/body weight in small children is higher. Necrosis at the envenomation site occurs in up to half of all patients. Despite extensive research, there is currently no cost- or time-effective, commercially available diagnostic test to confirm envenomation.

Treatment of Cutaneous Loxescelism

No definitive therapy exists although various interventions have been proposed: dapsone, surgical excision, steroids, hyperbaric oxygenenation (HBO), antivenom therapy (46) and, most recently, regional sympathetic blockade (47).

Polymorphonuclear Cell Inhibitors. Sulfones (i.e., dapsone) inhibit PMN degranulation, reducing local tissue inflammation and subsequent destruction caused by these cells. These inhibitors antagonize the intracellular calcium release that results in the expression of granule markers that occur with venom-induced endothelial cell activation. Dapsone has been investigated for loxoscelism in multiple animal and human studies (48), with inconclusive results. Because of its side effects (including cholestatic jaundice, hepatitis, leukopenia, methemoglobinemia, hemolytic anemia, and, rarely, peripheral neuropathy) and limited supporting data, the benefit-to-risk ratio of dapsone has been questioned. Nonetheless, its use is advocated in the USA as well as Brazil.

Surgical Excision. Surgical debridement and skin grafting was one of the first interventions used for cutaneous loxoscelism and has been employed as treatment alone or in conjunction with dapsone. Although preliminary results found improved outcome when the two were used together, early surgical management in general has been ineffective, and sometimes harmful, as an initial management technique. The poor cosmetic results that occurred in early interventions were due to increased levels of acute phase reactants secondary to surgery that exacerbate venom effects and prolong tissue injury.

A wound may take several days to reach maximum size (which is predictive of healing time). Surgical excision only after a delay of 2–8 weeks allows dissipation of venom and the subsequent acute phase reactants. Ultimately, 3% of all cutaneous loxoscelism patients require skin grafting once the acute phase of envenomation has passed and either the size of the lesion (>2 cm) or comorbidities, such as peripheral vascular disease or diabetes mellitus, make primary healing less likely. A delay of weeks is required for the wound to "declare itself" with stabilization of the area of necrosis or shrinkage. Prior to this, frequent evaluation is necessary to assess the wound and delayed surgical treatment should only be considered when a lesion fails to heal or complications occur.

Wound Care. Many topical wound treatments have been proposed. Although there are no prospective studies on decontamination, the most important intervention might be wound irrigation. Venom can remain in a wound for up to 5 days before elimination. A direct correlation between diffusion of venom from the wound and the degree of dermal inflammation has been described.

Corticosteroids. The controversy over systemic corticosteroids for both systemic and cutaneous loxoscelism started relatively early in the development of treatment modalities. Clinical studies are small and limited, hindered by lack of confirmation that lesions were actually *Loxosceles* envenomations. Various reviews indicate that while systemic corticosteroids, for the cutaneous form of loxoscelism, are not recommended, they might have a role for viscerocutaneous loxoscelism. Although corticosteroids are advocated in Brazil

for systemic illness, but not for simple necrotic ulcers, there is insufficient data to merit steroid use in either the cutaneous or the viscerocutaneous forms of *Loxosceles* envenomation. Nonetheless, the immunosuppression of corticosteroids early in the course of a systemic reaction might ameliorate immune-mediated morbidity.

Antibiotics. In the USA, necrotic lesions of any cause are usually treated with oral antibiotics to prevent infection, although this may be unnecessary if necrotic ulceration is highly likely to be due to envenomation. Since early envenomation alone can appear to be caused by infection, this might account for the high incidence of antibiotic use. Indeed, early *Loxosceles* bites are often misdiagnosed as infections until the characteristic necrotic lesion ensues. In a classical envenomation lesion, antibiotics are not indicated in the absence of evidence of infection.

Hyperbaric Oxygenation. HBO has been used for cutaneous loxoscelism. Its proposed efficacy is promotion of neovascularization with increased oxygen availability to ischemic tissue. However, there is no conclusive evidence to support the use of HBO in the treatment of cutaneous loxoscelism.

Antivenom Therapy. There are currently four sources of commercial *Loxosceles* antivenoms (Institute Butantan in São Paulo; Centro de Produção e Pesquisa em Imunobiológicos in Paraná, both in Brazil; The Institutos Nacionales de Salud in Lima, Peru; Instituto Bioclon in Mexico) but none are available in the USA. The Brazilian Ministry of Health has the most extensive use of antibody treatment and has developed guidelines for its use in large cutaneous lesions and extensive necrosis or systemic illness (46). Antivenom is also used to decrease the severity of reaction and shorten healing time, depending on how soon it is administered. However, no large-scale, prospective studies have been undertaken and administration is not without risk of allergic reactions.

In the majority of clinical investigations there is usually a significant delay between the actual bite and presentation for treatment. This delay previously had been considered to render antiserum administration ineffective, as the most damaging effects occur in the first 3–6 hours of the bite in animal studies and in vitro. However, recent work using a rabbit model suggests that intravenous equine anti-*Loxosceles* serum reduces the size of venom-induced lesions if used up to 12 hours after intradermal injection of venom. Taken together, all these studies suggest potential value of delayed use of antivenom in order to decrease lesion size and/or limit systemic illness, but more clinical trials are needed. In countries where antivenom is used, the usual indication is systemic loxoscelism, although there is a lack of clinical trial data.

Regional Sympathetic Blockade. As a potential adjunct to the aforementioned treatment modalities, clinicians from Missouri have recently suggested a possible role for a regional sympathetic block in managing cutaneous loxoscelism (47). This follows the successful management of a hitherto intractable case of neuropathic pain associated with probable and extensive loxoscelism affecting the lower limb. The possible more general application of this intervention was suggested on the basis of the value of the technique to increase blood supply to the extremity facilitating wound healing, and relief of a sympathetic mediated pain component.

Treatment of Viscerocutaneous Loxoscelism

Loxosceles species venoms vary in strength and are highly potent with an LD_{50} in the milligram per kilogram range in mice. A full envenomation can deliver up to 0.07 mg of venom. Rare deaths from loxoscelism may be secondary to renal failure and hemolysis as suggested by pediatric case reports. Such cases may be secondary, not only to renal failure from hemolysis, but also from direct nephrotoxic effect, which may be more pronounced in children. Children, particularly less than 7 years of age, are often more susceptible to the viscerocutaneous form of loxoscelism. Although relatively rare, once the systemic form of loxoscelism is fully manifested, it carries a significant morbidity and mortality.

A critically ill child without an obvious other cause of illness should prompt consideration of *Loxosceles* envenomation, particularly in an endemic area. A bite mark may be overlooked on physical exam. Measures such as fluid administration and vasopressor support to maintain renal perfusion and augment clearance of hemoglobin and myoglobin secondary to hemolysis and rhabdomyolysis can reduce the severity of renal damage.

The degree of hemolysis can be profound and may necessitate blood transfusion. Although the use of corticosteroids for viscerocutaneous loxoscelism is universally accepted as a means to help protect reticulocytes from the venom effect, there is a paucity of data to support this practice. Hemolysis may occur in delayed onset of a systemic reaction after development of a dermonecrotic lesion. Patients discharged home with an isolated dermal lesion discharged home should be instructed to watch carefully for a change in the color of the urine indicative of this complication.

SCORPION STINGS

Of 1500 known species of scorpions, about 30 cause serious and life-threatening illness. Annual world stings are estimated to exceed 1.2 million with 3250 deaths (0.27%) (1). Scorpions are nocturnally active creatures inhabiting areas with warm or hot dry climates within 45 degrees latitude either side of the Equator.

Venom

Scorpion venom is a complex mixture of mucopolysaccharides, hyaluronidase, serotonin, histamine, protease inhibitors, histamine releasers, and protein neurotoxins. In addition, the venom of some species contains potassium K channel inhibitors, ryanodine-type Ca^{2+} channel modulators as well as inhibitors of the inactivation of voltage-gated sodium channels (49) resulting in release of transmitters at sympathetic, parasympathetic, and neuromuscular receptors (50).

Envenomation

Distinctive syndromes of severe envenomation are caused by members of a scorpion genera in seven regions: Mexico, southern American States (Texas, Arizona, New Mexico), South America (Brazil, Venezuela, Colombia, Argentina), India, Near and Middle-East, north-Saharan Africa, Sahelian Africa, and South Africa (**Table 37.3**).

Life-threatening cardiovascular and neurotoxic effects are caused by most species except *Centruroides sculpturatus* whose effects are essentially confined to neurotoxicity. A systemic inflammatory response with cytokine release, kinin release, and complement activation may lead to multiorgan failure. Mortality is variable, for example, reported in Tunisia as 8.9% of 685 child victims over a 13-year period up to 2002 (51), as 1.3% of 1212 cases in Morocco (52) and in Egypt as 12.5% of 41 children (53). The effects of envenomation by Australian and European scorpions are confined to local pain and mild systemic effects.

TABLE 37.3

GENERA, SPECIES, DISTRIBUTION OF DANGEROUS SCORPIONS

■ GENUS	■ SPECIES	■ DISTRIBUTION
Androctonus	*aeneas*	North Africa, Saharan oases, African Sahel
	australis	North Africa, Saharan oases
	crassicauda	North Africa, Saudi Arabia, Turkey
	mauretanicus	Morocco
	hoggarensis	Saharan mountains
Hottenta	*franzwerneri*	Morocco
	tamulus (Indian Red Scorpion)	India
Buthus	*Occitanus*	East Mediterranean Rim, African Sahel
Leiurus	*Quinquestriatus*	Africa, Middle East
Parabuthus	*granulatus*	South Africa
	transvaalicus	South Africa, Zimbabwe
	villosus	South Africa, Namibia
	liosoma	Saudi Arabia
Hemiscorpius	*Lepturus*	Iran, Iraq
Mesobuthus	*Eupeus*	Turkey, Caucasus, Iran, Afghanistan
Centruroides	*sculpturatus*	South United States
	infamatus	South United States, Mexico
	elegans, noxius, suffuses, limpidus	Mexico
	gracilis	Columbia
Tityus	*pachyurus*	Columbia
	trinitatis	Trinidad
	bahiensis, brazilae,	Brazil
	discrepans, cambridgei, serrulatus, stigmurus,	Venezuela
	caripitensis, surorientalis, grellanoparrai	Argentina
	trivittatus	

Adapted from Chippaux JP, Goyffon M. Epidemiology of scorpionism: A global appraisal. *Acta Tropica* 2008;107:71–9.

Neurological Effects

Although pain is the universal feature of envenomation, a wide variety of other neurological symptoms and signs may constitute a syndrome as determined by the specific species. Generally, envenomation may cause the following: coma, convulsions, cerebral edema, external ophthalmoplegia, mydriasis, meiosis, agitation, rigidity, tremor, twitching, tongue and muscle fasciculation, respiratory failure, gastric and pancreatic hypersecretion, bradycardia, tachycardia, salivation, sweating, abdominal pain, vomiting, and priapism.

Cardiovascular Effects

Multiple toxicities may lead to acute cardiovascular failure. Myocardial ischemia or myocarditis with raised CPK-MB isoenzymes and cardiac troponin I levels may occur in children (53). Direct cardiotoxicity and release of endogenous catecholamines are responsible for high vascular resistance in both systemic and pulmonary circulations, low cardiac output, elevated left atrial pressure, and pulmonary edema.

Treatment

Antivenom Therapy

The efficacy of scorpion antivenoms, derived from various animals, has been debated. Numerous case series and retrospective reviews have cited beneficial effects and improvement in outcome. For example, coincident with introduction of antivenom and adjunctive therapy, the mortality among 24,000 patients in 18 health regions in Saudi Arabia was reduced from 4% to 6.8% to less than 0.05%. However, a meta-analysis of four randomized controlled trials and five observational studies (54) showed that the rate of clinical improvement associated with antivenom use was evident only for Arizona scorpion (Centruroides sculpturatus) envenomation while elsewhere neither clinical improvement nor mortality were altered by antivenom. Although there is little doubt that antivenom reduces the levels of free circulating venom antigenemia, the clinical relevance of this is questionable. In animal experiments, simultaneous administration of antivenom with venom is protective, but antivenom delayed even by 10 minutes after administration of venom fails to alter hemodynamic effects. Moreover, the incidence of acute and delayed adverse reactions to antivenom may be significant and must be weighed against the degree of envenomation, local knowledge of species, and their effects and duration since envenomation.

Supportive Therapy

Supportive cardiovascular therapy is important in severe envenomation. Intensive monitoring and titration of vasodilator and inotropic agents are required along with judicious mechanical ventilation. In early envenomation, catecholamine release causes hypertension but this later culminates in cardiac failure and hypotension. Vasodilators such as hydralazine, nifedipine, and oral prazocin (55) have been used successfully clinically while phentolamine has been proven experimentally. In 19 patients with pulmonary edema, of whom 11 required mechanical ventilation and 10 had peripheral circulatory failure, infusion of dobutamine markedly improved cardiac output, systemic arterial pressure, and right ventricular ejection fraction while decreasing pulmonary artery occlusion pressure (56). A titratable vasodilator would be beneficial at least in the hypertensive phase of the syndrome and possibly later in conjunction with an inotropic agent. The use of hydrocortisone has not influenced outcome.

BEE, WASP, AND ANT (HYMENOPTERA) STINGS

While most stings by Hymenoptera (insects) are mild and self-limiting, a life-threatening immediate hypersensitivity reaction (anaphylaxis) may occur for which the same treatment protocol should be adopted regardless of the responsible creature. Although anaphylaxis is more common in children, morbidity is greater in the elderly, due to greater comorbidities such as coronary atherosclerosis and medications such as beta-antagonists and angiotensin-converting enzyme (ACE) inhibitors. In Australia, annual deaths from anaphylactic reactions to insect stings are ~0.1 per million population, approximately equal to snakebite deaths (57). By contrast, in the USA, Hymenoptera stings account for about seven to eight times more deaths than snakebite (58).

The location of even a single sting may cause a significant problem. For example, a pharyngeal sting may obstruct the airway while a corneal sting may threaten vision. Multiple stings may also cause massive envenomation.

Bee Stings

Within the superfamily *Apoidea*, subfamilies include the social bumble bees (*Bombinae*) and honey bees (*Apinae*). The common honeybee (*Apis mellifera ligustica*) is well established throughout the world and is an important cause of Hymenopteran stings. It does not tend to attack in a swarm, unlike the aggressive "Africanized" honey bee (*Apis mellifera scutellata*) that is responsible for mass envenomations in the Americas. Cases of massive bee envenomation (venom toxicity) are rare outside of those areas where the Africanized strain is endemic. While the majority of bee stings are trivial, rapid death may follow either mass stings or from anaphylactic reactions in hypersensitive individuals (even after a single sting). Most bee sting-related deaths are among outdoor workers, especially farmers, truck drivers, and beekeepers (and their families, including children). Although uncommon, anaphylaxis can result from the sting of an Australian native bee (59).

Wasp Stings

The majority of social wasps belong to one of the two subfamilies of Vespidae: Vespinae and Polistinae. The subfamily Vespinae includes 4 genera: *Dolichovespula* "yellow jackets" (18 species); *Vespula* "common social wasps"—some species are also called "yellow jackets" (about 25 species); *Vespa* "hornets" (20 species; these large potentially very dangerous wasps inject more toxic venom, in larger quantities, than bees and smaller wasps); and *Provespa* (3 species). Within the subfamily *Polistinae*, some species of the paper wasps, genus *Polistes* (*P. anularis*, *P. exclamans*, *P. fuscatus*, *P. metricus*), are of medical importance. Vespinae are found in Eurasia, North America, and North Africa. The USA has 17 native species of yellow jacket, the exotic European hornet (*Vespa crabro*), and the European wasp (*Vespula germanica*). *Vespula* yellow jackets have spread and become well established in non-native regions such as Australia, New Zealand, South America, and South Africa. In northern Australia serious wasp stings are generally due to native paper wasps. In Asia, deaths frequently occur in children and young adults from stings of oriental and tropical *Vespa* wasps, which pose a particular hazard to persons climbing coconut palms, gathering fruit, working in coffee or rubber plantations, and cutting trees or bamboo.

Like bees, wasps are colony insects that construct large nests, often among the lower tree branches where they can be accidentally disturbed provoking an aggressive swarm attack. A wasp nest near a home or school should be destroyed (preferably at night when the wasps are less likely to attack) by experienced personnel wearing protective clothing.

Ant Stings

Ants (Family Formicidae) are widespread with ~8800 species worldwide. However, relatively few species are medically important and these can be divided into two major groups, distinguished by the development of a venom injection apparatus. The first group gives an irritating bite, which is then sprayed with secretions from their abdominal glands. The second group causes painful true stings injecting allergenic venom. These are typified by the *Myrmecia* ants in Australia and the Fire ants (*Solenopsis* species) in the Americas. Other groups also cause occasional allergic reactions.

The red fire ant, *Solenopsis invicta*, is of particular clinical significance. It forms super-colonies and is an aggressive, territorial species that swarms onto an intruder before stinging. Stings are multiple, usually in the tens or hundreds. Approximately one-quarter of patients stung will develop some degree of allergy. Numerous fatalities, but rarely among children, have occurred in the USA where it has become widespread since its introduction in the 1930s. It also now established in Australia (60). Fire ant venom contains alkaloids known as piperidines, which produce a very painful burning sensation, unlike that of other Hymenoptera, and cause a characteristic urticarious pustule at the sting site.

Venoms

In a typical wasp sting, 2–20 μg of venom is injected. It consists of active amines (serotonin, histamine, tyramine, and catecholamines), histamine-releasing peptides or mastoparans, wasp kinins, which are pain-inducing molecules, and antigen 5 (the most active allergen). In addition, venoms contain several enzymes, including phospholipases, hyaluronidases, and cholinesterases, which contribute to the allergic response. The venom of some wasp species contains neurotoxins and acetylcholine. Despite some common components, wasp venom components vary greatly among species with variable lethal doses. Hornets (*Vespa*) have potent venom (LD_{50} ranging from 1.6 to 4.1 mg/kg in 4 *Vespa* spp.) that can deliver lethal doses in as few as 50–200 stings. Social wasps (*Vespula* and *Dolichovespula*) have less-potent venom (LD_{50} ranging from 3.5 to 15 mg/kg) and deliver smaller quantities of venom per sting.

In contrast, a single bee sting typically contains about 50 μg of venom consisting of enzymes, small proteins, and peptides and amines. Melittin, which hydrolyzes cell membranes (changing cell permeability and inducing pain), is the primary component of bee venom, making up 50% of the venom dry weight. Another component, phospholipase A_2, is a major allergen that also causes pain and hemolysis. Additional components are hyaluronidase ("spreading factor" that allows venom components to permeate tissue), amines (histamine, dopamine, norepinephrine), and peptide 401 "mast-cell degranulating peptide" that triggers the inflammatory cascade. Honey bee venom has a median lethal dose in mice of 3 mg/kg body weight. In humans, the LD_{50} is estimated at 19 stings per kg, translating into roughly 500–1500 stings to deliver a lethal dose. Africanized honeybees deliver slightly less (but equally toxic) venom than European honeybees.

Deaths due to venom toxicity have occurred within 4 hours but may be delayed until 7–9 days after stinging. Secondary infection is a greater risk after wasp stings compared with bee

stings as the former are predators on insects and scavengers of sugar sources rather than being pure pollen and nectar feeders. Wasps also reuse their stings and may break the skin with their mandibles (mouth parts).

Envenomation by Bee, Wasp, and Ant Stings

Simple Stings

Bee, wasp, and ant stings in nonallergic individuals produce immediate burning pain, redness, and swelling at the sting site. Pain usually subsides over some hours, while redness and swelling resolve more slowly.

Multiple Stings

The effects are dramatically amplified and systemic effects include headache, vomiting, thirst, pain, edema, discolored urine (hematuria and/or myoglobinuria), jaundice, and confusion. Rhabdomyolysis with resultant acute renal failure may occur. Intravascular hemolysis, coagulopathy, thrombocytopenia, metabolic disturbances, encephalopathy, liver dysfunction, and myocardial damage have also been reported (57). The inflammatory response may precipitate an acute coronary syndrome. Deaths from venom toxicity have been recorded in many countries, generally when there are more than 200, and usually 500, bee stings but may also occur after as few as 25–30 wasp or hornet stings. Hospitalization is mandatory for anyone receiving more than 10 stings.

Systemic Allergy

Hypersensitive patients may develop rapid catastrophic anaphylaxis causing death in minutes. Severe systemic reactions are less common in children than adults but the risk of recurrence can persist for decades with a 30% chance of a similar reaction even 20 years later (61).

Large Local Reactions

In some patients venom allergy may cause large local reactions. These may involve the swelling of the whole limb within 24 hours.

Treatment for Bee, Wasp, and Ant Stings

Simple Stings

Remove the stinger as soon as possible (the method is unimportant) to limit the amount of venom injected. The majority of single bee stings do not require treatment, although cold packs and oral analgesia are valuable. Wasps and ants do not leave their stinger behind; therefore, each individual may sting multiple times.

Large Local Reactions

Large local reactions usually respond well to symptomatic treatment with nonsteroidal anti-inflammatory agents and topical steroid creams. Oral steroids and antihistamines are often used.

Anaphylaxis

Treatment is based on administration of epinephrine (adrenaline) as definitive therapy, supported by oxygen, β-agonists for bronchoconstriction, steroids, and intravenous fluid (for hypotension). Individuals at risk of anaphylaxis from insect stings must carry, and be taught to use, autoinjectable intramuscular epinephrine available in numerous proprietary preparations. An Australian study of Hymenoptera sting mortality (62) revealed that the majority of patients who died from anaphylaxis had a known insect sting allergy. Patients with a history of anaphylaxis to bee or wasp venom and a positive skin test should also have maintenance immunotherapy (injection of small quantities of pure bee or wasp venom) for at least 3–5 years. This provides 80% protection from further episodes of bee sting anaphylaxis and a 98% protection rate against wasp sting anaphylaxis. Long-term immune tolerance induced by venom immunotherapy is greater in children than adults (61).

Multiple Stings

Patients with serious systemic effects due to envenomation may require resuscitation. Renal function should be closely monitored. Prolonged hemofiltration or dialysis may be required. Permanent renal damage may necessitate long-term dialysis. Tetanus status should be checked and, in cases of multiple wasp stings, septicemia anticipated and antibiotic prophylaxis considered. Children are at greater risk of toxicity due to the higher dose of venom per unit of body mass.

TICK BITE

Ticks are arthropod ectoparasites, which feed on blood, piercing the skin of a host with a hypostome. A complex mixture of chemicals is secreted to enable long-term attachment to and maintain blood flow from the host. Such substances inhibit hemostasis, augment local blood flow, and suppress the inflammatory and immune responses of the host. Ticks cause a number of different illnesses including paralysis, allergy, and transmission of infection (zoonoses), secondary infection, and foreign body granuloma if not removed in entirety.

In North America, 40 species of indigenous soft ticks (*Argasidae*) and hard ticks (*Ixodidae*) parasitize humans but many foreign ticks are also discovered attached to victims returning from abroad (63). In the southern and Atlantic states, the soft tick *Amblyomma americanum* (Lone Star Tick) predominate, while in the eastern states *Demacentor variabilis* (American Dog Tick) and *Ixodes scapularis* (Blacklegged Tick) predominate while in Rocky Mountain and certain western states *Dermacentor andersoni* (Rocky Mountain Wood Tick) is common. In far western states, *I. pacificus* (Western Blacklegged Tick) is found. Parasitism by the soft ticks, *Ornithodoros* spp., occurs in western states. Paralysis and occasional death usually occur among children less than 8 years and *Dermacentor andersoni* is often the cause (64). In South Africa, a number of species are considered potentially dangerous, especially *Argas walkerae*. Mild cases have been reported in Europe and UK.

Tick paralysis occurs in several parts of the world. In Australia, this is caused by the female of *Ixodes holocyclus* (Australian Paralysis Tick) and to a lesser extent by *I. cornuatus* (27). At least 20 deaths occurred in New South Wales alone between 1900 and 1945 before availability of antitoxin. *I. holocyclus* is restricted to scrub and brush country in coastal regions from Cairns on the eastern coast of Queensland through New South Wales to the south-eastern parts of Victoria where its range overlaps *I. cornuatus*.

Zoonoses include rickettsial diseases, Lyme disease, and viral encephalitis (65). Polyinfection may occur. Worldwide, ticks are vectors of rickettsial diseases, which essentially consist of fever, rash, and myalgia. *Coxiella burnetii* causes Q Fever in Europe, Australia, and South Africa, while *Rickettsia australis* causes North Queensland tick typhus. Rickettsial spotted fevers occur in Victoria. In America, *Dermacentor andersoni* is the vector for *Rickettsia rickettsii* and *R. peacockii*, the causative agents of potentially lethal Rocky Mountain spotted fever and other spotted fevers (66).

Lyme disease, named after a town in Connecticut USA where it was first described, follows tick bite. It is a multisystem bacterial infectious disease caused by a spirochete *Borrelia burgdorferi*, which is carried by ixodid ticks. The principle features of the syndrome are a rash (erythema migrans), arthritis, various neurological manifestations (neuroborreliosis), and myocarditis. The disease is widespread in North America and Europe where *I. dammini*, *I. pacificus*, and *I. ricinus* are responsible. The presence of this condition in Australia remains uncertain; it is possible that sporadic cases occur and are transmitted by *I. holocyclus*. Other tick-borne bacterial zoonoses include tick-borne relapsing fever caused by *Borrelia persica* and infections by *Babesia*, *Ehrlichia/Anaplasma*, and *Francisella* species.

In Europe, severe viral encephalitis and hemorrhagic fevers are caused by viruses of the genera *Flavivirus*, *Nairovirus*, and *Coltivirus*, which are transmitted by tick bite. The ticks mainly responsible are of the genera *Ixodes* (*ricinus*, *persulcatus*), *Haemaphysalis*, and *Dermacentor* (*reticulates*, *pictus*). Diseases such as tick-borne encephalitis (preventable via vaccination), Omsk hemorrhagic fever, louping ill, and Crimean-Congo hemorrhagic fever have mortality rates each of a few percent.

Envenomation

Human victims and their clinicians may be unaware of the presence of a tick until progressive muscle weakness and ataxia develop and, even then, unless a thorough search for an engorged tick is carried out, it may not be noticed. The tick may be above the hairline, in a skin fold, or in any body orifice. Local edema and inflammation may signal its presence but it may also make it difficult to see and extract. Regional lymphadenopathy may be present. If a hypersensitivity to tick secretions has developed, local changes may be dramatic.

Several protein neurotoxins of a molecular weight of about 5 kDa, which cause ascending paralysis in experimental animals, have been identified in *I. holocyclus* saliva (27). They probably inhibit release of neurotransmitters. Intoxication occurs after the tick has been feeding for three or more days. By this time, its weight will have increased from a mere 1 mg to some 450 mg. Significant illness is more common in children and the first obvious evidence of poisoning may be unsteadiness in walking or lethargy. Usually the child becomes subdued, sleepy, and refuses food. The paralysis commences as ascending symmetrical weakness progressing to involve the upper limbs and, terminally, the muscles involved with swallowing and breathing. Neurological examination will reveal a paralysis of a lower motor neuron type. The tendon reflexes are diminished or absent and the plantar response generally remains flexor in type. Early cranial nerve involvement particularly both internal and external ophthalmoplegia may occur. In older children and adults, the presenting complaint may be difficulty in reading. Double vision, photophobia, nystagmus, or pupillary dilation may be present.

Nerve paralysis may be limited to the vicinity of the engorging tick, as in, for example, unilateral facial nerve palsy caused by a tick embedded behind the ear, but in most cases it is general. neurophysiological studies that reveal general low-amplitude compound muscle action potentials with normal conduction velocities, normal sensory studies, and normal response to repetitive stimulation (67). Occasionally, cardiac failure due to toxic myocarditis may occur in humans.

Differential Diagnosis

The diagnosis may be difficult if the victim has travelled with the tick in situ to a different part of the country, from a rural to an urban environment or to another country where tick paralysis is unknown. Once the possibility of tick paralysis is considered, a careful search for the culprit(s) may confirm the diagnosis. General flaccidity or paralysis may be mistaken for poliomyelitis and vice versa (since they share some clinical similarities). Other diagnoses to be considered are diphtheria, myasthenia, Guillain–Barré syndrome, botulism, myopathies, and a variety of inflammatory and toxic neuropathies. A facial nerve palsy may be mistaken for a viral infection.

Treatment

Prompt and careful removal of the offending tick(s) is essential. The sprayed application of a personal insect repellent containing pyrethrins or synthetic pyrethroid rapidly kills the tick and causes the hypostome and chelicerae (mouth parts) to lose turgidity and shrink away from the host tissue. Extrication is then easily effected by use of curved forceps whose points are pressed into position on either side of the tick's mouth parts, pressing well down into the skin, avoiding any pressure on the tick's body and closing firmly on the hypostome before attempting to lift the tick out. The engorged body of the tick should not be grasped by the fingers or forceps since this may result in incomplete removal as well as the expression of toxin. An alternative method of extraction is by gentle upward traction of a thread encircling the mouth parts.

There is no need for surgical excision of the tick and there is no indication to apply a PIB after removal of the tick(s) since the onset of paralysis is gradual over several days.

If paralysis has occurred, mechanical ventilation may be required for several days. Due to delay in the onset of the effects of the toxin, the onset of paralysis may be delayed until after removal of a tick(s) in an asymptomatic victim, and the effects may worsen after the removal of the tick in an already poisoned victim. Adequate observation after tick removal is needed, even if the victim, particularly a child, is well at the time of its discovery and removal. Failure to recover should prompt a further search for additional ticks.

In Australia, a previously available antitoxin, introduced in 1936 and prepared from the serum of infested dogs, has been discontinued. Apart from neurotoxic effects, the likelihood of zoonosis and secondary infection must be considered and tetanus prophylaxis brought up to date. The possibility of renal damage should be borne in mind if rhabdomyolysis occurs. Tick-borne rickettsial infections and Lyme disease are treated with doxycycline.

Laboratory Investigations

Hematological investigations and lumbar puncture performed in several cases have not been helpful. Eosinophilia does not occur. However, plasma creatine kinase and troponin determinations should be made in suspected rhabdomyolysis.

JELLYFISH STINGS

All four classes of the Phylum Cnidaria (Hydrozoa, Scyphozoa, Cubozoa, Anthozoa) are characterized by possession of nematocysts (stinging cells) and cause human envenomation. Three of the classes are described as "Jellyfish" because of their gelatinous free-floating medusal life-cycle stage. Of these, Scyphozoa are true jellyfish, Cubozoa are "Box jellyfish," whereas Hydrozoa are hydroids. Large chirodropid (multi-tentacled) cubozoan jellyfish have killed or seriously injured numerous victims while small carybdeid (single tentacled) cubozoan jellyfish and some species of hydroids have caused occasional deaths.

Chirodropids

These are large jellyfish with a box-shaped bell from whose four corners arise numerous long tentacles. The most important is *Chironex fleckeri* (Australian "Box Jellyfish"). *C. fleckeri* inhabit waters of northern Australia and the Indo-Pacific region including Vietnam, The Philippines, Malaysia, Thailand, and Indonesia. It has caused more than 70 deaths in Australia. Chirodropid deaths in nearby countries may have been due to *C. fleckeri* or another closely related species *Chironex quadrigatus* (27). *C. fleckeri* and similar chirodropids have a white or translucent cubic or box-shaped bell as large as a two-gallon bucket (i.e., 20 × 30 cm) and weighing more than 6 kg. Four bundles of up to 15 translucent extensile tentacles stream out from 4 pedalia (fleshy arms) under the bell. Tentacles of mature specimens stretch 3 m. The wide ribbon-like tentacles are covered with millions of nematocysts ("spring loaded syringes"), which discharge toxins via a penetrating everting thread or tube upon contact. The threads have little denticles, which enable them to drill 1 mm into the dermis of human skin. As the tube everts and penetrates skin, it releases venom directly into any transfixed capillaries thus ensuring rapid toxicity.

Venom

Animals injected with a lethal venom dose die within 15 minutes from cardiorespiratory arrest. Toxic components include a hemolytic component (hemolysin) of a molecular weight of about 70 kDa, a dermatonecrotic factor, and a lethal protein component with probable direct cardiotoxicity induced by calcium influx as the result of membrane pore formation (68).

Envenomation

Chironex fleckeri is rarely noticed by a victim until contacting tentacles usually while wading or swimming in shallow water. The tentacles are easily torn from the jellyfish by the encounter and in adhering to the victim's skin resemble earthworms of a pink, gray, or bluish hue. During the first 15 minutes, pain increases in mounting waves, despite removal of the tentacles. The victim may scream and become irrational. The lesions are distinctive and resemble marks made by a whip 8–10 mm wide on which is a "frosted ladder pattern," which matches the bands of nematocysts on the tentacles. Whealing is prompt and massive. Edema, erythema, and vesiculation soon follow, and when these subside (after some 10 days), patches of full-thickness necrosis leave permanent scars. Severity of injury is related to size of the jellyfish and the extent of tentacle contact. Most stings are quite minor. The mechanism of death in humans is not known with certainty but case reports suggest a consequence of combined cardiovascular and respiratory failure. A recent study has suggested a contributory role of hyperkalemia but this has yet to be confirmed clinically (69).

Antivenom

Chironex fleckeri antivenom is the only jellyfish antivenom manufactured worldwide and has been in use since 1970. It is a concentrated immunoglobulin derived from the serum of sheep injected with *C. fleckeri* venom. Each vial contains sufficient activity to neutralize 20,000 intravenous LD_{50} mouse doses. Antivenom is used in about 10% of envenomations. It may not be effective against Australian *Chiropsalmus* sp. venom.

Treatment of Envenomation

The severity and rapidity of envenomation necessitate decisive action of which the mainstays are:

- First aid: Retrieval of victim from the water to avoid further contact with the creature(s) and to prevent drowning; basic life support; inactivation of undischarged nematocysts by pouring vinegar (4%–6% acetic acid) over adhering tentacles for at least 30 seconds to prevent further envenomation. (Alcohol in any form, which discharges nematocysts, must not be used this purpose). Vinegar-treated tentacles are harmless but if vinegar is not available, tentacles may nonetheless be picked off safely by rescuers since only a harmless prickling may occur on their fingers.
- Advanced cardiopulmonary resuscitation on the beach, during transportation and in hospital. Extracorporeal life support may be required.
- Administration of diluted CSL antivenom (3 vials of <10% ovine whole Ig). This is available in Australia but has a limited distribution internationally.

Calcium-Channel Blockade. The role of verapamil has been a controversial issue. No successful clinical uses have been reported and combined evidence from animal studies contraindicates its use (70). *C. fleckeri* venom causes a large elevation of cytosolic Ca^{++} in rat myocytes not prevented by verapamil (68). On an overall evidentiary basis, verapamil cannot be recommended. Indeed, it is harmful and contraindicated because of its hypotensive effect.

Magnesium. Magnesium may prove to be an important adjunctive therapy in envenomation since it improved the effectiveness of antivenom from 40% to 100% (70) but prophylactically did not prevent cardiovascular collapse in animal studies. The possible adjunctive use of magnesium is also supported by in vitro cardiovascular pharmacological studies (71).

Ice Packs. Mildly painful stings respond well to application of ice packs after dowsing with vinegar.

Indications for Antivenom

Antivenom should be administered as soon as possible in the following circumstances:

- unconsciousness, cardiorespiratory arrest, hypotension, dysrhythmia, or hypoventilation;
- difficulty with breathing, swallowing, or speaking;
- severe pain (parenteral analgesia is also usually required);
- possibility of significant skin scarring.

The initial dose is 3 vials infused intravenously diluted 1 in 10 with a crystalloid solution.

Laboratory Diagnosis

The simplest and quickest way to confirm *Chironex* envenomation is detection of characteristic nematocysts on microscopic examination of a 4–8-cm-long piece of ordinary transparent sticky tape, which has been applied to the sting site. The tape is applied to a lesion, stroked several times, removed, and with its sticky side up affixed onto a glass slide. Microscopic examination of skin scrapings is an alternative. Nematocysts of *C. fleckeri* and *Chiropsalmus* sp. are difficult to distinguish.

Prevention

People should never swim, wade, or paddle in the subtropical waters of Australia (beaches, estuaries) when a "jellyfish alert" has been issued. Swimming should be restricted to the safe months of the year and to beaches enclosed by jellyfish-resistant nets ("stinger enclosures"). If water must be entered because of a person's occupation or hobby, protective clothing (i.e., a "stinger suit" or diving gear) should be worn.

Other Chirodropids

Lesions produced by another highly dangerous Australian chirodropid jellyfish, *Chiropsalmus* sp., are narrower and milder and the tentacular contact is far less than that of *C. fleckeri*. Lethal chirodropids are found elsewhere in the world including the Gulf of Mexico where a fatality was attributed to *Chiropsalmus quadrumanus*. Another, *Chiropsalamus quadrigatus* (Habu-kurage), inhabits Japanese waters.

Carybdeids

Carybdeids (Order Carybdeidae, Class Cubozoa) are also "box" jellyfish: the bell is cubic but from each four corners arises an arm (pedalium) usually bearing only a single tentacle in contrast to those of chirodropids, which bear many tentacles. Species of medical importance are *Carybdea rastoni* (the "Jimble"), Carybdeids causing "Irukandji syndrome," and *Carybdea alata* (Hawaiian "Box jellyfish").

Carybdea rastoni

Carybdea rastoni is a small jellyfish often found in swarms with a very wide distribution in the Western Pacific Ocean and most Australian and Japanese waters. The bell is around 2 cm diameter and its tentacles trail 30 cm.

Venom and Envenomation. Purified protein toxins cause vasoconstriction (perhaps by release of catecholamines), release of prostaglandins, and contraction of smooth muscle (27). Tentacles bear ovoid nematocysts. Stings cause immediate pain with four linear lesions 10–20 cm in length and may blister. No specific management exists.

Carybdeid Jellyfish Causing "Irukandji" Syndrome

Numerous small Australian Carybdeid jellyfish (72) cause a distinct syndrome observed geographically from Exmouth in Western Australia, across northern Australia and down the Queensland coast as far south as Bundaberg. The envenomation was initially attributed to the sting of a near-invisible jellyfish named *Carukia barnesi*. Its squarish bell is barely 12 mm wide with 4 tentacles up to 35 cm. "Irukandji syndrome," attributed to other carybdeids, has been reported from Papua New Guinea, Hawaii, Fiji, Japan, China, Quatar, Thailand, Malaysia, and Florida (72).

Venom and Envenomation. *C. barnesi* venom contains a potent neuronal sodium-channel modulator, which releases high levels of catecholamines causing tachycardia, increased cardiac output, and systemic and pulmonary hypertension (73). This hyperadrenergic state may explain some clinical features of the "Irukandji syndrome." The victim rarely sees the offending jellyfish but is often aware of a slight sting to the upper body. Although the sting may be unnoticed, the onset of symptoms forces the victim to leave the water. The sting is merely an oval area of barely perceptible erythema measuring about 5 cm × 7 cm. Irregularly spaced papules ("goose pimples") up to 2 mm in diameter develop within 20 minutes and then fade but erythema may last several days.

From 5 minutes to 2 hours after the sting, but usually after about 30 minutes, a distinctive severe syndrome develops.

Severe low back pain, cramping muscle pains, nausea, vomiting, profuse sweating, headache, restlessness, and agitation almost invariably occur, sometimes with hypertension. Abdominal pain is associated with spasm of the muscles of the abdominal wall and cramps occur in limb muscles. Occasionally cerebral edema causes loss of consciousness. Occasionally, acute cardiac failure occurs and manifests as pulmonary edema, poor contractility, low cardiac output, and raised cardiac enzymes (74). The onset of pulmonary edema is delayed, occurring after several to many hours.

The mechanism of cardiac failure is speculative but may be secondary to hypertension or direct myocardial depression. Although hypertension may have been brief, it may cause "stress cardiomyopathy" (Takotsubo cardiomyopathy) secondary to catecholamine release. Alternatively, toxins may cause "membrane poration" with disruption of membrane function and accompanying rises in serum troponin levels.

Most stings do not cause serious illness but two fatalities have been attributed to unseen jellyfish causing the "Irukandji syndrome" in northern Australia. In both, intracerebral hemorrhage was associated with severe hypertension.

Treatment. Pain relief is important in mild-moderate cases. Repeated doses of IV or IM opiates may be required with care not to cause hypotension. In a series of 10 victims with "Irukandji syndrome," intravenous magnesium salts provided pain relief and a reduction in blood pressure (75). However, such treatment did not reduce the need for other analgesia in a small randomized trial (76). Otherwise, treatment is oxygen, diuretics, vasodilators, inotropic support, and mechanical ventilation or application of CPAP. Antihypertensive therapy may be required initially. Although infusions of phentolamine have been used successfully, a "titratable" nitrate is preferable.

Carybdea alata (Hawaiian Box Jellyfish)

This species has a bell ~8 cm high and 5 cm wide and tentacles about 0.5 m. Stinging causes moderate pain and it may cause "Irukandji syndrome" (77). Immersion of the sting in hot water is analgesic (78).

Physalia physalis (Portuguese Man-o'-War); *Physalia utriculus* (Bluebottle)

These easily identifiable "jellyfish" are the most frequent cause of significantly painful stings. Three deaths have been attributed to Atlantic *P. physalis* on the south east coast of the United States but no fatalities have been attributed to *Physalia utriculus* in Australia (27).

Species of *Physalia* are found in all hot and temperate world waters. Each is a colony of hydrozoans grouped into four specific roles. One group (the "sail") forms a gas-filled float maintaining buoyancy and enabling wind-assisted travel. The float of *P. physalis*, the multitentacled species, measures up to 25 cm in length, while that of *P. utriculus* is smaller up to 10 cm. Another group involves reproduction, while another has polyps and tentacles with nematocysts, acting as a "keel" or "sea anchor" and also collects food. A fourth group performs digestion. The multiple fishing tentacles of *P. physalis* may be 13 m long while the single tentacle of *P. utriculus* is 2–3 m. *Physalia* is a significant hazard to swimmers and when beach stranded may cause stings if handled.

Venom and Envenomation. The main lethal toxin, physalitoxin, is a glycoprotein with cardiovascular toxicity. It causes nonselective channels or pores in membranes ("poration") (79). Upon contact, contracted tentacles produce a linear lesion, like a row of beans or buttons, while uncontracted tentacles cause fine linear stings. Undischarged nematocysts are spherical.

Treatment. Most stings are minor. Immersion of a stung limb in hot water provides pain relief (80). In the few deaths, victims were in cardiac arrest within minutes of contacting tentacles. Death in one case was attributed to respiratory arrest. No antivenom exists.

FISH STINGS

Numerous fish have dorsal or pectoral spines, which may inflict a traumatic wound made worse by deposition of venom (27).

Stonefish

Species of the stonefish genus *Synanceia* (*Synanceja*) are found throughout the whole Indo-Pacific region and, in Australia, from Brisbane to 500 km north of Perth. Stonefish are easily mistaken for a piece of rock or dead coral, which has become encrusted with marine growth. The venom apparatus is purely defensive, and plays no role in the capture of prey. Stonefish have 13 dorsal spines, each of which carries two basal venom glands. When disturbed, the spines become erect. When trodden upon, venom is forced out the tips of the spines into the victim's foot.

Venom

Venoms of all three species (*S. verrucosa, S. horrida, and S. trachynis*) depress the cardiovascular and neuromuscular systems and have a direct effect on muscle. Less-dangerous effects are hemolysis, an increase in vascular permeability, and effects due to a host of enzymes including hyaluronidase. Experimentally, venom injected intravenously causes hypotension, respiratory distress, and paralysis by direct myotoxicity. Various protein toxins have been isolated, which are cytotoxins, release acetylcholine and other transmitters, cause myolysis, and cause cardiovascular collapse by negative inotropic actions and vasodilation.

Envenomation

Stings are extremely painful causing the victim to become irrational. The severity of the signs and symptoms is usually in direct proportion to the depth of penetration of the spine(s) and the number of spines involved. As well as local swelling and pain, muscle weakness and paralysis may develop in the affected limb and shock may occur. Fatalities have occurred in Indo-Pacific regions, and one in Australia.

Antivenom

Stonefish antivenom, a pure equine F(ab)$_2$ preparation, is manufactured by CSL Ltd in Australia. It neutralizes the venoms of *S. trachynis, S. verrucosa*, and *S. horrida*. Vials contain ~2 mL, which will neutralize 20 mg of venom in vitro.

Treatment

The initial priority is pain relief. No attempt should be made to retard the movement of venom from the stung area, which would only enhance local pain and tissue damage. Relief in minor cases may be achieved by bathing or immersing the sting with warm-to-hot water. In severe cases, pain relief may only be obtained by the combined use of antivenom and opiate drugs. A local anesthetic agent may be injected into the track of the sting and the surrounding area. A regional nerve block should be considered.

Antivenom is recommended for all cases, except those involving only a single puncture wound with moderate discomfort. The initial dose of antivenom is determined by the number of spines and depth of penetration. One vial (2000 units of antivenom in 2 mL) is sufficient for each 1–2 spine punctures. Antivenom is usually given intramuscularly. In very severe cases, three or more vials may be required and the use of the intravenous route should be considered, particularly if the pain is widespread or the patient is shocked. Antivenom should not be injected in or around the area of the sting. Due to lack of antivenom availability in much of the Indo-Pacific, stonefish stings are frequently managed with fastidious wound toilet, regional analgesia, and appropriate antibiotics. Delayed presentation and suboptimal care may be associated with poor wound healing and problematic infection (81).

The injured limb should be comfortably immobilized. Administration of an antibiotic (e.g., trimethoprim-sulfamethoxazole, third-generation cephalosporins, or imipenem) active against pathogens found in salt or brackish water (*Vibrio* spp., *Aeromonas* spp., *Plesiomonas* spp.) is recommended. Tetanus prophylaxis should be given according to the victim's immune status. Severe injuries may require early surgical debridement of dead tissue and drainage. Skin grafting may be necessary when antivenom has been delayed and considerable ulceration exists. Sometimes a sting remains painful for months or recurrent inflammation or discharge occurs. This is usually due to a spine fragment, which being semitransparent and deeply embedded may be undetectable except by ultrasound examination and subsequent surgical exploration.

Other Stinging Fish

Numerous other fish with stinging spines of the families Scorpaenidae (Scorpion Fish), Synanceiidae, and Trachinidae are to be found in the world's oceans and fresh waters. The mechanical penetration or laceration by their spines is painful and many also envenomate. Examples are the Butterfly Cod (*Pterois volitans*), Waspfish (*Apistops caloundra*), Scorpion Cod (*Scorpaenia cardinalis*), South Australian Cobbler (*Gymnapostes marmoratus*), Fortescue (*Centropogon australis*), Bullrout (*Notesthes robusta*), Gurnard perch (*Neosebastes pandus*), Goblinfish (*Glyptauchen panduratus*), Ghoul (*Inimicus caledonicus*), and numerous Catfish, Weeverfish, Rabbitfish, and Spinefeet (*Siganus lineatus* and *spinus*). Many envenomations occur among amateur collectors of *Pterois volitans*.

Treatment

Little is known about the nature of the venoms associated with the dorsal spines of the many stinging fish. There are no antivenoms, except for the possibility of using stonefish antivenom for Lionfish and other closely related Scorpaenidae based on analogous venom pharmacology (82). Otherwise the management of a wound is as for stonefish.

Stingrays

Stingrays have barbed tails, which may inflict serious leg, abdominal, or chest wounds. Direct damage by penetration of the stinging barb is usually of greater importance than the introduction of the venom or a marine pathogen. A swimmer cruising the ocean floor is at risk of a serious chest wound when disturbing settled rays, as is the occupant of an open small boat when a ray leaps from the water surface.

Significant wounds require exploratory surgery because the wound track may contain a trail of glandular and integumentary sheath material as well as necrotic tissue. Penetrating wounds to the chest or abdomen, however minor, should be imaged or explored, because of likely damage to internal organs. Tetanus and introduction of marine bacterial infection is possible.

OCTOPUS BITE

At least six species of *Hapalochlaena*, the Blue-ringed or Blue-lined octopuses, are found around the coast of Australia. Species also exist in the Indo-Pacific waters including Papua New Guinea, New Zealand, and southern Japan. These small creatures, rarely larger than 20 cm from the tip of one arm to the tip of another, have characteristic dark brown or ochre bands over the body and arms with irregularly shaped blue circles, lines, or figures of eight superimposed. When the animal is disturbed, these markings become brilliant iridescent peacock blue. The saliva of three species, *H. lunulata*, *H. fasciata*, and *H. maculosa*, is highly venomous and is delivered when the octopus bites. The toxin, tetrodotoxin, is distributed throughout the body of the octopus and probably produced by bacteria. It causes flaccid paralysis by reversibly blocking neuronal sodium channels.

13 ## Envenomation

Most bites occur when an octopus is brought into contact with human skin. Fatalities and near fatalities follow a fairly similar pattern: the octopus, having been found in a rock pool, is caught and placed usually on the back of the hand or arm of a victim while being shown to interested parties. The victim is generally unaware of any actual bite, but symptoms of envenomation occur within 5 or 10 minutes and commence with weakness and numbness about the face and neck, combined with difficulty in breathing and nausea. Vomiting often occurs. In severe cases, a state of complete flaccid paralysis and apnea may progress rapidly. Cardiac function remains unaltered until hypoxemia occurs.

Treatment

No specific therapy is available. The pressure-immobilization method of first aid should be applied immediately to the bitten area, if accessible. Rescue breathing (expired air resuscitation) followed by a form of mechanical ventilation must be instituted and continued until recovery, usually after several hours. From a clinical viewpoint, the syndrome of envenomation differs from tetrodotoxic fish poisoning only because of the route of absorption of the toxin: after an effective bite by *Hapalochlaena* spp., death could occur within 30 minutes due to the sudden onset of a flaccid paralysis, but ingestion of tetrodotoxic fish flesh may lead to vomiting, hypotension, severe abdominal pain, and the onset of paralysis over several hours.

14 # CONE SNAIL STING

Cone snails are molluscs, which inhabit conical-shaped shells, prized by collectors. They fire a venom-laden miniature harpoon to rapidly paralyze prey, such as fish. They inhabit the floor of tropical and subtropical seas. Venoms contain numerous small proteins, which target voltage-sensitive sodium, calcium, potassium, N-methyl-D-aspartate (NMDA)-glutamate, and nicotinic acetylcholine receptor channels. These conotoxins cause rapid disruption of neuronal transmission, neurotransmitter release (particularly acetylcholine), and neuroreceptor activation. Several conotoxins are antinociceptive and at least one (ziconotide), derived from *Conus magus*, is commercially available for intrathecal treatment of chronic pain.

Treatment

The unwary human who handles a live cone shell is at risk of serious illness or death, although deaths have been few. A sharp stinging pain is followed by local numbness or paresthesia. In serious envenomation, weakness and incoordination of voluntary muscles occur rapidly and are accompanied by difficulties with vision, swallowing, and speech. Respiratory failure due to paresis or paralysis may eventuate. Apart from mechanical ventilation, no specific treatment exists. Spontaneous recovery of full neuromuscular function may take days to weeks.

FISH AND SHELLFISH POISONOUS TO EAT

Toxins produced by bacteria or microalgae (dinoflagellates) are known as phycotoxins (83) and may accumulate in fish flesh. Particular fish may contain tetrodotoxin or ciguatoxin (CTX) and related toxins causing syndromic illnesses on consumption. Filter-feeding shellfish (oysters, scallops, mussels, etc.) also accumulate phycotoxins, namely brevetoxins, saxitoxins, okadaic acid, or domoic acid, which also cause specific illnesses. Fish flesh may also be contaminated by bacteria.

Tetrodotoxin Poisoning

Hundreds of species of tetrodotoxic fish exist in sea waters. Characteristic features are absence of scales, large eyes, and teeth arranged as four plates (tetraodontiformes). Many have spikes and most, when threatened, inflate themselves into spheres, using either air or water, and thus have common names such as Puffer fish, Toad fish, Globe fish, Toado, Swell fish, and Balloon fish. Tetrodotoxin is concentrated in the fish liver, ovaries, intestine, and skin but easily contaminates flesh being prepared for consumption. In Japan, the flesh of selected Toad fish, "fugu," is a culinary delight, as traces of tetrodotoxin produce a pleasant tingling gustatory sensation.

Tetrodotoxin

This toxin (TTX) is one of the most potent known, originally extracted from the eggs of Puffer fish. The most important effects are upon nerve fibers, where blockage of excitability occurs causing flaccid paralysis. Because of the unique action of TTX, sodium-channel blockade, it has been extensively studied. Passage of action potentials along nerves is prevented by selective inhibition of the sodium-carrying mechanism, while the movement of potassium is not disturbed. The effect is selective for some sodium channels, not sodium ion. This nerve-blocking potential is greatest in peripheral nerves, but it also affects sensory and autonomic nerve fibers. Skeletal and smooth muscle and, to a lesser extent, cardiac muscle have their excitability reduced by TTX. The central effects are depression of spinal reflex paths, induction of vomiting, and hypothermia. Hypoventilation is due to paralysis of peripheral nerves, while hypotension is due to blockade of vasomotor nerves and direct suppression of vascular smooth muscle causing vasodilation. The medullary vasomotor and respiratory centers are not affected. Cardiac cells are relatively insensitive to tetrodotoxin.

Tetrodotoxin has also been isolated from the skin of Central American frogs of the genus *Atelopus*, from skin glands of the Californian newt of the genus *Taricha*, from the posterior salivary glands and from other parts of the Blue-ringed octopus, *Hapalochlaena maculosa*, from the Pacific Goby fish, from certain flatworms, and from a variety of other creatures including starfish and crabs. This widespread distribution has yet to be satisfactorily explained but the toxin is probably produced by bacteria present in these species (27).

Poisoning

Signs and symptoms of poisoning develop within 10–45 minutes of consumption (the toxin is not destroyed by cooking). Most victims have some nausea, but vomiting is uncommon. Mildly poisoned victims usually experience only "tingling" sensations but the severely poisoned rapidly develop an alarming illness. Consciousness may remain unimpaired until near death; those who survive a near-fatal episode may recall careless comments made by relatives or hospital staff. Poisoning is classified into four grades:

Grade 1: Perioral numbness with or without gastrointestinal symptoms

Grade 2: Numbness of tongue, face, and other areas of skin. Early motor paralysis and incoordination. Slurred speech and ataxia but peripheral reflexes intact

Grade 3: Widespread paralysis, dyspnea, dysphonia, and hypotension but consciousness retained

Grade 4: Severe hypoxia, near-complete paralysis, and hypotension. Death due to rapid respiratory failure

Differential Diagnosis

The diagnosis is usually straightforward, especially when a number of individuals have shared a meal. Although Puffer fish are not ciguatoxic fish, the illness ciguatera may present in a similar fashion but later, usually 2–12 hours after consumption of fish, easily distinguished from Puffer fish. The ciguatera sufferer usually has reversed sensations, in particular hot objects feel cold and vice versa, whereas this phenomenon is absent in tetrodotoxic poisoning.

Treatment

Apart from gastric lavage, there is no antidote or specific treatment other than supportive. Vomiting should be induced, provided that there is no difficulty in swallowing or in protection of the airway. If aspiration is possible, gastric lavage should be performed after endotracheal intubation. If symptoms are confined to paresthesia and mild weakness without hypoventilation, light sedation with benzodiazepine or other sedative for anxious patients may be desirable, and close observation must be maintained until symptoms recede. If dysphagia is present, oral intake must be suspended and intravenous infusion started to maintain hydration and prevent hypotension.

Any difficulty in dealing with saliva or respiratory secretions is an indication for endotracheal intubation, as is increasing dyspnea, rising respiration rate, or progressive hypercapnia. The short natural course of intoxication makes tracheostomy unnecessary. As these patients are conscious (unless acutely hypoxic), adequate sedation is needed with full anesthesia for intubation.

Fluid administration should be regulated according to hemodynamic parameters. As tetrodotoxin causes vasodilatation as well as cardiac depression in severe toxicity, plasma volume replacement is needed along with an inotropic agent. Atropine may be ineffective in preventing bradycardia, which may respond to isoproterenol (isoprenaline). Complete atrioventricular dissociation may require temporary pacemaker insertion.

Anticholinesterases. Although anticholinesterases have been administered many times to victims of poisoning, with varied responses, there is neither theoretical grounds nor convincing experimental evidence why such drugs should be beneficial since the toxin causes paralysis not by an action at neuromuscular junctions but on motor axons and on muscle membranes. Anticholinesterases are not recommended but, if administered, should be in conjunction with an antimuscarinic agent to prevent bradycardia.

Laboratory Investigations

Although Japanese and Australian scientists have used mouse bioassay and various gas and liquid chromatography techniques to analyze gastric and intestinal contents of victims, these are not generally available.

Ciguatera

Ciguatera is a polymorphic illness contracted from consumption of fish contaminated with CTXs, one of a group of phycotoxins originating in microalgae (83). Gastrointestinal and neurological effects predominate but cardiovascular effects also occur. The name ciguatera is derived from "cigua," Spanish for a small poisonous Caribbean snail.

These toxins, probably produced by certain cyanobacteria (27), are passed up the food chain, reaching high concentration in the flesh of the larger carnivorous fish, such as Spanish mackerel (*Scomberomorus commersoni*). The toxins occur in various species of the dinoflagellate *Gambierdiscus*, notably *G. toxicus*, which are present in the benthic biodendritus. The organism is named after the Gambier Islands in French Polynesia where it was discovered. CTXs are tasteless, not destroyed by cooking and are potent ichthyotoxins, which may explain why human fatality is very low, i.e., only mildly affected fish survive to be caught and consumed.

Generally, ciguatera is confined to tropical and subtropical sea waters to 35 degree latitude. However, because of international and interstate commerce and tourism, the illness may occur virtually anywhere outside endemic areas. Approximately 50,000 cases occur annually. At least 400 species of tropical shore fish have been known to cause ciguatera. The numbers of the dinoflagellate increase dramatically after damage to coral reefs, either by natural phenomena or activities by man such as jetty construction.

Ciguatoxins

CTXs are a group of lipophilic polycyclic ethers (84), which bind to site five of the voltage-sensitive sodium channel, thereby increasing sodium permeability and triggering acetylcholine and norepinephrine release, and increased excitability in sensory neurons and potentiation of effects of norepinephrine on smooth muscle. Neuronal excitability is also increased by gambierol, a CTX, which blocks voltage-gated potassium channels. Nerve excitability in many parts of the autonomic nervous system alters visceral and thermoregulatory responses and causes smooth muscle contraction.

Experimentally, CTXs cause diarrhea, increased peristalsis (amenable to atropine), and increased mucus secretion. CTXs in low concentrations cause transient positive inotropy, which can be blocked with atropine and α- and β-adrenoceptor antagonists. In high concentrations, CTXs cause negative inotropy, which can be reversed with lidocaine. Repeated doses of CTXs cause cardiac necrosis, interstitial fibrosis, and bilateral ventricular hypertrophy. Arrhythmias including bradycardia, atrioventricular conduction disturbances, and transient hypertension precede terminal hypotension and cardiac failure. Death in unventilated experimental animals is due to respiratory depression and arrest.

Poisoning

Although there are many variations in this polymorphic illness, a typical case involves gastroenteritic symptoms for one or two days, weakness, myalgia, and arthralgia for several days to a week and paresthesias from several days to several weeks or longer.

The most common symptoms among 20,000 cases in French Polynesia (85) were grouped into four main categories: neurologic, digestive, cardiovascular, and generalized. From these, paresthesia, arthralgia, myalgia, vertigo, ataxia, diarrhea, vomiting, nausea, bradycardia, hypotension, pruritus, and asthenia account for the most frequent or typical with incidences from 15% to 90% in victims. Approximately 77% of patients developed symptoms within 12 hours of ingestion of fish. The recovery period varied from several days to months. The fatality rate was less than 1% with death occurring from cardiac rather than respiratory failure, but the latter has occurred secondary to prolonged central neurological depression. The paresthesias, numbness, and tingling are more often circumoral but may also involve the extremities. Other symptoms described include lacrimation, salivation, metallic taste, sweating, headache, neck stiffness, chills, shaking, dysuria, dyspnea, and abdominal pain.

There is usually no fever, and the victim shuns food and finds drinking water to be painful; indeed some 25% of cases complain of their teeth feeling painful or loose in their sockets. An erythematous rash is common and sometimes general desquamation occurs. By 10 hours after the meal, the acute symptoms have subsided. The patient is left weak and exhausted and still suffering from tingling and numbness that may last for 7 days or longer.

Some of the features of ciguatera poisoning are quite characteristic. Inability to discriminate temperatures and reversal of temperature perception (dysesthesias) are diagnostic. Victims often notice burning or pain on their skin when it is exposed to cold water. Often hot objects feel cold and *vice versa*. Such persons have to take great care not to scald themselves when bathing. The paradoxical reversal of temperature sensation, commonly described in ciguatera poisoning, is considered to be the result of an exaggerated and intense nerve depolarization in peripheral small A-delta myelinated and in C-polymodal nociceptor fibers. Ciguatoxin-1 depolarizes and contracts arterial smooth muscle. In New Caledonia, the illness is called "la grate" or "the itch." Pruritus and paresthesia may involve the soles of the feet and palms of the hands.

Recovery occurs from 48 hours to 7 days in mild cases, but takes several weeks or longer in severe cases. Sometimes a sensitivity to any kind of fish develops and in other cases vague tingling sensations, pruritus, and even ataxia may persist for years. In cases of death, it has occurred after 10 minutes but usually after several days. Should the patient survive a very severe poisoning, it may be a year or more before full recovery.

Differential Diagnosis. Sometimes the toxic fish is transported and eaten far from its place of origin and poses a diagnostic challenge for clinicians unless they make a connection with fish consumption. Ciguatera and bacterial contamination of seafood is usually easily distinguished from tetrodotoxin poisoning, which in contrast causes a very rapid onset of neurological effects.

Treatment

There is no specific treatment or antidote. Patients with marked gastrointestinal fluid loss will require parenteral fluid and electrolyte replacement. Severe cases may need tracheal intubation and mechanical respiration. Generally, milder cases need no special treatment other than attentive nursing. Sedation is usually required and opiates may be necessary.

Numerous drugs have been tried with limited success in the treatment of ciguatera poisoning. Among these are mannitol (*vide infra*), corticosteroids, analgesics, tricyclic antidepressants, antihistamines, calcium gluconate, atropine, phentolamine, pralidoxime, nifedipine, tiapride, and vitamins B$_6$ and B$_{12}$. No blinded controlled study of any drug, including mannitol, has been published. Gastric lavage would not be helpful (and possibly dangerous) unless the victim presented with severe signs soon (within an hour) after poisoning. The efficacy of activated charcoal is unknown but since appearance of symptoms is usually delayed at least several hours, it is unlikely to be helpful.

Mannitol. Intravenous mannitol has been extolled as an effective treatment, but there has yet to be convincing clinical evidence of its efficacy. Improvement in 24 patients was reported within minutes of treatment (86). The most notable improvements were in neurological symptoms and muscular dysfunction, whereas gastrointestinal symptoms disappeared more slowly. Recovery of two patients in coma was described: "One patient stood up and asked for orientation within ten minutes after mannitol therapy was started; the other patient, though confused, sat up after five minutes." Numerous other reports of case series have been published (27)—although all are suggestive of benefit, none are definitely conclusive. A randomized but unblinded trial compared mannitol to the standard treatment, which included calcium together with vitamins and glucose in selected patients (87). In that study, the mannitol group had significant reductions of paresthesia and gastrointestinal effects after 1 hour but no further improvement after 24 hours. There were no improvements in the other effects of ciguatoxicity in the mannitol-treated group. The efficacy of mannitol has been investigated in laboratory studies, with mixed results. In one study, mannitol reversed toxin-induced swelling of rat sensory dorsal root ganglia and prevented neuronal membrane depolarization and action potentials (88), suggesting that it acts both as an osmotic agent and reduces toxin binding to the nerve.

Laboratory Investigations in Ciguatera Poisoning

Although numerous methods of detecting CTX have been developed, none are readily available for diagnostic clinical use or for screening fish and all involve specialized laboratories in regional centers mostly using mouse bioassays.

Maitotoxin Poisoning

Maitotoxins are water-soluble, very-long-chain, polyether phycotoxins, distinct from CTXs, but also associated with the marine unicellular *Gambierdiscus toxicus* and other dinoflagellates. They were first recognized in the gut of the "maito," the surgeonfish *Ctenochaetus striatus*. Maitotoxins activate Ca^{++} channels. They probably contribute to the constellation of symptoms, particularly gastrointestinal, in ciguatera. Many of the in vitro effects of maitotoxin are prevented by calcium-channel blockers such as verapamil.

Treatment

No specific treatment exists. Since maitotoxicity is a possible contributory component of ciguatera, the same treatment may be appropriate along with calcium-channel blockade.

Neurotoxic Shellfish (Brevetoxin) Poisoning

A family of polyethers, similar to CTXs, are associated with worldwide "red tide" microalgae blooms, particularly with the dinoflagellate *Karenia* (formerly *Ptychodiscus*) *brevis*. Numerous blooms have occurred in the Gulf of Mexico. Toxins liberated into the water poison fish and other marine life and accumulate in filter-feeding shellfish, such as oysters. Toxins also become aerosolized with wave action and cause bronchoconstriction by mast-cell activation.

Brevetoxins activate voltage-sensitive sodium channels causing sodium influx and nerve membrane depolarization inducing release of acetylcholine and catecholamines from central and peripheral neuronal sites and possible acetylcholine from neuromuscular junctions. The clinical entity of "neurotoxic shell fish poisoning" is a cluster of gastrointestinal and neurological effects including nausea and vomiting, paresthesia of the mouth, lips and tongue, as well as distal paresthesias, ataxia, slurred speech, dizziness, and possibly partial paralysis (89). These toxins also cause bronchoconstriction by mast-cell activation resulting in respiratory distress and exacerbation of asthma. Experimentally, initial effects include bradycardia, hypotension, and bradypnea, followed by hypertension, tachycardia, cardiac arrhythmias, and respiratory arrest. Ventilated animals succumb to cardiovascular collapse. Interestingly, neurotoxicity is prevented by co-application of NMDA receptor antagonists such as ketamine, dextromethorphan, and dextrorphan. No specific treatment is available.

Paralytic Shellfish (Saxitoxin) Poisoning

Blooms (red-tides) of certain species of marine dinoflagellates (microalgae, plankton) genera including *Alexandrium, Pyrodinium,* and *Gymnodinium* and freshwater cyanobacteria ("blue-green algae") including *Lyngbya, Cylindrospermopsis,* and *Anabaena* produce a large group of small neurotoxins known collectively as saxitoxins. The toxins poison the water and are ingested by filter-feeding bivalve molluscs such as mussels, clams, oysters, scallops, and cockles, which in turn may be ingested by crabs and lobsters. Life-threatening illnesses may result from drinking poisoned fresh water but more frequently by ingesting the molluscs or other creatures, which have ingested the toxin-producing organisms. Outbreaks of poisoning occur in many parts of the world. The toxins are not destroyed by cooking.

The principal toxin, saxitoxin, is named after the butter clam *Saxidomus gigantea* from which it was isolated. It has a bicyclic guanidine structure and blocks sodium channels in a manner similar to but not identical to structurally unrelated tetrodotoxin. Tissues affected are neural, cardiac, and skeletal muscle and vascular smooth muscle. At such times, molluscs become heavily contaminated. Outbreaks of shellfish poisoning have occurred in many parts of the world.

Poisoning. Neurological, respiratory, and cardiovascular symptoms develop usually within 30 minutes. Experimentally, saxitoxin causes a rapid onset of respiratory and cardiovascular failure. The toxins are excreted by glomerular filtration.

Treatment. Only supportive treatment is available: airway protection, mechanical ventilation, and inotropic support. From animal studies of saxitoxin poisoning and their treatment, 4-aminopyridine holds promise. This drug selectively blocks potassium channels in excitable membranes and facilitates neurotransmitter release at synapses and has reversed saxitoxin-induced cardiorespiratory collapse.

Laboratory Investigations. Although numerous assays for saxitoxin and its derivatives have been devised, none are performed rapidly or easily.

Diarrhetic Shellfish (Okadaic Acid) Poisoning

This gastroenteritis is caused by ingestion of shellfish, in particular mussels, which have fed on blooms of marine dinoflagellates (phytoplankton) of the genera *Dinophysis* and *Prorocentrum,* which manufacture the polyethers okadaic acid and dinophysistoxins and their numerous derivatives, which inhibit serine/threonine phosphoprotein phosphatases. Symptoms of nausea, vomiting, diarrhea, abdominal pain, and fever occur within 30 minutes and last more than 8 hours. No specific treatment exists.

Amnestic Shellfish (Domoic Acid) Poisoning

Amnestic shellfish poisoning is a specific neurotoxic syndrome characterized by acute gastrointestinal symptoms and unusual neurological abnormalities occurring in persons who have eaten mussels, clams, or crabs. The agent responsible is domoic acid, an analog of the neuroexcitatory transmitter glutamic acid, which is produced by blooms of species of the diatom genus *Pseudo-nitzschia*. Severely poisoned patients have experienced hemiparesis, seizures, hypotension, ophthalmoplegia, and abnormalities of arousal ranging from agitation to coma and residual severe anterograde memory deficits. It poisons the water and threatens health of marine mammals and birds. No specific treatment is available.

Scombroid Poisoning

Scombroid poisoning occurs worldwide when scombroid fish, such as tuna or mackerel or other large oceanic fish, become contaminated with enteric bacteria. The toxin responsible is histamine converted from histidine in the flesh by bacteria. Large amounts of histamine, and other biogenic amines, may develop in dead fish if not promptly frozen or allowed to thaw too long before cooking—which does not destroy histamine. The illness may also be contracted from canned or smoked fish.

The contaminated fish is not putrefied, and although it has normal appearance and smell to the consumer, a sharpish or peppery taste is sometimes noted. *Proteus morgani* is the only bacterial species able to produce histamine in high-enough concentrations to cause human poisoning. Other substances present in spoiled fish may enhance the activity of histamine or facilitate its absorption or inhibit its inactivation since histamine is degraded in human intestines and the illness cannot be mimicked by ingestion of histamine alone.

Scombroid poisoning can be differentiated from "seafood allergy" and bacterial food poisoning by careful elucidation of the history of the illness. Typical symptoms in order of frequency are diarrhea, hot flushing or sweating, bright erythematous rash, nausea and vomiting, headache, abdominal pain, palpitations, burning in the mouth, fever, and dizziness. Sometimes facial edema is present and respiratory distress may occur. Occasionally cardiac dysrhythmias or hypotension occurs. Onset of illness is usually within 30 minutes of fish ingestion and lasts only 8–12 hours but is sometimes prolonged. The illness has been stated as the most significant cause of illness associated with seafood in USA and the most frequent in Canada. It may be worsened by certain classes of drugs (beta-adrenoreceptor antagonists, monoamine oxidase inhibitors, and antituberculous drugs such as isoniazid).

Treatment. Mild poisoning restricted to rash, flushing, sweating, tachycardia, palpitations, and headache may require a parenteral antihistamine (H_1 and H_2 antagonists). Moderate poisoning with additional gastrointestinal symptoms may require intravenous fluid replacement. Severe poisoning with additional bronchospasm, hypotension, or airway obstruction may require epinephrine (parenteral, inhaled), bronchodilator, and airway protection. No deaths have been reported.

Laboratory Tests. Contaminated fish contain large amounts of histamine, which along with its metabolite, N-methyl histamine, are excreted in urine of victims in high concentrations for ~24 hours after poisoning.

CONCLUSIONS AND FUTURE DIRECTIONS

Syndromes resulting from envenomation by terrestrial and marine creatures often need invasive treatment and monitoring, particularly of cardiac and respiratory function, which is well described in other chapters of this text. Although the toxins of some creatures and features of their envenomation syndromes are relatively well known, for example of some snake and spider bites, the nature of the toxins and envenomation syndromes resulting, for example, from scorpion and jelly-fish envenomation remain obscure. Basic scientific and clinical research is needed in many areas.

In addition to general therapy, numerous syndromes need specific therapy, which can only be anticipated from knowledge of the effects of toxins and poisons involved. Effective first aid also constitutes an important part of the management of some envenomations such as from elapid snake and funnel-web spider bites—in these instances first aid should not be neglected when the victim arrives in hospital as it serves to limit the amount of venom reaching the circulation of a victim. In several syndromes antivenom therapy is the key to successful treatment and good outcome. Unfortunately, antivenoms for the toxins of many creatures do not exist while some manufacturers of snake antivenoms around the world are ceasing or scaling back production because of lack of profitability.

References

1. Chippaux JP, Goyffon M. Epidemiology of scorpionism: A global appraisal. *Acta Tropica* 2008;107:71–9.
2. Mohapatra B, Warrell DA, Suraweera W. Snakebite mortality in India: A nationally representative mortality survey. *PLoS Negl Trop Dis* 2011;5:e1018.
3. Chippaux JP. Estimate of the burden of snakebites in sub-Saharan Africa: A meta-analytic approach. *Toxicon* 2011;57:586–99.
4. Williams D, Gutierrez JM, Harrison R, et al. The global snake bite initiative: An antidote for snake bite. *Lancet* 2010;375:89–91.
5. Ireland G, Brown SG, Buckley NA, et al. Changes in serial laboratory test results in snakebite patients: When can we safely exclude envenoming? *Med J Aust* 2010;193:285–90.
6. Sutherland SK, Coulter AR, Harris RD. Rationalisation of first aid measures for elapid snakebite. *Lancet* 1979;1:183–6.
7. Pearn J, Morrison J, Charles N, et al. First-aid for snakebite: Efficacy of a constrictive bandage with limb immobilization in the management of human envenomation. *Med J Aust* 1981;2:293–5.
8. Markenson D, Ferguson JD, Chameides L, et al. 2010 American Heart Association and American Red Cross International consensus on first aid science with treatment recommendations. *Circulation* 2010;122(suppl):S582–605.
9. Sutherland SK, Coulter AR. Early management of bites by the eastern diamond-back rattlesnake (*Crotalus adamanteus*): Studies in monkeys (*Macaca fascicularis*). *Am J Trop Med Hyg* 1981;30:497–500.
10. Sutherland SK, Harris RD, Coulter AR, et al. First aid for cobra (*Naja naja*) bites. *Indian J Med Res* 1981;73:266–8.
11. Pe T, Mya S, Myint AA, et al. Field trial of efficacy of local compression immobilization first-aid technique in Russell's viper (*Daboia russelii siamensis*) bite patients. *Southeast Asian J Trop Med Public Health* 2000;31:346–8.
12. Norris RL, Bush SP. North American venomous reptile bites. In: Auerbach PS, ed. *Wilderness Medicine*. 4th ed. St Louis, MO: Mosby, 2001:896–926.
13. Cumpston KL. Is there a role for fasciotomy in Crotalinae envenomation in North America? *Clin Toxicol* 2011;49:351–65.
14. Warrell D. Treatment of bites by adders and exotic venomous snakes. *BMJ* 2006;331:1244–7.
15. Lavonas EJ, Tomaszewski CA, Ford MD, et al. Severe puff adder (Bitis arietans) envenomation with coagulopathy. *J Toxicol Clin Toxicol* 2002;40:911–8.
16. Isbister GK, Scorgie FE, O'Leary MA, et al. Factor deficiencies in venom-inducedconsumption coaguloathy resulting from Australian elapid envenomation: Australian Snakebite Project (ASP-10). *J Thromb Haemost* 2010;8:2504–13.
17. Tibballs J. Fresh frozen plasma after brown snake bite—helpful or harmful? *Anaesth Intensive Care* 2005;33:13–5.

18. Dart RC, McNally J. Efficacy, safety, and use of snake antivenoms in the United States. *Ann Emerg Med* 2001;37:181–8.

19. Antonypillai CN, Wass JA, Warrell DA, et al. Hypopituitarism following envenoming by Russell's vipers (*Daboia siamensis* and *D. russelii*) resembling Sheehan's syndrome: First case report from Sri Lanka, a review of the literature and recommendations for endocrine management. *QJM* 2011;104:97–108.

20. Cheng AC, Currie BJ. Venomous snakebites worldwide with a focus on the Australia-Pacific region: Current management and controversies. *J Intensive Care Med* 2004;19:259–69.

21. Sinha R, Nandi M, Tullus K, et al. Ten-year follow-up of children after acute renal failure from a developing country. *Nephrol Dial Transplant* 2009;24:829–33.

22. Sutherland SK. Deaths from snake bite in Australia 1981–1991. *Med J Aust* 1992;157:740–6.

23. Chu ER, Weinstein SA, White J, et al. Venom ophthalmia caused by venoms of spitting elapid and other snakes: Report of ten cases with review of epidemiology, clinical; features, pathophysiology and management. *Toxicon* 2010;56:259–72.

24. Ong RK, Swindells K, Mansfield CS. Prospective determination of the specificity of a commercial snake venom detection kit in urine samples from dogs and cats. *Aust Vet J* 2010;88:222–4.

25. Sebat C, Ribet S, Barguil Y, et al. Envenimations sévères par serpents marins en Nouvelle-Calédonie: Deux tableaux cliniques différents. *JEUR* 2005;18:204–10.

26. Keating GM, Lyseng-Williamson KA. Crotalidae polyvalent immune Fab: A guide to its use in North American crotaline envenomation. *Clin Drug Investig* 2012;32:555–60.

27. Sutherland SK, Tibballs J. *Australian Animal Toxins*. 2nd ed. South Melbourne, Australia: Oxford University Press, 2001.

28. Sprivulis P, Jelinek GA, Marshall L. Efficacy and potency of antivenoms in neutralizing the procoagulant effects of Australian snake in dog and human plasma. *Anaesth Intensive Care* 1996;24:379–81.

29. Tibballs J, Sutherland SK. The efficacy of antivenom in prevention of cardiovascular depression and coagulopathy induced by brown snake (*Pseudonaja*) species venom. *Anaesth Intensive Care* 1991;19:530–4.

30. Allen GE, Brown SGA, Buckley NA, et al. Clinical Effects and Antivenom Dosing in Brown Snake (*Pseudonaja* spp.) Envenoming — Australian Snakebite Project (ASP-14). *PLoS One* 2012;7:e53188.

31. Schaeffer TH, Khatri V, Reifler LM, et al. Incidence of immediate hypersensitivity reaction and serum sickness following administration of Crotalidae polyvalent immune Fab antivenom: A meta-analysis. *Acad Emerg Med* 2012;19:121–31.

32. Habib AG. Effect of pre-medication on early adverse reactions following antivenom use in snakebite: A systematic review and meta-analysis. *Drug Saf* 2011;34:869–80.

33. Premawardhena AP, de Silva CE, Fonseka MM, et al. Low dose subcutaneous adrenaline to prevent acute adverse reactions to antivenom serum in people bitten by snakes: Randomised, placebo controlled trial. *BMJ* 1999;318:1041–3.

34. Fan HW, Marcopito LF, Cardoso JL, et al. Sequential randomized and double blind trial of promethazine prophylaxis against early anaphylactic reactions to antivenom for *Bothrops* snake bites. *BMJ* 1999;318:1451–2.

35. Watt G, Theakston RD, Hayes CG, et al. Positive response to edrophonium in patients with neurotoxic envenoming by cobras (*Naja naja philippinensis*): A placebo-controlled study. *N Engl J Med* 1986;315:1444–8.

36. Anil A, Singh S, Bhaila A, et al. Role of neostigmione and polyvalent antivenom in Indian common krait (*Bungarus caeruleus*) bite. *J Infec Pub Health* 2010;3:83–7.

37. Ferdinands M, Seneviratne J, O'Brien T, et al. Ophthalmoplegia in tiger snake envenomation. *J Clin Neurosci* 2006;13:385–8.

38. Isbister GK, Gray MR, Balit CR, et al. Funnel-web spider bite: A systematic review of recorded clinical cases. *Med J Aust* 2005;182:407–11.

39. Luch A. Mechanistic insights on spider neurotoxins. *EXS* 2010;100:293–315.

40. González Valverde FM, Gómez Ramos MJ, et al. [Fatal latrodectism in an elderly man]. *Med Clin (Barc)* 2001;117:319.

41. Nordt SP, Clark RF, Lee A, et al. Examination of adverse events following black widow antivenom use in California. *Clin Toxicol* 2012;50:70–3.

42. Hoyte CO, Cushing TA, Heard KJ. Anaphylaxis to black widow spider envenomation. *Am J Emerg Med* 2012;30:836.

43. Murphy CM, Hong JJ, Beuhler MC. Anaphylaxis with Latrodectus antivenin resulting in cardiac arrest. *J Med Toxicol* 2011;7:317–21.

44. Dart RC, Bogdan G, Heard K, et al. A randomized, double-blind, placebo-controlled trial of a highly purified equine F(ab)2 antibody black widow spider antivenom. *Ann Emerg Med* 2013;61:458–67.

45. Isbister GK, Brown SG, Miller M, et al. A randomised controlled trial of intramuscular vs. intravenous antivenom for latrodectism—the RAVE study. *QJM* 2008;101:557–65.

46. Hogan C, Barbaro KC, Winkel KD. Loxoscelism: Old obstacles, new directions. *Ann Emerg Med* 2004;44:608–24.

47. Yi X, AuBuchon J, Zeltwanger S, et al. Necrotic arachnidism and intractable pain from recluse spider bites treated with lumbar sympathetic block: A case report and review of literature. *Clin J Pain* 2011;27:457–60.

48. Manriquez JJ, Silva S. Cutaneous and visceral loxoscelism: A systematic review. *Rev Chilena Infectol* 2009;26:420–32.

49. M'barak S, Fajloun Z, Cestele S, et al. First chemical synthesis of a scorpion alpha-toxin affecting sodium channels: The Aah I toxin of *Androctonus australis hector*. *J Pept Sci* 2004;10:666–77.

50. Rodríguez de la Vega RC, Schwartz EF, Possani LD. Mining on scorpion venom biodiversity. *Toxicon* 2010;56:1155–61.

51. Bahloul M, Chabchoub I, Chaari A, et al. Scorpion envenomation among children: Clinical manifestations and outcome (analysis of 685 cases). *Am J Trop Med Hyg* 2010;83:1084–92.

52. Soulaymani-Bencheikh R, Soulaymani A, Semlali I, et al. Scorpion poisonous stings in the population of Khouribga. *Bull Soc Pathol Exot* 2005;98:36–40.

53. Meki AR, Mohamed ZM, Mohey El-deen HM. Significance of assessment of serum cardiac troponin I and interleukin-8 in scorpion envenomed children. *Toxicon* 2003;41:129–37.

54. Abroug F, Ouanes-Besbes L, Ouanes I, et al. Meta-analysis of controlled studies on immunotherapy in severe scorpion envenomation. *Emerg Med J* 2011;28:963–9.

55. Bawaskar HS, Bawaskar PH. Efficacy and safety of scorpion antivenom plus prazosin compared with prazosin alone for venomous scorpion (*Mesobuthus tamulus*) sting: Randomised open label clinical trial. *BMJ* 2011;342:c7136.

56. Elatrous S, Nouira S, Besbes-Ouanes L, et al. Dobutamine in severe scorpion envenomation: Effects on standard hemodynamics, right ventricular performance, and tissue oxygenation. *Chest* 1999;116:748–53.

57. Levick NR, Schmidt JO, Harrison J, et al. Bee and wasp sting injuries in Australia and the USA: Is it a bee or is it a wasp and why should we care? In: Austin AD, Dowton M, eds. *The Hymenoptera: Evolution, Biodiversity and Biological Control*. Canberra, Australia: CSIRO Publishing, 2000:437–47.

58. Forrester JA, Holstege CP, Forrester JD. Fatalities from venomous and nonvenomous animals in the United States (1999–2007). *Wilderness Environ Med* 2012;23:146–52.

59. Morris B, Southcott RV, Gale AE. Effects of stings of Australian native bees. *Med J Aust* 1998;149:109–10.

60. Solley GO, Vanderwoude C, Knight GK. Anaphylaxis due to red imported fire ant. *Med J Aust* 2002;176:518–9.

61. Golden DB. Insect allergy in children. *Curr Opin Allergy Clin Immunol* 2006;6:289–93.

62. McGain F, Winkel KD. Ant sting mortality in Australia. *Toxicon* 2002;40:1095–100.

63. Merten HA, Durden LA. A state-by-state survey of ticks recorded from humans in the United States. *J Vector Ecol* 2000;25:102–13.

64. Dworkin MS, Shoemaker PC, Anderson DE. Tick paralysis: 33 human cases in Washington State. *Clin Infect Dis* 1999;29:1435–9.

65. Elston DM. Tick bites and skin rashes. *Curr Opin Infect Dis* 2010;23:132–8.

66. Dantas-Torres F, Chomel BB, Otranto D. Ticks and tick-borne diseases: A One Health perspective. *Trends Parasitol* 2012;28:437–46.

67. Grattan-Smith PJ, Morris JG, Johnston HM, et al. Clinical and neurophysiological features of tick paralysis. *Brain* 1997;120:1975–87.

68. Bailey PM, Bakker AJ, Seymour JE, et al. A functional comparison of the venom of three Australian jellyfish—*Chironex fleckeri*, *Chiropsalmus sp.*, and *Carybdea xaymacana* on cytosolic Ca^{2+}, haemolysis and *Artemia sp.* lethality. *Toxicon* 2005;45:233–42.

69. Yanagihara AA, Shohet RV. Cubozoan venom-induced cardiovascular collapse is caused by hyperkalemia and prevented by zinc gluconate in mice. *PLoS One* 2012;7:e51368.

70. Ramasamy S, Isbister GK, Seymour JE, et al. The in vivo cardiovascular effects of box jellyfish *Chironex fleckeri* venom in rats: Efficacy of pre-treatment with antivenom, verapamil and magnesium sulphate. *Toxicon* 2004;43:685–90.

71. Hughes RJ, Angus JA, Winkel KD, et al. A pharmacological investigation of the venom extract of the Australian box jellyfish, Chironex fleckeri, in cardiac and vascular tissues. *Toxicol Lett* 2012;209:11–20.

72. Tibballs J, Li R, Tibballs HA, et al. Australian carybdeid jellyfish causing "Irukandji syndrome." *Toxicon* 2012;617–25.

73. Winkel KD, Tibballs J, Molenaar P, et al. The cardiovascular actions of the venom from the Irukandji (*Carukia barnesi*) jellyfish: Effects in human, rat and guinea pig tissues in vitro, and in pigs in vivo. *Clin Exp Pharmacol Physiol* 2005;32:777–8.

74. Little M, Pereira P, Mulcahy R, et al. Severe cardiac failure associated with presumed jellyfish sting. Irukandji syndrome? *Anaesth Intensive Care* 2003;31:642–7.

75. Corkeron M, Pereira P, Makrocanis C. Early experience with magnesium administration in Irukandji syndrome. *Anaesth Intensive Care* 2004;32,666–9.

76. McCullagh N, Pereira P, Cullen P, et al. Randomised trial of magnesium in the treatment of Irukandji syndrome. *Emerg Med Australas* 2012;24:560–5.

77. Yoshimoto CM, Yanagihara AA. Cnidarian (coelenterate) envenomations in Hawai'i improve following heat application. *Trans R Soc Trop Med Hyg* 2002;96:300–3.

78. Nomura JT, Sato RL, Ahern RM, et al. A randomised paired comparison trial of cutaneous treatments for acute jellyfish (*Carybdea alata*) stings. *Am J Emerg Med* 2002;20:624–6.

79. Edwards L, Luo E, Hall R, et al. The effect of Portuguese man-of-war (*Physalia physalis*) venom on calcium, sodium and potassium fluxes of cultured embryonic chick heart cells. *Toxicon* 2000;38:323–35.

80. Loten C, Stokes B, Worsley D, et al. A randomised controlled trial of hot water (45 degrees C) immersion versus ice packs for pain relief in bluebottle stings. *Med J Aust* 2006;184:329–33.

81. Lyon RM. Stonefish poisoning. *Wilderness Environ Med* 2004;15:284–8.

82. Church JE, Moldrich RX, Beart PM, et al. Modulation of intracellular Ca2+ levels by Scorpaenidae venoms. *Toxicon* 2003;41:679–89.

83. Rossini GP, Hess P. Phycotoxins: Chemistry, mechanisms of action and shellfish poisoning. *EXS* 2010;100:65–122.

84. Murata M, Legrand AM, Ishibashi Y, et al. Structures and configurations of ciguatoxin from moray eel *Gymnothorax javanicus* and its likely precursor from the dinoflagellate *Gambierdiscus toxicus*. *J Am Chem Soc* 1990;112:4380–6.

85. Bagnis RA. Clinical features on 19,890 cases of ciguatera (fish poisoning) in French Polynesia. *Toxicon* 1987;26:16.

86. Palafox NA, Jain LG, Pinano AZ, et al. Successful treatment of ciguatera fish poisoning with intravenous mannitol. *JAMA* 1988;259:2740–2.

87. Bagnis R, Spiegel A, Boutin JP, et al. Evaluation of the efficacy of mannitol in the treatment of ciguatera in French Polynesia. *Medicale Tropicale* 1992;52:67–73.

88. Birinyi-Strachan LC, Davies MJ, Lewis RJ, et al. Neuroprotectant effects of iso-osmolar D-Mannital to prevent Pacific ciguatoxin-1 induced alterations in neuronal excitability: A comparison with other osmotic agents and free radical scavengers. *Neuropharmacology* 2005;49:669–86.

89. Watkins SM, Reich A, Fleming LE, et al. Neurotoxic shellfish poisoning. *Marine Drugs* 2008;6:431–55.

CHAPTER 38 ■ **MECHANICAL VENTILATION**

MARK J. HEULITT, COURTNEY RANALLO, GERHARD K. WOLF, AND JOHN H. ARNOLD

KEY POINTS

1. The lung-ventilator unit can be thought of as a tube with a balloon network on the end, with the tube representing the ventilator tubing, endotracheal tube (ETT), and airways and the balloon network representing the alveoli.

2. To generate gas flow, the total forces must overcome the resistive forces of the airway, the ventilator tubing, and the ETT to allow gas to flow into or out of the lung, depending on driving pressure gradients.

3. The *equation of motion* for the respiratory system relates how volume (ΔV), pressure (ΔP), and flow ($\dot{V}$) interact to move gas into and out of the lung:

$$\Delta P = \Delta V/C + \dot{V} \cdot R + k$$

   where R is the airway resistance, C is the lung compliance, and k is a constant that defines end-expiratory pressure.

4. The manner in which each variable (pressure, volume, or flow) is controlled, described as the *mode of ventilation*, determines how the ventilator delivers the mechanical breath.

5. Compliance relates to the ease of inflation of lung units and is determined by

$$\text{Compliance} = \Delta \text{Volume}/\Delta \text{Pressure}$$

6. In pressure-control (PC) ventilation, the pressure pattern is "square," but flow increases rapidly at the beginning of the inspiratory phase to generate the set pressure limit and then decays exponentially over the inspiratory time. This flow pattern is described as *decelerating flow*.

7. Clinicians often choose PC ventilation in patients with poor compliance, although the true benefit of PC versus other modes has not been well established in animal or clinical studies.

8. If the clinician sets volume as a function of time, pressure then varies with compliance. Volume is the independent variable and pressure is the dependent variable.

9. Understanding the factors involved in tidal volume (VT) measurement and how they are determined in different ventilators and techniques is important in patient management.

10. The volume of gas that becomes compressed within the ventilator tubing and never reaches the patient is termed the *compressible volume of the circuit*.

11. When compression volume is accounted for in determination of patient VT, the resultant volume is termed the *effective tidal volume* (eVT), which means that this is the VT that reaches the patient's lungs.

12. Effective tidal volume (eVT) can be calculated as:

$$eVT = (VT_E) - [\text{Circuit compensation} \times (PI_{MAX}) - PEEP]$$

   where VT_E is the expired tidal volume, PI_{max} is the maximal inspiratory pressure, and PEEP is the positive end-expiratory pressure.

13. While measuring VT at the airway opening may give the best estimate of VT in the lungs, this can be associated with problems such as losing air around uncuffed ETTs, unreliable measuring sensors, and potential extubation from the weight of the measuring device.

14. The manner in which each variable (pressure, volume, or flow) is controlled, described as the *mode of ventilation*, determines how the ventilator delivers the mechanical breath.

15. *Control* variables are the independent variables, which arer pressure, volume, or flow. *Conditional* variables are determinants of a response to a preset threshold, which are both clinician set and influenced by dependent and independent variables. *Phase* variables are those that are used to start, sustain, and end the phase.

16. Most ventilators cannot directly measure volume; rather, they calculate volume delivered from flow that occurs over a period of time.

17. Studies have shown that the ventilator-displayed VT, without software compensation for circuit compliance, generally overestimates the true delivered VT. Conversely, when the circuit-compliance compensation feature is on, the ventilator-displayed VT generally underestimates the true delivered VT.

18. The neurally adjusted ventilatory assist approach to mechanical ventilation is based on the acquisition of the patient's neural respiratory output as it is transmitted through the phrenic nerve to the diaphragm.

19. In infants, the fact that lung volume may increase at a greater rate than airway diameter may be one reason why infants are especially prone to air trapping and hyperinflation.

20. The high compliance and low elastic recoil of the infant/young child's chest wall result in increased work of breathing to move the same VT as an adult.

21. Patient–ventilator asynchrony is a result of factors related to ventilator triggering, adequacy of flow delivery, adequate breath termination, and effects of PEEP and/or intrinsic PEEP ($PEEP_i$).

22. It is important to recognize that the goal of mechanical ventilatory support is not to normalize the patient's blood gases at the cost of ventilator-induced lung injury.

23. For patients with obstructive lung disease, lung protection may include a lower VT and prolonged exhalation times. A support mode with spontaneous breathing may also be useful.

24. In patients with poor compliance, maintaining lung recruitment without the use of excessive distending volume, changes in pressure to distend the alveoli, and end-expiratory pressure may limit ventilator-induced lung injury.

25. Lung injury prevention is directed toward reducing cyclic collapse and re-expansion of alveoli due to inadequate PEEP.

26 Widespread use of low VTs may result in reabsorption atelectasis in basal lung areas. This effect can be enhanced by the use of high-inhaled O_2 concentrations. PEEP may be protective in these circumstances.

27 It is important not to be misled by an improvement of oxygenation alone as a measure of lung recruitment. An increase in PEEP can reduce cardiac output and increase PaO_2 despite a decrease in O_2 delivery.

28 The effect of PEEP is as a distending pressure to increase the functional residual capacity (volume of gas at the end of exhalation in the lung).

29 The peak inspiratory pressure in PC ventilation is usually lower than in volume-control (VC) ventilation.

30 PC ventilation does not guarantee minute ventilation. Worsened compliance or resistance in the patient will result in decreased VT.

31 VT is assured in VC ventilation.

32 The constant-flow pattern in VC may not meet patient demands, especially in patients with poorly compliant lungs.

33 Airway-pressure-release ventilation (APRV) is a high-level continuous positive-airway pressure mode that is terminated for brief periods.

34 Dexamethasone, heliox, and noninvasive ventilation may be helpful in preventing intubation or reintubation in patients with respiratory illness.

35 Bulk convection, pendelluft, Taylor dispersion, convective dispersion, cardiogenic mixing, collateral ventilation, and molecular diffusion are distinct modes of gas exchange that interact with each other during high-frequency oscillation ventilation (HFOV).

36 Increasing the mean airway pressure increases alveolar recruitment and oxygenation during HFOV.

37 Alveolar ventilation during HFOV is a function of the rate of oscillations and the squared VT ($V_{CO_2} = f \times VT^2$).

38 In HFOV, VT delivery and CO_2 elimination are directly related to the peak-to-trough pressure amplitude, and negatively correlated with device frequency.

39 The presence of an ETT cuff leak in HFOV may further contribute to CO_2 clearance.

In simple terms, the lung-ventilator unit can be thought of as a tube with a balloon network on the end, with the tube representing the ventilator tubing, endotracheal tube (ETT), and airways and the balloon network representing the alveoli. During mechanical ventilation, the forces generated are a combination

1 of effort provided by the patient's muscles during spontaneous breathing attempts and support derived from the ventilator. The movement of gas is determined by forces, displacements, and the rate of change of component displacements, which are distensible. To generate a volume displacement, the total forces have to overcome both the elastic and resistive elements of the lung and airway/chest wall. To generate gas flow, the total forces must overcome the resistive forces of the airway, the ventilator tubing, and the ETT to allow gas to flow into or out of the lung, depending on driving pressure gradients.

This discussion of mechanical ventilation will first focus on an understanding of how the patient's physiologic changes occur to generate these forces, both by intrinsic patient effort and from forces generated by ventilator output. How the ventilator controls the variables of flow, volume, and pressure to

2 generate these forces and how these controllers interface with the patient will then be examined. Finally, the indications, settings, and modes of ventilatory support available to clinicians who care for infants and children will be discussed.

PHYSIOLOGY OF MECHANICAL VENTILATION

In physiology, force is measured as pressure [pressure = force / area], displacement is measured as volume (volume = area × displacement), and the relevant rate of change is measured as flow (e.g., average flow = Δvolume / Δtime; istantaneous flow = dv/dt, where d represents the derivative of volume with respect to time). The key components in positive-pressure mechanical ventilation are the pressure necessary to cause a flow of gas to enter the airway and increase the volume of gas in the lungs. The volume of gas (ΔV) going to any lung unit (the balloons in our simplified example) and the gas flow ($V^·$) may be related to the applied pressure (ΔP) by

$$\Delta P = \Delta V/C + \dot{V} \cdot R + k$$

where R is the airway resistance, C is the lung compliance, and k is a constant that defines end-expiratory pressure.

The above equation is known as the *equation of motion* for the respiratory system. The sum of the muscle pressures and the ventilator pressure is the applied pressure to the respiratory system. The muscle pressure represents the pressure generated by the patient to expand the thoracic cage and lungs. Unfortunately, this force is not able to be measured directly. In contrast, the ventilator pressure is the transrespiratory pressure (from the mouth to the alveolar space) generated by the ventilator during inspiration. Combinations of these pressures are generated when a patient is breathing on a positive-pressure ventilator. For example, when respiratory muscles are at complete rest, the muscle pressure is zero; thus, the ventilator must generate all of the pressure necessary to deliver the tidal volume (VT) and inspiratory flow. The reverse is also true—when the patient is making some respiratory effort and generating muscle pressure, the degree of support that must be supplied by the ventilator is less. Multiple modes of ventilator support can be used to assist the patient in this circumstance. With the basic principle behind the equation of motion defined, it must be applied to the forces that must be overcome to generate gas flow. The total pressure applied to the respiratory system (P_{RS}) of a ventilated patient is the sum of the pressure generated by the ventilator (measured at the airway, P_{AO}) and the pressure developed by the respiratory muscles (P_{MUS}).

$$P_{RS} = P_{A0} + P_{MUS} = \frac{V_T}{C_R} + \dot{V} \times R + PEEP_{total}$$

where V_T is the tidal volume, C_R the respiratory system compliance, (V_T/C_R) the elastic force, $\dot{V}$ the flow, R the airway resistance, ($\dot{V} \times R$) the resistive force, and $PEEP_{total}$ the total alveolar end-expiratory pressure.

P_{AO} and $\dot{V}$ can be measured by the pressure and flow transducers in the ventilator. Volume is derived mathematically from the integration of the flow waveform.

To generate a volume displacement, the total forces have to overcome elastic and resistive elements of the lung and airway/chest wall, represented by V_T/C_R and $\dot{V} \times R$, respectively. V_T/C_R (elastic force) depends on both the volume insufflated in excess of resting volume and on respiratory system compliance. To generate a flow of gas, the total forces must overcome the resistive forces of the airway and the ETT against the driving pressure gradients. Given the physics principle that any action has an opposing reaction, at any moment during inspiration, a balance is maintained of forces attempting to expand the lung and the chest wall and those opposing lung and chest wall expansion. We commonly measure the result of these forces as the airway pressure (P_{AWO}). Opposing pressures to lung and chest wall expansion are the sum of elastic recoil pressure ($P_{elastic}$), flow resistive pressure ($P_{resistive}$), and inertance pressure ($P_{inertance}$) within the respiratory system. Thus,

$$P_{AWO} = P_{elastic} + P_{resistive} + P_{inertance}$$

Inertial forces relate to the energy required for initiation of gas movement and are usually negligible during conventional ventilation; thus, this component is commonly ignored. For conventional ventilation, the forces exemplified in the equation of motion can be expressed as follows:

$$P_{AWO} = P_{elastic} + P_{resistive}$$

If the elastic forces are the product of elastance and volume ($P_{elastic} = E \times V$), and resistive forces are the product of flow and resistance (Resistive $= \dot{V} \times R$), and the formula can be written as:

$$P_{AWO} = (\text{Elastance} \times \text{Volume}) + (\text{Resistance} \times \text{Flow})$$

Elastance is the inverse of compliance. If compliance is substituted for elastance in the equation, the equation of motion results:

$$P_{AWO} = \frac{\text{Volume}}{\text{Compliance}} + \text{Resistance} \times \text{Flow}$$

It is important to note that the quotient of volume displacement over compliance of the respiratory system represents the pressure necessary to overcome the elastic forces above the resting lung volume (known as the functional residual capacity, FRC). The FRC represents the quantity of air remaining in the lungs at the end of a spontaneous expiration. Pressure, volume, and flow are all measured relative to their baseline values. Thus, for a patient on a ventilator, the pressure necessary to cause inspiration is measured as the change in airway pressure above positive end-expiratory pressure (PEEP), representing the change from baseline pressure to peak inspiratory pressure. For example, in a patient breathing spontaneously on continuous positive-airway pressure (CPAP), the ventilator pressure is zero; thus, the patient must utilize respiratory muscles to generate all of the work of breathing (WOB) and the force necessary to expand the lungs and chest, to enable forward gas flow into the alveoli. The same principle can be applied to the volume generated during inspiration (the VT), which is the change in volume in the lung during inspiration above FRC. The pressure necessary to overcome the resistive forces of the respiratory tract is the product of the maximum airway resistance (R_{max}) and the inspiratory flow. Flow is measured relative to its end-expiratory value and is usually zero at the beginning of an inspiratory effort, unless an intrinsic PEEP (PEEP$_i$) is present. In this circumstance, flow may still be occurring within the lung as alveoli attempt to achieve their baseline state—that is, due to time-constant differences, overfilled alveoli may be emptying into underfilled alveoli to help both to achieve their "best" resting volume. This effect is known as *pendelluft*. When PEEP$_i$ is present, it will take more "effort" from the patient and the ventilator to generate enough flow to move gas into the lung.

At this point in the discussion of mechanical ventilators, those factors that are directly clinician-controlled must be differentiated from those that occur indirectly. For example, pressure, volume, and flow are directly controlled variables, while other important factors such as resistance and compliance are dependent upon the resistive and elastic properties of the respiratory system and cannot be directly controlled.

VENTILATOR CONTROLLERS

Each ventilator is essentially a controller of pressure, volume, or flow in the equation of motion. The manner in which each variable is controlled, described as the *mode of ventilation*, determines how the ventilator delivers the mechanical breath. In the equation of motion, the form of any of the variables (pressure, volume, and flow are expressed as functions of time) can be predetermined. This principle serves as the theoretical basis for classifying ventilators as *pressure, volume,* or *flow* controllers (**Fig. 38.1**). The necessary and sufficient criteria for determining which variable is controlled are listed in **Table 38.1**. It is important to recognize that any ventilator can only directly control one variable—pressure, volume, or flow—at a time. Thus, a ventilator is simply a technology that controls the airway pressure waveform, the inspired volume waveform, or the inspiratory flow waveform, and pressure, volume, and flow are referred to in this context as *control variables*.

Most clinicians think of ventilators in terms of modes of ventilation. However, the mode of ventilation is meant to be a description of the way in which a mechanical breath is delivered. The determinants of how a mechanical breath is delivered are summarized not only in the control variables, but also in the phase and conditional variables (**Fig. 38.1**). Again, control variables are the independent variables that are either pressure, volume, or flow. *Conditional* variables are determinants of a response to a preset threshold, which are both clinician set and influenced by dependent and independent variables. Phase variables are those that are used to start, sustain, and end the phase. During inspiration, the phase variables include the trigger variable (determines the start of inspiration), limit variable (determines what sustains inspiration), and cycle variable (determines the end of inspiration).

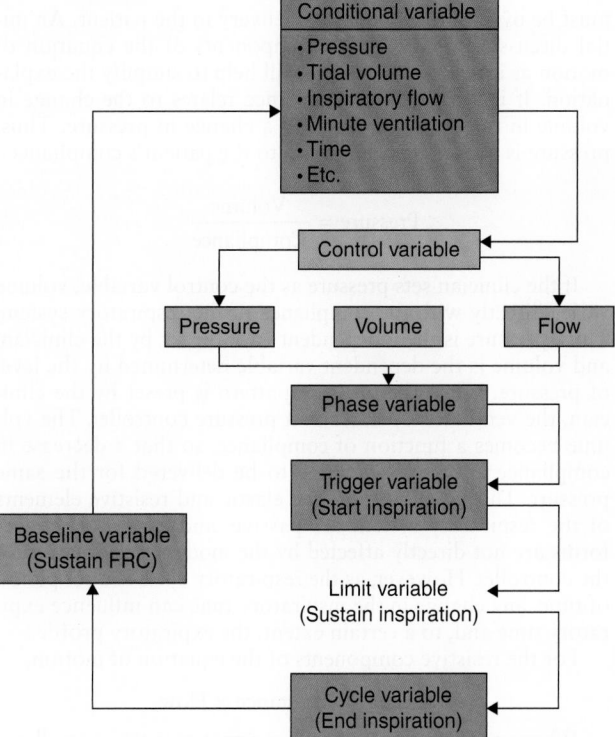

FIGURE 38.1. Flowchart to emphasize that each breath may have a different set of control and phase variables, depending upon the mode of ventilation. (From Chatburn RL. Classification of mechanical ventilators. *Respir Care* 1992;37:1009–25, with permission.)

TABLE 38.1

VENTILATOR CONTROLLERS

■ FLOW CONTROLLER (CONSTANT-FLOW CONTROLLER)	■ PRESSURE CONTROLLER (CONSTANT-PRESSURE CONTROLLER)	■ VOLUME CONTROLLER (VARIABLE FLOW CONTROLLER)
Modes VC, SIMV-VC Equation $Flow = \dfrac{Pressure}{Resistance}$	Modes PC, SIMV-PC, PRVC Equation $Flow = \dfrac{Volume}{Compliance}$ $Pressure = Resistance \times Flow$	Modes VC Equation $Flow = Pressure \times Compliance$
Independent variables Flow *Dependent variables* Pressure *Limiting variables* Volume *Trigger variables* Time Pressure Flow	*Independent variables* Pressure *Dependent variables* Volume Flow *Limiting variables* Pressure *Trigger variables* Time Pressure Flow	*Independent variables* Volume *Dependent variables* Pressure *Limiting variables* Volume *Trigger variables* Time Pressure Flow

VC, volume control; SIMV-VC, synchronized, intermittent mandatory ventilation-volume control; PC, pressure control; SIMV-PC, synchronized, intermittent mandatory ventilation-pressure control; PRVC, pressure-regulated volume control.

Control Variables

Control variables relate to the elastic and resistive forces that must be overcome to allow gas delivery to the patient. An initial discussion of the elastic components of the equation of motion as it relates to pressure will help to simplify the explanation. It is known that compliance relates to the change in volume in the lung as a result of a change in pressure. Thus, pressure is related to volume and to the patient's compliance.

$$Pressure = \frac{Volume}{Compliance}$$

If the clinician sets pressure as the control variable, volume varies directly with the compliance of the respiratory system. Thus, pressure is the independent variable set by the clinician, and volume is the dependent variable determined by the level of pressure. When the pressure pattern is preset by the clinician, the ventilator operates as a pressure controller. The volume becomes a function of compliance, so that a decrease in compliance allows less volume to be delivered for the same pressure. During expiration, the elastic and resistive elements of the respiratory system are passive, and expiratory waveforms are not directly affected by the modes of ventilation or the controller. However, as the respiratory cycle is a set period of time, any change in the inspiratory time can influence expiratory time and, to a certain extent, the expiratory profile.

For the resistive components of the equation of motion,

$$Pressure = Resistance \times Flow$$

When a ventilator operates as a constant-pressure controller—for example, in pressure-control (PC) mode, pressure-regulated volume-control (PRVC) mode, and synchronized, intermittent mandatory ventilation-pressure control (SIMV-PC) mode—pressure is an independent, or controlled, variable (**Table 38.1**). The set pressure will be delivered and maintained constant throughout inspiration, independent of what resistive or elastic

forces of the respiratory system might be. Even though pressure is constant, the delivered VT will vary as a function of compliance and resistance, and the flow will also vary exponentially with time.

A waveform from a ventilator operating as a pressure controller is displayed in **Figure 38.2**. Under this condition, volume and flow become the dependent variables, and their patterns will depend upon compliance and resistance. When a pressure pattern is preset (constant in a PC mode), flow-time and volume-time waveforms vary exponentially with time and are a function of compliance and resistance.

It is now clear that flow and resistance are associated only with the resistive components of the equation of motion. The elastic component refers to volume and compliance. Considering the resistive components of the equation of motion,

$$Pressure = Resistance \times Flow \ OR \ Flow = \frac{Pressure}{Resistance}$$

Thus, if the clinician sets flow as a function of time, pressure then varies with resistance. Flow is the independent variable and pressure is the dependent variable. When a flow pattern is preset, the ventilator operates as a flow controller; pressure is a function of resistance, and the inspiratory pressure–time waveform varies linearly with time. Volume increases linearly with time, although it does not have a direct relation to flow. Based on the equation of motion, volume does have an indirect relationship to flow, as volume is the integral of flow and flow is the derivative of volume. Again, expiration is passive, and the expiratory profile is not directly affected by mode of ventilation, but rather by compliance and resistance, even though the set inspiratory time can influence the expiratory time and, to a certain extent, the expiratory profile.

When a ventilator operates as a constant-flow controller (volume-controlled, VC, and SIMV-VC modes), flow is the independent variable. Regardless of the resistive or elastic forces of the respiratory system, the set flow will be delivered

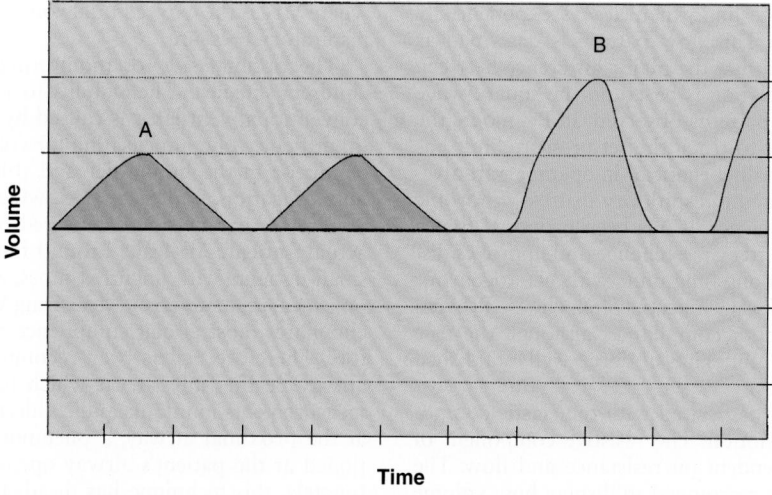

FIGURE 38.2. Volume–time wave form from a constant-pressure mode of ventilation. **A:** Increased resistance. With inspiration, an abnormal increase in tidal volume and decrease in inspired tidal volume occur, as compared to tracing B (normal resistance). Expiration has an abnormal linear decay to baseline. **B:** Normal resistance. During inspiration, a normal exponential increase in tidal volume occurs. Expiration has a normal exponential decay to baseline.

and maintained constant throughout inspiration. Pressure and VT will vary with time, depending on the compliance and resistance.

Waveforms from a ventilator operating as a flow controller are illustrated in **Figure 38.3.** Flow is the independent variable (controlled variable); pressure and volume are dependent variables. When a flow pattern is preset (constant in this case), pressure and volume are the dependent variables; they vary linearly with time and are functions of compliance and resistance. The modern ventilator can operate as a *flow controller* or as a *pressure controller.* As a flow controller, the most common pattern is *constant flow,* also referred to as a *square-wave* flow pattern. In this mode, the flow increases to a set level that is maintained for the duration of the inspiratory time. The pressure and volume that the patient receives are a function of compliance and resistance. When a ventilator is set as a pressure controller, the observed pressure pattern is constant and results in a *square-wave pressure* pattern.

From the equation of motion, it can be stipulated that, with the ventilator operating as a constant-flow controller, the pressure and volume are linear functions of time. The various ventilators are able to deliver various flow patterns. To have flow patterns different from the most common types, which are *constant* and *exponentially decelerating,* the ventilator must be controlled by a microprocessor, which performs a series of sequential adjustments dictated by an algorithm to produce various flow patterns, including *decelerating ramp, ascending ramp,* and *sinusoidal.* These flow patterns are used in various volume-cycled modes. Again, volume-cycled ventilation is still controlled by flow, and the independent variable set is flow. It is important to note that the decelerating rate of flow is controlled by an algorithm that does not reflect the elastic and resistive elements of the respiratory system. Abnormalities in these elements may result in flow-starvation asynchrony, as the flow from the ventilator may be inadequate to meet patient needs. Not all ventilators can provide novel flow patterns.

Describing the flow and pressure patterns observed in different modes of ventilation is often confusing jargon. To expand further, in PC ventilation, the pressure pattern is "square," but flow increases rapidly at the beginning of the inspiratory phase

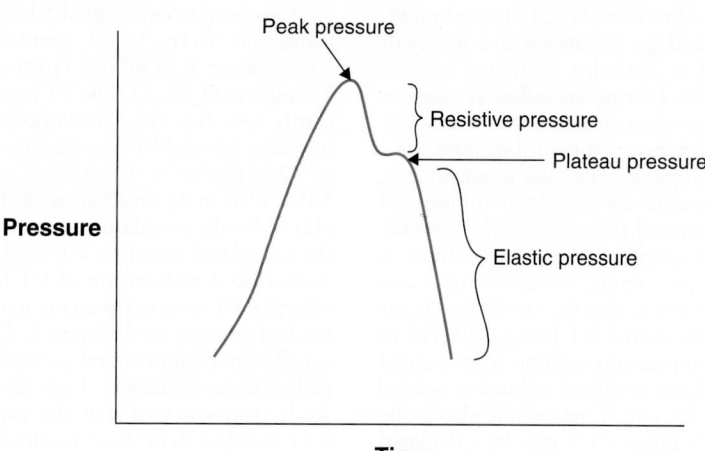

FIGURE 38.3. Pressure–time waveform from a constant-flow mode illustrating resistive and elastic elements of the respiratory system.

to generate the set pressure limit, then decays exponentially over the inspiratory time. This flow pattern is described as *decelerating flow*. It is said that the major difference between volume and pressure ventilation is based on the square-wave and the decelerating flow patterns observed. In PC mode, the **8** initial "snap" of high flow to reach the set pressure limit has been thought to be potentially beneficial in opening stiff alveoli in conditions such as acute respiratory distress syndrome (ARDS) or surfactant deficiency. It has been proposed that a decelerating flow favors better gas exchange and improves distribution of ventilation among lung units with heterogeneous time constants. For this reason, clinicians often choose PC ventilation in patients with poor compliance, although the true benefit of PC versus other modes has not been well established in animal or clinical studies.

Volume is most closely associated with the elastic component of the equation of motion. The resistive component of the equation is most dependent on resistance and flow. The **5** elastic components can be rearranged to display how volume is determined:

$$Volume = Pressure \times Compliance$$

If the clinician sets volume as a function of time, pressure then varies with compliance. Volume is the independent variable and pressure is the dependent variable.

Theoretically, when a ventilator sets a volume pattern, it operates as a volume controller. However, to be a true volume controller, the ventilator must measure volume directly in order to set the volume pattern. Most ventilators cannot directly measure volume; rather, they calculate volume delivered from flow that occurs over a period of time. Most ventilators use volume as a limiting variable, meaning that inspiration stops when the preselected volume is reached. When inspiration stops at the preset volume value, the ventilator is referred to as *volume cycled*, but it is really acting as a flow controller. That is, the ventilator is set to deliver a set VT at a certain number of breaths per minute and a specified inspiratory time, which determines the patient's minute ventilation. The ventilator gives a certain flow to meet the set requirements.

Understanding the delivery of a positive-pressure breath to a patient requires an understanding of the relationship of gas delivery to overcoming the resistive and elastic elements of the patient and the ventilator system.

Volume Measurement

The goals of modern mechanical ventilation in infants and children have focused on preventing overdistension of alveoli by limiting VT, thus reducing volutrauma (1,2,3). Exact knowledge of both inspired and expired gas volumes with a sufficient **6** level of precision is essential to optimize ventilator settings using lung-protective techniques. During the inflation phase of mechanical ventilation, pressure rises within the ventilator circuit, causing elongation and distension of the tubing and compression of the gas within the circuit. The volume of the gas, which becomes compressed within the ventilator tubing and never reaches the patient, is termed the *compressible volume of the circuit*. While in most circumstances, this volume is standard within different sizes of circuits, variation can occur. Knowing the compressible volume within the ventilator circuit is important in determining the actual VT being delivered to the patient's lungs. When compression volume is accounted for in determining patient VT, the resultant volume is termed **7** the *effective tidal volume* (eVT), which means that this is the VT that reaches the patient's lungs. eVT can be calculated thus:

$$eVT = (VTE) - [Circuit\ compensation \times (PI_{max} - PEEP)]$$

where VT_E is the expired tidal volume and PI_{max} is the maximal inspiratory pressure.

The optimal site for monitoring volumes in infants and children is unclear. The inability to accurately measure VT in a conventional ventilator is caused by several factors, including (a) difficulty of compensating for volume loss in the ventilator circuit or in the humidifier and (b) changes in temperature, humidification, and secretions, which may also influence the amount of gas that gets delivered from the ventilator to the actual patient. Air leaks around the ETT itself, especially in small patients with uncuffed tubes, are another source of volume measurement error. Measuring VT at the proximal airway eliminates most circuit compliance and other dead-space factors. Therefore, it has been recommended that the proximal airway be the only site at which to obtain accurate volume measurements in infants and children (4). To measure volumes at the proximal airway, a pneumotachograph must be positioned at the patient's airway opening or at the ETT. Unfortunately, this technique has disadvantages that are especially apparent in infants and children. A pneumotachograph placed at the proximal ETT opening creates dead space of its own, which can be detrimental in infants who already have small VTs (5). In addition, the proximally placed pneumotachograph may impair admittance to the ETT and airways and make suctioning more difficult. Secretions can also result in contamination of the pneumotachograph and distort observed measurements. Finally, the weight of the pneumotachograph at the proximal end of the ETT increases its overall weight and may result in an increased risk of extubation.

Given the importance of knowing the true VT delivered to a patient, it is essential to determine which is the most accurate, safe, and efficient site to monitor. It is also important to understand the reliability of conventional displays of VT generated by most ventilators. Three clinical studies have compared the ventilator-displayed VT (measured at the exhalation valve for exhaled VT displays) with the VT measured at the ETT. One group studied 98 ventilated infants and children using the Servo 300™ ventilator; 70 patients were ventilated with an infant circuit (compliance: 0.61 mL/cm H_2O), and 28 patients were ventilated with a pediatric circuit (compliance: 1.0 mL/cm H_2O) (6). In the patients with the infant circuit, poor correlation was noted between the expiratory VT measured with the pneumotachometer and the ventilator-displayed VT ($R^2 = 0.54$). Poor correlation ($R^2 = 0.58$) was also noted between the expiratory VT measured with the pneumotachometer and the calculated effective VT. In pediatric circuits, greater correlation occurred between the pneumotachometer-measured expiratory VT, the ventilator-displayed VT, and the calculated effective VT ($R^2 = 0.84$ and 0.85, respectively).

A second group studied 54 ventilated infants and children using the Servo 300™ ventilator with a pediatric circuit (compliance: 1.35 mL/cm H_2O) and adult circuit (compliance: 2.4 mL/cm H_2O) (7). The VT measured at the ETT was significantly less than the ventilator-measured tidal VT and varied between 2% and 91%, with a mean (standard deviation) error of 32% (20%) in 40 children with the pediatric circuit and 18% (6%) in 16 children with the adult circuit. The VTs displayed by the ventilator were also significantly different from the calculated effective VT (−63.3% to +29.1%), with substantial underestimation of VT from the VT displayed or the effective VT in many patients with small VTs. The third group studied 30 ventilated infants, 1–23 months old, on Servo 300™ ventilators with neonatal (compliance: 0.63 mL/cm H_2O) and pediatric (compliance: 1.13 mL/cm H_2O) circuits (8). This study demonstrated that the expiratory VT measured at the ETT was less than the expiratory VT displayed by the ventilator. When the ventilator was in the VC mode, the median difference was −36% (range: −5% to −2%), while the median was −35% (range: −6% to −60%) in the PC mode. The calculated effective VT was not statistically different from the ventilator-measured VT in PC mode; however, individual differences were large (range: –26% to +52%). The calculated effective VT was less than the VT measured at the ETT in the VC mode, with large individual differences (median: –23%, range: –48% to +21%). All of these clinical studies have recommended that the VT should be measured at the ETT in infants and small children. As stated previously, the effective VT can be calculated as the ventilator-measured expired VT. However, this method fails to take into account volume lost internally in the ventilator. Manufacturers have attempted to compensate for these volume losses by measuring compression volume loss in the system. The compliance factor can be calculated as

$$K_c = \frac{d_v}{(P_1 - P_0)} \, \text{mL/cm H}_2\text{O}$$

where K_c is the compliance factor, d_v is the total integrated volume, and P_0 and P_1 are the start and target pressures.

Data demonstrate good agreement in volume measured at the ventilator when compensation adjustment is on, as compared to volume measured at the proximal airway (9). The use of circuit-compliance compensation improved the agreement between the volume measured by the ventilator in an animal trial; pediatric pigs had improved agreement between the two volume methods attributable to circuit-compliance compensation (with circuit-compliance compensation "on," 0.97; with circuit-compliance compensation "off," 0.88; $p = 0.027$). It is essential for the clinician to understand the accuracy of the delivery of VT to their patients, especially in patients with small volumes, such as infants.

In a clinical study of 68 ventilated pediatric patients aged between 2 days and 18 years, the principal observation was that, when compression volume was compensated for by a computer algorithm, a negative bias occurred. Displayed volume was lower than that set by the clinician, but agreement was good when using compensation, with a concordance correlation between 0.90 and 0.98. Accuracy, expressed as percent difference, improved only in older patients (10). A limitation of this study, as well as previous studies that utilized an airway sensor or pneumotachograph as the reference value of volume, is the short time frame in which volumes were measured. A potential limitation of the airway sensor is the increased opportunity for the sensor to be contaminated by airway secretions and foreign substances, as compared to a pneumotachograph located within the ventilator. The potential for contamination, and thus degradation of the accuracy of the signal, of an airway sensor increases with increased length of time that the sensor is in place. In all of these studies, the airway sensor was only in place for a limited period. Caution must be used in extrapolating measurements from previously cited studies when the airway sensor is not left in place over a prolonged period.

When examining volume inaccuracies, the first source of error would be loss of volume within the ventilator circuit resulting from compression volume of the circuit. In the inflation phase, pressure rises within the ventilator circuit causing elongation and distention of the tubing and compression of the gas within the circuit. The volume stored in the circuit never reaches the patient but is instead released through the exhalation valve and is measured with the exhaled gases from the patient. The volume within the ventilator, circuit, and humidifier determines the magnitude of compression volume. The volume loss can theoretically be affected by a number of factors, including temperature and humidity of the circuit, and patient factors such as changes in the patient's compliance and resistance. In the above-mentioned study, it was found that the reported differences in the measured compliance of the circuit by the manufacturer and those measured by the ventilator with

differences were between 37% and 65% for the infant circuit and between 13% and 23% for the adult circuit. Because this factor is collected at startup of the ventilator and includes any compression volume in the ventilator and humidification system, this number will be higher. Subsequently, the compensation measured in the circuit and ventilator system was 51% and 18% higher, respectively, than could be expected from the compression volume calculated using the compliance factor alone. Thus, if only the circuit compliance factor is used, then the volume measurement at expiration, which accounts for both volume of the circuit and volume delivered to the patient, will be higher than the calculated effective volume.

Collectively, studies have shown that the ventilator-displayed VT, without software compensation for circuit compliance, generally overestimates the true delivered VT. Conversely, when the circuit-compliance compensation feature is on, the ventilator-displayed VT generally underestimates the true delivered VT.

Phase Variables

Discussion to this point has focused on the control variable required for a mechanical ventilator to deliver a breath to the patient and the interactions that occur with the delivery of that breath. The following discussion focuses on what have been described as *phase variables* (11). Phase variables control the ventilator during the period of time between the beginning of one breath and the initial phase of the next breath. In other words, phase variables are important in determining how a ventilator initiates, sustains, and ends inspiration and what it does between inspirations. Expiration, being passive, is not described in this terminology. In each phase, a particular variable is measured and used to initiate, sustain, and end the phase. The phase variables include the trigger variable (determines the initiation of inspiration), limit variable (determines what sustains inspiration), and cycle variable (determines the termination of inspiration).

Trigger Variables

Patient ventilator system interactions can be initiated under two settings: The ventilator can deliver a controlled breath independent of the patient's desire, or it can be coordinated with the patient's effort. Ventilators will measure one or more of the variables associated with the equation of motion (e.g., pressure, volume, flow, or time). Inspiration is initiated when one of these variables reaches a preset variable. A patient-triggered breath, sometimes known as *interactive ventilation*, provides patients with some autonomy to alter breathing patterns in response to their ventilatory demand. Such systems necessitate an interface between the ventilator and the patient to allow for rapid, measured responses from the ventilator to meet patient needs. For such systems to operate, they must sense a signal from the patient and recognize the beginning of inspiration. Second, they must pressurize the system to allow for delivery of the breath to the patient. Finally, the system must recognize the end of inspiration and thus termination of the breath. Ideally, if this interaction could be facilitated by direct interaction between the patient and mechanical ventilator, delays and patient discomfort created by the temporary or relative unavailability of the caregiver at the patient's bedside could be eliminated.

Initial recognition of the signal from the patient to begin inspiration is commonly referred to as *triggering*. Triggering can be subdivided into pretrigger and trigger phases (12). The pretrigger phase has been defined as the time from the onset of inspiration until triggering occurs. The trigger phase is the time from triggering until the maximum flow of gas occurs. The most common trigger variables are time and flow.

In *time triggering*, the ventilator initiates a breath according to a set frequency independent of the patient's spontaneous efforts. In flow triggering, the ventilator senses the patient's inspiratory effort as a change in flow from the baseline flow and begins inspiration independent of the set breath frequency. Ventilator features that affect the trigger phase include the response time of the ventilator and the presence of bias flow. *Bias flow* is a continuous delivery of fresh gas circulating through the inspiratory and expiratory limbs of the circuit. Theoretically, bias flow reduces the WOB by making flow available to satisfy the earliest demand of the patient during inspiration, before the flow is initiated during the pretrigger phase. Increased patient effort to trigger the ventilator and delayed response of the ventilator to the patient's effort can be translated directly into increased WOB.

Current ventilator designs have improved patient–ventilator interactions by improving both the signal sensed by the ventilator and the response time of the ventilator. Today, all ventilators have the capability to utilize a flow signal as the trigger signal from the patient to the ventilator. Flow triggering has the advantage of allowing the patient to trigger the ventilator with less effort, and it has a faster response time (13). The process of creating somewhat seemingly small amounts of negative pressure in pressure-triggered breaths is made increasingly more difficult when the patient has a smaller ETT and/or in the presence of $PEEP_i$.

Theoretically, patient-triggered ventilation could be improved if a signal could be acquired from the patient that represented the earliest attempt by the patient to acquire a breath and if that signal could represent the amount of effort or drive from the patient for that breath. This approach is represented in what has been termed *neurally adjusted ventilatory assist* (NAVA) (14). The NAVA approach to mechanical ventilation is based on the acquisition of the patient's neural respiratory output as it is transmitted through the phrenic nerve to the diaphragm. This signal is acquired via an esophageal catheter with an imbedded series of electrodes that capture the electrical activity signal of the diaphragm, known as E_{di}. NAVA responds by providing the requested level of ventilatory support to the patient from the E_{di}. The advantage of this system is the ability to acquire the patient's desire to trigger the ventilator quickly and to offer feedback between patient effort and ventilator output. At this writing, NAVA is being investigated in clinical trials in Europe in neonatal, pediatric, and adult patients.

Work of Breathing

Work is equal to the force applied to an object multiplied by the distance the object travels. That is, work = force $\times$ distance, or $W = F \times D$. If work is applied into the three dimensions of the respiratory system, work becomes the pressure applied to yield a change in the volume of the system and can be expressed as:

$$W = P \times V \quad \text{or} \quad W = \int_0^v P \times dv$$

where $\int_0^v P$ is the integral of the pressure across the respiratory system as a function of volume, and dv is the change in the volume of the respiratory system.

The concept of work associated with the functioning of the respiratory system has been known since the seminal analysis of Otis et al. (15). They elucidated that several forces were encountered while breathing, including the elastic forces of the chest wall and lungs, viscous and turbulent resistance of air, nonelastic tissue impedance, and inertia. Basically, motion requires work. Work is performed when pressure changes the volume of the respiratory system and is the product of pressure and volume integrated over time with respect to volume. Work is performed on the respiratory system by externally applied pressures from the ventilator via positive pressure, respiratory muscles, or both, as the lungs expand and contract. To achieve normal ventilation, the body performs work (WOB) to overcome the elastic and frictional resistance of the lungs and chest wall. Total work of breathing (WOB_T) is the sum of elastic work (WOB_E) and resistive work (WOB_R). Elastic WOB represents physiologic work to expand the lungs and chest wall. Resistive WOB is considered a measure of imposed WOB and includes work caused by the breathing apparatus, such as the ETT, breathing circuit, and ventilator demand-flow system. Artificial airways and physiologic resistive work of the airways are responsible for a large part of the imposed resistive work, with the mechanical ventilator also contributing some portion of resistive work (16).

Clinicians have long recognized that increased WOB occurs in patients being weaned from prolonged mechanical ventilation, when the patient begins to breathe spontaneously and take on more of the WOB. Patient-related factors, equipment factors, and decision making affect weaning of patients from mechanical ventilation and, thus, WOB. Equipment factors relate to the ability of the mechanical ventilator to meet the needs of the patient. It has been demonstrated in a lung model that the amount of WOB varies according to the device utilized (17). These equipment factors have an increased significance in patients with poor pulmonary reserve or high airway resistance, where the WOB associated with the equipment is increased (18,19). These factors also have an increased significance in pediatric patients, in whom equipment is often associated with increased WOB (20).

Limit Variable

The limit variable is the modality that sustains inspiration. Inspiration time is defined as the time interval from the beginning of inspiratory flow to the beginning of expiratory flow. During inspiration, pressure, volume, and flow increase above their end-expiratory values.

If one or more of these variables increases only as high as a preset value, this variable will be referred to as the *limit variable*. It is important to recognize that the limit variable determines what *sustains* inspiration but differs from the *cycle variable*, which determines the *end* of inspiration. Therefore, a limit value does not terminate inspiration but increases it to a preset value.

Cycle Variable

The cycle variable is the modality that terminates inspiration once a preset value is obtained, and this variable must be measured. The cycle variable also differs according to the mode of ventilation used. In *pressure-support ventilation* (PSV), the termination of the breath traditionally is triggered when either an absolute level of flow or a fixed percentage of peak inspiratory flow is reached. This gives the clinician little control over the ventilator cycling off as it relates to the patient's pathology. For example, in a patient with increased airway resistance and dynamic hyperinflation, it may be desirable to shorten the inspiratory phase and prolong the expiratory phase. By changing the cycle-off variable, the patient's inspiratory phase can be shortened, allowing the patient a longer expiratory phase.

The opposite is also true for patients with decreased pulmonary compliance. In this circumstance, the clinician might want to prolong the inspiratory phase and provide a shorter expiratory phase. Thus, delaying the beginning of expiration can extend termination of the breath.

PATIENT–VENTILATOR ASYNCHRONY

Patient–ventilator asynchrony is failure of two controllers to act in harmony (21). A patient on mechanical ventilation has the clinician-controlled mechanical pump of the ventilator and the patient's own respiratory muscle pump. Factors that affect patient–ventilator synchrony are listed in **Table 38.2** and can be subdivided into equipment factors, patient factors, and decision-making factors. Evaluation of patient–ventilator synchrony can also be subdivided into four phases that consist of issues of triggering, adequacy of flow delivery, adequate breath termination, and effects of PEEP and/or $PEEP_i$ (22).

Trigger Asynchrony

Trigger asynchrony is defined as the presence of muscular effort that results in a ventilator trigger (23). The incidence of patient–ventilator asynchrony is not well studied in pediatric patients. Clinical studies in adults have demonstrated trigger asynchrony in all of the common ventilator modes. Asynchrony occurs because of failure of the patient's drive to breathe, observed when additional support is provided by the base mode of the ventilator and the patient's drive to breathe

TABLE 38.2

VENTILATOR–PATIENT SYNCHRONY

Equipment factors
Trigger variables
Sensitivity settings
Response time of the ventilator
Inspiratory flow characteristics
Mode of ventilation
Expiratory valve design
Design of positive end-expiratory pressure valve and operation
External factors and equipment to the ventilator
Patient factors
Sedation and pain control
Patient's inspiratory effort and drive
Patient's disease process
Intrinsic positive end-expiratory pressure
Size of the airway
Presence of airway leak
Nutritional status
Patient homeostasis
Decision-making factors
Deleterious effects of patient–ventilator asynchrony
Patient fights the ventilator
Increased level of sedation
Higher work of breathing
Muscle damage
Ventilation–perfusion mismatch
Dynamic hyperinflation
Delayed or prolonged weaning
Prolonged intensive care or hospital stay
Higher costs

decreases. Trigger asynchrony is also associated with the development of auto-PEEP.

To trigger the ventilator, mechanically ventilated patients with obstructive lung disease who develop $PEEP_i$ must generate a negative intrapleural pressure to match the value of $PEEP_i$ plus the sensitivity threshold. When inspiratory effort by the patient is less than that threshold value, the ventilator will not deliver a breath, which causes effort by the patient without a response being generated from the ventilator. Thus, dynamic hyperinflation ($PEEP_i$) leads to frequent nontriggering of breaths in patients with obstructive lung disease. Such nontriggered breaths represent wasted breathing effort on the part of the patient and lead to patient–ventilator asynchrony, as the patient becomes distressed from the lack of ventilator response to their attempts to initiate a breath. In assist-control modes, the ventilator must be set to respond to the patient's breathing effort for the patient to receive any breathing assistance. In patients with obstructive lung disease or those in whom $PEEP_i$ is present, application of external PEEP may reduce nontriggered breaths by narrowing the difference between mouth pressure and alveolar pressure at end expiration. Similarly, in patients with high resistance to airflow from airway edema or constriction (such as asthma) who often also have air trapping and high levels on $PEEP_i$, application of external PEEP can help to "stent open" airways and improve flow during tidal expiration. Both of these conditions may have the elastic threshold load and WOB reduced by the use of extrinsic PEEP.

Flow Asynchrony

Flow asynchrony occurs whenever the ventilator flow does not match the patient's flow need. Flow delivered from the ventilator can be in either a fixed (such as in VC ventilation) or variable flow pattern (PC or PRVC). In VC mode, flow is fixed so that a set level of flow is delivered with each breath. As WOB is the sum of the work performed by the ventilator and the work performed by the patient, reduction in ventilator support or patient work will reduce the level of support. During ventilation with variable flow, the peak flow depends on a number of factors: set target pressure, patient effort, and the compliance and resistance of the respiratory system. In PC mode, the clinician can set the target pressure and the rate of flow acceleration or rise time. The control flow of acceleration varies according to the manufacturer, but the principles remain the same. A slower rise time may limit the ability of the ventilator to meet the patient's inspiratory demand. Studies of flow asynchrony during PC ventilation or PSV have implied that many patients require a rapid rise time to match increased ventilatory demand (24).

In a study that assessed whether adjustments in the initial flow or breath termination criteria affected patient–ventilator synchrony, the ventilator pattern response to PSV of 33 adult patients was studied under conditions with two parameters: seven different levels of delivered initial PSV flow, and during PSV termination that occurred when peak flow fell to 50% and 25%. It was found that an optimal initial flow could be defined for a given level of PSV, which resulted in the patient gaining a maximal pressure and volume from the ventilator. When the initial PSV flows were above and below this optimal flow, faster breathing rate, shorter inspiratory times, smaller VTs, and a tendency for airway pressure to fall short of the preset value occurred. Although increasing the inspiratory flow in PSV in adults may thus be useful, recommending the same maneuver in pediatric patients may be deleterious. Because pediatric patients have smaller ETTs, increased flow may lead to increased turbulence of gas and possible increased patient–ventilator asynchrony.

Termination Asynchrony

Termination asynchrony occurs when neural inspiratory time and ventilator inspiratory time do not coincide. The ability of the ventilator mode to terminate a breath when the patient desires constitutes an important factor in reducing the incidence of dyssynchrony. When the patient experiences high airway resistance, such as in bronchopulmonary dysplasia or chronic obstructive pulmonary disease, the inspiratory phase of a ventilator breath may be prolonged when a mode is selected that allows the patient to trigger spontaneous breaths. This situation can occur in PSV, resulting in early activation of expiratory muscles with premature termination of the ventilator breath.

Termination asynchrony can be caused by delayed termination or premature termination, with the most common being delayed termination. Generally, delayed termination results in dynamic hyperinflation, which then may result in missed trigger attempts as the patient is not able to overcome the effects of $PEEP_i$ and trigger the ventilator. Premature termination of a breath can also have deleterious effects with resultant asynchrony. In a 2001 study, premature termination led to substantially reduced V_T, increased respiratory rate, decreased inspiratory time, and increased WOB (25). A solution to help alleviate termination asynchrony has been incorporated into later-generation ventilators. This additional control allows for adjusting flow that causes the ventilator to cycle from the inspiratory phase to the expiratory phase (cycle-off) and allows for exhalation to be active. The effects of changing cycle-off when the ventilator begins exhalation as a function of peak inspiratory flow, in a ventilator with an active exhalation system, show that at a cycle-off set at 1%, the breath is terminated earlier than with the cycle-off set at 40%. In one study, WOB was not different between the two settings for cycle-off. However, considerable differences in the areas under both the time/flow and pressure/flow curves can be expected (26).

Expiratory Asynchrony

Expiratory asynchrony occurs due to a shortened or prolonged expiratory time, as well as patient efforts during expiration, when the ventilator is unresponsive. Shortened expiratory time creates the potential for hyperinflation secondary to air trapping and thus induces $PEEP_i$.

Historically, when patient effort signaled the ventilator to open the expiratory valve, the ventilator was no longer responsive to the patient's demands. Recently, manufacturers have introduced active exhalation valves that continue to sense patient effort during exhalation and respond to the patient effort. If the patient generates an effort during exhalation, the ventilator can terminate exhalation and respond to the patient effort. This mechanism is in contrast with systems that only allow the patient to attempt to pull flow from the bias flow in the system but require the patient to wait for expiration to terminate before another ventilator breath could be generated or triggered.

WHY ARE CHILDREN DIFFERENT?

Infants and children are both anatomically and physiologically different from adults, which limits the application of adult studies to the care of young children on mechanical ventilation. These differences decrease with the growth of the child. In a study of infants and children intubated for elective surgery, it was found that resistance of the respiratory system (R_{rs}) and airway resistance (R_{aw}) decreased as height increased (27).

A comparison of this relationship with the reported power function of lung volume changes suggests that R_{rs} is actually lower, relative to lung size, in infants than in older children. That is, increases in lung volumes are greater than decreasing resistance; therefore, specific resistance (resistance × volume) would increase with decreasing height. Thus, it is speculated that the airways do not grow at the same rate as the increase in lung tissue. In infants, lung volume may increase at a greater rate than the increase in airway diameter, which may be one reason why infants are especially prone to air trapping and hyperinflation in circumstances of airway narrowing or elevated resistance, such as in bronchiolitis.

It also appears that mechanical ventilation has detrimental effects on the airways of infants that include changes in the dimensions and mechanical properties of the airways. The extent of ventilation-induced deformation appears to be directly related to the compliance of the airway and inversely related to age. Anatomically, it has been demonstrated that the airways after mechanical ventilation have an increase in tracheal diameter, thinning of cartilage and muscle, disruption of the muscle-cartilage junction, and focal abrasions of the epithelium (28). In comparison to airways that have never been exposed to mechanical ventilation, airways that have been exposed are difficult to expand but easy to collapse (29). Also, these airways show greater resistance to airflow. These findings result clinically in patients with flow limitation, gas trapping, and increased dead space, airway resistance, and WOB (30).

Infants and young children are also at a mechanical disadvantage because of the high compliance and low elastic recoil of the infant and young child's chest wall. The child must perform more work to move the same VT than a more mature person, as part of the WOB is lost in distortion of the rib cage. The low elastic recoil of the chest wall places infants and young children at greater risk of lung collapse, as most tidal breathing takes place in the range of the closing capacity of the lung. Also, infants have a reduced ability to generate muscle force due to the shape of their rib cage, location of the insertion of their diaphragm, reduced muscle mass, and lower oxidative capacity (31).

INDICATIONS FOR MECHANICAL VENTILATION

No controlled studies have elucidated or evaluated the indications for the use of mechanical ventilation in pediatric patients. The use of mechanical ventilation in this population has evolved over the past 10 years as we have expanded our knowledge of lung injury caused by it (2,3). Also, the use of noninvasive intermittent mandatory ventilation (IMV) has increased, and the need for every patient to be intubated to offer positive-pressure mechanical ventilation is no longer absolutely necessary. The indications for the use of mechanical ventilation are diverse and include both primary respiratory and nonrespiratory causes. The decision to place a patient on positive-pressure mechanical ventilation is a combination of clinical judgment, assessing symptoms and signs of the need for mechanical ventilation, and laboratory tests. In essence, the decision to place a patient on either invasive or noninvasive positive-pressure mechanical ventilation represents the patient's inability to deal with increased inspiratory loads and maintenance of airway patency or inability to maintain gas exchange. Inspiratory loads consist of inertial (obesity, chest wall density), threshold (artificial loads placed on airway), resistive (upper-airway obstruction, asthma, artificial airway), and elastic (kyphoscoliosis, pulmonary restriction, chest wall trauma, pleural effusions, pneumonia, pulmonary edema, pulmonary fibrosis, hyperinflation) loads.

DETERMINING INITIAL SETTINGS FOR MECHANICAL VENTILATION

After the decision is made to place the patient on mechanical ventilatory support, it is essential that the settings of the mechanical ventilator be directed toward the indications for ventilatory support. Essentially, mechanical ventilatory support can be subdivided into three phases: acute, maintenance, and weaning. The acute phase of mechanical ventilation is the initial phase when the clinician matches the patient's disease process with the ventilatory mode and level of support. It is during the acute phase that the clinician must optimize mechanical ventilator support while minimizing potential deleterious effects. The initial settings of mechanical ventilatory support are dependent upon the patient's age and mode of support and can be subdivided into volume-targeted and pressure-targeted modes. The selection of ventilator settings is also directed by the clinician's desire to eliminate ventilator-induced lung injury. It is essential for the clinician to recognize that the goal of mechanical ventilatory support is not to normalize the patient's blood gases at the cost of ventilator-induced lung injury. For patients with obstructive lung disease, such as asthma, this lung protection strategy would include the prevention of high airway pressures and hyperinflation-associated complications. Initial settings would include a lower VT and prolonged exhalation times. Allowing such patients to breathe spontaneously in a support mode is ideal, as it allows the patient more control over the exhalation time. However, as some intubated asthmatics have elevated levels of $Paco_2$, this strategy may result in agitation in the patient and, therefore, an increase in sedation. The level of PEEP in patients with obstructive disease has traditionally been set at minimal levels, because of the development of auto-PEEP secondary to increased airway resistance and inadequate lung emptying during exhalation. However, some patients may require levels of PEEP to match the level of auto-PEEP to splint airways open, ensuring adequate oxygenation and improving exhalation.

Patients with decreased lung compliance must have ventilatory settings directed toward lung recruitment to reduce the severity of ventilator-induced lung injury. As discussed in previous sections, this lung protection strategy is primarily accomplished by

- limiting excessive distending volume (that would lead to disproportionate increases in alveolar pressure),
- limiting excessive change in alveoli distending pressure (that would lead to cyclic opening and closing of alveoli rather than relatively stable alveolar volume), and
- providing adequate level of end-expiratory pressure (to maintain alveolar recruitment during expiration).

This strategy is directed toward reducing the cyclic collapse and re-expansion of the alveoli due to inadequate levels of PEEP and thus the inability to maintain the alveoli open throughout the respiratory cycle.

LUNG RECRUITMENT

Lung recruitment is a strategy aimed at re-expanding collapsed lung tissue and maintaining high PEEP to prevent subsequent "derecruitment." The benefits of optimal lung recruitment and prevention of derecruitment involves (a) a reduction in the intrapulmonary shunt fraction with an improvement in arterial oxygenation, (b) an improvement in pulmonary compliance by shifting the compliance curve to the point where less pressure is required for the same change in volume, and (c) prevention of a cyclic opening, collapse, and reopening of

alveolar units with each breath associated with ventilator-induced lung injury. To recruit collapsed lung tissue, sufficient pressure must be imposed to exceed the critical opening pressure of the affected lung. Lung recruitment has gained widespread interest as a tool for opening closed lung units. The widespread use of low VTs may increase the risk of reabsorption atelectasis in the basal parts of the lung, which eventually may lead to consolidation of the affected areas. This atelectatic effect is further enhanced by high-inhaled O_2 concentrations. In certain patients, the use of a recruitment maneuver may provide a long-term improvement in oxygenation. If a proper PEEP level can be determined and set, the effect will stabilize and further protect the lung by avoiding cyclical opening and closing of lung units.

Ideal patients for recruitment maneuvers are those with putative ARDS in the early phase of the disease (before the onset of fibroproliferation). These patients will continue to be poorly oxygenated in spite of a high Fio_2. Preexisting focal lung disease that may predispose to barotrauma should be regarded as a relative contraindication to the maneuver (e.g., extensive apical bullous lung disease). Patients with "secondary" ARDS (e.g., following abdominal sepsis) are thought to be more likely to respond favorably to the maneuver than patients with "primary" lung disease and acute lung injury.

Several methods are used clinically to accomplish an opening of collapsed alveoli. The common denominator for most of these methods is to intermittently apply an increased positive pressure in the lung for a limited time. One method utilizes the graphical display of dynamic inspiratory compliance (C_{dyni}), which indicates the response of the patient's lung mechanics to each change in applied airway pressure and inspiratory VT (VT_i). For example, during a stepwise increase of the end-inspiratory pressure (EIP), a corresponding increase in VT will occur. C_{dyni} is defined as follows:

$$C_{dyni} = \frac{VT_i}{EIP - PEEP}$$

As long as the relative increase in EIP and VT is linear, the C_{dyni} will appear constant, reflecting the pressure–volume relation in the lung over time. With a continued stepwise increase in EIP, eventually less increase will occur in the corresponding VT, which is indicated by a slight decrease in C_{dyni}. Additional increase in EIP at this point may result in a gradually smaller increase in VT, accompanied by a decrease in C_{dyni}. This pattern may illustrate that the frequency of opening of collapsed alveoli is reduced relative to increase in pressure and that further increase in EIP may result in overdistension of already opened alveoli.

PEEP Titration

Although many different methods have been used to identify the "best" ("optimum" or "ideal") PEEP in patients with lung disease, none has been shown conclusively to improve survival. This section presents several of the more commonly used methods.

C_{dyni} may also be a useful parameter by which to find the appropriate level of PEEP that may prevent alveolar collapse during expiration, thereby helping to guide the titration of effective PEEP. This assessment may be performed by a stepwise decrease of the initial PEEP level and should be completed before the recruitment maneuver is performed. As PEEP is carefully decreased, the C_{dyni} will initially increase with each decrease of PEEP, indicating a relief of overdistended areas in the lung. Subsequently, the C_{dyni} will reach a plateau at which C_{dyni} no longer increases when the PEEP level is decreased. After further decrease in the PEEP level, the C_{dyni} will begin decreasing, indicating initial collapse of alveoli that can no longer be kept open at the current PEEP level. Effective PEEP should be set at 2–3 cm H_2O above the indicated collapse pressure as a safety margin after a preceding recruitment maneuver.

Another method is to identify the critical opening pressure of the airways by utilizing a static pressure–volume (P–V) loop to identify the lower inflection point (**Fig. 38.4**). As the lung is inflated from zero end-expiratory pressure, the clinician attempts to identify the point at which the compliance and hence volume abruptly increase. This point on the P–V loop is termed the *lower inflection point* (LIP). The pressure at LIP is also known as P_{flex}. It is thought to be the point at which alveolar recruitment occurs. As the lung is further inflated, another point is reached where the pressure–volume slope (i.e., compliance) abruptly decreases. This point is termed the *upper inflection point* (UIP). Ultimately, volume no longer changes with each change in pressure. This flattening of the pressure–volume loop is referred to as *beaking* (as in a bird's beak, referring to the pattern of the graphed pressure–volume loop) and represents overdistension of the lung. With this method, the ideal PEEP is thought to be 2–3 cm H_2O greater than the LIP pressure or P_{flex}. To avoid overdistension of the lung, the peak inflating pressure should be kept less than the UIP pressure.

The next phase of the pressure–volume loop occurs when expiration begins and the lung begins to deflate. A point on the deflation limb of the P–V loop is reached at which a more rapid loss of volume occurs per unit decrease in pressure indicating closure of a growing number of lung units. This point is called the *deflection point*. The pressure at the deflection point is called the critical closing pressure. After inflation, lung units are open and stabilized by surfactant. Once deflation begins, the lung volumes at any given pressure will be greater than the corresponding lung volume during inflation (a property known as hysteresis). Stated differently, the pressure needed to ㉑ maintain a given lung volume during deflation is less than the corresponding pressure during inspiration. Hence, the critical closing pressure (at the deflection point) is less than the critical opening pressure at the LIP. Some studies have suggested that titrating the PEEP just above the critical *closing* pressure

(deflection point) maintains alveolar volume during expiration with less risk of ventilator-induced lung injury (32).

Nearly 50 years ago, the observation was made that titrating PEEP for maximum O_2 delivery (the "optimum" PEEP) correlated with improved compliance, reduced dead space and, reduced shunt fraction (33). More recent studies have also confirmed that an oxygenation-based PEEP titration strategy is able to achieve lung recruitment, avoid overdistension, and maintain hemodynamic stability at lower FIO_2 (34). Clinicians may titrate PEEP to maximize O_2 delivery at lowest acceptable FIO_2 when P–V measurement is impractical.

Measures of Lung Recruitment

C_{dyni} can be used as a measure of improvement in lung compliance during lung recruitment; however, other measures should be utilized to ensure recruitment without overdistension of the recruited alveoli. If the lung is recruited, oxygenation, pulmonary compliance, and ventilation should improve. It is important not to be misled by an improvement of oxygenation alone as a measure of lung recruitment. An increase in PEEP can reduce cardiac output and increase PaO_2 despite a decrease in O_2 delivery. The CO_2 concentration in expired air depends on alveolar ventilation, cardiac output, and the metabolic state. The elimination of CO_2 via expired gas during normal conditions can be calculated using the *Brody formula*, which predicts CO_2 production during resting conditions:

$$\dot{V}CO_2(\text{elimination/minute}) = V/Q \times 10 \times BW^{0.75}$$

where BW is the body weight (kg).

A measure of CO_2 at the airway is the tidal elimination of CO_2 ($VTCO_2$), which can be calculated by dividing $\dot{V}CO_2$ by the respiratory rate. When a stepwise increase of EIP is applied to a collapsed lung, $VTCO_2$ will increase with each pressure step due to increased ventilation of already opened alveoli and recruitment of collapsed areas, allowing for additional diffusion of CO_2 from the blood into the alveolar space.

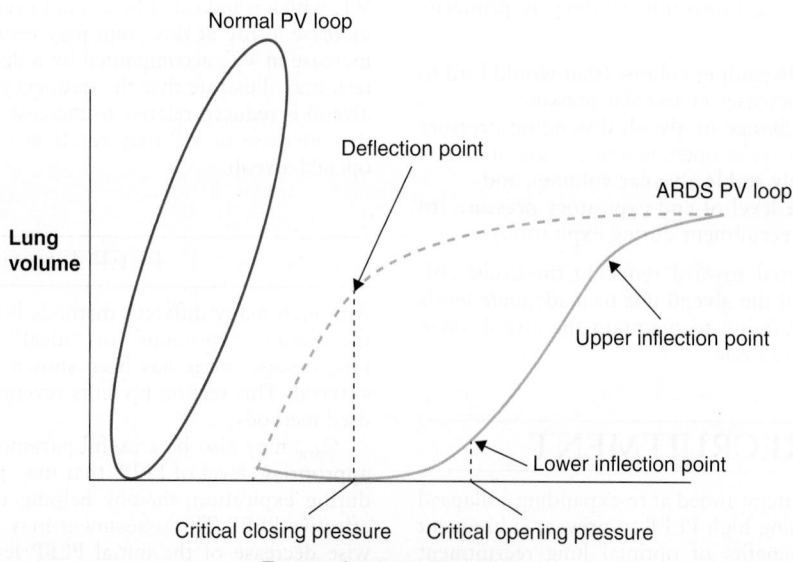

FIGURE 38.4. Pressure–volume (P–V) loop of the normal lung (green) and the acute respiratory distress syndrome (ARDS) lung (red) with solid inspiratory limb and dashed expiratory limb. Note that the lung volumes and compliance (slope of inspiratory P–V limb) are reduced in ARDS. During inflation of the ARDS lung, the lower inflection point is reached where lung units open and compliance increases until overdistension decreases compliance at the upper inflection point. During deflation, a point is reached (deflection point) where lung volume suddenly decreases as lung units close. Note that the critical closing pressure is lower than the critical opening pressure because of hysteresis. (See text.)

With a continued stepwise increase of EIP, VTCO$_2$ will continue to increase to a point at which no additional alveoli can be recruited without impeding alveolar blood supply. Alveoli already opened could also be overdistended, thus decreasing the diffusion of the CO$_2$ into the alveoli. Both circumstances will correspond to a drop in VTCO$_2$.

POSITIVE END-EXPIRATORY PRESSURE

PEEP can be added to any mode of mechanical ventilation and is produced by a number of devices that regulate the pressure in the expiratory limb of the ventilator circuit. The effect of PEEP is as a distending pressure to increase the FRC (volume of gas at the end of exhalation in the lung). By maintaining this pressure above the pressure in which the lungs collapse (closing pressure), atelectasis or alveolar collapse is minimized. The ultimate effect is decreased intrapulmonary shunting of blood and improved arterial oxygenation.

PEEP increases intrathoracic pressure and causes potential hemodynamic consequences by transmitting the applied PEEP to transmural capillary pressure, which affects the right and left heart. The most dramatic effect of increased PEEP is decreased venous return to the right heart. In children with normal cardiac function, compensation for this effect can easily be made by increasing intravascular volume with administration of isotonic crystalloids or colloids.

MODES OF VENTILATION

Intermittent Mandatory Ventilation

IMV is a mode of mechanical ventilation that allows the patient to breathe spontaneously between machine-cycled or clinician-controlled mandatory breaths. During IMV, a preset number of positive-pressure (mandatory) breaths are delivered between which the patient can breathe spontaneously. The mandatory breaths can control variables of volume (clinician-preset volume with flow limit, volume, or time cycled) or pressure (pressure limited, time cycled). IMV can be contrasted with single-control modes (assist control, PC, VC) because the patient is allowed to breath spontaneously between mandatory breaths. The most common mode of IMV is SIMV, in which mandatory, or machine, breaths are synchronized via a timing window to the patient effort at the patient's intrinsic respiratory rate rather than the breaths being evenly spaced over each minute (**Fig. 38.5**). Commonly, this mode is combined with PS, which provides support to nonmandatory breaths. The main disadvantage of SIMV, as compared to assist-control, is that the clinician may overestimate the amount of support, which leads to patient fatigue, as the WOB is increased (35). Another disadvantage in infants and children is that the support modes used during SIMV are not volume targeted but are usually limited by pressure. Thus, small changes in airway resistance or pulmonary compliance may lead to a decrease in VT obtained with the supported breaths, resulting in inadequate gas exchange and patient distress, especially if the mandatory breath rate is low.

Pressure-Controlled Ventilation

During PC ventilation, a pressure-limited breath is delivered during a preset inspiratory time at the preset respiratory rate (**Fig. 38.6**). The VT is determined by the preset pressure limit and the compliance and resistance of the respiratory system.

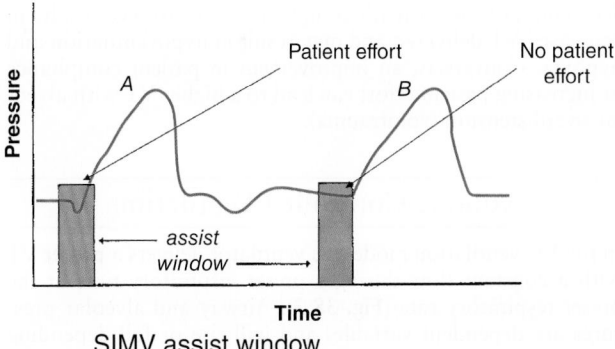

FIGURE 38.5. Two SIMV breaths. The first is patient triggered and the second is machine triggered. If the patient does not trigger a breath in the assist window, the ventilator will deliver a machine breath at the start of the next window. SIMV, synchronized, intermittent mandatory ventilation.

The flow waveform is always decelerating in PC. Gas flows into the chest along the pressure gradient. As the alveolar pressure rises with increasing alveolar volume, the rate of flow drops off (as the pressure gradient between the airway opening and the alveolar space narrows). The set pressure is maintained for the duration of inspiration.

PC ventilation has several advantages. The higher initial flow associated with PC ventilation more easily meets the patient's flow demands, especially in patients with "stiff" lungs. The peak inspiratory pressure during PC ventilation is usually less compared to VC ventilation for the same obtained VT. During PC breaths, the distribution of ventilation may be more even in a lung with heterogeneous mechanical properties. That is, the initial high flow opens alveoli, and the constant pressure maintained during inspiration may allow gas to flow from more well-distended alveoli to more collapsed areas and thus distribute gas more efficiently throughout the lung. PC is also useful in the patient with an air leak. Although volume is lost through the leak, the ventilator will continue to attempt to compensate by maintaining the airway pressure for the duration of the inspiratory phase.

PC ventilation also has several disadvantages. It does not guarantee minute ventilation, and therefore requires closer observation by the healthcare provider. The delivered VT will change as the patient's lung mechanics or effort changes.

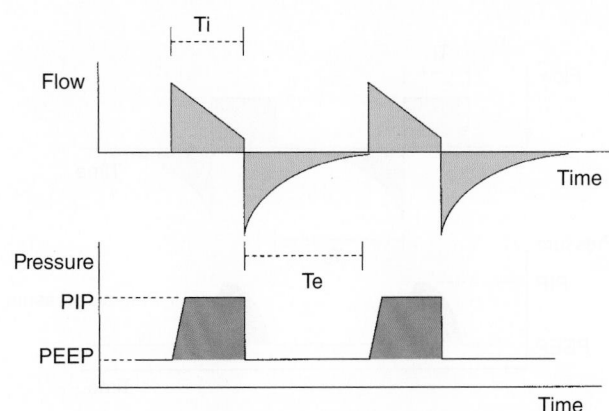

FIGURE 38.6. Pressure-controlled breath. Note that the flow pattern is rapidly decelerating from high initial flow to baseline. Ti, inspiratory time; Te, expiratory time.

Worsening of the patient's compliance or resistance results in decreased VT delivered and may result in hypoventilation and hypoxia. Conversely, an improvement in patient compliance or increasing patient effort can lead to a higher VT with alveolar overdistension (volutrauma).

Volume-Controlled Ventilation

In the VC ventilation mode, the ventilator delivers a preset VT with a constant flow during a preset inspiratory time at the preset respiratory rate (**Fig. 38.7**). Airway and alveolar pressures are dependent variables and will rise or fall depending upon changes in lung mechanics or patient effort. VC ventilation has some advantages. By setting the volume to be delivered and the breath rate, the clinician has control over the patient's minute ventilation and CO_2 clearance, provided only a small leak is present around the ETT. Ventilator-induced lung injury due to alveolar overdistension (volutrauma) can also be less in volume-control mode.

VC ventilation also has disadvantages. The constant-flow type of breath delivery in VC ventilation may not meet patient demands, especially if the patient has poorly compliant lungs that may benefit from the initial accelerated flow that occurs with PC ventilation, resulting in asynchrony between the patient's breathing efforts and the ventilator; this disadvantage leads to distress and often an increase in sedation requirements. The peak inspiratory pressure is higher in VC ventilation compared to PC ventilation for the same obtained VT.

Proportional-Assist Ventilation

Proportional-assist ventilation (PAV) is designed so that, theoretically, the level of ventilatory support is proportional to patient effort. This mode was designed to increase or decrease airway pressure by amplifying airway pressure proportional to inspiratory flow and volume. Unlike other modes in which a preset volume or pressure determines the level of support, in PAV, the level of support is determined in an interaction between the patient and the ventilator.

Most of the studies that utilized PAV have been observational, with limited reports in children. In patients supported with PAV, a greater variability was seen in VT than in PSV. However, PAV appears to be associated with better comfort. The current technology is associated with concerns regarding the interface with accurate measurements of elastance and resistance and regarding the issue of "runaway control" with changes in ETT resistance, presence of auto-PEEP, and a nonlinear relationship between elastance and resistance. Despite some potential advantages, no studies have demonstrated outcome benefits. PAV is currently not available in the US.

Airway-Pressure-Release Ventilation

Airway-pressure-release ventilation (APRV) is essentially a high-level CPAP mode that is terminated for a very brief period. The elevated baseline helps oxygenation, and the timed releases assist CO_2 removal. This mode allows the patient to spontaneously breathe during all phases of the cycle (**Fig. 38.8**). APRV is different from other modes of ventilation in that it is based on an intermittent decrease in airway pressure, rather than an increase. APRV has been successfully used in various forms of respiratory failure and acute lung injury in both adults and children.

In addition to F_{IO_2}, the operator-controlled parameters in APRV mode are P_{high}, T_{high}, P_{low}, and T_{low}, where P and T equate to pressure and time. P_{high} should be set at a level equivalent to the plateau pressure being used in a conventional mode when transitioning to APRV. If APRV is the first mode to be used, P_{high} is set at ~20–30 cm H_2O, P_{low} at zero, T_{high} at ~4–6 seconds, and T_{low} initially at ~0.2–0.6 seconds. T_{low} should then be adjusted based on the expiratory gas flow waveform so that the expiratory flow falls to ~25–75% of peak expiratory flow. Generally, T_{low} will be shortened in restrictive disease and lengthened in obstructive disease.

The P_{high} and T_{high} regulate end-inspiratory lung volume and provide a significant contribution to the mean airway pressure (MAP). MAP correlates to mean alveolar volume and is critical for maintaining an increased surface area of open air spaces for diffusive gas movement. As a result, these parameters control oxygenation and alveolar ventilation. Counterintuitive to conventional concepts of ventilation, the extension of T_{high} can be associated with a decrease in $PaCO_2$ as machine frequency decreases. P_{low} and T_{low} regulate end-expiratory lung volume and should be optimized to reduce airway closure/derecruitment and not as a primary ventilation adjustment. Generally, to maintain maximal recruitment, T_{high} should occur at the optimal P_{high} or CPAP level. To minimize derecruitment, the time (T_{low}) at P_{low} is brief. Partial assistance (PS or automatic tube compensation) can also be added to the spontaneous breaths. When the patient's underlying condition improves, APRV can gradually be weaned by lowering the P_{high} and extending the T_{high}. The goal is to arrive at straight CPAP.

APRV has several advantages. Clinical studies have shown that oxygenation and ventilation can be maintained at lower pressures with APRV when compared with conventional ventilatory management. Additionally, improvements in hemodynamic parameters and splanchnic perfusion have been reported. As the patient is able to breathe spontaneously throughout the entire respiratory cycle with this mode of ventilation, the need for heavy sedation and neuromuscular blockade is much less than with other modes of ventilation.

APRV, like all other modes, also has some disadvantages. APRV is a form of PC ventilation; therefore, mechanical VT varies according to lung mechanics. Also, the spontaneous breaths during the long inflation period can further increase end-inspiratory lung volume beyond that set by the inflation pressure; therefore, APRV may be less effective as a strategy to limit alveolar overdistension. APRV has not been well compared to other forms of conventional ventilation in a controlled fashion.

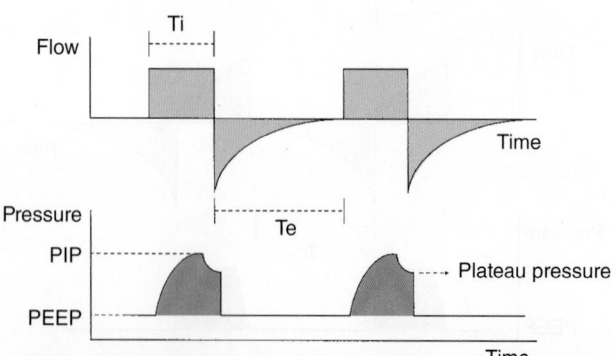

FIGURE 38.7. Volume-controlled breath. Note that the flow pattern is square with an initial high flow that is maintained during inspiration and then quickly terminated at expiration. Ti, inspiratory time; Te, expiratory time.

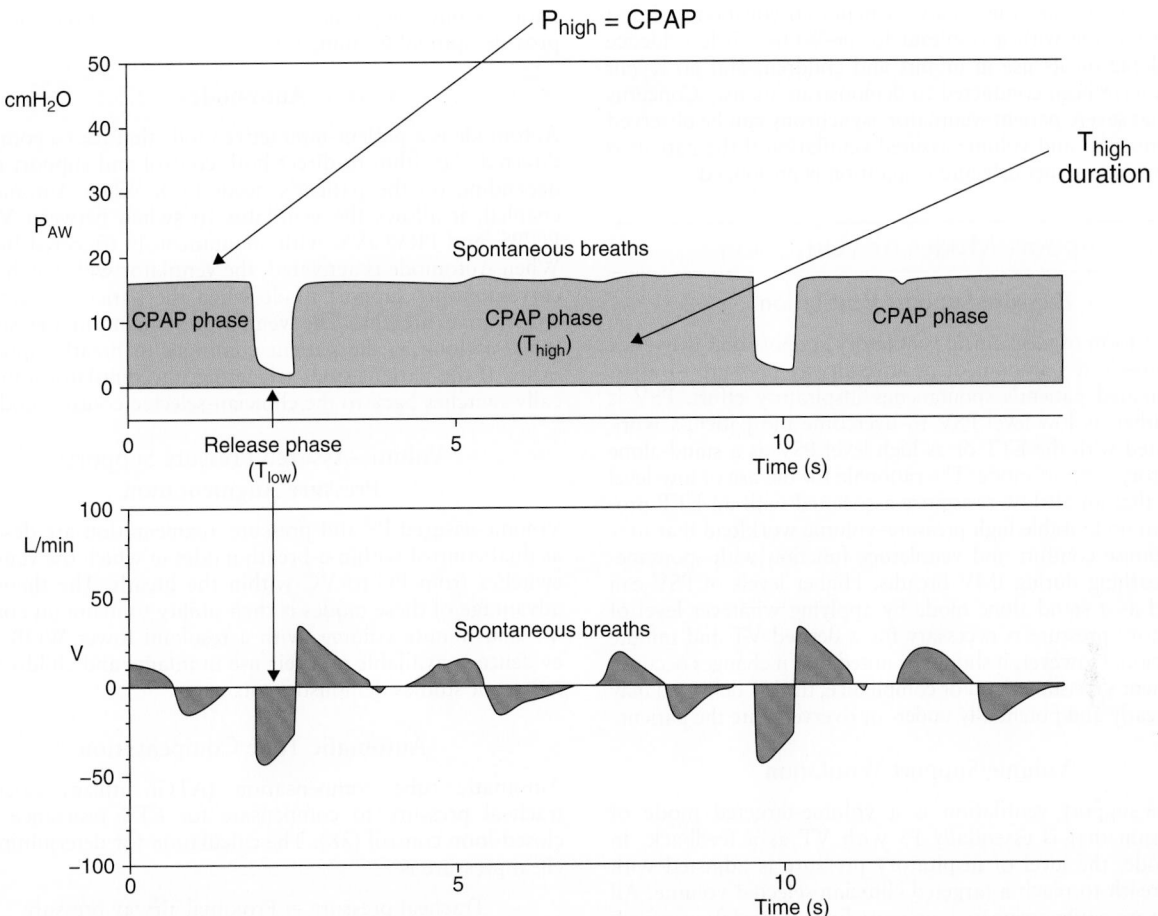

FIGURE 38.8. Patient breathing on APRV. The CPAP phase (P_{high}) is intermittently released to a P_{low} for a brief duration (T_{low}) reestablishing the CPAP level on the subsequent breath. Spontaneous breathing may be superimposed at both pressure levels and is independent of time-cycling. (Adapted from Slonim AD, Pollack MM. Mechanical ventilation. In Slonim AD, Pollack MM, Bell MJ, et al. eds. *Pediatric Critical Care Medicine.* Philadelphia, PA: Lippincott Williams & Wilkins, 2006.)

Hybrid Techniques

Hybrid techniques, also described as dual-controlled ventilation, are modes that allow the clinician to set a volume target while the ventilator delivers a PC breath. Dual control of the breath in these hybrid modes is designed to be either intrabreath (within a breath) or interbreath (breath to breath). Examples of dual-control *intrabreath* modes are volume-assured PS and pressure augmentation. In these modes, the ventilator switches from PC to VC during a single breath. Examples of dual-control *interbreath* modes are PRVC, adaptive pressure ventilation, variable PC, and Autoflow™. In these modes, the pressure limit is increased or decreased automatically to maintain a clinician-selected target volume. Frequently used hybrid modes are discussed in the following sections.

Pressure-Regulated Volume Control

PRVC (or adaptive pressure ventilation, variable PC, Autoflow™, or Volume Control Plus™) is a dual-control, breath-to-breath mode. PRVC has a variable decelerating flow pattern, with breaths time cycled. During PRVC, the pressure and volume are regulated. Thus, all breaths are volume targeted, with pressure adjusted to reach that volume target. PRVC often incorporates a "compliance curve" that is developed within the ventilator computer, as it gives several initial breaths at varying VTs that increase incrementally up to the set value.

From this information, the ventilator computes the pressure target required to deliver the desired VT. Depending on the respiratory system compliance, the pressure associated with the tidal breath can vary over time. If the patient's compliance decreases, the pressure required to ensure the volume breath can be increased up to within 5 mm Hg of the set pressure-alarm limit. If the patient's compliance improves, the pressure required to deliver the volume breath will be reduced. Thus, a specific VT and minute ventilation is assured, while pressure-induced lung damage is minimized. The proposed advantage of this mode is a constant $\dot{V}_E$ and VT with automatic weaning of the pressure limit as the patient's compliance improves.

Volume-Assured Pressure Support

Volume-assured PS and pressure augmentation are described as a dual-control-within-a-breath mode, where the ventilator switches from PC to VC within the breath. In this mode, the clinician chooses a volume target and the breath begins as a pressure-limited, flow-cycled breath, either spontaneously (PS) or mechanically. When inspiratory flow has decelerated to the minimum set level, delivered volume is measured. If the target volume has been met or exceeded, the breath ends. If the delivered volume has not met the target, the breath is transitioned to a volume-targeted breath by prolonging inspiration at the minimum flow and increasing the inspiratory pressure until the delivered volume has been obtained. The theoretical advantages of these modes are the ability to maintain constant VT and minute volume with a resultant lower WOB. Little evidence is available on its use in infants and children, and no recent studies have been conducted to demonstrate its use. Concerns exist that severe patient–ventilator asynchrony can be observed with pressure- and volume-assured ventilation if the patient is breathing spontaneously and inspiration is prolonged.

Support Modes of Ventilation

Pressure-Support Ventilation

PSV is a form of mechanical ventilatory support that delivers a clinician-selected amount of positive-airway pressure to assist an intubated patient's spontaneous inspiratory effort. PSV is used either as low-level PSV to overcome the patient's work associated with the ETT or as high-level PSV as a stand-alone ventilatory support mode. The rationale for the use of low-level PSV is that an airflow resistance associated with an ETT produces an undesirable high pressure–volume workload that may compromise comfort and ventilatory function with spontaneous breathing during IMV breaths. Higher levels of PSV can be used as a stand-alone mode by applying whatever level of inspiratory pressure is necessary for a desired VT and minute ventilation. However, it should be noted that if changes occur in the patient's resistance and/or compliance, the VT delivered may vary greatly and potentially under- or overventilate the patient.

Volume-Support Ventilation

Volume-support ventilation is a volume-targeted mode of ventilation that is essentially PS with VT as a feedback. In this mode, the level of inspiratory pressure is adjusted with each breath to reach a targeted clinician-selected volume. All breaths are patient triggered, pressure limited, and flow cycled.

As outlined in the weaning section, volume-support ventilation is utilized in patients once they demonstrate that they are ready to be weaned, which is best demonstrated when the patient begins to trigger the ventilator above the set rate. When the patient triggers the ventilator, the patient's set VT is reduced by 15%, and the pressure associated with maintaining adequate minute ventilation and gas exchange is followed over time. As the patient's compliance improves, the required pressure to deliver the VT will be diminished. Patients may be extubated from volume support (VS) once the required peak inspiratory pressure is ≤20 cm H_2O, PEEP is ≤6 cm H_2O, and standard extubation criteria are met (resolution of cause for intubation, ability to protect the airway, hemodynamic stability, etc.). By using the peak inspiratory pressure as a guide for extubation, the clinician is utilizing an indirect measure of improvement of pulmonary compliance to guide clinical improvement. Hybrid modes such as ventilator-support ventilation have an advantage in pediatric patients by maintaining a clinician-targeted volume even if changes occur in the patient's airway resistance (e.g., increased secretions) and/or pulmonary compliance. As the patient initiates all ventilator breaths, however, most hybrid modes will automatically alarm and switch to an assist-control or SIMV mode if the patient becomes apneic or breaths are inadequate to meet VT goals to prevent deleterious patient events.

Closed-loop Methods

An important factor in successful weaning of mechanical ventilation is the ability of the clinician to manipulate the ventilator so that it responds to the patient's physiologic respiratory demands by providing more or less support, as needed. If the ventilator itself could make these adjustments, based upon the patient's physiologic needs and ventilatory pattern, it would provide optimal weaning (36).

Automode

Automode is a patient-interactive mode that uses a computer-directed algorithm to direct both control and support modes depending on the patient's needs (37). When Automode is enabled, it allows the ventilator to switch between VC/VS, PC/PS, and PRVC/VS, with spontaneously triggered breaths. When Automode is activated, the ventilator will switch to the corresponding support mode when the patient triggers two consecutive breaths. The ventilator remains in the support mode as long as the patient continues to breathe spontaneously. If the patient stops triggering, the ventilator automatically switches back to the clinician-selected control mode.

Volume-Assured Pressure Support/ Pressure Augmentation

Volume-assured PS and pressure augmentation are described as dual-control-within-a-breath modes in which the ventilator switches from PC to VC within the breath. The theoretical advantage of these modes is their ability to maintain constant VT and minute volume, with a resultant lower WOB. Little evidence is available on their use in infants and children, and no recent studies demonstrate its use.

Automatic Tube Compensation

Automatic tube compensation (ATC) utilizes calculated tracheal pressure to compensate for ETT resistance via a closed-loop control (38). The calculation for determining tracheal pressure is

$$\text{Tracheal pressure} = \text{Proximal airway pressure} \\ - (\text{Tube coefficient} \times \text{Flow}^2)$$

Thus, the known resistive coefficients of the ETT and measurement of instantaneous flow are used to apply pressure proportional to the resistance of the entire respiratory cycle. Theoretically, ATC is designed to overcome the imposed WOB during inspiration. As discussed in the description of PRVC and VS, the use of ATC has theoretical advantages in pediatric patients with small ETTs. In the presence of airway secretions or kinking of the ETT, airway resistance may increase significantly such that ATC fails to adequately overcome the WOB. The theoretical advantages are (a) compensation for the WOB imposed by the artificial airway, (b) adjustment of the level of inspiratory flow to meet the patient's demand (similar to PAV), and (c) compensation for imposed expiratory resistance to reduce air trapping. However, the advantages are not always realized at the bedside. During expiration, the calculated tracheal pressure is greater than the airway pressure, and under those conditions, negative airway pressure could reduce expiratory resistance. However, as ATC cannot reduce PEEP to <0 cm H_2O during exhalation, expiratory resistance may not have complete compensation. Also, kinks, bends, or secretions in the ETT may lead to changes in airflow resistance, again causing incomplete compensation. The evidence for the advantages of ATC is strictly anecdotal, and its role in pediatric patients is yet to be determined.

HIGH-FREQUENCY VENTILATION

High-frequency ventilation (HFV) delivers minimal VTs that approximate the anatomic dead space at rates exceeding the normal respiratory rate. VTs of 1–3 mL/kg are delivered at rates from 3 to 20 Hz (180–1200 breaths/min). The main strategy of mechanical ventilation in patients with ARDS is to limit the delivered VTs and optimize alveolar recruitment in an effort to minimize atelectrauma (39) and volutrauma (40,41). At least theoretically, HFV provides lung-protective ventilation by applying maximal MAP and recruitment while delivering minimal VTs.

Classification of Devices

During HFV, an oscillating waveform is generated by rapidly altering gas flow. While inspiration during HFV is always active, depending on the device, expiration can be either active or passive. During passive expiration, the elastic recoil of the lungs generates a positive transpleural pressure and expiration. During active expiration, the air is actively withdrawn out of the lungs as the diaphragm or piston of an oscillator travels away from the airway opening in the ventilator circuit. The devices described differ by the technical modalities through which HFV is achieved. The nomenclature of devices is not entirely straightforward, and hybrid devices exist that combine HFV with conventional ventilation.

High-Frequency Oscillation Ventilation

A nearly square waveform is generated either by a diaphragm or by a piston (42). Inspiration and expiration are active. Gas is forced into the lungs and actively withdrawn from the airways, as the diaphragm or piston travels forward and backward. Fresh gas flow pressurizes the system to the required MAP. The magnitude of the oscillations (often referred to as ΔP) is controlled by the distance traveled by the piston or the diaphragm. The inspiratory time is set as a percentage of the respiratory cycle and determines the ratio of inspiratory-to-expiratory (I:E) time. An inspiratory time of 33% or 50%, resulting in an I:E ratio of 1:2 or 1:1, is frequently used in the clinical setting.

High-Frequency Jet Ventilation

During high-frequency jet ventilation, a jet ventilator is combined with a conventional ventilator. The gas flows from two sources: The jet ventilator is the source of the small delivered VTs, whereas the conventional ventilator is the source of the bias flow. Inspiration is active, whereas expiration is passive and driven by elastic recoil of the lungs and chest wall. Jet ventilation can be delivered during CPAP or conventional ventilation. The resulting VT of the jet ventilator is a result of the driving pressure of the jet, resistance of the ETT, and the set inspiratory time. Inspiratory and expiratory times are variable in most devices. High-frequency jet ventilation has been evaluated in a number of neonatal trials (43,44).

High-Frequency Flow Interrupters

With the use of high-frequency flow interrupters, a valve mechanism in the expiratory limb of the ventilator rapidly alters flow, causing a pulsating gas flow. Some conventional ventilators provide this mode as a back-up mode to transition to high-frequency flow interrupters without switching the ventilator. Due to their limited bias flow, high-frequency flow interruption devices are usually used in the neonatal setting.

Examples of Commercially Available Devices

Neonatal Devices

The Life Pulse High-Frequency Ventilator (Bunnell, Salt Lake City, UT) is a jet ventilator used in neonates. The ventilator is connected to a conventional ventilator at the patient's ETT with a special adapter. The jet ventilations are added to the conventional ventilation that the patient is receiving. The respiratory rate varies between 4 and 11 Hz (240–660 breaths/min), with airway pressure monitored at the ETT.

The Babylog 8000 plus (Draeger Medical, Telford, PA) is a conventional ventilator with the option to ventilate in a high-frequency mode (high-frequency flow interruption). Small delivered VTs are generated by rapidly switching the expiratory valve. The bias flow is up to 30 L/min. The ventilator can oscillate between 5 and 20 Hz (300–1200 breaths/min). HFV can be applied during CPAP or SIMV.

Pediatric and Adult Devices

The Sensormedics 3100 A/B (Viasys, Yorba Linda, CA) is a device used for high-frequency oscillation ventilation (HFOV). Oscillations are generated with a diaphragm. Fresh gas is provided by a bias flow system, with frequencies ranging from 3 to 15 Hz (180–900 breaths/min). The Sensormedics 3100 A is used for neonates and infants, with bias flow ranging from 0 to 40 L/min and MAPs ranging from 3 to 45 cm H_2O. The Sensormedics 3100 B is approved for adults and larger children who weigh >35 kg. In comparison to the 3100A, the 3100B has a more powerful diaphragm, can provide a larger bias flow (0–60 L/min), and can apply higher MAPs of up to 55 cm H_2O. The Sensormedics 3100 A/B generates effective gas exchange in neonates, infants, and adults. Such devices have been evaluated in large, multicentered trials (45,46,47).

Mechanisms of Gas Exchange

The mechanisms of gas exchange during HFV are different from conventional ventilation. While HFV is frequently used in the clinical setting, it seems counterintuitive that this modality of ventilation produces adequate oxygenation and removal of CO_2. Of interest, species such as dogs are capable of spontaneous respiratory rates of 5–6 Hz (240–300 breaths/min) while they are panting. Despite the fact that VTs approach the anatomic dead space, adequate gas exchange is still maintained (48). During HFV, gas exchange is achieved by a number of different mechanisms (Fig. 38.9). Although described as distinct modes in this chapter, all modes of gas exchange interact with each other during HFV of the architecturally unique human lung.

Ventilation of Alveolar Units with Short Path Lengths: Bulk Ventilation

When a small VT is delivered, it may reach the proximal alveolar units with short path lengths by bulk ventilation, resulting in direct ventilation of this fraction of lung units. This mode of gas exchange closely resembles conventional ventilation, but only the most proximal and most compliant alveoli are ventilated directly in this fashion during HFV.

Ventilation in the Conducting Airways: Taylor Dispersion and Convective Dispersion

In 1953, Taylor first described the dispersion of particles in the presence of laminar flow (49). When the velocity of gas flow increases, the initial planar surface of a gas column transforms into a parabolic surface, allowing a greater deal of longitudinal mixing and dispersion. The center of the gas column is believed to travel faster than the outer areas, allowing further diffusion and mixing downstream. Turbulence that occurs when this gas column reaches a bifurcation will partly replace laminar mixing, resulting in dispersion of gas molecules and further contributing to gas exchange. Convective dispersion occurs when a uniform column of air is transformed into a

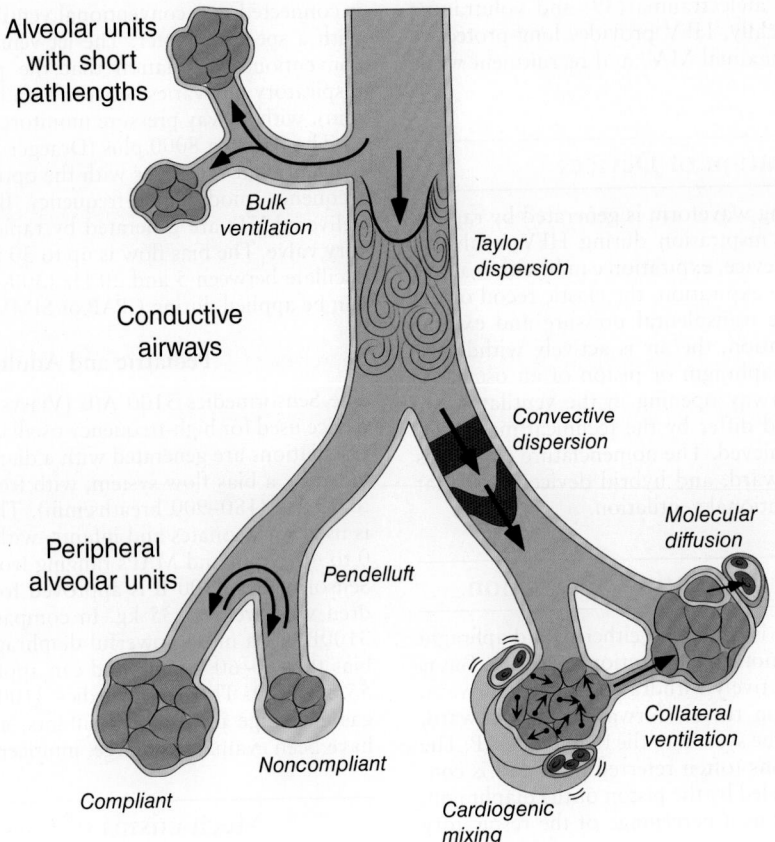

FIGURE 38.9. Mechanisms of gas exchange during high-frequency ventilation.

parabolic shape. Air molecules undergo mixing as molecules in the center of the gas column move to the tip of the parabolic shape and the molecules near the wall stay behind.

Ventilation of Peripheral Alveolar Units: Pendelluft and Collateral Ventilation

The heterogeneous nature of ARDS results in significant regional heterogeneity of lung mechanical properties: noncompliant, atelectatic areas are adjacent to compliant, overinflated areas. The regional time constant (τ = resistance × compliance) describes the rate of filling and emptying of a lung unit. Noncompliant areas fill and empty at a faster rate than compliant areas. Pendelluft (from the German: *pendel,* pendulum and *luft,* air) means that gas equilibrates between compliant and noncompliant lung units, resulting in regional mixing of gas. Pendelluft is an inspiratory and an expiratory phenomenon. At end expiration, air moves from the compliant to the noncompliant area, as the compliant area is still emptying when the noncompliant area is already empty. At end inspiration, air moves from the noncompliant area, which is already filled, to the compliant area, which is still filling (50). During HFV, this concept is believed to contribute to gas exchange, potentially ventilating areas otherwise not penetrated directly by HFV.

Collateral ventilation occurs between neighboring alveoli through collateral channels such as the interalveolar pores of Kohn. Collateral ventilation has been suggested as a mechanism of gas transport during HFV, although the high resistance of the collateral channels may limit the overall contribution to gas exchange during HFV (51).

Ventilation near the Alveolocapillary Membrane: Molecular Diffusion and Cardiogenic Mixing

Passive diffusion of gas molecules through the alveolocapillary membrane is the predominant form of gas transport during HFV and conventional ventilation in the peripheral lung units. Cardiac-induced pressure changes in the vascular bed add to gas mixing on the alveolar level. These mechanisms of gas exchange are not unique to HFV, as they also occur during conventional ventilation.

In summary, gas exchange during HFV is a function of several different mechanisms of gas transport in the conducting airways and alveolar units, which interact in a complex fashion. The various modes have a regional distribution: in the more proximal alveoli, direct ventilation of alveoli by bulk flow is predominant. In large airways such as the trachea and the left and right main stem, Taylor-type dispersion and convective dispersion take place. In the small peripheral airways and the alveoli, Pendelluft, collateral ventilation, molecular diffusion, and cardiogenic mixing play the main role (50).

Technical Description of High-frequency Ventilation

Alveolar Recruitment

Mean Airway Pressure. Alveolar recruitment is associated with improving gas exchange (52,53). Optimal lung volume during HFV has been described as the lowest MAP that achieves oxygenating efficiency and maintains lung volume (54). An increase in MAP during HFV is achieved by narrowing the orifice of the expiratory valve or by increasing the bias gas flow. MAP and pressure amplitude are significantly altered by the ETT (55). Decreasing the size of the ETT leads to a decrease of the peak-to-trough pressure amplitude. The diameter and length of the ETT also affect MAP.

Distal airway pressures vary in response to changes in the I:E ratio during HFV. Data from animal models using alveolar capsules indicate that MAP is nonhomogeneously distributed throughout the lung. Air trapping occurs if the inspiratory time is increased at the expense of the expiratory time. Data from animal models further suggest that distal alveolar pressures can exceed proximal MAPs during I:E ratios >1:2 (55,56,57). This phenomenon has led to the recommendation that I:E ratios be limited to 1:2 in the clinical setting.

Carbon Dioxide Elimination

Alveolar Ventilation. Several investigators have shown that alveolar ventilation is a function of the rate of oscillations and the squared V_T ($Vco_2 = f \times V_T^2$) (3,58). V_T contributes more to CO_2 elimination than frequency does, as V_T is squared in the formula. The relation between alveolar ventilation and V_T is further complicated by the branching generations of the tracheobronchial tree. In experimental studies using fluid models of branching tubes, the oscillatory diffusivity has been described as (50,59)

$$D_{osc} = f^{0.9} \times V_T^{2.2} \text{ and } D_{osc} = f^{1.4} \times V_T^{1.8}$$

In the clinical setting, it is appropriate to estimate alveolar ventilation as a product of the device frequency (f) and the square of the delivered V_T.

Any maneuver that alters V_T will alter CO_2 removal. Increasing the amplitude leads to increasing VTs and improves CO_2 elimination. Conversely, decreasing the amplitude decreases CO_2 elimination by directly decreasing delivered V_T.

Respiratory Frequency. During HFOV, the device frequency has a significant effect on delivered V_T. With an increasing respiratory rate, the inspiratory time is decreased and the oscillations of the diaphragm become less efficient, resulting in decreased delivered VTs. As VTs are more important than rate for CO_2 elimination, increasing the respiratory rate during HFV paradoxically diminishes CO_2 clearance. Conversely, decreasing the rate results in more efficient oscillations, larger VTs, and improved CO_2 clearance.

The following clinical example illustrates the described relationship. During HFOV with the Sensormedics 3100, the inspiratory time is set as a percentage of the total respiratory cycle. If the inspiratory time is set at 33% and the rate is decreased from 10 to 8 Hz, the inspiratory time increases from 33 to 42 milliseconds. The increased inspiratory time at a lower device frequency will lead to more efficient oscillations, increased delivered VTs (**Fig. 38.10**), and increased CO_2 elimination.

Effect of an Endotracheal Tube Leak. Creating an ETT cuff leak has been suggested as an alternative way to enhance CO_2 clearance in the setting of hypercarbia despite a maximized amplitude and a low rate. The clearance enhancement will occur by promoting a path of CO_2 egress via a path outside of the ETT. After the ETT cuff has been deflated to produce a cuff leak, the proximal MAP will decrease. The expiratory valve or bias flow should be adjusted to maintain the same MAP for this maneuver to be effective (60).

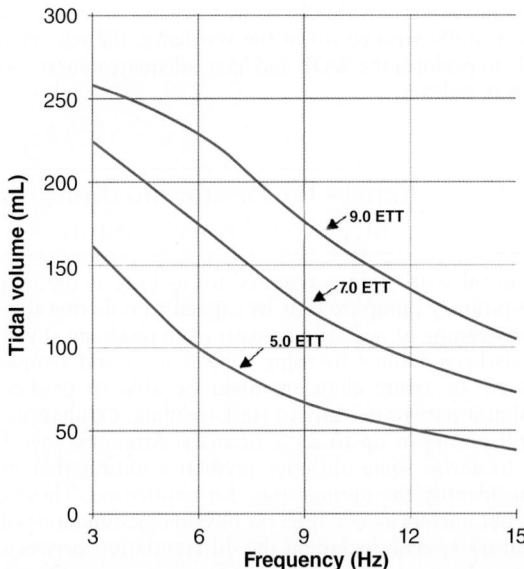

FIGURE 38.10. Tidal volumes (mL) and respiratory rate (Hz) during high-frequency oscillation ventilation with the Sensormedics 3100B (Viasys, Yorba Linda, CA). Increasing the rate leads to lower tidal volumes. Note the effect of the endotracheal tube size on tidal volumes. ETT, endotracheal tube. (From the Sensormedics 3100B user manual, with permission.)

WEANING FROM MECHANICAL VENTILATORY SUPPORT

Weaning of mechanical ventilatory support has traditionally been a mix of science and art. Although a relative consensus exists as to when mechanical ventilation should be initiated in the presence of respiratory insufficiency, the management of pediatric patients during recovery from respiratory failure remains largely subjective and is predominately determined by institutional or individual practices or preferences.

The median age of pediatric patients who receive mechanical ventilatory support is 1 year (61,62). The percentage of pediatric patients on mechanical ventilation for >12 hours was 35% in one study (61), while only 17% required ventilation for >24 hours in another report (62). The median duration of mechanical ventilation in these studies was 6–7 days. Of the patients who required mechanical ventilation, pneumonia (15%) and neurologic problems (14%) were reported as the underlying reason for initiation of mechanical ventilation.

As discussed earlier, mechanical ventilation in children can be subdivided into three phases: acute, maintenance, and weaning phases. The acute phase of mechanical ventilatory support includes primary lung recruitment. Once the lung is recruited and the patient's ventilatory support is decreased to levels that do not expose the patient to detrimental levels of inspired O_2 and distending volume ($F_{IO_2} \leq 0.6$; VT, 4–6 mL/kg; peak inspiratory pressure < 35 cm H_2O), the patient goes into the maintenance phase. The maintenance phase refers to that period spent waiting for improvement in the disease process that led to the need for intubation. Usually, only F_{IO_2} and PEEP are actively adjusted during this period. The patient moves from the maintenance phase to the weaning phase when the patient sends a signal (e.g., triggering the ventilator with spontaneous breathing efforts) to the clinician that weaning will be tolerated. Once weaning begins, the clinician must identify when the patient will tolerate removal of the ETT. The following discussion will review how weaning principles are applied to children.

The physiology of the WOB was discussed previously. To be successfully weaned off of the ventilator, the patient must be able to perform the WOB and have adequate neural control of airway reflexes.

Predictive Indices for Discontinuation from Mechanical Ventilatory Support

Mechanical ventilation is required for as long as the load on the respiratory pump exceeds its capacity. Predicting the success of weaning of pediatric patients from mechanical ventilation has been defined by using clinical signs and symptoms. Although an astute clinician might be able to predict the time that a patient is ready to start weaning, extubation failure still occurs in up to 24% of cases. Attempts have been made to devise some objective predictive indices that might help to identify the optimal time for extubation. These indices or parameters assess different physiologic functions of the respiratory system, including the differentiation between the elastic and resistive components of pulmonary dysfunction; defining alteration or limitation in inspiratory/expiratory airflow; determining the magnitude of driving pressure, work, and effort to maintain VT; and defining sequential changes to monitor the progression and resolution of the underlying disease process.

It is also likely that individual pulmonary mechanics or function-testing criteria per se might not have the same discriminatory power as composite parameters due to the multiple factors that influence successful withdrawal of mechanical ventilation. For this reason, it has been proposed that integrated indices that are a composite of two or more measurements may be more predictive of success. However, despite the inclusion of a variety of respiratory functions with good predictive value in adults, these integrated indices do not seem to be reliable predictors of success or failure in infants and children (63,64).

Clinical Trials of Weaning

A limited number of clinical trials of weaning from mechanical ventilation have been conducted in children. In adult patients, numerous studies, such as spontaneous breathing trials and respiratory therapist-driven protocols, have demonstrated the advantage of weaning strategies.

One trial studied 257 consecutive infants and children who received mechanical ventilation for at least 48 hours and were deemed ready to undergo a breathing trial by their primary physician (65). Patients were randomly assigned to undergo a trial of breathing with either PS of 10 cm H_2O or a T piece. Bedside measurements of respiratory function were obtained immediately before discontinuation of mechanical ventilation and within the first 5 minutes of breathing through a T piece. The decision to extubate a patient at the end of the breathing trial was made by the primary clinician, who was unaware of the results of respiratory function measurements. Of 125 patients in the pressure-support group, 99 (79.2%) completed the breathing trial and were extubated, and 15.1% required reintubation within 48 hours. Of the 132 patients in the T-piece group, 102 (77.5%) completed the breathing trial and were extubated, with 13 of them (12.7%) requiring reintubation within 48 hours. The percentage of patients who remained extubated for 48 hours after the breathing trial did not differ between groups (67.2% PS vs. 67.4% T piece, $p = 0.97$).

Process of Weaning

Weaning is a dynamic process that usually begins during patient recovery at some undefined point that is determined by the bedside physician. This subjective bias inevitably decreases the reproducibility of any study and makes results difficult to extrapolate to clinical practice. Standard indices for assessing patient weaning ability include (a) resolution of the etiology of respiratory failure and stable respiratory status; (b) decreased FIO_2 (usually to <50%) and decreased PEEP to 5 cm H_2O; (c) respiratory rate to <60 for infants <12 months of age, to <40 for preschool and school-aged children, and to <30 for adolescents; (d) no acidosis (pH < 7.35) or hypercapnia (PCO_2 > 60 torr). Other parameters that indirectly assess oxygenation and compliance include a P:F ratio of >267 (PaO_2 > 80 torr on FIO_2 of 0.3), SpO_2 >94% on FIO_2 ≤0.5, peak inspiratory pressure <20 cm H_2O, PEEP ≤5 cm H_2O, combined with adequate respiratory muscle function, and hemodynamic stability without evidence of shock. These criteria include good perfusion (e.g., capillary refill < 3 seconds), age-appropriate blood pressure (above –2 SD cutoff for age), and good cardiac function (e.g., no requirement of infusions of vasoactive and/or inotropic medications, with the exception of dopamine ≤5 μg/kg/min). Patients must be easily arousable to verbal or physical stimulation (e.g., pediatric Glasgow Coma Scale score of ≥11) and must be capable of moving an uninjured upper and lower extremity against gravity. Patients must also have acceptable serum potassium, magnesium, and phosphorous concentrations.

The individual who makes the decision to wean the patient may also have an impact on the length of mechanical ventilation. Decision making by respiratory care practitioners (RCPs) has long been felt to have the potential to reduce the length of mechanical ventilation because the respiratory therapist is more available to be at the bedside and perform frequent patient assessments. Respiratory therapist-driven weaning protocols are being examined as an alternative to current standard practices of weaning, which are physician-driven (35,66). RCPs classically perform diagnostic functions, such as blood gases, pulse oximetry, end-tidal CO_2 measurements, and airway function screenings; they also have the expertise to interpret these data. In a controlled trial of 300 adult patients who were randomized to daily screening and spontaneous breathing trials by RCPs, the intervention group had a 25% reduction in the median number of days of mechanical ventilation (66). A study of 223 pediatric patients demonstrated a decrease in total length of ventilation, weaning time, and time to extubation in patients weaned by an RCP-driven protocol versus physician-directed weaning (67).

Adjuncts to Weaning

Pharmacologic Agents

Routine administration of corticosteroids is a frequent adjunct for extubation. The anti-inflammatory effects of steroids form the basis of this approach. Two well-designed trials of dexamethasone therapy prior to extubation in children have unequivocally demonstrated that steroids reduce postextubation stridor (68,69). The inferences from these trials are strengthened because they were truly blinded studies. In contrast to the demonstrated effect on stridor, the effect of corticosteroids on reintubation is unclear. In one of the two studies, 7 of 32 patients who did not receive steroids required reintubation in contrast to 0 of 31 patients who received steroids. The trend in the second study was in the opposite direction, with 4 of 77 children who did not receive steroids and 9 of 76 who did receive steroids requiring reintubation. It is unclear why these studies demonstrated opposite results. Thus, while dexamethasone therapy may reduce stridor, no definitive evidence suggests that it reduces reintubation. Both of these trials found reintubation rates of >10% (68,69).

Heliox

After endotracheal extubation, upper and total airway resistances may frequently be increased, resulting in high inspiratory effort to breathe. A few patients, ranging from 5% to 16%, develop postextubation airway obstruction and frank respiratory distress (68). In addition, a substantial number of patients develop inspiratory distress after extubation, leading to reintubation (70,71). In these patients, an increase in upper airway and total inspiratory resistance may contribute to this respiratory distress. As discussed earlier, infants and children have both anatomic and physiologic differences from adults that predispose them to airway edema and dysfunction.

Helium-oxygen (HeO$_2$) mixture (heliox) has a low density and a high kinematic viscosity, allowing for a reduction in airway resistance. Some studies showed that it could have beneficial effects in the treatment of upper-airway obstruction (72). The use of HeO$_2$ mixture in adults (73) and in children (74) with upper-airway obstruction has been reported in several anecdotal series and a few studies, and it has become one of the more accepted indications for HeO$_2$ use (72). Although the effects of heliox have been shown predominantly by observational studies, the fact that the immediate improvement obtained with HeO$_2$ breathing was reversed when it was discontinued even briefly suggested an independent beneficial effect of the gas related to its physical properties.

Multiple studies have examined heliox delivery with commercially available ventilators and found that delivered VT was different from set VT in almost all ventilators tested (9,75–78). However, one ventilator, the Carefusion AVea (Carefusion Corp, San Diego, CA), has an internal blending system that allows for heliox delivery. The ventilator is different from other commercially available ventilators because it identifies and compensates for the low-density gas mixture of O$_2$ and helium, theoretically enhancing stability in delivered and monitored parameters. Recently, Clement et al demonstrated in utilizing the Carefusion with heliox that VT continued to be inaccurate (79). Clinicians should be vigilant in monitoring delivered VT using a commercially available ventilator equipped with an internal heliox blending system. Accuracy of delivered VT can vary greatly with the use of heliox in all available systems.

Noninvasive Mechanical Ventilatory Support

The process of discontinuing mechanical ventilation must balance the risk of complications due to unnecessary delays in extubation with the risk of complications due to premature discontinuation and the need for reintubation. The use of noninvasive positive-pressure ventilation is a promising therapy after failure of extubation but has not yet been shown to reduce the need for reintubation or reduce post-intubation mortality (80). In principle, as most pediatric patients require reintubation due to poor or excessive effort (81), noninvasive support may allow the patient to bridge to extubation.

Noninvasive ventilation (NIV) has well-established benefits in adult populations with COPD, neuromuscular diseases, obstructive sleep apnea, and immune deficiency. In pediatrics, NIV is less well studied beyond the use for chronic support in patients with neuromuscular disease. However, there are some small studies that support the use of NIV for acute respiratory failure even in a heterogeneous population of the pediatric intensive care unit. The advantages of NIV over invasive ventilation are the ability to maintain speech, cough, and gag reflexes, flexibility in the suspension of the therapy, lower sedation requirements especially among older children, avoidance of laryngeal damage/tracheal stenosis, and lower secondary pneumonia rates. Complications of NIV include skin breakdown, gastric distention, and interface discomfort. While NIV should not be considered in pending respiratory arrest or shock, other patients with acute or acute on chronic respiratory failure may benefit from a trial of NIV, especially those in whom intubation has high complication rates such as asthma or immunocompromised patients. Patient selection is difficult as studies that have tried to identify patients that will succeed with NIV have had mixed results. Bernet et al. prospectively followed 42 patients treated with NIV. Responders and nonresponders in their study did not differ in disease, Pediatric Index of Mortality 2 score, RR (respiratory rate), heart rate, Pco$_2$, pH, or secretions at baseline. However, responders did have a significantly lower RR and F$_{IO2}$ at 1 hour of NIV treatment. Thus, predicting NIV success is difficult and patient selection remains a process of careful institution, and not one selection variable. Thoughtful preparation and team skill are required prior to instituting NIV. Placement of an NG to avoid gastric distention and application of skin protectant barriers should be considered prior to initiation. A well-fitted interface is key to the success of NIV; whether that can be accomplished with a nasal or full face mask depends on the patient facial structure, tendency to mouth breath, and patient size. Ganu and colleges recently published results of their NIV experience in infants with bronchiolitis. They found an increase in NIV trial rates over a 10-year period, suggesting that team experience with this technology improves success. Although these patients were small (mean age 4.8 months), they trialed NIV in 285 of 399 infants with bronchiolitise, of which 237 (82%) had successful NIV trials and avoided invasive ventilation. They found an average length of stay of the NIV patients to be 2.38 days compared to 5.19 days for invasively ventilated infants (p < 0.001). Of those that failed NIV they were intubated 20% longer than the patients that received invasive ventilation from the beginning. Other studies have shown higher NIV failure rates. Dohna-Schwake et al. demonstrated 28% failure rate among a heterogeneous population of PICU patients with various diagnoses and 29% failure rate in a randomized controlled trial in patients with only pulmonary diseases (asthma, bronchiolitis, pneumonia). While NIV has been less studied in children, it is a viable option for some patients and should be considered by clinicians.

While NIV is a valuable technique for ventilatory support in pediatric patients, it has limitations that can cause it to fail. For noninvasive ventilatory support to function properly, the mask or nasal prongs must adequately seal to the patient. The varying physical sizes and the lack of tolerance of masks, or even prongs, can limit the utility of NIV in children. The variety of devices that are available for noninvasive support seems to be addressing some of these issues. Success with noninvasive techniques has been reported to avoid the need for tracheal intubation in some groups, such as immunosuppressed patients with asthma or respiratory insufficiency. However, no study to date has proven that NIV is superior to tracheal intubation and conventional mechanical ventilation. Some clinicians assert that the use of NIV in acute respiratory failure merely prolongs the time to tracheal intubation and thus may be of little benefit; these claims have also not been demonstrated. One form of NIV that seems to be increasing in popularity is the use of high-flow nasal cannula therapy. In studies of premature infants, use of support devices, such as Vapotherm, has shown equivalent changes in WOB and lower-airway pressure measurements as those provided by continuous positive-pressure ventilation using nasal prongs.

Recognition of Weaning Failure

Failure of weaning can be categorized by increased respiratory load or decreased respiratory capacity. Increased respiratory load is represented by increased elastic load (unresolved lung disease, secondary pneumonia, abdominal distension, and hyperinflated lungs), increased resistive load (thickened airway secretions, partially occluded ETT, upper-airway obstruction), or increased minute ventilation (pain and irritability, sepsis/hyperthermia, metabolic acidosis). Decreased respiratory capacity is represented by decreased respiratory drive (sedation, central nervous system infection, traumatic brain injury, hypocapnia/alkalosis), muscular dysfunction [muscular catabolism and weakness (malnutrition), severe electrolyte disturbances], and neuromuscular disorder (diaphragmatic dysfunction, prolonged neuromuscular blockade, cervical spinal injury).

Extubation failure with subsequent reintubation in pediatric patients ranges between 14% and 24% (18,43,66,70). It should be noted that it is not reasonable to expect the extubation failure rate to be 0% because this would represent that some patients could have been extubated earlier. In a study of 632 pediatric patients, the failure rate of planned extubation was 4.9%. This rate appears to be reasonable considering the above discussion. The rate of failure increased with the length of time patients received mechanical ventilation, with patients ventilated for >24 hours having a failure rate of 6.0% and those ventilated for >48 hours having a failure rate of 7.9% (82). Predicting extubation outcome in patients is usually based upon clinical judgment. However, attempts have been made to identify specific predictors of extubation failure. The success of these predictors has been mixed. Investigators adapted adult integrated indices to pediatric patients by normalizing the VT and dynamic compliance to body weight (31). Extubation failure was defined as reintubation within 24 hours and the failure rate was found to be 19%.

A study of 208 pediatric patients who were ventilated for at least 24 hours identified criteria for low risk (<10%) and high risk (25%) of extubation failure on the basis of direct measurements of pulmonary function (64). For this study, the rate of patients who required reintubation within 48 hours (excluding those who failed secondary to upper-airway obstruction) was 16.3%. Thirty-four of the 208 patients studied were reintubated, for an overall failure rate of 16.3%. Of the patients who failed extubation, 65% required reintubation secondary to poor or excessive effort. Extubation failure increased significantly with decreasing VT indexed to body weight of a spontaneous breath, increasing F_{IO_2}, increasing MAP, increasing oxygenation index, increasing fraction of total minute ventilation provided by the ventilator, increasing peak ventilatory inspiratory pressure, or decreasing mean inspiratory flow.

Advances in Weaning

To wean patients optimally and ensure patient comfort, ventilator adjustments must be made moment to moment in response to the patient's immediate physiologic needs. It is, of course, unrealistic for any member of the medical, nursing, or respiratory care staffs to perform in this manner. In response to this need for improved patient–ventilator interactions, some researchers have experimented (with promising results) with an interactive, computer-directed, closed-loop weaning system (83,84,85).

Weaning from mechanical ventilation remains a complex and poorly standardized area of respiratory care. Technical advancements in integration of patient effort and mechanical response have great potential to revolutionize this field to the benefit of patients.

CONCLUSIONS AND FUTURE DIRECTIONS

Mechanical ventilation can be considered as it relates to the issues of (a) equipment utilized to support the patient, (b) our understanding of what reduces potential iatrogenic lung injury and maintenance of the patients' normal physiology, and (c) how best to make decisions concerning the initiation, level of support, and removal of mechanical ventilatory support. The equipment used for mechanical ventilation continues to evolve, including new modes and interfaces between the patient and the ventilator. Traditionally, the site of the signal from the patient to the ventilator has been at either the patient's airway or at the ventilator. New technology is being evaluated that would allow the signal to be acquired as it moves from the patient's brain to the diaphragm. This technique will allow for a quantification of the patient's respiratory effort and thus regulate the level of support delivered by the ventilator to the patient's effort.

Further research is required to better understand the complex issues concerning how the lung is injured during positive-pressure mechanical ventilation. We have finally begun to understand what injures the lung, but it is still not clear how best to apply this knowledge to ventilation of critically ill patients to help prevent ongoing injury. The development of databases and collaborative groups such as the ARDSnet, the Pediatric Acute Lung Injury and Sepsis Investigators network, and the Pediatric Critical Care Research Network has great potential to enlist large groups of patients toward answering these many questions. Technically improved monitoring devices to study lung mechanics and the effects of treatment are also becoming available. Reliability and acceptance of research efforts will have an important impact on the use of mechanical ventilation in the future. Efforts at reducing or eliminating secondary lung damage from infection and other inciting causes may also change the landscape of the types of patients who require mechanical ventilation.

Before weaning from the ventilator can become more of a science and less of an art, more knowledge is required to define the optimal method of separating the patient from mechanical ventilation once their disease process improves.

References

1. Dreyfuss D, Saumon G. Barotrauma is volutrauma, but which volume is the one responsible? *Intensive Care Med* 1992;18:139–41.
2. Heulitt MJ, Anders M, Benham D. Acute respiratory distress syndrome in pediatric patients: Redirecting therapy to reduce iatrogenic lung injury. *Respir Care* 1995;40:74–85.
3. Heulitt MJ, Bohn D. Lung-protective strategy in pediatric patients with acute respiratory distress syndrome. *Respir Care* 1998;43:952–60.
4. Heulitt MJ, Holt SJ, Thurman TL, et al. Reliability of measured tidal volume in mechanically ventilated young pigs with normal lungs. *Intensive Care Med* 2005;31:1255–61.
5. Figueras J, Rodriguez-Miguelez JM, Botet F, et al. Changes in $TcPCO_2$ regarding pulmonary mechanics due to pneumotachometer dead space in ventilated newborns. *J Perinat Med* 1997;25:333–9.
6. Cannon ML, Cornell J, Tripp-Hamel DS, et al. Tidal volumes for ventilated infants should be determined with a

pneumotachometer placed at the endotracheal tube. *Am J Respir Crit Care Med* 2000;162:2109–12.

7. Neve V, Leclerc F, Noizet O, et al. Influence of respiratory system impedance on volume and pressure delivered at the Y piece in ventilated infants. *Pediatr Crit Care Med* 2003;4:418–25.

8. Brown MK, Willms DC. A laboratory evaluation of 2 mechanical ventilators in the presence of helium-oxygen mixtures. *Respir Care Med* 1999;160(1):354–60.

9. Ganu SS, Gautam A, Wilkins B, et al. Increase in use of non-invasive ventilation for infants with severe bronchiolitis is associated with decline in intubation rates over a decade. *Intensive Care Med* 2012;38(7):1177–83.

10. Alsaati BZ, Thurman TL, Holt S, et al. Reliability of measured tidal volume in mechanically ventilated pediatric patient in the PICU (abstract). *PAS* 2005;57:2421.

11. Chatburn RL. Classification of mechanical ventilators. *Respir Care* 1992;37:1009–25.

12. Sassoon CS. Mechanical ventilator design and function: The trigger variable. *Respir Care* 1992;37:1056–69.

13. Heulitt MJ, Torres A, Anders M, et al. Comparison of total resistive work of breathing in two generations of ventilators in an animal model. *Pediatr Pulmonol* 1996;22:58–66.

14. Allo JC, Beck JC, Brander L, et al. Influence of neurally adjusted ventilatory assist and positive end-expiratory pressure on breathing pattern in rabbits with acute lung injury. *Crit Care Med* 2006;34(12):2997–3004.

15. Otis AB, Fenn WO, Rahn H. Mechanics of breathing in man. *J Appl Physiol* 1950;2:592–607.

16. Beydon L, Chasse M, Harf A, et al. Inspiratory work of breathing during spontaneous ventilation using demand valves and continuous flow systems. *Am Rev Respir Dis* 1988;138:300–4.

17. Banner MJ, Downs JB, Kirby RR, et al. Effects of expiratory flow resistance on inspiratory work of breathing. *Chest* 1988;93:795–9.

18. Nishimura M, Hess D, Kacmarek RM. The response of flow-triggered infant ventilators. *Am J Respir Crit Care Med* 1995;152:1901–9.

19. Sanders RC, Jr., Thurman TL, Holt SJ, et al. Work of breathing associated with pressure support ventilation in two different ventilators. *Pediatr Pulmonol* 2001;32:62–70.

20. Carmack J, Torres A, Anders M, et al. Comparison of inspiratory work of breathing in young lambs during flow triggered and pressure triggered ventilation. *Respir Care* 1995;40:28–34.

21. Kondili E, Prinianakis G, Georgopoulos D. Patient-ventilator interaction. *Br J Anaesth* 2003;91:106–19.

22. Nilsestuen JO, Hargett KD. Using ventilator graphics to identify patient-ventilator asynchrony. *Respir Care* 2005;50:202–34; discussion, 32–4.

23. Chao DC, Scheinhorn DJ, Stearn-Hassenpflug M. Patient-ventilator trigger asynchrony in prolonged mechanical ventilation. *Chest* 1997;112:1592–9.

24. MacIntyre NR, Ho LI. Effects of initial flow rate and breath termination criteria on pressure support ventilation. *Chest* 1991;99:134–8.

25. Tokioka H, Tanaka T, Ishizu T, et al. The effect of breath termination criterion on breathing patterns and the work of breathing during pressure support ventilation. *Anesth Analg* 2001;92:161–5.

26. Heulitt MJ, Wankum P, Holt S, et al. Evaluation of the effects of an active exhalation valve and changing cycle offtime during pressure support ventilation in a neonatal animal model (abstract). *Pediatric Research* 2003;53:2711.

27. Lanteri CJ, Sly PD. Changes in respiratory mechanics with age. *J Appl Physiol* 1993;74:369–78.

28. Deoras KS, Wolfson MR, Bhutani VK, et al. Structural changes in the tracheae of preterm lambs induced by ventilation. *Pediatr Res* 1989;26:434–7.

29. Penn RB, Wolfson MR, Shaffer TH. Effect of ventilation on mechanical properties and pressure-flow relationships of immature airways. *Pediatr Res* 1988;23:519–24.

30. Wolfson MR, Bhutani VK, Shaffer TH, et al. Mechanics and energetics of breathing helium in infants with bronchopulmonary dysplasia. *J Pediatr* 1984;104:752–7.

31. Baumeister BL, el-Khatib M, Smith PG, et al. Evaluation of predictors of weaning from mechanical ventilation in pediatric patients. *Pediatr Pulmonol* 1997;24:344–52.

32. Hickling KG. Best compliance during a decremental, but not incremental, positive end-expiratory pressure trial is related to open-lung positive end-expiratory pressure: A mathematical model of acute respiratory distress syndrome lungs. *Am J Respir Crit Care Med* 2001;163:69–78.

33. Suter PM, Fairley B, Isenberg MD. Optimum end-expiratory airway pressure in patients with acute pulmonary failure. *NEJM* 1975;292:284–9.

34. Meade MO, Cook DJ, Guyatt GH, et al. Ventilation strategy using low tidal volumes, recruitment maneuvers, and high positive end-expiratory pressure for acute lung injury and acute respiratory distress syndrome: a randomized controlled trial. *JAMA* 2008;299:637–45.

35. Horst HM, Mouro D, Hall-Jenssens RA, et al. Decrease in ventilation time with a standardized weaning process. *Arch Surg* 1998;133:483–9.

36. Ranieri VM. Optimization of patient-ventilator interactions: Closed-loop technology to turn the century. *Intensive Care Med* 1997;23:936–9.

37. Holt SJ, Sanders RC, Thurman TL, et al. An evaluation of Automode, a computer-controlled ventilator mode, with the Siemens Servo 300A ventilator, using a porcine model. *Respir Care* 2001;46:26–36.

38. Guttmann J, Haberthur C, Mols G. Automatic tube compensation. *Respir Care Clin N Am* 2001;7:475–501, x.

39. Chu EK, Whitehead T, Slutsky AS. Effects of cyclic opening and closing at low- and high-volume ventilation on bronchoalveolar lavage cytokines. *Crit Care Med* 2004;32:168–74.

40. Hernandez LA, Peevy KJ, Moise AA, et al. Chest wall restriction limits high airway pressure-induced lung injury in young rabbits. *J Appl Physiol* 1989;66:2364–8.

41. Acute Respiratory Distress Syndrome Network. Ventilation with lower tidal volumes as compared with traditional tidal volumes for acute lung injury and the acute respiratory distress syndrome. *N Engl J Med* 2000;342:1301–8.

42. Pillow JJ. High-frequency oscillatory ventilation: Mechanisms of gas exchange and lung mechanics. *Crit Care Med* 2005;33:S135–41.

43. Engle WA, Yoder MC, Andreoli SP, et al. Controlled, prospective, randomized comparison of high-frequency jet ventilation and conventional ventilation in neonates with respiratory failure and persistent pulmonary hypertension. *J Perinatol* 1997;17:3–9.

44. Keszler M, Donn SM, Bucciarelli RL, et al. Multicenter controlled trial comparing high-frequency jet ventilation and conventional mechanical ventilation in newborn infants with pulmonary interstitial emphysema. *J Pediatr* 1991;119:85–93.

45. Arnold JH, Hanson JH, Toro-Figuero LO, et al. Prospective, randomized comparison of high-frequency oscillatory ventilation and conventional mechanical ventilation in pediatric respiratory failure. *Crit Care Med* 1994;22:1530–9.

46. Courtney SE, Durand DJ, Asselin JM, et al. High-frequency oscillatory ventilation versus conventional mechanical ventilation for very-low-birth-weight infants. *N Engl J Med* 2002;347:643–52.

47. Derdak S, Mehta S, Stewart TE, et al. High-frequency oscillatory ventilation for acute respiratory distress syndrome in adults: A randomized, controlled trial. *Am J Respir Crit Care Med* 2002;166:801–8.

48. Meyer M, Hahn G, Buess C, et al. Pulmonary gas exchange in panting dogs. *J Appl Physiol* 1989;66:1258–63.

49. Taylor GI. The dispersion of soluble matter in solvent flowing slowly through a tube. *Proc R Soc* 1953;223:446–68.

50. Chang HK. Mechanisms of gas transport during ventilation by high-frequency oscillation. *J Appl Physiol* 1984;56:553–63.

51. Armengol J, Jones RL, King EG. Collateral ventilation during high-frequency oscillation in dogs. *J Appl Physiol* 1985;58:173–9.

52. Maggiore SM, Jonson B, Richard JC, et al. Alveolar derecruitment at decremental positive end-expiratory pressure levels in acute lung injury: Comparison with the lower inflection point, oxygenation, and compliance. *Am J Respir Crit Care Med* 2001;164:795–801.

53. Ranieri VM, Eissa NT, Corbeil C, et al. Effects of positive end-expiratory pressure on alveolar recruitment and gas exchange in patients with the adult respiratory distress syndrome. *Am Rev Respir Dis* 1991;144:544–51.

54. Brazelton TB III, Watson KF, Murphy M, et al. Identification of optimal lung volume during high-frequency oscillatory ventilation using respiratory inductive plethysmography. *Crit Care Med* 2001;29:2349–59.

55. Gerstmann DR, Fouke JM, Winter DC, et al. Proximal, tracheal, and alveolar pressures during high-frequency oscillatory ventilation in a normal rabbit model. *Pediatr Res* 1990;28:367–73.

56. Allen JL, Frantz ID III, Fredberg JJ. Heterogeneity of mean alveolar pressure during high-frequency oscillations. *J Appl Physiol* 1987;62:223–8.

57. Allen JL, Fredberg JJ, Keefe DH, et al. Alveolar pressure magnitude and asynchrony during high-frequency oscillations of excised rabbit lungs. *Am Rev Respir Dis* 1985;132:343–9.

58. Berkenbosch JW, Grueber RE, Dabbagh O, et al. Effect of helium-oxygen (heliox) gas mixtures on the function of four pediatric ventilators. *Crit Care Med* 2003;31(7):2052–8.

59. Fletcher PR, Epstein RA. Constancy of physiological dead space during high-frequency ventilation. *Respir Physiol* 1982;47:39–49.

60. Van de Kieft M, Dorsey D, Morison D, et al. High-frequency oscillatory ventilation: Lessons learned from mechanical test lung models. *Crit Care Med* 2005;33:S142–7.

61. Farias JA, Frutos F, Esteban A, et al. What is the daily practice of mechanical ventilation in pediatric intensive care units? For the international group of mechanical ventilation in children. *Intensive Care Med* 2004;30:918–25.

62. Randolph AG, Meert KL, O'Neil ME, et al. Pediatric Acute Lung Injury and Sepsis Investigators Network. The feasibility of conducting clinical trials in infants and children with acute respiratory failure. *Am J Respir Crit Care Med* 2003;167:1334–40.

63. El-Khatib M, Jamaleddine G, Soubra R, et al. Pattern of spontaneous breathing: Potential marker for weaning outcome. Spontaneous breathing pattern and weaning from mechanical ventilation. *Intensive Care Med* 2001;27(1):52–8.

64. Khan N, Brown A, Venkataraman ST. Predictors of extubation success and failure in mechanically ventilated infants and children. *Crit Care Med* 1996;24(9):1568–79.

65. Farias JA, Retta A, Alía I, et al. A comparison of two methods to perform a breathing trial before extubation in pediatric intensive care patients. *Intensive Care Med* 2001;27(10):1649–54.

66. Ely EW, Baker AM, Dunagan DP, et al. Effects on the duration of mechanical ventilation of identifying patients capable of breathing spontaneously. *N Engl J Med* 1996;335(25):1864–9.

67. Schultz TR, Lin RJ, Watzman M, et al. Weaning children from mechanical ventilation: A prospective randomized trial of protocol directed versus physician directed weaning. *Respiratory Care* 2001;46(8):772–82.

68. Anene O, Meert KL, Uy H, et al. Dexamethasone for the prevention of postextubation airway obstruction: A prospective, randomized, double-blind, placebo-controlled trial. *Crit Care Med* 1996;24:1666–9.

69. Tellez DW, Galvis AG, Storgion SA, et al. Dexamethasone in the prevention of postextubation stridor in children. *J Pediatr* 1991;118:289–94.

70. Epstein SK, Ciubotaru RL, Wong JB. Effect of failed extubation on the outcome of mechanical ventilation. *Chest* 1997;112:186–92.

71. Epstein SK, Ciubotaru RL. Independent effects of etiology of failure and time to reintubation on outcome for patients failing extubation. *Am J Respir Crit Care Med* 1998;158:489–93.

72. Manthous CA, Morgan S, Pohlman A, et al. Heliox in the treatment of airflow obstruction: A critical review of the literature. *Respir Care* 1997;42:1034–42.

73. Barach A. The use of helium in the treatment of asthma and obstructive lesions in the larynx and trachea. *Ann Intern Med* 1935;9:739–65.

74. Duncan P. Efficacy of helium-oxygen mixtures in the management of severe viral and post-intubation croup. *Can Anaesth Soc J* 1979;26:206–12.

75. Benet V, Hug MI, Frey B. Predictive factors for the success of noninvasive mask ventilation in infants and children with acute respiratory failure. *Pediatr Crit Care Med* 2005;6:660–4.

76. Dohna-Schwake C, Stehling F, Tschiedel E, et al. Non-invasive ventilation on a pediatric intensive care unit: Feasibility, efficacy, and predictors of success. *Pediatr Pulmonol* 2011;46(11):1114–20.

77. Nava S, Navalesi P, Conti G. Time of non-invasive ventilation. *Intensive Care Med* 2006; 32:361–370.

78. Yanez LJ, Yunge M, Emilfork M, et al. A prospective, randomized, controlled trial of noninvasive ventilation in pediatric acute respiratory failure. *Pediatr Crit Care Med* 2008;9:484–9, 1182.

79. Clement KC, Thurman TL, Holt SJ, et al. Validation of volume delivery with the use of helix in mechanical ventilation. *J Pediatr Intensive Care* 2013;2(1):39–44.

80. Esteban A, Frutos-Vivar F, Ferguson ND, et al. Noninvasive positive-pressure ventilation for respiratory failure after extubation. *New Engl J Med* 2004;350(24):2452–60.

81. Randolph AG, Wypij D, Venkataraman ST, et al. Pediatric Acute Lung Injury and Sepsis Investigators (PALISI) Network. Effect of mechanical ventilator weaning protocols on respiratory outcomes in infants and children: A randomized controlled trial. *JAMA* 2002;288(20):2561–8.

82. Edmunds S, Weiss I, Harrison R. Extubation failure in a large pediatric ICU population. *Chest* 2001;119(3):897–900.

83. Strickland JH Jr, Hasson JH. A computer-controlled ventilator weaning system. *Chest* 1991;100:1096–9.

84. Strickland JH Jr, Hasson JH. A computer-controlled ventilator weaning system. A clinical trial. *Chest* 1993;103:1220–6.

85. Tong DA. Weaning patients from mechanical ventilation. A knowledge-based system approach. *Comput Methods Programs Biomed* 1991;35(4):267–78.

86. Boynton BR, Hammond MD, Fredberg JJ, et al. Gas exchange in healthy rabbits during high-frequency oscillatory ventilation. *J Appl Physiol* 1989;66:1343–51.

87. Castle RA, Dunne CJ, Mok Q, et al. Accuracy of displayed values of tidal volume in the pediatric intensive care unit. *Crit Care Med* 2002;30:2566–74.

88. Farias JA, Alia I, Retta A, et al. An evaluation of extubation failure predictors in mechanically ventilated infants and children. *Intensive Care Med* 2002;28(6):752–7.

89. Kamitsuka MD, Boynton BR, Villanueva D, et al. Frequency, tidal volume, and mean airway pressure combinations that provide adequate gas exchange and low alveolar pressure during high frequency oscillatory ventilation in rabbits. *Pediatr Res* 1990;27:64–9.

90. Leung P, Jubran A, Tobin MJ. Comparison of assisted ventilator modes on triggering, patient effort, and dyspnea. *Am J Respir Crit Care Med* 1997;155:1940–8.

91. Tassaux D, Joillet P, Thouret JM, et al. Calibration of seven ICU ventilators for mechanical ventilation with helium-oxygen mixtures. *Am J Respir Crit Care Med* 1999;160(1):22–32.

CHAPTER 39 ■ INHALED GASES AND NONINVASIVE VENTILATION

ANGELA T. WRATNEY, DONNA S. HAMEL, IRA M. CHEIFETZ, AND DAVID G. NICHOLS

KEY POINTS

Oxygen

1. There is no optimal target for oxygen saturation in the critically ill patient.
2. FIO_2 delivery varies depending upon the flow and entrainment of room air due to patient effort and/or system leaks.
3. Oxygen-mediated pulmonary toxicity is pathologically similar to acute respiratory distress syndrome (ARDS).

Nitric Oxide

4. Inhaled nitric oxide (iNO) is a selective pulmonary vasodilator.
5. Systemic uptake of iNO is limited by scavenging mechanisms that involve nitrosylation of plasma proteins, oxyhemoglobin, and heme iron.
6. Clinical application of iNO in hypoxemic respiratory failure due to ARDS has not improved clinical outcomes.
7. Rebound pulmonary hypertension or hypoxemia may occur during weaning or discontinuation of iNO.

Helium–Oxygen Mixtures

8. Heliox has a lower density than oxygen and therefore reduces work of breathing.
9. Work of breathing is improved due to increased laminar flow characteristics.
10. Stridor following viral croup or postextubation is usually relieved rapidly by heliox.

Bronchodilator Therapy

11. Nebulizers, metered-dose inhalers (MDIs), and dry-powder inhalers provide equally effective bronchodilation.
12. Systemic uptake, nonselective receptor binding, or dose- and bronchodilator-dependent patient variation may lead to unwanted side effects.
13. Small children will require a spacer during MDI use to ensure adequate delivery.

Inhalational Anesthetics

14. Inhaled general anesthesia in the PICU is used primarily to treat acute asthma that is refractory to all other therapies.
15. Use in settings outside of the operating room requires appropriate equipment, trained and licensed personnel, and specific scavenging and monitoring systems.
16. Prolonged isoflurane exposure can lead to fluoride ion nephrotoxicity.
17. Reversible neurologic changes can be unmasked when weaning or discontinuation after prolonged exposure.

Noninvasive Ventilation

18. Noninvasive positive-pressure ventilation and high-flow nasal cannula are the principal modes of noninvasive ventilation (NIV) support.
19. NIV supports spontaneous patient efforts to improve gas exchange, alveolar recruitment, and decrease work of breathing.
20. Patients receiving NIV support require frequent careful assessment to detect potential respiratory deterioration that might require intubation and invasive mechanical ventilation.

The provision of inhaled gases and the use of noninvasive respiratory support provide therapeutic resources fundamental to the management of critical care illness. The clinical and pathophysiologic processes associated with respiratory failure are directly targeted by medical gases used in the PICU (see also Chapters 46–50). Therefore, critical care personnel must be familiar with the following inhaled medical gases and medications: (a) oxygen (O_2), (b) inhaled nitric oxide (iNO), (c) helium–oxygen mixtures (heliox), (d) inhaled bronchodilators, and (e) inhalational anesthetics. In addition, noninvasive ventilation (NIV) offers a valuable alternative to intubation and mechanical ventilation for many critically ill patients. This chapter includes a discussion of the pharmacologic and therapeutic mechanisms of inhaled gases, the appropriate delivery system technology, and important safety considerations for each of these therapies used in the PICU.

HUMIDIFICATION

Humidification is an extremely important component of inhaled gas administration in the pediatric population. The nasal passages and upper airway warm, humidify, and filter air for the respiratory system. Thus, in the provision of inhaled gas therapies that bypass the upper airway or are administered with high pressure or flow, careful attention to temperature control, humidification, and infection control is warranted. Failure to do so may result in hypothermia, inspissated secretions, and airway injury and potentially contribute to the development of ventilator-associated pneumonia (1).

OXYGEN

The fraction of inspired oxygen (FIO_2) in ambient air is 0.21, which is commonly expressed as a percentage (21%). For medical use, 100% oxygen is mass produced from fractional distillation of atmospheric air. O_2 is provided to patients with impaired respiratory function to improve arterial O_2 saturation, to vasodilate the pulmonary capillary bed, and to enhance systemic oxygen delivery.

Energy Metabolism

O_2 is essential for cellular aerobic metabolism. Oxidative phosphorylation of NADH within the mitochondria generates 36 moles of ATP for every mole of glucose consumed. Under anaerobic conditions, glycolysis rapidly produces lactic acid as well as only 2 moles of ATP per mole of glucose. The resultant intracellular acidosis ultimately inhibits the enzymes involved in glycolysis.

Physiologic Mechanisms

Supplemental O_2 is administered to the hypoxemic patient to increase alveolar O_2 tension, which in turn raises arterial O_2 tension and saturation, thereby enhancing systemic O_2 delivery to the tissues. Arterial O_2 tension may fail to rise despite supplemental O_2 for the following reasons:

- Hypoventilation (e.g., oversedation).
- Decreased ventilation–perfusion ($\dot{V}/\dot{Q}$) matching in the lung (e.g., pneumonia, atelectasis). Low mixed venous O_2 saturation magnifies hypoxemia from decreased $\dot{V}/\dot{Q}$ ratios. The mixed venous O_2 saturation is reduced when systemic O_2 demand exceeds O_2 supply (e.g., shock, anemia).
- Anatomic right-to-left shunt (e.g., cyanotic congenital heart disease).

See Chapter 43 on Respiratory Physiology for more detail on these concepts.

Oxygen Delivery Systems

Depending on the desired FIO_2, a variety of devices exist for administering supplemental O_2 (Table 39.1). The flow provided by the O_2 delivery system will be either sufficient to meet the inspiratory flow demand of the patient (high-flow systems) or insufficient (low-flow systems), causing the patient to entrain additional room air flow. High-flow delivery systems provide a more stable, measurable delivery of the set FIO_2, independent of patient respiratory effort. High-flow delivery devices can be used with face masks with a reservoir (non-rebreather or partial rebreather), tracheostomy collars, nebulizers, O_2 hoods, and specialized high-flow nasal cannula (HFNC) systems. Low-flow systems include nasal cannulae or simple face masks (without reservoirs).

Nasal Cannulae

The nasal cannulae provide a comfortable, lightweight, and inexpensive method for low-flow O_2 delivery (0.1–6 L/min). FIO_2 delivery ranges between 24% and 50%. Although highly variable in practice, a general "rule of thumb" states that for each liter of supplemental O_2 flow, the inspired O_2 concentration increases by ~4% (2, 3). Rapid respiratory rates, higher tidal volumes, and shorter inspiratory times cause increased air dilution and reduce the actual inspired FIO_2. Two caveats bear mentioning for use of nasal cannulae in the infant: (a) when administering low flow (e.g., flow <1 L), the actual flow and FIO_2 provided may be highly inaccurate because of the frequent occurrence of system leaks, displaced nasal prongs, and the limitations in flow meter calibration; and (b) when administering higher flow (e.g., >2 L), the infant may receive significant positive end-expiratory pressure (PEEP) with the attendant risks of barotrauma (3, 4). Heating and humidification of the nasal cannula O_2 flow are *mandatory* with higher flow rates (>2 L/min) to prevent nasal drying, irritation, and heat loss.

Face Masks

Simple face masks fit over the patient's nose and mouth, providing an FIO_2 delivery of between 35% and 55% O_2. A *non-rebreathing face mask* consists of a simple face mask adapted with a reservoir bag and an inflow system for fresh gas infusion to increase FIO_2 delivery to close to 100% O_2. Two one-way valves, located between the mask and the reservoir and at one of the side exhalation ports, ensure that each inspiratory breath consists of fresh gas without entrainment of room air and that exhaled gas is eliminated into the environment rather than the reservoir bag. As a safety mechanism, the other side exhalation port is kept open to allow the entrainment of room air in the event that gas flow to the mask system is interrupted. Similarly, a *partial rebreathing mask* consists of a mask with an attached reservoir bag and an inflow gas source. However, the system lacks the unidirectional valve between the face mask and the reservoir. Thus, it allows the mixing of the exhaled CO_2 gas from the patient with the O_2 in the reservoir bag. To avoid rebreathing exhaled CO_2, the inspired gas flow rate should be maintained at or above 6 L/min.

Venturi masks are high-flow systems that provide fixed concentrations of 24%, 28%, 31%, 35%, 40%, or

TABLE 39.1

FRACTION OF INSPIRED OXYGEN PROVIDED BY VARIOUS DELIVERY SYSTEMS

	■ FIO_2 DELIVERY (%)	■ FLOW REQUIRED (L)
Nasal cannula	24–50	<6
Face mask	<60	6–10
Venturi mask	<60	Variable
Partial rebreather	<60	15
Non-rebreather	~100	15

TABLE 39.2

REACTIVE OXYGEN SPECIES AND THE ENDOGENOUS ANTIOXIDANT DEFENSE SYSTEMS

■ REACTIVE OXYGEN SPECIES	■ CHEMICAL SYMBOL	■ ANTIOXIDANT DEFENSE(S)
Superoxide anion	O_2^-	Superoxide dismutase
Hydrogen peroxide	H_2O_2	Glutathione peroxidase and catalase
Hydroxyl radical	$OH^\bullet$	Nonenzymatic mechanisms (e.g., vitamin C)

50% O_2. These concentrations are obtained by delivering manufacturer-recommended flow rates necessary to generate specific oxygen-to-air entrainment ratios. The flow velocity of O_2 entering the mask causes the entrainment of air through side ports in the device. Dependable O_2 concentrations are administered as long as total gas flow exceeds the patient's peak inspiratory flow rate.

Oxygen Hood and Tent

O_2 hoods and tents are transparent enclosures designed to surround the head or entire body of a small infant. Neither is commonly used today because they create access barriers to the infant, make observation of the infant more difficult, and may result in nonuniform (layered) O_2 distribution inside the enclosure (5). Hoods can provide 80%–90% FIO_2 with high flow of humidified O_2 (10–15 L/min), whereas tents typically achieve up to 50% FIO_2 with high O_2 flow.

Blow-by

"Blow-by" O_2 delivery involves wafting humidified O_2 at high flow rates through the corrugated tubing toward the face. This is especially useful for anxious toddlers who require <30% FIO_2 of fully humidified oxygen, because the caregiver can easily hold the child while directing the O_2 flow toward the child's face.

Risks

Oxygen Toxicity

The administration of O_2 is a universal practice in the PICU, but is not without risks. O_2-mediated pulmonary toxicity is pathologically very similar to acute respiratory distress syndrome (ARDS) (6). Clinically, the patient may complain of chest pain, cough, and tracheal inflammation. Physiologically, decreased pulmonary compliance and abnormal gas exchange result from impaired surfactant activity. Pathologically, inflammatory cell infiltrates contribute to proteolytic damage, loss of the alveolar–capillary membrane integrity, and pulmonary edema. Although an FIO_2 of 0.50 is commonly regarded as safe, the literature reports that toxicity may be seen with even brief periods of exposure to lower levels of O_2 (7). A safe level or duration of FIO_2 exposure has not been established. Therefore, clinicians should regularly review the indications for O_2 therapy for every patient.

The mechanism underlying oxygen toxicity involves the creation of reactive oxygen species (ROS), such as the superoxide anion (O_2^-), O_2 radical ($O_2^\bullet$), hydroxyl radical ($OH^\bullet$), and hydrogen peroxide (H_2O_2). ROS cause oxidative injury to proteins, DNA, and lipids. Organs rich in lipids and proteins, such as the pulmonary and central nervous system, are especially at risk. Endogenous antioxidant enzyme systems,

such as superoxide dismutase (SOD), glutathione peroxidase, and catalase, attempt to clear ROS to limit cellular injury (Table 39.2). SOD converts superoxide and hydrogen to O_2 and H_2O_2, whereas catalase detoxifies this product into H_2O and O_2. Glutathione peroxidase binds oxygen radicals with lipids to produce lipid hydroxides and water. Additional endogenous ROS scavengers include cholesterol, α-tocopherol (vitamin E), ascorbic acid (vitamin C), selenium, and bilirubin.

Antioxidant defense systems may be overwhelmed when exposed to high FIO_2 or during prolonged O_2 exposure. Individual patient susceptibility to O_2 toxicity may derive from variations in the duration and fractional percent of O_2 exposure, the underlying disease state, antioxidant availability, and individual genetic variations (7, 8).

Hypercapnia

Administering oxygen to patients with a chronically compensated respiratory acidosis may induce a mild increase in measured blood $PaCO_2$. A similar increase in $PaCO_2$ in response to exogenous oxygen administration has been seen in patients with neuromuscular disease, chronic asthma, and obesity hypoventilation syndrome. Hypercarbia is hypothesized to occur secondary to (a) loss of hypoxic pulmonary vasoconstriction, (b) decreased stimulation of peripheral chemoreceptors resulting in reduced ventilatory drive, and (c) the decreased CO_2-binding affinity of oxyhemoglobin (i.e., the Haldane effect) (9, 10). This effect is minimal in clinically hypoxemic patients and should never preclude the administration of oxygen. However, vigilance is always necessary because the underlying diseases may progress, necessitating assisted ventilation.

INHALED NITRIC OXIDE

Named "Molecule of the Year" by *Science* magazine in 1992, endogenous nitric oxide (NO) is an essential gaseous cell mediator in neurotransmission, inflammatory cell activation, and vascular smooth muscle relaxation. Therapeutically, inhaled NO (iNO) is used as a selective pulmonary vasodilator to reduce pulmonary vascular resistance and treat pulmonary arteriolar hypertension (see Chapter 80). Although iNO has also been used to treat hypoxemic respiratory failure by improving $\dot{V}/\dot{Q}$ matching, this therapeutic approach does not alter clinical outcomes and is very expensive.

Pharmacology

Endogenous NO is synthesized within most cells of the human body from arginine and O_2 by one of three isoforms of NO synthase (NOS): neural, inducible, and endothelial. Constitutive NO production is found in the vascular endothelium, neurons, platelets, adrenal medulla, and macula densa of the kidney. NO is also produced under pathologic conditions by the inducible NOS found within macrophages, hepatocytes, and airway epithelial and smooth muscle cells.

NO induces upregulation of cytosolic guanylyl cyclase, triggering the activation of cyclic guanosine 3',5'-monophosphate (cGMP)-dependent protein kinases (**Fig. 39.1**). Ultimately, this cascade results in smooth muscle cell relaxation and pulmonary arteriolar vasodilation due to decreased intracellular calcium levels. Phosphodiesterase enzymes cause cGMP levels within the smooth muscle cell to fall. Phosphodiesterase enzyme inhibitors (e.g., sildenafil, zaprinast, and dipyridamole) preserve the cGMP-dependent cascade and may provide a synergistic increase in the vasodilatory effects of iNO.

iNO provides a therapeutic, selective pulmonary vasodilator. This selectivity results from NO reactions that rapidly inactivate most iNO to nitrosylmethemoglobin before it enters the systemic circulation (11, 12). Systemic uptake of NO is also limited by two other scavenging mechanisms: (a) NO binding to plasma proteins (forming nitrosothiols, which potentially store NO activity and inhibit platelet aggregation), and (b) NO–heme iron binding. Ongoing research has focused on the potential for erythrocytes to store the vasodilatory properties of NO in the form of S-nitrosylated or SNO-Hb, formed during NO binding with oxyhemoglobin. SNO-Hb is a stable mediator with retained vasodilatory properties transported via erythrocytes to release NO peripherally in areas of low oxygen tension. Further, therapies targeting increased formation of S-nitrosylation of circulating proteins are under investigation (12).

NO can also react with free radicals when available (**Fig. 39.2**) to form nitrogen dioxide (NO_2) or peroxynitrite ($ONOO^-$). Protein nitration and oxidative lung injury can result from these toxic reactions and may underlie the pathologic mechanism for hyperoxic or ischemia–reperfusion injury (13). The biochemical fate of NO may depend upon the relative concentrations of the various blood components (oxyhemoglobin, iron, and plasma proteins), ROS, and antioxidants.

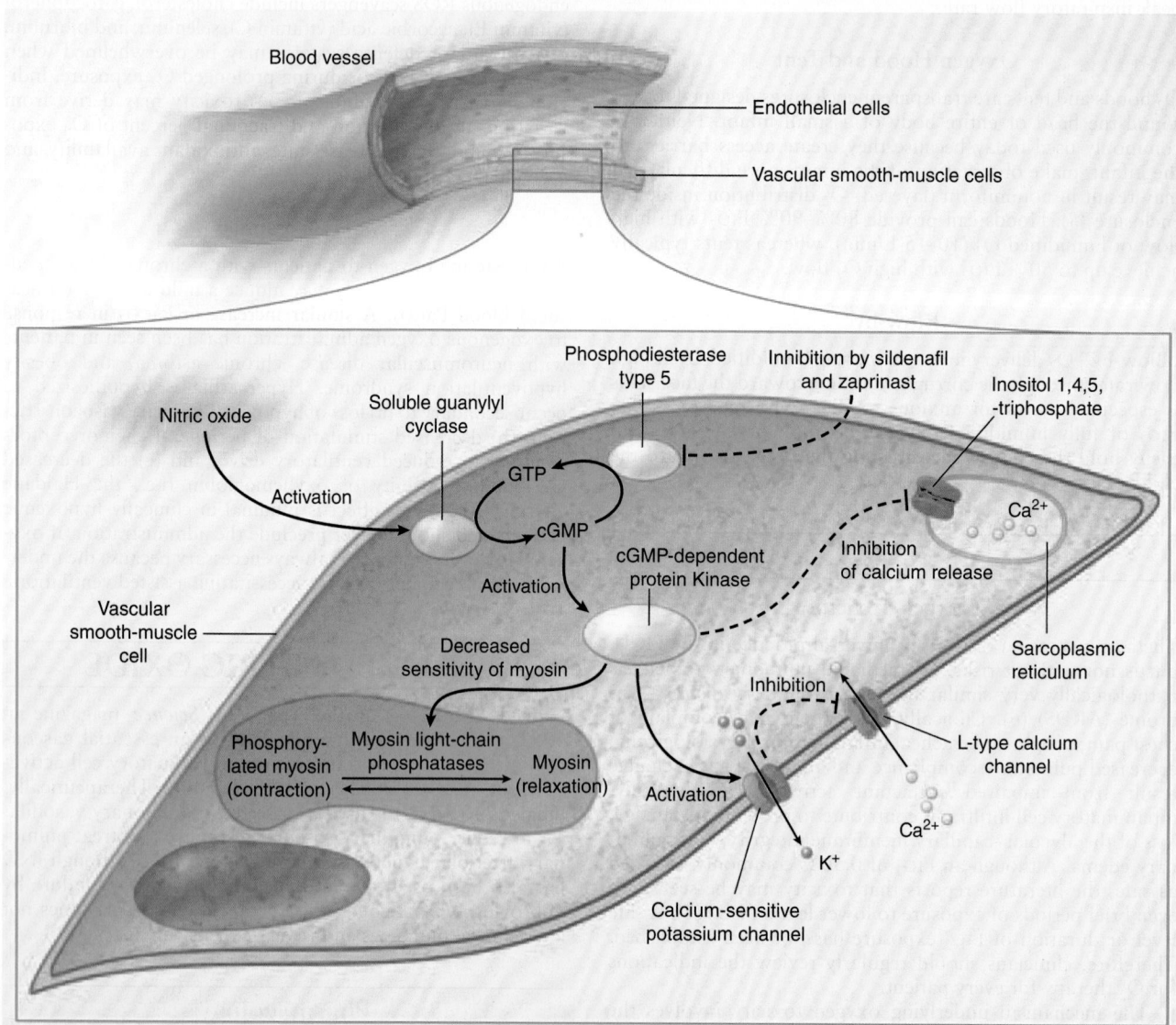

FIGURE 39.1. iNO causes pulmonary vascular endothelial smooth muscle cell relaxation, induces pulmonary capillary smooth muscle cell relaxation, and induces upregulation of guanylyl cyclase, resulting in cytosolic increase of cyclic guanosine 3',5'-monophosphate (cGMP). cGMP-dependent protein kinase (cGKI) ultimately lowers the intracellular calcium concentration and decreases the sensitivity of myosin to calcium-induced contraction. (Adapted from Griffiths MJD, TW Evans. Drug therapy: Inhaled nitric oxide therapy in adults. *N Engl J Med* 2005;353:2683–95.)

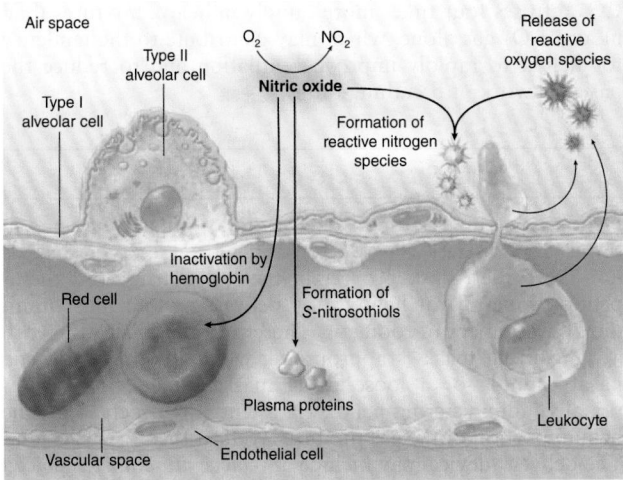

Air space

Type II
alveolar cell

O_2 NO_2

Nitric oxide

Type I
alveolar cell

Release of
reactive
oxygen species

Formation of
reactive nitrogen
species

Inactivation by
hemoglobin

Red cell

Formation of
S-nitrosothiols

Plasma proteins

Leukocyte

Vascular space   Endothelial cell

FIGURE 39.2. The biochemical fates of inhaled nitric oxide. Systemic uptake of iNO is limited by nitric oxide binding to oxyhemoglobin, heme iron, and plasma proteins. Depending upon the relative concentration of O_2 and free radicals (reactive oxygen species), nitrogen dioxide (NO_2) and reactive nitrogen species (i.e., peroxynitrite) may be produced. (Adapted from Griffiths MJD, TW Evans. Drug therapy: Inhaled nitric oxide therapy in adults. N Engl J Med 2005;353: 2683–95.)

Nitric Oxide Delivery Systems

NO gas is produced at high temperatures by a catalyst-induced oxidation of ammonia and is then stored with nitrogen as the balancing gas. iNO is generally delivered during mechanical ventilation, but can also be delivered to nonintubated patients via a tight-fitting face mask, transtracheal O_2 catheter, or nasal cannula. Effective iNO delivery via nasal cannula has been validated for flow rates as low as 1 L/min. iNO should not be administered via an O_2 hood owing to the potential for accumulation of toxic nitrogen dioxide byproducts within the hood.

During mechanical ventilation, a constant desired concentration of iNO is delivered to the patient, independent of ventilator mode or flow rate. An integrated iNO delivery unit and nitrogen dioxide–monitoring system, such as the Ohmeda INOvent Nitric Oxide delivery system (Datex-Ohmeda, Madison, WI), is generally used. With this system, the minimum delivered concentration of iNO is 0.1 ppm, at a flow rate between 4 and 120 L/min. iNO is injected directly into the inspiratory limb of the ventilator circuit in synchrony with each inspiratory breath. iNO has an effective half-life of 15–30 seconds. Therefore, to ensure that the iNO flow is not interrupted in the event the patient must be disconnected from the ventilator, a separate connector is used to facilitate iNO delivery via a manual bag system. iNO delivery with the Bunnell Life Pulse High-Frequency Jet ventilator has been used in the clinical setting for premature infants with respiratory distress syndrome and has been tested with infant lung models (14).

NO Metabolite Monitoring

During iNO administration, the appropriate monitoring and measurement of NO_2 and methemoglobin levels are necessary to prevent potential NO-induced toxicity. NO_2 results from the reaction of NO with O_2, and its level is continuously measured using electrochemical sensors. When administering iNO at doses <40 ppm, toxic levels of NO_2 (>2 ppm) rarely occur (15, 16).

Methemoglobin is produced from NO reaction with oxyhemoglobin, which converts the iron to the ferric or oxidized state (Fe^{3+}). Normally, methemoglobin is converted within the red cell by NADH–cytochrome b5 reductase to restore ferrous hemoglobin (Fe^{2+}). Methemoglobinemia may result in patients with inefficient methemoglobin reductase activity or in those who are exposed to high concentrations of iNO. Blood methemoglobin levels should be monitored within 4 hours of initiating iNO and after every 24 hours of continued treatment. Prilocaine local or topical anesthetics are contraindicated in patients receiving iNO because of the risk of methemoglobinemia.

NO Dosing

Dosing and duration of iNO therapy may depend on the therapeutic target defined for each patient (i.e., improved $\dot{V}/\dot{Q}$ matching versus decreased pulmonary arterial pressure). The effective dose of iNO may depend on the degree of reversible pulmonary arterial hypertension, the extent of $\dot{V}/\dot{Q}$ mismatching, and the concurrent level of alveolar recruitment. iNO doses between 5 and 20 ppm should produce a clinically apparent response in oxygenation and/or pulmonary vascular resistance. Continuous iNO of >40 ppm does not produce greater benefit; rather, it can produce increased measured levels of methemoglobin and nitrogen dioxide. In patients with hypoxemic respiratory failure, alveolar derecruitment has been associated with a poor response to iNO therapy at recommended doses. In patients with pulmonary hypertension, a decrease in pulmonary vascular resistance by 30% during a trial of 10 ppm iNO for 10 minutes has been predictive of those likely to derive a clinical response to oral agents (17). A systematic review of the literature fails to support the benefit of iNO on important clinical outcomes in ARDS, such as number of ventilator-free days or survival (18).

NO Weaning

Patients should be monitored for rebound pulmonary hypertension and hypoxemia when iNO therapy is being weaned. Nitration produced during exogenous iNO leads to impaired endothelial NOS activity (19). Therefore, abrupt discontinuation of iNO may precipitate $\dot{V}/\dot{Q}$ mismatch, pulmonary hypertension, and hemodynamic compromise. iNO must be steadily tapered, with concurrent clinical and hemodynamic evaluation, to safely identify the patient's response to weaning of iNO therapy. To facilitate weaning from iNO and to potentially prevent rebound pulmonary hypertension, patients may receive enteral pulmonary vasodilators such as sildenafil and/or bosentan. These agents have been successfully used in patients who have failed to wean from iNO, have congenital heart disease, or in infants with persistent pulmonary hypertension secondary to chronic lung disease or bronchopulmonary dysplasia (20–24). Sildenafil mediates vasodilation via its action as a phosphodiesterase type V inhibitor, thus increasing relative circulating concentration of cGMP. Bosentan augments pulmonary vasodilation as a receptor antagonist for the potent vasoconstrictor endothelin-1.

HELIUM–OXYGEN MIXTURES (HELIOX)

Helium is administered clinically as a helium–oxygen mixture, referred to as *heliox*. Although helium is biologically inert and provides no direct pharmacologic or biologic effects, heliox provides a medical gas therapy with unique therapeutic application to respiratory processes associated with high airways resistance or obstructive pathology (25). Owing to its low density, heliox can significantly decrease respiratory distress and work of breathing, and may improve the deposition of bronchodilator therapy to obstructed lower airways. Heliox provides a rapidly acting inhaled therapy that may afford the patient greater comfort and improved gas exchange while awaiting the therapeutic onset of slower, definitive medical therapies (e.g., corticosteroids).

Because of small sample sizes, variable helium concentrations, and poorly controlled effects of helium on other inhaled bronchodilators, the quality of the evidence for using heliox in specific diseases is generally poor. A recent systematic review of heliox therapy in *viral croup* concluded that heliox did not confer a significant benefit compared to humidified O_2 or racemic epinephrine, but did appear to benefit children short-term (90–24 min) while awaiting the onset of the effects of dexamethasone (26). One small study indicated an advantage of heliox over racemic epinephrine in the treatment of *postextubation stridor* (27). For *acute asthma exacerbations*, small studies have suggested enhanced bronchodilator deposition with heliox inhalation (28). The National Asthma Education and Prevention Program (NAEPP) 2007 guidelines indicate that heliox may be added to inhaled β-agonists for patients with impending respiratory failure who are refractory to other therapies (29). Heliox is not recommended for *bronchiolitis* therapy.

Pharmacology

Helium is an odorless, tasteless, and noncombustible gas. It is commercially produced from natural gas by liquefaction or by thermal release of helium from uranium ore. Helium (0.179 μP) is approximately one-seventh the density of air (1.293 μP) and O_2 (1.429 μP). The density of heliox is dependent on the relative percentage of helium compared with O_2. The higher the concentration of helium, the lower the concentration of O_2 and total density of the inhaled gas become. Premixed heliox provides 20% O_2 (80:20 mixture), 30% O_2 (70:30 mixture), or 40% O_2 (60:40 mixture).

Gas flow at high velocity through a relatively small cross-sectional area (e.g., gas flow within the upper airway or through partially obstructed air passages) is typically turbulent, whereas gas flow across a large cross-sectional area (e.g., in the lung periphery) is typically laminar. The lower density of heliox, as compared with O_2-enriched air, improves gas flow through high-resistance airways with turbulent gas flow. Turbulent gas flow is mathematically defined by the Bernoulli principle as:

$$\dot{Q} = (2\Delta P/p)^{1/2}$$

where $\dot{Q}$ = turbulent gas flow rate, ΔP = airway driving pressure, and ρ = gas density.

As gas flow becomes less turbulent in the affected airways, flow velocity is reduced, and the flow pattern may transition from turbulent to more laminar. This transitional zone is represented by the Reynolds number (Re). A lower Re indicates gas flow with greater laminar flow characteristics.

$$Re = 2Vrp/\eta$$

where V = gas velocity, r = airway radius, ρ = gas density, and η = gas viscosity.

The low density of heliox allows greater gas flow through airways with high resistance and decreases the Re in airways with transitional gas flow pattern to generate more laminar flow of gas delivery to the distal airways. Furthermore,

CO_2 diffuses four times more rapidly in heliox mixtures than in air or O_2 gas alone, which may contribute to the tendency for heliox to rapidly improve ventilation and to reduce the patient's work of breathing (30).

Heliox Delivery Systems

Heliox is normally administered to nonventilated patients in respiratory distress via a face mask with a reservoir bag or non-rebreather mask. To retain the low density and therapeutic properties of heliox, any delivery system must minimize entrainment of room air. Therefore, administration with a tight-fitting mask is appropriate, while administration via nasal cannula or a loose-fitting mask is ineffective. Additionally, administering heliox via a tent is impractical, as the helium portion of the gas mixture layers at the top of the tent. The delivery device may include a Y-piece attachment, placed between the mask and the reservoir bag, to add a nebulizer for concurrent bronchodilator administration. Owing to the production of less turbulent air flow, a minimum flow rate of 12 L/min is required to aerosolize the treatment (31). An O_2 analyzer should be placed in-line with the patient inspiratory limb when administering heliox to ensure that a known FIO_2 is being supplied to the patient.

Heliox delivery through mechanical ventilators may also be effective to reduce air trapping and airways resistance in partially obstructed airways (32). Most mechanical ventilators can be adapted to administer heliox, but calibration is required. Ventilators are designed and calibrated for a mixture of O_2 and air; thus, adding heliox gas, which is of a different density, viscosity, and thermal conductivity, can affect both the delivered and the measured tidal volumes (33). Some ventilators with in-line respiratory mechanics monitors have calibration settings for heliox. Otherwise, suggested correction factors are available for most ventilators in the United States and Europe (34). Heliox has only been thoroughly studied and clinically used when administered through a conventional mechanical ventilator. The use of heliox in conjunction with "nonconventional" ventilation, such as high-frequency oscillatory ventilation (HFOV) and high-frequency jet ventilation (HFJV), is based on laboratory evaluations and sporadic case reports (35). Routine use of heliox with nonconventional ventilation cannot be recommended at the current time.

Heliox administration can also alter the function of respiratory diagnostic and monitoring equipment. Unless appropriately calibrated for heliox use, diagnostic equipment, flow meters, gas blenders, and monitoring devices will erroneously report low flow and tidal volume readings. The delivered flow rate of an 80:20 heliox mixture is 1.8 times greater than the set flow rate, and the flow rate of a 70:30 heliox mixture is 1.6 times greater. Thus, for every 10 L/min flow of an 80:20 heliox mixture that is set, 18 L/min is actually delivered. One must account for the greater flow rate delivery when heliox is used.

Safety Considerations

Helium must always be administered with O_2. Although tanks of 100% helium are available, an interruption in O_2 delivery could result in the accidental administration of pure helium, which could be fatal. Continuous in-line monitoring of inspired O_2 concentration is essential to ensure adequate O_2 delivery to the patient. Consideration must be given to the patient's O_2 requirement. The higher the required FIO_2, the lower the helium concentration and the lower the therapeutic benefit derived. However, even those patients with high O_2 requirements ($FIO_2 \geq 0.80$) may have improved gas exchange with the administration of heliox, allowing for reduced O_2 therapy.

The effects of heliox on improved work of breathing are typically apparent within several minutes. A brief therapeutic trial can quickly assess for a clinical response, either by the patient's subjective report or on the basis of serial examination of respiratory effort, quality of air entry, and gas exchange.

Clinically, it is appropriate to forewarn the patient that, during heliox use, their voice may become high-pitched and their ability to generate an effective cough will be reduced. Coughing typically produces a high-velocity burst of turbulent expiratory air flow to expel upper airway irritants. When heliox is in use, air flow turbulence is minimized and coughing efficacy may be reduced. Removing the face mask briefly to wash out the heliox gas effects allows the patient to generate an effective cough.

INHALED BRONCHODILATOR THERAPY

Lower airway respiratory disease is often accompanied by bronchoconstriction, inflammatory cell activation, mucosal edema formation, and inspissated secretions. (See also Chapter 68 on Status Asthmaticus.) Inhaled bronchodilator therapy is provided to relieve lower airway bronchoconstriction, reduce airway resistance, and improve $\dot{V}/\dot{Q}$ matching. Inhaled bronchodilators are often given in combination with other pharmacologic agents, including anti-inflammatory agents, decongestants, mucolytic agents, and pulmonary vasodilators, to reverse multiple processes that limit effective gas exchange.

Pharmacology

Inhaled bronchodilator therapy may include the use of β-adrenergic receptor agonists and/or anticholinergic receptor blockade. The inhaled β-agonists (e.g., albuterol, metaproterenol, pirbuterol, levalbuterol, fenoterol, and salbutamol) interact with type 2 β-receptors (β_2) on the luminal surface of bronchial smooth muscle cells. β-Agonists can also bind β_2-receptors found on a variety of other cell types to decrease mast-cell mediator release, increase mucociliary transport, alter vascular tone, limit edema formation, and inhibit neutrophil, eosinophil, and lymphocyte functional responses (36). The inhaled anticholinergic agent ipratropium bromide competitively inhibits acetylcholine binding at the M_3 muscarinic receptor located on bronchial smooth muscle cells to decrease intracellular cyclic AMP (cAMP) and cause bronchodilation.

Although systemic uptake of inhaled agents is negligible, clinically notable side effects may result owing to receptor binding at nonpulmonary sites and nonselective receptor binding. Adverse effects of β_2 agents include vasodilation, decreased systemic vascular resistance, tremors, and decreased insulin release, which may become clinically evident with a widened pulse pressure, hyperglycemia, and hypokalemia. Rarely, prolonged administration of β-agonists can elevate creatine phosphokinase and lactate dehydrogenase. β-Adrenergic type 1 receptor binding causes tachycardia, palpitations, and/or arrhythmias. Nonselective binding by ipratropium at M_2 receptor sites located on sympathetic nerve terminals could theoretically provoke bronchoconstriction, but this effect is limited by the very poor systemic absorption of the inhaled drug.

Albuterol is a 1:1 racemic mixture of the R- and S-isomers. The R-isomer, levalbuterol, is responsible for the drug's bronchodilating activity, while the S-isomer has been proposed to contribute to a higher incidence of side effects, toxicity, and tolerance, which have been observed following chronic β-agonist use (37). Although often purported to decrease side effects, levalbuterol has not been shown to provide a significant advantage over albuterol in bronchodilator effect, side-effect profile, or in preventing hospital admission (38). Levalbuterol use should be reserved for those patients who have a known history of adverse effects to albuterol.

Delivery Systems

Three principal types of devices are used to generate therapeutic aerosols: nebulizers, metered-dose inhalers (MDIs), and dry-powder inhalers (DPIs). All three types of devices may be equally effective for aerosol administration to the spontaneously breathing patient, but the DPIs are ineffective devices for use in mechanically ventilated patients.

Nebulizers

Nebulizers physically "shatter" liquid into small particles to create an aerosol that can be effectively inhaled. Drug delivery to the distal airways is achieved by creating particle sizes between 1 and 5 μm. Particles that are too large (<10 μm) are deposited primarily in the oropharynx, and particles that are too small (<1 μm) are not effectively inhaled (28). To create the aerosol, a pressurized gas jet (air, O_2, or heliox) is forced through a small orifice above the medication reservoir, breaking the surface tension of the liquid to form large droplets. Typically, a baffle within the reservoir recycles larger droplets into the liquid reservoir to enable the formation of smaller particles, which can be entrained into the inspiratory gas stream that is inhaled by the patient. In place of a baffle, some nebulizers contain a vibrating mesh or plate with multiple apertures to produce a very fine-particle fraction. Alternatively, ultrasonic nebulizers create an aerosol by transmitting ultrasonic waves to the surface of the solution to create an aerosol. The aerosol is delivered to the patient during an inspiratory breath or by a fan operated within the nebulizer. Small-volume ultrasonic nebulizers are commercially available for delivery of inhaled bronchodilators; large-volume ultrasonic nebulizers are available for sputum induction in adult patients. Lastly, specialized small-volume nebulizers are equipped with filters, a scavenging system, and one-way valves and should be used for certain inhaled medications (e.g., pentamidine, ribavirin, rhDNase, and tobramycin) when it is necessary to prevent contamination of the ambient environment.

Three variables affect nebulizer output: initial fill volume (volume of medication and sterile diluent), nebulization time, and gas flow rate. An increase in any one of these variables increases the effective delivery of inhaled medication. During nebulization, water vapor evaporates and the aerosol becomes more concentrated, thus delivering a greater fraction of medication with each inspiratory cycle. A minimum driving gas flow rate of 8 L/min is required when using air or O_2; owing to the lower density of heliox and less turbulent gas flow properties, a gas flow rate >12 L/min is required to aerosolize the treatment when heliox is used as the driving gas (31).

Newer breath-actuated nebulizers significantly increase drug delivery by releasing aerosol only upon inhalation, rather than throughout the respiratory cycle. Inhaled aerosols can be effectively administered to the infant and pediatric patient using a face mask or a mouthpiece. The mask may not be well tolerated in the younger patient, and an improper fit can cause significant deposition of aerosol to the eyes, resulting in pupillary dilation. Hence, a mouthpiece may be more effective in the younger patient.

Metered-Dose Inhaler

An MDI consists of drug suspended in a mixture of propellants, surfactants, preservatives, flavoring agents, and dispersal agents within a pressurized canister. The mixture is released from the MDI canister through a metering valve and stem into an actuator boot. To improve effective delivery for the pediatric patient, a spacer (valved holding chamber) is commonly used. The MDI is actuated once every 15–20 seconds into the accessory device, to reduce the need to coordinate with inspiration. A spacer device is an open-ended tube or bag that allows the MDI plume to expand and the propellant to evaporate. A valved holding chamber incorporates a one-way valve to release aerosol from the chamber only during inspiration. Drug particle deposition on the inner surfaces of these devices can occur, resulting in less effective drug delivery. To avoid this particle deposition, the device must be washed prior to use to remove static charges on the plastic material of the chambers.

Dry-Powder Inhalers

A DPI creates aerosol by drawing air through a dose of powdered medication. The advantage of the DPI is that it is breath-actuated, thus delivering medication only upon inhalation, reducing the problem of coordinating inspiration with actuation. However, release of the drug requires high-inspiratory flow rates >50 L/min, which limit the use of the DPI in patients <6 years of age and in the neuromuscularly weak patient. The DPI is not effective for aerosol delivery during mechanical ventilation, as the high ambient humidity causes the dry powder to clump and create larger particles that do not aerosolize well.

Mechanically Ventilated Patients

Inhaled bronchodilators may be effectively administered and equally therapeutic in the mechanically ventilated patient using a nebulizer or MDI (39), and a recent systematic review concluded there was insufficient evidence to favor one technique over the other (40). To increase the effective drug delivery during mechanical ventilation, attention to several aspects of delivery is required: (a) location of delivery within the ventilator circuit, (b) humidity within the circuit, and (c) ventilator flow (Table 39.3). In terms of location of delivery, the nebulizer device or MDI (fitted with a chamber) provides optimum medication delivery when placed in the inspiratory limb of the ventilator circuit ~18–30 cm from the endotracheal tube Y-piece connector. Furthermore, the ventilator circuit distal to the device should have no kinks, elbow connectors, or other obstructions to gas flow. This location allows the circuit to act as a spacer reservoir and limits medication entrainment along plastic surfaces.

Humidity within the circuit significantly decreases aerosol deposition. Positioning the delivery device so that it bypasses the humidifier increases medication delivery by a factor of nearly 4 (41). Because of the high humidity, increased dosage of medication is often required to achieve a therapeutic effect in mechanically ventilated patients (42).

Required MDI actuations may range from 6 to 40 puffs (depending on patient age and size) to produce a therapeutic effect. In the neonatal and pediatric population, the required doses of specific aerosolized medications are not known. Attention to ventilator gas flow is important to affect drug delivery. Greater aerosol delivery occurs when MDI actuation is synchronized with a delivered inspired breath, a larger tidal volume, or the use of an end-inspiratory pause. Direct application of medication into the endotracheal tube is not recommended.

Using an MDI versus continuous nebulizer treatment for the intubated patient is associated with the relative advantages of decreased personnel time required for administration, no requirement to disconnect ventilator circuit (when an in-line MDI chamber is used), and no requirement to alter ventilator

TABLE 39.3

RECOMMENDED TECHNIQUES FOR METERED-DOSE INHALER AND NEBULIZER USE DURING MECHANICAL VENTILATION

Metered-Dose Inhaler

Agitate MDI and warm to hand temperature
Place MDI adaptor into inspiratory limb of circuit
  (18–30 cm from the Y-piece connector)
Attach MDI to adaptor in ventilator circuit
  (chamber-style is best)
Actuate ≥6 puffs at beginning of inspiratory cycle
Cycle each actuation with a spontaneous or ventilator
  inspiratory cycle
Wait ≥5 s between actuations
Assess patient response

Nebulizer

Establish dose to be administered
Place drug in nebulizer reservoir; fill with sterile water
  to ≥4 mL
Place nebulizer in inspiratory circuit ≥18–30 cm from
  the patient Y-piece connector
Initiate driving gas flow of oxygen ≥6 L/min; ≥12 L/min
  when heliox used
Turn off flow by or continuous flow during nebulization
Continue nebulization treatment until sputtering occurs,
  indicating end of treatment
Remove nebulizer and return ventilator to previous settings
Assure no leak in circuit
Assess patient response

Adapted with permission from Fink JB. Metered-dose inhalers, dry powdered inhalers, and transitions. Respiratory Care 2000.45 (6); 623-635.

settings during administration. Additionally, the disadvantages with an in-line nebulizer treatment include alteration of inspiratory flows, additional bias flow in the ventilator circuit that may interfere with patient-triggered modes of ventilation, and the possibility for aerosol particles to deposit and crystallize on the expiratory mechanisms, creating inadvertent expiratory resistance or intrinsic PEEP (43, 44).

INHALATIONAL ANESTHETICS

Inhalational anesthetics have been administered in the critical care unit to aid in the treatment of medically refractory bronchospasm (isoflurane, desflurane), for refractory pain (isoflurane, N_2O), refractory status epilepticus (isoflurane) (45), and for sedation (isoflurane, desflurane, sevoflurane) (46). The published literature suggests that few centers within the United States routinely use volatile anesthetic agents within the ICU, whereas, internationally, the use of volatile anesthetics is more common and is applied to broader clinical applications such as in pre hospital use for sedating trauma victims (47, 48). These agents have certain advantages for the mechanically ventilated over more traditional intravenous therapies, including (a) the rapid onset and titration of therapeutic effects, (b) limited metabolism that is independent of renal or hepatic function, and (c) the relief of bronchospasm. However, general anesthetics also have important disadvantages in the PICU. (See Safety Considerations below.) Inhaled anesthetics should be used only under the supervision of an anesthesiologist.

General Principles of Inhalation Anesthetics

To reach peak sedative effect, the inspired concentration must first reach equilibrium within the pulmonary alveolar capillary and subsequently reach equilibrium within the brain tissue. A low blood solubility (i.e., low blood:gas partition coefficient) establishes rapid equilibrium between the partial pressures of inspired gas within the alveolus, pulmonary capillaries, and brain tissue (Table 39.4). Clinically, this allows for rapid and easily titratable effects on the respiratory and central nervous systems. The end-tidal alveolar gas concentration is continuously monitored to determine the number of minimum alveolar concentration (MAC) of the volatile agent administered to the patient. For each inhaled anesthetic agent, 1 MAC refers to the concentration required to prevent movement in 50% of patients in response to surgical stimuli. On average, 1.3 MAC is typically required for any volatile anesthetic to provide sufficient anesthetic potency to allow for surgical incision and prevent movement in ~95% of patients. *MAC-hours* refers to the length of time (hours) the patient has been exposed to the anesthetic multiplied by the MAC exposure. For isoflurane, MAC exposure is derived by dividing the end-tidal concentration by 1.15 (46, 49). Notably, these references have not been established in ICU patients with multiple organ dysfunction or for long-term sedation.

Isoflurane

Isoflurane (1-chloro-2,2,2-trifluoroethyl difluoromethyl ether) is a fluorinated, nonflammable ether that is volatile at room temperature. It induces rapid anesthetic induction and recovery owing to a low blood:gas partition coefficient. In the ICU, isoflurane has been used to treat severe bronchospasm in cases refractory to conventional medical therapies. Published case reports suggest that administration produces therapeutic benefit within 1 hour and is associated with an improvement in alveolar minute ventilation, improved aeration on auscultation, and reduced intrinsic PEEP, obstructive physiology, and inspiratory and expiratory resistive indices (50–54). Of note, initial worsening of metabolic acidosis in the first 4 hours is frequently seen during the treatment of severe bronchospasm, and may reflect overall dehydration and $\dot{V}/\dot{Q}$ mismatch, which usually resolves as the patient responds to therapy. Fluid administration during isoflurane use in refractory status asthmaticus is common due to hypotension secondary to a combination of vasodilation from the volatile anesthetic and decreased left ventricular preload from massive hyperinflation

of the lungs in status asthmaticus. Treatment failure marked by progressive worsening respiratory acidosis, and persistent hypoxemia despite 4–6 hours of maximal therapy, may occur and should prompt consideration of extracorporeal membrane oxygenation.

Pharmacology

The mechanism of action for isoflurane's bronchodilatory properties is not well established. Isoflurane may affect multiple pathways involved in the relief of bronchospasm, and antagonize the actions of both histamine and acetylcholine although no direct effect on histamine levels or smooth muscle contraction is measurable. It is postulated that isoflurane activates the sympathetic system to cause elevated endogenous catecholamine levels, leading to bronchodilation. Isoflurane is eliminated almost completely from the lungs, with only 0.2% undergoing oxidative metabolism via cytochrome P450 2E1. Thus, elimination is dependent on exposure duration (MAC-hours), minute ventilation, and cardiac output. A higher minute ventilation with higher inspired oxygen concentration and higher cardiac output will enhance the gradient of volatile anesthetic in the pulmonary venous blood relative to the alveolus and lowers the alveolar partial pressure of the gas.

Isoflurane dosing in the ICU setting is initiated at 0.5% and titrated to clinical effect up to 2% (55). If oversedation occurs, the effects may be quickly reversed by temporarily discontinuing therapy and administering 100% F_{IO_2}. Dose-dependent side effects include systemic vasodilation and increased sympathetic stimuli, which result in increased cardiac output, skin flushing, and tachycardia. Isoflurane increases cerebral blood flow and may raise intracranial pressure, but it reduces cerebral O_2 consumption. Isoflurane is also a potent coronary vasodilator, the use of which results in improved coronary blood flow and decreased myocardial O_2 consumption. The bronchodilatory effect is usually immediate and is often sustained. Inhaled bronchodilator therapy and traditional intravenous sedatives and analgesics may be reduced or eliminated once the therapeutic effect of the inhalational anesthetic is maximized. Duration of use in the ICU setting varies according to clinical condition, but has been reported in several recent case series as a mean duration of 54.5 hours (range 1–181 hours), and the longest duration was reported as 13 days (170 MAC-hours) (52, 53). Slow weaning is recommended to evaluate patient recovery, to reinstitute intravenous sedation and analgesic agents as needed, and to prevent abstinence syndrome. Reducing isoflurane 0.1%–0.2% on average every 30 minutes to 1 hour is recommended.

TABLE 39.4

COMPARISON OF ANESTHETIC POTENCY FOR INHALATIONAL ANESTHETICS USED IN THE PICU

■ ANESTHETIC AGENT	■ MAC (%)[a]	PARTITION COEFFICIENT AT 37°C	
		■ ALVEOLAR GAS:BLOOD	■ BLOOD:BRAIN
Isoflurane	1.2	1.40	2.6
Desflurane	6.0	0.45	1.3
Sevoflurane	2.0	0.69	
N$_2$O	105.0[b]	0.47	1.1

[a]MAC, minimum alveolar concentration; MAC%, concentration of inhaled agent required to prevent movement in response to surgical stimuli in 50% of patients.
[b]Hyperbaric conditions are required to reach 1 MAC.

Delivery Systems

Use of inhalation anesthetics within the ICU requires proper facilities, personnel training, and equipment to ensure a safe environment for patients and staff. Direct collaboration and daily involvement with anesthesiologists is typical (given regulations imposed by hospital and state physician and nursing restricting those personnel who may administer, monitor, and adjust inspired concentration of the volatile anesthetic).

To safely administer isoflurane outside of the operative setting, specialized equipment for monitoring and scavenging the volatile anesthetic is needed. An anesthesia machine or adaptation of the ICU ventilator is required for delivery. The vapor pressure of each agent varies; thus, a vaporizer specific for each of the volatile anesthetics is required. In addition, an in-line volatile anesthetic gas analyzer for isoflurane is necessary as the delivered percentage of isoflurane may be different from what is set on the vaporizer when ventilators are adapted to deliver inhaled anesthetics.

The use of an anesthesia machine in the ICU allows the delivery of a set concentration of the inhalation anesthetic gas agent regardless of changes in ventilatory settings. For the mechanically ventilated ICU patient, the anesthesia machine may have limited ventilation modes and limited capacity to set inspiratory-to-expiratory ratios. Further, the anesthesia machine provides limited alarms monitoring, and the tidal volume provided is extrapolated by setting the minute ventilation and the respiratory rate. The ICU ventilator most commonly adapted for use with inhaled anesthetics is the Servo 900C anesthesia system (Siemens, Solna, Sweden), which includes a calibrated liquid injection vaporizer (Siemens vaporizer 952, Maquet Critical Care, Bridgewater, NJ) and an active scavenging system (Servo Evac 180). The gas flow from the air/oxygen blender is passed through the anesthetic vaporizer then into the low-pressure inlet on the Servo 900C. This allows for alterations in the ventilatory mode and tidal volume settings to be made without changing inspiratory gas content of anesthetic agent. Caution must be advised in administering an inhaled anesthetic with nontraditional equipment or when set up to add flow separately to the inspiratory flow limb as alterations in tidal volume or spontaneous patient breathing affects the minute ventilation and the inspired concentration of anesthetic gas.

Active scavenging systems and appropriate turnover of ambient air are required to protect patients and staff from inadvertent exposure. The ventilator exhalation port is connected to a self-inflating bag via a T-piece with the remaining limb connected to wall suction adjusted to allow the reservoir bag to both partially fill with each exhalation and to never fully collapse (11). Closed suctioning devices are used to prevent environmental contamination when the patients suctioned (46).

Continuous infrared monitoring equipment for both the inspired and the expired concentrations of O_2, CO_2, and the inhalational agent is necessary (Datex-Ohmeda Rascal II Mass spectrometer, Helsinki, Finland). The high- and low-concentration alarms are set within a narrow range to immediately detect variations from desired settings.

Safety Considerations

The safety of prolonged inhaled anesthetic administration, particularly in the critically ill patient, has not been established. Case reports suggest that prolonged administration can be associated with an abstinence syndrome (52, 56). Symptoms, which are reversible, include agitation, choreoathetoid movements, hypertension, tachycardia, diaphoresis, and diarrhea. These symptoms have been reported in patients who received >70 MAC-hours of isoflurane. The abstinence syndrome may be prevented or treated with the gradual withdrawal of the inhalation agent or use of IV sedation as the agent is withdrawn.

Fluoride ion nephrotoxicity is also associated with prolonged isoflurane exposure (57). Nephrotoxicity has been reported with serum fluoride levels ≥ 50 μM/L, resulting in decreased glomerular filtration rate and nephrogenic diabetes insipidus. A peak serum fluoride level of 26.1 μM was noted in 10 pediatric patients after 441 MAC-hours of isoflurane sedation (56). Periodic monitoring of renal function and ability to concentrate is warranted. Sevoflurane undergoes more rapid and different metabolism, causing no local renal release of fluoride, but does result in the production of compound A, which has been shown to variably react with the CO_2 absorbent in the anesthesia machine. No data are available regarding compound A in prolonged administration of sevoflurane in the PICU (46).

Acute concerns during use of inhalational anesthetics include the rare, but treatable, onset of malignant hyperthermia. Continuous temperature monitoring is necessary, and dantrolene sodium should be readily available for any patient receiving an inhaled volatile anesthetic.

Clinical side effects variably occur with the use of potent inhalational agents, such as hypotension and reflex tachycardia due to vasodilatation and decreased mean arterial pressure. Hypotension is typically volume responsive when treated with aggressive volume replacement with crystalloid. After 40–60 mL/kg, consider vasopressor of either epinephrine at 0.05 μg/kg/min or dopamine at 5 μg/kg/min titrated to maintain mean arterial blood pressure within range. Rarely, immune-mediated hepatitis may occur as a result of the metabolic byproduct of fluorinated anesthetics, trifluoroacetic acid, which produces a hapten that binds to hepatocytes.

The use of inhalational anesthetics in the PICU setting requires specific equipment and training, and remains a variable practice across ICU centers (47, 50). For the mechanically ventilated patient refractory to traditional escalating medical therapy targeted to bronchodilation and sedation, inhalational anesthetics may provide a therapeutic benefit. For those patients who do not respond within 4–6 hours of maximal anesthetic support, consideration for extracorporeal support is warranted.

Nitrous Oxide

Nitrous oxide (N_2O) has been used as an inhaled analgesic agent. N_2O is a relatively weak anesthetic agent such that only toxic concentrations (100% N_2O) produce anesthesia. However, N_2O may produce analgesia at low concentrations (20%). For this reason, N_2O is commonly administered in the operating room in combination with other inhalational agents. However, it is NOT recommended for use in the ICU because of the risks of administration of a hypoxic gas mixture. Furthermore, N_2O will enter any air-filled cavity faster than nitrogen can escape, thus increasing the volume and pressure within the cavity. Therefore, N_2O administration may result in expansion of an existing pneumothorax, pulmonary bullae, intracranial air, vascular air embolus, bowel obstruction, or intraocular air bubble.

NONINVASIVE VENTILATION

General Principles

NIV is a general term that describes the noninvasive interface. More specific terms such as noninvasive positive-pressure ventilation (NIPPV) and HFNC describe the NIV method. NIPPV applies to those modalities that can provide positive airway pressure such as continuous positive airway pressure (CPAP) or bi-level positive airway pressure (BiPAP). HFNC supply humidified, warmed air-oxygen mixtures, often with an ability to independently set flow and F_{IO_2}.

The use of noninvasive respiratory support has become increasingly popular in the treatment of acute respiratory failure, postextubation respiratory support, heart failure, and chronic respiratory failure. Noninvasive support avoids the potential complications of an endotracheal tube and the intubation procedure. These devices can achieve high oxygen flow rates and F_{IO_2}, creating a small amount of intrinsic PEEP, which can reduce work of breathing and promote increased alveolar ventilation (58). Thus, these devices are generally well-tolerated, and patients require less sedation than with traditional mechanical ventilation. As a result, patients may be more alert, interactive, and potentially better able to participate in rehabilitation, physical therapy, and enteral feeding.

Research supports clinical guidelines for use of NIPPV in specific patient populations and for the treatment of certain conditions leading to acute respiratory failure. Conversely, there are currently no established guidelines and/or decision-making pathways to guide the use of HFNC therapy for infants, pediatric, or adult patients with respiratory disease (58–60). These two forms of NIV will be discussed separately.

Noninvasive Positive-Pressure Ventilation (CPAP and BiPAP)

NIPPV requires optimization of each of the three components of the therapy: (a) a proper fitting mask interface and seal; (b) the inspiratory and expiratory pressures to obtain alveolar opening and reduce the patient's work of breathing; and (c) sufficient time to acclimate the patient with NIPPV.

The NIPPV interface may be nasal prongs, a nasal or full face mask, or helmet. The interface must fit comfortably and yet be of the smallest size to reduce dead space within the mask and to create a good seal to avoid pressure and/or flow leaks in the system. Mask accessories including choice of headgear, elasticity of the straps, cushions, foam spacers, and elastic chin straps may enhance the mask seal and patient comfort. Advantages of the nasal mask include smaller dead space, less claustrophobia, and fewer complications in the event of vomiting. Full face masks are used in acute respiratory failure to control dyspnea and mouth breathing. A helmet, or plastic cylinder that fits over the head and seals with the straps under the shoulders, may be helpful for smaller patients. Importantly, exhalation ports exist on the mask or within a separate attachment in the circuit (non-rebreathing valves or exhalation ports) to introduce an intentional small leak to flush the mask and circuit and prevent rebreathing of exhaled carbon dioxide. Because the ventilator algorithm takes into account leak flow, only circuit tubing and masks recommended by manufacturer should be used with a specific type of NIV ventilator. To further ensure patient safety, care must be taken with the skin sites in contact with the mask. A soft adhesive gelatin patch (Duoderm, Bristol-Myers-Squibb, New York, NY) is used to protect the nasal bridge. The skin in contact with the mask should be assessed routinely for breakdown. Many centers maintain the head-of-bed elevation raised to 30–45 degrees to prevent reflux, aspiration, and ventilator-associated pneumonia.

NIPPV may be applied in the mode of CPAP or BiPAP. BiPAP is a pressure-limited ventilatory mode that resembles the pressure support mode used in conventional (invasive) mechanical ventilation. Patients with neuromuscular disease, obesity hypoventilation syndrome, and acute respiratory failure may benefit from bi-level support (60–62). BiPAP permits the clinician to set the inspiratory positive airway pressure (IPAP) and expiratory positive airway pressure (EPAP) separately.

Much like PEEP with conventional mechanical ventilation, EPAP may improve gas exchange and decreases patient work of breathing by maintaining alveolar recruitment. EPAP also stabilizes upper airway patency during sleep and flushes dead space CO_2. IPAP supports the patient-initiated breath and thereby improves gas exchange and decreases work of breathing. The difference between the IPAP and EPAP is known as the pressure support, and should be at least 4 cm H_2O. EPAP is started for a brief period at 4 cm H_2O and increased to a maximum of 8–12 cm H_2O, with pressure support increased to generate an IPAP 4–6 cm H_2O above EPAP. Most modern BiPAP devices allow a backup ventilator frequency ("backup rate") to be set. The backup rate is typically set at 2 breaths below the patient's spontaneous rate in case the patient becomes apneic.

CPAP delivers a continuous level of positive airway pressure. There is no positive pressure above the CPAP level to initiate inspiration. Therefore, the inspiratory gas flow is achieved only by the patient's inspiratory effort creating a pressure gradient for gas flow from the upper airway to the alveoli. The most common indications for CPAP include obstructive sleep apnea and mild–moderate acute hypoxemic respiratory failure.

The third component of NIPPV involves engaging the patient in using the device and interface successfully. The following steps are recommended to acclimate the child to NIPPV:

- Begin with just a simple mask application without pressure for the initial use.
- Then apply EPAP at no more than 4 cm H_2O.
- Gradually increase EPAP by 2–3 cm H_2O at intervals.
- Apply the pressure support to target the desired IPAP if bi-level support is required.

Most patients tolerate NIPPV and will demonstrate improvement in work of breathing, dyspnea scores, and physiologic parameters such as respiratory rate (on average, a drop of 10–20 resp/min) and heart rate. Some patients receiving chronic daytime NIPPV may tolerate periods without NIPPV to allow for feeding, physical therapy, cough assist, and/or other nebulizer treatments as needed (59). Conversely, acute respiratory failure patients will require continuous application of NIPPV, with limited or no breaks in the initial 24–48 hours, to achieve target goals. These patients must be monitored carefully for any signs of worsening disease or refractory hypercarbia and/or hypoxemia. Aerosol medication can be administered without interruption using MDI or standard nebulizer through a T-piece connection.

NIPPV can be delivered by either a full-scale conventional mechanical ventilator that delivers a full range of ventilator modes or a lightweight, portable device designed only for NIPPV. Various conventional mechanical ventilators (e.g., Servo-i with NIV software, Bridgewater, NJ, Newport Wace, Newport E-500, Newport Medical Instruments, Newport, CA) and various portable mechanical ventilators (e.g., BIPAP STD 30 and VISION, Respironics, Murrysville, PA) may be used to provide NIPPV.

Conventional ventilators provide full monitoring functions, alarm settings, pressure-limited and volume-limited ventilation, and the ability to deliver precise F_{IO_2} at high levels with separate inhalation and exhalation circuit limbs to prevent rebreathing. Pressure-controlled breaths on conventional ventilators are delivered at set pressure and for a set inspiratory time. The advantage of the pressure-limited modes is compensation for leaks, which are common in patients receiving NIPPV. In the pressure-limited mode, the flow varies according to patient demand, making it easier for the patient to synchronize with the ventilator. Volume-limited ventilator modes, on the other hand, may have the advantage of providing a relatively constant tidal volume in the face of changing lung characteristics (increasing airways resistance/worsening lung compliance). However, a disadvantage to the volume-limited mode is that this mode may not come with a pressure limit, which may lead to gastric distension or barotrauma in susceptible patients. Also, the inspiratory flow rate is fixed in volume preset modes. Hence, if the flow demand of the patient exceeds the set flow rate, the patient will experience respiratory distress and ventilator dyssynchrony.

In contrast to the broad controls available on conventional mechanical ventilators, portable ventilators used for NIPPV will likely provide only the pressure support mode in which the pressure support breath is delivered and terminates when the flow rate decreases to a predetermined percentage of the initial flow. Therefore, the portable ventilators are very susceptible to leaks within the mask and inspiratory circuit, which may cause patient–ventilator dyssynchrony. Portable ventilators also have only a single tubing for inspiratory and expiratory gas mixtures with the potential for rebreathing expired gas. Finally, portable ventilators lack the ability to deliver precise control of oxygen–air mixture due to variations caused with the patient's respiratory pattern and by dilution of the FIO_2 by the base flow during the EPAP phase. Conversely, portable devices are much less expensive and can be used in the home, making them suitable for patients with mild–moderate disease.

Clinical Application

NIPPV is indicated in patients with acute respiratory failure (e.g., sickle cell acute chest syndrome, asthma, bronchiolitis, pneumonia, congestive heart failure), dynamic upper airway obstruction (e.g., obstructive sleep apnea), alveolar hypoventilation syndromes (e.g., congenital central hypoventilation syndrome, obesity hypoventilation syndrome), and chronic respiratory failure (e.g., cystic fibrosis). A favorable response to NIPPV is heralded by reduced heart rate, respiratory rate, and $PaCO_2$, as well as increased O_2 saturation and pH.

NIPPV has been used successfully in infants and children with poor systolic ventricular function after open-heart surgery (63). These patients are very sensitive to increased afterload to the heart, which is reflected by the left ventricular transmural pressure (LV_{TM}), where

$$LV_{TM} = \text{aortic pressure} - \text{pleural pressure}$$

Infants with cardiac disease and respiratory distress develop very negative pleural pressures, which lead to increased LV_{TM} and hence increased LV afterload. NIPPV is effective in relieving respiratory distress, lowering LV_{TM} and afterload, which allows (re)intubation to be avoided.

NIPPV is not suited for patients with severe hemodynamic instability, high risk of aspiration, or severe lung disease requiring higher levels of PEEP. These populations include patients with active or recent cardiorespiratory arrest, shock, multiorgan dysfunction, and severe neurologic dysfunction (lost protective airway reflexes, status epilepticus, persistent neonatal apnea, or Glasgow coma scale <10). NIPPV has demonstrated less efficacy for adults with a primary oncologic process or other primary extrapulmonary conditions (62,64,65). A full face mask is contraindicated in a patient with persistent vomiting and in patients with active upper GI/nasopharyngeal bleeding. Young children who are unable to pull the mask off in the event of blockage of the exhalation ports must be monitored closely in the ICU.

A randomized controlled trial (RCT) of NIPPV compared conventional oxygen therapy versus conventional therapy plus BiPAP in 50 pediatric patients with acute respiratory failure age 1 month to 15 years, and found a significant reduction in the need for endotracheal intubation and improved physiologic parameters (respiratory rate and heart rate) with the use of BiPAP (66). A number of other pediatric case–control studies document success of NIPPV in acute hypoxemic respiratory

failure and in higher risk groups such as patients with oncologic disease, status post bone marrow transplantation, and patients with ARDS (62,67–70).

Use of Noninvasive Positive-Pressure Ventilation Postextubation

NIPPV for postextubation respiratory support is either part of the planned transition from invasive mechanical ventilation to unassisted spontaneous breathing or a rescue application for patients who fail extubation (64,71). Elective application of NIPPV immediately after extubation appears to be more effective than rescue NIPPV (72). We have certainly seen an increase in the standard and broad use of NIPPV postextubation. We find it is helpful when applied to children thought to be at high risk. Although some children may have been extubated successfully without NIPPV, the risks of NIPPV are low.

Noninvasive Positive-Pressure Ventilation in Neuromuscular Disease

BiPAP can be used to support patients with chronic neuromuscular disease at baseline, during respiratory illness, for postoperative recovery, and in settings of acute illness. These patients additionally have chronic respiratory insufficiency and cough insufficiency, and may have swallowing dysfunction. Some neuromuscular disease patients require NIPPV only during sleep. Others (such as many spinal muscular atrophy patients) use NIPPV around the clock in conjunction with airway clearance devices such as cough assist.

Settings and duration of use are optimized to achieve adequate inspiratory chest wall expansion and air entry, improve work of breathing, and to normalize respiratory rate. The IPAP is often increased to 12–24 cm H_2O and EPAP to 3–8 cm H_2O. Patients who are unable to completely trigger will require a backup or minimum ventilatory rate. Clinicians should attempt to wean FIO_2 as tolerated. An increasing supplemental oxygen requirement may mask atelectasis owing to retained secretions in these patients. Desaturations may signal mucus plugging, atelectasis, or other V̇/Q̇ mismatch. Therefore, evaluation of chest x-ray or use of cough assist, and judicious use of increased pressure settings are the best interventions for desaturations rather than increased FIO_2. Weaning toward the prior baseline pressure settings should not occur until FIO_2 needs are at baseline levels of support.

Safety Considerations

20 One potential concern for NIPPV use is that it might give the clinical team a false sense of reassurance and delay a necessary intubation. In an adult prospective RCT, Esteban et al. (73) examined postextubation failure within 48 hours randomized to NIV versus standard treatment (supplemental O_2, physiotherapy, and bronchodilators). Although there was no difference in reintubation rate or mortality, the NIV group had a trend toward higher mortality (26% vs. 14%, $p = 0.48$). The median time from extubation to reintubation was longer in the NIV group (12 vs. 2.5 hours, $p = 0.02$), and a higher percentage of adults who required reintubation following NIV therapy died. A pediatric study compared elective NIV applied immediately after extubation of high-risk patients against rescue NIV applied after demonstrated failure of supplemental O_2 standard therapy. Elective NIV had a greater success rate of avoiding reintubation than rescue NIV (81% vs. 50%, $p = 0.037$) (72). Early initiation of NIV may be most successful when applied to the patient before muscle fatigue and progressive respiratory failure.

Early detection of clinical deterioration in patients receiving NIV therapy is important. This requires training to understand use of the devices and recognition of clinical deterioration requiring escalation. A higher likelihood of failed NIV therapy occurs in patients who have difficulty tolerating the device, hypoxemic respiratory failure, a higher severity of illness score, persistent tachypnea, or inability to wean F_{IO_2} in the presence of a high mean airway pressure (72, 74).

NIV allows enteral nutrition in most patients, which is associated with improved outcomes compared with parenteral nutrition. In general, there are no guidelines to favor a specific mode of enteral feeding (continuous vs. intermittent, gastric vs. postpyloric) (75–78). However, a recent meta-analysis revealed that jejuna feedings were associated with a lower relative risk of pneumonia (but no difference in vomiting or aspiration) compared with gastric feedings (79). In most cases, feeding is delivered via nasogastric tube, and the head of bed is elevated to at least 30 degrees to avoid aspiration. Enteral feedings are stopped for overt vomiting, suctioning material from mouth, higher residual gastric volumes, abdominal distension, or absent bowel sounds. Oral feedings may be offered when the patient is not receiving BiPAP based upon an assessment of the acuity of lung disease, work of breathing, or likelihood of intubation. Extra precautions must be taken if considering oral feedings in patients at high risk for aspiration, including patients with neuromuscular weakness, and gastroesophageal reflux disease and neonates with mouth breathing, poor oromotor coordination, and high palatal airway resistance.

High-Flow Nasal Cannula

Principles

HFNC oxygen therapy is a form of NIV and respiratory support that provides heated and humidified flow of air–oxygen mixtures to increase oxygen delivery, prevent the associated drying of upper airway mucosa, and increase patient comfort. The principle underlying HFNC is to set the air–oxygen flow rate from the flow meter greater than the child's inspiratory flow demand so that the child's inspired gas consists predominantly of air–oxygen mixture through the nasal cannulas without the need to entrain room air from the hypopharynx and thereby dilute the F_{IO_2}. HFNC systems offer independent adjustment of F_{IO_2} and humidified, warm gas flow titrated to match the inspiratory flow demands of tachypneic patients. HFNC flow may improve gas exchange via a number of proposed mechanisms including the following:

- An oxygen reservoir in the anatomic airways allowing for delivery of ~100% F_{IO_2} (higher than is achieved with non-rebreather or other high-flow sources);
- Bulk flow rinsing of airway dead space;
- Positive airway pressure effect;
- Greater patient tolerance of the device reducing anxiety and thoracoabdominal dyssynchrony;
- Ability of patients to expectorate to clear pulmonary secretions and to participate more actively in physical therapy.

Clinical Application

The advantages of HFNC as compared to NIPPV are the application of flow via nasal prongs similar to a routine nasal cannula to avoid the claustrophobic sensation of a face mask. This approach may allow patients to eat, drink, and speak during their use. Another advantage is the independent titration of flow and F_{IO_2}. Finally, the use of HFNC systems can be easily initiated in a variety of clinical settings such as emergency room, acute care units, and postsurgical care units. Although utilization of this NIV modality has increased and generated substantial literature, a recent systematic review concluded that there were no RCTs of sufficient quality to allow specific HFNC guidelines in respiratory support (80).

HFNC has been used clinically to provide higher F_{IO_2} for patients who present with persistent hypoxemia refractory to low-flow nasal cannula or face masks. Clinicians have applied HFNC as an alternative to NIPPV in the following settings (81–84):

- Neonatal respiratory distress syndrome (RDS);
- Neonatal apnea;
- Impending acute respiratory failure in pediatric and adult patients;
- Postextubation respiratory distress (impending respiratory failure);
- Comfort care for patients with do-not-intubate orders.

A positive response to HFNC is indicated by improved O_2 saturations, decreased dyspnea, improved thoracoabdominal synchrony, and improved comfort with decreased anxiety. Variable outcomes emphasize that HFNC may not be applicable as an alternative to positive-pressure ventilation in all situations of respiratory distress. Most notably, patients may require positive airway distending pressures that cannot be supplied by HFNC for respiratory distress secondary to obstructive upper airway disease, bronchomalacia, neuromuscular chest wall weakness or kyphoscoliosis, and for pediatric and adult patients with moderately significant atelectasis. Close clinical monitoring is required for patients receiving HFNC to detect early signs of progressive respiratory failure requiring escalation of therapy. There may be an unfortunate misperception among staff and clinicians that the device in use is a simple nasal cannula, thus failing to recognize the significant flow and oxygen support provided during HFNC use. Caution is also warranted in the neonatal population, where clinicians must recognize that NC flow or HFNC flow of >2 L has been associated with positive airway pressure and the risk of barotrauma. This risk is heightened because HFNC systems usually do not have accurate pressure alarms. Hyperoxia is an additional risk, particularly in the newborn if oxygen blenders are not used.

Delivery Systems

The HFNC device interface consists of short binasal prongs with manufacturer-recommended prong size that fit within the nares according to septum width without abrasion or pressure along the nare. Measuring patient septum width and avoiding indiscriminate use of prong size is important for two reasons. First, the larger the outer diameter of the prong, the more likely it will occlude the nostril, leading to the potential of positive airway pressure and barotrauma in the patient. Second, indiscriminate size of nasal prongs can cause pressure necrosis to delicate nasal tissues.

Several devices are available that combine a heated humidifier with an air/oxygen blender and a separate in-line oxygen analyzer. The Fisher & Paykel OptiFlow HFNC system uses a heated humidifier with hot-plate and single-use water chamber. Humidified gas mixtures exit the humidifier through large bore corrugated tubing that connects to the cannula with a 15-mm outer diameter adapter. A heated wire circuit is used to minimize condensation to prevent liquid water from obstructing the HFNC. Flow continues through an 18-cm length of 10-mm outer diameter flex tubing and finally to the cannula. The Vapotherm Precision high-flow humidification system uses a cartridge-like humidifier with an integrated air/O_2 blender and oxygen analyzer. The device has high-pressure sensors to detect downstream obstruction. Both devices allow for independent titration of flow and of F_{IO_2}.

F_{IO_2} and flow are adjusted to achieve target physiologic goals. HFNC is capable of delivering F_{IO_2} of 0.62, 0.82, 0.9, and 0.92 with flows of 10, 15, 20, and 30 L/min, respectively. A range of FIO_2 between 0.4 and 0.80 has been measured in infants receiving as little as 2 L/min flow on HFNC (85). Recommended flow rates are ≤2 L/min for premature or term infants: up to 12 L/min for older infants to toddlers, up to 30 L/min for children, and up to 40 L/min for adults. Although not validated, an estimate of HFNC for infants may be calculated using the formula HFNC flow = $0.92 + 0.68w$, where w = weight in kg (4, 86).

Positive airway pressures produced by HFNC vary by nasal prong selection, mouth breathing, and age and size of the patient, and have demonstrated large nonpredictable interpatient variability. For adults receiving 20, 40, and 60 L/min flow, mean pharyngeal pressures were 3.7, 7.2, and 8.7 cm H_2O, respectively, with a closed mouth. With mouth breathing, pressures fell to 1.4, 2.2, and 2.7 cm H_2O, respectively, at the same flow levels (87). Older patients have also been able to drop the inspiratory pressure to zero, which may be a key difference between HFNC and CPAP (87). During weaning support, flow is typically reduced in 10%–25% increments over time. Conversion to low-flow nasal cannula may be well tolerated for pediatric patients receiving ≤4 L/min and for adults receiving ≤6 L/min. If low-flow nasal cannula O_2 is not humidified (or humidified by standard bubble humidification), patients may still be more comfortable receiving the humidified and warmed airflow of the HFNC device.

Safety Considerations

HFNC devices provide a noninvasive, well-tolerated form of respiratory support that can provide several advantages for patient and respiratory care providers over NIPPV systems. However, close clinical monitoring is necessary, as failure to respond to HFNC therapy may indicate the need for intervention including intubation. Patients with sustained tachypnea, failure to tolerate weaning of FIO_2, and continued thoracoabdominal dyssynchrony or who develop alteration in mental status, respiratory acidosis, and/or progression to shock or multiorgan system failure are likely to fail HFNC and require invasive mechanical ventilation. Lost or absent airway protective reflexes mandate intubation.

When HFNC is well tolerated, patients are comfortable, require no sedation, may be able to participate in physical therapy, and are better able to tolerate eating, drinking, and speaking owing to maintained flow and oxygen than with BiPAP, where the O_2 supply through the mask must be removed to allow the patient to eat, drink, or speak.

Though no guidelines exist for enteral feeding regimens in patients receiving HFNC, we have found it useful to evaluate the following factors to guide introduction of enteral feedings:

- Tachypnea;
- Accessory muscle use;
- Agitation;
- Ability to clear secretions;
- Degree of lung aeration.

Clearly, if one or more of these factors suggest a moderate to high risk of intubation, enteral feedings will be withheld. Otherwise, patients are candidates for enteral feeding if they are within 1 standard deviation of age-appropriate vital signs and have only mild respiratory distress. We will maintain head-of-bed elevation to at least 30 degrees during gastric feedings. We generally recommend postpyloric feeds when older infants receive HFNC ≥8–10 L and in patients of any age who have reflux or a history of aspiration, or require the higher HFNC flows for age (75–78, 88).

Though HFNC has been successfully used in emergency departments, delivery rooms, hospital wards and perioperative areas, it is important to maintain training and education for all clinical staff on the use of HFNC. The importance of early recognition of respiratory failure is imperative. Further, the misidentification or unfortunate perception of this device as "a simple nasal cannula" can lead to underappreciation of the patient's severity of respiratory illness and current level of respiratory support.

CONCLUSIONS AND FUTURE DIRECTIONS

Inhaled medical gas therapies and medications provide a powerful therapeutic modality in patients with cardiorespiratory disease. Critical care personnel should understand the therapeutic potential and appropriate delivery and safe-handling practices of commonly used inhaled gas therapies. Careful patient selection, meticulous attention to the safe device setup, and close monitoring are the keys to successful application of these techniques. In the future, the spectrum of pharmacologic agents is expected to increase that target-specific disease processes via inhaled and noninvasive techniques.

References

1. Cook D, De Jonghe B, Brochard L, et al. Influence of airway management on ventilator-associated pneumonia: Evidence from randomized trials. JAMA 1998;279(10):781–7. Erratum in: JAMA 1999;281(22):2089.
2. Branson RD. The nuts and bolts of increasing arterial oxygenation: Devices and techniques. Respir Care 1993;38:672–86.
3. Ward JJ. High-flow oxygen administration by nasal cannula for adult and perinatal patients. Respir Care 2013;58:98–120.
4. Sreenan C, Lemke RP, Hudson-Mason A, et al. High-flow nasal cannula in the management of apnea of prematurity: A comparison with conventional nasal continuous positive airway pressure. Pediatrics 2001;107:1081–3.
5. McPherson SP. Gas regulation, administration and controlling devices. In: McPherson SP, ed. Respiratory Therapy Equipment. 4th ed. St. Louis, MO: CV Mosby, 1990:50–78.
6. Deneke SM, Fanburg BL. Normobaric oxygen toxicity of the lung. N Engl J Med 1980;303:76.
7. Budinger GR, Mutlu GM. Balancing the risks and benefits of oxygen therapy in critically ill adults. Chest 2013;143(4):1151–62.
8. Lodato RF. Oxygen toxicity. Crit Care Clin 1990;6:749–65.
9. Robinson TD, Freiberg DB, Regnis JA, et al. The role of hypoventilation and ventilation-perfusion redistribution in oxygen-induced hypercapnia during acute exacerbation of chronic obstructive pulmonary disease. Am J Respir Crit Care Med 2000;161:1524–9.
10. Sassoon CS, Hassell KT, Mahutte CK. Hyperoxic-induced hypercapnia in stable chronic obstructive pulmonary disease. Am Rev Respir Dis 1987;135:907–11.
11. Johnston RG, Noseworthy TW, Friesen EG, et al. Isoflurane therapy for status asthmaticus in children and adults. Chest 1990;97:698–701.
12. Moya MP, Gow AJ, Califf RM, et al. Inhaled ethyl nitrite gas for persistent pulmonary hypertension of the newborn. Lancet 2002;360:141–3.
13. Creagh-Brown BC, Griffiths MJD, Evans TW. Bench-to-bedside review: Inhales nitric oxide therapy in adults. Crit Care 2009;13:212–20.
14. Platt DR, Swanton D, Blackney D. Inhaled nitric oxide (iNO) delivery with high-frequency jet ventilation (HFJV). J Perinatol 2003;23:387–91.
15. Gerlach H, Keh D, Semmerow A, et al. Dose-response characteristics during long-term inhalation of nitric oxide in patients with severe

acute respiratory distress syndrome: A prospective, randomized, controlled study. *Am J Respir Crit Care Med* 2003;167:1008–15.

16. Griffiths MJD, TW Evans. Drug therapy: Inhaled nitric oxide therapy in adults. *N Engl J Med* 2005;353:2683–95.

17. Sitbon O, Brenot F, Denjean A, et al. Inhaled nitric oxide as a screening vasodilator agent in primary pulmonary hypertension. *Am J Respir Crit Care Med* 1995;151:384–9.

18. Afshari A, Brok J, Møller AM, et al. Inhaled nitric oxide for acute respiratory distress syndrome and acute lung injury in adults and children: A systematic review with meta-analysis and trial sequential analysis. *Anesth Analg* 2011;112(6):1411–21.

19. Pearl JM, Nelson DP, Raake JL, et al. Inhaled nitric oxide increases endothelin-1 levels: A potential cause of rebound pulmonary hypertension. *Crit Care Med* 2002;30:89–93.

20. Donohue PK, Gilmore MM, Cristofalo E, et al. Inhaled nitric oxide in preterm infants: A systematic review. *Pediatrics* 2011; 127:e414–22.

21. Goissen C, Ghyselen L, Tourneux P, et al. Persistent pulmonary hypertension of the newborn with transposition of the great arteries: Successful treatment with bosentan. *Eur J Pediatr* 2008;167:437–40.

22. Mourani PM, Sontag MK, Ivy DD, et al. Effects of long-term sildenafil treatment for pulmonary hypertension in infants with chronic lung disease. *J Pediatr* 2009;154:384:379–84.

23. Porta NFM, Steinhorn RH. Pulmonary vasodilator therapy in the NICU: Inhaled nitric oxide, sildenafil, and other pulmonary vasodilating agents. *Clin Perinatol* 2012;39:149–64.

24. Steinhorn RH, Kinsella JP, Pierce C, et al. Intravenous sildenafil in the treatment of neonates with persistent pulmonary hypertension. *J Pediatr* 2009;155:841–7.

25. Gupta VK, Cheifetz IM. Heliox administration in the pediatric intensive care unit: An evidence-based review. *Ped Crit Care Med* 2005;6:204–11.

26. Moraa I, Sturman N, McGuire T, et al. Heliox for croup in children. *Cochrane Database Syst Rev* 2013;12:CD006822.

27. Rodeberg DA, Easter AJ, Washam MA, et al. Use of a helium-oxygen mixture in the treatment of postextubation stridor in pediatric patients with burns. *J Burn Care Rehabil* 1995;16:476–80.

28. Anderson M, Svartengren M, Bylin G, et al. Deposition in asthmatics of particles inhaled in air or in helium-oxygen. *Am Rev Respir Dis* 1993;147(3):524–8.

29. National Asthma Education and Prevention Program. Expert panel report III: Guidelines for the diagnosis and management of asthma (NIH publication no. 08-4051). Bethesda, MD: National Heart, Lung, and Blood Institute, 2007. www.nhlbi.nih.gov/guidelines/asthma/asthgdln.htm. Accessed July 3, 2014.

30. Gluck EH, Onorato DJ, Castriotta R. Helium-oxygen mixtures in intubated patients with status asthmaticus and respiratory acidosis. *Chest* 1990;98:693–8.

31. Hess DR, Acosta FL, Ritz RH, et al. The effect of heliox on nebulizer function using a beta-agonist bronchodilator. *Chest* 1999;115:184–9.

32. Berkenbosch JW, Grueber RE, Dabbagh O, et al. Effect of helium-oxygen (heliox) gas mixtures on the function of four pediatric ventilators. *Crit Care Med* 2003;31(7):2052–8.

33. Myers TR. Therapeutic gases for neonatal and pediatric respiratory care. *Respir Care* 2003;48:399–422.

34. Tassaux D, Jolliet P, Thouret JM, et al. Calibration of seven ICU ventilators for mechanical ventilation with helium-oxygen mixtures. *Am J Respir Crit Care Med* 1999;27:1603–7.

35. Katz AL, Gentile MA, Craig DM, et al. Heliox does not affect gas exchange during high-frequency oscillatory ventilation if tidal volume is held constant. *Crit Care Med* 2003;31(7):2006–9.

36. Gern JE, Lemanske RF Jr. Beta-adrenergic agonist therapy. *Immunol Allergy Clin North Am* 1993;13:839.

37. Gibson P, Powell H, Ducharme F, et al. Long-acting beta2-agonists as an inhaled corticosteroid-sparing agent for chronic asthma in adults and children. *Cochrane Database Syst Rev* 2005;CD005076.

38. Carl JC, Myers TR, Kirchner HL, et al. Comparison of racemic albuterol and levalbuterol for treatment of acute asthma. *J Pediatr* 2003;143(6):731–6.

39. Duarte AG, Momii K, Bidani A. Bronchodilator therapy with metered-dose inhaler and spacer versus nebulizer in mechanically ventilated patients: Comparison of magnitude and duration of response. *Respir Care* 2000;45:817–23.

40. Holland A, Smith F, Penny K, et al. Metered dose inhalers versus nebulizers for aerosol bronchodilator delivery for adult patients receiving mechanical ventilation in critical care units. *Cochrane Database Syst Rev* 2013;6:CD008863.

41. Miller DD, Amin MM, Palmer LB, et al. Aerosol delivery and modern mechanical ventilation: In vitro/in vivo evaluation. *Am J Respir Crit Care Med* 2003;168:1205–9.

42. Georgopoulos D, Mouloudi E, Kondili E, et al. Bronchodilator delivery with metered-dose inhaler during mechanical ventilation. *Crit Care* 2000;4(4):227–34.

43. Hanhan U, Kissoon N, Payne M, et al. Effects of in-line nebulization on preset ventilatory variables. *Respir Care* 1993;38:474–8.

44. Hess D. Inhaled bronchodilators during mechanical ventilation: Delivery techniques, evaluation of response, and cost effectiveness. *Respir Care* 1994;39:105–22.

45. Kofke WA, Snider MT, Young RS, et al. Prolonged low flow isoflurane anesthesia for status epilepticus: A clinical series. *Anesthesiology* 1985;62:653–6.

46. Tobias JD. Therapeutic applications and uses of inhalational anesthesia in the pediatric intensive care unit. *Pediatr Crit Care Med* 2008;9:169–79.

47. Bratton SL, Odetola FO, McCollegan J, et al. Regional variation in ICU care for pediatric patients with asthma. *J Pediatr* 2005;147:355–61.

48. Curley MA, Molengraft JA. Providing comfort to critically ill pediatric patients: Isoflurane. *Crit Care Nurs Clin North Am* 1995;7:267–74.

49. Kong KL, Willats SM, Prys-Roberts C. Isoflurane compared with midazolam for sedation in the intensive care unit. *BMJ* 1989;298:1277–80.

50. Char DS, Ibsen LM, Ramamoorthy C, et al. Volatile anesthetic rescue therapy in children with acute asthma: Innovative but costly or just costly? *Pediatr Crit Care Med* 2013;14:343–50.

51. Maltais F, Sovilj M, Goldberg P, et al. Respiratory mechanics in status asthmaticus. Effects of inhalational anesthesia. *Chest* 1994;106:1401–6.

52. Shankar V, Churchwell K, Deshpande JS. Isoflurane therapy for severe refractory status asthmaticus in children. *Intensive Care Med* 2006;32:927–33.

53. Turner DA, Heitz D, Cooper M, et al. Isoflurane for life-threatening bronchospasm: A 15-year single-center experience. *Respir Care* 2012;57:1857–64.

54. Wheeler DS, Clapp CR, Ponaman ML, et al. Isoflurane therapy for status asthmaticus in children: A case series and protocol. *Pediatr Crit Care Med* 2000;1:55–9.

55. Kong KL. Inhalational anesthetics in the intensive care unit. *Crit Care Clin* 1995;11:887–902.

56. Arnold JH, Truog RD, Rice SA. Prolonged administration of isoflurane to pediatric patients during mechanical ventilation. *Anesth Analg* 1993;76:520–6.

57. Kong KL. Isoflurane sedation for patients undergoing mechanical ventilation: Metabolism to inorganic fluoride and renal effects. *Br J Anaesth* 1990;64:159–62.

58. Najaf-Zadeh A, Leclerc F. Noninvasive positive pressure ventilation for acute respiratory failure in children: A concise review. *Ann Intensive Care* 2011;1:15–25.

59. Baudouin S, Blumenthal S, Cooper B, et al. BTS Guideline: Non-invasive ventilation in acute respiratory failure: British Thoracic Society Standards of Care Committee. *Thorax* 2002; 57:192–211.

60. Marohn K, Panisello JM. Noninvasive ventilation in pediatric intensive care. *Curr Opin Pediatr* 2013;25:290–6.

61. Roper H, Quinlivan R, et al. Implementation of the "consensus statement for the standard of care in spinal muscular atrophy" when applied to infants with sever type I SMA in the UK. *Arch Dis Child* 2010;95:845–9.

62. Schettino G, Altobelli BA, Kacmarek RM. Noninvasive positive-pressure ventilation in acute respiratory failure outside clinical trials: Experience at the Massachusetts General Hospital. *Crit Care Med* 2008;36:441–7.

63. Gupta P, Kuperstock JE, Hashmi S, et al. Efficacy and predictors of success of noninvasive ventilation for prevention of extubation failure in critically ill children with heart disease. *Pediatr Cardiol* 2013;34:964–77.

64. Bersten AD, Holt AW, Vedig AE, et al. Treatment of severe cardiogenic pulmonary edema with continuous positive airway pressure delivered by face mask. *N Engl J Med* 1991;325:1825–30.

65. Masip J, Roque M, Sanchez B, et al. Noninvasive ventilation in acute cardiogenic pulmonary edema: Systematic review and meta-analysis. *JAMA* 2005;294:3124–30.

66. Yanez LJ, Yunge M, Emifork M, et al. A prospective, randomized, controlled trial of noninvasive ventilation in pediatric acute respiratory failure. *Pediatr Crit Care Med* 2008;9:484–9.

67. Dohna-Schwake C, Stehling F, Tschiedel E, et al. Noninvasive ventilation on a pediatric intensive care unit: Feasibility, efficacy, and predictors of success. *Pediatr Pulmonol* 2011;46:1114–20.

68. Fortenberry JD, Del Torro J, Jefferson LS, et al. Management of pediatric acute hypoxemic respiratory insufficiency with bilevel positive pressure (BiPAP) nasal mask ventilation. *Chest* 1995;108:1059–64.

69. Padman R, Lawless ST, Kettrick RG. Noninvasive ventilation via bilevel positive airway pressure support in pediatric practice. *Crit Care Med* 1998;26:169–73.

70. Pancera CF, Hayashi M, Fregnani JH, et al. Noninvasive ventilation in immunocompromised pediatric patients eight years of experience in a pediatric oncology intensive care unit. *J Pediatr Hematol Oncol* 2008;30:533–8.

71. Keenan SP, Powers C, McCormack DG, et al. Noninvasive positive pressure ventilation for postextubation respiratory distress: A randomized controlled trial. *JAMA* 2002;287:3238–44.

72. Mayordomo-Colunga J, Medina A, Rey C, et al. Noninvasive ventilation after extubation in pediatric patients: a preliminary study. *BMC Pediatrics* 2010;10:29–37.

73. Esteban A, Frutos-Vivar F, Ferguson ND, et al. Noninvasive positive pressure ventilation for respiratory failure after extubation. *N Engl J Med* 2004;350:2452–60.

74. Piastra M, De Luca D, Pietrini D, et al. Noninvasive pressure-support ventilation in immunocompromised children with ARDS: A feasibility study. *Intensive Care Med* 2009;35:1420–7.

75. Heyland DK, Drover JW, MacDonald S, et al. Effect of postpyloric feeding on gastroesophageal regurgitation and pulmonary micro-aspiration: Results of a randomized controlled trial. *Crit Care Med* 2001;29:1495–501.

76. Meert KL, Daphtary KM, Metheny NA. Gastric vs. small-bowel feeding in critically ill children receiving mechanical ventilation: A randomized controlled trial. *Chest* 2004;126:872–8.

77. Mehta NM. Approach to enteral feeding in the PICU. *Nutr Clin Pract* 2009;24:377.

78. Skillman HE, Mehta NM. Nutrition therapy in the critically ill child. *Curr Opin Crit Care* 2012;18:192–8.

79. Jiyong J, Tiancha H, Huiqin W, et al. Effect of gastric versus post pyloric feeding on the incidence of pneumonia in critically ill patients: Observations from traditional and Bayesian random-effects meta-analysis. *Clin Nutr* 2013;32:8–15.

80. Mayfield S, Jauncey-Cooke J, Hough HL, et al. High-flow nasal cannula therapy for respiratory support in children. *Cochrane Database Syst Rev* 2014;3:CD009850.

81. Chawla R, Khilnani GC, Suri N, et al. Guidelines for noninvasive ventilation in acute respiratory failure. *Indian J Crit Care Med* 2006;10:117–47.

82. Holets S, Gay P, Peters S. Nasal high flow (NHF) therapy in do-not-intubate patients with respiratory distress. *Respir Crit Care* 2013;58:597–600.

83. Lee JH, Rehder KJ, Williford L, et al. Use of high flow nasal cannula in critically ill infants, children, and adults: A critical review of the literature. *Intensive Care Med* 2013;39:247–57.

84. McKiernan C, Chua LC, Visintainer PF, et al. High flow nasal cannulae therapy in infants with bronchiolitis. *J Pediatr* 2010;156:634–8.

85. Kuluz JW, McLaughlin GE, Gelman B, et al. The fraction of inspired oxygen in infants receiving oxygen via nasal cannula often exceeds safe levels. *Respir Care* 2001;46:897–901.

86. Kubicka ZJ, Limauro J, Darnall RA. Heated humidified high-flow nasal cannula therapy: Yet another way to deliver continuous positive airway pressure? *Pediatrics* 2008;121:82–8.

87. Groves N, Tobin A. A high flow nasal oxygen generates positive airway pressure in adult volunteers. *Aust Crit Care* 2007;20:126–31.

88. Zamberlan P, Delgado AF, Leone C, et al. Nutrition therapy in a pediatric intensive care unit: Indications, monitoring, and complications. *JPEN J Parenter Enteral Nutr* 2011;35:523–30.

CHAPTER 40 ■ EXTRACORPOREAL LIFE SUPPORT

GRAEME MACLAREN, STEVEN A. CONRAD, AND HEIDI J. DALTON

KEY POINTS

1 Extracorporeal life support (ECLS) is the application of extracorporeal technology to facilitate gas exchange or circulatory support, including extracorporeal membrane oxygenation (ECMO) and related techniques.

2 ECLS can improve outcomes in children with refractory cardiac or respiratory failure.

3 The ECLS circuit compromises a blood pump, oxygenator, cannulas, tubing, a heater-cooler, and monitoring devices.

4 Venovenous (VV) ECLS is the most frequently used support for respiratory failure. Cardiac support is achieved with venoarterial (VA) ECLS, which provides partial cardiopulmonary bypass.

5 Percutaneous cannulation has largely replaced surgical cannulation for VV support, generally by using a dual-lumen catheter in the right internal jugular vein. Surgical cannulation is still required for most cardiac support in children, but percutaneous cannulation for partial support is used in selected cases.

6 Extracorporeal cardiopulmonary resuscitation (ECPR) is the emergent application of ECLS to support patients who have sustained refractory or recurrent cardiac arrest.

7 ECLS induces profound changes in cardiopulmonary physiology, coagulation, and inflammation, which require management in addition to that of the underlying disease.

8 The most common complications of ECLS are bleeding and thrombosis, requiring changes to anticoagulation management, blood component or factor replacement, and occasionally surgical intervention.

9 Data from the Extracorporeal Life Support Organization (ELSO) registry indicates that cumulative survival following ECLS is ~65% for pulmonary support in severe pediatric respiratory failure, ~65% following cardiac support, and 50% following ECPR. Contemporary outcomes are better in select situations.

Extracorporeal life support (ECLS) is the use of a modified cardiopulmonary bypass circuit to support children with refractory respiratory or circulatory failure. This form of life support technology, also known as extracorporeal membrane oxygenation (ECMO), has been used successfully in children since the 1970s and is now regarded as standard therapy in tertiary neonatal and PICUs. Venous blood is removed from the patient, pumped through an oxygenator where carbon dioxide removal and oxygenation occur, and then returned back into the venous (venovenous [VV] ECLS) or arterial circulation (venoarterial [VA] ECLS). Venovenous ECLS is used almost exclusively to provide respiratory support whereas VA ECLS is used for circulatory support or in combined cardiopulmonary failure.

In addition to providing oxygenation, carbon dioxide clearance, and potential circulatory support, another advantage to ECLS is facilitating a reduction in other forms of life support that can perpetuate organ dysfunction. For example, ECLS allows substantial reduction in (or even cessation of) mechanical ventilation and inotropic therapy, thus reducing the risks of ventilator-induced lung injury, myocardial dysfunction, and end-organ damage.

CIRCUIT COMPONENTS

The components of an ECLS circuit, although based on the traditional cardiopulmonary bypass circuit, have been developed or adapted for long-term support (**Fig. 40.1**). Vascular cannulas are placed for blood drainage and reinfusion. A small drainage reservoir (or bladder) helps to ensure continuous availability of blood for the pump. This reservoir is essential in roller-pump circuits and optional in centrifugal pump circuits. A roller or centrifugal pump provides blood flow through the circuit. An artificial lung (oxygenator) provides gas exchange and a heater-cooler provides precise temperature control. Other circuit components allow for infusion of medications, incorporation of a hemofilter or other adjunctive techniques such as plasmapheresis, and monitoring systems for blood gas, flow, and pressure.

Oxygenator

The oxygenator, also referred to as a membrane lung, provides gas exchange between the blood and the atmosphere. Although called an oxygenator, it is more appropriately called an artificial lung, as it transports CO_2 as well as O_2. The need to provide support for days to weeks imposes challenging requirements on oxygenator design.

The traditional oxygenator that has been used since the beginning of ECLS until recently is the spiral-wound solid silicone sheet membrane lung (**Fig. 40.2**). It consists of two long sheets of silicone sealed at the edges and wound on a polycarbonate support. Gas manifolds are attached at the ends and other manifolds provide blood distribution between the rolls. Sizes range from 0.6 to 4.5 m². The larger devices have integrated heat exchangers. Although they served well in the past,

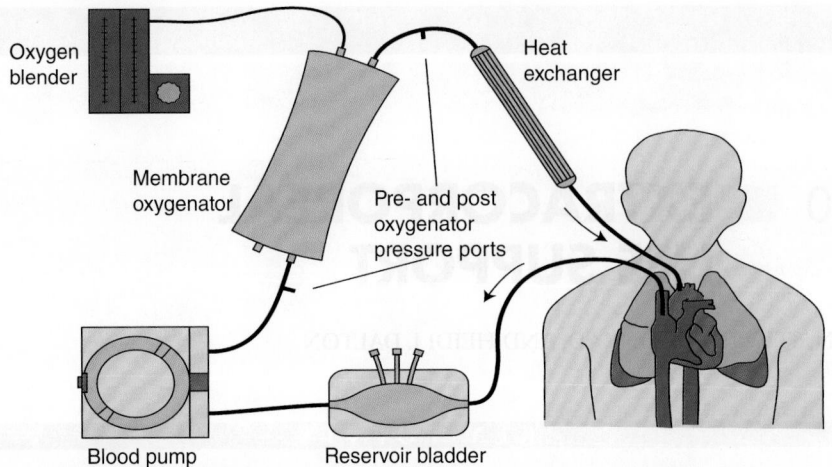

FIGURE 40.1. Components of a typical extracorporeal circuit. The circuit consists of a drainage reservoir (bladder), blood pump, membrane lung, heater-cooler, and connecting tubing. In many modern centrifugal pump circuits, the heater-cooler is integrated into the oxygenator and no reservoir is used (see Fig. 40.9).

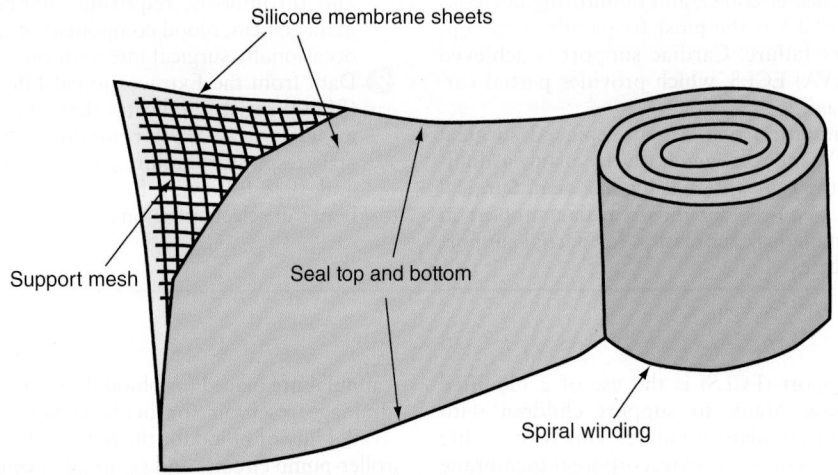

FIGURE 40.2. Solid silicone membrane lung used for ECLS. The silicone sheets are sealed at the edges and wound into a cylinder. The blood path is on the interior of the sheets, with the sweep gas on the exterior. ECLS, extracorporeal life support.

silicone membrane oxygenators had a number of problems compared with the latest generation of oxygenators, including higher resistance to flow, uneven distribution of flow, larger priming volumes, and a bulkier design that compounded the difficulties of ECLS patient transport.

The latest generation of artificial lungs is hollow-fiber oxygenators, constructed with polymethylpentene, which allows gas but not liquid transfer. Smaller than the old silicone membrane lungs, they may cause less platelet consumption and provide more effective gas exchange (1,2). Many of these devices are also coated with heparin to decrease the risk of clotting. Blood flows over the hollow fibers while fresh gas (100% oxygen or an air/oxygen mixture) runs through them, facilitating gas exchange (**Fig. 40.3**). The rate of fresh gas flow ("sweep") is the principal determinant of carbon dioxide clearance. Recent evaluation of data on oxygenator use from the Extracorporeal Life Support Organization (ELSO) shows that over 95% centers now use hollow-fiber oxygenators instead of solid membrane lungs.

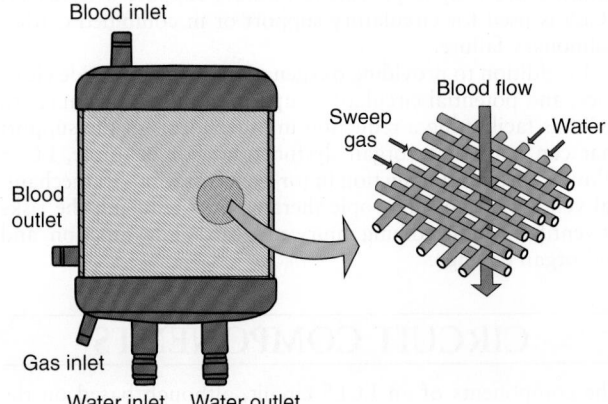

FIGURE 40.3. Hollow-fiber oxygenator. Fresh gas ("sweep") runs through the center of the hollow fibers while blood washes over them.

Blood Pump

Two types of blood pumps are currently used for ECMO. The traditional pump, still widely used throughout North America, is the roller pump, a positive-displacement pump in which a rotating roller head squeezes a length of blood-filled tubing against a backing plate as the roller head rotates (**Fig. 40.4**). This pump is used with gravity drainage, and thus it is necessary to use an assist reservoir (bladder) at the pump inlet to maintain a continuous supply of blood to the pump, as inlet occlusion can result in large negative pressures (-500 mm Hg or more). In the event of outlet tubing obstruction, the pump can generate pressures high enough to cause tubing rupture, requiring continuous monitoring of circuit pressures. When properly used and monitored, this type of pump has a low incidence of complications.

The centrifugal pump is a nonocclusive pump that generates flow via a rotating impeller (**Fig. 40.5**) and has been used for long-term support in many countries outside North America for over a decade. The impeller generates a constrained vortex, creating active suction at the pump inlet which siphons venous blood into the pump, and positive pressure at the pump outlet which propels blood through the oxygenator and back into the patient. These pumps have extremely low incidence of mechanical failure. The main risk with their use is hemolysis. When there is sudden inadequate inflow of blood into the pump (e.g., from hypovolemia or kinking of the venous cannula), the suction generated by the pump is strong enough to cause cavitation and red blood cell lysis (3). A second source of hemolysis in the absence of cavitation is the use of high pump speed in the face of reduced flow from the pump, continuously applying high shear rates with resultant shear injury, and hemolysis. These risks can be lowered by monitoring pump inlet pressure and plasma-free hemoglobin.

The choice of pump and oxygenator depends on product availability and institutional experience and resources. There is some evidence that the latest generation of ECLS equipment is associated with fewer mechanical complications and better patient outcomes than traditional circuitry (4).

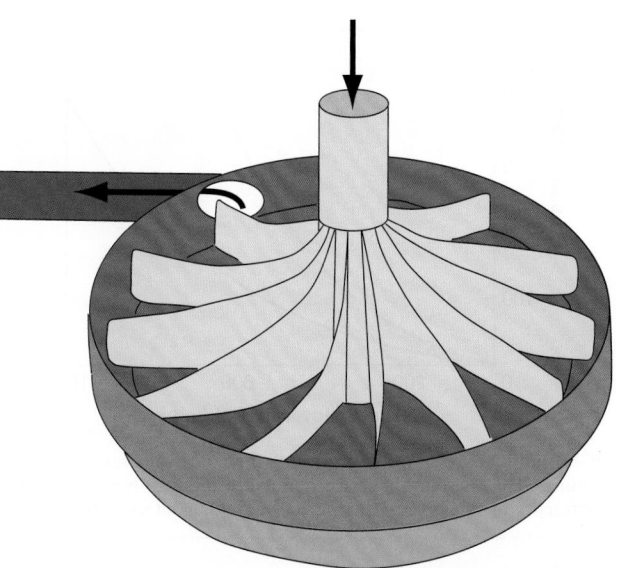

FIGURE 40.5. Centrifugal pump used in extracorporeal circulation. The tapered vanes on the roto create a centrifugal effect that forces blood from the central inlet port to the outer circumference, where it exits.

Vascular Cannulas

Extracorporeal life support requires high blood flows, often equal to cardiac output and occasionally higher. Cannulas of sufficient sizes to support this level of flow are necessary. The single-lumen cannulas used for vascular access are not unique to ECLS, having been developed for cardiovascular surgery. Most cannulas are constructed of polyurethane and may include wire reinforcement to prevent kinking. Cannulas that are placed percutaneously require appropriately sized tissue dilators.

Traditional cannulation employs two single-lumen cannulas, one for venous drainage and a second for return to the venous or arterial circulation. Single-lumen cannulas are used in all modes of support. The cannula size chosen is dictated by the size and flow requirements of the patient and the size of the vessel(s) available for cannulation. Neonates have vessels that range from ~6–10 French (Fr) (carotid artery) to 12–15 Fr (internal jugular vein), whereas adolescents can accommodate up to 20 Fr arterial and 24 Fr venous cannula (or larger).

Double-lumen cannulas have been developed specifically for VV ECLS (**Fig. 40.6**). Placed through the internal jugular vein, these cannulas have two drainage ports located near both atriocaval junctions and a reinfusion port located between these two, directed toward the tricuspid valve. Unlike single-lumen cannulation approaches, the double-lumen cannula is designed to reduce recirculation by capturing blood that returns via both vena cavas.

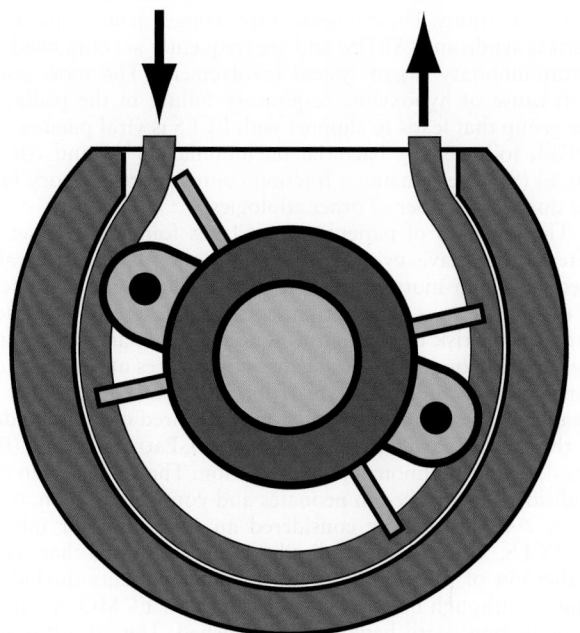

FIGURE 40.4. Roller pump used in extracorporeal circulation. The pump functions by having the rotor pinch and nearly occlude the raceway tubing against a backing plate, and the rotation forces blood through the tubing. The blood flow rate is linearly related to the size of the tubing and the rotational speed of the rotor.

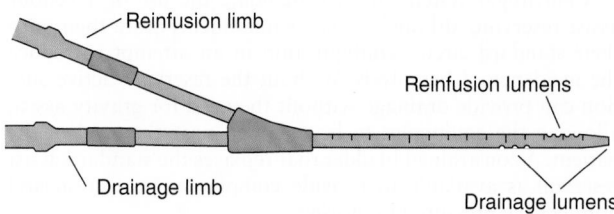

FIGURE 40.6. Double-lumen cannula for single-vessel (right internal jugular) access for venovenous extracorporeal life support.

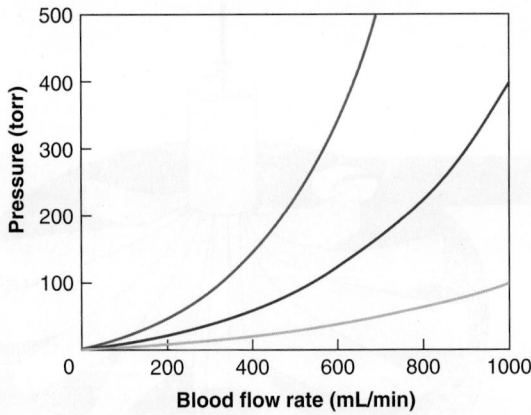

FIGURE 40.7. Pressure-flow curve for three different vascular access cannulas. The relationship between pressure and flow is nonlinear due to presence of side holes, tapering, and development of turbulence.

Blood flow through a vascular cannula is complex and not linearly dependent on pressure. In general, flow is generally not predictable from traditional hydraulic equations. The relationship between the pressure gradient applied to a cannula and the resultant flow is characterized and published as pressure-flow curves (**Fig. 40.7**). The M-number system was developed to characterize flow through ECLS cannulas and represents a single index of resistance based on a correlation between Reynolds numbers and friction factor. The number is experimentally determined for each catheter and allows comparison of expected flows among different cannulas. A higher M-number represents a higher resistance and thus a lower flow at a given driving pressure. An "updated" M-number system ("UM number") has recently been developed to simplify the application of these principles (5). Most centers have a cannulation chart for bedside use that lists cannula sizes alongside expected blood flow rates and patient weights.

OTHER COMPONENTS

Roller-pump systems require continuous availability of blood at the inlet to avoid development of large negative pressures and hemolysis. This availability is ensured by placing a small assist reservoir, or bladder, just before the pump inlet. Gravity assist is achieved by placing the reservoir and pump ~100 cm below the level of the cannula, providing a hydrostatic siphon for drainage and maintaining a positive pressure at the pump inlet. The reservoir also buffers against fluctuations in drainage. If drainage decreases, for example, due to hypovolemia, the reservoir will begin to empty, signaling the need for correction of the cause for poor drainage. Most roller-pump systems have the capability of servoregulation. A switch situated in the reservoir holder opens when the bladder empties, turning off the pump and allowing time for filling of the reservoir. With the pump off, the bladder refills and the pump resumes operation.

Centrifugal systems do not mandate the use of a venous assist reservoir, although some centers incorporate them into their standard circuit configuration in an attempt to reduce the incidence of hemolysis. Without the reservoir, active suction can provide drainage without the need for gravity assist, allowing the equipment to be operated near the level of the patient. A constrained bladder that replaces the standard assist reservoir is available to provide compliance protection and noninvasive pressure monitoring.

The tubing of ECLS circuitry is usually made from polyvinylchloride, although polyurethane and silicone rubber have also been used. Most contemporary ECLS circuits are lined with a surface coating designed to reduce either thrombosis or inflammation, although the effectiveness of these formulations is not well proven. Examples of the former are heparin-bonded coatings and the latter include phosphorylcholine or poly (2-methoxyethylacrylate). Regardless of the coating used, ECLS circuits bind many lipophilic drugs, including sedatives and antibiotics, necessitating increased dosing and careful monitoring (6–8).

The heater-cooler unit is essential in children on ECLS, especially infants. It provides extremely effective temperature control such that maintaining normothermia or inducing therapeutic hypothermia is literally done at the touch of a button.

An ECMO circuit is integrated with monitoring systems to ensure safe operation and effective gas transfer. Pressure monitors are used to monitor the development of excessive pressures across the membrane oxygenator, providing an indication of the development of clotting and impairment of blood flow. Inline monitors in the drainage and postoxygenator circuit provide real-time information on venous and arterial saturation, pH, and hemoglobin concentration. Temperature monitors are used to monitor circuit and patient temperatures.

PATIENT SELECTION

Indications

Hypoxemic Respiratory Failure

Children after the first 2 weeks of life have different physiology than that of younger infants and are susceptible to a different spectrum of lung disease. Most features of fetal cardiopulmonary physiology, such as flow through the ductus arteriosus and foramen ovale, have largely disappeared by the end of this period. Respiratory failure in the newborn due to persistent pulmonary hypertension and meconium aspiration is replaced by pulmonary infection, pulmonary aspiration, sepsis, and other conditions. These illnesses often trigger acute respiratory distress syndrome (ARDS) and are frequently accompanied by extrapulmonary organ system involvement. The most common cause of hypoxemic respiratory failure in the pediatric age group that leads to support with ECLS is viral pneumonia (19%), followed by bacterial pneumonia (11%) and ARDS (10%) (9). The remaining fraction comprises respiratory failure due to a number of other etiologies.

The selection of patients for ECLS is founded in a set of criteria that have evolved over time and have historically predicted high mortality (**Table 40.1**). The essential element of these criteria is to select patients with severe oxygenation impairment, risk of ventilator-induced pulmonary injury, and the capacity for pulmonary recovery. Measures of oxygenation impairment include the oxygenation index (OI: the product of mean airway pressure and fraction of inspired oxygen divided by the arterial partial pressure of oxygen), PaO_2/FiO_2 ratio (P/F ratio), or intrapulmonary shunt fraction. The OI has been the traditional index used in neonates and younger children, with levels >40 historically considered an indication for initiating ECLS. More recent studies have also identified that serial evaluation of OI may be useful in older patients (including adults), although no strict cut-off values for ECMO initiation or predicting death have been established. The P/F ratio and intrapulmonary shunt are two interrelated measures that do not include an inflation pressure component, but they have been most commonly applied in older children and adults.

The avoidance of ventilator-induced lung injury is a major goal of ECLS. Patients who require excessive inflation

TABLE 40.1

CRITERIA USED IN SELECTION OF PATIENTS FOR ECLS FOR PULMONARY SUPPORT IN HYPOXEMIC RESPIRATORY FAILURE

Severe, potentially reversible acute respiratory failure
Lack of response to conventional support measures[a]
Severe hypoxemia
    $Pao_2/Fio_2 < 80$
    Oxygenation Index > 40
    Qs/Qt > 0.5
Elevated inflation pressures
    MAP >20 on conventional ventilation, >30 on HFOV
    Persistent air leak or interstitial air
    Cardiovascular depression with shock (pH < 7.25)
Lack of irreversible ventilator-induced lung injury
    Duration of mechanical ventilation <14 d

[a]Conventional support may include measures such as high-frequency oscillation, inhaled nitric oxide, prone positioning, surfactant, or others.
Qs/Qt, intrapulmonary shunt; MAP, mean airway pressure; HFOV, high-frequency oscillatory ventilation.

pressures, even in the absence of life-threatening hypoxemia, should be considered for extracorporeal support. This is particularly important if lactic acidosis and shock result from high levels of ventilatory support. The presence of barotrauma (radiographic evidence of pneumomediastinum or pulmonary interstitial air, or persistent air leak) should lead to consideration of ECLS, especially if it is progressive and uncontrollable.

Even with these guidelines, the decision of whether to place a patient on extracorporeal support requires consideration of other factors, including comorbid conditions, contraindications to anticoagulation, duration of pre-ECLS cardiac arrest and quality of resuscitation and duration of mechanical ventilation prior to ECLS. The former contraindications to ECLS have given way to individualized decisions of risk assessment and potential benefit. It may be prudent to undertake high-risk or uncertain cases (e.g., uncertain neurologic status following cardiac arrest) with the provision that ECLS will be withdrawn if clinical information is discovered that would suggest futility.

VV support is the preferred ECLS mode for hypoxemic respiratory failure. The presence of inotropes, once used as an indication to proceed to VA support, is not a contraindication to VV support (10). In most cases, inotrope requirements are reduced as the myocardium recovers from hypoxemia and intrathoracic pressure is reduced by lowering mechanical ventilation. The presence of severe shock despite inotropes, however, is generally best supported with the VA approach. In other words, if the primary indication for ECLS is shock, VA should be regarded as the standard mode. If the primary indication is hypoxia, VV should be used irrespective of the inotrope dose. It is imperative to be able to rapidly change cannulation strategies in complex or uncertain cases and this should be factored into initial planning prior to cannulation.

Hypercapnic Respiratory Failure

Severe hypercapnia with respiratory acidosis, in particular severe asthma, is effectively managed by VV extracorporeal support. As CO_2 is more effectively exchanged in the oxygenator than O_2 (see below), blood flows lower than that required for oxygenation are effective in control of hypercapnia. The concept of low-flow extracorporeal CO_2 removal (ECCO$_2$R) was first described as an adjunct to enable lung-protective

ventilation in adult ARDS. An extracorporeal blood flow of $\leq 20\%$ of the cardiac output is sufficient for control of hypercapnia, although higher flows are required if hypoxemia is present. Another advantage of extracorporeal support of severe asthma is the ability to perform bronchoscopy to remove secretions and debris.

An alternative to using ECMO circuitry to provide VV ECCO$_2$R is pumpless AVCO$_2$R (11,12). Percutaneous cannulation of the femoral artery and vein can be rapidly performed, crystalloid priming of the circuit is simple, and there is no need for a specialized perfusion team. AVCO$_2$R can normalize pH and Pco_2, even in severe asthma. Decannulation is simple, as the small size of the arterial cannula permits hemostasis through direct pressure alone. However, its use requires a robust circulation to cope with the arteriovenous shunt and limb ischemia can be problematic. A new generation of standalone VV ECCO$_2$R pumps is becoming commercially available (3) and some manufacturers have designed specific pediatric cannulas for this purpose.

Circulatory Failure

Circulatory failure refractory to conventional treatment accounts for more than half of all pediatric ECLS cases beyond the neonatal period (9). Many of these cases required postoperative support after cardiac surgery, but cardiomyopathy and myocarditis are also frequent reasons for cardiac support with ECLS.

Early initiation of support following recognition of circulatory failure is essential. Patients who are placed on ECLS in the operating room following open heart surgery have better survival than those in whom it is delayed to the ICU (13,14), most likely due to prevention of shock, acidosis, and cardiac arrest. Prolonged low cardiac output and shock despite appropriate fluid, ventilator, and pharmacological management can result in neurologic injury and other organ dysfunction and should be avoided by early consideration of ECLS rather than repeated failed attempts at separation from bypass. One important caveat is that residual cardiac lesions should be repaired prior to the use of ECLS.

Venoarterial support is the mode of choice, as it provides cardiopulmonary bypass and maintains systemic circulatory flow at normal levels. Patients placed on ECLS in the operating room may be centrally cannulated, but the cervical approach with carotid and internal jugular cannulation is also commonly practiced in children who are not yet able to walk. In older children (>15 kg), the percutaneous femoral approach may be adequate but limb ischemia is a potential hazard. This risk can be reduced by surgically placing an anterograde perfusion cannula. If time allows, consideration can also be given to cannulation of the subclavian artery via a surgically placed end-to-side graft (see "Cannulation" below).

In cases of severe myocardial dysfunction in which the ventricle cannot empty against the afterload associated with ECLS-maintained arterial pressure, persistent elevation of end-diastolic pressure can result in pulmonary hypertension, pulmonary edema, pulmonary hemorrhage, and impairment of myocardial recovery. When required, the left heart can be decompressed via atrial septostomy, performed in the cardiac catheterization suite or at the bedside (15). If this is not technically possible, a surgeon can vent the systemic ventricle by inserting an atrial or ventricular drainage cannula via a small thoracotomy incision, which is then incorporated into the venous drainage of the ECLS circuit by means of a Y connector.

Primary severe myocardial dysfunction is also supported with ECLS. Cardiomyopathies differ from the postoperative causes of myocardial dysfunction in that recovery may take place after prolonged support. Fulminant myocarditis can be otherwise rapidly fatal, but the child can be supported with VA

ECLS until the inflammation resolves and the heart recovers. In a series of 15 patients with viral myocarditis and acute deterioration who were managed with mechanical support (12 with ECLS), survival was 80% (16). Support ranged in duration from 48 to 400 hours, with a median of 140 hours. Ventricular function in those recovering without transplantation was normal at follow-up periods up to 5.3 years. In another series of 14 patients with fulminant myocarditis managed with percutaneous femorofemoral VA ECLS, 10 patients (71%) survived. A smaller series reported survival in 4 of 5 patients with acute myocarditis, all but one of whom were managed with percutaneous femorofemoral bypass (17).

Venoarterial ECLS can also be used as a bridge to transplantation (18). Patients with cardiomyopathy have a better prognosis than those with congenital heart disease when bridged to transplantation. Acute viral myocarditis carries a good prognosis (19). However, long-term outcomes appear better when patients are bridged to cardiac transplantation with ventricular assist device (VAD) rather than ECMO (20–22).

Newer Indications

Septic shock was traditionally regarded as a contraindication to ECLS. However, a number of studies in the 1990s showed encouraging outcomes both in neonates and older children (23–26). The American College of Critical Care Medicine subsequently endorsed ECLS as rescue therapy in refractory pediatric septic shock and constructed a detailed algorithm of the steps recommended prior to instituting it (27). In brief, ECLS should be used as a last resort when all other attempts at goal-directed therapy with inotrope, fluid, ventilator, metabolic, and hormonal treatment are failing, but prior to cardiac arrest or prolonged periods of severe hypoperfusion (28). Pediatric septic shock, usually characterized by failure of one or both ventricles, is more amenable to temporary short-term support with VA ECLS than the distributive shock seen in adults.

Septic shock in children is often associated with early, severe circulatory failure, hypoxic respiratory failure, and evolving multiorgan dysfunction. This has an impact on cannulation strategies, which need to facilitate high circuit flows to meet increased metabolic demand while preventing differential cyanosis. This latter problem occurs when blood, deoxygenated from progressive respiratory failure, is ejected from the systemic ventricle and competes with distal, oxygenated blood returning from the ECLS circuit, potentially inhibiting myocardial recovery and leading to cerebral hypoxia (29,30). One strategy that fulfills both these requirements is central cannulation. Cannulating the right atrium and aorta allows the largest cannulas to be placed, which in turn facilitate the highest circuit flows. The proximal position of the arterial inflow cannula mitigates differential cyanosis. In one retrospective study, children with refractory septic shock treated with ECLS were more likely to survive to hospital discharge when cannulated centrally instead of peripherally (8 of 11 [73%] vs. 13 of 34 [38%], $p = 0.05$) (31). A follow-on study of 23 children who were all centrally cannulated reinforced these encouraging outcomes, with 17 (74%) patients surviving to hospital discharge. Predictors of death included high pre-ECLS lactate levels and lower circuit flows (32).

Another evolving use of ECLS is extracorporeal cardiopulmonary resuscitation (ECPR). Recognition of the poor rate of recovery from cardiac arrest following external chest compression has led to the expanded use of rapid-deployment ECLS. This technique involves the rapid institution of ECLS during cardiac arrest via percutaneous cannulation of the femoral vessels or through a reopened sternotomy and mediastinal cannulation. Many institutions keep one or more preprimed ECLS circuits on permanent standby to facilitate this. These circuits can be kept sterile for up to 30 days prior to use (33).

ECPR is the most rapidly growing application for ECLS and has been used more frequently in pediatrics than in neonates or adults (9). Nonetheless, ECPR requires considerable resources, coordination, and organization to perform effectively and should be regarded as one of the most challenging indications for ECLS. In many ECLS centers, survival rates are still well below 50%, irrespective of patient age (9). In the most experienced pediatric centers, approximately half the patients survive, with 75% of them having no or mild neurological impairment (34).

Contraindications

The list of contraindications to ECLS has shrunk over the last two decades, as a number of conditions previously regarded as unsuitable for ECLS support have been shown to be compatible with satisfactory long-term survival. Nonetheless, ECLS should not be offered if it is likely to be futile. A list of contemporary contraindications is shown in **Table 40.2**.

One additional consideration is the patient who has already survived one run of ECLS support. Offering ECLS a second time is often inadvisable because the complication rates during the second run are significantly higher (35). This is especially true in children who have received ECLS for circulatory support. Two studies in this population from experienced centers showed survival-to-discharge rates of approximately 25% (36,37). One of these studies provided long-term follow-up after a median time of 43 months (37). Of the seven (27%) patients who survived to discharge, six of them had subsequently died or had significant neurodevelopmental delay.

MODES

As ECMO evolved from cardiopulmonary bypass (e.g., VA bypass with intrathoracic vascular cannulation), the initial application mode of ECMO was also venoarterial. While VA support remains important, especially with cardiac dysfunction, VV support has supplanted the traditional VA mode, primarily for respiratory failure. A hybrid support mode that combines features of VA and VV has been described, known as venoarteriovenous (VAV). More recently, pumpless arteriovenous (AV) support has been shown to be clinically feasible for management of hypercarbic states. Each of these modes has particular advantages and disadvantages for different clinical situations (**Table 40.3**).

TABLE 40.2

POTENTIAL CONTRAINDICATIONS TO ECLS

Absolute contraindications

Extremes of prematurity or low birth weight (<32 wk gestational age or <1.5 kg)

Lethal chromosomal abnormalities (e.g., Trisomy 13 or 18)

Uncontrollable hemorrhage

Irreversible brain damage

Relative contraindications

Intracranial hemorrhage

Less extreme prematurity or low birth weight in neonates (<34 wk gestational age or <2.0 kg)

Irreversible organ failure in a patient ineligible for transplantation

Prolonged intubation and mechanical ventilation (>2 wk) prior to ECLS

TABLE 40.3

COMPARISON OF CARDIOPULMONARY BYPASS AND DIFFERENT MODES OF ECLS

	■ CPB	■ VA ECMO	■ VV ECMO	■ VAV ECMO	■ AVCO$_2$R
Setting	Cardiac surgery	Prolonged support	Prolonged support	Prolonged support	ED or ICU support
Support	Total cardiac and pulmonary	Cardiac and pulmonary	Pulmonary	Cardiac and pulmonary	Pulmonary
Cannulation	Intrathoracic (surgical)	Extrathoracic (surgical)	Extrathoracic (percutaneous)	Extrathoracic (percutaneous)	Extrathoracic (percutaneous)
Blood pump	Roller or centrifugal	Roller or centrifugal	Roller or centrifugal	Roller or centrifugal	None (pumpless)
ECMO blood flow (fraction of CO)	Total (100%)	Subtotal (70%–90%)	Subtotal	Subtotal (1/3–2/3 arterial, remainder venous)	Low (10%–20%)
Pulmonary flow	None	Low	Unchanged	Moderate decrease	Unchanged
Length of support	Hours	Days to weeks	Days to weeks	Days to weeks	Days
Anticoagulation	ACT >400	ACT 180–200	ACT 180–200	ACT 180–200	ACT 200–220
Reservoir	Large	Small or none[a]	Small or none[a]	Small or none[a]	None

[a]Reservoir used for roller pump, optional for centrifugal pump.

CPB, cardiopulmonary bypass; VA, venoarterial; ECMO, extracorporeal membrane oxygenation; VV, venovenous; VAV, venoarteriovenous; AVCO$_2$R, arteriovenous carbon dioxide removal; ED, emergency department; CO, cardiac output; ACT, activated coagulation time.

Venovenous

Venovenous ECLS effectively supports pediatric patients with isolated respiratory failure (38) and is the preferred mode for management of severe respiratory failure in children. One exception to this is in smaller neonates, where lack of suitably sized cannulas and the position of the ductus venosus may prohibit VV ECLS. This mode provides prepulmonary oxygenation by draining blood from the central venous circulation and returning it back into the venous circulation (**Fig. 40.8**). The reinfused blood elevates mixed venous saturation, diminishes the effect of intrapulmonary shunt, preserves pulsatile systemic blood flow, and delivers blood with a higher

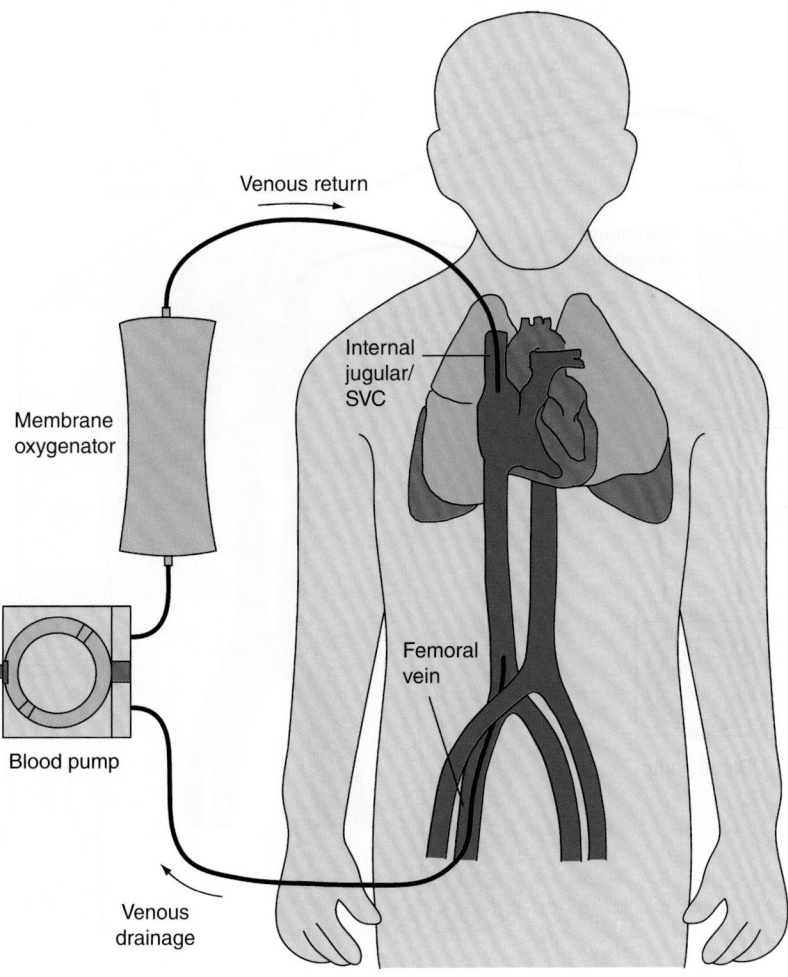

FIGURE 40.8. Venovenous mode of extracorporeal life support. Blood is drained from the inferior vena cava and returned to the proximal superior vena cava (SVC) or right atrium.

saturation to the coronary arteries. No direct cardiac support is delivered, although myocardial function commonly improves through elevation of myocardial oxygenation and reduction in intrathoracic pressures. Venovenous support may be successfully applied even in the presence of inotrope dependence (10).

An attractive aspect of VV support is the ability to cannulate the veins percutaneously, avoiding surgical vascular access and largely eliminating bleeding from the vascular access site. The carotid artery and jugular are spared from ligation, and venous return through the jugular vein can be maintained. Central nervous system (CNS) complications are lower with VV support (39), partially due to the less invasive nature of the vascular access technique. Cannulation was typically performed through the right internal jugular vein and the right common femoral vein but the recent manufacture of double-lumen cannulas for patients of all ages has allowed even simpler access, requiring only a single cannulation through the right internal jugular vein under echocardiography or fluoroscopic guidance. Recirculation, in which some of the return flow into the venous system is directed back into the drainage cannula, is present to a variable degree and reduces overall gas transfer.

Venoarterial

Venoarterial support is based on cardiopulmonary bypass, in which blood is drained from the right atrium via the central venous system and returned to the proximal arterial system (**Fig. 40.9**). Both ventricles and the intervening pulmonary system are bypassed. In most cases partial support is achieved, with some residual pulmonary blood flow present. Cardiac and pulmonary support is provided with this mode. Cannulation is usually performed by surgical access to the right internal jugular vein for right atrial drainage and to the right carotid artery for return to the aortic root. This mode provides high levels of systemic arterial saturation but may be associated with lower coronary oxygen saturation in patients with severe respiratory failure, as poorly saturated native cardiac output may be directed toward the coronary ostia (29). The advantages of VA support are offset by a higher potential for complications, such as cerebral embolism, reduction in pulmonary blood flow, increased ventricular afterload, and the loss of the right carotid circulation from ligation.

In place of the cervical approach, cannulation may be made through the femoral vessels (**Fig. 40.10**). This approach lends itself to percutaneous cannulation. Flow returning to the femoral artery will predominantly perfuse the lower half of the body, although retrograde flow up the aortic arch will also occur. The extent of retrograde flow is dependent on the adequacy of native cardiac output, with more flow reaching the upper aorta under conditions of poor intrinsic cardiac function. With good cardiac function, the heart and brain predominantly receive blood from the native cardiopulmonary system (29). Thus, in patients with severe pulmonary failure and good cardiac function, desaturated blood may perfuse the brain and heart (30). This is known as differential cyanosis (see below).

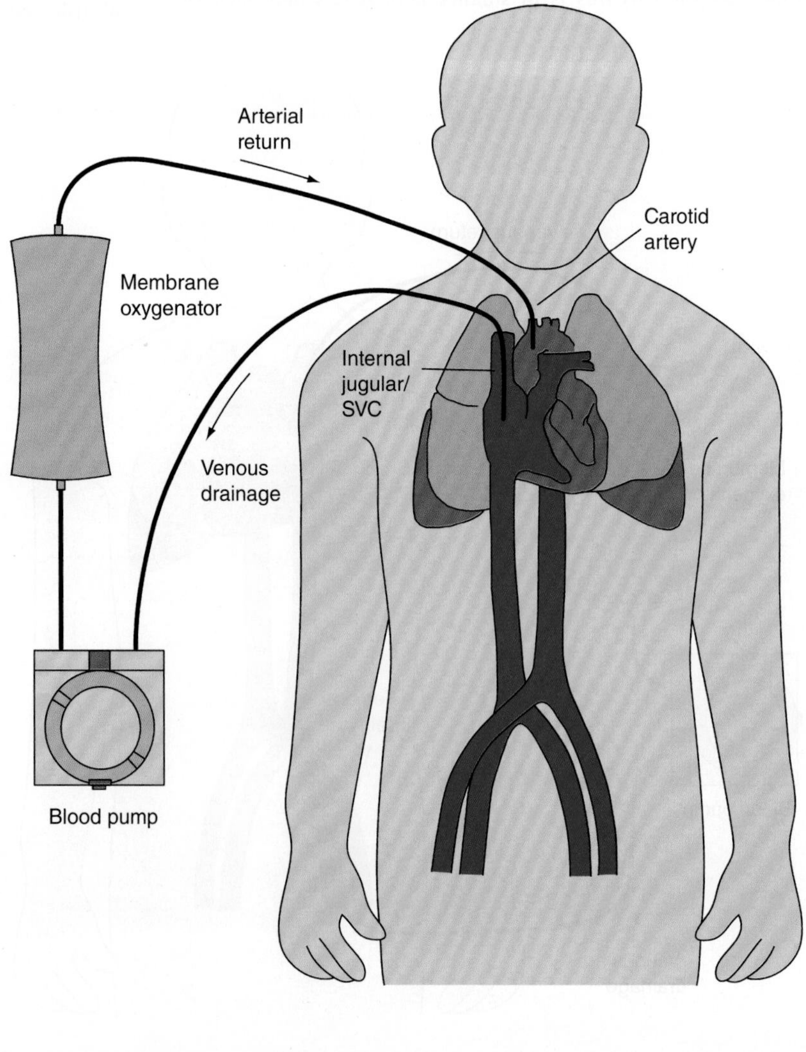

FIGURE 40.9. Venoarterial mode of extracorporeal life support via the cervical approach. Blood is drained from the right atrium and returned to the arterial system via the carotid artery into the proximal aorta. SVC, superior vena cava.

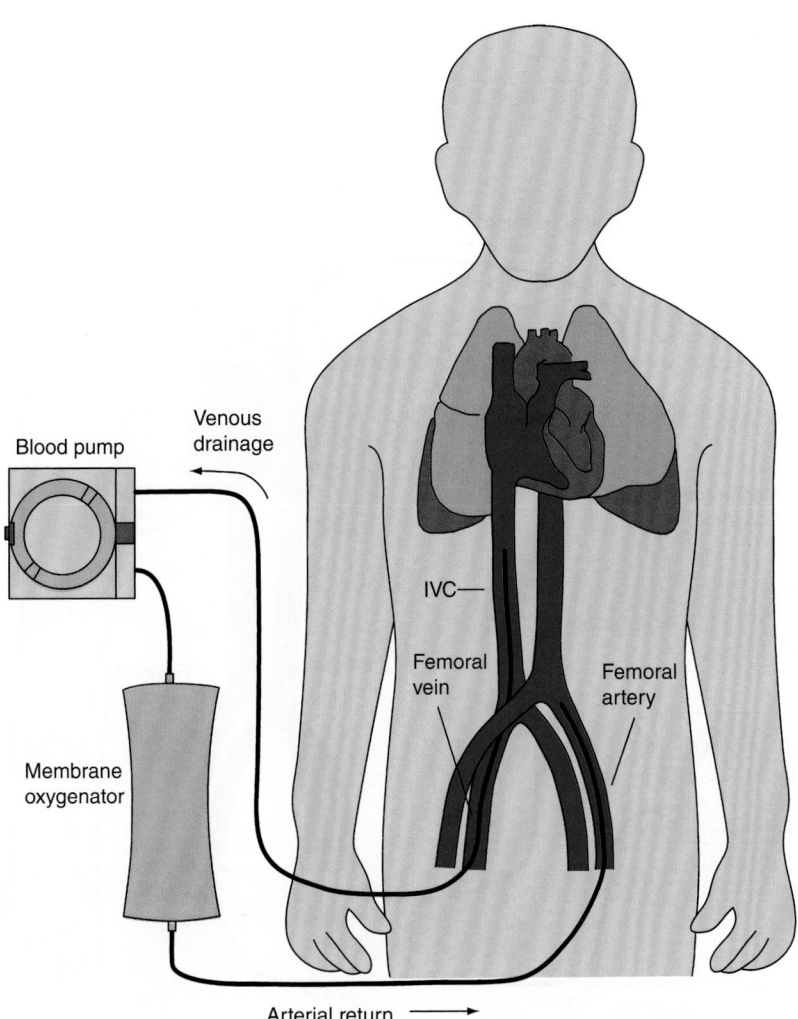

Blood pump

Venous drainage

Membrane oxygenator

IVC—

Femoral vein

Femoral artery

Arterial return ⟶

FIGURE 40.10. Venoarterial mode of extracorporeal life support via the femoral approach. Blood is drained from inferior vena cava and returned to the arterial system via the femoral artery into the distal aorta. IVC, inferior vena cava.

An alternative approach is subclavian artery cannulation, where the more proximal cannula position reduces the risk of differential cyanosis. Physiologically, it is similar to carotid cannulation but more suitable in older children (adolescents), who have less reliable collateral cerebral circulation than infants. Subclavian cannulation is best performed by anastomosing a temporary, artificial, end-to-side graft onto the artery and then cannulating the graft. The cannula can then be tunneled under the skin and brought out near the axilla. Venous drainage is provided by an internal jugular vein cannula on the same side of the patient. The catheters are secure and, being tunneled under the skin, are less prone to infection. This cannulation strategy is naturally time-consuming and not appropriate in emergent cannulation but is very suitable for older patients who are expected to require a long time on support because it facilitates extubation and ambulation.

Other Modes

Venoarteriovenous

The venoarteriovenous (VAV, sometimes also referred to as venovenoarterial) mode is a hybrid mode that combines VV support for pulmonary failure and partial VA support, with the advantage of percutaneous cannulation. The typical circuit consists of a drainage cannula in the right femoral vein and two return cannulae connected via a Y-connection, one in the right internal jugular vein and the second in a femoral artery (**Fig. 40.11**). Alternatively, a dual-lumen internal jugular venous cannula and carotid or subclavian arterial cannula can be used, which simplifies access. Blood flow between the two return limbs is controlled to achieve ~30%–70% flow into the arterial system by restricting the flow to the venous cannula (usually with a simple screw clamp). Venoarteriovenous support is ideally suited for larger pediatric patients who require partial cardiac support in addition to pulmonary support.

Arteriovenous

The concept of pumpless AV support of gas exchange was described over 40 years ago, but was not feasible until the development of low-resistance, high-efficiency membrane lungs. The arterial-venous pressure gradient drives flow through a membrane lung without the need for a pump. Because arterial blood is usually well oxygenated, oxygen transfer is limited, but CO_2 is readily removed. The applications of AV CO_2 removal ($AVCO_2R$) are identical to those of $ECCO_2R$, without the need for an extracorporeal pump, that is, reduction in mechanical ventilatory support and control of hypercapnia. A blood flow of 15%–20% of cardiac output is required and is well tolerated in the absence of significant cardiac depression.

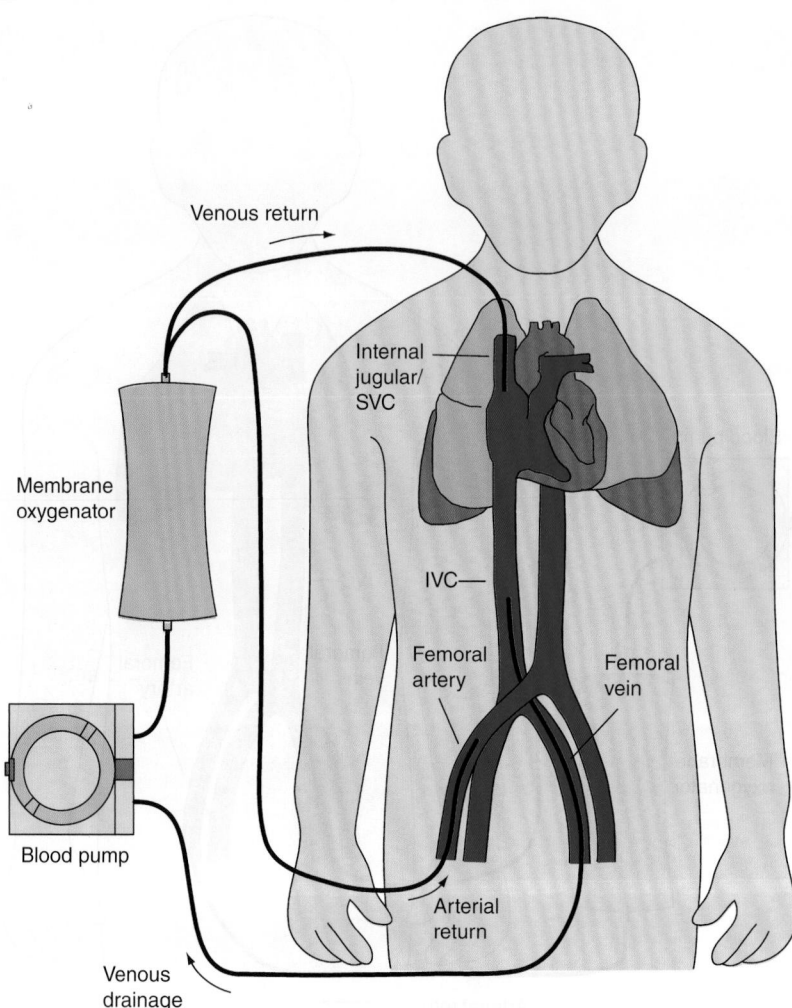

FIGURE 40.11. Hybrid venoarteriovenous mode of extracorporeal life support. Blood is drained from the inferior vena cava (IVC) and returned to the right atrium, as in venovenous support. In addition, some of the returning blood is diverted to the femoral artery.

CANNULATION

Vascular cannulation is one of the most challenging aspects of ECLS and can be the greatest constraint to providing adequate support. The traditional approach has been an open surgical approach with vessel ligation. Percutaneous approaches are replacing surgical approaches in some situations.

Percutaneous Cannulation

The trend in vascular cannulation is toward percutaneous or modified percutaneous techniques, as this approach is faster and is associated with less bleeding complications and simplified decannulation. Venovenous support is now almost exclusively approached percutaneously. One dual-lumen catheter (Avalon Elite, Maquet, Hirrlingen, Germany) is available in sizes ranging from 13 to 31 Fr, suitable for patients of all sizes from neonates to adults. This cannula has both drainage and reinfusion lumens. The catheter is placed by percutaneous puncture of the right internal jugular vein using the Seldinger technique and the tip is maneuvered into the inferior vena cava under ultrasound or fluoroscopic guidance. The drainage ports are located in both vena cavas while the reinfusion lumen returns blood into the right atrium adjacent to the tricuspid valve, minimizing recirculation. It is worthwhile noting that these new double-lumen cannulas are considerably more expensive than older models or single-lumen cannulas.

Other brands of double-lumen catheters are becoming commercially available.

A modified percutaneous technique for cannulation of the internal jugular vein in neonates has been described that uses a limited surgical exposure of the internal jugular vein with percutaneous cannulation under direct visualization of the vein (Semi-Seldinger technique) (40). The correct cannula size can then be determined.

Percutaneous arterial cannulation is limited to the femoral artery in larger children. As this vessel is usually too small to accommodate full VA support, this approach is limited to the provision of partial support. In the presence of concomitant respiratory failure, hybrid VAV support may be a suitable option.

Peripheral Surgical Cannulation

The open surgical technique is the original method of cannulation for ECLS and remains the approach of choice today for VA support through the common carotid artery and internal jugular vein. A transverse incision is made above the right clavicle over the vessels and dissection is performed to expose the carotid sheath (Fig. 40.12). The sheath is opened, and the vessels and vagus nerve identified. The vein is usually exposed first, with ligatures placed proximally and distally. The carotid is similarly exposed and prepared. An arteriotomy is made following distal ligation, and the arterial cannula is placed. Venotomy and venous cannulation follow next. The wound is closed and cannulas are secured in place.

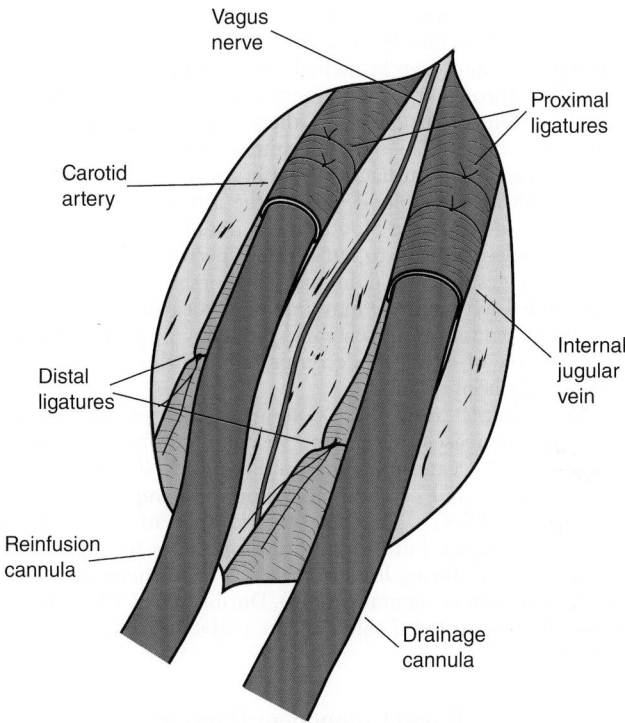

FIGURE 40.12. Open surgical approach to cervical cannulation. The carotid sheath is opened, the vessels are exposed, and ligatures are placed. An arteriotomy and venotomy provide access to the lumen for cannula insertion.

Labels: Vagus nerve; Carotid artery; Distal ligatures; Reinfusion cannula; Proximal ligatures; Internal jugular vein; Drainage cannula

Surgical placement of a dual-lumen venous cannula for VV bypass can be performed in a similar manner, although without the need for carotid ligation and arteriotomy. Inability to insert a dual-lumen cannula percutaneously is usually managed by conversion to an open surgical approach.

Central Cannulation

ECLS following failure to wean from cardiopulmonary bypass or sternotomy for resuscitation can be managed using the same cannulas placed for intraoperative support, although it may be preferable to use an arterial ECLS cannula in the aorta because it can be inserted farther in and secured. These cannulas are placed into the right atrium and ascending aorta and are secured with purse-string sutures. The chest is incompletely closed (allowing the cannulas to exit the wound) and dressed, usually with a Silastic membrane sutured over the defect. When feasible, the cannulas should be positioned at either end of the wound and the skin sutured around them to facilitate hemostasis.

PHYSIOLOGY OF EXTRACORPOREAL CIRCULATION

Venovenous

The principle aims of VV ECLS for isolated respiratory failure are oxygenation, CO_2 clearance, and lung rest. It is important to have sufficient extracorporeal gas exchange to minimize mechanical ventilation and lower the risk of ventilator-induced lung injury. Oxygenation and CO_2 clearance are

achieved through adjusting different parameters, just as they are with mechanical ventilation. Gas transfer by the oxygenator is determined by several factors. The membrane surface area, membrane diffusion coefficient, and thickness of the blood film in the oxygenator are determined by the manufacturer. An oxygenator can fully saturate blood only up to a certain flow, above which saturation falls off and total O_2 delivery reaches a plateau. The rated flow of an oxygenator is the amount of blood entering the oxygenator in a given time frame in which the oxyhemoglobin concentration is raised from 75% to 95%. Rated flow represents the maximal efficient flow for the device. Above the rated flow, O_2 transfer becomes diffusion limited and O_2 saturation diminishes.

Oxygenator design, intravascular gas transport, and the physico-kinetic properties of O_2 and CO_2 all tend to favor CO_2 clearance (41). Consequently, less blood flow (e.g., 10–15 mL/kg/min) is needed to effectively remove CO_2 than to oxygenate blood (generally >40–50 mL/kg/min). The principal means of achieving CO_2 clearance is adjusting the rate of fresh gas flow ("sweep"). Extracorporeal CO_2 removal with ECLS circuits is very efficient and it is important to measure arterial blood gases 10–15 minutes after any change to the rate of fresh gas flow to avoid overly rapid or extreme changes in $Paco_2$, which could have detrimental effects on cerebral blood flow.

The principal determinant of systemic oxygenation is the blood flow rate to the patient by the circuit. The blood path in the extracorporeal circuit includes the vascular cannulas, circuit tubing, oxygenator, and heat exchanger. The point of greatest impedance to blood flow is in the vascular cannulas, in particular the venous drainage cannula, as it depends upon gravity drainage (roller pump) or a low level of suction (centrifugal pump). Optimization of conditions for venous drainage, including selection of cannula size, is essential. The relationship between pressure and flow is not linear. At lower blood flows, laminar flow predominates and is approximately described by the Hagen-Poiseuille equation, with flow ($\dot{Q}$) directly related to pressure gradient (ΔP) and inversely related to catheter length (L):

$$\dot{Q} = \left(\frac{\pi r^4}{8\eta}\right)\frac{\Delta P}{L}$$

At higher flows, and as a result of catheter design (e.g., side holes), flow becomes nonlinearly related to pressure, and use of experimentally determined pressure-flow curves that are provided by manufacturers can be used. An alternative to published flow curves is the use of the M-number or more recent updated M (UM) system, which ascribes a single number to define flow impedance of a catheter or length of tubing (5,42).

As indicated by the Hagen-Poiseuille equation above, the catheter dimension that has greatest influence on blood flow is the diameter, followed by the length; thus, the goal is to place the catheter with the largest diameter and shortest length as allowed by the venous anatomy. As gravity-assisted drainage can yield up to ~100 cm H_2O, this pressure can be used to estimate maximal blood flow for a given catheter. Actual flow depends on adequate venous return as well as proper depth and intravascular positioning of the venous cannula.

Recirculation, in which some of the blood reinfused into the patient from the circuit is diverted back into the drainage cannula, is largely unavoidable in VV ECLS. The efficiency of extracorporeal support is reduced in proportion to the recirculation fraction (R), which can be theoretically calculated through the measurement of O_2 saturation in a fashion analogous to calculation of transpulmonary shunt fraction:

$$R = \frac{C_{pre}O_2 - C\overline{v}O_2}{C_{post}O_2 - C\overline{v}O_2}$$

where $C_{pre}O_2$ and $C_{post}O_2$ are the O_2 content of pre- and postoxygenator blood. $C\bar{v}O_2$ represents the true mixed venous blood O_2 content leaving the tissues and cannot be measured in the pulmonary artery (which is affected by the blood returned by the ECLS circuit). This value can be estimated by sampling venous blood proximal to the drainage cannula and out of the recirculation path.

The amount of recirculation is influenced by cannula placement and can sometimes be increased by attempts to compensate by increasing the flow. Dual-lumen cannulas minimize recirculation by draining from both vena cavas and returning venous inflow into the right atrium. With two-cannula support, drainage from the inferior vena cava via the femoral vein and reinfusion into the superior vena cava via the internal jugular vein usually results in less recirculation than flow in the reverse direction (43). A three-cannula technique (two short drainage and one long reinfusion) has been shown to improve extracorporeal blood flow and reduce recirculation (44).

Venoarterial

Venoarterial ECLS provides circulatory support by returning oxygenated blood under pressure into the arterial circulation. This blood flow is almost always nonpulsatile, although some newer diagonal blood flow pumps have the option of providing pulsatile flow. The oxygenator functions the same way as it does on VV ECLS and is needed to oxygenate the blood that bypasses the pulmonary circulation. Assuming the native heart has little effective output, the rate of blood flow through the ECLS circuit becomes analogous to cardiac output and (along with the oxygen content) determines systemic oxygen delivery. Historically, circuit blood flow rates were set to somewhat arbitrary norms on the basis of the weight of the child, such as achieving circuit flows equivalent to >2.4 L/min/m² in children >10 kg and >3.3 L/min/m² in children <10 kg. However, although these may provide some approximation of initial flow targets, such an approach does not take oxygen consumption into consideration and may be inadequate in advanced shock (28,31,32). In shock states, it is more appropriate to use the same time-critical, goal-directed principles as for shocked patients who are not receiving ECLS. For example, flows should be titrated to rapid normalization of lactate, achieving $SvO_2 > 70\%$, capillary refill time <2 seconds, age-appropriate mean arterial pressure targets, and improved end-organ function. As this approach may demand very high circuit flows, it is important to monitor for hemolysis using inlet-pressure measurement and plasma-free hemoglobin (32). If significant hemolysis is detected (e.g., plasma-free Hb > 0.5 g/L), larger or additional cannulas may need to be placed to improve venous drainage and the circuit changed.

In situations other than refractory shock, the native heart may remain an important contributor to global oxygen delivery. In these situations, systemic blood flow during VA ECLS is the sum of native cardiac output and blood flow through the circuit and thus systemic oxygen delivery is the total of that provided by fully saturated blood from the extracorporeal circuit mixed with that provided by the native lungs.

Adverse Effects

Nonpulsatile Flow

As circuit blood flow is progressively increased at the initiation of VA ECLS, less venous return becomes available to the native heart. As the proportion of systemic flow provided by the nonpulsatile blood pump increases, stroke volume diminishes and is recognized as a diminishing pulse pressure on the arterial waveform.

During total bypass, the left ventricle continues to receive some blood flow, mostly from the Thebesian veins (in the myocardial wall) and deep bronchial veins, and possibly intermittent flow through the pulmonary circulation. The ventricle slowly distends, particularly if there is concomitant regurgitant valve disease, so that intermittent pulsatile waveforms may appear. When cardiac contractility is sufficiently impaired and unable to eject blood against the afterload provided by the circuit, no pulsatile blood flow is noted. Distension of the left ventricle may lead to left atrial hypertension, pulmonary venous congestion, and pulmonary hemorrhage. Furthermore, a distended left ventricle may impair myocardial blood flow, precipitate endocardial ischemia, and delay or prevent recovery. The role of left-heart decompression in this circumstance has already been discussed.

Nonpulsatile flow has potentially deleterious effects, including increased peripheral vascular resistance through higher levels of catecholamines and reduced NO production, reduced renal and cerebral perfusion, and impaired release of cortisol (45–47). The clinical relevance of these effects has been debated, but nonpulsatile flow does not appear to be detrimental during long-term ECLS if adequate total systemic perfusion is maintained (48). During VV ECLS, systemic blood flow is provided solely by the native heart and remains pulsatile.

Blood Component Damage

The mechanical pumping of blood through a system that is recognized to produce high shear rates may result in injury to erythrocytes, platelets, and plasma proteins. Shear force represents a deforming force applied to blood components and is defined as the velocity gradient applied to the component. High shear rates can occur throughout the circuit, such as rapid directional changes at catheter side holes and edges, cavitation in the blood pump, and turbulence. The raceway of roller pumps and the rotating vanes of centrifugal pumps where they contact the blood are a known source of shear forces. High shear rates applied to erythrocytes induce membrane changes (altered deformability) or disruption (hemolysis). Roller pumps may cause more hemolysis than their centrifugal counterparts under proper operating conditions, but the rate of hemolysis is usually not clinically significant. Under improper operating conditions, however, both are capable of significant hemolysis. Elevated shear forces cause hemolysis, platelet deposition, and denaturation of plasma proteins and lipoproteins. Injury to plasma proteins, platelets, and white blood cells contributes to activation of coagulation and inflammation.

Activation of Coagulation

The extracorporeal circuit represents a large, nonendothelial contact surface that is known to induce profound effects on the coagulation system. The response is initiated during short-term support (e.g., during cardiopulmonary bypass) and during long-term support with ECLS, with activation of the intrinsic, extrinsic, and common pathways. The result is conversion of prothrombin to thrombin and of fibrinogen to fibrin. Fibrin polymers link to form a fibrin mesh and then cross-link.

Several serine protease inhibitors of coagulation (e.g., antithrombin III) are activated, along with procoagulant proteins, but this physiologic system is overwhelmed by the degree of activation of coagulation by the circuit. Systemic anticoagulation is thus mandatory. Heparin accelerates the action of antithrombin III but does not inhibit thrombin formation. As a result, it is not an ideal anticoagulant but remains the drug of choice for numerous reasons, including decades of familiarity.

Anticoagulation regimens, monitoring, and therapeutic interventions are not standardized between centers and vary dramatically, limiting the ability to extrapolate published reports to the wider community.

Systemic Inflammation

In addition to activation of coagulation, the extracorporeal circuit induces a systemic inflammatory response. Mediated by humoral and cellular components of the immune system, this response is complex, variable, and incompletely understood. Activation of macrophages and other immune system-related cells results in the production of proximal proinflammatory mediators, including tumor necrosis factor (TNF), interleukin-1 (IL-1), and IL-6. Proinflammatory cytokines have numerous actions that result in systemic inflammation, including increases in neutrophil adhesion and migration, stimulation of neutrophil phagocytosis, and degranulation and release of reactive O_2 species. Eicosanoids (e.g., thromboxanes) are more distal mediators of inflammation, particularly in the lungs, and are increased in extracorporeal circulation.

Neutrophils are activated by the introduction of extracorporeal circulation as well as the underlying disease state before initiation of ECLS. Hypoxemia, ischemia, and reperfusion contribute to pre-ECLS neutrophil priming. Neutrophils are activated by cytokine and bioactive lipids and, once activated, can also produce proinflammatory cytokines and additional arachidonic acid products that mediate inflammation. Neutrophil degranulation results in release of proteolytic and cytotoxic enzymes. Formation of reactive O_2 species ensues, which is important for normal microbial killing. When released systemically, however, reactive O_2 species can damage endothelial and other cells, resulting in endothelial activation, microvascular coagulation, organ dysfunction, and capillary leak syndrome.

CIRCUIT MANAGEMENT

Priming

The extracorporeal circuit volume is substantial relative to patient blood volume, mandating that the circuit prime consist of a solution that has normal electrolyte concentrations. In smaller children, especially neonates, this also necessitates using a blood prime. Priming begins with a balanced electrolyte solution (such as Normosol or PlasmaLyte). Albumin, packed red blood cells, or fresh frozen plasma may be added later. As citrated blood is acidic and depleted in calcium, bicarbonate and calcium chloride may be included.

ECPR circuits often have priming volumes that are small enough to allow initiation with a bloodless prime. Electrolytes (potassium and ionized calcium) and pH are measured and additional calcium and/or bicarbonate are added as needed.

Initiation of Support

Preparation of the patient prior to cannulation includes adequate sedation and analgesia. Activated clotting time (ACT) is measured as a baseline prior to heparin administration. If percutaneous cannulation is chosen, ultrasonographic measurement of vessel size and patency may be performed and used to guide needle insertion. Neuromuscular blockers can be administered just prior to cannulation to prevent inspiratory efforts during cannula insertion that could otherwise result in a large air embolism.

Cannulation takes place at the bedside under local or general anesthesia, or in a nearby procedure suite if fluoroscopy is used. An initial bolus of heparin (50–100 U/kg) is administered just prior to cannulation. After vascular access is achieved, the primed circuit is connected and flow is initiated at a low-flow rate, increased incrementally to the target rate over a short duration. Immediate initiation of high flow may result in sudden acid–base and electrolyte shifts, with resultant hypotension or arrhythmia.

Anticoagulation and Hematologic Management

The ECLS circuit is procoagulant, requiring continuous administration of a systemic anticoagulant. Inadequate anticoagulation leads to clot formation in the circuit, which can affect circuit performance, accelerate platelet deposition, and induce systemic fibrinolysis. At present, heparin remains the anticoagulant of choice. Newer agents, such as direct thrombin inhibitors, show promise but there is still insufficient experience or published data with their use in ECLS management. The level of heparin anticoagulation is measured with a bedside assessment of ACT. Maintaining the ACT between 180 and 200 seconds is a common target that may best balance the risk of bleeding complications and circuit clotting, but will vary according to institutional preference, clinical situation, type of ECLS circuit, and type of ACT machine being used (kaolin or celite). The ACT is a test that is influenced by factors other than heparin, such as thrombocytopenia, hypofibrinogenemia, and fibrin degradation products, so supplementation of the ACT with other tests is sometimes required.

Platelet dysfunction is very common during ECLS support, possibly related to acquired von Willebrand syndrome (49), and daily transfusions are not uncommon during the early phase of support. A platelet count of 80,000–100,000 is maintained during the initial phase of support and during management of bleeding complications, but lower values may be accepted once transfusion requirements have stabilized and bleeding is not problematic, especially in older children. Red blood cell transfusions are often required, especially in the presence of overt bleeding. Even in the absence of bleeding, transfusion requirements are above normal, as red blood cell life span is shortened and erythropoietin deficiency or resistance are often present in critical illness. The target hemoglobin is generally 10–12 g/dL at the initiation of support, but later guided by assessment of oxygen delivery. Blood with a short storage life is preferred.

Troubleshooting

A comprehensive review of all aspects of troubleshooting ECLS is beyond the scope of this chapter and can be found in guidelines published by the ELSO (50). In order to conduct ECLS safely, it is vital to have a team of ECLS specialists and physicians who have had comprehensive practical training and regular recertification (51). Important issues to troubleshoot include circuit thrombosis, air embolism, equipment failure, and differential cyanosis.

Thrombi (clots) in the circuits are among the most common complications on ECLS (9). These clots are generally small and of little significance but need to be monitored closely by the ECLS specialist. Clots forming postoxygenator are of particular concern on VA ECLS, as they have the potential to cause systemic embolization to the patient. The detection of clots should prompt a review of anticoagulation strategies, circuit function, hematological management, and evaluation for hemolysis. If the clots appear to be affecting circuit function or causing hemolysis or pose the risk of embolizing into the patient, then part or all of the circuit should be changed urgently. Patient-related thromboses, especially cerebral infarcts or pulmonary emboli, also occur. The correlation between clinically suspected patient thromboses and those observed at autopsy has been reported as poor, with clinical thrombotic events noted in 35% of adult ECMO patients in one study, but 77% on postmortem exam (52).

Air embolism is a rare but potentially serious complication of ECLS. Although the oxygenator acts as a bubble trap, an enormous air embolus can still have fatal consequences. Thus, it is important to minimize the number of circuit access points, especially prepump, and limit breaches of the circuit to essential tests performed by trained staff. The servoregulator (bladder) of roller pumps also helps reduce the incidence of this complication. If it occurs, ECLS is temporarily discontinued by clamping the circuit and allowing the air to float through the circuit to the nearest access point (e.g., the oxygenator), where it can then be aspirated.

Equipment failure is a rare occurrence with contemporary ECLS. Nonetheless, having a backup plan in the event of pump failure is essential. This plan will depend on the type of pump. In some instances, this will necessitate using a handcrank until a new pump is primed or switching over to a backup pump that is kept in perpetual standby near the patient. All staff should be trained in crisis management, including the requisite steps to take in the event of sudden equipment failure.

Differential cyanosis may occur on VA ECLS when there is combined circulatory and respiratory failure. Blood passing through diseased, nonfunctioning lungs does not participate in effective gas exchange and enters the systemic ventricle where it is then ejected into the ascending aorta. Depending on the location of the arterial return cannula and the force of ventricular contraction, this can cause profoundly desaturated blood to enter the coronary and cerebral arteries, while the ECLS circuit merely perfuses the lower body. Differential cyanosis is most commonly seen with femoral cannulation and when there is a combination of significant ventricular ejection and profound lung disease. This can also occur as the myocardium recovers but the lungs remain poorly functioning. Adequate monitoring for this phenomenon must be used in all patients receiving VA ECLS. At the very least, this should include pulse oximetry on the right hand as a surrogate for right coronary and carotid oxygenation. Inserting a right radial arterial line prior to commencing ECLS and monitoring blood gases is ideal. Cerebral near-infrared spectroscopy (NIRS) may also have a role. If it is detected, the cannulation strategy should be reviewed. If blood passing through the lungs cannot be adequately oxygenated by modest increases in PEEP and FiO_2, then consideration should be given to changing to VV, VAV, or central VA ECLS, depending on the clinical scenario.

Weaning

Weaning from VV ECLS is very straightforward and can be initiated when there is improvement in clinical assessment, lung compliance, and radiographic appearance. The ventilator is set to moderate levels of support (e.g., PIP ≤ 30 cm H_2O, FiO_2 ≤50%, PEEP ≤ 10 cm H_2O, and rate <20–30) and the fresh gas flow to the oxygenator is turned off. If gas exchange is acceptable after 1–4 hours, the patient can be decannulated. It is not uncommon to see a slight rise in $PaCO_2$ after this, so patients with marginal lung function should remain longer on ECLS unless there is a clinical mandate to wean off.

Weaning from VA ECLS is initiated when signs of ventricular recovery are noted. An early manifestation of recovery is improvement in pulsatility, as evidenced by an increase in pulse pressure. Echocardiography permits serial noninvasive assessment of ventricular contractility and can assess the response to

changes in ventricular loading that are associated with reduction in flow. Once the decision to wean has been made, the patient is fully ventilated and extracorporeal flow is gradually reduced at discrete intervals over a period of 4–8 hours, with serial assessment of perfusion, myocardial function, and blood gases until a terminal flow of 25% of full support is achieved. Net circuit blood flow (mL/min) is also important to consider. Unless the surgical team is scrubbed in and ready to decannulate, it is inadvisable to lower the circuit flow to extremely low levels (e.g., <200 mL/min) because this may rapidly promote clot formation. Blood gas analysis and measurement of lactate, mixed venous O_2 saturation, and cardiac function by echocardiography ensure that native cardiac function is adequate. When the patient can tolerate low extracorporeal flow and maintain good perfusion, the ECLS circuit is discontinued and the cannulas are removed. Predictors of nonsurvival include persistent elevation of lactate, prolonged duration of support, progressive multiple organ dysfunction, and nosocomial pneumonia (53,54). In circuits with a bridge between the drainage and reinfusion lines, the bridge can be opened to maintain flow in the circuit while the patient cannulas are flushed and clamped. If successful, the patient is decannulated. The use of a bridge is decreasing, as it requires constant attention and can contribute to the formation of clots. In this case, patients are decannulated after the terminal flow is reached.

Decannulation

Termination of ECLS is followed by decannulation. If cardiopulmonary function is marginal after cessation of support, the decision may be made to maintain the cannulas in place for several hours or more. Provisions for maintaining anticoagulation and continuous flushing of the cannulas must be made.

Surgically placed cannulas are removed by opening the surgical site, partially withdrawing the cannulas, proximally ligating the vessels, and removing the cannula. Many surgeons will reconstruct the vessel. The wound is irrigated and closed. Percutaneous cannulas are removed by withdrawal and direct pressure over the site. At the venous site, a suture may be placed to close the tract just proximal to the insertion site. Removal of percutaneous arterial cannulas up to ~16 Fr can often be managed nonoperatively, but larger cannulas may require arterial repair.

PATIENT MANAGEMENT

Ventilator Management

Although the goal for ventilator management is to provide a protective ventilation strategy, no single strategy is universally practiced. The goal is to maintain alveolar recruitment, avoid overdistension and atelectasis, minimize cyclic shear stress associated with tidal ventilation, and reduce exposure to elevated concentrations of O_2. High-frequency oscillation with a mean airway pressure sufficient to minimize atelectasis may be used, although pulmonary toilet restrictions and need for sedation often negate any benefit. Use of pressure-limited ventilation, elevated levels of positive end-expiratory pressure (PEEP) (10–12 cm H_2O), low ventilator rates (6–10/min), and small tidal volumes (<6 mL/kg) will meet these goals. Recognition that patients on ECLS may be better served with less sedation and more interaction has led many centers to adopt pressure-support ventilation with modest levels of PEEP (10–12 cm H_2O). PEEP is usually less (5–10 cm H_2O) in patients with heart disease on VA ECLS. Spontaneous breathing with coughing better clears lower airway secretions. Adjuncts to mechanical ventilation include bronchoscopy to facilitate removal of airway secretions and prone positioning. New technologies are also leading to an increase in efforts to perform early tracheostomy or early extubation while on ECLS to allow more mobility of patients and facilitate spontaneous breathing.

Hemodynamic Management

The requirement for vasoactive agents is almost universal in patients about to undergo extracorporeal support. Patients with severe acute respiratory failure also have some degree of myocardial dysfunction. Right ventricular dysfunction due to acute pulmonary hypertension, myocardial depression from systemic inflammation, and altered ventricular filling due to high ventilation requirements are major contributors to myocardial dysfunction. Inotropic and vasopressor agents are weaned after initiation of support. Even patients on VV support can usually be weaned from high levels of pharmacologic support as a result of improved myocardial oxygenation and decreased right ventricular afterload. Most patients require some vasoactive agents initially while on ECLS, albeit at lower levels. After the initial period of support, vasoactive agents can often be weaned off completely. In patients on VA ECLS with severe cardiac dysfunction, it is common practice to enhance contractility with low-dose inotropes (e.g., ≤0.05 mcg/kg/min epinephrine or ≤5 mcg/kg/min dobutamine) in order to facilitate aortic valve opening and prevent stasis of blood in the systemic ventricle and aortic root.

Sedation and Analgesia

Provision of sedation and analgesia is part of the management of all critically ill children and ECLS is no exception. The same medications used for routine ICU sedation are also used in ECLS, usually consisting of a benzodiazepine (midazolam or lorazepam) and an opioid analgesic (morphine or fentanyl). Dosing requirements may be elevated, as drugs may be adsorbed by the circuit, tolerance can develop, and hemofiltration can remove administered drugs (8–10).

A major trend in extracorporeal support is to minimize sedation and allow spontaneous breathing, and even interaction with staff and family. Use of minimal doses of benzodiazepines and narcotics can be supplemented by other agents. Atypical antipsychotic agents are effective in reducing agitation and delirium without sedation, and dexmedetomidine provides sedation from which the patient can be easily aroused.

Fluids and Renal Replacement Therapy

Maintenance of normal intravascular volume is important during ECLS, as adequate venous return is necessary to maintain pump flow. Insufficient volume can be detected by poor filling of the bladder and downregulation of the pump. In centrifugal pump systems (without a bladder) blood flow variation at a constant pump speed heralds inadequate venous return and mandates prompt correction to avoid hemolysis. Volume can be replaced with crystalloid, colloid, or blood products. If blood products are required for other reasons, they are the first choice.

Excess interstitial edema leads to organ dysfunction, contributing to worsening pulmonary, cardiac, gastrointestinal, and renal function. Diuretics (intermittent or continuous infusion) are the first choice in reducing interstitial edema, but if response to diuretics is inadequate, hemofiltration can be incorporated into the ECLS circuit. However, there is evidence that patients on hemofiltration and ECLS have worse outcomes than those just receiving ECLS alone (55,56). Although

this may simply reflect more severe underlying disease, it is also possible that there is something intrinsically harmful about hemofiltration in this context.

Hemofiltration can be performed by inserting a hemofilter between high-pressure and low-pressure points in the circuit, such as preoxygenator and into the bladder, respectively. This configuration acts as a shunt, reducing blood flow to the patient; therefore, circuit flow must be monitored beyond the insertion point and compensated for the loss to the hemofilter. A better approach is to siphon postoxygenator blood into a dedicated pediatric continuous renal replacement therapy (CRRT) circuit and return the blood preoxygenator, where air or debris from the CRRT circuit can be trapped by the oxygenator. If a vascular access catheter is in place prior to ECLS, running two separate circuits, one for ECLS and one for CRRT, is the simplest way of avoiding detrimental interactions between the two systems (57).

Plasmapheresis for plasma exchange in the management of sepsis syndrome or immunologic disorders and extracorporeal liver support for hepatic failure can also be performed through the ECLS circuit without the need for additional vascular access.

Nutritional Support

It is well established that enteral nutrition has substantial benefits over IV nutrition in critically ill patients and is the preferred route of administration. Parenteral nutrition has given way to enteral nutrition as the route of choice, which is well tolerated in adults (58) and neonates (59) on ECLS. Initiation of enteral nutritional support should begin after resuscitation is complete and perfusion is restored, usually within 12–24 hours. The absence of bowel sounds does not predict intolerance and should not be used as a reason to withhold feeding. Postpyloric feeding may be better tolerated than gastric, but the addition of promotility agents such as erythromycin, allows successful gastric feeding in most patients. The reduction in intestinal edema that accompanies the achievement of euvolemia may facilitate tolerance of enteral feeds.

Contraindications to the enteral route include mechanical obstruction, ischemic bowel, and recent bowel resection. IV nutritional support is used when the enteral route is contraindicated or to supplement it when full support cannot be achieved by the enteral route alone. IV lipids administered to patients supported with a microporous, hollow-fiber oxygenator can result in plasma leakage. Newer hollow-fiber devices that have solid membranes or siloxane coating of the fibers are resistant to leakage.

Withdrawal of Care

The duration of support required for cardiac or pulmonary recovery is variable. The average duration of support for postoperative cardiac dysfunction is 3–5 days and slightly longer for myocarditis and nonoperative cardiomyopathy (7–9 days). Support duration is longer for pulmonary dysfunction (averages 11–13 days depending on the diagnosis). It had once been common practice to terminate support in apparently refractory cases if lung function had not returned after a period of time (2–3 weeks) under the assumption that organ damage was irreversible by this time. Recent experience, however, indicates that lung function can recover after extended periods of time, and support for 2–3 months or more with recovery is no longer uncommon. The decision to withdraw support is, therefore, an individualized one that includes underlying diagnosis, extent of organ dysfunction, complications, and perhaps further diagnostic tests to establish irreversibility (e.g., biopsy). Valid reasons to withdraw support include when complications that are incompatible with long-term survival or adequate functional outcome develop, or when the patient is ineligible for transplantation and does not recover (e.g., alveolar capillary dysplasia). As noted above, this latter issue is more commonly seen with heart disease and VA ECLS.

Withdrawal of care proceeds in the usual way following extensive family discussion, appropriate planning, and the administration of adequate anxiolysis and analgesia. However, as with other forms of withdrawal of life support, it is ethically important to make a distinction between withdrawing life support and hastening death by causing harm. In the case of patients on VA ECLS with some residual cardiac function, merely turning off the pump will create a large arteriovenous shunt that will hasten death. A more appropriate way is to place two short clamps on each cannula and cut in between them. This avoids creating a potentially harmful intravascular shunt and facilitates cradling of the child by its parents. The circuit can then be removed from the bedside.

COMPLICATIONS

Bleeding

Bleeding complications are among the most common problems associated with ECLS. Bleeding can occur at surgical (including cannulation) sites but can also be unrelated to procedures or trauma. Bleeding can be life-threatening, such as with intracranial hemorrhage. The initial approach to bleeding management is to identify causes that are surgically correctable (e.g., a bleeding vessel at a cannulation site). If no such treatable cause is found, the platelet count is increased and the level of anticoagulation is decreased. An ACT of 160–180 seconds, or perhaps 140–160 seconds, may be required for a period of time. If bleeding continues despite these efforts, pharmacologic agents may be helpful. Aminocaproic acid has historically been the predominant pharmacologic agent that helps to control bleeding on ECLS. Aminocaproic acid binds reversibly to plasminogen, blocking the binding of plasminogen to fibrin and its activation to plasmin, thus inhibiting thrombolysis. An IV loading dose of 100 mg/kg is administered, followed by a continuous infusion of 25–50 mg/kg. Tranexamic acid is another inhibitor of thrombolysis used in extracorporeal support. Recombinant factor VII has also been used for torrential bleeding but is associated with acute circuit thrombosis and cannot be recommended at present as standard rescue therapy. Life-threatening or uncontrollable bleeding may require the discontinuation of ECLS.

Heparin-induced thrombocytopenia (HIT) due to heparin-associated antibodies is an uncommon but potentially life-threatening complication of heparin use. A precipitous fall in platelet count 5 days or more after initiation of heparin in the presence of thrombotic complications mandates discontinuation of heparin and substitution of an alternative anticoagulant. Argatroban is a direct thrombin inhibitor that is gaining acceptance as the first alternative to heparin in cases of HIT (60,61).

Neurological

Neurological injury is the most potentially devastating complication of ECLS and can occur with both respiratory and cardiac ECLS (9). Assessment for potential neurological injury forms a regular and important part of clinical assessment. In children with an anterior fontanelle, it is normal practice to perform daily or second daily cranial ultrasound to monitor for cerebral thromboembolism, bleeding, or edema. Some centers also use continuous EEG monitoring to detect seizures in high-risk patients. Maintaining strict control over anticoagulation is probably among the most effective ways of preventing neurological injury, as is avoiding delays in instituting ECLS in severely hypoxic or hypotensive patients.

Vascular Injury

The procedure of cannulation entails placement of a large vascular cannula, imposing the risk of injury to the vessel or failure to complete cannulation. These complications may be more common in percutaneous cannulation as the vessels are not directly visualized, but they can occur during surgical approaches as well. Vascular injury can present as posterior perforation with extravascular placement, subintimal placement, or vessel transection. Failure to complete cannulation may result from an attempt to place a cannula larger than the vein can accommodate or from placement of the guidewire in a tributary rather than in the major vessel. These will usually require surgical exploration and management.

Ultrasonography can be used to measure vessel size prior to percutaneous cannulation to aid in selecting appropriately sized cannulas and in identifying abnormal venous anatomy prior to insertion. Ultrasonography is also helpful in guiding needle entry during vessel puncture, enhancing the chance of successful cannulation. Use of fluoroscopy during percutaneous catheter insertion can help to identify aberrant guidewire placement and reduce the chance of vascular injury.

Infection

The presence of sepsis or bacteremia at the institution of ECLS is not independently associated with worse outcomes (62,63). However, the acquisition of new infection while receiving ECLS is associated with a number of poor outcome measures, including longer duration of ECMO, increased mechanical ventilation time, and increased mortality (64). The most important risk factor for nosocomial infection on ECLS is the duration of support (65). Detecting new infection in ECLS patients is difficult, as conventional biomarkers such as leucocytosis are nonspecific and the heater-cooler masks fever. Clinicians have to rely on meticulous clinical examination and maintain a low threshold to institute therapy if new infection is suspected. There is little evidence to support routine surveillance cultures (66,67).

OUTCOMES FROM ECLS

Over 50,000 patients from all age groups who have undergone extracorporeal support have been reported to the ELSO registry as of June 2012 (9). Most were in the neonatal age group, but 12,995 were from the pediatric age group (**Table 40.4**). More than half of these were cardiac support cases, and most of the remaining were respiratory support cases. A small but growing experience with ECPR (1562 patients) was also reported.

Survival in pediatric ECLS for respiratory failure is 65%, with 56% surviving to hospital discharge. Although survival to hospital discharge in many centers appears to have been relatively static over the last two decades, there has been a steady increase in patient complexity (68). However, a recent single-center report examining outcomes in children with severe pneumonia requiring ECLS compared historical and modern cohorts (before and after 2005) and found improved survival in the modern era (60% vs. 88.2%, $p = 0.04$) (56). The survival in cardiac support is lower, with 65% surviving ECLS and 49% surviving to discharge. ECPR has the lowest survival

TABLE 40.4

OVERALL OUTCOMES IN ECLS AS REPORTED TO THE ELSO, ANN ARBOR, MICHIGAN, AS OF JUNE 2012 (9)

	TOTAL	SURVIVED ECLS (%)		SURVIVED TO DISCHARGE (%)	
Neonatal					
Respiratory	25,746	21,765	85	19,232	75
Cardiac	4797	2928	61	1912	40
ECPR	784	496	63	304	39
Pediatric					
Respiratory	5457	3556	65	3061	56
Cardiac	5976	3855	65	2913	49
ECPR	1562	843	54	630	40
Adult					
Respiratory	3280	2094	64	1808	55
Cardiac	2312	1243	54	891	39
ECPR	753	276	37	207	27

ECPR, extracorporeal cardiopulmonary resuscitation.

(40% to discharge), but considering the moribund condition of these children, this level of survival is remarkable.

Long-Term Outcomes

As noted above, one of the most devastating sequelae associated with ECLS is neurologic impairment. Unlike the neonatal experience, no large-scale outcome studies that focus on the pediatric age group have been reported. The ELSO registry reports complication rates, but with respect to neurologic complications these largely represent short-term complications. Clinically diagnosed brain death was reported in 5.2% of pediatric patients who were supported for respiratory failure and in 7.3% of children above 1 year of age supported for cardiac failure. Seizures, either clinically or electroencephalographically determined, were reported in 7.1% of respiratory support cases and 5.6% of cardiac support cases above 1 year of age. CNS infarction or hemorrhage was reported in 3.5%–6% of cases.

Studies examining long-term outcomes have reported severe disability rates in survivors of at least 4% (69–71). However, this varies with the population being studied, the duration of follow-up, and the methods used to analyze neurodevelopmental function. It is extremely likely that many of the adverse long-term effects are due to the underlying illness rather than ECLS (72). This issue deserves more robust, comprehensive study.

ORGANIZATION

Extracorporeal life support is complex medical therapy requiring a dedicated multidisciplinary team to provide it effectively. Recent data demonstrate a probable relationship between center volume and outcomes, with institutions managing fewer than 15–20 ECLS patients per year achieving poorer outcomes than higher volume centers (73,74). It is also likely that some regional or national coordination of ECLS services is economical and improves outcome (3).

The ELSO (Ann Arbor, MI) is a consortium of healthcare centers that use extracorporeal circulation for support of severe cardiopulmonary failure. These centers contribute detailed data to a registry on each ECLS case performed. The registry currently has data on more than 50,000 cases performed since the first neonatal case in 1975. The vast majority

of ECLS cases in the United States and a rapidly growing number of international cases are reported to ELSO. Thus, the registry data are highly representative of ECLS over the past four decades.

CONCLUSIONS AND FUTURE DIRECTIONS

Technical advances in ECLS have contributed to improvements in outcome and a reduction in complications. Further technical improvements have the potential to make ECLS safer and perhaps more effective. The availability of dual-lumen cannulas for patients of all sizes has reduced the complexity of support. Advances in centrifugal pump design have resulted in an increased use of these devices over traditional roller pumps for ECLS. Newer pump and oxygenator configurations that are more compact, safe, and efficient have expanded the ability of transport teams to move ECLS patients between hospitals or even countries. Investigation to identify and standardize optimal practice for anticoagulation management and other aspects of patient care to reduce complications such as bleeding may improve outcome. Fiscal analysis to monitor cost–benefit ratios and health care resource utilization is also required. Finally, research and development of implantable cardiac or pulmonary support devices in small patients may one day obviate the need for ECMO as we know it today.

References

1. Peek GJ, Killer HM, Reeves R, et al. Early experience with a polymethylpentene oxygenator for adult extracorporeal life support. *ASAIO J* 2002;48:480–2.
2. Khoshbin E, Roberts N, Harvey C, et al. Poly-methyl pentene oxygenators have improved gas exchange capability and reduced transfusion requirements in adult extracorporeal membrane oxygenation. *ASAIO J* 2005;51:281–7.
3. MacLaren G, Combes A, Bartlett RH. Contemporary extracorporeal membrane oxygenation for adult respiratory failure: Life support in the new era. *Intensive Care Med* 2012;38:210–20.
4. Sivarajan VB, Best D, Brizard CP, et al. Improved outcomes of paediatric extracorporeal support associated with technology change. *Interact Cardiovasc Thorac Surg* 2010;11:400–5.

5. Paulsen MJ, Orizondo R, Le D, et al. A simple, standard method to characterize pressure/flow performance of vascular access cannulas. *ASAIO J* 2013;59:24–9.

6. Preston TJ, Ratliff TM, Gomez D, et al. Modified surface coatings and their effect on drug adsorption within the extracorporeal life support circuit. *J Extra Corpor Technol* 2010;42:199–202.

7. Wildschut ED, Ahsman MJ, Allegaert K, et al. Determinants of drug absorption in different ECMO circuits. *Intensive Care Med* 2010;36:2109–16.

8. Shekar K, Roberts JA, McDonald CI, et al. Sequestration of drugs in the circuit may lead to therapeutic failure during extracorporeal membrane oxygenation. *Crit Care* 2012;16:R194.

9. Extracorporeal Life Support Organization. ECLS registry report. International Summary. Ann Arbor, July 2012.

10. Roberts N, Westrope C, Pooboni SK, et al. Venovenous extracorporeal membrane oxygenation for respiratory failure in inotrope dependent neonates. *ASAIO J* 2003;49:568–71.

11. Conrad SA, Zwischenberger JB, Grier LR, et al. Total extracorporeal arteriovenous carbon dioxide removal in acute respiratory failure: A phase I clinical study. *Intensive Care Med* 2001;27:1340–51.

12. Conrad SA, Green R, Scott LK. Near-fatal pediatric asthma managed with pumpless arteriovenous carbon dioxide removal. *Crit Care Med* 2007;35:2624–9.

13. Aharon AS, Drinkwater DC Jr, Churchwell KB, et al. Extracorporeal membrane oxygenation in children after repair of congenital cardiac lesions. *Ann Thorac Surg* 2001;72:2095—101.

14. Chaturvedi RR, Macrae D, Brown KL, et al. Cardiac ECMO for biventricular hearts after paediatric open heart surgery. *Heart* 2004;90:545–51.

15. Thiagarajan RR, Salvin JW. Cardiac catheterization procedures for ECMO patients. In: Annich GM, Lynch WR, MacLaren G, et al., eds. ECMO. *Extracorporeal Cardiopulmonary Support in Critical Care*. 4th ed. Ann Arbor, MI: Extracorporeal Life Support Organization, 2012:425–33.

16. Duncan BW, Bohn DJ, Atz AM, et al. Mechanical circulatory support for the treatment of children with acute fulminant myocarditis. *J Thorac Cardiovasc Surg* 2001;122:440–8.

17. Chen YS, Wang MJ, Chou NK, et al. Rescue for acute myocarditis with shock by extracorporeal membrane oxygenation. *Ann Thorac Surg* 1999;68:2220–4.

18. Goldman AP, Cassidy J, De Leval M, et al. The waiting game: Bridging to paediatric heart transplantation. *Lancet* 2003;362:1967–70.

19. Fiser WP, Yetman AT, Gunselman RJ, et al. Pediatric arteriovenous extracorporeal membrane oxygenation (ECMO) as a bridge to cardiac transplantation. *J Heart Lung Transplant* 2003;22:770–7.

20. Fraser CD, Jaquiss RD, Rosenthal DN, et al. Prospective trial of a pediatric ventricular device. *N Engl J Med* 2012; 367:532–41.

21. Jeewa A, Manlhiot C, McCrindle BW, et al. Outcomes with ventricular assist device versus extracorporeal membrane oxygenation as a brudge to pediatric heart transplantation. *Artif Organs* 2010;34:1087–91.

22. Imamura M, Dossey AM, Prodhan P, et al. Bridge to cardiac transplant in children: Berlin Heart versus extracorporeal membrane oxygenation. *Ann Thorac Surg* 2009;87:1894–1901.

23. McCune S, Short BL, Miller MK, et al. Extracorporeal membrane oxygenation therapy in neonates with septic shock. *J Pediatr Surg* 1990;25:479–82.

24. Hocker JR, Simpson PM, Rabalais GP, et al. Extracorporeal membrane oxygenation and early-onset group B streptococcal sepsis. *Pediatrics* 1992;89:1–4.

25. Beca J, Butt W. Extracorporeal membrane oxygenation for refractory septic shock in children. *Pediatrics* 1994;93:726–29.

26. Goldman AP, Kerr SJ, Butt W, et al. Extracorporeal support for intractable cardiorespiratory failure due to meningococcal disease. *Lancet* 1997;349:466–9.

27. Brierley J, Carcillo JA, Choong K, et al. Clinical practice parameters for hemodynamic support of pediatric and neonatal septic shock: 2007 update from the American College of Critical Care Medicine. *Crit Care Med* 2009;37:666–88.

28. MacLaren G, Butt W. Sepsis and ECMO. In: Annich GM, Lynch WR, MacLaren G, et al., eds. ECMO. *Extracorporeal Cardiopulmonary Support in Critical Care*. 4th ed. Ann Arbor, MI: Extracorporeal Life Support Organization, 2012:425–33.

29. Kinsella JP, Gerstmann DR, Rosenberg AA. The effect of extracorporeal membrane oxygenation on coronary perfusion and regional flow distribution. *Pediatr Res* 1992;31:80–84.

30. Shen I, Levy FH, Benak AM, et al. Left ventricular dysfunction during extracorporeal membrane oxygenation in a hypoxemic swine model. *Ann Thorac Surg* 2001;71:868–71.

31. MacLaren G, Butt W, Best D, et al. Extracorporeal membrane oxygenation for refractory septic shock in children: One institution's experience. *Pediatr Crit Care Med* 2007;8:447–51.

32. MacLaren G, Butt W, Best D, et al. Central extracorporeal membrane oxygenation for refractory pediatric septic shock. *Pediatr Crit Care Med* 2011;12:133–6.

33. Walczak R, Lawson DS, Kaemmer D, et al. Evaluation of a preprimed microporous hollow-fiber membrane for rapid response neonatal extracorporeal membrane oxygenation. *Perfusion* 2005;20:269–75.

34. Kane DA, Thiagarajan RR, Wypij D, et al. Rapid-response extracorporeal membrane oxygenation to support cardiopulmonary resuscitation in children with cardiac disease. *Circulation* 2010;122:S241–8.

35. Meehan JJ, Haney BM, Snyder CL, et al. Outcome after recannulation and a second course of extracorporeal membrane oxygenation. *J Pediatr Surg* 2002;37:845–50.

36. Shuhaiber J, Thiagarajan RR, Laussen PC, et al. Survival of children requiring repeat extracorporeal membrane oxygenation after congenital heart surgery. *Ann Thorac Surg* 2011;91:1949–55.

37. Bohuta L, d'Udekem Y, Best D, et al. Outcomes of second-run extracorporeal life support in children: A single-institution experience. *Ann Thorac Surg* 2011;92:993–6.

38. Pettignano R, Fortenberry JD, Heard ML, et al. Primary use of the venovenous approach for extracorporeal membrane oxygenation in pediatric acute respiratory failure. *Pediatr Crit Care Med* 2003;4:291–8.

39. Cengiz P, Seidel K, Rycus PT, et al. Central nervous system complications during pediatric extracorporeal life support: Incidence and risk factors. *Crit Care Med* 2005;33:2817–24.

40. Peek GJ, Firmin RK, Moore HM, et al. Cannulation of neonates for venovenous extracorporeal life support. *Ann Thorac Surg* 1996;61:1851–2.

41. Cove ME, MacLaren G, Federspiel WJ, et al. Bench-to-bedside review: Extracorporeal carbon dioxide removal, past present and future. *Crit Care* 2012;16:232.

42. Montoya JP, Merz SI, Bartlett RH. A standardized system for describing flow/pressure relationships in vascular access devices. *ASAIO Trans* 1991;37:4–8.

43. Rich PB, Awad SS, Crotti S, et al. A prospective comparison of atrio-femoral and femoro-atrial flow in adult venovenous extracorporeal life support. *J Thorac Cardiovasc Surg* 1998; 116:628–32.

44. Ichiba S, Peek GJ, Sosnowski AW, et al. Modifying a venovenous extracorporeal membrane oxygenation circuit to reduce recirculation. *Ann Thorac Surg* 2000;69:298–9.

45. Nakano T, Tominaga R, Nagano I, et al. Pulsatile flow enhances endothelium-derived nitric oxide release in the peripheral vasculature. *Am J Physiol Heart Circ Physiol* 2000;278:H1098–104.

46. Sezai A, Shiono M, Nakata K, et al. Effects of pulsatile CPB on interleukin-8 and endothelin-1 levels. *Artif Organs* 2005;29:708–13.

47. Undar A, Masai T, Yang SQ, et al. Effects of perfusion mode on regional and global organ blood flow in a neonatal piglet model. *Ann Thorac Surg* 1999;68:1336–42.

48. Bartlett RH. Physiology of extracorporeal life support. In: Annich GM, Lynch WR, MacLaren G, et al., eds. ECMO. *Extracorporeal*

Cardiopulmonary Support in Critical Care. 4th ed. Ann Arbor, MI: Extracorporeal Life Support Organization, 2012:11–31.

49. Heilmann C, Geisen U, Beyersdorf F, et al. Acquired von Willebrand syndrome in patients with extracorporeal life support (ECLS). *Intensive Care Med* 2012;38:62–8.

50. Extracorporeal Life Support Organization. *General Guidelines for all ECLS Cases.* http://www.elsonet.org/index.php/resources/guidelines.html. Accessed October 24, 2012.

51. Extracorporeal Life Support Organization. *ELSO Guidelines for Training and Continuing Education of ECMO Specialists.* http://www.elsonet.org/index.php/resources/guidelines.html. Accessed October 24, 2012.

52. Rastan AJ, Lachmann N, Walther T, et al. Autopsy findings in patients on postcardiotomy extracorporeal membrane oxygenation (ECMO). *Int J Artif Organs* 2006;29:1121–31.

53. Baslaim G, Bashore J, Al-Malki F, et al. Can the outcome of pediatric extracorporeal membrane oxygenation after cardiac surgery be predicted? *Ann Thorac Cardiovasc Surg* 2006; 12:21–7.

54. Montgomery VL, Strotman JM, Ross MP. Impact of multiple organ system dysfunction and nosocomial infections on survival of children treated with extracorporeal membrane oxygenation after heart surgery. *Crit Care Med* 2000;28:526–31.

55. Paden ML, Warshaw BL, Heard ML, et al. Recovery of renal function and survival after continuous renal replacement therapy during extracorporeal membrane oxygenation. *Pediatr Crit Care Med* 2011;12:153–8.

56. Smalley N, MacLaren G, Best D, et al. Outcomes in children with refractory pneumonia supported with extracorporeal membrane oxygenation. *Intensive Care Med* 2012;38:1001–7.

57. MacLaren G. Lessons in advanced extracorporeal life support. *Crit Care Med* 2012;40:2729–31.

58. Scott LK, Boudreaux K, Thaljeh F, et al. Early enteral feedings in adults receiving venovenous extracorporeal membrane oxygenation. *JPEN J Parenter Enteral Nutr* 2004;28:295–300.

59. Piena M, Albers MJ, Van Haard PM, et al. Introduction of enteral feeding in neonates on extracorporeal membrane oxygenation after evaluation of intestinal permeability changes. *J Pediatr Surg* 1998;33:30–4.

60. Young G, Yonekawa KE, Nakagawa P, et al. Argatroban as an alternative to heparin in extracorporeal membrane oxygenation circuits. *Perfusion* 2004;19:283–8.

61. Beiderlinden M, Treschan T, Gorlinger K, et al. Argatroban in extracorporeal membrane oxygenation. *Artif Organs* 2007;31:461–5.

62. Meyer DM, Jessen ME. Results of extracorporeal membrane oxygenation in children with sepsis. *Ann Thorac Surg* 1997;63:756–61.

63. Rich PB, Younger JG, Soles OS, et al. Use of extracorporeal life support for adult patients with respiratory failure and sepsis. *ASAIO J* 1998;44:263–6.

64. Bizzarro MJ, Conrad SA, Kaufman DA, et al. Infections acquired during extracorporeal membrane oxygenation in neonates, children and adults. *Pediatr Crit Care Med* 2011;12:277–81.

65. Hsu MS, Chiu KM, Huang YT, et al. Risk factors for nosocomial infection during extracorporeal membrane oxygenation. *J Hosp Infect* 2009;73:210–16.

66. Elerian LF, Sparks JW, Meyer TA, et al. Usefulness of surveillance cultures in neonatal extracorporeal membrane oxygenation. *ASAIO J* 2001;47:220–3.

67. Lynch W. Infections and ECMO. In: Annich GM, Lynch WR, MacLaren G, et al., eds. *ECMO. Extracorporeal Cardiopulmonary Support in Critical Care.* 4th ed. Ann Arbor, MI: Extracorporeal Life Support Organization, 2012:205–11.

68. Zabrocki LA, Brogan TV, Statler KD, et al. Extracorporeal membrane oxygenation for pediatric respiratory failure: Survival and predictors of mortality. *Crit Care Med* 2011;39:364–70.

69. Chow G, Koirala B, Armstrong D, et al. Predictors of mortality and neurological morbidity in children undergoing extracorporeal life support for cardiac disease. *Eur J Cardiothorac Surg* 2004;26:38–43.

70. Taylor AK, Cousins R, Butt W. The long-term outcome of children managed with extracorporeal life support: An institutional experience. *Crit Care Resusc* 2007;9:172–77.

71. Lequier L, Joffe AR, Robertson CM, et al. Two-year survival, mental, and motor outcomes after cardiac extracorporeal life support at less than five years of age. *J Thorac Cardiovasc Surg* 2008;136:976–83.

72. McNally H, Bennett CC, Elbourne D, et al. United Kingdom collaborative randomized trial of neonatal extracorporeal membrane oxygenation: Follow-up to age 7 years. *Pediatrics* 2006;117:e845–54.

73. Karamlou T, Vafaeezadeh M, Parrish AM, et al. Increased extracorporeal membrane oxygenation center case volume is associated with improved extracorporeal membrane oxygenation survival among pediatric patients. *J Thorac Cardiovasc Surg* 2013; 145:470–475

74. Freeman CL, Bennett TD, Casper TC et al. Pediatric and neonatal extracorporeal membrane oxygenation: does center volume impact mortality? *Crit Care Med* 2014; 42:512–519

CHAPTER 41 ■ EXTRACORPOREAL ORGAN SUPPORT THERAPY

WARWICK W. BUTT, PETER W. SKIPPEN, PHILLIPPE JOUVET, AND JIM FORTENBERRY

KEY POINTS

❶ Extracorporeal organ support therapy comprising peritoneal dialysis, intermittent hemodialysis (HD), various continuous renal replacement therapies (CRRTs), and therapeutic plasma exchange is a standard tool in the PICU.

❷ Common indications for renal replacement therapy (RRT) include acute or chronic renal failure, fluid overload, severe electrolyte disorders, and hyperammonemia.

❸ The standard components of the CRRT circuit consist of blood inflow tubing, a hemofilter, blood outflow tubing, and the ultrafiltrate drainage tubing from the hemofilter to the drainage bag. Roller head pumps control blood flow and ultrafiltrate flow. The hemofilter may also have infusion ports for replacement fluid and/or dialysis fluid depending on the CRRT technique.

❹ Pediatric CRRT requires either systemic anticoagulation with heparin or regional anticoagulation with citrate

infused pre-filter, the effect of which is then reversed with a calcium infusion post-filter to prevent filter clotting.

❺ Fluid removal during CRRT is caused by the hydrostatic pressure gradient (the transmembrane pressure) between the hemofilter inflow and the ultrafiltrate collection bag.

❻ Solute removal during RRTs occurs by osmosis (peritoneal dialysis), diffusion (all HD techniques), or convection (all continuous hemofiltration techniques).

❼ Careful monitoring for intake, output, serum chemistries, complete blood count, and coagulation profile is required during RRTs.

❽ Therapeutic plasma exchange is considered first-line therapy in the treatment of Guillain–Barrè syndrome (GBS), thrombotic thrombocytopenic purpura, antibody-mediated transplantation rejection, myasthenia gravis, and fulminant Wilson disease.

Extracorporeal *organ* support therapy (ECOST) is a standard and integral part of modern intensive care. It is distinguished from extracorporeal *life* support, which can maintain cardiac, cardiopulmonary, or pulmonary support for prolonged periods in a variety of diseases (see Chapter 40) (1).

❶ Various renal replacement therapies (RRTs) (2–4), liver support therapies (e.g., molecular adsorbent recirculating system [MARS]) (5–7), and total plasma exchange (TPE) (8) represent the most common forms of ECOST. Table 41.1 shows the general indications for the use of these therapies at the Royal Children's Hospital, Melbourne, Australia, over the past 25 years. Use of this technology is less common in children than in adults; in the four centers in which the authors work, the frequency is one to three patients per month. The many different modes of ECOST have reasonable alternatives that allow widespread international variation about the preferred mode for a given situation; this variation is reflected in Table 41.2 from centers in the United States and Australia.

All extracorporeal therapies have similar complications related to vascular access, infection, mechanical/equipment failure, thromboembolism, and bleeding. The principles that apply to all devices and circuit configurations in relation to blood flow and solute clearance are similar and depend on the nature and volume of the solute or protein that is to be removed. This chapter reviews the technical aspects of commonly performed adjunctive extracorporeal therapies such as dialysis, hemofiltration, plasma exchange, MARS, coupled plasma filtration and adsorption (CPFA) and their use in children with critical illness.

GENERAL CONCEPTS

Developmental Renal Physiology

Renal Blood Flow and Glomerular Filtration Rate

A newborn infant has a renal blood flow (RBF) of ~20% that of an adult. Consequently, the glomerular filtration rate (GFR) is also markedly reduced, as are tubular excretion and reabsorption. The normal age-related changes in GFR and RBF are given in Table 41.3.

Clearance

Renal clearance is a quantitative measure of the rate of removal of a substance from the blood by the kidneys. It is expressed in terms of the volume of blood that could be completely cleared of a substance in 1 minute (mL/min). Clearance is often normalized for body surface area (expressed as mL/min/m^2).

The ECOST Circuit Components

The basic ECOST filter circuit is shown in Figure 41.1. This consists of a double-lumen catheter, the hemofilter, as well as roller pumps for blood filtration, ultrafiltration, and replacement fluids. It is important to understand the technical functioning of these components for safe use in critical care (9,10).

TABLE 41.1

GENERAL INDICATIONS FOR ECOST AT ROYAL CHILDREN'S HOSPITAL (1987–2012)

INDICATION	PATIENTS (%)	FILTERS PER PATIENT (AVERAGE)
Fluid/electrolyte	39	2.15
Sepsis	27	2.1
Antibody removal	16	5.7
Renal failure	7	3
Elevated ammonia	6	2
Drug overdose	1	19
Other	4	8

TABLE 41.2

MODES OF ECOST USED: AN INTERNATIONAL COMPARISON (2010–2012)

ECOST	PATIENTS RCH	PATIENTS CHOA
CVVH	53	108
CVVP	18	90
CVVHD	5	0
ECMO/CVVH	11	75
ECMO/CVVP	1	9
CVVH (predilution)	0	108
CVVHDF	1	0
CVVH/CVVP	3	0
ECMO/CVVH/CVVP	2	8

CHoA, Children's Healthcare of Atlanta, Atlanta, Georgia, United States; RCH, The Royal Children's Hospital, Melbourne, Australia.

TABLE 41.3

NORMAL RENAL FUNCTION AT DIFFERENT AGES

AGE	GFR (mL/min/m²)	RBF (mL/min/m²)
Preterm	15	40
Term	20	90
1–2 wk	50	220
6 mo to 1 y	80	350
1–3 y	100	540
Adult	120	620

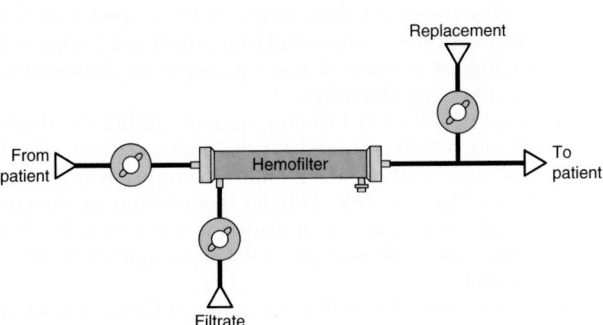

FIGURE 41.1. Basic ECOST circuit with catheters (from and to patient), hemofilter, filtrate, and replacement fluids. Roller pumps control flow rates for hemofilter blood, (ultra) filtrate, and replacement fluid.

Catheters

A large range of double-lumen, variable-length catheters is available. These catheters contain a proximal withdrawal lumen that has multiple side holes and a distal, single-end lumen for reinfusion to the patient. They are firm so that they will not collapse with suction applied by the system. Recommended sizes for hemofiltration/plasmafiltration catheters for children are listed in **Table 41.4**. The catheter is placed using the Seldinger technique, which requires introducing the dilator and catheter over a wire. Dilating the vessel using successively larger dilators reduces complications in small children and avoids puncturing a small vessel with a large needle (11).

Much debate surrounds the best vascular site for catheter placement, especially in small infants. The largest accessible percutaneous vessel is the subclavian vein, followed by the internal jugular and femoral veins. Ultrasound localization of vessels during placement may limit complications and improve success of catheter insertion. The closer the tip of the vascular catheter is to the right atrium, the better the flow obtained, although placing the catheter deep in the right atrium is associated with a greater risk of perforation. At high blood flow rates, high negative pressure can be generated in the dialysis circuit. Both blood drainage and blood return can be impaired. Alterations in circuit pressure (either too negative or too positive) outside the set alarm limits will cause a cessation of filtration. In situations in which drainage is inadequate, the filter connections can be reversed, so that the inflow (blood drainage) cannula is the single-end hole and the blood-return lumen is the side hole. Although this may increase recirculation of blood back into the circuit, the improved blood flow obtained may allow adequate filtration to continue.

Hemofilters

Two key elements determine filter function:

1. Size—The larger the surface area of the filter, the more effective is the filtration (i.e., the higher the filtration fraction [FF]) and also the less the hemoconcentration within the filter. However, larger filters require larger priming volumes (with potential hemodilution consequences) and slower blood flow within the filter.
2. The type of membrane—Filters may be composed of either microtubules or a plate membrane, and the material may be either polysulphone or polyacrylonitrile nitrate (see **Fig. 41.2**). The minor differences in FF and sieving coefficients (SCs) between these membranes are, for practical purposes, not relevant.

The continuous renal replacement therapy (CRRT) filters used for filtration vary around the world. In principle, large filters can be used even in small infants when venovenous circuits are used. The authors commonly use either 0.25 or 0.5 m² surface area filters in newborn infants, which allow for improved filter performance at lower blood flows but require more anticoagulation because of the slower blood flow.

TABLE 41.4

SUGGESTED SIZES OF CATHETERS FOR USE IN CVVH/CVVP

PATIENT AGE (y)	CATHETER SIZE (FRENCH)	FLOW (mL/min)
Neonate	Single-lumen 5 or Dual-lumen 6.5–7	25–40
1–4	Dual-lumen 7.0–8.5	40–80
5–10	Dual-lumen 8.5–11.5	50–100
>10	Dual-lumen 11.5–14	80–150

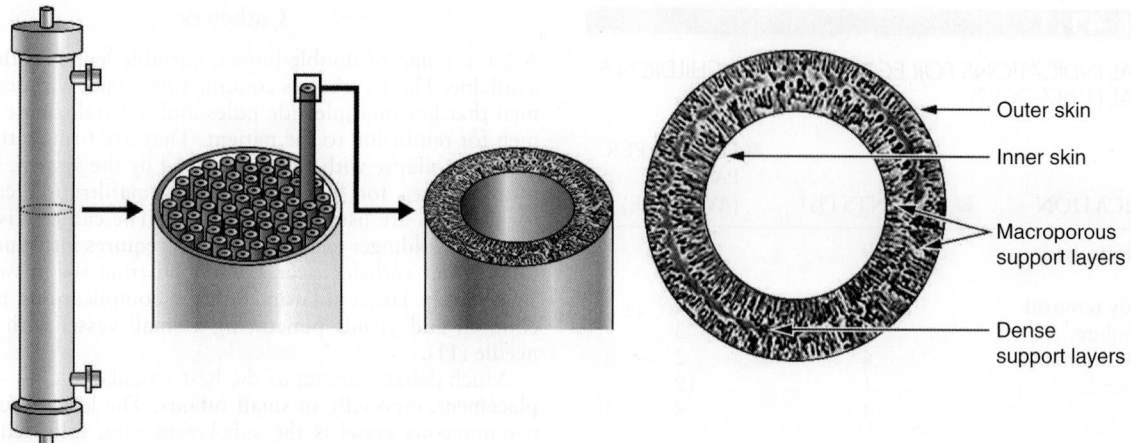

FIGURE 41.2. Cross-sectional view of a hemofilter.

Pumps

Almost all circuits use roller pumps to accurately control blood flow, ultrafiltrate flow, and replacement fluid. The tubing circuit diameter varies slightly, and the size of the pump head varies accordingly. These pumps vary in accuracy from 0.1 to 1 mL/min.

Heater

The use of extracorporeal circulation (ECC) and the infusion of solute with high flow rates can create substantial heat loss. Continuous monitoring of core temperature is necessary, and the use of heating systems is recommended. Newborns and small infants are kept warm with radiant incubators, and older children are warmed with warming blankets. Blood circuit and dialysate warmers are often used. The circuit may also be covered with aluminum foil (space blanket material) to minimize heat loss. If these procedures are unsuccessful, a heat exchanger can be added to the circuit.

Circuit Priming

With many modern continuous venovenous hemofiltration (CVVH) systems, circuit priming is automatic. In children who weigh >10 kg, circuit priming is often performed with the use of 0.9% saline or albumin with 5 U/mL of heparin. In children who weigh <10 kg, in children in whom the priming volume is >10%–15% of estimated patient blood volume (12), or in patients who are hemodynamically compromised, it is a common practice to use a blood prime. Hematocrit of the priming fluid should be >40%. The amount of albumin and packed red blood cells to be added to the circuit and tubing can be calculated as

$$(V_{prbc} \times Hct_{prbc}/P_{hct}) - V_{prbc} = V_{alb}$$

where

V_{prbc} = the volume of packed red blood cells for the prime
Hct_{prbc} = the hematocrit of the prime red blood cells
P_{hct} = the desired hematocrit of the prime
V_{alb} = the volume of 5% albumin to be added to the prime solution.

Small infants are also prone to hypotension when filtration is started, and the child's blood ionized calcium levels and hemodynamic parameters should be carefully monitored. Depending on the patient, vasoactive medications (e.g., epinephrine or norepinephrine) may need to be ready for administration to counteract hypotension during initiation of filtration, whereas for others increase in doses of vasoactive drugs may be needed to compensate for hemodilution and catecholamine adsorption to the circuit or filter.

Complications of Extracorporeal Therapy

1. Access—Large veins are needed for the large catheters, and the risk of complications of insertion are inevitable but may be minimized by use of an ultrasound-guided insertion by an experienced person. A systematic review involving 1014 critically ill children showed that pneumo- and hemothorax occurred most commonly with subclavian vein cannulation followed by internal jugular vein cannulation (13). Conversely, femoral vein cannulation had the highest rate of inadvertent arterial puncture (13). Arterial access is rarely used and is unnecessary. Avoiding arterial cannulation prevents potential limb ischemia and arterial bleeding complications.
2. Infection—Prevention of catheter-related infection requires good aseptic technique during catheter insertion and during access of circuit.
3. Technical—Equipment malfunction is always possible, so trained staff must be available, and adequate machine and patient monitoring is essential.
4. Clotting of blood vessel or membrane filter—Clotting of vessels is often related to catheter dysfunction (size of the catheter close to the size of the vessel). Clotting may also be increased in instances of infection. Despite the use of heparin, clots in the blood vessel used for cannulation can occur in 30%–50% of patients with large filtration catheters. Clotting of the filter is increased if there is a high FF (which causes hemoconcentration in the distal end of the filter), in instances of slow blood flow in large surface area filters, or if long microtubules with high resistance are used. Clotting is also increased with frequent interruption of flow (14), with poor anticoagulation, or in conditions with circulating procoagulants (e.g., sepsis or diffuse intravascular coagulopathy).
5. Bleeding—Patient bleeding may occur, but the degree of anticoagulation used for the dialysis circuit is fairly low and is often a regional technique, which minimizes bleeding risk. Platelet dysfunction or disseminated intravascular coagulation is much more likely to cause patient bleeding than the anticoagulants used for ECOST.
6. Embolism—Although uncommon, embolization of air, clots, or debris returning from the circuit can occur.

Complications of the different therapies and anticoagulation techniques are discussed in more detail in the respective sections.

Anticoagulation Use

Various factors affect the decision to anticoagulate a patient for CRRT, such as patient age, underlying condition, medications (coexisting heparin therapy), and platelet counts. Based on these considerations, different options are available to prevent clotting in the extracorporeal circuits. It is vital to remember that many factors lead to clotting within the circuit including

- kinking of catheters;
- high circuit resistance;
- obstruction to inflow (blood drainage from patient);
- obstruction of catheter (often by side-hole occlusion by the vessel wall);
- slow blood flow or stasis;
- high blood viscosity due to high hematocrit, high plasma proteins, or from hemoconcentration due to excess fluid filtration;
- fibrin-strand formation from binding to the plastic surface of tubing or the filter;
- circulating procoagulants (particularly in sepsis or systemic inflammatory response syndrome);
- inadequate anticoagulation.

Most pediatric filtration is performed with anticoagulation of some type. While one study in adults showed minimal difference in CRRT efficiency between the use of no anticoagulation, heparin, or regional anticoagulation, the blood flows used in adult patients are much higher than those used in children, making it questionable whether these same effects would be obtained in children (15). Although a wide variety of anticoagulants have been used in children (16), most PICUs follow one of the following schemes:

- Infusion of 10–20 U/kg **heparin** pre-filter and 1–2 U/kg heparin post-filter and maintenance of activated clotting time (ACT) at 1.5–2 times normal (to limit clots on the return line and tip of vascular-access catheter). **Figure 41.3** shows the corresponding circuit design for this option.
- Regional anticoagulation with **citrate**, which acts through calcium chelation. Trisodium citrate (0.5%) is infused *pre*-filter with the goal of maintaining a *post*-filter ionized Ca^{2+} (iCa^{2+}) of 0.3–0.4 mmol/L. (The pre-filter citrate infusion is *increased* if the post-filter iCa^{2+} is >0.4 mmoL/L and *decreased* if the iCa^{2+} is <0.3 mmol/L.) A *systemic calcium* infusion maintains the patient's iCa^{2+} of 1–1.2 mmol/L (17). Patients with

cardiovascular compromise may require higher levels of iCa^{2+} (1.2–1.4 mmol/L).

- Regional anticoagulation with **heparin** infused pre-filter with 10–20 U/kg/h and reversed post-filter with **protamine** (1 mg for every 100 U of heparin given pre-filter).
- The easiest form of anticoagulation is a simple unfractionated heparin infusion into the pre-filter limb of the circuit with regular monitoring of bedside ACTs and daily laboratory coagulation tests. The risk of hemorrhage rises significantly with activated partial thromboplastin time (aPTT) more than two to five times normal. An aPTT of 1.5–2 times normal appears to minimize the risk of filter clotting.

In situations of marked coagulopathy, such as sepsis, severe brain injury, trauma, liver failure, or active bleeding, it is logical to use regional anticoagulation, whereby the circuit is anticoagulated but the effect is reversed prior to blood return to the patient. Using some form of anticoagulation with these types of clinical situations is imperative because circulating procoagulants will often cause filter clotting if no anticoagulation is used. The most common method of regional anticoagulation used in the PICU is citrate/calcium, while the use of heparin/protamine predominates in adult patients. However, recent publications reflect a growing recognition of the safety of regional citrate anticoagulation in adults (18–22). Most clinicians who favor regional anticoagulation with citrate/calcium in the PICU argue that the heparin/protamine complex itself is an anticoagulant that prolongs the ACT, and the exact dose of protamine is not certain in children. Many use citrate as the standard form of anticoagulation, which incidentally avoids heparin-induced thrombocytopenia. This issue has been recently reviewed in a meta-analysis (23). Patients with severe liver failure are at risk for citrate toxicity because of inability to metabolize the citrate load (see below).

Citrate is provided differently in different countries. Citrate is not approved for use in CRRT by the FDA in the United States. There are commercial preparations that incorporate citrate into replacement fluids in Australia and Europe. Others centers use 3% anticoagulant citrate dextrose (ACD) or 0.5% trisodium citrate.

Anticoagulation Monitoring

The key to safe heparin anticoagulation is a systematic approach and adequate monitoring. There are two groups of tests that are used:

1. Bedside tests of "blood clotting" such as ACT with a goal level 1.5–2 times normal, depending on the patient's diagnosis, clinical condition, and risk for bleeding. A newer and more informative test, namely the Thrombo Elastogram (TEG), is now used in many centers instead of, or in addition to, the ACT.
2. Blood tests of clotting such as aPTT, D-Dimers, or Anti-Xa (for fractionated or low molecular heparins) or antithrombin III (ATIII). The preferred aPTT is 1.5–2 times normal.

The key to safe citrate anticoagulation is similarly a systematic approach and adequate monitoring of

1. post-filter iCa^{2+} to maintain levels 0.3–0.4 mmol/L
2. patient systemic iCa^{2+} levels 1–1.2 mmol/L
3. daily total calcium levels to monitor for citrate toxicity
4. avoiding excessive blood flow to minimize citrate flows and hence minimize risks of citrate toxicity

Each program should develop a specific anticoagulation protocol.

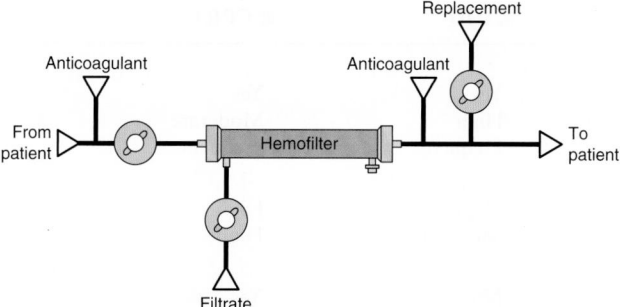

FIGURE 41.3. Location of pre- and post-filter anticoagulation ports for commonly used unfractionated heparin anticoagulation. Heparin 10–20 U/kg/h is infused pre-filter, whereas heparin 1–2 U/kg/h is infused post-filter. Heparin infusion rates are adjusted to keep ACT and aPTT 1.5–2 times normal.

TABLE 41.5

INDICATIONS FOR RENAL REPLACEMENT THERAPY

Renal
Oliguria (unresponsive to diuretics and/or fluid challenge)
Anuria (nonobstructive)
Metabolic acidosis
Hyperkalemia
Azotemia
Uremia symptoms (encephalopathy, myopathy, pericarditis, bleeding)
Hyperphosphatemia

Nonrenal
Fluid overload
Anticipated large transfusion in trauma or coagulopathy
Inborn errors of metabolism
Sepsis
Post-CPB systemic inflammatory response syndrome
Pancreatitis
Drug overdose

RENAL REPLACEMENT THERAPIES

This section reviews the technical aspects of the commonly performed RRTs in the PICU, the respective renal and nonrenal indications for each type of therapy (**Table 41.5**), and a guide to aid the determination of which type of RRT is most appropriate for the individual patient (**Table 41.6**) (24–26).

Indications

RRT is used in a variety of clinical situations to remove endogenous or exogenous toxins and to restore water, acid–base, or electrolyte balance (3,27,28). In children, RRT requires specific expertise owing to (a) the wide variation in the patient sizes (from 2 to 100 kg); (b) the variety of diseases necessitating RRT such as inborn errors of metabolism, cardiac failure, or sepsis; and (c) the variety of available techniques: peritoneal dialysis (PD), intermittent hemodialysis (iHD), and CRRTs (CVVH, continuous venovenous hemodialysis [CVVHD], and continuous venovenous hemodiafiltration [CVVHDF]).

The diseases that cause acute kidney injury (AKI) and that require RRT have been described in several large reviews (29–32) and a registry report (4). The frequency of use of RRT in the PICU varies between 2% and 7% of all patients admitted (29,32–34). The survival rate of children in the PICU who receive RRT is worse than that of children who do not receive it. Among 310 of 4104 children receiving RRT in the Royal Children's Hospital PICU in 2010–2012, the mortality was 12% compared with 3% for patients not receiving RRT. The average length of stay for RRT patients was 12.7 days (cardiac) to 14.5 days (noncardiac) compared with 4.5 days and 3.5 days, respectively, for patients without RRT. This reflects the severity and nature of the underlying diseases in the children who receive RRT, not the inherent safety of the procedure (35).

Contraindications

Very few absolute contraindications to CRRT exist. Even in the presence of intracranial hemorrhage or systemic bleeding, CRRT can be safely performed by using no anticoagulation, using small doses of heparin with close serial monitoring of anticoagulation by ACT, or using regional anticoagulation provided by citrate/calcium. Although some centers consider an intracerebral hemorrhage an absolute contraindication to CRRT, others would use a regional circuit anticoagulation technique (citrate/calcium).

Solute and Water Removal Mechanisms

Solute removal relies on one or more of the following mechanisms:

- *Osmosis* is the movement of *water* along a concentration gradient (from low solute concentration to high solute concentration). For example, the use of hypertonic PD fluid to remove fluid relies in part on osmosis.
- *Hydrostatic pressure* is the force a fluid under pressure exerts against the walls or edges of the area in which it is contained. This pressure tends to force fluid from an area of high pressure to an area of low pressure across a semipermeable membrane. The hydrostatic pressure gradient underlies the principle of *ultrafiltration* used in CRRTs (e.g., CVVH).
- *Diffusion* is the movement of a solute across a semipermeable membrane from a high to a low solute

TABLE 41.6

SPECIFICS OF THE THREE TECHNIQUES OF RRT IN THE PICU

	■ PD	■ IHD	■ CRRT
METHOD SPECIFICITIES			
Vascular access (ECC)	No	Yes	Yes
Complex method with specific expertise	Low	High	Moderate
Systemic or regional anticoagulation	No	Frequent	Frequent
DIALYSIS DOSE			
Efficacy to remove a toxin	Moderate	High	High
Efficacy to remove fluid	Moderate	Moderate	High
CLINICAL SITUATION INDICATION			
Hemodynamic instability	Yes	No	Yes
Intracranial hypertension	Yes	±	Yes
ARDS	±	Yes	Yes
Abdominal surgery	±	Yes	Yes

ARDS, acute respiratory distress syndrome.

TABLE 41.7

HEMOFILTRATION REPLACEMENT SOLUTION COMPOSITION

	■ mmol/L
Sodium	140
Calcium	2
Magnesium	1
Chloride	100
Acetate	23
Bicarbonate	25
Potassium	3
Phosphate	1
Dextrose	0.18%

concentration area. Infusion of dialysate fluid into the circuit in a countercurrent fashion promotes highly efficient removal of small solutes (e.g., urea) using the principle of diffusion. PD, hemodialysis (HD), and hemodiafiltration all rely on diffusion for removal of small molecules.

■ *Convection* (bulk flow, solvent drag) is the movement of solute that occurs in conjunction with, and linked to, fluid movement across a semipermeable membrane. Convection is facilitated by the infusion of replacement fluid into the circuit such that the greater the replacement fluid *flow rate*, the greater the clearance of solutes (small, medium, or large). Hemofiltration (e.g., slow continuous ultrafiltration [SCUF], CVVH) relies on the principle of convection.

Replacement (Substitution) Solution

6 Convection requires the infusion of a "replacement" solution (also known as the substitution solution) to solute removal. Commercial solutions usually include sodium, buffer, calcium, and magnesium, with concentrations similar to plasma. Some commercial solutions (outside of the United States) also are prepared with citrate as a special formulation for circuit anticoagulation. When prolonged CRRT is required, glucose and phosphorus may be present in the solution to limit depletion in the patient (**Table 41.7**). Many commercial solutions are available, each with its own advantages and disadvantages. Many also contain lactate as the buffer. In children with impaired lactate metabolism due to liver failure, critical illness, circulatory failure, or inborn errors of metabolism, significant lactic acidosis may occur with use of these solutions. Using a solution that contains a bicarbonate buffer rather than lactate can rectify this problem. The same solutions are often used for dialysate and replacement fluids in CRRT. The addition of albumin (40 g/L) allows this solution to be then used for plasma exchange (see below).

PERITONEAL DIALYSIS

Overview

PD is the oldest, simplest, and still the most commonly used form of RRT in children (36). PD requires the bidirectional exchange of fluid and solute between dialysis fluid and blood across the peritoneal membrane. The peritoneal membrane covers all loops of bowel and forms the peritoneal cavity by reflecting onto the anterior and posterior surfaces of the abdomen. Fenestrated capillaries, interstitial connective tissue, and a thin layer of mesothelial cells make up the membrane. Solute

and fluid move between gaps in the cells and between pores or channels in the interstitium.

The other major mechanism involved in fluid and solute clearance is peritoneal lymph drainage. Up to 50% of capillary ultrafiltrate can be reabsorbed via the lymphatics, which can limit fluid removal. The lymphatics can also absorb large molecules from the peritoneum, which then enter the vascular system via the thoracic duct, limiting the effectiveness of osmosis in PD.

PD is performed simply by allowing dialysis solution to run into the peritoneum, remain in situ ("dwell") for a time, and then drain for a period of time. This process completes one cycle, which can be repeated as desired. Similar to HD, PD corrects fluid and electrolyte abnormalities, metabolic acidosis, and azotemia through the processes of osmosis, diffusion, and filtration, but does so much more slowly than HD.

The ultrafiltration and solute clearance obtained during PD is dependent on the volume and osmolality of the dialysis fluid, the dwell time, and the permeability of the child's peritoneal membrane to a particular substance. Fluid is removed owing to an osmotic gradient, which diminishes over the time span of the cycle. Shortening the total cycle time or increasing the dialysate glucose concentration usually improves fluid removal by maintaining a larger osmotic gradient. Solute clearance is diffusion-related. Thus, the larger the volume of dialysis fluid instilled and the greater the available surface area covered, the greater the efficiency of PD. Although efficiency for solute removal can also be increased with longer dwell times, short dwell times of 20 minutes are adequate for smaller molecules.

Physiology of Peritoneal Dialysis

The surface area of the peritoneal cavity is directly proportional to the patient's body surface area (~0.6 m^2/m^2 of body surface area), and peritoneal permeability is similar in all patients from 2 years to adulthood (37–39). Infants and small children have a large surface area-to-body weight ratio, which may explain the better efficiency of PD in infants compared with that of adolescents or adults (**Fig. 41.4**). Both molecular size (weight and three-dimensional shape) and amount of charge affect passage through the peritoneal membrane: the larger the molecule, the lower the permeability; the more highly charged the molecule, the lower the permeability. Fluid

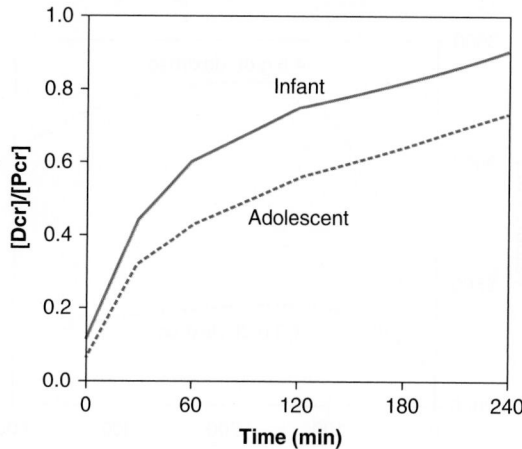

FIGURE 41.4. Ratio of dialysate creatinine (Dcr) to plasma creatinine (Pcr) as a function of duration of dwell time for infants and adolescents. Infants achieve greater PD efficiency because of the greater peritoneal surface area relative to body weight. (From Warady BA. *J Am Soc Nephrol* 1996;14:236–92, with permission.)

removal follows an osmotic gradient and is, therefore, more dependent on the concentration of the dialysis solution itself than on the peritoneal membrane. The peritoneal membrane is relatively impermeable to protein, unless diseases such as sepsis, systemic inflammatory response syndrome, cardiopulmonary bypass (CPB), pancreatitis, or shock have caused a marked increase in capillary permeability. Clearance achieved by PD depends on the following factors:

- size of the molecule (smaller molecules are cleared more quickly) (**Fig. 41.5**);
- dialysis fluid osmolality (the higher the glucose concentration, the more rapid the fluid removal) (**Fig. 41.6**);
- dwell time (most fluid removal occurs within the first 30 minutes, because the concentration gradients change the most during this period) (**Fig. 41.7**);
- volume of dialysis fluid (the larger the dialysate volume, the greater the clearance because more fluid is in contact with the peritoneal membrane and its large surface area) (**Fig. 41.8**) (40).

Indications for Peritoneal Dialysis

The standard indications for RRT (**Table 41.5**) also apply to PD. However, PD is especially indicated in newborns and small infants, where large bore vascular is difficult.

Contraindications for PD

There are absolute and relative contraindications to PD:

- Defect in peritoneal membrane or cavity, such as diaphragmatic hernia, gastroschisis, omphalocele, or postsurgical thoracoabdominal communication (absolute)
- Abdominal sepsis with adhesions (absolute)
- Fulminant necrotizing enterocolitis with perforation (absolute)
- Ventriculo-peritoneal shunt (relative)
- Profound shock or cardiac failure (relative)
- Massive rapid clearance required (relative)

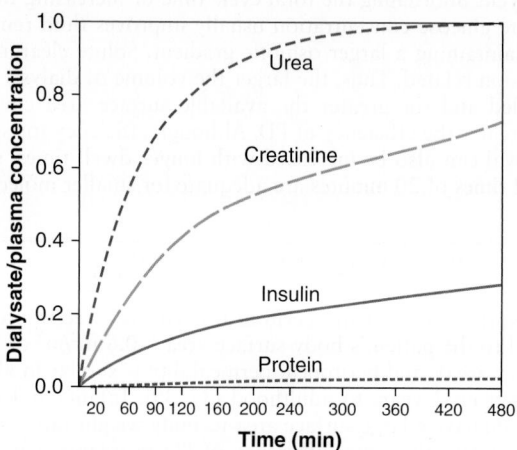

FIGURE 41.5. Solute clearances with PD (dialysate-to-plasma creatinine ratio) as a function molecular size. Note the extremely efficient clearance of urea (small molecule) with PD. (From Horl WH. *Replacement of Renal Function by Dialysis.* 5th ed. Dordrecht: Kluwer Academic, 2004, with permission.)

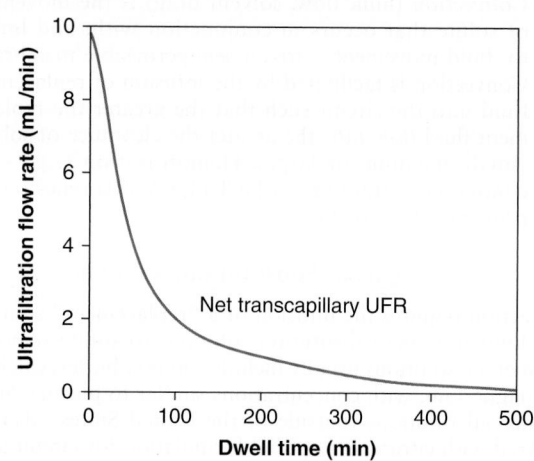

FIGURE 41.7. The effect of dwell time on fluid removal. (From Nolph KD. *Kidney Int* 1981;20:543–8, with permission.)

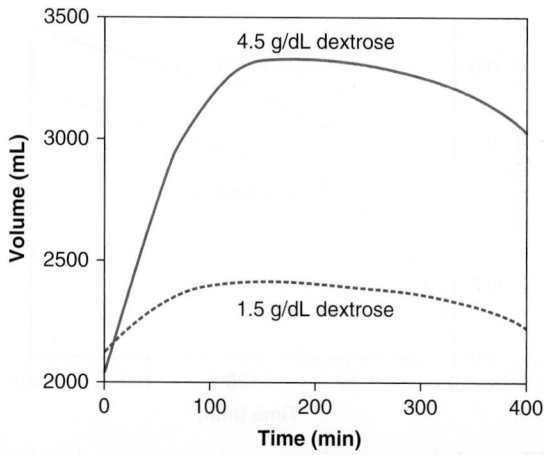

FIGURE 41.6. The effect of dialysis fluid osmolality on water removal over time. Higher dialysis fluid osmolality caused by increasing the glucose concentration leads to greater water removal. (From Mujias S. *Kidney Int* 2002;62:S17–22, with permission.)

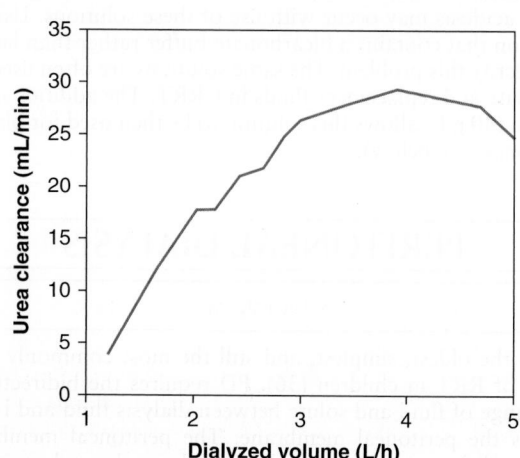

FIGURE 41.8. Volume of PD fluid and urea clearance in adults. (From Keshaviah P. *J Am Soc Nephrol* 1994;4:1820–6, with permission.)

Catheters Used for Peritoneal Dialysis

The Tenckhoff catheter is most commonly used for PD; it is available as either a straight or a curled catheter. It can be inserted by a surgeon in the operating theater (after CPB) or in the PICU. The catheters range in size and diameter. Larger patients require longer lengths and larger-diameter tubing. Typical sizes for infants and small children are 10, 12, and 14 French (fr), with 45-cm length for acute PD. Infection is minimized by the use of correct aseptic technique at the time of insertion, correct technique when dealing with the circuit or dialysis fluids, and a soft silicon catheter with a Dacron cuff near the skin entry site. At some centers, the catheter is inserted with a long, subcutaneous tunnel in both acute and chronic PD. Administration of a single dose of prophylactic antibiotics has also been recommended (41).

Manual versus Automated Peritoneal Dialysis

PD is a simple treatment to perform, and the process is easily automated. However, because automation involves substantial cost in establishing and training staff to be familiar with the technology and alarms, many ICUs use manual, nonmechanical therapy, which is managed by the bedside nurse.

Continuous-Flow Peritoneal Dialysis

When a higher clearance is required, continuous-flow PD has been used successfully. Urea clearances of 30–50 mL/min have been achieved with this technique (42). However, it is not routinely used because it necessitates the insertion of two catheters (one for fluid administration and one for removal) in the abdomen.

Complications of Peritoneal Dialysis

Similar to other methods of RRT, PD can be associated with fluid and electrolyte abnormalities, in particular, potassium, sodium, and, in small infants, lactate (if lactate dialysate solute is used). Significant potential also exists for fluid imbalance, with too much or too little fluid being removed. Overall fluid balance, daily weights, central filling pressures, and electrolyte balance of patients who receive PD must be closely monitored to avoid complications.

Peritonitis is an uncommon complication that is mainly related to poor aseptic insertion or poor aseptic handling of the circuit and stopcocks. Close monitoring for symptoms (cloudy dialysis effluent, abdominal pain, fever, poor function) and

signs (abdominal tenderness, fever, elevated white cell count) of peritonitis is essential to proper care. When peritonitis or sepsis is suspected, a daily sample of PD fluid is drawn for microbiologic microscopy and culture. Diagnosis of peritonitis is confirmed if the dialysate is cloudy, if the white blood cell count is >100/mm^3, and if >50% of the cells are polymorphonuclear cells. Early empiric therapy with intraperitoneal cefazolin and gentamicin is commenced. A single IV dose of vancomycin may also be given if the patient is clinically unstable.

Evidence of a pneumoperitoneum is also found in some patients with PD. Pneumoperitoneum usually results from air entrainment in the dialysis fluid, rather than from bowel perforation, although making the distinction between the two is obviously important. Bowel perforation at the time of insertion is rare but is always a potential concern.

Catheter-related problems with PD can occur frequently. Poor flow into the peritoneum can occur from kinking of the catheter, crystallization around the catheter installation/drainage holes, or infection. Poor drainage can occur with kinking, malposition of the catheter, or from omentum wrapped around catheter drainage holes. Leakage at the site of entry can also occur from excessive dwell volumes with a newly placed catheter, local irritation of the site of entry, or initial poor surgical technique. PD catheters placed in postoperative patients after cardiovascular surgery may also leak fluid into the thoracic cavity, especially if the catheter has been placed from the open thoracic cavity through the diaphragm into the abdomen. This approach to postoperative PD should be avoided, because instilled PD fluid frequently leaks out of the chest tubes, without spending enough time in the abdominal cavity to exchange solute and fluids.

Inguinal hernias can occur because of increased intra-abdominal pressure, and the development of scrotal fluid (hydrocele) is common in the neonate. Peritoneal fluid eosinophilia may occur owing to a reaction to the plastic tubing or may also be seen in fungal infection. Peritoneal sclerosis, in which thick, fibrinous tissue forms over the bowel and abdominal wall, occurs in rare circumstances and is often associated with repetitive episodes of peritonitis.

Peritoneal Dialysis Fluid Composition

The choice of PD solution depends on the amount of fluid to be removed, the age of the patient, and whether metabolic acidosis is present. Increased fluid removal usually involves the use of more hypertonic solutions. In the presence of metabolic acidosis, using a dialysis solution that does not contain lactate may be beneficial. Various solutions are given in **Table 41.8**. Depending on the measured electrolyte balance, potassium can be added. Some institutions also prefer to add heparin (usually 500 U/L) and/or antibiotics to the PD solution.

TABLE 41.8

VARIOUS PERITONEAL DIALYSIS SOLUTIONS USED IN THE PICU

	I	II	III	IV
Glucose (g/dL)	1.5	1.5	4.25	4.25
Sodium (mmol/L)	156	132	152	132
Chloride (mmol/L)	105	95	110	96
Magnesium (mmol/L)	0.28	0.25	0.29	0.25
Calcium (mmol/L)	2.0	1.25	2.1	1.8
Lactate (mmol/L)	0	40	0	40
Bicarbonate (mmol/L)	34	0	35	0
Acetate (mmol/L)	11.4	0	12	0

I, isotonic, lactate free; II, isotonic; III, hypertonic, lactate free; IV, hypertonic.

The volume of PD is an important decision point for the physician. Instillation of 10–20 mL/kg normally provides good clearance and minimal risk of intra-abdominal hypertension. Increased volume of dialysate to 30–40 mL/kg gives a better clearance of solutes, but an increased likelihood of intra-abdominal hypertension, respiratory embarrassment, or leakage from the insertion site of a newly placed catheter. Usually, a total time of 30–240 minutes (depending on diagnosis and clearance required) is provided for instillation, dwell time, and drainage, with dwell time providing 66%–85% of the total cycle time.

Cardiopulmonary Interactions

PD is the most common form of RRT in neonates and small children after receiving CPB (43). PD continues to be effective even in low cardiac output states, in hypotensive conditions, and in infants on vasoconstrictor infusions. However, increased PD volumes and abdominal muscle tone increases may impair ventilation, gas exchange, and cardiac performance. In a small study, dialysis volumes of up to 30 mL/kg did not result in intra-abdominal hypertension and had no negative effects on cardiac output, oxygen delivery, or respiratory function (44). In this study, cardiac index was highest with 10 mL kg, rather than with 0 or 20 mL/kg. Intra-abdominal pressure may be measured using a bladder catheter with a balloon filled to a volume of 1 mL/kg (45) and connected to a pressure-monitoring column or device. Debate exists over the exact pressures that constitute intra-abdominal hypertension and the "best" way to monitor intra-abdominal pressure. (See Chapter 100 on Abdominal Compartment Syndrome.) A recent review of intra-abdominal hypertension and abdominal compartment syndrome discusses potential problems that can arise (46).

Hemodialysis

HD is the extracorporeal exchange of fluid and solute that occurs across an artificial, semipermeable membrane between blood and dialysis fluid that are moving in opposite (countercurrent) directions. HD uses dialyzers with larger filter surface area, higher blood flow rates, and higher dialysis flow rates than CRRT. Thus, HD is much more efficient at removing solute than CRRT. The intermittent nature of the technique (sessions usually last 4–6 hours and are often repeated three times per week) lends itself to being used in stable children with chronic renal failure or acute renal failure (ARF) due to renal disease (such as hemolytic uremic syndrome [HUS] or glomerulonephritis). However, HD can be used in children in the PICU for indications of both renal failure and nonrenal failure. For instance, it can be effective in hemodynamically stable children with hyperammonemia (47), inborn errors of metabolism (48), and drug overdoses in which rapid substance removal may be desirable. Recent modifications and technical advances have allowed some critically ill children to receive more frequent and even daily HD (49,50) or sustained low-efficiency dialysis.

Physiology of Hemodialysis

Fluid Removal

Fluid removal is accomplished via the process of ultrafiltration along a pressure gradient called the transmembrane pressure (TMP) gradient, which is determined by the hydrostatic pressure difference across the semipermeable membrane minus

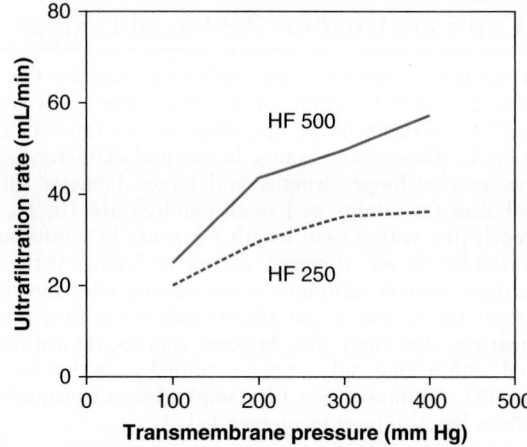

FIGURE 41.9. Relationship between UFR and TMP as a function of filter surface area. For any given TMP, the UFR increases with greater surface area. (From *Technical Specifications Manual*. Minneapolis, MN: Renal Systems, with permission.)

the plasma oncotic pressure (which tends to retain fluid in the blood) and is of the order of 20–30 mm Hg.

$$TMP = (Pb - Pd) - Po$$

where

   Pb = hydrostatic pressure on the blood side of the membrane
   Pd = hydrostatic pressure on the dialysis side of the membrane (often negative)
   Po = plasma oncotic pressure due to plasma protein concentration.

High-flux dialyzers are extremely permeable to water, whereas standard (low-flux) dialyzers are less permeable (**Fig. 41.9**). The permeability of a membrane is defined as Kuf, which is the amount of ultrafiltrate at a particular TMP, and is measured as mL/h × mm Hg. High-flux membranes permit high ultrafiltration rates, thereby allowing bulk flow of solute (also known as solute drag) to occur and larger middle molecules to be removed. Low-flux membranes remove less water and produce lower amounts of solute drag.

Solute Removal

Solute removal in HD occurs by diffusive transport along a concentration gradient, so that the larger the concentration gradient, the faster the removal (clearance) of solute or waste products.

$$Cl = \dot{Q}b \times (Ci - Co)/Ci$$

where

   Cl = clearance
   $\dot{Q}$b = blood flow (mL/min)
   Ci = concentration of solute at inlet
   Co = concentration of solute at outlet.

Solute removal also depends on the time allowed for dialysis, as well as the volume of distribution for the particular solute; their relationship to clearance is

$$Ci/Co \times e^{-(KT/V)}$$

where

   e = base of natural logarithm
   K = clearance at a given blood flow
   T = duration of dialysis
   V = volume of distribution for the solute.

Countercurrent flow is very important to improving the efficiency of solute removal because it maintains a continuous concentration gradient along the entire length of the dialyzer fibers.

Depending on the size of the solute molecule, transfer across the dialysis membrane may depend on blood flow rates (small molecules) and membrane characteristics (large molecules). Small molecules (<300 Da) move easily across the membrane. Increasing flow rates will increase solute transfer (increased blood flow brings more concentrated solute, whereas increased dialysate flow maintains low solute levels on the dialysate side of the membrane, thereby maintaining the concentration gradient); thus, small-molecule clearance is flow dependent. Large molecules do not diffuse as easily and, therefore, are not flow dependent, but they are dependent on physical characteristics (thickness, surface area, and type) of the plastic that constitutes the membrane dialyzer.

Catheters

In general, similar catheters are used in acute HD and in CRRT. A large range of catheters for acute HD are commercially available—from 6.5 to 7 French in the newborn, to 14 French in the large adolescent (**Table 41.4**). Currently, most centers use double-lumen catheters for acute HD. These are inserted into the femoral, internal jugular, or subclavian vein and must be large enough to obtain blood flow rates of 3–5 mL/kg/min to achieve adequate solute clearance. Some of the larger catheters also have an extra infusion lumen that can be used as a central venous access port.

Dialyzer Membrane

A large range of commercially available dialyzer membranes are used, and they have a number of features in common: small priming volume, biocompatibility (with minimal cytokine release), known sieving and filtration coefficients, known and consistent relationships between solute clearance and blood and dialysate flows, and low pressure drop across the membrane. Most centers use hollow-fiber (capillary) membranes. Modern membrane materials, such as polysulfone, polyamide, and polyacrylonitrile, are more biocompatible than the cellulose membranes of the past. Modern membranes have slightly different SCs, but the choice of membrane used is often a matter of local preference. Membrane permeability may be divided into diffusive (related to thickness, charge, and type of plastic) and hydraulic (related to Kuf) components. It is prudent to choose a membrane size that has a surface area that is less than the surface area of the patient and a priming volume that is less than 10% of the patient's circulating blood volume.

Choice of Dialysis Solution

It is important to remember that solute exchange in HD is a two-way process, so that the goals are removal of waste, normalization of electrolytes, and addition of buffer. In an excellent review article, the authors discuss the concept of "designer dialysate," in which dialysis fluid can be ordered to suit individual patient needs, and they discuss the components to be provided in the dialysate fluid (51). Removal of waste implies no urea, no creatinine, and minimal phosphate in the dialysis fluid. Normalization of electrolytes, in particular, focuses on key electrolytes of plasma, including sodium, potassium, calcium, magnesium, and chloride. Also, blood glucose should be maintained at a normal level. Finally, it is important to add buffer to prevent the metabolic acidosis that can be induced with dialysis. Buffering is usually accomplished by the addition of bicarbonate in concentrations of 30–35 mmol/L to the dialysis fluid—more is sometimes required.

Complications of Hemodialysis

Vascular-access risks in extracorporeal therapy are similar to those in CRRT, namely those associated with insertion of large catheters into central veins, including problems related to insertion, infection, thrombosis, embolism, and hemorrhage. Longer-term complications include vascular stenosis and vessel occlusion with clot. Catheter clots are fairly common and may be treated with clot lysis techniques using tissue plasminogen activator or urokinase, although the risk of bleeding with these medications must be recognized. (See Chapter 118 on Coagulation Issues.) Technical malfunction of equipment is always a potential risk, but proper care, training of staff, and troubleshooting algorithms can limit the effects of technical failure to the patient.

Disequilibrium syndrome occurs when the patients' plasma becomes hypotonic relative to their brain cells and water enters the brain. Initial symptoms include nausea, headache, dizziness, and vomiting but can rapidly progress to seizures or coma. Children most at risk are those with high serum sodium or urea and those in whom very rapid HD is performed. When disequilibrium syndrome is recognized or anticipated in high-risk patients, an attempt should be made to have slow changes of solute occur by using low blood flow rates to decrease the rate of clearance. Mannitol at doses of 0.25–1.0 g/kg may also be helpful.

Hemolysis can occur during dialysis from the use of a dialysate solution that is hypo-osmolar; hyperthermic; hyponatremic; or contaminated with formaldehyde, bleach, copper, or nitrates. Other causes of hemolysis include use of faulty blood pumps, which cause trauma to blood cells; inadequate anticoagulation leading to clot formation; and excess suction in the venous drainage line due to hypovolemia or kinking/obstruction of the dialysis catheter. The main danger that results from hemolysis is acute hyperkalemia (arrhythmia) and high plasma-free hemoglobin.

A variety of other complications may occur. Anaphylaxis reactions still occur, albeit much less frequently than with the older styles of cellulose/cuprophane membranes. Bacteremia/infection can occur with poor aseptic technique. Air embolism is also possible, as is a blood or dialysate leak. Hypothermia/hyperthermia can occur if heaters or temperature baths malfunction. Dosage adjustment of drugs, due to both renal failure and removal of drug by HD, is essential (51,52). These events are all potentially dangerous and require constant supervision of the procedure by vigilant, well-trained, specialist staff.

Recirculation can occur because of high blood flows and, especially in small children, the proximity of the two ends (the drainage and reinfusion holes) of the catheters. The percentage of recirculation can be calculated as

$$\% \text{ recirculation} \times 100 = (U_{\text{systemic}} - U_{\text{arterial line}})/(U_{\text{systemic}} - U_{\text{venous return line}})$$

where

U_{systemic} = urea concentration in peripheral blood
$U_{\text{arterial line}}$ = urea concentration in the predialyzer arterial line
$U_{\text{venous return line}}$ = urea concentration in the postdialyzer venous return line
No recirculation occurs when $U_{\text{arterial}} = U_{\text{systemic}}$
Some recirculation is occurring if $U_{\text{arterial}} < U_{\text{systemic}}$.

If recirculation is greater than 20%, the efficiency of HD is diminished and should be corrected.

Patient Monitoring During Dialysis

Blood pressure, heart rate, respiratory rate, O_2 saturation, electrocardiogram, and temperature should be continuously monitored. Laboratory values such as blood glucose, ACT, and hematocrit should be serially monitored. Technical parameters of the dialysis machine, such as arterial and venous pressures, TMP, and ultrafiltrate rate, must also be carefully watched. Some HD machines allow integrated blood volume monitoring based on hematocrit changes during iHD. Such monitoring seems to improve the safety of iHD (53). Clinical symptoms of headaches, nausea, dizziness, and muscle cramps should be assessed. Neurologic observations of mental status, and Glasgow Coma Scale score should be included as part of routine clinical assessment during dialysis.

CONTINUOUS RENAL REPLACEMENT THERAPY

CRRT is perceived to be a "gentler" form of removal of fluid and solute than iHD. It can be equivalent in efficiency to iHD and has the benefit of more hemodynamic stability. Several large series have reported the safety, efficacy, and outcome of children who were treated with CRRT. A study of 122 children with ARF found a higher mortality in those patients who received vasopressor therapy (54). Similar findings were noted in a series of 98 children (55). In a series that was corrected for patient severity of illness, it was noted that the amount of fluid overload present at the time of starting CRRT was related to outcome (56), suggesting that earlier use of CRRT to control fluid balance may improve outcome (57). Other authors have noted that outcome was related more to the underlying disease than to the treatment applied (28). A more recent study supported the harmful effects of fluid overload in critically ill children receiving extracorporeal membrane oxygenation (ECMO) and suggested improved outcome with earlier use of CRRT (58).

Goals of Pediatric Continuous Renal Replacement Therapy

The goals of CRRT include restoring fluid and electrolyte balance, improving lung function by decreasing lung water and capillary permeability, managing AKI by removing nitrogenous waste products and restoring acid–base balance, maintaining fluid balance while allowing nutrition or blood products to be given safely, purifying blood in conditions such as sepsis or metabolic disorders (e.g., hyperammonemia), and clearing ingested drugs or toxins. While many of these functions are still theoretical, the surge in use of CRRT in the ICU may provide data to further elucidate which indications are truly effective and beneficial.

Physiology of Continuous Renal Replacement Therapy

The filtration of blood during CRRT is analogous to native glomerular filtration and is determined by fluid movement across a semipermeable membrane down a pressure gradient. Bulk flow of solute (convection) also occurs concurrently. Simply stated, the filter acts as a sieve, allowing molecules dissolved in water to be carried along to the other side. Each filter is composed of many microtubules that act independently of each other but function with the same principles. The process of convective ultrafiltration is driven by three key factors: filter blood flow, TMP, and FF.

Filter Blood Flow

Poiseuille's law governs laminar flow through a tube and is defined by the following parameters:

$$\dot{Q}b = \Delta p - \pi r^4/8L\mu$$

where

$\dot{Q}b$ = blood flow
Δp = change in pressure across the tube
r = radius of the tube
L = length of the tube
μ = viscosity of the blood

Δp is the difference between the filter inlet and filter outlet pressure. The desired blood flow is set on the machine. Lower blood flow across the filter can result in a higher tendency for clotting to occur. As the filter clots, resistance to flow will increase, and filter pressure will increase as well. These parameters are monitored on the device.

Transmembrane Pressure

TMP is the major force that acts on water and solute clearance outside the microtubule. Fluid moves through the microtubule into the external chamber of the filter, where it is removed as ultrafiltrate. The relationship between ultrafiltrate production and TMP is shown in **Figure 41.9**. The amount of ultrafiltrate obtained varies with the surface area, length and type of material from which the filter is made, and the patient's blood viscosity.

In continuous arteriovenous hemofiltration (CAVH), the TMP is usually determined by the height difference between the filter and the continuous column of ultrafiltrate as it enters the collecting bag. All other forms of CRRT utilize a pump on the ultrafiltrate line to apply a precise amount of suction (negative pressure) to the ultrafiltrate line, thereby allowing precise determination of TMP to yield a controlled ultrafiltrate production.

Filtration Fraction

FF represents the efficiency of plasma water removal through filtration and is the ratio of ultrafiltration rate (UFR) to the plasma flow rate ($\dot{Q}_P$) through the filter.

$$FF\ (\%) = (UFR \times 100)/\dot{Q}_P$$

where $\dot{Q}_P$ (mL/min) = filter blood flow rate $\times$ (1 − Hct)
The FF depends on

- TMP
- Surface area of the filter
- Permeability of the membrane
- Plasma oncotic pressure (**Fig. 41.10**)
- Hematocrit

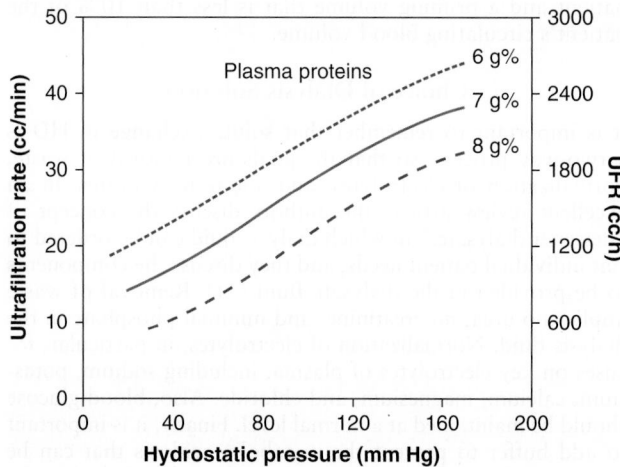

FIGURE 41.10. Effect of plasma protein concentration (oncotic pressure) on UFR at various hydrostatic pressures. (From *Technical Specifications Manual*. Minneapolis, MN: Renal Systems, with permission.)

An FF greater than 30% increases the risk of filter clotting.

The clearance of a substance in CRRT modes that involve HD depends on the dialysis flow rate, blood flow rate, the surface area of the filter, and the dialysis fluid composition. When using CRRT primarily for filtration, UFR/m² gives the approximate effective clearance that can be achieved. Clearance can be increased with higher blood flow, higher TMPs, and higher FFs. Thus, larger surface area and increased filter permeability will increase the efficiency of filtration, whereas higher hematocrit and high plasma protein concentration will decrease efficiency of filtration. It is important to note that use of post-filter fluid replacement provides more efficient clearance than pre-filter replacement. The duration of filtration that occurs over a 24-hour period is also an important determinant of total daily solute clearance.

Sieving Coefficient and Solute Removal

CRRT removes solute from the blood via filtration and adsorption (to the surfaces of the circuit tubing and filter). The substances that are removed by the filter vary, depending on the type of filter used and the modality of filtration. For example, the type of material used in the filter membrane (polysulfone or polyacrylonitrile) affects clearance.

The efficiency of solute transfer from the blood side of the membrane to the ultrafiltrate side is expressed by the SC, which is the concentration of a solute in the ultrafiltrate ($[Solute]_{UF}$) divided by the concentration of the same solute in the plasma ($[Solute]_{Plasma}$).

$$SC = [Solute]_{UF}/[Solute]_{Plasma}$$

Many small molecules have an SC of ~1, indicating free convective movement from plasma to ultrafiltrate. For example, the sodium concentration in patient's ultrafiltrate during SCUF is expected to be approximately the same as the patient's serum sodium concentration. Conversely, an SC of 0 indicates that no solute has been cleared into the ultrafiltrate. **Table 41.9** gives the SCs for many different solutes commonly cleared during CRRT.

Because solute clearance equals the ultrafiltrate flow times the SC, the ultrafiltrate flow rate determines the clearance of many solutes.

$$Solute\ clearance = UFR \times SC$$

7 **TABLE 41.9**

SIEVING COEFFICIENTS FOR CLEARANCE OF VARIOUS SOLUTES

■ SOLUTE	■ SIEVING COEFFICIENT
Bicarbonate	1.124
Blood urea nitrogen	1.048
Chloride	1.046
Phosphorus	1.044
Glucose	1.043
Creatinine	1.020
Uric acid	1.016
Sodium	0.993
Potassium	0.985
Citrate	0.9
Magnesium	0.879
Calcium	0.637
Total bilirubin	0.030
Direct bilirubin	0.030
Total proteins	0.021
Albumin	0.008

For example, creatinine clearance (Ccr, SC of 1) is the same as the UFR (Ccr = UFR).

The concept of the sieving coefficient and filtrate flow works well to determine the plasma clearance of many substances, especially when simple methods, such as SCUF, are used. However, at the higher flow rates used with CVVH, large amounts of replacement solutions may be required, which can also dramatically change plasma levels of solutes. Many commercial replacement solutions exist.

CRRT may clear a variety of "middle" molecules, including cytokines, complement, and tumor necrosis factor (TNF), interleukins (IL-1, IL-6, and IL-8), prostaglandin, myocardial depressant factor, interferon, and even Gram-positive bacterial exotoxins. These substances have molecular weights of up to 17–28 kDa. In addition to molecular weight, clearance of a substance depends on its charge, protein binding, and three-dimensional shape.

Drug clearance is also affected by the size, charge, and protein binding of the drug such that plasma and ultrafiltrate drug concentrations should be monitored closely where possible. For instance, CRRT clears only **un**bound drug. And the removal of certain antibiotics (penicillins, aminoglycosides, and cephalosporins) is especially affected by drug charge.

Pre- or Post-filter Infusion of Replacement Fluids

Views vary regarding location of replacement fluid within the CRRT circuit. The advantages of replacement fluid placement prior to the filter (predilution) are (a) increased urea clearance as diffusion of red cell urea into the plasma occurs, and (b) a theoretical increase in filter survival due to hemodilution of blood and clotting factors. Thus, predilution placement is preferred in some PICUs. However, predilution placement decreases the sieving coefficient of most solutes by lowering the filter inlet concentration of these substances. A study in adults that compared pre- and post-filter replacement showed increased filter survival with predilution from 13 to 18 hours (52). As most pediatric filter survival is >24 hours, with either pre- or post-filter replacement, factors other than location of delivery of replacement fluid within the circuit may be more important in determining filter life.

CRRT Mode and Solute Clearance

The effectiveness of solute clearance differs depending on the type of CRRT used (59). In a study that compared CVVH and CVVHD in 10 patients, little difference for urea and creatinine clearance was noted, a slight (4%) increase in uric acid clearance occurred with CVVH, and a significant (19%) increase in vancomycin clearance with CVVH occurred, suggesting that CVVH offers some advantage for the removal of middle molecules (60). This finding was confirmed in another study that showed that larger molecules, such as insulin, myoglobin, heparin, and vancomycin, are cleared well by CVVH (61). Other reviews of CVVH in the ICU environment have also supported these findings (62,63). A very interesting comparison of CVVHD and CVVH (with pre- and post-membrane dilution) found that CVVHD and postdilution CVVH gave similar urea and creatinine clearances that were 15% better than those achieved with predilution CVVH. Because low blood flow rates often used in pediatric CVVH might lead to filter clotting, the authors concluded that CVVHD is preferred over postdilution CVVH for small-molecule clearance during CRRT (64).

Modes of Continuous Renal Replacement Therapy

Continuous Arteriovenous Hemofiltration

In CAVH mode, the drainage catheter is placed in an artery, and the return catheter is placed in a vein (either peripheral or central). CAVH is simple to operate but has low ultrafiltrate production, especially in small patients or those with hypotension. It also provides a potential volume load to the heart in small infants that may not be well tolerated. In this mode, blood flows from artery to vein, and filtrate production depends on the patient's blood pressure, the filter surface area, and the height of the collecting system below the filter. Although CAVH is a standard in adults in the 1980s, it is inefficient in children (although could provide some SCUF) and is rarely used today.

Slow Continuous Ultrafiltration

SCUF uses a low volume of filtrate with no replacement solution and is useful in removing small amounts of fluid. Ideally, this can be done by using a pre-filter inflow pump, a small volume hemofilter, and post-filter return without replacement fluid. Although the difference between the height of the filter and the filtrate drainage bag can control the rate of ultrafiltrate flow, it is prudent to have a pump on the filtrate line to carefully control fluid loss. Note that the SCUF circuit design is analogous to CAVH except that the driving pressure in SCUF comes from the blood pump, whereas in CAVH it comes from the patient's heart creating an arterial pressure. SCUF is rarely used today.

Continuous Venovenous Hemofiltration

CVVH is the most common form of CRRT in many units. It is usually performed with a double-lumen catheter, which contains both a drainage and a return lumen that is placed in a central vein, although it can also be performed with separate catheters placed into two different peripheral or central veins. The critical difference between SCUF and CVVH is the addition of replacement fluid (Fig. 41.1), which drives convection (solute drag). Hence, CVVH allows solute removal in addition to fluid removal.

The physician must order the anticoagulation regimen (see above), the replacement fluid composition (Table 41.7), and infusion location (pre-or post-filter) as well as all the fluid rates that determine the net fluid loss in the patient. When a net fluid loss is desired in the fluid-overloaded patient, the replacement fluid rate (RFR) is set such that the sum of all outputs (ultrafiltrate, urine, chest tubes, etc.) exceeds the sum of all inputs (replacement fluid, IV fluids, nutrition, etc.) by a defined amount every hour. Expressed differently, the ultrafiltrate rate (UFR) must equal the sum of: (a) the desired fluid removal rate, (b) the net non-CRRT intake, and (c) the RFR. (No dialysis fluid is used in CVVH.)

$$\text{UFR (mL/h)} = \text{desired fluid removal rate (mL/h)} +$$
$$\text{net non-CRRT intake (mL/h)} + \text{RFR (mL/h)}$$

where

Net non-CRRT intake (or "fluid balance") = (all IV intake + nutritional intake) − (urine output + other outputs (stool, chest tubes, etc.))

Physician orders determine UFR, net non-CRRT intake, and RFR such that net fluid loss occurs when

UFR > net non-CRRT intake + RFR

Initial studies in adults suggested a survival benefit from higher UFRs (35–45 mL/kg/h) compared with standard rates (20 mL/kg/h) (65). However, more recent systematic reviews have not confirmed a benefit of higher UFRs (66). The typical range of ultrafiltration rates for PICU patients is 10–50 mL/kg/h (10–20 mL/min/1.73 m^2).

A careful balance between the blood flow rate, ultrafiltration rate, and RFR is required to achieve the desired goals of fluid and solute removal safely. Blood flow through the filter is maintained at a level that is at least three times the UFR. Inadequate blood flow risks clotting the filter, whereas excessive flow produces hemolysis. The faster the replacement fluid infusion rate, the greater the convective solute clearance. Commercially available replacement solutions have physiologic electrolyte concentrations and either lactate or bicarbonate buffer. Bicarbonate is the preferred buffer in hemodynamically unstable children, because lactate is a vasodilator and may not be metabolized effectively to bicarbonate in patients with liver failure.

Continuous Venovenous Hemodialysis

Continuous venovenous hemodialysis (CVVHD) is designed to achieve solute clearance and controlled fluid removal. CVVHD removes solute through diffusion rather than the convection mechanism seen in CVVH. CVVHD is more efficient than CVVH at removing small molecules such as urea, whereas CVVH can remove both small and larger molecules.

Dialysate is infused into the filter of the CVVHD circuit, but replacement fluid is not used. Dialysate (countercurrent) flow removes solute through diffusion. The greater hydrostatic pressure in the filter compared with the filtrate drainage bag results in fluid removal. The clinician orders the desired fluid removal rate and the dialysate flow rate. The UFR equals the sum of the desired fluid removal rate and the dialysate flow rate plus any net non-CRRT intake.

Instead of ordering replacement fluid, as is the case for CVVH, the physician must order dialysate infusion rate and composition. Commercially available dialysate solutions have physiologic electrolyte concentrations and also offer a choice of lactate or bicarbonate buffer. A calcium-free dialysate must be used for citrate anticoagulation. Because severe azotemia is the most common indication for CVVHD, formulas have been developed to calculate the dialysate flow rate based on urea clearance, volume of distribution, and intended duration of CVVHD. The typical dialysate flow rates of 1–2 L/h for CVVHD are much slower than for iHD.

Continuous Venovenous Hemodiafiltration

CVVHDF combines hemofiltration (through convection) and dialysis (through diffusion). It is therefore capable of achieving aggressive solute and fluid removal. Both dialysis and replacement fluids are infused into (and removed from) the filter. The clinician orders the desired patient fluid removal rate, the dialysate rate, and the RFR. The UFR is the sum of the rates for desired patient fluid removal, dialysate flow, and replacement fluid flow plus net non-CRRT intake.

Frequent monitoring of urea, electrolytes, and fluid balance is essential. Increased clearance of small molecules is obtained by increasing dialysis flow (and ultrafiltrate flow in an equal amount). Clearance of middle molecules requires an increase in the percentage of ultrafiltrate flow from hemofiltration and convection by increasing the filter blood flow rate and/or the RFR. When using citrate, a significant chloride loss can occur (or bicarbonate gain through citrate metabolism); this will require replacement of chloride through modification of the dialysate solution.

CRRT Mode Selection

The first decision to be made is the mode of CRRT to be used. Most centers usually have a single type of CRRT, which allows staff to develop expertise and safe systems of care for these patients and the machines. The following general principles apply when selecting a CRRT technique:

- SCUF: for slow fluid volume removal only
- CVVH, CVVDH: for solute and volume removal
- CVVHDF: for highly efficient solute (e.g., urea) removal and volume removal

Complications of Continuous Renal Replacement Therapy

Filter Clotting

Although filter clotting is common, effective anticoagulation strategies can increase filter survival. General factors that increase filter survival have already been highlighted, including unobstructed rapid laminar blood flow and avoidance of flow stasis. An increased TMP or a large rate of change of TMP substantially contributes to filter clotting. This causes an increase in fluid removal and thus concentration of blood with a rapid increase in viscosity and stasis of flow.

Fluid Imbalance

Hypo- or hypervolemia may occur from imbalances in fluid intake and filtration flow. In small infants, large volume changes may develop quickly and lead to hemodynamic compromise. Continuous monitoring of central venous filling pressures, blood pressure, and heart rate and use of venous saturation and lactate are helpful in monitoring patient status. Obtaining daily (or more frequent) patient weights (if the patient's condition allows) is also very important in the assessment of fluid balance.

Electrolyte Abnormalities

Changes in electrolytes may occur if nonstandard replacement or dialysis solutions are used or if large volume changes go undetected. *Phosphate losses can be expected and require replacement.* Some units add 1 mmol/L Na- or K-phosphate to replacement and dialysis solutions. A systemic calcium infusion is required to prevent systemic hypocalcemia when using citrate anticoagulation. Magnesium losses can also be expected when using citrate anticoagulation and should be replaced.

Metabolic Acidosis or Alkalosis

Either acidosis or alkalosis may occur during CRRT. Alkalosis is more common with citrate anticoagulation as citrate metabolism creates a large alkali load (see under Citrate Toxicity). High blood flow rates require increased citrate flow rates and increase the alkalosis. This often requires the replacement of chloride through manipulation of the dialysate solution. Use of dialysis or replacement solutions that contain lactate can lead to metabolic acidosis from hyperlactatemia.

Citrate Toxicity

High blood flow rates require increased citrate flow rates. This also increases the risk of systemic citrate toxicity by providing a citrate load that may not be able to be metabolized as quickly as it is delivered. Monitoring total patient calcium levels daily will help with early detection. Citrate toxicity should be suspected with rising systemic calcium infusion requirements, falling systemic *ionized* Ca levels, rising *total* serum calcium levels, and a total:ionized calcium ratio >2.25 (67). It can be managed by reducing the blood flow rate (and therefore citrate flow rate) and increasing clearance of the citrate load through increasing replacement fluid flow rates.

Other Solute Imbalances

CVVH leads to clearance of water-soluble vitamins and amino acids that must be replaced in long-term use. ACD (3%) solution provides an extra glucose load that should be factored into caloric requirements.

Hypothermia

Hypothermia occurs often from extracorporeal blood cooling and the infusion of large volumes of dialysate or replacement fluids at room temperature. Several complications are associated with hypothermia, including altered immune function, glucose and electrolyte imbalance, and prolonged clotting times. (See also Chapter 36, Thermoregulation.) Therefore, temperature monitoring is mandatory. When routine warming measures are not sufficient, an in-line heater or tube-warming device should be used. Modern CRRT devices have incorporated in-line heating devices and temperature monitors.

Thrombocytopenia

It is not uncommon to see a decrement in platelet count of up to 50% of baseline values every time a patient is placed on a new filter. The exposure to a new filter does not seem to affect white blood cell count or cause a rise in cytokines or inflammatory mediators.

Hypotension upon Initiation of CRRT

Hemodynamically unstable patients receiving vasopressors may experience hypotension and circulatory collapse upon initiation of CRRT. It is believed that this is not primarily due to volume shifts, but due to dilution and binding of catecholamine to the plastic of the circuit. Hence, it is important to have an adequate circulating blood volume prior to commencement of filtration; whether this is achieved with colloids or crystalloids appears not to be important (68). Thus, in patients on large doses of vasoconstrictors and inotropic drugs, an effective strategy may be to double drug infusion rates before starting CVVH and to begin with a slow blood flow that is gradually increased over 5–10 minutes to the desired rate. Once initiation of CVVH has safely occurred, filtration can begin. Some centers use either rapid infusion of volume or a vasoconstrictor, such as phenylephrine or norepinephrine, to treat the hypotension that often accompanies initiation of CVVH in patients receiving large amounts of vasoactive medications. Bradykinin release syndrome with the AN69 membrane is a potential problem in small infants, and, in general, these membranes are best avoided in small infants. Hypotension is less common when using smaller surface area filters (such as the HF 20) in children weighing <5 kg.

Hypoxemia

Neonates with severe lung disease who begin CRRT with a "blood-primed" circuit may experience hypoxemia from initial exposure to venous blood in the priming volume. This may be avoided by increasing the F_{IO_2} up to 100% before beginning CRRT in such patients. The F_{IO_2} is then weaned based on O_2 saturation and arterial blood gas analysis.

How to Choose the Type of Renal Replacement Therapy

Three main types of RRT—PD, iHD, and CRRT—are available at most modern PICUs. Typically, the staffs will select a few principal RRT methods to address the common clinical scenarios. In general, PD is used in small infants (<10 kg) after cardiac surgery and in those patients with early-onset chronic renal failure. The choice between iHD and the various modes of CRRT is more difficult and often depends on personal preference. However, in general, CRRT tends to be used in the very sick or unstable patient with multiorgan failure, whereas iHD tends to be used in hemodynamically stable patients with acute or chronic renal failure (**Table 41.6**). Some units will use only one type of CRRT in the PICU to avoid confusion among staff members and to facilitate training in a particular type of CRRT. Some units use mainly CVVH in the PICU, while others use primarily CVVHD.

A number of meta-analyses have been performed to identify whether one form of CRRT is better than another. One analysis showed a benefit to treatment with CRRT compared with iHD (relative risk, 0.72; $p < 0.01$) (17), while an analysis of six trials showed no difference in mortality or outcome of renal failure when either dialytic mode was used (69). Clearly, intensivists and nephrologists should work together to provide effective RRT, irrespective of which mode is chosen.

Prognosis in Acute Renal Failure

Over the last 20 years, CRRT has become a standard treatment in the PICU (70). Although some technical limitations have had to be overcome and randomized, controlled trials are lacking, increasing animal and human experience continues to document the efficacy of the technique. The first multicenter outcome trial of children who received CRRT in multiorgan dysfunction syndrome reported lower central venous pressure and less fluid overload in survivors, as compared with nonsurvivors. The investigators hypothesized that early use of CRRT might be expected to improve survival (30). Similar findings confirmed that less fluid overload occurred in survivors, especially with three or more organ system failures (57). Both of these studies help to confirm the role of CRRT in critically ill children, although controversy remains regarding when and how it should be implemented.

Renal Replacement Therapy in the Newborn

A large review of the causes of renal failure in newborn infants and available RRT for these babies was published in 2004 (71). The type of RRT offered to newborn infants depends on two key factors: local preference and the indication for RRT. After cardiac surgery, many centers would prefer PD. Catheters can be placed in the operating theater in a sterile and safe manner. PD enables controlled hypothermia for arrhythmia management, and RRT is likely to be needed for a relatively brief duration. PD avoids the need for anticoagulation and does not require specialized vascular-access catheters, with their attendant risks of infection, emboli, and vascular thrombosis, which can be a very important factor for future management of the patient with heart disease who may need further surgery or cardiac catheterizations.

In neonates and small infants with inborn errors of metabolism, all forms of extracorporeal RRT (CVVH, CVVHD, and CVVHDF) have been used, with rapid decrease in branched chain amino acids, keto-acids, lactate, and ammonia, aiming to minimize cerebral injury (12,72–74). In newborns with sepsis, CVVH has been used alone or in combination with ECMO with encouraging results; the reasons quoted have included cytokine clearance, maintenance of fluid balance, and renal support during ARF. In infants with chronic renal failure, nephrologists must determine the long-term plan, and a combination of modalities may be required.

Extracorporeal Membrane Oxygenation and CRRT

Fluid overload or ARF often develops in patients with sepsis or cardiogenic shock receiving ECMO for hemodynamic support. Given that these patients have all of the risks of extracorporeal therapy and are already anticoagulated, there is no additional access or bleeding risk associated with adding CVVH, CVVHDF, or CVVHD to the ECMO circuit. In 35 patients who received both therapies, 43% survived to hospital discharge, and renal function returned to normal in 93% (75). The CVVH circuit usually runs from the higher-pressure to the lower-pressure end of the oxygenator, representing a small shunt. It can also be run separately from the ECMO circuit in the usual fashion by using a CRRT machine (58). HD can also be performed while patients are on ECMO by means of connecting to the ECMO circuitry. When run through the ECMO circuit, the setup of the CRRT machine requires the CRRT circuit to recognize positive pressures and not negative pressures.

Cardiopulmonary Bypass and CRRT

CPB presents a unique situation in which it is known beforehand that a patient will suffer a significant insult that leads to a systemic inflammatory response with a marked cytokine response. Much effort is directed toward limiting this response with the use of pre-bypass corticosteroids, heparin-bonded circuits, albumin priming of circuits, and modified ultrafiltration at the end of CPB. A preliminary study from Vienna in 1984 showed improvement in postoperative ventricular function in 27 adults who received hemofiltration at the end of surgery. An unpublished, randomized, controlled trial of prophylactic PD for 24 hours in 160 children who weighed <10 kg after cardiac surgery, conducted in 1986–1987, showed a nonsignificant trend to improvement with the dialysis group. A 1996 study, in which PICU staff members were blinded, examined the effect of high-volume (5 L/m^2), zero-balanced hemofiltration in 20 children who underwent CPB (76). Significant differences were noted in postoperative bleeding, decreased time to extubation, and improved oxygenation in patients who received hemofiltration. Decreased TNF, IL-10, C3a, and myeloperoxidase were noted after filtration, while 24 hours later, IL-1, IL-6, IL-8, and myeloperoxidase were decreased. A 1997 report on the use of PD in 32 children with ARF after cardiac surgery noted improved fluid removal along with improved cardiac and pulmonary function (32). Only minor complications were encountered and reported, reflecting on the overall safety of the technique. In 2001, a prospective randomized, controlled trial of modified ultrafiltration after CPB was conducted in 573 adults. Patients who received modified ultrafiltration had a slightly lower mortality, significantly lowered postoperative morbidity, and a decreased need for blood transfusion (77). It appears that modified ultrafiltration and early use of PD may be beneficial after pediatric cardiac surgery.

Therapeutic Plasma Exchange

Therapeutic plasma exchange (TPE), also known as plasmapheresis, is a technique for removing potentially harmful large molecules such as autoantibodies, immune complexes, or endotoxin from the circulation. Worldwide experience with TPE for a diverse range of medical conditions is rapidly increasing (78,79).

Background

A variety of terms describe various aspects of the process of removing large molecules or cells. *Apheresis* simply means "taking away" and describes the general process of removing a blood constituent and then infusing the remaining blood without the removed constituent back into the patient. The term apheresis is often modified by a term describing the constituent being removed. For instance, plasmapheresis refers to the removal and separation of plasma from the patient's blood with return of the blood cells and a (protein-containing) replacement fluid to the patient. Conversely, erythrocytapheresis and leukapheresis refer to the removal and separation of diseased red cells (e.g., sickle cells) or white cells (e.g., leukemic cells), respectively, from whole blood.

There are two main methods for separating plasma from the blood. *Centrifugation with* a centrifugal pump has been the conventional method to separate the blood into cellular and noncellular elements for apheresis. The noncellular plasma can be removed and replaced with an albumin/saline solution (or other solutions as desired). This technique is often used as part of an "apheresis program" directed by hematologists or blood banking experts for use in children with hematologic or oncologic conditions.

Filtration is a newer method for separation of blood components. This approach (also known as "membrane plasma separation") replaces the hemofilter of a simple CVVH circuit with a filter containing larger pore sizes to filter much larger (protein) molecules, up to 2 million Daltons in weight. The filtered plasma containing unwanted proteins is replaced with albumin or fresh frozen plasma.

Continuous Venovenous Plasmafiltration

Filtration or membrane plasma separation using the CVVH circuit design is well-suited to TPE in the ICU and has been called continuous venovenous plasmafiltration (CVVP, **Fig. 41.11**).

The basic principles of CVVP are similar to CVVH with a few important differences:

- The replacement fluid in CVVP must contain protein because large protein molecules have been removed. The typical choices are 5% albumin, an albumin/saline mixture, or fresh frozen plasma (FFP). Prolonged CVVP or large volume of CVVP will filter immunoglobulins and clotting factors, which may require specific replacement. FFP replacement fluid is specifically indicated for thrombotic thrombocytopenic purpura–HUS.
- Even small imbalances in CVVP intake and output will affect intravascular volume and risk of hypo- or hypertension.
  - Protein-bound drugs are also removed. Therefore, drug levels should be measured carefully so that dosing can be adjusted.
- Heparin or citrate anticoagulation each has advantages and disadvantages in CVVP. An increasing proportion of protein-bound heparin is removed at lower hematocrits, necessitating increased heparin administration in the anemic patient. Citrate anticoagulation combined with FFP replacement may lead to citrate toxicity because FFP consists of 14% citrate by volume.

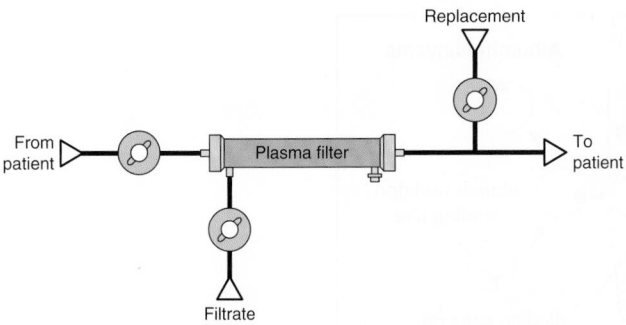

FIGURE 41.11. CVVP circuit design used to filter large proteins (e.g., immune complexes, antibodies). Note the "plasma filter" replaces the hemofilter used for CVVH.

Adsorption Techniques

Several techniques have been developed to augment filtration-aided removal of proteins with adsorption. Proteins (especially fibrinogen and albumin) and cytokines (such as TNF and IL) are adsorbed to the plastic surface of the circuit. However, such adsorption is probably small in amount, and unless circuits are changed frequently (every few hours), the adsorption effect is of minimal significance (29,80). However, if cartridges containing materials such as resin-coated fibers or beads targeting specific chemicals such as endotoxin or cytokines are included in the circuit, then substantial adsorption can occur. Small trials in Japan have shown safety and some improvement in survival with the use of Toramyxin (an endotoxin removal cartridge) (81).

Coupled Plasma Filtration Adsorption

CPFA (**Fig. 41.12**) incorporates adsorption into the circuit design. CPFA has a major advantage over plasma filtration in that much less albumin and other proteins are required, as recirculation of these proteins occurs after "cleansing" or removal of cytokines, etc. bound to albumin has occurred. This may allow more application or widespread use in ICU. Indeed, increasing numbers of units are publishing their experience with small numbers of patients having CPFA (38,82–84).

Indications for Therapeutic Plasma Exchange

Overview

The American Society for Apheresis (ASFA) divides the indications for TPE into four categories based on the evidence for clinical efficacy (85).

The following lists some of the more common PICU indications in each category.

Category I (TPE accepted as first-line therapy)

- GBS
- Thrombotic thrombocytopenic purpura
- HUS (atypical HUS due to autoantibody to factor H)
- Antibody-mediated transplantation rejection
- Myasthenia gravis
- Wilson disease (fulminant)

Category II (TPE accepted as second-line therapy)

- Acute disseminated encephalomyelitis
- Mushroom poisoning

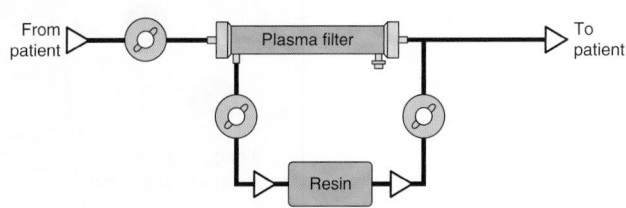

FIGURE 41.12. CPFA circuit design.

- Severe systemic lupus erythematosus (e.g., diffuse alveolar hemorrhage, cerebritis)
- Atypical HUS (due to complement factor gene mutation)
- Humoral renal transplant rejection

Category III (optimum TPE role not established)

- Dilated cardiomyopathy
- Henoch–Schonlein purpura (severe extrarenal disease)
- Acute liver failure (86)
- Sepsis with multiorgan failure
- Envenomation
- Refractory stem cell transplantation-associated thrombotic microangiopathy
- Refractory toxic epidermal necrolysis

Category IV (TPE ineffective or harmful)

- Dermatomyositis, polymyositis
- Shiga-toxin HUS
- Refractory immune thrombocytopenia

Liver Failure

TPE has been a useful temporizing therapy for patients with fulminant hepatic failure, and allows correction of coagulopathy, removal of hepatotoxins, and correction of abnormal liver function tests. Although viewed as a short-term supportive therapy, TPE has stabilized the patient to allow liver recovery or served as a bridge to liver transplantation. TPE for liver support can be performed as a simple CVVP. A modification of this technique with a continuous venovenous single-pass albumin hemodiafiltration in children with acute liver failure (4) has been successfully used in nine children. A further modification of CVVP, namely the MARS system (**Fig. 41.13**), has been commonly used in European centers, in adults with acute liver failure, as a bridge to recovery or transplantation (5,6,18,87,88). The use of MARS therapy in children is challenging, especially in infants (89), and needs further clinical studies before considering its use as routine in PICUs (90).

Guillain–Barrè Syndrome

Since 1985, children and adults with GBS have received plasma exchange. Despite some physiologic changes in patients with GBS, patient outcomes are excellent (91). Randomized control trials in France showed substantial long-term benefit in patients receiving five daily or twice daily plasma exchanges. Subsequent studies showed that treatment with immunoglobulin (IVIG) was equally efficacious. In a recent comparative study of TPE and IVIG, there was a small difference in ICU length of stay favoring TPE (91). This must be balanced with the safety of TPE in each hospital (92). Many children's hospitals that have experience with TPE use IVIG when children are admitted to the ward but TPE (plus IVIG immediately following TPE) when and if children develop respiratory failure.

Drug Overdose

TPE may be useful in overdose or poisoning with drugs/toxins that are highly protein bound with a low volume of distribution. It has been effectively used for theophylline (93,94),

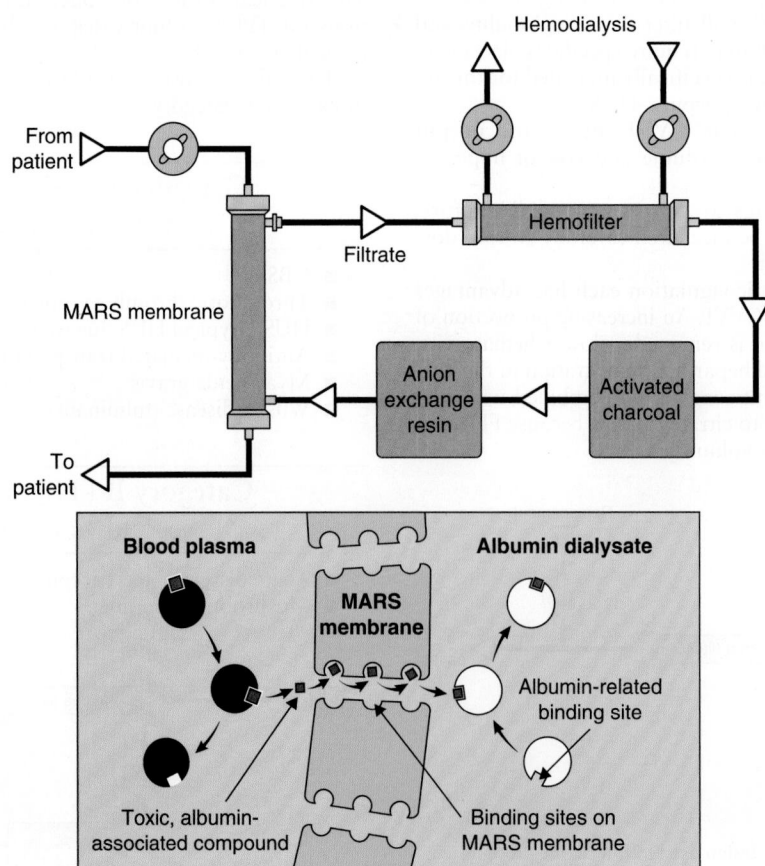

FIGURE 41.13. MARS for blood purification in severe liver failure.

vancomycin, colchicines (95), neonatal lead poisoning in association with chelation (96), and isobutyl nitrate–induced methemoglobinemia (97).

Sepsis with or without Thrombocytopenia-Associated Multiple Organ Failure

Sepsis remains one of the leading causes of death in children. Clinical derangements are thought to be due to the action of inflammatory and anti-inflammatory mediators. Several studies have demonstrated the safety and improved physiologic parameters from CVVH in sepsis (50,62,98–101). However, no clear and substantial survival benefit has been demonstrated with CVVH in sepsis.

The inhibition or removal of sepsis mediators by plasmapheresis or TPE is thought to be of possible benefit (102). However, results in clinical studies have been mixed (103). The postulated benefits of plasmapheresis include modulation or removal of contributing or causal factors, such as endotoxin from bacteria, antigens, antibodies, cell debris, activating enzymes, coagulation activating factors, cytokines, complement factors, removal of inhibitory factors, or a combination of these (50,103–105). Several clinical studies have shown minor benefits, depending on the stated treatment effects. A small study of 30 patients (adults and children) with sepsis syndrome demonstrated the removal of a wide variety of acute phase proteins and complement fragments, but did not influence IL-6 concentrations, thromboxane B_2, total white cell count, or platelet count. This study failed to show a difference in mortality or number of organs failing (106). A study of 106 consecutive adult patients with severe sepsis or septic shock randomized to either standard therapy or add-on plasmapheresis therapy reported a 28-day all-cause mortality of 33.3% (18/54) in the plasmapheresis group and 53.8% (28/52) in the control group (107). The number needed to treat was 4.9 for the benefit of plasmapheresis over control. However, the study was limited by comparability of treatment groups. Small pediatric studies have attempted to demonstrate an amelioration of the hemodynamic effects of sepsis, but lack of control of the volume and type of replacement solution given is a confounding variable (108). In 10 studies using CPFA, published between 2000 and 2009 (105) with 351 patients and a mixture of retrospective, prospective, and small randomized control trials, most showed improvements in hemodynamics and oxygenation, decreases in vasoactive drug requirements, and small survival benefit in some.

Interest in the use of TPE in sepsis has also focused on a subset of children with thrombocytopenia-associated multiple organ failure (TAMOF) (20,81,94,109). Nguyen et al. (20) have demonstrated that some patients with TAMOF have reduced or absent von Willebrand factor cleaving protease activity, now known as ADAMTS-13 (A Disintegrin And Metalloprotease with Thrombo-Spondin motifs), similar to thrombotic thrombocytopenia phenotypes that demonstrate excellent response to plasma exchange in adults. In a small prospective pediatric trial, plasma exchange (up to 11 days) restored ADAMTS-13 activity and was associated with an improvement in multiorgan failure in treated patients (20).

Interest in the use of extracorporeal therapies in sepsis in adults and children (81,110,111) continues to center on the concept of removal of bacteriotoxins and cytokines in sepsis (29). Successful use as a rescue therapy in 2009 in three children with H1N1 supports continued consideration of this therapy (64). In adult critical care, increasingly favorable experience with modifications of TPE with some form of CPFA shows promise (105,112).

The low mortality rate in pediatric sepsis (10%–15%) requires the recruitment of large patient numbers to demonstrate a survival benefit in a randomized control trial of these techniques in children. As a result, other outcome measures are being employed in pediatric studies, such as the pediatric logistic organ dysfunction scores (113). Use of ECMO for fulminant shock in children further complicates the assessment of these therapies. Individual centers have developed protocols of management for children with septic shock that includes some combination of these ECOSTs.

Training of Healthcare Providers in the PICU

The incidence of RRT in the PICU varies according to the specific case-mix of the hospital—from 0.7% to 7% (29,33,114). In the PICU, all modes of RRT (PD, iHD, and CRRT) are used, with increased use of CRRT in >50% of patients. Despite increased use, the multiple techniques available may make it difficult to maintain staff competency and expertise in all aspects of RRT with the same degree of proficiency. Attempts to address this dilemma have led to several options. The simplicity of manual PD allows the training of all nurses in this technique. The specific nature of the skills required and the low frequency of use of iHD in the PICU necessitate special training, and nephrology staff should be included in the care of patients while they receive iHD in the PICU. Among the staffing approaches for CRRT, patient management by both the nephrology staff and the PICU staff, with a pool of nurses on call, combines the expertise of both specialties and is promoted in many centers in the world.

CONCLUSIONS AND FUTURE DIRECTIONS

Since the effectiveness of PD is not hampered by low cardiac output or shock states, it can be used even in small infants with hemodynamic instability. The safety of PD is well known with minimal complexity and minimal effects on cardiorespiratory function. Complications with PD are usually minor and often involve difficulty with catheter placement or function (44). As children grow, the effectiveness of PD in critically ill children diminishes. The use of RRT and therapeutic plasma exchange is increasing in the PICU. These therapies are being applied to children with a wider range of nonrenal indications, as well as earlier in the course of renal insufficiency. The use of CRRT to diminish fluid overload and maintain fluid balance is an area of much interest. Other modes of filtration such as TPE and CPFA hold promise for substance removal that may improve outcomes of sepsis and other protein- or antibody-mediated illnesses. The structure of these support services varies among centers based on local expertise; clearly, cooperation between all concerned, including nephrologists and intensivists, is essential.

References

1. ECLS Registry Report: International Summary. Ann Arbor, MI: Extracorporeal Life Support Organization, January 2013.
2. John S, Eckardt K. Renal replacement strategies in the ICU. *Chest* 2007;132(4):1379–88.
3. Page M, Rimmele T. Filtration et adsorption plasmatiques couplees: principe et perspectives dans le traitement du chos septique (Coupled plasma filtration adsorption: Rational and perspectives in septic shock). *Can J Anaesth* 2008;55(12):847–52.
4. Reeves JH, Butt WW, Shann F, et al. Continuous plasmafiltration in sepsis syndrome. Plasmafiltration in Sepsis Study Group. *Crit Care Med* 1999;27(10):2096–104.

5. Abraham R, Szold O, Merhav H, et al. Rapid resolution of brain edema and improved cerebral perfusion pressure following the Molecular Adsorbent Recycling System in acute liver failure patients. *Transplant Proc* 2001;33:2897–99.

6. Koivusalo A, Vakkuri A, Hockerstedt K et al. Experience of MARS Therapy with and without transplantation in 101 patients with liver insufficiency. *Transplant Proc* 2005;37:3315–17.

7. Williams DM, Sreedhar SS, Mickell JJ, et al. Acute kidney failure: A pediatric experience over 20 years. *Arch Pediatr Adolesc Med* 2002;156:893–900.

8. Akodogan M, Camci C, Gurakar A. The effect of total plasma exchange on fulminant hepatic failure. *J Clin Apher* 2006;21:96–99.

9. Boyle M, Baldwin I. Understanding the continuous renal replacement therapy circuit for acute renal failure support. *AACN Adv Crit Care* 2010;21(4):367–75.

10. Cruz D, Bobek I, Lentini P, et al. Machines for continuous renal replacement therapy. The clinical application of CRRT. *Semin Dial* 2009;22:123–32.

11. Yilmazz AA, Can OS, Oral M, et al. Therapeutic plasma exchange in an intensive care unit (ICU): A 10-year single-center experience. *Transfus Apher Sci* 2011;45(2):161–6.

12. Jouvet P, Jugie M, Rabier D, et al. Combined nutritional support and continuous extracorporeal removal therapy in severe acute phase of maple syrup urine disease. *Intensive Care Med* 2001;27:1798–806.

13. Costello JM, Clapper TC, Wypij D. Minimizing complications associated with percutaneous central venous catheter placement in children: Recent advances. *Pediatr Crit Care Med* 2013;14:273–83.

14. Baldwin I, Bellomo R, Koch B. Blood flow reductions during continuous renal replacement therapy and circuit life. *Intensive Care Med* 2004;30(11):2074–9.

15. Thompson GN, Butt W, Shann FA, et al. Continuous venovenous hemofiltration in the management of acute decompensation in inborn errors of metabolism. *J Pediatr* 1991;118:879–84.

16. Brophy PD, Somers MJ, Baum MA, et al. Multi-center evaluation of anticoagulation in patients receiving continuous renal replacement therapy (CRRT). *Nephrol Dial Transplant* 2005;20(7):1416–21.

17. Dube S, Sharma VK. Renal replacement therapy in intensive care unit. *JAPI* 2009;57:708–712.

18. Balogun RA, Turgut F, Caldwell S, et al. Regional citrate anticoagulation in critically ill patients with liver and kidney failure. *J Nephrol* 2012;25(1):113–9.

19. Kreuzer M, Vester U, Homing A, et al. Regional anticoagulation with sodium citrate in pediatric patients on intermittent hemodialysis therapy with bleeding risks. *Hemodial Int* 2004;8(1):108.

20. Nguyen TC, Han YY, Kiss JE, et al. Intensive plasma exchange increases a disintegrin and metalloprotease with thrombospondin-13 activity and reverses organ dysfunction in children with thrombocytopenia-associated multiple organ failure. *Crit Care Med* 2008;36(10):2878–87.

21. Werner HS, Wensley DF, Lirenman DS, et al. Peritoneal dialysis in children after cardiopulmonary bypass. *J Thorac Cardiovasc Surg* 1997;113(1):64–8.

22. Woiff B, Machill K, Schumacher D, et al. MARS dialysis in decompensated alcoholic liver disease: A single-center experience. *Liver Transpl* 2007;13:1189–92.

23. My W, Yh H, Ch B, et al. Regional citrate versus heparin anticoagulation for continuous renal replacement therapy: A meta-analysis of randomized controlled trials. *Am J Kidney Dis* 2012;59(6):810–8.

24. Bock KR. Renal replacement therapy in pediatric critical care medicine. *Curr Opin Pediatr* 2005;17:368–71.

25. Ringe H, Varnholt V, Zimmering M, et al. Continuous venovenous single-pass albumin hemodiafiltration in children with acute liver failure. *Pediatr Crit Care Med* 2011;12(3):257–64.

26. Smoyer WE, McAdams C, Kaplan BS, et al. Determinants of survival in pediatric continuous hemofiltration. *J Am Soc Nephrol* 1995;6:1401–9.

27. Nandwani V, McCarthy P, Conrad S. Continuous renal replacement therapies: A brief primer for the neurointensivist. *Neurocrit Care* 2010;13:286–94.

28. Stickle S, Brewer ED, Goldstein SL. Pediatric (PED) acute renal failure (ARF) update: Epidemiology and outcome from a three and one-half year experience (Abstract). *J Am Soc Nephrol* 2002;13:649.

29. Bunchman TE, McBryde KD, Mottes TE, et al. Pediatric acute renal failure: Outcome by modality and disease. *Pediatr Nephrol* 2001;16:1067–71.

30. Goldstein SL, Currier H, Graf C, et al. Outcome in children receiving continuous venovenous hemofiltration. *Pediatrics* 2001;107:1309–12.

31. Selewski D, Cornell T, Blatt N et al. Fluid overload and fluid removal in pediatric patients on extracorporeal membrane oxygenation requiring continuous renal replacement therapy. *Crit Care Med* 2012;40(9):2694–9.

32. Warady BA, Bunchman T. Dialysis therapy for children with acute renal failure: Survey results. *Pediatr Nephrol* 2000;15:11–13.

33. Gong WK, Tan TH, Foong PP, et al. Eighteen years experience in pediatric acute dialysis: Analysis of predictors of outcome. *Pediatr Nephrol* 2001;16:212–5.

34. Lowrie LH. Renal replacement therapies in pediatric multiorgan dysfunction syndrome. *Pediatr Nephrol* 2000;14:6–12.

35. Miyamoto T, Yoshimoto A, Tatus K, et al. Zero mortality of continuous veno-venous hemodiafiltration with PMMA hemofilter after pediatric cardiac surgery. *Ann Thorac Cardiovasc Surg* 2011;17:352–55.

36. Bonilla-Felix M. Peritoneal dialysis in the pediatric intensive care unit setting. *Peritoneal Dial Int* 2009;29(2):S183–5.

37. Bouts AH, Davin JC, Groothoff JW, et al. Standard peritoneal permeability analysis in children. *J Am Soc Nephrol* 2000;11:943–50.

38. Esperanca M, Collins D. Peritoneal dialysis efficiency in relation to body weight. *J Pediatr Surg* 1996;1:162–9.

39. Morgenstern BZ. Equilibration testing: Close, but not quite right. *Pediatr Nephrol* 1993;7:290–1.

40. Kohaut EC. The effect of dialysate volume on ultrafiltration in young patients treated with CAPD. *Int J Pediatr Nephrol* 1986;7(4):13–9.

41. Patel P, Nandwani V, McCarthy P, et al. Continuous renal replacement therapies: A brief primer for the neurointensivist. *Neurocrit Care* 2010;13:286–94.

42. Amerling R, Glezerman I, Savransky E, et al. Continuous flow peritoneal dialysis: Principles and applications. *Semin Dial* 2003;16:335–40.

43. Veltri MA, Neu AM, Fivush BA, et al. Drug dosing during intermittent hemodialysis and continuous renal replacement therapy: Special considerations in pediatric patients. *Pediatr Drugs* 2004;1:45–65.

44. Morris KP, Butt W, Karl TR. Effect of peritoneal dialysis on intra-abdominal pressure and cardio-respiratory function infants following cardiac surgery. *Cardiol Young* 2004;14(3):293–8.

45. Davis PJ, Koottayi S, Taylor A, et al. Comparison of indirect methods of measuring intra-abdominal pressure in children. *Intensive Care Med* 2005;31:471–5.

46. Bradley-Stevenson C, Harish V. Intra-abdominal hypertension and the abdominal compartment syndrome. *Curr Pediatr* 2004;14:191–6.

47. Puliyanda DP, Harmon WE, Peterschmitt MJ, et al. Utility of hemodialysis in maple syrup urine disease. *Pediatr Nephrol* 2002;17:239–42.

48. McBryde KD, Kudelka TL, Kershaw DB, et al. Clearance of amino acids by hemodialysis in arginosuccinate synthetase deficiency. *J Pediatr* 2004;144(4):536–40.

49. Bradley A, Fischbach M, Geary D, et al. Frequent hemodialysis in children. *Adv Chronic Kidney Dis* 2007;14(3):297–303.

50. Venkataraman R, Subramanian S, Kellum J. Clinical review: Extracorporeal blood purification in severe sepsis. *Crit Care* 2003;7:139–45.

51. Ronco C, Ricci Z, Bellomo R. Importance of increased ultrafiltration volume and impact on mortality: Sepsis and cytokine story and the role of continuous venovenous haemofiltration. *Curr Opin Nephrol Hypertens* 2001;10(6):755–61.

52. Uchino S, Fealy N, Morimatsu H, et al. Pre-dilution vs. postdilution during continuous veno-venous hemofiltration: Impact on filter life and azotemic control. *Nephron* 2003;94(4):c94–8.

53. Merouani A, Kechaou W, Litalien C, et al. Impact of blood volume monitoring on fluid removal during intermittent hemodialysis of critically ill children with acute kidney injury. *Nephrol Dial Transplant* 2011;26:3315–9.

54. Maxvold NJ, Smoyer WE, Gardner JJ, et al. Management of acute renal failure in the pediatric patient: Hemofiltration versus hemodialysis. *Am J Kidney Dis* 1997;30:S84–8.

55. Sam R, Vaseemuddin M, Leong WH, et al. Composition and clinical use of hemodialysis. *Hemodial Int* 2006;10:15–28.

56. Goldstein SL, Somers MJ, Baum MA, et al. Pediatric patients with multiorgan dysfunction syndrome receiving continuous renal replacement therapy. *Kidney Int* 2005;67:653–8.

57. Foland JA, Fortenberry JD, Warshaw BL, et al. Fluid overload before continuous hemofiltration and survival in critically ill children: A retrospective analysis. *Crit Care Med* 2004;32:1771–6.

58. Ronco C, Tetta C, Mariano F, et al. Interpreting the mechanisms of continuous renal replacement therapy in sepsis: The peak concentration hypothesis. *Artif Organs* 2003;27(9):792–801.

59. Ratanarat R, Brendolan A, Ricci Z, et al. Pulse high-volume hemofiltration in critically ill patients: A new approach for patients with septic shock. *Semin Dial* 2006;19(1):69–74.

60. Jeffrey RF, Khan AA, Prabhu P, et al. A comparison of molecular clearance rates during continuous hemofiltration and hemodialysis with a novel volumetric continuous renal replacement system. *J Artif Organs* 1994;18(6):425–8.

61. Forni LG, Hilton PJ. Current concepts: Continuous hemofiltration in the treatment of acute renal failure. *New Engl J Med* 1997;336:1303–9.

62. Bellomo R. Continuous hemofiltration as blood purification in sepsis. *New Horiz* 1995;3:732–7.

63. Kellum JA, Angus DC, Johnson JP, et al. Continuous versus intermittent renal replacement therapy: A meta-analysis. *Intensive Care Med* 2002;28:29–37.

64. Parakininkas D, Greenbaum LA. Comparison of solute clearance in three modes of continuous renal replacement therapy. *Pediatr Crit Care Med* 2004;5(3):269–74.

65. Ronco C, Bellomo R, Homel P, et al. Effects of different doses in continuous veno-venous haemofiltration on outcomes of acute renal failure: A prospective randomized trial. *Lancet* 2000;356(9223):26–30.

66. Jun M, Heerspink HJ, Ninomiya T, et al. Intensities of renal replacement therapy in acute kidney injury: A systematic review and meta-analysis. *Clin J Am Soc Nephrol* 2010;5(6):956–63.

67. Meier-Kriesche JU, Gitomer J, Finkel K, et al. Increased total to ionized calcium ratio during continuous venovenous hemodialysis with regional citrate anticoagulation. *Crit Care Med* 2001;29:748–52.

68. Bayer O, Reinhart K, Kohl M, et al. Effects of fluid resuscitation with synthetic colloids or crystalloids alone on shock reversal, fluid balance, and patient outcomes in patients with severe sepsis: A prospective sequential analysis. *Crit Care Med* 2012;40(9):2543–51.

69. Symons J, Chua A, Somers M, et al. Demographic characteristics of pediatric continuous renal replacement therapy: A report of the prospective pediatric continuous renal replacement therapy registry. *Am Soc Nephrol* 2007;2:732–8.

70. Pugliese F, Novelli G, Poli L, et al. Hemodynamic improvement as an additional parameter to evaluate the safety and tolerability of the molecular adsorbent recirculation system in liver failure patients. *Transplant Proc* 2008;40:1925–8.

71. Andreoli SP. Acute renal failure in the newborn. *Semin Perinatol* 2004;28(2):112–23.

72. Jouvet P, Poggi F, Rabier JL, et al. Continuous venovenous hemodiafiltration in the acute phase of neonatal maple syrup urine disease. *J Inherit Metab Dis* 1997;20:463–72.

73. The CARI guidelines. Evidence for peritonitis treatment and prophylaxis: peritoneal dialysis-associated peritonitis in children. *Nephrology* 2004;9:S45–51.

74. Symons JM, Brophy PD, Gregory MJ, et al. Continuous renal replacement therapy in children up to 10 kg. *Am J Kidney Dis* 2003;41:984–9.

75. Meyer RJ, Brophy PD, Bunchman TE, et al. Survival and renal function in pediatric patients following extracorporeal life support with hemofiltration. *Pediatr Crit Care Med* 2001;2:238.

76. Journois D, Israel-Biet D, Pouard P, et al. High volume, zero-balanced hemofiltration to reduce delayed inflammatory response to cardiopulmonary bypass in children. *Anesthesiology* 1996;85(5):957–60.

77. Luciani GB, Menon T, Vecchi B, et al. Modified ultrafiltration reduces morbidity after adult cardiac operations: A prospective, randomized clinical trial. *Circulation* 2001;104(suppl 1):1253–9.

78. Kes P, Basic-Kes V, Basic-Jukic N. Therapeutic plasma exchange in the neurologic intensive care setting recommendation for clinical practice. *Acta Clin Croat* 2012;51(1):137–53.

79. Wu MY, Hsu YH, Bai CH, et al. Regional citrate versus heparin anticoagulation for continuous renal replacement therapy: A meta-analysis of randomized controlled trials. *Am J Kidney Dis* 2012;59(6):810–8.

80. Moretti R, Scarrone S, Pizzi B, et al. Coupled plasma filtration-adsorption in Weil's syndrome: Case report. *Minerva Anestesiol* 2011;77(8):846–9.

81. Fortenberry JD, Paden M. Extracorporeal therapies in the treatment of sepsis: Experience and promise. *Semin Pediatr Infect Dis* 2006;17:72–9.

82. Hu D, Sun S, Zhu B, et al. Effects of coupled plasma filtration adsorption on septic patients with multiple organ dysfunction syndrome. *Ren Fail* 2012;34(7):834–9.

83. Mao HJ, Yu S, Yu XB, et al. Effects of coupled plasma filtration adsorption on immune function of patients with multiple organ dysfunction syndrome. *Int J Artif Organs* 2009;32(1):31–8.

84. Oudemans–van Straaten HM, Kellum JA, Bellomo R. Clinical review: Anticoagulation for continuous renal replacement therapy—Heparin or citrate? *Crit Care* 2011;15(1):202.

85. Szczepiorkowski ZM, Winters JL, Bandarenko N, et al; Apheresis Applications Committee of the American Society for Apheresis. Guidelines on the use of therapeutic apheresis in clinical practice—Evidence-based approach from the Apheresis Applications Committee of the American Society for Apheresis. *J Clin Apher* 2010;25(3):83–177.

86. Chin C. Cardiac antibody-mediated rejection. *Pediatr Transplant* 2012;16(5):404–12.

87. Novelli G, Rossi M, Morabito V, et al. Pediatric acute liver failure with molecular adsorbent recirculating system treatment. *Transplant Proc* 2008;40:1921–4.

88. Patel P, Nandwani V, Vanchiere J, et al. Use of therapeutic plasma exchange as a rescue therapy in 2009 pH1N1 influenza A-An associated respiratory failure and hemodynamic shock. *Pediatr Crit Care Med* 2011;12(2):e87–9.

89. Zhang Z, Hongying N. Efficacy and safety of regional citrate anticoagulation in critically ill patients undergoing continuous renal replacement therapy. *Intensive Care Med* 2012;38(1):20–8.

90. Jouvet P, Litalien C, Phan V, et al. Epuration extra-rénale chez l'enfant. In: Bastien O, Honnoré P, Robert R, eds. *Circulations extra-corporelles en réanimation*. Paris, France: Elsevier, 2006:193–210.

91. Jayasena YA, Mudalige S, Manchanayake S, et al. Physiological changes during and outcome following 'filtration' based continuous plasma exchange in Guillain Barre Syndrome. *Transfus Apher Sci* 2010;42:109–13.

92. El-Bayoumi M, El-Refaey A, Abdelkader A, et al. Comparison of intravenous immunoglobulin and plasma exchange in treatment

of mechanically ventilated children with Guillain Barre syndrome: A randomized study. *Crit Care* 2011;15:R164.

93. Laussen P, Shann F, Butt W, et al. Use of plasmapheresis in acute theophylline toxicity. *Crit Care Med* 1991;19(2):288–90.

94. Nguyen TC, Carcillo JA. Bench to bedside review: Thrombocytopenia-associated multiple organ failure-a newly appreciated syndrome in the critically ill. *Crit Care* 2006;10:25.

95. Osborn HH, Henry G, Wax P, et al. Theophylline toxicity in a premature neonate-elimination of kinetics of exchange transfusion. *J Toxicol Clin Toxicol* 1993;31(4):639–44.

96. Mycyk MB, Leiken JB. Combined exchange transfusion and chelation therapy for neonatal lead poisoning. *Ann Pharmacother* 2004;38:821–4.

97. Jansen T, Barnung S, Mortensen CR, et al. Isobutyl-nitrate-induced methemoglobinemia; treatment with an exchange blood transfusion during hyperbaric oxygenation. *Acta Anaesthesiol Scand* 2003;47:1300–1.

98. Quan A, Quigley R. Renal replacement therapy and acute renal failure. *Curr Opin Pediatr* 2005;17:205–9.

99. Rajpoot DK, Gargus JJ. Acute hemodialysis for hyperammonemia in small neonates. *Pediatr Nephrol* 2004;19(4):390–5.

100. Reeves JH, Butt W. Blood filtration in children with severe sepsis: Safe adjunctive therapy. *Intensive Care Med* 1995;21(6):500–4.

101. Ronco C, Brendolan A, Bragantini L, et al. Treatment of acute renal failure in newborns by continuous arterio-venous hemofiltration. *Kidney Int* 1986;29(4):908–15.

102. Reeves JH, Butt W, Sathe AS. A review of venovenous haemofiltration in seriously ill infants. *J Paediatr Child Health* 1994;30(1):50–4.

103. McMaster P, Shann F. The use of extracorporeal techniques to remove humoral factors in sepsis. *Pediatr Crit Care Med* 2003;4:2–7.

104. Bellomo R, Honore P, Matson J, et al. Extracorporeal blood treatment (EBT) methods in SIRS/Sepsis. *Int J Artif Organs* 2005;26(5):450–8.

105. Kellum JA, Cellomo R, Mehta R, et al. Blood purification in non-renal critical illness. *Blood Purif* 2003;21:6–13.

106. Reeves JH, Butt WA. Comparison of solute clearance during continuous hemofiltration, hemodiafiltration, and hemodialysis using a polysulfone hemofilter. *ASAIO J* 1995;40(1):100–4.

107. Busund R, Kouklime V, Utrobin U. Plasmapheresis in severe sepsis and septic shock: A prospective randomized controlled trial. *Intensive Care Med* 2002;28:1434–9.

108. Berlot G, Gullo A, Fassiolo S, et al. Hemodynamic effects of plasma exchange in septic patients: Preliminary report. *Blood Purif* 1997;15(1):45–53.

109. Nguyen TC, Han Y, Fortenberry JD, et al. Plasma exchange for sepsis. *J Pediatr Infect Dis* 2010;4(2):137–45.

110. Butt W. Septic shock. *Pediatr Clin North Am* 2001;48(3):601.

111. Uchino S, Fealy N, Baldwin I, et al. Continuous venovenous hemofiltration without anticoagulation. *ASAIO J* 2004;50(1):76–80.

112. Bellomo R, Tetta C, Ronco C. Coupled plasma filtration adsorption. *Intensive Care Med* 2003:29:1222–8.

113. Letreutre S, Martinot A, Duhamel A, et al. Validation of the pediatric logistic organ dysfunction (PELOD) scores: Prospective multination, multicenter study. *Lancet* 2000;362:192–7.

114. Litalien C, Merouani A, Phan, et al. Thérapies Vasculaires D'épuration Extrarénale. In: Lacroix J, Gauthier M, Leclerc F, et al, eds. *Urgences et soins intensifs pédiatriques.* 2nd ed. Montreal and Paris: Éditions de l'Hôpital Sainte-Justine and Elsevier-Masson, 2007.

CHAPTER 42 ■ BLOOD PRODUCTS AND TRANSFUSION THERAPY

KARAM O, SPINELLA PC, WONG E, AND LUBAN N

KEY POINTS

1 Transfusions can be lifesaving; however, they are also associated with increased morbidity and mortality and should therefore be prescribed only to patients who will benefit from them.

Red Blood Cell Transfusion

2 No well-accepted physiologic parameter accurately indicates when a red blood cell (RBC) transfusion is indicated. While the use of hemoglobin is very common, the indication for an RBC transfusion should be based on physiologic and laboratory parameters, the risk of shock or oxygen debt, and the potential risks of transfusion.

3 A transfusion threshold of ≤7 g/dL for hemoglobin is as safe as one that is more liberal (≤9.5 g/dL) in critically ill, hemodynamically stable children based on a large randomized clinical trial in hemodynamically stable critically ill children.

4 A transfusion threshold of 9 g/dL for hemoglobin may be as safe as one that is more liberal (13 g/dL) in patients with cyanotic congenital heart disease (with the exception of stage 1 physiology), without hemodynamic instability or signs of shock based on a small randomized clinical trial in pediatric postoperative patients with univentricular physiology.

Plasma Transfusion

5 Plasma should not be used as a volume expander.

6 In massively bleeding patients with life-threatening hemorrhage, plasma transfusions should be given immediately, prior to the reporting of the results of coagulation tests. The appropriate ratio between RBC/plasma/platelets is still debated, but ranges between 1:1 and 1:2 for RBC to plasma or platelet units. This is based on evidence from adult observational studies.

7 In non-massively bleeding patients or patients undergoing procedures at risk for bleeding, plasma transfusion is appropriate in the presence of significantly abnormal coagulation tests (activated partial thromboplastin time [aPTT] ratio or prothrombin time [PT] ratio >1.5, International Normalized Ratio [INR] >2.0). This is based on evidence from adult observational studies. In critically ill nonactively bleeding patients, plasma transfusions do not seem to correct mild coagulation abnormalities. The evidence supporting this statement is two observational studies in critically ill adults.

Platelet Transfusion

8 Current guidelines for the use of prophylactic platelet transfusions are supported by expert opinion, adult retrospective studies, and a few randomized clinical trials. However, a recent study (PLAtelet DOse [PLADO]) examining prophylactic platelet transfusions in predominantly noncritically ill patients did not show an effect of three platelet dosing regimens on bleeding frequency in adults or children with malignancies.

9 Thresholds for platelet transfusion triggers are commonly used in certain patient populations, but there are no data to support any platelet concentration thresholds for transfusion of platelets in critically ill children.

Granulocyte Transfusion

10 Granulocyte transfusion should be considered for patients with protracted neutropenia (or dysfunctional neutrophils) and bacterial sepsis or fungal infections without response to antimicrobial or antifungal therapy.

BRIEF HISTORY OF TRANSFUSIONS

Perhaps the earliest recorded case of blood transfusion was that of Pope Innocent VIII (1432–1492). In April 1492, the Pope was in a coma after suffering a stroke and was given the blood of three boys through the mouth, as the concept of circulation was not yet discovered. Despite this treatment, the Pope (and all three boys) died. In 1628, William Harvey explained the circulatory system in humans. This knowledge permitted intravenous transfusion to be considered as a therapeutic option. In the early 1660s, Sir Christopher Wren used a quill-and-bladder syringe to inject fluid into the vein of a dog as a new method of administering medications. Richard Lower performed the first direct blood transfusion from one dog to another in 1665 by connecting an artery to a vein via a silver tube. In 1667, the French physician Jean Baptiste Denys used Lower's technique to successfully transfuse the blood of sheep into both a 15-year-old boy and a woman with postpartum hemorrhage. However, in 1668, Denys' fourth patient died after a transfusion and, although it was later established that the cause of death was arsenic poisoning by the patient's wife, transfusions were banned first in France and England.

In 1818, James Blundell, an obstetrician at Guy's Hospital in London, transfused a patient with blood taken from her husband's arm with a syringe. He went on to perform 10 transfusions over the next 12 years, 5 of which were beneficial for the patients. In 1900, Karl Landsteiner described the concept of different blood groups. In 1907, George Crile published the "Technique of Direct Transfusion of Blood," in which he described the interposition of a cannula between the donor's artery and the receiver's vein. In 1907, Ludvig Hektoen described hemolysis in incompatible transfusions, and in 1913, Ottenberg published the concept of blood group screening prior to transfusions. The major problem that remained was the preservation of blood, as it would coagulate if stored. In 1916, Rous and Turner published "The Preservation of Living Red Blood Cells in Vitro," in which they described sodium citrate as an anticoagulant. One of their students, Oswald Robertson, was sent to the battlefields in Europe, and transfused wounded soldiers with whole blood stored for up to 26 days. He published his work in 1918.

In 1943, Loutit and Mollison discovered that adding an acid to stored blood stabilized the glucose at high temperatures and allowed the stored blood to be sterilized with heat to prevent the transmission of infectious diseases. Since then, the ability to separate whole blood into individual components, the transition from the use of bottles to that of plastic storage containers, and alterations of storage solutions increasing the storage duration (and therefore availability of blood products) led to modern era blood banking.

TRANSFUSION

Constitution of Red Blood Cell Transfusions

Red blood cell (RBC) units are processed from whole blood or from apheresis collections. There are many different processing methods, and there are some recent data suggesting that quality is affected by the method used. Most frequently, whole blood is collected at the donation site into a plastic bag containing an anticoagulant-preservative solution. As soon as possible, the whole blood is centrifuged, the supernatant is used to prepare other blood products (frozen plasma, platelets, gamma globulin, and albumin), and the RBCs are resuspended in another anticoagulant-preservative solution. However, RBC units still contain a significant proportion of plasma and in most solutions (ACD-A, citrate phosphate dextrose [CPD], CPDA-1), the final hematocrit of 60% ± 10%. In many countries, RBC units are filtered to reduce leukocytes prior to storage (see below). After standard leukoreduction, the white blood cell count is decreased from 10^9 to $<1 \times 10^6$/unit of blood.

Scientific Foundation of Red Blood Cell Transfusion

Oxygen Transport

Oxygen transport requires extracting oxygen (O_2) from the atmosphere and then delivering it to cells, where it can be used for essential metabolic processes. Although some cells can temporarily produce energy in the absence of oxygen (anaerobic metabolism), other organs (such as the brain) are made up of cells that rely on continuous oxygen supply for their metabolism (aerobic metabolism). Physiologically, oxygen delivery (DO_2, in mL O_2/min) can be described with the following formula:

$$DO_2 = \text{cardiac output} \times \text{arterial } O_2 \text{ content}$$

The formula for the arterial O_2 content (CaO_2) is

$$CaO_2 = (SaO_2 \times Hb \times 1.34) + (0.003 \times PaO_2)$$

where CaO_2 and PaO_2 are expressed in millimeters of mercury (mm Hg), arterial saturation in oxygen (SaO_2) is expressed as a fraction, and hemoglobin (Hb) concentration is expressed in grams per deciliter (g/dL).

Not all the oxygen is used for the metabolism, and some returns to the lungs. The amount of oxygen utilized by the cells can be calculated by the oxygen consumption ($\dot{V}O_2$) equation:

$$\dot{V}O_2 = \text{cardiac output} \times 1.34 \times Hb \times (SaO_2 - SvO_2)$$

where arterial and venous saturations in oxygen (SaO_2 and SvO_2) are expressed as a fraction, and hemoglobin (Hb) concentration is expressed in grams per deciliter (g/dL).

Under normal circumstances, DO_2 exceeds $\dot{V}O_2$, indicating a physiologic reserve of oxygen delivery in excess of tissue O_2 requirements such that $\dot{V}O_2$ will remain constant even if there are mild to moderate reductions in DO_2. If DO_2 decreases progressively beyond a certain threshold, the physiologic DO_2 reserve is exhausted, and thereafter $\dot{V}O_2$ decreases linearly with further decreases in DO_2. This point in the $DO_2/\dot{V}O_2$ relationship is called the "critical threshold" and indicates the point at which $\dot{V}O_2$ is no longer governed by the metabolic need of the tissues but rather becomes limited by O_2 supply (DO_2). As DO_2 becomes inadequate, tissue hypoxemia occurs. Tissue hypoxia from low DO_2 may be due to a low Hb concentration (anemic hypoxia), low cardiac output (stagnant hypoxia), or low Hb saturation (hypoxic hypoxia). This is illustrated in **Figure 42.1**. It is important to recognize that calculation of $\dot{V}O_2$ is an indirect measure, which is susceptible to mathematical coupling errors. Direct measure of $\dot{V}O_2$ such as with direct calorimetry is more accurate but also more difficult to perform.

Adaptation to Anemia. Anemia is defined as Hb concentrations below the "normal" range for age. Approximately 50% of critically ill children treated in typical North American PICUs are anemic (1). The major physiologic consequence of anemia is a reduction in the DO_2 capacity of blood. The physiological adaptation to anemia is initially an increase in the other DO_2 variables or a decrease in $\dot{V}O_2$. These processes include increased extraction of available O_2, increased heart rate and stroke volume (i.e., cardiac output), redistribution of blood flow from nonvital organs toward the heart and brain (usually at the expense of the splanchnic vascular bed), and a shift to the left in the oxyhemoglobin dissociation curve (i.e., a decrease in O_2 affinity).

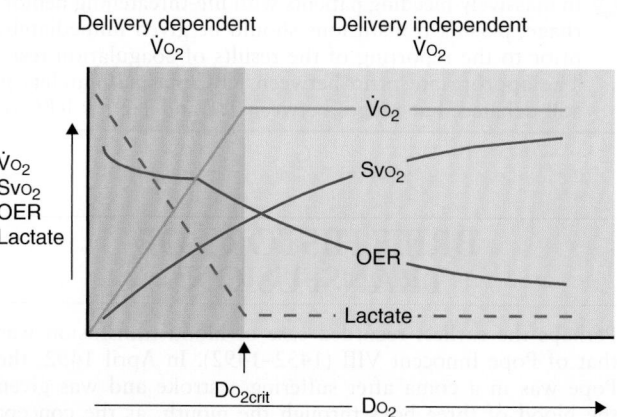

FIGURE 42.1. Effect of the oxygen delivery (DO_2) on the oxygen consumption ($\dot{V}O_2$), central venous oxygen saturation (SvO_2), oxygen extraction ratio (OER), and lactate levels.

Impairment in Adaptive Mechanisms. A number of diseases and host characteristics may impair the adaptive mechanisms to anemia in critically ill patients. The metabolic rate is increased, which decreases the Do_2 reserve in systemic inflammatory response syndrome (SIRS), sepsis, and multiple-organ dysfunction syndrome (MODS). Patients with sepsis and MODS may also have impaired left ventricular function and poor regulation of vascular tone due to impaired nitric oxide–mediated vasoregulation, restricting Do_2 and redistribution of blood flow, respectively.

A number of host characteristics specific to children and infants may impair their adaptive mechanisms. The energy requirements of young infants are much higher than those in adults. This difference is mostly attributable to growth, and it means that they need more substrates, including O_2 and nutrients. In addition to increased metabolic demands, major differences in O_2 transport also exist between adults and children in the first year of life. Fetal Hb has a left-shifted O_2 equilibrium curve, and the proportion of fetal Hb is significant during the first months of life. Physiologic anemia is expected during this period, partially explaining why the Hb concentration varies so much in the newborn and the infant. During the first weeks of life, myocardial compliance is decreased, significantly impairing diastolic filling, which limits increases in stroke volume. Moreover, in newborns and infants, the heart rate is already high, even at rest, which also limits the ability to increase cardiac output. Therefore, many characteristics specific to critically ill children alter their ability to physiologically adapt to low Hb concentrations.

Oxygen Kinetics and Transfusions. Do_2 exceeds resting O_2 requirements in healthy patients, but safety margins rapidly disappear during critical illness, where $\dot{V}o_2$ is often increased (e.g., burns, sepsis, ARDS) and Do_2 is often decreased (e.g., shock, sepsis). Some investigators have shown that patients with sepsis do indeed have some $Do_2/\dot{V}o_2$ dependence, which has led some to hypothesize that sepsis may increase the "critical threshold" Do_2 at which tissue oxygen consumption becomes limited by O_2 supply. The resultant tissue hypoxia contributes to the evolution of irreversible and often fatal MODS. However, RBC transfusion in critically ill patient groups has not been shown convincingly to increase Do_2 to the point that $\dot{V}o_2$ is independent of Do_2 and tissue hypoxia has been abolished. The potential reasons are multifactorial and may include (2) the following:

- Impaired tissue O_2 extraction in some critically ill patients;
- Decreased O_2 unloading due to reduced 2,3-diphosphoglycerate (2,3-DPG) in stored RBC;
- Decreased microcirculatory flow from increased blood viscosity after transfusion.

Furthermore, the $\dot{V}o_2$ calculation uses data from the central circulation, not the microcirculation. But Do_2 and $\dot{V}o_2$ occur in the microcirculation, and there is limited evidence that RBC transfusion improves either at the microcirculatory level. Therefore, it remains uncertain if RBC transfusion is the most useful method to achieve optimal Do_2. The effect of RBC storage duration may influence RBC transfusion oxygen kinetics. The clinical relevance of these effects is controversial and currently under intense investigation.

Microcirculatory Effects of Native and Transfused Red Blood Cells

The effects of transfused RBCs on the distribution of systemic blood flow to specific organs have been described. Despite investigation, the effect of transfused RBCs on systemic Do_2 is still controversial. For example, RBC transfusion may increase sublingual microcirculation without having an effect on global Do_2 (3). It remains unclear how transfused RBCs influence Do_2 in the microcirculation owing to the difficulty in obtaining in situ measurements of blood viscosity, microcirculatory flow, and $\dot{V}o_2$.

In theory, either too low or too high viscosity is associated with a risk of decreasing blood flow through small vessels. Capillaries collapse if the hematocrit is too low, and RBC transfusion may be viewed as a means of restoring blood viscosity (4). On the other hand, some have suggested that capillary resistance to blood flow increases rapidly if the hematocrit level increases (from 33% to 55%), which may result in microcirculatory stasis and impaired local Do_2 to the tissues (5).

The microcirculatory effects of transfused RBCs may also be related to the generation of inflammatory mediators as some cytokines may mediate vasoconstriction or thrombosis of small vessels, causing local ischemia.

Transfused RBCs differ from their endogenous counterparts. During storage, numerous changes occur to RBCs and the unit supernatant; these changes progress over time. Detailed mechanisms of these changes are reviewed in detail elsewhere (6). To summarize, RBC energetics alter during storage (principally from impaired glycolysis), which results in an adverse impact upon antioxidant systems and an increase in iron-based free radical generation. Consequently, intraerythrocytic 2,3-DPG is diminished, NO bioavailability is reduced, the RBC membrane loses deformability, RBC adhesion and aggregation are increased, and RBC membrane microparticles are generated. Combined, these effects reduce both perfusion and oxygen delivery. Moreover, RBC membrane microparticles generated during storage have immune suppressive and procoagulant properties. While these effects of storage have been demonstrated, their clinical relevance is unclear. The two-hit hypothesis, as applied to RBC storage duration, suggests critical illness (a state of immune, endothelial, and hemostasis dysregulation) increases vulnerability to impact from RBCs altered by storage and that the likelihood of adverse clinical effects from transfusion progresses with storage duration. A large, multicenter randomized controlled trial (RCT) is planned to examine this question in critically ill children. In summary, while RBC transfusions increase circulating oxygen content, donor RBCs may paradoxically decrease O_2 delivery to tissue, as well as disturb immune function and exacerbate thrombophilia in patients with critical illness, potentially increasing the risk of adverse clinical outcomes.

Hemolysis also occurs in packed RBC (PRBC) units over time. Free intravascular Hb as well as Hb within RBC membrane microvesicles may cause vasoconstriction, via the binding of NO. In summary, while RBC transfusions increase global Do_2, microcirculatory flow and O_2 availability may decrease in some tissues.

Immunologic Effects of Allogeneic Red Blood Cell Transfusions

❶ Transfused RBCs may adversely affect the immunologic responses. Some evidence suggests that transfused RBCs may result in clinically important immunomodulation in the recipient. For example, transfusions of packed RBCs decrease the number of rejection episodes and improve renal and cardiac allograft survival. Many proinflammatory molecules are detected in RBC units, including cytokines, complement activators, O_2 free radicals, histamine, lysophosphatidylcholine species, and other bioreactive substances such as RBC membrane microparticles that may initiate, maintain, or enhance an inflammatory process.

The white blood cells (WBCs) and the cytokines in unfiltered packed RBCs may trigger or maintain an SIRS in the RBC recipient. Giving an RBC transfusion to a critically ill patient with SIRS may stimulate their inflammatory syndrome, which may result in the development of MODS (second-hit theory of MODS). Some data suggest that the inflammatory risks of RBC transfusion decrease significantly if the packed RBC units are prestorage-leukocyte depleted. However, an in vitro study showed that even leukoreduced RBC units induced cytokine production in the host, and that this response varied according to the length of storage. A shorter storage time was associated with a mixed pro- and anti-inflammatory response, whereas a more prolonged storage time elicited an anti-inflammatory response (7). There are also some recent data suggesting that the preservative solution further modulates this response (8). The clinical effects of RBC transfusion on the immunologic responses of critically ill children remain to be determined. In summary, some evidence suggests that transfusion may cause immunosuppression, thereby increasing the risk of acquiring nosocomial infections. RBC transfusion can also reinforce SIRS, which can progress to MODS.

Transfusion of Red Blood Cells: Application to the PICU

Practice Pattern

2 The most frequent justification for prescribing an RBC transfusion is a low Hb concentration. Two surveys based on questionnaires and three observational studies demonstrated large variability in practice pattern with respect to an "acceptable" threshold Hb concentration. In two surveys of pediatric critical care practitioners designed to investigate RBC transfusion practices and clinical determinants that might alter transfusion thresholds in critically ill children, investigators reported a threshold Hb range from <7 to >13 g/dL (9,10). These results were confirmed by a bedside observational cohort study (11). In a third study completed in 2005 by the PALISI Network, the average Hb concentration before RBC transfusion given in 30 North American PICUs was >9 g/dL in children <5 years of age (1). The lack of data determining the appropriate indication for transfusion contributes to the striking variation in both the stated and the observed practice patterns among pediatric critical care practitioners.

Current Evidence

Transfusion in Severe Anemia. Some data suggest that severe anemia may increase the risk of mortality in critically ill mammals and human beings. In healthy animals undergoing acute hemodilution, evidence of heart dysfunction appears once the Hb concentration drops below 3.3–4 g/dL. However, animals with 50%–80% coronary artery stenosis can show evidence of ischemic insult to the heart with an Hb concentration as high as 7–10 g/dL (12).

Two studies undertaken in patients who refused blood products for religious reasons suggest that very low Hb levels may increase mortality (13,14). After bloodless surgery, the risk of death increased steadily once the postoperative Hb concentration dropped below 5–6 g/dL in healthy patients. A higher mortality risk was involved if heart disease was present, and the odds of mortality increased when Hb concentration dropped below 10 g/dL.

Few studies assess the relationship between anemia and mortality in acutely ill children. One group followed 2433 anemic African children who were hospitalized; 20% received a transfusion (15). Children with Hb 4.7 g/dL and respiratory distress who had received a whole blood transfusion had a lower mortality rate than those who did not receive a blood transfusion. Another prospective cohort study of 1269 Kenyan children hospitalized for malaria showed that whole blood

transfusion decreased mortality if anemia was severe (Hb level <4 g/dL) or if dyspnea was associated with an Hb level of <5 g/dL (16). These studies suggest that some benefit may be associated with keeping the Hb concentration of hospitalized children above 5 g/dL. This might also be true for critically ill children, although some of these African children had chronic anemia due to sickle cell disease or malaria, which could modify their response to acute anemia, and the transfusions were whole blood, not leukoreduced RBC units.

All of these data indicate that it is not the absolute Hb value that is the primary determinant of the risk of mortality, but instead it is the risk of inadequate oxygen delivery to meet demand. Since oxygen delivery is determined by both cardiac output and oxygen content and oxygen demand is governed by metabolic rate, the use of Hb alone to determine the risk of mortality is very imprecise.

Red Blood Cell Transfusion: Current Guidelines

In 1942, two anesthesiologists, Drs. Adams and Lundy, wrote: "When concentration of Hb is <8–10 g per 100 cubic centimeters of whole blood, it is wise to give a whole blood transfusion before operation." Thereafter, the "10/30" rule (Hb of 10 g/dL or hematocrit of 30%) was standard practice for more than 50 years, without support from high-quality clinical data. This concept also persisted despite the change from whole blood to the use of components and significant increase in the storage duration of RBC units. With recent publication of prospective RCT data, evidence-based medicine recommendations are now possible in some populations. Clinical situations requiring RBC transfusions can be divided into five categories: hemorrhagic shock, unstable patients, stabilized patients, patients with cyanotic heart disease, and chronic anemia.

Hemorrhagic Shock. Hemorrhagic shock is a specific clinical situation where shock is due partly to hypovolemia, which decreases cardiac output, and hence Do_2, and partly to RBC loss, which decreases HB and hence Do_2. Despite the high risk of mortality for this condition, no RCT has yet evaluated the proper RBC transfusion threshold in such a population. Therefore, physicians usually rely on expert recommendations. Both the Pediatric Advanced Life Support (PALS) and the Advanced Trauma Life Support (ATLS) recommend initiating volume resuscitation with 40–60 mL/kg of crystalloid solutions (normal saline or Ringer-Lactate) before transfusing RBC units. These current guidelines are based on animal data and very small human studies and are becoming more controversial with recent large observational studies of massive transfusion for hemorrhagic shock. (Massive transfusion is discussed elsewhere in this chapter.)

A recent trial in 921 adults with acute upper gastrointestinal bleeding demonstrated that, compared with a liberal transfusion strategy (Hb <9.0 g/dL), a restrictive strategy (Hb <7.0 g/dL) significantly improved mortality at 45 days (17). The percentage of patients who received a transfusion of *fresh frozen plasma* (FFP) or platelets and the total amount of fluid administered were similar in the two groups. These patients were not all in hemorrhagic shock, although the mean volume of fluid resuscitation was 5 L. This study suggests that trials on transfusion thresholds in hemorrhagic shock are needed.

Unstable Patients. An unstable patient can be defined as a patient with physical examination or laboratory evidence of shock (oxygen debt). Signs of shock include prolonged capillary refill, oliguria, abnormal level of consciousness, increased lactate levels, and decreased Svo_2 or Sto_2 (tissue oxygen saturation). While hypotension itself may not confer shock, it clearly increases the risk of it. It is reasonable to transfuse RBCs for a threshold >7g/dL in children who are unstable; however, no consensus defines the threshold. In addition, other methods of improving oxygen content or cardiac output should also be considered. How the oxygen delivery and consumption relationship is altered should be dependent upon the method that has the optimal risk to benefit ratio for the individual patient.

In an adult randomized clinical trial involving septic patients in an emergency room setting a rapid (<6 hours) and aggressive therapy-driven protocol with the specific goal of decreasing mortality in adults with severe sepsis and septic shock was studied (18). RBC transfusions to maintain the hematocrit over 30% were given to patients in the experimental group if the O_2 saturation in the central cava vein was lower than 70% after fluid challenge, vasopressors, and inotropes. Mortality was 46.5% in the standard treatment group ($n = 133$) versus 30.5% in the "early goal-directed therapy" group ($n = 130$, $p = 0.009$). Unfortunately, the isolated effect of RBC transfusions in these patients could not be evaluated. The applicability of this trial to children is debatable, but it is possible that the outcome of patients with severe sepsis may be better if the Hb concentration is kept over 10 g/dL if all other aspects of the sepsis bundle employed in the study are maintained, at least during the first hours following diagnosis. The extrapolation of these results to other unstable patients remains uncertain.

3 Stabilized Patients. Once the patient has been stabilized (the condition of patients can be considered stable if the mean systemic arterial pressure is not less than 2 SD below the normal mean for age and if cardiovascular treatments had not been increased for at least 2 hours), data show that critically ill children are able to tolerate Hb concentrations as low as 7 g/dL.

In critically ill adults, the transfusion requirements in critical care (TRICC) trial showed that in hemodynamically stable, critically ill patients, a restrictive transfusion strategy (RBC transfusions with non–leukocyte-depleted units given only if the Hb concentration dropped under 7 g/dL and maintained at 7–9 g/dL) was safer than a liberal transfusion strategy (RBC transfusions given if the Hb concentration dropped under 10 g/dL and maintained at 10–12 g/dL) (19). An adjusted multiple-organ dysfunction score and the hospital mortality rate were statistically lower in the restrictive transfusion group.

In 2007, the pediatric transfusion requirements in PICU (TRIPICU) study randomized 320 stabilized critically ill children to a hemoglobin threshold of 7 g/dL for red cell transfusion (restrictive-strategy group) and 317 patients to a threshold of 9.5 g/dL (liberal-strategy group) (20). The number of patients who developed new or progressive MODS (primary outcome) was similar in both groups: 38 (11.9%) in the restrictive versus 39 (12.3%) in the liberal group. No differences were reported in other major outcomes, including all-cause mortality (14 deaths after 28 days in both groups), nosocomial infection, and length of stay. This noninferiority trial suggests that hemodynamically stable critically ill children have similar outcomes with less exposure to RBCs when a restrictive (<7 g/dL) versus a liberal (<9.5 g/dL) transfusion approach is used. These results were consistent in subgroup analysis performed in noncyanotic cardiac surgery patients, general surgery patients, and septic patients. These subgroup analyses were, however, underpowered and need to be confirmed in larger trials.

4 Cyanotic Congenital Heart Disease. As a low arterial oxygen saturation proportionately decreases Do_2, the optimal Hb concentration may be even higher in cases of cyanotic congenital heart disease than in other kinds of congenital heart disease: non–evidence-based thresholds as high as 13 g/dL and even 16 g/dL are recommended in some textbooks. Cholette et al. (21) randomized 60 infants and children with variations of single-ventricle physiology (non–stage 1) presenting for cavopulmonary connection to a restrictive (hemoglobin of <9.0 g/dL) or liberal (hemoglobin of ≥13.0 g/dL) transfusion

strategy for 48 hours postoperation. There were no differences in the primary outcome measures mean lactate (1.4 ± 0.5 mmol/L [Restrictive] vs. 1.4 ± 0.4 mmol/L [Liberal]) or peak lactate (3.1 ± 1.5 mmol/L [Restrictive] vs. 3.2 ± 1.3 mmol/L [Liberal]). Clinical outcomes were also similar. Therefore, it might be reasonable to adopt a restrictive transfusion strategy (transfuse only when hemoglobin <9.0 g/dL) in non–stage 1 cyanotic congenital heart disease, although this needs to be confirmed in a larger trial.

Chronic Anemia. Patients with chronic anemia (i.e., anemia that is not the result of acute blood loss nor acute hemodilution) have usually increased their cardiac output (to maintain Do_2) or have decreased their $\dot{V}o_2$. No RCT has evaluated the transfusion threshold for these patients. The only data are from observational studies. In 61 adult Jehovah's Witnesses with an Hb <8 g/dL, deaths due to anemia increased only at an Hb below 5 g/dL (22). Although such a threshold seems reasonable to many physicians, no recommendation can be made until a proper trial is undertaken.

Red Blood Cell Products

Red Blood Cells. *RBCs* are prepared from blood collected into any approved anticoagulant-preservative solutions and separated from the plasma by centrifugation or sedimentation. Separation may occur at any time during the allowable shelf life of the product, which varies with the solution used. RBC may contain 160–275 mL of red cells (50–80 g of hemoglobin) suspended in varying quantities of residual plasma.

RBCs adenine saline added are prepared by centrifuging whole blood to remove as much plasma as possible, and replacing the plasma with 100–110 mL of an additive solution that contains some combination of dextrose, adenine, sodium chloride, and either monobasic sodium phosphate (AS-3) or mannitol (AS-1 and AS-5); the hematocrit of these products varies between 55% and 65%. RBCs in an additive solution have lower viscosity, and flow through administration systems rapidly. RBCs stored with an additive solution have an extended shelf life, dependent on the solution (42 days for RBCs in AS).

Leukocyte-Reduced Red Blood Cells. *RBCs leukocytes reduced* and *RBC adenine saline-added leukocytes reduced* are prepared from a unit of whole blood (collected in an approved anticoagulant-preservative solution) containing ≥1–10 × 10^9 white cells. Leukocyte reduction is achieved by filtration (a) soon after collection (prestorage) or (b) after varying periods of storage in the blood bank. Leukocyte reduction decreases the cellular content and volume of blood according to characteristics of the filter system used. *RBCs leukocytes reduced* have a residual content of leukocytes <5.0 × 10^6 in the United States and <1.0 × 10^6 in the EU and other countries; 85% of the original red cell content must be retained after filtration. The potential advantages of leukocyte reduction include decreased transmission of infections carried by leukocytes (cytomegalovirus [CMV]), decreased febrile transfusion reactions, and decreased transfusion-related immune modulation (TRIM) caused by residual white cells. Leukocyte-reduced preparations still contain leukocytes and should not be given to patients at risk for transfusion-associated graft-versus-host disease (TA-GVHD). If universal leukocyte reduction in all packed red cell units is not practiced, the intensivist should specifically order leukocyte-reduced blood for certain patient groups:

- Transplant patients;
- Patients with a history of febrile nonhemolytic transfusion reactions;
- CMV-seronegative patients for whom seronegative PRBC units are not available.

Washed Red Blood Cells. *Washed RBCs* are RBC units in which the plasma is removed and replaced with either normal saline or a plasma substitute, depending upon the institution. Washing removes between 98% and 99% of plasma constituents. They are used mainly for recurrent severe allergic reactions, or to deplete potassium.

Frozen Deglycerolized Red Blood Cells. *RBC frozen* and *frozen rejuvenated RBCs* are prepared by adding the cryoprotective agent glycerol to the RBCs before freezing. *Deglycerolized RBC* refers to the product that is made available postthaw and washing with successively lower concentrates of sodium chloride.

Deglycerolized RBCs contain 80% or more of the red cells present in the original unit of blood and have approximately the same expected posttransfusion survival as regular RBC units.

Deglycerolized RBCs provide the same physiologic benefits as RBCs, but their use is restricted to situations in which standard transfusion components are inappropriate or unavailable. Deglycerolized RBCs may be indicated for patients with previous severe allergic transfusion reactions, because the process efficiently removes plasma constituents. Intravascular hemolysis can occur in the recipient if deglycerolization has been inadequate. Deglycerolized RBCs must be transfused within 24 hours postthawing if prepared in an open system, within 2 weeks if a closed system has been used.

Irradiated Red Cells. GVHD is an extremely rare but potentially fatal complication of red cell transfusion in an immunosuppressed or immunodeficient patient. It is caused by the presence of donor T lymphocytes in the red cell unit, which subsequently divide in the transfusion recipient (host). Gamma irradiation of the PRBC unit inactivates T-lymphocyte proliferation and prevents transfusion-related GVHD in the susceptible recipient. Some authors recommend routine irradiation of all red cell units in infants, because of the possibility of an undiagnosed immunodeficiency state in this population. However, other experts do not recommend universal irradiation for infants, as the process per se increases the potassium in the PRBC, which could also have side effects in infants.

Prescription and Administration

Prescription of Red Blood Cell Transfusion. The physician must explain the benefits and risks of transfusion to the patient (or the patient's family) and obtain informed consent in accordance with institutional guidelines.

The transfusion process is initiated when a physician writes an order specifying the component and the volume to be given. In addition, pretransfusion medication (if indicated), rate and duration of administration, special processing needs (gamma irradiation, washed, etc.), and use of a blood warmer or electromechanical device should be specified.

The formula helpful in determining transfusion volumes is

$$\text{Volume (mL)} = [(\text{Hb}_{\text{targeted}} - \text{Hb}_{\text{observed}}) \times \text{weight} \times \text{blood volume}]/\text{Hb}_{\text{RBC}} \text{ unit}$$

where $\text{Hb}_{\text{targeted}}$ is the Hb concentration targeted posttransfusion (e.g., 10 g/dL), $\text{Hb}_{\text{observed}}$ is the most recently measured Hb concentration of the patient (g/dL), weight is expressed in kilograms, blood volume is expressed in mL/kg (80 mL/kg if the child is <2 years old and 70 mL/kg if the child is 2–14 years old), and Hb_{RBC} unit is the average Hb concentration in the packed RBC units (g/dL) prepared by the transfusion service.

For example, if the $\text{Hb}_{\text{observed}}$ in a 2-week-old baby weighing 3 kg is 6.5 g/dL, his or her blood volume is 80 mL/kg and the Hb_{RBC} unit is 19.5 g/dL (usual Hb for an AS-3 unit) and the desired Hb concentration ($\text{Hb}_{\text{targeted}}$) is 10 g/dL, the volume

of the RBC unit to be transfused would be determined by the following formula:

$$\text{Volume} = [(10.0 - 6.5 \text{ g/dL}) \times 3 \text{ kg} \times 80 \text{ mL/kg}] / 19.5 \text{ g/dL} = 43 \text{ mL}$$

Emergency-Release RBC Blood. In some situations, patients may require lifesaving transfusions before the usual compatibility tests can be performed. In a PICU, these situations are typically pediatric trauma, massive gastrointestinal bleeding, massive postoperative bleeding, bleeding on extracorporeal membrane oxygenation (ECMO), rupture of an extracorporeal circuit (ECMO or hemodiafiltration), etc. If the patient's blood type is known, type-specific un-crossmatched blood should be given in this situation. If the patient's blood type is unknown, most blood banks maintain an emergency-release blood for use when transfusion is required immediately and before ABO testing can take place.

Emergency-release universal donor blood:

- For females: Type O, Rh (D) Negative, un-crossmatched red cells
- For males: Type O, Rh (D) Negative *or* Positive, un-crossmatched red cells

Prior to administration of any blood, it is important to collect a blood sample from the patient for subsequent ABO testing.

Conclusions

An RBC transfusion is the only effective way to rapidly increase the Hb level of critically ill patients because their response to iron and erythropoietin is too slow. The risk–benefit ratio must be taken into account when transfusion is being considered.

Although most intensivists contend that transfusion should be based upon $\text{Do}_2/\dot{\text{V}}\text{o}_2$ adequacy and all methods of altering this relationship should be considered, in practice, the decision to prescribe an RBC transfusion is still predominantly based on Hb concentration. Improved methods of objectively determining RBC transfusion indications are needed.

According to the only large RCT, an RBC transfusion is not required if the Hb concentration remains above 7 g/dL, in critically ill stabilized children.

In unstable patients, a hemoglobin threshold above 7 g/dL may be appropriate, while also addressing all other determinants of oxygen delivery and consumption. In patients with non–stage 1 cyanotic congenital heart disease, a hemoglobin threshold of 9 g/dL may be appropriate. In chronically anemic patients, a hemoglobin threshold of 5 g/dL appears to be safe.

PLASMA

Constitution of Plasma

Plasma units contain the acellular portion of blood, that is the supernatant after centrifugation of whole blood, where the RBCs, WBCs, and platelets will have precipitated and been almost completely removed. Plasma contains many biologically active molecules, including coagulation factors, which are essential components of the coagulation system (23). One milliliter of plasma contains ~1 unit of each of the coagulation factors. There is, however, variability in coagulation factor levels. Labile coagulation factors, such as factors V and VIII, are unstable in plasma stored for prolonged periods at 1°C–6°C, which explains why plasma is usually stored frozen at or below −18°C.

Apart from coagulation factors, plasma contains fibrin, immunoglobulins, antithrombin, protein C, and protein S. It can also contain different allergens (24). Plasma contains significant amounts of glucose (535 mg/dL or 30 mmol/L), sodium (172 mEq/L), potassium (15 mEq/L), and proteins (5.5 g/dL with 60% albumin) (25). In addition, there are thousands of other proteins within plasma that have effects far beyond coagulation and immune function. The science of exploring the proteome of plasma is expanding, and there is much more to learn regarding the effects of plasma.

Scientific Foundation of Transfusion of Plasma

Effects of Plasma on Coagulation Disorders

In an adult critical care unit, Abdel-Wahab et al. (26) assessed the effect of plasma transfusions on the International Normalized Ratio (INR). Among 121 patients who received plasma for moderately abnormal coagulation tests (INR <1.85), only 1 (0.8%) was able to correct his INR (<1.1) after a plasma transfusion. The amount of transfused plasma was not associated with the INR after transfusion, whatever the volume. In another study, Holland and Brooks (27) showed that plasma transfusions did not correct INR levels <2.0–2.5. These studies suggest that plasma might not be appropriate to correct mildly abnormal coagulation tests.

Conversely the use of INR as an adequate measure of the hemostatic effect of plasma is currently debated. Prospective study of alternative measures of coagulation may provide useful information regarding the benefit (or not) of plasma for patients with mild to moderate coagulation deficits.

Immunologic Effects of Plasma Transfusions

As plasma contains many bioactive substances (cytokines, immunoglobulin and coagulation factors), it has been hypothesized that it could interact with the patient's immune system. The process of freezing and thawing plasma increases *per se* histamine and other bioactive products. Other studies have shown that plasma transfusions induce the production of TNF-alpha and IL-10 and increase lymphocyte count after plasma transfusion. Antithrombin, protein C, and protein S are present in plasma units and also seem to have immunomodulative properties.

This might explain why standard FFP transfusions can be associated with some adverse events, like MODS and TRIM, which might increase the risk of contracting nosocomial infections. Adult epidemiological studies have shown that patients who are transfused with plasma are indeed more prone to nosocomial infections (28) and acute respiratory distress syndrome (ARDS) (29). A pediatric retrospective study evaluated the association between plasma and mortality in 380 children with acute lung injury (ALI) (30). They showed a significant 8% increase in mortality for each mL/kg of plasma, after adjusting for severity at admission and coagulopathy. A recent prospective epidemiological study in 831 critically ill children evaluated the risks associated with plasma transfusions. The adjusted odds ratio for an increased incidence of new or progressive MODS was 3.2. There was also a significant difference in the occurrence of nosocomial infections and ICU length of stay (31).

All of these nonrandomized studies are subject to bias and may reflect the increased severity of illness in patients receiving plasma (confounding by indication bias). If these results are accurate, however, plasma transfusions may be associated with worse clinical outcome, perhaps due to their immunomodulative properties.

Other Effects of Plasma Transfusions

In animal models of hemorrhagic shock, plasma transfusions seem to improve capillary membrane permeability and reduce endothelial injury. Pati et al. (32) recently demonstrated that plasma had beneficial effects on endothelial permeability and vascular stability. On a molecular level, the glycocalyx, a network of soluble plasma components that projects from the endothelial cell surface and plays a key role in maintaining endothelial integrity, is disrupted by hemorrhagic shock. Plasma transfusions seem to preserve the glycocalyx and maintain endothelial integrity (33), or even to restore it (34).

Transfusion of Plasma: Application to PICU

Risk of Bleeding

A common use of plasma transfusion is to prevent or to stop bleeding. Therefore, one should be able to evaluate the risk of bleeding in order to guide this decision. Although classic coagulation tests should correlate with the risk of bleeding, this does not seem to be the case. Indeed, a recent meta-analysis evaluated whether a prolonged PT or elevated INR predicts bleeding during invasive diagnostic procedures. The authors concluded that clinicians should not assume that mild to moderate prolongation of the INR or PT predicts a higher risk of bleeding (35).

Thromboelastography, a method recently incorporated into ICU clinical practice, is performed with whole blood, and assesses the viscoelastic property of clot formation under low shear condition. Thromboelastography-based algorithms reduce both transfusion requirements and blood loss in cardiac surgery, liver transplantation, and massive trauma. However, there are currently no data on their adequacy to evaluate the risk of bleeding in other situations, especially in a PICU setting.

In conclusion, current coagulation tests, such as prothrombin time (PT) or activated partial thromboplastin time (aPTT), do not correlate with the risk of bleeding in a patient without active bleeding. As thromboelastography still requires prospective study in critically ill children, there are no current methods that adequately assess the risk of severe bleeding in this population.

Practice Pattern

In 2008, according to the US Department of Health and Human Services, 4,484,000 plasma units were transfused in the United States. More than 10% of critically ill patients, both adults and children, receive a plasma transfusion during their stay, making plasma transfusions a frequently used treatment modality (36).

In practice, plasma transfusions are administered to correct abnormal coagulation tests or to prevent or treat active bleeding. In a prospective study, Arnold et al. (37) showed that 60% of the plasma was prescribed to either nonbleeding patients or patients with normal coagulation tests. After deploying a multifaceted educational intervention in their 15-bed adult ICU, this proportion went down to 46%. No observational data have been published on the plasma transfusion practice pattern in PICU patients.

Current Evidence

In situations where active bleeding is attributable to a coagulation factor deficiency, plasma transfusions can constitute a lifesaving intervention by improving coagulation factor deficit, especially in patients requiring massive transfusion (38). However, in non–life-threatening situations, some authors have shown that transfusing plasma often fails to correct mild coagulation abnormalities (26,27).

Currently, there is no RCT that has evaluated the plasma transfusion thresholds in critically ill patients.

Current Guidelines

The following guidelines are based on observational studies and expert opinions (39,40).

⑤ Prophylactic. Current recommendations advise against the use of plasma for volume expansion. Prophylactic plasma transfusion is also not supported in nonbleeding patients, except in preparation for surgery or invasive procedures.

⑥ Therapeutic. In massive bleeding patients at risk for exsanguination, plasma should be transfused before the results of classic coagulation tests are made available (massive transfusion is further discussed elsewhere in this chapter). The use of rapid thromboelastography testing to guide plasma transfusion in massively bleeding patients, while still uncommon, is increasing over time.

⑦ In nonmassive bleeding patients, expert consensus is that plasma should be considered only if the PT ratio or aPTT ratio is higher than 1.5, or if the INR is above 2.0. No recommendations in this population currently include thromboelastography thresholds for plasma transfusion.

Prothrombin complex concentrates are the drug of choice for reversal of vitamin K antagonists. If these agents are not available, plasma is appropriate in the presence of major or intracranial hemorrhage or in preparation for surgery that cannot be delayed.

Plasma should be used only to replace single clotting factor deficiencies for which no fractionated product is available.

Plasma exchange therapy is currently indicated for treatment of thrombotic micro-angiopathies (e.g., thrombotic thrombocytopenic purpura, atypical hemolytic-uremic syndrome), as replacement fluid.

Plasma is also indicated as reconstitution of whole blood for exchange transfusions, as well as for hereditary angioedema in the case that C1-esterase inhibitor is not available.

Plasma Products

Fresh Frozen Plasma. FFP is prepared from whole blood or apheresis collection and frozen at −18°C or colder within the time delineated by the system in which it has been collected. Most units contain 200–250 mL, but apheresis-derived units may contain as much as 400–600 mL and some institutions repackage FFP into smaller aliquots for neonatal use. FFP contains plasma proteins including all coagulation factors. FFP contains normal levels of the labile coagulation factors V and VIII.

FFP is infused within 4 hours after thawing, or it can also be stored at 1°C–6°C. After 24 hours, the component must be discarded, or if collected in a functionally closed system may be relabeled as Thawed Plasma.

Frozen Plasma. *Plasma frozen within 24 hours after phlebotomy* (FP24) is prepared from a whole blood or apheresis collection. The product is stored at 1°C–6°C within 8 hours of collection and frozen at −18°C or below within 24 hours of collection. Another product, *plasma frozen within 24 hours after phlebotomy held at room temperature up to 24 hours after phlebotomy* (FP24RT24) is also available for use (kept at room temperature up to 24 hours rather than refrigerated at 1°C–6°C as for FP24). On average, units contain 200–250 mL, but apheresis-derived units may contain as much as 400–600 mL. Most plasma proteins are at levels similar to FFP. However, levels of factor VIII and protein C are reduced and levels of factor V and other labile plasma proteins are variable compared with FFP. FP24RT24 is different from FP24 in containing significantly less protein S and also should not be used for protein S–deficient patients. FP24RT24, however, contains comparable levels of protein C as FFP and can be used for protein C–deficient patients.

Thawed Plasma. *Thawed plasma* is derived from FFP, PF24, or PF24RT24 prepared using aseptic techniques. It is thawed at 30°C–37°C and maintained at 1°C–6°C for up to 5 days after the initial 24-hour postthaw period has elapsed. Thawed Plasma contains stable coagulation factors such as factor II and fibrinogen in concentrations clinically similar to those of FFP, but variably reduced amounts of other factors.

This component serves as a source of nonlabile plasma proteins. Levels and activation state of coagulation proteins in thawed plasma are variable and change over time. Thawed plasma is often used in the setting of massive transfusion protocols, especially in adult trauma settings.

Solvent/Detergent Plasma. As there is a high variability in coagulation factors between single-donor units of FFP (41), pooling plasma from many donors provides a method to maintain a constant concentration of these factors. However, pooling donors increases the risks of transmission of infectious diseases. To reduce this risk, multiple pathogen inactivation methods are used, such as solvent/detergent (S/D) treatment, methylene blue, ultraviolet light with riboflavin, and psoralens (amotosalen) (42). The S/D treatment process includes pooling of plasma, S/D treatment, lipid extraction, and sterile filtering.

The S/D method has been shown to inactivate enveloped viruses (such as HIV, hepatitis B virus, and hepatitis C virus) in a rapid and complete manner, but has no effect on nonenveloped viruses such as hepatitis A virus (HAV) and parvovirus B19. However, the presence of justified limits for neutralizing antibodies toward HAV and parvovirus B19 in the starting plasma and the final product results in immune neutralization and passive immunization, which both serve to limit or prevent virus replication in vivo and thereby infection in patients. Benefits of the S/D treatment process include the reduction of human leukocyte antibody (HLA) concentrations and the removal of bioactive lipids and lipoproteins. As a result, S/D treatment of plasma may have an increased safety profile regarding the immunologic adverse effects previously reported with FFP (41).

Limitations of S/D plasma are that it may increase the risk of nonenveloped virus and prion transmission as a result of pooling. These risks are mitigated by screening for nonenveloped viruses prior to use and filtering technology that removes prions. A safety concern with the use of S/D-treated plasma products is related to the low concentrations of protein S and plasmin inhibitor (alpha-2 antiplasmin) as a result of processing. Adequate safety regarding thrombotic risks is supported by clinical use of >10 million units in patients (41).

Absolute contraindications for S/D plasma include IgA deficiency with documented antibodies to IgA and severe protein S deficiency.

Prescription of Plasma Transfusions

Compatibility testing is not required before plasma transfusion, unless large volumes are given. Plasma must be ABO compatible with the recipient's RBCs. Type AB plasma can be administered in severe and acute situations as a universal donor type if necessary. If type AB plasma is unavailable and the patient's group is unknown, one might consider using type A plasma instead, as type A plasma has low anti-B titers. However, in such a situation, one must balance the risk of death from hemorrhage with the immunological risks.

Rh compatibility and crossmatching are not considered because there are virtually no RBCs in FFP.

Plasma dosing is calculated at 10–20 mL/kg, followed by repeat laboratory evaluation using a coagulation profile in nonmassively bleeding patients. In some cases, multiple repeat doses are necessary.

Normally, it takes 20–30 minutes to thaw FFP. Plasma can also be warmed in 7 minutes using a microwave oven;

however, only ovens specifically constructed for this task can be used, as standard microwaves will destroy the function of several coagulation factors.

Thawed plasma must probably be used within 4–6 hours after release. A macroaggregate filter (standard component filter, 170–260 µm) must be used. Centers with high-volume patients with traumatic injury and massive bleeding will prethaw AB (or A) plasma for immediate use for massive transfusion protocols, as some data suggest that thawed plasma can be stored at 1°C–6°C for 5 days, although its properties might decrease over that period (32).

Conclusions

Most clinical uses of plasma are not supported by evidence. Plasma is usually prescribed to prevent or stop bleeding, as it contains coagulation factors. However, the appropriate transfusion triggers are still not available, as abnormal classic coagulation tests in nonbleeding patients do not correlate with increased risk of bleeding. Furthermore, in critically ill patients, plasma transfusions do not seem to correct mild coagulation abnormalities based on INR testing.

In massively bleeding patients, plasma transfusions should be given before obtaining classic coagulation tests.

In nonmassively bleeding patients or patients undergoing procedures at risk of bleeding, plasma transfusions should probably not be given, except if coagulation tests are significantly abnormal.

Plasma should not be used as a volume expander.

PLATELETS

Constitution of Platelets

Platelet concentrates are manufactured from units of whole blood that have not cooled <20°C and are prepared within hours of collection or through apheresis from a single donor. Platelet concentrates derived from whole blood donors are often pooled prior to issue.

Platelets undergo irreversible activation when stored between 1°C and 8°C. Studies have shown that platelets stored between 20°C and 24°C have superior survival and are the current standard products. Normal platelet levels vary with age and gender for children. Normal levels for both adult females and males are $150,000–450,000/mm^3$ (conventional units) or $150–450 \times 10^9/L$ (SI units).

Scientific Foundation of Transfusion of Platelets

Thrombocytopenia

Thrombocytopenia and/or qualitative platelet defects increase the risk of bleeding, owing to impairment in the ability to form a platelet plug. Platelet concentrates are given to patients at risk of bleeding in order to increase their platelet count or to supply them with more functional platelets.

Thrombocytopenia is defined by a platelet count $<150 \times 10^9/L$ ($150,000/mm^3$). The prevalence of ICU-acquired thrombocytopenia is 44% in critically ill adults (43); no data seem to be available for critically ill children. Thrombocytopenia is observed when increased platelet consumption or decreased platelet production occurs. Increased platelet consumption in critically ill patients can result from non–immune-mediated

mechanisms (severe bleeding, disseminated intravascular coagulation, splenomegaly, and sepsis) or immune-mediated mechanisms (alloimmunization in patients undergoing chemotherapy who have received numerous blood products, patients with autoimmune thrombocytopenia purpura, and patients who develop heparin-induced thrombocytopenia or other drug-induced antiplatelet antibodies). Heparin-induced thrombocytopenia has a prevalence of about 1% following cardiovascular surgery for congenital heart disease. Decreased bone marrow platelet production can result from medications (most notably chemotherapy), sepsis, and viral infections, the latter of which can result in bone marrow histiocytic hyperplasia with hemophagocytosis (acquired hemophagocytosis syndrome) (44).

Qualitative platelet function defects are common in the ICU and result from toxins, drugs (salicylate, nitric oxide), exposure to extracorporeal circulation, and renal failure (uremia). Treatment of qualitative platelet function defects requires platelet transfusion, but can be aided with the administration of antifibrinolytic agents, cryoprecipitate or Desmopressin (DDAVP) to treat the platelet function defect associated with uremia. Certain rare inherited macrothrombocytopathies or other inherited qualitative platelet defects such as Bernard–Soulier disease and Glanzmann's thrombasthenia may require the use of recombinant factor VIIa, which avoids the potential alloimmunization of the foreign platelet glycoproteins (Ib/IX and IIb/IIIa, respectively) that these patients lack.

Efficacy of Platelet Transfusion

The ultimate test of efficacy of platelet transfusion is the cessation or slowing of bleeding in a patient with either thrombocytopenia or an inherited or acquired thrombocytopathy. In lieu of clinical response, adequate posttransfusion platelet increment (e.g., corrected count increment) is often used as a surrogate marker for efficacy.

Immunologic Effects of Platelet Transfusions

Platelet transfusions contain plasma or cellular elements (platelets and leukocytes) and can result in immunomodulation (via transfusion of cytokines or other immunomodulatory proteins, such as IL-1, IL-6, and IL-8, or soluble CD40 ligand) or development of antibodies directed against either histocompatibility (typically class I) antigens and/or specific platelet antigens. Prestorage leukoreduction can minimize the presence of cytokines in the product because cytokines are produced from metabolically active leukocytes remaining in concentrates stored between 20°C and 24°C in gas-permeable bags or containers. In addition, prestorage leukoreduction can reduce exposure to WBC-derived HLA antigens inhibiting the development of HLAs and decreasing the potential for platelet refractoriness (45). Furthermore, the levels of soluble CD40 ligand, an immunomodulatory molecule implicated in transfusion-related ALI, dramatically increase over storage time (46).

Transfusion of Platelets: Application to the PICU

Practice Pattern

There are several studies detailing platelet transfusion practice in both critically ill adults and neonates, but there is a paucity of data regarding platelet transfusion practice in critically ill children. Future studies are needed to address practice patterns in the PICU.

Current Evidence

Expert opinion along with data from adult retrospective studies and a few randomized clinical trials are used to support current guidelines for *prophylactic* platelet transfusion in critically ill children (47), whereas expert opinion and retrospective studies are used to support *therapeutic* platelet transfusion.

The PLAtelet DOse (PLADO) trial assessed the effect of three prophylactic platelets' transfusion strategies. They enrolled children (>10 kg) and adults with thrombocytopenia due to hematopoietic stem cell transplants (HSCTs) and/or chemotherapy for hematologic malignancy or solid tumor. The patients were randomized to three strategies: administration of 1.1×10^{11}, 2.2×10^{11}, and 4.4×10^{11} platelets/m^2 of body surface area (BSA) if morning platelet counts were <10,000/mm^3. Analysis of both the entire study population and the pediatric subgroup (198 children) found that mild to severe bleeding (WHO grade 2 and above) was similar in the three groups (48). Because of these results, an ongoing RCT of prophylactic versus no-prophylactic platelet transfusions (trial of prophylactic platelets study, the TOPPS trial) should yield valuable insights into whether therapeutic, rather than prophylactic, transfusions can be a safe and efficacious practice for some patients (49). It should be noted that a recent German open-label randomized clinical trial of prophylactic versus therapeutic platelet transfusions found that adults with acute myeloid leukemia appeared to benefit from prophylactic platelet transfusions, whereas prophylactic platelet transfusions were no different from therapeutic platelet transfusions in adult autologous HSCT patients in bleeding outcome measures (50). Further studies are needed to determine whether these results can be extrapolated to critically ill children.

Current Guidelines

There have been many guidelines from many different countries and organizations on the use of prophylactic and therapeutic platelet transfusion (40, 51–53). These guidelines typically stratify recommendations by age (e.g., neonatal vs. older child) and/or underlying clinical condition/situation.

8 Prophylactic. The purpose of platelet therapy is to stop an ongoing hemorrhage (therapeutic) or to prevent bleeding (prophylactic). There is evidence that correction of thrombocytopenia reduces mortality of critically ill patients (43). For example, in patients with hypoproliferative thrombocytopenia (such as seen in patients who have received chemotherapy), prophylactic platelet transfusion should be considered if the platelet count is <5–10×10^9/L (<5000–10,000/mm^3) or if there are additional risk factors for bleeding. Liumbruno et al. (40) recommend a prophylactic transfusion of platelets for a threshold of 10×10^9/L (10,000/mm^3) in the absence of disease. For ICU patients, they recommend a threshold of 50×10^9/L (50,000/mm^3) for surgical or invasive procedures, and 100×10^9/L (100,000/mm^3) for surgical interventions in critical sites (ocular or neurosurgery).

Platelet transfusion should not be used for the treatment of immune thrombocytopenic purpura (ITP) except in the presence of intracranial or life-threatening bleeding. Platelets are also contraindicated in cases of thrombotic thrombocytopenic purpura (TTP) and heparin-induced thrombocytopenia (HIT) because of increased thrombotic risk. However, in the case of life-threatening bleeding, it is permissible to transfuse platelets in patients with TTP (54). Alternatives to platelet transfusion, such as DDAVP or antifibrinolytic agents, the use of steroids, plasmapheresis, and avoidance of heparin should be considered as first-line therapies in patients with non-hypoproliferative thrombocytopenia.

It should be noted that platelet dysfunction is often associated with some thrombocytopenia in critically ill patients.

When a platelet dysfunction is suspected, platelet transfusion can be considered only if the patient is bleeding. However, some experts recommend keeping the platelet count over 100×10^9/L (100,000/mm^3) during the postoperative care of a pediatric cardiac surgery because platelet dysfunction is observed up to 4–6 hours post-cardiopulmonary bypass.

Although recent published guidelines for oncology and HSCT patients suggest that keeping platelet counts greater than 10–20×10^9/L (10,000–20,000/mm^3) may be helpful in preventing life-threatening hemorrhage, the PLADO pediatric subgroup analysis study suggests that the actual dose of platelets (within a wide range of possible appropriate dosing schemes) may be equally efficacious in prevention of bleeding; however, this study did not specifically address critically ill children (48).

9 Therapeutic. Well-designed randomized clinical trials do not exist for the support of therapeutic platelet transfusion guidelines. In general, bleeding patients should have their platelet counts maintained between $>50 \times 10^9$/L (50,000/mm^3) or higher, depending on the clinical situation and the location of the bleeding, while those bleeding patients on ventricular assist devices and ECMO should have platelet counts at least $>100 \times 10^9$/L (100,000/mm^3). Patients who have a qualitative platelet defect with life-threatening hemorrhage should also be considered for platelet transfusion, especially if hemostatic agents are ineffective.

Platelet Products

Apheresis. *Apheresis platelets* contain $\geq 3.0 \times 10^{11}$ platelets, equivalent to 4–6 units of random donor platelets (RDPs), but collected from a single donor. The number of leukocytes contained in this component varies. Apheresis platelets have one or more connected bags, which improve platelet viability by providing more surface area for gas exchange.

Apheresis platelets leukocytes reduced either are reduced during the collection process or may be prepared by further processing using leukocyte reduction filters. Apheresis platelets leukocytes reduced should contain $\geq 3.0 \times 10^{11}$ platelets and $<5.0 \times 10^6$ leukocytes. The volume, anticoagulant-preservative, and storage conditions for apheresis platelets leukocytes reduced are the same as those for apheresis platelets.

Apheresis platelet additive solution–added leukocytes reduced are platelets collected by apheresis and suspended in variable amounts of plasma and an approved platelet additive solution (PAS). One apheresis unit of platelets contains $\geq 3 \times 10^{11}$ platelets and $<5.0 \times 10^6$ leukocytes. Plasma proteins, including coagulation factors present in the plasma, are diluted in proportion to the PAS added. This component has a shelf life of 5 days.

Pooled Platelets. *Pooled platelets*, also called *random donor platelets*, are a concentrate of platelets, which have been separated from a single unit of whole blood. One unit of RDP derived from whole blood contains $\geq 5.5 \times 10^{10}$ platelets suspended in 40–70 mL of plasma. Pooled platelets are composed of RDP units combined by aseptic technique. The number of units of platelets in the pool is variable. The volume is indicated on the label and determined by the number of RDPs in the pool.

Platelets leukocytes reduced are made using either an open or closed system. One unit of platelets leukocytes reduced should contain $\geq 5.5 \times 10^{10}$ platelets and $<8.3 \times 10^5$ leukocytes. Components prepared using an open system expire 4 hours after preparation. Components prepared using a closed system have a shelf life as specified for the collection device. This product is usually provided as a pool.

Pooled platelets leukocytes reduced are prepared by pooling and filtering platelets or pooling leukocytes reduced platelets in an open system, which has a 4-hour shelf life. There should be $<5 \times 10^6$ leukocytes in the pool, and the label will indicate approximate volume. This component can also be prepared and pooled using an FDA-approved system to provide a product with a 5-day shelf life. In some countries, pooled platelets, depending on the system of pooling platelets, can also have a shelf life as long as 7 days.

Prescription of Platelets Transfusions

It is prudent to use ABO-matched platelets. The use of ABO-incompatible platelets requires that the transfusion service remove incompatible plasma. This additional procedure decreases the platelet content by 15%–20%, shortens the storage time to 4 hours, and delays platelet release by ~ 1 hour.

(One unit of pooled platelet concentrate usually contains 50–60 mL and 55×10^9 platelets; one unit of platelet-pheresis platelet concentrate usually contains 150–300 mL and 150,500 $\times 10^9$ platelets, so each contains ~ 1×10^9 platelets per mL.) Administering 10 mL/kg of platelet concentrate should increase the platelet count by 50×10^9/L (50,000/mm^3). Such an increase is not always observed, usually because platelet consumption is high, a frequent occurrence with disseminated intravascular coagulation or in patients on ECMO and cardiopulmonary bypass. Assessment of an adequate platelet count increment for number of platelets and patient size requires calculating a *1-hour post platelet transfusion corrected count increment* (CCI), which should be greater than 7500/mm^3 using the formula below:

$$CCI = \frac{\text{platelet count increment/mm}^3 \times \text{BSA [in m}^2]}{\text{total number of platelets transfused} \times 10^{11}}$$

where BSA = body surface area. For example, a 1-hour posttransfusion platelet count increment of 40,000/mm^3 (40×10^9/L) in the patient with a BSA of 0.9 m^2 who received 3 platelet units ($3 \times 5.5 \times 10^{10}$) platelets would have a CCI of 21,818/mm^3. The CCI varies with patient size; an adult with a BSA of 2 with the same observed increment (40,000) and the same number of platelets infused (1.65×10^{11}) would have a CCI of 48,485, while the CCI for this increment after that number of platelets in a 2-year old with a BSA of 0.5 would be 12,121. ABO identical platelet transfusions with CCIs <7500/mm^3 are suggestive of platelet refractoriness and require the use of crossmatched or HLA-matched platelets (55). For these specialized products, it is necessary to consult the transfusion medicine service.

Under certain circumstances, patients with renal failure may require volume-reduced platelets. Preparation of these platelets, much like ABO-incompatible platelets, also results in decreased storage life of platelets, decreases platelet content, delays release, and requires contacting the transfusion medicine service. An anti-D immunoglobulin preparation (WinRho SDR) may be given to avoid the development of anti-D if the patient is Rh negative and the donor is Rh positive and RBC contamination of the platelet product is known or expected. However, this practice is largely defined by the patient's underlying immunosuppression, patient gender and age, and the institution's defined clinical practice.

Despite the use of leukoreduction techniques, there are always some leukocytes in both RDP and apheresis platelets. Thus, leukoreduction is not a substitute for irradiation to prevent T-lymphocyte proliferation and eliminate the risk of *TA-GVHD*, in which activated donor lymphocytes attack an immune compromised recipient's tissues, including lymphoid tissue, after recognizing them as foreign. Immunocompetent recipients would neutralize the donor's lymphocytes on

transfusion. TA-GVHD is associated with a mortality of 90% despite treatment. TA-GVHD has been associated with most blood components, with the exceptions being FFP, frozen deglycerolized RBCs, and cryoprecipitate. Patients most at risk for TA-GVHD include patients with congenital cellular immunodeficiency, patients undergoing stem cell or solid organ transplantation or chemotherapy, and patients receiving HLA-matched products or directed donations from blood relatives. Irradiation of blood components to neutralize donor lymphocytes and prevent TA-GVHD is not sufficient to kill viruses and that irradiation alone will not prevent spread of CMV.

Platelets should be administered by either gravity or pump system through a filter (typically between 150 and 200 μm) that minimizes platelet loss. Microaggregate filters (20–40 μm) will remove a significant amount of platelets and should not be used. Approximately 10 mL/kg volume can be usually administered in 30 minutes and is usually well tolerated; however, slower administration and the possible use of a diuretic are advised for cardiac-compromised patients.

Conclusion

Current guidelines for the use of prophylactic platelet transfusions are supported by expert opinion, adult retrospective studies, and several randomized clinical trials. However, a recent study (PLADO) examining prophylactic platelet transfusions in predominantly noncritically ill patients did not show an effect of platelet dosing on the frequency of bleeding either in adults or in children with malignancies.

Thresholds for platelet transfusion triggers are commonly used in certain patient populations, but there are no data to support platelet concentration thresholds for transfusion of platelets in critically ill children.

GRANULOCYTES

Constitution of Granulocyte Concentrates

Granulocyte concentrates are collected using apheresis from donors who have undergone either steroid and/or growth factor (most commonly granulocyte colony-stimulating factor, G-CSF) stimulation. Steroid-only-stimulated granulocyte collections result in $1-2 \times 10^{10}$ granulocytes per unit, whereas steroid- and growth factor–stimulated collections can yield $4-8 \times 10^{10}$ granulocytes per unit. The volume of a granulocyte product is typically between 250 and 300 mL and expires within 24 hours of collection. The product contains RBCs and must be crossmatched to the recipient.

Scientific Foundation of Granulocyte Transfusion

The degree of neutropenia as the result of chemotherapy correlates with the risk of infection (56). As a result, transfusion of granulocytes may benefit neutropenic patients who are anticipated to be neutropenic for a protracted period. In fact, several studies have shown that transfused granulocytes have the ability to migrate to areas of infection. However, randomized and nonrandomized studies published from the 1970s and 1980s demonstrated lack of consistent efficacy of granulocyte transfusions in neutropenic patients. Factors possibly related to benefit included those patients that received at least three to four granulocyte transfusions, those patients with prolonged neutropenia, and those who received larger granulocyte doses.

Based on several randomized, controlled clinical trials, however, granulocyte use as a prophylactic measure in neutropenic patients in the setting of bone marrow transplantation or remission/induction chemotherapy for acute myelogenous leukemia is not recommended as there is no survival advantage over conventional therapy (57). Meta-analysis of these studies, however, revealed that granulocyte dose, leukocyte compatibility, and shorter duration of neutropenia were major determinants for prevention of bacterial infection (58). Thus, there is a need for randomized clinical trials to definitively determine the efficacy and adverse side effects of steroid- and G-CSF-stimulated granulocyte products. The future use of granulocytes will also depend on pharmacologic advances in antimicrobial and antifungal therapy, as a number of new antifungal agents are currently under investigation.

Granulocyte Transfusion: Application to PICU

Granulocyte transfusions might be considered in severely neutropenic patients with bacterial sepsis or fungal infections when poly antimicrobial and/or antifungal therapy appears to be ineffective and bone marrow recovery is expected to be delayed as long as 2–3 weeks. Granulocyte transfusions might also be considered in patients with granulocyte dysfunction syndromes with bacterial sepsis or fungal infection and lack of response to antimicrobial therapy. It is important that an infectious disease consult be obtained to ensure that optimal antimicrobial and/or antifungal therapy has been achieved prior to initiation of granulocyte transfusions.

Because it has been recommended that granulocyte transfusions of at least 1×10^{10} be transfused daily until clinical improvement, it is important to coordinate requests with the transfusion medicine service as granulocyte collection requires prior stimulation of donors who must undergo apheresis. It should be noted that there is a lack of consensus on dosing and frequency of granulocyte transfusion.

Current Evidence

Systematic reviews and meta-analyses have suggested a dose-dependent effect on efficacy (58,59). However, because of major logistical difficulties in the planning of large prospective RCTs, apheresis granulocyte transfusions from stimulated donors have not yet been evaluated for efficacy. The European RCT failed to establish the efficacy of granulocyte transfusion (60). This might be due to stimulation of granulocyte donors with only G-CSF and transfusion of granulocytes every other day.

To address these issues, the National Heart, Lung, and Blood Institute (U.S.A.) has opened the Resolving Infection in Neutropenia With Granulocytes (RING) trial. This study is designed to determine whether the benefits of daily G-CSF and dexamethasone-stimulated granulocyte transfusions outweigh the risks and side effects. The safety and efficacy of granulocyte transfusions with standard antimicrobial therapy will be compared with the safety and efficacy of standard antimicrobial therapy alone in increasing granulocyte numbers and in improving survival rates in patients with bacterial or fungal infection during neutropenia. Recently, the study has been closed to new participants, and a definitive answer may be forthcoming.

Thus, currently, the exact role of granulocyte transfusions remains unclear.

Indications

10 Therapeutic granulocyte transfusions are indicated for febrile neutropenic (absolute neutrophil count $<0.5 \times 10^9$/L) patients who have a severe bacterial or fungal infection that is refractory to antimicrobials (61,62). These patients have usually failed to respond to a trial G-CSF therapy. ABO, Rh-negative compatible donor granulocytes must be available.

Prescription of Granulocyte Concentrates

Because of the extremely high granulocyte count within a granulocyte product, granulocyte metabolic activity can rapidly deplete glucose, produce lactic acid, and increase cell death. This is accentuated because of the requirement to store granulocytes at room temperature as cold storage inactivates neutrophils. From a regulatory standpoint, granulocytes must be transfused within 24 hours; some even recommend transfusion as soon as possible. Because of this requirement, infectious disease testing cannot be completed prior to release; thus, there is a small, but not insignificant, risk of viral and protozoal disease transmission. Often CMV-seronegative or CMV "reduced risk" products are required in patients receiving granulocytes. As granulocytes cannot be leukoreduced, the risk of CMV transmission is higher than with other products if a CMV-seropositive donor with active viremia is inadvertently used. Selection of volunteer donors, therefore, can be a significant problem because donors have to endure the side effects of both steroids and possibly G-CSF. HLA matching and/or leukocyte crossmatching may be considered; however, this is not always possible.

A relative contraindication to granulocyte transfusions is if the recipient has anti-HLAs or antigranulocyte antibodies because of the possibility of developing transfusion-associated ALI.

Irradiation of the product is recommended to prevent the proliferation of T lymphocytes, given the immunocompromised state of the recipient and because of the possibility of HLA-matched (including related family member) donations that increases the risk of TA-GVHD.

Granulocytes should be transfused over 1–2 hours via a standard blood (150–200 μm) filter with intermittent agitation of the unit to avoid settling of the granulocytes. Transfusion of granulocytes is frequently accompanied by fever, chills, and allergic reactions and should be discontinued in the case of severe pulmonary reactions. Granulocyte transfusion should be separated by as much time as possible (at least 4 hours) from amphotericin transfusion as severe pulmonary reactions have been associated with the simultaneous infusion of both products. Overall efficacy of granulocyte transfusion can be ascertained either by clinical improvement or by assessment of absolute neutrophil counts.

Conclusions

Granulocyte transfusion should be considered in the treatment of bacterial sepsis or fungal infections in neutropenic patients or patients with dysfunctional neutrophils who may have protracted periods of neutropenia and in whom there appears to be no response to antimicrobial or antifungal therapy.

WHOLE BLOOD

Constitution of Whole Blood

Whole blood is stored after donation without any separation into individual components. A whole blood unit is typically between 450 and 500 mL with 63 mL of this volume containing CPD solution, and is licensed to be stored at 4°C for up to 21 days in CPD solution. The hematocrit, platelet, and plasma coagulation factor concentrations within each whole blood unit will be dependent upon the individual donor. Historically, whole blood units were not leukoreduced prior to storage, but with recently developed platelet sparring leukoreduction filters, some centers are providing leukoreduced whole blood.

Scientific Foundation of Transfusion of Whole Blood

Prior to the 1970s, whole blood was the predominant blood product transfused. Since then, the transition from whole blood to component therapy (RBCs, plasma, and platelet concentrates) occurred without prospective studies comparing the efficacy (increased oxygen use at the cellular level) and noninfectious safety between products. This transition occurred predominantly due to economic and logistic benefits of maintaining an inventory of single blood components used for patients with single-component deficiencies. In addition, the storage duration of products has increased since the 1970s without direct evidence demonstrating efficacy or noninfectious safety. Storage solutions are approved predominantly according to survival and recovery data, and not on direct evidence of function (in vivo oxygen use or hemostatic function) (63).

For patients with isolated anemia, thrombocytopenia, or coagulopathy due to coagulation factor deficiency or consumption, the use of single components is logical and appropriate. For patients with combined shock and coagulopathy secondary to massive blood loss, the use of whole blood may have advantages over the reconstitution of blood with components (64).

Two RCTs have been performed comparing whole blood to components with conflicting results that may be due to differences in methodology (65,66). Both trials included children requiring cardiac surgery. The trial by Manno randomized children to the use of either whole blood or RBCs, FFP, and platelets both intraoperatively and postoperatively in the ICU; the primary outcome was 24-hour postoperative blood loss, and multivariate regression analyses were performed to adjust for confounders. Their results indicated that patients transfused with whole blood had less 24-hour blood loss compared with patients receiving components. The decreased blood loss was associated with improved coagulation parameters to include improved platelet aggregation. The reduction in blood loss was more pronounced in children less than 2 years of age. The RCT by Mou compared the use of whole blood with RBCs and plasma intraoperatively within the cardiopulmonary bypass pump prime. Randomization of blood products transfused did not continue in the ICU. Their primary outcome was a composite morbidity score of ICU-related outcomes. Their results indicated no difference in morbidity, but did report an unadjusted increase in ICU length of stay and in fluid overload in the group receiving whole blood for the cardiopulmonary bypass pump prime.

Transfusion of Whole Blood: Application to PICU

Practice Pattern

Whole blood is currently transfused at a minority of pediatric tertiary care centers in the United States. A recent survey indicated that 15% of children's hospitals in the United States use whole blood (67), where it is primarily transfused for patients at high risk for hemorrhagic shock, such as patients requiring cardiac surgery or liver transplantation, or as a component of massive transfusion protocols.

Current Evidence

It is currently unknown whether these potential advantages of whole blood would improve outcomes for patients with life-threatening hemorrhagic shock. A controversial aspect of these proposed benefits centers around the "function" of platelets stored at 4°C. Platelet units are currently stored at 20°C–24°C on the basis of data indicating improved platelet survival over time compared with storage at 4°C (68). These same experiments and the Manno trial indicate that platelets or whole blood stored at 4°C have improved platelet activation and hemostatic function. Assessing platelet function related to circulation time or recovery instead of ability to become activated may have resulted in platelets being considered not to be "functional" when stored at 4°C past 48–72 hours. This has dramatically reduced the feasibility of providing whole blood clinically.

There is re-emerging interest in the concept that platelets containing blood products stored at 4°C might be beneficial for a patient with severe bleeding. Recent in vitro studies indicate improved hemostatic function of whole blood stored at 4°C versus 22°C for up to 10–14 days (69). Additional in vivo studies are needed in cohorts with severe hemorrhagic shock to determine whether whole blood is advantageous to transfusing reconstituted blood in high ratios similar to that of whole blood. The availability of platelet sparring leukoreduction filters for whole blood and the possibility of whole blood at 4°C maintaining hemostatic function for 10–14 days increase the feasibility of clinical trials and practical use in patients if well-designed trials indicate improved efficacy or safety compared with components for children with hemorrhagic shock.

Proposed benefits of whole blood for patients at risk for hemorrhagic shock or requiring massive transfusion include (a) increased concentration of hemoglobin, coagulation factors, and platelets relative to reconstitution with individual components; (b) limited impact of processing on function (with regard to both O_2 transport and coagulation); (c) avoidance of risk associated with extended storage duration; and (d) reduced donor exposure (64).

Current Guidelines

There are no current guidelines that advocate for the use of whole blood in critically ill children. Guidelines do exist for whole blood use in US Military facilities during combat that indicate ABO-specific whole blood is appropriate for the treatment of severe hemorrhagic shock if components are not available or if the patient is not responding to component therapy.

Conclusions

Clinical use of whole blood is limited to select pediatric tertiary centers. Current research regarding the safety and efficacy will assess the potential for whole blood use for patients with concomitant severe shock and coagulopathy.

MASSIVE TRANSFUSIONS

The definition of massive transfusion in children ranges between 40 and 80 mL/kg of RBCs transfused in a 24-hour period. The concept of defining massive transfusion according to only RBC transfusion and over a 24-hour period is controversial since death from hemorrhage often occurs within 6 hours of initiation of bleeding and current transfusion practice in patients with massive bleeding includes the use of plasma and platelets (70).

There is very little evidence in children to guide transfusion practice in a massively bleeding patient. Clinical guidelines are based upon low- to moderate-quality adult data from both military and civilian studies. For children with life-threatening bleeding, the classic approach taught within ATLS courses is being replaced with what is termed damage control resuscitation (DCR) (71). The traditional use of large volumes of crystalloid followed by the administration of only RBCs in a massively bleeding, hemodynamically unstable, patient promotes a dilutional coagulopathy. The use of classic laboratory measures of coagulation (PT/PTT and platelet count) to guide the use of plasma and platelets often requires at least 45 minutes to perform and report and delays the treatment of coagulopathy typically present in massively bleeding patients (including children).

DCR principles support the use of permissive hypotension (except in patients with severe traumatic brain injury), the rapid surgical control of bleeding, avoidance of hypothermia and acidosis, minimal use of crystalloids, treatment of hypocalcemia, and the use of empiric high unit ratios of plasma and platelets to RBCs to provide a balanced treatment of both shock and coagulopathy for patients with immediate life-threatening hemorrhagic shock. The development of shock and coagulopathy early after injury is strongly associated with mortality (72). DCR principles can be applied to children at risk for hemorrhagic shock and should be performed within a structured massive transfusion protocol (73).

Advantages of massive transfusion protocols include a proactive push of blood to the bedside instead of a reactive pull of blood to the patient that is slowed by the use of laboratory tests that require time to result. Disadvantages of an empiric use of ratios of blood products for massive transfusion include the use of blood products that might not necessarily be required for the patient, which then exposes them to the risk of the product without any potential benefit. To address this concern, the use of thromboelastographic methods of coagulation

monitoring is being studied to determine whether they can be used to provide a "goal-directed hemostatic resuscitation strategy" for patients with hemorrhagic shock (74–77). Massive transfusion protocols with or without the use of thromboelastographic monitoring in children are used for hemorrhagic shock secondary to trauma in addition to other etiologies such as intra- and postoperative bleeding.

Further research is required to determine whether the transfusion approach to hemorrhagic shock should be different based on the etiology. In addition, the use of adjunctive hemostatic agents such as fibrinogen concentrates, coagulation factor complex concentrates, and antifibrinolytics for massive bleeding in children requires study.

COMMON COMPLICATIONS OF BLOOD PRODUCT TRANSFUSIONS

Early Reactions

Early transfusion reactions can be life threatening or less serious, as seen in **Table 42.1**. The most common reactions include mild allergic and febrile nonhemolytic reactions, the latter of which is defined as an increase in temperature equal to or greater than 1°C that cannot be explained by the patient's clinical condition (i.e., other causes of fever must be ruled out). A febrile nonhemolytic transfusion reaction may be accompanied by dyspnea and/or anxiety. Some of the following symptoms can also be present: rigors, dyspnea, tachycardia, or headache. Mild allergic reactions are often characterized by the presence of hives without significant vital sign changes; however, these reactions include a spectrum of symptoms that can mimic anaphylactic reactions and may

TABLE 42.1

ACUTE AND DELAYED TRANSFUSION REACTIONS

Acute (<24 h): Immunologic	
Hemolytic	
ABO/Rh mismatched	1:40,000
Acute hemolytic transfusion reaction	1:76,000
Fatal	1:1.8 million
Febrile, nonhemolytic	0.1%–1% (universal leukoreduction)
Urticarial	1:100–1:33 (1%–3%)
Anaphylaxis	1:20,000–1:50,000
Transfusion-related ALI	1:1200–1:190,000
Acute (<24 h): Nonimmunologic	
Transfusion-associated sepsis	~<1:3000 (after implementation of platelet bacterial testing)
Hypotension associated with ACE inhibition	Depends on clinical situation
TACO	<1%
Nonimmunologic hemolysis	Rare
Air embolus	Rare
Hypocalcemia	Depends on clinical situation
Delayed (>24 h): Immunologic	
Alloimmunization, RBC antigens	1:100 (1%)
Alloimmunization, HLAs	1:10 (10%)
Hemolytic	1:2500–1:11,000
Graft-versus-host disease	Rare
Posttransfusion purpura	Rare
Delayed (>24 h): Nonimmunologic	
Iron overload	Typically after 100 RBC units
Viral and parasitic	See **Table 42.2**

ACE, angiotensin-converting enzyme; TACO, transfusion-associated circulatory overload.
Source: Modified from Mazzei CA, Popovsky MA, Kopko PM. Noninfectious complications of blood transfusion. In: Grossman BJ, Harris T, Roback JD, et al., eds. *AAB Technical Manual.* Bethesda, MD: American Association of Blood Banks Press, 2011.

include O_2 desaturation, decreased blood pressure, and airway closure, also known as "anaphylactoid" reactions. Patients with these reactions often require premedication with antihistamines and/or steroids, and if severe, may require the use of washed products or the avoidance of plasma containing blood products for future transfusions. Patients experiencing true anaphylactic reactions caused by the presence of anti-IgA antibodies require IgA-negative plasma containing blood products. This can be achieved by either obtaining blood products from IgA-deficient blood or apheresis donors (required in the case of cryoprecipitate or plasma transfusion) or using washed packed RBCs and platelet products. Febrile nonhemolytic transfusion reactions are typically caused by cytokines generated by leukocytes present within the blood product (most commonly in nonleukoreduced platelet products); however, given that many blood collection centers perform prestorage leukoreduction, the incidence of this reaction has been significantly reduced. Febrile nonhemolytic transfusion reactions typically present with fever and/or rigors and chills with often stable vital signs. Febrile nonhemolytic transfusion reactions must be distinguished from other serious less common, early transfusion reactions such as transfusion-related ALI, hemolytic transfusion reactions, and sepsis (bacterial contamination) as these often present with fever and treatment is much different from each other.

Hemolytic transfusion reaction is defined as hemoglobinuria or hemoglobinemia (measured as plasma-free hemoglobin above the normal range) with at least one of the following symptoms/signs: fever, dyspnea, hypotension and/or tachycardia, anxiety/agitation, and pain.

Major allergic and anaphylactic reaction, which may be fatal, is defined as at least one of the following symptoms/signs: (a) cardiac arrest; (b) generalized allergic reaction or anaphylactic reaction; (c) angioedema (facial and/or laryngeal); (d) upper airway obstruction; (e) dyspnea, wheezing; (f) hypotension, shock; (g) precordial pain or chest tightness; (h) cardiac arrhythmia; and (i) loss of consciousness. It is important to consult with the institutional transfusion medicine consultant when encountering these reactions.

It is very important to consider the risk of hyperkalemia and subsequent cardiac arrest in the transfusion of packed RBCs in children. Older units of RBCs, even more so if irradiated in order to avoid GVHD, are known to have elevated K^+ levels. Hyperkalemia can also result from exchange transfusion and after massive transfusion in cardiopulmonary bypass (78). Interestingly, a prospective study of 54 RBC transfusions found no adverse events or significant increases in posttransfusion potassium level in 28 critically ill children despite mean potassium levels of 16 mmol/L (one-third had potassium levels >25 mmol/L) in the blood units (79). Although the incidence of transfusion-associated hyperkalemia is unknown, it remains a risk that is associated with the patient's age and condition, the K^+ concentration in the plasma of the transfused unit, the volume and rate of transfusion, and the site of transfusion.

Late Reactions

Delayed reactions may occur and include transfusion-transmitted viral and parasitic infectious disease; TA-GVHD; and alloimmunization to RBC, platelet-specific (or HLA), or granulocyte antigens. The incidence of viral and parasitic disease transmission is seen in **Table 42.2**.

BLOOD BANKS AND ADMINISTRATION OF BLOOD PRODUCTS

Blood Banks and Transfusion Services

Blood banks and transfusion services are critical to the collection; processing; testing; labeling; dispensing; and monitoring of blood, blood products, and, in some institutions, blood derivatives, recombinant coagulation products, some biological agents, stem cells, and tissues for transplantation. They are staffed by individuals with knowledge of regulatory oversight and technical expertise to ensure safe collection, storage, and transfusion practices. Because of the risks to both donors and recipients, physicians with specialized training serve as transfusion medicine consultants; incorporating them into an ICU team can assist in maximizing blood management. Further, such individuals are knowledgeable about transfusion devices, including filters, warmers, and blood administration sets, and the appropriate and inappropriate use of both therapeutic apheresis and off-label products. In the United States, blood

TABLE 42.2

VIRAL AND PARASITIC INFECTIOUS RISKS

■ INFECTIOUS AGENT	■ INCIDENCE
HIV (with NAT)	1:1,467,000 (first-time donors)
HCV (with NAT)	1:1,149,000 (first-time donors)
HTLV	1:2,993,000
HBV	1:280,000
HAV	<1:1 million
Malaria	1:4 million
Chagas disease	Unknown (rare)
Cytomegalovirus	Unknown (presumed rare)
West Nile virus	Unknown (rare breakthrough despite NAT)
Epstein–Barr virus	Unknown (rare)

Note: Risks largely based on US data, risks in other countries may vary.
NAT, nucleic acid–based tests; HCV, hepatitis C virus; HIV, human immunodeficiency virus; HTLV, human T-lymphocyte viruses; HBV, hepatitis B virus.
Source: Based on Galel SA. Infectious disease screening. In: Roback JD, Grossman BJ, Harris T, et al., eds. *AABB Technical Manual*. Bethesda, MD: American Association of Blood Banks Press, 2011.

banks and transfusion services are overseen and/or inspected by local and state departments of public health through the U.S. Department of Health and Human Services, the FDA, College of American Pathology, American Association of Blood Banks, Joint Commission, and other national/international oversight organizations such as the Foundation for Accreditation of Cellular Therapies (FACT).

Administration of Blood and Blood Products

It is necessary to have a well-grounded understanding of the biology and physiology of the individual cellular and liquid components of whole blood in order to prescribe the proper component for patients. Transfusion should be undertaken only if the anticipated benefit outweighs the potential risk. Sound decision by the physician whether to transfuse a particular product can come only through knowledge of the characteristics and limitations of each product and appropriate indications.

The physician must explain the benefits and risks of transfusion to the patient and obtain informed consent in accordance with institutional guidelines. The transfusion process is initiated when a physician writes an order specifying the component, its attributes, the volume, and rate (and duration) of infusion.

The identity of the blood unit and the recipient must be verified at each step, starting from the collection of the sample for group, type, and cross-match, and continuing through release from the blood bank to the final infusion of the component. Verification may use a bar code or other identifier system such as radiofrequency identification (RFID) systems.

The patient's pretransfusion and posttransfusion vital signs must be recorded.

All blood components must be administered through a macroaggregate particulate filter (80–260 µm). Microaggregate filters can be used for RBCs to screen out microaggregates, which typically consist of degenerating platelets, leukocytes, and fibrin strands.

The transfusion must be completed within 4 hours of the time of release from the blood bank. In nonurgent situations, the infusion rate can be administered over 2–4 hours. In life-threatening situations, the infusion rate can be as fast as possible.

Special infusion sets for high flow typically have large filter surface areas and large-bore tubing. For massive transfusion, as in cases of trauma, rapid infuser/blood warmers are available. Other special sets include mechanical infusers, gravity drip sets, and, for transfusion of small volumes of blood products, syringe sets.

Solutions that can be coadministered with RBCs include normal saline (0.9% USP) and, under life-threatening circumstances, 5% albumin, lactated Ringer solution, ABO-compatible plasma, plasma protein fraction, and platelets. Although this is not evidence-based, it is common to avoid administering hypotonic or hypertonic saline, 5% dextrose, and medications with blood or blood components, to avoid hemolysis and loss of anticoagulation and to distinguish transfusion-mediated reactions from reactions mediated by other causes.

RBCs and whole blood can be safely warmed to 37°C, but not more than 42°C, using specifically designed devices. These devices are indicated for adults receiving rapid and multiple transfusions of RBCs or whole blood at a rate of >50 mL/kg/h, infants receiving rapid transfusions of >15 mL/kg/h, children or infants receiving exchange transfusions, and patients with cold agglutinin disease.

Blood or blood components can be modified in several ways to accommodate the patient's clinical situation. RBC and platelet products can be split into smaller amounts (60 mL) to reduce donor exposure by transfusing small amounts of blood from one donor, and storing the rest for another transfusion in the same patient. Washing of RBCs or platelets may be necessary to reduce anaphylactoid reactions from foreign plasma protein or bioactive lipid exposure, or to decrease the risk of hyperkalemia. For those patients with a history of anaphylactic reaction to blood or blood components and who have demonstrable anti-IgA antibodies, IgA-deficient blood or blood components can be obtained. Similarly, those patients with antibodies to RBC antigens must receive RBC units negative for the antigens to which the patient has developed antibodies. Consultation with a transfusion medicine physician may be necessary in these cases.

LIMITING BLOOD PRODUCT UTILIZATION

"Primum non nocere" (First, do no harm) holds as true with blood products as with any other medical therapy. Therefore, all possible steps must be taken to use blood conservation methods to limit blood loss and the need for transfusion. Common blood conservation methods include minimizing phlebotomy by limiting the number of blood tests and the volume of blood required. This often requires education of nursing and laboratory staff about the actual minimal amount of blood required to perform laboratory measures. Phlebotomy can also be decreased with the use of closed-system blood sampling techniques, pediatric blood collection tubes, microanalysis techniques that require small sample volumes, and in-line measurement of blood gas parameters. Reduction in operative blood loss can be achieved by prescribing erythropoietin and iron supplements (80).

The usefulness of erythropoietin in the PICU remains to be determined, and the risk of prothrombotic events must be taken into consideration prior to administration. In addition, the use of fibrin sealants, antifibrinolytics, and recombinant coagulation factor agents, and the judicious use of plasma and platelets instead of crystalloid-based resuscitation for patients with significant bleeding have the potential to reduce bleeding and the need for blood products. Viscoelastic measures of coagulation (thromboelastographic) can help guide the use of all of these prohemostatic products, although no prospective randomized data exist to indicate that outcomes are improved with their use. When possible, avoid the preoperative use of medications that can increase the risk of bleeding (e.g., anticoagulants and drugs that inhibit platelet function). Other blood conservation strategies include enforcing appropriate thresholds for transfusion and the use of cell saver technology for autotransfusion when appropriate. The efficacy of other blood-sparing strategies such as autotransfused blood products, acute normovolemic hemodilution, and hypervolemic hemodilution as adjunctive blood conservation strategies needs investigation (81).

CONCLUSIONS AND FUTURE DIRECTIONS

Transfusion of one or more blood products to critically ill children may be lifesaving, but can also cause clinically significant adverse events. The decision to proceed with transfusion of any blood product must be based on individualized indications, while weighing the risks and benefits.

In 1976, Beal (82) wrote "Blood transfusion is like marriage: it should not be entered upon lightly, unadvisedly or wantonly, or more often than absolutely necessary."

More clinical research is required to more accurately determine the cost and benefits of transfusion of blood products to improve clinical outcomes and safety in critically ill children.

ACKNOWLEDGMENT

We would like to thank Dr. Allan Doctor for his help on the RBC storage lesions, and Dr. Delphine Arni for her precious comments on this chapter.

References

1. Bateman ST, Lacroix J, Boven K, et al. Anemia, blood loss, and blood transfusions in North American children in the intensive care unit. *Am J Respir Crit Care Med* 2008;178(1):26–33.

2. Fernandes CJ, Akamine N, De Marco FV, et al. Red blood cell transfusion does not increase oxygen consumption in critically ill septic patients. *Crit Care* 2001;5(6):362–7.

3. Atasever B, van der Kuil M, Boer C, et al. Red blood cell transfusion compared with gelatin solution and no infusion after cardiac surgery: Effect on microvascular perfusion, vascular density, hemoglobin, and oxygen saturation. *Transfusion* 2012;52(11):2452–8.

4. Yuruk K, Almac E, Bezemer R, et al. Blood transfusions recruit the microcirculation during cardiac surgery. *Transfusion* 2011;51(5):961–7.

5. Vicaut E, Stucker O, Teisseire B, et al. Effects of changes in systemic hematocrit on the microcirculation in rat cremaster muscle. *Int J Microcirc Clin Exp* 1987;6(3):225–35.

6. Doctor A, Spinella P. Effect of processing and storage on red blood cell function in vivo. Seminars in perinatology2012;36(4):248–59.http://dx.doi.org/10.1053/j.semperi.2012.04.005.

7. Karam O, Tucci M, Toledano BJ, et al. Length of storage and in vitro immunomodulation induced by prestorage leukoreduced red blood cells. *Transfusion* 2009;49(11):2326–34.

8. Muszynski J, Nateri J, Nicol K, et al. Immunosuppressive effects of red blood cells on monocytes are related to both storage time and storage solution. *Transfusion* 2011;52(4):794–802.

9. Laverdière C, Gauvin F, Hébert PC, et al. Survey on transfusion practices of pediatric intensivists. *Pediatr Crit Care Med* 2002;3(4):335–40.

10. Nahum E, Ben-Ari J, Schonfeld T. Blood transfusion policy among European pediatric intensive care physicians. *J Intensive Care Med* 2004;19(1):38–43.

11. Armano R, Gauvin F, Ducruet T, et al. Determinants of red blood cell transfusions in a pediatric critical care unit: A prospective, descriptive epidemiological study. *Crit Care Med* 2005;33(11):2637–44.

12. Shander A. Anemia in the critically ill. *Crit Care Clin* 2004;20(2):159–78.

13. Carson JL, Duff A, Poses RM, et al. Effect of anaemia and cardiovascular disease on surgical mortality and morbidity. *Lancet* 1996;348(9034):1055–60.

14. Carson JL, Noveck H, Berlin JA, et al. Mortality and morbidity in patients with very low postoperative Hb levels who decline blood transfusion. *Transfusion* 2002;42(7):812–8.

15. Lackritz EM, Campbell CC, Ruebush TK, et al. Effect of blood transfusion on survival among children in a Kenyan hospital. *Lancet* 1992;340(8818):524–8.

16. English M, Ahmed M, Ngando C, et al. Blood transfusion for severe anaemia in children in a Kenyan hospital. *Lancet* 2002;359(9305):494–5.

17. Villanueva C, Colomo A, Bosch A, et al. Transfusion Strategies for Acute Upper Gastrointestinal Bleeding. *N Engl J Med* 2013;368(1):11–21.

18. Rivers E, Nguyen B, Havstad S, et al. Early goal-directed therapy in the treatment of severe sepsis and septic shock. *N Engl J Med* 2001;345(19):1368–77.

19. Hebert PC, Wells G, Blajchman MA, et al; Transfusion Requirements in Critical Care Investigators, Canadian Critical Care Trials Group. A multicenter, randomized, controlled clinical trial of transfusion requirements in critical care. *N Engl J Med* 1999;340(6):409–17.

20. Lacroix J, Hébert PC, Hutchison JS, et al. Transfusion strategies for patients in pediatric intensive care units. *N Engl J Med* 2007;356(16):1609–19.

21. Cholette JM, Rubenstein JS, Alfieris GM, et al. Children with single-ventricle physiology do not benefit from higher hemoglobin levels post cavopulmonary connection: Results of a prospective, randomized, controlled trial of a restrictive versus liberal red-cell transfusion strategy. *Pediatr Crit Care Med* 2011;12(1):39–45.

22. Viele MK, Weiskopf RB. What can we learn about the need for transfusion from patients who refuse blood? The experience with Jehovah's Witnesses. *Transfusion* 1994;34(5):396–401.

23. Stanworth SJ, Hyde CJ, Murphy MF. Evidence for indications of fresh frozen plasma. *Transfus Clin Biol* 2007;14(6):551–6.

24. Jacobs JF, Baumert JL, Brons PP, et al. Anaphylaxis from passive transfer of peanut allergen in a blood product. *N Engl J Med* 2011;364(20):1981–2.

25. Ewalenko P, Deloof T, Peeters J. Composition of fresh frozen plasma. *Crit Care Med* 1986;14(2):145–6.

26. Abdel-Wahab OI, Healy B, Dzik WH. Effect of fresh-frozen plasma transfusion on prothrombin time and bleeding in patients with mild coagulation abnormalities. *Transfusion* 2006;46(8):1279–85.

27. Holland LL, Brooks JP. Toward rational fresh frozen plasma transfusion: The effect of plasma transfusion on coagulation test results. *Am J Clin Pathol* 2006;126(1):133–9.

28. Sarani B, Dunkman WJ, Dean L, et al. Transfusion of fresh frozen plasma in critically ill surgical patients is associated with an increased risk of infection. *Crit Care Med* 2008;36(4):1114–8.

29. Pinkerton PH, Callum JL. Rationalizing the clinical use of frozen plasma. *CMAJ* 2010;182(10):1019–20.

30. Church G, Matthay MA, Liu K, et al. Blood product transfusions and clinical outcomes in pediatric patients with acute lung injury. *Pediatr Crit Care Med* 2009;10(3):297–302.

31. Karam O, Lacroix J, Robitaille N, et al. Association between plasma transfusions and clinical outcome in critically ill children: A prospective observational study. *Vox Sang* 2013;104(4):342–29.

32. Pati S, Matijevic N, Doursout MF, et al. Protective effects of fresh frozen plasma on vascular endothelial permeability, coagulation, and resuscitation after hemorrhagic shock are time dependent and diminish between days 0 and 5 after thaw. *J Trauma* 2010;69(suppl):S55–63.

33. Haywood-Watson RJ, Holcomb JB, Gonzalez EA, et al. Modulation of syndecan-1 shedding after hemorrhagic shock and resuscitation. *PLoS ONE* 2011;6(8):e23530.

34. Kozar RA, Peng Z, Zhang R, et al. Plasma restoration of endothelial glycocalyx in a rodent model of hemorrhagic shock. *Anesth Analg* 2011;112(6):1289–95.

35. Segal JB, Dzik WH. Paucity of studies to support that abnormal coagulation test results predict bleeding in the setting of invasive procedures: An evidence-based review. *Transfusion* 2005;45(9):1413–25.

36. Puetz J, Witmer C, Huang Y-SV, et al. Widespread use of fresh frozen plasma in us children's hospitals despite limited evidence demonstrating a beneficial effect. *J Pediatr* 2012;160(2):210–5.

37. Arnold DM, Lauzier F, Whittingham H, et al. A multifaceted strategy to reduce inappropriate use of frozen plasma transfusions in the intensive care unit. *J Crit Care* 2011;26(6):636.e7–636.e13.

38. Zink K, Sambasivan C, Holcomb J, et al. A high ratio of plasma and platelets to packed red blood cells in the first 6 hours of massive transfusion improves outcomes in a large multicenter study. *Am J Surg* 2009;197(5):565–70; discussion 570.

39. O'Shaughnessy DF, Atterbury C, Bolton Maggs P, et al. Guidelines for the use of fresh-frozen plasma, cryoprecipitate and cryosupernatant. *Br J Haematol* 2004;126(1):11–28.

40. Liumbruno G, Bennardello F, Lattanzio A, et al; Italian Society of Transfusion Medicine and Immunohaematology (SIMTI) Work

Group. Recommendations for the transfusion of plasma and platelets. *Blood Transfus* 2009;7(2):132–50.

41. Hellstern P, Solheim BG. The use of solvent/detergent treatment in pathogen reduction of plasma. *Transfus Med Hemother* 2011;38(1):65–70.

42. Klein HG. Pathogen inactivation technology: Cleansing the blood supply. *J Intern Med* 2005;257(3):224–37.

43. Strauss R, Wehler M, Mehler K, et al. Thrombocytopenia in patients in the medical intensive care unit: Bleeding prevalence, transfusion requirements, and outcome. *Crit Care Med* 2002;30(8):1765–71.

44. Gauvin F, Toledano B, Champagne J, et al. Reactive hemophagocytic syndrome presenting as a component of multiple organ dysfunction syndrome. *Crit Care Med* 2000;28(9):3341–5.

45. Seftel MD. Universal prestorage leukoreduction in Canada decreases platelet alloimmunization and refractoriness. *Blood* 2004;103(1):333–9.

46. Khan SY. Soluble CD40 ligand accumulates in stored blood components, primes neutrophils through CD40, and is a potential cofactor in the development of transfusion-related acute lung injury. *Blood* 2006;108(7):2455–62.

47. Bercovitz RS, Josephson CD. Thrombocytopenia and bleeding in pediatric oncology patients. *Hematology Am Soc Hematol Educ Program* 2012;2012:499–505.

48. Josephson CD, Granger S, Assmann SF, et al. Bleeding risks are higher in children versus adults given prophylactic platelet transfusions for treatment-induced hypoproliferative thrombocytopenia. *Blood* 2012;120(4):748–60.

49. Blajchman MA, Slichter SJ, Heddle NM, et al. New strategies for the optimal use of platelet transfusions. *Hematology Am Soc Hematol Educ Program* 2008;2008(1):198–204.

50. Wandt H, Schaefer-Eckart K, Wendelin K, et al. Therapeutic platelet transfusion versus routine prophylactic transfusion in patients with haematological malignancies: An open-label, multicentre, randomised study. *Lancet* 2012;380(9850):1309–16.

51. de Vries R, Haas F, on behalf of the working group for revision of the Dutch Blood Transfusion Guideline 2011. English translation of the Dutch Blood Transfusion guideline 2011. *Vox Sang* 2012;103(4):363–3.

52. Schiffer CA, Anderson KC, Bennett CL, et al. Platelet transfusion for patients with cancer: Clinical practice guidelines of the American Society of Clinical Oncology. *J Clin Oncol* 2001;19(5):1519–38.

53. British Committee for Standards in Haematology, Blood Transfusion Task Force. Guidelines for the use of platelet transfusions. *Br J Haematol*. 2003;122(1):10–23.

54. Swisher KK, Terrell DR, Vesely SK, et al. Clinical outcomes after platelet transfusions in patients with thrombotic thrombocytopenic purpura. *Transfusion* 2009;49(5):873–87.

55. Bishop JF, Matthews JP, Yuen K, et al. The definition of refractoriness to platelet transfusions. *Transfus Med* 1992;2(1):35–41.

56. Bodey GP, Buckley M, Sathe YS, et al. Quantitative relationships between circulating leukocytes and infection in patients with acute leukemia. *Ann Intern Med* 1966;64(2):328–40.

57. Strauss RG. Role of granulocyte/neutrophil transfusions for haematology/oncology patients in the modern era. *Br J Haematol* 2012;158(3):299–306.

58. Vamvakas EC, Pineda AA. Determinants of the efficacy of prophylactic granulocyte transfusions: A meta-analysis. *J Clin Apher* 1997;12(2):74–81.

59. Massey E, Paulus U, Doree C, et al. Granulocyte transfusions for preventing infections in patients with neutropenia or neutrophil dysfunction. *Cochrane Database Syst Rev* 2009;(1):CD005341.

60. Seidel MG, Peters C, Wacker A, et al. Randomized phase III study of granulocyte transfusions in neutropenic patients. *Bone Marrow Transplant* 2008;42(10):679–84.

61. Sachs UJH, Reiter A, Walter T, et al. Safety and efficacy of therapeutic early onset granulocyte transfusions in pediatric

patients with neutropenia and severe infections. *Transfusion* 2006;46(11):1909–14.

62. Hübel K, Carter RA, Liles WC, et al. Granulocyte transfusion therapy for infections in candidates and recipients of HPC transplantation: A comparative analysis of feasibility and outcome for community donors versus related donors. *Transfusion* 2002;42(11):1414–21.

63. Hess JR. An update on solutions for red cell storage. *Vox Sang* 2006;91(1):13–9.

64. Spinella PC, Sparrow RL, Hess JR, et al. Properties of stored red blood cells: Understanding immune and vascular reactivity. *Transfusion* 2011;51(4):894–900.

65. Manno CS, Hedberg KW, Kim HC, et al. Comparison of the hemostatic effects of fresh whole blood, stored whole blood, and components after open heart surgery in children. *Blood* 1991;77(5):930–6.

66. Mou SS, Giroir BP, Molitor-Kirsch EA, et al. Fresh whole blood versus reconstituted blood for pump priming in heart surgery in infants. *N Engl J Med* 2004;351(16):1635–44.

67. Spinella PC, Dressler A, Tucci M, et al. Survey of transfusion policies at US and Canadian children's hospitals in 2008 and 2009. *Transfusion* 2010;50(11):2328–35.

68. Murphy S, Gardner FH. Platelet storage at 22 degrees C; metabolic, morphologic, and functional studies. *J Clin Invest* 1971;50(2):370–7.

69. Jobes D, Wolfe Y, O'Neill D, et al. Toward a definition of "fresh" whole blood: An in vitro characterization of coagulation properties in refrigerated whole blood for transfusion. *Transfusion* 2011;51(1):43–51.

70. Levi M, Fries D, Gombotz H, et al. Prevention and treatment of coagulopathy in patients receiving massive transfusions. *Vox Sang* 2011;101(2):154–74.

71. Spinella PC, Holcomb JB. Resuscitation and transfusion principles for traumatic hemorrhagic shock. *Blood Rev* 2009;23(6):231–40.

72. Borgman MA, Maegele M, Wade CE, et al. Pediatric trauma BIG score: Predicting mortality in children after military and civilian trauma. *Pediatrics* 2011;127(4):e892–7.

73. Dressler AM, Finck CM, Carroll CL, et al. Use of a massive transfusion protocol with hemostatic resuscitation for severe intraoperative bleeding in a child. *J Pediatr Surg* 2010;45(7):1530–3.

74. Cotton BA, Faz G, Hatch QM, et al. Rapid thrombelastography delivers real-time results that predict transfusion within 1 hour of admission. *J Trauma* 2011;71(2):407–17.

75. Holcomb JB, Minei KM, Scerbo ML, et al. Admission rapid thrombelastography can replace conventional coagulation tests in the emergency department. *Ann Surg* 2012;256(3):476–86.

76. Schochl H, Cotton B, Inaba K, et al. FIBTEM provides early prediction of massive transfusion in trauma. *Crit Care* 2011;15(6):R265.

77. Schochl H, Nienaber U, Maegele M, et al. Transfusion in trauma: Thromboelastometry-guided coagulation factor concentrate-based therapy versus standard fresh frozen plasma-based therapy. *Crit Care* 2011;15(2):R83.

78. Smith HM, Farrow SJ, Ackerman JD, et al. Cardiac arrests associated with hyperkalemia during red blood cell transfusion: A case series. *Anesth Analg* 2008;106(4):1062–1069.

79. Parshuram CS, Joffe AR. Prospective study of potassium-associated acute transfusion events in pediatric intensive care. *Pediatr Crit Care Med* 2003;4(1):65–8.

80. Lavoie JEE. Blood transfusion risks and alternative strategies in pediatric patients. *Paediatr Anaesth* 2011;21(1):14–24.

81. Corwin HL, Gettinger A, Pearl RG, et al. Efficacy of recombinant human erythropoietin in critically ill patients: A randomized controlled trial. *JAMA* 2002;288(22):2827–35.

82. Beal RW. The rational use of blood. *Aust N Z J Surg* 1976; 46(4):309–13.

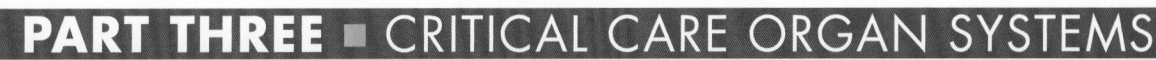

PART THREE ■ CRITICAL CARE ORGAN SYSTEMS

CHAPTER 43 ■ **RESPIRATORY PHYSIOLOGY**

FRANK L. POWELL, GREGORY P. HELDT, AND GABRIEL G. HADDAD

KEY POINTS

1 Most of the O_2 transported in blood is bound to hemoglobin, and this combination is sensitive to CO_2, pH, temperature, and phosphates. Developmental differences in O_2–hemoglobin binding are explained by differences between adult and fetal hemoglobin.

2 The first step in O_2 transport is alveolar ventilation ($\dot{V}A$), which is a function of respiratory rate, tidal volume, and dead space volume.

3 Oxygen diffusion from alveolar gas to pulmonary capillary blood is effective at equilibrating alveolar and arterial P_{O_2} ($P_{A_{O_2}} = P_{a_{O_2}}$) under most conditions.

4 The four major causes of arterial hypoxemia are hypoventilation, shunt, diffusion limitation, and ventilation–perfusion mismatch, which can be diagnosed by relatively simple tests and measuring the alveolar–arterial P_{O_2} difference ($P_{A_{O_2}} - P_{a_{O_2}}$).

5 Pulmonary mechanics is classically modeled as a capacitor (the elastance), a resistor (the airway and tissue resistance), and an inductor (primarily the inertia of the gas in the large airways) as a series circuit.

6 The elastic mechanical structure of the lungs, in conjunction with the surfactant system, makes the lung inflate uniformly and retain its end-expiratory volume to promote a good match of ventilation to perfusion. Mechanical ventilation of the immature lungs has special considerations, including surfactant replacement therapy.

7 Airflow limitation is a prominent feature of diseased lungs and is usually inferred from spirometric pulmonary function testing. Airflow limitation during mechanical ventilation may depend on the degree of inflation of the lungs, the resistance of the artificial airway, and the pattern of ventilation.

8 Recent developments of the forced oscillation technique have provided a deeper insight into the various mechanical components of the lung and may be applied clinically.

9 The pulmonary circulation has lower pressures and thinner vessel walls than the systemic circulation. Pulmonary vascular resistance is highly dependent on mechanical forces in the lungs and, in contrast to the systemic circulation, is increased by hypoxia.

10 Breathing is controlled by a negative feedback from chemoreceptors sensing arterial blood gas levels and mechanoreceptors from the lungs, airways, and chest wall acting on a respiratory rhythm generator in the brainstem.

11 The respiratory rhythm is generated by the integration of network, synaptic, and cellular properties of central neurons but it can be changed voluntarily, as well as being modulated by reflexes and being sensitive to the state of consciousness.

12 Developmental changes in respiratory control, and sensitivity to hypoxia, are explained by maturation of the central nervous system (CNS), peripheral sensory processes, the lung, and respiratory muscles.

PULMONARY GAS EXCHANGE

Pulmonary gas exchange describes the process of O_2 uptake and CO_2 elimination by the lungs to supply the metabolic demands of the body. This section of the chapter focuses on pulmonary gas exchange and how the lungs load adequate O_2 into the blood to meet tissue O_2 demand. It also covers the physiology of O_2 and CO_2 transport by the cardiovascular system and tissue gas exchange. Understanding pulmonary and tissue gas exchange also requires understanding O_2 and CO_2 blood dissociation curves. The general principles of respiratory physiology have been developed primarily in adults but the same principles apply to patients of any age. This chapter explains the general principles and highlights unique applications in pediatric and neonatal cases.

Normal O_2 values are shown as a so-called *oxygen cascade* in **Figure 43.1** as partial pressures (P_{O_2}) that can be measured in gas, blood, and tissue samples from a resting adult at sea level. Partial pressure (P_x) is calculated as the fraction of the total barometric pressure (P_{bar}) occupied by a given gas species:

$$P_x = F_x \times (P_{bar})$$

where F_x is the fractional concentration of gas "x" in a *dry* gas sample. Partial pressure is expressed in units of torr (1 torr = 1 mm Hg) or SI units of kilo Pascals (1 kPa = 7.5 mm Hg) in physiology.

The P_{O_2} decreases at every step in the O_2 cascade. The P_{O_2} drop between dry room air and inspired gas in the trachea ($P_{I_{O_2}}$) is due to humidification. Gas in the airways is saturated with water vapor at body temperature so that the total gas pressure available for O_2 and CO_2 inside the body is reduced. The water vapor pressure is 47 mm Hg at 37°C and 100% saturation. For a normal barometric pressure of 760 mm Hg at sea level:

$$P_{O_2} \text{ in dry ambient air} = 0.21 \times 760 \text{ mm Hg} = 160 \text{ mm Hg}$$

$$\begin{aligned} P_{I_{O_2}} \text{ in the airways} &= 0.21 \times (760 - 47) \text{ mm Hg} \\ &= 150 \text{ mm Hg} \end{aligned}$$

Further decreases in P_{O_2} along the O_2 cascade are explained by the physiology of gas exchange. The large drop in P_{O_2} between inspired and alveolar gas is a function of ventilation. Diffusion across the blood–gas barrier and other factors, such as shunts and the mismatching of ventilation and pulmonary blood flow, explains the relatively small decrease in P_{O_2} between

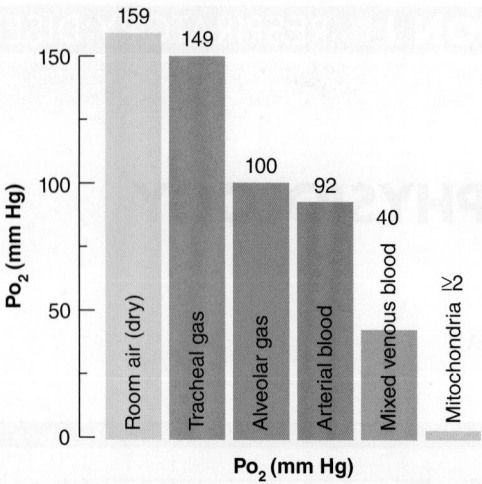

FIGURE 43.1. The "oxygen cascade" in a healthy subject breathing room air at sea level shows the pattern of P_{O_2} decrease between the different steps of O_2 transport. The difference between alveolar and arterial P_{O_2} occurs because of pulmonary gas exchange limitations. (From Powell FL. Pulmonary gas exchange. In: Johnson LR, ed. *Essential Medical Physiology*. 3rd ed. Boston, MA: Elsevier/Academic Press, 2003, with permission.)

alveolar gas and arterial blood. The circulation and O_2 diffusion from capillaries to tissues cause the large decreases in P_{O_2} between arterial and venous blood, and between blood and mitochondria in the tissues.

To quantify respiratory physiology for clinical diagnosis and research, standard symbols and conventions for reporting volumes and concentrations have been adopted. **Table 43.1** describes these symbols and gives examples of how they are used. Conditions of standard temperature and pressure and dry (STPD) are used for volumes of O_2 or CO_2 (e.g., metabolic rate, $\dot{V}_{O_2}$) while body temperate and pressure saturated (BTPS) conditions are used to report lung volumes and ventilation (e.g., expired ventilation, $\dot{V}_{E_2}$). For a normal pressure of 760 mm Hg and 37°C body temperature, $V_{BTPS} = 1.21 \times V_{STPD}$. Often, volumes are measured at ambient temperature and pressure, saturated conditions (V_{ATPS}) and at 760 mm Hg and 20°C, $V_{BTPS} = 1.086 \times V_{ATPS}$ and $V_{STPD} = 0.885 \times V_{ATPS}$.

Quantitative models of gas exchange are useful for diagnosing pulmonary disease. Generally, these models are based on the principle of conservation of mass, or *mass balance*, and they assume a steady state. *Steady state* means an equal and constant rate of gas transport at each step in the O_2 cascade, but it does not necessarily imply resting conditions. O_2 transport can be elevated but still equal at every step in the O_2 cascade (e.g., during steady-state exercise). However, non-steady-state conditions occur frequently (e.g., at the onset of exercise or in acute respiratory distress).

In an "ideal" model of alveolar gas exchange, arterial blood equilibrates with alveolar gas; therefore, the ideal alveolar–arterial P_{O_2} difference equals zero. In reality, the alveolar–arterial P_{O_2} difference exceeds zero, even in health (**Fig. 43.1**). Several factors, called *gas-exchange limitations*, increase the alveolar–arterial P_{O_2} difference. Gas-exchange limitations do not necessarily affect O_2 consumption at rest, but they can lower maximal O_2 consumption and decrease P_{O_2} values along the O_2 cascade in a steady state. The alveolar–arterial P_{O_2} difference is useful for diagnosing O_2 exchange limitations because different limitations respond differently to simple tests such as O_2 breathing.

TABLE 43.1

SYMBOLS IN RESPIRATORY PHYSIOLOGY

Primary variables (and units)

C	Concentration or content (mL/dL or mmol/L)
D	Diffusing capacity [mL O_2/ (min × mm Hg)]
F	Fractional concentration in dry gas (dimensionless)
P	Gas pressure or partial pressure (cm H_2O or mm Hg)
$\dot{Q}$	Blood flow or perfusion (L/min)
R	Respiratory exchange ratio (dimensionless)
T	Temperature (°C)
V	Gas volume (L or mL)
$\dot{V}$	Ventilation (L/min)

Modifying symbols

A	Alveolar gas
B	Barometric
DS	Dead space gas
E	Expired gas
$\overline{E}$	Mixed-expired gas
I	Inspired gas
L	Lung or transpulmonary
T	Tidal gas
aw	Airway
w	Chest wall
es	Esophageal
pl	Intrapleural
rs	Transrespiratory system (total system)
a	Arterial blood
b	Blood (general)
c	Capillary blood
c′	End-capillary blood
t	Tissue
v	Venous blood
$\overline{v}$	Mixed-venous blood

Examples

P_{AO_2} = Partial pressure of O_2 in alveolar gas

P_{aO_2} = Partial pressure of O_2 in arterial blood

$F_{\overline{E}CO_2}$ = Fraction of CO_2 in dry mixed, expired gas

$\dot{V}$ = O_2 consumption per unit time

$\dot{V}_A$ = Ventilation of the alveoli per unit time

Oxygen in Blood

The O_2 carriage by blood affects both O_2 uptake in the lungs and delivery in the tissues, so it is considered first. Blood–O_2 equilibrium curves (O_2 dissociation curves) quantify O_2 carriage as graphs of concentration versus partial pressure. It is necessary to consider both partial pressure and concentration because partial-pressure gradients drive diffusive gas transport in lungs and tissues, but concentration differences determine convective gas transport rates in lungs and the circulation (see the section, *Cardiovascular and Tissue Oxygen Transport*).

This topic would be much simpler to explain and understand if O_2 was physiologically inert and occurred in blood only as physically dissolved gas. There is a linear relationship between the concentration and partial pressure of a gas that is physically dissolved in a liquid according to Henry's law (C = αP, where α = solubility). However, O_2 also enters into chemical reactions with blood that result in a more

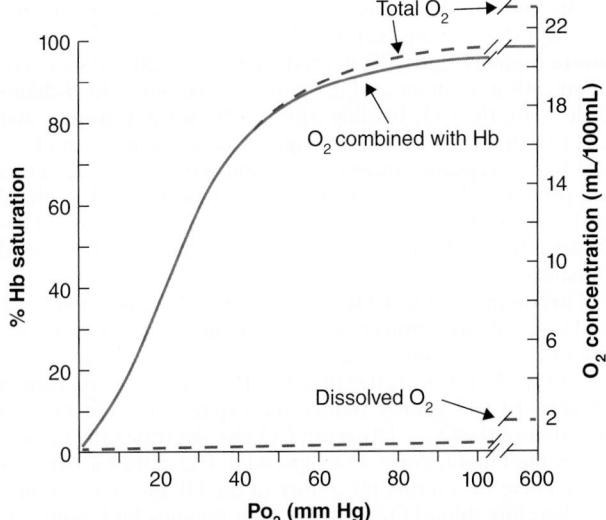

FIGURE 43.2. Standard human O_2–blood equilibrium (or dissociation) curve at pH = 7.4, P_{CO_2} = 40 mm Hg, and 37°C. Left ordinate shows O_2 saturation of hemoglobin (Hb) available for O_2 binding; right ordinate shows absolute O_2 concentration in blood. Most O_2 is bound to hemoglobin, and dissolved O_2 contributes very little to total O_2 concentration. (From Powell FL. Oxygen and CO_2 transport in the blood. In: Johnson LR, ed. *Essential Medical Physiology*. 3rd ed. Boston, MA: Elsevier/Academic Press, 2003, with permission.)

complicated, nonlinear relationship (**Fig. 43.2**) but this shape is essential for life as we know it. The normal O_2 concentration in arterial blood (Ca_{O_2}) is ~20 mL/dL but only 0.3 mL/dL is physically dissolved (note the usual units for O_2 and CO_2 concentration in blood are mL/dL, also called volume %, and 1 mL/dL ≈ 0.45 mmol/L for ideal gases). If arterial blood only contained dissolved O_2, then cardiac output would have to be 100 L/min to deliver enough O_2 to the tissues for a normal adult metabolic rate of 300 mL O_2/min!

Hemoglobin

Hemoglobin (Hb) is responsible for this dramatic increase in blood's O_2-carrying capacity. Hb consists of four polypeptide chains, each with a heme (iron-containing) protein that can bind O_2 with iron in the ferrous (Fe^{2+}) form. Methemoglobin results when iron is in the ferric form (Fe^{3+}) and cannot bind O_2. Small amounts of methemoglobin normally occur in blood and slightly reduce the amount of O_2 that can be bound to Hb. One gram of pure adult Hb can bind 1.39 mL of O_2 when fully saturated, but methemoglobin reduces this value to 1.34–1.36. The cellular packaging of Hb is important for the biophysics of the microcirculation, and it provides physiologic control of O_2 binding through cellular changes in the Hb microenvironment.

The four subunits of Hb include two α- and two β-chains, and variations in the amino acid sequence of these polypeptides explain the differences in Hb–O_2 affinity between species and at different stages of development. The three-dimensional shape of an Hb molecule, which is determined by the allosteric interactions of its four subunits, causes the O_2-equilibrium curve to be S-shaped, or sigmoidal (**Fig. 43.2**). O_2-equilibrium curves for individual α- and β-chains are not sigmoidal but simple convex curves similar to the O_2-equilibrium curve for myoglobin. Myoglobin occurs in muscle and has only a single polypeptide chain with one heme group. The sigmoidal shape of the O_2–Hb equilibrium curve facilitates O_2 loading into blood in the lungs and O_2 unloading from blood in the tissues.

Blood–Oxygen Equilibrium Curves

The two forms of the O_2 equilibrium curve are shown in **Figure 43.2**: (a) *saturation* of Hb with O_2 (S_{O_2}) versus P_{O_2}, and (b) O_2 *concentration* in blood (C_{O_2}) versus P_{O_2}. Saturation quantifies the amount of O_2 in blood as the percentage of the total Hb sites available for binding O_2 that actually bind O_2 at a given P_{O_2}. Therefore, saturation equilibrium curves are independent of Hb concentration in blood. In contrast, concentration curves quantify the absolute amount of O_2 in a volume of blood with a given P_{O_2}, and they depend on the amount of Hb available.

O_2 capacity (O_{2cap}) is defined as the O_2 concentration in blood when Hb is 100% saturated with O_2. Pure Hb binds 1.39 mL O_2/g Hb. **Figure 43.2** illustrates that the O_{2cap} for normal blood with Hb concentration of 15 g/dL is 20.85 mL/dL (1.39 × 15). Physically dissolved also contributes a small amount to O_2 concentration. Therefore, total O_2 concentration in blood (in mL O_2/dL blood) is calculated as:

$$C_{O_2} = (O_{2cap} \times [S_{O_2}/100]) + (0.003 \times P_{O_2})$$

where O_{2cap} is the O_2 capacity, S_{O_2} the saturation, and 0.003 is the physical solubility for O_2 in blood in (mL/dL)/mm Hg.

The shape of the O_2–Hb equilibrium curves is complex and can be generated only experimentally or by sophisticated mathematical algorithms. However, remembering only four points on the normal adult curve allows one to solve many common problems of O_2 transport:

    a. P_{O_2} = 0 mm Hg, S_{O_2} = 0% (the origin of the curve)
    b. P_{O_2} = 100 mm Hg, S_{O_2} = 98% (normal arterial blood, which is almost fully saturated)
    c. P_{O_2} = 40 mm Hg, S_{O_2} = 75% (normal mixed-venous blood)
    d. P_{O_2} = 26 mm Hg, S_{O_2} = 50% (i.e., P_{50})

The P_{50} quantifies the affinity of Hb for O_2 as the P_{O_2} at 50% saturation under standard conditions of partial pressure of CO_2 (P_{CO_2}) = 40 mm Hg, pH = 7.4, and 37°C. P_{50} is only 20 mm Hg in the human fetus, as discussed below. A decrease in P_{50} indicates an increase in O_2 affinity because S_{O_2} or C_{O_2} is greater for a given P_{O_2}.

Modulation of Blood–Oxygen Equilibrium Curves

The O_2-equilibrium curve can be physiologically modulated in three ways: (a) the vertical height of the concentration curve (but not the saturation curve) can change, indicating a change in O_{2cap}, (b) the horizontal position of saturation and concentration curves can change, indicating a change in Hb–O_2 affinity, and (c) the shape of saturation and concentration curves can change, indicating a change in the chemical reaction between O_2 and Hb. The maximum height of the saturation curve cannot change by definition; the maximum is always 100% when O_2 is bound to all available Hb sites. However, changes in Hb concentration [Hb] will change the maximum height of the concentration curve, according to the relationship between O_{2cap} and [Hb] as described previously. Mean corpuscular Hb concentration (MCHC) quantifies [Hb] in red blood cells and hematocrit (Hct) quantifies the percentage of blood volume that is red blood cells. Therefore, [Hb], in g/dL of blood, depends on both of these factors:

$$[Hb] = MCHC \cdot Hct$$

Typical adult values of MCHC = 0.33, Hct = 45%, and [Hb] = 15 g/dL are used in **Figure 43.2**, which shows normal Ca_{O_2} = 20 mL/dL and that Ca_{O_2} = 15 mL/dL in mixed-venous blood ($C\bar{v}_{oxygen}$). If [Hb] decreases, for example with decreased Hct in anemia, O_{2cap} and concentration decrease at any given P_{O_2}. The O_{2cap} increases when [Hb] increases by the stimulation of red blood cell production in bone marrow by the hormone erythropoietin or by transfusion. Erythropoietin transcription is regulated by hypoxia-inducible factors (HIF-1 and 2) released from cells in the kidneys in response to decreases in arterial O_2 levels. Polycythemia (increased Hct) occurs with chronic hypoxemia in healthy people (e.g., during acclimatization to altitude) and with disease.

The horizontal position of the Hb–O_2 equilibrium curves reflects the affinity of Hb for O_2, and changes in horizontal position are quantified as changes in P_{50}. A decrease in P_{50} is referred to as a *left shift* of the equilibrium curve and indicates increased Hb–O_2 affinity; So_2 or Co_2 is increased for a given Po_2. Similarly, increased P_{50}, or a *right shift*, reflects decreased Hb–O_2 affinity. The three most important physiologic variables that can modulate P_{50}—pH, Pco_2, and temperature—are shown in **Figure 43.3**.

The *Bohr effect* describes changes in P_{50} with changes in blood Pco_2 and pH. Decreased Pco_2 causes Hb–O_2 affinity to increase (decreased P_{50}), and increased Pco_2 causes Hb–O_2 affinity to decrease (increased P_{50}). As described later, pH decreases when Pco_2 increases and vice versa, and pH changes explain most of the Bohr effect with Pco_2 changes in blood. Hydrogen (H^+) binds to histidine residues in Hb molecules, thereby changing the conformation of Hb and the ability of heme sites to bind O_2. However, CO_2 also has a small, independent effect on Hb–O_2 affinity if pH is held constant. The physiologic advantage of the Bohr effect is that it facilitates loading in the lungs, where CO_2 is low and pH is high. In the tissues, the opposite occurs, and increased CO_2 causes pH to decrease and facilitates O_2 unloading from Hb to the tissues. The effect of temperature on Hb–O_2 affinity also has physiologic advantages. Warm temperatures in intensely exercising muscles will increase P_{50} and decrease Hb–O_2 affinity to facilitate O_2 unloading to tissues.

A physiologic O_2–blood equilibrium curve can be defined as the curve that shows the change in blood O_2 concentration when Po_2 decreases from arterial to venous levels in the tissues or increases in the opposite direction in the lungs. The increase in Pco_2, decrease in pH, and potential increase in temperature between arterial and venous points make the physiologic curve steeper than individual curves (**Fig. 43.3**). This is an advantage for gas exchange because it increases the change in O_2 concentration for a given change in Po_2, thereby increasing O_2 uptake or delivery (see the section, *Cardiovascular and Tissue Oxygen Transport*).

Hb–O_2 affinity is also affected by organic phosphates, with 2,3-diphosphoglycerate (2,3-DPG) being most important in humans. 2,3-DPG is produced during glycolysis in red blood cells and increases P_{50} by interacting with Hb β-chains to decrease their O_2-binding affinity. Physiologic stimuli that lead to enhanced O_2 delivery (e.g., chronic decreases in blood Po_2 levels) typically increase the concentration of 2,3-DPG and promote O_2 delivery to tissues. In blood stored in blood banks, 2,3-DPG is generally decreased, and the increased Hb–O_2 affinity can lead to problems in O_2 delivery after blood transfusion.

Carbon monoxide (CO) is a deadly gas that also modulates the Hb–O_2 dissociation curve by changing the shape and position of concentration or saturation curves. The affinity of Hb for CO is 240 times greater than it is for O_2, so even very small amounts of CO greatly reduce the capacity for Hb to bind O_2—that is, the O_{2cap}. However, CO also decreases the P_{50} and makes the Hb–O_2 curve less sigmoidal. CO causes a left shift of the curve by altering the ability of the Hb molecule to bind O_2; therefore, blood O_2 concentration remains high until Po_2 decreases to very low levels, which impairs O_2 unloading from blood to tissues. CO poisoning also has direct effects on cellular cytochromes, which contribute to its deadliness. CO is particularly dangerous because it is colorless and odorless, and the decrease it causes in arterial O_2 concentration is not sensed by respiratory control systems, which respond only to O_2 partial pressure, as explained in the *Respiratory Control* section. Hyperbaric O_2 exposure is used to treat CO poisoning because only very high Po_2 levels are effective at competing with CO for Hb-binding sites and driving CO out of the blood.

Oxygen Transport in Fetal Blood

The normal human fetus is exposed to a level of O_2 that would be considered severe hypoxia in adults, similar to the levels experienced on the summit of Mt. Everest! This is possible not only because the fetus is less sensitive to hypoxia than adults, but also because of fetal Hb (HbF). HbF has a P_{50} of 20 torr, compared to 26 torr for adults, thus facilitating O_2 transfer to the fetus in the placenta (**Fig. 43.4**). HbF is gradually replaced by adult Hb in the first year. O_2 delivery across the placenta is ~8 mL O_2/min/kg of fetal mass, which is approximately twice the rate for an adult, but blood O_2 stores in the fetus are sufficient for only a few minutes of metabolism. O_2 delivery across the placenta is limited by blood flow and Po_2 levels in the mother and fetus, but not by diffusion. For example, decreasing maternal Pao_2 below 70 torr can reduce placental O_2 transfer. Increasing maternal Pao_2 to 600 torr, with O_2 breathing, can increase fetal umbilical O_2 tensions by 3–5 torr, which can be important if the fetus is suffering any hypoxic stress. Both the left shift of fetal versus adult O_2–Hb equilibrium curves and the high fetal O_2 capacity facilitate O_2 unloading from the mother to the fetus (**Fig. 43.4**). It is also significant that O_2 capacity is decreased in the mother near term (11.5 vs. 14 g/dL Hb). The Bohr effect also contributes to placental O_2 transport, as pH decreases from 7.42 in the maternal artery to 7.35 in the maternal vein.

Carbon Dioxide in Blood

The general principles of CO_2 transport by blood are similar to those for O_2, i.e., blood carries much more CO_2 than would be possible if it was only physically dissolved, and the CO_2–blood equilibrium curve is modulated by physiologic factors. In addition, CO_2 carriage by blood has important effects on acid–base balance.

CO_2–blood equilibrium (or dissociation) curves are nonlinear, but they have a different shape and position than

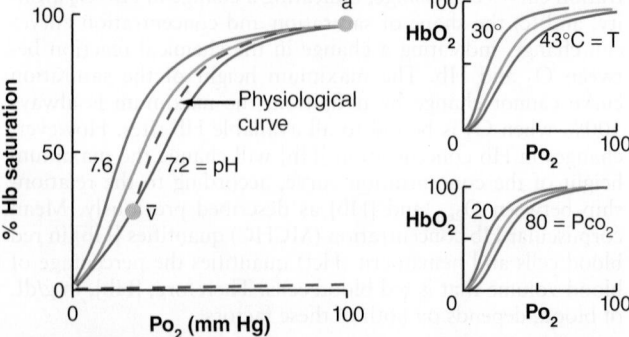

FIGURE 43.3. Effects of pH and Pco_2 (i.e., Bohr effect) and temperature on the position of the O_2–hemoglobin (HbO_2) equilibrium curve. The "physiological" curve connects the arterial (a) and mixed-venous points ($\bar{v}$), so that the in vivo curve is steeper than the standard curve at pH = 7.4 (green). (From Powell FL. Oxygen and CO_2 transport in the blood. In: Johnson LR, ed. *Essential Medical Physiology*. 3rd ed. Boston, MA: Elsevier/Academic Press, 2003, with permission.)

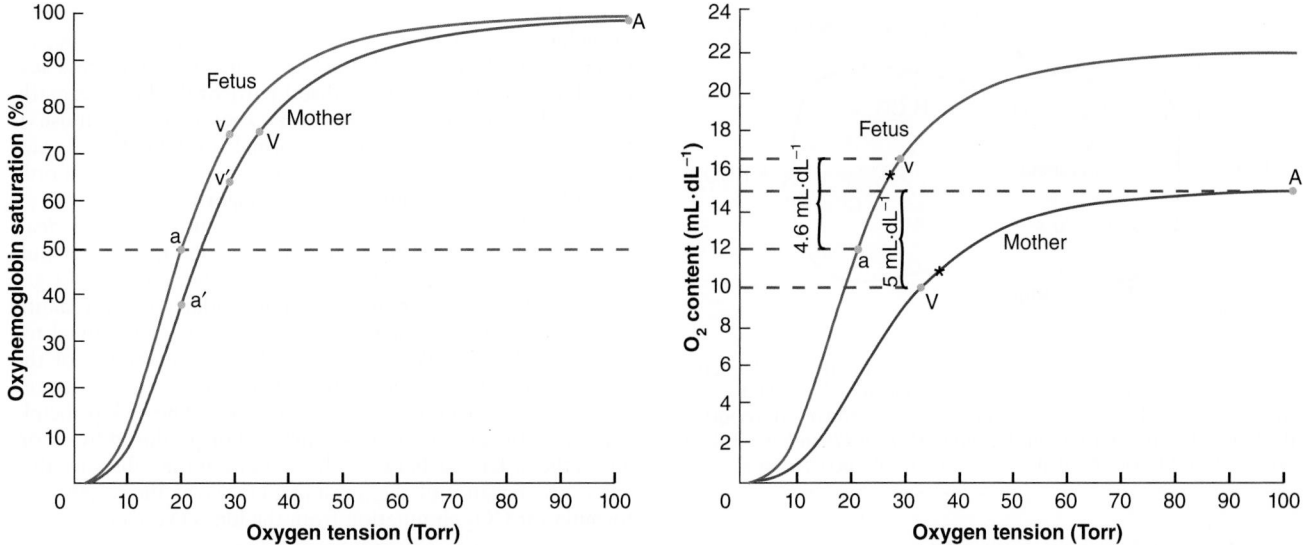

FIGURE 43.4. Oxygen–hemoglobin equilibrium curves for maternal and fetal hemoglobin. **A:** When P_{O_2} equilibrates between the fetal and maternal circulations, O_2 saturation is increased by 10% or more because of the lower P_{50} in fetal hemoglobin. **B:** Higher O_2 capacity of fetal compared to maternal blood further increases the amount of O_2 in blood for a given P_{O_2} and saturation. A, maternal arterial; V, maternal venous; a', umbilical (maternal) arterial; v', umbilical (maternal) venous; a, fetal arterial; v, fetal venous. (From Powell FL. Pulmonary gas exchange. In: Johnson LR, ed. *Essential Medical Physiology*. 3rd ed. Boston, MA: Elsevier Academic Press, 2003, with permission.)

O_2–blood equilibrium curves. Blood holds more CO_2 than O_2, in part because CO_2 is carried by blood in three forms (**Fig. 43.5**). Also, the CO_2–blood equilibrium curve is steeper than the O_2 curve, resulting in a smaller range of P_{CO_2} values in the body, compared with the range of P_{O_2} values, although the differences between arterial and venous concentrations are similar for CO_2 and O_2 (~5 mL/dL of blood). The resulting physiologic CO_2 dissociation curve between the arterial and venous points is much more linear than the physiologic O_2 dissociation curve (**Fig. 43.5**).

Carbon Dioxide and Blood Acid–Base

Physically dissolved CO_2 is a function of CO_2 solubility in plasma, which is 0.067 mL/(dL mm Hg) and 20 times more soluble than O_2. Still, dissolved CO_2 contributes only ~5% of total CO_2 concentration in arterial blood.

Carbamino compounds comprise the second form of blood CO_2. These compounds occur when CO_2 combines with amine groups in blood proteins, especially with the globin of Hb. However, this chemical combination between CO_2 and Hb is much less important than Hb–O_2 binding; therefore carbamino compounds comprise only 5% of the total CO_2 in arterial blood.

Bicarbonate ion HCO_3^- is the most important form of CO_2 carriage in blood. CO_2 combines with water to form carbonic acid, and this dissociates to HCO_3^- and H^+:

$$CO_2 + H_2O \leftrightarrow H_2CO_3 + HCO_3^- + H^+$$

Carbonic anhydrase is the enzyme that catalyzes this reaction, making it almost instantaneous. Carbonic anhydrase occurs mainly in red blood cells, but it also occurs on pulmonary capillary endothelial cells and accelerates the reaction in plasma in the lungs. The uncatalyzed reaction will occur in any aqueous medium, but at a much slower rate, requiring >4 minutes for equilibrium. The rapid conversion of CO_2 to bicarbonate results in ~90% of the CO_2 in arterial blood that is carried in that form and has important implications for acid–base balance.

Figure 43.6 shows the carbonic acid reactions in plasma and red blood cells and illustrates important ion fluxes that occur with CO_2 transport in blood. CO_2 rapidly enters red blood cells from the plasma because it is soluble in cell membranes. Carbonic anhydrase catalyzes the rapid formation of HCO_3^- and H^+ in the cells and an electrically neutral bicarbonate–chloride exchanger moves some of this HCO_3^- out of

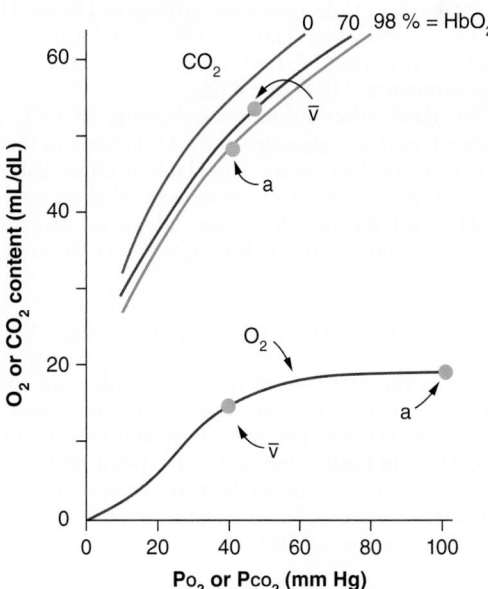

FIGURE 43.5. CO_2–blood equilibrium curve shown on same graph with O_2 equilibrium curve. Differences between the curves result in higher CO_2 concentrations in the blood and smaller P_{CO_2} differences between arterial (a) and venous ($\bar{v}$) blood. Hemoglobin–O_2 saturation affects the position of the CO_2 equilibrium curve (i.e., Haldane effect). (From Powell FL. Oxygen and CO_2 transport in the blood. In: Johnson LR, ed. *Essential Medical Physiology*. 3rd ed. Boston, MA: Elsevier/Academic Press, 2003, with permission.)

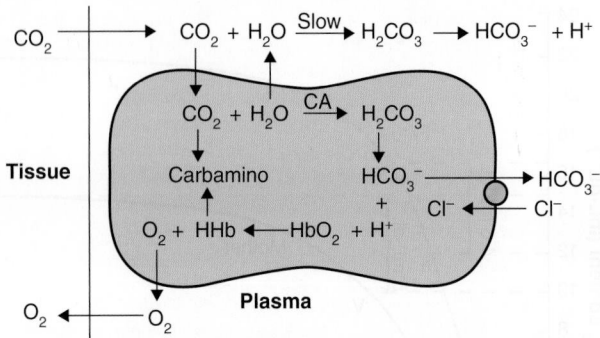

FIGURE 43.6. CO_2 and O_2 reactions in blood and tissues; the opposite reactions occur in the lungs. CA, carbonic anhydrase; HHb, protonated hemoglobin. (From Powell FL. Oxygen and CO_2 transport in the blood. In: Johnson LR, ed. *Essential Medical Physiology*. 3rd ed. Boston, MA: Elsevier/Academic Press, 2003, with permission.)

the cell. The chloride shift (*Hamburger shift*) is an increased intracellular chloride level with increased CO_2, or vice versa. The H^+ produced from CO_2 reacts with Hb and affects both the O_2 equilibrium curve (Bohr effect) and CO_2 equilibrium curve, as described next.

Modulation of Blood–Carbon Dioxide Equilibrium Curves

Hb–O_2 saturation is the major factor affecting the position of the CO_2 equilibrium curve. The *Haldane effect* increases CO_2 concentration when blood is deoxygenated or decreases CO_2 concentration when blood is oxygenated at any given PCO_2 (**Fig. 43.5**). The Haldane effect is actually another view of the same molecular mechanism that causes the Bohr effect on the O_2 equilibrium curve (described previously). H^+ ions from CO_2 can be thought of as competing with O_2 for Hb binding. Hence, increasing O_2 decreases the affinity of Hb for H^+ and blood CO_2 concentration (Haldane effect), and increased $[H^+]$ decreases the affinity of Hb for O_2 (Bohr effect). These interactions are summarized in **Figure 43.6**.

The Haldane effect promotes unloading of CO_2 in the lungs when blood is oxygenated and CO_2 loading in the blood when O_2 is released to tissues. The Haldane effect also results in a steeper physiologic CO_2–blood equilibrium curve (see **Fig. 43.5**), which has the physiologic advantage of increasing CO_2 concentration differences for a given PCO_2 difference.

❷ Alveolar Ventilation and Alveolar PO_2

Ventilation is the first step in the O_2 cascade, and the level of alveolar ventilation $\dot{V}A$ is the most important factor determining arterial PO_2 for any given PIO_2 and level of O_2 consumption ($\dot{V}O_2$) in healthy lungs. Total expired ventilation can be measured with a pneumotachometer or spirometer as the product of the volume of each breath, or tidal volume (VT), and respiratory frequency (fR):

$$\dot{V}E = VT \times fR$$

However, all the tidal volume is not effective for gas exchange because the lung consists of a conducting zone, which does not exchange gas, and a respiratory zone, in which all gas exchange occurs. The conducting zone includes the conducting airways from the trachea to the terminal bronchioles, which occur at the 16th order of bronchial branching. The gas volume of the conducting zone equals the *anatomic dead space*. The respiratory zone comprises the rest of the lung from the

17th to 23rd orders of bronchial branching (i.e., respiratory bronchioles to alveolar sacs), and all gas exchange occurs there. With 23 orders of bronchial branching, total cross-sectional area of the airways in distal parts of the lung is greatly increased; therefore, the respiratory zone comprises most of the lung volume. For example, a normal adult will have a total lung capacity (TLC) of 6 L but an anatomic dead space of only 175 mL (~1 mL per pound of body weight).

$\dot{V}A$ is the difference between total ventilation and dead space ventilation, and it is the effective conductance for pulmonary gas exchange. Total ventilation is not effective for gas exchange because part of the inspired tidal volume remains in the anatomic dead space (VDS). $\dot{V}A$ can be determined using the *Fick principle*, which is a physiologic version of the principle of conservation of mass that describes gas transport by convection or bulk flow of air or blood. The Fick principle states that the amount of gas consumed or produced by an organ is the difference between the amount of the substance that enters the organ and the amount that leaves the organ. The formula for CO_2 elimination from the lungs ($\dot{V}CO_2$) is:

$$(\dot{V}CO_2) = (\dot{V}A\ FACO_2) - (\dot{V}I\ FICO_2)$$

$\dot{V}CO_2$ is the difference between the CO_2 expired from the alveoli, and the amount of CO_2 inspired to the alveoli. $FICO_2$ is essentially zero; therefore, the equation can be simplified and rearranged to the *alveolar ventilation equation*:

$$\dot{V}A = (\dot{V}CO_2/PACO_2)K$$

where $\dot{V}A$ is expressed at body temperature and pressure saturated (i.e., LBTPS/minute), $\dot{V}CO_2$ is expressed at standard temperature and pressure dry (i.e., mLSTPD/minute), $PACO_2$ is substituted for $FACO_2$, and K is a constant (0.863).

In practice, arterial PCO_2 ($PaCO_2$) is substituted for alveolar PCO_2 ($PACO_2$) because the two values are equal in normal lungs, and an arterial blood sample is usually taken to evaluate gas exchange.

Alveolar *Ventilation* Equation Predicts Alveolar PCO_2

Rearranging the alveolar ventilation equation shows how $\dot{V}A$ and $PACO_2$ (or $PaCO_2$) are inversely related for any given metabolic rate:

$$PACO_2 = (\dot{V}CO_2/\dot{V}A)K$$

Hence, if $\dot{V}A$ is doubled, $PACO_2$ is halved, regardless of the exact values for either variable. *Hyperventilation* is defined by a decrease in $PaCO_2$ from the normal value, implying excess $\dot{V}A$ for a given $\dot{V}CO_2$. *Hypoventilation* is defined by an increase in $PaCO_2$, and this occurs when $\dot{V}A$ is lower than normal for a given $\dot{V}CO_2$.

As explained previously, $\dot{V}A$ is reduced from total ventilation by the amount of the dead space:

$$\dot{V}A = fR\ (VT - VDS)$$

Although anatomic dead space can be measured with gas analyzers and flow meters, it is more clinically relevant to estimate physiologic dead space, which is also called *Bohr dead space*. Physiologic dead space includes all "wasted ventilation" and can exceed anatomic dead space, as described next. Physiologic dead space can be calculated from another rearrangement of the Fick principle applied to CO_2 elimination by the lungs as:

$$VDS/VT = (PACO_2 - P\bar{E}CO_2)/PACO_2$$

where $P\bar{E}CO_2$ = *mixed-expired* PCO_2 that is measured by collecting all expired gas in a bag or a spirometer and includes gas exhaled from the alveoli *and* dead space. In practice, arterial PCO_2 is substituted for alveolar PCO_2 because it is easily measured.

Alveolar *Gas* Equation Predicts Alveolar P_{O_2}

Alveolar P_{O_2} ($P_{A_{O_2}}$) can be predicted from the *alveolar gas equation* that models an "ideal lung" with only physiologic dead space:

$$P_{A_{O_2}} = P_{I_{O_2}} - (P_{A_{CO_2}}/R) + F$$

where $P_{I_{O_2}}$ is inspired P_{O_2}, $P_{A_{CO_2}}$ is alveolar P_{CO_2}, R is the respiratory exchange ratio, and F is a constant that can be ignored under normal conditions (F = $P_{A_{CO_2}} \times F_{I_{O_2}}$ [1 − R]/R and increases $P_{A_{O_2}}$ only 2 mm Hg at normal O_2 and CO_2 levels).

In practice, arterial P_{CO_2} is substituted for alveolar P_{CO_2} because $P_{a_{CO_2}} = P_{A_{CO_2}}$ in normal lungs and arterial samples are easily obtained. The alveolar gas equation is only valid if inspired $P_{CO_2} = 0$, which is a reasonable assumption for room air breathing.

The *respiratory exchange ratio* (R) is the ratio of uptake to CO_2 elimination by the lungs:

$$R = \dot{V}_{CO_2}/\dot{V}_{O_2}$$

Under steady-state conditions, R equals the *respiratory quotient* (RQ), which is the ratio of CO_2 production to O_2 consumption in metabolizing tissues. RQ averages 0.8 on a normal, mixed, adult diet, but it can range from 0.67 to 1, depending on the relative amounts of fat, protein, and carbohydrate being metabolized. R can exceed this range in nonsteady states, for example, when R exceeds 1 during hyperventilation. CO_2 stores in the body are much greater than O_2 stores because of bicarbonate in blood and tissues. R can increase because it takes longer to wash out the CO_2 stores than it does to charge up the much smaller O_2 stores in the body.

Substituting normal adult values in the alveolar gas equation predicts that $P_{A_{O_2}}$ = 100 mm Hg in breathing room air ($P_{A_{O_2}}$ = 150 − 40/0.8). Increases in $\dot{V}_A$ (hyperventilation) increases $P_{A_{O_2}}$ by decreasing $P_{A_{CO_2}}$, whereas decreases in $\dot{V}_A$ (hypoventilation) decreases $P_{A_{O_2}}$. Why ideal alveolar P_{O_2} is greater than measured arterial P_{O_2} is explained in the next section.

Permissive Hypercapnia

Respiratory disease, and especially hypoventilation, is characterized by changes in blood gas homeostasis, namely, hypoxia and hypercapnia. Often, the only treatment that can be used is mechanical ventilation until the disease is resolved. While mechanical ventilation may be a lifesaver in certain conditions, this treatment can also injure the lungs with barotrauma. Epidemiologic data in the 1980s and 1990s showed that "permitting" an increase in $P_{a_{CO_2}}$ without imposing mechanical ventilation, or delaying mechanical ventilation, might have beneficial effects. Both animal and human studies have shown that therapeutic hypercapnia attenuates various measures of lung injury. For example, 8% CO_2 increases expression of genes encoding surfactant-associated proteins A and B, which contribute to host defense mechanisms in the lung.

In pediatrics, questions about this strategy have focused on bronchopulmonary dysplasia (BPD) in infants after prematurity. Higher $P_{a_{CO_2}}$ values are associated with lower BPD rates and large population-based studies in premature neonates show decreased BPD and death with permissive hypercapnia used before or during intubation and mechanical ventilation. Permissive hypercapnia also increased survival in neonates who have congenital diaphragmatic hernia. However, experiments in animal and human cell cultures also suggest some undesirable effects of elevated CO_2, such as suppressed immune function, increased oxidative lung injury, and impaired alveolar repair with potentiated tissue nitration. Summarizing, permissive hypercapnia is a ventilatory strategy that may reduce injury to the developing lung through a variety of mechanisms. Considering all of the evidence to date, permissive

hypercapnia appears to be safe and beneficial in neonates subject to barotraumas.

3 ## Diffusion

Diffusion of O_2 from alveoli to pulmonary capillary blood is the next step in the O_2 cascade after alveolar ventilation. It is important to note that blood leaving the pulmonary capillaries is in equilibrium with alveolar gas in healthy lungs under normal resting conditions. Hence, the small decreases between $P_{A_{O_2}}$ and $P_{a_{O_2}}$ shown in **Figure 43.1** are not caused by diffusion but by ventilation–perfusion mismatching in healthy lungs under normal conditions, as described in the next section.

O_2 moves from the alveoli to pulmonary capillary blood barrier according to Fick's first law of diffusion:

$$\dot{V}_{O_2} = \Delta P_{O_2} \times D_{O_2}$$

ΔP_{O_2} is the average P_{O_2} gradient across the blood–gas barrier and D_{O_2} is a "diffusing capacity" for O_2 across the barrier.

Diffusion of a gas always occurs down a partial-pressure gradient, for example, from alveolar gas to pulmonary blood. Some readers may find it helpful to note the analogy between Fick's law for O_2 flux and Ohm's law for the flow of electrons (current = voltage/resistance). $\dot{V}_{O_2}$ is analogous to current, and ΔP_{O_2} is analogous to the potential energy difference of voltage. However, D_{O_2} is analogous to a *conductance*, which is the inverse of resistance (current = voltage × conductance). Flux can be increased either by increasing the P_{O_2} gradient or increasing the conductance (D_{O_2}).

D_{O_2} depends on both the molecular properties of the gas and the geometric properties of that membrane:

$$D_{O_2} = (\text{solubility/MW}) \, O_2 \, (\text{area/thickness})_{\text{membrane}}$$

Solubility is important because gas molecules must "dissolve" in a membrane before they can diffuse across it, and once dissolved, low-molecular-weight (MW) molecules move more quickly by the random motions of diffusion. Large surface areas increase the probability that an O_2 molecule will come into contact with the membrane through random motion, but membrane thickness increases the distance that O_2 molecules must travel.

Blood–Gas Barrier

The pathway of an O_2 molecule diffusing from alveolar gas to Hb inside an erythrocyte (red blood cell) in an adult lung (**Fig. 43.7**) is the anatomic basis for D_{O_2}. The total area of the blood–gas barrier is nearly 100 m^2 in adult lungs; it is extremely thin but variable in thickness and consists of three different layers. The "thin" side of a pulmonary capillary (0.3 μm) separates gas from plasma with (a) thin cytoplasmic extensions from type I alveolar epithelial cells, (b) a thin basement membrane, and (c) thin cytoplasmic extensions from capillary endothelial cells. The thicker side of a capillary has collagen in the interstitial space to provide mechanical strength in the alveoli. Epithelial and endothelial cell bodies are in alveolar corners between capillaries to further minimize the thickness of the gas-exchange barrier. Finally, O_2 must diffuse through plasma and across the red blood cell membrane before it can combine with Hb. The diffusing capacity for O_2 between the alveolar gas and Hb is called the *membrane diffusing capacity for* O_2, or $D_{M_{O_2}}$.

After O_2 diffuses into red blood cells, the finite *rate of reaction between* O_2 *and Hb* (abbreviated with the symbol θ) offers an additional "resistance" to O_2 uptake. The magnitude of this chemical resistance depends on θ and the total amount of Hb, which is a physiologic function of pulmonary capillary volume (Vc). This chemical resistance is in series with the

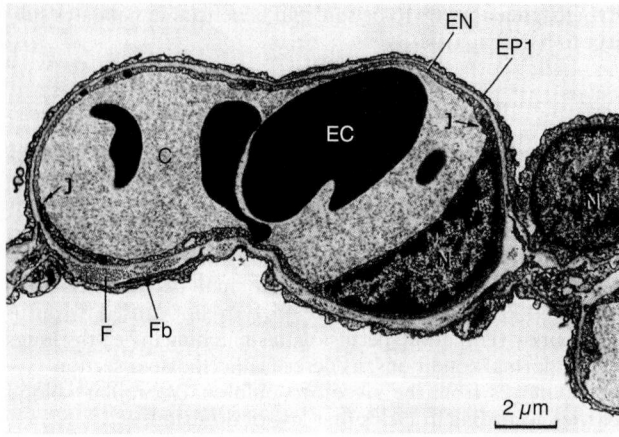

FIGURE 43.7. Electron micrograph of a pulmonary capillary showing the pathway for O_2 diffusion in the lung. O_2 diffuses from the alveolar space (open areas above and below capillary, C) through epithelial cell (*EP1*), interstitial space, endothelial cell (*EN*), and plasma before combining with hemoglobin in the erythrocyte (*EC*). Collagen fibers (*F*) and fibroblasts (Fb) thicken the interstitial space on one side of the capillary. N, nucleus; J, endothelial cell junctions. Scale marker = 2 μm. (From Weibel ER. Design and morphometry of the pulmonary gas exchanger. In: Crystal RG, West JB, Barnes PJ, et al., eds. *The Lung: Scientific Foundations.* 2nd ed. Philadelphia, PA: Lippincott Williams & Wilkins, 1997, with permission.)

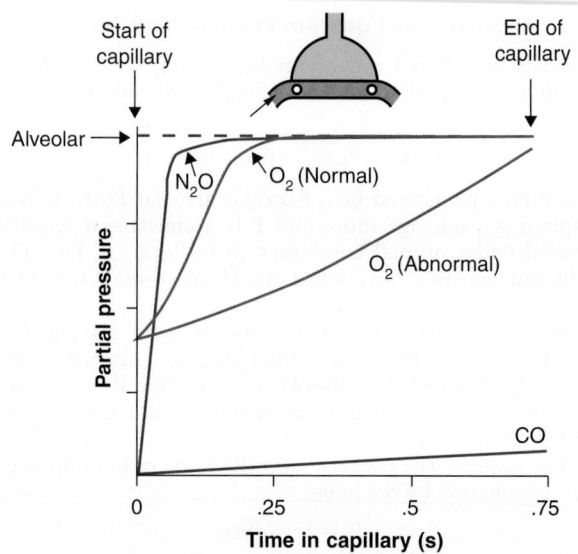

FIGURE 43.8. The time course of the increase in partial pressure for different gases diffusing from alveolar gas into pulmonary capillary blood. Nitrous oxide and O_2 under normal conditions equilibrate very quickly, but CO or O_2 under abnormal conditions do not equilibrate in the time it takes blood to flow through the capillary in adults (0.75 seconds). (From Powell FL. Pulmonary gas exchange. In: Johnson LR, ed. *Essential Medical Physiology.* 3rd ed. London, England: Elsevier Academic Press, 2003, with permission.)

membrane resistance, so that the total resistance to O_2 diffusion in the lung can be defined as:

$$1/D_{LO_2} = 1/D_{MO_2} + 1/(\theta V_c)$$

where D_{LO_2} *is the lung diffusing capacity for* O_2. (D_{LO_2} is a conductance; recall that conductance is the inverse of resistance, and resistors in series are additive.)

It is estimated that membrane and chemical reaction resistances to O_2 diffusion are approximately equal in normal lungs. Both D_{MO_2} and V_c are under physiologic control through pulmonary capillary recruitment and distension. Therefore, D_{LO_2} increases with exercise by recruitment of D_{MO_2} and θV_c. Methods for measuring D_{LO_2} are described below.

P_{O_2} Changes along the Pulmonary Capillary

The normal time course of P_{O_2} changes along the capillary in adult lungs at normal P_{O_2} levels, and the P_{O_2} in capillary blood increases from mixed-venous levels at the beginning to arterial levels at the end of the capillary (**Fig. 43.8**). Alveolar P_{O_2} is constant everywhere outside the capillary because diffusion is rapid in the gas phase. Any O_2 moving into the blood is instantly replaced by diffusive mixing in the small alveolar spaces. Hence, the gradient for O_2 diffusion changes along the length of the capillary, and the ΔP_{O_2} value used in Fick's law is an average value, corresponding to the mean partial-pressure gradient operating over the entire length of the pulmonary capillary.

The average capillary transit time of 0.75 seconds for adults (**Fig. 43.8**) is calculated from a cardiac output of 6 L/min and capillary volume of 75 mL (time = volume/flow rate). Note that diffusion equilibrium normally occurs between blood and gas in only 0.25 seconds, providing a threefold safety factor. However, if D_{LO_2} is decreased sufficiently with lung disease, capillary P_{O_2} may not equilibrate with P_{AO_2} during the transit time (see **Fig. 43.8**, abnormal O_2 curve). In the abnormal case, $P_{c'O_2} < P_{AO_2}$, which is defined as a *diffusion limitation for* O_2, where $P_{c'}$ is used to designate end-capillary partial pressure.

Only two conditions lead to diffusion limitation for O_2 in healthy adults. First, elite athletes at maximal exercise, with very high O_2 consumption and cardiac outputs, can have transit times that are too short for O_2 diffusion equilibrium. Capillary volume increases by recruitment and distension with elevated cardiac output, and this is sufficient to offset the increase in blood flow in most people. An exception is in elite athletes who have abnormally high cardiac outputs that can move blood through capillaries in less than 0.25 seconds, resulting in diffusion limitation. Second, normal adults exercising at altitude may not achieve diffusion equilibrium because transit time *and* P_{AO_2} decrease. Decreasing P_{AO_2} slows O_2 diffusion by decreasing the P_{O_2} gradient that is driving diffusion. Decreasing P_{AO_2} also slows the rate of rise in P_{O_2} because gas exchange is occurring on the steep portion of the O_2–blood equilibrium curve. This means that a given increase in O_2 concentration is less effective at increasing P_{O_2} than it is on the flat part of the O_2–blood equilibrium curve at high P_{O_2} levels.

Note that both of these types of diffusion limitation in healthy lungs are different than hypoxemia typically encountered in the ICU. In patients, metabolic rates and cardiac outputs may be depressed. Hypoxemia from a decrease in lung diffusing capacity (e.g., thickening of the blood–gas barrier from edema) may be corrected by increasing inspired O_2 levels.

Diffusion-limited and Perfusion-limited Gases

Dramatic differences in the time course of diffusion equilibrium for different gases in the lung are also shown in **Figure 43.8**. The anesthetic gas nitrous oxide (N_2O) achieves equilibrium rapidly, whereas CO never comes close to diffusion equilibrium. Understanding the differences between these gases is not only important for anesthesiology and emergency medicine, but it also helps in understanding the physiologic mechanisms for O_2 diffusion limitations.

The uptake of a gas that achieves diffusion equilibrium depends on the magnitude of pulmonary blood flow. For example, N_2O diffuses rapidly from the alveoli to capillary blood

(Fig. 43.8); therefore, the only way to increase its uptake is to increase the amount of blood flowing through the alveolar capillaries. N_2O is an example of a *perfusion-limited gas*. Changes in the diffusing capacity have no effect on the uptake of a perfusion-limited gas or its partial pressure in the blood and body. All anesthetic and "inert" gases that do not react chemically with blood are perfusion-limited. Under normal resting conditions, O_2 is also a perfusion-limited gas.

The uptake of a gas that does not achieve diffusion equilibrium could obviously increase if the diffusing capacity increased. CO is an example of such a *diffusion-limited gas* (Fig. 43.8). As Hb has a very high affinity for CO, the effective solubility of CO in blood is large. Therefore, increases in the CO concentration in blood are not effective at increasing partial pressure of carbon monoxide (P_{CO}), which keeps blood P_{CO} lower than alveolar P_{CO} and results in a large disequilibrium and diffusion limitation. In practice, the only diffusion-limited gases are CO and O_2 under hypoxic conditions. All other gases are perfusion-limited, including O_2 under normoxic conditions in healthy lungs.

Measuring Diffusing Capacity

The diffusing capacity of the lung can be measured from the uptake of a diffusion-limited gas such as CO. If very low levels of CO are inspired ($\sim 0.1\%$), Hb saturation with CO is very low, arterial oxygenation is not disturbed, and no toxic effects occur. Also, the amount of CO entering the capillary blood does not increase blood P_{CO} significantly because CO is so soluble in blood. Therefore, the lung-diffusing capacity for CO (D_{LCO}) can be defined by Fick's first law of diffusion as:

$$D_{LCO} = \dot{V}_{CO} / P_{A_{CO}}$$

where $\dot{V}_{CO}$ = CO uptake by the lung and the gradient driving CO diffusion equals $P_{A_{CO}}$ because average capillary $P_{CO} = 0$. In theory, although D_{LCO} could be used to calculate the D_L for O_2 by correcting for physical factors that determine diffusing capacity (MW and solubility), only D_{LCO} is reported clinically.

In the *steady-state D_{LCO} method*, the individual breathes a low level of CO for a couple of minutes. CO uptake is then calculated from the Fick principle using measurements of ventilation and inspired and expired P_{CO}. Alveolar P_{CO} can be estimated from expired P_{CO}. In the *single-breath D_{LCO} method*, an individual takes a breath with a low concentration of CO and holds the breath for 10 seconds. This method also requires a simultaneous measurement of lung volume (e.g., by helium dilution) to calculate $\dot{V}_{CO}$ from P_{CO} changes in the lung. Alveolar P_{CO} is estimated from expired P_{CO} and corrected for the change that occurs during the breath hold.

D_{LCO} in healthy adults is ~ 25 mL/(minute $\times$ mm Hg) and can increase twofold to threefold with exercise, as expected for capillary recruitment and distension. D_{LCO} also changes with O_2 level because the rate of chemical reaction between CO and Hb is deceased by Hb oxygenation, and D_{LCO} has a chemical reaction rate component (θV_c) similar to D_{LO_2}. In lung disease, D_{LCO} may be affected by other factors, such as unequal distributions of alveolar volume, pulmonary blood flow, and diffusing properties. Such factors explain why morphometric estimates of diffusing capacity, based on anatomic measurements of the blood–gas barrier surface area, thickness, and so on, are approximately twice as large as functional measurements of diffusing capacity. Because other factors can affect D_{LCO} measurement, it is sometimes referred to as a *transfer factor* instead of the diffusing capacity.

4   Four Causes of Hypoxemia

Hypoxemia is defined as a decrease in blood P_{O_2}, and arterial hypoxemia, or decreased $P_{a_{O_2}}$, indicates a limitation of pulmonary gas exchange. Gas-exchange limitations in the lungs

can reduce P_{O_2} throughout the O_2 cascade but they do not decrease resting oxygen consumption; maximal $\dot{V}_{O_2}$ during exercise may decrease however. In a steady state, P_{O_2} will adjust throughout the O_2 cascade to maintain $\dot{V}_{O_2}$. For example, $P_{\bar{v}_{O_2}}$ decreases as cardiac output ($\dot{Q}$) increases during exercise to satisfy the cardiovascular Fick equation.

Gas-exchange limitations not only decrease $P_{a_{O_2}}$, but some can increase the alveolar–arterial P_{O_2} difference. The concept of an "ideal" lung without limitations was introduced previously and, under such ideal conditions, the alveolar–arterial P_{O_2} difference is 0 mm Hg. However, in reality, $P_{A_{O_2}}$ calculated from the alveolar gas equation is greater than $P_{a_{O_2}}$ measured from an arterial blood sample, and the alveolar–arterial P_{O_2} difference increases with *most* (but not all) gas-exchange limitations.

The four kinds of pulmonary gas-exchange limitations are (a) hypoventilation, (b) diffusion limitations, (c) pulmonary blood-flow shunts, and (d) mismatching of ventilation and blood flow in different parts of the lung. The following sections explain how each of these limitations decreases $P_{a_{O_2}}$, and how the alveolar–arterial P_{O_2} difference is useful for diagnosing the causes of hypoxemia in a patient. A separate section is devoted to ventilation–perfusion mismatching because it is the most important cause of hypoxemia in healthy and diseased lungs.

Hypoventilation

By definition, hypoventilation occurs if arterial P_{CO_2} is greater than normal. Hypoventilation is the only pulmonary gas-exchange limitation that does not increase the alveolar–arterial P_{O_2} difference. Therefore, pure hypoventilation causes hypoxemia and increases arterial P_{CO_2}, but the alveolar–arterial P_{O_2} difference is normal. The magnitude of hypoxemia caused by hypoventilation is predicted by the alveolar gas equation:

$$P_{A_{O_2}} = P_{I_{O_2}} - (P_{A_{CO_2}}/R)$$

Hypoventilation increases $P_{A_{CO_2}}$, according to the inverse relationship between $\dot{V}_A$ and $P_{A_{CO_2}}$ described by the alveolar ventilation equation. If R = 1, then $P_{A_{O_2}}$ decreases 1 mm Hg for every 1 mm Hg increase in $P_{A_{CO_2}}$. Conceptually, $P_{I_{O_2}}$ represents the total amount of gas inspired because inspired CO_2 is negligible. Then gas exchange replaces each molecule of O_2 consumed with one molecule of CO_2. Hence, $P_{A_{O_2}}$ is simply the difference between $P_{I_{O_2}}$ and $P_{A_{CO_2}}$ when R = 1. However, a normal value for R is 0.8, and this magnifies the effects of hypoventilation and increased $P_{A_{CO_2}}$ on hypoxemia.

Two primary classes of problems that cause hypoventilation are (a) mechanical limitations and (b) ventilatory control abnormalities. Abnormal respiratory mechanics, such as increased airway resistance or decreased compliance with lung disease, may limit the effectiveness of the respiratory muscles in generating $\dot{V}_A$. Also, the respiratory muscles themselves may be damaged and ineffective at generating the pressures necessary for normal ventilation. In all of these cases, the ventilatory control system may be normal in terms of sensing $P_{a_{O_2}}$ and $P_{a_{CO_2}}$ changes and sending neural signals to the respiratory muscles to increase ventilation. However, abnormal control of ventilation can also occur.

Diffusion Limitation

Pulmonary diffusion limitation is defined as disequilibrium between the partial pressure of a gas in the alveoli and pulmonary capillaries. Therefore, diffusion limitations decrease $P_{a_{O_2}}$ by increasing the alveolar–arterial P_{O_2} difference, which occurs with (a) decreases in the pressure head driving O_2 diffusion across the blood–gas barrier ($P_{A_{O_2}}$), or (b) low diffusing capacity for O_2 (D_{LO_2}).

As described previously, diffusion limitations can occur in healthy adults when Pa_{O_2} is decreased at high altitude and O_2 demand is increased during hard exercise. With lung disease, the measured D_{LCO} can decrease with destruction of surface area and capillary volume (e.g., emphysema) or thickening of the blood–gas barrier (e.g., edema). However, D_{LCO} must decrease to <50% of normal before arterial hypoxemia is observed in resting patients. Ventilation–perfusion mismatching can also lower Pa_{O_2} (see below) and typically occurs with diseases that decrease D_{LCO} also. Arterial hypoxemia caused by a diffusion limitation can be relieved rapidly by increasing inspired O_2 (within several breaths); this increases the driving pressure for O_2 from the alveoli into the blood.

Shunt

The ideal models used to analyze alveolar ventilation and diffusion consider gas exchange as occurring in a single compartment so that arterial P_{O_2} equals P_{O_2} in the blood leaving the pulmonary capillaries ($Pa_{O_2} = Pc'_{O_2}$). In reality, arterial blood is not pure pulmonary capillary blood; it also includes shunt flow. *Shunt* is defined as deoxygenated venous blood flow that enters the arterial circulation without going through ventilated alveoli in the pulmonary circulation. This kind of shunt is also called *right-to-left shunt*, to distinguish it from left-to-right shunt, which shunts systemic arterial blood into pulmonary artery flow, for example with patent ductus arteriosus. Right-to-left shunt decreases Pa_{O_2} by diluting pulmonary end-capillary blood with deoxygenated venous blood.

Shunt is calculated by applying the principle of mass balance to a two-compartment model, which splits total cardiac output ($\dot{Q}t$) between a shunt flow to an unventilated compartment ($\dot{Q}s$) and flow to a normally ventilated alveolar compartment (**Fig. 43.8**) and defines shunt flow as a fraction of total cardiac output:

$$\dot{Q}s/\dot{Q}t = (Cc'_{O_2} - Ca_{O_2})/(Cc'_{O_2} - C\bar{v}_{O_2})$$

$\dot{Q}s/\dot{Q}t$ is calculated in practice by measuring arterial and mixed-venous blood samples in an individual during 100% O_2 breathing, which removes any diffusion limitation in ventilated alveoli; therefore, $Pc'_{O_2} = Pa_{O_2} - Ca_{O_2}$ and $C\bar{v}_{O_2}$ are measured directly. Cc'_{O_2} is estimated from Pa_{O_2} using an O_2–blood equilibrium curve, where Pa_{O_2} is calculated from the alveolar gas equation. (It should be noted, however, that $F_{I_{O_2}}$ appears in the constant "F" in the alveolar gas equation, and this constant should not be neglected when $F_{I_{O_2}} = 1.0$.)

The effect of shunt on Pa_{O_2} is illustrated in **Figure 43.9**. Alveolar and end-capillary Pa_{O_2} are predicted to be more than 600 mm Hg during pure O_2 breathing. However, shunt significantly decreases Pa_{O_2} because of the shape of the O_2–blood equilibrium curve. The large increase in P_{O_2} with O_2 breathing does not increase Cc'_{O_2} enough to offset the low level of $C\bar{v}_{O_2}$. Therefore, persistent hypoxemia during 100% O_2 breathing indicates a shunt. If Pa_{O_2} can be increased above 150 mm Hg during O_2 breathing, and cardiac output is normal, then 1% shunt increases the alveolar–arterial P_{O_2} difference by about 20 mm Hg.

In healthy adults, shunt during O_2 breathing averages <5% of cardiac output, including (a) venous blood from the bronchial circulation that drains directly into the pulmonary veins, and (b) venous blood from the coronary circulation that enters the left ventricle through the Thebesian veins. If shunt is calculated during room air breathing, it is called *venous admixture*. Venous admixture is larger than the shunt during O_2 breathing because it is an "as if" shunt, which includes the effects of low P_{O_2} from poorly ventilated alveoli. Hence, venous admixture occurs in healthy lungs because of ventilation–perfusion mismatching, as described in the next section.

Shunts in the newborn are common, especially during transition to air breathing. Most newborns with pulmonary

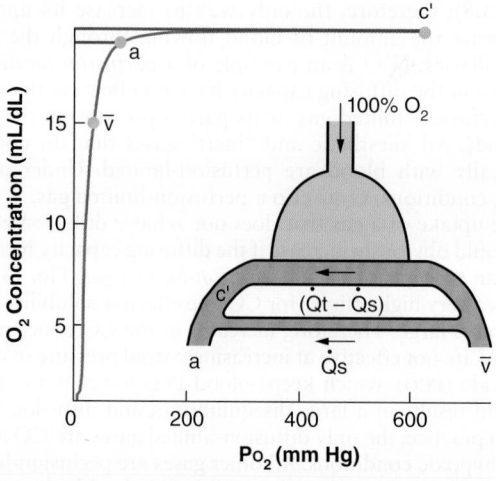

FIGURE 43.9. Two-compartment model for shunt flow ($\dot{Q}s$) and effective pulmonary blood flow ($\dot{Q}t - \dot{Q}s$). Oxygen–blood equilibrium curve illustrates how small shunt flows of mixed-venous blood ($\dot{Q}$) significantly decrease P_{O_2} in arterial blood (a) relative to P_{O_2} in end-capillary blood leaving the alveoli (c'). (From Powell FL. Pulmonary gas exchange. In: Johnson LR, ed. *Essential Medical Physiology*. 3rd ed. London, England: Elsevier/Academic Press, 2003, with permission.)

hypertension have a PDA if pulmonary arterial pressure exceeds systemic arterial pressure. Measuring Pa_{O_2} simultaneously from the preductal area (upper right chest or right radial artery) and the postductal area (umbilical artery, left radial artery, or legs) can measure this shunt. Dual pulse oximeters or transcutaneous electrodes are noninvasive methods to continuously monitor this shunt.

Ventilation–Perfusion Mismatching

Mismatching of ventilation and blood flow in different parts of the lung is the most common cause of hypoxemia and increased alveolar–arterial P_{O_2} differences in health and disease. It is also the most complicated mechanism of hypoxemia and will be approached in two steps. First, the effect of the alveolar ventilation–perfusion ratio ($\dot{V}A/\dot{Q}$) on Pa_{O_2} is described for an ideal lung. Second, the mechanisms that result in heterogeneity between $\dot{V}A/\dot{Q}$ ratios in different parts of lungs and the effect of this on Pa_{O_2} are considered. It is important to understand that only this second factor increases the alveolar–arterial P_{O_2} difference.

The $\dot{V}A/\dot{Q}$ Ratio

The effects of $\dot{V}A/\dot{Q}$ on Pa_{O_2} were introduced in the section on alveolar ventilation. Pa_{O_2} increases with $\dot{V}A$ according to the alveolar ventilation and alveolar gas equations. $\dot{V}A/\dot{Q}$ adds the concept of blood flow. If $\dot{Q}$ suddenly increases and removes more O_2 from the alveoli (recall that O_2 is normally a perfusion-limited gas), then Pa_{O_2} will decrease. However, if $\dot{V}A$ increases O_2 delivery to match increased O_2 removal (returning the $\dot{V}A/\dot{Q}$ ratio to normal), then Pa_{O_2} will return to normal.

The O_2–CO_2 diagram (**Fig. 43.10**) shows the effects of changing $\dot{V}A/\dot{Q}$ in an ideal lung, modeled as a single alveolus in a steady state, with no shunts or diffusion limitations. The $\dot{V}A/\dot{Q}$ line on the O_2–CO_2 diagram shows all of the possible combination of Pco_2 and P_{O_2} that can occur in this ideal lung with $\dot{V}A/\dot{Q}$ ratios ranging from 0 to infinity. When $\dot{V}A/\dot{Q} = 0$, a shunt is indicated. With shunt, alveolar P_{O_2} will equilibrate with mixed-venous blood so the $\dot{V}A/\dot{Q} = 0$ point corresponds to $P\bar{v}_{O_2}$ and $P\bar{v}_{CO_2}$. Dead space is indicated when $\dot{V}A/\dot{Q}$ is

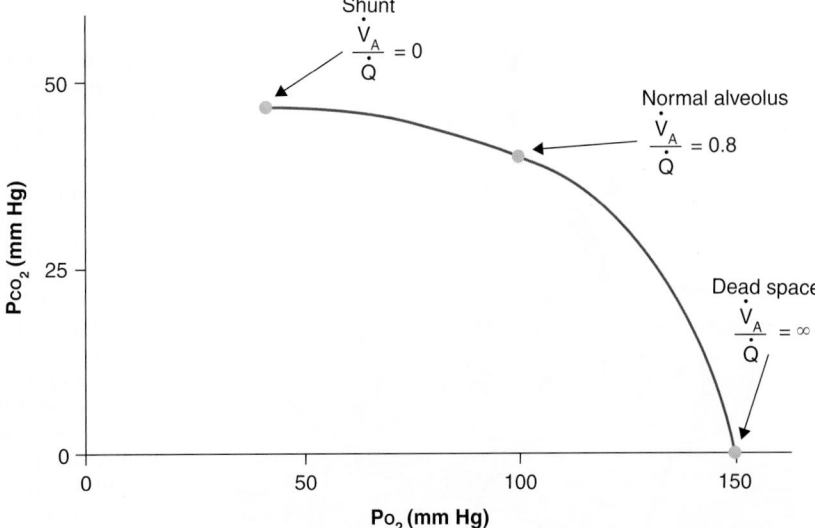

FIGURE 43.10. O_2–CO_2 diagram. The ventilation–perfusion curve describes all possible Po_2–Pco_2 combinations in the alveoli [in an ideal lung ($P_{AO_2} = P_{aO_2}$)]. Mixed-venous values occur in alveoli with no ventilation (shunt) and inspired values occur in alveoli with no perfusion (dead space). (From Powell FL. Pulmonary gas exchange. In: Johnson LR, ed. *Essential Medical Physiology*. 3rd ed. London, England: Elsevier/Academic Press, 2003, with permission.)

infinite. As dead space receives no blood flow, this alveolus equilibrates with inspired gas, and the infinite $\dot{V}_A/\dot{Q}$ point corresponds to P_{IO_2} and P_{ICO_2}, which = 0 in normal room air. "Normal" P_{ACO_2} and P_{AO_2} points are shown for $\dot{V}_A/\dot{Q} = 0.8$.

The important point to notice about the $\dot{V}_A/\dot{Q}$ line is that changes in $\dot{V}_A/\dot{Q}$ around the normal value affect P_{AO_2} more than they affect P_{ACO_2} (**Fig. 43.9**, note the scale for CO_2 is twice the scale for O_2). This generalization holds even if the $\dot{V}_A/\dot{Q}$ line is altered by changing mixed-venous or inspired gas (i.e., the end points), or by physiologic changes in the O_2–blood or CO_2–blood equilibrium curves (which determine the exact shape of the $\dot{V}_A/\dot{Q}$ line).

$\dot{V}_A/\dot{Q}$ Mismatching Between Different Lung Regions

In adult lungs, total alveolar ventilation and cardiac output must be distributed between some 300 million alveoli. Not surprisingly, these distributions are not perfect, resulting in $\dot{V}_A/\dot{Q}$ heterogeneity, or different $\dot{V}_A/\dot{Q}$ ratios in different parts of the lung. $\dot{V}_A/\dot{Q}$ mismatching refers to spatial $\dot{V}_A/\dot{Q}$ heterogeneity between functional units of gas exchange, which correspond anatomically to the *acinus*, or the collection of alveoli distal to a terminal bronchiole. This does not refer to a deviation in the overall $\dot{V}_A/\dot{Q}$ ratio from 1. Changes in the $\dot{V}_A/\dot{Q}$ ratio of an ideal lung (or a single alveolus) affect P_{AO_2} as described above (**Fig. 43.10**) and the alveolar–arterial P_{O_2} difference does not increase. In contrast, $\dot{V}_A/\dot{Q}$ mismatching *between* lung units *increases* the alveolar–arterial P_{O_2} difference.

Regional differences in alveolar ventilation occur because of the mechanical properties of the lung. In upright adults, gravity tends to distort the lung, and alveoli in the apex are more expanded than those in the base of the lung, resulting in basal alveoli operating on a steeper part of the lung's compliance curve, so that $\dot{V}_A$ is greater at the bottom than at the top of the lung. $\dot{V}_A$ per unit lung volume differs by a factor of 2.5 between the top and bottom of the upright adult lung (**Fig. 43.11**).

Regional differences in blood flow occur because of the effects of gravity on the pulmonary circulation, as described previously. Briefly, capillary pressure is greater at the bottom than at the top of the upright lung, which reduces local vascular resistance at the bottom of the lungs and increases regional blood flow. **Figure 43.10** illustrates that $\dot{Q}$ per unit lung volume changes by a factor of 6 between the top and bottom of the upright adult lung, or relatively more than $\dot{V}_A$. The net result is a large decrease in $\dot{V}_A/\dot{Q}$ between the top and bottom of upright adult lungs (**Fig. 43.11**). This $\dot{V}_A/\dot{Q}$ heterogeneity

between different regions of the lung leads to regional differences in P_{AO_2} and P_{ACO_2}, corresponding to differences predicted by the $\dot{V}_A/\dot{Q}$ line on the CO_2–O_2 diagram (**Fig. 43.10**).

Figure 43.12 illustrates how $\dot{V}_A/\dot{Q}$ heterogeneity leads to hypoxemia in a three-compartment model. End-capillary P_{O_2} equals P_{AO_2} in each functional unit of gas exchange, as determined by the local $\dot{V}_A/\dot{Q}$ ratio. O_2 concentration in the "mixed" arterial blood is a flow-weighted average from all three. The average arterial O_2 concentration is not increased significantly by "high" $\dot{V}_A/\dot{Q}$ units because the blood–O_2 equilibrium curve is flat at high O_2 levels. However, the "low" $\dot{V}_A/\dot{Q}$ units decreased average arterial O_2 concentration relatively more because the blood–O_2 equilibrium curve is steep at low P_{O_2}. Consequently, mixed arterial blood is weighted toward the level in the low $\dot{V}_A/\dot{Q}$ units and P_{aO_2} is lower than the numerical average of the P_{O_2} in blood from all three units. Conversely, mixed P_{AO_2} is greater than the numerical average of P_{O_2} from the three units because the high $\dot{V}_A/\dot{Q}$ contributes more volume to mixed alveolar gas. Hence, $\dot{V}_A/\dot{Q}$ heterogeneity increases the measured alveolar–arterial P_{O_2} difference without increasing the alveolar–arterial difference in any single gas exchange unit.

$\dot{V}_A/\dot{Q}$ heterogeneity increases the alveolar–arterial partial pressure difference for any gas, including CO_2 and anesthetic

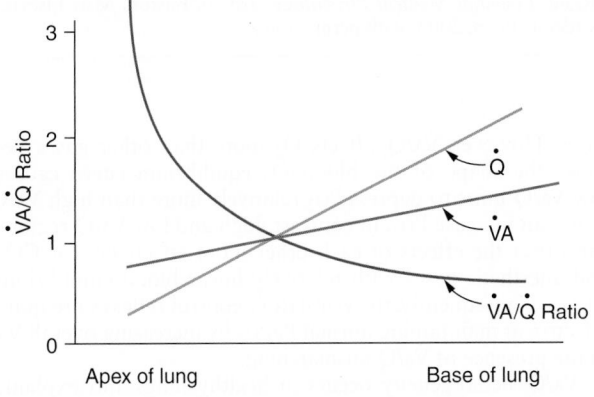

FIGURE 43.11. Gravity results in regional differences in alveolar ventilation ($\dot{V}_A$) and blood flow between the apex and base of adult lungs, which causes the $\dot{V}_A/\dot{Q}$ ratio to decrease ~2.5-fold from the top to the bottom of the lung. (From Powell FL. Pulmonary gas exchange. In: Johnson LR, ed. *Essential Medical Physiology*. 3rd ed. Boston, MA: Elsevier Academic Press, 2003, with permission.)

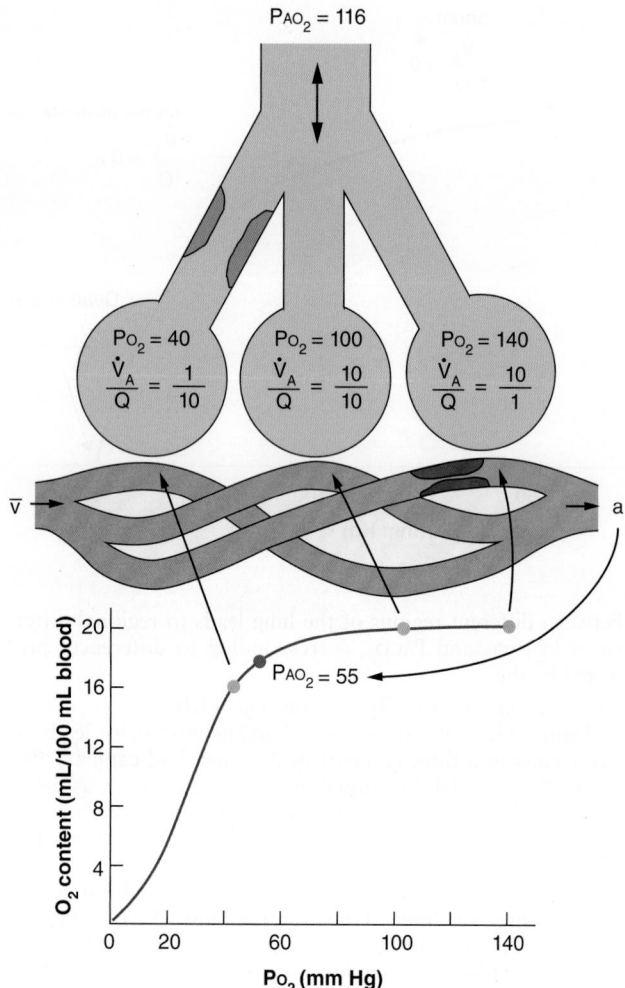

FIGURE 43.12. A three-compartment model showing how $\dot{V}_A/\dot{Q}$ differences between lung units can increase the difference between mixed-alveolar P_{O_2} ($P_{AO_2} = 116$ mm Hg) and mixed-arterial P_{O_2} ($P_{aO_2} = 55$ mm Hg). Inspired P_{O_2} is assumed normal (150 mm Hg). Alveolar P_{O_2} in any individual unit is assumed equal to the P_{O_2} in end-capillary blood from that unit (*open circles on O_2 dissociation curve in lower panel*). However, P_{O_2} in mixed arterial blood is weighted toward P_{O_2} in the low $\dot{V}_A/\dot{Q}$ units, and P_{O_2} in mixed alveolar gas is weighted toward P_{O_2} in the high $\dot{V}_A/\dot{Q}$ units. The shape of the O_2 dissociation curve also contributes to the large alveolar–arterial P_{O_2} difference. (From Powell FL. Pulmonary gas exchange. In: Johnson LR, ed. *Essential Medical Physiology.* 3rd ed. Boston, MA: Elsevier Academic Press, 2003, with permission.)

gases. However, $\dot{V}_A/\dot{Q}$ affects O_2 more than other gases because the shape of the blood–O_2 equilibrium curve causes low $\dot{V}_A/\dot{Q}$ units to depress P_{O_2} relatively more than high $\dot{V}_A/\dot{Q}$ units can increase P_{O_2}. In contrast, high and low $\dot{V}_A/\dot{Q}$ regions can offset the effects of each other more effectively for CO_2 and anesthetic gases with relatively linear blood equilibrium curves. Consequently, the ventilatory control reflexes are quite effective at maintaining normal P_{aCO_2} by increasing overall $\dot{V}_A$ in the presence of $\dot{V}_A/\dot{Q}$ mismatching.

$\dot{V}_A/\dot{Q}$ heterogeneity occurs in healthy lungs and explains the small but measurable alveolar–arterial P_{O_2} in young adults. About half of the normal $\dot{V}_A/\dot{Q}$ heterogeneity is caused by gravity-dependent differences in $\dot{V}_A$ and $\dot{Q}$ at different heights in the lung and intraregional $\dot{V}_A/\dot{Q}$ heterogeneity explains the rest.

The exact nature of $\dot{V}_A/\dot{Q}$ heterogeneity can be measured by several methods, but they are generally restricted to the

research laboratory and not useful clinically. $\dot{V}_A/\dot{Q}$ heterogeneity can be diagnosed clinically by eliminating other causes of hypoxemia. Hypoventilation can be ruled out if arterial P_{CO_2} is normal. Diffusion limitation can be ruled out if the measured D_{LCO} is at least 50% of normal or if breathing high inspired O_2 relieves hypoxemia and decreases the alveolar–arterial P_{O_2} difference. However, 100% O_2 breathing will also eliminate hypoxemia from $\dot{V}_A/\dot{Q}$ heterogeneity if all of the alveoli equilibrate with inspired P_{O_2}. With pure O_2 breathing, only O_2 and CO_2 (plus water vapor) are in the alveolar gas, and P_{AO_2} is at least 600 mm Hg in all alveoli. In practice, $\dot{V}_A/\dot{Q}$ heterogeneity includes poorly ventilated lung units; it may take up to 30 minutes to wash nitrogen out of all the alveoli during O_2 breathing. Consequently, O_2 breathing improves hypoxemia from $\dot{V}_A/\dot{Q}$ heterogeneity but not nearly as quickly as it does with a pure diffusion limitation (which requires <1 minute). If shunt is present, 100% O_2 breathing will never resolve the hypoxemia or decrease the alveolar–arterial P_{O_2} difference.

Other clinical measures of $\dot{V}_A/\dot{Q}$ heterogeneity include physiologic shunt and dead space. Low $\dot{V}_A/\dot{Q}$ gas exchange units and shunt have similar effects on P_{aO_2}. Therefore, physiologic shunt (or venous admixture) can be used to quantify $\dot{V}_A/\dot{Q}$ heterogeneity. Physiologic shunt is measured with the Berggren shunt equation (described previously) in an individual breathing less than 100% O_2 and usually room air (see the section, Shunts). $\dot{V}_A/\dot{Q}$ heterogeneity causes hypoxemia "as if" there were an increase in shunt, thereby increasing physiologic shunt. Similarly, the effects of high $\dot{V}_A/\dot{Q}$ units on P_{aO_2} resemble the effects of dead space. Therefore, physiologic dead space (see previous discussion) can be used to quantify the effects of $\dot{V}_A/\dot{Q}$ heterogeneity on P_{aO_2} and P_{aCO_2} "as if" there were an increase in anatomic dead space. Note that both physiologic shunt and dead space will be less than the actual amounts of blood flow or ventilation going to abnormal $\dot{V}_A/\dot{Q}$ units because shunt and dead space represent the extremes of the $\dot{V}_A/\dot{Q}$ ratio, and actual $\dot{V}_A/\dot{Q}$ ratios between 0 and infinity will have smaller effects on alveolar and arterial P_{O_2} and P_{CO_2} (**Fig. 43.10**).

Ventilation–perfusion inhomogeneities are common in clinical practice. The use of even small doses of supplemental O_2 is effective because the alveolar P_{O_2} is increased substantially by even small amounts of O_2. For example, the P_{AO_2} is raised by ~5–6 torr per percent supplemental O_2. In lung regions with low $\dot{V}_A/\dot{Q}$, supplemental O_2 dramatically reduces the venous admixture due to the shape of the oxyhemoglobin dissociation curve. Even an F_{IO_2} of 0.25 will produce an alveolar P_{O_2} that will saturate the blood in regions of the lung with a $\dot{V}_A/\dot{Q}$ ratio as low as 0.2. At an F_{IO_2} of 0.4, virtually all venous admixture due to ventilation–perfusion mismatch is eliminated, and the remainder of the alveolar–arterial gradient is due to pure shunt.

Carbon Dioxide Exchange

Physiologic CO_2 transport follows the same general principles described for O_2 in the previous sections. For example, the Fick principle was used previously to calculate P_{aCO_2}; the Fick principle can also be used to calculate the normal arterial–venous CO_2 concentration difference:

$$\dot{V}_{CO_2} = \dot{Q} \, (C_{aCO_2} - C\bar{v}_{CO_2})$$

For normal values of $\dot{V}_{CO_2} = 240$ mL of CO_2/min and $\dot{Q} = 6$ L/min, the arterial–venous CO_2 concentration difference is 4 mL/dL.

Differences between CO_2 and O_2 exchange result mainly from (a) differences in the O_2 and CO_2 dissociation curves, and (b) differences in the effects of CO_2 and O_2 on ventilatory control reflexes. P_{CO_2} differences are much smaller than P_{O_2} differences between arterial and venous blood, although the concentrations are similar because CO_2 is more soluble in blood. As explained later, Pa_{CO_2} is the most important value in determining the resting level of ventilation, and ventilatory reflexes tend to increase $\dot{V}_A$ as much as necessary to restore normal Pa_{CO_2} when gas exchange is altered.

Hypoventilation has almost the same effect on both O_2 and CO_2. The alveolar gas equation shows that decreases in Pa_{CO_2} are only 80% of the decrease in Pa_{O_2} when R = 0.8. Increases in Pa_{CO_2} with increased arterial O_2 concentration from diffusion limitation, shunt, or $\dot{V}_A/\dot{Q}$ heterogeneity are relatively small because the blood–CO_2 equilibrium curve is so steep (i.e., only small changes in partial pressure occur for a given change in concentration).

Normal ventilatory control will increase the overall $\dot{V}$ as necessary to restore Pa_{CO_2} toward normal. In fact, some patients with shunts and low $\dot{V}_A/\dot{Q}$ units may actually have decreased Pa_{CO_2} if hypoxemia is severe enough to override the normal control of Pa_{CO}. The extra ventilation necessary to compensate for shunt and low $\dot{V}_A/\dot{Q}$ units contributes to physiologic dead space calculated by the Bohr method. The difference between physiologic and anatomic dead space is sometimes called *alveolar dead space*, which represents an "as if" amount of wasted ventilation that could explain measured CO_2 exchange if no shunt or $\dot{V}_A/\dot{Q}$ mismatching were present in the lung.

Cardiovascular and Tissue Oxygen Transport

The mitochondria are the ultimate site of O_2 consumption and CO_2 production. Hence, gas exchange also occurs in the tissues as O_2 diffuses out of the circulation to meet metabolic demands. O_2 diffuses from the alveoli into pulmonary capillary blood; it is then pumped to the tissues in arterial blood by the heart and finally diffuses back out of the systemic capillaries to mitochondria in the tissues. The heart also pumps O_2-poor venous blood back to the lungs, where it is reoxygenated. The magnitude of the Po_2 decrease between arterial and venous blood (**Fig. 43.1**) depends on both the cardiovascular O_2 delivery and tissue O_2 demand.

O_2 delivery is the product of cardiac output and arterial O_2 concentration ($\dot{Q}$ Ca_{O_2}). The tissues will extract enough O_2 to meet their needs as long as O_2 supply is sufficient. Hence, O_2 supply and demand determine venous O_2 levels. These factors are related by the Fick principle, which describes O_2 transport by the cardiovascular system as:

$$\dot{V}_{O_2} = \dot{Q}\,(Ca_{O_2} - C\bar{v}_{O_2})$$

where $\dot{V}_{O_2}$ is O_2 consumption, $\dot{Q}$ is cardiac output, and the last term is the arterial–venous O_2 concentration difference. This equation can be used to calculate cardiac output from measurements of $\dot{V}_{O_2}$ and blood O_2 concentrations.

The Fick principle can predict the arterial–venous O_2 concentration difference from adult resting values for O_2 consumption ($\dot{V}_{O_2}$ = 300 mL/min) and cardiac output ($\dot{Q}$ = 6 L/min): (300 mL of O_2/min)/(6000 mL of blood/min) = 5 mL O_2/dL blood. If the normal value for Ca_{O_2} = 20 mL of O_2/dL of blood, $C\bar{v}_{O_2}$ = 15 mL/dL. Notice that the venous O_2 level is determined by (a) the ratio of metabolism to blood flow, and (b) arterial O_2 concentration, which is determined by alveolar Po_2 and the O_2–blood equilibrium curve. The O_2–blood equilibrium curve (see the previous section, *Oxygen in Blood*) is used to convert $C\bar{v}_{O_2}$ (15 mL/dL) to mixed-venous O_2 saturation (75%) and $C\bar{v}_{O_2}$ (40 mm Hg).

The cardiovascular Fick principle is graphically presented in **Figure 43.13** to illustrate the importance of the shape of the O_2–blood equilibrium curve. In the right panel, the height of the shaded rectangle represents the arterial–venous O_2 concentration difference, and its width represents cardiac output

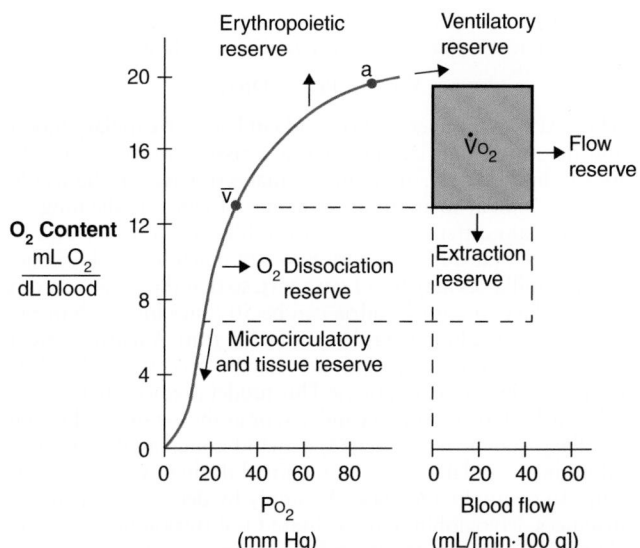

FIGURE 43.13. Graphic representation of O_2 transport by the cardiovascular system. (*Left*) O_2–blood equilibrium curve showing arterial (a) and mixed-venous ($\bar{v}$) points. (*Right*) Graphic representation of the Fick principle for cardiovascular O_2 transport. Horizontal axis is blood flow normalized to body mass; vertical axis is O_2 concentration from the left panel; shaded area is O_2 consumption. "Reserves," which can increase $\dot{V}_{O_2}$, are described in the text. (From Powell FL. Pulmonary gas exchange. In: Johnson LR, ed. *Essential Medical Physiology*. 3rd ed. London, England: Elsevier/Academic Press, 2003, with permission.)

(normalized to 100 g of body mass). The area of the rectangle is the product of these two factors, and represents $\dot{V}_{O_2}$.

Changes in $\dot{V}_{O_2}$ can be achieved by increasing cardiac output ("flow reserve") and/or increasing the arterial–venous O_2 difference. The dashed lines in **Figure 43.13** show the consequences of increasing $\dot{V}_{O_2}$ by increasing venous O_2 extraction ("extraction reserve"). Changes in $P\bar{v}_{O_2}$ are minimized with large decreases in venous O_2 concentration by the shape of the O_2–blood equilibrium curve. A right shift of the curve can increase $P\bar{v}_{O_2}$ for a given $C\bar{v}_{O_2}$ ("O_2-dissociation reserve"). Maintaining a high $P\bar{v}_{O_2}$ is important for tissue gas exchange and the "microcirculatory and tissue reserve," as discussed later. All these reserves are important mechanisms for meeting increased O_2 demands during exercise.

Increases in O_2 delivery are achieved primarily through increases in cardiac output in normoxic conditions. Increasing alveolar and arterial Po_2 is not effective at increasing Ca_{O_2} in normoxic conditions because the slope of the O_2–blood equilibrium curve is flat at normal Pa_{O_2} values ("ventilatory reserve"; Fig. 43.13). However, changes in Pa_{O_2} are much more effective at changing O_2 delivery when Po_2 is low and O_2 exchange occurs on a steeper part of the O_2–blood equilibrium curve. Changes in Hct and Hb concentration, which occur with chronic hypoxia, can increase O_2 delivery by increasing total O_2 concentration for any given Po_2 ("erythropoietic reserve"). The erythropoietic reserve is the physiologic basis for the questionable practice of "blood doping," which uses blood transfusions or artificial erythropoietin in attempts to increase maximal O_2 consumption and athletic performance.

Tissue Gas Exchange

Tissue gas exchange describes the process of O_2 moving out of systemic capillaries to the mitochondria in cells by diffusion. Therefore, O_2 consistency that is required for transport in tissues is described by Fick's first law of diffusion, similar to diffusion across the blood–gas barrier in the lung:

$$\bar{V}o_2 = \Delta Po_2 \times Dto_2)$$

where ΔPo_2 is the average Po_2 gradient between capillary blood and the mitochondria, and Dto_2 is a tissue-diffusing capacity for O_2. Interestingly, anatomic estimates of Dto_2 for the whole body are similar to anatomic estimates of Dmo_2 in the lung.

The main difference between O_2 diffusion in tissue and in the lung is that diffusion pathways are much longer in tissue. Tissue capillaries may be 50 μm apart, so that the distance from the capillary to mitochondria can be 50 times longer than the thickness of the blood–gas barrier ($<0.5\ \mu$m). A mathematical model called the *Krogh cylinder* can be used to predict Po_2 profiles in metabolizing tissue This model predicts that Po_2 in cells farthest away from a capillary, or at the venous end of the capillary, may be zero when O_2 demand is increased. However, additional capillaries may be recruited during exercise, which helps to maintain adequate O_2 supply by decreasing diffusion distances. Myoglobin may facilitate O_2 diffusion in muscle by shuttling O_2 to sites far away from a capillary also.

LUNG MECHANICS, RESPIRATORY, AND AIRWAY MUSCLES

The primary functions of the respiratory system are to transport O_2 from the environment to metabolizing cells and to remove CO_2 from the body. The first step in O_2 transport is ventilation of the lungs, which is a function of lung mechanics and the functioning of respiratory and airway muscles, as discussed in this section.

Pressure–Flow Relationships in the Respiratory System

The mammalian lung has a natural tendency to collapse. The respiratory muscles and the chest wall oppose this tendency and apply a continuous tension to the structure of the lungs to maintain lung volume at end-expiration. The tension within the lung is generated by its fibrous structure and by the gas–liquid interface in the distal airways and alveoli. The sum of the forces that make the lungs collapse is referred to as the *elastic recoil* (**Fig. 43.14**) and is reflected in the amount of pressure that must be applied across the lungs to produce both

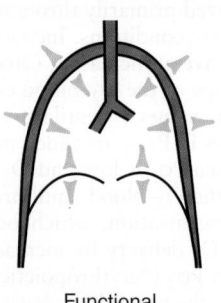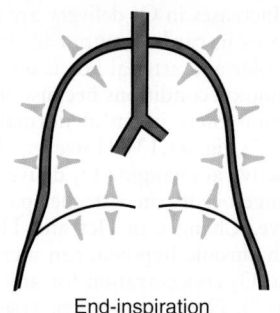

Functional residual capacity   End-inspiration

FIGURE 43.14. Elastic recoil, represented by the arrows, increases with increasing lung volume. It produces the negative pleural pressure at end-expiration. (From Heldt GP. The mechanics of breathing: developmental aspects and practical applications. In: Boynton BR, Carlo WA, Jobe AH, eds. *New Therapies for Neonatal Respiratory Failure.* Cambridge, England: Cambridge University Press, 1994, with permission.)

the end-expiratory lung volume (EELV) and changes in the lung volume with breathing. During mechanical ventilation, this pressure is predominantly the pressure applied to the endotracheal tube.

The basic relationships of pressures and flow in the respiratory system for a patient on a mechanical ventilator are shown in **Figure 43.15**. In panel A, the patient breathes spontaneously without positive end-expiratory pressure (PEEP). The respiratory muscles contract, and the pleural pressure (P_{pl}) decreases during inspiration from a negative value at end-expiration, which reflects the elastic recoil of the lungs. The transpulmonary pressure (P_{tp}), or the difference between the airway pressure (P_{aw}) and P_{pl}, also decreases, which produces the inspiratory flow (shown negative in the figure by convention). The elastic recoil of the lungs increases linearly with lung volume. The dashed lines on the P_{pl} record indicate the recoil pressure. The decrease in the transpulmonary pressure leads the elastic recoil pressure. This difference is the pressure that is needed to overcome the pulmonary resistance (P_{rs}) shown in the panel. The small decrease in P_{aw} reflects the resistance of the airway circuit. During expiration, the P_{pl} increases, and the elastic recoil of the lungs raises the alveolar pressure (PA) to produce expiratory flow. The pressure change again leads that of the elastic recoil pressure to overcome the expiratory resistance.

Panel B shows one respiratory cycle when 5 cm H_2O of PEEP is added. A small increase in the end-expiratory P_{pl} is seen, and the P_{tp} is more negative due to an increased lung volume with the addition of PEEP. Inspiratory and expiratory flows are generated by the same mechanism as the situation without PEEP. Panel C shows one respiratory cycle when a synchronized breath is given by the ventilator. The change in P_{tp} is greater, as the ventilator pressure is added to the P_{pl}, which produces a larger breath. The flow rates are higher, and P_{rs} is greater. Note that in these three breaths, the conventions for the pressures are equivalent.

The inset shows the flow–volume loops for breath A on no PEEP, B on PEEP, and on C that produced with the ventilator. The end-expiratory volumes are greater for B and C than for A. The slopes of the expiratory flow–volume curves are the same, even though shifted in volume. As discussed later, the expiratory flow limitation is independent of the effort made by either the patient or the ventilator.

In the clinical setting, measurements of pulmonary mechanics at the bedside in even the smallest infants can be made. Flow is measured with a pneumotachograph, which is a linear resistor of very low resistance that is placed on the endotracheal tube or on a face mask or nasal prongs. The P_{pl} is estimated by placing an esophageal pressure catheter in the lower thoracic esophagus. Proper measurement of esophageal pressure takes some experience, and the position of the pressure catheter is tested by performing an airway occlusion at end-expiration. The change in the airway occlusion pressure should be equal to the change in the esophageal pressure when the catheter is in proper position because, during occlusion, no resistive or elastic losses occur between the P_{pl} and the airway. Since the chest wall in infants is very compliant, it takes very little pressure to inflate it. Therefore, the airway pressure is used as the transpulmonary pressure for most clinical measurements. This must be remembered when results of the monitor on the ventilator in older children are interpreted or when the chest-wall compliance is significant, for example, in a very edematous patient.

Developmental Aspects of the Lung as They Affect Elastic Recoil

From a mechanical viewpoint, the embryology of the lung determines much of the nonsurfactant properties of the lung. Two major systems of elastic fibers distribute the stress on the

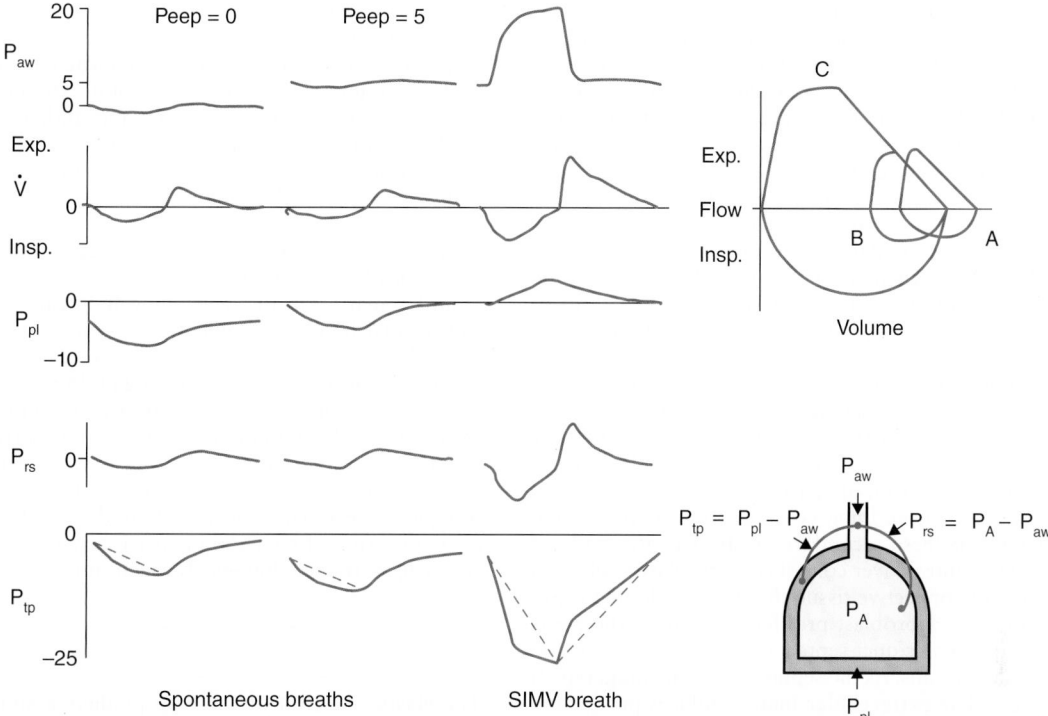

FIGURE 43.15. Recording of the airway pressure (P_{aw}), flow ($\bar{v}$), pleural pressure (P_{pl}), resistive pressure (P_{rs}), and transpulmonary pressure (P_{tp}) as defined in the diagram in the lower right corner. Three breaths are represented: two during spontaneous breathing with and without PEEP and one synchronized, intermittent, mandatory ventilator (SIMV) breath. Note that the P_{pl} is higher at end-expiration while on PEEP and that the P_{tp} is more negative. The elastic line (*dashed*) has been added to the P_{tp} and represents the pressure needed to overcome the elastic recoil. The fall in P_{tp} leads the elastic line during inspiration and lags during expiration. The difference is P_{rs}, or the pressure needed to overcome the resistance of the airways and the lung tissue. The flow–volume loops of the three breaths are shown in the upper right corner. Note that the end-expiratory volume is larger in breaths B and C and that the expiratory flow–volume relationship is parallel in all three breaths. This represents the intrinsic flow limitation of the lungs that is independent of effort and only dependent on elastic recoil.

lung that is induced by decreases in intrapleural pressure so as to evenly inflate the lung. The first system is that of the airways, and the second originates from the pleural surface that grows toward the hilum. The airway system provides the even distribution of gas to the alveolar ducts, and the second system provides the matrix to evenly distribute the tension from the pleural surface to the alveolar ducts. These two systems develop simultaneously as the lung bud grows centripetally into the pleural space.

Lung development begins with the formation of the respiratory diverticulum at 4 weeks from the ventral wall of the foregut. The location of the bud on the gut tube is determined by the transcription factor TBX4, and the epithelium of the lungs, larynx, and bronchi are of endodermal origin. The cartilaginous, muscular, and connective tissues are derived from the splanchnic mesoderm that surrounds the foregut. The respiratory diverticulum expands caudally, and the tracheoesophageal ridges grow to separate it from the foregut. The ridges close to form the tracheoesophageal septum. The lung bud then expands into the mesoderm, forming the pleural space.

The lung bud forms the tracheal and two lateral out-pouchings—the bronchial buds that become the main stem bronchi by the fifth week of gestation. Subsequent growth of the lung buds extends into the body cavity, forming the pericardioperitoneal canals, which are ultimately separated from the peritoneal and pericardial cavities by the pleuroperitoneal and pleuropericardial folds. The mesoderm, which covers the outside of the lungs, develops into the visceral pleura. The somatic mesoderm layer, covering the body wall in the inside, becomes

the parietal pleura. The secondary bronchi divide repeatedly in a dichotomous fashion, forming the 10 segmental bronchi on the right and left, which are completed by the 17th week of gestation.

Differentiation of the lungs is under the control of the extracellular matrix that is laid down in the mesenchyme, into which the developing lung bud grows. During the pseudoglandular stage (5–16 weeks), airway branching is complete to the level of primitive respiratory bronchioles. Each terminal bronchiole divides into two or more respiratory bronchioles, which in turn divide into three to six alveolar ducts by the end of the canalicular stage (16–24 weeks). The saccular stage then continues until birth, during which time the distal airways are differentiated until near term. Alveolarization occurs for many months after birth.

Much of the early branching is controlled by the presence of the proteoglycan syndecan, a molecule that is abundant in the mesenchyme and is critical to the formation of epithelial tubes. Epidermal growth factor supports the branching of the growing epithelium during the first 25 weeks of gestation. Fibronectin, a glycoprotein, directs the growth of the basement membrane and the formation of the collagen matrix. It ties the growth of the cells and the basement membrane via fibril formation, and it has three domains that bind to the collagen, heparin sulfate proteoglycans, and cells. The growth and branching of the epithelium into the airway structure are also under control of laminin, a large glycoprotein that is part of the basement membrane. Cellular interactions with laminin are mediated primarily through several molecules that bind to it: entactin for cell adherence; dystroglycan, which directs differentiation; and perlecan, which transduces stretching and is a signaling molecule for the action of dystroglycan. Cadherins are calcium-dependent molecules that direct the adherence of cells to each other, helping to form the cellular sheets and tubes of the alveolar ducts that will act as a vestibule for several additional generations of alveoli.

The terminal saccular stage, beginning at 25 weeks of gestation, is characterized by further widening of the airspaces and rearrangement of capillaries to form a more intimate air–blood interface. Airway extension and branching through the stage of alveolation is at least in part under the control of fibroblast growth factor 10 (FGF-10) that is produced by the mesenchymal cells, leading to thinning of the alveolar membrane and reduction in the mesenchymal mass. The process of thinning of the alveolar septae is associated with a highly organized deposition of elastin fibrils in the transitory alveolar ducts. Elastin is later deposited maximally in secondary crests, which protrude into future airspaces that form the foundation of future alveolation. Lung volume grows by protrusion and lengthening of these secondary crests that are made of three layers. The central layer consists of fibroblastic cells and is associated with connective tissue that has developing capillaries on both sides. Fibroblast proliferation causes the crests to develop into alveolar duct septae and produce elastin, collagen, and proteoglycans. As the septae are lengthening, type II cells proliferate. The extracellular matrix induces production of surfactant-associated proteins A, B, and C. As the septae thin out, the capillaries remodel to form a single capillary network. This fusion forms the central lamina densa of the basement membrane, which contains type IV collagen, which is extremely strong.

The main elastic elements of the lung are collagen and elastin. Collagen fibers are formed by binding fibrils together in a gel-like matrix with proteoglycans. Collagen is not very distensible but, when combined with elastin, forms interwoven strands similar to that of rubber and cotton, which are elastic with limited distensibility.

The central airways have two such collagen/elastin layers: one longitudinal and one circumferential, which grow out past the respiratory and terminal bronchioles and become thin fibers that spiral into the alveolar ducts. This network of fibers strengthens the mouth of the alveolar ducts and extends to several distal generations of alveoli. These fibers are continuous with the fibers of the blood vessels, airways, and the pleura.

Simultaneous with the development of the airways, the thick primary layer of the visceral pleura forms a system of fiber bags that grow toward the hilum from the pleural surface. These bags hold the developing subunits of the developing airways, of which the bottoms equally divide the pleural surface. The sides of each bag interdigitate with the fibers of the interlobular septae. The interlobular septae are fused with the alveolar septae they enclose. Tension developed at the pleural surfaces is thereby transmitted tangentially to the pleural surface and toward the hilum through the interlobular septae. This arrangement gives the lung isotropy, which makes each alveolar unit mechanically interdependent with its neighbors, so that the entire network is homogeneously self-inflating. In addition, spiral fibers at the level of the alveolar ducts maintain their patency when stretched during inspiration to enhance even entry of gas into each vestibule. The alveolar duct structure is especially important for maintaining alveolar expansion at low lung volumes. It is estimated that this system of fiber bags that originate from the pleura contributes 30% to the overall elastic recoil of the lung.

The airway and pleural systems may complement each other in distributing mechanical stress. They also form the continuous interstitial matrix, from the alveolar septae to both of the perivascular and pleural lymphatics, for transport of lymph to

keep the air–blood interface from flooding. Although collagen and elastin are virtually always found together throughout the lung, they have independent mechanical effects that depend on lung volume. Destruction of elastin experimentally causes increased lung compliance at low and middle volume ranges (25%–40% of TLC). Experimental destruction of collagen by collagenase results in an increase in compliance at high lung volumes. Together, elastin and collagen contribute to a smooth pressure–volume (PV) curve, with stabilization of stress from the pleural surface, down to the smallest unit of gas exchange, and centrally to the hilum.

Inflammation in the developing lung can dramatically affect normal lung development. The synthesis of FGF-10 that helps direct airway branching and alveolation can be inhibited in the saccular stage (beginning at 25 weeks gestation) by the activation of the NF-kB receptor by oxidant stress (hyperoxia), classical inflammation (chorioamnionitis or postnatal infection, and the proinflammatory environment of intensive care), and mechanical stress (mechanical ventilation). This is thought to be a major mechanism in the development of BPD, a complication of neonatal intensive care in up to 50% of the surviving extremely low–birth weight infants.

Surface Tension and Elastic Recoil

The elastic skeleton of the lung predicts a simple, linear relationship between the volume of the lung and the pressure applied across it. It has long been observed that pulmonary surfactant contributes greatly to the PV characteristics of the lungs. The observations just noted also demonstrate that the surfactant system of the lung contributes to this hysteresis in the PV curves.

In the first approximation, the PV relationship of an air–liquid interface can be modeled with a bubble on the end of a blow-tube, by the law of La Place (**Fig. 43.16**):

$$P = 2 \times \text{surface tension}/r$$

where P is the pressure inside the bubble (minus the pressure outside the bubble) and r the radius of the bubble.

The two theoretical alveoli presented in **Figure 43.16** have unequal radii. If the surface tension were the same in both alveoli, the alveolus with the smaller diameter would collapse into the larger one, as the pressure exerted by the surface-tension forces would be greater by this law. The fact that the pulmonary surfactant decreases on compression overcomes this problem and makes lung inflation more homogeneous.

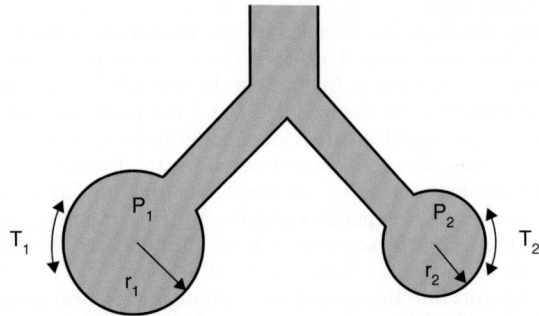

FIGURE 43.16. The distension pressure of two theoretical alveoli connected by a single airway is related by the law of La Place. In the larger alveolus, $P_1 = 2 \times \text{tension}_1/r_1$, and in the smaller alveolus, $P_2 = 2 \times \text{tension}_2/r_2$. If $\text{tension}_1 = \text{tension}_2$, the distending pressure of the smaller alveolus will be greater and will collapse into the larger alveolus. Alternatively, a greater pressure will be required to recruit the smaller alveolus, leading to overdistension and barotrauma to the larger alveolus.

Measurements of the alveolar septal stretch provide an estimate of the radius of the alveoli and the surface-area changes of the lung during inflation. The relationship of surface tension to area has been studied by three approaches in an effort to understand the in vivo behavior of the PV curve. The first was the study of surface-tension measurements in vitro on a Langmuir–Wilhelmy balance during compression of surface-active film from lung extracts. The second approach was to construct PV curves in air-filled lungs and compare them to curves obtained from lungs filled with liquids (perfluorocarbons and kerosene) with fixed interfacial surface tension. The third approach was by direct estimate of alveolar surface tension using a microdroplet, wherein a micropipette (diameter $\sim 2~\mu m$) was used to place a drop of fluorocarbon directly onto the alveolar surface through a micropuncture in the pleural surface. The fluorocarbon has a fixed low surface tension and spreads into a lens the diameter of which reflects the surface tension of the alveolar film.

Data from these three approaches are summarized in a plot of lung volume versus P_{tp} in **Figure 43.17**. Even though less hysteresis was seen in the PV curve in lungs inflated with liquids of fixed surface tension, it still represented several centimeters of H_2O, which may represent tissue "creep," as described in solid mechanics, or tissue remodeling. Inflation with liquids of increasing surface tension requires more pressure to open the lung, but lung inflation proceeds with equal ease until 80% of TLC is reached, when the compliance is markedly decreased. The equilibrium surface tension value of 25 dynes/cm, derived from the Langmuir–Wilhelmy balance data, has been added to the data interpolated from both the liquid-filled lung and micropipette measurements. The inflections in the PV curves for gas-filled lungs near 16 and 20 dynes/cm, by direct micropuncture measurements, coincide with this equilibrium

value of the surface tension. At lung volumes above this point, the film spreads and tissue forces become dominant due to the collagen in the elastic skeleton. The value of surface tension, measured at TLC (30 dynes/cm), is less than that of the fixed fluorocarbon (32 dynes/cm), corresponding to a considerably decreased transpulmonary pressure at TLC. At lung volumes below this point, film compression leads to marked lowering of the surface tension and collapse of the film. At 40% of TLC, values as low as 0.5 dynes/cm have been measured in cats.

The currently accepted model for the dynamics of the surfactant effect can be summarized as follows. Assuming that a sufficient amount of surfactant exists, surface-active material (SAM) is actively adsorbed to the surface film during lung inflation. Relatively bare areas of the air–liquid interface are filled from the subphase from the previously compressed packed film. During lung deflation, differential desorption of the SAM occurs. Areas with little SAM are squeezed out of the film by SAM-rich areas. At low lung volumes, the film is compressed far from the equilibrium state, becomes unstable, and is desorbed from the monolayer film. Saturated lipid, dipalmitoylphosphatidylcholine (DPPC), produces the most stable interfacial film, especially on compression. As the lipid is compressed, non-DPPC elements are squeezed out of the monolayer. Surfactant-associated proteins interact with the lipid monolayer to organize the process of adsorption–desorption from inspiration to expiration and stabilize the film under compression by decreasing the free energy of this transition. A number of synthetic peptides have been developed that can perform similarly to native surfactant-associated peptides. These peptides are being used to develop a new generation of totally synthetic replacement surfactant formulations. This process can explain much of the hysteresis of the PV curve.

The alveolar duct is pivotal to this process and is the point at which the interplay between the elastic skeleton and surfactant is most important. When lungs are washed of surfactant, the alveolar ducts increase in size, which suggests that alveolar collapse redistributes the stress to the more proximal airway. At 23–30 weeks gestation, the time when many infants are born prematurely, the elastic fibers are not yet developed and cannot bear the additional stress imposed by alveolar collapse. This effect is even greater during mechanical ventilation. Rupture of both the airways and the capillaries at this point causes the formation of edema and hyaline membranes, which are the primary pathologic precursor of BPD.

Surfactant replacement therapy is a well-established therapy for premature infants with respiratory distress syndrome (RDS). The surfactant is manufactured from the washings or homogenates of animal lungs and processed for separation of surfactant lipids and surfactant-associated proteins. The primary synthetic surfactant, Exosurf, is not as effective as natural surfactants and has fallen out of common clinical usage. Therapy is most effective if given either prophylactically at birth or within the first 2 hours after birth. Infants treated with surfactant have rapidly decreased O_2 and ventilatory requirements and can be weaned from mechanical ventilation more quickly. Surfactant therapy is most effective for infants of 26–32 weeks' gestation, probably because their primitive alveoli are smaller than the nonalveolated saccules of younger infants and because of unavoidable complications of extreme prematurity. The use of prenatal steroids accelerates the appearance of endogenous surfactant and makes extremely premature infants more responsive to replacement therapy. A number of surfactants are commercially available, and despite manufacturers' claims or individual preferences, they have not been shown to have different effects in clinical trials. Surfactant therapy has also been used in treatment of neonatal pneumonia and congenital diaphragmatic hernia in small studies that have demonstrated positive effects.

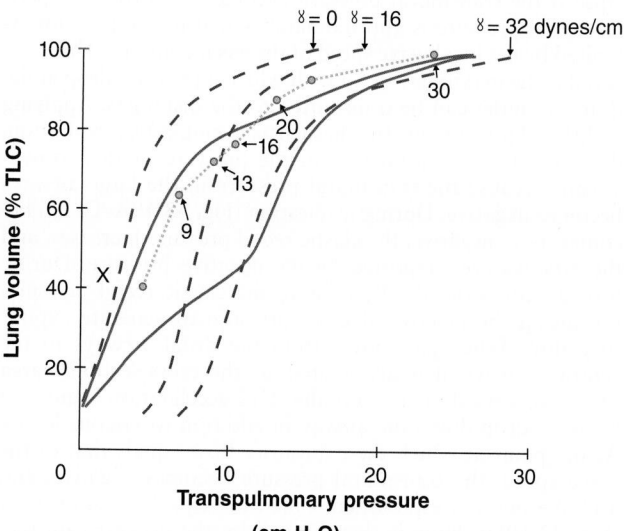

FIGURE 43.17. Summary of surface-tension effects on elastic recoil based on several types of experimental data. The solid curve shows the air inflation, with hysteresis. Dashed curves are deflation pressure–volume curves for lungs filled with perfluorocarbon liquids with fixed surface tensions of 0, 16, and 32 dyne/cm. Data points from direct alveolar surface-tension estimates using a micropuncture technique are shown joined by the dotted line. The X represents alveolar-wash surface tension in rat lungs. These four different techniques confirm the significant decrease in surface tension in vivo with lung inflation, which maintains lung stability at low lung volumes. TLC, total lung capacity. (From Heldt GP. The mechanics of breathing: Developmental aspects and practical applications. In: Boynton BR, Carlo WA, Jobe AH, eds. *New Therapies for Neonatal Respiratory Failure*. Cambridge, England: Cambridge University Press, 1994, with permission.)

7   ## Flow Limitation

The second element in the mechanics of breathing concerns where and how airflow limitation occurs. In purely elastic systems, the energy put into the system that causes deformation is released back to the system when the deformation is relieved. In purely resistive systems, the energy put into the system during deformation is lost, usually in the form of heat. This dissipation of energy in the lungs occurs both in the airways and tissue. The pulmonary resistance is usually thought to be that of the airways during spontaneous breathing, as most pathological states involve bronchoconstriction. Nevertheless, tissue resistive forces can more than equal those of the airways under certain pathologic states.

Airway resistance is usually modeled by the aerodynamics of flow through tubes. Flow through the airways is driven by a pressure drop between the alveoli and the atmosphere or the endotracheal tube in the case of ventilated patients. The decrease in the pressure in the direction of the gas flow represents a dissipation of the kinetic energy of the gas. The rate of this dissipation depends on the conditions of flow. In laminar flow, the gas has a precisely ordered velocity profile, with the flow in the center being the greatest, decreasing to zero at the walls (**Fig. 43.18**). A boundary layer of very low flow forms at the walls. Laminar flow was first described by Poiseuille and theoretically has the least possible pressure drop or energy dissipation for a given flow and tube diameter:

$$\text{Resistance} = (8 \times \text{viscosity} \times \text{length})/(\pi \times \text{radius}^4)$$

The resistance is dependent on the viscosity of the gas and is inversely proportional to the fourth power of the radius. This is an important consideration when endotracheal tubes are of very small radius, as in the premature infant (<3.5 mm internal diameter).

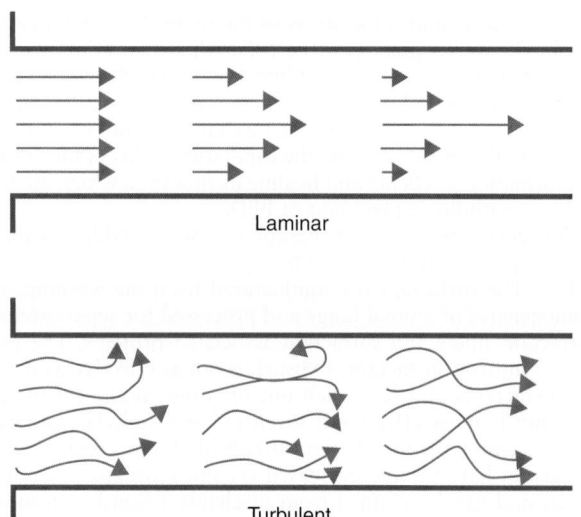

Laminar

Turbulent

FIGURE 43.18. Flow-velocity profiles for laminar and turbulent flow represented by velocity vectors during entry flow into a long, straight tube. In laminar flow, the profile is flat across the diameter of the tube but quickly attains a predictable parabolic profile. A balance is maintained between the convective force on the gas down the tube (related to density and velocity) and the viscous resistive forces developing the profile. In turbulent flow, random axial movement of the gas dissipates energy at a greater rate than during laminar flow, which is dependent on the density of the gas rather than on its viscosity. A very thin boundary layer forms next to the wall of the tube. Turbulent flow develops only at the peripheral airways, and laminar flow is characteristic of the larger airways.

A balance exists between the inertia of the gas and the viscous drag, which is expressed by the Reynolds number. This dimensionless number is proportional to the product of the gas density, the flow rate, and the diameter of the tube. When the Reynolds number is greater than ~2300, the inertial forces are greater than the viscous forces, and laminar flow cannot be established. Rather than moving in smooth lines straight down the tube, the gas is turbulent. The axial movement of the gas increases the pressure against the walls, and energy is dissipated at a greater rate than during laminar flow. During laminar flow, the pressure drop is proportional to the flow rate. During turbulent flow, the pressure drop is proportional to the square of the flow rate.

A third type of flow regime is that of unsteady flow. If the gas in a long, straight tube is moved in a laminar fashion by a sinusoidal pressure generator, the flow profile has to reverse with each cycle. The gas in the center of the tube must reverse velocity greater than that close to the wall, and the flow lags behind that of the gas close to the wall (asymmetric gas flow profiles), causing an underestimation of the pressure drop at points of maximal flow acceleration. This type of flow regime is most applicable during high-frequency oscillatory ventilation. It is also relevant in small endotracheal tubes for newborns during conventional ventilation of >60 breaths/min, when the inertia of the gas can cause an underestimation of airway pressure of several cm H_2O.

These simplified theoretical models can help to explain the pressure drop in the airways. The airways are not long, straight tubes, but branches. From estimates of the Reynolds number and the dimensions of the airways obtained from anatomic casts, flow in the large airways is turbulent. Laminar flow becomes established between the 4th and the 15th generation of airways, depending on the flow rate of the gas.

The airways are also flexible tubes. The airway will collapse if the transmural pressure becomes negative. The peribronchial pressure is approximately equal to the P_{pl}. Flow is limited by the local wave speed of the gas it contains. The wave speed is the maximum speed with which a pressure drop at the thoracic outlet can be transmitted to the distal gas. Applying additional pressure upstream, such as during active expiration, does not allow transmission of the pressure or flow downstream because the transmural pressure in the large airways becomes negative. During inspiration (**Fig. 43.19A–C**), P_{pl} becomes more negative, the elastic recoil pressure increases, and the airways are supported by the negative pressure. During forced expiration, the P_{pl} adds to the elastic recoil pressure, producing the positive alveolar pressure to generate expiratory flow. When gas moves from the distal airways to the central airways, it is accelerated, as the cross-sectional area of the airways decreases rapidly. This acceleration requires a pressure drop down the airway in addition to viscous losses. At the point at which the expiratory flow equals that of the wave speed, the transmural pressure becomes negative, and a choke point is established, called the *equal pressure point* (**Fig. 43.19D**). Flow is then limited by the downstream segment and is independent of the expiratory effort. The higher the flow, the greater the pressure required. Therefore, the transmural pressure primarily reflects the elastic recoil pressure of the lung, because the lung parenchyma is closely linked mechanically to the peribronchiolar space. Thus, at high lung volume, when recoil pressure is greatest, the flow limitation is in the second and third generation of bronchi. At lower lung volumes, flow decreases and the sites of flow limitation move peripherally. This phenomenon explains the linear shape of the expiratory flow–volume curve that is the basis of spirometric pulmonary function testing. Many measures applied to this curve, such as the fraction of the expired volume at one second, mid-expiratory flow, etc., are used to detect flow limitation at various points in the airways.

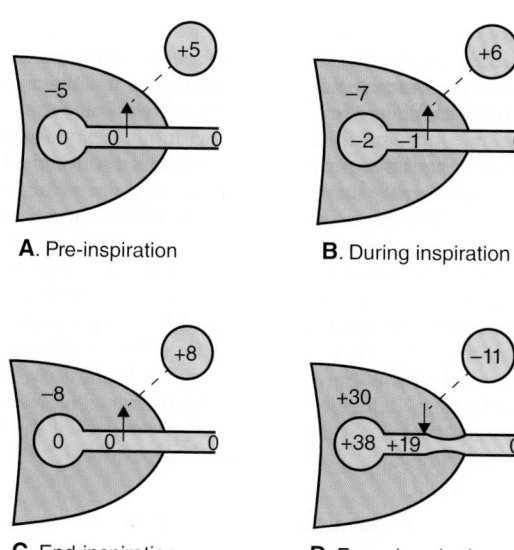

A. Pre-inspiration   **B.** During inspiration

C. End-inspiration   **D.** Forced expiration

FIGURE 43.19. Dynamic compression of the airways during forced expiration, caused by negative transmural airway pressure (**D**) beyond the equal pressure point. (From Powell FL. Mechanics of breathing. In: Johnson LR, ed. *Essential Medical Physiology*. 3rd ed. London, England: Elsevier/Academic Press, 2003, with permission.)

The P_{rs} is a mixture of laminar and turbulent flow. Flow in the large airways is turbulent, and the resistance in this flow regime is density dependent. In cases of extreme large-airway obstruction, the resistance can be reduced by reducing the density of the gas with the use of a mixture of helium and O_2 (Heliox). This reduction may help to relieve obstruction such that intubation of the patient is avoided. The primary limitation is the O_2 requirement of the patient that dilutes the helium in the mixture.

5   A Consolidated Model of the Dynamics of Breathing

The respiratory system has been classically modeled as a three-element physical system, consisting of an elastance, a resistance, and an inertial element (**Fig. 43.20**). The equation of motion for this system is as follows:

$$Ptp = [(l/C) \times V] + (R \times \dot{V}) + (I \times \dot{V})$$

where P_{tp} is the pressure inflating the lungs (transpulmonary pressure), C the compliance, or 1/elastance, R the resistance,

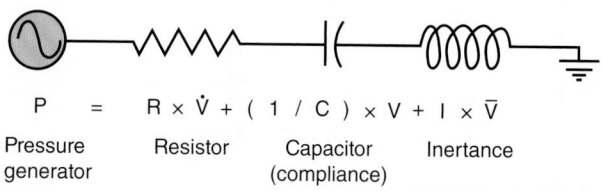

$$P = R \times \dot{V} + (1/C) \times V + I \times \overline{V}$$

Pressure generator   Resistor   Capacitor (compliance)   Inertance

FIGURE 43.20. Model of the respiratory system consisting of a pressure generator (the transpulmonary pressure) and a resistor, capacitor, and inertance connected in series. The values of the individual components are computed from the measurements of the pressure and flow into and out of the system, using the equation of motion to fit the experimental data. (From Heldt GP. The mechanics of breathing: Developmental aspects and practical applications. In: Boynton BR, Carlo WA, Jobe AH, eds. *New Therapies for Neonatal Respiratory Failure*. Cambridge, England: Cambridge University Press, 1994, with permission.)

I the inertance, V the lung volume, $\dot{V}$ the gas flow, and $\dot{V}$ the convective gas acceleration.

The compliance represents the elastic recoil of the lung, determined by the tissue elastic and surface-tension forces. The resistance consists of the dissipative forces of the airways and tissue. As described previously, the airway component is both laminar and turbulent, or transitional, as described by Röhrer's equation:

$$P_{resistive} = Kl \times (\dot{V} + K2) \times \dot{V}^2$$

where K1 and K2 are coefficients that represent the relative proportions of laminar and turbulent resistive drops.

It is also possible to describe the motion of the respiratory system using a mechanical model rather than the electrical model above. The pressure (P) that is required to deliver a tidal breath is given by:

$$P = V_T/C_R + (V_T/Ti * R_R) + PEEP_{total}$$
$$\downarrow \qquad \qquad \downarrow$$
$$P_{elastic} \qquad P_{resistive}$$

where V_T is the tidal volume, C_R the compliance of the respiratory system, $V_T/C_R = P_{elastic}$ is the elastic pressure, T_i the inspiratory time, V_T/T_i the flow, $(V_T/T_i * R_R) = P_{resistive}$ is the resistive pressure, R_R the resistance of the respiratory system, $PEEP_{total}$ the total positive end-expiratory pressure (i.e., alveolar pressure at end-expiration).

Clinical Implications

For most purposes, these parameters can be calculated by fitting these equations to the measured transpulmonary pressure and the resultant flow. These parameters are often displayed on ventilators and ventilator monitors and are of clinical usefulness in understanding and directing ventilator management. Infants who are treated with surfactant, for example, have increases in compliance, as would be expected from recruitment of alveoli. Infants who develop BPD have higher resistances in the first week of life and lower compliances. The use of steroids in BPD has been shown to yield improved gas exchange, reduced mechanical ventilatory requirements, and improvements in compliance. Bronchodilator therapy in infants with BPD results in statistically significant reductions in pulmonary resistance. Theophylline has been reported to reduce pulmonary and airway resistances in infants with BPD and, when used in conjunction with diuretics, appears to have a synergistic effect. The response to acute and chronic administration of furosemide has mixed results.

This classical model has limitations, which may explain why bedside measurement of mechanics tends to be nonspecific as a diagnostic test and why the parameters have a large coefficient of variation even within a diagnostic category. No standards have been established for the method of measurement, nor do age- or weight-related standard curves exist, as in spirometry. Ideally, both the compliance and resistance should be normalized for lung volume; however, lung volume is difficult or impossible to measure in mechanically ventilated infants or children due to leaks around the endotracheal tube. Finally, during mechanical ventilation, significant gas trapping occurs when either the resistance or compliance is high. The lung does not have adequate time to empty during the relatively short expiratory times. As mentioned previously, certain ventilator paradigms also lead to an underestimation of the airway pressure that is seen at the alveolar level due to turbulent flow in the proximal airway where the airway pressure is measured. Thus, these parameters can change due to changes in the pattern of mechanical ventilation and not due to changes in the mechanics of the lung.

Another limitation of the classical method of calculating mechanics is due to nonlinearities of both elastance and resistance. The elastic and resistive properties of the lung are coupled: At lung volumes above 50% TLC, elastic recoil increases with a decrease in the resistance because airway diameters are larger at higher lung volumes. This phenomenon explains why the flow–volume curves are straight over a large range of lung volumes during forced expiration in normal lungs and even in disease states. The time constant of the lungs, or the product of the compliance and resistance, remains constant even though both the compliance and resistance are changing in a complementary fashion.

The apparent complementary coupling between elastance and resistance has been studied by several methods in an effort to interpret these measurements. Several mechanisms are proposed, including interactions of the fiber network of the pleura and terminal airways; tissue "creep," or dissipative changes in lung tissue with large inflations; the cross-bridge dynamics of smooth airway muscle; and surface-active forces. The latter appears to be plausible, especially in young children. The alveolar duct is the site of the interaction of the elastic skeleton and the SAM. Although the alveolar duct does not impose a great contribution to total pulmonary resistance, it does interact with the process of alveolar recruitment. The act of cyclic recruitment (popping open) and derecruitment represents a resistive loss. By the same mechanism, recruitment and derecruitment would involve changes in the elastance. Both the patency of the alveolar ducts and stability of the alveoli are greatly under the influence of surfactant. Thus, this could be a single mechanism to explain this coupling.

8 The Forced Oscillation Technique

Another approach toward understanding the coupling of elastance and resistance is to measure the input impedance of the respiratory system with the forced oscillation technique (FOT). The measurement is made by applying a pressure signal composed of a range of frequencies using a loudspeaker at the airway opening. This method has the advantage that it does not involve the performance of any maneuver on the part of the patient and, in infants, takes advantage of the Hering–Breuer reflex. Impedance is a complex description of the resistance, elastance, and inertance of a system. It consists of resistive and reactive components when changes in pressure and flow are in phase or out of phase, respectively. The airway and tissue elastances and the inertia of the accelerated air in the airways determine the reactive components. The resistance

and reactance are computed as a function of the frequency as shown in **Figure 43.21**. The resulting spectra demonstrate different and separate mechanical properties of the airways and acinar tissues. At low frequencies, tissue resistance and reactance change in a curvilinear fashion with frequency. At higher frequencies, the tissue properties become less pronounced and the spectrum reveals the reactance and inertance primarily of the airways. The resonant frequency is where the reactance is zero, which represents the frequency at which the tissue-reactive and inertial components are equal. The parameters derived from fitting a model to these spectra include the airway resistance and inertance (R_{aw} and I_{aw}, respectively) and the tissue damping (G) and elastance (H). The coupling of the elastance and resistance of the tissues is the *hysteresity*, or the ratio of G to H. The use of these parameters gives a more complete description of the viscoelastic properties of the lung, as their coupling is significant and their separation is difficult.

Clinical Relevance of FOT

The FOT has provided unique insight into the pathophysiology of infants that has not been provided by classical calculation methods. The contribution of tissue viscoelasticity to total respiratory system impedance is significant, as demonstrated by studies both on surfactant-deficient lambs and human infants. The separation of the airway and tissue components using FOT is implied by the hysteresity, which is decreased after antenatal steroids, antenatal endotoxin exposure, postnatal surfactant treatment, and increasing postnatal size. The dependence of mechanics on the volume of the lungs is more dependent on the mechanical properties of the tissues, and the airway resistance measured by this method is relatively unchanged by increases in lung volume.

In older children, standards are available for some of these parameters based on height. The resistance at 10 Hz is concordant with spirometry obtained in most asthmatic children. The resistance at 5 or 8 Hz is significantly increased in children after maximal bronchodilation and is correlated with the clinical asthma score during acute asthmatic attacks. At age 8, significant increases in the resistance at 5 Hz and the decreases in the resonant frequency were found in children with BPD over a population of normal controls. Good agreement is also seen between the resistance at 5 Hz and airway resistance measured by body plethysmograph. Bronchodilator responsiveness can be demonstrated in children <7 years, with a cutoff value of an increase of 41% in the baseline resistance at 5 Hz. These

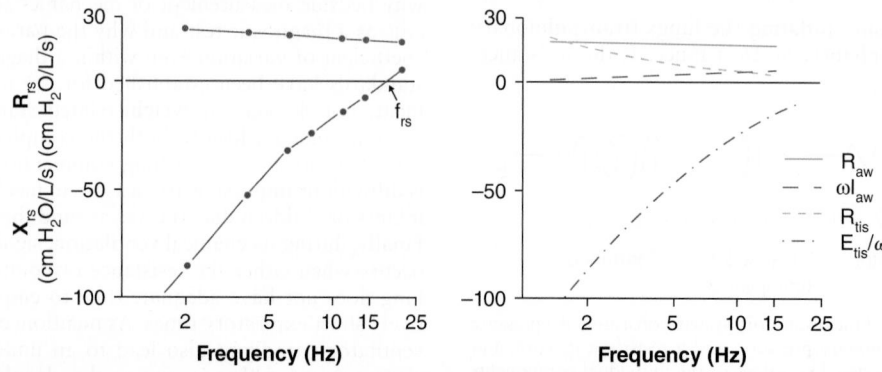

FIGURE 43.21. Impedance spectra measured by forced oscillation technique. **A:** The system resistance and reactance (X_{rs}) are plotted against frequency content of the forced pressure waveform. The point at which X_{rs} is zero is the resonant frequency (f_{rs}) of the system. **B:** The data are fit to a model that separates the contributions of the airway (R_{aw}) and tissue (R_{tis}) resistances, reactive elastance (E_{tis}/ω), and reactive inertance (ωI_{aw}) from the spectra in the left panel. (Adapted from Gappa M, Pillow JJ, Allen J, et al. Lung function tests in neonates and infants with chronic lung disease: Lung and chest-wall mechanics. *Pediatr Pulmonol* 2006;41:291–317.)

changes appear to be longer-lasting with the FOT method than with spirometry after the administration of short-acting bronchodilators. In methacholine bronchoprovocation testing, the reactance at 5 Hz is more sensitive than the FEV_1 or the specific airway conductance, especially in children aged 4–6 years.

The FOT is, in theory, easily applied to young children. It requires the patient to simply breathe quietly on the measurement system. The resistance and reactance at frequencies below 10 Hz correspond well with spirometric values for bronchodilation and bronchial challenge testing. In a recent study of asthmatics aged 2–4 years at high risk of developing asthma, it was possible to train them to perform both spirometry and the FOT with >80% success with one training session. The application of the method to intubated infants and children is surprisingly more difficult because the endotracheal tube imposes a very large resistance that masks the changes in the calculated parameters. The method, with more standardization, will be a valuable tool in the future for assessing the effects of therapies on mechanically ventilated patients.

PULMONARY CIRCULATION

Although the systemic and pulmonary circulations share many common features, they also exhibit important differences in structure and function, and further differences occur in the pulmonary circulation with developmental changes between the fetus, newborn, and adult.

The adult pulmonary circulation is unique because the lung is the only organ to receive the entire cardiac output. The systemic and pulmonary circulations are organized "in series," so the cardiac output from the right ventricle to the lung equals the cardiac output from the left ventricle to the entire rest of the body in children and adults (although this is different in the fetus and during parturition, see below). Hence, resistance to blood flow must be low in the lungs and this also allows lower pressures in the pulmonary circulation. Low pressure is beneficial for reducing the stress on the extremely delicate pulmonary capillaries, which are as thin as possible to enhance diffusion of O_2 and CO_2.

Fetal and Perinatal Pulmonary Circulation

The anatomy of the pulmonary circulation in the fetus differs from the adult because the placenta is the primary gas-exchange organ in utero (**Fig. 43.22**). Fetal blood flows into the placenta through the umbilical arteries. O_2 diffuses from the maternal circulation into the fetus. Diffusion is relatively inefficient in the placenta compared to the lungs, but O_2 transfer is enhanced by the high O_2 affinity of fetal, compared to adult, Hb (see the section Oxygen in Blood). The end result is a maximum PO_2 of 30 torr in the fetal circulation in blood leaving the placenta and entering the inferior vena cava. Some of the oxygenated blood in the inferior vena cava flows directly from the right into the left atrium via the foramen ovale, which is a normal connection between the right and left atria in the fetus. Hence, blood leaving the left ventricle in the aorta has a relatively high PO_2, diluted only by other systemic venous blood in the inferior vena cava to ~25 torr. The rest of the blood returning from the inferior vena cava mixes with blood returning from the superior vena cava in the right atrium, reducing the PO_2 to 19 torr in the right ventricle.

Blood is pumped from the right ventricle into the pulmonary artery, but only 10% flows into the lungs; the remainder goes into the aorta via the ductus arteriosus, which is a shunt vessel normally present in the fetus. Some pulmonary blood flow is important for the normal development of the lungs and the surfactant system. The ductus arteriosus joins the

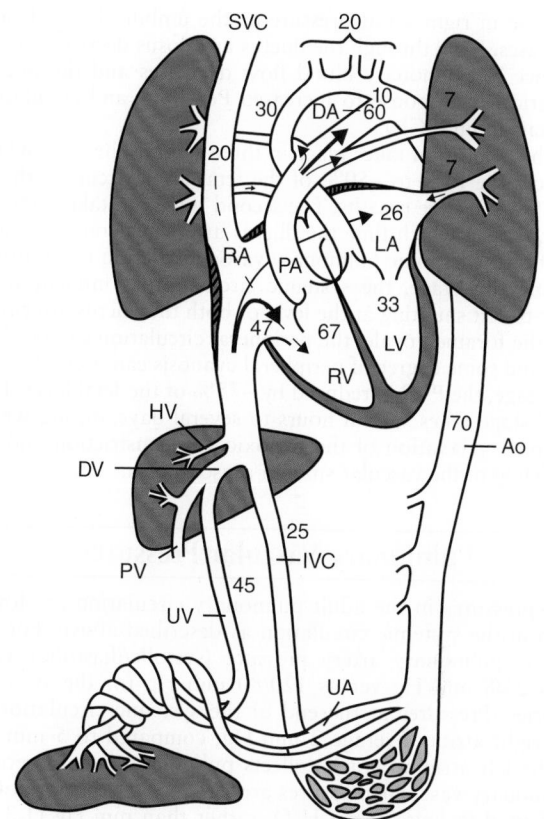

FIGURE 43.22. Schematic representation of human fetal circulation. Numbers refer to blood flow in milliliters per minute through the main vascular channels. SVC, superior vena cava; DA, ductus arteriosus; RA, right atrium; PA, pulmonary artery; LA, left atrium; RV, right ventricle, LV, left ventricle; Ao, aorta; HV, hepatic vein; DV, ductus venosus; PV, portal vein; UV, umbilical vein; IVC, inferior vena cava; UA, umbilical artery. (Adapted from Comroe JH. *Physiology of Respiration.* Chicago, IL: Year Book Medical Publishers, 1965.)

aorta distal to the carotid and coronary arteries. This anatomy maximizes the PO_2 in blood that perfuses the brain and heart because PO_2 is greater in the left ventricle than in the right ventricle (**Fig. 43.22**). It is important to note that the output of the left ventricle is only approximately half that of the right ventricle in the fetus, in contrast to being equal in adults, because the ductus arteriosus shunts blood from the pulmonary to systemic circulations.

The pressures in the fetal pulmonary circulation are high relative to adults because of the connection between the pulmonary arteries and the ductus arteriosus, which comes from the left ventricle, as well as high pulmonary vascular resistance (PVR) in the fetal lung. Hypoxic pulmonary vasoconstriction helps to keep the PVR high in the fetus. The high pressures, and perhaps hypoxia, produce a well-developed smooth muscle layer in the pulmonary circulation of the fetus, especially compared to the adult.

At birth at term, the first few breaths expand the lungs, filling them with a relatively high O_2 tension, which makes several dramatic changes in the physiology. Hypoxic pulmonary vasoconstriction is reduced, and the pulmonary capillaries are stretched, opening them so that pulmonary blood flow greatly increases. The infant breathes deeply and rapidly, lowering the PCO_2 and raising the pH, which enhances the effects of decreased hypoxic pulmonary vasoconstriction (described later).

With the increase in pulmonary blood flow, upon air breathing at birth, left atrial pressure increases, thus closing the flap-like foramen ovale. This closure is also aided by the decrease in right atrial pressure as the umbilical blood flow decreases. Flow through the ductus arteriosus decreases as resistance to pulmonary blood flow decreases and the ductus constricts in response to increased Po_2, NO, and circulating prostaglandin (PGI_2).

This transition takes place in three stages. The first, which reduces the PVR to ~50% of the fetal level, occurs with the first few effective breaths. The second stage can take up to ~1 hour, during which time the ductus arteriosus constricts, and relief of the hypoxic pulmonary vasoconstriction is stabilized. During this stage, the systemic circulation is influenced by right-to-left shunting at the level of both the ductus arteriosus and the foramen ovale; the peripheral circulation can be sluggish and some degree of peripheral cyanosis can occur. During this stage, the PVR is reduced by ~75% of the fetal level. This third stage takes several hours to several days, during which complete relaxation of the hypoxic vasoconstriction and remodeling of the vascular smooth muscle occur.

❾ Pulmonary Vascular Pressures

The pressures in the adult pulmonary circulation are lower than in the systemic circulation as described above. For example, pulmonary artery pressure (systolic/diastolic) averages 25/8 mm Hg versus 120/80 mm Hg for the systemic arteries. Pressures at the end of the systemic circulation in the right atrium average 2 mm Hg, compared to 5 mm Hg in the left atrium, which collects pulmonary venous return. Pulmonary vascular pressures are so low that they are often measured in units of cm H_2O, rather than mm Hg (1.3 cm H_2O = 1 mm Hg).

The pressure drop from artery to vein is more uniform in the adult pulmonary circulation than in the systemic circulation, and this is the same for the circulation in newborns. Direct and indirect measurements indicate that pulmonary capillary pressure is near the mean of the average pulmonary arterial and venous pressures. Pulmonary capillaries contribute to more of the total pressure drop from artery to vein than do systemic capillaries. Therefore, capillaries are more important determinants of total resistance in the pulmonary circulation as described later, compared with the systemic circulation.

Pulmonary vascular pressures can be altered by a variety of physiologic and pathologic conditions in adults. For example, mean pulmonary artery pressure can increase to more than 35 mm Hg during high levels of cardiac output with exercise, and pulmonary venous pressure can exceed 25 mm Hg in patients with congestive heart failure. Pressures in the pulmonary circulation also vary with normal breathing and especially with artificial ventilation because the heart is surrounded by the intrapleural space, in which pressure decreases during normal inspiration and increases during normal expiration (see the previous section on lung mechanics). During positive-pressure artificial ventilation, alveolar and intrapleural pressures may increase considerably during inflation, leading to large increases in pulmonary circulatory pressures. However, PVR can increase also, which may limit pulmonary blood flow and cardiac output, for example, during artificial ventilation with a bag connected to a facemask in neonatal resuscitation. Persistent pulmonary hypertension is common in most infants with pulmonary disease as a result of delayed transition to postnatal circulation. It is especially pronounced in larger infants whose pulmonary vasculature is more developed, but can significantly complicate RDS. Infants at greatest risk are those who have been asphyxiated in utero and have aspirated meconium, or who have congenital pneumonia. Increases in PVR, which is labile in these patients, increase right-to-left shunting through a patent ductus arteriosus or the foramen ovale.

Pulmonary Vascular Resistance

PVR is low compared to systemic vascular resistance, as described above. The hydraulic analogy of Ohm's law can be used to define PVR as:

$$\Delta P = \dot{Q} \times PVR$$

where ΔP is the pressure gradient between the inlet and outlet of a vessel (in mm Hg or cm H_2O) and $\dot{Q}$ is blood flow (L/minute). PVR is, by definition, the resistance for both lungs; in adults, it is ~1.7 (mm Hg × minute)/L for a normal cardiac output of 6 L/min, with an average pressure drop of 10 mm Hg from the pulmonary artery to left atrium.

The resistance to flow through a vessel obviously depends on its dimensions. The dimensions of pulmonary vessels are strongly influenced by several external forces, unlike the situation for rigid pipes in a plumbing system, or even in systemic arteries. The fundamental geometry of the pulmonary capillary network is also different from pipes or systemic capillaries. The numerous capillaries in the alveolar wall constitute an almost continuous sheet for blood flow between two flat membranes held together by numerous posts—called *sheet flow*; the resistance to sheet flow can be less than the resistance to flow through a network of tubes. Therefore, Poiseuille's law, which describes the resistance to laminar flow through a tube (resistance = 8 viscosity length/π radius^4), is not strictly correct for predicting the effects of pulmonary capillary dimensions on resistance. Still, PVR increases with length and decreases by a power function of the radius of pulmonary capillaries. Because the pulmonary capillaries are surrounded by the open air spaces of the alveoli, rather than solid tissue as in other organs, the primary determinant of vessel size in the lungs is the *transmural pressure*, which is the pressure difference between inside and outside the vessel:

$$P_{transmural} = P_{inside} - P_{outside}$$

Therefore, increasing pulmonary arterial pressure will increase flow by two mechanisms: (a) the pressure gradient for Ohm's law is increased, and (b) the transmural pressure is increased, which increases vessel size and decreases PVR (**Fig. 43.23**).

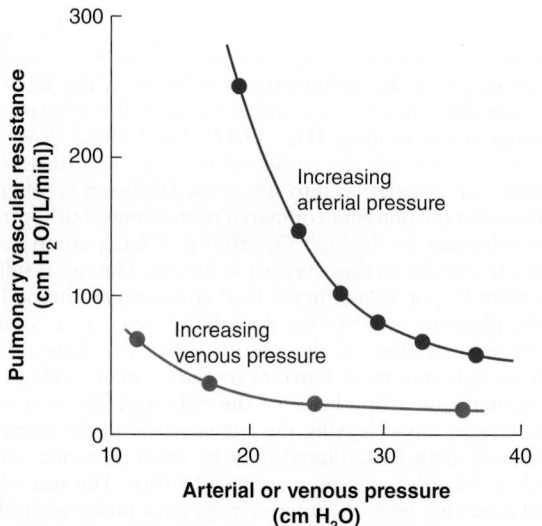

FIGURE 43.23. Pulmonary vascular resistance decreases with increasing pulmonary arterial or pulmonary venous pressure, while the other pressure is held constant. This is because increasing either pressure increases capillary pressure and causes recruitment and distention of pulmonary capillaries. (From Powell FL. Structure and function of the respiratory system. In: Johnson LR, ed. *Essential Medical Physiology*. 3rd ed. London, England: Elsevier/Academic Press, 2003, with permission.)

Increasing pulmonary venous pressure also decreases PVR, because some of this pressure increase is transmitted to the capillaries and dilates them. As discussed previously, capillary dimensions significantly affect PVR. Hence, pressure affects resistance and vice versa in the pulmonary circulation, in contrast to the systemic circulation, in which resistance primarily affects pressure.

Alveolar pressure is the outside pressure for calculating transmural pressure in most pulmonary vessels. Alveolar pressure varies with the ventilatory cycle, but it is generally near zero (i.e., atmospheric pressure). Therefore, vascular pressure is the primary determinant of transmural pressure in pulmonary vessels. However, large positive alveolar pressures can occur with some forms of artificial ventilation, as well as with PEEP and this will tend to collapse pulmonary capillaries. In other words, increased pulmonary arterial or venous pressures do not necessarily decrease vascular resistance unless they result in an increased transmural pressure, which dilates the capillaries.

Increasing transmural pressure can affect capillary dimensions by two mechanisms: recruitment and distention. At very low pressures, some capillaries may be closed, and increasing pressure will open them by recruitment. At higher pressures, capillaries are already open, but they may be distended or stretched by increased transmural pressure. Together, recruitment and distention increase the effective size of the pulmonary capillaries and reduce PVR. However, it is important to note that circulation in the fetal and neonatal lung is *not* as pliable because all of the capillaries are apparently fully recruited, even under resting conditions. Experiments on newborn lambs show no increase in pulmonary diffusing capacity with increased left atrial pressure, in contrast to the increase observed in adult sheep (and humans), as capillary recruitment and distention increase the surface area available for diffusion.

Another important determinant of pulmonary vessel size is lung volume, but this effect differs for different types of vessels. Extra-alveolar vessels are surrounded by lung parenchyma, which acts as a tether or support structure to hold the vessels open. Therefore, lung volume is more important than alveolar pressure for determining the dimensions of extra-alveolar vessels. At high lung volumes, above functional residual capacity (FRC), the extra-alveolar vessels are pulled open by tissues outside the vessels. At low lung volumes, below FRC, this tethering effect is reduced and the extra-alveolar vessels narrow. Also, extra-alveolar vessels have smooth muscle and elastic tissue that tend to collapse the vessels at low lung volumes. The effects of lung volume on alveolar vessels are generally opposite to those on extra-alveolar vessels. At high lung volumes, the alveolar wall is stretched and becomes thinner, reducing the size of pulmonary capillaries and alveolar vessels. At low lung volumes, the alveolar wall is not stretched and the capillaries relax open to a wider dimension. These factors account for why PVR is at its lowest at FRC—the lung volume at which normal tidal ventilation occurs. When EELV is greater or less than physiologic FRC, PVR is increased.

Hypoxic Pulmonary Vasoconstriction

Hypoxic pulmonary vasoconstriction is an important physiologic mechanism that actively controls PVR and blood flow in the lungs and is critical to the transition from the fetal to neonatal circulation during birth. The initiation of air breathing relieves hypoxic pulmonary vasoconstriction, so pulmonary blood flow increases and pulmonary vascular pressures drop, which promotes closing of the foramen ovale and ductus arteriosus. Since HPV was originally described by Von Euler and Lijestrand in 1946, researchers have determined

that it is a direct response of vascular smooth muscle in pulmonary arterioles to decreased alveolar P_{O_2}. Currently, the bulk of evidence suggests that the primary sensor is mitochondria in pulmonary artery smooth muscle cells, which increases production of ROS during hypoxia. However, several ion channels and signaling pathways have been suggested to explain the transduction and effector mechanisms of HPV. This includes several types of O_2-sensitive K^+ channels; the hypoxic inhibition of K^+ current induces membrane depolarization and thereby activates L-type Ca^{2+} channels with ensuing calcium influx and calcium-dependent vasoconstriction, as well as the voltage-gated K^+ channel (Kv) family, TASK, and Ca^{2+}-activated K^+ channel (BKca), which appears to be the most important mechanism in the fetus. The effects of PGI_2 and NO to vasodilate the lungs in neonates as oxygen increases during birth may involve their direct activation of BKca too.

Figure 43.24 shows the effect of P_{O_2} on PVR in a neonatal animal; the main effect of P_{O_2} occurs at very low levels, which are found in the fetus. However, blood pH has an effect even at high P_{O_2}; therefore, the increase in pH with the onset of air breathing will also reduce PVR as P_{O_2} increases with air breathing in the newborn. Other physiologic factors capable of influencing the adult pulmonary circulation include a weak vasoconstrictor effect from the sympathetic nervous system and potent vasoconstriction by endothelins, which are peptides released by pulmonary epithelial and endothelial cells (e.g., endothelin-1). The fetal and neonatal pulmonary circulations are also exquisitely sensitive to vasoconstrictors such as serotonin and vasodilators such as acetylcholine because the smooth muscle is more developed to support the higher pressures compared to adults.

In air breathing, hypoxic pulmonary vasoconstriction allows blood flow to be selectively diverted away from poorly ventilated regions of the lung. Hence, hypoxic pulmonary vasoconstriction is important for matching unequal distributions of ventilation and blood flow throughout the lungs and can improve gas exchange efficiency in lungs with $\dot{V}A/\dot{Q}$ mismatching (see above).

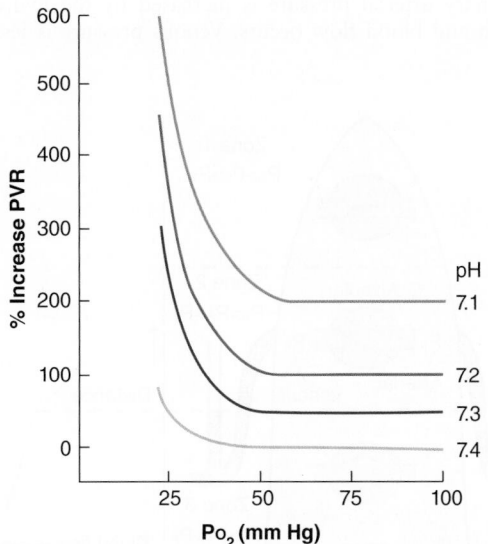

FIGURE 43.24. Deceasing O_2 in inspired gas (P_{O_2}) causes hypoxic vasoconstriction and increases pulmonary vascular resistance (PVR). Arterial acidosis exaggerates this effect in newborns and may be important in helping to establish the adult pattern of circulation. (From Powell FL. Pulmonary gas exchange. In: Johnson LR, ed. *Essential Medical Physiology*. 3rd ed. Boston, MA: Elsevier Academic Press, 2003, with permission.)

Distribution of Pulmonary Blood Flow

In the upright adult human lung, gravity affects the physical factors determining pulmonary capillary dimensions and PVR that were discussed above. As explained in more detail below, gravity increases vascular pressures in the bottom of the upright lung. This recruits and distends capillaries to decrease resistance and increase flow in the bottom, compared to the top, of the lung. Such effects are smaller in neonatal lungs because they are smaller but the principles are important and certainly apply as body and lung size increase.

The pulmonary vasculature can be considered a continuous hydrostatic column that is ~30 cm tall in the upright human lung, meaning that a hydrostatic pressure difference of 30 cm H_2O (or 23 mm Hg) exists between vessels at the top and bottom of the lung. As this pressure difference is nearly as large as the pulmonary artery pressure, it has profound effects on regional distribution of blood flow. Evidence for a gravitational mechanism includes (a) a reduction in the gradient for blood flow when in the erect posture and during exercise, when pulmonary arterial pressure increases, and (b) a reduction in the gradient of blood flow when in the supine posture. A dorsal–ventral gradient can be measured when the subject is supine, and the vertical gradient is reversed in those suspended upside down.

These effects using the zone model for pulmonary blood flow developed by West are illustrated in **Figure 43.25**. This model conceptually divides the lung into three zones to explain how gravity affects blood flow up the lung through alveolar vessels at different heights. Zone 1 occurs at the top of the lung, where the pulmonary arterial pressure is not sufficient to pump blood to the top. In this case, pulmonary arterial pressure is less than the hydrostatic pressure column between the heart and the top of the lung. Alveolar pressure, even if zero, is greater than arterial pressure; thus, the capillaries collapse. Zone 1 does not occur in the normal adult lung because the normal pulmonary arterial pressure (30 cm H_2O) is greater than the height of a water column between the heart and top of the lung (~15 cm).

Zone 2 describes the flow in most of the lung, where pulmonary arterial pressure is increased by the hydrostatic column and blood flow occurs. Venous pressure is less than alveolar pressure because these veins may be below the level of the heart. Intravascular pressure decreases from the arterial to venous level along the capillary, and at some point the alveolar pressure exceeds capillary pressure, which tends to collapse the capillary and reduce flow. If flow actually stops, pressure in the capillary rises toward the arterial level until the capillary is reopened and flow resumes. In zone 2, the relevant pressure gradient driving blood flow is the arterial–alveolar difference, and venous pressure is not important in determining zone 2 flow. Systems with flow determined by upstream and outside (instead of downstream) pressures are called *Starling resistors*. **Figure 43.25** shows flow progressively increasing down zone 2 because the hydrostatic column increases arterial pressure while alveolar pressure is constant. Both capillary recruitment and distention can contribute to increased flow in zone 2.

Zone 3 occurs near the bottom of the lung, where venous pressure is increased sufficiently by the hydrostatic column to exceed alveolar pressure. Therefore, the arterial–venous pressure difference determines blood flow in zone 3. **Figure 43.25** shows flow increasing down zone 3 because the hydrostatic column distends the capillaries.

Despite the success of the zone model at predicting regional differences in blood flow based on gravity, additional differences in blood flow occur, for example, between the center and the periphery of the lung at a given height up the lung. Local stresses and the anatomic details of vascular branching may contribute to such intraregional heterogeneity of blood flow. Local stresses may result from differences in vasoconstrictor influences (see next section) as well as bronchoconstriction, which affect pulmonary capillary dimensions through traction. Intraregional heterogeneity may explain up to half of the total heterogeneity of blood flow in the lungs.

The effect of mechanical ventilation on lung zones should also be considered. Clearly, elevating alveolar pressure will convert some zone 2 lung to zone 1 and some zone 3 lung to zone 2. Thus, the effect of mechanical ventilation could be to create more alveolar dead space (zone 1) and improve V/Q matching in zone 2.

Bronchial Circulation

The bronchial circulation is part of the systemic circulation and serves the metabolic needs of the large airways and blood vessels. The bronchial circulation does not extend to the gas-exchange zone, which is served by the pulmonary circulation. Bronchial arteries arise from the aorta and intercostal arteries, and the bronchial circulation returns blood to the heart by two pathways. Bronchial veins from large airways return approximately half of the bronchial blood flow to the right heart via the azygos vein. The other half of the bronchial circulation drains directly into the pulmonary circulation, which adds deoxygenated blood to the oxygenated blood returning to the left heart and constitutes an anatomic shunt. As blood flow through the bronchial circulation is only 1%–2% of cardiac output in normal adults, this anatomic shunt has a small effect on arterial O_2 levels. However, the anatomic shunt can increase with inflammatory airway disease and cause significant reductions in arterial O_2 levels.

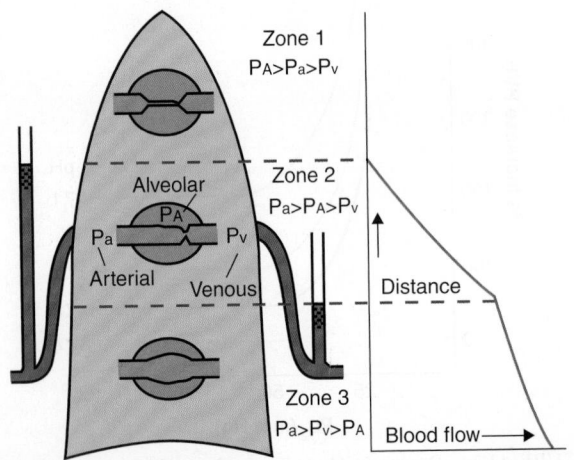

FIGURE 43.25. West's zone model for pulmonary blood flow predicts increasing blood flow down the lung because of the effects of gravity on pressures. Pa, arterial pressure; PA, alveolar pressure; Pv, venous pressure. (From Powell FL. Structure and function of the respiratory system. In: Johnson LR, ed. *Essential Medical Physiology*. 3rd ed. London, England: Elsevier/Academic Press, 2003, with permission.)

Lung Fluid Balance

The pulmonary capillaries are extremely thin and contain pores that allow fluid to move across their walls. Starling's law describes the forces that govern fluid flux across capillary walls, and an understanding of these forces is necessary to understand both normal and pathologic lung fluid balance. Starling's law states that the net fluid flux across the capillary depends on a balance of hydrostatic forces (P) and colloid osmotic (or oncotic) forces (π):

$$\text{Net fluid flux} = K_{fc}\,[(Pc - Pi) - \sigma(\pi c - \pi i)]$$

where K_{fc} is a filtration coefficient that depends on the total surface area of the capillary and the number and size of pores in the capillary. Hydrostatic pressure in the capillary (Pc) tends to move fluid out, and interstitial pressure (Pi) tends to move fluid into the capillary. Conversely, capillary osmotic pressure (πc) tends to hold fluid in the capillary, and interstitial osmotic pressure (πi) tends to draw fluid out of the capillary. The osmotic reflection coefficient (σ) describes the effectiveness of osmotic pressure at moving fluids and can range from 0 to 1. Conceptually, σ compares the size of the pore to the osmotically active solute: $\sigma = 0$ if the solute can move freely through the pore, and $\sigma = 1$ if the solute cannot move through the pore.

Normally, the balance of forces results in net filtration, or the movement of a few milliliters per hour of fluid out of the capillaries in adults. Normal Pc $\approx$ 10 mm Hg, and normal Pi in the lungs is subatmospheric, so that a positive hydrostatic force moves fluid out of the capillaries. The interstitial space around alveolar capillaries is not compliant, and filtration in this region tends to increase local interstitial pressure. This local pressure increase is thought to provide a gradient moving filtrate toward the interstitium around the extra-alveolar vessels. Filtrate in this extra-alveolar region can be reabsorbed by the bronchial circulation or collected by lymphatics, which also return the fluid to the vascular system.

Normal plasma protein concentration is ~7.5 g/dL (mainly albumin); this exerts an osmotic pressure of ~28 mm Hg. The interstitium contains only ~5 g/dL of protein with an osmotic pressure of 15–20 mm Hg. Therefore, the osmotic forces promote absorption. Also, osmotic forces provide a natural feedback system in which increased filtration dilutes the interstitial space, thus reducing the osmotic gradient pulling fluid out of the capillaries. The osmotic pressure depends on the number of molecules in solution.

When this normal balance of forces is disturbed, filtration can exceed the capacity of reabsorption and lymphatic drainage, and fluid accumulates in the interstitium. Edema is the accumulation of excess filtrate outside the capillaries. Pulmonary edema fluid accumulates first in the peribronchiolar and perivascular spaces; this is called *interstitial edema*. Interstitial edema can alter local ventilation and perfusion and make gas exchange inefficient by decreasing compliance, increasing the work of breathing, and ultimately leading to loss of lung volume. As interstitial fluid accumulates, it can enter into the alveolus causing alveolar edema. Only in severe pathologic states does fluid cross directly from the capillary lumen into the alveolus because the intact fused basement membrane between the endothelial and epithelial cells is quite impervious to water. When damaged, however, water (and, when damage is severe, protein and red blood cells) can flood the alveolus directly from the capillaries. Alveolar edema, or flooding of excess filtrate into the alveolar spaces, is more serious because it can totally block ventilation and cause blood-flow shunts in affected lung regions. The exact mechanisms that result in alveolar edema are not known, but they involve exceeding the lung's capacity for lymphatic drainage and changes in solute and fluid transport across airway epithelial cells. Alveolar type II epithelial cells normally transport sodium chloride to the basolateral surface, and water follows, keeping the alveoli dry.

Edema fluid can have low or high protein concentration. Hydrostatic edema, which may occur with elevated pulmonary capillary pressures in congestive heart failure, results in filtrate with low protein concentrations. Other lung injuries, such as acute RDS, may alter the permeability of the capillary endothelium and produce a protein-rich edema fluid. *Stress*

failure of pulmonary capillaries, in which high vascular pressures actually break the capillary wall, can lead to edema too. For example, this may contribute to high-altitude pulmonary edema with very high pulmonary artery pressures from global but patchy hypoxic pulmonary vasoconstriction.

The neonatal lung presents a unique situation for fluid balance as amniotic fluid must be cleared from the alveolar spaces. During the final stages of labor, a surge in maternal TSH and high levels of catecholamine reduce the lung fluid content. During vaginal delivery, the newborn's chest is compressed with pressures of up to 100 mm Hg, which squeezes out fluid. About one third of the lung fluid is cleared by these mechanisms and about half of the remaining fluid is cleared by direct absorption into the alveolar capillaries (cf. alveolar epithelial transport mechanisms that keep the alveoli dry in adults too). The remainder of the fluid in the neonatal lung is cleared through the interstitium over the next 24 hours.

RESPIRATORY CONTROL

General Concepts

In the past century, especially in the past two or three decades, we have learned a great deal about respiratory control. Using a series of "concepts" the following sections will detail our current understanding of respiratory control and explore some ideas related to it in early life and during human development, providing examples of aberrant or abnormal respiratory control and the consequences of tissue hypoxia.

Respiratory Control Concept 1

Respiration is controlled via a negative feedback system, using a controller in the CNS. The overall aim of the respiratory feedback loop is to keep blood gases in a normal range with the least possible energy expenditure and O_2 consumption. The afferent limb consists of receptors that send information to a central controller. For example, the carotid bodies inform the central controller of the O_2 level. Both airway and carotid body sensors compare actual and baseline (or programmed) "set" signals to generate error signals. The carotid sinus nerve fibers, which carry impulses generated by the carotid glomus cells, synapse in the medulla oblongata. The efferent limb is that part of the feedback loop that is responsible for the execution of the decision made centrally (i.e., the respiratory muscles and their innervation) after integrating afferent signals. The external intercostal and diaphragm muscles are the major muscles of respiration. Activity and timing of the airway muscles are very critical in determining airway resistance and patency.

Negative feedback resists change and occurs because the controller attempts to rectify deviations from normal. For example, if CO_2 increases because of lack of ability to remove CO_2 adequately (e.g., airway obstruction), the output of the controller is increased to increase alveolar ventilation and decrease CO_2. If O_2 is reduced in the blood (observed Po_2 is very different from a "programmed or set" Po_2 that carotid glomus cells detect as abnormal), these cells will fire to stimulate phrenic nerve activity via the CNS.

Respiratory Control Concept 2

Central neuronal processing and integration in the brainstem is hierarchical. Respiratory muscles are recruited to perform different tasks at different times, such as for respiration, jumping, splinting the abdomen, and doing Valsalva maneuvers. In other conditions, respiratory muscles can be totally inhibited, e.g., while one is delivering a speech, CO_2 responsiveness is decreased substantially because respiratory muscles are recruited mostly for speech at the expense of respiration. Another example relevant to infants is bottle- or breast-feeding, which is sometimes associated with a reduction in ventilation and Po_2 because respiratory muscles and breathing efforts are inhibited. If presented with a number of neurophysiologic signals (representing options about various needs), the central controller can enhance or reduce the response to certain stimuli at the expense of others. Therefore, a hierarchy is used by brainstem networks in determining the response of the respiratory system at any one time. Temporal and spatial summation of excitatory and inhibitory postsynaptic potentials will be critical in deciding the behavior of these neurons. In addition, their cellular and membrane properties will affect their output. Furthermore, changes in the state of consciousness modulate the ability of the brainstem to respond to afferent stimuli. Age is very important, as the response of the brainstem to stimuli varies with maturation and cortical input to brainstem structures.

A clinical correlation is the mechanical feedback that controls respiration in newborns. In addition to chemoreceptors, powerful mechanoreceptors in the lungs and chest wall function to preserve lung volume. Nowhere is this more evident than in the newborn, in whom the respiratory muscles are weak, whose lung mechanics are deranged, and whose oxygenation depends on maintenance of the FRC. The mechanoreceptors function to prolong inspiratory effort, shorten the expiratory time, and cause dynamic gas trapping. This tachypnea is commonly seen even in infants with normal gas exchange on mechanical ventilation. The mechanoreceptors are incorporated in the control of the airway muscles as well. Infants have expiratory grunting that can augment the expiratory transpulmonary pressure by several centimeters of H_2O to significantly increase their FRC.

Respiratory Control Concept 3

Brainstem neurons have cellular and membrane properties that allow them to beat (cycle) spontaneously. These properties play a role in generating rhythmic respiratory neuronal behavior. The central controller has two basic functions that are inherently linked: (a) integration of afferent information, and (b) generation and maintenance of respiration. These tasks are believed to be performed by different neuronal groups, but it is not known in precise mechanistic terms how each function takes place. The respiratory controller is probably a group of neurons that form a network. Respiratory neurons most likely do not have special inherent membrane properties (e.g., bursting, spontaneous depolarization properties) that would make their membrane potential spontaneously oscillate. Rather, the output of the network that they form oscillates because of the special interconnections and synaptic interactions among these respiratory neurons.

Data have suggested that the respiratory rhythm is generated by an oscillating neuronal network in the ventrolateral formation of the medulla. The region that seems to be essential for the rhythm is the pre-Botzinger complex (PBC), as all cranial nerve activities ceases after this region is separated from the lower brainstem. The properties of individual neurons in this area, how interconnected they are, and the nature of their synapses with neurons in the brainstem and other more rostral regions remain to be elucidated. Although the PBC is certainly a possible site for respiratory rhythm generation, the argument that this is the main site is unproven. Several experiments argue that the PBC is the rhythm generator: (a) drugs injected in the PBC alter breathing frequency, (b) lesions in the PBC do the same, and (c) respiratory afferents synapse in the PBC. However, it has not been shown that these types of experiments done in other areas have been negative. Data have delineated

other sites that may control expiratory rhythms rather than inspiratory rhythms, as hypothesized for the PBC.

Respiratory Control Concept 4

Respiratory rhythm generation in central neurons is most likely a result of integration between network, synaptic, cellular, and molecular characteristics. Rhythmic movements, such as locomotion or heart beat, are generally based either on the action of endogenous "burster" neurons (or conditional bursters) or on a network of neurons, which by virtue of their connections oscillate. In the case of networks, previous literature has suggested that central neurons can no longer be considered as just "followers." A very clear example of such an oscillating network is a set of neurons that have been well studied in Tritonia diomedea. In this animal, the central pattern generator responsible for escape swimming has been extensively studied and its properties well appreciated. The functional interaction of one set of synapses, for example, between C2 and ventral swim interneurons (VSIs) neurons is based on the fact that VSI-B neurons possess membrane properties that allow the excitation from C2 to be delayed, which is an important mechanism in the overall function of the Tritonia motor program. This current turns on with membrane depolarization but then quickly inactivates; hyperpolarization of the membrane potential removes this inactivation.

For dorsal and ventral medullary respiratory neurons, investigators have discovered a number of impressive membrane currents that can shape their repetitive firing. These include not only the classic sodium and K^+ currents responsible for the action potential, but also an A-current, two types of Ca^{2+} currents, Ca^{2+}-activated K^+ currents, inward-rectifier currents, ATP-sensitive K^+ currents, and others.

Data from studies of the cellular and membrane properties and synaptic efficiency of newborn neurons reveal differences in the integrated output from adult neural networks. For example, both active and passive cellular properties in newborn dorsal respiratory group cells are different from those in adults. Newborn brainstem neurons have less spike-frequency adaptation, less inward-rectifier currents, different afterhyperpolarization, a wider action-potential waveform, and no delayed excitation. Such electrophysiologic maturational changes are related to changes in a number of variables that pertain to cytosolic and membrane structure and function. For example, the distribution of ion channels and receptors on cell membranes, as well as the structural and functional nature and the regulation of ion channels, change with age in early life.

Respiratory Control Concept 5

Afferent information is not essential for generation of breathing, but modulates respiration. A multitude of afferent messages converge on the brainstem. Chemoreceptors and mechanoreceptors in the larynx and upper airways sense stretch, temperature, and chemical changes over the mucosa and relay this information to the brainstem. Afferent impulses from these areas travel through the superior laryngeal nerve and vagus. Changes in O_2 or CO_2 tensions are sensed at the carotid and aortic bodies, and afferent impulses travel through the carotid and aortic sinus nerves. Thermal or metabolic changes are sensed by skin or mucosal receptors or by hypothalamic neurons and are carried through spinal tracts to the brainstem. Afferent information is not a prerequisite for the generation and maintenance of respiration. When the brainstem and spinal cord are removed from the body and maintained in vitro, rhythmic phrenic activity can be detected for hours. Other in vivo experiments in chronically instrumented dogs in whom several sensory systems are simultaneously blocked indicate that afferent information is not necessary to stimulate the inherent respiratory rhythm in brainstem respiratory networks. However, both in vitro and in vivo studies demonstrate that, in the absence of afferent information, the inherent rhythm of the central generator (indexed by respiratory frequency) is slowed, and therefore, chemoreceptor afferents can play a role in modulating respiration and rhythmic behavior.

Among the many types of afferent information that affect the respiratory output of the CNS, CO_2 and O_2 are some of the most potent. If "afferent" is considered to be any information that converges on the brainstem respiratory network, CO_2 is certainly an important and powerful stimulus to respiration, even though it is sensed mostly in the CNS itself. Almost any change in CO_2 induces a change in ventilation and vice versa (for any given metabolic rate). A nearly normal ventilatory response to increased CO_2 can be observed in experimental animals that have no afferent input to the CNS from peripheral sensory nerves, e.g., removing the carotid bodies reduces the ventilatory response to CO_2 by a modest 20%. Chemoreceptors, in several specialized regions in the medulla, are particularly sensitive to changes in CO_2 and pH, although the exact mechanisms for responding to CO_2 and pH in these regions may not be understood. Furthermore, it is important to realize that nerve cells in the CNS, whether in these specialized regions or not, are responsive to CO_2 and pH as they do have either exchangers (e.g., Na/H exchanger) or ion channels (e.g., Na^+ channels) that are responsive to CO_2 and/or pH, and hence modulate cell excitability and neuronal output.

⑫ Developmental Aspects of Respiratory Control

Developmental studies have spanned a range of questions regarding such issues as the development of brainstem neurons, respiratory muscles, afferent receptors and systems (including the carotid bodies), and the end organs (lungs). These various aspects of respiratory control are not mature at birth.

Central Aspects of Respiratory Control

In vitro studies in the neonatal rat (whole brainstem preparation) have shed light on fundamental newborn issues. We know now that the young rat brainstem in vitro (which is very immature in the first week of postnatal life) does not require any peripheral drive for central oscillator discharge. The inherent respiratory rate is markedly reduced, however, and it is clear from these studies that peripheral and possibly central (rostral to the medulla and pons) input is necessary to maintain the respiratory output at a much higher frequency.

In that (a) the discharge of central neurons in the adult or neonate is affected by peripheral input, including input from the vagus nerve, and (b) the respiratory feedback system can operate on a breath-by-breath basis, the question has arisen as to whether the lack of myelination in the neonatal nerve fibers that subserve feedback affects function. Indeed, this is the case not only because of lack of myelination and potential delays in signaling, but also because inspiratory and expiratory discharges are so fast that they preclude the effect of peripheral input on the CNS *within* the same breath. Clearly, peripheral afferent may have effects on subsequent breaths. Therefore, whether breath-by-breath feedback is as effective in the young as in the adult remains an open question.

Differences between neonates and adults are also observed in response to endogenous stimuli such as responses to neurotransmitters or modulators. Young and immature animals respond differently to neurotransmitters, as documented by work in opossum. Glutamate injected in various locations in the brainstem, even in large doses, induces respiratory pauses, while it is clearly stimulatory in the older mature animal. Such inhibitory neurotransmitters as γ-aminobutyric acid have also been used, and they have age-dependent effects in the opossum. Indeed, a chloride (Cl^-)-mediated inhibition is noted in the adult but not in the neonate in the isolated brainstem.

Peripheral Sensory Aspects

The primary O_2 sensors in the body, the carotids, show major differences between the newborn and the adult. Recordings from both single-fiber afferents and sinus nerves show major differences between the fetus and newborn and between newborn and adult. For example, it has been demonstrated that fetal chemoreceptor activity is present in the normal fetus and that a large increase in activity may be evoked by decreasing P_{O_2} in the ewe. As would be predicted, the large increase in Pa_{O_2} at the time of birth virtually shuts off chemoreceptor activity in the newborn. However, this decreased sensitivity does not last long, and a normal adult-like sensitivity takes place by 1–2 weeks after birth.

A number of factors, both external and endogenous, play a role in this process. For example, arterial chemoreceptors are subject to external and hormonal influences, which may affect the sensor or alter tissue P_{O_2} within the organ. Neurochemicals may also play a major role as modulators of chemosensitivity. For example, endorphins are documented to decrease in the newborn period, and the effect of exogenous endorphin is inhibition of chemoreceptor hypoxia sensitivity. However, it has been shown that, even in the absence of external modulatory factors (hormonal or neural), chemosensitivity of the newborn chemoreceptor is less than in the adult. Nerve activity of rat carotid bodies in vitro following transition from normoxia to hypoxia is approximately fourfold greater in carotid bodies harvested from 20-day-old rats compared to 1- or 2-day-old rats. This finding corresponds well with the maturational pattern of the respiratory response to hypoxia in intact animals and suggests that major maturational changes occur within the carotid body itself. Histologic, biophysical, and neurochemical changes occur with development, but the significance of these changes is dependent on assumptions of how the organ senses P_{O_2}. For example, the maturational increase in chemosensitivity may be attributed to a maturational change in the biophysical properties of glomus cells. In one model, hypoxia inhibits a membrane-localized K^+ channel that is active at rest, and the resulting depolarization leads to calcium influx and increased neural activity in adult carotid cells. Support for this mechanism has been obtained from cultured, adult rabbit glomus cells, the outward (or K^+) current of which is apparently inhibited by hypoxia. In comparison, glomus cells harvested from immature animals (e.g., rats) show a decrease in whole-cell K^+ current during hypoxia, but the decrease in K^+ current is attributed to a decreased activation of a Ca^{+2}-dependent K^+ current and not to a specialized K^+ channel sensitive to P_{O_2}.

The ventilatory response to CO_2 also shows developmental changes. For example, premature infants and full-term newborns have a reduced response to CO_2 for several days (or weeks) in early life, which has been shown by studies to result from a complex integration of changes in neural control (maturation of the CNS or peripheral nerves) and respiratory mechanics (chest-wall mechanics and/or respiratory muscles).

In comparison to the adult, peripheral chemoreceptors assume a greater role in the newborn period. Although not essential for initiation of fetal respiratory movements, peripheral chemoreceptor denervation in the newborn results in severe respiratory impairment and high probability of sudden death. Lambs, following denervation, fail to develop a mature respiratory pattern and, more importantly, suffer a 30% mortality rate weeks or months following surgery. In other species, denervation leads to lethal respiratory disturbances. Denervated rats suffer from severe desaturation during REM sleep, and piglets suffer periodic breathing with profound apneas during quiet sleep. Of particular interest is the observation that these lethal impairments only occur during a fairly narrow developmental window, and denervation, before or after this period, results in minor alterations in respiratory function. This window of vulnerability, which is unmasked by denervation in the newborn period, supports the speculation that the sudden infant death syndrome may be due to immaturity or malfunction of peripheral chemoreceptors.

Oxygen Deprivation, Oxygen-sensing, and Cell Injury

Pathologic conditions cause respiratory failure. All cardiorespiratory diseases can potentially produce respiratory failure, and this may be deleterious to other organs because of the ensuing acidosis and hypoxia. It is the hypoxia that should be avoided at all cost, as human tissues, especially the CNS, have low tolerance to a microenvironment devoid of O_2.

A great deal is known about the effect of the lack of O_2 on tissues at various ages, including fetal, postnatal, and adult. The carotid bodies discharge and have an effect on ventilation when the PaO_2 reaches below 55–60 torr. In general, other tissues react to such levels of PaO_2 but in very different ways. For example, tissue growth may be affected if PaO_2 is at the level when carotids start discharging. The effect on most tissues, however, is that they develop remarkable dysfunction when PaO_2 is below 35–40 torr. For example, the brain, which is among the most sensitive to the lack of O_2, has a resting (no hypoxia-induced) interstitial O_2 tension in the range of 20–35 torr, depending on age, region (white vs. gray matter), neuronal metabolism, temperature, proximity to blood vessels, and so on.

Major questions remain about the mechanisms that lead to injury or that protect tissues from it. In the case of the nervous system, a number of mechanisms are activated during O_2 deprivation. Some events that take place during lack of O_2 are membrane biophysical events (e.g., those pertaining to Na^+ and K^+ channels); increased anaerobic metabolism; increased intracellular levels of H^+ and Ca^{2+}; increased concentrations in extracellular neurotransmitters (e.g., glutamate and aspartate); radical production; activation of kinases, protease, and lipase; injury and destruction of important cytoskeletal proteins; and gene regulation of a number of proteins (e.g., c-fos, NGF, HSP-70).

CONCLUSIONS AND FUTURE DIRECTIONS

From the point of view of the intensivist, the respiratory system is much more than the lung per se. It is the lung, the respiratory muscles, the chest cage, the blood and cardiovascular system, the brain (especially the brainstem), the endocrine system, and, often, the gastrointestinal tract. The respiratory system is indeed a reflection of the health and integrity of a number of systems in the body. Although many of the physiologic principles have been long described, a number of new ideas and discoveries presented in this chapter will no doubt affect our future thinking and allow us to better care for children. Some of these new ideas have been described: aquaporins and gas channels, the effect of CO_2 on lung development, the ion channels that control the smooth muscle contraction in the pulmonary vasculature and patent ductus arteriosus, and the ion channels that are important for ion flux in the absence of adequate oxygenation.

ACKNOWLEDGMENT

This work was supported by grants HL081823 (FLP), R41HL102940-01A1 (GPH), 5 P01 HD 32573–11 (GGH), and NIH/NHLB 1 P01 HL098053 (GGH and FLP).

Suggested Readings

Pulmonary Gas Exchange

1. Bauer C. Structural biology of hemoglobin. In: Crystal RG, West JB, Weibel ER, et al., eds. *The Lung: Scientific Foundations, Vol 1.* 2nd ed. Philadelphia, PA: Lippincott-Raven, 1997:1615–24.
2. Farhi LE, Tenney SM. Gas exchange. In: Geiger SR, ed. *Handbook of Physiology, Section 3, The Respiratory System.* Bethesda, MD: American Physiologic Society, 1987.
3. Longo LD, Nystrom GA. Fetal and newborn respiratory gas exchange. In: Crystal RG, West JB, Weibel WR, et al., eds. *The Lung: Scientific Foundations.* Vol 2. 2nd ed. Philadelphia, PA: Lippincott-Raven, 1997:2141–49.
4. Miller J, Carlo W. Safety and effectiveness of permissive hypercapnia in the preterm infant. *Curr Opin Pediatr* 2007;191:142–4.
5. O'Croinin D, Chonghaile M, Higgins B, et al. Bench-to bedside review: Permissive hypercapnia. *Crit Care* 2005;9:51–9.
6. Roughton FJW. Transport of oxygen and carbon dioxide. In: Fenn WO, Rahn H, eds. *Handbook of Physiology, Sec. 3, Respiration.* Bethesda, MD: American Physiological Society, 1964:767–826.
7. Wagner PD. Diffusion and chemical reaction in pulmonary gas exchange. *Physiol Rev* 1997;57:257–312.
8. West JB, Wagner PD. Ventilation-perfusion relationships. In: Crystal RG, West JB, Weibel WR, et al., eds. *The Lung: Scientific Foundations.* 2nd ed. Philadelphia, PA: Lippincott-Raven, 1997:1693–710.

Lung Mechanics, Respiratory and Airway Muscles

9. Benjamin JT, Carver BJ, Plosa EJ, et al. NF-kappaB activation limits airway branching through inhibition of Sp1-mediated fibroblast growth factor-10 expression. *J Immunol* 2010;185(8):4896–903. doi:10.4049/jimmunol.1001857
10. Boynton BR, Carlo WA, Jobe AH, eds. *New Therapies for Neonatal Respiratory Failure. A Physiological Approach.* New York, NY: Cambridge University Press, 1994.
11. Comroe JH. Retrospectroscope: Premature science and immature lungs. I. Some premature discoveries. *Am Rev Respir Dis* 1977;166:127–35.
12. Fredberg JJ, Stamenovic D. On the imperfect elasticity of lung tissue. *J Appl Physiol* 1989;67:2408–19.
13. Gappa M, Pillow JJ, Allen J, et al. Lung function tests in neonates and infants with chronic lung disease: Lung and chest-wall mechanics. *Pediatr Pulmonol* 2006;41:291–317.
14. Oostveen E, MacLeod D, Lorino H, et al. The forced oscillation technique in clinical practice: Methodology, recommendations, and future developments. *Eur Respir J* 2003;22:1026–41.
15. Wright CJ, Kirpalani H. Targeting inflammation to prevent bronchopulmonary dysplasia: Can new insights be translated into therapies? *Pediatrics* 2011;128(1):111–26. doi:10.1542/peds.2010-3875

Pulmonary Circulation

16. Bland R. Fetal lung liquid and its removal near birth. In: Crystal RG, West JB, Weibel WR, et al., eds. *The Lung: Scientific Foundations.* Vol 2. 2nd ed. Philadelphia, PA: Lippincott-Raven, 1997:2115–127.
17. Fishman AP, ed. Circulation and non-respiratory functions. In: Geiger SR. *Handbook of Physiology, Section 3, The Respiratory System, Volume I.* Bethesda, MD: American Physiological Society, 1985.
18. Sylvester JT, Shimoda LA, Aaronson PI, et al. Hypoxic pulmonary vasoconstriction. *Physiol Rev* 2012;92:367–520.

19. Tod ML, Cassin S. Fetal and neonatal pulmonary circulation. In: Crystal RG, West JB, Weibel WR, et al., eds. *The Lung: Scientific Foundations.* Vol 2. 2nd ed. Philadelphia, PA: Lippincott-Raven, 1997:2129–39.

Respiratory Control

20. Dekin MS, Haddad GG. Membrane and cellular properties in oscillating networks: Implications for respiration. *J Appl Physiol* 1990;69(3):809–21.
21. Donnelly DF, Haddad GG. Respiratory changes induced by prolonged laryngeal stimulation in awake piglets. *J Appl Physiol* 1986;61:1018–24.
22. Donnelly DF, Haddad GG. Prolonged apnea and impaired survival in piglets after sinus and aortic nerve section. *J Appl Physiol* 1990;68(3):1048–52.
23. Haddad GG, Donnelly DF. O$_2$ Deprivation induces a major depolarization in brainstem neurons in the adult but not in the neonatal rat. *J Physiol (London)* 1990;429:411–28.
24. Haddad GG, Donnelly DF, Getting PA. Biophysical properties of hypoglossal neurons in-vitro: Intracellular studies in adult and neonatal rats. *J Appl Physiol* 1990;69:1509–17.

CHAPTER 44 ■ THE MOLECULAR BIOLOGY OF ACUTE LUNG INJURY

TODD CARPENTER AND KURT R. STENMARK

KEY POINTS

Injury, Inflammation, and Edema Formation

1 Activation of the innate immune system by molecular patterns characteristic of pathogens and products released from damaged cells is a key mechanism of lung injury.

2 Many mediators—including transcription factors, signaling molecules, cytokines, chemokines, coagulation system proteins, and angiogenic mediators—amplify and extend the injury process in the lung.

3 Endogenous barrier-protective mediators also exist and may contribute to the pathophysiology of lung injury.

Regulation of the Alveolar–Capillary Barrier

4 Increased alveolar–capillary barrier permeability is a key feature of acute lung injury.

5 Endothelial permeability is largely determined by intercellular junctions and the endothelial cytoskeleton.

6 Calcium channels and Rho family GTPases are critical regulators of the endothelial barrier.

7 Impairment of innate alveolar liquid clearance mechanisms involving ENaC (epithelial sodium channel) and Na/K-ATPases contributes to pulmonary edema accumulation in acute respiratory distress syndrome (ARDS).

Control of Pulmonary Vascular Tone

8 Changes in vascular tone contribute to ventilation–perfusion matching as well as edema formation in the injured lung.

9 Vascular tone is determined by the balance of endogenous vasoconstrictors such as endothelin and endogenous vasodilators such as nitric oxide.

Fibroproliferation and Repair in the Injured Lung

10 Nonresolving inflammation contributes to poor outcomes in late ARDS.

11 Alveolar epithelial repair begins early in lung injury and is driven by a number of key growth factors and cytokines, including IL-1β (interleukin-1β), EGF (epidermal growth factor), and KGF (keratinocyte growth factor).

12 Fibroproliferation and scarring also begin early after injury, driven largely by TGF-β and the process of epithelial–mesenchymal transdifferentiation.

13 Progenitor cells also contribute to lung repair, and exogenous mesenchymal stem cells hold great promise as reparative and immune-modulating therapies.

Acute respiratory distress syndrome (ARDS) is an illness of great interest and importance in pediatric critical care. Children who suffer from ARDS are often among the sickest and most challenging patients in the PICU. In addition, an even greater proportion of the patients in pediatric critical care present with respiratory illnesses that have substantial mechanistic overlap with ARDS, even without cleanly fitting the clinical case definition of that condition. Understanding the cellular and molecular mechanisms that underlie ARDS, then, is important for understanding current and future approaches to treatment of many serious respiratory illnesses in the PICU.

The central derangement in ARDS is the disruption of the alveolar–capillary barrier, which allows protein-rich plasma components to cross into the airspaces. Once alveoli are flooded, surfactant is inactivated and a cycle of inflammation and local hypoxia leads to injury progression, augmented by mechanical forces from the use of artificial mechanical ventilation and oxidant stress from high inspired O_2 concentrations. These changes comprise the early, acute phase of ARDS, characterized by pulmonary edema, hypoxemic respiratory failure, poor lung compliance, and, often, some degree of pulmonary hypertension (Fig. 44.1). As the illness progresses, the disease enters a fibroproliferative phase, in which lung compliance improves but lung function remains poor as a result of progressive scarring and thickening of the lung interstitium. Ultimately, many patients recover lung function completely or nearly so, but substantial numbers of survivors have long-lasting pulmonary function deficits. These themes of injury, inflammation, fibroproliferation, and repair appear in almost every respiratory disease seen in the PICU. And while some studies have noted improvements in outcome for this illness in the last decade, specific therapies for ARDS remain unavailable and further progress will likely require a more detailed understanding of the complex molecular mechanisms contributing to lung injury.

670

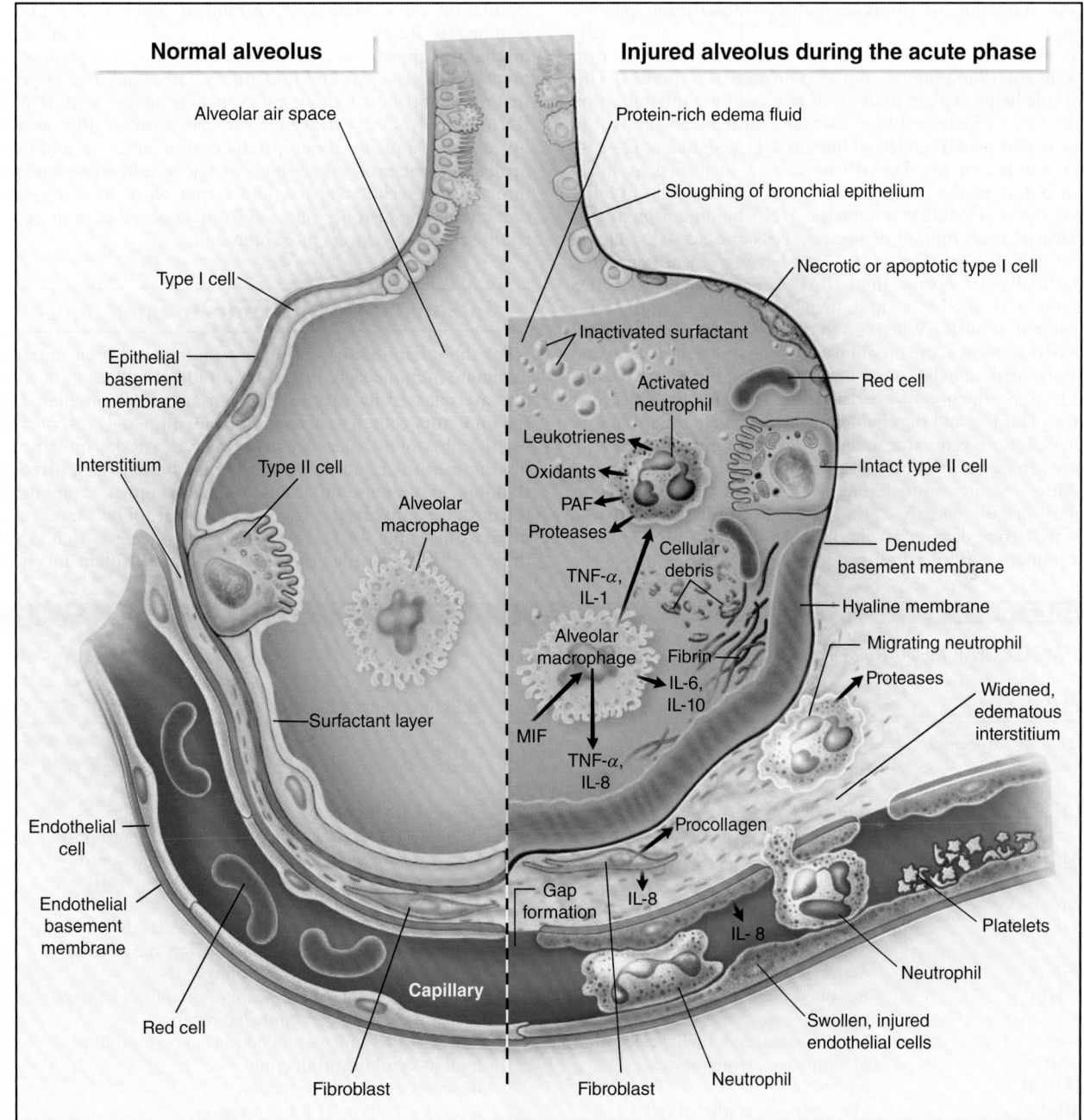

FIGURE 44.1. Cellular and molecular mechanisms of acute lung injury. Changes that occur as part of the early acute phase of lung injury are visible on the *right half* of the diagram in comparison to the *left*, including disruption of the endothelial and epithelial barriers, alveolar flooding, and influx of activated inflammatory cells into the alveolus and interstitium of the lung. PAF: Platelet Activating Factor.

INJURY, INFLAMMATION, AND EDEMA FORMATION

Toll-like Receptors/Mitochondrial DNA/ Danger-Associated Molecular Patterns and Pathogen-Associated Molecular Patterns

ARDS is initiated by either direct injury to the lung (respiratory infections, acid aspiration, or pulmonary contusion) or distant tissue injuries (sepsis or trauma). These initial injuries are sensed by the innate immune system, which then triggers

and amplifies inflammatory responses to the injury. Initial recognition of tissue injury occurs through pattern recognition receptors (PRRs), which include the Toll-like receptors (TLRs), NOD-like receptors (NLRs), and RIG-like receptors (RLRs) (1–4). As a general principle, PRRs recognize and bind specific molecular patterns, whether they are typical of pathogens (pathogen-associated molecular patterns [PAMPs]) or of damaged cells and tissues (danger-associated molecular patterns [DAMPs]). Examples of these interactions include sensing of bacterial lipopolysaccharide (LPS) by TLR4 and sensing of either viral RNA or endogenous RNAs released from damaged cells by TLR3 (3,5–8). Initiation of TLR signaling by specific PAMPs or DAMPs activates signaling cascades that result in the activation of proinflammatory transcription factors, most prominently nuclear factor-κB (NF-κB). Intriguingly, TLR signaling appears to activate not only inflammation in experimental lung injuries but also protective responses. This dual role helps explain findings of reduced lung inflammation in the face of increased lung damage and reduced survival in some experimental models of impaired TLR signaling (2–4,9).

A number of key DAMPs have been identified as likely contributors to the pathophysiology of ARDS. High-mobility group box 1 (HMGB1) is a nuclear DNA-binding protein that is released from injured or necrotic cells and acts as a ligand for both TLR2 and TLR4 (10,11). It has been identified in the bronchoalveolar lavage fluid (BALF) and plasma of ARDS patients and has been implicated in both sepsis and ARDS in animal models. When given intratracheally in animals, HMGB1 induces acute inflammatory lung injury, characterized by polymorphonuclear neutrophil (PMN) influx, lung edema, and local production of interleukin-1β (IL-1β), tumor necrosis factor (TNF)-α, and the chemokine macrophage-inflammatory protein 2. Both ventilator-induced and endotoxin-induced lung injury can be ameliorated using anti-HMGB1 antibodies.

More recently, mitochondrial DNA, which shares evolutionary origins with bacterial DNA, has been shown to be released from damaged cells in both experimental animals and humans suffering traumatic injuries (12–14). Once in the circulation, mitochondrial DNA binds to and activates TLR9, leading to inflammation and neutrophil activation. This mechanism appears to contribute to mortality in experimental models of both sepsis and lung injury. Other putative DAMPs that may contribute to lung injury include nucleic acids (DNA, RNA, microRNAs), extracellular matrix proteins (fibronectin, hyaluronin), and metabolic products (uric acid). In addition, nuclear histone proteins are highly toxic to cells when released into the extracellular space, and recent work has suggested that circulating histones released from damaged cells also contribute to the development of lung injury.

Inflammatory Mediators in Lung Injury

Once the inflammatory response to injury has been initiated by innate immune signaling, a multitude of additional mediators are released by various lung parenchymal, vascular, and inflammatory cells. These mediators are ultimately responsible for the physiologic derangements seen in ARDS, most notably the disrupted endothelial and epithelial barriers, alveolar flooding, and intense inflammation. While only a sampling of the mediators involved is discussed in what follows (and summarized in **Table 44.1**), the important concept is that while these multiple cascades of mediators likely explain much of

TABLE 44.1

KEY MOLECULAR MEDIATORS IMPLICATED IN ACUTE LUNG INJURY

■ MEDIATOR	■ SOURCE	■ EFFECTS IN ALI
Signaling Molecules		
PKC	Intracellular	Increases microvascular permeability
Transcription Factors		
HIF-1	Intracellular	Upregulates hypoxia-responsive genes
NF-κB	Intracellular	Regulates genes that control inflammatory responses
SMADs	Intracellular	Downstream of TGF-β; regulate genes that control endothelial and epithelial permeability, fibrosis
Cytokines		
TGF-β	Secreted by many cells	Increases endothelial and epithelial permeability, stimulates extracellular matrix production and fibrosis
TNF-α	Activated macrophages	Increases endothelial permeability
IL-1β	Activated macrophages	Increases endothelial permeability, amplifies immune responses, promotes epithelial repair
IL-6	Macrophages, endothelial cells, fibroblasts	Activates PKC, increases endothelial permeability
IL-10	Macrophages, lymphocytes	Inhibits cytokine production
HMGB1	Injured cells	Increases cytokine production
MIF-1	Macrophages, epithelial cells	Increases TNF-α, TLR4 expression
Chemokines		
IL-8	Alveolar macrophages	Neutrophil recruitment
GRO	Alveolar macrophages	Neutrophil recruitment
ENA-78	Alveolar macrophages	Neutrophil recruitment
Angiogenic Mediators		
VEGF	Epithelial cells, macrophages, smooth muscle	Increases endothelial permeability, involved in airway and vascular development and repair
Ang1	Vascular smooth muscle, endothelial cells	Reduces vascular permeability, decreases IL-8 expression
Ang2	Endothelial cells	Increases vascular permeability
Other Mediators		
Thrombin	Cleavage of prothrombin	Increases endothelial permeability, activates TGF-β
S1P	Platelets	Reduces endothelial permeability
TGF-α		Promotes epithelial repair
KGF	Fibroblasts	Promotes alveolar epithelial proliferation
HGF	Fibroblasts	Promotes alveolar epithelial proliferation

PKC, protein kinase C; HIF-1, hypoxia-inducible factor 1; NF-κB, nuclear factor-κB; TGF-β, transforming growth factor-β; TNF-α, tumor necrosis factor-α; IL, interleukin; HMGB1, high-mobility group box 1; MIF-1, macrophage migration inhibitory factor 1; GRO, growth-related oncogene; ENA-78, epithelial-derived neutrophil-activating peptide 78; VEGF, vascular endothelial growth factor; Ang, angiopoietin; S1P, sphingosine-1-phosphate; KGF, keratinocyte growth factor; HGF, hepatocyte growth factor.

the difficulty encountered in devising effective targeted therapies for ARDS, they also provide opportunities for the future development of more specific interventions.

Signaling and Transcriptional Mediators

Intracellular signaling pathways not only lead directly from cell surface receptors to intracellular targets but also cross-talk with each other, modulating and fine-tuning responses in complex networks. One of the best-described intracellular signaling pathways implicated in the development of ARDS involves the protein kinase C (PKC) family of serine/threonine kinases (15,16). These molecules contribute to many important cellular functions, including the control of endothelial permeability in the injured lung. Direct stimulation of PKC activity with diacylglycerol increases microvascular permeability, and PKC inhibitors reduce the increased lung vascular permeability caused by thrombin, vascular endothelial growth factor (VEGF), O_2 free radicals, TNF-α, and PMNs. While the specific downstream mediators responsible for the effect of PKC are still under investigation, PKC activation has been implicated in myosin light chain (MLC) phosphorylation in response to some agonists and in loosening of adherens junctions and focal adhesions in endothelial cells (**Fig. 44.2**).

As with signaling, the complexity of transcriptional regulation of protein expression seems to increase almost weekly. Among the many transcription factors currently thought to be involved in ARDS, hypoxia-inducible factor (HIF) 1, NF-κB, and SMAD transcription factors figure prominently (1,15).

HIF-1 is a ubiquitously expressed protein that is a critical regulator of cellular responses to hypoxia. The expression of many of the mediators involved in ARDS (including VEGF and endothelin 1 [ET-1], among others) is controlled, at least in part, by HIF-1. NF-κB is the most prominent transcriptional regulator of inflammatory responses and cytokine production and as a result plays a key role in controlling inflammation in the injured lung. In animal studies, for example, NF-κB inhibition or antagonism ameliorates experimental lung injury. SMAD transcription factors are a family of molecules that act downstream of TGF-β and have also been implicated in control of endothelial and epithelial permeability, as well as in fibrotic responses. While increasing evidence links the SMADs with these processes, the downstream targets of SMAD activation in the setting of lung injury remain uncertain.

Cytokine Mediators

Activation of the transcriptional regulators described earlier results in the production of a number of cytokine and chemokine mediators, which then recruit inflammatory cells to the injured lung and amplify the inflammatory response as well as regulate reparative responses.

Transforming growth factor (TGF)-β is one of the most important cytokines in the injured lung (5,17). It is secreted by most cells and stored in a latent form in the extracellular matrix. When enzymatically released from the latent form, active TGF-β binds to its receptors on the cell surface, phosphorylating and activating SMAD-family transcription

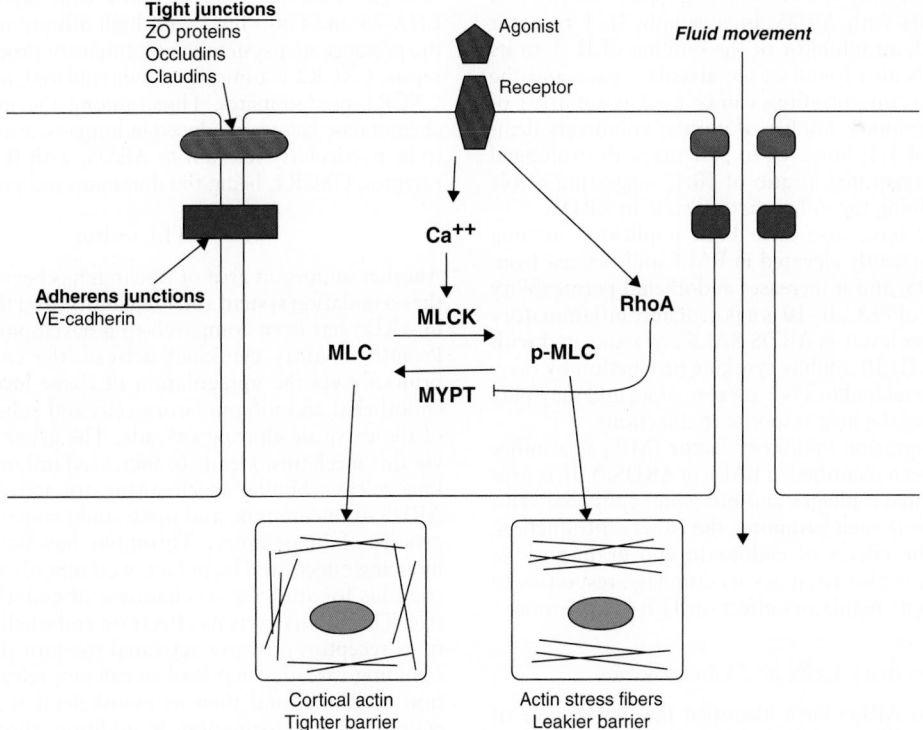

FIGURE 44.2. Molecular mechanisms that control endothelial permeability. Intact tight junctions and adherens junctions provide a barrier to paracellular fluid movement in unperturbed monolayers (*left side of figure*). Agonist stimulation leads to activation of myosin light chain kinase (MLCK) via calcium influx and to suppression of myosin phosphatase (MYPT) activity via RhoA activation, with the net result of rearrangement of the actin cytoskeleton and increased actin–myosin interactions, leading to endothelial cell contraction. Combined with additional mechanisms that lead to the breakdown of intercellular junctions (tight junctions, adherens junctions), these changes cause endothelial cells to contract away from each other, allowing paracellular fluid flux (*right side of figure*). ZO, zonula occludens; VE-cadherin, vascular/endothelial-cadherin; MLC, myosin light chain; p-MLC, phosphorylated myosin light chain.

factors, which then move into the nucleus and regulate the transcription of many other genes. TGF-β is nearly ubiquitously expressed and causes a plethora of conflicting effects. Relevant to ARDS, however, TGF-β activation increases both endothelial and epithelial permeability. Elevated lung TGF-β levels are found in both human ARDS and in animal models of lung injury, and TGF-β inhibition protects from experimental lung injury in animals. In cultured endothelial cells, TGF-β directly increases permeability through mechanisms that involve SMAD phosphorylation, activation of RhoA, and the disruption of adherens junctions. Recent evidence links the coagulation system (in the form of thrombin) with TGF-β activation and lung injury in the setting of both high tidal volume ventilation and bleomycin-induced lung injury (9,18,19). These findings suggest that TGF-β activation is one of the pivotal steps in the initiation and propagation of ARDS.

Many of the cytokines involved in systemic inflammatory responses to sepsis have also been implicated in ARDS. For example, TNF-α and IL-1β are cytokines predominantly produced by activated macrophages, and both are key elements of the systemic response to sepsis as well as to lung injury. TNF-α stimulation triggers the upregulation of adhesion molecules in human lung microvascular endothelial cells, which may lead to greater PMN attachment, cytoskeletal changes, and endothelial barrier dysfunction. TNF-α levels have been measured in the BALF of ARDS patients and are often elevated, although levels do not correlate well with outcomes. IL-1β increases the permeability of cultured endothelial cell layers and stimulates the production of a variety of chemotactic cytokines. This proinflammatory cytokine has been identified in BALF from patients with ARDS, and strong correlations exist between measures of IL-1β activity and clinical lung injury severity and outcome in patients with ARDS. Interestingly, IL-1 receptor antagonist (IL-1ra), an inhibitor of the binding of IL-1 to its primary receptor, is also found in the alveolar space and the ratio of IL-1:IL-1ra concentrations can be used as a marker of the severity of lung injury. Studies of normal volunteers demonstrated a ratio of 1:1; however, in patients with prolonged ARDS, BALF demonstrated a ratio of 10:1, suggesting a role for IL-1 in maintaining the inflammatory state in ARDS.

IL-6 and IL-10 have also have been implicated in lung injury. IL-6 is consistently elevated in BALF and plasma from patients with ARDS, and it increases endothelial permeability through activation of PKC. IL-10 is a potent anti-inflammatory cytokine, and higher levels in ARDS BALF are associated with improved survival. IL-10 inhibits cytokine production by macrophages, is closely related to TNF-α expression, and may play a role in modulating the host response to infections.

Macrophage migration inhibitory factor (MIF) is another cytokine that has been identified in BALF in ARDS. MIF is produced by alveolar macrophages and bronchial epithelial cells, and MIF and TNF-α each promotes the other's production. MIF potentiates the effects of endotoxin and gram-positive bacterial products; it also regulates macrophage responses to endotoxin through its regulatory effect on TLR4 expression.

Inflammatory Cells and Chemokines

Studies of BALF in ARDS have identified the importance of acute inflammatory cell populations, their evolution over time, and their impact on clinical outcomes. For example, neutrophils are abundant in the airspaces of patients with ARDS, and neutrophil numbers as well as their persistence after the first week of ARDS are associated with increased mortality. Despite these associations, the role of the neutrophil in lung injury remains a subject of some debate. For example, when neutrophils are recruited into the normal human lung simply by instilling the chemoattractant leukotriene B4 (LTB4), they can migrate without causing injury to the endothelial or epithelial barriers

of the lung. In addition, although it is clear that lung cellular injury and clinical ARDS can occur in neutropenic patients, it is also true that after the initial lung injury, lung dysfunction can acutely worsen during the resolution of neutropenia, as PMNs are recruited to the injured lungs. On balance, these observations suggest that while PMNs alone are neither necessary nor sufficient to cause lung injury in humans, activated PMNs contribute to the pathogenesis of the condition.

Neutrophils must be recruited from the bloodstream to gain access to the alveolar space and airways. Among the most important neutrophil chemoattractants in the injured lung are the CXC family chemokines, IL-8, epithelial-derived neutrophil-activating peptide-78 (ENA-78), growth-related oncogene (GRO), and granulocyte chemotactic peptide (GCP)-2, all of which are produced by human alveolar macrophages. IL-8, ENA-78, and GRO are present in biologically significant concentrations in BALF in ARDS, and their concentrations correlate with PMN concentrations. In general, as long as patients are ill enough to require continued mechanical ventilation, the concentrations of these CXC chemokines tend to remain logarithmically elevated above normal. Although GRO and ENA-78 concentrations are higher than IL-8 concentrations, IL-8 appears to be responsible for the majority of the PMN chemoattractant activity in human ARDS BALF. Several animal models of lung inflammation and injury also support the concept of IL-8 as the dominant PMN chemoattractant. For example, monoclonal antibodies to IL-8 significantly reduce lung injury and PMN migration in endotoxemia and acid-aspiration models (10,20).

Adding another level of complexity, two CXC chemokine receptors are found on human PMNs: CXCR1 and CXCR2. IL-8 can bind to either receptor with high affinity, whereas ENA-78 and GRO bind with high affinity only to CXCR2. In the presence of a systemic inflammatory process, such as severe sepsis, CXCR2 is tonically downregulated, and the function of CXCR1 predominates. Thus, among the multiple neutrophil chemotactic factors produced in humans, a small group appears to be particularly relevant to ARDS, with IL-8 and its cognate receptor, CXCR1, being the dominant receptor–ligand pair.

Thrombin

Another important area of research has been the links between the coagulation system and lung injury, and the injured alveolus in ARDS has been compared to a developing clot (12,14,21). Proinflammatory cytokines activate the coagulation system, primarily via the upregulation of tissue factor expression on endothelial and inflammatory cells and subsequent activation of the extrinsic clotting cascade. The generation of thrombin via this mechanism leads to increased inflammation and cytokine release. Similar mechanisms are active in the alveoli in ARDS or pneumonia, and these could contribute to the pathogenesis of lung injury. Thrombin has potent permeability-inducing effects and is, in fact, a commonly used experimental stimulus for studying mechanisms of endothelial barrier control. Thrombin exerts its effects on endothelial cells by binding to its receptor, protease-activated receptor (PAR) 1, activating signaling cascades that lead to calcium release and the activation of RhoA, and then to cytoskeletal rearrangements and endothelial gap formation. In addition, thrombin stimulation can lead to the disruption of adherens junctions via signaling that is dependent on PKC. Thrombin stimulation of PAR-1 has also been linked experimentally to integrin-mediated TGF-β activation and consequent lung injury.

Angiogenic Mediators

Many of the mediators involved in the formation of new blood vessels (angiogenesis) are activated by tissue injury, and many angiogenic mediators increase vascular permeability, both in the lung and in other vascular beds. Three major families of receptor tyrosine kinases and associated ligands have been implicated in the control of angiogenesis: the VEGFs, the angiopoietins, and the ephrins. Each of these groups has also been implicated in the pathophysiology of ARDS (15,22).

The VEGF family of receptors and ligands are perhaps the most potent regulators of blood vessel formation and vascular permeability and also play key roles in lung development and repair. VEGF is produced and secreted by many cell types in the lung, including alveolar epithelial cells, vascular smooth muscle cells, microvascular endothelial cells, and lung fibroblasts. Inflammatory cells such as neutrophils and monocytes can also produce VEGF, as can stimulated alveolar macrophages. VEGF in the normal lung is highly compartmentalized, with alveolar levels far exceeding plasma levels. This alveolar reservoir of VEGF plays a role in promoting epithelial integrity under normal conditions and may affect endothelial permeability if the epithelium is damaged, allowing the highly concentrated alveolar VEGF to reach the endothelial layer. VEGF expression in the lung is also strongly upregulated by hypoxia and by numerous cytokines and inflammatory mediators associated with lung injury, including TNF-α, TGF-β, IL-6, and ET. VEGF exerts its effects via several receptors, the two best characterized of which are VEGFR1 (also known as flt-1) and VEGFR2 (also known as flk-1). These receptors are able to initiate downstream phosphorylation cascades that activate numerous intracellular signaling molecules. Both VEGFR1 and VEGFR2 are expressed on pulmonary vascular endothelial cells and on airway and alveolar epithelial cells.

VEGF was originally named "vascular permeability factor" in view of its ability to dramatically increase endothelial permeability in vascular beds throughout the body. The effects of VEGF on vascular permeability typically involve the phosphorylation and activation of the intracellular signaling molecule Akt, which then causes the phosphorylation of endothelial NO synthase (eNOS), leading to increased NO production and increased cellular cGMP. The mechanism that connects NO and cGMP to increased permeability remains obscure, although it is likely linked to activation of RhoA and MLC phosphorylation.

A growing body of evidence implicates VEGF in the pathogenesis of lung injury, although considerable controversy remains regarding its exact roles. Overexpression of VEGF in the lungs of experimental animals leads to florid pulmonary edema, and VEGF antagonists reduce lung injury and edema formation in many lung injury models, including viral infection, high tidal volume ventilation, and LPS instillation. In addition, studies of ARDS patients generally show increased plasma levels of VEGF early in the course of the disease. Airway levels of VEGF, in contrast, appear to decrease during the early phases of human ARDS and increase during recovery, a finding that has led to speculation that VEGF is required for healing of epithelial injury. VEGF may thus play different roles at different times in the course of ARDS and in different anatomic compartments of the lung, promoting edema formation initially but promoting epithelial repair in the later phase of the illness.

The angiopoietin family consists of several known ligands, the most important of which appear to be angiopoietin 1 (Ang1) and angiopoietin-2 (Ang2), and two transmembrane receptor tyrosine kinases TIE-1 and TIE-2. Both receptors are expressed in endothelial cells during development, but only TIE-2 is expressed at high levels in the lung in adult animals. During development, Ang1 binding to endothelial TIE-2 receptors leads to maturation of the developing vessel and stabilization of cell–cell contacts. Ang2 also binds to TIE-2 but acts as an antagonist to the effects of Ang1, causing vessel destabilization and loosened cell–cell contacts. Postnatally, Ang1 stimulation reduces vascular permeability and improves the integrity of the vascular barrier, reduces PMN adhesion to the endothelium, and reduces endothelial IL-8 production. Mice exposed to LPS at doses sufficient to cause lung injury develop increased lung VEGF expression and reduced Ang1 expression, and Ang1 overexpression in those animals leads to reduced mortality and less lung injury (15,23). In contrast, circulating Ang2 levels are high in patients with sepsis and evidence of lung injury, and plasma from those patients leads to gaps in cultured endothelial cell monolayers (17,24). In addition, administration of Ang2 to healthy mice leads to pulmonary edema formation via increased capillary permeability, and Ang2 release from endothelial cells is stimulated by TNF-α and other cytokines. These findings suggest that the balance between Ang1 and Ang2 expression regulates endothelial barrier properties in the lung. The precise signaling mechanisms that underlie these effects of Ang1 and Ang2 are still under investigation, but again appear to involve Rho family GTPases, as Ang1 has been reported to block RhoA activation, and the effects of Ang2 on the endothelium appear to be mediated by activation of Rho kinase and MLC phosphatase.

Ephrin family ligands and receptors are important regulators of cell–cell interactions across a wide range of physiologic and pathophysiologic processes, including nervous system and vascular development, tissue morphogenesis, and cancer growth and metastasis. Ephrin signaling activates a number of downstream pathways, ultimately converging on Rho family GTPases and associated guanine nuclear exchange factors to exert their end effects. Ephrins have been implicated in the regulation of both vascular permeability and inflammation (18,19,25,26). For example, stimulation of the EphA2 receptor by ephrin-A1 ligand has been shown to increase vascular permeability both in cultured lung endothelial cells and in the intact lung. EphA2 expression is increased in models of acute lung injury, and either loss or antagonism of EphA2 reduces pulmonary vascular leak and inflammation in those models. EphA2 activation also increases endothelial chemokine transcription, and other ephrins have been implicated in regulation of leukocyte trafficking. Although these preclinical findings are highly intriguing, the role of ephrins in human lung injury is yet to be determined.

Barrier-Protective Mediators

In addition to mediators that degrade endothelial barrier function, other mediators are produced in the lung that can stabilize barriers and reduce permeability. The role of Ang1 as a barrier-stabilizer has already been discussed. Sphingosine-1-phosphate (S1P) is a lipid mediator released from activated platelets that exerts a protective effect on the lung endothelial barrier (20,27). S1P binds to a class of G-protein–coupled receptors; the net effect of activation of S1P receptors in the endothelium is to activate Rac-1, leading to the rearrangement of actin into a cortical pattern, which results in reduced permeability and to the assembly of focal adhesions and cadherins junctions. Studies in experimental animals demonstrate a protective effect of S1P infusion on several forms of lung injury, including those associated with LPS and with high tidal volume ventilation. Interestingly, S1P has effects on barrier function in vivo that far exceed its molecular half-life, suggesting that it may alter the expression of some cytokines and adhesion molecules, thus modulating the immune response to lung injury. Indeed, recent work has shown that synthetic S1P receptor ligands reduce endothelial chemokine generation in the setting of experimental pandemic influenza infection, suggesting a possible therapeutic role for these compounds in the future (21,28). S1P also has effects on other cell types in the lung that may limit its clinical application. Most importantly, the administration of S1P into the airways leads to pulmonary edema via disruption of epithelial adherens and tight junctions (22,29). These cell type–specific differences in S1P effect likely relate to S1P receptor expression patterns and to different downstream signaling mechanisms from those receptors.

Most recently, the Slit–Robo system has also been implicated in barrier regulation. Members of a family of neural guidance molecules, Slit ligands, are soluble proteins that are released by epithelial and endothelial cells in the lung and when bound by endothelial Robo4 receptors promote barrier stabilization. In cultured endothelial cells, Slit2 is able to block permeability increases caused by VEGF, LPS, TNF-α, or IL-1β. In animal models of sepsis and pandemic influenza infection, administration of Slit2 reduces vascular leak and mortality without altering cytokine levels (23,30). These results highlight the tantalizing possibility that barrier stabilization could provide a therapeutic approach to lung injury independent of modulation of inflammatory responses.

REGULATION OF THE ALVEOLAR–CAPILLARY BARRIER

Mechanisms of Increased Endothelial Permeability

These cascades of inflammatory mediators in the injured lung drive the primary early physiologic derangement in ARDS: disruption of the alveolar–capillary barrier, with subsequent interstitial and alveolar edema formation. While barrier dysfunction has long been thought to be a secondary consequence driven by inflammation and injury, recent experimental evidence suggests that molecular strategies aimed at improving barrier function may improve outcomes from lung injury even without altering markers of inflammation (24,31). In this light, understanding mechanisms of endothelial and epithelial barrier regulation assumes an even greater importance.

The movement of fluid across the injured pulmonary vascular endothelium is thought to occur primarily via paracellular channels between the cells. The permeability of endothelial cell layers is largely determined by the state of intercellular junctions between endothelial cells and by the cytoskeleton of the individual endothelial cells (**Fig. 44.2**). Loosening of the intercellular junctions and/or contraction of the actin–myosin cytoskeleton allows the cells to pull apart, opening paracellular gaps for fluid movement across the barrier. Several types of junctions contribute to regulation of the lung endothelial barrier: tight junctions, adherens junctions, and focal adhesions. Tight junctions, comprising a number of proteins, including occludens, claudins, and zonula occludens (ZO) proteins, are thought to be the major permeability-regulating element of the blood–brain barrier. Although some recent studies have implicated alterations in tight junction proteins in the control of lung vascular and epithelial permeability, the role of tight junctions and specific claudin proteins in this regard remains uncertain and is an area of active investigation.

Adherens junctions may be more important than tight junctions in controlling lung vascular permeability. In the pulmonary endothelium, adherens junctions are principally composed of vascular/endothelial-cadherin (VE-cadherin) and members of the catenin family of proteins. The adherens junctions connect extracellularly to neighboring cells and intracellularly to the actin cytoskeleton. The breakdown of adherens junctions has been observed in cultured lung microvascular endothelial cells in response to permeability-increasing stimuli (e.g., thrombin and oxidant stress), and VE-cadherin function-blocking antibodies have been demonstrated to disrupt the alveolar–capillary barrier in vivo (25,26,32). A third type of intercellular junction, focal adhesions, connects the endothelial cell to the extracellular matrix via integrin receptors and

a number of cytoplasmic focal adhesion proteins. The precise role of these junctions in ARDS also remains uncertain, but accumulating evidence suggests that they, too, are important regulators of barrier function. For example, rearrangement of focal adhesion complexes from the periphery of the cell to the ends of actin stress fibers has been observed in association with increases in endothelial permeability due to both cyclic stretch and vasoactive agonists such as thrombin (27,33).

Connected to these junctional complexes is the endothelial cytoskeleton, which has three principal components: actin fibers, microtubules, and intermediate filaments. Of these three types of fibers, the actin cytoskeleton is the best studied and appears to be the most important in controlling lung endothelial barrier function (28,34,35). Actin fibers in unstimulated endothelial cells assume a "cortical" pattern, lined up around the periphery of the cell. Agonists that increase endothelial permeability cause actin fibers to rearrange into a more linear pattern ("stress fiber formation") and to interact with nonmuscle myosin, allowing the cell to contract away from its neighbors and create intercellular gaps in the monolayer. Stress fiber formation and actin–myosin interactions occur principally as a result of phosphorylation of the MLC molecule. The extent of MLC phosphorylation, in turn, is regulated by a balance between the activity of two enzymes: MLC kinase (MLCK) and myosin phosphatase (MYPT). Many mediators with effects on endothelial barrier function exert their effects by modulating the activities of one or both of these enzymes.

Calcium handling is another key element in the control of the endothelial cytoskeleton. MLCK activation is a calcium-dependent process, and increased intracellular calcium generally leads to increased endothelial permeability. In nonexcitable cells like endothelial cells, calcium entry is mediated primarily by a class of channels known as store-operated calcium (SOC) channels. SOC channels are activated by the binding of an agonist to its receptor on the endothelial cell surface, leading to the release of calcium from sequestered intracellular stores. Depletion of the intracellular calcium stores triggers the opening of cell surface SOC channels, which further increases intracellular calcium, allowing calcium binding to calmodulin, activation of MLCK as well as RhoGTPases, which then reduce MYPT activity. The molecular identity of the endothelial cell SOC channels has yet to be conclusively determined, although the family of transient receptor potential channels (TRPCs) has been identified as one form of SOC channel (29,36). Evidence that links TRPC channels to lung injury includes the findings that lung microvessels from TRPC4 knockout mice show markedly reduced responses to permeability-increasing agonists such as thrombin, and that TRPC6 knockout mice are resistant to endothelial permeability increases caused by bacterial LPS (30,37). Intriguingly, TRPC6 knockout mice are also resistant to LPS-induced endothelial inflammation, suggesting that TRPC6 activation represents a molecular mechanism by which increased permeability promotes inflammation. The precise role of SOC calcium entry in acute lung injury remains uncertain, however, because other studies have suggested that SOC channels regulate permeability primarily in endothelial cells from larger conduit vessels and thus other mechanisms must provide the necessary intracellular calcium for microvascular permeability changes (31,38,39).

Rho family GTPases are important regulators of the actin cytoskeleton and of endothelial permeability (32,40). These molecules function as molecular switches, cycling between an active guanosine triphosphate (GTP)-bound form and an inactive guanosine diphosphate (GDP)-bound form. The best studied of these proteins, RhoA, moves to the cell membrane when activated and stimulates its downstream effectors, the Rho kinases, which then phosphorylate MYPT, reducing its activity. The net effect of RhoA activation, then, is increased

MLC phosphorylation, increased actin–myosin interaction, and increased endothelial cell gap formation. This mechanism of endothelial gap formation has been demonstrated to be important in endothelial permeability changes induced by mediators including thrombin, TNF-α, lysophosphatidic acid, and LPS. Interestingly, another member of the same Rho family of GTPases, Rac-1, appears to have more varied effects on permeability. In some settings, Rac-1 activation promotes a peripheral, cortical actin fiber pattern and increased barrier integrity, but Rac-1 is also a key mediator of pro-permeability effects as well, including those caused by VEGF and by dengue virus infection. The downstream mediators that are responsible for these divergent effects of Rac-1 are still uncertain.

While both calcium-dependent MLCK activation and Rho-mediated MYPT inactivation are clearly important in endothelial barrier regulation, the relative contributions of these two mechanisms remain incompletely understood. Nonetheless, most mediators implicated in ARDS appear to act, at least in part, via these mechanisms.

Epithelial Barrier Integrity and Function in the Injured Lung

Once plasma fluids have breached the endothelial barrier, they must cross the epithelial barrier to reach the alveolar airspace. By most estimates, the permeability of the epithelial barrier is ~10-fold lower than that of the endothelial barrier, suggesting that the epithelium is the greater barrier to edema formation. Despite this fact, much more research has been directed at understanding endothelial permeability than epithelial permeability, perhaps because of the difficulty until relatively recently of studying alveolar epithelial cells in vitro. In general, epithelial cells appear to form their barrier via intracellular junctions similar to those observed in the endothelium. Tight junctions exist in the alveolar epithelium and are composed of claudins, occludens, and ZO proteins, as in other cell types. The particular claudin isoforms expressed appear to vary substantially from those in the endothelium and change with different stimuli, leading to the suggestion that alterations in claudin expression pattern provide a level of regulation of epithelial barrier function. Adherens junctions are also important in the epithelial barrier, although the predominant cadherin protein expressed is E-cadherin, rather than VE-cadherin as in the endothelium. In addition, changes in epithelial permeability are sometimes associated with actin cytoskeleton rearrangements, although evidence that implicates MLCK and Rho kinase activity in those events is lacking.

Many mediators capable of altering epithelial permeability have been described. Certainly, direct epithelial cell death, as a result of bacterial or viral infection or direct injury by inhaled toxins, can alter permeability, as can mechanical injury to the epithelium from ventilator-induced lung injury. Airway LPS, presumably acting via TLRs, increases epithelial permeability via a mechanism that involves neutrophil influx, and it can be partially blocked by nitric oxide (NO). Other secondary mediators also contribute. For example, TGF-β1 has been shown to increase epithelial cell monolayer permeability via a mechanism that is dependent on oxidant stress but not on MLCK. Hypoxia leads to increased epithelial permeability and breakdown of epithelial tight junctions. Cytokines, including TNF-α, IL-8, and epidermal growth factor (EGF) can also increase epithelial permeability.

For edema fluid to result in alveolar flooding, the movement of fluid into the airspaces must overwhelm innate alveolar fluid clearance mechanisms (33,41) (**Fig. 44.3**). Alveolar liquid clearance is largely the result of active sodium transport. Both type 1 and type 2 alveolar epithelial cells express Na/K-ATPases on their basolateral membranes. These enzymes, comprising α and β subunits, actively pump sodium out of the epithelial cell and into the lung interstitium, exchanging three sodium molecules for two potassium molecules in the process. The epithelial cell also expresses epithelial sodium channels (ENaCs) on its apical (luminal) surface. Three distinct ENaC subunits exist in mammals: ENaC-α, ENaC-β, and ENaC-γ. The functional channel is composed of multimers of these subunits. ENaC channels allow sodium to move passively down the concentration gradient created by the basolateral pumps, out of the airspaces, and into the epithelial cell. The combined effect of the ENaC and Na/K-ATPases is to actively clear sodium from the airspaces across the epithelial barrier and into the interstitium, creating an osmotic gradient for water to follow. Water moves out of the alveolus along this osmotic gradient, both via specific water channels (aquaporins) and via paracellular routes.

A number of factors modulate the expression and activity of these molecules in ways relevant to lung injury. For example, both inflammation and infection impair alveolar liquid clearance by altering sodium channel expression

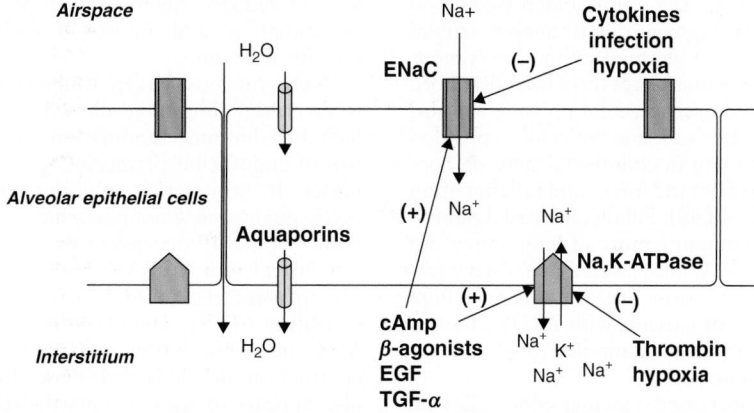

FIGURE 44.3. Molecular mechanisms regulating alveolar liquid clearance. Basolateral Na/K-ATPases (*pentagons*) pump sodium out of the epithelial cell and into the interstitium, creating a gradient for sodium movement out of the airspaces via apical ENaC sodium channels (*rectangles*). Water follows this gradient out of the airspaces via aquaporin channels (*cylinders*) and paracellular routes (*arrow between cells*). Stimuli, including cytokines, thrombin, hypoxia, and β-agonists, can increase or decrease ENaC and Na/K-ATPase function. ENaC, epithelial sodium channels; cAMP, cyclic adenosine monophosphate; EGF, epidermal growth factor; TGF-α, transforming growth factor-α.

and/or activity. ENaC subunit expression is downregulated by cytokines, such as TNF-α and IL-1β, and by infection with *Pseudomonas aeruginosa* bacteria (34,35,42). Influenza virus and respiratory syncytial virus (RSV) infections, in contrast, impair ENaC function without altering channel expression. In the case of RSV, this effect is mediated by uridine triphosphate (UTP) release from the epithelium and stimulation of purinergic receptors. Hypoxia also impairs epithelial sodium transport by reducing both ENaC and Na/K-ATPase activity. Thrombin reduces lung liquid clearance by promoting endocytosis of Na/K-ATPases (36,43,44). Mediators that can increase alveolar liquid clearance have also been described. β-adrenergic agents, such as isoproterenol and dopamine, act via cyclic adenosine monophosphate (cAMP) to promote alveolar liquid clearance by increasing Na/K-ATPase activity and upregulating ENaC expression. Corticosteroids and aldosterone also increase ENaC expression.

The physiologic importance of these sodium and water transport mechanisms is apparent from both animal and human studies. Targeted deletion of the ENaC-α subunit in mice leads to respiratory distress and death shortly after birth from inability to clear fluid from the airspaces, whereas overexpression of the Na/K-ATPase-β subunit leads to increased alveolar liquid clearance in rats that are subjected to high tidal volume ventilation. In adult patients with ARDS, alveolar fluid clearance rates are impaired and clinical outcome correlates inversely with the degree of impairment, suggesting that those patients whose alveolar epithelial liquid clearance mechanisms sustain the greatest damage do worse clinically. Unfortunately, recent clinical trials testing the strategy of using β-agonists to increase alveolar liquid clearance in adult ARDS patients found no benefit to that approach (37,45).

CONTROL OF PULMONARY VASCULAR TONE

The regulation of pulmonary vascular tone is also important to the pathophysiology and treatment of ARDS. Normal mechanisms of ventilation–perfusion matching are impaired in ARDS, and the resultant maldistribution in pulmonary blood flow and increase in intrapulmonary shunting contribute to the severe systemic hypoxemia in these patients. In addition, the movement of fluid out of the vasculature and into the airspaces depends both on the permeability of the endothelial barrier and on the hydrostatic forces that drive fluid movement. Increased microvascular pressure can occur as a result of increased blood flow through a given vascular segment due to uneven arterial vasoconstriction or as a result of elevated pulmonary venous pressure or resistance. Both circumstances have been described in ARDS (38,39,44). Increased microvascular pressure has also been demonstrated to upregulate adhesion molecule expression and increase intracellular calcium in endothelial cells, demonstrating a linkage between hydrostatic forces and inflammation in the lung microvasculature (40,46). Finally, increased pulmonary arterial pressure is a common feature of lung injury and correlates with worse outcome. While elevated pulmonary vascular pressures severe enough to cause overt right heart failure are present in only a minority of patients with ARDS, changes in vascular tone may contribute substantially to pulmonary edema formation in many more patients.

At the molecular level, increased vascular tone relies on molecular mechanisms similar to those involved in endothelial barrier function, although the key cell in this case is the vascular smooth muscle cell. Most vasoconstrictive agonists, such as angiotensin II and ET, bind G-protein–coupled receptors on the smooth muscle cell surface, stimulating phospholipase C, triggering diacylglycerol and inositol 1,4,5-triphosphate

(IP3) formation, and leading to release of intracellular calcium stores and a rise in intracellular calcium concentration. In contrast to endothelial cells, however, smooth muscle cells also express voltage-gated ion channels, and when the intracellular calcium concentration reaches a threshold level, the cell depolarizes and opens voltage-gated calcium channels, flooding the cell with calcium. Calmodulin is then activated and, in turn, activates MLCK, which phosphorylates MLCs, enabling the interaction of myosin with actin and cell contraction. Some agonists also stimulate Rho/Rho kinase signaling, which reduces MYPT activity, leading to "calcium sensitization," in which contractile tone is increased independently of increased intracellular calcium. Molecules that affect vascular tone in the lung can be released by the vascular endothelium, by adventitial cells, by interstitial cells in the lung parenchyma, and by circulating or inflammatory cells transiting the vascular bed. Recent work has increasingly focused on the role of those cells that surround the vessel as being key early mediators of many pulmonary vascular responses, in contrast to the previous concept of the endothelium as the primary controller of vascular tone.

Pulmonary vascular tone is the result of a balance between endogenous vasoconstrictors and vasodilators. ET is one of the most important endogenous vasoconstrictors. This small peptide is produced by many cells in the lung and acts via two G-protein–coupled receptors, ET_A and ET_B. Binding of ET to the ET_A receptor on smooth muscle cells leads to intense constriction of either the airway or blood vessel involved. Activation of the ET_B receptor leads to various consequences, depending on the cell type that expresses it. In vascular smooth muscle, ET_B receptor stimulation generally acts similarly to ET_A receptor stimulation. The stimulation of endothelial ET_B receptors, however, triggers the release of NO and causes vasodilation. In addition to its vascular effects, ET is a potent cytokine and contributes to both inflammatory responses and fibrosis. ET expression in the lung is upregulated both by hypoxia and by a host of inflammatory cytokines, including VEGF and TGF-β.

The ET system has been clearly implicated in both human and experimental lung injury. In both adults and children with ARDS, circulating ET levels are elevated and correlate with severity of illness. ET antagonists given via either the parenteral or inhaled routes ameliorate lung injury in experimental settings as diverse as endotoxin-mediated injury, acid injury, surfactant depletion, and viral infection coupled with hypoxia. Whether the beneficial effects of ET antagonism in these settings are primarily due to improved pulmonary hemodynamics and reduced microvascular pressures or due to reduced inflammation and improved endothelial barrier function remains uncertain.

NO is the most widely studied endogenous vasodilator and is also a signaling molecule with numerous roles in the lung, including immune modulation, epithelial function, and control of endothelial permeability. NO acts in vascular smooth muscle by stimulating soluble guanylate cyclase to produce cyclic guanosine monophosphate (cGMP). cGMP activates a family of cGMP-dependent protein kinases that reduce intracellular calcium levels via an effect on calcium flux out of the sarcoplasmic reticulum and reduce calcium sensitization by activating MYPT. The net effect of these events is to reduce MLC phosphorylation and reduce vascular smooth muscle contraction. In addition to these effects on vascular tone, NO also appears to regulate endothelial permeability, although it has been reported to both increase and decrease lung microvascular permeability depending on the experimental setting studied (41,47). NO is produced by a family of NO synthases (NOS). eNOS is constitutively expressed by endothelial cells, and neuronal NOS (nNOS) is expressed in neurons. Inducible NOS (iNOS) can be expressed by most mammalian cells as a response to inflammation or injury, in particular, by lung macrophages and neutrophils in the setting of lung injury.

Despite its widespread clinical use as an inhaled vasodilator to improve ventilation–perfusion matching in ARDS, the literature regarding the physiologic and molecular roles of NO in the injured lung remains a confusing field. For example, while much available evidence suggests that lung injury is accompanied by increased NO levels in the lung, studies of nonselective NOS inhibitors in ARDS have shown both improvement and worsening of edema formation. Similarly, the observed increase in local NO generation during lung injury would be expected to reduce vascular resistance and yet increased vascular resistance is more typical in patients with ARDS. The mechanisms that underlie this apparent insensitivity of the injured lung to increased NO production remain uncertain.

The role of hypoxia in the control of pulmonary vascular tone is also pertinent to a discussion of ARDS (48). Regional hypoxia is a characteristic of injured tissues and may be particularly evident in areas of dependent collapse in the injured lung, in which blood flow is reduced. Hypoxia can upregulate many of the transcriptional and signaling mechanisms that are active in the injured lung and may contribute to lung injury. Interestingly, despite this regional and global hypoxemia in the ARDS lung, high O_2 concentrations do little to improve pulmonary hemodynamics in these patients. This observation is consistent with the idea that the impaired ventilation–perfusion matching that is a prominent mechanism of hypoxemia in ARDS is in large part a result of blunted hypoxic pulmonary vasoconstriction in these patients. Thus, the increased pulmonary vascular resistance seen in ARDS appears to be predominantly attributable to the effects of vasoactive mediators rather than to O_2 tension per se.

Surfactant Biochemistry in the Injured Lung

The inflammation and loss of endothelial and epithelial barrier function in early ARDS lead to flooding of the alveolar space with plasma. A major consequence of this flooding and epithelial cell dysfunction is inactivation and loss of surfactant (42,49). Pulmonary surfactant reduces surface tension in the air–liquid interface, facilitates the stability of the expanded alveolus, and is essential for normal lung function. When surfactant activity is lost, the alveolus becomes unstable and prone to collapse, leading to dependent lung atelectasis and worsened V/Q matching. In addition to its biomechanical properties, surfactant also contributes to the host's innate defense system and possesses anti-inflammatory properties.

The composition of surfactant is similar among various species and consists of ~90% lipids and 10% surfactant-related proteins. The lipid portion of surfactant contains 90% phospholipid, 75% of which is phosphatidylcholine (PC). Approximately 40% of the PC exists in desaturated form as dipalmitoylphosphatidylcholine (DPPC), which is believed to be the main surface tension–reducing component at the air–liquid interface. Surfactant proteins (SP-A, SP-B, SP-C, and SP-D) also play an important role in these processes, especially the small, hydrophobic proteins SP-B and SP-C. SP-B enhances the adsorption of surfactant lipids to the interface and promotes the transformation of this lipid layer into a DPPC-rich surface film able to reduce the surface tension to very low values during exhalation. SP-C is the most hydrophobic of the surfactant-associated proteins. SP-C is more intimately associated with the surfactant film than is SP-B, although the exact role of SP-C is less defined than that of SP-B. The two other proteins associated with surfactant are designated SP-A and SP-D; their role appears predominantly related to host defense rather than to biophysical properties, although SP-A may contribute to surface tension reduction under stress conditions such as ARDS.

Deficiencies of either surfactant phospholipids or surfactant proteins can lead to impaired lung function, including poor compliance, atelectasis, inflammation, infection, and hypoxemia. Alterations of the endogenous surfactant system that contribute to the lung dysfunction associated with ARDS include changes in the lipid profile, altered concentrations of surfactant-associated proteins, and shifts in the relative amounts of surfactant aggregate forms within the airspace. These changes in lipid profile are due to altered synthetic and/or secretory pathways within the type II cell, as well as degradation of lipids within the airspace via phospholipase activity. In general, surfactant-associated protein concentrations are also decreased in BALF samples obtained from patients with ARDS compared with samples from control subjects. This decrease in protein concentration, like that in lipids, may be because of alterations in type II cell metabolism and/or increased proteolytic activity within the airspace. Increased levels of surfactant proteins have also been found in the serum of patients with ARDS, likely reflecting leakage of these proteins from the alveoli into the blood. Serum levels of SP-A and SP-B are inversely related to oxygenation values, and serum levels of SP-D correlate with patient survival. The potential use of these measurements as markers of disease severity is currently being investigated.

FIBROPROLIFERATION AND REPAIR IN THE INJURED LUNG

The pathophysiology of ARDS consists of overlapping acute inflammatory and delayed "repair/fibrotic" phases (43,44,50,51). As described earlier, loss of alveolar capillary barrier function occurs early in ARDS and allows influx of proteinaceous fluid, blood, and inflammatory cells into the alveoli. Activation of the coagulation system and complement and the release of cytokines amplify the inflammatory response and contribute to further injury. Overlapping with this acute exudative phase (rather than following it, as was previously thought) is a process of repair, markers of which have been identified as early as a few hours into the course of disease. This process is characterized by the presence of intraalveolar mesenchymal cells/fibroblasts, type II cell hyperproliferation, and extracellular matrix turnover. In many cases of ARDS, the process of repair proceeds normally, with complete resolution of inflammation and fibrosis and a reestablishment of normal alveolar architecture. In some instances, however, the resolution phase of lung injury results in disordered repair of the alveolus, a process characterized by impaired fibrinolysis of the inflammatory coagulum, fibrocellular proliferation, architectural distortion of the lung parenchyma, and abnormal angiogenesis. Clinically, the result of this fibroproliferation is a restrictive ventilatory defect and evidence of impaired alveolar membrane function, characterized by a prolonged reduction in the diffusing capacity for carbon monoxide (45,52).

Alveolar Epithelial Repair

Restoration of the normal airspace architecture requires reconstitution of the denuded type I alveolar epithelial cells that have undergone apoptotic and necrotic death during the exudative phase of ARDS. Regeneration of type II epithelial cells, in coordination with extracellular matrix turnover, is important in reestablishing surfactant production and ion transport, functions essential for maintaining open and dry alveoli. It is apparent that orderly reepithelialization suppresses fibroblast proliferation and matrix deposition after ARDS (44,53). Thus, efficient restoration of the alveolar epithelium in the early phase of ARDS may speed recovery by enhancing alveolar liquid clearance and preventing the development of pulmonary fibrosis. In addition, the endothelium plays a critical role in the repair and remodeling of the alveolar capillary membrane (46,54,55).

Several mechanisms have major roles in alveolar epithelial repair in vivo and in vitro. Proliferation of alveolar type II cells is the most obvious and easily measurable event in epithelial repair in vivo, but 1–2 days transpire before it becomes significant. Other mechanisms likely contribute to early alveolar epithelial wound repair, especially in those situations in which progression to severe fibroproliferative changes do not occur. For example, pulmonary edema fluid from patients with ARDS stimulates repair of epithelial monolayers that have been injured. One of the factors present in this edema fluid that helps support alveolar epithelial repair is IL-1β (47,56,57).

Evidence exists that EGF, TGF-α, and their common receptor, EGF receptor (EGFR), may also participate in epithelial repair following injury. TGF-α is elevated in edema fluid from patients with ALI (Acute Lung Injury)/ARDS and induces alveolar/epithelial repair in vitro. Further, blocking EGFR or its intracellular signaling through MAPK specifically inhibits the reparative effects of IL-1β in ARDS, suggesting that IL-1β acts, in part, by activating the EGF/TGF-α pathway (49,58). The potential value of using TGF-α or EGF to treat patients with ARDS has not yet been evaluated.

Animal studies suggest that keratinocyte growth factor (KGF) and hepatocyte growth factor (HGF) play a role in lung repair. KGF is produced primarily by fibroblasts and induces alveolar type II proliferation in vivo and in vitro. KGF has a protective effect against lung injury when administered before the injury, and elevated levels of KGF correlate with alveolar epithelial cell proliferation following bleomycin injury, again supporting a role for KGF in epithelial repair (50,51,59). Experiments using specific inhibitors of the EGF/TGF-α pathway suggest that the effects of KGF are mediated again

through the EGFR pathway. These findings, coupled with the previously mentioned role of IL-1β and TGF-α, suggest that EGFR may serve as a final common pathway in stimulating alveolar epithelial repair. HGF is another potent mitogen for alveolar type II cells and is upregulated in fibroblasts following inflammatory cytokine stimulation. HGF is elevated in pulmonary edema in ARDS, supporting a role for HGF in epithelial repair (52,60).

In summary, alveolar epithelial repair is extremely complicated and modulated by numerous growth factors and cytokines. These factors are secreted both from local cells, such as fibroblasts, and from inflammatory cells that accumulate in the alveolar space during lung injury. Proper communication must occur between the renewing epithelial cell populations, the underlying extracellular matrix, and the endothelial cells, which are undergoing constant changes in the setting of lung injury. Much additional work is needed, however, to determine whether the alveolar epithelial repair process can ultimately be manipulated with therapeutic strategies to heal the injured lung.

Mechanisms of Fibroproliferation

Either during or after the acute inflammatory response to injury, interstitial fibroblasts migrate into the alveolar space, marking the beginning of the fibroproliferative phase of ARDS (Fig. 44.4). These interstitial fibroblasts differentiate into myofibroblasts, which contain abundant α-smooth muscle actin and vinculin. This much more metabolically active myofibroblast proliferates in its new location and exhibits upregulated expression of important integrin receptors, including the fibronectin receptor $\alpha5\beta1$, CD44, and the receptor for hyaluronic acid–mediated motility (RHAMM), probably allowing for increased motility and specific interactions with the newly evolving microenvironment (53,61).

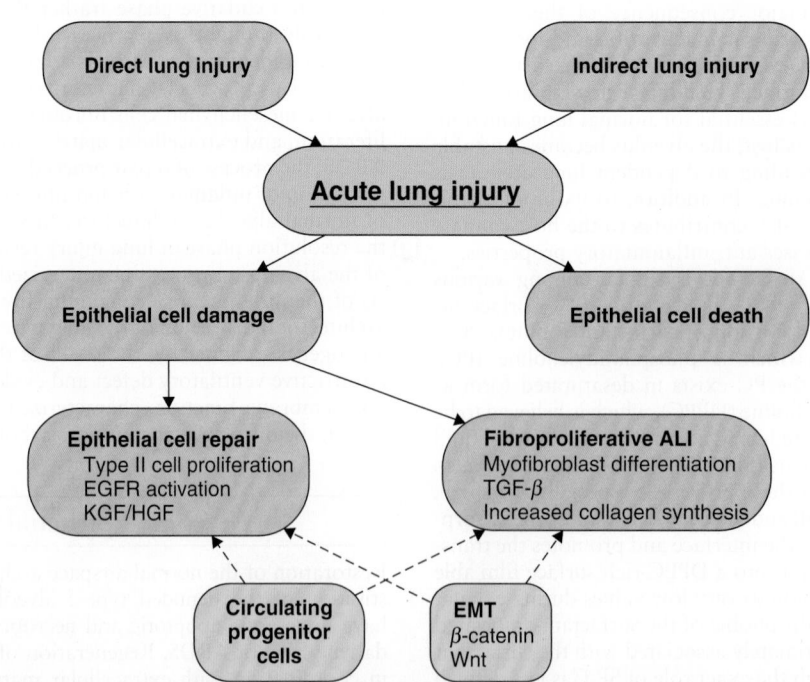

FIGURE 44.4. Fibroproliferation in lung injury. Direct and indirect triggers of acute lung injury lead to epithelial cell damage and death. Recovery from epithelial damage can proceed to normal regulated repair mechanisms or to dysregulated mechanisms of fibroproliferation. Circulating progenitor cells and epithelial–mesenchymal transitions (EMT) may contribute to both repair and fibroproliferation. EGFR, epidermal growth factor receptor; TGF-β, transforming growth factor-β; KGF, keratinocyte growth factor; HGF, hepatocyte growth factor.

Fibroproliferation is also seen in the microcirculation of the lung. In the airspace, fibroproliferation leads to shunt; in the microcirculation, it contributes to narrowing of the cross-sectional area, which contributes to pulmonary hypertension.

In addition to its roles in the acute phase of ARDS, TGF-β also has an important role in fibroproliferative responses (54,55,62). TGF-β is a major regulator of gene expression, particularly of extracellular matrix molecules, in mesenchymal cells and lung fibroblasts. It is a potent inducer of collagen synthesis, has the ability to directly cause differentiation of fibroblasts into myofibroblasts, and inhibits collagenase production (56,57,61,63). TGF-β also induces the proliferation of some fibroblast populations, most probably through the induction of other growth factors, such as platelet-derived growth factor. TGF-β can establish an apparent state of autocrine stimulation in structural cells, including fibroblasts, resulting in chronic activation and differentiation to a more aggressive phenotype, consistent with nonresolving or severe disease. Indeed, investigators have described a population of alveolar mesenchymal cells isolated from patients with nonresolving ARDS that exhibited constitutive activation of prosurvival signaling pathways (58,64). These observations are important because they support the theory that, during the resolution of the fibrotic phase of lung injury, apoptosis of mesenchymal cells is an essential component of normal repair and resolution. Conversely, they suggest that dysregulation of this process and the appearance of cells that are resistant to apoptosis may lead to persistent or nonresolving ARDS.

Additional support for the role of TGF-β in the fibroproliferative responses can be found in animal models of alveolar injury that lead to pulmonary fibrosis (e.g., bleomycin lung injury), as well as in human idiopathic pulmonary fibrosis. The steady-state expression of TGF-β transcripts increases at ~1 week after intratracheal installation of bleomycin (59,65). Increased expression of TGF-β precedes the increased matrix deposition in these experiments, supporting the involvement of this cytokine in the fibrotic process. An important source of TGF-β is the alveolar macrophage, which may be relevant to the controversy over the effect of corticosteroids on the late fibroproliferative stage of lung injury. Corticosteroids can inhibit macrophage secretion of IL-1, but they have very little effect on TGF-β1 (60,66,67). Thus, it is possible that the variable efficacy of corticosteroid therapy in patients in the late stages of ARDS is attributable to this divergence of effects, with corticosteroids causing a reduction in cytokine release but having little effect on TGF-β production by alveolar macrophages.

Epithelial–Mesenchymal Transdifferentiation

As accumulation of fibroblast- or myofibroblast-like cells is critical in the fibroproliferative state of ARDS, investigators have evaluated several pathways through which accumulation of these cells might occur. Work in other organ systems, especially the kidney, has suggested that transdifferentiation of epithelial cells into matrix-producing mesenchymal cells (fibroblasts and myofibroblasts) might be involved. Recent studies have suggested that transdifferentiation of epithelial cells into matrix-producing fibroblasts is one mechanism by which disordered epithelial repair promotes progression to the fibroproliferative stage of ARDS (61,68,69). Several pathways regulate this process of epithelial–mesenchymal transdifferentiation (EMT). TGF-β again seems especially important (62,68). Another important pathway in the EMT process is the Wnt signaling pathway. The Wnt pathway is a signaling pathway critical for precise temporal and spatial control of lung morphogenesis, which is interesting because several lines of investigation suggest that the mechanisms of resolution and

repair of ARDS in adults are controlled, in part, by regulatory pathways that are important in lung morphogenesis and development (61,63,70). Within the Wnt signaling pathway, β-catenin is a key regulatory protein. Targeted deletion of β-catenin from the alveolar epithelium of developing mouse embryos results in complete disruption of the peripheral terminal alveolar saccule formation and in disturbances of pulmonary vasculogenesis (64,71,72). Also, β-catenin signaling is upregulated in the reparative remodeling response to ARDS (65,73). These studies suggest a strong association between enhanced expression of the cadherin/catenin axis with epithelial regeneration and EMT. Thus, EMT could contribute to myofibroblast proliferation and collagen deposition in ARDS.

Stem Cells in the Injured Lung

Evidence in a number of experimental systems suggests that mobilization of progenitor cells from the injured tissue or from the bone marrow may repair damage caused by a variety of insults (66,67). Several experimental models confirm that, after lung damage, injured recipient lungs can become repopulated with cells of donor origins, including type I and II epithelial cells, endothelial cells, and fibroblast and interstitial monocytes. Engraftment of stem cells into the lung is most robust following injury and is minimal in uninjured animals (68,69). Intact, noninjured bone marrow may also be integral to protective responses. In one study, bone marrow ablation without transplantation caused changes in the lung reminiscent of emphysema in the absence of direct lung injury (68). Collectively, research suggests that when the lung is damaged by a variety of causes (chemicals, infection, radiation), progenitor cells are released from the bone marrow and attracted by as yet unidentified factors to the damaged lung. These cells act in a beneficial manner to repair the lung. For example, experiments in patients with ARDS demonstrated that they have an increased number of circulating endothelial progenitor cells compared to healthy controls. Further, a greater number of circulating endothelial progenitor cells is associated with improved outcomes in a multivariable analysis that corrected for the effects for age, gender, and severity-of-illness scores. It should be noted, however, that progenitor cells could also, under certain circumstances, contribute to ongoing fibroproliferative responses, as has been demonstrated following bleomycin injury. In that setting, a subset of circulating mesenchymal progenitor cells, termed *fibrocytes*, is recruited to the lung and contributes significantly to the fibroproliferative changes (4,70,74). Future studies will have to determine in more detail the role that these cells play in repair of the lung following injury.

The most promising stem cell work to date in the area of lung injury involves mesenchymal stem cells (MSCs). First described in 1974, these cells have received increasing attention in a number of clinical fields for their potential therapeutic effects (71,72,75). MSCs are multipotent cells derived from adult (usually) tissues that are capable of cell renewal and differentiation. They are a heterogeneous group of cells that can be isolated from many tissues including bone marrow, adipose tissue, fat, muscle, dermis, placenta, and lung. The derivation of MSCs from adult tissues, their relative ease of isolation and enormous expansion potential in culture as well as the fact that they are immunologically well tolerated and can be transplanted from one individual to another of the same species, makes them attractive therapeutic candidates (73,76,77).

Originally MSCs were thought to directly repair degenerative disease in the lung and other organs by engraftment and differentiation. More recent studies demonstrate that the direct engraftment rates of MSCs in lung injury models are low, suggesting that engraftment and differentiation are unlikely to be the mechanisms of therapeutic benefit and that the release by

MSCs of soluble factors that act in a paracrine manner to promote repair may be more important (2,4,6,7,11,13,16). The beneficial actions of MSCs encompass antiapoptotic and cytoprotective effects in the promotion of angiogenesis. Indeed, it is the multifactorial, coordinated, and targeted features of MSCs that make cell therapy approaches so intriguing and potentially superior to small molecule modalities. Perhaps the most important activity of MSCs, particularly in the setting of lung injury, is the fact that they are powerful modulators of the mammalian immune response.

In the past few years, there has been a rapid delineation of the mechanisms by which MSCs modulate different aspects of both the innate and adaptive immune response. An important characteristic of MSCs is the fact that both allogeneic and xenogeneic MSCs typically avoid acute and hyperacute rejection mechanisms that are normally mediated through complement. Protection from this deletional process is afforded by MSC expression of factor-H and other complement control proteins (4,74,78). MSCs are not only protected from host innate immune responses, but they may also contribute to shaping the processes of inflammation and repair. For instance, MSCs block neutrophil function by suppressing the neutrophil oxidative burst while preserving their phagocytic and chemotactic functions (75,79). MSCs also suppress inflammatory eosinophil localization in vivo, and "reprogram" the conventional myeloid dendritic cell (DC) response to activating stimuli, converting proinflammatory responses to anti-inflammatory cytokine production (IL-10) (76,77,80,81). DCs that have encountered MSCs suppress the proliferation of activated T-cells, influence the ratio of T-cell subsets, and promote regulatory T cells (T-reg) (78,79,81–83). MSCs decrease proinflammatory cytokine expression in neighboring cells, secrete anti-inflammatory agents (including IL-1 receptor antagonist, IL-10, and prostaglandin E_2, and may also augment the host immune response to infection by secreting antimicrobial peptides such as LL-37 (cathelicidin) (72,79). MSCs can also aid regenerative processes following injury, in part, via secretion of cytoprotective agents (80,81,84). MSC secretion of angiopoietin and KGF restores alveolar epithelial and endothelial permeability and enhances resolution of ARDS in preclinical models. Preclinical studies have demonstrated that MSCs can reduce lung injury caused by endotoxin, pneumonia, and systemic sepsis (79,81–83).

These observations of the potent immunomodulatory and reparative effects of MSCs and success in preclinical models suggest that MSCs might be beneficial in the treatment of human ARDS. However, gaps remain in our knowledge regarding mechanisms of action of MSCs as well as optimal administration routes and dosage regimens. Further, their safety in critically ill patients has not been thoroughly examined. In fact, safety concerns may represent a significant barrier to the successful translation of MSCs into an acceptable clinical therapeutic intervention. A recently published large meta-analysis has suggested, however, that based on recent clinical trials MSC therapy appears safe (72). This pooled analysis study found no association between MSCs and tumor formation, a concern which had been consistently raised, and no evidence of increased susceptibility to infection with MSC administration. Thus, while much work remains to be done, there is strong data to support further investigation regarding the use of these cells for the treatment of lung injury.

CONCLUSIONS AND FUTURE DIRECTIONS

The molecular biology of lung injury is a highly complex and incompletely explored topic. Nonetheless, these complex molecular interactions and signaling networks both form the basis for current treatment strategies and suggest possible avenues for developing new therapies. Current approaches to ARDS attempt to control the injury primarily by reducing inflammation, by treating the underlying or exacerbating conditions, and by limiting ventilator-induced damage to the alveolar–capillary barrier. Observed reductions in circulating cytokines in patients ventilated with "lung protective" strategies support the validity of this approach. Otherwise, very little modern medicine is directed specifically at reducing endothelial and epithelial permeability in the injured lung or at accelerating repair. Therapy directed at reducing microvascular pressures is generally reserved for patients in overt right heart failure, with the exception of inhaled NO (iNO), which is sometimes used to improve ventilation–perfusion matching in the injured lung. While iNO has gained much attention for its ability to improve oxygenation in some patients with ARDS, the effect is transient, and iNO treatment does not appear to alter the outcome of the illness, perhaps because of the multiple conflicting roles of NO in the injured lung. Efforts to reduce fluid intake and improve overall fluid balance have been suggested as a means of reducing microvascular pressures favoring edema formation. Corticosteroids have been studied for the prevention of late fibroproliferative changes in ARDS, but data in children do not yet exist and adult data demonstrate modest efficacy at best.

In terms of modulating epithelial function, the well-described surfactant lipid and protein changes in ARDS have led to trials of surfactant replacement as treatment for this condition. These trials have been generally disappointing, with the exception of a single pediatric study (84). Whether the lack of efficacy in most studies results from ineffective delivery methods or insufficient replacement of surfactant proteins (as opposed to surfactant lipids) remains to be determined.

Novel therapies directed at specific molecular mediators of lung injury have the potential to substantially improve the care of patients with ARDS. Treatments directed more specifically at the preservation of endothelial barrier integrity hold promise. Rho kinase inhibitors appear effective in experimental animals, and several compounds are being tested in human clinical trials for other indications. Similarly, S1P analogs and HMG-CoA-reductase inhibitors (statins) both act via Rac activation to improve endothelial barrier integrity and appear effective in ameliorating lung injury in animal models. Statins also prevent the posttranslational modifications necessary for RhoA activation and may prove helpful in both improving endothelial barrier function and controlling vascular tone.

Antiangiogenic therapies provide another possible avenue of investigation. VEGF antagonism may reduce endothelial permeability and edema formation, although this approach potentially could have detrimental effects on pulmonary vascular pressure and on epithelial regeneration. Available anti-VEGF agents are well tolerated as antineoplastic agents but have not yet been investigated for use in human ARDS. ET receptor antagonists are also well tolerated when used for pulmonary hypertension and may have beneficial effects in ARDS, both by reducing vascular pressures and by reducing the generation of excessive amounts of other mediators, such as VEGF, although they remain unstudied for this indication in humans. Some investigators have suggested targeting transcriptional mediators, such as HIF-1 or NF-κB, to reduce inflammation and injury in ARDS. Finally, as our understanding of the reparative processes in the lung improves, therapies targeted at improving epithelial cell regeneration and reducing fibroproliferation may ultimately reduce the long-term consequences of ARDS on lung function.

Clearly, many of the possible new approaches to interrupting the mechanisms that underlie lung injury are complicated by the fact that many of these key mediators appear to play important roles in the processes of both lung injury and repair.

VEGF is one example of such a molecule, as is NF-κB. Enthusiasm over the possibility that antagonizing these mediators early in the course of ARDS could alter its course and improve outcome is tempered by the possibility that such approaches could have deleterious effects on the recovery phase of lung injury. Devising strategies that reduce injury without reducing repair mechanisms remains a challenge and will require continued careful investigation of the molecular mechanisms that underlie both processes.

A final additional caveat in this discussion is the role of development. Most lung injury research has focused on adult animal models and adult patients, but data suggest that the developing lung may be more susceptible to some injuries and less susceptible to others as compared to the adult lung. The molecular mechanisms that underlie these differences remain largely unexplored and may have profound implications for the development of future treatments for ARDS in the PICU.

ACKNOWLEDGMENT

This work was supported by NIH SCOR Grant HL57144-10 and Program Project Grant HL14985-34 (KRS).

References

1. Shimoda LA, Semenza GL. HIF and the lung: Role of hypoxia-inducible factors in pulmonary development and disease. *Am J Respir Crit Care Med* 2011;183:152–6.
2. Caplan AI. Why are MSCs therapeutic? New data: New insight. *J Pathol* 2009;217:318–24.
3. Tolle LB, Standiford TJ. Danger-associated molecular patterns (DAMPs) in acute lung injury. *J Pathol* 2013;229:145–56.
4. English K, Mahon BP. Allogeneic mesenchymal stem cells: Agents of immune modulation. *J Cell Biochem* 2011;112:1963–8.
5. Morty RE, Königshoff M, Eickelberg O. Transforming growth factor-beta signaling across ages: From distorted lung development to chronic obstructive pulmonary disease. *Proc Am Thorac Soc* 2009;6:607–13.
6. Mei SHJ, McCarter SD, Deng Y, et al. Prevention of LPS-induced acute lung injury in mice by mesenchymal stem cells overexpressing angiopoietin 1. *PLoS Med* 2007;4:e269.
7. Ortiz LA, Dutreil M, Fattman C, et al. Interleukin 1 receptor antagonist mediates the antiinflammatory and antifibrotic effect of mesenchymal stem cells during lung injury. *Proc Natl Acad Sci USA* 2007;104:11002–7.
8. Karikó K, Ni H, Capodici J, et al. mRNA is an endogenous ligand for Toll-like receptor 3. *J Biol Chem* 2004;279:12542–50.
9. Jenkins RG, Su X, Su G, et al. Ligation of protease-activated receptor 1 enhances alpha(v)beta6 integrin-dependent TGF-beta activation and promotes acute lung injury. *J Clin Invest* 2006;116:1606–14.
10. Modelska K, Pittet JF, Folkesson HG, et al. Acid-induced lung injury. Protective effect of anti-interleukin-8 pretreatment on alveolar epithelial barrier function in rabbits. *Am J Respir Crit Care Med* 1999;160:1450–6.
11. Yanai H, Ban T, Taniguchi T. High-mobility group box family of proteins: Ligand and sensor for innate immunity. *Trends Immunol* 2012;33:633–40.
12. Ware LB, Camerer E, Welty-Wolf K, et al. Bench to bedside: Targeting coagulation and fibrinolysis in acute lung injury. *Am J Physiol Lung Cell Mol Physiol* 2006;291(3):L307–11.
13. Zhang Q, Raoof M, Chen Y, et al. Circulating mitochondrial DAMPs cause inflammatory responses to injury. *Nature* 2010;464:104–7.
14. Schultz MJ, Haitsma JJ, Zhang H, et al. Pulmonary coagulopathy as a new target in therapeutic studies of acute lung injury or pneumonia—A review. *Critical Care Med* 2006;34:871–7.
15. Karmpaliotis D, Kosmidou I, Ingenito EP, et al. Angiogenic growth factors in the pathophysiology of a murine model of acute lung injury. *Am J Physiol Lung Cell Mol Physiol* 2002;283:L585–95.
16. Siflinger-Birnboim A, Johnson A. Protein kinase C modulates pulmonary endothelial permeability: A paradigm for acute lung injury. *Am J Physiol Lung Cell Mol Physiol* 2003;284:L435–95.
17. Parikh SM, Mammoto T, Schultz A, et al. Excess circulating angiopoietin-2 may contribute to pulmonary vascular leak in sepsis in humans. *PLoS Med* 2006;3:e46.
18. Larson J, Schomberg S, Schroeder W, et al. Endothelial EphA receptor stimulation increases lung vascular permeability. *Am J Physiol Lung Cell Mol Physiol* 2008;295:L431–95.
19. Carpenter TC, Schroeder W, Stenmark KR, et al. Eph-A2 promotes permeability and inflammatory responses to bleomycin-induced lung injury. *Am J Respir Cell Mol Biol* 2011;46:40–7.
20. Wang L, Dudek SM. Regulation of vascular permeability by sphingosine 1-phosphate. *Microvasc Res* 2009;77:39–45.
21. Teijaro JR, Walsh KB, Cahalan S, et al. Endothelial cells are central orchestrators of cytokine amplification during influenza virus infection. *Cell* 2011;146:980–91.
22. Brinkmann V, Baumruker T. Pulmonary and vascular pharmacology of sphingosine 1-phosphate. *Curr Opin Pharmacol* 2006;6:244–50.
23. London NR, Zhu W, Bozza FA, et al. Targeting Robo4-dependent slit signaling to survive the cytokine storm in sepsis and influenza. *Sci Transl Med* 2010;2:23ra19.
24. Goldenberg NM, Steinberg BE, Slutsky AS, et al. Broken barriers: A new take on sepsis pathogenesis. *Sci Transl Med* 2011; 3:88ps25.
25. Corada M, Mariotti M, Thurston G, et al. Vascular endothelial-cadherin is an important determinant of microvascular integrity in vivo. *Proc Natl Acad Sci USA* 1999;96:9815–20.
26. Angelini DJ, Hyun SW, Grigoryev DN, et al. TNF-alpha increases tyrosine phosphorylation of vascular endothelial cadherin and opens the paracellular pathway through fyn activation in human lung endothelia. *Am J Physiol Lung Cell Mol Physiol* 2006; 291:L1232–95.
27. Birukova AA, Chatchavalvanich S, Rios A, et al. Differential regulation of pulmonary endothelial monolayer integrity by varying degrees of cyclic stretch. *Am J Pathol* 2006;168:1749–61.
28. Bogatcheva NV, Verin AD. The role of cytoskeleton in the regulation of vascular endothelial barrier function. *Microvasc Res* 2008;76:202–7.
29. Freichel M, Vennekens R, Olausson J, et al. Functional role of TRPC proteins in native systems: Implications from knockout and knock-down studies. *J Physiol* 2005;567(pt 1):59–66.
30. Tauseef M, Knezevic N, Chava KR, et al. TLR4 activation of TRPC6-dependent calcium signaling mediates endotoxin-induced lung vascular permeability and inflammation. *J Exp Med* 2012; 209:1953–68.
31. Stevens T. Functional and molecular heterogeneity of pulmonary endothelial cells. *Proc Am Thorac Soc* 2011;8:453–7.
32. Spindler V, Schlegel N, Waschke J. Role of GTPases in control of microvascular permeability. *Cardiovasc Res* 2010;87:243–53.
33. Matthay MA, Robriquet L, Fang X. Alveolar epithelium: Role in lung fluid balance and acute lung injury. *Proc Am Thorac Soc* 2005;2:206–13.
34. Roux J, Kawakatsu H, Gartland B, et al. Interleukin-1beta decreases expression of the epithelial sodium channel alpha-subunit in alveolar epithelial cells via a p38 MAPK-dependent signaling pathway. *J Biol Chem* 2005;280:18579–89.
35. Dagenais A, Gosselin D, Guilbault C, et al. Modulation of epithelial sodium channel (ENaC) expression in mouse lung infected with *Pseudomonas aeruginosa*. *Respir Res* 2005;6:2.
36. Vadász I, Morty RE, Olschewski A, et al. Thrombin impairs alveolar fluid clearance by promoting endocytosis of Na+, K+-ATPase. *Am J Respir Cell Mol Biol* 2005;33:343–54.
37. Gao Smith F, Perkins GD, Gates S, et al. Effect of intravenous β-2 agonist treatment on clinical outcomes in acute respiratory

distress syndrome (BALTI-2): A multicentre, randomised controlled trial. *Lancet* 2012;379:229–35.

38. Nunes S, Ruokonen E, Takala J. Pulmonary capillary pressures during the acute respiratory distress syndrome. *Intensive Care Med* 2003;29:2174–9.

39. Ganter CC, Ganter CG, Jakob SM, et al. Pulmonary capillary pressure. A review. *Minerva Anestesiol* 2006;72:21–36.

40. Kuebler WM, Ying X, Singh B, et al. Pressure is proinflammatory in lung venular capillaries. *J Clin Invest* 1999;104:495–502.

41. Durán WN, Breslin JW, Sánchez FA. The NO cascade, eNOS location, and microvascular permeability. *Cardiovasc Res* 2010;87:254–61.

42. Gregory TJ, Longmore WJ, Moxley MA, et al. Surfactant chemical composition and biophysical activity in acute respiratory distress syndrome. *J Clin Invest* 1991;88:1976–81.

43. Matthay MA, Ware LB, Zimmerman GA. The acute respiratory distress syndrome. *J Clin Invest* 2012;122:2731–40.

44. Ware LB, Matthay MA. The acute respiratory distress syndrome. *N Engl J Med* 2000;342:1334–49.

45. Neff TA, Stocker R, Frey HR, et al. Long-term assessment of lung function in survivors of severe ARDS. *Chest* 2003;123:845–53.

46. Orfanos SE, Mavrommati I, Korovesi I, et al. Pulmonary endothelium in acute lung injury: From basic science to the critically ill. *Intensive Care Med* 2004;30:1702–14.

47. Geiser T, Atabai K, Jarreau PH, et al. Pulmonary edema fluid from patients with acute lung injury augments in vitro alveolar epithelial repair by an IL-1beta-dependent mechanism. *Am J Respir Crit Care Med* 2001;163:1384–8.

48. Frohlich S, Boylan J, McLoughlin P. Hypoxia-induced inflammation in the lung: A potential therapeutic target in acute lung injury? *Am J Respir Cell Mol Biol* 2013;48:271–9.

49. Geiser T, Jarreau PH, Atabai K, et al. Interleukin-1beta augments in vitro alveolar epithelial repair. *Am J Physiol Lung Cell Mol Physiol* 2000;279:L1184–95.

50. Adamson IY, Bakowska J. Relationship of keratinocyte growth factor and hepatocyte growth factor levels in rat lung lavage fluid to epithelial cell regeneration after bleomycin. *Am J Pathol* 1999;155:949–54.

51. Atabai K, Ishigaki M, Geiser T, et al. Keratinocyte growth factor can enhance alveolar epithelial repair by nonmitogenic mechanisms. *Am J Physiol Lung Cell Mol Physiol* 2002;283:L163–95.

52. Verghese GM, McCormick-Shannon K, Mason RJ, et al. Hepatocyte growth factor and keratinocyte growth factor in the pulmonary edema fluid of patients with acute lung injury. Biologic and clinical significance. *Am J Respir Crit Care Med* 1998;158:386–94.

53. Zaman A, Cui Z, Foley JP, et al. Expression and role of the hyaluronan receptor RHAMM in inflammation after bleomycin injury. *Am J Respir Cell Mol Biol* 2005;33:447–54.

54. Dhainaut JF, Charpentier J, Chiche JD. Transforming growth factor-beta: A mediator of cell regulation in acute respiratory distress syndrome. *Critical Care Med* 2003;31:S258–95.

55. Fahy RJ, Lichtenberger F, McKeegan CB, et al. The acute respiratory distress syndrome: A role for transforming growth factor-beta 1. *Am J Respir Cell Mol Biol* 2003;28:499–503.

56. Kaminski N, Allard JD, Pittet JF, et al. Global analysis of gene expression in pulmonary fibrosis reveals distinct programs regulating lung inflammation and fibrosis. *Proc Natl Acad Sci USA* 2000;97:1778–83.

57. Broekelmann TJ, Limper AH, Colby TV, et al. Transforming growth factor beta 1 is present at sites of extracellular matrix gene expression in human pulmonary fibrosis. *Proc Natl Acad Sci USA* 1991;88:6642–6.

58. Horowitz JC, Cui Z, Moore TA, et al. Constitutive activation of prosurvival signaling in alveolar mesenchymal cells isolated from patients with nonresolving acute respiratory distress syndrome. *Am J Physiol Lung Cell Mol Physiol* 2006;290:L415–95.

59. Westergren-Thorsson G, Hernnäs J, Särnstrand B, et al. Altered expression of small proteoglycans, collagen, and transforming growth factor-beta 1 in developing bleomycin-induced pulmonary fibrosis in rats. *J Clin Invest* 1993;92:632–7.

60. Khalil N, Whitman C, Zuo L, et al. Regulation of alveolar macrophage transforming growth factor-beta secretion by corticosteroids in bleomycin-induced pulmonary inflammation in the rat. *J Clin Invest* 1993;92:1812–8.

61. Willis BC, Liebler JM, Luby-Phelps K, et al. Induction of epithelial-mesenchymal transition in alveolar epithelial cells by transforming growth factor-beta1: Potential role in idiopathic pulmonary fibrosis. *Am J Pathol* 2005;166:1321–32.

62. Okada H, Kalluri R. Cellular and molecular pathways that lead to progression and regression of renal fibrogenesis. *Curr Mol Med* 2005;5:467–74.

63. Shannon JM, Hyatt BA. Epithelial-mesenchymal interactions in the developing lung. *Annu Rev Physiol* 2004;66:625–45.

64. Mucenski ML, Wert SE, Nation JM, et al. Beta-Catenin is required for specification of proximal/distal cell fate during lung morphogenesis. *J Biol Chem* 2003;278:40231–8.

65. Douglas IS, Diaz del Valle F, Winn RA, et al. Beta-catenin in the fibroproliferative response to acute lung injury. *Am J Respir Cell Mol Biol* 2006;34:274–85.

66. Körbling M, Estrov Z. Adult stem cells for tissue repair—A new therapeutic concept? *N Engl J Med* 2003;349:570–82.

67. Kotton DN, Summer R, Fine A. Lung stem cells: New paradigms. *Exp Hematol* 2004;32:340–3.

68. Rojas M, Xu J, Woods CR, et al. Bone marrow-derived mesenchymal stem cells in repair of the injured lung. *Am J Respir Cell Mol Biol* 2005;33:145–52.

69. Yamada M, Kubo H, Kobayashi S, et al. Bone marrow-derived progenitor cells are important for lung repair after lipopolysaccharide-induced lung injury. *J Immunol* 2004;172:1266–72.

70. Lama VN, Phan SH. The extrapulmonary origin of fibroblasts: Stem/progenitor cells and beyond. *Proc Am Thorac Soc* 2006;3:373–6.

71. Friedenstein AJ, Chailakhyan RK, Latsinik NV, et al. Stromal cells responsible for transferring the microenvironment of the hemopoietic tissues. Cloning in vitro and retransplantation in vivo. *Transplantation* 1974;17:331–40.

72. Lalu MM, McIntyre L, Pugliese C, et al. Safety of cell therapy with mesenchymal stromal cells (SafeCell): A systematic review and meta-analysis of clinical trials. *PLoS ONE* 2012;7:e47559.

73. Prockop DJ, Kota DJ, Bazhanov N, et al. Evolving paradigms for repair of tissues by adult stem/progenitor cells (MSCs). *J Cell Mol Med* 2010;14:2190–9.

74. Tu Z, Li Q, Bu H, et al. Mesenchymal stem cells inhibit complement activation by secreting factor H. *Stem Cells Dev* 2010;19:1803–9.

75. Raffaghello L, Bianchi G, Bertolotto M, et al. Human mesenchymal stem cells inhibit neutrophil apoptosis: A model for neutrophil preservation in the bone marrow niche. *Stem Cells* 2008;26:151–62.

76. Kavanagh H, Mahon BP. Allogeneic mesenchymal stem cells prevent allergic airway inflammation by inducing murine regulatory T cells. *Allergy* 2011;66:523–31.

77. Zhang B, Liu R, Shi D, et al. Mesenchymal stem cells induce mature dendritic cells into a novel Jagged-2-dependent regulatory dendritic cell population. *Blood* 2009;113:46–57.

78. Ge W, Jiang J, Baroja ML, et al. Infusion of mesenchymal stem cells and rapamycin synergize to attenuate alloimmune responses and promote cardiac allograft tolerance. *Am J Transplant* 2009;9:1760–72.

79. Németh K, Leelahavanichkul A, Yuen PST, et al. Bone marrow stromal cells attenuate sepsis via prostaglandin E(2)-dependent reprogramming of host macrophages to increase their interleukin-10 production. *Nat Med* 2009;15:42–9.

80. Fang X, Neyrinck AP, Matthay MA, et al. Allogeneic human mesenchymal stem cells restore epithelial protein permeability in cultured human alveolar type II cells by secretion of angiopoietin-1. *J Biol Chem* 2010;285:26211–22.

81. Danchuk S, Ylostalo JH, Hossain F, et al. Human multipotent stromal cells attenuate lipopolysaccharide-induced acute lung

injury in mice via secretion of tumor necrosis factor-α-induced protein 6. *Stem Cell Res Ther* 2011;2:27.

82. Gupta N, Su X, Popov B, et al. Intrapulmonary delivery of bone marrow-derived mesenchymal stem cells improves survival and attenuates endotoxin-induced acute lung injury in mice. *J Immunol* 2007;179:1855–63.

83. Krasnodembskaya A, Song Y, Fang X, et al. Antibacterial effect of human mesenchymal stem cells is mediated in part from secretion of the antimicrobial peptide LL-37. *Stem Cells* 2010; 28:2229–38.

84. Willson DF, Thomas NJ, Markovitz BP, et al. Effect of exogenous surfactant (calfactant) in pediatric acute lung injury: A randomized controlled trial. *JAMA* 2005;293:470–6.

CHAPTER 45 ■ RESPIRATORY MONITORING

IRA M. CHEIFETZ, JAN HAU LEE, AND SHEKHAR T. VENKATARAMAN

KEY POINTS

❶ Technology augments physical examination. A physical examination is often the deciding factor between monitor error and a true change in a patient's status.

❷ Cardiorespiratory distress in infants and children is often associated with abnormalities in oxygenation and ventilation and, thus, requires diligent monitoring.

❸ Pulse oximetry is an integral part of all pediatric critical care monitoring systems. A key premise of pulse oximeters is that they are capable of early identification of changes in a patient's cardiorespiratory status, allowing for a rapid response. Recent software advances have helped to improve the clinical usefulness of this monitoring tool.

❹ Significant advances have occurred in transcutaneous monitor technology. The continuous monitoring and trending

of CO_2 and O_2 can be useful in critically ill patients, especially in neonates and infants.

❺ Capnography (both time- and volume-based) is playing an increasingly important role in the management of critically ill infants and children. Responses to changes in ventilatory strategies and cardiac function can be detected and trended with capnography.

❻ Waveform analysis can be used to optimize mechanical ventilation and to analyze ventilator incidents and alarm conditions. Using this technology, it is possible to shape the form of ventilatory support to improve patient–ventilator synchrony, reduce work of breathing, and calculate physiologic parameters related to respiratory mechanics.

WHY MONITOR?

Monitoring respiratory function is crucial in the management of critically ill children to (a) aid with diagnosis, (b) understand underlying pathophysiology, (c) assess status and progress of the disease, and (d) guide clinical management. In mechanically ventilated children, respiratory monitoring can also assist in understanding and optimizing patient–ventilator interactions, provide alerts and alarms, and aid in weaning.

Monitoring, which was once dependent solely on physical assessment and direct clinical observation, now includes elaborate automated surveillance of a tremendous number of variables related to cardiorespiratory physiology and ventilator performance. Noninvasive monitoring techniques assess gas exchange and pulmonary mechanics, supplement physical assessment, and provide a continuous data stream, with alarms to identify and alert caregivers to changes in the child's status. Although physical examination remains clinically relevant, the role of the clinician has evolved and now must include the incorporation of all aspects of cardiorespiratory monitoring into a comprehensive, responsive assessment system. The appropriate integration and interpretation of all data are essential for efficient, high-quality, cost-effective, pediatric critical care.

In this chapter, we focus our discussion on the monitoring of the main functions of the respiratory system: (a) removal of carbon dioxide (CO_2) and (b) facilitating oxygen (O_2) transport. The continuum of respiratory monitoring from basic physical assessment to complex, automated monitoring systems is addressed, and clinical indications, principles of operation, and functional limitations are discussed.

PHYSICAL ASSESSMENT

It is a concerning phenomenon of modern intensive care that physical examination is used with decreasing frequency.

Clinical scoring systems have been developed to evaluate the clinical parameters of skin color, nasal flaring, retractions, accessory muscle use, and presence and severity of an abnormal sound (e.g., rales, wheeze, or stridor). Scoring systems generally demonstrate that the more pronounced the abnormality, the worse the prognosis (1). As these parameters can only be discerned by visual and auditory assessments, physical examination and assessment should never be replaced by technology. Technology should be used to augment physical assessment. Physical examination is, in fact, often the deciding factor ❶ between monitor error and a true change in a child's status.

Respiratory Rate and Pattern

Physical examination remains the primary method by which respiratory rate is measured. However, through the evolution of technology, several techniques are now used for measuring respiratory movements. Impedance pneumography, the method used most often for spontaneously breathing children, requires the placement of at least three leads over the chest: one over the heart, and one each on the opposite sides of the lower lateral thorax. A small current is passed through one electrode, and the amount of current that passes through the chest is measured by the other electrode pair. The impedance to current flow varies with the fluid content of the chest, which in turn varies with the respiratory cycle. These differences can be converted by a microprocessor into a waveform and visually displayed on a monitor.

The respiratory rate and pattern of each child should be evaluated with reference to age-adjusted norms and pathophysiologic state. Respiratory patterns in children have generated debate, particularly in the definitions of respiratory pauses, periodic breathing, and apnea. In general, *respiratory pauses* last <5 seconds and occur in children who are <3 months of age. Pauses occur in groups of three or more, are separated by <20 seconds, and generally resolve by 6 months of age without medical intervention. The definition of apnea is even more troublesome because of the role of sudden infant death syndrome (SIDS) in infant mortality and the substantial effort underway to prevent this tragic occurrence. A National Institutes of Health Conference consensus statement on infantile apnea defined *apnea* as cessation of breathing for >20 seconds or any respiratory pause associated with bradycardia, pallor, or cyanosis. The relationship between infantile apnea and SIDS remains controversial (2).

GUIDELINES AND PRINCIPLES

Technologic advances of monitoring systems provide clinicians with reliable information regarding important physiologic variables and alert the patient care team to changes in these parameters, especially as they violate preset alarm limits. These monitors and systems generate trends so that changes in clinical condition can be more readily recognized.

Important management decisions are based on information provided by the monitor. The monitoring system must provide pertinent information that directly guides patient management. All data provided by the monitoring system must be easily and quickly interpretable both at the bedside and remotely. Additionally, the data must be accurate, and the technology must be sufficiently sensitive to detect absolute values and changes. The technology must be practical, easily attached to the patient, dependable, space efficient, and cost-effective. Patient safety must always be the primary goal.

The primary monitoring question is often, "What should be monitored?" (**Table 45.1**). Technology enables the monitoring of multiple parameters continuously or at various intervals. However, the fact that every cardiorespiratory parameter can be monitored does not mean that it should be monitored. Clinicians must address what is practical and clinically relevant to the management of each individual child, and keep in mind that the nature and intensity of monitoring may change over time. Physical assessment and observation should always be used to complement electronic surveillance.

TABLE 45.1

FUNDAMENTAL QUESTIONS REGARDING MONITORING

1. What should be monitored?
   a. What physiologic parameters do we want to monitor?
   b. Why should these parameters be monitored?
2. What is actually being measured?
   a. Are the parameters actually measured directly?
   b. Or, are inferences being made about the parameters based on measuring other variables?
3. If inferences are made, how do the monitors work?
   a. What are the assumptions behind the measurements, if any?
   b. Are assumptions being violated?
   c. How precise and accurate are the measurements?
4. What are the goals of monitoring?
   a. Diagnostic
      i. Type of physiologic impairment
      ii. Severity of physiologic impairment
   b. Therapeutic
      i. Selection of appropriate treatment
      ii. Measure effect of intervention(s)
   c. Prognostic
      i. Mortality
      ii. Morbidity
   d. Warning/alarms
      i. To alert about a change in patient status
      ii. To prevent catastrophic events

Assessment of Gas Exchange

Cardiorespiratory distress is often associated with abnormalities in oxygenation and ventilation and, thus, requires diligent monitoring. Monitoring of oxygenation includes an assessment of oxygen transfer in the lungs, oxygen transport to the tissues and organs by the circulatory system (O_2 delivery, Do_2), and oxygen transfer to and utilization by the tissues (**Figs. 45.1**

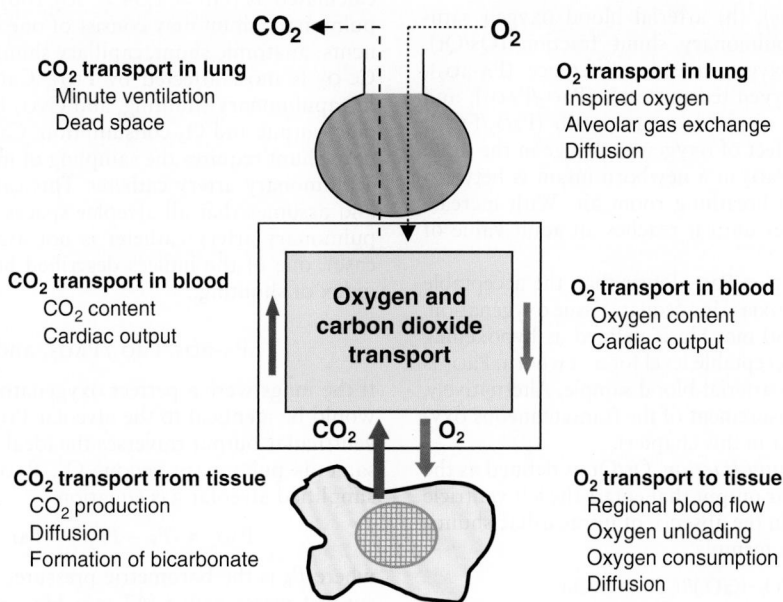

FIGURE 45.1. Physiology of oxygenation and ventilation. The primary functions of the cardiorespiratory system are to provide adequate O_2 to the tissues and to eliminate CO_2 via the lungs. This gas transfer process involves an elaborate interaction between the lungs, circulatory system, and the tissues throughout the body.

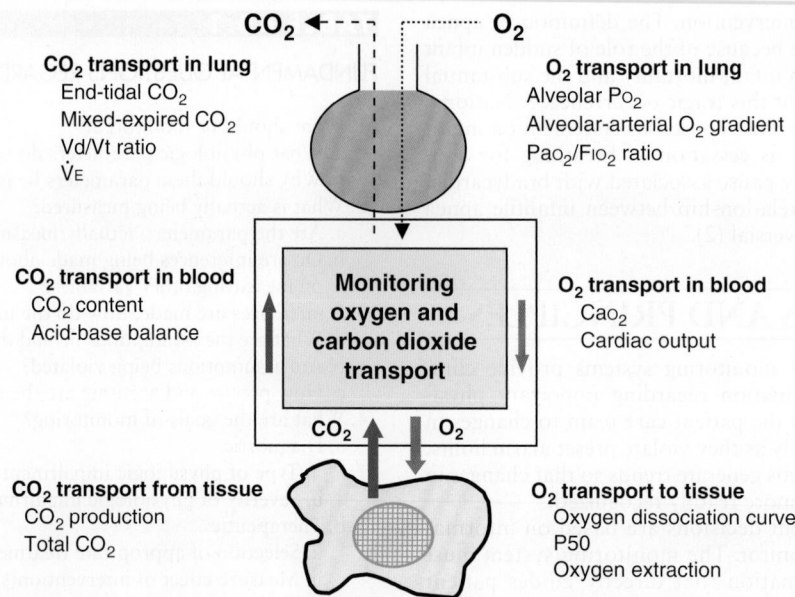

FIGURE 45.2. Variables associated with cardiorespiratory monitoring at each point in the transport of O_2 and CO_2. Monitoring of oxygenation includes an assessment of O_2 transfer in the lungs, O_2 transport to the tissues and organs by the circulatory system (i.e., O_2 delivery), and O_2 transfer to, and utilization by, the tissues. Elimination of CO_2 similarly involves CO_2 production by the tissues, transfer of CO_2 from the tissues to venous blood, transport of CO_2 by the circulatory system to the lungs, and elimination of CO_2 by alveolar ventilation in the exhaled gas. CO_2, carbon dioxide; Vd/Vt ratio, dead space-to-tidal volume ratio; $\dot{V}_E$, expired minute volume; Pa_{O_2}, arterial partial pressure of O_2; F_{IO_2}, fraction of inspired O_2; Ca_{O_2}, arterial O_2 content.

and **45.2**). Elimination of CO_2 similarly involves CO_2 production by the tissues, transfer of CO_2 from the tissues to venous blood, transport of CO_2 by the circulatory system to the lungs, and elimination of CO_2 by alveolar ventilation in the exhaled gas (**Figs. 45.1** and **45.2**).

Assessment of the Lung as an Oxygenator

Indices used to assess the lung as an oxygenator are (a) arterial oxygen tension (Pa_{O_2}), (b) arterial blood oxygen saturation (Sa_{O_2}), (c) intrapulmonary shunt fraction (Qs/Qt), (d) alveolar-to-arterial oxygen tension difference ($PA-a_{O_2}$), (e) arterial-to-alveolar oxygen tension ratio (Pa_{O_2}/PA_{O_2}), and (f) arterial-to-fraction of inspired oxygen ratio (Pa_{O_2}/F_{IO_2}). Pa_{O_2} represents the net effect of oxygen exchange in the lung. At sea level, the normal Pa_{O_2} in a newborn infant is between 40 and 70 mm Hg when breathing room air. With increasing age, the Pa_{O_2} increases until it reaches an adult value of 90–120 mm Hg.

Hypoxemia is defined as a Pa_{O_2} lower than the acceptable range for age, whereas hypoxia is inadequate tissue oxygenation. For a child, a Pa_{O_2} of <60 mm Hg is defined as hypoxemia, although that may be an acceptable level for a newborn. Pa_{O_2} is measured by obtaining an arterial blood sample. Alternatively, it can be estimated by measurement of the transcutaneous oxygen tension (discussed later in this chapter).

The *intrapulmonary shunt fraction*, Qs/Qt, is defined as the fraction of right ventricular output that enters the left ventricle without oxygen transfer. In the absence of intracardiac shunts, Qs/Qt is calculated by the formula

$$Qs/Qt = (Cc'_{O_2} - Ca_{O_2})/(Cc'_{O_2} - Cv_{O_2})$$

where Cc'_{O_2} is the oxygen content of the pulmonary venous blood, assuming the lung to be a perfect oxygenator, Ca_{O_2} is the arterial oxygen content, and Cv_{O_2} is the mixed venous oxygen content.

Oxygen content is the amount of O_2 carried by a unit volume of blood and is equal to the amount bound to hemoglobin (Hb) and dissolved in plasma. One gram per deciliter of Hb will carry 1.34 mL of O_2 when it is fully saturated. The amount dissolved in plasma depends on the solubility coefficient of O_2. For every millimeter of mercury increase in partial pressure of oxygen (P_{O_2}), the amount of dissolved O_2 increases by 0.003 mL. Therefore, the oxygen content of whole blood is calculated as $(Hb \times 1.34 \times S_{O_2}/100) + (0.003 \times P_{O_2})$. Intrapulmonary shunt may consist of one or more of three components: anatomic shunt, capillary shunt, and venous admixture. Cc'_{O_2} is most affected by F_{IO_2}, Ca_{O_2} is affected mostly by intrapulmonary shunting, and Cv_{O_2} is affected mostly by cardiac output and O_2 consumption. Calculation of intrapulmonary shunt requires the sampling of mixed venous blood using a pulmonary artery catheter. This calculation is cumbersome and assumes that all alveolar spaces behave equally. When a pulmonary artery catheter is not available (as is usually the case), one of the indices described below may be used as an index of shunting.

$PA-a_{O_2}$, Pa_{O_2}/PA_{O_2}, and Pa_{O_2}/F_{IO_2}

If the lungs were a perfect oxygenator, pulmonary venous O_2 would be identical to the alveolar P_{O_2} (PA_{O_2}), and if the right ventricular output traverses the ideal lung, Pa_{O_2} would be the same as pulmonary venous O_2. PA_{O_2} is calculated from the simplified alveolar gas equation

$$PA_{O_2} = (P_B - P_{H_2O}) \times F_{IO_2} - Pa_{CO_2}/RQ$$

where P_B is the barometric pressure, P_{H_2O} is the partial pressure of water vapor (47 mm Hg when fully saturated with H_2O) and RQ is the respiratory quotient (CO_2 production/O_2 consumption).

With intrapulmonary shunting, Pa_{O_2} is less than PA_{O_2}. $PA-a_{O_2}$, Pa_{O_2}/PA_{O_2}, and Pa_{O_2}/F_{IO_2} are indices that reflect the extent to which the PaO_2 deviates from PAO_2 as a measure of intrapulmonary shunting. The normal $PA\text{-}aO_2$ is usually <20 mm Hg in a child and <50 mm Hg in a newborn. A large $PA\text{-}aO_2$ represents intrapulmonary shunting or venous admixture. $PA\text{-}aO_2$ is affected not only by intrapulmonary shunting, but also by mixed venous oxygen saturation (SvO_2). A major limitation of this index is that it changes unpredictably with increasing FIO_2. To compare gradients over time, FIO_2 must remain constant. To be reliable, the arterial-to-mixed venous PO_2 difference must also be constant. Unlike $PA\text{-}aO_2$, PaO_2/PAO_2 changes much more predictably with increasing FIO_2. Thus, it is preferred over $PA\text{-}aO_2$ as an index of oxygen transfer in the lung and can be used to predict changes in PaO_2 when FIO_2 is altered. PaO_2/FIO_2 ratio is the easiest index to calculate and does not require calculation of PAO_2. The disadvantage is that it does not adjust for alveolar CO_2. At high FIO_2, this error becomes quite small. The normal PaO_2/FIO_2 in a child breathing room air at sea level is >400 mm Hg.

Oxygen Delivery

Oxygen delivery (DO_2) is the amount of O_2 delivered to the tissues every minute. It is calculated as:

$$DO_2 = CaO_2 \times CI$$

where CI is the cardiac index in $mL/min/m^2$.

A normal DO_2 in a child is ~650–750 $mL/min/m^2$. The major determinants of DO_2 are Hb and CI. Mild hypoxemia can be compensated by increasing Hb and/or CI. If DO_2 is adequate to meet the tissue O_2 demands, the absolute PaO_2 is not critical.

Assessment of Oxygen Utilization

Oxygen consumption ($\dot{V}O_2$) is the amount of O_2 utilized by the body in a minute, and it can be measured by analyzing the inspired and expired gases using a Douglas bag or calculated using the Fick equation, where $\dot{V}O_2 = CI$ ($CaO_2 - CvO_2$). Fever, thyrotoxicosis, and increased catecholamine release or administration increase $\dot{V}O_2$. Hypothermia and hypothyroidism tend to decrease $\dot{V}O_2$. Measurement of $\dot{V}O_2$ may be important in critically ill patients, especially those with moderately severe cardiorespiratory dysfunction. Under normal conditions, $\dot{V}O_2$ is independent of DO_2. In some critically ill patients, $\dot{V}O_2$ becomes DO_2 dependent. If clinically possible, DO_2 should be increased until $\dot{V}O_2$ is no longer DO_2 dependent.

Mixed Venous Oxygen Saturation

Mixed SvO_2 is commonly used as a measure of the balance between O_2 demand and supply. A low SvO_2 usually signifies that DO_2 is significantly decreased and the body is extracting more O_2 from the blood. This commonly occurs with hypovolemic and cardiogenic shock. In sepsis (where maldistribution of peripheral blood flow is present) and in inborn errors of metabolism (where O_2 utilization can be abnormal), SvO_2 may be normal or high despite O_2 deficits in the tissues. A high SvO_2 is often seen in hypothermia because of decreased O_2 demand and in brain death, as the brain usually constitutes a major site of the total body O_2 consumption.

The O_2 saturation of Hb reaches stability in the right ventricular outflow tract after the differences in saturation from the inferior vena cava, superior vena cava, coronary sinus, and Thebesian veins equilibrate. The normal saturation of Hb in the pulmonary artery is ~78% (range, 73%–85%).

Rearrangement of the terms of the Fick equation indicates that CvO_2 and, hence, SvO_2 are related to $\dot{V}O_2$ and cardiac

TABLE 45.2

COMMON CLINICAL CONDITIONS ASSOCIATED WITH CHANGES IN MIXED VENOUS O_2 SATURATION

Reduction in SvO_2
↓ O_2 delivery
↓ Cardiac output
↓ Arterial O_2 saturation
↓ Hemoglobin concentration
↑ O_2 consumption
Increase in SvO_2
↑ O_2 delivery
↓ O_2 consumption
↓ O_2 extraction
Left-to-right intracardiac shunt
Sepsis

SvO_2, venous oxygen saturation.

output ($\dot{Q}_T$) such that increases in $\dot{V}O_2$ or decreases in $\dot{Q}_T$ result in a reduction of SvO_2:

$$SvO_2 = CvO_2 - \text{Dissolved } O_2/(Hb \times 1.34)$$

$$CvO_2 = CaO_2 - (\dot{V}O_2/\dot{Q}_T)$$

where Hb is the hemoglobin concentration.

Additional causes of changes in SvO_2 are listed in **Table 45.2**.

Although continuous monitoring of mixed venous O_2 saturation is interesting, clear-cut clinical indications for this technique remain to be demonstrated in children. As most children in the intensive care setting do not have pulmonary artery catheters, pediatric intensivists usually use superior vena cava saturations as a surrogate for true mixed venous O_2 saturations. Although there is no clear relationship between central and mixed venous O_2 saturations and exact numerical values of mixed venous and central O_2 saturations are not equivalent in varying hemodynamic conditions, trends between these values were found to be reliable and presumably clinically valuable (3–5). While certain centers have utilized continuous central venous O_2 saturations successfully to guide management in pediatric septic shock, logistical barriers in obtaining such monitoring may prevent its routine use in children (6,7).

PULSE OXIMETRY

One of the most important advances in respiratory monitoring was the development of pulse oximetry (SpO_2), which provides a continuous, noninvasive measure of the percent O_2 saturation of arterial Hb. With the development of advanced microprocessor technology, pulse oximetry became widely available from the 1980s. Further technologic accomplishments (e.g., light-emitting diodes, plethysmography, and spectrophotometry) made pulse oximetry relatively inexpensive, very safe, reasonably accurate, and portable.

Oxygen-Dissociation Curve

The arterial O_2 saturation of Hb (SaO_2) is the percent oxyhemoglobin in the arterial blood. The O_2-dissociation curve describes the avidity with which O_2 binds to Hb. Acidemia, hypercarbia, increased temperature, and increased red-cell 2,3-diphosphoglycerate (2,3-DPG) level shift the curve to the right.

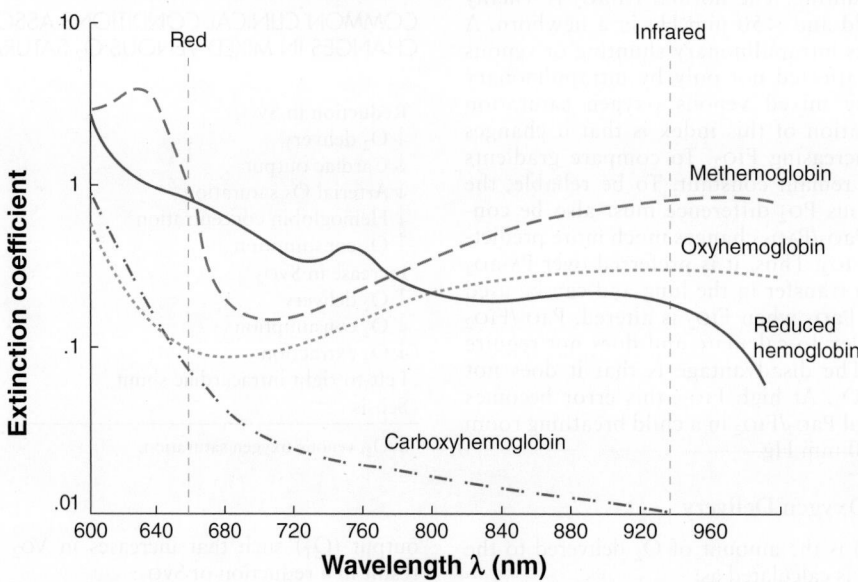

FIGURE 45.3. Hemoglobin extinction curves. The extinction curves of four hemoglobin species (oxyhemoglobin, reduced hemoglobin, methemoglobin, and carboxyhemoglobin) are displayed from red (660 nm) to infrared (940 nm). (Tremper KK, Barker SJ. Pulse oximetry. *Anesthesiology* 1989;70:98–108, with permission.)

Beer–Lambert Law

A discussion of the physics of pulse oximetry requires understanding of the Beer–Lambert law, which states that the concentration of a solute in a solvent can be determined by light absorption. The logarithmic relationship that exists between the transmission of light through a solution and the concentration of a given solute is expressed as

$$C = \frac{\log_{10}(I_0/I)}{\alpha d}$$

where C is the concentration, I_0 is the intensity of the incident light, I is the intensity of transmitted light, d is the distance the light travels through a solution, and α is the absorption coefficient of the solute and is wavelength dependent.

Pulse oximetry estimates arterial O_2 saturation by measuring the absorption of light in tissues. As pulse oximetry assesses whether or not O_2 is attached to Hb, the relevant solutes are reduced Hb and oxyhemoglobin and their respective absorption characteristics. Wavelengths of 660 nm (red) and 940 nm (infrared) are used because the absorption characteristics of these two Hbs are significantly different at these two wavelengths (**Fig. 45.3**).

Beer's spectrophotometric principle is applied using a light-emitting diode and optical plethysmography. A miniaturized light source is applied to an area of the body that is narrow enough to allow light to traverse a pulsating capillary bed and be sensed by a photodetector (optical plethysmography). When light passes through a pulsating vascular bed, the transmitted light has nonpulsatile and pulsatile components (**Fig. 45.4**). The nonpulsatile component is assumed to represent light transmitted through the tissues, capillaries, and veins. The pulsatile component is assumed to represent light transmitted through the arterial bed.

As each heartbeat physiologically produces arterial (i.e., O_2-saturated) blood, the increase in O_2 saturation of the Hb

results in an increased absorption of light. The pulse oximeter is empirically calibrated by comparing these ratios to direct arterial blood saturations obtained in healthy human volunteers. The O_2 saturation is calculated by comparing absorbencies at baseline (BA) and during the peak (PA) of a transmitted pulse at 660 nm (red) and 940 nm (infrared):

Red absorbance (R)/Infrared absorbance (IR)
$$= (PA_{660}/BA_{660})/(PA_{940}/BA_{940})$$

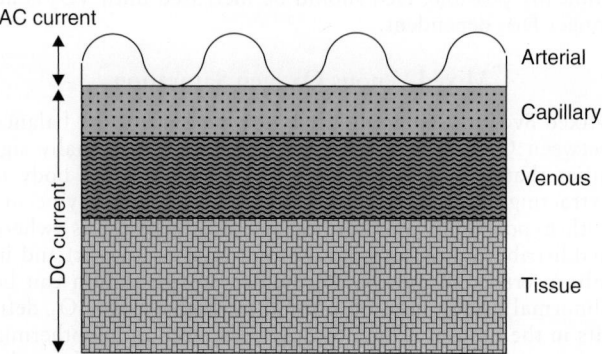

FIGURE 45.4. Spectrophotometric profile of transmitted light across a vascular bed. Pulse oximetry is characterized by a miniaturized light source applied to an area of the body that is narrow enough to allow light to traverse a pulsating capillary bed and be sensed by a photodetector. When light passes through a pulsating vascular bed, the transmitted light has nonpulsatile and pulsatile components. The pulsatile component is assumed to be due to arterial pulsations, while the nonpulsatile component represents light transmitted through the tissues, veins, and capillaries.

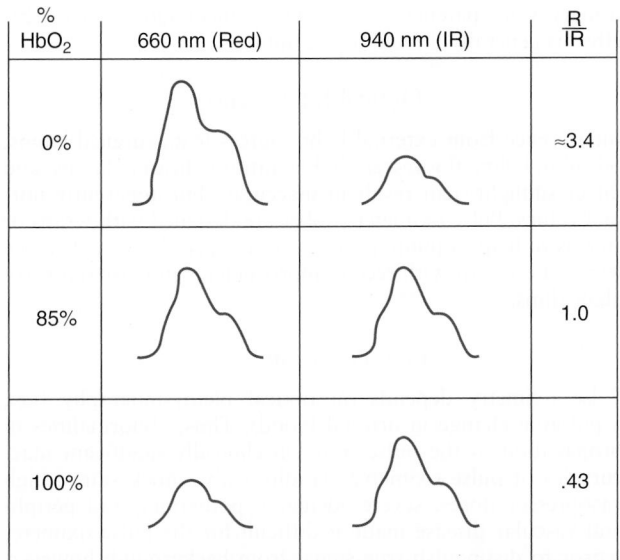

%HbO$_2$	660 nm (Red)	940 nm (IR)	$\frac{R}{IR}$
0%			≈3.4
85%			1.0
100%			.43

FIGURE 45.5. Relative plethysmographic (pulse-added) signal amplitudes, assuming that the transmission intensities are similar. (From Eisenkraft J. Pulse oximetry desaturation due to methemoglobinemia. *Anesthesiology* 1988;68:279–82, with permission.)

The oximetry-determined plethysmographic signal amplitudes at various saturations and the algorithm used by the microprocessor to determine the SpO$_2$ by the R/IR ratio are shown in **Figures 45.5** and **45.6**. By using the two wavelengths of light, the pulse oximeter determines "functional saturation."

$$\text{Functional SpO}_2 = \text{HbO}_2/(\text{HbO}_2 + \text{Hb})$$

where HbO$_2$ is the oxygenated Hb and Hb is the nonoxygenated Hb.

Functional SpO$_2$ is contrasted with fractional SpO$_2$ measured by co-oximetry on most blood gas analyzers. Fractional SpO$_2$ provides the ratio of oxygenated Hb to the sum of *all Hb types*, including carboxyhemoglobin (COHb) and methemoglobin (MetHb), which do not carry O$_2$:

$$\text{Fractional SpO}_2 = \text{HbO}_2/(\text{HbO}_2 + \text{Hb} + \text{COHb} + \text{MetHb})$$

The disadvantage of determining functional saturation is that other, possibly clinically significant Hb species will be missed. This shortcoming can be overcome in ambiguous clinical situations by using periodic co-oximetry that uses four to six wavelengths to determine the fractional saturation.

In a well-perfused, normothermic person, without any significant quantities of other Hb moieties, O$_2$ saturation determined by pulse oximetry correlates very closely with the O$_2$ saturation determined by the co-oximeter (correlation coefficient of 0.98) when the saturation is between 70% and 100% (8–10). Many of the differences that have been reported in the accuracy of pulse oximeters are a result of differences in the signal processing software and calibration curves for various brands of devices. Most manufacturers claim confidence limits ±2%–4% for readings >70%. During periods of desaturation <70%, the bias and precision are substantially worse and more variable, as a limited amount of calibration data exists for these low saturations. This issue primarily applies to children with cyanotic heart disease and those with oxygen saturation <70%.

Overall, pulse oximetry is based on three major assumptions: (a) only two forms of Hb are present: oxyhemoglobin and deoxyhemoglobin; (b) the pulsatile component of the spectrophotometric absorbance is only due to the arterial blood; and (c) the algorithms derived from human volunteers apply to all patients, including neonates. If any of these three assumptions are violated, then the pulse oximeter will not reflect the correct arterial O$_2$ saturation.

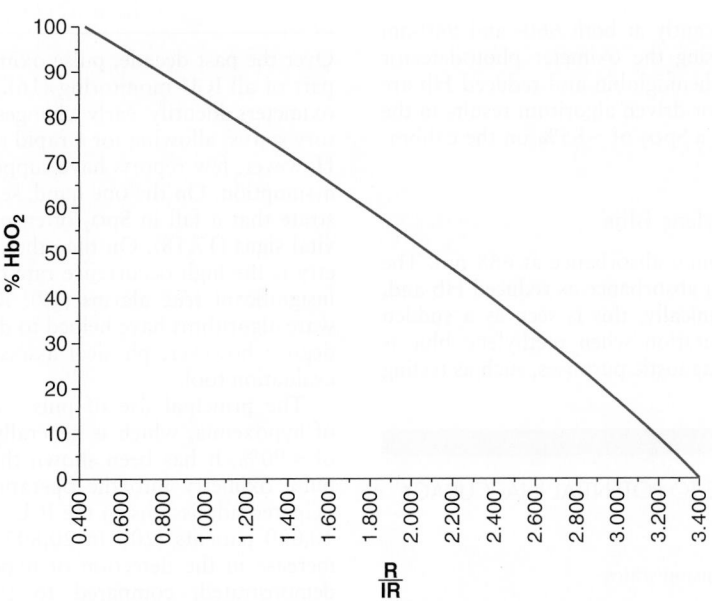

FIGURE 45.6. Algorithm relating % HbO$_2$ as *ordinate* to the ratio of the plethysmographic signal amplitudes and R/IR (or 660/940 nm) as *abscissa*. R, red absorbance; IR, infrared absorbance. (From Eisenkraft J. Pulse oximetry desaturation due to methemoglobinemia. *Anesthesiology* 1988;68:279–82, with permission.)

Factors That Affect the Performance of Pulse Oximeters

The limitations of the technology of pulse oximetry may affect the bias, precision, and applicability of the instrument (**Table 45.3**) (9). As with all monitoring systems, pulse oximetry should never replace physical examination and overall clinical assessment of a patient's respiratory status. Factors that affect the performance of pulse oximeters include artifacts introduced by patient motion, poor peripheral perfusion, and false alarms. Newer pulse oximeters have additional technology (generally advanced software algorithms) to improve performance during low-perfusion states and patient motion. Whether these newer technologies are superior is not clear (11–13).

Dyshemoglobinemia

Dyshemoglobinemia refers to an abnormal species of Hb that results in the reduced ability of the Hb molecule to carry O_2 to the tissues because of combination with substances other than O_2 (e.g., carbon monoxide) or molecular alterations that do not allow O_2 to combine with the Hb molecule in an efficient manner (e.g., MetHb and fetal Hb). The absorption spectra for the dyshemoglobins are shown in **Figure 45.3**.

Carboxyhemoglobin

Carboxyhemoglobin is interpreted as oxyhemoglobin by the photodetector of the two-light-source pulse oximeter. (Both carboxy- and oxyhemoglobin absorb similar amounts of light at 660 nm.) Thus, functional SpO_2 overestimates the true HbO_2, but fractional SpO_2 decreases dramatically in the presence of carboxyhemoglobin (9). Thus, in patients with known smoke inhalation or presenting with coma of uncertain cause (i.e., potential carbon monoxide poisoning), it is imperative to use co-oximetry (rather than pulse oximetry) to determine O_2 saturation.

Methemoglobin

MetHb absorbs light significantly at both 660- and 940-nm wavelengths, thereby confusing the oximeter photodetector into believing that both oxyhemoglobin and reduced Hb are increased. The microprocessor-driven algorithm results in the *R*/IR approaching unity and a SpO_2 of ~85% on the calibration curve (**Fig. 45.6**).

Methylene Blue

Methylene blue has a maximum absorbance at 668 nm. The oximeter interprets this extra absorbance as reduced Hb and, therefore, a lower SpO_2. Clinically, this is seen as a sudden (<30 seconds) drop in saturation when methylene blue is injected for therapeutic or diagnostic purposes, such as testing

urinary tract patency or treating methemoglobinemia. This effect is generally limited to ~2 minutes.

Optical Interference

Interference from external light sources (e.g., surgical lamps, bilirubin lights, fluorescent lights, infrared heating lamps, and direct sunlight) can result in inaccurate but apparently normal values. Pulse oximeter probes are designed with wraps or shields to help to minimize this interference. This has become less of a concern with recent improvements in pulse oximetry algorithms.

Low-Perfusion States

Pulse oximetry depends on optical plethysmography (i.e., a pulsatile change in arterial blood). Thus, abnormalities in propagation of the pulse result in clinically significant inaccuracies of pulse oximetry. Traditionally, shock states, high vasopressor doses, severe edema, hypothermia, and peripheral vascular disease made it difficult for the pulse oximeter sensor to distinguish true signal from background; however, improvements have enabled saturation monitoring despite decreased perfusion (14).

Motion Artifact

Excessive motion of the photosensor causes intermittent contact with the skin and mechanically modulates the path length of the transmitted light and the amplitude and intensity of the received light. This variance in light transmission and reception through the monitoring site can produce false arterial pulse waveforms that the oximeter may not be able to differentiate from the true arterial waveforms, thus producing spurious saturation values. Clinicians should verify pulse-rate accuracy in the assessment of pulse oximetry values to avoid misinterpretation in the face of motion artifact. Current-generation oximeters incorporate software algorithms to better minimize motion artifact (11,15).

Clinical Applications

Over the past decade, pulse oximetry has become an integral part of all ICU monitoring (16). A key premise is that pulse oximeters identify early changes in a child's cardiorespiratory status, allowing for a rapid response by the clinical team. However, few reports have supported this generally accepted assumption. On the one hand, several clinical studies demonstrate that a fall in SpO_2 often precedes any change in other vital signs (17,18). On the other, a concern with pulse oximetry is the high occurrence rate of false alarms and clinically insignificant true alarms (19). Recent advances in the software algorithms have helped to decrease this concern to some degree; however, physical assessment remains the definitive evaluation tool.

The principal use of pulse oximetry is in the detection of hypoxemia, which is generally defined as a SpO_2 reading of <90%. It has been shown that, with the introduction of pulse oximetry into the operating room, the rate of unanticipated admissions to the ICU decreased from 64 to 25 per 10,000 patients (20). In 20,802 surgical patients, a 19-fold increase in the detection of hypoxemia ($SpO_2 < 90\%$) was demonstrated, compared to the control (nonmonitored) group (21). There are an increasing number of studies that have examined the utility of SpO_2 as a noninvasive surrogate marker for PaO_2 in defining the severity of lung injury in acute respiratory distress syndrome (ARDS) (22–24). These studies demonstrated that indices utilizing SpO_2 (e.g., SpO_2/FIO_2 and oxygenation saturation index ($FIO_2 \times$ Mean Airway Pressure/

TABLE 45.3

FACTORS THAT CONTRIBUTE TO POTENTIAL INACCURACY OF PULSE OXIMETRY

Poor cardiac output/low-perfusion states
Motion artifact
Increased venous pulsations
Optical interference from environment
Dyshemoglobinemias: carbon monoxide, methemoglobinemia, fetal hemoglobin
Dyes and pigments: methylene blue, indocyanine green

SpO$_2$)) are reasonably specific and sensitive. Other uses of oximetry include (a) titration of FIO$_2$, (b) screening for cardiopulmonary disease, and (c) as a method to reduce unnecessary arterial blood gases in select patient populations.

TRANSCUTANEOUS MEASUREMENT OF GAS TENSION

Interest in transcutaneous measurement of gas tension (transcutaneous O$_2$ tension, P$_{Tc}$O$_2$, and transcutaneous CO$_2$ tension, P$_{Tc}$CO$_2$) began in neonatal intensive care units. With transcutaneous technology, the skin is warmed to facilitate hyperperfusion and to allow diffusion of gases through the dermal and epidermal layers. Monitors measure the PO$_2$ and CO$_2$ electrochemically. Electrodes are attached to the skin, by adhesive patches, to well-perfused, non-bony surfaces. The abdomen, inner thigh, lower back, and chest are desirable sites in neonates, as are the chest, abdomen, and lower back in larger children and adults. Perhaps the greatest benefit of this technology is continuous monitoring and trending that can reduce the frequency of blood gas measurement and, hence, potentially decrease blood transfusions, especially in neonates and infants.

Transcutaneous monitoring has been limited by the need for frequent calibration of electrodes, cost of supplies, occasional burns induced by the warming component, inaccuracy when the skin is not well perfused, reported inaccuracies in older patients, and the development of more advanced pulse oximetry technology. Recent improvements in technology have decreased the risks and limitations of transcutaneous monitoring.

Physiologic Basis for Transcutaneous Monitoring

To measure O$_2$ tension across the skin, O$_2$ must be able to diffuse through the capillaries to the skin surface. In 1851, Gerlach was able to demonstrate that O$_2$ and CO$_2$ could diffuse through the skin of animals and humans. The O$_2$ tension measured on the surface of unheated skin is ~0–5 mm Hg in adults, ~0–10 mm Hg in term infants, ~10–15 mm Hg in larger premature infants (birth weight, 1.5–2 kg), and ~15–25 mm Hg in smaller premature infants (birth weight, <1.5 kg). In 1951, Baumberger and Goodfriend reported that when a finger was immersed in a phosphate buffer solution heated to ~45°C, the partial pressure of the solution approached PaO$_2$ in adults. Subsequently, it was shown that PaO$_2$ can be measured through the skin in newborns and adults by vasodilating the skin blood vessels with drugs or heat. To determine the conditions under which P$_{Tc}$O$_2$ approximates PaO$_2$, an understanding of the structure and blood flow through the skin is essential.

Structure and Blood Supply of the Skin

The skin consists of the dermis and epidermis (**Fig. 45.7**). The dermis is supplied through a rich network of arteriovenous anastomoses in the subcutaneous tissue and through U-shaped capillary loops that arise from the arteriovenous plexus. The epidermis consists of a deep, "viable" layer that utilizes O$_2$ and a superficial, "dead" part that does not consume O$_2$. O$_2$ supply to the dermis occurs by diffusion of O$_2$ from the capillary to the tissues as blood traverses from the arterial to the venous side of the capillaries by diffusion. The epidermis is supplied with O$_2$ by diffusion from the dome of the capillary to the deep layers of the epidermis.

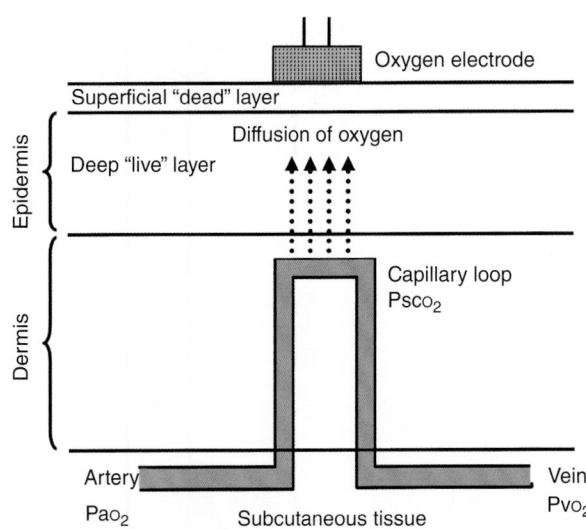

FIGURE 45.7. Schematic cross-section of the skin. The structure and blood supply of the skin, which consists of the dermis and epidermis, is displayed. O$_2$ diffuses out of the capillary into the tissues and can be measured by an electrode placed on the surface of the skin. PscO$_2$, skin capillary O$_2$ tension; PaO$_2$, arterial partial pressure of O$_2$; PvO$_2$, partial O$_2$ pressure in venous blood.

Gas Exchange in the Skin

O$_2$ tension decreases linearly along the skin capillaries due to O$_2$ consumption in the dermis, which results in an arteriovenous difference in PO$_2$, with the PO$_2$ in the capillary dome being intermediate. O$_2$ diffuses from the capillary dome to the deep part of the epidermis due the differences in PO$_2$ across the layer. O$_2$ consumption results in a further drop in O$_2$ tension across this layer (**Fig. 45.8**). As the superficial, "dead part" of the epidermis does not consume O$_2$, the PO$_2$ at the interface of the superficial and deep layers of the epidermis would be measured on the skin surface as transcutaneous O$_2$ tension.

Assuming that no change occurs in O$_2$ consumption as blood flow to the dermis increases, the difference between arterial and venous O$_2$ content decreases. As the flow becomes excessive, this difference becomes exceedingly small. The effect of increasing blood flow on P$_{Tc}$O$_2$ in the normal newborn infant is shown in **Figure 45.9**. As Hb concentration remains the same, the difference in the O$_2$ partial pressures between arterial and venous blood becomes negligible, and capillary dome PO$_2$, being intermediate between arterial and venous PO$_2$, reflects arterial O$_2$.

Principle of Operation

To ensure adequate blood flow, most transcutaneous monitors incorporate a heating element maintained at 42–44°C. Raising the temperature of blood has two opposing effects: (a) increased temperature shifts the O$_2$-dissociation curve to the right, causing the O$_2$ tension in the tissues to rise due to unloading of O$_2$, and (b) increased temperature raises O$_2$ consumption of the skin. As these effects act in opposite directions, they tend to offset each other, and the degree to which they offset each other determines any inaccuracy in P$_{Tc}$O$_2$.

The modern transcutaneous O$_2$ sensor consists of a heated electrode that has a platinum cathode and a silver reference anode encased in an electrolyte solution and separated from the skin by a membrane permeable to O$_2$. O$_2$ diffuses from the arterialized capillary bed through the epidermis and the membrane into the electrode, where it is reduced at the cathode,

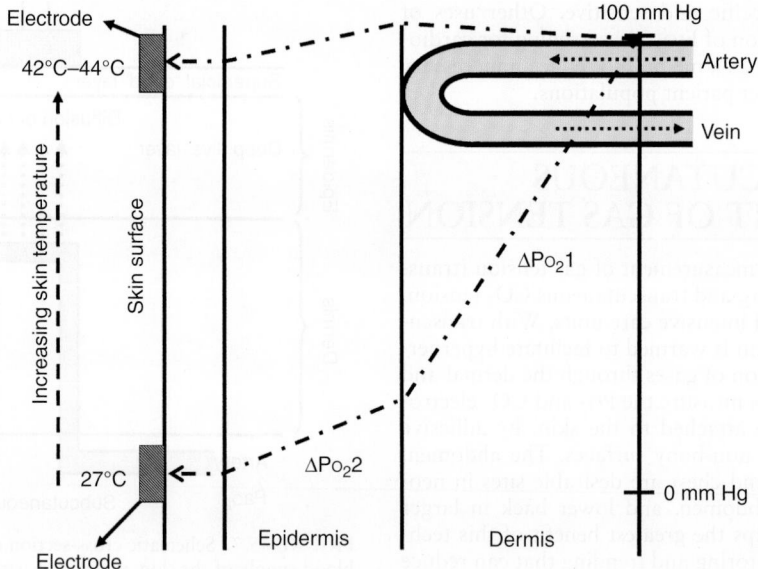

FIGURE 45.8. Schematic drawing of the O_2 profile in the skin. O_2 tension decreases along the skin capillaries due to O_2 consumption, predominantly in the dermis. PO_2, partial pressure of O_2. $\Delta PO_2 1$ represents the O_2 pressure drop in the dermis and $\Delta PO_2 2$ represents the drop in O_2 tension in the epidermis. When the skin is not heated, the surface O_2 is about 0–8 mm Hg in an infant. When the skin is heated to 42–44°C, the blood flow to the skin increases such that the supply of O_2 is in excess of the O_2 consumption of the underlying tissue. Then, the surface O_2 tension approximates arterial PO_2. (Adapted from Venkataraman SP. Assessment of oxygenation and ventilation. In: Singh NC, ed. *Manual of Pediatric Critical Care*. Philadelphia, PA: WB Saunders, 1997, with permission.)

thereby generating an electric current that is converted into the partial pressure measurements displayed by the monitor.

Clinical Applications

Transcutaneous O_2 monitoring has been used extensively in newborn infants with cardiorespiratory distress to estimate arterial O_2 tensions. The correlation between $P_{Tc}O_2$ and PaO_2 is excellent only when the blood pressure is within normal limits and peripheral circulation is normal. In circumstances where peripheral circulation is affected by hypotension, acidosis, or drugs, the correlation becomes less reliable (**Table 45.4**).

$P_{Tc}O_2$ monitoring in newborn infants has been traditionally used to closely follow PaO_2 to maintain normoxemia. Within the normal range, the correlation between $P_{Tc}O_2$ and PaO_2 is excellent. It is also important that $P_{Tc}O_2$ monitoring can detect hypoxemia ($PaO_2 < 50$ mm Hg) and hyperoxemia ($PaO_2 > 100$ mm Hg). $P_{Tc}O_2$ has been found to correlate with PaO_2 in the range between 30 and 200 mm Hg. $P_{Tc}O_2$ tends to underestimate O_2 tensions >200 mm Hg and to overestimate

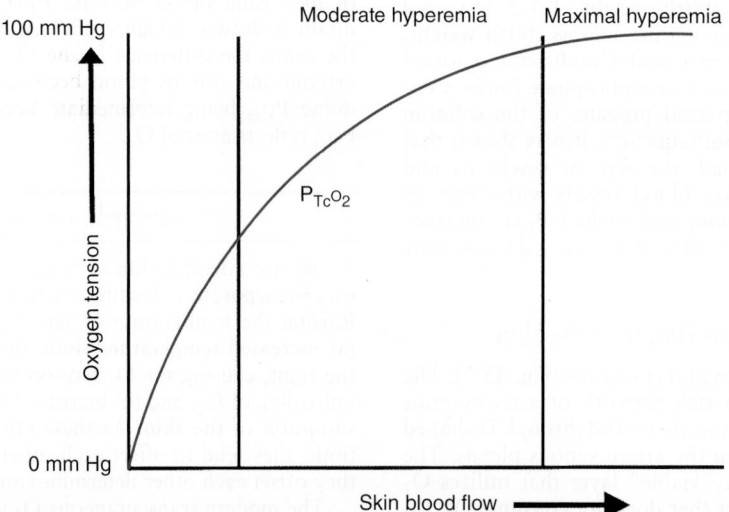

FIGURE 45.9. Influence of flow on the $P_{Tc}O_2$ with constant tissue respiration. The effect of increasing blood flow on $P_{Tc}O_2$ in the normal, newborn infant by hyperemia is displayed. If hemoglobin concentration remains the same, the difference in the O_2 partial pressures between arterial and venous blood becomes negligible, and capillary dome PO_2 reflects arterial O_2 as measured by transcutaneous technology. $P_{Tc}O_2$, transcutaneous partial pressure of O_2.

TABLE 45.4

CONDITIONS ASSOCIATED WITH POOR CORRELATION BETWEEN $P_{Tc}O_2$ AND PaO_2

1. Shock	<2 Standard deviations below mean for age
2. Acidosis	pH < 7.1
3. Hypothermia	Temperature < 35°C
4. Following cardiac surgery	Probably due to 1, 2, and 3
5. Skin edema	Severe
6. Cyanotic heart disease	PaO_2 < 30 mm Hg
7. Tolazoline infusion	Probably related to shunting in the skin blood vessels

$P_{Tc}O_2$, transcutaneous partial pressure of O_2; PaO_2, arterial oxygen tension.

PO_2 <30 mm Hg. The advantages and disadvantages of $P_{Tc}O_2$ monitoring are summarized in **Table 45.5**.

In critically ill newborns with mild circulatory failure, $P_{Tc}O_2$ can still reflect PaO_2, provided maximal hyperemia can be achieved. With moderate to severe circulatory failure, $P_{Tc}O_2$ no longer correlates with PaO_2. In these patients, $P_{Tc}O_2$ reflects skin perfusion more than PaO_2. The efficacy of various therapeutic maneuvers can be evaluated by their ability to restore the relationship between $P_{Tc}O_2$ and PaO_2.

There is an increasing clinical application of $P_{Tc}O_2$ in critically ill adults. In adults with peripheral vascular disease, $P_{Tc}O_2$ measurements have proven valuable in assessing adequacy of perfusion and in monitoring the effects of medical or surgical treatment. In adults with septic shock, the transcutaneous oxygen challenge test had been proposed. This oxygen challenge test documents the degree of change in $P_{Tc}O_2$ after 10 minutes at a F_{IO_2} of 1.0. A diminished response of $P_{Tc}O_2$ to an F_{IO_2} of 1.0 was associated with low cardiac output state and mortality (25,26).

TABLE 45.5

ADVANTAGES AND DISADVANTAGES OF $P_{Tc}O_2$ MONITORING

Advantages

Provides a reliably accurate measure of PaO_2 continuously and noninvasively

Accurate over a wide range of PaO_2 values

Very useful in neonates to maintain PaO_2 within a narrow range

Provides a trend of PaO_2 over time

Can detect variability and large changes in PaO_2 when SaO_2 is >95%

Provides a measure of circulatory dysfunction when $P_{Tc}O_2$ is <PaO_2

Disadvantages

Requires frequent calibration

Requires frequent site changes due to the possibility of local burns on the skin

Requires a warm-up time of 10 minutes

Underestimates PaO_2 in hyperoxic range (>150 mm Hg)

Overestimates PaO_2 in hypoxic range (<50 mm Hg)

Less useful with increasing age

$P_{Tc}O_2$, transcutaneous partial pressure of O_2; PaO_2, arterial oxygen tension; SaO_2, arterial blood oxygen saturation.

Accurate estimation of $PaCO_2$ with transcutaneous technology over a wide range of CO_2 values has been reported in infants and children with respiratory failure, including those who require high-frequency ventilation (27,28). Transcutaneous O_2 and CO_2 monitoring can be used to continuously evaluate tissue perfusion and serve as an early warning in critically ill children during resuscitation (29). In addition, this monitoring has also been used in other clinical scenarios such as apnea testing, noninvasive ventilation and diabetic ketoacidosis (30).

CAPNOGRAPHY

Capnography is the graphic waveform produced by variations in CO_2 concentration through the respiratory cycle as a function of time. Capnography can be either time- or volume-based (volumetric). Both time- and volume-based capnography respond to changes in ventilatory strategies and cardiac function. Time-based capnography is best known as end-tidal CO_2 ($ETCO_2$) monitoring. In addition to the E_TCO_2 measurements provided by time-based capnography, volumetric capnography has been used to measure anatomic dead space, pulmonary capillary perfusion, and effective ventilation.

Sampling Techniques

In clinical practice, capnometers use two sampling techniques: sidestream and mainstream. The sidestream sampler aspirates a small quantity of gas continuously from the ventilator circuit, or at the nares in spontaneously breathing patients (i.e., via a nasal cannula). This sampling method allows for the monitoring of respiratory gases without the additional dead space and weight associated with the more common mainstream adapters. However, several disadvantages exist, including (a) aspiration of mucous and water condensation into the sampling tubing, which can block flow of gas, and (b) excessive scavenging of gas flow, which may decrease minute ventilation in small children and infants. Slow aspiration rates can result in a significant time delay, and rapid aspiration rates can result in aspiration of fresh gas and an artifactual lowering of end-tidal CO_2 value.

Mainstream capnography incorporates a light-emitting source and detector on separate sides of an airway adaptor. This equipment does not aspirate gas but is occasionally susceptible to secretions and humidity that cover the light source or detector. Recent technologic advances have greatly reduced the weight of these connectors, which decreases traction and tension on the endotracheal tube (ETT). Dead space has been reduced to 1 mL in the neonatal sensor and it no longer poses a rebreathing problem in infants and children.

The two main techniques of capnography measurement are infrared spectroscopy and mass spectroscopy. Infrared spectroscopy requires three components: an infrared light source, a gas chamber, and a detector. Its success depends on the fact that each gas has unique absorption characteristics that can be used to quantify the amount (partial pressure) of a particular gas by application of the Beer–Lambert principle.

E_TCO_2 is defined as the peak CO_2 value during expiration and is dependent on adequate pulmonary capillary blood flow of CO_2-rich blood to alveoli, which in turn depends on adequate right and left heart function. The normal E_TCO_2 in healthy subjects is generally <5 mm Hg lower than the $PaCO_2$, representing normal anatomic dead space of the upper airway. Clinical conditions associated with alterations in E_TCO_2 are shown in **Table 45.6**.

TABLE 45.6

CLINICAL CONDITIONS ASSOCIATED WITH ALTERATIONS IN E_TCO_2

Increases in E_TCO_2
Increased pulmonary capillary blood flow
Increased cardiac output
Hypoventilation
Increased CO_2 production
Sudden release of a tourniquet
Sodium bicarbonate administration
Decreases in E_TCO_2
Decreased pulmonary capillary blood flow
Pulmonary hypertension
Pulmonary embolus (thrombus or air)
Decreased cardiac output
Hyperventilation
Ventilator circuit leak
Obstructed endotracheal tube
Hyperventilation
Decreased CO_2 production
Absent E_TCO_2
Esophageal intubation
Ventilator disconnect

Evaluation of Respiratory Pattern

The phasic changes in CO_2 concentration that occur during the respiratory cycle are demonstrated in **Figure 45.10.** Evaluation of the respiratory pattern is aided by noting the near-zero end-inspiratory CO_2 value in the normal capnogram, the plateau at end expiration, and the highest CO_2 recorded (E_TCO_2). The capnogram converts these phasic values of CO_2 into electrical signals and displays them as respiratory rate, inspiratory CO_2, and E_TCO_2, as a waveform and/or digitally, allowing analysis of changes that take place breath-to-breath and over longer periods of time.

Clinical Applications

Practical uses of E_TCO_2 monitoring in the ICU include adequacy of alveolar ventilation during mechanical ventilation, apnea monitoring, patient–ventilator system integrity, and

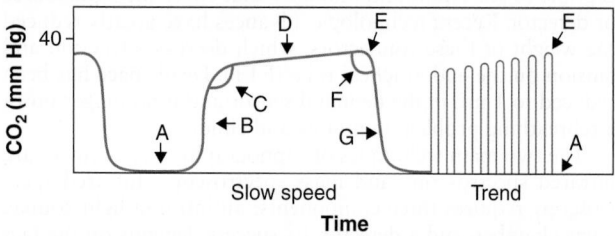

FIGURE 45.10. Normal features of a capnogram. *A,* baseline, represents the beginning of expiration and should start at zero. *B,* the transitional part of the curve, represents mixing of dead space and alveolar gas. *C,* the α angle, represents the change to alveolar gas. *D,* the alveolar part of the curve, represents the plateau average alveolar gas concentration. *E* is the end-tidal CO_2 value. *F,* the β angle, represents the change to the inspiratory part of the cycle. *G,* the inspiration part of the curve, shows a rapid decrease in CO_2 concentration. (From Thompson JE, Jaffe MB. Capnographic waveforms in the mechanically ventilated patient. *Respir Care* 2005;50(1):100–9, with permission.)

ETT patency and positioning. Many institutions use capnography at intubation for a rapid assessment of ETT placement by confirming the presence of CO_2 in the exhaled gas, and some centers use it for the duration of mechanical ventilation to monitor for inadvertent dislodgement of the ETT.

Esophageal intubation is one of the most serious and complications of attempted endotracheal intubation (31,32). Early detection of this inadvertent placement of the ETT can be lifesaving. Assessment of different methods of ETT placement verification found capnography to be the most rapid and reliable method for evaluation when compared to auscultation and transillumination (31).

While the validation of ETT placement in the trachea is improved with E_TCO_2 monitoring (31), limitations do exist (33). False-positive readings (i.e., the monitor displays an end-tidal CO_2 value when the ETT is not in the trachea) may occur following mouth-to-mouth ventilation, following ingestion of antacids or carbonated beverages, or when the tip of the ETT is in the pharynx. False-negative readings (i.e., no end-tidal CO_2 value is displayed when, in fact, the ETT is in trachea) may occur if the patient has severe airway obstruction, poor cardiac output, pulmonary emboli, or pulmonary hypertension. When discrepancies appear between the capnometer reading and the physical assessment, further investigation is necessary.

During cardiopulmonary resuscitation, capnography can be utilized to assess the quality of chest compressions and provide an early indication of return of spontaneous circulation. Effective chest compression should produce enough pulmonary blood flow to generate an exhaled CO_2 value of at least 10 mm Hg. The evidence for the use of capnography during cardiopulmonary resuscitation is slowly being established (34).

Capnography can be used to great advantage in mechanically ventilated patients if the waveform is displayed and analyzed along with the numeric data. Mechanical failures can be detected, the adequacy of respiratory support can be analyzed, and changes can be made in the mode of ventilation to maximize the efficiency of ventilation, decrease the patient's work of breathing (WOB), and improve patient–ventilator synchrony (**Figs. 45.11–45.13**).

Time-Based versus Volumetric Capnography

While both time-based and volumetric capnography provide the measurement and display of E_TCO_2, many differences exist between the techniques. It is important to determine (a) which values are pertinent to the specific patient population being monitored, and (b) the primary clinical objectives.

Time-based capnography is limited to the measurement and display of the respiratory waveform and E_TCO_2 value. The E_TCO_2 displayed represents the partial pressure of CO_2 end-exhalation (**Fig. 45.10**). E_TCO_2 can also be used to trend changes in $PaCO_2$ for patients in whom physiologic dead space is not significantly elevated or changing. However, this ability is weakened in conditions of increased physiologic dead space (e.g., impaired cardiac output). Optimization of mechanical ventilation may be better achieved with volumetric capnography than with time-based capnography, as described below (35).

Advances in technology allow the integration of flow and volume to be graphically displayed (**Fig. 45.14**), which is the basis of volumetric capnography. The display of measurements throughout the entire respiratory cycle is achieved providing a myriad of valuable information. Volumetric capnography provides a measurement of CO_2 production (VCO_2) and enables calculation of alveolar minute ventilation and the ratio of volume of dead space (Vd) to tidal volume (Vt), Vd/Vt. As many important management decisions are based on tidal volume determination and the resultant changes in gas exchange, accuracy of these values is essential (36,37).

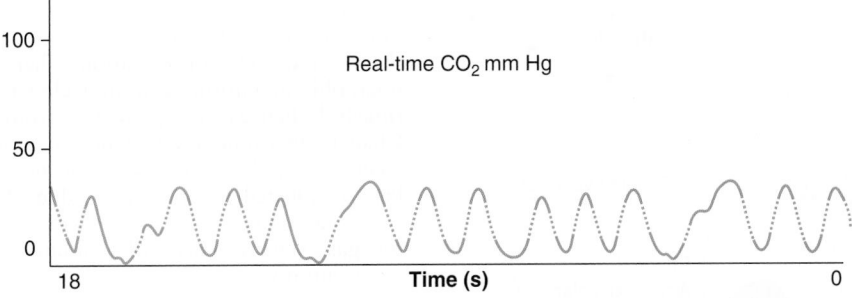

FIGURE 45.11. Chaotic respiratory pattern in a patient unable to tolerate spontaneous ventilation. (From Carlon GC, Ray C, Miodownik S, et al. Capnography in mechanically ventilated patients. *Crit Care Med* 1988;16:550–6, with permission.)

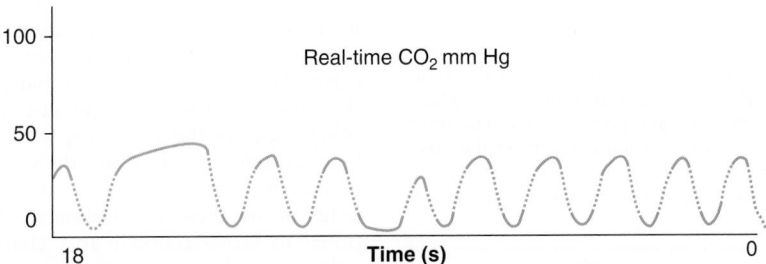

FIGURE 45.12. Intermittent mandatory ventilation without pressure support. Note irregular respiratory pattern, tachypnea, absence of alveolar plateau, low E_TCO_2, and high baseline CO_2. (From Carlon GC, Ray C, Miodownik S, et al. Capnography in mechanically ventilated patients. *Crit Care Med* 1988;16:550–6, with permission.)

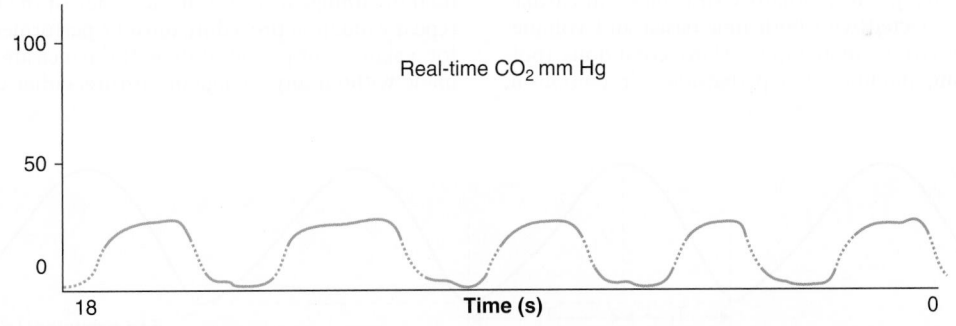

FIGURE 45.13. Same patient as in **Figure 45.12**, 15 minutes after addition of 20 cm H_2O pressure support. A normal capnogram and respiratory rate can now be observed. (From Carlon GC, Ray C, Miodownik S, et al. Capnography in mechanically ventilated patients. *Crit Care Med* 1988;16:550–6, with permission.)

Capnography is a very useful and sensitive clinical tool that reflects the cardiorespiratory status and metabolic state of the patient. The net volume of CO_2 eliminated through the lungs each minute (VCO_2) varies depending on CO_2 production, ventilation, circulation/perfusion, and, to a lesser degree, diffusion. VCO_2 signals future changes in $PaCO_2$, thus making VCO_2 a valuable marker for changes in the cardiorespiratory status of the ventilated patient (38). As CO_2 production varies between patients and within a patient over time, absolute values are not as significant as trends. As with O_2 consumption, CO_2 production and elimination comprise a continuous process. Therefore, VCO_2 rapidly reflects changes in ventilation and perfusion, regardless of the etiology, as well as the body's overall physiologic response to changes in mechanical ventilation.

The single-breath CO_2 waveform consists of three phases (**Fig. 45.14**). Phase 1 represents gas exhaled from the upper airways (i.e., gas exhaled from anatomic dead space), which is generally void of CO_2 (35). A prolongation of phase 1 indicates an increase in anatomic dead-space ventilation (Vd_{ana}). Phase 2 is the transitional phase from upper- to lower-airway ventilation. Changes in phase 2 generally reflect changes in perfusion. Phase 3 is the area of alveolar gas exchange, and represents changes in gas distribution. For example, when a maldistribution of gas exists, the slope of phase 3 increases.

When weaning from mechanical ventilation, it is important to ensure that the volume of gas delivered actually participates in gas exchange (i.e., effective ventilation). Volumetric capnography provides clinicians with a continuous numerical representation of effective ventilation. Pediatric studies

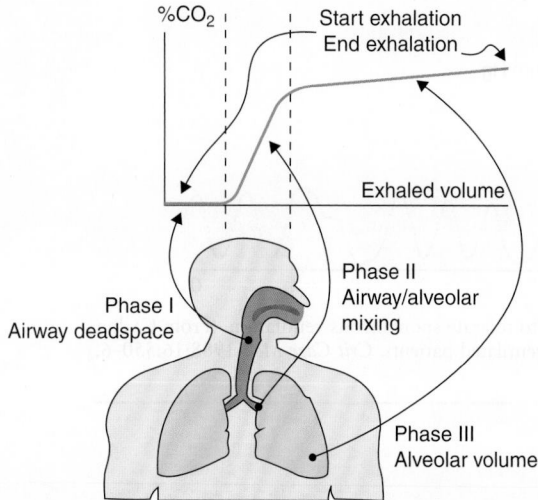

FIGURE 45.14. Volumetric capnogram. The initial portion of the volumetric capnogram (phase 1) represents the quantity of CO_2 eliminated from the large airways. Phase 2 is the transitional zone, which represents ventilation from both small and large airways. The third phase of the capnogram represents CO_2 elimination from the alveoli and, thus, the quantity of gas involved with alveolar ventilation. (Figure Courtesy of Respironics, Inc., and its affiliates, Wallingford, Connecticut.)

have examined the value of Vd/Vt in helping clinicians in the mechanical ventilation weaning process. Although there are no absolute cutoff values, Vd/Vt values of <0.5–0.55 and >0.65 have been proposed as predictive of extubation success and failure, respectively (39,40).

Responses to changes in ventilatory strategies and cardiac function can be detected with both time-based and volume-based (i.e., volumetric) capnography. Many conditions (pulmonary embolism, pulmonary hypertension, air embolism,

and severe cardiac dysfunction) increase dead-space ventilation, impair gas exchange, and cause a significant decrease in the expired CO_2 concentration. Therefore, continuous capnographic monitoring can alert clinicians to potentially detrimental changes in a patient's cardiorespiratory condition. Changes in capnography tend to occur more rapidly than changes in pulse oximetry. While no definitive studies have been conducted to prove the value of monitoring volumetric capnography on patient outcomes, monitoring the effective gas exchange effects of ventilator parameter adjustments seems intuitive.

MONITORING RESPIRATORY MECHANICS

Respiratory Inductive Plethysmography

Respiratory inductive plethysmography (**Fig. 45.15**) consists of two coils of insulated wires sewn in a sinusoidal pattern in elastic-fabricated bands. One band encircles the chest, with the upper level of the band just under the axillae, and the other encircles the abdomen, with the band located midway between the lower ribs and the upper edge of the iliac crests. Movement causes voltage changes, by generating magnetic fields in the chest and abdominal bands, which are proportional to cross-sectional area changes. These alterations in voltage can be interpolated to indicate changes in thoracic volume. Before obtaining measurements on a patient, a reference volume signal from a spirometer must be provided to the calibration unit.

Following calibration, the sum signal from the chest and abdominal sensors must be validated against a simultaneous spirometer (or an integrated pneumotachometer) during tidal breathing. To verify the accuracy of the measurements, a repeat validation procedure must be performed after recording for a significant period of time. If the measurements are being made without any change in posture, either the isovolume or

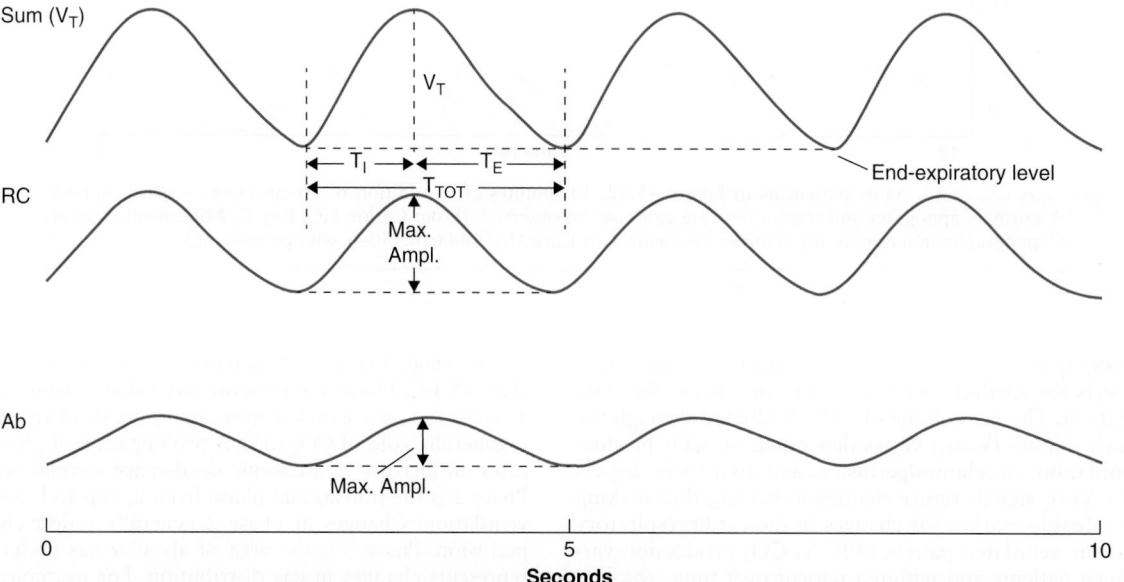

FIGURE 45.15. Schematic recording of the respiratory cycle obtained through a respiratory inductive plethysmograph. The algebraic sum of the ribcage (*RC*) and the abdominal (*Ab*) excursions equals Vt. T_i is the inspiratory time (seconds), T_e is the expiratory time, and T_{tot} is the total respiratory cycle (seconds). (From Tobin MJ. Respiratory monitoring in the intensive care unit. *Am Review of Respir Dis (Am J Resp Crit Care Med)* 1988;138:1625–42, with permission.)

multiple linear-regressions technique may be used for calibration without substantial loss of accuracy. If a change in posture is planned, only the least-squares method is likely to retain its accuracy over time.

Application in Critically Ill Patients

Minute ventilation is the product of Vt and respiratory frequency (f):

$$V = \text{Vt}/T_i \times T_i/T_{tot} \times 60$$

where V is the minute ventilation (L/min), T_i is the inspiratory time (seconds), and T_{tot} is the total respiratory cycle (seconds).

The parameter Vt/T_i is the mean inspiratory flow, and T_i/T_{tot} is the fractional inspiratory time.

Vt/T_i is a measure of respiratory drive and correlates well with other indices of respiratory drive such as $P_{0.1}$ and the ventilatory response to hypercapnia. $P_{0.1}$ is the pressure generated in the first 100 milliseconds after the onset of inspiratory effort against an occluded airway and provides a measure of respiratory drive as described later in this chapter.

Few pediatric studies have examined the utility of respiratory inductive plethysmography in critical illness. Use of this technique to diagnose bilateral diaphragmatic paralysis has been reported (41). In adults, an index of rapid, shallow breathing (f/Vt) >100 has been associated with a higher weaning failure. In children, however, f/Vt ratio does not predict extubation failure (42).

Monitoring of Respiratory Muscle Function

Maximal inspiratory pressure (P_{Imax}), often called negative inspiratory force, is defined as the maximal static pressure that can be generated with forceful efforts against an occluded airway. P_{Imax} may provide a noninvasive index of global muscle strength (43). P_{Imax} is usually measured after expiration to residual volume. In nonintubated patients, P_{Imax} is measured as the largest pressure sustained for at least 1 second. On the other hand, P_{Imax} in intubated patients is the peak pressure that can be generated. In intubated patients, a one-way valve and manometer are attached to the airway, which permits exhalation but not inspiration. As the patient breathes spontaneously through the one-way valve, the pressures become more and more negative. The period of occlusion is maintained for at least 10–20 seconds.

In normal infants, P_{Imax} during crying has been reported to be –118 ± 21 cm H_2O. In children 6–17 years of age, the P_{Imax} has been reported to be –70 to –110 cm H_2O, and pubertal children are capable of generating P_{Imax} of –80 to –120 cm H_2O (44,45). In adults, a P_{Imax} more negative than –30 cm H_2O has been reported to be associated with extubation success, and a value less negative than –20 cm H_2O has been associated with extubation failure. In children, P_{Imax} has poor discriminative capacity between extubation success and failure (46). Despite the poor discriminative capacity of P_{Imax}, it is common practice to measure P_{Imax} prior to extubation in children, especially those with neuromuscular weakness (e.g., Guillain–Barre syndrome, weakness from prolonged neuromuscular blockade) and to defer extubation unless the P_{Imax} is more negative than –20 cm H_2O. However, even if the P_{Imax} is more negative than –30 cm H_2O, successful extubation is not guaranteed. The clinician should use additional assessments of muscle strength such as hip flexion in the infant and head lift >5 seconds in the adolescent as well as careful observation of spontaneous breathing without distress, hypoxemia, or hypercapnia before deciding on readiness for extubation.

Monitoring Respiratory Mechanics in Ventilated Patients

In a relaxed patient during mechanical ventilation, measurements of respiratory mechanics can be obtained by rapid airway occlusion during constant-flow inflation, when the proximal airway pressure increases as the lung is inflated to a maximal pressure (P_{max}). Rapid airway occlusion at end-inspiration results in an immediate drop in both airway pressure and transpulmonary pressure (P_{tp}) from P_{max}, followed by a gradual decrease until a plateau (P_{plat}) is achieved after 3–5 seconds (**Fig. 45.16**). The pressure drop from P_{max} can be partitioned into an initial almost linear drop followed by a slower, multiexponential decrease to P_{plat}. P_{plat}, P_{tp}, and esophageal pressure (P_{es}) represent the static recoil pressure of the total respiratory system, lung, and chest wall, respectively.

Compliance and Elastance

Compliance is defined as a change in volume divided by a change in transmural pressure. *Elastance* is the reciprocal of compliance. Lung compliance is defined as the change in lung volume divided by the transalveolar pressure, which is equal to the difference between the alveolar pressure (P_{alv}) at the end of inflation and the pleural pressure (P_{pl} or P_{es}). At the bedside, the P_{plat} can be substituted for P_{alv} and tidal volume can be substituted for a change in lung volume.

$$C_{\text{lung}} = \text{Vt}/(P_{\text{plat}} - P_{\text{es}})$$

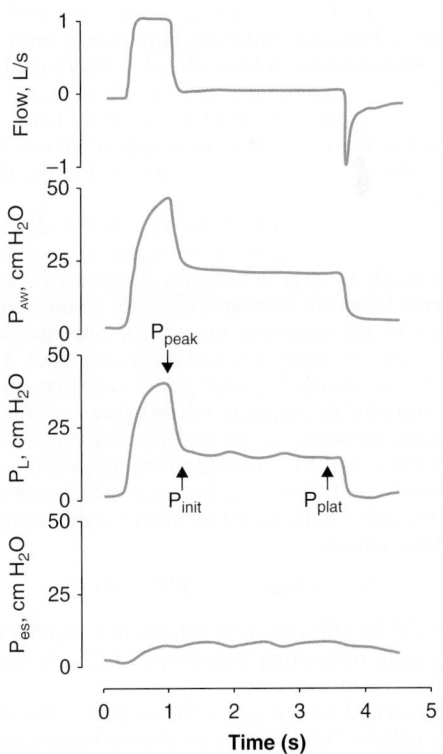

FIGURE 45.16. Flow (inspiration upward), airway pressure (P_{aw}), transpulmonary pressure (P_L), and esophageal pressure (P_{es}) tracings in a representative patient during passive ventilation. An end-inspiratory occlusion produced a rapid decline in both P_{aw} and P_{tp} from a peak value to a lower initial value, followed by gradual decrease until a plateau is achieved. (From Jubran A, Tobin MJ. Passive mechanics of lung and chest wall in patients who failed and succeeded in trials of weaning. *Am J Resp Crit Care Med* 1997;155:916–21, with permission.)

C_{lung} is also called *static lung compliance* (C_{stat}). Since esophageal pressure is often not measured in children, C_{lung} can be calculated by

$$C_{lung} = Vt_{(effective)}/(P_{plat} - PEEP)$$

where $Vt_{(effective)}$ is the tidal volume delivered to the patient (usually measured at the hub of the ETT or estimated by subtracting the compressible volume lost in the circuit from the ventilator-delivered tidal volume).

Chest-wall compliance is defined as the change in thoracic volume divided by the transthoracic pressure (atmospheric pressure (P_{atm}) $- P_{es}$). To compare among patients, compliance values should be indexed to body weight.

Dynamic Compliance

Dynamic compliance (C_{dyn}) is defined as the change in volume divided by the change in airway pressure from end expiration to end inspiration during a mechanical breath. It is commonly calculated by dividing the Vt by the difference between P_{max} and end-expiratory pressure.

$$C_{dyn} = Vt/(P_{max} - PEEP)$$

In patients without intrinsic PEEP ($PEEP_i$), the end-expiratory pressure to be used is the set PEEP. In patients with $PEEP_i$, the end-expiratory pressure to be used for the calculation of C_{dyn} is $PEEP_i$.

Tidal Volume Measurement

In adults, the inspiratory Vt displayed by the ventilator can generally be used for compliance calculations and for most aspects of mechanical ventilation. However, it must be noted that the delivered tidal volume (Vt_{del}) is distributed between the ventilator circuit and the patient. For infants and children, an accurate measurement of Vt is essential. Thus, the issue is determining the ideal location at which Vt measurements should be obtained, as Vt can be measured at the ETT or at the ventilator.

In children, the fraction of the Vt_{del} that is distributed to the ventilator circuit is substantially higher than in adults and can be as much as 70% in critically ill infants (47). Measuring delivered Vt at the ventilator does not compensate for the compliance of the ventilator circuit, for uncontrolled variations in the circuit setup or for changes over time. A Vt measured with a pneumotachometer positioned between the ETT and the ventilator circuit more reliably measures the Vt actually delivered to neonatal and pediatric patients (47–49). To determine the actual Vt delivered to the lungs without requiring additional equipment (i.e., a pneumotachometer), a mathematical formula can be used to correct for the compliance of the ventilator circuit:

$$Vt_{eff} = Vt_{del} - C_{vent}(PIP - PEEP)$$

where Vt_{eff} is the effective tidal volume that reaches the ETT, PIP is the peak inspiratory pressure, and C_{vent} is the compliance of the ventilator circuit.

This calculated Vt represents the ventilator-determined Vt minus the volume "lost" due to the distensibility (compliance) of the ventilator circuit. It should be noted that the calculated values can differ from those measured at the ETT (47–49). Additionally, it is preferable to index tidal volumes to body weight. When calculating compliances as described here, the Vt_{eff} should be used instead of the ventilator Vt.

Intrinsic PEEP

The static recoil pressure of the respiratory system at end expiration may be elevated in patients who receive mechanical ventilation, especially in those who have lower-airway disease and obstruction. With lower-airway obstruction, inspiration may begin before exhalation is complete, thus resulting in an end-expiratory alveolar pressure that remains elevated above the proximal airway pressure. This positive recoil pressure, or static $PEEP_i$, can be quantified in relaxed patients by using an end-expiratory hold maneuver on a mechanical ventilator immediately before the onset of the next breath. Patients who are spontaneously breathing may need to overcome $PEEP_i$ to trigger a ventilator. Thus, $PEEP_i$ increases muscle fatigue and WOB. Excessive $PEEP_i$ may also result in poor triggering because the patient is unable to generate the necessary negative pressure in the central airway. This problem can be largely overcome by flow triggering.

Static Pressure–Volume Curves

A static pressure–volume (PV) curve can be constructed in a paralyzed patient by measuring airway pressure as the lungs are progressively inflated and deflated with a graduated volumetric syringe, the "super-syringe technique." In small children, the aliquots of volume should be 1–2 mL/kg. The PV curve has both inflation and deflation portions. It should be noted that this technique is rarely used in clinical practice, especially in pediatrics.

The inspiratory phase of the PV curve consists of three sections. As the lung is inflated from low lung volumes, the initial lung compliance is low. With increasing airway pressure, lung compliance improves, which continues until the lung is fully inflated. Inflating the lung further results in a reduction in the lung compliance at the end of inflation (**Fig. 45.17**). The junction between the first and second portions of the curve is called the *lower inflection point* (LIP). The LIP can be discerned by visual inspection of the PV curve. More accurately, the LIP can be calculated by intersecting the lines from the first and second portions of the curve. Alternatively, the LIP can be calculated by measuring the steepest point of the second section and marking the LIP as the point of a 20% decrease in slope from this steepest point. The junction of the second and third portions of the curve is called the *upper inflection point* (UIP). The UIP can be measured in the same way as the LIP, except that the UIP would represent a 20% decrease from the point of the greatest slope. The LIP is thought to represent the point of alveolar recruitment, and the UIP is thought to represent overdistension. In patients with acute lung injury,

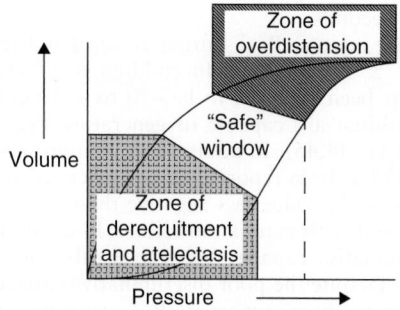

FIGURE 45.17. Pressure–volume curve. The inspiratory phase of the pressure–volume curve consists of three sections. As the lung is inflated from an initial low lung volume, the lung compliance is low. As airway pressure is increased, lung compliance improves, which continues until the lung is fully inflated. Inflating the lung further results in a reduction in the lung compliance at the end of inflation as the lung overdistends. The goal is to ventilate in the "safe window." (From Froese AB. High-frequency oscillatory ventilation for adult respiratory distress syndrome: Let's get it right this time! *Crit Care Med* 1997;25(6):906–8, with permission.)

some investigators have recommended that PEEP should be set at a pressure slightly above the LIP on a static PV curve.

Work of Breathing and Pressure–Time Product

WOB can be measured using esophageal manometry and measurement of Vt during spontaneous breathing. *Work* is defined as *force multiplied by displacement*. WOB can be estimated by integrating pressure and volume of a spontaneous breath.

A significant limitation of the measurement of WOB is that it may underestimate the total energy expenditure and O_2 consumption of the respiratory muscles. To overcome this problem, many have suggested the use of the pressure–time product for respiratory muscles. This also requires esophageal manometry but does not require simultaneous measurement of Vt. The pressure–time product is calculated as the time integral of the difference between P_{es} measured during assisted ventilation and the recoil pressure of the chest wall (50). The method of measuring the recoil pressure of the chest wall has been described previously.

Mechanical Ventilators and Airway Graphics Monitoring

Mechanical ventilators deliver gas at a pressure, which generates flow and results in a change in lung volume. Most mechanical ventilators in the PICU permit continuous monitoring of respiratory mechanics and include graphic display of Vt, gas flow (V), and airway pressure (P_{aw}).

Output waveforms are useful tools to study ventilator operation and provide a graphic display of the various modes of ventilation. Waveform analysis can be used to optimize mechanical ventilatory support and to analyze ventilator incidents and alarm conditions. Analysis of airway graphics can improve patient–ventilator synchrony, reduce WOB, and calculate a variety of physiologic parameters related to respiratory mechanics (50). The goal of this section is to provide clinicians with a clinical tool that can optimize their mechanical ventilation strategies through airway graphic analysis.

A primary goal of graphic analysis is to quantitate respiratory pathophysiology by evaluating tidal volume, airway pressures, compliance, airway resistance, and pressure–volume and flow–volume relationships. Airway graphic analysis can help to determine the effectiveness of various interventions. Additionally, adverse effects, including alveolar overdistension, air leak, dynamic hyperexpansion ("gas trapping"), and patient–ventilator asynchrony, can be diagnosed and corrected.

Airway Scalars

Airway scalars, the most commonly reported waveforms, comprise three distinct waveforms—flow, pressure, and volume (*y*-axis)—plotted against time (*x*-axis). Conventionally, in these waveforms, positive values correspond to inspiration events and negative values correspond to expiration. Simultaneous comparison of all three waveforms facilitates analysis of the patient–ventilator interface. Patient–ventilator asynchrony becomes evident when the timing and magnitude of flow, pressure, and volume are disproportionate or delayed. Additionally, each of these parameters (flow, pressure, and volume) can be plotted against each other. PV and flow–volume loops can be particularly helpful in assessing alterations in resistance, compliance, WOB, pulmonary overdistension, and premature termination of exhalation.

Optimal measurements are obtained when the pressure- and flow-monitoring device (pneumotachometer) is positioned between the ETT and ventilator circuit. Although resistance of the ETT is a component of the pressure graphic, pressures reported are generally considered to reflect proximal airway pressures. Volume is generally measured by integrating the flow signal over time. The upward deflection of the graphic represents the volume delivered to the patient, while the downward deflection represents the total expiratory volume. Inspiratory and expiratory volumes should be equal. However, it is not uncommon in patients with uncuffed ETTs or with cuffed ETTs that have inadequate cuff inflation for the expiratory volume to be less than the inspiratory volume. Percentage leak can be calculated and may aid in the decision to change the ETT size or to evaluate the adequacy of the cuff.

Scalar Display of Volume-Limited Ventilation

A typical airway graphic during time-cycled, volume-limited ventilation is displayed in **Figure 45.18**. The top graphic displays flow on the vertical axis and time on the horizontal axis. The bottom graphic displays airway pressure versus time. During volume-limited ventilation, the Vt is set, and the PIP is determined by lung compliance, airway resistance, inspiratory time (T_i), and flow characteristics.

Traditionally, this mode of ventilation is characterized by a square-wave, constant-flow inspiratory flow pattern. Constant inspiratory flow corresponds to a linear increase in airway pressure until the preset Vt is reached. When an unacceptable PIP occurs during volume-limited ventilation with a square-wave, constant-inspiratory flow pattern, consideration of increasing T_i, decreasing Vt (allowing permissive hypercapnia) (51), or changing the ventilation mode to a variable, decelerating inspiratory flow pattern (52) will decrease the PIP. It must be noted that many current-generation ventilators offer volume-limited ventilation with a variable, decelerating inspiratory flow pattern (e.g., pressure-regulated volume control).

In **Figure 45.18**, an inspiratory pause has been set and is represented by the lengthened T_i and the period of zero flow prior to exhalation. The plateau pressure corresponds to this zero-flow period during inspiration. The flow returns to zero during expiration, indicating the completion of exhalation.

Scalar Display of Pressure-Limited Ventilation

A typical airway graphic during pressure-limited ventilation with a variable, decelerating inspiratory flow pattern (i.e., pressure-control ventilation) is displayed in **Figure 45.19**. During pressure-limited ventilation, the PIP is set, and the Vt is determined by lung compliance, airway resistance, and delivered flow rate. In the following discussions, PIP refers to the total peak inspiratory pressure above zero and not a

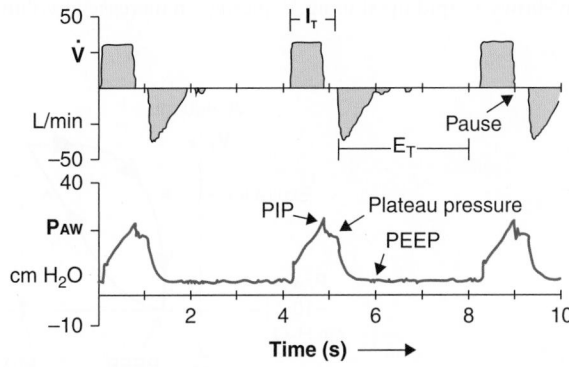

FIGURE 45.18. Normal scalar display of flow versus time and airway pressure versus time for volume-limited ventilation. P_{aw}, airway pressure; PIP, peak inspiratory pressure; PEEP, positive end-expiratory pressure. (Figure courtesy of VIASYS Healthcare Inc., Yorba Linda, CA.)

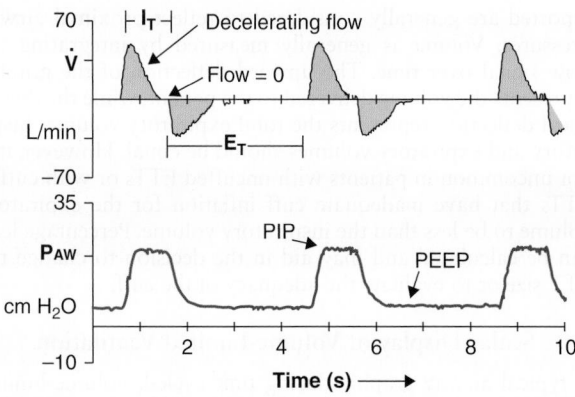

FIGURE 45.19. Normal scalar display of flow versus time and airway pressure versus time for pressure-limited ventilation. (Figure courtesy of VIASYS Healthcare, Inc., Yorba Linda, CA.)

set inspiratory pressure above PEEP. This characteristic flow pattern of pressure-control ventilation results in a curvilinear increase in airway pressure until the PIP is reached. Note the more rapid increase in pressure during the initial phase of a pressure-limited breath versus the linear increase in airway pressure that occurs with a volume-limited breath (Fig. 45.18). During pressure-limited ventilation, if Vt decreases, increasing the PIP limit, increasing the T_i, or optimizing the PEEP should be considered. At a similar Vt, the decelerating flow pattern of pressure-control ventilation results in a decrease in PIP (52) and an increase in dynamic compliance when compared to volume-limited ventilation with a square-wave, constant-inspiratory flow pattern.

In ARDS, pulmonary compliance is decreased. If PIP is held constant while compliance decreases, Vt will be reduced and gas exchange may be impaired, potentially resulting in respiratory acidosis. Approaches to the loss of Vt consist of allowing this to occur (i.e., permissive hypercapnia) (51) or increasing the airway pressures (PIP and/or PEEP) to recruit lung volume.

Pressure–Volume and Flow–Volume Loops

PV and flow–volume loops provide insight into the patient's pathophysiology and the response to therapeutic interventions. PV loops depict pressure on the horizontal axis and volume on the vertical axis. The first portion of inspiratory curve in Figure 45.17 shows a significant increase in pressure with little increase in volume (low compliance). The following portion shows a rapid up-sloping, depicting an increase in volume

per pressure delivered (high compliance). This point is termed the *LIP* and is created by a sudden opening of the alveoli. A sharp intersection is seen at the end of inspiration and the start of expiration. At the onset of expiration, a significant reduction in pressure with a smaller reduction in volume is seen. It should be noted that accurate inflection and deflection points can only be discerned with a static lung-inflation technique, using very low inspiratory flow, as previously described. The dynamic curves displayed on standard airway graphics monitors do not accurately detect inflection and deflection points, as gas flow is a significant variable.

The flow–volume loop depicts flow on the vertical axis and volume on the horizontal axis. Inspiration is seen on the upper portion of the loop, with exhalation depicted on the lower portion. Inspiratory volume is increased with increases in inspiratory flow. When flow terminates, expiration begins. Peak expiratory flow rate is reached when the expiratory flow rate begins to decay.

Pressure–Volume and Flow–Volume Loops in Volume-Limited Ventilation

The typical PV and flow–volume loops during volume-limited ventilation are displayed in Figure 45.20. As the ventilator delivers gas to the patient, airway pressure increases from the set PEEP level until the set Vt is reached and inspiration is terminated. During exhalation, both volume and pressure are reduced in the airways until exhaled flow reaches zero, signifying the termination of the breath. Alterations in the shape of the inspiratory limb of the PV loop provide insight into the compliance of the lung and the presence of various abnormalities, including alveolar atelectasis and overdistension. Dynamic compliance, which is the slope of the line connecting the PEEP with the PIP, is calculated as

$$Vt_{del}/(PIP - PEEP)$$

Note in Figures 45.20 and 45.21 that only a small quantity of gas volume is delivered during the initial phase of inspiration. As the inspiratory pressure increases, the critical opening pressure is achieved, and Vt is delivered. Hysteresis, which is a nonlinear change in the PV relationship over time, is present during both inspiration and expiration. A decrease in compliance (compare Fig. 45.20 with Fig. 45.21) results in higher airway pressures being required to achieve a similar Vt. As a result, the PV loop flattens, and the curvature of the inspiratory and expiratory limbs decreases (decreased hysteresis). Note that, during the initial phase of inspiration, airway pressure increases, with little gas being delivered to the patient, due to alveolar collapse and a decrease in lung volume during the expiratory phase. To re-expand the collapsed alveoli, the initial

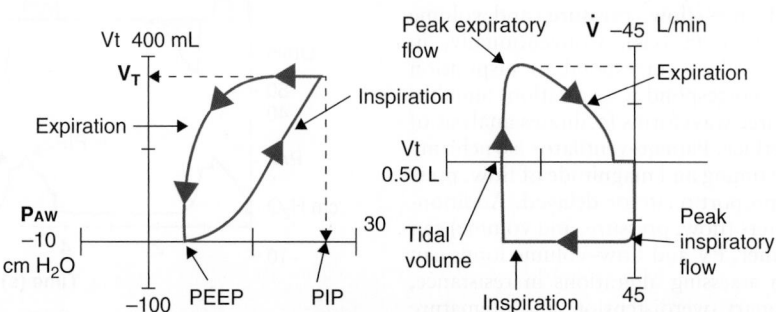

FIGURE 45.20. The pressure–volume graphic displays tidal volume on the vertical axis and airway pressure on the horizontal axis. The flow–volume graphic displays flow on the vertical axis and tidal volume on the horizontal axis. Note that in this flow–volume loop, the delivered inspiratory flow is represented during traditional volume-limited ventilation below the baseline as a square wave. (Figure courtesy of VIASYS Healthcare, Inc., Yorba Linda, CA.)

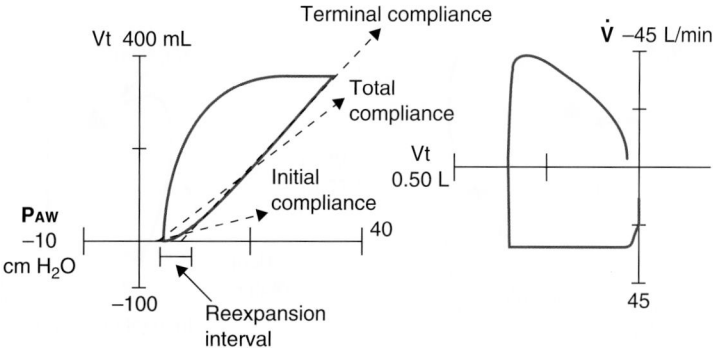

FIGURE 45.21. Pressure–volume and flow–volume loops for volume-limited ventilation during adult respiratory distress syndrome. (Figure courtesy of VIASYS Healthcare, Inc., Yorba Linda, CA.)

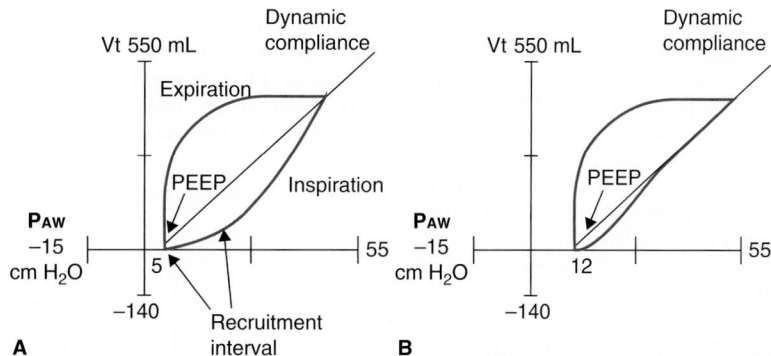

FIGURE 45.22. Pressure–volume loops indicating the optimization of PEEP during adult respiratory distress syndrome. **A:** Compliance at PEEP +5 cm H_2O. **B:** Compliance at PEEP +12 cm H_2O. (Figure courtesy of VIASYS Healthcare, Inc., Yorba Linda, CA.)

phase of inspiration requires an elevation of airway pressure prior to delivering a significant volume of gas. Therefore, the initial phase of the inspiratory limb (re-expansion interval) is less sloped than the later phase of inspiration. Subsequently, the PIP may be increased. Increasing the set PEEP may maintain improved alveolar patency during the expiratory phase and, thus, minimize this re-expansion interval (**Fig. 45.22**).

The evaluation of inspiratory and expiratory flow patterns can provide important information as to the presence of increased inspiratory or expiratory resistance (**Fig. 45.23**). In patients with elevated resistance, the response of these

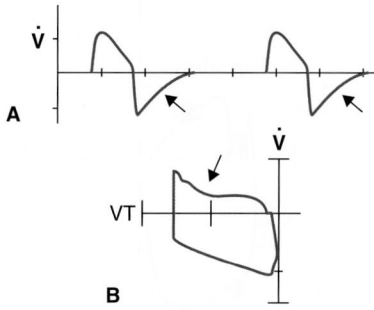

FIGURE 45.23. Increased expiratory resistance. **A:** Airway flow (V) is displayed over time. As noted by the arrows, exhalation is significantly prolonged, representing an increased expiratory resistance. **B:** Airway flow is graphed on the vertical axis and tidal volume (Vt) on the horizontal axis. The arrow again indicates that expiratory flow increases as the expiratory flow rate is greatly reduced early in exhalation.

abnormalities to various interventions, including suctioning, altering the inspiratory time, and/or bronchodilator therapy, can then be assessed.

Pressure–Volume and Flow–Volume Loops in Pressure-Limited Ventilation

The decelerating flow pattern of pressure-control ventilation results in a more rapid rise in airway pressure during the initial phase of inspiration, versus a traditional, volume-limited breath. The corresponding PV loop is demonstrated in **Figure 45.24**. During the initial phase of inspiration, the airway pressures are higher for a given Vt, and the PV loop demonstrates an initial "scooping." Although the initial airway pressures are higher for a given Vt, the Vt is delivered at a lower PIP, and dynamic compliance improves in this setting. This increase in dynamic compliance is demonstrated by the increased slope of the inspiratory loop (line connecting PEEP with PIP). The decelerating, variable inspiratory flow of pressure-control ventilation is higher than the fixed, constant flow of volume-limited ventilation. Thus, the peak inspiratory flow generated may better match the inspiratory demands of the patient.

Detection of Overdistension Using Pressure–Volume Loops

Pulmonary overdistension is defined as an abrupt decrease in compliance at the termination of a breath, demonstrated in the PV loop depicted in **Figure 45.25**. Overdistension occurs when the volume limit of some components of the lung is

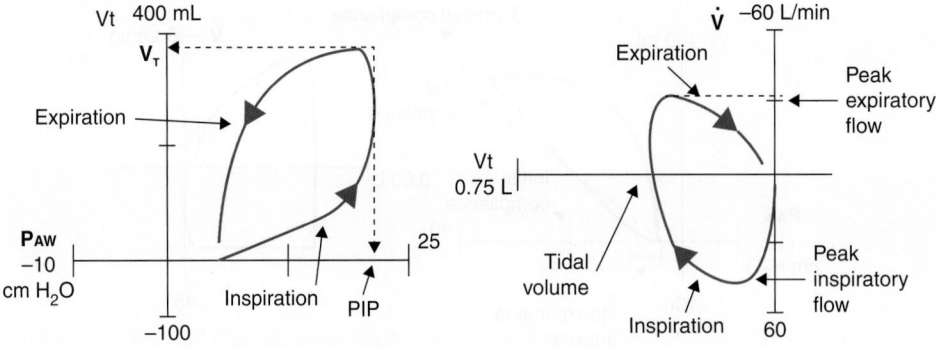

FIGURE 45.24. Normal pressure–volume and flow–volume loops for pressure-limited ventilation. Vt, tidal volume. (Figure courtesy of VIASYS Healthcare, Inc., Yorba Linda, CA.)

approached. As the ventilator attempts to provide gas to the patient, airway pressures increase, with little volume being delivered. Dynamic compliance is decreased, with the inspiratory loop having a reduced slope and terminal "beaking." Overdistension is clinically significant, as it can increase dead space, lead to volutrauma, and increase pulmonary vascular resistance. To eliminate overdistension, the set PIP or Vt should be decreased. Additionally, optimization of PEEP may be beneficial. Excessively high PEEP can lead to overdistension of the more compliant regions of lung. PEEP, therefore, should be titrated carefully, as outlined below.

Flow–Volume Loops Demonstrating Airway Obstruction

In **Figure 45.26A**, the delivered inspiratory flow is represented below the baseline as a decelerating wave. During early exhalation, near-complete obstruction to flow results in a high expiratory resistance. In **Figure 45.26B**, the airway obstruction is more severe, and both the inspiratory and expiratory phases are involved. In the inspiratory phase, the decelerating wave form is blunted and approaches a square wave, while in the expiratory phase, the peak flow is limited. Despite an increase in PIP, the Vt is reduced as a result of the severity of the obstruction. Both inspiratory resistance and expiratory resistance are elevated, indicating a fixed airway obstruction. Abnormalities of inspiratory and expiratory flow patterns can

provide important information as to the presence of airway obstruction and the response of the obstruction to various interventions. Flow abnormalities may be associated with a variety of conditions, including a kinked or blocked ETT, airway obstruction from anatomic causes, and bronchoconstriction.

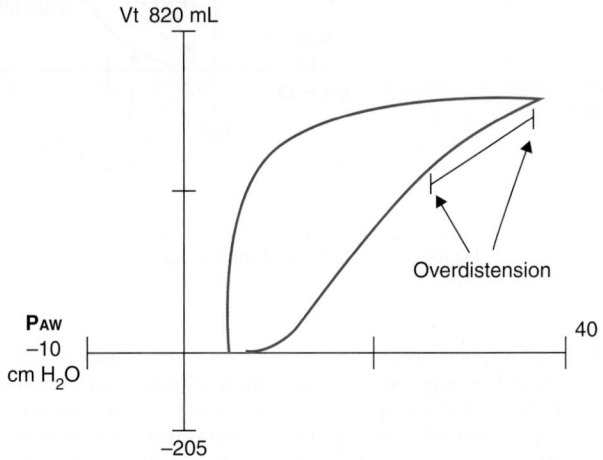

FIGURE 45.25. Pressure–volume loop demonstrating overdistension. (Figure courtesy of VIASYS Healthcare, Inc., Yorba Linda, CA.)

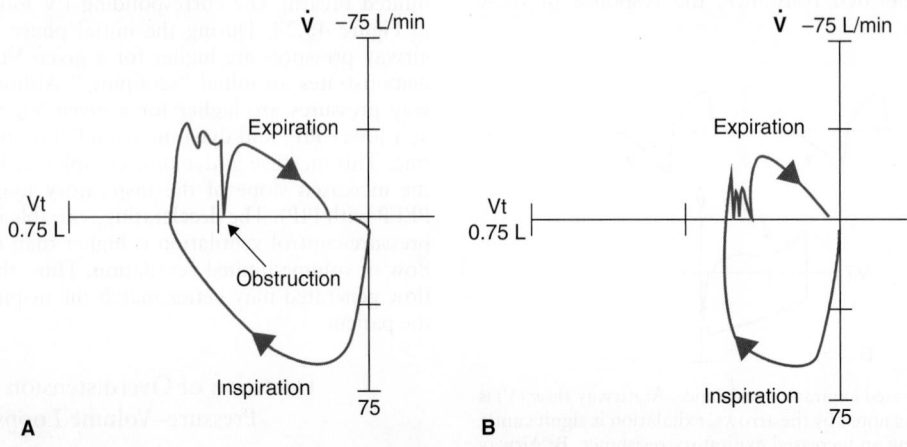

FIGURE 45.26. Flow–volume loops demonstrating airway obstruction. A: Mild airway obstruction, resulting in a high expiratory resistance. B: Severe airway obstruction that involves increased inspiratory and expiratory resistance. (Figure courtesy of VIASYS Healthcare, Inc., Yorba Linda, CA.)

Optimizing Positive End-Expiratory Pressure During Acute Respiratory Distress Syndrome

ARDS causes a loss of alveolar stability and the development of diffuse atelectasis. Alveolar collapse and a decreased end-expiratory lung volume may occur during the expiratory phase if the airway pressures are not adequate to maintain alveolar patency and an adequate opening volume. In **Figure 45.22A**, the PEEP is set at 5 cm H_2O, a setting that is inadequate to maintain alveolar patency and at which a significant amount of alveolar atelectasis and decreased lung volume occur during the expiratory phase. During the initial phase of inspiration, re-expansion of the collapsed alveoli is necessary, and the airway pressures increase before a volume of gas is delivered to the patient. Once the opening pressure is reached, the Vt is delivered.

The pressure cost of re-expansion is the amount of inspiratory airway pressure that is necessary to initiate the delivery of gas volume. The Vt can be delivered only after the critical opening pressure is reached. The development of a significant amount of alveolar atelectasis results in a high pressure cost of re-expansion, which elevates the opening pressure and the PIP that are required to deliver the same Vt.

Optimizing PEEP is an essential management strategy in patients with lung injury. By increasing the PEEP from 5 to 12 cm H_2O (**Fig. 45.22B**), a greater number of alveoli are maintained patent during the expiratory phase, and lung volume increases toward normal functional residual capacity. During the initial phase of inspiration, lower-airway pressures are required to achieve lung opening, and the pressure cost of re-expansion is less than in **Figure 45.22A**. As lung volume is restored toward functional residual capacity by optimizing PEEP, the PIP required to deliver the Vt may decrease over time. As a result, the lung is more compliant, and the Vt can be delivered with a smaller change in airway pressure. These effects may be more dramatic over time, as collapsed alveoli continue to be recruited. Additionally, the risk for ventilator-induced lung injury may decrease as PIP decreases.

Excessive levels of PEEP cause detrimental effects on cardiorespiratory function. These effects include (a) a reduction of venous return and cardiac output secondary to increased mean intrathoracic pressure and (b) overdistension of compliant lung units with redistribution of blood flow to the less-compliant lung units. To optimize PEEP using graphics, the level of PEEP is increased gradually until the best balance is achieved in the following variables: lowest PIP to deliver the desired Vt, highest compliance, and best O_2 delivery (requires a determination/estimate of cardiac output and a measurement of arterial oxygenation).

Dynamic Hyperexpansion/Intrinsic Positive End-expiratory Pressure

The square-wave, constant-flow pattern during inspiration is demonstrated in **Figure 45.27**, as in **Figure 45.18**. The respiratory rate and T_i have been increased, resulting in a dramatic increase in mean airway pressure. With inadequate time to complete exhalation before the next breath is initiated, dynamic hyperexpansion or "gas trapping" occurs. Dynamic hyperexpansion occurs with premature termination of exhalation. Prolongation of the T_i may be beneficial in certain clinical conditions (e.g., ARDS) by decreasing PIP and increasing mean airway pressure, which would be expected to improve oxygenation.

Dynamic hyperexpansion may result in $PEEP_i$, which elevates the baseline airway pressure (externally applied PEEP + $PEEP_i$). However, $PEEP_i$ is relatively uncontrolled compared to set PEEP, which can be more reliably titrated to achieve the desired oxygenation and ventilation endpoints. The increase in the baseline airway pressure secondary to $PEEP_i$ results in an increase in PIP that is required to maintain the set Vt during volume-limited ventilation or results in a decrease in Vt during pressure-limited ventilation (i.e., set total PIP).

The combination of an increased PIP and development of $PEEP_i$ will cause the mean airway pressure to rise. $PEEP_i$ may be desirable in the management of ARDS, as it results in improved oxygenation. However, careful monitoring of the amount of $PEEP_i$ is required to limit the development of secondary lung injury and hemodynamic compromise due to the increased mean intrathoracic pressure. While prolongation of the T_i may be beneficial, the resulting increase in intrathoracic pressure may compromise cardiac output by limiting venous return to the right side of the heart. Volume loading and/or the institution of inotropes may limit the adverse effects of dynamic hyperexpansion/$PEEP_i$ on cardiovascular performance.

Patient–Ventilator Asynchrony: Inaccurate Sensing of Patient Effort

Patient effort decreases airway pressure (arrows 1–3 in **Fig. 45.28**) and/or flow from baseline. Decreased airway pressure or flow (depending on the ventilator settings chosen)

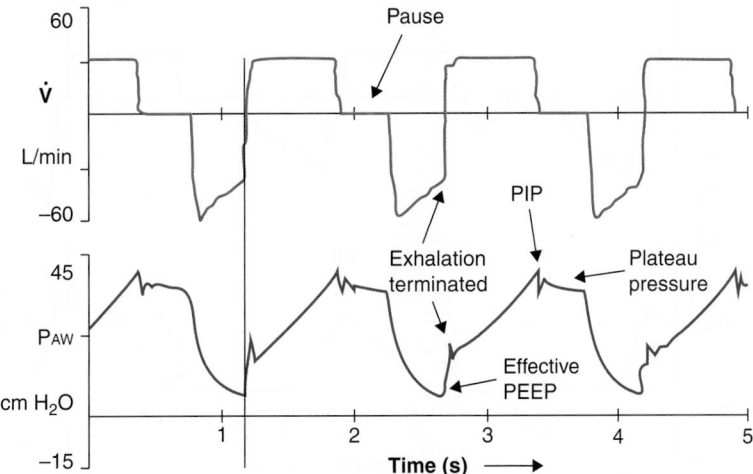

FIGURE 45.27. Scalar display of flow versus time and airway pressure versus time for volume-limited ventilation during adult respiratory distress syndrome. Premature termination of exhalation, which results in dynamic hyperexpansion (gas trapping), is shown. (Figure courtesy of VIASYS Healthcare, Inc., Yorba Linda, CA.)

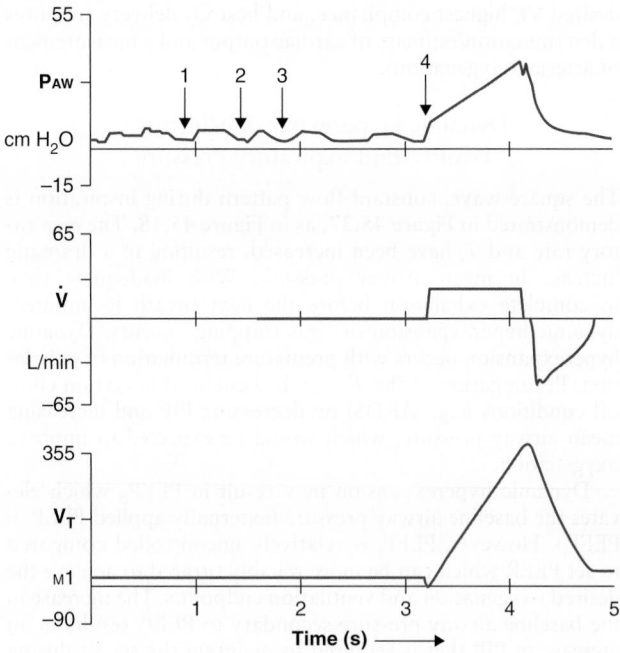

FIGURE 45.28. Scalar display of flow versus time, airway pressure versus time, and tidal volume versus time, representing patient–ventilator asynchrony to inadequate sensing of the patient effort. (Figure courtesy of VIASYS Healthcare, Inc., Yorba Linda, CA.)

Asynchrony may also occur when an air leak leads to the loss of PEEP, resulting in excessive ventilator triggering. This reduction in airway pressure or flow may be misinterpreted by the ventilator as a patient effort and result in a mechanical breath being triggered. This abnormality, commonly referred to as *autocycling*, may lead to frequent ventilator triggering without patient effort. In this case, the trigger sensitivity setting and/or the ETT air leak must be assessed.

Patient–Ventilator Asynchrony: Inadequate Ventilatory Support

Figure 45.29 reveals a patient effort that results in a decrease in airway pressure (arrows 1 and 2) and triggering of a mechanical breath. However, the constant inspiratory flow of the delivered mechanical breath is inadequate to meet the patient's inspiratory demands. The patient is not satiated by the constant inspiratory flow of the mechanical breath and, as a result, attempts to initiate a spontaneous breath during the mechanical breath (arrow 3), causing a transient reduction of airway pressure, which is signified by a decrease in the airway pressure tracing during inspiration (flow asynchrony). Inadequate ventilatory support to meet the patient's inspiratory needs leads to tachypnea, increased WOB, and patient discomfort ("fighting the ventilator").

In volume-limited ventilation, a reduction of the inspiratory airway pressure as a result of a patient effort (arrow 3) during the mechanical breath may result in an increase in peak inspiratory pressure (arrow 4) being required to achieve the set Vt. Increasing the flow rate during patient-assisted, volume-limited ventilation (i.e., constant, square-wave inspiratory flow) may eliminate flow asynchrony. The clinician should titrate the flow rate to reduce the drop in airway pressure (arrow 3) and return the airway pressure tracing to a more normal configuration. Additionally, decreasing the T_i or changing to another mode of ventilation with a variable, decelerating inspiratory flow is often beneficial. A variable flow mode may better meet the inspiratory demands of the patient. Such modes include pressure-support ventilation, pressure-assist/control ventilation, and pressure-regulated volume control. When increasing the flow rate or changing the inspiratory flow pattern is unsuccessful, inadequate ventilatory support should be considered as the cause of the patient–ventilator asynchrony.

should result in an assisted mechanical breath in supported ventilation modes. However, with inadequate trigger sensitivity, the ventilator is unable to determine that a patient effort has occurred (**Fig. 45.28**, patient breaths 1–3). During patient breath 4, the ventilator delivers the preset Vt at the preset rate without regard to patient effort. Inadequate sensing of patient effort leads to tachypnea, increased WOB, patient–ventilator asynchrony, and patient discomfort ("fighting the ventilator"). To ensure that the patient effort is not appropriately sensed, trigger sensitivity must be improved. Flow triggering is generally more sensitive than pressure triggering, as a small change in flow requires less inspiratory effort than a change in pressure.

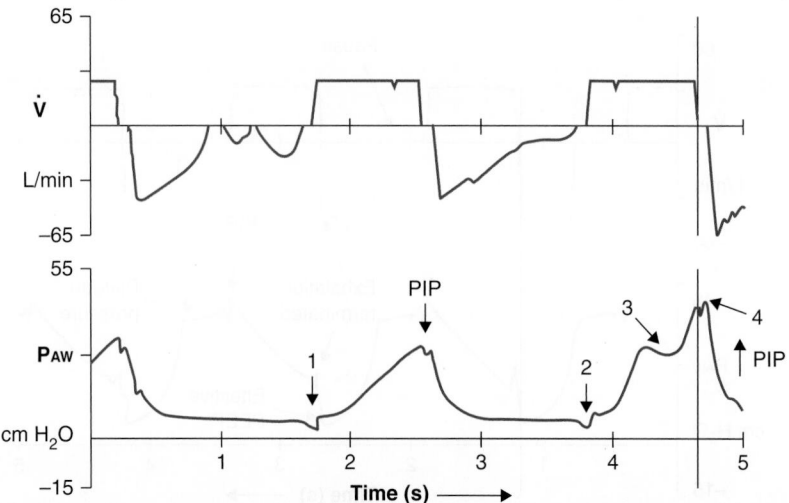

FIGURE 45.29. Scalar display of flow versus time and airway pressure versus time, representing patient–ventilator asynchrony secondary to inadequate ventilatory support. (Figure courtesy of VIASYS Healthcare, Inc., Yorba Linda, CA.)

Airway Graphics—Summary

With the many technical advances of current-day mechanical ventilators, multiple modes of ventilation and parameters must be set and monitored by the clinician. The use of airway graphics and continuous capnography provide invaluable tools to help design the most appropriate strategy for each child and to assess the efficacy of these management strategies (50). Airway graphics provide rapid assessment of the various respiratory parameters, help to generate and test hypotheses of patient management, and monitor for the presence of adverse effects of mechanical ventilation.

Esophageal and Gastric Manometry

Esophageal and gastric manometries are invasive methods by which to assess pressures generated during breathing. Esophageal manometry requires placement of an air-filled balloon attached to a catheter or a fluid-filled catheter in the lower third of the esophagus. In adults, polyethylene catheters with an internal diameter of 1.4 mm and a length of ~100 cm are commonly used. In children, fluid-filled catheters may be preferable, as their frequency response is high due to the noncompressibility of the fluid column in the catheter. The distal end of both systems should have multiple holes. Fluid-filled catheters must be constantly flushed to keep the catheter free of gas bubbles. Ideally, the tip of the catheter should be placed at the junction of the middle and lower third of the esophagus. To validate the position and measurement in spontaneously breathing patients, a dynamic occlusion test is employed. This requires breathing through an occluded airway, similar to the measurement for P_{Imax}. The change in proximal airway pressure should be the same as the change in the esophageal pressure. To validate the measurements in paralyzed patients, external pressure using a cuirass or a body plethysmograph can be used.

Constraints in measuring esophageal pressure include distortion of the esophagus, esophageal contraction, uneven distribution of pleural pressures, and displacement of the catheter tip. When combined with measurement of flow and volume at the airway, esophageal manometry can be used to measure WOB, as described later. It has been shown that esophageal pressure monitoring complements extubation readiness testing when patients are being weaned from mechanical ventilation (53).

Measurements of Diaphragmatic Function

Transdiaphragmatic Pressure

Transdiaphragmatic pressure (P_{di}) is defined as the difference between intrathoracic and abdominal pressures. It is usually calculated as the difference between P_{es} and gastric pressure (P_{ga}). Measurement of P_{di} is useful in the diagnosis of diaphragmatic strength, weakness, and fatigability, although few studies have been conducted in critically ill children.

Diaphragmatic Ultrasonography and Fluoroscopy

Diaphragmatic ultrasonography and fluoroscopy can be useful tools in detecting and diagnosing diaphragmatic paresis and paralysis. Diaphragmatic paresis and paralysis can occur from injury to the phrenic nerve or diaphragmatic muscle weakness. Diaphragmatic paresis is diagnosed by the reduction in diaphragm excursion during spontaneous breathing. Unilateral diaphragmatic paralysis can result in paradoxic movement of the diaphragm, when during inspiration, the normal diaphragm moves downward and the paralyzed diaphragm moves upward. It is important that testing be performed without positive pressure applied to the airway.

Measures of Inspiratory Drive

The pressure generated after the onset of inspiratory effort against an occluded airway in the first 100 milliseconds ($P_{0.1}$) provides a measure of respiratory drive. In adults, $P_{0.1}$ can be used to predict weaning outcome. For extubated children, $P_{0.1}$ can be measured by placing a tight-fitting mask over the face and attaching a one-way valve that allows exhalation but not inspiration. When the valve is activated, the patient makes an inspiratory effort against an occluded airway and the pressure can be recorded through a side port in the system. In children who are mechanically ventilated, $P_{0.1}$ can be measured using either a one-way valve attached to the ETT, similar to that used to measure P_{Imax}, and the pressure can be recorded through a side port. Alternatively, with ventilators that allow an expiratory hold maneuver, holding the expiratory "pause/hold" button causes the inspiratory valve to remain closed at expiration. When the patient initiates a spontaneous breath, the inspiratory effort occurs with the airway occluded, and the pressure generated can be recorded to measure $P_{0.1}$. It is important that there be no leak in the system. This maneuver cannot be performed with an uncuffed ETT.

Factors that influence the measurement of $P_{0.1}$ include chest-wall distortion (a problem in young children with compliant chest walls), alteration in expiratory lung volume, time constant of the respiratory system, expiratory muscle activity (such as in lower-airway obstruction), shape of the driving pressure wave, and pressure–flow phase lags.

An easier index to measure is the mean inspiratory flow (derived by dividing the Vt by the T_i), which can be determined in intubated patients by measuring spontaneous Vt and T_i using a pneumotachometer attached to the ETT without applying positive pressure to the airway. It can also be measured using respiratory inductive plethysmography, as previously described.

CONCLUSIONS AND FUTURE DIRECTIONS

As deterioration in respiratory status, including the need for mechanical ventilation, is the most common indication for admission to the PICU, monitoring of the respiratory system is of utmost importance to the pediatric intensivist. Respiratory monitoring is crucial to the optimal management of a critically ill child to aid with diagnosis, augment understanding of the pathophysiology, assess status and progress of a disease, and provide data for management. Methods of monitoring the respiratory system have improved immensely in recent years. While physical examination continues to have significant clinical relevance, the incorporation of all aspects of cardiorespiratory monitoring into a comprehensive, responsive assessment system is essential to the management of critically ill children.

The future of respiratory monitoring will clearly include continued hardware and software advances. More importantly, the future will likely bring an improved assessment of the available data, including smart prompts to help guide complex clinical decisions and closed feedback loops, in which the monitored data will be incorporated into management devices (i.e., ventilators) to affect routine patient care without the direct intervention of a clinician.

References

1. Wallach PM, Roscoe L, Bowden R. The profession of medicine: An integrated approach to basic principles. *Acad Med* 2002;77:1168–9.
2. Anonymous. VIII ESPID Conference (European Society for the Study and Prevention of Infant Death), the International Conference

on Prevention of Infantile Apnea and Sudden Infant Death on the Verge of the Millennium. *Pediatr Res* 1999;45:1A–52A.

3. Dueck MH, Klimek M, Appenrodt S, et al. Trends but not individual values of central venous oxygen saturation agree with mixed venous oxygen saturation during varying hemodynamic conditions. *Anesthesiology* 2005;103:249–57.

4. van Beest PA, van Ingen J, Boerma EC, et al. No agreement of mixed venous and central venous saturation in sepsis, independent of sepsis origin. *Crit Care* 2010;14:R219.

5. Varpula M, Karlsson S, Ruokonen E, et al. Mixed venous oxygen saturation cannot be estimated by central venous oxygen saturation in septic shock. *Intensive Care Med* 2006;32:1336–43.

6. de Oliveira CF, de Oliveira DS, Gottschald AF, et al. ACCM/PALS haemodynamic support guidelines for paediatric septic shock: An outcomes comparison with and without monitoring central venous oxygen saturation. *Intensive Care Med* 2008;34:1065–75.

7. Santschi M, Leclerc F. Management of children with sepsis and septic shock: A survey among pediatric intensivists of the Reseau Mere-Enfant de la Francophonie. *Ann Intensive Care* 2013;3:7.

8. Carter BG, Wiwczaruk D, Hochmann M, et al. Performance of transcutaneous PCO2 and pulse oximetry monitors in newborns and infants after cardiac surgery. *Anaesth Intensive Care* 2001;29:260–5.

9. Lee WW, Mayberry K, Crapo R, et al. The accuracy of pulse oximetry in the emergency department. *Am J Emerg Med* 2000;18:427–31.

10. Wouters PF, Gehring H, Meyfroidt G, et al. Accuracy of pulse oximeters: The European multi-center trial. *Anesth Analg* 2002;94:13–6.

11. Barker SJ. "Motion-resistant" pulse oximetry: a comparison of new and old models. *Anesth Analg* 2002;95:967–72. Table of contents.

12. Bohnhorst B, Peter CS, Poets CF. Detection of hyperoxaemia in neonates: Data from three new pulse oximeters. *Arch Dis Child Fetal Neonatal Ed* 2002;87:217–9.

13. Jopling MW, Mannheimer PD, Bebout DE. Issues in the laboratory evaluation of pulse oximeter performance. *Anesth Analg* 2002;94:62–68.

14. Durbin CG Jr, Rostow SK. More reliable oximetry reduces the frequency of arterial blood gas analyses and hastens oxygen weaning after cardiac surgery: A prospective, randomized trial of the clinical impact of a new technology. *Crit Care Med* 2002;30:1735–40.

15. Bohnhorst B, Peter CS, Poets CF. Pulse oximeters' reliability in detecting hypoxemia and bradycardia: comparison between a conventional and two new generation oximeters. *Crit Care Med* 2000;28:1565–8.

16. Aoyagi T, Miyasaka K. Pulse oximetry: its invention, contribution to medicine, and future tasks. *Anesth Analg* 2002;94:S1–3.

17. Jubran A. Pulse oximetry. *Intensive Care Med* 2004;30:2017–20.

18. Ochroch EA, Russell MW, Hanson WC, et al. The impact of continuous pulse oximetry monitoring on intensive care unit admissions from a postsurgical care floor. *Anesth Analg* 2006;102:868–75.

19. Poets CF, Urschitz MS, Bohnhorst B. Pulse oximetry in the neonatal intensive care unit (NICU): Detection of hyperoxemia and false alarm rates. *Anesth Analg* 2002;94:41–3.

20. Cullen DJ, Nemeskal AR, Cooper JB, et al. Effect of pulse oximetry, age, and ASA physical status on the frequency of patients admitted unexpectedly to a postoperative intensive care unit and the severity of their anesthesia-related complications. *Anesth Analg* 1992;74:181–8.

21. Moller JT, Johannessen NW, Espersen K, et al. Randomized evaluation of pulse oximetry in 20,802 patients: II. Perioperative events and postoperative complications. *Anesthesiology* 1993;78:445–53.

22. Khemani RG, Thomas NJ, Venkatachalam V, et al. Comparison of SpO2 to PaO2 based markers of lung disease severity for children with acute lung injury. *Crit Care Med* 2012;40:1309–16.

23. Rice TW, Wheeler AP, Bernard GR, et al. Comparison of the SpO2/FIO2 ratio and the PaO2/FIO2 ratio in patients with acute lung injury or ARDS. *Chest* 2007;132:410–7.

24. Thomas NJ, Shaffer ML, Willson DF, et al. Defining acute lung disease in children with the oxygenation saturation index. *Pediatr Crit Care Med* 2010;11:12–7.

25. He HW, Liu DW, Long Y, et al. The peripheral perfusion index and transcutaneous oxygen challenge test are predictive of mortality in septic patients after resuscitation. *Crit Care* 2013;17:R116.

26. He HW, Liu DW, Long Y, et al. The transcutaneous oxygen challenge test: A noninvasive method for detecting low cardiac output in septic patients. *Shock* 2012;37:152–5.

27. Berkenbosch JW, Lam J, Burd RS, et al. Noninvasive monitoring of carbon dioxide during mechanical ventilation in older children: End-tidal versus transcutaneous techniques. *Anesth Analg* 2001;92:1427–31.

28. Berkenbosch JW, Tobias JD. Transcutaneous carbon dioxide monitoring during high-frequency oscillatory ventilation in infants and children. *Crit Care Med* 2002;30:1024–7.

29. Tatevossian RG, Wo CC, Velmahos GC, et al. Transcutaneous oxygen and CO2 as early warning of tissue hypoxia and hemodynamic shock in critically ill emergency patients. *Crit Care Med* 2000;28:2248–53.

30. Tobias JD. Transcutaneous carbon dioxide monitoring in infants and children. *Paediatr Anaesth* 2009;19:434–44.

31. Knapp S, Kofler J, Stoiser B, et al. The assessment of four different methods to verify tracheal tube placement in the critical care setting. *Anesth Analg* 1999;88:766–70.

32. Nishisaki A, Turner DA, Brown CA III, et al. A National Emergency Airway Registry for children: Landscape of tracheal intubation in 15 PICUs. *Crit Care Med* 2013;41:874–85.

33. Li J. Capnography alone is imperfect for endotracheal tube placement confirmation during emergency intubation. *J Emerg Med* 2001;20:223–9.

34. Heradstveit BE, Sunde K, Sunde GA, et al. Factors complicating interpretation of capnography during advanced life support in cardiac arrest—A clinical retrospective study in 575 patients. *Resuscitation* 2012;83:813–8.

35. Johnson JL, Breen PH. How does positive end-expiratory pressure decrease pulmonary CO2 elimination in anesthetized patients? *Respir Physiol* 1999;118:227–36.

36. Hatzakis GE, Davis GM. Fuzzy logic controller for weaning neonates from mechanical ventilation. *Proc AMIA Symp* 2002;315–9.

37. Soo Hoo GW, Park L. Variations in the measurement of weaning parameters: A survey of respiratory therapists. *Chest* 2002;121:1947–55.

38. Manthous CA. The anarchy of weaning techniques. *Chest* 2002;121:1738–40.

39. Hubble CL, Gentile MA, Tripp DS, et al. Deadspace to tidal volume ratio predicts successful extubation in infants and children. *Crit Care Med* 2000;28:2034–40.

40. Riou Y, Chaari W, Leteurtre S, et al. Predictive value of the physiological deadspace/tidal volume ratio in the weaning process of mechanical ventilation in children. *J Pediatr (Rio J)* 2012;88:217–21.

41. Willis BC, Graham AS, Wetzel R, et al. Respiratory inductance plethysmography used to diagnose bilateral diaphragmatic paralysis: A case report. *Pediatr Crit Care Med* 2004;5:399–402.

42. Venkataraman ST, Khan N, Brown A. *Validation of predictors of extubation success and failure in mechanically ventilated infants and children.* *Crit Care Med* 2000;28:2991–6.

43. Dimitriou G, Greenough A, Rafferty GF, et al. Effect of maturity on maximal transdiaphragmatic pressure in infants during crying. *Am J Respir Crit Care Med* 2001;164:433–6.

44. Koechlin C, Matecki S, Jaber S, et al. Changes in respiratory muscle endurance during puberty. *Pediatr Pulmonol* 2005;40:197–204.

45. Matecki S, Prioux J, Jaber S, et al. Respiratory pressures in boys from 11–17 years old: A semilongitudinal study. *Pediatr Pulmonol* 2003;35:368–74.

46. Farias JA, Alia I, Retta A, et al. An evaluation of extubation failure predictors in mechanically ventilated infants and children. *Intensive Care Med* 2002;28:752–7.

47. Cannon ML, Cornell J, Tripp-Hamel DS, et al. Tidal volumes for ventilated infants should be determined with a pneumotachometer placed at the endotracheal tube. *Am J Respir Crit Care Med* 2000;162:2109–12.

48. Castle RA, Dunne CJ, Mok Q, et al. Accuracy of displayed values of tidal volume in the pediatric intensive care unit. *Crit Care Med* 2002;30:2566–74.

49. Chow LC, Vanderhal A, Raber J, et al. Are tidal volume measurements in neonatal pressure-controlled ventilation accurate? *Pediatr Pulmonol* 2002;34:196–202.

50. Tobin MJ, Jubran A, Laghi F. Patient-ventilator interaction. *Am J Respir Crit Care Med* 2001;163:1059–63.

51. Hemmila MR, Napolitano LM. Severe respiratory failure: Advanced treatment options. *Crit Care Med* 2006;34:278–290.

52. Kocis KC, Dekeon MK, Rosen HK, et al. Pressure-regulated volume control vs volume control ventilation in infants after surgery for congenital heart disease. *Pediatr Cardiol* 2001;22:233–7.

53. Jubran A, Grant BJ, Laghi F, et al. Weaning prediction: Esophageal pressure monitoring complements readiness testing. *Am J Respir Crit Care Med* 2005;171:1252–9.

CHAPTER 46 ■ STATUS ASTHMATICUS

MICHAEL T. BIGHAM AND RICHARD J. BRILLI

Definition

1 Status asthmaticus (also called acute severe asthma) is a condition of progressively worsening bronchospasm and respiratory dysfunction caused by asthma that is unresponsive to standard conventional therapy and may progress to respiratory failure and the need for mechanical ventilation.

Epidemiology

2 Asthma is the most common chronic disease of childhood.

3 Asthma mortality is associated primarily with cardiorespiratory arrest prior to presentation to medical care.

Mechanism of Disease: Core Pathophysiology

4 Asthma is an inflammatory disease that is characterized by airflow obstruction due to airway hyperresponsiveness, bronchospasm, airway inflammation, mucosal edema, and mucous plugging.

5 Gas-exchange abnormalities in status asthmaticus are primarily due to V/Q mismatch, resulting from distal airway obstruction due to mucous plugging, edema, and bronchoconstriction.

Clinical Presentation and Differential Diagnosis

6 For patients who first present for evaluation of new-onset wheezing, four disparate clinical entities—asthma, pneumonia, foreign-body aspiration, and congestive heart failure—must be distinguished, because each of these requires different diagnostic and therapeutic approaches.

7 Clinical interventions for spontaneously breathing children with status asthmaticus should be based primarily upon physical examination findings and not blood gas determinations.

8 The overriding physiologic derangement in asthma is airway inflammation, and corticosteroids are a mainstay in the management of both acute and chronic asthma. Sympathomimetic β-agonists cause direct bronchial smooth muscle relaxation and are key components in asthma therapy.

9 IV and subcutaneous administration of β-agonists are most beneficial for patients with severe status asthmaticus and limited respiratory airflow, in whom distribution of inhaled medications may be significantly reduced.

10 In status asthmaticus, tracheal intubation is indicated for patients with post-cardiorespiratory arrest, those with refractory hypoxemia, or those with significant respiratory acidosis unresponsive to pharmacotherapy.

11 When maximal medical therapy is failing, extracorporeal membrane oxygenation (ECMO) should be considered. The survival for patients with refractory status asthmaticus who are placed on ECMO is ~90%.

Asthma is the most common chronic disease of childhood and accounts for nearly 155,000 pediatric hospitalizations each year (1). Although the prevalence of asthma has reached a plateau, asthma-related mortality remains high. Consequently, national organizations continue to update guidelines that describe optimal treatment for this common childhood illness (2). A description of the pathophysiology, clinical presentation, and current treatment for children hospitalized in the PICU with status asthmaticus is the focus of this chapter.

DEFINITION

The word "asthma" is derived from the Greek verb "aazein," meaning to exhale with open mouth, to pant. The first recorded use of this word was 2700 years ago in Homer's *Iliad*, where it was used to describe hard breathing or the short-drawn breaths of a warrior who died after a furious battle.

Asthma was first used in a clinical context by Hippocrates (circa 460–360 BC) in describing respiratory findings, such as dyspnea, tachypnea, and orthopnea. The best clinical description of asthma in antiquity was by the Greek physician Areteus, ~500 years after Hippocrates. He devoted an entire chapter to detailed descriptions of asthma, suggesting that the cause of asthma was "a coldness and humidity of pneuma but the result was a thick viscid humor." Today, discussion does not include pneuma or viscid humor; rather, asthma is defined as "a chronic inflammatory disorder causing recurrent episodes of wheezing, breathlessness, chest tightness, (and) coughing associated with airflow obstruction that is often reversible" **1** (2). Status asthmaticus, also known as acute severe asthma, is a condition of progressively worsening bronchospasm and respiratory dysfunction due to asthma, which is unresponsive to standard conventional therapy and may progress to respiratory failure and the need for mechanical ventilation (3). For this review, status asthmaticus is defined as acute severe asthma that fails to respond to inhaled β-agonists, oral or IV steroids, and O_2, and that requires admission to the hospital for treatment.

EPIDEMIOLOGY

Worldwide, an estimated 300 million people suffer from asthma (4). In children, the prevalence of asthma varies significantly by country, with the highest rates in the United Kingdom, Australia, and New Zealand, and the lowest in Eastern Europe, China, and Indonesia. In the United States, asthma affects 9.1% (6.5 million) of children <18 years of age and is the leading cause of chronic illness in children (1). The economic burden of asthma is substantial, with ~10 million missed school days and $726 million (US dollars) lost because of missed work. Asthma accounts for 470,000 (adults and children) annual hospital admissions across the United States and is the leading cause of hospital admission for children <18 years of age (5). It is estimated that 13%–55% of all dollars spent on asthma care are hospital related, and status asthmaticus remains a leading cause of PICU admission (6).

Asthma-related death rates in American children nearly doubled between 1980 and 1995, but recently have stabilized or even decreased, though some of the apparent decrease after 1999 may reflect changes to the International Classification of Diseases between the ninth and tenth editions (7). The number of asthma deaths in all age groups in the United States is ~5000 per year, with 150–200 of those occurring in children <18 years of age (1). In a clinical review of ventilated asthmatics from eight different tertiary PICUs, mortality was 4% (8). Most of the deaths were associated with cardiac arrest prior to PICU admission (8). These data support prevailing experience that most asthma-related deaths in children occur as a result of respiratory failure or cardiopulmonary arrest that occurs prior to obtaining medical care. Models that seek to predict fatal asthma focus on identifying clinical, psychosocial, and ethnic risk factors (9). Clinical risks include a past history of ICU admission, respiratory failure, or rapid, sudden, severe deterioration. Psychosocial and ethnic risk factors include poor compliance with outpatient medical treatment, failure to perceive the severity of asthma attack, inner-city residence, denial of disease severity, and nonwhite race. African American children are four to six times more likely to die of asthma than are white children. Despite the aforementioned risk factors, nearly half of fatal asthma exacerbations occur in children with mild asthma. Some suggest that these deaths occur in a subpopulation of patients with decreased sensitivity to dyspnea or another group with "sudden asphyxial asthma" (10). This latter entity is characterized by rapid, sudden, severe airway obstruction that progresses to hypoxemic respiratory arrest over a short period, usually before presentation to medical care.

MECHANISM OF DISEASE: CORE PATHOPHYSIOLOGY

Genetics

No single asthma gene has been identified. It is likely that the disease is both polygenetic and environmentally influenced. More than 20 chromosomal regions have been linked to asthma. The most consistently linked regions have been on chromosomes 2q, 5q, 6p, 12q, and 13q (11). It is known that asthma inheritance is likely related to the inheritance of atopy. Studies in twins with asthma reveal significant genetic similarities but not identical phenotypic manifestations of

asthma. This variation in disease severity may occur because airway hyperresponsiveness may be genetically distinct from atopy and is further confounded by gene–gene and gene–environmental interactions. The gene polymorphisms of the β_2-adrenergic receptors at the amino acid positions 16 and 27 have been examined in depth in an effort to clarify the phenotypic variability of airway hyperresponsiveness. In a meta-analysis of pediatric asthmatic ADRB2 gene polymorphisms, the Arg16Arg was associated with favorable clinical response to β_2-adrenergic agonist therapy compared with Arg16Gly or Gly16Gly. No association was found between amino acid position 27 and clinical response in the same meta-analysis (12). In another study, critically ill pediatric patients with asthma who had improved β_2-adrenergic response and decreased ICU length of stay (LOS) were associated with Gly16Gly and Gln27Glu or Glu27Glu polymorphisms (13). The clinical application of specific genetic profiles for both asthma prevention and treatment remains uncertain.

Inflammation and Immunobiology

Asthma is an inflammatory disease characterized by airflow obstruction due to airway hyperresponsiveness, bronchospasm, and airway inflammation with mucosal edema and mucous plugging of the small airways. Airway inflammation is characterized by the submucosal cellular infiltrate of eosinophils, mast cells, and CD4 lymphocytes. The presence of these cells correlates with disease severity and is mediated by cytokines, chemokines, growth factors, lipid mediators, immunoglobulins, and histamine (14). The cascade of inflammation begins with degranulation of mast cells, usually in response to allergen exposure. Activated mast cells release histamine and leukotrienes, both activators of early airway smooth muscle spasm. The activated mast cells further activate T-lymphocytes, which produce inflammatory cytokines (TH2) and IL-4, -5, and -13 (15). In addition, chemokines (leukotriene B4) are released, which attract neutrophils and promote further activation of the proinflammatory cascade. Submucosal infiltration by eosinophils, neutrophils, and activated lymphocytes is responsible for late or delayed bronchospasm. The differentiation between "early" and "delayed" bronchospasm is important because early bronchospasm may be more sensitive to bronchodilating agents, whereas late bronchospasm is refractory to bronchodilation and more sensitive to antiinflammatory therapy. This inflammatory environment results in overproduction of mucus; injury to airway epithelium that exposes nerve endings, which augments airway irritability; hyperresponsiveness; and mucosal edema. The final common pathway for the inflammatory cascade is bronchoconstriction and mechanical airway obstruction by edema and mucus.

The autonomic nervous system also contributes to bronchoconstriction through parasympathetic activation of M_3 receptors by acetylcholine and excitatory nonadrenergic, noncholinergic pathways mediated by tachykinins. Similar parasympathetic pathways stimulate mucous production and concomitant airway obstruction.

Pulmonary Mechanics and Gas-Exchange Abnormalities

Pulmonary mechanical dysfunction occurs as a result of pathologic changes in bronchial smooth muscle contraction, mucosal edema, and increased mucous production, which cause decreased airway diameter and increased airflow resistance. During inspiration, negative pleural pressure causes physiologic intrathoracic airway dilation; however, during

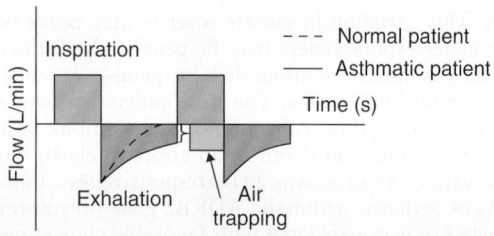

FIGURE 46.1. Flow–time waveform showing persistence of airflow at end expiration and resultant air trapping.

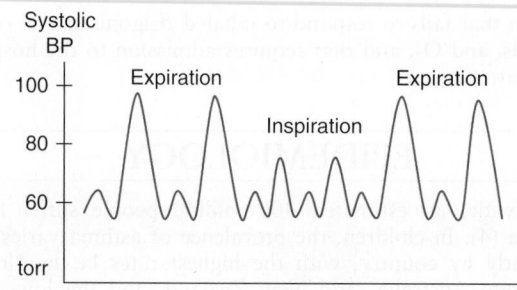

FIGURE 46.2. Pulsus paradoxus in status asthmaticus.

expiration, pleural pressure approaches zero, causing physiologic intrathoracic airway narrowing. In status asthmaticus, with pathologically narrowed and obstructed airways, these physiologic differences in airway diameter result in easier air entry during inspiration but airflow obstruction during expiration, causing air trapping with each breath and lung hyperinflation (**Fig. 46.1**). With higher end-expiratory lung volumes, coupled with bronchospasm leading to increased airway resistance and reduced expiratory flow, expiration becomes an active rather than a passive process, which results in high energy expenditure and increased work of breathing (WOB). Diaphragmatic flattening from hyperinflation causes additional mechanical disadvantages for the muscles of expiration and additional energy expenditure. Both forced expiratory volume and forced vital capacity are decreased in status asthmaticus as a result of high airway resistance. Total lung volumes are increased because of increased functional residual capacity.

5 Gas-exchange abnormalities in status asthmaticus are due to ventilation–perfusion (V/Q) mismatch, including increased intrapulmonary shunt (atelectasis) and increased dead space (airway overdistension) that result from small-airway obstruction due to mucous plugging, edema, and bronchoconstriction. Typically, these gas-exchange abnormalities initially manifest as hypoxemia and hypocarbia. Atelectasis from small-airway obstruction causes areas of decreased ventilation but adequate pulmonary blood flow, and the resultant shunt leads to arterial hypoxemia. As disease severity worsens, greater distal airway obstruction causes alveolar distension and increased pulmonary dead space. To compensate for this worsening V/Q mismatch, tachypnea occurs. Despite increasing dead space-to-tidal volume ratio (VDS/VT), hypocarbia persists because minute ventilation increases. Finally, intercostal and diaphragmatic muscles fatigue. Increased minute ventilation is unable to compensate for the greatly increased VDS/VT ratio and hypercarbia results. As fatigue worsens, progressive hypoxemia and hypercarbia ensue and result in respiratory failure.

Cardiopulmonary Interactions in Asthma

Dynamic hyperinflation in severe asthma can have significant cardiopulmonary consequences. First, high lung volumes stretch the pulmonary vasculature, increasing pulmonary vascular resistance and increasing right ventricular afterload, which compromises right ventricular function. In addition, fluctuations in pleural pressures produce significant effects on the intrathoracic vessels and right atrial venous return. During the large, negative intrathoracic pressure observed during inspiration, left ventricular afterload is increased and systolic blood pressure is decreased. Exaggerated variation in systolic blood pressure associated with intrathoracic pressure variation during inspiration is termed *pulsus paradoxus* (16) (**Fig. 46.2**). Inspiratory systolic blood pressure decreases of >10–15 torr are associated with declining respiratory function in children with status asthmaticus (16).

CLINICAL PRESENTATION AND DIFFERENTIAL DIAGNOSIS

Differential Diagnosis

Children with moderate-to-severe status asthmaticus have varying degrees of respiratory distress and gas-exchange abnormalities. Wheezing is the clinical hallmark of asthma; however, it is critical to consider the broad differential of the wheezing child prior to embarking on a diagnostic and therapeutic course to treat status asthmaticus. The differential diagnosis of wheezing is large, but the possibilities can be grouped into diagnoses that require differentiation at the time of first evaluation and those that may allow a more deliberative evaluation. Four disparate clinical entities must be distinguished when the patient is first evaluated because each of these entities results in different diagnostic and therapeutic approaches. These entities are asthma, pneumonia, foreign-body aspiration, and congestive heart failure (**Fig. 46.3**).

Other diagnostic considerations in the differential diagnosis of wheezing can be divided into upper and lower airway diseases. These clinical entities are more likely to present with

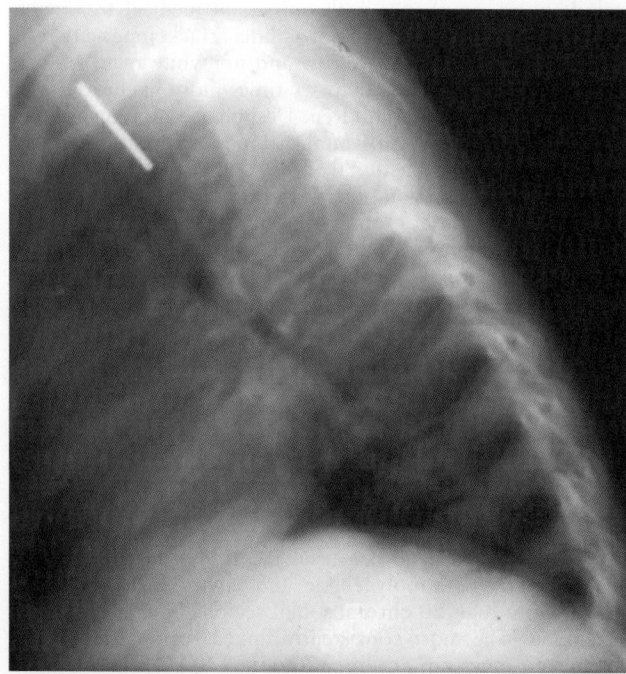

FIGURE 46.3. Chest radiograph of patient who presented with diffuse wheezing, revealing a coin in the esophagus.

chronic or recurrent symptoms, and, as such, a more contemplative evaluation may be appropriate. Upper airway obstruction, while usually presenting with stridor, can also present with wheezing. Diagnostic considerations include fixed anatomic lesions, such as vocal cord paralysis, anatomic webs, and airway hemangiomas, or dynamic airway obstruction, such as laryngomalacia, tracheomalacia, or bronchomalacia. Congenital anomalies, such as complete tracheal rings and bronchial slings, may also present with wheezing. Lower airway diseases that should be considered in addition to infection and congestive heart failure include cystic fibrosis and α_1 antitrypsin deficiency.

History

Children with status asthmaticus typically present with respiratory distress, cough, and wheezing that has progressed over 1–2 days. Allergen exposure and upper respiratory tract infection are often triggers for the onset of illness and are frequently identified by the child or family as inciting events. In contrast, foreign-body aspiration will usually present with an abrupt onset of clinical symptoms. Assessing the time course of a wheezing episode is important to help distinguish diagnostic considerations and to determine the urgency of required therapeutic interventions. The presence of fever suggests lower respiratory infection, though asthma and pneumonia can occur together. When time permits, it is important to determine the presence of high-risk factors for asthma severity and fatality, including previous severe sudden deterioration, past PICU admissions, and previous respiratory failure with the need for mechanical ventilation.

Physical Exam

The rapid assessment of a child with status asthmaticus should focus on determining the severity of airway obstruction. The "rapid 30-second cardiopulmonary assessment," as described by the American Heart Association, focuses on quick determination of general appearance, airway patency, effectiveness of respiratory effort, and adequacy of circulation (17). Children with severe status asthmaticus often appear lethargic and diaphoretic, are unable to phonate, and have severe retractions with paradoxical thoracoabdominal breathing. Poor air movement found on chest auscultation is an ominous sign of impending respiratory or cardiopulmonary failure.

Wheezing, which reflects turbulent airflow in obstructed airways, is usually equally audible on both hemithoraces. Asymmetric wheezing may imply unilateral atelectasis, pneumothorax, or foreign body. Expiratory wheezing alone is found in mild-to-moderate illness, whereas expiratory plus inspiratory wheezing is present in moderate-to-severe status asthmaticus. The "silent chest" is an ominous sign and may indicate either pneumothorax or the complete absence of

airflow due to severe airway obstruction and imminent respiratory failure. Hypoxemia, as estimated by measured pulse oximetry, is another sign of asthma severity. Several clinical asthma scores have been used to objectively assess the severity of status asthmaticus. The Becker asthma score (Table 46.1), modified by DiGiulio, determines severity by rating the acuity of four clinical characteristics—respiratory rate, wheezing, inspiratory:expiratory ratio, and accessory muscle use—and has the advantage of not requiring a PaO_2 measurement, which is used in the Wood/Downes score (18). A Becker score >4 is considered moderate status asthmaticus and has been used as entry criteria for several inpatient asthma treatment trials. Children with scores ≥7 should be admitted to the ICU. While such scores are valuable in clinical studies, they are not effective in predicting progression of clinical illness. Serial measurements allow an objective determination of disease progression, though significant interobserver variability is often associated with assigning clinical scores, which limits the usefulness of scoring systems in the active clinical environment.

Pulmonary Function Test and Exhaled Nitric Oxide

The fraction of exhaled nitric oxide (FeNO) is a noninvasive marker of acute eosinophilic airway inflammation and has been investigated as a tool in the diagnosis and management of childhood asthma (19). The pediatric data describing the use of FeNO to predict acute asthma exacerbations or to tailor inhaled corticosteroid therapy do not yet show convincing therapeutic value. Further, FeNO monitoring during acute asthma exacerbation in adults does not predict therapeutic response. At present, FeNO remains investigational and has no clinical role in the PICU patient with status asthmaticus.

Pulmonary function testing (PFT) is used to quantify the degree of airway obstruction primarily in the outpatient setting. The peak expiratory flow rate (PEFR) is an excellent measure of the degree of airway narrowing, and in children with severe asthma exacerbations can be less than 50% of normal values. PEFRs are currently recommended to monitor response to therapy although the role of PFTs or PEFRs in acute asthma exacerbation remains controversial (20). PEFR does not correlate with severity as measured by clinical asthma scoring systems, and as such has a limited role in the PICU (21).

Laboratory Evaluation

Laboratory tests commonly obtained in children with status asthmaticus include arterial or venous blood gas determination, complete blood count, and a basic metabolic panel. For spontaneously breathing children with status asthmaticus, clinical interventions should be primarily based upon the physical examination and not upon blood gas determinations.

TABLE 46.1

BECKER PULMONARY INDEX SCORE FOR ASTHMA

SCORE	RESPIRATORY RATE	WHEEZING	INSPIRATORY/ EXPIRATORY RATIO	ACCESSORY MUSCLE USE
0	<30	None	1:1.5	None
1	30–40	Terminal expiration	1:2.0	1 site
2	41–50	Entire expiration	1:3.0	2 sites
3	>50	Inspiration and entire expiration	>1:3.0	3 sites or neck strap muscle use

Typically, early in the course of severe asthma, arterial hypoxemia and hypocarbia are found as a result of V/Q mismatch and hyperventilation. As the air trapping worsens and V_{DS}/V_T increases, hypocarbia may be replaced by normal or elevated $PaCO_2$. Normal $PaCO_2$ in a tachypneic, hyperventilating child with status asthmaticus warrants close clinical observation and may be a sign of early respiratory muscle fatigue. Lactic acidosis is often present in status asthmaticus and usually reflects a combination of dehydration and excess lactate production from overuse of the respiratory musculature. Rarely, it can suggest poor perfusion from impaired cardiac function that is associated with the increased ventricular afterload caused by negative intrathoracic pressures (up to -60 to 100 cm H_2O). The presence of leukocytosis on complete blood count may suggest respiratory infection as the source of wheezing, though it can also represent a stress response to steroid administration or a response to β-agonist therapy. The white blood cell count in conjunction with chest x-ray and the presence or absence of fever will help determine the need for antibiotic therapy. A basic metabolic panel may be useful to assess the degree of dehydration and the level of electrolyte disturbance. Hypokalemia may result from intracellular potassium shifts from exposure to β-agonist therapy in children with status asthmaticus. Determining serum magnesium values may be important because the correction of relative hypomagnesemia in status asthmaticus may improve outcome.

Radiographic Evaluation

A chest x-ray may not be required at the time of hospital admission for all spontaneously breathing children with status asthmaticus; however, all children with first-time wheezing or patients who require PICU admission should receive a chest x-ray. Chest x-ray examination may reveal clinically relevant findings such as an infectious infiltrate, pneumothorax, cardiomegaly, pulmonary edema, or even unsuspected chest masses. For clinicians choosing not to obtain a chest x-ray at the time of hospital admission, a careful and meticulous examination looking specifically for signs and symptoms of occult pneumothorax, congestive heart failure, and foreign body is essential to prevent missing important clinical diagnoses other than asthma.

CLINICAL MANAGEMENT

Emergency Management in Anticipation of PICU Admission

Most children with asthma who are seen in the emergency department do not require hospital admission. Others with mild-to-moderate status asthmaticus require inpatient care and are usually treated with O_2, inhaled bronchodilators, and systemic corticosteroids. A small percentage of children require PICU admission. Clinical parameters that suggest the need for PICU admission are ill defined; however, children with past PICU admissions or a history of rapid clinical deterioration, children with severe distress (inspiratory and expiratory wheezing, limited air entry, air hunger, and inability to phonate) despite initial bronchodilator therapy, or those with a Becker asthma score ≥ 7 should be considered for PICU admission. Other indications for PICU admission include the child's sense of impending clinical doom, altered mental status, respiratory arrest, and a rising $PaCO_2$ coupled with clinical signs of fatigue (20). Recognizing the severely ill child with status asthmaticus and providing rapid aggressive care in the emergency department can interrupt a cycle of progressive air trapping, air hunger, and respiratory fatigue, and potentially prevent the onset of respiratory failure that may require mechanical ventilation.

Emergency-department management of a child with severe status asthmaticus should focus on the assessment of impending respiratory failure, followed by therapeutic interventions including, but not limited to, obtaining IV access, providing supplemental O_2 and continuous inhaled β-agonists, and administering IV methylprednisolone. Triage nurse-initiated oral corticosteroids in the emergency department can reduce time to discharge and reduce hospital admission rates (22). Some suggest that IV magnesium and/or IV β-agonists should be administered in the emergency department to aggressively treat severe status asthmaticus and prevent progression to the need for mechanical ventilation.

PICU Management

General-Care Issues

Children admitted to the PICU require IV access, continuous cardiorespiratory monitoring, and continuous pulse oximetry. For spontaneously breathing children in the PICU, frequent blood gas monitoring is not required. Such children can usually be managed with close clinical observation without indwelling arterial or central venous catheters. For children who require mechanical ventilation, a Foley catheter and arterial and central venous access are often required.

Standardized Care

Evidence-based clinical pathways are designed to reduce variation and standardize the delivery of high-quality care. Clinical pathways for the management of status asthmaticus are being used in both emergency-department and inpatient settings. PICU asthma pathway use can reduce ICU LOS and enhance adherence to national recommendations around asthma education and asthma specialist referral. We believe the routine critically ill child with status asthmaticus (exclude the intubated patient or one receiving multiple adjunct therapies) can be effectively managed using standardized clinical pathways based upon national management guidelines (20).

Fluids

Critically ill children with status asthmaticus are often dehydrated as a result of decreased oral intake prior to admission and increased insensible fluid losses from increased minute ventilation. Providing appropriate fluid resuscitation and ongoing maintenance fluid is essential; however, overhydration should be avoided because these children are at risk for pulmonary edema due to microvascular permeability, increased left ventricular afterload, and alveolar fluid migration associated with the inflammatory lung process in asthma.

Oxygen

Most children with severe status asthmaticus will have some degree of mucous plugging, atelectasis, V/Q mismatch, and hypoxemia. In those lung segments with atelectasis, compensatory hypoxic pulmonary vasoconstriction is often present. Treatment with inhaled β-agonists may induce generalized pulmonary vasodilatation and, as a result, exacerbate V/Q mismatch and worsen hypoxemia. O_2 should be a part of the management for *all* children with status asthmaticus.

Corticosteroids

The overriding physiologic derangement in asthma is airway inflammation, and corticosteroids are a mainstay in the management of both acute and chronic asthma. Among their many actions, glucocorticosteroids suppress cytokine production, granulocyte-macrophage colony-stimulating factor production, and inducible nitric oxide synthase activation, which are all important components of the inflammatory processes involved in the pathophysiology of asthma. As a result of their immunosuppressive activity, corticosteroids impede recruitment and activation of inflammatory cells, decrease airway mucous production, and attenuate microvascular permeability.

Systemically administered corticosteroids reduce asthma hospitalization rates and hospital LOS (23). Inhaled corticosteroids are of no clinical benefit in the treatment of status asthmaticus. While some emergency-department data suggest that enteral and parenteral administration of corticosteroids are of equal efficacy, the child in the PICU is less likely to tolerate oral medications, and therefore oral steroid administration is of limited value in these patients (24). Methylprednisolone is the most common agent used in the PICU and is preferred because of its limited mineralocorticoid effects. The initial IV dose is 2 mg/kg, followed by 0.5–1 mg/kg/dose administered IV every 6 hours. Other agents that are sometimes used include dexamethasone and hydrocortisone. Depending upon the agent used, systemic corticosteroids begin to exert their effect in 1–3 hours and reach maximal effect in 4–8 hours. Treatment duration depends upon the severity of illness, but generally continues until the asthma exacerbation is resolved. Short courses of steroid treatment are generally well tolerated. Side effects often observed in the critically ill child include hyperglycemia, hypertension, and, occasionally, agitation related to steroid-induced psychosis. These symptoms may be difficult to separate from those induced by β-agonist therapy. Prolonged steroid use may cause hypothalamic–pituitary–adrenal axis suppression, osteoporosis, myopathy, and weakness. The incidence of myopathy and weakness is increased when neuromuscular blocking agents are concomitantly administered in the mechanically ventilated asthmatic patient.

Inhaled β-Agonists

β-Agonists, as sympathomimetic agents, cause direct bronchial smooth muscle relaxation and are key components of acute and chronic asthma therapy. Bronchial smooth muscles express β_2-adrenergic receptors, which are activated by binding with β-agonists. Activation of the receptor, which is G-protein–coupled, results in activation of adenylate cyclase and increased cyclic AMP (cAMP) and cAMP-dependent protein kinase (protein kinase A, PKA). PKA promotes calcium (Ca^+) efflux and inhibits Ca^+ influx in the sarcolemma, while enhancing Ca^+ uptake in the sarcoplasmic reticulum. This PKA-dependent Ca^+ regulation results in decreased actin–myosin interactions and smooth muscle relaxation. In the treatment of status asthmaticus, inhaled β-agonists are a bridge to support ventilation and oxygenation until the anti-inflammatory effects of corticosteroids take effect.

In the United States, albuterol and terbutaline are commonly available, short-acting, selective β_2-agonists used for inhalation therapy. Terbutaline is less β_2 selective, compared with albuterol and, therefore, used less often for inhalation therapy than albuterol. Albuterol for inhalation is available in two forms: albuterol (salbutamol) and levalbuterol. Albuterol is a racemic mixture of two equal parts of mirror image forms: R-enantiomers and S-enantiomers. The R-enantiomer is the pharmacologically active enantiomer. The S-enantiomer is considered pharmacologically inactive, has a longer elimination half-life, and may contribute to airway irritation as a spasmogen. Levalbuterol consists solely of the R-enantiomer of albuterol, and some have suggested that levalbuterol has improved efficacy with fewer adverse effects compared with racemic albuterol. In comparison trials, the use of levalbuterol

has not proved superior to racemic albuterol. Currently, racemic albuterol remains the mainstay of inhaled β-agonist therapy in the ICU.

The delivery of albuterol in both acute and nonacute asthma has been studied extensively. The two primary delivery mechanisms are via small-volume nebulizer and metered-dose inhaler (MDI), usually with a vehicle-delivery device (i.e., spacer). Breath-actuated, inhaled β-agonist delivery devices are another relatively new delivery method; however, little data are available regarding the use of these devices in children with status asthmaticus. Intermittent MDI dosing is infrequently used in the critically ill child with status asthmaticus. Continuous albuterol nebulization is superior to intermittent dosing and is the primary delivery format for inhaled β-agonist therapy. With continuous inhalation, patients have more rapid clinical improvement than with intermittent administration. The usual dose of continuous albuterol nebulization is 0.15–0.5 mg/kg/h or 10–20 mg/h. During weaning from continuous albuterol inhalation, some practitioners transition children to intermittent albuterol MDI treatments—usually four to eight puffs per dose, with each puff delivering 90 μg.

Untoward side effects of continuous albuterol nebulization are common but relatively minor in severity. Sinus tachycardia is most common but rarely problematic. Other cardiovascular-related effects include palpitations, hypertension, diastolic hypotension, and, rarely, ventricular cardiac dysrhythmias. Excessive central nervous system (CNS) stimulation, including hyperactivity, tremors, and nausea with vomiting, are not uncommon. Hypokalemia and hyperglycemia are the most common metabolic derangements associated with albuterol use. Neither usually requires treatment although supplemental potassium beyond maintenance amounts is sometimes necessary. Periodic serum potassium levels should be monitored during inhaled β-agonist treatment.

Long-acting inhaled β-agonists (LABAs) are used predominately as controller medications for asthma and had previously been associated with serious asthma events and death in children (25). In a recent study, LABAs, when combined with inhaled corticosteroids use, were not associated with severe asthma events, increased risk for PICU admission, or death; however, there are no data to support the use of LABAs in the management of pediatric status asthmaticus (26).

Intravenous and Subcutaneous β-Agonists

IV and subcutaneous administration of β-agonists is most beneficial in children with severe status asthmaticus and limited respiratory airflow, when distribution of inhaled medications may be significantly reduced. Nonselective β-agonists, such as ephedrine, epinephrine, and isoproterenol, are rarely used because of their high side-effect profile and the availability of more selective IV or subcutaneous agents.

Terbutaline, a relatively selective β_2-agonist, is available in the United States for IV or subcutaneous administration. Because of its greater selectivity, terbutaline has largely supplanted the use of epinephrine for subcutaneous administration. Subcutaneous administration of β-agonists is primarily used for children with no IV access and as a rapidly available adjunct to inhaled β-agonists. Subcutaneous dosing for terbutaline is 0.01 mg/kg/dose, with a maximum dose of 0.3 mg. The dose may be repeated every 15–20 minutes for up to three doses. IV terbutaline therapy starts with a loading dose of 10 μg/kg over 10 minutes, followed by continuous infusion at 0.1–10 μg/kg/min. In the authors' experience, the usual range for effective IV terbutaline dosing is 1–8 μg/kg/min.

The side effects of subcutaneous or IV-administered terbutaline are similar to those of inhaled β-agonists. Some have suggested that the risk of myocardial ischemia is increased with the administration of relatively selective IV β-agonists.

Ten to fifty percent of pediatric asthmatics can have elevated troponin I levels during IV terbutaline therapy (27). To date, this concern remains small and data are limited. The authors believe that it is valuable to prospectively monitor ST analysis on continuous electrocardiography and cardiac-specific enzymes (creatine phosphokinase or troponin) in children who are receiving IV β-agonists, including terbutaline.

Methylxanthines

The role of methylxanthine therapy for critically ill children with status asthmaticus has changed as more selective β-agonists have become available. Methylxanthines promote relaxation of the bronchial smooth muscles; however, the exact mechanism of action remains controversial. Suggested mechanisms include increase of intracellular cAMP levels by blocking phosphodiesterase-4, control of intracellular calcium flux, inhibition of endogenous catecholamine release, and prostaglandin antagonism. In the 1970s, methylxanthines were a mainstay in the treatment of severe status asthmaticus, but some recent data have made their use in the ICU controversial. For children with status asthmaticus who are hospitalized on the general-care ward, theophylline adds little to O_2, intermittent inhaled β-agonist bronchodilators, and corticosteroids. Theophylline added to a regimen that includes inhaled and/or IV β-agonists, inhaled ipratropium bromide, and corticosteroids significantly improved clinical asthma score over time, but did not reduce PICU LOS in critically ill asthmatic children. In another randomized trial, no difference was observed in the rate of clinical asthma score improvement between three treatment groups—theophylline alone, terbutaline alone, or terbutaline plus theophylline—when these regimens were added to standard therapy with inhaled β-agonists, corticosteroids, and O_2 (28). Over half of pediatric critical care fellowship directors surveyed still use theophylline for status asthmaticus in those critically ill children who are not responsive to steroids, inhaled and IV β-agonists, and O_2.

Theophylline is administered by continuous IV infusion following a loading dose of 5–7 mg/kg infused over 20 minutes. In general, a loading dose of 1 mg/kg will raise the serum theophylline level by 2 μg/mL. For maximum therapeutic benefit, the goal serum theophylline level is 10–20 μg/mL. Serum theophylline levels should be measured 1–2 hours after the loading dose is completed. The continuous IV infusion should begin immediately after the bolus at a rate of 0.5–0.9 mg/kg/h. The infusion should be adjusted to maintain levels, as noted previously. Theophylline clearance is reduced in infants and adolescents. In these age groups, the usual dose for continuous infusion is closer to 0.5 mg/kg/h. Serum levels >20 μg/mL are associated with adverse effects that include nausea, jitters or restlessness, tachycardia (racing heart), and overall irritability. Serum levels >35 μg/mL have been associated with seizures and cardiac dysrhythmias. Careful attention to serum drug level measurements is required to minimize the risk of untoward side effects.

Anticholinergics

Ipratropium bromide is the most frequently used agent to provide anticholinergic effects in the treatment of status asthmaticus. Ipratropium promotes bronchodilation without inhibiting mucociliary clearance, as occurs with atropine. Acting as a parasympatholytic, aerosolized ipratropium antagonizes acetylcholine effects by blocking acetylcholine interactions with the muscarinic receptor on bronchial smooth muscle cells. By this mechanism, intracellular cyclic guanosine monophosphate levels are reduced, and bronchial smooth muscle contraction is impaired.

When administered in the emergency department, ipratropium bromide reduced both hospital admission rates and clinical asthma scores. For children hospitalized with mild-to-moderate status asthmaticus, ipratropium has no additional clinical benefit over inhaled β-agonists and corticosteroids alone. Inhaled ipratropium has not been evaluated in critically ill children with status asthmaticus. Although ipratropium therapy has no proven benefit in moderately ill children with asthma, the authors believe that it is prudent to add inhaled ipratropium therapy to the management of critically ill children who are not responding to other aggressive measures.

Ipratropium bromide can be delivered by either aerosol or MDI. Initial dose range is 125–500 μg (if nebulized) or four to eight puffs (if via MDI) administered every 20 minutes for up to three doses. The subsequent recommended dosing interval is every 4–6 hours. Ipratropium has few adverse effects because it has poor systemic absorption. The most common untoward effects are dry mouth, bitter taste, flushing, tachycardia, and dizziness. Tiotropium bromide, a long-acting selective anticholinergic compound with a higher affinity for the muscarinic receptors in the airway, has shown promising clinical benefits in chronic asthma management, but has not been tested in children with acute asthma exacerbation (29).

Magnesium Sulfate

Magnesium acts as a bronchodilator primarily through its activity as a calcium channel blocker and its role in activation of adenylate cyclase in smooth muscle cells. As a result of these mechanisms, magnesium inhibits calcium-mediated smooth muscle contraction and facilitates bronchodilation.

The value of magnesium administration in the treatment of status asthmaticus remains controversial. Some studies, completed in the emergency-department setting, demonstrate that magnesium administered either IV or by aerosol can reduce hospitalization rates, improve short-term PFT, and improve clinical asthma scores over time, whereas others have shown no benefit (30). No data are available regarding the efficacy of magnesium therapy in the ICU setting, though several studies report utilization rates of 6%–21%, with use varying by geographic region of the United States (8,31).

The usual dose of magnesium is 25–50 mg/kg/dose IV over 30 minutes, administered every 4 hours. Magnesium can also be given by continuous infusion at a rate of 10–20 mg/kg/h. With either dosing regimen, some have suggested a target magnesium level of 4 mg/dL to achieve maximal effect.

Side effects of magnesium administration include hypotension, CNS depression, muscle weakness, and flushing, though in the studies previously mentioned, no significant untoward effects were reported. Severe complications, such as cardiac arrhythmia including complete heart block, respiratory failure due to severe muscle weakness, and sudden cardiopulmonary arrest, may occur in the setting of very high serum magnesium levels (usually >10–12 mg/dL). Serum magnesium levels should be regularly monitored.

To date, magnesium therapy remains an unproven therapy in critically ill children with status asthmaticus. Nevertheless, given its low-risk profile and its demonstrated benefit in the emergency-department setting, it is appropriate to consider adding magnesium therapy to the treatment regimen of children in the PICU who are not responding to more conventional treatment measures.

Helium–Oxygen

Helium is a biologically inert, low-density gas that, when administered by inhalation in a mixture with O_2, reduces airflow resistance in small airways by reducing turbulent flow and enhancing laminar gas flow. These characteristics may also enhance particle deposition of aerosolized medications in distal lung segments. In aggregate, these characteristics make administration of a mixture of helium and O_2 (80% helium/20% oxygen—heliox) an attractive therapeutic option in the management of status asthmaticus, in which turbulent airflow and high airway resistance are common.

Clinical studies examining the efficacy of helium/oxygen administration in status asthmaticus have yielded conflicting results. A recent Cochrane review concluded that heliox was not beneficial in asthma, though most of the studies cited were in adults. A recent pediatric study of inpatients with moderate and severe asthma exacerbations showed no benefit in ICU/hospital LOS or time to improvement in clinical asthma score for patients receiving heliox-powered nebulized albuterol compared with air/oxygen powered albuterol (32). In contrast, some small studies in nonintubated children with moderately severe asthma have shown improvement in lung function and clinical asthma score with heliox therapy. For example, Kim et al. (33) demonstrated that the use of heliox to drive continuous albuterol nebulization treatments for children in the emergency department with moderately severe status asthmaticus was associated with significantly improved clinical asthma scores. In the PICU, the use of heliox in mechanically ventilated children reduces peak airway pressure by lowering airway resistance, and it may enhance weaning from mechanical ventilation. The use of heliox is sometimes limited by hypoxemia in the patient. If substantial supplemental O_2 is added to the two available mixtures of helium/oxygen (80/20 and 70/30), the salutary effect of low-density gas administration on reducing turbulent gas flow is lost.

Heliox remains unproven therapy in critically ill children with status asthmaticus. However, Pediatric Health Information System (PHIS) database reports show heliox use in 10% of critically ill asthmatic children (31). For children who are not improving with conventional therapy or children who are receiving high-pressure mechanical ventilatory support, heliox may be a reasonable adjunct therapy.

Noninvasive Mechanical Ventilation

Mortality rates in mechanically ventilated children with status asthmaticus are increased compared with those who do not require mechanical ventilation. Noninvasive positive-pressure ventilation (NIPPV) is an alternative to conventional mechanical ventilation in these patients and is used in 3%–5% of critically ill asthmatic children (34). A systematic review that examined data in these patients concluded that insufficient quality data are available to make recommendations about the use of NIPPV in patients with asthma. Other reports in small groups of adults suggest that NIPPV can prevent tracheal intubation. In one study, children were subjected to a crossover trial between NIPPV and standard therapy. The NIPPV group showed reduced WOB and dyspnea, compared with the standard therapy group (35). More recently, a study examining the use of early NIPPV showed improved clinical asthma scores within the first 24 hours, and decreased need for adjunct asthma therapies. NIPPV's safety profile and benefit are most apparent in the cohort of asthma patients weighing less than 20 kg (36). At this writing, noninvasive ventilation remains an unproven therapy for children with status asthmaticus; however, it is relatively easy to institute, and a trial may be warranted prior to tracheal intubation and conventional mechanical ventilation.

Mechanical Ventilation

10 In status asthmaticus, tracheal intubation is indicated for children following cardiorespiratory arrest, those with refractory hypoxemia, or those with significant respiratory acidosis unresponsive to pharmacotherapy. Mechanical ventilation is intended to provide support while the underlying pathology resolves. Currently, <1% of children with status asthmaticus require mechanical ventilation. Of the children admitted to the PICU, only 5%–12% require mechanical ventilation, and half of those patients are intubated prior to arrival in the PICU (34). In fact, children initially cared for at a community hospital were three times more likely to be intubated. Children who require mechanical ventilation are at increased risk for pulmonary barotrauma, nosocomial infection, pulmonary edema, circulatory dysfunction, steroid/muscle relaxant-associated myopathy, and death (**Fig. 46.4**).

Tracheal intubation of the asthmatic child with respiratory failure requires preparation and anticipation of patient deterioration. It should be performed by the most skilled individual available. Hypotension should be anticipated because many patients have relative hypovolemia that may be exacerbated by reduced preload as positive-pressure ventilation is initiated and by reduced vascular tone induced by anesthetic agents used for tracheal intubation. Histamine-producing agents, such as morphine or atracurium, must be avoided. Ketamine is an excellent anesthetic agent for induction because of its relatively long half-life, bronchodilating properties, and relative preservation of hemodynamic stability. A cuffed endotracheal tube with the largest diameter appropriate for the age of the child should be used, as high ventilatory pressures are typical when treating mechanically ventilated children in status asthmaticus.

Ventilatory support in status asthmaticus should maintain adequate oxygenation, allow for permissive hypercarbia (moderate respiratory acidosis), and adjust minute ventilation (peak pressure, tidal volume, and rate) to maintain an arterial pH of >7.2. Ventilator management strategies should attempt to minimize dynamic hyperinflation and air trapping (**Fig. 46.1**), which can usually be accomplished by employing slow ventilator rates with prolonged expiratory phase, minimal end-expiratory pressure, and short inspiratory time.

The ideal mode of mechanical ventilation has not been established for asthmatic children with respiratory failure. Most of these children will display disparate time-constant physiology, though slow time constants will predominate. Volume-control ventilation with constant or accelerating flow wave forms will provide stable tidal volumes from breath to breath but, in the setting of dynamic airway resistance, may result in high peak airway pressures, uneven distribution of tidal breaths, and increased risk for pulmonary barotrauma. Pressure-control ventilation with decelerating flow pattern results in lower peak pressure, higher mean airway pressure, and better distribution of gas into high-resistance, long time-constant airways. In pressure-control mode with preset peak inspiratory pressure, rapidly changing airway resistance can result in (a) significant variation in delivered tidal volume and (b) increased risk of pulmonary barotrauma if airway resistance changes abruptly. Pressure-regulated volume control is a relatively new mode of mechanical ventilation. Although experience is limited with this mode of ventilation in patients with asthma, the decelerating flow pattern combined with the option to independently adjust pressure with a preset tidal volume is appealing to enhance gas distribution and minimize risk of barotrauma.

The use of positive end-expiratory pressure (PEEP) is controversial. Most authors suggest minimal PEEP because most patients with status asthmaticus already have increased functional residual capacity. High PEEP is likely to further increase functional residual capacity and exacerbate hyperinflation. Others argue that these patients have dynamic collapse of small airways during forced exhalation, and PEEP may stent small airways open at the end of expiration and facilitate full expiration. Review of graphically displayed flow–time curves will demonstrate whether expiratory flow is completed prior

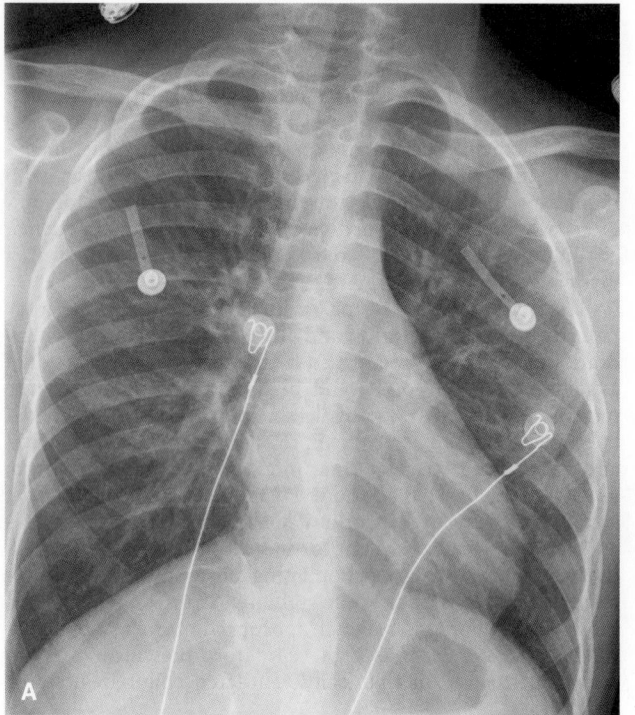

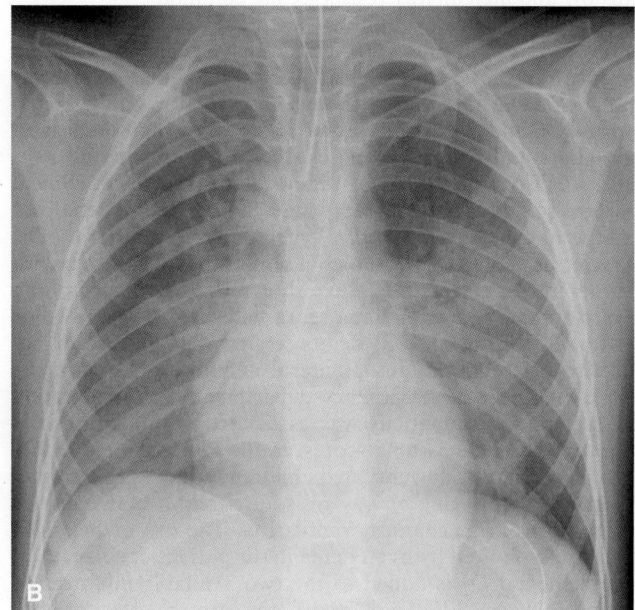

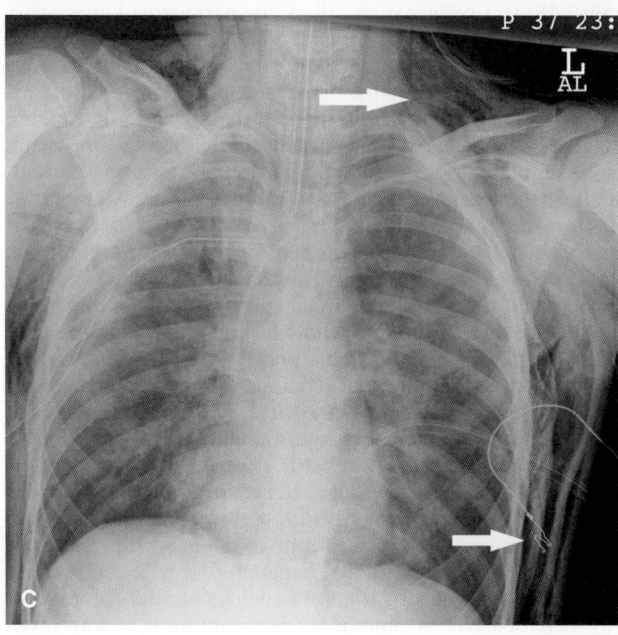

FIGURE 46.4. Pulmonary complications. **A:** Hyperinflation and air trapping. **B:** Pulmonary edema in patient receiving mechanical ventilation; note bilateral airspace disease. **C:** Significant barotrauma with bilateral pneumothoraces, requiring chest tubes and a large amount of subcutaneous air (*arrows*).

to the next breath (**Fig. 46.1**). Adjustments can then be made to the ventilator rate, inspiratory time, expiratory time, or PEEP to facilitate full expiration between breaths.

Other less conventional strategies have been used when standard mechanical ventilation approaches fail. The use of high-frequency ventilation has been described in a few case reports, though this mode of ventilation requires careful attention to the amplitude settings of the oscillator to avoid further hyperinflation. Some authors suggest using pressure-support ventilation without any preset rate and allowing the patient to breathe spontaneously. This strategy avoids complications associated with continuous or frequent use of muscle relaxants and has the further advantage of allowing the child to maintain forced exhalation while receiving support for

inspiration. Tracheal gas insufflation has also been used to facilitate expiratory gas flow and reduce severe hypercarbia. Careful attention to secretion accumulation around the insufflation tube is necessary to avoid the development of tracheal tube mucous plugging.

Tracheal extubation should occur as soon as possible. Rapid weaning from the ventilator should take place—"declare them well and pull the tube." The presence of the breathing tube, especially in awake children, may irritate the airway and stimulate further bronchospasm. Decreasing peak inspiratory pressure, adequate air movement by auscultation, and graphic evidence of full expiration of inspired tidal volume are sufficient criteria for tracheal extubation, even if expiratory wheezing is still present on clinical exam.

Bronchoscopy

The pathophysiologic hallmark of acute asthma includes mucosal edema, airway inflammation, and mucous production with associated worsening of airway obstruction. Bronchoscopy use in intubated children with status asthmaticus–induced respiratory failure can shorten the duration of mechanical ventilation and ICU LOS. Despite these data, bronchoscopy for intubated children with status asthmaticus is not recommended as routine care.

Chest Physiotherapy

Chest physiotherapy (CPT) may augment airway clearance and encourage resolution of mucous plugging; however, it should be considered only in children with clear segmental or lobar atelectasis. In all other populations of children with status asthmaticus, CPT has no therapeutic benefit. Some suggest that CPT is irritating to the severe asthmatic and may actually worsen clinical symptoms. CPT is not recommended as part of routine management in the critically ill patient with status asthmaticus.

Antibiotics

Most asthma exacerbations are associated with, or triggered by, viral infections and not bacterial infections. For this reason, empiric antibiotic treatment for children with status asthmaticus is not indicated. Influenza A, including pandemic H1N1 influenza A, was more commonly identified in children admitted with acute asthma exacerbations compared with influenza B. Pandemic H1N1 was more commonly associated with ICU admission and concomitant bacterial pneumonia compared with other seasonal influenza infections (37). Isolated lower respiratory tract bacterial infections do occur in children with status asthmaticus. The most commonly identified organisms are *Mycoplasma pneumoniae* and *Chlamydia pneumoniae*. When findings on chest x-ray, leukocytosis, and fever suggest pneumonia, appropriate antibiotics should be administered, especially targeted at the organisms previously noted. Sinusitis is a common nonpulmonary infection in children with status asthmaticus. When evidence of bacterial pneumonia is absent, and high fever and peripheral blood leukocytosis are present, the diagnosis of sinusitis should be considered, and, if found, antibacterial therapy should be instituted.

Sedation, Analgesia, Muscle Relaxants, Inhalational Anesthetics

Sedation of the unintubated asthmatic is generally not indicated. Some children who are excessively anxious and who are not hypoxemic or hypercarbic as a cause for their anxiety may benefit from sedation. Sedation should occur only in the closely monitored setting of the PICU. Ketamine is an excellent choice because it provides excellent sedation and bronchodilation with minimal risk of respiratory depression.

Mechanically ventilated children require sedation and, often, muscle relaxants to prevent ventilator–patient asynchrony and to reduce the risk of sudden cough-induced pulmonary barotrauma. Ketamine by continuous infusion is the first choice for sedation, usually combined with intermittent or continuous administration of benzodiazepines. Usual IV ketamine infusion dosing is 1 mg/kg/h and is adjusted to achieve sufficient sedation. Increased respiratory secretions occur with ketamine administration; however, these side effects are usually manageable. When opiates are used, fentanyl is preferred because morphine causes histamine release, which may exacerbate bronchospasm. Neuromuscular blocking agents are frequently required to facilitate mechanical ventilatory support. Vecuronium is a commonly used agent. The starting dose is 0.1 mg/kg/h, which should be titrated to train-of-four monitoring—usually one to two twitches. Drug holidays can be used to reduce the risk of overdose, prolonged paresis, and myopathy that are sometimes observed in children who receive continuous infusions of the nondepolarizing neuromuscular blocking agents.

Inhaled general anesthetics have been used when all other measures are failing, and their bronchodilating properties have proven beneficial in the management of the intubated asthmatic. Several small pediatric studies describe the safe use of isoflurane in the management of refractory status asthmaticus. These agents should be administered in conjunction with anesthesia services, and appropriate consideration should be made for delivery and scavenging strategies for inhaled volatile anesthetic agents. Hypotension, impaired renal perfusion, and cardiac dysrhythmias are associated with their use and are more likely to occur in hypoxemic children.

Extracorporeal Membrane Oxygenation Support

When maximal medical therapy is failing, ECMO should be considered. Numerous case reports demonstrate high survival rates, even in a gravely ill patient population. The survival rate for children with refractory status asthmaticus treated with ECMO is ~90%. Two reports describe the use of pumpless arteriovenous carbon dioxide removal in the context of refractory hypercapnia and metabolic acidosis and have shown favorable outcomes (38).

OUTCOMES

Mortality rates for children with severe status asthmaticus who arrive at the hospital intact are nearly zero (8). Sophisticated ventilatory strategies, the availability of more selective, less toxic bronchodilating agents, and the selective use of ECMO have contributed to this good prognosis. Nearly all asthma deaths occur in those children who suffer a cardiopulmonary arrest prior to arrival for emergency hospital care. Improved outpatient management strategies focused on prevention of acute life-threatening asthma exacerbations are likely necessary to eliminate these deaths (39).

CONCLUSIONS AND FUTURE DIRECTIONS

Asthma is a disease that is increasing in worldwide prevalence, and continues to have substantial clinical and financial impact on children and their families. Severe status asthmaticus is a life-threatening disorder that, if recognized and treated aggressively, has an extremely low mortality rate. It is incumbent upon the pediatric intensivist to rapidly diagnose and initiate therapy in these children. More work is required to recognize and provide earlier intervention options to those few asthmatics who suffer rapid-onset illness and resultant morbidity and mortality before they can receive emergent medical care.

Novel future therapies will likely involve modifying the inflammatory processes involved in the pathophysiology of asthma. Leukotriene modifiers and cytokine modulators may revolutionize asthma therapy, primarily in the outpatient arena, though these agents may also significantly impact ICU care as well. Other therapies on the horizon include phosphodiesterase inhibitors that are more specific than theophylline and anti-IgE monoclonal antibodies that reduce free IgE. Of these new asthma therapies, cytokine modulators and IgE inhibitors are receiving the most active research. Our understanding of viral-induced asthma is growing. Some suggest that an "asthma vaccine" to reduce viral-induced disease is at hand. Most experts are more realistic, suggesting that the multiple polymorphisms and interactions with environmental influences will preclude identification of an asthma cure.

Challenges exist in asthma research unique to critically ill children. Even within established pediatric critical care research networks, medication use and ventilation strategies are quite disparate (34). It is apparent that studying the impact of a novel therapeutic intervention may be limited because of this wide variability. Standardized care pathways including best evidence recommendations for escalation of adjunct therapies may strengthen efforts to answer the clinical questions that remain in the management of the critically ill asthmatic child.

References

1. Akinbami LJ, Moorman JE, Garbe PL, et al. Status of childhood asthma in the United States, 1980–2007. *Pediatrics* 2009;123: S131–45.

2. US Department of Health and Human Services, National Institutes of Health, National Heart, Lung, and Blood Institute. *Guidelines for the Diagnosis and Management of Asthma*. 2007. Pub No 08-5846.

3. Afzal M, Tharratt RS. Mechanical ventilation in severe asthma. *Clin Rev Allergy Immunol* 2001;20:385–97.

4. World Health Organization. *Global Surveillance, Prevention and Control of Chronic Respiratory Diseases: A Comprehensive Report*. Geneva, Switzerland: World Health Organization, 2007.

5. McCormick MC, Kass B, Elixhauser A, et al. Annual report on access to and utilization of health care for children and youth in the United States—1999. *Pediatrics* 2000;105:219–30.

6. Roberts JS, Bratton SL, Brogan TV. Acute severe asthma: Differences in therapies and outcomes among pediatric intensive care units. *Crit Care Med* 2002;30:581–5.

7. Szefler SJ. Advances in pediatric asthma in 2011: Moving forward. *J Allergy Clin Immunol* 2012;129:60–8.

8. Newth CJ, Meert KL, Clark AE, et al. Fatal and near-fatal asthma in children: The critical care perspective. *J Pediatr* 2012;161: 214–21.

9. Werner HA. Status asthmaticus in children: A review. *Chest* 2001;119:1913–29.

10. Kikuchi Y, Okabe S, Tamura G, et al. Chemosensitivity and perception of dyspnea in patients with a history of near-fatal asthma. *N Engl J Med* 1994;330:1329–34.

11. McCunney RJ. Asthma, genes, and air pollution. *J Occup Environ Med* 2005;47:1285–91.

12. Finkelstein Y, Bournissen FG, Hutson JR, et al. Polymorphism of the ADRB2 gene and response to inhaled beta- agonists in children with asthma: A meta-analysis. *J Asthma* 2009;46:900–5.

13. Carroll CL, Sala KA, Zucker AR, et al. Beta-adrenergic receptor polymorphisms associated with length of ICU stay in pediatric status asthmaticus. *Pediatr Pulmonol* 2012;47:233–9.

14. Hamid Q, Tulic M. Immunobiology of asthma. *Annu Rev Physiol* 2009;71:489–507.

15. Brightling CE, Symon FA, Birring SS, et al. TH2 cytokine expression in bronchoalveolar lavage fluid T lymphocytes and bronchial submucosa is a feature of asthma and eosinophilic bronchitis. *J Allergy Clin Immunol* 2002;110:899–905.

16. Jardin F, Farcot JC, Boisante L, et al. Mechanism of paradoxic pulse in bronchial asthma. *Circulation* 1982;66:887–94.

17. American Heart Association. Recognition of respiratory failure and shock. In: *Pediatric Advanced Life Support Provider Manual*. Dallas, TX: American Heart Association, 2002:23–42.

18. DiGiulio GA, Kercsmar CM, Krug SE, et al. Hospital treatment of asthma: Lack of benefit from theophylline given in addition to nebulized albuterol and intravenously administered corticosteroid. *J Pediatr* 1993;122:464–9.

19. Petsky HL, Cates CJ, Lasserson TJ, et al. A systematic review and meta-analysis: Tailoring asthma treatment on eosinophilic markers (exhaled nitric oxide or sputum eosinophils). *Thorax* 2012;67: 199–208.

20. National Institutes of Health. *Program NAEaP. Expert Panel Report 2: Guidelines for the Diagnosis and Management of Asthma*. 1997. NIH Pub No 55-4051.

21. Schneider WV, Bulloch B, Wilkinson M, et al. Utility of portable spirometry in a pediatric emergency department in children with acute exacerbation of asthma. *J Asthma* 2011;48:248–52.

22. Zemek R, Plint A, Osmond MH, et al. Triage nurse initiation of corticosteroids in pediatric asthma is associated with improved emergency department efficiency. *Pediatrics* 2012;129: 671–80.

23. Rachelefsky G. Treating exacerbations of asthma in children: The role of systemic corticosteroids. *Pediatrics* 2003;112:382–97.

24. Becker JM, Arora A, Scarfone RJ, et al. Oral versus intravenous corticosteroids in children hospitalized with asthma. *J Allergy Clin Immunol* 1999;103:586–90.

25. Weatherall M, Wijesinghe M, Perrin K, et al. Meta-analysis of the risk of mortality with salmeterol and the effect of concomitant inhaled corticosteroid therapy. *Thorax* 2010;65:39–43.

26. McMahon AW, Levenson MS, McEvoy BW, et al. Age and risks of FDA-approved long-acting beta(2)-adrenergic receptor agonists. *Pediatrics* 2011;128:e1147–54.

27. Chiang VW, Burns JP, Rifai N, et al. Cardiac toxicity of intravenous terbutaline for the treatment of severe asthma in children: A prospective assessment. *J Pediatr* 2000;137:73–7.

28. Wheeler DS, Jacobs BR, Kenreigh CA, et al. Theophylline versus terbutaline in treating critically ill children with status asthmaticus: A prospective, randomized, controlled trial. *Pediatr Crit Care Med* 2005;6:142–7.

29. Park HW. The role of tiotropium in the management of asthma. *Asia Pac Allergy* 2012;2:109–14.

30. Blitz M, Blitz S, Beasely R, et al. Inhaled magnesium sulfate in the treatment of acute asthma. *Cochrane Database Syst Rev* 2005;(3):CD003898.

31. Bratton SL, Odetola FO, McCollegan J, et al. Regional variation in ICU care for pediatric patients with asthma. *J Pediatr* 2005;147:355–61.

32. Bigham MT, Jacobs BR, Monaco MA, et al. Helium/oxygen-driven albuterol nebulization in the management of children with status asthmaticus: A randomized, placebo-controlled trial. *Pediatr Crit Care Med* 2010;11:356–61.

33. Kim IK, Phrampus E, Venkataraman S, et al. Helium/oxygen-driven albuterol nebulization in the treatment of children with moderate to severe asthma exacerbations: A randomized, controlled trial. *Pediatrics* 2005;116:1127–33.

34. Bratton SL, Newth CJ, Zuppa AF, et al. Critical care for pediatric asthma: Wide care variability and challenges for study. *Pediatr Crit Care Med* 2012;13:407–14.

35. Thill PJ, McGuire JK, Baden HP, et al. Noninvasive positive-pressure ventilation in children with lower airway obstruction. *Pediatr Crit Care Med* 2004;5:337–42.

36. Williams AM, Abramo TJ, Shah MV, et al. Safety and clinical findings of BiPAP utilization in children 20 kg or less for asthma exacerbations. *Intensive Care Med* 2011;37:1338–43.

37. Dawood FS, Kamimoto L, D'Mello TA, et al. Children with asthma hospitalized with seasonal or pandemic influenza, 2003–2009. *Pediatrics* 2011;128:e27–32.

38. Conrad SA, Green R, Scott LK. Near-fatal pediatric asthma managed with pumpless arteriovenous carbon dioxide removal. *Crit Care Med* 2007;35:2624–9.

39. Lee AY, Brilli RJ. Near-fatal asthma: An ounce of prevention may be worth more than a pound of cure. *J Pediatr* 2012;161: 182–4.

CHAPTER 47 ■ NEONATAL RESPIRATORY FAILURE

NARAYAN PRABHU IYER, PHILIPPE S. FRIEDLICH, ELISABETH L. RAAB,
RANGASAMY RAMANATHAN, AND ISTVAN SERI

KEY POINTS

1. Respiratory disorders in newborn infants are caused by diseases unique to the neonatal population and that often result in long-term respiratory complications.

2. Neonatal respiratory disorders could be developmental, congenital, or acquired; respiratory problems associated with prematurity are the most common cause for respiratory failure in newborn infants.

3. Management of respiratory distress syndrome (RDS) has changed significantly in the last two decades, with increasing emphasis on noninvasive respiratory support.

4. Current research has been focused on refining the indication for surfactant and postnatal steroids use and to identify the optimal pulse oximetry range for preterm infants that minimizes the risk for retinopathy of prematurity (ROP) without increasing the mortality.

5. Management of persistent pulmonary hypertension of newborn (PPHN) has improved dramatically after the introduction of inhaled nitric oxide. However, PPHN unresponsive to nitric oxide remains a challenge, and newer treatments such as sildenafil and bosantan are increasingly being used to improve outcomes in such patients.

Respiratory disease accounts for a significant proportion of admissions to the neonatal intensive care unit (NICU) and the pediatric intensive care unit (PICU). The unique aspects of neonatal respiratory physiology place the newborn at high risk for developing respiratory morbidity. Respiratory symptoms in the neonate, such as tachypnea, cyanosis, grunting, flaring, or retractions, may be due to a primary pulmonary process or may be the initial clinical manifestation of a nonrespiratory process, such as inborn errors of metabolism, polycythemia, congenital heart disease, and sepsis. Respiratory failure (due to RDS in the preterm neonate or due to a congenital infection, meconium aspiration syndrome, or congenital anomalies in the term infant) is a major cause of morbidity and mortality in the neonatal period and often has long-term implications for the health of the child. Causes of respiratory failure in a neonate can be categorized as respiratory problems associated with transition around the time of birth, respiratory diseases related to prematurity, cardiac causes, congenital conditions, and, finally, acquired respiratory problems.

DEVELOPMENTALLY REGULATED DISORDERS: RESPIRATORY CONDITIONS ASSOCIATED WITH PREMATURE LUNG

Respiratory Distress Syndrome

Respiratory distress syndrome (RDS) due to surfactant deficiency is a significant life-threatening condition that is seen primarily in preterm infants. The incidence and severity of RDS is inversely proportional to gestational age (GA) (Fig. 47.1). RDS occurs in about 50% of infants born at less than 29 weeks and in 25% of infants born after 29 weeks of gestation. Despite significant improvements in perinatal care practices, the incidence of prematurity has not decreased significantly over recent years. One out of eight babies is born preterm, and this translates into ~480,000 preterm births each year in the United States. Fortunately, with the maternal administration of prenatal steroids to accelerate fetal organ development in general and lung maturity and surfactant release in particular, the incidence and severity of RDS has decreased by nearly 50%. Neonatal outcomes in symptomatic infants with RDS have been significantly improved by the introduction of surfactant. The combination of prenatal steroid followed by postnatal surfactant therapy has resulted in a significant reduction in the mortality and morbidity in preterm infants with RDS (1).

Operational Definition of Respiratory Distress Syndrome

RDS is the collection of symptoms associated with deficiency of pulmonary surfactant. Surfactant deficiency leads to increased alveolar surface tension, subsequent alveolar collapse, decreased pulmonary compliance, and reduced functional residual capacity (FRC). The resultant symptoms include clinical findings of respiratory distress such as retractions, grunting, nasal flaring, and cyanosis. These clinical symptoms are nonspecific for surfactant deficiency. The need for supplemental oxygen, positive pressure ventilation (PPV), and use of radiographic criteria (diffuse haziness and air bronchograms) makes the definition more specific. Radiologic features may be altered by treatment of RDS such as provision of PPV and early surfactant administration. Recent trials have revealed a subgroup of premature infants, some very premature, who do not have "significant" surfactant deficiency (2–4). One of the arms of these randomized trials had infants, including

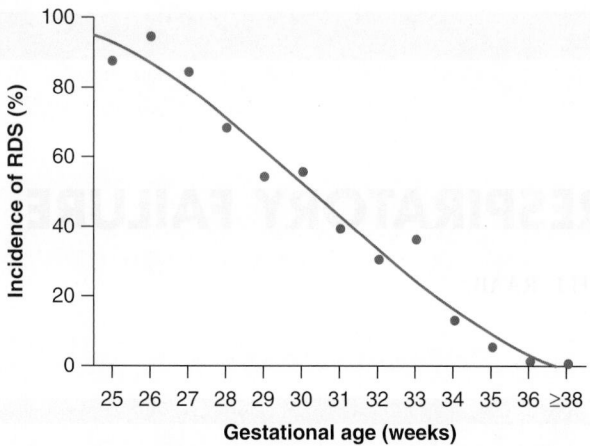

FIGURE 47.1. Incidence of RDS in relation to gestational age at birth (Reused from Robertson PA, Sniderman SH, Laros RK Jr, et al. Neonatal morbidity according to gestational age and birth weight from five tertiary care centers in the United States, 1983 through 1986. *Am J Obstet Gynecol* 1992;166(6, pt 1):1629–41; discussion 1641–5.)

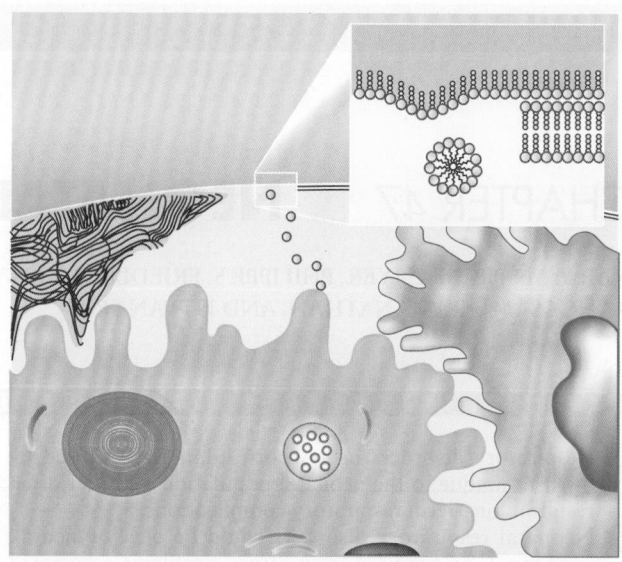

FIGURE 47.2. Surfactant physiology. Surfactant phospholipids and proteins are synthesized by alveolar type II cells lining the alveoli. Surfactant lipids and surfactant protein B (SP-B) precursor protein and surfactant protein C (SP-C) are transported to multivesicular bodies and, after proteolytic processing, stored in lamellar bodies. SP-B, SP-C, and surfactant lipids are secreted into the alveolar subphase and interact with surfactant protein A to form a tubular myelin reservoir from which multilayers and monolayers form a film, thus reducing surface tension at the air–liquid interface. Surfactant remnants are taken up and reutilized or catabolized by type II epithelial cells. Alveolar macrophages play a critical part in the clearance and catabolism of surfactant lipids and proteins. Formation of the active surface film is required to maintain lung volumes, thereby preventing atelectasis and respiratory failure. (Modified from Whitsett JA, Weaver TE. Hydrophobic surfactant proteins in lung function and disease. *N Engl J Med* 2002;347(26):2141–8.)

extremely premature infants (<28 weeks), being stabilized on CPAP after birth. In these trials, 33%–62% of the infants stabilized on CPAP completed the study without receiving surfactant. This finding suggests that these infants did not have "significant" surfactant deficiency but fulfill the clinical criteria for the diagnosis of RDS.

Pathophysiology of Respiratory Distress Syndrome

Surfactant Synthesis, Metabolism, and Function. The newborn lung provides an extensive surface area for gas exchange, ~1 m^2/kg body weight (70 m^2 in an adult lung). Pulmonary surfactant coats the lung surface at the air–liquid interface in the alveoli and maintains a very low surface tension that prevents collapse of the lung, especially at the end of expiration when the alveolar radius is at its lowest. Surfactant is primarily composed of phospholipids (80%–90%) and surfactant proteins (SP) SP-A, SP-B, SP-C, and SP-D. Dipalmitoyl phosphatidylcholine (DPPC) constitutes the major phospholipid. Surfactant is synthesized by the type II pneumocytes lining the alveoli and is stored as lamellar bodies. Lamellar bodies enter the alveoli by exocytosis and transform into tubular myelin. Under the influence of SP-A, which is cosecreted along with the lamellar bodies from type II pneumocytes, tubular myelin unravels to form mono- and multilayers of phospholipids rich in SP-B and SP-C. The spread and adsorption of phospholipids at the air–liquid interphase is dependent on SP-B and to a lesser extent on SP-C (**Fig. 47.2**) (5). Surfactant reduces surface tension at the air–liquid interphase, thereby improving pulmonary compliance. Deficiency of surfactant is associated with heterogeneous expansion of alveoli. According to the law of Laplace, the retractive forces are higher in the smaller alveoli compared with the bigger alveoli, resulting in further collapse of the smaller alveoli. Surfactant reduces surface tension independent of alveolar size, thereby equalizing surface tension forces across the lung, resulting in more uniform alveolar expansion (6). Catabolism of secreted surfactant is primarily regulated by lung macrophages and SP-A. Surfactant metabolism is highly regulated; remnants of phospholipids, SP-A, SP-B, and SP-C are taken up almost entirely and recycled or degraded by type II pneumocytes (7–9). The composition of surfactant across different mammalian species is fairly constant, making it possible to modify surfactant from one species and use it in another species.

Consequences of Surfactant Deficiency. Infants with RDS usually have surfactant lipid pools <10 mg/kg as compared with normal term infants, who have surfactant lipid pools of 100 mg/kg (10). In a preterm infant, this results in very low pulmonary compliance after delivery and an inability to maintain FRC. Because surfactant is responsible for uniform alveolar expansion, surfactant deficiency results in a heterogeneous disease with underaerated alveolus emptying into adjacent overdistended alveolus. The neonate has respiratory distress, hypoxemia, and may develop air leak syndrome. Introduction of PPV using high pressures in this setting, while lifesaving, causes lung injury and inflammation. Pulmonary edema inactivates and dilutes the remaining surfactant, which promotes a vicious cycle.

Management of Respiratory Distress Syndrome

❸ Management of RDS has revolved around the use of lung distending pressure and replacement of pulmonary surfactant. Below is a brief description of our current state of knowledge and practice.

Surfactant Therapy for Respiratory Distress Syndrome. Surfactant therapy has been extensively evaluated in randomized, controlled trials in neonatal medicine and has become the standard of care for preterm infants with RDS. Surfactant therapy has decreased the mortality and incidence of pneumothorax in preterm infants with RDS (11).

Timing of Surfactant. Surfactant therapy has been used *prophylactically* in all preterm infants at risk for RDS, as well as more selectively in infants with established RDS. In the 1990s, a time when antenatal steroids and stabilization of preterm infants on nasal continuous positive airway pressure (NCPAP) were not routine, many trials comparing prophylactic versus selective surfactant therapy were done. Meta-analysis of these trials supported the use of prophylactic surfactant (surfactant given within 15 minutes of birth), with 31% lower neonatal mortality in infants born before 32 weeks of gestation (12). With increasing evidence of lung injury associated with invasive mechanical ventilation, more recent trials have focused on the impact of avoiding routine intubation (and, therefore, avoiding routine surfactant) with initial stabilization of preterm infants on NCPAP at delivery in comparison with routine intubation and surfactant administration (2–4,13–17). A meta-analysis of two recent studies, where the use of antenatal steroids and postnatal CPAP was common, demonstrated a small but statistically significant increase in the risk of bronchopulmonary dysplasia (BPD) or death with the prophylactic administration of surfactant when compared with selective use of surfactant in infants stabilized on NCPAP after birth (relative risk 1.12; 95% CI: 1.02–1.24; number needed to treat 17) (12). Using slightly different inclusion criteria, two further meta-analyses have reported a benefit from the regular use of NCPAP in the delivery room with selective use of surfactant for infants with established RDS (18,19). However, once "significant" RDS is established and NCPAP is failing, *early rescue surfactant therapy* (given within 30 minutes to 120 minutes of age) has been shown to be better than *delayed rescue therapy*. Early rescue therapy has been shown to decrease the need for additional doses of surfactant as well as to allow for faster weaning of supplemental oxygen (20).

Types of Surfactant Preparations. Different surfactant preparations (natural modified surfactants derived from animal sources and synthetic surfactants) are available for the treatment of RDS. Synthetic surfactants that have been studied include colfosceril palmitate (Exosurf), pumactant (ALEC), Turfsurf, and lucinactant (Surfaxin). Of these four synthetic surfactants, the first three are no longer available for clinical use, and lucinactant was recently approved for prophylactic treatment of RDS by the Food and Drug Administration (FDA). Seven different natural, modified surfactant preparations have been used for the treatment of RDS globally. Natural surfactants that have been extensively studied include beractant (Survanta), calfactant (Infasurf), SF-RI 1 (Alveofact), and poractant alfa (Curosurf). They differ in composition, onset of

response, duration of action, dosing volume, and the need for additional doses (Table 47.1). Preterm infants with RDS are typically given 100–200 mg/kg of phospholipids as the initial dose, and subsequent doses are given at 6- to 12-hour intervals if the patient remains intubated and is receiving 30% or more oxygen. In patients who are on noninvasive ventilation, a higher F_{IO_2} threshold (>0.40) is used for retreatment with surfactant. Poractant alfa, one of the most concentrated surfactants available on the market, is given at an initial dose of 200 mg/kg, using a small volume (2.5 mL/kg) intratracheally. Many trials have compared natural versus synthetic surfactants as well as studies comparing different natural surfactants. In a meta-analysis, treatment with natural surfactants, in comparison with synthetic surfactants, was associated with a significant reduction in pneumothoraces (37%), mortality (13%), and BPD (5%) (21). In a meta-analysis of two other studies, synthetic surfactants with added peptides did not show any significant difference in outcome in comparison with the natural, modified surfactants (22).

Among natural surfactants, there has been controversy regarding the efficacy of different forms. In a meta-analysis of 529 patients from five different randomized controlled trials (RCTs), a high-dose (200 mg/kg) porcine-derived surfactant (poractant alfa) was associated with a reduction in mortality by 71% and a reduction in surfactant redosing by 36% when compared with a bovine-derived surfactant (Beractant) (23). Six randomized, controlled trials compared treatment using beractant and poractant alfa and found that treatment with poractant alfa was associated with faster weaning of oxygen, peak inspiratory pressure and mean airway pressure, less need for redosing, lower incidence of patent ductus arteriosus and air leaks, faster extubation, and less BPD. Three retrospective studies comparing different natural, modified surfactants have been published to date. Clark et al. (24) showed no difference in mortality between beractant and calfactant. Ramanathan et al. reported significant differences in mortality between beractant-, calfactant-, and poractant alfa–treated infants. Treatment with beractant was associated with a 37% higher likelihood of death (statistically nonsignificant) and a 49.6% higher likelihood of death with calfactant when compared with poractant alfa–treated infants (25). In the third retrospective study involving 51,282 infants, there were no differences in mortality between these three commonly used surfactants in the United States (26). However, in this study, unadjusted

TABLE 47.1

COMPOSITION OF ANIMAL-DERIVED SURFACTANTS COMMONLY USED IN PRETERM INFANTS WITH RESPIRATORY DISTRESS SYNDROME

■ SURFACTANT	■ PREPARATION	■ PHOSPHOLIPIDS (MG/ML)	■ DSPC (MG/ML)	■ TOTAL PROTEINS (MG/ML)	■ SP-B (MG/ML)	■ PLMGN (MOL% TOTAL PL)
Poractant alfa (Curosurf)[a]	Minced porcine lung extract—purified via liquid gel chromatography	76	30	1	0.45	3.8 ± 0.1[4]
Beractant (Survanta)[b]	Minced bovine lung extract/DPPC, palmitic acid, tripalmitin	25	11–15.5	<1	Not specified	1.5 ± 0.2[4]
Calfactant (Infasurf)[c]	Bovine lung lavage/DPPC, cholesterol	35	16	0.7	0.26	Not specified[229]

[a]Curosurf (poractant alfa) Intratracheal Suspension prescribing information, Cornerstone Therapeutics, Inc, April 2010.
[b]Survanta (beractant) Intratracheal Suspension prescribing information, Abbott Laboratories, Inc, March 2009.
[c]Infasurf (calfactant) Intratracheal Suspension prescribing information, ONY, Inc, June 2009.
DSPC, disaturated phosphatidylcholine; PLMGN, plasmalogens; PL, phospholipids; DPPC, dipalmitoyl phosphatidylcholine.

patient outcomes by surfactant preparation showed the lowest rate of all adverse outcomes among poractant alfa–treated infants, including air leaks, death, and death or BPD as a composite outcome. These authors also reported a statistical difference between poractant alfa versus calfactant or beractant in the simple logistic regression models (air leak syndromes: calfactant vs poractant OR = 1.25 [1.13, 1.40], and beractant vs poractant OR = 1.47 [1.35, 1.61] for BPD or death: calfactant vs poractant OR = 1.04 [0.95, 1.13], and beractant vs poractant OR = 1.35 [1.13, 1.51]) (26). Based on the results from RCTs and large retrospective studies, treatment with poractant alfa is consistently associated with improved outcomes. This is more likely due to the use of a higher initial dose (200 mg/kg). Studies have shown that use of a higher dose with any of the surfactants has been associated with better outcomes (27–30). More recently, use of a 200 mg/kg dose of poractant alfa has been shown to result in longer half-life (32 vs. 15 hours), less need for redosing (28.6% vs. 70%) and lower oxygenation index (4 vs. 6.9) in preterm infants (31). Based on these findings, European consensus guidelines recommend early rescue surfactant using 200 mg/kg for the first dose in infants <26 weeks' GA with FiO_2 >0.30 and in infants >26 weeks with FiO_2 >0.40 (32). In addition, early rescue surfactant is recommended in infants with evidence of RDS, infants <1000 g whose mothers had not received antenatal steroids, and infants needing intubation during delivery room stabilization. The European Association of Perinatal Medicine has also endorsed these guidelines. Since prophylactic surfactant therapy is no longer recommended, newer synthetic surfactants with better resistance to inactivation in a smaller dosing volume for early rescue treatment of RDS are needed to avoid use of animal-derived surfactant preparations. A new synthetic surfactant with SP-B and SP-C analogs showed improved survival in preterm lambs (33). The first human study using this synthetic surfactant is currently recruiting patients in Europe (ClinicalTrials.gov NCT 01651637).

Newer Approaches to Surfactant Administration. Recent trials on the selective use of surfactant have demonstrated that there are some very premature infants who will not need it. Nevertheless, infants less than 27 weeks' gestation, more often than not, will be symptomatic enough to need surfactant.

In order to minimize invasive mechanical ventilation while at the same time giving neonates the benefit of exogenous surfactant, attempts have been made to apply less invasive techniques of surfactant delivery including the Intubate-Surfactant-Extubate (INSURE) and techniques that avoid endotracheal intubation altogether (modified INSURE). The INSURE technique involves a very brief period (minutes) of intubation for surfactant administration. During this period, the neonate is provided with positive pressure ventilation. In appropriately selected patients, INSURE failure rate, defined as need for reintubation, is only 9% (34). A randomized trial failed to show any difference in BPD rates with INSURE when compared with NCPAP at delivery and selective surfactant and prophylactic surfactant and prolonged mechanical ventilation (2). Techniques for surfactant administration that avoid endotracheal intubation include the surfactant aerosols and surfactant administration using catheters or feeding tubes and a laryngeal mask airway (LMA). Aerosolized surfactant was first described in the 1960s, but multiple technical problems in preparation and administration led to a decline in its use. Recently, aerosolized lucinactant has been used in a pilot study with a plan for a larger RCT (35). Trials using LMAs are also ongoing, although these are generally only feasible in infants >800 g weight (36). Evidence has accumulated regarding the feasibility of using a catheter to instill surfactant in spontaneously breathing infants. This technique has been pioneered in Germany, where the first RCT using such a method was conducted (16). In this study (the Avoidance of Mechanical Ventilation – AMV trial), newborns between 26 and 28 weeks' GA and with birth weight <1500 g were enrolled. Need for mechanical ventilation at 2–3 days of age was significantly less in the experimental group with a number needed to treat (NNT) of 6 (95% CI: 3–20, $p = 0.008$). The procedure was well tolerated, and no differences were noted in serious adverse events between the groups. The impact of techniques that avoid intubation on the rate of BPD is still being evaluated.

Noninvasive Respiratory Support in the Management of Respiratory Distress Syndrome. Modes of noninvasive respiratory support in newborn infants include nasal continuous positive airway pressure (NCPAP), synchronized inspiratory positive airway pressure (Si-PAP), noninvasive positive pressure ventilation (NIPPV), heated humidified high-flow nasal cannula (HFNC), and nasal high-frequency oscillatory ventilation (HFOV) (**Table 47.2**).

Nasal Continuous Positive Airway Pressure. Since its introduction in 1971, NCPAP has led to a significant improvement in neonatal mortality and morbidity (37). Along with oxygen, NCPAP is considered to be an intervention with the greatest impact on neonatal mortality due to RDS (**Fig. 47.3**) (38). NCPAP provides a constant positive pressure in the airways and, in doing so, splints the airway open, diminishes the work of breathing by reducing resistance to air flow, and helps in preventing lung collapse. NCPAP can theoretically limit atelectrauma and reduce lung inflammation. Animal studies as well as more recent human studies have shown the benefit of NCPAP soon after birth (12,39,40). NCPAP can be safe and effective and is often the only therapeutic intervention needed in selected patients with RDS (41).

Devices Available for Continuous Distending Pressure (CDP). NCPAP devices vary by the source of pressure generated and type of flow. Devices for providing NCPAP include CPAP using an underwater seal (bubble CPAP) ventilator–driven constant flow CPAP, and infant flow–driven variable flow CPAP (such as Infant Flow, CareFusion, Yorba Linda, CA). The source for NCPAP delivery can be important, for instance, variable flow devices have been shown to decrease the work of breathing in infants (42). The type of nasal interface is equally important and adds a level of complexity to the care of an infant on noninvasive respiratory support. Results from a meta-analysis suggest that short binasal prongs are better than single-nasal or nasopharyngeal prongs (43).

Nasal Continuous Positive Airway Pressure Settings and Weaning. Few RCTs have been conducted to determine the optimal settings, with some authors considering 5 cm H_2O NCPAP to be the lowest setting below which CPAP is likely to be ineffective (44). Using respiratory inductance plethysmography, maximum increments in tidal volume and thoracoabdominal synchrony are found with 8 cm H_2O NCPAP (45). The major issue with NCPAP is the high extubation failures and no reduction in BPD. Seven RCTs using NCPAP from birth reported NCPAP failure rates of 29.8%–67% (46).

Nasal Intermittent Positive Pressure Ventilation. Nasal intermittent positive pressure ventilation provides noninvasive positive pressure breaths (synchronized or nonsynchronized) in addition to NCPAP. Nasal intermittent positive pressure ventilation is often used in preterm infants to augment CPAP and as a way to manage frequent apneas. In experimental models and in clinical studies, even short durations of invasive mechanical ventilation are associated with lung injury, inactivation of surfactant, and arrest of lung growth and development (47–49). In experimental models, less lung tissue inflammation and injury have been noted with nasal intermittent positive pressure ventilation in comparison with invasive mechanical ventilation (50). Provision of PPV support

TABLE 47.2

DIFFERENT MODES OF NONINVASIVE RESPIRATORY SUPPORT

■ MODE	■ MECHANISM	■ TYPICAL SETTINGS
Nasal continuous positive airway pressure (NCPAP)	Provides continuous distending pressure, improves functional residual capacity (FRC), and stents open upper airway. By preventing alveolar collapse NCPAP also helps conserve surfactant.	4–8 cm H_2O
Synchronized inspiratory positive airway pressure (Si-PAP)	Provides "biphasic" CPAP, allowing infant to breathe at two levels of pressure, further augmenting the FRC. Synchronized Si-PAP (not available in United States) can be used to synchronize the "high pressure" with inspiration.	PEEP: 4–8 cm H_2O Peak inspiratory pressure (PIP): 8–15 cm H_2O
Nasal intermittent positive pressure ventilation	Provides a peak inspiratory pressure in addition to CPAP, thereby, augmenting ventilation.	PEEP: 4–8 cm H_2O PIP: 15–30 cm H_2O
Heated humidified high-flow nasal cannula (HFNC)	Reduces work of breathing by "washout" of nasopharyngeal dead space. Also produces distending pressure comparable to NCPAP.	2–8 L/min Pressure generated cannot be measured or controlled by the user.
Nasal high-frequency oscillatory ventilation (HFOV)	Augmentation of FRC. Theoretically, does not require synchronization.	Mean airway pressure (MAP): 8–14 cm H_2O (usually 1–3 cm H_2O above the MAP used during conventional ventilation) Amplitude: 20–40 cm H_2O; Frequency:10–15 Hz
Noninvasive neurally adjusted ventilator assist (NIV-NAVA)	Provides noninvasive ventilation proportional to and synchronized with diaphragmatic electric activity. Support is not affected by leak conditions at nasal interface.	PEEP: 4–8 cm H_2O NAVA level: 0.5–3 cm $H_2O/\mu V$; Electrical activity of the diaphragm (Edi) peak goal is 5–15 and Edi minimum is <3 cm H_2O

noninvasively is, therefore, better than invasive mechanical ventilation.

Nasal intermittent positive pressure ventilation can be synchronized or nonsynchronized. Theoretically, synchronization could augment the patient's own tidal volume and reduce the

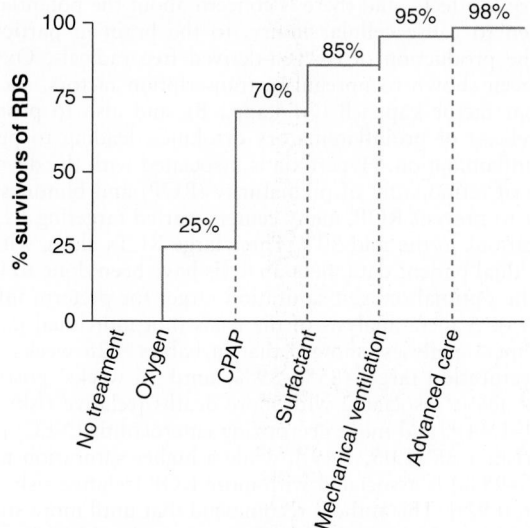

FIGURE 47.3. **Impact of different treatments on mortality related to respiratory distress syndrome (RDS):** Speculated increased percentage in RDS survivors with introduction of specific treatments. CPAP, continuous positive airway pressure. (Reused from Kamath BD, Macguire ER, McClure EM, et al. Neonatal mortality from respiratory distress syndrome: Lessons for low-resource countries. *Pediatrics* 2011;127:1139–46.)

work of breathing. Synchronization can be achieved by a variety of methods. The most common method used in clinical studies is a pneumatic capsule that detects abdominal movement to synchronize delivery of a breath (51–56). In one study, this capsule correctly detected an inspiration 88% of the time (56). Other methods of synchronization include flow trigger (affected significantly by leaks at patient interface), ventilator's inbuilt pressure trigger, respiratory inductance plethysmography, and diaphragmatic electromyogram (Neurally Adjusted Ventilatory Assist [NAVA]) (57–62).

Physiologic effects of synchronization include improvements in tidal volume delivery and work of breathing (51,60,62). One study showed improved thoracoabdominal synchrony with synchronized nasal intermittent positive pressure ventilation in comparison with nasal CPAP and CPAP, suggesting that synchronized nasal intermittent positive pressure ventilation provides better chest wall stabilization (63).

Outcomes Associated with Nasal Intermittent Positive Pressure Ventilation. While the long-term benefits of nasal intermittent positive pressure ventilation in humans are still being studied, in the short term, nasal intermittent positive pressure ventilation has been shown to decrease extubation failures in comparison with NCPAP (64). The effect of nasal intermittent positive pressure ventilation on apnea has not been well studied. When used as the initial form of respiratory support in RDS, nasal intermittent positive pressure ventilation is associated with a 40% reduction in intubation risk compared with NCPAP (65). Nasal intermittent positive pressure ventilation has also been used as postextubation support in order to reduce extubation failure rates. Use of synchronized nasal intermittent positive pressure ventilation in comparison with NCPAP has consistently been shown to reduce extubation failure rates in preterm infants, and a meta-analysis showed synchronized nasal intermittent positive pressure ventilation, in comparison with NCPAP, had 79% less reintubation rates (52–54,57,66) Another logical use of nasal intermittent positive pressure ventilation is in the prevention and treatment of apnea of prematurity. A meta-analysis of two trials suggested nasal intermittent positive pressure ventilation may augment the effects of NCPAP during severe apnea of prematurity (67). Regarding long-term effects, nasal intermittent positive pressure ventilation has been compared with NCPAP for the reduction of BPD, with one study showing reduced incidence of BPD with synchronized nasal intermittent positive pressure ventilation (52,54,57,59,68). The combination of early surfactant and early nasal intermittent positive pressure ventilation has been shown to reduce BPD in two studies (55,69).

Complications of Noninvasive Mechanical Ventilation.
Complications secondary to noninvasive ventilation are not uncommon. Nasal trauma and occasionally perforation of the nasal septum have been described (70). Pneumothorax has also been described when high pressures are applied (4). Gastric distension has been noted with both NCPAP and nasal intermittent positive pressure ventilation, but this has not affected feeding tolerance or time to full feeds (71,72). One report described an association between nasal intermittent positive pressure ventilation and gastric perforation, but this has not been replicated in the many trials where nasal intermittent positive pressure ventilation was used (68,73,74).

Heated Humidified High-Flow Nasal Cannula.
HFNC (flows >2 LPM) is increasingly being used due to its ease of use despite there being no documented benefits. With HFNC using heated and humidified gases, flows of up to 8 LPM have been used in newborn infants. The mechanism of action has been studied in humans and experimental models. HFNC is associated with an increase in transpulmonary pressure, and this effect is similar to the effect of CPAP (75). Pressure delivered by HFNC to the infant's pharynx, and possibly lungs, is associated with higher flow rates and possibly lower infant weight (76). Pressure delivery is not higher than NCPAP distending pressure in models where leak at the nasal interface was >50% (77).

Another proposed mechanism of action of HFNC is the reduction of dead space by nasopharyngeal washout. Because of relatively larger head size, infants have larger nasopharyngeal dead space compared with older children (78). In an experimental model, it was shown that HFNC causes flow-dependent improvement in oxygenation and carbon dioxide (CO_2) washout. These effects happened without an increase in tracheal pressure, supporting this hypothesis (77).

Clinically, HFNC has produced similar results to NCPAP in supporting infants less than or equal to 28 weeks' GA postextubation (79–82). The effects of HFNC on long-term outcomes, such as BPD are not known. There is also less nasal trauma with HFNC than with NCPAP (79,80). The major concern with the use of HFNC devices is the inability to control or measure the pressures delivered during HFNC use. In a study comparing two HFNC systems (Fisher and Paykel vs. Vapotherm), the pressures delivered were variable and unpredictable (83). At 8 LPM, mean pressures were between 4.1 and 4.9 cm H_2O with a standard deviation of 2.2 cm H_2O, meaning that 95% of the time, pressures were between 0 and 9 cm H_2O. In a meta-analysis of three RCTs comparing NCPAP with HFNC postextubation, there was no difference in extubation failures or BPD (84). In a study comparing noise levels during NCPAP versus HFNC, a trend toward increasing noise with increasing HFNC flow was reported (85). In a study comparing comfort levels using a neonatal pain and discomfort scale, there was no difference in comfort scores between NCPAP and HFNC in preterm infants (86). HFNCs are substantially more expensive than NCPAP systems. Complications, such as

air leaks, scalp emphysema, and pneumo-orbitis have been reported with HFNC (87). Nasal trauma can be minimized using a simple nasal interface, such as a modified nasal cannula (Neotech RAM nasal cannula) during NCPAP or nasal intermittent positive pressure ventilation. Until more studies are done, routine HFNC use in preterm infants should be considered experimental.

Noninvasive Ventilation with Neurally Adjusted Ventilator Assist NIV-NAVA.
NIV-NAVA is an interesting mode of ventilation that combines the benefits of NIV with true synchronization, where the patient controls initiation and termination of each breath as well as the rate and size of each breath. Significant reduction in BPD after implementation of NIV-NAVA has been reported. However, randomized, controlled trials are needed to evaluate the benefits of NIV-NAVA.

Nasal High-Frequency Ventilation.
Although first described in the 1990s, only the last few years have seen increasing evidence for the use of nasal high-frequency oscillatory ventilation (HFOV). Nasal HFOV has the theoretical advantage of not requiring synchronization with patient breaths. Nasal HFOV has been used with the same machines used to provide invasive HFOV, except that in the former, the interface is a nasal or nasopharyngeal prong. Small case series have elaborated the safety of short-term use of nasal HFOV in very low-birth-weight (VLBW) infants, while experimental models have shown better alveolarization with nasal HFOV in comparison with mechanical ventilation (88–91). Further trials are needed to establish the use of this novel form of noninvasive respiratory support.

Oxygenation and Ventilation Targets in Preterm Infants with Respiratory Distress Syndrome

Despite the advances attributable to prenatal steroids, surfactant, and newer modes of ventilation, RDS continues to be associated with significant morbidity, including the risk of BPD. New strategies have evolved over recent years to improve outcomes of preterm newborns with RDS. An aggressive approach to limiting exposure to hyperoxia is one of these widely adopted strategies. Oxygen is known to have numerous toxic effects, and there is concern about the potential for oxygen to cause cellular injury, to the brain in particular, via the production of oxygen-derived free radicals. Oxygen has been shown to upregulate transcription factors, such as nuclear factor kappa-B (NF-kappa B), and also to promote the release of proinflammatory cytokines, leading to persistent inflammation. Hyperoxia is associated with the development of retinopathy of prematurity (ROP) and blindness. In order to prevent ROP, many centers started targeting oxygen saturations in the mid-80's. Three large RCTs along with an individual patient data meta-analysis have been done to identify the optimal oxygen saturation target for preterm infants (92–95). A meta-analysis of the trials (not individual patient data meta-analyses) showed that in babies <28 weeks' GA, low saturation target (85%–89%) until 36 weeks' postmenstrual age is associated with more deaths [relative risk: 1.18 (1.04–1.34)], and more necrotizing enterocolitis (NEC) [relative risk: 1.25 (1.05, 1.49)], while a higher saturation target (91%–95%) is associated with more ROP [relative risk: 0.74 (0.59, 0.92)]. The authors recommend that until more studies are performed, oxygen saturation targets should be between 90% and 95% (96). However, these target ranges are arbitrary. Retinopathy of prematurity is clearly a biphasic disease with vaso-obliterative and vasoproliferative phases. Targeting low or high oxygen saturation during these two different phases of ROP may not be the optimal approach. Arora et al. (97) compared static (90%–94%) versus graded oxygen saturation (83%–89%) until 33 weeks' postmenstrual age (PMA) and 90%–94% until 36 weeks' PMA in a large retrospective study. They showed a significant reduction in severe ROP and BPD with no increase in mortality. Randomized, controlled trials using graded oxygen saturation targets during different phases of ROP are urgently needed to minimize the devastating impact of severe ROP and blindness globally.

Another recent change in neonatal practice is the adoption of permissive hypercapnia. Permissive hypercapnia involves allowing CO_2 levels in the blood to rise above the normal value of 40 mm Hg in order to minimize the pressures required for ventilation and thereby, hopefully, reduce the lung injury caused by ventilator-induced barotrauma. This practice also allows for infants to remain extubated who might have been reintubated in the past because of CO_2 retention. Although the range differs, CO_2 levels of 45–55 mm Hg are generally accepted, with some centers allowing higher CO_2 levels without changing ventilatory management. The side effects of this approach are unknown, but hypercapnia may decrease the autoregulatory capacity of cerebral vessels, resulting in a more-or-less pressure-passive cerebral circulation (98,99). This side effect is of concern primarily in the extremely low-birth-weight (ELBW; birth weight <1000 g) neonate during the immediate postnatal period. Therefore, the potential long-term neurodevelopmental effects of the hypercapnia-associated pressure-passive cerebral circulation need to be investigated.

Bronchopulmonary Dysplasia

Definitions and Epidemiology

Bronchopulmonary dysplasia (often referred to as chronic lung disease of prematurity) is the most common chronic lung disease of childhood. Northway et al. (100) first described the classic severe form of BPD in the late 60s. The BPD described in this publication (discussed in detail later in this section) was a disease that affected infants born at 30–35 weeks of gestation with a history of hyaline-membrane disease, significant ventilatory support, and prolonged oxygen exposure. Premature neonates born today are likely to be more immature and to have received antenatal steroids, postnatal surfactant, and a shorter period of mechanical ventilation than those born during the 1960s. In addition, with advances in neonatal care and technology, infants born at earlier and earlier gestational ages are surviving. Consequently, the chronic lung disease of prematurity has changed, and the classic severe form of BPD described by Northway is seen less frequently, if at all. An increasing number of small preterm infants are now surviving with a pathologically different form of chronic lung damage. This form has been described as "the new BPD."

The original description of BPD reported by Northway divides the process into four distinct stages. Stage 1 describes the early findings of hyaline-membrane disease, today referred to as RDS. Stage 2, occurring between the 4th and 10th day of progression of the disease, is characterized by atelectasis, alternating with areas of emphysema, and increasing opacification with air bronchogram on chest X-ray. In stage 3, typically present on days 11–30, permanent features of the disease appear, including bronchial and bronchiolar hyperplasia and cystic changes that were visible radiographically. The final stage (stage 4) presents after the first postnatal month and is characterized by the pathologic findings of extensive fibrosis and destruction of the airways and alveoli. At this last stage, radiographic findings consist of fibrosis and areas of both consolidation and overinflation.

In comparison with this "classic" form of BPD, the "new BPD" shows more uniform lung inflation on X-ray, and there is only minimal evidence of fibrosis. In ELBW infants, the lung is completing the canalicular phase of lung development at the

time of birth. It is believed that interference with the progress of alveolar development results in alveolar hypoplasia, the major abnormality described in the BPD of the premature infant seen today (47,101). In comparison with the classic form of BPD, characteristic features of the new BPD include the formation of alveoli that are *larger, more simplified, and fewer in number* and the presence of variable airway smooth muscle hyperplasia while there is a significant decrease in airway lesions and interstitial fibroproliferation (102). In addition, there is *arrest of vascular growth*, which in turn contributes to ventilation–perfusion mismatch and pulmonary hypertension. According to the "vascular hypothesis" proposed by Thebaud and Abman, lung angiogenesis, via the secretion of angiogenic growth factors, such as vascular endothelial growth factor (VEGF) and nitric oxide (NO), contributes to normal alveolar development (103). Noxious insults such as hyperoxia and inflammation cause a decrease in angiogenic factors, possibly contributing to reduced/arrested alveolarization (Fig. 47.4) (104–106). In experimental models, replacement with recombinant VEGF has been shown to improve alveolarization (107).

In addition to the changing pathophysiology of BPD, the definition of BPD has recently changed. The initial definition of BPD was a requirement for oxygen at 28 days after birth. At present, the definition has been revised to include the need for oxygen or ventilatory support at 36 weeks' corrected postmenstrual age (PMA) (108). In addition to this "clinical" definition of BPD, Walsh et al. proposed the use of the term "physiological BPD" to minimize variations of BPD rates between different centers. Physiologic BPD is diagnosed in infants, around 36 weeks of PMA, needing oxygen to maintain oxygen saturations > 90% (109). More recently, to describe respiratory status in infants who have passed the stage of surfactant deficiency and RDS but are not yet 36 weeks' PMA, the term "respiratory instability of prematurity" has been proposed by Bancalari and Jobe (110). These definitions are likely to be further refined as we learn more about the short- and long-term outcomes of new BPD.

Bronchopulmonary Dysplasia Incidence. Although severe BPD is now rare in infants born after 32 weeks of gestation, there is good evidence that the incidence of BPD is either staying the same or decreasing only minimally (111,112). In the

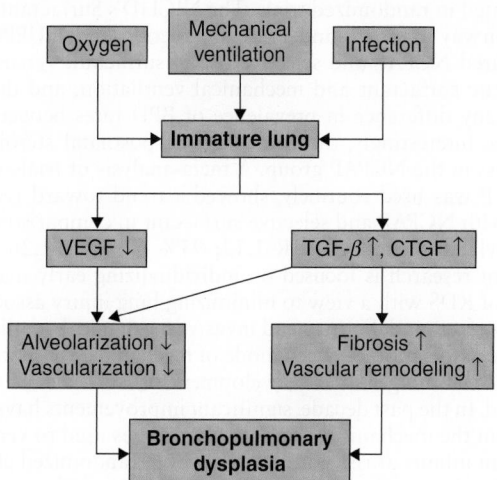

FIGURE 47.4. Bronchopulmonary dysplasia (BPD) pathogenesis. VEGF, vascular endothelial growth factor; TGF-β, transforming growth factor β; CTGF, connective tissue growth factor; ↑, increased; ↓, decreased. (Reused from Wu S. Molecular bases for lung development, injury, and repair. In: Bancalari E. *The Newborn Lung: Neonatology Questions and Controversies.* 2nd ed. Philadelphia, PA: Saunders/Elsevier, 2012.

National Institute of Child Health & Development (NICHD) network, the incidence of BPD at 36 weeks' PMA in ELBW infants has remained stubbornly unchanged at 40%–43%. Incidence of BPD is clearly associated with the younger GA, with 85% of infants born at 22 weeks having BPD, compared with 34% of infants born at 27 weeks having the diagnosis of BPD (112).

Etiology, Pathogenesis, and Prevention

Infants who are most commonly affected with the newer form of BPD are usually born very prematurely at less than 28 weeks of gestation. These infants typically receive antenatal corticosteroids and postnatal surfactant and initially do remarkably well, requiring low concentrations of supplemental oxygen and often only minimal ventilatory support for their initial RDS. However, subsequent complications thought to be due, at least in part, to the dysregulated production of inflammatory cytokines, shift the balance from developmentally regulated appropriate alveolar and vascular development to a process of premature maturation. This premature maturation of the lung is associated with an arrest in alveolar development and a loss of surface area for functional gas exchange. There is good scientific evidence that this disordered development of the lung parenchyma may lead to important abnormalities in lung function, which may persist throughout the first decade of life and beyond (113,114).

By far the most important factor in the pathogenesis of BPD is prematurity. In addition, intrauterine growth retardation places neonates at an increased risk (115). Evidence has been accumulating that suggests that prolonged mechanical ventilation plays a pivotal role in the pathogenesis of BPD. An inflammatory response can be triggered by mechanical ventilation–associated baro- and volutrauma, and free oxygen radicals. Invasive ventilation for 24 hours in newborn mice led to apoptosis, reduced alveolar septation (simplified alveoli), and blunting of vascular growth (116). Initial clinical evidence that noninvasive respiratory support might reduce rates of BPD came from a survey of centers that had variable rates of application of NCPAP in their units. NICU's that used NCPAP more than others had less incidence of BPD (117). In the current era of widespread surfactant and antenatal steroid use, such a clear benefit from NCPAP has not been replicated in randomized trials. The NICHD's Surfactant Positive Airway Pressure and Pulse Oximetry Trial (SUPPORT) compared NCPAP and selective use of surfactant versus prophylactic surfactant and mechanical ventilation, and did not show any difference in prevalence of BPD rates between the groups. Interestingly, the percentage of postnatal steroid use was less in the NCPAP group. A meta-analysis of trials where NCPAP was used routinely, showed a trend toward reduced BPD with NCPAP and selective surfactant in comparison with prophylactic surfactant (RR 1.12; 95% CI: 0.99–1.26) (12). Current research is focused on individualizing early management of RDS with a view to minimizing lung injury associated with surfactant deficiency and invasive mechanical ventilation.

The association between mode of mechanical ventilation of the preterm lung and the development of BPD has also been studied. In the past decade, significant improvements have been made in the mechanical ventilation strategies used to ventilate preterm infants at risk for BPD. However, randomized clinical trials have not yet identified the mechanical ventilation mode associated with the lowest incidence of BPD. Theoretically, HFOV, when compared with conventional ventilation, offers greater prospects for more uniform lung inflation, with fewer areas of lung overdistension and reduced atelectasis. Nevertheless, a reduction in BPD has not been found in a meta-analysis of randomized clinical trials comparing HFOV with conventional ventilation (118). This may be, at least in part, due to differences in HFOV strategy and the baseline incidence of BPD among the different trials (119–123).

The possible role of prenatal infection in increasing risk of BPD is still not convincing. The incidence of chorioamnionitis is as high as 50%–70% of very preterm births (124,125). Prenatal infection in the form of overt or subclinical chorioamnionitis was logically thought to expose the fetus to inflammation, which in turn could affect acinar and vascular growth in the fetal lung. In experimental models, such inflammation is associated with induction of fetal lung maturity, which in the short term has beneficial effects on lung compliance (126). In the longer term, such inflammation was associated with apoptosis and transient inhibition of alveolar septation (simplification of alveoli—a hallmark of "new BPD") and vascular growth (127,128). Prenatal exposure to steroids modifies the effect of chorioamnionitis on lung injury and repair. Betamethasone improved lung maturation in the presence of chorioamnionitis and allowed improved repair of alveolar epithelial cells following inflammatory injury (129–131). However, results are conflicting in clinical studies seeking to find an association between chorioamnionitis and BPD and are confounded by the lack of precise definitions of RDS, BPD, chorioamnionitis, and by inadequate history about the time of exposure and organism involved (132). An association between histologic chorioamnionitis and less severe RDS, but higher incidence of BPD has been reported (133). Lahra et al., (124) reported similar improvements in the severity of RDS with chorioamnionitis, but they reported a decrease in BPD incidence with histologic chorioamnionitis. Two large studies did not find any association between histologic chorioamnionitis and BPD (134,135). Van Marter et al. (136) reported a decrease in BPD unless there was prolonged ventilation (>7 days) or postnatal infection, thus showing the complex association between BPD and chorioamnionitis.

The association between oxygen toxicity and BPD has been known since the description of Northway and his colleague in the late 60s. Since that time, reports have continued to show an association between high supplemental oxygen exposure and lung damage in preterm infants receiving mechanical ventilation. The damage to the lung caused by oxygen toxicity appears to be mediated by reactive oxygen species such as superoxide anion, hydrogen peroxide, and hydroxyl radicals that are produced as molecular oxygen is reduced. In an elegant study, Vento et al. (137) showed that exposure to 90% oxygen in the delivery room, compared with 30% oxygen, increased the risk of developing BPD. The NICHD's SUPPORT trial found a lower incidence of BPD with the lower oxygen saturation group (oxygen saturation target 85%–89%) compared with the higher saturation group (oxygen saturation target 91%–95%) (93). In experimental models, the effect of hyperoxia on lung development is worsened by periods of hypoxia, a scenario very common in preterm infants (138).

Pharmacotherapy for Bronchopulmonary Dysplasia Prevention

Steroids for the Prevention of Bronchopulmonary Dysplasia. Dexamethasone was a key part of efforts to prevent and/or treat BPD for many years. Indeed, premature infants who receive postnatal corticosteroids demonstrated decreased levels of inflammatory markers, and clinicians have used corticosteroids in hopes of decreasing the incidence of BPD in high-risk populations. Although clinical trials have demonstrated short-term benefits, especially with respect to improving dynamic compliance and decreasing pulmonary resistance following treatment with corticosteroids, the overall impact on BPD remains controversial. Significant adverse effects of dexamethasone administration, especially when high cumulative doses are given to preterm neonates, include hypertension, hyperglycemia, adrenal suppression, decreased growth, and abnormal neurodevelopment. In addition, the concomitant use of hydrocortisone or dexamethasone and a prostaglandin synthesis inhibitor such as indomethacin has been associated with an increased risk of spontaneous intestinal perforation (SIP) during the first two postnatal weeks (139). As for the effect of postnatal administration of dexamethasone on neurodevelopmental outcome, early randomized trials showed that the administration of dexamethasone, in particular when given early and/or as a prolonged course, is associated with an increased incidence of adverse neurodevelopmental outcome (140–142). As a result, there was a significant decline in the use of dexamethasone during the neonatal period. Interestingly, use of less dexamethasone was also associated with increasing incidence of BPD (143,144). In a systematic review of 16 trials involving 1136 patients, higher dexamethasone dose reduced the relative risk of the combined outcome of BPD or mortality, with the largest effect in trials that used cumulative dose >4 mg/kg (145). In the moderately early treatment studies, the risk of mortality or cerebral palsy decreased by 6.2%, and the risk of a mental developmental index (MDI) below –2 SDs decreased by 6.6% for each incremental mg/kg cumulative dexamethasone dose. In a recent publication, Cheong et al. (146) reported a 15-year experience of using glucocorticoids (GC) and 2-year neurodevelopmental outcome. They concluded that despite the decreased rate of GC use (as well as total dose exposure) the rates of mortality or adverse neurodevelopmental outcomes remain unchanged, BPD rate over that time increased, and, therefore, factors other than GCs are likely to contribute to the persistent adverse outcomes. The adverse effect on the neurodevelopmental outcome seems to be modified by the underlying risk of developing BPD. In an update to their previous metaregression analysis, Doyle et al. (147) report that if there is a >68% chance of development of BPD, then there is more benefit than risk with the use of steroids (Fig. 47.5). In other words, in an infant who has a >68% chance of developing BPD, there is a greater likelihood of a poor neurodevelopmental outcome with not using steroids in comparison with using them. With validated models available for the prediction of BPD, clinicians should be able to make better evidence-based decisions regarding the use of steroids in an individual preterm infant (148). Dexamethasone is now reserved for patients with the most severe lung disease with

respiratory failure. Dexamethasone, if used at all, is now also given in lower doses and shorter courses than in the past. The American Academy of Pediatrics currently recommends that neonatologists counsel parents about the risks and benefits of dexamethasone prior to initiating treatment (149). Future studies need to be conducted to evaluate the effect, if any, of the newer treatment regimens on neurodevelopment outcome.

Hydrocortisone has also been used to prevent BPD. In a systematic review of 8 randomized trials in 800 patients using hydrocortisone in the prevention or treatment of BPD, there was no difference in BPD, mortality, or neurodevelopmental outcome. This review concluded that postnatal hydrocortisone cannot be recommended for the prevention or treatment of BPD (150). Currently, three large trials (ClinicalTrails.gov NCT00623740, NCT01353313, and NTR2768 from Netherlands) using hydrocortisone to prevent BPD (using doses ranging from 18.5 mg/kg to 72.5 mg/kg) are recruiting a total of 1986 patients in France, Netherlands, and United States. As for the side effects, the concomitant administration of hydrocortisone (just like that of dexamethasone) and indomethacin has been associated with an increased risk of SIP during the first two postnatal weeks (151). However, the findings of observational studies using MRI and neurodevelopmental and intelligence testing suggest that, contrary to dexamethasone, hydrocortisone given over three weeks in a cumulative dose over 50 mg/kg after the first postnatal week for the prevention and/or treatment of BPD in VLBW infants has no discernible effects at 7–8 years of age on cortical gray matter, white matter and hippocampal volumes, motor and sensorineural development, intelligence, and memory (152,153).

In summary, the use of steroids for the prevention of BPD requires careful risk–benefit analysis in each individual case. For infants most at risk for neurodevelopmental deficit associated with BPD, low-dose steroids may be considered beneficial, until the results from ongoing trials are available.

Nonsteroidal Agents. Many pharmacologic agents have been studied in randomized trials for the prevention of BPD. A recent systematic review has detailed these medications, and the reader is referred to the article for a detailed analysis of the benefits or lack thereof of these interventions (154). In brief, vitamin A, caffeine, dexamethasone, inositol, and clarithromycin have been shown to have a beneficial effect. Vitamin A requires

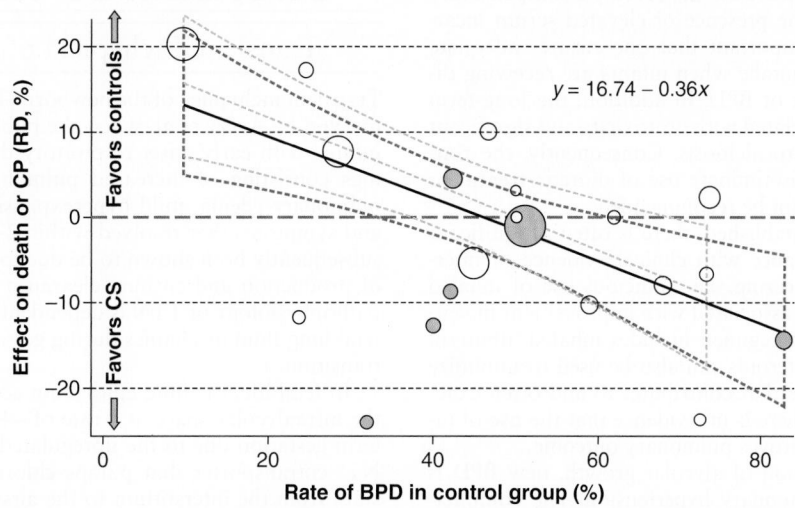

FIGURE 47.5. Association of corticosteroid and poor neurodevelopmental outcome modified by baseline risk of bronchopulmonary dysplasia (BPD). CP, cerebral palsy. (Reused from Doyle LW, Halliday HL, Ehrenkranz RA, et al. An update on the impact of postnatal systemic corticosteroids on mortality and cerebral palsy in preterm infants: Effect modification by risk of bronchopulmonary dysplasia. *J Pediatr* 2014;165:1258–60.)

intramuscular injection three times a week, which can be problematic in small infants. A beneficial effect of caffeine was found as a secondary outcome in the Caffeine for Apnea of Prematurity trial (155). Further studies are ongoing to understand further the effect of caffeine on BPD. Inositol and clarithromycin were studied in single-center randomized trials, and no other studies have been performed to confirm or refute these findings. Ibuprofen, a nonsteroidal anti-inflammatory drug, compared with placebo for patent ductus arteriosus (PDA) beyond 24 hours of life, is twice as likely to close the PDA compared with placebo, and was not associated with any benefit or harm on the short-term outcomes of NEC, any intraventricular hemorrhage (IVH), or death before discharge; however, ibuprofen use may be associated with an increase in the risk of BPD (~30% greater risk for BPD; RR 1.28; 95% CI: 1.03, 1.60) (156).

Management

The management and treatment of infants at risk for developing BPD should be directed toward (a) minimizing ventilatory support and alveolar overdistension, (b) supporting and maintaining adequate FRC with optimal positive end expiratory pressure, (c) optimizing growth, and (d) the judicious use of diuretics and bronchodilators. These goals can be achieved in part by employing optimal alveolar recruitment strategies to prevent atelectasis and sustain FRC, allowing as much as possible for synchrony between the infant and his or her ventilation and by embracing moderate permissive hypercapnia.

In addition, the optimization of growth and nutrition is essential to achieve early successful extubation. Careful attention to the infant's nutritional status is important for the promotion of lung growth. Diuretics have been used extensively to minimize pulmonary edema in the early stages of BPD. There is evidence that the use of loop diuretics such as furosemide improves lung mechanics and gas exchange in infants with established BPD. In addition, the use of thiazide diuretics, either alone or in combination with spironolactone, has been shown to improve short-term lung function and mortality in clinical studies and in a meta-analysis of these clinical studies, respectively (157,158). The major drawbacks to the long-term use of diuretics are the metabolic complications, including a diuretic-induced hypochloremic and hypokalemic metabolic alkalosis. The hypochloremic alkalosis induced by diuretics can be detected by evaluating the electrolytes and blood gases in chronic BPD patients. Over time, these infants develop a compensatory respiratory acidosis in the presence of elevated serum bicarbonate. It is therefore important that one ensures adequate chloride and potassium intake when infants are receiving diuretics for the treatment of BPD. In addition, the long-term use of furosemide is associated with ototoxicity and significant hypercalciuria and nephrocalcinosis. Consequently, the routine, prolonged, and indiscriminate use of diuretic treatment of infants with BPD cannot be recommended.

By the time BPD is established, there is often a significant increase in airway resistance with clinical evidence of intermittent or persistent wheezing. The judicious use of inhaled $\beta2$ adrenergic agonists is associated with improvement in ventilation. A common drug regimen includes inhaled albuterol therapy. Inhaled corticosteroids can also be used to minimize the inflammatory process that contributes to and often exacerbates BPD. However, there is no evidence that the use of inhaled corticosteroids improves pulmonary outcome.

In addition to inhibition of alveolar growth, new BPD is also associated with pulmonary hypertension. The combination of alveolar and vascular hypoplasia enhances ventilation–perfusion mismatch, leading to late-onset pulmonary hypertension in many ELBW infants. The management of this difficult problem is dealt with later in the section on *Pulmonary Hypertension*.

Implications for Long-Term Outcome

Fortunately, the mortality associated with BPD is significantly lower today than it was in the past (108,159). Nevertheless, it is estimated that the mortality rates associated with the most severe form of BPD and cor pulmonale can be as high as 40%. In addition, the morbidities are significant. BPD is a multisystem disorder that affects more than just the lungs and is likely to remain, for those infants afflicted, a life-long condition.

Long-term morbidities associated with BPD include airway damage as well as the cardiovascular complications such as pulmonary hypertension and cor pulmonale. Some patients with BPD require tracheostomy for long-term mechanical ventilation. Although alveolar growth accelerates in the first two years, infants with BPD often have a reduced pulmonary diffusion capacity and persistent impairment of expiratory flow in small airways (160,161). Unfortunately, there are reports of deterioration of lung function in adults who once had BPD (162). The implication of such reports is that infants with BPD need to be followed long into their adulthood.

In addition, in the long-term follow-up of preterm infants, BPD is one of the major conditions associated with poor neurodevelopmental outcome. However, it is not easy to separate the effects of BPD from the effects of immaturity and other complications associated with premature birth. It has been speculated that the recurrent episodes of hypoxia sustained by infants with significant respiratory disease and the effects of the dysregulated production of inflammatory cytokines on both the lungs and the brain explain, at least in part, the association between BPD and poor neurodevelopmental outcome. In addition, as previously described, the prolonged period of exposure to high concentrations of oxygen can lead to reactive oxygen species that may cause damage to the central nervous system again via triggering a dysregulated inflammatory response. Furthermore, infants with BPD are often exposed to several pharmacologic agents whose impact on the developing central nervous system has not been well established. Lastly, poor nutrition may also play a role in the poor developmental outcome of children with BPD; they are often challenging to feed, and their supraphysiologic caloric requirements are often difficult to consistently achieve.

DISORDERS OF TRANSITION

Transient Tachypnea of the Newborn

Transient tachypnea of the newborn (TTN) was first described in 1966 by Avery et al. when she published a series of 8 term infants with early-onset respiratory distress and X-rays findings consisting of increased pulmonary vascular markings, pulmonary edema, mild hyperexpansion, mild cardiomegaly, and symptoms that resolved within 2–5 days (163). TTN has subsequently been shown to be due to a delay in the cessation of production and ensuing clearance of fetal lung fluid. The pathophysiology of TTN is dependent on an understanding of fetal lung fluid mechanics during gestation and early neonatal transition.

In fetal life, the lung epithelium actively secretes fluid into the intraalveolar space at a rate of ~4–6 mL/kg/h by late preterm gestation due to the upregulated activity of the 2-Cl$^-$K$^+$Na$^+$ cotransporter that pumps chloride, sodium, and potassium from the interstitium to the airspaces. This rate of fluid secretion slows in the 1–2 days preceding the onset of labor due to increases in fetal catecholamine levels and the associated β-receptor mediated inhibition of the cotransporter in the lungs. The change in the hormonal milieu coincident with parturition changes the activity of other ion channels in the epithelium to actively absorb rather than secrete fluid primarily through activation of the Na-K-ATPase. Therefore, infants born by elective cesarean section (i.e., cesarean section without labor) are at a significantly higher risk of developing TTN and a significantly higher risk of overall pulmonary morbidity, most likely because they do not undergo the normal hormonal changes essential to the natural transition to extrauterine life, including a surge in epinephrine, norepinephrine, thyroid hormones, cortisol, etc (164,165).

Clinically, TTN presents with increased work of breathing, respiratory distress, hypoxemia, and CO_2 retention. The differential diagnosis includes sepsis, pneumonia, prematurity (RDS), pulmonary hypertension, congenital lung malformation, and congenital heart disease. The diagnosis of TTN is a diagnosis of exclusion. Early treatment is focused on supportive care with careful oxygen administration, positive pressure ventilation as needed, radiographs to rule out lung malformations, antibiotics while the infant is evaluated for sepsis, and an echocardiogram if indicated. TTN is, by definition, a transient disease, and although infants may appear clinically sick with moderate respiratory failure, initially they typically improve significantly within 8–24 hours. The initial chest radiograph findings of pulmonary edema, air bronchograms, and hyperexpansion also resolve within the same time frame, making X-rays an effective way to differentiate TTN from neonatal pneumonia as the X-ray findings in pneumonia will persist beyond the first 24–48 hours. There is a subset of infants presenting as TTN who may in fact have surfactant deficiency as well as abnormal surfactant function. In a recent study of term newborn infants with respiratory distress, surfactant deficiency was identified using lamellar body count in the gastric lavage fluid. If this finding is confirmed, surfactant assessment may become a useful tool in the management of TTN (166).

Persistent Pulmonary Hypertension of the Newborn

Persistent pulmonary hypertension of the newborn (PPHN) is a clinical syndrome characterized by failure of the normal pulmonary vascular transition to extrauterine life, resulting in increased pulmonary pressures, hypoxemia, and respiratory distress. Although the incidence is not precisely known, it is ~1–2/1000 live born births and continues to account for significant neonatal morbidity and mortality despite recent advances in available therapies.

In utero, the placenta, not the lungs, serves as the organ of gas exchange, and pulmonary resistance is maintained at or above systemic levels to maintain low pulmonary blood flow (estimated at 10% of combined ventricular output around midgestation and increasing to 20%–25% by term). Pulmonary vascular resistance is actively maintained despite a rapidly growing vascular surface area through constriction of the pulmonary vascular smooth muscle cells by a variety of pathways including hypoxia, endothelin-1, and thromboxane. As the fetus approaches term gestation, vasodilatory pathways are upregulated and become increasingly dominant. The most well studied and understood of these vasodilating pathways are the NO and prostacyclin pathways. NO is produced in vivo by the enzyme endothelial nitric oxide synthase (eNOS). NO then binds to soluble guanylate cyclase (sGC), which converts guanosine tri-phosphate (GTP) to cyclic guanosine monophosphate (cGMP). Increases in cGMP levels lead to vasorelaxation via a decrease in intracellular calcium. Cyclic GMP is inactivated by the phosphodiesterase (PDE) enzymes, specifically PDE5. Another pathway for pulmonary vasodilation is through prostacyclin. As an arachidonic acid metabolite, prostacyclin's rate limiting step involves the cyclooxygenase

enzymes, COX-1 and COX-2; however, the fate-determining step involves the enzyme prostacyclin synthase (PGIS). Prostacyclin activates adenylate cyclase to increase the production of cAMP from ATP, leading to decreased intracellular calcium concentration and thus vasorelaxation. The expression of eNOS, PGIS, and COX-1 are increased in the pulmonary endothelium as term gestation approaches, priming the vasculature to respond to vasodilatory stimuli (167–169).

At birth, multiple factors interact to regulate these pathways and dilate the pulmonary vasculature during the first few breaths, leading to an ~50% reduction in pulmonary resistance and a 5- to 10-fold increase in pulmonary blood flow. Critical signals for this transition are mechanical distension of the lung, falling carbon dioxide tension, and rising oxygen tension. Specifically, oxygen stimulates the activity of both eNOS and COX-1, leading to increased levels of the important vasodilators, NO and prostacyclin. Furthermore, the increased oxygen tension increases ATP release from red blood cells, which also activates COX-1 and eNOS. Significant derangements in metabolic homeostasis (i.e., acidosis, hypoxemia, or hypercarbia) will prevent the coordinated transition from vasoconstricting to vasodilating predominance from occurring normally, leading to the clinical syndrome of PPHN.

The most common precipitating diseases, most of which will be described in greater detail elsewhere in this chapter, are bronchopulmonary dysplasia, meconium aspiration syndrome, sepsis/pneumonia, perinatal depression/acidosis, abnormal pulmonary vascular development, pulmonary hypoplasia, and idiopathic "black lung" PPHN. In managing these patients, it is essential to have an understanding of the different etiologies of PPHN in order to tailor therapy appropriately. In congenital diaphragmatic hernia (CDH), both impaired alveolarization and arrest in pulmonary artery branching are noted. In addition, media and adventitia of pulmonary arterioles are thickened, contributing to pulmonary hypertension (170). Associated left ventricular hypoplasia and pulmonary venous hypertension make the prognosis worse. Finally, severity of pulmonary hypertension in CDH has also been linked to higher endothelin-1 levels (171). In BPD, pulmonary hypertension is considered a common complication, imparting a worse overall prognosis (170). The primary defect leading to pulmonary hypertension in BPD seems to be abnormal vascular development in an ELBW infant. In addition to impaired vascular growth, the vascular tone is also abnormal, and the high pulmonary vascular tone is worsened by recurrent hypoxia (172). In a cohort analysis, 11% of ELBW infants (birth weight ≤ 1000 g) who were >4 weeks of age were diagnosed with pulmonary hypertension, and 18% by 3–4 months (173).

The differential diagnosis of pulmonary hypertension includes congenital heart disease (most commonly obstructed total anomalous pulmonary venous return), sepsis/pneumonia, polycythemia, perinatal depression, and metabolic disease.

Initial treatment of the newborn with PPHN includes correction of metabolic derangements such as hypothermia, hypoglycemia, hypocalcemia, anemia, polycythemia, and hypovolemia. The use of alkalinizing agents is controversial, and induced alkalosis has been linked with adverse outcomes; however, correction of metabolic acidosis to physiologic pH is standard therapy (174). The appropriate use of vasopressor/inotropes (dopamine or epinephrine), inotropes (dobutamine) and lusitropes (milrinone) to support systemic perfusion (cardiac output) and myocardial function without inducing unwanted increases in the pulmonary vascular resistance (PVR) is important. However, the historical practice of using vasopressors/inotropes to drive the blood pressure to supraphysiologic levels in order to "force" the blood through the lungs cannot be recommended as concomitant increases in PVR may occur. Monitoring of the preductal (right arm or right side of the face) and postductal (lower extremities) saturations can provide a reasonable estimation of ductal level shunting and the severity of PPHN, assuming the ductus arteriosus is patent.

Specific Therapies for Persistent Pulmonary Hypertension of the Newborn

Oxygen. Oxygen is a specific, best known, and most commonly used pulmonary vasodilator in PPHN. Effectiveness of oxygen in vasodilating pulmonary arterial bed led to widespread use of 100% oxygen in PPHN. In the last decade, the problems associated with hyperoxia have been elucidated. In experimental models, hyperoxia does not result in additional benefit compared with normal oxygen levels. In fact, the best response was achieved with an oxygen saturation range of 90%–97% (175,176). Hyperoxia is associated with oxidant stress, which can cause alveolar damage and inactivate nitric oxide. It is therefore prudent to keep oxygen saturations in the normal range and avoid hyperoxia.

Mechanical Ventilation Strategy. The goal of mechanical ventilation is to achieve "optimal" lung volume and recruitment, tidal volume of 5–7 mL/kg or 9–10 ribs on chest X-ray, through the use of conventional or high-frequency oscillatory ventilation (HFOV) and to establish normal $PaCO_2$ levels and normal oxygenation. Failure to achieve lung recruitment at or above the FRC contributes to hypoxemia and high PVR. Conversely, hyperexpansion, particularly with the constant distending pressure of HFOV, may paradoxically worsen pulmonary hypertension by causing compression of capillaries and small arterioles and decrease cardiac output by interfering with venous return to the heart. There is some evidence that HFOV will improve lung recruitment in homogeneous lung disease and may improve delivery of nitric oxide to the alveolar surface (177).

Inhaled Nitric Oxide. Inhaled NO (iNO) has been shown in two large, multicenter RCTs to improve oxygenation and decrease the need for extracorporeal membrane oxygenation (ECMO) in term infants with hypoxemic respiratory failure and an oxygenation index (OI) of >25 when started at 20 ppm (178,179). Recent studies have looked at starting inhaled nitrous oxide (iNO) therapy earlier or at lower doses and have not shown any improvement in patient outcome when compared with this standard regimen.

Sildenafil. Sildenafil is an inhibitor of 5-phosphodiesterase (PDE5) and in doing so allows higher concentration of cyclic guanylate monophosphate (cGMP). cGMP is one of the most important vasodilators and is the target molecule for NO. Infants who have high concentrations of PDE5 are unresponsive to NO (173). Sildenafil use has been documented in case series in PPHN. These studies have shown sildenafil as having a good safety profile as well as being effective in improving oxygenation status (180,181). Sildenafil has also been used for the treatment of pulmonary hypertension in the setting of BPD and CDH (182–184). Long-term use of sildenafil in BPD became controversial after FDA issued a warning against its use in children aged 1–17 years (170). The basis of the warning was an increased mortality noticed in children with pulmonary hypertension (not due to lung pathology) receiving high-dose (around 8 mg/kg/d) sildenafil (185). Although the age group and underlying diagnosis are different than for infants with BPD, the warning led to uncertainty over the use of sildenafil in this disease. Later, the FDA clarified their stance on sildenafil use for children by stating that "health care professionals must consider whether the benefits of treatment with the drug are likely to outweigh its potential risks for each patient." Sildenafil has been used during the evolution of BPD in preclinical models to modify the severity of BPD or to prevent it altogether (186,187). Its use in refractory hypoxic respiratory failure in ELBW infants was associated with improved oxygenation, but also with pulmonary hemorrhage (188). The potential and limitations of sildenafil are likely to be determined in the coming years.

Other specific pulmonary vasodilators include prostanoids (PGI2, epoprostenol, treprostinil), milrinone (phosphodiesterase 3 inhibitor), and bosentan (endothelin receptor antagonist). These are currently used off label, and studies are underway to better describe their pharmacokinetics and utility in newborn infants with PPHN.

Extracorporeal Membranous Oxygenation (ECMO). ECMO remains the final rescue therapy for infants with PPHN. The United Kingdom ECMO trial published in 1996 was a randomized, controlled trial of conventional therapy with or without ECMO as rescue therapy. This trial was largely completed before the widespread use of iNO and showed a clear survival benefit with ECMO versus conventional therapy [RR of death 0.55 (0.39–0.77)] (189). More recent trials have looked at the effects of newer aggressive pre-ECMO therapy and not shown any changes in long-term outcome or time to discharge for infants who require ECMO despite aggressive pre-ECMO management (such as iNO, HFOV), at least as can be determined using the Extracorporeal Life Support Organization (ELSO) registry data (190).

Meconium Aspiration Syndrome

Approximately 13%–15% of all births in the United States are complicated by meconium stained amniotic fluid (MSAF) with about 3%–6% subsequently developing meconium aspiration syndrome (MAS). This translates to ~25,000–30,000 cases of MAS per year and makes MAS the most common cause of PPHN. Infants pass meconium in utero in response to stressful stimuli. A small subset of these infants that develop severe hypoxemia and acidosis and start gasping (second phase of apnea) will then aspirate the meconium stained fluid into their airway, setting up the scenario that can lead to MAS. MAS develops when an infant born through meconium stained fluid develops a subsequent pneumonitis leading to respiratory distress and PPHN. In infants who have significant MAS, it is important to consider the cause of the passage of meconium and to be alert to signs of perinatal depression.

The management of the delivery of infants born through MSAF has evolved over the last decade. The current Neonatal Resuscitation Program (NRP) guidelines no longer recommend (for infants born through MSAF) the routine suctioning of the oropharynx at the perineum (prior to delivery of the infant's body). It is, however, still recommended by the NRP that nonvigorous infants born through MSAF should be intubated and undergo tracheal suctioning by the neonatal team. It is also no longer recommended to intubate and suction vigorous infants. This recommendation is based on the study by Wiswell et al that showed that vigorous infants who had tracheal suctioning had no improvement in outcome but did have increased complications compared with those who were not intubated and suctioned (191).

Meconium appears to exert its toxic effect on the lung primarily through activation of the inflammatory cascade, resulting in the development of chemical pneumonitis. Meconium aspiration leads to the release of cytokines such as TNF-α, IL-1β, and IL-8 and activates the alternative complement pathway that directly injures the lung parenchyma, leading to vascular leak, pneumonitis, and pulmonary edema (192). There is evidence that meconium pneumonitis increases the postnatal release of endothelin-1 and thromboxane A2 and these potent vasoconstrictors worsen the pulmonary hypertension. Additionally, meconium can cause intermittent airway obstruction with a "ball-valve" effect. The combination of the inflammatory response, increase in vasoconstrictors, and the mechanical effect of meconium combine to make infants with MAS extremely sick, with increased need for support, decreased lung compliance, increased air trapping, and predisposed to pneumothoraces. The ensuing respiratory failure and the dysregulated production of vasoconstrictors prevent the normal drop in PVR required for the transition to extrauterine life and may result in severe pulmonary hypertension and hypoxia. The typical X-ray findings include patchy infiltrates with patchy areas of atelectasis and hyperinflation.

Initial management of infants with MAS includes supportive therapy with intubation, cardiovascular support, sedation, analgesia, and antibiotics. Corticosteroids have been studied extensively in these infants, and although it remains controversial, the evidence at this time does not support their routine use in MAS. Meconium has been shown in laboratory settings to inactivate surfactant and to displace it from the alveolar surface. Indeed, surfactant replacement therapy has been shown to be effective in improving lung compliance and oxygenation in infants with MAS and decrease the need for ECMO (193). Inhaled NO, the selective pulmonary vasodilator, is recommended for infants who do not respond to the above therapies. For further discussion, see the section on *Persistent Pulmonary Hypertension of the Newborn.*

CONGENITAL LUNG ANOMALIES

Congenital Diaphragmatic Hernia

Congenital diaphragmatic hernia (CDH) occurs in 1:2000 to 1:4000 live births and accounts for 1%–2% of infant mortality in the United States (194). The mortality for infants with CDH remains around 30% overall, although this is changing as the rate of antenatal diagnosis has increased and certain centers are currently reporting significant increases in survival. However, increased antenatal diagnosis is uncovering what Harrison refers to as the "hidden mortality" of CDH, i.e., a previously underappreciated rate of intrauterine fetal demise with CDH and an increasing rate of elective termination. CDH occurs due to a failure of closure of the pleuroperitoneal folds at around gestational week 5, resulting in a posterolateral diaphragmatic defect (Bochdalek hernia). The defect is most often on the left, although ~10% of the defects will be right sided and 2% bilateral. CDH is almost universally associated with lung hypoplasia primarily on the ipsilateral side (it is important to know that the contralateral side is typically hypoplastic as well).

CDH can occur as an isolated defect or, in ~40% of cases, in association with another major anomaly. CDH occurs as a feature of a number of syndromes that include Denys–Drash (mutations of Wilms tumor suppressor gene WT1), neonatal Marfan, Simpson–Golabi–Behmel syndrome (an x-linked recessive overgrowth syndrome), Beckwith–Wiedemann, Pallister–Killian (tetrasomy 12p), and Fryns. Animal models exist, but none completely mimic the human disease. The most studied animal model is the nitrofen-induced diaphragmatic hernia rodent model. Nitrofen, a pesticide, causes CDH in roughly 50% of the litter after feeding the toxin to the pregnant mouse or rat on embryonic days 8–11. The phenotype of this model includes CDH, pulmonary hypoplasia, conotruncal cardiac defects, and intestinal malrotation. Interestingly, some of the defects, pulmonary hypoplasia in particular, are seen in littermates who do not develop the diaphragmatic defects. The nitrofen model has been studied extensively to determine the genetics of the disease. Although the etiology remains unknown, there are interesting findings including increased expression of vascular cell adhesion molecule (VCAM), decreased expression of vascular endothelial growth factor

(VEGF), and downregulation of fibroblast growth factors 7 and 10 (195–197).

Antenatal screening has been useful to begin to stratify patients on the basis of risk. Important risk factors are the associated anomalies and the degree of pulmonary hypoplasia. In one series of 174 infants with CDH, 31 had major cardiac anomalies (including ventricular septal defect, aortic arch obstruction, Tetralogy of Fallot, and transposition of the great arteries), and only 4 of the 31 survived.(198) Currently, the best predictors of pulmonary hypoplasia are the lung-head ratio (LHR) and the presence or absence of liver herniated into the chest. The LHR compares the right lung volume at the level of the four-chamber view of the heart to the head circumference at 24–26 weeks' gestation, with LHR <0.6 predicting a 0% survival, 57% survival for LHR of 0.6–1.35, and 100% survival for an LHR >1.35 (199). Subsequent studies have confirmed a nearly universally fatal prognosis with an LHR <1 and a good outcome with LHR >1.4. Liver herniation into the chest, in comparison with liver in the abdomen is associated with a 9 times increase in mortality and >3 times increase in ECMO use (200). More recently, MRI of the chest has been used to assess fetal lung volume, and low fetal lung volumes are associated with increased mortality (201). The stratification of risk groups was developed for studies involving fetal intervention, the majority of which have looked at fetal tracheal occlusion. It is known that if the trachea is occluded in utero, the lungs become hyperplastic owing to the blockage of fluid egress from the lung, and the in utero intrapulmonary dynamics are altered. Wilson and DeFiore showed in separate studies using animal models of CDH that tracheal occlusion could lead to improved lung growth (202). Unfortunately, human studies using the in utero fetal tracheal occlusion strategy have failed to show benefit and have been complicated by an increased rate of premature deliveries. There is currently no role for fetal intervention for CDH outside of RCTs at experienced centers looking at novel fetal treatment strategies such as endoscopic intermittent tracheal obstruction.

When the presence of a CDH is known antenatally, the delivery room management focuses on immediate intubation and avoids bag and mask ventilation in order to minimize distension of the stomach and the proximal intestine that would add to compromised lung expansion and cardiac filling. The stomach should immediately be decompressed with a sump tube. Many centers will routinely paralyze and sedate the infants to prevent them from swallowing air and to limit activity during the initial stabilization. However, there is no evidence that the use of neuromuscular blockade in the delivery room (or later in the course) improves outcomes.

Even today, not all cases of CDH are diagnosed antenatally. A number of features should raise one's suspicion about the possibility of CDH in the newborn with early hypoxemic respiratory distress. On physical exam, breath sounds may be absent on the left side of the chest and the heart sounds shifted to the right, and the abdomen tends to be scaphoid because of some of the abdominal organs shifting to the thorax. It may be difficult to effectively ventilate and resuscitate the patient. A chest X-ray can confirm the diagnosis by demonstrating the presence of bowel loops in the chest.

Historically, it was felt that the infant with CDH constituted a surgical emergency and that the diaphragmatic defect should be repaired as soon as possible after delivery. The high operative mortality from early repair led to a shift in practice to provide time prior to surgery for the infant to be stabilized, the PVR to decrease, and associated defects or syndromes that are important in determining outcome to be assessed. The shift toward delayed surgery has occurred with little evidence other than the findings of two small studies that showed no change in outcome from surgery in the first 24 hours versus after the first 24 hours. However, in current practice, surgery is often delayed for weeks, not 1–2 days.

Ventilator management of CDH has also evolved on the basis of preclinical and clinical research data, but little evidence from RCTs. A major factor in the approach to providing ventilation for a CDH patient is pulmonary hypoplasia, and current judgment is to avoid barotrauma, limit peak inspiratory pressure to 24–26 cm H$_2$O, allow spontaneous ventilation, and allow permissive hypercarbia. It is well known that CDH patients have a high incidence of pulmonary hypertension; however, it is important to remember that the pulmonary vasculature in these patients is developmentally abnormal and hypoplastic and that attempts at aggressive ventilatory goals are likely to increase ventilator-induced injury rather than acutely lower the pulmonary pressures. Animal models of CDH show a relative surfactant insufficiency, but human studies of surfactant replacement demonstrate variable results, and data from the CDH registry at present do not support the use of surfactant in the term or near-term CDH infant (203).

As discussed earlier, selective pulmonary vasodilation with iNO has been studied and proven to be effective in patients with hypoxemic respiratory failure without CDH; however, its role in the CDH population is not as clear. The largest study of CDH patients with iNO was a subpopulation of the Neonatal Inhaled Nitric Oxide Study Group (NINOS) RCT of iNO. In that trial, there was no change in the combined outcome of death or need for ECMO with the use of iNO, but there was a trend toward an increase in ECMO utilization (204). These data have been interpreted in several ways, with some advocating that iNO stabilizes patients enough to allow for ECMO cannulation. Others question why patients with CDH did not have a sustained response and ask whether iNO actually made the infants less stable and thus more likely to require rescue therapy with ECMO. The answer remains unknown. Currently, iNO is widely used in the CDH population, and recent evidence from the ELSO registry supports the view that the pre-ECMO use of iNO does not worsen outcome (190). Given the lack of evidence of a sustained response, it is reasonable to restrict the use of iNO in the CDH patient to ECMO centers or to the stabilization of a patient for transport to the regional ECMO center. Late pulmonary hypertension remains a significant problem in the CDH population and is an active area of study. Researchers are looking at the role of pulmonary vasodilators such as sildenafil, inhaled prostacyclin, and chronic iNO therapy. However, there currently are insufficient data to recommend their routine use.

Congenital Cystic Adenomatoid Malformation and Bronchopulmonary Sequestration

Congenital Pulmonary Airway (Cystic Adenomatoid) Malformation

Congenital pulmonary airway malformation (CPAM), previously known as congenital cystic adenomatoid malformation (CCAM), is a relatively rare developmental abnormality. CPAM is believed to occur because of a failure of the normal bronchoalveolar development of the pulmonary mesenchyme between weeks 5 and 7 of gestation. The lesions are typically unilateral and isolated to one lobe, but can be bilateral in <10% of cases. Several classification systems exist for CPAM, but the most commonly used is the classification by Stocker:

Type 1: 50% of lesions, contains 1–4 large cysts, typically >3 cm
Type 2: 40% of cases, multiple small (<1 cm diameter) cysts
Type 3: 10% of cases, lesions appear solid due to multiple tiny cysts

CPAM is often diagnosed antenatally, and the information obtained from antenatal surveillance has helped to understand the natural progression of this lesion. The lesions typically grow significantly between 20 and 26 weeks of gestation and can lead to mediastinal shift and hydrops fetalis (most commonly seen with Type 3 CPAM or with a single dominant cyst). The development of hydrops is an extremely poor prognostic sign. Occasionally, the lesions regress as pregnancy develops. Routine ultrasound surveillance (approximately weekly during the period of active growth) is recommended for all types of CPAM.

Clinically, infants with CPAM present with a spectrum of illnesses ranging from severe respiratory failure to being asymptomatic. The severity of respiratory compromise cannot always be predicted antenatally. Initial management focuses on stabilizing the patient and confirming the diagnosis with a chest CT or MRI if possible. Surgical resection of the mass is recommended after stabilization. Timing of the surgery depends on the severity of the symptoms and ranges from 1 to 2 days to 4 to 6 months of age and asymptomatic cases are typically delayed. Eventual resection is recommended in all cases in view of the high likelihood of chronic infections within the lesion and a possibility of malignant transformation (reported to occur as early as 13 months of age).

Pulmonary Sequestration

Pulmonary sequestration is another cystic lesion of the lung differentiated from CPAM by the origin of its blood supply, which is systemic rather than pulmonary. In 15%–20% of cases, there are multiple feeding vessels. Sequestrations can be intrapulmonary or extrapulmonary. Sequestration is believed to occur due to development of an accessory lung bud. However, the exact etiology and timing are not known. Males are 4 times more likely to have sequestrations, which are typically unilateral and more commonly on the left. Many infants with sequestration are asymptomatic at birth, although sequestrations may be diagnosed early as part of an evaluation that is triggered by the presence of other congenital anomalies. Rarely, patients may be symptomatic due to enlargement of the lesion. Sequestrations present a significant risk for recurrent infections, which was how they came to medical attention before the availability of routine prenatal ultrasonography. Resection of the lesion is recommended in the first year of life, although exact timing depends on the case. Very rarely, a mixed lesion of CPAM and sequestration may present. The outcome and treatment of afflicted neonates usually do not significantly differ from those seen with CPAM or sequestration alone.

Pulmonary Hypoplasia

Pulmonary hypoplasia represents a broad spectrum of anatomic malformations ranging from total bronchial agenesis to mild parenchymal hypoplasia and may be either primary or secondary to other lesions. Primary pulmonary hypoplasia is typically unilateral and not associated with other malformations. Secondary pulmonary hypoplasia is, by definition, associated with other malformations such as CDH (as discussed earlier), skeletal or neuromuscular disease with decreased fetal movement (an important stimulus to lung growth), and oligohydramnios sequence. The latter will be the focus of this section.

Oligohydramnios is associated with either renal disease in the neonate or chronic amniotic fluid leak. Fetal urine output becomes the primary source of amniotic fluid after about 20–22 weeks of gestation; before that the amniotic fluid is primarily produced by the placenta. Infants with bilateral renal agenesis, bilateral dysplastic kidneys, or obstructive uropathies have severe oligohydramnios due to the lack of fetal urine output. These infants have characteristic facial features and limb contractures that were initially described in 1946 by Potter and are known by the eponym "Potter Syndrome" (205). These patients represent the most severely affected neonates and often have fatal lung hypoplasia and frequently suffer multiple pneumothoraces after birth. Fetal intervention in infants with obstructive uropathy usually involves a stent placed in the bladder to drain the urine into the amniotic cavity, restoring the amniotic fluid in the uterus and removing the pressure on the kidneys. Results to date have been mixed; however, it remains an active area of investigation and is a promising future therapy.

Oligohydramnios related to amniotic fluid leak appears to have a slightly different pathophysiology, and the degree of pulmonary hypoplasia is very difficult to assess antenatally. Although the difference in pathophysiology remains incompletely understood, it is postulated that because the infants are still creating urine, the amniotic fluid volume is variable, and therefore the effect on lung growth is also variable. In these infants, the degree of pulmonary hypoplasia must be assessed postnatally by the ability to oxygenate and ventilate the infant. Management is focused on limiting barotrauma while assessing the degree of lung hypoplasia and associated anomalies.

ACQUIRED DISEASE

Air Leak Syndrome

Air leak syndromes represent one of the most serious complications of assisted ventilation in the neonate. Air leaks begin with the rupture of alveoli or distal airways associated with high ventilation pressures and severe lung disease. They can occur suddenly (often complicating the treatment of RDS) and may be life-threatening if not rapidly identified and addressed.

Pulmonary Interstitial Emphysema (PIE)

PIE is a consequence of the overdistension of distal airways and usually occurs in the tiniest, most immature babies. Inspired gas distribution is not uniform in infants with severe parenchymal lung disease. The majority of the volume of each breath is preferentially distributed to more compliant lung units. As a consequence, the more compliant lung units become overdistended and rupture. The ruptured airways provide a pathway for leakage of air into the connective tissue sheets. It is this accumulation of air within those airway sheets that results in the radiographic findings of PIE (discussed below). As air moves within the connective tissue sheet around the airways, the free air can further track along the sheets toward the hilum of the lung. As the PIE increases, the volume of gas within the lung parenchyma causes a decrease in lung compliance. In addition, airway resistance increases as a result of air trapped within the interstitium. An increased need for ventilation typically occurs as the result of increased respiratory dead space and reduced minute ventilation. Hypoxemia results from the reduction in alveolar ventilation as well as from ventilation–perfusion mismatch secondary to obstruction of the airways by interstitial air. Death may occur secondary to an inability to achieve adequate ventilation and oxygenation.

The diagnosis of PIE is made radiographically based on the characteristic linear and cyst-like radiolucencies that reflect the accumulation of interstitial air (206). PIE may involve a single lobe, one lung or both lungs. The linear radiolucencies are coarse and rarely appear to branch. They must be differentiated from the smooth, branching, perihilar air bronchograms often seen with RDS. The cyst-like radiolucencies of PIE take the appearance of small bubbles, typically vary in size from ½ to 4 mm in diameter, and are often present in large numbers.

There is no precise treatment for PIE. Given the pathophysiology of the air leak, it is not surprising that neonatologists have used ventilatory techniques to minimize alveolar and airway distension in order to prevent PIE. When PIE is unilateral, it is often suggested that the infant be positioned with the affected side down. When PIE is bilateral or extensive, one can attempt to decompress the air leaks by using a short inspiratory time, low inflation pressures, and small tidal volumes. With the use of these techniques over time, the lungs will slowly deflate, and areas of overdistension should improve. One drawback of this approach is that it is often difficult to achieve optimal or even adequate oxygenation and ventilation while allowing for the collapse of the PIE-affected areas of lung. There is literature to suggest that high-frequency ventilation may allow for adequate ventilation and oxygenation in infants with PIE at lower peak and mean airway pressures than with conventional ventilation (207).

Pneumomediastinum and Pneumothorax

Although tightly associated with assisted ventilation and RDS (as is PIE), pneumothorax and pneumomediastinum may also occur spontaneously. Interestingly, 3%–5% of normal term newborns present with asymptomatic, spontaneous, nontension pneumothoraces during the first few postnatal hours. These pneumothoraces are thought to be a consequence of the large negative intrapleural pressure generated by the newborn at the first few breaths that are required to inflate the lungs immediately after delivery. In neonates with lung disease, it is believed that up to 10% develop an air leak syndrome as a result of poor lung compliance and the need for mechanical ventilation. Pneumomediastinum usually occurs when air tracks through the peribronchial cuffs to the hilum of the lungs, at which point air ruptures into the mediastinum. The accumulation of air through the mediastinum into the pleural space can produce a tension pneumothorax. When the collection of air is constrained to the mediastinum, it is unusual for the volume of air to primarily cause circulatory compromise. This is in part because the air can dissect from the mediastinum into the soft tissue, typically of the neck, producing subcutaneous emphysema. In contrast, tension pneumothorax can result in exceedingly high intrapleural pressures, collapse of the ipsilateral lung, hypoxia, hypercapnia, and mediastinal shift. The mediastinal shift of intrathoracic structures can impede cardiac output and lead to cardiovascular collapse. In the preterm neonate, the development of a tension pneumothorax is also associated with an increased incidence of peri/intraventricular brain hemorrhage.

The diagnosis of pneumothorax and/or pneumomediastinum is easily confirmed by clinical examination and chest radiograph. Isolated pneumomediastinum is often asymptomatic or associated with mild respiratory symptoms. With a pneumothorax, infants are usually symptomatic with signs of respiratory distress (tachypnea, retractions, grunting, flaring), cyanosis, and poor perfusion. Bedside evaluation may reveal tachycardia with a narrow pulse pressure. It is important to note that differential breath sounds are an unreliable marker for the diagnosis of pneumothorax in infants. An acute clinical deterioration in a mechanically ventilated infant should prompt an urgent search for the possibility of an air leak.

Transillumination of the chest can sometimes be used to make the diagnosis of an air leak, but if time allows, the diagnosis should be confirmed by chest radiograph. Nitrogen washout is a therapy used for stable, minimally symptomatic nonmechanically ventilated neonates with air leak. The infant is often placed on 100% inspired oxygen, typically delivered via an oxyhood, and monitored closely for resolution of the air leak. Recent studies of infants with spontaneous pneumothorax did not show any difference in time to resolution between room air and a 100% oxygen washout technique (208,209). Infants in room air remained so and did not require supplemental oxygen (209). Owing to the toxicity associated with the use of 100% oxygen, the risks of using it for the nitrogen washout technique may outweigh the risks associated with chest tube placement, especially in the unstable preterm infant where recurrence of the pneumothorax is likely. Tube thoracotomy is indicated in neonates with cardiorespiratory compromise or those receiving mechanical ventilation. Needle aspiration may be useful for acute relief of a tension pneumothorax, but is usually followed by chest tube placement, especially in the setting of high mean airway pressure, to allow for continued evacuation of the air leak while the lung tissue is healing. Expectant management with needle aspiration alone could be tried in infants on low ventilatory settings (210). The chest tube is typically connected to 10–20 cm H_2O of suction pressure, and drainage and radiographs are monitored to determine the timing of resolution of the air leak and readiness for removal of the tube.

Pulmonary Hemorrhage

Pulmonary hemorrhage has been associated with a wide range of predisposing conditions including prematurity, mechanical ventilation, sepsis, PDA, and asphyxia. Although commonly referred to as pulmonary hemorrhage, the process actually reflects a hemorrhagic pulmonary edema in most cases. Studies done more than 30 years ago compared the hematocrit and protein composition of the hemorrhagic fluid obtained from the lungs with arterial and venous samples of blood from infants with pulmonary hemorrhage, and concluded that the lung effluent was usually hemorrhagic edema rather than whole blood (211). The pathophysiology may involve acute injury to the left ventricle that results in left ventricular failure, increased filtration pressure, subsequent injury to the pulmonary capillaries, and marked capillary leak. Pulmonary hemorrhage in sepsis is likely related to endotoxin release and consequent increased pulmonary microvascular permeability. There is also a known association between pulmonary hemorrhage and surfactant administration, especially in the presence of a PDA. It is thought that the increased risk of developing hemorrhagic pulmonary edema after surfactant results from the rapid and significant decline in the PVR associated with surfactant administration and the subsequent increase in the left-to-right shunting through the PDA, resulting in severe pulmonary overcirculation.

The earliest clinical sign of pulmonary hemorrhage is usually the detection of blood-tinged secretions from the endotracheal tube. The amount of bloody fluid seen may be minimal or copious. On occasion, pulmonary hemorrhage can be dramatic, and fluid that resembles whole blood may egress in large volumes from the trachea. Chest radiograph may reveal fluffy infiltrates consistent with pulmonary edema, and there is often a clinical deterioration in the infant's respiratory status.

Treatment of pulmonary hemorrhage involves clearing the airway to prevent frank obstruction from the hemorrhagic fluid and adjusting support in order to provide adequate oxygenation and ventilation. However, every effort should be made to avoid unnecessary suctioning of the trachea, which may exacerbate the bleeding. Increasing the mean airway pressure, typically achieved by increasing the positive end-expiratory pressure (PEEP) on the ventilator, may help prevent the continued flow of blood into the trachea. Laboratory tests should be done to evaluate for the presence of coagulopathy or infection as well as to monitor the hematocrit. In most cases, packed red blood cell transfusion is unnecessary (the additional volume may worsen the pulmonary edema and hemorrhage). Therefore, volume administration in hypotensive neonates with pulmonary hemorrhage should be avoided

if possible, at least in the period immediately following the development of the hemorrhage. There is evidence to suggest that pulmonary hemorrhage causes increased surface tension and surfactant dysfunction and that there may be some benefit from administration of surfactant (212–214).

Pulmonary Edema

Pulmonary edema describes the abnormal accumulation of fluid in the pulmonary interstitium and alveolar spaces that can compromise oxygenation and ventilation. Fluid in the lungs normally flows from capillaries running in the alveolar septae into the pulmonary interstitium as a result of the gradient between the hydrostatic and oncotic pressures of the microvasculature and interstitium. The fluid is drained from the interstitium by lymphatic channels and thus returns to the intravascular space. Under normal conditions, fluid does not accumulate within the interstitium. However, if lymphatic drainage does not keep pace with filtration or if the alveolar membrane is injured, pulmonary edema can occur.

Pulmonary edema occurs in neonates in association with a variety of pathologic processes. Increased hydrostatic filtration pressure as a result of increased left atrial pressure is a common cause. Left atrial pressure may be elevated as a result of volume overload, presence of a PDA with left-to-right shunting, or obstruction to outflow due to congenital heart disease and abnormal anatomy. There is some evidence to suggest that increased filtration pressure from heart failure is the cause of the pulmonary edema seen with perinatal hypoxic ischemic injury. Pulmonary edema associated with sepsis likely results from increased capillary endothelial permeability caused by activated neutrophils and other inflammatory mediators.

Pulmonary edema may occur during either the acute or the chronic periods of a preterm infant's NICU course. During the early postnatal period, pulmonary edema is associated with both PDA and RDS. With the significant decreases in PVR following delivery, a left-to-right shunt of blood flow takes place at the level of the ductus; significantly increased pulmonary blood flow can cause an increase in fluid filtration that leads to edema. Studies have shown an association (but not causation) between PDA patency and BPD. In addition, there is evidence that implicates altered epithelial permeability in the pathogenesis of pulmonary edema in neonates with RDS (215).

Pulmonary edema also complicates the management of patients with BPD and may occur for a number of reasons. A diminished pulmonary capillary bed or hypoxia (both seen in patients with BPD) may cause increased PVR. In addition, there is evidence to suggest that patients with BPD have abnormal plasma oncotic pressure, perhaps due to inappropriate control of vasopressin secretion or to poor nutritional status (216). Capillary permeability may also be increased as a consequence of damage to the endothelium from the dysregulated release of proinflammatory cytokines and chemokines, infection, baro- and volutrauma, or oxygen toxicity. Long-term cardiac complications of BPD (cor pulmonale and left ventricular dysfunction) may contribute to and cause increased lymphatic and left atrial pressures.

Pulmonary edema may significantly complicate the respiratory management of the neonate. Every effort should be made to optimize nutrition and minimize barotrauma and excessive supplemental oxygen exposure during the patient's course. One must maintain a high degree of suspicion for persistent patency or reopening of the ductus arteriosus in VLBW neonates during the first days and weeks after delivery. Diuretics are frequently used as therapy for pulmonary edema to improve oxygenation and ventilation. Diuretics, especially furosemide, produce a diuresis of the water in the intravascular space, which causes fluid from the pulmonary interstitium to flow back into the intravascular space. Furosemide is typically used as the first-line agent of choice, but, as discussed earlier, chlorothiazide and spironolactone are frequently preferred for the management of the chronic phase of BPD, especially in the outpatient setting, in order to minimize the requirement for potassium and chloride supplementation, reduce the need for outpatient blood work to monitor electrolyte values, and to decrease the risk of sensorineural hearing loss associated with chronic furosemide administration.

Airway Injury

Despite the current trend toward early extubation and aggressive use of noninvasive mechanical ventilation, a prolonged duration of mechanical ventilation is often necessary for the survival of many of the sickest preterm infants. The impact of intubation and ventilation on lung development in the preterm neonate has been discussed earlier. Prolonged intubation carries the risk of significant upper airway complications. For instance, marked stridor following extubation or a history of repeated failure to successfully extubate in an infant may be due to airway injury secondary to the long-term intubation. Injury can occur due to mucosal irritation from the endotracheal tube over time or from damage at the time of intubation and can range from edema, ulcerations, and granulations to vocal cord paralysis and subglottic stenosis. Studies have reported ulceration and granulation in 44%–47% of infants surviving after prolonged intubation (217). There is also a risk of necrotic damage to the trachea or bronchi with high-frequency jet ventilation, especially if humidification of the inspired gas is inadequate.

Clinical subglottic stenosis was once reported to occur in as many as 9% of intubated neonates, but more recent reports estimate the incidence at <2% (218). Stenosis is thought to occur as a result of trauma or ischemia to the subglottis. The injury begins in areas where the tube compresses the airway mucosa and reduces blood flow. Eventually, areas of ischemia ulcerate, exposing the underlying cartilage. The cartilage can become infected, and scarring and stenosis result with healing of the ulcerated and infected areas. The posterior subglottis is the region most commonly affected in neonates.

Efforts should be made to minimize trauma to the airway during hospitalization, particularly during intubation attempts. Endotracheal tubes should be upsized only if a leak around the endotracheal tube is compromising adequate ventilation and the larger tube passes easily through the subglottis. A brief course of periextubation dexamethasone has been shown to decrease postextubation stridor in preterm neonates at high risk for subglottic edema (219). Nebulized racemic epinephrine also helps to reduce stridor in the acute setting after extubation although it carries the risk of rebound edema formation once the medication is discontinued. In some cases, these interventions are not enough to allow for safe, adequate gas exchange, and reintubation may be necessary. In such circumstances, the airway should be evaluated. Typically, the initial evaluation is at the bedside by flexible bronchoscopy, but rigid laryngoscopy in the operating room is often indicated to more completely visualize the extent and location of injury to the airway. Even when there is a history of numerous failed extubation attempts in the past, extubation is sometimes successful when reattempted after allowing time for growth and healing and if CPAP or nasal or nasopharyngeal intermittent assisted ventilation is used after extubation. Surgical intervention may be necessary when the laryngotracheal injury continues to impair oxygenation and/or ventilation. Surgical options include an anterior cricoid split or tracheostomy. Tracheostomy in infants chronically dependent on a ventilator due to BPD are associated with a high rate of neurodevelopmental

deficit or death (220,221). This is primarily related to underlying prematurity and severe BPD. Nevertheless, the timing of tracheostomy has been studied in relation to neurodevelopmental outcomes and death. The retrospective study by NICHD showed an association between early tracheostomy (<120 days) and improved neurodevelopmental outcome and survival (221).

Infection

Neonatal sepsis occurs in 1:1000 term and 1:4 preterm infants. Pneumonia, either congenital or acquired, frequently coexists with sepsis in the newborn period. The immature immune system puts the neonate at increased risk for infection, and pneumonia is a particularly significant cause of morbidity and mortality in the newborn. The preterm infant, whose immune system is markedly immature and who has diminished levels of serum immunoglobulin concentrations compared with the term newborn, is at very high risk for infection. Risk factors for early-onset sepsis include premature delivery, multiple pregnancy, prolonged rupture of amniotic membranes (>18 hours), maternal fever, maternal Group B Streptococcus (GBS) colonization, and chorioamnionitis. Nosocomial pneumonia, unfortunately a relatively common complication, is associated with mechanical ventilation and prolonged hospital stays. Both congenitally acquired and nosocomial pneumonias may have long-term ramifications for survivors. A growing body of evidence points to the connection between infection and the development of BPD (see earlier section on *Bronchopulmonary Dysplasia*).

Congenital Pneumonia. Congenital pneumonia frequently coexists with sepsis and is a significant source of morbidity and mortality in neonates. Infection is typically acquired when organisms ascend into the uterine cavity, either during or prior to labor, and come into contact with the fetus. Consequently, prolonged rupture of membranes is a significant risk factor for neonatal sepsis. The lungs may become infected when the fetus swallows infected amniotic fluid. Infection can occur even when membranes are intact until just prior to delivery. Transmission of bacteria can occur hematogenously, from the mother's blood via the placenta, or via aspiration of organisms at the time of delivery as the newborn passes through the birth canal.

GBS is the primary pathogen causing early-onset neonatal pneumonia in the United States. Premature infants are at increased risk for infection, and the mortality rate is higher than in term infants. In 1996, the Centers for Disease Control and Prevention (CDC) developed guidelines for screening pregnant women for GBS colonization at 35–37 weeks' gestation. The rate of GBS colonization is estimated to be 20%–30% for American women. It is currently recommended that colonized women and those with other risk factors for neonatal sepsis be given intrapartum antibiotic therapy beginning at least 4 hours prior to delivery. The incidence of early-onset GBS infection has been reduced by 65% in communities that have adopted the CDC GBS-prevention guidelines and is now reported to be as low as 0.37 per 1000 live births. A recent study indicates that the majority of cases of early-onset GBS infection in the era of intrapartum GBS prophylaxis occur in mothers who tested negative for GBS at the time of screening (222). Other organisms that may cause pneumonia in the neonate include gram-negative organisms, particularly *Escherichia coli*, group D streptococcus, listeria, pneumococci, staphylococcus species, and fungus. Chlamydia, although acquired congenitally, typically presents as pneumonia at several weeks of age rather than in the immediate postnatal period. Recently, there has been a renewed interest in the possibility that peripartum transmission of *Ureaplasma urealyticum* to the respiratory tract of the preterm neonate may contribute to the development of severe respiratory failure and/or BPD (223). Although more typically a cause of late-onset pneumonia in neonates, viruses (herpes simplex, enterovirus, adenovirus, in particular) can also cause congenital pneumonia and may have a severe and sometimes fatal course.

It can be difficult to make a definitive diagnosis of pneumonia in the neonate. Neonates may present with respiratory distress at birth (or shortly after birth) for a wide range of reasons unrelated to infection. Tachypnea, retractions, grunting, and cyanosis can all result from processes as varied as TTN, RDS, CDH, pneumothorax, and polycythemia. In addition, neonates with pneumonia can present without focal respiratory signs, demonstrating only temperature instability (typically hypothermia), glucose instability, or jaundice. Fever and cough, frequent findings in older patients, are uncommon in newborns with bacterial pneumonia.

It is often difficult to obtain bacterial confirmation of pneumonia in the neonate. Tracheal culture may not isolate the pathogen. However, the presence of many white blood cells on the aspirate may signal the presence of infection, and growth of an isolated organism can guide therapy. Blood cultures should be sent to evaluate for bacteremia and can help determine appropriate coverage when there is culture growth. A chest radiogram is indicated to evaluate for infiltrates, although it is often difficult to differentiate an infiltrate from atelectasis, RDS, retained lung fluid, or the edema seen with certain cardiac anomalies. Serial radiograms may be useful in differentiating the various processes. Appearance of an infiltrate may lag behind the onset of clinical symptoms by 24–48 hours. *Staphylococcus aureus* pneumonia is classically associated with empyema and pneumatocele formation. A decreased or elevated white blood cell count and/or a predominance of immature white blood cell forms are suggestive of infection. Although nonspecific, an elevated c-reactive protein (CRP) indicates the presence of an infectious or inflammatory process, and there are copious data to support the value of the CRP in the evaluation of infection in the neonate.

It is standard for antibiotic therapy to be started prior to the determination of a definitive diagnosis of pneumonia in the neonate. Treatment is usually begun as soon as respiratory symptoms develop or concerning lab findings in an infant at risk for sepsis are identified. Typical treatment pending identification of the pathogen is broad spectrum, consisting of a penicillin in addition to an aminoglycoside. Coverage should be narrowed if the causative organism is identified. The appropriate duration of antibiotic therapy for neonatal pneumonia has not been clearly established. Ten days of intravenous ampicillin and gentamicin is probably the most widely accepted treatment, but treatment duration varies. Given the high incidence of coexisting bacteremia, many neonatologists would treat a documented gram-negative pneumonia for a minimum of 14 days and rule out the possibility of meningitic involvement. Supportive care is also critical; intravenous nutrition, mechanical or assisted ventilation, and hemodynamic support are often required during the acute phase of the illness. Pneumonia may be complicated by PPHN, and patients should be monitored closely to ensure adequate oxygenation and ventilation.

Nosocomial Pneumonia. Nosocomial infection, including pneumonia, is rare in healthy newborns admitted to well-baby nurseries, but is a serious and frequent complication of prolonged intensive care admissions. Although not uniformly accepted, the CDC defines an infection as nosocomial if it occurs after admission to the ICU and was not vertically acquired from the mother. Nosocomial pneumonia is defined by the CDC in patients <1 year of age as the appearance of a new or progressive infiltrate on chest radiograph, increased respiratory secretions, or a change in sputum character, and isolation of the pathogen from a tracheal aspirate, bronchial washing, or biopsy specimen (224).

The risk of nosocomial infection during a NICU stay is inversely proportional to the patient's GA and birth weight. Data published in 2001 reported ventilator-associated pneumonia (VAP) per 1000 ventilator days stratified by birth weight. The rates of VAP per 1000 ventilator days were 3.5 at <1000 g birth weight, 4.9 at 1001–1500 g, 1.1 at 1501–2500 g, and 0.9 at >2500 g birth weight (225). A 2003 prospective single-center study showed a VAP rate of 28.3% in patients with a birth weight of 2000 g or less who were admitted to the NICU for >48 hours. The same study showed that VAP is an independent predictor of both mortality and prolonged length of hospital stay (226).

A prior bloodstream infection and the prolonged need for mechanical ventilation have both been shown to be predictors of a neonate's risk of acquiring a nosocomial pneumonia (226,227). Mechanical ventilation presents a risk because the respiratory tract of a patient receiving mechanical ventilation will, given time, become colonized with bacteria, typically gram-negative bacilli (*Pseudomonas aeruginosa*, *Klebsiella pneumoniae*, *E. coli*) or Staphylococcus species. Data supporting a correlation between time of intubation and colonization have been published (228). Bacterial colonization of the respiratory tract can occur as a result of contaminated respiratory equipment, the presence of bacteria in oral secretions that pool around the endotracheal tube, or via transmission of bacteria during labor and delivery. Fungus, typically candida, can also colonize the neonatal respiratory tract and potentially cause pneumonia and/or systemic disease. Viruses, particularly respiratory syncytial virus (RSV), may also cause nosocomial pneumonia in ICU patients.

Like congenital pneumonia, nosocomial pneumonia in the neonate can be difficult to diagnose. Nosocomial pneumonia should, in most cases, manifest with a clinical deterioration in the patient's respiratory status. The chest radiograph may show a focal infiltrate, but it is often difficult to clearly detect an infiltrate as many preterm infants have significant radiographic findings of lung disease at baseline and frequently develop areas of atelectasis. A tracheal aspirate should be sent for Gram stain and culture, but it is important to realize that most ventilated patients will have colonization of the respiratory tract with bacteria and subsequently will have growth of bacteria when tracheal aspirate cultures are sent. It is important to critically analyze tracheal aspirate results in an attempt to differentiate colonization from infection and determine the need for antibiotic therapy. The presence of many or a moderate amount of white blood cells has been used as an indicator that there is actual infection present. In addition, growth of a single or predominant organism that is a known pathogen may be helpful. Growth of mixed flora and the presence of only a few white blood cells are more consistent with colonization. Respiratory secretions can be sent for viral testing when a viral etiology is suspected. It is rare in infants to have additional samples such as bronchoalveolar lavage fluid or lung biopsy specimens to send for culture.

Given that the pathogens responsible for nosocomial infections differ somewhat from those responsible for early-onset infections, the antibiotics administered for nosocomial pneumonia prior to identification of the responsible organism vary from that used for early-onset infection. Vancomycin is often used in combination with an aminoglycoside for a suspected nosocomial infection in the NICU. Vancomycin is used in order to optimally cover staphylococcus species, particularly *Staphylococcus epidermidis*, which is frequently oxacillin resistant, and a common cause of infection in NICU patients. Some centers choose to treat neonates who develop nosocomial infections with double gram-negative antibiotic coverage while awaiting culture results, the theory being that gram-negative organisms typically cause more aggressive disease and vancomycin can always be added if there is continued clinical deterioration or significant growth of staphylococcus epidermidis from the cultures. Sometimes, antibiotic therapy is directed at the bacteria that are known colonizers in the infant based on growth seen on prior bacterial cultures and/or based on the pattern of unit-specific cultures and resistance panels.

CONCLUSION AND FUTURE DIRECTIONS

Although NICU survival has improved markedly over the years (owing to advances in knowledge and technology such as surfactant, iNO, and ECMO) many survivors have long-term sequelae from their neonatal illnesses that will result in further illness and hospital admissions during childhood and potentially beyond. Better understanding of diseases has led to studies that aim to individualize care of the sick newborn. Despite our improved understanding, the following challenges remain:

- Prevention or reduction of the incidence of premature delivery
- Development of well-informed guidelines for ideal target parameters for oxygen saturations and carbon dioxide levels in the preterm neonate
- A greater understanding of the optimal disease-specific approach to respiratory management in the neonate
- Development of safe and effective in utero interventions to improve outcomes of CDH, CPAM, and congenital heart disease
- Technologic advances in ECMO in the future that may reduce the need for anticoagulation and the chance of brain injury from hemorrhage
- Interventions that may decrease the risk of perinatal transmission of infection and reduce the incidence of hospital-acquired infection in the neonate

References

1. Effect of corticosteroids for fetal maturation on perinatal outcomes. NIH Consensus Development Panel on the Effect of Corticosteroids for Fetal Maturation on Perinatal Outcomes. *JAMA* 1995;273:413–8.
2. Dunn MS, Kaempf J, de Klerk A, et al. Randomized trial comparing 3 approaches to the initial respiratory management of preterm neonates. *Pediatrics* 2011;128:e1069–e1076.
3. Finer NN, Carlo WA, Walsh MC, et al. Early CPAP versus surfactant in extremely preterm infants. *N Engl J Med* 2010;362:1970–9.
4. Morley CJ, Davis PG, Doyle LW, et al. Nasal CPAP or intubation at birth for very preterm infants. *N Engl J Med* 2008;358:700–8.
5. Whitsett JA, Weaver TE. Hydrophobic surfactant proteins in lung function and disease. *N Engl J Med* 2002;347(26):2141–8.
6. Jobe AH. Pulmonary surfactant therapy. *N Engl J Med* 1993;328:861–8.
7. Jacobs H, Jobe A, Ikegami M, et al. The significance of reutilization of surfactant phosphatidylcholine. *J Biol Chem* 1983;258:4159–65.
8. Jacobs HC, Jobe AH, Ikegami M, et al. Reutilization of phosphatidylglycerol and phosphatidylethanolamine by the pulmonary surfactant system in 3-day-old rabbits. *Biochim Biophys Acta* 1985;834:172–9.
9. Jacobs HC, Ikegami M, Jobe AH, et al. Reutilization of surfactant phosphatidylcholine in adult rabbits. *Biochim Biophys Acta* 1985;837:77–84.
10. Jobe AH, Ikegami M. Biology of surfactant. *Clin Perinatol* 2001;28:655–69, vii–viii.
11. Soll RF. Prophylactic natural surfactant extract for preventing morbidity and mortality in preterm infants. *Cochrane Database Syst Rev* 2000:CD000511.
12. Rojas-Reyes MX, Morley CJ, Soll R. Prophylactic versus selective use of surfactant in preventing morbidity and mortality in preterm infants. *Cochrane Database Syst Rev* 2012;3:CD000510.
13. Rojas MA, Lozano JM, Rojas MX, et al. Very early surfactant without mandatory ventilation in premature infants treated with early continuous positive airway pressure: A randomized, controlled trial. *Pediatrics* 2009;123:137–42.
14. Sandri F, Plavka R, Ancora G, et al. Prophylactic or early selective surfactant combined with nCPAP in very preterm infants. *Pediatrics* 2010;125:e1402–e1409.
15. Tapia JL, Urzua S, Bancalari A, et al. Randomized trial of early bubble continuous positive airway pressure for very low birth weight infants. *J Pediatr* 2012;161:75.e1–80.e1.
16. Gopel W, Kribs A, Ziegler A, et al. Avoidance of mechanical ventilation by surfactant treatment of spontaneously breathing preterm infants (AMV): An open-label, randomised, controlled trial. *Lancet* 2011;378:1627–34.
17. Kanmaz HG, Erdeve O, Canpolat FE, et al. Surfactant administration via thin catheter during spontaneous breathing: Randomized controlled trial. *Pediatrics* 2013;131:e502–e509.
18. Schmolzer GM, Kumar M, Pichler G, et al. Non-invasive versus invasive respiratory support in preterm infants at birth: Systematic review and meta-analysis. *BMJ* 2013;347:f5980.
19. Fischer HS, Buhrer C. Avoiding endotracheal ventilation to prevent bronchopulmonary dysplasia: A meta-analysis. *Pediatrics* 2013;132:e1351–e1360.
20. Bahadue FL, Soll R. Early versus delayed selective surfactant treatment for neonatal respiratory distress syndrome. *Cochrane Database Syst Rev* 2012;11:CD001456.
21. Soll RF, Blanco F. Natural surfactant extract versus synthetic surfactant for neonatal respiratory distress syndrome. *Cochrane Database Syst Rev* 2001:CD000144.
22. Pfister RH, Soll RF, Wiswell T. Protein containing synthetic surfactant versus animal derived surfactant extract for the prevention and treatment of respiratory distress syndrome. *Cochrane Database Syst Rev* 2007:CD006069.
23. Singh N, Hawley KL, Viswanathan K. Efficacy of porcine versus bovine surfactants for preterm newborns with respiratory distress syndrome: Systematic review and meta-analysis. *Pediatrics* 2011;128:e1588–e1595.
24. Clark RH, Auten RL, Peabody J. A comparison of the outcomes of neonates treated with two different natural surfactants. *J Pediatr* 2001;139:828–31.
25. Ramanathan R, Bhatia JJ, Sekar K, et al. Mortality in preterm infants with respiratory distress syndrome treated with poractant alfa, calfactant or beractant: A retrospective study. *J Perinatol* 2013;33:119–25.
26. Trembath A, Hornik CP, Clark R, et al. Comparative effectiveness of surfactant preparations in premature infants. *J Pediatr* 2013;163:955.e1–60.e1.
27. Konishi M, Fujiwara T, Naito T, et al. Surfactant replacement therapy in neonatal respiratory distress syndrome. A multicentre, randomized clinical trial: Comparison of high- versus low-dose of surfactant TA. *Eur J Pediatr* 1988;147:20–5.
28. Speer CP, Robertson B, Curstedt T, et al. Randomized European multicenter trial of surfactant replacement therapy for severe neonatal respiratory distress syndrome: Single versus multiple doses of Curosurf. *Pediatrics* 1992;89:13–20.
29. Halliday HL, Tarnow-Mordi WO, Corcoran JD, et al. Multicentre randomised trial comparing high and low dose surfactant regimens for the treatment of respiratory distress syndrome (the Curosurf 4 trial). *Arch Dis Child* 1993;69:276–80.
30. Gortner L, Pohlandt F, Bartmann P, et al. High-dose versus low-dose bovine surfactant treatment in very premature infants. *Acta Paediatr* 1994;83:135–41.

31. Cogo PE, Facco M, Simonato M, et al. Dosing of porcine surfactant: Effect on kinetics and gas exchange in respiratory distress syndrome. *Pediatrics* 2009;124:e950–e957.

32. Sweet DG, Carnielli V, Greisen G, et al. European consensus guidelines on the management of neonatal respiratory distress syndrome in preterm infants—2013 update. *Neonatology* 2013;103:353–68.

33. Seehase M, Collins JJ, Kuypers E, et al. New surfactant with SP-B and C analogs gives survival benefit after inactivation in preterm lambs. *PLoS One* 2012;7:e47631.

34. Dani C, Corsini I, Bertini G, et al. The INSURE method in preterm infants of less than 30 weeks' gestation. *J Matern Fetal Neonatal Med* 2010;23:1024–9.

35. Finer NN, Merritt TA, Bernstein G, et al. An open label, pilot study of Aerosurf(R) combined with nCPAP to prevent RDS in preterm neonates. *J Aerosol Med Pulm Drug Deliv* 2010;23:303–9.

36. Trevisanuto D, Grazzina N, Ferrarese P, et al. Laryngeal mask airway used as a delivery conduit for the administration of surfactant to preterm infants with respiratory distress syndrome. *Biol Neonate* 2005;87:217–20.

37. Gregory GA, Kitterman JA, Phibbs RH, et al. Treatment of the idiopathic respiratory-distress syndrome with continuous positive airway pressure. *N Engl J Med* 1971;284:1333–40.

38. Kamath BD, Macguire ER, McClure EM, et al. Neonatal mortality from respiratory distress syndrome: Lessons for low-resource countries. *Pediatrics* 2011;127:1139–46.

39. Hillman NH, Nitsos I, Berry C, et al. Positive end-expiratory pressure and surfactant decrease lung injury during initiation of ventilation in fetal sheep. *Am J Physiol Lung Cell Mol Physiol* 2011;301:L712–L720.

40. Michna J, Jobe AH, Ikegami M. Positive end-expiratory pressure preserves surfactant function in preterm lambs. *Am J Respir Crit Care Med* 1999;160:634–9.

41. Finer NN, Carlo WA, Duara S, et al. Delivery room continuous positive airway pressure/positive end-expiratory pressure in extremely low birth weight infants: A feasibility trial. *Pediatrics* 2004;114:651–7.

42. Pandit PB, Courtney SE, Pyon KH, et al. Work of breathing during constant- and variable-flow nasal continuous positive airway pressure in preterm neonates. *Pediatrics* 2001;108:682–5.

43. De Paoli AG, Davis PG, Faber B, et al. Devices and pressure sources for administration of nasal continuous positive airway pressure (NCPAP) in preterm neonates. *Cochrane Database Syst Rev* 2008:CD002977.

44. Davis PG, Henderson-Smart DJ. Nasal continuous positive airways pressure immediately after extubation for preventing morbidity in preterm infants. *Cochrane Database Syst Rev* 2003:CD000143.

45. Elgellab A, Riou Y, Abbazine A, et al. Effects of nasal continuous positive airway pressure (NCPAP) on breathing pattern in spontaneously breathing premature newborn infants. *Intensive Care Med* 2001;27:1782–7.

46. Ramanathan R. Nasal respiratory support through the nares: Its time has come. *J Perinatol* 2010;30(suppl):S67–S72.

47. Jobe AJ. The new BPD: An arrest of lung development. *Pediatr Res* 1999;46:641–3.

48. Björklund LJ, Ingimarsson J, Curstedt T, et al. Manual ventilation with a few large breaths at birth compromises the therapeutic effect of subsequent surfactant replacement in immature lambs. *Pediatr Res* 1997;42:348–55.

49. Thomson MA, Yoder BA, Winter VT, et al. Delayed extubation to nasal continuous positive airway pressure in the immature baboon model of bronchopulmonary dysplasia: Lung clinical and pathological findings. *Pediatrics* 2006;118:2038–50.

50. Lampland AL, Meyers PA, Worwa CT, et al. Gas exchange and lung inflammation using nasal intermittent positive-pressure ventilation versus synchronized intermittent mandatory ventilation in piglets with saline lavage-induced lung injury: An observational study. *Crit Care Med* 2008;36:183–7.

51. Moretti C, Gizzi C, Papoff P, et al. Comparing the effects of nasal synchronized intermittent positive pressure ventilation (nSIPPV) and nasal continuous positive airway pressure (nCPAP) after extubation in very low birth weight infants. *Early Hum Dev* 1999;56:167–77.

52. Barrington KJ, Bull D, Finer NN. Randomized trial of nasal synchronized intermittent mandatory ventilation compared with continuous positive airway pressure after extubation of very low birth weight infants. *Pediatrics* 2001;107:638–41.

53. Friedlich P, Lecart C, Posen R, et al. A randomized trial of nasopharyngeal-synchronized intermittent mandatory ventilation versus nasopharyngeal continuous positive airway pressure in very low birth weight infants after extubation. *J Perinatol* 1999;19:413–8.

54. Khalaf MN, Brodsky N, Hurley J, et al. A prospective randomized, controlled trial comparing synchronized nasal intermittent positive pressure ventilation versus nasal continuous positive airway pressure as modes of extubation. *Pediatrics* 2001;108:13–7.

55. Bhandari V, Gavino RG, Nedrelow JH, et al. A randomized controlled trial of synchronized nasal intermittent positive pressure ventilation in RDS. *J Perinatol* 2007;27:697–703.

56. Chang HY, Claure N, D'ugard C, et al. Effects of synchronization during nasal ventilation in clinically stable preterm infants. *Pediatr Res* 2011;69:84–9.

57. Moretti C, Giannini L, Fassi C, et al. Nasal flow-synchronized intermittent positive pressure ventilation to facilitate weaning in very low-birthweight infants: Unmasked randomized controlled trial. *Pediatr Int* 2008;50:85–91.

58. Fischer HS, Roehr CC, Proquitté H, et al. Is volume and leak monitoring feasible during nasopharyngeal continuous positive airway pressure in neonates? *Intensive Care Med* 2009;35:1934–41.

59. Kugelman A, Feferkorn I, Riskin A, et al. Nasal intermittent mandatory ventilation versus nasal continuous positive airway pressure for respiratory distress syndrome: A randomized, controlled, prospective study. *J Pediatr* 2007;150:521.e1–526.e1.

60. Ali N, Claure N, Alegria X, et al. Effects of non-invasive pressure support ventilation (NI-PSV) on ventilation and respiratory effort in very low birth weight infants. *Pediatr Pulmonol* 2007;42:704–10.

61. Beck J, Reilly M, Grasselli G, et al. Patient-ventilator interaction during neurally adjusted ventilatory assist in low birth weight infants. *Pediatr Res* 2009;65:663–8.

62. Aghai ZH, Saslow JG, Nakhla T, et al. Synchronized nasal intermittent positive pressure ventilation (SNIPPV) decreases work of breathing (WOB) in premature infants with respiratory distress syndrome (RDS) compared to nasal continuous positive airway pressure (NCPAP). *Pediatr Pulmonol* 2006;41:875–81.

63. Kiciman NM, Andréasson B, Bernstein G, et al. Thoracoabdominal motion in newborns during ventilation delivered by endotracheal tube or nasal prongs. *Pediatr Pulmonol* 1998;25:175–81.

64. Lemyre B, Davis PG, De Paoli AG, et al. Nasal intermittent positive pressure ventilation (NIPPV) versus nasal continuous positive airway pressure (NCPAP) for preterm neonates after extubation. *Cochrane Database Syst Rev* 2014;9:CD003212.

65. Meneses J, Bhandari V, Alves JG. Nasal intermittent positive-pressure ventilation vs nasal continuous positive airway pressure for preterm infants with respiratory distress syndrome: A systematic review and meta-analysis. *Arch Pediatr Adolesc Med* 2012;166:372–6.

66. Davis PG, Lemyre B, de Paoli AG. Nasal intermittent positive pressure ventilation (NIPPV) versus nasal continuous positive airway pressure (NCPAP) for preterm neonates after extubation. *Cochrane Database Syst Rev* 2001:CD003212.

67. Lemyre B, Davis PG, De Paoli AG. Nasal intermittent positive pressure ventilation (NIPPV) versus nasal continuous positive airway pressure (NCPAP) for apnea of prematurity. *Cochrane Database Syst Rev* 2000:CD002272.

68. Kirpalani H, Millar D, Lemyre B, et al. A trial comparing noninvasive ventilation strategies in preterm infants. *N Engl J Med* 2013;369:611–20.

69. Ramanathan R, Sekar KC, Rasmussen M, et al. Nasal intermittent positive pressure ventilation after surfactant treatment for respiratory distress syndrome in preterm infants <30 weeks' gestation: a randomized, controlled trial. *J Perinatol* 2012;32:336–43.

70. Robertson NJ, McCarthy LS, Hamilton PA, et al. Nasal deformities resulting from flow driver continuous positive airway pressure. *Arch Dis Child Fetal Neonatal Ed* 1996;75:F209–F212.

71. Sai Sunil Kishore M, Dutta S, Kumar P. Early nasal intermittent positive pressure ventilation versus continuous airway pressure for respiratory distress syndrome. *Acta Paediatr* 2009;98:1412–5.

72. Dumpa V, Katz K, Northrup V, et al. SNIPPV vs NIPPV: Does synchronization matter? *J Perinatol* 2012;32:438–42.

73. Garland JS, Nelson DB, Rice T, et al. Increased risk of gastrointestinal perforations in neonates mechanically ventilated with either face mask or nasal prongs. *Pediatrics* 1985;76:406–10.

74. Bhandari V, Finer NN, Ehrenkranz RA, et al. Synchronized nasal intermittent positive-pressure ventilation and neonatal outcomes. *Pediatrics* 2009;124:517–26.

75. Lampland AL, Plumm B, Meyers PA, et al. Observational study of humidified high-flow nasal cannula compared with nasal continuous positive airway pressure. *J Pediatr* 2009;154:177–82.

76. Wilkinson DJ, Andersen CC, Smith K, et al. Pharyngeal pressure with high-flow nasal cannulae in premature infants. *J Perinatol* 2008;28:42–7.

77. Frizzola M, Miller TL, Rodriguez ME, et al. High-flow nasal cannula: Impact on oxygenation and ventilation in an acute lung injury model. *Pediatr Pulmonol* 2011;46:67–74.

78. Numa AH, Newth CJ. Anatomic dead space in infants and children. *J Appl Physiol* 1996;80:1485–9.

79. Fernandez-Alvarez JR, Gandhi RS, Amess P, et al. Heated humidified high-flow nasal cannula versus low-flow nasal cannula as weaning mode from nasal CPAP in infants ≤28 weeks of gestation. *Eur J Pediatr* 2014;173:93–8.

80. Yoder BA, Stoddard RA, Li M, et al. Heated, humidified high-flow nasal cannula versus nasal CPAP for respiratory support in neonates. *Pediatrics* 2013;131:e1482–e1490.

81. Collins CL, Holberton JR, Barfield C, et al. A randomized controlled trial to compare heated humidified high-flow nasal cannulae with nasal continuous positive airway pressure postextubation in premature infants. *J Pediatr* 2013;162:949. e1–954.e1.

82. Manley BJ, Owen LS, Doyle LW, et al. High-flow nasal cannulae in very preterm infants after extubation. *N Engl J Med* 2013;369:1425–33.

83. Collins CL, Holberton JR, König K. Comparison of the pharyngeal pressure provided by two heated, humidified high-flow nasal cannulae devices in premature infants. *J Paediatr Child Health* 2013;49:554–6.

84. Daish H, Badurdeen S. Question 2: Humidified heated high flow nasal cannula versus nasal continuous positive airway pressure for providing respiratory support following extubation in preterm newborns. *Arch Dis Child* 2014;99:880–2.

85. Roberts CT, Dawson JA, Alquoka E, et al. Are high flow nasal cannulae noisier than bubble CPAP for preterm infants? *Arch Dis Child Fetal Neonatal Ed* 2014;99:F291–F295.

86. Klingenberg C, Pettersen M, Hansen EA, et al. Patient comfort during treatment with heated humidified high flow nasal cannulae versus nasal continuous positive airway pressure: A randomised cross-over trial. *Arch Dis Child Fetal Neonatal Ed* 2014;99:F134–F137.

87. Jasin LR, Kern S, Thompson S, et al. Subcutaneous scalp emphysema, pneumo-orbitis and pneumocephalus in a neonate on high humidity high flow nasal cannula. *J Perinatol* 2008;28:779–81.

88. van der Hoeven M, Brouwer E, Blanco CE. Nasal high frequency ventilation in neonates with moderate respiratory insufficiency. *Arch Dis Child* 1998;79:F61–F63.

89. Colaizy TT, Younis UM, Bell EF, et al. Nasal high-frequency ventilation for premature infants. *Acta Paediatr* 2008;97:1518–22.

90. Carlo WA. Should nasal high-frequency ventilation be used in preterm infants? *Acta Paediatr* 2008;97:1484–5.

91. Null DM, Alvord J, Leavitt W, et al. High frequency nasal ventilation for 21 days maintains gas exchange with lower respiratory pressures and promotes alveolarization in preterm lambs. *Pediatr Res* 2014;75:507–16.

92. Schmidt B, Whyte RK, Asztalos EV, et al. Effects of targeting higher vs lower arterial oxygen saturations on death or disability in extremely preterm infants: A randomized clinical trial. *JAMA* 2013;309:2111–20.

93. Carlo WA, Finer NN, Walsh MC, et al. Target ranges of oxygen saturation in extremely preterm infants. *N Engl J Med* 2010;362:1959–69.

94. Stenson B, Brocklehurst P, Tarnow-Mordi W; U.K. BOOST II trial; Australian BOOST II trial; New Zealand BOOST II trial. Increased 36-week survival with high oxygen saturation target in extremely preterm infants. *N Engl J Med* 2011;364:1680-2.

95. Askie LM, Brocklehurst P, Darlow BA, et al. NeOProM: Neonatal Oxygenation Prospective Meta-analysis Collaboration study protocol. *BMC Pediatr* 2011;11:6.

96. Saugstad OD, Aune D. Optimal oxygenation of extremely low birth weight infants: A meta-analysis and systematic review of the oxygen saturation target studies. *Neonatology* 2014;105:55–63.

97. Arora V, Cayabyab R, Durand M, et al. Graded oxygen saturation targets in preterm neonates during the two phases of retinopathy of prematurity and outcomes. Pediatric Academic Society Meeting; 2013; Washington, DC; E-PAS2013:3355.4.

98. Kaiser JR, Gauss CH, Williams DK. The effects of hypercapnia on cerebral autoregulation in ventilated very low birth weight infants. *Pediatr Res* 2005;58:931–5.

99. Subramanian S, El-Mohandes A, Dhanireddy R, et al. Association of bronchopulmonary dysplasia and hypercarbia in ventilated infants with birth weights of 500-1,499 g. *Matern Child Health J* 2011;15(suppl 1):S17–S26.

100. Northway WH, Rosan RC, Porter DY. Pulmonary disease following respirator therapy of hyaline-membrane disease. Bronchopulmonary dysplasia. *N Engl J Med* 1967;276:357–68.

101. Husain AN, Siddiqui NH, Stocker JT. Pathology of arrested acinar development in postsurfactant bronchopulmonary dysplasia. *Hum Pathol* 1998;29:710–7.

102. Coalson JJ. Pathology of new bronchopulmonary dysplasia. *Semin Neonatol* 2003;8:73–81.

103. Thébaud B, Abman SH. Bronchopulmonary dysplasia: Where have all the vessels gone? Roles of angiogenic growth factors in chronic lung disease. *Am J Respir Crit Care Med* 2007;175:978–85.

104. Jakkula M, Le Cras TD, Gebb S, et al. Inhibition of angiogenesis decreases alveolarization in the developing rat lung. *Am J Physiol Lung Cell Mol Physiol* 2000;279:L600–L607.

105. Lassus P, Turanlahti M, Heikkilä P, et al. Pulmonary vascular endothelial growth factor and Flt-1 in fetuses, in acute and chronic lung disease, and in persistent pulmonary hypertension of the newborn. *Am J Respir Crit Care Med* 2001;164:1981–7.

106. Bhatt AJ, Pryhuber GS, Huyck H, et al. Disrupted pulmonary vasculature and decreased vascular endothelial growth factor, Flt-1, and TIE-2 in human infants dying with bronchopulmonary dysplasia. *Am J Respir Crit Care Med* 2001;164:1971–80.

107. Kunig AM, Balasubramaniam V, Markham NE, et al. Recombinant human VEGF treatment enhances alveolarization after hyperoxic lung injury in neonatal rats. *Am J Physiol Lung Cell Mol Physiol* 2005;289:L529–L535.

108. Jobe AH, Bancalari E. Bronchopulmonary dysplasia. *Am J Respir Crit Care Med* 2001;163:1723–9.

109. Walsh MC, Yao Q, Gettner P, et al. Impact of a physiologic definition on bronchopulmonary dysplasia rates. *Pediatrics* 2004;114:1305–11.

110. Bancalari EH, Jobe AH. The respiratory course of extremely preterm infants: A dilemma for diagnosis and terminology. *J Pediatr* 2012;161:585–8.

111. Stroustrup A, Trasande L. Epidemiological characteristics and resource use in neonates with bronchopulmonary dysplasia: 1993–2006. *Pediatrics* 2010;126:291–7.

112. Stoll BJ, Hansen NI, Bell EF, et al. Neonatal outcomes of extremely preterm infants from the NICHD Neonatal Research Network. *Pediatrics* 2010;126:443–56.

113. Jacob SV, Coates AL, Lands LC, et al. Long-term pulmonary sequelae of severe bronchopulmonary dysplasia. *J Pediatr* 1998;133:193–200.

114. Mitchell SH, Teague WG. Reduced gas transfer at rest and during exercise in school-age survivors of bronchopulmonary dysplasia. *Am J Respir Crit Care Med* 1998;157:1406–12.

115. Lal MK, Manktelow BN, Draper ES, Field DJ; Population-based study. Chronic lung disease of prematurity and intrauterine growth retardation: A population-based study. *Pediatrics* 2003;111:483–7.

116. Mokres LM, Parai K, Hilgendorff A, et al. Prolonged mechanical ventilation with air induces apoptosis and causes failure of alveolar septation and angiogenesis in lungs of newborn mice. *Am J Physiol Lung Cell Mol Physiol* 2010;298:L23–L35.

117. Avery ME, Tooley WH, Keller JB, et al. Is chronic lung disease in low birth weight infants preventable? A survey of eight centers. *Pediatrics* 1987;79:26–30.

118. Cools F, Askie LM, Offringa M, et al. Elective high-frequency oscillatory versus conventional ventilation in preterm infants: A systematic review and meta-analysis of individual patients' data. *Lancet* 2010;375:2082–91.

119. Courtney SE, Durand DJ, Asselin JM, et al. High-frequency oscillatory ventilation versus conventional mechanical ventilation for very-low-birth-weight infants. *N Engl J Med* 2002;347:643–52.

120. Johnson AH, Peacock JL, Greenough A, et al. High-frequency oscillatory ventilation for the prevention of chronic lung disease of prematurity. *N Engl J Med* 2002;347:633–42.

121. Moriette G, Paris-Llado J, Walti H, et al. Prospective randomized multicenter comparison of high-frequency oscillatory ventilation and conventional ventilation in preterm infants of less than 30 weeks with respiratory distress syndrome. *Pediatrics* 2001;107:363–72.

122. Thome U, Kössel H, Lipowsky G, et al. Randomized comparison of high-frequency ventilation with high-rate intermittent positive pressure ventilation in preterm infants with respiratory failure. *J Pediatr* 1999;135:39–46.

123. Van Reempts P, Borstlap C, Laroche S, et al. Early use of high frequency ventilation in the premature neonate. *Eur J Pediatr* 2003;162:219–26.

124. Lahra MM, Beeby PJ, Jeffery HE. Intrauterine inflammation, neonatal sepsis, and chronic lung disease: a 13-year hospital cohort study. *Pediatrics* 2009;123:1314–9.

125. Goldenberg RL, Culhane JF, Iams JD, et al. Epidemiology and causes of preterm birth. *Lancet* 2008;371:75–84.

126. Bry K, Lappalainen U. Intra-amniotic endotoxin accelerates lung maturation in fetal rabbits. *Acta Paediatr* 2001;90:74–80.

127. Kallapur SG, Bachurski CJ, Le Cras TD, et al. Vascular changes after intra-amniotic endotoxin in preterm lamb lungs. *Am J Physiol Lung Cell Mol Physiol* 2004;287:L1178–L1185.

128. Kramer BW, Kramer S, Ikegami M, et al. Injury, inflammation, and remodeling in fetal sheep lung after intra-amniotic endotoxin. *Am J Physiol Lung Cell Mol Physiol* 2002;283:L452–L459.

129. Newnham JP, Moss TJ, Padbury JF, et al. The interactive effects of endotoxin with prenatal glucocorticoids on short-term lung function in sheep. *Am J Obstet Gynecol* 2001;185:190–7.

130. Moss TJ, Knox CL, Kallapur SG, et al. Experimental amniotic fluid infection in sheep: Effects of Ureaplasma parvum serovars 3 and 6 on preterm or term fetal sheep. *Am J Obstet Gynecol* 2008;198:122.e1–122.e8.

131. Been JV, Zimmermann LJ, Debeer A, et al. Bronchoalveolar lavage fluid from preterm infants with chorioamnionitis inhibits alveolar epithelial repair. *Respir Res* 2009;10:116.

132. Jobe AH. Effects of chorioamnionitis on the fetal lung. *Clin Perinatol* 2012;39:441–57.

133. Watterberg KL, Demers LM, Scott SM, et al. Chorioamnionitis and early lung inflammation in infants in whom bronchopulmonary dysplasia develops. *Pediatrics* 1996;97:210–5.

134. Soraisham AS, Singhal N, McMillan DD, et al. A multicenter study on the clinical outcome of chorioamnionitis in preterm infants. *Am J Obstet Gynecol* 2009;200:372.e1–372.e6.

135. Laughon M, Allred EN, Bose C, et al. Patterns of respiratory disease during the first 2 postnatal weeks in extremely premature infants. *Pediatrics* 2009;123:1124–31.

136. Van Marter LJ, Dammann O, Allred EN, et al. Chorioamnionitis, mechanical ventilation, and postnatal sepsis as modulators of chronic lung disease in preterm infants. *J Pediatr* 2002;140:171–6.

137. Vento M, Moro M, Escrig R, et al. Preterm resuscitation with low oxygen causes less oxidative stress, inflammation, and chronic lung disease. *Pediatrics* 2009;124:e439–e449.

138. Ratner V, Slinko S, Utkina-Sosunova I, et al. Hypoxic stress exacerbates hyperoxia-induced lung injury in a neonatal mouse model of bronchopulmonary dysplasia. *Neonatology* 2009;95:299–305.

139. Paquette L, Friedlich P, Ramanathan R, et al. Concurrent use of indomethacin and dexamethasone increases the risk of spontaneous intestinal perforation in very low birth weight neonates. *J Perinatol* 2006;26:486–92.

140. O'Shea TM, Kothadia JM, Klinepeter KL, et al. Randomized placebo-controlled trial of a 42-day tapering course of dexamethasone to reduce the duration of ventilator dependency in very low birth weight infants: Outcome of study participants at 1-year adjusted age. *Pediatrics* 1999;104:15–21.

141. Yeh TF, Lin YJ, Huang CC, et al. Early dexamethasone therapy in preterm infants: A follow-up study. *Pediatrics* 1998;101:E7.

142. Shinwell ES, Karplus M, Zmora E, et al. Failure of early postnatal dexamethasone to prevent chronic lung disease in infants with respiratory distress syndrome. *Arch Dis Child Fetal Neonatal Ed* 1996;74:F33–F37.

143. Shinwell ES, Lerner-Geva L, Lusky A, et al. Less postnatal steroids, more bronchopulmonary dysplasia: A population-based study in very low birthweight infants. *Arch Dis Child Fetal Neonatal Ed* 2007;92:F30–F33.

144. Yoder BA, Harrison M, Clark RH. Time-related changes in steroid use and bronchopulmonary dysplasia in preterm infants. *Pediatrics* 2009;124:673–9.

145. Onland W, Offringa M, De Jaegere AP, et al. Finding the optimal postnatal dexamethasone regimen for preterm infants at risk of bronchopulmonary dysplasia: A systematic review of placebo-controlled trials. *Pediatrics* 2009;123:367–77.

146. Cheong JL, Anderson P, Roberts G, et al.; Victorian Infant Collaborative Study Group. Postnatal corticosteroids and neurodevelopmental outcomes in extremely low birthweight or extremely preterm infants: 15-year experience in Victoria, Australia. *Arch Dis Child Fetal Neonatal Ed* 2013;98:F32–F36.

147. Doyle LW, Halliday HL, Ehrenkranz RA, et al. An update on the impact of postnatal systemic corticosteroids on mortality and cerebral palsy in preterm infants: Effect modification by risk of bronchopulmonary dysplasia. *J Pediatr* 2014;165:1258–60.

148. Laughon MM, Langer JC, Bose CL, et al. Prediction of bronchopulmonary dysplasia by postnatal age in extremely premature infants. *Am J Respir Crit Care Med* 2011;183:1715–22.

149. Watterberg KL; American Academy of Pediatrics; Committee on Fetus and Newborn. Policy statement—Postnatal corticosteroids to prevent or treat bronchopulmonary dysplasia. *Pediatrics* 2010;126:800–8.

150. Doyle LW, Ehrenkranz RA, Halliday HL. Postnatal hydrocortisone for preventing or treating bronchopulmonary dysplasia in preterm infants: A systematic review. *Neonatology* 2010;98:111–7.

151. Watterberg KL, Gerdes JS, Cole CH, et al. Prophylaxis of early adrenal insufficiency to prevent bronchopulmonary dysplasia: A multicenter trial. *Pediatrics* 2004;114:1649–57.

152. Lodygensky GA, Rademaker K, Zimine S, et al. Structural and functional brain development after hydrocortisone treatment for neonatal chronic lung disease. *Pediatrics* 2005;116:1–7.

153. Rademaker KJ, Rijpert M, Uiterwaal CS, et al. Neonatal hydrocortisone treatment related to 1H-MRS of the hippocampus and short-term memory at school age in preterm born children. *Pediatr Res* 2006;59:309–13.

154. Beam KS, Aliaga S, Ahlfeld SK, et al. A systematic review of randomized controlled trials for the prevention of bronchopulmonary dysplasia in infants. *J Perinatol* 2014;34:705–10.

155. Schmidt B, Roberts RS, Davis P, et al. Caffeine therapy for apnea of prematurity. *N Engl J Med* 2006;354:2112–21.

156. Jones LJ, Craven PD, Attia J, et al. Network meta-analysis of indomethacin versus ibuprofen versus placebo for PDA in preterm infants. *Arch Dis Child Fetal Neonatal Ed* 2011;96:F45–F52.

157. Stewart A, Brion LP, Ambrosio-Perez I. Diuretics acting on the distal renal tubule for preterm infants with (or developing) chronic lung disease. *Cochrane Database Syst Rev* 2011:CD001817.

158. Stewart A, Brion LP. Intravenous or enteral loop diuretics for preterm infants with (or developing) chronic lung disease. *Cochrane Database Syst Rev* 2011:CD001453.

159. Rojas MA, Gonzalez A, Bancalari E, et al. Changing trends in the epidemiology and pathogenesis of neonatal chronic lung disease. *J Pediatr* 1995;126:605–10.

160. Balinotti JE, Tiller CJ, Llapur CJ, et al. Growth of the lung parenchyma early in life. *Am J Respir Crit Care Med* 2009;179:134–7.

161. Balinotti JE, Chakr VC, Tiller C, et al. Growth of lung parenchyma in infants and toddlers with chronic lung disease of infancy. *Am J Respir Crit Care Med* 2010;181:1093–7.

162. Doyle LW, Faber B, Callanan C, et al. Bronchopulmonary dysplasia in very low birth weight subjects and lung function in late adolescence. *Pediatrics* 2006;118:108–13.

163. Avery ME, Gatewood OB, Brumley G. Transient tachypnea of newborn. Possible delayed resorption of fluid at birth. *Am J Dis Child* 1966;111:380–5.

164. Ramachandrappa A, Jain L. Elective cesarean section: Its impact on neonatal respiratory outcome. *Clin Perinatol* 2008;35:373–93, vii.

165. Tutdibi E, Gries K, Bücheler M, et al. Impact of labor on outcomes in transient tachypnea of the newborn: Population-based study. *Pediatrics* 2010;125:e577–e583.

166. Machado LU, Fiori HH, Baldisserotto M, et al. Surfactant deficiency in transient tachypnea of the newborn. *J Pediatr* 2011;159:750–4.

167. Bloch KD, Filippov G, Sanchez LS, et al. Pulmonary soluble guanylate cyclase, a nitric oxide receptor, is increased during the perinatal period. *Am J Physiol* 1997;272:L400–L406.

168. Morin FC, Egan EA. Pulmonary hemodynamics in fetal lambs during development at normal and increased oxygen tension. *J Appl Physiol* 1992;73:213–8.

169. Shaul PW, North AJ, Wu LC, et al. Endothelial nitric oxide synthase is expressed in cultured human bronchiolar epithelium. *J Clin Invest* 1994;94:2231–6.

170. Steinhorn RH. Diagnosis and treatment of pulmonary hypertension in infancy. *Early Hum Dev* 2013;89:865–74.

171. Keller RL, Tacy TA, Hendricks-Munoz K, et al. Congenital diaphragmatic hernia: Endothelin-1, pulmonary hypertension, and disease severity. *Am J Respir Crit Care Med* 2010;182:555–61.

172. Mourani PM, Ivy DD, Gao D, et al. Pulmonary vascular effects of inhaled nitric oxide and oxygen tension in bronchopulmonary dysplasia. *Am J Respir Crit Care Med* 2004;170:1006–13.

173. Bhat R, Salas AA, Foster C, et al. Prospective analysis of pulmonary hypertension in extremely low birth weight infants. *Pediatrics* 2012;129:e682–e689.

174. Walsh-Sukys MC, Tyson JE, Wright LL, et al. Persistent pulmonary hypertension of the newborn in the era before nitric oxide: Practice variation and outcomes. *Pediatrics* 2000;105:14–20.

175. Lakshminrusimha S, Russell JA, Steinhorn RH, et al. Pulmonary arterial contractility in neonatal lambs increases with 100% oxygen resuscitation. *Pediatr Res* 2006;59:137–41.

176. Lakshminrusimha S, Swartz DD, Gugino SF, et al. Oxygen concentration and pulmonary hemodynamics in newborn lambs with pulmonary hypertension. *Pediatr Res* 2009;66:539–44.

177. Kinsella JP, Truog WE, Walsh WF, et al. Randomized, multicenter trial of inhaled nitric oxide and high-frequency oscillatory ventilation in severe, persistent pulmonary hypertension of the newborn. *J Pediatr* 1997;131:55–62.

178. Neonatal Inhaled Nitric Oxide Study Group. Inhaled nitric oxide in full-term and nearly full-term infants with hypoxic respiratory failure. *N Engl J Med* 1997;336:597–604.

179. Clark RH, Kueser TJ, Walker MW, et al. Low-dose nitric oxide therapy for persistent pulmonary hypertension of the newborn. Clinical Inhaled Nitric Oxide Research Group. *N Engl J Med* 2000;342:469–74.

180. Steinhorn RH, Kinsella JP, Pierce C, et al. Intravenous sildenafil in the treatment of neonates with persistent pulmonary hypertension. *J Pediatr* 2009;155:841.e1–847.e1.

181. Baquero H, Soliz A, Neira F, et al. Oral sildenafil in infants with persistent pulmonary hypertension of the newborn: A pilot randomized blinded study. *Pediatrics* 2006;117:1077–83.

182. Mourani PM, Sontag MK, Ivy DD, et al. Effects of long-term sildenafil treatment for pulmonary hypertension in infants with chronic lung disease. *J Pediatr* 2009;154:379–84, 384.e1–384.e2.

183. Bialkowski A, Moenkemeyer F, Patel N. Intravenous sildenafil in the management of pulmonary hypertension associated with congenital diaphragmatic hernia [published online ahead of print on October 25, 2013]. *Eur J Pediatr Surg*.

184. Noori S, Friedlich P, Wong P, et al. Cardiovascular effects of sildenafil in neonates and infants with congenital diaphragmatic hernia and pulmonary hypertension. *Neonatology* 2007;91:92–100.

185. Barst RJ, Ivy DD, Gaitan G, et al. A randomized, double-blind, placebo-controlled, dose-ranging study of oral sildenafil citrate in treatment-naive children with pulmonary arterial hypertension. *Circulation* 2012;125:324–34.

186. de Visser YP, Walther FJ, Laghmani el H, et al. Sildenafil attenuates pulmonary inflammation and fibrin deposition, mortality and right ventricular hypertrophy in neonatal hyperoxic lung injury. *Respir Res* 2009;10:30.

187. Ladha F, Bonnet S, Eaton F, et al. Sildenafil improves alveolar growth and pulmonary hypertension in hyperoxia-induced lung injury. *Am J Respir Crit Care Med*. 2005;172:750–6.

188. Steiner M, Salzer U, Baumgartner S, et al. Intravenous sildenafil i.v. as rescue treatment for refractory pulmonary hypertension in extremely preterm infants. *Klin Padiatr* 2014;226:211–5.

189. UK collaborative randomised trial of neonatal extracorporeal membrane oxygenation. UK Collaborative ECMO Trail Group. *Lancet* 1996;348:75–82.

190. Fliman PJ, deRegnier RA, Kinsella JP, et al. Neonatal extracorporeal life support: Impact of new therapies on survival. *J Pediatr* 2006;148:595–9.

191. Wiswell TE, Gannon CM, Jacob J, et al. Delivery room management of the apparently vigorous meconium-stained neonate: Results of the multicenter, international collaborative trial. *Pediatrics* 2000;105:1–7.

192. Wiswell TE. Handling the meconium-stained infant. *Semin Neonatol* 2001;6:225–31.

193. Lotze A, Mitchell BR, Bulas DI, et al. Multicenter study of surfactant (beractant) use in the treatment of term infants with severe respiratory failure. Survanta in Term Infants Study Group. *J Pediatr* 1998;132:40–7.

194. Langham MR, Kays DW, Ledbetter DJ, et al. Congenital diaphragmatic hernia. Epidemiology and outcome. *Clin Perinatol* 1996;23:671–88.

195. Unemoto K, Sakai M, Shima H, et al. Increased expression of ICAM-1 and VCAM-1 in the lung of nitrofen-induced congenital diaphragmatic hernia in rats. *Pediatr Surg Int* 2003;19:365–70.

196. Chang R, Andreoli S, Ng YS, et al. VEGF expression is down-regulated in nitrofen-induced congenital diaphragmatic hernia. *J Pediatr Surg* 2004;39:825–8; discussion 8.

197. Teramoto H, Yoneda A, Puri P. Gene expression of fibro-blast growth factors 10 and 7 is downregulated in the lung of nitrofen-induced diaphragmatic hernia in rats. *J Pediatr Surg* 2003;38:1021–4.

198. Cohen MS, Rychik J, Bush DM, et al. Influence of congenital heart disease on survival in children with congenital diaphragmatic hernia. *J Pediatr* 2002;141:25–30.

199. Laudy JA, Van Gucht M, Van Dooren MF, et al. Congenital diaphragmatic hernia: An evaluation of the prognostic value of the lung-to-head ratio and other prenatal parameters. *Prenat Diagn* 2003;23:634–9.

200. Hedrick HL, Danzer E, Merchant A, et al. Liver position and lung-to-head ratio for prediction of extracorporeal membrane oxygenation and survival in isolated left congenital diaphragmatic hernia. *Am J Obstet Gynecol* 2007;197:422.e1–422.e4.

201. Victoria T, Bebbington MW, Danzer E, et al. Use of magnetic resonance imaging in prenatal prognosis of the fetus with isolated left congenital diaphragmatic hernia. *Prenat Diagn* 2012;32:715–23.

202. Wilson JM, DiFiore JW, Peters CA. Experimental fetal tracheal ligation prevents the pulmonary hypoplasia associated with fetal nephrectomy: Possible application for congenital diaphragmatic hernia. *J Pediatr Surg* 1993;28:1433–9; discussion 9–40.

203. Van Meurs K; Congenital Diaphragmatic Hernia Study Group. Is surfactant therapy beneficial in the treatment of the term newborn infant with congenital diaphragmatic hernia? *J Pediatr* 2004;145:312–6.

204. Neonatal Inhaled Nitric Oxide Study Group. Inhaled nitric oxide and hypoxic respiratory failure in infants with congenital diaphragmatic hernia. *Pediatrics* 1997;99:838–45.

205. Potter EL. Facial characteristics of infants with bilateral renal agenesis. *Am J Obstet Gynecol* 1946;51:885–8.

206. Campbell RE. Intrapulmonary interstitial emphysema: A complication of hyaline-membrane disease. *Am J Roentgenol Radium Ther Nucl Med* 1970;110:449–56.

207. Keszler M, Donn SM, Bucciarelli RL, et al. Multicenter controlled trial comparing high-frequency jet ventilation and conventional mechanical ventilation in newborn infants with pulmonary interstitial emphysema. *J Pediatr* 1991;119:85–93.

208. Clark SD, Saker F, Schneeberger MT, et al. Administration of 100% oxygen does not hasten resolution of symptomatic spontaneous pneumothorax in neonates. *J Perinatol* 2014;34:528–31.

209. Shaireen H, Rabi Y, Metcalfe A, et al. Impact of oxygen concentration on time to resolution of spontaneous pneumothorax in term infants: A population based cohort study. *BMC Pediatr* 2014;14:208.

210. Litmanovitz I, Carlo WA. Expectant management of pneumothorax in ventilated neonates. *Pediatrics* 2008;122:e975–e979.

211. Cole VA, Normand IC, Reynolds EO, et al. Pathogenesis of hemorrhagic pulmonary edema and massive pulmonary hemorrhage in the newborn. *Pediatrics* 1973;51:175–87.

212. Bozdag S, Dilli D, Gökmen T, et al. Comparison of two natural surfactants for pulmonary hemorrhage in very low-birth-weight infants: A randomized controlled trial [published online ahead of print on September 21, 2014]. *Am J Perinatol*.

213. Aziz A, Ohlsson A. Surfactant for pulmonary haemorrhage in neonates. *Cochrane Database Syst Rev* 2012;7:CD005254.

214. Amizuka T, Shimizu H, Niida Y, et al. Surfactant therapy in neonates with respiratory failure due to haemorrhagic pulmonary oedema. *Eur J Pediatr* 2003;162:697–702.

215. Jefferies AL, Coates G, O'Brodovich H. Pulmonary epithelial permeability in hyaline-membrane disease. *N Engl J Med* 1984;311:1075–80.

216. Hazinski TA, Blalock WA, Engelhardt B. Control of water balance in infants with bronchopulmonary dysplasia: role of endogenous vasopressin. *Pediatr Res* 1988;23:86–8.

217. Hoeve LJ, Eskici O, Verwoerd CD. Therapeutic reintubation for post-intubation laryngotracheal injury in preterm infants. *Int J Pediatr Otorhinolaryngol* 1995;31:7–13.

218. Walner DL, Loewen MS, Kimura RE. Neonatal subglottic stenosis—incidence and trends. *Laryngoscope* 2001;111:48–51.

219. Couser RJ, Ferrara TB, Falde B, et al. Effectiveness of dexamethasone in preventing extubation failure in preterm infants at increased risk for airway edema. *J Pediatr* 1992;121:591–6.

220. Overman AE, Liu M, Kurachek SC, et al. Tracheostomy for infants requiring prolonged mechanical ventilation: 10 years' experience. *Pediatrics* 2013;131:e1491–e1496.

221. DeMauro SB, D'Agostino JA, Bann C, et al. Developmental outcomes of very preterm infants with tracheostomies. *J Pediatr* 2014;164:1303.e2–1310.e2.

222. Puopolo KM, Madoff LC, Eichenwald EC. Early-onset group B streptococcal disease in the era of maternal screening. *Pediatrics* 2005;115:1240–6.

223. Kotecha S, Hodge R, Schaber JA, et al. Pulmonary *Ureaplasma urealyticum* is associated with the development of acute lung inflammation and chronic lung disease in preterm infants. *Pediatr Res* 2004;55:61–8.

224. Garner JS, Jarvis WR, Emori TG, et al. CDC definitions for nosocomial infections, 1988. *Am J Infect Control* 1988;16:128–40.

225. Stover BH, Shulman ST, Bratcher DF, et al. Nosocomial infection rates in US children's hospitals' neonatal and pediatric intensive care units. *Am J Infect Control* 2001;29:152–7.

226. Apisarnthanarak A, Holzmann-Pazgal G, Hamvas A, et al. Ventilator-associated pneumonia in extremely preterm neonates in a neonatal intensive care unit: Characteristics, risk factors, and outcomes. *Pediatrics* 2003;112:1283–9.

227. Suara RO, Young M, Reeves I. Risk factors for nosocomial infection in a high-risk nursery. *Infect Control Hosp Epidemiol* 2000;21:250–1.

228. Friedland DR, Rothschild MA, Delgado M, et al. Bacterial colonization of endotracheal tubes in intubated neonates. *Arch Otolaryngol Head Neck Surg* 2001;127:525–8.

229. Rudiger M, Tolle A, Meier W, et al. Naturally derived commercial surfactants differ in composition of surfactant lipids and in surface viscosity. *Am J Physiol Lung Cell Mol Physiol* 2005;288:L379–L383.

CHAPTER 48 ■ PNEUMONIA AND BRONCHIOLITIS

WERTHER BRUNOW DE CARVALHO, MARCELO CUNIO MACHADO FONSECA,
CINTIA JOHNSTON, AND DAVID G. NICHOLS

KEY POINTS

Pneumonia

1. The pathogenesis of pneumonia is dependent on host defense and microorganism virulence.
2. Bacterial pneumonia is not common in previously healthy children; it usually occurs after a viral infection or in the presence of an underlying chronic disease.
3. Diagnosis is clinical and based on history, physical examination, and epidemiologic data.
4. Admission criteria of children with community-acquired pneumonia (CAP) are not fully defined and accurate; many patients are hospitalized without adequate justification.
5. Pneumonia associated with mechanical ventilation is the second highest cause of nosocomial infections.
6. Important components of pneumonia therapy include nutrition; fluid-, electrolyte-, and acid–base balance; temperature control; heated and humidified O_2; and secretion management (chest physiotherapy, suctioning).
7. Antimicrobial therapy is guided by epidemiologic and clinical data, the patient's age, the infective microorganism, and antimicrobial resistance.

Acute Bronchiolitis

8. Acute bronchiolitis (AB) is the most frequent and severe respiratory system syndrome involving children <2 years of age. It has an epidemic pattern and increased prevalence during the fall and winter. In winter, AB is one of the most frequent causes of infant hospitalization.
9. Respiratory syncytial virus (RSV subtypes A and B) is the most frequently involved agent, although other viral pathogens may be clinically indistinguishable.
10. Comorbidities associated with increased severity of AB include
    a. Prematurity
    b. Chronic lung disease
    c. Immunodeficiency
    d. Hemodynamically significant heart disease
11. Apnea may be a presenting sign of AB and warrants admission to a pediatric intensive care unit (PICU) because of the risk of recurrence.
12. Clinical or diagnostic signs of impending respiratory failure despite adequate O_2 therapy are indications for admission to the PICU.
13. Treatment of AB is supportive, as neither bronchodilators nor antibiotics have proven effective.
14. Adequate hydration and oxygenation remain the backbone of AB treatment, and respiratory support is indicated in patients with refractory and recurring episodes of apnea, progressive hypoxia, refractory hypercapnia, or increasing respiratory distress secondary to severe AB.
15. Careful hand-washing and other infection control measures are necessary to prevent the spread of RSV.
16. The monoclonal antibody palivizumab provides passive immunization against RSV in select populations of high-risk children.

PNEUMONIA

Introduction

Pneumonia is an inflammatory condition of the lung parenchyma, which distinguishes it from inflammatory conditions of the airways such as bronchiolitis, bronchitis or tracheitis. The etiology may be associated with infection, aspiration, hypersensitivity to inhaled materials (hydrocarbon and lipoid pneumonia), or drug- or radiation-induced pneumonitis. Pneumonia usually presents with clinical signs of alveolar compromise and radiographic opacification without lung volume loss. The term *bronchopneumonia* refers to characteristic clinical findings with multiple opacities on radiologic examination, generally poorly defined, without clear segmental limits, and associated with a more serious clinical presentation.

Classification

There are several approaches to the classification of pneumonia.
The World Health Organization (WHO) (1) classifies pneumonia into three stages based on clinical criteria:

■ Stage I, fever (≥38°C) and tachypnea (>50 bpm for ages 2–11 months, and >40 bpm for ages 1–5 years)
■ Stage II includes chest retractions
■ Stage III includes difficulty with breastfeeding or drinking and/or central cyanosis

Additional classification based on age and the underlying infectious agent is common in pediatrics, which reflects the distinct clinical findings associated with various age groups and organisms. The radiographic classification is based on anatomic location (lobar, lobular, alveolar, or interstitial).

The infection control classification distinguishes between community-acquired and nosocomial pneumonia, which are associated with different causative agents and hence different therapeutic decisions. Classification based on underlying chronic disease occurs in special populations because these children experience recurrent pneumonias with distinctive features. Examples include acute chest syndrome in sickle cell disease, gram-negative pneumonia in cystic fibrosis, or aspiration pneumonia in tracheoesophageal fistula or cleft palate patients.

When a child presents with recurrent pneumonia, the possibility of an underlying disease (e.g., acquired or congenital lung anatomical abnormalities, immunodeficiency, prematurity, lung sequestration, tracheoesophageal fistula, foreign body, cystic fibrosis, heart failure, cleft palate, bronchiectasis, ciliary dyskinesia, neutropenia, or increased pulmonary blood flow) should be considered. Other predisposing factors are lower socioeconomic status, parental smoking, and prolonged critical illness.

Epidemiology

Pneumonia is one of the most frequent infections in children and one of the main causes of hospitalization. More than 95% of the episodes of pneumonia in the world occur in developing countries. UNICEF maintains current statistics on pneumonia in the developing world (http://data.unicef.org) and provides links to a WHO integrated management plan for resource-limited environments.

It is estimated that 150 million cases of pneumonia occur annually in children who are <5 years old (2). Although the introduction of the pneumococcal vaccine has reduced hospitalization rates in developed countries, ~50% of young children (<5 years old) with community-acquired pneumonia (CAP) still require hospitalization. The wealth of the society and the availability of medical resources impact the mortality rate, and pneumonia is the leading cause of mortality in developing countries.

Pathogenesis

Pneumonia typically occurs either by colonization of the upper airway followed by invasion of the lower respiratory tract or, less commonly, through hematogenous spread to pulmonary parenchyma (e.g., *Streptococcus pneumoniae* and *Staphylococcus aureus*). Lower respiratory tract invasion usually begins with population of the nasopharynx by a serotype, against which the patient lacks immunity. The child may experience cough, coryza, or pharyngitis. Subsequently, the virulent organism is either inhaled or aspirated into the trachea and distal airway. Once microorganisms inoculate the respiratory tract, a normal inflammatory response (including antibodies, complement, phagocytes, and cytokines) begins and causes injury to the functioning pulmonary tissue (3). The mobilization of immunoglobulins (IgG and IgM) and complement facilitates opsonization of microorganisms. Macrophages and polymorphonuclear leukocytes then phagocytize the antibody-coated microorganisms. The inflammatory response associated with this normal immune response leads to increased airway reactivity, transudation of plasma into the air spaces, and excess mucus production. The bronchiolar and alveolar epithelia may become necrotic in severe cases. The accumulation of fluid and cellular debris in the alveoli may lead to decreased ventilation relative to perfusion in the affected lung segments, which in turn leads to hypoxia.

Protection against respiratory pathogens includes the airway defense barriers, mainly the mucous membrane and the mucociliary layer, which are responsible for the clearance of foreign material or microorganisms. The bacteria that cause pneumonia may have specific virulence factors that increase their survival and reproduction and result in more extensive lesions.

Frequent histopathologic findings in viral pneumonia are congestion, inflammation, bronchial epithelium necrosis, and hemorrhage. Viral pneumonia also affects the lung through direct invasion, causing mucosal inflammation and respiratory cilial injury, allowing the possibility of secondary bacterial infection. Globally, viruses are responsible for ~30%–67% of CAPs and are more frequently identified in children <1 year compared to those >2 years old (77% vs. 59%) (4).

Neonatal Pneumonia

It is estimated that 800,000 deaths occur worldwide due to respiratory infections during the neonatal period. Neonatal pneumonia may be either early-onset or late-onset depending on the route and mechanism of acquiring the pathogen. Early-onset neonatal pneumonia (<3 days of life) is classified as follows:

- Congenital: acquired by transplacental (hematogenous) transmission
- Intrauterine: caused by maternal chorioamnionitis and fetal aspiration of infected amniotic fluid
- Intrapartum: due to aspiration of organisms colonizing the maternal genital tract

Clinical Presentation of Neonatal Pneumonia

The newborn with bacterial pneumonia usually presents with tachypnea, grunting, nasal flaring, and chest wall retractions. Other nonspecific signs, including poor feeding, vomiting, irritability, lethargy, and apnea, are also seen with bacteremia and meningitis, which makes the diagnosis of pneumonia difficult without a chest radiography. In preterm newborns, lower respiratory tract infection may present as apnea without fever or tachycardia. Infants with *Chlamydia trachomatis* pneumonia usually present between 3 weeks and 3 months of age with staccato cough, tachypnea, and rales.

Early-Onset Neonatal Pneumonia

Group B streptococcus (GBS) is the most common cause of early-onset pneumonia in developed countries. Vaginal colonization in the mother, prematurity, and premature or prolonged (>18 hours) rupture of membranes are major risk factors for early-onset GBS pneumonia. GBS pneumonia usually occurs as part of GBS sepsis. Diffuse alveolar infiltrates mimic hyaline membrane disease. Severely affected infants may develop persistent pulmonary hypertension of the newborn. Maternal screening for GBS colonization and the use of intrapartum antibiotic prophylaxis have decreased the incidence and severity of GBS pneumonia, although racial and ethnic disparities persist, with greater incidence and severity among black newborns.

Although microbiologic studies from newborns with pneumonia in developing countries are more limited, gram-negative enteric organisms (especially *Klebsiella* spp.) as well as *Staphylococcus aureus* and *Streptococcus pneumoniae* appear to be responsible for most early-onset neonatal pneumonia. These organisms may produce significant lung damage, including abscess, empyema, and pneumatocele.

Among viral etiologies of neonatal pneumonia, herpes simplex virus (HSV) is most common and carries a high mortality rate. Approximately half of newborns with disseminated

HSV infection will exhibit pneumonia as part of the disease. Because the presentation of disseminated HSV with pneumonia is often indistinguishable from early-onset neonatal sepsis, acyclovir should be included in empiric therapy until HSV can be excluded.

Empiric treatment of early-onset neonatal pneumonia takes the earlier microbiologic patterns into account. Parenteral antibiotics are necessary and should cover microorganisms known to colonize or infect the mother. Ampicillin, gentamicin, and acyclovir are a useful antibiotic combination until cultures and polymerase chain reaction (PCR) studies are available to tailor therapy.

Early-onset pneumonia may also be noninfectious in origin as when fetal asphyxia and gasping respirations result in *meconium aspiration syndrome* (MAS) (5). MAS is usually readily distinguished from infectious early-onset pneumonia based on clinical and radiographic criteria:

- Meconium staining of the amniotic fluid, newborn skin, and airway secretions
- Respiratory distress immediately at birth
- History of fetal distress (Apgar score < 8)
- Small for gestational age or postmaturity
- Linear ("streaky") infiltrates and hyperinflation on chest radiograph

Late-Onset Neonatal Pneumonia

Late-onset neonatal pneumonia is defined as pneumonia occurring 48–72 hours after birth but within the first month of life and usually reflects a postpartum nosocomial infection. The newborn acquires the infectious agent from fomites, contaminated devices, or caregivers who are carriers. The microorganisms gain access to the lung via either the respiratory tract or the circulation. Prolonged mechanical ventilation represents the most important risk factor for late-onset pneumonia and often leads to ventilator-associated pneumonia (VAP) with *Pseudomonas aeruginosa* as a common pathogen. *Staphylococcus* spp. (*S. aureus*, *S. pyogenes*, or *S. epidermidis*) are also common agents especially in newborns with vascular access devices or other invasive devices. Late-onset GBS usually presents with bacteremia or meningitis rather than pneumonia. Respiratory syncytial virus (RSV) is the most common cause of late-onset neonatal pneumonia of viral origin (see later).

Community-Acquired Pneumonia

The British Thoracic Society (BTS) defines community-acquired pneumonia (CAP) as the presence of signs and symptoms in previously healthy children with an infection that has been acquired outside the hospital. The Infectious Diseases Society of America and the BTS have published clinical practice guidelines recently in an attempt to streamline the management of pediatric CAP (6–8). Most CAP in children >6 months of age can be managed on an outpatient basis. This section focuses on severe CAP requiring hospitalization and pediatric intensive care unit (PICU) admission.

Microbiology Based on Age Group and Symptoms

Among infants <2 months old, the bacterial etiologies are more frequent, including *Streptococcus pneumoniae*, group B streptococci, gram-negative bacilli (from maternal genital tract or hospital flora), *Staphylococcus aureus*, and *C. trachomatis*. Even though the introduction of routine vaccination against *Haemophilus influenzae* type B (Hib) and pneumococcal disease in developed countries has significantly lowered infection rates among children <2 years old, infants <6 months old will not have completed the primary vaccination series against

these agents. Young infants with "typical" bacterial pneumonia are usually highly febrile (>39°C) and tachypneic, and appear toxic. *C. trachomatis* (or less commonly *Mycoplasma hominis*, or *Ureaplasma urealyticum*) may cause a syndrome of "afebrile pneumonia of infancy" among infants 2 weeks to 4 months old.

Pertussis ("whooping cough") is making resurgence worldwide, but especially in developed countries, where introduction of universal vaccination against *Bordetella pertussis* was once thought to have nearly eradicated the disease (9). Young infants are at greatest risk for complications of the disease. The presentation is characteristic with prolonged staccato cough, followed by an inspiratory "whoop." Many infants will vomit after the coughing spasm. Infants with pertussis pneumonia are critically ill with extreme leukocytosis (WBC > 50,000–60,000 cells/μL), pulmonary hypertension, hypoxia, apnea (15%–30% incidence), and seizures (1% incidence). A high index of suspicion is needed to diagnose pertussis early when an upper respiratory tract infection does not resolve after a week, but instead progresses with worsening cough. The diagnosis should be made based on clinical grounds but confirmed with culture and PCR. The American Academy of Pediatrics Committee on Infectious Disease ("Redbook") recommends azithromycin for treatment of young infants with pertussis. The US Food and Drug Administration (FDA) has not approved azithromycin for infants <6 months old. The risk of infantile hypertrophic pyloric stenosis should be considered with the use of erythromycin in infants <1 month of age. The risk of cardiac electrical abnormalities should be considered with azithromycin use in infants with prolonged QT syndrome, those on antiarrhythmic therapy, and those with abnormal potassium or magnesium levels. Strict use of droplet precautions (e.g., caregiver mask) avoids nosocomial spread of pertussis.

Among infants 6–12 months old, viruses are the main pneumonia-causative pathogens (10). RSV and influenza are most common, but parainfluenza, adenovirus, rhinovirus, coronavirus, measles, rubella, varicella, cytomegalovirus, or herpes may also cause pneumonia. A viral etiology (as opposed to a bacterial one) is more likely if the infant with tachypnea has a temperature <38.5°C, WBC < 20,000, and no evidence of lobar infiltrates on chest radiograph.

Among children 1–5 years, viruses remain the predominant cause of pneumonia. To date, *S. pneumonia* remains the most common cause of bacterial pneumonia in this age group, although further reductions in prevalence of pneumococcal disease are expected following the conversion from a 7-valent pneumococcal vaccine to a 13-valent vaccine in 2009. The incidence of community-acquired methicillin-resistant *Staphylococcus aureus* (MRSA) has increased in many regions of the world, but especially in the United States (US). MRSA is more commonly associated with necrotizing pneumonia and empyema than other organisms. The knowledge of local and regional antibiotic resistance patterns is critically important for the treating intensivist. Clinical deterioration in a young child with influenza or varicella may arise because of secondary infection with *Staphylococcus aureus* or *Staphylococcus pyogenes*, respectively.

Less common pathogens include helminths (*Ascaris lumbricoides*, *Strongyloides stercoralis*, Toxocara kennels), human metapneumovirus (hMPV), *B. pertussis*, *Mycobacterium tuberculosis*, *Listeria monocytogenes*, *Legionella pneumophila*, Hantavirus, *Coxiella burnetii*, protozoa (e.g., *Toxoplasma gondii*), fungi (including *Pneumocystis jiroveci*), and physical and chemical agents.

Among children >3–5 years of age, *Streptococcus pneumoniae*, *Chlamydophila pneumoniae*, and *Mycoplasma pneumoniae* are the most common bacterial causes of pneumonia. The relative incidence of *Mycoplasma* pneumonia increases with age, and it accounts for approximately half of all pneumonias among college students. Viral pneumonia is verified based on laboratory investigations in ~8% of older children with pneumonia. Diagnostic studies will be negative in 50%–60% of older children with clinical pneumonia (11).

Specific Pneumonia Treatment

❼ The Pediatric Infectious Diseases Society and the Infectious Diseases Society of America have developed evidence-based recommendations for CAP antibiotic therapy that are based on the child's immunization status (Table 48.1).

For the treatment of infections caused by *C. trachomatis* and *M. pneumoniae*, a macrolide is the drug of choice. Data suggest the use of azithromycin for 5 days for the treatment of *C. pneumoniae* pneumonia (12).

For patients with suspicion for *S. pneumoniae* pneumonia, therapy is driven by the local antimicrobial susceptibility pattern, and IV ampicillin or ceftriaxone (in cases with probability of penicillin resistance) is used. Vancomycin is rarely necessary for the treatment of suspected *S. pneumoniae* pneumonia (may depend on incidence of cephalosporin resistance in the community), but should be added if MRSA is prevalent in the community. When infection due to Hib is suspected (e.g., unimmunized child), ceftriaxone, cefotaxime, or ampicillin–sulbactam should be used because of the presence of β-lactamase–mediated resistance to ampicillin in several Hib strains. The optimal duration of the antimicrobial therapy for complicated or uncomplicated pneumonia has not been established for the majority of pathogens. However, most pneumonia are treated for 10 days, although shorter courses may be indicated in mild disease in order to minimize microbial selection for resistance. Conversely, MRSA or pneumonia complicated by effusion or empyema is guided by clinical response and may extend to 2–4 weeks. Initial empiric therapy can be modified after the identification of the etiologic agent (Table 48.2).

Pneumonia in the Immunocompromised Host

❶ In the immunocompromised child, pulmonary infection leads to increased morbidity and mortality from a wide spectrum of microorganisms, including opportunistic agents. The pathogenesis is similar to that of the healthy host, except that the impaired host defense allows ready spread of the organism from the upper respiratory tract. The clinical manifestations in an immunocompromised child are highly variable. Several chronic immune deficiency states are associated with characteristic pneumonia syndromes, which are discussed in detail in Chapter 50 (Chronic Respiratory Failure), Chapter 86 (Primary Immune Deficiency Disorders), Chapter 95 (Opportunistic Infections), Chapter 115 (Oncologic Emergencies), Chapter 117 (Stem Cell Transplantation), and Chapter 119 (Sickle Cell Disease). The radiologic pattern in immunocompromised children may indicate the probable pathogens:

- Focal consolidation (*Streptococcus pneumoniae*, *H. influenzae*, *Legionella* sp., mycobacteria, and fungi)
- Micronodular pattern (viruses, mycobacteria, *Histoplasma*, *Candida* sp., and *Cryptococcus*)
- Nodular pattern (*Aspergillus* sp., other fungi, mucormycosis, *Nocardia* sp., and Epstein-Barr Virus (EBV)—lymphoproliferative disease)
- Diffuse interstitial pattern (viruses, *M. pneumoniae*, Chlamydia, and *P. jiroveci*).

Children with immunodeficient conditions and presenting with tachypnea or hypoxia require immediate hospitalization, empiric antibiotics (pending the outcome of diagnostic tests), and close monitoring. Aggressive interventions (e.g., bronchopulmonary lavage or lung biopsy) may be needed to determine a definitive microbiologic diagnosis (13).

TABLE 48.1

EMPIRIC THERAPY FOR PEDIATRIC COMMUNITY-ACQUIRED PNEUMONIA (CAP)

■ SITE OF CARE	EMPIRIC THERAPY		
	■ PRESUMED BACTERIAL PNEUMONIA	■ PRESUMED ATYPICAL PNEUMONIA	■ PRESUMED INFLUENZA PNEUMONIA
Inpatient (all ages)			
Fully immunized with conjugate vaccines for *Haemophilus influenzae* type b and *Streptococcus pneumoniae*; local penicillin resistance in invasive strains of pneumococcus is minimal	Ampicillin or penicillin G; alternatives: ceftriaxone or cefotaxime; addition of vancomycin or clindamycin for suspected CA-MRSA	Azithromycin (in addition to β-lactam, if diagnosis of atypical pneumonia is in doubt); alternatives: clarithromycin or erythromycin; doxycycline for children >7 years old; levofloxacin for children who have reached growth maturity, or who cannot tolerate macrolides	Oseltamivir or zanamivir (for children ≥7 years old; alternatives: peramivir, oseltamivir and zanamivir (all intravenous) are under clinical investigation in children; intravenous zanamivir available for compassionate use
Not fully immunized for *H. influenzae* type b and *S. pneumoniae*; local penicillin resistance in invasive strains of pneumococcus is significant	Ceftriaxone or cefotaxime; addition of vancomycin or clindamycin for suspected CA-MRSA; alternative: levofloxacin; addition of vancomycin or clindamycin for suspected CA-MRSA	Azithromycin (in addition to β-lactam, if diagnosis in doubt); alternatives: clarithromycin or erythromycin; doxycycline for children >7 years old; levofloxacin for children who have reached growth maturity or who cannot tolerate macrolides	As above

See **Table 48.2** for dosages.
CA-MRSA, community-acquired methicillin-resistant *Staphylococcus aureus*.
Reproduced with permission from Bradley JS, Byington CL, Shah SS, et al. The management of community-acquired pneumonia in infants and children older than 3 months of age: Clinical practice guidelines by the Pediatric Infectious Diseases Society and the Infectious Diseases Society of America. *Clin Infect Dis* 2011;53(7):e25–76.

TABLE 48.2

ETIOLOGY-SPECIFIC THERAPY

■ AGENT	■ ANTIMICROBIALS
Chlamydia trachomatis	Azithromycin (10 mg/kg/day for 2 days, then 5 mg/kg/day), clarithromycin (15 mg/kg/day in 2 doses), oral erythromycin (40 mg/kg/day in 4 doses), or intravenous erythromycin lactobionate (20 mg/kg/day every 6 hours); for children >7 years old, doxycycline (2–4 mg/kg/day in 2 doses
	Levofloxacin 16–20 mg/kg/day every 12 hours for children 6 months to 5 years old and 8–10 mg/kg/day once daily for children 5–16 years old; maximum daily dose, 750 mg
Chlamydophila pneumoniae	Azithromycin (10 mg/kg/day for 2 days, then 5 mg/kg/day), clarithromycin (15 mg/kg/day in 2 doses), oral erythromycin (40 mg/kg/day in 4 doses), or intravenous erythromycin lactobionate (20 mg/kg/day every 6 hours); for children >7 years old, doxycycline (2–4 mg/kg/day in 2 doses
	Levofloxacin 16–20 mg/kg/day every 12 hours for children 6 months to 5 years old and 8–10 mg/kg/day once daily for children 5–16 years old; maximum daily dose, 750 mg
Mycoplasma pneumoniae	Azithromycin (10 mg/kg/day for 2 days, then 5 mg/kg/day), clarithromycin (15 mg/kg/day in 2 doses), oral erythromycin (40 mg/kg/day in 4 doses), or intravenous erythromycin lactobion-ate (20 mg/kg/day every 6 hours); for children >7 years old, doxycycline (2–4 mg/kg/day in 2 doses
	Levofloxacin 16–20 mg/kg/day every 12 hours for children 6 months to 5 years old and 8–10 mg/kg/day once daily for children 5–16 years old; maximum daily dose, 750 mg
Group B β-hemolytic streptococcus	Ampicillin (100–200 mg/kg/day) plus gentamicin (5 mg/kg/day)
	OR
	Plus amikacin (15 mg/kg/day)
Streptococcus pneumoniae	
Sensitive to penicillin	Crystalline penicillin (100,000–250,000 units/kg/day) or ampicillin (150–200 mg/kg/day)
Intermediate sensitivity	Penicillin (200,000–250,000 units/kg/day)
Resistant to penicillin	Cefotaxime (200 mg/kg/day) or ceftriaxone (100 mg/kg/day)
Resistant to penicillin and cephalosporins	Vancomycin (40–60 mg/kg/day) or clindamycin (30–45 mg/kg/day)
With MICs for penicillin ≤2.0 µg/mL or resistant to penicillin, with MICs ≥4.0 µg/mL	Levofloxacin 16–20 mg/kg/day every 12 hours for children 6 months to 5 years old and 8–10 mg/kg/day once daily for children 5–16 years old; maximum daily dose, 750 mg
Haemophilus influenzae	
β-Lactamase negative	Ampicillin (100–200 mg/kg/day)
β-Lactamase positive	Cefotaxime (200 mg/kg/day), ceftriaxone (100 mg/kg/day), or levofloxacin (16–20 mg/kg/day every 12 hours for children 6 months to 5 years old and 8–10 mg/kg/day once daily for children 5–16 years old; maximum daily dose, 750 mg)
Staphylococcus aureus	
Methicillin sensitive	Oxacillin (200 mg/kg/day)
Methicillin resistant	Vancomycin (40–60 mg/kg/day) or teicoplanin (10 mg/kg/day) plus clindamycin (30–35 mg/kg/day)
Simian retrovirus, influenza B, parainfluenza	Ribavirin (15–20 mg/kg/day) (orally or IV; IV not approved in US) for immunocompromised patients, premature babies, those with chronic pulmonary diseases, congenital heart disease, or pulmonary hypertension, or critically ill patients
Influenza A and B	Oseltamivir 3 mg/kg/dose PO/NG bid × 5 days (2 weeks–1 year old)
	Oseltamivir 30 mg PO/NG bid × 5 days (>1 year old and <15 kg body weight)
	Oseltamivir 45 mg PO/NG bid × 5 days (15–23 kg body weight)
	Oseltamivir 60 mg PO/NG bid × 5 days (23–40 kg body weight)
	Oseltamivir 75 mg PO/NG bid × 5 days (>40 kg body weight)
Herpes simplex or zoster	Acyclovir (250 mg/m^2/8 h) (IV)
	(20 mg/kg/8 h)
	OR
	Foscarnet (60 mg/kg/8 h) (IV)
Cytomegalovirus	Ganciclovir 2.5 mg/kg/8 h initial (IV)
	5 mg/kg/12 h (2–3 weeks) or foscarnet
Fungi	Amphotericin B (1 mg/kg/day)
	Liposomal amphotericin B (3 mg/kg/day) or fluconazole (6 mg/kg/day)

MIC, minimum inhibitory concentration.

Nosocomial Pneumonia

5 Pneumonia is a frequent nosocomial infection. According to the National Nosocomial Infections Surveillance System, pneumonia associated with mechanical ventilation is the second leading cause of nosocomial infection (20%). Nosocomial pneumonia occurs more frequently in children between 2 and 12 months of age, and the most frequent microorganism recovered is *P. aeruginosa* (22%) (14). The European multicentered study group found a nosocomial infection rate of 23.6% in children, and the most frequent infection was pneumonia (53%), with *P. aeruginosa* (44%) being the most frequent pathogen (15). Another study in PICU patients found a nosocomial infection prevalence of 12%, and in this group, pneumonia was associated with mechanical ventilation in 22.7% (16).

Pneumonias acquired after 48 hours of hospitalization are considered nosocomial. Nosocomial pneumonia can occur in mechanically ventilated patients (*ventilator-associated pneumonia, VAP*) or in hospitalized patients breathing through a natural airway (*health care-associated pneumonia, HCAP*) (17). Tracheobronchitis may be part of the nosocomial respiratory infection and is characterized by an increasing volume of respiratory secretions, fever, and leukocytosis without radiologic evidence of pulmonary infiltrates or consolidation.

Identification and reduction of VAP in the PICU is a current focus of infection control efforts at many centers (see Chapter 92). The airways may be colonized by pathogens originating from pharyngeal, intestinal, or hospital flora. A systematic review of VAP in children from 1947–2010 has identified *P. aeruginosa* followed by *S. aureus* as the predominant microorganisms in pediatric VAP (18). *Pseudomonas* is more common in pediatric ICUs, whereas *S. aureus* is more common in neonatal ICUs. Polymicrobial infections occur in 38% and 58% of PICU and Neonatal Intensive-Care Unit (NICU) VAP, respectively (19,20). Other gram-negative organisms such as *Klebsiella* spp., *Escherichia coli*, *Enterobacter* spp., *Serratia marcescens*, and *Acinetobacter* spp. are the next most common VAP organisms. *S. pneumonia* and *Candida albicans* each account for 3%–12% of VAP isolates (18). Patients with leukemia, lymphoma, acquired immunodeficiency syndrome (AIDS), or post–organ transplant may develop VAP due to viral infections or *P. jiroveci*.

Empiric Treatment of Nosocomial Pneumonia

Based on the above etiologic considerations, potential empiric antibiotic regimens for bacterial nosocomial pneumonia include any one of the following combinations for children >6 months of age:

- Gentamicin* 2.5 mg/kg/dose IV q8h *plus* meropenem 20 mg/kg/dose IV q8h
Or
- Gentamicin* 2.5 mg/kg/dose IV q8h *plus* piperacillin–tazobactam 75 mg/kg/dose IV q8h
Or
- Gentamicin* 2.5 mg/kg/dose IV q8h *plus* ticarcillin–clavulanate 50 mg/kg/dose IV q4h
Or
- Gentamicin* 2.5 mg/kg/dose IV q8h *plus* clindamycin 10 mg/kg/dose IV q6h (Note: useful for anaerobic coverage)
Or
- Gentamicin* 2.5 mg/kg/dose IV q8h *plus* ceftazidime 50 mg/kg/dose IV q8h (Note: does not offer any anaerobic coverage)

If MRSA is suspected, add vancomycin to any of these combinations.

If extended-spectrum β-lactamase–producing gram-negative bacilli are prevalent in the hospital, these combinations should be replaced with:

- Amikacin* 5 mg/kg/dose IV q8h *plus* meropenem 20 mg/kg/dose IV q8h

---

*After the first gentamicin or amikacin dose, subsequent dosing should be adjusted based on the measurement of peak and trough serum concentrations to avoid neuro- and ototoxicities.

TABLE 48.3

PNEUMONIA CLINICAL MANIFESTATIONS AND ETIOLOGIC AGENTS

■ CLINICAL MANIFESTATIONS	■ ETIOLOGIC AGENT
High fever	Bacterial pneumonia
Cyanosis	All pneumonia pathogens
Wheezing	Virus (especially respiratory syncytial virus)
Myalgia	Virus (especially influenza), *Mycoplasma. pneumoniae*
Upper airway distress	Virus (especially parainfluenza)
Conjunctivitis	*Chlamydia*, adenovirus
Cutaneous abscesses	*Staphylococcus aureus*
Purpura	*Pseudomonas aeruginosa*
Paroxysmal cough	*Chlamydia trachomatis, Bordetella pertussis*
Acute otitis	*Streptococcus pneumoniae*/type B *Haemophilus influenzae*
Effusion/empyema	*S. pneumoniae/S. aureus*
Sudden onset	*S. aureus*

Aspiration Pneumonia

Aspiration pneumonia occurs when airway protective reflexes are either inadequate or overwhelmed. Obtundation or other neurologic disability represents the most common predisposing factor for aspiration pneumonia in the PICU. Gastroesophageal reflux, swallowing incoordination, protracted vomiting, and instrumentation involving the upper airway (e.g., nasogastric tube) represent other risks for aspiration. The nature of the resulting pneumonia depends on whether the aspirate consists of gastric acid (chemical pneumonitis), upper airway flora (bacterial pneumonia), or particulate matter (airway obstruction).

Prevention constitutes the most effective approach to the risk of aspiration pneumonia. Older children can be cared for with the head elevated to 30 degrees. Patients with altered levels of consciousness should have serial assessments of cough and gag reflexes so that prophylactic endotracheal intubation can be performed before aspiration occurs. Dental hygiene decreases the bacterial load available for aspiration. Treatment is primarily supportive once aspiration pneumonia has developed and involves suctioning of the trachea and escalation of ventilator support. Large particulate matter may require bronchoscopic removal. Corticosteroids have not been demonstrated to improve outcome. Aspiration of oral secretions, especially in neurologically impaired children, should be directed at anaerobic organisms. A commonly used empiric coverage regimen for aspiration of oral secretions includes ampicillin and clindamycin. Gastric acid aspiration does not require antibiotic coverage; however, vigilance is needed because of the risk of bacterial superinfection.

---

3 ## Diagnosis

Clinical Manifestations

The clinical features of pneumonia vary according to the etiologic agent (**Table 48.3**), and the child's nutritional status, immunologic competence, and comorbidities. A careful history provides valuable clues to the etiology and hence guides therapy. A fully immunized child is unlikely to present with pneumonia from influenza, *B. pertussis*, Hib, or an *S. pneumoniae* serotype covered by the current vaccine. A history of a choking episode should prompt evaluation for aspiration. Headache or photophobia may suggest *M. pneumonia*. Recent or prolonged antibiotic usage raises the concern of antibiotic resistance.

The individual signs of pneumonia are nonspecific, but taken together and combined with a careful history, they are valuable in arriving at the correct diagnosis. Fever, lethargy, poor appetite (~75%), pallor or cyanosis, toxemia, agitation, vomiting (30%–45%), abdominal distension, abdominal pain (>20%), and dehydration (25%) represent some of the signs of pneumonia. While most children with infectious pneumonia develop fever, children with *C. trachomatis* or viral pneumonia may have minimal or no fever. Lung auscultation findings include crackles, diminished breath sounds, or bronchial breath sounds. Wheezing can be observed in children with bacterial pneumonia, but it is more common in children with bronchiolitis.

Tachypnea is the most sensitive parameter in children with pneumonia (21). The WHO defines tachypnea based on the age of the child:

- <2 months old: >60 breaths/minute
- 2–12 months old: >50 breaths/minute
- 1–5 years old: >40 breaths/minute
- >5 years old: >20 breaths/minute

Tachypnea in a child should trigger measurement of O_2 saturation. Hypoxia, defined as O_2 saturation <92% while breathing room air, is an indication for hospitalization. The extent of respiratory distress (nasal flaring, intercostal and subcostal retractions, grunting, and chest pain) and lethargy suggest whether PICU care will be required (22).

Laboratory Studies

In the presence of bacterial pneumonia, the white blood cell count is elevated >25,000/mm^3 or even >35,000/mm^3 (23). Other inflammatory markers, such as C-reactive protein, procalcitonin, and erythrocyte sedimentation rate, are usually elevated. Bacterial blood cultures are recommended for the diagnosis and management of pneumonia, particularly when a bacterial etiology is suspected (24). Bacterial isolation in blood cultures varies from 3%–11%, but this rarely modifies the patient's management (25). Although uncommon, the identification of a specific organism (*S. pneumoniae* or *S. aureus*), along with the antimicrobial activity, can be especially useful in more serious cases or when pleural effusions are present. Viral diagnosis (culture, PCR, or antigen detection using direct fluorescence) is important in guiding therapy (especially for immunocompromised children) and in establishing infection control precautions. PCR has high sensitivity and specificity for *Mycoplasma* infections, which can also be identified using serology (positive IgM indicates an acute infection). When *Legionella* infection is suspected, the pathogen urinary antigen is the diagnostic test of choice. The test remains positive for weeks after acute infection. When chest x-ray suggests a mycobacterium disease (mediastinal enlargement) or when epidemiologic risk factors increase the probability of tuberculosis infection, a purified protein derivative of tuberculin skin test should be performed.

Imaging

A chest radiography is indicated in any child with suspected pneumonia exhibiting any one of the following conditions:

- Room air O_2 saturation <92%
- Moderate–severe respiratory distress
- History of apneic episodes
- Altered mental status
- Hemodynamic instability
- Temperature >39°C in a child <36 months old with WBC > 20,000/μL
- Planned hospitalization
- Failure to respond to therapy
- Suspected complication (e.g., pleural effusion, empyema)

There are limitations to the radiographic examination. Radiographic findings cannot distinguish viral, bacterial, and atypical pneumonia. Furthermore, the radiographic findings may lag behind the clinical examination, especially in the presence of dehydration. The presence of large pleural effusions, necrotizing pneumonia, and abscesses support a high suspicion of bacterial infection, but in the absence of complications, radiographic findings should not be used to differentiate bacterial from viral etiology. There is high reliability among the radiologists' analyses of the radiographic findings of alveolar infiltrates and pleural effusions. The interpretations of radiographic interstitial infiltrates appear to be less reliable (26). The radiologic changes resolve in a few weeks, and complete resolution varies depending on the pneumonia extent, etiology, and other host factors.

Lung ultrasound is a nonionizing, real-time procedure that is easy and fast using handheld systems. It can be accomplished without the need for sedation. The nonionizing aspect is important in newborns and children due to the risk of cancer associated with ionizing radiation (27,28). Recent studies suggest that in the hands of a skilled sonographer, lung ultrasound is at least as accurate as chest radiography in diagnosing bronchiolitis (29) and pneumonia (30,31). It is useful in early identification of a cavitation and in the differentiation of a pneumonic process in relation to another intrathoracic event. Thoracic ultrasound requires an acoustic window (usually through the intercostal region) because bone and gas densities interfere with the sound beam. Ultrasound is suitable for injuries located peripherally (chest wall borderline processes, diaphragm). In patients with peripheral lesions, chest ultrasound allows differentiation between the lung and pleural involvement, and is also useful to guide biopsies, needle aspiration, or drainage.

High-resolution computed tomography (HRCT) shows all anatomical structures, including bones and aerated lungs, and is more sensitive than chest x-ray for the detection of pneumonia. It may be especially useful in immunosuppressed patients, in whom the image pattern may suggest fungal or *P. jiroveci* pneumonia. HRCT may also be useful in defining the optimal location for lung biopsy or evaluating suppurative complications such as empyema or lung necrosis.

Differential Diagnosis

A diagnosis of pneumonia is possible in children who present with fever, cough, tachypnea, and an infiltration on chest x-ray. However, several other diseases can have a similar presentation, such as AB, tracheobronchitis, pulmonary embolism, and thoracic tumors. One should also consider nonpulmonary diseases such as leukemia infiltrates, congestive heart failure, metabolic acidosis with compensatory tachypnea, malaria, or inflammatory diseases (systemic vasculitis).

The diagnosis is essentially clinical, based on history, physical examination, radiologic interpretation, and epidemiologic data (**Table 48.3**). When the symptoms persist despite empiric therapy, fiberoptic bronchoscopy with bronchoalveolar lavage is a diagnostic option. Early bronchoscopy may be indicated in immunocompromised children in whom the selection of antibiotics is otherwise difficult.

Management

Hospital Admission Criteria

There is no validated scoring system for hospitalization of children with pneumonia and specific risks indicating the need for hospitalization (32). However, guidelines for the assessment of pneumonia severity are available from the BTS (7). The Pediatric Infectious Diseases Society and the Infectious Diseases Society of America have assigned levels of evidence to its recommendations for hospitalization of children >3 months of age with pneumonia (33). Hospitalization is recommended under the following conditions:

- Moderate-to-severe CAP including respiratory distress and hypoxemia (SpO$_2$ < 90 at sea level); strong recommendation, high-quality evidence
- Age <3–6 months with suspected CAP; strong recommendation, low quality of evidence
- CAP due to highly virulent microorganisms (e.g., MRSA); strong recommendation, low quality of evidence
- Parental inability to comply with therapy or follow-up; strong recommendation, low quality of evidence

PICU Admission Criteria

The Pediatric Infectious Diseases Society (33) outlined seven recommendations for PICU admission (or for admission to a unit with continuous cardiorespiratory monitoring):

- Need for invasive ventilation via a nonpermanent artificial airway (i.e., endotracheal intubation, not tracheostomy) requires admission to PICU; strong recommendation, high-quality evidence
- Need for noninvasive positive pressure ventilation; strong recommendation, very low-quality evidence
- Progressive respiratory failure; strong recommendation, moderate evidence
- Sustained tachycardia, inadequate blood pressure, or need for pharmacological support to maintain blood pressure or perfusion; strong recommendation, moderate evidence
- Pulse oximetry is <92% with FIO$_2$ ≥ 0.50; strong recommendation, low quality of evidence
- Altered level of consciousness due to hypercarbia or hypoxemia resulting from pneumonia; strong recommendation, low quality of evidence
- Disease severity scores should not be used as the sole criteria for PICU admission, but should be considered in the context of other clinical, laboratory, and radiologic data; strong recommendation, low-quality evidence

Supportive Therapy

Supportive therapy is an essential component of the care of the critically ill child with pneumonia. Proper nutritional support is vital, especially if the pneumonia presents in the context of chronic nutritional deficiency states (see Chapter 97). Children with severe respiratory distress or needing assisted ventilation will require nasogastric or nasojejunal feedings. If possible, the child's head and upper body should be elevated 30 degrees to minimize the risk of aspiration. Dehydration and hyponatremia due to the syndrome of inappropriate antidiuretic hormone secretion (SIADH) represent two possible fluid and electrolyte disorders associated with pneumonia that require correction (see Chapter 107). Respiratory therapy with heated and humidified O$_2$ therapy, suctioning of the airway, chest physiotherapy, and assisted ventilation represent the cornerstones of supportive care in severe pneumonia and are discussed in Chapters 38 and 39.

Prevention (Including Vaccines)

Primary prevention measures such as infection control (hand hygiene, use of mask), immunization, and avoidance of exposure of the airways and lungs to irritants (cigarette, pollution) help reduce the susceptibility to infection by microorganisms in the respiratory tract. Chemoprophylaxis is indicated for some types of pneumonia in immunocompromised patients and in children with heart disease or asplenia.

The current resurgence of vaccine-preventable disease in the US and the persistence of vaccine-preventable disease in many developing countries make full immunization of every child a global health priority (34). Vaccination against Hib, *B. pertussis*, and the pneumococcal strains included in 13-valent *S. pneumonia* vaccine provide the best protection of every child against pneumonia.

Although there has been an increased prevalence of pneumococcal strains that are not present in the vaccine, the current vaccine remains highly effective in reducing invasive pneumococcal disease. The antipneumococcal conjugated vaccine reduces by 30% the episodes of radiographically confirmed pneumonia in young children (7). Children older than 2 years and who are at high risk for pneumococcal disease (sickle cell disease, chronic heart and lung disease, HIV, and diabetes mellitus type 1) should also receive the 23-valent vaccine against pneumococcus. Viral infections cause pneumonia or predispose children to infection due to typical or atypical pathogens; therefore, immunization against influenza should be performed. In Ontario, Canada, the introduction of universal immunization against influenza was compared with the immunization program in other provinces and showed a decrease in mortality in all age groups, as well as a reduction in the rate of hospitalization, emergency department visits, and outpatient visits in patients aged <5 years and between 5 and 19 years (35).

Complications

Pneumonia complications include pleural effusions, empyema, extrapulmonary infection, sepsis, acute respiratory distress syndrome, shock, lung abscess, pneumothorax, atelectasis, and multiple organ system dysfunction. These conditions are discussed in other chapters of this book. Pleural effusion and empyema are the most frequent acute complications and are collectively known as parapneumonic effusions.

Pleural Effusion

Pleural effusion represents a fluid collection within the pleural cavity in association with pneumonia. It develops in 1% of patients with CAP, but in hospitalized children, this rate can be as high as 40% (36). The pathogenesis of pleural effusion involves the spread of the inflammatory mediators from the lung to adjacent pleura. Inflammation of the pleura results in leakage of plasma and white cells into the pleural cavity. The fluid in pleural effusion is usually sterile.

Pleural effusions can occur associated with many etiologic agents. *S. pneumoniae* is responsible for most of the cases, although *S. aureus* and *S. pyogenes* are also associated with high incidence of pleural effusion and empyema (37). Tuberculosis is also a frequent cause of pleural effusion, and it should be considered in the differential diagnosis of certain patients. Pleural effusions are classified as transudates or exudates depending on the laboratory analysis of the pleural fluid (**Table 48.4**). Exudates have low pH (<7.2), low glucose (<40 mg/dL), and high lactate dehydrogenase (LDH; >1000 IU). Additional data include a positive microbiologic study (Gram test, culture, or other diagnostic tests, such as PCR).

Chest x-ray is indispensable for the correct diagnosis and follow-up of pleural effusion, demonstrating the magnitude and the evolution of this complication. The Pediatric Infectious Disease Society grades the magnitude of the effusion based on the width of the opacified rim from the inner margin of the ribs to the outer surface of the lung in a lateral decubitus (LD) chest x-ray (33):

- Small effusion: Rim < 10 mm (or <25% of hemithorax) in LD position
- Moderate effusion: Rim > 10 mm but <50% of hemithorax in LD position
- Large effusion: Rim > 50% of hemithorax in LD position

The risk of long-term sequelae of an effusion is directly proportional to its size. Chest ultrasonography is also useful in the diagnosis and follow-up. CT findings have not been reliable in predicting the effusion that will fulfill empyema criteria (38).

All children with a diagnosis of pleural effusion should have a diagnostic and sometimes therapeutic thoracentesis performed. The management algorithm depends on the size of the effusion and the degree of respiratory compromise in the child (**Fig. 48.1**). Conservative treatment of pleural infection consists of either isolated antibiotic therapy or antibiotic therapy and simple drainage (39). Most small parapneumonic effusions respond to antibiotic therapy without additional intervention. However, the pleural effusions that increase in volume or compromise breathing in an ill, feverish child must

TABLE 48.4

PLEURAL FLUID CHARACTERISTICS

	■ TRANSUDATE	■ EXUDATE
pH	>7.20	<7.20
Proteins (pleural fluid/serum level rate)	<0.5	≥0.5
LDH (pleural fluid/serum level rate)	<0.6	≥0.6
LDH (IU/L)	<200	≥200
Glucose (mg/dL)	>40	<40
Red cells (mm^3)	<5000	>5000
Leukocytes (mm^3)	<10,000 (PMN)	>10,000 (PMN)

LDH, lactate dehydrogenase; PMN, polymorphonuclear neutrophil.

Management of pneumonia with parapneumonic effusion

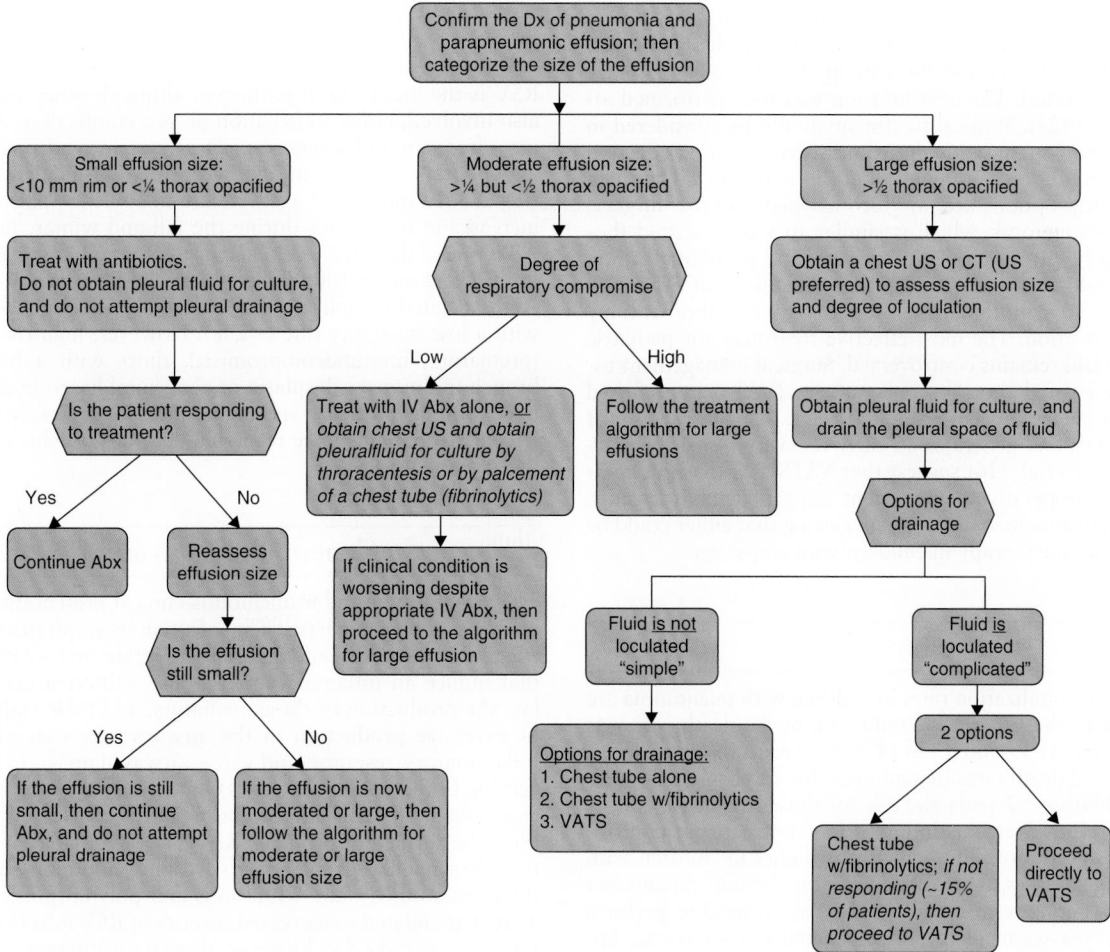

FIGURE 48.1. Management algorithm for parapneumonic effusion in children. Abx, antibiotics; CT, computed tomography; Dx, diagnosis; IV, intravenous; US, ultrasound; VATS, video-assisted thoracoscopic surgery. (From Bradley JS, Byington CL, Shah SS, et al. Executive summary: The management of community-acquired pneumonia in infants and children older than 3 months of age: Clinical practice guidelines by the Pediatric Infectious Diseases Society and the Infectious Diseases Society of America. *Clin Infect Dis* 2011;53(7):617–30, with permission.)

be drained. If the child has a significant pleural infection, a thoracostomy tube should be inserted. Repeated thoracentesis punctures are not recommended.

The initial empiric IV antibiotic therapy should cover *S. pneumoniae*. Broad-spectrum antibiotics are necessary for nosocomial infections, as well as for those secondary to surgery, trauma, and aspiration. The antibiotic choice should be guided by the microbiologic results.

Empyema

Pneumonia with pleural fluid containing pus is termed empyema (40). One should suspect empyema in a child with persistent fever, beyond 7 days, despite appropriate antibiotic treatment. The best method to estimate the amount of fluid in the pleural space is ultrasound examination (41). Chronic complications include bronchial wall thickening, bronchiectasis, predisposition to asthma, constrictive bronchiolitis, fibrothorax, mediastinal fibrosis, constrictive pericarditis, and pleural thickening.

Intrapleural fibrinolytics may shorten hospital length of stay and are recommended by some for complicated parapneumonic effusions (loculated thick fluid) or empyema; however, only urokinase was analyzed in randomized controlled trials (TCTs) involving children (42). Urokinase should be administered twice per day for three consecutive days: 10,000 units in 10 mL of normal saline for children <1 year of age and 40,000 units in 40 mL of normal saline in those ≥ 1 year old. In the original urokinase clinical trial, the chest tube was clamped for 4 hours and the patient stimulated to mobilize during this period. The next infusion was then performed after 8 hours (42a). Surgical treatment should be considered in patients who remain septic due to persistent pleural collection despite chest thoracostomy and antibiotic therapy. The three main surgical options are (a) video-assisted thoracic surgery; (b) minithoracotomy, which is similar to video-assisted thoracic surgery but is an open procedure; and (c) decortication, a more prolonged and complicated procedure. An organized empyema in a symptomatic child may require a thoracotomy and decortication. The most effective treatment for pediatric empyema still remains controversial. Surgical management using video-assisted thoracoscopic surgery (VATS) is preferred because it is least invasive, safe, efficient, decreases length of hospital stay, and generates an early recovery (43–45). However, St Peter et al. (46) suggest that VATS as a therapy, compared to nonoperative management using fibrinolytic agents, offers no advantage in recovery, suggesting that either could be used as first-line therapy in children with empyema.

Outcome

Although hospitalization rates in children with pneumonia are increasing in the US, a 97% reduction in the death rate was seen between 1939 and 1996 (47). Between 1995 and 1997, the estimated death rates (not adjusted for comorbidities) were 4% for children <2 years and 2% for those between 2 and 17 years (48). Improvements in intensive care treatment contributed to reduced mortality, which was higher in children with underlying diseases. Most children who develop pneumonia do not have long-term sequelae. There is no need to perform radiologic reassessment in uncomplicated cases showing improvement after 48 hours of antibiotic therapy (7).

Children who have noncomplicated parapneumonic effusions respond well to conservative treatment, without any residual lung lesion. Usually, the pleural disease due to virus or *Mycoplasma* resolves spontaneously. In contrast to adult patients, infants and children have a better ability to resolve pleural thickening without any subsequent detrimental effect in lung growth and function. The increased incidence of MRSA and organisms with increasing virulence factors may result in an increase in the occurrence of pneumonia and septic shock precipitated by these infections.

BRONCHIOLITIS

⑧

Definition and Overview

Acute bronchiolitis (AB) is a respiratory illness in infants and toddlers <24 months of age typically caused by viral infection and manifested by respiratory distress, wheezing, and crackles (rales) after a 1–3-day history of an upper respiratory tract infection (49). Approximately 5% of infants with bronchiolitis will experience life-threatening manifestations of the disease. The diagnosis of AB is primarily clinical; however, there is substantial heterogeneity among countries in diagnosing AB. In US the presence of expiratory wheezing is the main clinical sign, while in the United Kingdom it is crackling. Most AB cases are mild and self-limited and symptoms persist between 3 and 7 days. The majority of the cases can be managed at home with symptomatic measures. Transmission of pathogens is likely for hospitalized patients; hence, selective control measures are needed.

Epidemiology

RSV is the main causal pathogen, although other viruses are also involved, either in isolation or as a coinfection. AB is the most frequent and severe respiratory system syndrome involving children <2 years of age, with the peak incidence occurring at <12 months of age. AB has an epidemic pattern, with increases in prevalence during the fall and winter. In winter, AB is one of the most frequent causes of infant hospitalization. In the US, 2 out of 100,000 live-birth children die as a result of AB-associated complications (50). AB is generally self-limited, with a low mortality rate (<2%). However, high-risk infants (premature, immunocompromised, those with a history of bronchopulmonary dysplasia or congenital heart disease) may have prolonged disease and higher mortality rates. More than half of AB patients have recurring episodes of wheezing until 7–11 years of age.

Genetic Predisposition

The variability in the bronchiolitis clinical presentation probably has a polygenic basis. The infection by respiratory viruses triggers an event cascade that releases inflammatory mediators that induce an inflammatory response. Different genes regulate the production of these mediators, and their malfunction or excessive production in the airways may exacerbate the inflammatory response and cause airway damage (51). Concerning bronchiolitis, the genes containing the instructions for assembling the Toll-like receptor (TLR), the CX3C chemokine, the surfactant proteins, RANTES (Regulated on Activation, Normal T Cell Expressed) cytokine, and interleukins are the most studied ones. Mutations and polymorphisms in the TLR-4 are related to increased severity of RSV infections in infants <1 year (52,53); however, these results have not been reproduced in other populations. Polymorphisms of the CX3CR receptor gene (54), of the surfactant proteins (SP-B and SP-A2) (55,56) genes, and of the gene of CCR5 receptor of RANTES are associated with more severe bronchiolitis. Likewise, polymorphisms of interleukins IL-4, IL-8, IL-10, IL-13, and IL-18 are also associated with severe RSV infection (57). Some of these genetic variations (TLR, IL-4, IL-10) have their effect linked to the age of the patients. Janssen et al. (58) demonstrated that the greatest association between genetic variation and RSV infection occurs in the genes of innate immunity such as those of the vitamin D receptor and nitric oxide synthase, JUN oncogene, and the gene IFNA5 (58).

Pathogenesis

Viral infection of the distal bronchiolar epithelial cells leads to cellular swelling, excess mucus production, and, ultimately, cellular necrosis and sloughing. Peribronchiolar infiltration of inflammatory cells (lymphocytes, plasma cells, and macrophages) produces submucosal and adventitial edema. In parallel, goblet cells proliferate and produce excessive mucus that is poorly eliminated by the nonciliated (regenerating) epithelial cells. Subsequent to these changes, plugs of mucus laden with cellular debris are formed, leading to areas of narrowing and blocking of the bronchioles, causing the airway obstruction, hyperinflation, increased airway resistance, atelectasis, and ventilation–perfusion mismatch that characterize AB. In young infants, atelectasis may be hastened by the scarcity of collateral channels and by the supplementation of oxygen in high concentrations. Note that bronchial smooth muscle constriction appears to have little part in the disease course and has not been described. Infants' lungs are particularly sensitive to this pathology because of their small airways, high closing volumes, insufficient collateral ventilation, increased airway smooth muscle reactivity, and the absence of active immunity against RSV as well as to other respiratory viruses. The recovery stage of the disease begins after a few days with the regeneration of the epithelial cells from the basal membrane. The ciliated epithelium takes 13–17 weeks to be restored.

Studies indicate that the immune response can have a major impact on the disease. The infection triggers the immune system and increases secretion of various mediators that prompt and activate neutrophils, eosinophils, and activated T cells. However, the inflammatory response seen in the airway of AB children is different from that in children with asthma and allergies. Neutrophils are the prominent cells in the respiratory tract of children with RSV, while eosinophils are prominent in asthma. Also, neutrophil inflammation, not eosinophil inflammation, is related to the severity of a first AB in infants. The release of cytokines and chemokines (interferon and IL-4, IL-8, and IL-9 are found in high concentrations in respiratory secretions of AB patients) increases cellular recruitment into infected airways and amplifies the immune response. Damage to the bronchiolar epithelium is associated with recurrent wheezing later in childhood.

Microbiology Overview

A wide range of pathogens (parainfluenza, adenovirus, influenza, M. pneumoniae, rhinovirus, hMPV, and coronavirus) may cause AB. However, RSV (subtypes A and B) is by far the most frequently involved agent (59). Coinfection rates particularly in hospitalized young children may reach up to 30%. The most common concomitant infections are RSV combined with hMPV or rhinovirus. The relationship between disease severity and multiple-virus coinfection is not clear (60,61).

Specific Pathogens

Respiratory Syncytial Virus

RSV is the most common agent to cause AB. It is a single-stranded RNA virus member of the Paramyxoviridae family, and it is divided into two large subtypes mostly based on the surface G glucoproteins: A (dominant strain) and B. Subtype A causes the most severe cases. Generally, in a given season there is predominance of one over the other subtype.

Transmission of RSV occurs after contact with contaminated surfaces followed by inoculation into the nasopharynx or eye. RSV may persist for several hours on surfaces. Because direct contact is the major route for transmission, careful hand-washing forms the main infection control measure.

Prior infection with RSV generates serum antibodies which only offer partial protection. Hence it is possible to become infected with RSV more than once and even within the same season. Subsequent infections usually produce milder symptoms. High maternal antibody levels are associated with lower infection rates in infants. Prophylactic administration of antibodies has been effective in reducing, but not eliminating, severe RSV disease. In humans and animals with deficient T cells, the infection is more severe and RSV replication lasts longer (62).

Rhinovirus

The rhinovirus is typically associated with the common cold, but is also the second most common cause of bronchiolitis after RSV. The greater than 100 serotypes of rhinovirus have single-stranded RNA and are members of the Picornavirus family. Transmission occurs by self-inoculation into nasopharynx or conjunctiva and by aerosol droplets.

Influenza Virus

The Centers for Diseases Control report the child hospitalization rate associated with influenza virus as similar to that in the adult population (63). RSV and influenza lower respiratory tract infections cannot be distinguished based on clinical grounds alone in children <3 years of age (64). Current (2013–2014) isolates in the US are predominantly Influenza A H1N1 (65). Among patients with fatal influenza, the most frequent diagnosis before death was pneumonia (49%), followed by sepsis or shock (34%), laryngotracheobronchitis or croup (20%), disseminated intravascular coagulation (12%), AB (8%), and encephalopathy (6%). Studies conducted in Japan showed that ceasing influenza virus vaccination was associated with increased child mortality in those between 1 and 4 years of age (66).

Although influenza infection is self-limited, it may cause complications, such as pneumonia, Reye syndrome, myositis, febrile convulsion, and acute encephalopathy. Hospitalization, an increased disease severity, and complications are more frequent in children <2 years and in those with risk factors (asthma or other chronic pulmonary disease, severe heart disease, immunocompromise, hemoglobinopathies, and diabetes mellitus) (67).

Human Metapneumovirus

hMPV was first described in 2001 in 28 Dutch children with RSV-like disease (68). A paramyxovirus was isolated in these children and identified as a new metapneumovirus family member based on viral data, gene sequence, and constellation. This serologic study showed that all children >5 years old had anti-hMPV antibody, suggesting a high transmission level. This virus has probably been circulating in humans for the last 50 years.

The hMPV virus has universal distribution, especially during fall and winter seasons in temperate climates (69). It is associated with several clinical presentations, such as upper respiratory tract infection, AB, asthma exacerbation, pneumonia, and, occasionally, severe infections in immunocompromised patients (70). Severe AB can be caused by combined infection with hMPV and RSV (71).

Of the new metapneumovirus types, hMPV is the first known to infect humans (Paramyxoviridae family) (68). RSV belongs to a separate genus in the same family. hMPV has been identified in the nasopharynx aspirate of children and adults with respiratory system infection in several countries. The clinical syndrome of infected children ranges from mild respiratory symptoms to AB and pneumonia (72). The signs and symptoms of hMPV are fever (67%), cough (100%), rhinorrhea (92%), retractions (92%), wheezing (83%), vomiting (25%), and diarrhea (8%). Infection with hMPV causes AB (67%), pneumonia (17%), and acute otitis (50%). Average hospitalization time is 4.5 days, and one-third of the patients were in the hospital for >7 days. PCR studies indicate that hMPV is found in 1.5%–10% of children who had previously unexplained infection in the respiratory system (73).

The hMPV mostly affects children <2 years of age, predominantly those between 3 and 5 months. Epidemics of hMPV occur at different times than do those of other viruses. Due to its heterogeneity, multiple reinfections of hMPV may occur in the same patient, particularly in the aged and immunocompromised (69). In a prospective study that evaluated 208 children <3 years old hospitalized due to acute respiratory system infection, hMPV was identified in 12 (6%), RSV in 118 (57%), and influenza A in 49 (24%) (74). Of the hMPV-infected children, AB was diagnosed in 8 (68%), and pneumonia was diagnosed in 2 (17%). Of the RSV-infected children, AB was diagnosed in 99 (84%) and pneumonia was diagnosed in 30 (25%). In another prospective study (75), hMPV was found in 14% of a sample of 749 children <2 years of age and was second only to RSV (76%) in frequency. The hMPV infection occurs more frequently in infants. Recurrent wheezing was noted in 49.3% of children, followed by AB (46.4%). O₂ therapy was necessary in 58% of the patients, although mechanical ventilation was required for only one child. Mean hospital length of stay was 5 ± 3 days.

Coronavirus

Clinical manifestations of coronavirus infection are milder in young children than in adolescents and adults (76). The incubation period ranges from 2–7 days but may be >10 days, with fever higher than 38°C (100.4°F), dry cough, and dyspnea progressing to hypoxemia. Chest x-ray demonstrates early focal infiltration, progressing to generalization with interstitial infiltration in the majority of patients. Radiologic features are not distinct from bronchopneumonia caused by other pathogens. Laboratory changes include leukopenia or moderate lymphopenia with liver enzyme elevation.

A causal relationship between febrile respiratory disease and a new coronavirus (other than human coronavirus) was initially shown in China in 2003 (77); this disease was named severe acute respiratory syndrome (SARS). Infants and young children were not detected as a risk group, and only a few cases were found in children <15 years old.

Adenovirus

Adenovirus is so named because it is frequently isolated from adenoid and other lymphatic tissues; 51 serotypes are currently identified. Adenovirus is a DNA virus, has no lipid viral envelope, is highly stable outside of host cells, and may remain infectious at room temperature for 2 weeks. It is destroyed by heat (54°C, 129.2°F, for 30 minutes), usual disinfectants and detergents, and hand-cleansing agents. It is one of the most frequent causes of acute respiratory infection and conjunctivitis, and may be latent and cause later relapse. Adenovirus is transmittable between individuals by respiratory and eye drops and, in case of enteric adenovirus, by stools. The incubation period ranges from 5–10 days. It is not common in the first 6 months of life, suggesting protection by maternal antibodies. By 5 years, 75% of children have positive serology for adenoviruses. Serotypes 1–7 are responsible for acute respiratory diseases. Approximately 2%–3% of acute respiratory infections are caused by adenoviruses, with >8% caused in children <2 years old (78). Lower respiratory system infections include pneumonia, AB, laryngotracheobronchitis, or a pertussis-like cough (Table 48.5).

Parainfluenza

The seasonal pattern of types 1, 2, and 3 parainfluenza viruses is curiously interactive. Every second year, type 1 parainfluenza virus causes a defined epidemic, with a larger number of croup cases than AB. Type 2 parainfluenza virus epidemic is erratic and comes just after a type 1 epidemic; a type 3 parainfluenza virus epidemic occurs yearly (mostly in spring and summer) and has a prolonged duration in relation to types 1 and 2 (79). Parainfluenza viruses cause a disease similar to RSV with a lower hospitalization rate. Generally, these infections involve upper airways, and 30%–50% of cases are complicated with acute otitis. Type 3 parainfluenza virus pneumonia and AB occur mainly in the first 6 months of life, with a lower incidence when compared to RSV.

Risk Factors

There are several risk factors in AB associated with increased severity of illness and need for admission. They include a history of chronic lung disease (bronchopulmonary dysplasia), congenital heart disease, prematurity (risk values dependent on the gestational age), immunodeficiency, and neurologic disease. In a few studies symptomatic infection in early infancy (<3 months) has also been considered a medium-to-high risk factor. Other factors present in few studies are breastfeeding

TABLE 48.5

ADENOVIRUS CLINICAL SYNDROMES

SYSTEM	CLINICAL MANIFESTATIONS
Respiratory	*Upper respiratory tract*
	Pharyngitis
	Coryza
	Lower respiratory tract
	Laryngotracheobronchitis
	Cough
	Acute bronchiolitis
	Pneumonia
Ocular	Conjunctivitis with respiratory disease
	Acute follicular conjunctivitis
	Epidemic keratoconjunctivitis
	Pharyngoconjunctival fever
Gastrointestinal	Diarrhea
	Hepatitis (immunocompromised host)
Urinary	Hemorrhagic cystitis
Nervous	Aseptic meningitis
	Meningoencephalitis, encephalitis
	Myelitis, acute flaccid palsy
	Myositis
Skin	Rash
Disseminated infections (immunocompromised newborns)	Multiple-organ failure

for less than 2 months, low birth weight or intrauterine growth retardation, day care attendance, cystic fibrosis, Down syndrome, cerebral palsy, and congenital neurological problems (80). Hospitalization due to AB has increased in the last 20 years, perhaps reflecting the increased survival of infants with comorbid conditions that may predispose them to contracting AB and the expanded use of pulse oximetry to identify hypoxemia and severity of illness. **Table 48.6** summarizes the risk factors for severe AB.

DIAGNOSIS

Clinical Manifestations and Typical Clinical Course

AB usually occurs in winter but, as noted, can be observed in any season. Parents usually report that affected infants had contact with people with cold symptoms. In the beginning of the disease, infants have abundant rhinorrhea and typically a "tight" cough, along with poor food intake (4–6 days after symptoms start). The degree of fever in infants depends on the infecting organism. Children experiencing AB caused by RSV are frequently mildly febrile by the time of consultation (≤38.3°C), and those with adenovirus, influenza, or parainfluenza may have a fever ≥ 39°C. Because *apnea* may be a presenting sign of RSV infection, physicians should specifically question parents about episodes of irregular breathing or "blue spells."

Examination of infants with AB often reveals fever, significant tachypnea, tachycardia, and signs of respiratory distress, such as nasal flaring and respiratory accessory muscle use. The modified Wood score has been validated to grade AB severity (**Table 48.7**) (81,82). Pulmonary examination frequently demonstrates audible fine wheezing, fine rales, or rhonchi (apical ventilatory pattern), and a prolonged expiratory phase. Other common findings are rhinitis, otitis media, and conjunctivitis. Pulmonary hyperinflation may produce a distended abdomen or a hyperexpanded chest with increased anterior–posterior diameter and resonance to percussion. Mild-to-moderate hypoxia, which is detected by perioral cyanosis, pulse oximetry, or arterial blood gases, correlates with

tachypnea (>50 breaths/minute) and is a predictor of severe disease.

Laboratory Testing: Overview

Laboratory studies are not necessary to diagnose AB when the history and the physical examination are consistent. Therefore, afebrile infants in low-risk groups with mild disease do not need routine laboratory testing. However, high-risk patients or those presenting with severe disease do require laboratory testing to assess disease severity, specific viral etiology, or potential complications.

Bacterial Cultures in Febrile Young Infants with Bronchiolitis

The indication for bacterial cultures and complete blood count (CBC) in febrile young infants with bronchiolitis has been controversial. The American Academy of Pediatrics Pediatric Emergency Medicine Collaborative Research Committee RSV-SBI study group reported a 1.1% rate of coexisting bacteremia in febrile infants <60 days old with RSV bronchiolitis (83). None of the infants had coexisting meningitis, and 5.4% had coexisting urinary tract infections (83). The value of CBC in identifying bronchiolitis patients with coexisting bacterial infection has not been adequately studied. A 2011 systematic review examined the risk of serious occult bacterial infections in young (<3 months old) febrile (>38.3°C) infants with presumed bronchiolitis (84). Among the 11 studies reviewed, the weighted rate for urinary tract infections was 3.3%. No cases of meningitis were reported. The bacteremia rate ranged from 0.2% to 1.4% (84).

In summary, the yield of bacterial cultures in febrile infants (<3 months old) with bronchiolitis will be very low, with the urinary tract being the most likely site of any bacterial infection (although asymptomatic bacteriuria was not excluded in these studies). These studies were not focused on high-risk populations (e.g., prematurity, immunodeficiency) or infants destined for PICU admission. Neonates (<30 days old) represent a special population with increased risk of occult serious bacterial infection that is not modified by the presence of bronchiolitis.

TABLE 48.6

RISK FACTORS FOR CLINICAL WORSENING OF ACUTE BRONCHIOLITIS

Initial presentation
  Tachypnea (RR > 60–70 bpm) or retractions
  Hypoxia (SaO$_2$ < 90%–92%)
  Feeding difficulty or dehydration
Age
  Age <10–12 weeks at the onset of the epidemic
Comorbidities
  Bronchopulmonary dysplasia
  Congenital heart disease
  Pulmonary hypertension
  Immunodeficiency
Prematurity
  Gestational age <32 weeks
Other
  Malnutrition
  Poverty
  Siblings attending school/day care
  Parents and/or family members who smoke
  Mutations and polymorphisms in the genes that regulate the production of inflammatory mediators involved in AB

RR, respiratory rate; bpm, breaths per minute; SaO$_2$, arterial oxygen saturation; RSV, respiratory syncytial virus; AB, acute bronchiolitis.

TABLE 48.7

WOOD–DOWNES SCORE

■ SCORE	■ WHEEZING	■ RETRACTION	■ RESPIRATORY RATE	■ HEART RATE	■ VENTILATION	■ CYANOSIS
0	No	No	<30	<120	Good symmetrical	No
1	End expiratory	Subcostal/ intercostal		>120	Regular symmetrical	Yes
2	All expiration	Supraclavicular + nasal flaring	31–45		Very reduced	
3	Inspiration and expiration	Intercostal + suprasternal	40–60		Silent thorax	

The highest scores from each column are summed to attain the total severity score: 1–3, mild; 4–7, moderate; 8–14, severe.
Adapted from Wood DW, Downes JJ, Lecks HI. A clinical scoring system for the diagnosis of respiratory failure. Preliminary report on childhood status asthmaticus. *Am J Dis Child* 1972;123(3):227–8, with permission.

Therefore, we recommend the following approach in an attempt to balance the desire to detect all infants with a serious bacterial infection while avoiding overtesting and unnecessary antibiotics:

- Febrile neonates (>38°C) with or without bronchiolitis should receive CBC, urinalysis, chest radiography, blood-, urine-, and cerebrospinal fluid (CSF) cultures, followed by the initiation of empiric antibiotics pending culture results.
- Febrile infants with bronchiolitis who belong to a high-risk population, appear toxic, or are being considered for PICU admission should receive CBC, urinalysis, chest radiography, blood-, urine-, and CSF cultures, followed by the initiation of empiric antibiotics pending culture results.
- Febrile infants (>1 to <6 months old) with bronchiolitis who do *not* belong to a high-risk population, do *not* appear toxic, and are *not* being considered for PICU admission should receive CBC, urinalysis, chest radiography, and blood and urine cultures. Empiric antibiotics are *not* administered pending culture results *unless*:

  - WBC is >15,000 or <5,000. (An abnormal WBC should also trigger lumbar puncture for CSF culture.) Or
  - Urinalysis has >10 WBC/high power field (hpf)

Viral Testing

Viruses may be detected from nasopharyngeal samples, bronchoalveolar lavage fluid, or lung tissue by direct immunofluorescent antibody staining, enzyme-linked immunosorbent assay (ELISA), PCR, or direct culture. Virus-diagnosing test results may be used to limit inappropriate use of antibiotics as well as to properly cohort patients and apply other infection control measures. If the resources are available, we recommend that all infants with severe bronchiolitis undergo rapid antigen testing and real-time quantitative polymerase chain reaction (RT-PCR) to detect possible influenza virus infection, for which oseltamivir treatment would be indicated.

Imaging Studies

Chest x-rays often show nonspecific findings, including hyperinflation, gross infiltrates that are typically migratory and attributable to post–obstructive atelectasis, and peribronchial filling. Because AB is not an alveolar space disease, secondary bacterial pneumonia should be suspected if a true alveolar infiltrate is seen. Chest x-rays are not usually required for mild bronchiolitis in the outpatient setting. However, all high-risk infants with severe bronchiolitis should receive a chest x-ray to assess possible coexisting disease (e.g., congenital heart disease, lobar pneumonia, congestive heart failure, or foreign-body aspiration) and serve as a baseline if respiratory failure develops.

Differential Diagnosis

The typical respiratory signs and symptoms described above in the context of an epidemic outbreak are highly suggestive of AB. Other diagnoses that may mimic AB include congenital heart disease, gastroesophageal reflux, aspiration pneumonia, *Mycoplasma* pneumonia, other bacterial pneumonias, or foreign-body aspiration.

Severity Assessment

Scoring Systems

The scarcity of reliable clinical tools to assess AB severity in clinical practice is evident. A number of parameters have been proposed to identify the presence of a severe form of AB (need for oxygen support or assisted ventilation) or to predict respiratory failure, apnea, or other complications that justify hospitalization and PICU admission. A clinically isolated parameter probably has less value than a group of factors combined to predict the severity of a disease. A clinical score for AB may have a threefold objective: to discriminate the severity of bronchiolitis, to predict hospitalization, or to allow the evaluation of the effectiveness of a proposed treatment (85). The currently available bronchiolitis scoring systems use subjective and objective parameters, and variable levels of validation and reliability (many of them are not validated yet). Most of the practice guidelines do not recommend their use to assess disease severity or predict hospital admission (86–88). Although McCallum et al. (89) recently found the Tal and Modified-Tal scoring systems to be valid and reliable, their clinical utility in identifying a severe form of the AB (i.e., prediction of oxygen requirement) is uncertain.

Hospital Admission

Clinical judgment remains the gold-standard criterion for hospital admission and cannot be replaced by objective criterion. Several parameters should be considered rather than a set of criteria. Hospital admission is recommended in the following patients (86–88):

- Younger than 4–6 weeks
- Oral intake below 50% of usual
- Dehydration
- Lethargy
- Apnea
- Tachypnea for age
- Increased work of breathing: grunting, nasal flaring, retractions
- Cyanosis
- Oxygen saturation <90%–92% on room air
- Presence of comorbidities: clinically significant heart disease, pulmonary hypertension, neuromuscular disease, immunodeficiency, chronic lung disease, history of prematurity, or Down syndrome
- When the diagnosis is doubtful
- Rapid progression of the symptomatology
- Uncertain follow-up care
- Doubtful competence of parents or caregivers to assess the severity of the child

Arterial O_2 saturation (SaO_2) is the most consistent clinical predictor of a worsening clinical condition (the cutoff point ranging from <90% ≤92%).

The diagnosis of bronchiolitis and its severity is anchored in the clinician's assessment of the history and physical examination and is not dependent on any specific clinical finding or diagnostic test. Therefore, *repeated* clinical evaluation is important.

PICU Admission Criteria

PICU admission is indicated if:

- SaO_2 < 92% despite supplemental O_2
- Rapidly worsening condition
- Increasing respiratory distress
- Lethargy or fatigue
- Recurrent apneas

Management

Supportive Therapy

Most supportive measures lack consistent scientific evidence and represent extrapolations of the management for other respiratory diseases. Adequate monitoring, hydration, and oxygenation are the backbone of AB treatment. Supportive measures include the following:

1. Careful monitoring and the timely introduction of ventilatory support.
2. Adequate oxygenation—supplemental O_2 is offered for SaO_2 < 90%–92% in room air (86,87).
3. Maintenance of hydration and nutrition. Intravenous fluid therapy is indicated if significant tachypnea or respiratory distress is judged to increase the risk of aspiration or if the patient presents with significant dehydration (86,90–92).
4. Removal of mucous obstruction to nasal airways with instillation of saline drops followed by gentle suction.
5. Avoidance of excess stimulation or painful procedures which increase work of breathing.

The importance of supportive care is underscored by the systematic review and meta-analysis that showed that no specific therapy clearly improves outcomes among critically ill infants with bronchiolitis (93).

Physiotherapy

A 2012 systematic review involving 9 trials and 891 patients found that chest physiotherapy did not improve severity of illness, oxygen requirement, or outcome compared to the no intervention in bronchiolitis children <24 months old (94). Therefore, routine chest physiotherapy (percussion, vibration, or passive expiratory maneuvers) is not recommended in bronchiolitis.

Medications

β_2 **Bronchodilators (Albuterol, Salbutamol, and Epinephrine).** A 2014 meta-analysis of 30 trials involving nearly 2000 infants with bronchiolitis determined that inhaled β agonists (e.g., albuterol, salbutamol) did not improve oxygen saturation, reduce hospital admission, or shorten length of stay (95). A 2011 Cochrane Collaboration review (96) concluded that, compared to placebo, inhaled epinephrine decreased the need for hospital admission, but did not shorten the length of stay. Among studies that compared epinephrine to salbutamol inhalation in hospitalized infants, there was a significant reduction in the length of stay in the epinephrine group compared to the salbutamol group. Short-term outcome variables for hospitalized infants such as clinical score, oxygen saturation, or respiratory rate did not differ between the epinephrine and placebo groups. Most epinephrine studies used the racemic mixture of epinephrine.

All bronchodilator studies in bronchiolitis suffer from the limitation that it is clinically almost impossible to distinguish bronchiolitis from acute asthma triggered by a viral infection. Taken together, the current evidence supports the current American Academy of Pediatrics (AAP) recommendation of offering two options regarding the use of inhaled bronchodilators (86):

RECOMMENDATION A
"Bronchodilators should not be used routinely in the management of bronchiolitis (recommendation: evidence level B; RCTs with limitations; preponderance of harm of use over benefit)."
RECOMMENDATION B
"A carefully monitored trial of α- or β-adrenergic medication is an option. Inhaled bronchodilators should be *continued only if there is a documented positive clinical response to the trial using an objective means of evaluation* (option: evidence level B; RCTs with limitations and expert opinion; balance of benefit and harm)."

We believe the second option (B) is an acceptable approach as long as the medical team is willing to discontinue further inhaled bronchodilator administration if the single dose does not result in documented improvement. Racemic epinephrine is the preferred bronchodilator for a trial among closely monitored hospitalized patients (but is not a safe therapy in the home).

Anticholinergics. There are only limited data on the use of anticholinergics (ipratropium bromide) in AB. The Cochrane Collaboration systematic review published by Everard et al. (2005) (97) found a lack of effect of anticholinergics, alone or in combination with β_2 agonists, to improve objective variables (SaO_2, respiratory rate, or length of hospital stay). In summary, anticholinergics were not superior to β_2 agonists alone and did not improve the results when used in combination.

Inhaled and Systemic Steroids. The most recently updated systematic review involving 17 trials and nearly 2600 patients found no benefit from inhaled or systemic steroids in bronchiolitis (16,98).

Inhaled Epinephrine and Corticosteroid Combination. Owing to a possible synergy between inhaled epinephrine and corticosteroid administration, this combination was examined in a large Canadian study in emergency departments using nebulized epinephrine and 6 days of oral dexamethasone. The authors showed a significant reduction in hospitalization by the seventh day and an earlier discharge from medical care (99). However, the result was not significant when adjusted for multiple comparisons and has not been replicated in other studies. Therefore this combination therapy cannot be recommended without further investigation (100).

Aerosolized Recombinant Human DNAse. RCTs evaluating the effects of aerosolized recombinant human DNAse for treatment of children with RSV infection could not demonstrate significant differences between intervention and placebo groups concerning length of hospital stay, duration of supplemental oxygen, rate of improvement of the symptom score, and number of intensive care admissions (101). As DNAse may be effective in infections complicated by atelectasis, bronchial secretions, and mucous plugs that have high DNA concentration, there is the opportunity to study aerosolized DNAse in AB patients complicated by atelectasis.

Ribavirin. Ribavirin is an antiviral drug that inhibits the structural protein synthesis of the virus, reducing viral replication and immunoglobulin (Ig) E response. Following the initial excitement regarding this drug, problematic issues arose related to its high cost, logistic issues, possible teratogenicity, and low clinical efficacy. Cochrane Collaboration reviews published in 2004 (102) and 2007 (103) by Ventre et al. found studies with conflicting results and insufficient power to support conclusions. There is a predominance of risks over benefits in the use of ribavirin for AB. The AAP recommends avoiding ribavirin for routine use in RSV bronchiolitis. If ribavirin is to be considered, it should be reserved for immunosuppressed infants with severe disease who are also under the care of infectious diseases specialists (100).

Antibiotics. In infants with AB and fever, the risk of coexisting bacteremia is lower (0%–3.7%) than in a comparable population of febrile young infants without recognizable viral infection (see earlier section Bacterial Cultures in Febrile Young Infants with Bronchiolitis). Hence, the AAP recommends that young infants with AB receive antibiotics only if there are specific indications of a coexisting bacterial infection (86). Routine antibiotic use is not recommended (104). Documented secondary bacterial infections, such as urinary tract infection (the most frequently documented bacterial infection in these patients) (86), pneumonia, sinusitis, or acute otitis media, must be treated appropriately. Otitis media is present in more than 50% of patients in some series (105,106), although RSV itself can be the cause of acute otitis media. The potential antiinflammatory and immunomodulatory effects of macrolides in AB due to RSV has been studied (107); however, the beneficial effect of clarithromycin and azithromycin (108) seems to be marginal and could be related to the coexistence of atypical bacteria (109).

Nebulized 3% hypertonic saline solution. Hypertonic (3%) saline may improve mucociliary clearance of airway secretions (110). Mechanisms include reducing viscosity, breaking the ionic bonds within mucus, rehydrating mucus, absorbing water from the mucosa and submucosa, reducing wall edema, inducing sputum production and cough, and inducing cilial mobility by releasing prostaglandin E_2.

In 2008 Zhang et al. (111) published a Cochrane Database systematic review of the use of hypertonic saline (3%). It was used along with bronchodilators in three of the four included RCTs. The authors showed a reduction in the length of stay and improvement in the clinical score compared to the control groups (nebulized 0.9% saline). The effect was more pronounced for outpatients than for hospitalized patients. There were no significant adverse events associated with hypertonic saline use. Hypertonic saline (3%) was nebulized at a dose of 4 mL (in three studies) (112,113) or 2 mL (one study) (114). Except for one study (Kuzik et al.), hypertonic saline (3%) was nebulized with bronchodilators—1.5 mg of adrenaline or terbutaline 5 mg using a jet nebulizer with O_2 (three studies) or an ultrasonic nebulizer (113). The doses were repeated every 6–8 hours (113,115). The duration of treatment ranged from 5 days to until discharge. Unfortunately there are methodologic concerns around these studies because the length of stay for both the intervention and control groups was longer than the known median length of stay for bronchiolitis in the US. Furthermore, hypertonic saline may increase histamine release and bronchoconstriction in patients with asthma (116). Therefore, although hypertonic saline may be an option, more study is needed before it can be recommended for routine use in bronchiolitis.

Heliox. Heliox is a gas mixture containing 70%–80% helium, with the balance consisting of oxygen. Helium has a density seven times lower than nitrogen and results in a reduction of the Reynolds number, allowing a more laminar airflow, less airway resistance, less mechanical energy requirement, and hence reduces the patient's work of breathing (117). A meta-analysis found that heliox improved the clinical score only in the first hour after starting treatment without decreasing the rate of intubation, days of mechanical ventilation, or length of ICU stay (118). Therefore, heliox cannot be recommended as routine therapy for bronchiolitis.

Surfactant. Type II pneumocytes produce surfactant, a four-component tensioactive substance (phospholipids >85%, surfactant proteins A, B, C, and D 5%, and other neutral lipids and albumin 5%–10%), whose components (surfactant proteins A and D) bind bacteria and virus surface markers facilitating their elimination by macrophages (119). The surfactant of infants with severe AB has qualitative and quantitative alterations. The supplementation of exogenous surfactant was studied in infants requiring intensive care and mechanical ventilation. In a systematic review, the infants who received surfactant had lower duration of mechanical ventilation and PICU length of stay; they also experienced positive effects on oxygenation and ventilation. Even though the existing evidence on surfactant therapy suggests clinical and blood gas benefits, it is not sufficient to provide an estimate of its effectiveness in mechanically ventilated infants with bronchiolitis (120).

Nitric Oxide. Some bronchiolitis patients may have elevated pulmonary arterial pressure (>25 mm Hg), which is associated with prolonged hospital stay (74). However, there is no evidence that nitric oxide is beneficial either as a pulmonary vasodilator (121,122) or as a bronchodilator in this population.

Complications

Apnea

Apnea is linked to several different respiratory tract infections in infants exhibiting clinical syndromes analogous to AB (123–126). The mechanism of apnea in AB is uncertain, but may resemble that of prematurity and upper airway reflex apnea. There are reports suggesting that RSV has direct effect on CNS (127,128). As already noted, apnea may be an AB presenting symptom, a marker of a severe form of AB, and an indication for hospital admission. The incidence of apnea in patients with bronchiolitis who are referred to the hospital or intensive care unit ranges between 1.2% and 23.8% (126), and it affects patients who are generally less than 2 months old and have a history of prematurity (129,130). Although bronchiolitis-related apnea usually resolves within 48 hours (131), recurrent apnea spells may occur. An apnea spell should be considered a risk factor for recurrent apneic spells during the course of bronchiolitis.

In order to stimulate breathing and reduce apnea and its effects in preterm infants, methylxanthines (such as caffeine, theophylline, or aminophylline) have been used (132). Caffeine and theophylline have proven short-term efficacy in reducing the incidence of apnea of prematurity and bradycardia (132). Compared to theophylline, caffeine would be the preferred drug for the treatment of apnea (132), as it presents better longer-term outcomes, has lower rates of toxicity, and a more favorable therapeutic index. However, there are no RCTs justifying the use of methylxanthines in AB. However, a small retrospective series suggests that caffeine may decrease the need for intubation in infants with bronchiolitis and apnea (133).

Premature infants with bronchiolitis or young infants with apnea spells due to bronchiolitis should be admitted to a PICU for close monitoring and possible assisted ventilation. Possible noninvasive respiratory support modalities include continuous positive airway pressure (CPAP), bilevel positive airway pressure (BiPAP) (134), or heated humidified high-flow nasal cannula (HFNC) therapy (see Chapter 39 on Inhaled Gases). Preliminary data suggest that HFNC may decrease the need for intubation and length of stay in children with bronchiolitis (135).

Respiratory Failure

Beyond patients with refractory apnea, respiratory support may be necessary for those patients experiencing respiratory failure. Respiratory support is indicated in patients with progressive hypoxia or hypercapnia and increasing respiratory distress secondary to severe AB. A recent prospective multicenter study (136) identified some factors independently associated with the need for respiratory support (CPAP or intubation): young age (<2 months), low birth weight (<2.26 kg), maternal smoking history, onset of respiratory symptoms <1 day before admission, presence of apnea, severe retractions, room air oxygen saturation <85%, and insufficient oral intake.

Different types of respiratory supports have been used in AB, but they have not been studied in RCTs; thus, there is no clear evidence on which ventilation mode to select. CPAP or BiPAP is generally used as an alternative before invasive ventilation. CPAP helps reduce the work of breathing by preventing dynamic airway collapse during the respiratory cycle, avoids atelectasis, and improves gas distribution in the obstructed airways.

Conventional Mechanical Ventilation

Patients with refractory hypoxemia and hypercapnia will require intubation and mechanical ventilation (see Chapter 38). Patients with a hyperinflated chest, profound wheezing, and severe hypercapnia are best managed with pressure-controlled ventilation using low respiratory rates, short inspiratory and prolonged expiratory times, and low peak inspiratory pressure. Conversely, if the patient has severe atelectasis, pulmonary infiltrates, and hypoxemic respiratory failure, longer inspiratory times and positive end-expiratory pressure (PEEP) will be needed.

High-Frequency Oscillatory Ventilation

High-frequency oscillatory ventilation (HFOV) has been successfully used in infants with bronchiolitis and severe hypoxemia (137,138). There is a risk of air trapping with the use of

HFOV in obstructive lung disease such as bronchiolitis. Berner et al. (139) describe the successful application of HFOV for bronchiolitis-induced respiratory failure with hypercapnia. The authors used higher mean airway pressure and larger pressure swings than for respiratory distress syndrome and were able to avoid paralysis and preserve spontaneous breathing. Additional research is needed before HFOV can be recommended for routine management of hypercapnic respiratory failure in AB.

Extracorporeal Membrane Oxygenation

As with other forms of life-threatening respiratory failures that are refractory to all other interventions, extracorporeal membrane oxygenation may be employed (see Chapter 40).

Discharge Criteria

As with hospital admission, careful clinical judgment is needed when deciding on hospital discharge. A personalized discharge plan should be proposed on admission and agreed to with the parents or caregivers. At discharge, they should be properly informed about the evolution of AB and be warned of when and why they should return for a health care. To ensure clinical stability before hospital discharge, pulse oximetry should be continued after the removal of oxygen support for about 8–12 hours, including a sleep period, to verify the infant is able to maintain normal Sao$_2$ in room air.

Discharge is considered when (86–88)

- Respiratory rate is appropriate for the patient's age, without clinical evidence of increased respiratory distress.
- Oxygen saturation is adequate (>90%–94%) in room air.
- Oral intake is adequate (>75% of usual intake).
- Parents/caregivers are able to clear airway secretions and mucus.

Prevention

Infection Control Measures

RSV is highly contagious and can survive for more than 24 hours on surfaces. Therefore, prevention of nosocomial transmission using various infection control measures is the cornerstone of infection control. Standard infection control measures include the following (86,88):

- For all patients (universal precautions):
  - Careful hand-washing (soap or alcohol-based solutions) before and after patient contact
  - Alcohol wipe of stethoscope and other devices before and after patient contact
- For suspected bronchiolitis:
  - Gloves during handling of affected patients
- For bronchiolitis with high concern of aerosol transmission:
  - Contact precautions (gloves, masks, protective eye wear, disposable gowns)
- For bronchiolitis outbreaks with large numbers of hospitalized patients:

  - Private isolation rooms (ideal)
  - Cohorting of infected patients
  - Limited intrahospital patient transport

Patient Education

Parents should be educated to avoid secondhand smoke exposure, promote breastfeeding, practice careful hand-washing, and consider the risks of day care during bronchiolitis outbreaks in the community.

Immunoprophylaxis (Palivizumab)

16 Immunoprophylaxis for RSV has relied on two potential approaches: vaccines (active immunization) and monoclonal antibodies. Efforts to obtain an effective vaccine have not been successful to date. Passive immunization against RSV using humanized monoclonal antibodies, palivizumab, was approved by the US FDA in 1998. Palivizumab is administered intramuscularly at a dose of 15 mg/kg once per month for a maximum of 5 months, during the epidemic months. The first dose should be given before the onset of RSV season. Among different high-risk groups, hospitalization rates due to RSV are reduced by 39%–82%, compared to control groups. Updated guidelines for palivizumab use were published by the American Academy of Pediatrics in 2014 (140,141), which suggest administering palivizumab to the following patient groups:

- Preterm infants (<29 weeks gestation)
- Preterm infants (<32 weeks) with chronic lung disease of prematurity and a requirement for >21% oxygen for at least 28 days after birth
- Infants with hemodynamically significant heart disease
- Children in the second year of life who required ≥28 days of supplemental oxygen after birth and who continue to require supplemental oxygen, chronic corticosteroid, or diuretic therapy

Depending on clinical judgment, palivizumab is optional for:

- Infants unable to clear airway secretions due to pulmonary or neuromuscular disease
- Immunocompromised children <24 months

Other special considerations apply to palivizumab. Administration should be discontinued if the child requires hospitalization due to breakthrough RSV infection. It is not indicated for prevention of nosocomial spread in the health care setting.

Outcome

It is estimated that RSV infects ~70% of children; 22% develop symptoms (87), 2%–5% of these need to be hospitalized, and 5–16% of those hospitalized may require admission to PICU (142). Overall mortality in developed countries from RSV bronchiolitis is <2%, although high-risk groups are at greater risk. Symptoms typically persist for up to 12 days, but up to 9% remain symptomatic for up to 28 days. Breathing and feeding difficulties usually last for 6–7 days. Most children with AB, regardless of severity, recover without sequelae. It is not known whether recurrent wheezing and asthma after AB are secondary to the damage caused by the infection that causes AB, or whether there is a previous genetic or environmental predisposition.

CONCLUSIONS AND FUTURE DIRECTIONS

Although AB is a frequent cause of consultation and hospitalization among young children, only a small number—those with underlying diseases—have a high risk of developing a more severe disease. Treatment is limited to supportive care, including fluid replacement and O_2 therapy. Other therapeutic modalities are controversial and the subject of additional studies. Future studies are necessary to further investigate the therapies that show early promise and to continue the search for more effective acute therapies. Macrolides are the drugs of choice for atypical pneumonia caused by bacteria, but their use is not safe in pneumonia due to pneumococcus. Novel antiviral treatments and vaccines are needed to advance treatment and prophylaxis.

The incidence of nosocomial and community-acquired pneumonia and their complications remain elevated, with a high morbidity mainly in developing countries. Early diagnosis and improved access to care are needed for this population. The emergence of resistant microorganisms perpetuates the need for continuous research for new antimicrobials.

References

1. World Health Organization. Pneumonia. Fact sheet No. 321. 2009. http://www.who.int/mediacentre/factsheets/fs331/en/index.html. Accessed November 28, 2012.
2. Rudan I, Tomaskovic L, Boschi-Pinto C, et al. Global estimate of the incidence of clinical pneumonia among children under five years of age. *Bull World Health Organ* 2004;82(12):895–903.
3. Wijnands GJ. Diagnosis and interventions in lower respiratory tract infections. *Am J Med* 1992;92:91–7S.
4. Cilla G, Oñate E, Perez-Yarza EG, et al. Viruses in community-acquired pneumonia in children aged less than 3 years old: High rate of viral coinfection. *J Med Virol* 2008;80(10):1843–9.
5. Duke T. Neonatal pneumonia in developing countries. *Arch Dis Child Fetal Neonatal Ed* 2005;90(3):F211–9.
6. Principi N, Esposito S. Management of severe community-acquired pneumonia of children in developing and developed countries. *Thorax* 2011;66(9):815–22.
7. Harris M, Clark J, Coote N, et al. British Thoracic Society guidelines for the management of community acquired pneumonia in children: Update 2011. *Thorax* 2011;66(suppl 2):ii1–23.
8. Bradley JS, Byington CL, Shah SS, et al. Executive summary: The management of community-acquired pneumonia in infants and children older than 3 months of age: Clinical practice guidelines by the Pediatric Infectious Diseases Society and the Infectious Diseases Society of America. *Clin Infect Dis* 2011;53(7):617–30.
9. Greenberg DP, von König CH, Heininger U. Health burden of pertussis in infants and children. *Pediatr Infect Dis J* 2005;24(5 suppl):S39–43.
10. McIntosh K. Community-acquired pneumonia in children. *N Engl J Med* 2002;346(6):429–37.
11. Wubbel L, Muniz L, Ahmed A, et al. Etiology and treatment of community-acquired pneumonia in ambulatory children. *Pediatr Infect Dis J* 1999;18(2):98.
12. Harris JA, Kolokathis A, Campbell M, et al. Safety and efficacy of azithromycin in the treatment of community-acquired pneumonia in children. *Pediatr Infect Dis J* 1998;17(10):865–71.
13. McIntosh K, Harper MB. Pneumonia in the imunocompromised host. In: *Principles and Practice of Pediatrics Infectious Disease.* 4th ed. Philadelphia, PA: Elsevier Saunders, 2012:252–6.
14. Richards MJ, Edwards JR, Culver DH, et al. Nosocomial infections in pediatric intensive care units in the United States. National Nosocomial Infections Surveillance System. *Pediatrics* 1999;103(4):e39.
15. Raymond J, Aujard Y; European Study Group. Nosocomial infections in pediatric patients: A European, multicenter prospective study. *Infect Control Hosp Epidemiol* 2000;21(4):260–3.
16. Garrett DA, McKibben P, Levine G, et al. Prevalence of nosocomial infections in pediatric intensive care unit patients at US children's hospitals. 4th Decennial International Conference on Nosocomial and Healthcare-Associated Infections; March 5–9, 2000; Atlanta, Georgia.
17. Zilberberg MD, Shorr AF. Healthcare-associated pneumonia: The state of evidence to date. *Curr Opin Pulm Med* 2011;17(3):142–7.

18. Venkatachalam V, Hendley JO, Willson DF. The diagnostic dilemma of ventilator-associated pneumonia in critically ill children. *Pediatr Crit Care Med* 2011;12:286–96.

19. Srinivasan R, Asselin J, Gildengorin G, et al. A prospective study of ventilator-associated pneumonia in children. *Pediatrics* 2009;123:1108–15.

20. Apisarnthanarak A, Holzmann-Pazgal G, Hamvas A, et al. Ventilator-associated pneumonia in extremely preterm neonates in a neonatal intensive care unit: Characteristics, risk factors, and outcomes. *Pediatrics* 2003;112:1283–9.

21. Lucero MG, Tupasi TE, Gomez ML, et al. Respiratory rate greater than 50 per minute as a clinical indicator of pneumonia in Filipino children with cough. *Rev Infect Dis* 1990;12(8):S1081–3.

22. Esposito S, Bosis S, Cavagna R, et al. Characteristics of Streptococcus pneumoniae and atypical bacterial infections in children 2–5 years of age with community-acquired pneumonia. *Clin Infect Dis* 2002;35(11):1345–52.

23. Mazur LJ, Kline MW, Lorin MI. Extreme leukocytosis in patients presenting to a pediatric emergency department. *Pediatr Emerg Care* 1991;7(4):215–8.

24. Mandell LA, Bartlett JG, Dowell SF, et al. Update of practice guidelines for the management of community-acquired pneumonia in immunocompetent adults. *Clin Infect Dis* 2003;37(11):1405–33.

25. Campbell SG, Marrie TJ, Anstey R, et al. The contribution of blood cultures to the clinical management of adult patients admitted to the hospital with community-acquired pneumonia: A prospective observational study. *Chest* 2003;123(4):1142–50.

26. Neuman MI, Lee EY, Bixby S, et al. Variability in the interpretation of chest radiographs for the diagnosis of pneumonia in children. *J Hosp Med* 2012;7(4):294–8.

27. Miller RW. Special susceptibility of the child to certain radiation-induced cancers. *Environ Health Perspect* 1995;103(suppl 6):41–4.

28. Coley BD. Chest sonography in children: Current indications, techniques, and imaging findings. *Radiol Clin North Am* 2011;49(5):825–46.

29. Caiulo VA, Gargani L, Caiulo S, et al. Lung ultrasound in bronchiolitis: Comparison with chest X-ray. *Eur J Pediatr* 2011;170(11):1427–33.

30. Iuri D, De Candia A, Bazzocchi M. Evaluation of the lung in children with suspected pneumonia: Usefulness of ultrasonography. *Radiol Med* 2009;114(2):321–30.

31. Copetti R, Cattarossi L. Ultrasound diagnosis of pneumonia in children. *Radiol Med* 2008;113(2):190–8.

32. Sandora TJ, Harper MB. Pneumonia in hospitalized children. *Pediatr Clin North Am* 2005;52(4):1059–81.

33. Bradley JS, Byington CL, Shah SS, et al. The management of community-acquired pneumonia in infants and children older than 3 months of age: Clinical practice guidelines by the Pediatric Infectious Diseases Society and the Infectious Diseases Society of America. *Clin Infect Dis* 2011;53(7):e25–76.

34. Cherry JD. Epidemic pertussis in 2012—the resurgence of a vaccine-preventable disease. *N Engl J Med* 2012;367(9):785–7.

35. Kwong JC, Stukel TA, Lim J, et al. The effect of universal influenza immunization on mortality and health care use. *PLoS Med* 2008;5(10):e211.

36. Bharti B, Bharti S, Verma V. Role of Acute Illness Observation Scale (AIOS) in managing severe childhood pneumonia. *Indian J Pediatr* 2007;74(1):27.

37. Hardie WD, Roberts NE, Reising SF, et al. Complicated parapneumonic effusions in children caused by penicillin-nonsusceptible Streptococcus pneumoniae. *Pediatrics* 1998;101(3):388–92.

38. Donnelly LF, Klosterman LA. CT appearance of parapneumonic effusions in children: Findings are not specific for empyema. *Am J Roentgenol* 1997;169(1):179–82.

39. Balfour-Lynn IM. Paediatric Pleural Diseases Subcommittee of British Thoracic Society Standards of Care Committee. Some consensus but little evidence: Guidelines on management of pleural infection in children. *Thorax* 2005;60(2):94–6.

40. Jaffe A, Balfour-Lynn IM. Management of empyema in children. *Pediatr Pulmonol* 2005;40(2):148–56.

41. Byington CL, Spencer LY, Johnson TA, et al. An epidemiological investigation of a sustained high rate of pediatric parapneumonic empyema: Risk factors and microbiological associations. *Clin Infect Dis* 2002;34(4):434–40.

42. Balfour-Lynn IM, Abrahamson E, Cohen G, et al. BTS guidelines for the management of pleural infection in children. *Thorax* 2005;60(1):i1–21.

42a. Thomson AH, Hull J, Kumar MR, et al. Randomised trial of intrapleural urokinase in the treatment of childhood empyema. *Thorax*. 2002;57(4):343-7.

43. Pappalardo E, Laungani A, Demarche M, et al. Early thoracoscopy for the management of empyema in children. *Acta Chir Belg* 2009;109(5):602–5.

44. Oak SN, Parelkar SV, Satishkumar KV, et al. Review of video-assisted thoracoscopy in children. *J Minim Access Surg* 2009;5(3):57–62.

45. Meier AH, Hess CB, Cilley RE. Complications and treatment failures of video-assisted thoracoscopic debridement for pediatric empyema. *Pediatr Surg Int* 2010;26(4):367–71.

46. St Peter SD, Tsao K, Spilde TL, et al. Thoracoscopic decortication vs tube thoracostomy with fibrinolysis for empyema in children: A prospective, randomized trial. *J Pediatr Surg* 2009;44(1):106–11.

47. Dowell SF, Kupronis BA, Zell ER, et al. Mortality from pneumonia in children in the United States, 1939 through 1996. *N Engl J Med* 2000;342(19):1399–407.

48. Feikin DR, Schuchat A, Kolczak M, et al. Mortality from invasive pneumococcal pneumonia in the era of antibiotic resistance, 1995–1997. *Am J Public Health* 2000;90(2):223–9.

49. McConnochie KM. Bronchiolitis. What's in the name? *Am J Dis Child* 1983;137(1):11–3.

50. Holman RC, Shay DK, Curns AT, et al. Risk factors for bronchiolitis-associated deaths among infants in the United States. *Pediatr Infect Dis J* 2003;22:483–90.

51. Oshansky C, Zhang V, Moore E, et al. The host response and molecular patogenesis associated with respiratory syncytial virus infection. *Future Microbiol* 2009;4:279–97.

52. Tal G, Mandelberg I, Dalal K, et al. Association between common Toll like receptor 4 mutations and severe respiratory syncytial virus disease. *J Infect Dis* 2004;189:2057–63.

53. Puthothu B, Forster J, Heinzmannn A, et al. TLR-4 and CD14 polymorphism in respiratory syncytial virus associated disease. *Dis Markers* 2006;22:303–8.

54. Amanatidou V, Sourvinos G, Apostoilakis S, et al. T280M variation of the CX3C receptor gene is associated with increased risk for severe respiratory syncytial virus bronchiolitis. *Pediatr Infect Dis J* 2006;25:410–4.

55. Puthou B, Forster J, Heinze J, et al. Surfactant protein B polymorphisms are associated with severe respiratory syncytial virus infection, but not with asthma. *BMC Pulm Med* 2007;7:6.

56. Logfren J, Ramet M, Renko M, et al. Association between surfactante protein A gene locus and severe respiratory syncytial virus infection in infants. *J Infect Dis* 2002;185:283–9.

57. Miyairi I, De Vicenzo JP. Human genetic factors and respiratory syncytial virus disease severity. *Clin Microbiol Rev* 2008;21:686–703.

58. Janssen R, Bont L, Siezen C, et al. Genetic susceptibility to respiratory syncytial virus bronchiolitis is predominantly associated with innate immune genes. *J Infect Dis* 2007;196:826–34.

59. Wright AL, Taussig LM, Ray CG, et al. The Tucson Children's Respiratory Study. II. Lower respiratory tract illness in the first year of life. *Am J Epidemiol* 1989;129(6):1232–46.

60. Hall CB, Weinberg GA, Iwane MK, et al. The burden of respiratory syncytial virus infection in young children. *N Engl J Med* 2009;360(6):588–98.

61. Paranhos-Baccalà G, Komurian-Pradel F, Richard N, et al. Mixed respiratory virus infections. *J Clin Virol* 2008;43(4):407–10.

62. McCarthy CA, Hall CB. Respiratory syncytial virus: Concerns and control. *Pediatr Rev* 2003;24:301–9.

63. Centers for Diseases Control. Prevention and control of influenza. *Morb Mortal Wkly Rep* 2005;54:1–40.

64. Peltola V, Reunanen T, Ziegler T, et al. Accuracy of clinical diagnosis of influenza in outpatient children. *Clin Infect Dis* 2005;41(8):1198–200.

65. Epperson S, Blanton L, Kniss K, et al; Influenza Division, National Center for Immunization and Respiratory Disease, CDC. Influenza activity—United States, 2013-14 season and composition of the 2014-15 influenza vaccines. *Morb Mortal Wkly Rep* 2014;63(22):483–90.

66. Sugaya N, Takeuchi Y. Mass vaccination of schoolchildren against influenza and its impact on the influenza-associated mortality rate among children in Japan. *Clin Infect Dis* 2005;41:939–47.

67. Hillenbrand K. Ativiral therapy for influenza infections. *Pediatr Rev* 2005;26(11):427–8.

68. van den Hoogen BG, Bestebroer TM, Osterhaus AD, et al. Analysis of the genomic sequence of a human metapneumovirus. *Virology* 2002;295(1):119–32.

69. Pelletier G, Dery P, Abed Y, et al. Respiratory tract reinfections by the new human Metapneumovirus in an immunocompromised child. *Emerg Infect Dis* 2002;8(9):976–8.

70. van den Hoogen BG, De Jong JC, Groen J, et al. A newly discovered human pneumovirus isolated from young children with respiratory tract disease. *Nat Med* 2001;7:719–24.

71. Semple MG, Cowell A, Dove W, et al. Dual infection of infants by human metapneumovirus and human respiratory syncytial virus is strongly associated with severe bronchiolitis. *J Infect Dis* 2005;191:382–86.

72. Jartti T, van den Hoogen B, Garofalo RP, et al. Metapneumovirus and acute wheezing in children. *Lancet* 2002;360(9343):1393–4.

73. Nissen MD, Siebert DJ, Mackay IM, et al. Evidence of human metapneumovirus in Australian children. *Med J Aust* 2002;176(4):188.

74. Bardi-Peti L, Ciofu EP. Bronchiolitis and pulmonary hypertension. *Pneumologia* 2010;59(2):95–100.

75. García-Garcia ML, Calvo C, Martín F, et al. Human metapneumovirus infections in hospitalised infants in Spain. *Arch Dis Child* 2006;91:290–5.

76. Hon KL, Leung CW, Cheng WT, et al. Clinical presentations and outcome of severe acute respiratory syndrome in children. *Lancet* 2003;361(9370):1701–3.

77. Ksiazek TG, Erdman D, Goldsmith CS, et al. A novel coronavirus associated with severe acute respiratory syndrome. *N Engl J Med* 2003;348(20):1953–66.

78. Langley JM. Adenoviruses. *Pediatr Rev* 2005;26(7):244–9.

79. Hall CB. Respiratory syncytial virus and parainfluenza virus. *N Engl J Med* 2001;344(25):1917–28.

80. Murray J, Bottle A, Sharland M, et al. Medicines for neonates investigator group. Risk factors for hospital admission with RSV bronchiolitis in England: A population-based birth cohort study. *PLoS One* 2014;9:e89–186.

81. Wood DW, Downes JJ, Lecks HI. A clinical scoring system for the diagnosis of respiratory failure. Preliminary report on childhood status asthmaticus. *Am J Dis Child* 1972;123(3):227–8.

82. Duarte-Dorado DM, Madero-Orostegui DS, Rodriguez-Martinez CE, et al. Validation of a scale to assess the severity of bronchiolitis in a population of hospitalized infants. *J Asthma* 2013;50:1056–61.

83. Levine DA, Platt SL, Dayan PS, et al. Risk of serious bacterial infection in young febrile infants with respiratory syncytial virus infections. *Pediatrics* 2004;113:1728–34.

84. Ralston S, Hill V, Waters A. Occult serious bacterial infection in infants younger than 60 to 90 days with bronchiolitis: A systematic review. *Arch Pediatr Adolesc Med* 2011;165:951–6.

85. Chevallier B. Bronchiolitis in infants. Clinical criteria of severity for hospital admission. *Arch Pediatr* 2001;8(suppl 1):39–45S.

86. American Academy of Pediatrics (AAP). Subcommittee on Diagnosis and Management of Bronchiolitis. Diagnosis and management of bronchiolitis. *Pediatrics* 2006;118(4):1774–93.

87. SIGN. Bronchiolitis in children. A national clinical guideline. http://www.sign.ac.uk. 2006.

88. Bronchiolitis Guideline Team. Cincinnati Children's Hospital Medical Center. *Evidence-based care guideline for management of bronchiolitis in infants 1 year of age or less with a first time episode, Bronchiolitis Pediatric Evidence-Based Care Guidelines, Cincinnati Children's Hospital Medical Center. Guideline 1,* 2010, 1–16. www.cincinnatichildrens.org/workarea/linkit.aspx?linkidentifier=id&itemid=87885&libid=87573. Accessed December 2, 2012.

89. McCallum GB, Morris PS, Wilson CC, et al. Severity scoring systems: Are they internally valid, reliable and predictive of oxygen use in children with acute bronchiolitis? *Pediatr Pulmonol* 2013;48(8):797–803.

90. Kennedy N, Flanagan N. Is nasogastric fluid therapy a safe alternative to the intravenous route in infants with bronchiolitis? *Arch Dis Child* 2005;90:320–1.

91. Sammartino L, James D, Goutzamanis J, et al. Nasogastric rehydration does have a role in acute paediatric bronchiolitis. *J Paediatr Child Health* 2002;38:321–2.

92. Vogel AM, Lennon DR, Harding JE, et al. Variations in bronchiolitis management between five New Zealand hospitals: Can we do better? *J Paediatr Child Health* 2003;39:40–5.

93. Davison C, Ventre KM, Luchetti M, et al. Efficacy of interventions for bronchiolitis in critically ill infants: A systematic review and meta-analysis. *Pediatr Crit Care Med* 2004;5:482–9.

94. Roque i Figuls M, Gine-Garriga M, Granados Rugeles C, et al. Chest physiotherapy for acute bronchiolitis in paediatric patients between 0 and 24 months old. *Cochrane Database Syst Rev* 2012;2:CD004873.

95. Gadomski AM, Sribani MB. Bronchodilators for bronchiolitis. *Cochrane Database Syst Rev* 2014;6:CD001266.

96. Hartling L, Bialy LM, Vandermeer B, et al. Epinephrine for bronchiolitis. *Cochrane Database Syst Rev* 2011;(6):CD003123.

97. Everard ML, Bara A, Kurian M, et al. Anticholinergic drugs for wheeze in children under the age of two years. *Cochrane Database Syst Rev* 2005;3:CD001279.

98. Fernandes RM, Bialy LM, Vandermeer B, et al. Glucocorticoids for acute viral bronchiolitis in infants and young children. *Cochrane Database Syst Rev.* 2013;6:CD004878.

99. Plint AC, Johnson DW, Patel H, et al. Epinephrine and dexamethasone in children with bronchiolitis. *N Engl J Med* 2009;360:2079–89.

100. Schuh S. Update on management of bronchiolitis. *Curr Opin Pediatr* 2011;23(1):110–4.

101. Boogaard R, Hulsmann AR, Van Veen L, et al. Recombinant human deoxyribonuclease in infants with respiratory syncytial virus bronchiolitis. *Chest* 2007;131:788–95.

102. Ventre K, Randolph A. Ribavirin for respiratory syncytial virus infection of the lower respiratory tract in infants and young children. *Cochrane Database Syst Rev* 2004;4:CD000181.

103. Ventre K, Randolph AG. Ribavirin for respiratory syncytial virus infection of the lower respiratory tract in infants and young children. *Cochrane Database Syst Rev* 2007;1:CD000181.

104. Spurling GK, Doust J, Del Mar CB, et al. Antibiotics for bronchiolitis in children. *Cochrane Database Syst Rev* 2011;(6):CD005189.

105. Andrade MA, Hoberman A, Glustein J, et al. Acute otitis media in children with bronchiolitis. *Pediatrics* 1998;101(4 pt 1):617–4.

106. Shazberg G, Revel-Vilk S, Shoseyov D, et al. The clinical course of bronchiolitis associated with acute otitis media. *Arch Dis Child* 2000;83:317–9.

107. Tahan F, Ozcan A, Koc N. Clarithromycin in the treatment of RSV bronchiolitis: A double-blind, randomised, placebo-controlled trial. *Eur Respir J* 2007;29:91–7.

108. Kneyber MC, van Woensel JB, Uijtendaal E, et al. Azithromycin does not improve disease course in hospitalized infants with respiratory syncytial virus (RSV) lower respiratory tract disease: A randomized equivalence trial. *Pediatr Pulmonol* 2008;43:142–9.

109. Korppi M. Macrolides and bronchiolitis in infants. *Eur Respir J* 2007;29(6):1283–4.

110. Mandelberg A, Amirav I. Hypertonic saline or high volume normal saline for viral bronchiolitis: Mechanisms and rationale. *Pediatr Pulmonol* 2010;45:36–40.

111. Zhang L, Mendoza-Sassi RA, Wainwright C, et al. Nebulized hypertonic saline solution for acute bronchiolitis in infants. *Cochrane Database Syst Rev* 2008;(4):CD0064586.

112. Mandelberg A, Tal G, Witzling M, et al. Nebulized 3% hypertonic saline solution treatment in hospitalized infants with viral bronchiolitis. *Chest* 2003;123:481–7.

113. Tal G, Cesar K, Oron A, et al. Hypertonic saline/epinephrine treatment in hospitalized infants with viral bronchiolitis reduces hospitalization stay: 2 years experience. *Isr Med Assoc J* 2006;8:169–73.

114. Sarrell EM, Tal G, Witzling M, et al. Nebulized 3% hypertonic saline solution treatment in ambulatory children with viral bronchiolitis decreases symptoms. *Chest* 2002;122:2015–20.

115. Kuzik BA, Al-Qadhi SA, Kent S, et al. Nebulized hypertonic saline in the treatment of viral bronchiolitis in infants. *J Pediatr* 2007;151:266–70, 270.e1.

116. Ratnawati, Morton J, Henry RL, et al. Mediators in exhaled breath condensate after hypertonic saline challenge. *J Asthma* 2009;46(10):1045–51.

117. Reuben AD, Harris AR. Heliox for asthma in the emergency department: A review of the literature. *Emerg Med J* 2004;21:131–5.

118. Liet JM, Ducruet T, Gupta V, et al. Heliox inhalation therapy for bronchiolitis in infants. *Cochrane Database Syst Rev* 2010 14;(4):CD006915.

119. LeVine AM, Elliott J, Whitsett JA, et al. Surfactant protein-d enhances phagocytosis and pulmonary clearance of respiratory syncytial virus. *Am J Respir Cell Mol Biol* 2004;31(2):193–9.

120. Jat KR, Chawla D. Surfactant therapy for bronchiolitis in critically ill infants. *Cochrane Database Syst Rev* 2012;9:CD009194.

121. Fitzgerald D, Davis GM, Rohlicek C, et al. Quantifying pulmonary hypertension in ventilated infants with bronchiolitis: A pilot study. *J Paediatr Child Health* 2001;37:64–6.

122. Patel N, Hammer J, Nichani S, et al. Effect of inhaled nitric oxide on respiratory mechanics in ventilated infants with RSV bronchiolitis. *Intensive Care Med* 1999;25:81–7.

123. Mitchell I, Barclay RP, Railton R, et al. Frequency and severity of apnoea in lower respiratory tract infection in infancy. *Arch Dis Child* 1983;58:497–9.

124. Jofre ML, Luchsinger FV, Zepeda FG, et al. Apnea as a presenting symptom in human metapneumovirus infection. *Rev Chilena Infectol* 2007;24:313–8.

125. Simon A, Volz S, Hofling K, et al. Acute life-threatening event (ALTE) in an infant with human coronavirus HCoV-229E infection. *Pediatr Pulmonol* 2007;42:393–6.

126. Ralston S, Hill V. Incidence of apnea in infants hospitalized with respiratory syncytial virus bronchiolitis: A systematic review. *J Pediatr* 2009;155(5):728–33.

127. Ng YT, Cox C, Atkins J, et al. Encephalopathy associated with respiratory syncytial virus. *J Child Neurol* 2001;16:105–8.

128. Sweetman LL, Ng YT, Butler IJ, et al. Neurologic complications associated with respiratory syncytial virus. *Pediatr Neurol* 2005;32:7–10.

129. Al-balkhi A, Klonin H, Marinaki K, et al. Review of treatment of bronchiolitis related apnoea in two centres. *Arch Dis Child* 2005;90(3):288–91.

130. Anas N, Boettrich C, Hall CB, et al. The association of apnea and respiratory syncytial virus infection in infants. *J Pediatr* 1982;101:65–8.

131. Sajit NT, Steggall M, Padmakumar B. Apnoeas in bronchiolitis: Is there a role for caffeine? *Arch Dis Child* 2005;90(4):438.

132. Henderson-Smart DJ, De Paoli AG. Methylxanthine treatment for apnoea in preterm infants. *Cochrane Database Syst Rev* 2010;(12):CD000140.

133. Cesar K, Iolster T, White D, et al. Caffeine as treatment for bronchiolitis-related apnoea. *J Paediatr Child Health* 2012;48:619.

134. Donlan M, Fontela PS, Puligandla PS. Use of continuous positive airway pressure (CPAP) in acute viral bronchiolitis: A systematic review. *Pediatr Pulmonol* 2011;46(8):736–46.

135. McKiernan C, Chua LC, Visintainer PF, et al. High flow nasal cannulae therapy in infants with bronchiolitis. *J Pediatr* 2010; 156:634.

136. Mansbach JM, Piedra PA, Stevenson MD, et al. Prospective multicenter study of children with bronchiolitis requiring mechanical ventilation. *Pediatrics* 2012;130(3):e492–500.

137. Medbo S, Finne PH, Hansen TWR. Respiratory syncytial virus pneumonia ventilated with high frequency oscillatory ventilation. *Acta Paediatr* 1997;86:766–8.

138. Duval ELIM, Leroy PLJM, Gemke RJBJ, et al. High frequency oscillatory ventilation in RSV bronchiolitis patients. *Respir Med* 1999;93:435–40.

139. Berner ME, Hanquinet S, Rimensberger PC. High frequency oscillatory ventilation for respiratory failure due to RSV bronchiolitis. *Intensive Care Med* 2008;34(9):1698–702.

140. Committee on Infectious Diseases. From the American Academy of Pediatrics: Policy statements—Modified recommendations for use of palivizumab for prevention of respiratory syncytial virus infections. *Pediatrics* 2009;124(6):1694–701.

141. Committee on Infectious Diseases and Bronchiolitis Guidelines Committee. Updated guidance for Palivizumab prophylaxis among infants and young children at increased risk of hospitalization for respiratory syncytial virus infection. *Pediatrics* 2014;134:415–20.

142. Working Group of the Clinical Practice Guideline on Acute Bronchiolitis. Clinical practice guideline on acute bronchiolitis. http://www.guiasalud.es/GPC/GPC_475_Bronchiolitis_AIAQS_compl_en.pdf. Accessed on December 8, 2014.

CHAPTER 49 ■ ACUTE LUNG INJURY AND ACUTE RESPIRATORY DISTRESS SYNDROME

KATHLEEN M. VENTRE AND JOHN H. ARNOLD

KEY POINTS

1. Acute lung injury (ALI) and acute respiratory distress syndrome (ARDS) have multiple potential causes. The host inflammatory response is a key feature in the pathogenesis of these diseases.

2. Recent randomized controlled trials using explicit supportive care protocols indicate that mortality in ALI/ARDS is decreasing.

3. The mainstay of therapy in ALI/ARDS is supportive care. Low tidal volume mechanical ventilation and prone positioning are the only components of supportive therapy that have been associated with a significant mortality benefit in ALI/ARDS.

4. Steroids, fluid restriction, surfactant, prone positioning, and inhaled nitric oxide (NO), although theoretically beneficial, will not benefit all children with ALI/ARDS when applied indiscriminately.

5. We have entered a new era compelling further refinement of ARDS diagnostic criteria and the identification of relevant subgroups of patients who stand to benefit from novel therapies.

INTRODUCTION AND DEFINITIONS

In 1967, Ashbaugh et al. described a syndrome of tachypnea, hypoxia, and decreased pulmonary compliance in a series of 11 adults and 1 child with respiratory failure. The pathologic features included interstitial and intra-alveolar edema and hemorrhage as well as hyaline membrane formation. On its face, this condition seemed to have many features in common with the previously described infant respiratory distress syndrome. Although the syndrome had been widely recognized and reported in the years that followed, it was not until 1994 that a consensus definition entered the scientific literature (1). The American–European Consensus Conference (AECC) proposed that the "adult" respiratory distress syndrome be renamed the "acute" respiratory distress syndrome (ARDS) to acknowledge the existence of this condition in children. The panel defined ARDS as a severe form of acute lung injury (ALI) characterized by acute, noncardiogenic pulmonary edema with bilateral pulmonary infiltrates on chest x-ray and a ratio of PaO_2 to FIO_2 of <200. The AECC designated ALI as a term comprehensively including all patients with PaO_2/FIO_2 <300 who otherwise meet criteria for ARDS (**Table 49.1**). This consensus document set the stage for a highly productive couple of decades in which the application of consistent diagnostic criteria facilitated the conduct of large-scale cohort studies and clinical trials that have shed considerable light on the epidemiology and pathophysiology of ALI and ARDS, creating many opportunities to rigorously evaluate the impact of novel therapeutic approaches.

Published incidence estimates for ALI and ARDS vary, and are best interpreted in the context of the study design, case ascertainment methods, population demographics, and mechanical ventilation practices that were used at the time patients were identified as meeting criteria for either condition. The data that are available suggest that there are striking differences in the incidence of ALI and ARDS in children as compared to adults. Population-based cohort studies in which

investigators used AECC criteria to identify cases estimate that ALI occurs at a rate of 2.95–12.8 cases per 100,000 children per year, compared to as many as 78.9 cases per 100,000 adults per year (2–9). ARDS is estimated to occur at a rate of 2.2–9.5 cases per 100,000 children per year (2,5) compared to as many as 58.7 cases per 100,000 adults per year in adults (8). Among individuals at least 15 years old, the incidence of both ALI and ARDS increases dramatically with advancing age, reaching a peak incidence of 306 cases per 100,000 adults per year among individuals between 75 and 84 years of age (8). A recent downward trend in the incidence of adult ARDS is suggested by a carefully validated population-based cohort in suburban Minnesota. This study indicated that the incidence of ALI and ARDS among hospitalized adults appears to have declined between 2001 and 2008 from 81 to 38.3 cases per 100,000 adults per year (10).

Recent data indicate that ARDS occurs in 1%–4% of PICU admissions and as many as 8%–10% of children requiring mechanical ventilation (5,11,12). Historically, mortality for pediatric ARDS has varied between 20% and 75%, depending on the presence of coexisting risk factors such as immune compromise, the criteria that are used to identify cases, and the presence of nonpulmonary organ failures (11). The highest mortality rates tend to be reported in small, single-centered, retrospective studies from the 1980s and early 1990s, before consensus diagnostic criteria were developed. Data from contemporary epidemiologic investigations and the control groups of multicentered clinical trials conducted during the past decade indicate that mortality in the pediatric ALI/ARDS population ranges between 8% and 36% (11,13,14), although among immunocompromised children it may be as high as 60% (14–16). As is the case in the adult literature, the lowest mortality rates are reported in trials that evaluate the efficacy of a particular therapy while introducing it in the context of contemporary, evidence-based supportive care protocols (13,17,18). As supportive care improvements continue to drive down mortality rates, it is becoming increasingly challenging to design clinical trials that are adequately powered to

TABLE 49.1

AMERICAN–EUROPEAN CONSENSUS CRITERIA FOR ALI AND ARDS

	■ ALI	■ ARDS
Timing	Acute onset	Acute onset
Chest radiography	Bilateral pulmonary infiltrates	Bilateral pulmonary infiltrates
Edema	Pulmonary artery occlusion pressure ≤18 mm Hg or no clinical evidence of left atrial hypertension	Pulmonary artery occlusion pressure ≤18 mm Hg or no clinical evidence of left atrial hypertension
Oxygenation impairment	Pao_2/Fio_2 ratio ≤300[a,b]	Pao_2/Fio_2 ratio ≤200[a,b]
Estimated incidence		
Adults	17.9–78.9[c] cases per 100,000/year (8,147,148)	14–58.7[d] cases per 100,000/year (8,147)
Children	2.95–12.8[e] cases per 100,000 children/year (4,9,149)	2.2–9.5[e] cases per 100,000 children/year (2,5,6,9)

[a]At altitudes exceeding 1000 m, Pao_2/Fio_2 should be adjusted for local barometric pressure [$Pao_2/Fio_2 \times$ (barometric pressure/760)].
[b]In children with a Spo_2 ≤97%, a Spo_2/Fio_2 of ≤253 has been proposed as a noninvasive approximation of ALI oxygenation criteria. A Spo_2/Fio_2 of ≤212 would correspond to ARDS (150).
[c]Incidence of ALI/ARDS in adults depends on age. Among adolescents, the incidence has been reported as low as 16/100,000 (8).
[d]Recent evidence indicates that the incidence of ARDS among adults may be decreasing to as low as 38.9/100,000 (10).
[e]High estimate for pediatric ALI and ARDS incidence comes from a cohort assembled between 1999 and 2000 who were ventilated with a mean (± SD) VT of 9.3 ± 1.5 cc/kg (9). The most recent large, population-based cohort, including children receiving lung-protective mechanical ventilation, suggests an ARDS incidence of 3.9/100,000 children per year (6).
Adapted from Bernard GR, Artigas A, Brigham KL, et al. The American-European Consensus Conference on ARDS: Definitions, mechanisms, relevant outcomes, and clinical trial coordination. *Am J Respir Crit Care Med* 1994;149:818–24.

evaluate the impact of novel therapies on clinically meaningful outcome measures.

This chapter reviews what we have learned from more than 20 years of scholarly work on ALI and ARDS, as these conditions were defined by the AECC. For all that the AECC criteria have accomplished to date, it is important to recognize that the ALI/ARDS continuum does not represent a single disease. These terms in fact describe a diverse group of conditions for which the final common pathway involves the acute onset of permeability edema, parenchymal opacification, and marked oxygenation impairment. Having reached a point where large-scale clinical trials are consistently unable to demonstrate outcome benefits for even the most scientifically promising new ARDS therapies, we have entered a new era obligating further refinement of diagnostic criteria with an eye toward identifying relevant subgroups who may stand to benefit from interventions whose merits may not be apparent in unselected populations of lung-injured patients. The ARDS Definition Task Force has recently proposed a revised definition for the *acute respiratory distress syndrome* (Table 49.2). The updated definition addresses various aspects of the AECC consensus criteria that clinicians now recognize as potentially problematic. For instance, the Pao_2/Fio_2 can be manipulated by altering the ventilator settings, ALI can sometimes coexist with hydrostatic pulmonary edema, and there can be considerable variability among radiologists in interpreting chest radiographs (19). It is evident from its final form that the new "Berlin Definition" forecloses the possibility that ARDS can be diagnosed in a patient not requiring mechanical ventilation—a change that seems appropriate in light of the many lines of evidence suggesting a major role for mechanical ventilation in the pathogenesis of this disease. The task force has proposed eliminating the term *acute lung injury* in favor of simply classifying the degree of oxygenation impairment in ARDS patients as "mild," "moderate," or "severe." Using a large validation cohort assembled from observational studies and several clinical trials, the investigators empirically determined that patients in the "severe" category have higher mortality (45%; 95% CI, 42%–48%) than those in the "moderate" and "mild" categories (mortality 32% for "moderate" ARDS; 95% CI, 29%–34% vs. mortality 27% for "mild" ARDS; 95% CI, 24%–30%) (20). Provided with refined diagnostic criteria, the scientific community is now poised to face the complicated challenge of how best to evaluate novel therapies in specific subpopulations of ARDS patients while designing clinical trials that are adequately powered to provide reliable estimates of their effects.

MECHANISM OF DISEASE: CORE PATHOPHYSIOLOGY

Host Genetic Factors

Our present understanding of the pathophysiology of ALI and ARDS comes from postmortem histopathologic data and careful study of its clinical course in animal models and affected humans. Over the past decade, much effort has been extended to apply techniques from molecular genetics to understanding the role of host factors by linking the presence of specific genetic polymorphisms to the development and/or severity of ARDS. In particular, specific polymorphisms in genes that govern endothelial barrier function, proinflammatory and anti-inflammatory cytokine production, the transcription regulator nuclear factor-κB (NF-κB) and its inhibitor NF-κB1A, pattern recognition receptors (PRRs) of the innate immune system, oxidant mediated injury, surfactant protein B production, angiotensin-converting enzyme, and the coagulation cascade have all been associated with either susceptibility to ARDS or the severity of its presentation (21–24). To date, many of these associations have been reported in case-control studies using candidate gene-based approaches to confirm a relationship between the ALI/ARDS phenotype and allelic variations in genes already acknowledged to have a role in disease pathogenesis. Not all of these associations have been replicated in follow-up studies (21).

One of the problems with candidate gene-based association studies is that they are not able to address the role of noncoding DNA sequences in disease expression. This is one reason why the portrait of disease pathogenesis that emerges from these types of studies can be somewhat reductive (25). Additionally, the strength of the inferences drawn from candidate gene-based studies tends to be limited by their small sample size and the difficulty of accounting for posttranslational modifications and other interactions that could alter the relationship between genotype and disease phenotype in the affected host (26). When interpreting these studies, careful attention must be given to their design, as erroneous associations between the candidate gene and the phenotype of interest can result if the study is not adequately powered to detect a true positive association, if inappropriate controls are selected, if cases and controls are not adequately matched, or if the finding is not replicated in an independent validation cohort (27). In the future, greater attention must be given to understanding the genetic epidemiology

TABLE 49.2

THE ACUTE RESPIRATORY DISTRESS SYNDROME (BERLIN DEFINITION)

Timing	Onset within 1 wk of a known clinical trigger, or new/worsening respiratory symptoms
Chest imaging (x-ray or CT)	Bilateral opacities not fully explained by effusion, regional atelectasis, or nodules
Origin of edema	Respiratory failure not fully explained by cardiac failure or fluid overload[a]
Oxygenation impairment	
Mild ARDS	$200 < \text{Pao}_2/\text{Fio}_2 \leq 300$ with PEEP or CPAP ≥ 5 cm H_2O[b]
Moderate ARDS	$100 < \text{Pao}_2/\text{Fio}_2 \leq 200$ with PEEP ≥ 5 cm H_2O
Severe ARDS	$\text{Pao}_2/\text{Fio}_2 \leq 100$ with PEEP ≥ 5 cm H_2O

[a]Objective assessment, such as echocardiography, is needed to exclude hydrostatic edema in the absence of specific risk factor(s).
[b]Noninvasive positive pressure ventilation may be provided in mild ARDS.
Adapted from Ranieri VM, Rubenfeld GD, Thompson BT, et al.; ARDS Definition Task Force. Acute respiratory distress syndrome: The Berlin Definition. *JAMA* 2012;307(23):2526–33.

of ALI and ARDS in ethnic groups that have been underrepresented in published studies. In addition, more widespread use of high-throughput, genome-wide association studies should broaden our understanding of the genetic basis for ARDS. Genome-wide investigative approaches stand to elucidate novel aspects of the pathogenesis of ALI and ARDS, and they will likely accelerate the pace at which we discover host genetic factors that have a role in determining disease phenotype.

In theory, ongoing efforts to understand the genetic signature of ALI and ARDS could help define clinically important subgroups of patients with either of these conditions, but it is not certain whether this work will translate into a way to use a patient's genetic profile to help guide strategic approaches to therapy. In conditions like ALI and ARDS in which multiple possible pathways converge on a nonspecific phenotype, clinical heterogeneity among patients may impede efforts to distinguish "normal" from "abnormal" patterns of gene expression (21). Regulatory pathways in the sequence of genetic events beginning with RNA and ending with the proteome (and beyond) will need to be elucidated over time. Incorporating all of this additional information into a validated, more comprehensive model of disease pathogenesis will require sophisticated new statistical approaches (25). Finally, intriguing new evidence suggests that the human immunologic response to critical illness involves a massive, genome-wide, reordering of cellular functions (28) and may compel a reexamination of the premise that specific polymorphisms can be manipulated in ways that would have a meaningful impact on the incidence or outcomes of ALI and ARDS.

Initiating Factors

ARDS develops following either "direct" or "indirect" lung injury. Pneumonia and pulmonary aspiration are among the most common conditions with the potential to inflict direct lung injury and ARDS, but traumatic pulmonary contusion, fat embolism, submersion injury, and inhalational injury are other relatively common causes of direct lung injury. The most common forms of indirect lung injury include systemic conditions, such as sepsis, shock, exposure to cardiopulmonary bypass, and transfusion-related lung injury. One of the more important reasons for attempting to distinguish between direct and indirect injury is that these pathways are associated with distinct pathologic changes in respiratory system mechanics, and these differences appear to be associated with distinctly different clinical outcomes (4,29,30). For example, direct injury is suspected of causing regional consolidation from destruction of the alveolar architecture, while indirect injury is believed to be associated with pulmonary vascular congestion, interstitial edema, and less severe alveolar involvement (29). Patients with direct forms

of lung injury tend to dominate enrollment in clinical trials, in keeping with the current predominance of pneumonia as the inciting factor for ARDS. However, careful appraisal of study outcomes in other subgroups may reveal differences in the response to particular therapies. For example, subgroup analyses from several recent randomized controlled trials (RCTs) that evaluated surfactant for treatment of ALI and ARDS have shown an outcome benefit associated with the use of surfactant in patients with direct forms of lung injury and not in those with indirect forms (13,31,32). Ongoing efforts to understand the relative contribution of direct versus indirect lung injury to the development of ALI and ARDS will be an important step in allowing future clinical trials to test novel therapies among more homogeneous subgroups of affected patients.

Phases of Disease

Regardless of the inciting factors, ARDS commonly progresses through stages defined by clinical, radiographic, and histopathologic features. The first, or *exudative phase*, is characterized by the acute development of decreased pulmonary compliance and arterial hypoxemia. The alteration in pulmonary mechanics leads to tachypnea. Arterial blood gas analysis typically reveals hypocarbia at this stage, and the chest x-ray usually reveals diffuse alveolar infiltrates from pulmonary edema. The proinflammatory events that occur during the exudative phase create the setting for transition into the *fibroproliferative stage* of ARDS, during which an increased alveolar dead-space fraction and refractory pulmonary hypertension may develop as a result of chronic inflammation and scarring of the alveolar–capillary unit. The fibroproliferative phase then gives way to a *recovery phase*, with restoration of the alveolar epithelial barrier, gradual improvement in pulmonary compliance and resolution of arterial hypoxemia, and eventual return to premorbid pulmonary function in many patients (33).

Alveolar–Capillary Barrier Dysfunction and Edema Formation

By definition, the edema in ARDS is not caused by cardiac failure but results from disruption of the structural components that regulate alveolar fluid balance under normal conditions. Normally, integrity of the gas–blood barrier is maintained by junctional complexes between adjacent pulmonary capillary endothelial cells and between adjacent alveolar epithelial cells. Adjacent pulmonary capillary endothelial cells are connected by adherens junctions, which are protein complexes (e.g., cadherins) that interlink with actin filaments of the cellular cytoskeleton on the cytoplasmic surface of the cell membrane. Attachments between endothelial cells allow some movement of fluid, but no movement of proteins or other solutes, into the interstitial space. Alveolar epithelial cells, on the other hand, are connected by adherens junctions and also by tight junctions, which are apical multiprotein complexes that connect neighboring cell membranes tightly enough to hinder molecular diffusion between adjacent cells. As a result of its robust intercellular attachments, the epithelial layer normally resists transalveolar movement of fluid, proteins, or other solutes (34). The rate of fluid movement into the interstitium is therefore governed by the net difference between hydrostatic pressure and osmotic pressure in the pulmonary capillaries, relative to the pulmonary interstitium. Generally, fluid movement across a semipermeable membrane, such as the pulmonary capillary endothelial layer, is characterized by the well-known Starling formula:

$$Q = K_f [(P_c - P_{is}) - \sigma(\pi_{pl} - \pi_{is})]$$

where Q is the filtration rate across the semipermeable membrane, K_f is the membrane filtration coefficient, P_c is the capillary hydrostatic pressure, P_{is} is the interstitial hydrostatic pressure, σ is the membrane reflection coefficient, π_{pl} is the plasma oncotic pressure, and π_{is} is the interstitial oncotic pressure.

Usually, the small amount of fluid that accumulates in the interstitial space can be cleared easily by the pulmonary lymphatic system. The key pathophysiologic event that distinguishes the orderly regulation of alveolar fluid balance in the normal state from the dysfunction typified by ALI and ARDS is injury to the alveolar epithelium and/or pulmonary capillary endothelium. This injury can occur directly as the result of parenchymal injury or following a distant or systemic disease process that provokes the host immune response, causing neutrophil activation and elaboration of proinflammatory cytokines. Either pathway results in the opening of intercellular connections, which causes unregulated leakage of fluid, protein, cytokines, and other solutes into the interstitium and the alveolar space. Impairment of gas exchange, through multiple potential mechanisms, soon ensues.

Surfactant Dysfunction and Alteration of Pulmonary Mechanics

Injury to the pulmonary surfactant system is one of the more serious consequences of damage to the alveolar epithelium and subsequent alveolar flooding. Surfactant is produced mainly by alveolar epithelial type II cells and contains phospholipid and protein components. Its major function is to promote alveolar and small airway stability by lowering surface tension, although its principal protein constituents also have an important role in facilitating clearance of infectious organisms (35,36). The Laplace equation illustrates the relationship between surface tension (T), cavity radius (r), and the pressure (P) required to maintain the patency of a spherical structure:

$$P = 2T/r$$

In reality, alveoli are polygonal rather than spherical, and their patency is facilitated by outward traction forces that are generated by the pulmonary interstitial matrix (37). Notwithstanding the inherent assumptions, application of Laplace formula to explain alveolar inflation makes it easy to see that an increase in surface tension in a small cavity, such as an alveolus, will require elevated transalveolar pressures to achieve and maintain patency.

Following lung injury, surfactant production declines because of damage to alveolar epithelial cells, and the surface activity of any surfactant remaining in the alveolar space is impaired because of alterations in its phospholipid constituents

and inactivation by alveolar exudates (38). It is important to appreciate how the loss of surfactant integrity dramatically alters the mechanical properties of the entire lung. In the nondiseased state, the interaction of surfactant with the elastic properties of the lung and chest wall produce *pulmonary hysteresis*, which allows for the maintenance of lung volume at lower transpulmonary pressures ($P_{transpulmonary} = P_{airway} - P_{pleural}$) during expiration than are required during inspiration. One way to demonstrate the volume–pressure relationships throughout the respiratory cycle is to perform a static inflation maneuver, in which discrete gas volumes are introduced into the lung up to total lung capacity, using a calibrated syringe ("super syringe"). Carefully measured volumes are similarly withdrawn from the lung to plot the volume–pressure relationships during lung emptying (**Fig. 49.1**). During inspiration, increasing transpulmonary pressure produces little change in lung volume until the patient reaches a lower inflection point on the inspiratory limb of the curve (lower Pflex) (**Fig. 49.2**). At that point, the change in lung volume produced by each upward increment of pressure (i.e., compliance) increases quickly, and then more slowly, until reaching an upper inflection point (upper Pflex) (**Fig. 49.2**) where compliance again decreases. The upward and leftward displacement of the expiratory limb relative to the inspiratory limb (**Fig. 49.1**) illustrates the difference in the transpulmonary pressures needed to maintain lung volume as the lung recoils and empties. This difference is potentiated by the properties of surfactant. In the injured lung, hysteresis is less pronounced, and the entire curve is displaced downward and rightward, reflecting the higher pressures required to achieve and maintain lung recruitment, and an overall decrease in lung compliance that is evident throughout the respiratory cycle (**Figs. 49.1** and **49.2**).

The effect of alveolar and small airways collapse on overall airway resistance can be explained by the Hagen–Poiseuille equation describing laminar flow in straight circular tubes:

$$R = (8\eta l)/\pi r^4$$

where R is resistance to flow, η is gas viscosity, l is tube length, and r is airway radius.

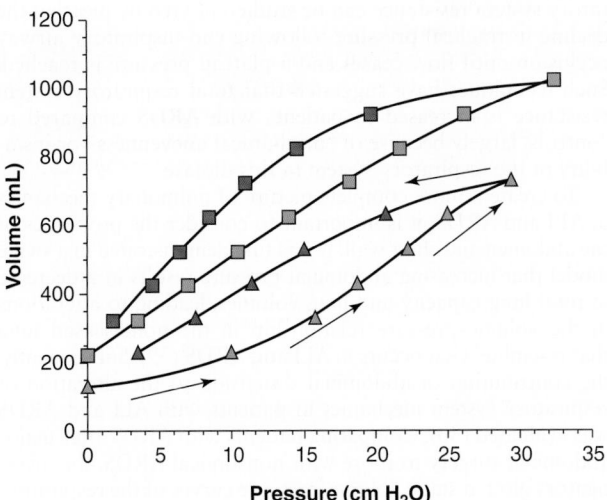

FIGURE 49.1. Pulmonary hysteresis: volume–pressure relationships before and after lung injury. Inflation (*green symbols*) and deflation (*red symbols*) volume–pressure data in a canine model before (*squares*) and 60 minutes after (*triangles*) oleic acid-induced ALI. During deflation (expiration), higher lung volumes are maintained at lower transpulmonary pressures. Original experimental data are fitted with a sigmoidal equation to construct the curves ($R^2 > 0.9997$). (From Venegas JG, Harris RS, Simon BA. A comprehensive equation for the pulmonary pressure-volume curve. *J Appl Physiol* 1998;84:389–95, with permission.)

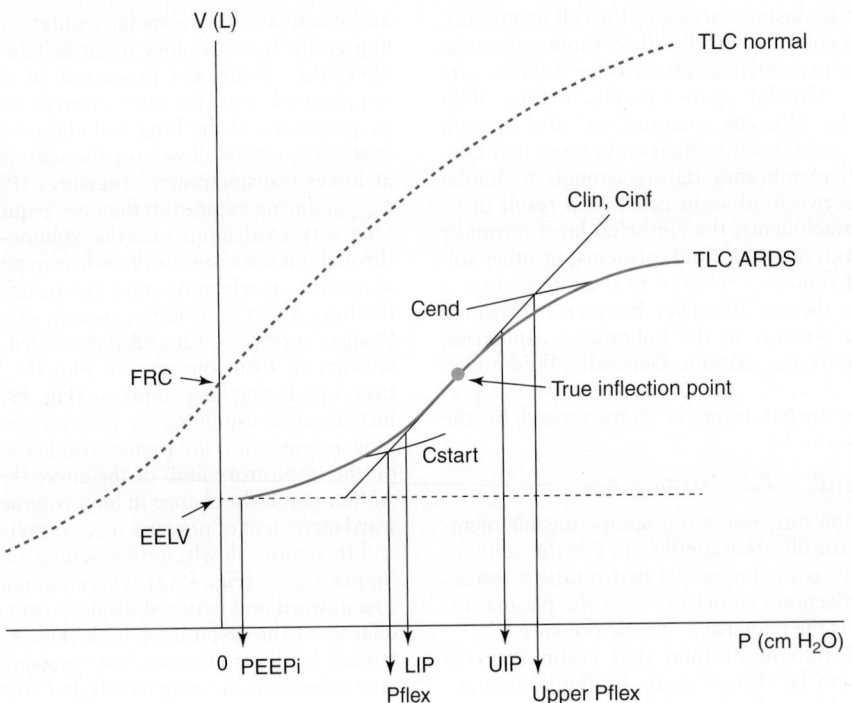

FIGURE 49.2. Volume–pressure curve in absence of disease (*dashed lines*) and in ARDS (*solid line*). Inspiratory curves are shown. Important transitions during lung inflation are indicated on the ARDS curve. Note that in ARDS, total lung capacity (TLC) is reduced, compared to TLC in the normal lung. In this example, a small amount of positive end-expiratory pressure (intrinsic PEEP [PEEPi]) is present at EELV in the ARDS lung. EELV in the ARDS lung is below FRC. Compliance is indicated at various points as the slope of the volume–pressure curve. Pflex is indicated on the curve as the intersection of the low-compliance portion of the curve obtained at low lung volume (Cstart). Upper Pflex is indicated at the transition between the nearly linear zone of maximal compliance (Clin) and the zone of low compliance at high lung volume (Cend). The lower inflection point (LIP) and upper inflection point (UIP) are points at which the volume pressure curve begins to depart from Clin at the extremes of lung volume. The "true inflection point" marks the actual change in concavity of the volume–pressure curve. (From Harris RS. Pressure-volume curves of the respiratory system. *Respir Care* 2005;50:78–98, with permission.)

From this equation it follows that a reduction in airway caliber, from peribronchiolar edema or outright airway collapse, produces a marked increase in airways resistance. Respiratory system resistance can be studied in vivo by plotting the decline in tracheal pressure following end-inspiratory airway occlusion until flow ceases and a plateau pressure is reached. Such techniques have suggested that total respiratory system resistance is increased in patients with ARDS compared to controls, largely because of "mechanical unevenness" or instability of the respiratory system in this disease.

To create a more complete picture of pulmonary mechanics in ALI and ARDS, it is important to consider the properties of the abdomen and chest wall. It was first demonstrated in a swine model that increasing abdominal pressure results in a decrease in total lung capacity and lung volumes, leading to alterations in the volume–pressure relationship in the nondiseased lung that resemble what occurs in ALI and ARDS (39). Subsequently, the contribution of abdominal distension to the alteration of respiratory system mechanics in patients with ALI and ARDS was evaluated (30). Comparing patients with ARDS after major abdominal surgery to those with nonsurgical ARDS, the investigators plotted static volume–pressure curves of the respiratory system, chest wall, and lung by relating calibrated changes in lung volume to end-inspiratory plateau pressures obtained at the airway opening and in the esophagus. Static abdominal pressure was obtained by relating end-inspiratory gastric plateau pressure to gastric plateau pressure measured at end-expiratory lung volume (EELV). This study was able to identify clear differences in the shape of the volume–pressure curves obtained from patients with ARDS related to abdominal pathology in the postoperative setting versus "medical" ARDS. Specifically, the volume–pressure relationship of the chest wall among surgical ARDS patients was shifted downward and rightward relative to curves obtained from nonsurgical ARDS patients (**Fig. 49.3**). The differences in curve morphology between these two groups correlated with differences in static abdominal pressures, indicating a decrease in chest wall compliance in surgical ARDS that is attributable to increases in intra-abdominal pressure. In comparison, the nonsurgical ARDS group demonstrated chest wall compliance curves that resembled those produced by the preoperative surgical controls (30). These observations suggest that ARDS impairs respiratory system mechanics in different ways depending on the underlying etiology, a finding that has significant implications for understanding clinical outcomes in ALI and ARDS and for defining subgroups within a large and heterogeneous disease population that may benefit from specific therapies or alternative management strategies.

Mechanisms of Alveolar Fluid Clearance

Once fluid accumulates in the alveolar space, its clearance is regulated by ion channels in distal airway Clara cells and in alveolar epithelial type I and type II cells. Type I cells make up about 95% of the alveolar epithelial lining (40) and are highly permeable to water, owing, in part, to their expression of the lung's principal water transport protein, aquaporin-5, on their apical surface. While they account for a much smaller share of the alveolar lining, alveolar type II cells can be isolated under experimental conditions and thus, have been studied in great detail. Besides producing pulmonary surfactant, type II cells are also responsible for transepithelial ion transport (41). Sodium is taken up by channels on the apical surface of type II cells. These channels can be classified

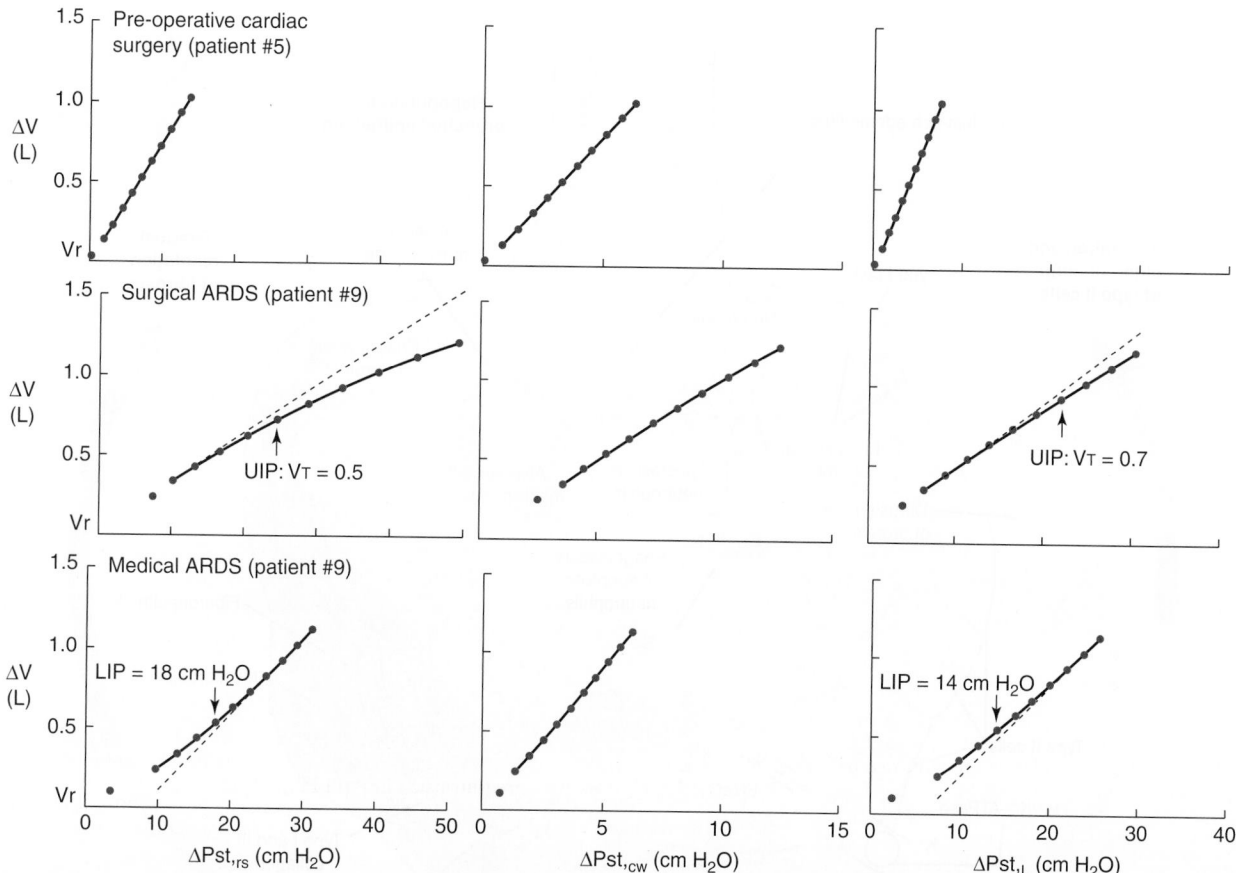

FIGURE 49.3. Static inflation volume–pressure curves of the respiratory system (rs), chest wall (cw), and lung (L) in one preoperative cardiac surgery patient (**top**), one surgical ARDS patient (**middle**), and one medical ARDS patient (**bottom**). *Closed symbol* indicates intrinsic positive end-expiratory pressure, with the corresponding increase in EELV. *Dashed lines* indicate zone of lowest elastance (highest compliance), as determined by regression analysis. Note that in the nonsurgical ARDS patient, the chest wall compliance curve resembles the corresponding curve in the preoperative surgical control patient. The chest wall compliance curve in the surgical ARDS patient is shifted downward and rightward by comparison (see text). ΔPst, changes in end-inspiratory static pressure; ΔV, changes in lung volume relative to equilibrium volume; UIP, upper inflection point; LIP, lower inflection point. (From Ranieri VM, Brienza N, Santostasi S, et al. Impairment of lung and chest wall mechanics in patients with acute respiratory distress syndrome: Role of abdominal distension. *Am J Respir Crit Care Med* 1997;156:1082–91.)

according to whether or not their activity can be suppressed by the diuretic amiloride. The critical role of the amiloride-sensitive epithelial sodium channel (ENaC) in regulating sodium influx at the apical type II cell membrane has been confirmed using knockout mouse models. Inactivation of particular ENaC subunits appears to result in the development of respiratory distress syndrome in the neonatal period whose severity ranges from relatively mild to rapidly lethal, depending on which subunits remain intact (40).

Once sodium enters through apical channels, Na^+/K^+-ATPases located on the basolateral cell membrane actively transport sodium back into the interstitial space, which creates the gradient for passive movement of water across the alveolar epithelium and back into the interstitium (**Fig. 49.4**) (42). The alveolar epithelial damage that occurs in ALI creates conditions that compromise the capacity of membrane proteins to effectively regulate alveolar fluid balance. Moreover, in vitro and in vivo experimental models have shown that exposure of alveolar epithelium to hypoxia inhibits transepithelial sodium transport and decreases overall alveolar fluid clearance (43). The permeability edema that is the defining feature of early ARDS sets the stage for reduced compliance and an EELV that decreases below functional residual capacity (FRC) to a point approaching closing capacity, creating conditions that favor the development of regional atelectasis, intrapulmonary shunt, and alveolar hypoxia.

Alteration of Gas Exchange in ALI and ARDS

There are many potential sources of hypoxia in ALI and ARDS. It is easy to understand that edema in the interstitial compartment or in the alveolar space will inhibit gas exchange and that pulmonary blood flowing past compromised or collapsed lung units will be poorly oxygenated, lowering the oxygen content of pulmonary venous blood and reducing systemic oxygen content. The fraction of pulmonary blood flow that ultimately enters the systemic circulation without being oxygenated (the "shunt fraction," or venous admixture) can be approximated using the equation:

$$\dot{Q}_S/\dot{Q}_T = (Cc'_{O_2} - Ca_{O_2})/(Cc'_{O_2} - C\bar{v}_{O_2})$$

where $\dot{Q}_S/\dot{Q}_T$ is the shunt fraction, $\dot{Q}_S$ is the amount of shunt flow and $\dot{Q}_T$ the total flow, Cc'_{O_2} is the end-pulmonary capillary oxygen content, Ca_{O_2} is the arterial oxygen content, and $C\bar{v}_{O_2}$ is the mixed venous oxygen content.

Shunted blood is low in oxygen and high in carbon dioxide, but intrapulmonary shunt does not tend to elevate systemic $Paco_2$ because chemoreceptors sensitive to acute increases in $Paco_2$ stimulate respiratory drive, eliminating CO_2 before an increase would be detectable by blood gas analysis. Therefore, the arteriovenous CO_2 gradient under normal conditions is ~4–6 mm Hg.

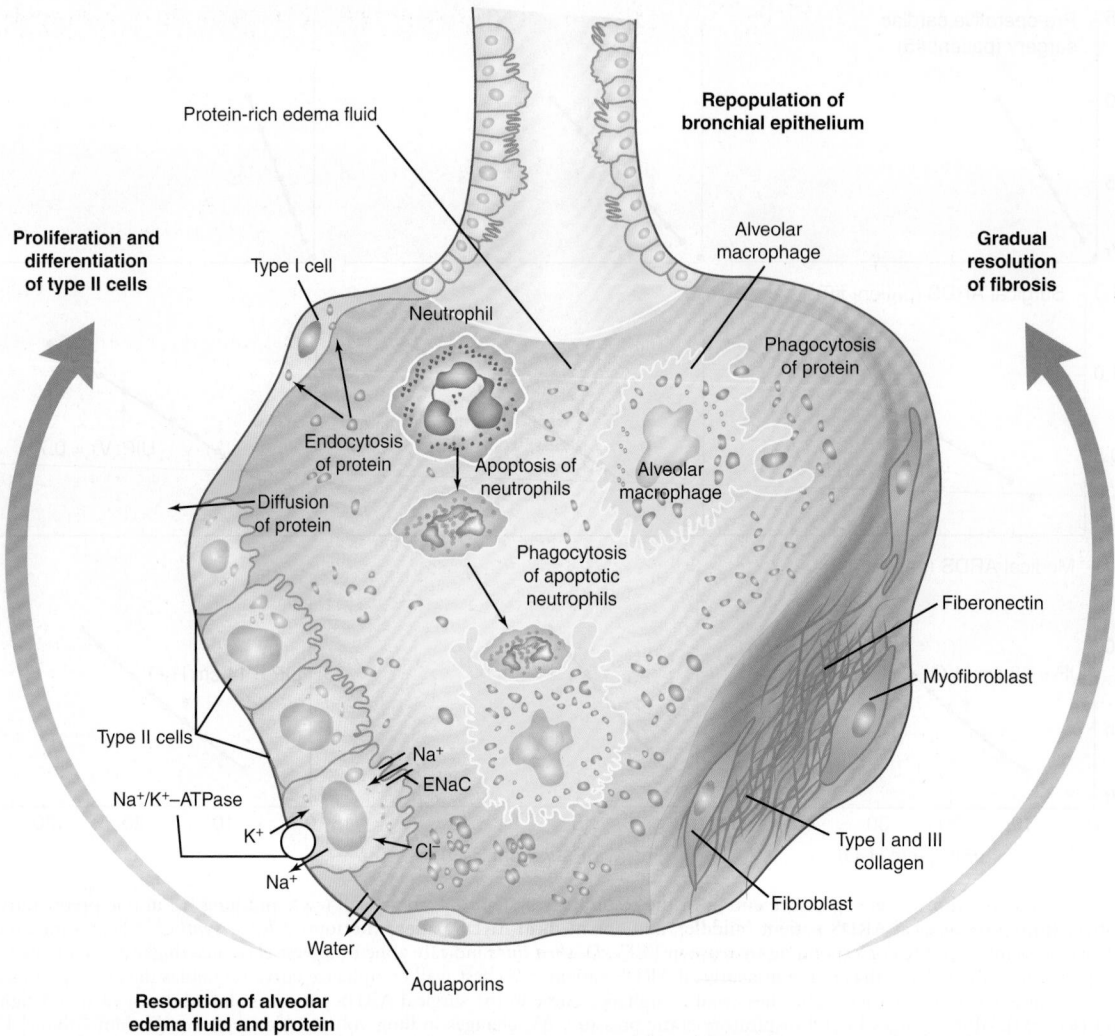

FIGURE 49.4. Cellular mechanisms of ARDS resolution. Repopulation of the alveolar epithelial barrier is shown on the left side of the figure. It is now believed this process may involve endogenous stem cell proliferation (see text). Within the alveolus, neutrophils are undergoing apoptosis and phagocytosis by alveolar macrophages. Structural elements governing fluid transport across the alveolar epithelium are illustrated. (From Ware LB, Matthay MA. The acute respiratory distress syndrome. *N Engl J Med* 2000;342(18):1334–49, with permission.)

The phenomenon of "right-to-left" intrapulmonary shunt is ameliorated to some degree by pulmonary vasoconstriction, which redirects blood toward better ventilated lung units. The pulmonary vascular bed is unique in human physiology for containing smooth muscle that *contracts* in response to hypoxemia.

The relationship of alveolar ventilation ($\dot{V}$) to perfusion ($\dot{Q}$) is not anatomically fixed. Even in the absence of disease, the distribution of inspired gas is subject to gravitational forces acting on the lung (44). In the upright human lung, spontaneous breathing creates a decreasing gradient of transpulmonary pressure from lung apex to lung base. In other words, the driving pressure for alveolar filling is greater in the (nondependent) apex than it is at the (dependent) lung base. Consequently, the less distended, dependent alveoli are positioned on a more compliant portion of the volume–pressure curve, compared to the more distended nondependent alveoli (**Fig. 49.5**). Therefore, dependent alveoli collectively account for a greater portion of alveolar ventilation than do nondependent alveoli (**Fig. 49.6**). The effects of gravity on the distribution of pulmonary blood flow are perhaps less straightforward. In the upright, isolated, and perfused canine lung, detection of blood flow using simple radiolabeled gas techniques has indicated that blood flow is greater in dependent regions than that in nondependent regions. On a global level, gravity does have a role in creating higher pulmonary vascular hydrostatic pressure in dependent lung regions, which should theoretically produce a favorable matching of ventilation to perfusion, at least in the upright, nondiseased lung. However, high-resolution experimental techniques have demonstrated that local variability in pulmonary blood flow distribution cannot be completely explained by gravity and is more likely related to the pulmonary vascular architecture. Studying anesthetized dogs in the prone and supine position, investigators were able to characterize pulmonary blood flow distribution using inert, radiolabeled microspheres injected under low lung volume conditions (45). After injection, microspheres embolize within pulmonary capillaries, and sectioning of the lung into small segments reveals the spatial distribution of pulmonary blood flow. In the supine position, pulmonary blood flow was distributed preferentially to the dorsal (dependent) region, but marked heterogeneity of perfusion existed within tissue planes that were subject to identical gravitational forces (46). In the prone position, pulmonary blood flow was also preferentially distributed to the dorsal (now nondependent) region, and flow within isogravitational planes was more uniform (45,46).

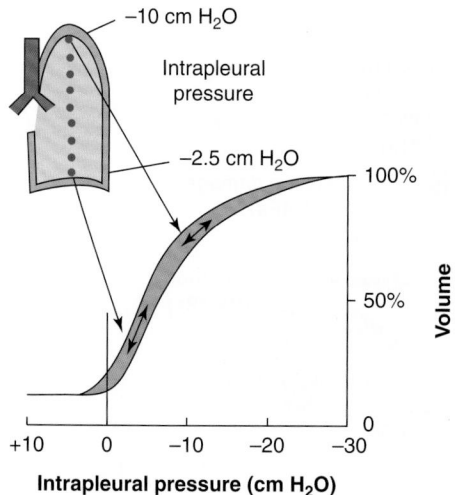

FIGURE 49.5. Regional differences in ventilation in the upright lung. The weight of the lung creates less negative intrapleural pressure at the lung base, while more negative intrapleural pressure is created at the apex. These differences translate into a decreasing transpulmonary pressure gradient in the dependent lung regions (see text). (From West JB. Mechanics of breathing. In: *Respiratory Physiology: The Essentials.* 4th ed. Baltimore, MD: Williams and Wilkins, 1990:87–113, with permission.)

Imbalances in the distribution of ventilation and perfusion create alveolar–capillary units that vary in their gas-exchanging efficiency according to the local distribution of alveolar gas flow relative to pulmonary blood flow. In healthy patients, ~10% of cardiac output does not come into contact with alveolar gas. This "physiologic shunt" fraction includes baseline $\dot{V}/\dot{Q}$ inequality, as well as blood from the bronchial, pleural, and thebesian veins, which returns to the systemic circulation without passing through the pulmonary vascular bed. The influence of $\dot{V}/\dot{Q}$ imbalance on blood gas tensions is magnified in ALI and ARDS, conditions in which consolidation and collapse of lung units are widespread and fluid-filled alveoli act as low $\dot{V}/\dot{Q}$ lung units with the potential to create measurable elevations in $PaCO_2$ and decreases in PaO_2. Consolidation of diseased alveoli creates radial traction forces on neighboring lung units that result in alveolar overdistension and pulmonary capillary narrowing, creating high $\dot{V}/\dot{Q}$ areas and adding to alveolar

dead space. Addition of positive pressure ventilation adds to distension of nondependent alveoli and can displace local pulmonary blood flow, creating even more pronounced $\dot{V}/\dot{Q}$ inequality, particularly in supine patients in whom positive alveolar pressure enhances the gradient between gas distribution and pulmonary blood flow distribution. Use of the multiple inert gas elimination technique in experimental animals and human subjects has confirmed that, although both intrapulmonary shunt and $\dot{V}/\dot{Q}$ inequality contribute to impairment of gas exchange in ALI and ARDS, intrapulmonary shunt is the dominant cause of arterial hypoxemia in these conditions.

Host Immune Response: Role of Cytokines and Alteration of Hemostasis

The host immune response plays a crucial role in the pathogenesis of ALI and ARDS. The ALI sequence can be initiated by any number of infectious and noninfectious environmental pathogens, as well as by endogenous substances that are liberated after cellular injury. The redundancy of potential triggering mechanisms all but assures that exposure to one or more inciting factors reliably produces a swift and robust response from the host's innate immune system that upsets the precarious balance between proinflammation and anti-inflammation, and procoagulation and anticoagulation.

The cascade of events that characterizes the innate immune response to alveolar injury begins with the engagement of intra- and extracellular PRRs. PRRs are a family of molecules expressed in alveolar macrophages, epithelial cells, and intraepithelial dendritic cells that recognize pathogen-associated molecular patterns (PAMPs) or cellular damage-associated molecular patterns (DAMPs) and activate the synthesis of proinflammatory cytokines in response (47). Clinically, it is often not possible to distinguish whether the host inflammatory response was incited by molecular motifs expressed on invading pathogens or by motifs expressed on fragments of injured native cells. Zhang et al. (48) have proposed that similarities between a PAMP-triggered and a DAMP-triggered inflammatory phenotype may be attributable to similarities between bacterial DNA and host mitochondrial DNA, both of which can activate the innate immune response through the Toll-like receptor (TLR) signaling pathway. Among the most widely recognized PRRs, TLRs are a series of cell surface or endosomal membrane structures that can recruit intermediary adapter molecules to assemble a signaling pathway that

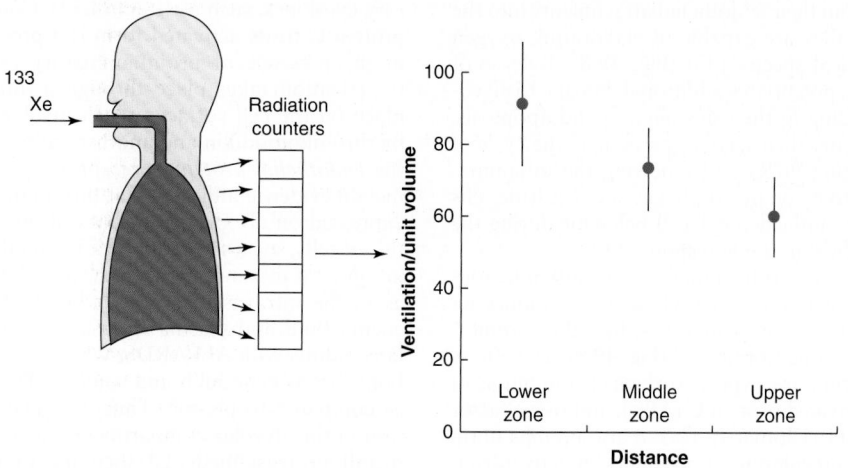

FIGURE 49.6. Regional differences in lung ventilation. Distribution of inhaled radiolabeled xenon gas is recorded by external radiation counters in a series of normal subjects. The ventilation per unit lung volume is greatest near the lung base ("lower zone") and is smallest toward the lung apex ("upper zone"). (From West JB. Ventilation. In: *Respiratory Physiology: The Essentials.* 4th ed. Baltimore, MD: Williams and Wilkins, 1990:11–20, with permission.)

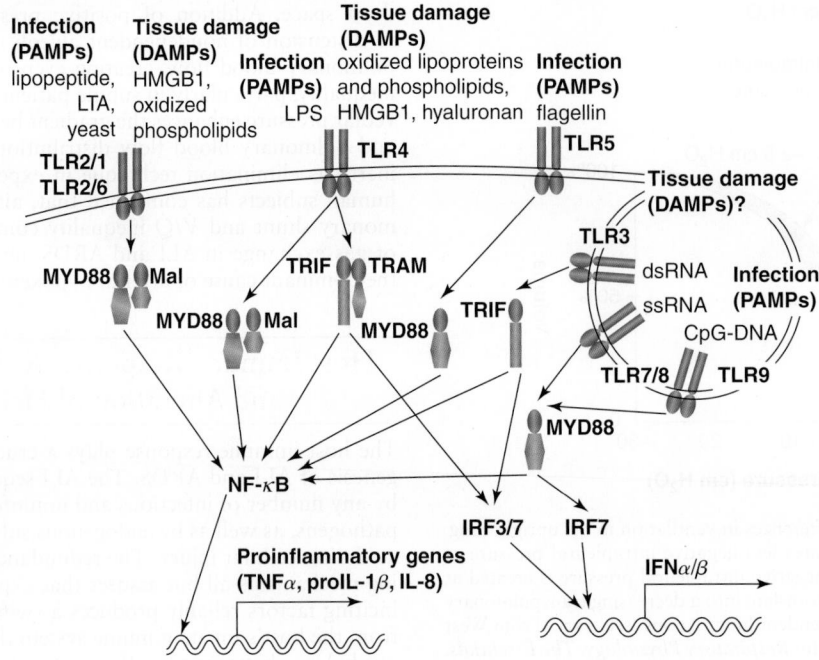

FIGURE 49.7. PRRs and cytokine synthesis following cellular injury. TLRs are shown on the outer cell membrane and endosomal surfaces. Like other PRRs, TLR subtypes (1–10) recognize specific PAMPs or DAMPs. PAMP- or DAMP-mediated activation of TLRs initiates signaling pathways involving recruitment of intermediary adapter molecules and culminating in NF-κB–dependent proinflammatory cytokine transcription. LTA, lipoteichoic acid; HMGB1, high-mobility group protein B1; LPS, lipopolysaccharide; MYD88, myeloid differentiation primary response gene 88; TRIF, Toll/IL-1 receptor homology domain–containing adapter inducing interferon (IFN)-β; TRAM, TRIF-related adapter molecule; IRF, interferon regulatory factor. (From Opitz, van Laak V, Eitel J, et al. Innate immune recognition in infectious and noninfectious diseases of the lung. *Am J Respir Crit Care Med* 2010;181(12):1294–309.)

ultimately triggers interferon α and β expression and/or NF-κB activation (Fig. 49.7) (47). NF-κB is a transcription factor that controls the expression of proinflammatory cytokines tumor necrosis factor-α (TNF-α), IL-1β, and IL-8, a few of the earliest response agents of the innate immune system. Once expressed, TNF-α and IL-1β subsequently stimulate the production of other proinflammatory interleukins, such as IL-6, and potentiate the interaction between β2 integrins on neutrophils and intercellular adhesion molecule-1 (ICAM-1) on vascular endothelial cells. This interaction attaches the neutrophil to the endothelium. Thereafter, IL-8 works together with the complement system (factors 3a and 5a), leukotriene B4, and platelet-activating factor (PAF) to establish a chemotactic gradient that recruits neutrophils from their endothelial attachments into the alveolar space, where they are capable of elaborating oxygen and nitrogen free radical species (33) (Fig. 49.8). Release of reactive oxygen species potentiates additional damage to alveolar epithelial cells, leading to their dysfunction and apoptosis. Products of cellular injury then serve to perpetuate the cycle of tissue injury by engaging PRRs and renewing the inflammatory response. PRR activity on macrophages and dendritic cells ultimately has a role in influencing T cell behavior during the adaptive phase of the host immune response (47).

TNF-α and IL-6 play a part in connecting the inflammatory response with the coagulation cascade. These two cytokines act in a complementary fashion on hemostasis, by either promoting coagulation or impairing fibrinolysis (Fig. 49.9). The effects of TNF-α on coagulation are expressed through inhibition of antithrombin (AT), activated protein C (APC), and tissue factor pathway inhibitor (TFPI). Ultimately TNF-α also inhibits fibrin degradation through upregulation of plasminogen activator inhibitor (PAI) (49). IL-6 stimulates the extrinsic coagulation pathway through interaction with tissue factor, which is expressed on the surface of alveolar epithelial cells, activated macrophages, and vascular endothelial cells, and is upregulated in response to

inflammatory stimuli (50). In addition, Bastarache et al. (51) recently reported the intriguing finding that the pulmonary edema fluid, of mechanically ventilated patients with ALI, is enriched with TF-bearing, highly procoagulant microparticles, which appear to have arisen from alveolar *epithelial* cells. Tissue factor binds and activates factors VII and X, and the TF-factor VIIa–factor Xa complex initiates a cascade of events culminating in the increased conversion of fibrinogen to fibrin (52).

Experimental evidence has emerged over the past several years emphasizing a key role for APC in attenuating the inflammatory response. Long acknowledged as a coagulation inhibitor, APC also possesses an important capacity to inhibit neutrophil chemotaxis and to downregulate production of proinflammatory cytokines, such as IL-6 (53,54). Conversely, conversion of protein C to its activated form is a process that is suppressed in the presence of proinflammatory cytokines (34). Protein C activation takes place through a multistep process taking place on the cell surface, which involves proteolytic cleavage by thrombomodulin and another entity traditionally known as the *endothelial protein C receptor* (EPCR). The latest experimental evidence indicates that thrombomodulin and EPCR are expressed on alveolar epithelial cells as well as vascular endothelial cells, suggesting that APC is intended to modulate coagulation (and inflammation) in the alveolar compartment as well as in the intravascular space (34,52). Examining pulmonary edema fluid and plasma from a series of mechanically ventilated adults with ALI/ARDS, Wang et al. found higher levels of both thrombomodulin and soluble EPCR in the alveolar fluid as compared to plasma. Thus, coagulation and fibrin deposition in the alveolar compartment may owe their origins to the metalloprotease-mediated shedding of thrombomodulin and EPCR from injured epithelia and the resulting reduction in protein C activation capacity (34,52). In theory, the procoagulant milieu of the alveolar compartment in ALI might be modifiable through the strategic administration of APC, although it is not

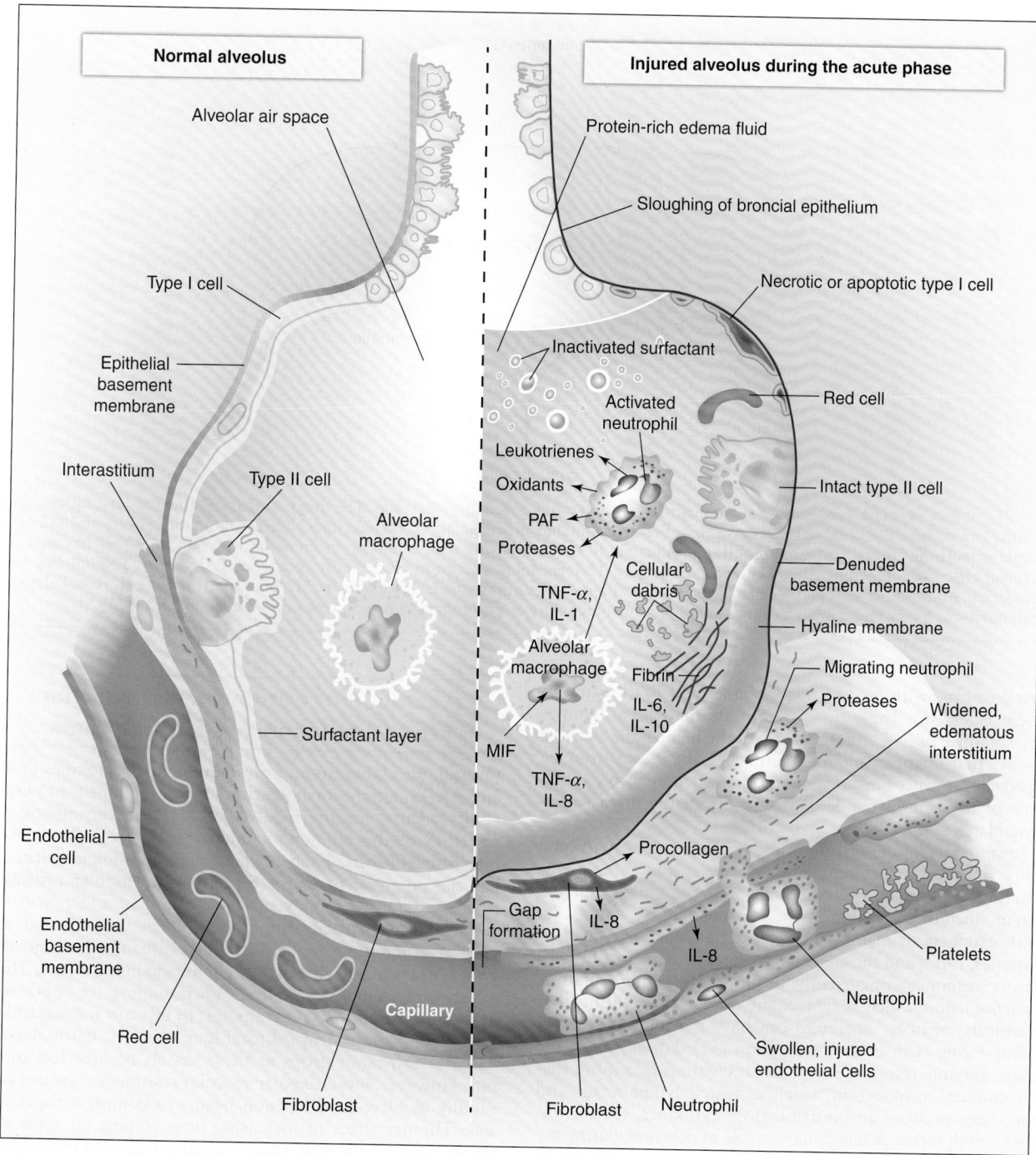

FIGURE 49.8. Cellular and molecular mechanisms of inflammation and alteration of hemostasis in ALI and ARDS. The normal alveolus is shown on the left, and the injured alveolus is shown on the right (see text). (From Ware LB, Matthay MA. The acute respiratory distress syndrome. *N Engl J Med* 2000;342(18):1334–49, with permission.)

known whether this approach might have the collateral effect of suppressing critical aspects of the host immune response.

Whether the individual patient with ALI and/or ARDS expresses, on balance, a predominantly procoagulant or anticoagulant phenotype seems likely to be a function of the interaction between host genetics and the specific inciting factors that lead to disease development. However, data from the laboratory as well as the clinical setting indicate that the supportive strategy selected by the clinician can potentially modify this process. For example, mechanical ventilation using large tidal volumes seems to be associated with release of PAI-1 and reduced fibrinolytic activity in a small animal

model of lung injury (55). In another model, rats ventilated with 20 cc/kg tidal volumes after receiving priming doses of intratracheal thrombin and fibrinogen exhibited amplified increases in alveolar PAI-1 activity, as compared to control animals that were similarly primed but were ventilated with 6 cc/kg tidal volumes (52). Another group of investigators has reported that patients who were ventilated for 5 hours with high (12 cc/kg) tidal volumes and zero positive end-expiratory pressure (PEEP) following elective surgery demonstrated significant elevation in levels of thrombin–antithrombin complexes, tissue factor, and factor VIIa in bronchoalveolar lavage (BAL) fluid, as compared to those who were ventilated over the same

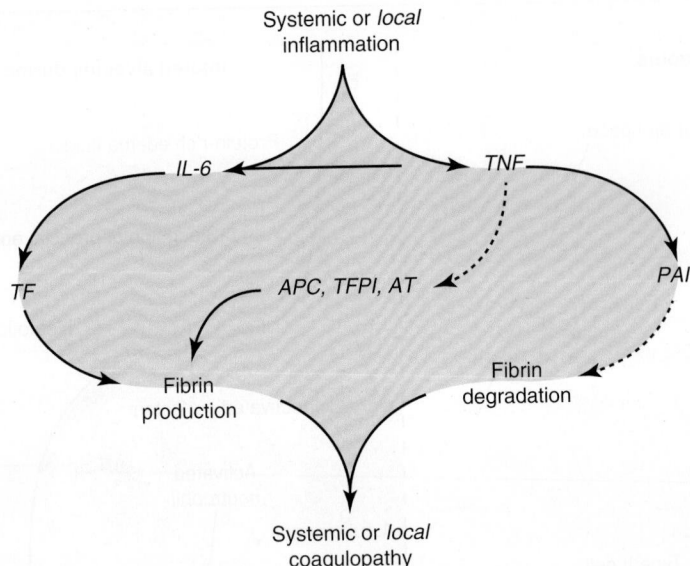

FIGURE 49.9. Cross talk between pro-inflammatory cytokines and coagulation cascade. The diagram depicts how the host inflammatory response can disrupt the usual balance between anticoagulation and procoagulation. *Dashed lines* indicate inhibitory effects and *solid lines* indicate stimulating effects. TNF promotes IL-6 production. IL-6 interacts with tissue factor to promote fibrin production. TNF has dual anti-coagulant effects. By inhibiting APC, TFPI, and AT activity, TNF encourages fibrin production. By promoting PAI activity, TNF inhibits fibrin degradation. Abbreviations: TFPI, tissue factor pathway inhibitor; AT, antithrombin. (From Schultz MJ, Haitsma JJ, Zhang H, et al. Pulmonary coagulopathy as a new target in therapeutic studies of acute lung injury or pneumonia: A review. *Crit Care Med* 2006;34(3):871–7.)

period of time with 6 cc/kg tidal volumes and PEEP equal to 10 cm H_2O (56). These findings indicate that the inflammatory response in ALI and ARDS alters the hemostatic balance in ways that might be modifiable through the use of strategic approaches to mechanical ventilation. They may also explain some of the hemodynamic consequences of the disease, discussed later.

In summary, amplification of the immune response to lung injury is a product of multiple redundancies and complex interactions among various components of the innate immune system, including cytokines, the complement system (C3a, C5a), products of membrane phospholipid metabolism (leukotrienes, PAF), and the coagulation cascade. The host inflammatory response concurrently produces its own regulators, a phenomenon which may account for the observation that "anti-inflammatory" therapies can have the undesired effect of interfering with disease resolution (57). For instance, the innate immune response eventually transitions to a more specific immune response in which activated lymphocytes and monocytes produce anti-inflammatory cytokines, such as tumor growth factor-β, which have a role in downregulating the effects of their proinflammatory counterparts on neutrophils and endothelial cells. Elaboration of extracellular matrix eventually takes place, giving way to the fibroproliferative stage of disease. Successful containment of exogenous and/or endogenous triggers of the inflammatory response induces a distinct "proresolution" program in host tissues, allowing egress and apoptosis of infiltrating cells and a return to premorbid levels of cellular homeostasis (**Fig. 49.4**) (57). Dysregulation of this process can actually set the stage for chronic inflammation (28,57), an observation which may open new avenues for future therapeutic approaches. Optimally, resolution of acute inflammation in ALI/ARDS is mediated by IL-10, an anti-inflammatory cytokine that attenuates fibrosis and the activity of NF-κB (58). Its impact on NF-κB helps to induce neutrophil apoptosis and allow for repopulation of bronchial and alveolar epithelium, a process that may involve endogenous stem cell proliferation rather than multiplication of any differentiated cells that remain (58,59).

Alteration of Cardiovascular Function: Effects on Pulmonary Hemodynamics

Overall, the elaboration of proinflammatory cytokines in ALI and ARDS initiates or potentiates the development of permeability edema, leading to alveolar hypoxia, thrombotic obstruction of the pulmonary microvasculature, and eventual interstitial fibrosis. Each of these pathophysiologic elements has the potential to increase pulmonary vascular resistance (PVR), adding to right ventricular afterload and potentially compromising cardiac output. Studies in open-chested and excised canine lung models established many years ago that PVR is dramatically affected by changes in lung volume. These experiments demonstrated that PVR is minimal (or "optimal") at the lung volume that corresponds to FRC, or normal EELV. As EELV increases toward total lung capacity, extra-alveolar vascular resistance drops as these vessels become less tortuous. However, intra-alveolar vascular resistance escalates very rapidly as alveolar distension begins to compress these vessels. The net effect of increasing lung volume on these two components of the pulmonary vascular bed is an exponential increase in PVR. As EELV drops toward residual volume, resistance of the extra-alveolar vessels increases as they become more tortuous. In addition, collapse of small airways as lung compliance falls results in alveolar hypoxia and reflex pulmonary vasoconstriction. Collectively, the effects of lung volume on PVR produce a parabolic curve whose nadir occurs at FRC (**Fig. 49.10**). Increases in PVR and right ventricular afterload at the extremes of lung volume can ultimately reduce systemic cardiac output, as increased end-diastolic volume in the highly compliant right ventricle (RV) shifts the interventricular septum toward the left, resulting in decreased left ventricular (LV) compliance and poor LV filling. These cardiopulmonary interactions suggest that strategies that emphasize the maintenance of alveolar volume while avoiding alveolar overdistension are not only necessary to improve gas exchange but also likely to have a favorable effect on cardiovascular performance in ALI and ARDS.

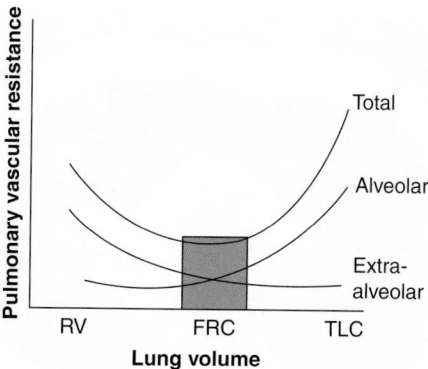

FIGURE 49.10. Effect of lung volume on PVR. "Optimal" or nadir PVR occurs at FRC. As lung volume increases toward total lung capacity (TLC), extra-alveolar resistance drops, while intra-alveolar vascular resistance escalates. As lung volume drops toward residual volume (RV), extra-alveolar vascular resistance increases as these vessels become tortuous, while alveolar hypoxia results in intra-alveolar vasoconstriction. The "total" or net effect of these findings on overall PVR is represented by the uppermost curve. (From Shekerdemian L, Bohn D. Cardiovascular effects of mechanical ventilation. *Arch Dis Child* 1999;80(5):475–80.)

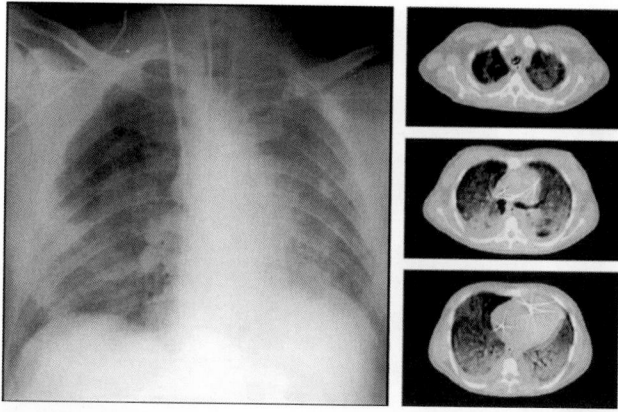

FIGURE 49.11. Nonuniform parenchymal involvement in ARDS. Chest x-ray and CT scans corresponding to lung apex, hilum, and base from a patient with sepsis and ARDS. Images are taken with the patient in supine position, at a positive end-expiratory pressure of 5 cm H_2O. The CT scans illustrate the influence of the gravitational axis on the pattern of alveolar consolidation in ARDS: nondependent regions are aerated, while dependent regions remain consolidated. (From Gattinoni L, Caironi P, Pelosi P, et al. What has computed tomography taught us about the acute respiratory distress syndrome? *Am J Respir Crit Care Med* 2001;164:1701–11, with permission.)

CLINICAL PRESENTATION

Diffuse alveolar disease that meets criteria for ALI and ARDS produces a predictable sequence of clinical changes. When fluid accumulation in the interstitial space exceeds the absorptive capacity of the pulmonary lymphatics, lung compliance declines and tachypnea ensues as the patient attempts to generate adequate minute ventilation in the face of lower tidal volumes. The eventual leakage of proteinaceous fluid into the alveolar spaces interferes with native surfactant function, creating conditions that favor regional atelectasis and small airways closure, as well as a decrease in EELV to a point near or below closing capacity, especially in small infants and those with highly compliant chest walls (e.g., patients with neuromuscular disease). At this point, hypoxia rapidly worsens and breathing becomes more labored in an effort to generate transpulmonary pressures sufficient to maintain alveolar patency. Hypocarbia is often present early in the disease process, when the patient first manifests tachypnea. However, as the work of breathing escalates, the $PaCO_2$ will further rise as respiratory muscle fatigue ensues. At this stage, positive pressure ventilation is required to open a sufficient number of atelectatic lung units for adequate gas exchange. On auscultation, the patient will typically demonstrate rales over areas of atelectasis or alveolar congestion, and decreased air entry over areas that are largely consolidated. Occasionally, it is possible to appreciate wheezes over areas in which intermittent small airways closure is occurring.

Imaging Studies

Clinical changes of early ALI and ARDS manifest on chest x-rays as diffuse alveolar infiltrates and air bronchograms that may be accompanied by pleural effusion and widespread atelectasis (**Fig. 49.11**). Areas of lung injury that are evolving into fibrosis may appear as prominent reticular opacities. Studies that have evaluated patients with ALI and ARDS using CT have facilitated an understanding that lung consolidation occurs along a gradient corresponding to the gravitational axis. The spatial distribution of ALI has been demonstrated in anesthetized and paralyzed dogs that were rotated while being injected with oleic acid in divided doses to encourage a diffuse pattern of lung injury (60). The animals were then exposed to high tidal volume ventilation while they were in either the supine or the prone position. At the end of the experiment, all animals developed lung edema distributed, for the most part, to dependent areas. However, regardless of body position, histologic abnormalities were more severe in dorsal lung regions, in a pattern reflecting the preferential distribution of pulmonary blood flow, the pathway by which lung injury was initiated in this model.

Development of dependent atelectasis in any patient oriented horizontally is not a new concept; CT images obtained in supine, anesthetized patients without lung disease who were administered neuromuscular blockade have identified the same phenomenon. However, serial CT imaging in patients with ALI and ARDS has revealed that, in later stages of the disease, fibrosis begins to be identifiable in nondependent areas that seemed to be relatively free of disease earlier in the course (**Figs. 49.12** and **49.13**). The reticular pattern of infiltration that appears in these areas seems to be associated with lengthy and aggressive strategies of mechanical ventilation (61). Lung regions in which this pattern develops also correspond to zones in which every breath subjects local alveoli to repetitive cycles of expansion and collapse. The implications of the CT changes seen in mechanically ventilated patients with ALI led to management strategies recognizing that cyclic alveolar deformation can actually trigger an inflammatory response (discussed later). Thus, the past 10 years has seen the "natural history" of ALI and ARDS reframed as the combined inflammatory effects of the initial biologic insult and the process of mechanical ventilation.

PRINCIPLES OF CLINICAL MANAGEMENT

As more of the pathophysiologic elements involved in ALI and ARDS have been elucidated in the laboratory, considerable effort has been given toward translating them into innovative targets for therapeutic intervention. At the moment, therapeutic drug trials in this area have not identified an agent that improves clinically important outcome measures in a way that

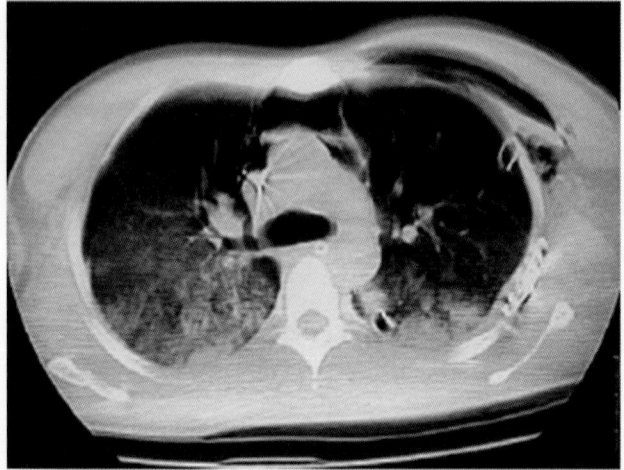

FIGURE 49.12. CT scan of a patient with ARDS, 5 days after multiple trauma. A view at the level of the carina shows diffuse alveolar opacification, with areas of consolidation located in dependent regions. (From Gattinoni L, Caironi P, Pelosi P, et al. What has computed tomography taught us about the acute respiratory distress syndrome? *Am J Respir Crit Care Med* 2001;164:1701–11, with permission.)

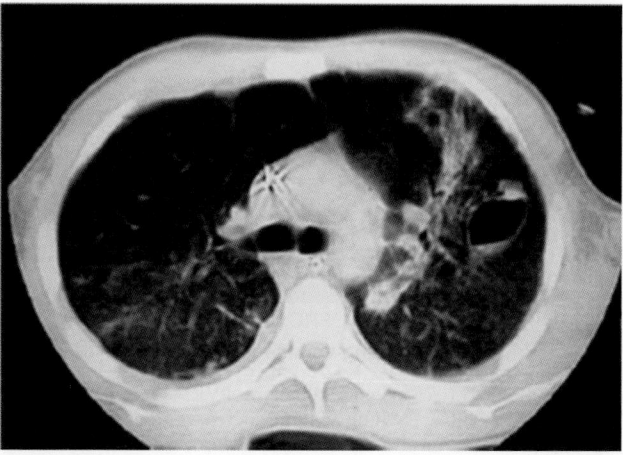

FIGURE 49.13. CT scan of same patient (as in **Figure 49.12**) 12 days after onset of ARDS. Alveolar opacities have largely cleared, giving way to reticular infiltrates. A pneumatocele is evident on the left, and an area of atelectasis is seen medial to it. (From Gattinoni L, Caironi P, Pelosi P, et al. What has computed tomography taught us about the acute respiratory distress syndrome? *Am J Respir Crit Care Med* 2001;164:1701–11, with permission.)

warrants its routine use in the management of all patients with ALI and ARDS (**Table 49.3**). The mainstay of therapy remains supportive care, of which a critically important component is the application of positive pressure ventilation (**Table 49.4**).

Positive Pressure Ventilation

Hypoxia is an essential feature of ALI and ARDS; the basis for its development is the breakdown of the alveolar–capillary barrier. Once this occurs, pulmonary compliance and EELV tend to decline dramatically and $\dot{V}/\dot{Q}$ imbalance ensues, which explains why hypoxia in ALI and ARDS is typically refractory to the provision of supplementary oxygen alone. Moreover, exposing animals to high concentrations of supplemental oxygen without effectively reversing atelectasis can bring about a form of lung injury that is remarkably similar to ALI and ARDS. Humans begin to consistently manifest this type of lung injury when they are exposed to an $FiO_2 > 0.5$. To stabilize consolidated or collapsed alveoli to a degree that is sufficient to provide oxygenation without the use of high FiO_2, positive pressure ventilation is necessary. In Ashbaugh's original description of ARDS, he reported that the hypoxemia associated with this disease could be reversed with PEEP. In the decade that followed publication of this initial case series, a study conducted in a small number of patients with severe hypoxic respiratory failure demonstrated that upward titration of PEEP from 0 to 15 cm H_2O resulted in similar linear increases in EELV, PaO_2, and static compliance (62). A few years later, the effects of PEEP were evaluated in an oleic acid model of canine lung injury. In that study, increasing PEEP from 3 to 13 cm H_2O decreased intrapulmonary shunt fraction without altering pulmonary blood flow; alveolar septa were thicker and a greater portion of alveoli were flooded in the lungs ventilated without PEEP, as compared to those that were ventilated with PEEP. In lungs ventilated with PEEP, edema was confined to the perivascular space (63). It is tempting to conclude from these observations that PEEP reverses hypoxemia in ALI and ARDS by simply redistributing extravascular lung water and restoring EELV toward FRC. However, it is useful to look at these results in light of Webb and Tierney's study from the mid-1970s, in which they demonstrated that a

pattern of injury resembling ARDS could be created in healthy lungs by mechanically ventilating with high peak inflation pressures (PIP), and applying PEEP in this context similarly limited edema formation. Taken together, these studies shed light on the possibility that besides restoring an interface for adequate gas exchange, stabilizing alveolar volume through the application of PEEP might also limit the development of ventilator-associated injury. While the salutary effects of PEEP have been well established, it is important to recognize the potential for PEEP to augment anatomical dead space by distending large airways, and potentially adding to alveolar dead space as well.

When managing a patient with hypoxic respiratory failure, it is important to appreciate the effects of positive pressure ventilation on cardiovascular function. During normal breathing, negative intrathoracic pressure lowers intracavitary pressure in the right atrium and, together with positive intra-abdominal pressure, creates a gradient that promotes right atrial filling. In ARDS, lung inflation toward FRC is associated with a decrease in PVR, which lowers right ventricular afterload, and pulmonary venous return proceeds unimpeded to the left heart and systemic circulation. Although, positive pressure ventilation is required to restore lung volume toward FRC and achieve adequate gas exchange in hypoxic respiratory failure, it also increases right atrial pressure, diminishing the pressure gradient for systemic venous return and lowering right ventricular stroke volume. On the other hand, positive pressure ventilation tends to enhance LV function because of its favorable effects on LV afterload, as determined by transmural pressure (P_{tm}). P_{tm} is defined as the intracavitary pressure (P_{ic}) minus the surrounding, or pleural pressure (P_{pl}):

$$P_{tm} = P_{ic} - P_{pl}$$

This formula illustrates that LV transmural pressure (or afterload) is reduced in the setting of positive pressure ventilation and increased in the setting of negative pressure ventilation. Although the gradient for cardiac filling can be manipulated by intravascular volume loading and the use of vasoactive infusions, the effects of positive pressure ventilation on overall cardiac output have much to do with the relationship between alveolar volume and pulmonary blood flow. It has been known for many years that the sensitivity of RV contractile function

TABLE 49.3

RESULTS OF SELECTED CLINICAL TRIALS EVALUATING VENTILATION STRATEGIES OR PHARMACOLOGIC THERAPIES FOR ALI AND ARDS

■ INTERVENTION	■ YEAR	■ NUMBER OF PATIENTS	■ FINDINGS	■ STUDY
Low tidal volume mechanical ventilation	2000	861	*22% relative mortality benefit*	NIH Acute Respiratory Distress Syndrome Network (2)
Increased recruitment vs. minimal alveolar overdistension in ALI and ARDS *(PEEP titrated to Pplat 28–30 cm H_2O vs. PEEP 5–9 cm H_2O)*	2008	767	No mortality benefit	Mercat et al. (78)
Recruitment maneuvers, low tidal volumes, and high PEEP in ALI and ARDS *(higher PEEP, Pplat ≤40 cm H_2O, VT 6 cc/kg, and recruitment maneuvers vs. "conventional" PEEP, Pplat ≤30 cm H_2O, and VT 6 cc/kg)*	2008	983	No mortality benefit	Meade et al. (77)
HFOV at maximal Hz vs. conventional ventilation with higher PEEP, VT 6 cc/kg, and Pplat ≤35 cm H_2O *"OSCILLATE" trial*	2013	548 (of 1200)	Increased in-hospital mortality with HFOV[a]	Ferguson et al. (82)
HFOV vs. "usual" conventional ventilation *(~8 cc/kg ideal body weight)* *"OSCAR" trial*	2013	795 (of 1006)	No mortality benefit[b]	Young et al. (151)
Prone positioning	2001	304	No mortality benefit[c]	Gattinoni et al. (87)
	2004	791	No mortality benefit[d]	Guerin et al. (152)
	2005[e]	102	No mortality benefit	Curley et al. (13)
	2006	136	No mortality benefit[f]	Mancebo et al. (153)
	2009	342	No mortality benefit[g]	Taccone et al. (88)
	2013	237	*51% relative mortality benefit[h]*	Guerin et al. (89)
Conservative vs. liberal fluid administration strategy	2006	1000	No mortality benefit[i]	NIH Acute Respiratory Distress Syndrome Network (84)
Activated Protein C	2008	75	No mortality benefit	Liu et al. (112)
Inhaled β-agonist	2011	282	No mortality benefit	Matthay et al. (17)
IV β-agonist	2012	324	No mortality benefit[j]	Gao Smith et al. (121)
Surfactant	1996	725	No mortality benefit	Anzueto et al. (92)
	2004	448	No mortality benefit	Spragg et al. (32)
	2005[e]	152	Mortality benefit seen in surfactant group[k]	Willson et al. (14)
	2009	418	No mortality benefit[l]	Kesecioglu et al. (31)
	2011	419	No mortality benefit[m]	Spragg et al. (94)
	2012[e]	165	No mortality benefit[m,n]	Thomas et al. (95)
Corticosteroids	1998	24	Mortality benefit[o]	Meduri et al. (98)
	2006	180	No mortality benefit	NIH Acute Respiratory Distress Syndrome Network (99)
Inhaled nitric oxide	1998	177	No mortality benefit	Dellinger et al. (102)
	1999[e]	108	No mortality benefit	Dobyns et al. (104)
	2004	385	No mortality benefit	Taylor et al. (103)
Early trophic vs. full enteral feeding	2012	1000	No mortality benefit	Rice et al. (18)
Omega-3 fatty acid, γ-linoleic acid, and antioxidant supplementation vs. isocaloric control supplement	2012	272	No mortality benefit	Rice et al. (134)

[a]Trial terminated prematurely for potential harm. Enrolled patients had Pao_2/Fio_2 ≤200 with an Fio_2 ≥0.5, and had ≤2 weeks of symptoms. HFOV delivered using the SensorMedics 3100B ventilator (CareFusion, San Diego, CA).
[b]Target enrollment reduced from 1006 at interim analysis. Enrolled patients had Pao_2/Fio_2 ≤200 on PEEP ≥5 cm H_2O. HFOV delivered using Novalung R100 ventilator (Metran, Kawaguchi, Japan).
[c]Patients ventilated using (approximate) average VT 10 cc/kg predicted body weight.
[d]Trial enrolled patients with acute hypoxic respiratory failure, a portion of whom had ALI/ARDS. They were proned for median 8 h/day and ventilated with (approximate) average VT 8 cc/kg measured body weight. Concern for increased position-related adverse events in prone group.
[e]Pediatric trial.
[f]Patients proned for average of 17 h/day, and VT of up to 10 cc/kg and PIP up to 40 cm H_2O were allowed. ICU mortality 58% in control arm; study ultimately underpowered.
[g]Trial enrolled patients with moderate (Pao_2/Fio_2 100–200) and severe (Pao_2/Fio_2 < 100) ARDS. Patients proned for ≥20 h/day; ventilated using VT limited to ≤8 cc/kg and Pplat ≤30 cm H_2O.
[h]Absolute mortality reduction 16.8% (see text).
[i]Patients who received a fluid-conservative strategy had an improved oxygenation index and a significant increase in ventilator-free days during the first 28 days of therapy.
[j]Trial terminated prematurely at interim analysis; patients in intervention arm had higher mortality rate than controls.
[k]Study ultimately underpowered (see text).
[l]Nonsignificant trend toward increased mortality and increased adverse effects in treatment arm.
[m]Trial enrolled patients with severe direct lung injury, a portion of whom met all criteria for ALI/ARDS.
[n]Phase II trial.
[o]Small study; crossover design (see text).
Adapted from Ware LB, Matthay MA. The acute respiratory distress syndrome. *N Engl J Med* 2000;342:1334–49.

TABLE 49.4

SUGGESTED THERAPY GUIDELINES FOR ALI/ARDS

	■ PULMONARY	■ CARDIOVASCULAR	■ OTHER
Resuscitation	■ Supplemental O_2 ■ Early arterial access for disease identification (PaO_2/FiO_2, OI) and early implementation of therapy ■ Consider early NPPV for alveolar recruitment in alert, cooperative patient ■ Endotracheal intubation and positive pressure ventilation for respiratory failure failing noninvasive therapy ■ Titrate PEEP to achieve $FiO_2 \leq 0.5$–0.6/ SpO_2 88%–95% ■ Limit tidal volume (6 cc/kg *ideal* body weight) and alveolar plateau pressure (≤ 30 cm H_2O)[a] ■ Permissive hypercapnia unless contraindicated (coexisting increased intracranial pressure, etc.)	■ Crystalloid, colloid, or blood to optimize intravascular volume and support hemodynamics[b] ■ Anticipate potentially adverse hemodynamic consequences of transition to positive pressure ventilation in setting of intravascular volume depletion ■ Titrate supportive therapy to correct perfusion abnormalities and optimize urine output	■ Cultures ■ Broad-spectrum antimicrobial agents ■ Consider antifungal, antiviral, atypical agent coverage in immunocompromised population ■ Consider early bronchoalveolar lavage in immunocompromised population
Escalation	■ Titrate PEEP upward if ongoing hypoxemia in setting of alveolar derecruitment ■ Early transition to HFOV if high inflation pressures are necessary ■ Consider prone positioning in selected cases ■ Short-term administration of neuromuscular blocking agents to facilitate mechanical ventilation may benefit patients with severe disease[c]	■ Titrate fluid and vasoactive infusions to achieve age-appropriate blood pressure parameters and adequate end-organ function	■ Sedation/analgesia ■ Neuromuscular blockade if necessary
Maintenance	■ Follow OI to track response to therapy ■ Wean ventilator as allowable	■ Monitoring: CVP, serial clinical examination, and review of organ function[d] ■ Maintain euvolemia ■ Diuretics	■ Nutrition: Implement enteral nutrition as early as feasible. Avoid excess glucose administration. Careful attention to nitrogen balance ■ Neuromuscular blockade: Daily infusion interruption and discontinue as soon as feasible ■ Sedation and analgesia: Daily infusion interruption and wean during plateau phase of illness
Advanced therapy	■ OI not improving on optimal ventilator strategy/HFOV: Consider ECMO	■ Consider early renal replacement therapy for persistent hypervolemia and oliguria despite diuretics	

[a]Optimal tidal volume and plateau pressure are not known, but use of 6 cc/kg has been associated with a 22% relative mortality benefit compared to 12 cc/kg (2). High tidal volumes are also associated with proinflammatory cytokine release (65,67,149).
[b]Optimal hemoglobin concentration is not known. In physiologically stable critically ill children, hemoglobin of 7 g/dL is probably adequate and may avert adverse effects of red cell transfusion (154).
[c]Short-term administration of *cis*-atracurium early in the course of severe ARDS improved 90-day survival in a multicenter clinical trial (91). The mechanism behind this observation is not clear and may involve direct anti-inflammatory effects and/or mitigation of transalveolar pressure swings during spontaneous breathing (155). Clinicians should take steps to minimize the risk of increasing muscle weakness if pursuing such a strategy.
[d]Published evidence suggests pulmonary artery catheter use in ALI/ARDS is not associated with improved outcomes and may be associated with increased incidence of catheter-related complications (156). CVP must be interpreted in the context of surrounding compartment pressure (e.g., intrathoracic pressure for SVC lines) and/or myocardial compliance. In absence of coexisting intracardiac shunt, mixed venous oxygen saturation may clarify adequacy of cardiac output.
OI, oxygenation index [100 x mean airway pressure x FiO_2]/PaO_2; NPPV, noninvasive positive pressure ventilation; PEEP, positive end-expiratory pressure.
Adapted from Fackler JC, Arnold JH, Nichols DG, et al. Acute respiratory distress syndrome. In: Rogers M, ed. *Textbook of Pediatric Intensive Care*. 3rd ed. Baltimore, MD: Williams and Wilkins, 1996:197–233.

to RV afterload is such that acute changes in lung volume can produce increases in PVR capable of precipitating RV failure. The effects of this phenomenon on systemic cardiac output may outweigh any reduction in LV afterload that occurs with the transition to positive pressure ventilation. Moreover, because gas distribution in mechanically ventilated patients is preferentially distributed to nondependent, high $\dot{V}/\dot{Q}$ areas, PEEP can exacerbate the tendency toward alveolar overinflation, adding to alveolar dead space and possibly escalating PVR. In summary, a sound physiologic basis supports the expectation that titrating positive pressure (or PEEP) in a way that achieves alveolar recruitment, avoids alveolar overdistension, and optimizes the relationship of ventilation to perfusion will provide adequate gas exchange, while limiting the possibility for exposure to additional lung injury and potentially adverse cardiovascular effects.

Therapeutic goals for the use of positive pressure in the management of ALI and ARDS have evolved considerably over the past several decades. "Adequate gas exchange" was once defined as normal blood gas tensions, without regard for the level of mechanical support that was required to produce them. For the many reasons outlined earlier, mechanical ventilation has come to be regarded as a legitimate source of injury important enough to impact survival in patients with ALI and ARDS. Comparison of CT images of the lung in mechanically ventilated patients during inspiration and expiration illustrates that gravitational forces likely create zones of differential susceptibility to mechanical injury, as tidal volumes are preferentially delivered to unconsolidated, nondependent lung units (64). In heterogeneous conditions such as ALI and ARDS, it is difficult to know what level of PEEP will open enough alveoli to produce adequate oxygenation without creating conditions for ongoing stress-induced lung injury. Expert opinion has always varied when it comes to specifying precise algorithms for achieving adequate oxygenation. Recognizing the prudence of limiting a patient's exposure to high concentrations of supplementary oxygen and high transpulmonary pressures, a logical strategy suggests stepwise escalation of PEEP in 3- to 5-cm H_2O increments, until arriving at the minimum PEEP that allows for a Pao_2 in the range of 55–80 mm Hg, with peripheral oxygen saturation (Spo_2) of 88%–95%, using an Fio_2 of 0.5–0.6 (65).

The tidal volume selected by the clinician also deserves careful consideration, because multiple lines of evidence indicate that limiting phasic changes in lung volume and preventing alveolar overdistension at end-inspiration will reduce the risk of ventilator-associated lung injury (66–68). Exposure to large tidal volume ventilation strategies have been associated with the development of ALI in patients with previously normal pulmonary mechanics, and exposure to high-volume/low PEEP strategies has been associated with rapid enhancement of inflammatory cytokine expression in plasma or BAL fluid samples in adults with and without ARDS (67,69,70). Both observations implicate physical forces imposed by mechanical ventilation in the pathogenesis of ALI.

Acute injury makes the lung particularly susceptible to ventilator-induced stress and strain wounds. Mechanical stress, as experienced by the human lung, can be described as the force per unit area that develops in response to a force applied in the opposite direction (71). Strain is related to the ratio of a structure's change in length (in response to an applied force) to its length at rest. In the mechanically ventilated lung, "stress" is analogous to transalveolar distending pressure, which is determined by PEEP and plateau pressure. "Strain" amplitude is analogous to phasic alveolar stretch, which is determined by end-inspiratory lung volume (referenced to EELV). In the homogeneously inflated lung, these forces are borne more or less equally by all lung regions. When the lung is heterogeneously inflated, as in the anesthetized supine state,

or most dramatically, in ALI and ARDS, some lung units remain collapsed throughout the respiratory cycle. This shifts a greater than usual share of stress and strain forces onto adjacent, more compliant lung units, making them vulnerable to structural deformation. Over 40 years ago, Mead et al. (72) first proposed that alveoli positioned at the interface between lung units that open and those that remain closed bear a disproportionate amount of mechanical stress. More recent experimental work has helped elucidate how this phenomenon connects with the host inflammatory response. We now know that in an attempt to prevent "stress failure," alveolar cells respond to deformation by fortifying their cell membranes with additional lipids. At the same time however, "mechanosensors" (e.g., integrin proteins on the cell surface and structural elements of the cytoskeleton) detect and translate deformation forces into NF-κB–mediated signaling pathways that culminate in the production of the cytokine IL-8 and neutrophil recruitment (71,73,74).

In 2000, the ARDS Clinical Trials Network (ARDSnet) demonstrated conclusively in a multicentered RCT that limiting tidal volumes could result in significantly decreased mortality in ARDS. The trial was stopped early, after investigators found that patients randomized to receive tidal volumes of 6 cc/kg ideal body weight had a 22% relative reduction in mortality, compared to those randomized to receive tidal volumes of 12 cc/kg ideal body weight (65). The experimental arm of the study called for limitation of plateau pressures to ≤30 cm H_2O, while the control arm had plateau pressure limited to ≤50 cm H_2O. Management in both study arms also allowed for development of a respiratory acidosis, down to a pH of 7.15. Remarkably, the investigators were also able to demonstrate a significant reduction in plasma levels of the proinflammatory cytokine IL-6 among patients in the low tidal volume group. This study was the first of several investigations to establish that reducing the magnitude of phasic stretch during mechanical ventilation influences patient outcomes by attenuating the systemic inflammatory response (75,76).

Mechanically, the salutary effects of limiting transalveolar pressure (i.e., plateau pressure) and limiting phasic stretch through tidal volume reduction may be related to a reduction in alveolar stress and strain forces. EELV is another important determinant of alveolar stress and strain, but it is not yet clear how best to mitigate ventilator-associated injury through strategic manipulation of PEEP. In 2008, two multinational RCTs enrolling a total 1750 adults with ALI/ARDS examined the question of whether stabilizing EELV through routine recruitment maneuvers and/or applied PEEP could enhance the outcome benefits of a ventilating with a tidal volume of 6 cc/kg predicted body weight (Table 49.3) (77,78). Neither trial was able to demonstrate a mortality benefit. A recent systematic review and meta-analysis of three high-quality clinical trials examining the effects of higher versus lower PEEP used on adults with ALI found no significant in-hospital mortality benefit, which was the primary outcome (79). The trials collectively enrolled 2299 patients whose disease was defined according to AECC criteria. In each trial, a 3 cm H_2O mean difference in PEEP level was maintained between the study groups for the first 3 days after randomization. Apart from the PEEP strategy, patients were managed using the lung-protective strategy that had been applied in the experimental arm of the ARDSnet trial (65). Among the 1892 patients in the three trials that met criteria for ARDS however, higher PEEP conferred a 4%-absolute reduction in mortality (95% CI, 0.81–1.00; number needed to treat is 25).

Ongoing interest in the lung-protective merits of low tidal volume ventilation has led to the expectation that high-frequency oscillatory ventilation (HFOV) would have an important role in the management of patients with ALI and

ARDS. HFOV is an attractive mode of ventilation because of its unique ability to provide adequate gas exchange using tidal volumes below dead-space volume in the setting of continuous alveolar recruitment. Theoretically, high-frequency ventilation should provide the ultimate "open-lung" strategy of ventilation. HFOV offers the promise of mitigating dynamic alveolar strain forces by preserving EELV, minimizing cyclic stretch, and avoiding parenchymal overdistension at end-inspiration so that the patient is ventilated on the most compliant portion of the volume–pressure curve (**Fig. 49.1**). The first and largest multicentered, randomized trial to evaluate the effect of HFOV versus conventional ventilation in children used a crossover design and enrolled children with diffuse alveolar disease and/or air leak (80). The investigators randomized 70 patients (a) to receive conventional ventilation with limitation of peak inspiratory pressure, or (b) to HFOV using a strategy that targeted a lung volume at which optimal oxygenation occurred ($Sao_2 \geq 90\%$ and $Fio_2 < 0.6$). The mean age ($\pm$ SD) of the patients was 2.5 ± 2.5 years in the HFOV group and 3.1 ± 3.3 years in the conventional ventilation group. For patients with air leak, airway pressure was further limited, while Fio_2 was preferentially increased to achieve saturations of $\geq 85\%$ and pH ≥ 7.25 until the air leak resolved. The study found no difference in survival or duration of mechanical ventilation between the two groups, but significantly fewer children randomized to receive HFOV remained dependent on supplemental oxygen at 30 days. Post hoc analysis revealed that outcome benefits were not as great in those that crossed over to the HFOV arm, supporting the suggestion by numerous studies that use of HFOV will be more successful if employed early in the course of disease. Across the age spectrum of pediatric patients with diffuse alveolar disease, the outcome advantages for HFOV over a well-executed lung-protective conventional ventilation protocol may vary. One recent multicenter randomized clinical trial has demonstrated that preterm surfactant-deficient infants who were managed with HFOV at 10–15 Hz successfully extubated earlier than infants randomized to receive conventional ventilation calibrated to deliver a tidal volume of 5–6 cc/kg, and demonstrated a reduced need for supplemental oxygen at 36 weeks corrected gestational age (81). For adult-sized patients, there is new evidence suggesting that HFOV may not confer a mortality advantage over a lung-protective conventional strategy. The multicenter **Oscill**ation for **ARDS** **T**reated **E**arly ("OSCILLATE") trial randomized 548 adults with acute ARDS ($Pao_2/Fio_2 \leq 200$ on standardized ventilator settings) to receive either conventional ventilation targeting a tidal volume of 6 mL/kg predicted body weight and plateau pressure ≤ 35 cm H_2O, or HFOV using a "maximally protective" strategy emphasizing alveolar recruitment and oscillating at the highest possible frequency that would allow maintenance of an arterial pH > 7.25 (82). This trial was terminated before reaching its goal of recruiting 1200 patients, after a planned interim analysis revealed that the HFOV group had an in-hospital mortality rate of 47% compared to 35% for the conventional ventilation group (RR for mortality with HFOV, 1.33; 95% CI, 1.09–1.64; $p = 0.005$). Whether or not these data provide "definitive" information regarding the relative benefits and potential harms of HFOV, they could be pointing toward the possibility that HFOV may be a technique better suited for patients with diffuse alveolar disease that is coupled with increased chest wall compliance—conditions that commonly coexist in infants and young children with ALI/ARDS. Developing additional insights into this question would likely depend on future research that is designed to evaluate therapies in ALI/ARDS subpopulations defined according to their lung mechanics.

Fluid Management

When managing ALI and ARDS, clinicians often face a dilemma regarding how best to support hemodynamics without potentiating alveolar fluid accumulation and ongoing pulmonary dysfunction. Decades ago, laboratory evidence from large animal models of ALI indicated that lower cardiac filling pressures and intravascular pressures could limit extravascular lung water accumulation without impairing tissue oxygenation. Case series from the 1970s through the early 1990s also identified a relationship between fluid-restrictive management strategies and improved pulmonary compliance, as well as actual improvements in survival. Recent laboratory evidence offers new insights into the mechanism behind this observation, by suggesting that hydrostatic pressure elevations in postcapillary pulmonary venules may in fact be capable of triggering (or exacerbating) the inflammatory response. Using fluorescence imaging of an isolated blood-perfused rat lung, Ichimura et al. (83) observed that 10 cm H_2O increases in hydrostatic pressure, sustained for 10 minutes, produced definite margination of rhodamine-labeled leucocytes. This phenomenon appeared to be mediated by P-selectin, a leucocyte attachment receptor expressed on the surface of activated endothelial cells and activated platelets (83).

Contemporary lung-protective strategies of mechanical ventilation that have recently proven to reduce mortality in ALI and ARDS (65) often call for high levels of PEEP to stabilize alveolar volume, and intravascular volume supplementation may be necessary in this context to optimize $\dot{V}/\dot{Q}$ relations and improve overall cardiac output. With this in mind, the ARDSnet designed a multicentered RCT to evaluate the effects of various fluid management protocols on outcomes in ALI and ARDS using a contemporary "open-lung," low tidal volume strategy. This trial randomized 1000 intubated adults with evidence of ALI or ARDS for <48 hours to receive either conservative or liberal administration of IV fluids (crystalloid, colloid, or blood), with hemodynamic monitoring by pulmonary artery catheter or central venous catheter, according to a two-by-two factorial design (84). The protocol called for frequent hemodynamic assessment, with administration of a specified amount of fluid, furosemide, dobutamine, or a vasopressor, according to cardiac filling pressures, urine output, mean arterial blood pressure, and cardiac index or clinical perfusion. Patients in the liberal treatment arm received therapies targeting higher filling pressures (central venous pressure [CVP] of 10–14 mm Hg or pulmonary artery occlusion pressure of 14–18 mm Hg). Those in the conservative arm were assigned to receive therapies targeting lower filling pressures (CVP <4 mm Hg or pulmonary artery occlusion pressure of <8 mm Hg). In the final analysis, the investigators reported no interaction between the assigned fluid strategy and the assigned catheter. Mortality (the primary outcome) was similar between the conservative group (25.5%) and the liberal group (28.4%; $p = 0.30$). However, review of the secondary outcome measures revealed that the conservative strategy was associated with an improvement in oxygenation index and a significant increase in ventilator-free days during the first 28 days of therapy (14.6 ± 0.5 vs. 12.1 ± 0.5; $p < 0.001$), although it did not seem to increase the incidence of renal failure or need for dialysis (84). Interestingly, the "liberal" fluid management strategy produced cumulative fluid balances in study subjects that are comparable to both pre-study baseline cardiac filling pressures and published data reflecting "best practice" almost 20 years earlier (84). It is important to emphasize that the results of this study are relevant to patient management during the "maintenance" phase of therapy—after adequate initial resuscitation. Patients entered this study after hemodynamic variables were "optimized" (CVP 11.9 ± 0.3 and cardiac index 4.2 ± 0.1 L/min/m² in the conservative group; CVP 12.2 ± 0.3 and cardiac index 4.3 ± 0.1 L/min/m² in the liberal group), and patients with renal failure were excluded.

Adjuvant Therapies in ALI and ARDS

Prone Positioning

Because alveolar consolidation occurs along the gravitational axis in ALI and ARDS and because pulmonary blood flow is distributed preferentially to dorsal lung regions, it is logical to speculate that ventilation–perfusion relationships in the mechanically ventilated injured lung can be improved by manipulating body position. Animal models demonstrating attenuation of lung injury by prone positioning offer support for this expectation (60,85). Specifically, one could also imagine that placing a patient prone might reduce chest wall compliance, thus transmitting airway pressure to the alveoli more efficiently, stabilizing alveolar volume, and distributing stress and strain forces over a larger portion of previously nonaerated lung units. Large animal experiments have confirmed that prone positioning improves oxygenation and $\dot{V}/\dot{Q}$ matching, allows for the generation of transpulmonary pressure sufficient to open previously consolidated areas, and actually attenuates ventilator-associated lung injury (60,85,86). Prone positioning was first offered to adults with ALI/ARDS as part of a multicentered RCT published in 2001 (87). In this study, patients randomized to the intervention arm received an average of 7 hours of prone positioning per day. All patients were managed using an average tidal volume of ~10 cc/kg based on predicted body weight. The majority showed an increase in PaO_2/FiO_2 of at least 10, with greatest effect occurring during the first hour prone. Interestingly, responders also manifested a favorable change in $PaCO_2$. Nonetheless, mortality at the end of the 10-day period was comparable [prone, 21.1%, vs. supine, 25%; relative risk, 0.84; 95%,CI 0.56–1.27] (87). The investigators' post hoc analysis revealed several intriguing findings. First, patients in the lowest PaO_2/FiO_2 quartile and highest simplified acute physiology score (SAPS) II quartile saw a significant mortality benefit from prone positioning. Second, the subgroup of patients exposed to tidal volumes >12 cc/kg predicted body weight saw a particularly dramatic mortality benefit from prone positioning, as compared to the cohort randomized to supine positioning (18.2% vs. 41%; relative risk of death, 0.44; 95% CI, 0.2–1.0). In follow-up, these investigators performed another multicentered RCT, limiting enrollment to adults with moderate (PaO_2/FiO_2 100–200) or severe (PaO_2/FiO_2 <100) ARDS, and increasing the "dose" of prone positioning to 20 hours per day (88). This trial, too, was unable to demonstrate a significant mortality benefit (28-day mortality 31% in prone group vs. 32.8% in supine group; $p = 0.72$), and prone positioning was associated with significantly higher complication rates. Prone positioning did not alter 28-day mortality for those with moderate ARDS (25.5% in prone group vs. 22.5%; $p = 0.62$) or those with severe ARDS (37.8% in prone group vs. 46.1%; $p = 0.31$).

Twelve years after publication of the first prone positioning trial, Guerin et al. (89) released the results of a major multicentered RCT that was designed to evaluate the effect of early prone positioning on all-cause 28-day mortality among adults with severe ARDS. Taking an approach informed by the outcomes of preceding trials, the investigators designed a protocol to randomize 466 adults who had been intubated <36 hours and who demonstrated a PaO_2/FiO_2 ≤150 on standardized ventilator settings to receive either prone or supine (i.e., semirecumbent) positioning. In both

arms of the trial, patients were mechanically ventilated in a manner that targeted a tidal volume of 6 mL/kg predicted body weight, plateau pressure ≤30 cm H_2O, PaO_2 55–80 torr (guided by prespecified combinations of PEEP and FiO_2), and arterial pH 7.20–7.45. Importantly, all patients were recruited from 27 ICUs with extensive experience in the use of prone positioning, and no patient officially entered the trial until investigators confirmed that each eligible patient continued to meet oxygenation criteria after 12–24 hours of mechanical ventilation. This feature resulted in the exclusion of patients whose oxygenation parameters improved very early in their course. Prone positioning was initiated within 1 hour of randomization, and continued for at least 16 consecutive hours per session. The study protocol is particularly notable for incorporating numerous evidence-based "best practices" that had emerged over the preceding 15 years, including "low stretch" ventilation (65), goal-directed sedation management (90), and endorsement of neuromuscular blockade administration during the first 48 hours of patient management (91). The trial proceeded to completion and remarkably, 28-day mortality was 16.0% among patients in the prone group, compared to 32.8% in the supine group ($p < 0.001$). The incidence of adverse events did not differ between the study groups, except the incidence of cardiac arrests was higher in the supine group (31 arrests vs. 16 arrests; $p = 0.02$).

The first group to systematically evaluate prone positioning in infants and children with ALI and ARDS conducted a multicentered trial that randomized patients to receive 20 hours of prone positioning each day during the acute phase of illness for a maximum of 7 days (13). Customized cushions were used to stabilize the most compliant portion of the chest wall during prone positioning. This study protocolized almost every aspect of supportive care, including delivery of lung-protective mechanical ventilation as well as explicit algorithms to guide sedation, hemodynamic management, nutrition, and skin care. The vast majority (>80%) of the patients enrolled in each study arm had direct pulmonary injury as the etiology of ALI or ARDS. In the end, this trial was stopped according to predetermined futility criteria, after enrolling 102 of an expected 180 patients. The investigators reported a very low mortality rate of 8% in each arm of the study. Despite favorable changes in PaO_2/FiO_2 and oxygenation index among patients who were randomized to use of the prone position, no difference in the number of ventilator-free days between the prone group and the supine group was observed (mean difference, −0.2 days; 95% CI, −3.6 to 3.2 days; $p = 0.91$) (13).

In the interest of future clinical trial development, perhaps it is useful to speculate about why such a thoughtfully designed clinical trial was unable to demonstrate an outcome benefit. First, while the strikingly low mortality rate in the control arm may have made it particularly difficult for the investigators to demonstrate an outcome benefit from prone positioning, it also suggests that the protocols guiding supportive care in this trial were highly efficacious and may be worthy of incorporation into "standard care" algorithms. A second issue to consider is that prone positioning may still be useful for specific subpopulations of pediatric patients, such as children with increased chest wall compliance from baseline neuromuscular weakness or patients in whom chest wall compliance is increased as a result of pharmacologic neuromuscular blockade. Although existing data do not support the routine use of prone positioning for infants and young children with ALI/ARDS, the strong scientific basis for this intervention may prompt clinicians to use it in individual patients whose specific underlying physiology suggests that their gas exchange efficiency may improve as a result. In such cases, improvements in gas exchange are occasionally substantial enough to allow weaning from potentially injurious inflation pressures and/or fractional inspired oxygen concentrations.

Surfactant

Ten years after ARDS was described, dysfunction of the surfactant system was described in this disease, which helped to explain why its histopathologic features seem so similar to the respiratory distress syndrome associated with neonatal surfactant deficiency. Analysis of BAL fluid from postmortem lung specimens and from adult patients with respiratory failure demonstrated alterations in the lipid-to-protein ratio of endogenous surfactant and an overall increase in surface tension in ARDS, compared to healthy controls (38). Surfactant was thereafter approached as a potential therapy in ARDS, and the first multicentered RCT to evaluate its use in ARDS was published in 1996 (92). The investigators randomized patients with ALI or ARDS (Pao_2/Fio_2 <250), including only those with *indirect* lung injury referable to sepsis. In all, 725 adults received (a) synthetic surfactant (Exosurf, Glaxo-Wellcome), aerosolized for delivery into the inspiratory limb of the ventilator circuit, or (b) 0.45% aerosolized saline placebo for a maximum of 5 days. Both groups showed similar changes in the alveolar–arterial oxygen gradient and Pao_2/Fio_2 throughout the study period, and no difference in survival (the primary outcome measure) was noted between the two groups; 30-day survival in each group was ~60%. A potential explanation for the lack of benefit in this study was the difficulty of delivering aerosolized surfactant to the lower airways in the intubated patient. Subsequent trials evaluating the use of surfactant replacement in ALI and ARDS delivered the drug by intratracheal instillation. One small, open-label study used semisynthetic bovine surfactant (Survanta) (93). Two other larger multicentered trials used either a surfactant containing recombinant surfactant protein C (SP-C) (Venticute) (32) or a porcine surfactant named HL 10, respectively (31). Each demonstrated the feasibility of administering intratracheal surfactant in the adult ALI and ARDS population, and each demonstrated some short-term improvement in oxygenation among patients in the intervention arm. However, none of the three trials demonstrated a survival benefit. In fact, one was terminated after enrolling 300 of the expected 1000 patients, because a planned interim safety analysis suggested a trend toward higher mortality and increased adverse events in the surfactant group (31). In both of the large multicenter trials that evaluated intratracheal surfactant in adult ALI/ARDS patients, post hoc analysis suggested that among patients who received surfactant, those with direct lung injury experienced a pronounced mortality benefit as compared to those with indirect lung injury (31,32). This observation was replicated in a pediatric trial and went on to inform the design of subsequent surfactant trials, as discussed in what follows.

Evidence on the use of surfactant in children comes in large part from a multicentered RCT that compared administration of modified bovine surfactant (Calfactant) with air placebo in 152 infants and children with ALI and ARDS (14). The study was notable for attempting to blind study personnel and clinicians to the treatment and for its inclusion of immunocompromised patients, who are traditionally excluded from such studies. Participating centers agreed to ventilator management guidelines specifying a tidal volume ≤8 cc/kg, PIP ≤40 mm Hg, Fio_2 ≤0.6, and maintaining $Paco_2$ between 40 and 60 torr. Other aspects of patient care apart from the study intervention were not protocolized. The original power calculations called for recruiting 300 patients, but the pace of enrollment was slower than expected and the study closed after enrollment of 152 patients. Despite this, the authors reported

a significant reduction in mortality in the surfactant patients, compared to the placebo patients (19% vs. 36%; $p = 0.03$), as well as significant improvements in oxygenation index. However, it should be emphasized that the risk-adjusted analysis that accounted for the asymmetric randomization of patients with immune compromise eliminated the statistically significant mortality benefit from surfactant (adjusted odds ratio of mortality for placebo compared to surfactant, 2.11; 95% CI, 0.93–4.79; $p = 0.07$). The results suggest a possible benefit of surfactant in this population, but it is not clear if this finding is due to the intrinsic superiority of Calfactant compared to other preparations, or to other issues with the study design. In the Calfactant trial as well, post hoc analysis revealed that patients with direct forms of lung injury experienced a greater mortality benefit than those with indirect forms of injury.

Efforts to identify a population with acute hypoxic respiratory failure (apart from preterm infants) who might benefit from surfactant administration are ongoing. The most recently published surfactant trials show a shift in focus from enrolling patients with documented ALI/ARDS to enrolling critically ill patients with severe direct lung injury who do not necessarily meet all AECC criteria (1). In a large multicenter phase III trial, a group of investigators randomized 419 adult patients with pneumonia, Pao_2/Fio_2 ≤170 mm Hg, and no extrapulmonary source of sepsis to receive usual care plus intratracheal recombinant SP-C–based surfactant or usual care only (94). "Usual care" included lung-protective mechanical ventilation as administered in the experimental arm of the ARDSnet trial (65). This recombinant surfactant trial was not able to demonstrate an outcome benefit (28-day mortality 22.7% in surfactant group vs. 23.8% for usual care alone; $p = 0.26$). In a phase II trial, another group of investigators randomized 165 infants ≤2 years of age with acute hypoxic respiratory failure (sustained Pao_2/Fio_2 ratio ≤300 or Spo_2/Fio_2 ≤250) to receive intratracheal lucinactant or air placebo (95). Lucinactant is a synthetic form of surfactant composed of phospholipids and a 21–amino acid synthetic peptide that simulates the action of surfactant protein B. Importantly, the investigators did not enforce adherence to a ventilator management protocol or a weaning protocol. This trial was not able to demonstrate a benefit from surfactant therapy with regard to its primary efficacy endpoint, the duration of mechanical ventilation (geometric least square means 4.0 days for lucinactant; 4.5 days for placebo; $p < 0.25$).

It is difficult to draw meaningful conclusions from the surfactant trials because they differ so greatly with respect to the study population, surfactant composition, and surfactant dosing regimen. Each of the surfactant preparations studied differs in its protein and phospholipid ingredients, and these differences may translate into distinct clinical effects. It is also important to acknowledge the differences in mechanical ventilation strategy among these studies because both animal and human data indicate that response to exogenous surfactant seems to be diminished in the setting of mechanical ventilation using large tidal volumes, while surfactant function seems to be enhanced when strategies are used that promote alveolar stability throughout the respiratory cycle (96). Despite the evidence for surfactant dysfunction in ALI and ARDS, outcome benefits associated with the use of surfactant in this relatively heterogeneous patient cohort have not come close to those reported in association with its use in surfactant-deficient neonates with the neonatal respiratory distress syndrome. It is logical to speculate that the mechanical ventilation strategy used for ALI and ARDS may confound the effects of exogenous surfactant in these diseases, because such patients generally require mechanical ventilatory support for a longer period of time than do newborn infants with neonatal respiratory distress syndrome. Although the data have yet to identify a clear indication for the use of surfactant in ALI and ARDS, arriving at the "ideal" surfactant dose and composition, as well as the timing of its administration, will ultimately depend on understanding its interaction with the chosen mechanical ventilation strategy.

Corticosteroids

Numerous clinical trials have attempted to establish a role for corticosteroids in modulating the role of the immune response to improve clinical outcomes in patients with ALI and ARDS. Using corticosteroids is appealing for several reasons. First, these agents are understood to limit transudation of plasma across the capillary endothelium. Second, they exert anti-inflammatory effects by downregulating expression of steroid-responsive genes coding for proinflammatory cytokines. Third, they upregulate genes encoding for anti-inflammatory cytokines, such as IL-10 (97). Compelling as these mechanisms appear to clinicians seeking to influence the course of ALI, it has proven quite challenging for investigators to demonstrate conclusively that corticosteroids are ultimately beneficial to patients with ALI/ARDS. Studies that evaluated short courses of high-dose corticosteroids administered early in ARDS were not able to demonstrate an outcome benefit, although the data on the use of corticosteroids in persistent ARDS are thought to be more encouraging. In actuality, the evidence cited by many clinicians to support administration of corticosteroids to patients with persistent ARDS is based on one single-centered trial that included only 24 patients, of whom 16 received methylprednisolone for ARDS with a lung injury score that failed to improve by day 7 of illness (98). The study found that patients in the methylprednisolone group had improved oxygenation and other indices of lung injury and reduced mortality (12% vs. 62%; $p = 0.03$).

In 2006, the ARDSnet investigators published a multi-centered RCT evaluating the use of methylprednisolone versus placebo in 180 patients who continued to meet consensus criteria for ARDS 7–28 days after onset of disease (1). As in the prior study, the methylprednisolone was administered and tapered over several weeks. The mechanical ventilation strategy varied according to year of enrollment, with tidal volumes decreasing over time, in accordance with evidence favoring the use of low tidal volume ventilation that emerged during the 7-year span of the trial. Explicit criteria were used to govern ventilator weaning and subsequent extubation. Overall, the investigators did not find an interaction between time of enrollment, tidal volumes, and outcomes with regard to methylprednisolone administration. Mortality at 60 days (the primary outcome) did not differ between the placebo group (28.6%) and the methylprednisolone group (29.2%; $p = 1.0$), despite the fact that corticosteroids were associated with an improvement in short-term measures, such as oxygenation and respiratory system compliance and shorter duration of vasoactive infusions. Finally, methylprednisolone was not associated with an increase in infectious complications, but the investigators did identify a higher incidence of neuromuscular weakness in the treatment group (99). However, it is important to note that, among patients who entered the study on or after day 14 of ARDS, methylprednisolone was associated with a significant increase in both 60- and 120-day mortality.

Although, a much stronger study than its predecessors in many respects, this most recent corticosteroid trial leaves open a number of questions, including how best to address hyperglycemia and other collateral effects of corticosteroid administration in critically ill patients. The intuitive appeal of leveraging the host immune response to improve outcomes in inflammatory conditions, such as ALI and ARDS, is likely to endure, although the redundancy and complexity of the immune response will make it challenging to develop more precise immunomodulatory interventions. Prospects of future studies to translate corticosteroids or other anti-inflammatory therapies into an outcome benefit in ALI and ARDS will likely depend on developing additional insights into the role of inflammation, anti-inflammation, and recovery programs in the pathogenesis and resolution of lung injury. Moreover, future studies must incorporate the evolving evidence base of "best practices" with regard to mechanical ventilation strategy and metabolic, hemodynamic, and sedation management.

Inhaled Nitric Oxide

Nitric oxide (NO) has been known for some time as the endogenous "endothelium-derived relaxing factor" that couples with the cyclic 3′,5′-monophosphate (cGMP) system to mediate vasodilation by local smooth muscle relaxation and to modify immune function and platelet aggregation. In the lung, NO is produced by the endothelium, airway smooth muscle cells, inflammatory cells, platelets, epithelial cells, and fibroblasts as a product of the conversion of L-arginine to citrulline by the enzyme NO synthase. NO binds readily with hemoglobin, resulting in its own inactivation and the production of nitrosyl-hemoglobin and methemoglobin. NO can also interact with oxygen to form nitrogen dioxide (NO_2), which has been associated with provoking the host inflammatory response in laboratory animals exposed to ambient concentrations as low as 1.5 parts per million (ppm).

Considering that its exceedingly short half-life limits its effects to the immediate local environment, it follows that NO could serve as a selective pulmonary vasodilator if administered exogenously. Clinical trials of inhaled NO (iNO) in persistent pulmonary hypertension of the newborn demonstrated significant improvement in oxygenation and a decrease in the need for extracorporeal membrane oxygenation (ECMO) (100). Subsequently, iNO was investigated for its therapeutic potential in ALI and ARDS, with the goal of reversing pulmonary vasoconstriction, relieving microvascular obstruction by reducing platelet aggregation, improving gas exchange by improving the ratio of ventilation to perfusion in diseased lung units, and potentially reducing neutrophil adhesion and local inflammation. Results were promising in experimental animal models of ARDS (101), but in the clinical arena it has been difficult to demonstrate a benefit from iNO with respect to clinically relevant outcomes in ALI and ARDS.

In 1998, the multicentered Inhaled Nitric Oxide in ARDS Study Group published the results of a prospective RCT to evaluate safety and dose–response relationships in a total of 177 adults with ARDS from causes other than sepsis (102). The study found that iNO delivered in concentrations ranging from 1.25 to 40 ppm was well tolerated. Administration of iNO was associated with early but nonsustained increases in PaO_2 and transient decreases in oxygenation index. These short-term physiologic improvements did not translate to a measurable difference in mortality between the two groups. A few years later, the same group of investigators published a follow-up multicentered, blinded, RCT that evaluated the use of low dose iNO (5 ppm) in nonseptic adults with ALI and ARDS (PaO_2/FIO_2 ≤250) (103). Subgroup analysis in the former study had indicated that this dose was associated with an increase in ventilator-free days and decreased short-term mortality. As in their prior study, the investigators suggested guidelines for mechanical ventilation that emphasized limiting peak inspiratory pressures and titrating PEEP to optimize pulmonary compliance and reduce FIO_2, but no specific supportive care protocols were included. The study found that, despite association with transient increases in PaO_2, iNO at 5 ppm did not increase the number of days during which patients were alive and free of mechanical ventilation (mean difference, −0.1 day; 95% CI, −2.0 to 1.9 days; $p = 0.97$).

Data on the use of iNO in pediatric ALI/ARDS are for the most part limited to one multicentered RCT that randomized 108 children (mean PaO_2/FIO_2 84 ± 33 in control arm; 78 ± 30 in intervention arm) to treatment with mechanical ventilation alone or in combination with iNO at 10 ppm over at least 72 hours (104). An "open-lung" strategy of mechanical ventilation was used, and the study protocol allowed for permissive hypercapnia. Patients were allowed to exit the study if they met predetermined treatment failure criteria. This feature did not allow the study to identify a mortality benefit from iNO therapy. This study also showed acute but nonsustained improvements in oxygenation associated with iNO, and the number of treatment failures did not differ between study groups. Improvement in oxygenation was more prevalent and more sustained in children with an oxygenation index >25 at enrollment. In 2012, a systematic review and meta-analysis summarized the evidence from 3 pediatric and 11 adult trials evaluating iNO as a supplemental therapy for children and adults with ALI/ARDS (105). Included trials enrolled a total of 1303 patients. The criteria used to identify ALI/ARDS cases varied among the trials, as did the supportive care strategies. The meta-analysis found no significant mortality benefit from iNO (combined longest follow-up mortality 40.2% among iNO patients vs. 38.6% among control patients; RR 1.06 [95% CI, 0.93–1.22; $I^2 = 0\%$]).

In summary, the data do not support routinely offering iNO to nonseptic patients with ALI and ARDS, but of course, some individuals suspected of having particularly reactive pulmonary vasculature may yet benefit from this therapy. In cases in which the clinician elects to use iNO as adjuvant therapy in ALI and ARDS, its dose–response behavior should be considered. After a few days of exposure to iNO at a constant dose, ARDS patients appear to become more sensitive to its effects. Using a randomized, controlled study protocol, Gerlach et al. (106) demonstrated that among ARDS patients inhaling NO over several days, the improvement in PaO_2/FIO_2 that they demonstrate upon initial exposure to 10 ppm of iNO can be achieved using as little as 1 ppm after 96 hours of iNO therapy. In fact, several days of ongoing exposure to 10 ppm caused the PaO_2/FIO_2 to fall in some patients, whereas a lower iNO dose, which once had no effect in those individuals, was capable of producing a favorable change in oxygenation several days into therapy. Clinicians should also consider potential strategies for optimizing iNO delivery to the alveoli. Because existing clinical trials do not incorporate specific protocols for mechanical ventilation, one can speculate that the collective results cannot control for a potential interaction between the effect of iNO and the ventilation strategy. Post hoc analysis of the original iNO study data (discussed earlier) reported that delivering iNO in combination with HFOV appeared to produce greater improvement in oxygenation than either therapy alone (107). These findings suggest that ventilation strategies that incorporate sustained alveolar recruitment may be more likely to potentiate any favorable effect of iNO.

Activated Protein C

Much evidence has accumulated over the past 15 years that has helped to elucidate the complex relationship between the inflammatory response and the coagulation system. We now know that the two systems interact to alter the hemostatic balance in inflammatory states. APC is a naturally occurring anticoagulant that reduces the tendency toward thrombosis by inhibiting coagulation factors Va and VIIIa, which decreases thrombin formation (49). It is also capable of downregulating production of proinflammatory cytokines, such as IL-6, and inhibiting neutrophil chemotaxis (53,54). Protein C activation has long been known to take place through the actions of the thrombin–thrombomodulin complex and the protein

C receptor (EPCR), both located on the surface of vascular endothelial cells. This process is impaired during the systemic inflammatory response, owing, in part, to widespread endothelial injury.

APC was first approached as a potential therapy for sepsis. One large, multicentered RCT was able to show a significant mortality benefit from the administration of recombinant APC to adults with severe sepsis, a portion of whom also met criteria for ARDS (108). The trial actually ended before completing its enrollment goals, when a planned interim analysis showed a compelling reduction in mortality among patients in the experimental arm. This outcome suggested therapeutic potential in manipulating the systemic hemostatic balance in the context of inflammatory disease, although the mortality benefit from APC was confined to a subgroup of the most gravely ill patients. Unfortunately, other trials conducted in follow-up to the first APC trial were not able to replicate its promising findings in patients with severe sepsis (109–111). One of them was terminated early for meeting futility criteria (109). Moreover, at least two of the follow-up APC trials, including one pediatric trial, reported troubling increases in serious central nervous system bleeding events among patients randomized to the intervention arm (110,111).

Evidence supporting a role for APC in the mitigation of both local (alveolar) and systemic coagulation and fibrin deposition in ALI/ARDS (34,50) makes a compelling case for designing a clinical trial examining whether APC might be a beneficial therapy for ALI. A key development during the last 10 years has been the discovery that protein C is likely activated on the surface of alveolar epithelial cells, and not just vascular endothelial cells (50,52). Interpreting the adult APC trials in light of this information raises the possibility that APC exerts important local effects, rather than generalized systemic effects in patients with severe sepsis, and one such benefit includes modulation of fibrin turnover in the lung (49).

A phase II, multicenter randomized clinical trial of APC in adults with ALI and ARDS was published in 2008 (112). The trial randomized 75 critically ill adults with ALI to receive a 96-hour infusion of either APC or placebo in addition to usual supportive care, including lung-protective, low tidal volume ventilation (65). Although the trial demonstrated significantly increased levels of APC in plasma among patients who received the drug, the trial was stopped early when a planned interim analysis revealed no difference between study groups in the number of ventilator-free days (median, 19 days in each group; 95% CI, −3 to 4 days; $p = 0.78$). However attractive the protein C pathway appears as a therapeutic target for conditions characterized by a proinflammatory/ procoagulant host response, novel approaches will be needed in the future. At this point, it appears that the APC chapter may have closed with the withdrawal of recombinant human APC from the market in 2011.

Modifying Alveolar Fluid Clearance

Laboratory and clinical evidence has demonstrated at least short-term benefits from limiting fluid replacement and accumulation in order to potentiate improvement in pulmonary compliance in ALI and ARDS (84,113). Studies that related impairment of alveolar fluid clearance to increased mortality in ALI and ARDS suggest that attention to this aspect of care in these conditions should, in theory, offer the promise of reduced mortality. However, the potential for restrictive fluid strategies to translate into an overall clinical outcome benefit may be limited by the possibility of contributing to the development of hypoperfusion and organ dysfunction. Since the local cellular mechanisms of alveolar fluid accumulation and clearance in lung injury have been elucidated, these pathways have attracted interest as potential therapeutic targets with less apparent risk of provoking unwanted systemic effects. As described earlier, airway epithelial ion and fluid transport is reduced by alveolar hypoxia, and recent data indicate that this phenomenon can be reversed by reoxygenation, as well as through stimulation of $\beta1$ and $\beta2$ adrenergic receptors found on alveolar epithelial cells (43). For instance, alveolar fluid clearance appears to be stimulated by β-receptor agonists administered IV or instilled directly into the alveolar space (41). The β-agonist–mediated increase in alveolar fluid clearance is reversible by amiloride, suggesting that β-agonists are upregulating transepithelial sodium transport (41). It appears that the adrenergically mediated increase in sodium flux is triggered by intracellular movement of chloride through the cystic fibrosis transmembrane regulator (CFTR) located on the apical surface of alveolar type II cells (114–116). In fact, it has been demonstrated in a small animal model of lung injury that exposing the alveoli of hypoxic animals to terbutaline at a dose previously demonstrated to provide therapeutic alveolar fluid concentrations in critically ill humans quickly reversed the hypoxia-related decrease in alveolar fluid clearance (68). In addition, β-agonists are suspected of having other potentially favorable effects, such as inhibiting endotoxin-induced proinflammatory cytokine release, endotoxin-related coagulation, and proinflammatory neutrophil activity (117,118). Attempts to use β-agonists in patients with ALI began with small preclinical experiments and a single-centered placebo-controlled phase II trial of intravenous salbutamol (albuterol) (119,120). These studies demonstrated a reduction in extravascular lung water in the intervention group, attributed to accelerated alveolar fluid clearance. In follow-up, two multicentered, randomized trials were conceived to evaluate the effects of $\beta2$ agonists on clinical outcomes of adults with ALI/ARDS. The first of these was conducted by the ARDSnet investigators (17). This trial randomized 282 mechanically ventilated adults with ALI to receive either aerosolized albuterol or saline placebo every 4 hours for a maximum of 10 days. Mechanical ventilation and hemodynamic management were governed by modified versions of previously published lung-protective and fluid-conservative protocols (65,84). Although patients in the experimental arm achieved plasma albuterol levels that should have been sufficient to enhance alveolar fluid clearance, they did not differ significantly from patients in the control arm with regard to the primary outcome measure (ventilator-free days: 14.4 days in albuterol group and 16.6 days in placebo group; 95% CI, −4.7 to 0.3 days; $p = 0.087$). This trial was terminated before completing enrollment of an expected 1000 patients, for meeting predefined futility criteria at a planned interim analysis. The second of the multicentered $\beta2$ agonist trials was a pragmatic trial that randomized 324 mechanically ventilated adults with ARDS to receive an infusion of either IV salbutamol or normal saline placebo for a maximum of 7 days (121). Apart from the intervention, no aspect of supportive care was protocolized. This trial was stopped before completing the target enrollment of 1334 patients, when a planned interim analysis revealed that patients who received salbutamol had a higher mortality rate than those who received placebo (28-day mortality 34% vs. 23%; risk ratio, 1.47; 95% CI, 1.03–2.08; $p = 0.02$). Tachycardia, arrhythmias, and lactic acidosis were common enough among patients in the salbutamol arm that the study drug infusion was discontinued more often among salbutamol patients than placebo patients. Together these two trials illustrate the difficulties of navigating the competing challenges of delivering $\beta2$ agonist agents to injured alveoli while avoiding systemic toxicity. Even if $\beta2$ agonists could be delivered reliably to injured alveoli, the alveolar epithelium in some lung units may be so denuded as to be unable to respond to them (122,123). Ultimately the outcomes from these trials raise questions as to whether the experimental models in which $\beta2$ agonists were successful in

accelerating alveolar fluid clearance are somehow not entirely reflective of the complex pathophysiology seen critically ill ALI/ARDS patients.

Nutritional Support in ALI and ARDS

Much attention has been given to the ideal method of delivering nutrition to critically ill patients, and over the past several years, a number of reports support the concept that enteral, rather than parenteral, nutrition can preserve functional integrity of the gastrointestinal mucosal barrier and decrease the potential for intestinal bacterial translocation and systemic infection. Moreover, at least one study has shown that providing enteral nutrition early in the ICU course can potentially reduce mortality and duration of hospital stay in patients with ARDS (124). Nonetheless, a substantial amount of practice variation exists with regard to timing, volume, and composition of enteral feeding in critically ill patients, and no clear consensus guidelines exist to guide clinician practice in this area. A recent multicentered, randomized trial examined whether mechanically ventilated patients with ALI would benefit more from receiving low volume enteral feedings as compared to full volume enteral feedings for the first 6 days of supportive care (18). This trial originally had a factorial design, as it originally intended to evaluate (a) full versus trophic enteral feedings and (b) omega-3 enriched feedings versus feedings containing an isocaloric control supplement. The omega-3 enrichment was later dropped from the factorial design, and is discussed later in this section. The trial enrolled 1000 adult ALI patients whose care teams were ready to initiate enteral feedings within 72 hours of intubation. Mechanical ventilation and hemodynamic management were governed by modified versions of previously published lung-protective and fluid-conservative protocols (65,84), and strict glucose control was maintained using insulin administration protocols. This trial was unable to demonstrate a benefit of trophic enteral feedings relative to full enteral feedings, with respect to the primary outcome measure (ventilator-free days: 14.9 days vs. 15.0 days; 95% CI, −1.4 to 1.2 days; $p = 0.89$).

There is evidence supporting a critical role for fatty acid metabolism in the inflammatory cascade. Specifically, linoleic and α-linolenic acid are essential fatty acids that are converted after ingestion to cell membrane–associated lipids, such as arachidonic acid, eicosapentaenoic acid (EPA), and docosahexaenoic acid (DHA), which possess a central role in host immunity. In inflammation, the activity of phospholipases release membrane lipid, and the breakdown products of these compounds participate in the potentiation of the host immune response (**Fig. 49.14**). For example, lipoxygenases and cyclooxygenases acting on the arachidonic acid pathway release leukotrienes, prostaglandins, and thromboxanes, while metabolism of other membrane lipids, such as EPA and DHA, release far less active compounds, and the metabolic pathways that lead to their release seem to be inhibited by downregulation of required enzyme systems (125). The central role of the arachidonic acid pathway in inflammation results from the ubiquity of its parent compound, linoleic acid, in the human diet, leading to its over-representation as a cell membrane constituent relative to compounds in the α-linolenic acid family (126). Not surprisingly, increases in arachidonic acid metabolites have been documented in ALI and ARDS; leukotrienes, prostaglandins, and thromboxanes have been identified in plasma, urine, and BAL fluid and are believed to be accountable for many undesired collateral effects of the host immune response, such as vasoconstriction, platelet aggregation, and increased airways resistance. Administration of arachidonic acid precursors to patients with ALI and ARDS seems to increase thromboxane A_2 production, while inhibiting cyclooxygenase activity seems

788   Section I: Respiratory Disease

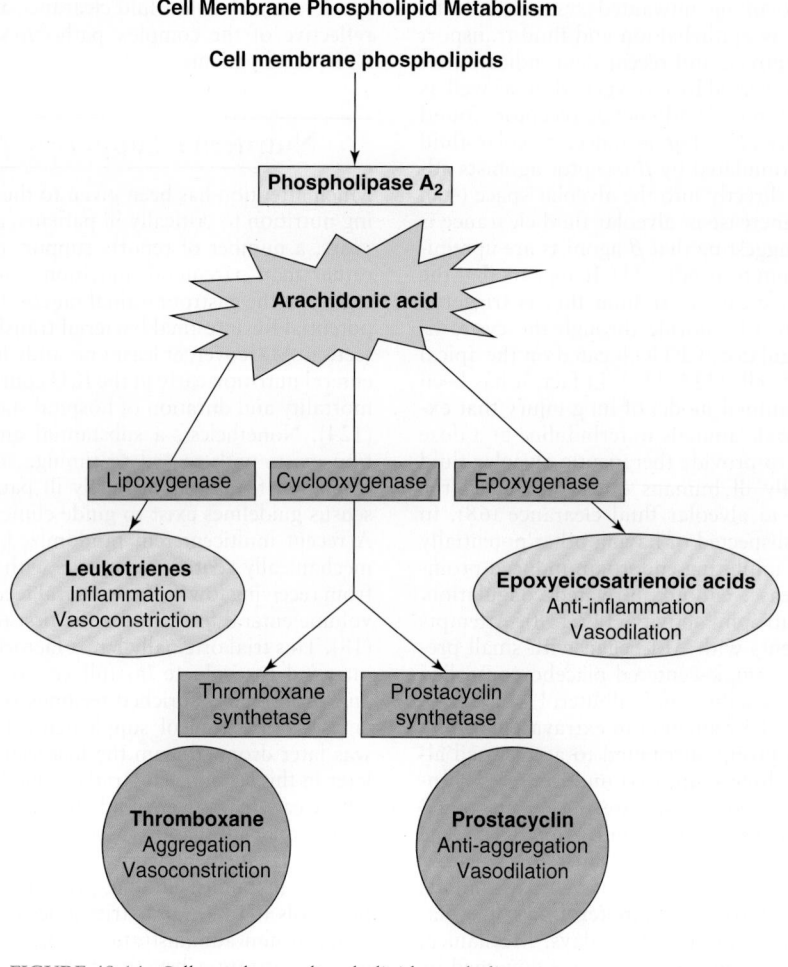

Cell Membrane Phospholipid Metabolism

Cell membrane phospholipids

Phospholipase A₂

Arachidonic acid

Lipoxygenase   Cyclooxygenase   Epoxygenase

Leukotrienes
Inflammation
Vasoconstriction

Epoxyeicosatrienoic acids
Anti-inflammation
Vasodilation

Thromboxane
synthetase

Prostacyclin
synthetase

Thromboxane
Aggregation
Vasoconstriction

Prostacyclin
Anti-aggregation
Vasodilation

FIGURE 49.14. Cell membrane phospholipid metabolism.

to improve gas exchange, relieve vasoconstriction, and decrease airways resistance (127,128). Thus, the ultimate constituents of cell membranes reflect the balance of ingested fatty acids, and dietary manipulations can influence the characteristics of the host inflammatory response.

Experience with providing alternative ratios of fatty acids in an attempt to repopulate host cell membranes has demonstrated that feedings enriched with "omega-3" fatty acids, such as EPA and DHA, decrease proinflammatory cytokine concentrations in plasma and BAL fluid in animal models of ALI and ARDS (129). Data in humans include studies of omega-3 fatty acids in populations with chronic inflammatory conditions (130,131) and ALI/ARDS (132,133). Early results indicated that such dietary manipulations are well tolerated and result in favorable short-term improvements in relevant physiologic parameters within days of their administration. One of these early studies was a prospective RCT in 146 ARDS patients that showed an increased EPA-to-AA ratio in plasma and reductions in BAL fluid neutrophil content, intensive care unit stay, development of new organ failures, and duration of mechanical ventilator support among patients receiving enteral feeds supplemented with the omega-3 fatty acid EPA, γ-linolenic acid, and antioxidants (132). Importantly, outcomes for only 98 of the 146 patients could be evaluated, because of incomplete data and protocol violations. These findings set the stage for a follow-up trial conceived by the ARDSnet investigators to evaluate the effect on ALI outcomes of twice daily

supplementation with omega-3 fatty acids EPA and DHA, γ-linolenic acid, and antioxidants (134). The trial used a factorial design to examine the impact of enriched versus unenriched enteral feedings, and early initiation of trophic versus full feedings. After enrolling 272 of an expected 1000 patients, the dietary supplements were dropped from the factorial design when a planned interim analysis revealed that patients who received omega-3 fatty acids, γ-linolenic acid, and antioxidant supplementation had fewer ventilator-free days (14.0 vs. 17.2; $p = 0.02$) than those who received control supplements. One of the more disappointing findings from this trial was that the active dietary supplements dramatically increased plasma EPA-to-AA ratios without altering plasma levels of IL-6, IL-8, or leukotrienes E₄ (a product of arachidonic acid metabolism) and E₅ (a product of EPA and DHA metabolism). Previous work in animal models suggests that the magnitude of the plasma EPA increase should have been enough to influence a change in cell membrane phospholipid constituents (135,136). However, in this trial and the preceding trial (132), it is unclear whether the intervention succeeded in altering membrane composition, because the investigators did not conduct an analysis of participants' membrane fatty acids during the course of the trial. At this time it remains uncertain whether enteral supplementation with less inflammatory fatty acids can reliably produce a shift in cell membrane phospholipid in critically ill ALI/ARDS patients to a degree that would produce a mortality benefit.

Role of Extracorporeal Membrane Oxygenation in Pediatric ALI and ARDS

Existing data indicate that ECMO is an effective therapy for hypoxemia associated with pulmonary hypertension in newborns. In the nearly 40-year history of using ECMO for this purpose, tens of thousands of neonates with diverse etiologies of respiratory failure have been supported with this technology. Data from the Extracorporeal Life Support Organization (ELSO) registry indicate an average overall survival to discharge of 75% in this cohort (137). Looking at annual survival figures over the past 20 years shows a gradual decrease in overall survival from a peak of 86% in 1989, to 67% in 2010 (137). As of 2010, the highest survival rates occur among infants with the meconium aspiration syndrome (97%), and lowest survival is found among infants with congenital diaphragmatic hernia (43%) (138). These temporal trends likely indicate that the neonatal ECMO population demographics are gradually shifting to reflect greater numbers of infants with more complex disease. Outcome trends among children who require ECMO for pediatric respiratory failure appear to show a similar phenomenon. Current ELSO registry data indicate that overall survival for this cohort is 57% (139). At the present time, an increasing proportion of children who receive ECMO for acute respiratory failure have concurrent extrapulmonary organ failures, a circumstance which appears to reduce their prospects for survival (139). Survival figures for pediatric patients with acute respiratory failure are lower than those reported in the neonatal population, perhaps because children who fail "conventional therapy" for ALI and ARDS represent a much more clinically heterogeneous group, with more protracted clinical courses and a higher likelihood of having important comorbidities. Increasingly, pediatric critical care specialists have come to recognize the potential for lung-protective ventilation strategies to limit the development of excess lung injury and cytokine-mediated dysfunction of distant organs. As protective ventilation protocols are more commonly implemented in clinical practice, "conventional therapy" is expected to produce an increasing number of survivors of more and more complex varieties of critical illness, and identifying a role for ECMO in this population is likely to become increasingly difficult. In any case, the best outcomes can be expected from patients with reversible lung injury who are identified as failing conventional therapy before they begin to develop nonpulmonary organ failures. Early recognition of the patient with hypoxic respiratory failure who is destined to fail even the most strategic mode of mechanical ventilation is difficult but necessary to maximize the patient's prospects for survival. A growing amount of data indicate that the trend in oxygenation index, a measurement that characterizes oxygenation as a function of the intensity of ventilatory support, is a reliable indicator of a patient's prospects for responding to a course of mechanical ventilation for severe ALI and ARDS, and serial measures may assist the clinician in identifying patients who may benefit from ECMO, before they transition into a syndrome of irreversible multiorgan dysfunction (16,80).

OUTCOMES IN PEDIATRIC ALI AND ARDS

Recent data indicate that mortality in pediatric ALI and ARDS seems to be decreasing. While retrospective case series published 15–20 years ago documented mortality rates of 50%–75% (140–143), at least one recent and carefully controlled clinical trial has documented a mortality rate of <10% for pediatric ALI/ARDS (12,13). Outcome improvements over the past 15 years extend even to immunocompromised children

with ALI/ARDS, a subgroup that has historically demonstrated particularly high mortality rates. Fifteen years ago, the mortality rate among children with allogeneic hematopoietic stem cell transplants and ALI/ARDS was as high as 70%–80%, while more recent studies are consistently reporting that it has improved to 55%–60% (15,16,143). Although these outcome improvements have accrued in the era of lung-protective ventilation, the data are conflicting as to whether tidal volume reduction or other supportive care advances are responsible for this encouraging trend.

It has long been suspected that death from ALI and ARDS rarely occurs as a result of refractory impairment of gas exchange, but that it more often occurs in association with the development of multiorgan dysfunction. In fact, current outcomes data support the fact that the presence of one or more nonpulmonary organ failures correlates with a six- to eightfold increase in the likelihood of mortality (11,16), which may explain why ECMO has been used as rescue therapy with somewhat limited success in this population. Several potential mechanisms have been proposed by which multiorgan system failure could follow from single organ failure, including disordered systemic thrombosis, and elaboration of proinflammatory cytokines as a result of ALI. Systemic administration of the anticoagulant APC to adults with ALI/ARDS did not impact organ failure–free days in a recent clinical trial (112). However, in animal models and adult humans, investigators have been able to demonstrate that low tidal volume ventilation promotes less proinflammatory cytokine release than a high tidal volume strategy (63,65,144). Thus, one mechanism by which a noninjurious mechanical ventilation strategy impacts ALI/ARDS outcomes may involve its interference with the development of nonpulmonary organ dysfunction.

CONCLUSION AND FUTURE DIRECTIONS

ALI and ARDS can be conceptualized as the combined inflammatory consequences of a variety of potential insults to the lung. Rapid translation of core physiologic principles and laboratory observations to the clinical arena over the past 15 years has produced a number of high-quality trials in which the benefits of targeted therapies and supportive care strategies have been rigorously evaluated. The pediatric intensivist is faced with the challenge of providing supportive therapies that are carefully titrated to limit their potential for inflicting additional injury and exacerbating the host inflammatory response. Although mortality rates in ALI/ARDS seem to be decreasing, it is not clear which specific "advances" are responsible for this finding. Despite significant progress in understanding the pathophysiology of these diseases, attempts to translate novel medical therapies into clinically meaningful outcome benefits have been unsuccessful (Table 49.3). The only interventions that have proven to result in a significant mortality benefit among patients with ARDS are simple variations on a form of therapy that is applicable to all patients with this disease, regardless of etiology; namely, low tidal volume ventilation, and mechanical ventilation in the prone position (65,89). As long as operational definitions for ALI and ARDS remain nonspecific, there may be some value in developing trials to evaluate the impact of standardizing specific supportive care strategies that are otherwise applied in a nonsystematic fashion across the spectrum of pediatric or adult ALI/ARDS patients. As well, there is an emerging evidence base that could make the case for designing clinical trials to evaluate ALI/ARDS prevention strategies for patients requiring extended courses of mechanical ventilation (12,70,145,146). Going forward, it appears that evaluating novel therapies that target specific facets in the pathogenesis of conditions arising from a broad array of potential insults will depend on refining the diagnostic criteria in ways that make them capable of distinguishing clinically relevant subgroups of ARDS patients.

References

1. Bernard GR, Artigas A, Brigham KL, et al. The American-European Consensus Conference on ARDS. Definitions, mechanisms, relevant outcomes, and clinical trial coordination. *Am J Respir Crit Care Med* 1994;149:818–24.

2. Bindl L, Dresbach K, Lentze MJ. Incidence of acute respiratory distress syndrome in German children and adolescents: A population-based study. *Crit Care Med* 2005;33:209–312.

3. Dahlem P, van Aalderen WM, Hamaker ME, et al. Incidence and short-term outcome of acute lung injury in mechanically ventilated children. *Eur Respir J* 2003;22:980–5.

4. Erickson S, Schibler A, Numa A, et al. Acute lung injury in pediatric intensive care in Australia and New Zealand: A prospective, multicenter, observational study. *Pediatr Crit Care Med* 2007; 8:317–23.

5. Kneyber MC, Brouwers AG, Caris JA, et al. Acute respiratory distress syndrome: Is it underrecognized in the pediatric intensive care unit? *Intensive Care Med* 2008;34:751–4.

6. Lopez-Fernandez Y, Azagra AM, de la Oliva P, et al. Pediatric Acute Lung Injury Epidemiology and Natural History Study: Incidence and outcome of the acute respiratory distress syndrome in children. *Crit Care Med* 2012;40:3238–45.

7. Randolph AG. Management of acute lung injury and acute respiratory distress syndrome in children. *Crit Care Med* 2009; 37:2448–54.

8. Rubenfeld GD, Caldwell E, Peabody E, et al. Incidence and outcomes of acute lung injury. *N Engl J Med* 2005;353:1685–93.

9. Zimmerman JJ, Akhtar SR, Caldwell E, et al. Incidence and outcomes of pediatric acute lung injury. *Pediatrics* 2009;124:87–95.

10. Li G, Malinchoc M, Cartin-Ceba R, et al. Eight-year trend of acute respiratory distress syndrome: A population-based study in Olmsted County, Minnesota. *Am J Respir Crit Care Med* 2011;183:59–66.

11. Flori HR, Glidden DV, Rutherford GW, et al. Pediatric acute lung injury: Prospective evaluation of risk factors associated with mortality. *Am J Respir Crit Care Med* 2005;171:995–1001.

12. Randolph AG, Meert KL, O'Neil ME, et al. The feasibility of conducting clinical trials in infants and children with acute respiratory failure. *Am J Respir Crit Care Med* 2003;167: 1334–40.

13. Curley MA, Hibberd PL, Fineman LD, et al. Effect of prone positioning on clinical outcomes in children with acute lung injury: A randomized controlled trial. *JAMA* 2005;294:229–37.

14. Willson DF, Thomas NJ, Markovitz BP, et al. Effect of exogenous surfactant (calfactant) in pediatric acute lung injury: A randomized controlled trial. *JAMA* 2005;293:470–6.

15. Tamburro RF, Barfield RC, Shaffer ML, et al. Changes in outcomes (1996–2004) for pediatric oncology and hematopoietic stem cell transplant patients requiring invasive mechanical ventilation. *Pediatr Crit Care Med* 2008;9:270–7.

16. Trachsel D, McCrindle BW, Nakagawa S, et al. Oxygenation index predicts outcome in children with acute hypoxemic respiratory failure. *Am J Respir Crit Care Med* 2005;172:206–11.

17. Matthay MA, Brower RG, Carson S, et al. Randomized, placebo-controlled clinical trial of an aerosolized beta(2)-agonist for treatment of acute lung injury. *Am J Respir Crit Care Med* 2011;184:561–8.

18. Rice TW, Wheeler AP, Thompson BT, et al. Initial trophic vs full enteral feeding in patients with acute lung injury: The EDEN randomized trial. *JAMA* 2012;307:795–803.

19. Rubenfeld GD, Caldwell E, Granton J, et al. Interobserver variability in applying a radiographic definition for ARDS. *Chest* 1999;116:1347–53.

20. Ranieri VM, Rubenfeld GD, Thompson BT, et al. Acute respiratory distress syndrome: The Berlin Definition. *JAMA* 2012; 307:2526–33.

21. Gao L, Barnes KC. Recent advances in genetic predisposition to clinical acute lung injury. *Am J Physiol Lung Cell Mol Physiol* 2009;296:L713–25.

22. Gong MN, Wei Z, Xu LL, et al. Polymorphism in the surfactant protein-B gene, gender, and the risk of direct pulmonary injury and ARDS. *Chest* 2004;125:203–11.

23. Marshall RP, Webb S, Bellingan GJ, et al. Angiotensin converting enzyme insertion/deletion polymorphism is associated with susceptibility and outcome in acute respiratory distress syndrome. *Am J Respir Crit Care Med* 2002;166:646–50.

24. Ye SQ, Simon BA, Maloney JP, et al. Pre-B-cell colony-enhancing factor as a potential novel biomarker in acute lung injury. *Am J Respir Crit Care Med* 2005;171:361–70.

25. Sznajder JI, Ciechanover A. Personalized medicine: The road ahead. *Am J Respir Crit Care Med* 2012;186:945–7.

26. Mehta NM, Arnold JH. Genetic polymorphisms in acute respiratory distress syndrome: New approach to an old problem. *Crit Care Med* 2005;33:2443–5.

27. Vitali SH, Randolph AG. Assessing the quality of case-control association studies on the genetic basis of sepsis. *Pediatr Crit Care Med* 2005;6:S74–7.

28. Xiao W, Mindrinos MN, Seok J, et al. A genomic storm in critically injured humans. *J Exp Med* 2011;208:2581–90.

29. Gattinoni L, Pelosi P, Suter PM, et al. Acute respiratory distress syndrome caused by pulmonary and extrapulmonary disease. Different syndromes? *Am J Respir Crit Care Med* 1998;158:3–11.

30. Ranieri VM, Brienza N, Santostasi S, et al. Impairment of lung and chest wall mechanics in patients with acute respiratory distress syndrome: Role of abdominal distension. *Am J Respir Crit Care Med* 1997;156:1082–91.

31. Kesecioglu J, Beale R, Stewart TE, et al. Exogenous natural surfactant for treatment of acute lung injury and the acute respiratory distress syndrome. *Am J Respir Crit Care Med* 2009;180:989–94.

32. Spragg RG, Lewis JF, Walmrath HD, et al. Effect of recombinant surfactant protein C-based surfactant on the acute respiratory distress syndrome. *N Engl J Med* 2004;351:884–92.

33. Ware LB, Matthay MA. The acute respiratory distress syndrome. *N Engl J Med* 2000;342:1334–49.

34. Wang L, Bastarache JA, Wickersham N, et al. Novel role of the human alveolar epithelium in regulating intra-alveolar coagulation. *Am J Respir Cell Mol Biol* 2007;36:497–503.

35. Wright JR. Pulmonary surfactant: A front line of lung host defense. *J Clin Invest* 2003;111:1453–5.

36. Wu H, Kuzmenko A, Wan S, et al. Surfactant proteins A and D inhibit the growth of Gram-negative bacteria by increasing membrane permeability. *J Clin Invest* 2003;111:1589–602.

37. Prange HD. Laplace's law and the alveolus: A misconception of anatomy and a misapplication of physics. *Adv Physiol Educ* 2003;27:34–40.

38. Hallman M, Spragg R, Harrell JH, et al. Evidence of lung surfactant abnormality in respiratory failure. Study of bronchoalveolar lavage phospholipids, surface activity, phospholipase activity, and plasma myoinositol. *J Clin Invest* 1982;70:673–83.

39. Mutoh T, Lamm WJ, Embree LJ, et al. Abdominal distension alters regional pleural pressures and chest wall mechanics in pigs in vivo. *J Appl Physiol* 1991;70:2611–8.

40. Matthay MA, Folkesson HG, Clerici C. Lung epithelial fluid transport and the resolution of pulmonary edema. *Physiol Rev* 2002;82:569–600.

41. Folkesson HG, Matthay M. Alveolar Epithelial ion and fluid transport: Recent progress. *Am J Respir Cell Molec Biol* 2006;35(1):10–19.

42. Ware LB, Matthay MA. Clinical practice. Acute pulmonary edema. *N Engl J Med* 2005;353:2788–96.

43. Vivona ML, Matthay M, Chabaud MB, et al. Hypoxia reduces alveolar epithelial sodium and fluid transport in rats: Reversal

by beta-adrenergic agonist treatment. *Am J Respir Cell Mol Biol* 2001;25:554–61.

44. Newman JH. Pulmonary hypertension. *Am J Respir Crit Care Med* 2005;172:1072–7.

45. Glenny RW, Lamm WJ, Albert RK, et al. Gravity is a minor determinant of pulmonary blood flow distribution. *J Appl Physiol* 1991;71:620–9.

46. Hlastala MP, Glenny RW. Vascular structure determines pulmonary blood flow distribution. *News Physiol Sci* 1999;14:182–6.

47. Opitz B, van Laak V, Eitel J, et al. Innate immune recognition in infectious and noninfectious diseases of the lung. *Am J Respir Crit Care Med* 2010;181:1294–309.

48. Zhang Q, Raoof M, Chen Y, et al. Circulating mitochondrial DAMPs cause inflammatory responses to injury. *Nature* 2010;464:104–7.

49. Schultz MJ, Haitsma JJ, Zhang H, et al. Pulmonary coagulopathy as a new target in therapeutic studies of acute lung injury or pneumonia: A review. *Crit Care Med* 2006;34:871–7.

50. Bastarache JA, Wang L, Geiser T, et al. The alveolar epithelium can initiate the extrinsic coagulation cascade through expression of tissue factor. *Thorax* 2007;62:608–16.

51. Bastarache JA, Fremont RD, Kropski JA, et al. Procoagulant alveolar microparticles in the lungs of patients with acute respiratory distress syndrome. *Am J Physiol Lung Cell Mol Physiol* 2009;297:L1035–41.

52. Ware LB, Camerer E, Welty-Wolf K, et al. Bench to bedside: Targeting coagulation and fibrinolysis in acute lung injury. *Am J Physiol Lung Cell Mol Physiol* 2006;291:L307–11.

53. Esmon CT. The anticoagulant and anti-inflammatory roles of the protein C anticoagulant pathway. *J Autoimmun* 2000;15:113–6.

54. Nick JA, Coldren CD, Geraci MW, et al. Recombinant human activated protein C reduces human endotoxin-induced pulmonary inflammation via inhibition of neutrophil chemotaxis. *Blood* 2004;104:3878–85.

55. Dahlem P, Bos AP, Haitsma JJ, et al. Alveolar fibrinolytic capacity suppressed by injurious mechanical ventilation. *Intensive Care Med* 2005;31:724–32.

56. Choi G, Wolthuis EK, Bresser P, et al. Mechanical ventilation with lower tidal volumes and positive end-expiratory pressure prevents alveolar coagulation in patients without lung injury. *Anesthesiology* 2006;105:689–95.

57. Serhan CN, Brain SD, Buckley CD, et al. Resolution of inflammation: State of the art, definitions and terms. *FASEB J* 2007;21:325–32.

58. Shimabukuro DW, Sawa T, Gropper MA. Injury and repair in lung and airways. *Crit Care Med* 2003;31:S524–31.

59. Chapman HA, Li X, Alexander JP, et al. Integrin alpha6beta4 identifies an adult distal lung epithelial population with regenerative potential in mice. *J Clin Invest* 2011;121:2855–62.

60. Broccard AF, Shapiro RS, Schmitz LL, et al. Influence of prone position on the extent and distribution of lung injury in a high tidal volume oleic acid model of acute respiratory distress syndrome. *Crit Care Med* 1997;25:16–27.

61. Desai SR, Wells AU, Rubens MB, et al. Acute respiratory distress syndrome: CT abnormalities at long-term follow-up. *Radiology* 1999;210:29–35.

62. Falke KJ, Pontoppidan H, Kumar A, et al. Ventilation with end-expiratory pressure in acute lung disease. *J Clin Invest* 1972;51:2315–23.

63. Malo J, Ali J, Wood LD. How does positive end-expiratory pressure reduce intrapulmonary shunt in canine pulmonary edema? *J Appl Physiol* 1984;57:1002–10.

64. Gattinoni L, Caironi P, Pelosi P, et al. What has computed tomography taught us about the acute respiratory distress syndrome? *Am J Respir Crit Care Med* 2001;164:1701–11.

65. The Acute Respiratory Distress Syndrome Network. Ventilation with lower tidal volumes as compared with traditional tidal volumes for acute lung injury and the acute respiratory distress syndrome. *N Engl J Med* 2000;342:1301–8.

66. Chu EK, Whitehead T, Slutsky AS. Effects of cyclic opening and closing at low- and high-volume ventilation on bronchoalveolar lavage cytokines. *Crit Care Med* 2004;32:168–74.

67. Ranieri VM, Suter PM, Tortorella C, et al. Effect of mechanical ventilation on inflammatory mediators in patients with acute respiratory distress syndrome: A randomized controlled trial. *JAMA* 1999;282:54–61.

68. Slutsky AS, Tremblay LN. Multiple system organ failure. Is mechanical ventilation a contributing factor? *Am J Respir Crit Care Med* 1998;157:1721–5.

69. Gajic O, Dara SI, Mendez JL, et al. Ventilator-associated lung injury in patients without acute lung injury at the onset of mechanical ventilation. *Crit Care Med* 2004;32:1817–24.

70. Mascia L, Pasero D, Slutsky AS, et al. Effect of a lung protective strategy for organ donors on eligibility and availability of lungs for transplantation: A randomized controlled trial. *JAMA* 2010;304:2620–7.

71. Gattinoni L, Carlesso E, Cadringher P, et al. Physical and biological triggers of ventilator-induced lung injury and its prevention. *Eur Respir J* 2003;47(suppl):15s–25s.

72. Mead J, Takishima T, Leith D. Stress distribution in lungs: A model of pulmonary elasticity. *J Appl Physiol* 1970;28:596–608.

73. Belperio JA, Keane MP, Burdick MD, et al. Critical role for CXCR2 and CXCR2 ligands during the pathogenesis of ventilator-induced lung injury. *J Clin Invest* 2002;110:1703–16.

74. Razinia Z, Makela T, Ylanne J, et al. Filamins in mechanosensing and signaling. *Annu Rev Biophys* 2012;41:227–46.

75. Parsons PE, Eisner MD, Thompson BT, et al. Lower tidal volume ventilation and plasma cytokine markers of inflammation in patients with acute lung injury. *Crit Care Med* 2005;33:1–6; discussion 230–2.

76. Parsons PE, Matthay MA, Ware LB, et al. Elevated plasma levels of soluble TNF receptors are associated with morbidity and mortality in patients with acute lung injury. *Am J Physiol Lung Cell Mol Physiol* 2005;288:L426–31.

77. Meade MO, Cook DJ, Guyatt GH, et al. Ventilation strategy using low tidal volumes, recruitment maneuvers, and high positive end-expiratory pressure for acute lung injury and acute respiratory distress syndrome: A randomized controlled trial. *JAMA* 2008;299:637–45.

78. Mercat A, Richard JC, Vielle B, et al. Positive end-expiratory pressure setting in adults with acute lung injury and acute respiratory distress syndrome: A randomized controlled trial. *JAMA* 2008;299:646–55.

79. Briel M, Meade M, Mercat A, et al. Higher vs lower positive end-expiratory pressure in patients with acute lung injury and acute respiratory distress syndrome: Systematic review and meta-analysis. *JAMA* 2010;303:865–73.

80. Arnold JH, Hanson JH, Toro-Figuero LO, et al. Prospective, randomized comparison of high-frequency oscillatory ventilation and conventional mechanical ventilation in pediatric respiratory failure. *Crit Care Med* 1994;22:1530–9.

81. Courtney SE, Durand DJ, Asselin JM, et al. High-frequency oscillatory ventilation versus conventional mechanical ventilation for very-low-birth-weight infants. *N Engl J Med* 2002;347:643–52.

82. Ferguson ND, Cook DJ, Guyatt GH, et al. High-frequency oscillation in early acute respiratory distress syndrome. *N Engl J Med* 2013;368:795–805.

83. Ichimura H, Parthasarathi K, Issekutz AC, et al. Pressure-induced leukocyte margination in lung postcapillary venules. *Am J Physiol Lung Cell Mol Physiol* 2005;289:L407–12.

84. Wiedemann HP, Wheeler AP, Bernard GR, et al. Comparison of two fluid-management strategies in acute lung injury. *N Engl J Med* 2006;354:2564–75.

85. Broccard A, Shapiro RS, Schmitz LL, et al. Prone positioning attenuates and redistributes ventilator-induced lung injury in dogs. *Crit Care Med* 2000;28:295–303.

86. Lamm WJ, Graham MM, Albert RK. Mechanism by which the prone position improves oxygenation in acute lung injury. *Am J Respir Crit Care Med* 1994;150:184–93.

87. Gattinoni L, Tognoni G, Pesenti A, et al. Effect of prone positioning on the survival of patients with acute respiratory failure. *N Engl J Med* 2001;345:568–73.

88. Taccone P, Pesenti A, Latini R, et al. Prone positioning in patients with moderate and severe acute respiratory distress syndrome: A randomized controlled trial. *JAMA* 2009;302:1977–84.

89. Guerin C, Reignier J, Richard JC, et al. Prone positioning in severe acute respiratory distress syndrome. *N Engl J Med* 2013;368(23):2159–68.

90. Brook AD, Ahrens TS, Schaiff R, et al. Effect of a nursing-implemented sedation protocol on the duration of mechanical ventilation. *Crit Care Med* 1999;27:2609–15.

91. Papazian L, Forel JM, Gacouin A, et al. Neuromuscular blockers in early acute respiratory distress syndrome. *N Engl J Med* 2010;363:1107–16.

92. Anzueto A, Baughman RP, Guntupalli KK, et al.; Exosurf Acute Respiratory Distress Syndrome Sepsis Study Group. Aerosolized surfactant in adults with sepsis-induced acute respiratory distress syndrome. *N Engl J Med* 1996;334:1417–21.

93. Gregory TJ, Steinberg KP, Spragg R, et al. Bovine surfactant therapy for patients with acute respiratory distress syndrome. *Am J Respir Crit Care Med* 1997;155:1309–15.

94. Spragg RG, Taut FJ, Lewis JF, et al. Recombinant surfactant protein C-based surfactant for patients with severe direct lung injury. *Am J Respir Crit Care Med* 2011;183:1055–61.

95. Thomas NJ, Guardia CG, Moya FR, et al. A pilot, randomized, controlled clinical trial of lucinactant, a peptide-containing synthetic surfactant, in infants with acute hypoxemic respiratory failure. *Pediatr Crit Care Med* 2012;13:646–53.

96. van Kaam AH, Haitsma JJ, Dik WA, et al. Response to exogenous surfactant is different during open lung and conventional ventilation. *Crit Care Med* 2004;32:774–80.

97. Rhen T, Cidlowski JA. Antiinflammatory action of glucocorticoids—New mechanisms for old drugs. *N Engl J Med* 2005;353:1711–23.

98. Meduri GU, Headley AS, Golden E, et al. Effect of prolonged methylprednisolone therapy in unresolving acute respiratory distress syndrome: A randomized controlled trial. *JAMA* 1998;280:159–65.

99. Steinberg KP, Hudson LD, Goodman RB, et al. Efficacy and safety of corticosteroids for persistent acute respiratory distress syndrome. *N Engl J Med* 2006;354:1671–84.

100. Roberts JD Jr, Fineman JR, Morin FC III, et al.; The Inhaled Nitric Oxide Study Group. Inhaled nitric oxide and persistent pulmonary hypertension of the newborn. *N Engl J Med* 1997;336:605–10.

101. Fratacci MD, Frostell CG, Chen TY, et al. Inhaled nitric oxide. A selective pulmonary vasodilator of heparin-protamine vasoconstriction in sheep. *Anesthesiology* 1991;75:990–9.

102. Dellinger RP, Zimmerman JL, Taylor RW, et al.; Inhaled Nitric Oxide in ARDS Study Group. Effects of inhaled nitric oxide in patients with acute respiratory distress syndrome: Results of a randomized phase II trial [comment]. *Crit Care Med* 1998;26:15–23.

103. Taylor RW, Zimmerman JL, Dellinger RP, et al. Low-dose inhaled nitric oxide in patients with acute lung injury: A randomized controlled trial. *JAMA* 2004;291:1603–9.

104. Dobyns EL, Cornfield DN, Anas NG, et al. Multicenter randomized controlled trial of the effects of inhaled nitric oxide therapy on gas exchange in children with acute hypoxemic respiratory failure. *J Pediatr* 1999;134:406–12.

105. Afshari A, Brok J, Moller AM, et al. Inhaled nitric oxide for acute respiratory distress syndrome (ARDS) and acute lung injury in children and adults. *Cochrane Database Syst Rev* 2010;(7):CD002787.

106. Gerlach H, Keh D, Semmerow A, et al. Dose-response characteristics during long-term inhalation of nitric oxide in patients with severe acute respiratory distress syndrome: A prospective, randomized, controlled study. *Am J Respir Crit Care Med* 2003;167:1008–15.

107. Dobyns EL, Anas NG, Fortenberry JD, et al. Interactive effects of high-frequency oscillatory ventilation and inhaled nitric oxide in acute hypoxemic respiratory failure in pediatrics. *Crit Care Med* 2002;30:2425–9.

108. Bernard GR, Vincent JL, Laterre PF, et al. Efficacy and safety of recombinant human activated protein C for severe sepsis. *N Engl J Med* 2001;344:699–709.

109. Abraham E, Laterre PF, Garg R, et al. Drotrecogin alfa (activated) for adults with severe sepsis and a low risk of death. *N Engl J Med* 2005;353:1332–41.

110. Nadel S, Goldstein B, Williams MD, et al. Drotrecogin alfa (activated) in children with severe sepsis: A multicentre phase III randomised controlled trial. *Lancet* 2007;369:836–43.

111. Vincent JL, Bernard GR, Beale R, et al. Drotrecogin alfa (activated) treatment in severe sepsis from the global open-label trial ENHANCE: Further evidence for survival and safety and implications for early treatment. *Crit Care Med* 2005;33:2266–77.

112. Liu KD, Levitt J, Zhuo H, et al. Randomized clinical trial of activated protein C for the treatment of acute lung injury. *Am J Respir Crit Care Med* 2008;178:618–23.

113. Long R, Breen PH, Mayers I, et al. Treatment of canine aspiration pneumonitis: Fluid volume reduction vs. fluid volume expansion. *J Appl Physiol* 1988;65:1736–44.

114. Brochiero E, Dagenais A, Prive A, et al. Evidence of a functional CFTR Cl(−) channel in adult alveolar epithelial cells. *Am J Physiol Lung Cell Mol Physiol* 2004;287:L382–92.

115. Matthay MA, Ware LB, Zimmerman GA. The acute respiratory distress syndrome. *J Clin Invest* 2012;122:2731–40.

116. O'Grady SM, Jiang X, Ingbar DH. Cl-channel activation is necessary for stimulation of Na transport in adult alveolar epithelial cells. *Am J Physiol Lung Cell Mol Physiol* 2000;278:L239–44.

117. Maris NA, de Vos AF, Dessing MC, et al. Antiinflammatory effects of salmeterol after inhalation of lipopolysaccharide by healthy volunteers. *Am J Respir Crit Care Med* 2005;172:878–84.

118. Zhang H, Kim YK, Govindarajan A, et al. Effect of adrenoreceptors on endotoxin-induced cytokines and lipid peroxidation in lung explants. *Am J Respir Crit Care Med* 1999;160:1703–10.

119. Matthay MA, Abraham E. Beta-adrenergic agonist therapy as a potential treatment for acute lung injury. *Am J Respir Crit Care Med* 2006;173:254–5.

120. Perkins GD, McAuley DF, Thickett DR, et al. The beta-agonist lung injury trial (BALTI): A randomized placebo-controlled clinical trial. *Am J Respir Crit Care Med* 2006;173:281–7.

121. Gao Smith F, Perkins GD, Gates S, et al. Effect of intravenous beta-2 agonist treatment on clinical outcomes in acute respiratory distress syndrome (BALTI-2): A multicentre, randomised controlled trial. *Lancet* 2012;379:229–35.

122. Frank JA, Pittet JF, Lee H, et al. High tidal volume ventilation induces NOS2 and impairs cAMP-dependent air space fluid clearance. *Am J Physiol Lung Cell Mol Physiol* 2003;284:L791–8.

123. Modelska K, Matthay MA, Brown LA, et al. Inhibition of beta-adrenergic-dependent alveolar epithelial clearance by oxidant mechanisms after hemorrhagic shock. *Am J Physiol* 1999;276:L844–57.

124. Stapleton R, Stainberg D, Rubenfeld G, et al. Early versus delayed enteral feeding in medical ICU patients with acute lung injury. *Proc Amer Thor Soc* 2005;2:A36.

125. Kumar KV, Rao SM, Gayani R, et al. Oxidant stress and essential fatty acids in patients with risk and established ARDS. *Clin Chim Acta* 2000;298:111–20.

126. Simopoulos AP. Omega-3 fatty acids in health and disease and in growth and development. *Am J Clin Nutr* 1991;54:438–63.

127. The ARDS Network. Ketoconazole for early treatment of acute lung injury and acute respiratory distress syndrome: A randomized controlled trial. *JAMA* 2000;283:1995–2002.

128. Bernard GR, Wheeler AP, Russell JA, et al.; The Ibuprofen in Sepsis Study Group. The effects of ibuprofen on the physiology and survival of patients with sepsis. *N Engl J Med* 1997;336:912–8.

129. Endres S, Ghorbani R, Kelley VE, et al. The effect of dietary supplementation with n-3 polyunsaturated fatty acids on the synthesis of interleukin-1 and tumor necrosis factor by mononuclear cells. *N Engl J Med* 1989;320:265–71.

130. MacLean CH, Mojica WA, Newberry SJ, et al. Systematic review of the effects of n-3 fatty acids in inflammatory bowel disease. *Am J Clin Nutr* 2005;82:611–9.

131. Simopoulos AP. Omega-3 fatty acids in inflammation and autoimmune diseases. *J Am Coll Nutr* 2002;21:495–505.

132. Gadek JE, DeMichele SJ, Karlstad MD, et al.; Enteral Nutrition in ARDS Study Group. Effect of enteral feeding with eicosapentaenoic acid, gamma-linolenic acid, and antioxidants in patients with acute respiratory distress syndrome. *Crit Care Med* 1999;27:1409–20.

133. Singer P, Theilla M, Fisher H, et al. Benefit of an enteral diet enriched with eicosapentaenoic acid and gamma-linolenic acid in ventilated patients with acute lung injury. *Crit Care Med* 2006;34:1033–8.

134. Rice TW, Wheeler AP, Thompson BT, et al. Enteral omega-3 fatty acid, gamma-linolenic acid, and antioxidant supplementation in acute lung injury. *JAMA* 2011;306:1574–81.

135. Palombo JD, DeMichele SJ, Lydon E, et al. Cyclic vs continuous enteral feeding with omega-3 and gamma-linolenic fatty acids: Effects on modulation of phospholipid fatty acids in rat lung and liver immune cells. *JPEN J Parenter Enteral Nutr* 1997;21:123–32.

136. Palombo JD, DeMichele SJ, Lydon EE, et al. Rapid modulation of lung and liver macrophage phospholipid fatty acids in endotoxemic rats by continuous enteral feeding with n-3 and gamma-linolenic fatty acids. *Am J Clin Nutr* 1996;63:208–19.

137. Suttner DM, Short BL. Neonatal respiratory ECLS. In: Annich G, Lynch W, MacLaren G, et al., eds. *ECMO: Extracorporeal Cardiopulmonary Support in Critical Care.* 4th ed. Ann Arbor, MI: Extracorporeal Life Support Organization, 2012.

138. Van Meurs K, Hintz S, Sheehan A. ECMO for Neonatal respiratory failure. In: Van Meurs K, Lally K, Peek G, et al., eds. *ECMO: Extracorporeal Cardiopulmonary Support in Critical Care.* 3rd ed. Ann Arbor, MI: Extracorporeal Life Support Organization, 2006:273–306.

139. Zabrocki LA, Brogan TV, Statler KD, et al. Extracorporeal membrane oxygenation for pediatric respiratory failure: Survival and predictors of mortality. *Crit Care Med* 2011;39:364–70.

140. Davis SL, Furman DP, Costarino AT Jr. Adult respiratory distress syndrome in children: Associated disease, clinical course, and predictors of death. *J Pediatr* 1993;123:35–45.

141. DeBruin W, Notterman DA, Magid M, et al. Acute hypoxemic respiratory failure in infants and children: Clinical and pathologic characteristics. *Crit Care Med* 1992;20:1223–34.

142. Timmons OD, Dean JM, Vernon DD. Mortality rates and prognostic variables in children with adult respiratory distress syndrome. *J Pediatr* 1991;119:896–9.

143. Bojko T, Notterman DA, Greenwald BM, et al. Acute hypoxemic respiratory failure in children following bone marrow transplantation: An outcome and pathologic study. *Crit Care Med* 1995;23:755–9.

144. Imai Y, Parodo J, Kajikawa O, et al. Injurious mechanical ventilation and end-organ epithelial cell apoptosis and organ dysfunction in an experimental model of acute respiratory distress syndrome. *JAMA* 2003;289:2104–12.

145. Serpa Neto A, Cardoso SO, Manetta JA, et al. Association between use of lung-protective ventilation with lower tidal volumes and clinical outcomes among patients without acute respiratory distress syndrome: A meta-analysis. *JAMA* 2012;308:1651–9.

146. Spragg RG, Bernard GR, Checkley W, et al. Beyond mortality: Future clinical research in acute lung injury. *Am J Respir Crit Care Med* 2010;181:1121–7.

147. Bersten AD, Edibam C, Hunt T, et al. Incidence and mortality of acute lung injury and the acute respiratory distress syndrome in three Australian States. *Am J Respir Crit Care Med* 2002;165:443–8.

148. Luhr OR, Antonsen K, Karlsson M, et al.; The ARF Study Group. Incidence and mortality after acute respiratory failure and acute respiratory distress syndrome in Sweden, Denmark, and Iceland. *Am J Respir Crit Care Med* 1999;159:1849–61.

149. Altemeier WA, Matute-Bello G, Frevert CW, et al. Mechanical ventilation with moderate tidal volumes synergistically increases lung cytokine response to systemic endotoxin. *Am J Physiol Lung Cell Mol Physiol* 2004;287:L533–42.

150. Thomas NJ, Shaffer ML, Willson DF, et al. Defining acute lung disease in children with the oxygenation saturation index. *Pediatr Crit Care Med* 2010;11:12–7.

151. Young D, Lamb SE, Shah S, et al. High-frequency oscillation for acute respiratory distress syndrome. *N Engl J Med* 2013;368:806–13.

152. Guerin C, Gaillard S, Lemasson S, et al. Effects of systematic prone positioning in hypoxemic acute respiratory failure: A randomized controlled trial. *JAMA* 2004;292:2379–87.

153. Mancebo J, Fernandez R, Blanch L, et al. A multicenter trial of prolonged prone ventilation in severe acute respiratory distress syndrome. *Am J Respir Crit Care Med* 2006;173(11):1233–9.

154. Lacroix J, Hebert PC, Hutchison JS, et al. Transfusion strategies for patients in pediatric intensive care units. *N Engl J Med* 2007;356:1609–19.

155. Forel JM, Roch A, Marin V, et al. Neuromuscular blocking agents decrease inflammatory response in patients presenting with acute respiratory distress syndrome. *Crit Care Med* 2006;34:2749–57.

156. The National Heart Lung, and Blood Institute Acute Respiratory Distress Syndrome (ARDS) Clinical Trials Network. Pulmonary-artery versus central venous catheter to guide treatment of acute lung injury. *N Engl J Med* 2006;354:2213–24.

CHAPTER 50 ■ CHRONIC RESPIRATORY FAILURE

THOMAS G. KEENS, SHEILA S. KUN, AND SALLY L. DAVIDSON WARD

KEY POINTS

1. The respiratory system in children is immature and vulnerable to chronic respiratory failure. With respiratory disorders, ventilatory muscle power and/or central respiratory drive may not be adequate to overcome the respiratory load, resulting in respiratory failure.

2. Chronic respiratory failure requires a different philosophy and strategy to treat optimally. As these children will not wean quickly from mechanically assisted ventilation, their ventilatory needs should be fully supported by the ventilator, and weaning (if possible) requires optimizing the function of the lungs, ventilatory muscles, and central drive.

3. Children with chronic respiratory failure can often be cared for at home. Candidates for home mechanical ventilation (HMV) must have a stable respiratory disorder that does not require frequent changes in ventilator settings.

4. HMV is most commonly provided using positive-pressure ventilation via tracheostomy. However, some children are able to use noninvasive techniques (noninvasive positive-pressure ventilation via mask, negative-pressure ventilation, or diaphragm pacing), which may permit removal of their tracheostomies.

5. Prior to hospital discharge, children using HMV and their families require thorough education, complete equipment including safety monitors, and arrangements for ancillary health care needs and community resources (school).

6. Once at home, children using HMV require ongoing medical care from an interdisciplinary team who can address medical, developmental, psychosocial, and equipment needs.

7. An integrated health delivery system, breaking the barriers of ICU, inpatient, outpatient, and home health services will improve the care of our HMV patients.

Advancements in pediatric critical care medicine have increased survival from catastrophic childhood illnesses and injuries. However, this improved survival has come at a price. Sometimes, children survive, but with chronic illnesses (1–4). Children treated in the PICU for acute respiratory failure may emerge with chronic lung disease. A smaller proportion of survivors develop chronic respiratory failure (CRF), and may require long-term ventilatory support (2,5–7). Many children already had significant chronic disease when they were admitted to the PICU (5). Thus, their reserve was likely already compromised, making it more likely that these patients may develop CRF (5). Rather than being maintained as long-term residents in the PICU, most of these children can now be cared for in the home, even if ventilatory support is required. Home mechanical ventilation (HMV) is often performed with a relatively good quality of life for many children (8–12). However, children requiring ventilatory support for CRF are, by definition, fragile, have little reserve, and face a 20% mortality rate in the first 5 years after discharge (13). This chapter reviews CRF, including what can be done to attempt to wean patients from long-term assisted ventilation in the PICU, and how to care for the child who requires HMV.

The ability to sustain spontaneous ventilation requires adequate mechanisms that control ventilation, ventilatory muscle function, and lung mechanics. Significant dysfunction of any of these three components of the respiratory system may impair a child's ability to breathe spontaneously. Respiratory failure occurs when central respiratory drive and/or ventilatory muscle power are inadequate to overcome the respiratory load (Fig. 50.1). For some children, severe lung disease alone (i.e., acute respiratory distress syndrome [ARDS]) may impose a respiratory load so high that it cannot be overcome by normal ventilatory muscles and central respiratory drive. For others, decreased ventilatory muscle power

(i.e., neuromuscular diseases) and/or central respiratory drive (i.e., central hypoventilation syndromes or pharmacologic central nervous system depression) may be inadequate to overcome even a normal respiratory load. CRF occurs if the cause of this imbalance is not reversible, and chronic ventilatory support will be required. Once the decision has been made to institute long-term mechanical ventilation in an infant or child with a stable or progressive disorder, a disposition plan is required since the child cannot reside indefinitely in a PICU (8–12,14).

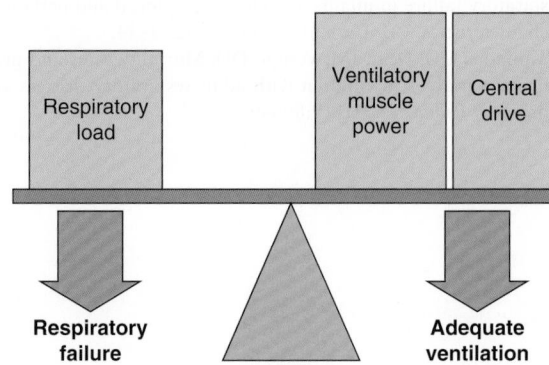

FIGURE 50.1. The respiratory balance. In normal individuals, ventilatory muscle power and central drive are more than adequate to overcome the respiratory load, tipping the balance to the right, which results in adequate ventilation. However, when ventilatory muscle power and/or central drive are decreased and/or the respiratory load is increased, or some combination thereof, ventilatory muscle power and central drive may not be sufficient to overcome the respiratory load. The balance will tip to the left, and respiratory failure will result.

Thus, the approach to managing CRF must be appropriate for home or chronic care facility settings. Chronic ventilatory support in the home is, for many patients, a safe and relatively inexpensive alternative.

The goals of ventilatory support in the home for children with CRF are quite different from the goals of assisted ventilation for children with acute respiratory failure in the PICU (9,15–17). The support at home goals include (a) ensure medical safety of the child, (b) prevent or minimize complications, (c) optimize the child's quality of life, (d) maximize rehabilitative potential, and (e) reintegrate with the family. Medical safety is ensured by attempting to normalize respiratory function. The child's quality of life is optimized by rehabilitation to as normal a lifestyle as possible and by reintegration into the family. To achieve these goals, it is necessary to adopt a different approach from that employed in the care of children with acute respiratory failure.

RESPIRATORY SYSTEM IN CHILDREN

① Neurologic control of breathing must ensure adequate ventilation to meet the metabolic needs of the body during sleep, rest, and exercise. Ventilation varies with the state of the individual. It becomes less adequate during sleep, and it is less responsive to modulation by chemoreceptor input during rapid eye movement (REM) or active sleep. It is not surprising that sleep is the most vulnerable period for the development of inadequate ventilation in disorders of respiratory control (15,17,18). Immaturity of the respiratory control systems in the infant and young child predispose to apnea and hypoventilation. Furthermore, the infant spends ~50% of sleep time in REM sleep (in contrast to 15%–20% spent by the adult), and an infant sleeps for a longer portion of the day. Active sleep is associated with greater variation in respiratory timing and amplitude, resulting in periods of inadequate gas exchange. Thus, CRF always includes inadequate gas exchange during sleep.

The diaphragm must perform the work of breathing. Ventilatory muscles of normal strength and endurance may fatigue in the face of increased respiratory loads (19,20). On the other hand, weak ventilatory muscles may successfully perform the work of breathing when pulmonary mechanics are optimal, yet fail when mechanics worsen, as during respiratory infections (21). The factors that predispose to ventilatory muscle fatigue include hypoxia, hypercapnia, acidosis, malnutrition, hyperinflation, changes in pulmonary mechanics that cause increased work of breathing, and disuse. The infant diaphragm also has

a significantly smaller proportion of fatigue-resistant muscle fibers and is weaker than the diaphragm of older children and adults (22,23). Consequently, the infant is predisposed to ventilatory muscle fatigue. Underlying muscle pathology will further limit ventilatory muscle endurance. Therefore, infants and children are predisposed to respiratory failure compared with adults, because of differences in the control of sleep and breathing, and decreased ventilatory muscle strength and endurance.

ACUTE RESPIRATORY FAILURE

The clinical picture, etiology, pathophysiology, medical management, and ventilator management of acute respiratory failure are discussed in detail in other chapters of this text. However, aspects of CRF can be contrasted with acute respiratory failure as follows. Acute respiratory failure is most commonly seen in children who experience the abrupt onset of a severe respiratory disorder, such as severe pneumonia or ARDS. This is accompanied by an increase in the respiratory load, which exceeds the ability of the child's physiology to continue performing that level of work. The ventilatory muscles fatigue while attempting to exert increased effort for breathing (24,25). Thus, the child breathes inadequately, resulting in hypoxia, hypercapnia, and acidosis. If work of breathing is plotted on the ordinate, the fatigue threshold indicates the highest level of work that a subject can sustain indefinitely without fatigue (**Fig. 50.2**). In adults, this limit for diaphragmatic work is at about 40% of the maximal diaphragm strength, and 60%–70% of combined inspiratory muscle strength (24,25). If the work of breathing that is associated with a respiratory illness remains below the fatigue threshold, a child can continue to breathe spontaneously and acute respiratory failure may not occur. In a typical episode of acute respiratory failure, the work of breathing rapidly exceeds the child's fatigue threshold.

Most children with acute respiratory failure can be weaned from mechanically assisted ventilation when the work of breathing decreases with recovery from the lung disease. Usually, in the PICU, ventilator settings for children with acute respiratory failure are adjusted to provide the minimal level of support necessary to achieve adequate gas exchange. Weaning is performed in such a way that the patient assumes increasing proportions of the work of breathing. As the primary objective in a child with acute respiratory failure is to wean from assisted ventilation, settings are adjusted so that the child expends all available energy as work of breathing, leaving little or no reserve for other activities. However, this strategy is successful only if the underlying cause of respiratory failure is subsiding.

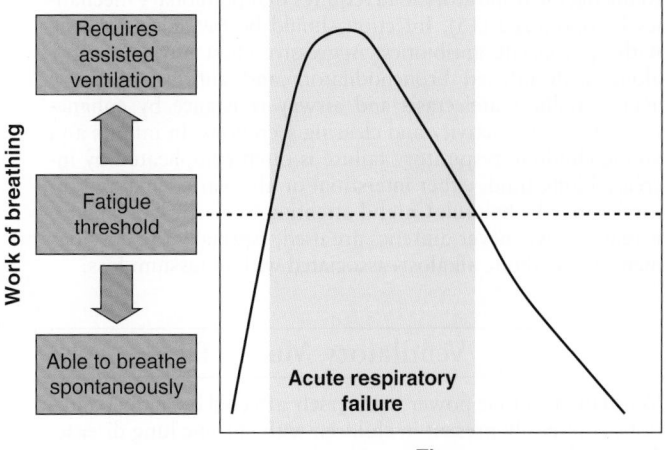

FIGURE 50.2. **Acute respiratory failure.** Work of breathing (Y axis) increases with worsening lung disease until it exceeds the fatigue threshold, at which point, mechanically assisted ventilation is required (shaded area) until the lung disease improves to the point at which work of breathing falls below the fatigue threshold. Then, the child is able to perform the work of breathing required to breathe spontaneously and he/she can be weaned from mechanical ventilation.

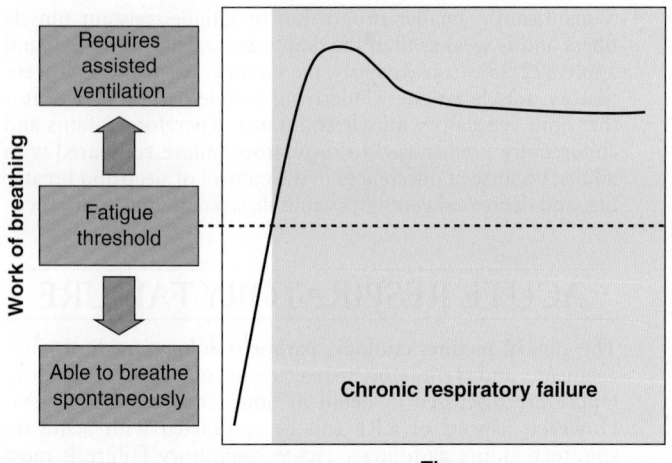

FIGURE 50.3. **Chronic respiratory failure.** Work of breathing (Y axis) increases with worsening lung disease until it exceeds the fatigue threshold. Mechanically assisted ventilation is required at this point (shaded area). However, the lung disease does not improve to the point that work of breathing falls below the fatigue threshold. Thus, the child is not able to perform the work of breathing required to breathe spontaneously and remains ventilator dependent.

❷ CHRONIC RESPIRATORY FAILURE

CRF implies that a chronic, perhaps irreversible, underlying respiratory disorder is causing respiratory insufficiency that results in inadequate ventilation or hypoxia (16). The diagnosis of CRF is traditionally made once repeated attempts to wean from assisted ventilation have failed for at least 1 month in a patient without superimposed acute respiratory disease or a patient who has a diagnosis with no prospect of being weaned from the ventilator, such as high spinal cord injury (16) (**Fig. 50.3**).

For purposes of this discussion, the term "prolonged respiratory failure" will be used for children who are difficult to wean from mechanically assisted ventilation but have not yet satisfied the time criteria for the diagnosis of "CRF," defined as at least 1 month of ventilator dependence. Some patients with prolonged respiratory failure will develop CRF if appropriate therapeutic interventions fail, but others may be able to be weaned from mechanically assisted ventilation. The proper approach to a patient with prolonged respiratory failure must include addressing all barriers to weaning. Keeping the respiratory system balance in mind (**Fig. 50.1**), therapy should be directed toward reducing the respiratory load, improving ventilatory muscle power, and increasing central respiratory drive as much as possible.

Reduce the Respiratory Load

Reducing the respiratory load requires that pulmonary mechanics be optimized (15). Infection should be treated vigorously with appropriate antibiotics. Aggressive chest physiotherapy, along with inhaled bronchodilators and anti-inflammatory agents, reduces atelectasis and airway resistance by enhancing mucociliary activity and clearing secretions. In infants and young children, respiratory failure is often complicated by increased lung fluid, either interstitial or alveolar edema and diuretics may be helpful. Careful attention to electrolyte balance is required whenever diuretics are used, especially the development of metabolic alkalosis associated with potassium loss.

Increase Ventilatory Muscle Power

Ventilatory muscle power is adversely affected by many conditions commonly present in children with chronic lung disease. The work output of the ventilatory muscles is measured as

the generated pleural, airway, or transdiaphragmatic pressures (21). Fatigue of the ventilatory muscles occurs when muscle energy production is hindered (22,24–26). Ventilatory muscles cannot perform work if they cannot produce energy. Hypoxia, hypercapnia, and acidosis all decrease the efficiency of muscle energy production, predisposing the muscle to fatigue. Malnutrition decreases oxidative energy-producing enzymes in muscle. Hyperinflation places the diaphragm at a mechanical disadvantage, so that the same amount of muscle tension develops less pressure. Infants have decreased strength and endurance of the ventilatory muscles compared with adults or older children (22,23). If the child has received assisted ventilation for some time, muscle changes may occur from disuse (26). Thus, even a child who does not have a diagnosis of a neuromuscular disorder may have ventilatory muscle dysfunction or fatigue, contributing to respiratory failure. Bronchopulmonary dysplasia, for example, is a primary lung disease associated with hypoxia, hypercapnia, hyperinflation, malnutrition, and infancy, all of which decrease ventilatory muscle endurance. Thus, therapy should be directed toward adequate oxygenation and ventilation, removal of airway obstruction and hyperinflation, adequate nutrition, and ventilatory muscle training (26). Pharmacologic neuromuscular blockade, sedation, and pain medications also decrease ventilatory muscle function. When possible, these medications should be weaned as tolerated. Attention to the optimization of ventilatory muscle function is an important adjunct to the treatment of any child with prolonged respiratory failure.

The approach to weaning from the ventilator should be designed to improve ventilatory muscle power in an attempt to raise the child's fatigue threshold (**Fig. 50.4**). The desired approach is similar to athletic training of any other skeletal muscle (26). Athletes train for performance by bursts of muscle activity (training stress) followed by rest periods. "Sprint weaning" is analogous to this form of athletic training, and ventilatory muscle training may result. Intermittent mandatory ventilation (IMV) weaning imposes a gradually increasing functional demand on the ventilatory muscles, but it does not provide the alternating stress and rest training pattern. In our experience, some children who have not been weaned from mechanically assisted ventilation by traditional IMV weaning approaches were able to be weaned by sprint weaning, though this may take several weeks.

In a child with prolonged respiratory failure, sprint weaning, or sprinting, is instituted in the following way. Ventilator settings are adjusted to completely meet the child's ventilatory demands by the use of a physiologic ventilator rate for age and the attainment of normal noninvasive monitoring of gas

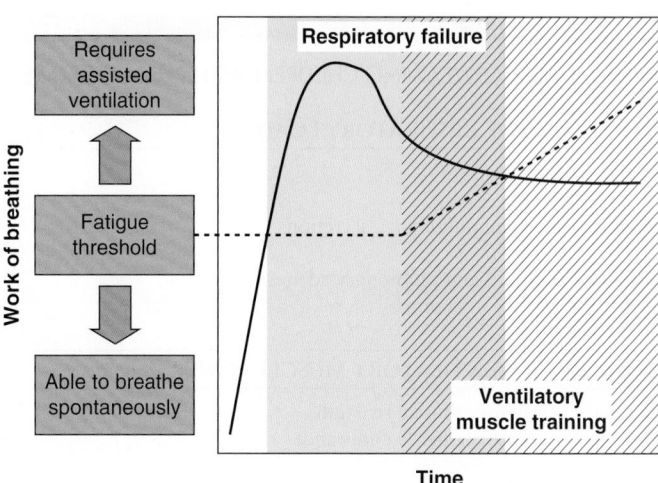

FIGURE 50.4. Ventilatory muscle training. Work of breathing (Y axis) increases with worsening lung disease until is exceeds the fatigue threshold. Mechanically assisted ventilation is required at this point (shaded area). The lung disease does not improve to the point that work of breathing falls below the fatigue threshold. However, ventilatory muscle training may increase the work of breathing that the patient can perform (hatched area), raising the fatigue threshold until it exceeds the work of breathing required. Respiratory failure overlaps ventilatory muscle training until the fatigue threshold exceeds the required work of breathing. Then, the child is able to perform the work of breathing required to breathe spontaneously and can be weaned.

exchange ($SpO_2 \geq 95\%$ and end-tidal PCO_2 [$ETCO_2$] of 30–40 torr). The goal is to provide total ventilatory muscle rest. The patient is then removed from the ventilator for short periods of time during wakefulness approximately two to four times per day. In some cases, these initial sprints may last only 1–2 minutes. The child is carefully monitored noninvasively during sprints to identify hypoxia or hypercapnia, using pulse oximetry and $ETCO_2$ monitoring. Increased supplemental oxygen, above that required on the ventilator, may be required during sprinting. Guidelines for terminating sprints, such as SpO_2 <95% or $ETCO_2$ >45–50 torr, should be provided as written orders. In addition, if the child develops signs of distress such as tachypnea, retractions, diaphoresis, tachycardia, hypoxia, or hypercapnia, the sprint should be stopped. Note that the child with a respiratory control disorder may not exhibit these signs of distress. The length of each sprint is increased daily as tolerated. The physicians should avoid the temptation to increase the sprint length too rapidly, as this often hinders the progress of weaning. Initially, sprinting should be performed only during wakefulness, as ventilatory muscle function and central respiratory drive are more intact during this period than during sleep. Usually a child is weaned off the ventilator completely during wakefulness, before attempting to reduce sleeping ventilatory support. It is important to remember that sprint weaning requires that the child receives complete ventilatory support during rests (27). Because sprint weaning simulates athletic training, better success has been observed with this form of ventilator weaning in prolonged respiratory failure when ventilatory muscle fatigue is thought to be a component. In effect, this technique raises the fatigue threshold, so that a child can perform an increased level of work of breathing, and sustain adequate spontaneous ventilation (26) (Fig. 50.4).

Improve Central Respiratory Drive

Central respiratory drive can be inhibited by metabolic imbalance (15,17,18,28). Chronic metabolic alkalosis, for example, decreases central respiratory drive. Thus, electrolyte balance should be maintained, with careful attention to maintaining serum chloride concentrations >95 mEq/dL and avoiding alkalosis. Chronic hypoxia and/or hypercapnia may cause habituation of chemoreceptors, leading to a decrease in respiratory center stimulation, and decreased central respiratory drive. Although methylxanthines have been used to stimulate drive by some clinicians, Swaminathan et al. (29) demonstrated no effect of theophylline on

ventilatory responses to hypercapnia or hypoxia in normal subjects. Furthermore, children with central hypoventilation syndrome have chemoreceptor dysfunction, which does not respond to pharmacologic stimulation (15,17,18,28). In general, pharmacologic respiratory stimulants have not been shown to be effective in the treatment of prolonged respiratory failure (29).

This three-pronged approach to children with prolonged respiratory failure may result in successful weaning from mechanically assisted ventilation (summarized in **Table 50.1**). However, when children remain ventilator dependent for at least 1 month despite appropriate use of the above techniques and the respiratory load has been reduced, ventilatory muscle power has been improved, and central respiratory drive has been increased as much as possible, the cause of respiratory failure may be irreversible, or weaning the child from assisted ventilation may take several months to years. In either case, the diagnosis of "CRF" is made, and chronic ventilatory support will be required (16).

DECISION TO INITIATE CHRONIC VENTILATORY SUPPORT

The decision to initiate chronic ventilatory support may be made electively or nonelectively (30–32). In the past, most decisions to begin chronic ventilatory support were made nonelectively. Typically, a child with a preexisting respiratory disorder developed acute respiratory failure from a respiratory infection or pneumonia and progression of underlying disease. The child was intubated, and mechanically assisted ventilation was initiated as a life-saving measure. Subsequently, it was not possible to wean the child from mechanical ventilation. Because it is often emotionally difficult to abruptly stop this therapy in an alert child who might experience severe distress without it, the transition to chronic ventilatory support was made. In this setting, the child and family often did not have the opportunity to discuss this therapeutic option in advance. Thus, the child and family were not really given an informed choice about whether or not to initiate chronic ventilatory support (30,32).

Increasingly, the decision to initiate chronic ventilatory support is being made electively to preserve physiologic function and improve the quality of life. Using this decision-making approach, the health care team begins the discussion of options for long-term care, including the varying approaches to chronic ventilatory support, in patients who

TABLE 50.1

APPROACHES TO WEANING CHILDREN WITH PROLONGED RESPIRATORY FAILURE

■ REDUCE THE RESPIRATORY LOAD

Relieve bronchospasm	Aerosolized bronchodilator
	Aerosolized corticosteroids or other anti-inflammatory agents
Remove excessive pulmonary secretions	Chest physiotherapy
	If ventilatory muscle weakness, cough assist device
Reduce lung fluid and pulmonary edema	Diuretics with careful attention to electrolyte balance
Treat pulmonary infections	Antibiotics
	Consider aerosolized antibiotics for chronically colonized patients

■ INCREASE VENTILATORY MUSCLE POWER

Increase ventilatory muscle strength	Eliminate or reduce hyperinflation
Increase ventilatory muscle endurance	Adequate oxygenation
	Avoid hypercapnia
	Avoid acidosis
	Achieve optimal nutrition
	Reduce respiratory load (as above)
Train ventilatory muscles to improve strength and endurance	Sprint weaning

■ IMPROVE CENTRAL RESPIRATORY DRIVE

Avoid hypochloremic alkalosis	Maintain serum $[Cl^-] \geq 95$ mEq/dL
	Avoid alkalosis
Reset chemoreceptors	Ventilate to adequate oxygenation ($Spo_2 \geq 95\%$) and ventilation ($ETCO_2 \leq 40$ torr)
Avoid respiratory depression	Reduce or avoid central nervous system-depressant medications

can be expected to develop CRF (30–32). The most obvious example is the child with a progressive neuromuscular disorder, such as spinal muscular atrophy or muscular dystrophy (33,34). Discussion begins long enough before the anticipated need to allow the child and family to thoroughly evaluate the options, discuss their feelings, and reach a decision. Families need to be informed that a home ventilator is not a guarantee that the child will survive. We found that children receiving HMV via tracheostomy face a 20% mortality rate in the first 5 years after discharge home (13). If the family opts for chronic ventilatory support, then noninvasive ventilatory support is usually initiated first, or a tracheostomy is performed and positive-pressure ventilation (PPV) is started electively before the patient develops major complications of CRF (27,33–35). Since hypoventilation is more severe during sleep than during wakefulness, nocturnal assisted ventilation often prevents the development of pulmonary hypertension and other complications of chronic intermittent hypoxia (35). Nocturnal ventilation allows ventilatory muscle rest and improves endurance for spontaneous breathing while awake; therefore, it is actually associated with an enhanced quality of life (27,35). Further, with this approach, the child and family do have the opportunity to make a truly informed decision about whether or not to initiate chronic ventilatory support (30,32). Preemptive initiation of assisted ventilation prior to sleep related alveolar hypoventilation has not been shown to be helpful in Duchene muscular dystrophy, and is not indicated.

Consensus has not been reached regarding the length of time that a child can remain intubated before airway damage from prolonged intubation occurs. Therefore, an "outside limit" has not been reached on the length of time intubation is permitted before performing a tracheostomy. In practice, if a child requires PPV via tracheostomy, a tracheostomy should be surgically placed when the diagnosis of CRF is made.

CANDIDATES FOR HOME MECHANICAL VENTILATION

Children with CRF and relatively stable ventilator settings are candidates for HMV (15–17,36). The pulmonary component of the disorder is usually the most likely to provide instability. Therefore, the pulmonary disease must be such that the child does not require frequent adjustments in ventilator settings to maintain adequate gas exchange. Generally, the Fio_2 should be 40% or less. The requirement for peak inspiratory pressure (PIP) should be less than 40 cm H_2O. Although higher Fio_2 and PIP can be delivered by portable ventilators, patients requiring these settings are often too unstable to be successfully ventilated at home. Portable ventilators are increasingly sophisticated and can provide positive end-expiratory pressure (PEEP), pressure support, and various other modes of ventilatory support. Children with CRF fall into three basic diagnostic categories: ventilatory muscle weakness and neuromuscular diseases, central hypoventilation syndromes, and chronic pulmonary disease.

Ventilatory Muscle Weakness and Neuromuscular Diseases

Ventilatory muscle weakness has three physiologic consequences. Inspiratory muscle weakness prevents children from inspiring deeply, resulting in atelectasis. Expiratory muscle weakness prevents effective coughing, resulting in decreased removal of pulmonary secretions and foreign material from the lungs, both of which increase the incidence and severity of pneumonia, which is the leading cause of morbidity and mortality in children with neuromuscular disease. Frequent or severe pneumonias in a child with neuromuscular disease indicate that ventilatory muscle weakness is significant, and should prompt an investigation of the adequacy of spontaneous ventilation, especially during sleep. Once weakness of the ventilatory muscles progresses sufficiently, hypoventilation and inadequate gas exchange result (24,25). Two basic types of ventilatory muscle weakness are seen in neuromuscular disease: progressive and nonprogressive. In progressive neuromuscular disease, such as spinal muscular atrophy and Duchene muscular dystrophy, muscle weakness worsens with time, resulting in the inevitable development of CRF (27,32,33–35,37). In nonprogressive neuromuscular diseases, such as a congenital myopathy, while muscle weakness does not progress, there may be a relative progression because muscle strength cannot increase to meet the increasing functional demands of somatic growth. Many children with static neuromuscular disorders become nonambulatory and ventilator dependent at or near puberty, because of the increase in body mass associated with the pubertal growth spurt. The development of neuromuscular scoliosis can also tip the respiratory balance toward respiratory failure.

Often, children with chronically elevated PCO_2 greater than 55–60 torr, due to ventilatory muscle weakness, will develop progressive pulmonary hypertension. Although oxygen administration improves the PaO_2 and relieves hypoxia, this treatment alone is inadequate, as hypoventilation persists resulting in complications including atelectasis, recurrent respiratory infections, and pulmonary hypertension. These children will then require HMV (27,33–35).

Children with ventilatory muscle weakness make good candidates for HMV. Because the cause of their respiratory failure is primary muscle weakness, these patients usually do not have significant lung disease, which would require the need for frequent changes in ventilator settings. They are usually much more stable on HMV and have less frequent pneumonias and hospital admissions than they did before it was initiated (27,32–35,37). Some children will require full-time ventilatory support, whereas others may require only nocturnal ventilation.

Central Hypoventilation Syndromes

The cause of CRF in children with central hypoventilation syndrome is inadequate central respiratory drive (15,17,18,28, 38–42), and it can be congenital or acquired. The congenital form may be idiopathic (congenital central hypoventilation syndrome [CCHS] or Ondine's curse) or due to an identifiable brainstem lesion (Chiari malformation Type II in myelomeningocele). Acquired forms of central hypoventilation syndrome may be due to brainstem trauma, tumor, hemorrhage, stroke, infection, etc. In children with respiratory control disorders, usually little can be done to augment central respiratory drive (18,28). However, it can be further inhibited by metabolic imbalance, such as chronic metabolic alkalosis. Thus, serum chloride concentrations should be maintained at >95 mmol/L, and alkalosis should be avoided. Pharmacologic respiratory stimulants are not helpful (32). Sedative medications and central nervous system depressants should be avoided, as these may cause apnea or hypoventilation. Children with respiratory control disorders are generally good candidates for chronic HMV (15,17,18,28,38–42). While central respiratory drive is impaired, the lungs and ventilatory muscles may be nearly normal, permitting reasonably stable ventilator settings to achieve adequate gas exchange. Some of these children will require full-time ventilatory support, whereas others will require ventilatory support only while sleeping (15,17–19,28). Because of this and the fact that respiratory load is not substantially increased, this group of patients can be offered a variety of modalities for ventilatory support, including positive-pressure ventilators via tracheostomy, noninvasive positive-pressure ventilatory support, negative-pressure ventilators, and diaphragm pacing (15,17,18,19,28,38,41,43,44). In general, children with central hypoventilation syndrome make good candidates for HMV. However, some children may have neurologic problems due to the underlying disorder, which may affect the long-term prognosis.

Chronic Pulmonary Disease

Chronic pulmonary disease may increase the work of breathing to a level higher than that can be sustained by the child. Often, the underlying lung disease is intrinsically unstable, requiring frequent adjustments in ventilator settings, but some children with chronic pulmonary disease will stabilize to the point where HMV is possible (8–11,16,45). No consensus has been reached on the PCO_2 level at which a child with chronic lung disease is considered to be in CRF and to require chronic ventilatory support. However, in our experience, children with PCO_2 consistently ≥ 60 torr have a better clinical outcome if chronic ventilatory support is used to keep $PCO_2 \leq 45$–50 torr. The improvement is seen primarily in improved growth, decreased hospitalization time, and avoidance of pulmonary hypertension. However, some patients with chronic lung disease may require very high ventilator settings to achieve $PCO_2 \leq 45$–50 torr. In this instance, rather than risk of ventilator-induced lung injury, one may have to accept a higher level of PCO_2.

Many of these children requiring HMV because of chronic lung disease will be able to wean from chronic ventilatory support with time (13). The most common chronic lung disease for which home ventilation has been used in children is chronic lung disease of infancy, or bronchopulmonary dysplasia. Newer, continuous-flow home ventilators have also permitted successful HMV in children with restrictive lung disease, such as hypoplastic lungs from thoracic restriction (i.e., skeletal dysplasias, congenital diaphragmatic hernia) or interstitial lung diseases. HMV has also been used in children with advanced obstructive lung disease, such as cystic fibrosis as a bridge to lung transplantation (45). Children with unstable lung disease, requirements for significant support (high FIO_2 and PIP), or the need for frequent changes in ventilator settings are poor candidates for HMV.

PHILOSOPHY OF CHRONIC VENTILATORY SUPPORT

For most children on HMV, weaning is not a realistic goal in the short term. In order to optimize quality of life, these children must have energy available for other physical activities. Thus, ventilators are adjusted to completely meet their ventilatory demands, leaving much of their energy available for other activities. For children without significant lung disease, ventilators are adjusted to provide an $ETCO_2$ of 30–35 torr and an $SpO_2 \geq 95\%$. For those who do not require assisted ventilation while awake, ventilating to $PCO_2 \leq 35$ torr during sleep is associated with better spontaneous ventilation while awake (46). Optimal ventilation also avoids atelectasis and the development of coexisting lung disease. It has also been our experience that children who receive chronic ventilatory support actually have fewer complications and generally do better clinically, with some degree of hyperventilation during assisted ventilation (15–18,35,40,46).

For the child who requires HMV, mobility and quality of life are maximized if the child can breathe unassisted for portions of the day. Even if a child cannot be weaned completely from assisted ventilation, nocturnal ventilation preserves waking quality of life and allows the ventilatory muscles a recovery period during the time when the patient is at highest risk for hypoventilation. In our experience, the weaning of daytime-assisted ventilation is best accomplished by sprint weaning. From the perspectives of the patient, parent, and caregiver, it is preferable to have a child who can be away from a ventilator for several hours a day rather than to have a child who must remain on the ventilator at all times, even if the ventilator rate or settings are lower.

MODALITIES OF HOME MECHANICAL VENTILATION

4 The ideal ventilators for home use are different from those used in hospitals for the treatment of acute respiratory failure (36,47). Because many children who require HMV do not have severe lung disease, a number of different techniques are available for providing chronic ventilatory support at home, including (a) portable positive-pressure ventilator via tracheostomy; (b) noninvasive PPV via a mask or other interface; (c) negative-pressure chest shell (cuirass), wrap, or portable tank ventilator; or (d) diaphragm pacing.

Portable Positive-Pressure Ventilator via Tracheostomy

Portable PPV via tracheostomy is the most common method of providing assisted ventilation for infants and children in the home (8,10–12,15–18,27,35,40,47,48). Commercially available electronic positive-pressure ventilators have the capability for battery operation, are relatively portable, and maximize mobility. Portable positive-pressure ventilators are not as powerful, technologically sophisticated, or as versatile as hospital ventilators. Consequently, when infants and children acquire a superimposed respiratory infection, these may not be capable of adequately ventilating the child and hospitalization may be required. Most ventilator-assisted infants and small children are subject to frequent respiratory infections, which often require hospitalization and ventilation with higher settings. A tracheostomy offers the advantage of providing ready access to the airway for hospital ventilators without the need for endotracheal intubation.

For HMV, small, uncuffed tracheostomy tubes are preferred, as the work of breathing required to overcome the increased resistance is performed by the ventilator, not the child. The rationale for the small uncuffed tracheostomy tube is to (a) minimize the risk of tracheomalacia or tracheal mucosal damage, (b) allow an expiratory leak so that the child may speak, and (c) provide a margin of safety because the child may still be able to ventilate around the tracheostomy tube. Furthermore, the use of a one-way, positive-closure speaking valve when the child is not receiving ventilatory support enables the child to phonate from early childhood and thus to speak relatively normally in childhood and adolescence (16). These valves may not be required when using mechanical ventilation, because current home ventilators provide continuous gas flow and PEEP, which facilitates vocal sound production when being ventilated.

Small, uncuffed tracheostomy tubes are associated with leaks, which can be large and variable, especially in small children. If the same PIP is achieved on each breath, the lungs are inflated to the same tidal volume, dependent on pulmonary mechanics, regardless of the amount of leak around the tracheostomy. Because of this, pressure ventilation is preferred, and it can be easily utilized on newer portable home ventilators with continuous flow (49). A significant portion of the ventilator-delivered breath escapes in the leak around the uncuffed tracheostomy. In some older children and adolescents, this leak is relatively constant and a higher tidal volume setting can be used to compensate for the leak and achieve adequate ventilation at home. However, this tidal volume setting must be derived empirically, as it is not possible to predict the portion of a ventilator-delivered breath that escapes through the tracheostomy leak. In infants and smaller children, the tracheostomy leak is large and variable and can rarely be compensated for by a single tidal volume setting. In this situation, the tracheostomy leak can be compensated for by using the ventilator in a pressure-limited modality. It is important to note that the ventilator's high-pressure alarm, useful in detecting an occluded tracheostomy tube, will not function when pressure control, pressure limit, or pressure plateau is used. Thus, a backup alarm on the patient, such as a pulse oximeter, is required. Pressure plateau controlled ventilation is very successful in-home ventilation of infants and small children, and it has allowed us to ventilate these patients without the use of cuffed tracheostomy tubes or cumbersome continuous-flow devices. It is also useful in older children or adolescents who have large or variable tracheostomy leaks (49).

The development of newer portable ventilators with continuous flow has allowed more sophisticated adjustments of ventilation settings to minimize patient asynchrony and has allowed more medically complicated patients to be ventilated at home. A second ventilator is required for those who require ventilatory support ≥20 h/day or who live a long distance from respiratory home care vendors who can provide emergency service in the event of malfunction (16).

Tracheostomy

A tracheostomy is performed when a diagnosis of CRF is established. As previously discussed, a small size, uncuffed tracheostomy tube is preferred. After the procedure, it usually takes 7–10 days for the tract to establish and mature. The first tracheostomy tube change is performed by an otolaryngologist to avoid complications that may arise with granulation tissue or false tract and to document easy reinsertion.

One of the most common complications for a child with a tracheostomy is mucous plugging, which can obstruct the airway within minutes following suctioning. No standard scheduled time for suctioning is defined, as each child is different, and tracheal suctioning needs vary. Hence, vigilance for airway obstruction must be keen and constant. Ventilator alarms and backup monitoring devices are not optimally designed to respond to mucous plugs, nor are they sensitive enough to signal airway obstruction quickly. Therefore, caregivers should be taught not to rely on alarms alone as an indication for the need to suction. Rather, they should be trained to observe early signs of airway obstruction. For a child who is ventilator dependent, the tubing and the noise from the ventilator may make it difficult to discern the problem. Mucous plugging is reportedly more prevalent at night time, when bedside observation is less rigorous. As the consequences of this complication can be serious, caregivers should be trained to routinely triage "a breathing problem" by inspecting the airway for its patency. When in doubt, caregivers should suction and then change the entire tracheostomy tube.

The weight of ventilator tubing pulling on the tracheostomy can cause erosion, laceration of the skin, and an exacerbation of granulation tissue growth. Bleeding from aggressive suctioning is another common problem, which occasionally may lead to potential life-threatening bleeding in extreme situations. Granulation tissue forms from persistent irritation from suctioning and can obstruct the airway, compromising ventilation. Granulation tissue formation is an indication for bronchoscopy and possible laser removal. Tracheitis is also a common complaint, which requires medical attention. When systemic signs and symptoms of infection are not present, inhaled antibiotics are helpful to reduce upper respiratory infection and prevent pneumonia.

If a tracheostomy tube is dislodged accidentally, an immediate replacement is recommended to ensure adequate ventilation and airway access. Tracheostomy stomas can constrict and close in a very short time. A spare tracheostomy tube is necessary as a backup at all times.

While we advocate a small, uncuffed tracheostomy tube, some patients require a customized length or an extension from the stoma site. Newly developed types allow choices. A few children, especially the older ones, might need cuffed tubes to decrease the leak and allow better ventilation during sleep, when upper airway resistance decreases. Cuffed tubes, which are inflated during sleep, can almost always be deflated during wakefulness, permitting speech. Sometimes, cuffed tubes do not even require inflation to decrease the air leak and to improve ventilation. Choice of cuffed tubes should be made according to the needs of the patient. Recommended cuffs can be tight to the shaft or with light, soft sleeves. In summary, the type, length, and size of the tracheostomy tube may need to be individualized to the patient, as these can influence ventilator parameters. As the patients grow, the tracheostomy tube must be periodically upsized to provide adequate ventilation. Autocycling is a sign that the leak has increased to the extent that the ventilator can no longer compensate by increasing flow to deliver the desired inspiratory pressure.

Ventilator Circuits

A circuit is required to deliver air from a positive-pressure ventilator to the patient. Gas from the ventilator goes through a heated humidification system, which is essential in infants and children. The desired temperature range is 26°C–29°C (80°F–85°F). Heat moisture exchange (HME) humidifiers are not as effective for infants and small children as heated humidifiers, but they can be used for travel or for short periods of time. The circuit is usually connected to the tracheostomy with a swivel adapter. Dead space between the tracheostomy and exhalation valve should be minimized, to avoid an elevated Pco_2. Two to three circuits are generally provided for home care, and they are changed each day. The circuit (tubing, valve, and cascade) not in use should be cleaned with mild soap and water, then rinsed in a disinfectant (such as 10% alkyl dimethylbenzol ammonium chloride), and air dried (16).

Monitoring and Alarm Systems

Infants and children who require HMV have very little respiratory reserve. These children may have rapid changes in their clinical condition, which affects the adequacy of both spontaneous and assisted ventilation. These require constant awareness of the child's respiratory status. Caregivers should be trained to assess color change, chest excursion, respiratory distress, tachycardia, tachypnea, diaphoresis, edema, lethargy, and tolerance for spontaneous ventilation off the ventilator (16). Changes in these parameters may be clinical signs that ventilation is inadequate. These children can be checked by noninvasive blood gas monitoring, if available. In some cases, when in-home nursing care is used, nursing personnel can assist in the continual evaluation of the child's clinical condition. Alarm systems are crucial, but they do not take the place of a trained and attentive caregiver.

All positive-pressure ventilators have a low-pressure alarm, which sounds in the event that a minimally acceptable pressure level is not being achieved. These alarms are important to detect a sudden disconnect of the ventilator from the tracheostomy or other very large leak in the circuit and are usually set to alarm if the maximal airway pressure achieved on a breath is less than the desired PIP minus 10 cm H_2O. However, if an infant or small child with a small tracheostomy is decannulated with the small tracheostomy still connected to the ventilator, sufficient resistance from the small tracheostomy tube alone may keep the low-pressure alarm from sounding (50). Ventilators also have high-pressure alarms, which sound if the pressure required to deliver a breath is too high. Very useful in detecting a plug or occlusion of the tracheostomy tube, these alarms are usually set to sound if the maximal airway pressure achieved on a breath is greater than 10 cm H_2O above the desired PIP. As mentioned above, high-pressure alarms will not sound if a ventilator is being used in a pressure plateau or pressure-controlled mode. Therefore, an additional monitoring system that is external to the ventilator and monitors the child directly is required. Currently, a pulse oximeter, which can alarm for low SpO_2 or low heart rate, is the recommended patient monitor. Alarms are usually set to sound for SpO_2 <85% or heart rate below 60 bpm for ages 1–12 months and 50 bpm for those over 1 year of age. High heart rate alarms are not used. The pulse oximeter alarm should be used at all times during sleep and when a ventilator-dependent patient is not being observed.

More sophisticated home ventilators have low- and high-minute ventilation alarms. For those, which monitor inspired minute ventilation ($\dot{V}I$), low-minute ventilation alarms will sound for airway occlusion, and they should be set to alarm for $\dot{V}I$ below the measured $\dot{V}I$. High-minute ventilation alarms will sound an alarm for a disconnection, and they should be set for $\dot{V}I$ above the measured $\dot{V}I$, assuming it will alarm if the ventilator is completely disconnected. High- and low-minute ventilation alarms, which monitor exhaled minute ventilation, are not useful with uncuffed tracheostomy tubes and variable leaks. Although these alarms may improve patient safety, they are not a substitute for the use of pulse oximetry as an additional alarm system.

Noninvasive Positive-Pressure Ventilation by Mask or Nasal Prongs

Noninvasive intermittent positive-pressure ventilation (NIPPV) is delivered via a nasal mask, nasal prongs, or face mask using a noninvasive positive-pressure ventilator (13,18,19,37,38,42,44,45,51). This technique is commonly used in older children but has also been used successfully in infants and small children. NIPPV can be used in children who require ventilatory support only during sleep and who have relatively mild intrinsic lung disease. Thus, NIPPV is most frequently used in children with neuromuscular disorders and central hypoventilation syndromes (19,33,34,38,42,44,51). NIPPV has also been used for children with chronic lung disease who require ventilatory muscle rest (45). NIPPV ventilators are smaller, less expensive, and generally easier to use than conventional ventilators. Newer models have pressure and apnea alarms and adjustable rise times. NIPPV ventilators can provide variable continuous flow via a blower (fan), have a fixed leak (which prevents CO_2 retention), and can compensate for leaks around the mask. Inspiratory positive airway pressure (I-PAP) and expiratory positive airway pressure (E-PAP) can be adjusted independently. The I-PAP to E-PAP difference is proportional to tidal volume. When NIPPV ventilators are used for ventilatory assistance rather than for obstructive sleep apnea, a large I-PAP to E-PAP difference is desirable. Tidal volume increases linearly, with I-PAP to E-PAP difference up to ~14 cm H_2O (19). Higher differences may increase tidal volume with stiff lungs. The lowest E-PAP that can be used without CO_2 accumulation at the interface is 4 cm H_2O. The highest I-PAP that can be used is generally 24 cm H_2O, but some NIPPV ventilators can go to an I-PAP of 30 cm H_2O. However, most children need to begin with lower I-PAP in the range of 10–14 cm H_2O and increase slowly as tolerated and as is necessary (19). For infants with neuromuscular diseases, one can start with an I-PAP of ~15 cm H_2O, and increase as required. Humidification and supplemental oxygen can be added to the circuit, though they are not always necessary.

Four modes of NIPPV can be used: (a) continuous positive airway pressure, (b) spontaneous mode—only assists spontaneously generated breaths, (c) timed mode—controls ventilation at a set rate, and (d) spontaneous/timed mode—assists generated breaths as long as the patient breathes at least the set backup rate and adds control breaths if the patient does not breathe at the minimum backup rate. Only the timed mode guarantees breath delivery and should be used in children with respiratory control disorders because these patients cannot be trusted to generate their own adequate respirations or, with very weak ventilatory muscles, because the ventilator cannot sense a spontaneous breath. It is important to set the rate to at least that which is physiologic for the patient's age. For example, normal infants usually breathe at least 30 bpm. Therefore, the NIPPV rate should be set at this value. NIPPV is not usually used 24 hours/day, because the mask interferes with daily activities and social interaction and the risk of skin breakdown increases significantly. Because of the risk of aspiration, children who are unable to remove their own masks should not have full-face masks unless they are closely observed. Most side effects related to bi-level ventilation are minimal, such as rhinitis, aerophagia, conjunctival injection, and skin breakdown, most of which can be avoided by proper fitting of the mask. Mask ventilation has been associated with some mid-face hypoplasia, although it is not clear if the mask was causative.

NIPPV is not as powerful as PPV via tracheostomy. Using this mode, children may require intubation and more sophisticated ventilatory support during acute exacerbations, such as respiratory syncytial virus (RSV) infections, the risk of which is higher in young children. The major benefit of NIPPV is that a tracheostomy is not required. In general, children successfully managed with NIPPV have less severe respiratory failure than those who require PPV via tracheostomy. Therefore, nonadherence with prescribed NIPPV is more common than with PPV via tracheostomy. A comfortable well-fitting interface and ventilator settings that minimize ventilator–patient asynchrony are key to enhancing adherence.

Negative-Pressure Ventilation

Negative-pressure ventilators (NPVs) apply a negative pressure outside the chest and abdomen to generate inspiration (15–18,47). A chest NPV uses a dome-shaped shell that is fitted over the anterior chest and abdomen. The negative-pressure wrap ventilator is a "jump suit" that fits snugly around the neck, wrists, and ankles to minimize leaks. A metal "cage" inside the jump suit creates a space where negative pressure can be generated during inspiration. A portable tank is a negative-pressure ventilator into which the child's torso is placed, with the head outside. The ventilator rate and the negative pressure to be developed inside the chest shell, wrap, or portable tank can be controlled. The pressure is proportional to the tidal volume, but may be limited by leaks around the chest shell or wrap. These ventilators can provide effective ventilation in children and adolescents, sometimes without a tracheostomy. However, airway occlusion can occur when breaths are generated by an NPV during sleep because synchronous activation of the upper airway muscles does not occur as it does with spontaneous breathing. This asynchrony can be improved if the negative-pressure breath is triggered by a sensor that detects breath initiation by the patient via a fall in pressure

measured either by a nasal cannula placed at the nares or by pressure changes within the cuirass.

In order for negative-pressure chest shell ventilators to provide adequate ventilation, the chest shell must be closely fitted to the chest to avoid large leaks. Further, chest shells must be changed and refitted as the child grows. The adequacy of gas exchange produced by negative-pressure chest shell ventilation must be checked frequently to ensure that the fit and ventilator settings are optimal. Negative-pressure wrap ventilators or portable tanks need not conform exactly to the chest configuration. Thus, they are better suited for small children or some children with scoliosis or chest wall deformities. However, the effectiveness of negative-pressure ventilation depends on the ability to move the chest wall. Children with marked scoliosis or chest wall deformities, which restrict chest wall motion, are not good candidates for NPV.

NPVs can be used to enhance airway clearance by high-frequency chest oscillation and compression, to simulate a cough. Skin irritation may occur when the chest shell rubs the skin, although this can usually be avoided by having the child sleep with a T-shirt under the chest shell and with the use of baby powder or corn starch on the skin. In general, children complain that NPVs are quite cool, because of the continuous movement of air. Thus, wearing a warm shirt is sometimes necessary for comfort, even during warm weather.

NPV may permit decannulation of a tracheostomy. Children with CCHS have been successfully transitioned from PPV via tracheostomy to NPV without tracheostomy after 5–6 years of age. Upper airway obstruction can be minimized by tonsillectomy and adenoidectomy. Reducing the inspiratory negative pressure and/or increasing the inspiratory time may also reduce episodes of obstructive apnea.

Negative-pressure ventilation is not as powerful as PPV via tracheostomy. Thus, children may require intubation and more sophisticated ventilatory support during acute exacerbations (e.g., RSV infections), the risk of which is higher in young children. The major benefit of negative-pressure ventilation is that a tracheostomy may be avoided.

Diaphragm Pacing

Diaphragm pacing generates breathing using the child's own diaphragm as the respiratory pump (Fig. 50.5) (17,18,20,28,43). Commercially available diaphragm pacing systems have battery-operated external transmitters. An antenna is taped on the skin over subcutaneously implanted receivers. The transmitter generates a train of pulses for each breath, which is transmitted through the antenna to the receiver under the skin, similar to radio transmission. The receiver converts this energy to standard electrical current, which is directed to a phrenic nerve electrode by lead wires. The electrical stimulation of the phrenic nerve causes a diaphragmatic contraction, which generates the breath. The amount of electrical voltage is proportional to the diaphragmatic contraction, which generates tidal volume. In children, simultaneous bilateral diaphragm pacing is generally required to achieve optimal ventilation. In older children or adolescents who have a stable chest wall, adequate ventilation may be achieved by pacing only one side. In general, bilateral implantation of diaphragm pacer electrodes and receivers is recommended. But, if one side fails, adequate ventilation can often be achieved using only unilateral pacing (43).

Use of pacers requires that the phrenic nerves and the diaphragm function appropriately to enable effective ventilation. Therefore, ventilatory muscle myopathy and phrenic neuropathy are contraindications to pacer use. Obstructive apnea can be a complication of pacing during sleep, because synchronous upper airway skeletal muscle contraction does not occur with inspiration. However, this can often be overcome by adjusting

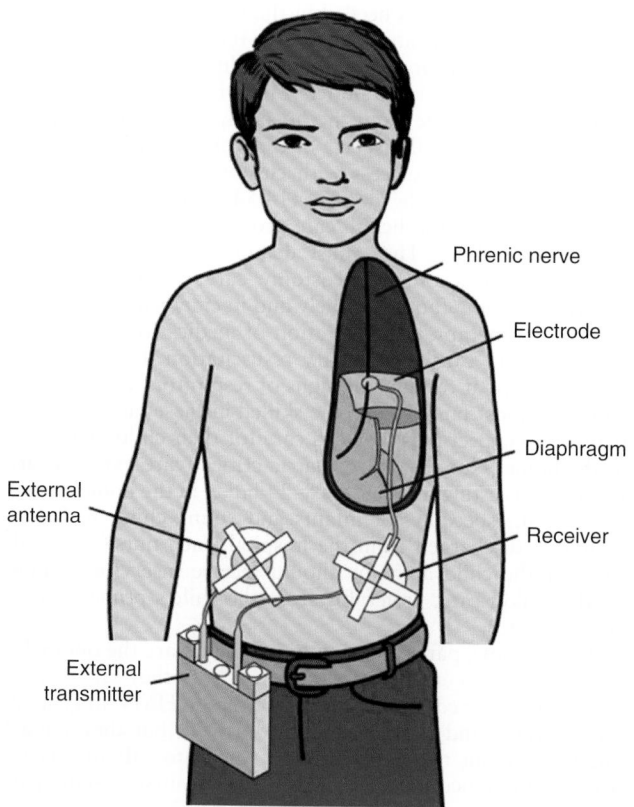

of breathing, substantially increase the patient's ability to breathe spontaneously, and may allow weaning from assisted ventilation for some portion of the day, significantly improving mobility and quality of life.

Nearly all infants and young children who receive HMV develop chronic lung disease with elements of bronchoconstriction, chronic inflammation of the airway, and impaired mucociliary clearance. Therapy should be directed toward relief of bronchospasm, clearance of pulmonary secretions, reduction in lung water, treatment of pulmonary infections, and prevention of aspiration. These children usually benefit from aerosolized bronchodilators followed by intensive pulmonary physiotherapy on a routine basis. Patients should receive the routine immunizations and annual split virion influenza vaccine.

The patient's respiratory status must be stable on the child's home ventilator for at least 1–2 weeks prior to discharge (**Table 50.2**). Eighty percent of children who had a change in management (such as a change in ventilator settings) within a week of discharge required an unplanned readmission within 1 month (52). Therefore, it is important that the child's respiratory status be stable prior to discharge. If the condition changes and multiple changes in management are required, discharge should be delayed until the child is stable. It is important to emphasize that settings on a home ventilator do not provide the same ventilation in the child as the same settings on a hospital ventilator. Therefore, the child must be tested on home

FIGURE 50.5. Diaphragm pacing. Diaphragm pacing provides ventilatory support using the child's diaphragm as the respiratory pump. A phrenic nerve electrode is implanted thoracoscopically, and connected to a receiver in a subcutaneous pocket in the abdomen by a lead wire. When pacing, an external antenna is taped on the skin over the receiver and connected to a battery-operated transmitter. Electrical energy form the transmitter is transferred to the receiver similar to radio transmission. The receiver converts this to electrical current, which stimulates the phrenic nerve, causing a diaphragmatic contraction.

settings on the pacers to lengthen inspiratory time and/or decrease the force of inspiration. In general, diaphragm pacers can be used only up to ~14 hours a day, and cannot be used for 24 hours continuously. Thus, patients who require ventilatory support 24 h/day should have an alternate form of ventilation for part of the day if pacers are used. They can be used for daytime support of ambulatory children who require full-time ventilatory support, in combination with PPV at night (20,43).

Diaphragm pacing has the advantage that the diaphragm pacer system is small, light, battery operated, and easily portable (20,43). Some adolescents believe diaphragm pacing is a "more natural way to breathe" than a ventilator and thus derive psychologic benefit. However, the surgical technique is difficult, and use of the pacers once implanted requires a fair amount of experience. Therefore, diaphragm pacing should generally be performed in centers with experience in the technique. This may provide benefit to select groups of children with central hypoventilation syndrome or high cervical spinal cord injury (18,20,28,43).

HOSPITAL MANAGEMENT PRIOR TO DISCHARGE

5 The underlying conditions that result in the need for HMV are not reversible with specific treatment (15–17). However, improvement in pulmonary mechanics will reduce the work

TABLE 50.2

NEEDS OF THE VENTILATOR-ASSISTED CHILD PRIOR TO HOSPITAL DISCHARGE

1. Medical stability of the child's condition, permitting relatively constant ventilator settings
2. Family commitment to care for the ventilator-assisted child at home, including at least one backup care giver
3. Realistic assessment of the medical care requirements and arrangement for the family's ability to meet them, including in-home nursing assistance, if necessary
4. Thorough education of the family and other caregivers in technical aspects of medical care, equipment operation, and response to emergencies. Allow independent 24-h practice for each primary caregiver. Rehearse "out-of-room" activities, practice transport activities. Use the "teach back" approach to verify competency of all home procedures
5. Selection of a respiratory equipment vendor with ability to supply and service the desired equipment and 24-h emergency availability
6. Selection of a local primary pediatrician to provide well child care, emergency care, and liaison with community resources
7. Informing community emergency medical systems of the ventilator-assisted child and his/her needs
8. Notification of telephone and power companies to provide priority service in the event of interruption of service and medical discount utility rate
9. Arrangement for routine and emergency transport from home to the medical center responsible for medical care. Assist with application for handicapped parking
10. Arrangement for other medical, psychosocial, and developmental support, such as physical and occupational therapy, respite care, community assistance program, and school
11. Preparation of discharge medication and description of the refill procedures

equipment before discharge (16). Invariably, ventilator settings must be increased on the home ventilator to achieve the same level of gas exchange achieved on a hospital ventilator. In the hospital near discharge, it is important to use the actual ventilator and circuits that the child will use in the home (16,36).

Patients tolerate a $PaCO_2$ slightly lower than physiologic, 30–35 torr, which provides a margin of safety and eliminates any subjective feeling of dyspnea. In the home, ventilator settings cannot be changed frequently to maintain perfect blood gas values. Thus, settings should not be changed in response to minor variations in blood gas values, but only to correct persistent trends or major abnormalities (14–16,36,47,48,53).

The equipment essential for home care of the ventilator-assisted child is listed in **Table 50.3** (16,36). Service contracts for the maintenance of the ventilator and other respiratory equipment must be arranged. The respiratory equipment vendor should make home visits every month to verify proper operation of equipment, troubleshoot problems, and provide preventive maintenance. Prompt 24-hour emergency availability of the vendor is essential in the event of equipment malfunction. A backup ventilator and other essential equipment should be provided to all families, but *must* be provided for children who are ventilator dependent ≥20 h/day or when they live long distances from medical or technical assistance (16,36,47). A resuscitation bag is necessary for resuscitation and to permit manual ventilation in the event of power failure or ventilator malfunction. An appropriate size mask made for

the resuscitation bag is needed in the event the tracheostomy is decannulated and cannot be readily reinserted. The physical environment of the home should be evaluated for adequacy of space, grounded electrical outlets, and wiring (16,36,48,53).

Prior to discharge from the hospital, the family must become familiar with all aspects of their child's care. Many institutions have had success with chronic ventilator units on hospital wards outside the ICU (14,54). These are safe, cost less, and often permit health care professionals to focus more on home teaching. They must demonstrate competency in equipment operation, tracheostomy care, ability to change the tracheostomy (both routinely and in emergencies), pulmonary physiotherapy, administration of medications (including aerosols), and cardiopulmonary resuscitation. Families must become adept at recognizing signs of respiratory compromise. Although most families become skilled in these tasks, it is not realistic to expect that they can care for their child unassisted in the home. Nurses with pediatric critical care expertise are helpful in assisting families for 8–24 h/day in the home care of their child, especially for infants and young children. Before a child is discharged from the hospital, each nurse who will care for the child at home should receive inservice training on the child's care, preferably from the child's primary nurse (16,36,48,53).

In the home, parents and in-home nurses are the ones who must respond to emergencies; how much do they know? Kun et al. (55) surveyed caregivers of children on HMV. In general, both parents and in-home nurses did well, but they missed questions about the significance of ventilator alarms. There was no difference in knowledge between nurses versus parents, English versus Spanish speakers, caregivers of part-time versus full-time ventilator-dependent children, or those who had responded to an emergency at home versus those who had not. The length of time their child had been on HMV did correlate with knowledge. This study demonstrated that training for caregivers of children on HMV should focus on technical aspects of ventilator alarms and emergency responses (55).

Children who are ventilator assisted in the home must be closely linked to a medical center capable of providing the subspecialty care required. Prior to home care, arrangements should be made for transportation to the hospital from the home or local emergency department in the event of an emergency. Currently available portable ventilators usually permit the families to transport their ventilator-assisted child for routine visits. When possible, a local primary pediatrician should be recruited to provide routine pediatric care. The local emergency department or paramedics should be familiar with the child and be able to provide emergency care or transport to the medical center when necessary. The local telephone and utility companies must be notified in writing of the patient's location and condition. In the event of a power outage or other interruption of service, the home ventilator patient should be given priority for restoration of service (16,36).

TABLE 50.3

HOME RESPIRATORY EQUIPMENT FOR HOME MECHANICAL VENTILATION (POSITIVE-PRESSURE VENTILATION VIA TRACHEOSTOMY)

1. Electronic portable positive-pressure ventilator with:
   1 humidifier with humidifier jar
   1 heater and thermometer, water trap
   2 circuits with bleed in adapter/connector
   Flex tubing
   Automobile cigarette lighter adaptor for car use, if available
2. Backup ventilator: Absolutely essential for patients who require 20 h/d of assisted ventilation or who are living long distances from medical and technical support
3. Deep-cycle marine gel battery with case and cables for operation of the ventilator and battery charger (unless built into the ventilator)
4. E-cylinder of oxygen with stand and regulator for emergency use supplemental oxygen system, if necessary
5. Aerosol delivery system with:
   2 aerosol setups
   2 trach adapters
   2 connector/adapters of 22/15 cm
6. Portable suction machine with battery pack, connecting tubing, appropriately sized tracheal suction catheters, and tonsil fine-tip catheters
7. Resuscitation bag with appropriate size mask
8. Pulse oximeter as an alarm system (alarm settings: SpO_2 <85%; low heart rate <60 bpm age 1–12 months, <50 bpm age ≥1 year); high heart rate off; probes/sensors
9. Other essential accessories are:
   Tracheostomy tube holder
   Artificial nose HME
   In-line speaking valve
   Bacterial filter
10. Stationary suction machine—for bedside use
11. Backup/Emergency trach tubes

HOME MANAGEMENT OF THE VENTILATOR-ASSISTED CHILD

Routine evaluation of ventilator settings should be performed on a regular basis, so that ventilation meets the changing requirements of the growing child. Although no consensus is available on the minimum frequency of evaluations, they are generally required more frequently in the first year of life (15,16). Older children, who are medically stable, probably only need such evaluations yearly. Following any change in the respiratory system (severe infection, hospitalization, etc.), settings should also be checked and readjusted. These evaluations are usually performed by polysomnography, and it is important to monitor $ETCO_2$ as an indication of the adequacy of ventilation. Sleep studies during daytime naps may also be adequate for the evaluation of ventilator settings if the child's clinical course is reasonably stable. Sleep studies may also be used to predict the success of sprint weaning during sleep when sprinting schedules are advancing in the home. In the absence of the availability of a sleep laboratory, an overnight hospital admission with continuous recording of SpO_2 and $ETCO_2$ may be required to assess the adequacy of ventilator settings.

Some ventilator-assisted children will also require supplemental oxygen. This may be required during spontaneous breathing and/or during mechanically assisted ventilation. Oxygen requirements must be assessed at regular intervals using noninvasive monitoring of oxygenation. Supplemental oxygen is not a replacement for home ventilation in those patients with chronic hypoventilation.

Because HMV may not completely meet the ventilatory requirements at all times, even the most successfully managed patients may be exposed to periods of alveolar hypoxia and hypoventilation (Table 50.4). Thus, all ventilator-assisted children are at risk for the development of pulmonary hypertension and cor pulmonale. The usual clinical findings of right heart failure may not be present until late in the course. Echocardiography may be a more sensitive method for following right heart function and should be used to measure right ventricular dimensions, pulmonic valve systolic time intervals, septal morphology, pulmonic valve "a dip," pulmonic valve early systolic closure, and acceleration time of pulmonary artery flow (Doppler). Echocardiography should be obtained annually and more often if clinically indicated. When signs of pulmonary hypertension are discovered, it should be assumed that an inadequate level of mechanical ventilation is the cause until proven otherwise. The patient should be hospitalized for continuous noninvasive monitoring of gas exchange and ventilator adjustments. Some patients who require assisted ventilation only while sleeping may hypoventilate intermittently while breathing spontaneously during wakefulness. If this occurs frequently, pulmonary hypertension may result, even if mechanical ventilation at night is adequate.

Physicians have tended to categorize CRF patients as those who are full-time ventilator dependent and those who require ventilatory support only while sleeping. This view oversimplifies the problem. There is a continuum of the need for ventilatory support. Some children may require support at all times while asleep and sometimes while awake, but not all the time. It is probably better to think of the hours per day of ventilatory support required. Some children may require 16, 18, or 20 hours of ventilatory support per day.

Growth failure can result from chronic hypoxemia and/or inadequate ventilation. If patients fail to grow normally, caloric intake and the adequacy of ventilatory support should be assessed. Some patients, especially those with ventilatory muscle weakness, may have a decreased caloric expenditure due to decreased body movement. These patients do not expend calories as work of breathing, since this is being performed by the ventilator. Growth and weight gain should be monitored carefully, and too rapid weight gain may mean that caloric intake is excessive.

Common childhood illnesses pose a unique threat to the ventilator-assisted child. A number of normal host defenses against disease are either lost or impaired in these patients. For example, breathing via tracheostomy bypasses the normal humidifying and filtering functions of the upper airway, predisposing to inspissated secretions and tracheobronchitis. Ineffective cough leads to decreased clearance of pulmonary secretions. An inability to increase respiratory rate in response to fever may lead to dyspnea and hypoxia. Despite the use of preventive and therapeutic measures directed at these problems, even a relatively trivial upper respiratory infection may compromise the ventilator-assisted child. Ventilator adjustments, with an increased level of support, are usually needed. Patients ordinarily requiring ventilation only during sleep often need 24 h/day support during illnesses. Because of these changes in the ventilatory requirements, they may require hospitalization for blood gas monitoring and frequent ventilator changes. Hospital ventilators with greater flexibility than portable electronic ventilators, are usually required to ensure adequate ventilation during these events. After recovery, patients should demonstrate adequate ventilation on their home ventilator for at least a day or two prior to discharge.

Placement of a ventilator-assisted child in the school system poses unique challenges to the teachers and the school district. Nevertheless, many can attend regular school, especially if they require assisted ventilation only during sleep. Whenever possible, it is desirable that a ventilator-assisted child receive education in as normal a school setting as possible. When the discharge team works closely with school district personnel, the optimal educational setting for the child can often be arranged. Educating school officials about the true nature of the child's disorder often eases fear and facilitates school placement and acceptance. Obviously, some children are better served in special schools, but this is usually dependent on disease involvement in bodily systems other than the respiratory system (15,16,36).

Even with sophisticated management at home, ventilator-assisted children may succumb to a catastrophe stemming from

TABLE 50.4

MANAGEMENT OF COMPLICATIONS OF HOME MECHANICAL VENTILATION

■ MEDICAL PROBLEM	■ MANAGEMENT
Hypoxia	Evaluate oxygenation by noninvasive monitoring
	If SpO_2 is <95%, add supplemental oxygen or increase ventilatory support
Hypoventilation	Evaluate ventilator settings by noninvasive monitoring
	If $ETCO_2$ is >35 torr, increase ventilatory support
Chronic lung disease	Have a high index of suspicion
	The diagnosis of chronic lung disease is often missed in ventilator-assisted children
	Treatment includes aerosolized bronchodilators, pulmonary physiotherapy, and diuretics
Pulmonary hypertension	Ensure adequate oxygenation and ventilation
	Periodically monitor electrocardiogram and echocardiogram for signs of pulmonary hypertension
Pulmonary infections	Complete immunizations, including influenza A/B split virion vaccine
	Treat respiratory infections aggressively with antibiotics, chest physiotherapy, and possibly increased ventilator settings
Growth delay	Ensure adequate caloric quantity and quality
	Growth delay can be a complication of chronic hypoxia or hypercapnia. Assess oxygenation and ventilation

a simple problem, such as a disconnected ventilator or plugged tracheostomy, emphasizing the need for compulsive care (56). The 5-year mortality rate for children on HMV is ~20% (13). However, home ventilator equipment failure is uncommon, occurring only approximately once every 1.3 patient-years, and Srinivasan et al. (56) found no serious sequelae to equipment failure in a home care program with careful attention to detail.

The first month after discharge is a critical time for unplanned readmission of children on HMV (52). Thus, families require close follow-up and support from the hospital health care team working in collaboration with home nursing and respiratory care vendors. Communication between these two groups of health care professionals is crucial during this critical period of time. Home care professionals should be alert to signs of distress, inability to provide needed care, confusion, or lack of knowledge on the part of caregivers, and to communicate early signs of these to the hospital health care professionals. Similarly, hospital health care professionals should alert home care professionals of potential problems with specific patients and their families. When barriers between hospital and home care professionals are removed, truly comprehensive and supportive care for the family can occur. Many hospitals have policies governing the care of their patients by using a multidisciplinary action plan (MAP). We propose that the MAP should include the plans and management strategies post discharge. As the first month post discharge is a critical period for readmission, the activities that need monitoring include communication to the entire team (inpatient and outpatient): status report from home health services within 48 hours post-discharge, the first clinic visit, the psychosocial adaptation, barriers to return appointments, the completion of application to community resources for outpatient therapies and successful refill of all home medication.

OUTCOME

⑦ Children with CRF are, by definition, fragile, and they have limited reserve. While many children do well at home, HMV is a high risk situation. Edwards et al. (13) found a 20% mortality rate in the first 5 years after discharge, and a 35% mortality rate in the first 10 years. The mortality rates did not differ significantly by the cause of CRF. Not all deaths were predictable. While 30% of deaths were due to progression of the child's baseline disease, nearly 20% of them were due to unexpected tracheostomy accidents (13). This emphasizes the importance of rigorously training caregivers to recognize and respond to emergency situations in the home (13,55).

Because we anticipate many chronic lung diseases to improve with age, half of children on HMV due to chronic lung disease were able to wean off ventilatory support by 5 years after discharge (13). Understandably, children requiring ventilatory support due to ventilatory muscle weakness or central hypoventilation syndromes were less likely to wean, since these conditions rarely improve. Only ~5%–10% of these patients were able to wean from ventilatory support in 5 years. In all cases, this was due to an improvement in the child's underlying condition.

In a series of 109 children discharged on HMV, Kun et al. (52) found that 40% required unplanned readmissions within a year after discharge, 4%–6% occurred in the first 3 months. The most common causes were pneumonia, tracheitis, and tracheostomy related complications (such as decannulation and mucous plugs). The most important predictor of unplanned readmission was a change in medical care (such as a change in ventilator settings) within a week prior to discharge, and 80% of these children were re-admitted all within 1 month of discharge (52). To minimize the chance of hospital readmission, patients should be medical stable, not requiring changes in medical care, prior to discharge.

CONCLUSIONS AND FUTURE DIRECTIONS

Successful care of the ventilator-assisted child at home demands compulsive attention to detail on the part of medical personnel, the child, and the family. However, the potential rewards are great. Many ventilator-assisted children do quite well at home, and home care of these patients is a safe and relatively inexpensive management technique. The high motivation of parents for the care of their children in the home often results in a high quality of care. After the transition from hospital to home, parent–child relationships and child development are enhanced. Potential for rehabilitation in all aspects of daily living is increased, and many children will experience a near-normal lifestyle. Future technologic improvements are likely to improve portability, effectiveness of ventilation, versatility of ventilation modalities, and, potentially, the ability to care for more severely affected children at home. Caregiver knowledge and abilities to handle emergencies in the home still require improvement. Increased attention should be paid to educating caregivers about technical aspects of ventilator function and in recognizing and responding to emergencies. Taking advantage of the digital age, future educational materials could be more animated and readily available through the Internet. Simulation practice to promote critical thinking in a more practical way will be one of the ways to improve caregiver knowledge of emergency care. The prompt recognition of tracheostomy emergencies, and response, may reduce hospital readmissions and mortality.

References

1. Ben Abraham R, Efrati O, Mishali D, et al. Predictors of mortality after prolonged mechanical ventilation after cardiac surgery in children. *J Crit Care* 2002;17:235–9.
2. Ben-Abraham R, Weinbroum AA, Roizin H, et al. Long-term assessment of pulmonary function tests in pediatric survivors of acute respiratory distress syndrome. *Med Sci Monit* 2002;8:153–7.
3. Tibby SM, Taylor D, Festa M, et al. A comparison of three scoring systems for mortality risk among retrieved intensive acre patients. *Arch Dis Child* 2002;87:421–5.
4. Welton JM, Meyer AA, Mandelkehr L, et al. Outcomes of and resource consumption by high-cost patients in the intensive care unit. *Am J Crit Care* 2002;11:467–73.
5. Randolph AG, Meert KL, O'Neil ME, et al. The feasibility of conducting clinical trials in infants and children with acute respiratory failure. *Am J Respir Crit Care Med* 2003;167:1334–40.
6. Slater A, Shann F, Pearson G. PIM2: A revised version of the Pediatric Index of Mortality. *Intensive Care Med* 2003;29:278–85.
7. Weiss I, Ushay HM, DeBruin W, et al. Notterman. Respiratory and cardiac function in children after acute hypoxic respiratory failure. *Crit Care Med* 1996;24:148–54.
8. Appierto L, Cori M, Bianchi R, et al. Home care for chronic respiratory failure in children. *Paediatr Anaesth* 2002;12:345–50.
9. Fauroux B, Sardet A, Foret D. Home treatment for chronic respiratory failure in children: A prospective study. *Eur Respir J* 1995;8:2062–6.
10. Jardin E, O'Toole M, Paton JY, et al. Current status of long-term ventilation of children in the United Kingdom. *BMJ* 1999;318:295–9.
11. Kamm M, Burger R, Rimensberger P, et al. Survey of children supported by long-term mechanical ventilation in Switzerland. *Swiss Med Wkly* 2001;131:261–6.
12. Sasaki M, Sugai K, Fukumizu M, et al. Mechanical ventilation care in severe childhood neurological disorders. *Brain Dev* 2001;23:796–800.
13. Edwards JD, Kun SS, Keens TG. Outcomes and causes of death in children on home mechanical ventilation via tracheostomy. *J Pediatr* 2010;157:955–9.

14. Ambrosio IU, Woo MS, Jansen MT, et al. Safety of hospitalized ventilator-dependent children outside of the intensive care unit. *Pediatrics* 1998;101:257–9.

15. Keens TG, Davidson Ward SL. Central hypoventilation syndromes. In: Marcus CL, Loughlin GM, Carroll JL, et al, eds. *Breathing During Sleep in Children.* 2nd ed. New York, NY: Informa Healthcare, 2008:363–82.

16. Make BJ, Hill NS, Goldberg AI, et al. Mechanical ventilation beyond the intensive care unit: Report of a consensus conference of the American College of Chest Physicians. *Chest* 1998;113:289S–344S.

17. Witmans MB, Chen ML, Davidson Ward SL, et al. Congenital syndromes affecting respiratory control during sleep. In: Lee-Chiong T, ed. *Sleep: A Comprehensive Handbook.* Hoboken, NJ: John Wiley and Sons, 2006:517–27.

18. Chen ML, Keens TG. Congenital central hypoventilation syndrome: Not just another rare disorder. *Paediatr Respir Rev* 2004;5:182–9.

19. Marcus CL. Ventilator management of abnormal breathing during sleep: Continuous positive airway pressure and nocturnal noninvasive intermittent positive pressure ventilation. In: Loughlin GM, Marcus CL, Carroll JL, eds. *Sleep and Breathing in Children: A Developmental Approach. Lung Biology in Health and Disease Series.* New York, NY: Marcel Dekker, 2000:797–811.

20. Chin AC, Shaul DB, Patwari PP, et al. Diaphragm pacing in infants and children with congenital central hypoventilation syndrome. In: Keirandish-Gozal L, Gozal D, eds. *Sleep Disordered Breathing in Children.* New York, NY: Springer Science + Business Media, 2012:553–73.

21. Gozal D, Shoseyov D, Keens TG. Inspiratory pressures with CO_2 stimulation and weaning from mechanical ventilation in children. *Am Rev Respir Dis* 1993;147:256–61.

22. Keens TG, Bryan AC, Levison H, et al. Developmental pattern of muscle fiber types in human ventilatory muscles. *J Appl Physiol* 1978;44:909–13.

23. Scott CB, Nickerson BG, Sargent CW, et al. Developmental pattern of maximal transdiaphragmatic pressure in infants during crying. *Pediatr Res* 1983;17:707–9.

24. Nickerson BG, Keens TG. Measuring ventilatory muscle endurance in humans as sustainable inspiratory pressure. *J Appl Physiol* 1982;52:768–72.

25. Roussos CS, Macklem PT. Diaphragmatic fatigue in man. *J Appl Physiol* 1977;43:189–97.

26. Keens TG, Chen V, Patel P, et al. Cellular adaptations of the ventilatory muscles to a chronic increased respiratory load. *J Appl Physiol* 1978;44:905–8.

27. Gilgoff RL, Gilgoff IS. Long-term follow-up of home mechanical ventilation in young children with spinal cord injury and neuromuscular conditions. *J Pediatr* 2003;142:476–80.

28. Weese-Mayer DE, Berry-Kravis EM, Checcherini I, et al. An official ATS clinical policy statement: Congenital central hypoventilation syndrome: Genetic basis, diagnosis, and management. *Am J Respir Crit Care Med* 2010;181:626–44.

29. Swaminathan S, Paton JY, Davidson Ward SL, et al. Theophylline does not increase ventilatory responses to hypercapnia or hypoxia. *Am Rev Respir Dis* 1992;146:1398–401.

30. Edwards JD, Kun SS, Graham RJH, et al. End-of-life discussions and advance care planning for children on long-term assisted ventilation with life-limiting conditions. *J Palliat Care* 2012;28:22–8.

31. Gilgoff IS, Prentice W, Baydur A. Patient and family participation in the management of respiratory failure in Duchenne's muscular dystrophy. *Chest* 1989;95:519–24.

32. Sritippayawan S, Kun SS, Keens TG, et al. Initiation of home mechanical ventilation in children with neuromuscular diseases. *J Pediatr* 2003;142:481–5.

33. Finder JD, Birnkrant D, Carl J, et al. American Thoracic Society: Respiratory care of the patient with Duchenne muscular dystrophy. ATS consensus statement. *Am J Respir Crit Care Med* 2004;170:456–65.

34. Lyager S, Steffensen B, Juhl B. Indicators of need for mechanical ventilation in Duchenne muscular dystrophy and spinal muscular atrophy. *Chest* 1995;108:779–85.

35. Gilgoff IS, Kahlstrom E, MacLaughlin E, et al. Long-term ventilatory support in spinal muscular atrophy. *J Pediatr* 1989;115:904–9.

36. Holecek MS, Nixon M, Keens TG. Discharge of the technology dependent child. In: Levine DL, Morriss FC, eds. *Essentials of Pediatric Intensive Care.* 2nd ed. New York, NY: Churchill Livingston, 1997:1537–48.

37. Simonds AK, Ward S, Heather S, et al. Outcome of paediatric domiciliary mask ventilation in neuromuscular and skeletal disease. *Eur Respir J* 2000;16:476–81.

38. Kerbl R, Litscher H, Grubbauer HM, et al. Congenital central hypoventilation syndrome (Ondine's curse syndrome) in two siblings: Delayed diagnosis and successful noninvasive treatment. *Eur J Pediatr* 1996;155:1059–64.

39. Lesser DJ, Davidson Ward SL, Kun SS, et al. Congenital hypoventilation syndromes. *Sem Respir Crit Care Med* 2009;30:339–47.

40. Marcus CL, Jansen MT, Poulsen MK, et al. Medical and psychosocial outcome of children with congenital central hypoventilation syndrome. *J Pediatr* 1991;119:888–95.

41. Perez IA, Keens TG, Davidson Ward SL. Central hypoventilation syndromes. In: Keirandish-Gozal L, Gozal D, eds. *Sleep Disordered Breathing in Children.* New York, NY: Springer Science + Business Media, 2012:391–407.

42. Villa MP, Dotta A, Castello D, et al. Non-invasive positive pressure (BiPAP) ventilation in an infant with central hypoventilation syndrome. *Pediatr Pulmonol* 1997;24:66–9.

43. Chen ML, Tablizo MA, Kun S, et al. Diaphragm pacers as a treatment for congenital central hypoventilation syndrome. *Exp Rev Med Dev* 2005;2:577–85.

44. Teague WG. Non-invasive positive pressure ventilation: Current status in paediatric patients. *Paediatr Respir Rev* 2005;6:52–60.

45. Hodson ME, Madden BP, Steven MH, et al. Non-invasive mechanical ventilation for cystic fibrosis patients—a potential bridge to transplantation. *Eur Respir J* 1991;4:524–7.

46. Gozal D, Keens TG. Passive nighttime hypocapnic hyperventilation improves daytime eucapnia in mechanically ventilated children. *Am J Respir Crit Care Med* 1989;157(3):A779.

47. Davidson Ward SL, Keens TG. Home mechanical ventilators and equipment. In McConnell MS, ed. *Guidelines for Pediatric Home Health Care.* Evanston, IL: American Academy of Pediatrics, 2002:177–86.

48. DeWitt PK, Jansen MT, Davidson Ward SL et al. Obstacles to discharge of ventilator assisted children from the hospital to home. *Chest* 1993;103:1560–5.

49. Gilgoff IS, Peng R-C, Keens TG. Hypoventilation and apnea in children during mechanical assisted ventilation. *Chest* 1992;101:1500–6.

50. Kun S, Nakamura CT, Ripka JF, et al. Home ventilator low pressure alarms fail to detect accidental decannulation with pediatric tracheostomy tubes. *Chest* 2001;119:562–4.

51. Paditz E. Nocturnal nasal mask ventilation in childhood. *Pneumologie* 1994;48:744–9.

52. Kun SS, Edwards JD, Davidson Ward SL, et al. Hospital readmissions for newly discharged pediatric home mechanical ventilation patients. *Pediatr Pulmonol* 2011;47:409–14.

53. Noyes J. Barriers that delay children and young people who are dependent on mechanical ventilators from being discharged from the hospital. *J Clin Nurs* 2002;11:2–11.

54. Edwards JD, Rivanis C, Kun SS, et al. Costs of hospitalized ventilator-dependent children: Differences between a ventilator ward and intensive care unit. *Pediatr Pulmonol* 2011;46:356–61.

55. Kun SS, Davidson Ward SL, Hulse LM, et al. How much do primary caregivers know about tracheostomy and home ventilator emergency care? *Pediatr Pulmonol* 2010;45:270–4.

56. Srinivasan S, Doty SM, White TR, et al. Frequency, causes, and outcome of home ventilator failure. *Chest* 1998;114:1363–7.

CHAPTER 51 ■ SLEEP AND BREATHING

SALLY L. DAVIDSON WARD AND THOMAS G. KEENS

KEY POINTS

1 Obstructive sleep apnea occurs when the upper airway is functionally or anatomically narrowed. Sleep predisposes to airway instability and obstruction.

2 Most children with obstructive sleep apnea syndrome (OSAS) can be treated with adenotonsillectomy (T&A) in the ambulatory surgery center. However, those who are at very high risk for severe OSAS and for postoperative complications will need PICU care.

3 In addition to adenotonsillectomy, OSAS can be successfully treated with other surgical approaches and by the use of positive airway pressure. Children with obesity-related OSAS will often require continuous positive airway pressure (CPAP) or bi-level positive airway pressure (BPAP) to control OSAS.

4 Children who present to the PICU for other reasons may have unrecognized OSAS. Screening for sleep-related breathing disorders should be a part of the preoperative evaluation of all children who are to undergo elective surgical procedures. CPAP can be used both before and after surgery for stabilization.

5 The respiratory system in infancy is immature and intrinsically unstable. Infants may suffer an apparent life-

threatening event (ALTE) owing to a number of etiologies that perturb the respiratory system. A targeted diagnostic evaluation and therapy directed at the underlying cause is indicated. Home monitoring is needed for infants at risk for subsequent events.

6 Sudden infant death syndrome (SIDS) is the most common cause of death in infants between the ages of 1 month and 1 year. The etiology of SIDS remains unknown, but the risk has been significantly reduced by the promotion of safe infant sleep practices. The parents of SIDS babies suffer overwhelming grief and need education and emotional support, which are best provided by SIDS parent organizations.

7 Sleep fragmentation and deprivation occur in the PICU setting, and may interfere with physiologic responses to stress and add to the discomfort of being a patient in the PICU. Many medications, therapies, and the PICU environment negatively impact sleep. A consideration of the importance of sleep in the PICU may enhance patient outcomes and satisfaction.

Sleep-related breathing disorders (SRBDs) may be severe enough to warrant admission to the ICU setting for management or require PICU monitoring following surgical therapy. In addition, previously unrecognized SRBD may complicate the course of patients admitted to the PICU for other reasons. This chapter will summarize the reasons why sleep represents a period of vulnerability for the respiratory system and how this results in an array of breathing disorders unique to sleep, discuss the common forms of SRBD that may be found in an ICU setting, outline the postoperative challenges in caring for patients affected by SRBD, document the presentation and differential diagnosis of infants with apparent life-threatening events (ALTEs), and review the impact of poor sleep quality on patients cared for in ICUs.

RESPIRATORY CONTROL AND SLEEP

Breathing is under both voluntary and involuntary control during wakefulness. Chemoreceptor activity ensures that minute ventilation is appropriately matched to metabolic needs, whereas voluntary control of ventilation allows the integrated performance of complex behavioral activities. The muscles of

even an anatomically narrowed upper airway are usually able to maintain sufficient tone such that breathing can occur without compromise during wakefulness. However, respiratory control and upper airway muscle tone are state specific, and are entirely different during sleep, thus predisposing to upper airway obstruction and instability. As sleep commences in normal individuals, the arterial P_{CO_2} rises by several mm Hg. The proposed mechanism is "withdrawal of the wakefulness stimulus," suggesting that the sum total of the sensory input of wakefulness is a nonspecific stimulus to the neurologic centers of respiratory control that is lost with sleep onset (1). Similarly, the wakefulness stimulus has an influence on the resting muscle tone of the upper airway, which when withdrawn at the onset of sleep may favor airway obstruction. Behavioral control of ventilation is absent during non–rapid eye movement (NREM) sleep. Thus, adequate ventilation is critically dependent on chemical control. However, the ventilatory responses to hypoxemia and hypercapnia, both potent stimuli of chemoreceptor activity during wakefulness, are blunted during sleep. Important respiratory reflexes such as coughing and swallowing are inhibited by sleep. The changes in lung volumes that occur with moving from the upright to the supine position reduce the caudal traction on the upper airway, thus increasing airway collapsibility (2). The respiratory pattern becomes irregular during rapid eye movement (REM) sleep with a variable rate and tidal volume and frequent respiratory pauses. Finally, during REM sleep, the skeletal muscle atonia that is characteristic of this state affects all of the muscles of the upper airway and all of those involved in respiration except the diaphragm. This leads to increased collapsibility of the upper airway and a decrease in functional residual capacity of the lungs, predisposing to upper airway obstruction or obstructive sleep apnea (OSA) and impaired gas exchange. REM accounts for about 20% of normal sleep time in adults and children and 50% of sleep time in newborn infants; thus, the importance of REM sleep is not trivial. In addition, there are important maturational differences that affect sleep and breathing in infancy that will be discussed in the context of ALTEs and apnea of infancy (3).

OBSTRUCTIVE SLEEP APNEA SYNDROME

The most common form of sleep-disordered breathing in childhood is obstructive sleep apnea syndrome (OSAS). OSA is defined as an absence of airflow at the nose and mouth despite continued respiratory efforts. Discrete events that are partial in nature (reduced, but not absent airflow) are termed obstructive hypopneas. Obstructive apneas and hypopneas are often accompanied by hypoxemia, hypercapnia, and sleep disruption. Continuous partial airway obstruction can result in the obstruction or hypoventilation. Children with OSAS present with snoring and difficulty breathing during sleep. Parents may describe gasping, choking, or observed apneas during their child's sleep. Because OSAS and snoring are often worse in the supine position, parents may reposition their children several times during the night. Nocturnal symptoms may be accompanied by impaired quality of life as well as behavioral or neurocognitive impairment during the day (4–7).

The patency of the upper airway during sleep is determined by the bony and soft tissue anatomy of the airway and the upper airway muscle tone. The latter is influenced both by state (wakefulness vs. sleep and REM vs. NREM sleep) and by neural and chemical controls. The pharyngeal airway serves more than one purpose. To propel boluses of food, forceful constriction of the pharyngeal muscles is required, whereas speech requires rapid and dynamic changes in structure and rigidity of the pharynx and larynx. Although respiration would be best served by a rigid airway, these other functions require the pharynx to be collapsible. Thus, the neuromuscular function of the upper airway is critical to maintaining airway patency. If neural inputs maintaining airway patency during sleep are inadequate and/or the airway is anatomically narrowed, OSAS may result. Implicit in this feature is the fact that physical exam during wakefulness does not accurately predict the presence of OSAS during sleep nor does correction of the anatomic defect by surgery invariable relieve all of the symptoms. The significant familial pattern to the risk of OSAS is likely related to both heritable anatomic and central nervous system factors (2–4).

There are a number of conditions that predispose to OSAS; the most common are listed in **Table 51.1**. Common to all these etiologies is the feature of an anatomically or functionally narrowed upper airway (5,6,8,9). With the onset of the obesity epidemic in children, the landscape of sleep-disordered breathing has changed dramatically, with many children and adolescents now at risk for severe obesity-related OSAS (5,6,10–12). Obstructive apneas and hypopneas can result in continuous or episodic hypoxemia and/or hypoventilation during sleep, as well as repetitive arousals. These stimuli alter the function of the autonomic nervous system. Thus, both systemic and pulmonary hypertension are recognized

TABLE 51.1

CONDITIONS THAT PREDISPOSE TO OBSTRUCTIVE SLEEP APNEA SYNDROME IN CHILDREN

- Adenotonsillar hypertrophy
- Obesity
- Craniofacial abnormalities
- Down syndrome
- Sickle cell disease
- Cerebral palsy

complications of OSAS. Because the protective response to OSA includes arousal from sleep, sleep can be fragmented, and in the most severe cases, results in excessive daytime sleepiness. This sleepiness is the most common presenting feature in adults with OSAS, but is not nearly as common in children because they are less likely to arouse following each obstructive event. An exception to this is the morbidly obese child in whom excessive daytime sleepiness is often severe. Although children with OSAS may not have daytime sleepiness, they may suffer from other neurobehavioral complications, including school failure, hyperactivity, and mood or conduct disorders. It is plausible that the sleep disruption and hypoxemia of OSAS are responsible for the neurologic and behavioral complications, and one large population-based study found a correlation between the severity of OSAS and the extent of these complications (13). A recent randomized trial of early adenotonsillectomy (T&A) versus watchful waiting as therapy for mild to moderate pediatric OSA found that the surgical group had improvements in quality of life and measures of behavior, but not in neuropsychological estimates of attention and executive function (7). Primary snoring (snoring without findings of OSA on formal testing) has been found by others to result in neurobehavioral difficulties (14). Further study is required to explore these relationships. Other complications of OSA include failure to thrive, nocturnal enuresis, and worsening of parasomnias such as sleepwalking (6,9). Recent evidence implicates sleep disruption and hypoxemia as contributors to abnormalities of glucose homeostasis in obese children with SRBD (10,12).

Because neither history nor physical exam is sufficient to firmly establish the diagnosis of OSAS, a polysomnogram (PSG; sleep study) is required to reliably make the diagnosis (5,6). Normative PSG values have been established for children and are quite different from those used in adults with normal children having only one to two obstructive apneas or hypopneas per hour of sleep. Normal adults may have as many as five obstructive events per hour of sleep and be considered normal (5,6,9,15,16).

The first approach to therapy for OSAS is generally adenotonsillectomy. This should be performed following documentation of the syndrome by polysomnography, and usually is completed in the ambulatory surgery center. Some children are at higher risk, and one night of observation postoperatively on the pediatric inpatient unit is indicated (5,6). At least one study has demonstrated that pediatric patients with *mild* OSAS will do well postoperatively from the respiratory standpoint, irrespective of the use of opiates for analgesia. Polysomnography was performed on the first postoperative night, revealing decreased obstructive events and oxygenation compared with the preoperative PSG, although sleep efficiency was decreased (17). However, there are groups of patients who are at higher risk for postoperative complications who will benefit from a higher level of care. Immediate complications of T&A include postoperative bleeding, upper airway obstruction secondary to airway edema, pulmonary edema, or respiratory failure

TABLE 51.2

CONDITIONS WITH A HIGHER RISK OF COMPLICATIONS
FOLLOWING ADENOTONSILLECTOMY

- Age less than 3 y
- Severe OSAS (profound hypoxemia, AHI >10, significant hypoventilation)
- Morbid obesity
- Neuromuscular disease
- Pulmonary hypertension
- Down syndrome
- Craniofacial anomalies

(5,6,18–21). Diagnostic groups at the highest risk for postoperative complications are listed in **Table 51.2** (5,6,20,22).

Children at higher risk for postoperative complications should be admitted for overnight observation and may benefit from the intensive cardiorespiratory monitoring afforded by a PICU (18,23). In a retrospective series of 69 patients who were observed postoperatively in the PICU following T&A, 23% had respiratory compromise—defined as oxygen saturation less than 70% and/or hypercapnia. The patients with compromise were younger (3.4 vs. 6.1 years); had higher numbers of obstructive events per hour on pre-op PSGs (49 vs. 19); and were more likely to have failure to thrive, to have abnormalities of cardiac function, or to have craniofacial abnormalities. Multiple regression analysis revealed that age less than 3 years and more than 10 obstructive events per hour of sleep were the most significant risk factors for postoperative respiratory compromise (22). Another retrospective study of 83 children admitted after T&A because of severe OSA revealed that just more than 19% had postoperative airway complications. The authors identified age less than 2 years, apnea hypopnea index (AHI) >24, intraoperative laryngospasm requiring treatment, SpO_2 <90% in the postanesthesia care unit (PACU), and a prolonged PACU stay (>100 minutes) as predictors of postoperative airway complications (22,24). Finally, Kieran and coworkers performed a multicenter, retrospective review of over 4000 patients who underwent T&A in order to identify risk factors for postoperative hypoxemia. This study included patients who had the surgery for OSA or for other indications. Most did not have a preoperative PSG. Almost 300 patients had hypoxemia, and these were compared with a matched comparison group without hypoxemia. They identified Down syndrome, a clinical diagnosis of OSA, neurologic, cardiac or pulmonary disease, young age, and extremes of weight as risk factors (25). Therefore, a preoperative review of the history and the PSG results accompanied by scrutiny of the immediate postoperative course can aid in the identification of which patients can be safely scheduled for same-day surgery and those who will require postoperative hospital observation or care in the PICU. Omitting the PSG and performing surgery simply on the basis of a history of snoring and the presence of adenotonsillar hypertrophy has the potential to place children at risk for unanticipated complications (5,6,22).

Increasingly, patients with morbid obesity are presenting with OSAS, and it is often severe in this group with frequent obstructive events, profound hypoxemia, and significant hypoventilation. Similar to adults with OSAS, both systemic and pulmonary hypertension may be present (11). Unlike the majority of children with OSAS, respiratory control can be altered with resetting of the chemoreceptor function, resulting in daytime hypoventilation. In this instance, ventilation may be dependent on hypoxic drive, requiring that supplemental oxygen be used judiciously and necessitating close monitoring both preoperatively and postoperatively. In a retrospective

review of 957 children undergoing T&A, 543 were admitted to the hospital after surgery. Fourteen of these were identified as morbidly obese and were admitted to the PICU for observation (26). Three (20%) required assisted ventilation in the postoperative period. Another retrospective review of 26 morbidly obese patients, all of whom were sent to the ICU following T&A as per routine, found that 14 patients (54%) had an uncomplicated postoperative course, but a significant proportion (45%) required respiratory intervention, including one intubation and two with a need for bi-level positive airway pressure (BPAP) support.

Infants and children with craniofacial abnormalities including micrognathia or mid-facial hypoplasia can have severe OSAS. It has been reported that surgery for OSAS in patients with craniofacial malformations is less likely to succeed in infants <12 months of age, and can result in long hospital stays and difficulty with extubation as compared to older infants and children undergoing similar procedures. Although older children with craniofacial abnormalities are more likely to have improvement in OSAS by surgical intervention, they are still at risk for postoperative complications (27). Craniosynostosis with associated midface hypoplasia can result in severe OSAS and a coexisting Chiari malformation can add an element of abnormal central respiratory control, further adding to the risk of complications. Children with Down syndrome have multiple reasons for OSAS, including midface hypoplasia, relative macroglossia, hypotonia, obesity, and occasionally hypothyroidism. Severe OSAS is therefore not uncommon in these children. A series of 16 patients with Down syndrome found that 25% required PICU care postoperatively. In addition, the authors commented that persistent symptomatic apnea and hypoxemia were common following T&A (28).

Therapy to support children with respiratory compromise following T&A or other airway surgery can include prolonged intubation or a nasopharyngeal airway. The use of noninvasive ventilation, either continuous positive airway pressure (CPAP) or BPAP is attractive as it avoids intubation and can sometimes be performed on a pediatric unit after the patient is stable. However, some practitioners have questioned the safety of BPAP in the immediate postoperative period with concerns regarding subcutaneous emphysema dissecting at the surgical site, bleeding, and uncomfortable drying of the upper airway. A study of 1321 patients following T&A described that nine patients managed postoperatively with BPAP. Four patients were obese, four had underlying neurologic disease, three had asthma, and three were younger than 3 years of age. All tolerated positive-pressure therapy without complications. Two of the obese patients were eventually discharged home with BPAP therapy. Thus, there appears to be a role for noninvasive ventilation in the management of complicated patients immediately following adenotonsillectomy. Careful attention to the selection of the mask interface to avoid skin breakdown and for adequate humidification is critical (29).

Most children with OSAS will be treated with adenotonsillectomy as first-line therapy, even if there are other anatomic or functional abnormalities that are likely contributing to the upper airway obstruction. However, some will undergo a more extensive procedure, uvulopalatopharyngoplasty, which includes not only removal of the tonsils, but the tonsillar pillars and uvula as well. This procedure is most often reserved for patients with cerebral palsy or Down syndrome where there is a high probability that there will be residual obstruction following T&A alone (1,30–32). The use of mandibular distraction osteogenesis is being used with increasing frequency for infants and children with syndromes that include micrognathia. Among them are Robin sequence, Treacher–Collins syndrome, and conditions with hemifacial microsomia (33–35). This procedure represents a considerable therapeutic advance, as previously many of these patients would have required a tracheostomy. Studies evaluating infants with upper airway obstruction treated by internal mandibular distraction osteogenesis have documented success and avoidance of tracheostomy in the majority of infants. The infants are kept intubated for several days postoperatively (34,35). Treatment of OSAS in patients with Beckwith–Wiedemann (and occasionally Down syndrome) may require tongue reduction surgery (30). As a whole, the group of children requiring complex surgical treatment for OSAS tends to have more severe sleep-disordered breathing and other risk factors for postoperative difficulties. Thus, they should be observed for a period of time in the PICU and may require several days of intubation following surgery. Despite surgical therapy, some will have only minimal improvement in OSAS and will need transition to long-term positive-pressure therapy (CPAP or BPAP) or will require tracheostomy placement.

Occasionally, the initial presentation of patients with OSAS will be as acute respiratory failure. This is less common in the current era, where the recognition of sleep-disordered breathing has increased, and the literature contains little evidence to guide treatment. These patients may be otherwise normal or have one of the risk factors listed in **Table 51.2**. Unlike the majority of patients with OSAS, they may have experienced long-term hypercapnia with resulting blunting of their respiratory drive necessitating extreme caution in the use of supplemental O_2. Injudicious application of high flow O_2 in this situation can precipitate a respiratory arrest (9). Intubation and ventilation or continuous noninvasive ventilation to correct respiratory acidosis may be indicated. Intubation may be technically difficult. Less severe patients may be managed with placement of a nasopharyngeal tube (36). Pulmonary hypertension with right heart failure and pulmonary edema may be present and will require treatment with diuretics and referral to a cardiologist. Long-standing upper airway obstruction may have prevented adequate clearance of pulmonary secretions, and treatment with antibiotics may be indicated. Systemic steroids may be administered to attempt to acutely decrease the size of adenoidal and tonsillar tissue (37). The patient should be stabilized before definitive surgical therapy is considered. In this instance, PSG documentation of OSAS is not required preoperatively, but it is necessary following therapy as residual breathing difficulties during sleep are common following this presentation (5,6).

OSAS is estimated to affect about 3% of all children. Therefore, unrecognized cases of OSAS can present to the PICU following other surgical procedures, trauma, or other medical illnesses. Unrecognized sleep apnea can adversely affect surgical outcomes (38). Changes in respiratory control following anesthesia can worsen symptoms of OSAS. They are likely to have a greater degree of respiratory depression (lower minute ventilation, hypercapnia, and central apnea) associated with anesthesia and worsened by opiates, as compared with children without sleep-disordered breathing (32). The stress of surgery has important effects on sleep architecture that can result in sleep fragmentation and deprivation and REM sleep reduction. Studies in adults have revealed that although REM sleep may be inhibited on the first postoperative night, there is a rebound of REM sleep on the second or third night. While potentially important for all postoperative patients, in the presence of OSAS, this can result in more opportunity for REM-related hypoxemia or obstructive apneas, at a time when the intensity of monitoring may have been relaxed. In addition, the sleep fragmentation inherent in hospitalization may change upper airway neuromuscular function, favoring airway obstruction and apnea. Studies of adults with OSAS who underwent orthopedic procedures document cardiorespiratory complications in one-third of patients, including unplanned ICU transfers and reintubation (39). Therefore, careful screening of surgical patients for OSAS and its recognition in postoperative patients is essential (40).

The adult OSAS literature contains evidence that stabilization by positive airway pressure (CPAP or BPAP) therapy prior to elective surgery significantly reduces the operative risk and improves the postoperative course as compared with untreated OSAS (39,41). Positive-pressure therapy can be administered continuously postoperatively with a gradual wean to nighttime use only, allowing the use of adequate sedation and analgesia with less concern regarding respiratory depression. With the advent of the pediatric obesity epidemic, more patients who have coexisting OSAS will require intensive care for various reasons. Some will suffer from the metabolic syndrome with insulin resistance and systemic hypertension. A significant number will have OSAS that may not be recognized until extubation, which will require transition to positive-pressure therapy and long-term follow-up by a pulmonary or sleep medicine specialist.

As discussed previously, the perioperative use of positive-pressure therapy has been reported to reduce complications in adult patients with OSAS. Certainly, if this therapy has been used at home, arrangements must be made to continue this after surgery. Although patients with untreated OSAS may benefit from positive-pressure support after surgery, pressure titration and adaptation of the patient to the mask may be difficult when the child is recovering from surgery. Judicious use of narcotics in pain management, avoiding or minimizing sedation, and careful respiratory monitoring with frequent assessment of airway status are required with OSAS (36,39).

SUDDEN INFANT DEATH SYNDROME

Sudden infant death syndrome (SIDS) is defined as the sudden unexpected death of an infant, under 1 year of age, with onset of the fatal episode apparently occurring during sleep, that remains unexplained after a thorough investigation, including performance of a complete autopsy and review of the circumstances of death and the clinical history (42,43). SIDS is the most common cause of death in infants between the ages of 1 month and 1 year, yet its cause remains unknown (44,45). The typical scenario is that parents or caregivers place their apparently healthy baby for an overnight sleeping period or a daytime nap. They return later to find the baby lifeless. In some cases, the parents or caregivers have been within hearing distance of the baby, and they have come back within 30 minutes of putting their baby down, to find that the baby has died during that short period of time. Yet no sounds suggested that struggling occurred. Thus, SIDS appears to occur swiftly and silently.

Most SIDS infants are without vital signs when found. However, many receive cardiopulmonary resuscitation by emergency responders, and these infants are often transported from the place of death to a nearby hospital by emergency medical personnel. Most SIDS infants are not able to be resuscitated in the Emergency Department. However, in a small percentage of babies, resuscitation successfully restores a heartbeat, though spontaneous ventilation does not return, and the infant is transported to a PICU on life support. Thus, pediatric intensivists care for "SIDS" infants in these situations. These cases are frequently referred to as "aborted" or "interrupted" SIDS.

For those babies presenting with a sudden severe cardiorespiratory arrest, and who were only able to be resuscitated to the point that a heartbeat returns, the outlook is poor. These babies usually deteriorate and develop signs of brain death within 24–48 hours. Most often, these babies are pronounced death by neurologic criteria (brain death) using appropriate clinical expertise and/or testing. In some infants, this may be problematic because agonal or gasping respiration is preserved as the open fontanelle prevents downward brainstem coning. Presumably, the initial event was so severe that neurologic damage occurs despite the brief success at regaining a heartbeat. However, these babies should be evaluated for disorders that can cause rapid death. These would include sepsis, trauma (particularly head trauma), cardiac lesions (particularly serious arrhythmias or anomalous coronary arteries), metabolic disorders, and respiratory disorders (particularly pneumonia, or craniofacial abnormalities predisposing to OSAS). If child abuse or neglect is suspected, the intensivist should notify appropriate legal authorities. It is not the primary job of the intensivist to make the case of child abuse or to rule it out. Rather, trained professionals specializing in evaluation for child abuse are likely to be more successful at making these determinations (46).

All states in the United States and most Western countries require a thorough postmortem investigation, including an autopsy with toxicology screen, to determine the cause of death of babies who died suddenly at home, in child care, or outside a hospital setting. By definition, the autopsy does not reveal an identifiable cause of death in SIDS deaths (42,43). In most jurisdictions, babies treated in the ICU still fall under the legal mandate for the Coroner or Medical Examiner to determine the cause of death. In these cases, the death should most appropriately be viewed as occurring where the baby was discovered in arrest (where the death process began), rather than in the hospital. Thus, an examination of the death scene by trained coroner's investigators and a complete autopsy by skilled pathologists should be performed.

Infrequently, a baby diagnosed with brain death, but having a heartbeat on life support, may be a suitable donor for organ transplantation. Usually, the "SIDS" event is accompanied by such severe hypoxemia that organs are not useful for transplantation. However, if the intensivist believes that organs may be suitable for transplantation, permission of the medical examiner is usually required before organs can be harvested. A potential conflict exists between examination of vital organs by the medical examiner to determine the cause of death, and using these organs for transplantation to save the life of other infants. If some organs do seem potentially useful for transplantation, most coroners and medical examiners will permit this after discussion. Organs that function as successful transplants in another child are not likely to have been the cause of death of the "SIDS" baby.

An important aspect of the intensivist's care of such "SIDS" infants is to provide the surviving family members with information about SIDS and resources for support (47–50). If the infant does not have gross evidence of trauma or another cause of death, SIDS is most likely to emerge as the cause of death after the postmortem evaluation. Increasingly, many sudden deaths in infants during sleep occur with epidemiologic risk factors, such as prone sleeping, overheating, pillow and soft blankets in the crib, bed-sharing, and smoking in the home (51,52).

The death scene investigation is the most useful to distinguish SIDS from accidental causes of death (42). Babies requiring treatment in the PICU have been transported from the scene where the death process began, and death was pronounced later at the hospital. Often, a death scene investigation has not been performed at the location where the process began, and therefore valuable information about environmental contributors to the death can be lost. Hence, it is not always possible to know whether the death represents a "true SIDS" or whether it has had some contribution by accidental causes.

The intensivist is not in a position to investigate the cause of death. When speaking with the parents, the intensivist can indicate that this looks like it was a SIDS death, if appropriate, although further investigations and autopsy are needed to

confirm this. Parent grief following a SIDS death is complicated by the fact that no one can tell parents why their baby died. They tend to blame themselves, and their guilt is even greater than that of parents whose babies died from other causes (47–50). SIDS parent support groups are the single best source of support and information for them and parents of infants dying from other causes. SIDS parents from these groups are available 24 hours per day to speak with newly bereaved parents and to provide comfort and support. In the United States, the national SIDS parent support organization is First Candle/SIDS Alliance. In the United Kingdom, the national SIDS parent support organization is the Foundation for the Study and Prevention of Infant Deaths (47–50).

By definition, SIDS occurs in the first year of life. It is most common between 2 and 4 months of age. It is less common in the first month of life, and approximately 95% of SIDS deaths occur before 6 months of age (44,45). SIDS is slightly more common in males. The risk of SIDS is higher in infants born prematurely or with low birth weight. Babies born to mothers who smoked cigarettes, drank alcohol, or used illicit drugs during pregnancy also face an increased risk. African American and Native American babies also have an increased risk. Although the cause of SIDS is unknown, most researchers believe that it results from an interaction of a developmental window of vulnerability (age 2–4 months), extrinsic environmental risks, and intrinsic infant vulnerability (infants have immature protective responses to environmental and physiologic challenges) (3,51,53,54).

The sleeping environment plays an important role in SIDS (44). Sleeping in the prone position, on soft bedding, with soft items in the bed, overheating, and bed-sharing are all associated with an increased risk of SIDS. In 2010, the most recent year where we have complete data, the incidence of SIDS in the United States was 0.50 SIDS deaths per 1000 live births, or 1 in every 2000 babies born. The SIDS rate has fallen dramatically since 1992 owing to the "Back to Sleep" and "Safe to Sleep" campaigns, which seek to educate parents to place their babies to sleep in a safe sleeping environment (44,45). However, even babies whose parents have followed all of these recommendations continue to die of SIDS.

APPARENT LIFE-THREATENING EVENTS

An apparent life-threatening event (ALTE) is defined as an event, which is frightening to the observer, where the infant is witnessed to have color change (cyanosis or pallor), tone change (limpness, rarely stiffness), or apnea, and vigorous stimulation, mouth-to-mouth breathing, or resuscitation are required to revive the infant (55–57). In most cases, observers feared that the infant was in the process of dying. Sometimes, they appear to respond quickly and may appear entirely normal when medically examined at a later time. Other infants appear to require intensive intervention or resuscitation, and they may still exhibit signs of a serious hypoxic event several minutes later (57). It is this latter group, with persistent respiratory distress or a continued need for ventilatory support, who will usually be admitted to an ICU for observation and/or treatment.

Initial Evaluation

ALTE is a clinical diagnosis based on a good history of the event by an observer (55,57). There are no diagnostic tests that can be used to determine whether a child experienced an ALTE. However, the presence of laboratory evidence for severe hypoxia (increased acidosis, lactate, liver enzymes, or urinary hypoxanthines) can contribute to the assessment of the severity of the event. In order for a diagnosis of ALTE to be made, most clinicians require that significant intervention was required to revive the baby (57). For those infants with a history of some serious event, who have signs and/or persistent symptoms suggesting a major hypoxic episode, there is little doubt that something serious has occurred. These infants will require a diagnostic evaluation to discover the etiology of the event. This is necessary both to properly treat the underlying etiology and to reduce the chance of a recurrence (58). In a series of infants presenting with an ALTE, those who had recurrent events and were less than 1 month of age had subsequent events, required subsequent intervention, or had a diagnoses for which hospitalization was required (58). Therefore, these infants should always be admitted to the hospital.

Relationship Between Apparent Life-Threatening Event and Sudden Infant Death Syndrome

Clinically, there is concern about infants who present with an ALTE because it has been believed to be associated with an increased risk for SIDS. However, there is no scientific evidence that ALTE confers an increased risk for SIDS (55,57,59–61). The Collaborative Home Infant Monitoring Evaluation (CHIME) study monitored over 1000 babies during sleep in their homes for 6 months (61). They did not find that ALTE babies had a higher risk of recurrent apneic events than healthy term control infants (61). Further, the peak incidence of apnea in babies occurred at a much younger age than when SIDS occurs, suggesting that apnea is not related to SIDS (60,61). In addition, relatively few SIDS parents report that their babies had any serious apneas prior to death (62). The most important difference between ALTE and SIDS is that ALTE babies survive their episodes, whereas SIDS babies die. SIDS babies die after a single event. ALTE babies often survive, many even before treatment. Thus, ALTE babies do not all die of SIDS, and the two conditions should not be equated

(55,57,60,61). Nevertheless, the cardiorespiratory physiology of infants is rapidly undergoing change, and is intrinsically unstable. Therefore, a number of diseases and stresses can cause cardiorespiratory collapse. These infants deserve a careful diagnostic evaluation and appropriate treatment.

Diagnostic Evaluation

Infants who experienced an ALTE and are admitted to an ICU may have evidence of ongoing cardiorespiratory instability, metabolic acidosis (presumably from a prolonged hypoxic event), or evidence of some other potentially life-threatening event. They must first be evaluated for adequate cardiorespiratory status. An arterial blood gas, blood sugar, and chest x-ray are first-line diagnostic procedures. If the infant appears to be septic, then a diagnostic evaluation for sepsis will be necessary, including a lumbar puncture. Other diagnostic evaluations should be performed as indicated by the clinical history of the event and physical examination (57). There is no cookbook series of diagnostic tests for all infants with ALTE. Testing should be guided by the specific circumstances of the ALTE infant and event (57,63). A list of possible etiologies for ALTE, and appropriate diagnostic testing, is shown in Table 51.3. It should be emphasized that not all of these diagnostic studies are required for evaluating an ALTE; only those indicated by the history and physical examination should be performed (63). In a series of 243 infants presenting with ALTE, only 17% of the diagnostic tests performed were positive, and only 6% contributed to making a diagnosis (63). Tests most likely to be positive include blood count, blood gases, chest x-ray, and an evaluation for gastroesophageal reflux (63).

Sleep studies are frequently used to evaluate infants with ALTE. Generally, these are not useful in predicting the recurrence risk for subsequent events (57). Therefore, they should not be used to decide if an infant will or will not have other severe ALTE. However, they are extremely useful in diagnosing sleep-disordered breathing that may have contributed to or caused an ALTE, such as OSAS, hypoxia due to chronic lung disease, or central hypoventilation syndromes.

TABLE 51.3

DIAGNOSTIC EVALUATION FOR APPARENT LIFE-THREATENING EVENT INFANTS

■ POTENTIAL DIAGNOSIS/ETIOLOGY	■ DIAGNOSTIC TESTS
Infection, sepsis	Complete blood count. Blood, urine, and cerebrospinal fluid cultures
Hypocalcemia	Serum calcium
Electrolyte imbalance	Serum electrolytes
Dehydration	BUN, creatinine
Hypoglycemia	Blood sugar
Asphyxia	Arterial blood gas (pH)
Pneumonia, chronic lung disease	Chest x-ray
Congenital heart disease, cardiomyopathy	Electrocardiogram, echocardiogram
Cardiac arrhythmia, prolonged QT interval syndrome	Electrocardiogram, 24-h Holter monitoring
Trauma, child abuse	Skeletal series, skull x-ray, head CT scan, retinal examination
Seizures	Electroencephalogram
GERD	Barium swallow, gastric scintiscan
Sleep-disordered breathing	Overnight polysomnography
OSA	
Central hypoventilation syndrome	
Upper airway obstruction, craniofacial abnormality, congenital airway anomaly	Laryngoscopy, bronchoscopy
Inborn errors of metabolism	Serum ammonia level, urine organic acids, plasma amino acids
Drug ingestion, toxic exposure	Serum and urine toxicology

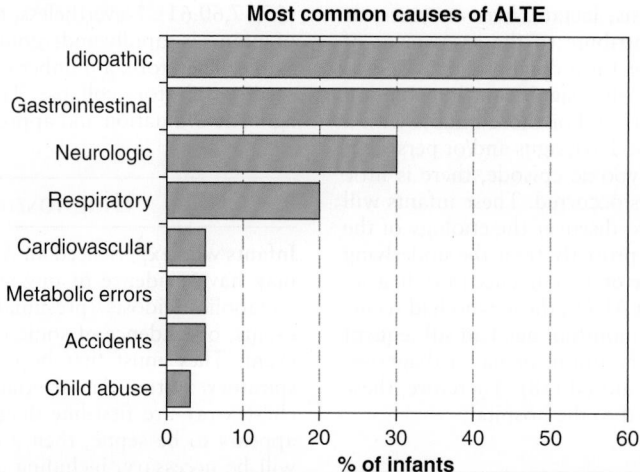

FIGURE 51.1. The most common etiologies of ALTE. The approximate proportion of ALTE infants (X-axis) who have ALTE caused by the listed diagnoses. (Data modified from Kahn A. Recommended clinical evaluation of infants with an apparent life-threatening event. Consensus document of the European Society for the Study and Prevention of Infant Death, 2003. *Eur J Pediatr* 2004;163:108–15.)

Etiology

As many as 50%–70% of ALTE can be explained by an identified diagnosis (9,44). The most common causes of ALTE are shown in **Figure 51.1**. In some series, as much as 50% of ALTEs are caused by gastrointestinal disorders (57). Although gastroesophageal reflux disease (GERD) is frequently found on diagnostic testing for ALTE, it should not be assumed that this is the cause of the event (57,64). Apneas have not temporally correlated with gastroesophageal reflux events on polysomnography (65). ALTEs of gastrointestinal origin usually occur during or shortly after feeding, and they are more likely to occur during wakefulness. They may be accompanied by choking, vomiting, or coughing. Neurologic problems account for up to 30% of ALTE in some series (57,63). Seizures are the most common neurologic etiology of an ALTE. Electroencephalograms should be performed when seizures are suspected, but they may not be diagnostic. The diagnosis of seizures is based on a typical history. Congenital brainstem anomalies, especially Arnold Chiari type I or II, may cause apnea. When neurologic causes of ALTE are suspected, a brainstem MRI may be helpful.

Approximately 20% of ALTE may be due to respiratory disorders (57,63). OSA can occur with viral infections, such as CMV, RSV, or influenza. Craniofacial anomalies predispose to obstructive apnea in infants (66). Central nervous system depressant medications enhance susceptibility to OSAS. OSAS can be idiopathic in infants, especially if premature and exacerbation by anemia (67). A history of noisy breathing, snoring, or excessive sweating during sleep should prompt a further evaluation for OSAS (57,66). Cardiovascular problems account for only ~5% of ALTE (57).

It has been estimated that inborn errors of metabolism account for 2%–5% of ALTE (57,68). These are associated with fasting, fever, or vomiting. Inborn errors of β-oxidation of fatty acids have been described in ALTE babies with severe recurrent events, those that persist beyond a year of age, and in babies with a family history of previous infant deaths and/or severe apneas (68).

Less than 3% of ALTE appear to be due to child abuse (57,69). The diagnosis of child abuse is clear when there are signs of trauma, abuse, previous fractures, or neglect (failure to thrive) (46,69). A family history of previous SIDS, infant deaths, or ALTE, especially if there are unusual associated circumstances, may increase suspicion for child abuse. However, it is not the primary role of the intensivist to rule the diagnosis of child abuse in or out. Rather, they should refer suspicious cases to experts in the field who are trained to deal with these issues (46).

Management

Medical management of the ALTE infant in the ICU is primarily directed toward stabilizing the cardiorespiratory status of the infant following the event. Once this is achieved, a diagnostic evaluation, directed by the history and physical examination, should be performed. If an identifiable cause explains the ALTE, the treatment should be directed toward that diagnosis. However, in as many as 50% of ALTE infants, a specific etiology will not be determined (57). The appropriate post-PICU treatment of these infants is controversial. Although home apnea-bradycardia monitoring has been used to manage infants with ALTE and no identified etiology, few of these infants will have recurrent events, and infants have died while home apnea–bradycardia monitoring was in use (61,70).

SLEEP IN THE INTENSIVE CARE UNIT

The purpose of sleep is not fully understood, but the consequences of sleep deprivation are well described. Addressing the impact of sleep deprivation on health care providers is one of the most important aims of improving health care safety. However, sleep deprivation also affects the hospitalized patients we care for, particularly in the PICU. Inadequate sleep can cause neurocognitive and psychological deficits. Sleep deprivation is a physiologic stressor and can affect autonomic, immunologic, metabolic, and hormonal function. Finally, patients have identified poor sleep as one of the greatest hardships endured during their ICU stays (71–73).

Sleep in critically ill patients is characterized by an abnormal distribution with sleep times scattered throughout a 24-hour period, rather than consolidated at night. Thus, total sleep time may not be affected, but because it is fragmented, the restorative properties may be lacking. The organization, or architecture, of sleep stages is also affected with an increase in "light sleep" (Stage N1) and decreased time in deeper sleep (Stages N2, N3, and REM). Sleep in the ICU is disrupted by frequent arousals and awakenings. Over one-third of adult patients recall poor sleep during their ICU stay, and the vast majority rate poor sleep as being moderate or extremely bothersome. In one study, only an inability to communicate by ventilated patients was rated as more stressful than the inability to sleep (74).

All hospitalized children are at risk for poor sleep from illness, pain, medications, therapies, and an unfamiliar sleep environment. However, the ICU environment is believed to be the most important factor in sleep disruption for the critically ill patient. Noise and light levels are high and are not conducive to sleep (75). Although monitors, alarms, ventilators, pagers, etc. contribute to the ambient noise, talking appears to be the biggest culprit. Mechanical ventilation poses an additional challenge to a good night's sleep. Intubation, the ventilator mode, intermittent suctioning, and an inability to communicate may all contribute to sleep disruption. Patient-ventilator asynchrony with noninvasive positive-pressure ventilation also appears to interfere with sleep (76). The need for assisted ventilation may also be a marker for greater disease severity with inherently poor sleep. The presence of sepsis alters sleep architecture and interferes with the normal circadian pattern of melatonin secretion (73,77,78).

The medications used in the ICU often impact sleep, both during use and after discontinuation. Benzodiazepines and opioids cause REM suppression, and consequently there is a REM rebound effect following discontinuation, which can result in nightmares or disturbing dreams. Sedation has some of the properties of natural sleep (decreased awareness of surroundings, decreased motor activity), but it is not known whether, or how well, sedation mimics the proposed function and purpose of sleep, which likely includes restoration and maintenance of neural and somatic function. One study followed two children receiving continuous sedation and neuromuscular blockade following laryngotracheoplasty by continuous polysomnography for 96 hours. The PSG records revealed that sleep did occur under these conditions, but it was fragmented and occurred both during the day and the night (79). Another study of ventilated children who received continuous sedation and opiate analgesia found that sleep was severely fragmented and that REM sleep accounted for only 3% of total sleep time (75). A study of fentanyl withdrawal in neonates revealed that a reduction in sleep time was the most frequent troublesome sign (80). The use or discontinuation of many other classes of medications can also affect sleep. For example, an abrupt discontinuation of a β-blocker can fragment sleep dramatically. Therefore, a review of all medications, both current and recent, should be performed whenever sleep disturbance or deprivation affects children in the PICU (72,73).

Sleep deprivation results in a number of neurologic and behavioral complications. Reduced vigilance and reaction time are the impairments most relevant for sleep deprivation in health care providers. For patients, mood alterations (irritability) and organic brain dysfunction (delusions and hallucinations) are probably more important. Delirium can occur in the PICU setting and has serious negative prognostic implications. The possible link between sleep disturbance and delirium clearly makes this an important area for future research (81,82).

Sleep deprivation in critically ill patients may impair immunologic function (83,84). While it is true that the clinical significance of these findings is unknown, when a patient's survival may depend on their ability to mount adequate immune response to multiple challenges, it seems prudent to enhance sleep quality whenever possible. Sleep loss affects the secretion of hormones that can play a role in the body's response to stress, including increases in cortisol, norepinephrine, and thyroid hormone. Critical illness can also alter these same hormones. Both sleep deprivation and critical illness cause insulin resistance that can be clinically significant. As the presence of sleep deprivation is potentially more amenable to change than the severity of the underlying illness, efforts to enhance sleep in the PICU are a worthwhile endeavor (72,73,78).

Monsen et al. reported their efforts to reduce noise and sleep disturbance in a neurointensive care unit. Sleep disturbances were documented in subsets of patients in a total of fourteen 24-hour periods before the intervention. The purpose of the study was to target efforts before and after the intervention to evaluate effectiveness. Investigators found that routine nursing care activities were the most disturbing. Also implicated were inhalational treatments, CPAP, and ambient noise. A behavioral modification program was introduced for the staff that included education about the concept of healthy sleep, or sleep hygiene, and how to structure activities to minimize sleep disruption. The findings of the study emphasized the need to limit care activities between the hours of midnight and 05:00 to provide time with consolidated sleep as well as engaging the ICU staff in continuous efforts to reduce noise levels (77). Controlling light exposure with open blinds during the day and decreased light at night has also been recommended. Melatonin therapy may have a role in entraining circadian rhythm-based results from a small trial in critically ill adults (85). Kamdar and colleagues implemented a comprehensive quality improvement project directed at improving sleep and reducing delirium in an adult ICU. While significant differences in perception of sleep quality were lacking following the intervention, there were improvements in noise levels and in the incidence of delirium and coma (71).

CONCLUSIONS AND FUTURE DIRECTIONS

Sleep is a period of vulnerability for the respiratory system. OSAS, ALTE, and SIDS are manifestations of this vulnerability. The perturbations of the pathophysiology inherent in critical illness do not spare the process of sleep, and the typically healing environment of the PICU disturbs rather than enhances sleep. Goals for the future include identifying more exact methods of predicting the infants and children at the greatest risk for OSAS and its attendant complications, understanding the etiologies of ALTE and SIDS, and establishing preventative strategies and developing approaches to minimize the effects of sleep disruption in the PICU setting.

References

1. Krimsky WR, Leiter JC. Respiratory control during sleep. In: Lee-Chiang T, ed. *Sleep: A Comprehensive Handbook*. Hoboken, NJ: John Wiley and Sons, 2006:663–7.
2. Woodson BT. Physiology of sleep-disordered breathing. In: Lee-Chiong T, ed. *Sleep: A Comprehensive Handbook*. Hoboken, NJ: John Wiley and Sons, 2006:211–22.
3. Carroll JL, Agarwal A. Development of ventilatory control in infants. *Paediatr Respir Rev* 2010;11(4):199–207.
4. Isono S. Upper airway muscle function during sleep. In: Loughlin GM, Caroll JL, Marcus CL, eds. *Sleep and Breathing in Children: A Developmental Approach*. New York, NY: Marcel Dekker, 2000:261–92.
5. Marcus CL, Brooks LJ, Draper KA, et al; American Academy of Pediatrics. Diagnosis and management of childhood obstructive sleep apnea syndrome. *Pediatrics* 2012;130(3):576–84.

6. Marcus CL, Brooks LJ, Ward SD, et al; American Academy of Pediatrics. Diagnosis and management of childhood obstructive sleep apnea syndrome. *Pediatrics* 2012;130(3):e714–55.

7. Marcus CL, Moore RH, Rosen CL, et al; Childhood Adenotonsillectomy Trial (CHAT). A randomized trial of adenotonsillectomy for childhood sleep apnea. *N Engl J Med* 2013;68(25):2366–76.

8. Balbani APS, Weber SAT, Montovani JC. Update in obstructive sleep apnea syndrome in children. *Rev Bras Otorrinolaringol* 2005;71(1):74–80.

9. Marcus CL. Sleep-disordered breathing in children. *Am J Respir Crit Care Med* 2001;164:16–30.

10. Kelly A, Dougherty S, Cucchiara A, et al. Catecholamines, adiponectin, and insulin resistance as measured by HOMA in children with obstructive sleep apnea. *Sleep* 2010;33(9):1185–91.

11. Kessler R, Chaouat A, Schinkewitch P, et al. The obesity–hypoventilation syndrome revisited: A prospective study of 34 consecutive cases. *Chest* 2001;120:369–76.

12. Lesser DJ, Bhatia R, Tran H, et al. Sleep fragmentation and intermittent hypoxemia are associated with decreased insulin sensitivity in obese adolescent Latino males. *Pediatr Res* 2012;72:293–8.

13. Kaemingk KL, Pasvogel AE, Goodwin JL, et al. Learning in children and sleep-disordered breathing: Findings of the Tucson Children's Assessment of Sleep Apnea (TuCASA) prospective cohort study. *J Int Neuropsychol Soc* 2003;9:1016–26.

14. O'Brien LM, Mervis CB, Holbrook CR, et al. Neurobehavioral implications of habitual snoring in children. *Pediatrics* 2004;114:44–9.

15. Marcus CL, Omlin KJ, Basinki DJ, et al. Normal polysomnographic values for children and adolescents. *Am Rev Respir Dis* 1992;146:1235–9.

16. Witmans MB, Keens TG, Davidson Ward SL, et al. Obstructive hypopneas in children and adolescents: Normal values. *Am J Respir Crit Care Med* 2003;168:1540.

17. Helfaer MA, McColley SA, Pyzik PL, et al. Polysomnography after adenotonsillectomy in mild pediatric obstructive sleep apnea. *Crit Care Med* 1996;24:1323–7.

18. Helfaer MA, Wilson MD. Obstructive sleep apnea, control of ventilation, and anesthesia in children. *Pediatr Clin North Am* 1991;41:131–51.

19. Paradise JL, Bluestone CD, Colborn DK, et al. Tonsillectomy and adenoidectomy for recurrent throat infections for moderately affected children. *Pediatrics* 2002;110:7–15.

20. Rosen GM, Muckle RP, Mahowald MW, et al. Postoperative respiratory compromise in children with obstructive sleep apnea syndrome: Can it be anticipated? *Pediatrics* 1994;93:784–8.

21. Sher AE. Upper airway surgery for obstructive sleep apnea. In: Lee-Chiong T, ed. *Sleep: A Comprehensive Handbook*. Hoboken, NJ: John Wiley and Sons, 2006:211–22.

22. McMolley SA, April MM, Carroll JL, et al. Respiratory compromise after adenotonsillectomy in children with obstructive sleep apnea. *Arch Otolaryngol Head Neck Surg* 1992;118:940–3.

23. Walker P, Whitehead B, Rowley M. Criteria for elective admission to the paediatric intensive care unit following adenotonsillectomy for severe obstructive sleep apnoea. *Anaesth Intensive Care* 2004;32:43–6.

24. Hill CA, Litvak A, Canapari C, et al. A pilot study to identify pre- and peri-operative risk factors for airway complications following adenotonsillectomy for treatment of severe pediatric OSA. *Int J Pediatr Otorhinolaryngol* 2011;75(11):1385–90. doi:10.1016/j.ijporl.2011.07.034.

25. Kieran S, Gorman C, Kirby A, et al. Risk factors of desaturation after tonsillectomy: Analysis of 4,092 consecutive pediatric cases. *Laryngoscope* 2013;123(10):2554–9.

26. Spector A, Scheid S, Hassink S, et al. Adenotonsillectomy in the morbidly obese child. *Int J Pediatr Otolaryngol* 2003;67:359–64.

27. Januskiewicz JS, Cohen SR, Burstein FD, et al. Age-related outcomes of sleep apnea surgery in infants and children. *Ann Plast Surg* 1997;38:465–77.

28. Bower CM, Richmond D. Tonsillectomy and adenoidectomy in patients with Down syndrome. *Int J Pediatr Otorhinolaryngol* 1995;33:141–8.

29. Friedman O, Chidekel A, Lawless SL, et al. Postoperative bilevel positive airway pressure ventilation after tonsillectomy and adenoidectomy in children—A preliminary report. *Int J Pediatr Otorhinolaryngol* 1999;51:177–80.

30. Kennedy DJ, Waters KA. Investigation and treatment of upper-airway obstruction: Childhood sleep disorders I. Obstructive sleep apnea syndrome is common and is associated with significant childhood morbidities. *MJA Pract Essent* 2005;182(8):419–23.

31. Magardino TM, Tom LW. Surgical management of obstructive sleep apnea in children with cerebral palsy. *Laryngoscope* 1999;109:1611–5.

32. Waters KA, McBrien F, Stewart P, et al. Effects of OSA, inhalational anesthesia, and fentanyl on the airway and ventilation of children. *J Appl Physiol* 2002;92:1987–94.

33. Chigurupati R, Massie J, Dargaville P, et al. Internal mandibular distraction to relieve airway obstruction in infants and young children with micrognathia. *Pediatr Pulmonol* 2004;37:230–35.

34. Hammoudeh J, Bindingnavele VK, Davis B, et al. Neonatal and infant distraction as an alternative to tracheostomy in obstructive sleep apnea. *Cleft Palate Craniofac J* 2012;49(1):32–8.

35. Izadi K, Yellon R, Mandell DL, et al. Correction of upper airway obstruction in the newborn with internal mandibular distraction osteogenesis. *J Craniofac Surg* 2003;14:493–9.

36. Moos D, Cuddeford J. Implications of obstructive sleep apnea syndrome for the peri-anesthesia nurse. *J Perianesth Nurs* 2006;21:103–18.

37. Al-Ghamdi SA, Manoukian JJ, Morielli A, et al. Do systemic corticosteroids effectively treat obstructive sleep apnea secondary to adenotonsillar hypertrophy? *Laryngoscope* 1997;107(10):1382–7.

38. Warwick JP, Mason DG. Obstructive sleep apnoea syndrome in children. *Anaesthesia* 1998;53:571–79.

39. Kaw R, Michota F, Jaffer A, et al. Unrecognized sleep apnea in the surgical patient: Implications for the perioperative setting. *Chest* 2006;129:198–205.

40. Kaw R, Gali B, Collop NA. Perioperative care of patients with obstructive sleep apnea. *Curr Treat Options Neurol* 2011;13(5):496–507.

41. Rennotte MT, Baele P, Aubert G, et al. Nasal continuous positive airway pressure in the perioperative management of patients with obstructive sleep apnea submitted to surgery. *Chest* 1995;107:367–74.

42. Krous HF, Beckwith JB, Byard RW, et al. Sudden infant death syndrome (SIDS) and unclassified sudden infant deaths (USID): A definitional and diagnostic approach. *Pediatrics* 2004;114:234–8.

43. Willinger M, James LS, Catz C. Defining the sudden infant syndrome (SIDS): Deliberations of an expert panel convened by the National Institute of Child Health and Human Development. *Pediatr Pathol* 1991;11:677–84.

44. Moon RY, Darnall RA, Goodstein MH, et al; American Academy of Pediatrics. Task Force on Sudden Infant Death Syndrome: SIDS and other sleep-related infant deaths: Expansion of recommendations for a safe infant sleeping environment. *Pediatrics* 2011;128:1030–9.

45. Moon RY, Darnall RA, Goodstein MH, et al. Technical report: American Academy of Pediatrics Task Force on Sudden Infant Death Syndrome: SIDS and other sleep-related infant deaths: Expansion of recommendations for a safe infant sleeping environment. *Pediatrics* 2011 Nov;128(5):e1341-67. doi: 10.1542/peds.2011-2285. Epub 2011 Oct 17.

46. Hymel KP; The Committee on Child Abuse and Neglect; American Academy of Pediatrics. Distinguishing sudden infant death syndrome from child abuse fatalities. *Pediatrics* 2006;118:427–31.

47. DeFrain J. Learning about grief from normal families: SIDS, stillbirth, and miscarriage. *J Marital Fam Therapy* 1991;17:215–32.

48. Dyregrov K, Nordanger D, Dyregrov A. Predicting psychosocial distress after suicide, SIDS, and accidents. *Death Stud* 2003;27:146–65.

49. Ostfeld BM, Ryan T, Hiatt M, et al. Maternal grief after sudden infant death syndrome. *Develop Behav Pediatr* 1993;15:156–62.

50. Wender E; The Committee on Psychosocial Aspects of Child and Family Health; American Academy of Pediatrics. Supporting the family after the death of a child. *Pediatrics* 2012;130:1164–9.

51. Fleming PJ, Tsogt B, Blair PS. Modifiable risk factors, sleep environment, developmental physiology, and common polymorphisms: Understanding and preventing sudden infant deaths. *Early Hum Dev* 2006;82:761–6.

52. Ostfeld BM, Esposito L, Perl H, et al. Concurrent risks in sudden infant death syndrome. *Pediatrics* 2010;125:447–53.

53. Filiano JJ, Kinney HC. A perspective on neuropathological findings in victims of the sudden infant death syndrome: The triple risk model. *Biol Neonate* 1994;65:194–7.

54. Kinney HC, Thach BT. The sudden infant death syndrome. *N Engl J Med* 2009;361:795–805.

55. Blackmon LR, Batton DG, Bell EF, et al; American Academy of Pediatrics Policy Statement. Apnea, sudden infant death syndrome, and home monitoring. *Pediatrics* 2003;111:914–7.

56. Kahn A, Rebuffat E, Franco P, et al. Apparent life-threatening events and apnea of infancy. In: Beckerman RC, Brouillette RT, Hunt CE, eds. *Respiratory Control Disorders in Infants and Children.* New York, NY: Williams & Wilkins, 1992:178–89.

57. Kahn A. Recommended clinical evaluation of infants with an apparent life-threatening event. Consensus document of the European Society for the Study and Prevention of Infant Death, 2003. *Eur J Pediatr* 2004;163:108–15.

58. Claudius I, Keens T. Do all infants with apparent life-threatening events need to be admitted? *Pediatrics* 2007;119:679–83.

59. Esani N, Hodgman JE, Ehsani N, et al. Apparent life-threatening events and sudden infant death syndrome: Comparison of risk factors. *J Pediatr* 2008;152:365–70.

60. Mitchell EA, Thompson JMD. Parent reported apnoea, admissions to hospital and sudden infant death syndrome. *Acta Paediatr* 2001;90:417–22.

61. Ramanathan R, Corwin MJ, Hunt CE, et al. Cardiorespiratory events recorded on home monitors: Comparison of healthy infants with those at increased risk for SIDS. *J Am Med Assoc* 2001;285:2199–207.

62. Hoffman HJ, Damus K, Hillman L, et al. Risk factors for SIDS: Results of the National Institute of Child Health and Human Development SIDS Cooperative Epidemiological Study. *Ann N Y Acad Sci* 1988;533:13–30.

63. Brand DA, Altman RL, Purtill K, et al. Yield of diagnostic testing in infants who have had an apparent life-threatening event. *Pediatrics* 2005;115:885–93.

64. Arad-Cohen N, Cohen A, Tirosh E. The relationship between gastroesophageal reflux and apnea in infants. *J Pediatr* 2000;137:321–6.

65. Kahn A, Rebuffat E, Sottiaux M, et al. Arousals induced by proximal esophageal reflux in infants. *Sleep* 1991;14:39–42.

66. Guilleminault C, Pelayo R, Leger D, et al. Apparent life-threatening events, facial dysmorphia and sleep disordered breathing. *Eur J Pediatr* 2000;159:444–9.

67. DeMaio JG, Harris MC, Deuber C, et al. Effect of blood transfusion on apnea frequency in growing premature infants. *J Pediatr* 1989;114:1039–41.

68. Arens R, Gozal D, Williams JC, et al. Recurrent apparent life-threatening events during infancy: A manifestation of inborn errors of metabolism. *J Pediatr* 1993;123:415–8.

69. Samuels MP, Southall DP. Alarms during apparent life-threatening events. *Am J Respir Crit Care Med* 2003;167:A677.

70. Davidson Ward SL, Marcus CL. Obstructive sleep apnea in infants and young children. *J Clin Neurophysiol* 1996;13(3):198–207.

71. Kamdar BB, Needham DM, Collop NA. Sleep deprivation in critical illness: Its role in physical and psychological recovery. *J Intensive Care Med* 2012;27(2):97–111.

72. Kamdar BB, King LM, Collop NA, et al. The effect of a quality improvement intervention on perceived sleep quality and cognition in medical ICU. *Crit Care Med* 2013;41(3):800–9.

73. Weinhouse GL, Schwab RJ. Sleep in the critically ill patient. *Sleep* 2006;29:707–16.

74. Nelson JE, Meier DE, Oei EJ, et al. Self-reported symptom experience of critically ill cancer patients receiving intensive care. *Crit Care Med* 2001;29:277–82.

75. Al-Samsam RH, Cullen P. Sleep and adverse environmental factors in sedated mechanically ventilated patients. *Pediatr Crit Care Med* 2005;6:562–7.

76. Roche Campo F, Drouot X, Thille AW, et al. Poor sleep quality is associated with late noninvasive ventilation failure in patients with acute hypercapnic respiratory failure. *Crit Care Med* 2010;38(2):477–85.

77. Monsén MG, Edéll-Gustafsson UM. Noise and sleep disturbance factors before and after implementation of a behavioral modification programme. *Intensive Crit Care Nurs* 2005;212:201–19.

78. Venkateshiah SB, Collop NA. Sleep and sleep disorders in the hospital. *Chest* 2012;141(5):1337–45.

79. Carno MA, Hoffman LA, Henker R, et al. Sleep monitoring in children during neuromuscular blockade in the pediatric intensive care unit. *Pediatr Crit Care Med* 2004;5:224–9.

80. Dominguez KD, Lomako DM, Katz RW, et al. Opioid withdrawal in critically ill neonates. *Ann Pharmacother* 2003;37:473–7.

81. Ely EW, Shintani A, Truman B, et al. Delirium as a predictor of mortality in mechanically ventilated patients in the intensive care unit. *J Am Med Assoc* 2004;291:1753–62.

82. Figueroa-Ramos MI, Arroyo-Novoa CM, Lee KA, et al. Sleep and delirium in ICU patients: A review of mechanisms and manifestations. *Intensive Care Med* 2009;35:781–95.

83. Faraut B, Boudjeltia KZ, Vanhamme L, et al. Immune, inflammatory and cardiovascular consequences of sleep restriction and recovery. *Sleep Med Rev* 2012;16(2):137–49. doi:10.1016/j.smrv.2011.05.001.

84. Vgontzas AN, Zoumakis E, Bixler EO, et al. Adverse effects of modest sleep restriction on sleepiness, performance, and inflammatory cytokines. *J Clin Endocrinol Metab* 2004;89(5):2119–26.

85. Bourne RS, Mills GH, Minelli C. Melatonin therapy to improve nocturnal sleep in critically ill patients: Encouraging results from a small randomized controlled trial. *Crit Care* 2008;12(2):R52.

CHAPTER 52 ■ ELECTRODIAGNOSTIC TECHNIQUES IN NEUROMUSCULAR DISEASE

MATTHEW PITT

KEY POINTS

1. Electromyography (EMG) and nerve conduction studies (NCS) should be possible in any PICU.
2. EMG and NCS data are useful to direct evaluation and provide a diagnosis in children with neuromuscular disorders.
3. EMG and NCS can help identify disorders of the peripheral nervous system acquired during intensive care.
4. Providing EMG and NCS, while possible in any PICU, requires the availability of both equipment and expertise.

This chapter is about the use of neurophysiological techniques for the investigation of disorders of the peripheral nervous system (PNS) in the pediatric intensive care unit (PICU). The PNS is defined as the motor nervous system from the anterior horn cell to the muscle and the sensory pathways up to and including the dorsal root ganglia. Discussion will be limited to the use of electrodiagnostic techniques (nerve conduction studies [NCS] and needle electromyography [EMG]). With recent developments in both machines and consumables, it is possible to do NCS and EMG in any PICU. The primary function of these techniques is the diagnosis of neuromuscular disorders (which may have resulted in the need for ventilatory support) as well as the diagnosis of unexplained weakness that develops during the PICU admission. The chapter will not cover somatosensory evoked potentials and transcranial magnetic stimulation as their primary function is to diagnose abnormality of the central nervous system, in particular, the spinal cord.

When we consider investigation of the PNS, we first need a framework for considering the neuromuscular conditions that may have resulted in admission or ventilator dependence. These conditions can be divided anatomically into those affecting the anterior horn cell, the peripheral nerves, neuromuscular junction (NMJ), and, finally, the muscle itself (see Chapters 53 and 54). These conditions may be hereditary or acquired. The pertinent *hereditary neuromuscular conditions* for pediatric intensivists include the severe forms of spinal muscular atrophy, hypomyelinating and Dejerine Sottas neuropathies, congenital myasthenic syndromes, myotonic dystrophy, and nemaline and centronuclear myopathies. The relevant *acquired neuromuscular conditions* include poliomyelitis, acute inflammatory demyelinating polyneuropathy, infantile botulism, Tick paralysis, autoimmune myasthenia gravis, and acute myositis. Conditions acquired while children are in the PICU include critical care neuromyopathy and the mononeuropathies that result from pressure or ischemia.

SIGNAL RECORDING

Equipment

Recent advances and the transition to digital technology have resulted in neurophysiological recording equipment that is smaller, more reliable, and more portable. Typical EMG and NCS recording equipment is capable of amplifying signals that are a few microvolts (μV) up to 100 mV and a bandwidth from 1 or 2 Hz up to 20 Hz. Modern construction techniques shield most electrical activity effectively, such that it is rare to encounter an electrical supply artifact due to the use of an alternating current (AC) power supply in the PICU. Current systems simultaneously display multiple traces so that sequential acquisitions can be examined in the same investigation (e.g., superimposed displays are frequently used for F-wave recordings, see below). Computerized algorithms are available that measure the latency and amplitude of signals.

Electrodes

Surface electrodes, concentric needle electrodes, and single fiber needle electrodes are used in EMG and NCS (**Fig. 52.1**). *Surface electrodes* are used to record compound muscle action potentials (CMAP) and are placed over the muscle of interest. Similarly, electrodes used to record nerve action potentials are placed over the nerve being investigated. **Table 52.1** summarizes the commonly used upper limb stimulation and recording sites. The *concentric needle electrode* has its recording surface at the tip. When placed into a muscle, it allows the recording of activity from fibers that lie within a hemisphere of its radius (~0.5 mm). Since muscle fibers have diameters of between 25 and 100 μM, the needle records activity from about 20 fibers. The total number of motor units recorded depends on the muscle, the anatomic arrangement of fibers within the motor unit, and the state of contraction. The *single fiber needle electrode* has its recording surface on the side of the needle (behind the tip), and it has a much smaller range of activity recording because of the arrangement of muscle fibers in a normal motor unit. The single fiber needle allows recording from only 1–3 single muscle fibers from the same motor unit.

Definitions and Diagnostic Findings

The *American Association of Neuromuscular & Neurodiagnostic Medicine* has developed practice guidelines, professional consensus statements, and recommendations about conducting and reporting EMG and NCS data (Available at their website: http://www.aanem.org/).

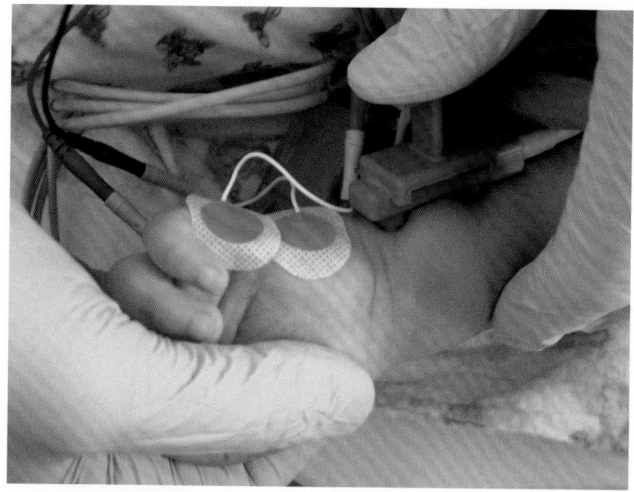

FIGURE 52.1. Stimulation of the left ulnar nerve at the wrist in a neonate recording from adductor digiti minimi showing the position of the stimulating electrodes and the stick on electrodes used for recording the compound muscle action potential.

Electromyography Patterns

At rest, muscle is electrically inactive. On first piercing the muscle with a recording needle, there may be transient (<1 second) bursts of activity due to mechanical stimulation or injury of muscle fibers. After this activity ceases, the EMG should be electrically silent except at the NMJ. Action potentials appear when the muscle is made to contract. At full contraction (complete recruitment of the muscle), there is a disorderly group of action potentials of varying rates and amplitudes. The EMG can be used to diagnose neuropathies, NMJ diseases, and myopathies. Table 52.2 summarizes typical EMG characteristics of neuropathic and myopathic conditions. The other phenomena that are sometimes recorded include muscle fibrillations, fasciculations, and jitter.

Fibrillations. These biphasic potentials can be recorded only with needle electrodes and are often regarded as the key feature of denervation when demonstrated at more than one site in a muscle.

Fasciculations. These variably shaped waveforms of high amplitude can be recorded with needle or surface electrode recordings. Fasciculations can be seen with lower motor neuron

---

TABLE 52.1

SOME OF THE PLACEMENT SITES FOR SURFACE ELECTRODES USED IN RECORDING PERIPHERAL ELECTROPHYSIOLOGY

■ PHYSIOLOGY	■ MUSCLE OR NERVE RECORDING	■ INNERVATION
Compound muscle action potential (CMAP)	*Upper limb* ■ Abductor digiti minimi ■ First dorsal interosseous ■ Abductor pollicis brevis ■ Extensor indicis *Lower limb* ■ Extensor digitorum brevis ■ Flexor halluces brevis ■ Abductor digiti minimi	■ Ulnar ■ Ulnar ■ Median ■ Radial ■ Deep peroneal ■ Tibial ■ Tibial
Sensory action potential	*Upper limb* ■ Median ■ Ulnar ■ Superficial radial *Lower limb* ■ Sural ■ Plantar ■ Saphenous	
Compound nerve action potential	*Upper limb recording* ■ Flexor surface at elbow ■ Ulnar groove behind elbow *Lower limb recording* ■ Fibular neck	*Wrist stimulation* ■ Median ■ Ulnar *Ankle stimulation* ■ Common peroneal

---

TABLE 52.2

TYPICAL EMG FINDINGS IN NEUROPATHIC AND MYOPATHIC DISEASE

	Typical EMG Features		
■ DISEASE	■ ACTION POTENTIAL AMPLITUDE	■ ACTION POTENTIAL DURATION	■ MOTOR UNIT NUMBER ESTIMATES
Neuropathic	Increased (×2) due to more fibers per motor unit	Increased	Decreased
Myopathic	Reduced area to amplitude ratio of the action potential	Reduced	Decreased in severe cases

200 µV

1 ms

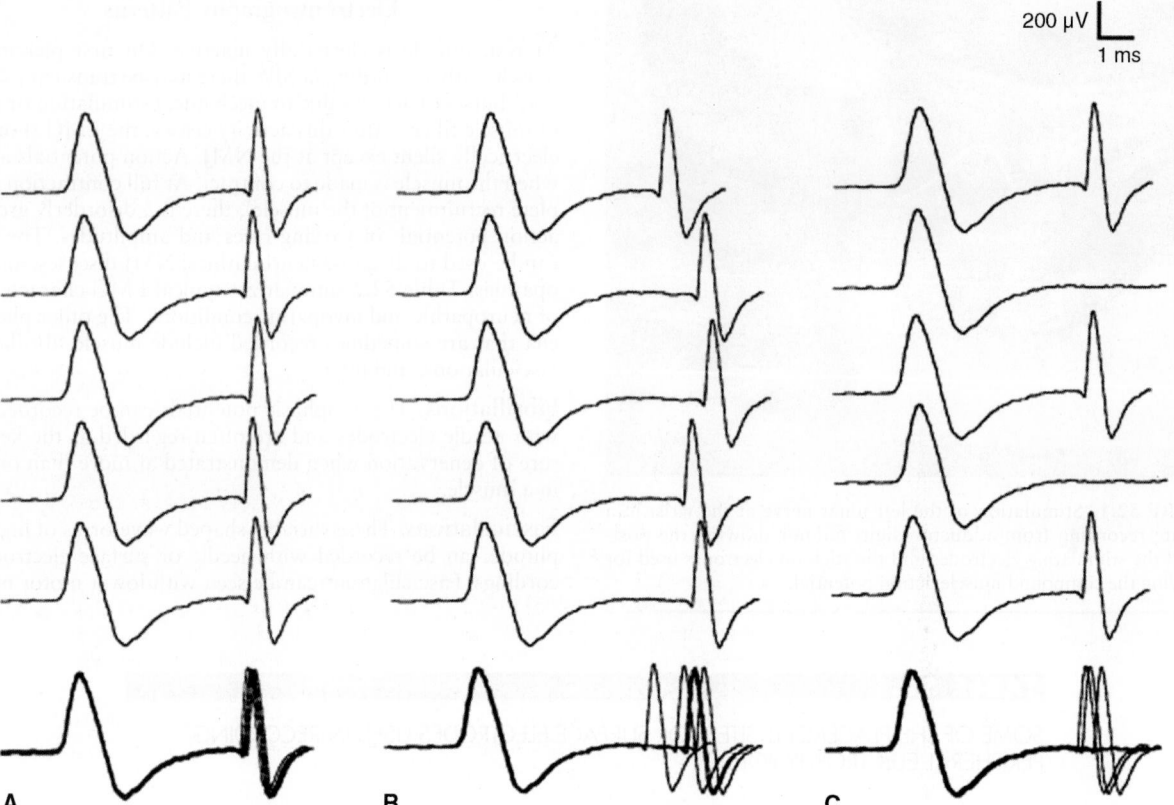

FIGURE 52.2. Single fiber electromyography recordings. **A:** Normal. **B:** Increased *jitter*, note temporal variation in F-waves. **C:** *Blocking*, note absent response in traces 2 and 4. In each set, five rastered traces (**top**) and superimposed traces (**bottom**) are shown. Both increased jitter and blocking are seen in neuromuscular junction disorders. (From Preston DC, Shapiro BE. *Electromyography and Neuromuscular Disorders: Clinical–Electrophysiologic Correlations*. 3rd ed. Philadelphia, PA: Elsevier, 2013.)

disease (poliomyelitis, spinal muscular atrophy), medications (stimulants, succinylcholine), and hypomagnesemia.

Jitter and Blocking. Single muscle fiber needle EMG (SFEMG) is a sensitive method for recording two muscle fiber action potentials from the same motor unit. When these action potentials are simultaneously recorded, small variations in the timing of the action potentials can be assessed by various calculations, and this variation is called *jitter* (**Fig. 52.2B**). Most of this variability relates to small differences in the time required for an endplate potential to reach threshold. Jitter can be thought of as a measure of the safety factor of neuromuscular transmission (NMT). When the safety factor is small (i.e., the endplate potential is just above the threshold for generation of muscle fiber action potential), jitter values are very large, reflecting high variability in muscle fiber action potential discharge (as seen in myasthenia, see below). If NMT is sufficiently impaired, an individual endplate potential may not reach the threshold, and a muscle fiber action potential is not generated. This phenomenon is referred to as *blocking* (**Fig. 52.2C**). The decremental response recorded in patients with myasthenia gravis during repetitive motor nerve stimulation is related to blocking of individual muscle fiber action potentials.

Nerve Conduction Study Results

Nerve Conduction Velocity. Motor and sensory NCS data are obtained from electrical stimulation of the appropriate peripheral nerve. Motor NCS are performed with recording from a muscle supplied by the nerve being stimulated (**Table 52.1**). The time it takes for the electrical impulse to travel from the stimulation to the recording site (i.e., *latency*) is measured in

milliseconds, the height of the response (i.e., *amplitude*) is measured in millivolts, and the length of the response (*duration*) is measured in milliseconds (**Fig. 52.3A,B**). Stimulation of two or more sites along the same nerve and using the difference in latencies and distance between stimulating electrodes allows calculation of motor nerve conduction velocity (NCV). Sensory NCV can be calculated on the basis of latency and distance between stimulating and recording electrodes from a purely sensory portion of the nerve being stimulated. Sensory nerve amplitudes are much smaller than motor nerve amplitudes (in the microvolt rather than millivolt range).

M-wave. The M-wave is recorded in the muscle and represents a response to a stimulus that travels in an orthodromic direction down the motor neuron to the muscle. The M-wave usually occurs with an onset of 3–5 ms and increases in amplitude as the stimulus intensity increases (see **Fig. 52.4** for representation of M-, F-, and H-waves).

F-wave. The *F-wave study* involves a supramaximal stimulation of the motor nerve and recording of action potentials from the muscle supplied. In this recording the action potential from the motor nerve stimulation travels from the site of stimulation to the anterior horn of the spinal cord (antidromic) and back to the limb (orthodromic) through that same nerve. The F-wave latency can be used to calculate the NCV of the nerve between the limb and spine, which cannot be assessed by the methods described above. The F-wave is measured in the muscle and usually occurs with an onset that is 25–32 ms after the stimulus. Since the F-wave increases slightly with stimulus intensity, a higher intensity stimulus helps differentiate the F-wave from the H-wave (see next page).

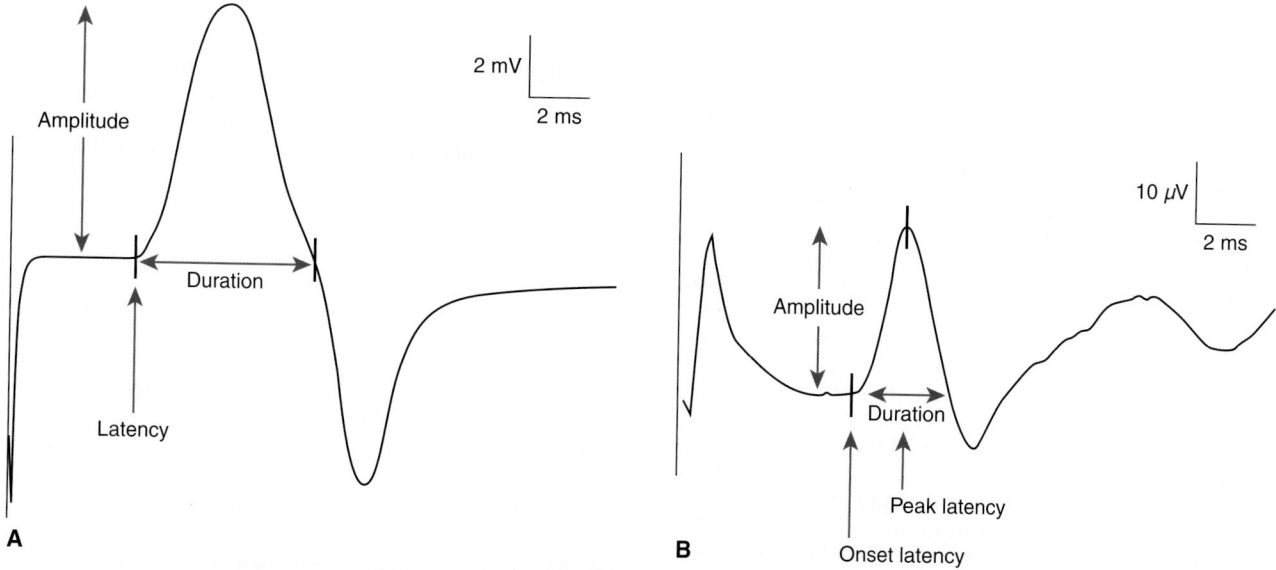

FIGURE 52.3. Basic nerve conduction studies. Components and shapes of (A) compound muscle action potential (CMAP) and (B) sensory nerve action potential (SNAP). (From Preston DC, Shapiro BE. *Electromyography and Neuromuscular Disorders: Clinical–Electrophysiologic Correlations.* 3rd ed. Philadelphia, PA: Elsevier, 2013.)

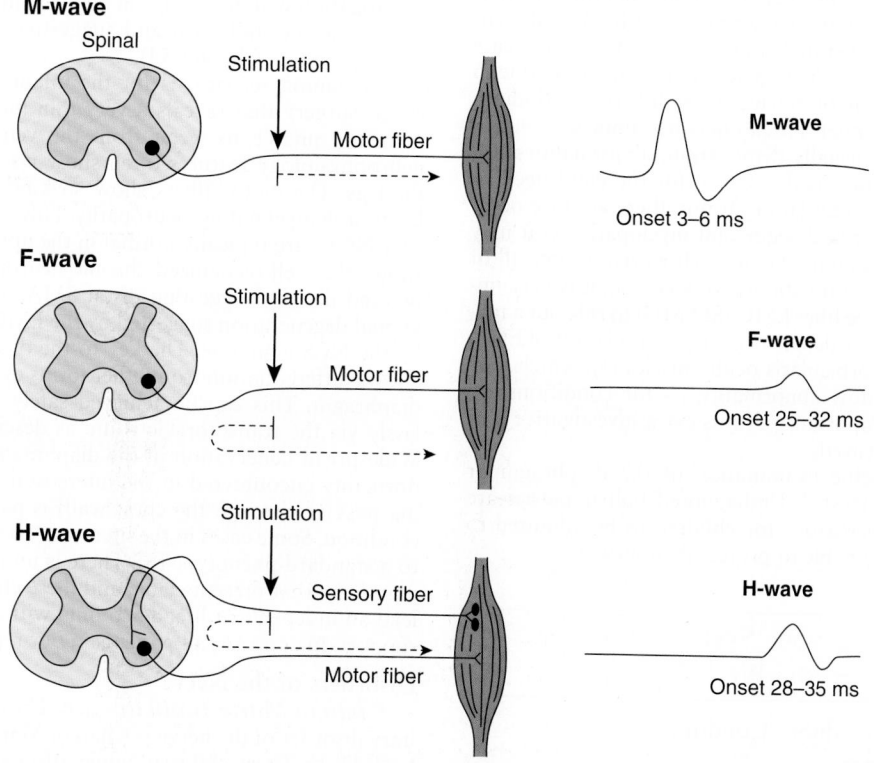

FIGURE 52.4. **M-wave:** Excitement is conducted along motor neuron from stimulus to recording at muscle fiber (orthodromic); M-wave increases as stimulus increases. **F-wave:** Excitement is conducted along motor neuron from stimulus to nerve body (antidromic) before returning along the motor neuron to the muscle fiber (orthodromic); F-wave increases slightly as stimulus increases. **H-wave:** Excitement is conducted along the sensory neuron to the motor neuron (antidromic), then travels down motor neuron to muscle (orthodromic); H-wave decreases as stimulus increases. (Modified from Kai S, Nakabayashi K. Evoked EMG makes measurement of muscle tone possible by analysis of the H/M ratio. In: Turker H, ed. *New Frontiers of Clinical Research.* Croatia: Intech, 2013.)

H-reflex. The *H-reflex study* uses the stimulation of a sensory nerve and records the reflex muscle activity in the limb. This reflex also assesses conduction between the limb and the spinal cord, but in contrast to the F-wave, the afferent and efferent impulses are from sensory and motor nerves, respectively.

The H-wave that is measured in the muscle during the H-reflex usually occurs with an onset that is 28–35 ms after the stimulus. Since the H-wave decreases with stimulus intensity and the F-wave increases slightly with stimulus intensity, the H-wave can be more readily identified at lower stimulus intensity.

Performing Electromyography and Nerve Conduction Studies in the PICU

In most circumstances, children with disorders of the PNS have generalized abnormalities, and an EMG protocol can be standardized. The first test is determination of the sensory nerve action potential (SNAP) amplitude and velocity in the leg. In the smallest babies, the medial plantar nerve is used, because a greater distance between the stimulating and recording electrodes reduces the stimulus artifact. In older children, either the superficial peroneal or the sural nerve is used. If results are normal, a sensory or sensorimotor neuropathy is excluded, and the arms do not need to be tested.

Motor nerve stimulation follows with recording either the peroneal nerve from extensor digitorum brevis, or the ulnar nerve from adductor pollicis (**Table 52.1**). In the presence of abnormalities of the sensory nerve, it may be possible to document motor nerve involvement and indicate whether this might be due to demyelination or axonal degeneration. Since effective reinnervation may cause the CMAP to be only slightly reduced, or not at all, EMG should be performed to look for signs of chronic denervation (**Table 52.2**).

EMG is always performed with the smallest gauge (30 g) needles, the so-called "facial needles." These are placed first in the tibialis anterior, which is easily activated by stimulating the sole of the foot. If abnormal, and motor neuronopathy is suspected, the tongue should be sampled next by the submental route. This is well tolerated, and if abnormal, will indicate that the motor neuronopathy is generalized rather than due to segmental spinal cord involvement. Depending on the findings in these two muscles, other muscles may be sampled.

This protocol will usually demonstrate abnormalities if a neuromuscular condition is the reason for the child needing supportive mechanical ventilation. If not, there are rare occasions when, with a cervical segmental myelopathy, you may specifically wish to examine the arm. However, if after all of these investigations, still no abnormality is seen, it is very important to include single fiber EMG (SFEMG) to rule out a myasthenic syndrome. Our department uses stimulation SFEMG (StimSFEMG) of the orbicularis oculi muscles (1), which may be the only test to show abnormality. As the conditions are often treatable, the importance of this extra investigative step cannot be overemphasized.

On occasion, specific examination of the diaphragm or bulbar muscles is requested. Undiagnosed bulbar palsies are increasingly common reasons for children to be admitted to the PICU as they are unable to protect their airway.

Peripheral Nervous System Disorders in the PICU

Hereditary Conditions

Anterior Horn Cell Disease

Spinal Muscular Atrophy. The most common anterior horn cell disease is a spinal muscular atrophy (SMA) due to mutations on the 5q chromosome (see Chapter 54). It is the most common genetic neuromuscular disorder of childhood (2), and its presentation is well known. It is classified according to severity, with SMA 0 the worst affected and presenting as a floppy neonate, and SMA 3 the least affected and often not recognized until adulthood. It is only the very severest forms (SMA 0 and 1) that will present diagnostic difficulties in the PICU. Diagnosis of an infant born with these severe forms of SMA is not straightforward with EMG and NCS. First, it is quite common to find that the sensory nerve fibers are affected, as the condition is associated with a dorsal

root ganglionopathy (3), and distinction from an early onset neuropathy is difficult. Furthermore, while the reduction in the CMAP gives an indication that there has been a severe loss of muscle fibers, occasionally, the EMG is not classically abnormal in the neuropathic sense (**Table 52.2**). The reinnervated motor units (an expected feature of anterior horn cell disease) may not yet have developed. Fibrillation potentials are regarded as an important sign, but these can be seen in conditions such as acute myositis, or severe myopathies, and their presence alone does not indicate that the condition is an SMA. It is fortunate that despite the diagnostic difficulties presented with EMG and NCS, the genetic test in severe cases is almost invariably positive and can be rapidly obtained in most parts of the world. Interestingly, before the genetic testing was well established, pathology laboratories also encountered difficulty in diagnosing the underlying motor neuron disorder.

Spinal Muscular Atrophy with Respiratory Distress (SMARD). In addition to 5q SMA, another anterior horn cell condition that may result in a child needing intensive care is spinal muscular atrophy with respiratory distress (SMARD). SMARD is an exceedingly rare condition associated with the immunoglobulin mu-binding protein 2 (IGHMBP2) gene abnormality (4). In its most common form, affected babies have intrauterine growth retardation (usually a birth weight less than the third centile), go home normally after the delivery, and return at 3 months of age with respiratory compromise. Investigation will then show an abnormality of the diaphragm, which may be unilateral and suggestive of a diaphragmatic eventration (see Chapter 53).

A common scenario is for the infant to have diaphragm repair surgery that reveals a very thin muscle and to be permanently unable to wean from the ventilator. The clinical neurophysiology features often show no sensory response in the legs. The motor fibers show strikingly slow NCVs similar to a demyelinating neuropathy. However, motor and sensory NCVs are typically normal in the upper limbs. The EMG shows the well-recognized chronic neuropathic change, most marked distally suggesting distal SMA. This combination of axonal degeneration suggested by the EMG but demyelination by the NCS is unique. The key to the diagnosis and one that allows differentiation from other forms of SMA is EMG of the diaphragm. This can be achieved safely and relatively painlessly via the transthoracic route as described by Bolton (5). Widespread denervation in the diaphragm, often with no abnormality encountered in the intercostal muscles (found during passage through the chest wall) is pathognomonic of the condition. Some cases in the literature do not seem to conform to a standard phenotype (6). There is undoubtedly a more benign form that presents later, and these children, while able to lead an independent life, do so only with constant respiratory support. In contrast, all patients in our report died.

Disorders of the Nerve

Charcot Marie Tooth disease. The most common hereditary disorder of the nerve is Charcot Marie Tooth disease type I (CMT 1). These children, while affected to varying degrees, are rarely likely to be weak enough to need PICU. There are instances where exposure to neurotoxins (vincristine) may cause a profound weakness and unmask undiagnosed CMT 1 (7).

The mutations that cause CMT are also associated with more severe forms of hereditary neuropathy (8), which can present with sufficient weakness for a newborn to require ventilation. The two forms that cause this are Dejerine Sottas disease (DSD) and congenital hypomyelinating neuropathy. The clinical presentation for these two conditions is similar, with the child born very floppy and requiring immediate mechanical ventilation. The neurophysiological findings are striking. One of the most characteristic features of this condition is that the intensity of the stimulus needed to provoke any response from the nerve may be exceedingly high. Often, one has to use the longest duration and maximum intensity of stimulation available. Even then the responses may be missed because the time base on the recording screen is not long enough to allow the very long distal motor latency to be captured. It is not uncommon to have distal motor latencies exceeding 20 ms (normal is around 3 ms). With the correct set-up and level of stimulation, it is possible to record NCVs as slow as 1 m/s (a normal neonate has velocities in excess of 25–30 m/s). The EMG may show fibrillation potentials indicating that there is some associated secondary axonal degeneration. Genetic confirmation then follows.

NMJ Disorders

Congenital Myasthenic Syndromes. The congenital myasthenic syndromes (CMS) are hereditary disorders of the proteins in and around pre-and postsynaptic areas of the NMJ that cause abnormalities of NMT (9). They are exceptionally rare, but, most importantly, with regard to pediatric neurological disease in general (and neuromuscular disease in particular), they may be treatable. It is for this reason that almost any amount of effort and expense is justifiable to recognize the rare, unsuspected case. The use of StimSFEMG has revolutionized our ability to pick up this unusual condition. Over the years, we have seen the age at which the diagnosis is made significantly drop because of this technique's increased use (one recent case of fast channel CMS was diagnosed at the age of 14 months). These conditions can be fatal, but with effective treatment, a child may have a near to normal life expectancy if they can avoid the life-threatening episodes early in life. Regrettably, it has still been our experience to diagnose myasthenia in an infant who has lost older siblings that were erroneously thought to have a myopathy. Our most recent case had a Rapsyn mutation (a gene that codes for a 43 kDa receptor-associated protein of the synapse), which was present in two deceased siblings' blood post–mortem. This regrettable sequence of events should be a thing of the past.

While there are many different types of CMS, few are likely to present as diagnostic dilemmas in the PICU. The commonest cause of CMS is due to a mutation of the epsilon subunit of the acetylcholine receptor and is associated with less significant weakness, certainly not requiring ventilation. Because these patients will continue to produce the fetal form of the acetylcholine receptor (containing a gamma subunit), the weakness is less profound. CMS will enter into the differential diagnosis of any floppy infant needing ventilation and include those associated with apnea. The particular conditions that should be considered include CMS with episodic apnea (CMS-EA, previously called infantile myasthenic syndrome), which is associated with a presynaptic abnormality of the choline acetyltransferase enzyme (CHAT) (10). Some mutations of Rapsyn (11) may also be associated with apnea. Finally, the conditions that present with stridor and require ventilatory support can be associated with the newly identified Dok7 mutation (Dok7 CMS) (12).

We perform StimSFEMG based on the method described by Trontelj (13) and use the orbicularis oculi as the target muscle. Even in cases with limb girdle weakness (some cases of Dok 7) or stridor, this muscle appears to be exquisitely sensitive and will show abnormalities irrespective of the distribution of weakness. Its sensitivity is not matched by its specificity, which is relatively low. Other (nonmyasthenic) conditions may show abnormalities of StimSFEMG such as central hypoventilation syndrome due to PHOX2B, Prader Willi syndrome, and some myopathies. If the StimSFEMG is entirely normal, with its very high negative predictive value, the likelihood of myasthenia being present is very low, although it cannot be ruled out completely. Repetitive nerve stimulation is easy to perform in the PICU, but we do not use this routinely as it has a significantly reduced sensitivity in comparison with StimSFEMG.

Muscle Disease

Myotonic Dystrophy. The babies with myotonic dystrophy, who are sufficiently weak to need mechanical ventilation, will all have inherited it from the mother, in whom it will often have been undiagnosed. On careful examination and EMG testing of the mother, it is often determined that they have the condition (14). EMG testing of the neonate in these circumstances is unnecessary, and examination of CTG trinucleotide (cytosine-thymine-guanine) repeats on the DMPK gene (code for myotonic dystrophy protein kinase) quickly secures the diagnosis. If the mother does not clearly have the condition, EMG examination of the newborn looking for myotonic discharges may not be helpful because the myotonic discharges, seen in older children and adults, may not be seen in babies. The use of a long-duration electrical stimulation of the muscle (up to one second) can produce a train of myotonic discharges (15). This, unfortunately, is not an easy technique to apply as many commercial EMG/NCS machines do not allow stimulator duration to be extended to that extent. However, looking for CTG repeats is routine and should present no diagnostic difficulties.

Other Myopathies. Nemaline rod myopathy and minitubular (centronuclear) myopathy are among the few myopathies that are sufficiently devastating at onset to require ventilatory support from birth (16). EMG is usually clearly abnormal, indicating a myopathic process, but further delineation of the exact condition requires other tests such as muscle biopsy or genetic analysis. It is worth remembering that some myopathies can have large fibers and also splitting of the muscle fibers with reinnervation, both pathologies presenting some neurogenic features on an EMG. However, the clue to their separation from primary neurogenic abnormalities is that in all instances they still have in their interference patterns, short duration, low amplitude, units that are pathognomonic of myopathy and point toward the correct diagnosis of myopathy.

Acquired Disorders of the PNS

Anterior Horn Cell Disease

Poliomyelitis. Historically, the commonest infection causing anterior horn cell disease, and a need for supportive ventilation, was poliomyelitis due to poliovirus. Polio vaccination has effectively eradicated this except for three or four areas worldwide. Additionally, poliomyelitis as a complication of the vaccination now does not occur because of vaccination with the killed virus. There are enteroviruses, other than poliovirus, which have been implicated in a poliomyelitis-like *acute flaccid paralysis (AFP)* (17). Even common viruses such as Coxsackie or Echoviruses may exhibit anterior horn cell involvement. The most commonly implicated virus varies according to region. For example, enterovirus 71 is particularly common in certain parts of Southeast Asia. West Nile virus is seen perhaps more commonly in the United States. Other causes of AFP include the viruses causing Japanese B encephalitis, Murray Valley encephalitis, St Louis encephalitis, Russian Spring encephalitis, tick-borne viruses, and the herpes virus. When AFP occurs in epidemics, it is not difficult to recognize affected children. The greater diagnostic challenge is when it occurs as isolated cases. AFP should be considered in the child who has respiratory illness, becomes overly weak, requiring ventilation, but does not have Guillain–Barre syndrome (GBS).

Disorders of the Peripheral Nerve

Guillain–Barre Syndrome. GBS is the most common cause of acute nontraumatic paralysis in children and has been linked to antibodies cross-reacting against neuronal gangliosides. These children usually present with prodromal symptoms of gastrointestinal or respiratory illness preceding the development of the ascending weakness. Irritability caused by neuropathic pain is another hallmark of the disease.

GBS is now recognized to encompass several variants, which can be identified by clinical, laboratory, and neurophysiological characteristics. *Acute Inflammatory Demyelinating Polyneuropathy (AIDP)* is the most common variant (18). *Acute Motor Axonal Neuropathy (AMAN)* is a GBS variant involving only motor neurons that is more common in Northern China and rarely occurs in children in the United States or Europe. Respiratory failure is more common in AMAN than in AIDP. See Chapter 53 for a detailed discussion of GBS variants.

The diagnosis of GBS variants is aided by information from NCS. Most of the recognized changes of GBS are regularly encountered in children, such as increase in the distal motor latency, temporal dispersion, and slowing of the main nerve trunk velocity. However, sometimes the changes are subtle and may only manifest as absent F-waves. This can present problems in infants as F-waves are difficult to obtain in normal subjects of that age, especially when on the PICU, and it may be difficult to know whether their absence is significant. Fortunately, in difficult cases, computed tomography (CT) scans or magnetic resonance imaging (MRI) often show inflammatory changes around the nerve roots, and cerebrospinal fluid (CSF) results show elevated protein levels (see Chapter 53). Both of these changes may take some time to develop, and there may be a delay between the appearance of the neurophysiologic abnormalities and the onset of the condition. Antiganglioside antibodies may also be found, but this is not common, in our experience.

NMJ Abnormalities

Botulism. Botulinum toxin is one of the most potent poisons known. It has several classical presentations (See Chapter 94, Toxin Related Diseases) (19). The most important presentation for the PICU specialist is infantile botulism. Infantile botulism usually occurs in children under 6 months of age and is due to colonization of the intestine and production of toxin by *Clostridium botulinum* (20). Constipation, when noted, is rapidly followed by paralysis, which starts cranially and descends (in contrast to the ascending paralysis in GBS). One of the mysteries about the condition is that while *C. botulinum* is widely distributed, infantile botulism occurs only in certain parts of the world. In the United States, the condition is common in California and Utah (21). It is possibly related to a particular climatic environment that allows the spores to develop. Interestingly, in Utah, it has a seasonal presentation and has been related to construction work which releases spores into the air (22). It is well recognized that children can have the organism in their bowels and yet be asymptomatic (23). The time of particular sensitivity is when the infant changes from breast feeding to the first formula feed (24).

The classic changes described in clinical neurophysiological literature (25) are rarely seen in this author's experience. It is most likely that the well-recognized finding of a small CMAP, with a significant increment on rapid repetitive nerve stimulation (up to a 200% increase at stimulation rates of 20 and above) occurs only at a particular level of NMJ involvement. Clearly, when all NMJs are paralyzed, no abnormality will be seen; in fact, no responses will be seen. At the other end of the spectrum, if there is minimal infection, then only a small proportion will be able to demonstrate abnormalities. It is unequivocal that NMJ function will be affected (demonstrated by StimSFEMG) and jitter reduced at faster rates of stimulation (26). The development of human botulism immune globulin (BIG), which neutralizes unbound toxin, has revolutionized treatment and can reduce PICU stay (27). If given too late, recovery can occur only by regrowth of the NMJ; this usually takes nearly 3 months and makes BIG administration both preferred and cost-effective.

It is necessary to be aware and alert to the diagnosis of infant botulism in areas where it is not common. Indeed, in Utah, the diagnosis is often made clinically with no recourse to neurophysiology or seeking confirmation from demonstration of the spores in the stool (28). The United Kingdom's experience is quite different, and our first case in 2004 was the first in London for 12 years. After this case, and the awareness it generated, several more cases were recognized within the next few years. None of them demonstrated the full neurophysiological signature. It is important to realize that there are variants of the *Clostridium* toxin, and it is possible to have a less aggressive form, which may not necessitate intensive care support.

Tick Paralysis. Ticks are obligate hematophagous ectoparasites of both animals and humans, and are abundant in temperate and tropical zones around the world. Paralysis from the toxins of the tick is well recognized by veterinarians (29). Similar to infantile botulism, despite the ubiquitous presence of ticks, paralysis in humans occurs only in certain parts of the world (30). The author, working in the United Kingdom, has never seen a case, but colleagues in the United States have had such experience. In areas where tick paralysis is seen, GBS should not be diagnosed without looking very carefully for a tick. The removal of the tick immediately restores the child to normal strength (a most rewarding intervention).

Autoimmune Myasthenia Gravis. Whether this condition should appear as a hereditary condition or an acquired disease is a matter of debate, but for the purposes of this section, we will consider it among the acquired phenomena. Autoimmune myasthenia gravis (AIMG) may present in the congenital form when a mother with myasthenia gravis gives birth to a floppy baby who has been paralyzed by the transplacental diffusion of antibodies against the mother's NMJ. After birth, this transfer stops, and the child recovers over a period of weeks. It is rare for the mother not to have been known to be myasthenic, and therefore the condition should present no diagnostic difficulties.

A more confusing situation occurs when a child is born with arthrogryposis and the Pena-Shokeir phenotype, which may occur in utero from lack of movement (31). Once again, the antibodies are against the adult form of the NMJ (against its alpha subunit). There is a further form of congenital myasthenia gravis, where the mother produces antibodies against the gamma subunit of the NMJ (the gamma subunit is seen only in the fetal NMJ and is replaced by the epsilon subunit in the adult NMJ). These children also may be born with arthrogryposis, and the mother will have had a succession of miscarriages (32). The diagnosis is often delayed because this is an exceedingly rare disorder, and most routine testing for acetylcholine receptor antibodies looks only for those against the adult and not the fetal form. All these children should have abnormalities demonstrable on StimSFEMG.

Outside of the neonatal period, AIMG can be caused either by receptor antibodies or by antibodies against the muscle specific kinase (MuSK) receptors. It is uncommon for children with myasthenia gravis to need intensive care. On occasion, a child may take a long time to recover from the neuromuscular blocking agent (NMBA) used in standard treatment. The most common reason for this is that the NMBA has taken longer to be neutralized because of concomitant renal or liver problems, but if this is not the case, undiagnosed myasthenia gravis or even a CMS may be present. We have had several occasions when this proved to be the case.

Acute Muscle Disease.
It is very rare that an acute muscle disease is sufficiently severe for a child to need intensive care. When it presents, an extremely elevated CPK and markers such as rhabdomyolysis with the concomitant renal changes facilitate diagnosis. EMG and NCS usually have no role in their diagnosis.

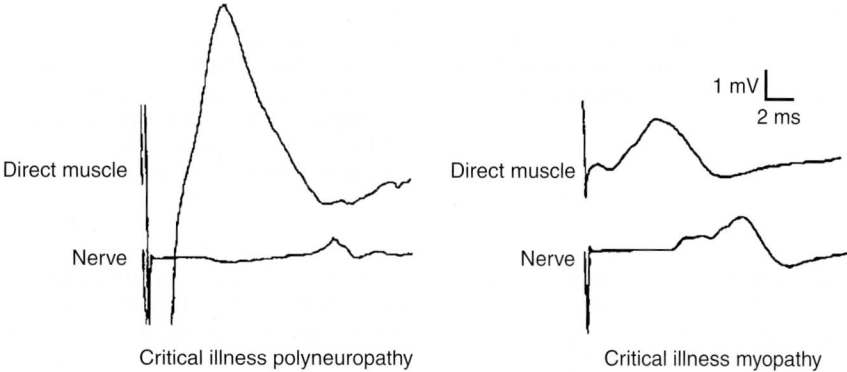

FIGURE 52.5. Studies showing critical illness polyneuropathy and critical illness myopathy. Compound muscle action potentials from the tibialis anterior muscle of a patient with critical illness neuropathy (**left**) and critical illness myopathy (**right**). Note the higher amplitude with direct muscle stimulation compared with nerve stimulation in the patient with critical illness neuropathy, whereas there is little difference in amplitude between direct muscle and nerve stimulation in the patient with critical illness myopathy. (From Preston DC, Shapiro BE. *Electromyography and Neuromuscular Disorders: Clinical–Electrophysiologic Correlations.* 3rd ed. Philadelphia, PA: Elsevier, 2013.)

Conditions Acquired in the PICU Affecting the Peripheral Nervous System

Critical Illness Neuromyopathy

Weakness in the context of critical illness can be considered to have occurred from one of three causes: a critical illness neuropathy, a critical illness myopathy, or a combination of two (critical illness polyneuropathy and myopathy). It is considered that these conditions may affect up to 85% of critically ill adult patients (33). However, proportions of this level may be due to a selection bias as only those cases with sepsis, multiorgan failure, or prolonged intensive care admission were selected. When unselected cohorts of adults are studied, the prevalence is much lower, varying between 0.2% and 0.5% (34). The neuropathy is usually an axonal neuropathy, with the motor nerve affected more than the sensory. This assumption is based on the marked reduction in the CMAP amplitude in the context of usually preserved or only slightly affected sensory nerve action potentials (**Fig. 52.5**). If present, this indicates a slow and prolonged recovery. Reports vary regarding the prevalence of this condition in children (35). Personal experience suggests that it is exceedingly rare (3–4 cases over 20 years) and most were teenagers or older. One study has suggested that only 1.7% of children troubled by muscle weakness would have this (36).

Critical illness myopathy may be more common both generally and in children. Some of this evidence arises from the studies of the nerve endpoints and noticing the differences in the evoked responses from the muscle according to whether you stimulate the nerve or the muscle itself (37). Other studies include those looking at muscle fiber conduction velocity or at muscle fiber excitability (38). Most of the studies have been reported only in adults, which is hardly surprising given the invasive nature of these tests. Fortunately, it has been discovered that the duration and the configuration of the CMAPs have a very close relationship to the muscle conduction velocity, and even though no study has been performed in children, there is potential for a prospective study.

In conclusion, there is a great deal that is unknown about the generalized acquired affections of the nerves and muscles in critically ill children. It seems likely that the incidence is lower than in adults for a variety of reasons. First, and foremost, it is likely that the child's nervous system has a greater potential for recovery than the adults. Another consideration is that the

condition has simply not been investigated or sought assiduously enough.

Mononeuropathies That Develop in the PICU

The mononeuropathies that occur in the PICU are usually the result of pressure or inadvertent damage from resuscitation or monitoring procedures. Certain nerves are more susceptible than others, and within those more susceptible nerves, certain parts are more vulnerable to pressure. Our experience has been that we do not tend to see upper limb involvement. As an example, although it is well recognized that the ulnar nerve can be affected by pressure at the elbow, we have not seen any cases. The lower limb nerves seem much more susceptible, and in particular the sciatic nerve. Children with sciatic nerve injury often present with a foot drop. Although a common peroneal palsy is the most likely cause of this in general, in the PICU setting, this is most uncommon. Instead, it is often the sciatic nerve that has been damaged. We have seen this in children returning from surgery to the PICU, particularly if they are cachectic and the surgery prolonged. This is despite the anesthesiologist being fully aware of this complication and taking what normally are adequate precautions against it. It is possible there may be a vascular element to this, rather than being the result solely of pressure. The sciatic nerve's blood supply comes from the femoral artery and can be compromised by femoral artery cannulation. One such setting is when the Berlin heart, a bypass machine used to allow recovery from infective myocarditis, is connected by a large cannula in the femoral artery.

The neurophysiologic findings of sciatic nerve palsy require the demonstration of abnormalities not only in the peroneal but also in the tibial element of the nerve. It is well recognized that the peroneal fascicle is more susceptible to pressure and therefore those elements of sensory and motor served by that fascicle often show more abnormality than those from the tibial nerve fascicle. However, it is inevitable that even with a very clear predominance of peroneal abnormality, you will find some abnormality in the tibial nerves. This may be loss or reduction in the medial plantar sensory response, a pure tibial sensory nerve, or perhaps denervation in one of the calf muscles. Unfortunately, when sciatic nerve palsies do occur, because of the long distance required for the nerve to regrow, if there is axonotmesis, prognosis for full recovery can be poor.

The other mononeuropathy that we have seen is involvement of the femoral nerve. This is also particularly susceptible, perhaps more so than the sciatic nerve, when the femoral artery is cannulated. With increasing use of cardiovascular support (particularly in the cardiac PICU) often using large cannulae, one must be aware of these complications, which if diagnosed promptly, allow early intervention that may prevent significant damage.

Recent EMG and NCS Findings From Our PICU

The discussion above has considered those well-recognized conditions that occur in the PICU affecting the PNS and for which EMG and NCS data may be an important diagnostic intervention. The cases and conditions described are recognizable from other reviews of the subject (39). In addition, personal cases have been added. However, our recent experience in the PICU has shown that with ready access to neurophysiology, other uses are emerging.

In order to understand the likely trends in EMG and NCS use in the PICU, we reviewed our experience over a period of 4 years from July 2007. In our PICU, 141 EMGs were performed in 111 children, representing 5% of the 3000 EMG and NCS performed during that period. The referrals for EMG and NCS do not reflect the actual number of children coming to the PICU with neuromuscular abnormalities as many have been diagnosed before admission and do not need EMG. Not surprisingly, our children tended to be very young, with 104 EMGs (74%) performed in children under one year of age, many of whom were neonates. In fact, 77 (55%) studies were performed in children aged less than 6 months.

The documented reasons for these referrals varied. **Table 52.3** compares the referring diagnosis and the EMG diagnosis in the 91 patients examined once. These data show some interesting patterns: First, the wide range of neuromuscular diagnoses, particularly true when a specific condition is not suspected (e.g., neuromuscular disorder, floppy infant). Next, the high frequency

with which a motor neuronopathy is diagnosed, often not suspected by clinicians. Finally, within this group fell some of the children referred with bulbar palsy, but isolated bulbar palsy was also found in a significant number.

Investigation of bulbar palsy became a frequent reason for EMG referral as pediatricians realized that bulbar function can be determined by simple tongue EMG. Affected children are admitted to PICU, not because of generalized respiratory weakness but because of failure to protect their airway and recurrent aspiration. More important still is the realization that some of the neurodegenerative conditions that present with a bulbar palsy, such as Brown–Vialetto–Van Laere (BVVL) syndrome, may be treatable. Recent discoveries that these children may have an abnormality of riboflavin metabolism and therefore can be treated with vitamin B_6 have heightened clinicians' awareness of the importance of diagnosing these early. EMG demonstration of a bulbar palsy offers a very sensitive and early method of detecting these children.

An important reason for referral for EMG was failure to wean from mechanical ventilation (12 children). In half the cases, we found no abnormality, but four of them had evidence of neuromuscular transmission disorder (NMTD). A proportion of these were slow to wean because of altered pharmacokinetics of administered NMBAs, usually the result of impairment of renal function. It is recognized that some children who are slow to wean have a coexisting myopathy, and these will show myopathic potentials on EMG, although we saw no cases. It may also be the presentation of a myasthenic syndrome, and it is important to consider this within the differential diagnosis.

The second part of our analysis considered children who had multiple EMG examinations while in the PICU (**Table 52.4**). In many ways, these 15 children are the most interesting of the whole group. Many of them were very young, and the fact that they had multiple examinations demonstrates the difficulties of making diagnoses with EMG and NCS in the youngest children.

TABLE 52.3

REFERRAL AND EMG DIAGNOSIS MADE IN 91 PATIENTS EXAMINED ONCE

■ REFERRAL DIAGNOSIS	Motor Neuronopathy		■ NERVE	■ NMT	■ MYOPATHY	■ NORMAL	■ TOTALS
	■ BULBAR	■ GENERALIZED					
Apnea		1	1	1		1	4
Arthrogryposis		4		2	1		7
Axonal neuropathy			2				2
Botulism				3			3
Bulbar palsy	6	3	1		1	5	16
Failure to wean		1	1	4		6	12
Cervical segmental myelopathy		1					1
Critical illness neuropathy			2		1		3
Floppy infant		1	1		1	3	6
Diaphragmatic palsy	1	3				2	6
GBS			1			1	2
Leukodystrophy						2	2
Mononeuropathy			4			1	5
Myotonia					1		1
Neuromuscular disorder		4	2		7	5	18
Rhabdomyolysis				1			1
Stridor	2						2
Total	9	18	15	11	12	26	91

NMT, Neuromuscular transmission.

TABLE 52.4

REFERRAL TYPES AND DIAGNOSES MADE BEFORE AND AFTER EMG AND NCS DATA IN 15 PICU CASES EXAMINED MORE THAN ONCE

■ CASE NUMBER	■ AGE IN MONTHS	■ NUMBER OF STUDIES	■ REFERRAL TYPES	■ INITIAL DIAGNOSIS	■ FINAL DIAGNOSIS
1	1	2	Floppy baby Failure to wean	NMT disorder	NMT disorder
2	1	2	Failure to wean × 2	NMT disorder	Bulbar palsy
3	1–3	2	Floppy baby Axonal neuropathy	Axonal neuropathy	Axonal neuropathy
4	13	2	Rhabdomyolysis Diaphragm palsy	Motor neuronopathy	Normal diaphragm function
5	8	2	Congenital myasthenia	NMT disorder	NMT disorder (agrin abnormality)
6	2	2	Apnea Bulbar palsy	Bulbar palsy	Bulbar palsy
7	4	3	Stridor × 3	Uncertain	NMT disorder (Dok7 mutation)
8	0	2	Floppy baby × 2	Motorneuronopathy	Uncertain
9	1–2	3	Failure to wean × 3	Bulbar palsy	Motor neuronopathy
10	0–2	7	Failure to wean × 7	NMT disorder	NMT disorder
11	1–3	2	Apnea Bulbar palsy	Equivocal	Bulbar palsy
12	19	2	Bulbar palsy × 2	Normal	Motor neuronopathy
13	3	2	Failure to wean CMS	NMT disorder	NMT disorder (Probable CMS)
14	3	2	Floppy baby Diaphragm palsy	Motor neuronopathy	Diaphragm normal
15	2	2	Failure to wean Bulbar palsy	Neuropathy	Motor neuronopathy

NMT, Neuromuscular transmission; CMS, congenital myasthenic syndrome.

Here, distinction between various neuromuscular conditions from normal findings can be exceptionally difficult.

CONCLUSIONS AND FUTURE DIRECTIONS

There have been several developments in the use of EMG and NCS in the PICU. These techniques can now be used even in the youngest children (<1 year). A child presenting with an undiagnosed neuromuscular disorder (floppy infant) is a common reason for investigation. In patients with suspected anterior horn cell disease, EMG and NCS will become increasingly important for diagnosis and treatment, especially for neurodegenerative conditions such as Brown–Vialetto–Van Laere. Within the anterior horn cell conditions, those affecting the bulbar nuclei can be quickly identified with studies of the tongue, and those children at risk of aspiration can be determined. Children failing to wean from mechanical ventilation may include those with an underlying NMTD such as myasthenia, and electrophysiology is highly effective in identifying these conditions and differentiating them from drug-induced neuromuscular blockade. The single biggest barrier to further development is the sufficiency of neurophysiological expertise, which will likely change with demand for availability.

References

1. Pitt M. Neurophysiological strategies for the diagnosis of disorders of the neuromuscular junction in children. *Dev Med Child Neurol* 2008;50:328–33.

2. Wee CD, Kong L, Sumner CJ. The genetics of spinal muscular atrophies. *Curr Opin Neurol* 2010;23:450–8.

3. Rudnik-Schoneborn S, Goebel HH, Schlote W, et al. Classical infantile spinal muscular atrophy with SMN deficiency causes sensory neuronopathy. *Neurology* 2003;60:983–7.

4. Pitt M, Houlden H, Jacobs J, et al. Severe infantile neuropathy with diaphragmatic weakness and its relationship to SMARD1. *Brain* 2003;126:2682–92.

5. Bolton CF, Grand'Maison F, Parkes A, et al. Needle electromyography of the diaphragm. *Muscle Nerve* 1992;15:678–81.

6. Guenther UP, Handoko L, Varon R, et al. Clinical variability in distal spinal muscular atrophy type 1 (DSMA1): Determination of steady-state IGHMBP2 protein levels in five patients with infantile and juvenile disease. *J Mol Med* 2009;87:31–41.

7. Chauvenet AR, Shashi V, Selsky C, et al. Vincristine-induced neuropathy as the initial presentation of charcot-marie-tooth disease in acute lymphoblastic leukemia: A Pediatric Oncology Group study. *J Pediatr Hematol Oncol* 2003;25:316–20.

8. Baets J, Deconinck T, De VE, et al. Genetic spectrum of hereditary neuropathies with onset in the first year of life. *Brain* 2011;134:2664–76.

9. Palace J, Beeson D. The congenital myasthenic syndromes. *J Neuroimmunol* 2008;201-202:2–5.

10. Ohno K, Tsujino A, Brengman JM, et al. Choline acetyltransferase mutations cause myasthenic syndrome associated with episodic apnea in humans. *Proc Natl Acad Sci U S A* 2001;98:2017–22.

11. Engel AG, Sine SM. Current understanding of congenital myasthenic syndromes. *Curr Opin Pharmacol* 2005;5:308–21.

12. Jephson CG, Mills NA, Pitt MC, et al. Congenital stridor with feeding difficulty as a presenting symptom of Dok7 congenital myasthenic syndrome. *Int J Pediatr Otorhinolaryngol* 2010;74:991–4.

13. Trontelj JV, Khuraibet A, Mihelin M. The jitter in stimulated or-bicularis oculi muscle: Technique and normal values. *J Neurol Neurosurg Psychiatry* 1988;51:814–9.

14. Rutherford MA, Heckmatt JZ, Dubowitz V. Congenital myotonic dystrophy: Respiratory function at birth determines survival. *Arch Dis Child* 1989;64:191–5.

15. Renault F, Fedida A. [Early electromyographic signs in congenital myotonic dystrophy. A study of ten cases]. *Neurophysiol Clin* 1991;21:201–11.

16. Polat M, Tosun A, Ay Y, et al. Central core disease: Atypical case with respiratory insufficiency in an intensive care unit. *J Child Neurol* 2006;21:173–4.

17. Solomon T, Willison H. Infectious causes of acute flaccid paralysis. *Curr Opin Infect Dis* 2003;16:375–81.

18. Ryan MM. Guillain-Barre syndrome in childhood. *J Paediatr Child Health* 2005;41:237–41.

19. Brook I. Botulism: The challenge of diagnosis and treatment. *Rev Neurol Dis* 2006;3:182–9.

20. Koepke R, Sobel J, Arnon SS. Global occurrence of infant botulism, 1976-2006. *Pediatrics* 2008;122:e73–e82.

21. Morris JG Jr, Snyder JD, Wilson R, et al. Infant botulism in the United States: An epidemiologic study of cases occurring outside of California. *Am J Public Health* 1983;73:1385–8.

22. Long SS. Epidemiologic study of infant botulism in Pennsylvania: Report of the Infant Botulism Study group. *Pediatrics* 1985;75:928–34.

23. Chin J, Arnon SS, Midura TF. Food and environmental aspects of infant botulism in California. *Rev Infect Dis* 1979;1:693–7.

24. Long SS, Gajewski JL, Brown LW, et al. Clinical, laboratory, and environmental features of infant botulism in Southeastern Pennsylvania. *Pediatrics* 1985;75:935–41.

25. Cornblath DR, Sladky JT, Sumner AJ. Clinical electrophysiology of infantile botulism. *Muscle Nerve* 1983;6:448–52.

26. Chaudhry V, Crawford TO. Stimulation single-fiber EMG in infant botulism. *Muscle Nerve* 1999;22:1698–703.

27. Arnon SS, Schechter R, Maslanka SE, et al. Human botulism immune globulin for the treatment of infant botulism. *N Engl J Med* 2006;354:462–71.

28. Brook I. Infant botulism. *J Perinatol* 2007;27:175–80.

29. Hall-Mendelin S, Craig SB, Hall RA, et al. Tick paralysis in Australia caused by *Ixodes holocyclus* Neumann. *Ann Trop Med Parasitol* 2011;105:95–106.

30. Diaz JH. A 60-year meta-analysis of tick paralysis in the United States: A predictable, preventable, and often misdiagnosed poisoning. *J Med Toxicol* 2010;6:15–21.

31. Brueton LA, Huson SM, Cox PM, et al. Asymptomatic maternal myasthenia as a cause of the Pena-Shokeir phenotype. *Am J Med Genet* 2000;92:1–6.

32. Vincent A, Newland C, Brueton L, et al. Arthrogryposis multiplex congenita with maternal autoantibodies specific for a fetal antigen. *Lancet* 1995;346:24–5.

33. Pati S, Goodfellow JA, Iyadurai S, et al. Approach to critical illness polyneuropathy and myopathy. *Postgrad Med J* 2008;84:354–60.

34. Lacomis D, Petrella JT, Giuliani MJ. Causes of neuromuscular weakness in the intensive care unit: A study of ninety-two patients. *Muscle Nerve* 1998;21:610–7.

35. Williams S, Horrocks IA, Ouvrier RA, et al. Critical illness polyneuropathy and myopathy in pediatric intensive care: A review. *Pediatr Crit Care Med* 2007;8:18–22.

36. Banwell BL, Mildner RJ, Hassall AC, et al. Muscle weakness in critically ill children. *Neurology* 2003;61:1779–82.

37. Lefaucheur JP, Nordine T, Rodriguez P, et al. Origin of ICU acquired paresis determined by direct muscle stimulation. *J Neurol Neurosurg Psychiatry* 2006;77:500–6.

38. Allen DC, Arunachalam R, Mills KR. Critical illness myopathy: Further evidence from muscle-fiber excitability studies of an acquired channelopathy. *Muscle Nerve* 2008;37:14–22.

39. Darras BT, Jones HR Jr. Neuromuscular problems of the critically ill neonate and child. *Semin Pediatr Neurol* 2004;11:147–68.

CHAPTER 53 ■ ACUTE NEUROMUSCULAR DISEASE

SUNIT C. SINGHI, NAVEEN SANKHYAN, AND ARUN BANSAL

Guillain–Barré Syndrome

1. Guillain–Barré syndrome (GBS) is the major cause of acute flaccid paralysis. Its annual incidence in children under 9 years of age is 0.62 per 100,000.

2. GBS characteristically presents as a progressive, ascending, symmetric, areflexic weakness of more than one limb, with autonomic dysfunction.

3. The proportion of various subtypes of GBS varies with the geographical regions. Acute inflammatory demyelinating polyradiculopathy accounts for 85%–90% of cases of GBS in Europe and North America.

4. The diagnosis is based on a characteristic clinical picture, nerve-conduction abnormalities, and the cerebrospinal fluid, which shows dissociation in albumin level and cell count.

5. Indications for PICU admission include rapid progression of motor weakness involving respiratory muscles, ventilatory insufficiency, pneumonia, severe bulbar weakness, autonomic instability, arrhythmia, or bradycardia. Autonomic dysfunction is an important cause of death due to hemodynamic instability and arrhythmias.

6. Autonomic instability and risk for succinylcholine-induced hyperkalemia/arrhythmia complicate the intubation of these patients.

7. Treatment involves either plasma exchange (50 mL/kg) or intravenous immunoglobulin (IVIG) 400 mg/kg/day for 5 days. IVIG may be preferable for young children whose line access for plasmapheresis is likely to be difficult.

8. Plasmapheresis may be preferable for (a) patients with immunoglobulin A (IgA) deficiency who would be at risk for anaphylaxis with IVIG administration, (b) patients with congestive heart failure, or (c) those at risk of volume overload.

Myasthenia Gravis

9. Myasthenia gravis (MG) is characterized by fluctuating weakness and fatigability, especially of ocular muscles.

10. Diagnosis of MG is made with positive Tensilon/Neostigmine test, acetylcholine receptor antibodies (in 85% of cases), decremental response to repetitive nerve stimulation, and abnormal single-fiber electromyogram.

11. Myasthenic crisis, defined as respiratory failure (which occurs in 15%–20% patients), must be differentiated from cholinergic crisis.

12. Cholinesterase inhibitors are the first-line treatment for MG. Immunotherapy or steroids are generally second-tier treatment, and plasmapheresis or IVIG is third-tier treatment. Thymectomy is considered in indicated patients.

Acute Intermittent Porphyria

13. The porphyrias comprise a group of disorders caused by enzymatic defects in heme the biosynthesis that leads to an overproduction and accumulation of 5-aminolevulinic acid and porphobilinogen.

14. Clinical features of acute pophyria include a triad of abdominal pain, changes in mental state, and peripheral neuropathy; respiratory paralysis and failure occur in up to 20% patients.

15. Precipitating factors of acute intermittent porphyria are drugs, starvation, hormonal factors, and infections.

16. Treatment of an acute attack includes stopping offending drug(s), control of, pain using opiate analgesics, hypertension using propranolol, seizures using diazepam, and gastrointestinal symptoms using promethazine. Specific therapy is IV 10% glucose and hemin infusion (3–4 mg/kg, once daily for 4 days). One needs to be alert to the increased risk of hyponatremia with use of large volumes of 10% glucose.

17. Clinical improvement with hemin therapy is rapid, often noticeable within 2–4 days. Motor weakness usually resolves; occasionally, footdrop and wasting of the hand muscles are seen.

ICU-Acquired Weakness

18. In adults, intensive care unit–acquired weakness is common and adds to hospital length of stay and cost of care.

19. The disorder is broadly categorized into three subcategories: critical illness polyneuropathy (CIP), critical illness myopathy (CIM), and critical illness neuromyopathy.

20. No specific treatments are recommended. Strict glycemic control using intensive insulin therapy has been shown to significantly reduce the incidence of CIP/CIM in adults.

21. Patients with CIM may recover faster and have better prognosis than will patients with CIP.

Diaphragmatic Paralysis

22. Diaphragmatic palsy can be bilateral or unilateral. Unilateral palsy is more common in infants and children. Most common causes are birth trauma and cardiac surgery.

23. Unilateral palsy is often asymptomatic in older children, but in newborn infants and young children, it can cause severe respiratory compromise.

24. Fluoroscopy on sniffing is a traditional method of diagnosis. Sonographic assessment of diaphragmatic motion can be used for diagnosis and to follow the progression.

25. Surgical plication is accepted as the effective treatment. Diaphragmatic palsy secondary to phrenic nerve injury in the newborn invariably requires surgery. Older children, if asymptomatic, may be managed conservatively.

26. Prognosis of unilateral diaphragmatic paralysis depends on the etiology and age.

A child with acute neuromuscular disease (NMD) may require critical care for respiratory assistance, including intubation of the trachea and mechanical ventilation. The common indications for intensive monitoring or critical care include when the patient is at risk of aspiration pneumonia because of poor airway protection, inadequate oxygenation and/or ventilation because of failed mechanics of breathing, or cardiovascular instability because of autonomic nervous system involvement. Endotracheal intubation may be necessary for airway protection if bulbar muscle dysfunction is present. Mechanical ventilation, either noninvasively or with endotracheal intubation, may be necessary if respiratory failure develops. Occasionally, children with acute NMDs will require airway management solely to facilitate pulmonary toilet. Typically, more than one of these needs is present when a child with an acute NMD requires respiratory assistance.

Acute NMD can be the primary reason for admission to the pediatric intensive care unit (PICU). However, such disorders may also develop de novo during the PICU stay and result in increased morbidity, prolonged hospital length of hospital stay, excess healthcare costs, and mortality. In adults, the so-called critical care–acquired neuromuscular weakness, comprising critical illness polyneuropathy (CIP) and critical illness myopathy (CIM), occurs more often than primary NMDs such as Guillain–Barré syndrome (GBS), motor neuron disease, or myopathies (1). The incidence of these secondary illnesses (CIP/CIM) in children is much less common than in adults, which may, in part, be due to underrecognition and underreporting (see Chapter 52) (2).

REGULATION OF RESPIRATION

Respiration is regulated by both voluntary and involuntary neural mechanisms. The cerebral cortex is responsible for voluntary control of breathing, whereas the brainstem, mainly the medulla oblongata with additional inputs from the pons and vagus, provides involuntary control. Spontaneous breathing is generated by rhythmic discharge of motor neurons innervating the respiratory muscles under the control of the brainstem and is regulated by alterations in arterial partial pressure of carbon dioxide ($PaCO_2$), oxygen (PaO_2), and pH. The afferent limb of the respiratory feedback system is composed of input from the tissues and airways with receptor endings and chemoreceptors in the carotid bodies, which send information to the central nervous system (CNS). The efferent limb involves signals sent from the CNS via cranial and peripheral nerves to the respiratory muscles, which produce an increase or decrease in respiratory activity. This feedback system optimizes airway patency, work of breathing, and gas exchange.

NMDs can be classified according to the site of primary pathology: brain, spinal cord, peripheral nerve, neuromuscular junction, or the skeletal muscle (Table 53.1). In primary NMDs, ineffective motor nerve input to muscles may originate from diseases of the brain (central hypoventilation), spinal cord (trauma), anterior horn cells (poliomyelitis, spinal muscular atrophy), peripheral nerve (GBS), neuromuscular junction (botulism, myasthenia gravis [MG]), or skeletal muscle system (muscular dystrophy).

RESPIRATORY MECHANICS

The lungs and surrounding chest-wall muscles form the ventilatory apparatus, which is similar in function to a pump. The integrity of this "respiratory pump" and the central control from brain and nerves is essential for maintaining normal breathing. Inspiratory effort is mainly driven by the diaphragm and muscles of the chest wall. The abdominal muscles are important for expiratory function and coughing. The accessory muscles of

TABLE 53.1

ANATOMIC CLASSIFICATION AND EXAMPLES OF CONDITIONS WITH NEUROMUSCULAR WEAKNESS THAT REQUIRE PEDIATRIC INTENSIVE CARE

Brain
  Intracranial hemorrhage
  Hypoxic ischemic encephalopathy
  Meningoencephalitis
  Acute demyelinating encephalomyelitis
Spinal cord
  Trauma
  Epidural abscess
  Myelitis
  Acute poliomyelitis
  Spinal muscular atrophy
Peripheral nerve
  Guillain–Barré syndrome
  Critical illness polyneuropathy
  Toxic (lead, arsenic) neuropathy
  Drug-induced neuropathy, e.g., vincristine
  Diphtheric polyneuropathy
  Acute porphyria
  Phrenic nerve injury—diaphragmatic paralysis
Neuromuscular junction
  Myasthenia gravis and congenital myasthenic syndromes
  Prolonged neuromuscular blockade
  Antibiotic (aminoglycoside, D-penicillamine) therapy
  Snake bite and scorpion sting
  Organophosphorus poisoning
  Botulism
  Tick paralysis
  Hypermagnesemia
Muscle
  Critical illness myopathy
  Hypokalemia
  Muscular dystrophies
  Congenital myopathies
  Acute rhabdomyolysis
  Inflammatory myopathies, e.g., dermatomyositis

breathing are located in the neck and the upper chest wall and include the sternocleidomastoid, trapezius, intercostal, and rhomboid muscles. Inspiration is an active process during which an increase in intrathoracic volume is produced by chest and lung expansion, resulting from contraction that causes a downward movement of the diaphragm. The intercostal muscles stabilize the chest wall during changes in intrathoracic pressure. Expiration is a passive process during quiet breathing that results from elastic recoil of the lungs as the diaphragm relaxes to resume its resting configuration. The alternating inspiratory and expiratory activity moves gases in and out of the lung for gaseous exchange. As breathing becomes vigorous with increased activity (exercise) or in the presence of an airway obstruction, the accessory muscles of breathing augment ventilation.

Brain and brainstem diseases cause respiratory depression, characterized by central patterns of respiration, including hyperventilation; irregular, ataxic (or cluster) breathing; hiccups, hypopnea, and apnea. Bulbar involvement may cause impaired clearance and aspiration of oropharyngeal secretions. Children unable to clear secretions are more prone to pulmonary infection, which can lead to further deterioration of their clinical condition. Malfunction of a motor nerve unit (i.e., anterior horn cell, axon of anterior horn cell with its myelin covering, neuromuscular junction, and the muscle innervated by the anterior horn cell) may result in an inability to protect the airway, dysfunction of respiratory muscles, or both.

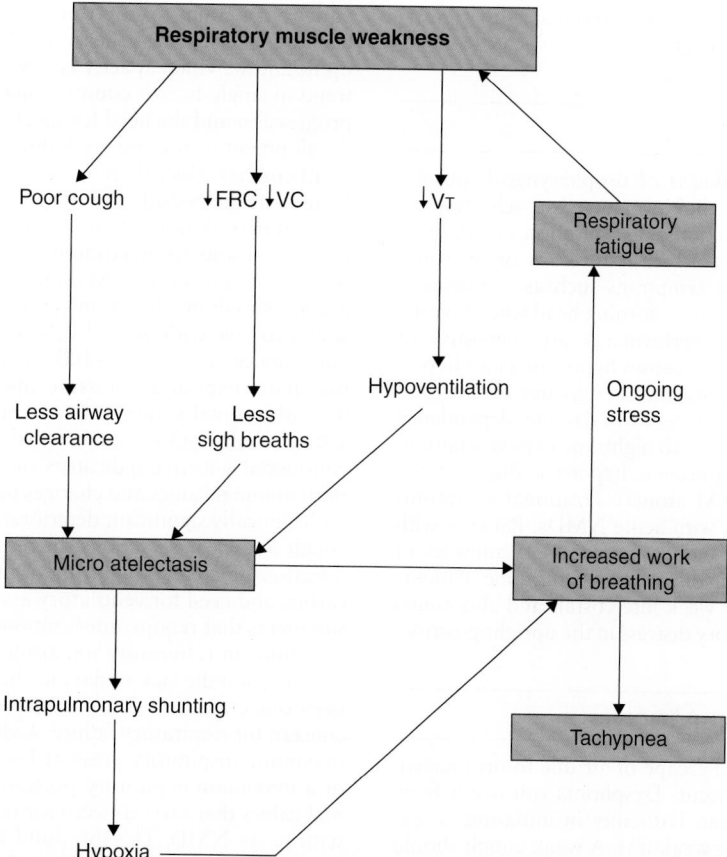

FIGURE 53.1. Pathophysiology of respiratory failure in neuromuscular disorders. FRC, functional residual capacity; VC, vital capacity; VT, tidal volume.

In neuromuscular weakness, a combination of abnormalities often contributes to ineffective gas exchange (**Fig. 53.1**). Unable to generate normal inspiratory effort, these patients have rapid shallow breathing—they take breaths of decreased tidal volume and increase their respiratory rate in order to maintain adequate alveolar ventilation. This pattern of breathing can lead to a decrease in lung compliance, an increase in work of breathing, and a decrease in respiratory reserve. The decrease in tidal volume and minute ventilation contributes to hypoxemia and hypercapnia. An ineffective cough results in retention and aspiration of secretions and microatelectasis. Lack of muscle tone also leaves the recoil pressure of the lung relatively unopposed, resulting in decreased functional residual capacity and impairment in gas exchange. The development of respiratory symptoms may be relatively insidious or sudden. Most of these patients are not very active and may not complain of shortness of breath, but a minor respiratory infection can precipitate sudden respiratory collapse.

EVALUATION OF RESPIRATORY DYSFUNCTION IN A PATIENT WITH A NEUROMUSCULAR DISORDER

Respiratory muscle weakness and fatigue frequently contribute to ventilatory failure in patients with NMD. Monitoring of clinical parameters that indicate the severity and progression of weakness is very important (**Table 53.2**). Respiratory dysfunction at night, increased risk of chest infection, and need

TABLE 53.2

CLINICAL AND LABORATORY PARAMETERS THAT ARE USEFUL IN ASSESSMENT OF ADEQUATE RESPIRATORY FUNCTION IN PATIENTS WITH NEUROMUSCULAR WEAKNESS

Clinical
    Respiratory rate—Good index of response to hypoventilation caused by muscular weakness; tachypnea is the earliest response
    Swallowing and handling of secretions
    Quality of cough
    Volume of speech
    Single-breath count
    Chest expansion
    Presence of tachycardia/diaphoresis (nonspecific)
    Use of accessory muscles
    Orthopnea
    Inward movement of abdomen during inspiration
    Breathing pattern alternates between accessory and major respiratory muscles, signifying weakness of major respiratory muscles
    Change in status when sleeping—accessory muscle tone decreases
    Rate of progression of generalized weakness
Laboratory
    Vital capacity
    Maximum inspiratory pressure
    Maximum expiratory pressure
    Sao_2, Pao_2, $Paco_2$, pH
    Chest radiograph

for respiratory support have all been correlated with significant reductions in clinical parameters.

History

Patients with significant weakness of oropharyngeal muscles may present with intermittent choking, slurred speech, dysphonia, difficulty in clearing secretions, or aspiration pneumonia. Patients may exhibit shortness of breath at rest or on exertion, or they may have nonspecific symptoms such as restlessness, difficulty sleeping, or fatigue. Early morning headache, daytime somnolence, and poor school performance are suggestive of nocturnal hypoventilation, which causes hypoxemia and hypercapnia. Weakness of the diaphragm, to a greater extent than weakness of the intercostals, can result in daytime dependency on accessory muscles and can lead to nighttime hypoventilation, as the intercostal muscles can become hypotonic during rapid eye movement sleep (i.e., REM atonia). Positional symptoms may be described by patients with acute NMDs. Patients with diaphragmatic weakness commonly use accessory muscles of breathing and report becoming distressed when supine. Patients with an intact diaphragm but weak intercostals and abdominal muscles may develop respiratory distress in the upright position.

Examination

Speech may be slurred. Nasal escape of air due to oropharyngeal muscle weakness may occur. Dysphonia can result from laryngeal muscles involvement. Difficulty in initiating an explosive cough suggests glottic weakness. A weak cough should alert the examiner that the patient is at high risk of decompensation from retained secretions. Respiration may be rapid and shallow and fail to increase in response to the patient's activity. Patients may present in respiratory failure with a normal or decreased respiratory rate, which is a late and ominous sign for exhaustion and decompensation. A scaphoid appearance in the abdomen may relate to an isolated diaphragm weakness, with the diaphragm drawn up into the chest during inspiration.

In many neuromuscular conditions, patients demonstrate so-called *paradoxical breathing*. Early in the disease, weakness of the intercostal muscles is relatively greater than weakness of the diaphragm. The intercostal muscles usually stabilize the chest wall during inspiration. Paradoxical breathing occurs when, during inspiration, the chest wall is pulled inward due to weak intercostal muscles while the abdomen expands outward as the diaphragm contracts downward; this appears as a rocking motion of chest and abdomen. The pattern differs from normal inspiration in which contraction of diaphragm results in abdominal expansion and intercostal contraction causes chest expansion (i.e., synchronized motion of the abdomen and chest).

Blood Gases

Abnormalities or progressive deterioration in blood gas values indicate respiratory failure. Arterial blood gas monitoring may not be the optimal method for determining when a patient with NMD has a significant problem, since changes in blood gases and oxygen-hemoglobin saturation tend to occur late, at a time when patients can no longer compensate for increasing weakness.

Spirometry

A simple, single-breath counting test may be used at the bedside in older children and adolescents to assess severity and follow progression of weakness due to acute NMD. If the patient can count up to 10 in one breath, the forced vital capacity is likely to be at least 15–20 mL/kg. If they can count up to 25, the vital capacity is ~30–40 mL/kg. Monitoring the trend in single-breath counting may help to determine disease progression and the need for mechanical ventilation before the development of respiratory failure.

In children older than 5 years, a spirometric assessment can be used at the bedside to monitor the severity and progression of weakness. A normal vital capacity is measured from maximum inspiration to maximum expiration (normal values range from 55 to 80 mL/kg). Maximum static respiratory pressures are measured: maximum inspiratory pressure (measured at residual volume with normal values of –100 to –120 cm H_2O for adult males and –80 to –100 cm H_2O for adult females) and maximum expiratory pressure (measured at total lung capacity with normal values 150–240 cm H_2O for adult males and 108–160 cm H_2O for adult females). These measurements are considered sensitive indicators of respiratory muscle strength. Both minimal values and changes in values have been associated with clinically significant deterioration, including an inability to cough and clear secretions, increased incidence of pulmonary infections, increased nighttime ventilatory insufficiency, hypercarbia, and need for ventilatory assistance. Exact minimal measurements that require intervention are not available because of variations in respiratory impairment among NMDs or among patients, and the lack of data in children. A "20/30/40 rule" has been suggested for adult patients for minimal values that raise concern for respiratory failure. A vital capacity of ~20 mL/kg, a maximum inspiratory pressure less negative than –30 cm H_2O, or a maximum expiratory pressure of <40 cm H_2O are minimal values that raise concern for respiratory problems in adults with acute NMD. The threshold for all the three values may also be lower in children. Values that fall by 50% from baseline or >30% in a 24-hour period are of concern. It has been observed that life-threatening respiratory failure occurs when vital capacity drops below 20 mL/kg or 30% of predicted values (3).

Radiologic Studies

Radiographic findings are often late or nonspecific. Helpful findings on chest x-ray may include an elevated hemidiaphragm, in fixed position during inspiration and expiration, suggestive of hemidiaphragmatic weakness or paralysis. A bell-shaped thoracic cage indicates long-standing intercostal muscle weakness. Nonspecific findings include patchy atelectasis or areas of consolidation in patients with aspiration or infection of the respiratory tract.

MANAGEMENT

Respiratory management is one of the most critical aspects common to all NMDs. It includes airway protection and supportive ventilation, which take priority over the investigation of the underlying cause and precipitating factors. Nonspecific or supportive management of respiratory failure and the problems that result from generalized weakness will be discussed in this section. Specific management will be discussed with the discussion of specific disorders.

Respiratory Monitoring and Care

Ventilatory muscle insufficiency and diaphragmatic weakness may not correlate with general neuromuscular weakness. Respiratory function may be compromised even before clinical signs of ventilatory insufficiency are obvious. Because of concomitant pulmonary infection, progression to respiratory failure may be more rapid than that predicted by the underlying condition. Respiratory status, therefore, must be closely and carefully monitored.

Airway protection should be assessed. Nasal speech, gurgling sounds, difficulty in swallowing, or protrusion of the tongue indicates significant bulbar muscle involvement and imminent airway obstruction and ventilatory failure. Clinical manifestations of respiratory muscle weakness include increased respiratory rate, decreased tidal volume, paradoxical inward chest movement during inspiration, and frequent change in breathing pattern. Active use of accessory muscles of respiration, acidosis, mechanical airway obstruction, and pneumonitis indicate weakness of major muscles of respiration. Hypercapnia is a late finding. Whenever possible, bedside spirometry should be performed. A forced vital capacity that falls below 15–20 mL/kg indicates increased risk of ventilatory failure. Patients unable to generate –20 to –30 cm H_2O of negative inspiratory force (NIF) on manometer testing are also at higher risk for respiratory insufficiency. These assessments should be conducted every 2–4 hours. Once admitted to the PICU, these patients should be monitored closely and oral fluids and feeds should be discontinued to prevent aspiration. There should be a low threshold for intervening with endotracheal intubation and mechanical ventilation in patients exhibiting declining respiratory function.

Endotracheal Intubation

Endotracheal intubation is important because (a) the oropharyngeal muscles are weak and there is risk of severe aspiration into the lungs via an unprotected airway; (b) the thoracic pump is weak and there is risk of declining tidal volumes, hypoxemia, and hypercapnia; and (c) the cough and clearance of airway secretions may be poor and there is risk of inadequate pulmonary toilet. An elective endotracheal intubation may prevent sudden respiratory arrest and its consequences (4).

Mechanical Ventilation

If in doubt, early initiation of ventilator support should be preferred in order to ensure adequate minute ventilation. In severe cases, endotracheal intubation and controlled mechanical ventilation may be required. If the patient is able to generate some respiratory muscle effort, synchronized intermittent mandatory ventilation (SIMV), pressure-support ventilation (PSV), or combination of both is appropriate. With SIMV, unassisted, spontaneous breathing may burden the accessory ventilatory muscles, but in PSV, inability to trigger breaths or unanticipated changes in lung compliance can result in insufficient ventilation. If fatigue, hypoxemia, or hypercapnia is encountered, the support from either mode must be increased. Available data are limited regarding the use of noninvasive ventilation (NIV) for children with acute NMDs. NIV is a safe and effective first-line therapy for hypoxemic acute respiratory failure (ARF) in children and infants with NMD (5). In a prospective study of 15 children (aged 3 months to 18 years) with NMD and ARF due to pneumonia, 6 cases refused intubation; in these cases a combination of NIV and assisted coughing by mechanical in-exsufflator was a safe and effective method for rapidly hypercarbia and acidosis (6). However, at present, there are no generally accepted guidelines for the use of NIV in children.

Weaning

Weaning from mechanical ventilation should be started when ventilatory muscle strength begins to return, provided the chest x-ray does not show atelectasis or infiltrates and oxygenation is adequate. A vital capacity >10 mL/kg and a maximum NIF of at least –20 cm H_2O are useful indicators of ability to wean. Weaning from SIMV can be accomplished by gradually reducing ventilation breaths or by increasing the duration of spontaneous breathing time off of the ventilator. Weaning from PSV can be accomplished by gradually decreasing the inspiratory pressure support. During weaning, the patient should not be allowed to become significantly tachypneic and end-tidal CO_2 should be monitored to confirm that Pco_2 is maintained within the normal range. Ventilatory support may be maintained at preweaning levels at night in order to provide rest. During sleep, some level of PSV is required to prevent loss of lung volume and hypoxemia.

Generally, if a pressure support of 5 cm H_2O is well tolerated, or the patient is maintaining minute ventilation without intermittent mechanical ventilation breaths, ventilation can be discontinued. A high-flow T-piece system with an end-expiratory pressure of 2.5–7.5 cm H_2O can be added to the endotracheal tube to prevent atelectasis during nonventilated periods. With increasing muscle strength, patients can be kept off the ventilator for increasing periods using either continuous positive airway pressure or a T-piece circuit. Before considering endotracheal tube extubation, clinical assessment of bulbar muscle weakness is very important, as upper airway difficulties may compromise breathing after extubation.

Complications of Mechanical Ventilation

Complications of mechanical ventilation in children with acute NMD depend on the duration of ventilation. Nosocomial pneumonia and atelectasis are the most common complications. Long-term, invasive ventilation may result in tracheomalacia, tracheoesophageal fistula formation, or tracheal stenosis. Practicing sterile techniques during suctioning of the airway may decrease the incidence of nosocomial pneumonia.

Tracheostomy

Advantages of early tracheostomy include increased comfort, airway safety, and help in weaning from ventilation. No guidelines exist for tracheostomy in children with these disorders. Some disease-specific data suggest that children are less likely to require tracheostomy than are adults.

General Supportive Care

General care is directed toward preventing complications that arise as a result of prolonged immobilization. It should include regular physiotherapy, provision of splints to prevent joint contractures, prevention of deep vein thrombosis, and keeping conscious patients comfortable by careful positioning and repositioning. Enteral nutrition should be started early; parenteral nutrition should be reserved for patients with ileus. Handwashing, strict policies regarding intravenous and urinary catheter asepsis and antimicrobial procedures, avoidance of gastric alkalization, and infection surveillance are needed to prevent nosocomial sepsis.

Physiotherapy

Chest physiotherapy is believed to prevent mucus retention and segmental pulmonary collapse. To maintain joint mobility and prevent deep vein thrombosis in the limbs, early occupational and physical therapy and use of heparin and support stockings are recommended for nonambulatory adult patients, but no specific recommendations exist for children.

Frequent Changes in Position

Patients supported by mechanical ventilation require frequent and gentle posture changes. The use of water or air mattresses to prevent pressure sores and positioning and padding of limbs to prevent secondary nerve damage are advised. Inflamed nerves are more susceptible to pressure injury. Frog positioning (i.e., knees flexed and apart, elbows partially flexed, and shoulders extended) may prevent pressure injury. A trochanteric roll may help to prevent peroneal nerve compression and footdrop. In patients with facial nerve palsy, eye care is imperative to prevent eye desiccation and corneal injury.

Bowel Care

The risk of constipation is increased by prolonged immobilization and use of opiates for analgesia. Daily monitoring of bowel sounds by auscultation for early detection of ileus is recommended.

Bladder Care

Bladder catheterization is performed as a part of general nursing care, in order to maintain body hygiene and prevent distension. Whenever urinary retention is encountered, a sterile, closed, urinary drainage system should be used or manual decompression should be performed with close monitoring for the development and treatment of urinary tract infections (7). The risk of infection should be balanced against the benefit of catheterization.

Nutrition

Critical illness is a hypercatabolic state. To meet the patient's need for increased energy, enteral feeding should be started as soon as possible. It will also reduce the risk of gastric mucosal atrophy and of nosocomial infection. Full-strength formula should be used to meet high-protein and high-caloric need. Inadequate intake of calories and protein may result in ventilator dependence.

Pain Relief

Pain relief may be tried, initially, with paracetamol or nonsteroidal analgesics. Carbamazepine or gabapentin (5 mg/kg/dose TID PO) can be added for neurogenic pain. Opioids may be needed in some patients.

Psychological and Emotional Support

Psychological and emotional disturbances may require attention. In patients with quadriparesis or cranial nerve dysfunction who require mechanical ventilation, continuous psychological support and psychopharmacologic measures may be useful.

GUILLAIN–BARRÉ SYNDROME

GBS is an acute, autoimmune (often postinfectious), disorder of the peripheral nervous system characterized by areflexic weakness of limbs. Recent work on the pathogenesis of the GBS suggests that the disease encompasses a group of acute peripheral-nerve disorders. Each of the variants is characterized by its pathophysiology and clinical distribution of weakness in the limbs and/or cranial nerve innervated muscles. The disease derives its name from two French neurologists Georges Guillain and Jean Alexandre Barré who, in association with Andre Strohl, an electrophysiologist, described the clinical, electrophysiologic, and cerebrospinal fluid (CSF) characteristics of the syndrome. The first modern description of an illness similar to GBS is credited to Jean Landry in 1859. The diagnostic criteria for GBS were reported by the National Institute of Neurological and Communicative Disorders and Stroke in 1978 and revised by Asbury and Cornblath in 1990 (8).

Epidemiology

With the eradication of paralytic poliomyelitis, GBS has become the most common cause of acquired, nontraumatic, generalized motor paralysis. The disease can occur at any age, in any race, and in all climates (seasonal variation from China). The incidence increases with age. In children under 9 years of age, the incidence is 0.62 per 100,000, whereas the overall median annual incidence is ~1.3 (range 0.5–4.0) per 100,000 population (9). The average age of presentation in children ranges between 4 and 8 years, though children as young as 1 year may be affected. Males have a slight predilection for GBS (male-to-female ratio, 1.2:1).

Etiology and Pathogenesis

As many as 70% of the patients with GBS have experienced an infectious illness in the 28 days preceding the onset of neurologic symptoms. Minor respiratory infections account for ~60%, followed by gastrointestinal ailments and nonspecific febrile illnesses. Various infections and other events implicated in the development of GBS are listed in Table 53.3.

The neurophysiologic and pathologic processes that underlie GBS are classified into several subtypes (or variants), and the more common of those subtypes include acute inflammatory demyelinating polyradiculopathy (AIDP), acute motor axonal neuropathy (AMAN), and acute motor and sensory

TABLE 53.3

INFECTIONS AND EVENTS REPORTED TO PRECEDE GUILLAIN–BARRÉ SYNDROME

Infections
  Common cold
  Gastrointestinal illness
  Epstein–Barr virus
  Cytomegalovirus
  Viral hepatitis
  Varicella (in 3%–4% children)
  Campylobacter jejuni infection
  Human immunodeficiency virus infection
  Mycoplasma pneumoniae (in 1%–5%)
  Japanese encephalitis virus
  Falciparum malaria
  Haemophilus influenzae
Immunization
  Rabies vaccine (sample rabbit brain, suckling mouse)
  Influenza vaccination
  Hepatitis B
  ? Typhoid, tetanus
Minor surgery

axonal neuropathy (AMSAN). The Miller Fisher syndrome, another variant of GBS, is characterized by a triad of signs—ophthalmoplegia, ataxia, and areflexia. AIDP is the most prevalent form of GBS and accounts for 85%–90% of cases in Europe and North America, whereas in China, Japan, Bangladesh, and Mexico, the frequency of AMAN ranges from 30% to 65% and the frequency of AIDP ranges from 22% to 46%.

It is believed that GBS results from an antibody against a protein from an infecting organism that cross-reacts with patients' gangliosides (10). Molecular similarity of certain endogenous myelin and ganglioside antigens to constituents of the infecting organism results in hyperimmune responses being mounted by T-cell lymphocytes and macrophages directed against peripheral nerve fibers. Antibodies against anti-peripheral nerve neutral glycolipids have been found in patients with GBS. Antibodies to GQ1b, a minor glycoside in peripheral nerves have been detected in 90% of patients with Miller Fisher syndrome. AMAN is frequently associated with anti-ganglioside antibodies (e.g., GM1, GM1b, GD1a) and evidence of preceding *Campylobacter jejuni* infection. For AIDP, no specific autoantigens or autoantibodies have yet been identified. However, it is believed that autoantibodies bind to myelin antigens and activate complement. This is followed by the formation of *membrane-attack complex* on the outer surface of Schwann cells and the initiation of vesicular degeneration. Macrophages subsequently invade myelin and act as scavengers to remove myelin debris (11). However, it is not yet known as to why some individuals are at risk of developing GBS.

The pathogenesis of the axonal variant of GBS is better defined. An animal model of AMAN has been proposed to be the first proof of molecular mimicry in a human autoimmune disorder (12). Myelinated axons are divided into four functional regions: the nodes of Ranvier, paranodes, juxtaparanodes, and internodes. Gangliosides GM1 and GD1a are strongly expressed at the nodes of Ranvier, where the voltage-gated sodium (Nav) channels are localized. Contactin-associated protein (Caspr) and voltage-gated potassium (Kv) channels are respectively present at the paranodes and juxtaparanodes. Immunoglobulin G (IgG) anti-GM1 or anti-GD1a autoantibodies bind to the nodal axolemma, leading to the formation of the membrane-attack complex. This results in the disappearance of Nav clusters and the detachment of paranodal myelin, which can lead to nerve-conduction failure and muscle weakness. Axonal degeneration may follow at a later stage. Macrophages subsequently invade from the nodes into the periaxonal space, scavenging the injured axons (11).

Pathology

Demyelinating lesions are seen along the entire length of the peripheral nerve in GBS, including the nerve roots. All nerve types may be involved, including those serving autonomic, motor, and sensory systems. Generally, the motor nerve involvement is more than the sensory nerve involvement. AIDP typically shows segmental demyelination along with perivenular mononuclear cell infiltrate. At an early stage, the infiltrate is composed of small- and medium-sized lymphocytes that are subsequently replaced by macrophages involved in active phagocytosis of myelin. The immune target in AIDP appears to be within the Schwann-cell surface membrane or myelin.

The cytoplasmic projection of macrophages that penetrate through myelin gaps insinuate themselves between myelin lamellae and peel away layers of myelin from the axon (10). Macrophages have also been observed within axonal cylinders; this may explain some cases of GBS with axonal degeneration in the absence of severe demyelination. During the recovery phase, Schwann-cell proliferation with imperfect

remyelination is seen. AMAN typically shows axonal degeneration of motor fibers with little or no demyelination. The immune response in AMAN seems to be directed primarily against the axonal membrane.

Clinical Features

A common initial symptom of GBS is paresthesia of the toes and fingers or limb pains, followed by progressive weakness of the lower limbs and/or unsteadiness in gait. Fever, upper respiratory or gastrointestinal symptoms may be reported by two-third of patients in preceding 3 weeks (9,13). As the disease progresses over a period of a few hours to days and weeks, weakness of the upper limbs occurs and cranial nerve palsies develop. This ascending weakness or paralysis is usually symmetrical. In half of the children, pain may be the initial complaint, resulting in the diagnosis being missed or delayed. Ataxia, limb pain, and back pain are more frequent in children than in adults. Urinary retention is seen in 10%–15% of children. Dysautonomia, presenting with symptoms and signs of dizziness, hypertension, excessive sweating, and tachycardia may also occur. The symptoms progress for a median of 7 days. Thereafter the disease plateaus for a variable period and then improvement begins (13).

The hallmark of GBS on physical examination is ascending motor weakness, along with areflexia. Lower-limb, deep-tendon reflexes are usually absent at presentation, but the upper limb reflexes may still be elicited, although with difficulty. Motor weakness may ascend the body to involve respiratory muscles. The progression may occur slowly or rapidly, or in "fits and starts." Cranial nerve involvement (35%–50%), autonomic instability (26%–50%), ataxia (23%), or dysesthesia (20%) may occur. The most common signs of autonomic dysfunction are either sinus tachycardia or bradycardia or hypertension. In severely affected patients, arrhythmias and changes in peripheral vasomotor tone are seen, manifesting as hypotension and lability of blood pressure. Dysautonomia usually correlates with the muscle weakness and more than two-thirds of hospitalized children may display dysautonomia. Loss of normal vasoregulation has been associated with exaggerated hemodynamic responses to drugs and anesthetic agents. Loss of autonomic control of either systemic blood flow distribution or renin–aldosterone release and fluid loss from sweat glands commonly result in volume and electrolyte disturbances. Hyponatremia is common in GBS and has often been attributed to syndrome of inappropriate antidiuretic hormone, but excess antidiuretic hormone in these patients may also be caused by hypovolemia, hypotension, or positive-pressure ventilation.

Variant clinical features include fever at onset of neurologic symptoms, severe sensory loss with pain (myalgias and arthralgias, meningismus, radicular and back pain), sphincter dysfunction (urinary retention), ileus, CNS involvement (cerebellar ataxia, extensor planter response, absent pupillary response, and rarely, loss of all brainstem reflexes), and papilledema. Studies show that adults with GBS may experience abnormal mental state, as evidenced by vivid dreams, hallucinations, delusions, and psychosis. Autonomic dysfunction, mechanical ventilation, and increased CSF proteins are risk factors for developing an abnormal mental state (14).

Variants of GBS may be seen in pediatric patients, although this is a rare finding. These variants include descending GBS (facial or bulbar muscles are first to be involved), Miller Fischer syndrome (characterized by ophthalmoplegia, ataxia, and areflexia with relatively little weakness), and the less common variants of polyneuritis cranialis, pharyngocervicobrachial syndrome, acute sensory neuropathy of childhood, and acute pandysautonomia (Table 53.4) (11).

TABLE 53.4

SELECTED SUBTYPES OF GUILLAIN–BARRÉ SYNDROME

■ SUBTYPE	■ PATHOLOGICAL AND IMMUNOLOGICAL FEATURES	■ CLINICAL FEATURES
Guillain–Barré Syndrome		
Acute inflammatory demyelinating polyneuropathy	Multifocal demyelination, pathological antibodies unknown	Progressive, ascending, symmetrical, areflexic, or hyporelexic weakness
Facial diplegia	Pathological antibodies unknown	Bilateral facial weakness
Acute motor axonal neuropathy	Antibodies against gangliosides GM1, GD1a, GNalNAc-GD1a, and GD1b affecting motor axons only	Acute motor neuropathy of variable severity, reflexes may be preserved in a few patients
Acute motor conduction blocks neuropathy	Antibodies against gangliosides GM1, GD1a, affecting motor axons only	Milder form of acute axonal neuropathy, does not progress to axonal degeneration
Acute motor sensory axonal neuropathy	As above; additionally sensory axons are also affected	Sensory symptoms predominate
Pharyngo-cervico-brachial weakness	Antibodies against gangliosides GT1a, GQ1b, GD1a	Prominent pharyngeal, neck, and shoulder weakness
Miller Fisher Syndrome		
Miller Fisher syndrome	Demyelination, antibodies against gangliosides GQ1b, GT1a, GD3	Ophthalmoplegia, ataxia, areflexia, incomplete forms can occur, can overlap with generalized weakness
Acute ataxic neuropathy	Antibodies against gangliosides GQ1b, GT1a, GD1b	Acute ataxia, no ophthalmoplegia, considered an incomplete form of Fisher syndrome
Acute oropharyngeal palsy	Antibodies against gangliosides GQ1b, GT1a	Acute oropharyngeal weakness
Others		
Acute autonomic neuropathy	Pathological antibodies unknown	Acute autonomic failure, symptoms generally due to cardiovascular involvement

Adapted from Yuki N, Hartung HP. Guillain–Barré syndrome. *N Engl J Med* 2012;366:2294–304.

Diagnosis and Differential Diagnosis

The diagnosis of GBS may be difficult because of variable symptomatology and the apparent lack of etiology. The possibility of GBS as a diagnosis should be considered in any patient with rapid onset of acute neuromuscular weakness. In its evolving phase, GBS must be differentiated from other conditions that cause progressive symmetric weakness including transverse myelitis, acute polyneuropathies caused by toxins/heavy metals, organophosphorus poisoning, tick paralysis, acute porphyria, diphtheria polyneuropathy, myelopathies (poliomyelitis and other enteroviral infections of anterior horn cell), Myasthenia gravis (MG), and electrolyte disturbances (especially hypokalemia). Evidence of neurotoxic conditions, marked or persistent asymmetric involvement, preserved or brisk reflexes, severe sensory signs or distinct sensory level should suggest a diagnosis other than GBS. MG presents with intact tendon reflexes, no dysautonomia, and a normal CSF examination. Enteroviral infections usually cause CSF pleocytosis, and motor neuronal injury is found on electromyogram. Transverse myelitis causes a sensory-deficit level, urinary incontinence, and CSF pleocytosis. Botulism may mimic GBS but these patients have ophthalmoplegia with pupillary involvement, dry mouth, and ileus. Tick paralysis can cause an acute ascending paralysis with areflexia and is seen in North America and Australia. These patients have complete ophthalmoplegia but preserved sensation. A tick is usually found on the scalp or behind the ear. Certain laboratory tests seem particularly valuable in differentiating GBS from other conditions.

Lumbar Puncture

4 If lumbar puncture is performed a week after onset of weakness, the CSF findings typically reveal elevated protein (>45 mg/dL) without CSF pleocytosis (<10 cells/mm³) (often

referred to as albuminocytologic dissociation). Repeat spinal taps may be required if the initial findings are normal. Occasionally, the protein level may not rise throughout the illness, and a mildly elevated cell count (10–50 cells/mm³) is all that is seen. More than 50 cells/mm³ should prompt a reconsideration of the diagnosis of GBS. The decision to do an early lumbar puncture is governed primarily by the need to exclude differentials like infectious myelitis.

Electrodiagnostic Studies

At least three sensory and motor nerves should be tested for neurophysiologic studies (see Chapter 52) (15).

Imaging

The primary use of imaging is to exclude myelitis. In GBS, 2 weeks after the onset of symptoms, lumbosacral magnetic resonance imaging (MRI) with gadolinium contrast may reveal enhancement of the cauda equina nerve roots. This finding has a diagnostic sensitivity for GBS of 83% and is present in 95% of typical cases (16).

Management

Children with GBS are at risk for life-threatening respiratory complications and autonomic disturbance. Indications for
5 PICU admission include rapid progression of motor weakness involving respiratory muscles, ventilatory insufficiency, pneumonia, severe bulbar weakness, autonomic instability, arrhythmia, or bradycardia. Complications related to therapy that require intensive care include fluid overload or anaphylaxis

from intravenous immunoglobulin (IVIG) administration or hemodynamic instability related to plasmapheresis. These factors may exist alone or in combination.

Respiratory Monitoring and Care

It is reported that about 15%–25% of children with GBS develop respiratory failure that requires supportive mechanical ventilation (13,17). It is more likely to occur in children with rapid progression, upper limb weakness, autonomic dysfunction, and cranial nerve involvement. Close observation with serial assessment of ventilatory parameters is essential for early diagnosis of respiratory failure.

Endotracheal Intubation

Endotracheal intubation may be required in children with GBS to protect the airway from aspiration, overcome obstruction from loss of airway tone, or facilitate supportive mechanical ventilation. In GBS, rapid disease progression, presence of bilateral facial nerve palsy, and autonomic dysfunction have been associated with increased likelihood of intubation (18). Planning for early intubation to minimize pulmonary complications has been encouraged to prevent inherent risks of emergency intubation.

Dysautonomia may increase the risks of endotracheal intubation in patients with GBS. Dysautonomia may exaggerate the hemodynamic responses to the drugs used to induce anesthesia during intubation. Patients without full stomachs or ileus may benefit from topical/local anesthetic administration to blunt airway response, and short-acting benzodiazepine sedation and atropine decrease sudden hypotension and arrhythmia induced by airway manipulation. For patients who require emergency intubation (with full stomachs or ileus), a classic or modified rapid-sequence technique, including preoxygenation, cricoid pressure, atropine, lidocaine, a titrated (when possible) or reduced dose of a sedative, and short-acting nondepolarizing muscle relaxants should be used; use of muscle relaxant must be weighed against the risk of a difficult airway. Succinylcholine should be avoided since there is a potential risk of drug-induced hyperkalemia. When feasible, careful titration of drugs with monitoring of heart rate, oxygen saturation, blood pressure, and electrocardiogram during intubation is preferred to prevent catastrophic responses.

Mechanical Ventilation

Independent predictors of the need for ventilation in adults with GBS are interval between the onset of symptoms to admission of <7 days, inability to cough, inability to stand, inability to flex arms or head, increasing liver enzymes, and vital capacity <60% of predicted (19). Clinical signs that indicate the need for mechanical ventilation include ventilatory muscle insufficiency, an increasing oxygen requirement to maintain SpO_2 >92%, or signs of alveolar hypoventilation (e.g., $Pco_2 > 50$ torr). Other indications for initiating mechanical ventilation in GBS are forced vital capacity <15 mL/kg, rapid decline in vital capacity by 50% from baseline, and inability to generate a maximum NIF more negative than –20 cm H_2O. In GBS, recovery from respiratory failure is to be expected, even though some residual motor weakness may remain in the recovering phase.

Tracheostomy

No definitive guidelines exist for tracheostomy in children with GBS. Early tracheostomy may benefit patients who have severe GBS with clinical and electrophysiologic evidence of axonal involvement together with respiratory failure and autonomic dysfunction. With studies that report mean duration of ventilation ranging between 15 and 43 days, some patients can be spared tracheostomy. Tracheostomy may be deferred until the end of the second week of illness, when definitive treatment is completed and potential for recovery can be predicted. If the pulmonary function test tends to improve above baseline, tracheostomy could be deferred for an additional week, allowing the patient to attempt weaning from the ventilator (7).

Autonomic Dysfunction

Autonomic failure is a major factor in mortality from GBS. Fatal cardiovascular collapse due to autonomic dysfunction occurs in 2%–10% of seriously ill patients. Risk of dysautonomia is high in patients with respiratory failure, quadriplegia, or bulbar involvement. Heart rate, blood pressure, and electrocardiographic monitoring should be continued until patients are off respiratory support. A reduction or absence of normal "beat to beat" variation in the heart rate suggests vagal involvement and may be an indicator for risk of arrhythmia in patients with GBS. Transcutaneous cardiac pacing may be used for symptomatic bradycardia. Hypotension should be treated with volume repletion, and if refractory to fluids, a pure α-agonist such as phenylephrine should be preferred to avoid potential arrhythmogenic effects from combined α- and β-agonists. When hemodynamic instability is severe, continuous arterial blood pressure recording should be performed to guide volume therapy. Hypertension may occur but this complication does not need specific treatment unless it is associated with signs of end-organ damage (i.e., pulmonary edema, encephalopathy, or subarachnoid bleed). A high index of suspicion for other medical complications (e.g., pulmonary embolism, pneumothorax, sepsis) should be considered before attributing cardiovascular complications to dysautonomia alone.

General Supportive Care

The patient with GBS who requires intensive care usually has a lengthy stay; hence, the general care in the PICU is as important as mechanical ventilation and specific therapy. Constipation is seen in more than 50% of patients with GBS as a result of adynamic ileus with or without other features of autonomic instability. Prokinetic bowel motility drugs are contraindicated in patients with dysautonomia. Pain relief may be necessary, with acetaminophen usually the first choice. Opioids may be needed in addition, and carbamazepine or gabapentin may be used in case of neurogenic pain.

Specific Therapy—Immunomodulation

Various immunomodulatory therapies have been attempted in GBS. The Cochrane Neuromuscular Group has reviewed evidence regarding the use of steroids, plasma exchange, and IVIG in children and adults (20,21).

Corticosteroids

A recent Cochrane review concluded that corticosteroids should not be used in the treatment of GBS; corticosteroids given alone do not hasten recovery from GBS or affect the long-term outcome. A combination of methylprednisolone and IVIG also does not offer any additional advantage (21).

Plasma Exchange (Plasmapheresis)

Plasma exchange is believed to remove or dilute the antibodies implicated in the pathogenesis of GBS. During each exchange, 40–50 mL/kg of plasma is replaced with a mixture of normal saline and albumin. The value of plasma exchange in younger children (<12 years old) is not clear, but in adults, it is beneficial. A review of 6 randomized trials that comprised 649 patients found plasma exchange to be beneficial (22). The plasma-exchange group showed reduced time to recover to walking, reduced need for artificial ventilation, decreased duration of ventilation, and lower rate of severe sequelae at 1 year. These advantages are best obtained if the plasma exchange is performed within 2 weeks of onset of illness. At least four exchanges have been found to be optimal for moderate to severely affected patients (i.e., unable to walk unsupported or worse), and two exchanges are sufficient for mildly affected patients (22). Relapses are seen in ~10% of patients within 3 weeks of plasmapheresis.

Complications associated with plasmapheresis include hematoma at vascular puncture site, pneumothorax following central venous catheterization, and sepsis. Mild hypotension that is responsive to fluid administration is common in children who undergo plasma exchange. Plasmapheresis is contraindicated in patients with severe hemodynamic instability, bleeding diathesis, and septicemia. Plasma exchange has been compared to CSF filtration (5–6 cycles of daily filtration of 30–50 mL of CSF) in a small trial with no significant difference in outcome (23).

Intravenous Immunoglobulin. IVIG has been shown to be of equivalent benefit to plasma exchange in GBS in children. It is therefore indicated in severely affected patients (i.e., unable to walk unaided or disability grade 3) within 2 weeks from onset. There is moderate quality evidence that, in severe disease, IVIG started within 2 weeks from onset hastens recovery as much as plasma exchange. Adverse events are not significantly more frequent with either treatment, but IVIG is easier to manage and significantly much more likely to be completed than plasma exchange (20,24). In patients with severe GBS, IVIG reduces the need for mechanical ventilation and reduces the average length of PICU stay by 50%. Early recovery from muscle weakness and decreased duration of endotracheal intubation and mechanical ventilation contribute to reducing the incidence of pulmonary complications such as pneumonia and atelectasis (25). The mechanism of action of IVIG is likely multifactorial and is believed to involve modulation of complement activation, binding and neutralization of idiotypic antibodies, saturation of Fc receptors on macrophages, and suppression of various inflammatory mediators, such as cytokines, chemokines (26). There are no controlled studies of IVIG in milder forms of GBS and the Miller Fisher syndrome. A combination of plasmapheresis and IVIG is not superior to either treatment alone.

IVIG is given as daily infusion (0.4 g/kg/day) for 5 days in the first 2 weeks of illness. Systematic data are inadequate to support the use of 1 g/kg/day for 2 days. A second course of IVIG (2 g/kg in 2–5 days) may be given to 5%–10% of patients who deteriorate after initial improvement (so-called treatment-related clinical fluctuation) (27). Minor side effects of IVIG include headache, myalgia, and arthralgia; flu-like symptoms; fever; and vasomotor reactions. IgA-deficient patients may develop anaphylaxis after the first course of IgA-containing IVIG. Rarely, aseptic meningitis, congestive heart failure, vascular complications, and renal failure have been reported; therefore, IVIG should not be used in patients with congenital IgA deficiency, hyperviscosity syndromes, and congestive heart failure. In all of these conditions plasma exchange is the treatment of choice.

Outcome

GBS remains a severe disease despite the availability of current treatment. In comparison with adults, children may have a more favorable outcome—which may be complete rather than partial. The estimated mortality in childhood GBS is <5%; higher rates are seen in medically disadvantaged areas. Causes of death due to GBS include respiratory failure and cardiac arrest secondary to dysautonomia. Death may occur because of complications associated with immobility and mechanical ventilation, such as pneumonia, sepsis, acute respiratory distress syndrome, and thromboembolic events. Recovery usually begins 2–4 weeks after plateau of symptom progression. The median time from the onset of symptoms to full recovery was 66 days, with 90%–95% of full recoveries occurring in children by 3–12 months. Recurrence of symptoms, though less common in children, can be encountered within the first 2–3 weeks after IVIG therapy. Literature regarding the long-term outcome of children with GBS is limited; 75%–80% of children recover fully (10). About 20% of patients are still unable to walk after 6 months (28). In a prospective long-term follow-up study, at the end of the observation period (288 days), 75% of patients were free of symptoms. Twenty-one percent suffered residual symptoms, having no effect on daily functioning. The more severely disabled 4% either suffered from either chronic inflammatory demyelinating polyneuropathy or concurrent myelitis (13).

Younger age group (<9 years), rapid progression to maximal weakness (within 10 days), and need for mechanical ventilation are important predictors of long-term deficits (29). Early presence of IgG or IgA anti-GM1 antibodies and serologic evidence of *C. jejuni* infection are laboratory features predictive of severe disease and poor outcome.

MYASTHENIA GRAVIS

Myasthenia gravis (literally *grave muscle weakness*) is a disorder of the neuromuscular junction characterized by fluctuating weakness and fatigability of the voluntary skeletal muscles that result from autoimmune destruction of acetylcholine receptors (AChRs) at the postsynaptic end plate. Erb first reported the childhood onset of this condition in 1879. In childhood, MG is categorized by age or immunological involvement as (a) autoimmune MG or juvenile MG (JMG), (b) congenital MG or genetic MG, or (c) transient neonatal MG (TMG).

Epidemiology

The population-based incidence of MG is 3–30 per million per year (30). MG is rare during childhood. The incidence in children (0–19 years) is 1–5 per million per year, which may be an underestimate as mild cases may have been missed. No epidemiologic data exist regarding children who have AChR autoantibodies, muscle-specific kinase (MuSK) antibodies, or the genetic form of the disease without antibody involvement. Some demographic differences are seen in the epidemiology. The incidence is higher in African American than in Caucasian children. In general, female preponderance is seen, but before puberty both sexes are equally affected in the Caucasian population. This demographic difference may be the result of genetic differences or different predisposing environmental triggering factors.

Pathogenesis

The pathogenesis usually involves polyclonal IgG autoantibodies that are directed against AChR. Autoantibodies against nicotinic AChR are detectable in 85%–90% of cases of MG, and the remaining cases include either antibodies against other targets (e.g., MuSK) or a genetic basis for abnormal neuromuscular transmission at the neuromuscular junction. The production of the AChR autoantibodies requires both autoreactive T cells (i.e., failure of T-cell tolerance) and subsequent failure of B-cell tolerance. The autoantibodies cause disease at the neuromuscular junction by both blocking the Ach-binding sites on the receptors and inducing local deposition of complement, which causes destruction of the receptors. This results in a reduction in the number of functional AChRs with disruption of normal neuromuscular transmission, manifesting as weakness of skeletal muscles. Severity of weakness is proportional to the reduction in functional AChRs.

Patients with increased levels of autoantibodies against AChRs are termed *seropositive*. *Seronegative* (no AChR antibodies) patients may have autoantibodies against other antigens, such as MuSK, acetylcholine premembrane receptor (PremRab), or other neighboring postsynaptic proteins. Alternatively, seronegative patients may have some genetic mutation of AchRs (or its associated protein) or a congenital absence of acetylcholine esterase. A lot (40%–50%) of seronegative MG patients with generalized weakness have antibodies against MuSK. These patients have atypical illness characterized by involvement of facial, bulbar, neck, shoulder, and respiratory muscles, with less involvement of ocular muscles. They have variable response to first-line treatment, i.e., cholinesterase inhibitors (CEIs) (31).

The mechanism that triggers autoimmune destruction of AchRs is still unclear. Microbial infections have been implicated. Strong evidence suggests that the thymus gland plays a central pathophysiologic role as thymic hyperplasia is found in ~70% of cases. Thymomas and myasthenic thymus contain abundant AchR-reactive T cells.

Clinical Features

Juvenile Myasthenia Gravis

Juvenile myasthenia gravis (JMG) can be separated into three broad subtypes: AChR antibody-positive JMG, MuSK antibody-positive JMG, and seronegative JMG. JMG (autoimmune MG of childhood) has an age of onset between 3 months and 16 years, mostly before 3 years (32), and a clinical picture that is similar to MG in adults. Symptoms are least apparent on awakening, and they become more evident later in the day. Weakness may remain localized to the eye muscles or it may progress to be generalized. Ocular involvement is present in most children with JMG, taking the form of intermittent drooping of eyelids with a persistent upward gaze or double vision, especially while reading. This weakness is variable and often asymmetric. In 10%–15% of children, weakness may be limited to the extraocular muscles, a condition known as *ocular MG*. Seventy-five percent of children who present initially with ocular symptoms develop progressive disease that results, within 4 years, in bulbar weakness or generalized weakness.

Almost 75% of patients have bulbar weakness at the time of initial presentation; for example, weakness of tongue and soft palate that results in nasal or slurred speech, especially after prolonged talking, or difficulty in chewing during meals due to weakness of muscles of mastication. Pharyngeal and laryngeal muscle weakness leads to dysphonia and choking on food and secretions. Facial muscle weakness results in a flattened, expressionless face and in drooling. Diminished strength of neck muscles may cause the tendency of the head to fall forward or backward, requiring manual assistance for holding up the head. Involvement of muscles of the legs results in fatigability and weakness while climbing stairs or running. This weakness tends to be symmetrical and proximal; distal weakness is an atypical presentation of MG.

Systemic weakness that involves diaphragm and muscles of respiration may also occur and may be so severe as to cause respiratory failure. *Weakness of respiratory muscles, in combination with bulbar weakness, warrants hospitalization for immediate evaluation and management.*

On physical examination, findings are confined to the motor system, with no loss of sensation or coordination. Ptosis may be asymmetric, but extraocular muscle weakness is symmetric and fluctuating. Pupillary responses are not affected. Various maneuvers can be performed to unmask the underlying fatigability, including repetitive trips up and down the staircase, repetitive fun exercises in young children, having the patient count to 100 or chew for 30 seconds, and may provide a rough assessment of fatigable weakness. An adaptation of a scale devised by Osserman is commonly used to grade strength and fatigability:

- Grade I: Weakness restricted to extraocular muscles
- Grade IIa: Generalized mild weakness
- Grade IIb: Generalized moderate weakness
- Grade III: Generalized severe weakness
- Grade IV: Life-threatening weakness of respiratory muscles.

The clinical state of the patient during the examination may not show correlation with the level of antibodies (32).

MuSK Antibody-Positive JMG

The prevalence of MuSK antibodies in AChR-negative JMG patients shows geographical and racial differences. The frequency of juvenile cases ranges between 0% and 24% (33,34). JMG with MuSK antibodies is rare in young children, while it is relatively more common in the second decade of life; females are predominantly affected, irrespective of age of onset. In AChR-negative MG the thymus is usually normal or harbors only mild alterations; a thymoma has never been reported in these children. Worldwide studies confirm three major phenotypes in MuSK antibody-positive MG patients: (1) A phenotype indistinguishable from AChR antibody–positive patients, (2) A phenotype with prominent faciopharyngeal weakness, usually with marked muscle atrophy, and (3) A phenotype with relatively isolated neck extensor and respiratory weakness. MuSK antibody–positive MG predominates in women and weakness is typically more severe, with more frequent respiratory crises than non-MuSK MG (35). It is uncertain how MuSK antibody–positive MG results in neuromuscular transmission failure since MuSK antibodies alter neuromuscular junction morphology without altering AChR numbers or turnover (36).

Seronegative JMG

The frequency of seronegative MG is higher in childhood (seronegative JMG). This is partly explained by the higher frequency of ocular myasthenia, although a real increase in prevalence is also possible. The main differential diagnosis from seronegative children is congenital myasthenic syndrome (CMS), which usually presents in the first year of life (JMG is most common after the first year), but can also occur later in childhood or adolescence.

Transient Neonatal MG

Transient neonatal MG presents shortly after birth, occurring in 10%–20% of babies born to mothers with autoimmune MG. Passive transplacental transfer of circulating AchR antibodies is the cause. Correlation exists between the occurrence and severity of neonatal MG and AchR antibody titers in the mother and newborn. However, the condition may occur in babies of mothers in clinical remission or without elevated AchR antibody titers. A high ratio of anti-embryonic muscle AchR antibodies to anti-adult muscle AchR antibodies correlates very well with the occurrence of neonatal MG.

The features of TMG may develop within a few hours of birth. Infants may show a range of symptoms from mild hypotonia to a generalized weakness, feeble cry, difficult feeding, ptosis, facial weakness, or life-threatening respiratory distress. The syndrome usually resolves within 3 weeks but will occasionally persist for months. Every newborn of myasthenic mothers should be observed during the neonatal period for signs of muscle weakness, respiratory failure, and any impairment of bulbar muscles. Treatment includes anticholinesterase and, if indicated, ventilatory support. Very severe cases may require plasmapheresis (37).

Lambert–Eaton Myasthenic Syndrome

This is an exceedingly rare myasthenic syndrome in children. It presents with the classic clinical triad of proximal weakness, autonomic dysfunction, and areflexia. Diagnosis is based on repetitive nerve stimulation (see Chapter 52). The presence of serum antibodies to the P/Q-type voltage-gated calcium channel supports the diagnosis in doubtful cases. In adults, the most common association is the small-cell lung cancer. Both immune-mediated and tumor-associated (neuroblastoma, Wilms tumor) Lambert–Eaton myasthenic syndrome have been described in children. Hence, recognition of this syndrome is important to initiate a search for malignancy or another immune-mediated process (38).

Congenital Myasthenic Syndromes

Congenital myasthenic syndromes (CMS) are genetic disorders of neuromuscular transmission produced by mutations that alter the expression and function of ion channels, receptors, enzymes, or other accessory molecules necessary to maintain neuromuscular transmission. Most cases present at birth, but some may present later in childhood or adolescence; severe cases present in infancy or early childhood. The presenting features include any combination of ptosis, ophthalmoparesis, dysphagia, dysarthria, poor feeding, weak cry, hypotonia, motor delay, respiratory distress, chronic respiratory and limb weakness, and arthrogryposis multiplex. CMS must be differentiated from myopathies, muscular dystrophies, and JMG. Anticholinesterase agents, such as pyridostigmine, are the first-line therapy, except for slow-channel CMS, COLQ, and DOK7 mutations (3,4-diaminopyridine is a useful option in the later) (39). Ephedrine, quinidine, and fluoxetine are other options. Immunotherapy does not have a role in treatment. Some disorders (slow-channel CMS, congenital acetylcholinesterase deficiency) progressively worsen over years due to progression of end-plate myopathy and degeneration of the postsynaptic region because of cationic overload. If patients with other abnormalities (AchR deficiency, fast-channel congenital MG, congenital choline acetyltransferase deficiency) survive infancy and childhood, they may show some improvement with age or develop static or slowly progressive weakness.

Emergencies in Myasthenia Gravis

Myasthenic crisis and cholinergic crisis are two emergencies in MG associated with acute, life-threatening respiratory failure. *Myasthenic crisis* is an acute exacerbation of the disease process that results in severe weakness from dysfunction of the neuromuscular junctions. Myasthenic crisis is characterized by respiratory failure due to weakness of either the upper airway muscles or of the diaphragm and other respiratory muscles. Myasthenic crisis can be precipitated by a number of factors, including respiratory infection, sepsis, aspiration, surgical procedures, rapid tapering off of corticosteroid or immunotherapeutic drugs, initiation of corticosteroid therapy, and

exposure to drugs. Myasthenic crisis may be the initial presentation of undiagnosed MG; 20% of patients with MG suffer from myasthenic crisis within the first year of illness, and approximately one-third of them experience another episode.

Cholinergic crisis is a severe weakness usually caused by overtreatment with cholinergic medication, resulting in overstimulation and blockade of the already functionally compromised neuromuscular junction by acetylcholine. The weakness due to cholinergic crisis may be indistinguishable from myasthenic crisis. The muscarinic effects of CEIs increase bronchopulmonary secretions, which can obstruct the airway and cause aspiration. Patients show features of cholinergic excess, including excessive salivation, excessive lacrimation, diarrhea, sweating, pupillary constriction, and, possibly, muscle fasciculation. Patients with compromised renal function are more susceptible to cholinergic crisis. Patients in crisis should be observed and monitored in the PICU.

Cholinergic crisis and myasthenic crisis may be difficult to distinguish. CEI treatment should be withheld initially to avoid contributing to cholinergic overload in cholinergic crisis. CEI treatment is potentially harmful in patients with myasthenic crisis if they have significant weakness, as it may cause increased secretions and thus hasten respiratory failure. Supportive care is generally required for both crises. CEI is withheld and atropine is used to treat cholinergic crisis. Removal of triggers and institution of plasmapheresis or administration of IVIG may be necessary to treat myasthenic crisis. Steroids, immunotherapy, and thymectomy are not immediately useful for myasthenic crisis, as they may take weeks to be effective.

Diagnosis

The diagnosis of MG is based on clinical history, neurologic examination, and pharmacologic, electrophysiologic (see Chapter 52), and serologic testing.

Pharmacologic Testing

Edrophonium chloride (Tensilon) is an IV CEI agent with rapid onset (30 seconds) and short duration (15 minutes) of action. It acts by inhibiting the enzyme acetylcholinesterase, thereby allowing acetylcholine to diffuse widely throughout the synaptic cleft and to interact with AchRs, resulting in a larger and longer end-plate potential. The dose that produces improvement cannot be predicted, as the response is variable. A Tensilon test (for children >2 years old) involves administration of edrophonium intravenously in incremental doses, beginning with 0.01 mg/kg up to a maximum of 0.1 mg/kg and observing for improvement in function. Bradycardia can be a significant side effect; therefore, patients should be on a cardiac monitor, and atropine should be available. Relative contraindications to this test are a history of bronchial asthma or cardiac dysrhythmias. Any group of muscles can be tested, but it is considered more sensitive and useful when improvement in ptosis and double vision are used as the diagnostic end points. The key is to identify precisely which muscle or muscle group is to be tested. Objective improvement in muscular strength is more important than the perception of improvement. The result of the test is influenced by the patient's maximal exertional effort prior to and after administration of the drug. The test is reasonably sensitive but not specific for MG. False-positive results can occur in other neuromuscular conditions (e.g., botulism, GBS, motor neuron disease, and lesions of brainstem). Edrophonium is not recommended in infants because of its brief action, which precludes objective assessments and secondly due to an increased risk of arrhythmias. In children below 2 years of age, Neostigmine is used and administered intramuscularly at a dose of 0.04 mg/kg.

The peak effect is seen in 20–40 min. A video of the test is often helpful in recording, and later comparing, before and after drug effects.

Other CEIs

Some patients may not show a response to edrophonium, but they may show improvement to neostigmine or pyridostigmine. These agents have an onset of action 5–15 minutes after intramuscular administration, and their effect may last for up to 4 hours. This longer duration of action (compared to edrophonium) may make neostigmine and pyridostigmine more useful in the evaluation of children. A therapeutic trial of oral pyridostigmine may have a subjective benefit on strength and fatigability that is not apparent after a single dose of edrophonium.

Serologic (Immunologic) Tests

Measurement of antibodies to AchR by radioimmunoprecipitation assay is one of the most specific diagnostic tests for MG. These antibodies are present in about 85% of patients with JMG (40). Normal levels do not exclude the diagnosis. Because seronegative patients can become seropositive, monitoring of serology is helpful. The level may be raised in other conditions, such as autoimmune liver disease, systemic lupus erythematosus, inflammatory myopathies, and first-degree relatives of patients with acquired MG. Approximately 40%–60% of seronegative patients with JMG may have serum antibodies to MuSK. Other antibodies that are useful in the diagnosis of MG include low-affinity anti-AChR, anti-titin, anti-ryanodine receptor antibodies. CD-cell examination may be abnormal in 85% of cases, mostly because of reduced levels of CD4$^+$ or CD3$^+$ and CD8$^+$ (32).

Management

MG is no longer the uniformly fatal illness that it was in the past. It can now be managed with safe and effective therapies. Management in a PICU is indicated in patients with respiratory compromise or bulbar weakness and in those at risk for deterioration during initiation of therapy, myasthenic or cholinergic crisis, or perioperative management, including thymectomy.

Patients in myasthenic crisis have intact respiratory drive; hence, the reduction in tidal volume in evolving ventilatory failure is initially countered by increasing respiratory rate. Diaphragmatic weakness and excessive use of accessory muscles of respiration becomes evident. A weak cough or low, single-breath counting performance, denoting significant expiratory muscle weakness, also occurs. Respiratory compromise due to oropharyngeal and laryngeal muscle weakness may have normal tidal volume and vital capacity. With diaphragm and accessory muscle weakness, vital capacity will be reduced, as will maximum inspiratory pressure measurements. An inability to produce an NIF more than −20 cm H_2O suggests the need for urgent intubation. Vocal cord weakness may be demonstrated by direct laryngoscopy.

Endotracheal Intubation

At the time of intubation, careful consideration should be given to the use of neuromuscular-blocking agents (NMBAs) because of prolonged and unpredictable duration of action. Resistance to the effects of succinylcholine is possible due to relative deficiency of AchRs, and higher doses may be needed to induce paralysis. Once the patient is paralyzed with succinylcholine,

prolonged paralysis is highly likely, as is increased sensitivity to nondepolarizing NMBAs, which causes marked and prolonged paralysis. Short-acting, nondepolarizing agents may be less likely to result in unwanted prolonged paralysis, but prolongation of any paralytic should be anticipated.

Mechanical Ventilation

Initially, patients may be too weak to trigger the ventilator and will require controlled ventilation. Administration of pyridostigmine can be discontinued to facilitate mechanical ventilation and improve airway toilet and suctioning. No particular mode of mechanical ventilation is superior. If Pco_2 is not >50 mm Hg, NIV with bilevel positive-pressure ventilation may obviate the need for endotracheal intubation in ARF due to myasthenic crisis (41). In adults, proactive and thorough respiratory care reduces the risk of prolonged respiratory complications and the duration of mechanical ventilation (42).

General PICU Care

Some medications exacerbate muscle weakness, and these should be avoided or stopped (Table 53.5).

Specific Therapies

The management of MG involves a graded approach in which the choice of treatment depends on the patient's age, severity, and rate of disease progression.

Cholinesterase Inhibitors

In patients with moderately severe muscle weakness but no evidence of respiratory failure, it is reasonable to increase the

TABLE 53.5

PHARMACEUTICAL AGENTS WITH THE POTENTIAL TO AGGRAVATE MYASTHENIA GRAVIS

Antibiotics
Ampicillin, aminoglycosides (gentamicin, kanamycin, streptomycin, tobramycin), clindamycin, colistin, erythromycin, fluoroquinolones (e.g., ciprofloxacin, norfloxacin), lincomycin, neomycin, penicillin, polymyxin B, sulfonamides, tetracycline, trimethoprim-sulfamethoxazole, vancomycin

Anticonvulsants
Barbiturates, carbamazepine, gabapentin, phenytoin, trimethadione (no longer available in the US)

Antirheumatic drugs
Chloroquine, penicillamine (could cause myasthenia gravis or elevation of antibodies)

Cardiovascular drugs
Bretylium, calcium-channel blockers (nifedipine, verapamil), lidocaine, oxprenolol, procainamide, propranolol, and other β-blockers, quinidine

Psychotropic agents
Chlorpromazine, diazepam, lithium, promazine

Replacement hormones
Adrenocorticotropic hormone, corticosteroids, estrogens, oral contraceptives, thyroid hormones

Other drugs
Diuretics (lower serum potassium), interferon-α, iodinated radiographic contrast agents, muscle relaxants, magnesium, opioids, neuromuscular-blocking agents, quinine

dose of pyridostigmine every few days until a satisfactory response is apparent. In patients in ARF, one approach is to gradually increase the dose of pyridostigmine while undertaking a course of plasma exchange. These drugs cross the blood–brain barrier poorly and, therefore, no CNS side effects are seen. Rather, side effects are related to increased peripheral cholinergic activity and include bronchospasm, excessive salivation, bradycardia, nausea, diarrhea, and miosis.

ACh Release Promoters

Guanidine and 4-aminopyridine have been reported to improve ocular muscle and limb muscle strength in some patients, without any benefit for respiratory paralysis. These two drugs enhance the release of ACh from nerve terminals.

Immunosuppressive Therapy

If no improvement in weakness is seen despite adequate CEI therapy, immunosuppressive drugs can be added. These include corticosteroids, azathioprine, cyclophosphamide, cyclosporine, and methotrexate. These drugs suppress the immune system by inhibiting both cellular and humoral mechanisms and reducing the damage due to autoimmunity. Limited evidence from randomized, controlled trials suggests that corticosteroid treatment offers short-term benefit in MG. However, corticosteroids are not better than azathioprine or IVIG (43,44). Pulsed, high-dose methylprednisolone has been used, with sustained response lasting for months.

Prednisolone, the most commonly used immunosuppressive agent, is added at a once-daily dose of 1.5–2 mg/kg PO in patients with moderate-to-severe disease that is refractory to CEIs. Improvement can occur within 2–3 weeks, but transient paradoxical deterioration in weakness may occur in ~50% of cases, and 10% may need mechanical ventilation (45). After maximum improvement is achieved, a slow tapering off of steroids is required. Some patients will need maintenance of low-dose steroids for years, or for life.

Other agents are used in individuals who relapse on corticosteroids or in those with disabling steroid side effects (e.g., osteoporosis, psychosis, hypertension, myopathy, glaucoma, and infection). In adults, oral prednisolone combined with azathioprine results in fewer relapses, more remission, and less steroid usage. Other, newer immunosuppressants used in MG are mycophenolate mofetil and tacrolimus (45). Patients with disabling but stable symptoms with concerns about high-dose steroids may receive mycophenolate mofetil. If these fail, azathioprine or cyclosporine is the next option. Recently, rituximab has emerged as a promising treatment for seronegative JMG including MuSK antibody–positive patients refractory to other immunosuppressive medications.

Plasmapheresis

Plasmapheresis removes AchR antibodies from the circulation and has been advocated as an effective treatment for MG because it brings about improvement within a few days that lasts for several weeks (46). However, to date, only case series of plasma exchange in myasthenic crisis are available. Guidelines have not been established regarding number, volume, or frequency of exchanges. Five or six single-volume exchanges are performed on alternate days until an adequate response is obtained, which is usually seen after two to five exchanges. Plasmapheresis is used to prevent crises prior to thymectomy or any surgery. It is also used in very weak patients who are admitted for initiation of corticosteroid therapy and in cases that are refractory to CEIs and other immunomodulatory therapies. Two controlled trials that included only a small number of patients failed to demonstrate a cumulative long-term effect of plasma exchange (47).

Intravenous Immunoglobulin

IVIG is considered to be as effective as plasmapheresis. In one randomized trial that compared IVIG to plasmapheresis, both treatments were equally effective (48). An evidence-based review of available randomized studies concluded that IVIG is probably effective and should be considered for treating moderate-to-severe MG (49). With 2 g/kg given over 5 days (0.4 g/kg/day), 60%–70% of patients are expected to show response within days to weeks, and the response lasts up to 60 days. In patients with ARF or who are in myasthenic crisis, IVIG is used if plasmapheresis is not available or cannot be done (e.g., in young children with difficult venous access or in whom sepsis is the trigger for myasthenic crisis). IVIG may also be useful in patients who are refractory to other immunosuppressants.

Thymectomy

Some studies suggest that early removal of the thymus may adversely affect the patient's immune status. Usually, thymectomy is recommended in moderate and severe MG that is inadequately controlled on CEIs. Studies show that the subgroup of MG patients that most benefit from thymectomy includes those with early-onset, AchR antibody-positive MG. A consensus group concluded that the benefit of thymectomy in nonthymomatous autoimmune MG has not been established. They were unable to determine whether the observed association between thymectomy and improved outcome was a result of thymectomy or because of differences in severity at baseline before therapy. Thus, for patients with nonthymomatous autoimmune MG, thymectomy should only be considered as an option to increase the probability of remission or improvement (50). In children who have undergone thymectomy, thymus hyperplasia has been found with high frequency, especially in postpubertal cases (51). In contrast, thymoma is very uncommon in adolescents and exceedingly rare in prepubertal children.

Patients selected for thymectomy should have pulmonary function testing, including vital capacity and maximum expiratory force, both before and after cholinergic inhibition. If the patient is already on CEIs and can tolerate withdrawal of drug for 6–8 hours, preoperative low NIF off CEIs indicates the risk of postoperative respiratory complications. In such cases, plasmapheresis for 5 days or IVIG is recommended. If the maximum NIF off CEIs is satisfactory, early postoperative extubation is expected. CEIs are discontinued on the morning of surgery to avoid interactions and side effects in the operating room. Atropine is recommended to reduce secretions, and in patients on corticosteroids, preoperative, stress-dose, hydrocortisone is used for 3 days postoperatively.

Natural Course and Outcome of MG

The natural history of MG is highly variable. Weakness tends to be limited to ocular muscles in 10%–15% of patients. Approximately 50% of those who present with ocular features develop systemic or bulbar weakness within the first 2 years of onset, with 75% progressing within 4 years (24). Spontaneous remission can occur, especially in younger children. In a large pediatric series, collected over 44 years, spontaneous remission was found in 7.6% within 3 years of onset of the disease and in 30.1% within 15 years (52). Seventy-five percent of children and adolescents with JMG who undergo thymectomy have complete remission, with improvement in up to 95% of cases (53). The course of congenital MG is more static or slowly progressive. A subset of congenital MG patients who do not respond to CEIs worsen over years with a progressive motor end-plate myopathy.

ACUTE INTERMITTENT PORPHYRIA

The word *porphyria* is derived from the Greek *porphuros*, which means red or purple. The porphyrias are a group of disorders caused by defects in the enzymes of heme biosynthesis. Four of these defects may present as acute porphyria, which is characterized by acute, life-threatening attack of neurovisceral symptoms (54). Acute intermittent porphyria (AIP) is the most common among all acute porphyrias; the average worldwide prevalence is 1 per 20,000, with an incidence of 1 new case per 100,000 per year. AIP has its highest incidence in people of Swedish descent. The annual incidence is 1.5 per 100,000 in the US Swedish population and 1 per 1000 in Lapland, Sweden (55). Other acute porphyrias are hereditary coproporphyria, variegate porphyria, and 5-aminolevulinic acid (ALA) dehydratase-deficient porphyria. These conditions are either inherited as autosomal dominant (except AIP, which is autosomal recessive) with weak penetrance.

Pathophysiology

The porphyrias are classified as hepatic or erythroid types, based on the site of expression of the enzyme defect, from which most of the heme biosynthetic inhibitors arise and where most of them accumulate, i.e., liver or erythrocytes. They are also classified as either acute or cutaneous, based on the predominant clinical presentation. The enzyme defect associated with each type of porphyria and the metabolic by-products that are likely to accumulate are shown in **Figure 53.2**. The abnormal functioning of enzymes may occur because of a defective gene or a toxin, which results in overproduction and accumulation

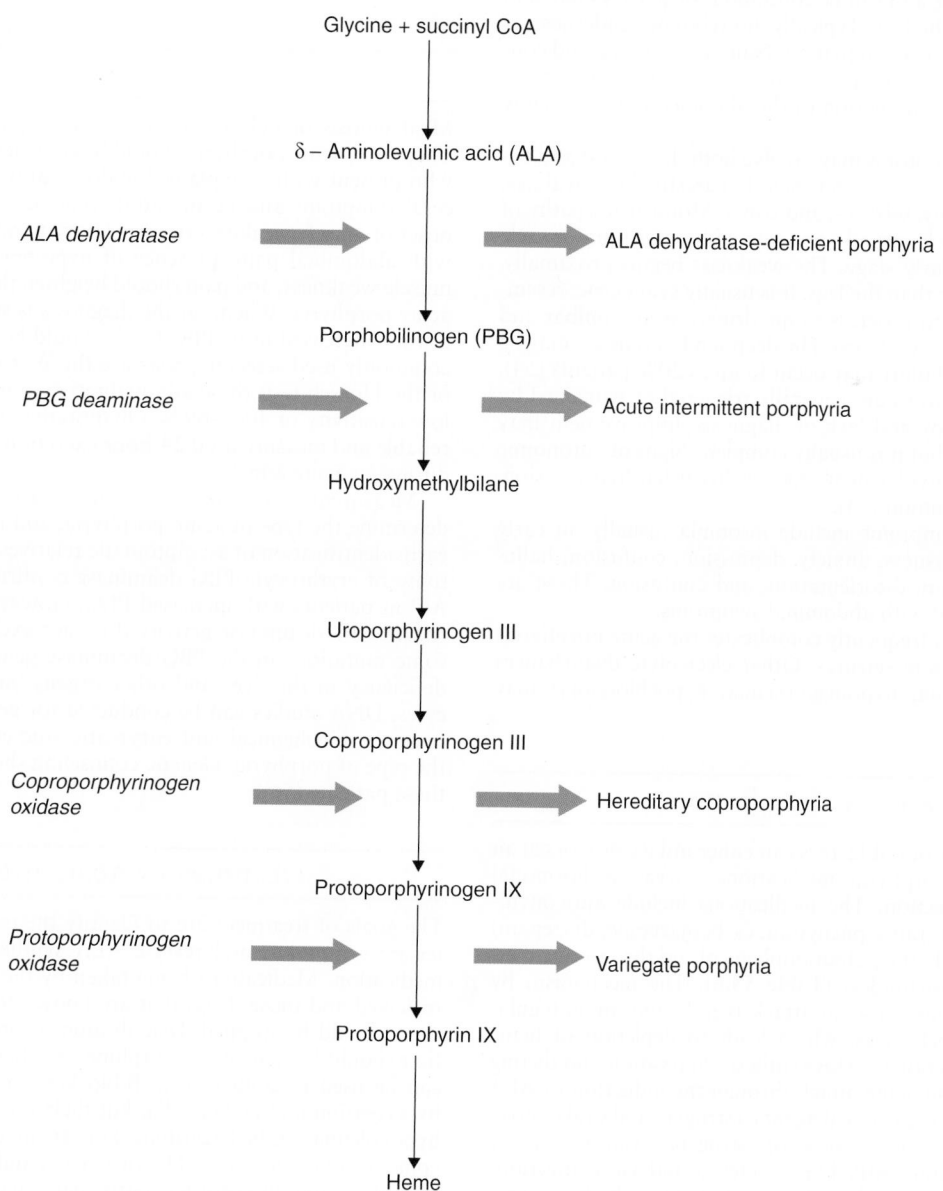

FIGURE 53.2. Heme biosynthetic pathway showing the enzyme defect causing acute hepatic porphyrias.

of intermediates that are known as *porphyrins* or *porphyrin* **13** *precursors*. Common to all acute porphyrias is overproduction and accumulation of ALA and porphobilinogen (PBG). AIP is due to reduced activity of PBG deaminase, the enzyme that catalyzes the conversion of PBG to hydroxymethylbilane. The neurovisceral symptoms are due to the neurotoxic effect of PBG and ALA and interaction of ALA with γ-aminobutyric acid receptors (55).

Clinical Features

The classic features of acute porphyrias are abdominal pain, **14** altered mental state, and peripheral neuropathy. Abdominal pain is present in most patients (14). Clinical presentation without abdominal pain is unusual. Pain in the limbs, back, neck, and chest occur in up to 70% of cases. A similar proportion have weakness and paresis (54). Patients may have different types of episodes because of a varied response to precipitating factors.

Abdominal pain is likely to be due to visceral neuropathy. It is usually diffuse and can be continuous or paroxysmal, and it can radiate to the legs. Typically, no rebound tenderness or guarding is found on examination. Nausea, vomiting, and constipation accompany the pain, but occasionally, diarrhea occurs. Radiologic examination of the abdomen does not show any abnormality.

Neurologic symptoms may involve both the central and peripheral nervous systems and include paresthesias, myalgias, paresis, neuropathy, seizures, and coma. Motor neuropathy of acute, severe attacks usually presents with paresis and muscle weakness at an early stage. The weakness begins proximally, in the arms rather than the legs. It is usually symmetric, resembling GBS, and can progress to quadriparesis and bulbar and respiratory muscle weakness. The deep-tendon reflexes may be lost. Respiratory failure may occur in up to 20% patients (54). Neurologic symptoms are generally triggered or worsened by inadequate therapy and lack of diagnosis. Improvement may take a long time, but it is usually complete. Signs of autonomic nervous system involvement (e.g., tachycardia, hypertension, sweating) are common (54).

Psychiatric symptoms include insomnia (usually an early symptom), restlessness, anxiety, depression, confusion, hallucinations, delirium, disorientation, and confusion. These are usually associated with abdominal symptoms.

Hyponatremia frequently complicates the acute porphyrias and may precipitate seizures. Other electrolyte disturbances (e.g., hypokalemia, hypomagnesemia, hypochloremia) may also occur (55).

Precipitating Factors

Four main categories of factors can either induce or worsen an **15** attack of acute porphyria: medications, starvation, hormonal factors, and infection. The medications include anticonvulsants (i.e., barbiturates, phenytoin, carbamazepine, diazepam) and antibacterials (i.e., chloramphenicol, erythromycin, metronidazole, sulfonamides) (Table 53.6). The mechanism by which medications cause an attack is induction or upregulation of the cytochromes, which leads to depletion of heme stores, and induction of ALA synthesis. Starvation and dieting can precipitate an acute attack through the induction of ALA synthetase. Use of hormonal agents, estrogen, and oral contraceptives or endogenous excess of estrogen during pregnancy can also precipitate AIP. Both bacterial and viral infections induce an acute attack by catabolizing heme, which, in turn, induces ALA synthetase and the accumulation of porphyrin precursors.

TABLE 53.6

COMMONLY USED DRUGS THAT ARE UNSAFE IN PORPHYRIA

Analgesics	Diclofenac and other nonsteroidal anti-inflammatories, pentazocine
Antihypertensives	α-methyl dopa, captopril, diltiazem, hydralazine, nifedipine
Antiepileptics	Phenytoin, barbiturates, carbamazepine, clonazepam (high dose), primidone, succinimides
Antibiotics and antibacterials	Sulfonamides, griseofulvin, chloramphenicol, doxycycline, erythromycin, ciprofloxacin, pyrazinamide, rifampicin
Diuretics	Furosemide, hydrochlorothiazide
Hormones and endocrine agents	Estrogens (oral contraceptives), progesterone and synthetic progestins, sulfonylureas
Miscellaneous	Ergot compounds, imipramine, lidocaine, metoclopramide, cimetidine

Diagnosis

Misdiagnosis or delayed diagnosis of porphyria is common. Therefore, acute porphyria should be considered in all patients who present with unexplained abdominal pain and neurovisceral symptoms and in any adolescent or female with acute onset of muscle weakness or respiratory paralysis. In a patient with abdominal pain, presence of hypertension, dark urine, muscle weakness, and pain should heighten the suspicion of an acute porphyria. Whenever the diagnosis is suspected, a rapid test for increased urine PBG levels should be undertaken. The commonly used screening tests are the Watson–Schwartz test or the Hoesch test; these are qualitative in nature and have a low sensitivity of 40%–69%. Quantitative methods are more reliable and measure total 24-hour excretion of PBG and ALA during an acute attack.

Measurement of enzyme activity and genetic testing can determine the type of acute porphyria, and may be helpful in early identification of asymptomatic relatives. Half-normal activity of erythrocyte PBG deaminase confirms a diagnosis of AIP in patients with increased PBG. However, normal erythrocyte PBG deaminase activity does not exclude AIP because some mutations in the PBG deaminase gene lead to enzyme deficiency in the liver and other organs but not in erythrocytes. DNA studies can be conducted for genetic localization once the biochemical and enzymatic studies have confirmed the type of porphyria. Genetic counseling should be offered to these patients (56).

Treatment of Acute Attack

The goals of treatment are to identify the triggering event, alleviate symptoms, and reverse ALA synthetase activity with **16** medication. Medications being taken by the patient should be reviewed and those drugs that are known to aggravate symptoms should be stopped. Dehydration, malnutrition, or infection should be managed. Morphine or other opiate analgesics can be used to control pain. β-blockers can be used to treat hypertension and tachycardia, but their use in the presence of hypovolemia can be hazardous. For seizure control benzodiazepines can be safely used. Hyponatremia and hypomagnesemia should be carefully corrected, particularly in those with seizures. Symptoms like nausea, vomiting, anxiety, and restlessness can be treated with chlorpromazine or other phenothiazines (54).

Enzyme activity is reversed by administering 10% glucose and hemin infusion; these act by directly suppressing ALA synthetase activity (56). Sucrose, glucose polymers, or carbohydrate-rich foods may be given to patients without abdominal distention or ileus, who are able to tolerate oral nutrition. The standard intravenous regimen is 10% glucose for a total of at least 300 g daily. Higher total daily doses may be needed. One needs to be alert to the increased risk of hyponatremia with use of large volumes of 10% glucose. Saline dextrose solutions may be safer (57). Severe or prolonged attacks should be treated with hemin and may also require more thorough nutrition support. Hemin infusion is given in a dose of 3–4 mg/kg once daily for 4 days. Excessive production of porphyrin precursors is decreased within hours of hemin infusion and clinical improvement is seen within 2–4 days. Many studies, mostly uncontrolled, have shown that early initiation of hemin is associated with improved outcome. Use of the tin protoporphyrin has been shown to prolong remission induced by heme arginate. Hemin infusion may cause abnormality of coagulation and a bleeding diathesis and, rarely, transient renal insufficiency.

Monitoring should include regular assessment of vital capacity, respiratory and skeletal muscle weakness, serum sodium, potassium, magnesium, and creatinine. Prevention is best achieved with counseling about avoiding precipitating drugs, maintaining a high-carbohydrate diet, and promptly treating infection (56).

Outcome

Clinical improvement with hemin therapy occurs within 1–2 days. However, if treatment is delayed, neurologic damage may be slow to recover and may occasionally leave residual weakness. Motor weakness usually resolves; occasionally, footdrop and wasting of intrinsic muscles of the hand are seen. The overall outcome has greatly improved over recent years, with better diagnosis, availability of hemin treatment, and prevention. Since the introduction of hemin therapy in 1971, case fatality rates have fallen from 10%–52% before 1970 to up to 10% currently (54).

INTENSIVE CARE UNIT–ACQUIRED WEAKNESS

Intesive Care Unit–acquired weakness (ICUAW) refers to clinically detected weakness in critically ill patients in whom there is no plausible etiology other than critical illness. The spectrum of illness varies from isolated nerve entrapment, which presents with focal pain or weakness, to severe myopathy or neuropathy with associated severe and prolonged weakness (58). Study of these entities has been hampered by the varying terminologies and definitions used by researchers. Recently, a classification of *ICUAW and related disorders* using clinical and electrophysiological criteria has been proposed (59). Patients with ICUAW and documented polyneuropathy and/or myopathy are classified in three subcategories. CIP refers to patients with ICUAW who have electrophysiological evidence of an axonal polyneuropathy, and CIM indicates patients with ICUAW who have electrophysiologically and/or histologically defined myopathy. The term *critical illness neuromyopathy* (CINM) is reserved for patients who have electrophysiological and/or histologic findings of coexisting CIP and CIM.

Initially, CIP was considered an uncommon condition, but it is now considered to be one of the most common and severe complications in critically ill adults. ICUAW is infrequent in children (58).

Incidence and Prevalence

The prevalence of ICUAW is likely to be higher than generally recognized. Clinical assessment alone may not be sufficient to provide the true incidence. A systematic review showed CIP/CIM to occur in nearly 50% of critically ill adults, with sepsis, multiple-organ failure, or protracted mechanical ventilation (60).

Risk Factors

In adults, a number of factors increase the risk of ICUAW, including sepsis, systemic inflammatory response, multiorgan failure, mechanical ventilation, corticosteroids, neuromuscular-blocking drugs, aminoglycosides, hyperosmolality, parenteral nutrition, and hyperglycemia (61,62).

Pathogenesis

The pathogenesis of ICUAW is not fully understood. CIP is likely to be another end-organ manifestation of multiple-organ dysfunction. In this regard, various cytokines and inflammatory mediators may have a role in pathogenesis by damaging myelin, oligodendrocytes, and even axons. For example, nitric oxide maintains vascular tone and may contribute to paralysis of arteriolar vasoreactivity in septic shock. As blood vessels supplying peripheral nerves lack autoregulation, impaired microcirculation may cause nerve energy failure. Both hypoxia and ischemia impair axonal transport of proteins. An alternative mechanism involves hyperglycemia and hyperosmolality, both of which increase endovascular resistance. Microvascular permeability may aggravate endoneural edema (58). It is of interest that in the adult studies of glycemic control in critical illness, tight glycemic control using insulin is associated with a reduction in CIP (63).

In CIM, both a depolarization of the resting potential and a hyperpolarized shift in the voltage dependence of sodium channel gating contribute to muscle membrane inexcitability (64). Second, changes in the excitation–contraction coupling at the level of sarcoplasmatic calcium release seem to be involved in CIM. Contributing to this pathophysiology is a rapid decrease in muscle protein and a lack of parallel increase in protein synthesis. The proapoptotic pathways leading to programmed cell death seem to be stimulated. Finally, oxidative stress results from nitric oxide overproduction and antioxidant (glutathione) depletion. This is accompanied by multifactorial mitochondrial dysfunction and decreased adenosine triphosphate concentrations resulting in a state termed as "bioenergetic failure" (65). All these mechanisms possibly interplay in an individual patient to result in CIM (66).

Clinical Features

Prolonged Neuromuscular Transmission Blockade

Prolonged neuromuscular transmission blockade has been described in those who receive muscle relaxants for several days or weeks. These patients become ventilator-dependent and have persistent paralysis and areflexia long after the drug is discontinued. Renal failure or dysfunction is an important factor, as many commonly used NMBAs have significant clearance via the kidney. In a patient with renal failure, only a few hours of high-dose NMBA can result in several days of neuromuscular blockade. Hypermagnesemia and metabolic acidosis are other risk factors in prolonging neuromuscular blockade.

Critical Illness Polyneuropathy

CIP is characterized by acute, generalized neuropathy occurring after overwhelming sepsis and multiorgan dysfunction. Approximately 70% of adults with sepsis demonstrate peripheral nerve dysfunction on electrophysiologic studies, but only 30% of these develop clinical symptoms. Clinical signs usually develop 2–3 weeks after the onset of sepsis. Rapid development of flaccid quadriparesis or paraparesis with hyporeflexia/areflexia occurs. The symptoms of polyneuropathy are usually not identified early because these patients are usually sedated during mechanical ventilation. The problem is recognized when an obvious difficulty is encountered in weaning from mechanical ventilation. During recovery, some patients may complain of painful paresthesia and some may develop weakness after discharge. Loss of sensation in a glove-and-stocking distribution is seen. These patients fail to grimace or move their limbs in response to a painful stimulus. Clinically, the cranial nerves appear to be spared, but they may show abnormal electrophysiology. Bladder and bowel function is usually preserved. Limb edema, a common occurrence in critically ill patients, may obscure distal atrophy.

Critical Illness Myopathy

Terms used to describe CIM include acute quadriplegic myopathy, floppy-person syndrome, necrotizing myopathy of intensive care, thick-filament myopathy, and steroid-induced quadriparesis. CIM is a more common cause of ICUAW weakness than CIP (67). It was first described as acute myopathy in individuals with acute severe asthma treated with corticosteroids. Exposure to corticosteroids or NMBAs appears to be the major risk factors for developing CIM. Other risk factors include sepsis and multiorgan failure. Irrespective of age, the clinical features of CIM appear to be the same. Patients have flaccid tetraparesis or tetraplegia. Deep-tendon reflexes are either normal or diminished but, usually, are not completely lost. The cranial nerves are intact on examination, although facial weakness may be mild. Sensation is preserved. Painful stimulation elicits facial grimacing without limb withdrawal, unlike the finding in CIP. Weaning from mechanical ventilation is difficult.

Diagnosis

The diagnosis of ICUAW is not easy, mainly because of limitations imposed by concurrent therapy and because the patient is usually deeply sedated and immobile. The laboratory findings are unhelpful, as these may merely reflect critical illness. Elevated creatine phosphokinase may suggest a possible toxic or inflammatory cause of myopathy. The diagnosis begins with a thorough history and examination followed by diagnostic testing (e.g., neuroimaging, CSF analysis). If no alternative etiology is plausible, a diagnosis of ICUAW can be considered. In severely affected patients, electrophysiological testing should be obtained (**Table 53.7**) (see Chapter 52).

Tissue Biopsy

Nerve biopsy in patients with CIP shows acute axonal degeneration that involves both sensory and motor nerve fibers, which is more pronounced in distal rather than proximal segments. No features of inflammation are seen. In the chronic stage, the nerve shows severely reduced numbers of myelinated large-diameter fibers, thin myelin in almost all fibers, and cluster formation of myelinated small-diameter fibers, which indicates primary axonal degeneration with regeneration (68). Muscle biopsy from patients with CIP shows chronic denervation and myopathic changes. In CIM, atrophy of type II fibers

is seen with occasional atrophy of type I fibers. Muscle fiber necrosis is also seen. Electron microscopy and immunohistochemical studies demonstrate the loss of thick myosin filaments. The differences between CIP and CIM are summarized in **Table 53.8**.

Treatment and Prevention

No specific treatments have been recommended for CINMA. Early physiotherapy and good nutrition should help recovery. Studies have shown that glutamine and glutathione supplementation and branched-chain amino acid supplementation are associated with improved survival and shorter intensive care unit stay. Strict glycemic control, using intensive insulin therapy (maintaining normoglycemia at 80–110 mg/dL), reduces the incidence of CIP/CIM in critically ill adults but the treatment is associated with significant increase in hypoglycemia (63). Other preventive measures include avoidance of prolonged immobilization and oversedation and minimization of dosages and duration of corticosteroids and NMBAs.

Outcome

The development of CIP/CIM affects both the short- and long-term outcomes of critical illness, with increased duration of mechanical ventilation, prolonged hospitalization, and increased healthcare cost (61,69). Much of the data on outcome in CINMA are related to patients with CIP. Mortality is high in adults (50%–60%) and much lower in children (70). Chronic disability is a common finding in many patients after discharge from hospital. Forty percent of pediatric cases had persistent neurologic sequelae (56). In adults, 68% recovered to the extent of being able to breathe spontaneously and walk without support. However, 28% were tetraplegic or paraplegic. Milder disabilities have been reported in patients with full functional recovery and include hyporeflexia or areflexia, sensory abnormalities, muscle atrophy, and footdrop (70). The time course of recovery varies greatly. Neuromuscular abnormalities may continue for 5 years after illness (61). Weakness and/or neuropsychologic changes may also persist for 5 years (71). Some patients may never become fully functional, which will have a major impact on their quality of life. Limited data are available regarding the outcome of CIM. If weakness occurs as a complication of severe asthma treated with steroids and NMBAs, recovery occurs within days to weeks. It is generally thought that patients with CIM recover faster and have better prognosis than do those patients with CIP (67).

DIAPHRAGMATIC PALSY

Diaphragmatic palsy can be bilateral or unilateral. Bilateral palsy is usually due to systemic illnesses, while unilateral palsy is due to injury to phrenic nerve (cervical motor neurons C3–C5) and is more common in infants and children than in adults.

Incidence and Causes

The most common causes of unilateral diaphragmatic palsy in children are birth trauma (due to difficult or breech delivery), congenital diaphragmatic eventration, and cardiothoracic surgery. The incidence of diaphragmatic palsy in children who underwent cardiac surgery in a large, prospective study was 4.9%, 5.4% following open surgery and 3.3% following closed heart surgery (72). Apart from this cause, attention is

TABLE 53.7

PROPOSED DIAGNOSTIC CRITERIA FOR ICU-ACQUIRED WEAKNESS (ICUAW) AND ITS SUBTYPES

ICU-ACQUIRED WEAKNESS
1. Generalized weakness developing after the onset of critical illness
2. Weakness is diffuse (involving both proximal and distal muscles), symmetric, flaccid, and generally spares cranial nerves
3. Muscle power assessed by the MRC sum score <48, or mean MRC score <4 in all testable muscle groups noted on ≥2 occasions separated by >24 h
4. Dependence on mechanical ventilation
5. Causes of weakness not related to the underlying critical illness have been excluded
Minimum criteria for diagnosing ICUAW: 1, 2, 5, and either 3 or 4

CRITICAL ILLNESS POLYNEUROPATHY (CIP)
1. Patient meets criteria for ICUAW
2. Compound muscle action potential amplitudes are decreased to <80% of lower limit of normal in ≥2 nerves
3. Sensory nerve action potential amplitudes are decreased to <80% of lower of normal in ≥2 nerves
4. Normal or near-normal nerve-conduction velocities without conduction block
5. Absence of a decremental response on repetitive nerve stimulation

CRITICAL ILLNESS MYOPATHY (CIM)
1. Patient meets criteria for ICUAW
2. Sensory nerve action potential amplitudes are >80% of the lower limit of normal in ≥2 nerves
3. Needle electromyogram in ≥2 muscle groups demonstrates short-duration, low-amplitude motor unit potentials with early or normal full recruitment with or without fibrillation potentials
4. Direct muscle stimulation demonstrates reduced excitability (muscle/nerve ratio >0.5 in ≥2 muscle groups)
5. Muscle histology consistent with myopathy
Probable CIM: criteria 1, 2, 3, or 4; or 1 and 5
Definite CIM: criteria 1, 2, 3 or 4, 5

CRITICAL ILLNESS NEUROMYOPATHY (CINM)
1. Patient meets criteria for ICUAW
2. Patient meets criteria for CIP
3. Patient meets criteria for probable or definite CIM
4. CINM is diagnosed when all three criteria are present

PROLONGED NEUROMUSCULAR BLOCKADE
1. Patient meets criteria for ICUAW with cranial nerve involvement
2. Exposure to a nondepolarizing neuromuscular-blocking agent, usually administered in multiple doses or as an infusion, in the last 10 d
3. Decreased or absent compound muscle action potential amplitudes
4. Presence of a >10% decremental response on 2–3-Hz repetitive nerve stimulation
5. Recovery of motor function over a period of <14 d

MRC, Medical Research Council; ICUAW, intensive care unit–acquired weakness; CIP, critical illness polyneuropathy; CIM, critical illness myopathy, CINM, critical illness neuromyopathy.
Adapted from Stevens RD, Marshall SA, Cornblath DR, et al. A framework for diagnosing and classifying intensive care unit-acquired weakness. *Crit Care Med* 2009;37(10 suppl):S299–308, with permission.

TABLE 53.8

DIFFERENCES BETWEEN CRITICAL ILLNESS POLYNEUROPATHY AND CRITICAL ILLNESS MYOPATHY

	■ CRITICAL ILLNESS POLYNEUROPATHY	■ CRITICAL ILLNESS MYOPATHY
Predisposing factor	Preceding systemic inflammatory response syndrome, sepsis, or multiorgan failure	Often received nondepolarizing muscle blocking agent, high-dose corticosteroid, or both
Clinical features	Sensory deficits present	No sensory deficit
	Weakness distal > proximal	Weakness proximal > distal
	Tendon reflexes normal or ↓	Tendon reflexes ↓ or absent
		Weakness of muscles supplied by the cranial nerves may occur
Electrophysiology	Low amplitude/absent sensory action potentials	Retained sensory nerve action potentials
	Normal motor unit potentials	Small motor unit potentials
	Reduced motor unit recruitment	Early motor unit recruitment
	Normal muscle excitability	Absent/reduced muscle excitability
	Features of axonopathy without demyelination	
Pathology	Axonal loss (sensory and motor nerve)	Loss of thick myosin filament
	Acute and chronic denervation of muscle	Type II fiber atrophy (type I less common) or severe muscle fiber necrosis

Adapted from Khan J, Burnham EL, Moss M. Acquired weakness in the ICU: Critical illness myopathy and polyneuropathy. *Minerva Anestesiol* 2006;72:401–6.

now being drawn to diaphragmatic contractile dysfunction secondary to prolonged mechanical ventilation. For example, in laboratory animals and humans, a period of mechanical ventilation as short as 18 hours can result in diaphragmatic atrophy. The mechanisms involved overlap with the pathophysiology of CIM (73).

Pathophysiology

Unilateral palsy is often asymptomatic in older children but can cause severe respiratory compromise in newborn infants and young children because older children use the accessory muscles of respiration, while infants have a horizontal rib cage and weak intercostal muscles. A significant alteration in respiratory mechanics that occurs following diaphragmatic palsy is paradoxical movement of the diaphragm on the affected side, with mediastinal shifting to the contralateral side during inspiration. This alteration causes decreased lung volumes, alveolar collapse, and atelectasis, which leads to dyspnea, failure to clear secretions, and pneumonia.

Clinical Features

Children with diaphragmatic palsy present with varied manifestations depending on their age and the underlying lung condition. Immediately after birth and during the first hours of life, tachypnea, increasing need for oxygen, hypercapnia, atelectasis, pneumonia, and a mediastinal shift are present. Over the next few days, the clinical condition may stabilize, only to recur days to weeks later; progression is often provoked by atelectasis or infection. In older children, uncomplicated diaphragmatic palsy may present as tachypnea, dyspnea on exertion, or orthopnea. Patients with postsurgical phrenic nerve palsy experience pleural effusion, pneumonia, and difficulty in weaning from the ventilator or mechanical ventilation.

Diagnosis

After exclusion of cardiac disease, diaphragmatic palsy should be suspected in any child who has decreased breath sounds, fails to wean from a ventilator, and who has a raised hemidiaphragm on chest x-ray. However, the chest x-ray sign lacks sensitivity and specificity in the diagnosis of unilateral paralysis (74). Fluoroscopy on sniffing is a traditional method of diagnosing diaphragmatic movements. The normal diaphragm descends during a sniff. In the presence of unilateral diaphragmatic palsy, the affected diaphragm ascends. The sniff test is positive if a 2-cm or longer excursion is present and the whole leaf of the hemidiaphragm is involved. The sniff test is difficult to interpret if the hemidiaphragm is not completely paralyzed or when a child is on positive airway pressure support. Electrical stimulation of the phrenic nerve that demonstrates delayed conduction time is more specific than fluoroscopy. Unilateral magnetic phrenic nerve stimulation is a reliable and sensitive alternative for diagnosing diaphragm paralysis (75). Sonographic assessment of diaphragmatic motion can be used for diagnosis and to follow the progression of diaphragmatic function at the bedside. M-mode sonography has better results than the more commonly performed real-time, B-mode sonography. In a retrospective study of 278 children with diaphragmatic palsy and 742 hemidiaphragm elevations, M-mode ultrasound detected palsy correctly in all of the right-sided lesions and missed it in only 0.71% of the left-sided lesions (74).

Computed tomography scanning of the chest may be indicated in patients who have diaphragmatic palsy due to mediastinal pathology. MRI of the neck is advised in those who are suspected to have involvement of the spinal column or nerve roots that is causing diaphragmatic paralysis.

Management

The management of eventration of the diaphragm secondary to phrenic nerve injury in the newborn period invariably requires surgery. Plication of the diaphragm is also usually required in very young children with diaphragmatic palsy following cardiac surgery. Plication is required in diaphragmatic palsy as follows: due to arterial switch operation in almost all cases, due to Blalock–Taussig shunt in 58%, and due to correction of tetralogy of Fallot in 10% (72). In older children, phrenic nerve paralysis is thought to be potentially reversible; if the patient is asymptomatic, it may be managed conservatively, as spontaneous recovery of the affected hemidiaphragm has been reported in up to 90% of children.

Surgical plication is accepted as the effective treatment, but controversy exists regarding its timing. Some authors advocate a proactive approach; others recommend surgical plication after 30 days of ineffective conservative therapy or if a child cannot be weaned from the ventilator after 2 weeks (76). Some authors believe that the time between the diagnosis and surgical management of diaphragmatic palsy in children who have undergone cardiac surgery should not exceed 10 days, especially in infants (72).

Usual surgical procedures in diaphragmatic palsy are (a) open transthoracic plication of the noncontractive part of the paralyzed and elevated diaphragm, or (b) the thoracoscopic repair and fixation of the diaphragm. Some authors have used the laparoscopic approach, as it is minimally traumatic. The long-term outcome in these children is the same as with the conventional approach. The aim of diaphragmatic plication is to decrease lung compression, stabilize the thoracic cage and mediastinum, and strengthen the respiratory action of intercostal and abdominal muscles, resulting in improved diaphragmatic recruitment that leads to better ventilation and lung volumes and improved respiratory functions (77). Diaphragmatic pacing through the placement of electrodes in the diaphragm to stimulate it to contract is being used in children with spinal cord injury or phrenic nerve injury. This procedure can be performed transthoracically, transabdominally, laparoscopically, or through thoracoscopy.

Outcome

Unless a potentially fatal comorbid illness threatens the prognosis of the patient with unilateral diaphragmatic paralysis, death from respiratory insufficiency does not occur if good ventilatory support is provided. Prognosis of unilateral diaphragmatic paralysis depends on etiology; it is usually excellent unless the patient has significant underlying pulmonary disease. The beneficial effect of diaphragmatic plication has been shown to be long-lasting and does not interfere with return of diaphragmatic function, which may occur within 18 months to 3 years (78).

CONCLUSIONS AND FUTURE DIRECTION

Improving our understanding of pathogenesis and pathophysiology of GBS, specifically with respect to bacterial and viral proteins, which share homologous epitopes to components of the peripheral nerves, may help in developing more effective specific therapies. The role of immunomodulatory therapies particularly in those who do not respond to the first therapeutic intervention needs to be better defined to optimize the long-term outcome.

The place for various immunosuppressants and immunomodulatory therapies in childhood MG is far from clear. In the future, the respective roles of various therapies in long-term management (especially of IVIG and newer immunosuppressants, mycophenolate mofetil and tacrolimus) should be clearly defined, and consensus should be reached on the role and timing of thymectomy in children with JMG.

With the advantage of well-understood pathogenesis of the porphyrias and an effective way to overcome the enzyme deficiencies, a cure for this disabling disease may be possible in the future using gene therapy.

We are in the early stages of understanding ICUAW in children, or even whether it occurs; therefore, consensus should be developed regarding the terminology used and the diagnostic criteria. Interventions to prevent and treat ICUAW should result from a better understanding of the epidemiology.

References

1. Maramattom BV, Wijdicks EF. Acute neuromuscular weakness in the intensive care unit. *Crit Care Med* 2006;34:2835–41.
2. Williams S, Horrocks IA, Ouvrier RA, et al. Critical illness polyneuropathy and myopathy in pediatric intensive care: A review. *Pediatr Crit Care Med* 2007;8(1):18–22.
3. Lawn ND, Fletcher DD, Henderson RD, et al. Anticipating mechanical ventilation in Guillian Barré syndrome. *Arch Neurol* 2001;58:893–8.
4. Wijdicks EF, Henderson RD, McClelland RL. Emergency intubation for respiratory failure in Guillain-Barré syndrome. *Arch Neurol* 2003;60(7):947–8.
5. Piastra M, Antonelli M, Caresta E, et al. Noninvasive ventilation in childhood acute neuromuscular respiratory failure: A pilot study. *Respiration* 2006;73(6):791–8.
6. Chen TH, Hsu JH, Wu JR, et al. Combined noninvasive ventilation and mechanical in-exsufflator in the treatment of pediatric acute neuromuscular respiratory failure. *Pediatr Pulmonol* 2013; 49(6):589–96.
7. Hughes RAC, Wijdicks EF, Benson E, et al. Supportive care for patients with Guillian Barré syndrome. *Arch Neurol* 2005; 62:1194–8.
8. Asbury AK, Cornblath DR. Assessment of current diagnostic criteria for Guillain-Barré syndrome. *Ann Neurol* 1990;27:S21–4.
9. Sejvar JJ, Baughman AL, Wise M, et al. Population incidence of Guillain-Barre syndrome: A systematic review and meta-analysis. *Neuroepidemiology* 2011;36(2):123–33.
10. McGrath TM, Percy AK. Guillain-Barré syndrome. In: Scheld WM, Whitley RJ, Marra CM, eds. *Scheld's Infections of Central Nervous System*. Philadelphia, PA: Lippincott Williams & Wilkins; 2004:287–304.
11. Yuki N, Hartung H-P. Guillain–Barré syndrome. *N Engl J Med* 2012;366:2294–304.
12. Shahrizaila N, Yuki N. Guillain-Barré syndrome animal model: The first proof of molecular mimicry in human autoimmune disorder. *J Biomed Biotech* 2011;2011:829129.
13. Korinthenberg R, Schessl J, Kirschnerl J. Clinical presentation and course of childhood Guillain-Barré syndrome: A prospective multicentre study. *Neuropediatrics* 2007;38:10–17.
14. Cochen V, Arnulf I, Demeret S, et al. Vivid dreams, hallucinations, psychosis and REM sleep in Guillain-Barré syndrome. *Brain* 2005;128:2535–45.
15. Hughes RA, Cornblath DR. Guillain-Barre syndrome. *Lancet.*2005;366(9497):1653–66.
16. Gorson KC, Ropper AH, Muriello MA, et al. Prospective evaluation of MRI lumbosacral nerve root enhancement in acute Guillain-Barré syndrome. *Neurology* 1996;47:813–7.
17. Sladky JT. Guillian-Barré syndrome in children. *J Child Neurol* 2004;19:191–200.
18. Lawn ND, Fletcher DD, Henderson RD, et al. Anticipating mechanical ventilation in Guillian Barré syndrome. *Arch Neurol* 2001;58:893–8.
19. Sharshar T, Chevret S, Bourdain F, et al. Early predictors of mechanical ventilation in Guillian Barré syndrome. *Crit Care Med* 2003;31:278–83.
20. Hughes RA, Swan AV, van Doorn PA. Intravenous immunoglobulin for Guillain-Barré syndrome. *Cochrane Database Syst Rev* 2012;7:CD002063.
21. Hughes RA, van Doorn PA. Corticosteroids for Guillain-Barré syndrome. *Cochrane Database Syst Rev* 2012;8:CD001446.
22. Raphaël JC, Chevret S, Hughes RA, et al. Plasma exchange for Guillain-Barré syndrome. *Cochrane Database Syst Rev.* 2012;7: CD001798.
23. Wollinsky K, Huiser P, Brinkmeier H, et al. CSF filtration is an effective treatment of Guillain-Barré syndrome: A randomized clinical trial. *Neurology* 2001;57:774–80.
24. Korinthenberg R, Schessl J, Kirschner J, et al. Intravenously administered immunoglobulin in the treatment of childhood Guillian Barré syndrome: A randomized trial. *Pediatrics* 2005;116: 8–14.
25. Singhi SC, Jayshree M, Singhi P, et al. Intravenous immunoglobulin in very severe childhood Guillain-Barré syndrome. *Ann Trop Paediatr* 1999;19:167–74.
26. Dalkas MC. Mechanism of action of IVIG and therapeutic consideration in treatment of acute and chronic demyelinating neuropathy. *Neurology* 2002;59:S13–21.
27. Hughes RA, Swan AV, Raphael JC, et al. Immunotherapy for Guillain-Barre syndrome: A systematic review. *Brain* 2007;130: 2245–47.
28. van Doorn PA. Diagnosis, treatment and prognosis of Guillain-Barré syndrome (GBS). *Presse Med* 2013;42(6, pt 2):e193–201.
29. Vajsar J, Fehlings D, Stephens D. Long term outcome in children with Guillian Barré syndrome. *J Pediatr* 2003;142:305–9.
30. McGrogan A, Sneddon S, de Vries CS. The incidence of myasthenia gravis: A systematic literature review. *Neuroepidemiology* 2010;34(3):171–83.
31. Sanders DB, El-Salem K, Massey JM, et al. Clinical aspects of MuSK antibody positive seronegative MG. *Neurology* 2003;60: 1978–80.
32. Zhou SZ, Li WH, Sun DK. Myasthenia gravis in children: Clinical study of 77 patients. *Zhonghua Er Ke Za Zhi* 2004;42:256–9.
33. Lavrnic D, Losec M, Vujic A, et al. The features of myasthenia gravis with autoantibodies to MuSK. *J Neurol Neurosurg Psychiatry* 2005;76:1099–102.
34. Evoli A, Tonali P, Padua L, et al. Clinical correlates with anti-MuSK antibodies in generalized seronegative myasthenia gravis. *Brain* 2003;126:2304–11.
35. Guptill JT, Sanders DB. Update on muscle-specific tyrosine kinase antibody positive myasthenia gravis. *Curr Opin Neurol* 2010; 23:530–5.
36. Farrugiaa ME, Vincent A. Autoimmune mediated neuromuscular junction defects. *Curr Opin Neurol* 2010;23:489–95.
37. Ciafaloni E, Massey JM. The management of myasthenia gravis in pregnancy. *Semin Neurol* 2004;24:95–100.
38. Morgan-Followell B, de Los Reyes E. Child neurology: Diagnosis of Lambert-Eaton myasthenic syndrome in children. *Neurology* 2013;80(21):e220–2.
39. Eymard B, Stojkovic T, Sternberg D, et al. Membres du reseau national Syndromes Myastheniques Congenitaux Congenital myasthenic syndromes: Difficulties in the diagnosis, course and prognosis and therapy – The French National Congenital Myasthenic Syndrome Network experience. *Rev Neurol (Paris)* 2013; 169(1):S54–5.
40. Castro D, Derisavifard S, Anderson M, et al. Juvenile myasthenia gravis: A twenty year experience. *J Clin Neuromuscul Dis* 2013; 14(3):95–102.

41. Rabinstein A, Wijdicks EF. BIPAP in acute respiratory failure due to myasthenic crisis may prevent intubation. *Neurology* 2002; 59:1647–9.

42. Varelas PN, Chua HC, Natterman J, et al. Ventilatory care in myasthenia gravis crisis: Assessing the baseline adverse event rate. *Crit Care Med* 2002;30:2663–8.

43. Schneider-Gold C, Gajdos P, Toyka KV, et al. Corticosteroids for myasthenia gravis. *Cochrane Database Syst Rev* 2005;2: CD002828.

44. Hart IK, Sathasivam S, Sharshar T. Immunosuppressive agents for myasthenia gravis. *Cochrane Database Syst Rev* 2007;(4): CD005224.

45. Romi F, Gilhus NE, Aarli JA. Myasthenia gravis: Clinical, immunological, and therapeutic advances. *Acta Neurol Scand* 2005; 111:134–41.

46. Batocchi AP, Evoli A, Palmisani MT, et al. Early onset myasthenia gravis: Clinical characteristics and response to therapy. *Eur J Pediatr* 1990;150:66–8.

47. Gajdos P, Chevret S, Toyka K. Plasma exchange for myasthenia gravis. *Cochrane Database Syst Rev* 2002;4:CD002275.

48. Gajdos P, Chevret S, Clair B, et al. Clinical trial of plasma exchange and high-dose intravenous immunoglobulin in myasthenia gravis. *Ann Neurol* 1997;41:789–96.

49. Patwa HS, Chaudhry V, Katzberg H, et al. Evidence-based guideline: Intravenous immunoglobulin in the treatment of neuromuscular disorders: Report of the Therapeutics and Technology Assessment Subcommittee of the American Academy of Neurology. *Neurology*. 2012;78(13):1009–15.

50. Gronseth GS, Barohn RJ. Practice parameter: Thymectomy for autoimmune myasthenia gravis (an evidence-based review). Report of the Quality Standards Subcommittee of the American Academy of Neurology. *Neurology* 2000;55:7–15.

51. Chiang LM, Darras BT, Kang PB. Juvenile myasthenia gravis. *Muscle Nerve* 2009;39:423–31.

52. Rodriguez M, Gomez MR, Howard FM Jr, et al. Myasthenia gravis in children: Long-term follow-up. *Ann Neurol* 1983;13: 504–10.

53. Seybold ME. Thymectomy in childhood myasthenia gravis. *Ann NY Acad Sci* 1998;841:731–41.

54. Anderson KE, Bloomer JR, Bonkovsky HL, et al. Recommendations for the diagnosis and treatment of the acute porphyrias. *Ann Intern Med* 2005;142:439–50.

55. Dombeck AT, Satonik RC. The porphyrias. *Emerg Med Clin N Am* 2005;23(3):885–99.

56. Chemmanur AT, Bonkovsky HL. Hepatic porphyrias: Diagnosis and management. *Clin Liver Dis* 2004;8:807–38.

57. Puy H, Gouya L, Deybach JC. Porphyrias. *Lancet* 2010;375: 924–37.

58. Petersen B, Schneider C, Strassburg HM, et al. Critical illness neuropathy in pediatric intensive care patients. *Pediatr Neurol* 1999;21:749–53.

59. Stevens RD, Marshall SA, Cornblath DR, et al. A framework for diagnosing and classifying intensive care unit-acquired weakness. *Crit Care Med* 2009;37(10 suppl):S299–308.

60. Stevens RD, Dowdy DW, Michaels RK, et al. Neuromuscular dysfunction acquired in critical illness: A systematic review. *Intensive Care Med* 2007;33:1876–91.

61. De Jonghe, Sharshar T, Lefaucheur JP, et al. Paresis acquired in the intensive care unit: A prospective multicenter study. *JAMA* 2002;288:2859–67.

62. Banwell BL, Mildner RJ, Hassal AC, et al. Muscle weakness in critically ill children. *Neurology* 2003;61:1779–82.

63. Hermans G, De Jonghe B, Bruyninckx F, et al. Interventions for preventing critical illness polyneuropathy and critical illness myopathy. *Cochrane Database Syst Rev* 2014;1:CD006832.

64. Teener JW, Rich MM. Dysregulation of sodium channel gating in critical illness myopathy. *J Muscle Res Cell Motil* 2006;27: 291–6.

65. Brealey D, Brand M, Hargreaves I, et al. Association between mitochondrial dysfunction and severity and outcome of septic shock. *Lancet* 2002;360:219–23.

66. Hermans G, Vanhorebeek I, Derde S, et al. Metabolic aspects of critical illness polyneuromyopathy. *Crit Care Med* 2009;37(10 Suppl):S391–7.

67. Khan J, Burnham EL, Moss M. Acquired weakness in the ICU: Critical illness myopathy and polyneuropathy. *Minerva Anestesiol* 2006;72:401–6.

68. Ohto T, Iwasaki N, Ohkoshi N, et al. A pediatric case of critical illness polyneuropathy: Clinical and pathological findings. *Brain Dev* 2005;27:535–8.

69. Garnecho-Montero J, Amaya-Villar R, Garcia-Garmendia JL, et al. Effect of critical illness neuropathy on the withdrawal from mechanical ventilation and the length of stay in septic patients. *Crit Care Med* 2005;33:349–54.

70. van der Schaaf M, Beelen A, de Vos R. Functional outcome in patients with critical illness polyneuropathy. *Disabil Rehabil* 2004;26:1189–97.

71. Fletcher SN, Kennedy DD, Ghosh IR, et al. Persistent neuromuscular and neurophysiologic abnormalities in long term survivors of prolonged critical care illness. *Crit Care Med* 2003;31: 1012–6.

72. Akay TH, Ozkan S, Gultekin B, et al. Diaphragmatic paralysis after cardiac surgery in children: Incidence, prognosis and surgical management. *Pediatr Surg Int* 2006;22:341–46.

73. Powers SK, Kavazis AN, Levine S. Prolonged mechanical ventilation alters diaphragmatic structure and function. *Crit Care Med* 2009;37(10 suppl):S347–53.

74. Epelman M, Navarro OM, Daneman A, et al. M-mode sonography of diaphragmatic motion: Description of technique and experience in 278 pediatric patients. *Pediatr Radiol* 2005;35:661–7.

75. Luo YM, Harris ML, Lyall RA, et al. Assessment of diaphragm paralysis with oesophageal electromyography and unilateral magnetic phrenic nerve stimulation. *Eur Respir J* 2000;15:596–9.

76. Simansky DA, Paley M, Refaely Y, et al. Diaphragm plication following phrenic nerve injury: A comparison of paediatric and adult patients. *Thorax* 2002;57:613–6.

77. Freeman RK, Wozniak TC, Fitzgerald EB. Functional and physiologic results of video-assisted thoracoscopic diaphragm plication in adult patients with unilateral diaphragm paralysis. *Ann Thorac Surg* 2006;8:1853–57.

78. Huttl TP, Wichmann MW, Reichart B, et al. Laparoscopic diaphragmatic plication: Long-term results of a novel surgical technique for postoperative phrenic nerve palsy. *Surg Endosc* 2004;18:547–51.

CHAPTER 54 ■ CHRONIC NEUROMUSCULAR DISEASE

ELENA CAVAZZONI, JONATHAN GILLIS, AND MONIQUE M. RYAN

KEY POINTS

Clinical Management in Intensive Care

1 Neuromuscular diseases (NMDs) are a common cause of significant chronic neurologic morbidity in childhood. Recent advances have improved clinical and genetic characterization of many of these conditions.

2 Chronic NMDs are a common cause of admission to the pediatric intensive care unit. Most acute complications of pediatric NMDs relate to respiratory insufficiency.

3 It is important to consider the natural history in managing children with chronic NMDs. While some disorders are progressive, inevitably causing increasing weakness and respiratory insufficiency, in many children, strength and ventilatory function stabilize (and even improve) with increasing age.

Ongoing Ventilatory Support

4 Most children recover from their acute episode and are discharged. In some cases, however, respiratory decompensation heralds a more permanent deterioration in the child's condition and should trigger consideration of more aggressive respiratory support in the form of noninvasive ventilation or ventilation via tracheostomy.

5 Supportive care of children with chronic NMDs includes physical therapy for stretching and maintenance of range of motion, optimization of upper-limb function with occupational therapy, orthopedic management of contractures and scoliosis, and monitoring of swallow and nutrition.

6 A case manager should be assigned to each patient early in his/her admission in order to coordinate the multidisciplinary team and provide consistent, clear, and comprehensive care.

Children with chronic neuromuscular diseases (NMDs) may have recurrent admissions to the pediatric intensive care unit (PICU) and may have a disproportionate impact on use of healthcare resources. For the staff, these admissions often engender discussion about the appropriate use of intensive care support and the patient's quality of life. Management of these patients also highlights one of the major shortcomings of contemporary PICU practice: lack of continuity in care and long-term follow-up. In managing these patients, it is critical that the intensivist works with a neuromuscular neurologist who provides up-to-date information on diagnosis, disease trajectory, and prognosis, and who is able to develop a long-term care plan with the child and family. In most instances, this neurologist will remain the primary physician or an ongoing consultant to the general pediatrician after the child's discharge from the PICU.

OVERVIEW OF CHRONIC NEUROMUSCULAR DISEASES

Clinical Presentation and Differential Diagnosis

The presentation of chronic NMDS relates largely to their pathophysiology (**Table 54.1**). Diagnosis is based on clinical findings and ancillary investigations (e.g., serum creatine kinase, neurophysiology, and muscle and nerve biopsy). In this chapter, chronic NMD will be discussed under the categories of disorders primarily affecting nerves, the neuromuscular junction, or muscles.

Nerve Disorders

Spinal Muscular Atrophy

Spinal muscular atrophy type 1 (SMA 1), the most common motor neuronopathy of childhood, is a devastating disease of childhood, with an incidence of 1 in 5000 live births. SMA is caused by recessive mutations in the survival motor neuron gene on chromosome 5. The four clinical subtypes of SMA are defined on the basis of disease severity and progression. Infants with SMA 1 never sit unsupported, children with SMA type 2 sit but never stand, those with SMA type 3 are able to walk without assistance, and SMA type 4 is of adult onset (1). All forms of SMA have the same genetic basis. The variable rate of disease progression relates to differential expression of modifying genes.

Children with SMA type 1 present in the first months of life with hypotonia and decreased spontaneous movement. Progressive weakness causes loss of antigravity strength and increasing difficulty in breathing and feeding. Without ventilatory support, death from chronic respiratory insufficiency before the age of 2 is virtually universal (2,3). In some cases, noninvasive ventilatory support by nasal prongs or face mask has been successful in prolonging survival into the second

TABLE 54.1

CHRONIC NEUROMUSCULAR DISORDERS OF CHILDHOOD

	■ ETIOLOGY	■ AGE OF ONSET	■ COURSE
Anterior Horn Cell			
Spinal muscular atrophy	Genetic (AR)	Variable (infancy–adulthood)	Progressive
Poliomyelitis	Infectious	Variable	Static
Acid maltase deficiency	Genetic (AR)	Variable (infancy–adulthood)	Progressive
Peripheral Nerve			
Congenital hypomyelinating neuropathy	Sporadic/genetic (AD/AR)	Neonatal	Static
Dejerine–Sottas disease	Sporadic/genetic (AD/AR)	Infancy	Static
Charcot–Marie–Tooth disease	Genetic (AD, AR, XL)	Childhood	Slowly progressive
Chronic inflammatory demyelinating polyneuropathy	Autoimmune	Variable (childhood)	Relapsing–remitting or progressive
Neuromuscular Disorders			
Congenital myasthenic syndromes	Genetic (AR, AD)	Neonatal or infancy	Static
Myasthenia gravis	Autoimmune	Variable (childhood)	Relapsing–remitting
Myopathies			
Congenital myopathies	Genetic (AR, AD, XL)	Variable (infancy–adulthood)	Static or slowly progressive
Congenital muscular dystrophies	Genetic (AR)	Infancy–childhood	Static or slowly progressive
Myotonic dystrophy	Genetic (AD)	Variable (neonatal–adulthood)	Static or slowly progressive
Duchenne and Becker muscular dystrophies	Genetic (XL)	Childhood	Progressive
Other muscular dystrophies	Genetic (AD, AR)	Variable (infancy–adulthood)	Progressive

AR, autosomal recessive; AD, autosomal dominant; XL, X-linked recessive.

decade of life (3), although others report less success (4,5). Invasive mechanical ventilation via tracheostomy does lead to long-term survival in SMA 1, and this form of support is used in Asia, Europe, and the United States (5–7).

Congenital Neuropathies

The congenital hypomyelinating or demyelinating neuropathies generally present in the first few years of life with hypotonia, weakness, and absent deep-tendon reflexes, often in association with congenital or acquired joint contractures. Complications include respiratory insufficiency, gastroesophageal reflux, and vocal cord paresis (8). These rare disorders are most often related to dominant or recessive mutations in genes for myelin proteins and represent an extreme of the Charcot–Marie–Tooth disease spectrum. Classification into congenital hypomyelinating neuropathy, Déjerine–Sottas syndrome, or other forms of Charcot–Marie–Tooth disease is contingent on age at presentation and findings on nerve biopsy.

Neuromuscular Junction Disorders

Myasthenic Syndromes

The myasthenic syndromes are discussed in Chapter 53.

Muscle Disorders

Congenital Myopathies

The congenital myopathies are a heterogeneous group of rare disorders defined by distinctive histochemical or ultrastructural changes in muscle (9). The number of morphologically and genetically distinct congenital myopathies has grown

rapidly in recent decades (**Table 54.2**). Clinical severity varies widely within each form of myopathy, and marked clinical overlap with other chronic NMDs is observed. All may be associated with early-onset weakness, hypotonia and hyporeflexia, poor muscle bulk, dysmorphic features secondary to muscle weakness (e.g., pectus carinatum, scoliosis, foot deformities, high-arched palate, and elongated facies), and a distinguishing morphologic abnormality on muscle biopsy. Affected patients may present later in life with delayed motor milestones, frequent falls, or disease complications such as contractures, scoliosis, and respiratory insufficiency.

Muscle weakness in the congenital myopathies is generally static. Facial weakness is common. Distal as well as proximal weakness may be present. The respiratory muscles are usually involved, but cardiac involvement is rare (10,11). Respiratory muscle involvement in the congenital myopathies generally parallels the extent of limb weakness. Some disorders (e.g., myotubular myopathy and nemaline myopathy) may present at birth with severe hypotonia, little spontaneous movement, and respiratory insufficiency. In severely affected infants, death from respiratory insufficiency, aspiration, or pneumonia is common during the first weeks or months of life (11). However, some severely hypotonic infants survive with little residual disability (12). Increasing weakness of the axial musculature may cause spinal deformities, which can progress rapidly during periods of rapid skeletal growth, particularly adolescence. Paraspinal muscle rigidity and kyphoscoliosis frequently result in significant restriction of lung capacity and respiratory insufficiency (10).

Congenital Muscular Dystrophies

Muscle disorders include the congenital muscular dystrophies, some of which affect only muscle. Others are associated with structural abnormalities of the brain and eyes (**Table 54.3**). The muscular dystrophies are generally caused by genetic

TABLE 54.2

CONGENITAL MYOPATHIES

	■ INHERITANCE	■ MUSCLE BIOPSY FINDINGS	■ NATURAL HISTORY	■ ADDITIONAL FINDINGS
Central core disease	AD	Type 1 fiber predominance Cores in type 1 muscle fibers	Weakness static or slowly progressive Most patients remain ambulant	Scoliosis Congenital hip dislocation Predisposition to malignant hyperthermia
Nemaline myopathy	Variable: AD, AR, sporadic	Type 1 fiber predominance Nemaline bodies on trichrome stain	Weakness static or slowly progressive Variable severity Respiratory insufficiency common Bulbar involvement common	Scoliosis Acquired joint contractures
Myotubular myopathy	X-linked	Central nuclei in all muscle fibers	Severe congenital weakness Most patients are ventilator-dependent Significant early mortality	Ptosis Ophthalmoplegia Macrocephaly Pyloric stenosis
Centronuclear myopathy	AD, AR	Central nuclei in all muscle fibers	Variable weakness in childhood or later Most patients remain ambulant	Ophthalmoplegia in some Respiratory insufficiency may present late
Minicore myopathy	AR	Type 1 fiber predominance Multiple small cores in type 1 muscle fibers	Moderate weakness Most patients are ambulant Respiratory insufficiency in those with spinal rigidity	Ophthalmoplegia in some Spinal rigidity Hand involvement Cardiomyopathy in minority Predisposition to malignant hyperthermia
Congenital fiber-type disproportion	AD, AR, XL	Type 1 fiber predominance Type 1 fibers small	Variable weakness Respiratory insufficiency in some	Ophthalmoplegia in some Scoliosis common

AD, autosomal dominant; AR, autosomal recessive; XL, X-linked recessive.

abnormalities of the muscle membrane. These conditions are associated with progressive weakness, elevated serum creatine kinase, and dystrophic changes in muscle. Respiratory insufficiency is common. Some congenital muscular dystrophies are associated with a characteristic pattern of axial weakness, spinal rigidity, and early respiratory insufficiency with relative sparing of the limb muscles.

Myotonic Dystrophy

Myotonic dystrophy is caused by an abnormal expansion of a CTG trinucleotide repeat sequence in the myotonic protein kinase gene (DMPK) at 19q13. The size of the expanded repeat sequence corresponds with the severity of peripheral and respiratory muscle weakness. Normal individuals have 5–37 repeats; 50–350 repeats are seen in childhood- and adult-onset myotonic dystrophy, and infants with severe congenital myotonic dystrophy may have more than 2000 repeats. The mother is the affected parent in cases of congenital myotonic dystrophy.

Infants with congenital myotonic dystrophy have congenital contractures, generalized hypotonia, and weakness. Facial weakness causes the characteristic tented upper lip and scaphoid temporal fossae. Swallowing difficulties are common; most children require gavage feeding. Respiratory insufficiency is common in children who present in the first few weeks of life and relates to lung hypoplasia caused by reduced intrauterine breathing movements, poor intercostal muscle action, and diaphragmatic hypoplasia (13). Bulbar weakness predisposes to aspiration. Preterm birth and asphyxia may exacerbate neonatal pulmonary hypertension and failure of central respiratory

control. Approximately 50% of patients with congenital myotonic dystrophy require ventilation at birth (14). Poor prognostic factors include continued requirement for ventilatory support at 30 days of age, prematurity, pulmonary hypertension, and a large number of CTG repeats (15). Children who require ventilation beyond the first month of life have a 25% mortality in their first year (15). Most survivors eventually become ambulant, with improved respiratory function with increasing age, but remain at risk of later respiratory deterioration, cardiac arrhythmia, complications of poor gastrointestinal motility, diabetes, and mental retardation (9,15).

Duchenne Muscular Dystrophy

Duchenne and Becker muscular dystrophies are related muscle disorders caused by mutations in the gene for dystrophin at Xp21. Duchenne muscular dystrophy (DMD) affects 1 in 5000 boys and is the most common muscular dystrophy of childhood. DMD usually presents between 3 and 5 years of age with an abnormal ("waddling") gait and frequent falls. Progressive muscle weakness causes loss of independent ambulation between ages 8 and 13. Becker muscular dystrophy is less common (affecting approximately 1 in 30,000 boys), generally presents between 5 and 15 years of age, and is more slowly progressive. Long-term corticosteroid treatment slows the progression of DMD (16). Loss of ambulation is followed by the development of scoliosis and muscle contractures. Other findings in DMD include muscle pseudohypertrophy, which most commonly affects the calves, and static intellectual impairment in 30% of patients. Most young men with DMD die before the age of 30, because of respiratory insufficiency

TABLE 54.3

CONGENITAL MUSCULAR DYSTROPHIES

■ SITE OF DEFECT	■ PROTEIN DEFECT	■ DISORDER/ INHERITANCE	■ NATURAL HISTORY	■ ADDITIONAL FINDINGS
Extracellular matrix protein	Laminin α_2 (merosin)	Merosin-deficient CMD (CMD type 1A) (AR)	Severe muscle weakness Respiratory insufficiency common	Leukodystrophy Demyelinating neuropathy
	Collagen VI	Ullrich (AD, AR) and Bethlem (AR) CMDs	Mild-to-moderate muscle weakness Respiratory insufficiency by late childhood–adolescence	Proximal joint contractures Distal hyperlaxity Follicular keratosis
Sarcolemmal proteins	Integrin α_7 (AR)		Congenital muscular dystrophy	
Glycosyltransferase enzymes	Fukutin (AR)	Fukuyama CMD (AR) Walker–Warburg disease (AR)	Severe muscle weakness Early respiratory insufficiency	Cerebellar dysgenesis Cobblestone lissencephaly Severe mental retardation
	POMGnT1	Muscle–eye–brain disease (AR)	Severe muscle weakness Early respiratory insufficiency	Cerebellar dysgenesis Cobblestone lissencephaly Severe mental retardation
	POMT1	Walker–Warburg disease (AR) LGMD with mental retardation (AR)	Severe muscle weakness Early respiratory insufficiency	Cerebellar dysgenesis Cobblestone lissencephaly Severe mental retardation
	Fukutin-related protein	CMD type 1C (AR) LGMD type 2I (AR)	Variable muscle weakness	Macroglossia Calf hypertrophy Cardiomyopathy
	LARGE	CMD type 1D (AR)	Moderately severe muscle weakness	Severe mental retardation Leukodystrophy
Endoplasmic reticulum protein	Selenoprotein 1 (SEPN1)	CMD with spinal rigidity (AR) Multiminicore disease (AR) Congenital fiber-type disproportion (AR)	Axial rigidity Axial weakness Respiratory insufficiency	Characteristic facies

CMD, congenital muscular dystrophy; AR, autosomal recessive; AD, autosomal dominant; LGMD, limb-girdle muscular dystrophy.

(90%) or cardiomyopathy (10%) (17). Long-term survival is reported in men who are supported with mechanical ventilation via tracheostomy (18).

Other Muscular Dystrophies

The limb-girdle muscular dystrophies (LGMDs) usually present in adulthood. These relatively uncommon neuromuscular conditions cause characteristic patterns of muscle weakness, preferentially affecting the pectoral and pelvic girdle muscles and generally sparing the face (Table 54.4). Respiratory muscle involvement is generally seen late in the disease course, but some LGMDs are associated with preferential involvement of the axial musculature and early respiratory insufficiency.

CLINICAL MANAGEMENT IN INTENSIVE CARE

Presentation to the PICU

❷ Most presentations to the PICU by children with chronic NMDs will be for the management of respiratory compromise because of intercurrent illness, surgery, or disease progression. The severity of pulmonary compromise in such

patients depends on the pattern and severity of involvement of respiratory muscles, the development of secondary thoracic wall abnormalities, and resultant changes in lung compliance (19).

Inspiratory muscle weakness limits the ability to take deep breaths, which leads to peripheral airway collapse. Respiratory muscle weakness may also make coughing ineffective. The cough reflex involves an initial inhalation of gas followed by closure of the glottis, then generation of an expiratory force against a closed glottis and, finally, rapid expiratory flow once the glottis reopens (20). These steps require, in turn, inspiratory, bulbar, and expiratory muscles. Impairment of the cough reflex because of poor function of any of these muscles results in the inability to clear secretions and the development of atelectasis. Superimposed upper respiratory tract infections also increase the volume of secretions, leading to frequent and rapid development of pneumonia (21).

In children with DMD and congenital myopathies, weakness of the diaphragm develops at the same rate as weakness of the intercostal and abdominal muscles. Significant respiratory compromise may occur, although paradoxical breathing is absent. Diaphragmatic weakness may be accentuated by supine positioning, exacerbating respiratory compromise in sleep (22).

In children with SMA, the intercostal muscles are more affected than the diaphragm. As the descent of the diaphragm during inspiration generates negative intrathoracic pressure,

TABLE 54.4

THE LIMB-GIRDLE MUSCULAR DYSTROPHIES

■ MUSCULAR DYSTRO-PHY (INHERITANCE)	■ SYMBOL	■ GENE LOCATION	■ PROTEIN PRODUCT	■ CLINICAL FINDINGS
Autosomal dominant	LGMD1A	5q22–q34	Myotilin	Dysarthria, neuropathy, cardiomyopathy
	LGMD1B	1q11–q23	Lamin A/C	Cardiomyopathy, conduction defects, proximal contractures
	LGMD1C	3p25	Caveolin 3	Muscle cramps, calf hypertrophy
	LGMD1D	6q23	?	
	LGMD1E	7q	?	
Autosomal recessive	LGMD2A	15q15.1–q21.1	Calpain 3	Scapular winging, calf hypertrophy, thigh abductors spared
	LGMD2B	2p13	Dysferlin	Distal weakness, wasting posterior compartment calf
	LGMD2C	13q12	γ-Sarcoglycan	Duchenne phenocopy, cardiomyopathy
	LGMD2D	17q12–q21.33	α-Sarcoglycan (adhalin)	Duchenne phenocopy, cardiomyopathy
	LGMD2E	4q12	β-Sarcoglycan	Duchenne phenocopy, cardiomyopathy
	LGMD2F	5q33–44	δ-Sarcoglycan	Duchenne phenocopy, cardiomyopathy
	LGMD2G	17q11–q12	Telethonin	Rare, marked clinical variability
	LGMD2H	9q31–34.1	E3 ubiquitin ligase (*TRIM32*)	Seen only in Manitoba Hutterites
	LGMD 2I	19q13.3	Fukutin-related protein	Calf and tongue hypertrophy, variable course, cardiomyopathy
	LGMD2J	2q	Titin	Rare, wasting posterior compartment calf
Emery–Dreifuss (X-linked)	EDMD	Xq28	Emerin	Early proximal contractures, cardiac conduction defects
Emery–Dreifuss (AD)	EDMD-AD	1q11–q23	Lamin A/C	Early proximal contractures, cardiac conduction defects
Facioscapulohumeral muscular dystrophy (AD)	FSHD1	4q35	?	Facial weakness, scapular winging, foot drop

LGMD, limb-girdle muscular dystrophy; EDMD, Emery–Dreifuss muscular dystrophy; AD, autosomal dominant.

the thoracic cage will collapse (because of weaker intercostal muscles) at a time when the abdomen is expanding. This abnormal pattern—"paradoxical" breathing—can lead to chest-wall deformity and abnormal lung development.

Young children with chronic NMDs have abnormally high chest-wall compliance because of hypotonia and loss of muscle bulk. Intercostal muscle weakness makes the rib cage less able to withstand the elastic recoil of the lungs, leading to low end-expiratory volume and atelectasis. With increasing age, cartilaginous ossification causes a reduction in chest-wall compliance and increased chest-wall rigidity. Thoracic kyphoscoliosis may develop because of weak paraspinal musculature. Scoliosis further reduces chest-wall compliance and may lead to asymmetrical chest expansion. Together, these factors contribute to the development of ventilation/perfusion mismatch, increased work of breathing, and respiratory muscle fatigue.

Sleep apnea and episodes of hypoxemia are the usual initial manifestations of respiratory muscle compromise in children with chronic NMDs, with later development of alveolar hypoventilation and respiratory failure. Two types of respiratory failure are seen. Type 1 respiratory failure is characterized by hypoxemia and a low-to-normal arterial partial pressure of carbon dioxide ($Paco_2$). It is corrected by supplemental inspired oxygen. Hypoxemia and CO_2 retention characterize

type 2 respiratory failure. Patients in type 2 respiratory failure may adapt to chronic hypercapnia, relying on hypoxic drive to breathing. Administration of supplemental oxygen in this instance may lead to respiratory depression. Children with type 2 respiratory failure often require ventilatory support to improve gas exchange (14,23).

Disease-Specific Aspects of Respiratory Care

Spinal Muscular Atrophy

Patients with SMA types 1 and 2 are at risk of respiratory complications, at an early stage, which may present as recurrent chest infections or failure to thrive (4,5). Ventilatory support during acute infectious exacerbations of this condition may be complicated by disease progression and may hence be difficult to withdraw.

Congenital Myopathies and Muscular Dystrophies

Respiratory problems are the primary cause of death in chronic NMDs. The degree of skeletal muscle weakness usually, but not always, reflects the severity of respiratory muscle involvement (11). Bulbar muscle involvement increases the risk of aspiration, and poor nutritional state may increase the susceptibility to respiratory infection (10). Most patients, even those who are asymptomatic, have restricted respiratory capacity and are at risk of insidious nocturnal hypoxemia (23). Sleep-related symptoms include sleep disturbance, nightmares, morning headache, daytime tiredness, and weight loss. Sudden respiratory failure may be precipitated by intercurrent infection or anesthesia and can occur at any age (11,14).

All patients with congenital myopathy should have baseline evaluation of their respiratory function as part of routine clinical and preoperative care. Any child with a vital capacity (VC) <60% of the predicted value for age should be reviewed annually with lung-function testing (forced vital capacity in the sitting and supine positions, forced expiratory volume in 1 second, and maximal inspiratory and expiratory pressures), pulse oximetry, $Paco_2$ when awake and when asleep, and an assessment of bulbar function (14). Regular chest physiotherapy, postural drainage, and assisted coughing techniques may improve respiratory toilet in patients with bulbar weakness, reduced VC, and recurrent aspiration. Respiratory infections should be treated early and aggressively (14,20).

Duchenne Muscular Dystrophy

3 The natural history of respiratory muscle involvement in DMD follows a characteristic pattern. First, an increase occurs in VC that parallels somatic growth until the age of 10–12 years. After this age, during the next 2–4 years, most patients lose the ability to walk unaided and their respiratory function gradually declines, with a fall in VC of 8.5% per year. Slower rates of deterioration, on the order of ~4.5% per year, are seen in children who achieve a maximum VC above 2.5 L (24). DMD is associated with characteristic patterns of respiratory dysfunction (24). Sleep-disordered breathing is associated with a VC <60% of that predicted for age. Sleep-disordered breathing and hypoventilation are associated with a VC <40% of that predicted for age. In adults, a VC of <1.5 L or cough peak flow of <160 L/min predicts risk of respiratory failure, and a VC of <1 L is terminal unless respiratory support is offered (25).

Practical Issues during PICU Admission

Children with chronic NMD are particularly vulnerable to influenza, other viral respiratory infections, and aspiration. Pneumococcal and influenza vaccinations should be given routinely (21). Most children with chronic NMD who are admitted to PICU will recover and be discharged without **4** needing prolonged invasive mechanical ventilation. At least 25%, however, will require noninvasive respiratory support (26). Sometimes, the episode that necessitates admission signifies the inevitable decline in the underlying illness. The major issue, therefore, is to decide when such ongoing respiratory support is required. On admission, the child's primary physician should be contacted and the following questions should be asked of both the family and the physician: What is the child's present level of respiratory and bulbar function? What is the present level, if any, of respiratory support? Have there been discussions about prognosis, and have previous decisions been made about the level of mechanical ventilation to be offered? Are other long-term providers, such as neurologists or pulmonologists, involved for respiratory management? Is a case-worker providing the coordination of respiratory care and other multidisciplinary care involving physiotherapy, occupational therapy, social work, and home nursing staff?

ONGOING VENTILATORY SUPPORT

The indications for ongoing ventilatory support include CO_2 retention ($Paco_2$ > 50 mm Hg), chronic hypoxia (arterial partial pressure of oxygen, Pao_2 < 90 mm Hg), VC <1 L, and recurrent pneumonia (14). The preferred method of home mechanical ventilation will depend on the clinical state of the patient and the rate of progression of the underlying disorder. The mode of support includes bilevel positive-airway pressure by nasal mask or mechanical ventilation via tracheostomy if noninvasive support is not feasible (14). Domiciliary oxygen is rarely indicated but may be necessary if oxygen saturation remains <90% once hypoventilation has been corrected. Home ventilation requires a large and ongoing support network for the patients and their families and may not be appropriate for all patients (27). Aggressive management is appropriate for the older child for whom assisted ventilation may result in marked improvement in quality of life (27).

During the PICU admission it is important to have a clear plan for weaning from mechanical ventilation that incorporates best practice in multidisciplinary care.

Long-term, Noninvasive Ventilation for Chronic NMD

Home noninvasive ventilation (NIV) is used increasingly in children with chronic NMD because it decreases hospitalization rates (26–28) and improves respiratory function (29). NIV is not curative and does not prevent progression of the underlying neuromuscular disorder, but it may improve quality of life (27). The optimal time for introduction of NIV is controversial. In boys with DMD, daytime hypercapnia predicts death within 9 months unless ventilatory support is given (18). NIV should be considered in children with DMD and recurrent desaturation to <90%, an increase in transcutaneous CO_2 by >15 mm Hg in REM (rapid-eye movement) sleep, symptoms of sleep-disordered breathing, or more than three admissions per year for respiratory distress (14). The benefit of NIV before the development of respiratory insufficiency is unproven.

Delivery of Respiratory Support

NIV can be delivered by a nasal mask, face mask, or mouthpiece connected to bilevel, pressure-targeted ventilators. Most bilevel pressure-targeted ventilators include a continuous positive-airway pressure (CPAP) mode in addition to spontaneous and timed bilevel support modes (30). In the CPAP mode, the ventilator delivers a flow of gas set at a constant positive pressure. CPAP is not helpful in the patient with frequent central apneas or hypoventilation. Bilevel positive-airway pressure ventilators also provide CPAP but allow independent control of expiratory and inspiratory muscles. NIV is contraindicated in patients with upper airway obstruction and uncontrollable airway secretions. Severe swallowing impairment secondary to bulbar involvement is a relative contraindication. Complications of NIV include pneumothorax, facial irritation, gastric distension, and, in the long-term, midface hypoplasia (31).

Bulbar Dysfunction

Chronic NMDs that cause significant facial and bulbar weakness may result in feeding difficulties in infancy and, in older children, lead to recurrent aspiration, dysarthria, poor articulation, and poor control of secretions (9). In the PICU, poor control of oral secretions may delay extubation.

Feeding problems in the newborn period often necessitate gavage feeds. Insertion of a gastrostomy tube should be considered if problems persist after the first few months of life. Careful attention to nutrition is important, particularly during acute illnesses. Malnutrition can cause slow recovery after surgery or intercurrent illnesses (11). Accelerated weight gain and improvement of respiratory function may follow gastrostomy placement.

Treatments for sialorrhea, such as anticholinergic agents and salivary gland botulinum toxin injections, may be effective but may cause increased viscosity of secretions and other side effects (11,32) (Table 54.5).

Orthopedic Complications

❺ Scoliosis and kyphosis are common complications of chronic NMDs and can impact upon mobility and respiratory function. Thoracic bracing does not prevent or reverse spinal curvature but can improve stability during sitting. Spinal fusion halts progressive spinal deformity and preserves lung function. The introduction of segmental spinal instrumentation, with sublaminar wire fixation (incorporating Luque rods), has greatly eased postoperative management in the PICU. The posterior surgical approach is considered best for preventing progression of spinal deformity. An anterior approach in patients reliant on anterior abdominal muscles and the diaphragm for respiration can lead to postoperative respiratory difficulty and long-term respiratory compromise. Postoperative complications are more common in children with VC of <30% predicted for age (33) and those with a spinal curve of >100 degrees (34). The development of a multidisciplinary care pathway for neuromuscular patients undergoing spinal surgery was associated with shorter length of stay and a reduction in perioperative complications compared to case-matched retrospective controls (35).

Orthopedic surgery may also be needed for congenital and acquired contractures and pathologic fractures secondary to disuse osteopenia. Orthotics, splinting, and serial plaster casting may be necessary in children who are immobilized for long periods by illness or surgery, particularly for prevention of Achilles tendon and long finger flexor contractures. Splinting must be undertaken in combination with passive stretching exercises to optimize benefit (36).

Cardiac Function

Symptomatic cardiac involvement is uncommon in the congenital myopathies and myasthenic syndromes, but cor pulmonale may be seen in those with advanced respiratory disease. Several of the congenital and LGMDs (particularly CMD1C/LGMD 2I, LGMD 1A, and Emery–Dreifuss muscular dystrophy) are associated with cardiomyopathy and conduction defects. Patients with these conditions should undergo annual cardiac review.

Advanced DMD is commonly associated with cardiac conduction defects, resting tachycardia, and cardiomyopathy. Mitral valve prolapse and pulmonary hypertension may also occur. Subclinical or clinical cardiac involvement is present in ~90% of Duchenne or Becker muscular dystrophy patients but is the cause of death in only 10% of men with DMD and 50% of patients with Becker muscular dystrophy. Progression of cardiomyopathy in DMD or Becker muscular dystrophy is prevented or slowed by early treatment with angiotensin-converting enzyme inhibitors (17).

Myotonic muscular dystrophy is rarely associated with cardiomyopathy, but children with myotonic dystrophy commonly develop symptomatic or subclinical conduction disturbances that may cause left ventricular dysfunction. Patients with myotonic dystrophy require monitoring of cardiac conduction and may require a cardiac pacemaker (37).

Anesthesia

Patients with congenital myopathies and muscular dystrophies usually tolerate general anesthesia, but the potential exists for decompensation of respiratory function and rapid loss of muscle conditioning. Subclinical respiratory insufficiency may be unmasked by anesthesia and exacerbated by postoperative atelectasis and spinal instrumentation. For example, in a series of 143 patients with nemaline myopathy, 5 patients developed unexpected postoperative respiratory failure, 1 child had an unexpected respiratory arrest 24 hours after fundoplication, and another developed persistent lobar collapse (11). Preoperative assessment of respiratory state is important in helping to decide the timing of surgery. Patients should receive intensive preoperative physiotherapy, and must be mobilized as soon as possible after surgery, as prolonged immobility often exacerbates muscle weakness.

Children with myotonic dystrophy may be extremely sensitive to anesthetics and analgesics, especially barbiturates and opiates, with a prolonged response to non-depolarizing muscle relaxants and a tendency to postoperative apnea and sedation (38).

Malignant hyperthermia is an autosomal-dominant, pharmacogenetic disorder characterized by an increase in skeletal muscle metabolism in response to certain inhalation anesthetics (particularly halothane) and depolarizing muscle relaxants (particularly succinylcholine). The triggering agent increases sarcoplasmic calcium concentrations, resulting in uncontrolled muscle contraction and hyperthermia, which may be fatal if untreated. Central core disease and minicore myopathy are associated with an increased risk of malignant hyperthermia. Malignant hyperthermia is less commonly associated with other congenital myopathies (39) and has only very rarely been reported in DMD and other muscular dystrophies, but DMD is associated with a risk of life-threatening hyperkalemia after exposure to volatile anesthetics. Malignant hyperthermia precautions should be undertaken in all patients who are to undergo muscle biopsy for diagnostic purposes. Triggering anesthetics should be avoided.

QUALITY OF LIFE IN CHILDREN VENTILATED FOR CHRONIC NMD

It is a common, if unstated, concern of PICU staff that, once intubated for an acute episode of respiratory compromise, children with chronic NMD will not be able to be extubated and weaned from full ventilation (20,40). This concern is not supported by the literature. In a 15-year review of children with chronic NMD who were admitted to the PICU, most were discharged without the need for prolonged invasive ventilation, and only 9% of unplanned admissions ended in death (26). Nocturnal respiratory support was started in the PICU and continued after discharge in 23% of admissions. The authors concluded that "all children with underlying NMD should be provided with acute respiratory support in the anticipation that they are likely to recover. However, repeat admissions and chronic respiratory failure are likely and should be anticipated."

TABLE 54.5

MANAGEMENT OF CHILDREN WITH CHRONIC NEUROMUSCULAR DISORDERS

■ PROBLEM IDENTIFIED	■ REFERRAL	■ POSSIBLE INTERVENTIONS
Skeletal muscle involvement ■ Hypotonia ■ Weakness ■ Contractures	Physiotherapy Occupational therapy	Objective testing of muscle strength Regular exercise program Active and passive stretching Standing frame Orthotics/splinting—upper and lower limb Serial plaster casting Enhance mobility—walking frames or wheelchair Liaison with local services prior to discharge
Respiratory muscle involvement ■ Reduced respiratory capacity ■ Recurrent chest infections ■ Aspiration ■ Nocturnal hypoxia ■ Respiratory failure	Physiotherapy Lung-function tests Sleep study Respiratory physician Occupational therapy	Breathing exercises Chest physiotherapy to clear secretions Seating assessment Influenza and pneumococcal vaccination Aggressive management of acute infections Nocturnal/daytime ventilation Liaise with local services
Bulbar involvement ■ Feeding and swallowing difficulties ■ Failure to thrive	Speech pathologist Dietitian Gastroenterologist	Speech therapy Modified barium swallow Caloric supplementation/thickened feed Gavage feeding or gastrostomy feeding
Bulbar involvement ■ Dysarthria ■ Excessive drooling	Speech pathologist Surgeon	Speech therapy Anticholinergic medications Pharyngoplasty Salivary duct surgery/botulinum toxin injections
Developmental or psychosocial delay	Occupational therapy Physiotherapy Speech pathology Psychologist Developmental physician	Developmental stimulation Home programs Reassessment if deterioration
Scoliosis	Physiotherapy Orthopedic surgeon	Spinal x-ray Monitoring of degree of curve Bracing Corrective surgery
Foot deformities	Physiotherapy Orthopedic surgeon	Splinting/serial casting Corrective surgery
Cardiac involvement ■ Conduction defects ■ Cardiomyopathy ■ Cor pulmonale	Cardiologist	Electrocardiogram, Holter monitor, echocardiogram Medication if indicated
Inability to perform activities of daily living ■ Inability to achieve independence with bathing, toileting, dressing, feeding ■ Difficulties with access ■ Handwriting difficulties	Occupational therapy Community nurse	Aides for individual activities of daily living Wheelchair assessment Home nursing assistance Home and school modifications Typing and computer programs Car modifications Liaise with local services
Excessive weight gain ■ Limits mobility and exacerbates weakness	Dietitian Physiotherapy	Calorie-controlled diet Exercise program
Inability to participate in sport/leisure activities	Physiotherapy Occupational therapy	Liaison with/visit schools Sporting organizations for people with disabilities Hydrotherapy
Constipation	Dietitian Physician Gastroenterologist	High-fiber diet Laxatives/enemas
Depression or behavioral problems	Psychologist	Individual or family therapy Medication
Family financial and social difficulties	Social work Muscular Dystrophy Association Government assistance bodies	Disability allowance/pension Support groups Financial assistance with equipment and home modifications Transport and travel assistance
Planning future pregnancies	Geneticist Genetic counselor	Genetic counseling Planning prenatal diagnosis

■ PROBLEM IDENTIFIED	■ REFERRAL	■ POSSIBLE INTERVENTIONS
Planning surgery	Consult with anesthesiologist Respiratory physician	Malignant hyperthermia precautions Lung-function tests and presurgical physiotherapy
Planning future employment	Vocational counseling service Occupational therapy	Planning school studies Vocational planning Training, work placement and support
Coordination of care	Pediatrician, pediatric neurologist, or rehabilitation specialist	Contact with general practitioner via telephone and letter Liaise with local services Arrange case conferences when necessary Determine timing of respiratory, orthopedic, and palliative interventions

Most ventilator-dependent adults consider that their quality of life is reasonable (41,42). Relatively few studies have been undertaken in children ventilated long term, but the information that is available suggests that their quality of life is considered good (27,43).

CONCLUSIONS AND FUTURE DIRECTIONS

The complex ethical issues involved in the use of long-term ventilation in children with chronic NMD have been reviewed (44). While the clinical management of these children varies within and between countries, some fundamental guidelines should be followed:

1. A specialist in chronic NMDs should be involved so that the most up-to-date information on prognosis, function, and quality of life is available. This physician should be the one who usually cares for the child and family and who has discussed ventilatory options and negotiated a proposed plan of care.
2. The difficulty of prediction of the exact clinical course should be acknowledged.
3. Palliative care principles should always be followed, because most of these diseases cannot be cured. The treatment strategy should be to maintain the highest quality of life for as long as possible. It is important to stress to the child and family that their care will be actively continued even if they choose not to pursue artificial ventilation. The primary aim of treatment is maintenance of an acceptable quality of life.

Advances in the PICU management of children with chronic NMD should be focused on improved management of respiratory impairment and better monitoring and prevention of complications.

References

1. Zerres K, Rudnik-Schoneborn S. Natural history in proximal spinal muscular atrophy. Clinical analysis of 445 patients and suggestions for a modification of existing classifications. *Arch Neurol* 1995;52:518–23.
2. Iannaccone ST, Browne RH, Samaha FJ, et al. Prospective study of spinal muscular atrophy before age 6 years. *Pediatr Neurol* 1993;9:187–93.
3. Bach JR, Baird JS, Plosky D, et al. Spinal muscular atrophy type 1: Management and outcomes. *Pediatr Pulmonol* 2002;34:16–22.
4. Birnkrant DJ, Pope JF, Martin JE, et al. Treatment of type I spinal muscular atrophy with noninvasive ventilation and gastrostomy feeding. *Pediatr Neurol* 1998;18:407–10.
5. Ioos C, Leclair-Richard D, Mrad S, et al. Respiratory capacity course in patients with infantile spinal muscular atrophy. *Chest* 2004;126:831–7.
6. Bach JR. There are other ways to manage spinal muscular atrophy type 1. *Chest* 2005;127:1463–4.
7. Chung BH, Wong VC, Ip P. Spinal muscular atrophy: Survival pattern and functional status. *Pediatrics* 2004;114:e548–53.
8. Ouvrier RA, Geevasingha N, Ryan MM. Autosomal-recessive and X-linked forms of hereditary motor and sensory neuropathy in childhood. *Muscle Nerve* 2007;36:131–43.
9. North KN, Ryan MM. The congenital myopathies. In: Noseworthy J, ed. *Neurological Therapeutics, Principles and Practice.* Rochester, NY: Martin Dunitz, 2006.
10. Jungbluth H, Sewry C, Brown SC, et al. Minicore myopathy in children: A clinical and histopathological study of 19 cases. *Neuromuscul Disord* 2000;10:264–73.
11. Ryan MM, Schnell C, Strickland CD, et al. Nemaline myopathy: A clinical study of 143 cases. *Ann Neurol* 2001;50:312–20.
12. Banwell BL, Singh NC, Ramsay DA. Prolonged survival in neonatal nemaline myopathy. *Pediatr Neurol* 1994;10:335–7.
13. Sarnat HB, O'Connor T, Byrne PA. Clinical effects of myotonic dystrophy on pregnancy and the neonate. *Arch Neurol* 1976;33:459–65.
14. Wallgren-Pettersson C, Bushby K, Mellies U, et al. 117th ENMC workshop: Ventilatory support in congenital neuromuscular disorders—congenital myopathies, congenital muscular dystrophies, congenital myotonic dystrophy and SMA (II). 4–6 April 2003, Naarden, The Netherlands. *Neuromuscul Disord* 2004;14:56–69.
15. Campbell C, Sherlock R, Jacob P, et al. Congenital myotonic dystrophy: Assisted ventilation duration and outcome. *Pediatrics* 2004;113:811–6.
16. Biggar WD, Gingras M, Fehling DL, et al. Deflazacort treatment of Duchenne muscular dystrophy. *J Pediatr* 2001;138:45–50.
17. Finsterer J, Stollberger C. The heart in human dystrophinopathies. *Cardiology* 2003;99:1–19.
18. Vianello A, Bevilacqua M, Salvador V, et al. Long-term nasal intermittent positive pressure ventilation in advanced Duchenne's muscular dystrophy. *Chest* 1994;105:445–8.
19. Bach JR, Niranjan V, Weaver B. Spinal muscular atrophy type 1: A noninvasive respiratory management approach. *Chest* 2000;117:1100–5.
20. Birnkrant DJ. The assessment and management of the respiratory complications of pediatric neuromuscular diseases. *Clin Pediatr* 2002;41:301–8.
21. Keren R, Zaoutis TE, Bridges CB, et al. Neurological and neuromuscular disease as a risk factor for respiratory failure in children hospitalized with influenza infection. *JAMA* 2005;294:2188–94.
22. Fromageot C, Lofaso F, Annane D, et al. Supine fall in lung volumes in the assessment of diaphragmatic weakness in neuromuscular disorders. *Arch Phys Med Rehab* 2001;82:123–8.
23. Smith PE, Edwards RH, Calverley PM. Mechanisms of sleep-disordered breathing in chronic neuromuscular disease: Implications for management. *Q J Med* 1991;81:961–73.

24. McDonald CM, Abresch RT, Carter GT, et al. Profiles of neuromuscular diseases: Duchenne muscular dystrophy. *Am J Phys Med Rehab* 1995;74(5 suppl):S70–92.

25. Seddon PC, Khan Y. Respiratory problems in children with neurological impairment. *Arch Dis Child* 2003;88:75–8.

26. Yates K, Festa M, Gillis J, et al. Outcome of children with neuromuscular disease admitted to paediatric intensive care. *Arch Dis Child* 2004;89:170–5.

27. Young HK, Lowe A, Fitzgerald DA, et al. Non-invasive ventilation in children with neuromuscular disease. *Neurology* 2007;68(3):198–201.

28. Katz S, Selvadurai H, Keilty K, et al. Outcome of non-invasive positive pressure ventilation in paediatric neuromuscular disease. *Arch Dis Child* 2004;89:121–4.

29. Simonds AK, Ward S, Heather S, et al. Outcome of paediatric domiciliary mask ventilation in neuromuscular and skeletal disease. *Eur Respir J* 2000;16:476–81.

30. Teague WG. Noninvasive ventilation in the pediatric intensive care unit for children with acute respiratory failure. *Pediatr Pulmonol* 2003;35:418–26.

31. Villa MP, Pagani J, Ambrosio R, et al. Mid-face hypoplasia after long-term nasal ventilation. *Am J Respir Crit Care Med* 2002;166:1142–3.

32. Brei TJ. Management of drooling. *Semin Pediatr Neurol* 2003;10:265–70.

33. Jenkins JG, Bohn D, Edmonds JF, et al. Evaluation of pulmonary function in muscular dystrophy patients requiring spinal surgery. *Crit Care Med* 1982;10:645–9.

34. Grossfeld S, Winter RB, Lonstein JE, et al. Complications of anterior spinal surgery in children. *J Pediatr Orthop* 1997;17:89–95.

35. Miller NH, Benefield E, Hasting L, et al. Evaluation of high-risk patients undergoing spinal surgery: A matched case series. *J Pediatr Orthop* 2010;30:496–502.

36. McDonald CM. Limb contractures in progressive neuromuscular disease and the role of stretching, orthotics, and surgery. *Phys Med Rehabil Clin N Am* 1998;9:187–211.

37. English KM, Gibbs JL. Cardiac monitoring and treatment for children and adolescents with neuromuscular disorders. *Dev Med Child Neurol* 2006;48:231–5.

38. White RJ, Bass SP. Myotonic dystrophy and paediatric anaesthesia. *Paediatr Anaesth* 2003;13:94–102.

39. Asai T, Fujise K, Uchida M. Anaesthesia for cardiac surgery in children with nemaline myopathy. *Anaesthesia* 1992;47:405–8.

40. Gillis J, Rennick J. Affirming parental love in the pediatric intensive care unit. *Pediatr Crit Care Med* 2006;7:165–8.

41. Bach JR, Barnett V. Ethical considerations in the management of individuals with severe neuromuscular disorders. *Am J Phys Med Rehabil* 1994;73:134–40.

42. Hotes LS, Johnson JA, Sicilian L. Long-term care, rehabilitation, and legal and ethical considerations in the management of neuromuscular disease with respiratory dysfunction. *Clin Chest Med* 1994;15:783–95.

43. Frates RC Jr, Splaingard ML, Smith EO, et al. Outcome of home mechanical ventilation in children. *J Pediatr* 1985;106:850–6.

44. Simonds AK. Ethical aspects of home long-term ventilation in children with neuromuscular disease. *Paediatr Respir Rev* 2005;6:209–14.

CHAPTER 55 ■ **DEVELOPMENTAL NEUROBIOLOGY, NEUROPHYSIOLOGY, AND THE PICU**

LARRY W. JENKINS AND PATRICK M. KOCHANEK

KEY POINTS

1 Important biochemical, molecular, physiologic, and structural differences in central nervous system (CNS) development influence treatment of brain injury in newborns, infants, children, adolescents, and adults.

2 A unique aspect of programmed cell death (PCD) in the developing brain versus the adult brain is an imbalance between pro-death and pro-survival pathways induced by decreases in trophic and neurotransmitter neuronal input. Thus, the developing brain may be more sensitive to injuries that mimic regional developmental changes in trophin and neurotransmitter levels. It may also be sensitive to anesthetics and/or sedatives as suggested by recent studies in primates. This is a vital area for current and future research to define the potential risks for infants in the PICU.

3 Synaptogenesis is an active process that has a high rate of occurrence until puberty.

4 Myelination persists longer than most other CNS developmental processes, continuing through adolescence.

5 Around the time of birth, the neurotransmitter γ-aminobutyric acid (GABA) switches from being excitatory to inhibitory in the CNS. The developing brain prior to this switch has enhanced sensitivity to excitotoxic injury.

6 The lower limits of blood pressure autoregulation of cerebral blood flow (CBF) for infants and adults are similar, putting the developing brain at risk for ischemia, as normal mean arterial pressure is age dependent.

7 CBF and cerebral metabolic rate increase from birth and plateau between 3 and 9 years of age. This developmental progression mirrors synapse formation in the brain.

8 Cerebrovascular tight junctions prevent movement of hydrophilic substances, osmotic agents, and proteins across the blood–brain barrier (BBB).

The field of pediatric neurointensive care is challenged with designing and implementing optimal therapies for complex insults, such as traumatic brain injury (TBI), asphyxial arrest, stroke, refractory status epilepticus, and infections, for the most complex organ system—the central nervous system (CNS). The challenge is magnified in pediatrics by the need to accomplish this goal in an optimal manner, whether the patient is a newborn, infant, child, or adolescent. Salient differences in structural, biochemical, physiologic, and behavioral components of the brain from infancy to adolescence have been recognized, and an understanding of these factors may be important to the clinician when appropriately defining prognosis and/or guiding therapy. This chapter provides fundamental insights into this complexity and is organized around key concepts and developmental milestones that should provide useful constructs for understanding both developmental brain function and pathology in clinical practice. It provides basics in developmental neurobiology and neurophysiology that will help the reader navigate the chapters that follow. We recognize that, in several areas, a complete picture of developmental differences in neurobiology and neurophysiology across the PICU-relevant age spectrum is lacking—and extrapolation from data on newborns or adults is necessary. In some cases, only data from experimental animal models are available. Nevertheless, certain stages of development may be particularly resistant or vulnerable to PICU-relevant insults that may interfere with subsequent normal developmental progression. Key factors germane to pediatric intensive care that differentiate the newborn, infant, child, adolescent, and adult brain are discussed whenever possible. For more details, the reader is referred to several excellent reviews (1–20) to which much of this chapter is indebted.

CENTRAL NERVOUS SYSTEM DEVELOPMENT

Brain Development Timeline

CNS development occurs through the process of neurulation during embryogenesis. The neural plate is formed by ectodermal tissue at ~2 weeks of gestation. By the 18th day of gestation, the neural plate forms the neural groove, which in turn eventually fuses by the 3rd gestational week, giving rise to the neural tube. Completed human neural tube formation occurs between 26 and 28 gestational days (18). Throughout the first month of human gestation, specific CNS regions, such as the forebrain, midbrain, and hindbrain, form because of neurogenesis and cellular migration. Concomitant with regional CNS development, neurogenesis and proliferation, migration, differentiation, synaptogenesis, apoptosis, and myelination occur and continue postnatally up to 10 years of age (Fig. 55.1). Major CNS developmental milestones in gestational weeks are as follows (12):

- 3–4 weeks—Formation of the neural tube occurs.
- 5–10 weeks—Hemispheres form.
- 8–18 weeks—Neuronal proliferation is ongoing.

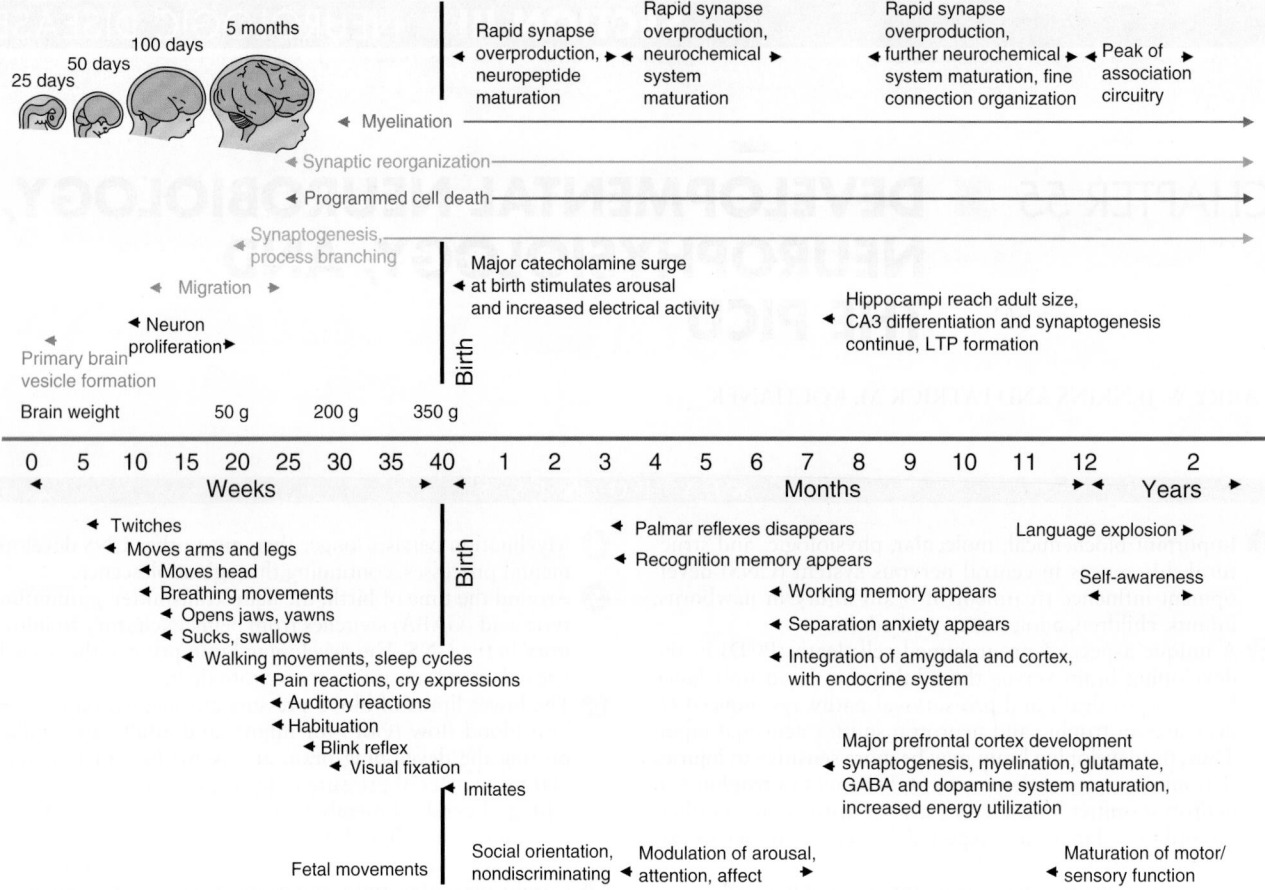

FIGURE 55.1. The key events of the human developmental timeline. The appearance of specific structural and functional developmental events is shown for the human fetus, infant, and young child up to 2 years of age. LTP, long-term potentiation; GABA, γ-aminobutyric acid. (Modified from Lagercrantz H, Ringstedt T. Organization of the neuronal circuits in the central nervous system during development. *Acta Paediatr* 2001;90:707–15; additional data from Levitt P. Structural and functional maturation of the developing primate brain. *J Pediatr* 2003;143:S35–45; and from Herschkowitz N. Neurological bases of behavioral development in infancy. *Brain Dev* 2000;22:411–16.)

- 12–24 weeks—Neuronal migration proceeds.
- 25+ weeks—Neuronal arborization, synaptogenesis, programmed neuronal death, and neural connectivity occur.
- 40+ weeks—Myelination is ongoing.

Aberrations in any of these brain developmental processes may produce congenital CNS defects, many of which can be life threatening (18).

Development of Specific Brain Regions

Human brain size increases dramatically, beginning from early gestation and continuing for at least 2–3 postnatal years. CNS growth, based on changes in gross brain size, peaks at around 4 months postnatally. However, specific brain regions have different growth time windows (**Fig. 55.2**) and periods of genetic and environmental vulnerabilities before and after birth (18). In general, the forebrain develops slower than the hindbrain, with the medial aspects of the hindbrain developing faster than the lateral. The neocortical and hippocampal structures grow mostly during the fetal period but do have some continuing neuronal and glial postnatal development. In contrast, the thalamus and hypothalamus develop during the early fetal and late embryonic periods, as does the mesencephalon. The pons and medulla of the hindbrain develop

primarily during the embryonic period, which in humans encompasses weeks 3–7.5 of gestation (21).

Neurogenesis and Proliferation

The neural tube is formed by the neuroectoderm, with neuroepithelial cells differentiating into various types of neurons and glia. The mature human brain contains an estimated 10^{10} neurons (22). Neural precursor cells from the epithelium form the developing CNS and undergo mitotic arrest at various times during development. Prior to becoming postmitotic cells, these cells determine their position within the embryonic axis and either reenter the cell cycle to increase the precursor pool or enter mitotic arrest (7). During development, neuronal populations within each brain region are highly regulated along a structured timetable. This regional variability appears conserved across species with regard to neuronal developmental patterns, but with species-specific timelines. For example, neurogenesis occurs within days in the rat compared to weeks in human. Environmental or genetic stress during neurogenesis is a particularly vulnerable time for regional brain development. However, the CNS is more resistant to such stressors following neurogenesis. Fetal alcohol syndrome is a classic example of environmental stress that can interfere with the developmental process of neurogenesis (18).

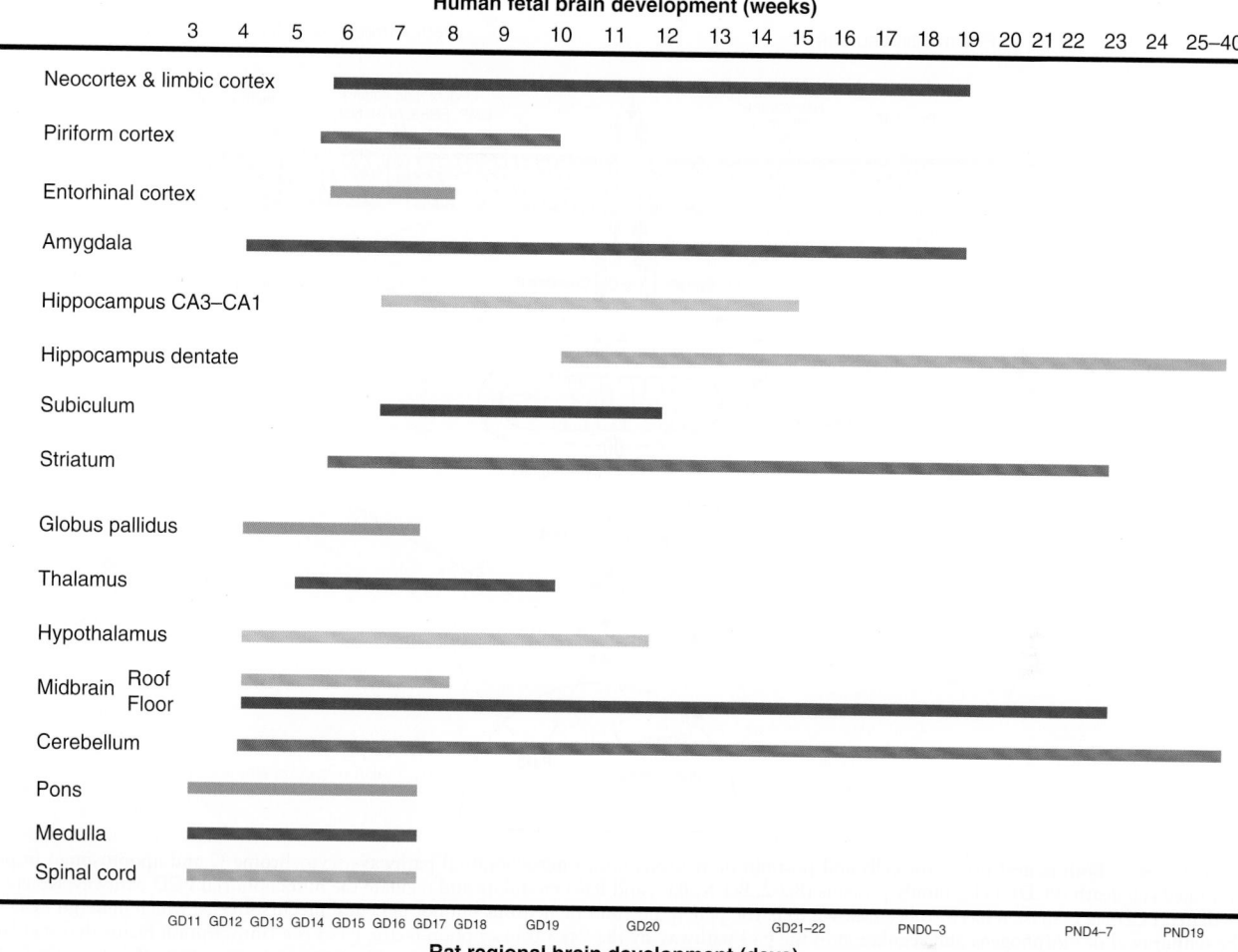

FIGURE 55.2. Human fetal brain development. The developmental timeline of selected human brain regions is shown in comparison with rat development timeline. The rat is the most commonly used species to study both normal and injury-related CNS development and thus has the most extensive normative database. GD, gestational day; PND, postnatal day. (Modified from Rice D, Barone S, Jr. Critical periods of vulnerability for the developing nervous system: Evidence from humans and animal models. *Environ Health Perspective* 2000;108(suppl 3):551–33, with permission.)

The prenatal stage of brain development is characterized by rapid cell division under the control of the cell cycle and, in turn, numerous cell signaling pathways, including at least nine different growth factor cascades (4). Cells also must duplicate their organelles and cellular molecules to maintain their size; thus, growth processes must also be coordinated with cellular replication. It has been estimated that ~200,000 new neurons are produced each minute at between 8 and 18 weeks of gestation. In contrast, it has been proposed that little neurogenesis occurs after birth, except in some select brain regions that continue into adulthood (12).

Programmed Cell Death

Neuronal cell type and number are regulated by apoptotic cell death during CNS development, which occurs in waves. Programmed cell death (PCD) begins in zones of proliferation and recurs as CNS remodeling proceeds based on the kind and number of connections made by each individual neuroblast and neuron (4). Furthermore, PCD persists postnatally owing to continued CNS development. Two types of developmental PCD have been classified: (a) a proliferative apoptosis

that affects morphogenetic processes involving neural precursor cells and postmitotic neuroblasts, and (b) a neurotrophic-related apoptosis that affects postmitotic neurons that fail to establish appropriate synaptic connections. Apoptotic regulation of neurons that undergo PCD prior to developing synaptic contacts (proliferative apoptosis) has been proposed to differ from target-dependent neuronal death pathways (neurotrophic-related apoptosis) (7) (**Fig. 55.3**). Proliferative neuronal apoptosis prevents premature and dysfunctional neurogenesis from occurring secondary to premature differentiation signals.

Interference in normal developmental neuronal death cascades by environmental or genetic stress can result in a number of different pathologies (4). In contrast to the trophin-mediated signals that promote growth and survival, extracellular signaling proteins inhibit these processes. These survival and death signals, as will be seen in Chapter 56, appear to play a key role in the evolution of neuronal death after CNS injuries such as asphyxia, TBI, seizures, infections, and other PICU-relevant insults.

The Bcl-2 protein family, the adaptor protein Apaf1, and the cysteine protease caspase family are the principal regulators of PCD (7). PCD pathways involve both intrinsic and extrinsic

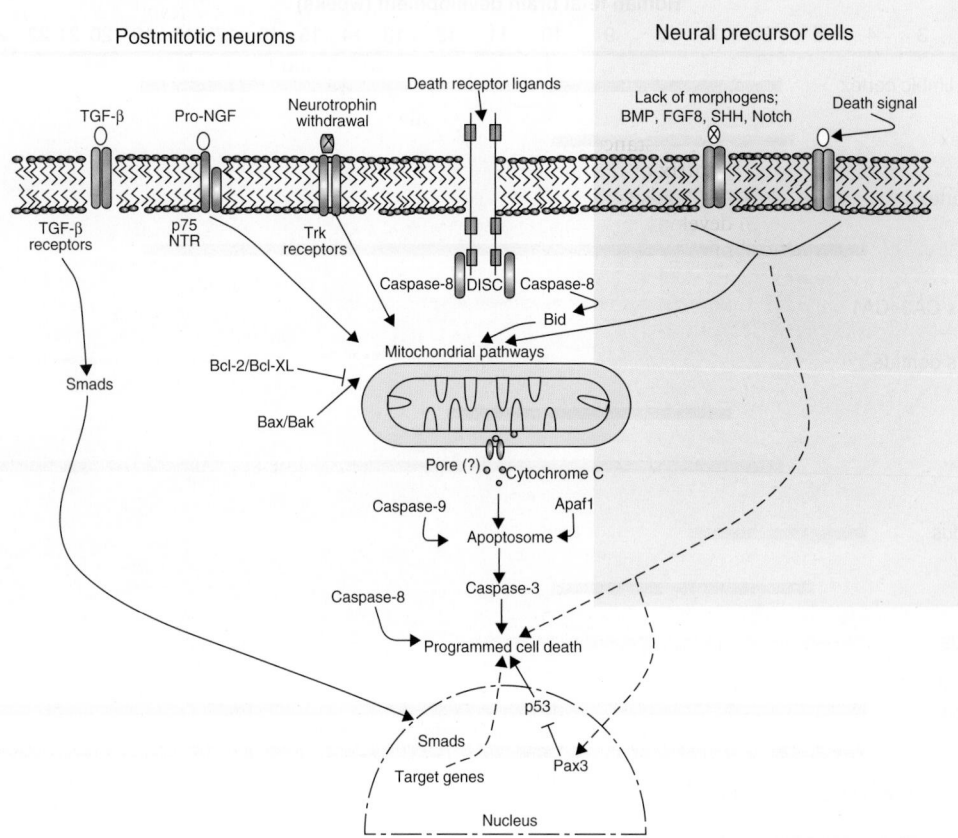

FIGURE 55.3. Both neural precursor cells and postmitotic neurons utilize mitochondrial pathways (cytochrome C and apoptosome) in programmed cell death (PCD). Bcl-2 family proteins (Bcl-2, Bcl-X, Bax, and Bak) modulate and regulate the mitochondrial PCD pathway. Receptor-mediated PCD via caspase 8 has also been shown to participate in postmitotic neurons but not in neural precursor cells, which undergo PCD via the withdrawal of morphogens and regulation of the p53 pathway by the Pax3 transcription factor. Pax3 is a transcription factor that regulates neural development at the transcriptional level and can modulate the cell cycle via p53 to modulate PCD pathways. TGF-β and proNGF also stimulate PCD in postmitotic neurons. Smad proteins are regulators of transcription that are phosphorylated by activated TGF-β receptors and, in turn, activate gene expression patterns that modulate PCD and survival. (Modified from De Zio D, Giunta L, Corvaro M, et al. Expanding roles of programmed cell death in mammalian neurodevelopment. *Semin Cell Dev Biol* 2005;16:281–94, with permission.)

types of neuronal death. Intrinsic PCD signaling pathways involve a reduction in mitochondrial membrane potential, resulting in the release of cytochrome C by the activation of Apaf1 and caspase 9, with ultimate activation of caspase 3. Bcl-2 family proteins Bcl-2 and Bcl-XL are pro-survival molecules that inhibit the release of mitochondrial cytochrome C, whereas pro-death molecules, such as Bax and Bad, can directly affect mitochondrial membrane integrity.

In the extrinsic pathway, removal of neurotrophic factors leads to activation of the protein kinase c-Jun kinase (JNK). JNK can phosphorylate different substrates, including c-Jun, which, in turn, activates transcription of Fas-L by binding to AP-1 sites in the gene promoter site (23). Fas modulates various effectors to activate caspases directly, to activate the stress-activated JNK pathway, or to inhibit the protein kinase B (PKB or Akt) survival pathway (23). Other receptor-coupled pro-death pathways also exist in developmental CNS PCD, but the mitochondrial apoptotic pathway is the most important (7) (**Fig. 55.3**). As many as 70% of developing neurons die via PCD during embryogenesis to eliminate excess cell numbers and to assist in neural tube closure. Due to the upregulation of PCD machinery during development, the developing CNS may be more prone to injury-related PCD than is the adult brain. An especially sensitive age for injury-induced CNS PCD is in newborn infants in the PICU environment, discussed in greater detail in Chapter 56.

Migration, Differentiation, and Axonal Guidance

Neuronal migration occurs at between 12 and 24 gestational weeks in humans and is modulated by neurotransmitters such as glutamate. Importantly, glutamate N-methyl-D-aspartate (NMDA) receptor antagonists can inhibit neuronal migration and affect developmental neuronal apoptosis (12), which may have important effects on developing CNS recovery and plasticity and, therefore, great relevance to the PICU.

The developmental processes responsible for the progression of neural lineages from stem cells to progenitors to postmitotic precursors and, ultimately, to mature neurons are controlled by multiple pathways (24). Stem cell commitment to neuronal lineage and neuronal progenitor specification to a specific neural subtype are two distinct steps of neurogenesis. However, they are linked mechanistically by the same genes that regulate both processes (24). Both extracellular and intracellular signals modulate new gene expression that, in large part, determines neuronal and glial phenotypes. Differentiated neurons possess unique and characteristic sizes, shapes, polarities, and expressions of neurotransmitters, neurotrophins, and receptors, to name but a few differentiation attributes. Knowledge of this area of research is important, as both positive and negative experimental results have been reported concerning the potential of stem cells as therapy after brain injury, and this is sure to remain an active field of inquiry in the future.

Four primary types of signals guide axonal growth and target contact: chemoattractant, chemorepellent, contact attractive, and contact repellent. The first two classes of molecules are diffusible molecules that act over longer distances, while the latter two are within the extracellular matrix or membrane. Axonal pathfinding is most dependent on repulsive cues and pioneer axons that reach targets early in development. Some of these guidance molecules also affect cell migration, as both developmental processes tend to share common mechanisms (12).

Synaptogenesis, Gliogenesis, and Myelination

Synaptogenesis is one of the most important developmental processes that occur during childhood and is an important potential mechanism of CNS injury and recovery in PICU-relevant injuries. Based on nonhuman primate studies, a tentative timetable composed of five temporally distinct phases of synaptogenesis has been proposed for human development (12) (Figs. 55.1 and 55.4). At ~6–8 weeks of gestation, phase 1 of synaptogenesis is limited to the subplate. Beginning at ~12–17 weeks of gestation, synaptogenesis phase 2 remains somewhat limited to the cortical plate, with most new synapses on neuronal dendritic shafts. Phase 3 is more rapid and dynamic; with up to 40,000 new synapses made per second, it begins at ~20–24 weeks of gestation and lasts up to 8 months postnatally. Similarly, phase 4 has a high rate of synaptogenesis, lasting until puberty. The third and fourth phases are more influenced by use-dependent experience. Lastly, phase 5 levels of synaptogenesis persist throughout adulthood to age 70, but with significant synapse loss during this period as well (12).

As a developing neuron reaches its destined position in the CNS, it extends dendrites and axons to distant targets via growth cones, which are guided by numerous extracellular molecules. On making target contact, presynaptic neurotransmitters or other secreted molecules diffuse and bind to the postsynaptic membrane and, along with other signals, induce postsynaptic receptor clustering and other elements of the synapse. Consequently, numerous proteins, molecules, and signal cascades play a role in synaptogenesis (22). Synaptic vesicle accumulation in the presynaptic terminal of a brain region

is a helpful hallmark of the level of synapse maturation (25). A tremendous amount of synaptogenesis is ongoing in young children that could have important implications for injury response and recovery in the PICU.

Glia are not passive participants in CNS development; rather, they exert significant influence over neuronal development. Glia include astrocytes, oligodendrocytes, radial glia, and microglia. Astrocytic development occurs well after neuronal migration and differentiation, and oligodendrocytic development occurs after that of axonogenesis (18). Astrocytes have a multitude of functions in the CNS aside from the structural support of neurons. These functions include K^+ buffering, H^+ and Ca^{2+} ion homeostasis, ammonia detoxification, free radical scavenging, metal sequestration, growth factor production, immune response participation, and neuronal metabolic support functions (pH regulation, neurotransmitter uptake, supply of glycogen and tricarboxylic acid cycle intermediates, and provision of neurotransmitter precursors). Astrocytes also participate in synaptogenesis and neurogenesis in CNS development as well as in cognitive function (17). Protoplasmic astrocytes occur in gray matter, and fibrous astrocytes in white matter. An important feature of astrocytes is the use of the energy-dependent Na^+ gradient to uptake glutamate and K^+ and to regulate H^+ ions. As a result, excessive release of glutamate, energy failure, neuronal depolarization, or tissue acidosis in brain injury result in astrocytic swelling in both the perivascular and perineuronal astrocytic compartments, which can increase diffusion distances in the brain for metabolic gases (O_2 and CO_2), substrates, and waste products. It has been proposed that severe glial swelling may compress capillaries to reduce cerebral blood flow (CBF) and distort synaptic contacts, resulting in neuronal synaptic deafferentation. These changes can become important in a variety of CNS insults (see Fig. 56.12).

Microglia are CNS immune cells of myeloid origin that are similar to macrophages and represent 10% of the CNS cell populations in adults (19). They are normally in a resting state in normal brain, but with activation in response to infection or CNS injury, they morphologically (enlarge) and functionally change, resulting in the upregulation of cytokines and chemokines, as well as surface antigens. They have been implicated in the response to encephalitis, ischemia, TBI, and demyelinating diseases.

Oligodendrocytes produce myelin, modulate axonal function in the CNS, and are vulnerable to excitotoxic injury, decreased trophin levels, and oxidative stress conditions. Neurons and oligodendrocytes signal each other during myelination to modulate neurofilament spacing, phosphorylation, and axonal diameter. As myelination continues to occur until 10 years of age, injury to oligodendrocytes and altered myelination is an important consideration in the PICU in children who suffer brain injuries.

Myelination persists longer than most other CNS developmental processes, continuing through adolescence, making it, like synaptogenesis, another aspect of CNS development of special relevance to the PICU infant or child (18) (Fig. 55.1). In fact, myelination continues in humans until at least 30 years of age, and new evidence suggests that myelination may even be an important mechanism of activity-dependent plasticity (defined as both short- and long-term changes in synaptic strength stimulated by altered neural electrical activity via altered synaptic protein levels, protein posttranslational modifications, and nerve conduction velocity) (26). Several lines of evidence suggest that myelination is a process that is influenced by environmental factors. Neural activity also affects myelination. White matter development in children correlates with motor skill and increased cognitive function. MRI has shown a strong correlation between white matter development and cognitive function (intelligence quotient) in children and

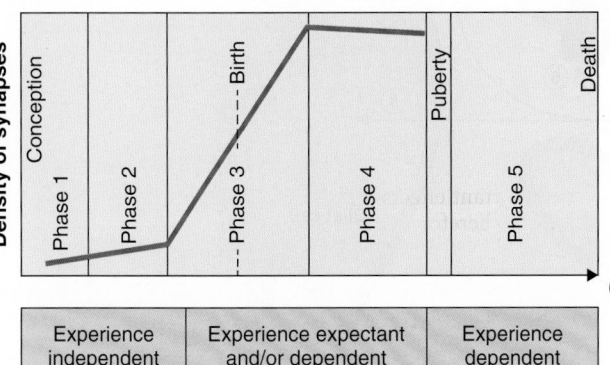

FIGURE 55.4. Synaptic changes (shown as relative densities based on a logarithmic scale) from data of the macaque monkey that has been extrapolated to humans. Phases of synaptogenesis that are predominately experience dependent (require neural activity and are epigenetically regulated) or independent (genetically programmed) are indicated by the boxes along the X-axis. (Modified from Lagercrantz H, Ringstedt T. Organization of the neuronal circuits in the central nervous system during development. *Acta Paediatr* 2001;90:707–15, with permission.)

adolescents (26). While such data are correlative and do not prove an underlying relationship, it has been postulated that increased white matter conduction speed may have as strong an influence on synaptic amplitude as do changes in pre- and post-synaptic elements and neurotransmitter function in plasticity paradigms, such as long-term potentiation (LTP), an electrophysiologic model of memory formation (26). Furthermore, neural activity may produce activity-dependent interactions between myelinating glia, neurons, and myelinated axons (26).

NEUROTRANSMITTER AND NEUROTROPHIN DEVELOPMENT

The synapse serves as the anatomical substrate for information flow between neurons and the point at which the release and response to neurotransmitters predominately occur within the nervous system (**Fig. 55.5**). The release of neurotransmitters from within presynaptic vesicles occurs by fusion with the presynaptic plasma membrane due to electrical depolarization and the influx of Ca^{2+} into the presynaptic bouton, which contains synaptic vesicles. Receptors in the postsynaptic membrane couple directly to ion channels or second messengers to mediate downstream effects. The removal of neurotransmitters that have been released occurs by glial uptake, enzymatic degradation, or transport proteins coupled to the Na^+ gradient established by synaptic and glial sodium and potassium adenosine triphosphate translocase enzymes (Na/K-ATPase). Neurotransmitter levels and receptor expression serve critical roles in synapse formation and in the circuitry and networks

necessary for behavioral function in the immature and mature CNS. Furthermore, synaptic activity mediated by neurotransmitters is a requirement for the survival of developing synaptic contacts in the immature brain (9). It is well documented that neurotransmitters both mediate synaptic transmission and have trophic functions (5,9,18). Neurotransmitters and neuromodulators that have been shown to play important roles in development include glutamate, γ-aminobutyric acid (GABA), acetylcholine, catecholamines, serotonin, and opioids. The human developmental neurotransmitter timeline displays considerable regional and temporal variation for various transmitter systems (18) (**Figs. 55.6 and 55.7**). These variations come into play when considering age- and regional-dependent injury, manipulations of the transmitter systems, and the possible effects of the transmitter systems on recovery. Insults to the brain at vulnerable developmental periods can produce long-term structural and functional CNS changes. Given the important neurotransmitter functions during CNS development, it is not surprising that a number of recent studies have implicated age-dependent adverse effects with the manipulation of neurotransmitter systems, especially the glutamatergic and GABAergic systems, using either commonly employed sedative and anesthetic agents or treatments with such agents after ischemia, status epilepticus, or TBI (5,27,28).

Preterm fetuses and newborn infants appear to be at particularly critical periods of developmental neurotransmitter vulnerability. Before birth, the majority of neuromodulators and neurotransmitters increase during synaptogenesis. At birth, increased brain activity and a surge of catecholaminergic activity are associated with arousal. A decrease in adenosine occurs, along with a desensitization of adenosine receptors during the

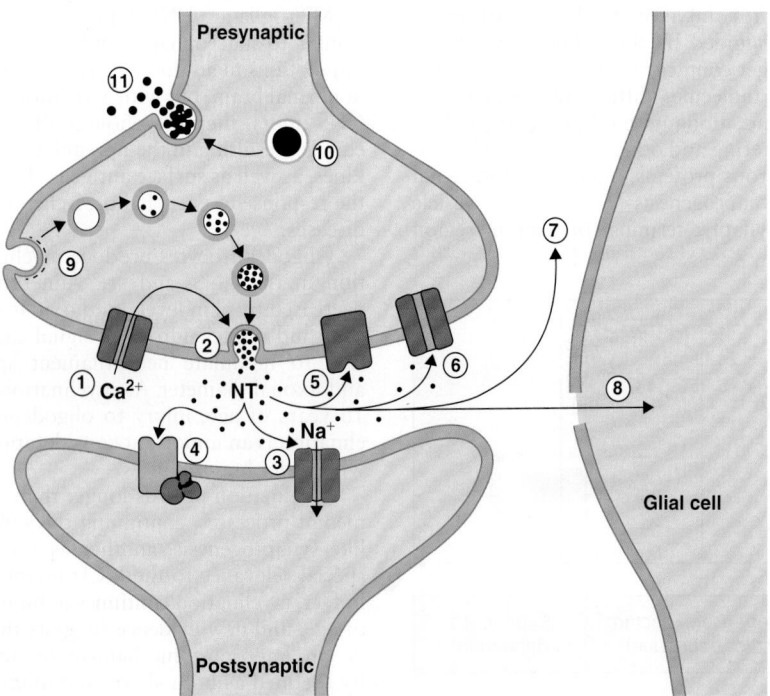

FIGURE 55.5. Schematic of a typical axodendritic synapse as seen at a dendritic spine. Calcium entry triggered by presynaptic terminal depolarization (*1*) induces neurotransmitter (*NT*)-containing synaptic vesicle exocytosis (*2*), which in turn, releases neurotransmitters into the synaptic cleft. NTs bind to their receptors at the postsynaptic density (concentration of postsynaptic proteins involved in synaptic function) of the postsynaptic membrane. These receptors modulate either ion channels (*3*) or G-proteins that stimulate second-messenger production (*4*). Similar NT presynaptic receptors (*5*) are also activated, which can modulate subsequent NT presynaptic release. The uptake of many NTs occurs via a transport protein coupled to the sodium gradient at the presynaptic terminal (e.g., dopamine, norepinephrine, glutamate, and GABA) (*6*) or by degradation (acetylcholine) (*7*) or uptake by glia (glutamate) (*8*). Synaptic vesicle membranes are recycled by clathrin-mediated endocytosis (*9*). Large, dense core vesicles (*10*) that store protein and neuropeptides are released by repetitive stimulation at a more distant site from the postsynaptic density (*11*). (From Holz RW, Fisher SK. *Basic Neurochemistry*. 6th ed. Philadelphia, PA: Lippincott Williams & Wilkins; 1999, with permission.)

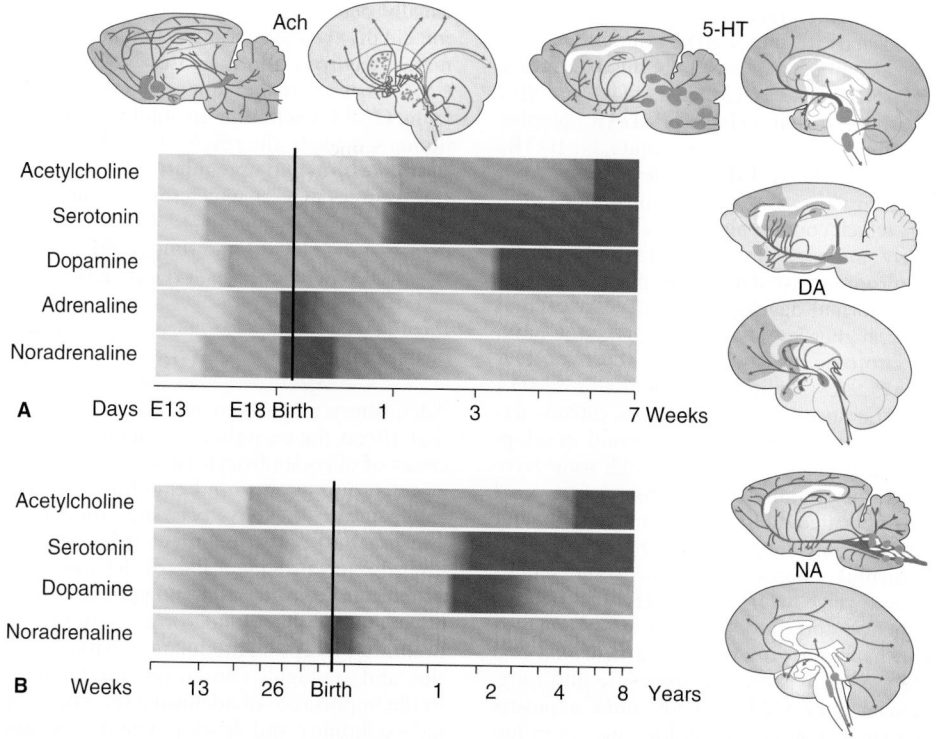

FIGURE 55.6. Comparison of rat (**A**) and human brain (**B**) timelines of the regional and temporal distribution of several major neurotransmitter levels during development. Ach, acetylcholine; 5-HT, serotonin; DA, dopamine; NA, noradrenaline. (From Herlenius E, Lagercrantz H. Development of neurotransmitter systems during critical periods. *Exp Neurol* 2004;190(suppl 1):S8–21. with permission.)

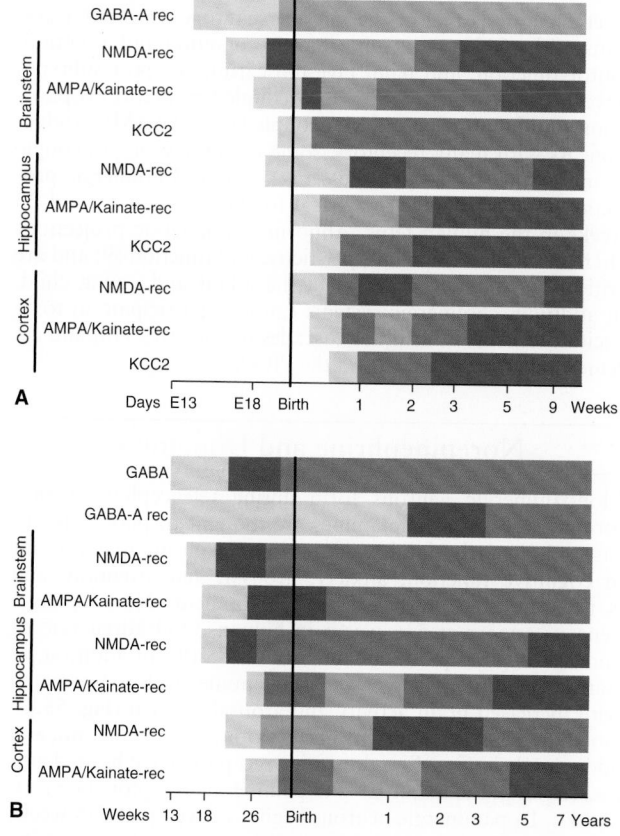

FIGURE 55.7. Comparison of rat (**A**) and human brain (**B**) timelines of the regional and temporal distribution of several major neurotransmitter receptor levels during development. rec, receptor. (From Herlenius E, Lagercrantz H. Development of neurotransmitter systems during critical periods. *Exp Neurol* 2004;190(suppl 1):S8–21, with permission.)

first postnatal days (9). In addition, periods of developmental "switches" in neurotransmitter function occur at birth, and sensitivity to glutamate toxicity may be especially high and vulnerable at this time.

Glutamate and GABA

Amino acids are the most abundant neurotransmitters in the CNS and have important functions in brain development regarding neural networks, CNS structure, and plasticity. Glutamatergic and GABAergic neurotransmission play major roles in brain development. In fact, many of the CNS behavioral and functional milestones during development can be correlated with the maturation of these systems and their receptors (29).

Glutamate Receptor Development

Almost half of the synapses of the forebrain are glutamatergic, and excessive glutamate synapse creation occurs during the most active period of synaptogenesis in the first 2 years of postnatal human brain development. Each of the five types of major glutamate receptors contains various subtypes (9). Three general types of glutamate ionotropic receptors exist that couple to Na$^+$ and Ca^{2+}, namely, four alpha-amino-3-hydroxy-5-methyl-4-isoxazolepropionic acid (AMPA) receptor subtypes (GluR$_{1-4}$), five kainate receptor subtypes (GluR$_{5-7}$, KA$_{1-2}$), and seven NMDA receptor (NMDAR) subtypes (NR$_{1-3B}$). Eight G-protein–coupled metabotropic glutamate receptors (mGluR$_{1-8}$) exist, which positively or negatively couple to phosphoinositide and cyclic nucleotide second messengers to varying degrees with pre- and post-synaptic and regional CNS distributions. AMPA receptors (which normally activate NMDARs) mature more slowly than NMDARs; thus, the NMDAR must depend on other systems (the immature GABA_A receptor) to help depolarize immature neurons and activate the NMDA-coupled calcium channel. NMDARs are composed of four subunits from three related families: NR1 (NR1-1–4), NR2 (NR2A–D), and NR3 (NR3A–B). Evidence suggests that a single NMDAR complex contains two NR1 subunits and two NR2 subunits. NMDARs regulate not only neuronal survival during development but axon and dendrite arborization as well as synaptogenesis (30). Immature NMDARs, which contain higher levels of the NR2B subunit, are relatively more excitable during early phases of development, to promote use-dependent plastic changes that are necessary for normal development and learning and memory (9). However, higher levels of NR2B make the brain more sensitive to excitotoxic insults, such as ischemia, TBI, and status epilepticus (5,9,28). In addition, the use of NMDA antagonists or anesthetic agents (e.g., ketamine), nitrous oxide, and isoflurane may also increase experimental developmental neuronal PCD in rodents (31,32), although some have challenged these laboratory findings (33). Subsequent animal studies have further implicated anesthetic agents that modify NMDAR function in not only enhancing PCD but also altering normal developmental synapse development and sculpting, dendritic branching via NMDA cytoskeletal interactions (34,35), synaptic function and mitochondrial morphogenesis (36). Two studies in neonatal primates found neuronal and glial cell death after a 5-hour isoflurane exposure and long-term behavioral deficits after a 24-hour ketamine exposure (37,38). It is not yet clear if similar pathology occurs in humans and what the functional consequences might be, but it does appear that either too much or too little NMDAR activation can result in abnormal developmental processes and even neuronal death (9). A practical clinical example would be the use of nitrous oxide or ketamine (both NMDAR antagonist) in newborn infants. Although presently no definitive evidence indicates that NMDAR anesthetic modulation triggers neural apoptosis or neuronal cytoskeletal modifications in human infants, the aforementioned studies, particularly the work in primates support the considerable ongoing research that is necessary in this area (39), as it could have broad implications in the PICU, particularly with regard to the long-term use of sedatives and anesthetic agents in infants.

GABA and the GABA Switch

In addition to its neurotransmitter role on neuronal excitability, GABA has trophic actions on synaptic and neuritic outgrowth, as well as neuronal viability during development. An estimated 25%–40% of all CNS synapses contain GABA, and its deficiency is fatal to infants (9). GABAergic inhibition of excitatory synaptic CNS activity occurs by neuronal hyperpolarization via postsynaptic GABA_A (outward chloride channel) and GABA_B (G-protein–coupled inward potassium channel) receptors in the adult brain. The inhibitory actions of GABA are also mediated by a reduction of presynaptic excitatory neurotransmitter release via presynaptic GABA_B receptors (5). In contrast, GABA is an excitatory neurotransmitter during prenatal development prior to birth in humans. The GABA_A receptor binds barbiturates, benzodiazepines, and ethanol, which alter chloride (Cl⁻) flux through the channel (9). Thus, GABA is mainly excitatory during the fetal period but becomes inhibitory around birth in humans. The so-called "GABA switch" marks the point at which GABA becomes an inhibitory rather than excitatory neurotransmitter (9,12,40) (Fig. 55.8).

As discussed previously, glutamate synaptic transmission is initially based on NMDAR function at developmental stages when the CNS lacks functional AMPA receptors, and the GABA_A receptor stimulates NMDAR calcium influx, a role

usually performed in the mature brain by the AMPA receptor. GABA_A receptor stimulation induces depolarization of immature neurons and increases NMDA-mediated intracellular Ca²⁺ during late human prenatal development. The switch from GABA excitation to inhibition that occurs at birth in humans is likely the result of a GABA-mediated induction of the expression and upregulation of the potassium–chloride cotransporter (KCC2), which serves to decrease the high Cl⁻ content of immature neurons (9,41). Several types of brain injury downregulate KCC2 and thus could affect the development of the GABA switch of the developing brain (9).

Adenosine

Adenosine is a neuronal, glial, and cerebrovascular transmitter that affects the excitability of neurons and the functional processes of oligodendrocyte progenitor proliferation and myelination during infancy and childhood (9). Four receptors—A₁, A_{2a}, A_{2b}, and A₃—have been identified with different regional and pre- and post-synaptic distributions. A₁ receptors are inhibitory and provide a line of defense against developmental excitotoxic cascades and, along with GABA, may be the most important inhibitory neurotransmitter receptor system in the brain. A_{2a} receptors modulate dopaminergic D₂ receptor function and are highly concentrated in the basal ganglia (9). Due to the importance of adenosine receptor modulation of neuronal excitability and developmental processes, this system may be an important therapeutic target in brain injury (9).

Acetylcholine

Acetylcholine is one of the major excitatory transmitter systems of the CNS and is important in cognition and attention, motor function, and pain. Five muscarinic receptor subtypes have been identified, with M_{1,2,5} coupled primarily to phosphoinositide turnover and M_{2,4} coupled to cyclic AMP production. As with many receptors, some receptor subtypes couple to more than one second messenger system. Cholinergic projections to the cortex from basal forebrain occur around 20 weeks in the human fetus. Abnormal cholinergic projections alter cortical development, plasticity, and function (9) and are critical to cognitive function in the infant and young child. In addition, cholinergic systems can also participate in toxic excitatory neurotransmitter cascades in epilepsy, TBI, and cerebral ischemia in children in the PICU.

Norepinephrine and Dopamine

Monoaminergic neurons form during telencephalic vesicle formation, and catecholamines are thought to play a significant role in early development. Norepinephrine is important in cognitive function, anxiety, arousal, and attention, and is necessary for normal brain development. Noradrenergic neurons appear at 5–6 weeks in humans, and adrenergic α₂ and β₁ receptors predominate in the CNS (9). In addition, as stated previously, a surge of catecholamine levels is associated with increased brain activity and arousal at birth (Fig. 55.1). Dopamine is also important in cognition, motor function, and addiction behavior. Five dopamine receptors have been identified (D₁–D₅), the major CNS dopaminergic receptors being D₁ and D₂. Dopaminergic neurons begin to develop at 6–8 weeks in humans. D₁ receptors, in particular, are critical for working memory function during the first year of life (9) (Fig. 55.1). The use of catecholamines for blood pressure support in the PICU in infants with immature or injury-altered blood–brain barrier (BBB) function warrants consideration owing to the

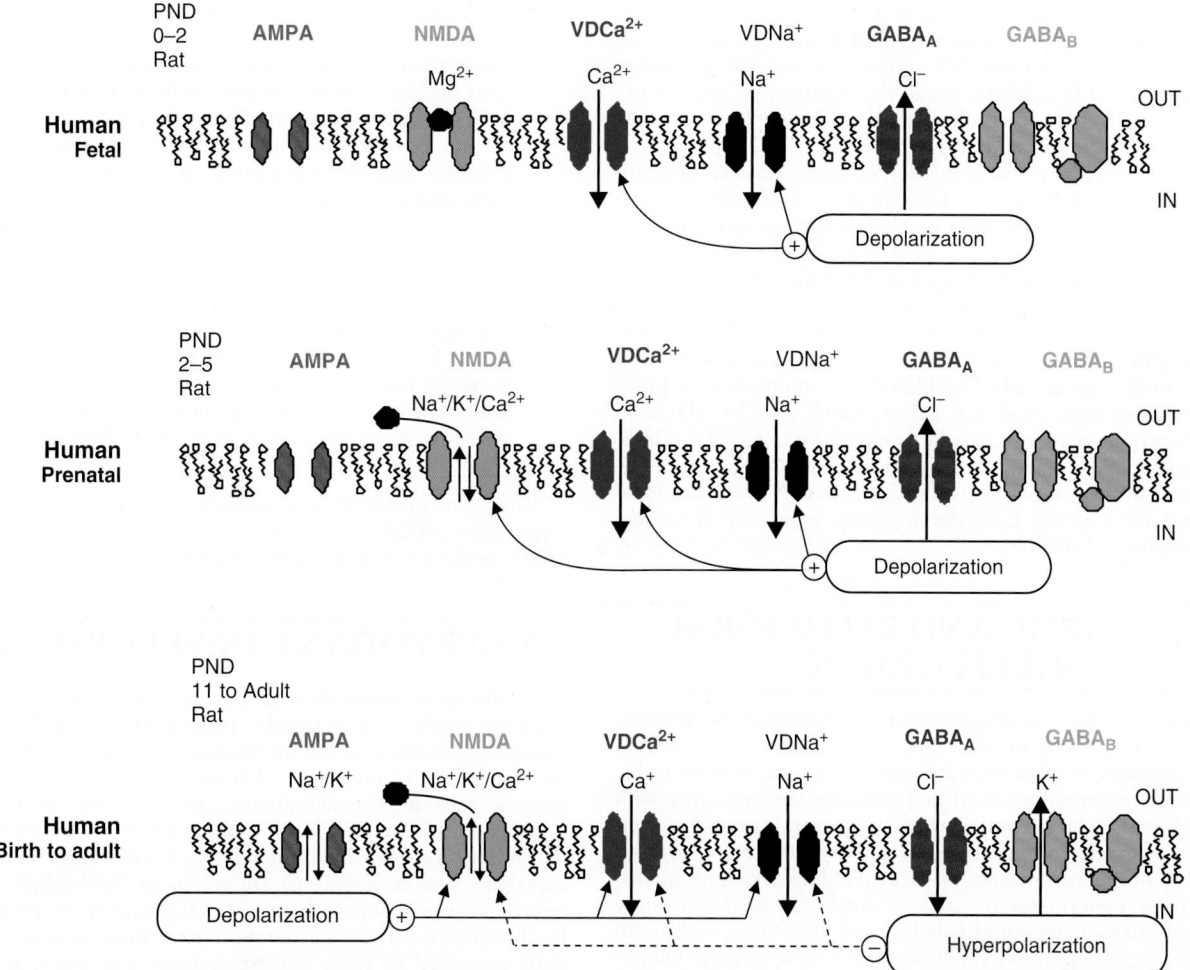

FIGURE 55.8. Comparison of the GABA switch in the human and the rat, which is well-documented in the rat and thought to occur in humans at birth. Prior to the switch of $GABA_A$ receptors from an outward gating depolarizing Cl^- current to an inward hyperpolarizing Cl^- current (**upper 2 panels**), the receptor is excitatory and helps to remove the magnesium (Mg^{2+}) block of the NMDAR channel, allowing calcium influx. Thus, $GABA_A$ receptors assume the excitatory role of nonfunctioning AMPA receptors during the developmental period prior to the switch. However, once AMPA receptors mature and the high Cl^- content of developing neurons is reduced owing to the upregulation of the potassium–chloride cotransporter (KCC2) (not shown), the $GABA_A$ receptor becomes inhibitory by gating an inward hyperpolarizing Cl^- current (**lower panel**). Prior to the switch, GABA tone may contribute to excitotoxic glutamate cascades during brain injury (see Chapter 56). PND, postnatal day. (Modified from Ben-Ari Y, Khazipov R, Leinekugel X, et al. $GABA_A$, NMDA and AMPA receptors: A developmentally regulated "menage a trois." *Trends Neurosci* 1997;20:523–29, with permission.)

potent catecholinergic excitatory actions at birth, which in theory could be potentially excitotoxic at this critical developmental time. High dopamine concentrations have even been shown to exacerbate brain edema in adult animals after experimental TBI (42).

Serotonin

Serotonin (5-HT) neurons have extensive contacts and synchronize complex motor and sensory information, and at least fifteen 5-HT receptors are identified. The $5-HT_1$ receptors, in general, inhibit cyclic AMP formation and open K^+ channels, while $5-HT_2$ receptors stimulate phosphoinositide second messengers, release intracellular calcium, and are generally excitatory. Serotonin also modulates developmental proliferation, differentiation, migration, and synaptogenesis. Aberrations in serotonin levels during development and early childhood result in CNS connectivity malformations and may contribute to later psychiatric disorders (9).

Neurotrophins

Growth factors, both intrinsic and extrinsic to the CNS, play a major role in normal brain function, developmental processes, and in the injury and repair process. Nerve growth factor (NGF), brain-derived neurotrophic factor (BDNF), and neurotrophins 3–5 (NT3, NT4/5) are diffusible peptides that compose the neurotrophin family of trophic factors in mammalian brain. Receptors for the neurotrophin peptides are the tropomyosin kinase receptors (TrkA, TrkB, and TrkC) and the p75 neurotrophin receptor (p75 NTR), a member of the transforming growth factor (TGF) receptor family. NTs are critical for neuronal survival, and the loss of NT activity after CNS injury can contribute to neuronal death and loss of function. The role of neurotrophins in response to CNS injury is discussed in more detail in Chapter 56. NT precursors are called proneurotrophins and are cleaved by proteases to produce mature NTs. Proneurotrophins can also activate NT receptors and appear to be the preferred ligand for p75 NTR.

ProNGF induces apoptosis via p75 NTR, and proNGF and NGF produce opposite responses—cell death and cell survival, respectively (7,25,43,44). NT receptors couple to a number of protein and lipid kinase intracellular pathways, such as the mitogen-activated proteins kinase (MAPK), the phosphoinositide 3-kinase (PI3K), and the PKB pathways. This coupling is extremely important to the regulation of neural survival or death after ischemia, TBI, or other CNS insults (see Chapter 56).

The regional distribution of NGF is highest in regions innervated by the cholinergic system of the basal forebrain, such as the neocortex and the hippocampus. Lower but significant levels are also seen in other brain regions (43). BDNF has a wider distribution than NGF, having been detected in the hippocampus, amygdala, thalamus, neocortex, cerebellum, and other brain regions (44). The adult hippocampus has the highest levels of both NGF and BDNF, which may be related to its important plasticity role in cognitive function (43). Obviously, any major change in neurotrophin systems during development by disease, injury, or treatment can have a dramatic impact on ongoing CNS development, especially at critical developmental periods.

SYNAPTIC AND BEHAVIORAL DEVELOPMENT

Because of ongoing developmental synaptogenesis, connectivity, wiring, and myelination, an associated increase and development of CNS electrical activity occurs. A measurable electrical encephalogram (EEG) develops and matures with gestational and postnatal age (29). However, birth is the point of significantly increased neural activity due to the arousal effects of neurotransmitters, neuromodulators, and neurotrophins. Preterm infants at ~32 weeks of gestation show quantitative changes in EEG before and after birth, with up to a 30% increase in EEG amplitude and a 60% increase in continuity over the first postnatal weeks (45). Consistent changes are seen in quantitative EEG neurophysiologic measures over the first week after birth and, particularly, in measures of continuity over the first 4 days in normal preterm infants (46). Such behavioral and functional milestones also correlate with the development of glutamatergic and GABAergic neurotransmission and synaptic maturity (21). As NMDA, AMPA, and GABA receptor (47) and neurotrophin (25) systems mature, LTP (an increase in synaptic strength of a population of neurons that may be an electrophysiologic and biochemical correlate of memory storage) and long-term depression (LTD) (a decrease in synaptic strength of a population of neurons that may also be an electrophysiologic and biochemical correlate of memory storage) are established. Thus, LTP and LTD are likely associated with cognitive function and definitively occur in cortical and hippocampal circuits within 2–3 weeks in the postnatal rat (48) and have been proposed to occur at 7–10 months in infants (10).

Primary behavioral and functional developments in the infant (**Fig. 55.1**) over the first 2 years:

- The cortical inhibition of brainstem reflexes due to maturation of GABA inhibition and myelination occurs postnatally at ~3 months. Excessive cortical inhibition of brainstem nuclei, such as respiratory centers, may increase the risk for the sudden infant death syndrome (10).
- The development of recognition memory also takes place near the postnatal age of 3 months, which requires adequate hippocampal and cortical visual development (10).
- Working memory (recent past memory that enables one to solve a current cognitive task) develops in the infant over the latter half of the first year; it is dependent on prefrontal cortical function and is modulated by

glutamate, GABA, and dopamine (10). Between 7 and 10 months, infant prefrontal cortices undergo dramatic maturation in synaptic density and neurotransmitter systems and have increased glucose utilization required for both growth and activity-dependent processes. Similarly, the hippocampus reaches adult size, and synaptogenesis, coupled with the maturation of neurotransmitter systems, makes LTP development possible. During this time of rapid growth and activity-dependent synaptogenesis and maturation, the infant brain is especially vulnerable to injury, resulting in either short- or long-term changes in behavioral function (10). For example, at 2 years of age, rapid language development and acquisition occur, which has been further linked to increased connections between prefrontal cortex and associational cortical regions with the limbic and motor systems. Significant synaptogenesis also occurs in many of these same brain regions (10).

These functions can be extremely vulnerable to injury and represent a critical period of developing brain vulnerability to injury-mediated, long-term dysfunction.

ANTIOXIDANT DEVELOPMENT

Free radicals are molecules that contain one or more unpaired electrons, such as superoxide, peroxynitrite, and hydroxyl radicals. Enzymes and low-molecular-weight antioxidants are the major brain antioxidant defense systems. Major enzyme systems include peroxyredoxins, thioredoxins, superoxide dismutase, catalase, and peroxidases that vary in concentration depending on species and brain regions. Glutathione, vitamin E, ascorbate, and coenzyme Q are water- or lipid-soluble low-molecular-weight antioxidants (49). Oxidative stress, produced by abnormal free radical generation in the brain, is at least partially quenched by these defense systems. The levels of these antioxidant enzymes and molecules in the brain vary with developmental age (49,50). In general, lower levels occur during fetal development but increase at birth, as the transition from a low- to high-oxygen environment occurs (50). Based on enzyme levels, catalase appears to be more of a contributor to antioxidant defenses in the immature brain, which may influence the choice of antioxidant interventions in the developing brain after injury (49). Based on the antioxidant enzyme profile during brain development, the immature CNS may be at greater risk than the adult brain for oxidative injury (49).

CEREBROVASCULAR AND METABOLISM DEVELOPMENT AND FUNCTION

Vascular Development

The CNS vascular system develops in three phases: vasculogenesis, angiogenesis, and barrier genesis (51). Not surprisingly, the first functional organ developed in the human embryo is the cardiovascular system, with blood vessels generated by mesodermal differentiated endothelial cells. These cells give rise to new blood vessels by a process called *vasculogenesis*, as compared to the generation of new blood vessels from existing vessels, called *angiogenesis* (52). The CNS developmental rate of angiogenesis is maximal around birth and early infancy and decreases thereafter (51). A major role for vascular endothelial growth factor and its endothelial receptors has been documented for developmental CNS angiogenesis (51,52). Other trophic factors, especially some of the components of the TGF-β family, may also influence developmental CNS angiogenesis. These factors have been implicated in sprouting, vascular remodeling, and perivascular cell recruitment (51). In addition, platelet-derived growth factor, as well as numerous adhesion molecules and factors/receptors that provide axonal cues, modulates CNS vascularization (51,52). Immature blood vessels are stabilized by vascular mural cells, called *pericytes*, which are recruited to endothelial cells via some of these aforementioned factors (51,52). Tissue oxygen levels are very important in developing CNS vasculature, as low levels stimulate angiogenesis and high oxygen levels inhibit this process (52).

Cerebral Blood Flow and Vascular Reactivity

Vascular reactivity of the cerebral circulation is an important neuroprotective mechanism whereby the CNS vessel diameter adjusts to physiologic changes (i.e., perfusion pressure, PaO_2, $PaCO_2$) to regulate CBF so that metabolic demands of the brain can be met. The ability of the cerebrovascular system to dilate or constrict has limits that are defined physiologically as the upper and lower limits of autoregulation. Impaired CBF autoregulation and vascular reactivity are considered potential candidates in the etiology of secondary injury across the spectrum of age. For example, loss of pressure autoregulation could underlie, in part, the marked vulnerability of the acutely injured brain in a child to otherwise tolerable hypotension (see Chapter 56). Similarly, it is believed to contribute to periventricular hemorrhagic venous infarction in preterm infants. Most developmental studies of CBF and vascular reactivity have occurred in newborn infants and near-term and early postnatal laboratory animals.

Perfusion Pressure Autoregulation of Cerebral Blood Flow

Pressure autoregulation is the major cerebrovascular response to acute changes in perfusion pressure, changes that result, at the extreme range, either in hypotension with hypoperfusion and tissue ischemia or in hypertension and possible hyperemia and BBB disruption. Vascular tone in the cerebral circulation compensates for changes in cerebral perfusion pressure (CPP) over a range of pressures to maintain CBF constant (between a CPP of ~40–160 mm Hg in adults) (**Fig. 55.9**). CPP is equal to the difference between mean arterial pressure and intracranial pressure. Autoregulation occurs instantaneously and is believed to be mediated by changes in vascular smooth muscle tension by a direct myogenic mechanism; a review of this topic is available (14). Developmental studies of pressure autoregulation of CBF in newborns suggest a narrower perfusion pressure range, with a similar lower limit to that seen in adults—but an upper limit that is only ~90–100 mm Hg (8) (**Fig. 55.10**). Note that, for most of the studies in the normal state, intracranial pressure is generally assumed negligible, and CPP is thus approximated by mean arterial blood pressure, which is obviously not the case in the clinical setting of raised intracranial pressure or elevated central venous pressures. In both the term and preterm newborn lamb, the lower limit of pressure autoregulation is between 40 and 50 mm Hg. In contrast, the resting mean arterial blood pressure is substantially lower in the preterm than in the term newborn, demonstrating that the autoregulatory vascular reserve is much less in premature than in term lambs (53). This finding suggests a greater risk for the preterm brain to a reduction in blood pressure. In addition, evidence suggests that, in critically ill infants, the autoregulatory responses may be absent or significantly impaired (54,55) and that early postnatal hypercapnia may further impair pressure autoregulation (56). Finally, pressure autoregulation of CBF is often disturbed after brain injury (6).

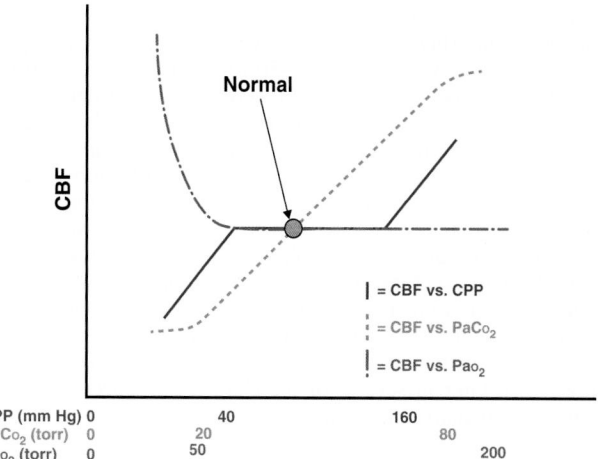

FIGURE 55.9. Relationships between CBF and CPP, $PaCO_2$, and PaO_2 across therapeutic ranges generally encountered in the PICU. These values are provided based on normative data from adults. Pressure autoregulation maintains CBF constant between a CPP of between ~40 and 160 mm Hg. CBF is linearly related to $PaCO_2$, with an approximate 4% change in CBF per torr change in $PaCO_2$ between ~20 and 80 torr. Below 20 torr, this curve dramatically flattens. Above ~80–100 torr, this relationship also more gradually flattens. The relationship between CBF and PaO_2 is relatively flat until a PaO_2 of ~50 mm Hg is reached, below which, a dramatic increase in CBF is observed.

The occurrence and consequences of impaired CBF autoregulation will be addressed in several of the following chapters across the spectrum of disorders in pediatric neurointensive care.

Cerebrovascular Response to PaO_2

The cerebrovascular response to changes in PaO_2 is mediated locally and results in vasodilation under reduced oxygen conditions (hypoxic) and in vasoconstriction under high oxygen

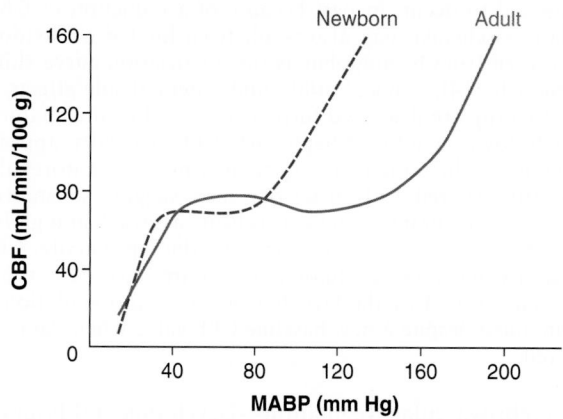

FIGURE 55.10. Comparison of the relative pressure: CBF autoregulatory curves from studies of subhuman primate newborns and adults. In the adult, CBF is maintained relatively constant when arterial blood pressure is between 50 and 160 mm Hg, while in newborns, CBF is maintained over a narrower range owing to a reduced upper limit of CBF autoregulation. CBF autoregulation of newborns makes them more vulnerable to both hypotensive and hypertensive episodes. MABP, mean arterial blood pressure. (From Hardy P, Varma DR, Chemtob S. Control of cerebral and ocular blood flow autoregulation in neonates. *Pediatr Clin North Am* 1997;44:137–52, with permission.)

conditions (hyperoxia) to maintain CBF constant over a range of Pao_2 values (**Fig. 55.9**). This curve is relatively flat, except at reduced Pao_2 levels (less than ~50 torr), at which a steep rise in CBF curve occurs to maintain cerebral oxygen delivery. At the end ranges of hypoxia and hyperoxia, the cerebrovascular response occurs in parallel with carotid body sensors that may also adjust systemic blood pressure and respiration to compensate for changes in blood oxygen levels. Consequently, the cerebrovascular response to oxygen and blood pressure interact and may not occur in isolation at the outermost values. The dramatic increase in CBF (and cerebral blood volume) when Pao_2 is reduced to levels below 50–60 torr is the basis for meticulously avoiding even mild or moderate levels of hypoxemia in patients with reduced intracranial compliance (discussed later in several of the chapters on specific disease entities in pediatric neurointensive care).

Cerebrovascular Response to $Paco_2$

The cerebrovascular response to changes in $Paco_2$ is mediated locally by changes in perivascular pH (57). However, in contrast to changes in perfusion pressure and Pao_2, a nearly linear relationship between $Paco_2$ and CBF exists between the range of $Paco_2$ values of 20 and 80 torr, with an approximate 4%/mm Hg change in $Paco_2$ (6,14) (**Fig. 55.9**). At the ends of the spectrum (either hypocapnia or hypercapnia), the response is blunted, and these curves flatten. Consequently, vasodilation is seen with increasing arterial CO_2 concentration (hypercapnia), and vasoconstriction is seen with low arterial CO_2 concentration (hypocapnia). This vasoreactivity is the basis of hyperventilation-mediated reduction in CBF and the resultant reduction in cerebral blood volume that serves therapeutically to reduce intracranial hypertension. The CBF response to changes in $Paco_2$ is generally related to the level of CBF at rest in a given brain region; thus, hyperventilation tends to equalize CBF throughout the brain (57). In addition, the CBF response to changes in $Paco_2$ is transient, lasting less than 24 hours for a given change (57) and is believed to be mediated by compensatory changes in brain interstitial bicarbonate concentration, which take time to manifest. When a hyperventilation-mediated reduction in $Paco_2$ is used to reduce intracranial pressure, despite flattening of the CBF response to reduction in $Paco_2$, relative ischemia has been suggested to occur, in part because of a reduction in CBF. Relative ischemia may also result from limited off-loading of oxygen from hemoglobin as the dissociation curve shifts to the left (14). Clinical utility and potential side effects of this therapy are discussed further in several of the chapters that follow, including Chapter 61. CO_2 reactivity appears to be less vulnerable to injury than is pressure autoregulation (6). Altered CO_2 reactivity may suggest substantial damage to the brain region that is being assessed, and global loss of CO_2 reactivity is a concerning finding. Finally, CO_2 reactivity and pressure autoregulation are separate entities, as demonstrated by the fact that pressure autoregulation is maintained despite a new baseline CBF value when $Paco_2$ is altered.

Cerebrovascular Regulation—Developmental Issues

Given that the most dramatic change facing the developing child is birth, going from a relatively hypoxic to an oxygen-rich environment, it is intuitive that the cerebrovascular system would normally be ready to respond to such challenges. However, even in normal term infants, it appears that several days are required for such vascular responses to further mature. Experimental studies in piglets have shown that CO_2 reactivity and pressure autoregulation are present but poorly developed at birth; however, both autoregulation

and CO_2 reactivity mature rapidly over the first postnatal days. Resting CBF levels also increase over the first few postnatal days (58), and studies in preterm human infants have confirmed that CBF increases over the first 3 postnatal days (54,55). Similarly, CO_2 reactivity increases from birth to early postnatal age (54), as do EEG amplitude (46) and arterial blood pressure. However, during this postnatal period, CBF in infants is still lower than in adults. CBF further increases in children until 5–6 years of age, when it may be as much as 50%–85% higher than in adults, then decreases to adult levels by 15–19 years of age (15) (**Fig. 55.11**). **Figure 55.11** shows the developmental changes in cerebral metabolic rate for glucose (CMRg) and CBF for both human and rat. Because of the higher fat content of rodent maternal milk, the growing rat fuels a large percentage of cerebral metabolism during the synthetic work related to early postnatal developmental growth spurts by utilizing ketone oxidation (15). In humans, CBF parallels glucose metabolism, and peak CBF and glucose metabolism occur between 3 and 9 years of age, corresponding to a very active growth period. However, it has been estimated that human infants also may utilize up to 20% of their energy needs from ketones during the postnatal period, when nourishment is based primarily on maternal milk.

Cerebral Blood Flow–Metabolism Coupling

In adults, a tight coupling of CBF to brain metabolism normally occurs and is termed "flow–metabolism coupling," as described previously. It has been shown that CBF–metabolism coupling appears intact in normal newborn infants (56). The peak in cerebral glucose utilization during development correlates with the density of glucose transport proteins (59). Postnatal changes in regional CBF and cerebral metabolism occur in parallel in the human infant, with the highest rates of local cerebral metabolic rate for glucose (LCMRg) and CBF occurring at between 3 and 9 years of age during the well-recognized period of rapid cognitive development (**Fig. 55.11**). Glucose is normally the lone cerebral substrate fueling active growth during this same period (15).

Cerebral Metabolism

Glucose serves as the major energy source for the developing brain. Glucose utilization through glycolytic and oxidative decarboxylation pathways parallels the energy demand of the developing brain. Consequently, LCMRg increases with developmental maturation and critical periods of growth and functional activity (20). Glucose entry into brain occurs via glucose transporter proteins (GLUTs). Of the five GLUTs (GLUT1–5), two (GLUT1 and GLUT3) are located in the brain, with GLUT1 found in the BBB and choroid plexus and GLUT3 found in neurons. GLUT5 is located in activated brain microglia. GLUT expression in the developing brain is proportional to energy demand, increases during maturation, and is highest during peak synaptogenesis (20). Peak GLUT protein expression correlates with glutamate receptor maturity and learning and memory development in the developing CNS.

Germane to the PICU is the fact that cerebral energy metabolism and blood flow peak between 3 and 8 years of age in humans (15). Glucose utilization in 5-week-old infants in most brain regions is 71%–93% of that in the adult brain. LCMRg increases over the next 3 months, especially in the basal ganglia and parietal, temporal, and occipital cortices. Frontal cortex LCMRg further increases by 8 months—at which time, cognitive function is rapidly developing (15). Adult levels of

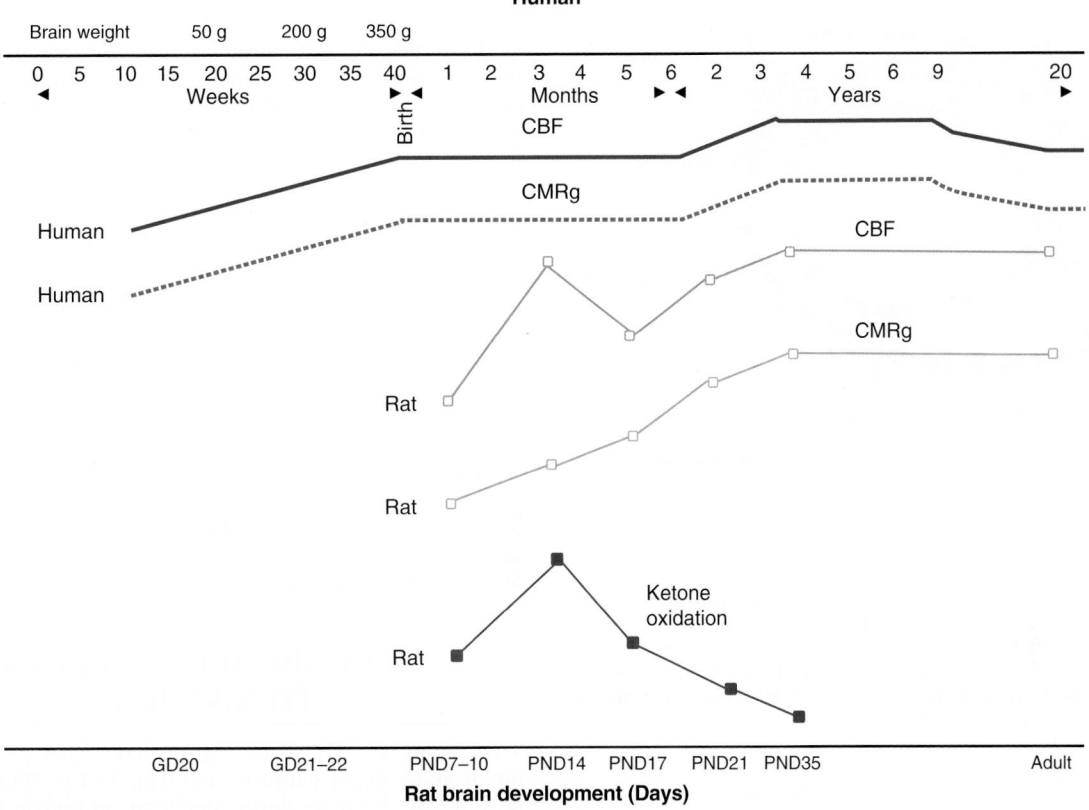

FIGURE 55.11. Developmental changes in CMRg and CBF for both human and rat. The rat fuels a large percentage of cerebral metabolism during the synthetic work related to early postnatal developmental growth spurts with ketone oxidation. In humans, peak CBF and CMRg occur between 3 and 9 years of age, corresponding to a very active growth period. GD, gestational day; PND, postnatal day. (From Nehlig A. Cerebral energy metabolism, glucose transport and blood flow: Changes with maturation and adaptation to hypoglycaemia. *Diabetes Metab* 1997;23:18–29, with permission .)

LCMRg are found by the time children are 2 years of age. LCMRg increases further until it reaches its highest levels, which are maintained until age 9 (**Fig. 55.11**). From this point forward, LCMRg declines until about age 20 (15). Thus, the child's brain has considerable metabolic demand compared to adults.

In addition to the metabolism of glucose by the developing brain, the immature brain can utilize lactic acid, ketone bodies, and a large number of other metabolites, such as amino acids and free fatty acids (20). Monocarboxylate transporters for lactate and pyruvate develop over the midgestation period in the human brain, providing another significant energy source, using both extracellular lactate and pyruvate as substrates (60). Lactate and pyruvate have also been shown to modulate the LTP and LTD that may be involved in synaptic plasticity critical to cognitive development at later stages of brain maturation (21). Due to the high fat ingestion of infants secondary to milk intake, more ketones are available in infant blood than in adult blood and can represent up to 20% of the carbon skeletons used in energy production in infants (20). The BBB is quite permeable to ketones, and coupled with enhanced developmental brain enzymatic activity for ketone use compared to adults, ketones play a more important role in bioenergetics of the immature CNS (15). CNS substrate use of ketones may also be linked to amino acid and lipid biosynthetic pathway precursors, which are subsequently used in developmental membrane and myelin formation (15). However, as has been shown in rats (**Fig. 55.11**), once the child is no longer dependent on maternal milk, the use of ketones as a metabolic fuel decreases as well.

BLOOD–BRAIN BARRIER AND CHOROID PLEXUS DEVELOPMENT

Primary BBB functions serve to isolate brain blood compartments; provide selective transport of metabolites, ions, and molecules; and either metabolize or modify many blood- or brain-borne substances (3) (**Fig. 55.12**). The BBB is impermeable to hydrophilic molecules, ions, and proteins, while key metabolic substrates (e.g., glucose) enter via transport proteins (e.g., GLUT1) and water passes through the BBB via aquaporin-4 channels (11). In addition, numerous metabolic barriers block the passage of molecules from blood to brain via the BBB, including P-glycoprotein (which involves energy-dependent movement of hydrophobic drugs out of the CNS) and enzymes (such as monoamine oxidase to metabolize catecholamines), which protect synaptic function (1,2).

The BBB is commonly thought to be "leaky" during fetal development and in the newborn infant. However, this issue remains a matter of debate (based on experimental technical approaches), as evidence suggests that the fetal BBB is highly developed during the developmental period, including some mechanisms not found in the adult BBB (61). Tight junctions develop early during CNS maturation, and most proteins do not gain access to the extracellular compartment via the BBB during development. Cerebrospinal fluid (CSF) protein concentration is higher during early brain development and is thought to result from an immature choroid plexus; however,

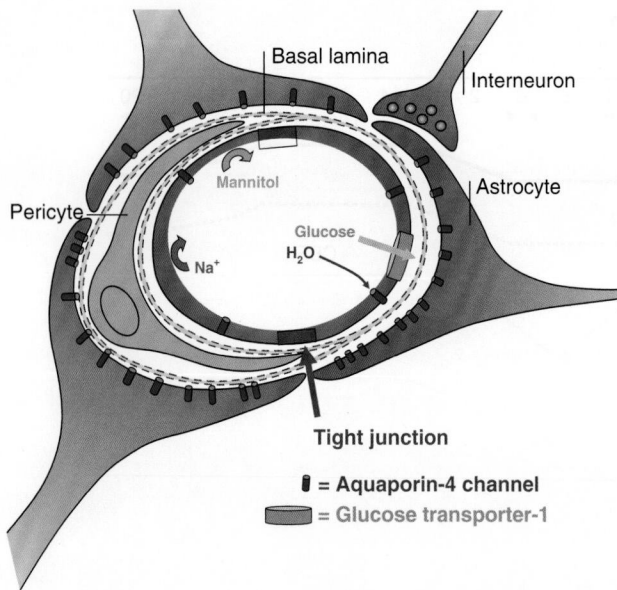

FIGURE 55.12. The structure of the mature BBB consists of endothelial cells connected by tight junctions, specialized supportive cells called pericytes, a basal lamina, and perivascular astrocytic end feet. (Modified from Abbott NJ, Ronnback L, Hansson E. Astrocyte-endothelial interactions at the blood–brain barrier. *Nat Rev Neurosci* 2006;7:41–53, with permission.)

high CSF protein concentrations during development are not reflected in the extracellular space because of junctional complexes forming barriers at the CSF–brain interfaces that are not found in the adult brain (61). The BBB's permeability to ions and amino acids develops as transport systems mature in the brain; however, lipid-insoluble molecules are more permeable in the immature brain than in the adult brain (61). The majority view suggests that fetal BBB permeability to macromolecules is similar to adults, but small molecules enter the fetal brain more readily than in the adult CNS. Ion permeability decreases just before birth in large animal experiments (51).

Small lipophilic molecules, such as CO_2, O_2, and ethanol, can readily pass through the BBB (1). However, the mature BBB is impermeable to many molecules and substances that are provided by cerebrovascular endothelial cell tight junctions, which form the complete zona occludens (11) (**Fig. 55.12**). Small polar molecules needed for brain function, such as glucose and amino acids, are transported across the barrier by carrier proteins (e.g., GLUT1 for glucose and the L-system carrier L1 for large neutral amino acids, such as leucine) (1). Some small molecules and lipids are transported across the BBB by receptor-mediated endocytosis. The BBB is also able to remove hydrophobic molecules via P-glycoprotein—the energy-dependent, broad-spectrum efflux carrier, which plays a key role in BBB transport of a number of drugs. Finally, the cerebrovascular endothelial cells have an important metabolic function that is an integral component of the BBB. They contain monoamine oxidase and can defend brain synaptic function against circulating catecholamines (1). Abbott and Romero (2) have characterized the BBB as having important "static and dynamic properties." In addition, the barrier is surrounded by astrocyte foot processes, and these astrocytes can further modulate the entry and egress of substances across the BBB via their possession of various channels and transporters (such as the GLUTs previously discussed and the aquaporins discussed later) and through intracellular metabolism (11).

A complete discussion of astrocyte metabolic function is beyond the scope of this chapter.

A number of specific proteins mediate barrier functions at tight junctions (11). Germane to pediatric critical care medicine, cerebrovascular tight junctions effectively prevent the movement of hydrophilic substances, such as cations (Na^+, K^+) and osmolar agents (e.g., mannitol), along with proteins, among other molecules (11) (**Fig. 55.12**). Thus, the intact BBB is impermeable to salts and proteins, making osmolar gradients rather than oncotic gradients critical to water movement across the barrier (62) and serving as the theoretical basis for the use of hypertonic saline and mannitol in the treatment of intracranial hypertension (discussed in several later chapters). Water movement across the BBB is mediated via special water channels, termed *aquaporins*. In the BBB and astrocyte foot processes, water movement is facilitated specifically by aquaporin-4 channels (1). These are in relatively low concentration in the vascular endothelial cells and in higher concentration in the astrocytes, which use them for their rapid astrocytic influx of water during uptake of potassium, glutamate, and other substances (**Fig. 55.12**). The role of the BBB and astrocytes in CNS injury is discussed in detail in Chapter 56, as it relates to excitotoxicity and cellular swelling.

CEREBROSPINAL FLUID DYNAMICS

Two pathways of CSF circulation have been proposed—a minor and a major pathway (16) (**Fig. 55.13**). While the details of CSF dynamics during development remain unclear, it is classically thought that they differ in the developing brain compared to the adult. The major pathway of CSF absorption is via the arachnoid villi (arachnoid granulation) into the venous sinuses. The minor pathway includes drainage via ventricular ependyma, the interstitial and perivascular space, and perineural lymphatics (16). In adult humans, CSF production is around 500 mL/24 hours, and the turnover may be three to four times a day. Interplay between the two drainage pathways maintains normal homeostasis and the neurochemical milieu in balance (16). The CSF circulation begins in development, with choroid plexus formation at around 40–60 days of gestation, depending on the ventricle. The arachnoid granulation appears just before birth, and CSF reabsorption occurs at later ages (**Fig. 55.13**). The minor CSF pathway is the primary route for CSF dynamics in the developing immature human brain because arachnoid granulation function does not occur until the late infant stages. Radiologic evidence for the arachnoid granulation as a gross structure occurs around age 7 and continues to develop until age 20 (16).

CONCLUSIONS AND FUTURE DIRECTIONS

Fundamental aspects of normal brain biology and physiology have been reviewed in this chapter, with a focus on developmental issues. A number of important developmental differences exist in the immature versus the adult brain relevant to pediatric neurointensive care. These differences span the gamut of biochemical, molecular, physiologic, and structural factors that influence current therapy on a daily basis and are likely to have an even greater impact on the future development of novel therapies that target brain injury in infants and children. This information also provides a foundation for the chapters that follow, which focus on the molecular biology of brain injury and the pathophysiology and treatment of key disorders in pediatric neurointensive care.

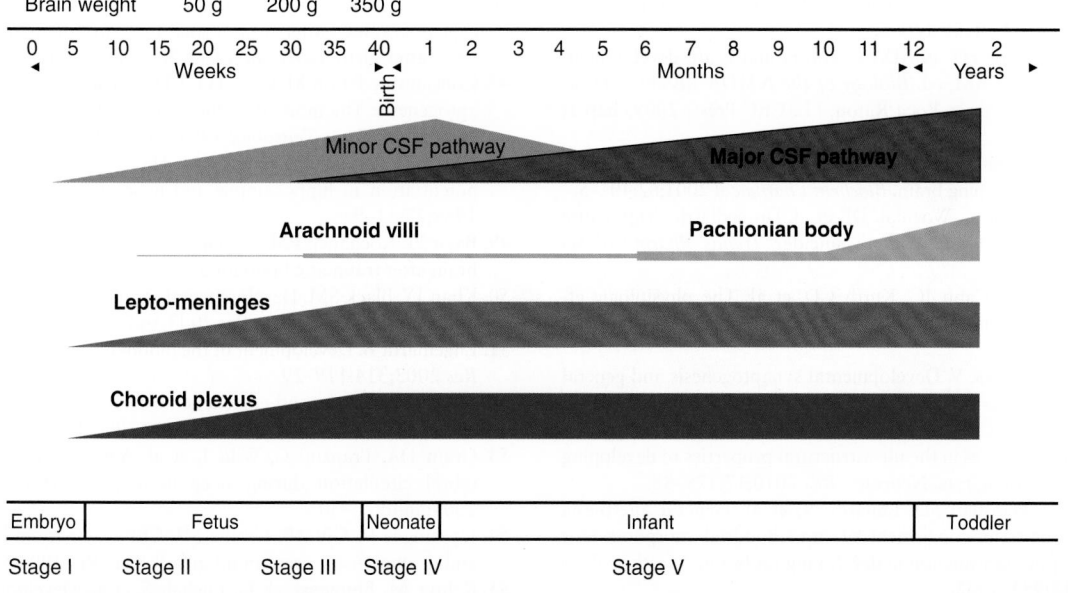

FIGURE 55.13. CSF dynamics differ in the developing brain, compared to the adult. CSF absorption via the arachnoid villi (arachnoid granulation) into the venous sinuses is the major pathway. The minor pathway includes drainage via the ventricular ependyma, the interstitial and perivascular space, and the perineural lymphatics. In the developing immature human brain, the minor CSF pathway is the primary route for CSF dynamics, because arachnoid granulation function does not occur until the late infant stages. (From Oi S, Di Rocco C. Proposal of "evolution theory in cerebrospinal fluid dynamics" and minor pathway hydrocephalus in developing immature brain. *Childs Nerv Syst* 2006;22:662–9, with permission.)

References

1. Abbott NJ. Astrocyte-endothelial interactions and blood–brain barrier permeability. *J Anat* 2002;200:629–38.
2. Abbott NJ, Romero IA. Transporting therapeutics across the blood–brain barrier. *Mol Med Today* 1996;2:106–13.
3. Abbott NJ, Ronnback L, Hansson E. Astrocyte-endothelial interactions at the blood–brain barrier. *Nat Rev Neurosci* 2006;7:41–53.
4. Altshuler K, Berg M, Frazier LM, et al. Critical periods in development: OCHP Paper Series on Children's Health and the Environment 2003; Paper 2.
5. Ben-Ari Y, Khazipov R, Leinekugel X, et al. GABA$_A$, NMDA and AMPA receptors: A developmentally regulated "menage a trois." *Trends Neurosci* 1997;20:523–9.
6. Bouma GJ, Muizelaar, JP. Cerebral blood flow, cerebral blood volume, and cerebrovascular reactivity after severe head injury. *J Neurotrauma* 1992;9(suppl 1):S333–48.
7. De Zio D, Giunta L, Corvaro M, et al. Expanding roles of programmed cell death in mammalian neurodevelopment. *Semin Cell Dev Biol* 2005;16:281–94.
8. Hardy P, Varma DR, Chemtob S. Control of cerebral and ocular blood flow autoregulation in neonates. *Pediatr Clin North Am* 1997;44:137–52.
9. Herlenius E, Lagercrantz H. Development of neurotransmitter systems during critical periods. *Exp Neurol* 2004;190(suppl 1):S8–21.
10. Herschkowitz N. Neurological bases of behavioral development in infancy. *Brain Dev* 2000;22:411–6.
11. Kimelberg HK, Water homeostasis in the brain: Basic concepts. *Neuroscience* 2004;129:851–60.
12. Lagercrantz H, Ringstedt T. Organization of the neuronal circuits in the central nervous system during development. *Acta Paediatr* 2001;90:707–15.
13. Levitt P. Structural and functional maturation of the developing primate brain. *J Pediatr* 2003;143:S35–45.
14. Michenfelder JD. *Anesthesia and the Brain*. New York, NY: Churchill, Livingstone; 1988:chap 1.
15. Nehlig A. Cerebral energy metabolism, glucose transport and blood flow: Changes with maturation and adaptation to hypoglycaemia. *Diabetes Metab* 1997;23:18–29.
16. Oi S, Di Rocco C. Proposal of "evolution theory in cerebrospinal fluid dynamics" and minor pathway hydrocephalus in developing immature brain. *Childs Nerv Syst* 2006;22:662–9.
17. Panickar KS, Norenberg MD. Astrocytes in cerebral ischemic injury: Morphological and general considerations. *Glia* 2005;50:287–98.
18. Rice D, Barone S, Jr. Critical periods of vulnerability for the developing nervous system: Evidence from humans and animal models. *Environ Health Perspective* 2000;108(suppl 3):511–33.
19. Town T, Nikolic V, Tan J. The microglial "activation" continuum: From innate to adaptive responses. *J Neuroinflammation* 2005;2:24.
20. Vannucci RC, Vannucci SJ. Glucose metabolism in the developing brain. *Semin Perinatol* 2000;24:107–15.
21. Yang B, Sakurai T, Takata T, et al. Effects of lactate/pyruvate on synaptic plasticity in the hippocampal dentate gyrus. *Neurosci Res* 2003;46:333–7.
22. Munno DW, Syed NI. Synaptogenesis in the CNS: An odyssey from wiring together to firing together. *J Physiol* 2003;552:1–11.
23. Raoul C, Pettmann B, Henderson CE. Active killing of neurons during development and following stress: A role for p75(NTR) and Fas? *Curr Opin Neurobiol* 2000;10:111–7.
24. Guillemot F. Cellular and molecular control of neurogenesis in the mammalian telencephalon. *Curr Opin Cell Biol* 2005;17:639–47.
25. Lessmann V, Gottmann K, Malcangio M. Neurotrophin secretion: Current facts and future prospects. *Prog Neurobiol* 2003;69:341–74.
26. Fields RD. Myelination: An overlooked mechanism of synaptic plasticity? *Neuroscientist* 2005;11:528–31.
27. Johnston MV. Neurotransmitters and vulnerability of the developing brain. *Brain Dev* 1995;17:301–6.
28. Johnston MV, Nakajima W, Hagberg H. Mechanisms of hypoxic neurodegeneration in the developing brain. *Neuroscientist* 2002;8:212–20.
29. Klebermass K, Kuhle S, Olischar M, et al. Intra- and extrauterine maturation of amplitude-integrated electroencephalographic

activity in preterm infants younger than 30 weeks of gestation. *Biol Neonate* 2006;89:120–5.

30. Ewald RC, Cline HT. NMDA receptors and brain development. In: Van Dongen AM, ed. *Biology of the NMDA Receptor, Frontiers in Neuroscience*. Boca Raton, FL: CRC Press; 2009:chap 1; 1–16.

31. Ikonomidou C, Bittigau P, Koch C, et al. Neurotransmitters and apoptosis in the developing brain. *Biochem Pharmacol* 2001;62:401–5.

32. Olney JW, Young C, Wozniak DF, et al. Do pediatric drugs cause developing neurons to commit suicide? *Trends Pharmacol Sci* 2004;25:135–9.

33. Loepke AW, McCann JC, Kurth CD, et al. The physiologic effects of isoflurane anesthesia in neonatal mice. *Anesth Analg* 2006;102:75–80.

34. Jevtovic-Todorovic V. Developmental synaptogenesis and general anesthesia: A kiss of death? *Curr Pharm Des* 2012;18:6225–31.

35. Lunardi N, Ori C, Erisir A, et al. General anesthesia causes long-lasting disturbances in the ultrastructural properties of developing synapses in young rats. *Neurotox Res* 2010;17:179–88.

36. Sanchez V, Feinstein SD, Lunardi N, et al. General anesthesia causes long-term impairment of mitochondrial morphogenesis and synaptic transmission in developing rat brain. *Anesthesiology* 2011;115:992–1002.

37. Brambrink AM, Back SA, Riddle A, et al. Isoflurane-induced apoptosis of oligodendrocytes in the neonatal primate brain. *Ann Neurol* 2012;72:525–35.

38. Paule MG, Li M, Allen RR, et al. Ketamine anesthesia during the first week of life can cause long-lasting cognitive deficits in rhesus monkeys. *Neurotoxicol Teratol* 2011;33:220–30.

39. Reddy SV. Effect of general anesthetics on the developing brain. *J Anaesthesiol Clin Pharmacol* 2012;28:6–10.

40. Herlenius E, Lagercrantz H. Neurotransmitters and neuro-modulators during early human development. *Early Hum Dev* 2001;65:21–37.

41. Rivera C, Voipio J, Kaila K. Two developmental switches in GABAergic signalling: The K^+-Cl^- cotransporter KCC_2 and carbonic anhydrase CAVII. *J Physiol* 2005;562:27–36.

42. Beaumont A, Hayasaki K, Marmarou A, et al. Contrasting effects of dopamine therapy in experimental brain injury. *J Neurotrauma* 2001;18:1359–72.

43. Connor B, Dragunow M. The role of neuronal growth factors in neurodegenerative disorders of the human brain. *Brain Res Brain Res Rev* 1998;27:1–39.

44. Das KP, Chao SL, White LD, et al. Differential patterns of nerve growth factor, brain-derived neurotrophic factor and neurotrophin-3 mRNA and protein levels in developing regions of rat brain. *Neuroscience* 2001;103:739–61.

45. Olischar M, Klebermass K, Kuhle S, et al. Reference values for amplitude-integrated electroencephalographic activity in preterm infants younger than 30 weeks' gestational age. *Pediatrics* 2004;113:e61–6.

46. West CR, Harding JE, Williams CE, et al. Quantitative electroencephalographic patterns in normal preterm infants over the first week after birth. *Early Hum Dev* 2006;82:43–51.

47. Constantine-Paton M, Cline HT. LTP and activity-dependent synaptogenesis: The more alike they are, the more different they become. *Curr Opin Neurobiol* 1998;8:139–48.

48. Teyler TJ, Perkins AT, Harris KM. The development of long-term potentiation in hippocampus and neocortex. *Neuropsychologia* 1989;27:31–9.

49. Bayır H, Kochanek PM, Kagen VE. Oxidative stress in immature brain after traumatic brain injury. *Dev Neurosci* 2006;28:420–31.

50. Khan JY, Black SM. Developmental changes in murine brain antioxidant enzymes. *Pediatr Res* 2003;54:77–82.

51. Engelhardt B. Development of the blood–brain barrier. *Cell Tissue Res* 2003;314:119–29.

52. Ribatti D. Genetic and epigenetic mechanisms in the early development of the vascular system. *J Anat* 2006;208:139–52.

53. Grant DA, Franzini C, Wild J, et al. Autoregulation of the cerebral circulation during sleep in newborn lambs. *J Physiol* 2005;564:923–30.

54. Jayasinghe D, Gill AB, Levene MI. CBF reactivity in hypotensive and normotensive preterm infants. *Pediatr Res* 2003;54:848–53.

55. Kehrer M, Blumenstock G, Ehehalt S, et al. Development of cerebral blood flow volume in preterm neonates during the first 2 weeks of life. *Pediatr Res* 2005;58:927–30.

56. Taga G, Asakawa K, Hirasawa K, et al. Hemodynamic responses to visual stimulation in occipital and frontal cortex of newborn infants: A near-infrared optical topography study. *Early Hum Dev* 2003;75(suppl):S203–10.

57. Todd M, Shapiro HM, Obrist WD. Cerebral blood flow measurements and the critically ill patient. In: Grenvik A, Safar P, eds. *Brain Failure and Resuscitation*. New York, NY: Churchill Livingstone, 1981:135.

58. Haaland K, Karlsson B, Skovlund E, et al. Postnatal development of the cerebral blood flow velocity response to changes in CO_2 and mean arterial blood pressure in the piglet. *Acta Paediatr* 1995;84:1414–20.

59. Pereira de Vasconcelos A, Ferrandon A, Nehlig A. Local cerebral blood flow during lithium-pilocarpine seizures in the developing and adult rat: Role of coupling between blood flow and metabolism in the genesis of neuronal damage. *J Cereb Blood Flow Metab* 2002;22:196–205.

60. Fayol L, Baud O, Monier A, et al. Immunocytochemical expression of monocarboxylate transporters in the human visual cortex at midgestation. *Brain Res Dev Brain Res* 2004;148:69–76.

61. Saunders NR, Habgood MD, Dziegielewska KM. Barrier mechanisms in the brain, II. Immature brain. *Clin Exp Pharmacol Physiol* 1999;26:85–91.

62. Zornow MH, Todd MM, Moore SS. The acute cerebral effects of changes in plasma osmolality and oncotic pressure. *Anesthesiology* 1987;67:936–41.

CHAPTER 56 ■ MOLECULAR BIOLOGY OF BRAIN INJURY

PATRICK M. KOCHANEK, HÜLYA BAYIR, LARRY W. JENKINS, AND ROBERT S.B. CLARK

KEY POINTS

1 The two distinct types of secondary injury are (a) evolution of damage mediated by endogenous secondary injury cascades and (b) damage that results from secondary insults (e.g., hypotension) in the field, emergency department, or ICU.

2 Ischemia is an important injury mechanism that plays varying roles across the spectrum of PICU-relevant central nervous system (CNS) insults.

3 Cell death pathways after CNS injury include necrosis, apoptosis, autophagy, and necroptosis. Some cells display mixed phenotypes with characteristics of two or more of these pathways.

4 Key initiators of damage in the evolution of secondary injury include energy failure, excitotoxicity, oxidative stress, and trophic factor withdrawal.

5 Apoptosis after CNS injury can result from activation of a number of mechanisms, including (a) an intrinsic (mitochondrial) pathway, (b) an apoptosis-inducing factor pathway, (c) an endoplasmic reticulum stress pathway, and

(d) an extrinsic (extracellular signaling) pathway. Age-related differences in the cell death response to brain injury could be highly important.

6 An endogenous neuroprotectant response to CNS injury occurs and includes a variety of pathways: adenosine, heat shock proteins, and a variety of antiapoptotic proteins such as Bcl-2.

7 Brain swelling after CNS injury results from cellular swelling, vasogenic edema, osmolar swelling, mixed edema patterns, and/or an increase in cerebral blood volume.

8 Inflammation after CNS injury plays an important role in exacerbation of secondary damage and in initiating signals for repair and regeneration.

9 Axonal injury involves a process that includes secondary axotomy after axonal stretch and/or ischemia.

10 Key secondary extracerebral insults that adversely impact outcome across CNS injury etiologies include hypotension, hypoxemia, hyperthermia, and hypoglycemia/hyperglycemia.

Knowledge of the pathophysiology of central nervous system (CNS) injury, such as intracranial and cerebrovascular dynamics, has guided brain-oriented therapy since the inception of critical care medicine. In the chapters of Section III, the pathophysiology of each disease process is described, along with how it influences outcome and guides therapy. Although therapy that is based solely on physiologic parameters, such as intracranial pressure (ICP) and cerebral blood flow (CBF), is important, it has limitations. For example, some patients with well-controlled cerebral hemodynamics still have poor outcome. Indeed, some recent studies in the field of neurocritical care have questioned the relative importance of control of raised ICP to outcome (1). For example, the standard medical care group had significantly better long-term outcome in the recent randomized controlled trial (RCT) of decompressive craniectomy in adults with severe traumatic brain injury (TBI) despite substantially better control of ICP in the surgery group. Many explanations have been suggested to explain this finding, and the authors of this chapter do not suggest discounting the importance of ICP in severe TBI; however, one possibility is that the rapid weaning of other neurocritical care therapies such as osmolar therapy, sedation, barbiturates, etc., led to a relative deficit in therapies targeting other mechanism of secondary injury in brain such as excitotoxicity in the patients treated with decompression. We, thus, are working in an exciting era in which knowledge of the pathobiology of CNS injury is gaining importance for the intensivist and can augment pathophysiology-based therapy. Insight into secondary brain injury at the biochemical, cellular, and molecular levels

has finally begun to yield dividends, with efficacy shown for several new therapies in ICU-relevant CNS injuries (2–5). This chapter builds on the material in the preceding chapter that addresses developmental issues of the CNS relevant to critical care. Where possible, this information on the bedside care of critically ill patients is linked with clinical data. It is hoped that this chapter and its counterpart (Chapter 55) aptly set the stage for the following chapters that discuss the individual CNS disorders encountered in the practice of pediatric critical care medicine.

INJURY RESPONSE IN THE IMMATURE BRAIN

Most research on developmental brain injury suggests that the immature brain is more resistant to injury and more capable of recovery than is the adult brain due to enhanced plasticity (ability to rewire or repair). For example, despite similar impact parameters, the immature brain exhibits less neuronal death than the adult brain in experimental TBI. Similarly, tolerance of the immature brain to status epilepticus (SE) is greater than in the adult in experimental models (6). Classic studies of ablative brain lesions in laboratory models, such as hemispherectomy in cats, show that the earlier the brain lesion occurs in development, the better the outcome (7). Unfortunately, critical windows in development represent periods of the brain's enhanced vulnerability to specific developmental processes (8) (see Chapter 55). Some developmental aspects predispose the immature brain to greater injury than the adult. For example, the small size of the infant skull may predispose to a more diffuse pattern of injury from a traumatic impact than does the adult skull (9). An injury that is more global than focal may yield a more profound disruption of function. Much of the controversy on this point results from the fact that outcomes from brain injury in infants and young children are often poorer than in adults (10). For example, outcome from out-of-hospital cardiac arrest is worse in children than in adults. However, the mechanism that underlies the cardiac arrest in children—asphyxia—is particularly injurious to the brain, compared with ventricular fibrillation (VF) (11). Similarly, reported outcomes in infants from severe TBI can be as bad as or worse than those in adults (10). This finding likely results from the contribution of abusive head trauma (AHT) to severe TBI in infancy. Thus, although most data suggest that the developing brain exhibits both resistance and resilience to injury versus the adult, the mechanisms of injury are often more severe in children. Our challenges for developing new therapies are no less than in adults.

PATHWAYS AND APPLICATIONS TO PEDIATRIC INTENSIVE CARE

Secondary Injury

The essence of neurointensive care is the prevention of secondary injury. Two distinct types of secondary injury are frequently lumped into a single concept. First, endogenous secondary injury cascades evolve in the minutes to days after the initial insult. Processes such as excitotoxicity, oxidative stress, and delayed neuronal death cascades kill neurons and injure other components of the CNS at varying rates. Emerging evidence supports the concept that, in some cases, these cascades may be able to be abrogated, resulting in salvage of injured tissue and improved recovery of function. Efficacy in large RCTs has been reported for mild hypothermia after both cardiac arrest from VF in adults and perinatal asphyxia (2,3,5). Similarly, thrombolytics have shown efficacy in large, randomized, controlled clinical trials in stroke in adults (4). Although these therapies are being further evaluated and only beginning to be integrated into standard care, it is likely that additional therapies will follow. This chapter is focused on those events in injury evolution that may represent therapeutic targets.

In contrast to the endogenous cascades, a parallel form of secondary injury involves critically ill patients who suffer secondary insults in the field, emergency room, or ICU. These secondary insults produce adverse consequences on a CNS with enhanced vulnerability after cardiac arrest, stroke, TBI, SE, or CNS infection. For example, hypoxemia, at a level tolerated by the normal brain, can have detrimental effects after TBI. (Why the injured brain is highly vulnerable to secondary insults is

discussed later.) Thus, the biochemical, cellular, and molecular aspects of endogenous damage evolution are discussed, followed by a discussion of the mechanisms that underlie enhanced vulnerability of the injured brain to secondary insults in the PICU.

Evolution of Secondary Injury

Presenting a complete synthesis of the mechanisms involved in the evolution of secondary damage after CNS injury is challenging, particularly when one considers that the concepts discussed in this chapter serve as the basis for all PICU-relevant CNS insults. It is necessary to consider studies in models of CNS injury and, where possible, the relevant clinical conditions. We will focus on global cerebral ischemia/cardiac arrest, focal cerebral ischemia/stroke, and TBI. Where possible, insight into the relevance of these mechanisms in epilepsy and CNS infection will be included.

Studies have begun to unravel those mechanisms producing secondary damage that are relevant to cardiac arrest, stroke, TBI, SE, CNS infection, and other insults. Five categories of mechanisms can be defined (Fig. 56.1): those associated with (a) ischemia and energy failure and (b) excitotoxicity, both initiating cell death cascades; (c) inflammation; (d) cerebral swelling; and (e) axonal injury. Within each category, a constellation of mediators of secondary damage is involved (12). The quantitative contribution of each mediator to outcome and the interplay between these mediators remains unclear and varies with the insult. A sixth component of the response to brain injury will be briefly discussed, namely, the role of endogenous neuroprotectants, repair, and regeneration. The ultimate result of the primary injury from TBI, which sets into motion these six cascade initiators, is summarized in Figure 56.2. The details of these initiators represent the crux of information to follow.

Study of the acute biochemical and molecular aspects of human brain injury has been limited, particularly in infants and children; however, several methods have been used, most commonly in TBI and occasionally in asphyxia. These include (a) the analysis of brain biochemistry and molecular biology using ventricular cerebrospinal fluid (CSF); (b) assessment of brain interstitial fluid by cerebral microdialysis; (c) imaging-related tools, such as positron emission tomography (PET) and MR spectroscopy; and (d) the assessment of molecular markers in brain tissue obtained from patients treated with surgical decompression. Assessment of postmortem brain tissue has provided molecular clues in some cases. We will discuss these clinical studies supporting proposed mechanisms whenever possible.

Ischemia

Global Cerebral Ischemia. The brain is exquisitely vulnerable to ischemia, which represents a unifying mechanism involved in the evolution of secondary damage across CNS insults. When CBF globally ceases, such as in cardiac arrest,

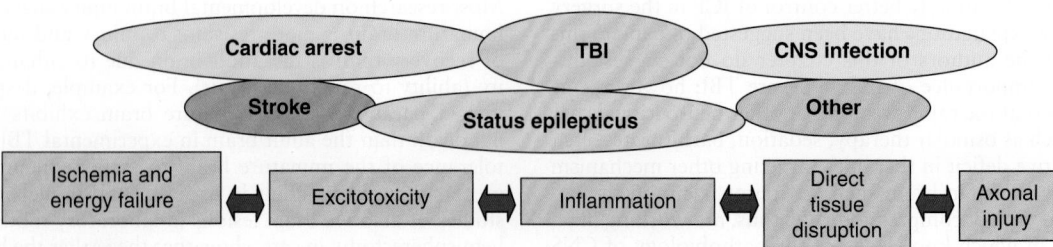

FIGURE 56.1. Overview of the major pathways of secondary injury after PICU-relevant insults to the CNS. Five categories of injury include ischemia and energy failure, excitotoxicity, inflammation, direct tissue disruption, and axonal injury.

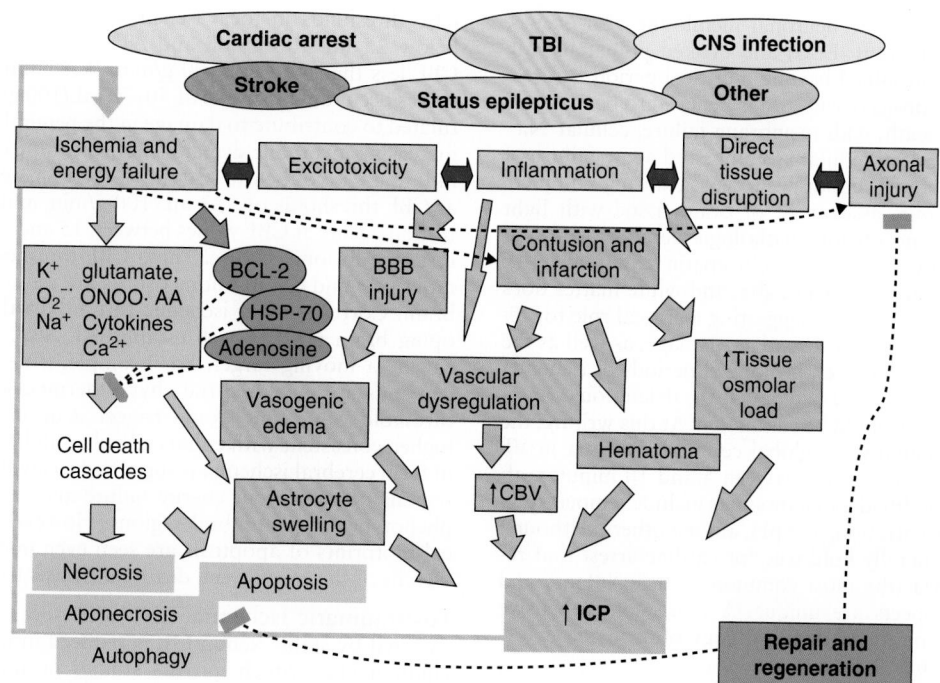

FIGURE 56.2. Secondary cascades triggered by the five initiators of secondary damage identified in **Figure 56.1** are shown for cell death cascades (*gray*), and for brain swelling–related process (*stippled gray*). In addition, a sixth category of endogenous neuroprotectants and repair and regeneration is initiated; the components of this cascade are shown in *black*. TBI, traumatic brain injury; O$_2^-$, superoxide anion; ONOO, peroxynitrite; AA, arachidonic acid; HSP-70, heat shock protein 70; ICP, intracranial pressure.

a stereotypic time course of events occurs that is initiated by acute cellular energy failure. These changes are outlined in **Figure 56.3**. Phosphocreatine is depleted in 1 minute, and the adenylate energy charge is depleted in ~5 minutes. After this time, no useful energy can be made available to ATP-requiring reactions (13). Membrane failure follows, with loss of ionic gradients, increases in intracellular calcium (Ca^{2+}) and sodium (Na$^+$), and a decrease in intracellular potassium (K$^+$). Free

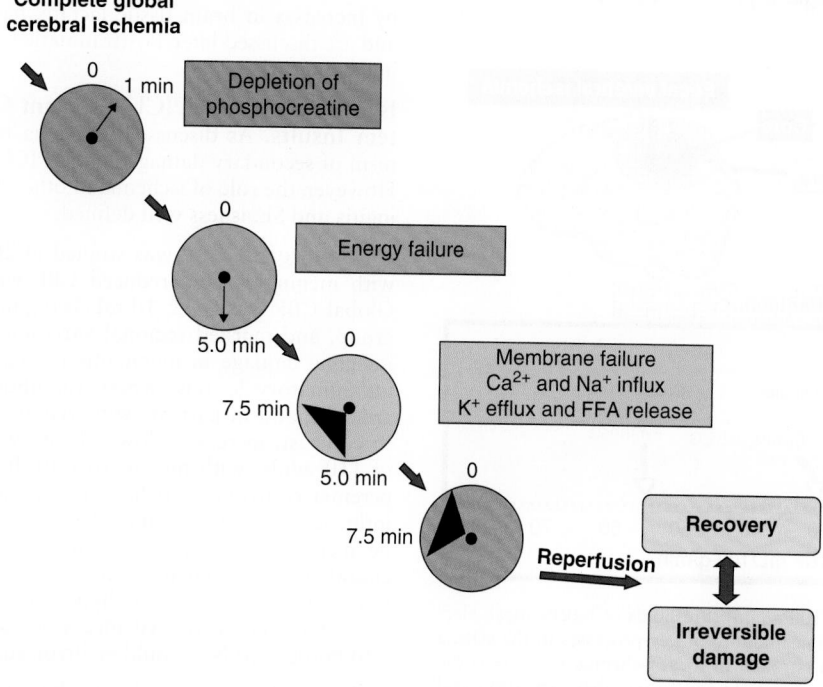

FIGURE 56.3. Temporal sequence of events that occurs in global cerebral ischemia, as seen with a "square-wave" ischemic brain insult, such as VF cardiac arrest. Although ischemia rapidly sets the stage for damage, histology—even by electron microscopy—reveals little damage during the period of ischemia. With ischemic durations beyond 10 minutes at normothermia, considerable damage is manifest with reperfusion. FFA, free fatty acid.

fatty acid release from the neuronal membrane also occurs, and electroencephalogram (EEG) and evoked potentials fail. If energy failure is sustained beyond a critical period, an irreversible insult to neurons occurs and is believed to be manifest by acute necrotic death, with membrane failure, cellular Na^+ and Ca^{2+} accumulation, cellular swelling, and acute failure of organelles, such as mitochondria. However, during complete global brain ischemia, assessment of brain tissue with light microscopy reveals no obvious pathologic derangement, and electron microscopy reveals only chromatin clumping (14). The resultant damage to neurons, glia, and white matter does not manifest until reperfusion, suggesting a critical role for reperfusion in the evolution of secondary damage, as well as the intriguing possibility that even prolonged periods of ischemia might be survived with good outcome if the deleterious consequences of reperfusion could be eliminated. At this writing, the duration of irreversibility for global cerebral ischemia in VF cardiac arrest is believed to be between 5 and 10 minutes, although it can be modified by factors that include temperature, blood glucose concentration, and pH, among others. Although these principles generally hold true for cardiac arrest that results from asphyxia (the most common form in infants and children), some aspects are unique. A more comprehensive discussion of the specific pathophysiology of asphyxia is discussed in Chapter 65.

Focal Cerebral Ischemia. Unlike global brain ischemia, focal ischemic insults (strokes) produce brain regions with different degrees of blood flow reduction related to the vascular anatomy surrounding the area of occlusion. The typical result is an ischemic core, in which flow reductions are profound, surrounded by penumbral brain regions that have less severe but still compromising CBF reductions. The consequences of penumbral CBF reductions on brain metabolism have been reviewed (15). The most sensitive biochemical or molecular event to CBF reduction in the ischemic penumbra is protein synthesis, which is inhibited by ~50% at a CBF of 55 mL/100 g/min and generally fails below 35 mL/100 g/min (**Fig. 56.4**). Other homeostatic processes that fail at decreasing

CBF thresholds in focal ischemia include glucose utilization below 25 mL/100 g/min and ATP depletion, beginning at a CBF less than ~20 mL/100 g/min. Peri-infarct depolarization waves occur at CBF levels of 50–70 mL/100 g/min and are postulated to contribute to damage in the penumbra by transiently increasing metabolic demands in this compromised zone. EEG fails at a CBF of below ~30 mL/100 g/min, hemiparesis is seen at CBF thresholds of ~23 mL/100 g/min, and anoxic depolarization occurs at CBF values between 15 and 20 mL/100 g/min, resulting in ionic failure. These CBF thresholds for failure of molecular and cellular homeostasis are estimates for the adult brain. Corresponding ischemic threshold values in the developing brain are less well established. Also, threshold values can be a moving target. For example, if neuronal metabolic demands are increased (i.e., hyperthermia, seizures), the CBF threshold value that would trigger neuronal death could be higher, consistent with enhanced vulnerability. Neuronal death in focal cerebral ischemia is suggested to involve necrosis in the regions of permanent energy failure and mixed or apoptotic phenotypes in penumbral regions. However, some biochemical footprints of apoptosis are seen even in core regions (16). Details of the specific cell death pathways are provided later.

Posttraumatic Ischemia. Early after severe TBI, the CBF, as assessed by stable xenon CT, is reduced in infants and young children (12), which mirrors studies in adults and suggests that early posttraumatic ischemia might represent a therapeutic target. Further supporting this possibility, early hypoperfusion or ischemia (CBF <20 mL/100 g/min) after severe TBI in infants and children was associated with poor outcome. Regional hypoperfusion is also commonly seen in contused brain regions. Mechanisms that underlie the early posttraumatic hypoperfusion may include a reduced vasodilatory response to nitric oxide (NO), cyclic guanosine monophosphate (cGMP), cyclic AMP (cAMP), and prostanoids, reduced NO production by endothelial NO synthase (NOS), and/or release of vasoconstrictors, such as superoxide anion or endothelin-1 (12). After TBI in children, increases in metabolic demands related to uptake of the excitatory neurotransmitter glutamate, as reflected by increases in brain tissue lactate, have been reported (17) and are discussed later. Posttraumatic CBF is further discussed in Chapter 61.

Ischemia in Other PICU-Relevant Central Nervous System Insults. As discussed, ischemia is one unifying mechanism of secondary damage across PICU-relevant CNS insults. However, the role of ischemia in other disorders, such as meningitis and SE, is less well defined.

Meningitis. CBF was studied in 20 seriously ill children with meningitis, and reduced CBF was reported in 7 (18). Global CBF was 26 ± 10 mL/100 g/min in the reduced flow group, and marked regional variability was seen. A role for ischemic damage in meningitis is suggested in focal cortical inflammatory lesions, where vasculitis and local infarction are seen, and in patients with venous sinus thrombosis (19). In contrast, increased flow velocity was reported in a study of 110 adults with meningitis (20). It is unclear if acute hyperemia contributes to herniation, which could importantly influence therapy. Vascular dysregulation in meningitis may be mediated by superoxide anion and the vasoconstrictor endothelin (19) and by disturbed regulation of NO production (21). The causes of hyperemia remain to be defined but inflammation-related mediators, such as inducible NOS (iNOS)-derived NO, could be involved.

Status Epilepticus. In SE, clinical studies of CBF are limited; however, experimental work shows the anticipated early increases in CBF—as much as fourfold—in an attempt to meet increased metabolic demands (22). Although ischemic blood flows are generally not seen, in some models, the marked

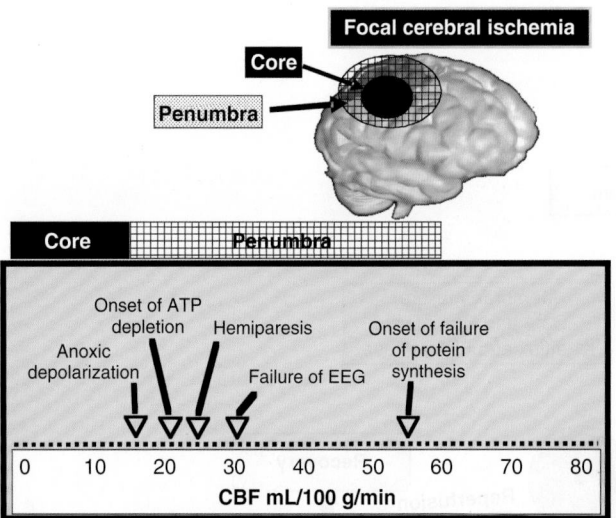

FIGURE 56.4. CBF (mL/100 g/min) thresholds of biochemical, electrophysiologic, and the clinical failure of key processes in the setting of focal cerebral ischemia (stroke). In focal ischemia, the core is the area with CBF below the threshold for anoxic depolarization and energy failure, while the penumbra has moderately reduced CBF, with levels above the threshold for energy failure. However, many processes are compromised in the penumbra (15). ATP, adenosine triphosphate; EEG, electroencephalogram.

increase in CBF is not sustained (23), which might lead to relative ischemia and resultant neuronal injury, given that cerebral metabolic rate for oxygen and glucose are markedly increased during SE (13). Increases in CBF during SE likely result from metabolic coupling.

Cell Death Pathways

Selective Vulnerability. Neurons in certain regions are exceptionally vulnerable to injury in global brain ischemia, including the CA1 region of the hippocampus; cerebral cortex layers 3, 5, and 6; cerebellar Purkinje cells; and in infants, some brainstem nuclei (12,24, also reviewed in 25). Approximately ≥5 minutes of complete global brain ischemia can result in neuronal death in these regions when they are examined at or beyond 72 hours after the insult. The mechanisms that underlie selective vulnerability of these neurons have been the topic of considerable research; however, a definitive answer remains elusive. These neurons do not have a unique vascular distribution; thus, intrinsic vulnerability is suggested. Nevertheless, insight has been gained from these studies into the question of how neurons die in cerebral ischemia.

A process known as *delayed neuronal death* causes these highly vulnerable neurons to die after threshold insults. During ischemia, cellular membrane failure occurs, with Ca^+ and Na^+ accumulation and K^+ efflux. However, in threshold insults, these ionic disturbances can be reversed, and ionic gradients reestablished. In delayed neuronal death of selectively vulnerable neurons after global brain ischemia, electrophysiologic studies have revealed neuronal hyperexcitability in these regions after reperfusion, followed by a second wave of irreversible Ca^{2+} accumulation at~48 hours (22). The molecular cascades involved in delayed neuronal death in selectively vulnerable neurons are discussed in what follows.

Although much has been written about selective vulnerability of the CA1 hippocampus after cardiac arrest, different neurons are selectively vulnerable after TBI. After experimental TBI, hippocampal neurons in the dentate hilus and the CA3 region of the hippocampus are most vulnerable (26) **(Fig. 56.5)**. This pattern of neuronal vulnerability is shared with that seen in experimental models of epilepsy, as produced by systemic injection of the proconvulsant agent kainic acid. This finding suggests an important role for posttraumatic excitation in mediating neuronal death in CA3 and, consistent with that notion, neurons in the dentate gyrus and CA3 region of the hippocampus show regional excitation after TBI and mediate early posttraumatic seizures (27). In experimental SE, limbic structures, including hippocampus, the piriform cortex, temporal cortex, and amygdala, are vulnerable (28). Thus, which specific cells are most vulnerable after CNS insult depends on the type of insult; the intrinsic mechanisms involved in this vulnerability may differ. The optimal approach to treatment could thus differ in cardiac arrest, stroke, TBI, and other insults. The pattern of neuronal death is also unique in meningitis. In experimental meningitis, the granular layer of the dentate gyrus of the hippocampus is highly vulnerable, particularly in regions closest to the CSF ventricular compartment (29). Selective vulnerability of the dentate was shown in acute bacterial meningitis in humans and may underlie learning deficits seen in this condition (30).

Necrosis and Apoptosis. Neuronal death can occur through multiple pathways including necrosis, programmed cell death (PCD) or apoptosis, and mixed phenotypes. Necrosis, which is characterized by denaturation and coagulation of cellular proteins, results from a progressive reduction in cellular ATP (12,25). Necrosis involves progressive derangements in energy and substrate metabolism, followed by a series of morphologic alterations, including swelling of cells and organelles,

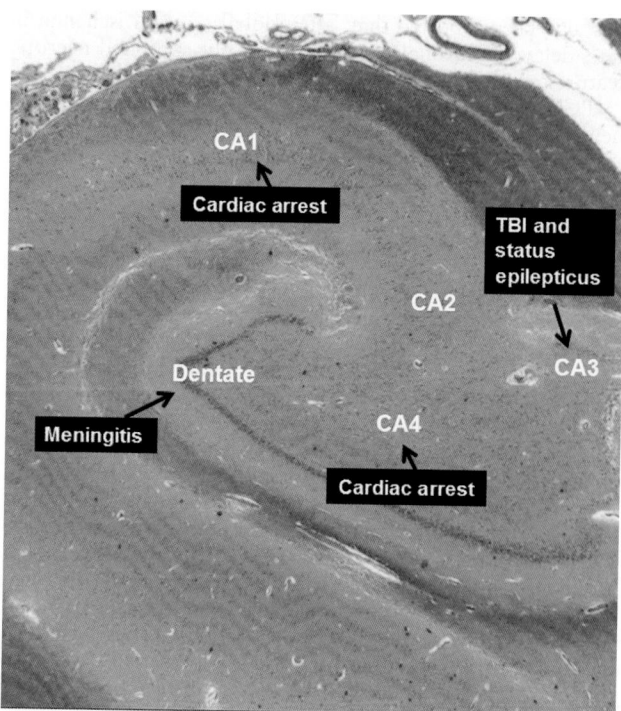

FIGURE 56.5. Horizontal section through the hippocampus of the human brain showing neuronal degeneration in the various hippocampal subfields, namely, CA1, CA2, CA3, CA4 (hilus), and dentate gyrus. The hippocampal subfields are some of the most selectively vulnerable brain regions to ischemic, traumatic, and infectious insults relevant to pediatric neurointensive care. The *black boxes* show the insults generally associated with damage in a given hippocampal subfield. The CA1 and CA4 regions are highly vulnerable to global ischemic insults, such as cardiac arrest. In contrast, the dentate gyrus is vulnerable in meningitis, while CA3 is vulnerable in TBI and SE. This figure is not to suggest that all of these regions cannot be damaged by a given injury (for example, a prolonged cardiac arrest); rather, these injury patterns represent those seen with threshold insults. Hippocampal injury is important to disturbances in learning and memory, among other cognitive processes.

subsurface cellular blebbing, amorphous deposits in mitochondria, condensation of nuclear chromatin, and, finally, breaks in plasma and organellar membranes. It was assumed that all ischemic cell death occurred via this process and that selective vulnerability represented a predilection for the development of necrosis in certain neurons. However, neuronal death after hypoxic–ischemic insults can also occur through PCD or apoptosis. More recently, it has been suggested that mixed phenotypes of neuronal death exist that have features of both necrosis and apoptosis. And, as discussed later, two additional forms of neuronal death, necroptosis and pyroptosis, also participate in delayed cell death (31,32). The development of PCD involves new protein synthesis and the activation of endonucleases, with a characteristic cleavage of DNA into nucleosomal fragments of double-stranded DNA, called "DNA laddering" on Southern blot analysis. PCD was classically described as being associated with cell death during embryogenesis (11,25). However, PCD occurs across insults. Some reports indicate that selective vulnerable cell death in brain regions, such as the CA1 hippocampus after transient global brain ischemia, occurs by an apoptotic mechanism. Delayed cell death of selectively vulnerable neurons was attenuated by inhibition of protein synthesis (33), and DNA extracted from the hippocampus of gerbils at 4 days after a threshold global ischemic insult showed a characteristic laddering pattern consistent with apoptosis (34). In contrast, it has also been reported that, after global cerebral ischemia in rats, delayed neuronal death occurred but exhibited necrotic features on electron microscopy (35).

PCD in the postischemic brain is not limited to scattered neuronal death in what have been traditionally deemed to be "selectively vulnerable regions," but it is also seen in penumbral regions around evolving cerebral infarcts (36). Apoptosis was evident in injured brain regions of infants who died from perinatal asphyxia between 3 and 7 days after birth, and was common in cortical layers I, II, and III, while necrosis was seen in deeper layers (37). Finally, cells with mixed phenotypes were seen in rat brain after experimental CNS injury that resulted from injection of excitatory amino acids (EAAs) (38). These cells showed features of both apoptosis and necrosis.

It is likely that the severity of the ischemic insult and other local factors determine whether an injured neuron recovers or dies from PCD or necrosis. After cardiac arrest, stroke, TBI, epilepsy, and CNS infections, a continuum from recovery to necrosis may exist in neurons; progress through this continuum depends on the severity and duration of the insult, the local milieu, and the given brain region. It is thus likely that an understanding of the mechanisms involved in all neuronal death pathways will be necessary for development of novel therapies in CNS injury. The next section discusses the key initiators of neuronal death, followed by a brief discussion of the many cell death effector pathways that have been defined to date.

Autophagy. Autophagy, a term from the Greek that means "self-eating," is a process that mediates normal turnover of cellular constituents, such as organelles and membranes in autophagic vacuoles (39). It is associated with cell death during starvation. However, after ischemia and TBI, disruption of this process may lead to "autophagic stress" with an accumulation of autophagic vacuoles resulting in cell death. The mechanisms by which accumulation of autophagic vacuoles leads to cell death remain unclear, but vacuole overload may enhance vulnerability to injury. This pathway operates in brain ischemia and TBI, and may be able to be inhibited by novel therapies.

Key Initiators

Energy Failure. Energy failure sustained beyond a critical period produces neuronal membrane failure, Na^+ and Ca^{2+} accumulation, K^+ efflux, cellular swelling, and acute failure of organelles such as mitochondria and the endoplasmic reticulum (ER). Increases in intracellular Ca^{2+} mandate its sequestration, notably in mitochondria. Increases in intracellular Ca^{2+} result in mitochondrial dysfunction and ER stress. (See review of mitochondrial failure in CNS injury in reference (40).) Three pathways are involved. First, Ca^{2+} activates several degradative enzymes (including calpain proteases and phospholipases) that modify mitochondrial proteins and lipids. Second, oxidative stress further modifies mitochondrial constituents. Finally, unchecked Ca^{2+} sequestration in mitochondria leads to mitochondrial permeability transition, which involves the formation of a large conductance pore in the inner mitochondrial membrane and produces uncoupling of oxidative phosphorylation, osmotic swelling, release of matrix metabolites, and ultimately, physical rupture. These processes can lead to neuronal necrosis, apoptosis, or mixed cellular phenotypes. Links between mitochondrial failure, excitotoxicity, and oxidative stress likely play a key role, as shown in **Figure 56.6**. Support for this hypothesis includes efficacy for cyclosporine-A in experimental cerebral ischemia and TBI. Cyclosporine-A blocks formation of the mitochondrial permeability transition pore and is neuroprotective in these models when its passage across the blood–brain barrier (BBB) is facilitated.

Parallel mechanisms underlying the role of disturbed Ca^{2+} homeostasis in the evolution of secondary damage after CNS injury involve the ER (41). The ER normally sequesters Ca^{2+}, and the resultant high concentration is important to its normal function in activating enzymes that control protein folding. Ischemia induces Ca^{2+} release from the ER when it is

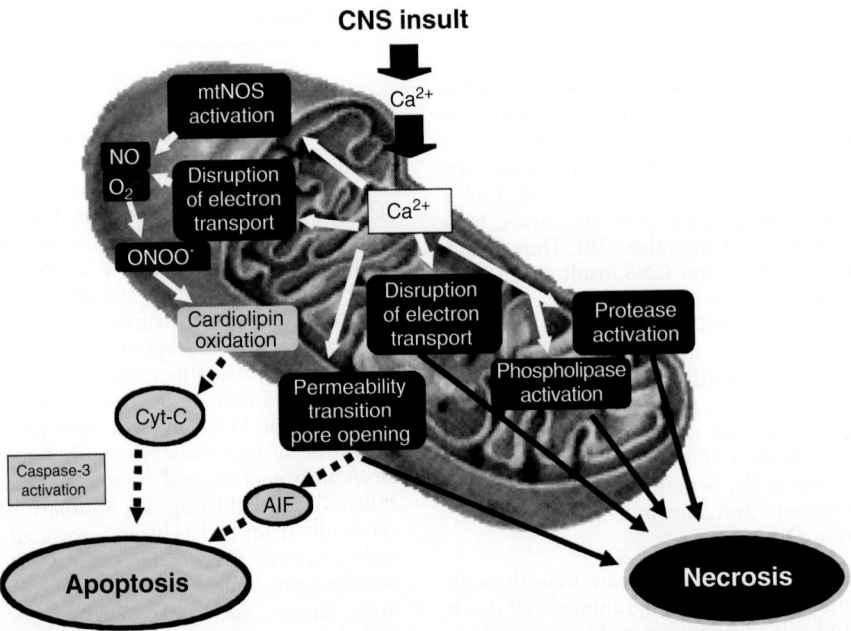

FIGURE 56.6. Mitochondrial cell death pathways resulting from calcium overload. Mitochondrial injury is one of the key pathways leading to either necrotic cell death (as a result of energy failure) or apoptotic cell death (as a result of release of apoptogenic factors [cytochrome-c and AIF] from the mitochondrial membrane), along with death in cells with mixed necrotic and apoptotic phenotypes. mtNOS, mitochondrial nitric oxidase synthase; NO, nitric oxide; O_2^-, superoxide anion; $ONOO^-$, peroxynitrite; Cyt-c, cytochrome-c; AIF, apoptosis-inducing factor.

stimulated by inositol 1,4,5-triphosphate (IP3) or via activation of ryanodine receptors. IP3 is produced in the activation of metabotropic glutamate receptors in the excitotoxic process. Reduced ER Ca^{2+} concentration can trigger apoptosis, as discussed later.

An interesting biochemical finding that appears consistent across PICU-relevant CNS insults is the presence of sustained increases in brain tissue levels of lactate. Clinical studies that use MR spectroscopy have shown that brain tissue lactate levels are increased even at 1–2 weeks after cardiac arrest or TBI in infants and children, with poor outcome (17). The mechanisms involved may include chronic mitochondrial dysfunction/failure, sustained excitotoxicity, occult ischemia, or macrophage accumulation. This finding suggests chronic energy failure.

Excitotoxicity. Excitotoxicity is the process by which glutamate and other EAAs cause neuronal damage. Several cell injury mechanisms are linked to glutamate toxicity, which is also associated with neuronal damage in cardiac arrest, stroke, TBI, epilepsy, CNS infection, and hypoglycemia. Glutamate is the predominant excitatory neurotransmitter in the brain and acts through receptor types that are characterized according to specific EAA agonists. Glutamate levels increase in the brain early after ischemia or TBI as a result of release and/or failure of reuptake (12,42). The three main ionotropic glutamate receptors are the N-methyl-D-aspartate (NMDA), kainate, and α-amino-3-hydroxy-5-methyl-4-isoxazoleproprionic acid (AMPA) receptors. NMDA receptors act primarily by allowing Ca^{2+} influx, both directly and through voltage-gated channels, whereas the non-NMDA receptors mediate Na^+ influx with secondary action on voltage-gated Ca^{2+} channels and reverse action of the Na^+/Ca^{2+} transporter. Glutamate also

acts at metabotropic receptors, which trigger second messenger systems and increase intracellular Ca^{2+} levels by causing a release of intracellular stores. Increased intracellular Ca^{2+} triggers processes that can lead to cellular injury or death, including oxidative and nitrative stress, mitochondrial or ER failure, and activation of Ca^{2+}-dependent proteases. However, it is well known that physiologic levels of glutamate are essential to neuronal survival whereas excessive levels are neurotoxic (31,32). In addition, it is also known that NMDA receptors are localized at both synaptic and extrasynaptic sites, and that at those sites there are NMDA receptor subunits that may have very different roles, namely, the NR2A and NR2B subunits (31). One construct, that has some support, suggests that at synaptic or extrasynaptic sites, activation of NR2A is neuroprotective because it is coupled to activation of the cell survival protein kinase B (PKB), cAMP response element–binding protein (CREB), and extracellular signal–regulated kinase (ERK) pathways (31,32). In contrast, activation of NR2B is neurotoxic related to classical excitotoxicity. Indeed, it has been suggested that developmental differences in these two receptor subtypes may underlie the age-related differences in neuronal vulnerability to anesthetics previously discussed (31). However, it should be recognized that some studies have disputed the specific death versus survival linkage between NR2B and NR2A receptor activation (32) (**Fig. 56.7**). EAAs other than glutamate may also mediate excitotoxicity, and regional effects may depend on the local transmitter systems involved.

Two bodies of evidence link excitotoxicity to secondary brain injury: (a) demonstration of pathologic levels of glutamate after CNS insults at levels that are known to cause cell death in vitro and (b) improvement in outcome with the use of EAA receptor antagonists in experimental models. Increased levels of EAAs in

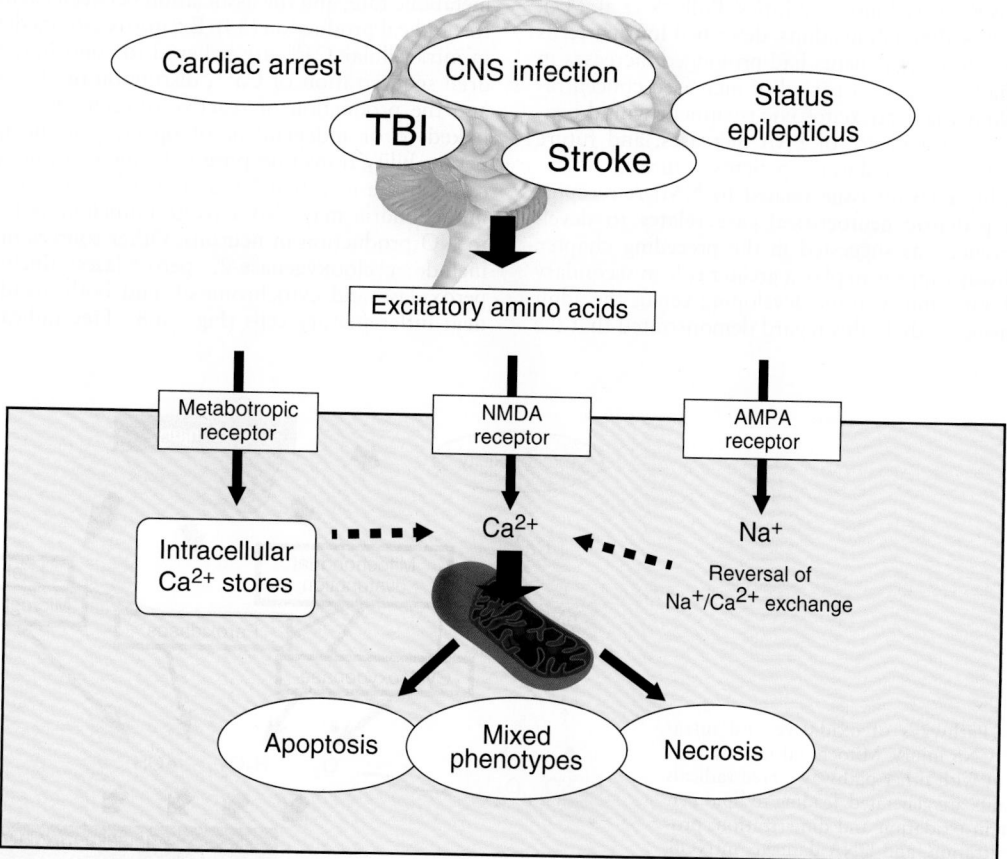

FIGURE 56.7. Receptors and key intracellular events resulting from excitotoxicity in neurons after PICU-relevant CNS insults. TBI, traumatic brain injury; NMDA, N-methyl-D-aspartate; AMPA, α-amino-3-hydroxy-5-methyl-4-isoxazoleproprionic acid.

ventricular CSF from adult patients with TBI were first reported in 1994 (43). Glutamate levels were as high as 7 μM—sufficient to cause neuronal death in cell culture. Other investigators studied CSF and reported a dramatic excitotoxic response to TBI in infants and children (44). Victims of AHT had particularly high and sustained increases in CSF glutamate.

Several therapies have antiexcitotoxic properties, including hypothermia, barbiturates, inhaled anesthetics, calcium channel blockers, and anticonvulsants. Most clinical documentation of the antiexcitotoxic properties of these therapies has been in patients with severe TBI. In adults with severe TBI, researchers used intracerebral microdialysis and reported that induction of barbiturate coma was associated with a 59% reduction of glutamate and a 37% reduction of lactate concentration (45). Adults with severe TBI had lower CSF levels of glutamate when treated with 24 hours of hypothermia (32°C) versus normothermia (46). It remains unclear if the antiexcitotoxic properties of these agents confer benefit. Other contemporary drugs that have specific actions on glutamate physiology have been developed, including NMDA- and AMPA receptor antagonists, glutamate release inhibitors, NMDA channel blockers, NMDA glycine-site antagonists (glycine is a co-agonist at the NMDA receptor), magnesium (which regulates NMDA receptor activation), and gamma-amino butyric acid (GABA) agonists (which reduce glutamate release). More recently, selective antagonists of the NR2B receptor have been studied, such as Ro-25-6981 (31).

Although excitotoxicity is important after cardiac arrest, stroke, and TBI, differences exist that likely influence the effect of therapies. Excitotoxic damage seems to be largely mediated by NMDA receptor stimulation after stroke and TBI. However, clinical trials have been performed to evaluate glutamate antagonists after stroke and TBI in adults, and none have proven successful. A limitation to studies of antiexcitotoxic therapies in human TBI is the variability of injuries. Bullock et al. (47), using microdialysis after TBI in adults, described four patterns of EAAs. Although many patients had prolonged increases in EAAs, others had only a brief period of increased concentrations. It is unlikely that antiexcitotoxic treatment would benefit patients without evidence of EAA increases, and future trials may need to be tailored to the patients' injuries.

Another highly relevant issue related to NMDA receptor antagonists in pediatric neurocritical care relates to developmental differences, as suggested in the preceding chapter. Apoptotic pathways appear to play a greater role in secondary neuronal death after injury in the developing versus the adult brain. A promising study in this regard demonstrated that the combination of xenon gas (an NMDA antagonist) with mild hypothermia was highly effective in preventing damage after a hypoxic–ischemic insult in developing rat pups (48). Some caution may be in order, as apoptotic neuronal degeneration was seen in neonatal rats and primates after treatment with NMDA antagonists (49–51). Whether strategies such as selective NR2B receptor blockade could allow antiexcitotoxic benefit to be facilitated without exacerbating apoptotic neuronal death remains to be determined. Also, this issue could have important implications to the neurocritical care of infants in the PICU both after neurologic insults and in routine sedation for other disease processes. This represents an active and extremely important area of current research.

Contrasting stroke and TBI, AMPA receptor antagonists have been suggested to represent an effective antiexcitotoxic strategy after experimental global ischemia. However, in a model of neonatal asphyxia in newborn piglets, the AMPA antagonist 2,3-dihydroxy-6-nitro-7-sulfamoyl-benzo[f]quinoxaline-2,3-dione (NBQX) was detrimental rather than efficacious, suggesting developmental differences (52). Inhibition of plasticity by antiexcitotoxic therapies may also limit their efficacy, especially during subacute periods. If antiexcitotoxic therapies are shown to be efficacious in clinical CNS injury, it is likely to be with early application.

Oxidative Stress. Free radicals are generated during normal cerebral metabolism, with the normal reducing environment being maintained by a myriad of endogenous antioxidant systems. After cardiac arrest, stroke, TBI, and in CNS infection, a number of biochemical pathways contribute to a marked increase in free radical production. Oxidative stress-mediated injury is of heightened importance in the CNS because of the high level of polyunsaturation of lipids, high metabolic rate, and the association between excitotoxicity and free radical production (53). Excitotoxicity-mediated increases in intracellular Ca^{2+} are believed to contribute to mitochondrial sequestration of Ca^{2+}, disruption of electron transport, and the production of reactive oxygen species (ROS) either linked to or independent of opening of the mitochondrial permeability transition pore (54). Increases in cytosolic Ca^{2+} can activate neuronal NOS. Similarly, Ca^{2+} sequestration by mitochondria may also activate mitochondrial NOS, leading to NO production in neurons. Other sources of free radicals include cyclooxygenase-2, peroxidases (including myeloperoxidase and cytochrome-c), and both invading and resident inflammatory cells (**Fig. 56.8**). Free radicals cause lipid

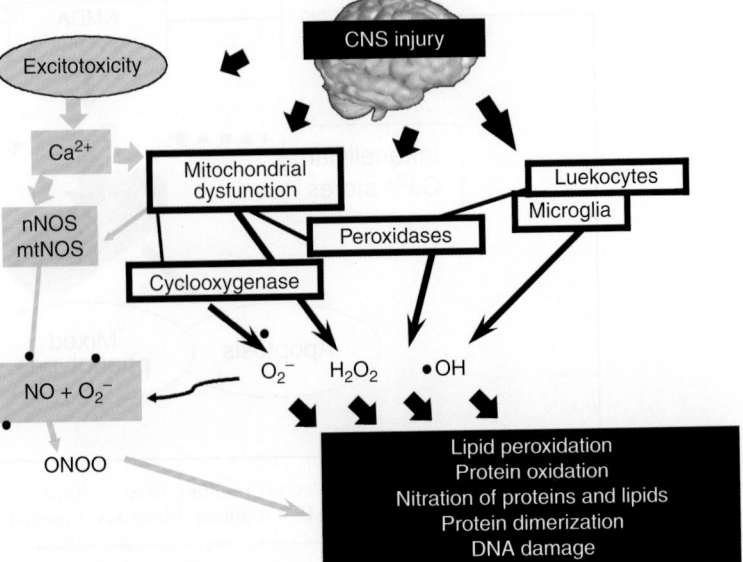

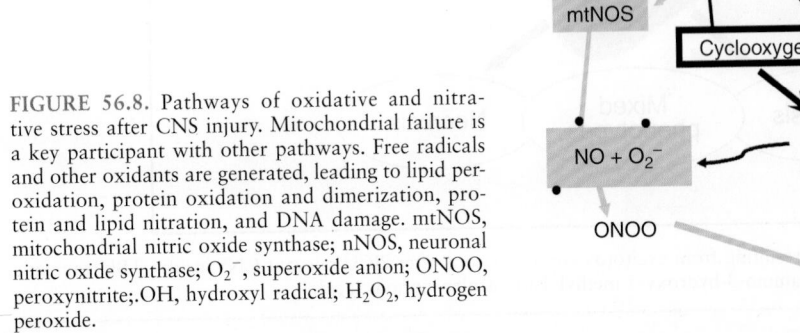

FIGURE 56.8. Pathways of oxidative and nitrative stress after CNS injury. Mitochondrial failure is a key participant with other pathways. Free radicals and other oxidants are generated, leading to lipid peroxidation, protein oxidation and dimerization, protein and lipid nitration, and DNA damage. mtNOS, mitochondrial nitric oxide synthase; nNOS, neuronal nitric oxide synthase; O_2^-, superoxide anion; ONOO, peroxynitrite; .OH, hydroxyl radical; H_2O_2, hydrogen peroxide.

peroxidation, protein and DNA oxidation, protein dimerization, and activation of transcription factors with dysregulation of neuronal homeostasis. Free radicals can be grouped into ROS and reactive nitrogen species. ROS include superoxide anion, hydrogen peroxide, and hydroxyl radicals, the latter of which is highly reactive with almost every molecule in living cells. Among the reactive nitrogen species is NO, which is lipid soluble and readily crosses cell membranes. NO reacts with other free radicals and can inhibit lipid peroxidation and, in some settings, act as an endogenous antioxidant. However, the reaction of NO with superoxide anion leads to peroxynitrite formation, a highly reactive radical species that can produce lipid, protein, and DNA nitration. The final oxidation product of NO is nitrite, which is increased in the CSF of children with acute bacterial meningitis (55) and in adults after severe TBI and is associated with injury severity and death.

Oxidative stress may serve as a key initiator of cell death cascades in cardiac arrest, stroke, TBI, epilepsy, and CNS infection. Oxidation of the abundant mitochondrial lipid cardiolipin leads to the release of cytochrome-c from the mitochondrial membrane and may serve as a seminal event that links oxidative stress and the intrinsic pathway of apoptosis (56,57). DNA damage from peroxynitrite in both the nucleus and mitochondria may also serve to activate the enzyme poly(ADP-ribose) polymerase (PARP), which can result in energy failure via the PARP-mediated cellular suicide pathway.

CNS insults are associated with evidence of free radical production and loss of antioxidant defenses. After experimental asphyxia, decreases are seen in a variety of antioxidants, including ascorbate, glutathione, thiols, and α-tocopherol in hippocampus at 10 minutes after reperfusion (58). In experimental cardiac arrest, hyperoxic resuscitation plays a critical role in the level of oxidative stress (59). Oxidation of the key enzyme pyruvate dehydrogenase was dramatic, with resuscitation on F$_{IO_2}$ of 1.0 but minimal after room air resuscitation, and a beneficial effect on hippocampal neuronal death was seen with room air resuscitation. Hyperoxia has been recently shown to be associated with unfavorable outcome after cardiac arrest in adults (60). Marked depletion of endogenous antioxidants, including ascorbate, glutathione, protein thiols, and total antioxidant reserve, was seen in the CSF from infants and children with severe TBI (61). A novel mitochondrial-targeting antioxidant strategy recently demonstrated marked benefit in an experimental model of TBI in developing rat pups (57). Studies on experimental cerebral ischemia indicate that mild hypothermia blocks cytochrome-c release (62). Finally, increases in the concentrations of markers of oxidative stress in CSF have also been reported in infants and children with both acute bacterial meningitis and seizures (55,63).

Trophic Factor Withdrawal. Another important trigger for neuronal death is trophic factor withdrawal, and this process likely has relevance in the evolution of secondary damage after CNS insults in pediatric neurointensive care. Neurotrophins, such as nerve growth factor, brain-derived neurotrophic factor, basic fibroblast growth factor, and others, are constitutively produced by neurons and glia, bind to receptors on target neurons, and are essential to survival and plasticity. Loss of trophic input to a target neuron via death of, or damage to, neuronal input from another brain region can trigger death of the target neurons. This process has been reported in experimental CNS injury models and is often manifest by apoptotic death of neurons in a brain region remote from the injury site at several days after injury. Neuronal death is mediated by loss of endogenous neuroprotectant signals, such as phosphoinositide 3-kinase (PI3K) and PKB, which are otherwise constitutively produced. The details of these pathways are discussed in the section Cellular Signaling Pathways in this chapter.

❺ Neuronal Death Effector Pathways. In mature tissues, PCD requires initiation by either intracellular or extracellular signals. These signals have been characterized in vitro and are becoming better characterized in vivo (12,42,64,65) (**Fig. 56.9**).

Intrinsic (Mitochondrial) Pathway of Apoptosis. Intracellular signaling appears to be initiated in mitochondria, triggered by disturbances in cellular homeostasis, such as ATP depletion, oxidative stress, or calcium fluxes. Mitochondrial dysfunction leads to egress of cytochrome-c from the inner mitochondrial membrane into the cytosol. As discussed, oxidation of the mitochondrial lipid cardiolipin appears to play an important role in cytochrome-c release (56). Cytochrome-c release can be blocked by antiapoptotic members of the bcl-2 family (bcl-2, bcl-XL, Mcl-1) and promoted by proapoptotic bcl-2 family members (bax, bad, bid) (65). Cytochrome-c in the presence of dATP and a specific apoptotic protease–activating factor (Apaf-1) in cytosol activates the initiator cysteine protease caspase-9. Caspase-9 then activates the effector cysteine protease caspase-3, a key apoptosis effector that cleaves cytoskeletal proteins, DNA repair proteins, and activators of endonucleases (64). Evidence that supports a role for this pathway can be found across CNS insults, including global and focal ischemia, TBI, meningitis, and SE (65–69). Caspase inhibitors and mild hypothermia can attenuate neuronal death in experimental paradigms across these CNS insults (62,65,70).

Apoptosis-inducing Factor Pathway. An additional intracellular cascade of PCD linked to mitochondrial injury is the apoptosis-inducing factor (AIF) pathway (65). This caspase-independent pathway is activated by mitochondrial permeability transition and results in the release of AIF from the mitochondrial membrane. AIF release leads to large-scale DNA fragmentation (50–700 Kbp in size). The AIF pathway is activated in experimental ischemia and TBI. A unique pathway for the induction of neuronal death via AIF release has been reported in experimental pneumococcal meningitis. This organism releases the toxin pneumolysin, which creates membrane pores in lipid bilayers and triggers AIF release (71). To date, specific pharmacologic inhibitors of this pathway are lacking; however, this form of delayed neuronal death may represent an important therapeutic target.

Endoplasmic Reticulum Stress-triggered Apoptosis. Another intracellular pathway that can trigger apoptosis independent of mitochondrial failure is through synthesis of unique proapoptotic factors associated with ER stress. The aforementioned reduction in ER Ca^{2+} concentration that results from IP3-mediated Ca^{2+} release from the ER leads to induction of proteins such as CCAAT/enhancer-binding protein homologous protein (CHOP) in neurons, which mediate apoptosis (72). Although additional details of this pathway remain to be clarified, selectively vulnerable CA1 hippocampal neurons are rich in IP3 receptors.

Extrinsic Pathway Apoptosis. Extracellular signaling of apoptosis occurs through the tumor necrosis factor (TNF) superfamily of cell surface death receptors, which include TNFR1 and Fas/Apo1/CD95 (reviewed in 65). Receptor–ligand binding of TNFR1-TNF-α or Fas-Fas-L promotes formation of a trimeric complex of TNF- or Fas-associated death domains, respectively. These death domains facilitate caspase recruitment. The proximity of multiple caspases (in this case, caspase-8) allows for activation of the effector cysteine protease, followed by activation of caspase-3, where the mitochondrial and cell death receptor pathways converge. Clinical studies suggest that this mechanism may play a role in stroke and TBI. Fas and caspase-8 levels are increased in human cerebral contusions (73). Caspase-8 was seen predominantly in neurons.

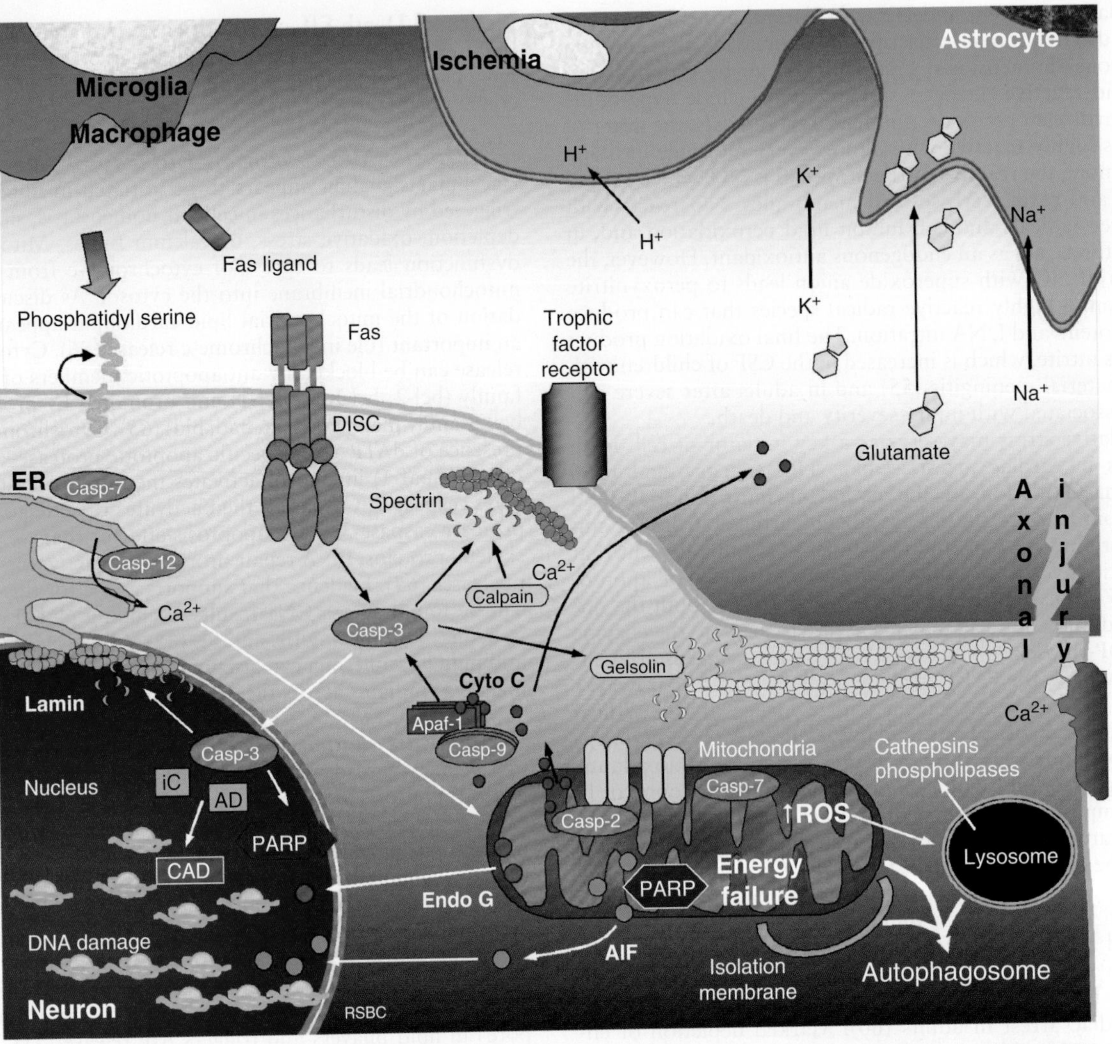

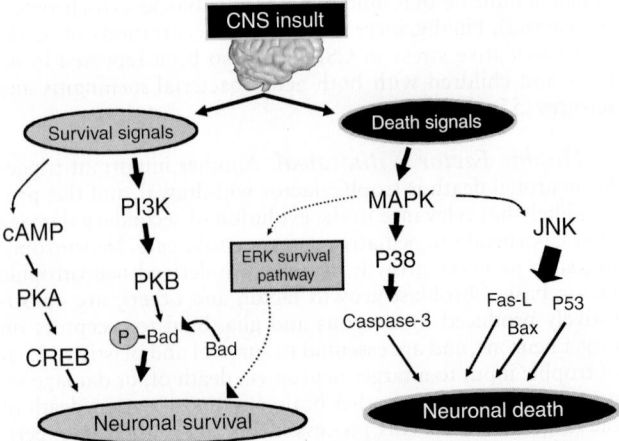

FIGURE 56.9. Neuronal death cascades resulting from necrosis, apoptosis (intrinsic, extrinsic, and apoptosis-inducing factor [AIF] pathways), and autophagy in CNS injury. Also see references 25, 42, and 65 for additional details. ER, endoplasmic reticulum; Casp, caspase; CAD, caspase-activated deoxyribonuclease; Endo G, endonuclease G; ROS, reactive oxygen species; PARP, poly(ADP-ribose) polymerase; DISC, death-inducing signaling complex; iC/AC, inhibitor of caspase-activated deoxyribonuclease.

Cellular Signaling Pathways. Neurotrophic factors, neurotransmitters, cytokines, and ROS activate multiple upstream signaling pathways linked to either pro-survival or pro-death activities (42). These receptors couple to signal transduction pathways, involving interactions and cross talk between multiple serine/threonine and tyrosine protein kinase cascades. Many kinases involved in the cell death process are serine/threonine protein kinases. Important participants in the cell death cascades include the mitogen-activated protein kinases (MAPKs). MAPK cascades are complex and are mediated by successive protein kinases that sequentially activate each other by phosphorylation. They are linked to two key components of the cell death cascade: c-Jun kinase (JNK) and p38 MAPK (**Fig. 56.10**). JNK and p38 MAPK pathways activate caspase-3 (74). Activation of JNK leads to induction of pro-death genes, including Fas-L. The JNK increases p53 and Bax levels, which increase cell death. JNK and p38 function in different stress-signaling pathways, and both target similar nuclear transcription factors that can be activated by pro-death stimuli such as ROS (75). Studies in various injury models have documented changes in both JNK and p38 MAPK that may be related to cell death and functional impairment. MAPKs are also linked to survival signals through the ERK pathway, highlighting the complex cross talk between these cascades.

FIGURE 56.10. Cell survival and death signals in CNS injury. The protein kinase A and B pathways are associated with neuronal survival, while the MAPK pathway is associated generally with neuronal death. cAMP, cyclic adenosine monophosphate; PKA, protein kinase A; CREB, cAMP response element–binding protein; PI3K, phosphoinositide 3-kinase; JNK, c-Jun kinase; Fas-L, Fas ligand; ERK, extracellular signal–regulated kinase.

Several protein kinase cascades have a major survival role (**Fig. 56.10**). PI3-K, PKB, and protein kinase A (PKA) pathways are prototypic examples. PKB is also called akt; the complex nomenclature of these kinases has evolved across many disease processes. PI3K responds to neurotrophins and other prosurvival signals and activates PKB (76); PKB affects survival by a number of mechanisms, including the phosphorylation and inactivation of several pro-death mediators such as Bad. Bad, a member of the Bcl-2 family, is phosphorylated by PKB, resulting in Bad dissociation from Bcl-XL and binding to 14-3-3 proteins (a family of phosphoserine-binding molecules involved in survival signaling), thereby inhibiting cell death (77). cAMP-mediated activation of PKA can also lead to formation of the transcription factor CREB, which is similarly associated with cell survival (78). Survival signals are exemplified by growth factors, cytokines, hormones, cell–cell interactions, and extracellular matrix adhesion molecules. Of course, inactivation of two pro-death members of the MAPK family, p38 and JNK/stress activated protein kinase (SAPK), has also been proposed as promoting survival by extracellular stimuli. Finally, activation of some PKC isoforms by PI3K can transduce pro-death signals, again highlighting the complexity of these kinase cascades. Thus, complex but important kinase pathways control neuronal death and plasticity. Recently, moderate hypothermia has been shown to preserve PKB activity in the brain after experimental cerebral ischemia (79), suggesting that this may mediate hypothermic neuroprotection. Further insight into these cascades may lead to the development of new therapies. As previously discussed, NR2A receptor activation appears to be coupled to these neuronal survival pathways.

Poly(ADP-Ribose) Polymerase Activation. Research has uncovered a unique cell death pathway related to activation of the enzyme PARP that plays a role in neuronal death in ischemia and TBI (80, reviewed in 11). PARP is found in both mitochondria and the nucleus and plays a homeostatic role in DNA repair in these two organelles. When activated by DNA damage, PARP catalytically adds poly(ADP-ribose) units onto proteins in mitochondria and the nucleus, such as histones, to help direct DNA repair enzymes to sites of damage. However, a deleterious consequence of PARP activation in CNS injury is the consumption of large quantities of nicotine adenine dinucleotide (NAD), thus depleting mitochondrial energy stores. This paradoxic consequence of PARP activation has been labeled the "PARP cell suicide theory" and leads to mitochondrial failure and cell death, from either overwhelming energy failure or delayed neuronal death through release of cytochrome-c and/or AIF. This pathway may have clinical relevance, as PARP knockout mice are highly protected from neuronal damage in experimental models of stroke and TBI (80, reviewed in 11).

Protease Activation. In addition to the many consequences of Ca^{2+} homeostasis loss that have been discussed, increase in intracellular Ca^{2+} in neurons activates calpain proteases, which sets into motion a cascade of protease activation that has been referred to as the "calpain–cathepsin cascade" (81). Calpains (both mu and m isozymes) are located in dendritic regions and in axons and, when activated, cleave key cytoskeletal targets, such as spectrin, kinases, phosphatases, membrane receptors, and, importantly, lysosomes. Lysosomal rupture, believed to be mediated in part by calpains, leads to release of over 80 hydrolytic enzymes, of which cathepsins B, D, H, and L are believed to play a role in executing neuronal death. These pathways could have special importance in necrotic cascades. As discussed, failure or dysfunction of lysosomal degradation pathways may lead to an accumulation of autophagic vacuoles and result in cell death by autophagy.

Necroptosis. Recently, a novel form of programmed neuronal necrosis was discovered that has been called necroptosis.

In this pathway, TNF-α or Fas can activate necrosis, as evidenced by loss of neuronal membrane integrity, via a receptor-mediated process (82). This novel neuronal death pathway can be inhibited by the drug necrostatin, which has been shown to confer benefit in experimental TBI (82).

Endogenous Neuroprotectant Pathways. Studies have begun to define, in infants and children with CNS injury, the endogenous retaliatory response to these ischemic and excitotoxic insults. Due to space constraints, we focus here on selected examples of this cascade. The most extensive amount of clinical work on these pathways has been conducted in TBI (12,42) (**Fig. 56.2**).

Adenosine is an endogenous neuroprotectant produced in response to both ischemia and excitotoxicity. Adenosine antagonizes a number of events thought to mediate neuronal death (12). Breakdown of ATP leads to formation of adenosine, a purine nucleoside that decreases neuronal metabolism and increases CBF, among other mechanisms. Adenosine binding to A_1 receptors decreases excitation by increasing K^+ and Cl^- and decreasing Ca^{2+} conductances in the neuronal membrane. A_1 receptors are located on neurons in brain regions that are susceptible to injury (e.g., hippocampus) and are spatially associated with NMDA receptors. Thus, released adenosine minimizes excitotoxicity. Binding of adenosine to A_2 receptors (on cerebrovascular smooth muscle) causes vasodilation, although binding to A_{2a} receptors on neurons may be detrimental. In clinical studies, marked increases in CSF levels of adenosine have been shown in children with severe TBI, and brain interstitial levels of adenosine in adults with TBI were seen during episodes of jugular venous desaturation (secondary insults), thus supporting a role of adenosine as a "retaliatory" metabolite (12). Adenosine A_1 receptor knockout mice develop lethal SE after experimental TBI, supporting an endogenous neuroprotectant effect (83).

Another endogenous neuroprotectant is heat shock protein 70 (HSP70), which is induced as part of the classic preconditioning response in brain and is increased in both CSF and brain tissue after severe TBI in children (42). HSP70 is believed to play an important role in optimizing protein folding as a molecular chaperone. It also inhibits proinflammatory signaling.

Bcl-2 is an important endogenous inhibitor of PCD in vitro (42). It is induced in experimental TBI and reduces cortical tissue loss. Bcl-2 is increased in injured brain after severe TBI in children (12). CSF levels of bcl-2 were increased approximately fourfold in TBI patients and associated with survival. Recent studies also suggest that nitrite may be a powerful cytoprotective molecule. Hypoxia-dependent bioactivation of nitrite reduces it to NO, S-nitrosothiols, N-nitrosamines, and iron-nitrosylated heme proteins within 1–30 minutes of reperfusion. These mediators appear to confer their protective effects on a number of systems (84). Thus, the brain mounts an important endogenous defense response to injury. Therapies designed to augment these pathways deserve further study.

Brain Injury without Neuronal Death

It would be remiss to suggest that neuronal death is required for insults relevant to pediatric neurointensive care to produce important or even permanent impairment of neurologic function. Several processes that result from injury may lead to substantial functional impairments without cell death. These include synaptic damage, disturbances in cell signaling and glial–neuronal cross talk, and alterations in neurotransmitter balance. Although these mechanisms are of principal importance to cognitive dysfunction in mild TBI, they are likely operating in damaged brain regions in severe TBI and may contribute to impaired recovery. For example, substantial synaptic loss in injured hippocampus and fiber degeneration remote from the impact has been reported in experimental models of TBI (85,86). These mechanisms may represent novel therapeutic targets in both the acute and chronic phases after injury. It is possible that these types of damage may be highly responsive to therapeutic interventions.

Brain Swelling

A unifying concept in brain injury is the occurrence of brain swelling. Cerebral swelling invariably develops, resulting from edema and/or increased cerebral blood volume (CBV), and can contribute to secondary ischemia from raised ICP, local compression, or the devastating consequences of herniation, as discussed in Chapter 61 (Traumatic Brain Injury). Brain edema develops via three mechanisms: cellular swelling, BBB injury (vasogenic edema) (11,12,42,64), and/or osmolar swelling (**Fig. 56.11**).

Cellular Swelling

Astrocyte Swelling. Cellular swelling, a term that has supplanted the traditional "cytotoxic edema," occurs predominantly in astrocyte foot processes and is less representative of a "toxic" rather than a homeostatic or mediator-driven process. For example, astrocyte-mediated reuptake of glutamate from the extracellular space is coupled to Na^+ and water accumulation. Similarly, acidosis, K^+, cytokines, and arachidonic acid mediate astrocyte swelling. The traditional concept of cytotoxic edema in neurons resulting from energy failure (the pump-leak model) is incomplete. Both perivascular and perineuronal astrocytes are involved (see Chapter 55). Cellular swelling is an important form of brain edema across insults but particularly so in ischemia and TBI. Cellular swelling may predominate after secondary insults. Using a model of diffuse TBI in rats, diffusion-weighted MRI was used to localize the increase in brain water (87). A decrease in the apparent diffusion coefficient after injury suggested predominantly cellular swelling, rather than vasogenic edema, in the development of intracranial hypertension.

Aquaporins. An additional molecular aspect of brain edema formation germane to astrocyte swelling that has recently been uncovered is the role of endogenous water channels called *aquaporins*. Aquaporins 1–9 represent a ubiquitous family of water channels that are integral membrane proteins that serve as water transport pathways. For example, aquaporin-1 is involved in membrane transport of water across osmotic gradients, while aquaporins 4 and 9 are localized in astrocyte end-feet. Aquaporins also play an important role in production of CSF. Aquaporin-1 knockout mice had markedly reduced ICP and improved survival after experimental brain injury (88). Astrocyte swelling may also play an important role in the pathogenesis of brain edema in CNS infections. Studies in experimental meningitis have shown marked swelling of astrocyte foot processes that is mediated by aquaporin-4 (89). Aquaporin-4 knockout mice exhibited substantially lower brain water content and ICP versus wild-type mice in experimental pneumococcal meningitis, supporting an important contribution of cellular swelling and water movement across the BBB even in meningitis. Thus, these water channels may represent a key new therapeutic target for control of raised ICP after TBI, ischemia, and CNS infections.

Vasogenic Edema

BBB permeability, with resultant vasogenic edema, can also contribute to secondary brain swelling; this is particularly true in CNS infections (90), stroke and, to some extent, in TBI. This mechanism is likely of less importance after cardiac arrest, although some studies of cardiac arrest in developing animals have suggested a role for BBB injury (91). Unfortunately, clinical study of BBB permeability in pediatric neurointensive care has been limited.

In acute bacterial meningitis, the acute inflammatory cascade also contributes to BBB damage and includes cytokine-mediated induction of leukocyte adhesion molecules, neutrophil accumulation, and related oxidative injury

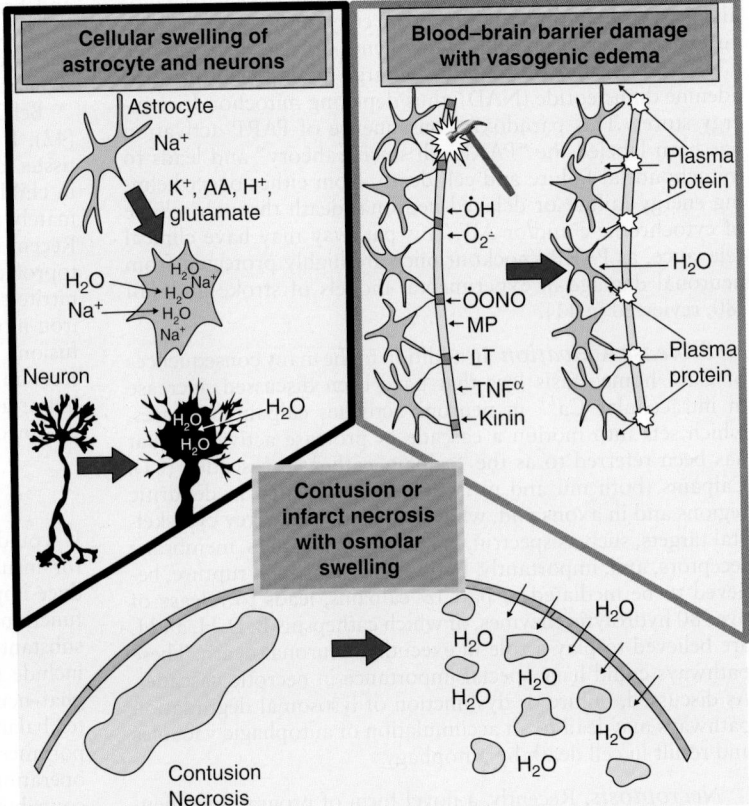

FIGURE 56.11. Three major mechanisms underlying the development of cerebral edema, including cellular swelling, BBB injury with vasogenic edema, and osmolar swelling that develops in both contusions and infarcts. AA, arachidonic acid; O_2^-, superoxide anion; ONOO, peroxynitrite; OH, hydroxyl radical; MP, metalloproteinase; LT, leukotriene; TNF-α, tumor necrosis factor α.

to vascular endothelium (90). In addition, an important role for matrix metalloproteinases (MMPs) has been reported in experimental meningitis. MMPs are endoproteases that can degrade the extracellular matrix. CSF levels of MMPs were markedly upregulated and associated with poor outcome in children with acute bacterial meningitis (92). Similar increases in MMPs were not seen in viral meningitis (93). Hyaluronidase and pneumolysin also contribute to endothelial damage and BBB permeability.

Osmolar Swelling. A mechanism that appears to contribute greatly to the development of edema, particularly in TBI, is osmolar swelling in areas of contusion necrosis. Ironically, reconstitution of the injured BBB and/or development of an osmolar barrier around a necrotic focus may contribute to marked focal edema as the local osmolar load of the tissue increases, as macromolecules are degraded to constituents. This mechanism has been shown in adult TBI (94) and likely represents one of the underpinnings for the beneficial effects of osmolar therapy in the setting of cerebral contusion (**Fig. 56.12**). Osmolar swelling also likely underlies the development of compromising or potentially fatal mass lesions in the evolution of hemispheric stroke.

Mixed Edema Pictures. Vasogenic edema, cellular swelling from glutamate and hydrogen ion (H^+) uptake and opening of aquaporin channels, and tissue swelling from increased local osmolality all lead to brain edema in TBI. In asphyxial cardiac arrest, it is probably astrocyte swelling and vasogenic edema that predominate. In stroke, all three of these mechanisms likely operate, depending on the timing and location. For example, in stroke, early astrocyte swelling may occur in the infarct core, followed by vasogenic edema in injured but perfused penumbral regions, and then delayed osmolar swelling of the infarct as the macromolecules are degraded. In meningitis, vasogenic edema and cellular swelling likely contribute.

Cerebral Blood Volume. A role of increased CBV in brain swelling has long been suggested (12), particularly in pediatric brain injury. However, this notion was challenged in a comprehensive study in adult patients with severe TBI (95). Brain tissue water was increased in 76 adults with severe TBI; however, CBV was generally reduced. It is possible that increases in CBV contribute to secondary cerebral swelling in some patients; however, based on this study, the predominant mechanism of posttraumatic brain swelling is most likely edema rather than vascular engorgement. Similar studies should be conducted in children in pediatric neurointensive care, as hyperemia has been suggested to play a greater role in pediatric versus adult brain injury (12). A role for hyperemia in the pathogenesis of cerebral swelling in meningitis is controversial but is suggested in some studies. When an increase in CBV is seen after CNS injury, it may contribute to raised ICP and result from local increases in cerebral glycolysis—"hyperglycolysis" (an absolute increase in glucose metabolism by two standard deviations or a relative increase in glucose metabolism compared to a decreased oxygen metabolic rate) (96). In regions with increases in glutamate levels, such as in contusions, increased glycolysis is seen because astrocyte uptake of glutamate is coupled to glucose utilization. Hyperglycolysis may also mediate a coupled increase in CBF and CBV and resultant local brain swelling. As glutamate uptake by astrocytes is coupled to Na^+ and water uptake, local cellular swelling is also seen (**Fig. 56.13**).

Additional clinical studies of brain swelling, BBB permeability, and CBV are needed in infants and children with critical CNS insults. Also, as MRI and MR spectroscopy methods continue to develop and become applied to critically ill patients, our knowledge of the mechanisms involved in cerebral swelling should greatly advance. Although neuronal death is the key downstream event in insults relevant to pediatric neurointensive care, brain swelling (and the resultant raised ICP) is still the principal target for titration of therapy.

Inflammation and Regeneration

Except in the setting of CNS infections, inflammation traditionally was thought to be limited in the brain, as it was considered an immunologically privileged organ. However, that notion has changed greatly over the past 20 years. Currently, three major components are involved in the CNS inflammatory response to PICU-relevant insults: leukocytes, microglia, and regeneration. Contributions to secondary damage in the evolution of injury can be mediated by circulating leukocytes in the inflammatory response. However, an endogenous inflammatory response mediated by microglia—the macrophages of the CNS—along with neurons and astrocytes has been recognized. Finally, the inflammatory response appears to have a delayed beneficial role, across insults, in the signaling of regenerative processes and neurogenesis. The contribution of each of these

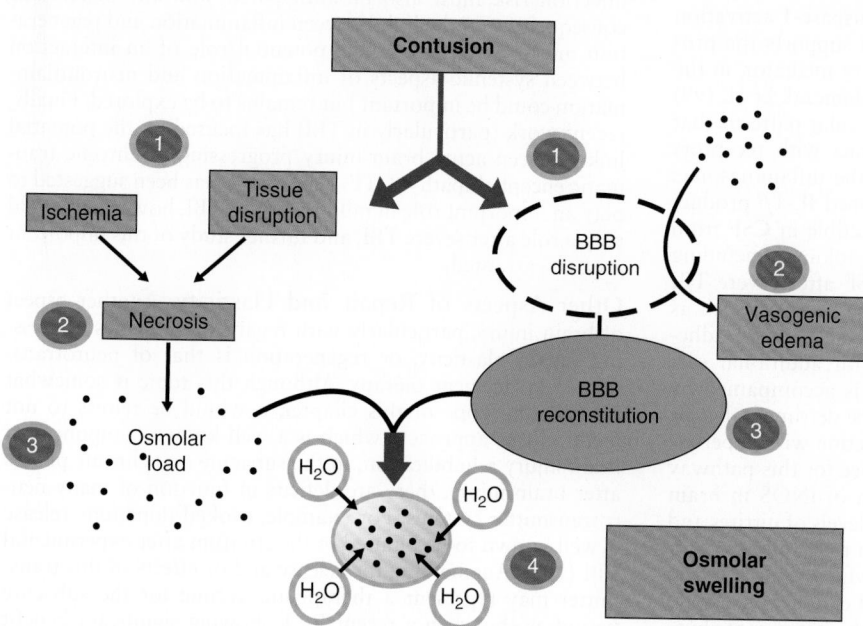

FIGURE 56.12. Temporal pathway involved in osmolar swelling in brain contusions or infarcts. Temporal profile shown by numbers 1–4. Necrotic brain regions generate a large osmolar load as they are degraded to constituent molecules. Early after the insult, BBB damage allows influx of additional proteins. With time, usually within 24–72 hours, an osmolar barrier re-forms, and water is then osmotically drawn from the surrounding brain regions into the contused or infarcted area, resulting in expansion of the mass lesion, an event often appreciated on follow-up CT of the head in affected patients. BBB, blood–brain barrier.

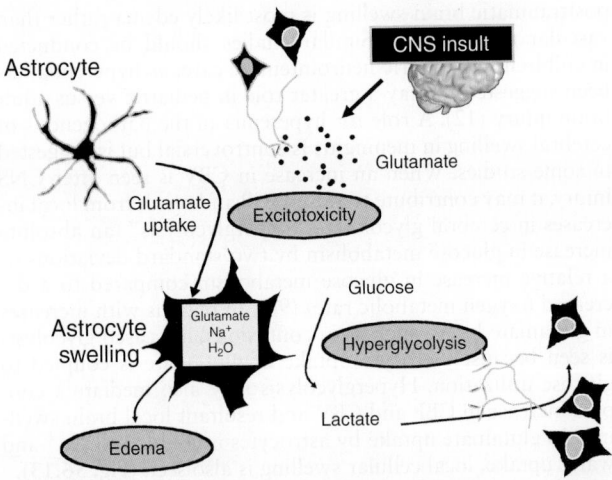

FIGURE 56.13. Cartoon depicting the phenomenon of "hyperglycolysis" and its potential relationship to brain swelling. In injured brain regions, astrocyte uptake of glutamate is coupled to Na$^+$ and water uptake and resultant astrocyte swelling. This process is exclusively dependent on glucose utilization by astrocytes, with local lactate generation. This lactate either may serve as a fuel for neurons or is washed out. If this local increase in glucose utilization is coupled to perfusion, it can result in an increase in CBV and thus exacerbate brain swelling by two mechanisms—astrocyte swelling and increased CBV.

components to the evolution of damage and recovery appears to vary importantly with the specific insult.

Role of Inflammation in Secondary Injury. CNS infections are associated with robust acute inflammation, as discussed previously in the section on vasogenic edema. However, the inflammatory process also makes important contributions in stroke and TBI (12,42,97). Nuclear factor (NF)-κB activation, TNF-α, IL-1β, eicosanoids, neutrophils, and macrophages contribute to both secondary damage and repair. Clinical evidence for inflammatory cascade participation in PICU-relevant CNS injury has been shown best in TBI. Consistent with a role for IL-1β in the evolution of tissue damage in human TBI, Western analysis was performed on brain samples surgically resected from adults with refractory raised ICP secondary to severe contusion (98). Caspase-1 was activated, as evidenced by specific cleavage in patients with TBI. Caspase-1 activation is critical to the production of IL-1β. This supports the production of IL-1β, a pivotal proinflammatory mediator, in the injured brain in humans. More recently, Adamczak et al. (99) demonstrated that damage-associated molecular patterns that initiate the innate immune response interact with receptors that form a multiprotein complex called the inflammasome, which ultimately leads to the aforementioned IL-1β production, and that this pathway is readily detectible in CSF from adults with severe TBI. A number of cytokines, including IL-6, IL-8, and IL-10, also increase in CSF after severe TBI in children (12). Contusion and local tissue necrosis, such as infarction in stroke, trigger upregulation of leukocyte adhesion molecules and neutrophil influx, with additional secondary tissue damage. Neutrophil influx is accompanied by increases in brain iNOS levels which can be detrimental early after injury via NO production and its reaction with superoxide anion to produce peroxynitrite. Evidence for this pathway in the human brain includes upregulation of iNOS in brain tissue in stroke (100) and increases in CSF levels of nitrites and nitrates after TBI. Macrophage infiltration then follows, with activation of resident microglia, both of which peak between 24 and 72 hours (12). The circulating and endogenous, acute and subacute, inflammatory processes in the brain contribute

to oxidative and nitrative stress and protease activation, with resultant BBB and neuronal injury.

The contribution of inflammation to injury due to cardiac arrest is more speculative. Traditional inflammatory pathways, such as leukocyte influx, do not appear to play an important role. However, endogenous inflammatory pathways may be important. NF-κB is activated in selectively vulnerable CA1 neurons after experimental global cerebral ischemia (101), and administration of an NF-κB decoy attenuates neuronal damage. However, hippocampal neurons from mice that lack the p50 subunit of NF-κB show enhanced excitotoxic injury (102), suggesting a protective role. Similarly, although TNF-α is rapidly upregulated in mouse hippocampus after transient global cerebral ischemia, TNF-α gene–deficient mice do not have reduced damage (69).

Role of Inflammation in Repair and Regeneration. As indicated, possible beneficial aspects of inflammation have been observed in the CNS, particularly during the subacute or chronic injury phases. Two prototypic examples of the biphasic role of inflammation in CNS injury are seen when examining the role of TNF-α in experimental TBI (103). Mice deficient in TNF-α exhibit reduced brain edema and improved functional outcome (vs. wild type) early after TBI, supporting a detrimental role of this proinflammatory cytokine early after injury. However, the long-term consequences of TNF-α deficiency on functional and histologic outcome are detrimental, supporting a beneficial role for TNF-α in recovery and repair. For TNF-α, the transition from a beneficial to detrimental role occurs between 2 and 7 days after injury. Similarly, despite a detrimental role for iNOS early after cerebral ischemia (104), iNOS-deficient mice show impaired long-term outcome, versus controls, in experimental TBI (12). iNOS is important in neurogenesis and wound healing (105).

Regeneration and plasticity play important roles in mediating beneficial long-term effects on recovery, and these responses are linked to inflammation. Macrophage infiltration and differentiation of endogenous microglia into resident macrophages may link inflammation and regeneration, with elaboration of a number of trophic factors (e.g., nerve growth factor among others). A link has been reported between IL-6 and nerve growth factor production (106).

It remains unclear whether anti-inflammatory therapies will improve outcome in clinical CNS injury. If inhibition of the inflammatory response is considered, exacerbation of infection risk must also be anticipated, and any deleterious consequences on the link between inflammation and regeneration must be addressed. The potential role of an interaction between systemic aspects of inflammation and neuroinflammation could be important but remains to be explored. Finally, recent work (particularly in TBI) has focused on the potential link between acute brain injury progressing to chronic traumatic encephalopathy (CTE) (107). CTE has been suggested to play an important role in mild repetitive TBI, however, it could play a role after severe TBI, and further study of this important area is warranted.

Other Aspects of Repair and Plasticity. Another aspect of brain injury, particularly with regard to strategies addressing repair, plasticity, or regeneration is that of neurotransmitter replacement therapy. Although this topic is somewhat beyond the scope of this chapter, it would be remiss to not mention this approach, which is a well-known component of brain injury rehabilitation. In the subacute and chronic phases after brain injury, there are deficits in function of many neurotransmitter systems. For example, evoked dopamine release is well known to be blunted in the striatum after experimental TBI (108). Augmenting the release and/or effects of this transmitter may represent a therapeutic avenue for the subacute period as shown in a recent RCT showing significant benefit on functional recovery in adults after moderate or severe TBI by treatment with the dopaminergic agonist amantadine (109). Augmenting other transmitter systems such as cholinergic or glutamatergic pathways may also have merit, and combinations of acute therapies to minimize secondary damage with neurotransmitter augmenting approaches to maximally utilize the remaining circuitry in the injured brain are logical to pursue.

Axonal Injury

Axonal injury plays an important role in TBI, and perinatal brain injury and white matter injury may also be important in stroke. Traumatic axonal injury (TAI) is the most established type of white matter damage in PICU-relevant CNS insults. The classic view that TAI occurs because of immediate physical shearing is represented primarily in severe injury, in which frank axonal tears occur. However, experimental studies suggest that TAI also occurs by a delayed process termed "secondary axotomy" (**Fig. 56.14**) (110). Two hypothetical sequences have attempted to explain secondary axotomy, one attributing axolemmal permeability and calcium influx as the initiating event, the other suggesting a direct cytoskeletal abnormality that impairs axoplasmic flow (110,111). It has been posited that both forms of reactive axonal swelling take place but in different proportions, depending on the severity of injury. Superimposed on these theories is the finding that hypoxic–ischemic insults can also produce axonal swelling that resembles retraction balls. As a result, differing as well as unifying theories for axonal injuries in brain injury have been proposed (42). Common mechanistic features include focal ion flux, calcium dysregulation, and mitochondrial and cytoskeletal dysfunction. TAI contributes to the morbidity after TBI. Studies in experimental TBI models have shown that hypothermia and cyclosporin A can reduce TAI (112,113). Whether or not these therapies can minimize axonal damage

in other CNS insults is uncertain. Another form of injury to white matter relates to the vulnerability of oligodendrocytes to excitotoxic injury from glutamate or other EAAs. However, the contribution of this pathway remains to be determined. New imaging modalities such as high definition fiber tracking could enhance our ability to understand the role of axonal injury in acute CNS insults in children, and in defining the effects of targeted therapies (114).

Mechanisms of Enhanced Vulnerability of Injured Brain

Hypotension and Hypoxemia

The injured brain is extremely vulnerable to secondary physiologic derangements that occur in the field, emergency department, or ICU, and hypotension and hypoxemia have received the most investigation (105). For example, hemorrhagic shock exacerbates intracranial hypertension early after experimental TBI and worsens long-term functional outcome. The blood pressure threshold varies, depending on the injury severity and duration, but some reports suggest that hemorrhage with even minimal blood pressure reductions can be deleterious (115). Similarly, hypoxemia to Pao_2 levels between 40 and 50 mm Hg for periods as short as 30 minutes can exacerbate neuronal death in experimental models of TBI. The period of enhanced vulnerability of the injured brain is not clearly defined; however, it is well described along the entire continuum of care in the critically ill. The mechanisms that underlie enhanced vulnerability are likely multifactorial and may differ over time. In the initial minutes to hours after cardiac arrest, TBI, and stroke, CBF is compromised, while metabolic demands are increased. Mechanical factors (e.g., thrombosis, vascular disruption, or vascular compromise from glial swelling), biochemical/molecular mechanisms (e.g.,

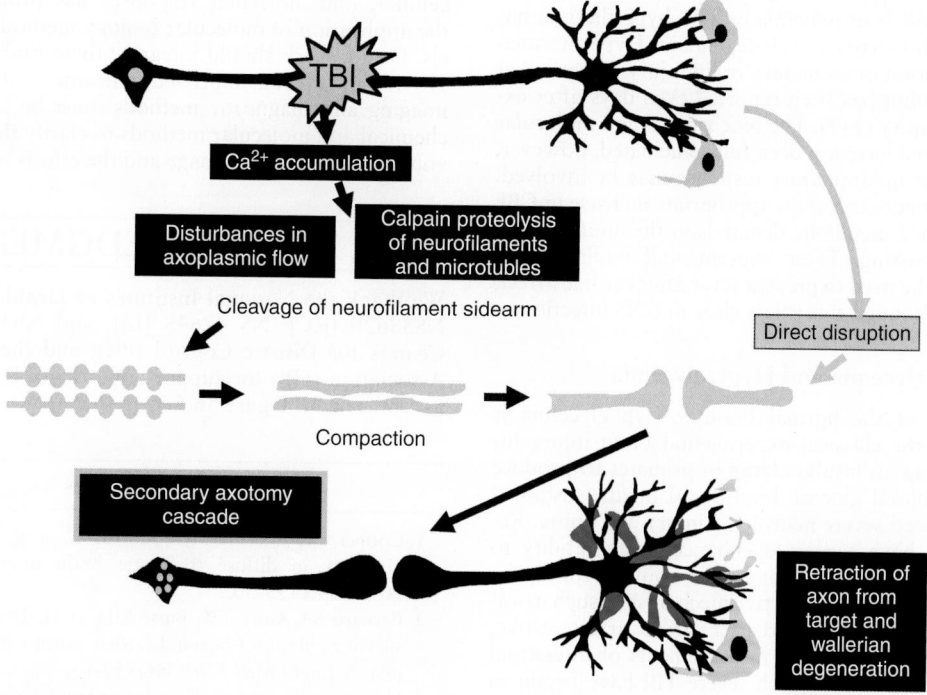

FIGURE 56.14. Cascades of axonal injury seen in either TBI or cerebral ischemia. Direct disruption of axons can occur in TBI, as shown on the *right side* of the figure. Believed to be more important, however, are two cascades of secondary axotomy related to either disturbances in axoplasmic flow or calcium-mediated proteolytic events, resulting in neurofilament compaction. These cascades may be responsive to some therapies, similar to those used to target neuronal death.

loss of endothelial NOS), or increases in levels of vasoconstrictors (e.g., endothelin-1) may mediate the inability of the vasculature to respond to additional challenges such as hypotension or hypoxemia. Similar mechanisms may also underlie the frequently observed loss of CBF blood pressure autoregulation that is seen in some insults (e.g., TBI). Increased metabolic demands early after these insults are substantial and result from both direct excitation of neurons, clinical or subclinical seizures, and increases in glucose utilization from glycolytic demands of astrocytes in EAA reuptake and mitochondrial dysfunction. During more delayed periods, such as in the ICU, the enhanced vulnerability of injured brain to secondary insults is typified by studies showing that a single jugular venous desaturation to <50% in adults with severe TBI doubled mortality rate (116). Enhanced vulnerability of the injured brain in the ICU may result from mechanisms other than those seen during acute injury, as cerebral metabolic demands several days after the insult are generally reduced. The most likely candidate for enhanced vulnerability during this phase is concomitant brain swelling, which generally peaks between 24 and 72 hours. Hypotension or hypoxemia, even within the autoregulatory range, results in compensatory vasodilation with an increase in CBV, further increasing ICP and potentially leading to a vicious cycle. Compromised CBF can also impair protein syntheses as regeneration is beginning. Other mechanisms may also be important. Progressive loss of endogenous antioxidant defenses in CSF was shown over several days in children with severe TBI (61). This loss would place the injured brain at heightened risk for oxidative damage from an ischemia–reperfusion event. Finally, persistently increased levels of lactate, seen even weeks after brain injury in infants and children, may reflect chronic mitochondrial dysfunction or failure, which may represent an important underpinning for enhanced vulnerability of the brain to second insults in the PICU.

Hyperthermia

In experimental models of ischemia or TBI, hyperthermia has consistently been shown to exacerbate damage. Hyperthermia-mediated exacerbation of secondary brain injury is marked at the time of injury, but has been reported even days after experimental brain injury (117). The biochemical and molecular mechanisms involved have not been fully elucidated; however, exacerbation of the inflammatory response may be involved. An inability to compensate for an appropriate increase in CBF related to heightened metabolic demands in the injured brain could also be occurring. These experimental findings have served to support the need to prevent fever after cardiac arrest, stroke, and TBI, although this is less clear in CNS infections.

Hypoglycemia and Hyperglycemia

The vulnerability of the normal brain to hypoglycemia is well described in the classical experimental brain injury literature (118). Using an insulin clamp in primates to produce hypoglycemia, a blood glucose level of 20 mg/dL sustained for 5 hours produced severe neurologic injury and coma. Recent clinical data have suggested enhanced vulnerability to hypoglycemia in the injured brain; this would certainly be anticipated, as endogenous protective mechanisms, such as vasodilation, are often compromised after cardiac arrest, stroke, and TBI. Regional microdialysis measurements of interstitial brain glucose levels in adults with severe TBI have begun to shed some light on this issue. Brain glucose levels can reach critically low values after TBI (119). This finding may be particularly true in pericontusional brain regions in TBI, where astrocyte uptake of glutamate and mitochondrial dysfunction occur (96). Astrocyte-dependent homeostatic processes, such as uptake of excitatory neurotransmitters and pH regulation,

are dependent on glycolytic rather than oxidative metabolism. Tight glucose control using insulin to achieve a serum glucose level between 90 and 120 mg/dL was associated with more frequent, critically low brain interstitial glucose levels than when serum glucose concentration was more loosely maintained at <150 mg/dL. Also concerning was the fact that tight glucose control was associated with increases in brain interstitial levels of glutamate and the lactate/pyruvate ratio, suggesting exacerbation of metabolic failure. Thus, it might be advisable to avoid tight glucose control in patients with brain injury, in favor of a more conservative approach.

Although care must be taken to avoid hypoglycemia after CNS insults, it is also well recognized that hyperglycemia can exacerbate CNS injury. This event has been most thoroughly investigated in experimental global cerebral ischemia, in which blood glucose concentrations >180 mg/dL achieved before the insult substantially exacerbate damage (120). The mechanisms involved in this exacerbation of ischemic brain injury by hyperglycemia include worsened brain swelling by lactate-mediated osmolar effects, along with greater local brain tissue acidosis following enhanced iron-catalyzed lipid peroxidation. It appears that before or after brain injury, marked hyperglycemia (>180 mg/dL) should be avoided or treated. Recently, Smith et al. (121) reported that although early and delayed severe hyperglycemia could be seen in children with severe TBI, only delayed hyperglycemia beyond 48 hours after injury was associated with unfavorable outcome. Further study of this issue is needed across insults in pediatric neurocritical care.

CONCLUSIONS AND FUTURE DIRECTIONS

Mechanisms involved in the evolution of secondary brain injury after CNS insults relevant to pediatric critical care medicine have been reviewed. Particular attention has been paid to studies at the bedside. Our understanding of the biochemical, cellular, and molecular responses has progressed following the application of molecular biology methods to human models. Future work should integrate these findings with bedside physiology and an improved assessment of outcome. Novel imaging and diagnostic methods must be coupled with biochemical and molecular methods to clarify the mechanisms involved in secondary damage and the effects of novel therapies.

ACKNOWLEDGMENTS

We thank the National Institutes of Health (NS38087 [PK], NS38620 [RC], NS 42648 [LJ], and NS30318 [PK, RC]), Centers for Disease Control (PK), and the American Heart Association (HB) for support. We thank Dr. R. Garman for assistance with **Figure 56.5**.

References

1. Cooper SD, Rosenfeld JF, Murray L, et al. Decompressive craniectomy in diffuse traumatic brain injury. *N Engl J Med* 2011;364:1493–502.
2. Bernard SA, Gray TW, Buist MD, et al. Treatment of comatose survivors of out-of-hospital cardiac arrest with induced hypothermia. *N Engl J Med* 2002;346:557–63.
3. Hypothermia after Cardiac Arrest Study Group. Mild therapeutic hypothermia to improve the neurologic outcome after cardiac arrest. *N Engl J Med* 2002;346:549–56.
4. Lees KR, Zivin JA, Ashwood T, et al. Stroke-acute ischemic NXY treatment (SAINT I) trial investigators. *N Engl J Med* 2006;354:588–600.

5. Shankaran S, Laptook AR, Ehrenkranz RA, et al. Whole-body hypothermia for neonates with hypoxic-ischemic encephalopathy. *N Engl J Med* 2005;353:1575–84.

6. Holmes GL, Ben-Ari Y. The neurobiology and consequences of epilepsy in the developing brain. *Pediatr Res* 2001;49:320–5.

7. Villablanca JR, Burgess JW, Olmstead CE. Recovery of function after neonatal or adult hemispherectomy in cats. I. Time course, movement, posture and sensorimotor tests. *Behav Brain Res* 1986;19:205–26.

8. Giza CC, Maria NS, Hovda DA. N-methyl-D-aspartate receptor subunit changes after traumatic injury to the developing brain. *J Neurotrauma* 2006;23:950–61.

9. Margulies SS, Thibault KL. Infant skull and suture properties: Measurements and implications for mechanisms of pediatric brain injury. *J Biomech Eng* 2000;122:364–71.

10. Levin HS, Aldrich EF, Saydjari C, et al. Severe head injury in children: Experience of the Traumatic Coma Data Bank. *Neurosurgery* 1992;31:435–44.

11. Kochanek PM, Clark RSB, Ruppel R, et al. Cerebral resuscitation after traumatic brain injury and cardiac arrest in infants and children in the new millennium. *Pediatr Clin North Am* 2001;48(3):661–81.

12. Kochanek PM, Clark RSB, Ruppel RA, et al. Biochemical, cellular and molecular mechanisms in the evolution of secondary damage after severe traumatic brain injury in infants and children: Lessons learned from the bedside. *Pediatr Crit Care Med* 2000;1:4–19.

13. Rehncrona S, Siesjö BK. Metabolic and physiologic changes in acute brain failure. In: Grenvik A, Safar P, eds. *Brain Failure and Resuscitation*. New York, NY: Churchill Livingstone, 1981:11–33.

14. Jenkins LW, Povlishock JT, Lewelt W, et al. The role of postischemic recirculation in the development of ischemic neuronal injury following complete cerebral ischemia. *Acta Neuropathol* 1981;55:205–20.

15. Hossman KA. Pathophysiology and therapy of experimental stroke. *Cell Mol Neurobiol* 2006;26:1055–81.

16. Sharp FR, Lu An, Tang Y, et al. Multiple molecular penumbras after focal cerebral ischemia. *J Cereb Blood Flow Metab* 2000;20:1011–32.

17. Ashwal S, Holshouser BA, Shu SK, et al. Predictive value of proton magnetic resonance spectroscopy in pediatric closed head injury. *Pediatr Neurol* 2000;23:114–25.

18. Ashwal S, Stringer W, Tomasi L, et al. Cerebral blood flow and carbon dioxide reactivity in children with bacterial meningitis. *J Pediatr* 1990;117:523–30.

19. Nau R, Bruck W. Neuronal injury in bacterial meningitis: Mechanisms and implications for therapy. *Trends Neurosci* 2002;25:38–45.

20. Haring HP, Rotzer HK, Reindl H, et al. Time course of cerebral blood flow velocity in central nervous system infections. A transcranial Doppler sonography study. *Arch Neurol* 1993;50:98–101.

21. Hauck W, Samlalsingh-Parker J, Glibetic M, et al. Deregulation of cyclooxygenase and nitric oxide synthase gene expression in the inflammatory cascade triggered by experimental group B streptococcal meningitis in the newborn brain and cerebral microvessels. *Semin Perinatol* 1999;23:20–6.

22. Pereira de Vasconcelos A, Ferrandon A, Nehlig A. Local cerebral blood flow during lithium-pilocarpine seizures in the developing and adult rat: Role of coupling between blood flow and metabolism in the genesis of neuronal damage. *J Cereb Blood Flow Metab* 2002;22:196–205.

23. Engelhorn T, Doerfler A, Weise J, et al. Cerebral perfusion alterations during the acute phase of experimental generalized status epilepticus: Prediction of survival by using perfusion-weighted MR imaging and histopathology. *AJNR Am J Neuroradiol* 2005;26:1563–70.

24. Kirino T. Delayed neuronal death in the gerbil hippocampus following ischemia. *Brain Res* 1982;239:57–69.

25. Clark RSB, Lai Y, Hickey RW, et al. Hypoxic-ischemic encephalopathy: Pathobiology and therapy of the postresuscitation syndrome in children. In: Fuhrman BP, Zimmerman J, eds. *Pediatric Critical Care*. 3rd ed. Philadelphia, PA: Mosby-Elsevier, 2006;904–28.

26. Lowenstein DH, Thomas MJ, Smith DH, et al. Selective vulnerability of dentate hilar neurons following traumatic brain injury: A potential mechanistic link between head trauma and disorders of the hippocampus. *J Neurosci* 1992;12:4846–53.

27. Golarai G, Greenwood AC, Feeney DM, et al. Physiological and structural evidence for hippocampal involvement in persistent seizure susceptibility after traumatic brain injury. *J Neurosci* 2001;21:8523–37.

28. Weise J, Englehorn T, Dörfler A, et al. Expression time course and spatial distribution of activated caspase-3 after experimental status epilepticus: Contribution of delayed neuronal cell death to seizure-induced neuronal injury. *Neurobiol Dis* 2005;18:582–90.

29. Braun JS, Novak R, Herzog KH, et al. Neuroprotection by a caspase inhibitor in acute bacterial meningitis. *Nature Med* 1999;5:298–302.

30. Nau R, Soto A, Bruck W. Apoptosis of neurons in the dentate gyrus in humans suffering from bacterial meningitis. *J Neuropathol Exp Neurol* 1999;58:265–74.

31. Lui Y, Wong TP, Aarts M, et al. NMDA receptor subunits have differential roles in mediating excitotoxic neuronal death both in vitro and in vivo. *J Neurosci* 2007;27:2846–57.

32. Martel MA, Wyllie DJA, Hardingham GE. In developing hippocampal neurons, NR2B-containing N-methyl-D-aspartate receptors (NMDARs) can mediate signaling to neuronal survival and synaptic potentiation, as well as neuronal death. *Neuroscience* 2009;159:334–43.

33. Shigeno T, Mima T, Takakura K, et al. Amelioration of delayed neuronal death in the hippocampus by nerve growth factor. *J Neurosci* 1991;11:2914–9.

34. Nitatori T, Sato N, Waguri S, et al. Delayed neuronal death in the CA1 pyramidal cell layer of the gerbil hippocampus following transient ischemia is apoptosis. *J Neurosci* 1995;15:1001–11.

35. Colbourne F, Sutherland GR, Auer RN. Electron microscopic evidence against apoptosis as the mechanism of neuronal death in global ischemia. *J Neurosci* 1999;10:4200–10.

36. Li Y, Chopp M, Jiang N, et al. Temporal profile of in situ DNA fragmentation after transient middle cerebral artery occlusion in the rat. *J Cereb Blood Flow Metab* 1995;15:389–97.

37. Edwards AD, Yue X, Cox P, et al. Apoptosis in the brains of infants suffering intrauterine cerebral injury. *Pediatr Res* 1997;42:684–9.

38. Portera-Cailliau C, Price DL, Martin LJ. Non-NMDA and NMDA receptor-mediated excitotoxic neuronal deaths in adult brain are morphologically distinct: Further evidence for an apoptosis-necrosis continuum. *J Comp Neurol* 1997;378:88–104.

39. Chu CT. Autophagic stress in neuronal injury and disease. *J Neuropathol Exp Neurol* 2006;65:423–32.

40. Starkov AA, Chinopoulos C, Fiskum G. Mitochondrial calcium and oxidative stress as mediators of ischemic brain injury. *Cell Calcium* 2004;36:257–64.

41. Paschen W, Doutheil J. Disturbance of endoplasmic reticulum functions: A key mechanism underlying cell damage? *Acta Neurochir Suppl* 1999;73:1–5.

42. Kochanek PM, Clark RSB, Jenkins LW. Traumatic brain injury: Pathobiology. In: Zafonte R, Zasler N, eds. *Brain Injury Medicine*. New York, NY: Demos Medical Publishing, 2006.

43. Palmer AM, Marion DW, Botscheller ML, et al. Increased transmitter amino acid concentration in human ventricular CSF after brain trauma. *Neuroreport* 1994;6:153–6.

44. Ruppel RA, Kochanek PM, Adelson PD, et al. Excitotoxicity amino acid concentrations in ventricular cerebrospinal fluid after severe traumatic brain injury in infants and children: The role of child abuse. *J Pediatrics* 2001;138:18–25.

45. Goodman JC, Valadka AB, Gopinath SP, et al. Lactate and excitatory amino acids measured by microdialysis are decreased by pentobarbital coma in head-injured patients. *J Neurotrauma* 1996;13:549–56.

46. Marion DW, Penrod LE, Kelsey SF, et al. Treatment of traumatic brain injury with moderate hypothermia. *N Engl J Med* 1997;336:540–6.

47. Bullock R, Zauner A, Woodward JJ, et al. Factors affecting excitatory amino acid release following severe human head injury. *J Neurosurg* 1998;89:507–18.

48. Ma D, Hossain M, Chow A, et al. Xenon and hypothermia combine to provide neuroprotection from neonatal asphyxia. *Ann Neurol* 2005;58:182–93.

49. Ikonomidou C, Bosch F, Miksa M, et al. Blockade of NMDA receptors and apoptotic neurodegeneration in the developing brain. *Science* 1999;283:70–4.

50. Zou X, Lui F, Zhang X, et al. Inhalation anesthetic-induced neuronal damage in the developing rhesus monkey. *Neurotoxicol Teratol* 2011;33:592–7.

51. Brambrink AM, Back SA, Riddle A, et al. Isoflurane-induced apoptosis of oligodendrocytes in the neonatal primate brain. *Ann Neurol* 2012;72:525–35.

52. Brambrink AM, Martin LJ, Hanley DF, et al. Effects of the AMPA receptor antagonist NBQX on outcome of newborn pigs after asphyxic cardiac arrest. *J Cereb Blood Flow Metab* 1999;19:927–38.

53. Bayır H. Reactive oxygen species. *Crit Care Med* 2005;33 (suppl 12):S498–501.

54. Chinopoulos C, Adam-Vizi V. Calcium, mitochondria and oxidative stress in neuronal pathology. Novel aspects of an enduring theme. *FEBS J* 2006;273:433–50.

55. Tsukahara H, Haruta T, Todoroki Y, et al. Oxidant and antioxidant activities in childhood meningitis. *Life Sci* 2002;71:2797–806.

56. Bayır H, Tyurin VA, Tyurin YY, et al. Selective early cardiolipin oxidation after brain trauma: A lipidomics analysis. *Ann Neurol* 2007;62:154–69.

57. Ji J, Kline AE, Amoscato A, et al. Lipidomics identifies cardiolipin oxidation as a mitochondrial target for redox therapy of brain injury. *Nat Neurosci* 2012;10:1407–13.

58. Katz L, Callaway C, Kagan V, et al. Electron spin resonance measure of brain antioxidant activity during ischemia/reperfusion. *Neuroreport* 1998;9:1587–93.

59. Vereczki V, Martin E, Rosenthal RE, et al. Normoxic resuscitation after cardiac arrest protects against hippocampal oxidative stress, metabolic dysfunction, and neuronal death. *J Cereb Blood Flow Metab* 2006;26:821–35.

60. Kilgannon JH, Jones AE, Shapiro NI, et al. Association between arterial hyperoxia following resuscitation from cardiac arrest and in-hospital mortality. *JAMA* 2010;303:2165–71.

61. Bayır H, Kagan VE, Tyurina YY, et al. Assessment of antioxidant reserve and oxidative stress in cerebrospinal fluid after severe traumatic brain injury in infants and children. *Pediatr Res* 2001;51:571–8.

62. Zhao H, Yenari MA, Cheng D, et al. Biphasic cytochrome c release after transient global ischemia and its inhibition by hypothermia. *J Cereb Blood Flow Metab* 2005;25:1119–29.

63. Kawakami Y, Monobe M, Kuwabara K, et al. A comparative study of nitric oxide, glutathione, and glutathione peroxidase activities in cerebrospinal fluid from children with convulsive diseases/children with aseptic meningitis. *Brain Dev* 2006;28:243–6.

64. Kochanek PM, Forbes ML, Ruppel R, et al. Severe traumatic brain injury in infants and children. In: Fuhrman BP, Zimmerman J, eds. *Pediatric Critical Care*. 3rd ed. Philadelphia, PA: Mosby-Elsevier, 2006:1595–617.

65. Zhang X, Chen Y, Jenkins LW, et al. Bench-to-bedside review: Apoptosis/programmed cell death triggered by traumatic brain injury. *Crit Care* 2005;9:66–75.

66. Chan PH. Mitochondria and neuronal death/survival signaling pathways in cerebral ischemia. *Neurochem Res* 2004;29:1943–9.

67. Gianinazzi C, Grandgirard D, Imboden H, et al. Caspase-3 mediates hippocampal apoptosis in pneumococcal meningitis. *Acta Neuropathol* 2003;105:499–507.

68. Henshall DC, Clark RS, Adelson PD, et al. Alterations in bcl-2 and caspase gene family protein expression in human temporal lobe epilepsy. *Neurology* 2000;55:250–7.

69. Murakami Y, Saito K, Hara A, et al. Increase in tumor necrosis factor-α following transient global cerebral ischemia do not contribute to neuron death in mouse hippocampus. *J Neurochem* 2005;93:1616–22.

70. Narkilahti S, Nissinen J, Pitkanen A. Administration of caspase 3 inhibitor during and after status epilepticus in rat: Effect on neuronal damage an epileptogenesis. *Neuropharmacology* 2003;44:1068–88.

71. Braun JS, Sublett JE, Freyer D, et al. Pneumococcal pneumolysin and H₂O₂ mediate brain cell apoptosis during meningitis. *J Clin Invest* 2002;109:19–27.

72. Tajiri S, Oyadomari S, Yano S, et al. Ischemia-induced neuronal cell death is mediated by the endoplasmic reticulum stress pathway involving CHOP. *Cell Death Differ* 2004;11:403–15.

73. Zhang X, Graham SH, Kochanek PM, et al. Caspase-8 expression and proteolysis in human brain after severe head injury. *FASEB J* 2003;17:1367–9.

74. Cross TG, Scheel-Toellner D, Henriquez NV, et al. Serine/threonine protein kinases and apoptosis. *Exp Cell Res* 2000;256:34–41.

75. Ono K, Han J. The p38 signal transduction pathway: Activation and function. *Cell Signal* 2000;12:1–13.

76. Nunez G, del Peso L. Linking extracellular survival signals and the apoptotic machinery. *Curr Opin Neurobiol* 1998;8:613–18.

77. Coffer PJ, Jin J, Woodgett JR. Protein kinase B (c-Akt): A multifunctional mediator of phosphatidylinositol 3-kinase activation. *Biochem J* 1998;335:1–13.

78. Kaplan DR, Miller FD. Neurotrophin signal transduction in the nervous system. *Curr Opin Neurobiol* 2000;10:381–91.

79. Zhao H, Shimohata T, Wang JQ, et al. Akt contributes to neuroprotection by hypothermia against cerebral ischemia in rats. *J Neurosci* 2005;25:9794–806.

80. Eliasson MJ, Sampei K, Mandir AS, et al. Poly(ADP-ribose) polymerase gene disruption renders mice resistant to cerebral ischemia. *Nat Med* 1997;3:1089–95.

81. Yamashima T. Ca²⁺-dependent proteases in ischemic neuronal death. A conserved "calpain–cathepsin cascade" from nematodes to primates. *Cell Calcium* 2004;36:285–93.

82. You Z, Savitz SI, Yang J, et al. Necrostatin-1 reduces histopathology and improves functional outcome after controlled cortical impact in mice. *J Cereb Blood Flow Metab* 2008;28:1564–73.

83. Kochanek PM, Vagni VA, Janesko KL, et al. Adenosine A1 receptor knockout mice develop lethal status epilepticus after experimental traumatic brain injury. *J Cereb Blood Flow Metab* 2006;26:565–75.

84. Duranski MR, Greer JJ, Dejam A, et al. Cytoprotective effects of nitrite during in vivo ischemia-reperfusion of the heart and liver. *J Clin Invest* 2005;115:1232–40.

85. Hall ED, Sullivan PG, Gibson TR, et al. Spatial and temporal characteristics of neurodegeneration after controlled cortical impact in mice: More than a focal brain injury. *J Neurotrauma* 2005;22:252–65.

86. Scheff SW, Price DA, Hicks RR, et al. Synaptogenesis in the hippocampal CA1 field following traumatic brain injury. *J Neurotruama* 2005;22:719–32.

87. Barzo P, Marmarou A, Fatouros P, et al. Contribution of vasogenic and cellular edema to traumatic brain swelling measured by diffusion-weighted imaging. *J Neurosurg* 1997;87:900–7.

88. Oshio K, Watanabe H, Song Y, et al. Reduced cerebrospinal fluid production and intracranial pressure in mice lacking choroid plexus water channel Aquaporin-1. *FASEB J* 2005;19:76–8.

89. Papadopoulos MC, Verkman AS. Aquaporin-4 gene disruption in mice reduces brain swelling and mortality in pneumococcal meningitis. *J Biol Chem* 2005;280:13906–12.

90. Meili DN, Christen S, Leib SL, et al. Current concepts in the pathogenesis of meningitis caused by *Streptococcus pneumoniae*. *Curr Opin Infect Dis* 2002;15:253–7.

91. Schleien CL, Koehler RC, Shaffner DH, et al. Blood–brain barrier disruption after cardiac resuscitation in immature swine. *Stroke* 1991;22:477–83.

92. Shapiro S, Miller A, Lahat N, et al. Expression of matrix metalloproteinases, sICAM-1 and IL-8 in CSF from children with meningitis. *J Neurol Sci* 2003;206:43–8.

93. Kolb SA, Lahrtz F, Paul R, et al. Matrix metalloproteinases and tissue inhibitors of metalloproteinases in viral meningitis: Upregulation of MMP-9 and TIMP-1 in cerebrospinal fluid. *J Neuroimmunol* 1998;84:143–50.

94. Katayama Y, Kawamata T. Edema fluid accumulation within necrotic brain tissue as a cause of the mass effect of cerebral contusion in head trauma patients. *Acta Neurochir Suppl* 2003; 86:323–7.

95. Marmarou A, Barzo P, Fatouros P, et al. Traumatic brain swelling in head injured patients: Brain edema or vascular engorgement? *Acta Neurochir Suppl (Wien)* 1997;70:68–70.

96. Bergsneider M, Hovda DA, Shalmon E, et al. Cerebral hyperglycolysis following severe traumatic brain injury in humans: A positron emission tomography study. *J Neurosurg* 1997;86: 241–51.

97. Barone FC, Feuerstein GZ. Inflammatory mediators and stroke: New opportunities for novel therapeutics. *J Cereb Blood Flow Metab* 1999;19:819–34.

98. Clark RSB, Kochanek PM, Chen M, et al. Increases in Bcl-2 and cleavage of caspase-1 and caspase-3 in human brain after head injury. *FASEB J* 1999;13:813–21.

99. Adamczak S, Dale G, De Rivero Vaccari JP, et al. Inflammasome proteins in cerebrospinal fluid of brain-injured patients as biomarkers of functional outcome. *J Neurosurg* 2012;117:1119–25.

100. Forster C, Clark HB, Ross ME, et al. Inducible nitric oxide synthase expression in human cerebral infarcts. *Acta Neuropathol* 1999;97:215–20.

101. Clemens JA, Stephenson DT, Dixon EP, et al. Global cerebral ischemia activates nuclear factor-kappa B prior to evidence of DNA fragmentation. *Brain Res Mol Brain Res* 1997;48:187–96.

102. Yu Z, Zhou D, Bruce-Keller AJ, et al. Lack of the p50 subunit of nuclear factor-kappaB increases the vulnerability of hippocampal neurons to excitotoxic injury. *J Neurosci* 1999;19:8856–65.

103. Scherbel U, Raghupathi R, Nakamura M, et al. Differential acute and chronic responses of tumor necrosis factor-deficient mice to experimental brain injury. *Proc Natl Acad Sci USA* 1999;96:8721–6.

104. Wada K, Chatzipanteli K, Kraydieh S, et al. Inducible nitric oxide synthase expression after traumatic brain injury and neuroprotection with aminoguanidine treatment in rats. *Neurosurgery* 1998;43:1427–36.

105. Chesnut RM, Marshall LF, Klauber MR, et al. The role of secondary brain injury in determining outcome from severe head injury. *J Trauma* 1993;34:216–22.

106. Kossmann T, Stahel PF, Lenzlinger PM, et al. Interleukin-8 released into the cerebrospinal fluid after brain injury is associated with blood–brain barrier dysfunction and nerve growth factor production. *J Cereb Blood Flow Metab* 1997;17:280–9.

107. Dekosky ST, Ikonomovic MD, Gandy S. Traumatic brain injury—football, warfare, and long-term effects. *N Engl J Med* 2010;1293–6.

108. Wagner AK, Sokoloski JE, Ren D, et al. Controlled cortical impact injury affects dopaminergic transmission in the rat striatum. *J Neurochem* 2005;95:457–65.

109. Giacino JT, Whyte J, Bagiella E, et al. Placebo-controlled trail of amantadine for severe traumatic brain injury. *N Engl J Med* 2012;366:819–26.

110. Povlishock JT. Traumatically induced axonal injury: Pathogenesis and pathobiological implications. *Brain Pathol* 1992;2:1–12.

111. Fitzpatrick MO, Maxwell WL, Graham DI. The role of the axolemma in the initiation of traumatically induced axonal injury. *J Neurol Neurosurg Psychiatry* 1998;64:285–7.

112. Buki A, Koizumi H, Povlishock JT. Moderate posttraumatic hypothermia decreases early calpain-mediated proteolysis and concomitant cytoskeletal compromise in traumatic axonal injury. *Exp Neurol* 1999;159:319–28.

113. Buki A, Okonkwo DO, Povlishock JT. Postinjury cyclosporin A administration limits axonal damage and disconnection in traumatic brain injury. *J Neurotrauma* 1999;16:511–21.

114. Shin SS, Verstynen T, Pathak S, et al. High-definition fiber tracking for assessment of neurological deficit in a case of traumatic brain injury: Finding, visualizing, and interpreting small sites of damage. *J Neurosurg* 2012;116:1062–9.

115. Matsushita Y, Bramlett HM, Kuluz JW, et al. Delayed hemorrhagic hypotension exacerbates the hemodynamic and histopathologic consequences of traumatic brain injury in rats. *J Cereb Blood Flow Metab* 2001;21:847–56.

116. Gopinath SP, Robertson CS, Contant CF, et al. Jugular venous desaturation and outcome after head injury. *J Neurol Neurosurg Psychiatry* 1994;57:717–23.

117. Baena RC, Busto R, Dietrich WD, et al. Hyperthermia delayed by 24 hours aggravates neuronal damage in rat hippocampus following global ischemia. *Neurology* 1997;48:768–73.

118. Kahn KJ, Myers RE. Insulin-induced hypoglycaemia in the nonhuman primate. I. Clinical consequences. In: Brierley JB, Meldrum BS, eds. *Brain Hypoxia*. London: Spastics International Medical, 1971:185–94.

119. Vespa P, Boonyaputthikul R, McArthur DL, et al. Intensive insulin therapy reduces microdialysis glucose values without altering glucose utilization or improving the lactate/pyruvate ratio after traumatic brain injury. *Crit Care Med* 2006;34:850–6.

120. Li PA, Siesjö BK. Role of hyperglycaemia-related acidosis in ischaemic brain damage. *Acta Physiol Scand* 1997;161:567–80.

121. Smith RL, Lin JC, Adelson PD, et al. Relationship between hyperglycemia and outcome in children with severe traumatic brain injury. *Pediatr Crit Care Med* 2012;13:85–91.

CHAPTER 57 ■ EVALUATION OF THE COMATOSE CHILD

NICHOLAS S. ABEND AND DANIEL J. LICHT

Coma is a not a specific diagnosis but instead describes an altered state of consciousness which may be the consequence of a range of insults to the brain. The estimated incidence of nontraumatic coma is 30/100,000 children per year (1), and the estimated incidence of severe traumatic coma is 5.6/100,000 (2). Morbidity and mortality are highly dependent on the coma etiology (1,3). The comatose child requires immediate evaluation and medical stabilization, followed by a history and physical examination directed at identifying the underlying etiology of coma, which will direct specific management. Coma is the most severe form of the acute encephalopathy spectrum. All types of acute encephalopathy are serious disorders that involve the same differential diagnosis and management approach. This chapter aims to (a) define coma and distinguish it from other states of encephalopathy and altered consciousness; (b) review coma pathophysiology; (c) discuss a differential diagnosis of etiologies; and (d) outline an approach to evaluation of a comatose child.

DEFINITIONS

Consciousness, as defined by Plum and Posner (4), is a state of wakefulness and awareness of self and surroundings. Coma is a state of altered consciousness with loss of both wakefulness

(arousal, vigilance) and awareness of self and environment. Sleep–wake cycles are absent. Coma is characterized by sustained, pathologic, eyes-closed, unarousable unresponsiveness (4). Coma is a transitory state that can evolve toward recovery of consciousness, a minimally conscious state, a vegetative state, or brain death.

Between normal consciousness and coma is a spectrum of diminished consciousness, conventionally subdivided into lethargy, obtundation, and stupor. *Lethargy* is a state of reduced wakefulness with attentional deficits. *Obtundation* is characterized by blunted alertness and diminished interaction with the environment. *Stupor* is a state of unresponsiveness with little or no spontaneous movement, resembling deep sleep, but differs from coma because vigorous stimulation induces temporary arousal. The descriptive terms listed above are not defined uniformly in the literature, nor are they defined consistently by the physicians involved in a given patient's care. Thus, since tracking changes in the patient's state is important in the acute setting, a description of the patient's examination along with these terms may convey more information than these one word descriptors alone.

Other chronic states of altered neurologic function may resemble coma but must be differentiated from coma (Table 57.1). A patient in the *persistent vegetative state* has sleep–wake cycles but is unaware of self and environment.

TABLE 57.1

STATES OF ALTERED CONSCIOUSNESS

■ STATE	■ AROUSAL	■ AWARENESS	■ SLEEP–WAKE CYCLING	■ MOTOR FUNCTION	■ RESPIRATORY FUNCTION
Brain death	–	–	–	None or Spinal reflexes	–
Coma	–	–	–	Non-purposeful	Variable
Vegetative state (unresponsive wakefulness syndrome)	+	–	+	Non-purposeful	+
Minimally conscious state	+	Partial	+	Intermittently purposeful or Absent but nonmotor evidence of responsiveness	+

Although such patients may make sounds, facial expressions, or body movements, detailed testing does not demonstrate reproducible purposeful responses to stimulation. Since patients in whom coma is due to head trauma may recover consciousness after a longer period than those in whom coma is nontraumatic, the diagnosis of a persistent vegetative state may be made 3 months following nontraumatic brain injury, but not until 12 months following traumatic brain injury (5,6). Of children in the vegetative state 1 month after head injury, 1-year outcome was death (9%), persistent vegetative state (29%), and recovery of consciousness (62%). However, outcome was worse when the etiology was nontraumatic, with death (22%), persistent vegetative state (65%), and recovery of consciousness (usually with severe cognitive disabilities) in only 13% (7). A patient in a *minimally conscious state* has severely altered consciousness but has behavioral evidence of self or environmental awareness, such as following simple commands or making simple nonreflexive gestures. Recent functional neuroimaging and electrophysiological studies have indicated that some patients considered to be in the vegetative state demonstrate reproducible physiologic changes in response to tasks, indicating there may be some awareness despite the absence of behavioral signs of responsiveness (8–10). These findings have prompted the use of more neutral and descriptive terms (11,12). The vegetative state may be referred to as the *unresponsive wakefulness syndrome*. The minimally conscious state may be subdivided into the minimally conscious positive state (high-level behavioral responses, such as following commands or intelligible verbalizations) and the minimally conscious negative state (lower level behavioral responses, such as visual pursuit or contextually-appropriate crying or smiling) (11).

Akinetic mutism is a condition of extreme slowing or absence of bodily movement with loss of speech. Wakefulness and awareness are preserved, but cognition is slowed. Causes include extensive bihemispheric disease and lesions involving the bilateral inferior frontal lobes, paramedian mesencephalic reticular formation, or the posterior diencephalon. Frontal release signs may be evident, and electroencephalogram (EEG) may show background slowing. The *locked-in syndrome* is a state of preserved cognition with complete paralysis of the voluntary motor system. Cortical function is intact as indicated by normal EEG patterns. Eye movements, most commonly vertical eye movements, may be preserved, allowing for some communication. It may result from lesions of the corticospinal and corticobulbar pathways at or below the pons or severe peripheral nervous system disease such as Guillain–Barré syndrome, botulism, and critical illness polyneuropathy. *Psychogenic unresponsiveness* may also mimic coma. Coma must also be distinguished from *brain death*, which is the permanent absence of all brain activities, including brainstem function (13). *Delirium* is an acute confusional state characterized by changes in level of consciousness, impaired attention, and a fluctuating course.

ANATOMY

Maintaining consciousness depends on interactions between the reticular activating system (RAS), thalamus, posterior hypothalamus, and cerebral hemispheres (**Fig. 57.1**). The RAS constitutes the central core of the brainstem and extends from the caudal medulla to the thalamus and the basal forebrain. The RAS receives input stimulation from all sensory pathways and projects to vast areas of the cerebral cortex. The RAS activates the cortex and participates in feedback control that regulates incoming signals. This may account for the ability of certain signals to cause more arousal than other signals of equal electrical intensity. The RAS can be

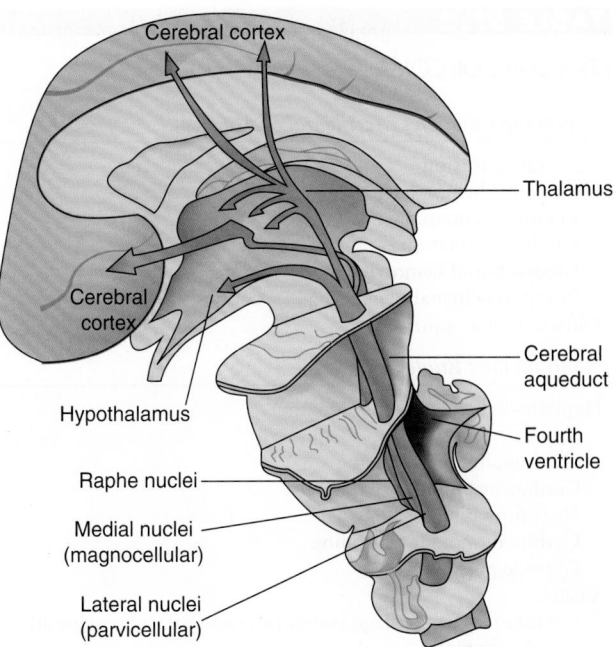

FIGURE 57.1. Key structures in maintaining an awake and alert state.

partitioned into medial and lateral zones. The medial RAS contains a mixture of large and small neurons. The most prominent cells in this region are the giant neurons that have long ascending and descending axons. The ascending portions of the medial RAS emanate from the Raphe nuclei, which regulate sleep cycles and utilize *serotonin* as their major neurotransmitter. The descending pathways regulate automatic motor functions, including the automatic rhythms of breathing. The lateral RAS projects to the reticular nucleus of the thalamus, which relays signals to the cortex, forming the ascending RAS, which maintains wakefulness. These projections are both *cholinergic* and *noradrenergic*. A second *cholinergic* pathway ascends through the hypothalamus to influence basal forebrain structures, including the *limbic system*, which influences conscious behavior. *Noradrenergic* pathways originating in the *locus ceruleus* have an excitatory effect on most of the brain, mediating arousal and priming the brain's neurons to be activated by stimuli. The RAS extends to the posterior portion of the hypothalamus and the thalamus. The thalamus (intralaminar and medial nuclei) rely information from the RAS diffusely throughout the cerebral hemispheres via thalamocortical projections. In general, wakefulness is maintained by the RAS and thalamus, whereas awareness is dependent on the cortex.

ETIOLOGIES OF COMA

The main causes of coma are listed in **Table 57.2**. Coma subdivisions have occurred along several lines including (a) traumatic or nontraumatic and (b) structural or nonstructural. A population-based study of 600,000 children evaluated 345 episodes of coma (1). Infection was the most common cause of nontraumatic coma, accounting for 38% of cases. Intoxication, epilepsy, and complications of congenital abnormalities each accounted for 8%–10% of cases. Nontraumatic accidents (such as smoke inhalation and drowning) and metabolic

TABLE 57.2

ETIOLOGIES OF COMA

Traumatic Etiologies (Accidental or Abusive)

Cerebral contusion
Intracranial hemorrhage
  Epidural hematoma
  Subdural hematoma
  Subarachnoid hemorrhage
  Intraparenchymal hematoma
Diffuse axonal injury

Nontraumatic Etiologies

Hypoxic–ischemic encephalopathy
  Shock
  Cardiopulmonary arrest
  Cardiac or pulmonary failure
  Near drowning
  Carbon monoxide poisoning
  Cyanide poisoning
Vascular
  Intracranial hemorrhage (subdural, epidural, subarachnoid, parenchymal)
  Arterial ischemic infarct
  Venous sinus thromboses
  Vasculitis
  Carotid or vertebral artery dissection (cervical or intracranial)
Mass lesions
  Primary neoplasms
  Brain metastases
  Abscess
  Granuloma
Hydrocephalus
Infections
  Meningitis and encephalitis: bacterial, viral, rickettsial, fungal, protozoal
  Abscess
Inflammatory/Autoimmune/Postinfectious
  Acute disseminated encephalomyelitis
  Multiple sclerosis
  Sarcoidosis
  Sjogren disease
  Cerebritis (e.g., systemic lupus erythematosus)
  Sepsis-associated encephalopathy
  Autoimmune-mediated encephalitis

Paroxysmal neurologic disorders
  Seizures, status epilepticus, nonconvulsive seizures, postictal state
  Acute confusional migraine
Hypertensive encephalopathy
Posterior reversible encephalopathy syndrome
Systemic metabolic disorders
  Substrate deficiencies
    Hypoglycemia
    Cofactors: thiamine, niacin, pyridoxine, folate, B12
  Electrolyte and acid–base imbalance: sodium, magnesium, calcium
  Hypoglycemia
  Diabetic ketoacidosis
  Endocrine
    Acute hypothyroidism
    Addison disease
    Acute panhypopituitarism
  Uremic encephalopathy
  Hepatic encephalopathy
  Reye syndrome
  Sepsis-associated encephalopathy
  Porphyria
  Inborn errors of metabolism
    Urea cycle disorders
    Aminoacidopathies
    Organic acidopathies
    Mitochondrial disorders
Toxins
  Medications: narcotics, sedatives, antiepileptics, antidepressants, analgesics, aspirin, valproic acid encephalopathy
  Environmental toxins: organophosphates, heavy metals, cyanide, mushroom poisoning
  Illicit substances: alcohol, heroine, amphetamines, cocaine, and many others
Drug induced
  Neuroleptic malignant syndrome
  Serotonin syndrome
  Malignant hyperthermia
Psychiatric
  Conversion disorder
  Catatonia
Other
  Hypothermia

causes each accounted for 6% of cases. Approximately one-quarter of children with traumatic brain injury present with coma (2). Importantly, multiple interrelated factors crossing these subdivisions may be present in one patient. For example, status epilepticus may occur in the setting of encephalitis; infection inducing a catabolic state may produce decompensation in a child with an inborn error of metabolism; and hyponatremia or other electrolyte dysfunctions may accompany brain injury and contribute to cerebral dysfunction.

EVALUATION OF THE COMATOSE CHILD

Coma is often a manifestation of life-threatening condition. The initial evaluation of the child begins with evaluation and stabilization of vital functions and identification of immediately

reversible etiologies. Medical stabilization must occur as the coma etiology is being investigated to prevent development of secondary brain injury. An algorithm for initial evaluation of coma is outlined in **Table 57.3** and discussed below. The Pediatric Accident and Emergency Research Group of the Royal College of Paediatrics and Child Health and the British Association for Emergency Medicine have published guidelines for practice on the basis of an extensive literature review and expert consensus (www.nottingham.ac.uk/paediatric-guideline) (14). Other literature reviews are also available (15–17).

Patient History

Historical information must be gathered as quickly as possible since it may be crucial in identifying the cause of coma. The history must include a detailed description of events leading

TABLE 57.3

INITIAL EVALUATION OF COMA

- Resuscitation and medical stabilization
  - Airway, breathing, and circulation assessment and stabilization
  - Ensure adequate ventilation and oxygenation
  - Determine whether hypertension is reactive (maintaining cerebral perfusion pressure) or problematic
- Bedside glucose assessment
- Draw blood for glucose, electrolytes, ammonia, arterial blood gas, liver and renal function tests, complete blood count, lactate, pyruvate, and toxicology screen
- Neurological assessment
  - GCS (modified for children) or FOUR score or coma description
  - Assess for evidence of raised intracranial pressure and herniation
  - Assess for abnormalities suggesting focal neurologic disease
- Head CT scan (and possibly MRI when stable)
- Identify and treat critical elevations in intracranial pressure
  - Neutral head position, elevated head by 20 degrees, sedation
  - Consider hyperosmolar therapy (mannitol or hypertonic saline)
  - Hyperventilation as temporary measure
  - Consider need for intracranial monitoring and/or neurosurgical intervention
- Lumbar puncture if concern for infection or coma etiology unknown
  - Generally head CT scan first and defer lumbar puncture if concern for elevated intracranial pressure
  - If there is concern for infection and lumbar puncture must be delayed, then provide broad-spectrum infection coverage (including bacterial, viral, and possibly fungal)
  - If infection suspected, also draw blood and urine cultures
- Consider clinical and electrographic seizures
  - Treat seizures with anticonvulsants
  - Consider EEG monitoring to identify persisting nonconvulsive seizures
- Give specific antidotes if toxic exposures are known
  - Opiates = naloxone; benzodiazepine = flumazenil; anticholinergic = physostigmine
- Investigate source of fever and use antipyretics and/or cooling devices to reduce cerebral metabolic demands
- Detailed history and examination
- Consider additional metabolic, autoimmune, and endocrine testing

to coma, with particular attention to timing, exposures, and accompanying symptoms. Preceding somnolence or headaches suggests metabolic, toxic or infectious etiologies, hydrocephalus, or expanding mass lesions. Sudden onset of coma without trauma suggests seizure, intracranial hemorrhage, or hypoxic–ischemic encephalopathy caused by a cardiac event. A slowly progressive loss of consciousness suggests hydrocephalus, an expanding mass lesion, or indolent infection. Fluctuations in mental status may occur with metabolic etiologies, seizure, or subdural hemorrhage. Preceding headache aggravated with positional changes or Valsalva maneuver implies increased intracranial pressure from hydrocephalus or a mass lesion. Headache with neck pain or stiffness suggests meningeal irritation from inflammation, infection, or hemorrhage. Fever suggests infection but its absence does not rule it out,

particularly in infants younger than 3 months of age, or immunocompromised children. Recent fevers or illnesses suggest autoimmune processes such as acute disseminated encephalomyelitis (ADEM) or possibly Reye-like illness although this is uncommon. Questions about possible toxic ingestions should include a survey of medications and poisons kept in the places that the child has been.

The child's past medical history may be valuable. A history or multiple episodes of coma, developmental delay, or other prior neurologic abnormalities suggests inborn errors of metabolism but are also risk factors for epilepsy, which may present with coma due to nonconvulsive seizures or a postictal state. Toxic ingestions or inflicted childhood neurotrauma are also suggested by multiple episodes of coma. Recent weight changes or other constitutional abnormalities suggest endocrine dysfunction. Previously existing cardiac disease raises the possibility of dysrhythmia or cardiac failure leading to hypoxic–ischemic encephalopathy. Travel history may explain exposure to infections prevalent in certain areas, such as Lyme in the northeastern Unites States. Exposure to kittens in a patient with axillary or inguinal lymphadenopathy may be a clue to infection with *Bartonella henselae*, which causes cat-scratch encephalopathy.

Physical Examination

Numerically scored rating scales of conscious level allow objective description of a patient's degree of impairment and allow the patient's state to be tracked over time and conveyed quickly to other caregivers. Although these scores permit efficient standardized communication of a child's state, more detailed description of the child's clinical findings is often more useful for relaying detailed information and detecting changes over time. The most widely used instrument is the Glasgow Coma Scale (GCS) score, which was initially developed to evaluate adults with head injury (18). Pediatric adaptations to the GCS, more developmentally appropriate for infants and children, include the Pediatric Coma Scale, the Children's Coma Scale, and the GCS-Modified for Children (Table 57.4) (19–21). The GCS and the pediatric adaptations categorize the patient on the basis of measures of verbal response, eye opening, and movement. The Full Outline of UnResponsiveness (FOUR) score was developed for use in adults with coma (Table 57.5) (22). Each of the four functional categories (eye response, motor response, brainstem reflexes, and respiration) receives a score of 0 (nonfunctioning) to 4 (normal functioning). While developed for adults, one study has evaluated the interrater reliability and predictive value of the GCS-Modified for Children and FOUR score in critically ill children. In a study of 60 children aged 2–18 years in an ICU with both traumatic and nontraumatic brain injury, the FOUR score had better interrater reliability than the GCS-Modified for Children (excellent for FOUR score and good for GCS) and both predicted outcome similarly (23).

Consideration of vital signs is essential for resuscitation and may also help identify the coma etiology. Hyperthermia suggests an infectious etiology, a lesion impacting temperature control mechanisms, heat stroke, or anticholinergic ingestion. The absence of fever does not rule out infection, especially in infants or children who are immunosuppressed. Hypothermia may also be due to intoxication, sepsis, hypothyroidism, adrenal insufficiency, chronic malnutrition, or environmental exposure. Hypotension may be due to sepsis, cardiac dysfunction (which may be secondary to severe neurologic injury in neurogenic stunned myocardium), toxic ingestion, or adrenal insufficiency. Hypotension may lead to poor cerebral perfusion, resulting in diffuse or watershed hypoxic–ischemic injury. Hypertension may cause or result from coma-related

TABLE 57.4

GLASGOW COMA SCALE AND MODIFICATION FOR CHILDREN (27,64)

■ SIGN	■ GLASGOW COMA SCALE	■ MODIFICATION FOR CHILDREN	■ SCORE
Eye opening	Spontaneous	Spontaneous	4
	To command	To sound	3
	To pain	To pain	2
	None	None	1
Verbal response	Oriented	Age appropriate verbalization, orients to sound, fixes and follows, social smile	5
	Confused	Cries, but consolable	4
	Disoriented—inappropriate words	Irritable, uncooperative, aware of environment—irritable, persistent cries, inconsistently consolable	3
	Incomprehensible sounds	Inconsolable crying, unaware of environment or parents, restless, agitated	2
	None	None	1
Motor response	Obeys commands	Obeys commands, spontaneous movement	6
	Localizes pain	Localizes pain	5
	Withdraws	Withdraws	4
	Abnormal flexion to pain	Abnormal flexion to pain	3
	Abnormal extension	Abnormal extension	2
	None	None	1
Best total score			15

TABLE 57.5

FOUR SCORE (22)

Eye response	4	Eyelids open or opened, tracking or blinking to command
	3	Eyelids open but not tracking
	2	Eyelids closed but opens to loud voice
	1	Eyelids closed but opens to pain
	0	Eyelids remain closed with pain
Motor response	4	Thumbs up, fist, or peace sign to command
	3	Localizing to pain
	2	Flexion response to pain
	1	Extensor posturing
	0	No response to pain or generalized myoclonus status epilepticus
Brainstem reflexes	4	Pupil and corneal reflexes present
	3	One pupil wide and fixed
	2	Pupil or corneal reflexes absent
	1	Pupil and corneal reflexes absent
	0	Absent pupil, corneal, and cough reflex
Respiration	4	Not intubated, regular breathing pattern
	3	Not intubated, Cheyne–Stokes breathing pattern
	2	Not intubated, irregular breathing pattern
	1	Breathes above ventilator rate
	0	Breathes at ventilator rate or apnea

conditions. Hypertension can be a physiologic response to increased intracranial pressure that functions to maintain cerebral perfusion pressure. In such a case, acutely lowering blood pressure may worsen the neurologic injury by reducing cerebral perfusion pressure. Hypertension with bradycardia and a change in breathing pattern (Cushing triad) is a sign of elevated intracranial pressure and may signal impending herniation. Management may require temporary emergent measures to lower intracranial pressure such as hyperventilation (to reduce carbon dioxide and induce vasoconstriction) and hyperosmolar therapy followed by more definitive neurosurgical therapy. Hypertension in the setting of coma may also be the product of nonspecific sympathetic response or of stimulant intoxication. Primary or secondary hypertension may cause hypertensive encephalopathy that can manifest as coma. Primary hypertensive

encephalopathy is suggested by a history of hypertension or renal disease, or by preceding headache, visual complaints, or seizures. Differentiating reactive/compensatory hypertension from a primary hypertensive encephalopathy may be difficult but is crucial in determining how to manage blood pressure. Bradycardia may occur with intracranial hypertension, cardiac disease, hypothermia, toxin exposure (sedating drugs), uremic coma, or myxedema coma. Tachycardia may occur with hypovolemic or cardiogenic shock, sepsis, pain, toxin exposure (amphetamines, cocaine, nicotine, and caffeine), malignant hyperthermia, anemia, heart failure, hyperthyroidism, pheochromocytoma, or pulmonary embolism. Abnormalities in respiratory rate and pattern of breathing may indicate pathology originating in the lungs, acid–base derangement, or nervous system dysfunction (**Fig. 57.2**). *Cheyne–Stokes respiration*

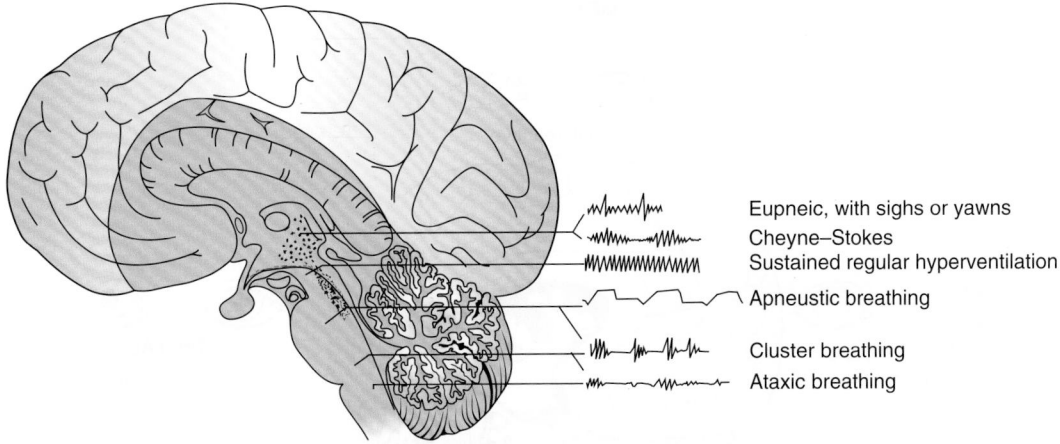

Eupneic, with sighs or yawns
Cheyne–Stokes
Sustained regular hyperventilation
Apneustic breathing
Cluster breathing
Ataxic breathing

FIGURE 57.2. Respiratory patterns characteristic of specific lesion locations. (From Brazis PW, Masdeu JC, Biller J. *Localization in Clinical Neurology.* 6th ed. Philadelphia, PA: Wolters Kluwer/Lippincott Williams & Wilkins, 2011, with permission.)

describes a rhythmic pattern of accelerating hyperpnea followed by fall in amplitude of breathing culminating in decelerating rate of breathing and apnea. It is a nonspecific pattern seen with extensive bihemispheric cerebral dysfunction, diencephalic (thalamic and hypothalamic) dysfunction, or cardiac failure. Pontine or midbrain tegmental lesions may result in central neurogenic hyperventilation. *Apneustic breathing*, in its most common form, is characterized by a pause at the end of inspiration and reflects damage to respiratory centers at the mid- or lower pontine levels, at or below the level of the trigeminal motor nucleus. Apneusis occurs with basilar artery occlusion (leading to pontine infarction), hypoglycemia, anoxia, or meningitis. *Ataxic breathing* is completely irregular in rate and tidal volume, and occurs with damage to the reticular formation of the dorsomedial medulla (4).

A complete general examination is important in elucidating the coma etiology and identifying medical issues requiring management. Involuntary hip flexion with passive flexion of the neck (*Brudzinski sign*) and resistance to knee extension with hips flexed (*Kernig sign*) indicate meningeal inflammation/irritation. Skin examination provides information about accidental or abusive trauma (bruises, lacerations), systemic medical disease (jaundice in liver failure, uremic frost, hyperpigmentation in adrenal insufficiency), and infection (superficial lacerations in cat-scratch fever, erythema migrans in Lyme disease, petechiae and purpura in meningococcemia). Clear fluid emanating from the nose or ears may indicate a cerebrospinal fluid (CSF) leak due to skull fracture. Organomegaly raises suspicion of metabolic, hematologic, and hepatic diseases. Abusive head trauma is suggested by retinal hemorrhages, metaphyseal fractures, rib fractures, and subdural hemorrhages.

The neurologic examination is directed toward localizing brain dysfunction, identifying coma etiology, and determining early indicators of prognosis. In a comatose child, much of the examination that requires patient cooperation (such as mental status and sensory testing) cannot be performed. Thus, it is aimed as assessing response to stimuli and function of the brainstem and motor systems. Evaluation of responsiveness must include vigorous auditory and sensory stimulation. Nail-bed pressure, pinching, and sternal rubbing may be required. Responsiveness must be evaluated in terms of lack of verbal, motor, and cranial nerve responses.

Fundoscopic examination yields information about the retina and optic nerves. Papilledema may be seen with increased intracranial pressure. However, papilledema may take hours or days to develop, so the absence of papilledema does not confirm that intracranial pressure is normal. Retinal hemorrhages may be seen in inflicted childhood neurotrauma. Flame shaped hemorrhages and cotton-wool spots are seen in hypertensive encephalopathy.

Pupils (**Fig. 57.3** and **Table 57.6**) are examined first by observing the size of both pupils in dim light, and then by assessing reactivity to a bright light shined in each eye. Asymmetric pupils are caused by either oculomotor nerve (cranial nerve III) disruption or impairment of sympathetic fibers (Horner syndrome). Because the oculomotor nerve innervates the pupil constrictors, oculomotor nerve impairment results in an abnormally dilated pupil. Oculomotor nerve palsy also results in ptosis and ophthalmoparesis and may be a sign of uncal herniation. Horner syndrome describes disruption of the sympathetic innervation to the face, characterized by mild ptosis over an abnormally small pupil (meiosis). In traumatic coma, Horner syndrome may be an important clue to dissection of the carotid artery, along which the sympathetic fibers travel, or an injury to the lower brachial plexus (C8–T1). Anisocoria (asymmetric pupils) is an important physical finding, and differentiating whether a pupil is abnormally large or abnormally small is crucial to identifying underlying pathology; asymmetric pupils in bright light indicate pathology in the larger pupil, which is most likely the result of oculomotor palsy (cranial nerve III). Investigations to rule out uncal herniation or an aneurysm of the posterior communicating artery should follow. Pupils that are more asymmetric in darkness suggest the pathology lies with the smaller pupil. Investigation of the carotid artery, the low cervical–high thoracic spinal cord or brachial plexus roots should follow to find causes of the Horner syndrome.

Abnormalities of eye position and motility may be signs of cortical, midbrain, or pontine dysfunction. Conjugate lateral eye deviation may be caused by destructive lesion of the ipsilateral cortex, or pons, or focal seizures in the contralateral hemisphere. Rarely thalamic lesions may cause "wrong-way eyes," in which the eyes deviate away from the side of the destructive lesion (24). Tonic down gaze suggests dorsal midbrain compression. The complete dorsal midbrain syndrome of Parinaud (usually associated with pineal gland or midbrain tumors in children) includes pupillary light-near dissociation, lid-retraction, and convergence-retraction nystagmus.

Dysconjugate gaze suggests extraocular muscle weakness or, more commonly, abnormalities of the third, fourth, or sixth cranial nerves or nuclei. Unilateral or bilateral abducens nerve

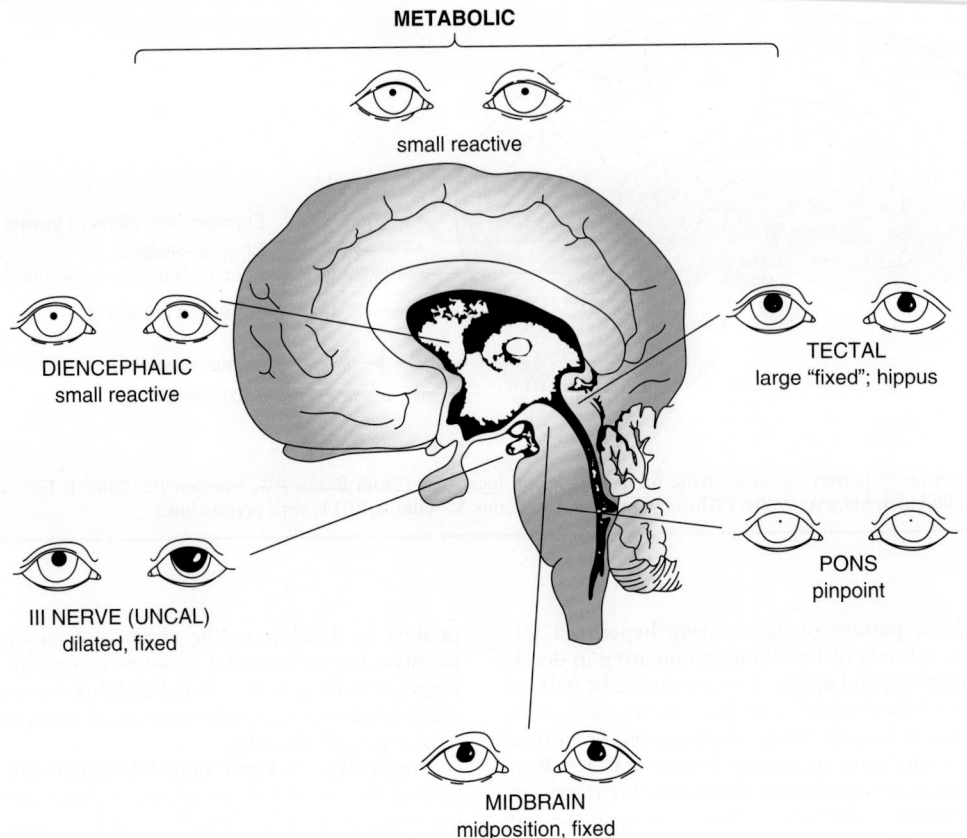

METABOLIC

small reactive

DIENCEPHALIC
small reactive

TECTAL
large "fixed"; hippus

III NERVE (UNCAL)
dilated, fixed

PONS
pinpoint

MIDBRAIN
midposition, fixed

FIGURE 57.3. Pupil abnormalities characteristic of specific lesion locations.

TABLE 57.6

PUPIL ABNORMALITIES IN COMA

■ ETIOLOGY/LOCALIZATION	■ PUPIL APPEARANCE
Metabolic	Small, reactive
Hypothalamic	Small, reactive
Tectal	Large, nonreactive, hippus
Pontine	Pinpoint
Midbrain	Midposition, fixed
Oculomotor nerve, uncal herniation	Ipsilateral pupil dilated, fixed
Severe hypoxic–ischemic encephalopathy	Bilateral dilated, fixed
Opiate intoxication	Pinpoint
Anticholinergic poisoning	Dilated and fixed, unreactive to 1% pilocarpine

(cranial nerve VI) palsies are commonly seen in increased intracranial pressure (causing diplopia), presumably because the nerve is stretched. This is therefore considered a "false localizing sign" since it suggests a focal brainstem lesion but in fact represents a more diffuse intracranial pressure change. An eye with oculomotor nerve (cranial nerve III) palsy is ptotic, depressed, and abducted, and has a dilated pupil. As discussed above, oculomotor nerve palsy in a comatose patient suggests uncal herniation with midbrain compression, and thus requires urgent intervention. Trochlear nerve (cranial nerve IV) palsy causes hypertropia (one eye has higher visual axis) in the affected eye.

Roving eye movements are seen in comatose patients with intact brainstem function. Their disappearance may signal the onset of brainstem dysfunction. Periodic alternating gaze

(ping-pong gaze) describes conjugate horizontal eye movements back and forth with a pause at each end. It may be seen with extensive bilateral hemispheric, basal ganglia, or thalamic–midbrain damage with an intact pons, and is thought to result from disconnection of cortical influences on oculovestibular reflex generators. It has also been reported in reversible coma from monoamine oxidase and tricyclic antidepressant toxicity.

Oculocephalic and oculovestibular reflexes are useful for assessing the integrity of the midbrain and pons in a comatose patient without spontaneous eye movements. To test oculocephalic reflexes, the examiner holds the patient's eyelids open and quickly moves the head to one side. In a comatose patient with an intact brainstem, the eyes will move in the direction opposite the head motion. For example, if the head is moved to the right, the eyes will move conjugately to the left. After several seconds, the eyes may return to a neutral position. The head should be tested in both horizontal and vertical directions. Oculocephalic reflexes should not be tested if the patient has sustained cervical spine trauma or if the spine has not been cleared.

The oculovestibular reflex, commonly referred to as cold calorics, tests the function above the pontomedullary junction. The child must have an open external auditory canal with an intact tympanic membrane (including the absence of pressure equalization tubes), so visual inspection of the canal is an important first step. With the head elevated at 30 degrees, up to 120 cc of ice water is introduced in the ear canal with a small catheter. A conscious patient would experience nystagmus with slow deviation of the eyes toward the irrigated ear and a fast corrective movement away from the ear (the mnemonic COWS, Cold Opposite, Warm Same, applies to the fast phase). In a comatose patient, the fast correction mediated by the cortex is not seen. Instead, the eyes will deviate slowly toward the irrigated ear and remain fixed there. If the brainstem vestibular nuclei (located at the pontomedullary junction) are impaired, no movement will be seen. In brain death, where there is no brainstem function, no eye movement is seen with both ears tested. Five minutes should be allowed before the second ear is tested to allow return of temperature equilibrium between the two ears. Vertical eye movements may be tested by simultaneously irrigating both auditory canals with cold water, producing downward deviation in the comatose patient. Warm water irrigation produces up gaze.

The corneal reflex is tested by tactile stimulation of the cornea, which should elicit bilateral eyelid closure. The afferent (sensory) signal is carried by the trigeminal nerve (cranial nerve V), and the efferent (motor) pathway is carried by the facial nerve (cranial nerve VII). Completion of the reflex loop requires intact trigeminal and facial nerve nuclei in the mid- and lower pons. The cough reflex, which may be seen with stimulation of the carina when a patient is intubated or undergoes suctioning, is mediated by medullary cough centers; sensory and motor signals are carried by glossopharyngeal (cranial nerve IX) and vagus (cranial nerve X) nerves. When the soft palate is stimulated, the gag reflex is elicited, manifested as elevation of the soft palate. As in the cough reflex, afferent and efferent signals are carried by the glossopharyngeal and vagus nerves, with processing in the medulla.

A comatose child may be flaccid, or may display an abnormal flexor or extensor posture. The term decorticate posturing describes flexion of the arms and extension of the legs. Decerebrate posturing describes extension and internal rotation of the arms and legs. Traditionally, decorticate posturing has been considered by relating to dysfunction primarily in the supratentorial compartment, whereas decerebrate posturing has been considered to relate to brainstem dysfunction. Plum and Posner (4) describe the following guidelines to interpreting abnormal postures: flexor arm responses reflect more rostral and less severe supratentorial damage; extensor responses in the arm and leg correlate best with more severe but still supratentorial dysfunction; arm extension with leg flexion suggests pontine damage; and diffuse flaccidity correlates with brainstem damage below the pontomedullary level.

Testing

Investigation should continue with laboratory, neuroimaging, and electrophysiological testing. This area has been reviewed (16) and is summarized in **Table 57.7**. Guidelines have also been published online by the Pediatric Accident and Emergency Research Group of the Royal College of Paediatrics and Child Health and the British Association for Emergency

Medicine on the basis of an extensive literature review and expert consensus (14). This guideline can be printed and can provide detailed and easy-to-access flowcharts of the evaluation and management of a child with decreased consciousness. The guideline initially points out the importance of airway, breathing, and circulation and the importance of continuous cardiopulmonary monitoring and frequent GCS assessment. Hypoxia, hypotension, hypoglycemia or hyperglycemia, hyperthermia or hypothermia, and anemia worsen the prognosis of coma and must be treated aggressively and quickly. Hypotonic fluids should not be administered since this can worsen cerebral edema.

Core investigations should then occur. All children should have a finger-stick blood glucose measurement at the initial evaluation, and even if normal, laboratory testing of glucose should occur since hypoglycemia alone may cause coma and hypoglycemia in association with other etiologies may worsen outcome. Hypoglycemia must be treated urgently with intravenous dextrose. Hyperglycemia may occur in diabetic ketoacidosis or as a manifestation of the sympathetic response to systemic illness/injury. All patients should have a blood gas performed. All patients should have electrolytes measured since abnormalities may cause coma, or may occur secondary to intracranial abnormalities. Liver function tests should be performed since hepatic encephalopathy may cause coma, and liver injury can occur in the setting of systemic hypoxic–ischemic injury. A complete blood count with differential is indicated in all patients to detect infection, anemia, disseminated intravascular coagulopathy, lead encephalopathy, or sickle cell disease. Blood, urine, and stool cultures should be obtained in most patients to investigate infectious etiologies. Toxin screens (urine and expanded plasma testing) should be performed if the etiology of coma is unknown. Specific tests for medications found in the home should be carried out as indicated. Ammonia, lactate, and pyruvate may be performed to screen for metabolic disorders. If abnormal or the history is suggestive of metabolic disease, then measurement of organic acids, amino acids, very long chain fatty acids, and acylcarnitine profile may be indicated. Some patients may require endocrine testing, including cortisol levels and thyroid function studies.

After resuscitation, a head computed tomography (CT) scan should be performed in all children. A normal head CT scan does not rule out all structural intracranial processes. Thus, once the patient has been stabilized and if the etiology of coma remains unclear, then a brain magnetic resonance imaging (MRI) should be performed. MRI is superior to CT in assessing the subcortical structures, brainstem, and spinal cord and in detecting ischemic stroke and venous disease, early hypoxic–ischemic injury, hypertensive encephalopathy, demyelinating disease, toxic leukoencephalopathies, encephalitis, and diffuse axonal injury (see Chapter 59, Neuroimaging).

If the patient is febrile, infection is suspected, or no other etiology can be determined, then a lumbar puncture should be performed. If there is clinical or radiological evidence for intracranial hypertension, then lumbar puncture should be deferred and treatment should be initiated for possible infections (bacterial and viral). CSF should be tested for cell count (both the first and the last tubes need to be tested to help differentiate true findings in the case of a traumatic tap), glucose, protein, Gram stain, bacterial culture, viral polymerase chain reaction (PCR), and additional cultures when suspected clinically (fungal or tuberculosis). If the cause of coma remains unknown, additional studies may be directed at uncommon causes of coma in pediatrics such as Hashimoto encephalitis (thyroid function tests and thyroid autoantibodies), cerebral vasculitis (erythrocyte sedimentation rate, antinuclear antibody panel, and possibly angiography), or paraneoplastic disorders.

An EEG may be useful for several reasons. Although most EEG findings are etiologically nonspecific, they may help

TABLE 57.7

INVESTIGATION OF NONTRAUMATIC COMA (16)

INVESTIGATIONS	INDICATION/CLINICAL CLUES	POSSIBLE ABNORMALITY	FURTHER INVESTIGATION IF ABNORMAL	POSSIBLE DIAGNOSES	ACTION
Dextrostix	All	Low	Blood glucose Liver function tests Blood ammonia Blood lactate Blood and urine amino acids Urine organic acids	Hypoglycemia secondary to: ■ Fasting ■ Severe illness ■ Reye syndrome ■ Organic aciduria ■ Fatty acid oxidation defect ■ Hemorrhagic shock and encephalopathy	IV dextrose
Blood glucose		High		Diabetic ketoacidosis	Fluids/insulin
Blood sodium	Previous polydipsia/polyuria	Low/high	Urinary sodium	Hypo/hypernatremia ± dehydration	Appropriate fluids
Blood urea	All	High	Blood creatinine Blood film	Dehydration Hemolytic uremic syndrome	Rehydrate Dialysis, plasmapheresis
Aspartate transaminase	All	High	Blood ammonia	Reye syndrome Hypoxia–ischemia	
Blood ammonia	All (unless cause known)	High	Blood orotic acid Urine organic acids	Urea cycle defect Organic acidemia	Sodium benzoate Hemodialysis
Full blood count and film	All	Low Hb High WBC Low platelets Sickle cells Burr cells	Hb electrophoresis	Anemia Infection DIC infection Sickle cell disease Hemolytic uremic syndrome	Transfusion Third-generation cephalosporin Dialysis, plasmapheresis
	Residence in endemic area	Parasites on thick/thin films		Malaria	Quinine
	Pica	Basophilic stippling	Wrist x-ray—lead line	Lead encephalopathy	Chelation
Blood culture	All			Infection	Appropriate antibiotics
Stool culture	All	Shigella, enteroviruses			
Mycoplasma IgG, IgM	All (unless cause known)		Chest x-ray	Mycoplasma encephalitis	Azithromycin, prednisolone
Viral titers	Analyze if unexplained		Repeat at discharge		
Urine for toxin screen	Analyze if unexplained			Poisoning	Antidote
Blood lead	Analyze if unexplained		Blood film—basophilic stippling, wrist x-ray—lead line		Chelation
Head CT scan without contrast	All (after resuscitation, afebrile patients should ideally be transferred for CT scan to a unit with neurosurgical facilities)	Blood: Subdural Extradural Intracerebral Space-occupying lesion Hydrocephalus: Obstructive Communicating	Skull x-ray/skeletal survey/clotting screen CSF examination	Nonaccidental injury Tumor Space-occupying lesion Meningitis, especially tuberculous	Neurosurgical referral Child protection Neurosurgical referral Antituberculosis coverage Neurosurgical referral

INVESTIGATIONS	INDICATION/CLINICAL CLUES	POSSIBLE ABNORMALITY	FURTHER INVESTIGATION IF ABNORMAL	POSSIBLE DIAGNOSES	ACTION
		Abscess	Culture aspirate		Neurosurgical referral Anaerobic coverage
		Swelling	Contrast CT/MRI		Mannitol hypertonic saline
		Focal low density		Cerebral abscess, herpes simplex, stroke, ADEM	
		Abnormal basal ganglia	Plasma/CSF lactate, blood gas	Leigh syndrome, hypoxic-ischemic, striatal necrosis	
Lumbar puncture	In febrile patient if no clinical or radiologic evidence of raised ICP (delay and treat if doubt)	Gram stain, CSF cultures, PCR for viruses, TB			
		Pressure measurement: High	CT scan		Hypertonic therapy, hyperventilate
		Microscopy: High WBC		Meningitis/encephalitis	Third-generation cephalosporin, acyclovir
		Microscopy: High RBC	CT (traumatic tap should clear by third bottle)	Hemorrhage/encephalitis/nonaccidental injury	Neurosurgical referral, acyclovir, child protection
		Glucose: Low		Tuberculous meningitis	Immediate and prolonged antituberculosis therapy
		Protein: High		Tuberculous meningitis	Immediate and prolonged antituberculosis therapy
Prolonged search for acid-fast bacilli, culture for TB on Lowenstein–Jensen agar	Prodrome >7 days, optic atrophy, focal signs, abnormal movements, CSF polymorphs <50%, hydrocephalus and/or basal enhancement on contrast CT			Tuberculous meningitis	Immediate and prolonged antituberculosis therapy
Antibodies; e.g., herpes simplex, mycoplasma				Encephalitis	Acyclovir, Azithromycin
Lactate	Abnormal breathing/eye movements, basal ganglia lucencies		Muscle biopsy	Leigh syndrome	
EEG	All, especially if ventilated or evidence of subtle seizures (nystagmus, tonic deviation of eyes, clonic jerking limbs)	Epileptiform discharges		Status epilepticus	IV benzodiazepines, fosphenytoin, barbiturates
		Asymmetrical foci of spikes or periodic lateralizing epileptiform discharges on slow background		Herpes simplex encephalitis (many patients do not have characteristic EEG)	High-dose IV acyclovir for 2 wk
MRI	Unexplained encephalopathy	Frontotemporal abnormality	CSF for herpes simplex, PCR	Herpes simplex encephalitis	High-dose IV acyclovir for 2 wk
		Thalamic abnormality	CSF for EBV (arboviruses in endemic area)		

hb, hemoglobin; WBC, white blood cell; RBC, red blood cell; TB, tuberculosis; EBV, Epstein–Barr virus. From Kirkham FJ. Non-traumatic coma in children. *Arch Dis Child* 2001;85:303–12, with permission.

distinguish between focal and diffuse etiologies. Focal abnormalities suggest focal dysfunction. An unexpectedly normal or only mildly abnormal EEG may raise concern for psychogenic, neuromuscular, or locked-in conditions. Additionally, an EEG may identify nonconvulsive seizures or nonconvulsive status epilepticus, which may cause encephalopathy and occur in response to other acute encephalopathies that are also contributing to producing altered mental status. Studies have indicated that 10%–40% of children with acute encephalopathy experience nonconvulsive seizures or status epilepticus (25–29).

Continuous EEG monitoring has a much higher yield than a standard EEG when aiming to identify nonconvulsive seizures. Continuous EEG monitoring or serial standard EEGs may be useful for following the evolution of encephalopathic states and identifying abrupt changes that could require evaluation and intervention. Tracking EEG features over time may help determine the depth of encephalopathy and can help establish whether brain dysfunction is improving, stable, or worsening. Finally, serial EEGs may help with prognostication, particularly if the coma etiology is known (30–32).

Because the child's systemic and neurologic function will evolve over time, continuous monitoring, including and frequent serial neurologic examinations, is essential. Related chapters address the most common etiologies for neurocritical illness leading to encephalopathy and coma, and appropriate condition-specific management.

CONCLUSIONS

Coma refers to a severe abnormality in consciousness in which both wakefulness and awareness are disturbed. Coma and related forms of acute encephalopathy are medical emergencies since some causes are reversible and secondary neurological injury must be prevented. The history, examination, laboratory, imaging, and electrophysiological evaluation may disclose the etiology of coma, allowing specific treatment. The prognosis in coma is more dependent on the specific etiology than any other factor, and thus prognostic information cannot be provided for the family until the etiology is determined.

References

1. Wong CP, Forsyth R, kelly T, et al. Incidence, aetiology, and outcome of non-traumatic coma: A population based study. *Arch Dis Child* 2001;84(3):193–9.
2. Parslow RC, Morris KP, Tasker RC, et al. Epidemiology of traumatic brain injury in children receiving intensive care in the UK. *Arch Dis Child* 2005;90(11):1182–7.
3. Michaud LJ, Rivara FP, Grady MS, et al. Predictors of survival and severity of disability after severe brain injury in children. *Neurosurgery* 1992;31(2):254–64.
4. Plum F, Posner JB. *The Diagnosis of Stupor and Coma.* 3rd ed. Philadelphia, PA: FA Davis, 1980.
5. Ashwal S, Bale JF Jr, Coulter DL, et al. The persistent vegetative state in children: Report of the Child Neurology Society Ethics Committee. *Ann Neurol* 1992;32(4):570–6.
6. Practice parameters: Assessment and management of patients in the persistent vegetative state (summary statement). The Quality Standards Subcommittee of the American Academy of Neurology. *Neurology* 1995;45(5):1015–8.
7. Kriel RL, Krach LE, Jones-Saete C. Outcome of children with prolonged unconsciousness and vegetative states. *Pediatr Neurol* 1993;9(5):362–8.
8. Owen AM, Coleman MR. Detecting awareness in the vegetative state. *Ann N Y Acad Sci* 2008;1129:130–8.
9. Owen AM, Schiff ND, Laureys S. A new era of coma and consciousness science. *Prog Brain Res* 2009;177:399–411.
10. Landsness E, Bruno MA, Noirhomme Q, et al. Electrophysiological correlates of behavioural changes in vigilance in vegetative state and minimally conscious state. *Brain* 2011;134(pt 8):2222–32.
11. Bruno MA, Vanhaudenhuyse A, Thibaut A, et al. From unresponsive wakefulness to minimally conscious PLUS and functional locked-in syndromes: Recent advances in our understanding of disorders of consciousness. *J Neurol* 2011;258(7):1373–84.
12. Gosseries O, Bruno MA, Chatelle C, et al. Disorders of consciousness: What's in a name? *NeuroRehabilitation* 2011;28(1):3–14.
13. Nakagawa TA, Ashwal S, Mathur M. Guidelines for the determination of brain death in infants and children: An update of the 1987 task force recommendations. *Crit Care Med* 2011;39(9):2139–55.
14. Schmitt FC, Buchheim K, Meierkord H, et al. Anticonvulsant properties of hypothermia in experimental status epilepticus. *Neurobiol Dis* 2006;23(3):689–96.
15. Michelson DJ, Ashwal S. Evaluation of coma and brain death. *Semin Pediatr Neurol* 2004;11(2):105–18.
16. Kirkham FJ. Non-traumatic coma in children. *Arch Dis Child* 2001;85(4):303–12.
17. Seshia SS, Bingham WT, Kirkham FJ, et al. Nontraumatic coma in children and adolescents: Diagnosis and management. *Neurol Clin* 2011;29(4):1007–43.
18. Teasdale G, Jennett B. Assessment of coma and impaired consciousness. A practical scale. *Lancet* 1974;2(7872):81–4.
19. Reilly PL, Simpson DA, Spord R, et al. Assessing the conscious level in infants and young children: A paediatric version of the Glasgow Coma Scale. *Childs Nervous System* 1988;4(1):30–3.
20. Raimondi AJ, Hirschauer J. Head injury in the infant and toddler. Coma scoring and outcome scale. *Child's Brain* 1984;11(1):12–35.
21. Hahn YS, Chyung C, Barthel MJ, et al. Head injuries in children under 36 months of age. Demography and outcome. *Childs Nervous System* 1988;4(1):34–40.
22. Wijdicks EF, Bamlet WR, Maramattom BV, et al. Validation of a new coma scale: The FOUR score. *Ann Neurol* 2005;58(4):585–93.
23. Cohen J. Interrater reliability and predictive validity of the FOUR score coma scale in a pediatric population. *J Neurosci Nurs* 2009;41(5):261–7; quiz 268–9.
24. Messe SR, Cucchiara BL. Wrong-way eyes with thalamic hemorrhage. *Neurology* 2003;60(9):1524.
25. Abend NS, Gutierrez-Colina AM, Topjian AA, et al. Nonconvulsive seizures are common in critically ill children. *Neurology* 2011;76(12):1071–7.
26. Williams K, Jarrar R, Buchhalter J. Continuous video-EEG monitoring in pediatric intensive care units. *Epilepsia* 2011;52(6):1130–6.
27. Jette N, Claassen J, Emerson RG, et al. Frequency and predictors of nonconvulsive seizures during continuous electroencephalographic monitoring in critically ill children. *Arch Neurol* 2006;63(12):1750–5.
28. Saengpattrachai M, Sharma R, Hunjan A, et al. Nonconvulsive seizures in the pediatric intensive care unit: Etiology, EEG, and brain imaging findings. *Epilepsia* 2006;47(9):1510–8.
29. McCoy B, Sharma R, Ochi A, et al. Predictors of nonconvulsive seizures among critically ill children. *Epilepsia* 2011;52(11):1973–8.
30. Kessler S, Topjian AA, Gutierrez-Colina AM, et al. Short-term outcome prediction by electroencephalographic features in children treated with therapeutic hypothermia after cardiac arrest. *Neurocrit Care* 2011;14(1):37–43.
31. Mandel R, Martinot A, Delepoulle F, et al. Prediction of outcome after hypoxic-ischemic encephalopathy: A prospective clinical and electrophysiologic study. *J Pediatr* 2002;141(1):45–50.
32. Mewasingh LD, Christophe C, Fonteyne C, et al. Predictive value of electrophysiology in children with hypoxic coma. *Pediatr Neurol* 2003;28(3):178–83.

CHAPTER 58 ■ NEUROLOGIC MONITORING

ROBERT C. TASKER, MATEO ABOY, ALAN GRAHAM, AND BRAHM GOLDSTEIN

KEY POINTS

1 Increasing evidence suggests that neuromonitoring with various modalities can improve diagnosis, treatment, and outcome in critically ill and injured children.

2 To understand the current and future applications of neuromonitoring in the pediatric intensive care unit, it is necessary to understand the basic engineering and physiologic principles that underlie different monitoring technologies.

3 Because digital signal processing algorithms generally use a moving window of the physiologic signal to generate estimates, the clinical parameters displayed on the bedside monitor represent an average over past values of the signal and cannot respond instantaneously to alarm conditions. Thus, in a deteriorating patient, monitors typically generate alarms after the alarm condition has persisted for several seconds and following resuscitation typically lag a few seconds after the patient's condition improves.

4 Our management of three disease states necessitates advanced neuromonitoring. These include continuous electroencephalogram coupled with digital video monitoring for status epilepticus in diagnosing nonconvulsive seizures, intracranial pressure monitoring in patients with severe traumatic brain injury, and intraoperative and postoperative neurophysiologic monitoring of children who undergo repair of congenital cardiac disease with near-infrared spectroscopy technology.

5 Multimodality neuromonitoring may have the potential to improve overall patient outcome, but definitive pediatric studies are required.

Increasing evidence demonstrates tangible benefits from neurologic monitoring in a variety of PICU patients. Continuous **1** electroencephalogram (EEG) coupled with digital video monitoring for status epilepticus (SE) is routinely applied with good results in diagnosing and managing nonconvulsive seizures. Intracranial pressure (ICP) monitoring is the mainstay of our management in patients with severe traumatic brain injury (TBI). Near-infrared spectroscopy (NIRS) technology is used increasingly in the neonatal, cardiac surgical, and extracorporeal membrane oxygenation populations. Last, the practice of transcranial Doppler (TCD) insonation of intracranial vessels with determination of cerebral blood flow (CBF) velocity is a **2** practice being translated from neurocritical care in adults to PICU practice. Thus, it is important for PICU personnel to understand the underlying engineering and physiologic principles of such neuromonitoring.

SCIENTIFIC FOUNDATIONS

General Engineering Aspects of PICU Monitoring

Medical instrumentation systems are often composed of sensors, signal conditioning hardware and software, output displays, and auxiliary signals. Sensors are used to convert a physical measurement (i.e., a quantity, property, or condition of interest) into an electrical signal output. The sensors used for medical instrumentation purposes are designed to be minimally invasive and to respond to the source of energy present in the measure, while excluding all other sources as much as possible. Generally, the electrical signal produced by these sensors cannot be connected directly to the output display device. Signal conditioning and processing, such as amplification and analog filtering, are typically required (1). Additionally, the sensor outputs are analog signals and must be converted to digital form before they can be processed using more advanced digital signal processing techniques. Analog-to-digital (A/D) conversion involves signal conditioning, antialiasing filtering, uniform sampling, and quantization. **Table 58.1** provides definitions for the engineering terms used in this chapter. For an in-depth discussion of medical instrumentation, such as sensors, biopotential electrodes and amplifiers, blood pressure, flow, and volume measurement equipment, chemical biosensors, and imaging systems, the reader is referred to a general textbook on biomedical engineering (1).

Most signals are filtered with analog integrated circuits before A/D conversion. These frequency-selective filters are usually linear bandpass or highpass filters used to remove drift, prevent aliasing, and reduce noise; they can distort the waveform morphology due to nonlinear phase in the passband or removal of signal frequencies.

During A/D conversion, analog signals are sampled at a rate determined by the manufacturer (i.e., the sampling rate or sampling frequency). To accurately represent the signal on the patient's monitor display, the sampling rate must be high enough so that a linear interpolation between the sample points results in a visually smooth and representative signal. To achieve this, the sampling rate should be at least 10 times higher than the highest-frequency component of the prefiltered signal. For most physiologic signals that vary with the cardiac and respiratory cycles, a sampling rate of 100 Hz is sufficient. Due to the impulsive nature of the QRS complex, electrocardiogram (ECG) signals have a higher bandwidth than most other physiologic signals encountered in the PICU and require a higher sampling rate of at least 250 Hz to accurately represent different segments of the ECG waveform. EEGs also require a higher sampling rate, although this signal is infrequently displayed directly on PICU patient monitors.

TABLE 58.1

ENGINEERING TERMS AND DEFINITIONS

Aliasing—The apparent conversion of high-frequency signals to low-frequency signals due to an insufficient sample rate

Analog-to-digital (A/D) conversion—The electrical conversion of an analog signal (often a voltage) to a digital representation that enables manipulation and processing by computers

Bandpass filter—A filter that eliminates low- and high-frequency components of a signal, but retains an intermediate range

Bandwidth—The range of frequencies spanned by a signal. When applied to bandpass filters, it describes the range of frequencies that are allowed to pass through the filter

Capacitance—A measure of the ability of a circuit element to store electrical charge. Elements with a large capacitance dampen or resist rapid fluctuations in voltage

Demodulation—The process of extracting an information-bearing signal from another signal; analogous to extracting a file of interest from a compressed or encrypted file

Hertz (Hz)—A measure of frequency; equivalent to cycles per second (cps)

High-frequency noise—Many types of artifact in physiologic signals contain significant power at high frequencies. This noise is often emitted by medical equipment near the patient

Highpass filter—A filter that eliminates low-frequency components of a signal but retains high-frequency components

Inductance—A measure of the ability of a circuit element to store energy in a magnetic field. Elements with a large inductance dampen or resist rapid fluctuations in current

Linear interpolation—The process of estimating a value of a signal or function between two intermediate values using a line between the two points

Low-frequency noise—Some types of artifact in physiologic signals contain significant power at low frequencies. This noise is often caused by patient movement

Lowpass filter—A filter that eliminates high-frequency components of a signal but retains low-frequency components

Modulation—The process of embedding an information-bearing signal in another signal; analogous to creating an encrypted or compressed file that contains a file of interest

Moving window—A technique for estimating an average quality of a signal continuously by averaging over period of the preceding 3–5 s. For example, the systolic blood pressure is usually calculated by averaging the systolic peaks over a moving window of 3–5 s

Nonlinear—Any system or device the behavior of which is governed by a set of nonlinear equations

Signal power—The power contained in a signal is generally defined as the square of the signal; often averaged over a moving window to create a smoothly varying continuous estimate

In addition to the sampling rate requirements, quantization requirements must be met to avoid *quantization error*. Each sample of the digital signal is represented by B bits and can only take one of 2^B levels. The quantization error is the error that results from using the quantized signal rather than the true signal amplitude.

Once the physiologic signals have been converted to digital form, more advanced digital signal processing algorithms are used to process these physiologic digital signals and extract clinically significant parameters. For instance, heart rate is estimated from the ECG signal using automatic QRS detection algorithms, and diastolic and systolic pressures are obtained from pressure signals. It is important for the clinician to understand that digital signal processing algorithms generally use a moving window of the physiologic signal to generate estimates. These moving-window segments (signal frames) range from 3 to 10 seconds in duration. Consequently, the clinical parameters obtained represent an average over past values of the signal and monitors do not respond instantaneously to alarm conditions. Thus, patient monitors typically generate alarms *after* the alarm condition has persisted for several seconds. The obverse is also true. For example, after a successful resuscitation from cardiopulmonary arrest, the arterial oxygen saturation value will typically lag a few seconds after the patient's cyanosis has resolved.

Common Clinical Questions

Specific problems in assessing the neurological state of PICU patients arise when sedative and muscle relaxant medications have been used as part of supportive care. Some of the typical questions that clinicians have about patients at risk of brain injury are:

- Is the unresponsive and immobile patient awake or aware of pain from procedures?
- Are repetitive movements purposeful responses, reflexes, or seizures?
- Is this patient at risk of ongoing subclinical or nonconvulsive seizures?
- Is the patient at risk of cerebral edema and intracranial hypertension?
- Is the patient at risk of cerebral ischemia?
- Is the brain functionally intact or irreversibly damaged?

These questions fall into two categories, *diagnostic* versus *monitoring* requirements. Both of these requirements are essential and usually complimentary. Diagnostic assessment focuses on documentation of a certain event, such as nonconvulsive seizures using the EEG or middle cerebral artery vasospasm using TCD. Theoretically, monitoring acquires continuous information that allows accurate detection of intracranial changes that will lead to more precise treatment. In this regard, monitoring should be undertaken if the following three conditions are satisfied:

- Significant changes in the signal provide ongoing diagnostic information or occur at the stage of reversible injury.
- Criteria are well established for identifying significant changes in the signal.
- Identification of *diagnostic* information or new signal from *monitoring* results in a change of practice. In regard to information from *monitoring*, there is some intervention that bedside caregivers can correct so as to minimize injury.

Clinically Important Physiologic Systems and Signals

A limited number of physiologic systems may be monitored within the central nervous system (CNS). **Table 58.2** provides a list of commonly used monitoring modalities, according to frequency of usage in the PICU.

The EEG has been widely available for decades to record and quantitatively measure brain electrical activity. Technology for monitoring ICP has also been widely available for decades, and now is accomplished with more accurate fiber-optic technology. Additional techniques involve the surrogates of CBF and include ultrasound and TCD, brain tissue oxygenation using NIRS, and jugular venous oxyhemoglobin saturation ($SjvO_2$). Additionally, monitoring of cellular and extracellular processes includes local brain tissue oxygen tension ($PbtO_2$) and extracellular fluid concentrations of glutamate, glucose, lactate, and pyruvate using microdialysis. Finally, the term *multimodality neuromonitoring* refers to the simultaneous use of different combinations of these methods to provide a more complete physiologic picture of CNS activity from cellular, to tissue, to organ level.

APPLICATIONS IN THE PICU

The most commonly used forms of monitoring in the PICU are EEG and ICP. Of the other modalities described in **Table 58.2**, NIRS and TCD have ongoing clinical evaluations in the pediatric critical care literature. The focus of this chapter will be on these four forms of monitoring.

Diagnostic EEG and Evoked Potentials

The EEG monitors the electrical activity of the brain observed via scalp electrical potentials. The sources of this electrical activity are the neurons located predominantly in the outermost layers of the cerebral cortex. Thus, the EEG follows the spatial

TABLE 58.2

MONITORING SYSTEMS

■ SYSTEM	■ TYPE	■ FEATURES	■ MEASURE	■ APPLICATIONS	■ USAGE
Clinical	Coma scale scores	Noninvasive Regional or global Intermittent	Change in clinical parameters	Very sensitive in awake, non-intubated patients	*Common* in all cases
ICP	Invasive pressure transducer	Invasive Regional Continuous	Change in pressure with known norms	Guides treatment in intracranial hypertension algorithm	*Common* in severe TBI
EEG	Brain activity (focal and global)	Noninvasive Focal or global Intermittent or continuous	Seizure detection, depth of anesthesia, and severity of injury	Guides treatment and prognostic	*Common* in seizure cases and encephalopathy
NIRS	Light absorption in near-infrared range	Noninvasive Regional Continuous	Estimate of frontal region cerebral venous oxygen saturation	Identification of unappreciated cerebral hypoxia; desaturation associated with outcome	*Less common* with most data in cardiac cases
TCD	Ultrasound of cerebral arteries	Noninvasive Regional Intermittent or continuous	Assessment of CBF-velocity; assessment of vasospasm	Noninvasive assessment of CBF-velocity, ICP and autoregulation	*Rarely used* in pediatrics since lack of norms
$PbtO_2$	Intraparenchymal electrode measurement	Invasive Focal Continuous	Focal assessment of oxygen tension	Level III recommendation in adult severe TBI, with certain thresholds	*Rarely used* in pediatrics
$SjvO_2$	Assessment of cerebral venous oxygen saturation	Invasive Global Intermittent or continuous	Global assessment of cerebral oxygen extraction	Level II recommendation in adult severe TBI, with certain thresholds	*Rarely used* in pediatrics
Pupillometry	Pupil assessment with standardized light source	Noninvasive Regional Intermittent	Quantified pupillary diameter and reactivity	Detects pupillary constriction even in small pupils	*Rarely used* in pediatrics
Cerebral microdialysis	Measurement of cerebral analytes	Invasive Focal Intermittent	Focal assessment of bioenergetics and tissue glutamate	Some recommendation for use in adults with severe TBI or poor-grade SAH	*Rarely used* in pediatrics

CBF, cerebral blood flow; EEG, electroencephalography; ICP, intracranial pressure; $PbtO_2$, partial pressure of oxygen in brain tissue; NIRS, near-infrared spectroscopy; SAH, subarachnoid hemorrhage; $SjvO_2$, oxygen-hemoglobin saturation in jugular vein (bulb); TBI, traumatic brain injury; TCD, transcranial Doppler.

topography of the cortex. The information provided can sometimes be diagnostic of certain forms of encephalopathy (e.g., hepatic) or indicative of the severity of encephalopathy (2–5).

Vision, hearing, sensory, and motor functions may all be discretely monitored to assess peripheral and CNS damage in patients with suspected injury. The integrity of the complete neural pathways may be assessed using evoked potentials, with abnormalities assigned to specific levels or sites of injury. As a diagnostic test, the information from evoked potential studies may help with prognostication after severe brain injury, but as with any diagnostic test the risk of false positives and false negatives need to be considered. For example, a recent systematic review of the literature (1981–2007) on the prognostic value of somatosensory evoked potentials (SEPs) in comatose children identified 14 studies covering 732 patients (6). The authors concluded that the use of SEPs was supported in an integrated process of outcome prediction after acute brain injury in children. However, they advised caution when predicting unfavorable outcomes in patients with an absence of SEPs in cases of severe TBI and cases of hypoxic–ischemic encephalopathy or postresuscitation disease.

Continuous EEG Monitoring

While a 1-hour EEG is often used in most clinical circumstances, continuous 24-hour EEG or video-EEG monitoring is increasingly used in the ICU. The various clinical indications in which 24-hour EEG monitoring has proven useful include the surveillance for subclinical seizures, the effectiveness of therapy in refractory SE, the achievement of electrical silence in the severe treatment of TBI, metabolic encephalopathies, and neurologic conditions that limit a patient's ability to respond (e.g., brainstem injuries or severe peripheral neuropathic syndromes). The depth of impaired consciousness or coma can be immediately assessed, as can the degree to which ongoing electrographic seizures contribute to that state.

The most common pediatric EEG is a 20-lead EEG with continuous recording and simultaneous digital video recording, with clinical annotations made by bedside observers, usually the PICU nurse or parent. A variety of channel configurations (i.e., bipolar or reference montages) can be used, depending on the area of interest. A *channel* is simply a representation of the potential difference between two recording electrodes. Additional electrodes may include eye leads to discern ocular movements, electromyography, ECG, and a measurement of respiratory frequency.

Current digital acquisition systems record continuous EEG data to computer hard drives (1–1.5 GB/24 h/patient). These systems can acquire 32, 64, 128, or more channels, with higher numbers used for large arrays of electrodes, usually in patients who are undergoing intracranial recording for epilepsy surgery (**Figs. 58.1** and **58.2**). Most patients require 32 or fewer channels. Sampling rates vary from 60 to 257 Hz, and data can be instantly remontaged to allow better localization and interpretation of focal or generalized abnormalities.

A variety of software packages are available to interpret EEG data, often in real time. Specialized software can identify numerous epileptiform abnormalities and detect electrographic seizure activity. The parameters of these detection algorithms can be adjusted to increase yield and decrease false detections. Special software packages are available for the detection of neonatal seizures, while other packages can identify sleep stages. Some software systems include the ability to trigger alarms when a seizure or abnormality of interest is detected.

Most digital EEG monitoring systems also acquire simultaneous digital video and audio signals. Temporal resolution is excellent, far surpassing analog video modalities. Data can be recorded from cart-mounted cameras and microphones in the patient's room, or remotely via wall- or ceiling-mounted devices. Digital video files can be large and the storage and transmission of data across hospital networks can be expensive and difficult. Programs can automatically prune files, saving portions of every hour or time period and computer-detected abnormalities and use compression algorithms to create small files for storage, transmission, or review via cable linkage to workstations in the neuroepileptologist's laboratory.

The amount of useful clinical information gained through prolonged recordings (including simultaneous video monitoring) has proven superior to routine EEGs. Prognostic information can be gained in patients with hypoxic–ischemic encephalopathies. Using continuous recording or serial studies, EEG monitoring can also be used to confirm the diagnosis of brain death.

Useful technology includes quantitative and graphic techniques (e.g., compressed spectral arrays and voltage maps) that transform the EEG signal using frequency and amplitude modulations and aid in the interpretation and source localization of abnormalities of interest. The spatial information obtained from EEG data collected with standard electrode arrays is confounded by spatial aliasing error. However, a dense-array EEG allows sensors to be placed at more than 100 sample locations, making possible accurate measurement of the EEG as a time-varying, spatially distributed, electrical potential. Advantages of dense-array EEGs are that the time for electrode placement and removal is minimal, as the sensor net is only soaked in a solute bath, and the smell and potential skin irritation from collodion glue are eliminated.

Limitations of continuous EEG monitoring primarily involve the level of expertise required for data interpretation. In many cases, PICU staff can be taught to identify seizures and patterns of interest, but full review and analysis usually require a neurophysiologist or neurologist. The time required for interpretation remains significant but has been reduced by technologic advances in digital acquisition, the use of spike- and seizure-detection algorithms, and networked systems. Limitations persist, automatic detection software remains error prone, delays in analysis reduce the benefits of anticipatory care, the application and maintenance of electrodes requires trained technologists and prolonged electrode placement using collodion can cause scalp breakdown.

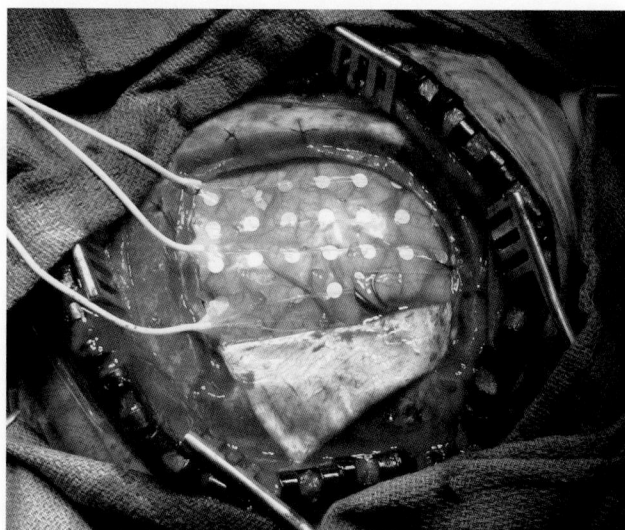

FIGURE 58.1. High-density subdural electrode grid placed intraoperatively over the frontotemporal region in a patient with intractable focal seizures. (Photo courtesy N. Selden, PhD, MD, Oregon Health & Science University, Portland, OR).

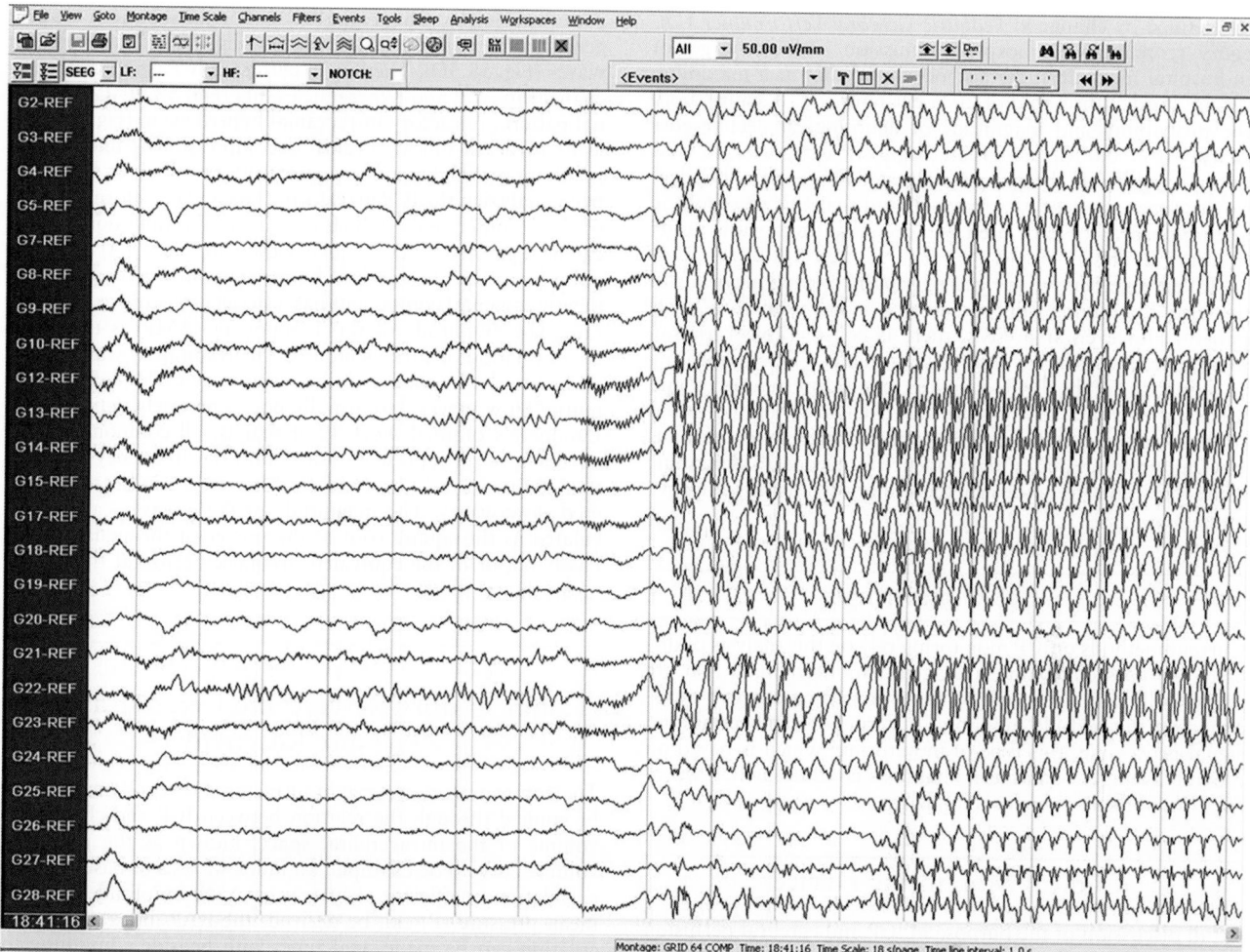

FIGURE 58.2. Intracranial EEG showing focal onset of a seizure with regional spread after 10 seconds. (Photo courtesy N. Selden, PhD, MD, Oregon Health & Science University, Portland, OR).

Clinical Reports of Continuous EEG Monitoring in the PICU

Most of the recent reports of continuous EEG monitoring in the PICU are focused on the problem of seizure detection. Seizures may be difficult to detect in comatose children, especially if the episodes are subtle or if neuromuscular blocking agents are being used. In these situations, there is increased emphasis on detecting brief electroencephalographic seizure (ES) activity or more prolonged episodes of electroencephalographic SE (ESE). Typically, ES activity is described as an abnormal paroxysmal event that differed from background activity "lasting longer than 10 seconds with a temporal–spatial evolution in morphology, frequency, and amplitude, and with a plausible electrographic field." ESE is defined as "either a single 30 minute ES or a series of recurrent independent ES totaling more than 30 minutes in any one hour" (7,8).

In recent PICU series of such monitoring, ES has been identified in 7%–46% of the cases and ESE in 18%–35% of the cases (8–21). The wide range in the prevalence of ES and ESE in the recent PICU literature reflects the case mix in different series. Groups at high risk for ES are patients with epilepsy (17), CNS infection (11,16), structural brain lesions (12,18), encephalopathy after cardiac arrest (10), and TBI (8). When therapeutic hypothermia is used after cardiac arrest, it is common for seizures to occur during the period of rewarming because treatments that suppressed or treated the EEG activity (neuromuscular blockade, sedation, and hypothermia) are discontinued (9,10). Topjian et al. (50) recently reported the PICU prevalence of ES or ESE to be 56% in cases of epilepsy, 45% in cases of encephalitis, 36% in cases of hypoxic–ischemic encephalopathy after cardiac arrest, and 31% in cases of severe TBI.

The clinical significance (relationship to etiology or need for treatment) of ES and ESE was, until recently, largely unknown. In the 2013 report by Topjian et al. (50) of a PICU series of 200 patients undergoing continuous EEG monitoring during acute encephalopathy, the presence of ESE rather than ES alone was associated with increased mortality and worsened neurologic outcome at discharge. In the past, there has been much debate about the significance of ES and ESE in comatose, sedated, and paralyzed, possibly postictal patients (21) and, as a consequence, there is substantial variation in treatment in the PICU (7). The presence of ESE may merely serve as a biomarker of disease pattern, and the link with severity in underlying pathology having the major effect on outcome. Kirkham et al. (16) recently described that larger numbers and total duration of ES/ESE was related to worsening outcome in a population of 204 critically ill comatose children. Last, Payne et al. in 2014 (22) prospectively evaluated 259 critically ill infants and children admitted at a single center who underwent continuous EEG monitoring over a 3-year period. By relating seizure burden to worsening neurological decline (as defined by change in *Pediatric Cerebral Performance Category* score between hospital admission and discharge, or in-hospital mortality), the authors found that at a maximum seizure burden threshold of 20% per hour (i.e., 12/min), both the probability and magnitude of neurological decline rose sharply ($p < 0.0001$) across all diagnostic categories. In view of this association, the authors suggested that early antiepileptic drug management is warranted, and that this threshold in seizure burden could be used as a potential therapeutic target in future studies.

Taken together, we are getting closer to knowing what to do with continuous EEG monitoring in the comatose PICU patient. However, at present, there is considerable variation in this practice (7). Instituting continuous EEG monitoring as a service in the PICU requires significant resources and needs to be available nights and weekends. While the recent studies show the added information provided by continuous EEG monitoring, additional evidence is needed to determine if the interventions guided by the use of this therapy improve outcomes.

ICP Monitoring

Current methods of ICP monitoring rely on the analysis of discrete 3- to 5-second, time-averaged, parametric data that are numerically displayed next to the averaged parametric waveforms on the bedside monitors. In terms of engineering and signal processing, this type of monitoring, which is based on moving averages, is not as valuable as continuous ICP waveform monitoring at high sampling rates.

Clinical Monitoring Devices

A full discussion of the purpose in ICP and cerebral perfusion pressure (CPP, defined as the difference between the mean arterial blood pressure [ABP] and the mean ICP) monitoring is found in Chapter 61. Raised ICP is the most common cause of death in neurosurgical patients, and is extremely common in patients who suffer from severe TBI. Elevated ICP following TBI often results in secondary injury due to ischemia secondary to decreased CPP. The major aim of monitoring and managing elevated ICP is the prevention of cerebral ischemia.

ICP monitoring devices are categorized according to the site of placement and the way in which the pressure signal is transduced. Standard approaches for the measurement of ICP rely on manometry of catheters placed in the lateral ventricles. Alternatively, pressure sensors may be placed within the brain. Overall, an intraventricular drain connected to an external pressure transducer is considered the gold standard for measuring ICP because the transducer can be adjusted to zero externally. Modern, catheter-tipped ventricular, subdural, or intraparenchymal microtransducers have less infection rate and risk of hemorrhage, but cannot be recalibrated to zero after insertion, and considerable zero drift can occur in long-term monitoring. For example, a cumulative drift up to ± 6 mm Hg over 5 days has been described (23).

ICP Trend and Waveform Data

When monitored continuously, changes in the time-averaged mean ICP may be classified into relatively few patterns (**Fig. 58.3**) (24). The first pattern, low and stable ICP (below 20 mm Hg), is seen after uncomplicated TBI (**Fig. 58.3A**). Such a pattern is also seen commonly in the initial period after brain trauma before brain swelling evolves. The second pattern, high and stable ICP (above 20 mm Hg), is the most common

pattern to follow TBI (**Fig. 58.3B**). The third pattern is vasogenic waves and includes B waves (**Fig. 58.3C**) and plateau waves (**Fig. 58.3D**). The fourth pattern is ICP waves related to changes in ABP and hyperemic events (**Fig. 58.3E–G**). The final pattern, refractory intracranial hypertension (**Fig. 58.3H**), leads to death unless surgical decompression is undertaken. In addition to these patterns, more information can be gained from analyzing the ICP waveform. The ICP waveform consists of three components, which overlap in the time domain but can be separated in the frequency domain (**Fig. 58.4**) (24). The pulse waveform has several harmonic components; of these, the fundamental component has a frequency equal to the heart rate. The amplitude of this component (AMP) is useful for the evaluation of various indices. The respiratory waveform is related to the frequency of the respiratory cycle (8–20 cycles/min). "Slow waves" are usually not as precisely defined as in Lundberg's original work (25); that is, all components that have a spectral representation within the frequency limits of 0.05–0.0055 Hz (20-second to 3-minute period) are considered slow waves. The magnitude of these waves can be calculated as the square root of the power of the signal, of the passband, or of the equivalent frequency range at the output of the digital filter.

Assessment of Pressure–Volume Compensatory Reserve and Cerebrovascular Pressure Reactivity

The compensatory reserve in intracranial hydrodynamics can be studied through the relation between ICP and changes in volume of the intracerebral space, known as the pressure–volume curve. For example, an index of reserve based on the correlation coefficient (R) between AMP amplitude (A) and mean pressure (P) can be derived (the RAP index). This calculation can be made, real time, with bedside computing to calculate the linear correlation between consecutive, time-averaged data points of AMP and ICP (usually 40 such samples) acquired over a reasonably long period to average over respiratory and pulse waves (usually 6- to 10-second epochs). The RAP index indicates the degree of correlation between AMP and mean ICP over short periods (~4 minutes). A RAP index close to zero indicates lack of synchronization between changes in AMP and mean ICP. This index denotes good pressure–volume compensatory reserve at low ICP (i.e., a change in volume produces little or no change in pressure) (**Fig. 58.5**) (26). When the RAP index rises to +1, AMP varies directly with ICP and indicates that the "working point" of the intracranial space shifts to the right toward the steep part of the pressure–volume curve. Here compensatory reserve is low; therefore, any further rise in volume may produce a rapid increase in ICP. After TBI and subsequent brain swelling, the RAP index is usually close to +1. With any further increase in ICP, AMP decreases and RAP values fall below zero. This phenomenon occurs when cerebral autoregulatory capacity is exhausted; the pressure–volume curve bends to the right, the capacity of cerebral arterioles to dilate in response to a fall in CPP is exhausted, and the arterioles tend to collapse passively. This phenomenon indicates terminal cerebrovascular derangement with a decrease in pulse pressure transmission from the arterial bed to the intracranial compartment.

Another ICP-derived index is the pressure-reactivity index (PRx), which incorporates the idea of assessing cerebrovascular reaction by observing the response of ICP to slow spontaneous changes in ABP (27). For example, when the cerebrovascular bed is normally reactive, any change in ABP produces an inverse change in cerebral blood volume and thus ICP. When cerebrovascular reactivity is disturbed, changes in

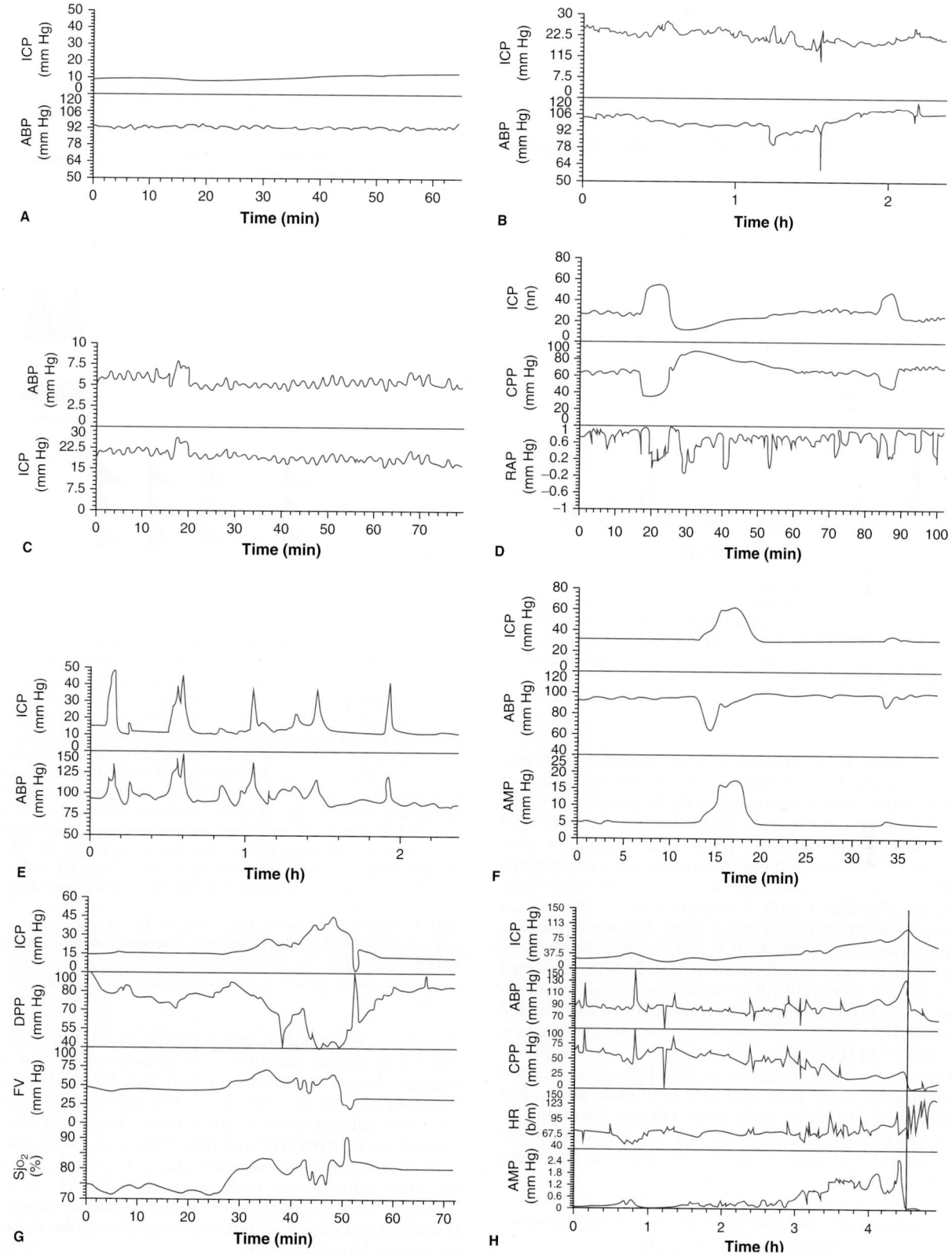

FIGURE 58.3. Examples of intracranial pressure (ICP) recording in various clinical scenarios after head trauma (34); note the different scales. **A:** Low and stable ICP: mean arterial blood pressure (ABP) is plotted in the *bottom panel.* **B:** Stable and elevated ICP: such a picture can be seen most of the time in patients with head injuries. **C:** B waves of ICP: these are seen both in mean ICP and spectrally resolved pulse amplitude of ICP (AMP). They are also usually seen in a plot of time-averaged ABP, but not always. **D:** Plateau waves of ICP: cerebrospinal compensatory reserve is usually low when waves are recorded (the correlation coefficient between AMP and mean ABP, RAP, is close to +1). At the top of the waves, during maximal vasodilatation, integration between pulse amplitude and mean ICP fails, as indicated by a fall in RAP. After the plateau wave, ICP usually falls below the baseline level and cerebrospinal compensatory reserve becomes better. CPP, Cerebral perfusion pressure. **E:** High, spiky waves of ICP caused by sudden increases in ABP. **F:** Increase in ICP caused by temporary decrease in ABP. **G:** Increase in ICP of hyperemic nature: both blood flow velocity (FV) and jugular bulb oxygen saturation (SjO2) increase in parallel with ICP. **H:** Refractory intracranial hypertension: ICP increases within a few hours to 100 mm Hg. The *vertical line* denotes the likely moment when the vasomotor centers in the brainstem became ischemic. At this point the heart rate (HR) increased and CPP decreased abruptly. Note that pulse amplitude of ICP (AMP) disappeared around 10 minutes before this terminal event. (Taken from Kirkham FJ, Wade AM, McElduff F, et al. Seizures in 204 comatose children: Incidence and outcome. *Intensive Care Med* 2012;38:853–62.)

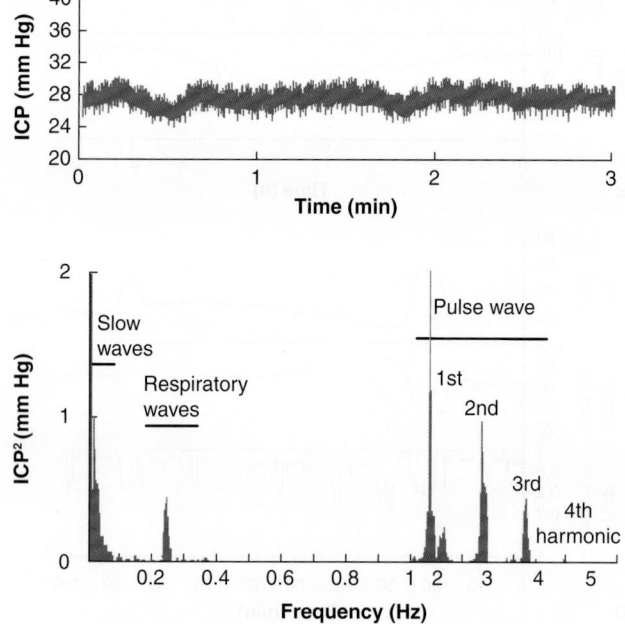

FIGURE 58.4. Example of intracranial pressure (ICP) recording showing pulse, respiratory waves, and "slow waves" overlapped in the time domain (*top panel*) and separated in the frequency domain (*bottom panel*). (Taken from Kirkham FJ, Wade AM, McElduff F, et al. Seizures in 204 comatose children: Incidence and outcome. *Intensive Care Med* 2012;38:853–62.)

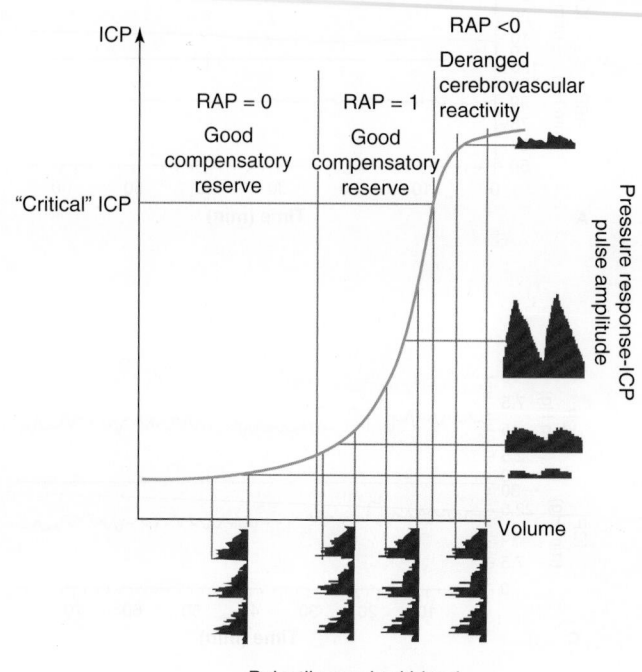

FIGURE 58.5. In a simple model, pulse amplitude of intracranial pressure (ICP) (AMP, expressed along the y axis on the right side of the panel) results from pulsatile changes in cerebral blood volume (expressed along the x axis) transformed by the pressure–volume curve. This curve has three zones: a flat zone, expressing good compensatory reserve; an exponential zone, depicting poor compensatory reserve; and a flat zone again, seen at very high ICP (above the "critical" ICP), depicting derangement of normal cerebrovascular responses. The pulse amplitude of ICP is low and does not depend on mean ICP in the first zone. The pulse amplitude increases linearly with mean ICP in the zone of poor compensatory reserve. In the third zone, the pulse amplitude starts to decrease with rising ICP. RAP, index of compensatory reserve.(Taken from Abend NS, Dlugos DJ, Hahn CD, et al. Use of EEG monitoring and management of non-convulsive seizures in critically ill patients: A survey of neurologists. *Neurocrit Care* 2010;12:382–9; Kirkham FJ, Wade AM, McElduff F, et al. Seizures in 204 comatose children: Incidence and outcome. *Intensive Care Med* 2012;38:853–62)

BP are transmitted passively to ICP. Again, with the use of computational methods similar to those used for the calculation of the RAP index, PRx is determined with the calculation of the correlation coefficient between 40 consecutive, time-averaged data points of ICP and BP. A positive PRx signifies a positive slope of the regression line between the slow components of BP and ICP and signifies a loss of cerebral pressure autoregulation (**Fig. 58.6A**) (28). A negative value of PRx reflects a normally reactive vascular bed, because ABP waves provoke inversely correlated waves in ICP and signifies the presence of cerebral pressure autoregulation (**Fig. 58.6B**). Abnormal values of both PRx and RAP are indicative of poor autoregulation or deranged cerebrospinal compensatory reserve, and have been shown to be predictive of a poor outcome in adults with severe TBI (29).

There are few data on the use of these hydrodynamic indices in children. Brady et al. (27) used continuous monitoring of the PRx in 21 children with severe TBI and found this parameter to be associated with outcome. In addition, impaired cerebrovascular pressure reactivity was evident at low levels of CPP.

Transcranial Doppler

TCD allows for portable, invasive, and repeatable measures of regional CBF. Although not strictly a continuous signal in terms of 24-hour availability, a multidirectional ultrasound probe has been constructed for simultaneous TCD of the middle cerebral artery, ophthalmic artery, and/or posterior cerebral artery (**Fig. 58.7**). The middle cerebral artery is the most commonly studied in children in a number of pediatric critical care conditions.

Technically, insonation of the middle cerebral artery is readily accessible to the ultrasonographer; it is the most convenient for probe fixation and long-term monitoring, and it delivers

the largest percentage of supratentorial blood. Although the blood flow velocity cannot express a baseline volume of flow, dynamic changes of CBF are usually reflected in TCD readings. Increased baseline flow velocity (>100 cm/s in adult vasculature) may indicate cerebral vasospasm or hyperemia (30,31). Uncoupling between CBF and flow velocity in vasospasm has been documented experimentally (32). For example, if the ratio of flow velocity in the insonated artery to the velocity in the ipsilateral internal carotid artery is greater than 3, vasospasm is likely. A ratio below 2 indicates hyperemia as the cause for accelerated blood flow (33).

Assessment of Autoregulation

There is a range of assessments that can be conducted at the bedside using TCD, such as:

- **Static test:** measurement of middle cerebral artery blood flow velocity during vasopressor infusion–induced changes in mean ABP. The static rate of pressure autoregulation is the percentage increase in vascular resistance divided by the percentage rise in ABP. Fully intact

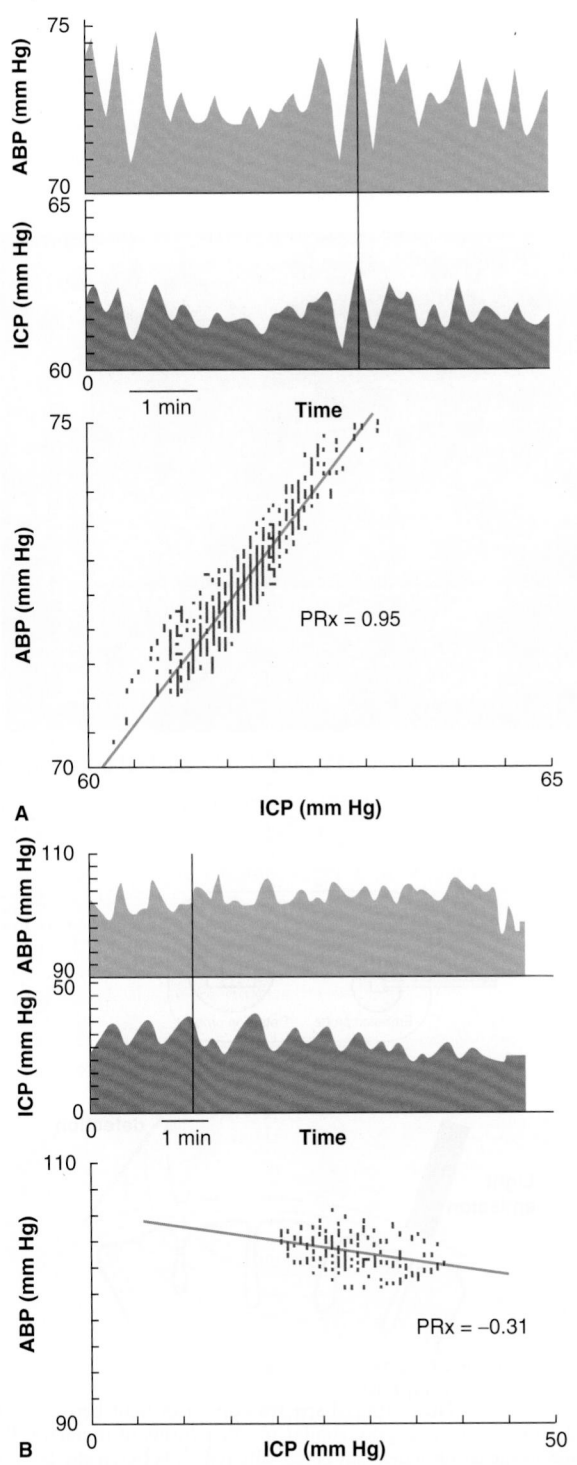

FIGURE 58.6. Relation between slow waves of arterial pressure (ABP) and intracranial pressure (ICP). **A:** Slow waves in ICP and ABP produce a positive correlation (*lower left panel*), giving a positive value of the pressure-reactivity index (PRx), which indicates loss of cerebrovascular reserve. **B:** Coherent waves both in ABP and ICP produced a negative correlation coefficient when plotted on the regression graph (*lower right*), giving values of PRx that were clearly negative. (Taken from Kirkham FJ, Wade AM, McElduff F, et al. Seizures in 204 comatose children: Incidence and outcome. *Intensive Care Med* 2012;38:853–62.)

autoregulation is indicated by a value of 100%, and fully depleted autoregulation is indicated by values close to zero.

- **Vascular reactivity to changes in carbon dioxide (CO_2):** cerebral vessels are reactive to changes in the partial pressure of CO_2 when cerebral pressure autoregulation is impaired.
- **Dynamic test:** an index of pressure autoregulation describing how quickly cerebral vessels react to fall in BP. When performed in a formal manner with stepwise changes in BP induced by deflation of compression leg cuffs, the dynamic rate of pressure autoregulation is considered to express autoregulatory reserve (34).
- **Continuous analysis:** in patients undergoing ICP monitoring, mean blood flow velocity samples can be correlated with simultaneously acquired CPP samples. The correlation coefficient (named mean index) may be positive or negative, and the regression line describing the relationship between the systolic-, mean-, and diastolic-flow velocity and CPP may be used for the assessment. A positive correlation coefficient signifies positive association of flow velocity with CPP; a negative correlation signifies a negative association.

Clinical Context of TCD in Pediatric TBI

Some data on TCD assessments of cerebral autoregulation in children with TBI are now available. For example, in a series of 36 children, the incidence of impaired cerebral pressure autoregulation was greatest following moderate-to-severe TBI (35). Impaired autoregulation was associated with poor outcome, and hyperemia was associated with both impaired autoregulation and poor outcome. In severe cases, cerebral autoregulation often changes over the course of a critical illness, with worsening autoregulation that mirrors progression of worsening injury (36). Importantly, in children, bilateral assessment of cerebral autoregulation is required because hemisphere differences are common in those with an isolated focal injury (37). (Inflicted TBI is a special case: in a small case series, Vavilala et al. (38) found that none of their critically ill cases had intact autoregulation.) Recently, Vavilala et al. (37) reported the relationship between CPP and CBF in 46 severe pediatric TBI cases. The main finding was that there was considerable variability in the blood flow velocity (low, high, or normal for age and gender) despite CPP within a normal range (i.e., >40 mm Hg). Interestingly, patients with high mean blood flow velocity had lower hematocrit than patients with normal mean blood flow velocity, reflecting both the sensitivity of the technique to physiologic change and potential target for optimization of hemoglobin level.

More recently, there have also been studies of intracranial vasospasm in pediatric TBI (39,40). In a single-center, prospective observational study of 69 children with Glasgow Coma Scale score ≤12 (in the setting of moderate-to-severe TBI and abnormal imaging), TCD was performed to follow the presence of vasospasm. Vasospasm was defined as an elevation in velocity ≥2 standard deviations above age and gender normal values for the middle cerebral and basilar arteries, or a middle cerebral artery to internal carotid ratio in flow ≥3 (see above). In those with moderate TBI, the prevalence of vasospasm in the middle and basilar cerebral arteries was 8.5% and 3%, respectively. In those with severe TBI, the prevalence of vasospasm in the middle and basilar cerebral arteries was 33.5% and 21%, respectively. Mean time to onset of vasospasm was

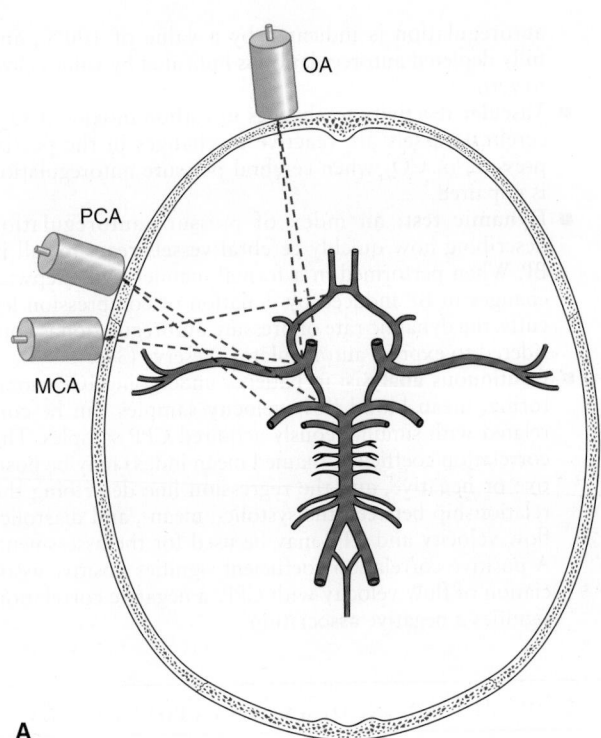

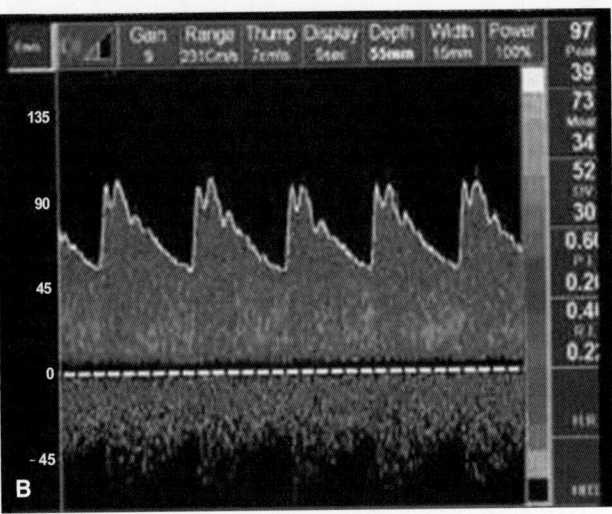

FIGURE 58.7. A: Position of TCD probes of posterior cerebral artery (PCA), ophthalmic artery (OA), and middle cerebral artery (MCA). **B:** A sample tracing of normal MCA waveform.

4–5 days in the middle cerebral and basilar arteries. Mean duration of vasospasm was ~2 days in both the middle cerebral and basilar arteries. Future studies should establish the relationship between vasospasm and long-term functional outcomes and should also evaluate potential preventative or therapeutic options for vasospasm in these children.

Monitoring by NIRS

NIRS uses a modification of the Beer–Lambert Law, which describes the relationship between absorption of light and the concentration of intravascular chromophores, such as deoxyhemoglobin (Hb), oxyhemoglobin (HbO$_2$), and the intracellular chromophore cytochrome aa3. Key factors in the Beer–Lambert calculation are the absorption coefficient, tissue concentration of chromophore, distance between optodes, differential path length factor (described below), and scattering losses. NIRS technology differs from pulse oximetry in that it does not require a pulse; therefore, cerebral NIRS monitoring can be used during cardiopulmonary bypass.

The distance that the light travels, known as the optical path length, must be determined to obtain quantitative concentration changes from the light absorption data. The path length varies due to tissue scattering, which is reflected by the differential path length factor (DPF). The DPF is a correction factor that is multiplied by the inter-optode distance to obtain the true path length.

NIRS can be accomplished by three mechanisms. A continuous-wave spectrometer is most commonly used in clinical devices. Investigational devices exist that measure "time-of-flight," which has the added benefit of accurately measuring the path length of the light. Phase-resolved spectroscopy emits light that is modulated at a known frequency and assesses the phase shift of the transmitted light to derive the path length.

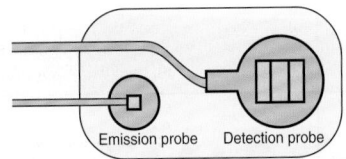

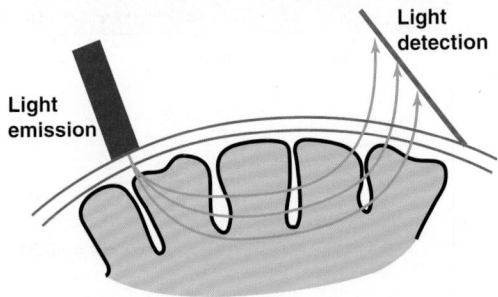

FIGURE 58.8. Near-infrared spectroscopy uses light between 700 and 1000 nm wavelengths, similar to other forms of oximetry. The tissue oxygenation index can detect differences between the left and right frontal hemispheres of the brain at a tissue depth of 2–3 cm. (Illustration courtesy L. Ibsen, MD, MediaLab@Doernbecher).

Commercially available NIRS monitors use two detector optodes at fixed distances (**Fig. 58.8**). The shorter inter-optode distance is designed to represent extracerebral (scalp and bone) tissue infrared absorption. In an effort to better represent intracranial brain tissue infrared absorption, the extracerebral component is subtracted from the absorption data received by the longer inter-optode distance (41). From the light absorption data generated, via absorption at the 730-nm (Hb) and 805-nm wavelengths (Hb + HbO$_2$), regional cerebral oxyhemoglobin saturation (rSO_2) is calculated. A measurement of scaled absolute hemoglobin concentrations (oxygenated hemoglobin to total hemoglobin ratio), as the tissue oxygenation index, is also available (42).

The range of baseline rSO_2 values is very wide. In healthy children, rSO_2 was reported to be 68% ±10%, while in children with cyanotic heart disease, baseline values range from 38% to 57% (43). Current clinical usage of NIRS includes detection of superior vena cava occlusion during cardiopulmonary bypass (44) and assessing the effect of carotid ligation during initiation of venoarterial extracorporeal life support (45).

Some limitations of NIRS technology are its inability to account for patients' varying ratios of brain and extracerebral tissues and the fact that DPF values vary with age and pathologic state (41). Icteric patients have depressed cerebral rSO_2 values, presumably due to absorption of light by bilirubin (46). Ongoing blood loss is associated with a decrease in rSO_2, despite $SjvO_2$, which may indicate that a changing Hb level confounds cerebral oximetry measurement (47). Furthermore, the reproducibility of cerebral oxygenation measurements in infants is poor (48). However, the major limitation is that no "gold standard" exists with which to compare NIRS-derived rSO_2. Poor to moderate correlation is seen in comparing rSO_2 to global cerebral oxygenation measures, such as $SjvO_2$ (49), central venous saturation (50,51), and invasively monitored cortical brain tissue $PbtO_2$ (52). A pediatric pilot study reported good agreement between NIRS and $SjvO_2$ in a normal pediatric brain (53).

Clinical Context of NIRS in the PICU

The most robust data for the use of NIRS and outcome in critically ill children has been from the cardiac surgical population, typically in children undergoing complex repairs under deep hypothermic circulatory arrest.

In 2009, Hirsch et al. (54) reported a systematic literature review of the use of NIRS in congenital heart disease, from 1950 to April 2007. There were 47 case series, 4 randomized trials, and 3 retrospective studies. Two studies had postdischarge follow-up, one incorporating neurologic testing. Neither of these studies demonstrated a benefit. One retrospective study, which included NIRS and other intraoperative measures of cerebral perfusion, demonstrated a decrease in neurologic dysfunction using this combination of monitors. Three small studies were able to correlate NIRS with other clinical and radiologic findings.

Three recent studies since the above review have attempted to tackle the question of correlating NIRS findings with indirect measures of neurologic outcome or mortality. Two sequential studies from the same center found, first, that at 2 years of age (in those who had undergone cardiac surgery before 1 year of age) receptive communication was influenced by rSO_2 nadir (55); second, that at 2 years of age (in those who had undergone cardiac surgery in the first 2 months of age) worse receptive communication and cognitive outcome correlated with the intraoperative percentage decrease in rSO_2 below the baseline (measured during induction of anesthesia) and a postoperative rSO_2 nadir of 56%, respectively (56). Third, Hoffman et al. (57) reported neurological outcome in a sequential cohort of patients who had undergone stage 1 palliation for hypoplastic left heart syndrome and received postoperative NIRS monitoring. In contrast to the studies reported by Simons et al. (55) and Sood et al. (56), Hoffman et al. (57) used a protocol that included targeting rSO_2 >50%. Generally, this cohort had good outcome, with 4 of 21 patients showing deficits in visual motor integration. The authors found that these outcomes were better than their historical controls managed without the use of NIRS (58).

Taken together, it is possible that targeting rSO_2 >50% may improve outcome. However, the key question is whether a multicenter, prospective, goal-directed therapy protocol improves outcome. Unfortunately, it may be too late to test this hypothesis because many centers, and even entire countries, have adopted NIRS monitoring as standard of care.

Multimodality Neuromonitoring

Multimodal neuromonitoring refers to a practice most described in adult neurocritical care that involves combined use of the multiple monitoring systems described in Table 58.2.

Regional Brain Tissue Oxygen ($PbtO_2$) Monitoring

A tissue-monitoring catheter (0.5 mm diameter) may be placed alongside the ICP catheter in the frontal cortex to a depth of 1.5–3 cm to measure regional brain partial pressure tissue oxygen ($PbtO_2$) changes (59). The technology uses a fluorescent dye that responds to O_2, or it can be used with a Clark electrode for measurements of partial pressure in O_2. A temperature probe may be added to obtain continuous brain tissue temperature measurements. Some limitations of this technology are that measurements reflect regional rather than global changes and a lack of correlation with other metabolic measures, such as $SjvO_2$. Adult studies in TBI have suggested that differences in $PbtO_2$ are associated with outcome. For example, with normal CPP and ICP, threshold values in $PbtO_2$ are usually 25–30 mm Hg; measurements <15 mm Hg likely represent tissue at significant risk of hypoxia and <10 mm Hg suggests ongoing ischemia; therefore, a threshold of <20 mm Hg may provide a margin of safety to prevent ischemia.

In PICU practice, recent reports on the use of $PbtO_2$ in severe TBI have been limited to the experience from two centers, one in South Africa (60,61) and one in the USA (62). In the recent USA experience, 46 children with severe TBI were described who underwent monitoring between September 2004 and June 2008. $PbtO_2$ was measured in the uninjured frontal cortex. Hourly recordings and calculated daily means of various variables including $PbtO_2$, ICP, CPP, mean BP, partial pressure of arterial O_2, and fraction of inspired O_2 were compared using several statistical approaches. A $PbtO_2$ of 30 mm Hg was associated with the highest sensitivity/specificity for favorable neurological outcome at 6 months after TBI, yet CPP was the only factor that was independently associated with favorable outcome.

Brain Tissue Microdialysis

A microdialysis catheter may be inserted into brain tissue and connected to a microdialysis pump, which delivers a perfusion fluid that equilibrates with extracellular brain tissue fluid through the dialysis membrane of the catheter. Fluid samples are collected hourly and analyzed at the point of care with a special microdialysis analyzer. Changes in levels of glucose, lactate, pyruvate, glutamate, and various amino acids in the interstitial fluid may be measured. Extracellular concentrations of lactate and glutamate are increased during episodes of jugular venous desaturation. Recent adult studies have suggested that changes in these levels may precede the onset of symptomatic vasospasm in subarachnoid hemorrhage, may signal ischemia before detection by changes in either ICP or CPP, and may be predictive of outcome in TBI. Studies also show that increasing the fraction of inspired O_2 results in decreased levels of lactate and glucose, suggesting a potential role for hyperoxygenation as an early therapy. A pediatric catheter is available, but clinical experience is limited and it is difficult to make useful conclusions (63,64).

Clinical Context of Multimodal Monitoring in the PICU

Overall, high-quality pediatric studies or case series on the use of multimodal monitoring are lacking. In future we will need to examine critical thresholds for each neuromonitoring modality (singularly and in combination) and determine the risk-to-benefit ratio and impact of such monitoring on patient outcome.

CONCLUSIONS AND FUTURE DIRECTIONS

In conclusion, the past decade has seen significant technologic advances in the depth and breadth of neurologic monitoring of the PICU patient. However, caution must be exercised before widespread adoption of any new monitoring technology, as excessive or indiscriminate use may prove less effective and potentially detrimental if misinterpreted or acted on inappropriately. Whether these advances in neuromonitoring technology will affect clinical outcome remains to be studied and demonstrated, and careful evaluations, including risk to the patient, cost, avoidance of incorrect interpretations, and a clear association with improved outcome, must precede widespread adoption. Understanding the pathophysiologic correlates of these neuromonitoring modalities, including the complex interrelationships between CBF, cerebral metabolism, cerebral autoregulation, and tissue and cellular states, will prove vital to fully utilizing these technologies in the PICU to their best advantage.

References

1. Pethig R, Smith S. *Introductory Bioelectronics: For Engineers and Physical Scientists.* Chichester, UK: Wiley, 2013.
2. Aoki Y, Lombroso CT. Prognostic value of electroencephalography in Reye's syndrome. *Neurology* 1973;23:333–43.
3. Janati A, Erba G. Electroencephalographic correlates of near-drowning encephalopathy in children. *Electroencephalogr Clin Neurophysiol* 1982;53:182–91.
4. Pampiglione G, Harden A. Resuscitation after cardiocirculatory arrest. *Lancet* 1968;291:1261–5.
5. Tasker RC, Boyd S, Harden A, et al. Monitoring in non-traumatic coma. Part II: Electroencephalography. *Arch Dis Child* 1988;63:895–9.
6. Carrai R, Grippo A, Lori S, et al. Prognostic value of somatosensory evoked potentials in comatose children: A systematic literature review. *Intensive Care Med* 2010;36:1112–26.
7. Abend NS, Dlugos DJ, Hahn CD, et al. Use of EEG monitoring and management of non-convulsive seizures in critically ill patients: A survey of neurologists. *Neurocrit Care* 2010;12:382–9.
8. Tortoriello TA, Stayer SA, Mott AR, et al. A noninvasive estimation of mixed venous oxygen saturation using near-infrared spectroscopy by cerebral oximetry in pediatric cardiac surgery patients. *Paediatr Anaesth* 2005;15:495–503.
9. Abend NS, Topjian A, Ichord R, et al. Electroencephalographic monitoring during hypothermia after pediatric cardiac arrest. *Neurology* 2009;72:1931–40.
10. Abend NS, Gutierrez-Colina AM, Topjian AA, et al. Nonconvulsive seizures are common in critically ill children. *Neurology* 2011;76:1071–7.
11. Carrera E, Claassen J, Oddo M, et al. Continuous electroencephalographic monitoring in critically ill patients with central nervous system infections. *Arch Neurol* 2008;65:1612–8.
12. Greiner HM, Holland K, Leach JL, et al. Nonconvulsive status epilepticus: The encephalopathic pediatric patient. *Pediatrics* 2012;129:e748–e755.
13. Hosain SA, Solomon GE, Kobylarz EJ. Electroencephalographic patterns in unresponsive pediatric patients. *Pediatr Neurol* 2005;32:162–5.
14. Hyllienmark L, Amark P. Continuous EEG monitoring in a paediatric intensive care unit. *Eur J Paediatr Neurol* 2007;11:70–5.
15. Jette N, Claassen J, Emerson RG, et al. Frequency and predictors of nonconvulsive seizures during continuous electroencephalographic monitoring in critically ill children. *Arch Neurol* 2006;63:1750–5.
16. Kirkham FJ, Wade AM, McElduff F, et al. Seizures in 204 comatose children: Incidence and outcome. *Intensive Care Med* 2012;38:853–62.
17. McCoy B, Sharma R, Ochi A, et al. Predictors of nonconvulsive seizures among critically ill children. *Epilepsia* 2011;52:1973–8.
18. Saengpattrachai M, Sharma R, Hunjan A, et al. Nonconvulsive seizures in the pediatric intensive care unit: Etiology, EEG, and brain imaging findings. *Epilepsia* 2006;47:1510–8.
19. Schreiber JM, Zelleke T, Gaillard WD, et al. Continuous video EEG for patients with acute encephalopathy in a pediatric intensive care unit. *Neurocrit Care* 2012;17:31–8.
20. Shahwan A, Bailey C, Shekerdemian L, et al. The prevalence of seizures in comatose children in the pediatric intensive care unit: A prospective video-EEG study. *Epilepsia* 2010;51:1198–204.
21. Walker M, Cross H, Smith S, et al. Nonconvulsive status epilepticus: Epilepsy Research Foundation workshop reports. *Epileptic Disord* 2005;7:253–96.
22. Payne ET, Zhao XY, Frndova H, et al. Seizure burden is independently associated with short term outcome in critically ill children. *Brain* 2014;137:1429–38.
23. Crutchfield JS, Narayan RK, Robertson CS, et al. Evaluation of a fiberoptic intracranial pressure monitor. *J Neurosurg* 1990;72:482–7.
24. Czosnyka M, Pickard JD. Monitoring and interpretation of intracranial pressure. *J Neurol Neurosurg Psychiatry* 2004;75:813–21.
25. Lundberg N. Continuous recording and control of ventricular fluid pressure in neurosurgical practice. *Acta Psychiatr Scand Suppl* 1960;36(suppl 149):1–193.
26. Balestreri M, Czosnyka M, Steiner LA, et al. Intracranial hypertension: What additional information can be derived from ICP waveform after head injury? *Acta Neurochir* 2004;146:131–41.
27. Brady KM, Schaffner DH, Lee JK, et al. Continuous monitoring of cerebrovascular pressure reactivity after traumatic brain injury in children. *Pediatrics* 2009;124:e1205–e1212.
28. Czosnyka M, Smielewski P, Kirkpatrick P, et al. Continuous assessment of the cerebral vasomotor reactivity in head injury. *Neurosurgery* 1997;41:11–9.
29. Steiner LA, Czosnyka M, Piechnik SK, et al. Continuous monitoring of cerebrovascular pressure reactivity allows determination of optimal cerebral perfusion pressure in patients with traumatic brain injury. *Crit Care Med* 2002;30:733–8.
30. Aaslid R, Huber P, Nornes H. Evaluation of cerebrovascular spasm with transcranial Doppler ultrasound. *J Neurosurg* 1984;60:37–41.
31. Compton JS, Teddy PJ. Cerebral arterial vasospasm following severe head injury: A transcranial Doppler study. *Br J Neurosurg* 1987;1:435–9.
32. Nelson RJ, Perry S, Hames TK, et al. Transcranial Doppler ultrasound studies of cerebral autoregulation and subarachnoid hemorrhage in the rabbit. *J Neurosurg* 1990;73:601–10.

33. Lindegaard KF, Grolimund P, Aalid R, et al. Evaluation of cerebral AVM's using transcranial Doppler ultrasound. *J Neurosurg* 1986;65:335–44.

34. Aaslid R, Lindegaard KF, Sorteberg W, et al. Cerebral autoregulation dynamics in humans. *Stroke* 1989;20:45–52.

35. Vavilala MS, Lee LA, Boddu K, et al. Cerebral autoregulation in pediatric traumatic brain injury. *Pediatr Crit Care Med* 2004; 5:257–63.

36. Tontisirin N, Armstead W, Waitayawinyu P, et al. Change in cerebral autoregulation as a function of time in children after severe traumatic brain injury: A case series. *Childs Nerv Syst* 2007;23:1163–9.

37. Vavilala MS, Tontisirin N, Udomphorn Y, et al. Hemispheric differences in cerebral autoregulation in children with moderate and severe traumatic brain injury. *Neurocrit Care* 2008;9:45–54.

38. Vavilala MS, Muangman S, Waitayawinyu P, et al. Impaired cerebral autoregulation in infants and young children early after inflicted traumatic brain injury: A preliminary report. *J Neurotrauma* 2007;24:87–96.

39. O'Brien NF, Reuter-Rice KE, Khanna S, et al. Vasospasm in children with traumatic brain injury. *Intensive Care Med* 2010;36:680–7.

40. O'Brien NF, Maa T, Yeates KO. The epidemiology of vasospasm in children with moderate-to-severe traumatic brain injury [published online ahead of print December 4, 2014]. *Crit Care Med.* 2015;43:674–85.

41. Thavasothy M, Broadhead M, Elwell C, et al. A comparison of cerebral oxygenation as measured by the NIRO 300 and the INVOS 5100 near-infrared spectrophotometers. *Anaesthesia* 2002;57:999–1006.

42. Taillefer MC, Denault AY. Cerebral near-infrared spectroscopy in adult heart surgery: Systematic review of its clinical efficacy. *Can J Anaesth* 2005;52:79–87.

43. Kurth CD, Steven JL, Montenegro LM, et al. Cerebral oxygen saturation before congenital heart surgery. *Ann Thorac Surg* 2001;72:187–92.

44. Ing RJ, Lawson DS, Jaggers J, et al. Detection of unintentional partial superior vena cava occlusion during a bidirectional cavopulmonary anastomosis. *J Cardiothorac Vasc Anesth* 2004; 18:472–4.

45. Ejike JC, Schenkman KA, Seidel K, et al. Cerebral oxygenation in neonatal and pediatric patients during veno-arterial extracorporeal life support. *Pediatr Crit Care Med* 2006;7:154–8.

46. Madsen PL, Skak C, Rasmussen A, et al. Interference of cerebral near-infrared oximetry in patients with icterus. *Anesth Analg* 2000;90:489–93.

47. Zauner A, Doppenberg EM, Woodward JJ, et al. Continuous monitoring of cerebral substrate delivery and clearance: Initial experience in 24 patients with severe acute brain injuries. *Neurosurgery* 1997;41:1082–91; discussion 91–3.

48. Dullenkopf A, Kolarova A, Schulz G, et al. Reproducibility of cerebral oxygenation measurement in neonates and infants in the clinical setting using the NIRO 300 oximeter. *Pediatr Crit Care Med* 2005;6:344–7.

49. Nagdyman N, Fleck T, Schubert S, et al. Comparison between cerebral tissue oxygenation index measured by near-infrared spectroscopy and venous jugular bulb saturation in children. *Intensive Care Med* 2005;31:846–50.

50. Topjian AA, Gutierrez-Colina AM, Sanchez SM, et al. Electrographic status epilepticus is associated with mortality and worse short-term outcome in critically ill children. *Crit Care Med* 2013;41:215–23.

51. Weiss M, Dullenkopf A, Kolarova A, et al. Near-infrared spectroscopic cerebral oxygenation reading in neonates and infants is associated with central venous oxygen saturation. *Paediatr Anaesth* 2005;15:102–9.

52. Brawanski A, Faltermeier R, Rothoerl RD, et al. Comparison of near-infrared spectroscopy and tissue Po_2 time series in patients after severe head injury and aneurysmal subarachnoid hemorrhage. *J Cereb Blood Flow Metab* 2002;22:605–11.

53. Shimizu N, Gilder F, Bissonnette B, et al. Brain tissue oxygenation index measured by near infrared spatially resolved spectroscopy agreed with jugular bulb oxygen saturation in normal pediatric brain: A pilot study. *Childs Nerv Syst* 2005;21:181–4.

54. Hirsch JC, Charpie JR, Ohye RG, et al. Near-infrared spectroscopy: What we know and what we need to know—a systematic review of the congenital heart disease literature. *J Thorac Cardiovasc Surg* 2009;137:154–9, 159e1–159e12.

55. Simons J, Sood ED, Derby CD, et al. Predictive value of near-infrared spectroscopy on neurodevelopmental outcome after surgery for congenital heart disease in infancy. *J Thorac Cardiovasc Surg* 2012;143:118–25.

56. Sood ED, Benzaquen JS, Davies RR, et al. Predictive value of perioperative near-infrared spectroscopy for neurodevelopmental outcomes after cardiac surgery in infancy. *J Thorac Cardiovasc Surg* 2013;145:438.e1–445.e1; discussion 444–5.

57. Hoffman GM, Brosig CL, Mussatto KA, et al. Perioperative cerebral oxygen saturation in neonates with hypoplastic left heart syndrome and childhood neurodevelopmental outcome. *J Thorac Cardiovasc Surg* 2013;146:1153–64.

58. Hoffman GM, Mussatto KA, Brosig CL, et al. Systemic venous oxygen saturation after the Norwood procedure and childhood neurodevelopmental outcome. *J Thorac Cardiovasc Surg* 2005;130:1094–100.

59. Martini RP, Deem S, Treggiari MM. Targeting brain tissue oxygenation in traumatic brain injury. *Respir Care* 2013;58:162–72.

60. Figaji AA, Zwane E, Graham Fieggen A, et al. The effect of increased inspired fraction of oxygen on brain tissue oxygen tension in children with severe traumatic brain injury. *Neurocrit Care* 2010;12:430–7.

61. Figaji AA, Zwane E, Kogels M, et al. The effect of blood transfusion on brain oxygenation in children with severe traumatic brain injury. *Pediatr Crit Care Med* 2010;11:325–31.

62. Stippler M, Ortiz V, Adelson PD, et al. Brain tissue oxygen monitoring after severe traumatic brain injury in children: Relationship to outcome and association with other clinical parameters. *J Neurosurg Pediatr* 2012;10:383–91.

63. Charalambides C, Sgouros S, Sakas D. Intracerebral microdialysis in children. *Childs Nerv Syst* 2010;26:215–20.

64. Richards DA, Tolias CM, Sgouros S, et al. Extracellular glutamine to glutamate ratio may predict outcome in the injured brain: A clinical microdialysis study in children. *Pharmacol Res* 2003;48:101–9.

CHAPTER 59 ■ NEUROLOGIC IMAGING

DAVID J. MICHELSON AND STEPHEN ASHWAL

KEY POINTS

❶ Cranial computed tomography (CT) can be obtained with less time and need for sedation than magnetic resonance imaging (MRI).

❷ MRI provides greater anatomic and metabolic detail of the brain than CT, without exposing patients to ionizing radiation and iodinated contrast.

❸ CT visualizes large traumatic hemorrhages that may need surgical intervention, and is ideal for identifying cervical spine fractures.

❹ MRI of the cervical spine can show traumatic soft tissue and cord injury not visible on CT.

❺ MRI with diffusion-weighted imaging (DWI) detects cytotoxic edema within hours of ischemic injury and can differentiate abscesses from necrotic tumors.

❻ MRI with susceptibility-weighted imaging (SWI, which is sensitive to venous blood) is superior for identifying and quantifying traumatic diffuse axonal injury and microhemorrhage.

❼ MRI with proton spectroscopy can identify metabolic properties of tissues and improves the accuracy of prognosis in children with traumatic and ischemic brain injury.

❽ CT may be normal up to 24 hours after focal or global ischemic brain injury.

❾ MRI can identify patterns of abnormalities associated with inborn errors of metabolism.

Care for children with critical central nervous system (CNS) injuries has been substantially improved by advances in neuroimaging. Cranial computed tomography (CT) and magnetic resonance imaging (MRI), the two most commonly used techniques, provide images with increasingly specific diagnostic and prognostic anatomical and functional information. This chapter discusses these techniques and their use in common pediatric critical care applications.

TECHNIQUES

Computed Tomography

CT images, generated by the collection and analysis of x-ray beams as they are sent through tissues from multiple angles, are more than adequate for the identification of surgically remediable forms of acute neuropathology, such as fractures, tumors, large hemorrhages, and obstructive hydrocephalus. One major factor in favor of CT in comparison with MRI is that it can be quickly and easily obtained. Helical (spiral) scanners have so substantially shortened the acquisition times required ❶ for high-quality images that sedation for CT is unnecessary in the vast majority of infants and children who can refrain from moving briefly or who can be lightly restrained (1). One of the drawbacks of CT is radiation exposure, particularly of concern for young patients and those who require repeated studies, given the known dose-related risk of radiation-associated neoplasia (2) and possible risk of developmental impairment (3). Considering this, alternative studies, such as ultrasound, MRI, or CT of lower resolution (and thus lower radiation dose) may be preferable. Also, while the radiodense, iodinated contrast agents used in CT scanning are well tolerated by most children, acute allergic reactions can occur, particularly in older children and in children with a history of asthma. Portable CT machines

have been developed that make it possible to safely acquire images of reasonable resolution in patients who might otherwise be too unstable for transport to a fixed scanner. Studies have shown clinical efficacy and cost-effectiveness for use of such devices in patients who are receiving critical monitoring or therapies in NICU, PICU, ER, and operating room settings (4).

Conventional Anatomic Imaging

Axial images of the head are routinely obtained with a slice thickness of 5 mm, although thinner slices can be obtained if greater detail is required, and images can be reformatted into other planes or into three dimensions. The brightness of each voxel (a pixel representing a three-dimensional [3-D] volume) on a CT image reflects tissue density. Fatty tissue, water, and air appear dark; soft tissues appear as intermediate shades of gray; and mineralized bone, concentrated blood, iodinated contrast, and metallic objects appear bright. CT is limited by streaking artifacts in areas around metal prostheses, fragments (such as dental fillings or gunshot pellets), and dense bone (such as the temporal petrous bones in the posterior fossa). Areas of abnormal signal on CT can be characterized as hypodense, isodense, or hyperdense, relative to the normal neural tissue. The differential for hypodense parenchymal lesions includes edema, infarction, neoplasia, demyelination, inflammation, and cyst formation. Hyperdensity is found in areas of contrast enhancement, hemorrhage, calcification, and hypercellularity. Abnormal calcification can be seen with congenital or chronic infections, tumors and hamartomas, abnormal blood vessels, areas of ischemia, metabolic disorders, and endocrine disorders (5). Calcification of subependymal nodules in a patient with tuberous sclerosis complex is shown in **Figure 59.1**. Isodense lesions may be recognizable by their replacement of, or effect on, normal structures, unless they show abnormal contrast enhancement.

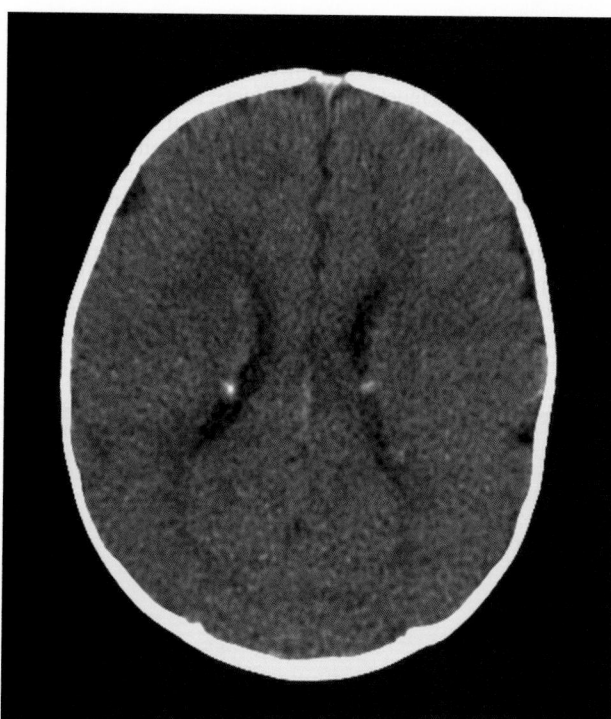

FIGURE 59.1. Four-month-old boy presenting with infantile spasms. Axial CT shows multiple bright nodules along the surface of the lateral ventricles due to subependymal hamartomas associated with tuberous sclerosis complex.

CT Angiography

CT angiography allows the vascular anatomy of the brain to be imaged fairly well by high-resolution CT scanning that is closely timed with an intravenous bolus of an iodinated contrast agent. A test bolus is initially given so as to determine the time delay required to capture images within either the arterial or the venous phase, depending on the study desired. Thinly cut source images can be reformatted into 2- and 3-D images that are nearly as detailed as MR angiograms. As with anatomic imaging, the choice of CT depends on the constraints of radiation exposure, contrast sensitivity, and timing. CT angiography is faster than MR angiography and can usually be done without sedation in older children.

Magnetic Resonance Imaging

MR images are generated by analysis of signals produced by hydrogen nuclei of molecules in varying tissues as the spins of the nuclei are aligned in a strong external magnetic field and then perturbed by radiofrequency pulses. MRI is the modality of choice when resolution of fine anatomic detail is desired. Moreover, this technology also offers several specialized sequences that highlight metabolic changes within the brain and are applicable to a wide variety of diagnostic situations. MRI is also the imaging test of choice for spinal cord injury when neurologic deficits are present, as CT images of the spine, while superior for visualizing fractures and dislocations, do not allow for adequate assessment of the cord. MRI also allows for far more precise imaging of posterior fossa structures, as it is not subject to the artifact produced by the dense temporal petrous bones on CT.

The principal drawback of MR imaging is the long acquisition time, which frequently necessitates procedural sedation for most children less than 8 years old and for some older

children. An audiovisual system within the scanner greatly reduces the need for sedation in children over 3 years old. When intravenous propofol is used for sedation, fractional inspired concentrations of supplemental O_2 above 0.60 can cause artifactual cerebrospinal fluid (CSF) hyperintensity within the sulci and cisterns that can be mistaken for subarachnoid hemorrhage (6). Another drawback of MRI is the incompatibility of ferromagnetic materials with the strong electromagnetic field within the imaging suite. Plastic and aluminum MR-compatible monitors, ventilators, and anesthesia machines are available, but patients with metallic bullet fragments or implants, including cardiac pacemakers and neurostimulators, may not be able to undergo MRI safely. Information regarding the MRI compatibility of implanted medical devices is maintained at http://www.MRIsafety.com (7). Even metallic objects that pose no safety risk (tracheostomy tubes with spiral metal reinforcement) may create artifacts and distortions in the surrounding tissues. Gadolinium contrast for MRI studies is safe for most patients but does pose a risk of nephrogenic systemic fibrosis for patients with severely impaired renal function. Detailed guidelines regarding the safe use of contrast agents for CT and MRI are published online by the American College of Radiology (http://www.acr.org/quality-safety/resources/contrast-manual).

Conventional Anatomic Imaging

As with CT, MR images are gray-scale maps, with the shade of each voxel reflecting the composition of the tissue it represents. The shade of a voxel on an MR image is referred to as its *intensity*, rather than its *density*, because it is determined by factors beyond proton density, including proton mobility (T1 relaxation) and local magnetic effects (T2 relaxation). Various sequences, such as spin echo (SE), gradient-recalled echo (GRE), and fluid-attenuated inversion recovery (FLAIR), use programmed pulses of radiofrequencies and gradient magnetic fields to produce images that highlight T1 or T2 signal effects. On T1-weighted images, fat, methemoglobin, and gadolinium-containing contrast agents appear bright (or hyperintense), while CSF, muscle, deoxyhemoglobin, and hemosiderin appear dark. On T2-weighted images, CSF, edema, extracellular methemoglobin, and areas of hypercellularity, infarction, and demyelination appear bright, while muscle, cortical bone, deoxyhemoglobin, and hemosiderin appear dark.

Routine brain imaging in most institutions begins with a sagittal T1-weighted sequence that serves as a localizer for subsequent sequences and allows evaluation of the corpus callosum, pituitary gland, cerebellar vermis, and other midline structures. Axial T1- and T2-weighted images are also routinely acquired, although coronal images may be particularly helpful for investigation of the cerebellum, temporal lobes, and skull base. FLAIR sequences have improved sensitivity in older children for areas of abnormal intracranial T2 brightness in close proximity to CSF-filled spaces, such as the ventricles and sulci, which are bright on conventional T2 studies but dark on FLAIR images. High-resolution volumetric 3-D T1-weighted scans are particularly useful for patients who undergo evaluation of developmental abnormalities and patients undergoing surgical planning.

Diffusion-weighted Imaging

The diffusion of water molecules can be measured along any 2-D plane to which a strong magnetic field gradient has been applied. Diffusion reflects random (Brownian) motion, capillary flow, and transcellular active transport. In standard diffusion-weighted imaging (DWI), bright areas reflect decreased or restricted movement of water along the studied plane. The apparent diffusion coefficient (ADC) map is an additional sequence that summarizes the diffusion in all three dimensions with the coloring reversed, such that areas in which all water movement is restricted appear dark. DWI is particularly useful in the early evaluation of ischemia, as diffusion restriction becomes apparent within minutes after cytotoxic injury is sustained (8). DWI is also used in the evaluation of brain tumors, helping to distinguish cystic tumors from epidermoid tumors and recurrent tumors from areas of peritumoral edema. Diffusion restriction is also seen within cerebral abscesses and empyemas, and this methodology is helpful in the evaluation of an intracranial cystic lesion that may be an abscess but that cannot otherwise be distinguished from a tumor with central necrosis (9).

Susceptibility-weighted Imaging

Deoxygenated blood and certain blood breakdown products are weakly paramagnetic. The artifacts that these materials produce on T2-weighted MR sequences can be exploited in the evaluation of patients for vascular abnormalities and small hemorrhages. Gradient echo T2-weighted imaging has been used for this purpose for some time but is not nearly as sensitive as the increasingly available susceptibility-weighted imaging (SWI) which makes these same paramagnetic artifacts far more apparent (10) (**Fig. 59.2**). SWI can also potentially show areas of cerebral ischemia, with more prominent (darker)

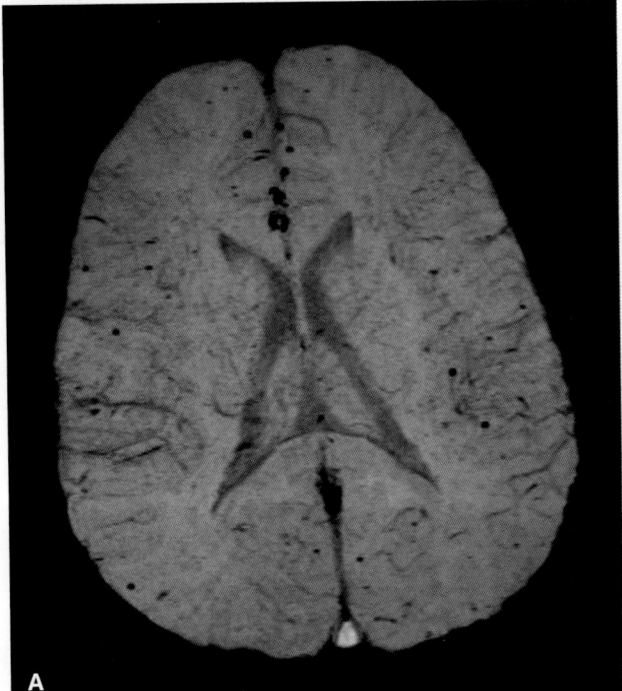

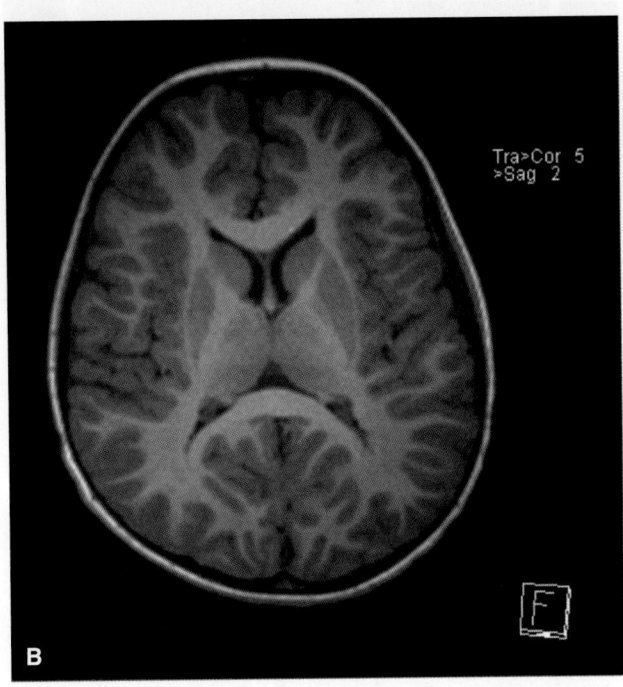

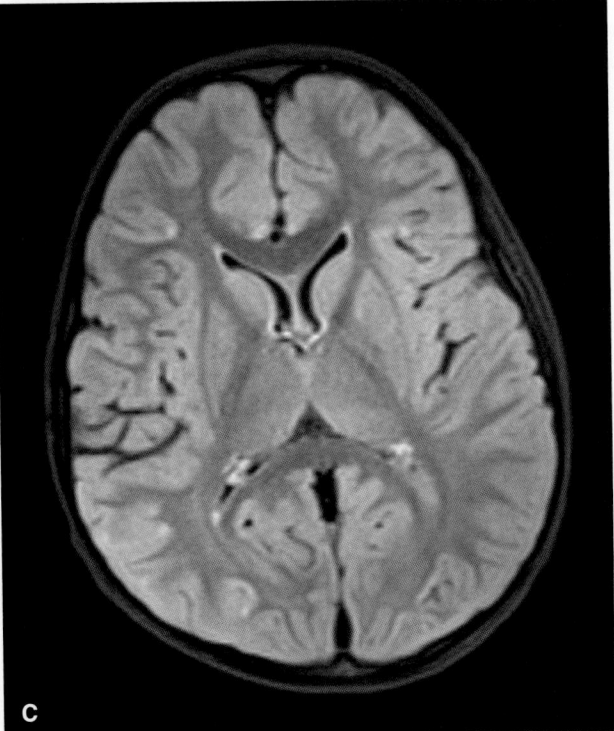

FIGURE 59.2. Four-year-old boy with a history of complex congenital heart disease (including a double outlet right ventricle) who underwent cardiac bypass for an arterial switch procedure. Diffusely scattered punctate hemorrhages at the cortical–subcortical junction are visible on MRI using the SWI sequence (**A**) that would not have been identified using T1-weighted (**B**) and FLAIR (**C**) sequences.

veins from increased deoxyhemoglobin concentrations due to greater oxygen extraction in areas with slowed or diminished blood flow (11).

Diffusion Tensor Imaging (DTI)

Because water will diffuse more freely parallel to white matter fiber tracts, DWI using multiple planes can be used to create color-coded maps of the fiber tracts and to allow visualization of tract disruption by mass lesions, traumatic shearing, and ischemic injury. These images are sometimes called fractional anisotropy (FA) maps, as each voxel of the image is assigned a color based on the portion of its water diffusion that is directional (anisotropic) as opposed to free to diffuse equally in all directions (isotropic) (12). The direction of the diffusivity of each voxel can also be represented as a sum of vectors which are described by their eigenvalues (length) and eigenvectors (directions). The diffusivity of each voxel can be summarized graphically by an ellipsoid with more or less radial (perpendicular) and axial (parallel) diffusivity. Clinical applications currently include presurgical planning for resection of brain tumors and epileptic regions of cortex, although some studies show a benefit in the identification of subtle cortical and subcortical abnormalities in patients with medically intractable epilepsy (13) (**Fig. 59.3**).

MR Angiography/Venography

Reconstructions of the arterial supply and venous drainage of the brain can be obtained from maximum intensity projections (MIPs) from 2-D or 3-D time-of-flight images. The images created by this process represent blood flow better than luminal diameter, however, and can overstate the degree of stenosis present in a vessel. As the process of generating MIP images may also produce artifacts, any suspected abnormality should be confirmed in the source images. Gadolinium infusion is rarely used for MR angiography as higher resolution non-contrast techniques have come into use (14).

MR Spectroscopy

Spectroscopic imaging most often analyzes the signals generated by protons from a number of clinically important neuronal and glial metabolites, including N-acetyl aspartate (NAA), choline and phosphatidylcholine (Cho), creatine and phosphocreatine (Cre), myoinositol (mI), and lactate. Images can be generated using short, medium, or long echo relaxation times. The short echo images demonstrate a wider variety of metabolites and are useful for assessing inborn errors of metabolism (15). Longer echo times provide more accurate quantification of the principal brain metabolites, useful in the assessment of prognosis in the setting of trauma (16), global anoxic injury (17), or neoplasia (18).

MR Perfusion

A number of MR methods have been developed for measuring cerebral perfusion. Fast imaging during paramagnetic contrast injection provides a purely qualitative picture of blood volume, relative regional blood flow, and perfusion delay (mean transit time). Alternatively, the protons within the blood entering the brain through the carotid arteries can be used as an endogenous contrast via spin labeling, particularly with higher-resolution machines that can deliver higher signal-to-noise ratios (19). Applications for perfusion imaging include assessing the risk of ischemia in tissues with decreased perfusion, identifying the decreased perfusion in primary and secondary vasculopathies, and grading the vascularity of tumors (20).

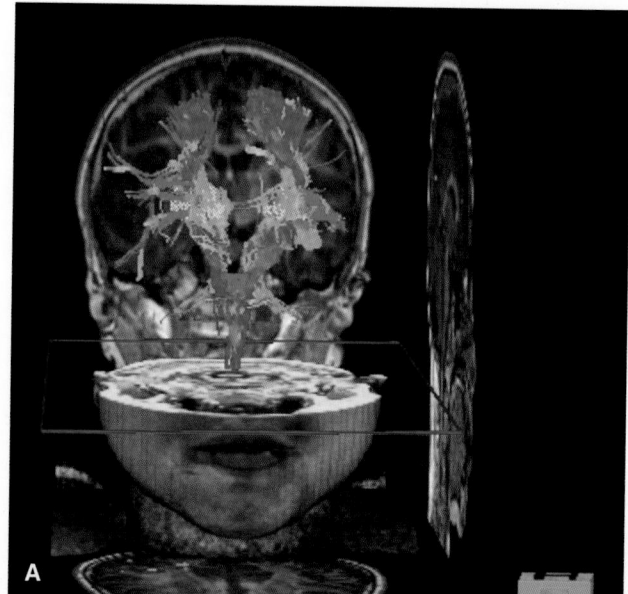

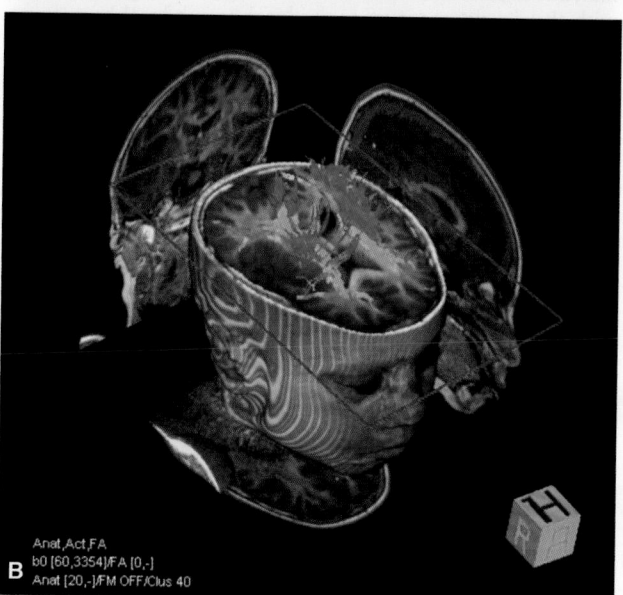

FIGURE 59.3. Eight-year-old boy who presented with focal seizures. DTI images with 3-D fiber tractography showing disruption of white matter tracts of the right external capsule and right sylvian-insular regions from an anterior view (**A**) and oblique view (**B**).

SELECTED CLINICAL APPLICATIONS

Trauma

The initial workup of children with known or suspected head trauma will usually begin with a CT of the head and neck, looking for evidence of acute hemorrhage, fracture, or displacement of vertebrae out of their normal alignment. Young children who suffer traumatic brain injury are at particular risk of upper cervical spine injury because of the relative weight of the cranium, weakness of the paraspinous muscles, elasticity and redundancy of the interspinous ligaments, and horizontal orientation of the incompletely ossified facet joints (21). Children younger than 8 years have such mobility of their cervical spine as to have a normal atlantodental space as wide as 5 mm and anterior movement of C2 on C3 and of C3 on C4 of up to 4 mm. Alignment of the spinolaminar line is disrupted in true subluxation.

Spinal MRI should be considered in children even when no evidence of misalignment or fracture of the vertebrae is seen on plain imaging in a neutral position, as soft tissue and cord edema, ischemia, and hemorrhage may only be visible on spinal MRI. The tendency of children to develop soft tissue and spinal cord injury without radiologic abnormality (SCIWORA) refers only to plain-film and CT imaging (22). As children reach adolescence, they are increasingly likely to sustain bony injuries with spinal trauma, but less severe injuries can still occur without plain-film evidence of fractures. Adolescents are also more likely than young children to present with lower cervical injuries and traumatic disc herniation.

MRI of the brain provides greater sensitivity than CT for brainstem injury, edema and petechial hemorrhages from axonal shearing, small extra-axial fluid collections, and older blood products and is, therefore, the study of choice once a patient has been stabilized (23).

Imaging may find traumatic hemorrhage that is parenchymal, due to contusion or axonal shearing, or extraparenchymal, with the development of an epidural or subdural hematoma. On CT, hemorrhages appear hyperdense in the first week, isodense to brain between 1 and 3 weeks, and increasingly hypodense thereafter. The outline of the hematoma may enhance with intravenous contrast as it becomes organized. On MRI, hyperacute blood appears dark on T1-weighted images and bright on T2-weighted images, while acute blood appears bright on T1-weighted images and dark on T2-weighted images. Table 59.1 summarizes the evolution of the appearance of hemorrhage on CT and MRI. With layering of blood cells within a hematoma, the upper layer of fluid appears bright on T1- and T2-weighted images, while the bottom layer appears isointense to brain on T1-weighted images and dark on T2-weighted images. Finding signs of both old and new traumatic brain injury adds to the suspicion for abusive head trauma in infants, in whom this mechanism is 10–15 times more common than accidental trauma (24).

Subarachnoid blood due to trauma is most commonly seen layering along the falx cerebri in the posterior interhemispheric fissure or the tentorium cerebelli and is best detected in the acute stage by CT. Subacute hemorrhage can be detected by FLAIR sequences on MRI, although high signal intensity on FLAIR can also be caused by rapid CSF flow, normally seen around the ventricular foramina, the aqueduct of Sylvius, and the prepontine cistern (6).

Children may have normal-appearing CT and MRI in the first 12 hours after even severe traumatic brain injury, with severe cerebral edema becoming evident thereafter. Diffusion-weighted MRI can show areas of restricted diffusion due to cytotoxic edema within hours of injury. Proton spectroscopy is useful in determining the prognosis of children who are in a coma after head trauma, with poor outcome associated with decreased NAA levels and increased lactate and glutamate/glutamine levels in the first 2–4 days (25). The amount and depth of hemorrhage seen on SWI has also been shown to correlate with the duration of coma and long-term outcome in patients with severe diffuse axonal injury (26).

Hypoxic–Ischemic Injury

Stroke is increasingly recognized as a significant cause of morbidity and death in childhood. The imaging characteristics of infarctions depend more on the vascular distribution, degree, and duration of substrate deprivation than on the particular etiology and risk factors involved.

Infarctions and hemorrhages occur in nearly half the number of children with cerebral sinovenous thrombosis (27). Presenting symptoms depend on the age of the child and the severity of the injury but range from signs of focal injury such as neurologic deficits and seizures to diffuse signs of increased intracranial pressure such as depressed consciousness, headache, and vomiting. Superior sagittal sinus thrombosis can result in parasagittal infarction; transverse sinus and vein of Labbé thrombosis can result in temporal lobe infarction; and thrombosis of the deep cerebral veins, the straight sinus, or vein of Galen can result in thalamic infarction. Greater degrees of venous outflow reduction progressively cause vasogenic edema, infarction, and hemorrhage, all of which appear differently on neuroimaging. A CT scan may show areas of subcortical white matter hypodensity due to cerebral edema and areas of hyperdensity due to hemorrhage. Intravenous contrast is often necessary for detection of the venous thrombosis, with the flow of contrast around the thrombus described as the empty delta sign. MRI will show corresponding changes on routine T1- and T2-weighted images and is likely to visualize the thrombosis within the venous system, even without the use of contrast. MR venography can be useful when the diagnosis is suspected but uncertain. DWI may show reduced, normal, increased, or mixed water movement, depending on the relative contributions of vasogenic (bright on ADC map) and cytotoxic (dark on ADC map) edema.

Focal arterial infarction appears on CT as a wedge-shaped area of hypodensity that involves the cortex and white matter supplied by the occluded artery (Fig. 59.4A). Posterior circulation infarctions may be particularly difficult to appreciate in infants whose temporal and occipital white matter normally appears hypodense owing to hypomyelination. Gyriform contrast enhancement along the cortical injury is apparent between 5 days and 5 weeks following injury and thus is indicative of a subacute stage of the infarction. MRI is even more sensitive than CT for the detection of early ischemia-related cerebral edema (Fig. 59.4B), although both modalities may appear normal within the first 24 hours after the appearance of clinical symptoms. DWI, on the other hand, can show

TABLE 59.1

THE EVOLVING APPEARANCE OF HEMORRHAGE ON CT AND MR IMAGING

Timing	Hyperacute (<1 d)	Acute (1–3 d)	Early subacute (3–7 d)	Late subacute (7–14 d)	Chronic (>14 d)
Blood Product	OxyHb (intracellular)	DeoxyHb (intracellular)	MetHb (intracellular)	MetHb (extracellular)	Hemosiderin (extracellular)
CT Image	Hyperdense	Hyperdense	Isodense	Isodense	Hypodense
MR Image					
T1-weighted	Dark or gray	Dark or gray	Bright	Bright	Dark or gray
T2-weighted	Bright	Dark	Dark	Bright	Dark

Data from Bradley WG Jr. MR appearance of hemorrhage in the brain. *Radiology* 1993;189:15–26.

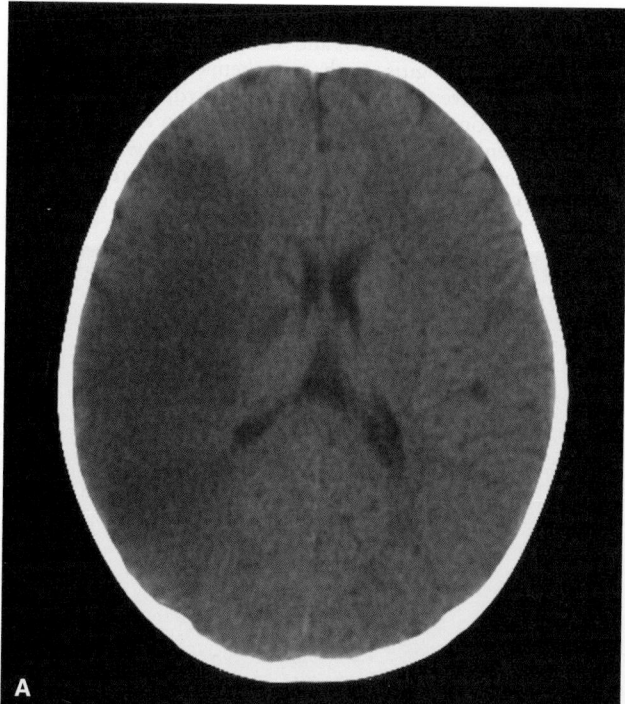

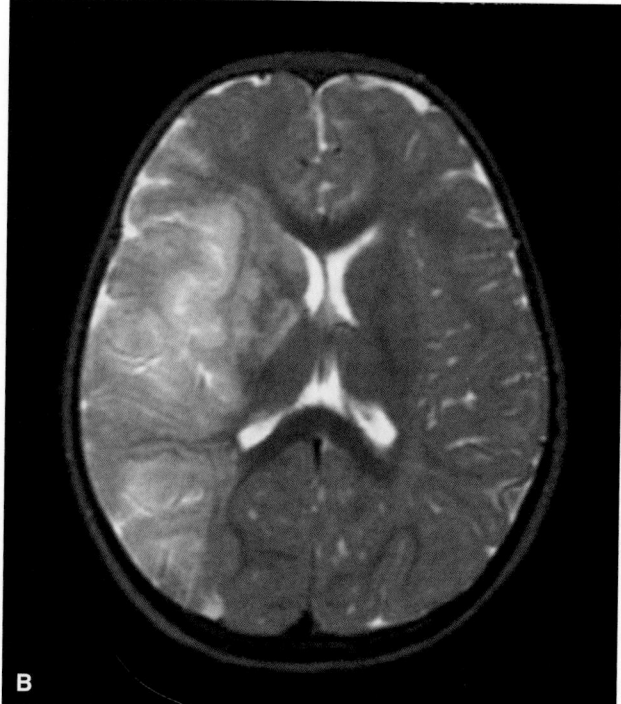

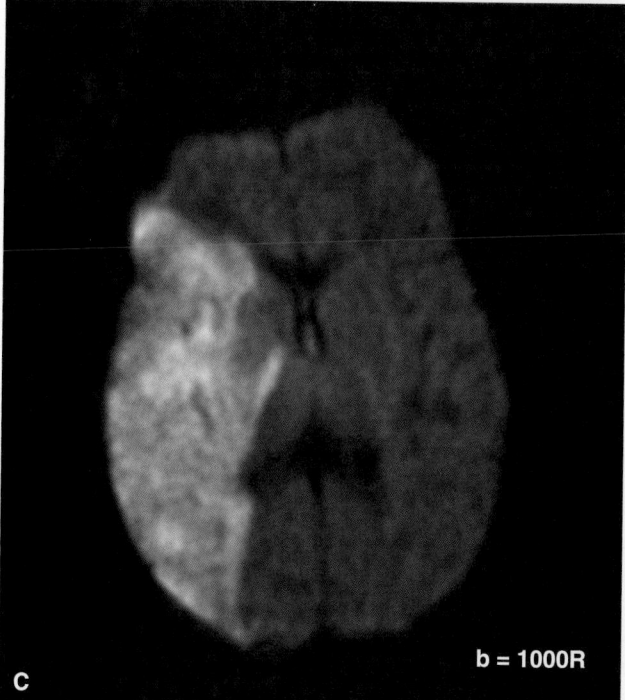

b = 1000R

FIGURE 59.4. Two-year-old girl who awoke with left hemiparesis and right gaze preference. A: A wedge-shaped area of hypodensity is seen on axial CT. MRI shows (B) T2 hyperintensity and (C) corresponding diffusion restriction, indicative of an ischemic stroke in the distribution of the right middle cerebral artery.

restricted water movement from cytotoxic edema (Fig. 59.4C) in as little as 1 hour after injury (28). Angiography, using either CT or MR, can be used to assess the possibility of medium-to-large vessel abnormalities, such as occlusion, thrombosis, dysplasia, inflammatory vasculopathy, or dissection (Fig. 59.5). Neither method is likely to detect narrowing of arterioles and smaller vessels, as might typically be seen in association with inflammatory diseases such as systemic lupus erythematosus.

Diffuse hypoxic–ischemic injury can result from cardiopulmonary arrest or from severe hypotension or hypoxemia. A decrease in cerebral perfusion will initially cause shunting of blood flow to the posterior circulation, protecting the brainstem. The cortical areas supplied by branches of the carotid artery, especially the intervascular boundary zones, are vulnerable to ischemic injury, often resulting in a pattern referred to as a "watershed" distribution (Fig. 59.6A–C). More profound decreases in cerebral blood flow do not allow for preferential shunting and put regions with the highest basal metabolic rates (including the thalami, basal ganglia, and sensorimotor cortex) at the highest risk of injury.

CT can be used for initial imaging of unstable patients, although scans within the first 24 hours may be read as normal even when severe ischemic injury has occurred. The earliest appreciable changes, such as basal ganglia hypodensity and effacement of the perimesencephalic cisterns, may be very subtle, with poor interobserver reliability (28). Later CT scans will

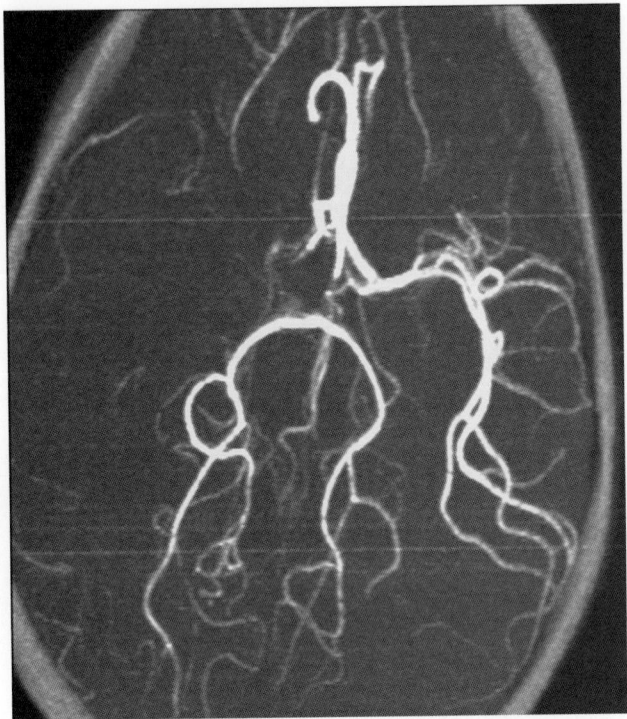

FIGURE 59.5. MIP from the MR angiogram of the patient with a right hemispheric stroke described in **Figure 59.2**, showing absent flow through the right middle cerebral artery.

show clearer evidence of cerebral edema, with decreased differentiation between the cortex and white matter, effacement of the sulci and cisterns, and hypodensity of the deep and cortical gray matter. Particularly ominous for prognosis is the "reversal sign," with white matter appearing denser than cortex, possibly owing to congestion from impaired venous drainage (29).

Early changes of global ischemia can be as subtle with conventional MRI sequences as with CT, although diffusion restriction can usually be seen in areas of infarction and proton MR spectroscopy can show a rise in glutamate and glutamine, with or without the presence of lactate. However, very early DWI can significantly underestimate the complete extent of ischemic injury (30). Prognosis is best assessed by the presence of lactate or of significantly reduced NAA-to-Cre ratios on MR spectroscopy obtained from 3 to 5 days after injury (**Fig. 59.7**).

Infection and Inflammation

Visualization of CNS infections is important for prompt diagnosis and treatment, as well as for monitoring the response to treatment and for possible complications. When CNS infection is clinically suspected and a lumbar puncture is being contemplated, it is common practice to first obtain a CT of the head to determine whether a mass lesion is present that might predispose to cerebral herniation. Studies in adults have suggested that imaging prior to a lumbar puncture is unlikely to be abnormal in patients with normal neurologic examinations (31) and that the presence of a mass lesion on CT is poorly predictive of the risk of imminent cerebral herniation, whether or not lumbar puncture is performed.

Meningitis

CT in patients with meningitis may show meningeal contrast enhancement, especially in later stages, and is important for

investigating possible sources of local spread of infection such as mastoiditis, sinusitis, and skull-based fractures. Complications of meningitis, such as ischemic stroke from vasculitis, obstructive and communicating hydrocephalus, and hemorrhage from venous thrombosis, are also evaluated well by contrast-enhanced CT. Scans from a patient with obstructive hydrocephalus from tuberculous meningitis are shown in **Figure 59.8A and B**. MRI is more likely to show meningeal

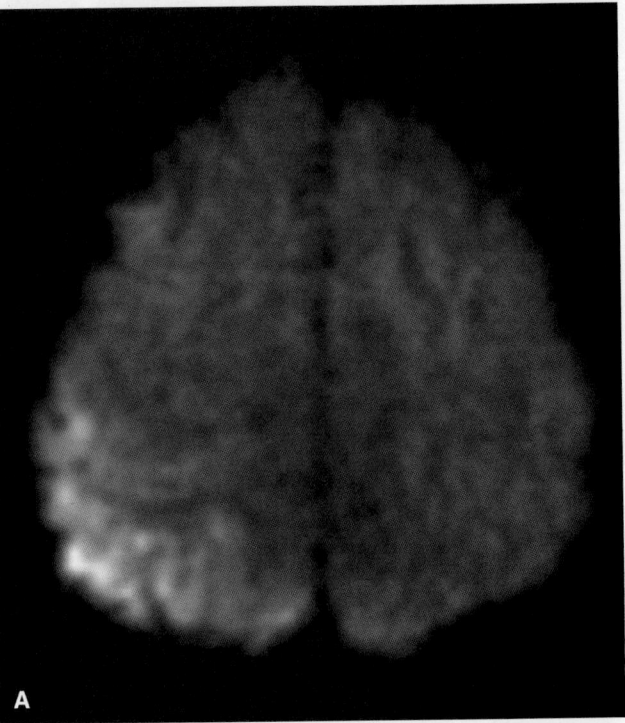

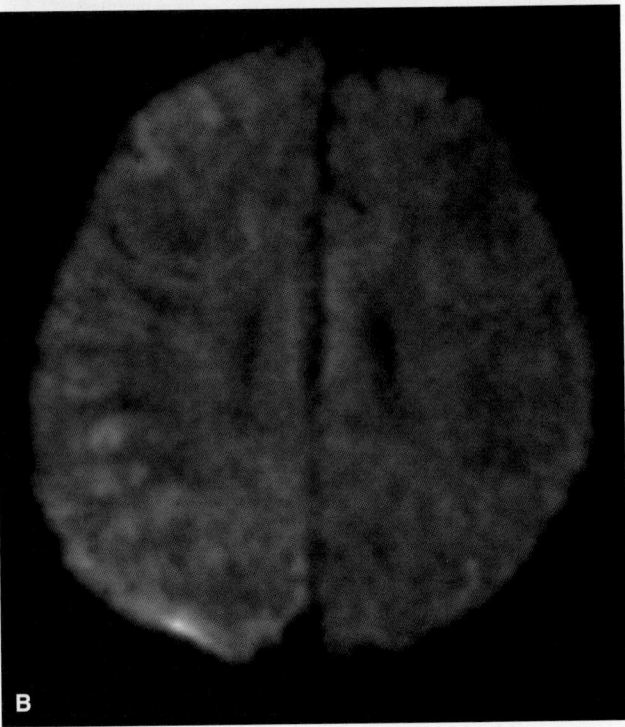

FIGURE 59.6. **A–C:** Thirteen-month-old boy presenting with pneumococcal meningitis and mild left-sided weakness. DWI shows restriction within the interarterial or watershed regions of the right frontal and parietal cortex.

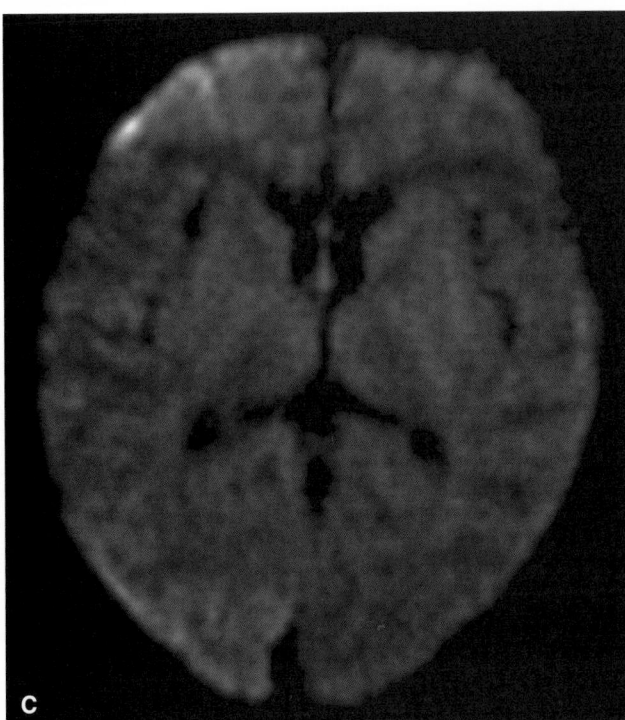

FIGURE 59.6. (*continued*)

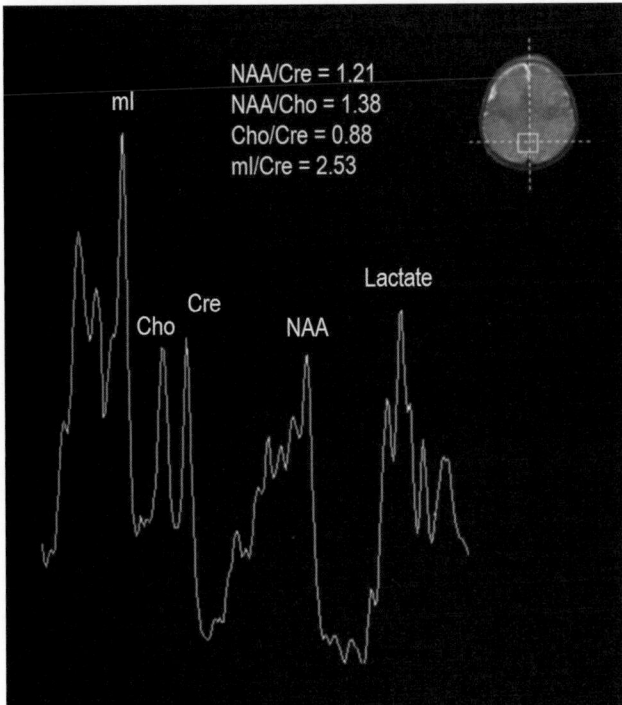

FIGURE 59.7. Two-year-old boy who underwent prolonged resuscitation after a near-drowning. The short echo proton MR spectroscopy of a voxel of cortex shows a very high myoinositol (*mI*) peak, an elevated choline (*Cho*) peak, a normal creatine (*Cre*) peak, a very low *N*-acetyl aspartate (*NAA*) peak, and a very large lactate peak. The metabolites are best described relative to Cre (as shown). The MR spectroscopy findings seen in this patient are highly predictive of a poor neurologic outcome.

contrast enhancement in uncomplicated meningitis, and MRI with DWI is superior to CT in demonstrating some infectious and vasculitic complications of meningitis, including encephalitis, cerebritis, abscess, empyema, ventriculitis, and ischemia (**Fig. 59.9**).

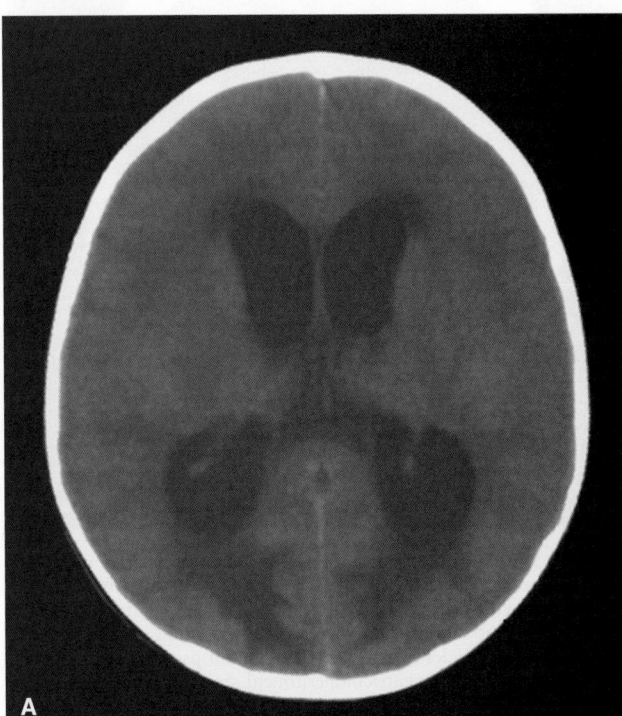

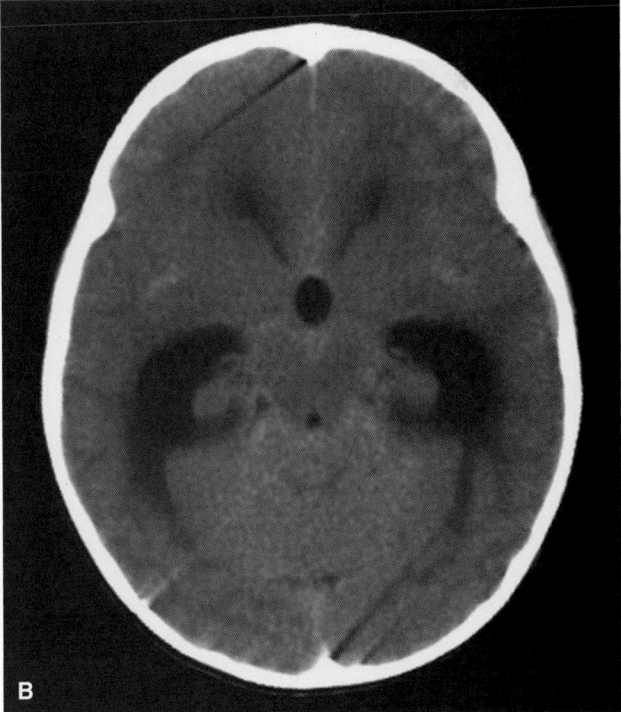

FIGURE 59.8. Eighteen-month-old boy with tuberculous meningitis who presented with obstructive hydrocephalus. Axial CT images show (**A**) marked enlargement of the lateral ventricles, periventricular hypodensity from transependymal edema, and effacement of the cerebral sulci and (**B**) hyperdense, purulent CSF within the basal cisterns surrounding the midbrain.

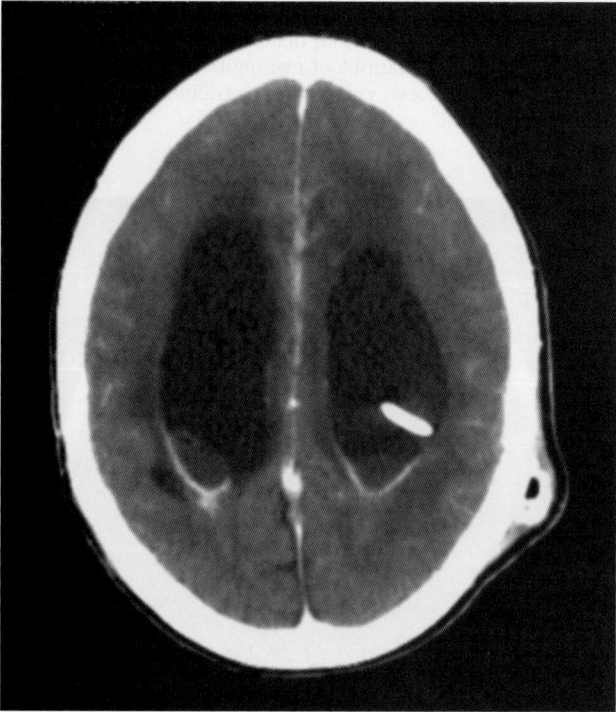

FIGURE 59.9. Thirteen-year-old boy with lumbar myelomeningocele and congenital hydrocephalus presenting with fever and obtundation. Brain MRI with contrast shows expanded lateral ventricles due to shunt failure and contrast enhancement of the lining of the posterior horns of the ventricles due to ventriculitis and pseudomonas meningitis. A portion of the ventriculoperitoneal shunt is visible in the left lateral ventricle.

Meningoencephalitis

CSF analysis is the principal method employed for diagnosing viral meningoencephalitis, but in children infected with the most common etiologic agents, the herpes simplex viruses (HSVs), false-negative polymerase chain reaction (PCR) results are not uncommon when testing is done within the first 72 hours of illness (32). MRI with DWI is highly sensitive for the cytotoxic edema and necrosis associated with this infection and predictive of the long-term neurologic prognosis (33). **Figure 59.10A–C** shows an infant with evolving necrosis from HSV encephalitis. Imaging findings in encephalitis due to other viral agents, including enteroviruses and arboviruses, are often nonspecific and may be limited to subtle T2 hyperintensity within the cortical and subcortical gray matter. Ring-enhancing lesions should raise the possibility of unusual causes of meningoencephalitis, including fungi (*Cryptococcus*, *Aspergillus*, *Candida*), parasites (toxoplasmosis, cysticercosis, amoebae), and *Mycobacterium tuberculosis*. The differential is expanded in patients who are immunocompromised. A case of subacute amoebic meningoencephalitis is illustrated in **Figure 59.11A–C**.

Spinal Infections

Spinal CT with contrast enhancement has a higher detection rate for paraspinal infection than that of plain x-ray, which may only detect bony erosion and vertebral destruction, but it is insufficiently sensitive to exclude the presence of an early discitis or epidural abscess and does not directly assess the integrity of the spinal cord. Given the urgency with which surgical intervention might be needed to avoid permanent spinal cord injury from cord compression, MRI should be performed early in the evaluation of all patients with suspected spinal infections if no contraindication exists (**Fig. 59.12**). In patients with spinal

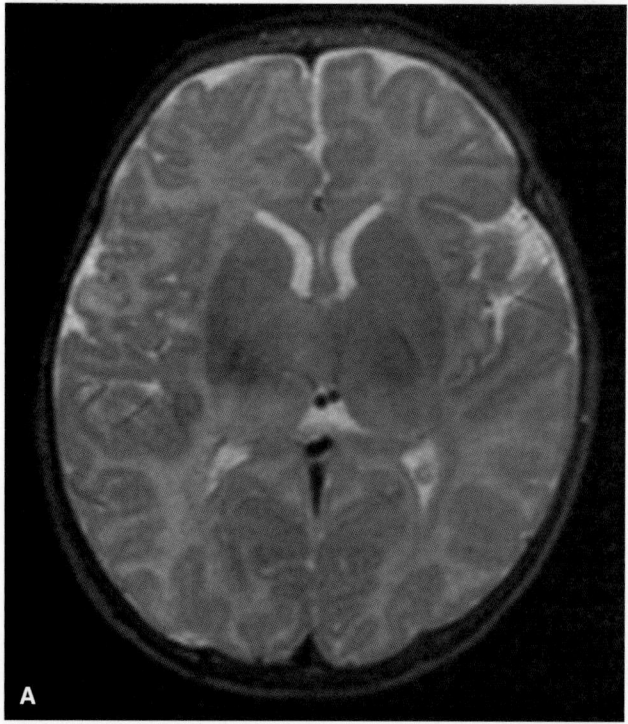

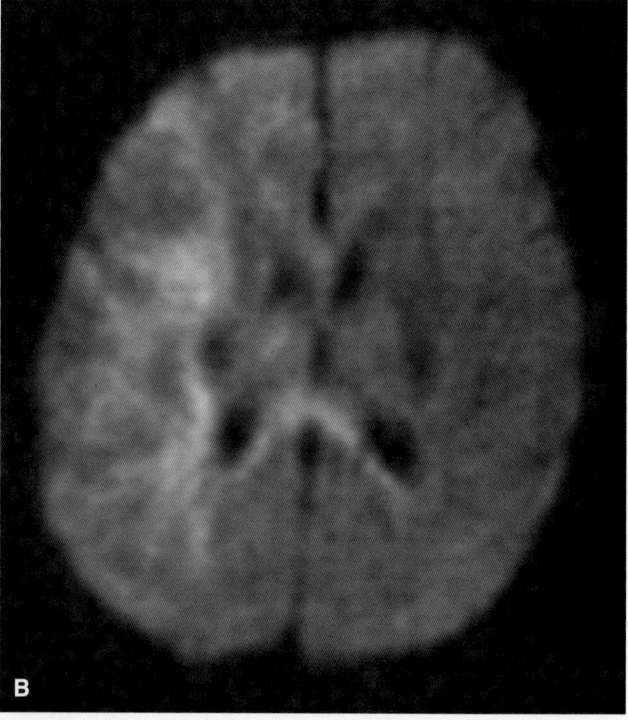

FIGURE 59.10. Ten-week-old girl who presented with focal seizures and hemiparesis due to HSV meningoencephalitis. MRI obtained on admission shows (**A**) normal signal characteristics on T2-weighted images but (**B**) widespread right hemispheric diffusion restriction. MRI obtained 3 weeks later shows (**C**) corresponding extensive right hemispheric encephalomalacia on axial FLAIR image.

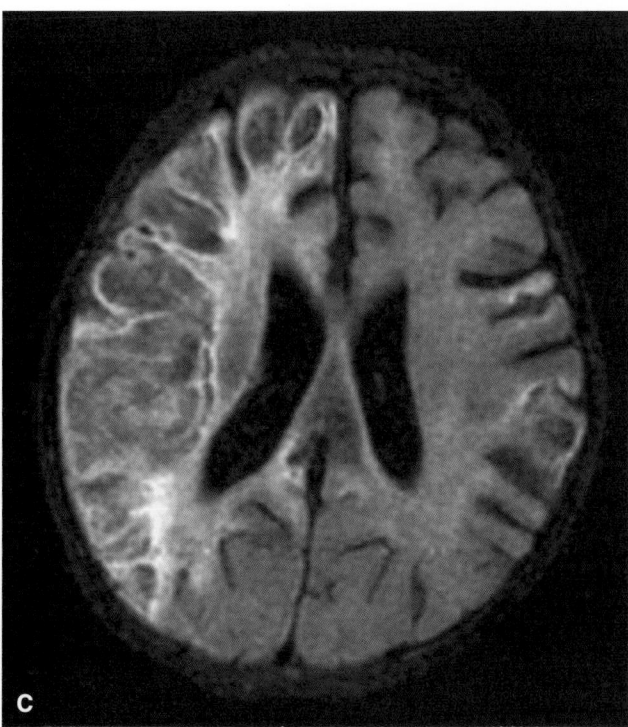

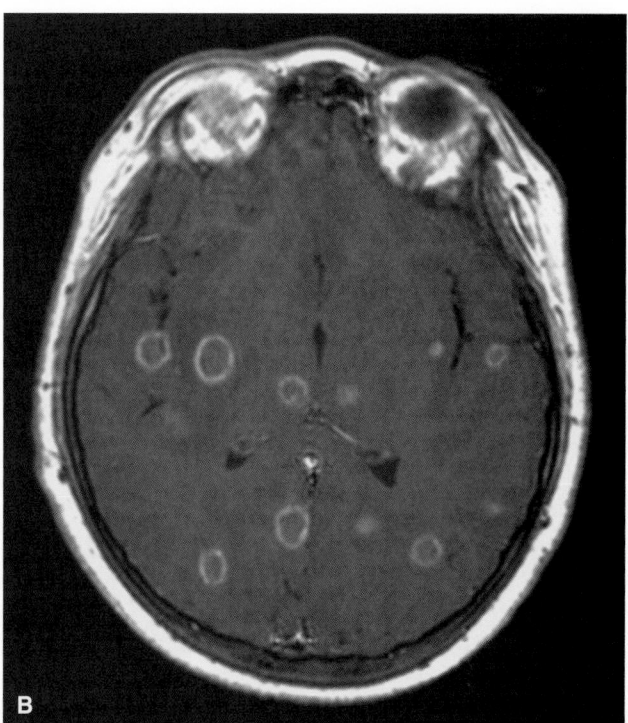

FIGURE 59.10. (continued)

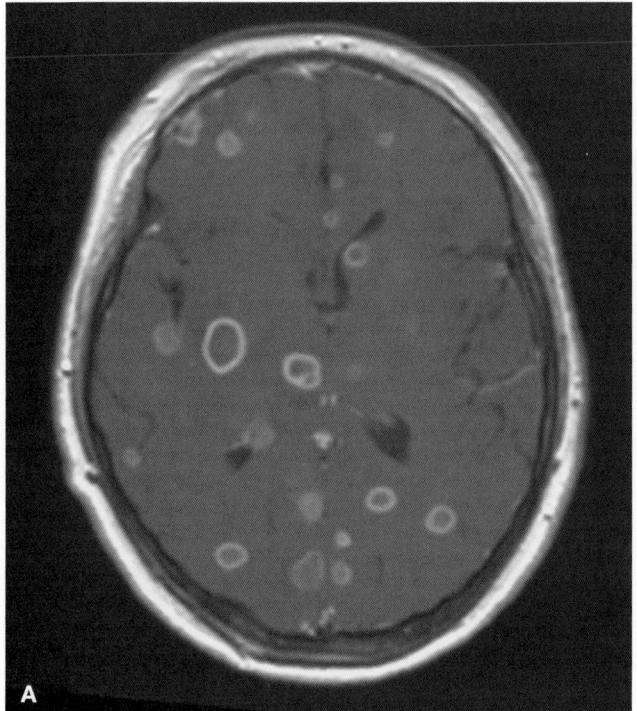

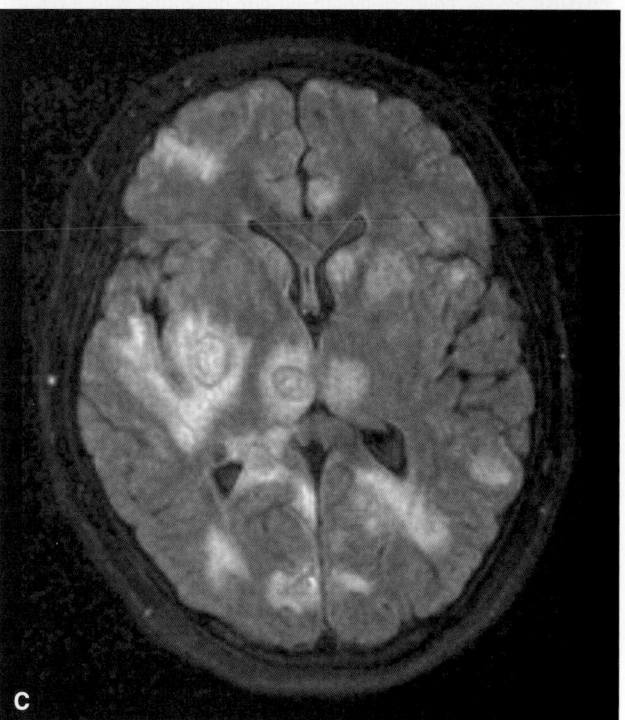

FIGURE 59.11. (continued)

FIGURE 59.11. Twelve-year-old boy who presented with headaches and lethargy due to subacute amoebic meningoencephalitis from *Balamuthia mandrillaris*. **A** and **B**: Axial T1-weighted MR images with gadolinium contrast demonstrate multiple ring-enhancing lesions that show (**C**) surrounding T2 hyperintensity from vasogenic edema on axial FLAIR image.

epidural abscesses that show no cord compression but have signs of severe neurologic impairment, neuroimaging can reveal cord ischemia due to vessel compression or thrombosis (34).

Postinfectious Encephalomyelitis

Autoimmune inflammatory neuropathies appear in most cases to follow infections, vaccinations, and traumatic

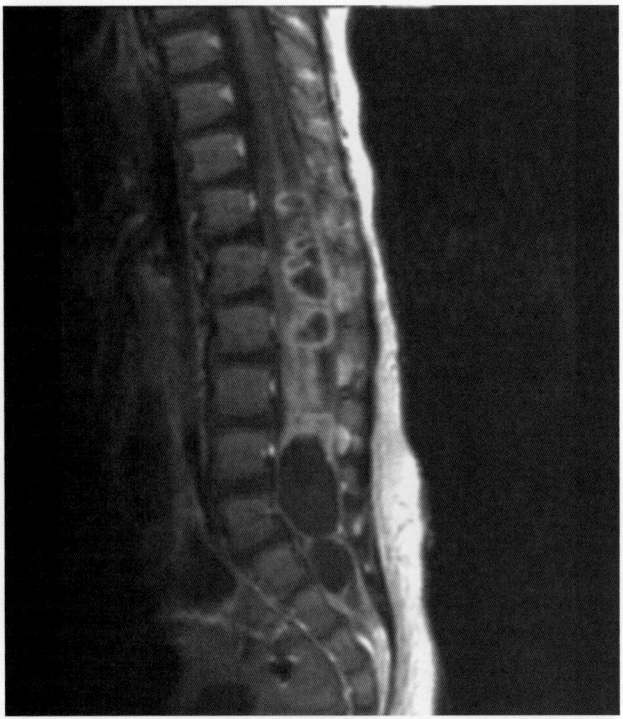

FIGURE 59.12. Fourteen-month-old boy presenting with fever, irritability, and sudden refusal to walk. MRI of the thoracolumbar spine shows multiple loculated ring-enhancing abscesses within the spinal epidural space. Imaging also revealed a dural sinus tract associated with a small conus medullaris lipoma and tethering of the spinal cord.

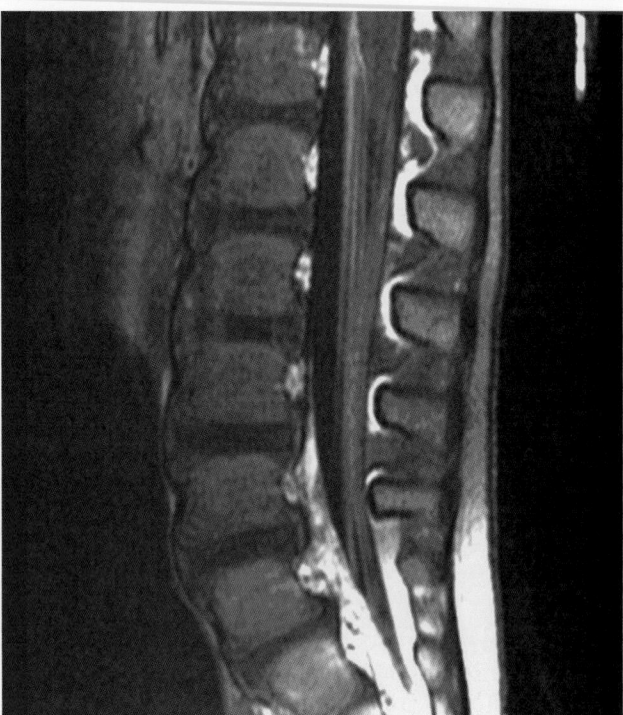

FIGURE 59.13. Eighteen-month-old boy who presented with refusal to walk and absent deep tendon reflexes 1 week after the resolution of a bout of infectious gastroenteritis. Sagittal T1-weighted MRI of the lumbar spine shows intense contrast enhancement of the dorsal and ventral nerve roots, consistent with his electrophysiologic diagnosis of Guillain–Barré syndrome.

injuries. Any portion of the central or peripheral nervous system can be involved individually, as in such isolated syndromes as optic neuritis, acute cerebellar ataxia, transverse myelitis, and Guillain–Barré syndrome. **Figure 59.13** shows the cauda equina enhancement sometimes found in patients with Guillain–Barré syndrome. Alternatively, multiple areas of the nervous system can undergo autoimmune demyelination at once in cases of acute disseminated encephalomyelitis (ADEM). MRI is well suited for the detection of ADEM lesions within the brain and spinal cord, although patients may have severe optic neuritis without radiologic evidence of optic nerve involvement. The differential considered in cases of ADEM often includes atypical infection (e.g., cryptococcal meningitis), neoplasia (e.g., lymphoma), ischemia (e.g., vasculitis), and demyelination from multiple sclerosis (MS). An aggressive case of demyelination from MS or ADEM can mimic the ring enhancement, surrounding vasogenic edema, and central necrosis of an anaplastic astrocytoma or glioblastoma multiforme (GBM). Such cases of tumefactive demyelination (TD) pose difficult decisions about whether to pursue tissue biopsy for diagnosis. Non-contrast CT imaging showing hypodensity in areas that had shown contrast enhancement on MRI has been shown to correlate well with a diagnosis of TD. Other cases of TD have been identified by minimal metabolic changes on Positron Emission Tomography (PET) scanning or by resolution over time with corticosteroid therapy and serial imaging over weeks and months (35,36). A fulminant case of ADEM is presented in **Figure 59.14A–C.**

Toxic and Metabolic Injury

A wide variety of metabolic disorders, from inborn errors of metabolism to acquired endogenous or exogenous toxins, can show similar, nonspecific patterns of injury on neuroimaging. From an imaging perspective, these patterns can be characterized by whether they affect gray matter, white matter, or both (**Tables 59.2–59.4, Fig. 59.15**). Although CT is sometimes useful for the detection of the calcifications that can occur in these disorders, MRI is superior for identifying the pattern of injury and can, in some instances, provide a specific diagnosis, as with T2-weighted imaging in pantothenate kinase–associated neurodegeneration (PKAN) (**Fig. 59.16**) and with MR spectroscopy in leukodystrophies such as Canavan disease (15). While nonspecific, detection of otherwise unexplained deep gray matter lactate contributes to the diagnosis of mitochondrial disorders (**Figs. 59.17 and 59.18**).

Posterior Reversible Encephalopathy Syndrome (PRES, RPLS)

This syndrome of vasogenic edema, also known as reversible posterior leukoencephalopathy syndrome (RPLS), is usually reversible and usually seen in the parietal and occipital cortical and subcortical regions, and has been associated not only with hypertensive crisis but also with a number of other factors seen in critically ill children, including sepsis, multiorgan dysfunction, anemia, and exposure to cytotoxic medications, all of which may cause endothelial injury or impair cerebral autoregulation (37). MRI using FLAIR sequences is particularly sensitive for this condition, which most often presents with headaches, seizures, and visual disturbances. **Figure 59.19** shows a typical case of PRES diagnosed by head CT, MRI, and MR Perfusion. MRI with SWI and DWI sequences can also identify more atypical or complex cases in which there is an unusual distribution of lesions or associated hemorrhage or ischemia (38).

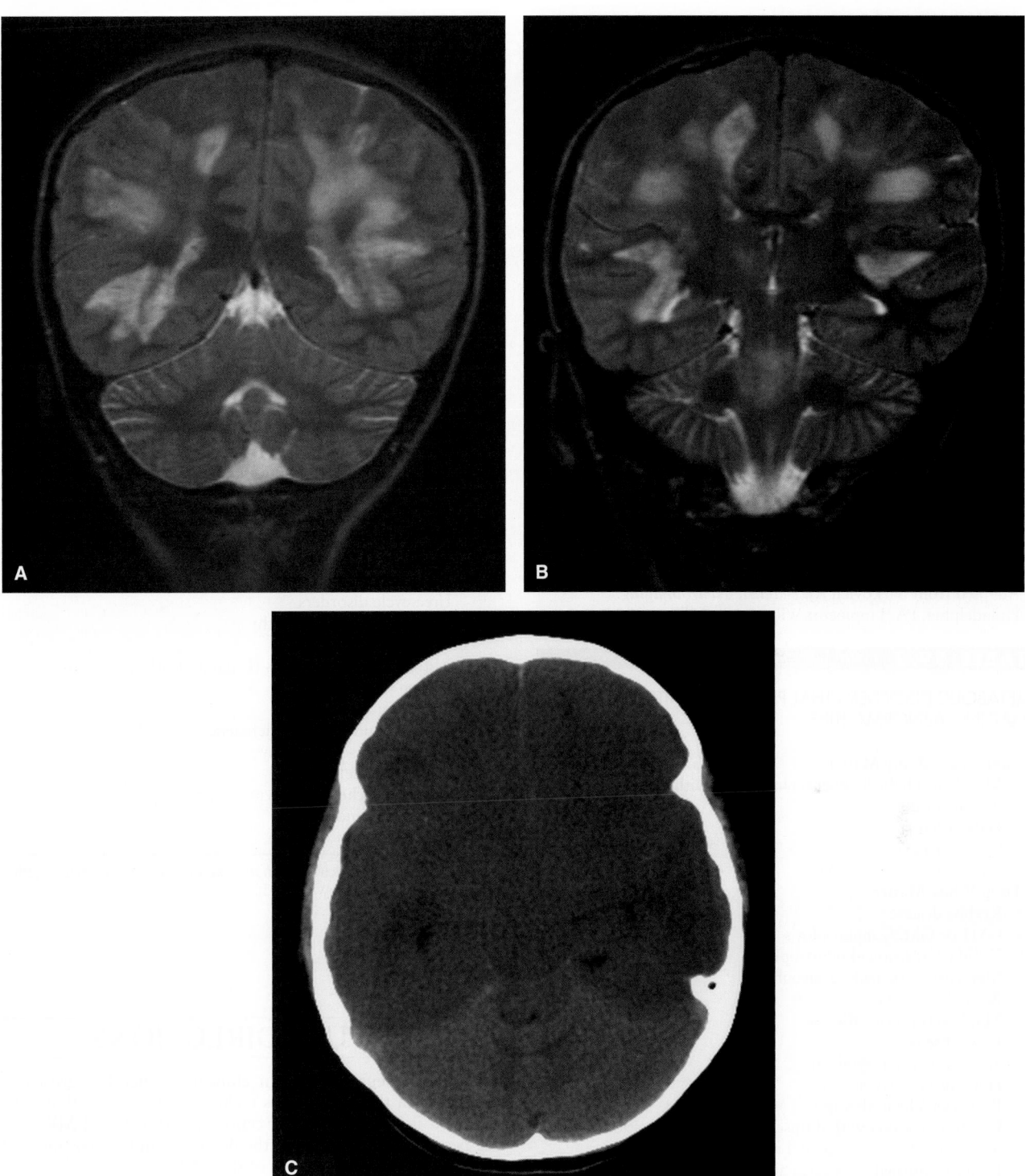

FIGURE 59.14. Seven-year-old girl who presented with hallucinations and obtundation due to ADEM. A and B: T2-weighted coronal MR images show diffuse T2 hyperintensity within the subcortical white matter, right thalamus, and pons. The patient deteriorated clinically despite aggressive immunomodulatory therapy. C: CT shows diffuse hypodensity of the supratentorial tissues with obliteration of the perimesencephalic cisterns. Autopsy showed diffuse cerebral edema and transtentorial herniation.

TABLE 59.2

METABOLIC DISORDERS THAT PRODUCE GRAY MATTER IMAGING ABNORMALITIES

Cortical Gray Matter
  Neuronal ceroid lipofuscinoses
  Mucolipidosis I
Deep Gray Matter
  Striatal T2 Hyperintensity
    Mitochondrial disorders (Leigh and Mitochondrial
      Encephalomyopathy, Lactic Acidosis, and Stroke-like
      episodes (MELAS) syndromes)
    Juvenile Huntington disease
    Organic acidopathies
    Hypoxia–ischemia or hypoglycemia
  Globus Pallidus T2 Hypointensity
    PKAN
    Oculodigital dental dysplasia
  Globus Pallidus T2 Hyperintensity
    Methylmalonic academia
    Toxins (carbon monoxide, manganese, cyanide)
    Kernicterus
    Succinate semialdehyde dehydrogenase deficiency
    Guanidoacetate methyltransferase deficiency
    Isovaleric academia

Adapted from Barkovich AJ. *Pediatric Neuroimaging.*
Philadelphia, PA: Lippincott Williams & Wilkins, 2005.

TABLE 59.3

METABOLIC DISORDERS THAT PRODUCE WHITE MATTER IMAGING ABNORMALITIES

Subcortical White Matter
  Megalencephalic leukoencephalopathy with subcortical cysts
  Alexander disease
  Galactosemia
  Salla disease
  4-Hydroxybutyric aciduria
Deep White Matter
  Krabbe disease
  GM1 or GM2 gangliosidosis
  X-linked adrenoleukodystrophy
  Metachromatic leukodystrophy
  Phenylketonuria
  Maple syrup urine disease
  Lowe disease
  Sjögren–Larsson syndrome
  Hyperhomocysteinemia
  Radiation/chemotherapy
  Childhood ataxia with diffuse CNS hypomyelination
  Merosin-deficient congenital muscular dystrophy
  Dentatorubropallidoluysian atrophy
Lack of Myelination
  Pelizaeus–Merzbacher disease
  Trichothiodystrophy
  18q-syndrome
  Salla disease
Nonspecific Pattern of Involvement
  Nonketotic hyperglycinemia
  Urea cycle disorders
  3-Hydroxy-3-methylglutaryl-coenzyme A lyase deficiency
  Collagen vascular diseases
  Demyelinating diseases
  Viral infections

Adapted from Barkovich AJ. *Pediatric Neuroimaging.* Philadelphia, PA:
Lippincott Williams & Wilkins, 2005.

TABLE 59.4

METABOLIC DISORDERS THAT PRODUCE GRAY AND WHITE MATTER IMAGING ABNORMALITIES

Cortical Gray Matter Only
  Cortical Dysgenesis
    Congenital CMV infection
    Congenital muscular dystrophy
    Peroxisomal disorders
  No Cortical Dysgenesis
    Mucopolysaccharidoses
    Lipid storage disorders
Deep Gray Matter
  Early Thalamic Involvement
    Krabbe disease
    GM1 or GM2 gangliosidosis
    Wilson disease
    Profound neonatal hypotensive encephalopathy
  Early Globus Pallidus Involvement
    Canavan disease
    Kearn–Sayre syndrome
    Methylmalonic academia
    Toxins (carbon monoxide and cyanide)
    Maple syrup urine disease
    L-2-hydroxyglutaric aciduria
    Dentatorubropallidoluysian atrophy
    Urea cycle disorders
    Cree leukoencephalopathy
  Early Striatal Involvement
    Mitochondrial disorders (Leigh and MELAS syndrome)
    Wilson disease
    Organic acidurias
    Molybdenum cofactor deficiency
    β-Ketothiolase deficiency
    Biotinidase deficiencies
    Hypoxia–ischemia or hypoglycemia
    Cockayne syndrome
    Toxins

Adapted from Barkovich AJ. *Pediatric Neuroimaging.* Philadelphia, PA:
Lippincott Williams & Wilkins, 2005.

FUTURE DIRECTIONS

The role of neuroimaging in clinical practice has grown in parallel with the tremendous technical innovations that have occurred in the last quarter century, with CT and MR having become indispensable to the diagnosis and management of most patients with disorders of the CNS.

MR spectroscopy can be performed on entire brain regions either in 2-D (e.g., an axial slice through the basal ganglia and thalami for a patient with hypoxic–ischemic injury) or in 3-D (e.g., the whole brain) to provide far more information about the degree and distribution of injury than a single-voxel study. Ongoing research is successfully correlating these chemical-shift imaging (CSI) maps to short- and long-term clinical outcomes. DTI is also proving to be a useful clinical tool, with recent research showing that the degree of fiber tract disruption (caused by traumatic, metabolic, and toxic injuries) correlates with cognitive outcomes (39).

The diagnostic and prognostic utility of imaging studies will continue to expand as further innovations allow us an ever more detailed view of the physiologic underpinnings of neurologic diseases.

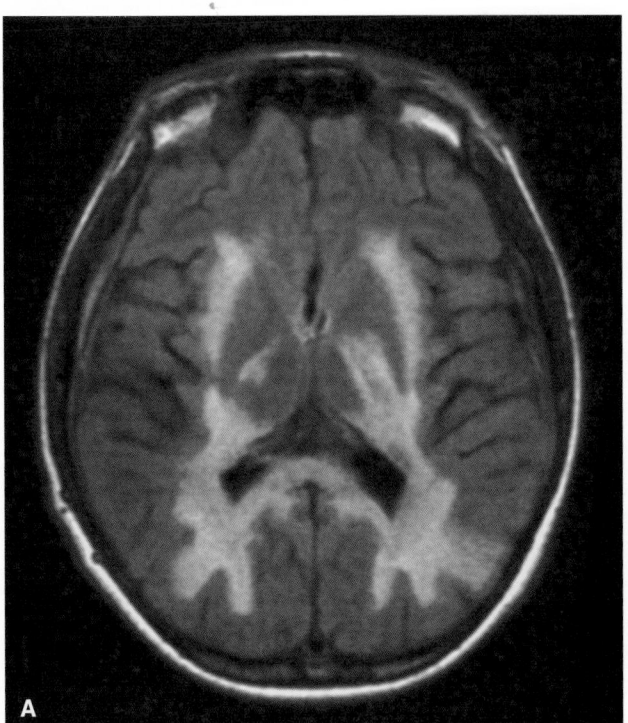
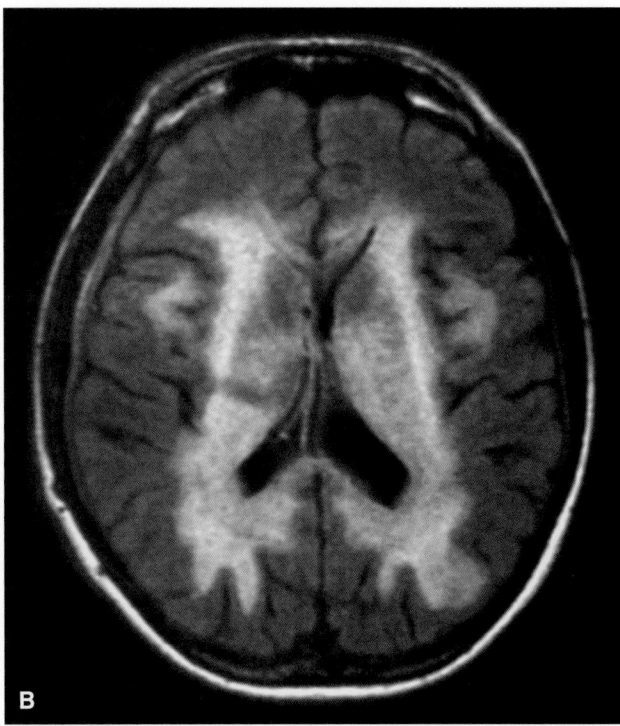

FIGURE 59.15. **A** and **B:** Seventeen-year-old boy with fulminant presentation of X-linked adrenoleukodystrophy, with MRI showing posteriorly predominant and confluent areas of hyperintensity within the periventricular and subcortical white matter on FLAIR imaging.

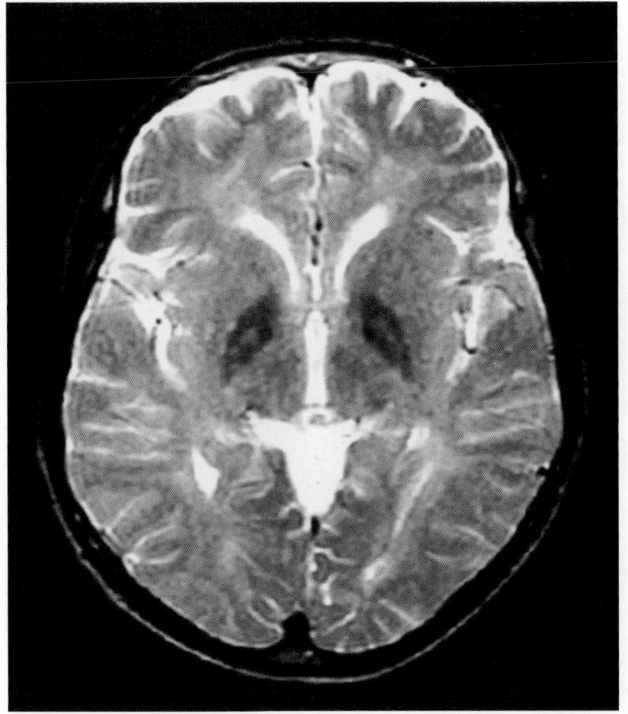

FIGURE 59.16. Fifteen-year-old boy presenting with tremor, dystonia, and dysarthria, diagnosed with PKAN associated with mutation of the gene for pantothenate kinase 2. MR imaging was obtained using a 1.5 Tesla scanner. Axial T2-weighted image shows characteristic hypointensity within the globus pallidi bilaterally with a central high signal intensity focus, often described as the eye-of-the-tiger sign. (Image courtesy of Dr. R. Nuri Sener of the Department of Radiology, Ege University Hospital, Bornova, Izmir, Turkey.)

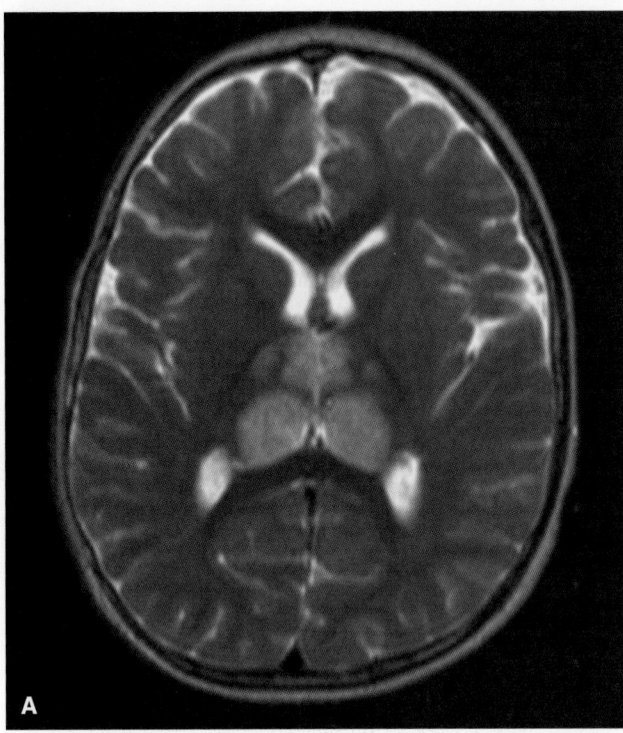
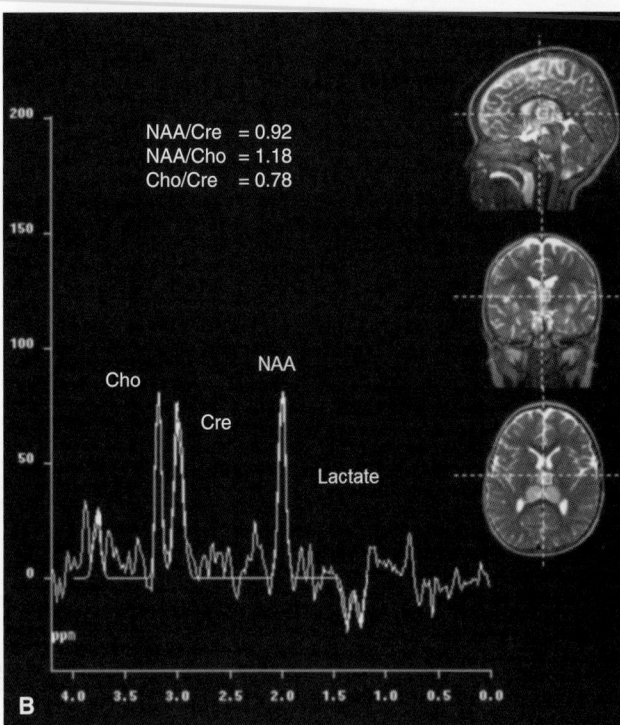

FIGURE 59.17. Eighteen-month-old boy who presented with coma after influenza vaccination. A: MRI of the brain shows symmetrical bright T2-weighted signal within the thalami, and (B) long echo proton MR spectroscopy of a voxel centered in the left thalamus shows a markedly low NAA-to-Cre ratio, indicating neuronal loss or dysfunction, and a high concentration of lactate, indicative of ischemia, consistent with a diagnosis of acute necrotizing encephalopathy.

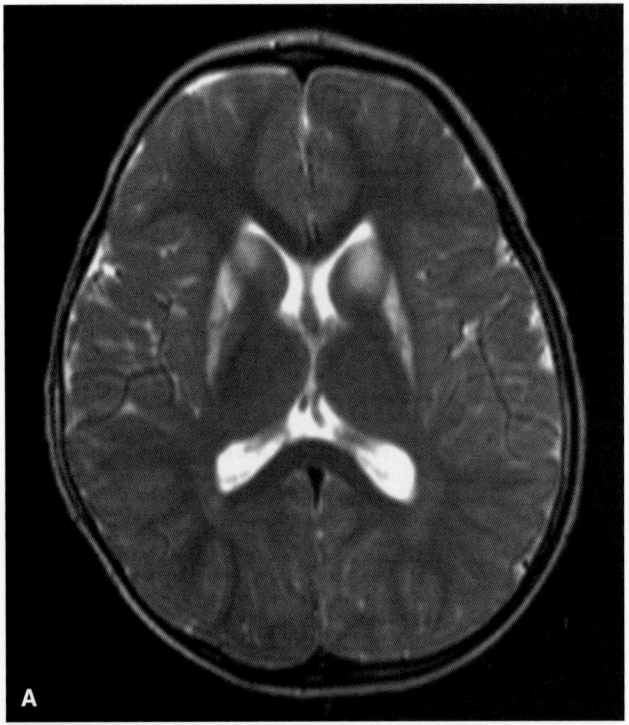
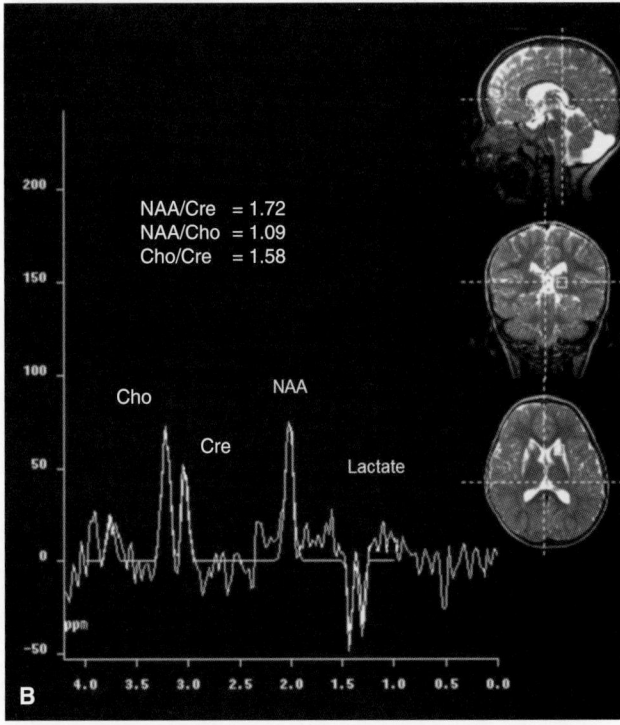

FIGURE 59.18. Sixteen-month-old boy who presented with slowly progressive ophthalmoplegia that acutely worsened during an otherwise mild febrile gastroenteritis. A: MRI of the brain 9 months later shows persistent T2 hyperintensity within both caudate nuclei, and (B) long echo proton MR spectroscopy of a voxel centered in the left caudate nucleus shows a low NAA-to-Cre ratio and a high concentration of lactate, consistent with a diagnosis of Leigh syndrome.

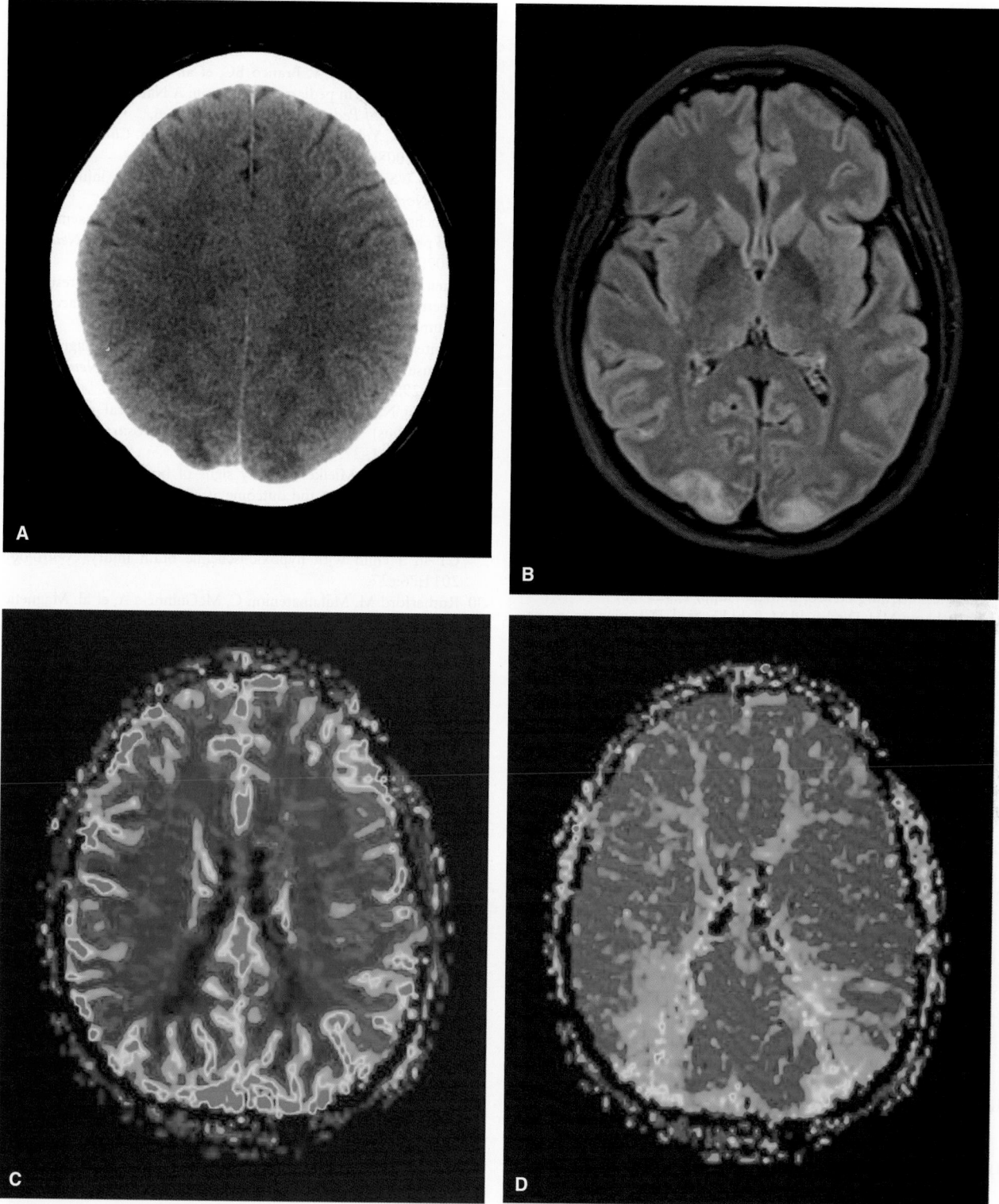

FIGURE 59.19. Twenty-two-year-old woman with hypertensive crisis in the postpartum period, presenting with a severe headache, transient loss of vision, and a generalized tonic–clonic seizure. Subcortical edema is visible as subtle hypodensity in the occipital cortex on head CT (**A**) and is more evident as hyperintensity on the FLAIR sequence of a head MRI (**B**). An MR perfusion study showed a slightly increased cerebral blood volume (**C**) but a clearly delayed mean transit time (**D**) in the occipital region.

References

1. Rao P, Bekhit E, Ramanauskas F, et al. CT head in children. *Eur J Radiol* 2013;82(7):1050–8.
2. Pearce MS, Salotti JA, Little MP, et al. Radiation exposure from CT scans in childhood and subsequent risk of leukaemia and brain tumours: A retrospective cohort study. *Lancet* 2012;380:499–505.
3. Hall P, Adami HO, Trichopoulos D, et al. Effect of low doses of ionizing radiation in infancy on cognitive function in adulthood: Swedish population-based cohort study. *BMJ* 2004;328:19.
4. LaRovere KL, Brett MS, Tasker RC, et al. Head computed tomography scanning during pediatric neurocritical care: Diagnostic yield and the utility of portable studies. *Neurocrit Care* 2012;16:251–7.
5. Erdem E, Agildere M, Eryilmaz M, et al. Intracranial calcification in children on computed tomography. *Turk J Pediatr* 1994;36:111–22.
6. Stuckey SL, Goh TD, Heffernan T, et al. Hyperintensity in the subarachnoid space on FLAIR MRI. *AJR Am J Roentgenol* 2007;189:913–21.
7. Shellock FG, Spinazzi A. MRI safety update 2008: Part 2, screening patients for MRI. *AJR Am J Roentgenol* 2008;191:1140–9.
8. Kanekar SG, Zacharia T, Roller R. Imaging of stroke: Part 2, Pathophysiology at the molecular and cellular levels and corresponding imaging changes. *AJR Am J Roentgenol* 2012;198:63–74.
9. Lai PH, Hsu SS, Ding SW, et al. Proton magnetic resonance spectroscopy and diffusion-weighted imaging in intracranial cystic mass lesions. *Surg Neurol* 2007;68(suppl 1):S25–36.
10. Beauchamp MH, Ditchfield M, Babl FE, et al. Detecting traumatic brain lesions in children: CT versus MRI versus susceptibility weighted imaging (SWI). *J Neurotrauma* 2011;28:915–27.
11. Chalian M, Tekes A, Meoded A, et al. Susceptibility-weighted imaging (SWI): A potential non-invasive imaging tool for characterizing ischemic brain injury? *J Neuroradiol* 2011;38:187–90.
12. Niogi SN, Mukherjee P. Diffusion tensor imaging of mild traumatic brain injury. *J Head Trauma Rehabil* 2010;25:241–55.
13. Lerner A, Mogensen MA, Kim PE, et al. Clinical applications of diffusion tensor imaging. *World Neurosurg.* 2013 Aug 3. pii:S1878-8750(13)00897-8.
14. Miyazaki M, Akahane M. Non-contrast enhanced MR angiography: Established techniques. *J Magn Reson Imaging* 2012;35:1–19.
15. Iles RA. Nuclear magnetic resonance spectroscopy and genetic disorders. *Curr Med Chem* 2008;15:15–36.
16. Ashwal S, Holshouser B, Tong K, et al. Proton MR spectroscopy detected glutamate/glutamine is increased in children with traumatic brain injury. *J Neurotrauma* 2004;21:1539–52.
17. Aragão Mde F, Law M, Netto JP, et al. Prognostic value of proton magnetic resonance spectroscopy findings in near drowning patients: Reversibility of the early metabolite abnormalities relates with a good outcome. *Arq Neuropsiquiatr* 2006;67:55–7.
18. Steffen-Smith EA, Shih JH, Hipp SJ, et al. Proton magnetic resonance spectroscopy predicts survival in children with diffuse intrinsic pontine glioma. *J Neurooncol* 2011;105:365–73.
19. Dahmoush HM, Vossough A, Roberts TP. Pediatric high-field magnetic resonance imaging. *Neuroimaging Clin N Am* 2012;22:297–313.
20. Huisman TA, Sorensen AG. Perfusion-weighted magnetic resonance imaging of the brain: Techniques and application in children. *Eur Radiol* 2004;14:59–72.
21. Mohseni S, Talving P, Branco BC, et al. Effect of age on cervical spine injury in pediatric population: A National Trauma Data Bank review. *J Pediatr Surg* 2011;46:1771–6.
22. Yucesoy K, Yuksel KZ. SCIWORA in MRI era. *Clin Neurol Neurosurg* 2008;110:429–33.
23. Kubal WS. Updated imaging of traumatic brain injury. *Radiol Clin North Am* 2012;50:15–41.
24. Trenchs V, Curcoy AI, Navarro R, et al. Subdural haematomas and physical abuse in the first two years of life. *Pediatr Neurosurg* 2007;43:352–57.
25. Aaen GS, Holshouser BA, Sheridan C, et al. Magnetic resonance spectroscopy predicts outcomes for children with nonaccidental trauma. *Pediatrics* 2010;125:295–303.
26. Hunter JV, Wilde EA, Tong KA, et al. Emerging imaging tools for use with traumatic brain injury research. *J Neurotrauma* 2012;29:654–71.
27. Dlamini N, Billinghurst L, Kirkham FJ. Cerebral venous sinus (sinovenous) thrombosis in children. *Neurosurg Clin N Am* 2010;21:511–27.
28. Wardlaw JM, Mielke O. Early signs of brain infarction at CT: Observer reliability and outcome after thrombolytic treatment – Systematic review. *Radiology* 2005;235:444–53.
29. Iyer RS, Thomas B. Teaching neuroimages: Reversal sign on CT in a child with hypoxic-ischemic brain injury. *Neurology* 2011;76:e27.
30. Rutherford M, Malamateniou C, McGuinness A, et al. Magnetic resonance imaging in hypoxic-ischaemic encephalopathy. *Early Hum Dev* 2010;86:351–60.
31. Hasbun R, Abrahams J, Jekel J, et al. Computed tomography of the head before lumbar puncture in adults with suspected meningitis. *N Engl J Med* 2001;345:1727–33.
32. Adler AC, Kadimi S, Apaloo C, et al. Herpes simplex encephalitis with two false-negative cerebrospinal fluid PCR tests and review of negative PCR results in the clinical setting. *Case Rep Neurol* 2011;3:172–8.
33. Dhawan A, Kecskes Z, Jyoti R, et al. Early diffusion-weighted magnetic resonance imaging findings in neonatal herpes encephalitis. *J Paediatr Child Health* 2006;42:824–6.
34. Wang VY, Chou D, Chin C. Spine and spinal cord emergencies: Vascular and infectious causes. *Neuroimaging Clin N Am* 2010;20:639–50.
35. Hardy TA, Chataway J. Tumefactive demyelination: An approach to diagnosis and management. *J Neurol Neurosurg Psychiatry* 2013;84(9):1047–53.
36. Saini J, Chatterjee S, Thomas B, et al. Conventional and advanced magnetic resonance imaging in tumefactive demyelination. *Acta Radiol* 2011;52:1159–68.
37. Raj S, Overby P, Erdfarb A, et al. Posterior reversible encephalopathy syndrome: Incidence and associated factors in a pediatric critical care population. *Pediatr Neurol* 2013;49(5):335–9.
38. Stevens CJ, Heran MK. The many faces of posterior reversible encephalopathy syndrome. *Br J Radiol* 2012;85(1020):1566–75.
39. Tournier JD, Mori S, Leemans A. Diffusion tensor imaging and beyond. *Magn Reson Med* 2011;65:1532–56.

CHAPTER 60 ■ NEUROSURGICAL AND NEURORADIOLOGICAL CRITICAL CARE

MICHAEL L. MCMANUS, CRAIG D. MCCLAIN, AND ROBERT C. TASKER

KEY POINTS

❶ The PICU should be considered an extension of the neurosurgical operating room and interventional neuroradiology suite. As such it is imperative that all practitioners in the continuum of perioperative care communicate plans, concerns, and strategies.

❷ It is important to have familiarity with current and potential neuromonitoring for children with neurosurgical and cerebrovascular disease.

❸ It is important to be cognizant of special problems that occur in this population in the postoperative period, in particular the dysnatremias.

❹ Special issues arise in the management of cases undergoing brain tumor surgery, hydrocephalus treatment, cerebrovascular surgery, epilepsy surgery, or craniosynostosis repair.

Critical care in neurosurgical and neuroradiological cases spans a continuum that begins with the operating theater or neuroradiology suite and continues through the PICU. In addition, good patient care often requires the intensivist to provide expertise outside the PICU, in the emergency department, the radiology suite, and even into general or rehabilitative care settings. It is important, therefore, for a critical care physician to maintain a "systems" perspective and good working knowledge of the specialties and practices comprising this continuum of care. The focus of this chapter is upon close coordination of neurosurgery, neuroradiology, anesthesia, and critical care practices in this population of critically ill children. We begin with an overview of considerations important to our colleagues in anesthesiology, neurosurgery, and neuroradiology; continue with discussion of routine postoperative care; and then proceed with more detailed discussion of specific surgical entities. We conclude with discussion of a few specific postoperative challenges that are common in neurointensive care.

CLINICAL SCIENTIFIC FOUNDATIONS

Procedural and Operating Room Issues

The fundamental principles of postoperative and postprocedural neurocritical care include knowledge of the patient's pre-procedure neurologic status, of the details of the procedure, of the patient's post-procedure neurologic status, of the potential ongoing concerns, and whether there are interventions that will optimize outcome.

General Anesthetic Considerations

The general goal of anesthetic management is to maintain stable hemodynamics and adequate gas exchange while providing analgesia and, when needed, sedation. In neuroanesthesia, this translates to maintenance of oxygenation, provision of appropriate carbon dioxide levels, preservation of adequate cerebral blood flow (CBF), and avoidance of exacerbations of intracranial hypertension. Hyponatremia, hypo-osmolarity, and hyperglycemia can contribute to cerebral swelling and neurological injury and are avoided. Anesthetic agents and depth are managed so as to permit a crisp wakeup and immediate neurological assessment once surgery is complete. Despite these seemingly straightforward goals, hypotension (1), hyperglycemia (2), and inadvertent hyperventilation (3) are persistent, but modifiable, risk factors in the perioperative period.

Induction of anesthesia usually involves premedication followed by titration of intravenous or inhaled agents at a rate that minimizes the hemodynamic consequences of transition from waking to anesthetic states. Premedication is administered with caution to avoid respiratory depression and is often avoided when significant intracranial hypertension is present. Induction agents are carefully titrated to avoid hypotension and decreased CBF. Thiopental (not available in United States), propofol, etomidate, and ketamine are common induction agents, and their effects on blood pressure (BP), intracranial pressure (ICP), CBF, and cerebral metabolic rate for oxygen ($CMRO_2$) are considered prior to use. Recently, concerns about these deleterious effects of ketamine have been questioned (4,5). To minimize vasodilation that accompanies volatile agents, anesthetic maintenance classically involves a "balanced" technique using nitrous oxide, a narcotic, and low-dose volatile agent. The effect of volatile agents on CBF can vary with the dose of agent (increased vasodilation at higher dose), the region of brain studied (more pronounced on surface vessels), and the use of hyperventilation to cause vasoconstriction (often requested by neurosurgeons, to shrink brain tissue, even when ICP is normal). All volatile agents cause dose-dependent increases in CBF that can be attenuated with controlled ventilation. There is longstanding debate around the use of nitrous oxide since it can cause some degree of cerebral vasodilation, it may contribute to postoperative vomiting, as well other limitations (6). In addition, nitrous oxide is relatively contraindicated when air collections are present (such as after recent craniotomy) since its diffusion may cause their expansion. Increasingly, there is addition or substitution of ultra-short-acting agents such as remifentanil or dexmedetomidine for anesthetic maintenance. The general effects of commonly used anesthetics on $CMRO_2$, CBF, pressure autoregulation, and ICP are summarized in **Table 60.1**.

Pre- and Intraoperative Fluid Management

Euvolemia is preferred before induction of anesthesia because the associated loss of sympathetic tone produces hypotension. The primary intraoperative fluids are exclusively isotonic as vasodilation and acute blood loss can necessitate sudden infusion of large volumes. Of the available solutions, normal saline is often the fluid of choice since it is slightly hypertonic to plasma and is compatible with all medications (including phenytoin). Fluid replacement is best guided by heart rate, BP, and perfusion since urine output can be profoundly influenced by stress-related changes in antidiuretic hormone (ADH) secretion. In addition, general anesthesia and prone positioning can interfere with urine production and urinary catheter drainage. Overall, urine output is an unreliable marker of volume status since oliguria can arise from many unrelated sources. Nonetheless, maintenance of euvolemia is critically important both to support CBF and to avoid venous air embolism via skull dural sinuses. A special situation arises in cerebrovascular cases that receive 1.5 times maintenance fluid requirements as preoperative preparation (see section on *Cerebrovascular Surgery*); in these cases intrinsic homeostasis will lead to excretion of the excessive salt load in the postoperative period, which may be mistakenly interpreted as postoperative "cerebral salt wasting" (CSW; see section on *Dysnatremia*).

In regard to the use of intraoperative glucose-containing fluids, the stress response should maintain normal serum glucose levels without exogenous glucose administration. However, in postoperative infants and small children, particularly if there has been an effective fast of 6–12 hours, there is the risk of perioperative hypoglycemia. Therefore, glucose-containing fluids can be used to meet baseline demands for neonates and susceptible infants. In general, older children and adolescents can tolerate 18–24 hours of fasting before requiring glucose-containing fluid administration. One risk of giving exogenous glucose is that along with the stress of critical illness (and resulting insulin resistance) hyperglycemia may be induced and, in turn, may be associated with neurologic injury and poor outcome. Concern persists that hyperglycemia can worsen injury due to ischemia, but it remains unclear if tight glycemic control offers significant benefits to children.

Hemodynamic Management

As a general rule, intravenous anesthetics agents preserve CBF and autoregulation while volatile agents cause some degree of vasodilation and autoregulatory impairment (**Table 60.1**). As depth of anesthesia increases, so too does the impact on the circulation and CBF. To closely monitor and direct the control of mean BP and cerebral perfusion during anesthetic administration, an intra-arterial catheter is used. Especially in cerebrovascular surgery, vasoactive medications are always kept immediately available if needed to manipulate the circulation. Although α-2 agonists have direct constrictive effects on cerebral vasculature, all agents that increase mean BP will increase CBF when the limits of autoregulation are exceeded.

There are interactions between anesthetic agents and vasopressors. In short time frames, BP and cerebral autoregulation vary with anesthetic depth (i.e., as depth of anesthesia increases, BP and the ability to autoregulate CBF decrease). Over longer time frames, vasopressors can impact their effectiveness. In animal models, catecholamine infusion produces circulatory changes that increase the distribution of propofol and reduce its anesthetic effects (7,8). A similar phenomenon can be demonstrated with remifentanil (9). The practical implication of this phenomenon is that hemodynamics and depth of anesthesia must be continuously balanced both in the operating room and throughout the transition to the PICU.

Surgical Considerations

Cranial surgeries require rigid skull fixation and pins may be placed prior to positioning. Complications of the use of pins include sudden increases in heart rate, BP, and ICP, as well as pin-related skull fractures and intracranial hemorrhages in infants and small children. The patient position carries risks and the sitting position is associated with an increased risk of venous air embolism. In pediatric neurosurgery, the sitting position is infrequently necessary and many adult neurosurgeons often choose to avoid it. Perioperative antibiotics are routinely administered. Blood loss varies widely among procedures and

---

TABLE 60.1

EFFECTS OF ANESTHETICS, BENZODIAZEPINES, AND OPIOIDS ON CEREBRAL METABOLISM, CIRCULATION, AND ICP

■ AGENT	■ $CMRO_2$	■ CBF	■ PRESSURE AUTOREGULATION	■ ICP
Inhaled anesthetic ■ Sevoflurane ■ Isoflurane ■ Desflurane	↓↓	↑	Absent	↑
Inhaled nitrous oxide	↑ or no change	↑	Present	↑
Intravenous anesthetic ■ Propofol ■ Thiopental	↓↓	↓↓	Present	↓↓
Dissociative anesthesia ■ Ketamine	No change	↑↑	?	↑↑
Sedative benzodiazepines	↓↓	↓	Present	↓
Analgesic opioids	No change	No change	Present	No change

See Chapter 58 for pressure autoregulation. The direction of arrows indicates increased or decreased, and the number of arrows indicates the strength of the derangement above "no change" qualitatively.

can be particularly challenging in hemispherectomies and craniofacial reconstruction. In addition, chronic and even short-term anticonvulsant use may predispose to platelet dysfunction, thrombocytopenia, and factor deficiencies that can lead to increased blood loss.

Cranial Imaging Considerations

Imaging for neurosurgical patients presents many challenges. Cranial computed tomographic (CT) and magnetic resonance (MR) imaging may require transport and sedation of unstable patients. Complex imaging and interventional procedures may require prolonged immobility, controlled ventilation, and manipulation of the circulation. The neuroradiology and imaging suites can be "unfriendly" environments, in the sense that many of the supports routinely available in the operating room and PICU are either unavailable or difficult to secure. Full monitoring, safe positioning, access to the patient, and help during emergencies may all present challenges to anesthesia and PICU staff.

In some centers, portable CT devices have been introduced to mitigate transport hazards and decrease barriers related to the imaging of critically ill patients. Although the resolution and versatility of portable scanners are below those of fixed machines, their diagnostic utility is similar (10). The radiation doses attendant to portable machines is approximately 15% higher than fixed machines, so extra precautions are necessary to limit patient exposure and assure radiation safety of staff.

MR imaging is an indispensable tool in neurosurgery and neurocritical care, but MR safety is an important concern since the behavior of ferromagnetic materials in the MR suite can be dangerous. The terms "MR conditional," "MR safe," and "MR unsafe" have been proposed to clarify discussion of these hazards (11), and the MR suite itself has been divided into four zones of varying risk (12). *MR unsafe* materials must be excluded from the suite. *MR safe* equipment presents no threat when its operating instructions are followed. *MR conditional* refers to an object that has been demonstrated to pose no known problems under specified MR conditions (i.e., the magnetic field strength, its spatial gradient, its time rate of change, the radiofrequency field strength, and its specific absorption rate). For critically ill patients, special monitors, infusion pumps, and *MR safe* or *MR conditional* anesthesia machines may all be required. Historically, cardiac pacemakers have been considered a contraindication to MR imaging, but compatible devices are now available. Programmable cerebrospinal fluid (CSF) shunts may be altered by magnetic fields, so those devices should always be interrogated following an MR examination. To prevent malfunctions or thermal injury, manufacturers of nerve stimulators offer strict guidelines regarding radiofrequency and gradient fields.

Intraoperative MR imaging has been developed to improve surgical navigation and resections. First-generation facilities employed an "open" configuration wherein both patient and magnet are stationary and surgery is conducted with limited access but real-time imaging capabilities. In later configurations, either the patient or magnet is mobile, permitting better access but requiring repositioning between scan sequences. In open systems, all anesthesia and surgical equipment must be *MR safe*. Unfortunately, some important equipment found in conventional operating rooms (e.g., precordial Doppler ultrasonography, core temperature probes, fluid warmers) do not yet have *MR safe* or *MR conditional* counterparts. Nevertheless, numerous neurosurgical procedures have been safely performed in children in suites with combined MR and operating room capability, and the equipment for these procedures is rapidly evolving (13).

Emergence

Regardless of the anesthetic technique used during the procedure, quick postoperative emergence is a basic requirement by neuroanesthesia. Awakening, extubation, and a screening neurological examination are important before transfer to the PICU in order to ensure that the patient has experienced no occult injury and is following the expected postoperative trajectory. When extubation is not possible, as in the patient with multiple trauma, respiratory impairment, or other comorbidities, it is prudent to confirm some level of responsiveness upon arrival in the PICU.

There are, potentially, two interlocking viscous cycles in pathophysiology that may lead to hemodynamic instability, cerebral edema, and intracranial hemorrhage in the immediate postoperative period (**Fig. 60.1**). Hence, in some high-risk children, there might be a plan for postoperative mechanical ventilation or deep sedation (**Table 60.2**). Emergence agitation may be due to pain, a full bladder, dysnatremia (see later), drug reaction (e.g., paradoxical reaction to midazolam or diphenhydramine), or emergence delirium (e.g., reaction to sevoflurane). Treatable causes will have been identified and dealt with, or even anticipated, by the anesthesiologist. For example, pain and agitation can be anticipated and treated with bolus doses of opioids, propofol, clonidine, or dexmedetomidine. The stress response with emergence hypertension can be treated with low-dose fentanyl infusion (1–1.5 mcg/kg/h) and an antihypertensive. In regard to the antihypertensive, the choice is between a β-blocker (labetalol or esmolol) and a calcium channel antagonist (nicardipine). There is no ideal vasodilator: β-blockers have the risk of bradycardia and cardiac conduction delays; the calcium channel antagonists cause cerebral vasodilatation, impaired autoregulation, and risk of

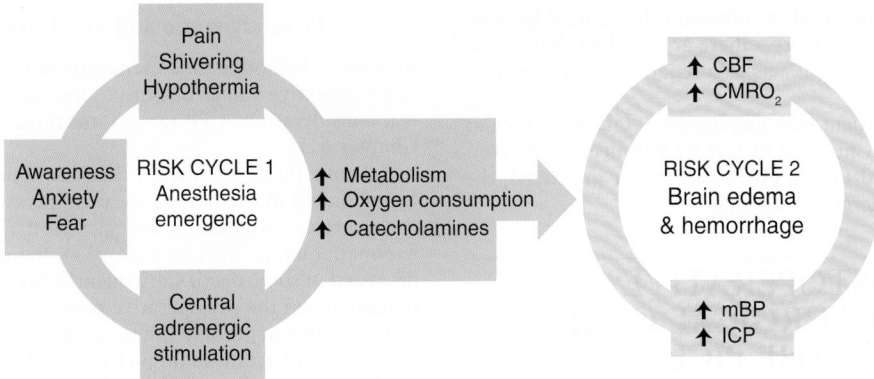

FIGURE 60.1. Potential stress-induced pathophysiology during emergency from anesthesia. mBP, mean blood pressure.

TABLE 60.2

LIKELY CANDIDATES FOR DELAYED EMERGENCE AND DELAYED ENDOTRACHEAL EXTUBATION AFTER NEUROSURGERY

■ CAUSES FOR CONSIDERATION OF DELAYED EXTUBATION AND EMERGENCE FROM ANESTHESIA

- Preoperative altered level of consciousness
- Surgery lasting >6 h
- Large tumor resection with preoperative midline shift
- Injury to cranial nerves IX, X, XI
- Complications during surgery
- Intraoperative brain swelling
- Hypothermia
- Coagulopathy
- Acid–base abnormality
- Dysnatremia (see text for details)

TABLE 60.3

FACTORS TO CONSIDER IN THE PATIENT FAILING TO WAKE UP AT THE END OF NEUROSURGERY

■ FACTOR	■ INTERVENTION
Neuromuscular blockade	Impaired hepatic and/or renal metabolism may prolong the effect
Altered drug metabolism	Consider drug dosing and drug clearance of continuous infusions used (also see hypothyroid)
Seizure	Assess and treat accordingly
Intracranial bleeding	Imaging required and surgery
Intracranial pressure/ischemia	Imaging required
Hypothermia	Warm patient
Hypoglycemia	Check blood glucose and treat accordingly
Hypercapnia	Check blood gas and support ventilation as needed
Hypo-osmolality	Check serum electrolytes and treat accordingly
Hypothyroidism	Thyroid hormone required for benzodiazepine metabolism; support patient until full emergence and thyroid function tests available

hypotension. Dexmedetomidine infusion is being used increasingly in pediatric neurosurgery—there are no data, but its use is gaining popularity since it acts as a sedative, sympatholytic, and analgesic.

Occasionally, a patient may unexpectedly fail to awaken at the end of surgery. A number of factors will need to be considered and corrected (**Table 60.3**) and, if not improved, the patient may need emergency imaging.

POSTOPERATIVE NEUROSURGICAL CARE IN THE PICU

The overall goal of postoperative neurosurgical care is to manage the patient with optimal management of physiology and pharmacology for the best expected outcome for the child's

underlying condition. In order to achieve these objectives, there must be clear documentation in the patient's medical record and good communication between all team members. All hospitals have their own *Policy and Procedures Manual* that covers the detail of what is expected of medical practitioners, and what is considered best care practices in preparing a child for a neurosurgical procedure. Clinical assessment, coma scale scores, neuromonitoring, mechanical ventilation, and head and spinal cord injury are covered elsewhere in this textbook.

Initial PICU Care

Patient Hand-Off

Table 60.4 outlines a checklist for the general neurosurgical admission to the PICU. After the operation, those caring for the child will also need information in a systematic manner. We use the *Formula One* hand-off technique (14). This idea addresses the limited time to transfer information and the necessary details need to be conveyed to the next team caring for the child. **Table 60.5** outlines a checklist for the postoperative transition of care. The neurosurgeon and anesthesiologist need to convey succinctly what happened in the operating room and what they want to happen in the immediate postoperative period. The postoperative attendants need to be cognizant of any concerns about bleeding, compromised tissue, derangements in homeostasis, and requirements for postoperative antibiotics, steroids, etc. We find that this process is best served by attending-to-attending sign-out. The critical care team examines every patient on arrival, documenting physiological stability, level of consciousness, and the presence or absence of focal neurological findings.

Mechanical Ventilation

Most cases requiring PICU care will not require mechanical ventilation (15). However, when prolonged mechanical ventilation is necessary, the aim is to support gas exchange while permitting ongoing neurosurgical assessment. End-tidal carbon dioxide monitoring helps prevent inadvertent hyper- or hypoventilation and positive end-expiratory pressure is delivered as necessary to support oxygenation (16,17). When inflation pressures are high, care is taken to avoid falls in mean BP and cerebral perfusion pressures (CPP, the difference between mean BP and mean ICP). High-frequency oscillatory ventilation may be used without significant impact on ICP (18). ICP monitoring may be necessary in cases in which the sedation needed to tolerate intubation and ventilation interferes with the ability to follow neurologic examination or in which the administration of PEEP may contribute to increasing ICP.

Hemodynamic and Fluid Management

In general, hemodynamic management targets BP within 20% of preoperative values or normal for age. When increased ICP is a consideration, CPP targets are those used in trauma (see Chapter 61).

Isotonic fluids are always used intraoperatively and should be continued in the immediate postoperative period. Since the neurosurgical population has increased risk of postoperative hyponatremia, as high as 12% (19), the dysnatremias will be discussed in some detail subsequently. Because of the risk of hyponatremia in the perioperative period, many clinicians choose to avoid using hypotonic solutions altogether. It should be noted that Ringer's Lactate sodium (130 mmol/L) might also result in a fall in serum sodium. This fluid is sometimes used intraoperatively as it is a balanced solution with a physiologic amount of base, calcium and potassium, and will limit the hyperchloremic acidosis that occurs with large volumes of normal saline.

TABLE 60.4

INFORMATION REQUIRED AT TIME OF NEUROSURGICAL ADMISSION TO THE PICU

■ ACTIVITY	■ DETAILS	■ ACTION
History	■ Presenting complaint ■ Previous medical history ■ Developmental level ■ Previous anesthetics ■ Medications ■ Allergies ■ Seizures	■ Documented
Examination	■ Central and peripheral nervous systems ■ Presence of raised ICP ■ Cardiopulmonary ■ General level of hydration	■ Documentation of neurologic deficits ■ May need preoperative resuscitation and treatment
Comorbidities	■ Intercurrent illness ■ Any cardiopulmonary disease ■ Any gastroesophageal reflux ■ Endocrinopathy	■ Discuss with anesthesiologist
Blood testing	■ Hemoglobin ■ Urea and electrolytes ■ Blood cross-matched	
Fasting period[a]	■ Solid food ■ Formula ■ Breast milk ■ Clear fluids	■ 6–8 h ■ 6 h ■ 4 h ■ 2 h
Preoperative anesthesia review		■ IV access ■ Premedication
Special preoperative interventions required	■ Cerebrovascular cases ■ Endocrine-risk cases	■ Intravascular euvolemia ■ Stress hormone and other HPA-axis assessment
Medications	■ All medications including route	■ Discussion of route of administration and whether they can be withheld
Seizure plan	■ Current AEDs, if any	■ Review with pediatric epilepsy/neurology AEDs

AEDs, antiepileptic drugs; HPA, hypothalamic–pituitary–adrenal.
[a]Varies by institution.

3 Postoperative Dysnatremia. Disorders of salt and water homeostasis are common in postoperative neurosurgical patients. The four main renal salt and water-handling problems that occur in such children are inappropriate intravenous fluid administration, euvolemic state of ADH excess (i.e., syndrome of inappropriate ADH [SIADH]), CSW, and diabetes insipidus (DI).

In the postoperative setting pain, stress, nausea, vomiting, narcotics, and volume depletion may all have the potential to stimulate vasopressin production and induce a state of euvolemic hyponatremia not dissimilar to SIADH. However, it is also clear that hypotonic fluid administration or fluid restriction may also result in hyponatremia (serum sodium concentration <135 mmol/L). The few trials of intravenous fluid administration in postoperative neurosurgical patients in the PICU indicate that urine tonicity is almost always fixed in the postoperative period (i.e., children receiving normal saline at maintenance rate have a urine tonicity of ~200 mOsm/L, while those receiving any other prescription have lower urine tonicity of ~160 mOsm/L) and urine output is constant at ~1 mL/kg/h (20–23). What this indicates is that isotonic fluids prevent postoperative falls in serum sodium concentration and that hypotonic fluids may result in falls in serum sodium concentration because of renal desalination. In none of these studies was fluid overload or significant hypernatremia a complication.

Also, before embarking on detailed analysis of salt and water balance, when an abnormally low serum sodium level is received from the laboratory an assessment of salt losses should be made (e.g., via CSF drainage). Consideration as to whether the cause of hyponatremia is pseudohyponatremia due to the use of perioperative radiologic nonionic hyperosmolar contrast medium should be made.

Syndrome of Inappropriate ADH Secretion

Postoperative hyponatremia, euvolemia, and ADH excess define the SIADH. As a screening approach we often use the following parameters: serum sodium concentration <135 mmol/L, minimal or normal urine output <2 mL/kg/h, variable urinary sodium concentration (spot urine sodium >20 mmol/L), and variable urine osmolarity. Therefore, monitoring of intravascular volume, urine output and tonicity, and serum electrolytes is needed during the period of intravenous fluid administration. The other causes of hyponatremia that need to be excluded are volume depletion, edematous states (congestive heart failure, cirrhosis, and nephrosis), renal dysfunction, adrenal insufficiency, and hypothyroidism. If the cause is perioperative SIADH, it has occurred because of free water retention at the same time as natriuresis that maintains fluid balance at the expense of serum osmolality. The ADH excess leads to increased water permeability in the collecting duct, water

TABLE 60.5

"FORMULA ONE" SIGN-OUT TECHNIQUE FOR POSTOPERATIVE HAND-OFF

■ ITEM	■ DETAILS
Operation	■ Procedure ■ Complicated or uncomplicated ■ Concerns ■ Wound drains ■ External ventricular drain (e.g., where and what head-of-pressure being used
Anesthesia	■ Premedication used ■ Laryngoscopy and whether the airway is difficult ■ Anesthesia ■ Emergence ■ Postoperative pain management ■ Whether sedation is required (e.g., neurovascular child needing dexmedetomidine for deep sedation to prevent early postoperative agitation, crying, and hypocapnia)
Intraoperative fluids	■ Intravenous fluids used ■ Estimated blood loss and use of blood products; final hematocrit ■ Urine output ■ Any intraoperative laboratory tests
Surgical plan	■ Head-of-bed positioning required ■ Blood pressure targets ■ Perioperative antibiotics ■ Use of antiemetics and steroids ■ Laboratory tests ■ In those who return with an endotracheal tube in situ, the plan for extubation ■ Frequency of neurologic observations and special instructions on signs to watch for ■ Seizure plan ■ Postoperative imaging plan ■ What has been discussed with the family ■ Any other consultants required (e.g., infectious disease, neuro-oncology)
Postoperative fluids	■ Volume required (maintenance or more) ■ Serum sodium target ■ Strategy for cerebral edema, if required
Organ system review	■ Detailed presentation of preoperative neurologic abnormalities or significant findings ■ Presentation of postprocedure neurologic findings or changes from preoperative neurologic evaluation ■ Special concerns, particularly in regard to comorbidities and when other therapies are required (e.g., asthma treatment) ■ When feeding can be restarted

retention, and subclinical volume expansion, with an increase in total body water of 7%–10%. Volume expansion also triggers hemodynamic regulatory mechanisms to maintain plasma volume at the expense of sodium, which is in part due to a pressure natriuresis and a secondary release of natriuretic peptides.

The treatment of SIADH is to reduce free water excess by fluid restriction and diuretics. If a hyponatremic seizure occurs, then hypertonic saline should be used to correct serum sodium to a target of ≥130 mmol/L, which often provides seizure control. Taking 0.6 L/kg as the apparent volume of distribution for sodium, one should anticipate an increase of 3–5 mmol/L in serum sodium concentration with a rapid intravenous bolus of 4–6 mL/kg of 3% saline.

Cerebral Salt Wasting

CSW is a diagnosis of exclusion on the basis of clinical criteria and it is overdiagnosed. The essential features of the syndrome are renal sodium and chloride wasting in a patient with a *contracted effective arterial blood volume*, where other causes of excess sodium excretion have been excluded. Volume contraction is likely to be present when there is a deficit of sodium that exceeds 2 mmol/kg. Hyponatremia is a nonspecific clue. Patients with SIADH also present with hyponatremia, but exhibit *mild hypervolemia*.

The literature suggests that this condition is common in children after all types of neurosurgical procedures and that it results from excessively high atrial or brain natriuretic peptide levels. **Table 60.6** lists some of the diagnoses that should be excluded before concluding that the patient has CSW. (It should be noted that the atrial natriuretic peptide level is high in cerebrovascular patients who have received perioperative hypervolemic fluid management, and natriuresis is a response to volume control as part of homeostasis, and not CSW.)

The incidence of CSW is on the order of 1%–5% of neurosurgical procedures (24), and it has been reported in association with calvarial remodeling, tumor resection, and hydrocephalus. Parameter used for screening approach, when concerned about possible CSW, is hyponatremia (<135 mmol/L) with brisk diuresis (>3 mL/kg/h), elevated urine sodium (>120 mmol/L) when available, or elevated urinary osmolarity (>300 mOsm/L water). The physiology involves inappropriate and excessive release of natriuretic peptides that leads to a primary natriuresis and volume depletion. A secondary hormonal response occurs with an increase in the renin–angiotensin system and arginine vasopressin production. The median onset of CSW is on postoperative day 3, lasting a median of 3 days. In contrast to hyponatremia due to SIADH, the fractional excretion of urate is elevated but *does not* improve when hyponatremia is corrected. Patients with CSW are more

TABLE 60.6

DIFFERENTIAL DIAGNOSIS OF SALT WASTING

- Physiologic extracellular fluid volume expansion (e.g., hyperhydration with 1.5 times maintenance followed by abrupt decreases in intake)
- Diuretics
- Hypoaldosteronism (Note: aldosterone stimulates sodium reabsorption.)
- Adrenocortical insufficiency
- Renal tubular disorders (including congenital salt-losing disorders—Bartter or Gitelman syndrome)
- Presence of an inhibitor of renal reabsorption of sodium such as osmotic agents, high concentration of ligands for the calcium receptor in the loop of Henle (e.g., hypercalcemia, gentamicin)
- Obligatory excretion of sodium by the excretion of anions other than chloride
- High-output renal failure (renal tubular damage such as obstructive uropathy, interstitial nephritis, and acute tubular necrosis)
- Sodium wasting from cerebrospinal fluid drainage
- Pressure natriuresis from adrenergic agents
- Downregulation of renal sodium transport by chronic hypervolemia

likely to have suffered postoperative stroke, have chiasmatic or hypothalamic tumors, or are younger than patients with normal postoperative sodium concentration. Almost half of the patients with CSW have postoperative hyponatremic seizures (serum sodium <130 mmol/L). The treatment of CSW involves sodium administration to match urinary losses and correction of intravascular volume contraction. In some instances, more rapid resolution of hyponatremia after volume expansion has been achieved with fludrocortisone.

Diabetes Insipidus

DI results from a deficiency of vasopressin and it is an expected complication of surgical procedures near the pituitary or hypothalamus. It is most frequently seen in association with craniopharyngioma, where it can be a presenting symptom in 40% of cases. In most patients, DI is transient, but ~6% develop permanent DI. The diagnosis should be suspected when serum sodium rises above 145 mmol/L in association with urine output above 2.5 mL/kg/h for 3 consecutive hours, or more than 4 mL/kg/h in any 1 hour. The urine osmolality should be hypotonic (<300 mOsm/L) in the face of increased plasma osmolality (>300 mOsm/L), in the absence of glycosuria, mannitol use, and renal failure. An important consequence of this condition is severe dehydration and hypovolemia since urine output is driven by lack of vasopressin.

Knowledge of the patterns of DI that can occur following surgery in the hypothalamic–pituitary area is important. The most common pattern is associated with local edema as a result of traction or manipulation of the pituitary stalk. This lesion usually results in transient polyuria that begins 2–6 hours after surgery and resolves as edema diminishes in 1–7 days. A "triphasic pattern" has also been described (25–27). Transection of the pituitary stalk or destruction of the hypothalamic median eminence will result in permanent DI. Frequently, permanent DI, either partial or complete, develops without interphase changes.

There are a variety of successful approaches to treating DI. It is useful to have a neuroendocrine assessment preoperatively, with a perioperative care plan, since deficiencies of thyroid and/or adrenocortical hormones can coexist. In the child with known DI, preoperatively, some endocrinologists prefer not to replace vasopressin and to restrict total fluid intake to approximately twice-normal maintenance (scaling to body surface area rather than weight, i.e., 3 L/m^2/d), recognizing that this can result in mild hypernatremia and thirst but minimizing the more dangerous risk of water intoxication with vasopressin administration. Others prefer to withhold long-acting 1-desamino-8-d-arginine vasopressin (DDAVP, desmopressin acetate, the synthetic analogue of ADH) in the perioperative period and instead manage DI with intermittent injections of intramuscular (or continuous infusions of intravenous) vasopressin. Administration of excessive fluids in this setting, as with the perioperative maintenance of DDAVP, can result in hyponatremic seizures.

When new-onset, postoperative DI is recognized, the following strategy should lead to serum sodium concentrations between 130 and 150 mmol/L (28). These patients respond to an infusion of aqueous vasopressin (20 Units/500 mL). Aqueous vasopressin is used because of its rapid onset of action and brief duration of effect. However, its potential vascular effect (i.e., hypertension) means that close observation in a monitored setting is required. The infusion is started at 0.5 mUnits/kg/h and titrated upward in 0.5 mUnits/kg/h increments every 5–10 minutes until urine output decreases to less than 2 mL/kg/h. It is rare to require more than 10 mUnits/kg/h. Once urine output is less than 2 mL/kg/h, the vasopressin infusion is not adjusted downward. Neither is fluid administration adjusted according to urine output. Antidiuresis with vasopressin is essentially an "all-or-none" phenomenon and the aqueous infusion is being used to produce a "functional SIADH" state. This strategy recognizes that renal blood flow remains normal in the normovolemic, but maximally antidiuresed, child. Because urine output is then minimal (0.5 mL/kg/h), other clinical markers of volume status must be followed closely. For example, anuria together with increased heart rate or decreased BP may be evidence of hypovolemia. Vasopressin infusion does not induce acute tubular necrosis, and severe oliguria or anuria is an indication for additional fluid and not for decreasing or discontinuing the infusion. When using vasopressin infusion, fluids should be carefully restricted because in the presence of full antidiuresis, excessive fluids (oral or intravenous) can lead to intravascular volume overload. In addition, administration of hypotonic fluids (oral or intravenous) can result in dangerous hyponatremia. Restricting fluids to replacement of insensible losses, which is generally considered to be about two-thirds usual maintenance rates, may prevent this complication.

In children at risk for developing permanent DI, in whom adequate oral intake has been established, intravenous fluids and the vasopressin infusion can be discontinued while permitting free oral intake. Subsequent treatment of DI is withheld until the child demonstrates polyuria. At that time, treatment with DDAVP rather than restarting a vasopressin infusion is recommended. DDAVP is a synthetic vasopressin with duration of action of 12–24 hours. It is usually administered intranasally at a dose of 5–10 μg. Oral DDAVP can be used at 10–20 times the nasal dose. Antidiuresis generally begins within 1 hour. In children with known DI, DDAVP treatment can be resumed once an intact thirst mechanism has returned and oral intake without vomiting.

Analgesia and Sedation

Pain control and sedation present unique challenges in the postoperative neurosurgical patient needing mechanical ventilation. They need to be comfortable, awake, and cooperative with their care. While the ideal sedation regime would include short-acting or reversible agents that can be withdrawn intermittently to permit neurologic assessment, a single agent suitable for children has yet to be developed. Some agents suitable for adults are unsuitable in children and some agents used widely in pediatrics are less useful in adults.

For example, propofol is a potent, ultra-short-acting, sedative–hypnotic that is extremely useful in adult neurocritical care but has only limited utility in pediatrics. This is because of its association with a fatal syndrome of bradycardia, rhabdomyolysis, metabolic acidosis, and multiple organ failure when infused over extended periods in children (29,30). While the mechanism remains unclear, it appears related to both the duration of therapy and the cumulative dose. These difficulties are much less common in adults. While some centers have advocated pediatric use under strict controls, propofol is generally limited to operative anesthesia, procedural sedation, and continuous infusions of limited duration.

Dexmedetomidine, an α-2 agonist, offers many of the advantages of propofol as an ultra-short-acting, single-agent, postoperative sedative. Unlike propofol, apnea is not a problem and spontaneous breathing is maintained. In children, the drug appears to be safe and its population pharmacokinetics are similar to adults (31). Cross-tolerance with other sedatives can make it a useful agent for treatment of opioid or benzodiazepine withdrawal (32,33). Because dexmedetomidine is both an α-2a and α-2b agonist, its central effects cause sympatholysis while its peripheral effects cause vasoconstriction. As a result, transient increases in BP can be seen with boluses followed by hypotension and bradycardia as sedation deepens. In our experience, both hypo- and hypertension can occasionally be observed with long-term infusions, and a withdrawal syndrome results when extended infusions are discontinued. Hence, by far, the mainstay of sedation in the PICU remains a combination of opioid and benzodiazepine administered via continuous infusion. Titration to a validated sedation score is advised and regular "drug holidays" help insure that excessive sedation is avoided. If neuromuscular blocking agents must be used to control ICP or facilitate mechanical ventilation, use of a neuromuscular blockade monitor helps avoid prolonged blockade and weakness. Infants and children receiving sedative infusion for more than 3–5 days are subject to tolerance and experience symptoms of withdrawal when infusions are discontinued.

❹ SURGERY-SPECIFIC PICU MANAGEMENT

Brain Tumors

Brain tumors are the most common solid tumors in children, exceeded only by the leukemias as the most common pediatric malignancy. There are 1500–2000 new brain tumors diagnosed annually in children in the United States. The majority of brain tumors in children are infratentorial, in the posterior fossa; thus, obstruction of CSF flow occurs frequently with increased ICP occurring early. Symptoms include early morning vomiting and irritability or lethargy. Cranial nerve palsies and ataxia are common early findings, with respiratory and cardiac irregularities usually occurring late.

Perioperative seizures are a significant problem. Hardesty et al. (34) recently reviewed all patients between 0 and 19 years of age without prior seizures who underwent intracranial tumor resection at their institution over a 5-year period. About 7.4% of 223 patients experienced at least one clinical seizure during the surgical admission, yet only ~4% of patients received prophylactic anticonvulsants. Independent factors associated with perioperative seizures included supratentorial tumor, age <2 years, and hyponatremia due to SIADH or CSW. Tumor type, lobe affected, operative blood loss, and length of surgery were not independently associated

with seizure incidence. Because of the low incidence of seizures in this series in patients more than 2 years old with normal serum sodium, the authors recommended that pediatric patients with brain tumors did not routinely receive perioperative prophylactic anticonvulsants. However, the role for prophylaxis in patients younger than 2 years of age deserves further study.

Posterior Fossa Surgery

Childhood tumors of the posterior fossa will frequently present with increased ICP and supratentorial symptoms due to hydrocephalus secondary to aqueductal obstruction. Posterior fossa surgery deserves special consideration since it involves a high density of critical structures within a relatively small space. Procedures are conducted in the prone or sitting position, the latter carrying increased risk of venous air embolism. Postoperative bleeding or edema can rapidly bring severe consequences, including apnea, hypertension, bradycardia, and death. Associated cranial nerve injury may bring hoarseness, stridor, and loss of protective airway reflexes. On occasion, delayed awakening is the first sign of ongoing brainstem injury. In all cases, outcome depends on swift recognition and management of postoperative complications.

Tumors of the posterior fossa may be approached via suboccipital craniotomy, and Chiari decompression may consist of craniectomy with or without laminectomy. In most cases, blood loss is modest. At the conclusion of surgery, the goal is to awaken, extubate, and assess the patient before leaving the operating room. Because of the potential for sudden deterioration, admission to the PICU is essential. Initial evaluation after hand-off includes a careful neurologic examination and baseline laboratory studies. Complications of posterior fossa surgery include mutism, oculomotor palsies, hearing loss, ataxia, and hemiparesis. Vomiting is very common and hydrocephalus or CSF leak can also occur. The *posterior fossa syndrome* consists of a wide range of symptoms including aphasia, mutism, dysphagia, weaknesses, oculomotor palsies, and neurobehavioral abnormalities. Symptoms may appear hours or days (typically 24 hours to 4 days) after surgery and be of unpredictable duration. Although most symptoms are transient, long-term cognitive sequelae have been documented (35). Posterior fossa syndrome is more commonly described in children but is also seen in adults (36).

Hydrocephalus

Eighty percent of CSF is produced in the choroid plexus of the lateral and fourth ventricles. The remainder is produced in the interstitial space and ependymal lining. In the adult, normal CSF volume is 150 mL (50% intracranial and the rest intraspinal). In the neonates, CSF volume is 50 mL. The rate of CSF production across all ages is 0.15–0.30 mL/min (up to ~450 mL/d). There are two pathways for CSF circulation: a major, *adult*, pathway with CSF absorption through arachnoid villi (arachnoid granulation) into the venous sinuses; and a minor, *infantile*, pathway with CSF drainage through the ventricular ependyma, the interstitial and perivascular space, and perineural lymphatics.

Hydrocephalus reflects a mismatch of CSF production and absorption, resulting in an increased intracranial CSF volume. It can be caused by a variety of pathologic processes, including arachnoid cysts. Except for rare instances of excess CSF production, such as in choroid plexus papillomas, the majority of cases of hydrocephalus are secondary to some type of obstruction or inability to absorb CSF appropriately. Commonly, this is a result of hemorrhage (neonatal intraventricular or subarachnoid), congenital problems (aqueductal stenosis), trauma, infection, or tumors (especially in the posterior fossa).

Hydrocephalus can be classified as nonobstructive/communicating or obstructive/noncommunicating based on the ability of CSF to flow around the spinal cord in its usual manner.

Although "balanced" hydrocephalus can occur whereby ventricular dilation may be static and asymptomatic, intracranial hypertension or a decrease in intracranial compliance almost always accompanies untreated hydrocephalus in children. The rapidity with which hydrocephalus develops and the remaining degree of intracranial compliance determine the severity of symptoms. In the young infant, if hydrocephalus develops slowly, the skull will expand and the cerebral cortical mantle will stretch until massive craniomegaly (often with irreversible neurologic damage) occurs. However, if the cranial bones are fused or the cranium cannot expand fast enough, neurologic signs and symptoms appear quickly. In these cases, the child may become progressively more lethargic and develop vomiting, cranial nerve dysfunction ("setting sun" sign), bradycardia, and, ultimately, brain herniation and death.

The perioperative plan in a child with hydrocephalus should be directed at controlling ICP and relieving the obstruction as soon as possible. In the presence of increased ICP, children are at risk for emesis and pulmonary aspiration and usually require rapid-sequence intubation. The use of ketamine as an induction agent has been thought to exacerbate intracranial hypertension, but growing evidence indicates that it may actually offer some relief of elevated ICP (4,5). Although an intravenous, rapid-sequence induction is usually preferred, this must be balanced against other risks and benefits (acute ICP rise with stress, difficult venous access, etc.). Intraoperatively, the possibility of venous air embolism during placement of the distal end of a ventriculoatrial shunt should always be kept in mind. Postoperatively, children should be observed carefully to confirm that CSF diversion has been successful and symptoms do not recur. Since anesthesia and peritoneal incisions decrease gut motility, children may be at risk for ileus, vomiting, and pulmonary aspiration until bowel sounds return.

Children who develop a shunt infection usually have their entire system removed and external ventricular drainage established. They then return to the operating room for insertion of a new shunt after infection has resolved. While an external drain is in place, care must be taken to not dislodge the ventricular tubing. In addition, the height of the drainage bag should not be significantly changed in relation to the child's head to avoid sudden alterations in ICP. For example, suddenly lowering an open drainage bag can siphon CSF rapidly from the head, resulting in collapse of the ventricles and rupture of cortical veins. When transporting children with CSF drainage, or when moving them from a stretcher to the CT scanner, it is often best to close off the ventriculostomy tubing during these brief periods.

Slit Ventricle Syndrome

Intensivists should be aware of a condition known as slit ventricle syndrome (SVS) (37). First described in 1982 as consisting of headache, small ventricles, and slow refill of pumping chambers in shunted children (38), SVS has an incidence of ~5% and is one of the most important long-term complications in patients with ventriculoperitoneal shunts. Although many hypotheses have been offered (39), it appears to result from chronic CSF overdrainage, low CSF volume, and diminished compensation for acute alterations in brain or cerebrovascular volumes. Preoperatively and postoperatively, special attention should be paid to patients in whom CT scans indicate the presence of this condition. In particular, it is important to avoid the administration of excess or hypotonic fluids and minimize any potential for brain swelling. Some of these children appear unable to accommodate to situations that otherwise healthy children would easily tolerate. Episodes of

postoperative cerebral herniation have been reported after uneventful surgical procedures.

Cerebrovascular Surgery

Vascular anomalies are uncommon in childhood but usually present early in life. When large, complex malformations are discovered, they require careful planning and, often, multimodal therapy for resolution. It is not uncommon for a child to require multiple procedures to isolate and devascularize a single lesion. Seizure, stroke, hemorrhage, and cerebral edema are the primary perioperative concerns. The corresponding PICU goals are straightforward (euvolemia, normocapnea, normotension, prompt seizure control, and maintenance of the neurological examination) but can be extremely challenging in small children.

Arteriovenous Malformations

Arteriovenous malformations (AVMs) are the most common cause of spontaneous intracerebral hemorrhage in children. These lesions are primarily congenital, arising during vasculogenesis in the third week of gestation. Though usually isolated and sporadic, familial cases can exist as in hereditary hemorrhagic telangiectasia (HHT or Osler–Weber–Rendu disease). AVMs consist of arterial feeding vessels, dilated communicating vessels, and draining veins carrying arterialized blood. Large malformations, especially those involving the posterior cerebral artery and vein of Galen, may present with congestive heart failure (high-output heart failure, often with pulmonary hypertension) in the neonatal period.

As vascular shunting grows, blood follows the path of least resistance and cerebrovascular territories served by feeder vessels become ischemic. This vascular steal brings local vasodilation that, over time, becomes fixed. As a consequence, areas surrounding high-flow lesions may become pressure-passive and subject to severe postoperative hyperemia, edema, and hemorrhage. At the same time, obstruction of venous outflow may occur during surgery and small feeder vessels may be disrupted. Taken together, these mechanisms may precipitate a phenomenon termed "normal perfusion pressure breakthrough" that carries severe consequences, including massive brain swelling, brainstem herniation, and death (40–42). Treatment is controversial but generally involves therapy for increased ICP (diuretics, moderate hyperventilation, 30 degrees head-of-bed elevation) in addition to judicious use of moderate hypotension (while maintaining CPP) and moderate hypothermia. It remains to be determined whether staged reduction offers any advantage in this regard.

Malformations not large enough to produce congestive heart failure usually remain clinically silent unless they cause seizures or stroke. Overall, intracranial hemorrhage is the most common presentation in children, with an associated mortality of up to 25% (43). Subarachnoid or intracerebral hemorrhage usually results from acute rupture of a communicating vessel. After hemorrhage, seizure is the second most common presentation of AVMs. Other, less common, presentations include macrocephaly, headaches, and altered mental status. Occasionally, presentation relates to mass effect as in vein of Galen dilation manifesting as hydrocephalus secondary to obstruction of the aqueduct of Sylvius. Increasingly, AVMs are discovered as incidental findings or even on prenatal ultrasound.

Nonemergent intervention often involves multimodal therapy beginning with an endovascular neuroradiological approach. Embolization may offer either definitive treatment or substantial flow reduction before surgery or radiotherapy. Platinum coils and/or ethylene–vinyl alcohol copolymer can serve as embolic agents once the malformation is accessed. A percutaneous transfemoral approach is most common, with the child anesthetized and heparinized for the procedure. Angiographic localization and endovascular navigation may require high contrast loads and long operative times. Care should be taken to limit contrast dose (<7 mL/kg, see above section on *Dysnatremia*) and copolymer vehicle (dimethyl sulfoxide). Intraoperative complications include perforation, hemorrhage, vessel dissection, unintentional occlusion, and cerebrovascular end-artery "territorial" infarction. Tight BP control and heparinization is usually continued in the PICU for a minimum of 24 hours postoperatively and low-molecular-weight heparin is maintained thereafter. In our institution, complex high-flow lesions are usually treated with staged embolization, leaving 6 weeks between procedures (44,45).

Emergency evaluation usually begins with a noncontrast CT identifying the presence and location of hemorrhage, followed by MR imaging and angiography. Treatment may consist of embolization or stereotactic radiation for deep malformations, surgical excision of superficial ones, or a combination of modalities. For endovascular procedures, mild hyperventilation may actually enhance visualization of abnormal blood vessels that do not respond with vasoconstriction. Anticonvulsant therapy is routine and neonates in cardiac failure may require inotropic agents. Because these children may be critically ill following their acute event, all of the aforementioned risks are magnified. Bleeding, including that from the femoral arterial puncture site, is an even greater concern. Visualization may be difficult and large amounts of contrast may be used. Fluid overload and renal injury are significant concerns, especially in a young infant who may already be in high-output cardiac failure. In some centers, stereotactic radiosurgery is favored because of its low morbidity and mortality. However, this must be weighed against an obliteration delay of 2–3 years, an annual re-hemorrhage rate of 6% and success rates that are highly variable due to differing treatment protocols (46).

Aneurysms

Intracranial aneurysms among children can be traumatic, infectious, or most often of unknown etiology (likely due to congenital malformations of an arterial wall) (47). Children with coarctation of the aorta, polycystic kidney disease, fibromuscular dysplasia, Ehlers–Danlos syndrome, or systemic vasculopathy have an increased incidence. Aneurysms usually remain asymptomatic during childhood, but the ruptures that do occur in childhood are frequently lethal. Symptoms of subarachnoid or intracerebral hemorrhage appear suddenly, usually with intense headache, neurological deficit, or unconsciousness in a previously healthy child. Occasionally aneurysms may present with symptoms related to ischemia within the distribution of the parent vessel or giant lesions may present with symptoms of mass effect. Seizure and hydrocephalus have also been reported (48). Surgical ligation or clipping has historically been the treatment of choice, but recent trends have been more toward endovascular therapy (49).

Anatomic diagnosis presents many challenges, especially if imaging is recently preceded by subarachnoid hemorrhage and vasospasm. As general rules, saccular aneurysms occur at vessel bifurcation points and fusiform dissecting aneurysms are found in posterior circulations. Once a lesion is identified, both open surgical and endovascular approaches may exclude it from the circulation while preserving the parent vessel. Preoperative preparations include arterial access for continuous monitoring, central venous access for administration of vasoactive agents, and blood available in the room should emergent transfusion be required.

Intraoperatively, a brief period of controlled hypotension has been used in order to reduce vessel wall tension and the risk of surgical manipulation. It is not clear, however, that the potential benefits of controlled hypotension outweigh its risks, particularly in small children. Certainly, controlled hypotension should not be used in the presence of increased ICP when support of CPP is critical. Although the absolute limits of acceptable hypotension are unknown, a mean BP greater than 40 mm Hg (for infants) and 50 mm Hg (for older children) generally appears safe while teenagers should have a target mean BP no lower than 55 mm Hg. At the conclusion of the procedure, BP is returned to normal and the operative site is carefully inspected for bleeding before dural closure. Hemodynamic stability is then maintained during emergence and bucking, coughing, or straining is avoided prior to extubation. Although excessive hypertension can result in postoperative bleeding, a slightly increased BP may be desirable to minimize the risk of vasospasm. When surgery is completed, it is particularly important that children are able to cooperate with a neurologic examination and that there is careful control of BP in the PICU. This is most easily accomplished with light sedation, reduction of external stimuli, and titration of mild antihypertensives such as labetalol.

In patients with severe subarachnoid hemorrhage and vasospasm, treatment is controversial (50,51). Historically, many adult centers have considered hemodynamic augmentation therapy to be the mainstay of treatment (the so-called "Triple-H" or "Hyper" approach of hemodilution, hypervolemia, and induced hypertension with catecholamines used to produce a hyperdynamic circulation). Evidence-based consensus recommendations, however, now call for nimodipine (Class I recommendation, Level A evidence), euvolemia (Class I, Level B), induced hypertension (Class I, Level B), transcranial Doppler monitoring for vasospasm (Class IIa, Level B), advanced imaging to detect delayed cerebral ischemia (Class IIa, Level B), and cerebral angioplasty or intra-arterial vasodilators for symptomatic vasospasm (Class IIa, Level B) (52–54). To what extent any or all of these recommendations are transferable to pediatrics is unclear.

Moyamoya Disease

Moyamoya disease is a steno-occlusive disease that results in progressive and life-threatening obstruction of intracranial vessels, primarily the internal carotid arteries near the circle of Willis (55). A dense vascular network of tiny collaterals subsequently develops at the base of the brain giving rise to the Japanese name (translated roughly as "puff of smoke") associated with the angiographic appearance of this condition. In its congenital form, the dysplastic process may also involve systemic (especially renal) arteries. The acquired variety may be associated with meningitis, neurofibromatosis, chronic inflammation, connective tissue diseases, certain hematologic disorders, Down syndrome, or prior intracranial radiation. Some patients with sickle-cell disease, even in the absence of neurologic symptoms, may also have moyamoya (56). For reasons that are unknown, this disease appears to be more common in children of Japanese ancestry. Associated intracranial aneurysms are rare in children but may occur in more than 10% of affected adult patients. Abnormal electrocardiographic findings have also been described in adults with this syndrome. In children, moyamoya disease usually manifests as transient ischemic attacks progressing to strokes and fixed neurologic deficits. The attacks may begin in infancy (57) and can be precipitated by crying with hyperventilation (58). There is a high morbidity and mortality rate if the condition is left untreated.

Medical management consists of antiplatelet therapy (such as aspirin) or calcium channel blockers. Surgical interventions aim to restore blood flow by bypassing obstructions or stimulating angiogenesis. In adults, extracranial to intracranial vascular bypass procedures, usually with anastomosis of the superficial temporal and middle cerebral arteries, are common (59). In children, the most common surgical intervention is pial synangiosis, wherein a scalp artery (usually the superficial temporal artery) is sutured directly onto the pial surface of the brain to enhance growth of new vessels into the brain and remove obstruction to growth by the arachnoid layer (55). Because neovascularization requires months, post-operative stroke remains a high concern.

Careful and continuous monitoring of end-tidal carbon dioxide is essential to anesthetic management because children with moyamoya disease have decreased hemispheric blood flow bilaterally. Inadvertent hyperventilation can be catastrophic, critically reducing regional CBF to cause significant electroencephalographic (EEG) and neurologic changes (60). It is crucial, therefore, that normocapnia be maintained throughout all phases of the procedure, including induction and emergence phases of anesthesia. Adequate hydration and maintenance of baseline BP are also extremely important. To avoid dehydration during the perioperative period, we elect to insert an intravenous catheter the night before surgery and provide 1.5 times maintenance fluids until surgery (see section on *Dysnatremia*). Normothermia must also be maintained, particularly at the end of the procedure, to avoid postoperative shivering and an exaggerated stress response. There may also be some benefit in EEG monitoring to detect and potentially guide treatment of ischemia resulting from the cerebral vasoconstriction that can accompany direct surgical manipulation (60). As with most neurosurgical procedures, a smooth extubation without hypertension or crying is desirable.

Although very little literature exists regarding intraoperative and postoperative complications during moyamoya surgery, it appears that most complications (strokes) occur postoperatively and are associated with dehydration and crying (hyperventilation) episodes. PICU care must therefore strive to minimize extremes of BP and maintain hydration while providing sufficient analgesia and sedation to prevent crying with hyperventilation. Treatment of nausea and prevention of vomiting is also important. In addition, some centers elect to quickly restart antiplatelet therapy (61) and to begin or continue calcium channel blockers.

Epilepsy Surgery

Epilepsy is one of the most common neurologic disorders of childhood. It is estimated that 30% of children continue to have seizures after starting medication. Despite the development of new drugs and regimens, polypharmacy is common, side effects frequently limit drug use, and the prevalence of pharmacologically intractable seizures remains high (62). Fortunately, advances in neuroimaging and EEG monitoring now provide epileptologists with anatomic targets from which seizures originate. Modern pediatric neurosurgery has exploited these technologies and dramatically improved the outcome in infants and children.

Children presenting for surgical management of seizures usually do so after chronically receiving anticonvulsants. These agents often carry significant side effects and multiple agents are often used to reduce the untoward effects of any single drug. Some antiepileptics, like topiramate and zonisamide, induce a metabolic acidosis that varies from patient to patient and can be significant (63). Others, like felbamate and carbamazepine, can cause bone marrow suppression with anemia or thrombocytopenia. Valproic acid is well known to affect hepatic function and can occasionally cause pancreatitis. Specific anticonvulsant concentrations should be determined preoperatively to detect subtherapeutic or toxic concentrations. It is also worth noting that many anticonvulsants enhance metabolism of nondepolarizing neuromuscular blocking drugs and opioids, thereby leading to an increase (up to 50%) in the amount of these drugs needed during a surgical procedure.

Postoperative care in this population (hemispherectomy— partial or functional; seizure focus excision or isolation) focuses on limiting the risks of intracranial fluid shifts and seizures.

Craniosynostosis and Craniofacial Surgery

Craniosynostosis, the premature fusion of one or more cranial sutures, results in cranial deformities that carry both cosmetic and physiological consequences. These deformities may be syndromic or non-syndromic in nature and can frequently involve elevated ICP, obstructive sleep apnea (OSA), malocclusion, and neurobehavioral impairment. Premature closure of the sagittal sutures results in anterior–posterior elongation of the skull referred to as scaphocephaly or dolichocephaly. Closure of the metopic suture fixes forehead growth, resulting in a triangular pattern or trigonocephaly. Fusion of a single coronal suture skews skull growth anteriorly or posteriorly to produce plagiocephaly while fusion of both results in foreshortening of the skull or brachycephaly. Taken together, these anomalies are relatively common, affecting approximately 1 in 2000 live births.

To avoid physiological consequences and optimize aesthetic results, repair of craniosynostosis is best undertaken as early in life as possible. Up to about 6 months of age, endoscopic strip craniectomy with subsequent helmet modeling offers a minimally invasive solution for children with uncomplicated anomalies. Routinely, strip craniectomy involves only minimal blood loss, few complications, and a brief hospital stay. Beyond infancy, however, or when larger, more complex craniofacial reconstructive procedures are required, there are numerous challenges that necessitate postoperative PICU care. In looking after these patients, the intensivist must have an appreciation both for the magnitude of the procedure at hand and for its associated complications. Clinical practice guidelines for management of craniosynostosis have been proposed (64) that outline five major categories of perioperative concern:

- Airway management,
- Management of associated defects,
- Intraoperative monitoring,
- Fluid and blood product management, and
- Postoperative care.

Among children with syndromic craniosynostosis, approximately half present with OSA, and for many of these, progressive airway obstruction is the primary indication for surgery. Patients with Apert, Pfeiffer, Crouzon, and related syndromes can present challenges for intubation, with some requiring tracheostomy to see them safely through surgery. In many cases, even mask ventilation can be difficult due to associated facial anomalies. While a full discussion of difficult airway management is beyond the scope of this chapter, the intensivist must remain ever mindful of the airway, particularly when considering the timing of endotracheal tube extubation. In our institution, return to the operating room for a trial of extubation under controlled conditions is common among postoperative patients with difficult airways. We also institute a "Critical Airway" policy within the PICU.

In contrast to endoscopic strip craniectomy, blood loss during craniofacial reconstruction and remodeling procedures can be significant. Depending upon the nature of the procedure, scalp incision, bone flap elevation, and continuous oozing may combine to produce losses totaling 50%–100% (or more) of the circulating blood volume. In addition, massive blood loss and cardiac arrest have been reported to occur over just a few minutes, even without inadvertent sagittal sinus entry. The potential for this catastrophic complication mandates secure venous access (two large bore IVs at minimum), arterial access, and blood products available in the operating room prior to incision. Many anesthesiologists may also elect to secure central access and others will begin transfusing as soon as the incision is made.

Because the operative site involves noncollapsible veins positioned above the level of the heart, there is increased risk for venous air embolism during cranial remodeling. Precordial ultrasound is a sensitive monitor for this (Grade I: microbubbles detected by precordial Doppler or transesophageal echocardiography), followed by falls in end-tidal nitrogen or carbon dioxide (Grade II), and ultimately by arterial BP decline (Grade III). Early detection alerts the surgeon to flood the field and the anesthesiologist to immediately place the patient in Trendelenburg (head-down) position. Aspiration of air via an in situ central venous line confirms massive embolism, but the benefit of this in resuscitation is unclear. Standard resuscitation involves vasopressors, volume, and repositioning.

Blood Loss

Brisk blood loss and associated coagulopathy have fueled a variety of blood conservation strategies. Preoperative erythropoietin, cell saver, and anti-fibrinolytics have all been employed with different degrees of success (65,66).

When blood loss reaches 50%–75% of the preoperative blood volume (or 40–60 mL/kg), some derangement in coagulation is likely. At this level, serum prothrombin and partial thromboplastin times are obtained and fresh frozen plasma given if necessary. The derangements in the balance between coagulation and anticoagulation may be complex (e.g., hypercoagulability, which may be related to hemodilution versus coagulopathy, due to factor depletion as hemorrhage approaches 100% of blood volume) and advice from the blood bank and transfusion service is often required. Each hospital should have a *Massive Transfusion Protocol* and for certain procedures blood loss should be anticipated and a special protocol used. This strategy may include anticipatory use of tranexamic acid, fresh frozen plasma, platelets, cryoprecipitate, and calcium gluconate. Tranexamic acid offers the benefit of decreasing ongoing blood loss in the postoperative period (67). With a 2-hour half-life, loading doses of 10 mg/kg followed by infusions of 5 mg/kg/h are sufficient to support hemostasis and can be continued in the PICU (68). In addition to blood products, crystalloid resuscitation may need to be so vigorous that saline-induced metabolic acidosis may occur. In this regard, buffered solutions such as lactated ringers may offer advantages over normal saline (69).

In the postoperative period, blood loss via drains should be followed closely, and signs of significant blood loss (tachycardia, hypotension, hypocapnia, and respiratory variation in systolic BP) should be recognized and acted upon.

PICU and Airway Care

Initial PICU care may involve mechanical ventilation; sedation; thermoregulation; and correction of any residual volume deficits, acidosis, or coagulopathy (70). When surgery is long or blood loss is great, the endotracheal tube is routinely left in place until fluid shifts complete. Continued loss of fluid into the third space and oozing may necessitate ongoing fluid replacement for several hours. Coagulopathy may be consumptive or dilutional in nature and frequently requires specific correction. Suspicion of coagulopathy should be raised when the estimated blood loss exceeds 1.5 blood volumes or when substantial and persistent oozing is present (71). Once hemostasis is secure and fluid shifts have completed, attention moves to the airway.

Oropharyngeal and laryngotracheal edema may exacerbate preexisting obstructive apnea or critically worsen an already

difficult intubation. Timing of extubation is therefore critical, and great care must be taken to avoid obstruction or premature displacement of the endotracheal tube. Traditionally, extubation is safely accomplished when edema has begun to resolve, tongue swelling is minimal, and an air leak is present around the endotracheal tube. Since the sensitivity of these measures is questionable, earlier extubation may also be possible. Following extubation, noninvasive ventilatory support (continuous positive airway pressure, CPAP, or bilevel positive airway pressure, BiPAP) may be useful in selected cases if operative considerations and facial morphology permit.

CONCLUSIONS AND FUTURE DIRECTIONS

The patient admitted to the PICU following a neurosurgical or interventional neuroradiological procedure presents some special considerations for the intensivist. Awareness of pre- and intraoperative exposures as well as any special issues related to the underlying condition is paramount for effective and efficient care. These patients are at significant risk of postoperative pain, infection, and intracranial bleeding.

In the postoperative period, clinicians are often faced with the problem of trying to achieve neuroprotection. In this regard, the BP target that we should use in the perioperative neurosurgical and neurovascular patient is far from clear. There are few data and there are too many factors to consider—not least is the fact that the measured variable (driving pressure) is not our main interest (flow, which can only be inferred), but BP is the best surrogate that we have.

Questions about hemoglobin, carbon dioxide, BP, and their respective effects on cerebral blood volume and CBF are the topics discussed at the bedside; in the future, we may have better data to assist our understanding and management.

References

1. Miller P, Mack CD, Sammer M, et al. The incidence and risk factors for hypotension during emergent decompressive craniotomy in children with traumatic brain injury. *Anesth Analg* 2006; 103:869–75.
2. Sharma D, Jelacic J, Chennuri R, et al. Incidence and risk factors for perioperative hyperglycemia in children with traumatic brain injury. *Anesth Analg* 2009;108:81–9.
3. Curry R, Hollingworth W, Ellenbogen RG, et al. Incidence of hypo- and hypercarbia in severe traumatic brain injury before and after 2003 pediatric guidelines. *Pediatr Crit Care Med* 2008;9:141–6.
4. Bar-Joseph G, Guilburd Y, Tamir A, et al. Effectiveness of ketamine in decreasing intracranial pressure in children with intracranial hypertension. *J Neurosurg Pediatr* 2009;4:40–6.
5. Chang LC, Raty SR, Ortiz J, et al. The emerging use of ketamine for anesthesia and sedation in traumatic brain injuries. *CNS Neurosci Ther* 2013;19:390–5.
6. Baum VC, Willschke H, Marciniak B. Is nitrous oxide necessary in the future? *Paediatr Anaesth* 2012;22:981–7.
7. Kurita T, Morita K, Kazama T, et al. Influence of cardiac output on plasma propofol concentrations during constant infusion in swine. *Anesthesiology* 2002;96:1498–503.
8. Myburgh JA, Upton RN, Grant C, et al. Epinephrine, norepinephrine and dopamine infusions decrease propofol concentrations during continuous propofol infusion in an ovine model. *Intensive Care Med* 2001;27:276–82.
9. Kurita T, Uraoka M, Jiang Q, et al. Influence of cardiac output on the pseudo-steady state remifentanil and propofol concentrations in swine. *Acta Anaesthesiol Scand* 2013;57:754–60.

10. LaRovere KL, Brett MS, Tasker RC, et al. Head computed tomography scanning during pediatric neurocritical care: Diagnostic yield and the utility of portable studies. *Neurocrit Care* 2012; 16:251–7.

11. Kanal E, Borgstede JP, Barkovich AJ, et al. American College of Radiology. American College of Radiology White Paper on MR Safety: 2004 update and revisions. *AJR Am J Roentgenol* 2004;182:1111–4.

12. Practice advisory on anesthetic care for magnetic resonance imaging: A report by the Society of Anesthesiologists Task Force on Anesthetic Care for Magnetic Resonance Imaging. *Anesthesiology* 2009;110:459–79.

13. McClain CD, Rockoff MA, Soriano SG. Anesthetic concerns for pediatric patients in an intraoperative MRI suite. *Curr Opin Anaesthesiol* 2011;24:480–6.

14. Dunn W, Murphy JG. The patient handoff: Medicine's Formula One moment. *Chest* 2008;134:9–12.

15. Mekitarian Filho E, Brunow de Carvalho W, Cavalheiro S, et al. Perioperative factors associated with prolonged intensive care unit and hospital length of stay after pediatric neurosurgery. *Pediatr Neurosurg* 2011;47:423–9.

16. Caricato A, Conti G, Corte Della F, et al. Effects of PEEP on the intracranial system of patients with head injury and subarachnoid hemorrhage: The role of respiratory system compliance. *J Trauma* 2005;58:571–6.

17. Cooper KR, Boswell PA, Choi SC. Safe use of PEEP in patients with severe head injury. *J Neurosurg* 1985;63:552–5.

18. David M, Markstaller K, Depta AL, et al. Initiation of high-frequency oscillatory ventilation and its effects upon cerebral circulation in pigs: An experimental study. *Br J Anaesth* 2006; 97:525–32.

19. Williams CN, Belzer JS, Riva-Cambrin J, et al. The incidence of postoperative hyponatremia and associated neurological sequelae in children with intracranial neoplasms. *J Neurosurg Pediatr* 2014;13:283–90.

20. Choong K, Arora S, Cheng J, et al. Hypotonic versus isotonic maintenance fluids after surgery for children: A randomized controlled trial. *Pediatrics* 2011;128:857–66.

21. Coulthard MG, Long DA, Ullman AJ, et al. A randomised controlled trial of Hartmann's solution versus half normal saline in postoperative paediatric spinal instrumentation and craniotomy patients. *Arch Dis Child* 2012;97:491–6.

22. Foster BA, Tom D, Hill V. Hypotonic versus isotonic fluids in hospitalized children: A systematic review and meta-analysis. *J Pediatr* 2014;165:163.e2–169.e2.

23. Neville KA, Sandeman DJ, Rubinstein A, et al. Prevention of hyponatremia during maintenance intravenous fluid administration: A prospective randomized study of fluid type versus fluid rate. *J Pediatr* 2010;156:313–9.e1–2.

24. Hardesty DA, Kilbaugh TJ, Storm PB. Cerebral salt wasting syndrome in post-operative pediatric brain tumor patients. *Neurocrit Care* 2012;17:382–7.

25. Finken MJJ, Zwaveling-Soonawala N, Walenkamp MJE, et al. Frequent occurrence of the triphasic response (diabetes insipidus/ hyponatremia/diabetes insipidus) after surgery for craniopharyngioma in childhood. *Horm Res Paediatr* 2011;76:22–6.

26. Hoorn EJ, Zietse R. Water balance disorders after neurosurgery: The triphasic response revisited. *NDT Plus* 2010;3:42–4.

27. Pratheesh R, Swallow DMA, Rajaratnam S, et al. Incidence, predictors and early post-operative course of diabetes insipidus in paediatric craniopharyngioma: A comparison with adults. *Childs Nerv Syst* 2013;29:941–9.

28. Wise-Faberowski L, Soriano SG, Ferrari L, et al. Perioperative management of diabetes insipidus in children. *J Neurosurg Anesthesiol* 2004;16:220–5.

29. Fudickar A, Bein B. Propofol infusion syndrome: Update of clinical manifestation and pathophysiology. *Minerva Anestesiol* 2009; 75:339–44.

30. Kam PCA, Cardone D. Propofol infusion syndrome. *Anaesthesia* 2007;62:690–701.

31. Su F, Nicolson SC, Gastonguay MR, et al. Population pharmacokinetics of dexmedetomidine in infants after open heart surgery. *Anesth Analg* 2010;110:1383–92.

32. Oschman A, McCabe T, Kuhn RJ. Dexmedetomidine for opioid and benzodiazepine withdrawal in pediatric patients. *Am J Health Syst Pharm* 2011;68:1233–8.

33. Tobias JD. Dexmedetomidine to treat opioid withdrawal in infants following prolonged sedation in the pediatric ICU. *J Opioid Manag* 2006;2:201–5.

34. Hardesty DA, Sanborn MR, Parker WE, et al. Perioperative seizure incidence and risk factors in 223 pediatric brain tumor patients without prior seizures. *J Neurosurg Pediatr* 2011;7:609–15.

35. De Smet HJ, Baillieux H, Wackenier P, et al. Long-term cognitive deficits following posterior fossa tumor resection: A neuropsychological and functional neuroimaging follow-up study. *Neuropsychology* 2009;23:694–704.

36. Mariën P, De Smet HJ, Wijgerde E, et al. Posterior fossa syndrome in adults: A new case and comprehensive survey of the literature. *Cortex* 2013;49:284–300.

37. Rekate HL. The slit ventricle syndrome: Advances based on technology and understanding. *Pediatr Neurosurg* 2004;40:259–63.

38. Hyde-Rowan MD, Rekate HL, Nulsen FE. Reexpansion of previously collapsed ventricles: The slit ventricle syndrome. *J Neurosurg* 1982;56:536–9.

39. Jang M, Yoon SH. Hypothesis for intracranial hypertension in slit ventricle syndrome: New concept of capillary absorption laziness in the hydrocephalic patients with long-term shunts. *Med Hypotheses* 2013;81:199–201.

40. Pennings FA, Ince C, Bouma GJ. Continuous real-time visualization of the human cerebral microcirculation during arteriovenous malformation surgery using orthogonal polarization spectral imaging. *Neurosurgery* 2006;59:167–71; discussion 167–71.

41. Spetzler RF, Wilson CB, Weinstein P, et al. Normal perfusion pressure breakthrough theory. *Clin Neurosurg* 1978;25:651–72.

42. Young WL, Kader A, Ornstein E, et al. Cerebral hyperemia after arteriovenous malformation resection is related to "breakthrough" complications but not to feeding artery pressure. The Columbia University Arteriovenous Malformation Study project. *Neurosurgery* 1996;38:1085–93; discussion 1093–5.

43. Rubin D, Santillan A, Greenfield JP, et al. Surgical management of pediatric cerebral arteriovenous malformations. *Childs Nerv Syst* 2010;26:1337–44.

44. Greene AK, Orbach DB. Management of arteriovenous malformations. *Clin Plast Surg* 2011;38:95–106.

45. Thiex R, Williams A, Smith E, et al. The use of Onyx for embolization of central nervous system arteriovenous lesions in pediatric patients. *AJNR Am J Neuroradiol* 2010;31:112–20.

46. Zadeh G, Andrade-Souza YM, Tsao MN, et al. Pediatric arteriovenous malformation: University of Toronto experience using stereotactic radiosurgery. *Childs Nerv Syst* 2007;23:195–9.

47. Agid R, Jonas Kimchi T, Lee S-K, et al. Diagnostic characteristics and management of intracranial aneurysms in children. *Neuroimaging Clin N Am* 2007;17:153–63.

48. Rao VY, Shah KB, Bollo RJ, et al. Management of ruptured dissecting intracranial aneurysms in infants: Report of four cases and review of the literature. *Childs Nerv Syst* 2013;29:685–91.

49. Vasan R, Patel J, Sweeney JM, et al. Pediatric intracranial aneurysms: Current national trends in patient management and treatment. *Childs Nerv Syst* 2013;29:451–6.

50. Adamczyk P, He S, Amar AP, et al. Medical management of cerebral vasospasm following aneurysmal subarachnoid hemorrhage: A review of current and emerging therapeutic interventions. *Neurol Res Int* 2013;2013. doi:10.1155/2013/462491

51. Siasios I, Kapsalaki EZ, Fountas KN. Cerebral vasospasm pharmacological treatment: An update. *Neurol Res Int* 2013;2013. doi:10.1155/2013/571328

52. Connolly ES Jr, Rabinstein AA, Carhuapoma JR, et al. Guidelines for the management of aneurysmal subarachnoid hemorrhage: A guideline for healthcare professionals from the American Heart Association/American Stroke Association. *Stroke* 2012; 43:1711–37.

53. Steiner T, Juvela S, Unterberg A, et al. European Stroke Organization guidelines for the management of intracranial aneurysms and subarachnoid haemorrhage. *Cerebrovasc Dis* 2013;35:93–112.

54. Vivancos J, Gilo F, Frutos R, et al. Clinical management guidelines for subarachnoid haemorrhage. Diagnosis and treatment. *Neurologia* 2014;29:353–70.

55. Scott RM, Smith ER. Moyamoya disease and moyamoya syndrome. *N Engl J Med* 2009;360:1226–37.

56. Lin N, Baird L, Koss M, et al. Discovery of asymptomatic moyamoya arteriopathy in pediatric syndromic populations: Radiographic and clinical progression. *Neurosurg Focus* 2011;31:E6.

57. Amlie-Lefond C, Zaidat OO, Lew SM. Moyamoya disease in early infancy: Case report and literature review. *Pediatr Neurol* 2011;44:299–302.

58. Tagawa T, Naritomi H, Mimaki T, et al. Regional cerebral blood flow, clinical manifestations, and age in children with moyamoya disease. *Stroke* 1987;18:906–10.

59. Han JS, Abou-Hamden A, Mandell DM, et al. Impact of extracranial-intracranial bypass on cerebrovascular reactivity and clinical outcome in patients with symptomatic moyamoya vasculopathy. *Stroke* 2011;42:3047–54.

60. Vendrame M, Kaleyias J, Loddenkemper T, et al. Electroencephalogram monitoring during intracranial surgery for moyamoya disease. *Pediatr Neurol* 2011;44:427–32.

61. Schubert GA, Biermann P, Weiss C, et al. Risk profile in EC-IC bypass surgery; The role of antiplatelet agents, disease pathology and surgical technique in 168 direct revascularization procedures. *World Neurosurg* 2013;82:672–7.

62. Crepeau AZ, Moseley BD, Wirrell EC. Specific safety and tolerability considerations in the use of anticonvulsant medications in children. *Drug Healthc Patient Saf* 2012;4:39–54.

63. Mirza NS, Alfirevic A, Jorgensen A, et al. Metabolic acidosis with topiramate and zonisamide: An assessment of its severity and predictors. *Pharmacogenet Genomics* 2011;21:297–302.

64. Warren SM, Proctor MR, Bartlett SP, et al. Parameters of care for craniosynostosis: Craniofacial and neurologic surgery perspectives. *Plast Reconstr Surg* 2012;129:731–7.

65. Dadure C, Sauter M, Bringuier S, et al. Intraoperative tranexamic acid reduces blood transfusion in children undergoing craniosynostosis surgery: A randomized double-blind study. *Anesthesiology* 2011;114:856–61.

66. Krajewski K, Ashley RK, Pung N, et al. Successful blood conservation during craniosynostotic correction with dual therapy using procrit and cell saver. *J Craniofac Surg* 2008;19:101–5.

67. Goobie SM, Meier PM, Pereira LM, et al. Efficacy of tranexamic acid in pediatric craniosynostosis surgery: A double-blind, placebo-controlled trial. *Anesthesiology* 2011;114:862–71.

68. Goobie SM, Meier PM, Sethna NF, et al. Population pharmacokinetics of tranexamic acid in paediatric patients undergoing craniosynostosis surgery. *Clin Pharmacokinet* 2013;52:267–76.

69. Zunini GS, Rando KA, Cox RG, et al. Fluid replacement in craniofacial pediatric surgery: Normal saline or ringer's lactate? *J Craniofac Surg* 2011;22:1370–4.

70. Tamburrini G, Caldarelli M, Massimi L, et al. Complex craniosynostoses: A review of the prominent clinical features and the related management strategies. *Childs Nerv Syst* 2012;28:511–23.

71. Williams GD, Ellenbogen RG, Gruss JS. Abnormal coagulation during pediatric craniofacial surgery. *Pediatr Neurosurg* 2001;35:5–12.

CHAPTER 61 ■ HEAD AND SPINAL CORD TRAUMA

ROBERT C. TASKER AND P. DAVID ADELSON

KEY POINTS

1. Hypotension and hypoxemia are strongly associated with poor outcome; the focus should be on these targets in resuscitation.

2. Hypoventilation due to lung or neurologic causes is common in traumatic brain injury and spinal cord injury.

3. The mechanism and pattern of head and brain injury will help to anticipate meningitis, carotid dissection, and hypopituitarism.

4. Optimal brain and spinal cord trauma care requires multidisciplinary expertise.

The practicalities of critical care in children with traumatic brain injury (TBI) or traumatic spinal cord injury (TSCI) are discussed in this chapter. The developmental neuroscience of acute neurotoxicity, vascular control, and cerebral hemodynamics and physiology is discussed in other chapters within this section of the book. The principal aim of this chapter is to review the recent clinical literature (in the main, between 2005 and 2014) toward informing the practice of neurocritical care.

Central to our understanding and treatment of TBI is the fact that mechanical forces at the time of accident—direct or contact force, acceleration and deceleration forces, and rotational or torsional forces—are responsible for primary injury. As a consequence of these forces, a variety of primary and secondary brain injuries occur (**Table 61.1**). The pathophysiology of these forms of injury is dealt with in other chapters.

EPIDEMIOLOGY

Traumatic Brain Injury

TBI is a major public health problem. Worldwide, TBI is the leading cause of death and disability for children (>1 year old) and young adults. In 2009, the US Centers for Disease Control and Prevention estimated that at least 2.4 million emergency department visits, hospitalizations, or deaths were related to a TBI, either alone or in combination with other injuries (1). Approximately 75% of TBIs are mild concussions. Children, adolescents, and older adults are most likely to sustain a TBI. Nearly one third of all injury deaths included a diagnosis of TBI. In addition, an estimated 5.3 million people in the US are living with TBI-related disabilities, including long-term cognitive and psychologic impairments. A severe TBI not only affects a person's life and family, but also has a large societal and economic toll. The economic costs of TBIs in 2010 were estimated at $76.5 billion, including $11.5 billion in direct medical costs and $64.8 billion in indirect costs (e.g., lost wages, lost productivity, and nonmedical expenditures).

Spinal Cord Injury

The burden of acute TSCI among US children and adolescents (≤17 years) using emergency department data from the Nationwide Emergency Department Sample (2007–2010) is, on average, 17.5 per million population (2). The median age at presentation in this sample of over 6000 cases was 15 years, with the majority males (72.5%). Children ≤5 years are more likely to have been injured from a road traffic accident (RTA) (50.9%), present with cervical spine C1–C4 injuries (47.4%), and have concurrent TBI (24%) compared to older children and adolescents.

In this chapter we will focus on the intensive care management of infants, children, and adolescents with severe TBI and those with acute TSCI. The prevalence rate for severe TBI in children (0–14 years of age) who are subsequently admitted to intensive care (the majority of whom are intubated and ventilated) is 5.4 per 100,000 population annually (3).

HEAD INJURY PATTERNS

3. In general, head injuries conform to one of three types: *blunt* head injury, *sharp* head injury, or *compression* injury.

TABLE 61.1

PRIMARY AND SECONDARY BRAIN INJURY

■ PRIMARY BRAIN INJURY	■ SECONDARY BRAIN INJURY
Diffuse and focal axonal injury	Diffuse and focal hypoxic-ischemic injury
Diffuse and focal vascular injury	Diffuse and focal brain swelling
Focal brain contusion	Intracranial hypertension
Focal brain laceration	Hydrocephalus
	Infection and fever
	Seizures
	Metabolic disturbance, e.g., hyponatremia

Blunt Head Injury

A blunt injury occurs when the head comes into forcible contact with a flat, smooth surface. This injury can be caused by a fall when the head hits the ground or a blow to the head by a blunt object. In both instances, the curvature of the skull at the point of impact tends to flatten. The area of impact is therefore spread over an area proportional to the deformation of the skull. If the deformity produces a fracture, its direction and extent will be related to the thickness of the scalp, the elasticity of the bone, and local weaknesses in the skull. In addition, the head and its contents will be subjected to either significant deceleration in the case of a fall or significant acceleration in the case of a blow.

When the deformity of the skull exceeds the limit of tolerance, fracture lines begin. In children, the unfused cranial sutures may be involved and produce the "bursting fracture" of childhood. When the distorting force is spent, the elasticity of the skull causes it to move back toward its original shape. The acceleration and deceleration produced by the changes in speed and direction of motion of the head are important factors in the production of brain damage. An immediate and steep rise in pressure occurs at the point of impact, while a fall in pressure that can equal a negative pressure of one atmosphere occurs at the opposite pole. The increased positive pressure may have little effect on the brain, but the negative pressure, if it exceeds one atmosphere, may produce small areas of cavitation and focal hemorrhages in the superficial cortex. The injury combinations that are likely to follow blunt head injury to the vault are summarized in **Table 61.2**.

Sharp Head Injury

The area of impact and extent of skull distortion are small in sharp head injury. Laceration of the scalp, local depression or fragmentation of the skull, tearing of the dura, and bruising and laceration of the underlying brain may be seen. An example of this injury is a blow by a thrown hard ball. When the area of impact is small, the effect upon the underlying bone is almost explosive; fragments may be sprayed out into the brain beneath. Intracerebral hemorrhage in these injuries usually arises from torn superficial vessels of the cortex.

Compression Head Injury

A compression or crush injury is unusual. Severe injuries may occur without initial loss of consciousness. Fractures tend to involve the foramina at the base of the skull, producing cranial nerve (CN) palsies (**Table 61.3**). Occasionally, the internal carotid artery is torn as it passes through the base of the skull, and fatal hemorrhage may occur. Less-severe cases may be associated with vessel dissection and cerebrovascular stroke (see Chapter 64). Side-to-side compression causes fractures through the middle fossa across the sella turcica to the opposite side. In these cases, the pituitary is at risk from direct trauma.

Penetrating/Blast Injuries

Given the recent military conflicts and the proliferation of guns and other weapons, there has been a rise in children injured from blast injuries and/or penetrating cranial and/or spinal trauma. Although not as common as closed head injuries, pediatric penetrating craniocerebral injuries account for significant morbidity and mortality within the pediatric population. As would be expected, the extent of brain tissue damage as well as compromise of vascular supply may lead to worsened secondary mechanisms and injury and increased morbidity and mortality. Many neurosurgical techniques and principles apply to the management of these injuries including evacuation of mass lesions, debridement of devitalized tissue, and decompression. For blast injuries, the pressure wave and forces applied to the tissues can be disruptive of connections and lead to significant distortion creating several unique factors that require further consideration and understanding.

Development and Head Injury Patterns

The stage of development of the skull, brain, and intracranial vasculature directly accounts for the types of injuries seen in different pediatric age groups. The infant's disproportionately large head and weaker neck muscles place them at more risk of rotational and acceleration–deceleration injuries. The relatively softer cranial vault, anatomy of the dura, and rich vascular supply of the subarachnoid space all place young children at risk for intracranial injury and bleeding—even when a skull fracture is not present. Last, the high water content and viscosity of the young brain means that it may be more at risk for axonal injury. With skull and brain maturation, adult patterns of intracranial injury are seen.

The developmental pattern of injury is reflected in the findings on brain imaging at presentation. The CT scan characteristics in moderate or severe pediatric TBI do differ from those identified in adult TBI (4). At one level, we might expect for a given severity of injury—as measured by the Glasgow Coma Scale (GCS) score (5,6)—similarity in CT scan findings in children and adults. However, from the perspective of biomechanics of TBI, there is evidence of unique age-dependent responses (7,8), which may be related to anatomical differences in skull thickness, overall mass of the skull and brain, the ratio of brain-volume-to-cerebrospinal-fluid-volume, and the physics of dissipating rotational forces to bridging veins (9,10). The net effect is that pediatric patients with thinner skull anatomy are more prone to skull fracture and epidural hematoma (EDH), whereas adult patients are more likely to demonstrate complex patterns such as subdural and intraparenchymal hemorrhages with >5 mm midline shift (4,11).

TYPES OF INTRACRANIAL INJURY

Blunt head injury is the most common reason for admission to the pediatric intensive care unit (PICU). The three main mechanisms by which such injury can cause intracranial damage are (a) focal hemorrhagic and nonhemorrhagic lesions that mainly involve the cortical gray matter, (b) diffuse traumatic axonal injury (TAI), and (c) secondary injury caused by edema and space-occupying hemorrhages (**Table 61.1**).

Hemorrhage and Other Focal Brain Tissue Effects

Focal injury is thought to occur when the brain impacts against the rigid inner table of the skull, with resulting areas of direct cortical contusion. Focal brain injury may also produce mass effects from hemorrhage, contusion, or hematoma that can induce herniation and brainstem compression.

EDHs complicate 2%–3% of all head injury admissions in children and are more frequent with advancing age; the peak is in the second decade. In infants, EDH of venous or bony

TABLE 61.2

FEATURES ASSOCIATED WITH VAULT FRACTURES IN BLUNT HEAD INJURY

■ SITE OF IMPACT	■ FEATURES ASSOCIATED WITH FRACTURE LINES

Mid-frontal	Clinical
	    CSF rhinorrhea
	    Meningitis, pneumocephalus
	    Anosmia
	Brain
	    General concussion
	    Direct bruising of underlying cortex
	    Laceration of subfrontal cortex
	Hemorrhage
	    SAH, SDH

Lateral-frontal or temporofrontal	Clinical
	    CSF rhinorrhea and meningitis in anterior fractures
	    Blindness in medial fractures
	    EDH in posterior fractures
	Brain
	    General concussion
	    Motor aphasia from a blow to the left side
	Hemorrhage
	    SAH, SDH, EDH

Lateral or temporoparietal	Clinical
	    Movement of the brain is restricted by dural folds, but their sharp edges may cut into the brainstem
	    If fracture lines involve the base of the skull, cranial nerves V, VI, VII, and VIII may be involved,
	    as well as the sella turcica
	    Involvement of middle meningeal vessels with EDH
	    Middle-ear involvement with CSF otorrhea and meningitis
	Brain
	    Concussion is not that severe in general
	    Local contusions beneath impact may cause aphasia or contralateral weakness if the Rolandic fissure
	    is involved
	Hemorrhage
	    SAH is uncommon
	    SDH follows small lacerations related to point of impact

Posterolateral or occipitoparietal	Clinical
	    CSF otorrhea, meningitis, and hearing loss when the petrous temporal bone is involved
	Brain
	    Concussion is severe
	    Distant injury with laceration of the frontal and temporal poles
	Hemorrhage
	    EDH may occur in fractures in the middle fossa or posterior fossa
	    High risk of tearing of vessels: SAH and SDH formation

Midline posterior or occipital	Clinical
	    Often associated fracture of cervical spine
	    Lower cranial nerve palsies
	Brain
	    Concussion is severe
	    Distant subfrontal or temporal contusions and laceration
	Hemorrhage
	    Subfrontal or temporal SAH and SDH

CSF, cerebrospinal fluid; SAH, subarachnoid hemorrhage; SDH, subdural hemorrhage; EDH, extradural hemorrhage.

TABLE 61.3

COMPRESSION FRACTURES

■ TYPE	■ CLINICAL PROBLEMS

Side-to-side
Fracture passes through the middle fossa across the sella turcica to the opposite side
	Injuries include:
	    Anterior group of cranial nerves may be involved, in particular, sixth nerve
	    Internal carotid artery may be torn

Front-to-back
Wide fissures through the frontal sinus extending back through the cribriform and ethmoid regions
	Disruption of:
	    Frontal sinus
	    Cribriform plate
	    Roof of the orbit

origin is found in the posterior fossa adjacent to the venous sinuses. These venous EDHs often have a delayed presentation because the infant has significant intracranial reserve from unfused sutures and open fontanelles. In older children, EDHs arise from arterial bleeding. Patients may have a short, lucid interval after injury, but they will deteriorate rapidly with an increasing intracranial mass.

Subdural hemorrhage (SDH) is a common problem in children, especially in those who suffer abusive TBI (see Chapter 62). The clinical presentation depends on the size and location of the hemorrhage and the presence of associated brain injuries. It is the associated brain injuries that account for immediate unconsciousness at the time of accident and any focal neurologic deficits (e.g., hemiparesis, pupillary abnormalities, and seizures).

Traumatic intraparenchymal hematomas, or contusions, are not common in children, but their frequency increases with age. These lesions most commonly involve white matter of the frontal and temporal lobes, the body and splenium of the corpus callosum, and the corona radiata. In the cortex, contusions frequently involve the inferior, lateral, and anterior aspects of the frontal and temporal lobes (12). These patterns and distribution of primary lesions are similar to those expected from mechanical modeling (13,14) and are found as well in children with severe TBI (15). It is likely that occult, diffuse white-matter changes may also be present—even in regions of the brain that appear normal on conventional imaging—and such findings are consistent with early generalized cellular injury (16) and later loss of white matter (17–19).

Involvement of the frontal lobes (as part of a focal frontal-lobe compartment syndrome) is suggested by reports of frontal hypoperfusion using single photon emission tomography (20) and subsequent white-matter loss in this brain region (17–19). This problem may also occur in children.

Diffuse Injury Involving Axons

Diffuse injury that involves axons results from shearing forces that act at interfaces of the brain with differing structural integrity, such as the gray-white-matter boundaries. The neuronal axons that cross multiple brain regions are particularly vulnerable. TAI may vary from small foci of axonal injury to a more severe form of diffuse TAI, in which injury is widespread throughout the brain, including the brainstem. In fatal injuries, the extent and distribution of TAI throughout the brain appears to be similar in children and adults (21,22). Lesser degrees of TAI may be seen in those patients with less-severe injury (23). In adults who survive 1–47 years after moderately severe TBI, diffuse TAI—but not of the severe type—was found in 6 of 20 patients (24). In recent imaging studies the identification of disrupted white-matter connectivity is now well documented, with particular involvement of the fornices—which are the major pathways projecting to the hippocampus. In more severe cases that survive in minimal states of awareness, this loss of connectivity results in abnormal brain network function. For example, in a group of 63 adult subjects surviving severe TBI, neural activity within what has been termed the fronto-parietal control network was abnormal in patients with impaired self-awareness. The dorsal anterior cingulate cortex—a key part of this network that is involved in performance monitoring—showed reduced functional connectivity to the rest of the fronto-parietal control network at "rest" (25). Overall, the impairment of self-awareness was not explained either by the location of focal brain injury, or the amount of TAI as demonstrated by diffusion tensor imaging. Rather, the results suggested that impairments of self-awareness after TBI resulted from breakdown of functional interactions between nodes within the fronto-parietal control network.

Cranial CT imaging of TAI is variable in children. The extent and distribution of TAI depends on injury severity and category. In one report, 14 out of 117 children had cranial CT evidence of TAI, as evidenced by small intraparenchymal and/or intraventricular hemorrhage; intradural or extradural cerebral mass lesion, including EDH or SDH; or an open skull fracture (26). MRI is more sensitive to the white-matter changes usually seen with TAI, and such studies are, increasingly, being performed during the acute period on the PICU. For example, in a recent prospective cohort study of 159 TBI patients (age range 5–65 years), diffuse TAI was found in almost three quarters of the patients with moderate and severe head injury who survived the acute phase (27). Diffuse TAI influenced the level of consciousness, and only in patients with TAI was the GCS score related to outcome (see below). Finally, TAI was a negative prognostic sign only when located in the brainstem.

Diffuse Swelling of the Cerebrum at Presentation

Diffuse swelling occurs in two forms—swelling of one cerebral hemisphere and swelling of both cerebral hemispheres. During the early phase of posttraumatic coma in children, cerebral swelling develops and generally peaks between 24 and 72 hours after injury. Diffuse swelling of one hemisphere may develop very rapidly, as was observed in 17 of 151 (11%) fatal nonmissile head injuries (21). The swelling was associated with acute SDH, even when this had been evacuated. Contusions in the ipsilateral hemisphere may also be related to such swelling. The incidence of diffuse brain swelling on initial head CT can be as high as 53% (28). However, the literature is inconclusive regarding the prognostic significance of this finding. A 1994 study found a mortality of 35% in adults and only 20% mortality in children (29).

In some instances, specific focal injury may occur in combination with diffuse injury. High-speed impact and acceleration–deceleration forces at the time of injury make the medial temporal lobe particularly vulnerable to mechanical deformation and contusion because of its position in the middle cranial fossa (30). Selective injury of the hippocampus may result from systemic vascular and metabolic perturbation—hypoxia, ischemia, seizures, and hypoglycemia—after injury (18,31). In TBI, the lesion found in the hippocampus most commonly consists of focal areas of selective neuronal loss in the CA1 subfield, similar to hypoxic insults. In the postacute period, hippocampal cell death may result from deafferentation or deefferentation caused by transneuronal degeneration.

Focal and global brain swelling can act as a mass leading to shifts in brain tissue across neighboring intracranial compartments (Fig. 61.1). These tissue herniation syndromes can exist despite normal global intracranial pressure (ICP) (Table 61.4).

Posttraumatic Ischemia, Tissue Oxygenation, and Metabolism

In adults seen early after injury, cerebral blood flow (CBF) is reduced and secondary insults such as hypotension and hypoxemia have devastating effect. Brain swelling and any accompanying intracranial hypertension can contribute to this early secondary ischemia. Problems in CBF and metabolism are not exclusive to adults and are observed in infants and children. Infants with severe TBI commonly have cerebral hypoperfusion, and a global CBF of <20 mL/100 g/min was associated with poor outcome (32). Following early posttraumatic hypoperfusion, CBF may increase to levels

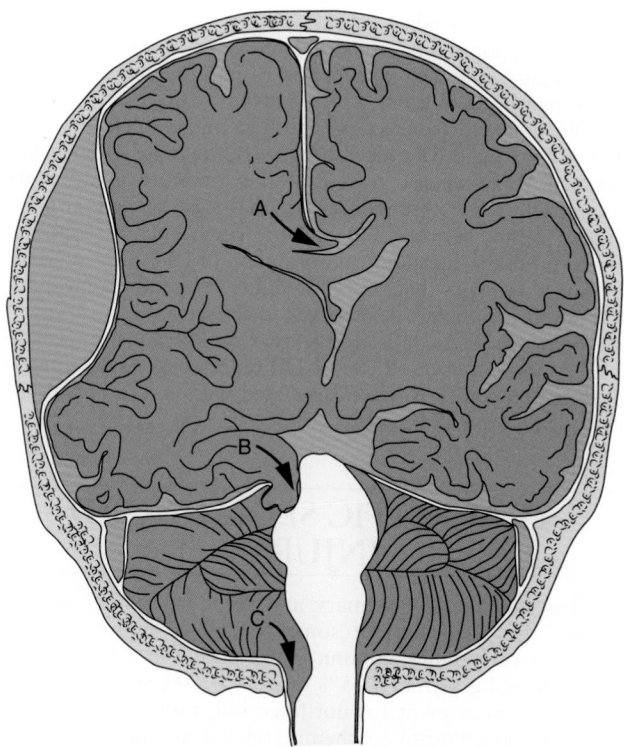

FIGURE 61.1. Herniation syndromes: (A) subfalcine and cingulate, (B) uncal, (C) foramen magnum (see **Table 61.4**). Subfalcine herniation occurs when one cerebral hemisphere is displaced under the falx cerebri across the midline (A). Uncal herniation refers to displacement of supratentorial structures inferiorly under the tentorium cerebelli, causing distortion and compression of the blood supply to infratentorial structures (B). Downward herniation of the cerebellum causes compression of the brainstem (C).

greater than metabolic demands, producing a state of relative hyperemia (33). Alternatively, a phase of increased cerebral metabolism of glucose may accompany posttraumatic hypoperfusion. In adults, the use of monitoring techniques that reflect the coupling between CBF and metabolism (e.g., using brain microdialysis and oxygen probes) is increasing, and the presence of key phenomena is influencing practice. In children, a recent report indicates a unique pattern of brain tissue oxygen tension with severe TBI: the best threshold for favorable outcome was noted at a level of 30 mm Hg, and high, rather than low, values were observed in some patients with refractory intracranial hypertension and compromised cerebral perfusion, likely reflecting failed uptake rather than failed delivery (34). Such impaired metabolism after severe TBI in children was recently confirmed in an MRI study of 17 children where the authors found variable CBF after injury, but hypoperfusion and low oxygenation predominating (35). Taken together, these findings are consistent with preclinical and adult clinical studies of brain metabolism suggesting mitochondrial dysfunction after TBI.

Hypothalamic–Pituitary Injury

The pituitary gland and its anatomic attachment to hypothalamic structures are vulnerable to injury following TBI, even though they are protected by the bony sella turcica. In blunt head injury, a lateral or temporoparietal fracture line may radiate down to the base of the skull and pass through the central area of the sella turcica to the opposite middle fossa (**Table 61.2**). In this instance, the pituitary stalk is at risk of trauma. In other forms of injury, the reason for pituitary vulnerability may be vascular or ischemic, as tissue swelling and edema cause compression of the hypophyseal blood vessels within the restrictive space of the sella turcica. The hypophyseal–pituitary portal circulation is a rich network of blood

TABLE 61.4

TYPES OF BRAIN TISSUE HERNIATION SYNDROMES

■ SYNDROME	■ MECHANISM	■ CLINICAL FEATURES
Foramen magnum	*Herniating tissue:* Downward mesial displacement of cerebellar hemispheres	Episodic tonic extension with opisthotonic posturing, leading to quadriparesis
	Compression: Unilateral or bilateral medulla by ventral parafollicular or tonsillae through foramen magnum	Changes in blood pressure, heart rate, and arrhythmias Ataxic breathing Small pupils and disturbance of conjugate gaze
Central tentorial	*Herniating tissue:* Downward displacement of one or both cerebral hemispheres	ICP is usually raised
	Compression: Diencephalon and midbrain through tentorial notch	Bilateral decorticate or decerebrate posturing An "upward" form of this syndrome may occur if supratentorial ventricles are decompressed in the presence of cerebellar mass
Uncal (lateral transtentorial)	*Herniating tissue:* Medial temporal lobe (uncus and parahippocampal gyrus) forced into the incisura	ICP is usually raised Contralateral hemiparesis Ipsilateral pupillary dilatation and ptosis Unilateral or bilateral occipital lobe infarction
	Compression: Midbrain and posterior cerebral artery	Obstructive hydrocephalus from compression of aqueduct or perimesencephalic cistern Regions of necrosis and hemorrhage in tegmentum, subthalamus, midbrain, and upper pons
Cingulate	*Herniating tissue:* Cingulate gyrus herniates under the anterior falx *Compression:* Anterior cerebral artery	Infarction of regional tissue seen on imaging Contralateral lower extremity paresis

ICP, intracranial pressure.

vessels, predominantly supplied by the superior hypophyseal arteries, which arise from the internal carotids. The long hypophyseal blood vessels and the dense network of capillaries are vulnerable to rupture and hemorrhage, leading to subsequent ischemia and infarction of the anterior lobe of the pituitary gland.

Few studies directly link TBI with disruption and damage to the hypothalamic–pituitary structures. However, they provide convincing histopathologic evidence that lesions do occur in this part of the brain in severe TBI. Autopsy in 106 fatal TBI cases revealed hypothalamic lesions in almost 43% of adults (36). Lesions were typically suggestive of infarction and ischemia and consistent with either shearing of small perforating blood vessels or with venous engorgement secondary to intracranial hypertension. In 28% of cases, pituitary lesions were also present and often associated with fracture of the middle cerebral fossa. Others have also reported traumatic infarction of the anterior pituitary gland, often in association with hemorrhage (37,38).

The key question is whether this form of injury is seen in nonfatal cases of TBI. The answer is yes, both acutely and on follow-up. A study of 50 adults admitted for intensive care following TBI found a high frequency of early posttraumatic endocrine abnormalities, in particular low basal cortisol levels with subnormal cortisol responses to a glucagon test, hypogonadism, and hyperprolactinemia (39,40). Another study confirmed the extent of these acute abnormalities, showing that 53% of patients demonstrate deficiency in at least one hormonal axis (18). Growth-hormone deficiency has also been demonstrated in the acute setting, although growth-hormone resistance would be expected in critical illness. Low plasma insulin-like growth factor-I level is also found in association with decreased growth-hormone secretion. On follow-up, hypothalamic–pituitary dysfunction is being recognized increasingly. The literature on adults has flourished since 2000, and more recent reviews describe this subject area in detail (41,42). It appears that in moderate or severe TBI, the frequency of hypopituitarism is high, and subnormal responses, in at least one hypothalamic–pituitary axis, occur in 23%–69% of cases (43,44). Dynamic tests of anterior pituitary function reveal a high prevalence of previously undetected deficiencies in the growth-hormone, adrenal, and thyroid axes. Serial

neuroendocrine studies suggest that the natural history of post-TBI hypopituitarism involves an acute phase of transient abnormality, followed by a period of late presentation of endocrinopathy, even up to several years.

The literature concerning children and adolescents with TBI-related hypothalamic–pituitary dysfunction is much less detailed. A systematic review of the literature up to 2008 found only a few case reports, or small case series that highlighted a link between TBI and the occurrence of hypothalamic–pituitary hormone abnormality (43,44). The current literature suggests that post-TBI–induced hypothalamic–pituitary dysfunction may be observed in children after a variety of mechanisms. RTAs, falls, and sport-related trauma appear to be the most common causes of TBI reported to have pituitary dysfunction, and it is often associated with loss of consciousness, SDH, or skull fracture.

TRAUMATIC SPINAL CORD INJURY

TSCI is the result of primary and secondary injury mechanisms. The occurrence of some neurologic injury in association with vertebral column injury occurs in <50%, while complete SCI is seen in <25% cases (45). At presentation, the damage from acute SCI is not fixed but, rather, evolves over hours or days. Post-SCI ischemia, related to failing autoregulation, blood pressure, cardiac output, and oxygenation, may contribute to worsening injury.

The clinician should be aware of the features and variety of spinal cord syndromes that may occur in the setting of trauma (Table 61.5). The pattern of SCI in children differs from that in adults in a number of ways because the child's spine is still developing. Children have wedge-shaped vertebral bodies, incomplete centers of ossification, and more lax ligaments (46). In children up to the age of 9 years, spinal injuries are more frequently seen in the atlas, axis, and upper cervical vertebrae (47). Ligamentous injuries that lead to atlanto-occipital dislocation (AOD) are also more common than are bone injuries. After this age, an adult pattern of injury is seen, i.e., less involvement of the cervical spine (~55%).

TABLE 61.5

SPINAL CORD SYNDROMES IN TRAUMA

■ SYNDROME	■ MECHANISM	■ FINDINGS
Complete cord transection	Trauma Secondary vascular	Loss of all motor function Loss of sensory function Above C3—apnea and death
Brown–Sequard (cord hemisection)	Penetrating trauma	Ipsilateral loss of proprioception Ipsilateral loss of motor function Contralateral loss of pain and temperature sensation Suspended ipsilateral loss of all sensory modalities
Central cord	Neck hyperextension	Motor impairment greater in upper limbs than in lower limbs Suspended sensory loss in cervicothoracic dermatomes
Anterior cord	Hyperflexion Anterior spinal artery occlusion	Variable motor impairment Pain and temperature loss with sparing of proprioception
Conus medullaris	Direct trauma	Extension to lumbosacral roots may produce both upper and lower motor neuron signs Spastic paraparesis Sphincter dysfunction Lower sacral "saddle" sensory loss

Spinal Cord Injury without Radiographic Abnormality

The anatomic characteristics of the younger child (i.e., lack of muscular development of the neck and the relatively large head size) also lead to the frequent occurrence of an entity known as spinal cord injury without radiographic abnormality (SCIWORA). That is, the elasticity of the immature spine may allow for significant distraction and flexion to injure the cord without resulting in either ligamentous or bone disruption and, hence, no apparent abnormalities on radiographic investigation. SCIWORA may occur in older children (even though bone maturity is reached by age 9 years) because ligamentous laxity continues into adolescence.

The possibility of SCIWORA should be considered in all pediatric TBI cases. The clinical features range from tingling dysesthesias or numbness to frank weakness or paralysis. MRI demonstrates five classes of post-SCIWORA cord findings: complete transection, major hemorrhage, minor hemorrhage, edema only, and normal (48–50). The neural findings are highly predictive of outcome. All patients with normal cord signals should make complete recovery (51). Patients with transection and major hemorrhage have very poor outcome, and intermediate outcomes are seen in the remaining grades of severity. A meta-analysis of 392 published cases found that complete recovery occurred in 39% of cases (52). A review of 1393 adult SCIWORA cases identified in 63 articles emphasized the prognostic significance of MRI findings (53). In children, thoracic SCIWORA has also been identified as an important clinical entity in a subset of children who are usually victims of accidents that involve high-speed, direct impact, distraction from lap belts, and crush injury by slow-moving vehicles (50,54).

Traumatic AOD

AOD is defined as disruption of the supporting ligaments such that displacement occurs in either the transverse or vertical direction. The diagnosis of AOD is often missed on spine plain radiographs. Hence, additional imaging of the craniocervical junction with either CT or MRI is recommended in patients suspected of having AOD. Neurological abnormalities including lower CN paresis (particularly CNs VI, X, and XII), monoparesis, hemiparesis, quadriparesis, respiratory dysfunction including apnea, and complete high cervical cord motor deficits in the setting of normal plain spinal radiographs should prompt additional imaging with CT or MRI (55).

AOD is rare in children and adolescents and, historically, most reported cases have been fatal, with the patient often not surviving initial cardiac arrest and apnea. However, the advent of modern prehospital care has led to an increase in survival following injury. Combined high-SCI and brainstem injuries must be suspected in this group (56).

Odontoid Epiphysiolysis

Fusion of the neurocentral synchondrosis of the second cervical vertebrum is not complete until the age of 7 years, which means that it is a vulnerable site for traumatic injury in young children. The lateral cervical spine radiograph is the imaging of choice and if injury is present it will show an anteriorly angulated (rarely posterior angulation) odontoid process. The injury occurs through the epiphysis and has a high likelihood of healing if closed reduction and immobilization—usually with halo—are used for ~10 weeks.

INITIAL CLINICAL MANAGEMENT

The clinical management of TBI cases requires a system and process that start at the scene of injury and run through to rehabilitation. In the initial phase, we favor a multidisciplinary approach where every team member understands their role and there are no gaps in patient management. Hence, there are multiple parallel activities. This section is somewhat artificial in that it assumes that there is time for a single individual to walk through each step when in reality these tasks are being performed by many individuals, e.g., airway management, history and evaluation, and so on. Within the first hour after injury, the imperative is to ensure the adequacy of the airway, keep systolic blood pressure at normal levels, protect the cervical spine, undertake cranial CT scan, and treat potential herniation syndromes. That said, we now present the essential components of assessment and information that are required for patient care. The more advanced reader is advised to explore the most up-to-date open-access *Guidelines* documents that are available from the *Brain Trauma Foundation* (https://www.braintrauma.org/coma-guidelines/).

History, Diagnosis, and Classification of TBI

It is important to know the mechanism of injury and anatomical status of the patient in cases of TBI because this information will help in anticipating potential patterns of injury and problems (**Tables 61.2** and **61.3**). The required details of an accident include the type of accident, the degree of force acting on the head, the position of the victim when found at the scene, and the victim's immediate state of consciousness. In some cases brain edema may have already evolved to life-threatening levels, and other superimposed secondary insults (e.g., seizures and apnea) may complicate full understanding of the primary injury.

Severe TBI is defined as TBI in a patient with an identified mechanism who is unconscious and has a GCS score <9 (**Table 61.6**). The GCS is a descriptive scoring system that evaluates performance in three areas: eye opening, which relates to the level of arousal; verbalization, which relates to content and mentation; and motor ability. The GCS score has not been validated in children, and in those <2 years of age it is almost impossible to use. The "Infant Face Scale" may be of use in this regard, but it remains to be seen whether a score of 9–12 on this scale is equivalent to (and has the same implications as) a score of 9–12 on the GCS (57). The motor component of the GCS score is the most important item to establish.

The *best motor response* in either the upper or lower limbs is rated on a scale of 1–6, with a score of 6 given when the patient obeys commands. If there is no response, or an incomplete reaction to verbal stimuli, it is necessary to apply a noxious stimulus. SCI must be excluded before this level of scoring. The preferred site for application of painful stimuli is the medial side of the arms or legs, since this will differentiate a localization of pain response as opposed to abnormal flexor or extensor posturing. If the patient moves the limb toward the noxious stimulus, the response is not consistent with localization because one would expect the patient to move their limb away from such a stimulus. The examiner should make sure that an adequate noxious stimulus has been applied before scoring 1 (i.e., no response). Other noxious stimuli include applying pressure to a fingernail-bed with a pen horizontally, or applying pressure to the supraorbital notch with your thumb. While applying the noxious stimulus, the observer

TABLE 61.6

GLASGOW COMA SCALE SCORE FOR CHILDREN AND INFANTS

■ ACTIVITY	■ CHILD RESPONSE	■ INFANT RESPONSE	■ SCORE
Eye opening (E)	Spontaneous	Spontaneous	4
	To verbal stimuli	To verbal stimuli	3
	To pain	To pain	2
	None	None	1
Verbal (V)	Oriented	Coos and babbles	5
	Confused	Irritable cries	4
	Inappropriate words	Cries to pain	3
	Nonspecific sounds	Moans to pain	2
	None	None	1
Motor (M)	Follows commands	Normal spontaneous movement	6
	Localizes pain	Withdraws to touch	5
	Withdraws in response to pain	Withdraws to pain	4
	Flexion in response to pain	Abnormal flexion	3
	Extension in response to pain	Abnormal extension	2
	None	None	1

Total Score: Minimum 1E + 1V + 1M = 3; Maximum 4E + 5V + 6M = 15.

should assess the patient's reaction and classify it into one of the following five categories: fending-off movements with localization of pain (score 5); fending-off movements without localization of pain (score 4); abnormal flexion (score 3); abnormal extension (score 2); and no response (score 1).

- A *localizing response* indicates that the stimulus at more than one site causes a limb to move so as to attempt to remove it.
- A *flexor response* in the upper limb may vary from rapid withdrawal associated with abduction of the shoulder to a slower decorticate posture with adduction of the shoulder.
- An *extensor response* is abnormal and usually associated with adduction, internal rotation of the shoulder, and pronation of the forearm.
- *No response* is usually associated with hypotonia.

It should be noted that the GCS score alone is not an adequate assessment of brainstem function. Neither does it assess vital signs (blood pressure, heart rate, body temperature, blood sugar); ability to protect the airway and clear any airway obstruction (cough and gag); and make an assessment as to what support or intervention is required to restore homeostasis. The GCS score should be calculated in the interval after any resuscitation and before any sedative or paralytic agents are used and when conveying information to other caregivers the individual components of the score are particularly helpful rather than a summed value alone.

Phase 1: Prehospital Care

The prehospital care of injured children is critical to outcome. Basic life support involves a rapid primary survey with an abbreviated, initial physical examination aimed at identifying and treating quickly any life-threatening injuries. The protection of the cervical spine and the identification and correction of airway obstruction, inadequate ventilation, and shock take priority over detailed neurologic assessment. In this context, general cardiopulmonary resuscitation takes precedence. **Table 61.7** outlines the hierarchy and initial priorities in prehospital management.

Airway

The initial evaluation begins by demonstrating the presence of a patent, maintainable airway; the patient must be conscious, alert, and breathing spontaneously. At the scene of an accident, the issues concerning recommendations for endotracheal intubation are complex and likely to include the expertise of attending paramedics and the distance for transport (58). The aim is to prevent hypoxia or hypercarbia, which may lead to secondary brain injury. Endotracheal intubation, if available, is the most effective procedure to maintain the airway. However, if prehospital endotracheal intubation is used within your system, then operators should have received specialized pediatric training in order to ensure that all intubated children have end-tidal carbon dioxide ($ETCO_2$) detectors to document correct tracheal tube placement.

The range of indications for endotracheal intubation is listed in **Table 61.8.** Beyond the prehospital setting, any children who are unable to open their eyes or verbalize must be considered candidates for intubation because of concerns about absent or impaired airway protective reflexes. Similarly, an unconscious patient must be assumed to have an obstructed airway that requires immediate evaluation. Intracranial hypertension with impending herniation may be inferred from the presence of dilated, unresponsive pupils or a triad of symptoms that includes systemic hypertension, bradycardia, and an abnormal breathing pattern.

The recommended route of airway control is orotracheal intubation; nasotracheal intubation should be avoided because of the possibility of base of skull fractures. Precautions to protect the cervical spine and minimize the rise in ICP associated with intubation should be undertaken. The patient's neck should be maintained in a neutral position, with axial traction applied by a person whose only role is to maintain the position of the neck. All trauma patients with supraclavicular injury should be assumed to have cranial and cervical spine injuries until proven otherwise.

Breathing and Ventilation

Several studies suggest that hypoxemia during prehospital care of children with severe TBI is common and that the proportion of patients with significant pulse oximetry oxygen–hemoglobin saturation (SpO_2) below 75% may be as high as 16% (59,60).

TABLE 61.7

PREHOSPITAL MANAGEMENT IN THE HEAD-INJURED CHILD

Spine
Spinal precautions maintained from time of first evaluation through to clearance
Neurology
Assess each component of the Glasgow Coma Scale score (see **Table 61.6**)
Examination of each pupil throughout resuscitation: asymmetry is present when there is >1 mm difference between the pupils; fixed pupil is defined as <1 mm response to bright light
Consider the signs of herniation remembering that eye trauma may mask the pupil signs
Airway
Basic and advanced care in order to maintain pulse oximetry measured oxygen-hemoglobin saturation (Spo_2) > 92%. Monitor Spo_2 continuously
Deliver supplemental oxygen by face-mask
Stabilize the airway in the spontaneously breathing patient while also maintaining cervical spine protection
If needed and tolerated use an oral airway to prevent airway occlusion by the tongue
Breathing
Endotracheal tube (ETT) intubation may be needed, but adhere to local Emergency Medical Systems recommendations.
Neuromuscular blockade to assist ETT intubation is not recommended unless appropriate training or personnel are in place.
If ETT intubation is used, check and maintain normal end-tidal carbon dioxide ($ETCO_2$) at 35–40 mm Hg
Hyperventilation to $ETCO_2$ <35 mm Hg can be used as a temporary measure if signs of herniation are present—titrate duration to resolution of signs
Circulation
Monitor blood pressure continuously using noninvasive arm-cuff and maintain systolic blood pressure above the fifth percentile for age (i.e., 70 mm Hg + [2 × Age in years])
Obtain intravenous access. If this is not possible, intraosseous access can be used
Monitor electrocardiogram continuously
Systolic hypotension should be treated with normal saline 20 mL/kg bolus doses
Check blood glucose level and correct hypoglycemia (<40–60 mg/dL) with intravenous dextrose: infant, dextrose 10%, 5 mL/kg; toddler, dextrose 25%, 2 mL/kg; older child, dextrose 50%, 1 mL/kg

In patients with SCI, the pattern of respiratory dysfunction depends on the level of injury (**Fig. 61.2**). A complete SCI above C3 causes respiratory arrest and death unless immediate ventilatory assistance is given. Injury at the C3–C5 level leads to respiratory failure, but the onset might be delayed. In severe TBI, supplemental oxygen (100%) should be provided in the resuscitation phase of care for all patients with moderate-to-severe injury in order to prevent, and immediately correct, hypoxia that could cause secondary brain injury. Monitoring oxygenation and ventilation should be assessed continuously by Spo_2 and, in intubated patients; $ETCO_2$ monitoring should also be used. Patients with physical findings suggestive of brainstem compression from brain tissue herniation should be hyperventilated with 100% oxygen as soon as possible to acutely lower ICP.

TABLE 61.8

INDICATIONS FOR INTUBATION IN THE HEAD-INJURED CHILD

Upper airway obstruction or loss of airway protective reflexes
Loss of pharyngeal muscle activity and tone
Inability to clear secretions
Foreign body
Direct trauma
Seizures
Abnormal breathing due to
Chest wall dysfunction
Respiratory muscle dysfunction
Pulmonary disease: aspiration, contusion, or neurogenic
Cervical spine injury
Apnea
Arterial partial pressure of carbon dioxide ($Paco_2$)
Hypercarbia: $Paco_2$ > 45 mm Hg
Hypocapnia: spontaneous hyperventilation, causing $Paco_2$ < 25 mm Hg
Pupils
Anisocoria > 1 mm
Glasgow Coma Scale (GCS) score
GCS < 9
Fall in GCS score of >3, irrespective of initial GCS

Circulation

After the airway and ventilation are confirmed as being ad-
1 equate, the next step is assessment and optimization of the circulation. The injured brain is at risk from hypotension and inadequate perfusion, problems that have a number of potential causes. Blood loss may be present. Generally, blood loss sufficient to cause hypotension is not due to bleeding in the cranium, except in small infants in whom subgaleal hematomas can be life-threatening. Cardiogenic shock and arrhythmia may be present due to cardiac contusion. Alternatively, neurogenic shock may be present in cases of SCI above T4. This hemodynamic syndrome reflects sympathetic denervation of the heart (T1–T4) and vasculature, with resulting decreased
2 inotropism, chronotropism, and arterial and venous dilation. It may be difficult to differentiate this syndrome from hypovolemia, but lack of compensatory tachycardia can be a useful diagnostic sign.

The initial assessment of circulatory function in patients with TBI includes the rapid determination of heart rate, blood pressure, quality of central and peripheral pulses, and capillary refill time. In children, hypotension is defined as systolic blood

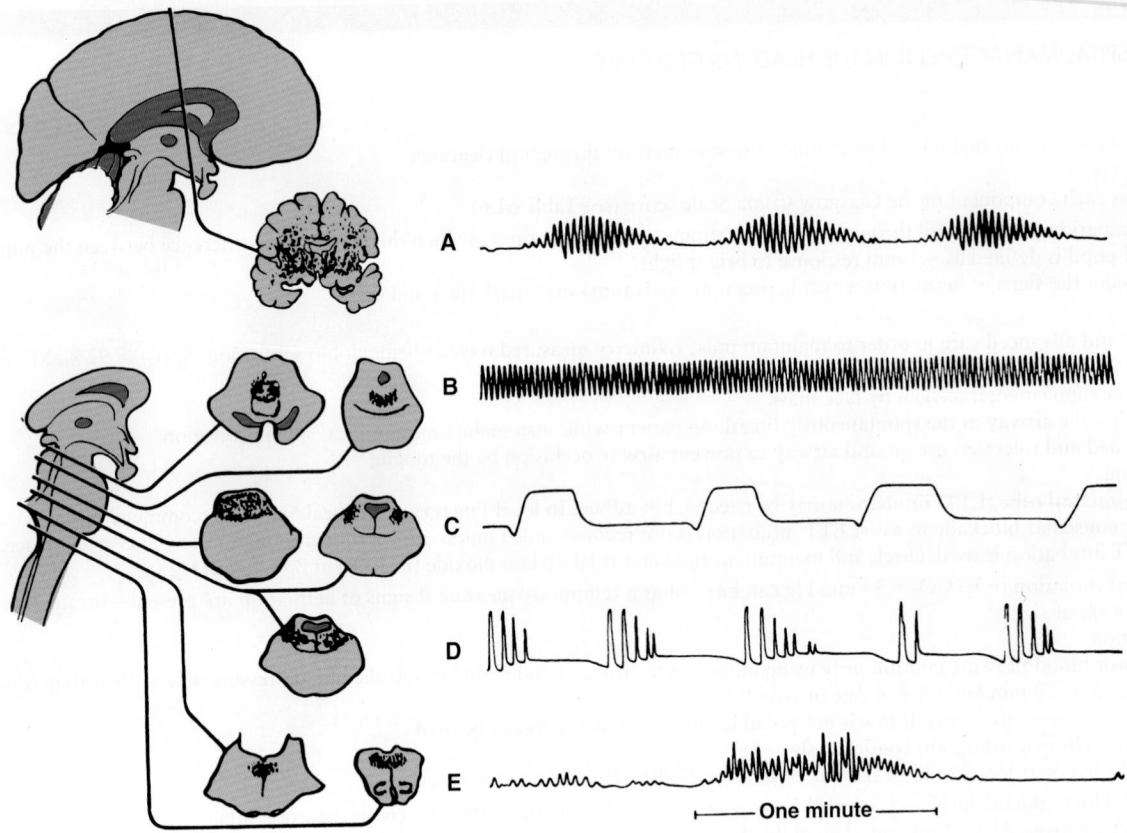

FIGURE 61.2. Abnormal breathing patterns due to lesions at different levels of the brain. Injury to different portions of the brain leads to distinctive abnormal breathing patterns that may help to localize the area of injury. **A:** Cheyne–Stokes respiration or alternating phases of hyperpnea indicate dysfunction deep within the cerebral hemispheres or diencephalon. **B:** Hyperventilation, or tachypnea, indicates damage in the rostral brainstem or tegmentum. **C:** Apneustic breathing or prolonged sustained end-inspiratory pauses indicate damage at the midpontine or caudal pontine level. **D:** Cluster breathing (periodic respirations that are irregular in amplitude) indicates lower pontine or high medullary injury. **E:** Ataxic respiration (completely random and irregular breathing) indicates medullary damage. See also text for explanation of each breathing pattern. (From Mettler FA. *Neuroanatomy.* St. Louis, MO: CV Mosby, 1948:816, with permission.)

pressure below the fifth percentile for age or by clinical signs of shock. The fifth percentile for age of systolic blood pressure can be estimated from the formula: 70 mm Hg + (2 × age in years). Hypotension should be identified and corrected as rapidly as possible with fluid resuscitation. If necessary, an intravenous bolus of 20 mL/kg 0.9% sodium chloride solution should be administered as soon as vascular access is obtained. Hypotonic fluid should not be used in the initial resuscitation phase, and subsequent doses of fluid should be guided by serial assessment of blood pressure, perfusion, and hematocrit.

Phase 2: Emergency Department and Hospital Management

At the time of arrival in the emergency department, the hierarchy and priorities for resuscitation and life support remain the same as those already outlined in **Table 61.7**. Rapid airway, breathing, and circulation assessment should be made and the patient intubated, if necessary, under the controlled conditions of a full resuscitation team and expert airway practitioners (**Table 61.8**).

Controlled Endotracheal Intubation

Rapid sequence intubation is the preferred method of securing the airway in children with suspected raised ICP, since it

provides protection against the reflex responses to laryngoscopy and rises in ICP. Coma does not signify the lack of a need to use pharmacologic agents for pretreatment, induction of anesthesia, and neuromuscular blockade. Problems associated with elevated ICP may be compounded by the techniques and drugs used in airway management, since they may further elevate ICP. Hence, throughout the procedure, attention should be given for minimizing risk of herniation and maintaining adequate cerebral perfusion with good blood pressure control. In practice this means optimizing body positioning before endotracheal intubation and avoiding hypoventilation. Keep the head of the bed up, with the patient's head in the midline, until you are ready to lay the patient flat in order to perform direct laryngoscopy. Pre-oxygenate the patient with 100% oxygen so as to maintain SpO_2 above 94%. When you are ready and the "intubation checklist" is complete, the medications we use are as below.

Airway Reflexes. When the airway is manipulated, two responses may occur and cause further increase in ICP: (a) the *reflex sympathetic response*, which results in tachycardia and hypertension and, in consequence, further increase in ICP; (b) the *direct laryngeal reflex*, which stimulates a patient response causing an increase in intrathoracic pressure, which is transmitted to the intracranial space and results in an increase in ICP independent of the reflex sympathetic response. In practice, pretreatment of the reflex sympathetic response is not needed in the hypotensive patient with suspected raised ICP.

However, elevation in ICP should be limited by minimizing airway manipulation—the most experienced operator should be performing this procedure and administering medication. Lidocaine, 1–1.5 mg/kg IV 60–180 seconds before intubation, is used by some operators to attenuate the direct laryngeal reflex, and it may limit the reflex sympathetic response.

Induction of Anesthesia.
Induction of anesthesia is carried out using an agent that will not affect maintenance of good cerebral perfusion. Again, local experience and expertise will dictate what medications are used. Commonly used agents include etomidate, propofol, or thiopental. Etomidate (0.3 mg/kg intravenous push) is a short-acting imidazole derivative that provides hypnosis with minimal hemodynamic effect. Its onset of action is 30–60 seconds and the duration of effect is 3–5 minutes. It is a good choice for patients with hypotension and suspected raised ICP. It decreases CBF and ICP, and preserves cerebral perfusion. Of concern is that it decreases seizure threshold and it decreases cortisol synthesis. Propofol (2 mg/kg intravenous push) is an alternative induction agent, but it has potent vasodilator and myocardial depressive actions such that hypotension is to be expected. Hence, simultaneous vasopressor and fluid administration may be needed to maintain cerebral perfusion. It reduces ICP and has anticonvulsive effects. Its onset of action is 10–50 seconds and the duration of effect is 3–10 minutes. Thiopental at a dose of 1–5 mg/kg (intravenous push) decreases the cerebral metabolic rate for oxygen, CBF, and ICP. However, it is a potent venodilator and negative inotrope with a strong tendency to cause hypotension and reduce cerebral perfusion. *A lower dose should be used in patients suspected of inadequate preload or hemodynamic compromise.* Its onset of action is 30–60 seconds and the duration of effect is 3–50 minutes. Although TBI has traditionally been considered a contraindication to ketamine, a recent systematic review in adults suggests that ketamine (2 mg/kg intravenous push) is an alternative induction agent for patients who are hypotensive and have suspected increased ICP (61).

Neuromuscular Blockade.
Succinylcholine (1.5–2 mg/kg intravenous), a depolarizing neuromuscular blocking agent, is the treatment of choice for emergency endotracheal intubation of the head-injured child with suspected raised ICP, because it has a rapid onset and short duration of action—30–60 seconds and 5–15 minutes, respectively. It should not be used in patients with hyperkalemia, known neuromuscular disease, or history of malignant hyperthermia. Its use in patients with eye injuries is controversial and the risk of extrusion of intraocular contents needs to be considered. Traditionally, we do not use succinylcholine in the TSCI patient; however, the risk of hyperkalemia from depolarization generally occurs after the first 48 hours of injury, once upregulation of acetylcholine receptors has occurred. In all of these instances, a nondepolarizing drug such as rocuronium (1.2–1.4 mg/kg, intravenous push) can be used. Its onset of action is 45–60 seconds and the duration of effect is 47–70 minutes.

Intubation for SCI

Every head trauma patient is presumed to have spinal cord trauma until proven otherwise. Hence, rapid sequence intubation as described above should always be accompanied by precautions to protect the cervical spine including in-line stabilization of the patient's neck by an assistant or use of a cervical collar.

The patient with suspected *isolated* cervical spine injury will also require specific spinal cord protective measures. For example, pre-intubation airway maneuvers (e.g., jaw tilt, bag-mask-valve ventilation, and direct laryngoscopy) can all be directly injurious to the spinal cord. Also, hypoxia or tracheal or laryngeal manipulation, at the time of intubation, can stimulate a bradycardic response, which will impair spinal cord perfusion.

An experienced operator can use an "awake" fiberoptic approach to intubate the trachea if (a) the patient has isolated spinal cord trauma without head trauma; (b) the patient is old enough to cooperate after topical anesthesia to the nasopharynx. This technique minimizes movement of the cervical spine and the risk of exacerbating SCI in the setting of ligamentous or fracture instability. The cervical collar should be removed while maintaining in-line stabilization. Extreme care must be taken to avoid hyperextension of the neck.

Aspiration is also a risk in patients with SCI. Trauma patients may have delayed gastric emptying. Therefore, large-bore suction devices should be immediately available in the event of vomiting even when airway protective reflexes remain intact.

Injury above upper thoracic spine levels may lead to loss of sympathetic tone and hypotension without the capacity to mount a compensatory increase in heart rate. Spinal shock results and is associated with a profound reduction in cardiac output. Anesthetic medications that diminish the catecholamine surge during intubation may also result in exacerbation of hypotension and bradycardia. Atropine should always be available.

Postintubation Procedures and Mechanical Ventilation

Immediately after endotracheal intubation the fractional inspired oxygen can be reduced to 0.5, or the lowest fraction that achieves adequate oxygenation. The head of the bed should be returned to the 30-degree-head-up position and the patient's head kept midline. A central venous line will need to be placed, but this should not involve placing the patient in the Trendelenburg position, turning the neck to one side, or compressing neck vessels—all of these maneuvers will lead to a rise in ICP and, possibly, evolution to herniation. Rather, a large-bore brachial venous line or other alternative is required in the acute setting.

The initial postintubation mechanical ventilator goals are:

- Normalization of oxygenation with the lowest fractional inspired oxygen in order to maintain SpO_2 >94%. In some instances, positive end-expiratory pressure (PEEP) will be required to maintain oxygenation. However, the ICP must be monitored during the application of PEEP in TBI patients, because the associated increase in intrathoracic pressure may decrease cerebral venous return and thereby raise ICP.
- Normalization of ventilation to achieve pH 7.35–7.45, with partial pressure CO_2 ($PaCO_2$) 35–45 mm Hg. The latter can be followed by $ETCO_2$ monitoring. Overventilation with large tidal volumes (>8 mL/kg) should be avoided so as to limit the risk of acute lung injury.
- Normalization of work of breathing, and avoidance of agitation and awareness. This will require optimization of patient–ventilator synchrony (or use of neuromuscular blockade) and use of sedative analgesic medications. In pediatric practice we use a benzodiazepine–opiate combination. In many countries, the adult practice of propofol by continuous infusion for sedation is not recommended in PICU patients.

When life-threatening raised ICP and brain herniation is suspected, intentional hyperventilation will be required temporarily until CT scan and definitive treatment (e.g., hematoma evacuation, decompressive craniectomy). In this circumstance, it is worth knowing that maximal cerebral vasoconstriction is achieved at $PaCO_2$ 20 mm Hg, so hyperventilation below this level will be ineffective and may even result in hypotension, which will further worsen cerebral hypoperfusion.

Survey of Other Injuries

After endotracheal tube intubation, if needed, it is appropriate to make a more extensive review of the immediate, life-threatening injuries beside those to the head and to make a more detailed review of the neurology. The aim of this survey is to identify all traumatic injuries and to begin to prioritize treatment. A thorough physical examination is required; the areas of this survey that are especially important in TBI are discussed here.

Head

Examination of the head entails careful inspection for surface depressions, swellings, lacerations, or ecchymoses that would indicate underlying injury. Evidence of skull-base fracture includes Battle sign (retro-auricular ecchymosis), raccoon eyes (periorbital ecchymosis), cerebrospinal fluid (CSF) otorrhea, CSF rhinorrhea, and hemotympanum. Evidence of facial fracture includes instability of facial bones and zygoma (i.e., LeFort fracture) and facial step-off abnormality (i.e., orbital rim fracture). Depending on mechanism of injury, if any lacerations are present, they should be explored with a gloved finger so that underlying open or depressed skull fracture or foreign material can be identified.

In infants, the fontanelles and sutures should be palpated. The tone of the fontanelle (bulging, soft, or sunken) is an indication of ICP level. If possible, the head circumference should be measured and recorded. The mouth should be examined, and notation should be made as to whether the frenulum is torn or not. Last, evidence of extracranial vascular injury should be sought. Abnormal carotid neck pulses, bruits, and Horner syndrome indicate traumatic carotid dissection. Eye globe bruit indicates traumatic carotid cavernous fistula.

Neck

Injury to the cervical spine must be assumed to have occurred in any head-injured patient until such time as neck soft tissue or bony injury has been ruled out. The neck should be immobilized in an appropriately sized collar, and manipulation should be kept to a minimum. If the collar is removed for any reason, the neck should be held in midline position and a single operator should apply gentle axial traction. Obvious deformity, swelling, or ecchymosis of the neck should be visible on inspection. Palpation of the neck may show a malalignment, step-off, or splaying of the spinous processes, suggesting a ligamentous and unstable injury.

Thorax

The chest wall should be observed for the pattern and adequacy of ventilation. Specific patterns of breathing are seen with head injury and may have important localizing value (Fig. 61.2). Posthyperventilation apnea indicates forebrain damage. Cheyne–Stokes respiration (Fig. 61.2A) or alternating phases of hyperpnea are caused by dysfunction deep within the cerebral hemispheres or diencephalon. Hyperventilation (Fig. 61.2B) or persistent, rapid breathing is caused by damage in the rostral brainstem or tegmentum. Apneustic breathing (Fig. 61.2C), or prolonged sustained end-inspiratory pauses, is caused by damage at the midpontine or caudal pontine level. Cluster breathing (Fig. 61.2D), periodic respirations that are irregular in amplitude, is seen with lower pontine or high medullary injury. Ataxic respiration (Fig. 61.2E), or completely random and irregular breathing, indicates damage to the medulla.

Spinal injury above the level of C4 results in paralysis of all muscles involved in breathing. These patients have poor-to-absent spontaneous respiratory effort. Injuries to the lower cervical spinal cord spare the diaphragm but abolish some of the accessory muscle strength, resulting in decreased vital capacity and retention of secretions. In adults, a direct relationship exists between the level of cord injury and the degree of respiratory dysfunction. With high lesions (i.e., C1 or C2) vital capacity is only 5%–10% of normal and cough is absent. With lesions at C3–C6, vital capacity is 20% of normal and cough is weak and ineffective. With high thoracic cord injuries (i.e., T2–T4), vital capacity is 30%–50% of normal and cough is weak. With lower cord injuries, respiratory function improves, and with injuries at T11, respiratory function, vital capacity, and cough should be near normal.

Detailed Neurology

The next step after adequate initial survey and stabilization is assessment of the neurologic examination. This process should be succinct and aimed primarily at diagnosing and treating life-threatening intracranial hypertension with imminent brain tissue herniation (Table 61.4), or a lesion needing emergency surgery.

Pupillary Response

The pupillary response to light should be assessed first. The pupillary size at rest and reaction to light (both direct and consensual) should be noted. The light reflex consists of an afferent pathway through the optic nerve (CN II) and an efferent pathway that involves both sympathetic and parasympathetic fibers. Transtentorial herniation causes compression of the parasympathetic fibers along CN III and results in ipsilateral pupillary dilation with no response to direct or consensual stimulation. Bilateral dilated pupils that are unresponsive indicate, in the absence of medication or poisoning, bilaterally compressed CN III or severe cerebral hypoxia–ischemia. The presence of unilateral or bilateral dilated, unresponsive pupil is an indication for emergency hyperventilation, brain imaging, and surgical evacuation of a hematoma, if present.

Pinpoint pupils are associated with pontine lesions. Unilateral pupil dilation unreactive to direct stimulation but consensually reactive is caused by absent light perception in that eye or a deafferentated pupil. Alternately shining the light into each eye reveals the paradoxical dilation on the affected side with direct stimulation; this is the Marcus Gunn pupil and represents dilation of the affected side after consensually stimulated constriction. When light is shone into the deafferentated eye, both eyes perceive darkness and both eyes dilate accordingly. Ipsilateral pupillary constriction associated with ptosis and anhidrosis (i.e., Horner syndrome) may be an early sign of transtentorial herniation, damage to the hypothalamus with interruption of sympathetic pathways, or disruption of the cervical sympathetics. Injury to the midbrain tectum may result in pupils that are at midposition and fixed to light but retain hippus, the ciliospinal reflex, and response to accommodation.

Ocular Responses

The position of the eyes at rest should be noted, and any deviation, conjugate, or disconjugate recorded. Spontaneous eye movements, including roving eye movements, ocular bobbing, or nystagmus, should be sought. Other noteworthy ocular phenomena are increased blinking, intermittent lid retraction, convergent or divergent spasms, and monocular nystagmus, most of which imply brainstem dysfunction. The corneal reflex should be tested, as its presence does relate to depth of coma.

Ocular motility should then be assessed with the "doll's eye maneuver" (also known as oculocephalic reflex) in comatose patients *but only if the cervical spine is known to be stable*. The child's eyelids are held open while the head is briskly rotated first to one side and then the other. A positive response, indicating an intact pathway in the brainstem, is obtained by full conjugate eye deviation to the opposite side (i.e., if the head is rotated to the right, the eyes deviate to the left). Vertical eye movements are tested by briskly flexing and extending the neck. A positive response is observed when the eyes deviate upward with neck flexion and downward with neck extension. Further assessment of brainstem function by the "caloric" or oculovestibular response may cause discomfort and should only be performed in the deeply unconscious child. It is important to ensure that the tympanic membranes are intact before starting to instill up to 60 mL of iced saline.

Examination of the fundi is best left until other ocular signs and responses have been documented. Adequate fundal examination is important, but sometimes it can only be achieved through the use of short-acting mydriatics. The clinician should consider this decision judiciously and, when employed, the patient must be labeled as having received these drugs and the fact must be clearly documented. When long-acting mydriatics are being used, consideration may be given to dilating one pupil and waiting until responsiveness has returned to dilate the other. In this way, one pupil can continue to be assessed for dilation and responsiveness at all times. Other intracranial hemorrhages should be strongly suspected if retinal hemorrhages are seen. Venous pulsations in the retinal vessels are a helpful sign, as their presence precludes any significant increase in ICP. Papilledema is the single most reliable sign of intracranial hypertension. With acute elevations in ICP, papilledema is rarely seen in the first 24–48 hours.

Motor System

Asymmetry of the face should be noted, and the gag reflex elicited. Assessment of power is best achieved by observing movement in response to supraorbital or sternal pressure. Responses to stimulation of the limbs may be reflex and serve to confuse the picture. Focal weakness usually implies a structural lesion. Tone should be assessed in all four limbs. Patterns of decerebration should be closely observed for, and not mistaken as, seizures. Whether they are unilateral or bilateral and whether they are spontaneous or occur only after stimulation must be assessed. In infants, "bicycling" movements of the upper and lower limbs may precede these episodes.

In comatose patients, the activity of the brainstem motor nuclei and their spinal projections may be used as indicators of the levels of brainstem impairment. Appropriate localizing and flexor responses in a comatose patient imply that sensory pathways are functioning and that the pyramidal tract from the cerebral cortex to effector is functioning, at least partially. When both sides are tested, unilateral absence of responses is consistent with interruption of the corticospinal tract somewhere along its length. Loss of response on both sides could reflect a lesion in the brainstem that interrupts the corticospinal tracts bilaterally, or injury to the pontomedullary reticular formation and associated extrapyramidal pathways.

Decorticate and Decerebrate Posturing. These inappropriate motor responses depend on the level of brainstem injury and are demonstrated by three main responses to a painful stimulus: *decorticate rigidity*, *decerebrate rigidity*, and *decerebrate changes in the arms combined with flexor responses in the legs*.

Decorticate rigidity consists of flexion of the arms, wrist, and fingers, with adduction in the upper extremity and extension, internal rotation, and plantar flexion in the lower extremity. This motor pattern occurs if the impairment of brainstem activity is located *above the level of the red nucleus*, as seen with lesions involving the corticospinal pathways at the internal capsule, cerebral hemisphere, or rostral cerebral peduncle. It occurs because the red nucleus has a strong influence on upper limb flexion.

Decerebrate rigidity consists of opisthotonus with the teeth clenched, the arms extended, adducted and hyperpronated, and the legs extended with the feet plantar flexed. This motor pattern occurs if the impairment of brainstem activity is located *between the levels of the rostral poles of the red nucleus and vestibular nuclei* (rostral midbrain to mid-pons), as seen during rostral-caudal deterioration with transtentorial herniation, expanding posterior fossa lesions, or neurotoxicity of the upper brainstem. It occurs because of the reduction in extensor inhibition normally exerted on the reticular formation by the cerebral cortex. As a result, the spinal extensor motor neurons are driven by extensor facilitation parts of the reticular formation that, during a painful stimulus, are activated by the pathways transmitting these impulses. The lateral vestibular nuclei are also intimately involved because, experimentally, extensor posturing is greatly reduced when the lateral vestibular nuclei are ablated.

Decerebrate rigidity or posturing in the arms combined with either flaccidity or weak flexor responses in the legs is a motor pattern that is found in patients with extensive brainstem damage extending down to or across the pons at the trigeminal level.

In extensor hypertonus, the lower limbs are extended with internal rotation and, often, plantar flexion and scissoring. Positioning in the upper limbs may be one of two distinct types. In decorticate rigidity, the arms are flexed across the chest, while in decerebrate rigidity, the elbows are extended. Such rigidity may result from structural lesions and is often associated with a rise in ICP. It is generally considered that decorticate posturing is associated with cortical or hemisphere dysfunction, whereas the brainstem is more often damaged in children in whom the upper limbs show decerebrate patterns.

The patient should be observed for seizures. Generalized tonic–clonic seizures or myoclonic jerks will be easily identified, but the more subtle phenomena seen in infants, such as cyanosis and chewing movements, are less readily recognized as ictal.

Finally, the deep tendon reflexes should be elicited. Areflexia in combination with flaccidity that is not due to muscle relaxants is grave. Asymmetric reflexes may be helpful in lateralizing the injury. Bilateral hyperactive reflexes may be associated with TBI or TSCI but should be symmetric and not associated with pathologic reflexes. Rapid, sustained dorsiflexion of each ankle to test for clonus should be performed. Stroking the sole of the foot with a firm object should cause a reflex of the great toe; a positive Babinski reflex occurs when the patient dorsiflexes his toe. Many infants retain this response and, in them, the test has little diagnostic value.

Functional Integrity of the Spine and Spinal Cord

The entire spine should be examined carefully. The patient should be log-rolled (with the head kept in-line) to perform this examination. Ecchymoses indicate trauma in the region and should be noted. The spinal column should be palpated, and widening of spaces between adjacent spinous processes, malalignment of the spine, or step-off of the spinous processes may indicate underlying distraction or dislocation.

The functional integrity of the spinal cord is evaluated by a thorough motor and sensory examination. The American

Spine Injury Association (ASIA at http://www.asia-spinalin-jury.org) has a new *International Standard for Neurological Classification of SCI* with a stepwise approach in determining lateralization of sensory levels, motor levels, the neurological level of injury, whether the injury is complete or incomplete, and the ASIA impairment scale grade. In the assessment of motor function grading, ASIA recommends use of the following scale of findings for the assessment of motor strength in TSCI:

0, total paralysis
1, palpable or visible contraction
2, active movement, full range of motion with gravity eliminated
3, active movement, full range of motion against gravity
4, active movement, full range of motion against gravity and moderate resistance in a muscle specific position
5, normal active movement, full range of motion against gravity and full resistance in a functional muscle position expected from an otherwise unimpaired person

5*, normal active movement, full range of motion against gravity and sufficient resistance to be considered normal if identified inhibiting factors (e.g., pain) are not present.

The systematic examination required for formal assessment in TSCI is best recorded using the charts that are available from the ASIA website (see above). However, by way of summary, **Figure 61.3** and **Table 61.9** provide general criteria for determining sensory and motor level. Superficial reflexes, such as abdominal, cremasteric, and anal reflexes, are also helpful in localizing the level of injury. Absent or diminished superficial reflexes suggest corticospinal lesions above the segmental innervation of this reflex. The sensory level is described according to the lowest dermatome in which sensation to light touch and pinprick is normal.

Complete injury is signified by loss of motor function, segmental reflexes, and sensation below a given level. The *zone of partial preservation* is an area adjacent to the neurologic level in which abnormal sensory and motor findings are noted.

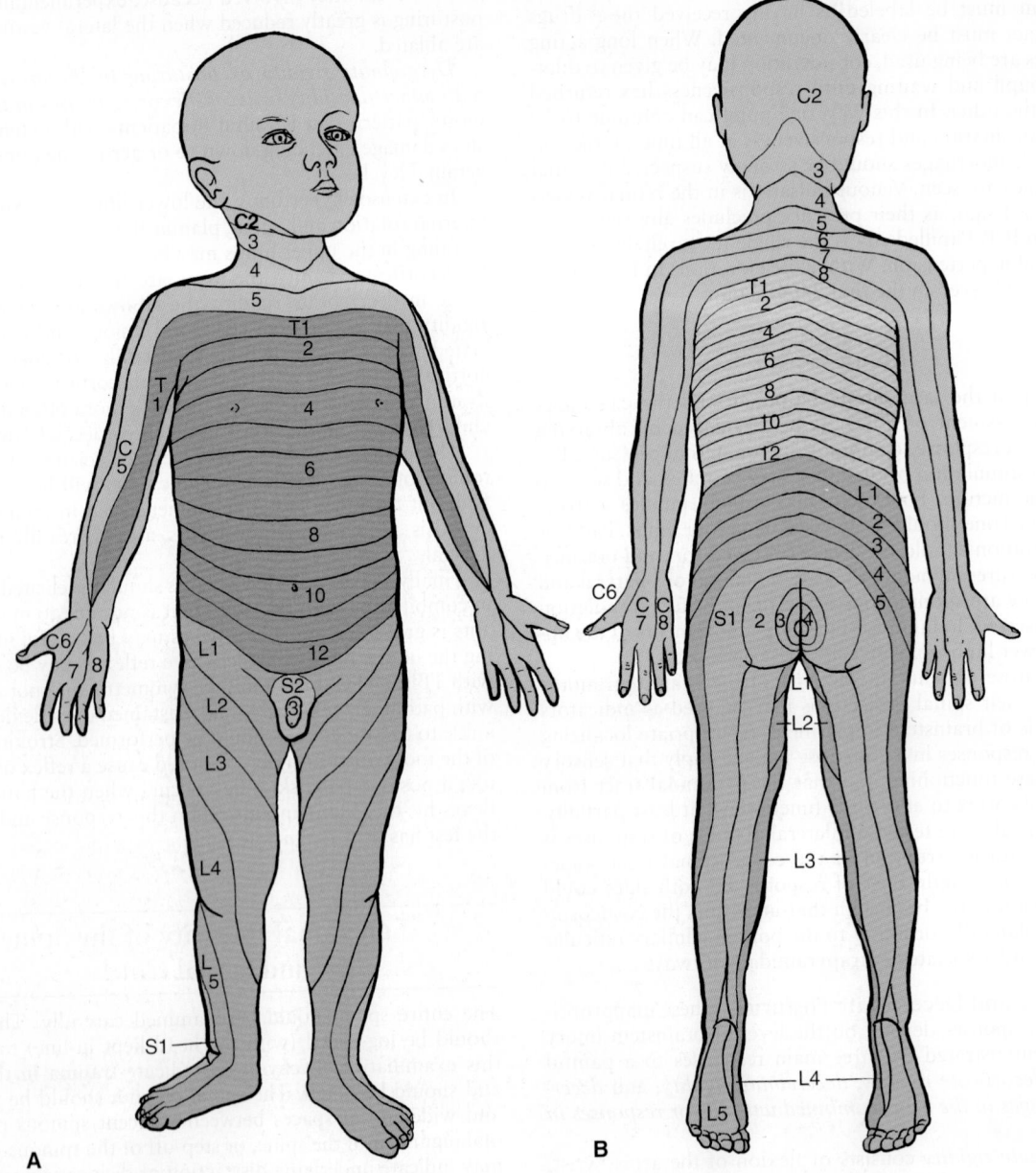

FIGURE 61.3. Segmental dermatomes are reproducible and helpful in identifying the level of spinal cord injury.

TABLE 61.9

NERVE ROOTS UNDERLYING MUSCLE FUNCTION AND REFLEXES

■ NERVE ROOT	■ MUSCLES AND FUNCTION	■ REFLEXES
C4	Diaphragm Inspiration	

C5	Deltoid
	  Shoulder flexion
	  Shoulder abduction
		Biceps (C5, C6)

C6	Biceps Elbow flexion	
C7	Extensor carpi radialis Wrist extension	Triceps (C7, C8)
C8	Flexor digitorum superficialis Finger flexion	

T1	Interossei
	  Finger abduction
	  Finger adduction	

T2–T7	Intercostals
	  Expiration
	  Forced expiration	

T8–T12	Abdominals
	  Expiration
	  Trunk flexion
		Superficial abdominals

L2	Iliopsoas Hip flexion	Cremasteric (L1, L2)
L3	Quadriceps Knee extension	Knee (L3, L4)
L4	Tibialis anterior Foot dorsiflexion	
L5	Extensor hallucis longus Great toe extension	Hamstring (L5, S1)
S1	Gastrocnemius Foot plantar flexion	Ankle (S1, S2)
S2–S5	Anal sphincter Fecal continence	Bulbocavernosus (S3, S4) Anal wink (S5)

An area of abnormal findings that is not contiguous with the postulated level qualifies as *incomplete injury*. As this lesion has the potential for improvement, a reassessment is vital. The function that is classically retained is that of the sacral nerves, which means that perianal sensation and reflexes must be tested and documented. The sacral roots are assessed using perineal sensation to light touch and pinprick, bulbocavernosus reflex (S3, S4), anal wink (S5) and rectal tone, and evidence of urine retention or incontinence. Flaccid areflexic paralysis and anesthesia to all modalities characterize *spinal shock*. This problem is found in half of TSCI patients and resolves within 24 hours in >90%. SCI above the seventh thoracic vertebra may mask the tenderness normally associated with an intra-abdominal injury. Therefore, a high index of suspicion is needed in these patients to diagnose intra-abdominal bleeding.

INITIAL INVESTIGATIONS

The purpose of emergency laboratory and neuroradiologic investigations in the child with TBI or TSCI is to be able to respond to four key questions:

- Do any systemic metabolic or acid–base derangements require correction?
- Does this patient have intracranial pathology that requires emergency surgery?

- Does this patient have an unstable spine that needs fixation?
- Does this patient require full investigation for suspected inflicted or abusive injury (see Chapter 62)?

Phase 3: Laboratory and Imaging Studies

A variety of baseline blood and serum tests are required in children with TBI or SCI. These include hemoglobin concentration and a saved sample for transfusion cross-matching; serum electrolytes, liver and renal function; and blood glucose level. Coagulation studies are usually checked in case ICP monitoring is needed. A full account of neuroradiologic investigation is discussed in Chapter 59. This section will focus on some of the issues related to the process of patient care and management.

Head CT

The head CT scan should be performed after respiratory and hemodynamic stabilization of the injured patient. Cardiorespiratory compromise within the scanner should be expected and avoided. This initial form of imaging is the diagnostic tool of choice in the acute phase of managing moderate and severe TBI. The CT scan serves primarily to detect life-threatening abnormalities requiring urgent neurosurgery, but in more severe cases it can also be used to decide whether to monitor ICP in the PICU. An unenhanced head CT scan is the test of choice because it reveals both hemorrhage and bony injury. The indications for head CT include GCS ≤14, progressive headache, decline in level of consciousness, seizure, unreliable history, vomiting, amnesia, signs of skull fracture or facial injury, penetrating skull injury, or focal or abnormal neurology. The initial head CT should include visualization of the craniocervical junction so that AOD, rotatory subluxation of C1 on C2, and other craniocervical disruptions can be evaluated.

Patients with negative CT scans and mild neurologic disturbances, such as posttraumatic seizures (PTS), vomiting, headache, irritability, or GCS score of 12–15, can be observed. Children with normal examination or minimal neurologic deficit and small EDH, SDH, or intraparenchymal hemorrhage may also be closely observed. In the child with a lower GCS score, the absence of abnormalities on initial CT does not rule out ICP elevation. A skull x-ray is only helpful if head CT scan is not available.

Prognostication Using Head CT. The head CT scan may also help with prognostication and optimizing treatments. In adults, there are two validated scales for rating CT scans acutely after TBI: the Traumatic Coma Databank (TCDB) CT classification (62) and the Rotterdam CT score (63). Both of these classification systems (**Table 61.10**) have significant correlation with Glasgow Outcome Score at 3 and 12 months after injury. The discriminating features of the TCDB-CT classification are (a) presence or absence of mass lesions,

(b) presence or absence of intracranial abnormalities, (c) CT signs of raised ICP (status of basal cisterns and midline shift), and (d) planned evacuation of mass lesions. However, this classification does not recognize the type of traumatic intracranial mass lesion and includes CT changes from impression fracture over contusions to extra-axial hematomas. The Rotterdam CT classification describes the severity of TBI on the CT in a similar manner to the TCDB-CT classification. The scale was originally investigated in the combined data sets of the International and North American Tirilazad trials conducted between 1991 and 1994; 2249 CT scans were available in 2269 patients with ages between 15 and 65 years, and the overall mortality was 22% at 6 months after injury. Recursive partitioning and logistic regression analyses were used to develop the model based on key predictors of 6-month mortality in this population. The main difference between the two systems is that the Rotterdam classification uses a scoring chart with CT characteristics (including type of mass lesion and hematoma or hemorrhage) to estimate outcome. The total scores in Rotterdam classification range from 1 to 6, where a score of 2 may represent no positive findings or a normal CT scan. A score of ≥3 represents complex intracranial findings. There is a direct correlation between Rotterdam score and mortality in children (4). A large series (>600 cases) of pediatric patients with moderate or severe TBI (4) shows that the adult risk-adjustment model for expected mortality using the Rotterdam score discriminates well the observed mortality in pediatric cases, but it had poor calibration (i.e., it overestimated mortality for Rotterdam scores of 2 and 3, and underestimated mortality for

---

TABLE 61.10

SCORING SYSTEMS FOR CT SCAN GRADING OF SEVERITY

■ SCORING SYSTEM	■ DEFINITION OF CT ABNORMALITIES IN TBI
TCDB grades (I–IV)	**Diffuse injury I** ■ No visible intracranial pathology on CT scan **Diffuse injury II** ■ Cisterns are present with midline shift 0–5 mm and/or lesion densities present ■ No high- or mixed-density lesion >25 cm³ that may include bone fragments and foreign bodies **Diffuse III (swelling)** ■ Cisterns compressed or absent with midline shift of 0–5 mm ■ No high- or mixed-density lesion >25 cm³ **Diffuse IV (shift)** ■ Midline shift >5 mm or high- or mixed-density lesion >25 cm³ **Evacuated mass lesion** Any lesion surgically evacuated **Nonevacuated mass lesion** ■ High- or mixed-density lesion >25 cm³ not surgically evacuated
Rotterdam CT score (total 1–6)	**Basal cisterns (scores 0–2)** ■ Normal = 0 ■ Compressed = 1 ■ Absent = 2 **Midline shift (scores 0 or 1)** ■ No shift or ≤5 mm = 0 ■ Shift >5 mm = 1 **Epidural mass lesion (scores 0 or 1)** ■ Present = 0 ■ Absent = 1 **Intraventricular blood or traumatic subarachnoid hemorrhage (scores 0 or 1)** ■ Absent = 0 ■ Present = 1 **Final score** = sum of the above scores +1

TBI, traumatic brain injury; TCDB, Traumatic Coma Databank.

scores of 4–6). These findings support an age-dependent bio-mechanical hypothesis (see above), since the authors found that 47% of their pediatric patients with moderate or severe TBI had Rotterdam CT score of 1 or 2, and only 9 of these cases died (mortality 0.03%).

Spinal Imaging and Assessment of Stability

Imaging of the spine should be obtained in all patients with pain or tenderness of the neck or back, sensory or motor deficits, an impaired level of consciousness, or with painful, distracting injuries outside of the spinal region. The goal of imaging is to rapidly identify injury of the spine that places neural tissue at risk. The majority of patients with TSCI are found to have associated spine injury. The standard practice for cervical radiographs includes anteroposterior, lateral, and odontoid views. Technically adequate films allow visualization of the entire cervical spine to the C7 through T1 intervertebral space. Lateral views should be screened for changes in vertebral alignment, bony structure, intervertebral space, and soft tissue. Flexion–extension views are useful for detecting occult instability that results from ligamentous injury. This procedure is safe only in patients who are neurologically intact and in whom there is no subluxation greater than 3.5 mm on lateral films. Spinal CT scan with three-dimensional reconstruction has become more common and has in many instances replaced plain radiographs because of the improved visualization and the ability to combine with the trauma head CT and reduce the radiation exposure in children. Spinal CT

is very sensitive in detecting bony injury. Spinal MRI is highly sensitive to changes in the soft tissues including spinal cord, hemorrhage, and ligamentous injury, and is indicated in the presence of cord-related neurologic findings.

Spinal stability is defined as the capacity of the spine to withstand physiologic loading without neurologic injury, deformity, or pain. In practice, this state is predicted by clinical examination and imaging. In the thoracolumbar spine, instability is defined as injury to more than two CT-based "columns": the *anterior column*, which consists of the anterior longitudinal ligament and the anterior half of vertebral body or disc; the *middle column*, which consists of the posterior half of the body or disc and the posterior longitudinal ligament; and, the *posterior column*, which consists of the posterior arch and ligaments.

Clearance of the cervical spine as being stable is controversial. The 2013 Imaging Guidelines from the American Association of Neurological Surgeons and the Congress of Neurological Surgeons are summarized in **Table 61.11** (47,54). In children with significant TBI or significant neck pain, a reasonable practice is to maintain cervical spine immobilization until an MRI can be performed to exclude ligamentous injury. However, no formal guidelines exist on this practice, and each unit should discuss its management strategy with neurosurgery, neuroradiology, and emergency medicine colleagues in the light of the recent guidelines. In the conscious child, immobilization can be discontinued when the pain has resolved and flexion and extension radiographs reveal no apparent injury.

TABLE 61.11

DIAGNOSTIC IMAGING RECOMMENDATIONS IN PEDIATRIC CERVICAL SPINE AND SPINAL CORD INJURIES

■ **LEVEL OF RECOMMENDATION**

Level I
CT imaging to determine the condyle-C1 interval for children with potential atlanto-occipital dislocation *is recommended*

Level II
If >3 years of age: Cervical spine imaging *is not recommended* in children who have experience trauma, and who:
■ Are alert
■ Have no neurological deficit
■ Have no midline cervical tenderness
■ Have no painful distracting injury
■ Do not have unexplained hypotension
■ Are not intoxicated

If <3 years of age: Cervical spine imaging *is not recommended* in children who have experienced trauma and who:
■ Have a GCS >13
■ Have no neurological deficit
■ Have no midline cervical tenderness
■ Have no painful distracting injury
■ Do not have unexplained hypotension
■ Are not intoxicated
■ AND do not have motor vehicle collision, a fall from height >10 feet, or abusive injury as a known mechanism of injury
If any of the above criteria are not met, then cervical spine radiographs or high-resolution CT *is recommended* for children who have experienced trauma

Level III
If >9 years of age: Anteroposterior (AP), lateral and open-mouth cervical spine radiography or high-resolution CT *is recommended* to assess the cervical spine
If <9 years of age: AP and lateral or high-resolution CT *is recommended* to assess the cervical spine
High-resolution CT scan with attention to the suspected level of neurological injury *is recommended* to exclude occult fractures or to evaluate regions not adequately visualized on plain radiographs
Flexion and extension cervical radiographs or fluoroscopy *are recommended* to exclude gross ligamentous instability when there remains suspicion of cervical spinal instability following static radiographs or CT scan
MRI of the cervical spine *is recommended* to exclude spinal cord or nerve root compression, evaluate ligamentous integrity, or possible information regarding neurological prognosis

NEUROCRITICAL CARE MONITORING OF INTRACRANIAL PRESSURE

This section will focus on the next phase, which is the use of ICP monitoring in the management of severe TBI. Children with severe TBI (GCS < 9) and a mass lesion should have the mass removed and, in many countries, an ICP monitor is inserted at the time of surgery. Nonsurgical children with GCS <9 or CT evidence of intracranial hypertension (e.g., swelling, shift, or cisternal compression) should, in our opinion, also have ICP monitoring. Children with moderate head injury (GCS 9–12) merit careful observation. In these children, an open fontanelle may be used as a proxy for invasive monitoring. Deterioration warrants repeat head CT to rule out interval development or enlargement of a mass lesion and consideration for placement of an ICP monitor.

Cerebrospinal Fluid and Intracranial Pressure

Eighty percent of CSF is produced in the choroid plexus of the lateral and fourth ventricles. The remainder is produced in the interstitial space and ependymal lining. In the adult, normal CSF volume is 150 mL (50% intracranial and the rest intraspinal). In the neonate, CSF volume is 50 mL. The rate of CSF production across all ages is 0.15–0.30 mL/min (up to ≈450 mL/day). There are two pathways for CSF circulation: a major, *adult*, pathway with CSF absorption through arachnoid villi (arachnoid granulation) into the venous sinuses; and a minor, *infantile*, pathway with CSF drainage through the ventricular ependyma, the interstitial and perivascular space, and perineural lymphatics. The need for CSF circulation begins early during intrauterine development because the choroid plexus is formed during the first trimester. Since arachnoid granulations do not appear until just before birth, it is unlikely that CSF reabsorption via the *adult* route of circulation is the major pathway during infancy. In fact, there is some evidence that arachnoid granulations continue to develop well into the second decade, and so the "infantile" route of circulation may be significant in childhood.

Normal CSF pressure in children at the time of lumbar puncture is positive in relation to atmospheric pressure, with 10th to 90th percentile of 11.5–28 cm H_2O, or 8.7–21.2 mm Hg, respectively (64). ICP is the pressure of CSF inside the cerebral ventricles, which is determined by CBF and CSF circulation. The Davson equation describes this relationship and states that ICP is the sum of sagittal sinus pressure and the product of CSF formation rate and resistance to CSF outflow (65). Normal values for sagittal sinus pressure, CSF formation rate, and resistance to CSF outflow are 5–8 mm Hg, 0.3–0.4 mL/min, and 6–10 mm Hg/mL/min, respectively. Measured ICP is often greater than the calculated value because of a vascular component, which is probably a result of pulsation in the arterial bed and the interaction between pulsatile arterial inflow and venous outflow curves, cardiac function, and cerebral vasomotor tone (66). Under usual conditions, ICP reflects the volume of three compartments: brain parenchyma (1200–1600 mL in the adult human), extracellular or CSF (100–150 mL), and CBV (100–150 mL). Since the intracranial vault is fixed in volume in the developed cranium, increases in the size of one component of the intracranial contents must be compensated by removal of an equivalent amount of another intracranial component or ICP will increase. The point at which perfusion-compromising ICP elevation occurs is dependent on brain elastance and potential displacement of intracranial contents.

All of the above interrelationships may be altered in critically ill comatose patients with TBI. These abnormalities may also be compounded by brain swelling, edema and increased cerebral blood volume, focal cerebral perfusion deficits around brain contusions, and variable levels of CBF and cerebrovascular CO_2 reactivity. The net result is raised ICP along with significant risk of brain tissue herniation and death.

Invasive Intracranial Pressure Monitoring

Traditionally, ICP monitoring is performed via a ventriculostomy. Newer technologies rely on fiberoptic monitoring, with the catheter sensor tip placed in the brain parenchyma. The advantage of the ventriculostomy is that it enables CSF drainage as a treatment. However, it can be difficult to place and maintain function in the child with small, compressed, or distorted ventricles. On reviewing the recent literature about ICP monitoring in severe TBI, three key observations emerge.

First, the use of invasive ICP monitoring in management of pediatric severe TBI is by no means universal around the world. In the United States there is variation in practice. For example, in a large multicenter database (2001–2011) of 4667 children with TBI there was significant between-hospital variation in ICP monitoring (67). Overall, 55% of patients (n = 2586) received ICP monitoring. Observed hospital ICP monitoring rates were 14%–83%. After adjustment for patient factors, 13% of the ICP monitoring variation was attributable to between-hospital variation. Hospitals with more observed ICP monitoring, relative-to-expected, and hospitals with higher patient volumes had lower rates of mortality or severe disability. After adjustment for between-hospital variation and patient severity of injury, ICP monitoring was independently associated with age 1 year and more (odds ratio, 3.1; 95% CI, 2.5–3.8) versus age less than 1 year. Another study, this time using the US National Trauma Data Bank of pediatric TBI cases managed in levels I and II centers (2001–2006), found that ICP monitoring was undertaken in few pediatric patients with severe TBI (68). Usage of ICP monitoring was associated with decreased mortality rate in only a small subset of the targeted population. In addition, children who received a monitoring device had longer hospital stay, longer PICU stay, and more ventilator days. These findings suggest that current use of ICP monitoring does not necessarily identify patients who are most likely to benefit from it.

Second, not all patients undergoing invasive ICP monitoring for severe TBI exhibit raised ICP. In a national study in the UK of all pediatric cases of severe TBI managed in the PICU (2001–2003), raised ICP was documented in only 49% (98 of 199 cases) of cases undergoing monitoring (69). The authors found that of the variables significantly associated with raised ICP in univariate analyses (emergency department GCS, pupil reactivity, age, and the findings on admission CT in relation to presence of subarachnoid hemorrhage, intracerebral hemorrhage or TAI, and lateral ventricle appearance), only the presence of TAI retained an independent association with development of raised ICP in multivariate logistic regression. GCS ≤8 predicted raised ICP with sensitivity 80% and specificity 55% (positive predictive value 59%, negative predictive value 77%). "Any abnormality on CT" predicted raised ICP with sensitivity 91% and specificity 38% (positive predictive value 58%, negative predictive value 82%). And, as also reported by others (70), the presence of raised ICP despite normal radiology and pupil responses likely reflects the known low sensitivity of CT for clinically significant TAI.

Third, it is now known that aggressive medical treatment of intracranial hypertension complicating severe TBI can be guided by one of two strategies, with no difference in outcome: use of ICP monitoring as a guide to therapy, or use of intensive clinical examination and serial CT scans to guide therapy (71,72). In this 2012 study from South America, 324 patients (13 years or older, 25% under 22 years of age) were randomly assigned to one of two specific protocols: guidelines-based management in which a protocol for monitoring intraparenchymal ICP was used or a protocol in which treatment was based on CT scans and clinical examination. The primary outcome was a composite of survival time, impaired consciousness, functional status at 3 and 6 months, and neuropsychological status at 6 months. There was no significant between-group difference in the primary outcome. Six-month mortality was not different between the groups (39% in the pressure-monitoring group and 41% in the imaging-clinical examination group). The median length of stay was similar in the two groups (12 days in the pressure-monitoring group and 9 days in the imaging-clinical examination group), although the number of days of brain-specific treatments (e.g., administration of hyperosmolar fluids and the use of hyperventilation) was higher in the imaging-clinical examination group than in the pressure-monitoring group.

Taking everything together, it is clear that there is still much to learn in how we select patients for invasive monitoring and how we use the information from monitoring to guide our therapies. Even so, it is our practice to use invasive monitoring to guide treatment, rather than to rely solely on serial clinical examinations and CT imaging.

Intracranial Pressure and Cerebral Perfusion Pressure Target Levels

Intracranial Pressure

In adults, the threshold for initiating treatment of intracranial hypertension is taken as 20–25 mm Hg. It is likely that the ICP threshold for poorer outcome is similar across all ages and the *Second Edition of the Brain Trauma Foundation Guidelines for the Acute Medical Management of Severe TBI in Infants, Children, and Adolescents* (73) concludes that treatment of raised ICP at a threshold of 20 mm Hg may be considered (Level III evidence). In this regard, brief increases in ICP that return to normal in <5 minutes may be insignificant; but, sustained increases of ≥20 mm Hg for ≥5 minutes likely warrant treatment. Despite this practice, it should be noted that the optimal ICP target or targets for pediatric TBI remain to be defined.

Cerebral Perfusion Pressure

Cerebral perfusion pressure (CPP) is calculated as the difference between mean arterial blood pressure and mean ICP. Normal values for mean arterial blood pressure and hence CPP are lower in children, particularly in infants and young children. Two assumptions are made when using calculated CPP to guide treatment. The first assumption is that the mean systemic arterial pressure is a good reflection of brain surface arteriolar pressure, and this may not be the case. The second assumption is that both pressures contributing to the calculation are calibrated to the same level. In the case of ICP monitoring via ventriculostomy, the point for zero calibration can be adjusted, although few reports discuss the exact details of calibration and zeroing. This adjustment is not possible with the fiber-tip intraparenchymal devices, for which the pressure is recorded at the tip of the sensor. If, in the case of ventricular monitoring, the zero point for ICP is taken as the level of the external auditory meatus and the zero point for blood pressure is taken as the level of the right atrium, then the actual CPP driving CBF would be lower than the simply calculated difference between the mean arterial blood pressure and the mean

ICP. The magnitude of this difference is related to the product of the sine of the angle of elevation of the bed and the distance between the two calibration points. In children, this difference is of the order of 5 mm Hg. However, if an intraparenchymal fiber-tip device is used and the bed is elevated beyond 30 degrees, the error could be doubled. We should, therefore, be cautious about how the data reporting exact critical CPP values are interpreted, particularly as few reports describe the methods of calibration in their practice. The 2012 Brain Trauma Foundation guidelines document (73) concludes the following Level III recommendation: a minimum CPP of 40 mm Hg may be considered in children with TBI; and a CPP threshold of 40–50 mm Hg may be considered—there may be age-specific thresholds with infants at the lower end and adolescents at the upper end of this range. In adult patients, with respect to CPP, it appears that the critical threshold for cerebral ischemia generally lies in the region of 50–60 mm Hg (74), and the Brain Trauma Foundation adult CPP guidelines therefore suggest "a general threshold in the realm of 60 mm Hg, with further fine-tuning in individual patients based on monitoring of cerebral oxygenation and metabolism and assessment of the status of pressure autoregulation" (75).

Most recently, in 2014, a report from the Brain Trauma Foundation trac-database of 317 pediatric severe TBI cases provided further insight into age-related CPP thresholds and survival in children and adolescents (76). The evidence suggests that CPP targets should be age specific: above 50 or 60 mm Hg in adults, above 50 mm Hg in 6–17-year olds, and above 40 mm Hg in 0–5-year olds. Furthermore, since systemic hypotension had an inconsistent relationship with events of low CPP, but elevated ICP did, the authors recommended that ICP should be controlled at all times, while also targeting systolic blood pressure in specific instances. We will discuss these ICP-directed therapies in the next section.

NEUROCRITICAL CARE TREATMENTS

Phase 4: Initial ICP-directed Therapies

In 2012, the second edition of the Guidelines for the Medical Management of Traumatic Brain Injury in Infants, Children and Adolescents was published (73), which included evidence-based recommendations. These guidelines indicate that the neurotrauma literature is insufficient to provide firm recommendations regarding a host of medical decisions that are important in caring for children with severe TBI. A major difference between the two editions of the guidelines is that the first edition provided an expert opinion in regard to a hierarchy in therapy—albeit with little or no evidence to support such an approach. It is our opinion that clinicians value such an approach and this section will summarize what we consider a reasoned strategy for controlling ICP and maintaining CPP at target levels. The advanced reader may, of course, come to different conclusions on what, when, and how to manage children under their care. Our view is that we all make decisions that are likely to have some effect on overall outcomes (77), and each center must decide on their strategy and ensure consistency in care.

Tier 1A: Sedation, Analgesia, and CSF Diversion Strategy

After endotracheal intubation and insertion of an ICP monitor, the first step used to reduce ICP is to ensure adequate sedation, analgesia, and neuromuscular blockade by using standard dosing of agents chosen by the treating physician.

Propofol should not be used in children with severe TBI. Both the Center for Drug Evaluation and Research of the US Food and Drug Administration and the UK Committee on Safety of Medicine have stated that "Propofol is not indicated for pediatric intensive care unit sedation, as safety has not been established."

The other "first-tier" therapies include elevation of the head of the bed to 30 degrees and positioning of the head in the midline, ensuring no obstruction to cerebral venous return. If ICP remains elevated and a ventriculostomy tube is in place, CSF can be drained. However, at present, there are no pediatric studies of sufficient quality to demonstrate the superiority of any CSF diversion strategy. The best available evidence supporting CSF diversion is derived from small series of children with refractory ICP (78,79).

Tier 1B: Hyperosmolar Therapies

If ICP is still elevated after the initial measures described above, mannitol or hyperosmolar therapy using hypertonic saline can be instituted. The 2012 pediatric guidelines (73) state that "hypertonic saline should be considered for the treatment of severe pediatric TBI associated with intracranial hypertension. The effective doses for acute use range between 6.5 and 10 mL/kg (Level II)." This dosage recommendation is based on a small randomized controlled trial (RCT) involving 18 children with TBI, where 3% hypertonic saline (6.5–10 mL/kg IV) lowered ICP compared to 0.9% saline and resulted in an average 7 mEq/L increase in serum Na (80). Furthermore, as a continuous infusion, "hypertonic saline should be considered for the treatment of severe pediatric TBI associated with intracranial hypertension" (Level III). The effective doses of 3% hypertonic saline are 0.1–1.0 mL/kg/h, given on a sliding scale. The minimum dose needed to maintain ICP <20 mm Hg should be used and serum osmolarity should be maintained <360 mOsm/L. Although mannitol is commonly used in the management of raised ICP in pediatric TBI, there are no studies of sufficient quality to support Level II/III evidence-based guidance. That said, typical doses of intermittent, intravenous infusions of mannitol, are usually in the range of 0.25–0.5 g/kg. Serum osmolality should be assessed before redosing, and the mannitol infusion withheld if the serum osmolality is above 320 mOsm/L, as dehydration induced by mannitol can precipitate renal failure.

Time Course of Action, Potential Treatment Failure, and Limits to Mannitol. Mannitol can reduce ICP by two distinct mechanisms. At high bolus dose, 1 g/kg, mannitol reduces blood viscosity. This effect is immediate, lasts <75 minutes, and results from a viscosity-mediated reflex vasoconstriction (when autoregulation is intact) that maintains a constant level of CBF and results in a reduction in cerebral blood volume and ICP (81–83). At all doses, mannitol reduces ICP by an osmotic effect on brain parenchyma, which develops over 15–30 minutes, as a result of the gradual movement of water from the brain parenchyma into the systemic circulation. The effect may persist up to 6 hours with regular dosing.

Mannitol has the potential to fail in treating cerebral edema. An intravenous bolus dose is distributed throughout the extracellular fluid within 3 minutes, except in areas protected by the intact blood–brain barrier (BBB). There is an acute rise in extracellular osmolality in body tissues (mannitol molecular weight is 182), which results in an influx of water from the intracellular compartment; this restores osmotic equilibrium between the intracellular and extracellular compartments, at a higher volume than before the drug was given. This water shift dilutes and lowers serum sodium concentration. Subsequent renal clearance of mannitol from the circulation produces an osmotic diuresis and elimination of free water, further raising total body osmolality and serum sodium concentration. The net effect of an initial, single dose of mannitol is no change or small net rise in total body osmolality. Practitioners should also be aware that "non-response" to intravenous mannitol is well described in adults. Non-response to intravenous mannitol after a single bolus dose may lead to hyponatremia or, over 48 hours of repeated treatment, failure to elevate serum sodium concentration by ≥1 mmol/L in at least 22% of neurocritical care adult cases receiving mannitol for cerebral edema and raised ICP (84).

Time Course of Action, Potential Treatment Failure, and Limits to 3% Hypertonic Saline. If we consider the apparent volume of distribution of sodium as 0.6 L/kg body weight, then one should anticipate an immediate increase of 3–5 mmol/L in serum sodium concentration with a rapid intravenous bolus of 4–6 mL/kg body weight of 3% hypertonic saline (0.5 mmol/mL). Hypertonic saline produces a 4-mm Hg decrease in ICP for 2 hours postinfusion and it has been associated with fewer required interventions to maintain an ICP of <15 mm Hg. The minimum dose required to maintain ICP <20 mm Hg should be used. Table 61.12 summarizes the data that better explain the effect of changes in serum sodium concentration during the course of treatment for cerebral edema.

TABLE 61.12

BLOOD–BRAIN BARRIER (BBB) PHYSIOLOGIC FUNCTION BASED ON THE STARLING EQUATION[a]

■ INTRAVENOUS SOLUTION	■ EFFECTIVE (mOsm/L)	■ REFLECTION COEFFICIENT		■ PERMEABILITY-SURFACE PRODUCT (mL[g × min]$^{-1}$)	■ HALF TIME ($t_{1/2}$)
		■ BBB	■ CP		
Saline 0.9%	285	1.00	1.00	2.4×10^{-4}	1 h
Mannitol 20%	1100	0.90	>0.53	1.0×10^{-3}	2.3 h
HS-3%	1026	1.00	1.00	2.4×10^{-4}	1 h
Albumin	–	1.00	–	1.5×10^{-6}	–

[a]$J_{cap} = L_{cap} [(P_{plasma} - P_{tissue}) - \sigma_{protein}(\pi_{protein,plasma} - \pi_{protein,tissue}) - \sigma_{salt}(\pi_{salt,plasma} - \pi_{salt,tissue})]$. Driving pressure $= (P_{plasma} - P_{tissue}) - \sigma_{protein}(\pi_{protein,plasma} - \pi_{protein,tissue}) - \sigma_{salt}(\pi_{salt,plasma} - \pi_{salt,tissue})$. Key: $P_{plasma} - P_{tissue}$ is the hydrostatic pressure difference between plasma and tissue; $\pi_{protein,plasma} - \pi_{protein,tissue}$ is the difference in protein osmotic pressure between plasma and tissue; L_{cap} is capillary hydraulic conductivity; J_{cap} is capillary water flow; and σ is the osmotic reflection coefficient; R is the universal gas constant (0.082 L atm/mol K); T is the absolute temperature (Kelvin); C_{solute} is the concentration of impermeant solute and $\pi_{solute,plasma}$ is the solute osmotic pressure in plasma.
BBB, blood–brain barrier; CP, choroid plexus; permeability-surface product, the capillary hydraulic conductivity; half times, approximate exchange half times of the intact BBB for various substances; HS-3%, 3% hypertonic saline. See text for details.

What is important is the state in serum-to-BBB extracellular space kinetics. For example, the half-life for equilibration of sodium across the intact BBB is 1 hour, but less if the barrier is disrupted. This means that change in serum sodium concentration as a strategy for treating cerebral edema will, theoretically, become less effective the longer one adopts this strategy—unless, of course, one is prepared to continue to escalate serum level to very high values. We should also note from **Table 61.12** that the choroid plexus behaves more like the peripheral circulation since it has a reflection coefficient to sodium of zero. Hence, changing serum sodium concentration will have no effect on limiting water flow across the endothelium within the choroid plexus, but mannitol would have such an effect. Similarly, in the case of vasogenic cerebral edema, as it worsens one would expect a fall in the reflection coefficient for sodium (decrease from 1 to 0.93 to 0). Therefore, prolonged and repeated dosing of intravenous 3% hypertonic saline is not without risk—it will have limited effect and may even worsen the edema as the BBB fails.

In comparison with mannitol, 3% hypertonic saline should be better tolerated than mannitol since the sodium loading should increase intravascular volume, rather than lead to diuresis and dehydration. However, hypertonicity is not without risk, particularly when it is used for a prolonged period. In a 2013 review of 88 children treated between 2004 and 2009 with ICP monitoring for at least 4 days and hypertonic saline infusion for elevated ICP, sustained (>72 hours) serum sodium levels above 170 mmol/L had a significantly higher occurrence of thrombocytopenia, renal failure, neutropenia, and acute respiratory distress syndrome after controlling for variables including age, gender, Pediatric Risk of Mortality score, duration of barbiturate-induced coma, duration of ICP monitoring, vasopressor requirements, and underlying pathology (85).

Taken together, in patients with cerebral edema, it seems reasonable to start treatment with 3% hypertonic saline to gain acute control, particularly when low volume status increases the risk of hypoperfusion. If the ICP becomes unresponsive to hypertonic saline, therapies for refractory intracranial hypertension must be considered (see below).

Phase 5: Therapies for Refractory Intracranial Hypertension

Second Tier: Surgical Options

Surgical therapy is considered for two reasons: (a) evacuation of mass lesion or debridement in the acute setting to prevent a second insult; or (b) intracranial hypertension from the secondary mechanisms. If the patient still continues to have raised ICP despite using all first-tier therapies, surgical "second-tier" therapies can be considered. At this stage further cranial CT scan imaging is required so as to determine surgical options (86,87). However, the risks associated with transporting the patient to the scanner at a time when they have refractory intracranial hypertension should not be underestimated and have to be weighed against the benefits of added information from the imaging—it is of note that some centers now use portable CT scanning in the intensive care unit (ICU) (88).

In regard to surgical treatment for refractory intracranial hypertension, there are two options that have been reported in the literature. When imaging shows open basal cisterns and no significant mass or midline shift, then some clinicians have reported using controlled lumbar CSF drainage (89,90). When imaging shows evidence of diffuse brain swelling, some clinicians use decompressive craniectomy to control ICP. However, the "best" available evidence for this intervention from a RCT in adults with severe TBI came to the conclusion that early bifrontotemporoparietal decompressive craniectomy for severe

diffuse injury and refractory intracranial hypertension merely decreased ICP and length of stay in the ICU, but was associated with more unfavorable outcomes (91). There has been much discussion of this study in the literature, as to differences in case mix and, in particular, those with fixed dilated pupils in each group in the study. We may gain more information from the ongoing RESCUE-ICP (Randomized evaluation of surgery with craniectomy for uncontrolled elevation of ICP, International Standard RCT number 66202560; projected completion date of December 2014) study, which includes subjects ≥12 years of age, and excludes those with fixed and dilated pupils. That said, it is interesting to note that there have been a number of recent pediatric case series reporting use of decompressive craniectomy during the course of treating severe TBI (92–96). To date, there has only been one RCT in children who were randomized to receiving either early (within 6 hours of enrollment), decompressive craniectomy, or standard medical management if the ICP was sustained >20 mm Hg for >5 minutes (97). ICP in the decompressive craniectomy group was significantly decreased, and the patients required substantially less medical intervention to control ICP after decompression. The control group of 14 patients had 2 patients with favorable outcomes (normal or mildly disabled at 6-month follow-up), while the decompression group had 7 out of 13 with favorable outcomes using the same outcome criteria.

Third Tier: Other Medical Therapies

Third-tier medical measures are the most aggressive level of management for cases of severe TBI and are associated with significant adverse events. Guidance as to how to manage patients who have failed to respond to tier 1 and 2 therapies is fraught with difficulty, since we do not have a significant number of valid and successfully completed RCTs to help us. Therefore, management is often guided by local experience or consensus. This tier includes use of barbiturate-induced coma, hypothermia, and hyperventilation.

If the patient has no medical contraindications to using barbiturates, barbiturates can be used to induce electrophysiological "burst suppression" and control elevated ICP by reducing cerebral metabolic activity. A commonly used protocol for pentobarbital is to use a loading dose of 10 mg/kg over 30 minutes, followed by 5 mg/kg every hour for three doses, and then a maintenance infusion of 1 mg/kg/h (98). The dose is titrated to the effect required (i.e., ICP control) while hypotension and unnecessary central nervous system depression are avoided. A recent, single-center report found that use of barbiturate coma led to control of refractory intracranial hypertension in almost one third of their cases with this severity of illness (99). The most common complication of this treatment is hemodynamic compromise and hypotension, but this did not appear to lead to worse outcome.

In regard to induced hypothermia, the weight of evidence in severe TBI, in adults, points to no effect in improving outcome after TBI (100). The 2012 edition of the Brain Trauma Foundation pediatric guidelines concluded that there are insufficient data to support a level I recommendation on the therapeutic use of induced hypothermia (73). In regard to level II, the recommendations are that moderate hypothermia (32°C–33°C) beginning early after severe TBI for only 24 hours should be avoided; moderate hypothermia (32°C–33°C) beginning within 8 hours after severe TBI for up to 48 hours duration should be considered to reduce intracranial hypertension; and, if hypothermia is induced for any indication, rewarming at a rate of >0.5°C per hour should be avoided. Since the publication of the second edition of the guidelines, the findings of the "Cool Kids" phase 3 RCT comparing hypothermia and normothermia after severe TBI in children has been reported (101), and Hutchison and Guerguerian have presented a meta-analysis of all five studies of induced hypothermia for pediatric severe TBI (102). The primary outcome in the "Cool Kids" study was all-cause mortality at 3 months, and other outcomes included global functional outcomes and adverse events. There were no statistically significant differences in mortality or functional outcomes between the two intervention groups, but the mortality was higher in the hypothermia group than it was in the normothermia group (6 of 39 patients vs. 2 of 38 patients; 15% vs. 5%, $p = 0.15$). Interestingly, given the discussion above about decompressive craniectomy, more patients in the normothermia group received decompressive craniectomy compared with the hypothermia group (17 of 38 patients vs. 7 of 39 patients; 45% vs. 18%, $p = 0.02$), which is one of those unavoidable confounders in such studies. In the meta-analysis that accompanied the publication of the "Cool Kids" report (102), there were five RCTs of hypothermia therapy for severe TBI in children that were reviewed (101,103–105). In these studies, there were 194 children that were treated with hypothermia and 206 that were assigned to normothermia management. Overall, the risk ratio of death in the hypothermia group compared with the normothermia group was not statistically significant, but there was a suggestion of increased risk of death with hypothermia therapy. The authors, therefore, concluded that "Because of the (these) safety concerns with hypothermia, we do not recommend further RCTs of the intervention in children with severe TBI. We are aware that some centers still use therapeutic hypothermia to treat intracranial hypertension refractory to other therapies. Data comparing the relative effectiveness of hypothermia therapy for intracranial hypertension could be obtained through alternative study designs such as comparative effectiveness research."

In regard to controlled hyperventilation ($PaCO_2$ 30–35 mm Hg), there are reports of its use in those with cerebral hyperemia. Generally, earlier in the course of therapy such management should be avoided (73), unless it is being used as a temporizing treatment before emergency surgery.

Individual PICU-ICP Strategy

Individual units should discuss their local strategy for ICP control. Such protocols often evolve over the years, and it is imperative that therapies are audited to identify whether any unusual practices or variances in care are occurring (77,106). In the literature, there are a number of protocols to be found. For example, there are useful flowcharts of sequential hierarchy in therapy to be found in the first edition of the Brain Trauma Foundation pediatric guidelines (59), and the recent report on use of barbiturate-induced coma (99). The most up-to-date iteration for this type of approach has been reported by Stocchetti and Maas, who describe escalating levels of therapeutic interventions (107). Based on the information we have provided, and for those seeking some guidance as to what is reasonable, the steps could include:

- Step One: Endotracheal intubation and mechanical ventilation with strict adherence a normocapnia target
- Step Two: Exclusion of need for surgery and consideration for ventricular CSF drainage and/or ICP monitoring
- Step Three: Nursing with head-of-bed up at 30-degree, head in the midline, and no kinking of the neck
- Step Four: Adequate sedation so as to limit coughing and dyssynchronous patient–ventilator interactions
- Step Five: Avoidance of hyperthermia and maintenance of normothermia target
- Step Six: Hyperosmolar therapy with mannitol or hypertonic saline
- Step Seven: Consideration of decompressive craniectomy
- Step Eight: Metabolic suppression with barbiturates

Whatever one's approach, it is important to review, document, and measure therapies used to control ICP, as well as outcomes. In this regard, Pineda et al. (108) recently reported the results of their pediatric neurocritical care program within their PICU focused on patients with severe TBI. The program was implemented on September 17, 2005, and involved "a coordinated communication and activity of PICU staff and physician faculty and trainees in several disciplines (critical care, neurosurgery, surgery, anesthesia, and radiology) and was implemented through a detailed training program, an explicit process for maintenance of pathway fidelity, and continuous quality improvement." The supplementary appendix to the paper describes the details of the pathway and the approach taken by this team. The center cares for 20–40 patients with severe TBI each year, and the report focused on a before-and-after analysis using data from 123 patients (~10 per year after excluding those with abusive head trauma, GCS score 3 and fixed and dilated pupils at presentation, preadmission cardiac arrest, and gunshot wounds to the head). By using an ordered probit statistical model to assess adjusted outcome as a function of initial severity, the authors came to the conclusion that outcomes for children with TBI can be improved by altering the system of care, that is, case review and iterative changes to one's protocol of management.

The "quantum" of treatment used in the care of individual patients can be summarized using the Pediatric Intensity Level of Therapy scale, which assigns scores to a variety of first- and second-tier treatments used in ICP control (**Table 61.13**) (109). The intensity of treatment in subgroups of patients and in different PICUs can be compared using this scale. It is the authors' experience that, in those patients in whom intracranial hypertension is a problem, the peak intensity of treatment occurs between days 3 and 4. Therefore, ICP treatments can be de-intensified in a stepwise process to ensure stability in adequate levels of ICP and CPP for at least 6–12 hours between each reduction in therapy. Most patients are able to leave the PICU by day 7 post-injury.

SEIZURES AND ANTICONVULSANTS

Acute symptomatic seizures may occur as a result of severe TBI (110). Such PTS are classified as *early* when they occur within 7 days of injury or *late* when they occur after 7 days following injury. After 7 days following injury, if seizures are recurrent, a label of posttraumatic epilepsy (PTE) is used.

A recent review of the literature from 1940 to 2013 revealed that the rate of early PTS in adult cases of TBI, of varying severity and in those not receiving seizure prophylaxis, was between 2.2% and 4.7% (111). In patients with severe TBI, the rate of clinical PTS may be as high as 12%, while that of subclinical seizures detected on electroencephalography may be as high as 20%–25%. In adults, the risk factors for early PTS include GCS score of ≤10; immediate seizures; posttraumatic amnesia lasting longer than 30 minutes; linear or depressed skull fracture; penetrating head injury; subdural, epidural, or intracerebral hematoma; cortical contusion; age ≤65 years or chronic alcoholism (112). A 2010 population-based study of hospitalized cases of civilian TBI in South Carolina, of varying severity, showed that the overall cumulative incidence of PTE in the first 3 years after discharge was 4.4 per 100 persons—the rate in severe TBI was 13.6 per 100 persons over 3 years (113). These rates of PTE are substantially higher than the risk of developing epilepsy in the general adult population, which has been estimated at 0.05 per 100 person-years (114). Those adults most at risk for PTE are individuals who have suffered the following: severe TBI and early PTS prior to discharge;

TABLE 61.13

PEDIATRIC INTENSITY LEVEL OF THERAPY (PILOT) SCALE

■ VARIABLE	■ SCORE	■ MAXIMUM SCORE
Individual daily scored components are denoted "a," "b," or "c" in the scoring section		
General (at any time in previous 24 h)		
Treatment of fever (>38.5°C) or spontaneous temperature (<34.5°C)	1a	1a + 1b + 2c = 4
Sedation (opiates, benzodiazepines: any dose)	1b	
Neuromuscular blockade	2c	
Ventilation (most frequently observed Paco$_2$ in 24 h)		
Intubated/normal ventilation (Paco$_2$ 35.1–40 mm Hg)	1a	4
Mild hyperventilation (Paco$_2$ 32–35 mm Hg)	2a	
Aggressive hyperventilation (Paco$_2$ < 32 mm Hg)	4a	
Osmolar therapy (total dose in 24 h)		
Mannitol ≤ 1 g/kg	1a	3a + 3b = 6
Mannitol 1.1–2 g/kg	2a	
Mannitol >2 g/kg	3a	
Hypertonic saline (any dose or rate, regardless of [Na])	3b	
Cerebrospinal fluid drainage (times in 24 h)		
0–11 times	1a	3
12–23 times	2a	
≥24 times or continuous	3a	
Barbiturates (total dose in 24 h; for score, 5 mg thiopental is equivalent to 1 mg pentobarbital)		
Pentobarbital ≤ 36 mg/kg	3a	4
Pentobarbital > 36 mg/kg	4a	
Surgery (at any time in 24 h)		
Evacuation of hematoma	4a	4a + 5b = 9
Decompressive craniectomy	5b	
Other treatments (at any time in 24 h)		
Induced mild hypothermia (≥35°C–37°C)	2a	4 + 2 + 2 = 8
Induced moderate hypothermia (<35°C)	4a	
Lumbar drain	2b	
Induced hypertension (≥95th percentile for age)	2c	
Total possible score		4 + 4 + 6 + 3 + 4 + 9 + 8 = 38

Data from Shore PM, Hand LL, Roy L, et al. Reliability and validity of the pediatric intensity level of therapy (PILOT) scale: A measure of the use of intracranial pressure-directed therapies. *Crit Care Med* 2006;34:1981–7.

acute intracerebral hematoma or cortical contusion; posttraumatic amnesia lasting longer than 24 hours; age > 65 years, or premorbid history of depression (113).

In the pediatric literature, the general incidence of early seizures varies between 12% and 19% (115,116). The risk of long-term seizures in these patients is ~15%. The more severe the injury, the higher the incidence of seizures becomes. Severe TBI has a risk of seizures between 19% and 68% (115,117,118). However, this literature is very much influenced by inclusion of infants who have suffered inflicted injuries often with SDH or a depressed skull fracture, and it is well known that these cases are at very high risk of developing epilepsy. Another factor that we have to consider is the new information from continuous electroencephalography (cEEG). For example, in a recent report of cEEG monitoring in 87 consecutive (mild to severe TBI) children admitted for PICU care, 42% of patients had seizures identified—with one third of these cases having subclinical episodes (119). Overall, we should therefore conclude that seizures are a significant problem in severe TBI; we need more prospective information on the prevalence; and, we need to better understand the significance of subclinical seizures in the early course of PICU management. We are, however, left with the problem of what to do about the risk of seizures and dysrhythmic episodes identified by cEEG.

In the acute period of hospital care, PTS may precipitate adverse events in the injured brain because of elevations in ICP, blood pressure changes, and changes in oxygen delivery and metabolism. The occurrence of seizures may also be associated with psychological effects, and loss of driving privileges in the adolescent. Antiseizure prophylaxis for PTS refers to the practice of administering anticonvulsants to patients following TBI in order to prevent the occurrence of seizures. The rationale for routine seizure prophylaxis is that there is a relatively high incidence of PTS in severe TBI patients, and there are potential benefits of preventing seizures following TBI (e.g., limiting derangement in acute physiology, preventing the development of chronic epilepsy). Prophylaxis should mean that anticonvulsant drug treatment prevents both early and late PTS. However, it is also desirable to avoid the neurobehavioral and other side effects of medications, particularly if they are ineffective in preventing seizures. It is therefore important to now evaluate the efficacy and overall benefit, as well as potential harms, of anticonvulsants used for the prevention of PTS.

Prophylactic anticonvulsants are recommended in adults with severe TBI, but their role in the management of children is controversial, as no prospective controlled trials have been conducted in children (120). In children, medications for seizure prophylaxis include phenytoin, phenobarbital, carbamazepine, and leviteracetam. It is the authors' observation that they and their colleagues now use leviteracetam in intubated, mechanically ventilated cases of severe TBI with abnormal CT scan on admission (121). There are no data to support this treatment over other therapies, but only that phenobarbital has sedative effects and will likely influence one's clinical examination, and phenytoin—although the most commonly prescribed anticonvulsant for this indication—requires hemodynamic monitoring during intravenous administration. In assessing this approach to treatment, readers should also be aware that in the adult TBI literature there is an argument that is emerging: antiseizure prophylaxis after TBI does not decrease seizure rates but may inhibit functional recovery, and therefore does more harm than good (111).

POSTTRAUMATIC MENINGITIS AND FEVER

Posttraumatic meningitis is a risk of mid-frontal, lateral-frontal, or temporofrontal fractures and posterolateral fractures (**Table 61.2**). It is best treated after an infective organism is cultured so that the antibiotic can be tailored appropriately. Initial empiric therapy after culture should cover *Streptococcus* and *Staphylococcus*. Ceftriaxone with or without vancomycin, depending on the local incidence of resistant Gram-positive organisms, is a reasonable choice until the specific organism is cultured.

Fever may be the earliest sign of meningitis but, in severe TBI, this is not always the cause. Early hyperthermia (i.e., temperature >38.5°C) within the first 24 hours of admission occurs in ~30% of children admitted to PICU post-TBI; this phenomenon appears to be a function of severity of injury (26) and is to be expected in children with moderate degrees of subarachnoid hemorrhage. Generally, a rise in temperature of >39°C demands investigation, and the presence of a compound fracture, either internal or external, should serve to focus attention immediately upon the possibility of meningitis. Extracranial causes of fever are also possible (e.g., chest infection, fat embolism, wound infection) and must be sought. Neurogenic hyperthermia may be due to primary brain lesions associated with TAI and dysautonomia with storming episodes (122). Another possibility is dehydration. In a review of 93 severely injured children, it was found that episodes of fever occurred in 52% and, of these cases, almost half were due to infection (123). Irrespective of the cause, a rise in temperature must be controlled, as it may worsen neurologic outcome.

FLUIDS AND NUTRITION

Discussion about IV fluids has been a topic of many debates, and the reader should refer to Chapter 97 for more details about the issues in children with critical illness. It is clear that the use of low-sodium-containing crystalloids is associated with mortality and morbidity in children with TBI. However, prolonged use of IV 0.9% sodium chloride will inevitably cause hyperchloremia and acidosis. IV saline-induced hyperchloremic acidosis causes reduced urine flow, confusion, and increased morbidity in adults who undergo major surgery. Alexis Hartmann (1894–1964), a pediatrician, introduced Ringer's solution in an effort to avoid the development of life-threatening hyperchloremic acidosis following saline administration.

Glucose-containing IV solutions are not used in adults who have suffered TBI. In fact, the emphasis is on limiting glucose in the insulin-resistant critically ill. Too few studies are available to consider the potential problems or merits of, respectively,

glucose or no glucose in children with TBI. Traditionally, glucose-containing fluids have been used, particularly in the very young. Until more is known about the relationship between blood glucose, brain glucose, and outcome, it is advisable to continue with one's current fluid strategy. An option that circumvents these issues is to initiate enteral nutritional support by 72 hours post-injury and aim for full nutritional replacement by day 7. In this regard, recently, Vavilala et al. (124) reported a retrospective cohort study in five regional pediatric trauma centers affiliated with academic medical centers, where she found that early ICU start of nutrition (within 72 hours) was associated with survival, with an adjusted hazard ratio of 0.06 (95% confidence interval 0.01–0.26). This report confirms previous single-center observations in severe pediatric TBI by others (125,126), but the questions that remain are how best to establish nutrition early in PICU management (enteral feeding via an orogastric/transpyloric tube *and not* nasal tube; or, parenteral nutrition), how many calories, and whether ketosis is good or detrimental to outcome. There are few data to guide our treatment at present and the reader is directed to general reviews of nutrition in the PICU populations. However, we do know that children with severe TBI are, in general, hypometabolic when patient metabolic studies using indirect calorimetry are compared with the calculated expected metabolism using equations such as the Harris–Benedict equation for resting energy expenditure——70% of what you would calculate as the requirement (127). In practice, one way of matching dietary energy provision to expenditure is to use a simplified equation for energy expenditure based on bedside volumetric carbon dioxide elimination measurement from the mechanical ventilator (128).

HYPOTHALAMIC–PITUITARY DYSFUNCTION

In adults with moderate to severe TBI, the endocrine changes within the first few hours and days immediately after injury share similarities with the changes in hypothalamic–pituitary-endocrine dysfunction observed in other critically ill patients (129,130). In particular, low basal cortisol levels with subnormal cortisol responses to stress test have been observed in adults and children (39–41,131–133). Posterior pituitary dysfunction that leads to abnormalities in water homeostasis and results in either cranial (central) diabetes insipidus or syndrome of inappropriate antidiuretic hormone (SIADH) secretion is also commonly observed in the acute period after TBI (39–41,134). In the majority of cases, perturbations in water balance are usually transitory and resolve within a few days or weeks of the event. SIADH is manifest as hyponatremia (serum sodium ≤ 130 mmol/L), which will exacerbate cerebral swelling, worsen ICP, and cause seizures. Cerebral salt wasting (CSW) may also cause hyponatremia (see below). SIADH is treated with volume restriction, and CSW is treated with volume and sodium repletion. The differentiation between these entities can be difficult to discern, but the single, clear, differentiating factor is the patient's volume state. Patients with high volume status have SIADH, while those with low intravascular volume have CSW. In that patients with SIADH tend to make smaller amounts of highly osmolar urine, careful documentation of urine volume and urinary sodium concentration may assist in the diagnosis (135).

CSW is a diagnosis of exclusion based on clinical criteria and it is overdiagnosed in our experience. The essential features of the syndrome are renal sodium and chloride wasting in a patient with a *contracted effective arterial blood volume*, where other causes of excess sodium excretion have been excluded. Volume contraction is likely to be present when there

TABLE 61.14

DIAGNOSIS OF CEREBRAL SALT WASTING IN A PATIENT WITH EXCRETION OF SODIUM AND CHLORIDE WITHOUT OBVIOUS CAUSE.

1. **Exclude:**
- A physiologic cause for the excretion of sodium chloride (e.g., an expanded extracellular fluid volume from hyperhydration with 1.5 times maintenance followed by abrupt decreases in intake)
- A non-cerebral cause for natriuresis:
  Diuretics
  States with low aldosterone (a stimulator for reabsorption of sodium)
  Adrenocortical insufficiency
  Congenital salt-losing renal tubular disorders (Bartter or Gitelman syndrome)
  Presence of an inhibitor of renal reabsorption of sodium such as osmotic agents, high concentration of ligands for the calcium receptor in the loop of Henle (e.g., hypercalcemia, gentamicin)
- Obligatory excretion of sodium by the excretion of anions other than chloride
- High-output renal failure (renal tubular damage such as obstructive uropathy, interstitial nephritis, and acute tubular necrosis)
- Sodium wasting from cerebrospinal fluid drainage

2. **Other explanations for salt wasting:**
- Natriuretic agents of cerebral origin
- Downregulation of renal sodium transport by chronic hypervolemia
- Pressure natriuresis from adrenergic agents
- Suppression of the release of aldosterone

is a deficit of sodium that exceeds 2 mmol/kg. Hyponatremia is a nonspecific clue. The literature suggests that this condition is common in children and that it results from excessively high atrial or brain natriuretic peptide levels. Table 61.14 lists some of the diagnoses that should be excluded before concluding that the patient has CSW. (It should be noted that atrial natriuretic peptide level is high in the patient who has been managed with hypervolemic fluid management. In this instance, natriuresis as a response to volume control is part of homeostasis, and not CSW.) A screening approach, when concerned about possible CSW, is hyponatremia (<135 mmol/L) with brisk diuresis (>3 mL/kg/h) and elevated urine sodium (>120 mmol/L) when available, or elevated urinary osmolarity (>300 mOsm/L water). The physiology involves inappropriate and excessive release of natriuretic peptides that leads to a primary natriuresis and volume depletion. A secondary hormonal response occurs with an increase in the renin–angiotensin system and arginine vasopressin production. In contrast to hyponatremia due to SIADH, the fractional excretion of urate is elevated but *does not* improve when hyponatremia is corrected. Patients with CSW are more likely to have suffered chiasmatic or hypothalamic injury, and be younger than patients

with normal sodium concentration. Almost half of the patients with CSW have hyponatremic seizures (serum sodium <130 mmol/L). The treatment of CSW involves sodium administration to match urinary losses and correction of intravascular volume contraction. In some instances, more rapid resolution of hyponatremia after volume expansion has been achieved with fludrocortisone.

In view of the neuroendocrine studies in adults with TBI and what is known about pediatric TBI, it seems likely that hypopituitarism is a neglected phenomenon in acute pediatric critical care. We, therefore, consider that, in the acute phase of illness, adrenal insufficiency should not be missed, because it can be life-threatening, and hypopituitarism must be identified early in the post-TBI period. An approach that is used in adults and is our practice in pediatric TBI cases with GCS scores 3–13 or cranial CT evidence of significant brain injury is summarized in Table 61.15 (43). A basal, early-morning cortisol concentration of <200 nmol/L suggests adrenocorticotropic hormone deficiency, and treatment with replacement doses of hydrocortisone is indicated until full endocrinologic assessment in the post-PICU phase. In patients with acute-phase basal cortisol concentrations between 200 and 400 nmol/L,

TABLE 61.15

SUGGESTED ALGORITHM FOR DIAGNOSIS OF ADRENAL INSUFFICIENCY IN PEDIATRIC TRAUMATIC BRAIN INJURY

Step 1	Consider testing in the following cases: Glasgow Coma Scale score 3–13 Cranial imaging that indicates significant brain injury Children who require inotropes or hyperosmolar therapy for intracranial pressure control
Step 2	Check morning cortisol daily for the first 7 d post-injury
Step 3	Treat patients with the following levels of replacement hydrocortisone: Morning cortisol < 200 nmol/L Morning cortisol ≥ 200 nmol/L but <400 nmol/L, and features of hypoadrenalism (i.e., hyponatremia, hypotension, or hypoglycemia)
Step 4	Refer patient to pediatric endocrinologist
Step 5	Endocrinologic assessment of anterior and posterior pituitary function in the postacute phase (usually 3–6 months)

Adapted from Acerini CL, Tasker RC. Traumatic brain injury-induced hypothalamic-pituitary dysfunction: A paediatric perspective. *Pituitary* 2007;10(4):373–80.

we consider replacement therapy if the child has features that could be due to adrenal insufficiency (e.g., hypotension, hyponatremia, or hypoglycemia). This indication may be difficult to assess in the patient who is receiving hyperosmolar therapy and inotropes for blood pressure support. Again, therapy is indicated until full endocrinologic assessment in the post-PICU phase. The reader should be aware that, at present, little prospective clinical evidence exists for this approach; therefore, replacement hydrocortisone should be viewed as an option.

Assessment of growth-hormone, gonadal, and thyroid axes is not necessary in the acute phase because, in adults, no evidence suggests that acute-phase replacement of these hormones in the deficient patient improves outcome. In children, there are now a number of studies that indicate that the endocrine axes should be assessed in the post-PICU period at 3, 6 months and 1 year after injury since there are abnormalities in up to 25% of patients (136–141).

OTHER ASPECTS OF TBI CARE

The content of this chapter is not exhaustive in regard to the full extent of patient care after severe TBI. There are areas of care that overlap with practices in other PICU neurocritical care populations. For example, is there a role for transcranial Doppler in severe TBI care? There is certainly a literature on its usefulness in identifying cases of subclinical traumatic carotid artery dissection and intracranial arterial vasospasm. At present, one main limitation is the absence of lack of normative data for the pediatric critical care population. However, there are two case series in the literature, together with over 130 cases described (142,143). There is also an emerging literature on *paroxysmal sympathetic hyperactivity* or *dysautonomia* complicating severe TBI. Much can be learned from case series in adults: pattern of MRI injuries that result in this condition, i.e., deep intraparenchymal pathology and TAI; impact on patient care, i.e., likely prolonged ICU stay and worse outcome; and, problems with management (144–146). There is one large pediatric TBI series published where 19 of 195 cases (~10%) exhibited dysautonomia (122). Last, there are few data on what to do about venous thromboembolism (VTE) prophylaxis in the pediatric trauma population (147). More studies are needed to assess overall incidence of VTE and whether mechanical and/or pharmacological prophylaxis impact outcomes. The concern when using pharmacological prophylaxis is the need for subsequent neurosurgery or the risk of hemorrhagic expansion of an intracranial contusion (148).

SCI-DIRECTED THERAPIES

In adults, high-dose methylprednisolone became the standard of care in the management of nonpenetrating acute SCI. This practice was based on the results of the National Acute Spinal Cord Injury Studies II and III, a Cochrane review of all RCTs and other published reports that verified significant improvement in motor function and sensation in patients with complete or incomplete SCI who were treated with high doses of methylprednisolone within 8 hours of injury. Since 1998, however, a number of authors have revisited these studies and questioned the validity of the results. Concerns have been raised about the study design, randomization, clinical endpoints, and statistical analysis. In addition, the risks of steroid therapy were not, in retrospect, considered inconsequential; an increased incidence of infection and avascular necrosis was noted.

Therefore, a number of professional organizations have revised their recommendations concerning steroid therapy in SCI. In 2013, the *American Association of Neurological Surgeons* and the *Congress of Neurological Surgeons* published comprehensive guidelines on the assessment and treatment of acute SCI (the whole document is open access at *Neurosurgery*, see http://journals.lww.com/neurosurgery/Fulltext/2013/03002/ Foreword.1.aspx). The guidelines conclude that the administration of methylprednisolone is not recommended for the treatment of acute SCI and that there is evidence that high-dose steroids are associated with harmful side effects including sepsis and death (149).

OUTCOMES AND PROGNOSIS OF BRAIN INJURY

Lethal and Fatal Injuries

Instances do occur when a child can be deemed to have sustained a lethal head injury and intensive care, as described in this chapter, is not appropriate. The types of brain damage in such children who are >2 years of age are remarkably similar to those seen in adults (150). Postresuscitant children with GCS score of 3 and bilateral, fixed, and dilated pupils (not due to medication) are in this category. The methods and protocols by which regional and local emergency systems deal with such patients should be decided locally. In our practice, we offer admission to the PICU to any child who has entered the emergency system; intensivists are best placed and best trained to deal with the issues surrounding brain death.

In any child with at least one pupil reactive to light, irrespective of the GCS score, all and full TBI-related interventions are offered. In our experience, it is impossible and inappropriate to use clinical features at the time of accident to predict survival. Such a child may well have sustained a fatal injury. If this should become evident over the course of intensive care, it should be assessed using appropriate technologies and discussed in an environment in which parents and the family can be supported.

Long-term Outcome

After intensive care, children with severe TBI often face challenges when living at home, at school, and in the community. The prognosis for recovery after severe TBI may be due to a number of ictal and postacute factors. It is not an exact science, but it is important that intensivists be aware of their outcomes, not least because it is the only way to inform our understanding of what works and what the therapeutic targets should be. At present, we work on the assumption that uncontrolled intracranial hypertension and inadequate cerebral perfusion cost brain tissue, function, and potential. The substrate for long-term deficits after TBI is undoubtedly the pathophysiologic problems that occur during the acute illness and how they impact on the white-matter architecture of the brain.

CONCLUSIONS AND FUTURE DIRECTIONS

The care of the child who suffers severe TBI or SCI is a continuum that starts with at-the-scene resuscitation by bystanders and the emergency services, followed by hospital transfer, neurosurgery, PICU care, and, lastly, rehabilitation in the community. This chapter has focused on one element within this continuum and the role of PICU therapies. The PICU aspect of head and spinal cord trauma care is summarized in **Table 61.16.**

TABLE 61.16

PICU SUMMARY POINTS ON HEAD AND SPINAL CORD TRAUMA

Resuscitation phase
  Quickly identify and treat life-threatening injuries
  Identify and correct airway obstruction, inadequate ventilation, and shock
  Assume that the cervical spine is unstable
  Identify intracranial hypertension with impending herniation, and use aggressive hyperventilation for a brief period if found
Secondary assessment phase
  Review all injuries and plan management with survey of head, neck, and thorax
  Assess ocular signs and responses
  Assess the motor system
  Assess the functional integrity of the spine and spinal cord
Investigation phase
  Head CT is the investigation of choice for bony and brain tissue injury
  Head CT should include visualization of the craniocervical junction
  Cervical radiographs include anteroposterior, lateral, and odontoid views; technically adequate films allow visualization
  of the entire cervical spine to C7–T1 intervertebral space
  Exclude metabolic or acid–base derangements that require correction
  Do not forget about inflicted TBI; a retinal examination is mandatory (Chapter 62)
PICU intensification phase
  After endotracheal intubation and insertion of ICP monitor target:
  ICP ≤ 20 mm Hg and CPP > 40 mm Hg
  Temperature 35°C–37°C
  Normoxia, normocarbia, normotension, normoglycemia
  Head in the midline and 30 degrees elevation position
  First-, second- and third-tier TBI therapies
  Other neurocritical care issues include:
  Seizures and anticonvulsants
  Posttraumatic meningitis and fever
  IV fluids and nutrition
  Repeat imaging to rule out interval development or enlargement of mass
  Cortisol for those with adrenal insufficiency
De-intensification phase
  Wean ICP- and CPP-directed therapies in reverse order of escalation (see above)
  Involve rehabilitation services at an early stage in cases of SCI and severe TBI
Postacute phase
  Follow-up investigation of anterior and posterior pituitary function in those treated with hydrocortisone replacement

TBI, traumatic brain injury; CSF, cerebrospinal fluid; SCI, spinal cord injury; ICP, intracranial pressure; CPP, cerebral perfusion pressure.

Possible topics for future studies include the type of IV fluids that should be used in TBI (lactate-containing or glucose-containing, or not), the role and risk of TBI-related hypothalamic–pituitary dysfunction in children and adolescents, and the individualization of patient care with the use of transcranial Doppler.

References

1. Centers for Disease Control and Prevention (CDC). CDC grand rounds: Reducing severe traumatic brain injury in the United States. *MMWR Morb Mortal Wkly Rep* 2013;62:549–52.
2. Selvarajah S, Schneider EB, Becker D, et al. The epidemiology of childhood and adolescent traumatic spinal cord injury in the United States: 2007–2010. *J Neurotrauma* 2014;31(18):1548–60.
3. Parslow RC, Morris KP, Tasker RC, et al. Epidemiology of traumatic brain injury in children receiving intensive care in the UK. *Arch Dis Child* 2005;90:1182–7.
4. Liesemer K, Riva-Cambrin J, Bennett KS, et al. Use of Rotterdam CT scores for mortality risk stratification in children with traumatic brain injury. *Pediatr Crit Care Med* 2014;15:554–62.
5. Gemke RJ, Tasker RC. Clinical assessment of acute coma in children. *Lancet* 1998;351:926–7.
6. Teasdale G, Jennett B. Assessment of coma and impaired consciousness. A practical scale. *Lancet* 1974;2:81–4.
7. Pinto PS, Poretti A, Meoded A, et al. The unique features of traumatic brain injury in children. Review of the characteristics of the pediatric skull and brain, mechanisms of trauma, patterns of injury, complications and their imaging findings, Part 1. *J Neuroimaging* 2012;22:e1–17.
8. Pinto PS, Meoded A, Poretti A, et al. The unique features of traumatic brain injury in children. Review of the characteristics of the pediatric skull and brain, mechanisms of trauma, patterns of injury, complications and their imaging findings, Part 2. *J Neuroimaging* 2012;22:e18–41.
9. El Sayed T, Mota A, Fraternali F, et al. Biomechanics of traumatic brain injury. *Comput Methods Appl Mech Eng* 2008;197:4692–701.
10. Ommaya AK, Goldsmith W, Thibault L. Biomechanics and neuropathology of adult and paediatric head injury. *Br J Neurosurg* 2002;16:220–42.
11. Sarkar K, Keachie K, Nguyen U, et al. Computed tomography characteristics in pediatric versus adult traumatic brain injury. *J Neurosurg Pediatrics* 2014;13:307–14.
12. Gentry LR, Godersky JC, Thompson B. MR imaging of head trauma: Review of the distribution and radiopathologic features of traumatic lesions. *AJR Am J Roentgenol* 1988;150:663–72.

13. Holbourn AHS. Mechanics of head injuries. *Lancet* 1943;2:438–41.
14. Holbourn AHS. The mechanics of brain injuries. *Br Med Bull* 1945;3:147–9.
15. Mendelsohn D, Levin HS, Bruce D, et al. Late MRI after head injury in children: Relationship to clinical features and outcome. *Childs Nerv Syst* 1992;8:445–52.
16. Garnett MR, Blamire AM, Rajagopalan B, et al. Evidence for cellular damage in normal-appearing white matter correlates with injury severity in patients following traumatic brain injury: A magnetic resonance spectroscopy study. *Brain* 2000;123:1403–9.
17. Slawik H, Salmond CH, Taylor-Tavares JV, et al. Frontal cerebral vulnerability and executive deficits from raised intracranial pressure in child traumatic brain injury. *J Neurotrauma* 2009;26:1891–903.
18. Tasker RC, Salmond CH, Gunn Westland A, et al. Head circumference and brain and hippocampal volume after severe traumatic brain injury in childhood. *Pediatr Res* 2005;58:302–8.
19. Tasker RC, Westland AG, White DK, et al. Corpus callosum and inferior forebrain white matter microstructure are related to functional outcome from raised intracranial pressure in child traumatic brain injury. *Dev Neurosci* 2010;32:374–84.
20. Prayer L, Wimberger D, Oder W, et al. Cranial MR imaging and cerebral 99mTc HM-PAO-SPECT in patients with subacute or chronic severe closed head injury and normal CT examinations. *Acta Radiol* 1993;34:593–9.
21. Adams JH, Graham DI, Scott G, et al. Brain damage in fatal non missile head injury. *J Clin Pathol* 1980;33:1132–45.
22. Gorrie C, Oakes S, Duflou J, et al. Axonal injury in children after motor vehicle crashes: Extent, distribution, and size of axonal swellings using beta-APP immunohistochemistry. *J Neurotrauma* 2002;19:1171–82.
23. Moen KG, Skandsen T, Folvik M, et al. A longitudinal MRI study of traumatic axonal injury in patients with moderate and severe traumatic brain injury. *J Neurol Neurosurg Psychiatry* 2012;83:1193–200.
24. Adams JH, Graham DI, Jennett B. The structural basis of moderate disability after traumatic brain damage. *J Neurol Neurosurg Psychiatry* 2001;71:521–4.
25. Ham TE, Bonnelle V, Hellyer P, et al. The neural basis of impaired self-awareness after traumatic brain injury. *Brain* 2014;137:586–97.
26. Natale JE, Joseph JG, Helfaer MA, et al. Early hyperthermia after traumatic brain injury in children: Risk factors, influence on length of stay, and effect on short-term neurologic status. *Crit Care Med* 2000;28:2608–15.
27. Skandsen T, Kvistad KA, Solheim O, et al. Prevalence and impact of diffuse axonal injury in patients with moderate and severe head injury: A cohort study of early magnetic resonance imaging findings and 1-year outcome. *J Neurosurg* 2010;113:556–63.
28. Feickert HJ, Drommer S, Heyer R. Severe head injury in children: Impact of risk factors on outcome. *J Trauma* 1999;47:33–8.
29. Lang DA, Teasdale GM, Macpherson P, et al. Diffuse brain swelling after head injury: More often malignant in adults than children? *J Neurosurg* 1994;80:675–80.
30. Adams JH, Graham DI, Gennarelli TA. Contemporary neuropathological considerations regarding brain damage in head injury. In: Becker DP, Povlishock JT, eds. *Central Nervous System Trauma Status Report*. Washington, DC: National Institutes of Health, 1985:65–87.
31. Tasker RC. Hippocampal selective regional vulnerability and development. *Dev Med Child Neurol* 2001;86:S6–7.
32. Adelson PD, Clyde B, Kochanek PM, et al. Cerebrovascular response in infants and young children following severe traumatic brain injury: A preliminary report. *Pediatr Neurosurg* 1997;26:200–7.
33. Kochanek PM, Clark RS, Ruppel RA, et al. Biochemical, cellular, and molecular mechanisms in the evolution of secondary damage after severe traumatic brain injury in infants and children: Lessons learned from the bedside. *Pediatr Crit Care Med* 2000;1:4–19.
34. Stippler M, Ortiz V, Adelson PD, et al. Brain tissue oxygen monitoring after severe traumatic brain injury in children: Relationship to outcome and association with other clinical parameters. *J Neurosurg Pediatr* 2012;10:383–91.
35. Ragan DK, McKinstry R, Benzinger T, et al. Alterations in cerebral oxygen metabolism after traumatic brain injury in children. *J Cereb Blood Flow Metab* 2013;33:48–52.
36. Crompton MR. Hypothalamic lesions following closed head injury. *Brain* 1971;94:165–72.
37. Daniel PM, Prichard MM, Treip CS. Traumatic infarction of the anterior lobe of the pituitary gland. *Lancet* 1959;2:927–31.
38. Harper CG, Doyle D, Adams JH, et al. Analysis of abnormalities in pituitary gland in non-missile head injury: Study of 100 consecutive cases. *J Clin Pathol* 1986;39:769–73.
39. Agha A, Sherlock M, Phillips J, et al. The natural history of post-traumatic neurohypophysial dysfunction. *Eur J Endocrinol* 2005;152:371–7.
40. Agha A, Sherlock M, Phillips J, et al. The natural history of post-traumatic hypopituitarism: Implications for assessment and treatment. *Am J Med* 2005;118:1416.
41. Agha A, Thompson CJ. Anterior pituitary dysfunction following traumatic brain injury (TBI). *Clin Endocrinol* 2006;64:481–8.
42. Popovic V, Aimaretti G, Casanueva FF, et al. Hypopituitarism following traumatic brain injury. *Growth Horm IGF Res* 2005;15:177–84.
43. Acerini CL, Tasker RC. Traumatic brain injury induced hypothalamic-pituitary dysfunction: A paediatric perspective. *Pituitary* 2007;10:373–80.
44. Acerini CL, Tasker RC. Neuroendocrine consequences of traumatic brain injury. *J Pediatr Endocrinol Metab* 2008;21:611–9.
45. Vogel LC, Betz RR, Mulcahey MJ. Spinal cord injuries in children and adolescents. *Handb Clin Neurol* 2012;109:131–48.
46. Bailey DK. The normal cervical spine in infants and children. *Radiology* 1952;59:712–9.
47. Rozzelle CJ, Aarabi B, Dhall SS, et al. Management of pediatric cervical spine and spinal cord injuries. *Neurosurgery* 2013;72(suppl 2):205–26.
48. Pang D, Wilberger JE. Spinal cord injury without radiographic abnormalities in children. *J Neurosurg* 1982;57:114–29.
49. Pang D, Pollack IF. Spinal cord injury without radiographic abnormality in children—The SCIWORA syndrome. *J Trauma* 1989;29:654–64.
50. Pang D. Spinal cord injury without radiographic abnormality in children, 2 decades later. *Neurosurgery* 2004;55:1342–3.
51. Mahajan P1, Jaffe DM, Olsen CS, et al. Spinal cord injury without radiologic abnormality in children imaged with magnetic resonance imaging. *J Trauma Acute Care Surg* 2013;75:843–7.
52. Launay F, Leet AI, Sponseller PD. Pediatric spinal cord without radiographic abnormality: A meta-analysis. *Clin Orthop Relat Res* 2005;433:166–70.
53. Boese CK1, Lechler P. Spinal cord injury without radiologic abnormalities in adults: A systematic review. *J Trauma Acute Care Surg* 2013;75:320–30.
54. Rozzelle CJ1, Aarabi B, Dhall SS, et al. Spinal cord injury without radiographic abnormality (SCIWORA). *Neurosurgery* 2013;72(suppl 2):227–33.
55. Theodore N, Aarabi B, Dhall SS, et al. The diagnosis and management of traumatic atlanto-occipital dislocation injuries. *Neurosurgery* 2013;72(suppl 2):114–26.
56. Meyer PG, Meyer F, Orliaguet G, et al. Combined high cervical spine and brain stem injuries: A complex and devastating injury in children. *J Pediatr Surg* 2005;40:1637–42.
57. Durham SR, Clancy RR, Leuthardt E, et al. CHOP Infant Coma Scale ("Infant Face Scale"): A novel coma scale for children less than two years of age. *J Neurotrauma* 2000;17:729–37.
58. Martinon C1, Duracher C, Blanot S, et al. Emergency tracheal intubation of severely head-injured children: Changing daily

practice after implementation of national guidelines. *Pediatr Crit Care Med* 2011;12:65–70.

59. Adelson PD, Bratton SL, Carney NA, et al. Guidelines for the acute medical management of severe traumatic brain injury in infants, children, and adolescents: Prehospital airway management. *Pediatr Crit Care Med* 2003;4:S9–S11.

60. Zebrack M1, Dandoy C, Hansen K, et al. Early resuscitation of children with moderate-to-severe traumatic brain injury. *Pediatrics* 2009;124:56–64.

61. Roberts DJ, Hall RI, Kramer AH, et al. Sedation for critically ill adults with severe traumatic brain injury: A systematic review of randomized controlled trials. *Crit Care* 2011;39(12):2743–51.

62. Marshall LF, Eisenberg HM, Jane JA, et al. A new classification of head injury based on computerized tomography. *J Neurosurg* 1991;75:S14–S20.

63. Maas AI, Hukkelhoven CW, Marshall LF, et al. Prediction of outcome in traumatic brain injury with computed tomographic characteristics: A comparison between computed tomographic classification and combinations of computed tomographic predictors. *Neurosurgery* 2005;57:1173–82.

64. Avery RA, Shah SS, Licht DJ, et al. Reference range for cerebrospinal fluid opening pressure in children. *N Engl J Med* 2010;363:891–3.

65. Davson H, Hollingsworth G, Segal MB. The mechanism of drainage of the cerebrospinal fluid. *Brain* 1970;93:665–78.

66. Tasker RC. Intracranial pressure: Influence of head-of-bed elevation, and beyond. *Pediatr Crit Care Med* 2012;13:116–7.

67. Bennett TD, Riva-Cambrin J, Keenan HT, et al. Variation in intracranial pressure monitoring and outcomes in pediatric traumatic brain injury. *Arch Pediatr Adolesc Med* 2012;166:641–7.

68. Alkhoury F, Kyriakides TC. Intracranial pressure monitoring in children with severe traumatic brain injury: National Trauma Data Bank-based review of outcomes. *JAMA Surg* 2014;149:544–48.

69. Forsyth RJ, Parslow RC, Tasker RC, et al. Prediction of raised intracranial pressure complicating severe traumatic brain injury in children: Implications for trial design. *Pediatr Crit Care Med* 2008;9:8–14.

70. Bailey BM, Liesemer K, Statler KD, et al. Monitoring and prediction of intracranial hypertension in pediatric traumatic brain injury: Clinical factors and initial head computed tomography. *J Trauma Acute Care Surg* 2012;72:263–70.

71. Chesnut RM, Temkin N, Carney N, et al. A trial of intracranial-pressure monitoring in traumatic brain injury. *N Engl J Med* 2012;367:2471–81.

72. Chesnut RM. Intracranial pressure monitoring: Headstone or a new head start. The BEST TRIP trial in perspective. *Intensive Care Med* 2013;39:771–4.

73. Kochanek PM, Carney N, Adelson PD, et al. Guidelines for the acute medical management of severe traumatic brain injury in infants, children, and adolescents—second edition. *Pediatr Crit Care Med* 2012;13(suppl 1):S1–82.

74. Clifton GL, Miller ER, Choi SC, et al. Fluid thresholds and outcome from severe brain injury. *Crit Care Med* 2002;30:739–45.

75. Bratton SL, Chestnut RM, Ghajar J, et al. Guidelines for the management of severe traumatic brain injury. IX. Cerebral perfusion thresholds. *J Neurotrauma* 2007;24(suppl 1):S59–64.

76. Allen BB1, Chiu YL, Gerber LM, et al. Age-specific cerebral perfusion pressure thresholds and survival in children and adolescents with severe traumatic brain injury. *Pediatr Crit Care Med* 2014;15:62–70.

77. Bell MJ, Adelson PD, Hutchison JS, et al. Differences in medical therapy goals for children with severe traumatic brain injury-an international study. *Pediatr Crit Care Med* 2013;14:811–8.

78. Jagannathan J, Okonkwo DO, Yeoh HK, et al. Long-term outcomes and prognostic factors in pediatric patients with severe traumatic brain injury and elevated intracranial pressure. *J Neurosurg Pediatr* 2008;2:240–9.

79. Topjian AA, Stuart A, Pabalan AA, et al. Risk factors associated with infections and need for permanent cerebrospinal fluid diversion in pediatric intensive care patients with externalized ventricular drains. *Neurocrit Care* 2014;21(2):294–9.

80. Fisher B, Thomas D, Peterson B. Hypertonic saline lowers raised intracranial pressure in children after head trauma. *J Neurosurg Anesthesiol* 1992;4:4–10.

81. Muizelaar JP, Wei EP, Kontos HA, et al. Mannitol causes compensatory cerebral vasoconstriction and vasodilation in response to blood viscosity changes. *J Neurosurg* 1983;59:822–8.

82. Muizelaar JP, Lutz HA III, Becker DP. Effect of mannitol on ICP and CBF and correlation with pressure autoregulation in severely head-injured patients. *J Neurosurg* 1984;61:700–6.

83. Muizelaar JP, Wei EP, Kontos HA, et al. Cerebral blood flow is regulated by changes in blood pressure and in blood viscosity alike. *Stroke* 1986;17:44–8.

84. Mortazavi MM, Romeo AK, Deep A, et al. Hypertonic saline for treating raised intracranial pressure: Literature review with meta-analysis. *J Neurosurg* 2012:116:210–21.

85. Gonda DD, Meltzer HS, Crawford JR, et al. Complications associated with prolonged hypertonic saline therapy in children with elevated intracranial pressure. *Pediatr Crit Care Med* 2013;14:610–20.

86. Figg RE, Stouffer CW, Vander Kolk WE, et al. Clinical efficacy of serial computed tomographic scanning in pediatric severe traumatic brain injury. *Pediatr Surg Int* 2006;22:215–8.

87. Schnellinger MG, Reid S, Louie J. Are serial brain imaging scans required for children who have suffered acute intracranial injury secondary to blunt head trauma? *Clin Pediatr (Phila)* 2010;49:569–73.

88. LaRovere KL, Brett MS, Tasker RC, et al. Head computed tomography scanning during pediatric neurocritical care: Diagnostic yield and the utility of portable studies. *Neurocrit Care* 2012;16:251–7.

89. Levy DI, Rekate HL, Cherny WB, et al. Controlled lumbar drainage in pediatric head injury. *J Neurosurg* 1995;83:453–60.

90. Tuettenberg J, Czabanka M, Horn P, et al. Clinical evaluation of the safety and efficacy of lumbar cerebrospinal fluid drainage for the treatment of refractory increased intracranial pressure. *J Neurosurg* 2009;110:1200–8.

91. Cooper DJ, Rosenfeld JV, Murray L, et al. Decompressive craniectomy in diffuse traumatic brain injury. *N Engl J Med* 2011;364:1493–502.

92. Bowers CA, Riva-Cambrin J, Hertzler DA II, et al. Risk factors and rates of bone flap resorption in pediatric patients after decompressive craniectomy for traumatic brain injury. *J Neurosurg Pediatr* 2013;11:526–32.

93. Csókay A, Emelifeonwu JA, Fügedi L, et al. The importance of very early decompressive craniectomy as a prevention to avoid the sudden increase of intracranial pressure in children with severe traumatic brain swelling (retrospective case series). *Childs Nerv Syst* 2012;28:441–4.

94. Desgranges FP, Javouhey E, Mottolese C, et al. Intraoperative blood loss during decompressive craniectomy for intractable intracranial hypertension after severe traumatic brain injury in children. *Childs Nerv Syst* 2014;30:1393–8.

95. Glick RP, Ksendzovsky A, Greesh J, et al. Initial observations of combination barbiturate coma and decompressive craniectomy for the management of severe pediatric traumatic brain injury. *Pediatr Neurosurg* 2011;47:152–7.

96. Khan SA, Shallwani H, Shamim MS, et al. Predictors of poor outcome of decompressive craniectomy in pediatric patients with severe traumatic brain injury: A retrospective single center study from Pakistan. *Childs Nerv Syst* 2014;30:277–81.

97. Taylor A, Butt W, Rosenfeld J, et al. A randomized trial of very early decompressive craniectomy in children with traumatic brain injury and sustained intracranial hypertension. *Childs Nerv Syst* 2001;17:154–62.

98. Eisenberg HM, Frankowski RF, Contant CF, et al. High-dose barbiturate control of elevated intracranial pressure in patients with severe head injury. *J Neurosurg* 1988;69:15–23.

99. Mellion SA, Bennett KS, Ellsworth GL, et al. High-dose barbiturates for refractory intracranial hypertension in children with severe traumatic brain injury. *Pediatr Crit Care Med* 2013;14:239–47.

100. Clifton GL, Miller ER, Choi SC, et al. Lack of effect of induction of hypothermia after acute brain injury. *N Engl J Med* 2001;344:556–63.

101. Adelson PD, Wisniewski SR, Beca J, et al. Comparison of hypothermia and normothermia after severe traumatic brain injury in children (Cool Kids): A phase 3, randomised controlled trial. *Lancet Neurol* 2013;12:546–53.

102. Hutchison JS, Guerguerian AM. Cooling of children with severe traumatic brain injury. *Lancet Neurol* 2013;12:527–9.

103. Adelson PD, Ragheb J, Kanev P, et al. Phase II clinical trial of moderate hypothermia after severe traumatic brain injury in children. *Neurosurgery* 2005;56:740–54.

104. Biswas AK, Bruce DA, Sklar FH, et al. Treatment of acute traumatic brain injury in children with moderate hypothermia improves intracranial hypertension. *Crit Care Med* 2002;30:2742–51.

105. Hutchison JS, Ward RE, Lacroix J, et al. Hypothermia therapy after traumatic brain injury in children. *N Engl J Med* 2008;358:2447–56.

106. Morris KP, Forsyth RJ, Parslow RC, et al. Intracranial pressure complicating severe traumatic brain injury in children: Monitoring and management. *Intensive Care Med* 2006;32:1606–12.

107. Stocchetti N, Maas AI. Traumatic intracranial hypertension. *N Engl J Med* 2014;370:2121–30.

108. Pineda JA, Leonard JR, Mazotas IG, et al. Effect of implementation of a paediatric neurocritical care programme on outcomes after severe traumatic brain injury: A retrospective cohort study. *Lancet Neurol* 2013;12:45–52.

109. Shore PM, Hand LL, Roy L, et al. Reliability and validity of the pediatric intensity level of therapy (PILOT) scale: A measure of the use of intracranial pressure-directed therapies. *Crit Care Med* 2006;34:1981–7.

110. Jennett B, Teasdale G. Trauma as a cause of epilepsy in childhood. *Dev Med Child Neurol* 1973;15:56–72.

111. Bhullar IS, Johnson D, Paul JP, et al. More harm than good: Antiseizure prophylaxis after traumatic brain injury does not decrease seizure rates but may inhibit functional recovery. *J Trauma Acute Care Surg* 2014;76:54–60.

112. Torbic H, Forni AA, Anger KE, et al. Use of antiepileptics for seizure prophylaxis after traumatic brain injury. *Am J Health Syst Pharm* 2013;70:759–66.

113. Ferguson PL, Smith GM, Wannamaker BB, et al. A population-based study of risk of epilepsy after hospitalization for traumatic brain injury. *Epilepsia* 2010;51:891–8.

114. Hirtz D, Thurman DJ, Gwinn-Hardy K, et al. How common are the "common" neurologic disorders? *Neurology* 2007;68:326–37.

115. Arango JI, Deibert CP, Brown D, et al. Posttraumatic seizures in children with severe traumatic brain injury. *Childs Nerv Syst* 2012;28:1925–9.

116. Chiaretti A, De Benedictis R, Polidori G, et al. Early post-traumatic seizures in children with head injury. *Childs Nerv Syst* 2000;16:862–6.

117. Ewing-Cobbs L, Kramer L, Prasad M, et al. Neuroimaging, physical, and developmental findings after inflicted and non-inflicted traumatic brain injury in young children. *Pediatrics* 1998;102:300–7.

118. Liesemer K, Bratton SL, Zebrack CM, et al. Early post-traumatic seizures in moderate to severe pediatric traumatic brain injury: Rates, risk factors, and clinical features. *J Neurotrauma* 2011;28:755–62.

119. Arndt DH, Lerner JT, Matsumoto JH, et al. Subclinical early posttraumatic seizures detected by continuous EEG monitoring in a consecutive pediatric cohort. *Epilepsia* 2013;54:1780–8.

120. Schierhout G, Roberts I. Prophylactic antiepileptic agents after head injury: A systematic review. *J Neurol Neurosurg Psychiatry* 1998;64:108–12.

121. Kirmani BF, Mungall D, Ling G. Role of intravenous levetiracetam in seizure prophylaxis of severe traumatic brain injury patients. *Front Neurol* 2013;4:170.

122. Kirk KA1, Shoykhet M, Jeong JH, et al. Dysautonomia after pediatric brain injury. *Dev Med Child Neurol* 2012;54:759–64.

123. Suz P, Vavilala MS, Souter M, et al. Clinical features of fever associated with poor outcome in severe pediatric traumatic brain injury. *J Neurosurg Anesthesiol* 2006;18:5–10.

124. Vavilala MS, Kernic MA, Wang J, et al. Acute care clinical indicators associated with discharge outcomes in children with severe traumatic brain injury. *Crit Care Med* 2014;42(10):2258–66.

125. Malakouti A, Sookplung P, Siriussawakul A, et al. Nutrition support and deficiencies in children with severe traumatic brain injury. *Pediatr Crit Care Med* 2012;13:e18–24.

126. Taha AA, Badr L, Westlake C, et al. Effect of early nutritional support on intensive care unit length of stay and neurological status at discharge in children with severe traumatic brain injury. *J Neurosci Nurs* 2011;43:291–7.

127. Mtaweh H, Smith R, Kochanek PM, et al. Energy expenditure in children after severe traumatic brain injury. *Pediatr Crit Care Med* 2014;15:242–9.

128. Mehta NM, Smallwood CD, Joosten KF, et al. Accuracy of a simplified equation for energy expenditure based on bedside volumetric carbon dioxide elimination measurement – A two-center study. *Clin Nutr* 2014. doi:10.1016/j.clnu.2014.02.008.

129. Olivecrona Z, Dahlqvist P, Koskinen LO. Acute neuro-endocrine profile and prediction of outcome after severe brain injury. *Scand J Trauma Resusc Emerg Med* 2013;21:33.

130. Woolf PD. Hormonal responses to trauma. *Crit Care Med* 1992;20:216–26.

131. Dupuis C, Thomas S, Faure P, et al. Secondary adrenal insufficiency in the acute phase of pediatric traumatic brain injury. *Intensive Care Med* 2010;36:1906–13.

132. Srinivas R, Brown SD, Chang YF, et al. Endocrine function in children acutely following severe traumatic brain injury. *Childs Nerv Syst* 2010;26:647–53.

133. Tanriverdi F, Senyurek H, Unluhizarci K, et al. High risk of hypopituitarism after traumatic brain injury: A prospective investigation of anterior pituitary function in the acute phase and 12 months after trauma. *J Clin Endocrinol Metab* 2006;91:2105–11.

134. Yang YH, Lin JJ, Hsia SH, et al. Central diabetes insipidus in children with acute brain insult. *Pediatr Neurol* 2011;45:377–80.

135. Berkenbosch JW, Lentz CW, Jimenez DF, et al. Cerebral salt wasting syndrome following brain injury in three pediatric patients: Suggestions for rapid diagnosis and therapy. *Pediatr Neurosurg* 2002;36:75–9.

136. Casano-Sancho P, Suárez L, Ibáñez L, et al. Pituitary dysfunction after traumatic brain injury in children: Is there a need for ongoing endocrine assessment? *Clin Endocrinol (Oxf)* 2013;79:853–8.

137. Khadr SN, Crofton PM, Jones PA, et al. Evaluation of pituitary function after traumatic brain injury in childhood. *Clin Endocrinol (Oxf)* 2010;73:637–43.

138. Norwood KW, Deboer MD, Gurka MJ, et al. Traumatic brain injury in children and adolescents: Surveillance for pituitary dysfunction. *Clin Pediatr (Phila)* 2010;49:1044–9.

139. Personnier C, Crosnier H, Meyer P, et al. Prevalence of pituitary dysfunction after severe traumatic brain injury in children and adolescents: A large prospective study. *J Clin Endocrinol Metab* 2014;99:2052–60.

140. Ulutabanca H, Hatipoglu N, Tanriverdi F, et al. Prospective investigation of anterior pituitary function in the acute phase and 12 months after pediatric traumatic brain injury. *Childs Nerv Syst* 2014;30:1021–8.

141. Wamstad JB, Norwood KW, Rogol AD, et al. Neuropsychological recovery and quality-of-life in children and adolescents with growth hormone deficiency following TBI: A preliminary study. *Brain Inj* 2013;27:200–8.

142. Melo JR, Di Rocco F, Blanot S, et al. Transcranial Doppler can predict intracranial hypertension in children with severe traumatic brain injuries. *Childs Nerv Syst* 2011;27:979–84.

143. O'Brien NF, Reuter-Rice KE, Khanna S, et al. Vasospasm in children with traumatic brain injury. *Intensive Care Med* 2010;36:680–7.

144. Baguley IJ, Heriseanu RE, Cameron ID, et al. A critical review of the pathophysiology of dysautonomia following traumatic brain injury. *Neurocrit Care* 2008;8:293–300.

145. Lv LQ, Hou LJ, Yu MK, et al. Prognostic influence and magnetic resonance imaging findings in paroxysmal sympathetic hyperactivity after severe traumatic brain injury. *J Neurotrauma* 2010;27:1945–50.

146. Lv LQ, Hou LJ, Yu MK, et al. Risk factors related to dysautonomia after severe traumatic brain injury. *J Trauma* 2011;71:538–42.

147. Thompson AJ, McSwain SD, Webb SA, et al. Venous thromboembolism prophylaxis in the pediatric trauma population. *J Pediatr Surg* 2013;48:1413–21.

148. Nickele CM, Kamps TK, Medow JE. Safety of a DVT chemoprophylaxis protocol following traumatic brain injury: A single center quality improvement initiative. *Neurocrit Care* 2013;18:184–92.

149. Hurlbert RJ, Hadley MN, Walters BC, et al. Pharmacological therapy for acute spinal cord injury. *Neurosurgery* 2013;72(suppl 2):93–105.

150. Graham DI, Ford I, Adams JH, et al. Fatal head injury in children. *J Clin Pathol* 1989;42:18–22.

CHAPTER 62 ■ ABUSIVE HEAD TRAUMA

RACHEL P. BERGER, DENNIS SIMON, JENNIFER E. WOLFORD, AND MICHAEL J. BELL

KEY POINTS

Epidemiology

1 Abusive head trauma (AHT) is a term that has evolved over the last 40 years to reflect brain injuries that occur as a result of child abuse.

2 AHT occurs in different cultures and ethnic groups.

3 Risk factors for AHT include the child's developmental stage as well as caregiver factors.

4 Mechanisms of injury include shaking, blunt force trauma, and hypoxia/ischemia.

Diagnosis

5 The history of present illness from the caregiver cannot be relied upon, as the perpetrator may not divulge accurately the circumstances around the events, and other caregivers may not be aware of the incident.

6 Careful documentation of the history is essential for reporting the incident to authorities.

7 A rapid, targeted physical examination is essential to begin resuscitative efforts and to document injuries as they are discerned.

8 The most common disorder mimicking AHT is noninflicted TBI, yet a number of other disorders must be considered.

Management

9 Rapid assessment and resuscitation to ensure a patent airway, effective breathing, and sufficient cardiovascular/circulatory support are essential for prevention of secondary injuries.

10 Intracranial pressure (ICP) and cerebral perfusion pressure (CPP) thresholds are believed to be age dependent, likely affecting clinical goals for young children with AHT.

11 Seizures are common after AHT and should be detected aggressively and treated.

Outcomes

12 Glasgow Outcome Scale Extended for Pediatrics (GOS E-Peds) is the newly established outcome measure for all pediatric TBI, including children with AHT.

13 Overall outcomes for AHT are significantly worse than noninflicted TBI in children in several series.

14 Developmental disabilities after AHT are extremely common and lifelong.

Reporting Legal Issues

15 In all the states of the United States, physicians are mandated to report suspected child abuse and are protected by law from the ramifications of doing so.

16 Although some institutions have designated Child Protection Teams to evaluate children with suspected abuse. Ultimately, it is the responsibility of the treating physician (often the pediatric intensivists) to ensure that state authorities are notified about any suspected child abuse or AHT.

The management of a critically ill child with abusive head trauma (AHT) is among the most challenging aspects of professional practice faced by the intensivist. Unlike almost any other disorder in clinical medicine, the children with AHT are generally brought to medical care with an unclear or patently false history of present illness, making the rapid diagnosis of the brain injury the first hurdle in a long series of challenges in managing these children. The nomenclature of this condition has evolved over the years since the 1974 publication in which Caffey (1) referred to "the whiplash shaken infant syndrome." There have been numerous terms used to describe the constellation of injuries that now is referred to as "abusive head trauma" (2). "Shaken baby syndrome" (3) is probably the most recognizable of these terms, although "inflicted traumatic brain injury," "inflicted childhood neurotrauma," "nonaccidental traumatic brain injury," and "intentional traumatic brain injury" are also used in the literature (4,5). The term AHT represents an improved understanding of the brain injuries that are not due to shaking alone, but can be the result of a combination of mechanisms including shaking, blunt impact, spinal cord injury, and hypoxic–ischemic injury. Use of the term AHT also changes the focus from the mechanism of injury to the abusive etiology of the injury. This review describes the necessary aspects of care of these children for the intensivist by focusing on the *brain injury* despite the fact that injuries to the abused child can include orthopedic, ophthalmologic, solid organ, and other injuries. For a comprehensive review of the multitrauma patient, the reader is referred to other chapters within this textbook.

EPIDEMIOLOGY

AHT is the leading cause of death from child abuse and the most common cause of severe traumatic brain injury (TBI) in infants. The incidence of AHT in the United States and Canada has been measured in multiple studies using different types of case ascertainment. Overall, the data demonstrate similar results regardless of the methodology, but suggest a lower rate of AHT in Canada than in the United States (6–11). Two active surveillance studies demonstrated an incidence of 29.7 (95% CI: 22.9–36.7) per 100,000 children less than 1 year of age in the United States and 14.1 (95% CI: 11.8–16.5) per 100,000 children less than 1 year of age in Canada. Small studies from Mexico and Estonia demonstrate that AHT is not unique to developed countries. All studies may ultimately underestimate the true incidence of the condition (12,13). Because of the vague nature of symptoms in mild cases of AHT, clinicians may miss the diagnosis of AHT in infants and young children who present without a history of trauma and with soft neurologic signs such as vomiting or fussiness(14). Even the most severe cases of AHT may only be diagnosed at autopsy (14), and of course, AHT may be misclassified as noninflicted TBI.

Risk Factors

Risk factors for AHT include those intrinsic to the child and to the caregiver. There is a unique age distribution for AHT, with peak incidence rates in the first year of life (mean age of 2–8 months in several reports) (7–8,11). Importantly, however, approximately 25% of children with AHT are older than 1 year of age, and it should be a part of the differential diagnosis in all young children because of the potentially grave consequences of misdiagnosis. AHT is thought to be associated with the peak period of crying during development, as this is the most commonly identified trigger (15,16). In addition to these child-based risk factors, circumstances related specifically to caregivers also contribute to the risk of AHT. Stress—both for communities as well as for individuals—may be the most pervasive of these risks. Studies have demonstrated that military deployment (17), natural disaster (18), and economic stress (8) can all affect the rate of AHT in communities. Specifically, there is an increased incidence of AHT in children on public insurance, which may integrate a number of these factors. On an individual basis, circumstances that decrease a parent's ability to deal with perceived stresses—including young parental age, poor impulse control, lower levels of maternal education, substance and alcohol abuse, and mental illness, including postpartum depression—can all increase the risk of AHT (19). While it is critically important to recognize these risk factors, the absence of these conditions does not remove the possibility, and hence concern for, AHT in one's clinical differential diagnosis.

Mechanisms of Injury

The mechanisms of injury in AHT are among the most controversial topics in pediatrics but likely include a combination of shaking, blunt force trauma, hypoxic–ischemic injury, and spinal cord injury. In his seminal paper, Caffey (1) described the unexplained occurrence of 23 long bone fractures in six children who also demonstrated subdural hematomas. In these cases, a nursemaid admitted to shaking the victims while holding them by the arms and trunk (1). Subsequently, there have been multiple studies to support the hypothesis that shaking is an important mechanism of injury in many cases of AHT (20–26). The effect of shear force is most observable within the orbit, as a study in neonatal pigs demonstrated that

extensive multilayer retinal hemorrhages and retinoschisis can be caused by shear forces on the retina and macula (27). Retinal hemorrhages rarely, if ever, occur in noninflicted TBI, and when present, do not have the same depth or affected area as retinal hemorrhages seen in AHT (27–29). Shaking injury may also explain some instances of subdural hematomas in AHT, with the proposed mechanism of tearing of bridging veins as the brain is rapidly moved within the cranial vault (14,30–32).

Blunt force trauma, either alone or in combination with shaking, is another potential mechanism of injury, with biomechanical studies demonstrating significantly greater rotational force when shaking is combined with blunt impact (3,33,34). Whether or not blunt force trauma is required to produce the forces necessary to cause severe (or fatal) brain injury has been the subject of much debate. An early biomechanical study suggested that shaking alone did not result in sufficient forces to cause such injuries (34)—findings supported by two postmortem studies (34,35). Geddes and colleagues (35) studied 14 cases of fatal AHT and found that while all cases had evidence of blunt force trauma, the evidence for this mechanism was only found in postmortem examination in half of the cases. In contrast, in two studies evaluating AHT cases where there were confessions by perpetrators, a significant proportion found no evidence of an impact (20,26). More contemporary experimental models (including porcine models of repetitive acceleration–deceleration and finite element model predictions) have suggested that previous models may have underestimated the complexity of the biomechanical forces in play as well as age-dependent differences in injury potential (36–38). Further evaluation of these and other models will likely improve our understanding of the complex interplay between the forces that are applied in AHT.

Hypoxic–ischemic damage to the brain in AHT has been widely observed. An intriguing study compared serum biomarkers of neuronal injury in patients with AHT, noninflicted TBI, and hypoxic–ischemic injury and found that the biochemical profile seen in AHT was more similar to that of patients with hypoxic–ischemic injury, demonstrating late peak biomarker concentrations that would be consistent with ongoing cell death (39,40). It has been theorized that hypoxia–ischemia may result from a delay in seeking medical attention after an incident of abuse by a perpetrator. However, the possible linkage between injury to the brain stem and upper spinal cord injury with the development of apnea and hypoxic injury has been proposed. A recent magnetic resonance imaging (MRI) study suggests that subdural hematomas within the cervical spinal cord are frequently observed with nonfatal AHT, but not in children with noninflicted TBI (41). Others have emphasized that damage to the respiratory centers in the cervicomedullary junction may play a role in the development of hypoxia-related injuries after AHT (41–44).

DIAGNOSIS

As mentioned earlier, the history provided by the caregiver in cases of AHT is almost never reliable, either because the informant is the perpetrator or because the informant is unaware that another person's actions caused the injuries. The challenge for clinicians is to recognize this lack of reliability as early as possible in the diagnostic process. In most cases of AHT, the historian does not provide any history of trauma (45–47). When obtaining a history in a case of possible AHT, it is critical to obtain detailed, time-focused information. For example, a chronology that includes the last time the child was observed to be healthy, the time at which the child became symptomatic, what prompted the seeking of medical attention, and exactly who was with the child when he or she became symptomatic. This information must be carefully documented so that any changes in the caregiver's account can be determined in subsequent investigations.

Physical examination, including assessment of the airway, adequacy of breathing, and appraisal of the cardiovascular/circulatory systems, is an essential part of the care of children with AHT. After the primary and secondary surveys are completed, additional aspects of the physical examination are essential. The neurologic symptoms in the child with AHT can range from asymptomatic to unresponsive. While most of the literature has focused on children with more severe injury, new data from a multicenter study of AHT demonstrated that just over half of the children with AHT had an initial Glasgow Coma Scale (GCS) score of 13–15 (Rachel Berger, personal communication). As a result, it is important to consider AHT even in cases in which an infant or young child appears well. In the classic study by Greenes and Schutzman (48), 19% of children younger than 2 years who had a subdural hemorrhage, cerebral edema, or cerebral contusions had a GCS score of 15. In the subacute stage of illness, additional information may be gleaned from brain MRI, including diffusion-weighted imaging sequences that highlight early changes of edema and ischemia. In addition to providing more complete information about diffuse axonal injuries and other forms of encephalomalacia, particularly the recently identified entity of *multifocal leukoencephalomalacia* or "big-black brain" (49), MRI may also be useful in determining the timing of injuries (50,51). Neuroimaging of the cervical spine may also be informative (41,42,52). As mentioned earlier, recent evidence from Choudhary and colleagues on the prevalence of spinal subdural hemorrhage in children with AHT compared with children experiencing noninflicted TBI showed that a spinal canal subdural hemorrhage was present in more than 60% of children with AHT compared to 1% of children with noninflicted TBI. Examples of common head computed tomography (CT) findings are provided in **Figures 62.1** and **62.2**.

This chapter focuses on the neurologic and neurocritical care aspects of AHT. However, it is essential to also discuss various ancillary aspects of the physical examination that are crucial to making the diagnosis, as evidence of other traumatic injuries can help differentiate AHT from alternative diagnoses (see what follows). The dermatologic exam may be more critical in AHT than most other diseases. Even though bruises, petechiae, and abrasions may have little clinical significance, meticulous documentation (including photodocumentation) is essential for future investigation into the circumstances surrounding the events. Orthopedic injuries are common, with some series describing 25%–85% of children with AHT as having either an acute or a healing noncranial fracture (53–55). In the majority of cases, these fractures cannot be diagnosed by physical examination alone and require comprehensive radiologic imaging at a time when the child has been stabilized. A postmortem skeletal survey should be part of the evaluation when any young child dies and AHT is in the differential diagnosis (56,57). An ophthalmologic examination should be performed as soon as feasible by an experienced pediatric ophthalmologist. Prudence, however, must be taken in judging when best to undertake the ophthalmologic examination. Topical mydriatics may nullify the value of the pupillary examination at a time when changes in pupil diameter may be a key sign of intracranial hypertension. It is important to identify patterns of retinal hemorrhages (multilayered and/or extend to the periphery of the retina) that are pathognomonic of AHT (29,58–60). Although rare, abdominal injuries must be considered in children with AHT. A multicenter study evaluating the use of screening laboratory tests (i.e., hepatic alanine aminotransferase and aspartate aminotransferase) suggested that a concentration of 80 IU/L should trigger diagnostic abdominal imaging (61); further study has validated this threshold value (62). As with fractures and dermatologic findings, the abdominal injuries most commonly seen in children with AHT often do not require medical or surgical intervention (e.g., grade 1 or 2 liver laceration), but provide important information for making a diagnosis of abuse and thereby being able to protect the child from further abuse. Importantly, in the study by Lindberg and colleagues (62), approximately one-third of subjects with abdominal injury due to abuse had no bruising, abdominal tenderness, or rebound on physical examination.

Differential Diagnosis

The challenge for the pediatric intensivist is to recognize that a child may have AHT when presented with a history that is inherently unreliable, and a dermatologic and neurologic examination that may be normal or nonspecific. In order to minimize the possibility of missing cases of AHT (which may prove fatal to the child), it is prudent to consider AHT in the

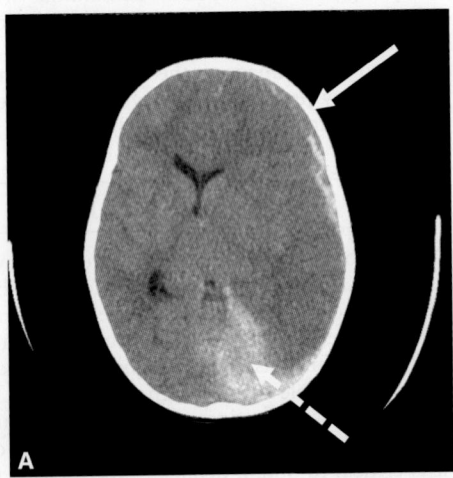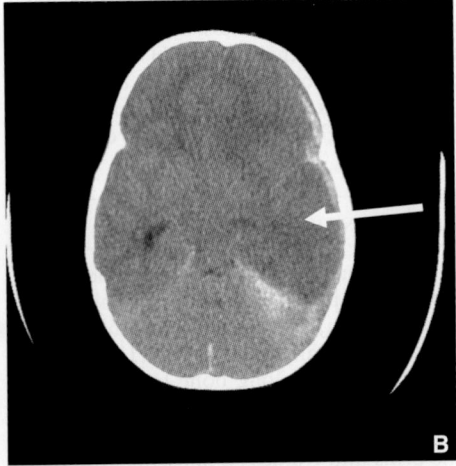

FIGURE 62.1. Head CT scan of a 3-month-old with AHT demonstrating acute subdural hematoma (**A**, *solid arrow*) with blood layering on tentorium (**A**, *dashed arrow*) and pronounced midline shift of cerebral contents. In **B**, early evidence of cerebral hypoperfusion and infarction is noted (*solid arrow*).

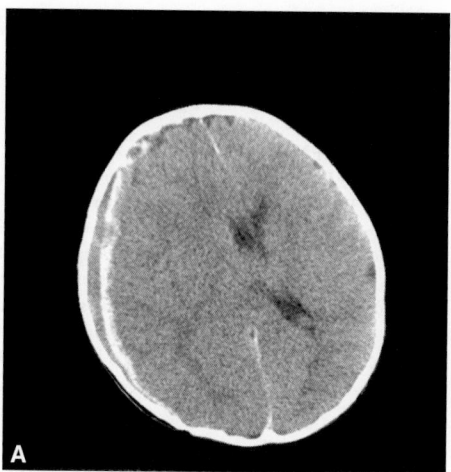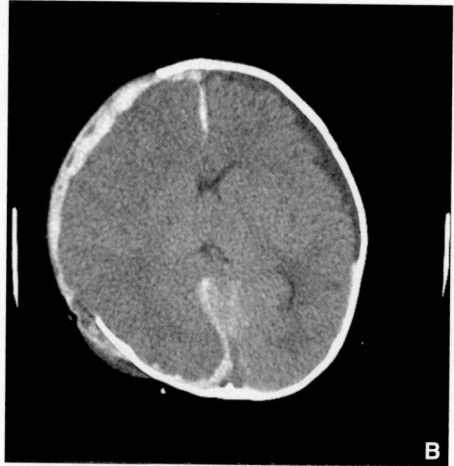

FIGURE 62.2. Head CT scan of a 9-month-old with AHT before (**A**) and after (**B**) decompressive craniectomy. In **A**, acute subdural hematoma on the right is prominent with diffuse cerebral edema, loss of gray–white matter differentiation, and marked midline shift of cerebral contents. In **B**, relief of midline shift is observed, along with resolution of much of the mass effect of the subdural hematoma on the right side. Of note, a chronic subdural fluid collection is observed on the left side, and bilateral edema is observed.

differential diagnosis of any young child: (a) with abnormal head CT imaging, where it is unclear whether the mechanism provided by the caretaker explains all of the child's injuries; and (b) with symptoms that may be neurologic in etiology and cannot be clearly explained by another disease process (e.g., infants with apnea and a negative respiratory syncytial virus test, or a young child with altered mental state and a normal urine toxicology screen). The evaluation of a child with possible AHT includes the evaluation for other diseases that can be confused with AHT (see **Table 62.1** for full list of recommended tests). These are often referred to as "mimics," meaning that there is some overlap between the clinical, radiologic, or other characteristics of the AHT and the mimic. The most common mimic is noninflicted TBI. Much less common are nontraumatic etiologies such as glutaric aciduria type I, hemophagocytic lymphohistiocytosis, hemorrhagic disease of the newborn, arteriovenous malformations, and bleeding disorders (63–69). While these diseases can resemble AHT, they rarely, if ever, share all of its characteristics. Every patient being evaluated for AHT should have a baseline set of hematologic labs (**Table 62.1**). Slight increases in PT/PTT are common after AHT as well as noninflicted TBI and do not represent an underlying bleeding disorder (70). In cases in which the only manifestation of abuse is bleeding (e.g., no fractures, no abdominal injury), when abnormalities of PT/PTT and/or platelets are persistent or more severe than one would expect from TBI alone, or when patient history or family history raises concern, it is important to consider the possibility of a bleeding diathesis. Consultation with a hematologist can be helpful in these cases. When a mimic is being considered and there are no other children in the home, filing a report with the proper authorities can sometimes wait for a few days until additional testing is performed. If there are other children in the home, however, reporting should not be delayed. The extent to which the pediatric intensivist becomes involved in the evaluation and diagnosis of suspected abuse varies among hospitals and often depends on the institutional choice of forming a separate service generally called a Child Protection or Child Advocacy Team. Nevertheless, the decision about whether to evaluate an infant or young child for AHT is often at the discretion of the intensivist, unless there are hospital protocols that dictate evaluation in specific circumstances.

Some data suggest that these protocols decrease the variability and bias in the evaluation for abuse (71,72).

MANAGEMENT/TREATMENT

The overall management of patients following AHT is similar to the management of all childhood TBI—as indicated by the inclusion of cases of AHT management manuscripts within the evidenced-based guidelines that have been published over the past decades. This chapter highlights AHT management decisions and challenges, as basic pediatric TBI management is reviewed elsewhere (Chapter 61). Mild and moderate AHT, defined as children with GCS score > 8, are generally treated expectantly with supportive measures to avoid secondary insults (e.g., hypoxia, hypotension, hyperthermia, hyponatremia, and seizures). However, reconsideration of this strategy for children with AHT may be warranted in the coming years. Specifically, this treatment strategy is largely based on the hypotheses within the overall TBI literature (including adult and childhood TBI victims) that mild decreases in consciousness after resuscitation are associated with: (a) a low incidence of intracranial hypertension; (b) decreased likelihood of deterioration or injury evolution; and (c) minimal mortality. In a recent study of over 300 AHT victims from four centers, however, the mortality rates of children with GCS scores of between 9 and 11 was 9.5%, which is similar to many published series for severe noninflicted TBI (GCS < 9) in children and in some adult series (73). Because of this higher than expected mortality rate for children with AHT who would be considered "moderate" injuries (based on GCS score alone), it may be prudent to consider more interventional approaches, possibly including intracranial pressure (ICP) monitoring to titrate neurocritical care therapies, with AHT victims with these slightly higher GCS scores when the clinical symptoms warrant concern. Of course, this novel approach would need to show efficacy in outcomes in future studies before it can be uniformly recommended.

Ideally, prehospital management of children with severe AHT should follow guidelines that emphasize early identification of injuries, establishment of a stable airway, and avoidance of secondary insults, including hypoxemia, hypotension,

TABLE 62.1

RECOMMENDED EVALUATION FOR A CHILD WITH AN INTRACRANIAL INJURY CONCERNING FOR AHT

■ TEST	■ REASON	■ SPECIALIST RECOMMENDED TO EVALUATE RESULTS	■ OTHER
Dilated ophthalmologic exam[a]	To evaluate for retinal hemorrhages	Pediatric ophthalmologist	Strongly recommend photodocumentation
Skeletal survey including oblique views of ribs[b]	To evaluate for fractures	Pediatric radiologist	This should not be done as portable films
Follow-up skeletal survey	To evaluate for fractures (especially metaphyseal and rib fractures) that were acute at the time of the initial skeletal survey and could not yet be visualized	Pediatric radiologist	To be done 10–14 d after the initial skeletal survey (pelvis and skull can be omitted)[c]
Screening for possible hematologic etiology of intracranial hemorrhage[d]	PT/PTT/platelets/INR, Factor VIII, Factor IX, d-dimer, fibrinogen	Pediatric hematology consultation recommended if any abnormalities on screening evaluation	
Urine organic acids and serum amino acids	To rule out glutaric aciduria type I as an etiology in children with isolated intracranial hemorrhage		Glutaric aciduria type I is very rare and its presentation does not overlap entirely with AHT, but should be ruled out as a mimic. A report to CPS should not be delayed until the results of the tests are known
Brain MRI with imaging of the spine	Brain MRI can provide improved information about injury to the brain parenchyma, hypoxia Spine MRI can provide important information about mechanism of injury	Pediatric neuroradiologist	
Screen for occult abdominal injury	Liver function tests, pancreatic enzymes		If AST or ALT >80 IU/L, recommend definitive testing (e.g., abdominal CT)

[a]In children who are too unstable to have their eye dilated, recommend initial evaluation without dilation and/or sequential dilation of eyes.
[b]In children who die prior to being able to complete a skeletal survey, the skeletal survey should be done postmortem. Any abnormalities need to be relayed to the coroner performing the autopsy.
[c]In children who are too unstable to undergo a skeletal survey until 1 w or more after admission, it is possible to perform a single skeletal survey 10–14 d after admission instead of both an initial and a follow-up.
[d]Measurement of Factors VIII and IX, fibrinogen, and d-dimer are not necessary in children who have other, nonhematologic manifestations of abuse as well (e.g., fractures).

hyperthermia, and seizures (74). However, since AHT or even traumatic injury on the whole may not be recognized at presentation to the health care system, this goal is often difficult to achieve. Additionally, since children with AHT tend to be younger than those who suffer from noninflicted injuries, tracheal intubation (while maintaining cervical spine precautions), establishing vascular access, airway management, and seizure recognition may be more challenging than in older children with noninflicted TBI. There are no specific adjuncts to the Advanced Trauma Life Support Guidelines for children with AHT, except considerations based on the young age of most victims (i.e., appropriate size for artificial airway, blood pressure norms, appropriate fluid volumes and drug doses). The "gold standard" for neurologic assessment is the GCS score. Although there are various adaptations of the GCS score to account for developmental age, none have been validated as measures of disease severity or as prognostic of outcome (75,76). If not already carried out by the Emergency Medical

Services, a protective cervical spine collar should be placed. Lastly, a CT scan should be obtained after resuscitation to guide medical and surgical therapies in the ICU.

Neurotrauma care within the ICU should be provided based on the best evidence available, generally outlined within the recent second edition of the evidence-based guidelines (77). The astute reader will note that the title of this document includes the inclusion of "infants, children, and adolescents," because all of these subgroups are represented within this guideline. The majority of studies include a subset of children with AHT within a larger population of children with noninflicted TBI. However, despite this limitation, this document represents the best current evidence to care for children with all types of TBI in the ICU. There are several aspects of the guideline that are most germane to the population of AHT children. First, although many children with AHT will have membranous fontanels, AHT can lead to intracranial hypertension and cerebral herniation in all ages if the compensatory mechanisms to maintain the volume/pressure relationship within the cranium are overcome. Therefore, minimizing ICP and maintaining cerebral perfusion pressure (CPP) (i.e., the difference between mean blood pressure and mean ICP) are as critical for the AHT population as for all other TBI populations. Second, while precise therapeutic thresholds for ICP and CPP have been sought for decades, the topic remains debated. In general, most studies suggest that an ICP target < 20 mm Hg is associated with best outcome, although some believe that a slightly lower ICP target may be best for young children (ICP of 15 or 18 mm Hg) (78). Third, a recent study in children with predominantly AHT (81% of all subjects) suggests that a threshold of CPP < 45 mm Hg is associated with poor outcome, which, if confirmed, may suggest a therapeutic target for a larger study (79). Fourth, the modality of partial pressure of brain tissue oxygen (Pbto$_2$) monitoring is likely unavailable to many AHT victims due to their age. The current commercially available monitor requires a crania fixation "bolt" or "screw" for stabilization of the catheter(s) within the brain parenchyma, and the placement of this apparatus can cause skull fractures in the nonossified skulls of young children (generally younger than 2 years of age). Fifth, children with AHT appear to have an increased risk of early posttraumatic seizures that may contribute to secondary injury and worsening outcomes. Seizures in infants may be difficult to discern and continuous electroencephalography (EEG) monitoring can be helpful for detection of significant events that require treatment (80,81). In a series of children with AHT, 296 of 404 (73%) presented with seizures, and in many of these cases seizures were refractory to first-line therapies (80). Moreover, subclinical status epilepticus was found in 25% of children. Prophylactic use of an anticonvulsant, therefore, appears warranted to reduce consequences from these early seizures, but evidence that such therapy improves overall outcome or the incidence of posttraumatic epilepsy is lacking.

Finally, in the only study, to our knowledge, that specifically examined a therapeutic intervention in AHT, Cho et al. (82) reported improved outcomes with decompressive craniectomy versus medical management in a small series of infants. However, the trial preceded the pediatric TBI guidelines and medical management included severe hyperventilation and was not randomized.

OUTCOMES

Outcome assessments after pediatric TBI, in general, have undergone standardization with the recent publication of common data elements for outcomes (83). In this effort, experts reviewed the various outcome tests available to clinicians and recommended "core," "supplemental," and "emerging" tests. The core outcome test identified to assess overall outcome after TBI was the recently validated Glasgow Outcome Scale Extended for Pediatrics (GOS E-Peds) (84), which is an expanded version of the previous GOS score that has been used for many years. While overall outcome after AHT differs between reported series, multiple studies demonstrate that mortality and morbidity after AHT is higher than after noninflicted TBI of similar severity (39,85). In a recent study by Shein and colleagues (73), mortality among children with AHT and an initial GCS score of 3 was 60% with stepwise decreases in mortality with increasing initial GCS score. Using composite scores of GOS (unfavorable outcome defined as GOS = 3−5 [severe disability + vegetative + dead]), a 50% rate of unfavorable outcome was observed 12 months after injury in a population of children <2 years of age with severe TBI (of which, 81% were diagnosed with AHT) (79). Greiner and colleagues (86) recently reported 71 children with AHT who underwent developmental testing at a mean of 12.4 months after injury and

found that 57% of survivors with the severest injuries had abnormal development (>2 standard deviations below the mean for the overall population). The reason for the increased mortality and morbidity in AHT compared with noninflicted TBI is not entirely clear, but is likely to be due to a combination of factors including: the characteristics of the injury as well any delay by caretakers in seeking medical care; a delay by medical providers in identifying trauma; the effect of prior maltreatment, particularly prior AHT; and, possibly, developmental factors. Additional studies are needed to determine the relative impacts of these various putative mechanisms.

REPORTING AND LEGAL ISSUES

In the United States, physicians are mandated to report suspected child abuse and are protected by law from any ramifications of reporting as long as the report is made in good faith. Each state has unique child abuse laws and different processes for filing a report of suspected child abuse. Many referring institutions have dedicated social services staff or other designated personnel who can assist physicians in making a report to Child Protective Services (CPSs), or the relevant investigative body for each state. Ultimately, it is the physician's responsibility to ensure that a report is made. Information about reporting is available online for each state at www.childwelfare.gov/systemwide/laws_policies/statutes. The physician's objective when making a report is to provide authorities with a statement of the medical facts in language that is as simple and as nonmedical as possible (e.g., use of the word "bruise" instead of "ecchymosis"), to inform them about the severity of these injuries (e.g., whether or not they are life-threatening), and to provide information about the strength of the diagnosis (e.g., there is concern for abuse vs. the injuries are diagnostic of abuse). A report is not a static document and more information including a change in the assessment of the likelihood of abuse can always be added as it becomes available (e.g., after a dilated eye exam or skeletal survey is performed). It is not the physician's responsibility to identify the perpetrator.

Ideally, whenever a report is made, the physician making the report will notify the parents at the time of the report. Failure to make parents aware of a report and of the content of that report can significantly jeopardize the doctor–parent relationship. When discussing the CPS report with the family, the discussion can be brief, respectful, and forthright. Throughout the conversation, the physician's focus should remain on the child's well-being. Including a hospital social worker or other support staff with expertise in the CPS system as part of the discussion with parents can be very helpful. While notification of parents is important, if no parent is available, physicians should not delay reporting. Reporting of child abuse serves the purpose of protecting the child, and alerting CPS to the presence of a potentially violent environment. This is important so that the safety of other children in the home as well as any adults who may be victims of domestic violence can be ensured.

PREVENTION

Unlike many conditions, measures to prevent AHT are generally societal in nature, and not in the realm of influence for the pediatric intensivist or within the scope of this review. The main way that an intensivist can prevent AHT is to have a high index of suspicion for possible cases, report them to the proper authorities for investigation, and work within this system to avert future cases of AHT from caregivers who are prone to this behavior.

CONCLUSIONS AND FUTURE DIRECTIONS

This review outlines the myriad of differences that exist between AHT and noninflicted injuries in children, and it is likely that these differences will continue to be clarified in the future. In the immediate future, it is possible that a better classification system for AHT—one that includes the use of biologic markers, imaging studies, and other factors—might allow for establishment of more homogeneous populations of children to study in interventional trials. In addition, specific therapies and clinical trials focused on AHT are desperately needed for these unfortunate children (e.g., those that might decrease intracranial hypertension, mitigate encephalomalacia, and improve outcome).

References

1. Caffey J. The whiplash shaken infant syndrome: Manual shaking by the extremities with whiplash-induced intracranial and intraocular bleedings, linked with residual permanent brain damage and mental retardation. *Pediatrics* 1974;54(4):396–403.
2. Christian CW, Block R. Abusive head trauma in infants and children. *Pediatrics* 2009;123(5):1409–11.
3. Duhaime AC, Christian CW, Rorke LB, et al. Nonaccidental head injury in infants—The "Shaken-baby syndrome." *N Engl J Med* 1998;338(25):1822–9.
4. Barlow KM, Milne S, Aitken K, et al. A retrospective epidemiological analysis of non-accidental head injury in children in Scotland over a 15 year period. *Scott Med J* 1998;43(4):112–4.
5. Sills MR, Libby AM, Orton HD. Prehospital and in-hospital mortality: A comparison of intentional and unintentional traumatic brain injuries in colorado children. *Arch Ped Adol Med* 2005;159(7):665–70.
6. Barr RG, Trent RB, Cross J. Age-related incidence curve of hospitalized shaken baby syndrome cases: Convergent evidence for crying as a trigger to shaking. *Child Abuse Negl* 2006;30(1):7–16.
7. Bennett S, Ward M, Moreau K, et al. Head injury secondary to suspected child maltreatment: Results of a prospective Canadian national surveillance program. *Child Abuse Negl* 2011;35(11):930–6.
8. Berger RP, Fromkin JB, Stutz H, et al. Abusive head trauma during a time of increased unemployment: A multicenter analysis. *Pediatrics* 2011;128(4):637–43.
9. Ellingson KD, Leventhal JM, Weiss HB. Using hospital discharge data to track inflicted traumatic brain injury. *Am J Prev Med* 2008;34(suppl 4):S157–62.
10. Fujiwara T, Barr RG, Brant RF, et al. Using international classification of diseases, 10th edition, codes to estimate abusive head trauma in children. *Am J Prev Med* 2012;43(2):215–20.
11. Keenan HT, Runyan DK, Marshall SW, et al. A population-based study of inflicted traumatic brain injury in young children. *JAMA* 2003;290(5):621–6.
12. Diaz-Olavarrieta C, Garcia-Pina, CA, Loredo-Abdala A, et al. Abusive head trauma at a tertiary care children's hospital in Mexico City. A preliminary study. *Child Abuse Negl* 2011;35(11):915–23.
13. Talvik I, Metsvaht T, Leito K, et al. Inflicted traumatic brain injury (ITBI) or shaken baby syndrome (SBS) in Estonia. *Acta Paediatr* 2006;95(7):799–804.
14. Jenny C, Hymel KP, Ritzen A, et al. Analysis of missed cases of abusive head trauma. *JAMA* 1999;281(7):621–6.
15. Lee C, Barr RG, Catherine N, et al. Age-related incidence of publicly reported shaken baby syndrome cases: Is crying a trigger for shaking? *J Dev Behav Pediatr* 2007;28(4):288–93.
16. Talvik I, Alexander RC, Talvik T. Shaken baby syndrome and a baby's cry. *Acta Paediatr* 2008;97(6):782–5.
17. Gibbs DA, Martin SL, Kupper LL, et al. Child maltreatment in enlisted soldiers' families during combat-related deployments. *JAMA* 2007;298(5):528–35.
18. Keenan HT, Runyan DK, Marshall SW, et al. Increased incidence of inflicted traumatic brain injury in children after a natural disaster. *Am J Prev Med* 2004;26(3):189–93.
19. Leventhal JM, Gaither JR. Incidence of serious injuries due to physical abuse in the United States: 1997 to 2009. *Pediatrics* 2012;130(5):e847–52.
20. Adamsbaum C, Grabar S, Mejean N, et al. Abusive head trauma: Judicial admissions highlight violent and repetitive shaking. *Pediatrics* 2010;126(3):546–55.
21. Bell E, Shouldice M, Levin AV. Abusive head trauma: A perpetrator confesses. *Child Abuse Negl* 2011;35(1):74–7.
22. Biron D, Shelton D. Perpetrator accounts in infant abusive head trauma brought about by a shaking event. *Child Abuse Negl* 2005;29(12):1347–58.
23. Eucker SA, Smith C, Ralston J, et al. Physiological and histopathological responses following closed rotational head injury depend on direction of head motion. *Exp Neurol* 2011;227(1):79–88.
24. Ibrahim NG, Ralston J, Smith C, et al. Physiological and pathological responses to head rotations in toddler piglets. *J Neurotrauma* 2010;27(6):1021–35.
25. Salehi-Had H, Brandt JD, Rosas AJ, et al. Findings in older children with abusive head injury: Does shaken-child syndrome exist? *Pediatrics* 2006;117(5):e1039–44.
26. Starling SP, Patel S, Burke BL, et al. Analysis of perpetrator admissions to inflicted traumatic brain injury in children. *Arch Ped Adol Med* 2004;158(5):454–8.
27. Coats B, Binenbaum G, Peiffer RL, et al. Ocular hemorrhages in neonatal porcine eyes from single, rapid rotational events. *Invest Ophthalmol Vis Sci* 2010;51(9):4792–7.
28. Levin AV. Retinal hemorrhage in abusive head trauma. *Pediatrics* 2010;126(5):961–70.
29. Morad YT, Wygnansky-Jaffe T, Levin AV. Retinal haemorrhage in abusive head trauma. *Clin Experiment Ophthalmol* 2010;38(5):514–20.
30. Case ME, Graham MA, Handy TC, et al. Position paper on fatal abusive head injuries in infants and young children. *Am J Forensic Med Pathol* 2001;22(2):112–22.
31. Geddes JF, Hacksaw AK, Vowles GH, et al. Neuropathology of inflicted head injury in children. I. Patterns of brain damage. *Brain* 2001;124(pt 7):1290–8.
32. Gilles EE, Nelson MD. Cerebral complications of nonaccidental head injury in childhood. *Pediatr Neurol* 1998;19(2):119–28.
33. Cory CZ, Jones BM. Can shaking alone cause fatal brain injury? A biomechanical assessment of the Duhaime shaken baby syndrome model. *Med Sci Law* 2003;43(4):317–33.
34. Duhaime AC, Gennarelli TA, Thibault LE, et al. The shaken baby syndrome. A clinical, pathological, and biomechanical study. *J Neurosurg* 1987;66(3):409–15.
35. Geddes JF, Vowles GH, Hacksaw AK, et al. Neuropathology of inflicted head injury in children: II. Microscopic brain injury in infants. *Brain* 2001;124(7):1299–306.
36. Coats B, Eucker SA, Sullivan S, et al. Finite element model predictions of intracranial hemorrhage from non-impact, rapid head rotations in the piglet. *Int J Dev Neurosci* 2012;30(3):191–200.
37. Ibrahim NG, Margulies SS. Biomechanics of the toddler head during low-height falls: An anthropomorphic dummy analysis. *J Neurosurg Pediatr* 2010;6(1):57–68.
38. Ibrahim NG, Natesh R, Szczesny SE, et al. In situ deformations in the immature brain during rapid rotations. *J Biomech Eng* 2010;132(4):044501.
39. Beers SR, Berger RP, Adelson PD. Neurocognitive outcome and serum biomarkers in inflicted versus non-inflicted traumatic brain injury in young children. *J Neurotrauma* 2007;24(1):97–105.
40. Berger RP, Adelson PD, Richichi R, et al. Serum biomarkers after traumatic and hypoxemic brain injuries: Insight into the biochemical response of the pediatric brain to inflicted brain injury. *Dev Neurosci* 2006;28(4–5):327–35.

41. Choudhary AK, Bradford RK, Dias MS, et al. Spinal subdural hemorrhage in abusive head trauma: A retrospective study. *Radiology* 2012;262(1):216–23.

42. Feldman KW, Avellino AM, Sugar NF, et al. Cervical spinal cord injury in abused children. *Pediatr Emerg Care* 2008;24(4):222–7.

43. Johnson DL, Boal D, Baule R. Role of apnea in nonaccidental head injury. *Pediatr Neurosurg* 1995;23(6):305–10.

44. King WJ, MacKay M, Sirnick A. Shaken baby syndrome in Canada: Clinical characteristics and outcomes of hospital cases. *CMAJ* 2003;168(2):155–9.

45. Ettaro L, Berger RP, Songer T. Abusive head trauma in young children: Characteristics and medical charges in a hospitalized population. *Child Abuse Negl* 2004;28(10):1099–111.

46. Hettler J, Greenes DS. Can the initial history predict whether a child with a head injury has been abused? *Pediatrics* 2003;111(3):602–7.

47. Keenan HT, Runyan DK, Marshall SW, et al. A population-based comparison of clinical and outcome characteristics of young children with serious inflicted and noninflicted traumatic brain injury. *Pediatrics* 2004;114(3):633–9.

48. Greenes DS, Schutzman SA. Occult intracranial injury in infants. *Ann Emerg Med* 1998;32(6):680–6.

49. Duhaime AC, Durham S. Traumatic brain injury in infants: The phenomenon of subdural hemorrhage with hemispheric hypodensity ("Big Black Brain"). *Prog Brain Res* 2007;161:293–302.

50. Kemp AM, Rajaram S, Mann M, et al. What neuroimaging should be performed in children in whom inflicted brain injury (iBI) is suspected? A systematic review. *Clin Radiol* 2009;64(5):473–83.

51. Vezina G. Assessment of the nature and age of subdural collections in nonaccidental head injury with CT and MRI. *Pediatr Radiol* 2009;39(6):586–90.

52. Kemp AM, Joshi AH, Mann M, et al. What are the clinical and radiological characteristics of spinal injuries from physical abuse: A systematic review. *Arch Dis Child* 2010;95(5):355–60.

53. Ghahreman A, Bhasin V, Chaseling R, et al. Nonaccidental head injuries in children: A Sydney experience. *J Neurosurg* 2005;103(suppl 3):213–8.

54. Maguire SA, Kemp AM, Lumb RC, et al. Estimating the probability of abusive head trauma: A pooled analysis. *Pediatrics* 2011;128(3):e550–64.

55. Reece RM, Sege R. Childhood head injuries: Accidental or inflicted? *Arch Pediatr Adolesc Med* 2000;154(1):11–5.

56. Hughes-Roberts Y, Arthurs OJ, Moss H, et al. Post-mortem skeletal surveys in suspected non-accidental injury. *Clin Radiol* 2012;67(9):868–76.

57. Weber MA, Risdon RA, Offiah AC, et al. Rib fractures identified at post-mortem examination in sudden unexpected deaths in infancy (SUDI). *Forensic Sci Int* 2009;189(1–3):75–81.

58. Bhardwaj G, Chowdhury V, Jacobs MB, et al. A systematic review of the diagnostic accuracy of ocular signs in pediatric abusive head trauma. *Ophthalmology* 2010;117(5):983–92.

59. Levin AV, Christian CW. The eye examination in the evaluation of child abuse. *Pediatrics* 2010;126(2):376–80.

60. Togioka BM, Arnold MA, Bathurst MA, et al. Retinal hemorrhages and shaken baby syndrome: An evidence-based review. *J Emerg Med* 2009;37(1):98–106.

61. Lindberg D, Makoroff K, Harper N, et al. Utility of hepatic transaminases to recognize abuse in children. *Pediatrics* 2009;124(2):509–16.

62. Lindberg D, Makoroff K, Harper N, et al. Utility of hepatic transaminases in children with concern for abuse: Validating the 80 IU/L threshold. *Pediatrics* 2013;131(2):268-75.

63. Fitzgerald NE, MacClain KL. Imaging characteristics of hemophagocytic lymphohistiocytosis. *Pediatr Radiol* 2003;33(6):392–401.

64. Hansen K, Frikke M. Dual and discrepant case publication in regard to hemophagocytic lymphohistiocytosis and child abuse. *Pediatr Radiol* 2007;37(8):846.

65. Jackson J, Carpenter S, Anderst J. Challenges in the evaluation for possible abuse: Presentations of congenital bleeding disorders in childhood. *Child Abuse Negl* 2012;36(2):127–34.

66. Anderst JD, Carpenter SL, Abshire TC. Evaluation for bleeding disorders in suspected child abuse. Pediatrics. 2013;131:e1314:22.

67. Reddy AR, Clarke M, Long VW. Unilateral retinal hemorrhages with subarachnoid hemorrhage in a 5-week-old infant: Is this nonaccidental injury? *Eur J Ophthalmol* 2010;20(4):799–801.

68. Rooms L, Fitzgerald N, McClain KL. Hemophagocytic lymphohistiocytosis masquerading as child abuse: Presentation of three cases and review of central nervous system findings in hemophagocytic lymphohistiocytosis. *Pediatrics* 2003;111(5 pt 1):e636–40.

69. Rutty GN, Smith CM, Malia RG. Late-form hemorrhagic disease of the newborn: A fatal case report with illustration of investigations that may assist in avoiding the mistaken diagnosis of child abuse. *Am J Forensic Med Pathol* 1999;20(1):48–51.

70. Hymel KP, Abshire TC, Luckey DW, et al. Coagulopathy in pediatric abusive head trauma. *Pediatrics* 1997;99(3):371–5.

71. Rangel EL, Cook BS, Bennett BL, et al. Eliminating disparity in evaluation for abuse in infants with head injury: Use of a screening guideline. *J Pediatr Surg* 2009;44(6):1229–34; discussion 1234–5.

72. Wood JN, Hall M, Schilling S, et al. Disparities in the evaluation and diagnosis of abuse among infants with traumatic brain injury. *Pediatrics* 2010;126(3):408–14.

73. Shein SL, Bell MJ, Kochanek PM, et al. Risk factors for mortality in children with abusive head trauma. *J Pediatr* 2012;161(4):716–22.

74. Badjatia N, Carney N, Crocco TJ, et al. Guidelines for prehospital management of traumatic brain injury. 2nd ed. *Prehosp Emerg Care* 2008;12(suppl 1):S1–52.

75. Holmes JF, Palchak MJ, MacFarlane T, et al. Performance of the pediatric glasgow coma scale in children with blunt head trauma. *Acad Emerg Med* 2005;12(9):814–9.

76. Massagli TL, Michaud LJ, Rivara FP. Association between injury indices and outcome after severe traumatic brain injury in children. *Arch Phys Med Rehabil* 1996;77(2):125–32.

77. Kochanek PM, Carney NA, Adelson PD, et al. Guidelines for the acute medical management of severe traumatic brain injury in infants, children and adolescents: Second edition. *Pediatr Crit Care Med* 2012;13(suppl 1):S1–82.

78. Chambers IR, Stobbart L, Jones PA, et al. Age-related differences in intracranial pressure and cerebral perfusion pressure in the first 6 hours of monitoring after children's head injury: Association with outcome. *Childs Nerv Syst* 2005;21(3):195–9.

79. Mehta A, Kochanek PM, Tyler-Kabara E, et al. Relationship of intracranial pressure and cerebral perfusion pressure with outcome in young children after severe traumatic brain injury. *Dev Neurosci* 2010;32(5–6):413–9.

80. Bourgeois M, Di Rocco F, Garnett M, et al. Epilepsy associated with shaken baby syndrome. *Childs Nerv Syst* 2008;24(2):169–72; discussion 173.

81. Lewis RJ, Yee L, Inkelis SH, et al. Clinical predictors of post-traumatic seizures in children with head trauma. *Ann Emerg Med* 1993;22(7):1114–8.

82. Cho DY, Wang YC, Chi CS. Decompressive craniotomy for acute shaken/impact syndrome. *Pediatr Neurosurg* 1995;23:192–8.

83. McCauley SR, Wilde EA, Anderson VA, et al. Recommendations for the use of common outcome measures in pediatric traumatic brain injury research. *J Neurotrauma* 2011;29(4):678–705.

84. Beers SR, Wisniewski SR, Garcia-Filion P, et al. Validity of a pediatric version of the glasgow outcome scale-extended. *J Neurotrauma* 2012;29(6):1126–39.

85. Adelson PD, Ragheb J, Kanev P, et al. Phase II clinical trial of moderate hypothermia after severe traumatic brain injury in children. *Neurosurgery* 2005;56(4):740–54.

86. Greiner MV, Lawrence AP, Horn P, et al. Early clinical indicators of developmental outcome in abusive head trauma. *Childs Nerv Syst* 2012;28(6):889–96.

CHAPTER 63 ■ STATUS EPILEPTICUS

KIMBERLY S. BENNETT AND COLIN B. VAN ORMAN

Status epilepticus (SE) is a medical emergency of varied etiologies that requires prompt recognition and intervention. Children with prolonged seizures are at risk for brain injury, respiratory or hemodynamic compromise due to both prolonged convulsions and high anticonvulsant dosing, and even multiorgan dysfunction. The pediatric intensivist must be familiar with the clinical presentation, causal pathophysiology, clinical evaluation, diagnostic monitoring techniques, potential complications, and goal-directed therapy of SE in infants and children.

DEFINITION

The *classical definition* of SE is seizure activity, either continuous or episodic, without complete recovery of consciousness, which lasts for at least 30 minutes. The evolution of SE can be conceptualized in stages (1,2): (a) *premonitory* or *prodromal SE*, characterized by an increasing frequency of serial seizures with recovery of consciousness between episodes; (b) *incipient SE*, defined as continuous or intermittent seizures that last up to 5 minutes without full recovery of consciousness; (c) *impending* or *early SE*, marked by seizure activity that persists 5–30 minutes; and (d) *established SE*, defined as seizures that last longer than 30 minutes. When SE lasts longer than 30–60 minutes, *subtle SE* usually develops. Subtle SE is characterized by progressive electromechanical dissociation, in which clinical signs diminish yet electroencephalographic (EEG) seizure activity persists. Finally, nonconvulsive SE (NCSE) refers to ongoing EEG seizure activity without associated clinical signs.

An *operational definition* that best helps to direct our treatment of SE, is to pragmatically define the condition as seizure activity lasting longer than 5 minutes. This duration also corresponds to initiation of therapy during impending or early SE, and recognizes the fact that prompt intervention is crucial. In children, unprovoked, afebrile seizures typically last less than 4 minutes, and seizures that last longer than 5 minutes are unlikely to remit spontaneously (3). Additionally, prolonged SE is associated with development of pharmacologic resistance and worse outcome (4). Indeed, children with SE that lasts longer than 30 minutes are less likely to respond to anticonvulsants (4). Consequently, treatment recommendations in this chapter will be based on a definition of SE as either continuous or intermittent seizure activity that lasts at least 5 minutes without full recovery of consciousness.

CLASSIFICATION

SE is commonly classified by seizure type. For the purpose of the pediatric intensivist, SE can be considered as convulsive or nonconvulsive (**Table 63.1**). Additionally, the pediatric intensivist should be familiar with the characteristics of *refractory SE* (RSE) and *neonatal SE*.

Generalized Convulsive Status Epilepticus

Generalized convulsive SE (GCSE) constitutes 73%–98% of pediatric SE (5) and is characterized by tonic, clonic, or tonic-clonic seizure activity that involves all extremities. In primary GCSE, seizure onset cannot be localized to one brain region by either clinical or EEG findings. In secondary GCSE, which is more common, seizures begin focally but spread to involve the entire brain. Early in the course, focal signs may persist on EEG; however, during prolonged GCSE, distinguishing secondary from primary GCSE often becomes difficult.

Focal motor SE, also called *simple complex SE*, *somatomotor SE*, or *epilepsia partialis continua*, is characterized by involvement of a single limb or side of the face. Focal motor SE

TABLE 63.1

CLASSIFICATION OF STATUS EPILEPTICUS

■ CONVULSIVE	■ NONCONVULSIVE
Generalized convulsive	Absence
Focal motor	Complex partial
Myoclonic	NCSE with coma

NCSE, nonconvulsive status epilepticus

TABLE 63.2

COMMON ETIOLOGIES OF FOCAL MOTOR STATUS EPILEPTICUS

Brain Tumor
  Astrocytoma
  Oligodendroglioma
  Glioblastoma
Infection
  Brain abscess
  Viral encephalitis
  Cysticercosis
  Tuberculosis
Vascular
  Cortical vein thrombosis
  Arteriovenous malformation
  Cerebrovascular accident
Trauma
  Posttraumatic cyst
  Chronic subdural hematoma
  Focal gliosis

is less common than GCSE and is frequently associated with focal brain pathology (**Table 63.2**).

Myoclonic SE is characterized by irregular, asynchronous, small-amplitude, repetitive myoclonic jerking of the face or limbs. Myoclonic SE is more common in comatose patients and is associated with several specific conditions, particularly anoxia or cardiac arrest (**Table 63.3**).

TABLE 63.3

COMMON ETIOLOGIES OF MYOCLONIC STATUS EPILEPTICUS

Anoxic Injury
  Cardiac arrest
  Cardiopulmonary bypass
  Carbon monoxide poisoning
  CO_2 narcosis
Infection
  Viral encephalitis
  Acute demyelinating encephalomyelitis
  Subacute sclerosing panencephalitis
  Opportunistic infection
Injury
  Heat stroke
  Lightning
  Intracranial hemorrhage
Metabolic
  Hepatic failure
  Renal failure
  Hypoglycemia
  Hyponatremia
  Nonketotic hyperglycemia
  Thiamine deficiency
Toxins
  Tricyclic antidepressants
  Anticonvulsants
  Antibiotics (β-lactam, carbapenem, quinolone)
  Opiates
  Lithium
  Heavy-metal poisoning
Genetic/Epilepsy Syndromes
  Juvenile myoclonic epilepsy
  Lennox-Gastaut syndrome
  Absence epilepsy
  Degenerative myoclonus epilepsy
  Angelman syndrome

Nonconvulsive Status Epilepticus

NCSE is characterized by continuous nonmotor seizures and requires EEG confirmation for diagnosis. NCSE may occur in ambulatory or comatose patients. The most common type of NCSE in ambulatory children is *absence SE*, which is characterized by altered consciousness and a generalized 3-Hz symmetric spike-and-wave pattern on EEG. In contrast, *complex partial SE* in ambulatory patients is marked by altered consciousness and focal activity on EEG, usually involving the temporal lobe. In comatose patients, NCSE may be difficult to diagnose and should be considered in any patient with prolonged obtundation after seizure cessation or with coma of unclear etiology (6,7).

The diagnosis of NCSE in critically ill patients requires a high degree of suspicion. Recognition is increasing as continuous EEG (cEEG) monitoring becomes more widely applied in critically ill patients. Pediatric-specific reports reveal nonconvulsive seizures in 16%–46% (8–12) and NCSE in 18%–33% (9,10,12,13) of critically ill children with unexplained alterations of consciousness and/or suspected SE. Nonconvulsive seizures and NCSE are more common among younger children, particularly those 1 month to 1 year of age, and are frequently associated with structural lesions (e.g., infarction, subdural hematoma, or intracerebral hemorrhage), anoxic injury, and acute infections (e.g., meningitis or encephalitis) (11,13). Although NCSE and nonconvulsive seizures occur in children with preexisting cerebral insults and epilepsy, more than 40% of children with nonconvulsive seizures are previously healthy (11).

Refractory Status Epilepticus

SE of any classification that fails to remit despite treatment with adequate doses of two anticonvulsants is termed refractory status epilepticus (RSE) (1). RSE develops in 30%–40% of adult patients and is associated with greater mortality than is more responsive SE (14,15). In children, 10%–40% of SE becomes refractory (4,16). Mortality for pediatric RSE is 13%–30%, and 33%–50% of survivors have neurologic sequelae (17,18). Almost half (46%) of neonates with SE develop RSE, and only 10% have good neurodevelopmental outcomes at 1 year of age (19).

Super-refractory SE is an important subtype of RSE. Super-refractory SE is defined as the persistence or recurrence of seizures despite at least 24 hours of pharmacologic coma, including the occurrence of breakthrough seizures during tapering of anesthetic medications (20). Super-refractory SE may occur in patients with severe brain injury or in those who are previously healthy with no apparent cause of SE. Super-refractory SE is important to recognize, as additional diagnostic testing and targeted therapy are often necessary.

Neonatal Status Epilepticus

SE presents differently in neonates than in older infants and children. Neonates are unlikely to demonstrate GCSE or continuous seizure activity; however, frequent, serial seizures without recovery of consciousness can occur. Neonatal seizures are frequently poorly organized and polymorphic and may involve rapid extensor or flexor posturing, tremor of extended extremities, apnea, eye deviation, or automatisms (2,17). Because of such atypical manifestations, most types of bizarre or unusual transient events in the neonatal period may be seizures, particularly if they are stereotypic, insensitive to stimuli, unaltered by restraint or limb displacement, and recur periodically. Neonatal SE is difficult to diagnose, and both clinical and EEG criteria are often required (17).

TABLE 63.4

COMMON ETIOLOGIES OF NEONATAL STATUS EPILEPTICUS

Perinatal or Acute Insults
  Hypoxia-ischemia
  Intracranial hemorrhage
  Cerebral vascular accident
Infection
  Meningitis
  Encephalitis
  Abscess
Metabolic
  Hypoglycemia
  Hypocalcemia
  Hyponatremia
  Hypomagnesemia
  Bilirubin encephalopathy
Inborn Errors of Metabolism
  Phenylketonuria
  Nonketotic hyperglycemia
  Pyridoxine deficiency
  Histidinemia
  Hyperammonemia
  Homocitrullinemia
  Maple syrup urine disease
  Leucine-sensitive hypoglycemia
Toxins
  Antibiotics (β-lactam, carbapenem, quinolone)
  Anesthetics
  Drug withdrawal
  Heavy-metal poisoning
Cerebral Malformations
  Neuronal migration defect
  Neurocutaneous syndrome
Degenerative Diseases
  Leigh encephalopathy
  Leukodystrophies
  Alpers' disease
  Sandhoff disease
  Tay-Sachs disease
Benign Familial Syndromes
  Benign familial neonatal seizures
  Benign neonatal sleep myoclonus

Conditions commonly associated with neonatal SE are presented in **Table 63.4.**

EPIDEMIOLOGY

Using the classic definition of continuous or intermittent seizure activity that lasts at least 30 minutes without recovery of consciousness, reported incidences for SE in children aged 1 month to 16 years are 17–38 per 100,000 individuals per year (4,16,21). More than 40% of pediatric SE occurs in children <2 years of age (22). Reported age-specific incidences for SE are 51 per 100,000 for children <1 year of age, 29 per 100,000 for those 1–4 years old, 9 per 100,000 for those 5–9 years old, and 2 per 100,000 for those 10–15 year old (16). Racial influences may be important in SE, with a greater incidence in nonwhites than in whites (21). Although mortality due to SE has decreased with improved supportive care, pediatric SE remains a medical emergency with overall mortality rates of 3%–7.2% (16,18,23).

Twenty-five percent to 40% of pediatric SE occurs in children with known epilepsy (24). In other words, 9.5%–27% of children with epilepsy will experience at least one episode of SE (5,25). Risk factors for SE in epileptic children include epilepsy induced by a known neurologic insult (symptomatic epilepsy) and previous episodes of SE (25). Other associated factors include use of multiple anticonvulsant medications, psychomotor retardation, generalized background abnormalities on EEG, and tapering of anticonvulsant medications. That being said, 60% of SE episodes among epileptic children occur despite therapeutic anticonvulsant drug levels and without any identifiable inciting event, such as fever or concurrent illness (26).

Conversely, more than half of SE occurs in patients without a prior diagnosis of epilepsy. In fact, 12% of children with new-onset unprovoked seizures present with SE (3,5). SE as the presentation of new-onset seizures is more common in younger children (22). Importantly, 17% of children with new-onset SE have associated, treatable inciting events, such as electrolyte abnormalities or central nervous system (CNS) infections (16).

Recurrent SE occurs in 13%–55% of pediatric patients, usually within 2 years of the first SE episode (5,16,18,27). The median interval between the first episode and recurrence is 25 days (range, 0–463 days) (16). Risk factors for recurrent SE are age <6 years, focal seizures, and an acute or remote CNS injury (5,18). In fact, children with a preexisting neurologic abnormality are 3–24 times more likely than previously healthy children to experience recurrence (16,18).

No population-based data are available to estimate the incidence of neonatal SE. Seizure type and brain maturation are influenced by gestational age, and studies suggest that neonatal SE is more common in full-term than preterm infants (17). In neonates with asphyxial injury, the duration of seizures has been "independently associated with brain injury" (17), emphasizing the need for prompt recognition and treatment in neonates.

ETIOLOGIES

Although initial supportive and anticonvulsant therapies are similar regardless of cause, diagnostic tests and adjunctive treatments are guided by suspected etiology. The etiologies of SE are commonly classified as cryptogenic, remote symptomatic, febrile, acute symptomatic, or progressive encephalopathic (Table 63.5) (22). Etiologies for pediatric SE vary by report: 30%–50% febrile, 24%–28% remote symptomatic, 8%–28% acute symptomatic, 15% cryptogenic, and 1%–5% progressive encephalopathies (22,28). The etiology of pediatric SE is age dependent (22), and variations likely reflect different age distributions or sampling biases of the studies.

Febrile or acute symptomatic etiologies are most common in younger children and account for more than 80% of SE among children <2 years of age (22). Two-thirds of episodes during the second year of life are due to febrile SE (22). In some cohorts, febrile SE continues to be a common etiology among children >3 years of age (28). However, cryptogenic and remote symptomatic etiologies account for more than 60% of SE in children >4 years of age (22). Tapering or withdrawal of anticonvulsant medications is a common inciting event among older children (23).

CNS infection, metabolic abnormalities, traumatic brain injury, and anoxic brain injury are the most common specific etiologies of acute symptomatic pediatric SE (22). Other reported inciting events are listed in Table 63.6. Meningitis is more frequent in infants. Anoxia is more common in children <5 years old. Among children who present with new-onset SE and fever, 12% have acute bacterial meningitis and 8% have viral CNS infections (16). Hypoxic-ischemic injury is the most prevalent cause of neonatal SE in developed countries, but electrolyte abnormalities continue to be more common in developing regions (17). Although rare, antibiotic-related SE is reported with the use of β-lactam antibiotics (particularly third- or fourth-generation cephalosporins and carbapenem), or quinolones in critically ill patients who have received high doses, have hepatic dysfunction, renal failure, or CNS lesions (29,30).

Identification and understanding of SE associated with fever and CNS inflammation in the absence of identified infection is increasing. Termed acute encephalopathy with inflammation-mediated status epilepticus (AEIMSE), the three most recognized disorders are idiopathic hemiconvulsive-hemiplegia syndrome in infancy (IHHS, age 0–4 years), fever-induced refractory epileptic encephalopathy in school-aged children (FIRES, age 4 years to adolescence and also known as acute encephalopathy with refractory, repetitive partial seizures [AERRPS]) and new-onset RSE (NORSE, age 20–50 years) (31,32). These disorders typically involve fever that may abate several days before seizure onset, often present as limbic encephalopathy (e.g., confusion or behavioral changes, movement disorders, and limbic seizures) and can be difficult to distinguish from other etiologies of RSE (31,32). Mortality is high (12%) and, among survivors, refractory epilepsy and

---

TABLE 63.5

ETIOLOGIC CLASSIFICATION OF STATUS EPILEPTICUS (SE)

■ ETIOLOGY	■ DEFINITION
Cryptogenic (idiopathic)	SE in the absence of an acute precipitating central nervous system insult or metabolic dysfunction in a patient without a preexisting neurologic abnormality
Remote symptomatic	SE in a patient with a known history of a neurologic insult associated with an increased risk of seizures (e.g., traumatic brain injury, stroke, static encephalopathy)
Febrile	SE provoked solely by fever in a patient without a history of afebrile seizures
Acute symptomatic	SE during an acute illness involving a known neurologic insult (e.g., meningitis, traumatic brain injury, hypoxia) or metabolic dysfunction (e.g., hypoglycemia, hypocalcemia, hyponatremia)
Progressive encephalopathy	SE in a patient with a progressive neurologic disease (e.g., neurodegeneration, malignancies, neurocutaneous syndromes)

Adapted from Shinnar S, Pellock JM, Moshe SL, et al. In whom does status epilepticus occur: Age-related differences in children. *Epilepsia* 1997;38:907–14.

TABLE 63.6

POTENTIAL ETIOLOGIES OF ACUTE SYMPTOMATIC STATUS EPILEPTICUS

	■ NEWBORN	■ 1–2 MONTHS OLD	■ INFANCY AND CHILDHOOD
Acute insult	Hypoxic-ischemic	CNS infection	CNS infection
	CNS infection	Subdural hematoma	Intracranial hemorrhage
	Intracranial hemorrhage	Anoxia	Anoxia
		VP shunt dysfunction	VP shunt dysfunction
Genetic and metabolic	Hypoglycemia	Hypoglycemia	Hypoglycemia
	Hypernatremia	Hypernatremia	Hypernatremia
	Hyponatremia	Hyponatremia	Hyponatremia
	Hypocalcemia	Hypocalcemia	Hypocalcemia
	Hypomagnesemia	Organic acidemia	Lysosomal defects
	Hyperbilirubinemia	Urea cycle defects	Urea cycle defects
	Organic acidemia	Phenylketonuria	Uremia
	Urea cycle defects	Riley-Day syndrome	Hepatic failure
	Nonketotic hyperglycemia		
	Congenital lactic acidosis		
	Pyridoxine dependency		
Malformation	Neuronal migration defect	Sturge-Weber syndrome	
	Chromosomal anomaly	Neurofibromatosis	
		Tuberous sclerosis	
Other	Toxins	Cocaine toxicity	Febrile convulsion
	Drugs	Drugs	Drugs
	Narcotic withdrawal	Narcotic withdrawal	Tricyclic antidepressants
			Anticonvulsants
			Calcineurin inhibitors
			Antibiotics (β-lactam,
			carbapenem, or quinolone)
			Opiates
			Narcotic withdrawal

significant cognitive disability are typical (31,32). Prompt recognition is important, as optimal diagnostic testing and treatment differ from other etiologies of SE.

MECHANISM OF DISEASE

The mechanisms of SE and the relationship between seizure activity, neuronal injury, and functional outcome are multifactorial and complex. Isolating the specific effects of seizures from those of underlying etiology and associated systemic influences remains difficult. Much of the current understanding of pathogenesis has been gleaned from experimental models. In many instances, experimental findings have been confirmed in patients with epilepsy.

Laboratory Models and Experimental Data

Experimental models of SE commonly use chemical convulsants or electrical stimulation to induce self-sustaining seizures. These models provide insight into the mechanisms of seizure initiation, propagation, and termination, as well as patterns of cerebral development that affect seizure development and SE.

Behavioral and Electroencephalographic Manifestations

The progression of both clinical and experimental convulsive SE (CSE) may be divided into five stages (33). The first stage is characterized by discrete seizures, which are typically focal with secondary generalization and manifest as generalized tonic-clonic convulsions. In the second stage, continued

discrete seizures merge to produce an EEG pattern of asymmetric sharp-and-spike waves with waxing and waning amplitude accompanied by either generalized convulsions or serial tonic or clonic seizures involving one or more extremities. The third stage is characterized by cEEG seizure discharges and either clonic jerks or subtle clonic convulsive activity. In the fourth stage, flat periods of EEG activity interrupt continuous seizure discharges, and behavioral clonic convulsions may be overt, subtle, or absent. During the fifth stage, the EEG shows monomorphic, repetitive, sharp waves, called *periodic lateralized epileptiform discharges* (PLEDS), on a flat background, and accompanying motor manifestations are absent. In the immature (vs. the adult) brain, the EEG progression through all five stages is less consistent and behavioral manifestations less discrete (34). Treatment with anticonvulsants can interrupt both EEG and behavioral progression of SE.

Seizure Initiation and Progression

Seizure initiation and propagation involve a failure of γ-aminobutyric-acid (GABA)-mediated inhibition and/or an increase in glutamate-mediated excitation. A seizure begins with an intrinsically firing neuron, which, facilitated by inadequate inhibition, recruits adjacent neurons (35). Aberrant neuronal excitation commonly originates near regions of cerebral injury or scarring but may arise from uninjured neurons (36). As adjacent neurons begin firing, excitatory mediators, including glutamate, are released. Glutamate activates N-methyl-D-aspartate (NMDA) receptors and is thought to facilitate local neuronal synchronization, as well as seizure spread. In experimental models, NMDA receptor antagonists block seizure progression (37).

The mechanisms that enable the self-sustained seizures necessary for SE remain poorly understood. Localized "feed-forward" excitatory circuits are identified in experimental models of self-sustaining hippocampal seizures (2). Aberrant excitatory circuits created by injury-induced axonal sprouting are associated with neuronal hyperexcitability and acquired epilepsy (36). The pathogenic contribution of such excitatory circuits to SE remains controversial, but they are unlikely to be a sufficient cause.

Other putative mechanisms that promote self-sustaining seizures include a reduction of inhibitory interneuron activity (36) and receptor trafficking changes that favor excitability (1). In seizure models, synaptic GABA_A receptors are downregulated, whereas NMDA receptors are upregulated, promoting neuronal excitability (1). These seizure-induced alterations of GABA and glutamate activity may facilitate seizure continuation and spread, as well as hinder seizure termination. A predominance of inhibition is required for seizure termination and may be achieved by augmenting inhibition or blocking excitation. Mechanisms implicated in seizure termination include a predominance of GABA activity, membrane stabilization by acidic extracellular pH, magnesium blockade of NMDA channels, activation of the sodium–potassium adenosine triphosphatase (Na/K-ATPase) pump system, and activation of potassium (K^+) conductance to allow membrane repolarization (38). Adenosine, an endogenous neuroprotectant, is thought to regulate basal neural inhibition (39) and may also prove important for seizure termination. Treatment with adenosine antagonists, such as caffeine or aminophylline, is proconvulsant. Conversely, adenosine-releasing stem cells attenuate seizure activity in epilepsy models (40).

Refractory Status Epilepticus

The mechanisms that underlie the pharmacologic resistance that characterizes RSE remain unclear and are likely multifactorial. Putative mechanisms include alterations in anticonvulsant drug targets and failure to achieve efficacious drug levels in the brain (1,41). Changes in receptor composition or membrane trafficking may be induced by prolonged seizure activity or chronic anticonvulsant therapy. For example, seizure-induced downregulation of GABA_A receptors may reduce the efficacy of benzodiazepines in RSE (1). Similarly, extrusion of anticonvulsants across the blood–brain barrier (BBB) may limit anticonvulsant activity. Overexpression of the transporter's multidrug resistance gene-1 P-glycoprotein (MDR1) and multidrug resistance–associated protein 1 (MRP1) has been implicated in refractory epilepsy (41). Rats with pharmacologic-resistant seizures show marked overexpression of MDR1 and lower brain levels of phenobarbital (41). In these models, co-administration of a P-glycoprotein inhibitor increases brain anticonvulsant levels and reduces pharmacologic resistance (41). Similarly, MDR1 and MRP1 are overexpressed in brain tissue from patients with refractory epilepsy (42); however, the relative contributions of MDR1 and MRP1 to RSE remain unknown. Still, modulation of P-glycoprotein activity may hold promise as adjunctive therapy. Case reports (one pediatric and one adult) suggest that verapamil, a nonselective P-glycoprotein inhibitor, may combat pharmacologic resistance in RSE (43,44); however, it also disrupts basal transporter activity, which may hinder endogenous neuroprotection (45). Cyclooxygenase-2 (COX-2) inhibitors (e.g., indomethacin and celecoxib) selectively inhibit seizure-induced P-glycoprotein upregulation and increase both brain levels of anticonvulsants and seizure control in experimental models (45), but clinical studies are needed.

Maturational Sequences in the Immature Brain

The immature brain is more susceptible to seizures than is the mature brain, likely due to maturational differences of excitatory and inhibitory systems (46). A predominance of excitatory activity guides early development. Consequently, the immature brain is more excitable, seizures generalize more rapidly, and the postictal refractory period is shorter. In rats, a mature balance of excitatory and inhibitory activity is achieved during the first 3 postnatal weeks (46). The corresponding timeline in humans is not clear; however, positron emission tomography studies suggest that functional GABA_A activity reaches adult-like patterns during the teenage years (47). Paradoxically, the immature brain is relatively resistant to seizure-induced cell death and synaptic reorganization (48). In contrast to the neuronal loss seen in adults, seizure-induced neurogenesis may occur in the immature brain (48). Despite a relative resistance to histologic injury, seizures during development can cause permanent, adverse effects, including cognitive impairment and lower seizure thresholds (46,48).

Cerebral Injury Induced by Status Epilepticus

Seizures that last 30–60 minutes are sufficient to cause neuronal injury (49). Importantly, both CSE and NCSE may be injurious, and both must be controlled as efficiently as possible. Neuronal injury induced by SE is predominantly due to prolonged seizure activity, not to systemic complications, such as hypoxia, hypoglycemia, or hyperthermia. Autopsy study of three adult patients dying of focal motor SE without any systemic complications revealed neuronal loss in the piriform and entorhinal cortex, hippocampus, amygdala, and cerebellum (50). Similar injury patterns are reported in experimental models of SE induced by glutamate receptor agonists and in humans who accidentally ingested mussels that were contaminated with domoic acid, a potent glutamate receptor agonist (49,50).

These findings corroborate the hypothesis that seizure-induced cerebral injury is mediated by excitotoxicity. Excessive glutamate activates NMDA receptors, causing excessive calcium influx with resultant activation of intracellular proteases, nitric oxide production, free-radical generation, oxidative injury, and ultimately cell death (49). Additionally, in cells that do not die, elevated intracellular calcium concentrations may alter calcium-dependent second-messenger effects, affecting neurogenesis, axonal sprouting, protein expression, gene regulation, and/or receptor-gated ion-channel recycling (37). These alterations may promote the development of epilepsy and cognitive deficits after SE.

Clinically, patterns of cerebral involvement after pediatric SE are not well defined and likely vary by etiology. Febrile SE, which is the best studied, has been linked to hippocampal abnormalities. In a prospective comparison of acute magnetic resonance imaging (MRI) findings in 35 children with febrile or afebrile SE, febrile SE was associated with acute, vasogenic, hippocampal edema, which resolved 3–5 days after SE (51,52). Additionally, 24% of children with febrile SE had other abnormal findings, such as hippocampal asymmetry, an arachnoid cyst, and subtle loss of gray–white differentiation in the left middle temporal gyrus. In contrast, children with afebrile SE had no hippocampal enlargement, but roughly 60% had nonhippocampal abnormalities (e.g., delayed myelination, cerebral infarction, cortical dysplasia, and cerebral vasculitis) (51). Follow-up MRI in 23 children with febrile SE, performed at a mean interval of 5.5 months, showed reduced hippocampal volumes and increased hippocampal asymmetry, compared with the initial scan (53). Furthermore, the expected age-dependent changes in hippocampal apparent diffusion coefficient measurements were not seen in children with febrile SE, which supports the hypothesis that they have underlying hippocampal abnormalities (52).

Increased Vulnerability with Concurrent Neurologic Insults

In the presence of an accompanying acute neurologic insult, the seizure duration necessary to cause neuronal injury may be shorter than 30–60 minutes. Seizures increase glucose metabolism and intracranial pressure (ICP), placing vulnerable cerebral tissue at greater risk for injury. In adult patients with stroke, seizures are associated with worsening of cerebral edema and midline shift (54), as well as a threefold increase in mortality, compared with patients who lack seizures (55). Similarly, seizures are an independent risk factor for poor outcome after severe traumatic brain injury (54,56). Posttraumatic seizures increase brain interstitial glutamate and glycerol concentrations, suggesting exacerbation of excitotoxicity, ischemia, and secondary neuronal injury (57,58). Among children <2 years of age, posttraumatic seizures portend a twofold increase in the risk of poor functional outcome (56). Importantly, subclinical seizures are common in patients with acute neurologic insults, yet diagnosis frequently requires a high degree of suspicion and cEEG monitoring (54). For example, cEEG monitoring detected nonconvulsive seizures in 14%–23% of critically ill acute pediatric stroke victims (59,60).

CLINICAL PRESENTATION AND DIFFERENTIAL DIAGNOSIS

Typical clinical presentations of CSE and NCSE are described here. Representative EEG tracings for the different classes of SE are shown in **Figure 63.1**.

Convulsive Status Epilepticus

Generalized Convulsive Status Epilepticus. GCSE may be tonic-clonic, clonic, or tonic in nature. Forty percent to 80% of GCSE in children presents as continuous seizures, most commonly with generalized tonic-clonic activity (24). In children with epilepsy, GCSE often starts as increasing frequency of serial seizures, with recovery of consciousness between episodes (premonitory SE), and prompt treatment during this stage may prevent progression (2). Serial seizures typically last 1–3 minutes but tend to shorten as time elapses. Between seizures, patients are obtunded, showing autonomic signs, such as salivation, bradypnea, cyanosis, and arterial hypotension. In some cases, cardiovascular collapse may occur. Neurologic examination may reveal abnormal cranial nerve function and unilateral or bilateral Babinski responses (2). Cerebrospinal fluid pleocytosis as a consequence of GCSE has been documented in all ages.

Clonic Status Epilepticus. Clonic SE may persist hours or even days, waxing and waning in intensity, and a persistent postictal hemiplegia is usually observed. The behavioral manifestations of clonic SE are variable. Seizures tend to be continuous and may be generalized, unilateral, or restricted to one limb or segment. Fluctuations between different patterns of involvement may occur during a single episode of clonic SE. Additionally, the rhythm of jerks is variable and may also fluctuate. Clonic seizures in young children are predominantly unilateral; however, they may shift from side to side (24). Approximately 75% of patients with unilateral clonic seizures are 3 years of age or younger (2,24). Consciousness may be preserved during clonic SE, and autonomic involvement is generally less pronounced than with tonic-clonic seizures.

Tonic Status Epilepticus. Tonic SE is less common than tonic-clonic or clonic SE and occurs almost exclusively in children and adolescents with known epilepsy (24). Importantly, tonic SE has been precipitated by intravenous or oral benzodiazepine treatment of absence SE in children with Lennox-Gastaut syndrome (2,24). Tonic SE can persist for several days, much longer than other CSE types (2,24). Serial tonic seizures are typical, and autonomic manifestations, particularly increased bronchial secretions, may be pronounced. Over time, behavioral manifestations become limited to slight eye deviation, respiratory irregularities, and marked tracheobronchial obstruction due to hypersecretion. Consciousness is moderately or severely impaired, and a postictal confusional state may persist for days. The initial behavioral manifestations of tonic SE may be attenuated or even subclinical (2,24). In these cases, polygraphic monitoring is necessary to demonstrate the tachycardia, altered respiratory rhythm, occasional hypertonus of the trunk or neck muscles, and EEG activity indicative of tonic SE.

Focal Motor Status Epilepticus. Focal motor SE may affect children with acute inciting insults (**Table 63.2**) or those with known epileptic disorders. Focal motor SE due to an acute illness, such as encephalitis, typically develops into secondary GCSE. Conversely, in children with epilepsy, focal motor SE tends to have a more restricted distribution and may be manifest only as jerking of the corner of the mouth or cheek, salivation, swallowing difficulties, and absent speech. Even with narrowly localized seizures, autonomic disturbances and some impairment of consciousness may be present. Children who appear to be in focal motor SE may be treated despite a lack of seizure activity on EEG (2,24).

Myoclonic Status Epilepticus. Myoclonic SE is characterized by the incessant repetition of massive myoclonic jerks. Acute hypoxic-ischemic encephalopathy is the most common cause of myoclonic SE among critically ill children. When associated with anoxic brain injury, myoclonic SE indicates severe diffuse brain damage and can be difficult to control. Myoclonic SE also occurs with metabolic insults, such as hypoglycemia, hepatic or renal failure, or heavy-metal intoxication (**Table 63.3**). Physical trauma or inflammatory disease rarely causes myoclonic SE. Importantly, myoclonic SE may be induced by high doses of β-lactam antibiotics, especially in patients with renal failure (2,24). Intrathecal administration of radiologic contrast agents is also associated with myoclonic SE, typically with a favorable prognosis (2,24). Finally, myoclonic SE also affects children with epilepsy (4,53) and has been described with Angelman syndrome (61).

Nonconvulsive Status Epilepticus

The diagnostic criteria for NCSE are in evolution, with no standard, uniformly accepted definitions or terminology. The classic definition of NCSE is tripartite: (a) prolonged (greater than 30 minutes) alteration of consciousness or complex partial seizures without full recovery of consciousness; (b) epileptiform changes on the EEG that are different from the preictal state; and (c) prompt observable improvement in both the EEG and clinical state after administration of an intravenous antiepileptic medication.

Whether generalized or focal, NCSE can present with a variety of clinical features, including agitation and aggression, lethargy, confusion, delirium, fugue-like state, decreased speech, mutism, echolalia, blank staring with or without blinking, chewing and picking, tremulousness, subtle facial or limb myoclonus, rigidity or waxy flexibility, or vegetative features. NCSE is seen in children with epilepsy (Landau-Kleffner syndrome) and ring chromosome 20 (17,24). Additionally, critically ill patients with unexplained coma or prolonged obtundation after CSE may have NCSE (7).

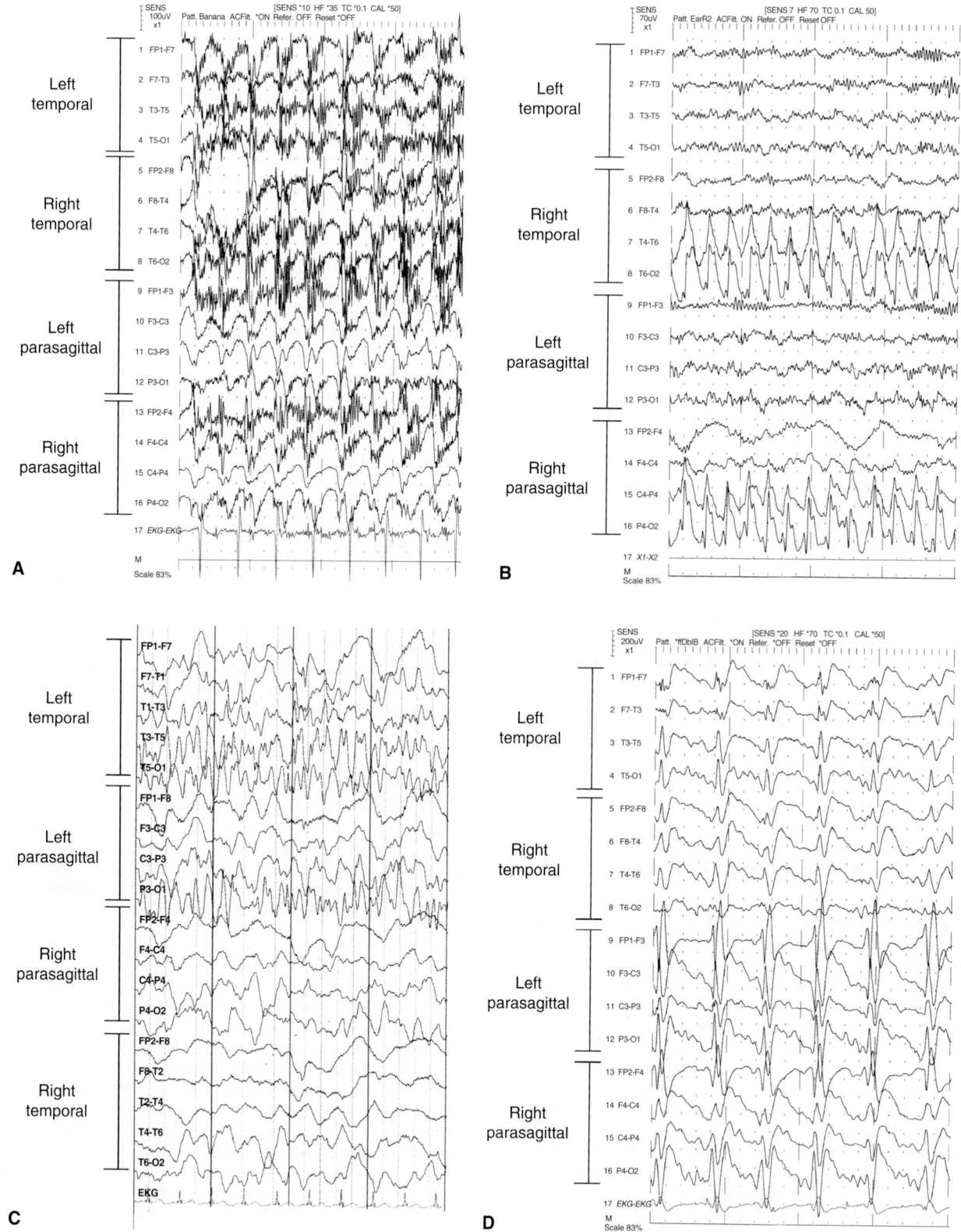

FIGURE 63.1. Representative EEG tracings that show status epilepticus. **A:** Generalized convulsive status epilepticus. Note the generalized spike-and-wave pattern, which is partially obscured by muscle artifact (heavy black tracings of fast activity), most prominent in the frontal and temporal leads. **B:** Focal motor status epilepticus in a patient with Sturge-Weber syndrome and a vascular lesion near the seizure focus. Note the repetitive spike and slow wave activity localized to the right posterior temporal and parietal leads. **C:** Complex partial status epilepticus arising from the left posterior temporal region. Note the rhythmic sharp wave activity in the left temporal leads with spread to the left occipital region. **D:** Nonconvulsive status epilepticus in a patient with Lennox-Gastaut syndrome. Note the bilateral symmetric spike and slow wave activity, which has maximal amplitude in the frontal leads.

Absence NCSE. Generalized NCSE is widely known as absence SE, although it has also been called *petit mal status* and *spike-wave stupor*. Absence SE typically occurs during the first decade of life, and 75% of cases occur before the age of 20 (24). Absence SE is characterized by a variable impairment of consciousness, ranging from mild slowing of higher cognitive functions to barely perceptible responsiveness. Complex automatisms may occur and motor manifestations (e.g., myoclonic eyelid and facial twitching, bilateral or unilateral limb myoclonus, and/or atonic phenomena that produce falls, head nods, knee buckling, or other alterations of posture) are seen in about half of the cases. Patients are totally or partially amnestic of these episodes. Of note, patients typically do not show the cycling in the clinical state that characterizes complex partial SE (24).

Complex Partial SE. Complex partial SE is also known as psychomotor status, focal NCSE, temporolimbic SE, or localized NCSE. It occurs less commonly in children but can be seen in the course of focal epilepsies (24). Complex partial SE can present as frequently recurring partial seizures without full recovery of consciousness between seizures or continuous long-standing episodes of mental confusion and behavioral disturbance with or without automatisms. Complex partial SE is often marked by cyclic alterations between unresponsive staring and partial responsiveness with quasipurposeful reactive automatisms (24).

Nonconvulsive SE in Comatose Patients. NCSE should be considered in children with prolonged "postictal state" or unexplained alterations in consciousness (e.g., confusion, stupor, coma). EEG monitoring of such children shows nonconvulsive seizures in 16%–46% and NCSE in 18%–33% (8–13). Continuous (vs. short-duration) EEG monitoring is often necessary, as reported detection rates increase from 43%–57% during the first hour to 71%–97% at 24 hours of monitoring (8,10,12). Localized EEG findings are common and typically correlate with neuroimaging abnormalities (11,13). Consultation with a neurologist is imperative, as EEG interpretation can be difficult and determining EEG activity that requires treatment remains controversial.

Refractory Status Epilepticus

RSE may occur with any classification or etiology of SE and is associated with greater morbidity and mortality than more responsive SE (38,62). Although RSE typically has motor manifestations, it may begin as NCSE. Even in patients who present with GCSE, RSE frequently becomes subtle or nonconvulsive (NCRSE). Risk factors for developing RSE include a family history of seizures, presence of electrographic seizures, and NCSE (62). Among children with a chronic seizure disorder, poorer baseline seizure control, and greater number of baseline anticonvulsant medications are additional risk factors (62). Patients with acute structural lesions are at higher risk for NCRSE (38). Poor outcomes after RSE are associated with age <5 years, acute symptomatic etiology, NCSE, and longer seizure duration (62). Encouragingly, better outcomes are associated with more aggressive treatment (62). A high degree of suspicion with cEEG monitoring is required for timely and accurate diagnosis (38), and cEEG monitoring is important to guide therapy in any patient with RSE.

Systemic Manifestations

Much of our knowledge of the systemic manifestations of SE comes from classic studies of GCSE in primates conducted during the early 1970s (63). GCSE can be divided into early and late phases. During early SE, compensatory mechanisms to attenuate seizure-associated injury are prominent (i.e., increased catecholamines, tachycardia, hypertension, increased cerebral blood flow). The transition from early to late SE occurs after ~30 to 45 minutes of continuous seizure activity. Late SE is marked by failure of compensatory mechanisms and seizure-associated injury (i.e., hyperthermia, hypotension, hypoglycemia, lost cerebral autoregulation). Additionally, once the transition from early to late SE has occurred, SE is more difficult to terminate.

Autonomic and Metabolic Changes

The autonomic and metabolic changes seen during GCSE differ between early and late SE. During early SE, increased catecholamine levels result in tachycardia, hypertension, increased central venous pressures, and hyperglycemia. Cerebral blood flow (CBF) increases in response to increased cerebral metabolic demands. Lactic acidosis commonly results from continued, rigorous muscle activity. Mild hypoxemia and modest hypercarbia may occur, but patients usually maintain sufficient oxygenation and ventilation if the airway remains patent. Other autonomic signs, including diaphoresis, hypersecretion, and mydriasis, are frequent.

During late SE, compensatory reserves are exhausted, and marked hyperthermia, hypotension, and hypoglycemia may occur. Cerebrovascular autoregulation is lost and CBF becomes pressure dependent, making prompt correction of hypotension crucial. Cerebral edema may accompany late SE and is more common in pediatric than in adult patients. Sustained motor convulsions may result in rhabdomyolysis and hyperkalemia. Hypoxia and hypercarbia are frequently more exaggerated during late SE. Respiratory compromise, associated with apnea or poor handling of secretions, is common. Pupillary and corneal reflexes may be absent in the ictal or postictal phases of both early and late SE.

Other Concerns

Rarely, disseminated intravascular coagulation and multiorgan failure may be induced by SE itself or by the inciting cause. Myoglobinuria or dehydration and shock may lead to renal failure. Hepatic insufficiency or failure may result from the underlying cause of SE, as a side effect of anticonvulsant therapy, or from hyperpyrexia. Finally, emesis is common, and patients with SE are at high risk for aspiration.

Differential Diagnosis

CSE is usually easy to diagnose and not readily confused with other disorders in a nonparalyzed patient. However, pseudostatus epilepticus can be confused with CSE on occasion, with disastrous results. Clinical signs suggestive of nonepileptic psychogenic seizures include motor movements that fluctuate in intensity, frequency, and/or distribution, with lack of facial muscle involvement and including pelvic thrusting. Vocalization, bizarre behavior, explosive emotional expression, and resistance to examination are common. Although urinary incontinence, tongue biting, and cyanosis can occur, they are less common than in CSE. In pseudostatus epilepticus, the EEG is often obscured by muscle and movement artifact, and no postictal EEG changes occur. A well-developed α rhythm can be discerned during brief moments of movement cessation or on termination of pseudoseizures. In contrast, patients with CSE have both ictal and postictal EEG changes. Furthermore, the muscle artifact associated with pseudoseizures lacks the repetitive characteristics seen in true CSE.

In contrast, the seizure behavior associated with NCSE is nonspecific and may produce diagnostic confusion. Two common conditions that may simulate the seizure behaviors of

NCSE are postictal drowsiness and anticonvulsant-induced sedation. Continuous EEG recordings may be necessary to accurately distinguish these disorders. Many toxic-metabolic (including drug intoxication and drug withdrawal) and infectious (including para- and postinfectious) encephalopathies present with altered mental status and may be clinically indistinguishable from NCSE. Additionally, altered mental status that mimics NCSE can be caused by acute structural lesions, including traumatic brain injury, tumors, and stroke. Neuroimaging studies are helpful in differentiating these etiologies. Finally, psychiatric disorders should be considered in patients with behavioral changes not associated with appropriate ictal and interictal EEG changes.

Clinical Management

SE is a medical emergency that requires prompt intervention, as seizure duration is inversely associated with treatment responsiveness and favorable outcome. Management of the critically ill child with SE is directed toward rapid cessation of seizures, supportive care of associated systemic derangements or complications, treatment of causal or underlying conditions, and prevention of seizure recurrence.

Initial Stabilization

As with any critically ill child, the first priority of initial stabilization is to ensure airway patency and control. The patient should be positioned so that ongoing seizure activity will not cause physical harm. Nothing should be placed into the patient's mouth due to the risk of aspiration. Supplemental oxygen should be provided and respiration assisted as needed. Precautions should be taken to prevent aspiration.

In patients with hypoxemia, hypoventilation, weakened airway protective reflexes, or a Glasgow Coma Scale score <8, rapid-sequence tracheal intubation should be considered for airway protection and respiratory support (see Chapter 24). Data regarding the preferred induction agents for intubation are lacking. Short-acting sedative-hypnotics are preferred, and dose-associated hypotension should be anticipated and avoided. If neuromuscular blockade is necessary to facilitate intubation, a short-acting agent allows more rapid evaluation of continued seizure activity. The risk of hyperkalemia associated with ongoing seizure activity should be considered if using succinylcholine. Repeated or continued neuromuscular blockade should also be avoided, as it may mask ongoing seizure activity.

Reliable intravenous access should be established as soon as possible. If placement of an intravenous catheter is difficult or prolonged, an intraosseous needle and catheter should be considered as an alternative for giving anticonvulsants and fluids. Hypotension or dehydration should be treated with isotonic fluid resuscitation. Due to concerns that cerebral hypoperfusion may exacerbate cerebral injury, some treatment guidelines advocate administration of vasopressor agents to assure and maintain normal blood pressure (64). Hypertension is common with ongoing seizure activity, and treatment should not be considered unless it persists after seizure activity has stopped.

Hypoglycemia should be considered as an inciting event, and the serum glucose level should be checked promptly. In the absence of rapid testing, empiric dextrose should be administered intravenously. Thiamine (50–100 mg IV) may be considered prior to dextrose administration in older children at risk of nutritional deficiencies. Pyridoxine (50–100 mg IV) should be given to neonates with persistent seizures and suspected pyridoxine-dependent seizure activity. Electrolyte abnormalities, such as hyponatremia or hypocalcemia, should also be considered. Serum electrolytes should be checked and replaced

appropriately. High-dose antibiotics should be administered empirically to all patients at risk of bacterial infection, as well as to those who present with new-onset SE and fever. Empiric acyclovir should also be considered for patients who present with new-onset SE and fever and who are at risk for herpetic infections.

Supportive Care for Associated Derangements

Prolonged seizure activity is associated with the development of metabolic acidosis, hyperthermia, and rhabdomyolysis. Metabolic acidosis usually corrects spontaneously after seizure cessation and appropriate hydration. Due to the potential for exacerbating cerebral injury, hyperthermia (>38.5°C) should be treated with antipyretic medications and, if needed, surface and/or systemic cooling to promptly achieve normothermia. Precautions should be taken to prevent shivering associated with active cooling. If neuromuscular blockade is required, cEEG monitoring is indicated to assess for ongoing seizure activity.

Other supportive care is determined by the cause of SE and side effects of necessary anticonvulsant therapies. Empiric therapies targeted to the cause of SE should be initiated concurrently with attaining seizure control. Among children admitted to the intensive care unit with SE, roughly 60% require intubation (65). The average duration of mechanical ventilatory support is 2 days (65). The typical ICU length of stay is 3 days; however, in patients with acute infectious etiologies, such as meningitis and encephalitis, length of stay is longer (65). For patients who require pharmacologically induced coma for RSE, continued respiratory, hemodynamic, and nutritional support are required. Vasoactive or inotropic agents are frequently needed to manage medication-induced hypotension or myocardial depression. Parenteral nutrition may be necessary due to development of ileus.

Nosocomial infections among SE patients, while not well studied, may be common and influence outcomes. Recently, ventilator-associated pneumonia was diagnosed in 13.6% of ventilated adults being treated for SE (66). Importantly, recognition of an infection during SE (whether community-acquired or nosocomial) has been associated with longer SE duration, 4.8-fold increased risk of RSE, 5.2-fold increased risk of death, and longer ICU and hospital lengths of stay (66). Rates and effects of nosocomial infections are not reported in children with SE; however, adherence to practices targeted toward prevention appears prudent.

Diagnostic Tests

Swift cessation of seizures is crucial, and anticonvulsant therapy should not be delayed to facilitate diagnostic testing. All patients with SE should have serum glucose and electrolyte levels measured. Further diagnostic tests are guided by probable or suspected etiology (Table 63.7). Serum anticonvulsant medication levels should be measured in children on chronic therapy. Blood and urine specimens should be obtained for culture, especially in febrile children. Serum and urine toxicology screening tests should be sent for patients with possible ingestions. After the seizures have stopped, a head computed tomography (CT) scan is appropriate in patients with new-onset seizures or those at risk for anatomic abnormalities, mass intracranial lesions (e.g., brain tumor, brain abscess, intracranial hemorrhage), or cerebral edema. Once a mass intracranial lesion or cerebral edema has been excluded, lumbar puncture is indicated in patients at risk for meningitis or those with a new-onset seizure disorder. Due to the risk of downward herniation, lumbar puncture should be avoided in patients with evidence of increased ICP. Serum ammonia, lactate, and serum

TABLE 63.7

INITIAL DIAGNOSTIC CONSIDERATIONS IN STATUS EPILEPTICUS

Laboratory tests	Serum glucose and electrolytes
	Anticonvulsant medication levels (if on chronic therapy)
	Complete blood count with differential and coagulation work-up
	Cultures and serology for bacterial, viral or fungal infections
	Serum and urine toxicology screens
	Serum lactate and ammonia levels
	Serum amino acids and urine organic acids (if suspected inborn error of metabolism)
Neuroimaging	Brain CT to evaluate for acute lesion or cerebral edema
	Brain MRI to evaluate for structural lesions or anomalies (if focal seizures or other concerns)
CSF evaluation (unless contraindicated)	Cell count with differential, glucose and protein levels
	Gram stain and culture
	Polymerase chain reaction (PCR) and antibody testing for viral infections[a]
Other	Nasopharyngeal swab testing for viral infections

[a]Please see Kneen et al. Management of suspected viral encephalitis in children: Association of British neurologists and British paediatric allergy, immunology and infection group national guidelines. *J Infect* 2012;65:449–77 for summary of potential pathogens.
Adapted from Wilkes R, Tasker RC. Pediatric intensive care treatment of uncontrolled status epilepticus. *Crit Care Clin* 2013;29:239–57.

TABLE 63.8

DIAGNOSTIC CONSIDERATIONS IN REFRACTORY OR SUPER-REFRACTORY STATUS EPILEPTICUS

Laboratory tests	Inflammatory markers (e.g., C-reactive protein, erythrocyte sedimentation rate)
	Autoimmune evaluation (e.g., immunoglobulin levels, complement levels, anti-nuclear antibodies, etc.)
	Carnitine and acyl-carnitine levels
	Very long chain fatty acids
	Heavy-metal testing
	Vitamin B12 and folate levels
	Repeat and/or expand serology for infectious agents
Neuroimaging	Brain MRI with and without gadolinium enhancement and with diffusion weighted imaging sequences
	Cerebral angiogram
CSF evaluation	Repeat cell count with differential, glucose and protein levels
	Repeat and/or expand PCR and antibody testing for infections[a]
	Oligoclonal banding
	Amino acids
	Neurotransmitters
	Neuronal and ion-channel antibodies
Genetic testing	Voltage-gated sodium channel subunit SCN1A mutations
Tissue	Brain biopsy to assess for microvascular vasculitis

[a]Please see Kneen et al. Management of suspected viral encephalitis in children: Association of British neurologists and British paediatric allergy, immunology and infection group national guidelines. *J Infect* 2012;65:449–77 for summary of potential pathogens.
Adapted from Wilkes R, Tasker RC. Pediatric intensive care treatment of uncontrolled status epilepticus. *Crit Care Clin* 2013;29:239–57.

amino and urine organic acid levels should be checked in infants and children at risk for inborn errors of metabolism. More specific metabolic testing may be appropriate for certain patients and should be considered in consultation with a pediatric neurologist or geneticist.

Evaluation for inflammation-induced or antibody-mediated SE should be considered in all cases of super-refractory SE not attributable to other causes (Table 63.8). Given the complexity and seriousness of these disorders, diagnostic testing will frequently be coordinated between intensivists, neurologists, infectious disease specialists, immunologists, and geneticists. Cerebral angiography or even brain biopsy may be necessary to accurately diagnose underlying microvascular cerebral vasculitis. The need for and extent of genetic testing should be reevaluated with each case, as more than 70 genes associated with epilepsy are currently identified and knowledge in this area is rapidly expanding.

Medications for Seizure Termination

Rapid cessation of SE is associated with improved response rates and clinical outcomes. Consequently, administration of anticonvulsants for SE should proceed along a defined timeline, with the goal of controlling SE within 30 minutes of presentation (Fig. 63.2). The progression of treatment includes administration of a first-line agent, administration of a second-line agent, and initiation of pharmacologic coma for treatment of RSE.

Randomized clinical trials that evaluate anticonvulsant efficacy in the pediatric population are lacking. Consequently,

anticonvulsant choice is guided largely by clinician experience, clinical reports, and expert opinion. Results of a comprehensive survey that investigated the anticonvulsant practices of ~40 pediatric neurologists who specialize in epilepsy (67) guide the first- and second-line anticonvulsant recommendations in this chapter. Treatment guidelines from the UK National Institute for Health and Clinical Excellence (NICE) (68), the Scottish Intercollegiate Guidelines Network (69), and the USA Neurocritical Care Society (64) are also incorporated. Recommendations for treatment of NCSE or RSE further incorporate findings from clinical cohort or case studies, extrapolation from adult practice, and clinical experience.

First- and Second-line Medications

First- and second-line medications for SE are determined by SE classification (Tables 63.9 and 63.10). Recommended medication doses are detailed in Table 63.11. Administration of levetiracetam, a newer anticonvulsant medication, is gaining interest and is discussed; however, there are insufficient evidence and experience to support incorporation as a preferred first- or second-line agent.

Benzodiazepines. Benzodiazepines bind the $GABA_A$ receptor complex and facilitate GABA action by increasing the frequency of channel opening, thereby increasing chloride permeability and leading to hyperpolarization. Commonly used benzodiazepines for SE include lorazepam, diazepam, and midazolam. In a retrospective, population-based study, 58% of children with convulsive seizures that lasted longer

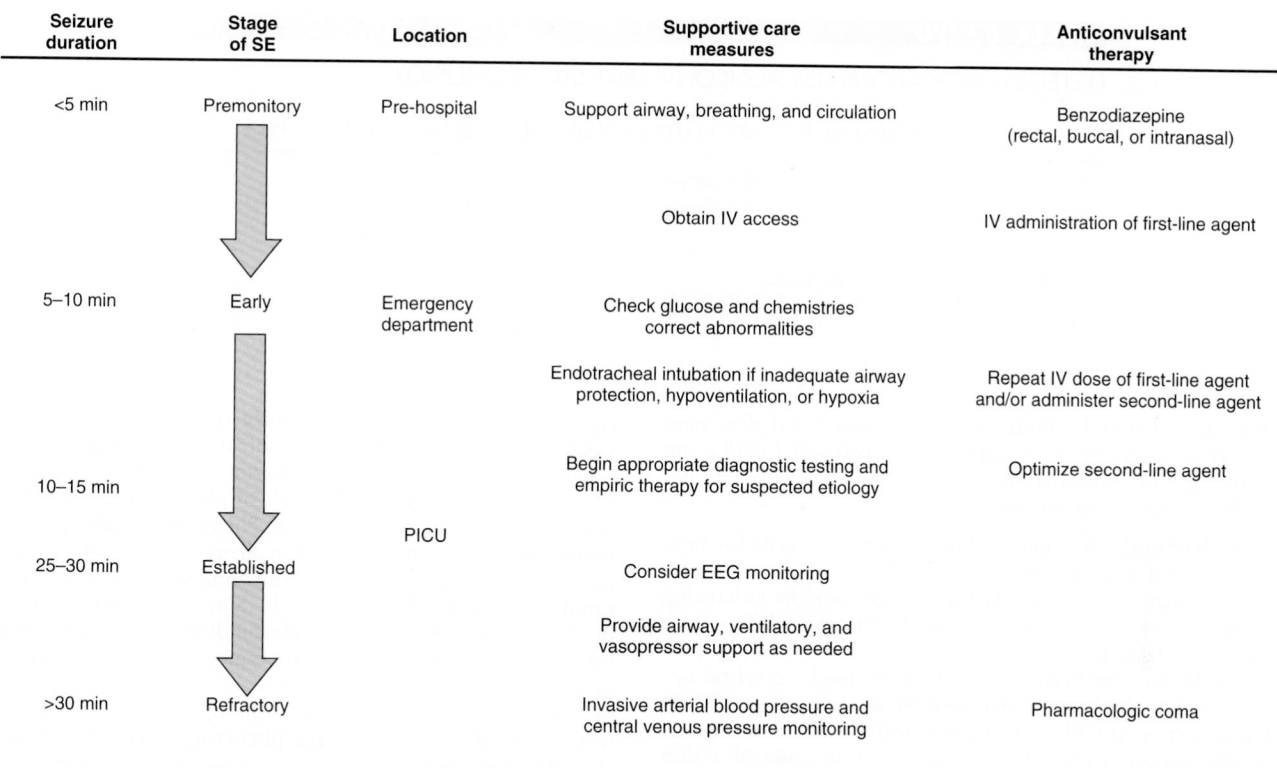

FIGURE 63.2. Suggested algorithm for the goal-directed treatment of pediatric status epilepticus. (Adapted from Chen JW, Wasterlain CG. Status epilepticus: Pathophysiology and management in adults. *Lancet Neurol* 2006;5:246–56 and Dhar R, Mirsattari SM. Current approach to the diagnosis and treatment of refractory status epilepticus. *Adv Neurol* 2006;97:245–54.)

than 5 minutes responded to benzodiazepines (70). However, benzodiazepines lose potency during prolonged SE (1,4,38), possibly related to seizure-induced GABA$_A$ receptor down-regulation (1). Additionally, benzodiazepines may precipitate myoclonus in a small percentage of neonates or tonic seizures in patients with Lennox-Gastaut syndrome.

The intravenous administration of lorazepam is the first-line treatment for all types of convulsive SE except neonatal SE, for which it is a second-line agent. The peak effect of intravenous lorazepam occurs 15 minutes after dosing, and the duration is 3–6 hours. If a single dose is not effective, a second dose is recommended before or concurrent with administration of a second-line agent. Both diazepam and midazolam may be administered intravenously as well, but they have less favorable pharmacokinetic profiles than lorazepam (1). Given intravenously, both diazepam and midazolam have shorter durations than lorazepam (roughly 15–30 and 30–80 minutes, respectively). Additionally, midazolam is metabolized by hepatic cytochrome P4503A4 enzymes and may have variable metabolism and more drug interactions.

For patients who do not have intravenous access, consider intramuscular, buccal, or intranasal routes of administration for midazolam (71–74). A recent prehospital randomized controlled trial showed equal or superior efficacy and similar safety for intramuscular midazolam compared with intravenous lorazepam (72). The bioavailability of intramuscular midazolam is ~90%, and it is rapidly absorbed, with an average onset of 2–3 minutes and peak plasma levels 30 minutes after dosing. The most recent NICE guidelines list buccal midazolam as the preferred treatment for prolonged seizures when unable to secure immediate intravenous access (68). Buccal administration of midazolam is easy and safe: an appropriate dose of the intravenous preparation of midazolam is placed between the gum and cheek. In a randomized trial that compared seizure cessation after equipotent doses of buccal midazolam and rectal diazepam, buccal midazolam was effective in twice as many patients and had better seizure control, shorter onset of action, less need for intravenous lorazepam dosing, and less seizure recurrence (71). Similarly, intranasal administration of midazolam has been shown to be safe in

TABLE 63.9

PREFERRED MEDICATIONS FOR CONVULSIVE STATUS EPILEPTICUS

	■ GCSE	■ FOCAL MOTOR	■ MYOCLONIC	■ NEONATAL
First-line	Lorazepam	Lorazepam	Lorazepam	Phenobarbital
Second-line	Fosphenytoin	Fosphenytoin	Fosphenytoin	Fosphenytoin
			Valproate	Lorazepam

GCSE, generalized convulsive status epilepticus.
Adapted from Wheless JW, Clarke DF, Carpenter D. Treatment of pediatric epilepsy: Expert opinion, 2005. *J Child Neurol* 2005;20(suppl 1):S1–56.

TABLE 63.10

PREFERRED MEDICATIONS FOR NONCONVULSIVE STATUS EPILEPTICUS

	■ ABSENCE	■ COMPLEX PARTIAL	■ NCSE WITH COMA
First-line	Lorazepam	Lorazepam	Lorazepam
Second-line	Valproate	Fosphenytoin	Fosphenytoin
			Pharmacologic coma

NCSE, nonconvulsive status epilepticus.
Adapted from Wheless JW, Clarke DF, Carpenter D. Treatment of pediatric epilepsy: Expert opinion, 2005.
J Child Neurol 2005;20(suppl 1):S1–56.

children and may be more efficacious than rectal diazepam (74). If rectal diazepam is used, the dose is 0.2–0.5 mg/kg (up to 10 mg), the bioavailability is 90%, and peak effect occurs 1.5 hours after administration.

Phenobarbital. Phenobarbital is the first-line agent for neonatal SE and a second-line agent for GCSE or complex partial SE. Phenobarbital is a barbiturate and acts by enhancing $GABA_A$ activity. The binding site for barbiturates differs from that of benzodiazepines, and reduced efficacy during prolonged SE has not been described. Interestingly, cerebral uptake of phenobarbital is increased by seizure activity, likely due to increased CBF and BBB permeability (2). Intravenous administration of phenobarbital results in an onset of action after roughly 5 minutes and peak levels after 15 minutes. Dose adjustment may be indicated in patients with severe renal or hepatic failure. Phenobarbital can cause dose-dependent respiratory and hemodynamic depression, and these potential side effects should be anticipated and avoided.

Fosphenytoin. Fosphenytoin is the second-line agent for GCSE, complex partial SE, and neonatal SE. Fosphenytoin is a pro-drug that is dephosphorylated to phenytoin. Phenytoin acts as an activity-dependent antagonist of voltage-dependent sodium (Na^+) channels. Fosphenytoin has similar efficacy and fewer administration side effects, such as local injection site irritation and arrhythmias, as compared with phenytoin. Still, electrocardiographic monitoring is indicated during administration of loading doses. Fosphenytoin is dosed as phenytoin

equivalents (PE units). To minimize risk of adverse cardiovascular events, the maximum intravenous administration rate should not exceed 3 mg PE/kg/min up to a maximum of 150 mg PE per minute. Peak levels of phenytoin are achieved roughly 20 minutes after IV dosing. Phenytoin is highly protein bound and, in patients on chronic phenytoin therapy, fosphenytoin may displace phenytoin from albumin binding sites and rapidly raise free phenytoin levels. Similarly, valproate may displace phenytoin from albumin-binding sites. Therapeutic total levels of roughly 20 mg/L are typically targeted, although in patients with hypoalbuminemia or concurrent valproate therapy, total levels may underestimate free plasma concentrations. In these patients, free phenytoin levels (1–2 mg/L) should be followed.

Valproate. Valproate is the second-line agent for absence SE and is advocated by some as a second-line agent for GCSE (64,75). Recent systematic review of valproate use in GCSE shows equal efficacy to phenytoin with fewer reported adverse effects (e.g., hypotension, respiratory compromise) (76). Valproate may also be useful as an adjunctive therapy for complex partial SE or myoclonic SE. The precise mechanism of action of valproate remains unclear, but it increases endogenous GABA levels, enhances GABA response, and may stabilize neuronal membranes. Larger loading doses may be required to achieve therapeutic levels in patients on liver enzyme-inducing drugs, such as phenobarbital, phenytoin, or carbamazepine. Therapeutic valproate levels are 50–150 mcg/mL; both efficacy and

TABLE 63.11

MEDICATION DOSING FOR STATUS EPILEPTICUS

■ MEDICATION	■ DOSE	■ DELIVERY RATE	■ COMMENTS
Lorazepam	0.05–0.15 mg/kg/dose IV (max 4 mg)	0.025 mg/kg/min	Repeat in 5 min
Midazolam	0.1–0.15 mg/kg/dose IM 0.3 mg/kg/dose buccal		McIntyre et al. (71) Silbergleit et al. (72), Towne, DeLorenzo (73)
	0.2–0.5 mg/kg/dose intranasal		Wolfe, Macfarlane (74)
Diazepam	0.2–0.5 mg/kg rectal (max 10 mg)		
Phenobarbital	15–20 mg/kg IV	1 mg/kg/min	Repeat 5-mg/kg dose PRN to ~40 mg/kg
Fosphenytoin	15–20 mg PE/kg IV	3 mgPE/kg/min (max 150 mg PE/min)	Repeat 5 mg/kg over 12 h
Valproate	15–20 mg/kg IV	5 mg/kg/min	Repeat 10-mg/kg dose PRN to ~40 mg/kg
Levetiracetam	5–30 mg/kg IV	5 mg/kg/min	Repeat 10-mg/kg dose PRN to ~60 mg/kg

PE, phenytoin equivalents.

toxicity may be increased at higher doses. Valproate is generally well tolerated but may rarely cause hypotension during acute administration. Hepatotoxicity and hyperammonemia are associated with valproate use, and transaminase levels and liver function should be monitored during treatment. Additionally, valproate has been associated with thrombocytopenia and coagulation disorders, possibly due to decreased hepatic production of clotting factors, as well as pancreatitis.

Levetiracetam. Levetiracetam is a newer anticonvulsant medication that is rapidly gaining favor as a second-line agent for GCSE (77,78). The mechanism of action of levetiracetam remains poorly understood, but it is independent of GABA or NMDA activity and likely involves modulation of synaptic vesicle protein 2A and N-type calcium channel activity (79). Growing favor is largely based on advantageous pharmacology (e.g., rapid onset of action, few drug interactions, minimal protein binding, lack of cardiorespiratory depression, similar bioavailability with enteral and intravenous dosing). Several retrospective studies and one systematic review describe levetiracetam as a first- or second-line agent for SE (80–83). Loading doses are 5–30 mg/kg given intravenously with a maximum infusion rate of 5 mg/kg/min followed by daily dosing of 20–60 mg/kg/day divided into two doses. Reported efficacy for seizure termination is 44%–75% (80,83). In adults, efficacy is reported to be similar to phenytoin but less than valproate (84). Adverse effects are seen in 12%–40% of patients (81,83). Sedation and aggression are most common; thrombocytopenia has been reported. Of note, levetiracetam accumulates in patients with renal failure, and dose adjustment is recommended for creatinine clearance <50 ml/min/1.73 m^2 (79).

Nonconvulsive Status Epilepticus

Treatment of NCSE in children is not well studied. Similar to CSE, medication choice is based on seizure type (**Table 63.9**). Treatment of NCSE in comatose children is identical to that used for RSE, with rapid progression to pharmacologic coma. Continuous EEG monitoring should be used to guide therapy; however, consensus regarding the optimal EEG end point is lacking. For example, should all seizure activity be stopped? Also, therapy for PLEDS in NCSE is controversial, and consultation with a pediatric neurologist is recommended. PLEDS are commonly seen with structural lesions or herpes simplex virus (HSV) encephalitis, and adjunctive therapies should target potential inciting insults.

Refractory Status Epilepticus

Due to the ongoing risk for seizure-induced cerebral injury and systemic complications, RSE, whether convulsive or nonconvulsive, should be treated urgently (**Table 63.12**). Regardless of the medication chosen for induction of pharmacologic coma in patients with RSE, invasive blood pressure and central venous pressure are generally indicated to guide titration of mechanical ventilation, fluids, and vasopressor support and to minimize systemic side effects of prolonged SE and high anticonvulsant dosing. Typically, pharmacologic coma is continued for 24–48 hours after seizure control. Tapering of coma-inducing medications typically occurs over 24 hours but may be more gradual, particularly with barbiturate-induced coma or in challenging cases (85). Prior to tapering coma-inducing medications, therapeutic levels of maintenance anticonvulsant medications should be assured in order to reduce the risk of seizure recurrence. Pharmacologic coma is typically achieved using benzodiazepine or barbiturate infusions, guided by cEEG monitoring. The end point of pharmacologic coma may be either cessation of EEG seizure activity or burst suppression. Unfortunately, a consistent association between EEG end point and outcome is lacking. Consequently, while

rapid seizure termination is desired, the most efficacious EEG end point remains controversial. Historically, benzodiazepines are targeted to seizure cessation, while barbiturates are titrated to burst suppression (86). Therapeutic goals should be identified for individual patients in consultation with a pediatric neurologist.

In cases of super-refractory SE, pharmacologic coma is typically reinstated for 1–5 days in order to provide time for development and initiation of a long-term treatment strategy. Prompt application of nonpharmacological therapies should be considered for super-refractory SE (see "Additional Treatment Options" later in this chapter).

Pharmacologic coma for pediatric RSE is not well studied and is based largely on clinical experience and extrapolation from adult practice. Randomized controlled trials of treatment efficacy in adults are also lacking; however, the three most common therapies—midazolam, pentobarbital, and propofol—have been compared by meta-analysis (86). Midazolam infusion, the most common therapy, is associated with the longest duration of therapy, the highest incidence of breakthrough seizures, and the greatest number of changes in therapy due to lack of efficacy, but with the least hemodynamic compromise. Conversely, pentobarbital is associated with the shortest duration of therapy, the lowest incidence of breakthrough seizures, the least changes in therapy, and the most hypotension. In the meta-analysis, outcomes were associated with etiology of RSE, not treatment choice, and were similar among therapies. Other studies link barbiturate use to longer duration of mechanical ventilation, higher frequency of vasopressor use, longer intensive care unit and hospital lengths of stay, and poorer functional outcomes (87). Perhaps largely as an effort to minimize potential adverse effects, several recent treatment guidelines advocate initial use of midazolam with transition to barbiturates should seizures persist (64,75,88).

Midazolam. Midazolam infusions have been used to treat neonatal and pediatric RSE. In neonates, midazolam infusions were efficacious for RSE resistant to phenobarbital and phenytoin, and hypotension was a rare side effect (19). In cohorts of pediatric patients, mean midazolam infusion rates of 8.7–15 mcg/kg/min were required (89,90). In comparison, the mean effective midazolam infusion rate in adults was 8 mcg/kg/min (91). Mild, transient hypotension occurred in treated children but responded to fluid administration and did not require initiation or escalation of vasopressor support (89,90).

Due to GABA$_A$ resistance, some authors advocate that midazolam infusions may not be efficacious for RSE, particularly if therapeutic doses of other benzodiazepines have already been given or if the duration of SE is quite prolonged (1). However, aggressive, goal-directed midazolam therapy may be efficacious, even for prolonged RSE. In one study, midazolam stopped SE in 65% of children, with higher efficacy when started within 3 hours of onset (92). Another study of 17 patients describes aggressive titration of high-dose midazolam using a goal-directed algorithm for RSE that lasted a median of 2.1 hours (range 0.5–63 hours): an initial intravenous loading dose of 0.5 mg/kg and an infusion rate of 2 mcg/kg/min, followed by an additional bolus dose of 0.5 mg/kg and escalation of the infusion to 4 mcg/kg/min if seizures persisted longer than 5 minutes (90). Persistent or recurrent seizures were then treated with repeated bolus doses of 0.1 mg/kg, with increases of 4 mcg/kg/min in the infusion rate every 5 minutes until seizures were controlled; most patients were treated with benzodiazepines before the midazolam algorithm and 12% (2/17) failed the high-dose strategy. The mean time to control of SE was 0.3 hour (range 0.1–1.5 hours). The median peak infusion rate was 4 mcg/kg/min (mean 8.7 mcg/kg/min; range 2–32 mcg/kg/min). The median duration of midazolam infusion was 16 hours (range 2–113 hours). Adverse effects were

TABLE 63.12

MEDICATION DOSING FOR REFRACTORY STATUS EPILEPTICUS

| ■ MEDICATION | Dose | |
	■ LOADING	■ INFUSION
Midazolam	0.2–0.5 mg/kg IV	0.05–4 mcg/kg/min[a]
Pentobarbital	10–15 mg/kg IV initially then 2–5 mg/kg q 5 min to stop seizure	1–3 mg/kg/h
Propofol	1–2 mg/kg IV	25–65 mcg/kg/min
Valproate	40 mg/kg IV	3 mg/kg/min
Ketamine	1.5 mg/kg IV	0.01–0.05 mg/kg/h
Topiramate	2–5 mg/kg NGT	Increase by 5–10 mg/kg/day NGT
Levetiracetam	15–70 mg/kg IV or NGT	20–70 mg/kg/day given in 2 doses
Lacosamide	2–2.5 mg/kg/dose IV (max 100–400 mg)	2–2.5 mg/kg/day (max 200–400 mg/day) given in 1 or 2 doses

NGT, nasogastric tube.
[a]Higher infusion rates may be used, as delineated in the text.

minimal. Transient mild hypotension, which responded to modest fluid resuscitation, occurred in 12%, breakthrough seizures occurred in 47%, and relapse of SE after discontinuation of midazolam therapy occurred in 6%. Endotracheal intubation was needed in 88% of the patients, all prior to beginning the high-dose midazolam algorithm. Because this approach has only been reported in a small series, we recommend vigilant monitoring with immediate ability for airway management if high-dose midazolam strategy is to be employed. Hypotension would be more likely in neonates, in patients with preexisting cardiovascular disease, and patients having received prior opioid administration.

Pentobarbital. Barbiturate coma is a common therapy for RSE. Fluid resuscitation and low-dose vasopressor or inotropic support are frequently required because of the adverse cardiovascular effects of high barbiturate doses. Although dosing is usually titrated to burst suppression, targeting the cessation of EEG seizure activity may provide similar efficacy with fewer side effects. Barbiturates suppress cerebral metabolism and may be beneficial for patients with increased ICP. In addition to cardiovascular toxicity, the adverse effects of high-dose barbiturates include hypothermia, ileus, and increased susceptibility to infections, especially ventilator-associated pneumonia (93).

Pentobarbital is the most commonly used barbiturate. Historically, thiopental has also been used, but it is not currently available in United States and will not be discussed in this chapter. Pentobarbital dosing is titrated to effect, and higher infusion rates than those listed in **Table 63.12** may be necessary. That said, administration of repeated, small bolus doses of pentobarbital is the most effective strategy to achieve burst suppression during coma induction and can facilitate the use of lower infusion doses (94,95). Pentobarbital tends to accumulate in fatty tissue, and recovery times may be prolonged because of the transition from first- to zero-order kinetics with continuous infusion. Due to the long elimination half-life, gradual tapering of pentobarbital is usually not necessary. Many clinicians will decrease the rate by half and then discontinue administration 8–12 hours later; however, some authors advocate tapering by 0.5 mg/kg/12 hours to minimize the risk of breakthrough seizures (85).

Other Medications. Propofol, valproate, ketamine, topiramate, levetiracetam, lacosamide, and volatile anesthetics have been used as adjunctive therapies for RSE.

Propofol administration is common in adults and has shown promise in children, controlling 64% of SE in one pediatric case series (93). However, the use of prolonged propofol infusions is associated with propofol infusion syndrome, which is characterized by metabolic acidosis, lipidemia, arrhythmias, and cardiovascular collapse (96). Risk factors for propofol infusion syndrome include lean body mass, high dose, and greater than 24 hours of administration (96). In response, propofol use for sustained sedation in children <16 years of age has been contraindicated in the United States, Canada, and the European Union. Consequently, the most recent NICE guidelines have removed propofol as a suggested therapy for children (68), and use of propofol for RSE in children remains controversial. Risks and benefits of propofol therapy must be carefully weighed for each patient. If used, the infusion duration should be as short as possible, and the dose should not exceed 67 mcg/kg/min (97). During propofol therapy, patients should be closely monitored for the development of metabolic acidosis or lipidemia, and therapy should be stopped at the first indication of toxicity.

Valproate has been added as adjunctive therapy in adults and children with RSE. Case series show efficacy, but larger therapeutic trials are lacking (98). When administered as a continuous infusion, the mean efficacious dose is roughly 3 mg/kg/min (98). Of note, valproate may be particularly helpful in patients with myoclonic SE, absence SE, or Lennox-Gastaut syndrome.

Ketamine is a noncompetitive NMDA receptor antagonist that is neuroprotective in experimental SE models and has been used in clinical RSE (1). Ketamine binds to a site within the ion-channel pore, close to the magnesium-binding site, and ketamine antagonism relies on release of the magnesium binding via partial depolarization. Consequently, the efficacy of ketamine is preserved during ongoing and prolonged RSE. Typically, ketamine has been added only after prolonged SE and failure of several other medications; however, some advocate that earlier use may be advantageous (31). Importantly, ketamine may increase ICP and should not be administered in the absence of neuroimaging that excludes mass intracranial lesions.

Topiramate is a newer anticonvulsant medication that potentiates GABA activity, reduces glutamate release, and provides activity-dependent blockade of voltage-gated sodium channels. Topiramate is typically used for chronic seizure control but has been given to adult and pediatric patients with RSE via nasogastric tube (99,100). In one series of adult patients, topiramate was added as adjunctive therapy at an initial dose of 25–100 mg twice daily, with rapid escalation to total doses of 300–1600 mg/day (100). In children, adjunctive topiramate therapy has been used at initial doses of 2–5 mg/kg/day and increased by 5–10 mg/kg/day, to a maximum dose of 25 mg/kg/day (99). For larger pediatric patients, care should be taken not to exceed the published total daily adult dose of 1,600 mg/day. Reported efficacy is as high as 70% for adults with RSE, typically within 3 days of starting therapy (101). High-dose topiramate is also efficacious for infantile spasms.

Levetiracetam use for RSE is described in one pediatric case series of 11 cases (102). All patients received concurrently 3–7 other anticonvulsants. Administration was via the enteral, rectal, or intravenous route and started at doses of 15–70 mg/kg (median 30 mg/kg), followed by daily titration to maximum dosing of 20–70 mg/kg/day divided into two doses. Levetiracteam was considered to be beneficial in 45% of cases. The median effective dose was 40 mg/kg/day, with all favorably responding patients receiving ≥30 mg/kg/day.

Lacosamide is a newer anticonvulsant that acts by enhancing slow inactivation of sodium channels. Lacosamide use in RSE shows promising efficacy with seizure termination reported in 38%–70% of adult patients (103,104). In all cases, lacosamide was used concurrently with at least one other anticonvulsant. In adults, typical intravenous loading doses of 100–400 mg (mean 180 mg) have been used, followed by intravenous 200–400 mg/day (mean 360 mg) were given as a single dose, or divided into two doses (103,104). In a pediatric case series, intravenous doses used were 2–2.5 mg/kg/dose (105). Adverse effects were rare, with only mild episodes of hypotension reported in 12.5% of patients (103,104). Lacosamide may be particularly helpful for focal RSE, but it has also been given for NCRSE and GCSE (104).

Finally, volatile anesthetics, such as isoflurane, may be used to treat RSE but these agents have not been subject to clinical trials (2). While use is typically effective for seizure cessation in both RSE and super-refractory SE, it is complicated by technical difficulties with safe administration outside of the operating room and potential toxicity with long-term use (106). Many pediatric intensive care units lack appropriate scavenging facilities and intensivists may have limited experience with inhalational anesthetic use. Collaboration with pediatric anesthesia is recommended.

Additional Treatment Options

RSE that fails to respond to high-dose suppressive therapy is associated with high morbidity and mortality in children. Most children are not surgical candidates; however, cerebral lobar resection or hemispherectomy can be considered in patients with discrete, localized seizure foci. In selected cases, surgical resection is effective and has low morbidity and mortality in experienced hands. The largest case series reports 10 children who underwent resection to treat RSE: 6 had functional hemispherectomy, and 4 had lobar or multilobar resection (107). All had acute control of SE, and 7 remained seizure-free at follow-up. Epilepsy syndromes commonly amenable to resection include hemimegalencephaly, Rasmussen encephalitis, prenatal cerebral artery infarction, tuberous sclerosis, malformations of cortical development, and Sturge-Weber syndrome. Other surgical options for patients without an identifiable discrete seizure focus may include multiple subpial transections, corpus callosotomy, and implantation of a vagal nerve stimulator (108–110). Surgical treatment for RSE requires specialist evaluation—often including functional neuroimaging and surgical implantation of subdural grids to localize seizure foci—that must be considered in consultation with experienced pediatric neurosurgeons, epileptologists, and neurologists.

Additional nonsurgical therapies for RSE include electroconvulsive therapy (ECT), immunomodulation, and ketogenic diet. ECT is not well studied in SE but it is known to elevate seizure threshold by promoting GABAergic transmission and to induce a refractory period that may "break" the cycle of RSE (111). A review of 11 published case reports (7 adult and 4 pediatric) describes several ECT approaches for SE and reports cessation of RSE in 80% of cases (111).

Immunomodulation may be helpful in cases of RSE due to inflammatory or autoimmune etiology (e.g., FIRES or antibody-mediated encephalitis) (31,32,112). Available immunomodulation therapies include steroids, intravenous immunoglobulins, and/or plasma exchange. Therapeutic responses are best when treatment is initiated early after symptom onset. For example, SE due antibody-mediated encephalitis responds best when immunomodulation is initiated within 4 weeks of seizure onset (31,32,113). Decisions to apply immunomodulation and the choice of therapy should be made in consultation with specialists in CNS inflammation, immunology, and neurology, as evidence-based guidelines regarding the most optimal choice are lacking.

Initiation of a ketogenic diet is less extreme and may be helpful, particularly if FIRES is the suspected etiology (31,32). In fact, in cases of RSE due to FIRES, prompt application of targeted treatment modalities, such as a ketogenic diet, is associated with better seizure control and improved cognitive outcomes (31,32,113). When providing a ketogenic diet, attention must be paid to avoid dextrose-containing carrier fluids, other medications containing dextrose, or concurrent treatment with steroids, and to provide water-soluble B-vitamin supplementation and kidney stone prevention with potassium citrate (114).

OUTCOMES

Prognosis after SE is largely dependent on etiology and age. In general, children with acute symptomatic or progressive encephalopathic etiologies have greater risk for mortality and morbidity (18,27,115). Conversely, children with febrile or cryptogenic etiologies tend to fare better. The risk of adverse outcome is particularly high among infants with perinatal difficulties or neurologic abnormalities prior to the development of SE (27).

Mortality is 3%–7% overall (1,23), but varies greatly according to the etiology of the SE. Reported mortality with cryptogenic or febrile SE is 0%–2% (18). Conversely, among children with acute symptomatic etiologies, mortality increases to 12.5%–16% (18,115). Anoxia and acute bacterial meningitis carry particularly high risks of mortality (18). Similarly, the risk of mortality is higher for younger children, ranging from 3% to 22.5% for those <2 years of age (18).

Risk of Developing Epilepsy

A greater risk of developing epilepsy may occur in children in whom new-onset seizures present as SE. In a prospective cohort study, the cumulative risk of epilepsy 5 years after new-onset seizures was 27% among children who presented with SE versus 3% among those who presented without SE (5). Additionally, afebrile, noncryptogenic etiologies of SE are associated with subsequent development of epilepsy (25,27). In fact, among children with acute or remote symptomatic SE, over half will develop epilepsy (18). Finally, intractable epilepsy is associated with young age at first SE episode, remote symptomatic etiology of SE, and AEIMSE (e.g., FIRES) (25,31,32).

Functional Disabilities

Cognitive or motor disabilities are reported after SE in 10%–35% of children (27,65,115). Risk factors for poor outcomes after SE include age <12 months, neuroimaging abnormalities, acute or remote symptomatic causes, progressive encephalopathy etiology or AEIMSE (27,31,32). While SE is associated with neurologic sequelae in many studies, other reports suggest a low incidence of morbidity after SE (70). Isolating the specific contributions of SE from those of seizure etiology is difficult, and similar functional outcomes are reported among epileptic children with or without SE (5). Additional longitudinal prospective studies are necessary to further clarify the specific effects of SE on cognitive and motor outcomes in children.

CONCLUSIONS AND FUTURE DIRECTIONS

SE is a medical emergency that responds best to prompt recognition and treatment. Treatment for SE will continue to evolve in the future because of the increased use of newer anticonvulsant medications as well as other targeted therapeutic modalities. Most episodes of SE will respond to prompt recognition and administration of first- or second-line anticonvulsants. However, in order to provide optimal care for the most difficult cases, it is important for the pediatric intensivist to remain aware of evolving understanding of pathophysiology and of advances in therapeutic modalities. Strong collaboration between pediatric intensivists, pediatric neurologists, and other relevant pediatric subspecialists is vital to promote prompt recognition and optimization of care for children with SE.

ACKNOWLEDGEMENTS

Drs. Bennett and Van Orman thank Dr. Susan Bratton for critical review of the manuscript.

References

1. Chen JW, Wasterlain CG. Status epilepticus: Pathophysiology and management in adults. *Lancet Neurol* 2006;5(3):246–56.
2. Shorvon S. *Status Epilepticus: Its Clinical Features and Treatment in Children and Adults*. Cambridge: Cambridge University Press, 1994:382.
3. Shinnar S, et al. How long do new-onset seizures in children last? *Ann Neurol* 2001;49(5):659–64.
4. Eriksson K, et al. Treatment delay and the risk of prolonged status epilepticus. *Neurology* 2005;65(8):1316–8.
5. Sillanpaa M, Shinnar S. Status epilepticus in a population-based cohort with childhood-onset epilepsy in Finland. *Ann Neurol* 2002;52(3):303–10.
6. Claassen J, et al. Detection of electrographic seizures with continuous EEG monitoring in critically ill patients. *Neurology* 2004;62(10):1743–8.
7. DeLorenzo RJ, et al. Persistent nonconvulsive status epilepticus after the control of convulsive status epilepticus. *Epilepsia* 1998;39(8):833–40.
8. Abend NS, et al. Nonconvulsive seizures are common in critically ill children. *Neurology* 2011;76(12):1071–7.
9. Hosain SA, Solomon GE, Kobylarz EJ. Electroencephalographic patterns in unresponsive pediatric patients. *Pediatr Neurol* 2005;32(3):162–5.
10. Jette N, et al. Frequency and predictors of nonconvulsive seizures during continuous electroencephalographic monitoring in critically ill children. *Arch Neurol* 2006;63(12):1750–5.
11. Saengpattrachai M, et al. Nonconvulsive seizures in the pediatric intensive care unit: Etiology, EEG, and brain imaging findings. *Epilepsia* 2006;47(9):1510–8.
12. Schreiber JM, et al. Continuous video EEG for patients with acute encephalopathy in a pediatric intensive care unit. *Neurocrit Care* 2012;17(1):31–8.
13. Tay SK, et al. Nonconvulsive status epilepticus in children: Clinical and EEG characteristics. *Epilepsia* 2006;47(9):1504–9.
14. Mayer SA, et al. Refractory status epilepticus: Frequency, risk factors, and impact on outcome. *Arch Neurol* 2002;59(2):205–10.
15. Rossetti AO, Logroscino G, Bromfield EB. Refractory status epilepticus: Effect of treatment aggressiveness on prognosis. *Arch Neurol* 2005;62(11):1698–702.
16. Chin RF, et al. Incidence, cause, and short-term outcome of convulsive status epilepticus in childhood: Prospective population-based study. *Lancet* 2006;368(9531):222–9.
17. Prasad AN, Seshia SS. Status epilepticus in pediatric practice: Neonate to adolescent. *Adv Neurol* 2006;97:229–43.
18. Raspall-Chaure M, et al. Outcome of paediatric convulsive status epilepticus: A systematic review. *Lancet Neurol* 2006;5(9):769–79.
19. Castro Conde JR, et al. Midazolam in neonatal seizures with no response to phenobarbital. *Neurology* 2005;64(5):876–9.
20. Shorvon S. Super-refractory status epilepticus: An approach to therapy in this difficult clinical situation. *Epilepsia* 2011;52 (suppl 8):53–6.
21. DeLorenzo RJ. Epidemiology and clinical presentation of status epilepticus. *Adv Neurol* 2006;97:199–215.
22. Shinnar S, et al. In whom does status epilepticus occur: Age-related differences in children. *Epilepsia* 1997;38(8):907–14.
23. KarasalIhoGlu S, et al. Risk factors of status epilepticus in children. *Pediatr Int* 2003;45(4):429–34.
24. Arzimangoglou A, Guerrini R, Aicardi J. *Aicardi's Epilepsy in Children*. 3rd ed. Philadelphia, PA: Lippencott, Williams, & Wilkins, 2004.
25. Berg AT, et al. Predictors of intractable epilepsy in childhood: A case-control study. *Epilepsia* 1996;37(1):24–30.
26. Maytal J, et al. Status epilepticus in children with epilepsy: The role of antiepileptic drug levels in prevention. *Pediatrics* 1996;98(6 pt 1):1119–21.
27. Barnard C, Wirrell E. Does status epilepticus in children cause developmental deterioration and exacerbation of epilepsy? *J Child Neurol* 1999;14(12):787–94.
28. Asadi-Pooya AA, Poordast A. Etiologies and outcomes of status epilepticus in children. *Epilepsy Behav* 2005;7(3):502–5.
29. Ekici A, et al. Nonconvulsive status epilepticus due to drug induced neurotoxicity in chronically ill children. *Brain Dev* 2012;34(10):824–8.
30. Misra UK, Kalita J, Chandra S, et al. Association of antibiotics with status epilepticus. *Neurol Sci* 2013;34(3):327–31.
31. Kramer U, et al. Febrile infection-related epilepsy syndrome (FIRES): Pathogenesis, treatment, and outcome: A multicenter study on 77 children. *Epilepsia* 2011;52(11):1956–65.
32. Nabbout R, et al. Acute encephalopathy with inflammation-mediated status epilepticus. *Lancet Neurol* 2011;10(1):99–108.
33. Treiman DM, Walton NY, Kendrick C. A progressive sequence of electroencephalographic changes during generalized convulsive status epilepticus. *Epilepsy Res* 1990;5(1):49–60.
34. Mikati MA, et al. Stages of status epilepticus in the developing brain. *Epilepsy Res* 2003;55(1–2):9–19.
35. Young GB. Status epilepticus and brain damage: Pathology and pathophysiology. *Adv Neurol* 2006;97:217–20.
36. Chang BS, Lowenstein DH. Epilepsy. *N Engl J Med* 2003;349(13):1257–66.
37. DeLorenzo RJ, Sun DA. Basic mechanisms in status epilepticus: Role of calcium in neuronal injury and the induction of epileptogenesis. *Adv Neurol* 2006;97:187–97.
38. Dhar R, Mirsattari SM. Current approach to the diagnosis and treatment of refractory status epilepticus. *Adv Neurol* 2006;97:245–54.

39. Boison D. Adenosine and epilepsy: From therapeutic rationale to new therapeutic strategies. *Neuroscientist* 2005;11(1):25–36.

40. Guttinger M, et al. Suppression of kindled seizures by paracrine adenosine release from stem cell-derived brain implants. *Epilepsia* 2005;46(8):1162–9.

41. Oby E, Janigro D. The blood-brain barrier and epilepsy. *Epilepsia* 2006;47(11):1761–74.

42. Sisodiya SM, et al. Drug resistance in epilepsy: Expression of drug resistance proteins in common causes of refractory epilepsy. *Brain* 2002;125(pt 1):22–31.

43. Iannetti P, Spalice A, Parisi P. Calcium-channel blocker verapamil administration in prolonged and refractory status epilepticus. *Epilepsia* 2005;46(6):967–9.

44. Schmitt FC, et al. Verapamil attenuates the malignant treatment course in recurrent status epilepticus. *Epilepsy Behav* 2010;17(4):565–8.

45. Potschka H. Modulating P-glycoprotein regulation: Future perspectives for pharmacoresistant epilepsies? *Epilepsia* 2010;51(8):1333–47.

46. Brooks-Kayal AR. Rearranging receptors. *Epilepsia* 2005;46 (suppl 7):29–38.

47. Chugani DC, et al. Postnatal maturation of human GABAA receptors measured with positron emission tomography. *Ann Neurol* 2001;49(5):618–26.

48. Holmes GL. Effects of seizures on brain development: Lessons from the laboratory. *Pediatr Neurol* 2005;33(1):1–11.

49. Fujikawa DG. Prolonged seizures and cellular injury: Understanding the connection. *Epilepsy Behav* 2005;7(suppl 3):S3–11.

50. Fujikawa DG, et al. Status epilepticus-induced neuronal loss in humans without systemic complications or epilepsy. *Epilepsia* 2000;41(8):981–91.

51. Scott RC, et al. Magnetic resonance imaging findings within 5 days of status epilepticus in childhood. *Brain* 2002;125(pt 9):1951–9.

52. Scott RC, et al. Prolonged febrile seizures are associated with hippocampal vasogenic edema and developmental changes. *Epilepsia* 2006;47(9):1493–8.

53. Scott RC, et al. Hippocampal abnormalities after prolonged febrile convulsion: A longitudinal MRI study. *Brain* 2003;126(pt 11):2551–7.

54. Vespa P. Continuous EEG monitoring for the detection of seizures in traumatic brain injury, infarction, and intracerebral hemorrhage: "to detect and protect". *J Clin Neurophysiol* 2005;22(2):99–106.

55. Waterhouse EJ, et al. Synergistic effect of status epilepticus and ischemic brain injury on mortality. *Epilepsy Res* 1998;29(3):175–83.

56. Keenan HT, et al. A population-based comparison of clinical and outcome characteristics of young children with serious inflicted and noninflicted traumatic brain injury. *Pediatrics* 2004;114:633–9.

57. Vespa P, et al. Delayed increase in extracellular glycerol with post-traumatic electrographic epileptic activity: Support for the theory that seizures induce secondary injury. *Acta Neurochir Suppl* 2002;81:355–7.

58. Vespa P, et al. Increase in extracellular glutamate caused by reduced cerebral perfusion pressure and seizures after human traumatic brain injury: A microdialysis study. *J Neurosurg* 1998;89(6):971–82.

59. Abend NS, et al. Seizures as a presenting symptom of acute arterial ischemic stroke in childhood. *J Pediatr* 2011;159(3):479–83.

60. Singh RK, et al. Seizures in acute childhood stroke. *J Pediatr* 2012;160(2):291–6.

61. Valente KD, et al. Epilepsy in patients with angelman syndrome caused by deletion of the chromosome 15q11-13. *Arch Neurol* 2006;63(1):122–8.

62. Lambrechtsen FA, Buchhalter JR. Aborted and refractory status epilepticus in children: A comparative analysis. *Epilepsia* 2008;49(4):615–25.

63. Meldrum BS, Brierley JB. Prolonged epileptic seizures in primates. Ischemic cell change and its relation to ictal physiological events. *Arch Neurol* 1973;28(1):10–17.

64. Brophy GM, et al. Guidelines for the evaluation and management of status epilepticus. *Neurocrit Care* 2012;17(1):3–23.

65. Lacroix J, et al. Admissions to a pediatric intensive care unit for status epilepticus: A 10-year experience. *Crit Care Med* 1994. 22(5):827–32.

66. Sutter R, et al. Associations between infections and clinical outcome parameters in status epilepticus: A retrospective 5-year cohort study. *Epilepsia* 2012;53(9):1489–97.

67. Wheless JW, Clarke DF, Carpenter D. Treatment of pediatric epilepsy: Expert opinion, 2005. *J Child Neurol* 2005;20(suppl 1):S1–56; quiz S59–60.

68. The epilepsies: The diagnosis and management of the epilepsies in adults and children in primary and secondary care. www.nice.org.uk. January 2012. Accessed October 1, 2012.

69. Guideline 81, Diagnosis and management of epilepsies in children and young people: A national clinical guideline. www.sign.ac.uk. 2005. Accessed April 3, 2006.

70. Metsaranta P, et al. Outcome after prolonged convulsive seizures in 186 children: Low morbidity, no mortality. *Dev Med Child Neurol* 2004;46(1):4–8.

71. McIntyre J, et al. Safety and efficacy of buccal midazolam versus rectal diazepam for emergency treatment of seizures in children: A randomised controlled trial. *Lancet* 2005;366(9481):205–10.

72. Silbergleit R, et al. Intramuscular versus intravenous therapy for prehospital status epilepticus. *N Engl J Med* 2012;366(7):591–600.

73. Towne AR, DeLorenzo RJ. Use of intramuscular midazolam for status epilepticus. *J Emerg Med* 1999;17(2):323–8.

74. Wolfe TR, Macfarlane TC. Intranasal midazolam therapy for pediatric status epilepticus. *Am J Emerg Med* 2006;24(3):343–6.

75. Friedman J. Emergency management of the paediatric patient with generalized convulsive status epilepticus. *Paediatr Child Health* 2011;16(2):91–104.

76. Brigo F, et al. IV Valproate in generalized convulsive status epilepticus: A systematic review. *Eur J Neurol* 2012;19(9):1180–91.

77. Cook AM, et al. Practice variations in the management of status epilepticus. *Neurocrit Care* 2012;17(1):24–30.

78. Riviello JJ, Jr., Claassen J, Laroche SM, et al. Treatment of status epilepticus: An international survey of experts. *Neurocrit Care* 2013;18(2):193–200.

79. Ulloa CM, Towfigh A, Safdieh J. Review of levetiracetam, with a focus on the extended release formulation, as adjuvant therapy in controlling partial-onset seizures. *Neuropsychiatr Dis Treat* 2009;5:467–76.

80. Abend NS, et al. Intravenous levetiracetam in critically ill children with status epilepticus or acute repetitive seizures. *Pediatr Crit Care Med* 2009;10(4):505–10.

81. McTague A, et al. Intravenous levetiracetam in acute repetitive seizures and status epilepticus in children: Experience from a children's hospital. *Seizure* 2012;21(7):529–34.

82. Ruegg S, et al. Intravenous levetiracetam: Treatment experience with the first 50 critically ill patients. *Epilepsy Behav* 2008;12(3):477–80.

83. Zelano J, Kumlien E. Levetiracetam as alternative stage two antiepileptic drug in status epilepticus: A systematic review. *Seizure* 2012;21(4):233–6.

84. Alvarez V, et al. Second-line status epilepticus treatment: Comparison of phenytoin, valproate, and levetiracetam. *Epilepsia* 2011;52(7):1292–6.

85. Kim S, Lee D, Kim JS. Neurologic outcomes of pediatric epileptic patients with pentobarbital coma. *Pediatr Neurol* 2001;25:217–20.

86. Claassen J, et al. Treatment of refractory status epilepticus with pentobarbital, propofol, or midazolam: A systematic review. *Epilepsia* 2002;43(2):146–53.

87. Kowalski RG, et al. Third-line antiepileptic therapy and outcome in status epilepticus: The impact of vasopressor use and prolonged mechanical ventilation. *Crit Care Med* 2012;40(9):2677–84.

88. Lee J, et al. Guideline for the management of convulsive status epilepticus in infants and children. *BCMJ* 2011;53(6): 279–85.

89. Igartua J, et al. Midazolam coma for refractory status epilepticus in children. *Crit Care Med* 1999;27(9):1982–5.

90. Morrison G, Gibbons E, Whitehouse WP. High-dose midazolam therapy for refractory status epilepticus in children. *Intensive Care Med* 2006;32(12):2070–6.

91. Ulvi H, et al. Continuous infusion of midazolam in the treatment of refractory generalized convulsive status epilepticus. *Neurol Sci* 2002;23(4):177–82.

92. Hayashi K, et al. Efficacy of intravenous midazolam for status epilepticus in childhood. *Pediatr Neurol* 2007;36(6):366–72.

93. van Gestel JP, et al. Propofol and thiopental for refractory status epilepticus in children. *Neurology* 2005;65(4):591–2.

94. Krishnamurthy KB, Drislane FW. Depth of EEG suppression and outcome in barbiturate anesthetic treatment for refractory status epilepticus. *Epilepsia* 1999;40(6):759–62.

95. Schreiber JM, Gaillard WD. Treatment of refractory status epilepticus in childhood. *Curr Neurol Neurosci Rep* 2011; 11(2):195–204.

96. Kumar MA, et al. The syndrome of irreversible acidosis after prolonged propofol infusion. *Neurocrit Care* 2005;3(3):257–9.

97. Cornfield DN, et al. Continuous propofol infusion in 142 critically ill children. *Pediatrics* 2002;110(6):1177–81.

98. Yu KT, et al. Safety and efficacy of intravenous valproate in pediatric status epilepticus and acute repetitive seizures. *Epilepsia* 2003;44(5):724–6.

99. Blumkin L, et al. Pediatric refractory partial status epilepticus responsive to topiramate. *J Child Neurol* 2005;20(3):239–41.

100. Towne AR, et al. The use of topiramate in refractory status epilepticus. *Neurology* 2003;60(2):332–4.

101. Hottinger A, et al. Topiramate as an adjunctive treatment in patients with refractory status epilepticus: An observational cohort study. *CNS Drugs* 2012;26(9):761–72.

102. Gallentine WB, Hunnicutt AS, Husain AM. Levetiracetam in children with refractory status epilepticus. *Epilepsy Behav* 2009;14(1):215–8.

103. Cherry S, et al. Safety and efficacy of lacosamide in the intensive care unit. *Neurocrit Care* 2012;16(2):294–8.

104. Mnatsakanyan L, et al. Intravenous lacosamide in refractory nonconvulsive status epilepticus. *Seizure* 2012;21(3):198–201.

105. Jain V, Harvey AS. Treatment of refractory tonic status epilepticus with intravenous lacosamide. *Epilepsia* 2012;53(4):761–2.

106. Wilkes R, Tasker R. Pediatric intensive care treatment of uncontrolled status epilepticus. *Crit Care Clin* 2013;29:239–57.

107. Alexopoulos A, et al. Resective surgery to treat refractory status epilepticus in children with focal epileptogenesis. *Neurology* 2005;64(3):567–70.

108. Greiner HM, et al. Corpus callosotomy for treatment of pediatric refractory status epilepticus. *Seizure* 2012;21(4):307–9.

109. Sierra-Marcos A, et al. Successful outcome of episodes of status epilepticus after vagus nerve stimulation: A multicenter study. *Eur J Neurol* 2012;19(9):1219–23.

110. Winston KR, et al. Vagal nerve stimulation for status epilepticus. *Pediatr Neurosurg* 2001;34(4):190–2.

111. Lambrecq V, et al. Refractory status epilepticus: Electroconvulsive therapy as a possible therapeutic strategy. *Seizure* 2012;21(9):661–4.

112. Kneen R, et al. Management of suspected viral encephalitis in children—Association of British Neurologists and British Paediatric Allergy, Immunology and Infection Group national guidelines. *J Infect* 2012;64(5):449–77.

113. Michael BD, Solomon T. Seizures and encephalitis: Clinical features, management, and potential pathophysiologic mechanisms. *Epilepsia* 2012;53(suppl 4):63–71.

114. Freeman JM, Kossoff EH. Ketosis and the ketogenic diet, 2010: Advances in treating epilepsy and other disorders. *Adv Pediatr* 2010;57:315–29.

115. Maytal J, et al. Low morbidity and mortality of status epilepticus in children. *Pediatrics* 1989;83(3):323–31.

CHAPTER 64 ■ CEREBROVASCULAR DISEASE AND STROKE

JOHN PAPPACHAN, ROBERT C. TASKER, AND FENELLA KIRKHAM

KEY POINTS

1. Morbidity and mortality are high for children who present with stroke in the context of critical illness.
2. Stroke and cerebrovascular disease are among the top 10 causes of childhood death.
3. In emergency stroke care, *time is brain*: any delays in appropriate interventions compromise tissue viability.
4. Emergency neuroimaging, ideally magnetic resonance imaging if time and the emergency permit, in order to

define the diagnosis and to direct diagnosis-specific intervention is good practice.
5. Optimal cerebrovascular disease treatment requires a multidisciplinary approach.
6. Intracranial hypertension is a common feature of stroke, and therapies targeted at cerebral perfusion should be considered.

Stroke and cerebrovascular disorders (CVD) are important causes of morbidity and mortality in children (1,2). Approximately 3200 cases of stroke occur per year in the population aged between 30 days and 18 years in the US alone. Although outcomes for stroke in children are significantly better than in adults, 20% of children who suffer a stroke die and 50%–80% are left with significant disability. The majority of children with acute stroke syndromes are now admitted to the pediatric intensive care unit (PICU) for endotracheal intubation, mechanical ventilation, and other emergency interventions (3). This chapter concentrates on presentation, pathophysiology, investigation, and treatment. The most recent epidemiologic data are reviewed, and the pathogenesis of hemorrhagic and ischemic stroke syndromes, their risk factors, and conditions that predispose to stroke are described.

PRESENTATION, EPIDEMIOLOGY, OUTCOME, AND COSTS

Overview of Childhood Presentation with Stroke and CVD

Acute focal signs of stroke in childhood can be symptomatic of a variety of pathologies (**Table 64.1**). The World Health Organization definition of stroke is *"rapidly developing clinical signs of focal (or global) disturbance of cerebral function, with symptoms lasting 24 hours or longer, or leading to death, with no apparent cause other than of vascular origin."* Patients whose signs resolve within 24 hours have transient ischemic attacks (TIAs) by definition, but many have recent cerebral infarction or hemorrhage on cerebral imaging (4). Coma is a well-recognized presentation in children with subarachnoid hemorrhage (SAH) or intracerebral hemorrhage (ICH), large middle cerebral artery (MCA) territory infarction, vertebro-basilar circulation stroke, sinovenous thrombosis, bilateral border-zone ischemia, and reversible posterior leukoencephalopathy syndrome (RPLS) (3). Seizures or headache may herald

stroke and CVD, particularly sinovenous thrombosis, in children (5). Silent infarction may be demonstrated in up to 25% of children with sickle cell disease (SCD) (6) on magnetic resonance imaging (MRI) and may affect other "at-risk" populations, such as those with congenital heart disease (CHD) (7).

Epidemiology

Stroke and CVD are relatively rare in children but cause disproportionate morbidity and mortality, particularly in those with critical illness (8). Already among the top 10 causes of childhood death, the prevalence is probably increasing as a consequence of increased recognition and improved sensitivity of diagnostic neuroimaging using MRI or cranial computed tomography (CT) angiography. In addition, therapeutic advances that now allow children with predisposing conditions such as SCD, CHD, and malignancy to survive may unfortunately increase the risk of stroke.

Neonatal stroke affects 25–30 per 100,000 live births, while epidemiologic data have suggested incidence rates of between 2 and 13 per 100,000 children/year, with one-half to two-thirds being arterial ischemic stroke (AIS) and the remainder being hemorrhagic or other diagnoses (e.g., sinovenous thrombosis without parenchymal involvement). The more conservative estimates predict 3200 cases of stroke per year in a population aged between 30 days and 18 years of age in the US alone. The prevalence of AIS peaks in the first year of life, while SAH is more common in teenagers. Boys are at higher risk, as are those of African heritage. Although childhood stroke is much more common in SCD, this condition does not entirely account for the disparity in rates of stroke by ethnic group.

Definitions, Costs, and Outcomes

Healthcare utilization is not adequately reflected by incidence figures. The socioeconomic costs of a disease are most appropriately described by disease outcome. Acute treatment costs

TABLE 64.1

DIFFERENTIAL DIAGNOSIS IN CHILDREN WHO PRESENT WITH ACUTE FOCAL NEUROLOGIC DEFICIT

- **Primary hemorrhagic stroke** +/– **mass effect**
- **Acute ischemic arterial stroke** +/– hemorrhage +/– **mass effect**
- **Acute venous stroke** +/– hemorrhage +/– venous infarction +/– **mass effect**
- **Postictal** (as Todd paresis is of short duration, if persistent, neuroimaging is essential; children with prolonged seizures may develop permanent hemiparesis)
- **Hemiplegic migraine** (but diagnosis of exclusion, as migrainous symptoms are commonly seen in cerebrovascular disease, e.g., dissection)
- **Acute disseminated encephalomyelitis**
- **Brain tumor**
- **Nonaccidental inflicted injury** (subdural hematoma, strangulation with compression of internal carotid artery)
- **Encephalitis** (e.g., secondary to herpes simplex—usually have seizures)
- **Rasmussen encephalitis**
- **Posterior leukoencephalopathy** (hypertension/hypotension or immunosuppression)
- **Unilateral hemispheric/focal cerebral edema**—e.g., secondary to metabolic
- **Alternating hemiplegia**

All stroke syndromes are potential neurosurgical emergencies and should always be discussed with a pediatric neurologist on presentation. Further management and any transfer must involve liaison with the nearest available PICU.

may be less than in adults because of the lack of proven acute interventions, but the long-term healthcare costs of rehabilitation and continued care and treatment of recurrent stroke might well be greater (9,10).

Ischemic stroke occurs commonly in an arterial distribution (i.e., AIS), but superficial infarcts in the parietal, occipital, or frontal lobes or the thalami may be venous in origin (**Figs. 64.1** and **64.2**). Mortality is 6%–20%, half of which is stroke related, and half is due to the underlying disease. In addition, 50%–80% of events result in permanent cognitive or motor disability (11–13). Importantly, prognosis in pediatric stroke is significantly better than in the adult population. However, children who do not die acutely will probably survive beyond middle age, making the treatment of any resulting comorbidity extremely expensive. Thus, the health burden of this disease entity is very large. Long-term disability may have decreased from ~85% to 40%–60%, probably due to the inclusion of children with a milder spectrum of disease due to increasing diagnostic sensitivity and perhaps related to the use of antithrombotic agents (11–15). Seizure disorders complicate 15%–20% of ischemic strokes. Predictors of poor outcome include the presence of multiple etiologic risk factors (16), seizures at onset (5,13), an arterial stroke rather than a sinovenous thrombosis (14), cortical and subcortical infarction (17), and for sinovenous thrombosis, the presence of venous infarcts (14).

The estimated rates of recurrent stroke for AIS are <5% for neonates and 6%–14% in older infants and children with a further 20% experiencing recurrent TIAs (7,18). Recurrence rates are lower for sinovenous thrombosis in older infants and children—~3%—although subsequent systemic thrombosis also occurs in a further 3% (19).

Hemorrhagic stroke includes ICH (**Fig. 64.1A**), most commonly due to arteriovenous malformation (AVM) (20), and SAH (often secondary to aneurysm) (21) but sinovenous thrombosis may cause either (13). Mortality of ICH and SAH is approximately twice that of ischemic stroke (22).

In summary, the available epidemiologic data indicate that stroke in children is increasingly recognized and it results in a significant long-term burden in terms of neurologic-cognitive disability and seizures. Such burden-of-illness for an individual child might last decades, as life expectancy is unaffected. Primary prevention is difficult but early recognition and referral at the time of the ictus is imperative.

MECHANISM OF DISEASE

Risk Factors

Numerous inherited conditions predispose to CVD and stroke but only 50% of children presenting with an AIS have a known predisposing condition, the commonest of which are heart disease (4,23,24) and anemias, including SCD (4,25) (**Figs. 64.2J–L,P–S**). Other acquired conditions such as leukemia, brain tumors (**Figs. 64.2H,I**), genetic disorders (including Trisomy 21 and neurofibromatosis), or single-gene disorders with a highly significant predisposition to stroke (e.g., homocystinuria, Fabry disease, and Menkes disease) are usually obvious at the time of presentation (7). Previously well children may have a recent history of trauma or infection (23,26) (e.g., with varicella—**Figs. 64.2A** and **64.3A**), otherwise investigations may reveal a vasculopathy (23) or hereditary coagulopathy (27).

Hemorrhagic stroke and sinovenous thrombosis may also occur in the context of acquired illnesses (13,26,28), and as in adult stroke, genes that control intermediate-risk factors such as hypertension and hyperhomocysteinemia may be important.

Stroke in Children with Recognized Diagnoses

Congenital Heart Disease

Embolization of air, thrombus, or infected vegetation may occur in children with CHD, particularly during interventions such as cardiac catheterization, or surgery, or secondary to infective endocarditis. Other causes of stroke also need to be considered including sinovenous thrombosis (**Figs. 64.1J,K** and **64.2M–O**) and primary cerebral arterial disease (**Figs. 64.3** and **64.4**) (4,13,23,24,29). Previously undiagnosed cardiac disease (e.g., a patent foramen ovale) may be diagnosed with contrast echocardiography (4,30,31), but there is currently no convincing evidence for treatment to prevent recurrence and investigation is therefore not essential. Asymptomatic abnormalities of the aortic valve are associated with primary CVD such as cervicocephalic dissection and moyamoya (**Figs. 64.3** and **64.4**) (4).

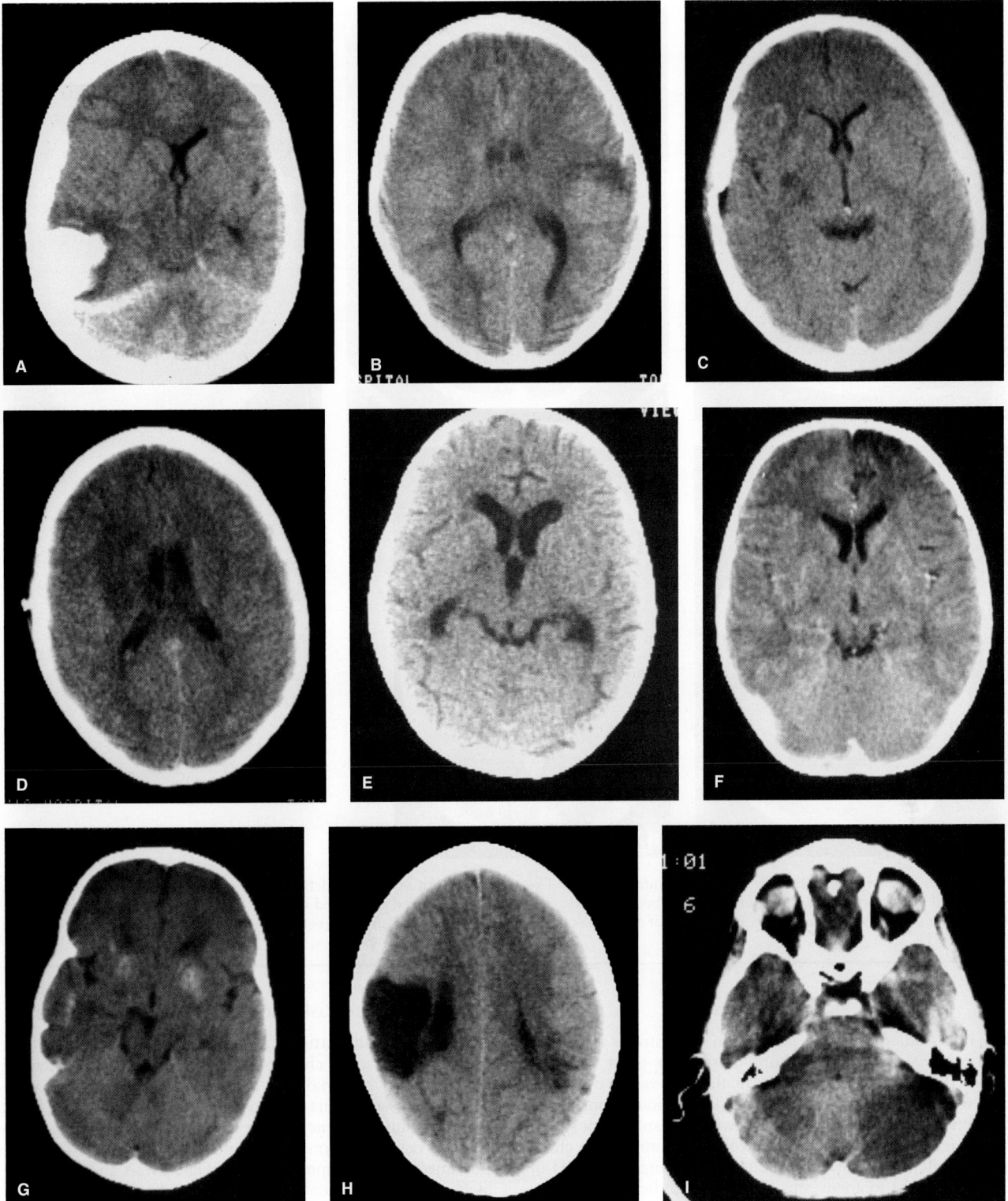

FIGURE 64.1. CT scans from children with hemorrhagic and ischemic (arterial and venous) stroke and its mimics. A: Spontaneous intracerebral hemorrhage with midline shift. B: Cortical ischemic stroke after minor head injury. C: Small infarct associated with middle cerebral artery stenosis. D: Larger infarct after recurrence of stroke in C. E: Hydrocephalus and basal ganglia infarct in tuberculous meningitis. F: Frontal infarction associated with moyamoya. G: Calcification associated with moyamoya. H: Old congenital infarct. I: Cerebellar infarction in an unconscious boy. (*Continued*).

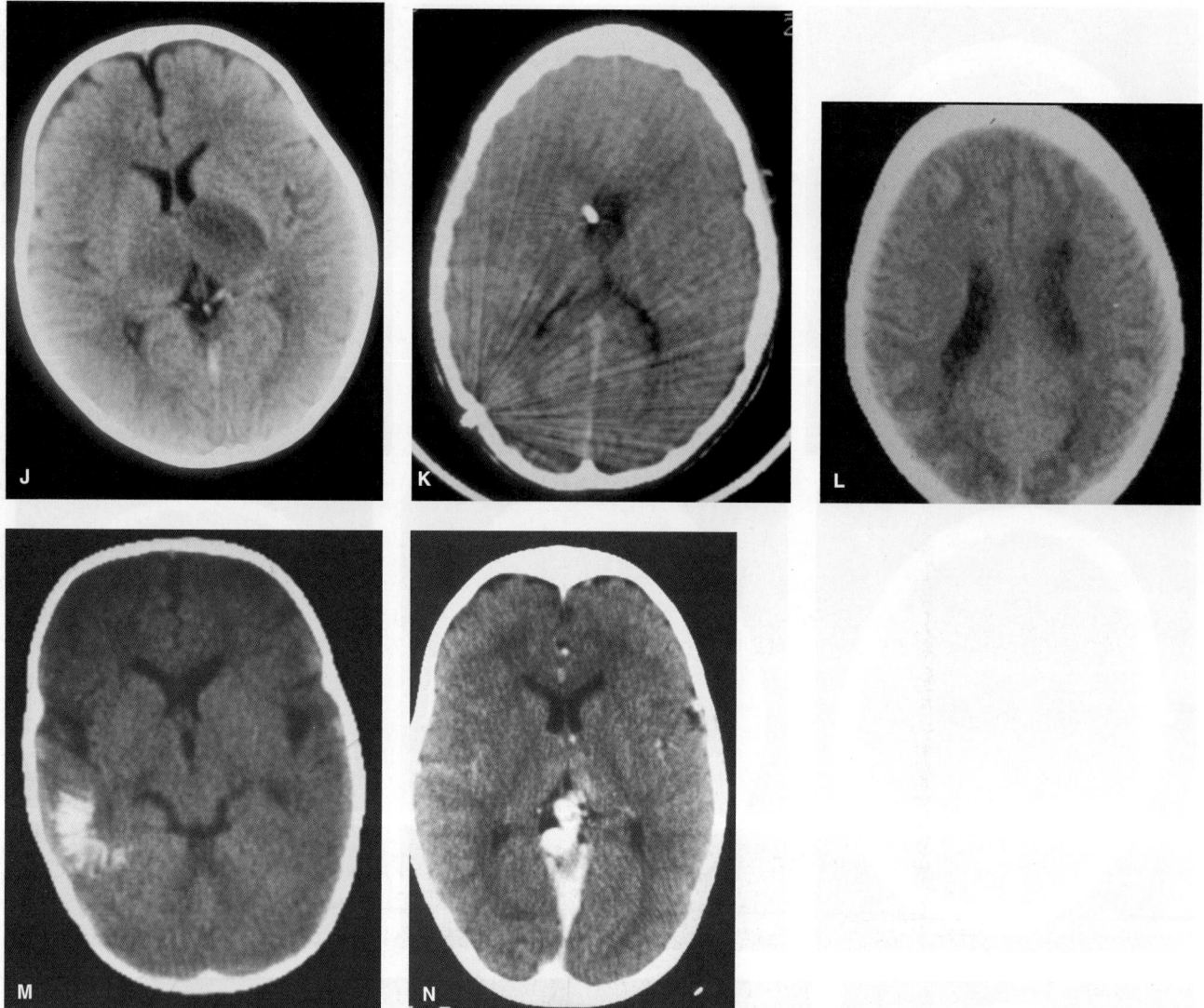

FIGURE 64.1. (*Continued*). **J:** Bilateral thalamic infarction in a 4-year-old girl with severe iron deficiency anemia and sinovenous thrombosis. **K:** Cerebral edema and dense straight sinus thrombosis in sickle cell disease. **L:** Bilateral watershed ischemia secondary to rapid blood pressure reduction in severe hypertension. **M:** Calcification of a parieto-occipital pial angioma in Sturge–Weber syndrome. **N:** Vein of Galen malformation (contrast CT).

Sickle Cell Disease

The best-studied pediatric population with stroke is in children with SCD, among whom most with overt ischemic stroke (**Fig. 64.2L**) have intracranial, large-vessel disease (-**Figs. 64.3D–F**) with intimal hyperplasia. Without prophylactic blood transfusion, 25% of patients will have suffered a stroke by the age of 45 years; ischemic stroke predominates in childhood, while the majority of adults have spontaneous ICH or SAH secondary to aneurysms (32), although hemorrhage secondary to hypertension and steroid use has also been well documented in children (33). Sinovenous thrombosis (**Figs. 64.1K and 64.2Q**), posterior leukoencephalopathy, watershed ischemia, and acute 'silent' infarction (**Figs. 64.2R,S**) have previously been under-recognized (34–37).

SCD is a complex, autosomal recessive inherited disease. The predisposition to large- and small-vessel disease, "silent" (covert) and clinical (overt) infarction, seizures, and cognitive deterioration may be, in part, related to genetic makeup (38) but is probably also linked to environmental factors, e.g., infection, poor nutrition, or hypoxemia (25,34,39,40).

Intermediate-Risk Factors for Childhood Stroke

Infection, Inflammation, and Immune Deficiency. At least one-third of cases of childhood stroke occur in the context of infection, and bacterial and tuberculous meningitis are well-recognized associations (**Figs. 64.1E, 64.2G,** and **64.3B**) (4,41). Overt immunodeficiency, either inherited or acquired, also appears to be an occasional association with stroke (4). Chickenpox infection is a common trigger (**Figs. 64.2A** and **64.3A**). In SCD, high leukocyte count is a risk factor for stroke, and cerebrovascular episodes are often precipitated by infections. This group of patients is also relatively immunodeficient, secondary to either splenic autoinfarction or surgical removal.

Anemia. Stroke syndromes are well described in the hemolytic anemias, including intermediate forms of thalassemia, hereditary spherocytosis, and paroxysmal nocturnal hemoglobinuria, as well as SCD (42). Iron deficiency appears to be a risk factor for stroke in children (43).

Hyperhomocysteinemia. Classic homocystinuria (deficiency of cystathionine β-synthase) has long been recognized

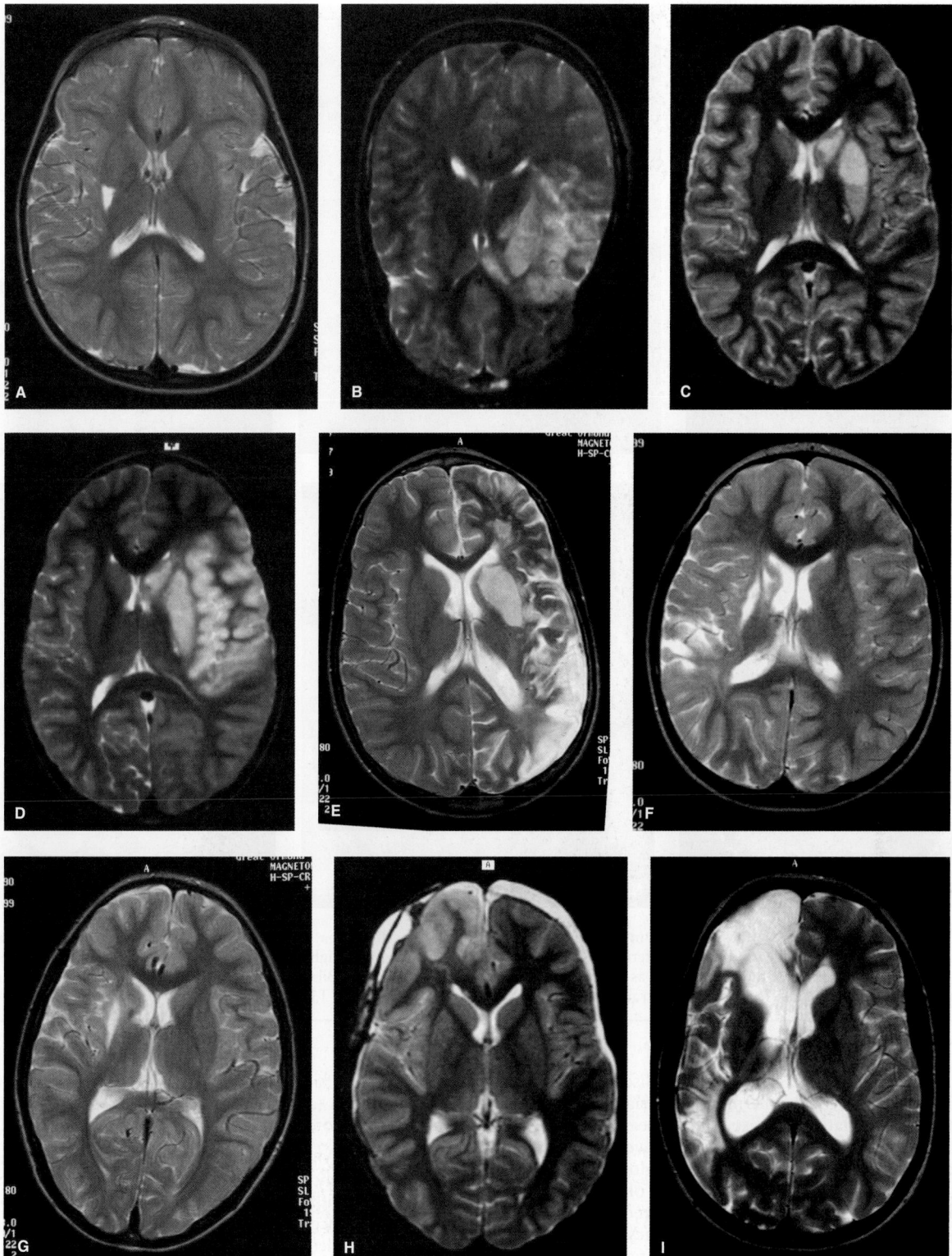

FIGURE 64.2. MRI scans from children with first and recurrent ischemic (arterial and venous) stroke and its mimics. **A:** Basal ganglia infarct associated with transient cerebral arteriopathy after varicella. **B:** Temporal infarction associated with dissection. **C:** Small infarct associated with middle cerebral artery stenosis. **D:** Larger infarct after recurrence of stroke in C. **E:** Recurrent infarction after dissection. **F:** "Silent" posterior watershed recurrent infarction after embolic occlusion. **G:** Deep white matter infarct in *Haemophilus influenzae* meningitis. **H:** Right frontal cortical edema after craniopharyngioma surgery. **I:** "Silent" recurrent infarction in the posterior watershed territory in the same patient as in **H**. (*Continued*).

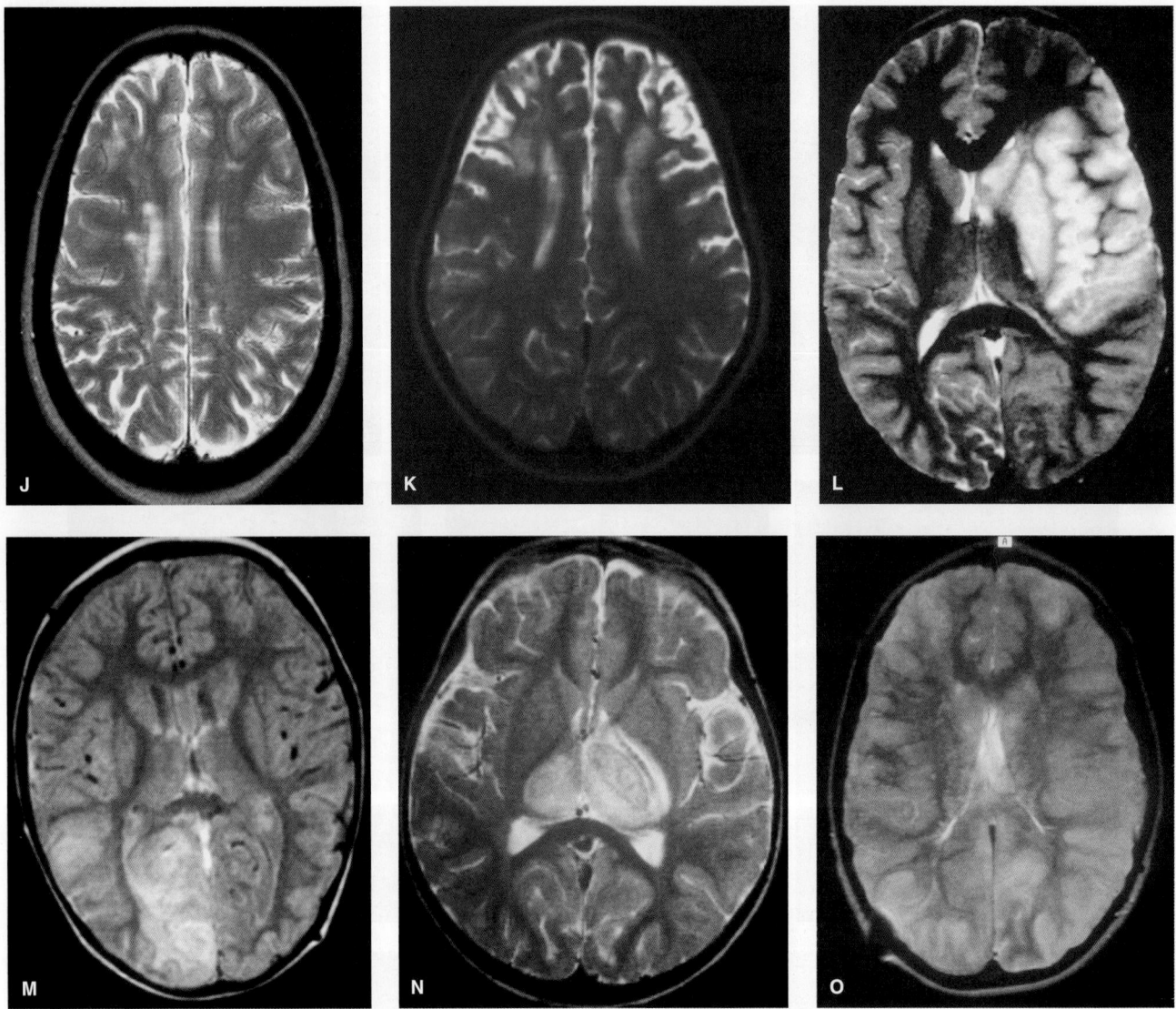

FIGURE 64.2. (*Continued*). **J:** "Silent" infarction in the deep white matter in sickle cell anemia. **K:** Bilateral frontal infarction in sickle cell anemia and moyamoya. **L:** Large middle cerebral artery territory infarct in sickle cell anemia. **M:** High signal in the right occipital lobe associated with straight sinus occlusion; subacute thrombus is seen as high signal on proton density images. **N:** Bilateral thalamic infarction in sinovenous thrombosis (same patient as **Fig. 64.1J**). **O:** Thrombus in the straight and left transverse sinuses on coronal T1-weighted MRI.

as an important cause of arterial vascular disease and infarction. Homozygosity for the thermolabile variant of the methylene tetrahydrofolate reductase gene appears to be a risk factor for neonatal and childhood AIS, sinovenous thrombosis, and recurrence in childhood AIS (27). Homocysteine levels are influenced by diet; supplementation of folate, vitamin B_{12}, and vitamin B_6 may reduce plasma homocysteine levels, although few available data support efficacy in stroke prevention, and a varied, healthy diet should provide adequate intake.

Hypertension. Hypertension is an important risk factor for stroke in young adults and in the elderly but has largely been ignored in the pediatric literature (44). In one series, 54% of children with cryptogenic stroke and 46% of children with symptomatic stroke had systolic blood pressure above the 90th percentile and there was a significant association with cerebral arterial abnormalities (4).

Lipid Abnormalities. In a series of childhood stroke, 9% of those in whom random cholesterol was measured had high

levels, while 31% had high triglyceride levels and 22% had high lipoprotein (a), a risk factor for atherosclerosis in adults (4). High lipoprotein (a) is a risk factor for stroke (27).

Disorders of Coagulation. Recognized disorders of coagulation occur acutely in a substantial proportion of children with stroke (27), but up to half resolve within 3 months of the ictus, and the prevalence of inherited coagulopathies is ~10% in previously well patients. Polymorphisms such as factor V Leiden (which is common in Caucasian populations and is the most frequent cause of activated protein C resistance) and Prothrombin 20210 may be associated with primary and recurrent neonatal and childhood sinovenous thrombosis and AIS (7,19,27,45).

Vascular Adhesion. Adhesion of red blood cells, white blood cells, or platelets appears to be an important mechanism of endothelial damage in SCD and may play a role in stroke of other etiologies, such as moyamoya. There is evidence that different molecular mechanisms are involved in the adhesion of blood cells and platelets to the vascular endothelium in SCD. These mechanisms include adhesive ligands (e.g., von Willebrand

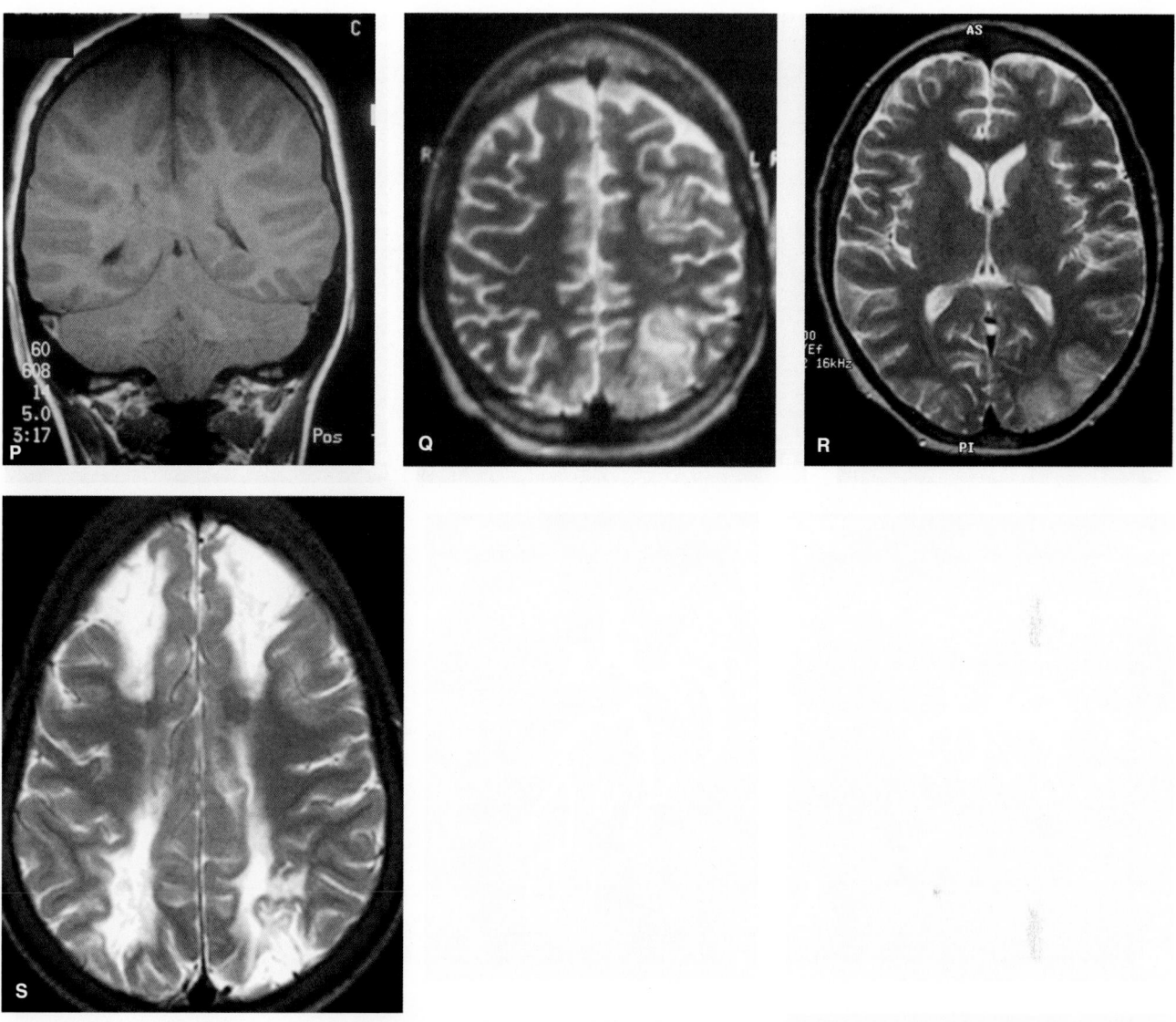

FIGURE 64.2. (*Continued*). **P:** Widespread cortical and basal ganglia hypersignal on T2-weighted axial MRI (same patient with sickle cell disease as shown in **Fig. 64.1K**). **Q:** T1-weighted coronal images showing marked swelling of the cerebral hemispheres and posterior fossa leading to tonsillar descent and brain death in same patient with sickle cell disease as shown in **Figs. 64.1K and 64.2P**. High signal is seen in the right transverse sinus (delta sign) due to sinovenous thrombus. **R:** Occipital edema in distribution compatible with reversible posterior leukoencephalopathy in sickle cell anemia and acute chest crisis. **S:** Bilateral watershed infarction in sickle cell anemia and facial infection.

factor) (45) and molecules on the red blood cells and endothelial cell surfaces (e.g., vascular cell adhesion molecule).

Arterial Disease

Between 30% and 80% of children with AIS have abnormal findings on cranial CT or MR angiographic studies (**Figs. 64.3 and 64.4**) (4,46). A less abrupt onset of stroke is characteristic of those with arteriopathy (47). Typical abnormalities include internal carotid artery (ICA) or vertebral dissection, stenosis or occlusion of the distal ICA or MCA, moyamoya syndrome (bilateral severe stenosis or occlusion of the internal carotid arteries with collateral formation), and, occasionally, patterns such as small-vessel vasculitis (4). A diagnosis of vascular disease predicts recurrent AIS (7,18) and moyamoya, and is associated with recurrent stroke and TIAs in patients with and without SCD (7). Stenoses commonly improve or stabilize [transient cerebral arteriopathy] but may progress (40). Spontaneous hemorrhage is most commonly secondary to an AVM

(20), but aneurysms and pseudoaneurysms are not unusual and may occur in association with underlying conditions, including trauma (21,26).

Extracranial/Intracranial Dissection. Among children, cervicocephalic dissections are reported in 6.5%–20% of any AIS, and in up to 50% of children with posterior circulation ischemic stroke. Statistics in the US estimate an annual caseload of 56–173 children with stroke due to cervicocephalic dissections, or 1–3 cases per week (48). Risk factors include major and minor trauma (including nonaccidental inflicted injury), infection, anatomical variants of the neck, migraine, hyperhomocysteinemia, and rare disorders such as fibromuscular dysplasia, Marfan or Ehlers–Danlos syndrome, and α_1-antitrypsin deficiency (48–50). The most frequently affected artery is the ICA, followed by the vertebral artery. In children, anterior circulation dissections are frequently intracranial (60%), affecting the intracranial ICA, MCA, and anterior cerebral artery, although circle of Willis involvement may be

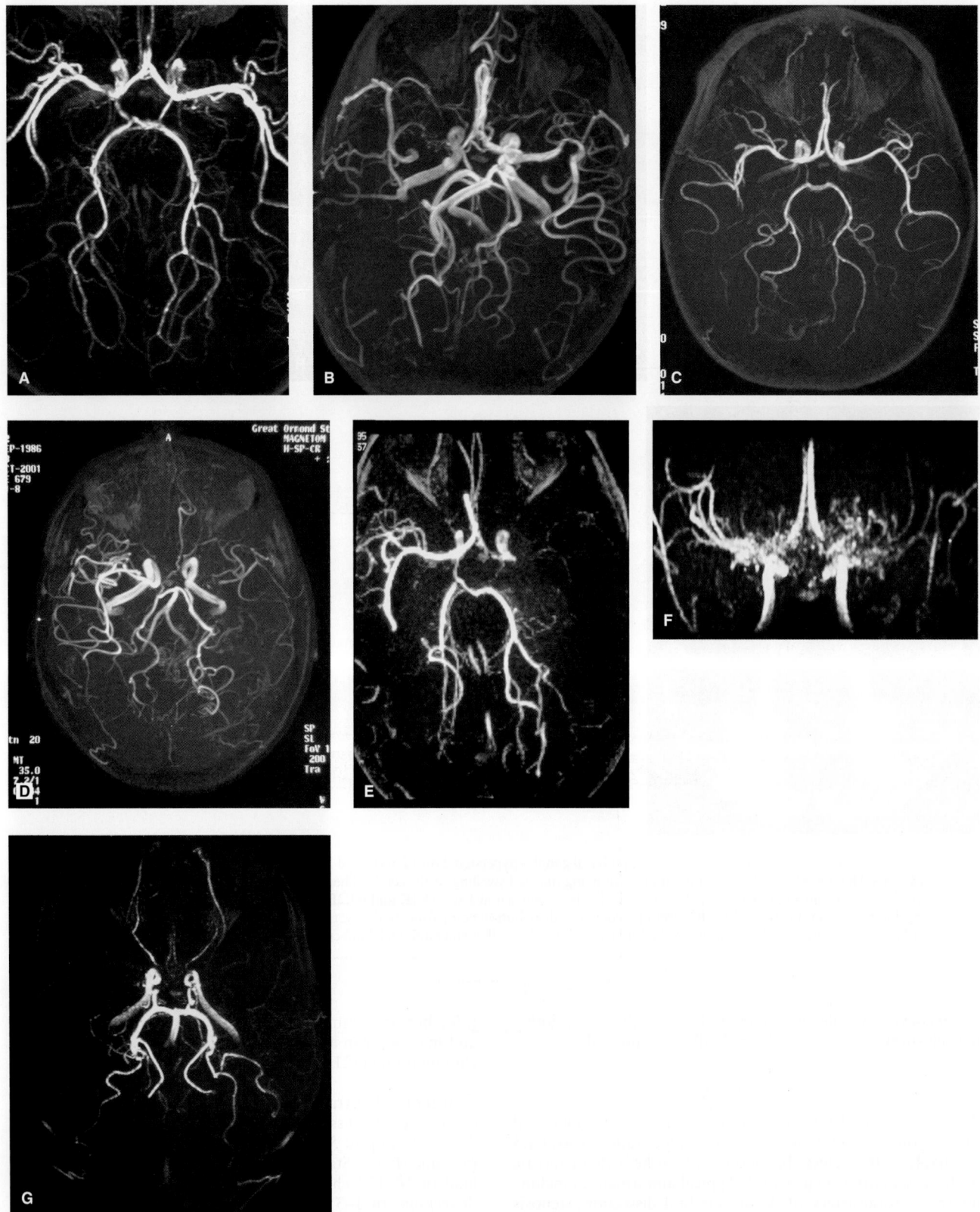

FIGURE 64.3. MRA from children with first and recurrent arterial ischemic stroke. A: "Transient" cerebral arteriopathy associated with basal ganglia infarct (Fig. 64.2A). B: Progressive arteriopathy associated with falloff in cognitive performance after *Haemophilus influenzae* meningitis and deep white matter infarction (Fig. 64.2G). C: Persistence of embolic arterial abnormality associated with "silent" recurrent infarction (Fig. 64.2F) in the posterior watershed territory. D: Unilateral arteriopathy associated with recurrent transient ischemic attacks in sickle cell anemia. E: Unilateral occlusion at the origin of the middle cerebral artery in sickle cell anemia with a large middle cerebral artery territory infarct (Fig. 64.2L). F: Bilateral moyamoya collaterals associated with severe stenosis of the distal internal carotid/proximal middle cerebral arteries. G: Bilaterally reduced flow in the middle cerebral artery without obvious moyamoya collaterals in sickle cell disease.

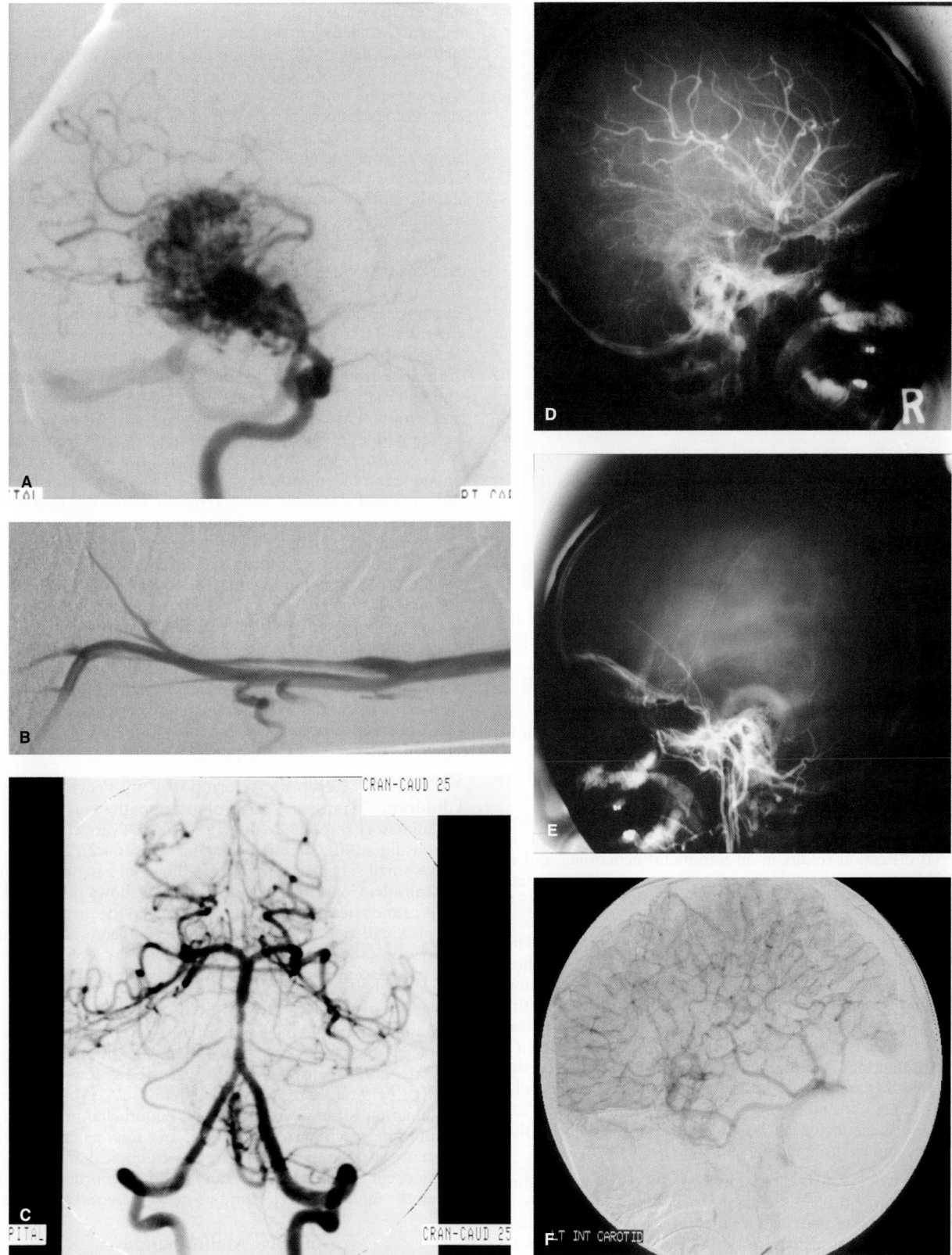

FIGURE 64.4. Conventional cerebral angiography from children with first and recurrent arterial and venous ischemic and hemorrhagic stroke. **A:** Arteriovenous malformation in an 11-year-old boy presenting with a spontaneous intracerebral hemorrhage. **B:** Typical "rat's tail" tapering occlusion in the internal carotid artery in dissection. **C:** Irregularity of the midsegment of the basilar artery and the origins of both anterior inferior cerebellar arteries. **D:** Right-sided moyamoya collaterals. **E:** Paucity of vessels on the left side in the patient in D with right-sided moyamoya. **F:** Venous phase demonstrating absence of flow in the occluded superior sagittal and straight sinus with multiple collateral vessels draining the hemisphere toward the cavernous sinus (**Fig. 64.2M**).

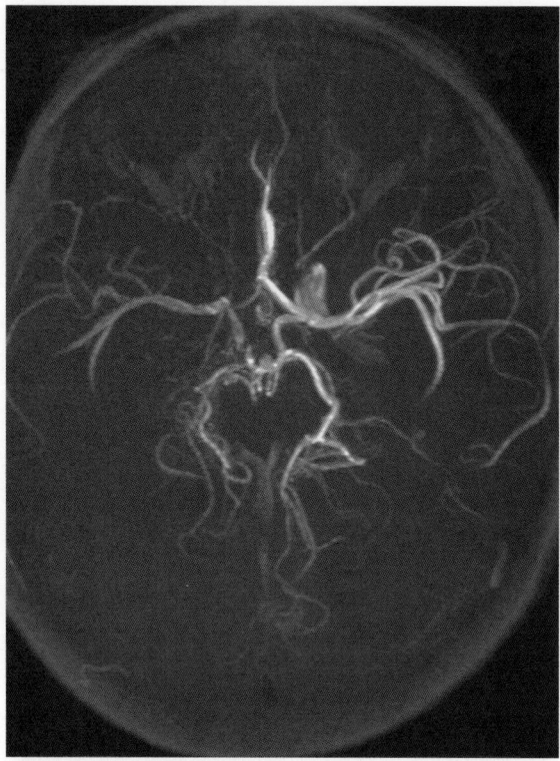

FIGURE 64.5. Axial fat-saturated, T1-weighted MRI of the neck in a patient presenting with an acute hemiparesis shows blood in the wall characteristic of dissection.

difficult to distinguish from transient cerebral arteriopathy (51). Approximately 80% of posterior circulation dissections are extracranial, and more than half are located within the vertebral artery at the level C1–C2 (52). Multiple dissections are common and are seen in 8%–28% of children.

The origin of the dissection is likely to be a small intimal tear or primary intramural hemorrhage of the vasa vasorum. Arterial dissection results in an intramural hematoma and its variable extension along the course of that artery. The magnetic resonance angiography (MRA) is not usually diagnostic (53), but a lesion in the neck vessels may be suggested by reduced flow in the intracranial vessels. In many cases, the intramural hematoma may be demonstrated using fat-saturated T1-weighted MRI of the neck (Fig. 64.5), although conventional arteriography may sometimes be required to demonstrate the tapering partial occlusion of the artery ("rat's tail") (Fig. 64.4B). Head or neck trauma is a well-recognized cause of dissection, and it is worth noting that intraoral injuries (e.g., from a pencil carried in the mouth) can contuse the carotid artery in the peritonsillar area. Although an underlying arteriopathy has long been suspected, no single factor has been identified, and a combination of genetic and environmental factors are probably involved.

Local Effects. The dissection may compress surrounding nerve structures, disrupting their nutrient blood supply. Subadventitial extension may lead to aneurysmal distension, which may either cause local compression or lead to thromboembolic phenomena. Extracranial aneurysms do not usually rupture, unlike intracranial dissections, which can lead to SAH. Subintimal dissection results in stenosis or occlusion of the arterial lumen and is a potent thrombogenic stimulus.

Distant Effects. Hemodynamic consequences of dissection may reduce oxygen delivery to neuronal tissue. However, arterial-to-arterial thromboembolism is probably the most important pathogenetic mechanism in dissection-related stroke.

The evidence that this is the case includes (a) the delay that often exists between the time of dissection and subsequent neurologic deficit; (b) angiographic evidence of distal embolization in 50% of children who present with cervicocephalic dissection; (c) patterns of stroke in ICA dissection that suggest the etiologic relevance of local hemodynamic effects in only 8% of cases (Fig. 64.3G); and (d) transcranial Doppler evidence that microemboli in the MCA downstream from the dissection correlate with stroke recurrence and are reduced with antithrombotic therapy (no randomized controlled trials have yet looked at reduction of microemboli or clinical stroke rate from antithrombolytic therapy).

Moyamoya. Moyamoya (**Figs. 64.3F and 64.4D,E**) derives from the Japanese word meaning "something hazy, like a puff of smoke drifting in the air" and describes the appearance of the collaterals seen in association with bilateral severe stenosis or occlusion of the terminal ICAs in childhood (54). Collaterals arise from the anterior and posterior ethmoidal arteries and external carotid system or the middle meningeal/superficial temporal arteries via transdural vessels. Moyamoya may be idiopathic (moyamoya *disease*) or occur in the context of other disorders (moyamoya *syndrome*) and is best considered an angiographic phenomenon rather than a pathologic entity. Ischemia and infarction occur typically in the border-zone regions between the major cerebral arteries.

Associations include SCD, where moyamoya syndrome predicts a higher recurrence risk, and Down syndrome, where a widespread vasculopathy may affect small and large vessels commonly associated with moyamoya collaterals. Moyamoya occurs in Williams syndrome, a disorder known to involve mutations in the elastin gene, suggesting that abnormal vessel distensibility may lead to hypoperfusion and promote development of collaterals. Other associations include neurofibromatosis, cranial irradiation, and arteriopathies. A genetic predisposition accounts for otherwise idiopathic, as well as familial, cases reported in Japan.

"Transient" Cerebral Arteriopathy in Previously Well Children. "Transient" cerebral arteriopathy may involve an inflammatory response to infections such as varicella, *Borrelia*, or tonsillitis (40). Cerebral imaging (**Figs. 64.2A and 64.3A**) shows small subcortical infarcts in the basal ganglia and internal capsule. Conventional arteriography shows multifocal lesions of the arterial wall with narrowing in the distal ICA, and the proximal anterior, middle, or posterior cerebral arteries. In many cases, the vasculopathy may stabilize or even disappear, and progression is associated with recurrent stroke.

Intracranial Arteriopathy in SCD. Narrowing of the distal ICA and proximal MCA and anterior cerebral artery is also characteristic of SCD (**Figs. 64.3D,E,G**), although in these patients, gradual progression to occlusion commonly occurs with or without moyamoya collaterals (25,34). Pathologic examination of these arteries shows endothelial proliferation, fibroblastic reaction, hyalinization, and fragmentation of the internal elastic lamina. The majority of clinical and silent infarcts occur in the MCA territory or in the border zones between the middle, anterior, and posterior cerebral territories.

Vascular Malformations

Arteriovenous Malformations. The prevalence of AVM is 10–500 per 100,000 children (55). AVMs are high-flow arteriovenous shunts through a nidus of abnormal thin-walled, coiled, and tortuous connections between feeding arteries and draining veins, without an intervening capillary network (**Fig. 64.4A**). AVMs represent abnormal vascular. In children, AVMs more commonly present with hemorrhage in deep areas of the brain (particularly basal ganglia and thalamus).

Capillary Telangiectasias. Capillary telangiectasias are collections of dilated ectatic capillaries with normal intervening neural tissue, without smooth muscle or elastic fibers; they are not commonly associated with ICH or SAH.

Cavernous Angioma. Cavernous angiomas (cavernomas) are vascular malformations that comprise thin-walled sinusoidal spaces lined with endothelial tissue and contain intravascular or intervascular calcifications, without any intervening parenchymal tissue. Multiple lesions are seen in 13% of sporadic cases and 50% of familial cases. It is thought that venous hypertension due to obstructed outflow results in the formation of the cavernoma. Cavernomas may present with symptoms related to frank ICH or with epilepsy, possibly secondary to intermittent leakage of blood around the cavernoma.

Venous Angioma. Venous angiomas are thin-walled venous channels with normal intervening neural tissue that are associated with a very low risk of bleeding.

Sturge–Weber Syndrome. Sturge–Weber syndrome (**Fig. 64.1M**) is a sporadic condition characterized by a venous angioma of the leptomeninges, a choroidal angioma, and a facial capillary hemangioma involving the periorbital area, forehead, or scalp that probably results from a failure of regression of a vascular plexus around the cephalic portion of the neural tube at between 6 and 9 weeks of gestation (55). Epilepsy, hemiplegia, and learning disability (often progressive) are probably the result of an ischemic mechanism. The patient may be relatively well between episodes of status epilepticus or acute hemiparesis, which may be triggered by trauma (56). Aspirin may reduce the frequency of stroke-like episodes. If intractable epilepsy cannot be controlled by medical means, hemispherectomy may be beneficial.

Vein of Galen Malformation. Vein of Galen malformation (**Fig. 64.1N**) is an embryonic choroidal AVM (57). It can be diagnosed antenatally, has a male preponderance but no known genetic predisposition, and usually presents in the neonatal period as heart failure or, in older children, with hydrocephalus, seizures, proptosis, or prominent scalp veins. Endovascular treatment is often offered at specialized centers and appears to provide good quality of life, particularly for older children not presenting in heart failure with mural, rather than choroidal, malformations (58).

Aneurysms

Arterial aneurysms are acquired lesions and are multiple in 2%–5% of pediatric cases (21). Three-quarters of patients with arterial aneurysms present with ICH. Approximately 10%–15% of arterial aneurysms are posttraumatic; a similar proportion are mycotic, and associated with infection (e.g., *Staphylococcus*, *Streptococcus*, Gram-negative organisms, and HIV). Mycotic aneurysms may also arise secondary to embolization of infective thrombi into the intracranial circulation in patients with subacute bacterial endocarditis. Other associations with arterial aneurysms in children are polycystic kidney disease, SCD, tuberous sclerosis, Marfan syndrome, Ehlers–Danlos syndrome type IV, pseudoxanthoma elasticum, and hypertension. No underlying systemic disorder is found in a substantial proportion.

Cerebral Sinovenous Thrombosis

The venous drainage of the brain occurs through the "superficial" or "deep" cerebral sinovenous systems, which consist of a network of sinuses and veins. Flow is highly responsive to changes in mean arterial pressure, reductions in which can result in stasis or reversal of blood flow within the dural sinuses. Also, a relative reduction of thrombomodulin in cerebral venous endothelium exaggerates the prothrombotic tendency. The

"superficial" venous system includes the cortical veins, which drain into the superior sagittal sinus and then mainly into the right lateral sinus. The "deep venous system" includes the inferior sagittal sinus and the paired internal cerebral veins, which join to form the vein of Galen and the straight sinus, draining predominantly into the smaller caliber left lateral sinus and jugular vein.

In neonates, pathogenesis of sinovenous thrombosis (**Figs. 64.1J,K** and **64.4F**) may be related to mechanical distortion of the cranial bones during birth. In older children, trauma, sepsis, and underlying illnesses such as malignancy or systemic inflammation play a larger role (13,59). Septic foci include the inner ear, mastoid, or air sinuses and lead to thrombophlebitic sinovenous thrombosis. Dehydration, anemia, and inherited prothrombotic disorders (congenital or acquired) are also recognized risk factors (59). Finally, positional alterations in flow dynamics can have a significant role in the pathogenesis of sinovenous thrombosis in neonates and older children with vascular malformations.

Sinovenous thrombosis leads to disruption of cerebrospinal fluid absorption within the superior sagittal sinus, resulting in diffuse cerebral swelling, communicating hydrocephalus, or pseudotumor cerebri (benign intracranial hypertension) (13).

Venous Infarction. Cerebral infarction results when perfusion to the affected area of the brain is reduced to critical level. In sinovenous thrombosis, "outflow" obstruction causes venous hypertension in the affected region of the brain, leading to focal cerebral edema (**Figs. 64.2M–Q**). When tissue hydrostatic pressure exceeds arterial inflow pressure, infarction, which may be hemorrhagic, ensues. Risk factors for venous infarction include rapid onset of sinovenous thrombosis, complete luminal occlusion, and thrombosis located at the entry points of cerebral veins into the sagittal sinus (**Fig. 64.6**).

Stroke Syndromes and Mimics

Posterior Circulation Arterial Stroke. Arterial disease in association with posterior circulation infarction in the cerebellum (**Fig. 64.1I**), brainstem, and parieto-occipital lobes is much more common in boys than in girls (52,60). A positive diagnosis of dissection may require conventional angiography in the acute phase, as MRI and angiography commonly miss the diagnosis in the posterior circulation (**Fig. 64.7**). Etiologic

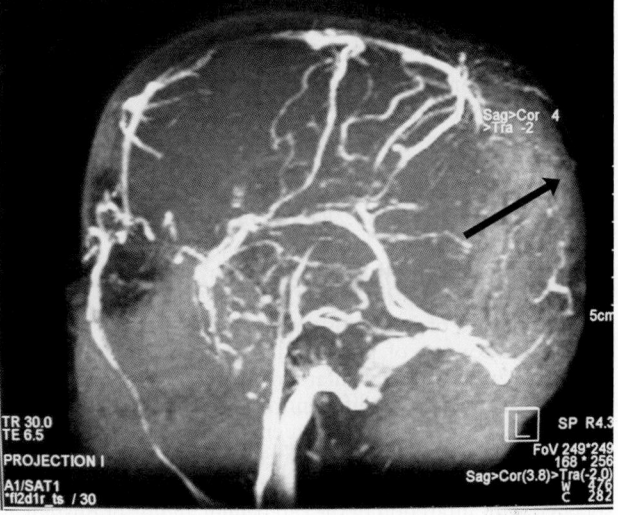

FIGURE 64.6. MR venogram in a teenager with systemic lupus erythematosus and a warm autoimmune hemolytic anemia showing chronic sagittal sinus thrombosis, with a flow void posteriorly.

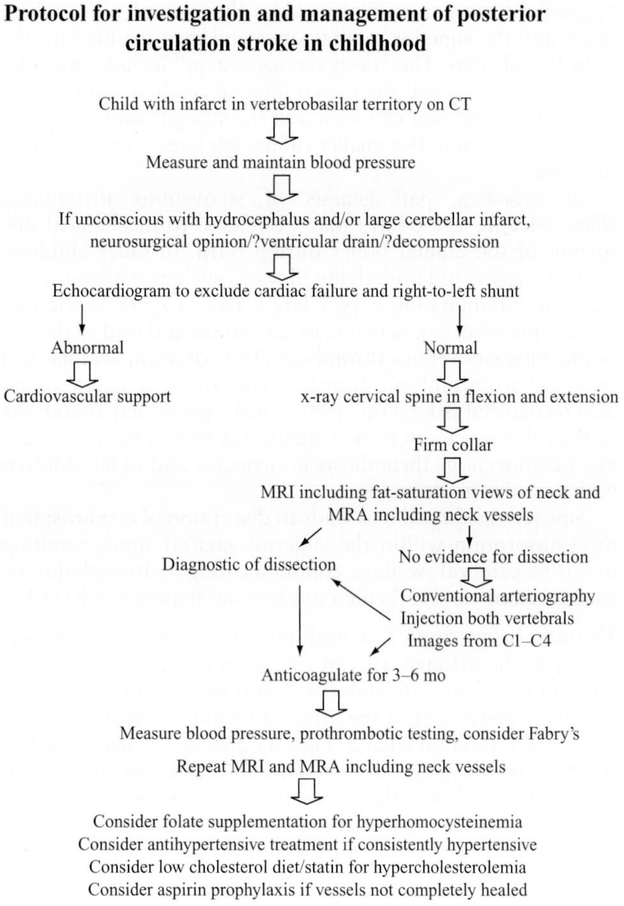

Protocol for investigation and management of posterior circulation stroke in childhood

Child with infarct in vertebrobasilar territory on CT

⇩

Measure and maintain blood pressure

⇩

If unconscious with hydrocephalus and/or large cerebellar infarct,
neurosurgical opinion/?ventricular drain/?decompression

Echocardiogram to exclude cardiac failure and right-to-left shunt

Abnormal   Normal

⇩   ⇩

Cardiovascular support   x-ray cervical spine in flexion and extension

⇩

Firm collar

⇩

MRI including fat-saturation views of neck and
MRA including neck vessels

Diagnostic of dissection   No evidence for dissection

Conventional arteriography
Injection both vertebrals
Images from C1–C4

Anticoagulate for 3–6 mo

⇩

Measure blood pressure, prothrombotic testing, consider Fabry's

Repeat MRI and MRA including neck vessels

⇩

Consider folate supplementation for hyperhomocysteinemia
Consider antihypertensive treatment if consistently hypertensive
Consider low cholesterol diet/statin for hypercholesterolemia
Consider aspirin prophylaxis if vessels not completely healed

FIGURE 64.7. Algorithm for the management of posterior circulation stroke.

factors include minor trauma, subluxation of the cervical spine at the extremes of flexion and extension, chiropractic manipulation, frequent neck movements (e.g., secondary to athetoid cerebral palsy), hypertension, cardiac anomalies, and perhaps Fabry disease. Some patients with conventional risk factors for stroke (hypertension, hypercholesterolemia, and hyperhomocysteinemia) have vascular imaging compatible with early atheroma (**Fig. 64.4C**) (52).

RPLS and Border-zone Ischemia. RPLS is a cliniconeuroradiologic syndrome characterized by seizures, altered mental state, visual abnormalities, and headaches, all of which are associated with predominantly posterior white matter abnormalities on CT and MRI examinations but without arterial or venous disease (**Fig. 64.2R**) (61). RPLS is a relatively common stroke mimic and has been recognized in an increasing number of medical settings, including hypertensive encephalopathy (44), eclampsia, after acute chest crisis in SCD (62), and during use of immunosuppression (61). Acute hypotension in the context of poor cardiac function and/or anemia may also cause occipital infarction without vascular disease (52). As treatments are different, it is essential to distinguish RPLS from posterior circulation embolic stroke secondary to vertebrobasilar dissection; the latter typically presents "out of the blue," is much more common in boys, and is typically associated with infarction in the cerebellum and/or brainstem as well as the occipitoparietal cortex, but MR and conventional arteriography may be required to make a positive diagnosis (52). It is also important to exclude sinovenous thrombosis, particularly of the sagittal and straight sinuses (**Figs. 64.1J,K**

and 64.2M–Q), which may be associated with venous infarction in the parietal and occipital lobes as well as the thalami (**Figs. 64.1J,K and 64.2M–Q**).

The rapid resolution of clinical and neuroradiologic abnormalities in the majority of cases of RPLS suggests vasogenic cerebral edema, which is thought to result from impaired cerebrovascular autoregulation and endothelial injury. Most patients make a full clinical and radiologic recovery after conservative measures, including slow reduction of blood pressure and maintenance of normal oxygenation. Some patients with otherwise typical RPLS have additional imaging abnormalities anteriorly and/or in the gray matter, often in a distribution suggestive of border-zone ischemia, and the changes are not necessarily reversible in all cases. Complications including status epilepticus, intracranial hemorrhage, and cerebellar herniation may be life-threatening (63). Patients with parietooccipital infarction may have visual problems and epilepsy in the long term.

Acute Disseminated Encephalomyelitis. Acute disseminated encephalomyelitis (ADEM) is an immune-mediated process resulting in inflammation and myelin damage in the brain and spinal cord that is usually associated with infection or immunization. MRI may reveal demyelination in children who present with acute focal neurologic signs (4). Evidence suggests that intravenous methylprednisolone reduces the duration of the illness and perhaps improves long-term outcome.

Metabolic Stroke. Diabetes and inborn errors of metabolism (now often treatable) can cause acute focal neurologic symptoms and signs (metabolic stroke) due to either vascular injury or direct tissue injury, which may be permanent or transitory (42).

Vascular Injury. Homocysteine is a highly chemically reactive thiol amino acid that can cause direct endothelial injury. Inborn errors that affect three enzymes (5,10-methylenetetrahydrofolate reductase, methionine synthase, and cystathionine β-synthase) or the synthesis of their vitamin cofactors are known to cause homocystinuria and may present with arterial or venous stroke in infancy or childhood.

Fabry disease is a lysosomal storage disorder that causes accumulation of the glycosphingolipid globotriaosylceramide in blood vessel endothelial cells and, to some extent, in the vascular smooth muscle. It is an X-linked disorder caused by deficiency of the lysosomal hydrolase α-galactosidase A and is an important cause of cryptogenic stroke in the young, particularly those with vertebrobasilar territory infarction. Proteinuria may be a useful screen, but if the clinician has a strong index of suspicion, exclusion should be by enzyme diagnosis, as replacement is available.

Menkes disease is an X-linked disorder of copper transport caused by deficiency of a copper-transporting adenosine triphosphatase, which in turn causes copper deficiency. Subdural hematomas, tortuosity, and obliteration of intracranial vasculature can result.

Nonvascular Injury. Some organic acidemias, urea cycle disorders, and other inborn errors of metabolism can cause metabolic stroke (42). Female carriers with ornithine carbamoyltransferase deficiency may present with focal signs. Mitochondrial disorders can cause stroke-like episodes (i.e., mitochondrial encephalopathy with lactic acidosis and stroke-like episodes). The exact mechanisms by which these occur are unknown. In the organic acidemias and urea cycle disorders, it is likely that accumulation of a toxic metabolite causes infarction of a selectively vulnerable area of the brain. By contrast, mitochondrial disorders are liable to cause infarction because of deficient energy supply and by the generation of oxygen free radicals. As arginine supplementation may be beneficial, it is important to exclude mitochondrial disorders.

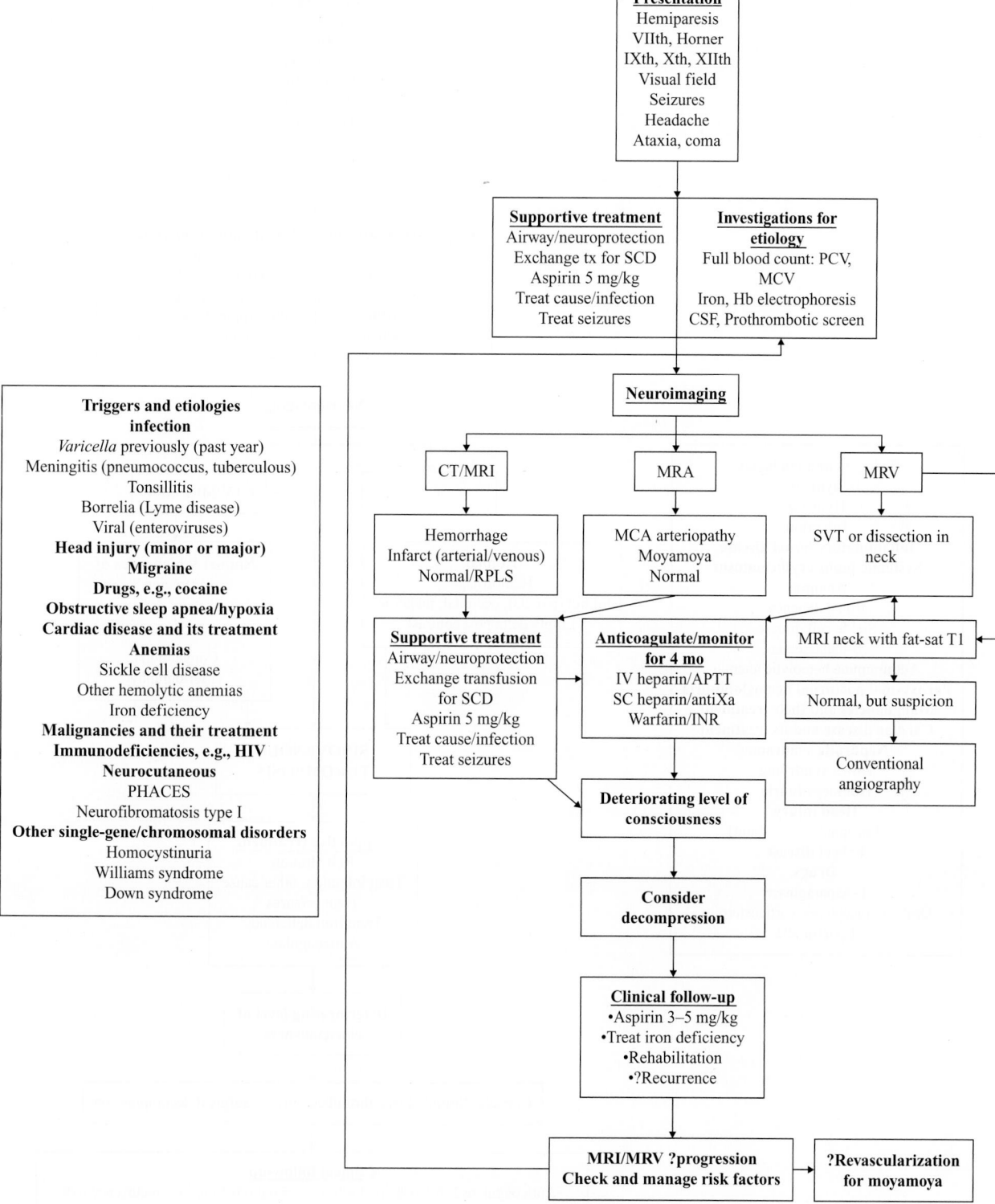

Presentation
Hemiparesis
VIIth, Horner
IXth, Xth, XIIth
Visual field
Seizures
Headache
Ataxia, coma

Supportive treatment
Airway/neuroprotection
Exchange tx for SCD
Aspirin 5 mg/kg
Treat cause/infection
Treat seizures

Investigations for etiology
Full blood count: PCV, MCV
Iron, Hb electrophoresis
CSF, Prothrombotic screen

Neuroimaging

CT/MRI   MRA   MRV

Hemorrhage
Infarct (arterial/venous)
Normal/RPLS

MCA arteriopathy
Moyamoya
Normal

SVT or dissection in neck

Supportive treatment
Airway/neuroprotection
Exchange transfusion for SCD
Aspirin 5 mg/kg
Treat cause/infection
Treat seizures

Anticoagulate/monitor for 4 mo
IV heparin/APTT
SC heparin/antiXa
Warfarin/INR

MRI neck with fat-sat T1

Normal, but suspicion

Conventional angiography

Deteriorating level of consciousness

Consider decompression

Clinical follow-up
•Aspirin 3–5 mg/kg
•Treat iron deficiency
•Rehabilitation
•?Recurrence

MRI/MRV ?progression
Check and manage risk factors

?Revascularization for moyamoya

Triggers and etiologies infection
Varicella previously (past year)
Meningitis (pneumococcus, tuberculous)
Tonsillitis
Borrelia (Lyme disease)
Viral (enteroviruses)
Head injury (minor or major)
Migraine
Drugs, e.g., cocaine
Obstructive sleep apnea/hypoxia
Cardiac disease and its treatment
Anemias
Sickle cell disease
Other hemolytic anemias
Iron deficiency
Malignancies and their treatment
Immunodeficiencies, e.g., HIV
Neurocutaneous
PHACES
Neurofibromatosis type I
Other single-gene/chromosomal disorders
Homocystinuria
Williams syndrome
Down syndrome

FIGURE 64.8. Algorithm for the diagnosis and management of arterial stroke. SCD, sickle cell disease; PCV, packed cell volume; MCV, mean corpuscular volume; CSF, cerebral spinal fluid; HIV, human immunodeficiency virus; PHACES, posterior fossa malformations–hemangiomas–arterial anomalies–cardiac defects–eye abnormalities–sternal cleft and supraumbilical raphe syndrome; RPLS, reversible posterior leukoencephalopathy syndrome; MCA, middle cerebral artery; SVT, sinovenous thrombosis; APTT, activated partial thromboplastin time; SC, subcutaneous; INR, international normalized ratio.

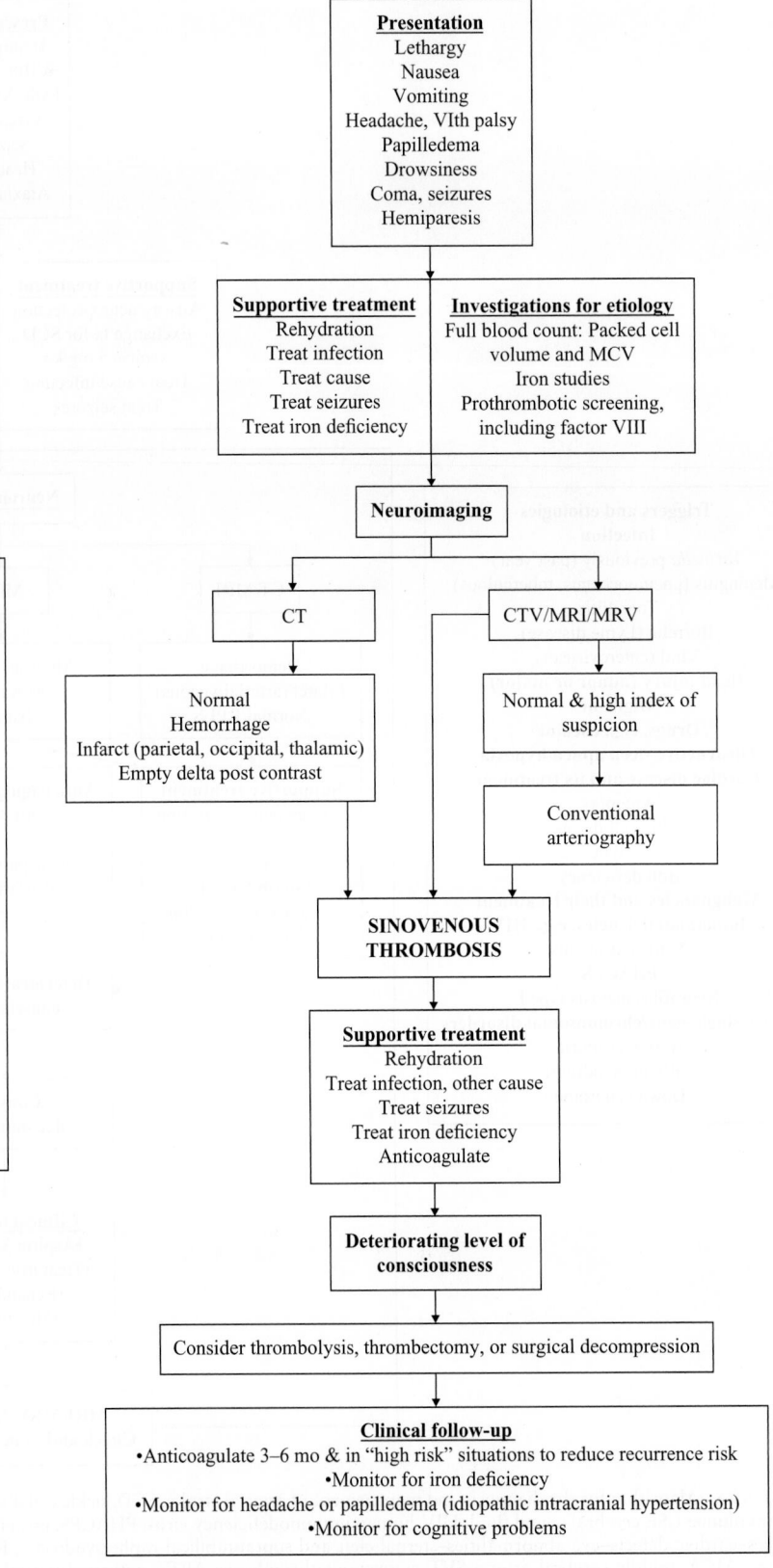

FIGURE 64.9. Algorithm for the management of sinovenous thrombosis. MCV, mean corpuscular volume.

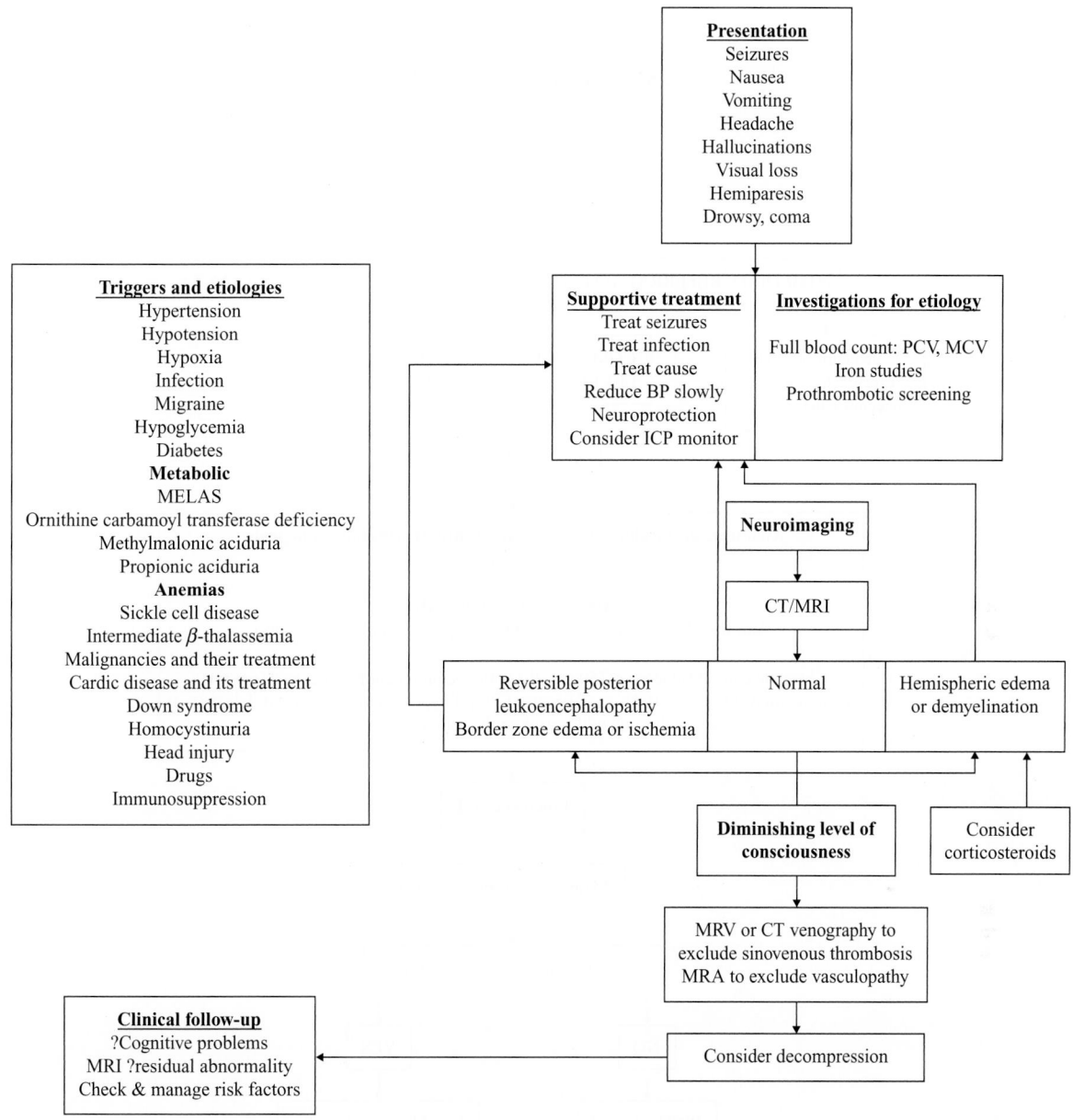

FIGURE 64.10. Algorithm for the management of stroke mimics. MELAS, mitochondrial encephalomyopathy, lactic acidosis, and stroke-like episode; BP, blood pressure; PCV, packed cell volume; MCV, mean corpuscular volume.

CLINICAL PRESENTATION AND DIFFERENTIAL DIAGNOSIS

Stroke and CVD can cause considerable anxiety to the pediatric intensivist at least in part because of the large number of individual conditions, each of which is relatively rare. The differential diagnosis includes a wide range of alternative pathologies (64), and protocols for investigation and treatment are not well defined. The important clinical clues for diagnosis are often (a) for symptomatic stroke, a preexisting diagnosis; and (b) for cryptogenic stroke, the trigger(s) (Figs. 64.7–64.10).

In adults, as a result of controlled trials of thrombolysis, increased awareness of the need for rapid assessment and appropriate management of acute stroke in stroke centers or units and the concept of "brain attack" have received widespread publicity. Thrombolysis for anterior circulation stroke must

begin within 4.5 hours. In contrast, few children are triaged this quickly. In many children, the correct diagnosis is not made for days or weeks. Currently, services for children are in the process of becoming organized, and it has not yet proved possible to conduct large randomized trials of treatment in groups of children with similar pathologies.

In regard to current management of children, the clinician should distinguish between the various "stroke mimics" that exist and are benign conditions, not requiring treatment, from those episodes where the viability of brain tissue is at risk (64). At presentation, patients may have potentially serious CVD, either venous or arterial, without infarction, and timely intervention may prevent stroke. Comprehensive radiologic investigation is essential, and increasing evidence suggests that in some settings emergency MRI provides information that may, in certain circumstances, guide management in the individual patient. Of course, in a time-limited emergency, where there may be consideration for the identification of intracranial

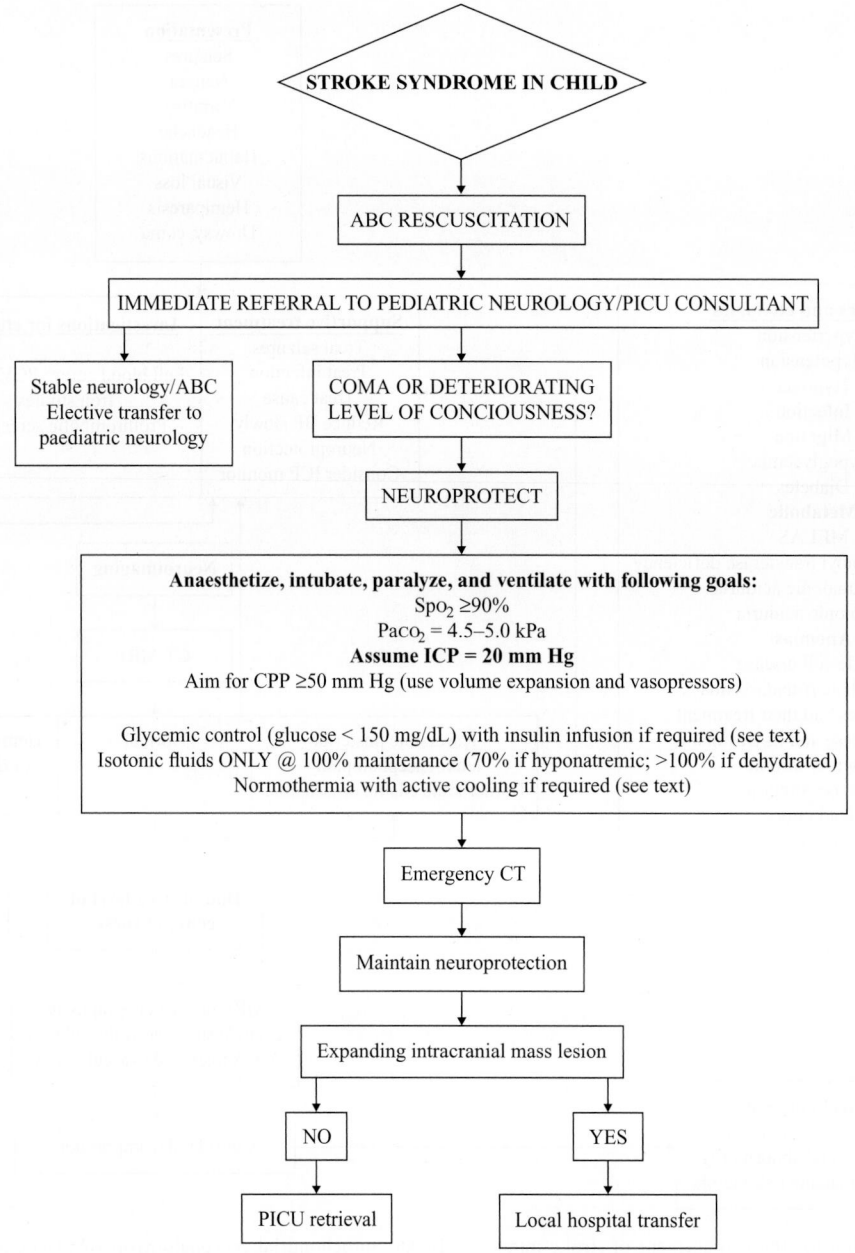

FIGURE 64.11. Emergency management of childhood stroke. ABC, airway, breathing, circulation; Spo_2, arterial oxygen saturation; $Paco_2$, arterial carbon dioxide pressure.

hemorrhage or need for neurosurgery, a CT scan as fast as possible is the investigation of choice.

Children with stroke syndromes can present to the pediatric intensivist in a variety of ways. Unlike adult stroke, the vast majority of pediatric stroke victims will either present to, or be rapidly referred to, a tertiary center. PICU involvement will thus commence at the stage of resuscitation and retrieval and will continue to facilitate elective or emergency intervention (Fig. 64.11). The common clinical presentations are presented in Table 64.1. The importance of recognizing these as a medical/surgical emergency cannot be overstated.

Children may present in coma (needing anesthesia and intubation for airway protection), with status epilepticus resistant to first-line therapy (requiring airway protection for second-line therapy, e.g., barbiturate coma) or with a reduced level of consciousness either requiring observation in the PICU or airway protection to facilitate further investigation.

Periprocedural admission to PICU may also be required for children who have known intracranial pathology that predisposes to stroke (e.g., embolization of AVM or aneurysm, extracranial–intracranial bypass for moyamoya). Children may also present with signs of intracranial hypertension or imminent central or uncal herniation (Fig. 64.12).

General Management

Emergency management of children who present with coma, altered level of consciousness, or status epilepticus must follow standard resuscitation algorithms targeted at the maintenance of airway, breathing, and circulation. No studies have specifically examined the effect of the loss of cardiorespiratory integrity on stroke outcome in children. However, based on principles that would be applied to the care of any acutely

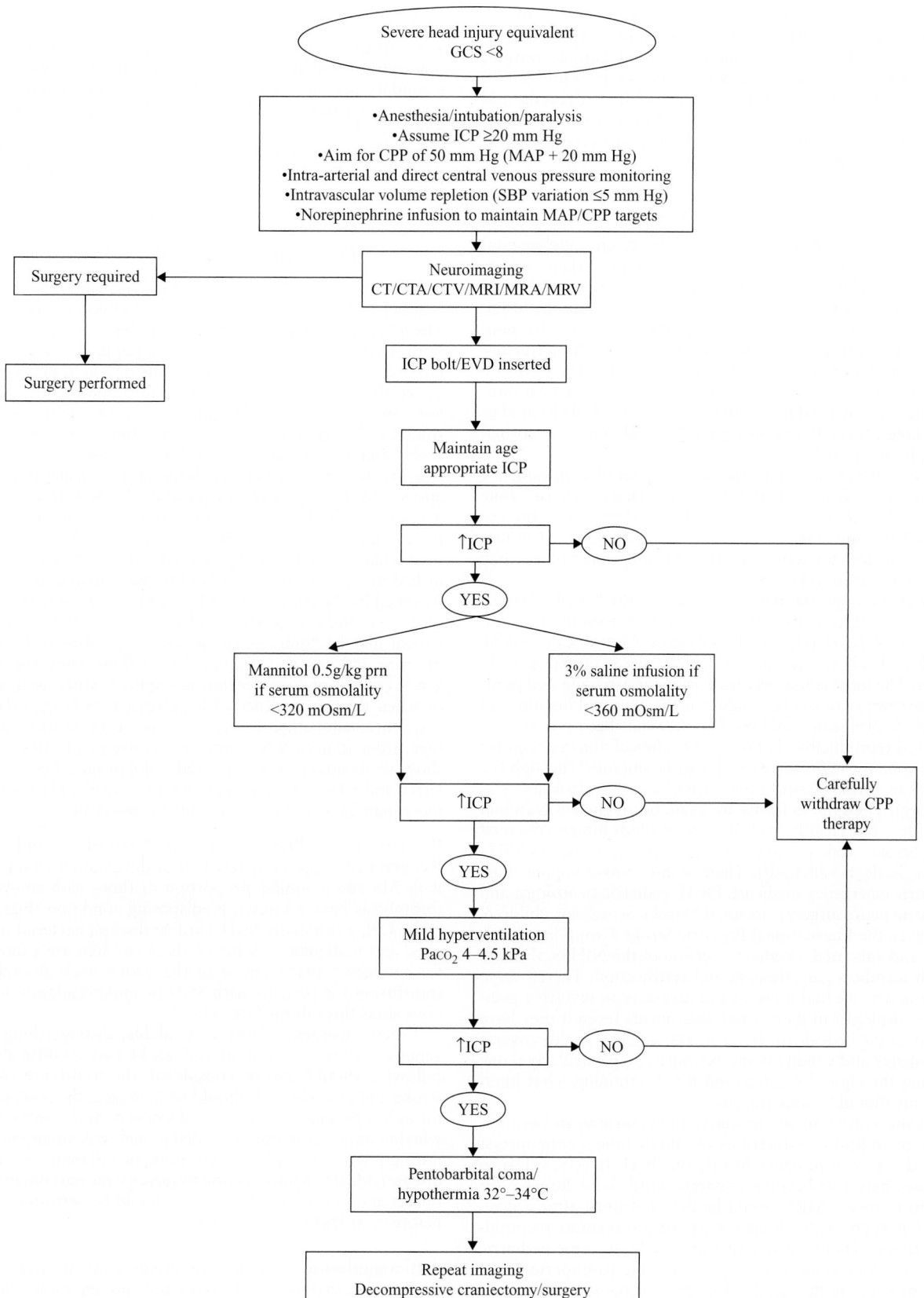

FIGURE 64.12. Neuroprotection in childhood stroke. GCS, Glasgow coma scale; MAP, mean arterial pressure; SBP, systolic blood pressure; CTA, CT angiography; EVD, external ventricular drain; Paco2, arterial carbon dioxide pressure.

ill child, as well as those from the evidence base in adults, the aim should be maintenance of normality, i.e., well-saturated oxygen-hemoglobin saturation, good cardiac output, optimized systemic and cerebral perfusion pressure (CPP), normothermia, and careful avoidance of hypoglycemia and hyperglycemia. This section provides an overview of emergent neuroprotection in this context, and the controversies are discussed in more detail later.

Stabilize, Assess, and Prepare

At presentation, all patients should be given supplemental oxygen via nasal cannula. If they cannot protect their airway, then endotracheal intubation is required. The head of the bed should be flat; this maneuver optimizes perfusion to the brain, but the cost may be the risk of aspiration in those with nausea and vomiting and compromised airway protection (further discussion about head-of-bed position below). Therefore, in the emergency setting, before imaging and endotracheal intubation, one may need to accept the head of the bed elevated to 15 degrees. If the blood pressure is low, administer a normal saline bolus (10 mL/kg).

In the history, determine the time of onset of symptom; ask the question "When was the child last seen as normal?" Take a focused history that will help in excluding stroke mimics (**Fig. 64.10**) and start on the *Airway, Breathing and Circulation* assessment for resuscitation and management of a stroke syndrome (Fig. 66.11).

Next, examine the patient and assess the "Stroke Score." There is no agreed cross-discipline score that should be used; many intensivists rely on the Glasgow Coma Scale (GCS), which is clearly not sensitive to the changes expected in acute stroke. The most commonly used scale for assessing and grading the severity of stroke in adults is the National Institutes of Health Stroke Scale (NIHSS). This scale has been proven reliable and reproducible, *but using it in clinical practice requires training and certification*, which can be obtained through the American Stroke Association's website (www.strokeassociation.org). The NIHSS forms are available at the US National Institutes of Health website (www.ninds.nih.gov/doctors/NIH_Stroke_Scale.pdf and www.ninds.nih.gov/doctors/NIH_Stroke_Scale_Booklet.pdf). There is no cross-discipline (i.e., pediatric emergency medicine, PICU, pediatric neurology, and pediatric neurosurgery)–accepted "Stroke Score" for children. However, the International Pediatric Stroke Group has developed and validated a pediatric version of the NIHSS, through which members gain training and certification. Therefore, in our practice, we find it useful and necessary to involve a pediatric neurologist in these serial assessments (even if they have to stay at the bedside for frequent assessments) as this ensures consistency and validity in the examination, particularly if one is using the clinical examination for determining what interventions should be undertaken.

At the same time as the above interventions and evaluations, the initial investigations should include a noncontrast cranial CT scan in order to rule out ICH. In AIS, CT scan changes may not become apparent until 3–24 hours after symptom onset. MRI should be deferred until after a decision has been made about the use of intravenous recombinant tissue plasminogen activator (rTPA). In some pediatric tertiary stroke centers, it may be possible to undertake the MRI as soon as the child enters the emergency system and this study is particularly useful (**Figs. 64.7–64.11**). Arrange for the following tests: an electrocardiogram, arterial blood gas, serum electrolytes, renal function tests, liver function tests, complete blood count including platelets, toxicology studies, and clotting studies (prothrombin time, international normalized ratio, and activated partial thromboplastin time).

The Four Targets of Early "Ischemic Stroke" Care

The four targets for ischemic stroke care are (a) acute therapy that optimizes neurological status; (b) etiological workup for secondary prevention; (c) prevention of neurological deterioration or medical complications; and (d) recovery and rehabilitation. The PICU team is involved in the first three of these targets. However, a multidisciplinary approach with pediatric neurology and neurosurgery is needed in order to deal with the full extent of the workup that is needed as well as to keep a focus on the recovery and rehabilitation phase of care.

Optimizing the Neurological Status

In instances where there is no hemorrhage, emergency therapy is about *getting the artery open* and reestablishing blood flow. The intensivist needs to be doing everything to optimize blood flow. Treatment with rTPA is rarely an option in our patients: rarely do they present within 4.5 hours of symptom onset and, as yet, there is no pediatric evidence to support its use (see below). Subsequent care will be informed by the results of imaging studies including head CT and angiography, MRI and angiography, and transcranial Doppler. Is there a dissection? Is there a stenosis? Is there an aneurysm? Is the circle of Willis intact? The answers to these questions then dictate the measures needed to maintain cerebral perfusion. For example, in order to maintain perfusion through stenoses and collateral vessels, we target intravascular euvolemia using normal saline and maintain head of bed in the flat position. Blood pressure management is determined by the patient's own level of pressure. If hypertensive (using age- and sex-specific standards), we do not treat since the patient may be "autoregulating" at a new set-point for blood pressure and regional cerebral blood flow. However, emergency control of hypertension is required when using rTPA, or when there is evidence of hypertensive end-organ damage (e.g., encephalopathy, dissection of the aorta, heart failure, or myocardial injury). When antihypertensive treatment is used, a short-acting intravenous agent (labetalol or nicardipine) is preferred and a 10%–15% reduction is the target, and certainly no more than 25% in the first 8 hours of treatment.

Prevention of Propagation of Thrombus and Early Recurrence. Approximately half of the children who present with AIS and a similar proportion of those with sinovenous thrombosis have a known predisposing condition (**Figs. 64.8 and 64.9**), particularly SCD, cardiac disease, bacterial meningitis, and malignancy. Some of these children are candidates for emergency management of the stroke, such as exchange transfusion for patients with SCD or anticoagulation for venous sinus thrombosis (see below).

Unless emergency MRI is available, distinguishing sinovenous thrombosis from arterial stroke may be difficult. The following should also be considered: the recurrence risk for stroke and how this risk should be managed; the potential for thrombus propagation in cases of sinovenous thrombosis; and whether anticoagulation is needed in high-risk situations (e.g., during relapse of nephritic syndrome or inflammatory bowel disease). Ideally, neuroimaging to identify the pathology of the infarct and of the vascular disease should be performed either before or as therapy commences.

Anticoagulation. The decision about acute anticoagulation is often deferred until 2–14 days after presentation when the underlying diagnosis has been determined. Anticoagulation is required for cardiac embolic disease, documented large artery occlusive clot (e.g., ICA, MCA, or basilar artery), arterial dissection, and venous thrombosis. Heparin or enoxaparin is used with the appropriate monitoring. The major concern and risk here is hemorrhagic transformation in the evolution of a large infarct (see below).

Several observational studies to date have suggested that anticoagulation therapy can be given safely in children with AIS and sinovenous thrombosis (59,65). Heparin-based anticoagulation is best monitored with anti-factor Xa activity with a therapeutic range of 0.3–0.7 anti-factor Xa activity (U/mL) for unfractionated heparin, and 0.5–1.0 U/mL for low–molecular weight heparin. For sinovenous thrombosis in adults, a small, controlled trial of intravenous unfractionated heparin showed reduction in mortality, and a larger controlled trial of subcutaneous low–molecular weight heparin showed a trend for benefit in terms of death and dependency. In children with sinovenous thrombosis, anticoagulation acutely and for 3–6 months thereafter in high-risk situations (e.g., relapse of the underlying disorder) is associated with a reduced risk of recurrent systemic or cerebral thrombosis (19). As children are probably less at risk of hemorrhage, a case may be made for anticoagulation in pediatric AIS, but cohort series so far show no advantage over aspirin. For AIS, the American College of Chest Physicians (ACCP) guidelines recommend anticoagulation with unfractionated or low–molecular weight heparin for 5–7 days or until cardioembolic stroke and dissection are excluded, and they offer a practical regimen (65). This is a reasonable approach, particularly if comprehensive emergency neuroimaging is not available. Providing no hemorrhage is seen on imaging, anticoagulation for 3–6 months should certainly be considered in children with confirmed extracranial arterial dissection associated with AIS or cerebral sinus venous thrombosis, as recommended in the ACCP guidelines. The use of anticoagulation in patients with cardiac disease is more controversial and may be influenced by the cardiac pathology and by neurologic and imaging findings, as embolism is often difficult to prove (4). Individual patient management should involve senior clinicians in cardiology and neurology. A case may also be made for anticoagulating patients with known prothrombotic abnormalities, as recurrence risk is higher in this group. However, no evidence suggests that the risk is reduced with anticoagulation compared with aspirin, which may be because pediatric studies involve cohorts in which the physicians were allowed to choose treatment, and no randomized data are available.

Antiplatelet Agents. In two very large controlled trials in adults, aspirin appeared to be associated with a modest improvement in outcome, probably because of a reduction in early recurrence and perhaps via its antipyretic effect. In adults, the risk of hemorrhage appears to be lower than with anticoagulants. No strong evidence has emerged for a benefit of using aspirin in childhood stroke, but the available data suggest that a dose of up to 5 mg/kg/d is safe. In a study from the UK, a trend for reduction of recurrence was seen, compared with no prophylaxis (7), and French data suggest that recurrence in cryptogenic anterior circulation stroke, where the pathology is likely to be inflammatory, is rare now that aspirin is widely used (66,67). Members of the International Pediatric Stroke Study have agreed to use a dose of 3–5 mg/kg/d of aspirin as short- and long-term prophylaxis if they do not choose anticoagulation.

Given the frequency of cardioembolism and dissection as etiologic factors in childhood AIS and the high prevalence of prothrombotic conditions, the ACCP guidelines recommend either unfractionated heparin or low–molecular weight heparin and continuing anticoagulation until cardioembolic sources and extracranial dissection have been excluded (65). The American Heart Association (AHA) guidelines support either anticoagulation or antiplatelet agents (68). Both guidelines support the use of anticoagulation in cardioembolism and extracranial dissection for the acute and subacute period after childhood-onset AIS. In fact, a recent retrospective analysis of 298 adults with carotid dissection suggested that aspirin may be as effective as anticoagulation in preventing recurrence (69). In addition, compliance with anticoagulation does not appear to prevent AIS in children with cardiac disease (70). Therefore, in AIS, both anticoagulation and antiplatelet agents are reasonable options. Our current practice, after comprehensive emergency neuroimaging to diagnose any sinovenous thrombosis or arteriopathy, is to use anticoagulation to prevent propagation in sinovenous thrombosis or recurrent embolic stroke in the context of cardiac disease or arterial dissection, and aspirin for other cryptogenic strokes (e.g., transient cerebral arteriopathy).

Workup for Secondary Prevention

During the PICU admission the child will require a screen for arterial stenosis or obstruction using a variety of imaging techniques (Table 64.2). In addition, a cardiac evaluation should be undertaken.

MR angiography is very useful either to exclude alternative pathology or confirm arterial disease. A guide to differential diagnoses in children who present with an acute focal neurologic deficit is provided in Table 64.1; many are obvious on MRI (Fig. 64.2, Table 64.2). In addition, it is important that the vascular pathology is defined so that conditions that require urgent management, such as arterial dissection, are not missed. Despite the need for general anesthesia in most cases, MRI has advantages over CT, as in addition to the essential exclusion of hemorrhage, ischemia may be documented within minutes (using diffusion-weighted imaging) or hours (using T2-weighted imaging) rather than days. The addition of MRA of the circle of Willis and of the neck vessels (Fig. 64.3), fat-saturated T1-weighted MRI of the neck (Fig. 64.5), and magnetic resonance venography (MRV) (Fig. 64.6) allows definition of the vascular pathology, which often guides management (Table 64.2).

Sinovenous thrombosis may be accompanied by hemorrhagic or bland infarction—typically occipital, parietal, frontal, or thalamic (Figs. 64.1J,K and 64.2M–Q); although often missed on CT (Fig. 64.1K), the occluded sinus may be seen on MRI (Fig. 64.2M) or computed tomography venography (CTV)/MRV (Fig. 64.6). Importantly, most of the conditions that mimic ischemic stroke, such as ADEM, metabolic disease, and posterior leukoencephalopathy (Fig. 64.2R), may be

---

TABLE 64.2

EMERGENCY IMAGING FOR CHILDHOOD STROKE

Magnetic resonance imaging (MRI) (including diffusion and perfusion), arteriography (MRA), venography (MRV)
Exclude hemorrhage
Define extent and territory of infarct
MRA to define vascular anatomy of circle of Willis and neck vessels
T1-weighted spin echo of the neck with fat-saturation sequence to exclude dissection
MRV to exclude sinovenous thrombosis
Diffusion imaging to differentiate acute from chronic infarction
Perfusion imaging to demonstrate areas of tissue larger than demonstrated on diffusion imaging of abnormal cerebral blood flow, blood volume, and mean transit time
CT scan to exclude hemorrhage if MRI not available acutely
Conventional angiography if:
Hemorrhage without coagulopathy and cause is not obvious on MRA or MRV
Ischemic stroke, MRA normal, and fat-saturated T1-weighted MRI of the neck does not demonstrate dissection

recognized on MRI, which may mean that a child is not exposed to the unnecessary risks of antithrombotic therapy but receives the appropriate evidence-based management strategy for the condition. Metabolic stroke is relatively rare, and clinical clues are often present (e.g., persistent vomiting; on neuroimaging, the infarcts are usually not in a typical vascular distribution). The demyelination associated with ADEM is usually obvious on MRI.

Approximately 30%–80% of children with an infarct in an arterial territory have large-vessel disease, e.g., stenosis, occlusion, or dissection, demonstrable on MRA or MRI. Thrombosis in the large venous sinuses (sagittal, lateral, or straight) may be diagnosed on MR (**Fig. 64.6**) or CTV, which is essential in patients with thalamic or cortical infarcts (particularly parietal and occipital) (**Figs. 64.1J,K** and **64.2M–Q**). Although a 1% risk of stroke exists, patients with a normal MRA and MRV and no evidence of dissection on fat-saturated MRI of the neck should undergo conventional angiography, which is usually required for the diagnosis of small-vessel vasculitis, cortical venous thrombosis, and, sometimes, for the diagnosis of dissection (**Fig. 64.4B**), particularly in the posterior circulation (52,53,60).

Prevention of Neurological Deterioration

Typically, stroke symptoms are maximal at presentation and the child shows gradual improvement over days to weeks. However, the intensivist will need to be vigilant with supervision of critical illness factors that impact on patient recovery. Each day of admission, a series of questions should be reviewed:

- Is the patient stable or improving?
- What are we doing to promote recovery?
- Is the patient dehydrated, and what should we be doing to avoid this?
- Is the patient receiving nutrition?
- In those who are hypertensive, is the blood pressure coming down?
- What is the mechanism of stroke, and is there anything else that we should be doing?
- Is temperature controlled? In adult stroke care there is a literature on the use of acetaminophen and cooling blankets (target temperature management) to maintain normothermia. We have no such studies in children, so our aim is to avoid fever and under rare circumstances use induced hypothermia, albeit rather idiosyncratically.

Having reviewed these questions, we also need to review general aspects of care that would prevent complications from developing. For example:

a. *Risk of deep vein thrombosis (DVT) prophylaxis.* This risk should be reviewed daily since the development of DVT will require anticoagulation, which may place the AIS patient at considerable danger for intracranial hemorrhage. In our unit we use a sequential compression device rather than subcutaneous heparin for prophylaxis.

b. *Gastrointestinal ulcer prophylaxis.* Patients with central nervous system (CNS) events are at increased risk of ulcers, and, again, the detrimental consequences of this complication should be avoided. In our unit we use a combination of histamine-H_2-receptor antagonists and proton-pump inhibitors for these patients.

c. *Aspiration precautions.* Pneumonia and fever are to be avoided since these factors impact on stroke outcome. Therefore, no oral feeding until a swallowing assessment has been carried out to confirm good function.

d. *Indwelling urinary (Foley) catheter.* The catheter should be removed as soon as possible, so as to prevent infection.

e. *Heparin therapy.* In those receiving heparin, this treatment will need to be monitored as well as the potential development of heparin-induced thrombocytopenia.

Neurological Deterioration in AIS

Deterioration in AIS can result from a number of mechanisms: recurrent stroke, enlargement of the stroke, or hemorrhagic transformation of the ischemic region; development of cerebral edema or midline shift with mass effect; a drop in perfusion pressure or fall in cardiac output; metabolic disturbance with change in hemoglobin and oxygenation, glucose control, or hyponatremia; seizures; or infection, inflammation, and fever.

The approach in managing deterioration is to both identify the cause and correct any abnormality. This process usually involves imaging and routine laboratory studies, and **Figure 64.12** provides a framework for practice. In cases with 'mass effect,' we do not give steroids. A bolus dose of mannitol to increase serum osmolarity by 10% ($\leq$320 mOsm/L) is used for acute control, followed by review for neurosurgery (see below).

Surgical Decompression in Acute Stroke

There are two instances where surgical decompression may be used: large MCA infarct and cerebellar/posterior fossa infarct. We have more information available for MCA infarction. For example, in adults, ~10% of MCA strokes have a malignant course, causing life-threatening cerebral edema (71). Clinical trials of decompressive craniectomy for adults with malignant ischemic stroke have shown increased survival and improved functional outcome when surgery is performed within 48 hours of stroke onset (72–75). The indications for surgery include an infarct volume of 145 mL on MRI; >50% MCA territory hypodensity within 5 hours from onset of stroke; complete MCA territory hypodensity within 48 hours from onset of stroke; midline shift >7.5 mm irrespective of symptoms or >4 mm in those with lethargy. There are no equivalent controlled trials in pediatric stroke, and the best available evidence comes from a recent review of 29 cases in the literature (76). The published reports suggest that a good outcome is possible even in the presence of signs of herniation, low preoperative GCS score, involvement of multiple vascular territories, or longer time to surgery. Importantly, one report indicates that the use of intracranial pressure (ICP) monitoring to guide the need for surgical intervention merely delays the timing of surgery rather than indicates when it should be used and, in consequence, can lead to significant morbidity (77,78).

Intracranial Hemorrhage and Hemorrhagic Stroke

Patients with intracranial hemorrhage or hemorrhagic stroke require immediate transfer to a PICU with on-site neurosurgery in the event that craniectomy is needed. A coordinated, multidisciplinary approach to investigation of the differential diagnosis is also required (65,79). Structural arterial disorders, specifically AVMs, aneurysms and cavernomas, sinovenous thrombosis, developmental venous anomalies, and coagulopathies such as hemophilia, are the most common pathologies. In the acute phase, the main priorities are to prevent cerebral herniation if the blood collection is space-occupying, reverse any coagulopathy, exclude sinovenous thrombosis, and to treat any associated vasospasm with volume expansion.

Underlying coagulopathy is particularly common in children <1 year of age. Hemorrhagic disease of the newborn should be treated with vitamin K, and disseminated intravascular coagulation should be treated with fresh Octaplas or Beriplex™ (a prothrombin complex containing a concentrate of factors II, VII, IX, and X). Fresh platelet transfusion is required if the hemorrhage has occurred in the context of thrombocytopenia or thrombocytopathy, and recombinant factor VIII is the treatment for hemophilia.

Emergency vascular imaging should include an MRV as well as an MRA, as 10% of hemorrhages in young adults are secondary to sinovenous thrombosis. The ability to undertake urgent and appropriate imaging is a prerequisite of critical care, because the conditions that underlie hemorrhagic stroke have a high mortality rate and may be treatable (e.g., the use of anticoagulation for sinovenous thrombosis) (13). Although such management of sinovenous thrombosis with hemorrhage in childhood is controversial, there are now two adult clinical trials where outcome overall was better in the treated group and new hemorrhage was not documented. Heparin should certainly be considered in the presence of deterioration in clinical status, e.g., intractable seizures, coma, or CTV/MRV evidence of propagation of thrombus (65,68).

If an underlying AVM is present, the recurrence risk for hemorrhage is 2%–3% per year for life if untreated, and a carefully considered decision regarding management (neurosurgery, neuroradiology with coils, or stereotactic radiotherapy) must be made once the patient has recovered from the acute phase. Although less common, aneurysms are associated with a significant rebleeding risk, particularly soon after presentation (21). A vascular team with considerable experience should evaluate these children so that an individualized management strategy, targeted at preventing recurrence, can be implemented (42,68).

Neurologic Deterioration and Surgical Clot Removal in Acute Hemorrhage

The principles of medical care for patients with intracranial hemorrhage or hemorrhagic stroke are similar to those described for AIS (see above). However, additional risks include hydrocephalus (with resultant impaired cerebral perfusion) and hematoma enlargement with deterioration due to tentorial herniation. Some of these patients will require ventricular drain insertion. Treatment of the unconscious patient, where no clinical examination is possible, may be aided by information from ICP and CPP monitoring. In patients with evolving hydrocephalus, head-of-bed elevation to 30 degrees is the usual positioning for cerebrospinal fluid drainage, but this positioning may compromise cerebral perfusion to ischemic regions. This issue of head-of-bed elevation causing worsened ischemia for children who may have suffered a stroke is under investigation and there is little data for recommendation. Head-of-bed elevation to 30 degrees is routine to prevent ventilator-associated pneumonia in intubated patients and to promote venous drainage in cases of suspected increased ICP. Since elevating the patient's head may reduce perfusion to an area at risk of cerebral ischemia, this practice may require individualization. Consideration should be given to the effects of bed position on hemodynamics, oxygenation, and neurologic status. If neurologic findings worsen with elevation of the head, the patient should remain flat. In patients whose neurologic status is unable to be monitored (e.g., coma, sedation, etc.), the effect of head elevation on transcranial Doppler flow studies is used in some institutions. The approach to head-of-bed elevation in pediatric stroke victims is under investigation and further guidance should be available in the near future (80).

The option of surgical clot removal should be reviewed by a neurosurgeon. In cases of cerebellar or posterior fossa hemorrhage, the indications for surgery include a displaced fourth ventricle, early obstructive hydrocephalus, compression of the brain stem, and decreased level of consciousness. In cases of supratentorial hemorrhage, the indications for surgery

include location close to the brain surface, hematoma volume >20 mL, and decreased level of consciousness.

Neuroprotection—Controversies

There are no neuroprotective therapies that are of proven benefit in pediatric stroke. Much of what we do uses evidence borrowed from adult stroke care. That said, there are some aspects of treatment that are controversial or, at best, variable between centers.

Intravenous Fluids. What type of fluids should we use and what volumes are required if we are trying to avoid edema formation? Neonates, infants, and smaller children are at risk of hypoglycemia if isotonic, glucose-free, maintenance fluids are used prior to the successful initiation of enteral nutrition. This group of children should receive isotonic normal saline with extra glucose added to achieve a final concentration of either 5% or 10%. For older children, glucose-free isotonic maintenance fluids using normal saline will normally suffice until enteral feeding is established.

Some centers chose to restrict fluids to 70% of calculated total requirements in anticipation of the patient developing a syndrome of inappropriate antidiuretic hormone secretion. Isotonic maintenance fluids greatly reduce the risk of hyponatremia. The risk of fluid restriction is to cause an inadequately filled circulation that may exacerbate ischemia by impaired perfusion.

Glycemic Control. Hyperglycemia is frequent in adults with stroke, and may be related to the prevalence of the prediabetic condition in this population. Hyperglycemia is also associated with worsened stroke outcomes. Glycemic control with insulin may well control serum glucose level (target blood glucose <150 mg/dL), but a potential danger is the development of low level of interstitial glucose in the brain, which may be injurious.

6 Intracranial Hypertension Management. ICP monitoring is used to guide CPP-directed therapy, particularly in traumatic brain injury. It is not clear whether such therapy is generally applicable to acute stroke care. In fact, if children require such therapy, it may be that they would have been better served by undergoing decompressive craniectomy (see above).

Thrombolysis with Tissue Plasminogen Activator

In adults with ischemic stroke, the main focus of recent studies has been in looking at the possibility of minimizing the effect of the initial stroke by promoting recanalization of the occluded artery using thrombolysis. No randomized evidence supports the use of rTPA in the acute treatment of stroke in children. Although some children with anterior circulation stroke present to a physician within 4.5 hours, the rarity of childhood stroke combined with the low sensitivity of CT for acute infarction and the wide differential in this age group result in a very low diagnostic rate in the time window described in adult thrombolytic trials. Due to the lower mortality in this age group, the lack of clinical trial data makes recommendations for the acute use of thrombolysis difficult to justify in risk–benefit terms.

After detailed counseling and consultation with the family, very occasionally, thrombolysis with intravenous rTPA within 4.5 hours or intra-arterial rTPA within 6 hours may be considered for anterior circulation stroke, or intra-arterial rTPA and/or mechanical embolectomy within 12 hours may be considered for basilar artery occlusion. Circumstances in which this practice may be justifiable include children known to be at risk and are in the hospital. Acute thrombolysis has also been used in children with propagation of venous sinus thrombosis when symptoms persist or deteriorate. In fact, despite the lack of evidence for efficacy and difficulties in recruiting to the Thrombolysis In Pediatric Stroke trial (81,82), use of rTPA in children with AIS is increasing (0.9% in 2001–2005, 2% in 2006–2010) and is associated with low rates of hemorrhage (83).

rTPA-Related Angioedema. When rTPA is used during acute stroke, there is risk of oropharyngeal angioedema. Therefore, all patients undergoing this stroke protocol should be observed and monitored in the PICU. If it is suspected, endotracheal intubation is needed—do not wait for the development of respiratory distress with airway edema. Medical treatments include epinephrine, diphenhydramine, methylprednisolone, and famotidine. This complication should resolve within 24 hours.

rTPA-Related Hemorrhage. Intracranial hemorrhage is a risk of rTPA. If this complication is suspected, then stop the infusion and arrange for CT scan. Therapies attempted include aminocaproic acid, vitamin K, cryoprecipitate, fresh frozen plasma (FFP), and platelet transfusion. One goal is to increase the fibrinogen level >100 mg/dL with immediate infusion of cryoprecipitate. Alternatively, FFP can be used if cryoprecipitate is not available since 1 Unit of cryoprecipitate is made from one bag of FFP. The reported outcome from rTPA-related hemorrhage is poor in adult patients and it is not clear that treatment of this complication improves outcome as the number of reports is small, levels of fibrinogen are often >100 mg/dL, and the half-life of rTPA is short (84,85).

DISEASE-SPECIFIC THERAPIES

Stroke Due to SCD

Children with SCD and high transcranial Doppler velocities (>200 cm/s) have a 40% stroke risk over the next 3 years. Primary prevention of stroke is possible if these children are screened appropriately and transfused indefinitely (86,87). However, therapy for acute stroke and secondary prevention has evolved through hematologic clinical experience rather than being subject to rigorous evaluation by randomized controlled trial (25). Hemoglobin and sickle hemoglobin percentages should be measured at presentation with any neurologic complication, and packed red blood cells (20 mL/kg) should be cross-matched as quickly as possible. The accepted goal is to begin transfusion within 2–4 hours of presentation, particularly if the deficit is persisting or progressing, although no randomized controlled data exist. If available, exchange (using a manual regime or an automated cell separator for erythrocytapheresis) transfusion is recommended rather than simple transfusion. In a retrospective analysis of this population, a fivefold increase in risk of recurrent stroke was observed in children who received initial and then chronic simple transfusion as opposed to exchange transfusion at the time of initial stroke (88), suggesting that exchange transfusion should be used for emergency management. Over the first 48 hours, the goal is to reduce the hemoglobin S percentage to <20% and raise the hemoglobin to 10–11 g/dL, with a hematocrit of >30%. Blood should be leukocyte-depleted and ABO, Rhesus D and K, Fy, Jk, and MNS red cell phenotype compatible with the recipient to minimize the risk of alloimmunization.

Patients with stroke in the context of SCD may have pathology that includes MCA territory and watershed infarction secondary to arterial stenosis, hemorrhage, sinovenous thrombosis, RPLS, acute necrotizing encephalitis, and arterial dissection. Emergency MRI, MRA, and MRV may guide management (**Table 64.2, Figs. 64.2, 64.3, 64.5, and 64.6**) (34). Controversy continues regarding the acute and long-term management of these alternative neurologic diagnoses, and the local hematologist and pediatric neurologist should be involved in decisions. Nevertheless, in the absence of clear contraindications, patients with SCD should be managed according to standard protocols for the pathology with which they present.

The most recent edition of the AHA management guidelines for stroke in SCD recommends the following acute management: optimal hydration, correction of hypoxemia and hypotension, exchange transfusion, and normoglycemia (68).

FUTURE DIRECTIONS

To date, it has not been possible to conduct a successful multicenter, randomized controlled trial of therapy in acute stroke in children. The recent rTPA trial funded by the US National Institutes of Health was stopped because of failure to recruit patients. However, multicenter and multinational epidemiological studies have been possible and it may be that prospective *comparative effectiveness research* is the more appropriate model for future investigations into effective critical care therapies. Areas of research priorities and challenges have been outlined in two recent reports, and neuromonitoring and critical care feature highly in the agenda (29, 68).

ACKNOWLEDGMENTS

This work has benefited from R&D funding received from the NHS executive. FJK was supported by the Wellcome Trust (0353521 B/92/2), Action Medical Research, the Stroke Association (PROG4), the National Institute of Health (USA), and the National Institute of Health Research (UK).

References

1. Mallick AA, Ganesan V, Kirkham FJ, et al. Childhood arterial ischaemic stroke incidence, presenting features, and risk factors: A prospective population-based study. *Lancet Neurol* 2014;13:35–43.
2. Mallick AA, Ganesan V, O'Callaghan FJ. Mortality from childhood stroke in England and Wales, 1921-2000. *Arch Dis Child* 2010;95:12–9.
3. Fox CK, Johnston SC, Sidney S, et al. High critical care usage due to pediatric stroke: Results of a population-based study. *Neurology* 2012;79:420–7.
4. Ganesan V, Prengler M, McShane MA, et al. Investigation of risk factors in children with arterial ischemic stroke. *Ann Neurol* 2003;53:167–73.
5. Fox CK, Glass HC, Sidney S, et al. Acute seizures predict epilepsy after childhood stroke. *Ann Neurol* 2013;74:249–56.
6. DeBaun MR, Gordon M, McKinstry RC, et al. Controlled trial of transfusions for silent cerebral infarcts in sickle cell anemia. *N Engl J Med* 2014;371:699–710.
7. Ganesan V, Prengler M, Wade A, et al. Clinical and radiological recurrence after childhood arterial ischemic stroke. *Circulation* 2006;114:2170–7.
8. Jordan LC, van Beek JG, Gottesman RF, et al. Ischemic stroke in children with critical illness: A poor prognostic sign. *Pediatr Neurol* 2007;36:244–6.
9. Lo W, Zamel K, Ponnappa K, et al. The cost of pediatric stroke care and rehabilitation. *Stroke* 2008;39:161–5.
10. Plumb P, Seiber E, Dowling MM, et al. Out-of-pocket costs for childhood stroke: The impact of chronic illness on parents' pocketbooks. *Pediatr Neurol* 2015;52:73–6.
11. Ganesan V, Hogan A, Shack N, et al. Outcome after ischaemic stroke in childhood. *Dev Med Child Neurol* 2000;42:455–61.
12. Lo WD, Hajek C, Pappa C, et al. Outcomes in children with hemorrhagic stroke. *JAMA Neurol* 2013;70:66–71.

13. Sebire G, Tabarki B, Saunders DE, et al. Cerebral venous sinus thrombosis in children: Risk factors, presentation, diagnosis and outcome. *Brain* 2005;128:477–89.

14. deVeber GA, MacGregor D, Curtis R, et al. Neurologic outcome in survivors of childhood arterial ischemic stroke and sinovenous thrombosis. *J Child Neurol* 2000;15:316–24.

15. Chung B, Wong V. Pediatric stroke among Hong Kong Chinese subjects. *Pediatrics* 2004;114:e206–e212.

16. Lanthier S, Carmant L, David M, et al. Stroke in children: The coexistence of multiple risk factors predicts poor outcome. *Neurology* 2000;54:371–8.

17. Westmacott R, Askalan R, MacGregor D, et al. Cognitive outcome following unilateral arterial ischaemic stroke in childhood: Effects of age at stroke and lesion location. *Dev Med Child Neurol* 2010;52:386–93.

18. Fullerton HJ, Wu YW, Sidney S, et al. Risk of recurrent childhood arterial ischemic stroke in a population-based cohort: The importance of cerebrovascular imaging. *Pediatrics* 2007;119:495–501.

19. Kenet G, Kirkham F, Niederstadt T, et al. Risk factors for recurrent venous thromboembolism in the European collaborative paediatric database on cerebral venous thrombosis: A multicentre cohort study. *Lancet Neurol* 2007;6:595–603.

20. Fullerton HJ, Achrol AS, Johnston SC, et al. Long-term hemorrhage risk in children versus adults with brain arteriovenous malformations. *Stroke* 2005;36:2099–104.

21. Jordan LC, Johnston SC, Wu YW, et al. The importance of cerebral aneurysms in childhood hemorrhagic stroke: A population-based study. *Stroke* 2009;40:400–5.

22. Jordan LC, Hillis AE. Hemorrhagic stroke in children. *Pediatr Neurol* 2007;36:73–80.

23. Fox CK, Sidney S, Fullerton HJ. Community-based case-control study of childhood stroke risk associated with congenital heart disease. *Stroke* 2015;46:336–40.

24. Dowling MM, Hynan LS, Lo W, et al. International Paediatric Stroke Study: Stroke associated with cardiac disorders. *Int J Stroke* 2013;8(suppl A100):39–44.

25. Kirkham FJ, DeBaun MR. Stroke in children with sickle cell disease. *Curr Treat Options Neurol* 2004;6:357–75.

26. Singhal NS, Hills NK, Sidney S, et al. Role of trauma and infection in childhood hemorrhagic stroke due to vascular lesions. *Neurology* 2013;81:581–584.

27. Kenet G, Lutkhoff LK, Albisetti M, et al. Impact of thrombophilia on risk of arterial ischemic stroke or cerebral sinovenous thrombosis in neonates and children: A systematic review and meta-analysis of observational studies. *Circulation* 2010;121:1838–47.

28. Ichord RN, Benedict SL, Chan AK, et al. Paediatric cerebral sinovenous thrombosis: Findings of the International Paediatric Stroke Study. *Arch Dis Child* 2015;100:174–9.

29. Sinclair AJ, Fox CK, Ichord RN, et al. Stroke in children with cardiac disease: Report from the International Pediatric Stroke Study Group Symposium. *Pediatr Neurol* 2015;52:5–15.

30. Benedik MP, Zaletel M, Meglic NP, et al. A right-to-left shunt in children with arterial ischaemic stroke. *Arch Dis Child* 2011;96:461–7.

31. Dowling MM, Ikemba CM. Intracardiac shunting and stroke in children: A systematic review. *J Child Neurol* 2011;26:72–82.

32. Ohene-Frempong K, Weiner SJ, Sleeper LA, et al. Cerebrovascular accidents in sickle cell disease: Rates and risk factors. *Blood* 1998;91:288–94.

33. Strouse JJ, Hulbert ML, DeBaun MR, et al. Primary hemorrhagic stroke in children with sickle cell disease is associated with recent transfusion and use of corticosteroids. *Pediatrics* 2006;118:1916–24.

34. Kirkham FJ. Therapy insight: Stroke risk and its management in patients with sickle cell disease. *Nat Clin Pract Neurol* 2007;3:264–78.

35. Dowling MM, Quinn CT, Rogers ZR, et al. Stroke in sickle cell anemia: Alternative etiologies. *Pediatr Neurol* 2009;41:124–6.

36. Dowling MM, Quinn CT, Plumb P, et al. Acute silent cerebral ischemia and infarction during acute anemia in children with and without sickle cell disease. *Blood* 2012;120:3891–7.

37. Quinn CT, McKinstry RC, Dowling MM, et al. Acute silent cerebral ischemic events in children with sickle cell anemia. *JAMA Neurol* 2013;70:58–65.

38. Kirkham FJ. Sickle cell disease. In: Rosenberg RR, Pascual J, eds. *Rosenberg's Molecular and Genetic Basis of Neurological and Psychiatric Disease*. 5th ed. London, UK: Academic Press, 2014:1237–52.

39. DeBaun MR, Armstrong FD, McKinstry RC, et al. Silent cerebral infarcts: A review on a prevalent and progressive cause of neurologic injury in sickle cell anemia. *Blood* 2012;119:4587–96.

40. Braun KP, Bulder MM, Chabrier S, et al. The course and outcome of unilateral intracranial arteriopathy in 79 children with ischaemic stroke. *Brain* 2009;132:544–57.

41. Hills NK, Johnston SC, Sidney S, et al. Recent trauma and acute infection as risk factors for childhood arterial ischemic stroke. *Ann Neurol* 2012;72:850–8.

42. Ganesan V, Kirkham F. *Stroke and Cerebrovascular Disease in Childhood*. 1st ed. London, UK: Mac Keith Press/International Child Neurology Series, 2011.

43. Azab SF, Abdelsalam SM, Saleh SH, et al. Iron deficiency anemia as a risk factor for cerebrovascular events in early childhood: A case-control study. *Ann Hematol* 2014;93:571–6.

44. Sharma M, Kupferman JC, Brosgol Y, et al. The effects of hypertension on the paediatric brain: A justifiable concern. *Lancet Neurol* 2010;9:933–40.

45. Kirkham FJ. Coagulopathies. In: Rosenberg RR, Pascual J, eds. *Rosenberg's Molecular and Genetic Basis of Neurological and Psychiatric Disease*. London, UK: Academic Press, 2014:1223–36.

46. Wintermark M, Hills NK, deVeber GA, et al. Arteriopathy diagnosis in childhood arterial ischemic stroke: Results of the vascular effects of infection in pediatric stroke study. *Stroke* 2014;45:3597–605.

47. Braun KP, Rafay MF, Uiterwaal CS, et al. Mode of onset predicts etiological diagnosis of arterial ischemic stroke in children. *Stroke* 2007;38:298–302.

48. Fullerton HJ, Johnston SC, Smith WS. Arterial dissection and stroke in children. *Neurology* 2001;57:1155–60.

49. Rafay MF, Armstrong D, deVeber G, et al. Craniocervical arterial dissection in children: Clinical and radiographic presentation and outcome. *J Child Neurol* 2006;21:8–16.

50. Sedney CL, Rosen CL. Cervical abnormalities causing vertebral artery dissection in children. *J Neurosurg Pediatr* 2011;7:272–5.

51. Dlamini N, Freeman JL, Mackay MT, et al. Intracranial dissection mimicking transient cerebral arteriopathy in childhood arterial ischemic stroke. *J Child Neurol* 2011;26:1203–6.

52. Ganesan V, Chong WK, Cox TC, et al. Posterior circulation stroke in childhood: Risk factors and recurrence. *Neurology* 2002;59:1552–6.

53. Tan MA, deVeber G, Kirton A, et al. Low detection rate of craniocervical arterial dissection in children using time-of-flight magnetic resonance angiography: Causes and strategies to improve diagnosis. *J Child Neurol* 2009;24:1250–7.

54. Rafay MF, Armstrong D, Dirks P, et al. Patterns of cerebral ischemia in children with moyamoya. *Pediatr Neurol* 2015;52:65–72.

55. Jagtap S, Srinivas G, Harsha KJ, et al. Sturge-Weber syndrome: Clinical spectrum, disease course, and outcome of 30 patients. *J Child Neurol* 2013;28:725–31.

56. Zolkipli Z, Aylett S, Rankin PM, et al. Transient exacerbation of hemiplegia following minor head trauma in Sturge-Weber syndrome. *Dev Med Child Neurol* 2007;49:697–9.

57. Chow ML, Cooke DL, Fullerton HJ, et al. Radiological and clinical features of vein of Galen malformations [published online ahead of print April 30, 2014]. *J Neurointerv Surg.* doi:10.1136/neurintsurg-2013-011005

58. Fullerton HJ, Aminoff AR, Ferriero DM, et al. Neurodevelopmental outcome after endovascular treatment of vein of Galen malformations. *Neurology* 2003;61:1386–90.

59. deVeber G, Andrew M, Adams C, et al. Cerebral sinovenous thrombosis in children. *N Engl J Med* 2001;345:417–23.

60. Mackay MT, Prabhu SP, Coleman L. Childhood posterior circulation arterial ischemic stroke. *Stroke* 2010;41:2201–9.

61. Chen TH, Lin WC, Tseng YH, et al. Posterior reversible encephalopathy syndrome in children: Case series and systematic review. *J Child Neurol* 2013;28:1378–86.

62. Geevasinga N, Cole C, Herkes GK, et al. Sickle cell disease and posterior reversible leukoencephalopathy. *J Clin Neurosci* 2014;21:1329–32.

63. Cordelli DM, Masetti R, Ricci E, et al. Life-threatening complications of posterior reversible encephalopathy syndrome in children. *Eur J Paediatr Neurol* 2014;18:632–40.

64. Braun KP, Kappelle LJ, Kirkham FJ, et al. Diagnostic pitfalls in paediatric ischaemic stroke. *Dev Med Child Neurol* 2006;48:985–90.

65. Monagle P, Chan AK, Goldenberg NA, et al. Antithrombotic therapy in neonates and children: Antithrombotic Therapy and Prevention of Thrombosis, 9th ed: American College of Chest Physicians Evidence-Based Clinical Practice Guidelines. *Chest* 2012;141(2, suppl):e737S–e801S.

66. Darteyre S, Chabrier S, Presles E, et al. Lack of progressive arteriopathy and stroke recurrence among children with cryptogenic stroke. *Neurology* 2012;79:2342–8.

67. Toure A, Chabrier S, Plagne MD, et al. Neurological outcome and risk of recurrence depending on the anterior vs. posterior arterial distribution in children with stroke. *Neuropediatrics* 2009;40:126–8.

68. Roach ES, Golomb MR, Adams R, et al. Management of stroke in infants and children: A scientific statement from a Special Writing Group of the American Heart Association Stroke Council and the Council on Cardiovascular Disease in the Young. *Stroke* 2008;39:2644–91.

69. Georgiadis D, Arnold M, von Buedingen HC, et al. Aspirin vs anticoagulation in carotid artery dissection: a study of 298 patients. *Neurology* 2009;72:1810–5.

70. Hoffman JL, Mack GK, Minich LL, et al. Failure to impact prevalence of arterial ischemic stroke in pediatric cardiac patients over three decades. *Congenit Heart Dis* 2011;6:211–8.

71. Moulin DE, Lo R, Chiang J, et al. Prognosis in middle cerebral artery occlusion. *Stroke* 1985;16:282–4.

72. Hofmeijer J, Kappelle LJ, Algra A, et al. Surgical decompression for space-occupying cerebral infarction (the Hemicraniectomy After Middle cerebral artery infarction with Life-treating Edema Trial [HAMLET]): A multicentre, open, randomised trial. *Lancet Neurol* 2009;8:326–33.

73. Juttler E, Schwab S, Schmiedek P, et al. Decompressive surgery for the treatment of malignant infarction of the middle cerebral artery (DESTINY): A randomized, controlled trial. *Stroke* 2007;38:2518–25.

74. Vahedi K, Vicaut E, Mateo J, et al. Sequential-design, multicenter, randomized, controlled trial of early decompressive craniectomy in malignant middle cerebral artery infarction (DECIMAL trial). *Stroke* 2007;38:2506–17.

75. Vahedi K, Hofmeijer J, Juettler E, et al. Early decompressive surgery in malignant infarction of the middle cerebral artery: A pooled analysis of three randomised controlled trials. *Lancet Neurol* 2007;6:215–22.

76. Shah S, Murthy SB, Whitehead WE, et al. Decompressive hemicraniectomy in pediatric patients with malignant middle cerebral artery infarction: Case series and review of the literature. *World Neurosurg* 2013;80:126–33.

77. Smith SE, Kirkham FJ, Deveber G, et al. Outcome following decompressive craniectomy for malignant middle cerebral artery infarction in children. *Dev Med Child Neurol* 2011;53:29–33.

78. Tasker RC. Paediatric neurointensive care and decompressive craniectomy for malignant middle cerebral artery infarction. *Dev Med Child Neurol* 2011;53:5–6.

79. Mackay MT, Chua ZK, Lee M, et al. Stroke and nonstroke brain attacks in children. *Neurology* 2014;82:1434–40.

80. Olavarria VV, Arima H, Anderson CS, et al. Head position and cerebral blood flow velocity in acute ischemic stroke: A systematic review and meta-analysis. *Cerebrovasc Dis* 2014;37:401–8.

81. Amlie-Lefond C, Chan AK, Kirton A, et al. Thrombolysis in acute childhood stroke: Design and challenges of the thrombolysis in pediatric stroke clinical trial. *Neuroepidemiology* 2009;32:279–86.

82. Rivkin MJ, deVeber G, Ichord RN, et al. Thrombolysis in pediatric stroke study. *Stroke* 2915;46:880–5.

83. Nasr DM, Biller J, Rabinstein AA. Use and in-hospital outcomes of recombinant tissue plasminogen activator in pediatric arterial ischemic stroke patients. *Pediatr Neurol* 2014;51:624–31.

84. Goldstein JN, Marrero M, Masrur S, et al. Management of thrombolysis-associated symptomatic intracerebral hemorrhage. *Arch Neurol* 2010;67:965–9.

85. Alderazi YJ, Barot NV, Peng H, et al. Clotting factors to treat thrombolysis-related symptomatic intracranial hemorrhage in acute ischemic stroke. *J Stroke Cerebrovasc Dis* 2014;23:e207–e214.

86. Adams RJ, McKie VC, Brambilla D, et al. Stroke prevention trial in sickle cell anemia. *Control Clin Trials* 1998;19:110–29.

87. Adams RJ, Brambilla D. Discontinuing prophylactic transfusions used to prevent stroke in sickle cell disease. *N Engl J Med* 2005;353:2769–78.

88. Hulbert ML, Scothorn DJ, Panepinto JA, et al. Exchange blood transfusion compared with simple transfusion for first overt stroke is associated with a lower risk of subsequent stroke: A retrospective cohort study of 137 children with sickle cell anemia. *J Pediatr* 2006;149:710–2.

CHAPTER 65 ■ HYPOXIC–ISCHEMIC ENCEPHALOPATHY

ERICKA L. FINK, MIOARA D. MANOLE, AND ROBERT S. B. CLARK

KEY POINTS

1 Hypoxic–ischemic encephalopathy (HIE) can be a consequence of multiple and diverse etiologies; the most common encountered in the PICU include cardiac arrest, severe shock, and stroke.

2 Poor outcomes, defined as death or severe neurologic disability, after cardiac arrest are disappointingly high. Children surviving with HIE have a wide spectrum of disability.

3 Characteristic cerebral blood flow (CBF) patterns occur after cardiac arrest and reperfusion. These include the "no-reflow," "hyperemic," "delayed hypoperfusion," and "recovery" phases. CBF data in animal models suggest that the depth and duration of "delayed hypoperfusion" correlates with the duration of ischemia.

4 Brain regions that are selectively vulnerable to HIE include the CA1 region of the hippocampus, cortical layers 3 and 5, basal ganglia, and cerebellar Purkinje cells.

5 High-quality cardiopulmonary (and cerebral) resuscitation and postresuscitation care are essential. Postresuscitation care should focus on the prevention of secondary brain insults (normoxia, normothermia, normocarbia, normotension).

6 There are no targeted therapies to prevent HIE, but early after resuscitation a therapeutic window exists for the testing of promising interventions such as hypothermia and other physiologic-based experimentally proven therapies.

Clinical hypoxic–ischemic encephalopathy (HIE) is a complex spectrum of brain injury due to diverse etiologies causing hypoxemia, and the brain injury results from hypoxemia and/or ischemia with or without reperfusion. In newborns, infants, and children, the management and prognostication of HIE is complicated by variability in developmental stage at the time of insult, regional vulnerability, and etiology. Consequently, gaining consensus on guidelines and standards for care remain elusive. Taken together, these daunting hurdles deserve special scientific attention, because HIE is a major cause of morbidity and mortality in pediatric patients, and carries a heavy burden for the patient and caregivers not only in terms of disability and quality of life in survivors but also in high costs associated with lifelong healthcare assistance. To date, there is no efficacious treatment for HIE. However, there has been progress in mitigating HIE, as demonstrated with postresuscitative hypothermia use for adults after ventricular tachycardia/fibrillation (VT/VF)-induced cardiac arrest and for neonates after birth asphyxia, and the early application of thrombolytics in adults after embolic stroke. The challenges remain to develop and optimize neuroprotective strategies to further improve outcomes for children at risk of HIE.

CORE PATHOPHYSIOLOGY AND PATHOBIOLOGY

Prolonged hypoxemia and/or ischemia lead to brain injury by triggering multiple pathologic cascades that can lead to cell death and loss of neurologic function. Interwoven with the pathologic cascades are endogenous neuroprotective responses to minimize damage. These cellular responses—with similarities to other types of acute brain injury, such as traumatic brain injury, central nervous system (CNS) infections, stroke,

and status epilepticus—are covered in detail in Chapter 56. However, a few fundamental aspects of particular relevance to HIE warrant further comment here.

Global and Focal Hypoxic–Ischemic Encephalopathy

HIE can result from multiple etiologies which cause either global or focal disease. Global HIE can result from respiratory arrest, cardiac arrest, strangulation, poisoning, sagittal sinus thrombosis, or profound shock states. Cardiac arrest due to asphyxia is the most common cause of global HIE in infants and children, while cardiac arrest due to arrhythmias is the most common cause in adults. Focal HIE can result from embolic or thrombotic stroke, or intracerebral hemorrhage. There are commonalities and important differences between HIE resulting from global and focal insults.

As outlined in Chapter 56, the principal commonality is the interruption of oxygen and blood flow to cells in the brain. Whether it is global due to cardiac arrest or focal due to vascular interruption of local cerebral blood flow (CBF), all parenchymal cells (neurons, astrocytes, oligodendrocytes, or microglia) will not tolerate prolonged durations of ischemia. The degree of brain damage is directly and strongly correlated with the duration of no-flow, and, as such, the clinical outcome is strongly and inversely correlated with the duration of no-flow. Thus the common clinical goal is to restore CBF as rapidly as possible, whether this is by return of spontaneous circulation (ROSC), in the case of cardiac arrest, or revascularization, in the case of stroke.

Final common pathways after critical global or focal ischemia include excitotoxicity from membrane failure with increased release and decreased reuptake of excitatory amino acids such as glutamate and glycine, oxidative stress,

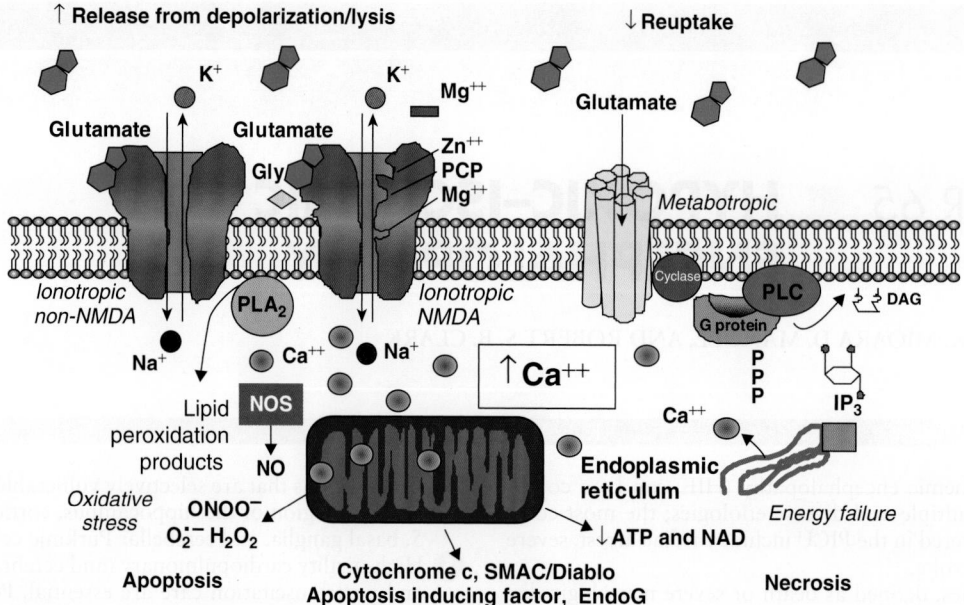

FIGURE 65.1. Cellular mechanisms resulting in cell death and hypoxic–ischemic encephalopathy. Prominent contributory mechanisms include excitotoxicity, disturbances in calcium homeostasis, oxidative stress, energy failure, and release of substances triggering cell death pathways. Gly, glycine; NMDA, N-methyl-D-aspartate; IP3, inositol 1,4,5-triphosphate; NO, nitric oxide; NOS, nitric oxide synthase; EndoG, endonuclease G; ATP, adenosine triphosphate. PCP, Phencyclidine; PLA, phospholipases A; PLC, Phospholipase C; DAG, diacyl-glycerol; SMA (second mitochondria-derived activator of caspases); C/Diablo, NAD, Nicotinamide adenine dinucleotide. From: Robert S. B. Clark.

mitochondrial dysfunction, energy failure, and initiation of cell death cascades (**Fig. 65.1**) (1). Neuronal and glial cell death can result from necrotic, apoptotic, and more recently described autophagic pathways (refer to Chapter 56). Each mechanism of cell death has a characteristic morphologic appearance and temporal pattern that can be observed at the microscopic and ultrastructural levels (2). Necrosis is a process characterized by immediate mitochondrial energy failure, leading to cellular swelling, loss of membrane integrity, and a prominent inflammatory response in surrounding tissues. Apoptosis is an energy-requiring process generally requiring new protein synthesis. Enzymatic degradation of cytoskeletal proteins results in cell soma and nuclear shrinkage, and nuclear deoxyribonucleic acid (DNA) is characteristically fragmented via endonucleases. In contrast to necrosis, apoptosis produces minimal inflammation. Autophagic stress can also result in cell death. Autophagy is an adaptive response to starvation, and results in autodigestion of cellular proteins and organelles to feed the cell. Triggering of autophagy after acute insults could potentially be beneficial or detrimental, likely depending on the degree and duration of injury. The role of autophagy after cerebral ischemia is only recently being investigated.

The obvious pathophysiologic difference between global and focal critical ischemia is whether systemic hypoxemia and ischemia occurred before, during, or after focal insults. Multiorgan system failure, particularly cardiovascular failure, can profoundly contribute to the pathologic evolution in the postresuscitative phase, making cardiovascular and systemic stabilization a priority after cardiac arrest. Induction of both pathologic and protective hypoxia-inducible cell-signaling pathways can occur prior to the insult in patients with cardiac arrest. These pathways can be triggered in all regions of the brain rather than in those downstream of vascular occlusion in cardiac arrest compared with stroke. Thus, cell-signaling pathways, both bad and good, represent global therapeutic targets after hypoxia–ischemia from cardiac arrest.

Cardiac Arrest

Epidemiology of Pediatric Cardiac Arrest

In one multicenter study, the incidence of out-of-hospital cardiac arrest per 100,000 person-years ranged from 73 for infants, 8 in children aged 1–11, 6 in those aged 12–19 years, to 127 in adults (3). In contrast, the incidence for in-hospital pediatric cardiac arrest was 1.06 per 1000 hospital admissions in a single-center study (4). Some pediatric centers have implemented special medical emergency teams that respond to pre-arrest and arrest events to address the frequency of in-hospital cardiac arrests and mortality (5).

Table 65.1 outlines several clinical studies examining cardiac arrest in children. In contrast to adults, where the majority of cardiac arrests are due to cardiac arrhythmia and intrinsic heart disease, the majority of cardiac arrests in children are due to asphyxia (6,7). This includes in-hospital and out-of-hospital arrests. Asphyxial cardiac arrest, accounting for ~80%–90% of pediatric cardiac arrests, begins with respiratory failure, followed by hypoxemia, hypercarbia and acidosis, hypotension, pulseless electrical activity (PEA), then, ultimately, asystole. The most common clinical entities associated with asphyxial cardiac arrest in an outpatient setting include sudden infant death syndrome, pneumonia, aspiration, and submersion injury (8) (Table 65.2). Notably, many of these events may be preventable. The most common etiologies in inpatients include respiratory failure and congenital heart disease complications (9). Cardiac arrhythmias account for ~10%–20% of pediatric cardiac arrest, with higher frequency occurring in inpatients. Reentrant arrhythmias, Wolff–Parkinson–White syndrome, long QT syndrome, congenital heart disease with postoperative arrhythmia, electrical injury, physical exertion, and trauma are the most frequent causes of arrhythmia in this cohort. Both adults and children who present with VT/VF as an initial rhythm have a higher incidence of good outcome compared with asphyxial arrest. For children with out-of-hospital cardiac arrest presenting

TABLE 65.1

REVIEW OF PEDIATRIC CARDIAC ARREST LITERATURE

AUTHORS (YEAR)	OH/IH	N	AGE[a]	MALE (%)	ROSC (%)	VT/VF (%)	SURVIVAL TO D/C (%)	GOOD OUTCOME (%)[b]	PREDICTORS OF GOOD OUTCOME	PREDICTORS OF POOR OUTCOME
Retrospective Studies										
de Mos et al. (2006)	IH	91	4 y		82	4	25	43	ECMO within 24 h	Renal failure; epinephrine gtt; calcium bolus during CPR
Engdahl et al. (2003)	OH	98	1 y	52		8	5	60		
Gerein et al. (2006)	OH	503	5.6 y	58	5	4	2			
Hickey et al. (1995)	OH	41	43 mo	68	56	22	27	73	ROSC in field; awake in ED	
Horisberger et al. (2002)	IH OH	89	6 mo		87 (IH) 57 (OH)		58	79		OH arrest; longer ROSC; trauma etiology
Kuisma et al. (1995)	OH	79	2.9 y	53	10	4		80	Witnessed arrest; near-drowning; bystander CPR; rapid ROSC	
Parra et al. (2000)	IH	32	3.5 mo		63		42	73	Mechanical support	
Pitetti et al. (2002)	OH	189	41 mo	64		4	2.6	0	Sinus rhythm in ED; fewer epinephrine doses	
Ronco et al. (1995)	OH	63	14 mo	65	39		9.5	17	Rapid ROSC	First ED rhythm non-VT/VF; ROSC > 20 min; >2 doses epinephrine
Schindler et al. (1996)	OH	80	1 y	50	63		7.5	0		
Slonim et al. (1997)	IH	205			24		13.7			Trauma etiology; longer ROSC; higher PRISM III
Suominen et al. (1997)	OH	50	1.2 y		26	8	16	12	CPR < 15 min	ROSC > 20 min
Prospective Studies										
Lopez-Herce et al. (2005)	OH	95	63 mo	64	47	9	28	82	ROSC > 20 min	ROSC > 20 min
Moler et al. (2009, 2011) and Meert et al. (2009)	IH/OH	353 / 138	0.9 y / 2.9 y	57 / 69	c	10 / 7	49 / 38	77 / 24	Both pupils reactive; postoperative CPR	More epinephrine doses; atropine, calcium, or sodium bicarbonate administered; preexisting diseases; electrolyte imbalance or drowning/asphyxia as etiology; low blood pH; duration of CPR
Nadkarni et al. (2006)	IH	880	5.6 y	54	63	14	27	65	Witnessed arrest; PEA or VF as first rhythm	No ROSC in field; >3 doses epinephrine; ROSC > 30 min; first rhythm asystole
Sirbaugh et al. (1999)	OH	300	9 mo	60	11	3	2	17		
Young et al. (2004)	OH	599		58	29	9	8.6	31		

[a]Mean or median age, depending on the study.
[b]Good outcome among survivors, defined as good outcome, mild disability, or unchanged from baseline at hospital discharge.
[c]ROSC was a study inclusion criteria.

OH, out-of-hospital; IH, in-hospital; ROSC, return of spontaneous circulation; VT/VF, ventricular tachycardia/fibrillation; D/C, discharge; ECMO, extracorporeal membrane oxygenation; CPR, cardiopulmonary resuscitation; ED, emergency department; PEA, pulseless electrical activity.

TABLE 65.2

COMMON ETIOLOGIES OF OUT-OF-HOSPITAL CARDIAC ARREST IN INFANTS AND CHILDREN, ADAPTED FROM YOUNG ET AL. (2004) (7)

■ ETIOLOGY	■ FREQUENCY (%)	■ SURVIVAL TO HOSPITAL DISCHARGE (%)
Sudden infant death syndrome	23	0
Trauma	20	5
Respiratory	16	21
Submersion	12	17
Cardiac	8	8
Central nervous system	6	3
Burn	1	0
Poisoning	1	17
Other	10	10
Unknown	3	6

with VT/VF, the survival to hospital discharge is significantly higher versus those presenting with asystole (30% vs. 5%, respectively) (10). This outcome, although less pronounced, appears similar for in-hospital cardiac arrest as children with VT/VF-associated cardiac arrest had the highest survival to hospital discharge (35%), followed by PEA/asystole (27%), and finally late onset VT/VF (11%) (11). Late onset VT/VF is considered a reperfusion arrhythmia (12). The incidence of asphyxial versus VT/VF cardiac arrest reverses with increasing age group. A recent study showed that 7.6% of children aged 1–7 years versus 27% aged 3–18 years presented with VT/VF (13).

Sudden cardiac arrest in children is rare (between 0.8 and 6.2 per 100,000 per year) but it is an important cause in the outpatient setting, especially in athletes (14). Hypertrophic cardiomyopathy accounts for approximately one-half of sudden cardiac deaths in children, and most occurred in previously well children (15). Other predisposing conditions include additional structural cardiac anomalies, electrical abnormalities in structurally normal hearts, and ingestion of medications or illicit substances. Most of these conditions are associated with ventricular tachyarrhythmias.

Outcome

Mortality after cardiac arrest in children is very high, and despite the potential for plasticity in the developing brain, neurologic outcomes can be dismal. These poor outcomes may be related to the prearrest hypoxemia and brain hypoperfusion prior to no-flow ischemia that is seen during asphyxial cardiac arrest (Fig. 65.2). Over half of the children who survive cardiac arrest develop some degree of HIE. A large meta-analysis showed that ROSC from all causes of cardiac arrest was achieved in 13% of pediatric patients. In this study, location of the cardiac arrest had a large impact on survival (24% for children with in-hospital cardiac arrest and 9% for out-of-hospital cardiac arrest) (7). Similarly, in a multicenter, prospective, observational study of children, the in- and out-of-hospital cardiac arrest survival was 49% and 38%, respectively (6). The leading cause of death was neurologic in 69% of the out-of-hospital arrest cohort and cardiovascular in the in-hospital arrest cohort (Table 65.1).

As mentioned earlier, deaths after successful ROSC are most often due to brain death, multi–organ system failure, or withdrawal of support (usually based on projected neurologic outcome). Patients that survive often develop HIE and can have single or multiple neurologic disabilities of varying severity that evolve after the insult. Common manifestations of HIE include cerebral palsy, mental retardation, dysphagia, cortical vision impairment or blindness, hearing impairment or deafness, microcephaly, temperature instability, chronic ventilator dependence, and seizures. Infants after hypoxic–ischemic injury may not demonstrate the clinical neurologic impairments

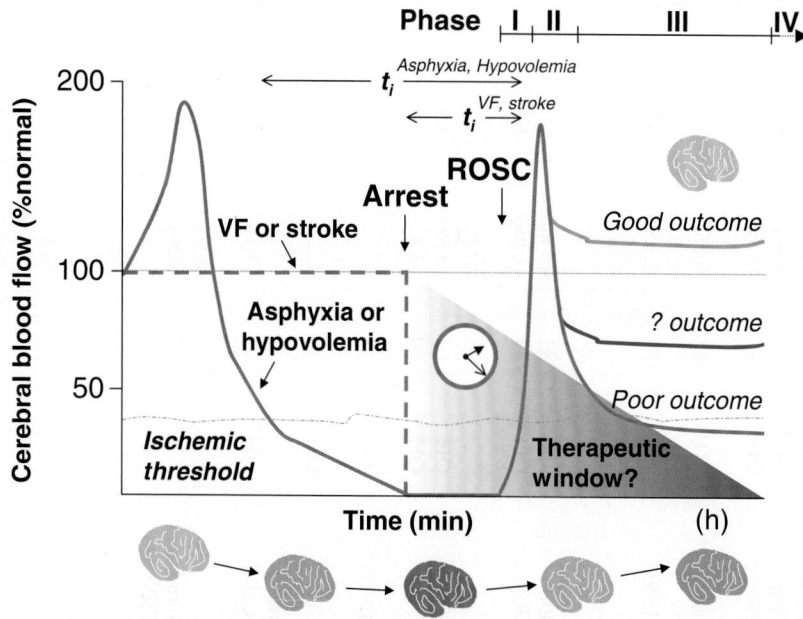

FIGURE 65.2. Typical patterns of cerebral blood flow (CBF) after cardiac arrest. There are differences between CBF after asphyxial arrest, more predominant in children, and cardiogenic arrest, more prominent in adults. Four typical phases of CBF have been described: no-flow (Phase I), hyperemia (Phase (II), hypoperfusion (Phase III), and recovery (Phase IV). ROSC, return of spontaneous circulation; VF, ventricular fibrillation. From: Robert S. B. Clark.

of HIE until later when developmental milestones are not met and should have long-term developmental screening. Although outcome after cardiac arrest is poor for any age, a Japanese study of out-of-hospital cardiac arrest found that adolescents, who were more likely to have a witnessed arrest and shockable rhythm, had a superior 1-month survival rate (11%) compared with younger children (1%–2%) (16).

Of the children who attain ROSC, prediction of survival and neurologic outcome after cardiac arrest is difficult at best. Precise data do not exist to aid in the delivery of timely and reliable information for clinicians and families involved in patient care or end-of-life decisions. The best scoring system, and timing of its performance, to definitively determine a child's outcome after cardiac arrest is not known. The Pediatric Overall Performance Category (POPC) score and Pediatric Cerebral Performance Category (PCPC) score can be used to quantify outcome in patients after brain injury in a simplified fashion (17). It is defined as follows: 1, *normal*; 2, *mild*; 3, *moderate disability*; 4, *severe disability*; 5, *coma or vegetative state*; and 6, *dead*. The POPC and PCPC provide a gross estimate of the degree of disability in patients after brain injury, and although they are used to assess therapeutic efficacy in clinical trials, they are not designed to discern specific neurologic diagnoses.

Data are available from large studies on the ability of clinical, radiologic, and/or other testing to predict poor neurologic outcome (**Table 65.1**). Survival rate to hospital discharge for children after out-of-hospital cardiac arrest is 9%, with two-thirds of survivors having neurologic impairment (7). Over half of patients are <1 year of age, with half of these being newly born and having the best survival rate (36%). Males comprise 50%–60% of pediatric cardiac arrest patients, and survival rates are equal between genders. The need for three or more doses of epinephrine or >30 minutes of resuscitation is associated with poor neurologic outcome in survivors (7). Patients with witnessed cardiac arrest have better outcomes than those with unwitnessed cardiac arrest, but the use of prehospital cardiopulmonary resuscitation (CPR) may not make a difference in overall survival rate. Based on data from the US National Registry of CPR (now called *Get with the Guidelines*), survival rate to hospital discharge was higher for in-hospital cardiac arrest patients (27%) versus out-of-hospital arrest patients (8%), with 65% of those survivors having good neurologic outcome. In that study, the mean time to initiation of CPR was <1 minute and was provided by trained healthcare personnel (12).

In a study of patients having cardiac arrests within a PICU, a hospital discharge rate of 13.7% was reported. For CPR durations of <15 minutes, 15–30 minutes, and >30 minutes, the survival rates were 19%, 12%, and 6%, respectively. Only 2 of 35 (5.7%) patients who had a cardiac arrest prior to their PICU cardiac arrest survived to discharge. Severity of illness, as measured by the Pediatric Risk of Mortality III score, was found to be a significant predictor of survival (18). Another study of cardiac arrest in PICU patients had a similar hospital discharge rate previously reported for inpatient pediatric cardiac arrest, and found that preexisting renal failure and requirement for epinephrine predicted poor outcome (19). One pediatric cardiac ICU reported successful CPR in 63% (24/38) of patients, with 20 having ROSC and 4 placed on mechanical cardiopulmonary support. All 4 of the mechanically supported patients and 10 ROSC patients survived to hospital discharge (37%) and 11 remained alive at 6 months, 3 with neurologic impairment (20). Using a large multi-center registry of in-hospital cardiac arrest, children with surgical-cardiac disease were found to have the best survival to discharge after cardiac arrest (37%), followed by those with medical cardiac disease (28%) and noncardiac disease (23%) (21).

A case series using extracorporeal support in the context of CPR (ECPR) showed that its implementation during CPR has utility for in-hospital cardiac arrest with surprisingly positive outcomes. Although patients had prolonged resuscitation times, good neurologic outcome was still possible, and survival

was better in patients with isolated cardiac disease (22). A larger, multicenter, cohort of children provided with ECPR after in-hospital cardiac arrest showed that 44% survived to hospital discharge and 99% of the survivors had favorable outcome (23). Having a cardiac etiology was associated with improved chance of survival.

Observational studies address the ability of clinical examination, laboratory findings, brain electrical activity, or radiologic tests to predict outcome. Absent pupillary and motor response had good predictive value when measured several days after ROSC (24). Children with an EEG that exhibited discontinuous activity and/or was nonreactive had worse outcome in the first 72 hours after ROSC (25). In children who drowned, presence of any hypoxic–ischemic abnormality on brain computed tomography (CT) at any time was associated with death or persistent vegetative state (26). Serum biomarkers of brain injury such as neuron specific enolase (NSE) from neurons and S100b from astrocytes show utility in preliminary studies(26a,101). Children with basal ganglia lesions on conventional brain magnetic resonance imaging (MRI) or in the brain lobes on diffusion-weighted MRI had poor outcome (27). Additional large studies with prospective data are needed to address the prognostic utility of clinical tests and markers in infants and children. The use of hypothermia has confounded much of the outcome prediction data gleaned from adults with cardiac arrest; however, somatosensory-evoked potentials (SSEPs) have demonstrated good reliability (28).

CBF after Cardiac Arrest in Experimental Models

Age-related changes in CBF during normal development and key facets of CBF regulation are presented in Chapter 55 and serve as important background information for the sections that follow. The temporal pattern of CBF after cardiac arrest has been ascertained predominately from experimental models using adult animals and VT/VF cardiac arrest, or global cerebral ischemia paradigms such as aortic or carotid occlusion. Recent studies describing CBF after asphyxial cardiac arrest in models of "pediatric"-relevant ages reveal a distinct pattern of cerebral reperfusion. These differences may be due to distinct pathophysiologic processes in asphyxial versus VF cardiac arrest and also due to dissimilarities in hemodynamic response in the early stages of postnatal brain development compared with the developed brain (29). Asphyxial cardiac arrest produces a physiologically different milieu compared with VT/VF arrest, because of the hypoxemia, acidosis, hypercarbia, and hypotension that precede cardiac arrest (**Fig. 65.2**). It has been reported that an asphyxial arrest of 7 minutes' duration produces severe impairment of neurologic function, comparable to a VT/VF arrest of 10 minutes' duration (30). Furthermore, asphyxial cardiac arrest, in comparison with VT/VF cardiac arrest of similar duration, in dogs resulted in more prevalent and prominent microinfarcts and petechial hemorrhage (31).

CBF during and after cardiac arrest is phasic in nature. During cardiac arrest, there is global ischemia, with no- or low-flow if CPR is being provided. Immediately following reperfusion, there can be heterogenous return of CBF in spite of normal or increased cerebral perfusion pressure (CPP, the difference between mean blood pressure and mean intracranial pressure), typically correlating with the duration of ischemia. Studies in adult animal models of cardiac arrest demonstrate that CBF in the postarrest period can be divided into four phases (**Fig. 65.2**): multifocal (regional) no-reflow (Phase I), hyperemia (Phase II), delayed hypoperfusion (Phase III), and restitution of normal blood flow (Phase IV) (32–34). Studies in pediatric asphyxial cardiac arrest demonstrate that CBF varies for different brain regions within each phase. In the setting of pediatric asphyxial cardiac arrest, progressively increased insult durations diminish the intensity of the hyperemia phase in all regions, with hypoperfusion predominating at longer insult durations (29).

The existence of a multifocal no-reflow phase is somewhat controversial, initially described by Ames et al. (32) in 1968, in a global cerebral ischemia model. Lin (35) and Fischer and Hossmann (33) demonstrated that the hetereogenous brain reperfusion, or the "no-reflow" phenomenon, can also occurr after VF cardiac arrest. This phase is characterized by regions of the brain that fail to reperfuse after ROSC. These areas are more extensive with increasing duration of cardiac arrest, and are observed at a macroscopic and microscopic level. At a microscopic level, there are areas of "no reflow" interspersed with areas of restored blood flow and microinfarcts. Brain regions that are selectively vulnerable include the thalamus, amygdala, hippocampus, and striatum. It is hypothesized that vasospasm, perivascular edema, and increased blood viscosity play a role in the development of this "no-reflow" phenomenon.

The second phase of CBF after cardiac arrest is characterized by increased global CBF immediately after ROSC and is often referred to as the "hyperemia" phase. This phase is present for ~15–30 minutes after ROSC. Global CBF during this phase is typically two to three times higher than baseline CBF. Kagstrom et al. (34) demonstrated that during the hyperemia phase, local CBF was extremely heterogeneous, with some areas of no-flow present. Some consider that this hyperemic phase is essential for neuronal functional recovery (36). This opinion is based on studies showing that hypertensive reperfusion improves neurologic outcome, whereas postarrest hypotension worsens neurologic outcome (36–38). In addition to hypertensive reperfusion, hemodilution and thrombolysis in this phase have been shown to improve outcome in animal models (39,40). Following resuscitation from asphyxial cardiac arrest in young rats, this phase is characterized by marked region-dependent and insult duration-dependent CBF alterations. Differing degrees of hypoperfusion are present in the cortex immediately after resuscitation, and the hypoperfusion increases proportionally with the duration of asphyxia. Hyperemia is present in the hippocampus, amygdala, and thalamus for 5–30 minutes after moderate durations of asphyxial cardiac arrest, and it is most pronounced in the thalamus, where CBF is two times higher than baseline CBF. Importantly, regional hyperemia is absent after prolonged asphyxial cardiac arrests, with CBF values similar to baseline values (29).

The third phase of CBF after cardiac arrest begins ~15–30 minutes after ROSC, can persist for several hours, and is often referred to as the "delayed hypoperfusion" phase. During this phase, there is regional heterogeneity of the CBF, with areas of high, normal, and low flow (32,33). The severity, or duration and degree, of delayed hypoperfusion is associated with more severe impairment of functional recovery, especially if not matched by a lower metabolic rate (30). Therefore, interventions that increase CBF and minimize the Phase III, delayed hypoperfusion after ischemia may improve neuorologic recovery. There is a spectrum of temporal and regional reperfusion patterns depending on the duration of cardiac arrest. After milder insults, the hypoperfusion phases are characterized by shorter duration and less impairment of CBF. After a 9-minute VF cardiac arrest in piglets, CBF was 10%–20% lower than baseline (41). In a global cerebral ischemia model in rats, ischemia of 3 minutes' duration produced a 23% reduction of CBF whereas ischemia of 20 minutes' duration produced a 50% reduction compared to baseline (42). Immature animals subjected to carotid artery ligation and hypoxia (Rice-Vannucci model) did not show hypoperfusion over the first 24 hours after ROSC (43). Delayed hypoperfusion seems to occur consistently with durations of ischemia over 15 minutes (44,45).

CBF after Cardiac Arrest in Humans

The normal level of whole brain CBF is ~50 mL/100 g/min and varies during development. For example, normal CBF in infants is less than in children and adults and peaks at age 7 years (46). Thresholds for CBF are associated with brain function: CBF

<18 mL/100 g/min results in loss of electrical activity while CBF <8–10 mL/100 g/min results in loss of cellular-ionic gradients. Most available data on CBF patterns after cardiac arrest in humans are recorded >6 hours after ROSC, since these patients need intensive stabilization during the initial first few hours. Furthermore, serial measurements of CBF have been rarely reported in these patients. To date, the objective of most studies has been to establish a relationship between CBF and outcome after cardiac arrest. There is even less information regarding CBF values after cardiac arrest in infants and children. In neonatal asphyxia, CBF velocities have been estimated by Doppler ultrasonography and have suggested that the development of high CBF velocities after 24 hours is predictive of poor prognosis (47). A study reporting CBF in nine children in a persistent vegetative state several days after cardiac arrest (Phase IV) of different etiologies (near-drowning, sudden infant death syndrome, postsurgery) showed CBF values ranging from 12 to 56 mL/100 g brain tissue/min. In this series, CBF in two children who were clinically brain dead at the time of the study were 0.2 and 2 mL/100 g brain tissue/min. CBF values of <10 mL/100 g brain tissue/min are thought to be reflective of brain death, and CBF >10–15 mL/100 g brain tissue/min is associated with potential for patient survival (48).

In adult patients, the CBF at 24 hours after ROSC can be low, normal, or high, and persistently high CBF values may be reflective of completely disrupted autoregulation (100–200 mL/100 g brain tissue/min) and indicate the onset of irreversible brain damage (49). Another study in adult patients showed that CBF below 20 mL/100 g brain tissue/min is associated with death within days (50). Hemispheric CBF in adult patients resuscitated from cardiac arrest was reported by Nogami et al. (51). These authors found that patients with favorable outcomes had CBF values of 39 mL/100 g brain tissue/min, whereas patients with poor outcome had CBF values of 25 mL/100 g brain tissue/min. In the same study, it was shown that low hemispheric CBF (<30 mL/100 g brain tissue/min) and low reactivity to acetazolamide—an indicator of intact reactivity to changes in $PaCO_2$—are associated with poor outcome in adults with HIE. The ischemic threshold is considered to be 18–20 mL/100 g brain tissue/min for all ages in humans, although the true ischemic threshold may vary by age and be relative to cerebral metabolism.

Cerebral Metabolism after Cardiac Arrest

Whether cerebral metabolism is coupled to CBF after cardiac arrest is controversial (52). Since Lassen (53) described the "luxury perfusion syndrome" in 1966, referring to a relative hyperemia in relationship to the brain's metabolic needs, several studies have determined whether CBF and metabolism are truly coupled. Michenfelder and Milde (54) compared cerebral metabolic rate for oxygen ($CMRo_2$) with CBF in a model of global cerebral ischemia without cardiac arrest. $CMRo_2$ increased immediately after ischemia during the hyperperfusion phase, and decreased to values lower than control during the delayed hypoperfusion phase. The same authors manipulated $CMRo_2$ by altering brain temperature and found that CBF increased parallel to $CMRo_2$ during hyperthermia (55). They concluded that CBF and metabolism are coupled and that delayed postischemic hypoperfusion is not an important determinant of neuronal injury, since CBF appears to be primarily determined by the cerebral metabolic demands. In contrast, Kofke et al. (56) found that $CMRo_2$ increased by 200% and remained at 160% of baseline values for several hours after ischemia, whereas CBF decreased by 40% compared to baseline. These results suggest that CBF is not coupled with $CMRo_2$ in the period of delayed hypoperfusion. Nonoxidative or anaerobic cerebral metabolism adds an additional level of complexity. Cerebral metabolic rate for glucose (CMRGlu) has been shown to decrease during the hypoperfusion phase and is considered to be coupled with CBF after potassium-induced cardiac arrest in rats (57,58). $CMRO_2$ and CMRGlu can be discordant after acute brain injury (59).

There are limited data on cerebral metabolic needs after cardiac arrest in humans. Brodersen (50) found that CBF and $CMRO_2$ were generally coupled in 11 patients resuscitated from cardiac arrest, when measurements were made >24 hours after arrest. In 14 patients resuscitated from cardiac arrest, Beckstead et al. (60) found that $CMRO_2$ and CBF were reduced, in proportion, to <50% of normal. In a study by Buunk et al. (61), nonsurviving patients gradually developed the "luxury perfusion syndrome," likely secondary to significant necrosis of brain tissue. In this study, the authors found coupling of CBF and $CMRO_2$ in survivors. CMRGlu is also generally felt to be reduced, in a magnitude similar to $CMRO_2$, after cardiac arrest in adults (62).

Systemic Variables Affecting CBF after Cardiac Arrest

As discussed in detail in Chapter 55, CBF is influenced by systemic physiologic variables, in particular, arterial partial pressure of carbon dioxide ($PaCO_2$), arterial partial pressure of oxygen (PaO_2), blood pressure, and temperature (Fig. 65.3). CBF is sensitive to changes in $PaCO_2$, referred to as CO_2 reactivity. Low $PaCO_2$ produces vasoconstriction and decreased CBF, and higher $PaCO_2$ produces vasodilatation and increased CBF. Typically, for every 1 mm Hg change in $PaCO_2$, CBF changes by 2%–6%. Cerebrovascular reactivity to CO_2 is often preserved in comatose patients resuscitated from cardiac arrest. Therefore, extreme hyperventilation and hypocarbia could exacerbate hypoperfusion, and should be avoided in the early postresuscitation period. Defining the optimal $PaCO_2$ early after resuscitation is complex, and issues such as profound acidosis and response to catecholamines must be considered. PaO_2 has little effect on CBF until it is less than ~55 mm Hg, in which case CBF dramatically increases. A major controversy exists regarding the target PaO_2 for resuscitation and during the postresuscitation period, since fractional inspired oxygen (FIO_2) of 1.0 does not appear to hold clinical advantages over room air resuscitation (63) and may actually be deleterious because of increased oxidative stress on reperfusion (64). A recent study suggests that pulse oxyhemoglobin saturation monitoring (SpO_2)-guided resuscitation may be optimal (65). At present, it appears most logical to target normocarbia and normoxia in patients during and after cardiac arrest.

In general, CBF is maintained constant with the brain's ability for autoregulation over a range of CPP, ~50–150 mm Hg in adults. Normal pressure autoregulation curves are age dependent, both in terms of lower and upper threshold limits, and baseline CBF (as discussed in Chapter 55). For CPP above or below threshold limits, CBF becomes directly correlative to

CPP (pressure passive). Adults resuscitated from cardiac arrest may have compromised autoregulation, with either absent pressure autoregulation or increased lower limits of autoregulation (range 80–120 mm Hg) (66,67). In experimental cardiac arrest studies, outcome was shown to be improved with induced arterial hypertension after ROSC (38). In humans, there is an association between blood pressure after ROSC and outcome. Patients with higher mean arterial pressure (MAP) in the first 2 hours after cardiac arrest are more likely to have better outcomes (36). The relationship between pressure autoregulation and outcome are not clear in infants and children after cardiac arrest.

Hypothermia, now a class IIb recommendation from the American Heart Association (AHA) for postresuscitation treatment of cardiac arrest, typically decreases CBF via a coupled reduction in cerebral metabolism (see Chapter 25). Hypothermia also has suppressive effects on excitatory neurotransmission and oxygen radicals. In animal studies, hypothermia and induced hypertension were associated with improved survival (68,69). The two randomized, multicenter, clinical trials in adult patients after primarily VT/VF cardiac arrest certainly support the use of hypothermia after cardiac arrest (70,71) and suggest that therapies that include metabolic suppression may have clinical utility.

Prolonged central hypoxia and depressed ventilation stimulate chemoreceptors and a vagal response that leads to bradycardia, PEA, or asystole (72). Oxygen stores are depleted ~20 seconds after cardiac arrest, and there is loss of consciousness. Glucose and adenosine triphosphate (ATP) stores are depleted within 5 minutes, whereupon the patient's brain crosses the threshold for cerebral ischemia (73). Following ROSC and reperfusion, there is typically a transient cerebral hyperemia lasting minutes that may be followed by global hypoperfusion. The duration and degree of postresuscitative hypoperfusion are proportional to the duration of the cardiac arrest, are related to ultimate severity of injury, and can last hours to several days (74). This is a period where the brain is at risk of secondary injury, and therefore may represent a therapeutic target.

Pathobiology after Reperfusion

With reperfusion after ROSC, a complex cascade of events is initiated that includes membrane depolarization, supraphysiologic accumulation of excitatory amino acids (primarily glutamate), calcium influx, acidosis, oxidative stress, mitochondrial dysfunction, and the activation of lipases, proteases, and nucleases (Fig. 65.1). A detailed discussion of the mechanisms of secondary injury in the postischemic brain was presented in Chapter 56. Reperfusion and restoration of oxygen delivery to injured brain leads to profound increases in oxygen and nitrogen radicals, free radical damage to cells, and initiation of redox-sensitive cell-signaling pathways (Fig. 65.4). Clinically, cellular hypoxia is

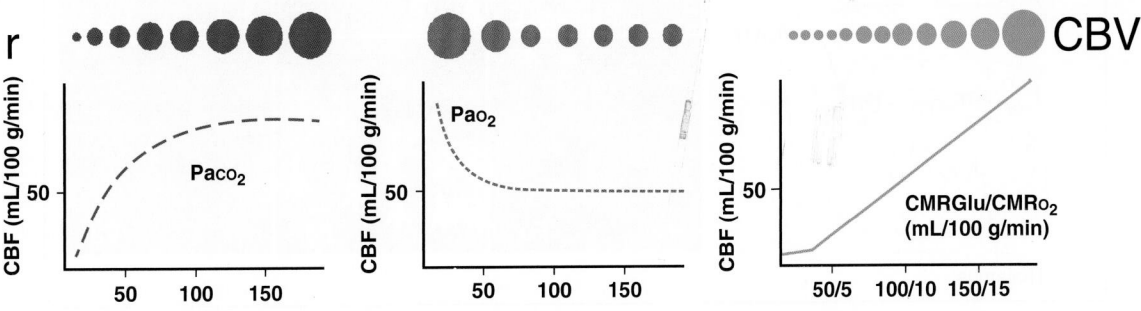

FIGURE 65.3. Physiologic factors affecting normal cerebral blood flow (CBF). Under a constant cerebral perfusion pressure CBF changes occur via changes in the diameter of the cerebral blood vessels (r = radius) resulting in changes in cerebrovascular resistance and cerebral blood volume (CBV). $PaCO_2$, partial pressure of carbon dioxide; PaO_2, partial pressure of oxygen; CMRGlu, Cerebral metabolic rate for glucose; $CMRO_2$, cerebral metabolic rate for oxygen, X-axis units are mmHg for each of the 3 graphs. From: Robert S. B. Clark.

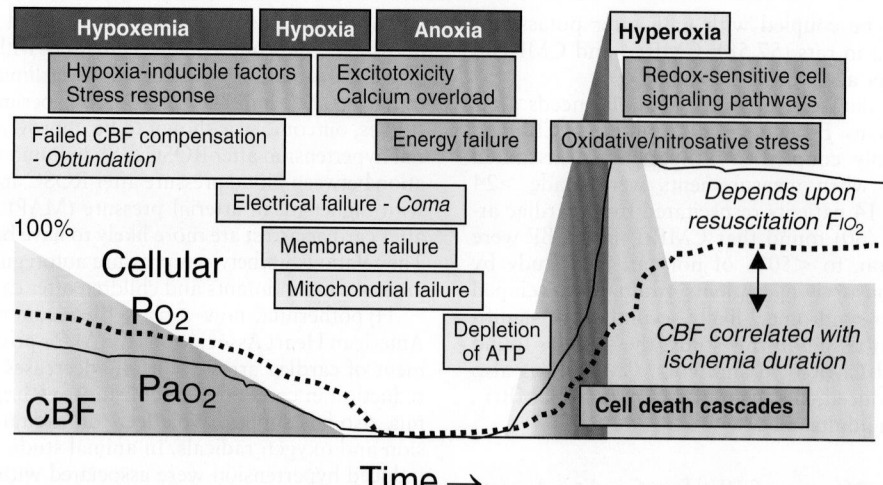

FIGURE 65.4. Pathobiology of asphyxial cardiac arrest. Hypoxemia triggers a stress response and induction of hypoxia-inducible factors, and manifests clinically as obtundation. Prolonged hypoxemia can result in tissue hypoxia and eventually anoxia, with cell membrane and mitochondrial failure, energy failure, electrical failure, and coma. Reperfusion triggers oxidative stress and redox-sensitive signaling pathways, and if sufficiently prolonged, initiation of cell death cascades in selectively vulnerable brain regions. CBF, cerebral blood flow; ATP, adenosine triphosphate; Pao$_2$, partial pressure of oxygen; Fio$_2$, fractional inspired oxygen. From: Robert S. B. Clark.

manifest as a depressed mental status that correlates with the depth and duration of hypoxia. The metabolic and electrical failure that is produced can result in coma despite restoration of CBF and oxygen and substrate delivery during reperfusion.

Although all parenchymal cells in brain are susceptible to hypoxia–ischemia, most attention has been directed toward neurons. Different neuronal populations are known to be selectively vulnerable to hypoxia–ischemia. These populations include neurons within the CA1 region of the hippocampus, cerebral cortical layers 3 and 5, amygdaloid nucleus, basal ganglia, and cerebellar Purkinje cells, which have a predilection to undergo delayed neuronal death—up to 5 days after injury (75). As discussed in Chapter 56, this hierarchy of neuronal vulnerability is of great importance in cardiac arrest, since the ischemic insult is global. Unique aspects in cellular energy metabolism and connectivity are thought to play a role in this susceptibility, since these regions in general do not have especially vulnerable microcirculatory patterns. That is not to say that watershed regions are not also selectively vulnerable to hypoxia–ischemia; although, interestingly, watershed infarcts appearing pathologically as laminar necrosis are more common after VT/VF versus asphyxial cardiac arrest (31). After asphyxial cardiac arrest, microinfarcts and petechial hemorrhage are more common. Selectively vulnerable regions prone to the development of HIE after cardiac arrest are similar in rats (**Fig. 65.5**) and humans (**Fig. 65.6**).

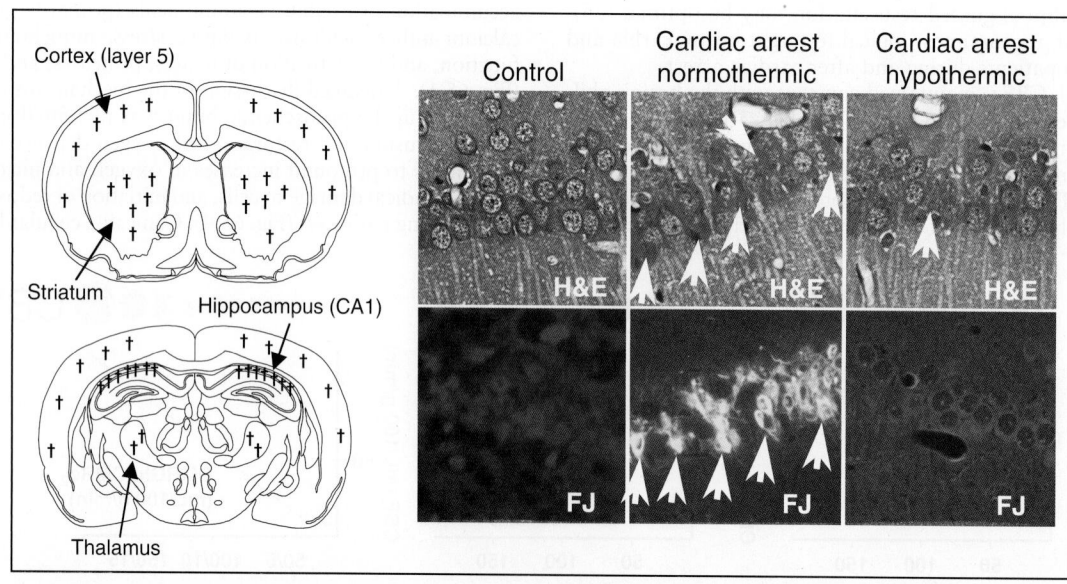

FIGURE 65.5. Selectively vulnerable brain regions after 8–9 minutes of cardiac arrest in rats (†). Neurons in the CA1 region of the hippocampus are particularly vulnerable. Dying neurons are identified as condensed cells using hemotoxylin and eosin (H&E) staining and using fluoro-jade B (FJ), which stains degenerating neurons (*arrows*). Photomicrographs depict coronal brain sections from postnatal day 17 rats after 8 minutes of asphyxial cardiac arrest under normothermic (37°C for 1 hour) or hypothermic (32°C for 1 hour) conditions. From: Robert S. B. Clark.

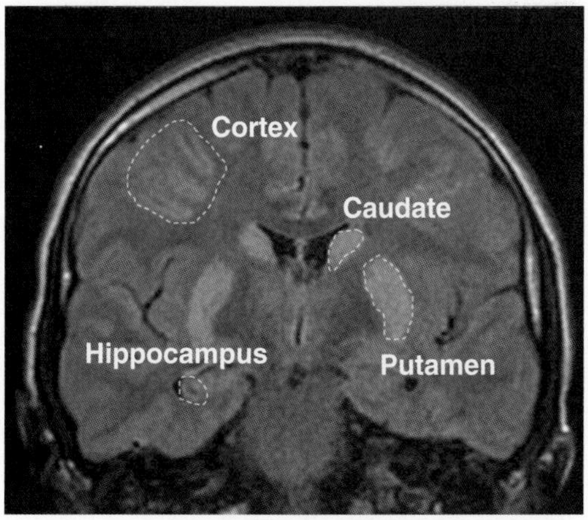

Structure	Function	Clinical consequence
Basal ganglia Putamen Caudate	Motor control, cognition Learning, memory, behavior	Dystonia Impairments in motivation, executive function, attention, memory, chorea & dystonia
Globus pallidus	Motor control	Akinetic-rigid syndrome, behavior
Cortex (esp. layers 3 and 5)	Cognition, learning, attention, consciousness, language/speech, higher- order processing, vision	Coma, persistent vegetative state, seizures, myoclonus, language, and executive impairment
Watershed areas ACA–MCA MCA–PCA		Brachial diplegia Cortical blindness
Cerebellum (esp. Purkinje cells)	Balance, gait, cognition	Dysmetria, fine movement disorder
Hippocampus (esp. CA1 region)	Learning, memory, visual- spatial organization	Seizure, amnesia, memory deficit

Selectively vulnerable brain regions after cardiac arrest in humans

FIGURE 65.6. Selectively vulnerable brain regions after cardiac arrest in humans. Table describes selectively vulnerable structures, their function, and clinical consequence. A T2 flair MRI image from a patient 1 week after asphyxial cardiac arrest due to anaphylaxis with bilateral enhancement and edema seen in the caudate and putamen, hippocampus, and cerebral cortex. ACA, anterior cerebral artery; MCA, middle cerebral artery; PCA, posterior cerebral artery. From: Robert S. B. Clark.

CLINICAL ASPECTS OF HYPOXIC–ISCHEMIC ENCEPHALOPATHY

Acute Management of Cardiac Arrest

The clinical goals for pediatric cardiac arrest are provision of effective and high-quality CPR, rapid ROSC, and prevention of secondary injury. Time to initiation of resuscitative efforts can strongly impact survival and neurologic outcome. Community education in bystander CPR may influence outcome after out-of-hospital arrests (76). Many hospitals have brought this concept to in-hospital cardiac arrest and organized dedicated rapid response teams (77,78). The AHA provides pediatric advanced life support guidelines with supporting scientific review (see Chapter 25). While CPR techniques and algorithms have been standardized and supported by agencies such as the AHA, American Academy of Pediatrics, International Liaison Committee on Resuscitation, etc., randomized controlled trials supporting these recommendations in children are lacking. A treatment guideline algorithm for in-hospital cardiac arrest that is based on the literature and protocols and practice at the Children's Hospital of Pittsburgh is provided in **Figure 65.7**. Chapter 25 thoroughly addresses the acute management of pediatric cardiac arrest. Establishment of an open airway for ventilation and oxygenation is especially imperative to the pediatric population, since most arrests in infants and children have an asphyxial etiology, most commonly respiratory failure or shock. Hyperventilation should be avoided unless there are signs and symptoms of brain herniation. Circulatory shock should be treated aggressively following published pediatric shock guidelines (refer to Chapter 28) (79).

After initial stabilization, it is useful to perform a quick neurologic assessment of the patient. At minimum, this should include an examination of pupillary responses and assignment of Glasgow Coma Scale (GCS) score. The GCS, although validated in patients with traumatic brain injury, may be useful in the assignment of severity of injury in the comatose patient after cardiac arrest as well. Problems with using the GCS in cardiac arrest patients can occur because sedatives and intubation

can hinder GCS interpretation given that the score is based on a patient's best verbal, motor, and eye opening abilities. In addition, an infant or younger child may not have the ability to understand and follow commands. The motor score was found to be a more sensitive predictor for brain injury severity after trauma than the full GCS (80), and deserves further study in children after cardiac arrest. Other groups have adapted the GCS for use in infants and children. One example is the Children's Hospital of Philadelphia infant coma scale ("Infant Face Scale"), validated for children <2 years of age (81).

Patients remain at significant risk of secondary brain injury after ROSC from hypotension, hypoxemia, seizures, hypoglycemia, and hyperthermia; so efforts should be made to prevent these conditions, or treat them promptly should they occur. Measurement of blood gas partial pressures, pH, serum electrolytes, and glucose should be performed if resources are available. It is our opinion that all surviving pediatric patients be transferred to a tertiary center that specializes in the care and rehabilitation of postarrest infants and children for further evaluation and treatment.

Pediatric Intensive Care Unit Management

PICU management of patients after cardiac arrest consists largely of supportive care and prevention of secondary insults. Maintenance of normoxia, normocapnia, and normotension are bedrocks of supportive care. While not proven to be effective, invasive cardiopulmonary monitoring can be useful in the prevention and identification of physiologic instability and reduce the incidence of, or minimize the effects of, secondary insults. Certainly, placement of an arterial catheter for continuous blood pressure measurement, a central venous catheter for central venous pressure measurement, and vasoactive drug delivery by continuous infusion are justified in patients who remain in coma after cardiac arrest. The AHA recommends titrating oxygen administration to maintain SpO$_2$ around 94%, to avoid hyperoxia, as a result of a large adult database study in which hyperoxia (PaO$_2$ > 300 mm Hg) was highlighted; however, hypoxia (PaO$_2$ < 60 mm Hg) was also associated

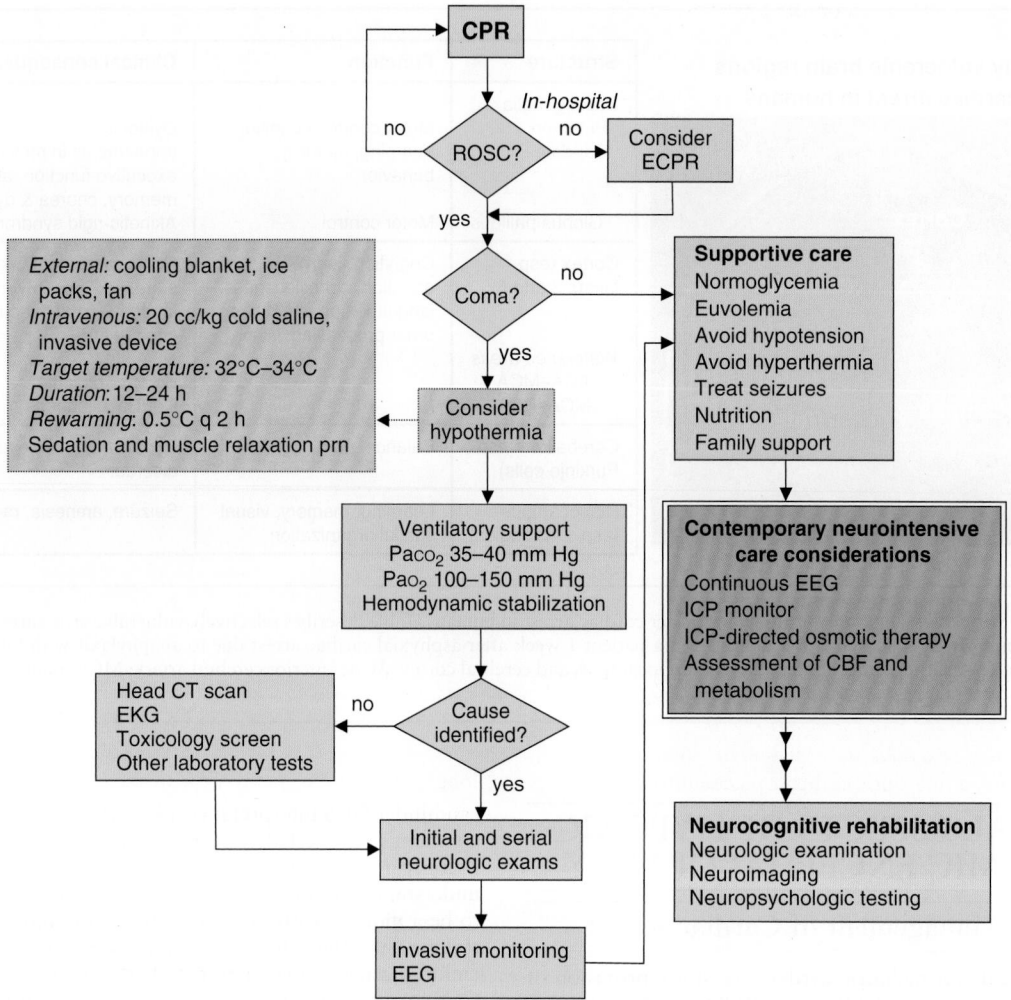

FIGURE 65.7. Algorithm for the management and treatment of post–circulatory arrest syndrome in infants and children. Guidelines based on medical literature and protocols and practice at the Children's Hospital of Pittsburgh. CPR, cardiopulmonary resuscitation; ROSC, return of spontaneous circulation; ECPR, extracorporeal cardiopulmonary resuscitation; EEG, electroencephalogram; ICP, intracranial pressure; CBF, cerebral blood flow; EKG, electrocardiogram; $Paco_2$, partial pressure of carbon dioxide; Pao_2, partial pressure of oxygen.

with increased risk of mortality in the multivariate analysis (82). Subsequently, hypoxia on ROSC was associated with increased risk of death in a large European pediatric cohort study (83).

The degree of cerebral edema is variable after cardiac arrest and reperfusion but is more common after asphyxial than VT/VF arrest. Morimoto et al. (84) noted that patients with respiratory arrest, followed by cardiac arrest, more frequently had evidence of cerebral edema on cranial CT scan on day 3 (and poorer outcome at 1 week) after arrest than did arrhythmia-induced cardiac arrest patients. In general, intracranial pressure is increased after global ischemia, and can be severe enough to cause intracranial hypertension and herniation syndrome if the period of ischemia is prolonged (68). However, intracranial pressure monitoring, which was once a standard measurement after cardiac arrest, is no longer considered standard practice. This is largely because of case series performed in the 1980s showing that aggressively treating intracranial hypertension in children after submersion injury increased the number of surviving patients with severe disability and vegetative state (85,86), and the fact that intracranial hypertension is often a consequence, rather than the cause, of cerebral ischemia. However, revisiting the use of such monitoring—particularly

in combination with concurrent monitoring of CBF, cerebral metabolism and brain tissue oxygenation—during evolving neurologic injury may be warranted.

An initial CT may be helpful in situations where the etiology of arrest is not clear or where there may be concomitant trauma. Serial head CT scans after cardiac arrest are indicated only if new or evolving pathology is suspected, such as hemorrhage, evolving mass lesion, or herniation.

Contemporary Neurointensive Care Monitoring

Cerebral Blood Flow and Estimation of Cerebral Perfusion

Currently, CBF can be measured directly, but intermittently, using techniques such as stable Xenon CT, positron emission tomography (PET), or perfusion MRI (87). While these measurements appear to have utility in that management of traumatic brain injury, little has been reported related to the use of these modalities in patients after cardiac arrest. The few available reports have focused on the relationship of temporal patterns of CBF to outcome rather than the use of CBF measurements to guide clinical management. Recently, surrogate measures reflecting CBF in humans have been evaluated, particularly those allowing continuous measurement.

Transcranial Doppler (TCD) ultrasonography is a noninvasive, bedside method for estimating CBF, and may also be used to extrapolate effects of cerebral edema and intracranial pressure on CBF velocity (88,89). TCD measures middle cerebral artery (MCA) blood flow velocity as a surrogate for CBF but does not provide a direct measurement. Another disadvantage of this method is that it provides no information about regional heterogeneity of CBF after cardiac arrest.

Cerebral Metabolic and Brain Activity Monitoring

Brain oxygenation can be measured using near-infrared spectroscopy (NIRS), which can be used to noninvasively and continuously estimate cerebral oxygen extraction. Current disadvantages of NIRS include limited depth of penetration—thus limiting interrogation to millimeters beneath the brain surface, focal rather than global information, and lack of definitions of target and critical values. However, theoretically, NIRS measurement of continuous oxyhemoglobin saturation on the brain surface can provide relative real-time alterations in brain oxygenation, which may be useful in titration of therapies. NIRS performed in the first 48 hours after neonatal asphyxia has been shown to be useful in predicting outcome at 3 months (90). Invasive brain tissue oxygenation can be determined using a fiberoptic catheter placed into brain parenchyma to measure the partial pressure of brain tissue oxygen ($Pbto_2$). The utility of $Pbto_2$ is being studied in patients with traumatic brain injury, and its use in patients after cardiac arrest remains investigational.

Global cerebral metabolism can also be measured directly if a jugular bulb catheter is placed and CBF is measured simultaneously. Cross-brain extraction of oxygen (arterial-venous difference of oxygen [$avDo_2$] content) and glucose (arterial-venous difference of glucose [AVDGlu]) can be used to calculate $CMRo_2$ and CMRGlu, respectively. There is also potential utility in examining jugular venous bulb oxygen saturation ($Sjvo_2$) as a reflection of cerebral metabolism, particularly if direct CBF measurements are not available and since Spo_2 is ~100%. $Sjvo_2$ is frequently employed to monitor patients with traumatic brain injury, with normal values reported to be 55%–71% and values below 50% considered the critical threshold for brain ischemia. Central venous saturation from the superior vena cava may not be a suitable substitute for $Sjvo_2$. In one study, $Sjvo_2$ was 10% lower than mixed venous saturation within 6 hours after cardiac arrest, and was later higher than the mixed venous saturation in nonsurvivors (61). Like $Pbto_2$ monitoring, $Sjvo_2$ monitoring in patients after cardiac arrest remains investigational.

EEG represents a real-time summation of an electrical signal from a pool of spatially related neurons displayed in 8 or 16 (or more) channels. EEG is a noninvasive bedside method increasingly being used after HIE to diagnose and monitor response to treatment of nonclinical seizures. The actual incidence of seizures in infants or children after cardiac arrest is unknown, but is as high as 30% in adults after cardiac arrest. A newer indication is continuous monitoring during periods of muscle relaxation, especially during the induction of hypothermia, which is increasingly being used for postresuscitation therapy in cardiac arrest patients (91). EEG alone, or in combination with other methods, has been used to predict outcome after pediatric cardiac arrest (92). Presence of discontinuous EEG activity, epileptiform spikes, or discharges correlated with poor outcome. SSEPs use electrical stimulation of peripheral nerves, and record the response of somatosensory pathways.

Absence of SSEPs may be more sensitive and specific in predicting unfavorable outcome after cardiac arrest (92).

Cerebral microdialysis uses intermittent or continuous sampling of extracellular fluid to measure changes in brain chemistry, and is based on the diffusion of small, water-soluble substances through a semipermeable membrane. It is invasive and involves insertion of a catheter equipped with a dialysis membrane into the brain parenchyma. Molecules that are diffusible—below 20,000 Da, and perhaps larger molecules up to 100,000 Da—may be measured depending on the cutoff size of the semipermeable membrane (93). Concentrations of glucose, lactate, neurotransmitters, drugs, and markers of tissue damage and inflammation can be measured. Currently, cerebral microdialysis is used as a research tool, and its place as a point-of-care monitor after cardiac arrest remains unclear (94).

Magnetic Resonance Imaging/Spectroscopy

MRI provides detailed information about ischemic brain injury, is noninvasive, and does not use ionizing radiation (95–97) (see Chapter 59). Diffusion-weighted imaging (DWI) uses differences in water diffusivity to acutely diagnose ischemia which may not be discernable on T2-weighted images, and to describe regions of brain at risk for HIE. The disadvantages of MRI are the relatively longer scanning time compared with CT, the increased need for sedation/muscle relaxant use to prevent motion artifact, and the restriction of metal objects (e.g., EEG leads if not MRI-compatible). Injury to cortical lobes and the basal ganglia have been associated with poor outcome after pediatric cardiac arrest. MRI, coupled with arterial spin labeling, can be used to trace arterial and venous blood supply to the brain and to quantify CBF and cerebral blood volume.

Brain magnetic resonance spectroscopy (MRS) has been used experimentally to demonstrate the relationship of metabolites (e.g., lactate, pyruvate, glutamate, N-acetylaspartate, and phosphocreatine) to outcome in patients with HIE. Elevated lactate and decreased N-acetylaspartate are associated with worse neurologic outcome in neonates with asphyxial injury (98,99). Increased lactate may persist up to 1 week after asphyxial injury (100). Currently, both MRI and MRS are used primarily for outcome prediction and not for minute-to-minute PICU management.

Biomarkers

There is currently no single clinical, laboratory, or imaging test to detect occult or evolving brain injury or predict neurologic outcome with certainty after cardiac arrest in children (or adults for that matter). Serum and urine biomarkers are surrogates of brain injury that present a promising approach to these problems (Fig. 65.8). Ideal serum or urine biomarkers would be uniquely found in the brain, be proportional to the degree of damage, and be readily detectable in a point-of-care fashion. Most work has focused on neuron-specific enolase (NSE, a glycolytic protein from neurons and neuroectodermal cells), S-100B (a calcium-regulated protein released by injured astrocytes to modulate differentiation of neurons and glia), and myelin basic protein (MBP). Serial cerebrospinal fluid sampling is an impracticable and possibly unsafe procedure for most cardiac arrest patients given the possibility of cerebral edema and increased intracranial pressure. A second prospective single center pediatric study found that serum NSE was associated with poor outcome and mortality at 24, 48, and 72 hours following ROSC(26a) in a pilot study in children (101). In adults, treatment with mild, induced hypothermia suppressed NSE concentration compared with normothermia, which was then associated with

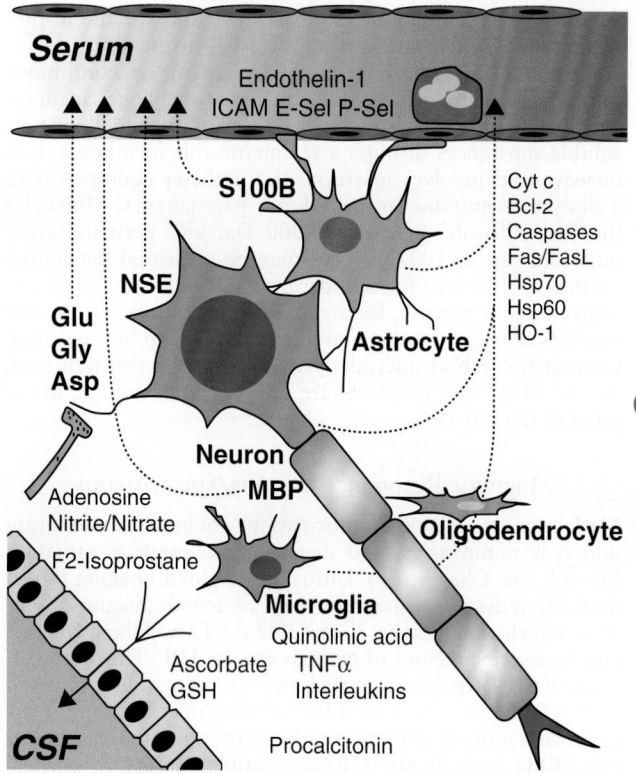

Serum

Endothelin-1
ICAM E-Sel P-Sel

S100B

NSE

Cyt c
Bcl-2
Caspases
Fas/FasL
Hsp70
Hsp60
HO-1

Astrocyte

Glu
Gly
Asp

Neuron
MBP

Oligodendrocyte

Adenosine
Nitrite/Nitrate
F2-Isoprostane

Microglia

Quinolinic acid

Ascorbate   TNFα
GSH   Interleukins

Procalcitonin

CSF

FIGURE 65.8. Potential biomarkers and biomediators for identifying and following brain injury, validating mechanisms of injury, and serving as targets for therapeutic drug monitoring. HSP60, heat shock protein 60; HSP70, heat shock protein 70; Gly, glycine; Glu, glutamate; Asp, aspartate; TNF, tumor necrosis factor; GSH, glutathione; MBP, myelin basic protein. ICAM, Intercellular adhesion molecule; E-Sel, E-selectin; P-Sel, P-selectin; CytC, cytochrome c; Fas, Fas (not an acronym); FasL, Fas-ligand; HO-1, heme-oxygenase-1; NSE, neuron specific enolase; CSF, cerebrospinal fluid. From: Robert S. B. Clark.

improved outcome after cardiac arrest (102). Decreased NSE levels were postulated to be due to the neuroprotective effects of hypothermia, and may be useful as a marker for future clinical trials. S-100B may have neuroprotective characteristics at low concentrations, but is associated with astroglial cell death at higher concentrations in animal models (103). A subsequent paper found that serum S100b was the most accurate biomarker after pediatric cardiac arrest with an area under the curve 0.955 for outcome and 0.908 for mortality (26a,101). Higher glucose concentrations in the first 24 hours after cardiac arrest were found to be an independent marker of poor outcome in one adult cardiac arrest study (104). Recently, Berger et al. (105) studied levels of NSE, S-100B, and MBP in serum in infants and children after the use of either rescue breaths or chest compressions. NSE was increased and showed a delayed peak over a period of days after the insult in many patients—suggesting the occurrence of delayed neuronal death. In contrast, S-100B was increased only early after the insult, consistent with the fact that delayed astrocyte death has not been reported. MBP was not increased, suggesting a limited role for axonal injury after asphyxia or asphyxial cardiac arrest (105).

Perhaps combining a panel of clinical findings with biomarkers will provide more powerful early prediction of long-term neurologic outcome. Pfeifer et al. (106) showed that a combination of GCS score, NSE, and S-100B could predict vegetative state or death in adults after cardiac arrest with 100% specificity. Another study found increased predictability for poor neurologic outcome when serum NSE levels were combined with SSEPs (107). Novel potential serum

biomarkers are also under investigation for their ability to predict outcome after cardiac arrest. For example, procalcitonin, the precursor for the hormone calcitonin, predicts survival but not neurologic outcome in adults after cardiac arrest (108). Inflammatory markers, such as interleukin-8, are also increased after adult cardiac arrest but are not predictive of neurologic outcome (109). Other biomarkers and biomediators have been found to be increased after traumatic brain injury and may be relevant to HIE as well (110).

Therapies Targeting the Prevention and Treatment of Hypoxic–Ischemic Encephalopathy

6

Temperature Management

Fever (>38°C) after acute brain insult from trauma or hypoxia–ischemia exacerbates injury and may lead to worse outcomes. Children with "persistent" hyperthermia, defined as a temperature ≥38°C for a 24-hour period post-ROSC, had worse outcomes when compared with children without persistent hyperthermia in a large cohort study. Therefore, the AHA recommends targeting normothermia (Class IIa, level of evidence [LOE] C) (Table 65.3).

Mild, induced hypothermia has come to the forefront as a promising strategy for improving survival and neurologic outcome after cardiac arrest in adult patients, but we still do not have the evidence to support what we should do in pediatric patients. Mechanisms of action for hypothermia include reduced brain metabolic needs, excitotoxicity, oxidative stress, and inflammation. In a pediatric model of asphyxial arrest in rats, brief (1 hour) application of mild hypothermia resulted in improved neuronal survival at 5 weeks after injury when compared with maintenance of normothermia (111) (Fig. 65.5). Thus far, pediatric data about the use of hypothermia after cardiac arrest are limited to nonrandomized, retrospective case series (112,113). A multicenter, randomized, controlled trial of hypothermia versus normothermia in pediatric cardiac arrest is currently enrolling subjects to examine the efficacy of hypothermia in this population. The AHA now endorses this therapy for comatose adult patients with VF/VT cardiac arrest after two multicenter, randomized, controlled studies demonstrated efficacy (70,71). Whole body hypothermia or selective head cooling is also endorsed in the neonatal population for reduction of morbidity and mortality after birth asphyxia (114,115). Whole body cooling may be the more effective modality given that deeper brain structures, as well as superficial brain structures, are cooled, and selective head cooling may not be as effective outside the neonatal period. On extrapolating these studies, the AHA recommends *considering* therapeutic hypothermia (32°C–34°C) for pediatric patients remaining comatose after cardiac arrest and ROSC (Class IIb recommendation, LOE C for children; Class IIa, LOE C for adolescents resuscitated from sudden, witnessed VF cardiac arrest) (82). Further, in children, the optimal method for inducing hypothermia, for maintaining hypothermia, and for rewarming after hypothermia are not clear. During induction of hypothermia, particular attention should be given to electrolyte abnormalities, volume state, shivering, coagulopathy, dysrhythmias, and any effects on drug metabolism (116). It is critical to realize that hypothermia decreases the systemic clearance of cytochrome P450 and CYP2E1-metabolized drugs commonly used in patients surviving cardiac arrest (117–120). Additionally, there is concern that the use of hypothermia requires a delay in the timing of clinical testing for accurate prognostication of neurologic outcome and brain death (24 hours of normothermia) (28,121). Previous concerns about the potential adverse effects of hypothermia

TABLE 65.3

IMPORTANT CHANGES IN RECOMMENDATIONS FOR PEDIATRIC RESUSCITATION FROM THE 2010 INTERNATIONAL CONSENSUS ON CARDIOPULMONARY RESUSCITATION AND EMERGENCY CARDIOVASCULAR CARE SCIENCE WITH TREATMENT: PEDIATRIC BASIC AND ADVANCED LIFE SUPPORT

■ RECOMMENDATION CHANGE	■ CLASSIFICATION[a]
For >1 rescuer CPR, continue to perform ABC's and activation of emergency response system simultaneously	IIa, C
For single-rescuer CPR, change order of interventions from ABC to CAB: chest compressions, airway, breathing/ventilation	IIa, C
Optimal CPR for infants and children includes both compressions and ventilations	I, B
However, compressions alone are preferable to no CPR	I, B
Compress at least one-third the anterior–posterior dimension of the chest during CPR (1½ inches (4 cm) for infants and 2 inches (5 cm) for children)	I, C
An initial energy dose of 2–4 J/kg is reasonable in children with VF/VT	IIa, C
Doses higher than 4 J/kg, not to exceed 10 J/kg, especially if delivered with a biphasic defibrillator, may be safe and effective in refractory VF	IIb, C
Both cuffed and uncuffed endotracheal tubes are acceptable in infants and young children	IIa, C
Application of cricoid pressure should be modified or discontinued if it impedes ventilation or speed or ease of intubation	III, C
Monitor capnography/capnometry to confirm proper endotracheal tube position	I, C
Once spontaneous circulation is restored, inspired oxygen concentration should be titrated to maintain the oxyhemoglobin saturation ≥94% to limit the risk of hyperoxemia	IIb, C
Rapid response systems in pediatric inpatient settings may be beneficial to reduce rates of cardiac and respiratory arrest and mortality	IIa, B
Protocol-driven or "goal-directed" therapy, with a target central venous (superior vena cava) oxygen saturation ≥70% appears to improve patient survival in severe sepsis	IIb, B
Refer families of patients with sudden cardiac arrest and no cause of death on autopsy to an arrhythmia referral center	I, C
Whenever possible, provide family members with the option of being present during resuscitation	I, B

[a]Class I: Evidence or general agreement that a procedure or treatment is useful and effective; Class II: Conflicting evidence or divergence of opinion exists; Class IIa: Weight of evidence or opinion favors utility or efficacy; Class IIb: Weight of evidence or opinion is less well established; Class III: Evidence or general agreement that the procedure or treatment is either not useful or effective, or in some cases may be harmful; LOE A: Data derived from multiple randomized clinical trials; LOE B: Data derived from a single randomized clinical trial; LOE C: Consensus expert opinion.

on successful defibrillation/cardioversion appear unfounded, as a recent laboratory study has shown that hypothermia increased the likelihood of successful cardioversion compared with normothermic arrest (122). Based on experimental studies, hypothermia is most effective when initiated as early as possible. The multicenter clinical studies cited show that hypothermia is effective even when applied up to 6 hours after the cardiac arrest. These studies used a range of duration of hypothermia (12–72 hours), of time to rewarming (12–24 hours), and of target temperatures (32°C–34°C). Pilot studies using intravenous cold saline infusion (not push) to more rapidly achieve target temperature in children with brain injury suggest that it is effective, feasible, and without obvious adverse effects (123). Further study is needed to define the optimal timing for initiation, duration, degree of cooling, rewarming interval, and to determine whether patients benefit from hypothermia.

Cutting-Edge Strategies

Certain centers with extracorporeal membrane oxygenation capabilities are now applying it as a rescue therapy for in-hospital pediatric cardiac arrest or imminent cardiac arrest (called ECPR), and for patients with impending heart failure post–cardiac surgery (22). ECPR reestablishes cardiac output, allows for heart–lung rest, and can be combined with hypothermia since bypass enables rapid cooling and temperature control and alleviates concerns for the arrythmogenicity or myocardial depression due to hypothermia. ECPR can be implemented during active CPR but requires significant resources and highly skilled personnel (22). Good neurologic outcome is sometimes possible even with prolonged resuscitation, and the survival rate is

higher in patients with isolated cardiac disease (22). It is likely that ECPR can be effective in select patients (124).

Other cutting-edge strategies to improve outcomes after prolonged cardiac arrest include high-volume continuous veno-venous hemofiltration, which improved neurologic outcome in a small nonrandomized trial in adults after cardiac arrest (125). Thrombolytics, one of the only proven treatments for stroke, has a narrow therapeutic time window but may be useful during CPR in patients with cardiac arrest from myocardial infarction or pulmonary embolus (126). Coenzyme Q administration, combined with mild, induced hypothermia, reduces mortality versus hypothermia alone after cardiac arrest in a pilot study (127). Failed clinical trials include magnesium with and without diazepam, calcium channel blockers, barbiturates, and corticosteroids (128–131).

Cognitive Rehabilitation

Experimentally, environmental enrichment and exercise have been shown to improve cognitive outcome in animal models of brain ischemia. There is scant literature on the effect of rehabilitation on pediatric neurocognitive outcome. Environmental enrichment increases the amount of dendritic branching and synapses (132) and may enhance neurogenesis (133). Since synaptogenesis occurs until late childhood (peaking around 4 years of age) (134), rehabilitation could make a significant impact, particularly in younger children with mild-to-moderate disability. Treatment in the form of therapies can help with muscle tone and control, oral muscle development, and vision in the case of cortical vision impairment. Even simple therapies can make a significant impact in the patient's quality of life.

FUTURE DIRECTIONS AND EMERGING THERAPIES

The first steps in improving outcome from cardiac arrest involve rapid achievement of ROSC and targeted post-resuscitation strategies. These include optimizing CPR and developing tailored practice parameters for the PICU management of blood pressure, temperature, PaO_2, $PaCO_2$, serum glucose, serum osmolality, and nutrition. Development of contemporary neurointensive care monitoring with the identification of treatment goals and thresholds is similarly imperative. Also vitally important and on the horizon is the tailoring of treatments based on the etiology of the insult, patient's age, gender, and, ultimately, genotype. Optimization of hypothermia and the use of ECPR also warrant further clinical evaluation, as do the development of several emerging therapies, some of which are discussed in what follows and shown temporally in **Figure 65.9**.

Reestablishment and Maintenance of Cerebral Blood Flow

It is well recognized that hypotension after ROSC can worsen cerebral ischemia. Studies assessing strategies to improve perfusion abnormalities after resuscitation from cardiac arrest have focused on the postischemic hypoperfusion phase. The mechanism of postischemic hypoperfusion is not well understood, but it is postulated to be the result of vasospasm, tissue edema, and cell aggregation. Hemodilution (hematocrit

to 25%) and hypertension in the immediate postresuscitation period can improve postischemic CBF and survival in animal models (39,68).

Pharmacologic agents for CBF promotion shown to be beneficial in animal studies include endothelin A antagonists, remifentanil, nitrous oxide, and nitric oxide (NO) donors. Studies in humans assessing improvement in neurologic function after treatment with these agents are lacking. The endothelin A receptor antagonist BQ485 administered shortly after ROSC improves CBF, functional activity, and neurologic outcome after cardiac arrest in rats (135). Nitrous oxide and remifentanil are cerebral vasodilators and increase regional CBF when used as anesthetics in healthy volunteers (136,137). Nitrous oxide increases CBF preferentially in the gray matter, whereas remifentanil has a more pronounced effect in the basal ganglia and subcortical structures. Anesthesia with remifentanil and/or nitrous oxide could increase CBF and perhaps be beneficial after cardiac arrest. Administration of the NO donor (diethylenetriamine NONOate) has also been shown to reduce neurologic injury following hypoxia–ischemia in the newborn rat (138).

Antiexcitotoxic Strategies

Many antiexcitotoxic therapies have been tried in patients after cerebral ischemia. This is logical given the pivotal influence of excitatory amino acid-induced neurotoxicity in the evolution of HIE (**Fig. 65.1**). Hypothermia, shown to be protective after adult VT/VF cardiac arrest and neonatal

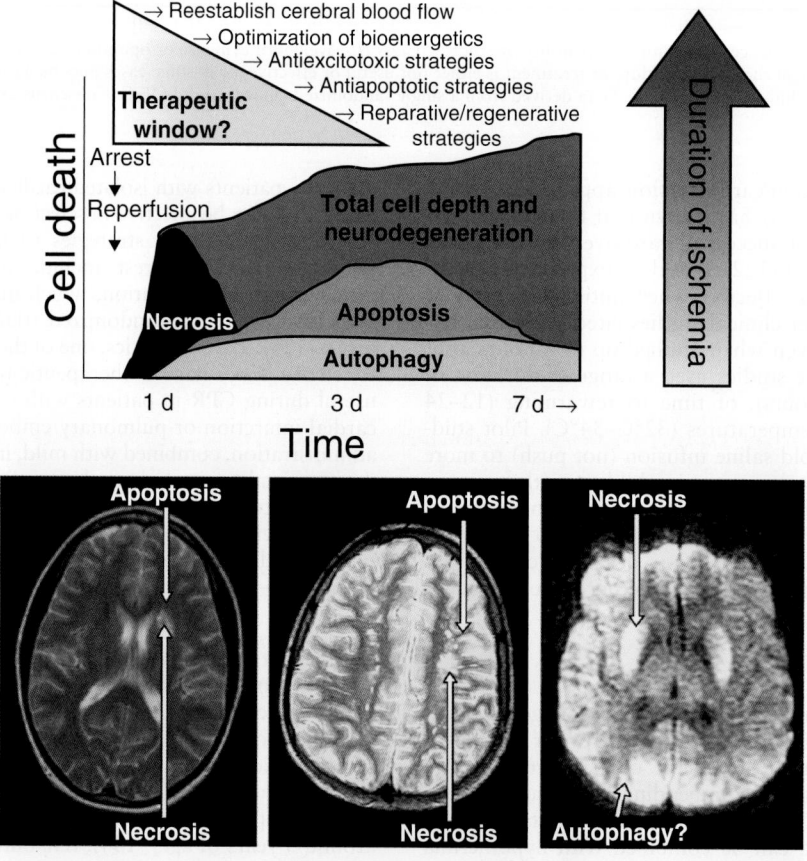

FIGURE 65.9. Futuristic treatment strategies targeting cell death pathways (apoptosis, necrosis, and/or autophagy) producing hypoxic–ischemic encephalopathy. The therapeutic windows for these novel strategies are likely temporally and regionally dependent. From: Robert S. B. Clark.

asphyxia, is thought to exert its effects at least in part by reducing excitotoxicity and cerebral metabolism. In contrast, pharmacologic antiexcitotoxic strategies have not shown benefit in preventing or reducing HIE. Pentobarbital given after VF in a cat model decreased the frequency of seizures but there was no overall difference in mortality or neurologic outcome (139). Thiopental given after global ischemia in monkeys also showed no difference in neurologic outcome or mortality, and many animals receiving thiopental had cardiac arrhythmias (140). However, barbiturates combined with halothane anesthesia improved neurologic outcome and reduced infarct size in a dog model of focal ischemia (141). *The Brain Resuscitation Clinical Trial I Study Group* has performed a randomized clinical trial of thiopental. This study of 262 comatose adult survivors of cardiac arrest, using otherwise identical postresuscitation protocols, showed no difference in mortality in patients receiving thiopental compared with controls; although patients receiving thiopental had double the incidence of hypotension (130). Novel antiexcitotoxic agents including those targeting N-methyl-D-aspartate and α-amino-3-hydroxy-5-methylisoxazole-4-propionic acid receptors, shown to be beneficial in animal models, have also failed in clinical trials. Many have showed not only lack of benefit but also undesirable side effects (142).

Optimization of Bioenergetics and Preventing Energy Failure

Energy stores and fuel preferences evolve during development and differ between neurons, astrocytes, and other cell types. Lust et al. (143) demonstrated that glycogen stores were decreased in the cerebral cortex of postnatal day 7 rats, compared with adult rats, and that, unlike adult rats, rat pups demonstrate a greater reliance on ketone bodies for energy correlating with their high-fat milk diet. Not surprisingly, the enzymes involved with ketone metabolism are maximal preweaning and decrease by 50% afterward and glycolytic enzymes reach adult levels after weaning, when the diet switches from high fat to primarily carbohydrates (144). A key enzyme in nonoxidative acetyl CoA metabolism, pyruvate dehydrogenase, matures during the weaning period, and its role in nonoxidative acetyl CoA can be inhibited by ketone and medium-chain fatty acid elements (145,146). The ability to metabolize fatty acids matures in parallel with glycolysis (147).

Cerebral metabolism is altered during brain ischemia. Within seconds of cessation of CBF, there is loss of consciousness and electrocerebral silence. ATP is depleted within 5 minutes, and lactate is produced as cells switch to anaerobic respiration to preserve energy stores (148). Repletion of energy substrates and oxidative metabolism after ROSC may restore function to vulnerable but irreversibly injured cells. After reperfusion, selectively vulnerable neurons may have a second wave of ATP depletion at 24 hours in the striatum and 48 hours in the hippocampus that coincides with cell death mainly by apoptosis (149). This may represent a window of opportunity where optimizing energy balance and restoring energy supply may be effective in reducing brain damage.

The administration of ketones has shown promise in preventing energy failure and lactic acidosis after global ischemia in juvenile mice (150). Fats are converted to the ketone bodies b-hydroxybutyrate, acetoacetate, and acetone, which cross the blood–brain barrier via monocarboxylic transporters. In a rat model of forebrain ischemia, treatment with ketone bodies decreased neuronal damage if the duration of ischemia was 10 but not 15 minutes (151). Ketogenic diets (composed of 80%–90% fat) have also been tested for neuroprotective effects in different models of brain injury (152,153).

Antiapoptotic Strategies

Developing neurons may be at higher risk of apoptotic cell death after brain injury, as demonstrated by their increased sensitivity to irradiation (154). Relative to adult rats, neonatal rats show increased apoptosis-inducing factor (AIF), caspase-3, and cytochrome c release from mitochondria after hypoxia–ischemia (155). In other words, the developing brain appears more primed for apoptosis after injury compared with the mature brain. Thus, antiapoptotic strategies may be more effective in infants and children compared with adults. In a model of neonatal hypoxia–ischemia, systemic injection of a pan-caspase inhibitor decreased infarction size in the striatum, hippocampus, and cortex versus vehicle treatment (156). Combining hypothermia (29°C) and intraventricular administration of a caspase inhibitor can also reduce histopathologic damage versus control groups (157). Interestingly, the degree of apoptosis after cerebral ischemia may be gender dependent. Female rats treated with a caspase inhibitor after neonatal hypoxia–ischemia had smaller stroke volumes whereas treatment was not effective in their male counterparts (158). This finding is consistent with both cell culture (159) and clinical studies (160) suggesting that gender may play a prominent role in apoptosis and therefore response to antiapoptotic treatments after brain injury in the developing brain.

Regeneration and Repair

As outlined in Chapter 55, the third trimester of human gestation through toddler age is a time of explosive brain growth and development due to neurogenesis, dendrite and synapse formation, axon lengthening, and myelination (161). The developing brain is more vulnerable to excitotoxicity and is biased toward programmed cell death as the brain is avidly pruning synapses and creating memories. That the adolescent brain continues to undergo modulation of cognitive function and anatomy is only recently being elicited (162,163). Studies in children have demonstrated superior adaptive plasticity (164), as seen in their ability to recover from epilepsy brain resection (165), ability to learn multiple languages, and the increased potential for gains in function with targeted rehabilitation versus adults. Experimental models have been developed to mimic appropriate developmental age and clinically relevant scenarios (166,167). The juvenile mouse brain has been postulated to have more potential for neurogenesis after hypoxia–ischemia than the neonatal brain, implying that the neonatal mouse is already at maximal capacity for regeneration at baseline (168). Consequently, the young brain may be at greater risk of injury, yet also have a greater potential for regeneration and repair (169).

Neurogenesis has been shown to occur postnatally in the dentate gyrus of the hippocampus and in the subventricular zones, peaking in the neonatal period (170,171). Stem cell proliferation and migration has been documented after hypoxia–ischemia in neonatal rats and mice in vivo (172), but there is limited survival of neuronal phenotypes versus supporting cells. Neural stem cells reproduce throughout life, but their ability to replicate, migrate, and survive in areas of injury declines with age. In addition, there is gradual change of the cellular environment with aging that does not favor regeneration. Cellular transplants and growth factor replacement remain potential adjuvant therapies after hypoxic–ischemic injury and require investigation. Agents such as erythropoietin are currently in clinical trials in traumatic brain injury in adults and in birth asphyxia studies in neonates. Finally, the disadvantages of these therapies are just beginning to be illuminated. For instance, abnormal axonal migration may cause seizures and promote the growth of tumors (171). Given that global cerebral ischemia causes extensive and diverse cellular injury in the brain, these therapies may not be tenable, although they may prove to be useful in more limited, focal brain injury. Further research is needed.

CONCLUSIONS

HIE in infants and children results in devastating consequences for the child and family. Certain etiologies are potentially preventable, such as submersion injuries and sudden infant death syndrome (back-to-sleep), and prevention strategies should be emphasized. Early recognition and urgent initiation of resuscitative efforts may prevent the development of HIE if ROSC is achieved before the irreversible ischemic threshold is reached. Future postresuscitation therapies and PICU management for pediatric patients at risk for the development of HIE should target outcomes with both increased survival and improved quality of life in mind.

ACKNOWLEDGMENTS

We thank the staff and our colleagues at the Children's Hospital of Pittsburgh for providing such excellent care of our patients. We also appreciate generous support from the NIH (K12 HD047349, ELF; K23 NS065132, MDM; R01 HD075760, HD04568, and NS30318, RSBC) and the Laerdal Foundation.

References

1. Liou AK, Clark RS, Henshall DC, et al. To die or not to die for neurons in ischemia, traumatic brain injury and epilepsy: A review on the stress-activated signaling pathways and apoptotic pathways. *Progr Neurobiol* 2003;69(2):103–42.

2. Harukuni I, Bhardwaj A. Mechanisms of brain injury after global cerebral ischemia. *Neurol Clin* 2006;24(1):1–21.

3. Atkins DL, Everson-Stewart S, Sears GK, et al. Epidemiology and outcomes from out-of-hospital cardiac arrest in children: The Resuscitation Outcomes Consortium Epistry-Cardiac Arrest. *Circulation* 2009;119(11):1484–91.

4. Tibballs J, Kinney S. A prospective study of outcome of in-patient paediatric cardiopulmonary arrest. *Resuscitation* 2006;71(3):310–8.

5. Tibballs J, Kinney S. Reduction of hospital mortality and of preventable cardiac arrest and death on introduction of a pediatric medical emergency team. *Pediatr Crit Care Med* 2009;10(3):306–12.

6. Moler FW, Meert K, Donaldson AE, et al. In-hospital versus out-of-hospital pediatric cardiac arrest: A multicenter cohort study. *Crit Care Med* 2009;37(7):2259–67.

7. Young KD, Gausche-Hill M, McClung CD, et al. A prospective, population-based study of the epidemiology and outcome of out-of-hospital pediatric cardiopulmonary arrest. *Pediatrics* 2004;114(1):157–64.

8. Moler FW, Donaldson AE, Meert K, et al. Multicenter cohort study of out-of-hospital pediatric cardiac arrest. *Crit Care Med* 2011;39(1):141–9.

9. Meert KL, Donaldson A, Nadkarni V, et al. Multicenter cohort study of in-hospital pediatric cardiac arrest. *Pediatr Crit Care Med* 2009;10(5):544–53.

10. Young KD, Seidel JS. Pediatric cardiopulmonary resuscitation: A collective review. *Ann Emerg Med* 1999;33(2):195–205.

11. Reis AG, Nadkarni V, Perondi MB, et al. A prospective investigation into the epidemiology of in-hospital pediatric cardiopulmonary resuscitation using the international Utstein reporting style. *Pediatrics* 2002;109(2):200–9.

12. Nadkarni VM, Larkin GL, Peberdy MA, et al. First documented rhythm and clinical outcome from in-hospital cardiac arrest among children and adults. *JAMA* 2006;295(1):50–7.

13. Smith BT, Rea TD, Eisenberg MS. Ventricular fibrillation in pediatric cardiac arrest. *Acad Emerg Med* 2006;13(5):525–9.

14. Pediatric sudden cardiac arrest. *Pediatrics* 2012;129(4):e1094–102.

15. Berger S, Utech L, Fran Hazinski M. Sudden death in children and adolescents. *Pediatr Clin North Am* 2004;51(6):1653–77, ix–x.

16. Nitta M, Iwami T, Kitamura T, et al. Age-specific differences in outcomes after out-of-hospital cardiac arrests. *Pediatrics* 2011;128(4):e812–20.

17. Fiser DH, Long N, Roberson PK, et al. Relationship of pediatric overall performance category and pediatric cerebral performance category scores at pediatric intensive care unit discharge with outcome measures collected at hospital discharge and 1- and 6-month follow-up assessments. *Crit Care Med* 2000;28(7):2616–20.

18. Slonim AD, Patel KM, Ruttimann UE, et al. Cardiopulmonary resuscitation in pediatric intensive care units. *Crit Care Med* 1997;25(12):1951–55.

19. de Mos N, van Litsenburg RR, McCrindle B, et al. Pediatric in-intensive-care-unit cardiac arrest: Incidence, survival, and predictive factors. *Crit Care Med* 2006;34(4):1209–15.

20. Parra DA, Totapally BR, Zahn E, et al. Outcome of cardiopulmonary resuscitation in a pediatric cardiac intensive care unit. *Crit Care Med* 2000;28(9):3296–300.

21. Ortmann L, Prodhan P, Gossett J, et al. Outcomes after in-hospital cardiac arrest in children with cardiac disease: A report from Get With the Guidelines—Resuscitation. *Circulation* 2011;124(21):2329–37.

22. Morris MC, Wernovsky G, Nadkarni VM. Survival outcomes after extracorporeal cardiopulmonary resuscitation instituted during active chest compressions following refractory in-hospital pediatric cardiac arrest. *Pediatr Crit Care Med* 2004;5(5):440–6.

23. Raymond TT, Cunnyngham CB, Thompson MT, et al. Outcomes among neonates, infants, and children after extracorporeal cardiopulmonary resuscitation for refractory in-hospital pediatric cardiac arrest: A report from the National Registry of Cardiopulmonary Resuscitation. *Pediatr Crit Care Med* 2010;11(3):362–71.

24. Abend NS, Topjian AA, Kessler S, et al. Outcome prediction by motor and pupillary responses in children treated with therapeutic hypothermia after cardiac arrest. *Pediatr Crit Care Med* 2012;13(1):32–8.

25. Nishisaki A, Sullivan J 3rd, Steger B, et al. Retrospective analysis of the prognostic value of electroencephalography patterns obtained in pediatric in-hospital cardiac arrest survivors during three years. *Pediatr Crit Care Med* 2007;8(1):10–17.

26. Rafaat KT, Spear RM, Kuelbs C, et al. Cranial computed tomographic findings in a large group of children with drowning: Diagnostic, prognostic, and forensic implications. *Pediatr Crit Care Med* 2008;9(6):567–72.

26a. Fink, EL, Berger, RP, Clark, RSB, et al. Serum Biomarkers of Brain Injury to Classify Outcome after Pediatric Cardiac Arrest. *Critical Care Medicine*, 2014;42(3):664–674.

27. Fink EL, Panigrahy A, Clark RS, et al. Regional brain injury on conventional and diffusion weighted MRI is associated with outcome after pediatric cardiac arrest. *Neurocrit Care* 2013;19(1):31–40.

28. Oddo M, Rossetti AO. Predicting neurological outcome after cardiac arrest. *Curr Opin Crit Care* 2011;17(3):254–9.

29. Manole MD, Foley LM, Hitchens TK, et al. Magnetic resonance imaging assessment of regional cerebral blood flow after asphyxial cardiac arrest in immature rats. *J Cereb Blood Flow Metab* 2009;29(1):197–205.

30. Cerchiari EL, Hoel TM, Safar P, et al. Protective effects of combined superoxide dismutase and deferoxamine on recovery of cerebral blood flow and function after cardiac arrest in dogs. *Stroke* 1987;18(5):869–78.

31. Vaagenes P, Safar P, Moossy J, et al. Asphyxiation versus ventricular fibrillation cardiac arrest in dogs. Differences in cerebral resuscitation effects—A preliminary study. *Resuscitation* 1997;35(1):41–52.

32. Ames A 3rd, Wright RL, Kowada M, et al. Cerebral ischemia. II. The no-reflow phenomenon. *Am J Pathol* 1968;52(2):437–53.

33. Fischer M, Hossmann KA. No-reflow after cardiac arrest. *Intensive Care Med* 1995;21(2):132–41.

34. Kagstrom E, Smith ML, Siesjo BK. Local cerebral blood flow in the recovery period following complete cerebral ischemia in the rat. *J Cereb Blood Flow Metab*. 1983;3(2):170–82.

35. Lin SR. Cerebral circulation after cardiac arrest. Angiographic and carbon black perfusion studies. *Radiology* 1975;117(3 pt 1):627–32.

36. Mullner M, Sterz F, Domanovits H, et al. Systemic and cerebral oxygen extraction after human cardiac arrest. *Eur J Emerg Med* 1996;3(1):19–24.

37. Safar P, Stezoski W, Nemoto EM. Amelioration of brain damage after 12 minutes' cardiac arrest in dogs. *Arch Neurol* 1976;33(2):91–5.

38. Sterz F, Leonov Y, Safar P, et al. Hypertension with or without hemodilution after cardiac arrest in dogs. *Stroke* 1990;21(8):1178–84.

39. Leonov Y, Sterz F, Safar P, et al. Hypertension with hemodilution prevents multifocal cerebral hypoperfusion after cardiac arrest in dogs. *Stroke* 1992;23(1):45–53.

40. Fischer M, Bottiger BW, Popov-Cenic S, et al. Thrombolysis using plasminogen activator and heparin reduces cerebral no-reflow after resuscitation from cardiac arrest: An experimental study in the cat. *Intensive Care Med* 1996;22(11):1214–23.

41. Nozari A, Rubertsson S, Gedeborg R, et al. Maximisation of cerebral blood flow during experimental cardiopulmonary resuscitation does not ameliorate post-resuscitation hypoperfusion. *Resuscitation* 1999;40(1):27–35.

42. Singh NC, Kochanek PM, Schiding JK, et al. Uncoupled cerebral blood flow and metabolism after severe global ischemia in rats. *J Cereb Blood Flow Metab* 1992;12:802–8.

43. Mujsce DJ, Christensen MA, Vannucci RC. Cerebral blood flow and edema in perinatal hypoxic-ischemic brain damage. *Pediatr Res* 1990;27(5):450–3.

44. Snyder JV, Nemoto EM, Carroll RG, et al. Global ischemia in dogs: Intracranial pressures, brain blood flow and metabolism. *Stroke* 1975;6(1):21–7.

45. Nemoto EM, Bleyaert AL, Stezoski SW, et al. Global brain ischemia: A reproducible monkey model. *Stroke* 1977;8(5):558–64.

46. Takahashi T, Shirane R, Sato S, et al. Developmental changes of cerebral blood flow and oxygen metabolism in children. *Am J Neuroradiol* 1999;20:917–22.

47. Ilves P, Lintrop M, Metsvaht T, et al. Cerebral blood-flow velocities in predicting outcome of asphyxiated newborn infants. *Acta Paediatr* 2004;93(4):523–28.

48. Ashwal S, Schneider S, Thompson J. Xenon computed tomography measuring cerebral blood flow in the determination of brain death in children. *Ann Neurol* 1989;25:539–46.

49. Cohan SL, Mun SK, Petite J, et al. Cerebral blood flow in humans following resuscitation from cardiac arrest. *Stroke* 1989;20(6):761–5.

50. Brodersen P. Cerebral blood flow and metabolism in coma following cardiac arrest. *Rev Electroencephalogr Neurophysiol Clin* 1974;4(2):329–33.

51. Nogami K, Fujii M, Kato S, et al. Analysis of magnetic resonance imaging (MRI) morphometry and cerebral blood flow in patients with hypoxic-ischemic encephalopathy. *J Clin Neurosci* 2004;11(4):376–80.

52. Buunk G, van der Hoeven JG, Meinders AE. Cerebral blood flow after cardiac arrest. *Neth J Med* 2000;57(3):106–12.

53. Lassen NA. The luxury-perfusion syndrome and its possible relation to acute metabolic acidosis localised within the brain. *Lancet* 1966;2:1113–5.

54. Michenfelder JD, Milde JH. Postischemic canine cerebral blood flow appears to be determined by cerebral metabolic needs. *J Cereb Blood Flow Metab* 1990;10(1):71–6.

55. Michenfelder JD, Milde JH. The relationship among canine brain temperature, metabolism, and function during hypothermia. *Anesthesiology* 1991;75:130–6.

56. Kofke WA, Nemoto EM, Hossmann KA, et al. Brain blood flow and metabolism after global ischemia and post-insult thiopental therapy in monkeys. *Stroke* 1979;10(5):554–60.

57. Blomqvist P, Wieloch T. Ischemic brain damage in rats following cardiac arrest using a long-term recovery model. *J Cereb Blood Flow Metab* 1985;5(3):420–31.

58. Nakashima K, Todd MM, Warner DS. The relation between cerebral metabolic rate and ischemic depolarization. A comparison of the effects of hypothermia, pentobarbital, and isoflurane. *Anesthesiology* 1995;82(5):1199–208.

59. Bergsneider M, Hovda DA, Shalmon E, et al. Cerebral hyperglycolysis following severe traumatic brain injury in humans: A positron emission tomography study. *J Neurosurg* 1997;86:241–51.

60. Beckstead JE, Tweed WA, Lee J, et al. Cerebral blood flow and metabolism in man following cardiac arrest. *Stroke* 1978;9(6):569–73.

61. Buunk G, van der Hoeven JG, Meinders AE. Prognostic significance of the difference between mixed venous and jugular bulb oxygen saturation in comatose patients resuscitated from a cardiac arrest. *Resuscitation* 1999;41(3):257–62.

62. Rudolf J, Ghaemi M, Ghaemi M, et al. Cerebral glucose metabolism in acute and persistent vegetative state. *J Neurosurg Anesthesiol* 1999;11(1):17–24.

63. Davis PG, Tan A, O'Donnell CP, et al. Resuscitation of newborn infants with 100% oxygen or air: A systematic review and meta-analysis. *Lancet* 2004;364(9442):1329–33.

64. Vereczki V, Martin E, Rosenthal RE, et al. Normoxic resuscitation after cardiac arrest protects against hippocampal oxidative stress, metabolic dysfunction, and neuronal death. *J Cereb Blood Flow Metab* 2006;26(6):821–35.

65. Balan IS, Fiskum G, Hazelton J, et al. Oximetry-guided reoxygenation improves neurological outcome after experimental cardiac arrest. *Stroke* 2006;37(12):3008–13.

66. Sundgreen C, Larsen FS, Herzog TM, et al. Autoregulation of cerebral blood flow in patients resuscitated from cardiac arrest. *Stroke* 2001;32(1):128–32.

67. Nishizawa H, Kudoh I. Cerebral autoregulation is impaired in patients resuscitated after cardiac arrest. *Acta Anaesthesiol Scand* 1996;40(9):1149–53.

68. Safar P, Xiao F, Radovsky A, et al. Improved cerebral resuscitation from cardiac arrest in dogs with mild hypothermia plus blood flow promotion. *Stroke* 1996;27:105–13.

69. Hachimi-Idrissi S, Corne L, Huyghens L. The effect of mild hypothermia and induced hypertension on long term survival rate and neurological outcome after asphyxial cardiac arrest in rats. *Resuscitation* 2001;49(1):73–82.

70. Hypothermia after Cardiac Arrest Study Group. Mild therapeutic hypothermia to improve the neurologic outcome after cardiac arrest. *N Engl J Med* 2002;346(8):549–56.

71. Bernard SA, Gray TW, Buist MD, et al. Treatment of comatose survivors of out-of-hospital cardiac arrest with induced hypothermia. *N Engl J Med* 2002;346(8):557–63.

72. Kaplan JL, Gao E, De Garavilla L, et al. Adenosine A1 antagonism attenuates atropine-resistant hypoxic bradycardia in rats. *Acad Emerg Med* 2003;10(9):923–30.

73. Siesjo BK. Cell damage in the brain: A speculative synthesis. *J Cereb Blood Flow Metab* 1981;1(2):155–85.

74. Edgren E, Enblad P, Grenvik A, et al. Cerebral blood flow and metabolism after cardiopulmonary resuscitation. A pathophysiologic and prognostic positron emission tomography pilot study. *Resuscitation* 2003;57(2):161–70.

75. Back T, Hemmen T, Schuler OG. Lesion evolution in cerebral ischemia. *J Neurol* 2004;251(4):388–97.

76. Wik L, Steen PA, Bircher NG. Quality of bystander cardiopulmonary resuscitation influences outcome after prehospital cardiac arrest. *Resuscitation* 1994;28(3):195–203.

77. Jones D, Bellomo R, Bates S, et al. Long term effect of a medical emergency team on cardiac arrests in a teaching hospital. *Crit Care* 2005;9(6):R808–15.

78. Tibballs J, Kinney S, Duke T, et al. Reduction of paediatric in-patient cardiac arrest and death with a medical emergency team: Preliminary results. *Arch Dis Child* 2005;90(11):1148–52.

79. Carcillo JA, Fields AI. Clinical practice parameters for hemodynamic support of pediatric and neonatal patients in septic shock. *Crit Care Med* 2002;30(6):1365–78.

80. Healey C, Osler TM, Rogers FB, et al. Improving the Glasgow Coma Scale score: Motor score alone is a better predictor. *J Trauma* 2003;54(4):671–8; discussion 678–80.

81. Durham SR, Clancy RR, Leuthardt E, et al. CHOP Infant Coma Scale ("Infant Face Scale"): A Novel Coma Scale for children less than two years of age. *J Neurotrauma* 2000;17(9):729–37.

82. Kleinman ME, Chameides L, Schexnayder SM, et al. Part 14: Pediatric advanced life support: 2010 American Heart Association Guidelines for Cardiopulmonary Resuscitation and Emergency Cardiovascular Care. *Circulation* 2010;122(18 suppl 3):S876–908.

83. Ferguson LP, Durward A, Tibby SM. Relationship between arterial partial oxygen pressure after resuscitation from cardiac arrest and mortality in children. *Circulation* 2012;126:335–42.

84. Morimoto Y, Kemmotsu O, Kitami K, et al. Acute brain swelling after out-of-hospital cardiac arrest: Pathogenesis and outcome. *Crit Care Med* 1993;21(1):104–10.

85. Biggart MJ, Bohn DJ. Effect of hypothermia and cardiac arrest on outcome of near-drowning accidents in children. *J Pediatr* 1990;117(2 pt 1):179–83.

86. Bohn DJ, Biggar WD, Smith CR, et al. Influence of hypothermia, barbiturate therapy, and intracranial pressure monitoring on morbidity and mortality after near-drowning. *Crit Care Med* 1986;14(6):529–34.

87. Robertson CL, Hlatky R. Advanced bedside neuromonitoring. In: Fink MP, Abraham E, Vincent JL, et al, eds. *Textbook of Critical Care.* 5th ed. Philadelphia, PA: Elsevier Saunders, 2005:287–94.

88. Lowe LH, Bulas DI. Transcranial Doppler imaging in children: Sickle cell screening and beyond. *Pediatr Radiol* 2005;35(1):54–65.

89. Saliba EM, Laugier J. Doppler assessment of the cerebral circulation in pediatric intensive care. *Crit Care Clin* 1992;8(1):79–92.

90. Toet MC, Lemmers PM, van Schelven LJ, et al. Cerebral oxygenation and electrical activity after birth asphyxia: Their relation to outcome. *Pediatrics* 2006;117(2):333–9.

91. Vespa PM, Nuwer MR, Nenov V, et al. Increased incidence and impact of nonconvulsive and convulsive seizures after traumatic brain injury as detected by continuous electroencephalographic monitoring. *J Neurosurg* 1999;91(5):750–60.

92. Mandel R, Martinot A, Delepoulle F, et al. Prediction of outcome after hypoxic-ischemic encephalopathy: A prospective clinical and electrophysiologic study. *J Pediatr* 2002;141(1):45–50.

93. Hutchinson PJ, O'Connell MT, Nortje J, et al. Cerebral microdialysis methodology—Evaluation of 20 kDa and 100 kDa catheters. *Physiol Meas* 2005;26(4):423–8.

94. Hillered L, Persson L. Neurochemical monitoring of the acutely injured human brain. *Scand J Clin Lab Invest Suppl* 1999;229:9–18.

95. Barber PA, Darby DG, Desmond PM, et al. Identification of major ischemic change. Diffusion-weighted imaging versus computed tomography. *Stroke* 1999;30(10):2059–65.

96. Bruce DA. Imaging after head trauma: Why, when and which. *Childs Nerv Syst* 2000;16(10–11):755–9.

97. Taylor SB, Quencer RM, Holzman BH, et al. Central nervous system anoxic-ischemic insult in children due to near-drowning. *Radiology* 1985;156(3):641–6.

98. L'Abee C, de Vries LS, van der Grond J, et al. Early diffusion-weighted MRI and 1H-Magnetic Resonance Spectroscopy in asphyxiated full-term neonates. *Biol Neonate* 2005;88(4):306–12.

99. Ashwal S, Holshouser BA, Tomasi LG, et al. 1H-magnetic resonance spectroscopy-determined cerebral lactate and poor neurological outcomes in children with central nervous system disease. *Ann Neurol* 1997;41(4):470–81.

100. Auld KL, Ashwal S, Holshouser BA, et al. Proton magnetic resonance spectroscopy in children with acute central nervous system injury. *Pediatr Neurol* 1995;12(4):323–334.

101. Topjian AA, Lin R, Morris MC, et al. Neuron-specific enolase and S-100B are associated with neurologic outcome after pediatric cardiac arrest. *Pediatr Crit Care Med* 2009;10(4):479–90.

102. Tiainen M, Roine RO, Pettila V, et al. Serum neuron-specific enolase and S-100B protein in cardiac arrest patients treated with hypothermia. *Stroke* 2003;34(12):2881–6.

103. Liu L, Li Y, Van Eldik LJ, et al. S100B-induced microglial and neuronal IL-1 expression is mediated by cell type-specific transcription factors. *J Neurochem* 2005;92(3):546–53.

104. Mullner M, Sterz F, Domanovits H, et al. The association between blood lactate concentration on admission, duration of cardiac arrest, and functional neurological recovery in patients resuscitated from ventricular fibrillation. *Intensive Care Med* 1997;23(11):1138–43.

105. Berger RP, Adelson PD, Richichi R, et al. Serum biomarkers after traumatic and hypoxemic brain injuries: Insight into the biochemical response of the pediatric brain to inflicted brain injury. *Dev Neurosci* 2006;28(4–5):327–35.

106. Pfeifer R, Borner A, Krack A, et al. Outcome after cardiac arrest: Predictive values and limitations of the neuroproteins neuron-specific enolase and protein S-100 and the Glasgow Coma Scale. *Resuscitation* 2005;65(1):49–55.

107. Meynaar IA, Oudemans-van Straaten HM, van der Wetering J, et al. Serum neuron-specific enolase predicts outcome in post-anoxic coma: A prospective cohort study. *Intensive Care Med* 2003;29(2):189–95.

108. Fries M, Kunz D, Gressner AM, et al. Procalcitonin serum levels after out-of-hospital cardiac arrest. *Resuscitation* 2003;59(1):105–9.

109. Mussack T, Biberthaler P, Kanz KG, et al. Serum S-100B and interleukin-8 as predictive markers for comparative neurologic outcome analysis of patients after cardiac arrest and severe traumatic brain injury. *Crit Care Med* 2002;30(12):2669–74.

110. Kochanek PM, Clark RS, Ruppel RA, et al. Biochemical, cellular, and molecular mechanisms in the evolution of secondary damage after severe traumatic brain injury in infants and children: Lessons learned from the bedside. *Pediatr Crit Care Med* 2000;1:4–19.

111. Fink EL, Marco CD, Donovan HA, et al. Brief induced hypothermia improves outcome after asphyxial cardiopulmonary arrest in juvenile rats. *Dev Neurosci* 2005;27(2–4):191–9.

112. Fink EL, Clark RS, Kochanek PM, et al. A tertiary care center's experience with therapeutic hypothermia after pediatric cardiac arrest. *Pediatr Crit Care Med* 2010;11(1):66–74.

113. Doherty DR, Parshuram CS, Gaboury I, et al. Hypothermia therapy after pediatric cardiac arrest. *Circulation* 2009;119(11):1492–500.

114. Gluckman PD, Wyatt JS, Azzopardi D, et al. Selective head cooling with mild systemic hypothermia after neonatal encephalopathy: Multicentre randomised trial. *Lancet* 2005;365(9460):663–70.

115. Shankaran S, Laptook AR, Ehrenkranz RA, et al. Whole-body hypothermia for neonates with hypoxic-ischemic encephalopathy. *N Engl J Med* 2005;353(15):1574–84.

116. Hovland A, Nielsen EW, Kluver J, et al. EEG should be performed during induced hypothermia. *Resuscitation* 2006;68(1):143–6.

117. Empey PE, de Mendizabal NV, Bell MJ, et al. Therapeutic hypothermia decreases phenytoin elimination in children with traumatic brain injury. *Crit Care Med* 2013;41(10):2379–87.

118. Tortorici MA, Kochanek PM, Poloyac SM. Effects of hypothermia on drug disposition, metabolism, and response: A focus of hypothermia-mediated alterations on the cytochrome P450 enzyme system. *Crit Care Med* 2007;35(9):2196–204.

119. Tortorici MA, Kochanek PM, Bies RR, et al. Therapeutic hypothermia-induced pharmacokinetic alterations on CYP2E1 chlorzoxazone-mediated metabolism in a cardiac arrest rat model. *Crit Care Med* 2006;34(3):785–91.

120. Empey PE, Miller TM, Philbrick AH, et al. Mild hypothermia decreases fentanyl and midazolam steady-state clearance in a rat model of cardiac arrest. *Crit Care Med* 2012;40(4):1221–8.

121. Webb AC, Samuels OB. Reversible brain death after cardiopulmonary arrest and induced hypothermia. *Crit Care Med* 2011;39(6):1538–42.

122. Boddicker KA, Zhang Y, Zimmerman MB, et al. Hypothermia improves defibrillation success and resuscitation outcomes from ventricular fibrillation. *Circulation* 2005;111(24):3195–201.

123. Fink EL, Kochanek PM, Clark RSB, et al. Induction of hypothermia and fever control using intravenous iced saline in pediatric neurocritical care. *CCM* 2009;37(12 suppl):A162.

124. Massetti M, Tasle M, Le Page O, et al. Back from irreversibility: Extracorporeal life support for prolonged cardiac arrest. *Ann Thorac Surg* 2005;79(1):178–183; discussion 183–174.

125. Laurent I, Adrie C, Vinsonneau C, et al. High-volume hemofiltration after out-of-hospital cardiac arrest: A randomized study. *J Am Coll Cardiol* 2005;46(3):432–37.

126. Abu-Laban RB, Christenson JM, Innes GD, et al. Tissue plasminogen activator in cardiac arrest with pulseless electrical activity. *N Engl J Med* 2002;346(20):1522–8.

127. Damian MS, Ellenberg D, Gildemeister R, et al. Coenzyme Q10 combined with mild hypothermia after cardiac arrest: A preliminary study. *Circulation* 2004;110:3011–16.

128. Machado C. Randomized clinical trial of magnesium, diazepam, or both after out-of-hospital cardiac arrest. *Neurology* 2003;60(11):1868; author reply 1868–9.

129. Brain Resuscitation Clinical Trial II Study Group. A randomized clinical study of a calcium-entry blocker (lidoflazine) in the treatment of comatose survivors of cardiac arrest. *N Engl J Med* 1991;324(18):1225–31.

130. Brain Resuscitation Clinical Trial I Study Group. Randomized clinical study of thiopental loading in comatose survivors of cardiac arrest. *N Engl J Med* 1986;314(7):397–403.

131. Jastremski M, Sutton-Tyrrell K, Vaagenes P, et al. Glucocorticoid treatment does not improve neurological recovery following cardiac arrest. Brain Resuscitation Clinical Trial I Study Group. *JAMA* 1989;262(24):3427–30.

132. Johansson BB. Functional outcome in rats transferred to an enriched environment 15 days after focal brain ischemia. *Stroke* 1996;27:324–6.

133. Kempermann G, Kuhn HG, Gage FH. More hippocampal neurons in adult mice living in an enriched environment. *Nature* 1997;386(6624):4935.

134. Rice D, Barone S Jr. Critical periods of vulnerability for the developing nervous system: Evidence from humans and animal models. *Environ Health Perspect* 2000;108(suppl 3):511–33.

135. Krep H, Brinker G, Schwindt W, et al. Endothelin type A-antagonist improves long-term neurological recovery after cardiac arrest in rats. *Crit Care Med* 2000;28(8):2873–80.

136. Lorenz IH, Kolbitsch C, Hormann C, et al. The influence of nitrous oxide and remifentanil on cerebral hemodynamics in conscious human volunteers. *Neuroimage* 2002;17(2):1056–64.

137. Lagace A, Karsli C, Luginbuehl I, et al. The effect of remifentanil on cerebral blood flow velocity in children anesthetized with propofol. *Paediatr Anaesth* 2004;14(10):861–5.

138. Wainwright MS, Grundhoefer D, Sharma S, et al. A nitric oxide donor reduces brain injury and enhances recovery of cerebral blood flow after hypoxia-ischemia in the newborn rat. *Neurosci Lett* 2007;415(2):124–9.

139. Todd MM, Chadwick HS, Shapiro HM, et al. The neurologic effects of thiopental therapy following experimental cardiac arrest in cats. *Anesthesiology* 1982;57(2):76–86.

140. Gisvold SE, Safar P, Hendrickx HH, et al. Thiopental treatment after global brain ischemia in pigtailed monkeys. *Anesthesiology* 1984;60(2):88–96.

141. Smith AL, Hoff JT, Nielsen SL, et al. Barbiturate protection in acute focal cerebral ischemia. *Stroke* 1974;5(1):1–7.

142. Muir KW, Lees KR. Excitatory amino acid antagonists for acute stroke. *Cochrane Database Syst Rev* 2003(3):CD001244.

143. Lust WD, Pundik S, Zechel J, et al. Changing metabolic and energy profiles in fetal, neonatal, and adult rat brain. *Metab Brain Dis* 2003;18(3):195–206.

144. Clark JB, Bates TE, Cullingford T, et al. Development of enzymes of energy metabolism in the neonatal mammalian brain. *Dev Neurosci* 1993;15(3–5):174–180.

145. Lai JC. Oxidative metabolism in neuronal and non-neuronal mitochondria. *Can J Physiol Pharmacol* 1992;70(suppl):S130–7.

146. Rust RS. Energy metabolism of developing brain. *Curr Opin Neurol* 1994;7(2):160–5.

147. Reichmann H, Maltese WA, DeVivo DC. Enzymes of fatty acid beta-oxidation in developing brain. *J Neurochem* 1988;51(2):339–44.

148. Siesjo BK, Wieloch T. Cerebral metabolism in ischaemia: Neurochemical basis for therapy. *Br J Anaesth* 1985;57(1):47–62.

149. Pulsinelli WA, Duffy TE. Regional energy balance in rat brain after transient forebrain ischemia. *J Neurochem* 1983;40(5):1500–3.

150. Suzuki M, Suzuki M, Sato K, et al. Effect of beta-hydroxybutyrate, a cerebral function improving agent, on cerebral hypoxia, anoxia and ischemia in mice and rats. *Jpn J Pharmacol* 2001;87(2):143–50.

151. Sims NR, Heward SL. Delayed treatment with 1,3-butanediol reduces loss of CA1 neurons in the hippocampus of rats following brief forebrain ischemia. *Brain Res* 1994;662(1–2):216–22.

152. Gasior M, Rogawski MA, Hartman AL. Neuroprotective and disease-modifying effects of the ketogenic diet. *Behav Pharmacol* 2006;17(5–6):431–9.

153. Yue Z, Horton A, Bravin M, et al. A novel protein complex linking the delta 2 glutamate receptor and autophagy: Implications for neurodegeneration in lurcher mice. *Neuron* 2002;35(5):921–33.

154. Shirai K, Mizui T, Suzuki Y, et al. Differential effects of x-irradiation on immature and mature hippocampal neurons in vitro. *Neurosci Lett* 2006;399(1–2):57–60.

155. Zhu C, Wang X, Xu F, et al. The influence of age on apoptotic and other mechanisms of cell death after cerebral hypoxia-ischemia. *Cell Death Differ* 2005;12(2):162–76.

156. Cheng Y, Deshmukh M, D'Costa A, et al. Caspase inhibitor affords neuroprotection with delayed administration in a rat model of neonatal hypoxic-ischemic brain injury. *J Clin Invest* 1998;101:1992–9.

157. Adachi M, Sohma O, Tsuneishi S, et al. Combination effect of systemic hypothermia and caspase inhibitor administration against hypoxic-ischemic brain damage in neonatal rats. *Pediatr Res* 2001;50(5):590–5.

158. Renolleau S, Fau S, Goyenvalle C, et al. Specific caspase inhibitor Q-VD-OPh prevents neonatal stroke in P7 rat: A role for gender. *J Neurochem* 2007;100:1062–71.

159. Du L, Bayir H, Lai Y, et al. Innate gender-based proclivity in response to cytotoxicity and programmed cell death pathway. *J Biol Chem* 2004;279(37):38563–70.

160. Satchell MA, Lai Y, Kochanek PM, et al. Cytochrome c, a biomarker of apoptosis, is increased in cerebrospinal fluid from infants with inflicted brain injury from child abuse. *J Cereb Blood Flow Metab* 2005;25(7):919–27.

161. Krageloh-Mann I. Imaging of early brain injury and cortical plasticity. *Exp Neurol* 2004;190(suppl 1):S84–90.

162. Luna B, Thulborn KR, Munoz DP, et al. Maturation of widely distributed brain function subserves cognitive development. *Neuroimage* 2001;13(5):786–93.

163. Huang H, Zhang J, Wakana S, et al. White and gray matter development in human fetal, newborn and pediatric brains. *Neuroimage* 2006;33(1):27–38.

164. Johnston MV. Clinical disorders of brain plasticity. *Brain Dev* 2004;26(2):73–80.

165. Boatman D, Freeman J, Vining E, et al. Language recovery after left hemispherectomy in children with late-onset seizures. *Ann Neurol* 1999;46(4):579–86.

166. Vexler ZS, Sharp FR, Feuerstein GZ, et al. Translational stroke research in the developing brain. *Pediatr Neurol* 2006;34(6): 459–63.

167. Fink EL, Alexander H, Marco CD, et al. An experimental model of pediatric asphyxial cardiopulmonary arrest in rats. *Pediatr Crit Care Med* 2004;5:139–44.

168. Qiu L, Zhu C, Wang X, et al. Less neurogenesis and inflammation in the immature than in the juvenile brain after cerebral hypoxia-ischemia. *J Cereb Blood Flow Metab* 2007;27(4): 785–94.

169. Hickey RW, Painter MJ. Brain injury from cardiac arrest in children. *Neurol Clin* 2006;24(1):147–58, viii.

170. Ong J, Plane JM, Parent JM, et al. Hypoxic-ischemic injury stimulates subventricular zone proliferation and neurogenesis in the neonatal rat. *Pediatr Res* 2005;58(3):600–6.

171. Lichtenwalner RJ, Parent JM. Adult neurogenesis and the ischemic forebrain. *J Cereb Blood Flow Metab* 2006;26(1):1–20.

172. Bartley J, Soltau T, Wimborne H, et al. BrdU-positive cells in the neonatal mouse hippocampus following hypoxic-ischemic brain injury. *BMC Neurosci* 2005;6(1):15.

CHAPTER 66 ■ METABOLIC ENCEPHALOPATHIES IN CHILDREN

LAURENCE DUCHARME-CREVIER, GENEVIEVE DUPONT-THIBODEAU, ANNE LORTIE, BRUNO MARANDA, ROBERT C. TASKER, AND PHILIPPE JOUVET

KEY POINTS

1. There are many causes of metabolic encephalopathy, so that a systematic investigation, including laboratory testing and neuroimaging, is essential.

2. The practitioner should not confuse a symptom or a syndrome (such as Reye-like illness) with an etiology.

3. Diseases that are amenable to treatment should be considered first.

4. Intracranial hypertension is frequent in metabolic encephalopathy and requires strict attention to whether hemodynamic support is needed.

5. Specific treatment of endogenous intoxication must be started as soon as possible and conducted simultaneously with diagnostic investigations.

Metabolic encephalopathy refers to a variety of disorders that result in global cerebral dysfunction in the absence of an underlying structural anomaly. These disorders can be divided into three groups, according to their pathophysiology (**Table 66.1**). In this chapter, we will review the pathophysiology, clinical presentation, acute neurology, and management of the metabolic encephalopathies commonly treated in the PICU (Status epilepticus caused by deranged metabolism is discussed in Chapter 63.) For details about specific diseases, the reader should refer to other sections in this textbook.

EPIDEMIOLOGY AND MECHANISM OF DISEASES

The mechanisms responsible for neurologic impairment in metabolic encephalopathy divide broadly into (a) endogenous intoxication due to accumulation of neurotoxic metabolite(s); (b) energy failure secondary to the lack of metabolites essential for brain function; and (c), acute water, electrolyte, and/or endocrine disturbances.

Encephalopathies with Endogenous Intoxication

Liver failure and several inborn errors of metabolism (IEM) in the catabolic pathway of amino acids have potential to induce metabolic encephalopathy by endogenous intoxication. In these diseases, intermediate products of amino acid catabolism are not detoxified by the liver (and/or the kidney), accumulate, and contribute to neurologic symptoms (**Fig. 66.1**). Cerebral edema, which is frequently associated with these disorders, is mainly due to cytotoxic mechanisms. As the encephalopathy is related to the accumulation of toxic metabolites, specific therapeutic strategies are required to decrease this accumulation and restore brain function.

Hyperammonemia and Liver Diseases

The neurotoxicity of ammonia has been studied extensively, but its relationship with endogenous intoxication is still not completely understood. Blood ammonia concentration higher than 300–500 μmol/L is associated with severe central nervous system (CNS) dysfunction, including cerebral edema and coma (1). The intestine and the muscles are the main sources of ammonia. When the hepatic urea cycle is nonfunctional, ammonia is not transformed into urea and, hence, ammonia free base (NH_3) crosses the blood–brain barrier (BBB). The BBB has a much lower permeability to the ammonium ion (NH_4^+), which implies that the diffusion of ammonia across the barrier depends partly on arterial blood pH (2–4). Once in the brain, ammonia is buffered by combining with glutamate in the formation of glutamine in the astrocytes via the action of the enzyme glutamine synthetase (GS). Once glutamine is formed in the astrocyte, it is released via the glutamine transporter SNAT5 into the extracellular space where it is taken up by neurons via SNAT1 and SNAT2 receptors. Glutamine in neurons is transformed into glutamate, and then γ-aminobutyric acid (GABA). Glutamate in brain tissue is in millimolar concentration (~1–2 mmol/L) and constitutes the metabolic pool of this amino acid. Glutamate packaged within synaptic vesicles is a very small fraction of this "metabolic" pool, and within these vesicles its concentration is ~20 mmol/L. Synaptic vesicle glutamate is released in a calcium-dependent manner on electrical stimulation, and its action is excitatory in neurotransmission. This metabolism illustrates the concept of the "Glutamate–Glutamine Cycle" in the brain (**Fig. 66.2**) (5). The enzyme GS functions at near maximal capacity during normal physiologic conditions (6). The brain's capacity to synthesize glutamine can be easily exceeded and hyperammonemia rapidly ensues. One of the hypotheses (extrapolated from animal studies) for the induction of brain edema during hyperammonemia is decreased expression of SNAT5 and the consequent trapping of glutamine inside the astrocyte, thereby resulting in cell swelling and brain edema. Glutamine is not only an osmotic agent but also a direct participant in the release of glutamate by surrounding

TABLE 66.1

CAUSES OF METABOLIC ENCEPHALOPATHIES CLASSIFIED ACCORDING TO PATHOPHYSIOLOGY

Endogenous Intoxication

Hyperammonemia and liver disease
   Urea cycle disorders
   Reye syndrome
   Hepatic encephalopathy
Organic acid disorders: MSUD, PA, MMA, IVA, 3HiB-uria, GA type I
Ketoacidosis
Wilson disease

Energy Failure

Hypoglycemia: hyperinsulinism, GSD
Mitochondrial defects: PDH deficiency, pyruvate carboxylase deficiency, respiratory chain deficiency
FAODs
Thiamine deficiency
BBGD

Water, Electrolyte, and Endocrine Disturbances

Disorders of osmolality: DKA and nonketotic hyperosmolar coma, hyponatremia, hypernatremia
Hypocalcemia
Hypercalcemia
Hypomagnesemia
Hypophosphatemia
Thyroid disorders
Intestinal diseases that induce encephalopathy
Burn encephalopathy

FAODs, fatty acid oxidation disorders; BBGD, biotin-responsive basal ganglia disease; MMA, methylmalonic aciduria; IVA, isovaleric aciduria; 3HiB-uria, 3-hydroxyisobutyric aciduria; GA type I, glutaric aciduria type I; MSUD, maple syrup urine disease; PA, propionic aciduria; GSD, glycogen storage disorders; PDH, pyruvate dehydrogenase; DKA, diabetic ketoacidosis.

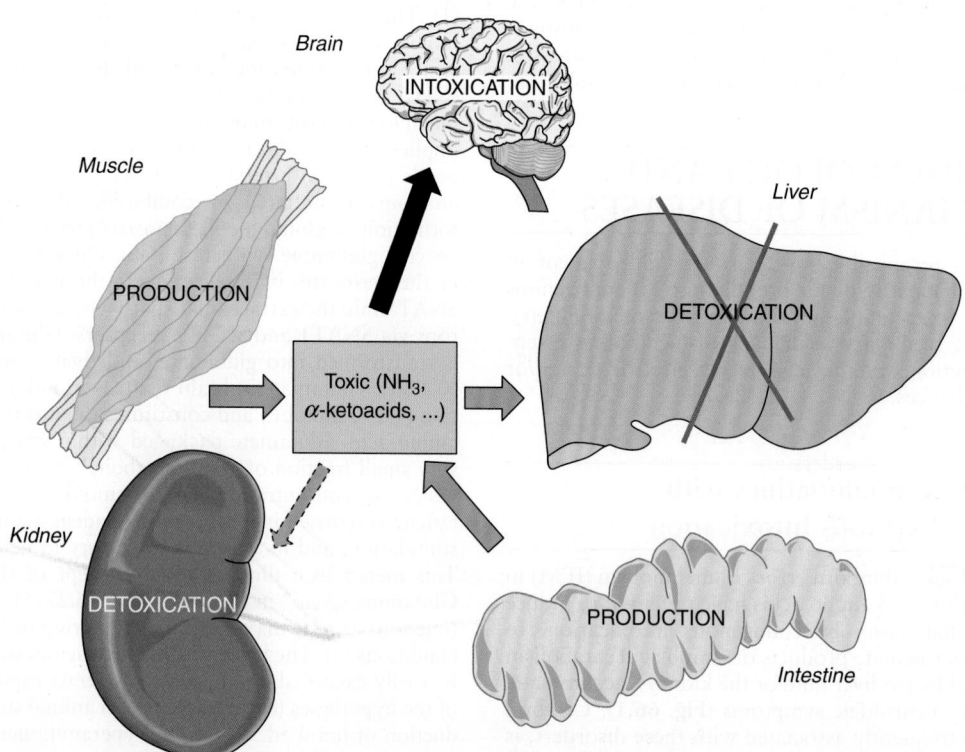

FIGURE 66.1. Endogenous intoxication model: impairment of nitrogen metabolism due to liver failure or inborn error of catabolic pathway of amino acids. The nitrogen produced by the intestine and muscle amino acid catabolism is not properly metabolized, resulting in toxic accumulation and brain damage. (Adapted from Rabier D [Biochemical Laboratory, Necker Hospital, France].)

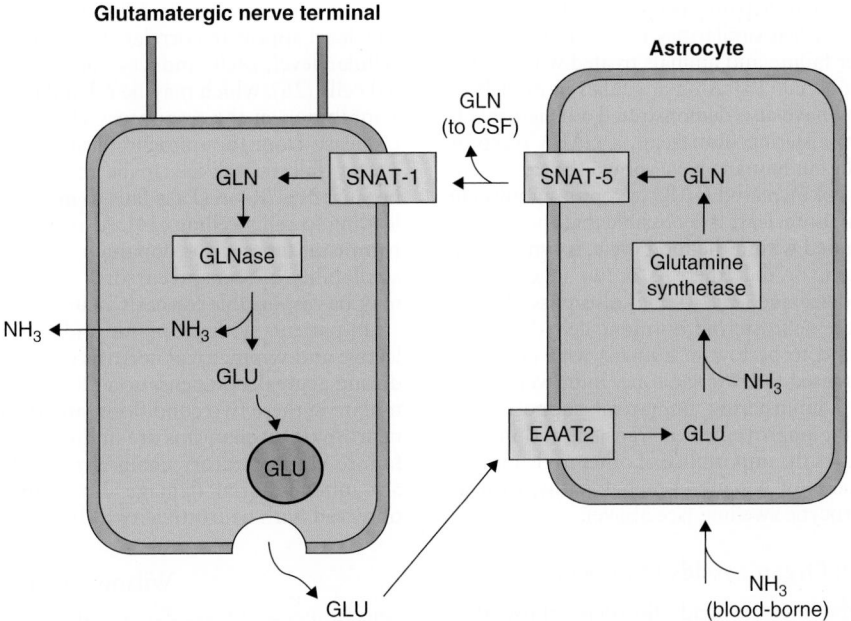

FIGURE 66.2. Schematic representation of a glutamate/glutamine cycle. The figure illustrates position of the astrocytic glutamine synthetase (GS), neuronal glutaminase (GLNase), the astrocytic glutamate transporter EAAT-2, and the astrocyte and neuron. (From Desjardins P, Du T, Jiang W, et al. Pathogenesis of hepatic encephalopathy and brain edema in acute liver failure: Role of glutamine redefined. *Neurochem Int* 2012;60(7):690–6, with permission.) Gln, glutamine; Glu, glutamate; NH_3, ammonia; CSF, cerebral spinal fluid.

neurons. The downregulation of SNAT5 can result in a decrease in excitatory neurotransmission in the brain and lead to excessive neuroinhibition, which is characteristic of encephalopathy in hyperammonemia (5–8). Glutamine is also thought to disrupt mitochondrial permeability by interference with the mitochondria-permeability-transition process and liberation of free radicals through hydrolysis of ammonia, all subsequently leading to mitochondrial swelling and dysfunction (9). Another hypothesis for hyperammonemia-induced encephalopathy is injury through the effect of increased production of glutamine that leads to an excess of extracellular glutamate, which induces neuronal hyperexcitability through activation of a subgroup of the glutamate family of receptors, the N-methyl-D-aspartate (NMDA) ionotropic receptors. Activation of NMDA receptors leads to depolarization and downstream changes in nitric oxide (NO) metabolism, disturbances in sodium/potassium adenosine triphosphatase (Na^+/K^+-ATPase) function, mitochondrial dysfunction, energy failure, and oxidative stress, together causing cell death (10). Finally, a high level of ammonia has the potential for participating in causing brain injury and cerebral edema by inducing hyperemia in cerebral blood flow (CBF) and by impairing cerebral autoregulation (11,12).

A number of human disorders are associated with hyperammonemia. IEM with hyperammonemia include primary urea cycle enzyme defects and secondary inhibition of urea cycle metabolism by organic acidurias (i.e., propionic, methylmalonic aciduria) (1).

Urea Cycle Disorders

The urea cycle is the final common pathway for the excretion of waste nitrogen in mammals. For more details on these diseases, please refer to Chapter 113.

Reye-Like Illness

Reye-like illness is characterized by the combination of liver disease and metabolic encephalopathy. In 1980, the Centers for Disease Control defined Reye syndrome as requiring the

each of the following criteria for diagnosis: an acute noninflammatory encephalopathy with microvesicular fatty metamorphosis of the liver, confirmed by biopsy or autopsy; a threefold increase of transaminases and/or ammonia; absence of cerebrospinal fluid (CSF) pleocytosis; and no other reasonable explanation for neurologic presentation with hepatic abnormality (13). The last criterion requires careful consideration and clinical expertise to identify other potential conditions. Therefore, whether *Reye syndrome* should be accepted as a diagnostic label before all other possible causes have been excluded is debatable (14). In this setting, we prefer to use the term "Reye-like illness."

The clinical features and electron microscopy of liver biopsy in patients with Reye syndrome are compatible with hepatotoxicity caused by acute, reversible mitochondrial failure. Mitochondria provide most of the energy for hepatic cell function via oxidative phosphorylation through the tricarboxylic acid cycle (15). Reye syndrome has a number of potential causes, and it is likely that these involve a mechanism in which mitochondrial failure results in impaired glucose homeostasis, ammonia metabolism, and hepatocyte function.

Hepatic Encephalopathy

The pathophysiology of hepatic encephalopathy is far from being understood. Its main mechanistic cause may be through ammonia-induced neurotoxicity, that is, astrocytic swelling and cytotoxic brain injury (see above for discussion) (16,17). However, hyperammonemia is certainly not the only mechanism at fault since some patients with severe encephalopathy continue to have normal ammonia levels. The other potential mechanisms are multiple and complex, involving (a) the combined toxic effects of accumulated ammonia and glutamine, mercaptans, fatty acids, and phenol; (b) increased "GABAergic tone"; (c) changes in BBB; and (d) disturbances in neurotransmission (18,19).

The "increased GABAergic tone" hypothesis, which is supported by the presence of increased benzodiazepine receptor ligand levels in patients with hepatic encephalopathy, was first considered a possibility when similarities between evoked potential in rats with liver failure and animals treated with GABA receptor agonists were noted (13). Animal studies in models of hepatic encephalopathy have also demonstrated a beneficial effect on arousal of administering flumazenil, a GABA receptor antagonist. A few studies in humans have shown the same benefit (20), but the origin of increased GABA receptor agonists in hepatic encephalopathy is unclear; it is possible that the agonist or a precursor is contained within the food cycle, is synthesized by gastrointestinal flora, or that there is occult ingestion of pharmaceutical benzodiazepine (21,22). It is also possible that endogenous levels of the neurosteroid hormone dehydroepiandrosterone sulfate, found to be low in humans with cirrhosis, may contribute to increased GABAergic tone. Improvement in encephalopathy after administering flumazenil supports this hypothesis. However, the improvement is transient and incomplete, which demonstrates the importance of other toxic mechanisms in the pathogenesis of hepatic encephalopathy, such as glutamine-induced astrocytic swelling (see above).

Amino and Organic Acids Disorders

Among the amino and organic acid disorders, those that most frequently cause patients to be admitted to the PICU for acute metabolic encephalopathy are maple syrup urine disease (MSUD), propionic aciduria (PA), and methylmalonic aciduria. Hyperammonemia and/or the accumulation of intermediate metabolites (due to downstream enzyme defects) are involved in the pathophysiology of acute encephalopathy and are reversible with specific treatment.

In MSUD, deficiency of branched-chain ketoacid dehydrogenase disrupts the normal breakdown of branched-chain amino acids (i.e., leucine, isoleucine, and valine) and leads to accumulation of branched-chain amino acids and branched-chain ketoacids. In acute encephalopathic crises, there is a high risk of cerebral edema and brain stem herniation (23,24). The mechanism of brain edema is not completely understood but is related to the neurochemical changes caused by the accumulation of leucine and α-keto isocaproic acid (αKIC, derivative product of leucine accumulation), with depletion of neurotransmitters (glutamate, GABA, and dopamine). Plasma

leucine concentration and duration of exposure to a high leucine level appear to correlate with encephalopathy (25). At the cellular level, αKIC induces apoptosis in rat glial and neuronal cells (26), which may be related to αKIC-induced complex 1 inhibition in the respiratory chain followed by cytochrome c release from the mitochondria in the cytosol (26,27). This energy failure is likely to be responsible for cerebral edema because Na^+/K^+-ATPase fails to maintain membrane gradients leading to cell swelling (24). Also, immediate depletion of neurotransmitters such as dopamine and serotonin, by limiting the availability of their precursors (i.e., tyrosine and tryptophan), may be responsible for early neurobehavioral changes (28).

In patients with propionic and methylmalonic aciduria, selective and symmetrical necrosis of the globi pallidi is observed during acute decompensation (29). Many toxic products accumulate in these two conditions, and their respective underlying neurotoxic mechanisms are unknown, but may involve energy failure via respiratory chain enzyme deficiencies and secondary mitochondrial damage. Hyperammonemia is frequently observed with neurotoxicity (30).

Wilson Disease

Wilson disease is associated with an initial neurologic presentation between the ages of 10 and 20 years in one-third of cases. In this disorder, oxidative damage may be caused by accumulation of copper in the basal ganglia (31).

Encephalopathies Associated with Energy Failure

Any mechanism that reduces brain energy supply may lead to encephalopathy. This process occurs in hypoxemia–ischemia, when energy substrates are decreased for other reasons. Cerebral energy is supplied by mitochondria, and the principal metabolic fuel in the brain is glucose (**Fig. 66.3**). As the encephalopathy is secondary to energy deprivation, specific therapeutic strategies that decrease cerebral energy demands and increase energy production, when possible, are required to restore brain function.

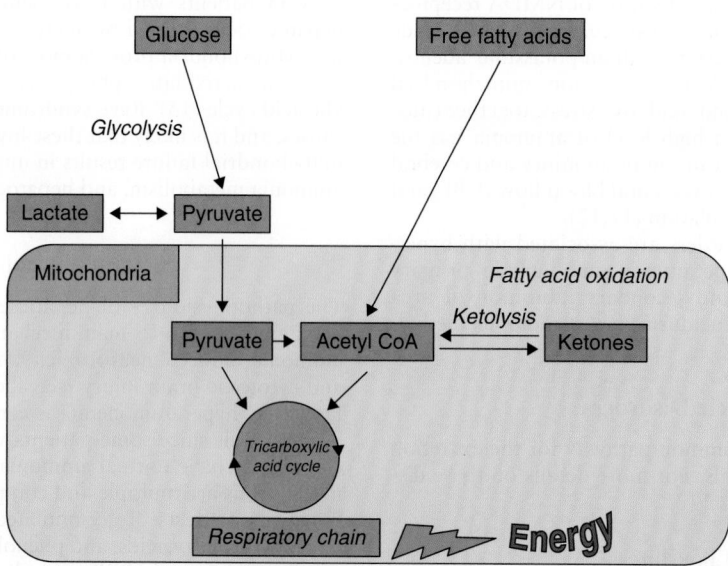

FIGURE 66.3. Energy failure model of metabolic encephalopathy. Hypoglycemia and any enzyme defect in mitochondrial energy production may result in metabolic encephalopathy. The pathophysiology of metabolic encephalopathy by fatty acid oxidation defect is multifactorial.

Hypoglycemia

Under normal conditions, the brain relies on a constant supply of glucose from the blood for oxidative metabolism and function. It stores only a little glycogen in astrocytes and does not perform gluconeogenesis. Glucose has to be transported across the BBB via glucose transporter proteins expressed in the brain, mainly as the GLUT-1 glucose transporter. Mutations in this gene are associated with hypoglycorrhachia without hypoglycemia. Disorder of carbohydrate metabolism, glycogen storage disease, hyperinsulinism, and fatty acid oxidation disorders (FAODs) and certain disorders of amino acid metabolisms may present with severe hypoglycemia. During prolonged fasting, the brain can switch to lactate oxidation and increase ketone body uptake to partially restore energy balance. At a critical glucose concentration, however, the brain receives inadequate glucose to support its needs (32). Specific neurons of the superficial cerebral cortex, basal ganglia, and hippocampus are most vulnerable, but lesions in white matter have also been reported.

The mechanism to explain the profound hypoglycemic effects on neurons appears to be mediated by both an early tetrotodo toxin–sensitive component and a more prolonged period of toxic NMDA receptor activation (33). Of importance, correction of plasma glucose concentration alone does not interrupt this cell death process. Oxidative DNA damage seems to be critical in the sequence of events leading to hypoglycemia-induced neuronal injury (34–37), but the source and mechanism of oxidant are not completely understood. Mitochondria have been implicated as a source of neuronal superoxide production in glutamate excitotoxicity and contribute to hypoglycemia-induced neuronal death. Furthermore, it has been proved that reactive oxygen species are generated in neurons at the time of glucose reperfusion. Oxidation of reduced nicotinamide adenine dinucleotide phosphate (NADPH) is the primary source of superoxide generation in the hypoglycemic reperfusion process. Reactive oxygen species can damage DNA, which in turn induces poly-(ADP ribose) polymerase 1 (PARP-1), which consumes much ATP and imposes further bioenergetic stress on the neuronal energy supply during hypoglycemia-induced neuronal death (38,39).

Primary Mitochondrial Energy Metabolism Defects

Mitochondria are essential in cellular energy metabolism and cellular homeostasis. They also play a key role in the mitochondrial pathway to apoptosis. Cellular respiration's first stage takes place in the inner mitochondrial membrane and consists of glycolysis of carbohydrates into pyruvate. The pyruvate is transported to the inner mitochondrial matrix, where it is converted to acetyl coenzyme A (acetyl CoA). The Krebs cycle achieves complete oxidation of acetyl CoA to produce two molecules of carbon dioxide and conserve free energy in the form of NADH (reduced form of nicotinamide adenine dinucleotide) and $FADH_2$ (reduced form of flavin adenine dinucleotide). Therefore, its major function is catabolic. Amino acids, fatty acids, and carbohydrates can enter mitochondria as intermediates of the Krebs cycle. Then, the reaction of oxidative phosphorylation takes place in the mitochondrial matrix, for which NADH and $FADH_2$ are the "substrates." The electron transport chain (a series of respiratory complexes) results in phosphorylation of the majority of cellular ADP to ATP.

Mitochondrial disorders result in impaired respiratory chain activity or impaired oxidative phosphorylation. Tissues with high-energy demand are most commonly involved in mitochondrial diseases: neurons, myocardial and skeletal muscles, liver, and kidneys. The brain is particularly vulnerable, given the neuronal requirement for ATP to maintain ionic gradients for electrical activity. The basal ganglia and their high metabolic needs are particularly at risk for insult. Primary defects in mitochondrial energy metabolism include pyruvate dehydrogenase (PDH) complex deficiency, tricarboxylic acid cycle deficiencies, and respiratory chain defects. These diseases can be caused by mutations in the mitochondrial DNA (maternal or sporadic transmission), mutations in nuclear DNA (Mendelian transmission), or defects of communication between the nuclear and mitochondrial genome. The term mitochondrial encephalomyopathies was first used in 1977 to describe the CNS implications in patients with mitochondrial alterations in their muscle biopsies (40). The clinical presentation of a mitochondrial disease in children is often nonspecific with myopathy associated with CNS involvement, such as cognitive impairment, ataxia, seizures, and impaired consciousness (somnolence to coma). These clinical problems may manifest early in life, in childhood, or later in life. Altered conscious state is particularly frequent in Leigh syndrome. Necrosis of the basal ganglia and brain stem nuclei, and stroke-like cortical lesions are often features of mitochondriopathies; nonspecific findings on brain imaging are also common (see Chapter 59) (41). Most of these diseases are currently untreatable.

FAODs comprise another group of diseases with impaired mitochondrial energy metabolism. The encephalopathy observed in these diseases is not fully understood and may result from multifactorial insults, including limited fuel for the brain due to hypoglycemia along with abnormally low ketones, hyperammonemia, and a decrease in CBF due to circulatory failure (42).

Thiamine Deficiency

Thiamine (vitamin B1) has an important role in several metabolic processes. It is an essential coenzyme in the pentose phosphate pathway and the tricarboxylic acid (Krebs) cycle. The pentose phosphate pathway contains the enzyme transketolase that requires thiamine diphosphate to function. In the tricarboxylic acid cycle, thiamine acts as a coenzyme, with magnesium as a cofactor, in the decarboxylation of pyruvate (the pyruvate dehydrogenate complex) and in the α-ketoglutarate dehydrogenase (α-KGHD) complex. It also participates in the conversion of five-carbon to six-carbon sugars by means of the enzyme transketolase (43). Thiamine deficiency, therefore, decreases the amount of energy available to the brain and increases the concentrations of several metabolites. Patients nourished with total parenteral nutrition are at risk for thiamine deficiency if they also have renal losses of thiamine (e.g., patients on chronic dialysis) or increased thiamine requirements because of systemic illness. Other causes of thiamine deficiency include organ transplant, gastrointestinal surgery, malignancy, and acquired immunodeficiency syndrome. In adults, thiamine deficiency is most often seen in chronic alcoholism. Administration of glucose to severely thiamine-deficient patients can deplete stores even further and acutely exacerbate an encephalopathy and heart failure. It is always more prudent to administer thiamine in the at-risk population before glucose administration and refeeding after starvation (11). The features are highly variable and may manifest by sudden collapse and death, or seizures, or by the classic, but extremely rare, triad of gait ataxia, confusion, and ocular abnormalities (44). If missed, it can lead rapidly to death.

Encephalopathies with Acute Water, Electrolyte, and/or Endocrine Disturbances

Disorders of Osmolality

The osmolality of a solution is determined by the particles in that solution. Sodium, glucose, and urea are the primary osmoles of the extracellular space. Potassium is the primary osmole of the intracellular space. Because cell membranes are permeable to water, an osmotic equilibrium is maintained. That is, the volume of intracellular fluid is determined by the osmolality of the extracellular space. Hypernatremia and hyperglycemia are the major causes of serum hyperosmolality, and hyponatremia is the major cause of serum hypo-osmolality. Any modification of brain water volume may result in acute encephalopathy.

Diabetic Ketoacidosis and Nonketotic Hyperosmolar Coma

Cerebral edema in diabetic ketoacidosis (DKA) typically occurs in the first 12 hours after the onset of treatment, but can be present before treatment initiation (45). The mechanism of cerebral edema is not well understood, but evidence points toward different mechanisms. Cerebral imaging and image-based calculations of water distribution and cerebral perfusion during treatment of uncomplicated DKA showed an expansion of the extracellular space relative to the intracellular space and increased CBF (46,47). These findings are consistent with a vasogenic process and a perturbed BBB (48) (increase in cerebral capillary endothelial permeability) function, rather than osmotic cell swelling, which is associated with expansion of the intracellular space. A mechanism leading to cerebral vasodilation and consequent vasogenic edema include an inflammatory process caused by the production of vasoactive cytokines by ketones; reperfusion injury of ischemic cerebral tissues during rehydration therapy; and loss of cerebral autoregulation (49). The accumulation of intracellular osmoles such as taurine and myoinositol may also play a role. These endogenous osmoles are generated in response to serum hyperosmolarity, to maintain adequate brain cell volume (50). They may induce cytotoxic edema as they take 12–24 hours to dissipate (51). Rehydration and insulin therapy cause a decrease in serum osmolarity and result in relative intracellular hyperosmolarity, and a shift of fluid from serum into brain cells. Regardless of the final mechanism, all authors agree that initial rehydration should be sufficient to restore hemodynamic stability and that the subsequent volume repletion should occur cautiously over a minimum of 48 hours.

PICU admission due to hyperosmolar hyperglycemic nonketotic coma is increasing in frequency because of the increasing problem of obesity in childhood. This condition shares a similar pathogenesis to the coma that can complicate DKA, but without the contribution from ketone body accumulation (52).

Hyponatremia

Osmotic disequilibrium between a low-osmolality plasma compartment and higher osmotic pressure within glial cells will result in astrocytic water accumulation and brain edema. Rapid decrease in sodium concentration (that develops within 12–24 hours) or level of sodium below 120 mEq/L is much more likely to cause severe edema. Hyponatremia may result from water retention, sodium loss, or both. Water retention is caused by inappropriate antidiuretic hormone secretion, inappropriate water intake with a low sodium diet, sodium loss from renal disease, vomiting, and diarrhea. Prolonged hyponatremia beyond 24–48 hours is associated with the loss of intracellular osmoles namely glutamate, whose purpose is to reequilibrate cellular osmolality but which are toxic to myelin. A too rapid correction of hyponatremia can induce central pontine myelinolysis (osmolar demyelination), a syndrome characterized by confusion, cranial nerve dysfunction, and, when severe, "locked-in" syndrome and quadriparesis (53).

Hypernatremia

Hypernatremia is associated with cellular dehydration, which affects brain function. Because the brain can compensate for slow or chronic changes in osmolality by producing intracellular idiogenic osmoles to retain water, acute changes, such as salt poisoning, should be treated quickly, whereas chronic changes should be treated slowly to avoid rebound cerebral edema. Hypernatremia is usually caused by dehydration (water loss exceeding sodium loss), diabetes insipidus, or overhydration with hypertonic saline solution. Patients with serum sodium greater than 160 mmol/L or serum osmolality greater than 350 mOsm/L may experience symptoms of lethargy, coma, and seizures. The most serious complication is dural sinus thrombosis, which happens with dehydration and hypovolemia but not saline toxicity (11).

Acute Uremic Encephalopathy—Dialysis Encephalopathy

Uremic encephalopathy typically occurs when renal glomerular function is less than 10%. It is worse in patients with acute rather than chronic renal failure and in patients with hepatorenal syndrome, given the kidney's inability to excrete ammonia. The severity of renal failure correlates with that of the uremic encephalopathy; however, the absolute level of urea and creatinine does not directly relate with the degree of encephalopathy (11). It is thought that many osmotically active toxins, which are not yet fully identified, participate in the pathogenesis of uremic encephalopathy. Organic compounds such as guanidine antagonize GABA receptors and are also agonists of NMDA receptors, thus leading to a disequilibrium between excitatory and inhibitory neurotransmission and increased cortical excitability. Disturbances in monoamine metabolism, decreased transport function, and increased permeability also participate in the neurologic disturbances in uremic encephalopathy. Hypertension, increased metabolites of drugs (like those of acyclovir), and elevated levels of opiates, all secondary to decreased kidney function, can also contribute to neurotoxicity (54,55). The treatment of uremic encephalopathy is dialysis (11). Dialysis encephalopathy is caused by the rapid shift of fluids and electrolytes between intracellular and extracellular spaces during and within 24 hours of dialysis, and may be associated with acute, transitory neurologic disturbances. Clinical symptoms consist of confusion, headache, nausea, vomiting, tremor, and myoclonus. Cerebral edema may be seen secondary to urea gradient between brain cells and blood.

Calcium, Magnesium, and Phosphate Disorders

Calcium is the major divalent cation in the extracellular fluid. It is an important regulator of cellular function and is essential for many cellular processes, especially neurotransmission. Severe hypocalcemia or hypercalcemia may induce encephalopathy.

Magnesium is the second most abundant intracellular cation in the body, and it is required for the maintenance of normal cellular activity. It is a cofactor of numerous enzymes that are vital for energy metabolism. Hypomagnesemia (usually in association with other electrolyte abnormalities, such as hypocalcemia) or hypermagnesemia may induce encephalopathy.

Hypophosphatemia may also cause neurologic dysfunction.

Other Causes of Encephalopathy

Autoimmune thyroid disorders, both hyperthyroidism (Grave disease) and hypothyroidism (Hashimoto thyroiditis), affect the CNS and may lead to encephalopathy and coma (56).

In terms of intestinal diseases that can induce encephalopathy, intestinal intussusception and abdominal surgery in children may be associated with altered levels of consciousness. The explanations for this clinical presentation include endogenous opioid poisoning caused by massive release of endorphins during paroxysms of pain; release of neurotoxic vasoactive peptides; and neuroactive gut hormones in reaction to gastrointestinal ischemia, dehydration, and electrolyte imbalance.

In burn encephalopathy, a few days after severe burn injury, awareness, and responsiveness may decline without any change in neurologic examination. The mechanism is not known. It may be related to an outpouring of stress hormones and cytokines after the massive inflammatory response, or to high doses of narcotics and/or sleep deprivation.

Sepsis-related encephalopathy is a common form of brain dysfunction. Its pathophysiology is not fully understood, but appears to involve the inflammatory cascade, direct mediator-induced cellular damage to the brain, mitochondrial and endothelial dysfunction, disturbed neurotransmission, and derangement in cerebral calcium homeostasis (57). CBF may also be affected (11).

DIAGNOSIS

In some circumstances, the patient's diagnosis is clear at the time of admission to the PICU, and specific treatment can be started almost immediately. This is the case in two-thirds of patients with IEMs who are admitted to the PICU (58). In the remainder of cases, the challenge is to quickly diagnose treatable disorders so as to ensure prompt treatment and reduce morbidity and mortality. In these cases, often infants, the clinical approach to diagnosis is based on a combination of careful history taking, complete physical examination and laboratory investigations. The possibility of metabolic encephalopathy must be considered in parallel with other common conditions, such as sepsis, hypoxic–ischemic encephalopathy, encephalitis, exogenous intoxication, and brain tumors.

General Clinical Presentation

Metabolic encephalopathy may present within hours or days with progressive confusion, diverse motor and sensory abnormalities, and rarely hallucinations. Patients must be assessed as soon as possible, and certainly before they deteriorate into coma (see Chapter 57). As the metabolic illness progresses, there may be increasing stupor or coma associated with progressive neurological abnormalities of tone, posture, and movements. At a more advanced state, problems with respiratory control and abnormalities such as hiccups, apnea, and bradypnea may occur. In addition, other autonomic and homeostatic functions may be lost and result in bradycardia and hypothermia.

A careful history may indicate the right diagnosis, in some circumstances, for example, the polyuria and polydipsia that precede the encephalopathy in DKA, or an infusion of hypotonic solutions in the perioperative hyponatremia-related encephalopathy. In other circumstances, especially in the case of IEM, the history is not obvious and requires specific details of the events that preceded any behavioral change. Drug exposure (see below), personal history and family history must be carefully reviewed. Acute encephalopathy may occur at any age from the neonatal period to adulthood. The following events may trigger acute encephalopathy.

Prolonged Fasting

Children with endogenous intoxication and FAODs may deteriorate with fasting, because during this state protein catabolism is increased and free fatty acid is the preferred fuel.

Anesthesia and Surgery

Both anesthesia and surgery induce metabolic stress and increased energy demand and, therefore, increased protein catabolism.

Infections

Infections also induce protein catabolism and increased energy demand (59). The typical cause of acute onset in infants is gastrointestinal infection, which combines the effect of infection on metabolism along with the effect of fasting on metabolism.

Prolonged Exercise

Patients with endogenous intoxication and FAODs may decompensate with prolonged exercise, because exercise promotes protein catabolism and increases free fatty acid use (42).

Drugs

Valproic acid may worsen the state of patients with urea cycle disorders (60) and respiratory chain disorders because of drug-induced enzyme inhibition. Steroids and adrenocorticotropic hormone increase protein catabolism.

High Protein Intake

Protein intake is restricted in patients with endogenous intoxication disorders, especially urea cycle disorders. Noncompliance to the diet, typically occurring during holidays and parties, may lead to acute attack.

An IEM should be suspected when the following history is found: (a) recurrent or episodic lethargy and coma; (b) unexplained death in the family or any neonatal death, even if it was attributed to another cause (e.g., sepsis, anoxia, etc.); and (c) consanguinity. Although most genetic disorders are hereditary and transmitted as recessive inheritance, the majority of cases appear sporadically in developed countries because of small family size and infrequent consanguinity.

The clinical features of metabolic encephalopathy are usually nonspecific and therefore IEM should be considered in the differential diagnosis of any sick neonate or infant presenting with poor feeding, lethargy, hypotonia, vomiting, or failure to thrive. There are a few classic presentations. In the comatose state, characteristic changes in muscular tone and involuntary movements appear in some diseases. In the classic form of MSUD, infants present at a few days of age with generalized hypertonic episodes, muscle rigidity, and opisthotonos. Boxing or pedaling movements in the limbs, and slow limb elevations (spontaneous or upon stimulation) are also observed. In organic aciduria, axial hypotonia and limb hypertonia with large amplitude tremors and myoclonic jerks, which are often mistaken for convulsions, are observed. Intracranial hypertension, secondary to cerebral edema and seizures, is a frequent presenting symptom in metabolic encephalopathies. Focal signs are sometimes seen, even in the context of a diffuse metabolic encephalopathy, such as hyponatremia or hypoglycemia. These focal signs can mimic a stroke in certain mitochondrial encephalopathies. Other patients with organic acidemias and urea cycle defects present with focal neurologic signs and cerebral edema. These patients can be mistakenly diagnosed as having cerebrovascular accident or cerebral tumor.

Hepatomegaly may be observed, especially in organic acidemia, FAOD, Wilson disease, hyperinsulinism, and glycogen storage diseases. An *abnormal urine or body odor* is present in some diseases in which volatile metabolites accumulate. In urine, an abnormal odor can be detected on a drying paper, or by opening a container of urine that has been closed at room temperature for a few minutes. The three most important examples are the fruity smell of ketoacids in DKA, the maple syrup odor of MSUD, and the sweaty feet odor of isovaleric acidemia.

TABLE 66.2

LABORATORY INVESTIGATIONS IN METABOLIC ENCEPHALOPATHY

	■ ROUTINE TESTS	■ STORAGE OF SAMPLES AND METABOLIC TESTS[a]
Urine	Smell (special odor) Look (special color) Acetone (Acetest) Ketoacids (DNPH)[b] pH Electrolytes (Na$^+$, K$^+$) Urea, creatinine	Fresh sample in the refrigerator, frozen sample at $-20°C$, for metabolic testing (AAC, OAC, orotic acid)
Blood	Electrolytes (Na$^+$, K$^+$, Cl$^-$, HCO$_3^-$) Glucose, Ca^{2+}, Mg^{2+}, phosphate Urea, creatinine Osmolality Blood gases Transaminases, bilirubin, GGT (Gamma Glutamyl Transferases) Ammonia Lactic acid Creatine kinase Blood cell count Prothrombin time	Plasma heparinized at $-20°C$ (5 mL) Whole blood (10 mL) collected on EDTA at $-20°C$ (for molecular biology studies) Plasma or blood on filter paper for acylcarnitine dosage Redox status if lactate >10 mmol/L (AAC, OAC, acylcarnitines)
Miscellaneous	CSF if no intracranial hypertension with concentration of lactate and pyruvate	CSF (1 mL) frozen for AAC *Other metabolic tests:* Skin biopsy for fibroblast culture; If death: liver and muscle biopsy

[a]Tests should be discussed with specialists in metabolic diseases.
[b]This test screens for the presence of α-keto acids, as occur in MSUD. It can be replaced by an AAC, if available, in an emergency situation.
DNPH, dinitrophenylhydrazine test; EDTA, ethylenediaminetetraacetic acid; OAC, organic acid chromatography; AA, amino acid chromatography; GGT, gamma glutamyl-transférases; CSF, cerebral spinal fluid.

Laboratory Investigations

General supportive measures and metabolic laboratory investigations should be initiated as soon as the possibility of metabolic encephalopathy is suspected. The initial approach for investigations is outlined in **Table 66.2**. It is important to perform these investigations as early as possible, and all laboratory tests should be obtained simultaneously, as most disorders may produce only intermittent abnormalities. If rapid metabolic and genetic analysis is impossible, a critical sample of blood and urine can be drawn and analyzed later on. Venous blood should be collected in an ammonia-free, heparinized blood tube, placed on ice at the bedside, and transferred quickly to the laboratory, where the plasma should be separated immediately. By conducting immediate laboratory investigations, the encephalopathies caused by acute water and electrolyte disturbances are rapidly evaluated. For further discussion on the causes of these disturbances, see Chapters 106–108 and 113. IEM are more difficult to diagnose, and some biologic signs should prompt consideration of such disorders (**Table 66.3**).

The determination of plasma ammonia concentration is crucial when metabolic encephalopathy is suspected because hyperammonemia is a life-threatening condition and necessitates urgent management. Moderate *hyperammonemia* (80–150 μmol/L) is frequently observed in IEM owing to a secondary blockade of the urea cycle. Severe hyperammonemia (>300 μmol/L) is observed in primary urea cycle defects, organic acid disorders, and FAOD. Hyperammonemia must be interpreted cautiously, as a falsely high level may be due to technical problems at the time of sampling and transfer to the laboratory. Two tests of ammonia level, obtained using the proper technique, are required to ensure the diagnosis. Hyperammonemia with abnormalities in liver function tests is seen in acute liver failure and Reye syndrome.

Metabolic acidosis with increased anion gap is observed in intermediate acid accumulation, such as organic acid disorders (propionic and methylmalonic acid). Metabolic acidosis also may be present in amino acid disorders, mitochondrial disorders, and disorders of carbohydrate metabolism. The anion gap results from the presence of abnormal metabolites, such as organic acid, ketoacids, or lactic acid.

Hyperlactatemia, elevated lactic acid, in the absence of sepsis or tissue hypoxia, is a significant finding. Moderate elevation (3–6 mmol/L or 270–550 mg/L) is often observed in organic acid disorders and glycogen storage disorders (GSDs). A level above 6 mmol/L (550 mg/L) is seen mainly in primary mitochondrial energy metabolism defects. In such circumstances, the simultaneous measurement of lactate-to-pyruvate ratio and 3-hydroxybutyrate-to-acetoacetate ratio (on a plasma sample that is immediately deproteinized at the bedside) is useful to assess the cytoplasmic and mitochondrial redox states, respectively (61). Ketones (acetoacetate and 3-hydroxybutyrate) are a product of fatty acid oxidation. *Hypoglycemia without ketonuria* is observed in FAOD and hyperinsulinism.

Neutropenia can be seen in organic acidemias. *Myoglobinuria* is an indicator of FAOD.

Neurophysiology and Neuroimaging

Neurophysiology

Regardless of etiology, electroencephalography (EEG) during an acute encephalopathic process usually shows varying degrees of slow activity. The severity of slowing usually correlates well with the severity of the encephalopathy. This slowing is nonspecific and reflects cortical and subcortical dysfunction. Triphasic waves were initially considered specific to hepatic coma but are now recognized in

TABLE 66.3

ALGORITHM FOR THE DIAGNOSIS OF IEM REVEALED BY ENCEPHALOPATHY

■ CLINICAL PRESENTATION	■ PREDOMINANT METABOLIC DISTURBANCE	■ ASSOCIATED METABOLIC/ NEUROLOGIC DISTURBANCE	■ MOST FREQUENT DIAGNOSES (DISORDER/ENZYME DEFICIENCY)	■ DIFFERENTIAL DIAGNOSIS
Metabolic coma without focal neurologic signs	Metabolic acidosis	With ketosis	**Organic aciduria (MMA, PA, IVA, GA I, MSUD)** PC MCD **Ketolysis, gluconeogenesis**	Diabetes Exogenous intoxication Encephalitis
		Without ketosis	PDH **Ketogenesis defect** FAO FDP	
	Hyperammonemia	Normal glucose	**Urea cycle defects**	Reye syndrome Encephalitis Exogenous intoxication
		Hypoglycemia	FAO HMG CoA lyase	
	Hypoglycemia	With acidosis	**Gluconeogenesis, MSUD, HMG CoA lyase** FAO	
		Without acidosis	FAO **Hyperinsulinism**	
	Hyperlactatemia	Normal glucose	PC MCD Krebs cycle PDH Respiratory chain disorder	
		Hypoglycemia	**Gluconeogenesis** FAO GSD	
Neurologic coma with focal signs, seizures, severe intracranial hypertension, strokes or stroke-like episodes	Biologic signs are variable, can be absent or moderate	Cerebral edema wo other lesions	MSUD OTC	Cerebral tumor Migraine Encephalitis
		Hemiplegia or hemianopsia	MSUD OTC MMA PA	
		Extrapyramidal signs	MMA GA I Wilson Homocystinuria	
		Caudate nucleus and putamen necrosis	BBGD Urea cycle defect MMA PA IVA	
		Stroke-like	Respiratory chain disorder CDG syndrome **Thiamine responsive megaloblastic anemia**	Moya moya syndrome, Vascular hemiplegia Cerebral sinus thrombosis Cerebral tumor

Treatable disorders appear in bold type.
MMA, methylmalonic academia; PA, propionic aciduria; IVA, isovaleric aciduria; GA I, glutaric aciduria type I; PC, pyruvate carboxylase; MCD, multiple carboxylase deficiency; FAO, fatty acid oxidation; FDP, fructose-1,6-diphosphatase; HMG CoA lyase, 3-hydroxy-3-methylglutaryl coenzyme A lyase; OTC, ornithine transcarbamylase; BBGD, biotin-responsive basal ganglia disease; CDG, carbohydrate-deficient glycoprotein.

different metabolic conditions. When clinical seizures occur, the EEG can provide information as to the severity of the epileptic condition. Seizures are easily recognized in metabolic encephalopathies, and, rarely, an EEG can also reveal subclinical epileptiform activity (62). A burst-suppression pattern that is not due to medication is associated with poor prognosis.

Neuroimaging

Cerebral computed tomography (CT) scan is essential when evaluating a comatose patient (see Chapter 57). If any clinical signs of intracranial hypertension are present, a CT scan should be obtained after the patient has been stabilized (i.e., adequacy of oxygenation and systemic perfusion, treatment of fluid and electrolyte imbalance, optimization of temperature control, etc.). The CT scan will help to evaluate the severity of cerebral edema. For example, the absence of CSF spaces above the tentorium and obliteration of the basal cisterns are associated with raised intracranial pressure. Also, some specific lesions may be observed in white matter or basal ganglia in organic acid disorders and mitochondrial disorders, respectively (63) (see Chapter 59).

Magnetic resonance imaging (MRI) of the brain is much more informative than CT scan, and specific abnormalities may suggest diagnosis of certain pathologies, such as mitochondrial encephalopathies (64). Magnetic resonance spectroscopy (MRS) can also provide clues to underlying neurologic processes by evaluating various brain metabolites, such as brain tissue lactate concentration, thus avoiding the risk of lumbar puncture, especially in cases with cerebral edema (65–67). Proton MRS can be useful in monitoring response to therapy (68,69).

Differential Diagnosis

The nonspecific clinical presentation, the many possible etiologies, and the presence of intermittent abnormalities may explain why metabolic encephalopathy is sometimes not diagnosed early. In clinical practice, it is not rare to find a history of previous unexplained coma in a patient hospitalized for a recurrent attack (70).

Infection/Sepsis

An infection may be responsible for acute encephalitis, or it may be the event that precipitates the acute metabolic deterioration.

Exogenous Intoxication: Poisons, Substance Abuse, and Drug Overdoses

Most accidental poisonings occur in small children younger than 2 years of age who ingest common household products. The ingestion is usually discovered quickly. The differential diagnosis may be difficult in cases of unrevealed intentional poisoning, such as in Munchausen syndrome by proxy.

The diagnosis of metabolic encephalopathy should be suspected when vaguely defined diagnoses (e.g., encephalitis, basilar migraine, intoxication, poisoning, or stroke) are suggested, especially in the presence of moderate ketoacidosis, hyperlactatemia, or hyperammonemia.

MANAGEMENT

General Management

The assessment and management of the infant or child with an altered level of consciousness is a pediatric emergency. A review of the appropriate clinical approach, including resuscitation and institution of initial therapy of the comatose child, is discussed in Chapter 57. Neurologic support includes attention to adequate oxygenation and perfusion, fluid and electrolyte balance, temperature control, seizure control, management of possible intracranial hypertension, and prevention of infection. The treatment of many of the diseases causing metabolic encephalopathy is covered in other chapters of this book. However, in the context of a child referred with presumed or identified metabolic encephalopathy, specific neurologic support is necessary, as discussed below.

Management of Intracranial Hypertension

The only circumstance in which the management of intracranial hypertension differs from the usual care in traumatic brain injury is in the presence of severe hyperammonemia (>300 μmol/L).

As explained in the Hyperammonemia and Liver Diseases section, the BBB has much lower permeability to NH_4^+ than to NH_3. For this reason, despite the lack of supportive clinical research, we recommend avoidance of respiratory alkalosis from excessive hyperventilation, and targeting of pH level at ~7.35 by titrating mechanical ventilation and sedation. This maneuver should be carried out until there is a sustained decrease in ammonia. In regard to spontaneous hypocapnia in the spontaneously breathing patient, some clinicians may be concerned about the risk of hypocapnia reducing CBF; however, it should be noted that in one experimental study hypocapnia did not decrease CBF during hyperammonemia (71).

Intracranial pressure monitoring is not routinely performed in metabolic encephalopathy because of the potential for rapid improvement with treatment. However, in some circumstances, intracranial pressure monitoring may be helpful in management to maintain an adequate cerebral perfusion pressure. No consensus exits on the indications of intracranial pressure monitoring in the PICU for patients with acute liver failure. In adults, such monitoring is considered for patients listed for orthotopic liver transplant with stage III/IV encephalopathy (72).

The use of near infrared spectroscopy for noninvasive cerebral oxygenation monitoring and the use of transcranial Doppler ultrasound (with assessment of pulsatility index, peak systolic flow minus end diastolic flow velocity divided by mean flow velocity) may help to detect changes in cerebral hemodynamics and guide management (73).

Seizure Control

In the case of hyperammonemia or suspicion of mitochondrial disorder, seizures should be treated to prevent secondary neurological insult; however, valproic acid is contraindicated.

Temperature Control

The use of therapeutic hypothermia in metabolic encephalopathy has not been studied extensively (74). Although the concept of reducing brain metabolism and secondary toxin production is appealing (72), the evidence for using such therapy in other pathologic brain conditions in children (e.g., traumatic injury and hypoxic–ischemic injury) has been discouraging. Fever should be prevented and treated.

Specific Treatment

Many of the specific metabolic therapies oriented toward the underlying process and etiology of encephalopathy are covered elsewhere in the book. This discussion is restricted to some key therapeutic considerations.

Diabetic Ketoacidosis

When patients with DKA have symptoms of cerebral edema, the rate of fluid administration should be reduced and rehydration should be carried out slowly over 48–72 hours. Mannitol (0.25–1 g/kg given intravenously over 20 minutes) or hypertonic saline (3% solution, 5–10 mL/kg over 30 minutes) may be used as an acute rescue for avoidance of cerebral herniation (75).

Initial Treatment of Suspected Inborn Error of Metabolism

If an IEM is suspected, then the aim is to reduce formation of toxic metabolites, by decreasing substrate availability, and to prevent catabolism, by providing adequate calories.

Concretely, the infant should be adequately hydrated. All oral intake should be stopped to eliminate protein, galactose, and fructose ingestion. Calories should be provided in the form of high-dose intravenous glucose to limit protein catabolism (which will treat endogenous intoxication). The rate of glucose infusion should be high, so that enough energy is generated via glycolysis. This therapy will also apply to FAODs and keto-acidosis. A central line is necessary to provide concentrated solutions of glucose, and the goal is to infuse 1000 kcal/m^2/d, which may require the addition of insulin infusion so as to avoid hyperglycemia.

As soon as an endogenous intoxication is diagnosed, nutritional support and other pharmacologic agents should be discussed with the specialist, and it can include the following:

- *Promotion of protein anabolism*: glucose and lipid, without proteins, preferably by enteral continuous feeding with a caloric intake of at least 1500 kcal/m^2/d. When the diagnosis is confirmed, special amino acid mixtures are used to supply nontoxic amino acids. For example, in MSUD, the enzyme defect involves the branched-chain amino acids (leucine, valine, and isoleucine) and feeds used initially are free of these three amino acids.
- Avoidance of any factor that promotes protein catabolism, including steroid therapy.
- *Metabolite excretion*: Small organic acids (e.g., methylmalonic, propionic, isovaleric, etc.) are excreted in urine, and hydration helps to decrease their concentration in blood and restore acid–base balance.
- *Specific medications in some IEM, such as ammonia removing drugs* (see **Table 66.4**): Sodium benzoate and sodium phenylacetate enhance alternative pathways for nitrogen excretion via the kidney. They are used for initial treatment of hyperammonemia related to urea cycle disorders. Once the patient is stabilized and tolerating the special amino acid mixture, the sodium benzoate and sodium phenylacetate combination is switched to oral phenylbutyrate, a prodrug, which is converted to phenylacetate.

- *Extrarenal removal therapy* (see Chapter 41): When high and/or prolonged toxic accumulation occurs, toxic removal by dialysis is necessary to prevent further brain damage. Extrarenal removal therapy can be indicated for treatment of hyperammonemia and intractable raised anion-gap metabolic acidosis. The criteria for dialysis and the optimal modality to use are not yet well established for each disease and are currently based on practices and experience at individual institutions. The decision is made using a multidisciplinary approach that involves intensivists, specialists in metabolic diseases, hepatologists, and nephrologists. The challenge is to quickly remove the toxins without worsening cerebral edema by hemodynamic compromise and/or osmotic shifts. The worse the cerebral edema is, the higher the risk of cerebral herniation during therapy, especially in cases of hyperammonemia. If neurologic deterioration is observed during extrarenal removal therapy, then the rate of toxin clearance should be reduced.

The efficacy of treatment is based on neurologic improvement, gastrointestinal tolerance showing that calories are being assimilated, and a decrease in blood level of toxics (e.g., amino acid chromatography [AAC] in MSUD, pH in organic aciduria, and ammonia in hyperammonemia, etc.). In some instances, additional tests may be helpful. For example, if urinary ketones are initially positive, then their later absence reflects improvement. Also, in MSUD and organic acid disorders, decrease in urinary urea-to-creatinine ratio reflects decrease in protein catabolism in the absence of renal failure and protein intake (25).

OUTCOMES

Morbidity and mortality of patients with metabolic encephalopathies who are admitted to the PICU are difficult to assess because of the many associated causes, each of which have incidence that varies according to the population concerned and the admission policy of the PICU. For example, the incidence

---

TABLE 66.4

SPECIFIC TREATMENTS OF INBORN ERRORS OF METABOLISM

■ DRUG	■ EFFECT	■ INDICATION(S)	■ DOSE	■ ADMINISTRATION ROUTE
Sodium benzoate	Ammonia removal	NH$_3$ >200 μmol/L	500 mg/kg/d	IV
Phenylbutyrate	Ammonia removal	NH$_3$ >200 μmol/L	600 mg/kg/d	IV or PO
Arginine	Ammonia removal	NH$_3$ >200 μmol/L	500 mg/kg/d	IVC
Carglumic acid	Ammonia removal	NAGS defect, MMA, PA, FAOD, and NH$_3$ >200 μmol/L	50 mg/kg/6 h	PO
Carnitine	Primary or secondary deficiency compensation	Organic aciduria, hyperlactatemia, FAOD	100 mg/kg/d	IVC or PO
Glycine	Increased urine excretion	IVA	500 mg/kg/4 h	IVC or PO
Vitamin B12	Enzyme cofactor	MMA	1–2 mg/d	IM
Metronidazole	Decreased toxin production by intestine bacteria	MMA, PA	20 mg/kg/d	PO
Biotin	PC cofactor	Hyperlactatemia, PA	10–20 mg/d	IV or PO
Riboflavin	Cofactor of acyl CoA dehydrogenase	FAOD	20–40 mg/d	IV or PO
Dichloroacetate or dichloropropionate	PDHk inhibitor	Hyperlactatemia >10 mmol/L	25 mg/kg/12 h	IV or PO

In suspected cases of IEM, the above specific treatments may be indicated in metabolic encephalopathy, after specialist consultation. Some therapies are specific for toxic accumulation (i.e., hyperammonemia) and some are specific for a particular disease.
IVC, continuous intravenous infusion; NAGS, *N*-acetylglutamate synthase; MMA, methylmalonic aciduria; PA, propionic aciduria; IVA, isovaleric aciduria; PC, pyruvate carboxylase; PDHk, pyruvate dehydrogenase kinase.

of cerebral edema in DKA in children is ~1% of acute episodes in the United Kingdom, with a mortality of 23%–24% and morbidity of 15%–35% in survivors (75). Metabolic encephalopathy due to IEM represented 2% of admissions to a PICU that was colocated with a national reference center for metabolic diseases. The mortality rate of these patients was 28.6% (76,77). Given that the incidence of metabolic encephalopathy due to IEM is probably lower in PICUs that do not have a national reference center, it is difficult for practitioners in those PICUs to develop expertise in treatment. Therefore, the development of a network among such referral centers may help to improve the outcome.

CONCLUSIONS AND FUTURE DIRECTIONS

In the infant or child with an acute encephalopathy, a variety of metabolic causes may account for acute brain dysfunction. Given the highly-selected population referred for PICU care, the intensivist should be aware of the more common differential diagnoses, necessary investigations, and therapeutic priorities. The future in the diagnosis and treatment of metabolic encephalopathy includes the following:

- Development of techniques that will speed the diagnosis of IEM, for example, tandem mass spectrometry is a specific and sensitive method that may improve diagnosis in an emergency (58).
- Development of neuroprotective strategies to limit secondary brain injury until specific treatment is obtained.
- Development of more precise neuromonitoring tools such as continuous EEG and transcranial Doppler to guide management and for prognostic purpose.
- Development of additional substitutive enzyme therapies for IEM. Only a few IEM can be treated with enzyme substitution. For example, carglumic acid (Carbaglu, Orphan Europe, France), an analog of N-acetylglutamate, treats hyperammonemia due to a defect in N-acetylglutamate synthase. The development of substitutive enzyme therapy for other IEM could prevent acute decompensation that requires intensive care.

References

1. Leonard JV, Morris AAM. Urea cycle disorders. *Semin Neonatol* 2002;7(1):27–35.
2. Carter CC, Lifton JF, Welch MJ. Organ uptake and blood pH and concentration effects of ammonia in dogs determined with ammonia labeled with 10 minute half-lived nitrogen 13. *Neurology* 1973;23(2):204–13.
3. Stabenau JR, Warren KS, Rall DP. The role of pH gradient in the distribution of ammonia between blood and cerebrospinal fluid, brain and muscle. *J Clin Invest* 1959;38(2):373–83.
4. Warren KS, Nathan DG. The passage of ammonia across the blood-brain-barrier and its relation to blood pH. *J Clin Invest* 1958;37(12):1724–8.
5. Desjardins P, Du T, Jiang W, et al. Pathogenesis of hepatic encephalopathy and brain edema in acute liver failure: Role of glutamine redefined. *Neurochem Int* 2012;60(7):690–6.
6. Cooper AJ, Plum F. Biochemistry and physiology of brain ammonia. *Physiol Rev* 1987;67(2):440–519.
7. Bachmann C, Braissant O, Villard A-M, et al. Ammonia toxicity to the brain and creatine. *Mol Genet Metab* 2004;81(suppl 1):S52–7.
8. Felipo V, Butterworth RF. Neurobiology of ammonia. *Prog Neurobiol* 2002;67(4):259–79.
9. Rama Rao KV, Jayakumar AR, Norenberg MD. Glutamine in the pathogenesis of acute hepatic encephalopathy. *Neurochem Int* 2012;61(4):575–80.
10. Auron A, Brophy PD. Hyperammonemia in review: Pathophysiology, diagnosis, and treatment. *Pediatr Nephrol* 2012;27(2):207–22.
11. Frontera JA. Metabolic encephalopathies in the critical care unit. *Continuum (Minneap Minn)* 2012;18(3):611–39.
12. Larsen FS, Gottstein J, Blei AT. Cerebral hyperemia and nitric oxide synthase in rats with ammonia-induced brain edema. *J Hepatol* 2001;34(4):548–54.
13. Schafer DF, Pappas SC, Brody LE, et al. Visual evoked potentials in a rabbit model of hepatic encephalopathy. I. Sequential changes and comparisons with drug-induced comas. *Gastroenterology* 1984;86(3):540–5.
14. Casteels-Van Daele M, Wouters C, Van Geet C, et al. Reye's syndrome revisited. Outdated concept of Reye's syndrome was used. *BMJ* 2002;324(7336):546.
15. Glasgow JF, Middleton B. Reye syndrome—Insights on causation and prognosis. *Arch Dis Child* 2001;85(5):351–3.
16. Kato M, Hughes RD, Keays RT, et al. Electron microscopic study of brain capillaries in cerebral edema from fulminant hepatic failure. *Hepatology* 1992;15(6):1060–6.
17. Traber PG, Dal Canto M, Ganger DR, et al. Electron microscopic evaluation of brain edema in rabbits with galactosamine-induced fulminant hepatic failure: Ultrastructure and integrity of the blood-brain barrier. *Hepatology* 1987;7(6):1272–7.
18. Butterworth RF. Pathophysiology of hepatic encephalopathy: A new look at ammonia. *Metab Brain Dis* 2002;17(4):221–7.
19. Mas A. Hepatic encephalopathy: From pathophysiology to treatment. *Digestion* 2006;73(suppl 1):86–93.
20. Ahboucha S, Butterworth RF. The neurosteroid system: Implication in the pathophysiology of hepatic encephalopathy. *Neurochem Int* 2008;52(4–5):575–87.
21. Baraldi M, Avallone R, Corsi L, et al. Natural endogenous ligands for benzodiazepine receptors in hepatic encephalopathy. *Metab Brain Dis* 2009;24(1):81–93.
22. Jones EA, Mullen KD. The role of natural benzodiazepines receptor ligands in hepatic encephalopathy. In: Mullen KD, Prakash RK, eds. *Hepatic Encephalopathy*. Totowa, NJ: Humana Press, 2012:71–93. http://rd.springer.com/chapter/10.1007/978-1-61779-836-8_6. Accessed October 15, 2012.
23. Riviello JJ Jr, Rezvani I, DiGeorge AM, et al. Cerebral edema causing death in children with maple syrup urine disease. *J Pediatr* 1991;119(1 pt 1):42–5.
24. Zinnanti WJ, Lazovic J. Interrupting the mechanisms of brain injury in a model of maple syrup urine disease encephalopathy. *J Inherit Metab Dis* 2012;35(1):71–9.
25. Jouvet P, Jugie M, Rabier D, et al. Combined nutritional support and continuous extracorporeal removal therapy in the severe acute phase of maple syrup urine disease. *Intensive Care Med* 2001;27(11):1798–806.
26. Jouvet P, Rustin P, Taylor DL, et al. Branched chain amino acids induce apoptosis in neural cells without mitochondrial membrane depolarization or cytochrome c release: Implications for neurological impairment associated with maple syrup urine disease. *Mol Biol Cell* 2000;11(5):1919–32.
27. Sgaravatti AM, Rosa RB, Schuck PF, et al. Inhibition of brain energy metabolism by the alpha-keto acids accumulating in maple syrup urine disease. *Biochim Biophys Acta* 2003;1639(3):232–8.
28. Zinnanti WJ, Lazovic J, Griffin K, et al. Dual mechanism of brain injury and novel treatment strategy in maple syrup urine disease. *Brain* 2009;132(pt 4):903–18.
29. de Sousa C, Piesowicz AT, Brett EM, et al. Focal changes in the globi pallidi associated with neurological dysfunction in methylmalonic acidaemia. *Neuropediatrics* 1989;20(4):199–201.
30. Wajner M, Goodman SI. Disruption of mitochondrial homeostasis in organic acidurias: Insights from human and animal studies. *J Bioenerg Biomembr* 2011;43(1):31–8.
31. Merker K, Hapke D, Reckzeh K, et al. Copper related toxic effects on cellular protein metabolism in human astrocytes. *Biofactors* 2005;24(1–4):255–61.
32. Herbel G, Boyle PJ. Hypoglycemia. Pathophysiology and treatment. *Endocrinol Metab Clin North Am* 2000;29(4):725–43.

33. Tasker RC, Coyle JT, Vornov JJ. The regional vulnerability to hypoglycemia-induced neurotoxicity in organotypic hippocampal culture: Protection by early tetrodotoxin or delayed MK-801. *J Neurosci* 1992;12(11):4298–308.

34. Ferrand-Drake M, Friberg H, Wieloch T. Mitochondrial permeability transition induced DNA-fragmentation in the rat hippocampus following hypoglycemia. *Neuroscience* 1999;90(4):1325–38.

35. Singh P, Jain A, Kaur G. Impact of hypoglycemia and diabetes on CNS: Correlation of mitochondrial oxidative stress with DNA damage. *Mol Cell Biochem* 2004;260(1–2):153–9.

36. Suh SW, Aoyama K, Chen Y, et al. Hypoglycemic neuronal death and cognitive impairment are prevented by poly(ADP-ribose) polymerase inhibitors administered after hypoglycemia. *J Neurosci* 2003;23(33):10681–90.

37. Wieloch T. Hypoglycemia-induced neuronal damage prevented by an N-methyl-D-aspartate antagonist. *Science* 1985;230(4726):681–3.

38. Bjørgaas MR. Cerebral effects of severe hypoglycemia in young people with type 1 diabetes. *Pediatr Diabetes* 2012;13(1):100–7.

39. Brennan AM, Suh SW, Won SJ, et al. NADPH oxidase is the primary source of superoxide induced by NMDA receptor activation. *Nat Neurosci* 2009;12(7):857–63.

40. Shapira Y, Harel S, Russell A. Mitochondrial encephalomyopathies: A group of neuromuscular disorders with defects in oxidative metabolism. *Isr J Med Sci* 1977;13(2):161–4.

41. Valanne L, Ketonen L, Majander A, et al. Neuroradiologic findings in children with mitochondrial disorders. *AJNR Am J Neuroradiol* 1998;19(2):369–77.

42. Saudubray JM, Martin D, de Lonlay P, et al. Recognition and management of fatty acid oxidation defects: A series of 107 patients. *J Inherit Metab Dis* 1999;22(4):488–502.

43. Lough ME. Wernicke's encephalopathy: Expanding the diagnostic toolbox. *Neuropsychol Rev* 2012;22(2):181–94.

44. Vasconcelos MM, Silva KP, Vidal G, et al. Early diagnosis of pediatric Wernicke's encephalopathy. *Pediatr Neurol* 1999;20(4):289–94.

45. Rewers A, Klingensmith G, Davis C, et al. Presence of diabetic ketoacidosis at diagnosis of diabetes mellitus in youth: The Search for Diabetes in Youth Study. *Pediatrics* 2008;121(5):e1258–66.

46. Glaser NS, Wootton-Gorges SL, Marcin JP, et al. Mechanism of cerebral edema in children with diabetic ketoacidosis. *J Pediatr* 2004;145(2):164–71.

47. Vavilala MS, Marro KI, Richards TL, et al. Change in mean transit time, apparent diffusion coefficient, and cerebral blood volume during pediatric diabetic ketoacidosis treatment. *Pediatr Crit Care Med* 2011;12(6):e344–9.

48. Vavilala MS, Richards TL, Roberts JS, et al. Change in blood-brain barrier permeability during pediatric diabetic ketoacidosis treatment. *Pediatr Crit Care Med* 2010;11(3):332–8.

49. Roberts JS, Vavilala MS, Schenkman KA, et al. Cerebral hyperemia and impaired cerebral autoregulation associated with diabetic ketoacidosis in critically ill children. *Crit Care Med* 2006;34(8):2217–23.

50. Cameron FJ, Kean MJ, Wellard RM, et al. Insights into the acute cerebral metabolic changes associated with childhood diabetes. *Diabet Med* 2005;22(5):648–53.

51. McManus ML, Churchwell KB, Strange K. Regulation of cell volume in health and disease. *N Engl J Med* 1995;333(19):1260–6.

52. Carchman RM, Dechert-Zeger M, Calikoglu AS, et al. A new challenge in pediatric obesity: Pediatric hyperglycemic hyperosmolar syndrome. *Pediatr Crit Care Med* 2005;6(1):20–4.

53. Kleinschmidt-Demasters BK, Rojiani AM, Filley CM. Central and extrapontine myelinolysis: Then...and now. *J Neuropathol Exp Neurol* 2006;65(1):1–11.

54. Rizzo MA, Frediani F, Granata A, et al. Neurological complications of hemodialysis: State of the art. *J Nephrol* 2012;25(2):170–82.

55. Seifter JL, Samuels MA. Uremic encephalopathy and other brain disorders associated with renal failure. *Semin Neurol* 2011;31(2):139–43.

56. Tamagno G, Celik Y, Simó R, et al. Encephalopathy associated with autoimmune thyroid disease in patients with Graves' disease: Clinical manifestations, follow-up, and outcomes. *BMC Neurol* 2010;10:27.

57. Zhan RZ, Fujiwara N, Shimoji K. Regionally different elevation of intracellular free calcium in hippocampus of septic rat brain. *Shock* 1996;6(4):293–7.

58. Jouvet P, Touati G, Lesage F, et al. Impact of inborn errors of metabolism on admission and mortality in a pediatric intensive care unit. *Eur J Pediatr* 2007;166(5):461–5.

59. Klose DA, Kölker S, Heinrich B, et al. Incidence and short-term outcome of children with symptomatic presentation of organic acid and fatty acid oxidation disorders in Germany. *Pediatrics* 2002;110(6):1204–11.

60. Honeycutt D, Callahan K, Rutledge L, et al. Heterozygote ornithine transcarbamylase deficiency presenting as symptomatic hyperammonemia during initiation of valproate therapy. *Neurology* 1992;42(3 pt 1):666–8.

61. Poggi-Travert F, Martin D, Billette de Villemeur T, et al. Metabolic intermediates in lactic acidosis: Compounds, samples and interpretation. *J Inherit Metab Dis* 1996;19(4):478–88.

62. Kaplan PW. The EEG in metabolic encephalopathy and coma. *J Clin Neurophysiol* 2004;21(5):307–18.

63. Tasker RC, Matthew DJ, Kendall B. Computed tomography in the assessment of raised intracranial pressure in non-traumatic coma. *Neuropediatrics* 1990;21(2):91–4.

64. Kölker S, Mayatepek E, Hoffmann GF. White matter disease in cerebral organic acid disorders: Clinical implications and suggested pathomechanisms. *Neuropediatrics* 2002;33(5):225–31.

65. Cecil KM. MR spectroscopy of metabolic disorders. *Neuroimaging Clin N Am* 2006;16(1):87–116, viii.

66. Faerber EN, Poussaint TY. Magnetic resonance of metabolic and degenerative diseases in children. *Top Magn Reson Imaging* 2002;13(1):3–21.

67. Xu D, Vigneron D. Magnetic resonance spectroscopy imaging of the newborn brain—A technical review. *Semin Perinatol* 2010;34(1):20–7.

68. Moats RA, Moseley KD, Koch R, et al. Brain phenylalanine concentrations in phenylketonuria: Research and treatment of adults. *Pediatrics* 2003;112(6 pt 2):1575–9.

69. Möller HE, Weglage J, Bick U, et al. Brain imaging and proton magnetic resonance spectroscopy in patients with phenylketonuria. *Pediatrics* 2003;112(6 pt 2):1580–3.

70. Bodman M, Smith D, Nyhan WL, et al. Medium-chain acyl coenzyme A dehydrogenase deficiency: Occurrence in an infant and his father. *Arch Neurol* 2001;58(5):811–4.

71. Barzilay Z, Britten AG, Koehler RC, et al. Interaction of CO_2 and ammonia on cerebral blood flow and O_2 consumption in dogs. *Am J Physiol* 1985;248(4 pt 2):H500–7.

72. Stravitz RT, Kramer AH, Davern T, et al. Intensive care of patients with acute liver failure: Recommendations of the U.S. Acute Liver Failure Study Group. *Crit Care Med* 2007;35(11):2498–508.

73. Abdo A, López O, Fernández A, et al. Transcranial Doppler sonography in fulminant hepatic failure. *Transplant Proc* 2003;35(5):1859–60.

74. Whitelaw A, Bridges S, Leaf A, et al. Emergency treatment of neonatal hyperammonaemic coma with mild systemic hypothermia. *Lancet* 2001;358(9275):36–8.

75. Dunger DB, Sperling MA, Acerini CL, et al. ESPE/LWPES consensus statement on diabetic ketoacidosis in children and adolescents. *Arch Dis Child* 2004;89(2):188–94.

76. Edge JA, Hawkins MM, Winter DL, et al. The risk and outcome of cerebral oedema developing during diabetic ketoacidosis. *Arch Dis Child* 2001;85(1):16–22.

77. Lawrence SE, Cummings EA, Gaboury I, et al. Population-based study of incidence and risk factors for cerebral edema in pediatric diabetic ketoacidosis. *J Pediatr* 2005;146(5):688–92.

CHAPTER 67 ■ THE DETERMINATION OF BRAIN DEATH

THOMAS A. NAKAGAWA AND MUDIT MATHUR

KEY POINTS

❶ The prerequisite conditions for the determination of brain death include correction of hypotension or shock, correction of hypothermia, correction of severe metabolic disturbances, and ensuring that sedative or neuromuscular blocking agents have had adequate time to be metabolized.

❷ The clinical criteria to determine brain death include deep unresponsive coma, loss of all brainstem reflexes (including apnea), and a lack of motor function (excluding spinal reflexes).

❸ The absence of brainstem function is defined by midposition, or fully dilated, nonreactive pupils; absent movement of bulbar musculature, including facial and oropharyngeal muscles; absence of cough, corneal, gag, sucking, and rooting reflexes; absence of spontaneous eye movements induced by oculocephalic or oculovestibular testing; and absent respiratory effort off ventilator support.

❹ The recommended intervals between brain death examinations are 24 hours for term newborns up to 1 month of age and 12 hours for children older than 1 month of age up to 18 years of age.

❺ The first examination determines whether the child meets neurologic criteria for brain death, and the second confirms brain death based on an unchanged and irreversible condition.

❻ Two apnea tests should be performed, one with each neurologic examination, unless a medical contraindication exists.

❼ During apnea testing, the threshold of 60 mm Hg is also valid in the newborn.

❽ The apnea test should be aborted if oxygen saturations fall below 85%, if hemodynamic instability occurs, or if a $Paco_2$ level of 60 mm Hg and a change of at least 20 mm Hg above the baseline $Paco_2$ cannot be safely achieved.

❾ Ancillary studies are not required unless a complete neurologic examination and apnea test cannot be completed, and should not be used as a substitute for the neurologic examination.

❿ Ancillary studies are indicated in the following circumstances: (a) when components of the neurologic examination and apnea test cannot be completed, (b) when conditions or confounding variables such as a medication effect interfere with the neurologic examination and apnea test, (c) when there are concerns about the validity of the neurologic examination, and (d) to reduce the observation period between examinations.

⓫ Recommendations for determination of brain death in preterm infants (<37 weeks gestational age) have not been described.

⓬ Apnea testing is difficult to perform if death occurs during VA ECMO (veno-arterial extracorporeal membrane oxygenation) and in children with cyanotic heart disease.

Advancements in medical treatments, technology, and the development of modern critical care units have improved outcomes and saved the lives of critically ill and injured patients. Mechanical ventilation, used for treatment of respiratory failure, and extracorporeal membrane oxygenation (ECMO), used to restore circulation, allow patients to survive injury and illness that might otherwise result in death. The administration of anesthetic and sedative agents allows patients to exist in a controlled, reversible state of unconsciousness. While these advances improve our care for critically ill patients, they also obscure the use of the usual neurologic, respiratory, and circulatory parameters to determine death. The development of these life-sustaining advances presented new challenges to physicians faced with the determination of death following a devastating brain injury in patients in whom recovery was unlikely (1). Advances in organ transplantation added to the need for changes in the determination of death in patients receiving critical care. The recovery of cadaveric kidneys from non–heart-beating donors had been occurring since the 1950s, but it was the first heart transplant from a neurologically devastated, heart-beating donor in 1967 that produced a different

set of challenges. These medical advancements required additional criteria to determine death based on irreversible coma, which came to be defined as brain death.

In 1967, a landmark article provided a foundation for the determination of death based on irreversible coma (2). The Harvard committee's definition of irreversible coma included patients who were unresponsive, who exhibited no movement or breathing, had no reflexes, and had an isoelectric electroencephalogram (EEG) (2).The criteria for the determination of death outlined by the Harvard committee were better defined in a report from the President's Commission for the Study of Ethical Problems in Medicine and Biomedical and Behavioral Research (3). This report clarified the determination of death in the modern era and stated, "[A]n individual who has sustained either (a) irreversible cessation of circulatory and respiratory functions or (b) irreversible cessation of all function of the entire brain, including the brainstem, is dead." These criteria differed from those used in other countries because they required the loss of function of the entire brain, not just the brainstem, in order to determine brain death. The guidelines of the 1981 President's Commission were intended for

1066

TABLE 67.1

RECOMMENDATIONS FOR THE DETERMINATION OF BRAIN DEATH IN INFANTS AND CHILDREN

1. Determination of brain death in term newborns, infants, and children is a clinical diagnosis based on the absence of neurologic function with a known irreversible cause of coma. Because of insufficient data in the literature, recommendations for preterm infants <37 wk gestational age are not included in this guideline.
2. Hypotension, hypothermia, and metabolic disturbances should be treated and corrected, and medications that can interfere with the neurologic examination and apnea testing should be discontinued, allowing for adequate clearance before proceeding with these evaluations.
3. Two examinations, including apnea testing with each examination, separated by an observation period are required. Examinations should be performed by different attending physicians. Apnea testing may be performed by the same physician. An observation period of 24 h for term newborns (37 wk gestational age) to 30 d of age, and 12 h for infants and children (31 d to 18 y) is recommended. The first examination determines whether the child has met the accepted neurologic examination criteria for brain death. The second examination confirms brain death based on an unchanged and irreversible condition. Assessment of neurologic function following cardiopulmonary resuscitation or other severe acute brain injuries should be deferred for 24 h or longer if there are concerns or inconsistencies in the examination.
4. Apnea testing to support the diagnosis of brain death must be performed safely and requires documentation of an arterial $PaCO_2$ 20 mm Hg above the baseline *and* 60 mm Hg with no respiratory effort during the testing period. If the apnea test cannot be safely completed, an ancillary study should be performed.
5. Ancillary studies (electroencephalogram [EEG] and radionuclide cerebral blood flow [CBF]) are not required to establish brain death and are not a substitute for the neurologic examination. Ancillary studies may be used to assist the clinician in making the diagnosis of brain death (a) when components of the examination or apnea testing cannot be completed safely because of the underlying medical condition of the patient, (b) if there is uncertainty about the results of the neurologic examination, (c) if a medication effect may be present, or (d) to reduce the interexamination observation period. When ancillary studies are used, a second clinical examination and apnea test should be performed and components that can be completed must remain consistent with brain death. In this instance, the observation interval may be shortened, and the second neurologic examination and apnea test (or all components that are able to be completed safely) can be performed at any time thereafter.
6. Death is declared when the above criteria are fulfilled.

Reused with permission from Nakagawa TA, Ashwal S, Mathur M, et al. Guidelines for the determination of brain death in infants and children: An update of the 1987 task force recommendations. *Crit Care Med* 2011;39:2139–55.

determining brain death in adults and did not address children other than recommending caution in applying neurologic criteria to determine death in children younger than 5 years (3). The need for recommendations for children led to the consensus-based guidelines developed by an expert panel "Report of Special Task Force. Guidelines for the Determination of Brain Death in Children" in 1987 (4). These guidelines emphasized the history and clinical examination to determine the etiology of coma so that remediable or reversible conditions were excluded. Age-related observation periods and specific neurodiagnostic testing were recommended for children younger than 1 year. For children older than 1 year, the diagnosis of brain death could be made solely on a clinical basis, and laboratory studies were optional. Still, little guidance was provided for the infant <7 days of age because of the lack of sufficient clinical experience and data in this age group.

The 1987 Special Task Force guidelines provided an important framework to determine brain death in children for almost 25 years. As therapies advanced in pediatric medicine, the limitations of these guidelines became apparent. These limitations include limited clinical information on which the guidelines are based, ancillary studies that rely heavily on EEG testing, and age-based criteria with little direction to address brain death in neonates. These limitations resulted in confusion and inconsistent application among physicians who determine brain death in children (5–11). These issues were not unique to infants and children or limited to the United States (12,13). Canadian guidelines for children and adults published in 2006 brought clarity to the definition and determination of brain death (13). The 1995 American Academy of Neurology guidelines to determine brain death in adults were updated in 2010 to address related issues (14,15). The most recent update of the pediatric brain death guidelines in 2011 clarifies issues such as observation intervals, determination of brain death for term

newborns, and use of ancillary studies for all age groups, and it provides a more uniform approach to determining brain death in infants and children. The 2011 guidelines also clearly define the age range for pediatric patients as 37 weeks (estimated gestational age) to 18 years of age, incorporate consideration for neonates and the pediatric trauma population, and provide minimum standards that must be satisfied for infants and children (16,17). **Table 67.1** lists current recommendations for the determination of brain death in infants and children.

Determination of death by neurologic criteria and consensus-based brain death guidelines have gained legal and medical acceptance in the United States. Despite the publication of guidelines, there are still physicians who feel that whole brain death criteria are flawed. A detailed discussion of the ethical issues related to this topic is beyond the scope of this chapter and interested readers are referred to a publication from the President's Council on Bioethics (18). It is important to recognize that no national brain death law exists. Physicians and healthcare providers are encouraged to become familiar with both the local and state laws and the policies within their respective institutions intended to provide consistency for the determination of brain death in infants and children.

PREREQUISITE CONDITIONS THAT MUST BE SATISFIED PRIOR TO BRAIN DEATH TESTING

There are specific preconditions that must be met prior to initiating brain death and/or neurodiagnostic testing. Evaluation of the neurologic criteria should be deferred until the prerequisites for brain death testing have been satisfied. Determination of brain death for any infant or child requires establishing and maintaining normal age-appropriate physiologic parameters. Certain conditions commonly seen in critically ill patients can influence the neurologic examination and must be corrected prior to examination and apnea testing. These prerequisite conditions include correcting hypotension or shock, correction of hypothermia, correction of severe metabolic disturbances, and ensuring that sedative or neuromuscular blocking agents have had adequate time to be metabolized.

The use of hypothermia as an adjunctive therapy for children with acute brain injury following trauma and cardiac arrest is increasing (19–25). Hypothermia depresses central nervous system (CNS) function and alters the metabolism and clearance of medications. These effects can interfere with the clinical examination or lead to a diagnostic error in the determination of brain death (26). Clinicians caring for critically ill children need to be aware of the potential impact of therapeutic modalities such as hypothermia when making a determination of brain death. The current pediatric guidelines specify that a minimum core body temperature of 35°C (95°F) should be maintained during the examination and testing period to determine brain death (16,17). Institutional guidelines may differ in the prerequisite hypothermia criteria.

In addition to maintaining temperature stability, other conditions capable of emulating brain death or factors that can alter the neurologic examination must be excluded. Reversible conditions such as severe hepatic or renal dysfunction, or inborn errors of metabolism, may play a role in the clinical presentation of the comatose infant or child. Organ system dysfunction can reduce metabolism of sedative and neuromuscular blocking agents affecting the neurologic examination. Severe metabolic disturbances capable of causing coma such as glucose, pH, and electrolyte disturbances should be treated and corrected prior to initiating brain death testing. Hypernatremia has been implicated as a potential cause for coma, resulting in recommendations to normalize serum sodium levels prior to determining brain death (27,28). The use of hypertonic sodium administration for the management of intracranial pressure (ICP) elevation produces elevated serum sodium levels and raises concern about the effect on the neurologic examination used to determine brain death. The use of osmolar therapy and its effect on actual neurologic function is unclear. A specific serum sodium threshold that can affect brain death testing is unknown and guidelines suggest correction of serum sodium levels to relatively normal limits (16,17). The use of mannitol can result in vascular volume depletion, reduced cardiac output, hypotension, and decreased cerebral blood flow (CBF).

Drug intoxication from barbiturates, opioids, sedative-hypnotics, anesthetic agents, antiepileptic agents, and alcohols can also affect the clinical examination and neurodiagnostic testing by imitating brain death. Administration of sedative agents should be discontinued for at least 24 hours in children and 48 hours in the neonate prior to neurologic examination. Observation periods may need to be extended following termination of continuous infusions of sedative agents for several elimination half-lives to allow adequate drug clearance prior to brain death testing. Serum levels of sedative agents or antiepileptic medications in the low- to mid-therapeutic range prior to testing should not interfere with the determination of brain death (16,17,29). Recent administration of neuromuscular blocking agents requires adequate clearance of these agents; this can be confirmed using a nerve stimulator to elicit a twitch response. Other unusual causes of coma such as neurotoxins and chemical exposure (i.e., organophosphates and carbamates) should be considered in rare cases when an etiology for coma has not been established (16,17).

Computed axial tomography (CAT) scan or magnetic resonance imaging (MRI) scan are routinely used in clinical practice to assist with evaluation of injury to the CNS. Neuroimaging studies usually demonstrate evidence of an acute CNS insult consistent with loss of brain function. Imaging studies performed immediately after presentation do not always demonstrate significant injury, and follow-up studies may be useful in these cases. CAT and MRI are not considered ancillary studies and should not be relied on to make a determination of death.

CLINICAL EXAMINATION CRITERIA TO DETERMINE BRAIN DEATH

Brain death determination is a clinical diagnosis that relies on the coexistence of coma and apnea during a period of observation after exclusion of confounding diagnoses. The foundation of brain death determination is the neurologic examination, which is consistent across the pediatric age spectrum. Table 67.2 lists the neurologic examination criteria, including motor, brainstem, and autonomic assessment that must be met to make a determination of brain death in infants and children. A detailed and specific neurologic examination must be performed for any patient being evaluated for brain death. The clinical examination to determine brain death should be pursued only after all prerequisite conditions have been satisfied. Clinical criteria to determine brain death are based on the absence of neurologic function that includes deep unresponsive coma, loss of all brainstem reflexes (including apnea), and a lack of motor function (excluding spinal reflexes). Noxious stimuli should not produce a motor response other than spinally mediated reflexes. Eye opening or eye movement should be absent as well. Absence of brainstem function is defined by the following findings on physical examination: midposition, or fully dilated, nonreactive pupils; absent movement of bulbar musculature, including facial and oropharyngeal muscles; absence of cough, corneal, gag, sucking, and rooting reflexes; absence of spontaneous eye movements induced by

---

TABLE 67.2

NEUROLOGIC EXAMINATION CRITERIA FOR BRAIN DEATH

1. **Coma.** The patient must exhibit complete loss of consciousness, vocalization, and volitional activity
2. **Apnea.** The patient must have the complete absence of documented respiratory effort (if feasible) by formal apnea testing demonstrating a $Paco_2 \geq 60$ mm Hg and ≥ 20 mm Hg rise above baseline
3. **Loss of all brainstem reflexes, including:**
   Mid-position or fully dilated pupils that do not respond to light
   Absence of movement of bulbar musculature, including facial and oropharyngeal muscles
   Absent gag, cough, sucking, and rooting reflexes
   Absent corneal reflexes
   Absent oculocephalic and oculovestibular reflexes
4. **Flaccid tone and absence of spontaneous or induced movements, excluding spinal cord events such as reflex withdrawal or spinal myoclonus**
5. **Reversible conditions or conditions that can interfere with the neurologic examination must be excluded prior to brain death testing**

See text for detailed information about the clinical examination. Reused with permission from Nakagawa TA, Ashwal S, Mathur M, et al. Guidelines for the determination of brain death in infants and children: an update of the 1987 task force recommendations. *Crit Care Med* 2011;39:2139-55.

oculocephalic or oculovestibular testing; and absent respiratory effort off ventilator support (15–17).

Testing for bulbar muscular activity should produce no grimacing or facial muscle movement when applying deep pressure on the mandibular condyles at the level of the temporomandibular joints and when applying deep pressure on the supraorbital ridge. Pharyngeal or gag reflex is tested by stimulation of the posterior pharynx with a tongue blade or suction device. Pushing or moving the endotracheal tube (ETT) posteriorly in the oropharynx can elicit the same response; however, care should be exercised not to dislodge the airway. The cough reflex can be reliably tested by examining the response to tracheal suctioning. The catheter should be inserted into the trachea and advanced to the level of the carina, followed by one or two suctioning passes. Testing for corneal reflexes is achieved by touching the edge of the cornea with a piece of tissue paper or a cotton swab, or using small squirts of water to stimulate a reflex response. No eyelid movement should be seen. Care should be taken not to damage the cornea during testing. The oculovestibular reflex is tested by irrigating each ear with ice water (caloric testing) after the patency of the external auditory canal is confirmed. The head is elevated to 30 degrees and each external auditory canal is irrigated separately with approximately 10–50 mL of ice water. Lack of movement of the eyes during at least 1 minute of observation means the reflex is absent (consistent with brain death criteria). Both ears should be tested, with an interval of several minutes separating each test. Oculocephalic testing may be performed in the absence of cervical fracture or instability. It is assessed by holding the eyes open and turning the head rapidly to each side and observing for eye movements. Absence of eye movement relative to movement of the head means the reflex is absent (consistent with brain death criteria). Caution is advised in patients with potential cervical spine injury to reduce risk of exacerbating a preexisting injury. Oculocephalic and oculovesibular testing evaluate the integrity of the medial longitudinal fasciculus. Either test is considered sufficient under the current pediatric brain death guidelines. The clinical diagnosis of brain death is highly reliable when made by experienced examiners using established criteria (11,30,31). There are no reports of children recovering neurologic function after meeting adult brain death criteria on neurologic examination when well-established physical examination criteria are applied (31).

Serial neurologic examinations are recommended to establish the diagnosis of brain death in children. Based on clinical experience and published reports, the current brain death guidelines recommend the performance of two neurologic examinations separated by an observation period (16,17). The 2011 guidelines recommend shorter observation periods than previously described for children. The recommended intervals between examinations are 24 hours for neonates (includes newborns of 37 weeks gestational age up to 1 month of age) and 12 hours for children older than 1 month of age up to 18 years of age. The first examination determines the child meets neurologic criteria for brain death. The second examination confirms brain death based on an unchanged and irreversible condition. These examination criteria are consistent with the currently accepted definition of death (3). If uncertainty about the examination exists, the time interval between observations and examinations warrants extension based on the physician's judgment of the child's neurologic status. The examination results should remain consistent with brain death throughout the observation and testing period. In contrast, the adult brain death guidelines recommend a single clinical examination (15). The recommendation for two examinations in children is based on experience declaring brain death in infants and children. Clinical experience determining brain death in infants and children is considerably less

than adults. Over an 11-year period, almost 80,000 adults have been declared brain dead compared with approximately 11,000 children, including 1264 children <1 year of age (32). We have gained more experience and knowledge determining brain death in children, but our experience remains limited compared with adults, thus the pediatric examination criteria remain more conservative.

Because of the profound clinical implications when determining brain death, the use of an indwelling arterial catheter to ensure that blood pressure remains acceptable throughout the testing period is reasonable and recommended (16,17). Many of these infants and children are critically ill, and continuous hemodynamic monitoring would be considered the standard of care. An indwelling arterial line also allows sampling of blood to accurately determine $PaCO_2$ levels during the apnea test.

Clinical criteria to determine brain death may not be present on ICU admission in all children; however, progression to brain death may evolve over the course of several days as a result of their underlying condition. Assessment of neurologic function may be unreliable immediately following resuscitation after cardiopulmonary arrest and in infants and children who have sustained acute hypoxic–ischemic brain injury (33–35). Additionally, initial stabilization may take several hours during which metabolic disturbances can be corrected and reversible conditions that mimic brain death can be identified and treated. Serial physical examinations are frequently indicated and it is a new recommendation that neurologic evaluation and testing for brain death be deferred for at least 24 hours or longer from admission as dictated by clinical judgment of the treating physician in such circumstances (cardiac arrest or severe acute brain injury) (16,17). If there are concerns about the validity of the examination (e.g., flaccid tone or absent movements in a patient with high spinal cord injury or severe neuromuscular disease) or if specific examination components cannot be performed because of medical contraindications (e.g., apnea testing in patients with significant lung injury or hemodynamic instability) or if examination findings are inconsistent and changing, continued observation and postponing further neurologic examinations until these issues are resolved are warranted to avoid improperly diagnosing brain death. An ancillary study can be pursued to assist with the diagnosis of brain death in situations where certain examination components cannot be completed.

The 2011 pediatric brain death guidelines recommend that two different attending physicians involved with the care of the child perform the neurologic examinations. This change in recommendations was made to reduce the chance of diagnostic error and avoid potential conflicts of interest in establishing the diagnosis of brain death if only one physician is involved in the determination of brain death. Moreover, two attending physicians involved with the care of the child provide consensus and greater medical certainty that brain death criteria are met. Apnea testing can be performed by the same physician who conducts the clinical examination, or by the attending physician who is managing ventilator support of the child (16,17).

APNEA TESTING

Testing for apnea associated with coma is an essential component of the brain death examination. The 2011 guidelines to determine brain death now recommend that two apnea tests be performed, one with each neurologic examination, unless a medical contraindication exists (16,17). Conditions that invalidate the apnea test or that raise safety concerns which prevent the apnea test to be completed safely include high cervical spine injury, excessive oxygen requirement, elevated ventilator settings, or the use of advanced ventilation modalities such as high frequency oscillatory or jet ventilation. The apnea test evaluates the ability of the respiratory center in the brainstem to respond to elevated levels of carbon dioxide (CO_2) and to stimulate respiration. The normal $PaCO_2$ threshold for establishing apnea in children ($PaCO_2 > 60$ mm Hg) has been assumed to be the same as adults (36,37). Neonatal studies reviewing $PaCO_2$ thresholds for apnea are limited. However, data from a series of neonates who were brain dead revealed a mean $PaCO_2$ of 65 mm Hg during apnea testing, suggesting that the threshold of 60 mm Hg is also valid in the newborn (38).

Apnea testing for infants and children is conducted in a manner similar to that for adults being evaluated for brain death. Testing for apnea must allow adequate time for $PaCO_2$ to increase from baseline to levels that would normally stimulate respiration. Apnea testing must be performed while maintaining normal oxygenation and stable hemodynamics. Additionally, adequate time for clearance of sedative and paralytic agents must be allowed prior to testing for apnea (16,17). Patients should be preoxygenated with 100% oxygen to prevent hypoxia during the apnea test. If it is safe to do, the $PaCO_2$ should be normalized and documented prior to initiating apnea testing. CO_2 rises in a linear fashion by approximately 3–5 mm Hg/min (36,37,39). However, the increase may be variable since the injured or dead brain may not contribute to CO_2 production. Mechanical ventilation is discontinued when apnea testing is initiated. The patient is then placed on continuous positive airway pressure (CPAP) ventilation, a T piece attached to the ETT, or a self-inflating bag valve system, such as a Mapleson circuit connected to the ETT. Ventilators that provide a backup ventilation rate when apnea is detected in the CPAP mode should not be used. Another concern is the report of the false appearance of spontaneous ventilation during CPAP administration due to trigger sensitivity problems on the mechanical ventilator (40). If a self-inflating bag valve system or Mapleson circuit is utilized, Positive end-expiratory pressure (PEEP) should be appropriately titrated to maintain oxygenation during apnea testing. Tracheal insufflation of oxygen using a catheter inserted through the ETT has also been used to provide supplemental oxygen during apnea testing. Care must be taken with this technique that the diameter of the insufflating catheter is small enough to allow adequate excursion of gas to prevent barotrauma. Additionally, the rate of rise of $PaCO_2$ can be affected if CO_2 washout occurs because of the use of a high gas flow with this technique. The physician(s) performing the apnea examination must continually observe the patient for any spontaneous respiratory movements over a 5- to 10-minute period after disconnecting the ventilator and ensure that hemodynamic parameters and oxygen saturations are maintained during the testing period. The $PaCO_2$ should be measured by arterial blood gas analysis prior to and during the apnea test. $PaCO_2$ should be allowed to rise to 60 mm Hg or greater *and* at least 20 mm Hg above the baseline $PaCO_2$. Achieving the increase of 20 mm Hg is especially relevant in infants and children with chronic respiratory disease or insufficiency who may already have supranormal $PaCO_2$ levels as their baseline. If no respiratory effort is noted during the apnea examination despite an adequate increment in $PaCO_2$, the test is consistent with brain death. The patient should be placed back on mechanical ventilation support until death is established with a repeat clinical examination, or ancillary testing. If the apnea test cannot be completed because of hemodynamic instability, desaturation, or an inability to reach a $PaCO_2$ of 60 mm Hg and a change of at least 20 mm Hg above the baseline $PaCO_2$, another apnea test can be attempted at a later time or an ancillary study must be pursued to assist in making the determination of brain death. Failure to complete that apnea test is more common

in patients with multitrauma prone to hemodynamic instability (41). If there is any concern regarding the validity of the apnea test, an ancillary study should be pursued. While some believe that a true spontaneous breath consists of abdominal or chest excursion that produces adequate tidal volumes, *any* respiratory effort is inconsistent with the current clinical definition of apnea and precludes the diagnosis of brain death.

Concerns regarding the safety of apnea testing have been raised by some authors (42,43). They have argued that apnea with its associated hypercarbia can be potentially harmful to a patient with recent brain injury and intracranial hypertension. Hypotension and hypoxemia can also have deleterious effects on an injured brain, affecting CBF and ICP. Furthermore, improper methods of oxygenation employed during the apnea test can result in barotrauma. Patient safety is imperative when apnea testing is being performed. Apnea testing should be undertaken only after the patient has met established clinical examination criteria for brain death testing with loss of all brainstem reflexes. Only a physician experienced in managing ventilator support of critically ill patients and capable of responding to acute hemodynamic or respiratory deterioration should perform apnea testing. In many cases, the intensive care specialist meets these criteria and is most capable to perform apnea testing. Preoxygenation prior to apnea testing can help to minimize potential complications and provide the greatest chance of successfully completing this test. Attention to pretest conditions such as hypovolemia can minimize potentially adverse circulatory effects during apnea testing (41,44). The apnea test should be aborted if oxygen saturations fall below 85%, if hemodynamic instability occurs, or if a $PaCO_2$ level of 60 mm Hg and a change of at least 20 mm Hg above the baseline $PaCO_2$ cannot be safely achieved (16,17). If apnea testing cannot be completed, the patient should be placed back on ventilator support with appropriate treatment to restore normal oxygenation and ventilation. Apnea testing may be repeated at a later time, or an ancillary study can be performed to assist with the determination of brain death if the apnea test cannot be safely completed.

ANCILLARY STUDIES USED TO ASSIST WITH THE DETERMINATION OF BRAIN DEATH

The emphasis on brain death as a clinical diagnosis has led healthcare providers to rely more heavily on repeated clinical examinations that demonstrate coma, apnea, and absent brainstem reflexes. The current guidelines for the determination of brain death in infants and children state that ancillary studies are not required unless a complete neurologic examination and apnea test cannot be completed (16,17). The current guidelines also emphasize that ancillary studies should not be used as a substitute for the neurologic examination.

There are situations when an ancillary study may assist with the determination of brain death. An ancillary study is indicated in the following circumstances: (a) when components of the neurologic examination and apnea test cannot be completed, (b) when conditions or confounding variables such as a medication effect interfere with the neurologic examination and apnea test, (c) when there are concerns about the validity of the neurologic examination, and (d) to reduce the observation period between examinations. An ancillary study can also help shorten the interval between examinations to determine brain death if the ancillary study is performed after the first neurologic examination and apnea test demonstrates brain death, and the ancillary test supports the diagnosis of brain death. The second neurologic examination and apnea test (or components that can be completed safely) can be performed and documented at any time thereafter to determine brain death for children of all ages. Ancillary studies can also be helpful for social and medical reasons. These studies may allow family members to better comprehend the diagnosis of brain death and may be important as additional supportive evidence in situations where death is the result of homicide. The most commonly used ancillary studies to assist with the diagnosis of brain death in infants and children include the documentation of electrocerebral silence (ECS) by EEG and the documentation of the absence of CBF by radionuclide CBF study. Four-vessel angiography evaluation of the anterior and posterior cerebral circulation remains the gold standard ancillary test, but the technical expertise to perform this test in children may not be available in every facility. For this reason, four-vessel angiography is an infrequently used ancillary study in children.

EEG can be easily performed at the bedside of a critically ill child in most institutions. Radionuclide CBF studies have been used extensively with good experience (45–47). Radionuclide CBF scan using a portable gamma camera is fairly easily accomplished at the bedside, without the need for extraordinary technical expertise. Some centers may not have portable technology, which requires transporting the patient to a nuclear medicine suite. In this situation, a decision is often necessary about whether the critically ill child can be safely transported outside the ICU. A preference for radionuclide CBF over EEG as an ancillary study to assist with the determination of brain death in infants and children has been shown, 74% versus 26%, but the reasons for this finding were not elucidated (7). Both of these ancillary studies remain acceptable to assist with the determination of brain death. Data suggest that EEG and CBF are of similar confirmatory value. However, the sensitivity of ancillary studies in newborns appears to be less than that in older children (16,17). Some experts believe that EEG may be more specific, although less sensitive, than the radionuclide CBF study. It is important to recognize that these studies evaluate different aspects of the CNS. EEG testing evaluates cortical and cellular function while radionuclide CBF testing evaluates flow and uptake into brain tissue. Each of these tests requires the expertise of appropriately trained and qualified individuals who understand the limitations of these studies to avoid misinterpretation. These tests must be performed in accordance with currently established medical standards (48–50).

The goal of radionuclide CBF study is to determine if CBF is present. Scintigraphic confirmation of brain death relies on planar imaging, with or without radionuclide angiography. Commonly used radiotracer agents for radionuclide CBF studies include nonspecific tracers such as Tc99m diethylenetriaminepentaacetic acid (DTPA), or brain-specific tracers such as Tc99m hexamethylpropylene-aminoxime (HMPAO) or Tc99m ethylene cysteine diethyl ester (ECD) (46). Tc99m DTPA does not cross the blood–brain barrier and is used for visualization of cerebral vasculature during the dynamic imaging phase. Two-dimensional Tc99m DTP images may show facial blood flow that prevents visualization of posterior fossa features. Tc99m HMPAO is lipid soluble and will cross the blood–brain barrier allowing for dynamic and static imaging during radionuclide scanning. Flow with multiprojection static planar imaging using Tc99m HMPAO can be used to evaluate the cerebral hemispheres, basal ganglia, thalamus, and cerebellum (46). Tc99m HMPAO has become the radiotracer agent of choice in many institutions performing radionuclide CBF studies because of its brain-specific uptake and ability to adequately visualize the posterior fossa on static imaging (46).

Prior to initiating neurodiagnostic testing, normal hemodynamic parameters based on age of the child must be attained, and a minimum core body temperature of 35°C (95°F) should be maintained during the testing period. Pharmacologic agents and clinically significant drug intoxications, including alcohol, barbiturates, opiates, and sedative-hypnotic agents, can affect EEG testing. Sedative agents should be discontinued for a minimum of 24 hours prior to EEG testing and clinical examination in the older patient, and a minimum of 48 hours in the neonate. Barbiturate levels in the low-to mid-therapeutic range should not preclude the use of EEG testing (51). While barbiturates reduce CBF, there is no evidence supporting that high-dose barbiturate therapy completely arrests CBF. Evidence suggests that a radionuclide CBF study can be utilized in patients with high-dose barbiturate therapy to demonstrate absence of CBF and establish brain death (52,53).

The use of Transcranial Doppler (TCD) and brainstem auditory evoked potentials as an ancillary study has been described in adults, but neither have been studied extensively or validated in children. Newer ancillary studies such as CT angiography have also been used in adults (53–55); however, there is no reported experience in children. Single-photon emission computed tomography (SPECT) is another technique that has been studied, but limited data exist for its use in confirmation of brain death (46). CT perfusion study measuring CBF, nasopharyngeal somatosensory evoked potentials (SSEPs), magnetic resonance angiography (MRA)-MRI, bispectral index, and perfusion MRI for infants and children lack sufficient studies or clinical experience to validate their use. None of these ancillary studies can be recommended to assist with determination of brain death in children at this time.

If the EEG study shows electrical activity or the radionuclide CBF study shows evidence of cerebral flow or cellular uptake, the patient cannot be pronounced dead. Observation of the patient should continue until death can be declared by clinical examination criteria and apnea testing, or a follow-up ancillary study is performed with results consistent with brain death. It is important to note that ancillary studies are an adjunct to the clinical examination and apnea testing. Continued coma and apnea during an extended observation period is ultimately the final determining factor to diagnose brain death. If a radionuclide CBF study is to be repeated, waiting at least 24 hours is recommended to ensure clearance of the radiotracer (48,56). While no evidence exists for a recommended waiting period between EEG examinations, the current pediatric brain death guidelines suggest a waiting period of 24 hours before repeating this examination as well (16,17).

DETERMINATION OF BRAIN DEATH FOR TERM NEWBORNS (37 WEEKS GESTATION) TO 30 DAYS OF AGE

The ability to diagnose brain death in newborns is still viewed with some uncertainty primarily due to limited clinical experience and the small number of neonates with brain death reported in the literature (32,57–59). Additionally, it is unclear whether there are intrinsic biologic differences in neonatal brain metabolism, blood flow, and response to injury. Anatomically, the newborn has patent sutures and an open fontanel, resulting in less dramatic increases in ICP after acute brain injury, compared with older patients. The cascade of events associated with increased ICP and reduced cerebral perfusion ultimately leading to herniation is less likely to occur in the neonate (16).

The physician declaring brain death in term newborns (37 weeks gestation) and older must be aware of the limitations of the clinical examination and ancillary studies in this age group. It is important to carefully and repeatedly examine term newborns, with particular attention to examination of brainstem reflexes and apnea testing. The recommended observation period between neurologic examinations is 24 hours for term newborns (37 weeks gestation) to 30 days of age (16,17). As for older children, the assessment of neurologic function may be unreliable immediately following an acute catastrophic neurologic injury or cardiopulmonary arrest. The metabolism of sedative agents may be prolonged in the newborn because of immature metabolism pathways or the therapeutic use of hypothermia. Brain death testing should be deferred for a period of 24 hours or longer in these situations (16).

As with any patient, a thorough neurologic examination must be performed in conjunction with the apnea test to make the determination of death. The limited neonatal data evaluating $Paco_2$ thresholds for apnea suggest that the threshold of 60 mm Hg is also valid in the newborn (38). Apnea testing in the term newborn may be complicated by the following issues: (a) treatment with 100% oxygen may inhibit the potential recovery of respiratory effort (60,61), and (b) profound bradycardia affecting hemodynamics may precede hypercarbia and limit apnea testing. If the apnea test cannot be completed as previously described, the examination and apnea test can be attempted at a later time, or an ancillary study may be performed to assist with determination of death. Ancillary studies in newborns are less sensitive than in older children (16). There are no reported cases of the resumption of respiratory effort in a neonate who fulfilled brain death criteria.

The experience with ancillary studies performed in neonates is limited (59). Ancillary studies in this age group are less sensitive in detecting the presence or absence of brain electrical activity or CBF than in older children. Comparison of the two studies shows that the detection of a lack of CBF (63%) was more sensitive than the demonstration of ECS (40%) in confirming the diagnosis of brain death; however, this sensitivity was low for both tests (59). Both EEG voltage and CBF levels can be low at baseline, and this raises concern about the accuracy of these tests in viable newborns (48). This greater level of uncertainty in using less sensitive ancillary studies to determine brain death contributes to the recommendations for a longer period of observation and repeated examinations.

There are also very limited data available regarding the preterm infant and the clinical examination for brain death (59). Determination of brain death of the infant <37 weeks gestation can be complicated by the lack of the development of all the brainstem reflexes at this age. It may also be difficult to assess the level of consciousness in a critically ill, sedated, and intubated preterm infant. Recommendations for determination of brain death in preterm infants <37 weeks gestational age have not been described owing to lack of sufficient data and clinical experience in this age group.

DIAGNOSTIC ERRORS AND DETERMINATION OF BRAIN DEATH

Several publications have suggested that brain death is a reversible condition (23,62,63).

After critical review of these case reports, it is apparent that these patients would not have fulfilled brain death criteria by currently accepted US standards. In these cases, it appears that apnea testing was not appropriately performed or completed, imaging studies did not reveal a significant intracranial injury, EEG testing did not reveal ECS, or radionuclide CBF study did not demonstrate absence of flow.

The use of therapeutic hypothermia after cardiac arrest may pose additional challenges. A case report describes an adult who was treated with induced hypothermia after cardiopulmonary arrest. That adult developed corneal reflexes, cough reflexes, and spontaneous respirations 24 hours after determination of brain death (23). In another study, time to awakening in adult patients receiving therapeutic hypothermia after cardiac arrest was highly variable, and often longer than 3 days (64). These cases highlight the importance of an adequate observation period following induced hypothermia and rewarming before initiating brain death testing. Hypothermia is known to depress CNS function and may lead to a false diagnosis of brain death if the patient is examined soon after being rewarmed. It is also important to consider that clearance of pharmacologic agents can be affected by the presence of organ dysfunction, total amount of medication administered, elimination half-life of the drug and any active metabolites, and other contributing factors such as hypothermia. The clinician caring for critically ill infants and children should be aware of the potential impact of cerebral protective therapies such as hypothermia and the effect it may have on the natural progression and diagnosis of brain death. Based on emerging literature and experience, the authors strongly suggest waiting at least 24 hours following rewarming to ensure adequate metabolism of pharmacologic agents before initiating brain death testing.

Another report that challenges the diagnosis of brain death in a 36-week-gestation newborn describes findings on TCD ultrasonography (63). Despite establishing brain death by clinical criteria, TCD ultrasonography showed persistent blood flow. Criteria to determine death by current US standards were also not met in this case based on the age of the neonate (<37 weeks) and use of TCD as an ancillary study. TCD ultrasonography has not been validated for use in children as an acceptable ancillary study to assist with the determination of brain death.

These examples of diagnostic errors highlight the importance of due diligence exercised by the clinician to ensure that any preexisting or confounding conditions that can impact brain death determination have been corrected prior to initiating brain death testing. The need to follow established guidelines is imperative to avoid diagnostic errors. None of the illustrated cases should be considered as "reversal" of brain death since the initial criteria for brain death were never met.

DETERMINATION OF BRAIN DEATH IN SPECIAL CIRCUMSTANCES

Extracorporeal support is utilized to provide circulatory and respiratory support when conventional therapies fail. Unfortunately, little information is available to guide the clinician in the determination of brain death when advanced therapies, such as ECMO, are utilized. A potential indicator of brain death on ECMO is an increase in mixed venous oxygen saturation that is suspicious for decreased brain oxygen consumption. Performing apnea testing to determine brain death in a patient supported by ECMO may present a challenge because the oxygenators used are highly efficient and may not allow the $Paco_2$ to rise to appropriate levels. Blending CO_2 into the oxygenator to elevate $Paco_2$ to required levels to demonstrate apnea has been suggested in a case report; however, the procedure could not be performed because of patient instability (65).

Apnea testing to determine brain death during VA ECMO has been successfully accomplished in our ICU (66). The CDI blood parameter monitoring system (Terumo Cardiovascular Systems Corp., Ann Arbor, MI, USA) continuously monitors oxygen saturation and blood gases inline in patients on ECMO. We recommend normalizing the $Paco_2$ before starting apnea testing by adjusting ECMO sweep gas flow. Preoxygenation on

VA ECMO can be accomplished by increasing sweep gas F_{IO_2} to 1.0. The patient should be removed from mechanical ventilation and placed on a flow-inflating or Mapleson anesthesia circuit using an F_{IO_2} 1.0 while maintaining adequate CPAP. ECMO sweep gas flow should be decreased to 0.1 L/min, and the CDI blood parameter monitoring system is used to indicate CO_2 rise. Arterial blood gas analysis should be obtained prior to and during apnea testing to confirm the $Paco_2$ level. In accordance with the guidelines, the child's hemodynamics and temperature must be maintained during apnea for brain death testing while supported on VA ECMO. These parameters can be easily achieved by increased ECMO flow and adjusting the heater temperature.

Determining brain death in a child with cyanotic heart disease poses another challenge, and there are no published reports to help the clinician tasked with this process. Current brain death guidelines recommend termination of the apnea test if hemodynamic instability occurs or oxygen saturations fall below 85%. These patients are already in a desaturated state compared with patients who is desaturating. In this situation, the apnea test cannot be completed as currently recommended in the brain death guidelines. An ancillary study should be pursued in this instance to assist with the determination of brain death. It is important to consider that many of these patients will be neonates in whom ancillary testing lacks sensitivity when compared with older children.

DOCUMENTATION AND DETERMINATION OF DEATH

In today's modern pediatric and neonatal ICUs, critical care practitioners and other physicians with expertise in neurologic injury are routinely called on to declare death in infants and children. Brain death examination should be carried out by experienced clinicians (attending physicians) who are familiar with neonates, infants, and children and have specific training in neurocritical care. Current guidelines in the United States recommend two examinations and apnea tests separated by an observation period in order to determine brain death (16,17). In most locations, death is declared after the second neurologic examination and apnea test confirm an unchanged and irreversible condition. This is in contrast to other countries where the time of death may be based on the first examination (13). When ancillary studies are used, documentation of components from the second clinical examination that can be completed, including a second apnea test, must remain consistent with brain death. The second clinical examination confirms continued coma and apnea during an extended observation period, which is ultimately the final determining factor to diagnose brain death. The diagnosis of brain death has profound medical and legal consequences. Care must be taken to ensure that all parts of the clinical examination, including the apnea test, are performed properly and appropriately documented. Current pediatric guidelines include a checklist in an attempt to standardize documentation of the clinical examination, apnea test, and ancillary studies to determine brain death (**Table 67.3**) (16). Standardization of the clinical examination and documentation to determine brain death in infants and children will help reduce and possibly eliminate confusion and variability in practice standards.

Diagnosing brain death should never be rushed or take a priority over the needs of the patient or the family. It should be the expectation of medical providers that patients will continue to be actively managed until a determination of death has been made or a decision to withdraw medical therapies is agreed on between the family and the healthcare team. Appropriate emotional support for the family should be provided during this process. State law in certain situations may require consultation or referral to the medical examiner or coroner when death occurs.

As critical care providers, we are obligated to provide support and guidance for the families as they face difficult end-of-life decisions and attempt to understand what has happened to their child. It is our responsibility to guide and direct families in the treatment of their child. We must be open and honest in our discussions with parents and families, and never allow a family to leave the hospital thinking they were responsible for allowing their child to die. Communication with families during end-of-life care should be done with compassion, empathy, and honesty. Clear, concise, and simple terminology should be used so that the parents and family members understand that their child has died. *Brain death* is a medical term and is poorly understood even by some healthcare professionals (11). The term *brain death* should be avoided, and discussions with parents and families should center on the death of the child, not the death of an organ. Allowing families to be present during the brain death examination and apnea test can assist families in understanding that their child has died. The family must understand that once brain death has been declared, the child is dead. Confusion or anger may result if discussions with the family regarding withdrawal of support or medical therapies are entertained after declaration of death. It should be made clear that once death has occurred, continuation of medical therapies, including mechanical ventilation, is no longer an option unless organ donation is planned. A reasonable grieving period should be allowed for family members to spend with their child before discontinuing mechanical ventilation and other supportive medical therapies.

CONCLUSIONS AND FUTURE DIRECTIONS

The clinical diagnosis of brain death is highly reliable when determined by experienced examiners using established criteria. Ancillary studies are no longer necessary unless the neurologic examination and apnea test cannot be entirely completed. We continue to gain more experience determining brain death in children, including infants. Ancillary studies are not as reliable or sensitive in infants, resulting in a great need to have more reliable and accurate ancillary studies in this age group. Current brain death guidelines continue to advise caution in the infant and support a longer observation period. Longer observation periods are also advised in patients who have received newer therapeutic modalities such as hypothermia, to ensure that all prerequisites have been met prior to brain death testing. The impact of cerebral protective strategies that may alter the natural course of brain death requires further review and investigation. The clinician caring for critically ill infants and children should be aware of the potential influence newer therapeutic modalities may have when making the determination of brain death.

Each state and institution may have specific guidelines to determine brain death in infants and children since no national law to determine death exists. National medical societies should work together to develop a uniform approach to determine death in all patients that can be adopted by all states and medical institutions. The medical and legal implications of determining brain death are profound and require a consistent approach during examinations and apnea testing. Diagnostic errors may result in an incorrect diagnosis of brain death and can be avoided by careful attention to potential confounding variables. The importance of accurately determining brain death is essential to the transplantation community to ensure that organ recovery is carried out within currently accepted medical standards. Research

TABLE 67.3

CHECKLIST FOR DOCUMENTATION OF BRAIN DEATH

Brain Death Examination for Infants and Children

Two physicians must perform independent examinations separated by specified intervals

Age of Patient	Timing of First Examination	Interexamination Interval
Term newborn 37 weeks gestational age and up to 30 days old	☐ First examination may be performed 24 hours after birth or following cardiopulmonary resuscitation or other severe brain injury	☐ At least 24 hours ☐ Interval shortened because ancillary study (Section 4) is consistent with brain death
31 days to 18 years old	☐ First examination may be performed 24 hours following cardiopulmonary resuscitation or other severe brain injury	☐ At least 12 hours OR ☐ Interval shortened because ancillary study (Section 4) is consistent with brain death

Section 1. PREREQUISITES for Brain Death Examination and Apnea Test

A. IRREVERSIBLE AND IDENTIFIABLE Cause of Coma (Please Check)

☐ Traumatic brain injury ☐ Anoxic brain injury ☐ Known metabolic disorder ☐ Other (Specify) _____

B. Correction of Contributing Factors That Can Interfere with the Neurologic Examination	Examination One		Examination Two	
a. Core body temperature is over 95°F (35°C)	☐ Yes	☐ No	☐ Yes	☐ No
b. Systolic blood pressure or MAP in acceptable range (systolic BP not less than two standard deviations below age-appropriate norm) based on age	☐ Yes	☐ No	☐ Yes	☐ No
c. Sedative/analgesic drug effect excluded as a contributing factor	☐ Yes	☐ No	☐ Yes	☐ No
d. Metabolic intoxication excluded as a contributing factor	☐ Yes	☐ No	☐ Yes	☐ No
e. Neuromuscular blockade excluded as a contributing factor	☐ Yes	☐ No	☐ Yes	☐ No

☐ If ALL prerequisites are marked YES, then proceed to Section 2, OR

☐ ———— confounding variable was present. Ancillary study was therefore performed to document brain death (Section 4)

Section 2. Physical Examination (Please Check) NOTE: SPINAL CORD REFLEXES ARE ACCEPTABLE	Examination One Date/Time: ——		Examination Two Date/Time: ——	
a. Flaccid tone, patient unresponsive to deep painful stimuli	☐ Yes	☐ No	☐ Yes	☐ No
b. Pupils are mid-position or fully dilated, and light reflexes are absent	☐ Yes	☐ No	☐ Yes	☐ No
c. Corneal, cough, gag reflexes are absent	☐ Yes	☐ No	☐ Yes	☐ No
Sucking and rooting reflexes are absent (in neonates and infants)	☐ Yes	☐ No	☐ Yes	☐ No
d. Oculovestibular reflexes are absent	☐ Yes	☐ No	☐ Yes	☐ No
e. Spontaneous respiratory effort while on mechanical ventilation is absent	☐ Yes	☐ No	☐ Yes	☐ No

☐ The ———— (specify) element of the examination could not be performed because ————.

Ancillary study (EEG or radionuclide CBF) was therefore performed to document brain death (Section 4)

Section 3. APNEA Test	Examination One Date/Time——	Examination Two Date/Time——
No spontaneous respiratory efforts were observed despite final Paco2 ≥ 60 mm Hg and a ≥ 20 mm Hg increase above baseline (Examination One) No spontaneous respiratory efforts were observed despite final Paco2 ≥ 60 mm Hg and a ≥ 20 mm Hg increase above baseline (Examination Two)	Pretest Paco2: —— Apnea duration: ——min Posttest Paco2: ——	Pretest Paco2: —— Apnea duration: ——min Posttest Paco2: ——

Apnea test is contraindicated or could not be performed to completion because ————. Ancillary study (EEG or radionuclide CBF) was therefore performed to document brain death (Section 4)

Section 4. ANCILLARY testing is required (a) when any components of the examination or apnea testing cannot be completed; (b) if there is uncertainty about the results of the neurologic examination; or (c) if a medication effect may be present. Ancillary testing can be performed to reduce the interexamination period; however, a second neurologic examination is required. Components of the neurologic examination that can be performed safely should be completed in close proximity to the ancillary test. Date/Time: ——

☐ EEG report documents electrocerebral silence, OR ☐ Yes ☐ No

☐ CBF study report documents no cerebral perfusion ☐ Yes ☐ No

Section 5. Signatures

Examiner One

I certify that my examination is consistent with cessation of function of the brain and brainstem. Confirmatory examination to follow

____ ____ ____ ____ ____ ____

(Printed Name) (Signature) (Specialty) (Pager #/License #) (Date mm/dd/yyyy) (Time)

Examiner Two

I certify that my examination ☐ and/or ancillary test report ☐ confirms unchanged and irreversible cessation of function of the brain and brainstem. The patient is declared brain dead at this time

Date/Time of Death: ————

____ ____ ____ ____ ____ ____

(Printed Name) (Signature) (Specialty) (Pager #/License #) (Date mm/dd/yyyy) (Time)

EEG, electroencephalogram; CBF, cerebral blood flow.

Reused with permission from Nakagawa TA, Ashwal S, Mathur M, et al. Guidelines for the determination of brain death in infants and children: an update of the 1987 task force recommendations. *Crit Care Med.* 2011;39:2139–55.

MAP = mean arterial pressure.

is needed to validate accuracy and safety of newer ancillary studies to assist with the determination of brain death. Additionally, more experience is needed to determine if a single brain death examination is sufficient to determine death in infants and children. Adherence to currently accepted guidelines is essential to ensure that testing and determination of brain death are performed in a standardized manner for all patients.

References

1. Mollaret P, Goulon M. Le coma dépassé. *Rev Neurol (Paris)* 1959; 101:3–15.

2. A definition of irreversible coma. Report of the Ad Hoc Committee of the Harvard Medical School to Examine the Definition of Brain Death. *JAMA* 1968;205:337–40.

3. Guidelines for the determination of death. Report of the medical consultants on the diagnosis of death to the President's Commission for the Study of Ethical Problems in Medicine and Biomedical and Behavioral Research. *JAMA* 1981;246:2184–6.

4. Report of special Task Force. Guidelines for the determination of brain death in children. American Academy of Pediatrics Task Force on Brain Death in Children. *Pediatrics* 1987;80:298–300.

5. Chang MY, McBride LA, Ferguson MA. Variability in brain death declaration practices in pediatric head trauma patients. *Pediatr Neurosurg* 2003;39:7–9.

6. Mejia RE, Pollack MM. Variability in brain death determination practices in children. *JAMA* 1995;274:550–3.

7. Mathur M, Petersen L, Stadtler M, et al. Variability in pediatric brain death determination and documentation in southern California. *Pediatrics* 2008;121:988–93.

8. Hornby K, Shemie SD, Teitelbaum J, et al. Variability in hospital-based brain death guidelines in Canada. *Can J Anaesth* 2006;53:613–9.

9. Joffe AR, Anton N. Brain death: Understanding of the conceptual basis by pediatric intensivists in Canada. *Arch Pediatr Adolesc Med* 2006;160:747–52.

10. Lynch J, Eldadah MK. Brain-death criteria currently used by pediatric intensivists. *Clin Pediatr (Phila)* 1992;31:457–60.

11. Harrison AM, Botkin JR. Can pediatricians define and apply the concept of brain death? *Pediatrics* 1999;103:e82.

12. Greer DM, Varelas PN, Haque S, et al. Variability of brain death determination guidelines in leading US neurologic institutions. *Neurology* 2008;70:284–9.

13. Shemie SD, Doig C, Dickens B, et al. Severe brain injury to neurological determination of death: Canadian forum recommendations. *CMAJ* 2006;174:S1–13.

14. Practice parameters for determining brain death in adults (summary statement). The Quality Standards Subcommittee of the American Academy of Neurology. *Neurology* 1995;45:1012–4.

15. Wijdicks EF, Varelas PN, Gronseth GS, et al. Evidence-based guideline update: Determining brain death in adults: Report of the Quality Standards Subcommittee of the American Academy of Neurology. *Neurology* 2010;74:1911–8.

16. Nakagawa TA, Ashwal S, Mathur M, et al. Guidelines for the determination of brain death in infants and children: An update of the 1987 task force recommendations. *Crit Care Med* 2011;39:2139–55.

17. Nakagawa TA, Ashwal, SA, Mathur M, et al; Committee for Brain Death in Infants and Children. Clinical report—guidelines for the determination of brain death in infants and children: An update of the 1987 task force recommendations. *Pediatrics* 2011;128:e720–40.

18. *Controversies in the Determination of Death: A White Paper by the President's Council on Bioethics.* Washington, DC: The President's Council on Bioethic, 2008. http://www.thenewatlantis.com/docLib/20091130_determination_of_death.pdf. Accessed August 3, 2011.

19. Hutchison JS, Ward RE, Lacroix J, et al. Hypothermia therapy after traumatic brain injury in children. *N Engl J Med* 2008; 358:2447–56.

20. Adelson PD, Ragheb J, Kanev P, et al. Phase II clinical trial of moderate hypothermia after severe traumatic brain injury in children. *Neurosurgery* 2005;56:740–54.

21. Azzopardi DV, Strohm B, Edwards AD, et al. Moderate hypothermia to treat perinatal asphyxial encephalopathy. *N Engl J Med* 2009;361:1349–58.

22. Hutchison JS, Doherty DR, Orlowski JP, et al. Hypothermia therapy for cardiac arrest in pediatric patients. *Pediatr Clin North Am* 2008;55:529–44.

23. Kochanek PM, Fink EL, Bell MJ, et al. Therapeutic hypothermia: Applications in pediatric cardiac arrest. *J Neurotrauma* 2009;26:421–7.

24. Doherty DR, Parshuram CS, Gaboury I, et al. Hypothermia therapy after pediatric cardiac arrest. *Circulation* 2009;119:1492–500.

25. Hoehn T, Hansmann G, Bührer C, et al. Therapeutic hypothermia in neonates. Review of current clinical data, ILCOR recommendations and suggestions for implementation in neonatal intensive care units. *Resuscitation* 2008;78:7–12.

26. Webb AC, Samuels OB. Reversible brain death after cardiopulmonary arrest and induced hypothermia. *Crit Care Med* 2011;39:1538–42.

27. Abend NS, Kessler SK, Helfaer MA, et al. Evaluation of the comatose child. In: Nichols DG, ed. *Rogers Textbook of Pediatric Intensive Care.* 4th ed. Philadelphia, PA: Lippincott Williams & Wilkins, 2008:846–61.

28. Michelson DJJ, Ashwal S. Evaluation of coma. In: Wheeler DS, Wong HR, Shanley TP, eds. *Pediatric Critical Care Medicine Basic Science and Clinical Evidence.* London: Springer-Verlag, 2007:924–34.

29. Wijdicks E. Confirmatory testing of brain death in adults. In: Wijdicks E, ed. *Brain Death.* Philadelphia, PA: Lippincott William & Wilkins, 2001:61–90.

30. Flowers WM Jr, Patel BR. Accuracy of clinical evaluation in the determination of brain death. *South Med J* 2000;93:203–6.

31. Ashwal S. Clinical diagnosis and confirmatory testing of brain death in children. In: Wijdick EFM, ed. *Brain Death.* Philadelphia, PA: Lippincott William & Wilkins, 2001:91–114.

32. Organ Procurement Transplantation Network. OPTN.transplant.hrsa.gov. Accessed February 2012.

33. Haque IU, Udassi JP, Zaritsky AL. Outcome following cardiopulmonary arrest. *Pediatr Clin North Am* 2008;55:969–87.

34. Mandel R, Martinot A, Delepoulle F, et al. Prediction of outcome after hypoxic-ischemic encephalopathy: A prospective clinical and electrophysiologic study. *J Pediatr* 2002;141:45–50.

35. Carter BG, Butt W. A prospective study of outcome predictors after severe brain injury in children. *Intensive Care Med* 2005;31:840–5.

36. Outwater KM, Rockoff MA. Apnea testing to confirm brain death in children. *Crit Care Med* 1984;12:357–8.

37. Rowland TW, Donnelly JH, Jackson AH. Apnea documentation for determination of brain death in children. *Pediatrics* 1984; 74:505–8.

38. Ashwal S. Brain death in the newborn. Current perspectives. *Clin Perinatol* 1997;24:859–82.

39. Paret G, Barzilay Z. Apnea testing in suspected brain dead children—Physiological and mathematical modelling. *Intensive Care Med* 1995;21:247–52.

40. Wijdicks EFM. Confirmatory testing of brain death in adults. In: Wijdick EFM, ed. *Brain Death.* Philadelphia, PA: Lippincott William & Wilkins, 2001:61–90.

41. Wijdicks EFM, Rabinstein AA, Manno EM, et al. Pronouncing brain death. Contemporary practice and safety of the apnea test. *Neurology* 2008;71:1240–4.

42. Joffe AR, Anton NR, Duff JP. The apnea test: Rationale, confounders, and criticism. *J Child Neurol* 2010;25:1435–43.

43. Tibballs J. A critique of the apneic oxygenation test for the diagnosis of "brain death." *Pediatr Crit Care Med* 2010;11:475–8.

44. Goudreau JL, Wijdicks EFM, Emery SF. Complications during apnea testing in the determination of brain death: Predisposing factors. *Neurology* 2000;55:1045–8.

45. Flowers WM Jr, Patel BR. Radionuclide angiography as a confirmatory test for brain death: A review of 229 studies in 219 patients. *South Med J* 1997;90:1091–6.

46. Sinha P, Conrad GR. Scintigraphic confirmation of brain death. *Semin Nucl Med* 2012;42:27–32.

47. Ruiz-García M, Gonzalez-Astiazarán A, Collado-Corona MA, et al. Brain death in children: Clinical, neurophysiological and radioisotopic angiography findings in 125 patients. *Childs Nerv Syst* 2000;16:40–5.

48. ACR Practice Guidelines for the Performance of Single Photon Emission Computed Tomography (SPECT) Brain Perfusion and Brain Death Studies, 2007. http://www.acr.org/~/media/ACR/Documents/PGTS/guidelines/CT_SPECT_Brain_Perfusion.pdf.

49. Donohoe KJ, Frey KA, Gerbaudo VH, et al. *Society of Nuclear Medicine Procedure Guideline for Brain Death Scintigraphy.* http://interactive.snm.org/docs/pg_ch20_0403.pdf. Accessed June 20, 2012.

50. Guideline three: Minimum technical standards for EEG recording in suspected cerebral death. American Electroencephalographic Society. *J Clin Neurophysiol* 1994;11:10–13.

51. LaMancusa J, Cooper R, Vieth R, et al. The effects of the falling therapeutic and subtherapeutic barbiturate blood levels on electrocerebral silence in clinically brain-dead children. *Clin Electroencephalogr* 1991;22:112–7.

52. López-Navidad A, Caballero F, Domingo P, et al. Early diagnosis of brain death in patients treated with central nervous system depressant drugs. *Transplantation* 2000;70:131–5.

53. Qureshi AI, Kirmani JF, Xavier AR, et al. Computed tomographic angiography for diagnosis of brain death. *Neurology* 2004;62:652–3.

54. Escudero D, Otero J, Vega P, et al. [Diagnosis of brain death by multislice CT scan: AngioCT scan and brain perfusion]. *Med Intensiva* 2007;31:335–41.

55. Frampas E, Videcoq M, de Kerviler E, et al. CT angiography for brain death diagnosis. *AJNR Am J Neuroradiol* 2009;30:1566–70.

56. Donohoe KJ, Frey KA, Gerbaudo VH, et al. Procedure guideline for brain death scintigraphy. *J Nucl Med.* 2003;44:846–51.

57. Ashwal S. Brain death in early infancy. *J Heart Lung Transplant* 1993;12(6 pt 2):S176–8.

58. Ashwal S, Schneider S. Brain death in the newborn. *Pediatrics* 1989;84:429–37.

59. Ashwal S. Brain death in the newborn. *Clin Perinatol* 1989;16:501–18.

60. Saugstad OD, Rootwelt T, Aalen O. Resuscitation of asphyxiated newborn infants with room air or oxygen: An international controlled trial: The Resair 2 study. *Pediatrics* 1998;102(1). http://www.pediatrics.org/cgi/content/full/102/1/e1.

61. Hutchinson AA. Recovery from hypopnea in preterm lambs: Effects of breathing air or oxygen. *Pediatr Pulmonol* 1987;3:317–23.

62. AR Joffe, Kolski H, Duff J, et al. A 10 month old with reversible findings of brain death. *Pediatr Neurol* 2009;41(5):378–382.

63. Mata-Zubillaga D, Oulego-Erroz I. Persistent cerebral blood flow by Transcranial Doppler ultrasonography in an asphyxiated infant meeting brain death diagnosis: Case report and review of the literature. *J Perinatol* 2012;32(6):473–5.

64. Grossestreuer AV, Aella BS, Leary M, et al. Time to awakening and neurologic outcome in therapeutic hypothermia-treated cardiac arrest patients. *Resuscitation.* 2013;84(12):1741–6. doi: 10.1016/j.resuscitation.2013.07.009. Epub 2013 Aug 1.

65. Muralidharan R, Mateen FJ, Shinohara RT, et al. The challenges with brain death determination in adult patients on extracorporeal membrane oxygenation. *Neurocrit Care* 2011;14:423–6.

66. Jarrah RJ, Ajizian SJ, Agarwal S et al. Developing a Standard Method for Apnea Testing in the Determination of Brain Death for Patients on Venoarterial Extracorporeal Membrane Oxygenation: A Pediatric Case Series. *Pediatr Crit Care Med* 2014;15:e38–e43.

CHAPTER 68 ■ **CARDIAC ANATOMY**

STEVEN M. SCHWARTZ, ZDENEK SLAVIK, AND SIEW YEN HO

KEY POINTS

1 The use of the segmental approach to describe the complex congenital heart disease systems allows a clear form of communication of all essential elements of the cardiac anatomy.

2 There are two primary systems that are used to describe the anatomy of congenital heart disease, one of which relies primarily on cardiac segments and their attachments, and the other invokes presumed embryologic events. Many clinicians use a combination of the two systems as well as additional colloquialisms.

3 The cornerstones of segmental anatomy are identification of the morphologic atria and ventricles with description of their connections and alignments to each other and of the ventricles to the great arteries.

4 Congenital cardiac defects are broadly classified into four categories: (a) *left-to-right shunts*, (b) cyanotic defects, (c) obstructive defects, and (d) other complex congenital heart defects.

Congenital heart disease is often simple to describe and understand, as in the case of an atrial or ventricular septal defect (VSD), but can also be quite complex and even forbidding to those not well versed in the subtleties of cardiac anatomy when there are more comprehensive defects. Significant controversies have persisted regarding the best overall approach to the nomenclature of complex congenital heart disease, and many cardiologists frequently use various shorthand designations or colloquialisms to describe these lesions, leading many noncardiologists to consider it an exercise in semantics or hairsplitting, best left to the pediatric cardiologist. In reality though, the intensive care physician must be familiar with the way in which such defects are described since anatomy often dictates physiology—physiology being the cornerstone of the clinical care of these patients. This chapter will review the common approaches to systematically and comprehensively categorizing the anatomy of congenital heart disease with the intended goal of familiarizing the pediatric critical care physician with the basic schemes used in assigning specific terms to specific defects. This chapter is not intended to resolve controversies where they exist, nor is it proffered as a comprehensive review of any one particular approach; rather, it will hopefully provide a practical framework for understanding how one goes about describing complex defects in an organized manner that helps the intensive care physician understand "how the blood goes 'round'" and sets the basis for better communication with cardiology and cardiac surgery colleagues.

SEGMENTAL APPROACH TO CONGENITAL HEART DISEASE

1 Even though many common lesions can be described directly, the underlying basis for complete description of any congenital heart lesion is a segmental approach. Segmental analysis of cardiac anatomy requires analysis of each cardiac segment, its morphology, and its relationship to adjoining cardiac segments. One can use this methodical approach to consider each part of the heart in turn: atria, ventricles, and great arteries. The connections between the segments (atrioventricular and ventriculo-arterial) are described, as are the atrial and ventricular septa, cardiac venous connections, and position of the heart within the thorax. Using a segmental approach, all congenital heart defects can be described in complete detail, and the physiology determined from the anatomy.

2 There are two primary systems in use today for describing complex cardiac defects. The merits of one system or the other have been the subject of numerous scholarly papers and debates (1,2), but in truth they have more similarities than differences, and many cardiologists and cardiac surgeons use terms derived from both systems at different times. Robert Anderson is the primary advocate of the concept of sequential segmental analysis emphasizing morphology, connections, and relations of segmental components as the basis for nomenclature. Richard and Stella Van Praagh, building substantially on work by Maurice Lev, have advocated a system also based on morphologic analysis of various segments, but with some significant differences in specific nomenclature, analysis, and definition of connections or junctions between segments. The use of this latter approach relies on cardiac embryology to understand the basic patterns of postnatal congenital heart disease and has inherent value, in that almost all lesions can be recognized to be the result of incomplete or inaccurate steps in the transition of the heart from the embryonic heart tube to the mature four-chamber heart. The value of the former system is that it allows description of any given situation, with no need to speculate about unobserved embryologic events.

Both of these systems are based on the principles (a) that specific cardiac chambers have unique, distinguishing characteristics that allow them to be clearly identified even when their left/right relationship to each other or connections to adjoining structures are altered or absent, and (b) that the precise nature of these relationships and connections should be carefully and fully described.

Atrial Situs

The terms "right" and "left" atria refer to specific, distinguishing morphologic characteristics of each atrium, not to the side of the heart on which they are located or their accompanying venous or ventricular connections. Features that identify the right atrium include (a) a blunt atrial appendage with a wide connection to the smooth-walled part of the atrium, (b) the limbus of the fossa ovalis, and (c) remnants of the valves of the sinus venosus such as the Eustachian valve of the coronary sinus. The left atrium is characterized by (a) a hooked appendage with a more narrow connection to the smooth-walled portion of the chamber, (b) the flap valve of the fossa ovalis, and (c) no remnants of venous valves. Note that venous connections are not used to designate the morphologic right and left atria since these connections can be variable in congenital heart disease (i.e., total anomalous pulmonary venous return, unroofed coronary sinus, bilateral superior vena cava). Additionally, the atrial appendages may be juxtaposed, wherein the morphologic left atrium has an appendage with the characteristics of a right atrial appendage or vice versa, so that use of this feature to identify which atrium is which is of limited value in certain cases.

Once the morphology of the atria has been identified, the atrial arrangement or situs can be defined. *Atrial situs* refers to the arrangement of the morphologic right and left atria within the heart. *Situs solitus* is the normal arrangement, wherein the right atrium is to the right and the left atrium is to the left. *Situs inversus* is the opposite arrangement; the right atrium is to the left and the left atrium is to the right. A major difference between the Anderson and Van Praagh approaches to nomenclature concerns the recognition of the possibility of atrial isomerism. *Atrial isomerism* is defined as having two morphologically left or right atria. Van Praagh contends that having two right or left atria is an impossibility and that atrial situs in all hearts can be described as solitus, inversus, or ambiguus, in which ambiguus refers to the situation where separate right and left atria cannot be differentiated (3). Using this approach, anatomic variants that would be considered cases of atrial isomerism are more generally defined in terms of heterotaxy syndromes since there are often extracardiac abnormalities of laterality that coexist with the congenital heart disease. *Polysplenia syndrome* is thus often used to mean the same thing as left atrial isomerism, and *asplenia syndrome* is often used to mean the same atrial arrangement as right atrial isomerism. Anderson argues that this approach is at times inaccurate, since not all patients with congenital heart disease congruent with polysplenia are actually polysplenic, and not all with cardiac anatomy consistent with asplenia are asplenic. Rather, the Andersonian system suggests that atrial situs can be identified in all cases as usual or solitus, mirror image or inversus, and right isomerism or left isomerism (4).

As suggested earlier, the assignment of atrial situs can be assisted by observation of other asymmetrically distributed structures, and the identification of atrial isomerism can lead to investigations for malposition of noncardiac structures. The bronchi can be particularly helpful in identifying atrial situs since the right and left bronchi have characteristic features readily seen on chest x-ray and since bronchial situs almost always reflects atrial situs (5). Specifically, the right mainstem bronchus is shorter, more vertically oriented and is located directly behind the mediastinal segment of the right pulmonary artery. The left mainstem bronchus is longer, more horizontally oriented and below the left pulmonary artery. When the atria are inverted, the left-sided bronchus will usually have the orientation of a typical right bronchus and the left lung may contain three lobes. The right-sided bronchus will then have a typical left mainstem bronchus anatomy. Isomeric

arrangement of the atria usually is reflected by a bilaterally symmetrical bronchial arrangement of either a right or a left type. In heterotaxy syndromes (atrial isomerism), abdominal structures in addition to the spleen can be abnormally distributed. Right atrial isomerism or asplenia can be thought of as bilateral right-sidedness and can be associated with a midline liver and intestinal malrotation. Left atrial isomerism or polysplenia syndrome can be thought of as bilateral left-sidedness and is also associated with an intestinal malrotation.

The finding of atrial isomerism is also typically accompanied by certain predictable, associated intracardiac defects. Right atrial isomerism or asplenia syndrome usually includes anomalies of pulmonary venous return, atrioventricular canal–type defects, double outlet right ventricle (DORV), and transposition (6–8). Left atrial isomerism tends to be more commonly associated with abnormalities of systemic venous connections (interrupted inferior vena cava) and DORV or normally related great arteries. Polysplenia can also be associated with atrioventricular canal defects and some abnormalities of pulmonary venous drainage, but usually not to the degree these are associated with asplenia. These associations are important for the cardiologist in that they prompt complete assessment for these types of lesions, but also for the intensivist in terms of providing a mental framework for understanding and description of these complex anatomic variants.

The Atrial Septum

The atrial septum, in its usual state, contains a foramen ovale on the right side and the flap valve of the foramen on the left. The foramen, when patent, allows right-to-left shunting of blood when the right atrial pressure exceeds the left, but is closed by the flap valve when left atrial pressure is higher. The foramen ovale is the remnant of the ostium secundum, and therefore, atrial septal defects (ASDs) in this area are referred to as *secundum ASDs*. The foramen primum is the embryologic opening between the early atrial septum (septum primum) and the area where the endocardial cushions ultimately form. The foramen primum is closed by endocardial cushion tissue, thus making *primum ASDs* a common component of atrioventricular canal (endocardial cushion) defects. The least common type of ASD is the *sinus venosus ASD*, which is found in the superior part of the atrial septum where the sinus venosus is incorporated into the embryonic atrium. This type of defect is often associated with partial anomalous venous connection of the right upper pulmonary vein.

Ventricular Morphology and Topology

As with the atria, the right and left ventricles are identified by certain constant morphologic patterns, not by their location within the heart or the body. The morphologic right ventricle (a) is heavily trabeculated, (b) contains the moderator band of the septum, and (c) has septal attachments of the associated atrioventricular valve. The left ventricle (a) is smooth walled, (b) is more bullet shaped, and (c) has no septal attachments of the atrioventricular valve. When there are two distinct atrioventricular valves, the tricuspid valve (TV) is *always* associated with the morphologic right ventricle, and the mitral valve is *always* associated with the left ventricle.

The topology of the ventricles refers to the spatial anatomy of the ventricle with regard to the inflow and outflow. Determination of the "handedness" of a ventricle is made by considering the relationship of the inflow and outflow tracts of the ventricle when looking at the septal surface (**Fig. 68.1**). One can imagine placing the palm of the hand on the septal

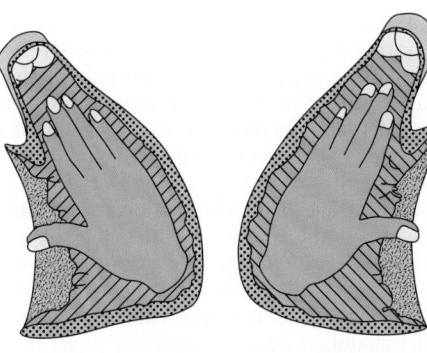

FIGURE 68.1. Ventricular topology is determined by imagining the palmer surface of the hand on the septal surface of the morphologically right ventricle with the thumb pointing toward the inlet and the fingers pointing toward the outlet. Right-hand topology is present if this can be accomplished with the right hand. Left-hand topology is present if this alignment requires use of the left hand. (From Anderson RH. Nomenclature and classification: Sequential segmental analysis. In: Moller JH, Hoffman JIE, eds. *Pediatric Cardiovascular Medicine*. Philadelphia, PA: Churchill Livingstone, 2000:263–74, with permission.)

surface of the morphologically right ventricle with the thumb extended toward the inflow and the fingers pointed toward the outflow. If this can be accomplished with the right hand, the ventricle is said to be "right handed"; if it can be accomplished with the left hand, the ventricle is "left handed." In general, a normal heart is said to have right-handed topology, but this terminology does not describe or identify the morphology of the ventricle, nor does it describe the location within the heart, although certain anatomic and morphologic arrangements are generally associated with specific handedness for the morphologic right and left ventricles.

Atrioventricular Connections, Junctions, and Alignments

The exact nature of the atrioventricular relationship can take many forms. Usually, there are two separate atrioventricular valves, one leading into each ventricle. Furthermore, the right atrium usually opens into the morphologic right ventricle, and the left atrium into the left ventricle. Of course, in complex congenital heart disease, this is not always the case and as such, it is important to precisely describe the way in which this part of the heart is arranged. For the purpose of clarity, it is helpful to consider both the type of atrioventricular connection and the mode of connection. The type of atrioventricular connection or alignment refers to the anatomic concordance or discordance of the atrium and ventricle. A normal heart has concordant atrial and ventricular connections or alignments, in that the morphologic right atrium opens to the morphologic right ventricle, and the left atrium does likewise with the left ventricle. A discordant connection or alignment is one in which the morphologic right atrium opens into the morphologic left ventricle and vice versa. When there is atrial isomerism or when both atria open into one ventricle, one can describe the relationship as ambiguous and refer to the topology of the ventricles (**Fig. 68.2**) or to the looping pattern. Also, a single common atrioventricular valve that guards the opening between right and left atria above and right and left ventricles below can still be referred to in terms of concordant and discordant connections or alignments.

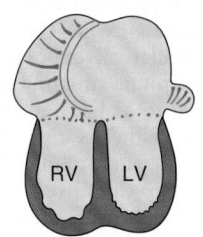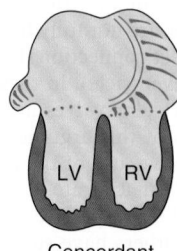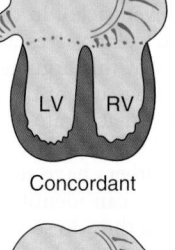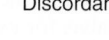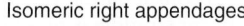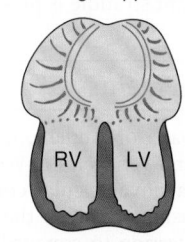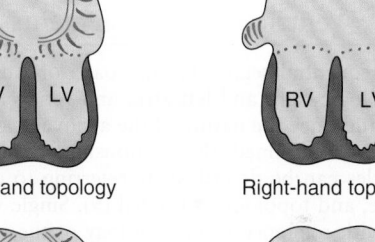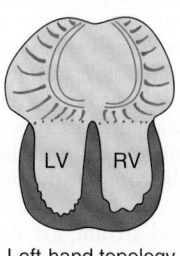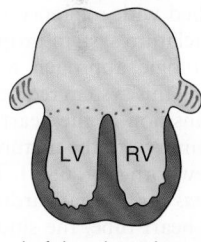

FIGURE 68.2. The atrioventricular connection can be described as concordant or discordant when there are two morphologically different atria (**A–D**). When there is atrial isomerism, the connection can be referred to by identifying the atrial morphology followed by the ventricular topology (**E–H**). RV, Right ventricle; LV, Left ventricle. (Modified from Anderson RH. Nomenclature and classification: Sequential segmental analysis. In: Moller JH, Hoffman JIE, eds. *Pediatric Cardiovascular Medicine*. Philadelphia, PA: Churchill Livingstone, 2000:263–74.)

The mode by which the atria open into the ventricles must also be described accurately. This refers to the precise morphology of the atrioventricular valve or valves. When there are two atria, two atrioventricular valves, and two ventricles, the TV is always associated with the morphologic right ventricle, and the mitral valve is always associated with the morphologic left ventricle. When one of the valves is atretic and/or the ventricle is hypoplastic, there are still considered to be two atrioventricular valves in terms of assignment of anatomic diagnosis (e.g., tricuspid atresia or hypoplastic left heart). Nomenclature is more complex when there is a single, common atrioventricular valve as in an atrioventricular canal type defect where the two valves are not fully formed and distinct, or when there is a double inlet connection (both atrioventricular valves open into the same ventricle). In these types of anatomic situations, the atrioventricular valves are often referred to as left and right. The basis of this argument is that since neither is a properly formed valve, use of the names "tricuspid" and/or "mitral" is technically inaccurate, and thus, referring to the valves on the basis of their respective position within the heart is most correct (1). Others have suggested that even under these circumstances one can identify the valves as mitral and/or tricuspid and should thus do so (2).

The nature of the atrioventricular connection can be further complicated when an *inlet VSD* is present. These types of VSDs often involve *override* or *straddle* the atrioventricular valve. Override occurs when the annulus of the atrioventricular valve overrides the ventricular septum and thus allows the atrium associated with the overriding valve to empty into both ventricles. A straddling atrioventricular valve is one in which the chordal attachments of the valve cross the plane of the septum to attach to the contralateral ventricle. The left atrioventricular valve, for example, may have chordal attachments to the right side of the ventricular septum. Override and straddle are not mutually exclusive, and straddle is the far more complex problem to repair, leading to consideration of single ventricle–type palliation when significant straddle is present.

Ventricular Arrangements

Using the sequential segmental approach of Anderson, once the morphologic right and left atria and ventricles have been identified, and once the nature of the atrioventricular connection has been ascertained, the relationships between the atria and ventricles can be described by referring to concordance, discordance, and topology as needed (9). Single ventricles are described with reference to morphology of the ventricle. The nomenclature system proposed by Van Praagh is based on an embryologic approach to segmental anatomy (10). Understanding this system requires one to have basic familiarity with the transition of the heart from the straight heart tube of the early embryo to the mature, four-chambered heart of the fetus and newborn (**Fig. 68.3**). The heart tube contains the *progenitor areas* for all four cardiac chambers. The most caudal areas of the heart tube, the sinus venosus and atrium, are destined to become the right and left atria. The embryologic atrium leads directly into the embryonic ventricle, which is the future left ventricle. Moving more rostrally, the ventricle opens into the bulbus cordis, destined to become right ventricle, which then gives rise to the outlet of the heart, the conus arteriosus and arterial trunk. Transition from the straight heart tube requires the tube to loop, usually with the apex of the loop being rightward, referred to as a *dextro* or *d-loop*. The apex occurs at the junction of the ventricle and bulbus cordis. When *d*-looping occurs, the embryologic ventricle ends up leftward of the bulbus cordis, thus placing the left ventricle to the left of the right ventricle. When looping occurs abnormally, with the apex of the loop to the left, one is faced with a situation in which the morphologic left ventricle ends up rightward of the morphologic right ventricle. This arrangement is referred to as a *levo* or *l-loop*.

Obviously, it is impossible to replay the exact sequence of embryologic development when it is necessary to make a precise anatomic diagnosis in a fetus or newborn. The power of this particular nomenclature system, however, lies in its ability to predict comprehensive patterns of abnormalities since much congenital heart disease represents incomplete or improperly finished incidents in embryologic heart

development. From a practical standpoint then, a heart in which the morphologic right ventricle is on the right and the morphologic left ventricle is on the left side of the heart is *d*-looped, and a heart in which the morphologic right ventricle is on the left and the morphologic left ventricle is on the right is *l*-looped. This nomenclature system further requires that the lower cardiac chamber have an inlet from an atrium to be called a ventricle. This inlet can be atretic, but must be present. Lower chambers with an outlet but not an inlet are referred to as *outlet chambers*; lack of both an inlet and an outlet is the hallmark of a *trabecular pouch*. A lower chamber with an inlet but no outlet is still considered a ventricle. Position of outlet chambers and/or trabecular pouches combined with the morphology of the ventricle can be used to determine the looping pattern in single ventricle anatomy. Recognize, however, that hypoplastic left heart syndrome, for example, has two anatomic ventricles so that it can be named using a system for biventricular hearts, even though the physiology is that of a single ventricle.

The Ventricular Septum

The ventricular septum is normally composed of an *inlet portion* formed by endocardial cushion tissue, a *trabecular* or *muscular portion* that represents the muscular area between the ventricle and bulbus cordis after looping is completed (sometimes described as having sinus and trabecular portions), and the *outflow* or *conal portion* of the septum. Malalignment defects such as those that occur in tetralogy of Fallot (TOF) or interrupted aortic arch are generally located in this area because they represent failure of proper alignment of the portions of the ventricular septum. The junction between all of these parts is the *membranous septum*, the most common site of VSDs. Inlet defects occur posteriorly in the plane of the atrioventricular valves, muscular VSDs occur anywhere in the trabecular septum, and outlet VSDs are found in the cono-truncal region. It is important to understand that the description of VSD location in many types of complex defects is more related to the position of the great arteries than to the VSD itself. In other words, two hearts with VSDs in the outlet septum may be called by different terms (e.g., subaortic vs. subpulmonary) based on the arrangement of the great arteries.

The Great Arteries

The great arteries have relationships with the ventricles and with each other. The ventricular relationships are defined and determined by outflow tract anatomy and alignments. The relationship of one great artery to the other is considered in terms of anterior–posterior and left–right positioning. Normally related great arteries occur when there are concordant ventriculo-arterial connections with the aorta posterior and slightly rightward of the pulmonary artery (**Fig. 68.4**A). In ventriculo-arterial concordance, the aorta arises from the morphologic left ventricle and the pulmonary artery arises from the morphologic right ventricle. Ventriculo-arterial discordance occurs when the aorta arises from the morphologic right ventricle and the pulmonary artery arises from the morphologic left ventricle. Concordance and discordance can thus be considered to be synonymous with normally related and transposed great arteries, respectively (11,12), although some have suggested the anterior–posterior relationship of the great arteries is the most definitive feature of transposition, at least from an historical perspective (1,13). Given the possibilities for confusion therefore, some have argued that the terms "concordant" and "discordant" should be used to

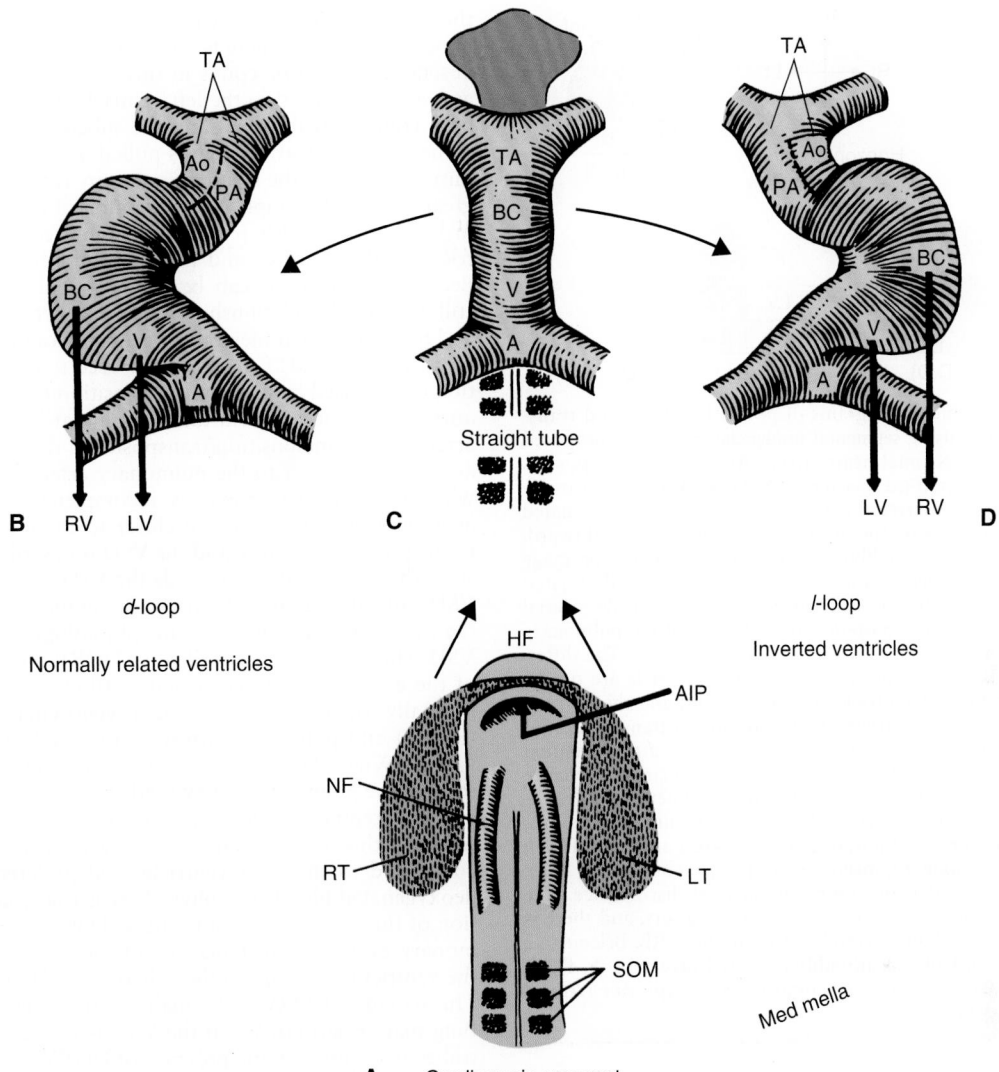

FIGURE 68.3. The embryologic cardiac crescent (**A**) contains the early precursors of the straight heart tube (**B**). The tube usually loops with the apex to the right forming a *d*-loop (**C**) and bringing the future right ventricle to the right of the future left ventricle. When the apex of the loop is to the left, or *l*-looped (**D**), the morphologic right ventricle ends up leftward of the morphologic left ventricle, so-called ventricular inversion. HF, Head fold; AIP, Anterior intestinal portal; NF, Neural fold; RT, Right side of cardiac crescent; LT, left side of cardiac crescent; som, somites; A, atrium; V, ventricle (future left ventricle); BC, Bulbus cordis (future right ventricle); TA, Truncus arteriosus; LV, Left ventricle; RV, Right ventricle; Ao, Aorta; PA, Pulmonary artery. (From Van Praagh R, Weinberg PM, Matsuoka R, et al. Malpositions of the heart. In: Adams FH, Emmanouilides GC, eds. *Moss' Heart Disease in Infants, Children and Adolescents.* 3rd ed. Baltimore, MD: Williams & Wilkins, 1983:422–58, with permission.)

describe all situations in which two ventricles connect individually to two great arteries (1). When there is a double outlet ventriculo-arterial connection, one of the ventricles gives rise to both great arteries. In this case, or in the case of only a single great artery arising from a discordant ventricle, the artery with improper orientation can be said to be *malposed* (11,12). The term *malposition* can also be used to describe anterior–posterior malposition in the presence of ventriculo-arterial concordance. The anatomic arrangement of the great arteries should be distinguished from their physiologic orientation, in that deoxygenated blood can course from right atrium to morphologic left ventricle to transposed pulmonary artery, resulting in a physiologically normal situation.

Using the nomenclature system proposed by Anderson, each great artery is assigned to the ventricle to which it is more than 50% committed (1). This approach offers the benefit of

simplicity that comes with the intuitiveness of the nomenclature. DORV, for example, occurs when both the great arteries are more than 50% committed to the right ventricle. One must also then describe the relationship of the great arteries to each other, such as DORV with the aorta rightward of the pulmonary artery. Accuracy of this schema for assigning ventriculo-arterial relationships is highly dependent on obtaining standard echocardiographic views, since some rotation from the standard plane can make a normally placed aorta appear to override a perimembranous VSD by more than 50%, thus leading to an incorrect anatomic diagnosis.

Using the more embryologically based approach of Van Praagh, one first describes the great arteries as normally related, transposed, or malposed. When there are normally related vessels, the aorta is posterior to the pulmonary artery, and the relationship between them can be noted as *situs solitus* (s)

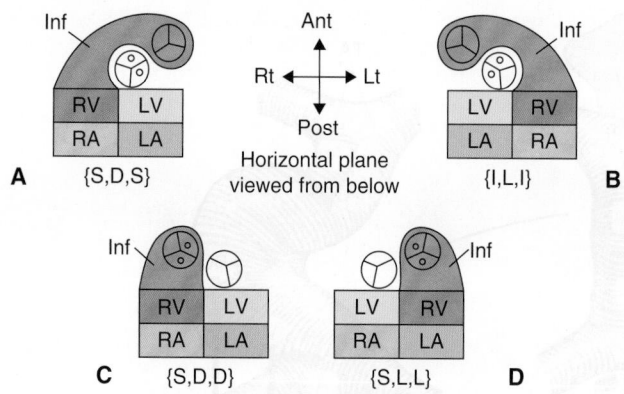

FIGURE 68.4. Schematic diagrams of normally related and transposed great arteries using segmental nomenclature scheme proposed by Van Praagh. (A) Normal heart: atrial situs solitus, *d*-loop, situs solitus normally related great arteries (S, D, S). There is atrioventricular and ventriculo-arterial concordance. The aorta (designated by the coronary orifices on the diagram) is posterior and rightward. There is subpulmonary infundibulum (Inf) or conus. (B) Mirror image normal: atrial situs inversus, *l*-loop, situs inversus normally related great arteries (I, L, I). There is atrioventricular and ventriculo-arterial concordance. The aorta is posterior and leftward of the pulmonary artery. There is a subpulmonary infundibulum or conus. The difference from normal is that the right atrium and ventricle are on the left, the left atrium and ventricle are on the right, and the aorta is leftward of the pulmonary artery. (C) Usual form of transposition of the great arteries (*d*-TGAs): atrial situs solitus, *d*-loop, *d*-transposition of the great arteries (S, D, D). There is atrioventricular concordance and ventriculo-arterial discordance. The aorta is anterior and rightward of the pulmonary artery, and there is subpulmonary conus. (D) Congenitally corrected transposition of the great arteries (*l*-TGA): atrial situs solitus, *l*-loop, *l*-transposition of the great arteries (S, L, L). There is atrioventricular and ventriculo-arterial discordance. The aorta is anterior and leftward of the pulmonary artery, and there is subpulmonary infundibulum. (Modified from Foran RB, Belcourt C, Nanton MA, et al. Isolated infundibuloarterial inversion (S, D, I): A newly recognized form of congenital heart disease. *Am Heart J* 1988;116:1337–50.)

when the aorta (aortic valve) is rightward of the pulmonary artery (pulmonary valve), or *situs inversus* (i) when the aorta is leftward of the pulmonary artery (**Fig. 68.4**). In transposition, the aorta is generally anterior to the pulmonary artery, and the relationship can be described as *dextro* (d) when the aorta is rightward, or *levo* (l) when the aorta is leftward. When the connection between one of the ventricles and a great artery is identifiable but the semilunar valve is atretic, one can still describe the relationship between that ventricle and the great artery in question. When the artery itself is atretic with no connection to the heart, as can occur in some forms of pulmonary atresia (PA), one cannot technically use the term "transposition" since only one artery arises improperly.

When there is a double outlet connection, the great artery (usually the aorta) that is committed to the improper ventricle is said to be malposed. The definition of a double outlet ventricle using this system is not based on the percentage override of the artery; rather, it is based on the precise anatomy of the infundibulum or conus of the outflow tracts. The *conus* is a remnant of the conus arteriosus of the embryonic heart that persists into the more mature heart. During normal cardiogenesis the great arteries each have subarterial conus separating the great arteries from the bulbus cordis. Since the bulbus cordis is the future right ventricle, both the outlets are initially aligned with the right ventricle. In the course of normal cardiac development, the subaortic conus is reabsorbed, and the aorta is brought down into continuity with the tricuspid and mitral valves. When seen in the echocardiographic long axis,

the continuity between the mitral and aortic valves can clearly be seen, even when there is a large perimembranous VSD. The absence of subaortic conus in this anatomy defines the aorta as being committed to the left ventricle. When the subpulmonary conus is reabsorbed and the subaortic conus persists, it is the pulmonary artery that is pulled into continuity with the mitral valve, and the resultant anatomy is transposition of the great arteries. Incomplete reabsorption of either conus results in both great arteries remaining committed to the right ventricle (bulbus cordis), and the anatomic diagnosis is DORV. Because either conus can be partially reabsorbed, one must still describe the relationship of the great arteries to each other and to the VSD that inevitably occurs in double outlet connections. The "*d*" and "*l*" terminology used to describe transposition can be used here, with *d*-malposition/transposition of the aorta describing an aorta that is rightward of the pulmonary artery and *l*-malposition/transposition defining a leftward aorta (with respect to the pulmonary artery). Physiologically, when the subaortic conus is incompletely reabsorbed, the aorta is generally positioned closer to the left ventricle than to the pulmonary artery and the VSD is described as subaortic since the aorta tends to override the VSD (when it is an outlet VSD) and the pulmonary artery is completely committed to the right ventricle. The resultant physiology is that of a large VSD. This anatomy is described as DORV with *d*-malposition of the aorta (the left ventricular outflow tract and aorta are normally rightward of the right ventricular outflow tract (RVOT) and pulmonary artery at the level of the semilunar valves). When the subpulmonary conus is incompletely reabsorbed, the pulmonary artery tends to override an outlet VSD and preferentially receive oxygenated blood from the left ventricle. In this arrangement, the aorta is generally completely committed to the right ventricle, and preferentially receives deoxygenated blood. The physiology is thus that of transposition of the great arteries, and the VSD is described as subpulmonary even though it may be in the same location within the ventricular septum as the subaortic VSD described earlier. This would be DORV with *l*-malposition of the aorta (Taussig-Bing malformation). When the VSD is located in the inlet or trabecular septum in the presence of DORV, the VSD is said to be remote, and the surgical course is usually that of single ventricle palliation due to an inability to baffle the two ventricles to separate outlets. In the rare circumstance that both parts of the embryologic conus are reabsorbed, the anatomy is double outlet left ventricle. Subaortic conus can also persist in the face of ventriculo-arterial concordance in the rare anatomy known as anatomically corrected malposition of the great arteries. In this case, great arteries arise from the morphologically appropriate ventricles, but the aorta is anterior to the pulmonary artery due to the persistent subaortic conus (14).

SYSTEMIC AND PULMONARY VENOUS CONNECTIONS

The systemic and pulmonary venous connections are often abnormal in complex lesions. The nomenclature is fairly intuitive, but it is important to specify these anomalies when they exist, since many have clinical implications for central line placement, surgical intervention, or physiologic shunts. Abnormalities of systemic venous connections include (a) bilateral superior vena cava, (b) left superior vena cava, (c) interrupted inferior vena cava, and (d) major alterations of venous connections to the heart from normal such that a right-to-left shunt occurs. Pulmonary venous connections may be either partially or totally anomalous, returning to sites other than the left atrium. Usually, the important aspects of description include noting which pulmonary veins are anomalous and categorizing the connection as supracardiac, cardiac, or infracardiac. Again, it is best to completely specify the exact nature of the connections when describing hearts with these anomalies.

CARDIAC POSITION

Chest x-ray is very helpful in making the diagnosis of an abnormally positioned heart, but usually a complete assessment requires echocardiography to identify the location of the cardiac apex. *Levocardia* is the normal positioning of the heart, and describes a situation in which the heart is on the left side of the thorax, *dextrocardia* occurs when the heart located predominantly in the right chest, and *mesocardia* is an intermediate situation with a more midline position. The position of the heart within the thorax does not automatically reveal the location of the apex of the heart. For example, one may find dextrocardia in which the apex of the heart still points toward the left side of the body and levocardia where the apex is to the right. In general, when describing cardiac position it is probably best to specify the position of the apex.

CLINICAL EXAMPLES

Using the segmental approach for the description of cardiac anatomy, one can see that a normal heart has atrioventricular concordance, two atrioventricular connections, and ventriculo-arterial concordance. Alternatively, this anatomy can be referred to as atrial situs solitus, *d*-loop ventricles, and arterial situs solitus (S, D, S). The most common form of transposition of the great arteries (*d*-TGA) has atrioventricular concordance and ventriculo-atrial discordance (**Fig. 68.4**C). This can be referred to as atrial situs solitus, *d*-loop ventricles, and *d*-transposition of the great arteries (S, D, D). Getting slightly more complex, congenitally corrected transposition (**Fig. 68.4**D), also called *isolated ventricular inversion*, is where the morphologic right atrium opens into the right-sided morphologic left ventricle which gives rise to the transposed pulmonary artery. The morphologic left atrium opens into the left-sided morphologic right ventricle which gives rise to the transposed aorta. The great arteries are considered anatomically transposed because they arise from the "wrong" morphologic ventricles, but they are in fact physiologically correct. The pulmonary artery still carries deoxygenated blood to the lungs, and the aorta brings oxygenated blood to the body. This anatomy can also be described as atrioventricular discordance and ventriculo-arterial discordance or as atrial situs solitus, *l*-looped ventricles, and *l*-transposition of the great arteries (S, L, L). The most common double inlet connection occurs when both the right and left atria open into a right-sided morphologic left ventricle which gives rise to the pulmonary artery. The aorta arises off an anterior and leftward chamber that lacks an atrioventricular inlet. The connection between the left ventricle and the chamber that gives rise to the aorta is through a VSD that can be referred to as a *bulboventricular foramen* since the lack of atrioventricular inlet might preclude referring to this outlet chamber as a ventricle. This heart can be referred to as having situs solitus atrial arrangement, a double inlet atrioventricular connection with single left ventricle, left-handed topology, and ventriculo-arterial discordance. It can also be designated as situs solitus atria, *l*-loop, and *l*-transposition of the great arteries (S, L, L) with double inlet left ventricle. A *Taussig–Bing heart*, in which there is a DORV, bilateral subarterial conus, and subpulmonary VSD (aorta completely committed to the right ventricle, pulmonary artery may override the septum), would be referred to as having atrioventricular concordance, ventriculo-arterial discordance with double outlet ventriculo-arterial connection, or as atrial situs solitus,

d-loop, *l*-malposition of the aorta (S, D, L) with DORV and subpulmonary VSD. Thus, any type of cardiac anatomy can be described using either school of segmental anatomy or even a combination of the two since both offer particular advantages in certain situations. Even the heterotaxy syndromes in which there is right or left atrial isomerism are initially described as above with appropriate modifications based on the ventricular and great artery relationships.

CONGENITAL CARDIAC DEFECTS

The incidence of congenital heart defects is 6–8 per 1000 live births (1 in 130–145 live births). Approximately 25% of congenital heart lesions can be considered complex, and one-third will require intervention during infancy (15) requiring intensive care. These figures do not include the clinically silent bicuspid, nonstenotic aortic valve or mitral valve prolapse and exclude the incidence of a patent ductus arteriosus (PDA) in those born prematurely. Congenital heart defects are the most common congenital malformations resulting in 10% of all infant deaths (16) and 50% of deaths due to congenital malformations (1). Twenty-five percent of neonates with congenital heart defects (16) have other associated congenital abnormalities. Thanks to advances in the evaluation and treatment of these fragile children by multidisciplinary teams of physicians led by pediatric intensivists and including cardiologists, surgeons, anesthesiologists, and other health care providers (nurses, respiratory therapists, nutritionists, etc.), up to 85% of neonates born with congenital heart disease survive to adulthood (17).

Congenital Heart Defects with Left-to-Right Shunts

Ventricular Septal Defects

VSDs are the most common congenital heart defect (30%). They are categorized depending on their location in various parts of the ventricular septum defects. VSDs are divided into (a) *inlet* (atrioventricular [AV] septal or endocardial cushion), (b) *muscular*, (c) *outlet* (doubly committed juxta arterial), and (d) *perimembranous* defects (**Fig. 68.5**). The surrounding semilunar (or AV) valves can be negatively affected by the jets through the VSD, resulting in aortic and/or pulmonary valve incompetence in doubly committed defects and aortic and TV incompetence associated with perimembranous defects. The size of the defect, the relative right and left ventricular pressures, the compliance, and the ratio of pulmonary and systemic vascular resistance are factors that influence the volume of left-to-right shunt. Multiple defects can be present (mainly in the muscular part of ventricular septum) and there is a frequent association with other congenital heart defects including complex congenital cardiac malformations (e.g., TOF). Eighty percent of VSDs are small (<3 mm diameter), with a high rate of spontaneous closure particularly in the muscular and membranous septums. If left unrepaired, a significant risk of infective endocarditis exists. Large unrepaired defects with increased pulmonary-to-systemic blood flow ratio (>2:1) are at risk of developing pulmonary vascular obstructive disease in later childhood and adolescence.

Atrial Septal Defects

ASDs are classified into (a) *ostium primum* ASD (part of atrioventricular septal defect [AVSD]), (b) *ostium secundum* (within oval fossa and around the foramen ovale), and (c) *sinus venosus* (superior or inferior adjacent to the orifice of superior or

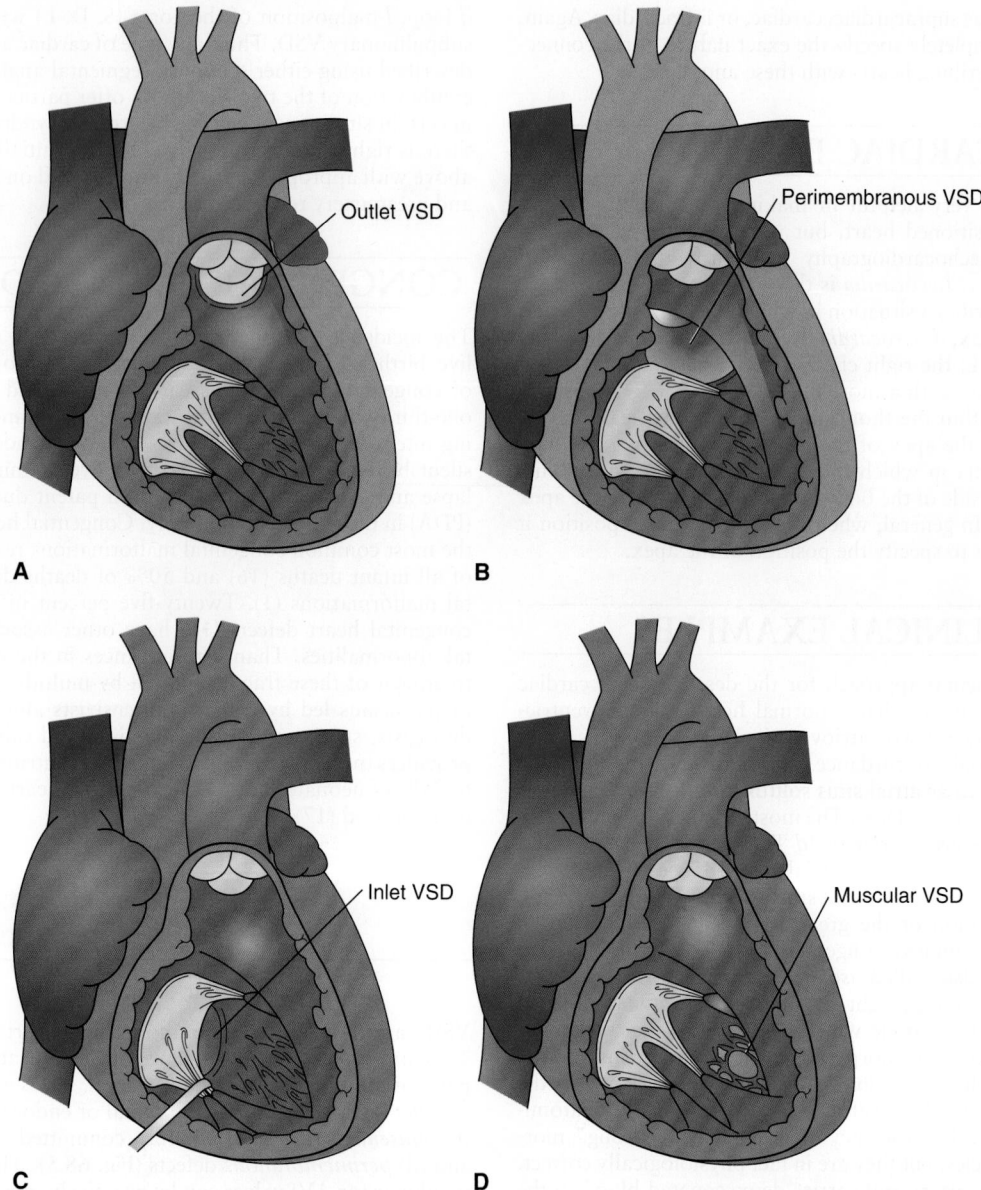

FIGURE 68.5. Types of ventricular septal defects. (A) outlet defect. (B) Perimembranous defect. (C) Inlet defect. (D) Muscular defect.

inferior caval vein, or at the coronary sinus [so-called unroofed coronary sinus into the left atrium]) (Fig. 68.6). The clinical spectrum of secundum defects exists dependent on the extent of missing septal tissue. Small secundum defects (<3–4 mm) are often considered a patent foramen ovale. Secundum ASDs are associated with other congenital heart defects (e.g., pulmonary valve stenosis). The superior sinus venosus defect is commonly associated with partial anomalous pulmonary venous drainage involving the right upper pulmonary vein joining the lateral wall of the superior vena cava. The volume of left-to-right shunt depends on the size of the defect and the relative compliance of the right and left ventricles. The low kinetic energy of blood reaching the pulmonary arteries makes the development of pulmonary vascular obstructive disease in childhood very rare. There is a risk of paradoxical emboli particularly in the face of atrial dysrhythmias, which occur more frequently in older children and adolescents. Pulmonary vascular obstructive disease from large defects can occur in adolescence and young adulthood.

Patent Ductus Arteriosus

The ductus arteriosus is part of the normal fetal circulation joining the main pulmonary artery (MPA) with the descending aorta. Prenatally, a PDA allows for the majority of blood reaching the MPA from the right ventricle (two-third of combined ventricular output) to bypass the lungs, with only 7% of combined output returning to the left atrium. The blood flow direction through the ductus arteriosus reverses postnatally, and the PDA undergoes functional closure in the majority of term neonates within the first few hours of postnatal life (Fig. 68.7). Patency beyond 1 month of age (3 months in premature infants) is considered abnormal. The PDA is mostly left-sided, but right-sided or bilateral PDAs can occur. The PDA can be the only source of pulmonary blood flow in some complex congenital heart defects (e.g., pulmonary valve atresia), but it can be absent in other defects (e.g., truncus arteriosus [TA]). Pulmonary vascular obstructive disease can occur when the PDA is left unligated in childhood. Subacute bacterial endocarditis is also fairly common in these uncorrected patients.

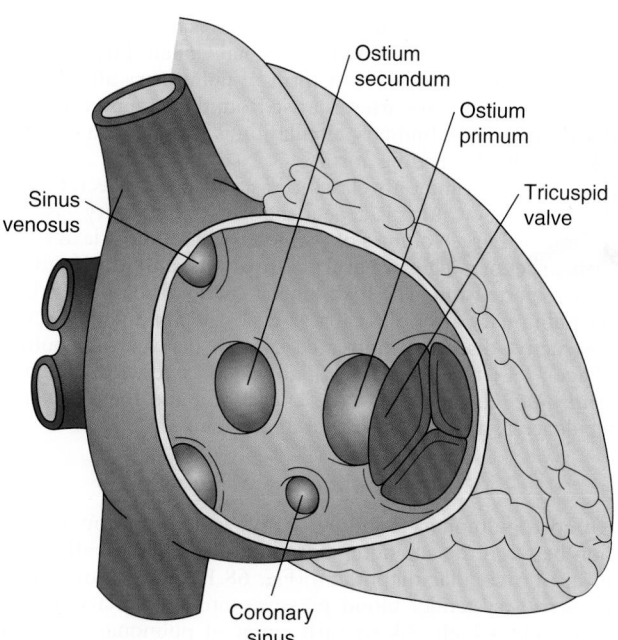

FIGURE 68.6. Types of atrial septal defects include ostium secundum, ostium primum, and sinus venosus.

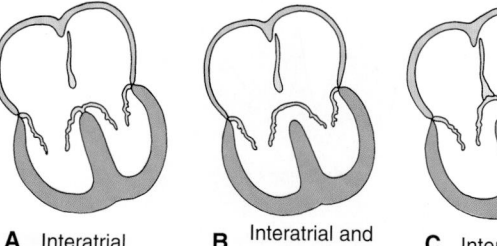

FIGURE 68.8. Types of atrioventricular septal defects (AVSD). (**A**) Partial AVSD with only atrial component. (**B**) Compete AVSD with atrial and ventricular components. (**C**) Partial AVSD with only ventricular component.

septum in isolation. Concomitant malformation of the single atrioventricular valve may produce variable degrees of valvar incompetence (**Fig. 68.8**). The complete form of AVSD is often associated with trisomy 21 and can lead to the early development of pulmonary vascular obstructive disease.

The relative size of the ventricles is an important consideration in the surgical repair of ASVD. If the left and right ventricles are approximately equal in size, the ASVD is considered "balanced" and a two-ventricle repair is possible. If one ventricle (more commonly the left ventricle) is hypoplastic, the ASVD is considered "unbalanced" and a single ventricle–staged palliation may be necessary.

Atrioventricular Septal Defects

The complete form of atrioventricular septal defect (AVSD) (also called *endocardial cushion defect*) is characterized by a single AV valve spanning across the inlet of both ventricles with septal deficiency in the primum atrial septum and the inlet part of ventricular septum with resultant interatrial and interventricular shunting (**Fig. 68.8**). Three subtypes (*Rastelli A–C*) are recognized based on the chordal attachments of the AV valve with regards to the septum. A partial AVSD is deficiency in either the interatrial or the interventricular

Common Truncus Arteriosus

Truncus arteriosus (TA) is a single arterial trunk guarded by a single truncal valve with multiple leaflets arising from the heart to divide into the ascending aorta and pulmonary arteries (**Fig. 68.9**). The truncal valve has a variable number of cusps, overrides a large, outlet VSD, and receives blood from

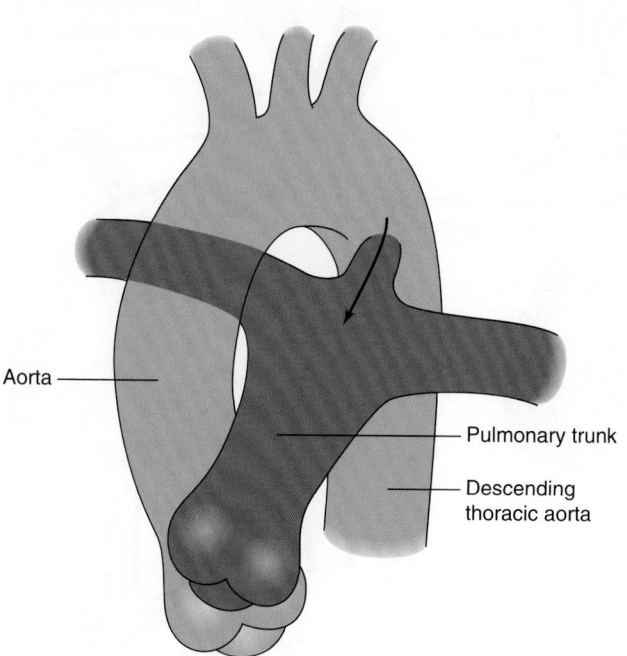

FIGURE 68.7. Patent ductus arteriosus.

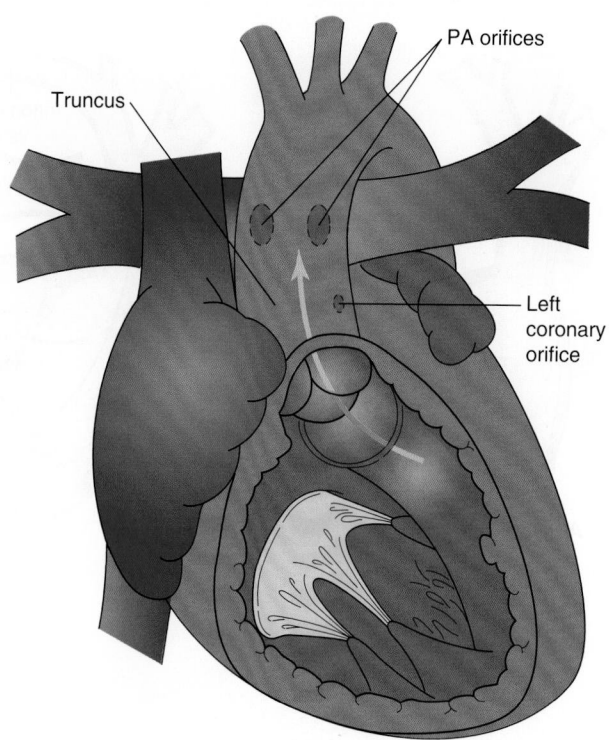

FIGURE 68.9. Common arterial trunk (truncus arteriosus).

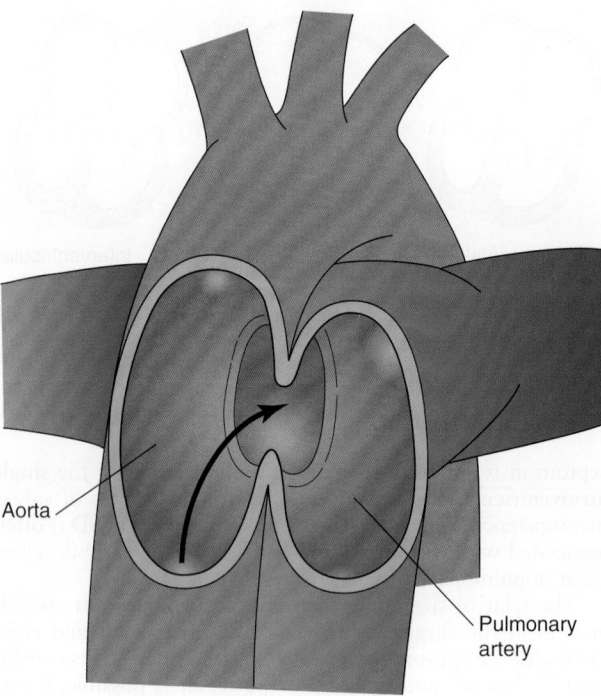

FIGURE 68.10. Aorta–pulmonary window.

TA, the right and left pulmonary arteries arise separately from the lateral walls of the TA. The original Collett–Edwards type IV TA is now classified as a form of pulmonary atresia (PA) where no pulmonary arteries arise from the common truncus, but rather, the pulmonary circulation is supplied via collaterals from the descending aorta.

TA is also commonly classified as a cyanotic defect, though the degree of cyanosis is dependent on the pulmonary vascular resistance. Large volumes of pulmonary blood flow lead to the early onset of congestive heart failure in the absence of pulmonary hypertension. The high kinetic energy of blood reaching the pulmonary arterioles causes very early pulmonary vascular obstructive disease in untreated patients (as early as a month of age). TA is the lesion most highly associated with *DiGeorge syndrome* (chromosome 22q11 deletion), and there is a high incidence of a right aortic arch in this lesion.

Aortopulmonary Window

An aortopulmonary window (APW) is a direct communication between the ascending aorta and the MPA usually in the form of a circular diaphragm (**Fig. 68.10**). Free transmission of aortic (systemic) blood pressure into pulmonary arteries represents a high risk of early onset of pulmonary vascular obstructive disease.

Partial or Total Anomalous Pulmonary Venous Connection

Between one and four pulmonary veins can connect anomalously with the systemic venous system, right atrium, or coronary sinus, resulting in partial or total anomalous pulmonary venous connection (PAPVC or TAPVC) (**Fig. 68.11**). The partial variety often involves the right upper pulmonary vein connected with the superior vena cava and is often associated with a superior sinus venosus ASD. The various forms of TAPVC are classified into (a) *supracardiac* (into the innominate vein; returns via superior vena cava), (b) *intracardiac*

both the left and right ventricles. Stenosis or incompetence of the truncal valve is common. The origin of the pulmonary arteries from the truncus above the truncal valve varies and describes the different subtypes of the defect (I–IV). In *type I TA*, the MPA arises from the common truncus and then divides into the left and right pulmonary arteries. In *type II TA*, both left and right pulmonary arteries arise together from the common truncus without a discernible MPA. In *type III*

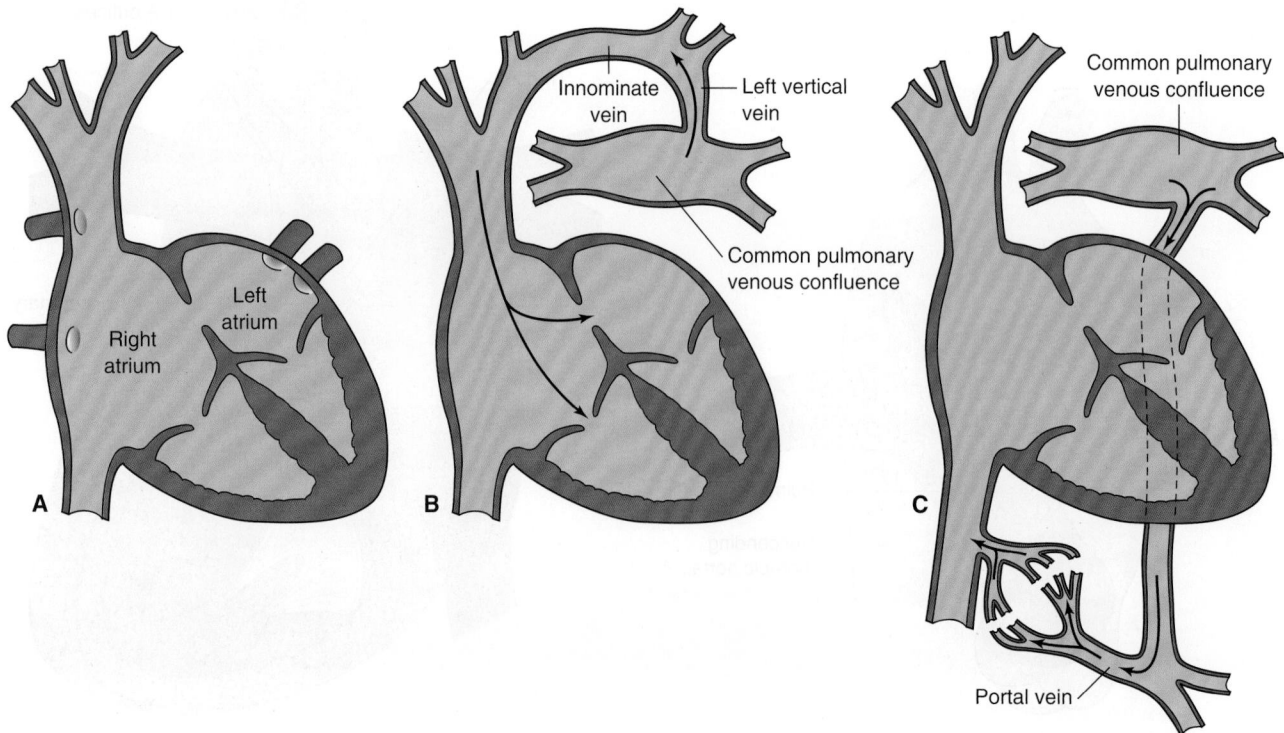

FIGURE 68.11. Variants of anomalous pulmonary venous connections. (**A**) PAPVC with return of the right upper pulmonary vein directly to the superior vena cava and the right lower pulmonary vein to the right atrium (cardiac). (**B**) Supracardiac TAPVC. (**C**) Infracardiac TAPVC.

(into the coronary sinus or directly to the right atrium), and (c) *infracardiac* (into the umbilical, hepatic, or portal veins; returns via the orifice of the inferior vena. An obligate right-to-left shunt at the atrial level is necessary through an unobstructed secundum ASD for survival. Obstruction of the vertical vein occurs most frequently in the infracardiac form and commonly in the supracardiac form, leading to severe hypoxia and pulmonary hypertension postnatally. Unobstructed forms present with congestive heart failure and mild cyanosis from a large left-to-right shunt once pulmonary vascular resistance drops postnatally. This lesion is commonly classified as a form of cyanotic heart disease. Atrial dysrhythmias are common and paradoxical embolic can occur.

Cyanotic Congenital Heart Defects

Tetralogy of Fallot

TOF is the most common cyanotic congenital heart defect and is made up of a combination of lesions, including (a) *outlet VSD* with (b) *overriding aorta* and (c) *RVOT obstruction (RVOTO)* with (d) right ventricular *hypertrophy* (**Fig. 68.12**). Interventricular septal malalignment involving superior and anterior shift of the outlet septum is the underlying anatomical malformation that ties these four components together and often contributes directly to subvalvar pulmonary stenosis. Some degree of pulmonary valve and supravalvar hypoplasia may be present. In severe forms, this may progress to pulmonary atresia (PA). Additional defects include muscular VSDs, ASDs, AVSD (5%), anomalous origin of the left anterior interventricular coronary artery from right coronary artery, and right-sided aortic arch. There is a significant incidence of DiGeorge syndrome (chromosome 22q11 deletion), especially if a right-sided aortic arch is present.

Pulmonary Atresia with Intact Ventricular Septum

Pulmonary atresia with intact ventricular septum (PA/IVS) includes the full spectrum from mild to severe of right ventricular hypoplasia due to outflow tract atresia with variable degrees of TV hypoplasia. The branch pulmonary arteries are usually of reasonable size in contrast to patients with TOF with PA. The PDA is typically the only source of pulmonary blood flow (**Fig. 68.13**) as it comes off the aorta in a reverse angle from

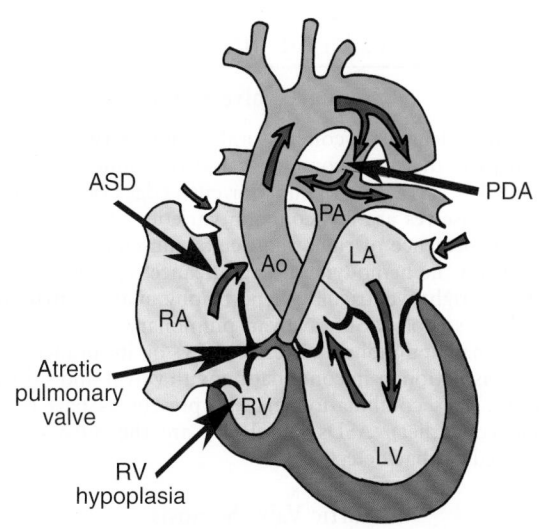

FIGURE 68.13. Pulmonary atresia with intact ventricular septum RA, Right atrium. RV, Right ventricle. LA, Left atrium. LV, Left ventricle. ASD, Atrial septal defect. Ao, Aorta. PA, Pulmonary artery. PDA, Patent ductus arteriosus.

normal. *Coronary arterial fistulae*, which are often stenotic, connect to the right ventricular cavity and are present in up to one-third of all cases. These coronary cameral connections can be fatal to the infant due to steal away from the coronary supply to the left ventricle with resultant left ventricular infarction.

Transposition of Great Arteries

Ventriculo-arterial discordance leads to aorta arising from the right ventricle and pulmonary artery from the left ventricle. Concomitant presence of atrioventricular concordance (right atrium connecting normally with right ventricle and left atrium with left ventricle) directs systemic and pulmonary blood flow as parallel circuits (**Fig. 68.14**). Postnatal mixing of blood depends on the presence of arterial duct and interatrial communication. VSD and subvalvar and/or valvar pulmonary stenosis are the most frequent associated cardiac defects. Coronary arterial anatomy (important for surgical treatment involving arterial switch procedure and coronary arterial transfer) varies with the most important anomaly represented by an intramural course of the coronary artery.

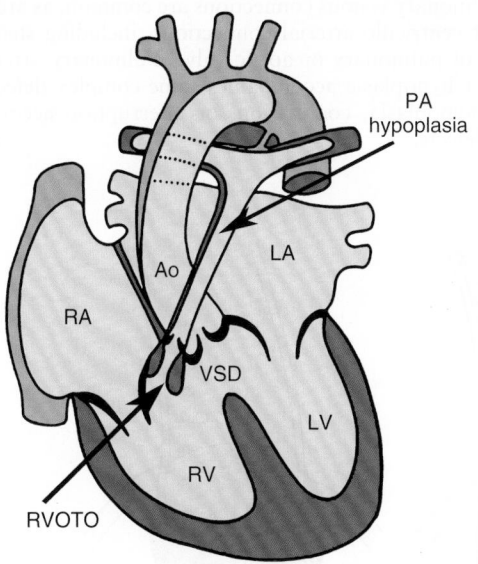

FIGURE 68.12. Tetralogy of Fallot. RA, Right atrium. RV, Right ventricle. LA, Left atrium. LV, Left ventricle. VSD, ventricular septal defect. Ao, Aorta. PA, pulmonary artery.

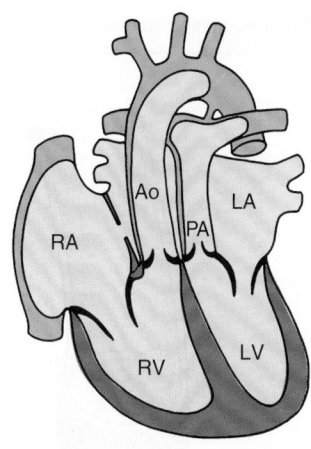

FIGURE 68.14. Complete transposition of the great arteries. RA, Right atrium. RV, Right ventricle. LA, Left atrium. LV, left ventricle. Ao, Aortal. PA, Pulmonary artery.

Obstructive Congenital Heart Defects

Pulmonary Valve Stenosis

A variable degree of commissural fusion between the valvar cusps is the most common cause of pulmonary stenosis (**Fig. 68.15**). Tethering of superior cusp edges or dysplasia of cusps themselves are less common varieties of stenosis. Concomitant presence of right ventricular muscular hypertrophy depends on the hemodynamic significance of stenosis. Severe forms of right ventricular hypertrophy may contribute to subvalvar stenosis. Supravalvar pulmonary stenosis affecting the main pulmonary artery (MPA) or its branches may occur in isolation or in combination with valvar and subvalvar stenoses. This combination may be present as part of TOF (discussed earlier). ASDs and VSDs are the most common associated cardiac defects.

Aortic Valve Stenosis

Stenotic aortic valves can be described as unicuspid, bicuspid, or tricuspid depending on the number of functional commissures between valvar cusps (**Fig. 68.16**). Unicuspid valves are usually the most severely stenosed. Bicuspid valves, on the other hand, may present without stenosis in childhood. Gross dysplasia of valvar cusps has been described in up to 10% of congenital aortic valve stenosis (AS). Concomitant aortic valve regurgitation is more common in previously treated valves. Aortic coarctation is the most common associated defect. Any malformed aortic valve is likely to undergo calcification in adulthood.

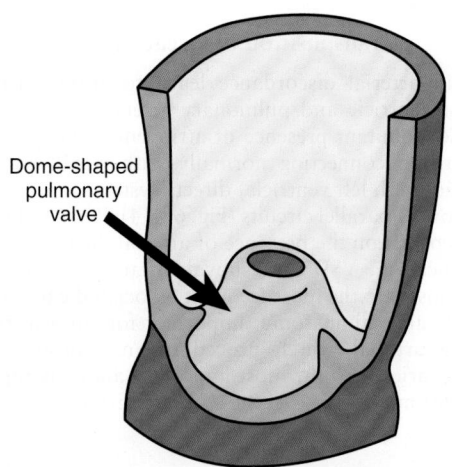

Dome-shaped pulmonary valve

FIGURE 68.15. Pulmonary valve stenosis.

Aortic Coarctation or Interruption of the Aortic Arch (IAA)

In aortic coarctation (CA), the narrowing in the distal part of aortic arch around the aortic isthmus may be accompanied by variable degree and extent of aortic arch hypoplasia (**Fig. 68.17, A and B**). Aortic coarctation is closely associated with arterial ductal insertion into the aortic wall, and a discrete shelf inside the aortic lumen may become obvious only on postnatal ductal closure. Arterial ductal patency plays an important role in the majority of cases with severe neonatal aortic coarctation as it allows for blood flow to reach lower part of the body. Collateral arteries bridging the narrow aortic segment develop gradually during childhood in untreated patients. VSDs, bicuspid aortic valve, and aortic and mitral valve stenoses are the most commonly associated anomalies. Systemic hypertension due to abnormal arterial wall structure and function and intracranial arterial aneurysms represent a long-term risk of severe complications even in successfully treated patients.

In aortic arch interruption, a segment of aortic arch is missing or replaced by a solid cord. Depending on the location of the missing aortic arch segment, the defect is divided into the following types: type A, interruption distal to the left subclavian artery; type B (most common), interruption between the common carotid and left subclavian arteries; and type C, interruption between the brachiocephalic and common carotid arteries (**Fig. 68.17, C-E**). Patent arterial ductus with right-to-left shunt is the only source of blood supply for lower part of the body postnatally. A VSD is the most common associated heart defect. Chromosome 22q11 deletion is strongly linked with type B interruption.

Complex Congenital Heart Defects

Univentricular Hearts

A wide variety of congenital heart defects involve hypoplasia of one ventricle and either absence of one atrioventricular connection (tricuspid or mitral) or both atrioventricular valves connecting to the dominant ventricle (double inlet ventricle) (**Fig. 68.18**). The hypoplastic ventricle may communicate with the dominant ventricle through a VSD. Anomalies of systemic and pulmonary venous connections are common, as are anomalies of ventriculo-arterial connections, including stenosis or atresia of pulmonary or aortic valve. Pulmonary arterial stenoses or hypoplasia accompanies some complex defects, and aortic hypoplasia, coarctation, or interruption accompanies other defects.

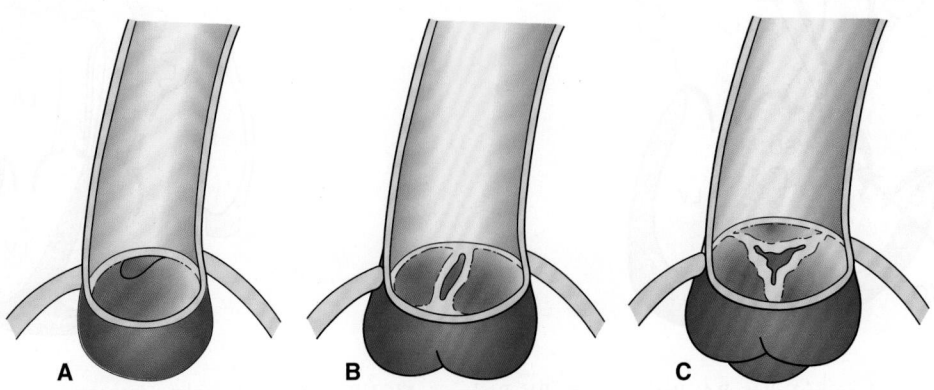

A   **B**   **C**

FIGURE 68.16. Aortic valve stenosis. (**A**) Unicuspid valve. (**B**) Bicuspid valve. (**C**) Tricuspid valve.

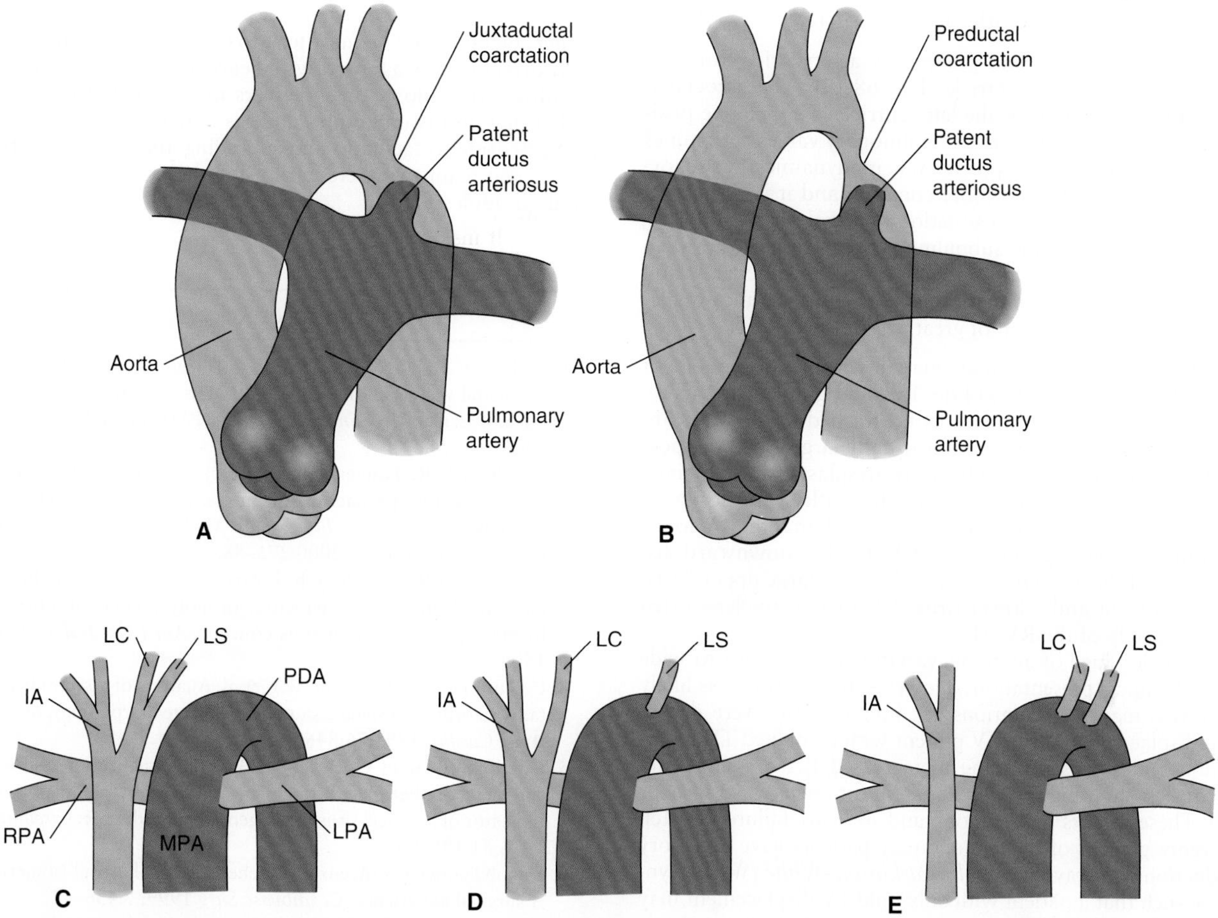

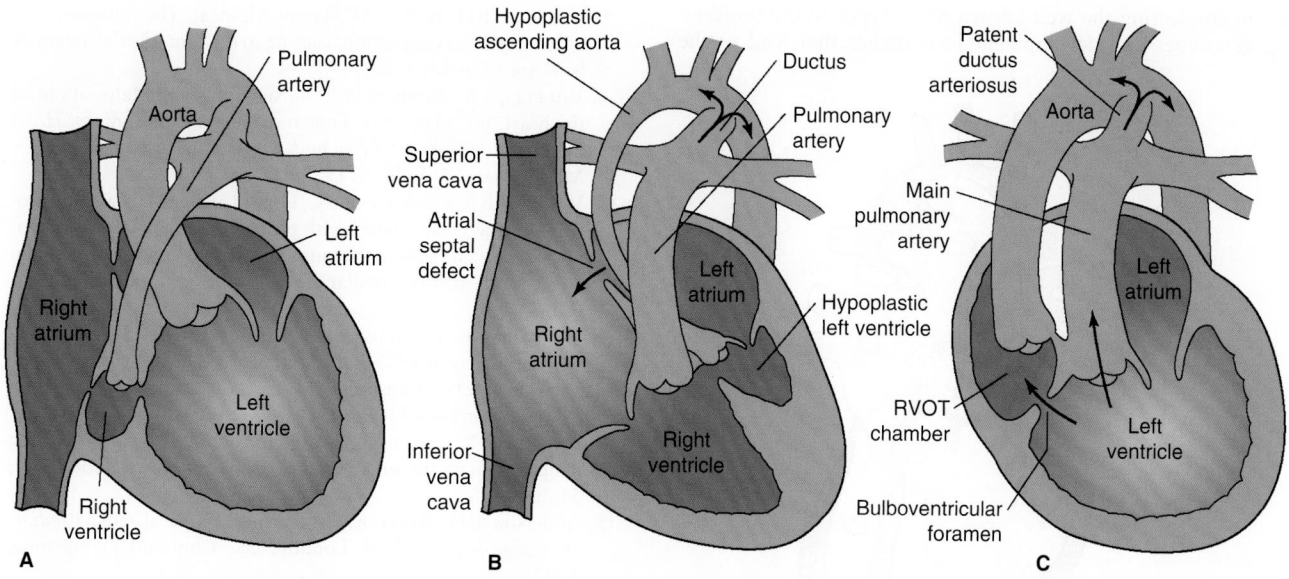

FIGURE 68.17. Coarctation and interruption of aortic arch. (A) Juxtaductal coarctation of the aorta. (B) Preductal coarctation of the aorta. (C) Interrupted aortic arch type A. (D) Interrupted aortic arch type B. (E) Interrupted aortic arch type C. MPA, Main pulmonary artery. RPA, Right pulmonary artery. LPA, Left pulmonary artery. PDA, Patent ductus arteriosus. IA, Innominate artery. LC, Left carotid artery. LS, Left subclavian artery.

FIGURE 68.18. Variants of hearts with one functional ventricle. (A) Hypoplastic right heart. There is severe tricuspid stenosis with a hypoplastic right ventricle, small ventricular septal defect, hypoplastic pulmonary artery and a patent ductus arteriosus that provide pulmonary blood flow. The great arteries are normally related. (B) Hypoplastic left heart syndrome. There is mitral and aortic stenosis with a hypoplastic left ventricle and ascending aorta. There is a ventricular septal defect and patent foramen ovale/secundum atrial septal defect. There is a patent ductus arteriosus that provides systemic blood flow. (C) Double inlet left ventricle with a ventricular septal defect or bulboventricular foramen providing flow to the right ventricle or outlet chamber. There is transposition of the great arteries. RVOT, right ventricular outflow tract.

Double Outlet Right Ventricle

In DORV, both aorta and pulmonary artery arise from the morphologically right ventricle (**Fig. 68.19**). The associated VSD is the only outlet for the left ventricle. The relative position of the VSD and the aortic or pulmonary valves determines associated anomalies and postnatal hemodynamics. A subaortic position of the VSD is more common and it is associated with pulmonary stenosis, a situation not dissimilar from TOF hemodynamically. In the subpulmonary position of the VSD, pulmonary stenosis is rare and associated aortic coarctation is more common. This situation is not hemodynamically dissimilar from transposition of great arteries with VSD.

Ebstein Anomaly. Ebstein anomaly involves a wide range of morphologic abnormalities of the TV and right ventricle (RV). In general, the TV anterior leaflet is attached to the valve annulus (or papillary muscle) and is usually larger than the posterior and septal leaflets, which are dysplastic and partially adherent to the RV endocardium. The leaflets are displaced downward toward the RVOT and apex such that the TV looks like a funnel pointing toward the RVOT. The downward displacement of the TV separates the RV into a large upper "atrialized" segment and a lower (true) RV that is smaller—often consisting only of the RVOT.

The wide range of anatomic variation corresponds to wide range of clinical presentations. However, the intensivist is likely to see two main presentations (9). Infants with severe downward displacement of the TV present with combined TV regurgitation and stenosis, leading to increased RA pressures and right-to-left shunting through a (patent foramen ovale) PFO or ASD. These infants are cyanotic and in heart failure (1). Ten to twenty percent of Ebstein anomaly patients have accessory conduction pathways and *Wolff–Parkinson–White (WPW)* syndrome such that a patient with only mild TV displacement may not present until the teenage years, when atrial fibrillation leads to heart failure or ventricular fibrillation and sudden death.

FUTURE DIRECTIONS

The future of understanding complex congenital heart disease lies in connecting the well-known phenotypes to the underlying genotypes and developmental anomalies that lead to the formation of the defect. Diagnosis of the cardiac defects into earlier stages of fetal life may lead to opportunities to intervene and correct or at least modify the cardiac defect. Advances in bioinformatics allow for caregivers in the PICU to visualize and review ultrasonographic images, MRI, and angiograms, at the bedside to facilitate understanding and communication among the team members caring for the critically ill infant, child, or adolescent.

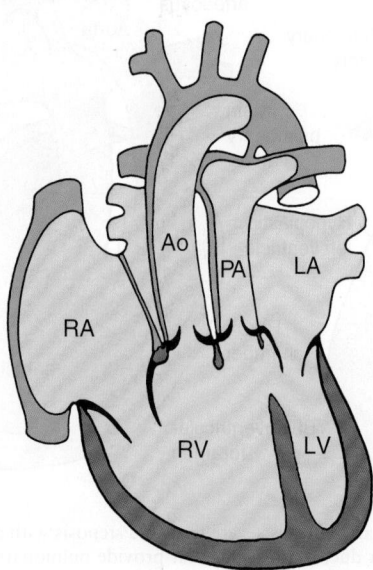

FIGURE 68.19. Double outlet right ventricle. RA, Right atrium. RV, Right ventricle. LA, Left atrium. LV, Left ventricle. Ao, Aorta. PA, Pulmonary artery.

References

1. Anderson RH. Nomenclature and classification: Sequential segmental analysis. In: Moller JH, Hoffman JIE, eds. *Pediatric Cardiovascular Medicine*. Philadelphia, PA: Churchill Livingstone, 2000:263–74.
2. Van Praagh R. Nomenclature and classification: Morphologic and segmental approach to diagnosis. In: Moller JH, Hoffman JIE, eds. *Pediatric Cardiovascular Medicine*. Philadelphia, PA: Churchill Livingstone, 2000:275–88.
3. Van Praagh R, Van Praagh S. Atrial isomerism in the heterotaxy syndromes with asplenia, or polysplenia, or normally formed spleen: an erroneous concept. *Am J Cardiol* 1990;60:1504–6.
4. Uemura H, Ho SY, Devine WA, et al. Analysis of visceral heterotaxy according to splenic status, appendage morphology, or both. *Am J Cardiol* 1995;76:846–9.
5. Partridge JB, Scott O, Deverall PB, et al. Visualization and measurement of the main bronchi by tomography as an objective indicator of thoracic situs in congenital heart disease. *Circulation* 1975;51:188–96.
6. Sinzobahamvya N, Arenz C, Brecher AM, et al. Atrial isomerism: A surgical experience. *Cardiovasc Surg* 1999; 7:436–42.
7. Uemura H, Ho SY, Devine WA, et al. Atrial appendages and venoatrial connections in hearts from patients with visceral heterotaxy. *Ann Thorac Surg* 1995;60:561–9.
8. Van Praagh S, Santini F, Sanders SP. Cardiac malpositions with special emphasis on visceral heterotaxy (asplenia and polysplenia syndromes). In: Fyler DC, ed. *Nadas' Pediatric Cardiology*. Philadelphia, PA: Hanley & Belfus, 1991:589–608.
9. Anderson RH, Becker AE, Tynan M, et al. The univentricular atrioventricular connection: Getting to the root of a thorny problem. *Am J Cardiol* 1984;54:822–8.
10. Van Praagh R, Weinberg PM, Matsuoka R, et al. Malpositions of the heart. In: Adams FH, Emmanouilides GC, eds. *Moss' Heart Disease in Infants, Children and Adolescents*. 3rd ed. Baltimore, MD: Williams & Wilkins, 1983:422–58.
11. Van Praagh R, Perez-Trevino C, Lopez-Cuellar M, et al. Transposition of the great arteries with posterior aorta, anterior pulmonary artery, subpulmonary conus and fibrous continuity between aortic and atrioventricular valves. *Am J Cardiol* 1971;28:621–31.
12. Van Praagh R. Transposition of the great arteries. II: Transposition clarified. *Am J Cardiol* 1971;28:739–41.
13. Van Mierop LHS. Transposition of the great arteries. I: Clarification of further confusion? [editorial]. *Am J Cardiol* 1971;28:735–8.
14. Van Praagh R, Durnin RE, Jockin H, et al. Anatomically corrected malposition of the great arteries {S, D, L}. *Circulation* 1975;51:20–31.
15. Anderson RH, Baker EJ, Macartney FJ, et al. eds. *Paediatric Cardiology*. 2nd ed. London, UK: Churchill Livingstone, 2005.
16. Peterson S, Peto V, Rayner M. *Congenital heart disease statistics 2003*. British Heart Foundation Statistics Database, 2003. http://www.heartstats.org.
17. Perloff JK, Warnes CA. Challenges posed by adults with repaired congenital heart disease. *Circulation* 2001;103:2637–43.

CHAPTER 69 ■ CARDIOVASCULAR PHYSIOLOGY

PETER E. OISHI, REBECCA J. KAMENY, JULIEN I. HOFFMAN, AND JEFFREY R. FINEMAN

KEY POINTS

1 Cardiovascular physiology is based on principles of hydrodynamics and fluid mechanics. Although the cardiovascular system does not conform precisely to simple physical models, a basic understanding of hemodynamic principles is essential in the care of critically ill patients with cardiovascular derangements.

Hemodynamic Principles

2 When Poiseuille's Law is applied, the resistance to flow is determined solely by the dimensions of the vessel and the viscosity of the fluid. Thus, in the cardiovascular system with constant blood viscosity, dynamic vascular resistance is mediated by vasoconstriction and vasodilation. Exceptions include alterations in surrounding pressure, such as compression of intra-alveolar capillaries with lung overdistension.

3 Precapillary arterioles (or equivalent vessels) are the site of maximal resistance in the cardiovascular circuit.

4 Venous capacitance is about 20 times greater than that of the arterial system; as a result, the majority of circulating blood volume at any one time resides in the venous system.

Interactions of the Cardiac Pump and Vasculature

5 The vascular function curve describes how changes in cardiac output affect central venous pressure (CVP), or venous return.

6 *Critical closing pressure* (P_{cc}) represents the lowest possible CVP and highest possible flow (Q) for any given blood volume.

7 The vascular function curve is affected by blood volume, undergoing a right shift with expansion of the circulating volume (e.g., transfusion) and left shift with volume depletion (e.g., hemorrhage).

8 The cardiac function curve is the reverse of the vascular function curve—it examines how changes in CVP affect Q.

9 At any given time, the cardiovascular system operates at one theoretical point of intersection between the vascular and cardiac function curves.

10 Pressure–volume loops provide information about total stroke work, myocardial efficiency, inotropic status of the heart, and diastolic function. Understanding alterations that occur in various disease states can help guide clinical management.

11 Improved ventricular-arterial coupling can improve cardiac efficiency; vasoactive medications may have competing effects on ventricular inotropy and vascular tone that may adversely affect this relationship.

Regulation of Vascular Resistance

12 Vascular endothelial cells produce factors, which interact with vascular smooth muscle cells to cause relaxation or contraction—and thus regulate dynamic changes in vascular resistance.

13 Neural, hormonal, myogenic, and local metabolic mechanisms are also integral to the regulation of vascular tone.

Fetal Circulation and Transition to Postnatal Life

14 In the fetus, the right ventricle supplies most of its blood via the ductus arteriosus and descending aorta to the placenta for oxygen uptake, and the left ventricle supplies most its blood to the brain and heart for oxygen delivery. Critical shunts within the fetal circulation enable this process.

15 The most important events in the transition from the fetal to the postnatal circulation are the rapid and large decrease in pulmonary vascular resistance, increase in pulmonary blood flow, and the disruption of the umbilical–placental circulation.

Regulation of Select Regional Circulations

16 The pulmonary vasculature is actively maintained in a dilated, low-resistance state. Alterations in this process are central to the pathophysiology of a number of pulmonary vascular disorders and can severely impact overall cardiovascular performance.

17 Hypoxic pulmonary vasoconstriction is an essential and unique feature of the pulmonary vasculature, as it allows for the matching of ventilation and perfusion.

18 The exact mechanism of pH-mediated pulmonary vascular reactivity is incompletely understood, but appears to be independent of Pa_{CO_2}.

19 West zones of the lung describe the relationship between pulmonary artery pressure, alveolar pressure, and pulmonary venous pressure. In addition to the three zones typically described (see text), an additional zone IV has been described in which pulmonary blood flow decreases at the extreme base (dependent portion) of the lung.

20 Alterations in coronary blood flow support cardiac work in a manner that allows myocardial performance (oxygen delivery) to match the overall needs (oxygen demand) of the entire body.

21 The left ventricle extracts an almost maximal amount of oxygen from blood passing through the myocardium such that increases in myocardial oxygen demand must be met by increases in coronary blood flow.

The chief function of the cardiovascular system is to deliver essential products to the tissues in order to maintain normal metabolic function and to remove metabolic waste products from them. Derangements in normal cardiovascular function are integral to the pathophysiology of a wide array of critical disease processes in children. In addition, many therapies employed in the intensive care setting directly or indirectly impact the cardiovascular system in ways that may either improve or impede its function. Complicating matters further, components within the cardiovascular system may be differentially or diametrically affected by specific therapies, requiring practitioners to reconcile these varying responses.

This chapter contains a review of the fundamental hemodynamic principles that govern flow through the circulation and measurements of cardiac performance, an examination of the basic mechanisms that regulate vascular tone, and a review of some specific regional circulations in detail. In addition, the special circumstance of the fetal circulation and the perinatal transition are reviewed. An understanding of these concepts should assist the intensivist in caring for patients with cardiovascular compromise and in arbitrating the various needs of the regional circulations.

THE CARDIOVASCULAR CIRCUIT AND VASCULAR ANATOMY

The cardiovascular system is composed of a pump and a large network of tubes that carry blood with all of its metabolic substances to and away from the tissues. The pump is the heart, which is actually two pumps in series: the right ventricle (RV) pumps blood through the pulmonary circulation, and the left ventricle (LV) pumps blood through the systemic circulation. The tubes are the arteries, arterioles, capillaries, venules, and veins that have differing anatomic compositions depending on their location and function within the circulation. Much of our understanding of cardiovascular physiology is based on principles of hydrodynamics and fluid mechanics. Although the cardiovascular system does not conform precisely to simple physical models, a basic understanding of hemodynamic principles is essential in the care of critically ill patients with cardiovascular derangements.

HEMODYNAMIC PRINCIPLES

Flow, Velocity, and Cross-Sectional Area

The velocity of blood flow through a segment of the circulation has units of distance and time (e.g., centimeters/second). The flow of blood through the circulation has units of volume and time (e.g., liters/minute). At a constant flow, the velocity of blood through a vessel relates to the cross-sectional area of the vessel, expressed by the equation:

$$v = Q/A$$

where v is velocity, Q is flow, and A is the cross-sectional area.

Therefore, velocity is proportional to flow and inversely proportional to the cross-sectional area. Thus, peak velocity occurs in the aorta and reaches its nadir in the capillary beds, which have tremendous cross-sectional areas. Velocity increases again as blood moves from the capillaries toward the central veins.

Pressure, Flow, and Resistance

The primary determinants of flow (Q) through a vascular segment are the inflow pressure (P_i), the outflow pressure (P_o),

and the vascular resistance (R). For Newtonian fluids moving with laminar flow through cylindrical tubes, the relationship of flow to various physical factors can be expressed by Poiseuille's Law, which is:

$$Q = \frac{(P_i - P_o)\pi r^4}{8\eta l}$$

where r is radius, η is viscosity, and l is length.

Thus, flow through a vessel will increase as the pressure difference across the vessel increases. Furthermore, as the diameter of the vessel increases, so too will flow at any given pressure difference ($P_i - P_o$). Conversely, increases in viscosity and vessel length result in a decrease in flow.

Alterations in blood vessel diameter, resulting from changes in the contractile state of vascular smooth muscle, are central to regulating blood flow, particularly in the regional vascular beds. The relationship of pressure and flow to resistance can be understood by examining the hydraulic equivalent of Ohm's Law:

$$R = \frac{P_i - P_o}{Q}$$

which states that the resistance to flow through a vessel is equivalent to the change in pressure across the vessel divided by the flow through the vessel. For Newtonian fluids moving through cylindrical tubes, this relationship can be expressed by a rearrangement of Poiseuille's Law to give the hydraulic resistance equation:

$$R = \frac{P_i - P_o}{Q} = \left(\frac{8}{\pi}\right)\left(\frac{1}{r^4}\right)\eta$$

Therefore, when Poiseuille law is applied, the resistance to flow is determined solely by the dimensions of the vessel and the viscosity of the fluid. Moreover, since resistance changes with the fourth power of the radius, even small changes in vessel caliber resulting from vascular contraction or relaxation have a profound impact on flow through a vessel.

Studies indicate that pressure within the vasculature decreases progressively from the aorta to the vena cava, with the largest drop at the level of the arterioles (1). Thus, it follows from the relationships above that resistance is greatest at the level of the arterioles if blood flow is constant through the circulation. How, then, do we reconcile this fact with the effect of vessel diameter on resistance, in that the internal diameter of a capillary is far less than an arteriole? These findings can be reconciled by understanding that capillary beds are vessels in parallel, while the arterial system feeding a particular capillary bed is in series. When calculating the resistance of a system composed of a set of resistors in series (e.g., aorta, large arteries, small arteries, and arterioles), the total resistance is equal to the sum of the individual resistances. Conversely, when calculating the resistance of a system composed of a set of resistors in parallel, such as a capillary network, the total resistance is equal to the sum of the reciprocals of the individual resistances ($1/R$). Thus, for a capillary network, the total resistance is less than the resistance in any individual capillary.

In addition, organs may have a number of resistance vessels in parallel proximal to the capillary bed. These vessels may be patent or may be recruited with increased flow. Increased pulmonary blood flow that occurs with exercise, for example, is in part accommodated by the recruitment of vessels that were previously closed. Thus, an additional factor, k, which represents these recruited vessels, can be added to the resistance equation:

$$R = \frac{P_i - P_o}{Q} = \left(\frac{8}{\pi}\right)\left(\frac{1}{kr^4}\right)\eta$$

From this equation, it can be seen that an increase in k will reduce resistance. In addition, the loss of these vessels—that is, a reduction in k—that may occur with disease (such as the obliteration of distal pulmonary arteries in advanced pulmonary arterial hypertension or the occlusion of vessels by intravascular emboli) will result in increased resistance.

Finally, changes in pressure that occur in response to changes in flow and resistance can be expressed when Ohm law is rearranged as:

$$P_i = QR + P_o$$

Thus, vascular inflow pressure may increase when vascular resistance, blood flow, or outflow pressure increases. These factors are not independent. Pressure may remain constant with increased blood flow because the increase in flow has caused vascular resistance to decrease, for example, by dilating or recruiting previously closed vessels; that is, if the product QR does not increase, neither will pressure.

Compliance

A change in intravascular pressure results in a proportional change in intravascular volume. The incremental change in volume (ΔV) per unit change in pressure (ΔP) defines the compliance (C) of a vessel, as indicated by the equation:

$$C = \Delta V / \Delta P$$

In addition, specific compliance can also be evaluated, since the implications of absolute volume changes are different between small and large structures. Specific compliance is calculated by dividing by the baseline volume, as in the equation:

$$C_{specific} = \frac{\Delta V / \Delta P}{V}$$

When calculations are made in this way, comparisons can be made more easily between patients of different sizes. For example, right ventricular compliance is of concern in atrial septal defects, as it is only when right ventricular compliance increases that a left-to-right shunt can develop. In order to measure right ventricular compliance, allowances must be made for the base volume. The same principle applies to measuring compliance of the aorta, the vena cava, and other fluid-filled structures.

The walls of veins are thinner, less well organized, and contain less elastic tissue than those of arteries, and thus are ~20 times more compliant. As a result, most of the circulating blood volume at any one time resides in the venous system, and therapeutic volume expansion has a disproportionate effect on venous, as opposed to arterial, volume.

Imprecision of Mathematical Models

The application of these mathematical relationships in the vasculature has important caveats. Blood is not a Newtonian fluid, although at normal hematocrits, this is probably of little consequence. The walls of small arteries are neither smooth nor straight; rather they branch, curve, and taper. Blood flow is pulsatile, so that additional energy (and therefore a higher pressure) is necessary to overcome inertia and to accelerate the blood at each ejection. Because of short distances between arterial branch points, laminar flow is unlikely in peripheral vascular beds, and viscous pressure losses would be greater than in a physical model. Arteries are also distensible, and continuously changing transvascular pressures alter their radii; therefore, pressure–flow relationships are not linear. Lastly, vascular beds are comprised of many blood vessels in parallel.

These vessels are not all open all the time, and their radii vary. Despite these differences, the general principles of changes in physical factors, such as viscosity and radius, apply (2).

INTERACTION OF THE CARDIAC PUMP AND THE VASCULATURE

Cardiac output is determined by heart rate, contractility, preload, and afterload. The precise mechanisms relevant to the control of heart rate and contractility, which are properties directly related to the heart, are reviewed in Chapter 71. Preload and afterload are related to both the heart and properties of the vasculature. These interactions can be understood by examining the vascular function curve, the cardiac function curve (otherwise known as the Starling curve) and their interactions.

Vascular Function Curve

The vascular function curve describes how changes in cardiac output affect central venous pressure (CVP), or venous return (**Fig. 69.1**). To understand this relationship, a conceptual model can be used to partition the circulation into components, including a pump, an arterial compartment with a given compliance (C_a), a resistor (which represents the resistance through the arterioles, capillaries, and venules), and a venous compartment with a given compliance (C_v) (**Fig. 69.2**). The pump displaces blood from the venous compartment into the arterial compartment at some rate (Q), which, in this model, is equivalent to the cardiac output. The compliance of the arterial compartment accommodates a portion of this volume before blood is propelled across the microvascular resistor into the venous compartment, which can accommodate a much larger volume than the arterial compartment owing to its greater compliance. Increases in Q will decrease the volume

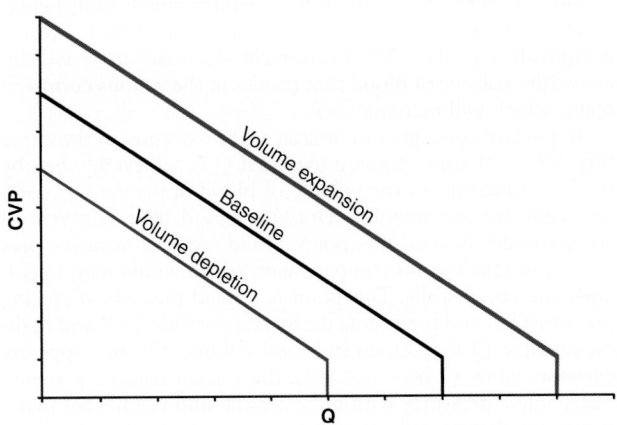

FIGURE 69.1. Vascular function curves shown at different intravascular volumes. The vascular function curve describes the effect of cardiac output (Q) on CVP, or venous return. Increases in Q decrease CVP, while decreases in Q increase CVP. Maximal Q occurs at the critical closing pressure of the venous circulation, whereby reductions in the volume of blood in the venous compartment are not possible, representing the lowest possible CVP and highest possible Q for any given blood volume (P_{cc}, critical closing pressure). At zero Q, the system reaches equilibrium, where pressures within the arterial and venous compartments are determined solely by compliance for any given blood volume. Volume expansion and depletion result in respective parallel increases and decreases in the vascular function curve.

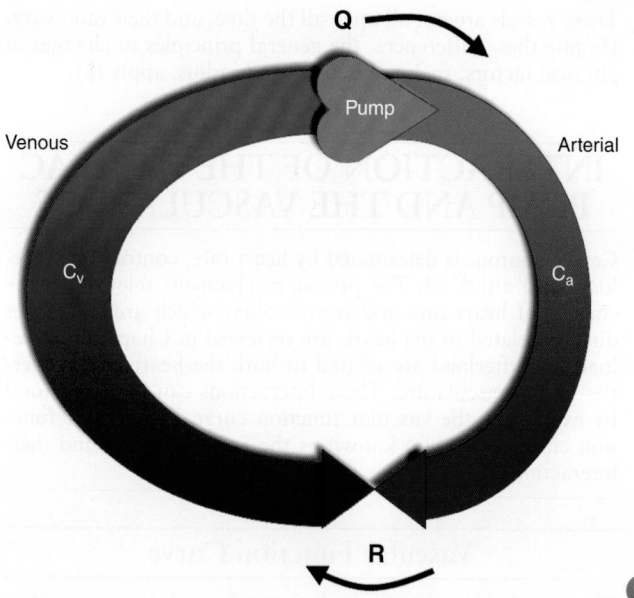

FIGURE 69.2. A conceptual model of the circulation. The circulation is partitioned into components, including a pump, an arterial compartment with compliance (C_a), a resistor (R), which represents the microvascular resistance of the arterioles, capillaries, and venules, and a venous compartment with compliance (C_v). The pump displaces blood from the venous compartment into the arterial compartment at rate (Q), which has units of volume and time (e.g., liters/minute). Increases in Q will decrease the volume of blood residing in the venous compartment and thus will decrease CVP. Conversely, decreases in Q will increase the volume of the venous compartment, which will increase CVP. CVP is determined by Q, R, and the ratio of C_a to C_v. As the compliance of the venous compartment is ~20 times that of the arterial compartment, the venous compartment contains a larger volume than the arterial compartment under normal conditions.

of blood that resides in the venous compartment and, hence, will decrease the pressure in the venous compartment, which is equivalent to the CVP. Conversely, decreases in Q will increase the volume of blood that resides in the venous compartment, which will increase CVP.

Important concepts can be seen at the extremes of the curve (Fig. 69.1). At some point, a maximal Q is achieved, whereby further reductions in the volume of blood in the venous compartment are not possible. Drawing blood from the venous compartment beyond this point would create a negative pressure within the venous compartment, which would tend to collapse the vessel walls. This point is termed the *critical closing pressure* (P_{cc}) and represents the lowest possible CVP and highest possible Q for any given blood volume. On the opposite extreme, when Q becomes zero, the system reaches a steady state, where pressures within the arterial and venous compartments are determined solely by compliance. In this situation, CVP would be at its maximum for any given blood volume. It is also important to note that the curve is affected by the blood volume, with parallel increases from baseline with expansion of the circulating volume (such that occur with blood transfusions) and decreases with volume depletion (such that occur with hemorrhage) (Fig. 69.1).

Cardiac Function Curve

The cardiac function curve is the reverse of the vascular function curve. It examines, how changes in CVP affect Q (Fig. 69.3). This relationship is based on Starling law

that describes increases in Q that result from augmented contractility due to increased stretch of the myocardium (see Chapter 71). On the steep portion of the curve, increases in CVP—through increased venous return—distend the RV (i.e., increased preload), which, in turn, augments right ventricular contractility and flow through the pulmonary circuit. This ultimately increases pulmonary venous return, which increases left ventricular preload and output. Although the cardiac function curve is directly related to CVP, it may also be affected by the other determinants of cardiac output, including afterload, contractility, and heart rate. For example, increases in systemic vascular resistance that increase afterload can result in a downward shift in the curve, whereas systemic vasodilation that decreases afterload shifts the curve upward (Fig. 69.3).

Interaction of Vascular and Cardiac Function Curves

At any given time, the cardiovascular system operates at one theoretical point of intersection between the vascular and cardiac function curves (Fig. 69.4). Deviations from this point are transient. For example, according to the simplified model presented here, if the pump suddenly ejected an increased volume of blood, volume and pressure would increase in the arterial compartment and decrease in the venous compartment, which would transiently shift the vascular function curve to the left. According to the cardiac function curve, subsequent ejection would decrease, as CVP was reduced. Over a short period of time, this decrease in Q would result in an increase in CVP in accordance with the vascular function curve, returning the system to the initial point of intersection.

The superimposition of these curves in various physiologic states is useful, as it illustrates relationships between contractility, preload (including blood volume), and afterload. For example, Figure 69.5 shows that alterations in vascular resistance might shift both the vascular and cardiac function curves, whereas a single cardiac function curve can intersect with several vascular function curves with changes in blood

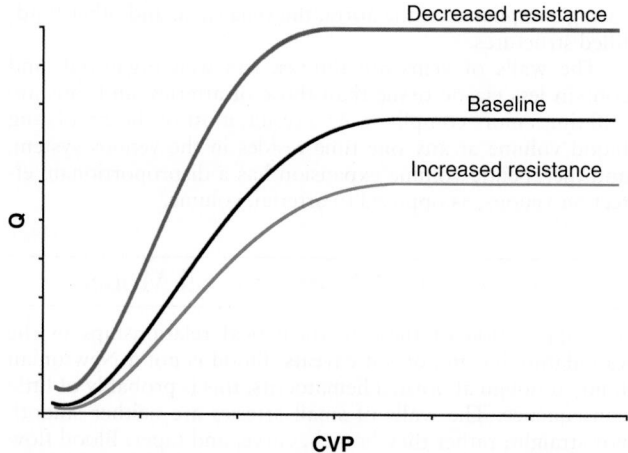

FIGURE 69.3. Cardiac function curves shown under conditions of varying degrees of systemic vascular resistance (afterload). The cardiac function curve describes how changes in CVP or venous return affect cardiac output (Q). On the steep portion of the curve, increases in CVP augment ventricular contractility. Increases in systemic vascular resistance (increased afterload) shift the curve downward, while decreases in systemic vascular resistance (decreased afterload) shift the curve upward.

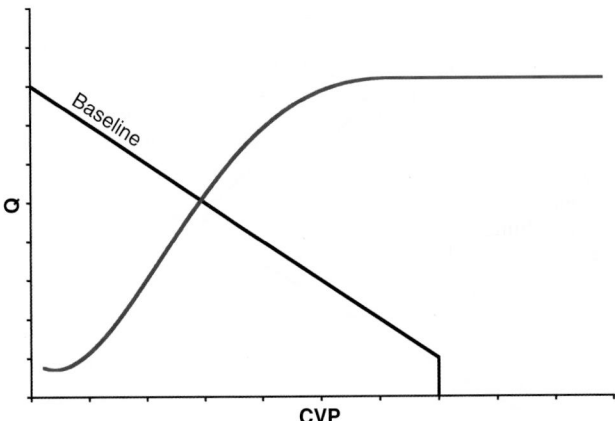

FIGURE 69.4. The cardiovascular system operates at one theoretical point of intersection between the vascular and cardiac function curves. Deviations from this point are transient when the curves are accurate.

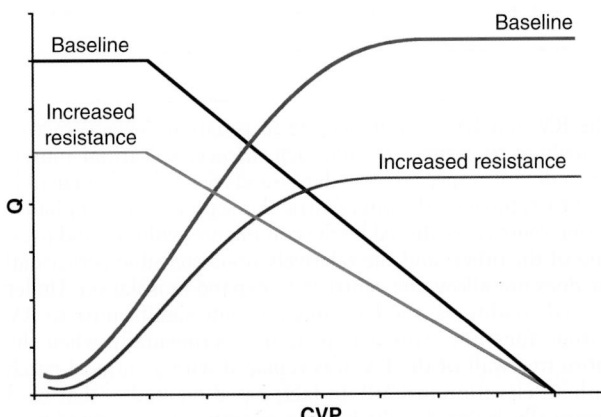

FIGURE 69.5. Effects of increased systemic vascular resistance on the vascular and cardiac function curves. Increased systemic vascular resistance (or afterload) shifts both curves downward, moving the operating state of the system that occurs at the point of intersection between the two curves downward. Increased systemic vascular resistance does not alter the vascular function curve at zero Q, as the CVP at this point is determined solely by the compliance of the venous compartment, at any given volume.

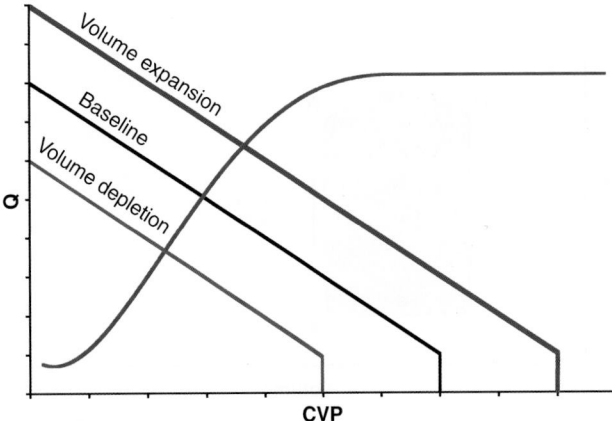

FIGURE 69.6. Effects of intravascular volume on the vascular and cardiac function curves. Intravascular volume expansion increases and intravascular volume depletion decreases the vascular function curve. The cardiac function curve is not altered by changes in intravascular volume. Because the cardiovascular system operates at the point of intersection between the two curves, the functional state of the system is affected by the volume status.

Pressure–Volume Loops

The hemodynamic and mechanical events of the cardiac cycle in the LV can be graphically represented by the instantaneous relationship of pressure and volume (Fig. 69.7). In this diagram, end-diastole is represented by point A; this is also the point in the cardiac cycle when the mitral valve closes. From points A to B, the ventricle undergoes isovolumic contraction. At point B, the aortic valve opens, and there is ejection with relatively little decrease in pressure until aortic valve closure (point C). Point C also represents end-systole. Then, diastole begins with isovolumic relaxation until point D, which represents mitral valve opening. From points D to A, there is filling of the ventricle.

By imposing a change in preload or afterload without altering cardiac contractility (e.g., transient vena caval occlusion or phenylephrine administration), an informative series of pressure–volume loops can be generated (Fig. 69.8). The end-systolic points of this family of loops will have a linear relationship, which defines the *end-systolic pressure–volume relationship* (ESPVR). The slope of this line is Ees, a load-independent index of the inotropic state of the myocardium. Interventions that affect inotropy (e.g., increase with epinephrine infusion or decrease with acute β-blockade) will alter the slope of the ESPVR. Thus, the ventricle has a different Ees for any given contractile state (Fig. 69.9); note that changes in inotropy (Ees) dramatically affect stroke volume at the same end-systolic pressure. In clinical practice, physiologic or pharmacologic states that alter Ees may also increase afterload, thus having competing effects on stroke volume. The total area enclosed by the pressure–volume loops represents *preload-recruitable stroke work* (PRSW) and can be used to extrapolate energy expenditure by the ventricle.

The *end-diastolic pressure–volume relationship* (EDPVR) is defined by connecting the end-diastolic points of the family of loops (Fig. 69.7). EDPVR reflects the pressure–volume relationship of the ventricle in its most relaxed state; it is inherently nonlinear as different muscle fibers are stretched at different points in the pressure–volume relationship. Constants can be derived from EDPVR to compare ventricular stiffness and diastolic function among individuals and between disease states. EDPVR is altered in patients with diastolic dysfunction, but, unlike ESPVR, EDPVR is less adaptable to changing physiologic states and altered hormonal control. Understanding the

volume (Fig. 69.6). Furthermore, whereas alterations in blood volume result in parallel changes in the vascular function curve (Figs. 69.1 and 69.6), alterations in resistance alter the slope of the curve but not the CVP at zero Q, because this point depends only on blood volume and compliance (Fig. 69.5). As the cardiovascular system operates at the point of intersection between the two curves, alterations in blood volume will shift the operative state of the system, even though it does alter intrinsic cardiac function (Fig. 69.6). However, adding an inotrope could shift the cardiac function curve, which explains the common practice of fluid administration and inotropic support in the setting of shock. Indeed, critical illnesses with their attendant physiologic derangements will variably affect the cardiovascular system and may differentially affect the vascular and cardiac function curves. Likewise, therapies may also have differential effects. Thus, although the theoretical model described by the vascular and cardiac function curves is overly simplified, it is useful as a foundation with which to rationalize a therapeutic approach to various cardiovascular derangements.

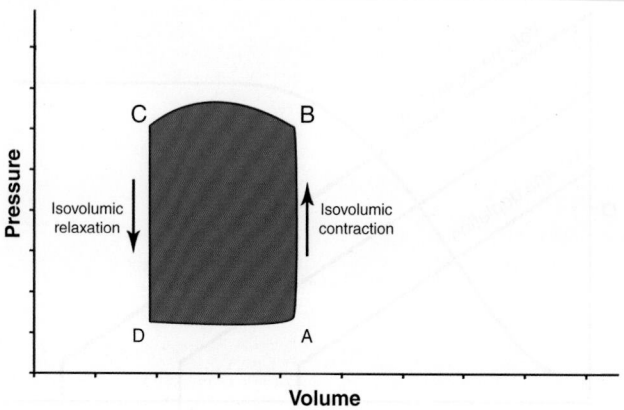

FIGURE 69.7. LV pressure–volume loop demonstrating the events of the cardiac cycle. Systole begins after point A with mitral valve closure. Then, the ventricle undergoes isovolumic contraction, followed by aortic valve opening (point B). Systole concludes after ejection and aortic valve closure (point C). Diastole begins with isovolumic relaxation, followed by mitral valve opening at point D. After filling of the ventricle, diastole ends at point A.

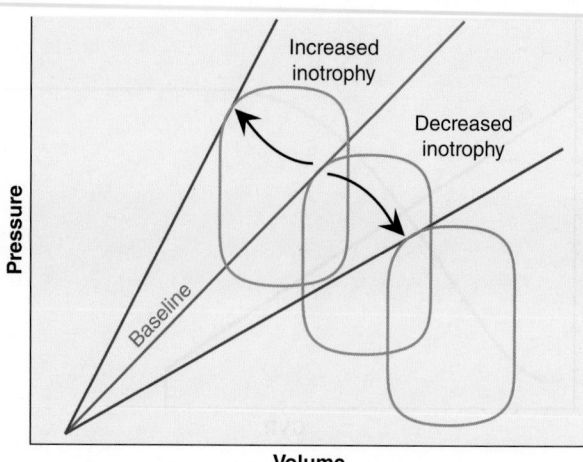

FIGURE 69.9. Changes in Ees occur as the inotropic status of the ventricle is altered. For example, an acute increase in inotropy (i.e., epinephrine administration) would shift the ESPVR line to the left (and increase Ees). Conversely, an acute decrease in inotropy, as would occur with β-blocker administration, would decrease Ees.

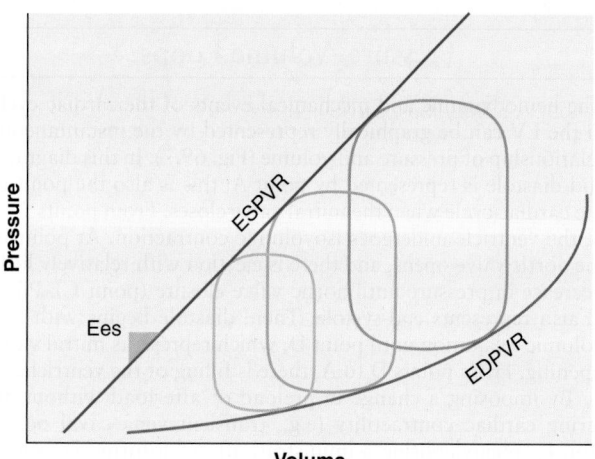

FIGURE 69.8. With acute alterations in preload (i.e., caval occlusion) or afterload (i.e., phenylephrine administration), a family of pressure–volume loops are generated. The linear ESPVR is defined by the connected end-systolic points of this group of curves; the slope of ESPVR is Ees. The nonlinear EDPVR describes the line generated by connecting the end-diastolic points of this group of loops.

Ventricular–Ventricular Interactions

The RV and LV do not operate in isolation. Several factors contribute to *ventricular interdependence*: epicardial muscle fibers do not respect ventricular boundaries but rather encircle the heart; through the interventricular septum, the compliance of one ventricle is altered by the compliance, volume, and pressure of the other; and the relatively nondistensible pericardial sac does not allow one ventricle to expand in isolation. Under normal conditions, the LV can contribute significantly to RV systolic function. This was proven experimentally when the entire free wall of the RV was replaced with a surgical patch without elevation in CVP. In fact, based on studies that used electrically isolated right heart preparations and experimental aortic constriction, it is estimated that 20%–40% of RV systolic pressure is due to LV contraction (3). Under normal conditions, the RV minimally effects LV function. However, in patients with pulmonary hypertension and resultant elevated RV pressures and end-diastolic volumes, septal position changes with flattening and eventual septal bowing into the LV. This affects LV diastolic function. Transmitted pressure from the RV interferes with left-sided filling, leading to diastolic dysfunction with a much greater dependence on active diastolic filling from atrial contraction.

differing effects of the EDPVR and ESPVR on stroke volume and the stroke work done by the heart provides unique insight into cardiovascular physiology in both disease and health.

Unlike pressure–volume loops obtained in the LV, RV pressure–volume loops under normal conditions do not contain an isovolumic relaxation or contraction phase, giving them a triangular shape. Additionally, the RV continues to eject after reaching peak pressure. This is due to the low-afterload state present in the pulmonary vasculature. Given the smaller total area of normal RV loops compared to LV pressure–volume loops at the same stroke volume, the RV is more efficient. These properties are load-dependent. With elevated RV afterload (i.e., pulmonary hypertension or stenosis), the RV pressure–volume loop becomes rectangular and looks more like the LV loop.
(10) Pressure–volume loops provide a powerful tool to assess cardiac performance and changes in loop characteristics give unique insight in physiologic and pathologic changes in the cardiovascular system.

Ventricular–Arterial Coupling

(11) The ventricles function as a unit with the vascular system; elevated vascular resistance increases afterload and thus will decrease stroke volume if contractility and preload remain constant. Pressure volume loops can be used to quantify this relationship. Ea is *effective arterial elastance* and is defined by the ratio of ESPVR to stroke volume (**Fig. 69.10**). Ea quantifies the composite factors of vascular load, including total vascular compliance, resistance, characteristic impedance, and intervals of the cardiac cycle. Ventriculovascular coupling is then described as the ratio of Ees to Ea; derangements in this relationship reveal inefficiencies in cardiac function, and may be present in patients before clinically overt heart failure becomes manifest. In critical care, this relationship is relevant to patients in shock who may have inappropriately elevated systemic vascular resistance in the face of myocardial dysfunction; consideration of ventriculovascular coupling can inform

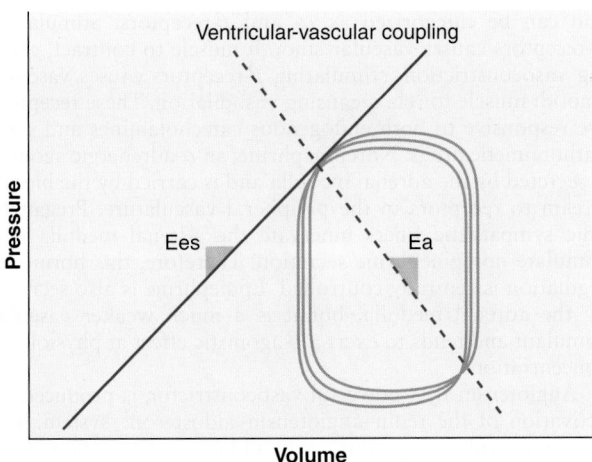

FIGURE 69.10. Relationship of Ees and Ea. Ea is defined by the ratio of ESPVR to stroke volume.

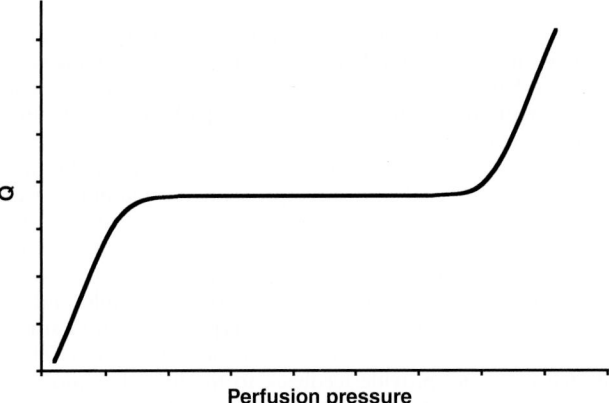

FIGURE 69.11. Autoregulation. Blood flow (Q) through most organs is maintained constant over a wide range of perfusion pressures. In general, decreases in perfusion pressure result in vasodilation, while increases in perfusion pressure result in vasoconstriction, thereby maintaining constant flow through alterations in vascular resistance. At the points of downward and upward inflection, maximal dilation or constriction have occurred, and constant blood flow can no longer be maintained in the face of decreased or increased perfusion pressures, respectively.

the most appropriate combination of inotropic and vasoactive agents for different pathophysiologic derangements.

REGULATION OF VASCULAR RESISTANCE

The contractile state of the vasculature is central to cardiovascular physiology because vascular resistance effects afterload and preload, two of the four main determinants of cardiac output, and because alterations in resistance within and between vascular beds dictate flow within organs as well as the distribution of blood flow throughout the body. The main site of resistance within the circulation occurs at the level of the arterioles. However, larger arteries and veins of varying sizes also affect resistance and may become a primary site of resistance under various conditions. Although, a number of anatomic factors contribute to the resistance imposed by a vessel, smooth muscle cell tone is the predominant regulating mechanism.

Several mechanisms control the contractile state of vascular smooth muscle and, thus, vascular resistance, including neural control, hormonal control, endothelial-derived factors, myogenic processes, and local metabolic products. Autoregulation is a more general phenomenon that may involve several of these specific mechanisms.

Autoregulation

Blood flow to tissues remains relatively constant over a wide range of arterial blood pressures owing to autoregulation (Fig. 69.11). The mechanisms of this phenomenon are largely unknown. Several hypothetical mechanisms exist, including local metabolic control, myogenic activity of vascular smooth muscle, and tissue pressure. These mechanisms may act alone or in combination. The metabolic hypothesis suggests that blood flow is closely linked to tissue metabolism. According to this theory, blood flow must be sufficient to support the metabolic demands of an organ. With increasing demands or with insufficient delivery of metabolic substrates, vasoactive substances are formed and/or released that result in vasodilation, which increases blood flow. As flow rises, the metabolites are washed out, restoring their concentration to normal. In organs with high oxygen consumption, autoregulation of blood flow is largely dependent on tissue oxygenation. However, a number of substances may contribute to this process,

including carbon dioxide, hydrogen ions, lactic acid, histamine, potassium ions, prostaglandin, endothelin (ET)-1, nitric oxide (NO), and adenosine. A second proposed mechanism of autoregulation is myogenic control (4). According to this theory, increased intravascular pressure stimulates vasoconstriction of vascular smooth muscle. A venous–arterial reflex has been described in which an increase in venous pressure causes arteriolar constriction, probably by a neurally mediated mechanism (4). Autoregulation seems to play a more significant role in control of resting blood flow in vital organs, such as the brain and heart, and becomes significant in other areas during times of increased metabolic demand. In addition, various mechanisms may be specific for a given organ, such as macula densa signaling in the kidney.

Whatever the mechanism, it is clear that intact autoregulation is essential for normal organ function, particularly for the heart, kidneys, and brain. For example, impaired cerebral autoregulation is central to the pathophysiology of traumatic brain injury, acute ischemic stroke, neonatal brain asphyxia, and acute hypertensive encephalopathy.

Neural Control

13 Neural control of the circulation allows rapid regulation and provides simultaneous control of various regions within the circulation. Neural regulation consists of feedback (afferent limb) information provided by *baroreceptors* and cardiac *stretch receptors* and neurologic control (efferent limb) through the autonomic nervous system, which is composed of the sympathetic and parasympathetic systems. Nearly all blood vessels in the body are innervated by the autonomic nervous system; the effect of this control varies from one vascular bed to another.

The afferent limb of the neural control mechanisms consists of *baroreceptors* in arterial walls and stretch receptors within heart muscle. Baroreceptors are found in each carotid sinus and in the aortic arch. Two types of baroreceptors have been identified. Type 1 receptors control dynamic changes in blood pressure; type 2 receptors are responsible for control of resting blood pressure (5). These receptors respond to stretch of the arterial wall and send nerve impulses to cardioinhibitory and vasomotor centers of the medulla. Stimulation of carotid sinus receptors results in slowing of heart rate, vasodilation, and a decrease in arterial blood pressure. Smooth muscle in the walls of these baroreceptor regions is innervated by vasoconstrictor efferent fibers, suggesting that sympathetic activity may modify baroreceptor responses.

Stretch receptors are also found in the walls of the atria and ventricles. Atrial stretch receptors are located in the walls of both atria at the venoatrial junctions. Two kinds of atrial receptors have been described. Type A receptors fire during atrial contraction and respond to changes in atrial pressure, and type B receptors fire during ventricular systole and respond to changes in atrial volume. Type A receptors stimulate and type B receptors inhibit sympathetic activity. These stretch receptors provide feedback to the hypothalamus and inhibit secretion of antidiuretic hormone (vasopressin). Atrial stretch causes secretion of atrial natriuretic factor (ANF), which is discussed in more detail later. Atrial receptors also alter sympathetic stimulation of the renal circulation (5). By these mechanisms, atrial stretch receptors play an important role in regulating intravascular volume. They are also responsible for stimulating increased heart rate by the *Bainbridge reflex* (tachycardia secondary to atrial distension).

Two types of stretch receptors are found in ventricular myocardium. The first type fires in a pulsatile manner in time with cardiac rhythm and are scarce. The second respond to mechanical stimulation and to various drugs and chemicals through nonmyelinated afferent nerves known as *C fibers*. Stimulation of C fibers, which are primarily located in the LV, causes hypotension and bradycardia from parasympathetic stimulation and sympathetic inhibition. Evidence suggests that carotid baroreceptors are more important for control of sympathetic regulation of muscle blood flow, whereas cardiac receptors are more important in control of sympathetic regulation of kidney blood flow.

The efferent limb of neural control of the circulation, the autonomic nervous system, is divided into the sympathetic and parasympathetic systems. Two different types of sympathetic nerve fibers exist: vasoconstrictor and vasodilator. Sympathetic stimulation of the arterioles by vasoconstrictor fibers increases vascular resistance; these vessels are called *resistance vessels*. The nerve endings of these sympathetic vasoconstrictor fibers contain the vasoconstrictor norepinephrine, which is released on nerve stimulation. Other substances present at the neurovascular junction, including monoamines, polypeptides, purines, and amino acids, can influence the release and the effects of norepinephrine (5). Impulses carried through vasoconstrictor fibers contribute the normal vascular tone or baseline constriction that is present at rest in most vascular beds. These vasoconstrictor fibers are more prevalent in skeletal muscles, where intrinsic tone is fairly high under resting conditions; they are much less prevalent in the cerebral and coronary beds. Sympathetic vasoconstriction of larger arteries and of veins changes their volume and thus changes the circulating volume; these vessels are known as *capacitance vessels*.

Hormonal Control

Hormonal control of the peripheral circulation can best be described as vascular constriction or dilation in response to circulating hormones. The vasculature in the peripheral circulation is responsive to various circulating substances, including catecholamines, angiotensin II, vasopressin, eicosanoids, NO, neurokinins, endothelin, bradykinin, and other peptide hormones.

Catecholamines are the hormones of the adrenergic system. Adrenergic receptors to catecholamines are present in the smooth muscle throughout the peripheral vascular system

and can be categorized as α- and β-receptors. Stimulating α-receptors causes vascular smooth muscle to contract, causing vasoconstriction; stimulating β-receptors causes vascular smooth muscle to relax, causing vasodilation. These receptors are responsive to both endogenous catecholamines and sympathomimetic drugs. Norepinephrine, an α-adrenergic agonist, is secreted by the adrenal medulla and is carried by the bloodstream to receptors in the peripheral vasculature. Preganglionic sympathetic fibers innervate the adrenal medulla and stimulate norepinephrine secretion. Therefore, this hormonal regulation is centrally controlled. Epinephrine is also secreted by the adrenal medulla, but it is a much weaker vascular stimulant and tends to exert a β-agonistic effect at physiologic concentrations.

Angiotensin II, a powerful vasoconstrictor, is produced by activation of the renin–angiotensin–aldosterone system. The juxtaglomerular apparatus in the kidney secretes renin in response to decreased renal arterial pressure or a decrease in extracellular fluid volume. Renin, in turn, cleaves angiotensinogen to angiotensin I, which is then converted to angiotensin II by angiotensin-converting enzyme (ACE) found in lung and renal endothelium. Angiotensin II has direct vasoconstrictor properties, acts centrally to stimulate the vasoconstrictor centers of the brain, and stimulates the secretion of antidiuretic hormone (vasopressin). In addition, renin can be formed locally in many organs, which partially explains why angiotensin-receptor blockade has an additive clinical effect with ACE inhibitors. Antidiuretic hormone is synthesized in the hypothalamus and secreted by the posterior pituitary. It is a very potent vasoconstrictor but plays a minimal role in regulation of the circulation under resting conditions.

Prostaglandins and other eicosanoids play a small role in regulating flow in the systemic circulation. ANF is another hormone that participates in regulating the systemic circulation. This peptide hormone is released from atrial myocytes of both atria, and in smaller amounts from the ventricular myocytes. Ventricular production of ANF decreases with maturation; large amounts of ANF are produced in fetal ventricular myocardium, whereas in adults, the ventricles produce small amounts. ANF is released in response to stretch of either atrium; increased circulating levels of ANF are detected when left atrial pressure is elevated, even when the right atrial pressure is normal. In the kidney, ANF decreases tubular reabsorption of sodium. In the circulatory system, ANF has vasodilator and cardioinhibitory effects. Circulating levels of ANF are increased in certain pathophysiologic conditions, such as congenital heart disease associated with elevated atrial pressures, congestive heart failure, valve disease, hypertension, coronary artery occlusion, and atrial arrhythmias. In addition, *B-type natriuretic peptide*, which is produced by the ventricular myocytes in response to stretch, has natriuretic, diuretic, and vasoactive properties. Measurements of B-type natriuretic peptide are used in the diagnosis, risk stratification, and management of adult cardiac disease and are increasingly used in the clinical management of pediatric patients as well.

Endothelial-Derived Factors

The vascular endothelial cells are capable of producing a variety of vasoactive substances, which participate in the regulation of normal vascular tone. These substances, such as NO and ET-1, are capable of producing vascular relaxation and/or constriction, modulating the propensity of the blood to clot, and inducing and/or inhibiting smooth muscle migration and replication (6,7) (**Fig. 69.12**). Increased understanding of the role of the vascular endothelium in regulating blood flow in health and disease has resulted in several treatment strategies

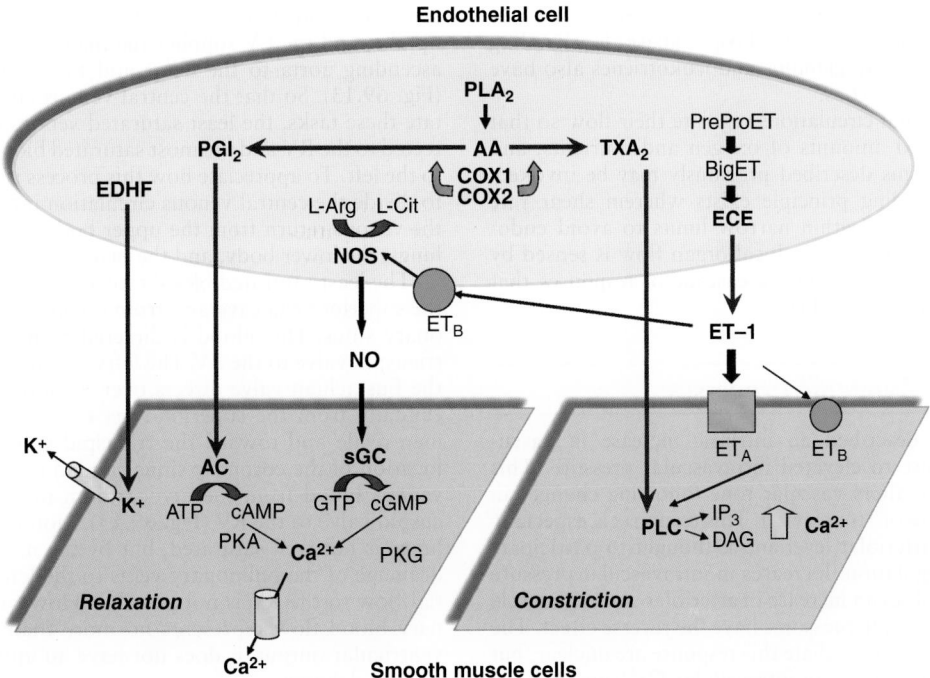

FIGURE 69.12. A schematic of some endothelial-derived factors, which may cause smooth muscle cell relaxation (**left**) and/or constriction (**right**). PGI$_2$, prostaglandin I$_2$; L-Arg, L-arginine; L-Cit, L-citrulline; PLA$_2$, phospholipase A$_2$; AA, arachidonic acid; COX1, cyclooxygenase-1; COX2, cyclooxygenase-2; TXA$_2$, thromboxane A$_2$; PrePro ET, PrePro endothelin; BigET, Big endothelin; NOS, nitric oxide synthase; ECE, endothelin-converting enzyme; ET$_B$, endothelin B receptor; NO, nitric oxide; ET-1, endothelin-1; K$^+$, potassium channels; AC, adenylate cyclase; sGC, soluble guanylate cyclase; ATP, adenosine-5′-triphosphate; cAMP, cyclic adenosine monophosphate; GTP, guanosine-5′-triphosphate; cGMP, cyclic guanosine-3′-5′ monophosphate; PKA, phosphokinase A; PKG, phosphokinase G; ET$_A$, endothelin A receptor; PLC, phospholipase C; IP$_3$, inositol triphosphate; DAG, diacylglycerol.

that target the endothelium. These include inhaled NO for pulmonary hypertension, L-arginine supplementation for coronary artery disease and the pulmonary vasculopathy of sickle cell disease, phosphodiesterase inhibitors [i.e., sildenafil, which prevents the breakdown of guanosine 3′,5′-monophosphate (cGMP)] for pulmonary hypertensive disorders, and endothelin-receptor antagonists (i.e., bosentan, ambrisentan) for pulmonary hypertensive disorders and subarachnoid hemorrhage. Indeed, many older therapies, such as nitrovasodilators, affect endothelial function.

NO is a labile humoral factor produced by NO synthase from L-arginine in the vascular endothelial cell. NO diffuses into the smooth muscle cell and produces vascular relaxation by increasing concentrations of cGMP, via the activation of soluble guanylate cyclase (**Fig. 69.12**). NO is released in response to a variety of factors, including shear stress (flow) and the binding of certain endothelium-dependent vasodilators (such as acetylcholine, ATP, and bradykinin) to receptors on the endothelial cell. Basal NO release is an important mediator of resting pulmonary and systemic vascular tone in the fetus, newborn, and adult, as well as a mediator of the reduction in pulmonary vascular resistance that normally occurs at the time of birth (8).

ET-1, a 21–amino acid polypeptide, is produced by vascular endothelial cells (9). The vasoactive properties of ET-1 are complex, and studies have shown varying hemodynamic effects on different vascular beds. However, its most striking property is its sustained hypertensive action. ET-1 is the most potent vasoconstricting agent discovered, with a potency 10 times that of angiotensin II. The hemodynamic effects of ET-1 are mediated by at least two distinctive receptor populations: ET$_A$ and ET$_B$. The ET$_A$ receptors are located on vascular smooth muscle cells

and mediate vasoconstriction, whereas the ET$_B$ receptors may be located on endothelial and smooth muscle cells and mediate both vasodilation and vasoconstriction (**Fig. 69.12**). Individual endothelins occur in low levels in the plasma, generally below their vasoactive thresholds, suggesting that they are primarily effective at the local site of release. Even at these levels, they may potentiate the effects of other vasoconstrictors, such as norepinephrine and serotonin. Nevertheless, alterations in ET-1 have been implicated in the pathophysiology of a number of disease states. ET-1 has emerged as a therapeutic target; endothelin-receptor antagonists are used in pulmonary hypertension (e.g., bosentan) and as additive therapies in refractory systemic hypertension (darusentan).

Endothelial-derived hyperpolarizing factors (EDHFs), diffusible substances that cause vascular relaxation by hyperpolarizing the smooth muscle cell, are another important group of endothelial factors. These are now known to be epoxyeicosatrienoic acids and perhaps hydrogen peroxide. The action of EDHF depends, at least in part, on potassium (K$^+$) channels (10) (**Fig. 69.12**). Activating K$^+$ channels in the vascular smooth muscle hyperpolarizes the cell membrane, closes voltage-dependent calcium (Ca^{2+}) channels, and ultimately causes vasodilation. K$^+$ channels are also present in endothelial cells. Activation within the endothelium results in changes in Ca^{2+} flux and may be important in releasing NO, prostacyclin (PGI$_2$), and EDHF. K$^+$ channel subtypes include ATP-sensitive K$^+$ channels, Ca^{2+}-dependent K$^+$ channels, voltage-dependent K$^+$ channels, and inward-rectifier K$^+$ channels (10).

The breakdown of phospholipids within vascular endothelial cells results in the production of the important byproducts of arachidonic acid, including PGI$_2$ and thromboxane (TXA$_2$). PGI$_2$ activates adenylate cyclase, resulting in increased cyclic

AMP production and subsequent vasodilation, whereas TXA_2 results in vasoconstriction via phospholipase C signaling (**Fig. 69.12**). Other prostaglandins and leukotrienes also have potent vasoactive properties.

In general, regional circulations regulate their flow so that they obtain required amounts of oxygen and nutrients, and all of the mechanisms described previously may be invoked. However, an overriding principle exists wherein shear rate must be kept constant within narrow limits to avoid endothelial damage. Any increase in local organ flow is sensed by endothelial integrins that trigger a cascade of responses that culminate in release of NO (11).

Myogenic Processes

In 1902, Bayliss described an intrinsic increase in vascular tone in response to elevated intravascular pressure. This myogenic response alters vascular tone following changes in transmural pressure or stretch (12). This response is especially important at the arteriolar level and is thought to participate in regional autoregulation. Increases in intravascular pressure and/or stretch result in an increase in arteriolar smooth muscle tone, whereas decreasing pressures have the reverse effect. The precise mechanisms that mediate this response are unclear, but a role for dynamic changes in intracellular Ca^{2+} and myosin light-chain phosphorylation has been documented (13). More recent work has focused on the role of tyrosine phosphorylation pathways in this response (14).

Local Metabolic Products

Tissues have the ability to regulate their own blood flow in response to changes in metabolic demands. The local chemical environment of arterioles can cause vasodilation or, to a lesser extent, vasoconstriction. For example, a decrease in Po_2, an increase in Pco_2, and an increase in hydrogen (H^+) or K^+ concentration will each cause arteriolar vasodilation. Many tissues will release adenosine, a potent vasodilator, in response to increased metabolism or decreased oxygen tension. Other mediators include lactic acid, histamine, prostaglandin, ET-1, and NO.

REGULATION OF REGIONAL CIRCULATIONS

Vascular resistance within each regional circulation dictates the distribution of blood flow to the individual organs. An understanding of the factors that regulate resistance within the specific regional vascular beds is essential in allowing the intensivist to combat cardiovascular derangements, while arbitrating the various, if not disparate, needs of the specific organs.

In addition, when caring for neonates, an understanding of the fetal circulation is critical, as a number of problems may occur when the normal transition from the fetal to postnatal circulation is compromised. Although not a regional circulation, the fetal circulation is marked by important differences in regional blood flow from the postnatal situation.

Fetal Circulation

⓮ The presence of central shunts allows the fetal circulation to be remarkably efficient at distributing oxygen and substrate. The fetal RV supplies the majority of its blood via the ductus

arteriosus and descending aorta to the placenta for oxygen uptake, and the LV supplies the majority of its blood via the ascending aorta to the heart and brain for oxygen delivery (**Fig. 69.13**). So that the central venous circulation can facilitate these tasks, the least saturated venous blood must be directed to the RV and the most saturated blood must be directed to the left. To appreciate how this process is achieved, it is best to divide the central venous circulation into five components: the venous return from the upper body, the myocardium, the lungs, the lower body, and the placenta.

The least saturated blood returns from the upper body via the superior vena cava and from the myocardium via the coronary sinus. This blood is directed appropriately across the tricuspid valve to the RV. The leftward and superior course of the Eustachian valve directs over 95% of the blood flowing caudally from the superior vena cava away from the foramen ovale and toward the tricuspid valve. In addition, the location of the coronary sinus caudad to the foramen causes venous blood from the myocardium to flow across the tricuspid valve to the RV (**Fig. 69.13**). Blood returning from the lungs is not well saturated, but by the nature of the normal drainage of the pulmonary veins to the left atrium, preferential flow to the RV is not possible. However, as fetal pulmonary blood flow represents no more than 8% of combined ventricular output, it does not have an appreciable effect on oxygen delivery.

Inferior vena caval return comes from the remaining two sources: the lower body and the placenta. The majority of lower body flow, except that from the liver, ascends the distal inferior vena cava. This stream of relatively desaturated blood enters the lateral margin of the right atrium and is directed primarily across the tricuspid valve. Placental (umbilical venous) and liver venous return is more complicated (**Fig. 69.14**). Under normal conditions in the fetal sheep, ~55% of the highly saturated umbilical venous return

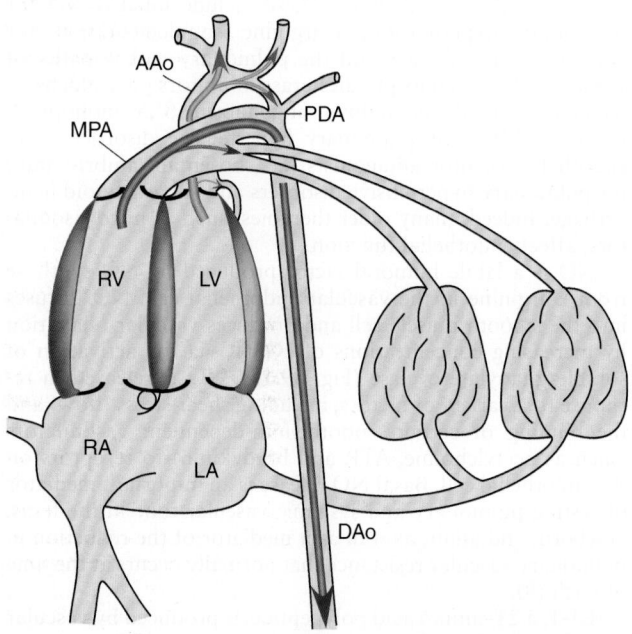

FIGURE 69.13. Preferential pattern of ventricular output. The LV receives blood from the left atrium (LA) and directs the majority via the ascending aorta (AAo) to the highly metabolic heart and upper body. The RV receives right atrial blood (RA) and ejects it via the main pulmonary artery (MPA) primarily down the ductus arteriosus (DAo) to the placenta for oxygen uptake. PDA, patent ductus arteriosus.

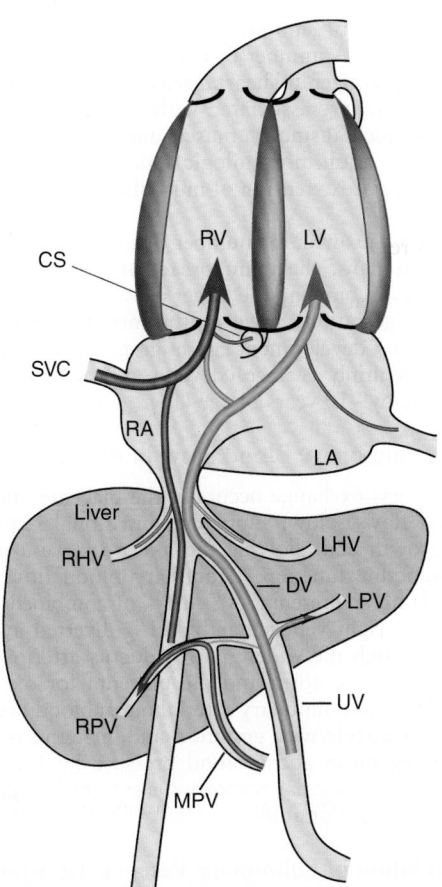

FIGURE 69.14. Preferential pattern of venous return to the right (RV) and left (LV) ventricles. Preferentially, higher-saturated blood from the umbilical vein (UV) passes via the ductus venosus (DV) and left hepatic vein (LHV) to the left atrium (LA) and LV. Less-saturated blood from the lower body via the inferior vena cava (IVC), the right hepatic vein (RHV) (via the right portal vein), the coronary sinus (CS), and the superior vena cava (SVC) passes to the right atrium (RA) and then the RV. MPV, main portal vein.

distribution to the myocardium and brain. Although the separation of fetal ventricular output is not as efficient as the postnatal separation, it is quite remarkable in its ability to allow the RV and LV to perform their normal postnatal functions of delivery of blood for oxygen uptake and oxygen supply, respectively.

Transition from the Fetal to the Postnatal Circulation

15 The changes in the central circulation at birth are primarily caused by external events. Most important of these external events are the rapid and large decrease in pulmonary vascular resistance and the disruption of the umbilical–placental circulation. The various mechanisms responsible for the decrease in pulmonary vascular resistance are discussed later. This decrease has profound effects on the central shunts in the systemic circulation. Abruptly at birth, the ductus arteriosus changes from a right-to-left conduit of blood to the descending aorta, to a left-to-right conduit of blood to the lungs (until it closes in the first hours or days of life). This shunt may be prolonged in the premature infant, causing a steal of blood from the regional vascular beds of greatest resistance.

As previously mentioned, the ductus venosus carries umbilical venous return primarily to the left heart. Although the amount of umbilical venous blood that enters the ductus venosus is variable and is greatly affected by stresses, such as hypoxemia, changes in flow do not appear to be caused by active vasoconstriction of the ductus venosus; rather they occur passively in accordance with changes in umbilical blood flow. At birth, portal venous flow through the ductus venosus increases dramatically. However, despite this increase in portal venous flow, total hepatic flow decreases because the placental circulation is removed. This shunt of portal venous blood through the ductus venosus is transient, generally lasting for 1 day to 2 weeks. The functional closure of the ductus venosus is probably passive, although the isolated ductus venosus can respond to adrenergic stimulation and prostanoids. In the intact newborn lamb, it can dilate in response to prostaglandin E_1. Thus, its closure may be partly induced by the same hormonal changes that are implicated in the closure of the ductus arteriosus.

Although vasoactive processes are involved in the closure of the ductus arteriosus and may be involved in closure of the ductus venosus, closure of the foramen ovale at birth is entirely passive, secondary to alterations in the relative return of blood to the right and left atria. Prior to birth, direct left atrial return via the pulmonary veins is only ~8% of combined venous return. Thus, the pressure gradient from right to left maintains a large flow of blood across the foramen ovale, and its flap appears as a windsock bulging into the left atrium. With the onset of oxygen ventilation, the proportion of combined venous return that directly enters the left atrium via the pulmonary veins increases dramatically, to >50% (15), because of the marked increase in pulmonary blood flow, which includes a transient left-to-right shunt through the ductus arteriosus. Left atrial pressure thus exceeds right, and the redundant flap of tissue of the foramen ovale that previously bowed into the left atrium is now pressed against the septum. Small left-to-right shunts may be visualized in the newborn by color Doppler ultrasonography, but these shunts are not hemodynamically significant. Although patency of the foramen ovale may be present for several years, shunts of any significance occur only when the primum septum is deficient, thus forming a secundum atrial septal defect, or when an ostium primum defect is present.

ascends via the ductus venosus to the inferior vena cava–right atrium junction, where it preferentially crosses the foramen ovale. Slightly less than half of the remaining umbilical venous return enters the left lobe of the liver, from whence it reaches the left hepatic vein. The left hepatic vein joins the ductus venosus near the inferior vena cava so that this highly saturated blood is also directed to the foramen ovale. The limbus of the foramen ovale helps to direct this blood into the left atrium. The remainder of the umbilical venous blood, along with over 95% of the poorly saturated portal venous blood, is directed to the right lobe of the liver. From the right lobe, this much-less saturated blood enters the right hepatic vein and tends to stream with the blood of the distal inferior vena cava to the tricuspid valve. In that the hepatic artery, which carries blood that is moderately well saturated, contributes <10% of hepatic blood flow in the fetus, it does not significantly contribute to oxygen supply. Hepatic arterial blood is distributed to both lobes of the liver, with the right lobe receiving somewhat more.

Thus, preferential streaming patterns among the various sources of venous return allow most of the poorly saturated blood from the upper body, myocardium, and lower body to reach the RV for return to the placenta and the more highly saturated umbilical venous return to reach the LV for

Interaction of the Systemic and Pulmonary Circulations

The simplified model of the circulation outlined in **Figure 69.2** describes resistance as a single resistor that lies between the large arteries and veins of the systemic circulation. In fact, total systemic vascular resistance represents the sum of the resistances of each regional vascular bed. The pulmonary vascular resistance, normally 10%–20% of the systemic vascular resistance, is distinct, as a separate pump (i.e., the RV) propels blood through the pulmonary circuit. Therefore, under normal conditions, only the total systemic resistance needs to be considered as a factor that affects cardiac output. However, if the RV fails, pulmonary vascular resistance is added in series to systemic vascular resistance. This effect is dramatically accentuated in the setting of right ventricular failure with elevated pulmonary vascular resistance. Thus, in various critical illnesses, consideration of the systemic and pulmonary vascular resistance is required.

Pulmonary Circulation

The exact mechanisms involved in intrinsic relaxation and constriction of the pulmonary vascular smooth muscle continue to be elucidated; the pulmonary vascular endothelium plays a critical role and derangements in endothelial function both precede and precipitate pulmonary arterial hypertension. Changes in pulmonary vascular resistance can occur at various levels within the circulation, and vasoactive substances and their properties may change during passage through the pulmonary vascular bed as a result of metabolism by the lung.

Morphologic Development

The stage of morphologic development of the pulmonary circulation affects vascular responses to various stimuli in the perinatal period. In the fetus and newborn, small pulmonary arteries have a thicker medial smooth muscle layer in relation to diameter than do similar arteries in adults. This increased muscularity is partly responsible for the increased vascular reactivity and pulmonary vascular resistance in the neonate immediately after birth.

Studies in human lungs identify the small pulmonary arteries by their relationship to the airways. Arteries follow the airways toward the alveoli. When these vessels are traced distally, a point is reached at which the medial smooth muscle coat no longer completely encircles the vessels; rather, it gives way to a region of incomplete muscularization. In these partially muscularized arteries, the smooth muscle is arranged in a spiral or helix. The nonmuscularized portions of these vessels contain precursor smooth muscle cells. Under certain conditions, such as hypoxia, these precursor cells may rapidly differentiate into mature smooth muscle cells. Moving distally, the muscle disappears altogether in arteries that are still larger than capillaries. In these arteries, an incomplete pericyte layer is found within the endothelial basement membrane.

In the near-term fetus, only approximately half the precapillary arteries (those associated with respiratory bronchioli) are muscularized or partially muscularized, and the vessels that are associated with alveoli are free of smooth muscle. In the first 4–6 weeks following birth, progressive involution of the circumferential medial smooth muscle occurs, with reduction in medial muscular thickness of the walls of the small pulmonary arteries. In adults, circumferential muscularization extends peripherally along the intra-acinar arteries so that most are completely muscularized, although with only a very thin layer of smooth muscle; this pattern is reached at about puberty. A number of neonatal pulmonary vascular disorders (e.g., congenital heart disease with increased pulmonary blood flow) are associated with a failure of the normal involution of medial smooth muscle and/or a precocious progression to the adult morphologic state, with a developmentally inappropriate extension of muscularized arteries toward the periphery.

During fetal growth, the number of small arteries increases greatly. In humans, the main preacinar pulmonary arterial branches that accompany the larger airways are developed by 16 weeks of gestation; however, the intra-acinar circulation follows alveolar development late in gestation and after birth, and arteries multiply as alveoli develop, a process that is generally complete by ~10 years of age (16).

Pulmonary Blood Flow in the Fetus

In the fetus, gas exchange occurs in the placenta and pulmonary blood flow is low, supplying nutritional requirements for lung growth and allowing the lung to serve a metabolic or paraendocrine function. Pulmonary blood flow in near-term fetal lambs represents ~8%–10% of combined ventricular output, as right ventricular blood is diverted away from the lungs through the widely patent ductus arteriosus to the descending thoracic aorta and the placenta for oxygenation (**Fig. 69.13**). Fetal pulmonary arterial mean blood pressure increases progressively with gestation and, at term, is ~50 mm Hg, exceeding mean aortic blood pressure by 1–2 mm Hg. Total pulmonary vascular resistance is extremely high relative to that in the infant or adult.

Regulation of Pulmonary Vascular Resistance in the Fetus

Pulmonary vascular resistance in the fetal lung is high and decreases slightly throughout the final third of gestation. Many factors, including mechanical effects, state of oxygenation, and the production of vasoactive substances, regulate the tone of the fetal pulmonary circulation. The most prominent factor associated with high fetal pulmonary vascular resistance is the low blood O_2 tension (pulmonary arterial blood Po_2, 17–20 torr). The exact mechanism and site of hypoxic pulmonary vasoconstriction in the fetal pulmonary circulation remain unclear. In addition to the low-oxygen environment, many substances, such as α-agonists, TXA_2, and leukotrienes, constrict the pulmonary circulation of the fetus. However, their role, if any, in maintaining the high fetal pulmonary vascular resistance does not appear prominent. In addition to the production of vasoconstrictors, the fetal pulmonary circulation produces vasodilating substances that modulate the degree of vasoconstriction under normal conditions and may play a more active role during periods of fetal stress. NO appears to be especially important. In fetal lambs, inhibiting NO synthesis produces marked increases in resting fetal pulmonary vascular resistance and inhibits the oxygen-induced decrease in pulmonary vascular resistance. In addition, studies of intrapulmonary arteries and isolated lung preparations of the sheep reveal maturational increases in NO-mediated relaxation during the late fetal and early postnatal period.

Regulation of Pulmonary Vascular Resistance during the Perinatal Transition

At birth, with initiation of pulmonary ventilation, pulmonary vascular resistance decreases rapidly and is associated with an 8- to 10-fold increase in pulmonary blood flow. By the first day of life, mean pulmonary arterial blood pressure is generally half systemic. After the initial abrupt decrease in pulmonary vascular resistance and pressure, a slow, progressive

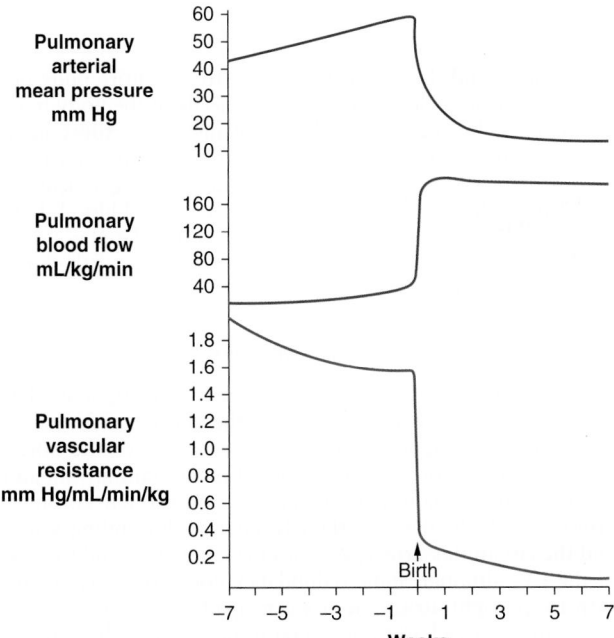

FIGURE 69.15. The changes in pulmonary arterial pressure, blood flow, and vascular resistance that occur around birth. (Data from Morin FC III, Egan E. Pulmonary hemodynamics in fetal lambs during development at normal and increased oxygen tension. *J Appl Physiol* 1992;73:213–8; Soifer SJ, FC Morin III, DC Kaslow, et al. The developmental effects of prostaglandin D2 on the pulmonary and systemic circulations in the newborn lamb. *J Dev Physiol* 1983;5:237–50.)

decrease follows, with adult levels reached after 2–6 weeks (**Fig. 69.15**).

The mechanisms that regulate the fall in pulmonary vascular resistance and increase in pulmonary blood flow after birth are in large part related to the increase in alveolar oxygen tension and the physical expansion of the lung. The role of oxygen is supported by increased pulmonary flow with hyperbaric oxygenation without ventilation. The role of physical expansion is supported by pulmonary vasodilation that occurs by inflating the lungs with a low-oxygen–containing gas mixture that does not change arterial blood gas composition. The exact mechanisms of oxygen-induced pulmonary vasodilation during the transitional circulation remain unclear. The increase in alveolar or arterial O_2 tension may decrease pulmonary vascular resistance, either directly via K^+ channel activation or indirectly by stimulating the production of vasodilator substances, such as PGI_2, bradykinin, adenosine, ATP, and NO. Lung inflation alone may lower pulmonary vascular resistance by either physical or chemical mechanisms. One mechanism operates through changes in alveolar surface tension. Another more important mechanism is the production and release of prostaglandins (predominantly PGI_2), which occurs either with mechanical stimulation of the lung or with rhythmic lung expansion (17).

NO has been implicated as an important mediator of the decrease in pulmonary vascular resistance at birth that is associated with increased oxygenation. For example, inhibition of NO synthesis attenuates the increase in pulmonary blood flow because of oxygenation of fetal lambs induced by either maternal hyperbaric oxygen exposure or in utero ventilation with oxygen. In utero ventilation without changing fetal blood gases increases endothelial NO synthase gene expression in lung parenchyma of fetal lambs; this is further increased by

ventilation with 100% oxygen. In vitro data reveal a maturational increase in NO production from late gestation to the early postnatal period that is modulated, in part, by oxygen. Moreover, both acute and chronic inhibition of NO synthesis prior to delivery significantly attenuate the normal increase in pulmonary blood flow at birth. These data suggest an important role for NO activity during the transitional circulation. However, the immediate decrease in pulmonary vascular resistance minutes after birth is not attenuated by NO inhibition. Therefore, the decrease in pulmonary vascular resistance is due to the initiation of ventilation and oxygenation. First, pulmonary vasodilation is caused by physical expansion of the lung and the production of prostaglandins (PGD_2 and PGI_2), which are probably independent of fetal oxygenation and result in a modest increase in pulmonary blood flow and decrease in pulmonary vascular resistance. Second, further maximal pulmonary vasodilation is associated with fetal oxygenation that is independent of prostaglandin production; it is most likely caused by the synthesis of NO, although the exact stimuli for NO production have not yet been defined. Both components are necessary for the successful transition to extrauterine life.

Regulation of Postnatal Pulmonary Vascular Resistance

16 The successful transition from the fetal to the postnatal pulmonary circulation is marked by the maintenance of the pulmonary vasculature in a dilated, low-resistance state. Evidence suggests that basal NO release and the subsequent increase in smooth muscle cell cGMP concentrations, in part, mediate the low resting pulmonary vascular resistance of the newborn (18). Other vasoactive substances, including histamine, 5-hydroxytryptamine, bradykinin, and metabolites of arachidonic acid by the cyclooxygenase and lipoxygenase pathways, have also been implicated in mediating postnatal pulmonary vascular tone. However, their roles are not well elucidated. Two of the most important factors affecting pulmonary vascular resistance in the postnatal period are oxygen concentration and pH. Decreasing oxygen tension and decreases in pH elicit pulmonary vasoconstriction. Alveolar hypoxia constricts pulmonary arterioles, diverting blood flow away from hypoxic lung segments, toward well-oxygenated segments, thus enhancing ventilation–perfusion matching. This response to hypoxia, unique to the pulmonary vasculature, is greater in the younger animal than in the adult. Indeed, in most vascular beds (e.g., cerebral vasculature), hypoxia is a potent vasodilator.

17 The exact mechanism of hypoxic pulmonary vasoconstriction remains incompletely understood but likely involves changes in the local concentration of reactive oxygen species that, in turn, regulate voltage-gated K^+ channels and Ca^{2+} channels (19). Acidosis potentiates hypoxic pulmonary vasoconstriction, whereas alkalosis reduces it (20). The exact **18** mechanism of pH-mediated pulmonary vascular reactivity also remains incompletely understood but appears to be independent of $Paco_2$. Data suggest that K^+ channels also play an important role in mediating these responses (21). Manipulating alveolar oxygen tension and systemic arterial pH are fundamental approaches to changing pulmonary vascular tone in the critical care setting. Alveolar hyperoxia and alkalosis are often used to decrease pulmonary vascular tone because they generally relieve pulmonary vasoconstriction with little effect on the systemic circulation as a whole. However, severe alkalosis is generally avoided due to the detrimental effects of severe hypocarbia or alkalosis on cerebral and myocardial blood flow (7).

Despite extensive innervation of the lung, neural input is not a major determinant of basal pulmonary vascular tone. However, given that pulmonary neurohumoral receptors are sensitive to α-adrenergic, β-adrenergic, and dopaminergic agonists, vasoactive agents that stimulate these receptors will affect the vascular tone of both the pulmonary and systemic circulations. As alterations in vascular tone in response to a given agent depend on the relative tone of the vascular bed at a given time, the response to these agents is difficult to predict in an individual critically ill patient.

Postnatal Pulmonary Blood Flow

Several other factors, unique to the lung, influence pulmonary blood flow in addition to pulmonary vascular tone. In a standing position, because of gravity, mean pulmonary vascular pressures increase from the apex to the base of the lung, but alveolar pressure is relatively constant throughout the lung. Therefore, the relationship between intravascular pressures and alveolar pressures is not uniform; rather, it is a function of the height within the lung. This relationship is further complicated by the variable effects of lung inflation on pulmonary vascular pressures, which depend on the spatial relationship between the alveoli and the vessels. Pulmonary vessels are termed extra-alveolar, corner, or intra-alveolar. Extra-alveolar and corner vessels increase their size with lung expansion because of radial traction placed on their walls by the lung parenchyma. However, intra-alveolar vessels are directly associated with alveoli and thus are subject to compression with alveolar expansion.

To characterize this relationship, West divided the lung into three theoretical zones that move down the lung from the apex to the base and are based on the relationship between pulmonary artery pressure (PAP), or inflow pressure, alveolar pressure (P_{av}), and pulmonary venous pressure (P_{ven}), or outflow pressure. In theory, no blood flows to zone I because P_{av} exceeds PAP, or $P_{av} > PAP > P_{ven}$. In this zone, intra-alveolar vessels would be collapsed. Clinically, zone I conditions probably do not exist in a healthy lung, as pulmonary blood flow does occur at the apex. The fact that extra-alveolar and corner vessels are patent in this zone may help to maintain blood flow. In zone II, PAP exceeds P_{av} and blood flow occurs independent of outflow pressures, or $PAP > P_{av} > P_{ven}$. In this zone, blood flow increases down the lung, as PAP, but not P_{av}, is influenced by gravity. In zone III, blood flow is dictated by the normal relationship of PAP to P_{ven}, or inflow pressure minus outflow pressure. In this zone, blood flow does not change dramatically down the lung as it does in zone II because gravity affects PAP and P_{ven} equally, or $PAP > P_{ven} > P_{av}$. Subsequently, an additional zone, zone IV, has been described in which pulmonary blood flow decreases at the extreme base of the lung. This decrease occurs due to the impact of the weight of the lung on the extra-alveolar and corner vessels, which causes compression that increases resistance to flow and the decrease in ventilation that occurs at the base, resulting in areas of relative hypoxia with resultant hypoxic pulmonary vasoconstriction.

Under normal conditions, pulmonary blood flow is largely determined by zone III conditions. However, with disease, less favorable conditions can predominate. Particularly pertinent to pediatric critical care are the effects of positive-pressure ventilation with high levels of peak end-expiratory pressure. Increased alveolar pressure may expand zone II and allow zone I conditions to be realized, resulting in mismatching of ventilation and perfusion and intrapulmonary shunting with hypoxia and hypercapnia. Likewise, pneumonia and pulmonary edema, along with other conditions, can increase zone IV conditions within the lung. Hypotension from multiple etiologies, such as hemorrhage, can expand zone I and II conditions. Finally, infants with small lungs and critically ill patients lying flat will have attenuated lung zones that exacerbate these pathologic conditions.

Coronary Circulation

Blood flow, and thus oxygen delivery, to the entire body depends on the cardiac pump. Increased needs of the body must be matched by increased delivery of metabolic substances, which often requires an increase in cardiac output and, thus, myocardial oxygen consumption. Myocardial oxygen demand is almost exclusively met by increased myocardial blood flow; in this way, coronary blood flow is, in fact, regulated not only by the needs of the heart but by the overall needs of the body at any given time.

Coronary Anatomy

Blood flow to the myocardium is supplied by the right and left coronary arteries, which arise from the sinuses of Valsalva, just behind the right and left coronary cusps of the aortic valve. The right coronary artery supplies the right atrium and ventricle, and usually part of the LV, and the left coronary artery, which divides into the left anterior descending artery and the circumflex artery, supplies the left atrium and the rest of the LV, although some redundancy does exist. Venous return to the right atrium occurs principally through the coronary sinus, with a lesser portion returning through the anterior coronary veins. In addition, arteriosinusoidal, arterioluminal, and thebesian vessels connect the coronary arterial system to the cardiac chambers, forming an extensive plexus of subendocardial vessels.

Regulation of Coronary Blood Flow

Coronary blood flow is regulated by physical forces that are related to the anatomic position of the coronary vessels within and around the dynamic myocardium, metabolic factors that couple coronary blood flow to oxygen demand, and neural factors. Because normally the perfusion, or inflow, pressure of the coronary circulation does not change dramatically, alterations in coronary blood flow are largely determined by alterations in vascular resistance, brought about by changes in luminal size.

Physical Factors That Regulate Coronary Blood Flow. Coronary perfusion pressure is directly related to aortic pressure. Blood flow within the coronary vasculature is dynamic as the vessels are exposed to the varying pressures generated within the cardiac cycle. At the end of diastole, when the ventricle is relaxed, pressures in the intramural coronary arteries are similar to each other and to aortic pressure. At the beginning of systole, subendocardial tissue pressure rises to equal intracavitary pressure but then falls off linearly across the wall to ~10 mm Hg in the outer subepicardium. These pressures are transmitted to the coronary vessels. Thus, intravascular pressures in the inner subendocardial arteries exceed aortic pressure but are lower than aortic pressure in the outer subepicardial arteries. In fact, during early left ventricular systole, flow is transiently reversed by extravascular compression of the subendocardial arteries that supply the LV. In early diastole, blood flows first into the subepicardial vessels that have not been compressed and then flows to the narrowed subendocardial vessels. Under normal conditions, subepicardial and subendocardial vessels are equally perfused during diastole. However, if diastole is excessively shortened, such as with severe tachycardia and/or if perfusion pressure is decreased, subendocardial ischemia can occur. On the other hand, flow within the coronary vessels that perfuse the right ventricular myocardium is normally maintained during systole and diastole because of the lower afterload induced by the pulmonary circulation that results in lower right ventricular intracavitary pressures (22). Perfusion of the hypertrophied RV of severe pulmonic stenosis or tetralogy of Fallot probably resembles that of the LV.

Myocardial Oxygen Demand–Supply Relationship.

The LV extracts an almost maximal amount of oxygen from the blood that passes through the myocardium, such that increases in myocardial oxygen demand must be met by increases in coronary blood flow. With maximal exertion, left ventricular oxygen consumption may increase fourfold, as does left coronary blood flow. Increased coronary perfusion pressures alone cannot increase flow to this extent, and thus the increased flow must be achieved by a decrease in coronary vascular resistance.

In fact, coronary blood flow is tightly coupled to the oxygen supply–to–oxygen demand ratio. Coronary blood flow increases when oxygen supply decreases and/or when oxygen demand increases. In this way, coronary blood flow is, in fact, linked to the overall oxygen needs of the body, as increases in cardiac output typically increase myocardial oxygen consumption. Likewise, when the body's metabolic needs decrease (e.g., during rest), myocardial oxygen consumption decreases, as does coronary blood flow. The mechanisms responsible for this coupling remain elusive. However, a number of substances known to influence vascular tone may participate, including adenosine, O_2, NO, H^+ ions, K^+, CO_2, and prostaglandins.

Coronary Reserve.

Under normal conditions, coronary blood flow is autoregulated such that if perfusion pressure is raised or lowered, there is a range over which almost no change in flow occurs; a rise in pressure evokes vasoconstriction, and a fall in pressure evokes vasodilatation (23). At perfusion pressures above some upper limit, flow increases, probably because the pressure overcomes the constriction. More importantly, at low perfusion pressures, flow decreases, indicating that the coronary vasculature is beginning to reach maximal vasodilatation and can no longer decrease resistance to compensate for the decreased perfusion pressure. A further decrease in perfusion pressure will cause ischemia.

Under normal conditions, when flow through the coronary circulation is autoregulated, maximal flow for any given inflow or perfusion pressure is limited by active vasoconstriction. The difference between this autoregulated flow and the maximal potential flow that would occur in the absence of any vasoconstriction (i.e., complete coronary dilation) is termed *coronary flow reserve* (24). Coronary flow reserve indicates the amount of extra flow that the myocardium can receive at a given pressure to meet increased demands for oxygen; insufficient reserve occurs when increases in myocardial oxygen demand cannot be matched with increased supply, which will result in ischemia. Coronary flow reserve is normally lower in the subendocardium than in the subepicardium such that decreases in coronary flow reserve are always more profound in the subendocardium than in the subepicardium.

Coronary reserve can be affected in a number of ways. For example, if autoregulation is normal but the maximal flow is decreased, then coronary flow reserve will be reduced. Such a change can occur with (a) marked tachycardia; (b) a decrease in the number of coronary vessels due to small-vessel disease, as in some collagen vascular diseases, especially systemic lupus erythematosus; (c) increased resistance to flow in one or more large coronary vessels because of embolism, thrombosis, atheroma, or spasm; (d) impaired myocardial relaxation due to ischemia; (e) myocardial edema; (f) a marked increase in left ventricular diastolic pressure; (g) marked increase in left ventricular systolic pressure if coronary perfusion pressure is not also increased, as in aortic stenosis or incompetence; and (h) an increase in blood viscosity, most commonly seen with hematocrits over 65%.

Coronary flow reserve can also be reduced if maximal flows are normal but autoregulated flows increase, which can occur with exercise, tachycardia, anemia, carbon monoxide poisoning, leftward shift of the hemoglobin–oxygen dissociation curve (as in infants with a high proportion of fetal hemoglobin), hypoxemia, thyrotoxicosis, acute ventricular dilatation (because of increased wall stress), inotropic stimulation by catecholamines, and acquired ventricular hypertrophy.

In addition, autoregulated flow and maximal flows may be reduced at the same time, such as with severe tachycardia or cyanotic heart disease with hypoxemia, ventricular hypertrophy, and polycythemia. Under these circumstances, coronary flow reserve can be drastically reduced. Furthermore, pericardial tamponade, a rise in right or left ventricular diastolic pressures, and α-adrenergic stimulation all raise the pressure at which autoregulation fails to compensate for decreased perfusing pressure.

Importantly, coronary reserve is also significantly reduced with ventricular hypertrophy. Myocardial wall stress is regulated within a fairly narrow range, with or without myocardial hypertrophy. Consequently, myocardial blood flow per unit mass is fairly constant. A close relationship exists between peak wall stress in systole and the ratio of left ventricular mass to volume (25,26). If hypertrophy does not occur, coronary flow reserve is normal, but it is reduced if the left ventricular mass is increased. If the heart dilates acutely, the mass-to-volume ratio decreases, wall stress and myocardial oxygen consumption increase, and coronary flow reserve falls. Decreasing ventricular dilatation by afterload and preload reduction reverses these unfavorable events and is another reason for the resulting improvement in ventricular function.

Right Ventricular Myocardial Blood Flow.

Right ventricular myocardial blood flow follows the general principles of coronary blood flow, but differences exist that are related to the low right ventricular systolic pressure and to the fact that alterations in aortic pressure change coronary perfusing pressure without altering right ventricular pressure work. For example, if the normal RV is acutely distended by pulmonary embolism, right ventricular failure will eventually occur; the increased wall stress increases oxygen consumption, but the raised systolic pressure reduces the coronary flow, so that when supply cannot match demand, right ventricular myocardial ischemia results. Raising aortic perfusing pressure mechanically or with a-adrenergic agonists or vasopressin increases right ventricular myocardial blood flow, relieves ischemia, and restores right ventricular function to normal. Improved coronary flow is not the only mechanism of this improvement; the increased left ventricular afterload moves the ventricular septum toward the RV and improves left ventricular performance (27). If right ventricular pressure is chronically elevated so that right ventricular hypertrophy occurs (as in pulmonic stenosis, many forms of cyanotic congenital heart disease, and some chronic lung diseases), right ventricular myocardial blood flow behaves in the same way as left ventricular blood flow, with one exception. If aortic pressure is lowered, left ventricular pressure also decreases, as does left ventricular work and oxygen consumption. However, in the RV, the workload may not be reduced (if no ventricular septal defect is present) so that an imbalance between myocardial oxygen supply and demand may occur. The worst imbalance occurs when aortic systolic pressure is maintained but coronary perfusing pressure decreases, and this can occur in a child with tetralogy of Fallot who has an aortopulmonary anastomosis (e.g., Blalock–Taussig shunt) that is too large. The high aortic and left ventricular systolic pressures mandate an equally high right ventricular systolic pressure, but the low diastolic aortic pressure reduces coronary perfusion pressure in diastole and can cause both left and right ventricular ischemia and failure.

Neural Factors. Coronary blood flow increases with sympathetic stimulation, but the mechanisms for this increase are not entirely straightforward. As sympathetic activation tends to increase myocardial oxygen consumption, in large part owing to increases in contractility and heart rate, coronary blood flow increases in order to increase oxygen supply, as described previously. However, experiments that isolate the effects of sympathetic stimulation on the coronary arteries from alterations in myocardial work indicate that, in fact, vasoconstriction is the predominant effect of sympathetic activation of the coronary arteries. Even though α-receptors and β-receptors are located on coronary vessels, these studies indicate that coronary blood flow is most strongly influenced by local metabolic processes that match oxygen supply and demand.

CONCLUSIONS AND FUTURE DIRECTIONS

An understanding of the various components and mechanisms that comprise the cardiovascular system is critical, but is only useful when placed in the total context of any given clinical scenario. Various pathophysiologic conditions, as well as therapies, result in alterations within the various components of the cardiovascular system that are synthesized into one clinical condition, albeit ephemeral. These conditions move the cardiovascular system away from its homeostatic baseline and evoke compensatory responses. For example, sepsis may cause vascular dilation, with a reduction in arterial blood pressure. This condition is detected by baroreceptors and chemoreceptors and through various central and local feedback loops that increase sympathetic discharge, heart rate, contractility, and vascular tone. Blood flow to the skin, muscle, and splanchnic circulations is reduced, and blood reserves from the splanchnic circulation and muscle are mobilized. Autoregulatory mechanisms are enacted to preserve blood flow through other vital organs, such as the brain and heart. Furthermore, renal mechanisms are set in motion to conserve salt and water in an effort to expand intravascular volume. These responses may transiently normalize the arterial pressure and may compensate for the initial insult. Of course, these mechanisms come at a physiologic cost and, with time, if the inciting stimulus remains, deleterious consequences may prevail. For example, with a prolonged reduction in flow, splanchnic ischemia may develop with subsequent translocation of enteric organisms into the bloodstream, myocardial oxygen demand may rise above supply with subsequent heart failure, and the renal compensatory mechanisms may result in renal failure. Thus, the clinician must consider the primary derangement, the compensatory responses, and the impact of therapy on all of these systems.

Furthermore, some clinical scenarios have the potential of placing portions of the cardiovascular system in conflict. For example, infants with tetralogy of Fallot who suffer severe right ventricular outflow tract obstruction with hypoxemia may be treated with α-agonists (e.g., phenylephrine) to increase systemic vascular resistance and pulmonary blood flow. This therapy increases left ventricular afterload and thus potentially decreases cardiac output. Whether oxygen delivery increases depends on an increase in arterial oxygen content sufficient to overcome the decrease in cardiac output. This situation requires a thorough understanding of the overarching physiology, the goals of therapy, and the effects of therapy on the various regional vascular beds.

A progressive expansion in our understanding of the cardiovascular system has led to an increasing ability to support patients with various ailments. This support comes in many forms, including mechanical support and pharmacologic agents that alter cardiac performance and vascular function. The massive literature on cardiovascular physiology belies the fact that many fundamental processes, such as the central role of the vascular endothelium in vascular biology, were only recently uncovered. Thus, it is probable that ongoing and future investigations will result in novel therapies that will allow more specific targeting of the various components within the cardiovascular system, maximizing therapeutic intentions while minimizing the unintended consequences.

References

1. Re Davis MJ, Ferrer PN, Gore RW. Vascular anatomy and hydrostatic pressure profile in the hamster cheek pouch. *Am J Physiol* 1986;250:H291–303.
2. Roos A. Poiseuille's law and its limitations in vascular systems. *Med Thorac* 1962;19:224–38.
3. Damiano RJ, La Follette P, Cox JL, et al. Significant left ventricular contribution to right ventricular systolic function. *Am J Physiol* 1991;261(5 Pt 2):H1514–24.
4. Johnson PC. Autoregulation of blood flow. *Circ Res* 1986;59:483–95.
5. Ebert TJ, Stowe DF. Neural and endothelial control of the peripheral circulation—Implications for anesthesia: Part I. Neural control of the peripheral vasculature. *J Cardiothorac Vasc Anesth* 1996;10:147–58.
6. Dinh-Xuan AT. Endothelial modulation of pulmonary vascular tone. *Eur Respir J* 1992;5:757–62.
7. Moncada S, Higgs A. The L-arginine-nitric oxide pathway. *N Engl J Med* 1993;329:2002–12.
8. Palmer RM, Ashton DS, Moncada S. Vascular endothelial cells synthesize nitric oxide from L-arginine. *Nature* 1988;333:664–6.
9. Yanagisawa M, Kurihara H, Kimura S, et al. A novel potent vasoconstrictor peptide produced by vascular endothelial cells. *Nature* 1988;332:411–5.
10. Faraci FM, Heistad DD. Regulation of the cerebral circulation: Role of endothelium and potassium channels. *Physiol Rev* 1998;78:53–97.
11. Shyy JY, Chien S. Role of integrins in endothelial mechanosensing of shear stress. *Circ Res* 2002;91:769–75.
12. Johnson PC. The myogenic response. In: Bohr DF, Somlyo AP, Sparks HV, eds. *Handbook of Physiology. The Cardiovascular System.* Bethesda, MD: American Physiologic Society, 1980.
13. Davis MJ, Hill MA. Signaling mechanisms underlying the vascular myogenic response. *Physiol Rev* 1999;79:387–423.
14. Murphy TV, Spurrell BE, Hill MA. Cellular signalling in arteriolar myogenic constriction: Involvement of tyrosine phosphorylation pathways. *Clin Exp Pharmacol Physiol* 2002;29:612–9.
15. Teitel DF, Iwamoto HS, Rudolph AM. Effects of birth-related events on central blood flow patterns. *Pediatr Res* 1987;22:557–66.
16. Reid LM. The pulmonary circulation: Remodeling in growth and disease. The 1978 J. Burns Amberson lecture. *Am Rev Respir Dis* 1979;119:531–46.
17. Leffler CW, Hessler JR, Green RS. The onset of breathing at birth stimulates pulmonary vascular prostacyclin synthesis. *Pediatr Res* 1984;18:938–42.
18. Rudolph AM, Yuan S. Response of the pulmonary vasculature to hypoxia and H$^+$ ion concentration changes. *J Clin Invest* 1966;45:399–411.
19. Moudgil R, Michelakis ED, Archer SL. Hypoxic pulmonary vasoconstriction. *J Appl Physiol* 2005;98:390–403.

20. Schreiber MD, Heymann MA, Soifer SJ. Increased arterial pH, not decreased $PaCO_2$, attenuates hypoxia-induced pulmonary vasoconstriction in newborn lambs. *Pediatr Res* 1986;20:113–7.

21. Cornfield DN, Resnik ER, Herron JM, et al. Pulmonary vascular K^+ channel expression and vasoreactivity in a model of congenital heart disease. *Am J Physiol Lung Cell Mol Physiol* 2002;283:L1210–9.

22. Berne RM, Levy MN. *Coronary Circulation, Cardiovascular Physiology.* Toronto, Canada: Mosby, 1986.

23. Hoffman JI. Transmural myocardial perfusion. *Prog Cardiovasc Dis* 1987;29:429–64.

24. Hoffman JI. Problems of coronary flow reserve. *Ann Biomed Eng* 2000;28:884–96.

25. Strauer BE. Significance of coronary circulation in hypertensive heart disease for development and prevention of heart failure. *Am J Cardiol* 1990;65:34G–41G.

26. Vogt M, Motz W, Strauer BE. Coronary haemodynamics in hypertensive heart disease. *Eur Heart J* 1992;13(suppl D):44–9.

27. Belenkie I, Horne SG, Dani R, et al. Effects of aortic constriction during experimental acute right ventricular pressure loading. Further insights into diastolic and systolic ventricular interaction. *Circulation* 1995;92:546–54.

CHAPTER 70 ■ CARDIORESPIRATORY INTERACTIONS IN CHILDREN WITH HEART DISEASE

RONALD A. BRONICKI AND LARA S. SHEKERDEMIAN

KEY POINTS

1 Ventilation is an important determinant of systemic cardiac output.

2 In healthy individuals, spontaneous breathing and positive pressure ventilation (PPV) primarily affect the right heart.

3 Ventilation has important effects on left ventricular afterload. A positive intrathoracic pressure can reduce afterload, and a negative intrathoracic pressure can increase it.

4 PPV may be beneficial for children with systolic heart failure, and it can be delivered by the noninvasive route.

5 Some unique cardiorespiratory interactions are present in children with congenital heart disease.

6 In children after right heart surgery, spontaneous respiration can have beneficial effects on cardiac output and systemic oxygen delivery.

INTRODUCTION AND HISTORICAL PERSPECTIVE

The term cardiorespiratory interaction describes the physiologic relationship between spontaneous or positive pressure ventilation (PPV) and the cardiovascular system. These interactions can be exaggerated or abnormal in certain disease states. The complex interactions that are present in congenital heart disease have formed the basis of extensive research, and ventilation is now routinely used as a hemodynamic tool in many circumstances. This chapter will include a brief overview of the evolution of our understanding of cardiopulmonary physiology and a discussion of the interactions between ventilation and the cardiovascular system, with particular reference to critically ill infants and children with congenital and acquired heart disease.

The Foundation of Our Current Knowledge

The ancient Greeks called the air that we breathe the "breath of life." Galen believed that the lungs served to provide the blood with heat from the inhaled air, which was then carried to the heart. He also described the functions of venous and arterial blood. The venous blood was responsible for nutrition, and arterial blood delivered vitality from the heart to the body's organs. The Galenic circulation did not recognize the pump function of the heart and the pulsatile nature of the arteries, or the passive pressure gradient for venous return, and therefore was based upon blood being "expended" at its destination and not returning to the heart. Thus, the heart constantly produced blood. In the early 1600s, William Harvey wrote that the "energy" from the right and left ventricles (LVs) drove blood in a pulsatile manner to the lungs and the body, and that the lungs enabled inspired air to be drawn into the blood that returns to the left heart (1). While this was correct, Harvey's theory of circulatory physiology did not connect the arteries to the veins. The "missing link" in the chain of the circulation was completed by Malpighi in the 1660s when he identified capillaries in the lungs and other organs.

With a better understanding of the cardiopulmonary circulation, scientists became interested in exploring the relationships between flow and pressure in blood vessels during respiration. In 1733, Reverend Stephen Hales, a veterinarian, observed the pulsatility of arterial blood through brass pipes that he inserted directly in the arteries of a live horse (2). Hales was the first to observe and measure blood pressure, and to show that this fell during inspiration and increased during expiration in healthy animals. In 1871, Kussmaul showed that the radial pulse was absent during inspiration but returned during expiration in patients with constrictive pericarditis due to tuberculosis (3). *Pulsus paradoxus*, which is in fact an exaggeration of normal physiology, was the first "pathologic" cardiopulmonary interaction to be described.

The Invasive Study of Cardiorespiratory Interactions: The Work of Cournand

A chapter on cardiopulmonary interactions, and our understanding of these, would be incomplete without discussion of the work of Cournand, Richards, and Forssmann who in the 1940s and 1950s conducted several hundred studies of cardiorespiratory physiology in healthy adults and in adults with cardiac failure, during spontaneous respiration and noninvasive ventilation. These studies were among the earliest to utilize cardiac catheterization and included measurements of intrathoracic (pleural) pressure, as well as intravascular pressures, stroke volume, and cardiac output. These comprehensive investigations provided important new insights into the

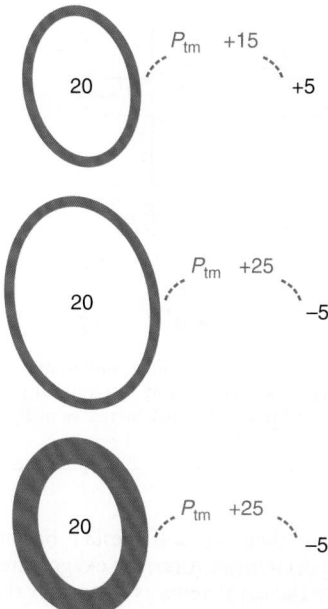

FIGURE 70.1. The pressure–volume relationships for a distensible/collapsible chamber. The degree to which a chamber undergoes deformation depends on its compliance and the magnitude and direction of the pressure exerted across its wall or its transmural pressure (P_{tm}). The pressure within each chamber is constant at 20. For the top chamber, the surrounding pressure of 5 produces a distending P_{tm} of +15. The middle chamber, with identical compliance to the top chamber (same thickness), distends to a greater extent because it is surrounded by a negative pressure of 5, resulting in a transmural pressure of +25. The bottom chamber is less compliant than the top two chambers. Even though its transmural pressure is identical to the middle chamber, its volume is less.

---

interrelationship between pleural pressure and cardiovascular performance, and provided explanations for many of the changes in hemodynamics that are observed during ventilation.

Pressure–Volume and Pressure–Flow Relationships

The study of the interactions between cardiovascular and pulmonary systems requires an understanding of pressure–volume and pressure–flow relationships applied to elastic structures, such as blood vessels, cardiac chambers, and alveoli. The fundamental property of an elastic structure is its ability to offer resistance to a distending or collapsing force and to return to its resting volume after the force has been removed. The extent to which a structure undergoes a change in volume depends on its compliance and the magnitude and direction of the pressure exerted across the wall—the transmural pressure (**Fig. 70.1**). The transmural pressure (P_{tm}) is equal to the difference between intra- and extracavitary pressures, where a positive transmural pressure distends the cavity and a negative transmural pressure causes the cavity to reduce in size.

$$P_{tm} = P_{intracavitary} - P_{extracavitary}$$

where P_{tm} is the transmural pressure, $P_{intracavitary}$ the intracavitary pressure, and $P_{extracavitary}$ the extracavitary pressure.

The physical principles that govern the flow of fluids (or air) through nonrigid conducting passages, such as vessels and airways, are derived from the general laws of hydrodynamics. **Figure 70.2** shows that the flow (Q) through a collapsible tube depends on the following:

- the "driving pressure" or "perfusion pressure," which is the inflow pressure (P_i) minus the outflow pressure (P_o);
- the pressure surrounding the tube (P_s);
- the transmural pressure ($= P_i - P_s$);
- the compliance of the structure (which is the change in intravascular volume per unit change in pressure).

When the tube has a positive transmural pressure throughout, the tube is widely patent and Q is proportional to the pressure gradient $P_i - P_o$. These conditions for the flow of fluid are also known as "zone III conditions." With a constant P_i, P_o, and compliance, as P_s increases, the transmural pressure decreases. As a result, the volume inside the tube decreases. Resistance to flow increases and flow is now proportional to the pressure gradient $P_i - P_s$. These conditions for the flow of fluid are also known as "zone II conditions." As P_s increases further, the transmural pressure becomes negative, the tube collapses, and resistance to flow increases further, producing "zone I conditions." The pressure at which P_i equals P_s is called the *critical closing pressure*. These different "zone" conditions may be created by changes not only in P_s but also as a result in changes in P_i, P_o, and compliance. The physiologic significance of these concepts is that changes in P_s are analogous to changes in intrathoracic, intra-abdominal, and intravascular pressures with corresponding effects on systemic and pulmonary blood flow, resistance, and intravascular volume. While these concepts apply to both veins and arteries, there are special features of venous versus arterial flow, which are described below.

INTRATHORACIC PRESSURE AND RIGHT VENTRICULAR PRELOAD

Systemic venous return to the right heart is driven by a pressure gradient between the systemic venous circulation and the right heart and opposed by resistance to systemic venous return (R_{VR}) or:

$$\text{Venous Return} = (P_{MS} - P_{RA})/R_{VR}$$

where P_{MS} is the mean systemic pressure and P_{RA} the right atrial pressure.

The mean systemic pressure (P_{MS}) defined as the circulatory pressure if the heart were arrested (i.e., zero cardiac output) represents the inflow pressure (P_i) for venous return. P_{MS} is a function of blood volume and capacitance of the systemic circulation (4). The systemic venous circulation is eighteen times more compliant than the systemic arterial circulation and therefore has much greater capacitance and holds the majority of intravascular volume (primarily within the splanchnic, splenic, and hepatic venous reservoirs) (5,6). The venous capacitance vessels, and not the arterial resistance vessels, are the principle determinant of P_{MS}. The volume and pressure within the systemic arterial circulation has little impact on the mean systemic pressure (7).

Right atrial pressure (P_{RA}) represents the outflow pressure (P_o) for venous return. An increase in P_{RA} causes systemic venous return and right ventricular output to decrease, unless there is a compensatory increase in P_{MS}. Vasoconstriction of venous capacitance vessels, primarily mediated by adrenergic activation, angiotensin, and vasopressin, may increase P_{MS} by reducing venous compliance and thereby mobilizing blood from the venous reservoirs to the central circulation (8–12).

Conversely, if venoconstriction increases the resistance to venous return *without* displacing venous blood volume from the periphery into the central circulation, the net effect will be to reduce venous return. Thus, the net effect of venoconstriction from sympatho-adrenergic discharge on venous return depends on whether it is accompanied by blood volume displacement into the central circulation (increasing P_{MS}) or not (increasing R_{VR}).

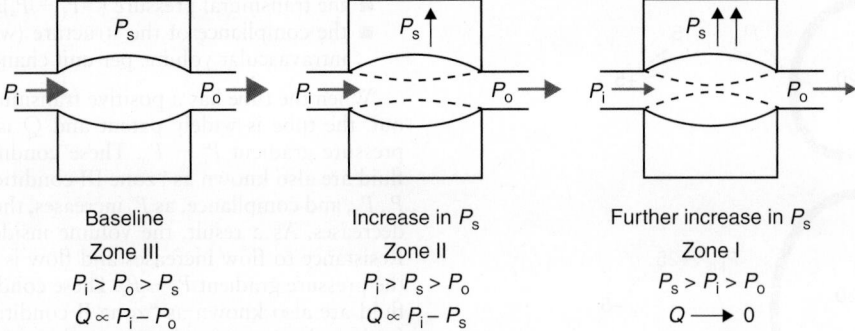

FIGURE 70.2. The pressure–flow relationships for a distensible/collapsible chamber. P_i, P_o, and P_s represent inlet, outlet, and surrounding pressure, respectively. With low P_s, the flow of fluid through the tube is governed by the difference between P_i and P_o (zone III conditions). If P_s is increased and rises above P_o, flow is governed by the difference between P_i and P_s (zone II conditions). Further increases in P_s to levels that rise above P_i result in cessation of flow.

Over time an increase in P_{MS} caused by increased central blood volume is complemented by the antidiuretic effects of vasopressin and by stimulation of the renin–angiotensin–aldosterone system (13,14). As P_{MS} decreases, venous return invariably decreases. Pharmacologic agents such as furosemide, nitric oxide donors, and angiotensin-converting enzyme inhibitors as well as pathologic conditions such as sepsis vasodilate venous capacitance vessels and cause a fall in venous return. (15–18). The fall in venous return leads to an equivalent fall in right ventricular output because the right heart can only eject the blood volume presented to it through systemic venous return.

Spontaneous Inspiration and Right Ventricular Preload

② In his landmark physiological investigations, Cournand demonstrated that the negative intrathoracic pressure (ITP) generated during spontaneous inspiration produced an increase in systemic venous return and hence right ventricular stroke volume and cardiac output (19). During spontaneous inspiration, the pleural pressure becomes negative and hence the transmural pressure of the right atrium increases.

Right atrial transmural pressure = Right atrial intracavitary pressure − Pleural pressure

The reduction in pleural pressure increases right atrial compliance, causing right atrial pressure to fall and thereby increasing the pressure gradient for venous return. Also, during inspiration, the descent of the diaphragm increases intra-abdominal pressure, decreasing the transmural pressure of the largest of venous reservoirs (20,21). Zone III conditions prevail in the abdomen if the abdominal transmural pressure remains positive (though reduced during inspiration). Hence, spontaneous inspiration in the euvolemic patient will displace abdominal blood volume into the central circulation and thereby contribute to venous return from the inferior vena cava. Alternatively, if diaphragmatic descent results in zero or negative abdominal transmural pressure (zone I and II conditions), the inferior vena cava becomes compressed and resistance to venous return is increased. Hence, a hypovolemic patient with decreased abdominal compliance will experience decreased venous return during inspiration. This is in contrast to venous return from the head and neck vessels, which are exposed to atmospheric pressure.

The increase in venous return as pleural pressure falls must not be limitless, otherwise during deep breathing the right heart would become overdistended. Guyton demonstrated that as right atrial pressure decreases venous return increases

and then plateaus (**Fig. 70.3**). If the ITP becomes excessively negative during deep inspiration, the exaggerated negative ITP is transmitted to the caval veins as they enter the thoracic cavity. When the transmural pressure for the caval veins becomes negative at the thoracic inlets, the veins collapse limiting venous return (i.e., zone I and II conditions are created) (22). Further decreases in right atrial pressure have no effect on venous return because flow is now a function of the difference between mean systemic pressure and atmospheric pressure or abdominal pressure. When the outflow or downstream pressure is elevated, as in heart failure, the transmural pressure of the vena cava remains positive and venous return is limited by the outflow pressure (i.e., zone III conditions are created).

Positive Pressure Ventilation and Right Ventricular Preload

Cournand demonstrated that during PPV, there was a fall in systemic venous return and hence right ventricular stroke volume and cardiac output, which was proportionate to increases in the mean airway pressure.

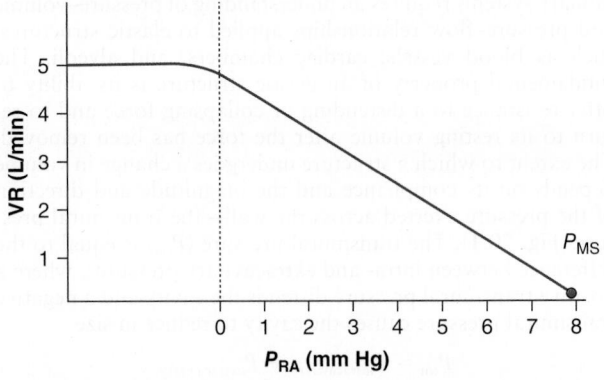

FIGURE 70.3. The relationship between right atrial pressure, mean systemic pressure, and venous return. Venous return (VR) increases as right atrial pressure (P_{RA}) decreases and then plateaus as P_{RA} falls below zero. The negative intrathoracic pressure is transmitted to the vena cava just outside the chest. As the transmural pressures for the vena cava become negative, they collapse at the thoracic inlet, creating zone I and II conditions, which limit or suspend venous return. Further decreases in P_{RA} have no effect on venous return because flow is now a function of the difference between the mean systemic pressure (P_{MS}) and atmospheric pressure or abdominal pressure.

As ITP becomes increasingly positive, right atrial pressure increases and the pressure gradient for venous return decreases, therefore reducing systemic venous return. It may seem counterintuitive that an increase in right atrial pressure causes venous return to decrease because the right atrial pressure is considered a surrogate for right ventricular volume. However, it is changes in the right atrial transmural pressure and the determinants of the pressure gradient for venous return that determine venous return (23). Further, it is the right ventricular diastolic transmural pressure, not the right ventricular diastolic pressure, and ventricular compliance that determine right ventricular stroke volume (see **Fig. 70.1**). A noncompliant ventricle, or one surrounded by elevated ITP, requires a higher-than-normal intracavitary pressure to maintain an adequate end-diastolic volume, which in turn is needed to maintain adequate right ventricular stroke volume.

The extent to which an increase in ITP affects venous return depends in large part on the degree to which airway pressure is transmitted to the cardiac fossa, a function of respiratory mechanics, and on the adequacy of compensatory circulatory reflexes. Given the intricate relationship between right ventricular preload and cardiac output, it would follow that intravascular volume administration should restore cardiac output in the presence of high ITP when the intrinsic circulatory response does not suffice. This strategy, however, may not maintain cardiac output, due to changes in right ventricular afterload.

INTRATHORACIC PRESSURE AND RIGHT VENTRICULAR AFTERLOAD

If venous return were the only determinant of cardiac output during PPV, one would expect that, in the presence of normal myocardial function, volume expansion would preserve cardiac output under conditions of increasing ITP without limit. This is not necessarily the case. In a landmark study in healthy dogs that were ventilated with an end-expiratory pressure of 20 cm H_2O, Henning observed that right ventricular stroke volume could not be normalized with volume administration despite complete restoration of right ventricular preload (24). The mechanism underlying this observation was that high ITP and lung volumes directly influenced pulmonary vascular resistance and right ventricular afterload and, hence, right ventricular output.

As lung volume is increased from residual volume to functional residual capacity, the radial traction provided by the pulmonary interstitium increases the diameter of the extra-alveolar vessels. In addition, alveolar recruitment improves gas exchange and thus reverses hypoxic pulmonary vasoconstriction, further decreasing the resistance of extra-alveolar vessels. Despite a concomitant increase in the resistance of alveolar vessels, resulting from an increase in alveolar transmural pressure, the net effect is reduction of right ventricular afterload as lung volume approaches functional residual capacity. As lung volumes increase above functional residual capacity, the caliber of alveolar vessels decreases as alveolar transmural pressure continues to increase. Ultimately, alveolar pressure becomes greater than pulmonary venous pressure, creating zone II conditions and further increases in the resistance to blood flow (see **Fig. 70.2**). As lung volumes increase further, zone I conditions are created, as alveolar pressure rises above pulmonary arterial pressure, resulting in collapse of alveolar vessels and the cessation of blood flow to these areas. The net effect as lung volumes approach total lung capacity is an increase in pulmonary vascular resistance.

In the absence of cardiopulmonary disease, zone I conditions do not exist in the lung; however, they may be present in a variety of clinical scenarios. In addition to increases in alveolar pressure, zone I conditions may be created when pulmonary arterial pressures are low. In either case, zone I conditions are initially created in non-gravity–dependent regions of lung. Conversely, increases in alveolar pressure may not create zone I conditions if pulmonary venous pressures are elevated, as in left-sided heart failure. When pulmonary arterial and venous pressures exceed alveolar pressure, as in congestive heart failure or in the more gravity-dependent regions of the lung, zone III conditions predominate and flow is proportional to the pressure gradient between pulmonary arterial and pulmonary venous pressures. In zone III regions, alveolar distension leads to the propulsion of pulmonary blood flow and pulmonary venous return (25).

It is important to appreciate that it is not changes in alveolar pressure per se but rather changes in the alveolar distending pressure (i.e., alveolar transmural or transpulmonary pressure), lung compliance, and the resulting changes in lung volume during ventilation that affect pulmonary vascular resistance.

Alveolar (airway) Distending (transmural) Pressure = Alveolar (airway) Pressure − Pleural Pressure

Changes in the inflow and outflow pressures of the pulmonary circulation (i.e., pulmonary arterial and venous pressures, respectively) also determine the extent to which changes in lung volume alter pulmonary blood flow.

INTRATHORACIC PRESSURE AND LEFT VENTRICULAR PRELOAD

As discussed previously, spontaneous inspiration increases systemic venous return and right ventricular diastolic volume and pressure. As the right ventricle fills, the interventricular septum, which normally bows into the right ventricle because left ventricular pressures exceed those in the right ventricle, occupies a more neutral position between the two ventricles during diastole (**Fig. 70.4**). This effectively decreases left ventricular compliance and cavitary volume resulting in reduced stroke volume during inspiration (26,27). The mechanism by which the filling of one ventricle affects the filling of the other is diastolic ventricular interdependence, and contributes to pulsus paradoxus, the fall in systemic arterial pressure that occurs during spontaneous inspiration (28). Over the next few cardiac cycles, the increase in systemic venous return leads to an increase in left ventricular filling and output.

PPV may also limit left ventricular filling as a result of its effects on the right heart. Whether PPV predominantly affects

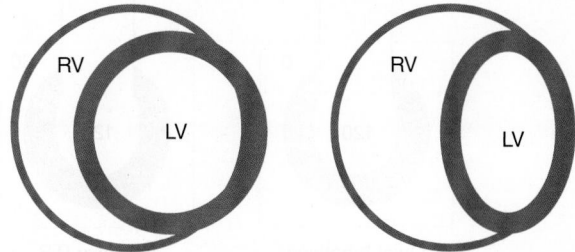

FIGURE 70.4. Ventricular interdependence. Cross-sectional view of ventricles from below. Under normal conditions (*figure on left*) the ventricular septum is oriented such that the left ventricle (*LV*) in its short axis is circular and the right ventricle (*RV*) is crescentic. Under conditions when the pressure in the RV is elevated (*figure on right*), the septum is displaced to the left, which decreases the effective compliance of the LV.

right ventricular preload or afterload depends on several factors including:

- the degree to which ITP is transmitted to the cardiac fossa (thereby reducing the pressure gradient for venous return);
- the intravascular volume and the function of venous capacitance vessels;
- the underlying right ventricular function;
- the effect of PPV on lung volumes and right ventricular afterload (lung recruitment vs. overdistension) (29,30).

If right ventricular afterload is elevated without a commensurate increase in systemic venous return and right ventricular filling, the ability of the right ventricle to generate pressure and overcome the increase in afterload (afterload reserve) is limited and right ventricular output falls. Further, right ventricular diastolic pressure is elevated and, as a result of ventricular diastolic interdependence, the effective compliance of the LV is reduced. In this instance, the LV is restrained not only by the deviated septum and right ventricular pressure but also its free wall is constrained by the pericardium and distended alveoli. Thus, left ventricular preload is reduced as a result of a decrease in right ventricular output and diastolic ventricular interaction. Further, as left ventricular operating volumes decrease, the pressure-generating capabilities of the LV are diminished. This adversely affects right ventricular output, as left ventricular contraction contributes substantially to right ventricular pressure generation as a result of systolic ventricular interdependence (31–33).

INTRATHORACIC PRESSURE AND THE LEFT VENTRICULAR AFTERLOAD

In healthy individuals, spontaneous and PPV primarily influences the right heart. However, ventilation also exerts subtle but important effects on left ventricular afterload that can have increased significance in certain pathologic states.

Changes in the transmural pressure of the intrathoracic arterial system alter the driving pressure for propelling blood from the LV and thoracic arterial circulation to the peripheral arterial circulation. While the right atrium and caval veins are much more compliant than the arterial vessels, it is the compliance and transmural pressure of the thoracic arterial vessels that determine the extent to which changes in ITP affect left ventricular afterload.

Spontaneous Ventilation and Left Ventricular Afterload

Left ventricular afterload is primarily determined by its systolic transmural pressure (aortic systolic pressure minus pleural pressure). Thus, an increase in afterload may result from an increase in aortic blood pressure or from a fall in pleural pressure (**Fig. 70.5**).

$$LV_{Afterload} \propto LV_{tm} = LV_{intracavitary} - P_{pl}$$

where LV stands for left ventricular, tm the transmural pressure, intracavitary the intracavitary pressure, and P_{pl} the pleural pressure.

During spontaneous respiration, the intrathoracic arterial pressure decreases as the transmural pressure and therefore volume of the intrathoracic arterial vessels increase (34). While intrathoracic arterial pressure decreases, pleural pressure falls to a greater extent, resulting in a net increase in the left ventricular systolic transmural pressure and hence an increase in left ventricular afterload.

With the generation of a negative ITP timed to ventricular diastole, the resulting increase in volume of the intrathoracic arterial vessels causes a decrease in the amount of anterograde flow runoff and an increase in intrathoracic arterial blood volume for the subsequent left ventricular ejection (35). With the generation of a negative ITP timed to ventricular systole, the egress of blood from the thorax as well as left ventricular ejection decreases, contributing to the fall in aortic systolic pressure. This represents the systolic component of pulsus paradoxus (35).

In health, the impact of spontaneous breathing on the left heart is minimal. However, the impact of changes in pleural pressure on the LV becomes much more significant in the presence of excessively negative pleural pressures, for example in severe airway obstruction, and particularly in patients with underlying left ventricular systolic dysfunction.

Positive Pressure Ventilation and Left Ventricular Afterload

During PPV, the decrease in transmural pressure of the intrathoracic arterial vessels decreases their effective compliance. As a result, their volumes decrease and their pressures increase relative to extrathoracic arterial vessels, creating a waterfall-like effect and driving blood into the extrathoracic circulation (34,35). An increase in ITP, therefore, unloads the

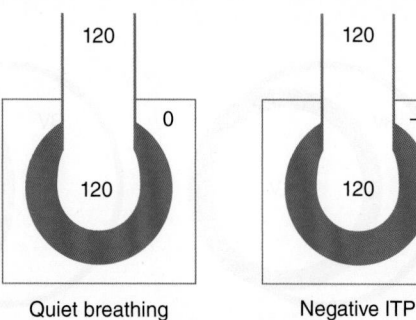
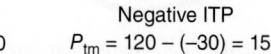
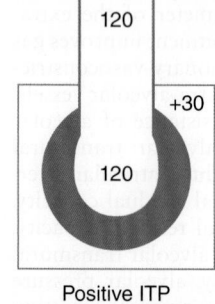
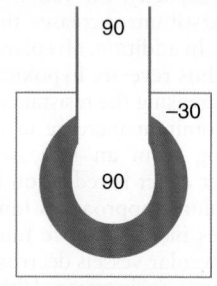

Quiet breathing	Negative ITP	Positive ITP	Vasodilator
$P_{tm} = 120 - 0 = 120$	$P_{tm} = 120 - (-30) = 150$	$P_{tm} = 120 - 30 = 90$	$P_{tm} = 90 - (-30) = 120$

FIGURE 70.5. The relationships between changes in intrathoracic pressure and aortic pressure on left ventricular afterload. During periods of quiet breathing in which intrathoracic pressure (ITP) is 0, the left ventricular (LV) transmural pressure (P_{tm}) is equal to the LV systolic pressure (120) (left-hand panel). When ITP is negative, the transmural pressure is increased (P_{tm} is now 150) and wall stress within the ventricle is elevated. The opposite occurs when ITP is positive (P_{tm} then becomes 90). The increase in transmural pressure imparted by a negative ITP can be reversed by vasodilator treatment, which restores transmural pressure to baseline levels (right-hand panel).

LV while increasing aortic pressure, so called "reverse pulsus paradoxus" (35,36).

Variation in Systolic Pressure and Pulse Pressure during the Respiratory Cycle

As discussed, changes in ITP affect venous return as well as induce changes in arterial blood pressure. The effect of changes in ITP during the respiratory cycle can be measured both as systolic pressure variation and as pulse pressure variation (37,38). Examination of the pressure variations that occur during PPV has been shown to predict fluid responsiveness. During the respiratory cycle of mechanical ventilation, the systolic arterial pressure and the pulse pressure increase during inspiration due to the effect of the increase in ITP on the thoracic arterial vessels. The greater the differences in systolic pressure values (or pulse pressure values) over a respiratory cycle the more likely the patient is to be responsive to volume administration. Increasing pulse pressure variation during a respiratory cycle correlated with volume responsiveness in septic patients receiving mechanical ventilation (39). In that study the variation in pulse pressure was a more reliable indicator of volume responsiveness than the variation in systolic pressure.

CARDIORESPIRATORY INTERACTIONS IN CHILDREN WITH HEART DISEASE

Ventilation is a valuable, though underutilized, hemodynamic tool in pediatric intensive care. When used carefully and tailored according to a clinical situation, ventilation is often far more effective in improving circulatory physiology than pharmacologic agents. Cardiopulmonary interactions should be considered in all patients in the intensive care unit, whether receiving mechanical ventilation or not, and in the presence or absence of structural or acquired heart disease. A number of common pediatric critical care scenarios in which ventilation can be used in this way are discussed below and are summarized in Table 70.1.

CARDIORESPIRATORY INTERACTIONS IN CHILDREN WITH SYSTOLIC HEART FAILURE

Cardiopulmonary interactions play a major role in the symptomatology, hemodynamic manifestations, and management of systolic heart failure in the intensive care unit. The term "systolic heart failure" covers a broad clinical spectrum of etiologies that includes transient ventricular dysfunction following repair of congenital heart disease; severe, acute decompensated heart failure secondary to myocarditis, sepsis, arrhythmia, or ischemia; and decompensated chronic heart failure, secondary to dilated cardiomyopathy or congenital heart disease with systemic ventricular failure.

Cardiorespiratory Interactions during Spontaneous Respiration

Children with systolic heart failure are very sensitive to the interactions between spontaneous breathing and the heart for several reasons. Even at rest, their work of breathing is increased due to pulmonary venous hypertension and an increase in extravascular lung water. This leads to a decrease in lung compliance and exaggerated negative pressure breathing,

TABLE 70.1

CARDIORESPIRATORY INTERACTIONS IN CHILDREN WITH HEART DISEASE DURING SPONTANEOUS AND POSITIVE PRESSURE VENTILATION

	■ KEY ISSUES	■ SPONTANEOUS RESPIRATION		■ POSITIVE PRESSURE VENTILATION/CPAP	
Heart failure (acute or chronic)	Elevated LV afterload Systolic LV dysfunction	Increased work of breathing Exaggerated negative intrapleural pressure swings	Increased LV afterload	Reduced work of breathing Obliterated negative swings in pleural pressure	Reduced venous return Reduced LV afterload Improved LV function
Postoperative— tetralogy of Fallot	Good systolic function Diastolic RV dysfunction Preload dependent	Increased RV preload Improved diastolic pulmonary artery flow	Improved cardiac output	Reduced RV preload Reduced diastolic pulmonary artery flow	Reduced cardiac output
Postoperative— Fontan/BCPS	Good systolic function Preload dependent Cardiac output depends on pulmonary blood flow	Increased preload Negative intrathoracic pressure improves pulmonary blood flow	Improved cardiac output	Reduced preload Reduced pulmonary blood flow	Reduced cardiac output
Duct-dependent systemic flow	Excessive pulmonary flow, leading to reduced systemic flow	Tachypnea and oversaturation are common Limited control of pulmonary flow	Possible excessive pulmonary flow and reduced systemic cardiac output	Better control of pulmonary flow, pH, and pulmonary resistance	Improved systemic cardiac output

CPAP, continuous positive airway pressure; BCPS, bidirectional cavopulmonary shunt; LV, left ventricle; RV, right ventricle.

which increases respiratory muscle oxygen consumption and therefore circulatory demand. As ITP becomes increasingly negative, left ventricular afterload and ventricular wall stress increase, further increasing myocardial oxygen demand. These interactions become even more pronounced with exertion, stress, or agitation—circumstances in which the work of breathing and vascular tone are elevated.

Positive Pressure Ventilation in Systolic Heart Failure

④ PPV may produce important beneficial hemodynamic effects in children with acute or chronic systolic heart failure through a number of mechanisms. PPV reduces right ventricular preload through its effects on the right heart and also reduces left ventricular afterload by eliminating exaggerated negative pressure breathing and decreasing the LV systolic transmural pressure. **⑥** As a result, myocardial oxygen demand is reduced. While systemic venous return may decrease with PPV in the heart failure patient, left ventricular stroke volume and cardiac output increase as a result of decreased left ventricular afterload. In addition, through its direct effects on the work of breathing, mechanical ventilation unloads the respiratory pump, decreasing respiratory muscle oxygen demand, allowing for a redistribution of a limited cardiac output to other vital organs.

Under normal conditions, the respiratory musculature is responsible for less than 3% of global oxygen consumption and receives less than 5% of cardiac output (40). However, with an increase in respiratory load, the oxygen demand of the respiratory pump may increase to values over 50% of the total oxygen consumption. In addition, oxygen extraction for the respiratory muscles under normal conditions is high (40). Thus, to meet these increased demands, perfusion of the respiratory musculature must increase, otherwise respiratory pump failure ensues (41). Viires and colleagues showed in an animal model of shock that respiratory muscle blood flow of spontaneously breathing dogs increased to 21% of total cardiac output, compared with only 3% in those receiving mechanical ventilation (42). As a result, vital organ perfusion, including the brain, was significantly greater in the mechanically ventilated group.

Several studies in patients with heart failure have demonstrated a beneficial impact of PPV on cardiac function (43–45). Rasanen and colleagues demonstrated that progressing from full ventilatory support to spontaneous breathing adversely affected myocardial oxygen transport balance and function in 5 of 12 patients with acute myocardial infarction complicated by respiratory failure (43). This subset of patients developed myocardial ischemia and a rise in left ventricular filling pressure immediately following extubation.

Approximately one third of adult patients receiving mechanical ventilation for respiratory failure accompanied by underlying ventricular dysfunction are unable to wean from mechanical ventilation due to a worsening of left ventricular function and respiratory muscle oxygen transport balance (46). With mechanical ventilation, substantial quantities of oxygen are released for other vital organs; meanwhile, respiratory muscle and myocardial oxygen demand are decreased significantly.

Positive Pressure Ventilation in Children with Post-cardiotomy Systolic Ventricular Dysfunction

Cardiac surgery inevitably results in a degree of myocardial injury due to intraoperative factors, including cardiopulmonary bypass-induced inflammation, myocardial reperfusion injury, and cardiotomy, which often lead to a degree of early postoperative systolic ventricular dysfunction. Most infants and children require PPV early after surgery, which in addition to providing respiratory support serves as an intrinsic part of their postoperative hemodynamic support through its effects on ventricular loading and work of breathing. Clinical scenarios where PPV may be particularly beneficial include infants early after reimplantation of an anomalous left coronary artery arising from the pulmonary artery in whom the preoperative myocardium was relatively deprived of oxygen delivery, and children following a late arterial switch operation in whom left ventricular deconditioning leads to early postoperative systolic ventricular dysfunction.

Positive Pressure Ventilation in the Nonsurgical Patient with Systolic Ventricular Dysfunction

Noninvasive positive pressure respiratory support, including ventilatory support with bilevel positive airway pressure (BiPAP) and continuous positive airway pressure (CPAP), is now a mainstay of therapy in hospitalized adults with acute cardiogenic pulmonary edema secondary to decompensated heart failure. In these patients, noninvasive respiratory support with CPAP or BiPAP has been shown to provide symptomatic improvement, a reduced need for endotracheal intubation, and lower early mortality (47,48). It has been recently demonstrated that the prolonged use of noninvasive ventilation leads to ventricular remodeling and improved ventricular diastolic and systolic function in adults with chronic heart failure (49). Long-term CPAP and BiPAP have also been shown to be effective in improving biventricular diastolic and systolic function in adults with obstructed sleep-disordered breathing associated with cardiac dysfunction (50–52).

CARDIORESPIRATORY INTERACTIONS IN CHILDREN WITH DIASTOLIC VENTRICULAR DYSFUNCTION

Diastolic ventricular dysfunction is relatively common in children with heart disease, in whom cardiac output may be compromised due to inadequate ventricular filling. So long as systemic ventricular systolic function is intact, the impact of changes in ITP on systemic venous return and ventricular filling predominates over the effects on ventricular afterload. Diastolic dysfunction can occur in the presence of primary myocardial disease, as well as in patients with congenital heart disease.

Diastolic Dysfunction in Children with Cardiomyopathy

Patients with restrictive cardiomyopathies typically have adequate if not normal systolic function, but as a result of diastolic disease are very sensitive to interventions that may decrease systemic venous return and right ventricular preload such as venodilators and PPV (53). The same is true of patients with hypertrophic cardiomyopathy who may not tolerate interventions that decrease systemic venous return. The interactions between PPV and the LV can also prove detrimental in these patients. By decreasing left ventricular preload and afterload, PPV may, if the substrate for an obstruction to left ventricular outflow is present, create or exacerbate this by reducing left ventricular operating volumes, resulting in reduced stroke volume and cardiac output (54,55). Based on the effects of respiration on left ventricular loading conditions, an emphasis should be placed on maintaining adequate ventricular preload and avoiding excessive PEEP in patients with diastolic dysfunction receiving PPV.

CARDIORESPIRATORY INTERACTIONS IN CHILDREN WITH CONGENITAL HEART DISEASE

In the field of pediatric intensive care, some unique cardiorespiratory interactions exist in children with congenital heart disease, which are of great importance to clinicians managing these patients during the perioperative period. The manipulation of these interactions impacts the clinical course of these patients, particularly early after surgery, either to their benefit or to their detriment. Discussed below are four specific patient groups for whom the application of mechanical ventilation has a well-described role in manipulating circulatory function.

Cardiorespiratory Interactions in a Functionally Univentricular Circulation

Young infants with a functionally univentricular circulation represent a large group with a spectrum of complex diagnoses. These include some with biventricular anatomy but functionally univentricular physiology as in critical aortic stenosis, interrupted aortic arch or truncus arteriosus; as well as those with single ventricle anatomy such as hypoplastic right or left heart. The unifying feature of the circulatory physiology of infants with these lesions is that the perfusion of the pulmonary and systemic circulations is from the output of a single or functionally single ventricle. Thus, the distribution of ventricular output to the systemic, and thus coronary, and pulmonary circulations depends on the relative resistances of the two circulations. The key to limiting morbidity and maximizing intact survival of infants with functionally univentricular circulations lies in maintaining a balanced ratio of pulmonary to systemic blood flow with adequate systemic oxygen delivery through attention to ventricular loading conditions and vascular resistances of the systemic and pulmonary vascular beds.

While the approach of utilizing ventilation to elevate pulmonary vascular resistance in order to limit pulmonary blood flow is now outdated, it is important for clinicians to avoid exacerbating pulmonary overcirculation through nonjudicious ventilatory maneuvers that result in respiratory alkalosis and pulmonary vasodilation such as hyperventilation and the excessive administration of supplemental oxygen. In patients with a functionally univentricular circulation, PPV should be used to optimize ventricular loading conditions and improving myocardial and global oxygen transport balance, as already described. Ventilation should be manipulated to provide a normal arterial pH (avoiding both acidosis and alkalosis) remembering that alveolar hypoxia and acidemia increase pulmonary vascular resistance while alkalosis and supplemental oxygen reduce it.

Cardiorespiratory Interactions after the Fontan Operation

The Fontan physiology presents intensivists with a unique set of challenges largely related to optimization of pulmonary blood flow and hence cardiac output, in a circulation that lacks a sub-pulmonary ventricle. As in the normal circulation, systemic venous return is dependent upon the maintenance of an adequate mean systemic venous pressure (56). In the Fontan circulation, however, the mean systemic pressure is also responsible for driving systemic venous return across the pulmonary circulation, rendering it much more susceptible to changes in pulmonary vascular resistance, and to ventricular dysfunction.

A low cardiac output state may complicate the early postoperative course following the Fontan procedure. When this occurs, it is much more likely to be due to diastolic dysfunction, as systolic function in typically preserved. As a result, the Fontan circulation is particularly sensitive to factors that affect systemic venous return and ventricular filling. Changes in ITP through its effects on systemic venous return, the ventricular diastolic transmural pressure, and pulmonary vascular resistance significantly impact cardiac output following the Fontan procedure. The function of the venous capacitance vessels and the maintenance of an adequate mean systemic pressure are integral to maintaining pulmonary blood flow in the Fontan circulation. This phenomenon is exemplified in the hemodynamic consequence of hemidiaphragmatic paralysis following the Fontan procedure. It has been demonstrated in Fontan patients with a plicated diaphragm that important inspiration-derived hepatic venous flow is suppressed, and portal venous flow loses its normal expiratory augmentation, both of which compromise venous return from the abdominal venous reservoirs (57,58). Further demonstrating the importance of the venous capacitance vessels in the Fontan circulation, studies have demonstrated neurohormonal activation causing decreased systemic venous compliance and increased intravascular volume, as well as over time elevated venous microvascular filtration pressures and filtration thresholds (59–61).

In the first reports in the literature of the atriopulmonary connection in three adults with tricuspid atresia, Fontan observed a clinical improvement after extubation and wrote that PPV should be "stopped early because positive pressure prevents central venous return" (62). Several years later, Laks wrote that extubation following the Fontan operation resulted in a fall in right atrial pressure, which was "in general accompanied by some improvement in clinical condition" (63).

In patients following the Fontan procedure, seemingly minor changes in ITP exert significant influences on pulmonary blood flow and hence cardiac output. The physiological manifestations of how these changes in ITP affect pulmonary blood flow have been extensively studied in spontaneously breathing patients after the Fontan operation. Redington and Penny observed that pulmonary blood flow increased by nearly two thirds during inspiration, as the pleural pressure becomes negative (**Fig. 70.6**) (64,65). Flow was reversed, implying a brief complete cessation of pulmonary blood flow when these patients performed a Valsalva maneuver (**Fig. 70.7**).

Following these observations, the question subsequently arose as to whether negative pressure ventilation might augment pulmonary blood flow and hence cardiac output by mimicking spontaneous respiration, and in doing so function as an adjunctive tool in the management of patients with low cardiac output. We performed a series of studies to explore this cardiopulmonary interaction further in children who were mechanically ventilated early after the Fontan operation. A brief period of cuirass negative pressure ventilation increased their pulmonary blood flow by 42% when compared with PPV (**Fig. 70.8**) (66,67). The actual utility of negative pressure ventilation as a hemodynamic tool is less relevant than the clear demonstration of the hemodynamic impact of ventilation in patients following the Fontan procedure. These studies highlight well the importance of minimizing airway pressures and establishing full spontaneous respiration as early as possible.

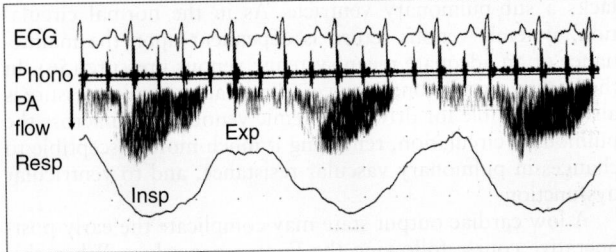

FIGURE 70.6. Pulsed-wave Doppler profile of pulmonary arterial flow in a spontaneously breathing Fontan patient. Pulmonary blood flow (*arrow*) bears no relationship to ventricular systole. Flow increases during spontaneous inspiration and is minimal during expiration. ECG, electrocardiogram; Phono, Phonocardiogram; PA, pulmonary artery; Resp, Respirometer trace; Insp, spontaneous inspiration; Exp, spontaneous expiration.

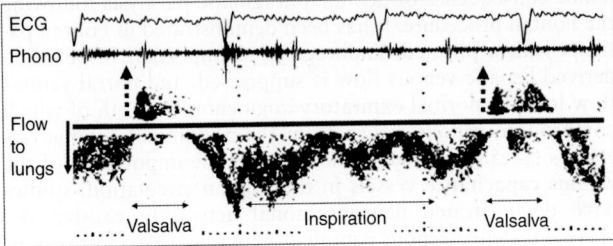

FIGURE 70.7. Pulsed-wave Doppler profile of pulmonary arterial flow during two brief Valsalva maneuvers in a Fontan patient. Blood flows toward the lungs during spontaneous inspiration (*solid arrow*). Flow is reversed (*dotted arrow*) during two brief Valsalva maneuvers. Thus, blood flows away from the lungs and cardiac output is lost during a sudden, substantial increase in intrathoracic pressure. ECG, electrocardiogram; Phono, Phonocardiogram.

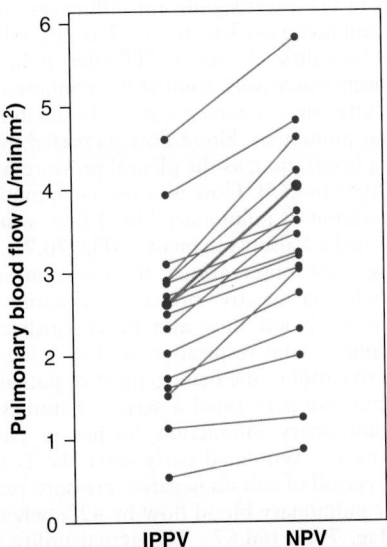

FIGURE 70.8. Pulmonary blood flow during intermittent positive pressure ventilation (IPPV) and after 15 minutes of cuirass negative pressure ventilation (NPV) in Fontan patients. Mean pulmonary blood flow increased from 2.4 to 3.5 L/min/m² after 15 minutes of NPV ($p < 0.001$).

Cardiorespiratory Interactions after the Bidirectional Cavopulmonary Shunt

The cardiopulmonary physiology following the bidirectional cavopulmonary shunt (or Glenn operation) resembles that of the Fontan circulation, in that the contribution of the subpulmonary ventricle to total pulmonary blood flow is at most limited if there is anterograde flow, and is often absent. In these patients, most, if not all, of pulmonary flow is derived directly from the upper body venous drainage, and is largely driven by the upper body peripheral venous pressure. Overall pulmonary flow is exquisitely sensitive to changes in cerebral vascular resistance, ITP, and pulmonary artery pressure.

The most common challenge following the bidirectional cavopulmonary shunt procedure is hypoxia due to inadequate pulmonary blood flow, and in turn this may be associated with reduced systemic oxygen delivery. Optimal ventilation early after a bidirectional cavopulmonary shunt is ideally aimed at providing a very careful balance between cerebral vasodilation and pulmonary arterial flow, which are impacted in directly conflicting ways by arterial acid–base balance and carbon dioxide tensions. There is little doubt, however, that routine postoperative ventilation after the bidirectional cavopulmonary shunt should be directed at early initiation of spontaneous respiration, and extubation as soon as it is feasible. In the event that pulmonary blood flow and oxygenation are inadequate, control of minute ventilation may be indicated to allow for a mild elevation of arterial carbon dioxide tension, which uncouples cerebral blood flow from cerebral blood metabolism by decreasing cerebral vascular resistance and increasing cerebral blood flow. The increase in superior caval return to the pulmonary artery directly results in increased pulmonary blood flow. Although in general, acidosis increases pulmonary vascular resistance, in these patients it appears that the effects of hypercapnia and mild respiratory acidosis on the cerebral vasculature outweigh those on the pulmonary vasculature (68).

Cardiorespiratory Interactions Following the Repair of Tetralogy of Fallot

Most infants have a relatively uncomplicated postoperative course following repair of tetralogy of Fallot. However, right ventricular diastolic dysfunction is common in these patients, and in a minority this may lead to a low cardiac output in the early postoperative period. Patients with a reduced cardiac output secondary to diastolic dysfunction typically have elevated right heart filling pressures, with a tendency to retain fluid and develop pleural effusions. Ventilation can significantly impact their hemodynamics and clinical course.

In 1995, Cullen demonstrated the echocardiographic features of diastolic right ventricular dysfunction in these patients. He demonstrated restrictive right ventricular physiology, which was characterized by diastolic anterograde flow in the pulmonary artery coincident with atrial systole. Although abnormal, this anterograde pulmonary arterial diastolic flow contributes to cardiac output by increasing forward pulmonary flow, and also by limiting the time available during the cardiac cycle for pulmonary regurgitation. Importantly, this flow was increased during spontaneous respiration (69).

Left ventricular systolic function is typically intact in patients following repair of tetralogy of Fallot; thus, changes in ITP impact primarily the right heart (69). Based upon the observations made by Cullen and colleagues, we hypothesized that negative pressure ventilation, by mimicking spontaneous respiration, would augment pulmonary blood flow and

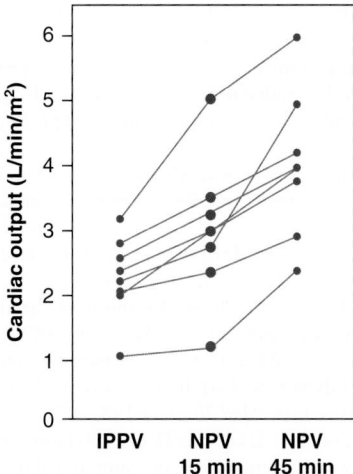

FIGURE 70.9. Cardiac output during intermittent positive pressure ventilation (IPPV), and during negative pressure ventilation (NPV) in children after tetralogy of Fallot repair. Cardiac output increased by 21% after 15 minutes of NPV and by a further 38% between 15 and 45 minutes. The total increase was 67% ($p < 0.0001$).

cardiac output in ventilated patients early after repair of tetralogy of Fallot. In a series of studies with a similar design to those discussed in Fontan patients, we showed that cuirass negative pressure ventilation increased cardiac output by 67% in children early after repair of tetralogy of Fallot (**Fig. 70.9**) (67,70). Echocardiographic studies confirmed that a significant contribution to this increase in cardiac output was the augmentation of anterograde pulmonary arterial diastolic flow as ITP became negative during inspiration (69).

A logical question that follows given the cardiopulmonary interactions in patients with diastolic dysfunction is whether or not global and regional oxygen transport balance improves when the respiratory pump is loaded during weaning from mechanical ventilation. We demonstrated that converting from PPV to spontaneous respiration resulted in improved global hemodynamics and cerebral oxygen delivery despite the potential confounder of increased metabolic demand with complete loading of the respiratory pump (71). In a subsequent study, we found that although extubation led to a significant increase in cardiac output and cerebral oxygenation, the metabolic cost of loading the respiratory musculature came at the expense of mesenteric perfusion, as mesenteric oxygenation fell significantly immediately following extubation (72). The implications of these findings remain to be determined but do underscore the importance of considering the metabolic cost of spontaneous breathing when cardiac output is limited.

Similar to patients following the Fontan procedure, ventilatory management of children with restrictive right ventricular physiology after repair of tetralogy of Fallot should be considered integral to their routine hemodynamic management. Indeed, many centers now utilize an approach to management that incorporates early postoperative extubation after uncomplicated tetralogy repair beyond the neonatal period. While on occasion therapeutic negative pressure ventilation has been used with success in children in a low–cardiac output state secondary to restrictive physiology, the key message of these investigations is that ventilation should always be tailored to the physiology of children with tetralogy of Fallot. Thus, efforts should be directed at minimizing airway pressures during PPV and establishing spontaneous respiration as early as feasible (73).

Cardiopulmonary Interactions during Cardiopulmonary Resuscitation

Effective cardiopulmonary resuscitation depends on adequate venous return to the chest after each compression cycle. Indeed, in patients with congenital heart disease who are highly dependent upon a low ITP for maintenance of pulmonary blood flow and systemic perfusion, adequate cardiac output during cardiopulmonary resuscitation can be difficult to achieve. The advent of mechanical devices that enhance venous return during cardiopulmonary resuscitation has been a topic of great interest in resuscitation science for the last several years (74). One such device is the inspiratory impedance threshold valve. During the decompression phase of cardiopulmonary resuscitation, a negative ITP is created as the chest wall recoils back to its resting position, thus enhancing the pressure gradient for systemic venous return. The impedance threshold valve prevents the inflow of ventilatory gases during the decompression phase, generating a more negative ITP with significant enhancement of cardiac output. Studies in animals have demonstrated a significant increase in stroke volume and cardiac output, including a significant increase in myocardial and cerebral perfusion, with the use of this device (75).

CONCLUSIONS AND FUTURE DIRECTIONS

Critically ill children with heart disease can present unique challenges to intensivists as we routinely consider in tandem their circulatory responses to ventilation, and vice versa. One cannot overstate how important it is for intensivists caring for cardiac patients to have an appreciation of the interactions between ventilation and the circulation, and that therapy must be tailored to the patient. Moreover, while there is a temptation to assume that "common things are common"—if there is any doubt as to the optimal way to manage ventilation in a critically ill child with heart disease—additional investigative modalities, particularly echocardiography, should be sought to assist in the assessment.

The primary goal in the intensive care of patients with heart disease is to ensure adequate systemic oxygen delivery. The manipulation of ventilation has a very clear role in this, and, in many cases, ventilation is far more effective in optimizing systemic hemodynamic than pharmacotherapy.

References

1. Harvey W. *Anatomical studies on the motion of the heart and blood in animals.* Springfield, IL: Charles C. Thomas, 1978.
2. Lewis O. Stephen hales and the measurement of blood pressure. *J Hum Hypertens* 1994;8:865–71.
3. Bilchick KC, Wise RA. Paradoxical physical findings described by kussmaul: Pulsus paradoxus and kussmaul's sign. *Lancet* 2002;359:1940–2.
4. Rothe CF. Mean circulatory filling pressure: Its meaning and measurement. *J Appl Physiol* 1993;74:499–509.
5. Karim F, Hainsworth R. Responses of abdominal vascular capacitance to stimulation of splanchnic nerves. *Am J Physiol* 1976;231:434–40.
6. Payen DM, Brun-Buisson CJ, Carli PA, et al. Hemodynamic, gas exchange, and hormonal consequences of lbpp during peep ventilation. *J Appl Physiol* 1987;62:61–70.
7. Gelman S. Venous function and central venous pressure: A physiologic story. *Anesthesiology* 2008;108:735–48.
8. Guyton AC, Richardson TQ. Effect of hematocrit on venous return. *Circ Res* 1961;9:157–64.

9. Greene AS, Shoukas AA. Changes in canine cardiac function and venous return curves by the carotid baroreflex. *Am J Physiol* 1986;251:H288–H296.

10. Guyton AC, Lindsey AW, Abernathy B, et al. Mechanism of the increased venous return and cardiac output caused by epinephrine. *Am J Physiol* 1958;192:126–30.

11. Hatanaka T, Potts JT, Shoukas AA. Invariance of the resistance to venous return to carotid sinus baroreflex control. *Am J Physiol* 1996;271:H1022–H1030.

12. Drees JA, Rothe CF. Reflex venoconstriction and capacity vessel pressure-volume relationships in dogs. *Circ Res* 1974;34:360–73.

13. Bark H, Le Roith D, Nyska M, et al. Elevations in plasma adh levels during peep ventilation in the dog: Mechanisms involved. *Am J Physiol* 1980;239:E474–E481.

14. Scharf SM, Ingram RH Jr. Influence of abdominal pressure and sympathetic vasoconstriction on the cardiovascular response to positive end-expiratory pressure. *Am Rev Respir Dis* 1977;116:661–70.

15. Jhund PS, Davie AP, McMurray JJ. Aspirin inhibits the acute venodilator response to furosemide in patients with chronic heart failure. *J Am Coll Cardiol* 2001;37:1234–8.

16. Chien S, Dellenback RJ, Usami S, et al. Blood volume and its distribution in endotoxin shock. *Am J Physiol* 1966;210:1411–8.

17. Rothe CF, Murray RH, Bennett TD. Actively circulating blood volume in endotoxin shock measured by indicator dilution. *Am J Physiol* 1979;236:H291–H300.

18. Tabrizchi R, Pang CC. Effects of drugs on body venous tone, as reflected by mean circulatory filling pressure. *Cardiovasc Res* 1992;26:443–8.

19. Lauson HD, Bloomfield RA, Cournand A. The influence of the respiration on the circulation in man; with special reference to pressures in the right auricle, right ventricle, femoral artery and peripheral veins. *Am J Med* 1946;1:315–36.

20. Takata M, Wise RA, Robotham JL. Effects of abdominal pressure on venous return: Abdominal vascular zone conditions. *J Appl Physiol* 1990;69:1961–72.

21. Lloyd TC Jr. Effect of inspiration on inferior vena caval blood flow in dogs. *J Appl Physiol* 1983;55:1701–8.

22. Guyton AC, Adkins LH. Quantitative aspects of the collapse factor in relation to venous return. *Am J Physiol* 1954;177:523–7.

23. Pinsky MR. Determinants of pulmonary arterial flow variation during respiration. *J Appl Physiol* 1984;56:1237–45.

24. Henning RJ. Effects of positive end-expiratory pressure on the right ventricle. *J Appl Physiol* 1986;61:819–26.

25. Jardin F, Farcot JC, Gueret P, et al. Cyclic changes in arterial pulse pressure during respiratory support. *Circulation*. 1983;68:266–74.

26. Santamore WP, Heckman JL, Bove AA. Right and left ventricular pressure-volume response to respiratory maneuvers. *J Appl Physiol* 1984;57:1520–7.

27. Belenkie I, Sas R, Mitchell J, et al. Opening the pericardium during pulmonary artery constriction improves cardiac function. *J Appl Physiol* 2004;96:917–22.

28. Peters J, Kindred MK, Robotham JL. Transient analysis of cardiopulmonary interactions. Part I. Diastolic events. *J Appl Physiol* 1988;64:1506–17.

29. Vieillard-Baron A, Loubieres Y, Schmitt JM, et al. Cyclic changes in right ventricular output impedance during mechanical ventilation. *J Appl Physiol* 1999;87:1644–50.

30. Jardin F, Vieillard-Baron A. Right ventricular function and positive pressure ventilation in clinical practice: From hemodynamic subsets to respirator settings. *Intensive Care Med* 2003;29:1426–34.

31. Santamore WP, Gray L Jr. Significant left ventricular contributions to right ventricular systolic function. Mechanism and clinical implications. *Chest* 1995;107:1134–45.

32. Woodard JC, Chow E, Farrar DJ. Isolated ventricular systolic interaction during transient reductions in left ventricular pressure. *Circ Res* 1992;70:944–51.

33. Feneley MP, Gavaghan TP, Baron DW, et al. Contribution of left ventricular contraction to the generation of right ventricular systolic pressure in the human heart. *Circulation* 1985;71:473–80.

34. Robotham JL, Rabson J, Permutt S, et al. Left ventricular hemodynamics during respiration. *J Appl Physiol* 1979;47:1295–303.

35. Peters J, Kindred MK, Robotham JL. Transient analysis of cardiopulmonary interactions. Part II. Systolic events. *J Appl Physiol* 1988;64:1518–26.

36. Massumi RA, Mason DT, Vera Z, et al. Reversed pulsus paradoxus. *N Engl J Med* 1973;289:1272–5.

37. Magder S. Clinical usefulness of respiratory variations in arterial pressure. *Am J Respir Crit Care Med* 2004;169:151–5.

38. Feihl F, Broccard AF. Interactions between respiration and systemic hemodynamics. Part II: Practical implications in critical care. *Intensive Care Med* 2009;35:198–205.

39. Michard F, Boussat S, Chemla D, et al. Relation between respiratory changes in arterial pulse pressure and fluid responsiveness in septic patients with acute circulatory failure. *Am J Respir Crit Care Med* 2000;162:134–8.

40. Rochester DF, Briscoe AM. Metabolism of the working diaphragm. *Am Rev Respir Dis* 1979;119:101–6.

41. Roussos C, Macklem PT. The respiratory muscles. *N Engl J Med* 1982;307:786–97.

42. Viires N, Sillye G, Aubier M, et al. Regional blood flow distribution in dog during induced hypotension and low cardiac output. Spontaneous breathing versus artificial ventilation. *J Clin Invest* 1983;72:935–47.

43. Rasanen J, Nikki P, Heikkila J. Acute myocardial infarction complicated by respiratory failure. The effects of mechanical ventilation. *Chest* 1984;85:21–8.

44. Lemaire F, Teboul JL, Cinotti L, et al. Acute left ventricular dysfunction during unsuccessful weaning from mechanical ventilation. *Anesthesiology* 1988;69:171–9.

45. Scharf SM, Bianco JA, Tow DE, et al. The effects of large negative intrathoracic pressure on left ventricular function in patients with coronary artery disease. *Circulation* 1981;63:871–5.

46. Epstein SK. Etiology of extubation failure and the predictive value of the rapid shallow breathing index. *Am J Respir Crit Care Med* 1995;152:545–9.

47. Masip J, Roque M, Sanchez B, et al. Noninvasive ventilation in acute cardiogenic pulmonary edema: Systematic review and meta-analysis. *JAMA* 2005;294:3124–30.

48. Winck JC, Azevedo LF, Costa-Pereira A, et al. Efficacy and safety of non-invasive ventilation in the treatment of acute cardiogenic pulmonary edema—a systematic review and meta-analysis. *Crit Care* 2006;10:R69.

49. Haruki N, Takeuchi M, Kaku K, et al. Comparison of acute and chronic impact of adaptive servo-ventilation on left chamber geometry and function in patients with chronic heart failure. *Eur J Heart Fail* 2011;13:1140–6.

50. Shivalkar B, Van de Heyning C, Kerremans M, et al. Obstructive sleep apnea syndrome: More insights on structural and functional cardiac alterations, and the effects of treatment with continuous positive airway pressure. *J Am Coll Cardiol* 2006;47:1433–9.

51. Arias MA, Garcia-Rio F, Alonso-Fernandez A, et al. Obstructive sleep apnea syndrome affects left ventricular diastolic function: Effects of nasal continuous positive airway pressure in men. *Circulation* 2005;112:375–83.

52. Kaneko Y, Floras JS, Usui K, et al. Cardiovascular effects of continuous positive airway pressure in patients with heart failure and obstructive sleep apnea. *N Engl J Med* 2003;348:1233–41.

53. Bengur AR, Beekman RH, Rocchini AP, et al. Acute hemodynamic effects of captopril in children with a congestive or restrictive cardiomyopathy. *Circulation* 1991;83:523–7.

54. Braunwald E, Oldham HN Jr, Ross J Jr, et al. The circulatory response of patients with idiopathic hypertrophic subaortic stenosis to nitroglycerin and to the valsalva maneuver. *Circulation* 1964;29:422–31.

55. Buda AJ, MacKenzie GW, Wigle ED. Effect of negative intrathoracic pressure on left ventricular outflow tract obstruction in muscular subaortic stenosis. *Circulation* 1981;63:875–81.

56. Mace L, Dervanian P, Bourriez A, et al. Changes in venous return parameters associated with univentricular fontan circulations. *Am J Physiol Heart Circ Physiol* 2000;279:H2335–43.

57. Hsia TY, Khambadkone S, Redington AN, et al. Effects of respiration and gravity on infradiaphragmatic venous flow in normal and fontan patients. *Circulation* 2000;102:III148–III153.

58. Hsia TY, Khambadkone S, Bradley SM, et al. Subdiaphragmatic venous hemodynamics in patients with biventricular and fontan circulation after diaphragm plication. *J Thorac Cardiovasc Surg* 2007;134:1397–405; discussion 1405.

59. Krishnan US, Taneja I, Gewitz M, et al. Peripheral vascular adaptation and orthostatic tolerance in fontan physiology. *Circulation* 2009;120:1775–83.

60. Myers CD, Ballman K, Riegle LE, et al. Mechanisms of systemic adaptation to univentricular fontan conversion. *J Thorac Cardiovasc Surg* 2010;140:850–6, 856. e851–6.

61. Kelley JR, Mack GW, Fahey JT. Diminished venous vascular capacitance in patients with univentricular hearts after the fontan operation. *Am J Cardiol* 1995;76:158–63.

62. Fontan F, Baudet E. Surgical repair of tricuspid atresia. *Thorax* 1971;26:240–8.

63. Laks H, Williams WG, Hellenbrand WE, et al. Results of right atrial to right ventricular and right atrial to pulmonary artery conduits for complex congenital heart disease. *Ann Surg* 1980;192:382–9.

64. Penny DJ, Redington AN. Doppler echocardiographic evaluation of pulmonary blood flow after the fontan operation: The role of the lungs. *Br Heart J* 1991;66:372–4.

65. Redington AN, Penny D, Shinebourne EA. Pulmonary blood flow after total cavopulmonary shunt. *Br Heart J* 1991;65:213–7.

66. Shekerdemian LS, Bush A, Shore DF, et al. Cardiopulmonary interactions after fontan operations: Augmentation of cardiac output using negative pressure ventilation. *Circulation* 1997;96:3934–42.

67. Shekerdemian LS, Shore DF, Lincoln C, et al. Negative-pressure ventilation improves cardiac output after right heart surgery. *Circulation* 1996;94:II49–II155.

68. Hoskote A, Li J, Hickey C, et al. The effects of carbon dioxide on oxygenation and systemic, cerebral, and pulmonary vascular hemodynamics after the bidirectional superior cavopulmonary anastomosis. *J Am Coll Cardiol* 2004;44:1501–9.

69. Cullen S, Shore D, Redington A. Characterization of right ventricular diastolic performance after complete repair of tetralogy of fallot. Restrictive physiology predicts slow postoperative recovery. *Circulation* 1995;91:1782–9.

70. Shekerdemian LS, Bush A, Shore DF, et al. Cardiorespiratory responses to negative pressure ventilation after tetralogy of fallot repair: A hemodynamic tool for patients with a low-output state. *J Am Coll Cardiol* 1999;33:549–55.

71. Bronicki RA, Herrera M, Mink R, et al. Hemodynamics and cerebral oxygenation following repair of tetralogy of fallot: The effects of converting from positive pressure ventilation to spontaneous breathing. *Congenit Heart Dis* 2010;5:416–21.

72. Bronicki RA, Checchia PA, Anas NG, et al. Cerebral and somatic oxygen saturations after repair of tetralogy of Fallot: Effects of extubation on regional blood flow. *Ann Thorac Surg* 2013;95:682–6.

73. Walsh MA, Merat M, La Rotta G, et al. Airway pressure release ventilation improves pulmonary blood flow in infants after cardiac surgery. *Crit Care Med* 2011;39:2599–604.

74. Lurie K, Zielinski T, McKnite S, et al. Improving the efficiency of cardiopulmonary resuscitation with an inspiratory impedance threshold valve. *Crit Care Med* 2000;28:N207–N209.

75. Lurie KG, Voelckel WG, Zielinski T, et al. Improving standard cardiopulmonary resuscitation with an inspiratory impedance threshold valve in a porcine model of cardiac arrest. *Anesth Analg* 2001;93:649–55.

CHAPTER 71 ■ HEMODYNAMIC MONITORING

RONALD A. BRONICKI AND NEIL C. SPENCELEY

KEY POINTS

1 An estimation of cardiovascular function based on the physical examination and standard hemodynamic data such as blood pressure, central venous pressure, and urine output may be discordant from measured values of cardiac function, cardiac output, and tissue oxygenation.

2 The complementary use of hemodynamic monitoring technology enables the clinician to make a more timely and accurate assessment of cardiovascular function.

3 It is imperative to know the advantages and limitations of the monitoring modalities deployed.

4 Hemodynamic monitoring enables the clinician to assess cardiopulmonary function and tissue oxygenation.

---

1 One of the tenets of critical care medicine is to ensure adequate tissue oxygenation. This determination is often based on the physical examination and the interpretation of standard hemodynamic parameters such as blood pressure, central venous pressure (CVP), and urine output. However, studies have demonstrated significant discordance between assessments based on these parameters and those based on measurements of cardiac function, cardiac output (CO), and tissue oxygenation (1–8). The pediatric intensivist must appreciate that no single observation or measurement taken in isolation can provide adequate hemodynamic monitoring. Rather, it is the application of a range of observations and measurements that allows the care team to balance oxygen delivery with the child's metabolic demands. The type and intensity of hemodynamic monitoring should be calibrated to prevent tissue hypoxia episodes and, when necessary, to document that adequate tissue oxygenation has been restored.

PHYSICAL EXAMINATION

The physical examination is an essential part of the clinical determination of cardiovascular function. Particularly pertinent are changes that occur over time or that occur in response to interventions. While individual physical examination tests may not correlate with measured CO, collectively these tests provide valuable guides to diagnosis, prognosis, and therapy for children during the acute presentation of an abnormal circulatory state (2–4). The predictive value of the cardiovascular examination depends on age, disease process (e.g., sepsis vs. post–cardiac surgery), and the phase of resuscitation (on presentation in the emergency department vs. in PICU). The following components of the circulatory exam deserve particular attention.

A **depressed or altered mental status** may signify that compensatory hemodynamic mechanisms are failing in the child with circulatory dysfunction. Irritability or agitation may reflect the catecholamine surge that accompanies impending shock. Lethargy or unresponsiveness suggests impaired cerebral oxygen delivery relative to cerebral oxygen demand.

Importantly, an abnormal mental status that implies inadequate cerebral oxygenation requires a rapid and broad response to restore adequate oxygen delivery before irreversible brain damage occurs.

A **capillary refill time** (CRT) ≤2 seconds is considered normal in the child. CRT is a measure of peripheral microvascular perfusion and therefore provides an indirect measure of CO and peripheral vascular resistance. Correct measurement of CRT requires the extremity to be slightly elevated above the level of the heart in order to determine arterial perfusion rather than venous stasis. The child should also be in a neutral thermic environment to avoid skin vasoconstriction. Skin vasoconstriction due to a cool ambient temperature is a common cause for delayed CRT in the otherwise well-appearing child.

The interpretation of CRT depends on the correlations being sought and the degree of prolongation of the CRT. A prolonged CRT (>2 seconds) does *not* correlate well with isolated hemodynamic measurements such as stroke volume index (SVI) or lactate concentration in a general PICU population (2). A very prolonged CRT (>6 seconds) has better correlation with low SVI (3). From a practical standpoint, a prolonged CRT on presentation of a sick child represents shock and increased mortality risk until proven otherwise (9). Prompt therapy directed at normalization of hemodynamics including the CRT is associated with improved outcomes (9).

Examination of **central and peripheral pulses** provides information on volume, rate, and regularity of the pulse. In particular, the pulse volume reflects the pulse pressure, which may be increased in high-output septic shock or decreased in hypovolemic or cardiogenic shock. An absent peripheral pulse after fluid resuscitation for severe diarrhea is a strong predictor of mortality (10).

The **core (rectal) to peripheral (great toe) temperature gradient** has been taken as an indicator of the adequacy of the peripheral circulation particularly in infants after cardiac surgery. As the patient rewarms and circulation improves, skin temperature rises to approach rectal temperature thereby diminishing the gradient. While many experienced cardiac intensivists will devote special attention to the infant who fails to exhibit this pattern, the core–peripheral temperature gradient neither correlates well with other hemodynamic measurements nor predicts circulatory collapse (2,11).

ELECTROCARDIOGRAM

The electrocardiogram (ECG) has progressed from a rather cumbersome tool in the early 1900s to a required, continuous monitor in today's management of critically ill patients. The major purpose of ECG monitoring in the PICU is to alert the bedside care team of deviations in the patient's heart rate and rhythm before they become life-threatening. In addition, ECG abnormalities may suggest dysrhythmias, ischemia, pain, inadequate sedation, or electrolyte abnormalities (i.e., hyperkalemia causing peaked T-waves).

Technique

Easily applied disposable electrodes use a combination of wet gel and silver/silver chloride sensors to detect electrical activity from the myocardium. This electrical activity is amplified and displayed continuously (it can also be printed or stored as a permanent record). In addition, variations in the electrical impedance are detected, which allows a respiratory rate to be calculated. Alarm parameters may be set on bedside monitors for extremes in heart rates or for subtle ST segment changes. The initial default lead viewed on the bedside monitor is usually lead II. The size (gain) is automatic but may be altered to allow the components of complexes to be more prominent.

Interpretation

This noninvasive, continuous modality identifies heart rate abnormalities, ischemic changes, and rhythm disturbances. Associated changes in blood pressure or atrial pressure tracings can lend additional weight to the interpretation of rhythm disturbances perhaps prompting an earlier investigation. Similarly, they may convey reassurance during technical problems such as dislodged ECG electrodes or electrical interference giving rise to a spurious visual display.

Deciphering any underlying rhythm abnormality with bedside monitoring may be difficult (see Chapter 77). High heart rates and limited monitor fidelity may conceal p waves, blur QRS morphology, and conceal A-V dissociation. Note that paying careful attention to invasive monitoring such as the CVP waveform or arterial pulse contour may help unmask these abnormalities. Running the ECG speed at 50 mm/s rather than 25 mm/s and altering the gain may be useful but ultimately any concerns should be investigated further with a 12-lead ECG. Additionally, interrogating atrial wires if present or using an esophageal probe may reveal a more accurate picture of the underlying rhythm.

A reduction in the size of the complexes may be significant. A fluid interface between the myocardium and chest wall (e.g., pericardial effusion) or poor electrical generation due to myocarditis or cardiomyopathy can reduce the size of the complexes and should prompt further investigation. ECG abnormalities should be promptly and thoroughly investigated and may be the first indication of impending circulatory dysfunction.

Technical Factors

Incorrect lead placement is the most common technical problem during ECG monitoring. Distortions or "noise" created by electrical interference from the power grid, adjacent equipment, or muscle movements are reduced by using high-frequency filters.

CAPNOGRAPHY

Capnography refers to the graphic display of the concentration or partial pressure of carbon dioxide measured continuously in both inhaled and exhaled gases over time (see Fig. 45.10). It is a required monitoring device in intubated patients to verify continued correct placement of the endotracheal tube in the airway. Furthermore, it provides important information on changes in pulmonary blood flow (see also Chapter 45).

Technique

The CO_2 concentration is measured by infrared spectroscopy and sampled by one of two methods: aspiration from the breathing circuit (sidestream analyzer) or measured inline (mainstream analysis) by a flow-through adapter and sensor. The normal baseline on the capnogram should have a CO_2 concentration of zero, reflecting inspiratory as well as early expiratory (anatomic dead space) gas; this is followed by a sharp upstroke, reflecting mid-exhalation and increasing alveolar gas; this is followed by the plateau phase, which represents a leveling off of alveolar gas. The capnogram then abruptly falls to zero, as the expiratory phase is terminated and inspiratory gas dilutes out the remaining CO_2. The point on the capnogram plateau just prior to the abrupt fall-off is called the end-tidal CO_2 ($ETCO_2$) concentration and approximates the arterial PCO_2 ($PaCO_2$) under conditions of normal ventilation to perfusion matching in the lung.

Physiologic Considerations

Normally, the end-tidal CO_2 level approximates the arterial CO_2 level and the arterial to end-tidal CO_2 gradient ($PaCO_2$–$ETCO_2$) is <2–3 mm Hg. Hypercapnia that results from hypoventilation is associated with a normal arterial to $ETCO_2$ gradient. Hypercapnia that results from wasted or dead space ventilation is associated with an elevated arterial to $ETCO_2$ gradient. The arterial to $ETCO_2$ gradient rises because pulmonary perfusion (Q) is low compared to ventilation (V) (an increased $V:Q$ ratio). Diseases characterized by a decreased $V:Q$ ratio and intrapulmonary shunt (perfusion without ventilation) do not contribute significantly to the arterial to $ETCO_2$ gradient. These principles make $ETCO_2$ monitoring a useful hemodynamic monitor. Low CO (and therefore low pulmonary blood flow) or congenital heart disease with relatively low pulmonary perfusion will exhibit low $ETCO_2$ concentration and an increased end-tidal to arterial PCO_2 gradient. End-tidal CO_2 monitoring can also be used to assess the effectiveness of chest compressions and the return of circulatory function during cardiac arrest. A sudden reduction in pulmonary blood flow (e.g., Blalock–Taussig shunt obstruction or pulmonary embolus) will suddenly decrease the $ETCO_2$ concentration.

Technical Factors

Technical factors such as gas sampling method as well as the nature of the respiratory circuit can affect the accuracy of $ETCO_2$ measurements. The most common technical problem is a leak around the endotracheal tube, which lowers the $ETCO_2$ measurement and increases the arterial to $ETCO_2$ gradient.

ARTERIAL PRESSURE

Blood pressure is the product of CO and systemic vascular resistance (SVR). As with other hemodynamic parameters, blood pressure should be placed in its clinical context and used in conjunction with other monitoring modalities to create a comprehensive hemodynamic profile. Measuring blood pressure may be achieved in several ways; however, due to the frequency required in the critically ill setting, only two are practical: the noninvasive oscillometric method and invasive arterial monitoring.

Noninvasive Oscillometric Arterial Pressure Measurement

Noninvasive blood pressure monitoring is safe, simple, relatively reliable, reproducible, and inexpensive. It should be routinely performed in all children receiving inpatient care. The idea of sphygmomanometry was conceived by von Basch in the 1870s. However, the first indirect method, based on applying a known external pressure to occlude an artery, was developed in the 1890s. A cuff placed around the arm or leg abolishes the pulse when inflated above the patient's systolic blood pressure. Deflating the cuff slowly allows turbulent blood flow in the artery to develop, which can be appreciated either by auscultation or by observing the oscillations of a manometer reflecting pulsatile flow. Automated oscillometric technology with cuff pressure sensors and a microprocessor controlling the sequence of inflation and incremental deflation is now the standard of care in critical care units. Maximal oscillation amplitude corresponds to the mean arterial pressure. A microprocessor algorithm derives the systolic and diastolic pressure from the change in slope of oscillation amplitude. Oscillation frequency readily yields the heart rate.

The frequency of obtaining blood pressure measurement depends on the severity of disease. Frequent measurements (every 1–3 minutes) are advised during resuscitation or procedures such as intubation. During these occasions care must be taken to ensure that an inflated cuff will not interfere with the administration of drugs from a distal IV or interrupt pulse oximetry monitoring. Ulnar nerve palsy is a potential complication when pressures are measured frequently for a prolonged period.

Technical difficulties can occur if the patient is small, obese, edematous, agitated (moving), shivering (local muscle contraction causes pseudohypertension), extremely tachycardic, or suffering from burns. Error may arise with an inappropriate size cuff. The cuff should cover at least two thirds of the upper arm, and one too small may overestimate blood pressure and vice versa. Petechial rashes have been noted in the area under the cuff usually reflecting repeated external pressure but may reveal an underlying coagulation defect. Oscillometric blood pressure is not suitable for pressure measurement during nonpulsatile flow such as extracorporeal membrane oxygenation. Finally, the oscillometric-derived blood pressure tends to underestimate or show a lower-than-actual diastolic pressure (12).

Invasive Arterial Pressure Monitoring

Invasive arterial monitoring is the "gold standard" but is not without risk. Its higher degree of complexity increases the chance of technical errors and complications. However, a number of advantages over its noninvasive counterpart exist: improved accuracy, continuous beat-to-beat measurement, waveform analysis, and frequent arterial blood sampling.

The Reverend Stephen Hales first demonstrated invasive blood pressure monitoring in a horse, observing pressure as a column of blood in a glass tube connected to an artery.

The principle for today's measurement systems consists of a column of fluid that directly connects the arterial system to a strain gauge transducer, or Wheatstone bridge, which alters resistance to electron flow with variable pressure. Modern transducers utilize silicon crystals within a semiconductor that change electrical resistance in proportion to applied pressure.

To ensure accuracy and to counteract baseline drift, the transducer must regularly be zeroed to atmospheric pressure at the level of the right atrium (RA), which corresponds to the mid-axillary line. If the transducer is placed below the reference level, the arterial pressure reading will be falsely elevated and vice versa.

A transmitted arterial pressure waveform is converted into an electrical signal, amplified, and displayed continuously. The arterial pressure waveform represents the summation of a series of sine waves of different frequency, amplitude, and phase. It primarily consists of a fundamental wave (the pulse rate) and a series of further harmonics. Harmonics are smaller waves whose frequencies are multiples of the fundamental frequency. Fourier analysis, described by Lord Kelvin as "a great mathematical poem," allows the waveform to be examined in terms of its constituent parts then reconstructed and displayed on the bedside monitor in a manner that is simple to interpret.

Monitoring systems are designed to have dynamic response characteristics brisk enough to ensure accurate reproduction of these waveforms across the wide range of heart rates and frequencies encountered in clinical practice. However, every substance has its own natural frequency at which it will oscillate freely. Any component sine wave of the arterial waveform close to that of the monitoring system's natural (or resonant) frequency will cause resonance, which accentuates the waveform. This is of particular importance in pediatrics, because high heart rates can approach the system's natural frequency resulting in an exaggerated and distorted signal, falsely elevating the systolic pressure.

In addition to the frequency response, the optimal dynamic capability and accuracy of a system also depends on its damping coefficient. All monitoring systems produce natural energy at rest through oscillation, which can create artifact and therefore possible distortion of the resultant waveform. This is counteracted by an inherent damping capability, dissipating this natural energy by frictional forces in the system. The degree of damping is rarely perfect. Too much (overdamping) or too little (underdamping) may falsely lower or elevate systolic pressures, which, if unrecognized, could influence therapeutic decision-making (Fig. 71.1). Overdamping is most commonly encountered in the ICU and occurs with obstruction or excessive compliance in the system resulting in a narrow pulse pressure and a flattened appearance on the displayed waveform. The mean arterial pressure is usually unaffected. Causes include large bubbles; clots; compliant, cracked, lengthy, or kinked tubing; soft transducer diaphragm; three-way taps; or a poorly secured transducer. If this picture emerges then it is worth examining the system for air bubbles and aspirating and flushing the cannula. Smaller-diameter cannula cause overdamping but this cannot be avoided in younger children. Underdamping has the opposite effect. Again, the mean pressure remains largely unchanged. Accurate invasive systems can be achieved by using a short length of wide, stiff tubing, filled with low-viscosity fluid, and free of air bubbles and clot. This ensures that the natural frequency is usually sufficiently high to overcome the problem of resonance and optimal energy dissipation and damping. The system is continuously flushed to reduce the chance of clotting. The ideal solution for this is dextrose due to its nonconducting properties; however; with children, and especially small babies, there is the risk of administering relatively large volumes of free water, which may lead to hyponatremia. Therefore, line patency is maintained by using saline (with or without heparin), which is driven by a 500-mL bag that is pressurized to 300 mm Hg, delivering ~1–2 mL/h/lumen. A syringe driver (pump) is the

An optimally damped arterial trace

Small overshoot of 7% of the step change with no oscillations then follows arterial trace

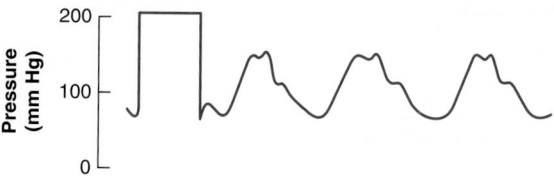

An under-damped arterial trace

Rapid response with overshoot and supermposed oscillations
Overestimates systolic and underestimates diastolic pressure

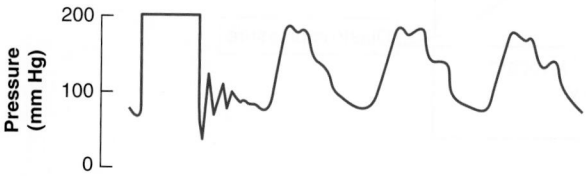

An over-damped arterial trace

Slow response with no overshoot
Phase shift as response gets slower

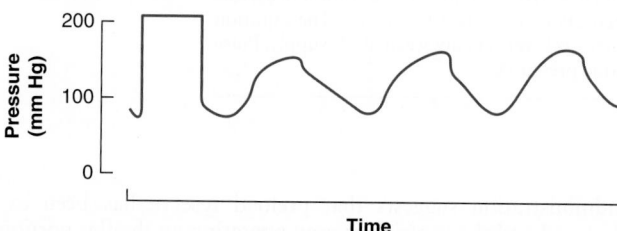

Time

FIGURE 71.1. Quantification of the degree of damping via the fast-flush test. Reproduced from Anaesthesia UK web site http://www.frca.co.uk/article.aspx?articleid=100382, with permission. Accessed October 12, 2014.

preferred method in smaller children due to improved accuracy of volume infused, which should be taken into account when calculating fluid balance. Infusion sets should be renewed every 72 hours to minimize line infections.

Placement and Complications

There are a number of places to insert an arterial line in the infant and child. Placement of the tip in or near the aorta, either by the umbilical or femoral route, may give a more consistent reading for a longer period. Both can increase the chance of line infections and both could potentially impinge blood flow down the celiac and mesenteric axis. Aortic waveforms usually appear slightly damped because of the impedance and harmonic resonance properties of the aorta. Further down the arterial tree the pressure wave reflection from the extremities augments the waveform resulting in a higher systolic pressure, a lower diastolic pressure, and a later appearance of the dicrotic notch. The mean arterial pressure remains fairly constant regardless of measurement site.

Complications of invasive arterial monitoring include bleeding, infection, nerve damage, arterial–venous fistulae, and vascular compromise. Risk factors for limb ischemia are low CO, preexisting vascular injury, and large catheter size relative to the dimension of the artery. The radial artery is selected for catheterization most commonly. The femoral, dorsalis pedis,

tibial arteries are also considered acceptable sites. Most clinicians avoid the brachial and ulnar arteries because of decreased collateral circulation in the event of vascular injury. The temporal artery is contraindicated because of the risk of intracranial embolization. The axillary artery may be cannulated when access at other sites has failed, but the care team must consider the increased risks of retrograde embolization (resulting in stroke) compared to more distal sites.

Interpretation

Invasive blood pressure monitoring provides a continuous display of the arterial waveform and additional information not available with the noninvasive modality (**Fig. 71.2**). The slope of the upstroke of the arterial waveform may be proportional to myocardial contractility. A slow upstroke can be indicative of poor cardiac function but is also seen in aortic stenosis and elevations in SVR. The area under the systolic portion of the waveform is proportional to the stroke volume. A low pulse pressure may reflect a low stroke volume. A widened pulse pressure due to elevated systolic and depressed diastolic pressures is seen in states characterized by poor systemic vascular tone, in patients with an aorta-to-pulmonary artery runoff (e.g., patent ductus arteriosus and aortopulmonary artery window), and in patients with aortic insufficiency.

CENTRAL VENOUS AND ATRIAL PRESSURES

A central venous catheter (CVC) is essential for managing a critically ill patient. The CVC provides secure intravenous access for the administration of volume and medications and to sample blood for analysis. It also provides valuable information by monitoring CVP and central venous oxygen saturations (SvO_2).

Placement and Complications

The CVC may be inserted in the subclavian, femoral, basilic, or jugular veins using the Seldinger technique or by way of a cut-down procedure. An additional site in the newborn is the umbilical vein. There are substantial risks associated with the use of CVCs, and most important are the risks of infectious and thrombotic complications. There are extensive recommendations for maintaining CVCs and minimizing the incidence of catheter-related bloodstream infection (see Chapter 9). The placement of a subclavian CVC has the inherent risk of causing a pneumothorax. In the event that arterial or venous bleeding occurs, the subclavian vessels are inaccessible to direct pressure for control of bleeding, which is a significant concern in coagulopathic patients. Inadvertent arterial placement is a frequent complication that is detected by checking the catheter for venous pressure waveforms and venous saturation of a blood sample. A "central" venous catheter does not need to reside near or within the RA to accurately measure right heart filling pressures. Several studies have demonstrated excellent correlation between pressures measured in the inferior vena cava and RA, so long as there is a continuous column of fluid between the tip of the catheter and the RA allowing for equilibration of pressure (13).

Interpretation

A normal central venous or right atrial pressure in the spontaneously breathing patient is −2 to 5 mm Hg. The atrial pressure waveform (**Fig. 71.3**) normally demonstrates three

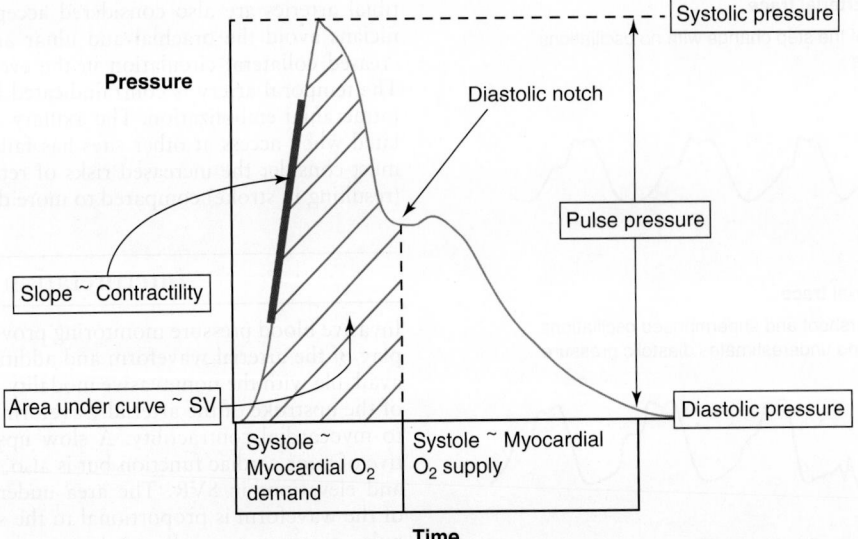

FIGURE 71.2. Arterial pulse waveform. Inspection of the arterial pulse waveform provides a *first approximation* of various aspects of hemodynamic function. The slope of the systolic upstroke may be proportional to myocardial contractility and inversely proportional to systemic vascular resistance. The area under the systolic curve approximates stroke volume. The duration of systole relative to the duration of the entire cardiac cycle reflects myocardial O_2 demand. The duration of diastole relative to the duration of the entire cardiac cycle reflects myocardial O_2 supply. Pulse pressure is the difference between systolic and diastolic pressures.

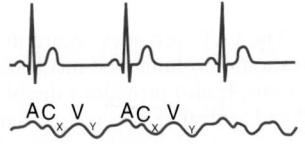

FIGURE 71.3. Central venous pressure trace with corresponding ECG. See text for explanation. From O'Rourke RA. The measurement of systemic blood pressure: Normal and abnormal pulsations of the arteries and veins. In: Hurst JW, ed. *The Heart*. New York: McGraw-Hill, 1990:159, with permission.

positive and two negative waves: the "*a*" wave follows the p wave on the ECG and is produced by atrial contraction; the "*c*" wave is produced by ventricular contraction and bulging of the tricuspid valve upward into the RA; the "*x*" descent results from atrial relaxation; the "*v*" wave results from right atrial filling and occurs in late systole before opening of the tricuspid valve; and the "*y*" descent results from opening of the tricuspid valve and passive filling of the right ventricle (RV). The CVP is the mean right atrial pressure, which approximates the right ventricular end-diastolic pressure, when right ventricular compliance and tricuspid valve function are normal. When ventricular function and compliance are diminished, atrial systole generates an end-diastolic pressure (reflected in the "*a*" wave) that is disproportionately higher than the mean pressure (14). Cannon "*a*" waves are produced when right atrial contraction occurs against a closed tricuspid valve, as in atrioventricular disassociation. Prominent "*v*" waves may be seen in tricuspid insufficiency and rapid "*x*" and "*y*" descents are suggestive of pericardial disease and restraint.

The relationship between CVP (ventricular filling pressure) and stroke volume is curvilinear. So long as volume administration produces an increase in stroke volume, the ventricle resides on the ascending portion of its Frank–Starling curve. The lack of a further increase in stroke volume after fluid administration suggests that preload reserve has been exhausted and the ventricle is now operating on the flat portion of its Frank–Starling curve (see Chapter 69). Any increase in stroke volume at this point would require inotropic support or afterload reduction.

Ventricular compliance is the ratio of the change of ventricular pressure (ΔP) to the change in ventricular volume (ΔV). One of the challenges of relying on the central venous (or ventricular filling) *pressure* as an indication of ventricular *volume* is that the relationship between volume and pressure (i.e., compliance) for a distensible chamber varies considerably from moment to moment in patients with cardiopulmonary disease (15). The effective compliance of the ventricle is affected by pericardial pressure and intrathoracic pressure. Thus, the end-diastolic transmural pressure (ventricular pressure–pericardial pressure) and ventricular compliance are the determinants of ventricular end-diastolic volume (**Fig. 71.4**). With a decrease in compliance, a greater distending pressure is needed to maintain ventricular filling. Ventricular compliance may be diminished as result of:

- myocardial disease (hypertrophic or ischemic myocardium);
- elevated operating volumes, as occurs in systolic heart failure and elevated afterload;
- pericardial disease;
- an increase in intrathoracic pressure, as occurs with positive pressure ventilation, lower airway disease, and excessive lung volumes;
- large pleural effusions.

Ventricular compliance may also be affected as a result of diastolic ventricular interdependence. Ventricular interdependence defines a circumstance where changes in the volumes and pressures of one ventricle alter the volumes and pressures of the other ventricle. Under normal ventricular loading conditions and function, the interventricular septum deviates into the RV throughout the cardiac cycle because left ventricular

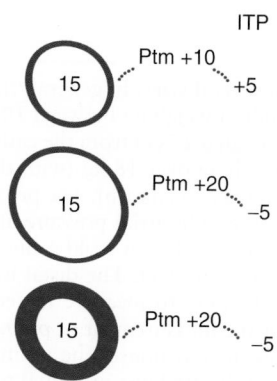

FIGURE 71.4. The pressure–volume relationship for a distensible/collapsible chamber. The degree to which a chamber undergoes deformation depends on its compliance and the magnitude and direction of the pressure exerted across its wall or its transmural pressure (Ptm). The pressure within each chamber is constant at 15. For the top chamber, the surrounding pressure of 5 produces a distending Ptm of +10. The middle chamber, with identical compliance to the top chamber (same thickness), distends to a greater extent because it is surrounded by a negative pressure of 5, resulting in a transmural pressure of +20. The bottom chamber is less compliant than the top two chambers. Even though its transmural pressure is identical to the middle chamber, its volume is less.

pressures exceed right ventricular pressures. If the interventricular septum shifts from its normal position, either due to an increase in right or left ventricular diastolic pressure, the compliance and therefore pressure and volume (filling) of the contralateral ventricle is altered.

Left Atrial Pressure Monitoring

The same principles used to interpret central venous and right atrial pressures are applied to left atrial pressures. In addition to the limitations that exist in relying on a ventricular filling pressure as an indication of ventricular volume, it cannot be overstated that in the presence of underlying cardiopulmonary disease there is no correlation between right and left atrial pressures (16,17). The exception to this rule occurs in patients with single-ventricle anatomy and a nonrestrictive interatrial communication, where the CVP is a measurement of the systemic ventricular filling pressure. A left atrial pressure obtained from a transthoracic line placed during cardiac surgery or a pulmonary arterial catheter (PAC) (discussed below) also enables measurement of left-sided filling pressures. If air or clot is dislodged from a left atrial catheter, the consequences may include stroke or myocardial infarction. Therefore, it is safest to use the left atrial catheter strictly for pressure monitoring and avoid aspiration of blood or intermittent flushing of the line.

PULMONARY ARTERIAL CATHETER

In 1970, Swan and Ganz first described the use of a flow-directed, balloon-tipped, catheter inserted into the pulmonary artery for the measurement of the pulmonary artery occlusion pressure (PAOP) (18). This was soon followed by the implementation of a triple-lumen catheter with a thermistor tip by Forrester and colleagues that allowed for the measurement of CO by the thermodilution technique (19). Heralded as a breakthrough in hemodynamic monitoring, the PAC enabled the clinician to readily measure a number of hemodynamic variables that were not previously obtainable at the bedside (Table 71.1). Ventricular filling pressures (right atrial pressure or CVP and PAOP), pulmonary artery pressures, mixed venous oxygen saturation, and temperature are directly measured. With the addition of heart rate and systemic arterial blood pressure, a number of hemodynamic parameters may be derived including CO, stroke volume, systemic and pulmonary vascular resistance, oxygen delivery, and oxygen consumption. Other uses of the PAC have included cardiac pacing, segmental pulmonary artery angiography, and the diagnosing of left-to-right intracardiac shunting.

TABLE 71.1

COMMON HEMODYNAMIC VARIABLES

■ PARAMETER	■ FORMULA	■ NORMAL RANGE	■ UNITS
Cardiac index	$CI = CO/\text{body surface area}$	3.5–5.5	$L/min/m^2$
Stroke index	$SI = CI/\text{heart rate}$	30–60	mL/m^2
Systemic vascular resistance index	$SVRI = 79.9 \times (MAP - CVP)/CI$	800–1600	$dyne\text{-}sec/cm^5/m^2$
Pulmonary vascular resistance index	$PVRI = 79.9 \times (MPAP - PAOP)/CI$	80–240	$dyne\text{-}sec/cm^5/m^2$
Left ventricular stroke work index	$LVSWI = SI \times MAP \times 0.0136$	50–62 (adult)	$g\text{-}m/m^2$
Right ventricular stroke work index	$RVSWI = SI \times MPAP \times 0.0136$	5.1–6.9 (adult)	$g\text{-}m/m^2$
Arterial oxygen content	$Cao_2 = (1.34 \times Hb \times Sao_2) + (Pao_2 \times 0.003)$		mL/L
Oxygen delivery index	$Do_2I = CI \times Cao_2$	570–670	$mL/min/m^2$
Fick principle	$CI = Vo_2I/(Cao_2 - Cvo_2)$	160–180 (infant Vo_2I)	$mL/min/m^2$
		100–130 (child Vo_2I)	$mL/min/m^2$
Mixed venous oxygen saturation		65%–75%	
Oxygen extraction ratio[a]	$O_2ER = (Sao_2 - Svo_2)/Sao_2$	0.24–0.28	

CI, cardiac index; CO, cardiac output; SI, stroke index; SVRI, systemic vascular resistance index; MAP, mean systemic arterial pressure; CVP, central venous pressure; PVRI, pulmonary vascular resistance index; MPAP, mean pulmonary arterial pressure; PAOP, pulmonary artery occlusion pressure; LVSWI, left ventricular stroke work index; RVSWI, right ventricular stroke work index; Cao_2, arterial oxygen content; Hb, hemoglobin concentration (g/L); Sao_2, arterial oxygen saturation; Pao_2, partial pressure of dissolved oxygen; Do_2I, oxygen delivery index; Vo_2I, oxygen consumption index; Cvo_2, mixed venous oxygen content; O_2ER, oxygen extraction ratio; Svo_2, mixed venous oxygen saturation.
[a]The equation given for O_2ER is only valid if the contribution from dissolved oxygen is minimal. If this is not the case, oxygen content (Cao_2, Cvo_2) must be substituted for saturation (Sao_2, Svo_2).

With its incredible capacity to provide a comprehensive evaluation of the cardiovascular system while enhancing our understanding of pathophysiological derangements, the PAC was perceived to be an unrivaled monitoring tool, leading to its widespread and unbridled use in the critical care population. However, over time, significant concerns began to emerge regarding its use (20). Randomized clinical trials performed in high-risk patients uniformly documented that the routine use of the PAC is not beneficial and may be associated with increased morbidity and mortality (21–28). The PAC came under an unusual amount of scrutiny and some authors rightly noted that the weight of evidence attributing improved outcomes to any modality of hemodynamic monitoring is virtually absent. This led the Society of Critical Care Medicine to publish a consensus statement on the use of the PAC (29). This document suggests that the PAC should be used as infrequently as possible in children, but may be used to clarify cardiopulmonary physiology in selected patients with the following characteristics: (a) pulmonary hypertension; (b) shock refractory to fluid resuscitation and/or low-to-moderate doses of vasoactive agents; and (c) severe respiratory failure requiring high airway pressure. There are no randomized controlled trials (RCTs) on the use of PAC in children. However, a systematic review of 13 RCTs in adults revealed that the use of the PAC did not alter mortality, length of hospital stay, or length of ICU stay (30).

Placement and Complications

The PAC comes in several sizes. In general, the 5-French catheter is used for children weighing between 10 and 18 kg (with the proximal port located 15 cm from the catheter tip) and it is used in patients weighing over 18 kg (with the proximal port located 30 cm from the catheter tip). The proximal lumen port is used to measure the right atrial pressure and allows for the injection of an indicator solution (cold saline in the thermodilution method) to measure CO. The distal lumen port allows for the sampling of blood to measure mixed venous oxygen saturations and for the measurement of pulmonary artery and PAOP. The thermistor port houses the wiring to the thermistor. The thermistor is located just proximal to the balloon and measures changes in the temperature of pulmonary arterial blood, which is used for thermodilution-derived CO measurements. And the fourth lumen allows for the inflation and deflation of the balloon (located 1 cm proximal to the catheter tip).

The catheter is introduced through an introducer sheath and advanced by inflating the balloon with CO_2 or air and "floating" the tip while continuously monitoring the distal port pressures and waveforms (**Fig. 71.5**), as well as the ECG for dysrhythmias. Whenever withdrawing the catheter, the balloon should be deflated to avoid valvular and vessel rupture. After

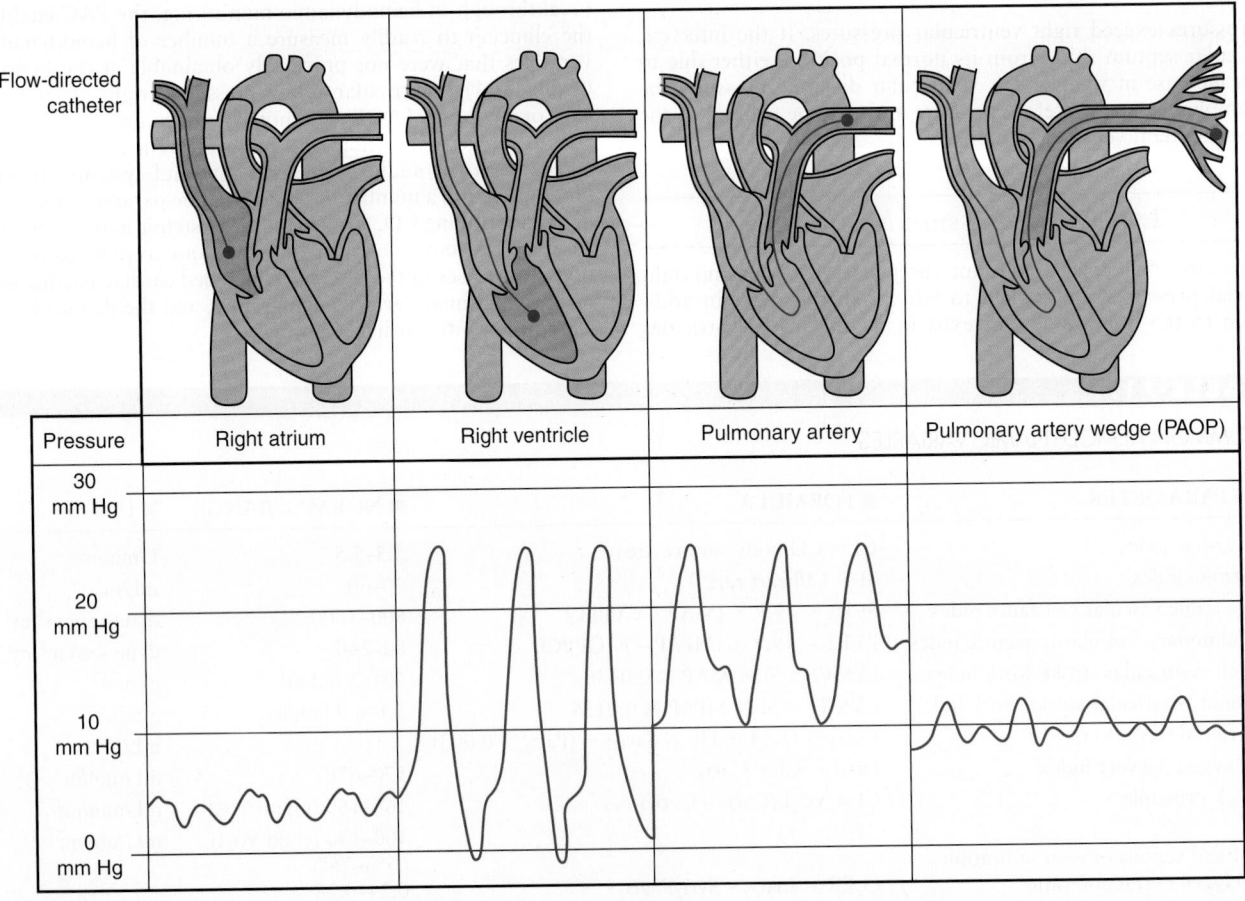

FIGURE 71.5. Pulmonary artery catheter waveforms. When the balloon is inflated and the catheter is advanced, a series of characteristic waveforms appear. As the catheter passes from the right atrium (RA) through the tricuspid valve into the right ventricle (RV), the low-amplitude RA waveform suddenly changes to a high-amplitude (high pulse pressure, high systolic pressure, low diastolic pressure) RV waveform. Further advancement through the pulmonary valve into the pulmonary artery (PA) yields a waveform with a higher diastolic pressure than in the RV while the systolic pressure is unchanged. Ultimately a position is reached where the systolic and mean pressures decrease, the tracing becomes damped, and the appearance of an "a" and "v" venous waves become more pronounced. This is the PA occlusion (or wedge) pressure (*PAOP*). When the balloon is deflated, the tracing should immediately return to a PA waveform.

placement, the balloon should be deflated and pulmonary artery pressures should be monitored continuously in order to identify inadvertent migration of the catheter tip into the pulmonary capillary bed or "wedged" position. The catheter should be allowed to "float" (i.e., the balloon is inflated) into the wedged position *only* when actively obtaining a PAOP in order to minimize the risk of pulmonary infarction or rupture. For the PAOP to approximate left atrial and left ventricular end-diastolic pressure, a continuous column of blood must exist between the catheter tip and the left atrium (zone III conditions). Ideally, a portable lateral chest film should be obtained to confirm placement of the catheter tip in a zone III area (below the level of the left atrium). Other indications that the tip resides in the correct (zone III) area include a tracing with "*a*" and "*v*" waves during wedging as well as the absence of marked variation with inspiration and expiration. There are several complications associated with the placement and use of the PAC including arrhythmias, pulmonary artery rupture, pulmonary infarction, air embolus, catheter knotting (most likely in patients with large atrial or ventricular cavities and low flow), valvular damage, as well as thrombotic and infectious complications.

Interpretation of Thermodilution-derived CO

Perhaps the PAC's greatest asset is the ability to measure CO and, despite its reduction in use over the years, it still remains the gold standard by which newer monitoring modalities are compared. A thermodilution-derived measurement of CO is based on the indicator dilution principle, which was first described by Stewart in the late 1800s and later refined by Hamilton. This involves injecting a volume of indicator into a central vein and observing the resultant change in concentration downstream over time. Thermodilution involves injecting a known quantity (volume) of cold saline into the RA and measuring the resultant temperature change with the thermistor located near the catheter tip. CO is determined by the amount of indicator divided by the change in concentration over time. Using the *Stewart Hamilton equation*, analysis of the temperature change from baseline allows the calculation of blood flow with the area under the curve being inversely proportional to the CO.

Studies have demonstrated that thermodilution-derived CO measurements are reliable in children and adults over a wide range of flow (31–33). Accuracy of the technique relies on very rapid injection rates, accurate measurements of the injectant temperature and volume, thorough mixing of the injectant in the systemic venous return, and no loss of injectant. Conditions in which the thermodilution method may prove unreliable are those that have backward flow of blood on the right side, such as tricuspid and pulmonary valve regurgitation and ventricular or atrial septal defects (with left-to-right and/or right-to-left shunting). In small children, the proximal port may not reside in the RA, which may affect the accuracy of thermodilution CO and CVP determinations (34).

Interpretation of Other Hemodynamic Measurements from the PAC

Additional information obtained from the PAC includes ventricular filling pressures. The PAOP may be used as an indication of left ventricular end-diastolic volume; however, there are significant limitations to this approach, as described above. In patients with poor ventricular compliance and function, the PAOP will underestimate the left ventricular end-diastolic pressure, which is reflected in the "*a*" wave (14). In any case, it is the ventricular diastolic transmural pressure and compliance that determine

ventricular end-diastolic volume. The PAOP may also be used to distinguish between cardiogenic (PAOP >18 mm Hg) and permeability pulmonary edema (PAOP <12 mm Hg). Right ventricular afterload and the response of the pulmonary vasculature to vasodilators can be assessed by deriving pulmonary vascular resistance using measurements of CO and pulmonary arterial pressures. Similarly, CO measurements and *systemic* arterial pressures allow for the derivation of SVR and an assessment of systemic vascular function. Finally, as described in detail under venous oximetry, the PAC allows for the measurement of the mixed venous oxygen saturation and a determination of global oxygen transport balance (the relationship between systemic oxygen supply and oxygen demand).

THE FICK EQUATION AND INDIRECT CO MEASUREMENTS

The Fick principle is an indirect method for determining CO and is based on the law of conversation of mass. It relies on the observation that the total uptake of a substance by an organ is equal to the product of the blood flow to the organ and the arterial–venous concentration difference of the substance. In Fick's original work, the substance (or indicator) used for the determination of CO was oxygen. Oxygen uptake from the lung was measured with a spirometer, and the difference in oxygen content between the pulmonary artery and pulmonary vein allowed for the calculation of flow across the pulmonary circulation. Fick made two other very important assumptions: (a) the amount of oxygen taken up by the lungs during breathing was equal to the amount of oxygen extracted by the body from the blood and (b) the flow of blood through the lungs must equal the flow of blood to the remainder of the body in the absence of a shunt.

Thus, the Fick equation states that:

$$V_{O_2} = Q \times Ca_{O_2} - Q \times Cv_{O_2} = Q(Ca_{O_2} - Cv_{O_2}) \quad [71.1]$$

or rearranging

$$Q = V_{O_2}/(Ca_{O_2} - Cv_{O_2}) \quad [71.2]$$

where V_{O_2} is the O_2 consumption (mL O_2/min), Q the CO (L/min), Ca_{O_2} the arterial O_2 content (mL O_2/dL blood), Cv_{O_2} the *mixed* venous O_2 content (mL O_2/dL blood), and (Ca – Cv) O_2 = arteriovenous O_2 content difference.

The O_2 content in blood is directly proportional to hemoglobin concentration and oxygen saturation. The dissolved O_2 in blood is a function of the partial pressure of O_2 (dissolved O_2 = 0.003 × P_{O_2}) and is negligible under most circumstances. Therefore,

$$Ca_{O_2} \text{ (mL } O_2\text{/dL plasma)} = [1.34 \text{ (mL/g)} \times \text{hemoglobin concentration (g/dL)} \times [Sa_{O_2} (\%)/100]] + [0.003 \text{ (mL/dL/mm Hg)} \times Pa_{O_2} \text{ (mm Hg)}] \quad [71.3]$$

$$Cv_{O_2} \text{ (mL } O_2\text{/dL plasma)} = [1.34 \text{ (mL/g)} \times \text{hemoglobin concentration (g/dL)} \times [Sv_{O_2} (\%)/100]] + [0.003 \text{ (mL/dL/mm Hg)} \times Pv_{O_2} \text{ (mm Hg)}] \quad [71.4]$$

where Sa_{O_2} is the arterial O_2 saturation and Sv_{O_2} the *mixed* venous O_2 saturation.

The estimated or measured V_{O_2} and arteriovenous oxygen content difference becomes hemodynamic monitoring tools because they permit calculation of CO (Q). It is possible to determine V_{O_2} by measuring the O_2 concentration difference between inhaled and exhaled gas in a metabolic hood or through a cuffed endotracheal tube. However, in practice, V_{O_2} is usually retrieved from published tables based on age, gender, and size. Ca_{O_2} is measured via co-oximetry from an arterial blood gas. Although the pulmonary artery is the ideal location for measurement of mixed venous O_2 saturation and content, most pediatric patients will not have a PAC in place and therefore measurements obtained from the superior vena cava or RA via a central venous line are taken as an approximation of Svo_2 and Cvo_2. With estimated or measured values for Vo_2 and $(Ca - Cv) O_2$, CO (Q) may be calculated using Equation 71.2.

Calculation of the Q_p/Q_s Ratio

Another benefit of the Fick principle is that it allows separate calculations of systemic (Q_s) and pulmonary (Q_p) blood flow. Q_p and Q_s are nearly equal ($Q_p/Q_s = 1$) in the child with a structurally normal heart (except for the very small right-to-left shunt from the Thebesian and bronchial veins). Conversely, Q_p and Q_s diverge in children with many forms of congenital heart disease. Children with right-to-left shunts have $Q_p/Q_s < 1$ (pulmonary undercirculation and hypoxemia), whereas those with left-to-right shunts have $Q_p/Q_s > 1$ (pulmonary overcirculation and heart failure). The magnitude of the shunt is described by the $Q_p:Q_s$ ratio, such that:

$$Q_p = Vo_2/(Cpvo_2 - Cpao_2) \qquad [71.5]$$

$$Q_s = Vo_2/(Cao_2 - Cvo_2) \qquad [71.6]$$

$$Q_p/Q_s = (Cao_2 - Cvo_2)/(Cpvo_2 - Cpao_2) \qquad [71.7]$$

$$Q_p/Q_s \approx (Sao_2 - Svo_2)/(Spvo_2 - Spao_2) \qquad [71.8]$$

where $Cpvo_2$ is the pulmonary vein O_2 content, $Cpao_2$ the pulmonary artery O_2 content, $Spvo_2$ the pulmonary vein O_2 saturation, and $Spao_2$ the pulmonary artery O_2 saturation.

Technical Factors

Technical factors affect the measurement of Q_p/Q_s. Pulmonary venous blood is very difficult to sample. Therefore, the pulmonary venous O_2 saturation is presumed to be 100% in the patient without significant lung disease who is receiving supplemental O_2. The Fick method of Q_p/Q_s determination is more likely to be inaccurate in patients with severe lung disease unless pulmonary venous O_2 saturation is measured directly.

Direct measurement of oxygen consumption is impractical and is seldom used in the critical care setting. The use of an assumed value for Vo_2 from standardized tables is the most common method used during cardiac catheterization. This approach is not useful in the critical care setting as oxygen demand and consumption vary considerably over time as a result of several factors, including the dynamic nature of pathophysiological processes and therapeutic interventions among others. If the assumed value for Vo_2 is greater than actual, the calculated CO will be overestimated, and therefore the calculated vascular resistance will be underestimated. And the converse is true if the assumed value for Vo_2 is less than actual.

PULSE CONTOUR ANALYSIS

Another method for measuring CO is pulse contour analysis (35). This technology is based on the principle that the area under the systolic portion of curve of a central arterial waveform correlates with the stroke volume (**Fig. 71.2**). Many different systems are now available commercially, but they can be divided into calibration-dependent systems (e.g., Pulse Contour Cardiac Output [PiCCO], LiDCO, and PulseCO) and noncalibration systems (e.g., FloTrac/Vigileo, PRAM, and LiDCOrapid).

The PiCCO system (Pulsion Medical Systems, Munich, Germany) serves as a prototype for the calibration-dependent systems. It requires placement of a CVC and a thermistor-tipped 3F or 4F femoral artery catheter for *transpulmonary thermodilution* measurement of CO. Proprietary algorithms analyze the femoral artery waveform continuously to derive the CO based on the pulse contour. The thermodilution-derived measurement of CO allows for initial and periodic calibrations of the pulse contour-derived CO measurement. Studies have found the bias and precision for transpulmonary thermodilution to be very good compared with the Fick and pulmonary artery thermodilution methods (36–38). Other systems rely on lithium dilution as the indicator for CO calibration (LiDCO and PulseCO manufactured by LiDCO, London, UK).

Technical Factors

Pulse contour analysis–derived measurements of CO are less reliable than those derived by pulmonary arterial thermodilution. Therefore, it is necessary to recalibrate the pulse contour CO frequently with transpulmonary thermodilution-derived COs to insure accuracy of pulse contour COs (39,40). This is especially true in hemodynamically unstable patients. The lower correlation coefficients with important bias and wider limits of agreements suggest that the pulse contour-derived CO values might be more useful for trend monitoring than in the determination of an isolated value. The presence of an intracardiac shunt renders the pulse contour-derived measurement of CO inaccurate.

ECHOCARDIOGRAPHY

Echocardiography is an essential diagnostic tool in the critical care setting, providing information about cardiovascular function that is not available from other monitoring modalities. Limited transthoracic echocardiograms are increasingly being performed and interpreted by noncardiologists, including pediatric and adult intensivists, anesthesiologists, and emergency medicine physicians. The advent of portable ultrasound platforms has contributed to the evolving use of echocardiography as an acute monitoring modality, readily enabling critical care physicians to perform a timely and accurate study in order to establish a diagnosis and to monitor responses to interventions. Studies have shown that with adequate training the accuracy of these studies performed by noncardiologists is very good (41–44).

Ventricular Shortening Fraction and Ejection Fraction

Several hemodynamic parameters can be readily assessed by performing a limited transthoracic echocardiogram. Left ventricular systolic function can be assessed by determining the *fractional shortening* (FS), which is a determination of the change in left ventricular short-axis diameter based on one-dimensional wall motion analysis or M-mode echocardiography:

$$FS = (\text{End-Diastolic Dimension} - \text{End-Systolic Dimension})/\text{End-Diastolic Dimension} \qquad [71.9]$$

Normal Values = 0.28–0.40.

The primary limitation of this technique is that the contraction of the left ventricle cannot be assumed to be entirely uniform or symmetric and M-mode interrogation may not capture regional differences in wall motion and wall thickening. Similarly, a flattened interventricular septum nullifies the measurement.

Calculation of the *ejection fraction* (EF) is based on two-dimensional imaging of the left ventricular systolic function by quantifying changes in ventricular volume during the cardiac cycle:

$$EF = (\text{End-diastolic Volume} - \text{End-Systolic Volume})/\text{End-diastolic Volume}. \quad [71.10]$$

Normal values: LVEF = 0.68 ± 0.09. This technique relies on the modified Simpson rule method for measuring volumes. Because of its complex geometric shape and the motion of the interventricular septum during systole, an assessment of right ventricular systolic function is most often qualitative and based on the inward motion of right ventricular free wall toward the ventricular septum.

An assessment of ventricular systolic function with either technique is sensitive to ventricular loading conditions and heart rate. The presence of tricuspid or mitral valve insufficiency allows the ventricle(s) to eject retrograde into a low-pressure atrium. In addition, ventricular end-diastolic volumes are elevated leading to enhanced contractility and ejection. Based on these factors an index of systolic function should be normal or elevated (45). The same is true for those patients with elevated operating volumes resulting from other lesions, such as semilunar valve insufficiency (45). For those with experience reading echocardiograms, there is a very good correlation between visually estimated and measured EFs (46). Ventricular wall thickness and volume can be assessed, giving some indication of diastolic function and operating volumes, respectively.

Doppler techniques enable clinicians to estimate intracardiac and vascular pressures by measuring the velocity of blood in relation to the ultrasound beam. Based on a modified *Bernoulli's equation*, the pressure gradient that exists across an obstructive lesion is equal to:

$$\text{Pressure gradient} = 4V^2 \quad [71.11]$$

where "V" is the velocity of blood as it accelerates across a narrowed orifice. Right ventricular systolic pressure may be estimated by interrogating the tricuspid regurgitant jet from the RV to the RA. For instance, if the tricuspid regurgitant jet velocity is 3 m/s, then the modified Bernoulli equation states:

$$\text{RV} - \text{RA pressure} \approx 4 \times 3^2 = 36 \text{ mm Hg}. \quad [71.12]$$

The addition of 36 mm Hg to the RA or CVP during systole yields the RV systolic pressure. In the absence of a right ventricular outflow tract obstruction, RV pressure also approximates the pulmonary artery systolic pressure. Another method for assessing RV or pulmonary artery pressures is to evaluate the position and orientation of the interventricular septum during ventricular systole. The transseptal pressure gradient determines the position and orientation of the septum throughout the cardiac cycle. Under normal conditions, left ventricular pressures exceed right ventricular pressures. As a result, the interventricular septum bows into the RV throughout the cardiac cycle. Studies have shown that with systolic flattening of the interventricular septum, right ventricular systolic pressure is at least half systemic (47). Similarly, the orientation of the septum during ventricular diastole gives some indication of biventricular filling pressures. A midline position during diastole indicates that right and left ventricular filling pressures are similar. In this instance, deviation of the septum from its normal position toward the left ventricle reduces the effective compliance of the left ventricle. The Bernoulli equation may be used to assess the pressure gradients across valves, septum, and coarctations.

Other uses of echocardiography include a qualitative assessment of valvar regurgitation, pericardial effusion, and intracardiac shunting. The earliest indication of tamponade physiology is collapse of the RA. Echocardiography can be used to delineate causes of hypoxemia from right-to-left shunting. Interrogation of the atrial and ventricular septum may be used to detect right-to-left shunting, and the appearance of left-sided saline contrast detects the presence of extracardiac physiologic right-to-left shunting resulting from pulmonary arteriovenous malformations and systemic venous collaterals (48–51).

VENOUS OXIMETRY

The routine use of CVCs in the management of critically ill patients enables the clinician to assess oxygen extraction, the relationship between oxygen consumption and delivery, and hence the adequacy of tissue oxygenation. Accurately interpreting and appreciating the use and limitations of venous oximetry requires an understanding of the determinants of tissue oxygenation, the relationship between oxygen consumption and oxygen delivery, and global and regional compensatory circulatory responses to alterations in oxygen demand and delivery.

Basic Principles

According to the Fick equation (Equation 71.1), total body oxygen consumption (V_{O_2}) is equal to the product of CO and the difference in arterial–venous oxygen content ($Ca_{O_2} - Cv_{O_2}$). Total body oxygen delivery (D_{O_2}) is simply the product of CO and arterial oxygen content or:

$$D_{O_2} = Q \times Ca_{O_2} \quad [71.13]$$

Hence, the *ratio* of oxygen demand to oxygen delivery (V_{O_2}/D_{O_2}) can be expressed as (52):

$$V_{O_2}/D_{O_2} = Q(Ca_{O_2} - Cv_{O_2})/Q(Ca_{O_2}) = (Ca_{O_2} - Cv_{O_2})/(Ca_{O_2}). \quad [71.14]$$

This is known as the oxygen extraction ratio (O_2ER):

$$\text{Oxygen extraction ratio } (O_2ER) = (Ca_{O_2} - Cv_{O_2})/(Ca_{O_2}). \quad [71.15]$$

Assuming minimal amounts of dissolved oxygen in blood and constant hemoglobin levels, the equations for V_{O_2}/D_{O_2} and O_2ER can be simplified to:

$$V_{O_2}/D_{O_2} = O_2ER \cong Sa_{O_2} - Sv_{O_2}/Sa_{O_2}. \quad [71.16]$$

Sv_{O_2} is the pulmonary artery oxygen saturation or mixed venous oxygen saturation and is the weighted average of venous return from all viscera. Under normal circumstances, the Sa_{O_2} is ~100% and Sv_{O_2} is ~75%. Therefore, the normal $Sa_{O_2} - Sv_{O_2}$ difference is ~25%. Because Sa_{O_2} (the denominator in the O_2ER equation) is usually ~100%, clinicians often use the $Sa_{O_2} - Sv_{O_2}$ difference as a surrogate for O_2ER and refer to it as "oxygen extraction." An increased $Sa_{O_2} - Sv_{O_2}$ difference suggests a reduction in D_{O_2}, an increase in V_{O_2}, or both (**Table 71.2**).

The body is able to preserve constant oxygen consumption (V_{O_2}) over a wide range of oxygen delivery (D_{O_2}) by adjusting oxygen extraction ratio (O_2ER). This phenomenon is reflected in the "oxygen supply *independent*" portion of the V_{O_2}/D_{O_2} curve (**Fig. 71.6A**). However, the ability of tissues to extract oxygen has a limit such that a drop of D_{O_2} below a certain critical level may overwhelm the body's ability to compensate for falling D_{O_2}, through increased oxygen extraction. This "critical D_{O_2}" represents the point at which oxygen demand exceeds oxygen supply, anaerobic metabolism ensues, and lactate begins to accumulate (the beginning of the "oxygen supply *dependent*" portion of the V_{O_2}/D_{O_2} curve). The critical D_{O_2} is the same regardless of whether the decrease in D_{O_2} results from anemia, hypoxemia, and/or low CO (53). The

TABLE 71.2

OXYGEN EXTRACTION RATIO^a

A. Oxygen extraction ratio (O_2ER)

$$O_2ER = \frac{Sao_2 - Svo_2}{Sao_2}$$

Sao_2, arterial O_2 saturation; Svo_2, mixed venous O_2 saturation.

B. Interpretation of oxygen extraction ratio values

25%	Normal
30%–40%	Increased
40%–50%	Impending shock
>50%–60%	Shock, lactic acidosis

^{a}Based on mixed venous O_2 saturation.

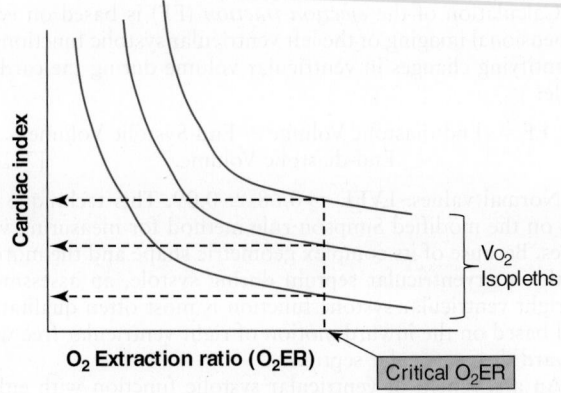

FIGURE 71.7. The curvilinear relationship between cardiac index and oxygen extraction ratio as oxygen consumption (Vo_2) varies. The critical oxygen extraction ratio remains the same; however, the critical delivery increases as O_2 demand increases.

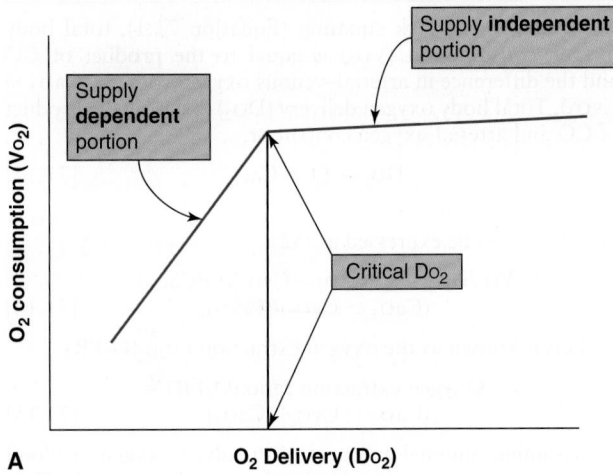

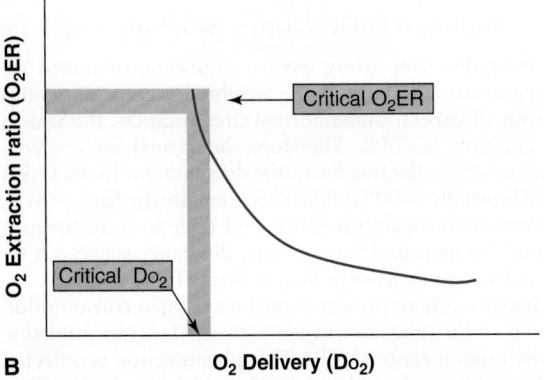

FIGURE 71.6. The relationship between oxygen delivery (Do_2), oxygen consumption (Vo_2), and oxygen extraction. A: Initially, as Do_2 decreases, Vo_2 remains constant as a result of an increase in O_2 extraction ratio (O_2ER), i.e., Vo_2 is independent of Do_2. As Do_2 decreases further, O_2ER increases further but not enough to maintain a constant Vo_2 (i.e., Vo_2 becomes dependent on Do_2). Without a change in O_2 demand, the critical Do_2 is defined when Vo_2 begins to fall. B: The critical Do_2 corresponds to a critical oxygen extraction ratio (O_2ER), where O_2ER has reached a maximum and cannot increase further to maintain Vo_2.

corresponding percent oxygen extraction represents the critical (i.e., maximal) O_2ER (Fig. 71.6B and Table 71.2). If oxygen demand were to change, the critical Do_2 would change in parallel; however, the indicator of the adequacy of tissue oxygenation, the critical O_2ER, remains constant between 50% and 60% (Fig. 71.7) (54,55,56).

Systemic Compensatory Circulatory Responses to Maintain Adequate Tissue Oxygenation

There are several different scenarios involving alterations in oxygen consumption, delivery, and extraction:

1. As oxygenation falls acutely, chemoreceptors are stimulated, which leads to neurohormonal activation and a compensatory increase in CO to maintain Do_2 and a normal oxygen extraction ratio. Over time, hemoglobin production increases to compensate for the decrease in oxygenation.

2. With an acute decrease in oxygen-carrying capacity (anemia), the resistance to ventricular ejection and venous return decreases, allowing for a compensatory increase in CO. Anemia also stimulates aortic chemoreceptors, leading to neurohormonal activation and increases in heart rate and contractility. Do_2 is maintained and the O_2ER remains normal. Over time, this acute response is complemented by an increase in intravascular volume.

3. With a decrease in oxygen content, the result of either arterial hypoxemia or anemia, there is a compensatory increase in CO, which preserves adequate Do_2 and a normal O_2ER. If the decrease in oxygen content is so large as to result in reduced Do_2 despite increased CO, then the O_2ER will begin continue. If the O_2ER exceeds the critical O_2ER (50-60%), anaerobic metabolism ensues.

4. Increases in oxygen demand are met by a commensurate increase in CO and the O_2ER remains stable unless the increase in oxygen demand is severe and/or the compensatory circulatory response is limited.

5. Vincent and De Backer have argued that the relationship between Do_2 and Vo_2 is highly individualized, especially in patients with ARDS or sepsis (57). Some

patients may develop supply-dependent Vo_2 at higher (or even normal) levels of Do_2. Hence, O_2ER (reflected by Svo_2) should be closely monitored in these critically ill patients, so that judicious therapies (e.g., fluid volume expansion, inotropic support, ventilator manipulations) may be targeted to return oxygen extraction to normal when supply-dependent Vo_2 is suspected.

Regional Compensatory Circulatory Responses to Maintain Adequate Tissue Oxygenation

A redistribution of CO is another mechanism by which the systemic circulation attempts to maintain oxygenation of the most vital organs. Organs that are less vital, such as the mesentery and dermis, and organs with considerable flow reserve, such as the kidneys, experience an increase in vascular resistance and a reduction in perfusion, as a result of activation of neurohormonal pathways. Vital organs such as the brain, myocardium, and diaphragm have sparse sympathetic innervation and are thus less responsive to sympathetic control and flow is maintained, if not augmented, as a result of a redistribution of CO. This represents an important compensatory mechanism, because these vital organs have high resting O_2ER, necessitating a relatively large percentage of CO under normal conditions, and an increase in flow as oxygen demand increases.

All organs are capable of microcirculatory adjustments that attempt to maintain regional perfusion and tissue oxygenation despite systemic circulatory influences. For most viscera, flow is tightly coupled to metabolism. Local metabolic regulation of vasomotor tone provides the homeostatic mechanism by which metabolic demand influences perfusion, producing stable O_2ERs despite modest changes in the determinants of oxygen delivery and consumption (52,58,59). When regional perfusion becomes limited, tissues compensate further by recruiting previously closed capillaries. The accumulation of adenosine, a byproduct of adenosine-5′-triphosphate utilization, and a decrease in tissue oxygen tension, as examples, lead to vascular recruitment, which enables tissue to extract a greater amount of oxygen. Vascular recruitment increases capillary density, shortening the diffusion distance for oxygen while increasing the capillary surface area available for gas exchange. In addition, the cross-sectional area of the individual vessel and that of the vascular bed increases. Because the linear velocity of blood is inversely related to the cross-sectional area, red blood cell velocity decreases and its transit time increases, increasing oxygen diffusion times and oxygen extraction.

There are some situations in which a normal or even reduced O_2ER is associated with a pathological state of impaired oxygen utilization. In cases such as in cyanide poisoning or in some patients with septic shock, tissues are unable to utilize oxygen even though adequate volumes of oxygen are delivered. Cyanide poisoning leads to impaired oxygen utilization and decreased O_2ER because of direct inhibition of mitochondrial respiration. Septic shock may lead to impaired oxygen utilization as peripheral vascular shunt channels are opened in muscle and other tissues thereby diverting Do_2 from tissue capillaries. Measured O_2ER decreases because of an admixture of shunted arterial blood into the venous circulation. In these states, serum lactate levels rise despite normal or reduced O_2ER.

The Oxygen–Hemoglobin Dissociation Curve

The shape and position of the oxygen–hemoglobin dissociation curve relate the partial pressure of oxygen to the percent oxygen bound to hemoglobin or the affinity of oxygen for hemoglobin

at varying partial pressures of oxygen. The P50 is the partial pressure of oxygen at which 50% of hemoglobin is saturated. A shift in the curve to the right, or an increased P50, represents a decrease in the affinity of oxygen for hemoglobin, whereas a shift to the left is reflective of an increase in affinity. The affinity of oxygen for hemoglobin is frequently altered, which may affect the loading and unloading of oxygen and the interpretation of venous oximetry. A decrease in the affinity of oxygen for hemoglobin is thought to be teleological in shock because it increases the efficiency of oxygen extraction. If this were true, an increased P50 would increase the critical O_2ER, while a decreased P50 would decrease the critical O_2ER. However, this does not appear to be the case. Regardless of the P50, the O_2ER increases in proportion to decreases in CO and Do_2. Whether the P50 is reduced (60) or increased (61), the efficiency of oxygen extraction and the critical O_2ER remains unchanged. At the critical O_2ER, the venous partial pressure of oxygen will be lowest in those with a reduced P50, intermediate in those with a normal P50, and highest in those with an increased P50. However, the critical O_2ER remains the same across all groups.

Central Venous Oximetry

Mixed venous oximetry may not be available, as placement of a pulmonary artery catheter is often not feasible. Alternative "central venous" sites for monitoring the global/systemic oxygen supply–demand relationship include the RA, which are close to and track changes in mixed venous O_2 saturation (62–64). The superior vena cava, jugular vein, and the inferior vena cava–right atrial junction have also been used for Svo_2 measurement. The normal oxygen extraction ($Sao_2 - Svo_2$) for the superior vena cava is 25%–30%, 30%–35% for the jugular vein, and 15%–20% for the right atria–inferior vena cava junction (65,66). As CO decreases, inferior vena cava O_2 saturations fall first, which is accompanied by a less severe drop in the pulmonary artery O_2 saturations, as blood flow is redistributed away from less vital organs. As CO falls further, superior vena cava and jugular O_2 saturations begin to decrease (62,66).

Advantages and Limitations of Venous Oximetry

There are several advantages and limitations of venous oximetry. It is not until the critical O_2ER is reached and the production of lactate exceeds its clearance that the serum lactate level may begin to rise. Therefore, a rising O_2ER provides an indication of impending shock while a lactic acidosis usually signifies a shock state. It should be noted that sepsis may lead to lactate accumulation for reasons other than inadequate oxygen supply relative to demand, including altered lactate clearance, abnormal pyruvate metabolism, and increased glycolysis (see below).

A determination of CO and Do_2 does not provide an indication of whether they are adequate to meet metabolic demand. Conversely, the O_2ER assesses the adequacy of Do_2 *relative* to Vo_2. However, the O_2ER does not necessarily reflect underlying cardiac function, CO, and Do_2, because Vo_2 varies considerably between and within disease states over time. Vo_2 is impractical to measure and there are several factors, which may increase it (**Table 71.3**). These factors must have remained constant in between O_2ER measurements before the clinician can conclude that an increase in O_2ER is likely caused by a decrease in Do_2.

The relationship between CO and O_2ER is curvilinear. Thus, for a given Vo_2, the O_2ER is relatively insensitive at detecting changes in CO as it falls from normal values. It is

TABLE 71.3

FACTORS THAT INCREASE OXYGEN CONSUMPTION

Catecholamines, endogenous and exogenous
Systemic inflammatory response
Fever
Pain or anxiety
Spontaneous respiration
Enteral nutrition

when CO becomes low that further decreases produce a large increase in the O_2ER (**Fig. 71.7**).

Just as systemic hemodynamic parameters (e.g., CO) do not necessarily reflect regional perfusion, systemic or global indicators of oxygen transport balance do not necessarily reflect the adequacy of regional tissue oxygenation (67–71). For example, the critical O_2ER for the splanchnic circulation is similar to the global or systemic critical O_2ER. However, as CO falls, the splanchnic O_2ER increases first and becomes critical sooner than does the global O_2ER (68).

Special considerations may apply to the use of venous oximetry after surgery for congenital heart disease. Right atrial oximetry is rendered useless in the presence of left-to-right intracardiac shunting. Because of streaming in the inferior vena cava, venous oximetry from this site should be obtained from the right atrial junction. For superior vena cava and jugular venous oximetry, changes in the arterial PCO_2 will, in the absence of changes in systemic perfusion, alter the cerebral O_2ER, as cerebral blood flow is uncoupled from cerebral metabolism.

Clinical Studies

Studies in children and adults have demonstrated improved outcomes in patients managed with venous oximetry. Venous oximetry has been studied extensively in severe sepsis and septic shock with the seminal study published by Rivers and colleagues in 2001 (72). Adults with severe sepsis and septic shock were randomized in the emergency department to receive either 6 hours of standard therapy, interventions based on CVP, blood pressure, and urine output, or "early goal-directed therapy" (EGDT), which included the targeting of an Svo_2 of ≥70%. The group randomized to EGDT had significantly less severe organ dysfunction and improved survival with an in-hospital mortality of 30.5% (vs. 46.5%, $p = 0.009$) and 28-day mortality of 33.3% (vs. 49.2%, $p = 0.01$). Of note, although the EGDT group had a significantly higher mean blood pressure during the initial 6 hours, all patients in both groups reached the goal mean blood pressure and there was no difference between groups for heart rate or CVP. Several studies since the original report by Rivers and colleagues have evaluated the impact of EGDT on outcomes in adults with severe sepsis and septic shock (73–76). These studies differed from the study by Rivers and colleagues in that they relied on historical controls; nonetheless, several single-center studies and one national study demonstrated a significant reduction in mortality following implementation of EGDT, whereas two inadequately powered studies did not demonstrate improved outcomes.

A study similar to that conducted by Rivers and colleagues was carried out by de Oliveira and colleagues in children with severe sepsis (77). Patients were recruited from the emergency department, inpatient unit, and ICU. The duration of the resuscitation protocol was 72 hours and the intervention group targeted an Svo_2 of ≥70%, which was obtained from the RA, or superior vena cava–right atrial or inferior vena cava–right

atrial junction. Those children in whom a Svo_2 of ≥70% was targeted had significantly less mortality at 28 days (11.8 vs. 39.2%, $p = 0.002$) and less organ dysfunction than the control group. And as was the case in the study by Rivers and colleagues, there was no difference in heart rate, mean blood pressure, or CVP between groups.

NEAR-INFRARED SPECTROSCOPY

Cerebral oximetry relies on the relative transparency of biological tissue such as skin and bone to near-infrared light, where oxy- and deoxyhemoglobin have distinct absorption spectra. The oximeter relies on the differential absorption of at least two light wavelengths of light and a dual-detector system that can subtract the effects of shallow signals, enabling the oximeter to estimate tissue oxygenation (78). The depth of the optical field is approximately half the source–detector distance, which is 4 cm in most devices. The source–detector distance and the subtraction algorithm allow the device to estimate oxygen saturations in a tissue sample ~1 cm^3 beneath the sensor. The algorithm evaluates the nonpulsatile signal of the microcirculation where 75%–85% of the blood volume is venous (79). Thus, the oxygen saturation is a surrogate for tissue venous oxygen saturation. Studies have demonstrated a very good correlation between cerebral oxygen saturations and jugular bulb and superior vena cava saturations (80–84). However, as with pulse oximeters, NIRS oximeters rely on a complex algorithm to convert the change in absorbance of at least two wavelengths of light to an absolute saturation value (85). Thus, while the correlation of pulse and NIRS oximetry with measured values is very good, these derived values may vary from measured values (85). Due to technical constraints such as these, the technology is limited to relative quantitation but is useful for tracking changes for a given patient (79).

Cerebral NIRS Oximetry

As indicated above, cerebral NIRS values correlate very well with superior vena cava and jugular saturations. Based on studies in humans and animals using venous and cerebral oximetry, the normal cerebral O_2ER is 35% and the critical cerebral O_2ER, corresponding to the onset of neurologic deficits and a rise in brain lactate levels, is similar to the global critical O_2ER at ~50%–60% (86–89). Slater and colleagues demonstrated in adults undergoing cardiac surgery that the duration of time with intraoperative cerebral saturations less than 50% was significantly associated with the development of neurocognitive decline (90). Dent and colleagues found a significant association between prolonged postoperative cerebral saturations less than 45% and the development of new or worsened ischemic lesions on magnetic resonance imaging following the Norwood procedure (91). While studies thus far are limited, intervention protocols based on intraoperative cerebral oximetry have been found to lessen the incidence and severity of neurologic injury and overall morbidity in adults and children following cardiac surgery (92–94).

Cerebral oximetry may also be used as an indicator of systemic or global oxygen transport balance (95). Li and colleagues found cerebral oxygen saturations to closely and negatively correlate with the systemic O_2ER (based on superior vena cava measurements). There are however important factors to consider when using cerebral oxygen saturations as indicator of systemic oxygenation. As CO becomes limited, blood flow is redistributed from less vital organs to maintain perfusion of the most vital organs, rendering cerebral oximetry a relatively late indicator of a falling CO. In addition, changes in the arterial P_{CO_2} uncouple cerebral blood flow from metabolism, confounding the relationship between cerebral and systemic hemodynamics. No study thus far has evaluated the use of postoperative cerebral oximetry and intervention protocols on outcomes following pediatric or adult cardiac surgery.

Renal and Mesenteric NIRS Oximetry

The rationale for monitoring renal and mesenteric oximetry is to provide an earlier indication of a falling CO than that provided by systemic/global parameters of tissue oxygenation (central or mixed venous oximetry and serum lactate levels) or cerebral oximetry. The normal mesenteric oxygen extraction is ~25%–35% and the critical O_2ER is similar to the global O_2ER at roughly 50%–60% (68). However, as CO falls and blood flow is redistributed, the mesenteric O_2ER increases first and becomes critical sooner than global parameters (67,68,71,96). Studies on mesenteric NIRS oximetry thus far have been limited. Kaufman and colleagues found a good correlation between intramural gastric pH (using gastric tonometry) and mesenteric NIRS (97). Additional studies are needed to evaluate the accuracy and utility of mesenteric oximetry. The kidneys are second only to the heart in terms of V_{O_2}. The vast majority of renal V_{O_2} occurs with active reabsorption of filtrate. Because renal sodium transport is coupled to renal blood flow, changes in renal V_{O_2} are met by corresponding changes in renal oxygen delivery (98,99). In addition, relative to metabolic demand, the kidneys receive a very high blood flow (~20% of CO), which results in a low oxygen extraction of ~10%–15% under normal conditions. As a result, the renal O_2ER increases appreciably only with significant decreases in renal D_{O_2} (100,101). Multisite oximetry (combined renal and cerebral) may provide a more sensitive indication of a falling CO than isolated cerebral oximetry (102,103). Additional studies are needed however to determine the accuracy and clinical utility of renal oximetry.

LACTATE

Measurement of lactate concentration does not readily conform to the ideals of hemodynamic monitoring: it is usually only intermittently available, requires invasive access, and is a relatively late indicator of tissue hypoxia. As a monitoring biomarker it adds useful information and has good clinical availability, but lacks a suitably high specificity, sensitivity, or predictive value (104). Irrespective of these drawbacks, it is considered to be a downstream surrogate of oxygen supply–demand balance, and an elevated level is abnormal. Some studies have suggested lactate levels associated with poor outcomes (105,106). To that end, it is routinely used as a tool to assess the adequacy of tissue perfusion.

It is increasingly recognized that an elevated lactate level may be due to either anaerobic (Type A) or aerobic (Type B) mechanisms acting alone or in combination. This is in keeping with situations in which hyperlactatemia fails to correlate with other indicators of inadequate oxygen delivery. In some cases, it may actually reflect a beneficial adaptive response to disease, facilitating energy distribution and conserving crucial glucose stores in cells where oxygen availability is reduced while preserving the redox state (105). Therefore, correctly interpreting the underlying mechanism of lactate elevation is important, ensuring that any intervention is timely and appropriate. In some cases, aggressive resuscitation may be unnecessary.

The final product in the glycolytic pathway (oxidation of glucose) is pyruvate, from which lactate is generated continuously under fully aerobic conditions according to the following reaction:

$$Pyruvate + NADH + H^+ = Lactate + NAD^+.$$

Predominantly favoring lactate production, the normal lactate/pyruvate ratio is around 10:1. Although the amount of lactate produced is around 1500 mmol/L/d, the normal circulating level is less than 2 mmol/L, reflecting the continuous balance between production and consumption (liver and kidneys) (105). The majority of lactate is produced in muscle, skin, brain, intestine, and red blood cells. In severe illness, the lungs and leucocytes can be a significant source, even in the absence of hypoxia. Lactate clearance principally occurs in the liver and to a lesser extent the kidney. Once the renal threshold is exceeded (usually around 5 mmol/L), renal excretion occurs. Therefore, hepatic or renal dysfunction in any disease state can contribute to a lactatemia.

Under hypoxic conditions, pyruvate production from glycolysis, irrespective of cause, exceeds the oxidative capacity of the mitochondria. Hypoxia blocks oxidative phosphorylation by halting the donation of electrons. ATP production falls, NADH fails to regenerate, and proton numbers overwhelm the mitochondrial capacity for their consumption. With demand now exceeding supply, alternative (nonmitochondrial) ATP turnover is utilized, further increasing proton numbers that cannot be reused by mitochondrial respiration. The result is a lowering of the cytosolic pH and an alteration of the cell's redox state by reducing the $NAD^+/NADH$ ratio. This promotes pyruvate accumulation and decreases pyruvate utilization because of the inhibition of pyruvate carboxylase and dehydrogenase. As a consequence, lactate dehydrogenase (LDH) is induced, converting significant quantities of pyruvate into lactate.

The term "lactic acidosis" is a sloppy term. It erroneously suggests that the production of a lactate molecule is accompanied by the generation of a proton. It should be very clear that glycolytic ATP production produces lactate and not lactic acid. In hypoxic conditions, H^+ is produced as a result of nonmitochondrial regeneration of ATP decreasing the cytosol redox, which collectively shifts the LDH equilibrium toward lactate production. Therefore, it is a consequence rather than a cause of acidosis. Lactate functions as a strong ion in the human body and is fully dissociated irrespective of how it enters the system. The unequal accumulation and/or removal of cations and anions directly contribute to an increase in H^+. This may also include ketone bodies resulting from the effects of epinephrine on free fatty acid flux.

With causes extending beyond that of hypoxia, hyperlactatemia is now viewed as more than just a waste product or an end point for resuscitation. With our increased, though incomplete, understanding of its role, it is perhaps evident why the prognostic value of lactate has never been completely clear. A raised level is still abnormal but, as suggested, may be a beneficial response to stress. Therefore, distinguishing between hypoxic and nonhypoxic causes could potentially prevent detrimental effects of over-resuscitation when striving for normalization of a number in isolation. Elevated lactate levels are used to activate adult goal-directed therapy protocols or identify high-risk postoperative pediatric cardiac patients on admission. A targeted reduction in arterial lactate may be beneficial. A rising or persistent level is a poor sign. More recently, it has been shown that lactate can act as a biomarker, identifying patients with presumed sepsis who have a higher likelihood of mortality even without any evidence of organ dysfunction (106). Perhaps early resuscitation in this group may improve outcome. An abnormal lactate should alert the physician to a probable inadequacy of oxygen delivery. Lactate levels should never be acted upon alone and other parameters should be assessed to determine any accompanying disturbance in oxygen transport balance.

CONCLUSIONS AND FUTURE DIRECTIONS

The physical examination and the use of routine hemodynamic monitoring are essential for determining a patient's cardiovascular status. However, it is imperative to have an acute appreciation of the limitations to this approach. The complementary use of additional monitoring modalities provides a much more robust and objective assessment of cardiovascular function and tissue oxygenation. This approach enables the clinician to make a more timely and accurate determination of the patient's clinical status and overall clinical trajectory, a strategy much more likely to lead to proactive rather than reactive therapeutic interventions.

References

1. Connors AF Jr, McCaffree DR, Gray BA. Evaluation of right-heart catheterization in the critically ill patient without acute myocardial infarction. *N Engl J Med* 1983;308:263–7.
2. Tibby SM, Hatherill M, Murdoch IA. Capillary refill and core-peripheral temperature gap as indicators of haemodynamic status in paediatric intensive care patients. *Arch Dis Child* 1999;80:163–6.
3. Tibby SM, Hatherill M, Marsh MJ, et al. Clinicians' abilities to estimate cardiac index in ventilated children and infants. *Arch Dis Child* 1997;77:516–8.
4. Lobos AT, Lee S, Menon K. Capillary refill time and cardiac output in children undergoing cardiac catheterization. *Pediatr Crit Care Med* 2012;13:136–40.
5. Steingrub JS, Celoria G, Vickers-Lahti M, et al. Therapeutic impact of pulmonary artery catheterization in a medical/surgical icu. *Chest* 1991;99:1451–5.
6. Eagle KA, Quertermous T, Singer DE, et al. Left ventricular ejection fraction. Physician estimates compared with gated blood pool scan measurements. *Arch Intern Med* 1988;148:882–5.
7. Mattleman SJ, Hakki AH, Iskandrian AS, et al. Reliability of bedside evaluation in determining left ventricular function: Correlation with left ventricular ejection fraction determined by radionuclide ventriculography. *J Am Coll Cardiol* 1983;1:417–20.
8. Stevenson LW, Perloff JK. The limited reliability of physical signs for estimating hemodynamics in chronic heart failure. *JAMA* 1989;261:884–8.
9. Carcillo JA, Kuch BA, Han YY, et al. Mortality and functional morbidity after use of PALS/APLS by community physicians. *Pediatrics* 2009;124:500–8.
10. Christi MJ. *Acta Pediatr* 2011;100:e27–e79.
11. Seear MD, Scarfe JC, LeBlanc JG. Predicting major adverse events after cardiac surgery in children. *Pediatr Crit Care Med* 2008;9(6):606–11.
12. Papadopoulos G, Mieke S, Elisaf M. Assessment of the performances of three oscillometric blood pressure monitors for neonates using a simulator. *Blood Press Monit* 1999;4:27–33.
13. Fernandez EG, Green TP, Sweeney M. Low inferior vena caval catheters for hemodynamic and pulmonary function monitoring in pediatric critical care patients. *Pediatr Crit Care Med* 2004;5:14–8.
14. Raper R, Sibbald WJ. Misled by the wedge? The swan-ganz catheter and left ventricular preload. *Chest* 1986;89:427–34.
15. Reuse C, Vincent JL, Pinsky MR. Measurements of right ventricular volumes during fluid challenge. *Chest* 1990;98:1450–4.
16. Forrester JS, Diamond G, McHugh TJ, et al. Filling pressures in the right and left sides of the heart in acute myocardial infarction. A reappraisal of central-venous-pressure monitoring. *N Engl J Med* 1971;285:190–3.
17. Toussaint GP, Burgess JH, Hampson LG. Central venous pressure and pulmonary wedge pressure in critical surgical illness. A comparison. *Arch Surg* 1974;109(2):265–9.
18. Swan HJ, Ganz W, Forrester J, et al. Catheterization of the heart in man with use of a flow-directed balloon-tipped catheter. *N Engl J Med* 1970;283:447–51.
19. Forrester JS, Ganz W, Diamond G, et al. Thermodilution cardiac output determination with a single flow-directed catheter. *Am Heart J* 1972;83:306–11.
20. Dalen JE, Bone RC. Is it time to pull the pulmonary artery catheter? *JAMA* 1996;276:916–8.
21. Chatterjee K. The swan-ganz catheters: Past, present, and future. A viewpoint. *Circulation* 2009;119:147–152.
22. Sandham JD, Hull RD, Brant RF, et al. A randomized, controlled trial of the use of pulmonary-artery catheters in high-risk surgical patients. *N Engl J Med* 2003;348:5–14.
23. Rhodes A, Cusack RJ, Newman PJ, et al. A randomised, controlled trial of the pulmonary artery catheter in critically ill patients. *Intensive Care Med* 2002;28:256–64.
24. Harvey S, Harrison DA, Singer M, et al. Assessment of the clinical effectiveness of pulmonary artery catheters in management of patients in intensive care (pac-man): A randomised controlled trial. *Lancet* 2005;366:472–7.
25. Connors AF Jr, Speroff T, Dawson NV, et al. The effectiveness of right heart catheterization in the initial care of critically ill patients. Support investigators. *JAMA* 1996;276:889–97.
26. Shah MR, O'Connor CM, Sopko G, et al. Evaluation study of congestive heart failure and pulmonary artery catheterization effectiveness (escape): Design and rationale. *Am Heart J* 2001;141:528–35.
27. Wheeler AP, Bernard GR, Thompson BT, et al. Pulmonary-artery versus central venous catheter to guide treatment of acute lung injury. *N Engl J Med* 2006;354:2213–24.
28. Binanay C, Califf RM, Hasselblad V, et al. Evaluation study of congestive heart failure and pulmonary artery catheterization effectiveness: The escape trial. *JAMA* 2005;294:1625–33.
29. Pulmonary Artery Catheter Consensus conference: Consensus statement. *Crit Care Med* 1997;25:910–25.
30. Rajaram SS, Desai NK, Kalra A, et al. Pulmonary artery catheters for adult patients in intensive care. *Cochrane Database Syst Rev* 2013;2:CD003408.
31. Sorensen MB, Bille-Brahe NE, Engell HC. Cardiac output measurement by thermal dilution: Reproducibility and comparison with the dye-dilution technique. *Ann Surg* 1976;183:67–72.
32. Wyse SD, Pfitzner J, Rees A, et al. Measurement of cardiac output by thermal dilution in infants and children. *Thorax* 1975;30:262–5.
33. Moodie DS, Feldt RH, Kaye MP, et al. Measurement of postoperative cardiac output by thermodilution in pediatric and adult patients. *J Thorac Cardiovasc Surg* 1979;78:796–8.
34. Borland LM. Allometric determination of the distance from the central venous pressure port to wedge position of balloon-tip catheters in pediatric patients. *Crit Care Med* 1986;14:974–6.
35. Proulx F, Lemson J, Choker G, et al. Hemodynamic monitoring by transpulmonary thermodilution and pulse contour analysis in critically ill children. *Pediatr Crit Care Med* 2011;12:459–66.
36. McLuckie A, Murdoch IA, Marsh MJ, et al. A comparison of pulmonary and femoral artery thermodilution cardiac indices in paediatric intensive care patients. *Acta Paediatr* 1996;85:336–8.
37. Tibby SM, Hatherill M, Marsh MJ, et al. Clinical validation of cardiac output measurements using femoral artery thermodilution with direct fick in ventilated children and infants. *Intensive Care Med* 1997;23:987–91.
38. Pauli C, Fakler U, Genz T, et al. Cardiac output determination in children: Equivalence of the transpulmonary thermodilution method to the direct fick principle. *Intensive Care Med* 2002;28:947–52.
39. Fakler U, Pauli C, Balling G, et al. Cardiac index monitoring by pulse contour analysis and thermodilution after pediatric cardiac surgery. *J Thorac Cardiovasc Surg* 2007;133:224–8.
40. Mahajan A, Shabanie A, Turner J, et al. Pulse contour analysis for cardiac output monitoring in cardiac surgery for congenital heart disease. *Anesth Analg* 2003;97:1283–8.

41. Weekes AJ, Quirke DP. Emergency echocardiography. *Emerg Med Clin North Am* 2011;29:759–87, vi–vii.

42. Manasia AR, Nagaraj HM, Kodali RB, et al. Feasibility and potential clinical utility of goal-directed transthoracic echocardiography performed by noncardiologist intensivists using a small hand-carried device (sonoheart) in critically ill patients. *J Cardiothorac Vasc Anesth* 2005;19:155–9.

43. Kobal SL, Trento L, Baharami S, et al. Comparison of effectiveness of hand-carried ultrasound to bedside cardiovascular physical examination. *Am J Cardiol* 2005;96:1002–6.

44. Spurney CF, Sable CA, Berger JT, et al. Use of a hand-carried ultrasound device by critical care physicians for the diagnosis of pericardial effusions, decreased cardiac function, and left ventricular enlargement in pediatric patients. *J Am Soc Echocardiogr* 2005;18:313–9.

45. Carabello BA, Crawford FA Jr. Valvular heart disease. *N Engl J Med* 1997;337(1):32–41.

46. Weekes AJ, Tassone HM, Babcock A, et al. Comparison of serial qualitative and quantitative assessments of caval index and left ventricular systolic function during early fluid resuscitation of hypotensive emergency department patients. *Acad Emerg Med* 2011;18:912–21.

47. King ME, Braun H, Goldblatt A, et al. Interventricular septal configuration as a predictor of right ventricular systolic hypertension in children: A cross-sectional echocardiographic study. *Circulation* 1983;68:68–75.

48. Buheitel G, Hofbeck M, Tenbrink U, et al. Possible sources of right-to-left shunting in patients following a total cavopulmonary connection. *Cardiol Young* 1998;8:358–63.

49. Fernandez-Martorell P, Sklansky MS, Lucas VW, et al. Accessory hepatic vein to pulmonary venous atrium as a cause of cyanosis after the fontan operation. *Am J Cardiol* 1996;77:1386–7.

50. Gatzoulis MA, Shinebourne EA, Redington AN, et al. Increasing cyanosis early after cavopulmonary connection caused by abnormal systemic venous channels. *Br Heart J* 1995;73:182–6.

51. McElhinney DB, Reddy VM, Hanley FL, et al. Systemic venous collateral channels causing desaturation after bidirectional cavopulmonary anastomosis: Evaluation and management. *J Am Coll Cardiol* 1997;30:817–24.

52. Vincent JL. Determination of oxygen delivery and consumption versus cardiac index and oxygen extraction ratio. *Crit Care Clin* 1996;12(4):995–1006.

53. Cain SM. Oxygen delivery and uptake in dogs during anemic and hypoxic hypoxia. *J Appl Physiol* 1977;42:228–34.

54. Dantzker DR, Foresman B, Gutierrez G. Oxygen supply and utilization relationships. A reevaluation. *Am Rev Respir Dis* 1991;143:675–9.

55. Baigorri F, Russell JA. Oxygen delivery in critical illness. *Crit Care Clin* 1996;12:971–94.

56. Ermakov S, Hoyt JW. Pulmonary artery catheterization. *Crit Care Clin* 1992;8:773–806.

57. Vincent JL, De Backer D. Oxygen transport—the oxygen delivery controversy. *Intensive Care Med* 2004;30:1990–6.

58. Woodson RD, Wills RE, Lenfant C. Effect of acute and established anemia on O_2 transport at rest, submaximal and maximal work. *J Appl Physiol* 1978;44:36–43.

59. Cain SM. Peripheral oxygen uptake and delivery in health and disease. *Clin Chest Med* 1983;4:139–48.

60. Schumacker PT, Long GR, Wood LD. Tissue oxygen extraction during hypovolemia: Role of hemoglobin p50. *J Appl Physiol* 1987;62:1801–7.

61. Curtis SE, Walker TA, Bradley WE, et al. Raising p50 increases tissue Po_2 in canine skeletal muscle but does not affect critical O_2 extraction ratio. *J Appl Physiol* 1997;83:1681–9.

62. Lee J, Wright F, Barber R, et al. Central venous oxygen saturation in shock: A study in man. *Anesthesiology* 1972;36:472–8.

63. Davies GG, Mendenhall J, Symreng T. Measurement of right atrial oxygen saturation by fiberoptic oximetry accurately reflects mixed venous oxygen saturation in swine. *J Clin Monit* 1988;4:99–102.

64. Perez AC, Eulmesekian PG, Minces PG, et al. Adequate agreement between venous oxygen saturation in right atrium and pulmonary artery in critically ill children. *Pediatr Crit Care Med* 2009;10:76–9.

65. Barratt-Boyes BG, Wood EH. The oxygen saturation of blood in the venae cavae, right-heart chambers, and pulmonary vessels of healthy subjects. *J Lab Clin Med* 1957;50:93–106.

66. Scheinman MM, Brown MA, Rapaport E. Critical assessment of use of central venous oxygen saturation as a mirror of mixed venous oxygen in severely ill cardiac patients. *Circulation* 1969;40:165–72.

67. Landow L, Phillips DA, Heard SO, et al. Gastric tonometry and venous oximetry in cardiac surgery patients. *Crit Care Med* 1991;19:1226–33.

68. Nelson DP, King CE, Dodd SL, et al. Systemic and intestinal limits of O_2 extraction in the dog. *J Appl Physiol* 1987;63:387–94.

69. Dahn MS, Lange MP, Jacobs LA. Central mixed and splanchnic venous oxygen saturation monitoring. *Intensive Care Med* 1988;14:373–8.

70. Uusaro A, Ruokonen E, Takala J. Splanchnic oxygen transport after cardiac surgery: Evidence for inadequate tissue perfusion after stabilization of hemodynamics. *Intensive Care Med* 1996;22:26–33.

71. Hamilton-Davies C, Mythen MG, Salmon JB, et al. Comparison of commonly used clinical indicators of hypovolaemia with gastrointestinal tonometry. *Intensive Care Med* 1997;23:276–81.

72. Rivers E, Nguyen B, Havstad S, et al. Early goal-directed therapy in the treatment of severe sepsis and septic shock. *N Engl J Med* 2001;345:1368–77.

73. Levy MM, Dellinger RP, Townsend SR, et al. The surviving sepsis campaign: Results of an international guideline-based performance improvement program targeting severe sepsis. *Intensive Care Med* 2010;36:222–31.

74. Micek ST, Roubinian N, Heuring T, et al. Before-after study of a standardized hospital order set for the management of septic shock. *Crit Care Med* 2006;34:2707–13.

75. Focht A, Jones AE, Lowe TJ. Early goal-directed therapy: Improving mortality and morbidity of sepsis in the emergency department. *Jt Comm J Qual Patient Saf* 2009;35:186–91.

76. Ferrer R, Artigas A, Levy MM, et al. Improvement in process of care and outcome after a multicenter severe sepsis educational program in spain. *JAMA* 2008;299:2294–303.

77. de Oliveira CF, de Oliveira DS, Gottschald AF, et al. ACCM/PALS haemodynamic support guidelines for paediatric septic shock: An outcomes comparison with and without monitoring central venous oxygen saturation. *Intensive Care Med* 2008;34:1065–75.

78. Ghanayem NS, Wernovsky G, Hoffman GM. Near-infrared spectroscopy as a hemodynamic monitor in critical illness. *Pediatr Crit Care Med* 2011;12:S27–S32.

79. MacLeod DB, Ikeda K, Vacchiano C, et al. Development and validation of a cerebral oximeter capable of absolute accuracy. *J Cardiothorac Vasc Anesth* 2012;26:1007–14.

80. Li J, Van Arsdell GS, Zhang G, et al. Assessment of the relationship between cerebral and splanchnic oxygen saturations measured by near-infrared spectroscopy and direct measurements of systemic haemodynamic variables and oxygen transport after the Norwood procedure. *Heart* 2006;92:1678–85.

81. Kirshbom PM, Forbess JM, Kogon BE, et al. Cerebral near infrared spectroscopy is a reliable marker of systemic perfusion in awake single ventricle children. *Pediatr Cardiol* 2007;28:42–5.

82. Abdul-Khaliq H, Troitzsch D. Cerebral oxygen monitoring during neonatal cardiopulmonary bypass and deep hypothermic circulatory arrest. *Thorac Cardiovasc Surg* 2003;51:52–3.

83. Daubeney PE, Pilkington SN, Janke E, et al. Cerebral oxygenation measured by near-infrared spectroscopy: Comparison with jugular bulb oximetry. *Ann Thorac Surg* 1996;61:930–4.

84. Ranucci M, Isgro G, De la Torre T, et al. Near-infrared spectroscopy correlates with continuous superior vena cava oxygen saturation in pediatric cardiac surgery patients. *Paediatr Anaesth* 2008;18:1163–9.

85. Fouzas S, Priftis KN, Anthracopoulos MB. Pulse oximetry in pediatric practice. *Pediatrics* 2011;128:740–52.

86. Kurth CD, Levy WJ, McCann J. Near-infrared spectroscopy cerebral oxygen saturation thresholds for hypoxia-ischemia in piglets. *J Cereb Blood Flow Metab* 2002;22:335–41.

87. Levy WJ, Levin S, Chance B. Near-infrared measurement of cerebral oxygenation. Correlation with electroencephalographic ischemia during ventricular fibrillation. *Anesthesiology* 1995;83:738–46.

88. Hou X, Ding H, Teng Y, et al. Research on the relationship between brain anoxia at different regional oxygen saturations and brain damage using near-infrared spectroscopy. *Physiol Meas* 2007;28:1251–65.

89. Schell RM, Cole DJ. Cerebral monitoring: Jugular venous oximetry. *Anesth Analg* 2000;90:559–66.

90. Slater JP, Guarino T, Stack J, et al. Cerebral oxygen desaturation predicts cognitive decline and longer hospital stay after cardiac surgery. *Ann Thorac Surg* 2009;87:36–44; discussion 44–5.

91. Dent CL, Spaeth JP, Jones BV, et al. Brain magnetic resonance imaging abnormalities after the Norwood procedure using regional cerebral perfusion. *J Thorac Cardiovasc Surg* 2006;131:190–7.

92. Murkin JM, Adams SJ, Pardy E, et al. Monitoring brain oxygen saturation during coronary bypass surgery improves outcomes in diabetic patients: A post hoc analysis. *Heart Surg Forum* 2011;14:E1–E6.

93. Murkin JM, Adams SJ, Novick RJ, et al. Monitoring brain oxygen saturation during coronary bypass surgery: A randomized, prospective study. *Anesth Analg* 2007;104:51–8.

94. Austin EH III, Edmonds HL Jr, Auden SM, et al. Benefit of neurophysiologic monitoring for pediatric cardiac surgery. *J Thorac Cardiovasc Surg* 1997;114:707–15, 717; discussion 715–6.

95. Li J, Zhang G, Holtby H, et al. The influence of systemic hemodynamics and oxygen transport on cerebral oxygen saturation in neonates after the Norwood procedure. *J Thorac Cardiovasc Surg* 2008;135:83–90, 90.e1–90.e2

96. Fiddian-Green RG, Baker S. Predictive value of the stomach wall pH for complications after cardiac operations: Comparison with other monitoring. *Crit Care Med* 1987;15:153–6.

97. Kaufman J, Almodovar MC, Zuk J, et al. Correlation of abdominal site near-infrared spectroscopy with gastric tonometry in infants following surgery for congenital heart disease. *Pediatr Crit Care Med* 2008;9:62–8.

98. Lassen NA, Munck O, Thaysen JH. Oxygen consumption and sodium reabsorption in the kidney. *Acta Physiol Scand* 1961;51:371–84.

99. Bradley SE, Halperin MH. Renal oxygen consumption in man during abdominal compression. *J Clin Invest* 1948;27:635–8.

100. Nitter-Hauge S, Brodwall EK. Influence of variations in blood flow on renal A-V oxygen difference and renal oxygen consumption in heart failure. A clinical study. *Am Heart J* 1975;90:445–50.

101. Gotshall RW, Miles DS, Sexson WR. Renal oxygen delivery and consumption during progressive hypoxemia in the anesthetized dog. *Proc Soc Exp Biol Med* 1983;174:363–7.

102. Chakravarti SB, Mittnacht AJ, Katz JC, et al. Multisite near-infrared spectroscopy predicts elevated blood lactate level in children after cardiac surgery. *J Cardiothorac Vasc Anesth* 2009;23:663–7.

103. Hoffman GM, Stuth EA, Jaquiss RD, et al. Changes in cerebral and somatic oxygenation during stage 1 palliation of hypoplastic left heart syndrome using continuous regional cerebral perfusion. *J Thorac Cardiovasc Surg* 2004;127:223–33.

104. Buijs EA, Zwiers AJ, Ista E, et al. Biomarkers and clinical tools in critically ill children: Are we heading toward tailored drug therapy? *Biomark Med* 2012;6:239–57.

105. Levy B. Lactate and shock state: The metabolic view. *Curr Opin Crit Care* 2006;12:315–21.

106. Mikkelsen ME, Miltiades AN, Gaieski DF, et al. Serum lactate is associated with mortality in severe sepsis independent of organ failure and shock. *Crit Care Med* 2009;37:1670–7.

CHAPTER 72 ■ HEART FAILURE: ETIOLOGY, PATHOPHYSIOLOGY, AND DIAGNOSIS

MARY E. MCBRIDE, JOHN M. COSTELLO, AND CONRAD L. EPTING

KEY POINTS

Introduction

1 An estimated 11,000–14,000 children are hospitalized for heart failure each year in the United States, approximately 7% of whom die prior to hospital discharge.

Etiology

2 Heart failure in patients with structural heart disease is often caused by ventricular volume or pressure overload.
3 Patients with single ventricle physiology are particularly prone to the development of heart failure.
4 Primary cardiomyopathies are the most common etiology of heart failure in patients with structurally normal hearts.

Pathophysiology

5 The common physiologic feature of heart failure is a shift in the diastolic pressure–volume relationship to preserve stroke volume at a higher end-diastolic volume (EDV) and filling pressure.
6 Neurohormonal compensation is critical early in heart failure, yet it becomes maladaptive when sustained.

Classification and Evaluation

7 For patients with acute heart failure, initial diagnostic testing should be individualized on the basis of the clinical scenario.

The clinical features of heart failure, including dyspnea and edema, have been recognized since Greco-Roman times when they were thought to originate in the brain, and the heart was presumed to be a heater. In the 17th century, Harvey discovered the pumping capacity of the heart and also found that valvar abnormalities could produce clinical symptoms of heart failure (1). Our modern understanding of heart failure appreciates the associated clinical features in the context of their underlying genetic, biochemical, and cellular mechanisms. Heart failure is now recognized as a clinical syndrome encompassing various signs and symptoms, and an array of cardiovascular structural and functional abnormalities, which lead to increased intracardiac filling pressures, elevation of neurohormonal mediators, systemic inflammation, and premature myocyte death.

Heart failure contributes substantially to morbidity and mortality in children. The annual incidence of heart failure in the United States alone has been estimated, by extrapolated data from several studies, to between 12,000 and 35,000 cases (2). Administrative data suggest that 11,000–14,000 children are hospitalized for heart failure each year in the United States, approximately 7% of whom die prior to hospi-

1 tal discharge (3). A growing number of adults surviving with congenital heart disease are also afflicted with heart failure (4).

This chapter will review our contemporary understanding of the etiology, pathophysiology, classification, and evaluation of infants and children with acute heart failure. Management of these patients is reviewed in Chapters 74 and 75, and the evaluation and treatment for acute, transient myocardial dysfunction after cardiopulmonary bypass are covered in Chapter 79.

ETIOLOGY

The underlying causes of pediatric heart failure are diverse and, most simply, can be broadly divided into structural and myocardial heart diseases (**Table 72.1**). This list of etiologies is quite different from that seen in adults and includes both cardiac and noncardiac causes. More common conditions are briefly reviewed below.

Structural Heart Disease

Many infants and children with congenital and acquired structural heart disease are at risk for developing heart failure. Broadly speaking, heart failure in patients with structural heart disease is often caused by chronic ventricular volume or
2 pressure overload. Volume overload may be caused by left-to-right shunting or valvar regurgitation. Pressure overload may be due to left or right ventricular outflow tract obstruction or high systemic or pulmonary vascular resistance (PVR). Less commonly, coronary ischemia or incessant arrhythmias may be the fundamental problem. In some cases, a combination of the above factors may be present.

Volume Overload

Significant left-to-right shunts lead to left ventricular volume overload and clinical signs and symptoms of heart failure. The pulmonary blood flow is a combination of systemic venous return as well as flow across the shunt, the entirety of

TABLE 72.1

ETIOLOGY OF PEDIATRIC HEART FAILURE

I. Structural heart disease
  a. Volume overload
    i. Left-to-right shunts
      1. Ventricular septal defect
      2. Atrioventricular septal defect
      3. Patent ductus arteriosus
      4. Aortopulmonary window
      5. Systemic arteriovenous malformation
    ii. Valvular regurgitation
      1. Aortic regurgitation
      2. Mitral regurgitation
      3. Tricuspid regurgitation
      4. Pulmonary regurgitation
  b. Pressure overload
    i. Right ventricular outflow tract obstruction
      1. Pulmonary stenosis
      2. Peripheral pulmonary stenosis
    ii. Left ventricular outflow tract obstruction
      1. Critical aortic stenosis
      2. Critical coarctation
  c. Complex congenital heart disease
    i. Congenitally corrected transposition of the great arteries
    ii. Common arterial trunk (truncus arteriosus)
    iii. VSD with IAA
    iv. Functionally single ventricle
      1. Fontan physiology

II. Myocardial heart disease
  a. Cardiomyopathy
    i. Dilated cardiomyopathy
    ii. Hypertrophic cardiomyopathy
    iii. Restrictive cardiomyopathy
    iv. Tachycardia-induced cardiomyopathy
    v. Arrhythmogenic right ventricular cardiomyopathy
    vi. Left ventricular noncompaction
    vii. Myocardial ischemia
  b. Systemic disease
    i. Sepsis/septic shock
    ii. Postarrest myocardial dysfunction
    iii. Systemic hypertension
    iv. Pulmonary hypertension
    v. Thyrotoxicosis
    vi. Transient dysfunction after cardiopulmonary bypass

which returns to the left ventricle. The resultant increase in left ventricular size results in muscle fiber lengthening, thereby increasing myocardial contractility and stroke volume (5). Tachycardia and increased stroke volume serve to augment cardiac output. A classic example is the young infant with a large ventricular septal defect. As the PVR drops in the weeks following birth, the degree of left-to-right shunting increases. Such patients typically present with tachypnea, tachycardia, poor weight gain, and diaphoresis with feeds (2). Increased return to the left side eventually results in remodeling, leading to an elevation of diastolic pressure, and contributing to left atrial hypertension. Increased pulmonary venous pressures, coupled with increased pulmonary blood flow, contribute to interstitial lung water and pulmonary edema and result in tachypnea. Chronic tachycardia contributes to preservation of cardiac output, and the constant exercise (tachycardia, tachypnea) drives up caloric consumption contributing

to failure to thrive. Ventricular systolic function is typically preserved, and thus in the overwhelming majority of cases, a low cardiac output state does not exist. Other commonly encountered left-to-right shunt lesions are listed in **Table 72.1**.

Atrioventricular and semilunar valve regurgitation may also result in a volume-overloaded state that can present with signs and symptoms of heart failure. Patients at risk for developing left-sided heart failure include those with severe aortic or mitral insufficiency or atrioventricular septal defects with important valvar regurgitation (2). Endocarditis or rheumatic heart disease are examples of acquired conditions that may result in significant left-sided valvar disease. Right-sided heart failure may also be caused or exacerbated by regurgitation of the tricuspid or pulmonary valves. Severe cases of Ebstein's anomaly and patients with long-standing pulmonary regurgitation after tetralogy of Fallot repair are classic examples.

Pressure Overload

Infants and children with ventricular outflow tract obstruction may develop heart failure. Significant obstruction to systemic or pulmonary blood flow leads to ventricular myocyte hypertrophy, eventually reducing end-diastolic volume (EDV), increasing ventricular wall stress, decreasing ventricular compliance, subendocardial ischemia from insufficient coronary blood flow, and, ultimately, poor cardiac output. This physiology may be seen in neonates with critical aortic stenosis, in whom cardiac output is dependent on ductal flow and the work of the right ventricle (2). Such patients may become symptomatic shortly after birth if the ductus arteriosus constricts and the right ventricle is no longer able to adequately provide systemic cardiac output. Right ventricular failure may develop in neonates with critical pulmonary stenosis, who also may have hypoxemia related to right-to-left shunting at the atrial level. Right ventricular failure in the setting of pressure overload may also be seen in pulmonary artery stenosis, conduit stenosis, and pulmonary hypertension.

Right ventricular pressure load can ultimately affect left ventricular performance due to the effects of interventricular dependence. As the right ventricle ejects against significant right ventricular outflow tract obstruction or increased PVR, the trans-septal pressure gradient reverses. The interventricular septum begins to flatten and then bow into the left ventricle. This in turn decreases left ventricular compliance, which may ultimately lead to a state of biventricular failure (6).

Complex Congenital Heart Disease

Select patients with complex cardiac lesions are at particular risk for developing heart failure. A combination of volume and pressure overload, reduced ventricular muscle mass, as well as primary myocardial dysfunction may be present. For example, in patients with congenitally corrected transposition of the great arteries, the left-sided morphologic right ventricle functions to support the systemic circulation. The right ventricle is not morphologically designed to perform this task and is intrinsically prone to failure if chronically operating at systemic pressures. Furthermore, the Ebsteinoid-like tricuspid valve is prone to regurgitation (7). Some patients with corrected transposition also have a ventricular septal defect, which may be the source of additional ventricular volume load (8). Approximately 30% of such patients will develop advanced heart block during the first several decades of life, leading to atrioventricular dysynchrony and worsening myocardial function. Long-term survivors after complex congenital heart surgery are at risk of developing heart failure. Fifty percent of patients with a systemic right ventricle will develop heart failure symptoms by age 20 (9).

Patients with single ventricle physiology are particularly prone to the development of heart failure. Due to the fact that the single ventricle must support both the systemic and pulmonary circulations at systemic pressure, both volume and pressure overload are initially present in all cases. Variable degrees of systemic or pulmonary outflow obstruction are often present, along with atrioventricular valve regurgitation and intrinsic myocardial dysfunction (8). Repeated periods of myocardial ischemia-reperfusion injury may occur during staged surgical palliation. The Fontan circulation is a unique framework for heart failure. Pulmonary blood flow is passive and can lead to under filling of the systemic ventricle. Patients at greater risk include those with a systemic right ventricle, significant atrioventricular valve regurgitation, or a nonsinus rhythm (8). These patients typically develop exercise intolerance (10).

Myocardial Heart Disease

Cardiomyopathy

In patients with structurally normal hearts, primary cardiomyopathies are the most common etiology of heart failure (2). A multidisciplinary writing group recently proposed the following definition:

Cardiomyopathies are a heterogeneous group of diseases of the myocardium associated with mechanical and/or electrical dysfunction that usually (but not invariably) exhibit inappropriate ventricular hypertrophy or dilatation and are due to a variety of causes that frequently are genetic. Cardiomyopathies either are confined to the heart or are part of generalized systemic disorders, often leading to cardiovascular death or progressive heart failure–related disability (11).

Traditionally, cardiomyopathies have been classified into dilated, hypertrophic and restrictive subtypes. However applying this scheme rigidly is a challenge because nearly 10% of patients have features of more than one subtype (12).

The Pediatric Cardiomyopathy Registry was developed in 1994 to study and follow the epidemiology and course of pediatric cardiomyopathy patients (13). This registry obtains data from 11 pediatric cardiology centers in North America. Data from this registry have been used to generate insight into the epidemiology, clinical presentations, and outcome of cardiomyopathies in children (12,14).

Dilated Cardiomyopathy

Of pediatric cardiomyopathies, the dilated phenotype is most commonly encountered, present in approximately one-half of cases. The incidence of dilated cardiomyopathy in the United States has been estimated at 0.56 cases per 100,000 children per year (14). Risk factors for the development of dilated cardiomyopathy include male gender, African American heritage, and an age less than 1 year (14,15). Dilated cardiomyopathy is characterized by a dilated and poorly functioning left ventricle without compensatory left ventricular wall hypertrophy. In approximately two-thirds of cases, the cause cannot be readily identified and thus are deemed idiopathic (14). Of cases with known etiologies, myocarditis and neuromuscular disorders are most common. One well-known example is mutations in dystrophin, which cause Duchenne muscular dystrophy (15). Dilated cardiomyopathy can also be seen with toxic, nutritional and endocrine-related etiologies, as well as inborn errors of metabolism (15).

While some cases of myocarditis and idiopathic dilated cardiomyopathy appear to be on a continuum clinically, there is prognostic value in distinguishing the two because there is a better chance for recovery in patients with myocarditis.

Currently, no single clinical test exists to reliably make this distinction. However, laboratory markers of inflammation, myocardial biopsy, microbiological tests, and cardiac MRI may have a role in the diagnostic process (15).

Hypertrophic Cardiomyopathy

Hypertrophic cardiomyopathy is characterized by a hypertrophied, nondilated ventricle in the absence of other disease processes (16). Approximately one-third of pediatric cardiomyopathy patients have a hypertrophic phenotype (12). The incidence of pediatric hypertrophic cardiomyopathy is 0.47 per 100,000 children per year, with most cases diagnosed in the first year of life (13). The vast majority of cases of hypertrophic cardiomyopathy are idiopathic in nature, but others are the result of inborn errors of metabolism (e.g., Pompe disease), malformation syndromes (e.g., Noonan or Costello syndrome), and neuromuscular disorders (e.g., Friedrich ataxia) (17). Pediatric patients with hypertrophic cardiomyopathy can present with classic symptoms of congestive heart failure but more commonly present with chest pain, arrhythmias, or exercise intolerance. Infants are more likely to die from congestive symptoms, whereas older children are at greater risk for sudden cardiac death. The risk of sudden death has been reported in the range of 1%–8% per year, depending on age and other factors (18).

Restrictive Cardiomyopathy

Restrictive cardiomyopathy is defined by its unique physiology, which presents largely with significant diastolic dysfunction. Ventricular size, systolic function, and wall thickness are all typically normal, as are atrioventricular valve morphology and function (19). Marked bi-atrial enlargement is present due to chronically elevated ventricular filling pressures. Restrictive cardiomyopathy can be a primary or secondary disease process. Restrictive cardiomyopathies may have genetic (e.g., sarcomeric mutations), acquired (e.g., sarcoidosis), and mixed (e.g., amyloidosis) etiologies (19). Restrictive cardiomyopathy is very rare, with an estimated incidence in the United States of 0.04 per 100,000 children per year (19). Approximately 3% of pediatric cardiomyopathies have a restrictive phenotype (12). Of note, restrictive cardiomyopathy is more commonly encountered in selected areas of Africa, South America, and Asia in the setting of endomyocardial fibrosis (20). Children afflicted with restrictive cardiomyopathy can present with signs and symptoms of congestive failure, failure to thrive, or syncope (21). These patients are at risk for sudden death due to ischemia and ischemia-related complications (21). Pulmonary hypertension may also be a significant issue.

Tachycardia-Induced Cardiomyopathy

The presence of a prolonged rapid heart rate can result in a phenotypic presentation that mimics dilated cardiomyopathy. Supraventricular tachycardias, such as atrial flutter or orthodromic reciprocating tachycardia, are most commonly encountered. Sustained ventricular arrhythmias may occasionally precipitate heart failure. Ion channelopathies, including catecholaminergic polymorphic ventricular tachycardia, and Brugada syndrome are examples of genetic disorders resulting in mutations in myocardial ion channels. These patients can present with sudden death or malignant ventricular arrhythmias resulting in acute myocardial dysfunction (11). The presence of a nonsinus tachycardia in the setting of a cardiomyopathy is an important finding regarding prognosis. If an arrhythmia is the primary disease process, conversion to sinus rhythm or rate control almost always improves cardiac function (22).

Arrhythmogenic Right Ventricular Cardiomyopathy/Dysplasia

Arrhythmogenic right ventricular cardiomyopathy/dysplasia (ARVC/D) is characterized by fatty infiltration of the right ventricular free wall. Roughly one-third of cases are familial, and several gene mutations have been identified (22). Making the diagnosis of ARVC/D can be difficult, but the electrocardiogram, cardiac MRI, and a high index of suspicion are helpful (22). The electrocardiogram can show T-wave inversions, an epsilon wave and QRS duration greater than 110 ms in V_1–V_3. A cardiac MRI may show fibrous and fatty changes in the right ventricle (23). Afflicted patients may present with decreased right ventricular function, arrhythmias, and sudden death (22).

Ventricular Noncompaction

Left ventricular noncompaction was recently categorized as a unique form of cardiomyopathy (11). The incidence is unknown but thought to be quite rare (24). Noncompaction refers to the pathologic finding of a developmental failure to form compact ventricular myocardium. In afflicted patients, the normal developmental process of myocardial compaction is arrested *in utero*, leading to excessive and unusual trabeculation, typically most evident in the apical aspect of the left ventricle (24). Noncompaction cardiomyopathy may exist in isolation or in association with congenital heart disease, specifically AV septal defects, pulmonary stenosis, and hypoplastic left heart syndrome (24). Noncompaction may present as an incidental finding, or with heart failure or arrhythmias. The diagnosis may be established by echocardiogram or cardiac MRI. Noncompacted left ventricles may have decreased systolic function, chamber dilation, and hypertrophy with characteristic heavy trabeculations (24).

Myocardial Ischemia

Ischemic cardiomyopathy is a common disorder among adults but is relatively rare in children. In patients with an anomalous left coronary artery from the pulmonary artery, myocardial ischemia often develops as PVR falls and coronary blood flow runs off into the low-resistance pulmonary circulation. Although uncommon with current surgical techniques, coronary ischemia may develop after any operation involving the aortic root or coronary arteries. In patients with Kawasaki disease who develop coronary aneurysms, luminal stenosis or thrombosis may occur, either of which may cause myocardial ischemia (25). Ischemic cardiomyopathy can present with congestive symptoms as well as arrhythmias, chest pain, syncope, and sudden death. Echocardiographic evaluation may demonstrate regional wall motion abnormalities and papillary muscle dysfunction with mitral regurgitation.

Rejection of the Transplanted Heart

The transplanted heart is at risk for rejection. Rejection is an immune response against the myocytes and endothelial cells resulting in a myocardial inflammation, cytokine release, and cell death from necrosis (26). The incidence of rejection is higher in the first 3 months after transplantation with an incidence of 0.8 rejections per month. Subsequently, the rejection rate is approximately 0.1 rejection episodes per month (26). When compared with adults, rejection in children is twice as likely to cause hemodynamic compromise (26).

Systemic Diseases

A number of systemic diseases may result in heart failure. Of children with severe sepsis or septic shock, nearly one-half have secondary myocardial dysfunction (27). Septic patients may exhibit systolic and diastolic dysfunction, thought to be due to mitochondrial dysfunction as well as infiltration of immune cells into the myocardium (27). This is a reversible process, with recovery of myocardial function expected within a week of the onset of sepsis (27).

Postresuscitation myocardial dysfunction is a well-described phenomenon (28). The postarrest state is characterized by myocardial edema, which results in decreased contractility, reduced left ventricular EDV, and impaired relaxation. The catecholamine surge that occurs after a cardiac arrest increases afterload and decreases microcirculatory blood flow. Postresuscitation myocardial dysfunction typically improves over several days.

Patients with significant systemic or pulmonary hypertension may develop heart failure. Systemic hypertension may be the result of medications, renal disease, arteriopathies (e.g., Williams syndrome), or essential hypertension. Pulmonary hypertension may be primary in nature or secondary to a multitude of diseases (see Chapter 80).

High output cardiac failure may be seen in patients with arteriovenous malformations or large coronary-cameral or arteriovenous fistulae. Thyroid disorders can cause heart failure at any age. Thyrotoxicosis of the newborn can present with tachycardia, tachypnea, and cardiomegaly (29). Less than 2% of fetuses from mothers with Graves disease will show signs of maternal thyrotoxicosis (30). Other endocrinopathies, such as Addison disease, various drugs, and several toxins can result in heart failure.

PATHOPHYSIOLOGY

Cellular Adaptations in the Heart Failure Syndrome

The mechanisms underlying heart failure include disturbances in cellular organization, energetics, and compensatory pathways. It should be recognized that this topic is vast and has been extensively reviewed (24,31,32). Below is a brief summary of the fundamental cellular adaptations and neurohormonal responses that occur in adults and children with heart failure.

Contractile Apparatus

Myocardial contractility involves excitation–contraction coupling. Calcium-dependent calcium release from the sarcoplasmic reticulum triggers the actin–myosin contractile elements, leading to cross-linkage of myosin–actin filaments sliding under dynamic inhibition from the troponin complex. The system is critically dependent upon the temporal-spatial regulation of intracellular calcium, which is achieved largely by the sarcoplasmic reticulum and the actions of the ryanodine receptor (33). Two critical energy-dependent phases are the pumping (efflux) of calcium from the cytoplasm back into the sarcoplasmic reticulum calcium via the ATPase pump (SERCA), and reloading of the actin–myosin cross-bridges with adenosine triphosphate (ATP) during diastole in preparation for the next contractile cycle. Myocyte calcium handling becomes dysregulated in the failing heart, leading to a depletion of sarcoplasmic reticulum calcium stores, desensitization of the contractile apparatus, and ultimately decreasing the amplitude and duration of calcium release and reducing contractile force generation. A myriad of cytoskeletal proteins, including dystrophin, various intermediate filaments, troponin members, and the contractile complex, may be critically involved in the etiology of heart failure (34,35). These proteins, when mutated genetically, placed under chronic stress, or subjected to the adaptation of regulatory gene networks, often contribute directly to heart failure progression.

In patients with ventricular dilation, as the myocardial fibers become excessively stretched, force generation becomes less efficient, as defined by the Frank Starling relationship (**Fig. 72.1**) (36,37). The common physiologic feature of heart failure is a shift in the diastolic pressure–volume relationship to preserve stroke volume at a higher EDV and filling pressure. With progressive increases in the EDV, the wall tension in the ventricle increases, driving up myocardial energy consumption and increasing stroke work during systole (Laplace's law). The failing heart, which even under normal conditions has high oxygen consumption, now contributes to the progressive exercise intolerance of the patient, one hallmark of chronic heart failure. At rest, cardiac output and stroke volume may be preserved in heart failure, yet with exertion or stress, unfavorable filling pressures can rapidly compromise the host, transforming compensated into uncompensated heart failure (38). The resting state in compensated heart failure is maintained by a series of cellular and systemic compensatory responses, which collectively, along with cardiac remodeling, help define the "heart failure syndrome" (39).

Neurohormonal Response

In a graded response to decreased perfusion, a variety of chemo- and baroreceptors in the brain, kidney, and vasculature signal for increases in circulating hormonal mediators. The neurohormonal adaptation to stress is initially adaptive, yet maladaptive in the chronic state (40). The sympathetic nervous system is activated, leading to elevated levels of circulating epinephrine and norepinephrine, which promote tachycardia, myocardial contractility (via β_1 adrenergic receptors), and arterial and venous vasoconstriction (via α adrenergic receptors). This surge in catecholamines, while critical and lifesaving in a "flight-or-fight" response, when sustained contributes to tissue injury, including myocyte apoptosis. Renin–aldosterone–angiotensin system (RAAS) outflow collectively increases sodium and water retention, thus increasing the circulating volume. Angiotensin specifically augments afterload through vasoconstriction and promotes cardiac hypertrophy. Systemic cortisol, vasopressin, and endothelin-1 are also increased, further enhancing vasoconstriction. This collective neurohormonal response increases myocardial oxygen demand and promotes hypertrophy, oxidative stress, apoptosis, and systemic inflammation (40,41). Globally, vascular and cardiac nitric oxide production is increased through eNOS and iNOS, which acutely decreases preload, reduces afterload,

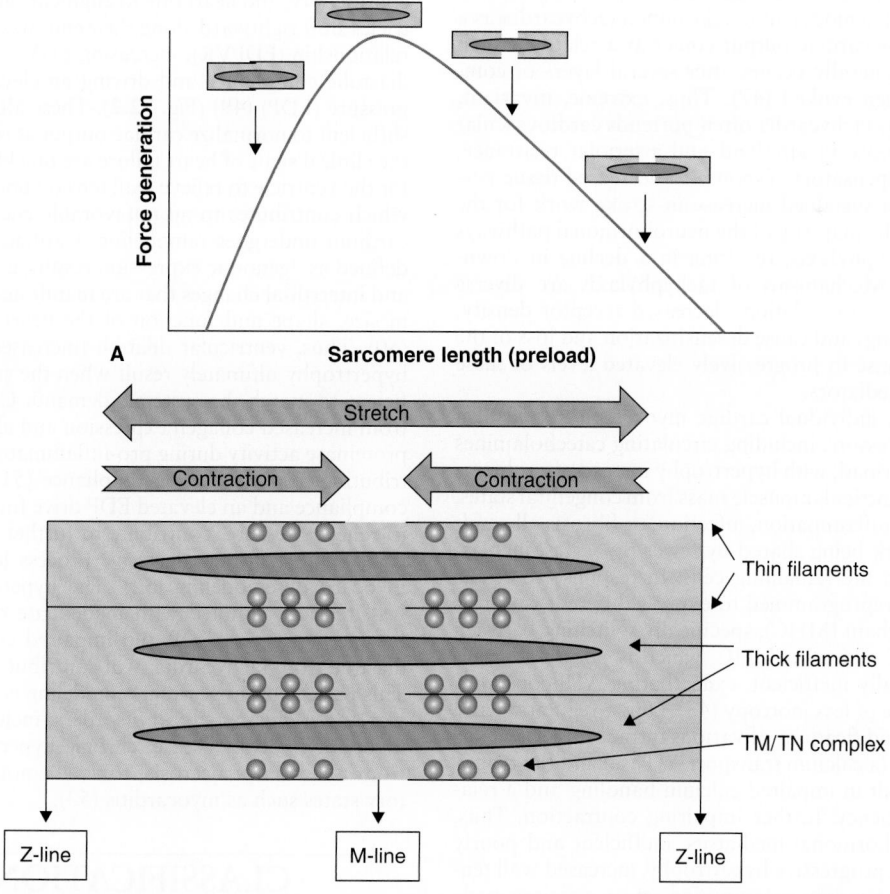

FIGURE 72.1. Frank Starling relationship. A: As the sarcomere stretches, potential force generation increases, peaks, and diminishes with overstretch. Small stylized sarcomeric units demonstrate progressive stretch from left to right. **B:** A sarcomeric unit, demonstrating thick filaments (myosin heavy/light chains) and thin filaments (actin complexed with their associated tropomyosin/troponin [TM/TN] proteins). Lateral movement of the sarcomere during contraction brings the Z-lines closer together in systole. Excessive stretch in diastole, with progressive increases in EDV, decreases maximal force generation.

and augments end-organ perfusion through vasorelaxation. However, chronic elevations in NO promote apoptosis and inflammation, decrease inotropy, and contribute to adrenergic desensitization (42). Thus in the compensatory response for the failing heart, pathophysiologic changes with immediate benefit leading to later harm is a recurring theme in heart failure.

Various natriuretic peptides, some released in response to myocardial wall tension, such as *B-type natriuretic peptide*, counteract the RAAS and promote sodium natriuresis, contributing to chronic hyponatremia. Natriuretic peptides also cause transient vasodilatation, suppress inflammation, and may promote lusitropy (43). Innate immunity and systemic inflammation are widely recognized for their significant contribution to heart failure. Tumor necrosis factor, IL-1, IL-6, are endogenously produced by cardiomyocytes and are produced systemically in heart failure patients. These cytokines, among others, trigger further pro-inflammatory cascades, which have negative inotropic effects and contribute to cardiotoxicity, apoptosis, hypertrophy, extracellular matrix remodeling, and altered calcium homeostasis (44,45). The important contribution of inflammation to heart failure may help explain the benefit derived from medical therapies with significant immunomodulatory properties, such as the angiotensin-converting enzyme inhibitors (46).

Cellular Adaptation and Energetics

As cardiac failure develops and the graded compensatory mechanisms escalate, the heart has relatively few options to improve its overall hemodynamics. Sustained tachycardia as a strategy to increase cardiac output comes at a relatively high energy cost and generally occurs after several layers of compensation have been evoked (47). Thus, extreme, invariant, and sustained sinus tachycardia often portends cardiovascular collapse. The increase in afterload and arteriolar resistance, driven by the compensatory response to decreased tissue perfusion, results in a sustained increase in stroke work for the failing ventricle. The majority of the neurohormonal pathways also undergo tachyphylaxis, resulting in a decline in downstream response. Mechanisms of tachyphylaxis are diverse (transcriptional down-regulation, decreased receptor density, and altered signaling) and cause desensitization and loss of the finely tuned response to progressively elevated levels of these neurohormonal mediators.

After fetal life, individual cardiac myocytes respond to a wide variety of stressors, including circulating catecholamines and increased afterload, with hypertrophy instead of proliferation. The loss of ventricular muscle mass from congenital states, chronic ischemia, inflammation, infection, or fibrosis all result in the cardiac work being shared by fewer myocytes, increasing the burden on the remaining cells. In response to stress, the myocytes are reprogrammed to express different isoforms of myosin heavy chain (MHC), specifically switching between the adult β-MHC to fetal α-MHC, which is poorly contractile and energetically inefficient, exacerbating ATP consumption at the expense of less inotropy (48). Down-regulation and posttranslation modifications of various intracellular proteins, such as SERCA2a (a calcium transport ATPase) and the ryanodine receptor, result in impaired calcium handling and a relative calcium deficiency, further impairing contraction. Thus, tachyphylaxis to hormonal mediators, inefficient and poorly contractile MHC, progressive hypertrophy, increased wall tension, and increased energy consumption set up a vicious cycle contributing to the heart failure syndrome.

Ventricular Remodeling

In response to decreased perfusion of critical tissues (e.g., brain, kidneys), the body signals the heart to increase stroke volume,

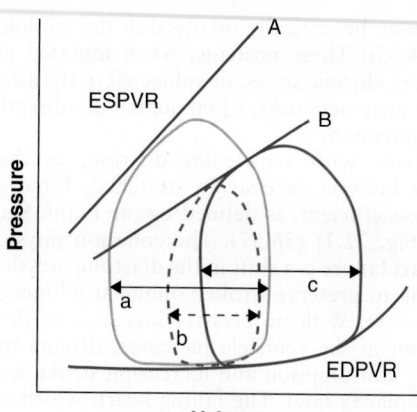

FIGURE 72.2. Compensation during systolic heart failure. Decreased inotropy (systolic failure) shifts the PV-loop along its end-systolic pressure volume relationship (ESPVR) from *line A* to *line B*, resulting in a decreased stroke volume (SV, *arrow a* to *arrow b*). During compensation, the ventricle restores SV (*arrow c*) by increasing its end-diastolic volume (EDV), which necessitates operating at a higher filling pressure secondary to the shape of the end-diastolic pressure–volume relationship (EDPVR). Worsening diastolic compliance shifts the EDPVR upward or increases its slope, resulting in a similar decrease in SV (not shown), forcing the ventricle to increase inotropy to preserve SV, and drives tachycardia to preserve cardiac output.

contractility, and heart rate to augment cardiac output. The ventricles shift rightward along their end-diastolic pressure–volume relationship (EDPVR), increasing EDV and eventually reduced diastolic compliance and driving an elevation in end-diastolic pressure (EDP) (49) (**Fig. 72.2**). These alterations are generally sufficient to normalize cardiac output at rest, but with exertion, the clinical signs of heart failure are quickly unmasked. In order for the ventricle to relieve wall tension under loaded conditions, which contributes to an unfavorable energetic state, the myocardium undergoes remodeling. Cardiac remodeling has been defined as "genomic expression resulting in molecular, cellular, and interstitial changes that are manifested clinically as changes in size, shape and function of the heart after cardiac injury" (50). Thus, ventricular dilation (increased EDV) and myocyte hypertrophy ultimately result when the stroke volume is insufficient to match the systemic demand. Cardiac fibrosis results from increased collagen expression and altered matrix metalloproteinase activity during pro-inflammatory states, further contributing to diastolic noncompliance (51). Decreased diastolic compliance and an elevated EDP drive further increases in EDV to relieve pressure, contribute to further increases in wall tension, and set up a progressive process leading to detrimental myocardial remodeling (52). The hypertrophy and increased wall tension, coupled with inadequate coronary perfusion in the face of a high EDP and impaired coronary filling during diastole from tachycardia, will contribute to ongoing ischemia. This pattern of myocardial remodeling is a final common pathway for a wide variety of disorders, including primary cardiomyopathy, valvar disease, chronic hypertension, myocyte loss from ischemia or necrosis, toxic chemotherapy, or inflammatory states such as myocarditis (53).

CLASSIFICATION AND EVALUATION

Patient History

The assessment of a child with suspected heart failure begins with a careful history, the focus of which will vary depending upon the age of the patient. In a neonate or young infant, parents should be queried about problems with increased work of breathing, cyanosis, feeding, and weight gain. The feeding history should include an assessment of the volume of feeds, diaphoresis with feeding, and time to completion of feeds. Irritability with feeding may be a sign of underlying coronary ischemia or gut hypoperfusion. Failure to thrive is common in infants with heart failure.

A careful maternal history should also be taken. Maternal diabetes and lithium and alcohol exposure are associated with an increased risk of congenital heart defects or cardiomyopathy. A maternal viral illness in late gestation may be associated with subsequent viral myocarditis in the neonate. Maternal nonsteroidal anti-inflammatory drug use may lead to premature closure of the fetal ductus arteriosus, manifesting with pulmonary hypertension and right heart failure soon after birth (54). The perinatal course should be reviewed, including a review of any evidence for perinatal asphyxia, which may be associated with variable degrees of myocardial dysfunction.

In older children and adolescents, the most common symptoms of acute heart failure, listed in order of decreasing frequency, are fatigue, dyspnea, cough, nausea or vomiting, diarrhea, abdominal pain, chest pain, and diaphoresis (55). Of note, the vast majority of children presenting with acute heart failure have signs or symptoms attributable to the respiratory or gastrointestinal systems, which may distract the initial evaluating clinicians from considering a cardiac diagnosis (55). Reports of wheezing or a recent diagnosis of asthma may be cardiac in nature due to pulmonary congestion or bronchial compression from left atrial hypertension. Uncommonly, children may also present with seizures or syncope due to underlying arrhythmias. In patients of any age, signs of muscular weakness or developmental delay may suggest an underlying neuromuscular or metabolic disorder. Patients should be queried for drug ingestions or toxin exposures, such as prior use of anthracyclines for the treatment of malignancies. Heart failure in children may be unmasked by the stress of an intercurrent illness. Note that the typical adult risk factors for heart failure, such as hypercholesterolemia, tobacco use, obesity, hypertension, and diabetes are rarely relevant to children with underlying heart failure. The frequent nonspecific presentation of heart failure in infants and children, which may often include poor growth, respiratory complaints, or gastrointestinal symptoms, may be associated with multiple prior healthcare encounters and a delay in diagnosis.

A careful family history should be taken in all children with suspected heart failure. An inquiry should be made regarding relatives with congenital heart disease, cardiomyopathies, arrhythmias, sudden death, or muscular disease, all of which are associated with a variety of hereditary transmission patterns. Nearly one-quarter of pediatric cardiomyopathy patients will have a family history of a cardiomyopathy (12). Screening of first-degree relatives by echocardiogram and/or genetic testing may be indicated following a diagnosis of a cardiomyopathy in an index case.

Physical Examination

The initial physical examination in a child with suspected heart failure includes not only a careful cardiovascular assessment, but a thorough examination of all other organ systems. The clinician must be aware that many of the classic signs of heart failure seen in adults, such as jugular venous distension, crackles on lung auscultation, and edema of the lower extremities, are not commonly found in infants and young children with heart failure.

A general assessment is made of the child's overall appearance, including nutritional state, activity level, and color. The child's growth chart should be carefully inspected. In infants, poor weight gain is commonplace. Older children may have either weight loss due to excessive catabolism (mismatched caloric intake to demand) and/or weight gain due to accumulation of edema.

The vital signs should be carefully reviewed (55). The heart rate is commonly elevated in children with heart failure as a compensatory response to limited stroke volume. The pulse pressure may be widened with low diastolic blood pressure in children with run-off lesions, such as a large ductus arteriosus, unrepaired common arterial trunk (truncus arteriosus), or an arterial-venous malformation. The systolic blood pressure is typically preserved except in patients with cardiogenic shock. Four extremity blood pressure measurements should be obtained in neonates with heart failure to assess for evidence of aortic arch obstruction. Note that an arm–leg gradient may be undetectable in such patients with coarctation of the aorta if an aberrant right subclavian artery or shock is present. Tachypnea is a common finding in children with heart failure, often related to pulmonary congestion and elevated left atrial pressure. The systemic oxygen saturation should be measured via pulse oximetry. An infant with an unrepaired complete atrioventricular septal defect, for example, may have mild systemic desaturation due to intracardiac mixing. Neonates with unrepaired common arterial trunk, total anomalous pulmonary venous return, or single ventricle heart defects may have complete intracardiac mixing and hypoxemia.

A detailed cardiac examination begins with an assessment of the precordium. Bulging just to the left of the sternum suggests underlying long-standing cardiomegaly. A prominent right ventricular impulse may occur in children with right ventricular hypertrophy from pulmonary hypertension. A palpable thrill may suggest significant systemic ventricular outflow tract obstruction. In older children and adolescents, the neck should be assessed for signs of jugular venous distention. Careful cardiac auscultation for murmurs, gallops, a single second heart sound, or other abnormalities is then performed. A loud second heart sound suggests pulmonary hypertension. The heart rhythm should be determined by both auscultation and palpation. The volume of peripheral pulses in all four extremities should be assessed, with careful attention to differential in pulse intensity between the right arm and lower extremities. The lower extremities should be examined for evidence of peripheral edema, although this finding is uncommon in infants with heart failure.

The assessment of the respiratory system begins with a visual inspection for tachypnea, retractions, nasal flaring, or tracheal tugging. Older children and adolescents with heart failure may have crackles or rales on auscultation of the lungs, although these findings are uncommon in neonates and infants. The abdomen should be inspected for hepatomegaly (common) or abdominal masses (rare; e.g., related to pheochromocytoma or medulloblastoma). In infants, the head and liver should be auscultated for bruits that may suggest an underlying arteriovenous malformation. Patients who have abnormal facial features may have underlying genetic conditions. A neurological examination should include an assessment of muscle strength, bulk, and tone in order to screen for neuromuscular disorders. Any signs of global developmental delay should be noted.

Laboratory, Radiographic, and Cardiac Evaluation

The evaluation of children with suspected heart failure may be performed in a stepwise fashion. The initial evaluation for all patients includes a chest x-ray, electrocardiogram, echocardiogram, and basic laboratory studies as discussed further below. Advanced testing may then be indicated in a subset of patients based on the clinical scenario and findings of these initial

TABLE 72.2

DIAGNOSTIC TESTING FOR CHILDREN WITH SUSPECTED HEART FAILURE

		■ ALL PATIENTS	■ SELECTED PATIENTS
Imaging		Chest radiograph	Cardiac magnetic resonance imaging
		Echocardiogram	
Blood tests		Electrolytes	Blood gases
		Renal function	Troponin
		Liver function tests	Viral serology
		Complete blood count	ESR, CRP
		Thyroid function tests	Lactate, pyruvate
		Brain natriuretic peptide	Ammonia
			Amino acids
			Carnitine/acylcarnitine
			Selenium
			Chromosomal analysis
			Genetic testing for cardiomyopathies
Other		Electrocardiogram	Cardiac catheterization
			Myocardial biopsy
			Urine (carnitine, ketones, amino and organic acids)
			Muscle biopsy

screening tests (**Table 72.2**). For patients being evaluated for heart transplantation, additional testing will be required (see Chapter 76).

A chest radiograph should be obtained and carefully inspected, starting with the size and shape of the cardiac silhouette. A cardiac-to-total-thoracic ratio of greater than 0.55 in infants or greater than 0.5 in older children is abnormal and suggests cardiomegaly. Note that the cardiac silhouette size may be normal in some patients with fulminant viral myocarditis and severe cardiac dysfunction, as the chambers have not had time to dilate in the acute setting. In a minority of cases, a chest x-ray will give specific clues to the type of underlying cardiac disease. For example, the pulmonary artery shadow may be prominent in patients with long-standing left-to-right atrial shunts, such as a secundum atrial septal defect, or a box-shaped heart may suggest corrected transposition of the great arteries. The lung fields should be assessed for increased pulmonary vascular markings and perihilar congestion. Retrocardiac atelectasis, if present, may be due to left atrial compression of the left main stem bronchus.

Children with suspected heart failure should have an electrocardiogram. Attention is given to the rhythm, as incessant arrhythmias, such as ectopic atrial tachycardia, occasionally present with heart failure. The QRS axis and voltage should be inspected. Patients with complete atrioventricular septal defects typically have left axis deviation. Those with acute viral myocarditis may have low voltage, ST segment changes, repolarization abnormalities, Q-waves, or arrhythmias. Signs of ventricular hypertrophy may be present, such as is commonly found in patients with hypertrophic cardiomyopathy or Pompe disease. Patients with restrictive cardiomyopathy typically have prominent P waves. Symptomatic patients with an anomalous left coronary artery from the pulmonary artery often have a deep, wide Q wave in leads I, AVL, or V5–V7 (56).

A complete echocardiogram is an important component of the evaluation of infants and children with suspected heart failure. The cardiac anatomy can be definitively established in most cases. An assessment of left and right ventricular function is obtained. The normal left ventricular shortening fraction is 28%–40% and the ejection fraction 56%–78%. Note that shortening and ejection fractions are dependent on cardiac loading conditions. Gradients across the atrioventricular or semilunar valves and intracardiac shunting may be assessed

using color Doppler interrogation. Intracardiac clots, which may develop due to stasis of blood flow in patients with poor myocardial function, may also be identified (57).

In patients with dilated cardiomyopathy, the echocardiogram will demonstrate an enlarged and globally dysfunctional left ventricle, often associated with left atrial enlargement. Occasionally, the right ventricle and right atrium also are dilated. The severity of any valvar regurgitation may be assessed by color Doppler. In children with hypertrophic cardiomyopathy, echocardiographic findings include asymmetric hypertrophy of the interventricular septum, and less commonly hypertrophy of the free wall and apex. The left ventricular outflow tract may or may not have a pressure gradient related to this hypertrophy. There may be systolic anterior motion of the mitral valve leaflets leading to dynamic left ventricular outflow tract obstruction. Evidence of diastolic function based on mitral inflow and tissue Doppler patterns may exist. In restrictive cardiomyopathy, the most striking finding on the echocardiogram is marked dilatation of both atrial chambers. The ventricular size and systolic function are typically normal, although dilation, hypertrophy, and/or systolic dysfunction may evolve over time in a subset of these patients. Patients with noncompaction cardiomyopathy have a thin epicardial band of ventricular myocardium. The endocardial noncompacted layer is typically at least two times the thickness of the epicardial layer. Color flow by Doppler may be seen into the trabeculations of the noncompacted myocardium. The noncompacted regions typically localize to the mid lateral apical and mid inferior segments of the left ventricle. In children with noncompaction cardiomyopathy, congenital heart disease may be coexistent.

Initial laboratory studies include basic chemistries and a complete blood count. Hyponatremia and hypochloremia may be present due to free water retention. Renal function is a simple yet sensitive marker of the adequacy of cardiac output and renal perfusion pressure. The blood urea nitrogen (BUN) and creatinine may be elevated in patients with inadequate renal perfusion. The hemoglobin level should be assessed as an adequate hemoglobin level is essential for oxygen-carrying capacity. Anemia is present in approximately one-half of children with new onset acute heart failure (55). Polycythemia may suggest an unrecognized long-standing cyanotic heart defect. Severe anemia or polycythemia may also cause heart failure in the neonate. Thyroid function tests should be obtained as thyrotoxicosis may cause heart failure. Plasma brain natriuretic peptide (BNP) levels are typically elevated in patients with heart failure (58), and the trend of BNP may be a useful prognostic indicator of both disease progression and response to therapy. Blood gases and lactate levels may be warranted depending on the severity of illness.

Additional laboratory studies may be obtained in selected patients based on the clinical scenario. For example, in patients with Fontan physiology and heart failure, serum albumin and stool alpha-1 antitrypsin levels should be measured to assess for concurrent protein-losing enteropathy. In patients with suspected myocardial ischemia or viral myocarditis, measurement of troponin levels may be useful to screen for acute myocardial injury (59). In those with suspected myocarditis, serum and respiratory specimens can be sent for viral testing.

Second-tier testing for many cardiomyopathy patients is warranted (12). Those with suspected inborn errors of metabolism should have blood tests for amino acids, a carnitine/acylcarnitine profile, lactate, pyruvate, and ammonia. Urine may be sent for carnitine, ketones, and amino and organic acids. A skeletal muscle biopsy may provide useful information in children with suspected mitochondrial or neuromuscular disorders, although often musculoskeletal disease is identified before the development of cardiomyopathy. Genetic testing is available for a number of specific gene mutations known to cause dilated and hypertrophic cardiomyopathy. Genetic testing may also be useful for patients with a suspected malformation syndrome (e.g., Noonan syndrome). Consultation with a geneticist or neurologist with expertise in neuromuscular disorders and metabolic disorders is often helpful.

Cardiac MRI has a growing role in the assessment of children with heart failure, although indications in critically ill children are less well established. Right and left ventricular function and shunts can be precisely quantified and chamber volumes tracked serially. Tissue characteristics of the myocardium may be useful in some cases for underlying diagnosis. For example, myocardial tissue edema may be detected by T2-weighted imaging in patients with viral myocarditis (60). Hyperemia may be identified using special sequences to detect early gadolinium enhancement. The presence of late gadolinium enhancement is suggestive of myocardial necrosis or fibrosis.

Cardiac catheterization may be useful in a subset of children with heart failure. Hemodynamics may be obtained, including the left ventricular EDP and pulmonary arterial wedge pressure. Cardiac index and central venous pressure are also obtained. The pulmonary artery pressure and PVR should be noted. In children with heart failure, cardiac catheterization is associated with a number of risks related to the procedure itself and the use of sedation or anesthesia and thus must be used judiciously.

Patients with palliated or repaired congenital heart disease who present with acute heart failure warrant consideration for a diagnostic catheterization if noninvasive evaluation fails to establish a definitive diagnosis. In patients with suspected coronary artery abnormalities for whom the noninvasive imaging is inadequate, coronary angiography may be obtained. This information may be invaluable in patients with coronary ostial stenosis and/or atresia, or for clarifying the diagnosis in patients with suspected anomalous origin of the left main coronary artery from the pulmonary artery.

In heart transplant candidates with an elevated transpulmonary gradient (>15 mm Hg), assessment of the reactivity of the pulmonary vascular bed may be determined by vasodilator testing with oxygen, inhaled nitric oxide, and other drugs. Traditionally, those with a pretransplant baseline PVR greater than 6 Wood units per m² or greater than 4 Wood units per m² with vasodilator testing are at significant risk for posttransplant right ventricular failure (61). With the availability of selective pulmonary vasodilators such as inhaled nitric oxide, children with higher PVR may successfully undergo cardiac transplantation, albeit with an increased risk of early postoperative right ventricular failure (62). Patients with significantly elevated and fixed PVR who are otherwise candidates for heart transplantation may benefit from hemodynamic unloading with a ventricular assist device, followed by a reevaluation of their PVR (63).

In patients with suspected myocarditis, a myocardial biopsy may be obtained for histology, viral polymerase chain reaction and electron microscopy. In heart transplantation patients who present with acute heart failure, a myocardial biopsy should generally be obtained to evaluate for rejection. Samples should be assessed for cellular and antibody-mediated rejection. Heart transplant patients with myocardial dysfunction may also warrant coronary angiography to assess for graft vasculopathy, although this is typically not performed in the setting of acute rejection.

CONCLUSIONS AND FUTURE DIRECTIONS

Given the diverse etiologies and the nonspecific signs and symptoms of heart failure in children, even in advanced cases, establishing a timely diagnosis remains a challenge. Improvements in the education of pediatricians, emergency room physicians, and other clinicians who care for children at risk for heart failure are needed. In addition, further understanding and application of screening tests, such as pulse oximetry screening for congenital heart disease in seemingly healthy neonates and the measurement of BNP levels in children presenting with respiratory distress, are desirable. Such changes may facilitate the recognition of cardiomyopathies and other conditions at risk for heart failure in earlier stages. This can result in more timely diagnosis and initiation of therapy, prior to the onset of acute decompensation that leads to hospitalization and, in many cases, the need for intensive care. Advances in noninvasive imaging technology and application, particularly echocardiography and MRI, are occurring rapidly and will add further clarity to our understanding of the pathophysiology of children afflicted with heart failure.

References

1. Katz AM. Evolving concepts of heart failure: Cooling furnace, malfunctioning pump, enlarging muscle—Part I. *J Card Fail* 1997;3:319–34.
2. Hsu DT, Pearson GD. Heart failure in children: Part I: History, etiology, and pathophysiology. *Circ Heart Fail* 2009;2:63–70.
3. Rossano JW, Kim JJ, Decker JA, et al. Prevalence, morbidity, and mortality of heart failure-related hospitalizations in children in the United States: A population-based study. *J Card Fail* 2012;18:459–70.
4. Rodriguez FH 3rd, Moodie DS, Parekh DR, et al. Outcomes of heart failure-related hospitalization in adults with congenital heart disease in the United States. *Congenit Heart Dis* 2013;8(6):513–9.
5. Rudolph AM. Pulmonary stenosis and atresia with ventricular septal defect (tetralogy of Fallot). In: Rudolph AM, ed. *Congenital Diseases of the Heart: Clinical-Physiological Considerations.* 2nd ed. Armonk, NY: Futura Publishing Company, 2001:538.
6. Bronicki RA, Anas NG. Cardiopulmonary interaction. *Pediatr Crit Care Med* 2009;10:313–22.
7. Hraska V, Duncan BW, Mayer JE Jr, et al. Long-term outcome of surgically treated patients with corrected transposition of the great arteries. *J Thorac Cardiovasc Surg* 2005;129:182–91.

8. Kantor PF, Redington AN. Pathophysiology and management of heart failure in repaired congenital heart disease. *Heart Fail Clin* 2010;6:497–506.

9. Verheugt CL, Uiterwaal CS, Grobbee DE, et al. Long-term prognosis of congenital heart defects: A systematic review. *Int J Cardiol* 2008;131:25–32.

10. McCrindle BW, Zak V, Sleeper LA, et al. Laboratory measures of exercise capacity and ventricular characteristics and function are weakly associated with functional health status after Fontan procedure. *Circulation* 2010;121:34–42.

11. Maron BJ, Towbin JA, Thiene G, et al. Contemporary definitions and classification of the cardiomyopathies: An American Heart Association scientific statement from the Council on Clinical Cardiology, Heart Failure and Transplantation Committee; Quality of Care and Outcomes Research and Functional Genomics and Translational Biology Interdisciplinary Working Groups; and Council on Epidemiology and Prevention. *Circulation* 2006;113:1807–16.

12. Cox GF, Sleeper LA, Lowe AM, et al. Factors associated with establishing a causal diagnosis for children with cardiomyopathy. *Pediatrics* 2006;118:1519–31.

13. Wilkinson JD, Sleeper LA, Alvarez JA, et al. The pediatric cardiomyopathy registry: 1995–2007. *Prog Pediatr Cardiol* 2008;25:31–6.

14. Towbin JA, Lowe AM, Colan SD, et al. Incidence, causes, and outcomes of dilated cardiomyopathy in children. *JAMA* 2006;296:1867–76.

15. Hsu DT, Zak V, Mahony L, et al. Enalapril in infants with single ventricle: Results of a multicenter randomized trial. *Circulation* 2010;122:333–40.

16. Colan SD. Hypertrophic cardiomyopathy in childhood. *Heart Fail Clin* 2010;6:433–44.

17. Colan SD, Lipshultz SE, Lowe AM, et al. Epidemiology and cause-specific outcome of hypertrophic cardiomyopathy in children: Findings from the pediatric cardiomyopathy registry. *Circulation* 2007;115:773–81.

18. Moak JP, Kaski JP. Hypertrophic cardiomyopathy in children. *Heart* 2012;98:1044–54.

19. Denfield SW, Webber SA. Restrictive cardiomyopathy in childhood. *Heart Fail Clin* 2010;6:445–52.

20. Mocumbi AO, Ferreira MB, Sidi D, et al. A population study of endomyocardial fibrosis in a rural area of Mozambique. *N Engl J Med* 2008;359:43–9.

21. Mogensen J, Arbustini E. Restrictive cardiomyopathy. *Curr Opin Cardiol* 2009;24:214–20.

22. Berger S, Dubin AM. Arrhythmogenic forms of heart failure in children. *Heart Fail Clin* 2010;6:471–81.

23. Azaouagh A, Churzidse S, Konorza T, et al. Arrhythmogenic right ventricular cardiomyopathy/dysplasia: A review and update. *Clin Res Cardiol* 2011;100:383–94.

24. Towbin JA. Left ventricular noncompaction: A new form of heart failure. *Heart Fail Clin* 2010;6:453–69.

25. Tulloh RM, Wood LE. Coronary artery changes in patients with Kawasaki disease. *Acta Paediatr Suppl* 2004;93:75–9.

26. Dodd DA, Cabo J, Dipchand AI. Acute rejection: Natural history, risk factors, surveillance and treatment. In: Canter CE, Kirklin JK, eds. *ISHLT Monograph Series Volume 2: Pediatric Heart Transplantation*. Philadelphia, PA: Elsevier, 2007.

27. Smeding L, Plotz FB, Groeneveld AB, et al. Structural changes of the heart during severe sepsis or septic shock. *Shock* 2012;37:449–56.

28. Chalkias A, Xanthos T. Pathophysiology and pathogenesis of post-resuscitation myocardial stunning. *Heart Fail Rev* 2012;17:117–28.

29. Farrehi C, Mitchell M, Fawcett DM. Heart failure in congenital thyrotoxicosis. *Pediatrics* 1966;37:460–6.

30. Lesser J. Heart failure in a neonate. *Clin Pediatr (Phila)* 2005;44:637.

31. van Berlo JH, Maillet M, Molkentin JD. Signaling effectors underlying pathologic growth and remodeling of the heart. *J Clin Invest* 2013;123:37–45.

32. Madriago E, Silberbach M. Heart failure in infants and children. *Pediatr Rev* 2010;31:4–12.

33. Cheng H, Lederer WJ, Cannell MB. Calcium sparks: Elementary events underlying excitation-contraction coupling in heart muscle. *Science* 1993;262:740–4.

34. Chen J, Chien KR. Complexity in simplicity: Monogenic disorders and complex cardiomyopathies. *J Clin Invest* 1999;103:1483–5.

35. Towbin JA, Bowles NE. The failing heart. *Nature* 2002;415:227–33.

36. Shiels HA, White E. The Frank-Starling mechanism in vertebrate cardiac myocytes. *J Exp Biol* 2008;211:2005–13.

37. Solaro RJ. *Regulation of Cardiac Contractility*. San Rafael, CA: Morgan & Claypool, 2011.

38. Borlaug BA, Melenovsky V, Russell SD, et al. Impaired chronotropic and vasodilator reserves limit exercise capacity in patients with heart failure and a preserved ejection fraction. *Circulation* 2006;114:2138–47.

39. Maciver DH, Dayer MJ, Harrison AJ. A general theory of acute and chronic heart failure. *Int J Cardiol* 2012;165:25–34.

40. Dube P, Weber KT. Congestive heart failure: Pathophysiologic consequences of neurohormonal activation and the potential for recovery: Part I. *Am J Med Sci* 2011;342:348–51.

41. Yndestad A, Damas JK, Oie E, et al. Systemic inflammation in heart failure—The whys and wherefores. *Heart Fail Rev* 2006;11:83–92.

42. Umar S, van der Laarse A. Nitric oxide and nitric oxide synthase isoforms in the normal, hypertrophic, and failing heart. *Mol Cell Biochem* 2010;333:191–201.

43. Clerico A, Recchia FA, Passino C, et al. Cardiac endocrine function is an essential component of the homeostatic regulation network: Physiological and clinical implications. *Am J Physiol Heart Circ Physiol* 2006;290:H17–29.

44. Kleinbongard P, Schulz R, Heusch G. TNFalpha in myocardial ischemia/reperfusion, remodeling and heart failure. *Heart Fail Rev* 2011;16:49–69.

45. Valen G. Innate immunity and remodelling. *Heart Fail Rev* 2011;16:71–8.

46. Watanabe K, Sukumaran V, Veeraveedu PT, et al. Regulation of inflammation and myocardial fibrosis in experimental autoimmune myocarditis. *Inflamm Allergy Drug Targets* 2011;10:218–25.

47. Yu X, Konstantinov IE, Kantoch MJ, et al. Dynamic changes of myocardial oxygen consumption at pacing increased heart rate—The first observation by the continuous measurement of systemic oxygen consumption. *Scand Cardiovasc J* 2011;45:301–6.

48. Swynghedauw B. Phenotypic plasticity of adult myocardium: Molecular mechanisms. *J Exp Biol* 2006;209:2320–7.

49. Cokkinos DV, Pantos C. Myocardial remodeling, an overview. *Heart Fail Rev* 2011;16:1–4.

50. Cohn JN, Ferrari R, Sharpe N. Cardiac remodeling—Concepts and clinical implications: A consensus paper from an international forum on cardiac remodeling. Behalf of an International Forum on Cardiac Remodeling. *J Am Coll Cardiol* 2000;35:569–82.

51. Bujak M, Frangogiannis NG. The role of TGF-beta signaling in myocardial infarction and cardiac remodeling. *Cardiovasc Res* 2007;74:184–95.

52. Andrew P. Diastolic heart failure demystified. *Chest* 2003;124:744–53.

53. Gajarsa JJ, Kloner RA. Left ventricular remodeling in the post-infarction heart: A review of cellular, molecular mechanisms, and therapeutic modalities. *Heart Fail Rev* 2011;16:13–21.

54. Manchester D, Margolis HS, Sheldon RE. Possible association between maternal indomethacin therapy and primary

pulmonary hypertension of the newborn. *Am J Obstet Gynecol* 1976;126:467–9.

55. Macicek SM, Macias CG, Jefferies JL, et al. Acute heart failure syndromes in the pediatric emergency department. *Pediatrics* 2009;124:e898–904.

56. Johnsrude CL, Perry JC, Cecchin F, et al. Differentiating anomalous left main coronary artery originating from the pulmonary artery in infants from myocarditis and dilated cardiomyopathy by electrocardiogram. *Am J Cardiol* 1995;75:71–4.

57. Law YM, Sharma S, Feingold B, et al. Clinically significant thrombosis in pediatric heart transplant recipients during their waiting period. *Pediatr Cardiol* 2013;34:334–40.

58. Law YM, Hoyer AW, Reller MD, et al. Accuracy of plasma B-type natriuretic peptide to diagnose significant cardiovascular disease in children: The Better Not Pout Children! Study. *J Am Coll Cardiol* 2009;54:1467–75.

59. Eisenberg MA, Green-Hopkins I, Alexander ME, et al. Cardiac troponin T as a screening test for myocarditis in children. *Pediatr Emerg Care* 2012;28:1173–8.

60. Friedrich MG, Sechtem U, Schulz-Menger J, et al. Cardiovascular magnetic resonance in myocarditis: A JACC White Paper. *J Am Coll Cardiol* 2009;53:1475–87.

61. Gajarski RJ, Towbin JA, Bricker JT, et al. Intermediate follow-up of pediatric heart transplant recipients with elevated pulmonary vascular resistance index. *J Am Coll Cardiol* 1994;23:1682–7.

62. Ofori-Amanfo G, Hsu D, Lamour JM, et al. Heart transplantation in children with markedly elevated pulmonary vascular resistance: Impact of right ventricular failure on outcome. *J Heart Lung Transplant* 2011;30:659–66.

63. Gazit AZ, Canter CE. Impact of pulmonary vascular resistances in heart transplantation for congenital heart disease. *Curr Cardiol Rev* 2011;7:59–66.

CHAPTER 73 ■ CARDIOMYOPATHY, MYOCARDITIS, AND MECHANICAL CIRCULATORY SUPPORT

WILLIAM G. HARMON, APARNA HOSKOTE, AND ANN KARIMOVA

KEY POINTS

1 Children with end-stage heart failure (either due to undiagnosed cardiomyopathy or myocarditis) often come to medical attention when an arrhythmia, infection, or injury results in an acute clinical decompensation that initiates a medical evaluation and subsequent disease recognition.

2 In small children and infants, the signs of decompensating heart failure might be nonspecific (masking as chest infection, gastrointestinal problem, and so on). Correct diagnosis of myocarditis and/or cardiomyopathy might prevent uncontrolled decompensation and sudden cardiac death.

3 The number of patients classified with idiopathic cardiomyopathy will decrease over time, as specific genetic diagnosis is increasing with the promise of more specific molecular-based therapies to treat individual diseases.

4 Aggressive early management involves stabilization of the airway, appropriate hemodynamic support, and antiarrhythmic agents with close monitoring for catastrophic decompensation and mechanical support.

5 Symptomatic supportive treatment is the mainstay in the management of acute viral myocarditis, rather than immunomodulatory treatment. If appropriately managed, outcome for fulminant myocarditis is excellent with full recovery.

6 Mechanical circulatory support is a life-sustaining therapy offered to children with severe circulatory failure refractory to conventional treatment, with the ultimate aim of bridging to recovery or heart transplantation.

Cardiomyopathy is a generalized term describing a disorder of cardiac myocyte structure or function. A cardiomyopathy can arise as a primary diagnosis, or result as a comorbidity from a wider systemic disease such as systemic hypertension, and infectious, rheumatologic, or metabolic disorders. This chapter will focus on primary childhood cardiomyopathies that are generally classified by phenotypic and functional characteristics into five disease categories: dilated (DCM), hypertrophic (HCM), restrictive cardiomyopathies (RCM), arrhythmogenic right-ventricular cardiomyopathy (ARVC), and left-ventricular noncompaction (LVNC). These five basic cardiomyopathy phenotypes are helpful in describing general patient characteristics and potential clinical courses, although wide heterogeneity does occur in terms of specific pathology, disease progression, and outcome. Among the acquired cardiomyopathies, the two most relevant ones, anthracycline and vitamin D deficiency–related cardiomyopathy, will be briefly covered. We will also discuss infectious myocarditis and review the developing practice of mechanical circulatory support (MCS) for children with decompensated heart failure.

CARDIOMYOPATHIES

Over the past 20 years, registry data have clarified many epidemiologic and clinical characteristics of childhood cardiomyopathy (1). In North America, the annual incidence of all pediatric cardiomyopathies approximates 1.13 cases/100,000 patient years, a rate similar to some childhood cancers and rheumatologic conditions. Cardiomyopathy in children is most commonly diagnosed during infancy, and those presenting with heart failure as infants have a 40% risk of death or cardiac transplantation within 2 years of their initial diagnosis (2). Older children with a long-standing cardiomyopathy often remain undiagnosed for long periods due to their remarkable ability to compensate for gradual decrements of cardiac function. Children with previously undiagnosed cardiomyopathy often come to medical attention when an arrhythmia, infection, or injury results in an acute clinical decompensation that initiates a medical evaluation and subsequent disease recognition. A diagnosis of cardiomyopathy has profound implications, as it is a lifelong illness with a significant morbidity and mortality, and has a major impact on the patient, their family, and the wider health-care system. These patients are often offered complex interventions, when available, such as MCS and cardiac transplantation.

Dilated Cardiomyopathy

Incidence, Etiology, and Classification

The North American Pediatric Cardiomyopathy Registry (PCMR) has provided epidemiologic and clinical descriptor data for all forms of primary pediatric cardiomyopathy over the past two decades (3). Beyond one year of life, DCM is the most common diagnosis leading to cardiac transplantation in both children and adult populations. DCM represents approximately half of diagnosed pediatric cardiomyopathy cases, with an estimated incidence rate of 0.57 cases/100,000 person years in the PCMR North American cohort. Boys were at a higher risk than girls, and African Americans showed a higher risk than whites. The PCMR data set found that DCM in children is most commonly diagnosed during the first year of life (41% of all patients), reflecting the large influence of genetic disease burden in this age group. Despite frequently aggressive diagnostic efforts, the majority of 1462 pediatric patients with primary DCM diagnosed mostly in the 1990s were ultimately classified as having idiopathic disease. Six etiologic classifications were used in this data set, which included (a) idiopathic DCM (66%), (b) myocarditis (16%), (c) neuromuscular disorders (9%), (d) familial DCM (5%), (e) inborn errors of metabolism (4%), and (f) malformation syndromes (1%) (**Table 73.1**). With the advent of clinical genetic testing, most children can now be placed into specific diagnostic categories, but such specialized services may not be universally available (4). Single-gene defects of sarcomeric proteins such as myosin and troponin are most commonly described in HCM, where some defect can now be detected in about 60% of affected individuals (5). Mutations in sarcomeric proteins (actin, myosin, troponins) as well as force-transducing molecules (titin [TTN], dystrophin), nuclear proteins (lamin A/C [LMNA]), RNA-binding proteins, and multiple other structural and metabolic molecules have been found to be either directly causative or implicated in the pathogenesis of DCM. Genetic analysis is most likely to identify specific mutations in the setting of familial DCM, where about 35% of families are found to have defects in TTN, LMNA, β-myosin heavy chain (MYH7) or cardiac troponin T (TNNT2). As there may be diagnostic uncertainty, incomplete penetrance, and a variable time course of illness, it is an important standard of care to screen first-degree family members, which allows for an earlier diagnosis of co-affected yet asymptomatic family members, and leads to better survival (6).

Pathophysiology of Heart Failure in Dilated Cardiomyopathy

DCM ultimately arises as a result of an intrinsic or extrinsic cardiomyocyte abnormality or cell injury. It is thought that postnatal cardiac myocytes do not regenerate, such that any insult that causes myocyte loss permanently decreases an individual's complement of myocardial cells. As a result, any acute myocardial insult may place a person at risk for the development of cardiomyopathy later in life. Anthracycline cardiotoxicity can lead to the late development of DCM post–cancer treatment and is considered a classic example of this construct.

Decreased ventricular function and progressive left-ventricular (LV) dilatation are the phenotypic hallmarks of DCM. On serial echocardiograms, the LV size is monitored as the LV end-diastolic dimension, whereas contractility is monitored as the LV ejection fraction or as the LV shortening fraction. Some patients will show a gradual thinning of the LV walls, which is tracked as the left-ventricular posterior wall thickness (LVPWT). Importantly, children show age- and size-related variation and hence comparative findings must be normalized for age and body surface area (BSA). This is done by reporting Z-values, which represent an individual's findings as the number of standard deviations away from normative mean values for age and size. Findings are considered abnormal for any Z-score that is greater than 2 (positive or negative). Of note, as this is normative data, roughly 2% of normal, unaffected, individuals may actually be considered to show abnormal findings using the $Z = \pm 2$ standard. Thus, it is always important to synthesize an entire data set with clinical data before classifying an individual based upon borderline echocardiographic results.

LV dysfunction is typically asymptomatic and subclinical in its early stages. Nevertheless, decreasing myocardial function and falling cardiac output (CO) initiate a variety of compensatory mechanisms targeted to maintain blood pressure and normal organ perfusion. The baroreceptor response is a primary mechanism, which combats a fall in CO. This results

TABLE 73.1

SELECTED CAUSES OF DILATED CARDIOMYOPATHY (DCM) IN CHILDREN

Gene defects (sarcomeric and other, often classified as familial DCM):
  Myosin (MYH7)
  Actin (ACTC)
  Titin (TTN)
  Troponin I (TNNI3)
  Troponin T (TNNT2)
  Taffazin mutations
Many others. Can be tested for using research and commercial sources, as guided by a cardiac geneticist.

Infectious/inflammatory:
  Previous viral myocarditis (acute and chronic)
  Nonviral infections (Chagas disease, and others)
  Inflammatory/toxic drug reactions (anthracycline, and others)

Neuromuscular:
  Duchenne muscular dystrophy
  Becker muscular dystrophy
  Emory-Dreifuss muscular dystrophy

Metabolic:
  Fatty acid oxidation defects (e.g., VLCAD, LCHAD, LCAD deficiency, others)
  Propionic aciduria
  Mitochondrial disorders
  Carnitine deficiency
  Nutritional deficiencies
  (Many others, metabolic consultation is generally recommended)

Syndromes associated with DCM:
  Barth syndrome
  Friedrich's ataxia
  Noonan's syndrome (HCM is more common)
  Kearns-Sayre syndrome
  Others—DCM is seen in many children with nonclassifiable syndromic features

Idiopathic:
A primary genetic abnormality is presumed for many of these children. In previous decades the majority of children were classified as having idiopathic disease. This is progressively decreasing and now an etiology is possible in the majority of children when thoroughly studied.

Note: Anatomical abnormalities (such as anomalous left coronary artery from pulmonary artery—ALCAPA or undiagnosed coarctation of the aorta) and arrhythmias (such as atrial ectopic tachycardia—AET) have to be excluded as underlying causes for left-ventricular dysfunction.

in catecholamine-mediated increases in heart rate, contractility, and systemic vascular resistance (SVR). Activation of the renin–angiotensin–aldosterone system augments preload by promoting fluid retention, and SVR is further increased via potent renin-induced peripheral vasoconstriction. These compensatory mechanisms are acutely adaptive and help maintain a stable physiology. However, over time and with progressive myocardial dysfunction, these normal physiologic responses become maladaptive and harmful to a failing heart. Increased SVR directly increases cardiac afterload and myocardial oxygen demand and decreases stroke volume. As heart failure progresses, increased intravascular volume raises filling pressures, which, in the extreme, can impede diastolic coronary perfusion and lead to systemic and pulmonary edema. These general mechanisms produce the clinical syndrome of congestive heart failure, where patients demonstrate a (a) subnormal CO, (b) volume overload, and (c) a high SVR state. One should remember that a dilated heart is a less efficient pump that requires more energy to function, has more oxygen demand, and increased wall tension. Afterload is also affected by cardiac geometry, and increases with progressive cardiac dilatation. This is explained by the law of Laplace, which describes the wall tension of a sphere under pressure:

$$Tension = Pressure \times Radius$$

A normal heart will hypertrophy when exposed to chronic volume load as a compensatory means to decrease the luminal radius, thereby lowering the wall stress and afterload. However, wall thinning is a pathophysiological hallmark of DCM, with many patients showing a progressively thinner LVPWT. Unfortunately, progressive LV dilation and wall thinning potentiate a worsening cycle of increasing afterload, worsening energy balance, and progressive heart failure.

Diagnostic Testing

The intensivist is often involved with DCM patients who present with uncompensated or fulminant heart failure. Initial efforts must be directed to stabilize the acidotic patient, but soon thereafter diagnostic issues must be addressed. Diagnostic emphasis is different depending on the age and the severity of presentation. Please see **Table 73.1** for a list of potential causes of DCM and **Table 73.2** for a summary of etiologic diagnostic testing suggestions for the newly presenting patient. A detailed family history is paramount for all patients, as inheritable conditions can present at any age. In neonates or young infants, there should be consideration of undiagnosed congenital defects such as an ALCAPA, coarctation of the aorta, aortic stenosis, or arteriovenous malformations, as these are surgically correctable conditions. Serum troponin should be measured, as elevated levels could indicate vascular compromise or ongoing inflammatory myocyte injury, as can be seen with acute myocarditis. Chronic arrhythmia, carnitine deficiency, or other inborn errors may also be seen more commonly in those presenting at less than 1 year of age (7). Children who present at older ages may be more likely to have an isolated gene defect or an acquired form of cardiomyopathy. Familial cardiomyopathies (with or without an identified gene defect), myocarditis, and ARVC seem to be more commonly diagnosed in older children and teens. In developing countries, Chagas disease is a common etiology of DCM. Muscular dystrophies (Duchenne and Becker) should be considered for boys presenting during the late school years and adolescence. Echocardiography, coronary CT imaging, cardiac magnetic resonance imaging (MRI), catheterization with myocardial biopsy, metabolic testing, and genetic analyses all play a role in the diagnosis of treatment of pediatric DCM, mandating careful coordination between multiple specialty services. MRI is taking on an increasing role in the diagnosis and long-term monitoring in many cases of cardiomyopathy. MRI can provide functional data and give insights into the presence and degree of acute myocardial inflammation, fibrosis, or ischemic injury. B-type natriuretic peptide (BNP) or the N-terminal-pro-BNP (NT-proBNP) levels can be used to help confirm a cardiac, as opposed to a respiratory source, of a patient's distress. Importantly, the serial monitoring of NT-proBNP levels has been shown to correlate with patient status, and can help guide drug therapy for patients with chronic DCM (8).

Therapeutic Strategies

The principles of treatment in children with DCM are similar to those with myocarditis, with the common goal of stabilizing progression of decompensated heart failure; the treatment strategies are described in a subsequent section of this chapter.

Hypertrophic Cardiomyopathy

Incidence and Etiology

HCM represents a diverse set of disorders, which lead to the development of a generalized diagnostic phenotype of inappropriate cardiac hypertrophy with its clinical impact spanning the spectrum that includes asymptomatic hypertrophy, clinical heart failure, arrhythmia, or early *sudden cardiac death* (SCD). Cardiac hypertrophy in HCM is not induced by or is secondary to any other cardiac or systemic disease, but is rather the result of primary sarcomeric mutations, identifiable syndromes (e.g., Noonan syndrome), inborn errors of metabolism, or similar genetic abnormalities (see **Table 73.3**). HCM is the most common inherited cardiac disease, and is thought to be found in 1 in 500 of the general population of young adults (9). HCM is now the preferred diagnostic term, but many names have been given to this condition, including idiopathic hypertrophic subaortic stenosis and hypertrophic-obstructive cardiomyopathy. HCM, often undiagnosed, is reported as the most common specific cause of SCD in children, being found in 36% of pediatric SCD. SCD in children is reported to occur at an annual incidence as high as 6.2/100,000 patient years (10). HCM represented ~42% of diagnosed pediatric cardiomyopathy cases in the PCMR cohort, which estimated incidence of *diagnosed* pediatric HCM to be 0.47/100,000 patient years in North America (1). These data suggest that the yearly incidence of HCM-associated pediatric SCD is nearly 5 times higher than the rate of diagnosed pediatric HCM cases. It appears that the majority of children with HCM, who may be at risk for SCD, remain undiagnosed, lack preventive care, and continue to participate in activities that may expose them to lethal arrhythmic risk.

Molecular Genetics

Genetic identification and testing for HCM has advanced from bench to bedside more quickly than for other types of cardiomyopathy. Hundreds of specific gene defects have been implicated as causative of HCM, typically involving 30 some genes encoding myofilaments (30%–50% of patients), Z-disc (~5% of patients), calcium-handling or mitochondrial proteins (11). Mutations of the MYH7 gene encoding the β-myosin heavy chain were first elucidated followed by a number of mutations involving the myosin light chain (MYL3) cardiac troponins (TNNTT2, TPM1, TNNI3) and other sarcomeric proteins. With these advances, gene testing of probands and first-degree relatives is rapidly becoming standard practice in the evaluation of patients and families with HCM.

Diagnosis and Screening

For the intensivist, HCM is often discovered in the PICU after a previously undiagnosed child has been resuscitated after a sports-related sudden cardiac arrest. During this time, the child is evaluated by a pediatric cardiologist, and appropriate echocardiographic and electrophysiologic testing is initiated. This is, often, an emotionally difficult time for the families, especially as they are being introduced to the presence of a previously unidentified genetic condition that could broadly affect their family unit. Many cases of HCM are subsequently identified by echocardiographic and genetic testing of family members following proband identification. Apart from those affected by SCD, HCM can be diagnosed by the general pediatrician during the evaluation of an outflow murmur (from the development of outflow tract obstruction), during evaluation for syncope, or from a patient's history that details risk factors such as sports-related syncope, and a family history of genetic heart disease or early sudden death. The American Academy of Pediatrics

TABLE 73.2

ETIOLOGIC AGENTS IN MYOCARDITIS

■ VIRUSES	■ NONVIRAL INFECTIOUS PATHOGENS	■ NONINFECTIOUS ETIOLOGIES
Adenovirus	**Bacteria**	**Pharmaceuticals**
Arbovirus	*Borrelia burgdorferi*	Acetazolamide
Cytomegalovirus	*Brucella melitensis*	Amphotericin B
Enterovirus	*Chlamydia pneumoniae*	Anthracyclines
Coxsackie A and B	*Chlamydia psittaci*	Cephalosporins
Echovirus	*Clostridium*	Cocaine
Poliovirus	*Klebsiella*	Cyclophosphamide
Epstein–Barr virus	*Legionella pneumophila*	Digoxin
Hepatitis A, B, and C	*Leptospira*	Diuretics
Herpes simplex virus	*Meningococcus*	Dobutamine
Human immunodeficiency virus	*Mycobacteria*	Indomethacin
Influenza A	*Mycoplasma pneumonia*	Isoniazid
Measles	*Salmonella*	Methyldopa
Mumps	*Streptococcus* species	Neomercazole
Parvovirus B19	*Treponema pallidum*	Penicillin
Rabies	Tuberculosis	Phenylbutazone
Respiratory syncytial virus	Typhoid	Phenytoin
Rhinovirus	**Rickettsial**	Sulfonamides
Rubella	*Rickettsia rickettsii*	Tetracycline
Rubeola	*Rickettsia tsutsugamushi*	Tricyclic
Vaccinia virus	**Fungi and yeasts**	Antidepressants
Varicella	Actinomyces	**Hypersensitivity/autoimmune**
	Aspergillus	Celiac disease
	Candida	Diabetes mellitus
	Coccidioides	Hashimoto's thyroiditis
	Cryptococcus	Mixed connective tissue disease
	Histoplasma	Myasthenia gravis
	Protozoa	Pernicious anemia
	Entamoeba histolytica	Rheumatoid arthritis
	Trypanosoma cruzi	Rheumatic fever
	Toxoplasma gondii	Scleroderma
	Parasites	Systemic lupus erythematosus
	Echinococcus granulosus	Takayasu arteritis
	Heterophyiasis	Thrombocytopenic purpura
	Plasmodium falciparum	Ulcerative colitis
	Schistosomiasis	Wegener granulomatosis
	Taenia solium (Cysticercosis)	Whipple disease
	Toxocara canis	**Toxins and others**
	Trichinella spiralis	Cornstarch
		Diphtheria
		Kawasaki disease
		Sarcoidosis
		Pertussis
		Scorpion venom
		Smallpox vaccine

addresses this issue by specifically recommending that all teen athletes undergo a focused history and exam before participating in organized sports activities (12).

Risk Stratification and Therapeutic Strategies

Once the diagnosis of HCM is made, the goals include alleviation of symptoms and the prevention of sudden death. Risk stratification and risk mitigation for the individual child remain topics of intense import, interest, and research (13,14). Factors such as a personal history of aborted SCD, detected episodes of sustained ventricular tachycardia, family history of HCM-related SCD, abnormal blood pressure response to stress exercise testing, and, increasingly, genetic results are interpreted to gage SCD risk. If the risk of SCD is thought to be high, then patients are typically targeted for automated implanted cardiodefibrillator

(ICD) placement. ICD placement, rather than antiarrhythmic medication, has been shown to be the only effective means to prevent arrhythmic SCD in the HCM population. Patients with ICDs inserted for HCM have shown a 4%–10% rate of yearly appropriate (and presumably life-saving) device discharge (15). However, ICD placement is an expensive undertaking in terms of the cost and potential complications. Complications include inappropriate discharge, lead fractures or dislodgement, device infections, bleeding, and thromboses. Inappropriate discharges and lead complications are thought to be more common in children due to growth and activity issues.

A number of interventions, including restrictions on physical activity, are mandatory as exercise-induced catecholamine release can exacerbate left-ventricular outflow tract (LVOT) obstruction, promote LV ischemia, and induce lethal arrhythmia. The American Heart Association (AHA) guidelines for exercise

TABLE 73.3

HYPERTROPHIC CARDIOMYOPATHY—SELECTED ETIOLOGIES AND ASSOCIATIONS

Gene defects found to be causative:
  Myosin heavy chain (MYH7)
  Myosin light chain (MYL3)
  Cardiac troponins (TNNTT2, TPMI, TNNI3)
  Titin
  Actin
  Mitochondrial proteins
  Calcium-handling proteins
  Z-disc proteins
  Others—specific gene defects are more commonly found in
HCM, as opposed to DCM.
Metabolic/storage disorders:
  Pompe disease
  Danon disease
  PRKAG2 familial glycogen storage disease
  Hunter's disease
  Hurler syndrome
  Fabry disease
Associated syndromes:
  Noonan syndrome
  Friedrich ataxia
  Barth syndrome
  LEOPARD (multiple lentigines) syndrome

LEOPARD, lentigines, electrocardiographic abnormalities, ocular hypertelorism, pulmonary stenosis, abnormal genitalia, retarded growth, deafness.

participation can direct clinician recommendations and provide objective information to families and often-resistant adolescent patients (16). Medical therapy is indicated in order to alleviate symptoms. Exercise intolerance generally stems from hypertrophy-related diastolic dysfunction, dynamic LVOT obstruction, or mitral valve insufficiency. Exertional symptoms are most commonly treated using β adrenergic (e.g., propranolol) or calcium-channel blocking agents (e.g., verapamil). These agents may provide multiple benefits, slow the heart rate to permit better diastolic filling, decrease dynamic LVOT obstruction through negative inotropic effects, improve angina symptoms by lowering myocardial oxygen demand, and in the case of calcium-channel blockers, improve microvascular perfusion. Vasodilators such as angiotensin-converting enzyme inhibitors (ACEi) should be avoided in patients with significant obstruction as afterload reduction could worsen dynamic LVOT narrowing. Digoxin is relatively contraindicated as increasing contractility could also worsen such an obstruction. Diastolic dysfunction can produce either systemic or pulmonary congestion, mandating the use of diuretic agents. These must be judiciously titrated in order to maintain sufficient preload because the stiff ventricle requires high filling pressures so as to not worsen dynamic outflow tract collapse. Similarly, affected children should be advised to maintain good fluid intake and avoid dehydration in order to maintain adequate cardiac preload.

In the intensive care setting, phenylephrine or norepinephrine is considered to be useful for the treatment of acute hypotension in the setting of obstructive HCM, similar to its use for tetralogy of Fallot "spells." Commonly used inotropic agents such as dopamine, dobutamine, and epinephrine remain relatively contraindicated in the setting of obstructive HCM. Patients with symptomatic or severe resting outflow tract obstruction, despite aggressive medication titration, should be considered for septal reduction surgery. Surgical myectomy is preferred in the younger populations, as opposed to alcohol

ablation, which is typically reserved for older patients with relatively higher operative risk. Experiential and evidence-based guidelines have been published for the management of HCM in adults; pediatric data are largely lacking, making this a necessary reference to help guide pediatric care (17).

Restrictive Cardiomyopathy

Incidence and Etiology

RCM is a relatively rare form of cardiomyopathy characterized by severe biventricular diastolic dysfunction, which leads to marked biatrial enlargement. Restrictive physiology can be part of a mixed type of cardiomyopathy, or present as a "pure" form with no associated ventricular hypertrophy, dilatation, or thinning. This "pure" RCM was classified in only 3% (101 children) in the PCMR cardiomyopathy cohort (18). Another 50 children were identified as having "mixed" RCM disease, which was commonly found in association with ventricular hypertrophic changes. RCM was initially identified as a state of severe diastolic dysfunction, rather than a specific cardiomyopathy. When found, efforts should be made to exclude alternative and treatable diagnoses such as pericardial disease (restrictive pericarditis) or other conditions with cardiac involvement such as glycogen storage diseases or amyloidosis. Restrictive physiology has also been described following cancer treatment with chest radiation or anthracycline agents. Echocardiographically, patients demonstrate small to normal ventricular dimensions, with profound atrial dilation, which creates a so-called "Mickey Mouse" appearance on apical four-chamber imaging. Gene defects in troponin (TTNI3) and the sarcomeric protein desmin have been implicated in familial cases (19).

Pathophysiology and Treatment Strategies

RCM leads to pulmonary venous congestion with children often coming to medical attention with nonspecific respiratory symptoms. High filling pressures can lead to rapid progression of pulmonary vascular disease; SCD can be the presenting sign of RCM. Echocardiography remains the major diagnostic tool. Cardiac catheterization can further define hemodynamics, and MRI is playing an increasing role in terms of ruling out pericardial disease and can further define and trend diastolic filling parameters.

RCM is thought to be a high-risk diagnosis, with many centers opting for early transplantation. PCMR data report that 40% of patients undergo transplantation while 20% die without transplant within 2 years of diagnosis. There is only a 20% transplant-free survival demonstrated in the PCMR cohort 6 years following the diagnosis of RCM. Advocates of early transplantation point to a relatively high incidence of SCD and progressive pulmonary hypertension to support this choice. Atrial enlargement also raises the risk of embolic stroke. Prior to transplantation, symptoms can be treated with careful diuresis, but no specific convincing therapy is currently promoted to treat diastolic dysfunction. With such an absence of specific therapy, a careful symptomatic approach to medical therapy is currently applied to these children, with much of their care focused upon the timing of transplant listing. PCMR data could only identify decreased LV function and signs of CHF as risk factors for early death, making risk stratification and transplant timing topics worthy of further research.

Arrhythmogenic Right-Ventricular Cardiomyopathy

ARVC is increasingly recognized as a cause of SCD in children (20). It represents an important group of genetic heart diseases caused by several gene abnormalities that make up the desmosomal complex, which lead to fibro-fatty infiltration of either ventricle, but is more classically seen affecting the right side. Most cases are inherited in an autosomal dominant manner, with ventricular arrhythmias typically occurring during adolescence or young adult years. Arrhythmia and a family history of SCD are the most common factors leading to the diagnosis of ARVC. Isolated right heart failure has also been described as the presenting sign in some children. ARVC is classically suspected during arrhythmia evaluation with the ventricular tachycardia in ARVC typically showing left bundle branch block morphology. *Epsilon waves*—low-amplitude signals between the end of the QRS complex to the onset of the T wave—are perhaps the most characteristic ECG findings in ARVC. Specific diagnostic criteria for ARVC were first published in the 1990s and have been recently updated to be more inclusive and reflect advances in imaging and clinical experience (21). The AHA task force utilizes cardiac imaging, biopsy, ECG, presence of ventricular tachycardia, and family history to define a series of major and minor criteria in order to come to a diagnosis of ARVC. Of note, current diagnostic criteria do not rely upon the presence of fatty infiltration as detected on MRI imaging, as this has been found to be a nonspecific finding. Definitive diagnosis of ARVC may be confounded in children who may develop phenotypic changes over time, and child-specific diagnostic criteria await further genetic and clinical progress.

Similar to other forms of genetic heart disease, once a patient is diagnosed with ARVC, a risk assessment must be performed and other family members must be evaluated. Many patients, particularly those with history of resuscitated sudden cardiac arrest, benefit from ICD placement. Sports restriction, genetic testing, and regular cardiac evaluation (including ambulatory ECG and echocardiographic monitoring) become lifelong measures for ARVC patients and families.

Left-Ventricular Noncompaction

LVNC is a state of abnormal myocardial morphogenesis characterized by diffuse LV trabeculations and deep intertrabecular recesses (22). It is thought to represent an interruption of the normal fetal process of myocardial structural compaction and has previously been descriptively referred to as "spongy myocardium." LVNC has recently been identified as a relatively frequent cause of LV dysfunction, being reported at least as a phenotypic component in up to 9% of childhood cardiomyopathies. The etiology of LVNC is highly heterogeneous and has been described as resulting from single-gene defects, syndromic disorders, and neurologic, metabolic, mitochondrial, and neuromuscular disease. One study from Italy reported LVNC in association with syndromic children such as Turner, DiGeorge, and LEOPARD syndromes (23). Approximately 20% of LVNC cases show an associated congenital heart defect, from simple septal defects, through to complex lesions such as Ebstein's anomaly or the hypoplastic left heart syndrome. LVNC can be readily diagnosed by echocardiography where deep intertrabecular recesses can be seen, with most patients demonstrating reduced LV function. Often layers of compacted versus noncompacted myocardium can be distinguished, and these ratios have been used as one measure of severity. MRI imaging can also assist with this diagnosis in children with poor acoustic windows that do not allow for complete echocardiographic imaging. The majority of patients will demonstrate ECG changes that include biventricular hypertrophy, extremely increased QRS voltages, and diffuse T wave changes.

As LV noncompaction can be seen in association with a wide variety of conditions and associations, it is difficult to generalize a specific prognosis for a given patient. Many children do demonstrate progressive LV dysfunction, with other manifestations including arrhythmia, thromboembolism, and eventual decompensated heart failure. Patients who develop heart failure should be treated similar to those with DCM, with attention to arrhythmia and thromboembolic prevention. As is true with all types of cardiomyopathy, it is important to rule out causative primary metabolic or neuromuscular disorders. This construct may be even more crucial in the setting for LVNC, which is more commonly a component of a more global pathologic process.

Acquired Cardiomyopathies

This chapter focuses upon primary pediatric cardiomyopathies, which result largely as consequences of inborn sarcomeric or metabolic abnormalities. This is in direct contrast to adults, in whom cardiomyopathies typically occur as secondary to insults such as atherosclerosis-induced coronary ischemia or chronic hypertension. Unfortunately, issues such as obesity, drug use, chronic hypertension, diabetes, and renal disease seem to be increasing in western cultures and may lead to earlier onset of cardiomyopathy in a progressively younger population. There are several groups of children such as those with Kawasaki disease, renal disease, vitamin D deficiency, and cancer survivors for whom pediatricians should be on guard for LV dysfunction. Data are particularly clear that essentially all childhood cancer survivors should be considered at risk for the development of long-term cardiac complications. Long-term data show that at 15–25 years after diagnosis, childhood cancer survivors have an eightfold higher rate of cardiac death as compared to age-matched controls (24).

Anthracycline-induced Cardiomyopathy

Anthracyclines are thought to injure the myocardium by a variety of mechanisms, including free radical generation leading to cardiocyte mitochondrial damage. Clinical cardiotoxicity can be both acute or of late onset thereby mandating echocardiographic monitoring throughout all stages of care. Acute DCM can occur, but is rare, occurring in only 1%, of treated patients. Late-onset disease is more common, with increased risk with longer-term follow-up (as high as 16% in longer-term studies) (25). It is important to note that cardiovascular risk following cancer treatment is not unique to anthracycline exposure, as wide-reaching effects of many differing drugs, radiation, dysautonomia, and endocrine responses also contribute to this complex pathological milieu. Current pediatric chemotherapy protocols tend to limit anthracycline exposure to a cumulative dosing of <300 mg/m². Regardless of the specific regimen applied, an intensivist should be aware of the association between cancer treatment and potential cardiomyopathy.

Vitamin D Deficiency–induced Cardiomyopathy

DCM related to hypocalcemia associated with vitamin D deficiency and rickets has been described in infants belonging to the dark-skinned ethnic minority groups, who are typically exclusively breastfed and not on any calcium or vitamin D supplements. Biochemistry on admission shows low serum calcium/ionized calcium level, elevated parathormone level, and low vitamin D level. There may be radiological evidence of rickets. The first reported case of rickets cardiomyopathy in the United States was published in 2003 as an "unusual cause of pediatric cardiomyopathy" (26). These children can often develop severe acute heart failure and present in extremis, but can fully recover with appropriate intensive care support and metabolic management of rickets. Maiya et al. (27) in their series of affected infants reported slow improvement on serial echocardiograms with normalization of LV fractional shortening over an average period of 12.4 (8.0–16.7) months after presentation.

MYOCARDITIS

Myocarditis is defined as an inflammatory disease of the myocardium associated with lymphocytic infiltrate and cardiomyocyte degeneration, which is not ischemic in origin. The definition does not include the etiology as it may be caused by a variety of infective and noninfective agents, but does include the histopathological diagnosis obtained from an endomyocardial biopsy. However, as an endomyocardial biopsy diagnosis may not always be available, a clinical definition would involve presentation of new-onset heart failure associated with ventricular dysfunction with positive markers of inflammation, with or without positive virology in a previously well child, with no structural heart disease. Acute fulminant myocarditis is a specific entity of particular interest to the intensivist; it is characterized by rapid progression of clinical symptoms after a distinct short viral prodrome with significant hemodynamic compromise and risk of cardiovascular collapse.

Etiology

Myocarditis may be caused by a number of infective and noninfective agents (see **Table 73.4**). Worldwide, the most common cause of myocarditis is Chagas disease caused by *Trypanosoma cruzi*, which is endemic in South and Central America (28). In the United States and Western Europe, viral infections account for most cases: the common viruses include enteroviruses (coxsackievirus B, serotypes 1–6), adenovirus (serotypes 2, 5), parvovirus B19, and influenza (29). In a large series investigating a viral cause for biopsy- or autopsy-proven acute viral myocarditis ($n = 624$) and DCM ($n = 149$), Bowles et al. (30) reported on positive viral polymerase chain reaction (PCR) in 38% of patients with acute viral myocarditis and 20% with DCM; and the commonest virus identified were adenovirus (23%) and enterovirus (14%) in patients of all ages. The epidemiology of viral myocarditis has undergone a shift over time with enteroviruses, being the predominant responsible viral agent in the 70s and 80s, to adenovirus in the 90s, and to parvovirus B19 in the last decade (29–34). Most recently, fulminant myocarditis has been reported as part of the pandemic outbreak caused by the H1N1 influenza A in children (35). Also, in many cases, the etiology may remain unidentified, even after detailed investigations.

Eosinophilic and Giant cell Myocarditis

There are two other distinct forms of myocarditis, which will be briefly mentioned here. Eosinophilic myocarditis is a rare entity characterized by eosinophilia and myocardial inflammation with infiltrating eosinophils. It is attributed to eosinophilic syndromes, allergic reactions, autoimmune diseases, and parasitic infections, and has been seen post-vaccination in children. The patients present with congestive cardiac failure, ventricular arrhythmias, heart block, or myocardial infarction and have a characteristic endomyocardial biopsy. Steroid treatment may be helpful (36–39).

Idiopathic giant cell myocarditis is a rare disease, where the patients present with congestive cardiac failure, ventricular arrhythmias, or heart block and have a characteristic endomyocardial biopsy with giant cells and active inflammation. Despite institution of medical therapy, patients continue to have poorly controlled heart failure and arrhythmias that may respond to aggressive immunosuppressive therapy (40).

Epidemiology

The estimated annual incidence of acute myocarditis in children worldwide is around 1/100,000 (1,3,41). However, the

---

TABLE 73.4

SELECTED ETIOLOGIC TESTING FOR A CHILD PRESENTING WITH ACUTE MYOCARDIAL DYSFUNCTION

Immediate evaluation:
- Clinical and family history
- Basic chemistries (including total and ionized calcium, magnesium, glucose, renal profile, liver function tests including aminotransferases, lactic acid)
- Complete and differential blood count (neutropenia, lymphocytosis), coagulation profile
- Chest x-ray (cardiomegaly, pulmonary congestion/edema, persistent left lower lobe collapse from compression of left main bronchus by enlarged left atrium)
- 12-lead ECG (voltage changes, ST-T changes)
- Echocardiogram (to rule out anatomic abnormalities, assess degree of ventricular dysfunction)
- C-reactive protein, erythrocyte sedimentation rate
- Troponin, creatine kinase isoenzyme (CK-MB), B-type natriuretic peptide (BNP), N-terminal fragment (NT-proBNP)

Further etiologic testing:
- **Microbiological studies:** Viral IgM, PCR virology in serum, urine, stool, nasopharyngeal, tracheal aspirate (Enterovirus, Adenovirus, Parvovirus and then extended panel), Viral IgM, bacterial tests
- **Metabolic studies:** Urine organic acids, serum amino acids, ammonia, urine glycosaminoglycans, carnitine levels/acylcarnitine profile/cholesterol/triglycerides, RBC transketolase, red cell folate, transferrin, thiamine, selenium, vacuolated lymphocytes on peripheral smear
- (Amino acid and organic metabolism, disorders of fatty acid metabolism, disorders of glycogen metabolism, glycoprotein metabolism, lysosomal storage disorders, mitochondrial disorders)
- **Endocrine:** Thyroid studies, parathyroid hormone, vitamin D levels
- **Autoimmune:** Autoantibody screen, antinuclear antibodies, anti-DNA antibodies, anti-Ro
- **Genetic testing:** Barth syndrome

Testing for further management or diagnosis in selected cases:
- Metabolic and genetic consultation
- Cardiac MRI
- Cardiac catheterization
- Endomyocardial biopsy (for both electron microscopy and viral PCR testing)
- Peripheral muscle biopsy
- Electrophysiologic studies and 24-hour Holter monitoring when primary arrhythmia suspected

---

true incidence is underestimated, with a significant number of clinical presentations being diagnosed as the "flu" because of the lack of specific cardiac symptoms. In addition, a significant number of missed diagnoses occur because of the incomplete investigation of sudden death, especially in young children. Acute viral myocarditis accounts for 7.5%–28% of SCD in children and young adults, without previously diagnosed heart disease as reported from different parts of the world (42–48), and is as high as 42% in infants with SCD (49). In another study of sudden infant death, enterovirus was identified in 50% of infants, who had clinical signs of viral illness (50).

Myocarditis may evolve into cardiomyopathy in ~10% of children and young adults on follow-up (1,41). The incidence of DCM due to acute viral myocarditis, confirmed at either biopsy or autopsy, is 14% in an Australian study of children less than 10 years of age during a 10-year period (41) and is

9% in an American study of children 1–18 years of age during a 4-year period (1). Even though these studies are not comparable, more than 10% of children presenting with heart failure and DCM will have underlying viral pathology, which may be an underestimate due to the lack of biopsy confirmation in many cases and an unknown number of subclinical cases.

The reason for the predisposition to progress to DCM instead of resolution, in some cases after an enteroviral infection, is difficult to explain. It is speculated that host genetic factors and molecular mechanisms, such as expression of the *coxsackie B virus and adenovirus receptor* (CAR) and dystrophin deficiency, may have a role to play (51–53).

Pathogenesis and Histology

The pathogenesis of myocarditis involves direct invasion by the cardiotropic virus, which leads to local inflammation and activation of the humoral as well as the cell-mediated innate host immune response. The initial activation induces production of B cells, which results in myocytolysis and interstitial inflammation, and production of anti-heart antibodies. From an animal experimental model, three phases have been described—*acute myocarditis* lasting for up to 4 days with viremia leading to myocyte necrosis and macrophage activation, which in turn leads to release of cytokines; *subacute myocarditis* is the next phase with the proliferation of infiltrating mononuclear cells, cytotoxic T and B lymphocytes, and natural killer cells lasting between 4 and 14 days with clearing of the virus and finally *chronic myocarditis* with fibrosis and cardiac dilatation with the absence of the virus (54). Circulating autoantibodies that target the contractile, mitochondrial, and structural proteins have been described in murine and human myocarditis (55). With persistence of viremia and the accompanying immune response, acute myocarditis can progress to a more chronic DCM (56).

Histologic diagnosis involves identifying the presence of infiltrating cells—lymphocytes, mononuclear cells or eosinophils, or giant cells depending on etiology. The histological findings used to define myocarditis called the Dallas criteria are described in **Table 73.5** (57). The infiltrates may be of varying severity and are associated with myocyte cell necrosis and disorganization of myocardial cytoskeleton (**Fig. 73.1**). The inflammatory infiltrate has been described to be substantially less in adenoviral infection as compared to coxsackie B virus (29,31), and parvovirus B19 targets coronary endothelium, leading to myocardial ischemia and dysfunction (58). Viral particles are not routinely seen on histopathology; they may, however, be identified on electron microscopy. In giant cell myocarditis, endomyocardial biopsy shows characteristic giant cells and active inflammation. As the acute phase progresses into chronic myocarditis, interstitial fibrosis may replace fiber loss and myofiber hypertrophy may also be seen.

Clinical Manifestations

The spectrum of presentation of pediatric myocarditis ranges from minor flu-like illness with chest pain to acute cardiogenic shock and death in a previously healthy child.

Acute fulminant myocarditis, seen in about 20%–30% of all patients with myocarditis, is a distinctive entity, which has a very acute onset with hemodynamic instability, signs of congestive heart failure, and requirement for inotropic and even MCS. The patients typically have (a) a short viral prodrome with distinct onset of symptoms (<14 days), (b) significant cardiac dysfunction requiring at minimum inotropic support to maintain CO and perfusion, and (c) normal cardiac size to less than moderate cardiomegaly on chest radiography and normal LV end-diastolic volume by echocardiography (LV end-diastolic Z-score of <3) (59,60). On histology, an intense inflammatory response is seen with significant lymphocytic infiltration and myocyte necrosis.

Acute (nonfulminant) myocarditis, in contrast, has a longer prodrome and presentation is frequently insidious with a recent history of a nonspecific viral illness, associated at times

TABLE 73.5

CLINICAL PRESENTATION, HISTOPATHOLOGY, AND OUTCOME OF MYOCARDITIS IN CHILDREN

■ TYPE	■ CLINICAL PRESENTATION	■ HISTOPATHOLOGY	■ OUTCOME
Fulminant myocarditis	■ Viral prodrome ■ Distinct onset of illness within 2 wk of presentation ■ Severe cardiovascular compromise with ventricular dysfunction but not usually left-ventricular dilatation ■ Heart block or ventricular arrhythmias ■ Sudden death	■ Multiple foci of active inflammation and necrosis with lymphocytic infiltration, myocyte necrosis ± myocyte degeneration	■ Patients recover or die within 2 wk with complete histological and functional recovery of the myocardium in survivors
Acute myocarditis	■ Less distinct onset of illness, with established ventricular dysfunction	■ Lymphocytic infiltration ± myocyte necrosis	■ May progress to dilated cardiomyopathy
Chronic active myocarditis	■ Less distinct onset of illness with clinical and histologic relapses; development of moderate ventricular dysfunction	■ Active or borderline associated with chronic inflammatory changes	■ Chronic heart failure
Chronic persistent myocarditis	■ Less distinct onset of illness (despite symptoms, e.g., chest pain, palpitations) but without ventricular dysfunction	■ Persistent histologic infiltrate with foci of myocyte necrosis	■ Chronic heart failure

As per Dallas criteria, myocarditis is active if both myocyte degeneration or necrosis *and* definite cellular infiltrate with or without fibrosis is present, borderline if definite cellular infiltrate without myocyte injury and persistent if continued active myocarditis on repeat right-ventricular endomyocardial biopsy.

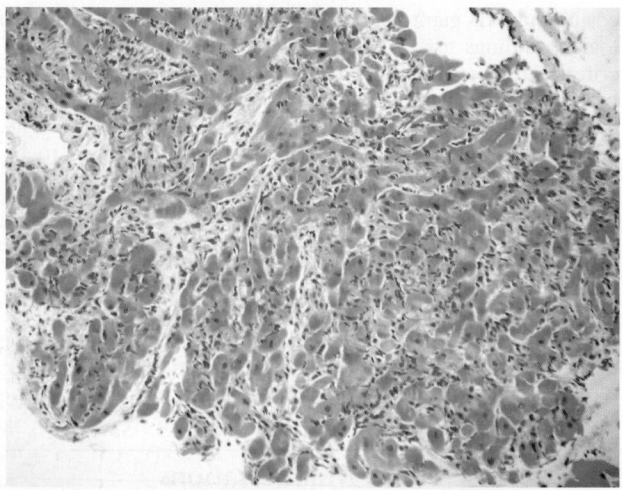

FIGURE 73.1. Endomyocardial biopsy of a child with acute viral myocarditis showing edema, inflammatory cell infiltration, myocyte destruction, and apoptosis. (Hematoxylin and eosin stain, text and image courtesy of Dr. Michael Ashworth, Consultant Histopathologist, Great Ormond Street Hospital for Children NHS Foundation Trust, London, UK.)

with abdominal pain, nausea and vomiting, and/or coryzal symptoms. It can often be mistaken for gastroenteritis or an upper respiratory tract infection in young children. Other presenting symptoms include chest pain in adolescents and young adults, congestive cardiac failure, and palpitations and syncope (from arrhythmias). Fever, rash, diarrhea, easy fatigability, and joint pains may be present as signs of viral illness. Importantly, the cardiovascular symptoms may be minimal and masked by the overlay of the gastroenterological or respiratory symptoms. Because of the relatively robust physiology in children and their ability to compensate for decreased heart function, the diagnosis frequently may not even be suspected until acute collapse or sudden death occurs.

The fulminant myocarditis, though severe, with more intense inflammatory response to viral infection usually recovers with supportive measures, in contrast to those with the nonfulminant variety, where the inflammation is less intense but the virus persists in a more indolent form. Only 45% in the nonfulminant group were alive without transplant up to 11 years after biopsy as compared to 93% in the fulminant group after an average follow-up of 5 years (61).

Chronic myocarditis from postinfectious immune or associated systemic autoimmune diseases manifests as persistent or progressive ventricular dysfunction, arrhythmias, and chronic congestive heart failure. The disease often presents as an acute form of DCM with symptoms and signs of chronic heart failure.

Age-specific Differences in Presentation

Differences in presentation are seen, depending on the age of the child (i.e., newborn/infant versus child or adolescent), making the diagnosis challenging.

Newborns or infants typically present with fever, poor feeding, vomiting, irritability or listlessness, periodic episodes of pallor, episodic cyanosis, tachypnea, or respiratory distress. The most common cause of myocarditis in neonates is enteroviral infection and can often present in the form of neonatal cardiovascular collapse. Sudden death may also occur. It is quite common to see signs of infarction on ECG, and severe ventricular dysfunction with mitral regurgitation on the echocardiogram (62,63). There may be associated meningoencephalitis and hepatitis with neonatal enterovirus infection.

Older children and adolescents commonly report a recent history of viral disease, generally 10–14 days prior to presentation. Initial symptoms are nonspecific and include lethargy and general malaise, diaphoresis, palpitations, rash, exercise intolerance, and low-grade fever; the child usually has decreased appetite and often complains of abdominal pain or chest pain suggestive of coronary ischemia (64). In particular, this may be more common with myocarditis due to parvovirus (33,58). Physical examination is consistent with the findings of congestive heart failure. Dysrhythmias are common. Syncope or sudden death may occur.

It is important to note that the diagnosis of myocarditis is commonly not made on the first presentation to a medical provider and hence increased awareness with a high index of suspicion should be maintained to ensure a good outcome (65,66). A differential diagnosis of myocarditis by age is listed in **Table 73.6**.

TABLE 73.6

DIFFERENTIAL DIAGNOSIS OF MYOCARDITIS BY AGE

■ NEWBORN AND INFANT	■ CHILD
Sepsis	Idiopathic DCM
Perinatal asphyxia	Familial DCM
Hypoglycemia	Sepsis
Hypocalcemia	Pneumonia
Inborn errors of metabolism including Pompe disease	
Structural heart disease (ALCAPA)	Structural heart disease (ALCAPA)
Endocardial fibroelastosis	Endocardial fibroelastosis
Left atrial myxoma	
Tachyarrhythmias	Chronic tachyarrhythmia
Hyperthyroidism	Pericarditis
Pneumonia	
Bronchiolitis	
Idiopathic DCM	
Barth syndrome	
Cerebral arteriovenous malformation	

Diagnostic Tests

Myocarditis should be suspected in any child presenting with new-onset heart failure, unexplained shortness of breath or fatigue, or a new arrhythmia on a background of structurally normal heart. In particular, tachycardia without a clearly defined cause is an important clue to the possibility of myocarditis. Timely diagnosis remains a challenge, as children do not present with specific signs and symptoms (67). The diagnosis is based on clinical symptoms and echocardiographic evidence of ventricular dysfunction in the setting of

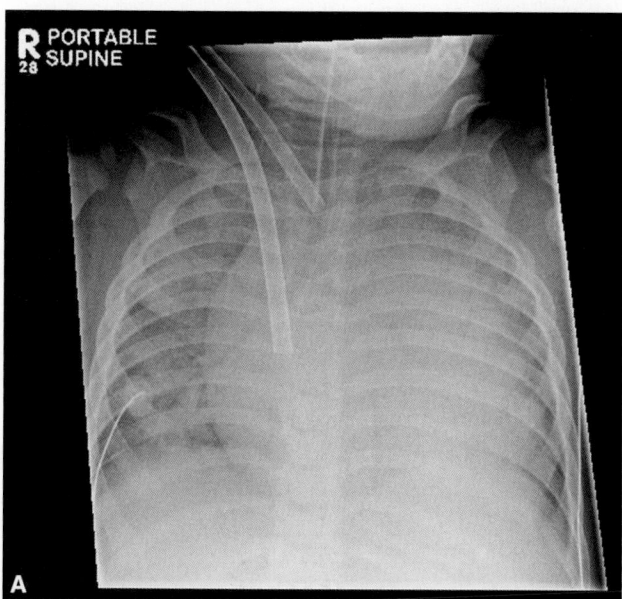

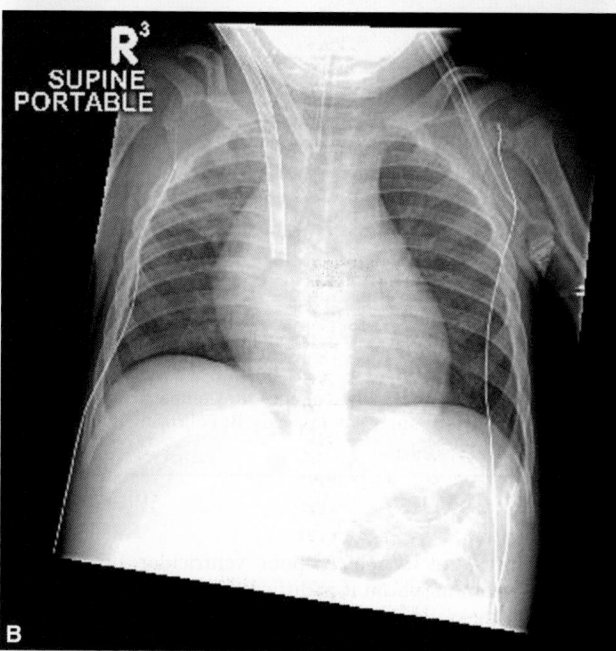

FIGURE 73.2. Chest x-ray of a 1-year-old child with acute fulminant myocarditis with severe congestive heart failure supported on ECMO. A: Shows cardiomegaly with prominent diffuse congestion of the lungs, which has improved dramatically after balloon atrial septostomy done by cardiac catheterization on ECMO support. B: The child was subsequently successfully decannulated off ECMO.

positive peripheral viral cultures (blood, nasopharyngeal, CSF, stool, or urine), serology, or histological evidence on biopsy. The cardiac silhouette on the chest x-ray is generally enlarged with acute viral myocarditis but may be normal in size and configuration in fulminant acute myocarditis. There may be pulmonary congestion present in variable degrees with pleural effusions and interstitial infiltrates (**Fig. 73.2A**). **Electrocardiogram** findings can be variable; however, they are commonly seen in 93%–100% of all cases with myocarditis with a reported sensitivity of 93% (66). The most common ECG findings are (a) sinus tachycardia; (b) low-voltage QRS complex in standard (total voltage <5 mm) and precordial leads, and low-amplitude Q waves in lateral precordial leads; and (c) ST-T wave changes—flattening or inversion of T waves in the standard or lateral precordial leads (41,65,66). In addition, signs of myocardial infarction such as marked elevation of the ST segment may be seen (**Fig. 73.3A**). Arrhythmias (supraventricular tachycardia, ventricular premature beats, atrial ectopic tachycardia, ventricular tachycardia, ventricular fibrillation, and variable degrees of atrioventricular block, including complete heart block) have been well described. Echocardiographic evaluation is essential for diagnosis. The most common finding is enlarged ventricular end-systolic and diastolic dimension and reduced shortening and ejection fractions (**Fig. 73.4**); atrioventricular valve regurgitation, especially mitral regurgitation, is also common. In fulminant myocarditis, the echocardiogram shows significant decrease in systolic function, thickened interventricular septum, and normal LV dimensions (LVEDV Z-score of <3) (68). Aspartate aminotransferase has been found to be a sensitive marker (reported sensitivity of 85%) (66). Creatine kinase isoenzyme (CK-MB) and cardiac troponin T, both markers for myocardial damage, may be elevated (69). NT-proBNP is a good marker for persistent LV dysfunction in children, who have had myocarditis, normalizing in children who show echocardiographic recovery (70). Viral studies including molecular (PCR) analyses of blood, nasopharyngeal aspirates, tracheal aspirates, and endomyocardial biopsy (when feasible and available taking into consideration hemodynamic condition permitting cardiac catheterization) should be performed to identify the viral agent. Tracheal aspirates have been shown to have a high yield for viral identification, particularly adenovirus (71). Endomyocardial biopsy used to be considered the gold standard for diagnosis of myocarditis. The Dallas criteria, established in 1986, for diagnosis in adults provide a histopathological categorization so as to minimize subjective discrepancies in interpretation (57). These criteria have not been modified for children. The optimal timing of the biopsy is within 3–6 weeks of onset of symptoms and may be taken from the right or the left ventricle by cardiac catheterization. However, false negatives may occur if performed early and diagnosis can be missed even if multiple samples are taken (72). There are major limitations, including sampling errors related to heterogeneity of the disease, the invasiveness of the procedure, low negative predictive value, and the inability of the pathologic result to reflect the physiologic effect of circulating mediators. Also, there may be complications with the biopsy, including perforation, hemothorax, dysrhythmia, and death, which may be increased in young patients with myocarditis particularly those requiring inotropic support (73). In view of the above factors, emphasis is placed on newer, less-invasive modalities of diagnosing myocarditis although biopsy may be essential if eosinophilic or giant cell myocarditis is suspected (28,74,75). In children, the use of MRI to diagnose myocarditis is not in widespread practice, because of the risks of anesthesia in poor hemodynamic status and other technical challenges. However, certain MRI image sequences in children can be correlated with biopsy-proven myocarditis (76).

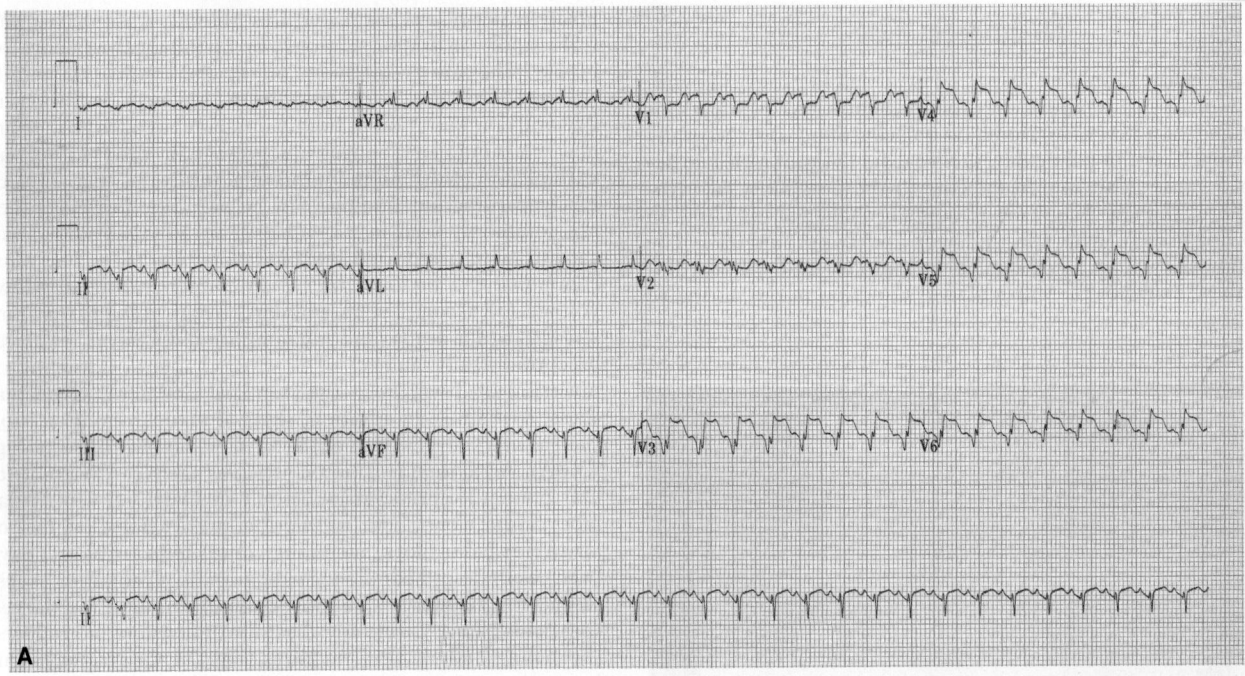

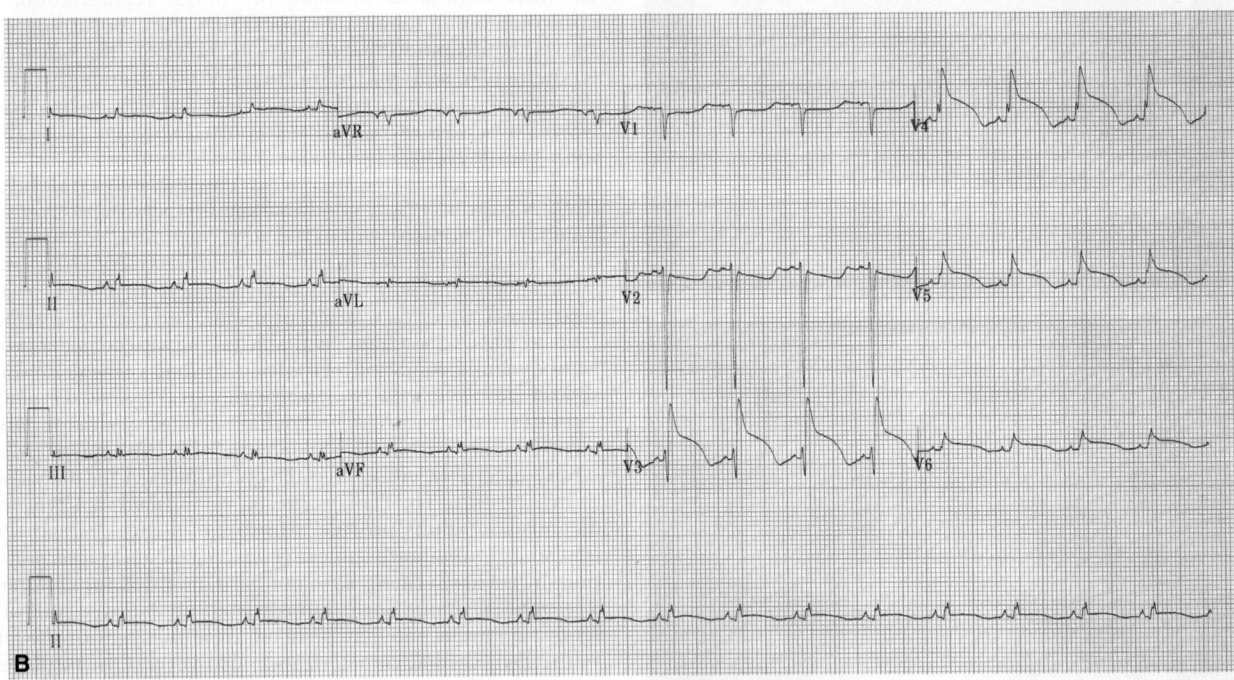

FIGURE 73.3. The 12-lead electrocardiogram in a child with acute fulminant myocarditis. **A:** Note the low-voltage QRS complexes (total voltage <5 mm) in standard limb and precordial leads. Note the significant elevation of ST-T segments in anterolateral leads. **B:** Following intensive care support and management, the rate has slowed but there is still evolving ischemic changes on ECG.

THERAPEUTIC STRATEGIES IN CHILDREN WITH CARDIOMYOPATHY OR MYOCARDITIS

Treatment of Acute Decompensated Heart Failure

It is not uncommon to have an acutely deteriorating patient admitted to ICU with severe heart failure, a structurally normal heart, and extremely poor ventricular function on echocardiogram in whom it is difficult to distinguish myocarditis from long-standing DCM with acute decompensation. It is therefore important to acknowledge that the principles of initial management of children with acute heart failure are essentially the same whether it is in the context of a patient with myocarditis or DCM.

DCM patients may present with decompensated heart failure, often around the time of their initial diagnosis or in a setting of progressive, long-standing disease. Patients with volume overload may exhibit hepatomegaly, orthopnea, tachypnea, dependent edema, and ascites, making diuresis a

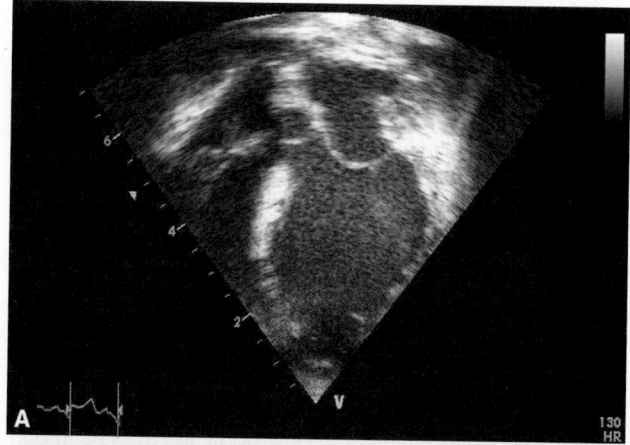

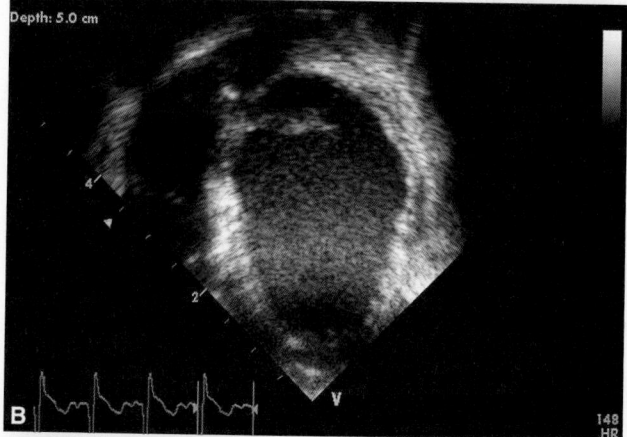

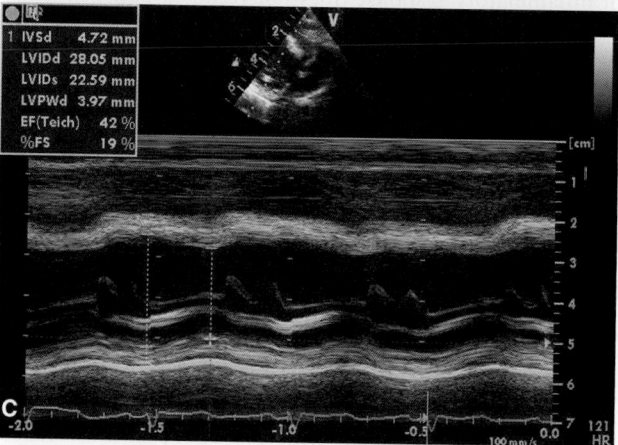

FIGURE 73.4. Echo images from a neonate with enteroviral myocarditis. (Text and image courtesy of Dr. Jan Marek, Consultant Cardiologist and lead for Echocardiography, Great Ormond Street Hospital for Children NHS Foundation Trust, London, UK). Two-dimensional parasternal long-axis view demonstrating left-ventricular dilatation axis view demonstrating left ventricle (LV) dilatation, which has progressed as shown in (**A**) (at presentation) and (**B**) (4 weeks later). **C**: Shows M mode demonstrating systolic dysfunction with flattened interventricular septal motion, fair LV posterior wall excursion, LV dilatation with increased LV end-diastolic dimension (LVEDD), and reduced systolic function.

mandatory part of therapy. Those with low perfusion generally show various degrees of tachycardia, poor feeding, narrow pulse pressure, or cool extremities; they may be irritable or show a decreased level of consciousness. Hypotension will eventually result, but may be a relatively late finding. Other signs of end-organ compromise will include prerenal azotemia,

elevated transaminase levels, and the ultimate development of a systemic lactic acidosis.

The acute treatment involves assessing the hemodynamic state of the patient and determining the need for intervention based upon the patient's perfusion (warm or cold) and volume status (wet or dry). These two characteristics combine to create four potential states, with restoration of the warm and dry state being the targeted goal of therapy. Once a low CO state is recognized, the intensivist must intervene in order to increase systemic oxygen delivery. This involves improving myocardial performance and modifying loading conditions using pharmacologic and nonpharmacologic therapies. The principles of management can be summarized by first, identifying the strategies that determine CO namely heart rate and stroke volume (the latter affected by the preload, afterload, and myocardial contractility) and second, optimization of the relationship of oxygen delivery (Do_2) and consumption ($\dot{V}o_2$) to improve and maintain tissue perfusion. The administration of diuretics (to reduce fluid overload) and afterload reduction (to reduce SVR) may be the first two therapeutic steps to stabilize the situation. Securing central venous access may be challenging, if respiration is not supported with mechanical ventilation. Dobutamine or milrinone infusions can be administered via peripheral venous access and are usually the first-line agents.

For the patient in extremis, the work of breathing is often greatly increased due to severe pulmonary congestion. A failing heart may not be able to meet the increased metabolic demand of distressed breathing, resulting in oxygen debt of the respiratory musculature. In this setting, endotracheal intubation and mechanical ventilation can be life-saving. Positive pressure ventilation provides the additional benefit of lowering the LV afterload, which may improve energy balance and increase LV stroke volumes. The process of stabilizing the airway and endotracheal intubation is in itself a high-risk procedure for children with worsening hemodynamic status and has to be carefully managed. It should be done in an intensive care environment by experienced staff with ready access to emergency extracorporeal membrane oxygenation (ECMO) cannulation in the event of cardiac arrest. It is important to bear in mind that there is no ideal agent for induction of anesthesia for these children who are in decompensating heart failure, and ideally, help from experienced anesthetist should be enlisted. The use of anesthetic induction agents that cause significant myocardial depression (thiopentone) or peripheral vasodilatation (inhalational agents, propofol) should be avoided. The attending intensivist should use the agent which he or she has most familiarity with, and smaller doses of medications may be appropriate in these often very compromised patients. Due to slower circulation, ample time should be allowed for medication effect as sequential, titrated agents are administered. Medications used are listed with caveats in brackets: fentanyl (offers less myocardial depression and has short duration of action), etomidate (has safe hemodynamic profile, however, risk of adrenocortical suppression and limited familiarity among intensive care physicians), ketamine (overall effect is increased heart rate and blood pressure provided the autonomic nervous system can compensate however, children with end-stage heart failure may not be able to mount a sympathetic response, and it can intrinsically depress myocardial contractility), and midazolam (to be used with caution in a conservative and supplemental manner in the hands of experienced anesthetist). However, once intubated, positive pressure ventilation with positive end-expiratory pressure augments CO, decreases transmural LV pressure, and reduces the afterload, thus supporting the impaired myocardial function. Additionally, positive pressure ventilation decreases right-sided venous return, which may alone necessitate judicious fluid administration surrounding endotracheal intubation.

In acute cardiogenic shock with acidosis, the use of β1 adrenoreceptor-targeted agents is often needed. Low-dose epinephrine (around 0.05 mcg/kg/min), dopamine (~5 mcg/kg/min), or dobutamine, all aim to increase CO by increasing the contractile state of the myocardium. $\beta1$ stimulation is also chronotropic, and may be pro-arrhythmic. In some patients, the heart rate may actually fall following vasopressor use as CO and blood pressure increase. Most vasoactive agents are readily titratable, as they have short half-lives of just a few minutes. As such, rapid titration of epinephrine may be life-saving for the acutely hypotensive patient, and short-term use of higher doses approaching the α agonism range may be acutely helpful. Although catecholamine use is often necessary and helpful for the acute treatment of heart failure, afterload reduction remains a primary therapeutic target in this setting. Milrinone represents the current standard agent, both acutely and for longer-term use, in severe pediatric heart failure (77). Milrinone can increase the cardiac index (CI), lower the capillary wedge pressure, and can prevent/lessen low CO syndrome after cardiac surgery (78). Milrinone is mainly renally eliminated, and in contrast to most catecholamine agents has complex and variable pharmacokinetics with a comparatively long and variable elimination half-life of 30 minutes to 3 hours. Clinicians must be aware that, in comparison to catecholamines, milrinone has a relatively delayed time to onset, and delayed clinical response after dose weaning. Loading doses of milrinone, while generally used in the operating room setting, are often avoided in patients with symptomatic heart failure due to hypotensive risk. Milrinone is administered as continuous infusion at 0.25–0.75 mcg/kg/min, with lower rates favored for early titration and in the setting of renal compromise. Milrinone use has been shown to be effective for the short- and medium-term treatment of severe heart failure in children. Levosimendan is an inotropic agent that increases the sensitivity of myofilaments to calcium and has been used outside of the United States as an alternative inotropic therapy in children with heart failure on prolonged catecholamine infusions that cannot be weaned. In acute heart failure, it may provide some improvement and allow weaning of catecholamines (79). However, there may be no benefit in the management of chronic heart failure or the long-term outcome. Diuretics help with reducing fluid overload and pulmonary congestion. Control of the heart rate by controlling temperature and reducing other causes of raised SVR improves filling and maintains preload. Vasoconstrictors in the presence of impaired ventricular function are potentially harmful. Higher doses of catecholamines are also likely to aggravate myocardial injury and are unlikely to improve outcome. One has to be careful that adrenergic agents do not contribute to the unwanted chronotropic effects with tachycardia, which can impair filling and increase in myocardial oxygen consumption and thus add to the low CO state.

In most settings, the goal is to treat an acute decompensation with intravenous vasoactive medications as needed, and then transition the patient to oral therapy using ACE inhibition, diuretics, β-blockade, and aldosterone antagonists. If a patient is not able to be transitioned to oral medications, this is considered to be end-stage, severe heart failure, and as such, mechanical support and cardiac transplantation should be considered as individually appropriate.

Patients with acute myocarditis, in particular fulminant myocarditis, are at high risk of cardiac arrest or progressive shock ending in cardiac arrest. Early consideration for mechanical support is important.

Specific Treatment for Myocarditis—Intravenous Immunoglobulin, Steroids, and Antiviral Agents

The use of immunotherapies for suspected or proven myocarditis is controversial. Multiple papers have reported varying successes with immunotherapies in the early stages of acute viral myocarditis in children (80–87) with early reports favoring the use of intravenous immunoglobulin (IVIG) and steroids (80,84). Drucker et al. (84) showed that the use of high-dose IVIG is associated with improved recovery of LV function with a tendency to better survival (though not statistically significant) during the first year after presentation. In some papers, the dose of IVIG administered was 2 g/kg infused over 24 hours (83–85), whereas in others, steroids were given over a length of time (80,82,88) and in one, a combination of IVIG and steroids was administered (82). Overall, the studies showed improvement in ventricular function but without a significant survival outcome benefit. Large controlled studies in adults have, similarly, shown no long-term survival benefit with immunoglobulin therapy (89,90). There are no multicenter, prospective, randomized controlled trials in children. A Cochrane systematic review of the use of IVIG in presumed viral myocarditis in children and adults did not find any evidence to support the use of IVIG (91). Thus, there is no evidence to support a standard for immunosuppressive therapy for viral myocarditis but there is some class II evidence to suggest that the use of immunoglobulin may improve long-term heart function without affecting mortality.

However, it is unclear whether immunotherapy would be beneficial in certain groups of patients, such as those with virus-negative autoantibody-positive myocarditis and possibly in certain phases of disease. Steroids may have beneficial results in myocarditis associated with autoimmune disorders, vasculitis, dengue myocarditis, eosinophilic syndromes, and giant cell myocarditis. Combination immunosuppression with monoclonal muromonab-CD3 (OKT3) has been used (92); however, efficacy of these agents has not been tested in randomized controlled trials. Despite the central pathogenic role of autoimmune injury in myocarditis, broad inhibition of inflammatory response does not result in patient benefit and hence there is no universal recommendation for the use of these in acute or chronic myocarditis.

Specific antiviral agents in children with myocarditis are of limited therapeutic value as patients present in the later stages when there is already significant cardiac involvement. Pleconaril showed promise in children with enterovirus myocarditis but a subsequent double-blind RCT in neonates has shown no significant differences in treated and untreated groups (93). Acyclovir has been used in myocarditis from EBV and varicella infections.

Management of Arrhythmias

Arrhythmias in the context of myocarditis or DCM have to be vigorously treated. Antiarrhythmic management includes correction of electrolytes and use of intravenous lidocaine, amiodarone, and direct current (DC) cardioversion. DC cardioversion has to be ideally performed in the setting of cardiac intensive care expertise when there is failing myocardial function. Complete AV block requires temporary pacing system and may be achieved in acute settings by transvenous pacing system.

Anticoagulation

Patients with myocarditis or DCM with LV fractional shortening of less than 20% are at risk of developing mural thrombi and systemic embolization. Systemic administration of heparin may be warranted in these high-risk cases followed by aspirin and/or warfarin.

Treatment of Chronic Heart Failure

Treatment is targeted at symptom control and modulating maladaptive renal and adrenergic responses, rather than correcting any underlying genetic or metabolic defect. With a general paucity of pediatric-specific data, children are treated similarly to adult-derived treatment protocols. In previous decades, outpatient anticongestive therapy in children has relied upon the widespread use of furosemide and digoxin, with very limited data to support the use of a wider pharmacopeia (94). More recently, and with recognition that chronic pediatric heart failure is modulated by the same compensatory mechanisms as found in adults, pediatric heart failure cardiologists are now advocating the broader use of ACEi, β-blockers, and aldosterone antagonists (95). These three agents, together with furosemide or similar diuretic, are the evidence-based standard for adult patients with chronic heart failure. β-Blockers, however, have to be used in children with caution in the context of severe ventricular dysfunction. A Cochrane review did not find enough evidence to recommend the use of β-blockers in children with congestive heart failure (96).

Progressive Heart Failure Unresponsive to Conventional Management

Heart transplantation remains the final therapeutic option for children with myocarditis and intractable severe heart failure, when all conventional medical management has failed (80,97). DCM is the most common primary diagnosis leading to heart transplantation for those transplanted beyond the first year of age. Transplantation is a good therapeutic option, but it does trade the disease process of chronic heart failure with that of chronic immunosuppression and eventual transplant organ failure. Patient selection and transplant timing are complex decision-making processes. In the setting of severe decompensated failure, pretransplant bridging using MCS may be indicated. The indications for instituting mechanical support are cardiogenic shock associated with dysrhythmias, severe hemodynamic compromise in fulminant myocarditis, and worsening end-organ function (59,97). The reversible nature of the disease and a short time frame for recovery in myocarditis make venoarterial ECMO a suitable mechanical support strategy (**Figs. 73.2A,B**). Early deployment before the development of end-organ dysfunction or cardiac arrest is essential for a good outcome. This is covered in detail in the next section of the chapter.

MECHANICAL CIRCULATORY SUPPORT

MCS is a life-sustaining therapy offered to children with severe circulatory failure refractory to conventional treatment. There are two technologies that are available for cardiac MCS in children: ECMO and ventricular assist devices (VADs); their use requires complex evaluations including a detailed knowledge of each technology, patient selection criteria, and optimal timing.

Devices

Extracorporeal Membrane Oxygenation

For many decades now ECMO has been the mainstay of pediatric cardiac MCS and thousands of children of all ages have been supported to date (98). ECMO has two main advantages: First, as a modification of cardiopulmonary bypass, ECMO is the most robust form of MCS suitable for patients with a cardiopulmonary failure; second, ECMO can be initiated rapidly, even during active cardiopulmonary resuscitation, by insertion of arterial and venous cannulae either peripherally (cervical or femoral vessels), or centrally via sternotomy. However, ECMO has number of limitations: Its use is limited to a few weeks before the risk of ECMO-related complications (particularly infective) increases and the design and complexity preclude ambulation and rehabilitation (patients on ECMO are typically sedated and mechanically ventilated). ECMO is, therefore, best suited to patients in whom the anticipated recovery of native cardiac function is within days to a few weeks.

Ventricular Assist Devices

Development of pediatric VADs has been slow compared to their use in adults and although VADs have been used alongside ECMO for decades, the outcomes in children have been frustratingly poor. The shortage of adequate pediatric devices was documented in a report analyzing outcomes of 99 children bridged to transplantation in the decade between 1993 and 2003; only 19% of patients were younger than 10 years and the rest were older children and adolescents treated "off label" with adult-type devices. The overall survival was satisfactory reaching 77%; however, there was a notable difference in survival depending on the age of the patient: less than 40% of children younger than 10 years were alive at 2 months after VAD implantation (99). Although the cause for this reduced survival seen in younger children is likely to be multifactorial, a key factor was the lack of pediatric pumps that could offer a lower range of flows suitable for different ages (unlike in adults, where "one size fits all"), combined with difficulties in anticoagulation related to a maturation of coagulation cascade during the first years of life. More recently, new VADs specifically designed for children have emerged, making VAD an excellent alternative. There is now a range of suitable devices, from which the Berlin Heart EXCOR VAD has been used most often and is approved for pediatric use in Europe, Canada, and the United States (100–102). This is a paracorporeal, pulsatile flow device, suitable for all ages from infants to adolescents, with a range of pump chamber volumes of 10–60 mL. Other new devices, including axial

TABLE 73.7

COMPARISON BETWEEN MECHANICAL SUPPORT WITH ECMO VERSUS VAD

	■ ECMO	■ VAD
Cardiac support	Yes (biventricular)	Yes (left or biventricular)
Respiratory support	Yes (oxygenator)	No
Decompression of left heart	Yes (septostomy or vent), can be suboptimal	Yes, optimal
Initiation	Emergency or elective (peripheral or transthoracic access)	Elective (transthoracic access)
Anticoagulation	Yes (heparin)	Yes (heparin plus antiplatelet)
Transfusion requirements	Frequent	Less frequent
Duration of support	Days–weeks	Days–months

and centrifugal pumps such as CentriMag or PediMag, Heart-Ware, and HeartMate II, have been used with good results for both short- and a long-term use (103,104).

VADs are classified according to (a) the mode of blood flow as pulsatile versus continuous flow (continuous flow may be driven by either centrifugal or axial pumps), (b) the relative position of the pump and patient as extra- or paracorporeal versus intracorporeal (fully implantable); and (c) the duration of intended use as temporary, short-term versus durable, long-term devices. Unlike venoarterial ECMO, patients supported with VAD are reliant on their own lung function, as a VAD provides pure cardiac support of either the left (or systemic) ventricle in case of LVAD or of both ventricles when BiVAD is applied (**Table 73.7**). The implantation of a VAD is typically performed on cardiopulmonary bypass and requires some planning, which precludes the use of VADs as a rapid form of support. Advantages of VADs include stable cannulae and excellent decompression of the left (systemic) atria, enabling extubation, discharge from ICU, and physical and nutritional rehabilitation. Compared to ECMO, VAD recipients have reduced transfusion requirements (105). Most importantly with long-term devices, patients can be supported for months, making VADs an ideal choice in children bridged to transplantation.

Choice of Device

Considerations when choosing between devices include (a) the expected end-point (bridge to recovery or to transplantation, or bridge to decision—also termed bridge to bridge); (b) the likely duration of support; (c) patient anatomy and pathophysiology of their circulatory failure; and (d) institutional experience (including device availability). It must be emphasized that during the course of a patient's illness, these end points may change and patients need to be frequently evaluated to ensure that the correct type of support is used (for example, a bridge to decision with ECMO can progress to a bridge to probable recovery and the patient converted to short-term VAD, which might later be converted to long-term VAD if a bridging to transplant becomes necessary). ECMO is typically reserved for: (a) the emergency institution of support for circulatory collapse when recovery is expected within days; (b) children with significant lung pathology requiring full cardiopulmonary support; or (c) to stabilize patients with unclear or severe end-organ dysfunction to determine reversibility with appropriate therapy. Typical clinical scenarios include post-cardiotomy support in patients who fail to wean from cardiopulmonary bypass after cardiac surgery, patients with severe refractory arrhythmias, patients who are in cardiac arrest or rapidly deteriorating as part of cardiopulmonary resuscitation, or as bridge to recovery in patients with fulminant myocarditis. Some patients with myocarditis might develop severe pulmonary congestion and an atrial septostomy on ECMO is needed to decompress the left side of the heart and assure lung recovery and smooth transition to VAD (**Fig. 73.2**). Most institutions consider transition from ECMO to VAD within 7–10 days of support, although this decision depends on an individual patient's potential for recovery and duration of support.

Short-term centrifugal VADs (CentriMag, PediMag, Deltastream) are suitable for acute processes such as myocarditis or acute cardiac allograft failure where recovery is expected within few weeks (106). They are also an attractive initial selection for unstable patients in multiorgan system failure (particularly coagulopathy secondary to hepatic dysfunction) awaiting stabilization and transition to a long-term device ("bridge to bridge"), or patients requiring frequent flow titrations, such as those patients with single ventricle physiology. Additionally, short-term VADs can be used for temporary right heart support in children with severe right heart dysfunction following LVAD implantation (107,108). Short-term VADs are

paracorporeal and patients on these pumps are usually ICU bound. A combination of centrifugal pump connected to long-term cannulae has been used in some units to enable a smooth conversion from a short-term to a long-term VAD (109).

Long-term VADs (Berlin Heart EXCOR, HeartWare HVAD and HeartMate II) have a unique role as a bridge to heart transplantation and their use has dramatically risen in the past decade. According to The Registry of the International Society for Heart and Lung Transplantation 2012 data, 25% of pediatric heart transplant recipients were mechanically bridged using VADs, with a sharp decline in ECMO use from 9.4% in 2005 to 2.6% in 2010 (110). The survival rates 75%–92% achieved with long-term VADs are superior to ECMO where only 45% children reaching transplant, thus making VADs a clear choice for a bridge to transplant (111). The actual VAD selection may be determined by the patient's size. For infants and small children with BSA <0.7 m^2, Berlin Heart EXCOR is currently used worldwide, while in bigger children and teenagers there is a wider choice, including implantable pumps such as HeartWare or HeartMate II.

Timing

The decision of when to commence MCS is a challenging one, balancing the ultimate goal, to prevent an uncontrolled circulatory decline with subsequent irreversible organ damage, against the risks inherent in mechanical devices. An analysis of adult data from the Interagency Registry for Mechanically Assisted Circulatory Support shows that optimal timing is critical for a successful outcome and a delayed start of MCS in adults who are either in a progressive circulatory decline or in shock is associated with a reduced survival (112). In children, Almond et al. (101) demonstrated that the presence of renal and hepatic dysfunction at the time of initiation of MCS was a risk factor for death during bridge to transplant. Similarly, children with myocarditis cannulated for ECMO had better outcome if their pH and blood pressure were preserved (113). It is likely that as the experience with pediatric VADs increases, the threshold for implantation will favor supporting patients in an earlier stage of heart failure.

Patient Selection

At present, MCS is considered in children who require more than one inotrope or who have clinical signs of heart failure with secondary organ dysfunction evidenced by need for a mechanical ventilation, feed intolerance, oliguria, or altered mental status and/or develop biochemical markers of low CO such as elevated serum lactate, significantly reduced mixed venous saturation, and signs of renal or hepatic dysfunction. Resting tachycardia and arrhythmias are additional warning signs of a progressive heart failure. An uncontrolled circulatory collapse must be avoided with individual patient candidacy for MCS as well as choice of device discussed and planned to avoid unnecessary delays.

There are few absolute contraindications to MCS, and those include irreversible severe brain damage, chromosomal abnormality, prematurity, or extremely small size and conditions that preclude systemic anticoagulation (including implantation of VAD on cardiopulmonary bypass) such as recent hemorrhagic stroke. In some patients with an incomplete history who present in shock, it is not feasible to fully assess their end-organ function. In most institutions, these patients are sustained on either ECMO or temporary VAD as "bridge to decision" until their clinical status is clarified. Another challenging scenario is managing those children with multisystem organ failure in whom the pre-implantation hepatic, pulmonary, and renal dysfunction might significantly complicate the peri-implantation period. In these patients, a recovery of organ function may occur once stable circulation is restored, and a period of MCS might be warranted to ascertain reversibility.

Principles of Management

Detailed description of the management of various devices is beyond the scope of this chapter and can be found elsewhere (114,115). The following are general principles of care in VAD patients.

Peri-implantation Management

Preoperative ECHO. All patients should have pre-implantation ECHO with the aim to exclude intracardiac thrombus, intracardiac shunts, and significant valvular regurgitation as these would need to be addressed at the time of implantation.

Cannulation. VAD implantation is performed on cardiopulmonary bypass and careful cannulae positioning is critical to achieve satisfactory pump flow. For LVAD, the cannulation is typically from the LV apex to the ascending aorta, while for RVAD the cannulae are from the right atrium into the pulmonary artery. Left atrial cannulation is reserved for selected cases with restrictive or HCM, in whom LV cannulation might not provide adequate drainage. The initial LVAD settings are set to produce a CI of 2.4–2.8 L/min/m². The cannulae position, right heart function, as well as the decompression of the left heart are verified on transesophageal ECHO.

LVAD versus BiVAD. There is great variability in practice in terms of LVAD or BiVAD use between pediatric centers. The majority of children can be supported with LVAD only and most centers would restrict use of right heart mechanical support for cases with most severe RV failure with preoperative CVP >20 mm Hg, ascites, severe hepatic dysfunction, and poor RV function on preoperative ECHO. Using the Berlin Heart EXCOR system, biventricular support is used in 20%–40% of patients and the use of BiVAD tends to decrease as the center's experience increases (100,115,116). With the advent of newer implantable pediatric continuous-flow devices, the correct selection of patients suitable for LVAD will become imperative and risk factors for biventricular support in children will need to be established.

Bleeding. Acute post-implantation bleeding is one of the most common complications and can be exacerbated by a coagulopathy due to pre-existing hepatic dysfunction and the effects of cardiopulmonary bypass. Complete reversal of heparin with protamine once the patient is off bypass and normalization of clotting profile with standard transfusions of blood products are targeted in the theater. If significant bleeding continues, an early re-exploration and surgical hemostasis are warranted. In the ICU, the benefit of multiple transfusions (particularly platelets) has to be carefully balanced against the risk of an early thrombus formation and a relatively conservative approach is advisable unless the bleeding compromises the VAD function.

Adequacy of Mechanical Support. The primary goal of MCS is to restore oxygen delivery to peripheral tissues and the usual markers of adequate CO including mixed venous oxygen saturation, lactate, peripheral perfusion, and urine output are followed. In the early post-implantation phase, direct arterial and central venous pressures are monitored and pump performance is optimized using volume expansion and vasodilators. The secondary aim of support is to rest the heart and provide an optimal physiological milieu for myocardial recovery. While on ECMO the decompression of the left ventricle is often problematic, on VAD the left ventricle is drained directly and optimal ventricular decompression can be achieved under ECHO guidance.

In the long term, the aim of support is to allow physical and nutritional rehabilitation with appropriate weight gain.

It is not uncommon to have to increase the device output in order to match growing metabolic demands once the patients become active and start growing.

Anticoagulation

Anticoagulation is particularly challenging in children. Different regimes exist for different devices and these are being constantly being refined with experience. Preoperative evaluation includes full clotting profile and thrombophilia screen. Coming off bypass, complete reversal of heparin with protamine and administration of blood products aim to prevent or limit postoperative bleeding. Once hemostasis has been achieved, an unfractionated heparin infusion is commenced and its effect monitored using anti-Xa levels and APTT. Long-term anticoagulation is maintained with warfarin or low–molecular weight heparin combined with antiplatelet agents. Most centers now use thromboelastogram and platelet function tests to ensure efficacy of anticoagulation. The frequency of monitoring depends on patient stability: frequent blood tests are required in the postoperative phases, which typically reduce to twice weekly, once the patient becomes stable. Heightened caution is advisable during infection and other inflammatory states that are known to affect coagulation and increase the risk of stroke. Similarly, diarrhea or vomiting can affect drug absorption, and in such cases, an increased frequency of testing or conversion from oral to intravenous agents is often needed (115,117,118).

Weaning

Children who demonstrate sufficient ventricular recovery should be considered for weaning from VAD. The weaning protocols vary depending on the underlying pathology, the anticipated potential for recovery, and the type of VAD, and their description can be found elsewhere (115). Generally, prolonged pump cessation or low flow should be avoided because of the risks of blood stagnation and thrombus formation. One of the most challenging questions in mechanical support is how to capture the subset of patients who are bridged to transplantation, but whose hearts have undergone sufficient recovery to come off mechanical support. While reverse remodeling of end-stage heart failure with subsequent myocardial recovery has been extensively studied in adult VAD recipients, data in children are scarce and the definition of "recovery" variable. In Almond's report of 204 children bridged to transplantation with Berlin Heart EXCOR, 6.2% "recovered" and survived >30 days after VAD explantation. The recovery data have to be interpreted with great caution, as clearly the potential for recovery will vary depending on the underlying pathology. In children with viral myocarditis, recovery of cardiac function after several months of support has been reported, justifying longer bridge to recovery before transplant listing (119,120). Interestingly, ventricular decompression with VAD combined with medical therapy might lead to a restoration of native heart function in children with end-stage heart failure due to cardiomyopathy (121). Thus, continuation of a heart failure medication on VAD with periodic checks of underlying ventricular function is common practice. Future research is aimed at understanding the mechanisms and markers of myocardial recovery and might open new therapeutic avenues for children in heart failure.

Complications

Neurological

Stroke is the leading cause of mortality and morbidity of mechanical support in children. In a prospective study of children supported with pulsatile VAD, the stroke rate was 29%, and in half of those, the neurological injury was lethal or severe enough to mandate a withdrawal of mechanical support (100). Similar results have been reported in other pediatric VAD series with the tendency for most neurological events to appear at an early stage of support (101,122,123). Despite aggressive anticoagulation regimens, the vast majority of strokes on pulsatile pumps are thromboembolic rather than hemorrhagic, and it is likely that future reduction of stroke rate will require further improvements in VAD technology. The newer implantable continuous-flow devices have encouragingly lower stroke rates of less than 10% in adults (103).

Hematological

Bleeding occurs frequently in the peri-implantation phase and can lead to tamponade with device malfunction. Major bleeding is reported in 20%–40% of VAD recipients and an early surgical re-exploration is advisable in such cases (101,124).

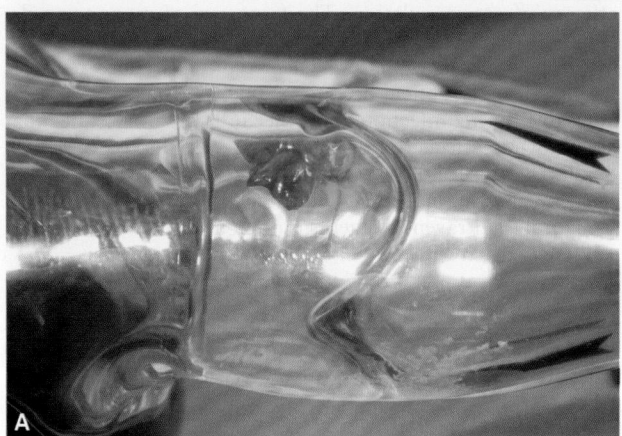

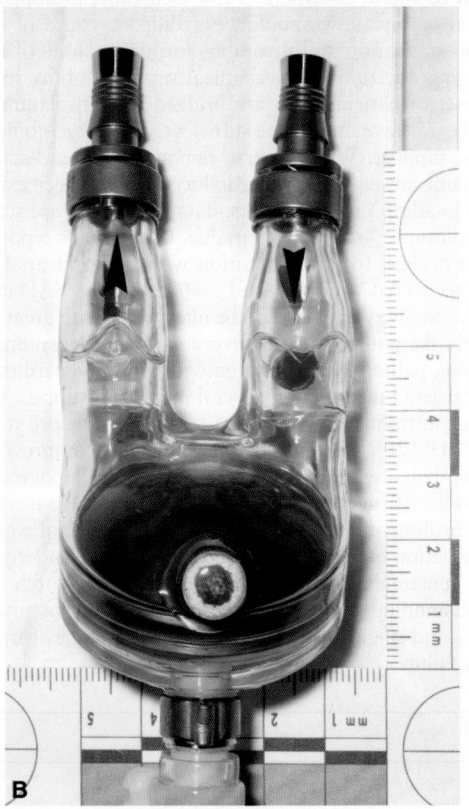

FIGURE 73.5. **A:** Thrombus on an inflow valve. **B:** Explanted Berlin Heart EXCOR L-VAD.

Balancing the risk of hemorrhage versus risk of thromboembolism is essential part of management and anticoagulation protocols are constantly being refined to address this. An early recognition of thrombus formation is essential as it can prevent a devastating systemic thromboembolic event, and if a significant thrombus in the pump is detected, the pump can either be replaced or pharmacological thrombolysis considered (**Fig. 73.5**). Intravascular hemolysis caused by mechanical stress is another recognized complication in continuous-flow devices, which can result into a detrimental release of free hemoglobin with subsequent renal dysfunction.

Right-Ventricular Failure

Deterioration of right-ventricular (RV) function is an acute phenomena observed in some patients after LVAD implantation, which can be difficult to predict. Several mechanisms have been postulated: deleterious effects of cardiopulmonary bypass, electromechanical dissociation of the right and left ventricles, and acute changes of loading conditions and RV geometry. Symptoms of RV failure include high CVP and impaired LVAD filling leading to reduced pump output and circulatory compromise. Aggressive pharmacological support of the RV with inotropes, pulmonary vasodilators, and diuretics, as well as rhythm control with pacing and/or antiarrhythmics, are often needed for a period of few days before the RV adapts (115). If mechanical support with RVAD is being considered in cases with refractory RV failure, an elective rather than emergency implantation has better outcomes (125).

Infection

Infection is a frequent complication reported in 30%–50% of pediatric VAD recipients and is known to be another risk factor for reduced survival (124,126). Device-related infection can originate and spread from the cannulation, pocket, or drive line sites into the blood stream. Both bacterial and fungal causes need to be considered when infection is suspected (127). Aseptic wound management, regular dressing changes, and promotion of skin healing around the cannulas and drive line and early recognition and aggressive treatment with antibiotics are essential aspects of management (128).

Other Adverse Events

Other adverse events in children supported with a pulsatile VAD include respiratory failure (defined as continuous need for respiratory support on VAD) in 29%, hepatic dysfunction in 9%, and renal dysfunction in 12% (101). Arrhythmias are reported in 9% of patients and are usually well tolerated once the left ventricle is mechanically supported and the heart rhythm can be controlled pharmacologically. Device malfunction is relatively rare and might be related to material fatigue or inappropriate handling; hands-on troubleshooting sessions for staff and families are an integral part of VAD training.

OUTCOMES FOR CHILDREN WITH MYOCARDITIS AND CARDIOMYOPATHIES (INCLUDING THOSE SUPPORTED WITH MECHANICAL CIRCULATORY SUPPORT)

Myocarditis

The outcomes range from spontaneous recovery with or without the development of DCM to heart transplant or death. Ejection fraction <30%, a shortening fraction <15%, and moderate to severe mitral regurgitation are all associated with ultimate development of severe cardiac failure (129). Mortality is high in newborns and infants and in those surviving with poor ventricular function (28–30). Patients with ventricular arrhythmias and heart block, suggestive of significant myocardial damage, have worse prognosis, and those surviving beyond 72 hours without the need for ECMO have better prognosis, and in one series had a 97% increased likelihood of survival (80). Foerster et al. (87) reported that lower LV fractional shortening Z-score at presentation predicted greater mortality (hazard ratio, 0.85; 95% CI, 0.73–0.98; p = 0.03) and greater LVPWT predicted transplantation (hazard ratio, 1.17; 95% CI, 1.02–1.35; p = 0.03). Certain viral etiologies, in particular, enterovirus (130) and parvovirus (34), are associated with worse prognosis. The outcome of acute lymphocytic myocarditis, in particular that of fulminant myocarditis, with appropriate advanced intensive care is excellent with 80%–90% survival with almost full recovery of ventricular function (59,61,80,131). The Extracorporeal Life Support Registry reported that the survival to hospital discharge was 61% in 255 children treated with ECMO for myocarditis over a 12-year period from 1995-2006. (113). These data have to be interpreted with caution, as in the current era, patients who failed to recover on ECMO and would have previously died can now be realistically converted to VAD and their support continued as a longer bridge to recovery or transplantation with survival chances of over 80% (102,103). However, about 20% of children with acute myocarditis go on to develop chronic heart failure. Recent reviews from Australia and North America have revealed that ~27%–46% of newly diagnosed nonidiopathic DCM were due to previous myocarditis (1,3,132).

Dilated Cardiomyopathy

It has long been known that some children with DCM recover. This is often quoted for perhaps one third of affected children. One recent case series reported on nearly 800 children with DCM for whom 2-year follow-up data were available. In this series, 22% of children recovered normal echocardiographic parameters measuring LV size and function, 51% died or were transplanted, and 27% survived with ongoing echocardiographic evidence of LV compromise (133). Younger children showed higher rates of improvement as compared to older children. This improvement was not always persistent, as 9% of children who improved went on to die or receive a transplant during these same two years of observation. Importantly, these data do not address physiologic markers such as ongoing diastolic function, do not include MRI markers, which may detect fibrotic change or ongoing inflammation, do not consider the possibility of arrhythmogenic foci, nor do they normalize cardiac mass to body size (which may be reduced following an episode of myocyte loss). Further data are required to decide which patients are "home free" versus those who are at risk for later development of recurrent heart failure. Similarly, it is unknown at this time which of these patients should be treated with long-term, preventive therapy with long-term ACE inhibition, β-blockade, or aldosterone antagonists.

Hypertrophic Cardiomyopathy

Registry data have examined outcomes for 1100 children diagnosed with HCM in North America over the past 20 years (13). As discussed previously, many affected children remain undiagnosed and present with near-miss or completed SCD. Risk of death or cardiac transplantation was broken down by a number of etiologic and clinical factors. Children who

developed HCM as a result of a known inborn metabolic defect had the worse outcomes, with a 57% risk of death or transplant by age 2 years. Children diagnosed during infancy (less than 1 year of age), who typically presented with clinical CHF, also appear to be at relatively high risk, showing a 21% risk of death or transplant by the age of 2 years. In contrast to these high-risk groups, relatively good outcomes can be expected for patients with HCM who were diagnosed at an older age with idiopathic (likely sarcomeric) HCM. These children with "typical" hypertrophic disease showed very low rates of death or transplant of 0.5% at 1 year, and 3% at 2 years following their diagnoses. These data, for children diagnosed outside of infancy, are somewhat consistent with the general teaching that pediatric HCM is associated with a 1% yearly rate of SCD, and supports more aggressive treatment and transplant listing for children with specific etiologic subtypes.

Outcome Following Mechanical Circulatory Support

There are now numerous reports in children supported with VAD or ECMO to recovery or transplantation emphasizing the impact of factors such as careful patient selection, timely initiation of support, and center experience on survival. In a series of 204 children bridged to transplantation with pulsatile Berlin Heart VAD between 2004 and 2010, the survival was 75% (101). A higher survival of 88%–92% in a cohort of 48 children was achieved in a prospective trial prior to FDA approval. These were a strictly selected subgroup with biventricular circulation without significant end-organ dysfunction, thus highlighting the importance of patient selection for outcome (100). An increasing experience in pediatric bridging has allowed the identification of risk factors for mortality. The need for BiVAD is a consistent risk factor in recent series, and is likely to reflect worse pre-implantation status and worse right heart function. Similarly, pre-existing hepatic and renal dysfunction with elevated bilirubin and reduced creatinine clearance are also associated with reduced survival, highlighting the critical impact of end-organ dysfunction on outcomes (101,113).

With the new pediatric VADs, patients of all age categories can be supported, and children <1 year have become the dominant age group in bridging. Several series looked at the outcomes of smaller children and reported their outcomes and complication rates to be comparable to older children when new pulsatile devices such as Berlin Heart EXCOR were used (116,123). The patient group that remains a major challenge includes neonates and infants <5 kg as their complication rates and subsequent mortality on bridge to transplant are still relatively high, exceeding 50% (101). This is probably due to a combination of reasons including longer waiting times, lower pump rates with slow blood flow, and immature hemostasis (134).

Timing of Transplant and Outcome

This has been investigated systematically for DCM patients, where death or transplantation was considered as competing outcomes (135). On analyzing the 5-year outcomes for 1711 children with DCM, divided into etiologic subsets of (a) idiopathic disease, (b) neuromuscular disease, (c) familial isolated DCM, and (d) myocarditis, best overall outcomes were seen in patients with myocarditis with a 5-year death rate of 9%, transplant rate of 22%, and survival (with their own native heart) of 70%. All deaths in the myocarditis cohort occurred in the first 6 months following initial presentation, with no reported interval mortality in the subsequent 4.5 years of reporting. In contrast, patients with idiopathic disease showed worse outcomes at 5-year follow-up, with interval, progressive mortality reaching 16%, transplant rate of 33%, and a transplant-free survival of 51%. Myocarditis patients are hypothesized to have better outcomes due to the acute and self-limiting nature of a specific inflammatory insult, as opposed to those with idiopathic DCM, which typically arise from intrinsic genetic disease. Transplantation decisions are based upon the complex summation of the patients' current status, expected prognosis, ongoing risk of sudden death, and transplant risk factors. Longer-term PCMR data show an estimated 45% transplant-free survival for their entire cohort of 1803 children with DCM at 15-year follow-up (136). Transplantation rates approach 35% by 15 years post-diagnosis, with cumulative rates of unexpected sudden death occurring in 2.7% of this large cohort. These data can be roughly summarized to predict that half of the children with DCM will stabilize over time on oral anti-heart failure medications. Nearly one third will go on to cardiac transplantation over the decade following their diagnosis, and ~20% will die without reaching or being eligible for transplantation.

SUMMARY

A diagnosis of cardiomyopathy has profound implications, as it is a lifelong illness with significant morbidity and mortality, and major impact on the patient, their family, and the wider health-care system. A history of acute viral prodrome supports the diagnosis of myocarditis; however, viral illness can also precipitate heart failure in a previously stable patient with cardiomyopathy and the distinction is difficult to make at the time of presentation. These children usually present to the ICU in decompensating heart failure and with a fragile hemodynamic state. Skilled management at the bedside with a spectrum of modalities that advanced cardiac intensive care can offer, and the backup of MCS may be needed with the option of cardiac transplantation, if all conventional management fails and suitability for cardiac transplant is agreed. DCM remains the most common reason for cardiac transplantation beyond infancy. New-onset heart failure may also be caused by other cardiomyopathies, which are less common, but need to be investigated and managed, although the final pathway for these children may be heart transplantation.

FUTURE DIRECTIONS

Main areas of future research include newer diagnostic modalities (MRI and genetics), therapies that facilitate recovery/remodeling of a failing heart with end-stage heart failure (stem-cell therapy, newer pharmacotherapies), and advances in MCS (miniaturized pumps, mechanical unloading of the heart with VAD).

MRI is taking on an increasing role in the diagnosis and long-term monitoring of myocarditis and cardiomyopathy. MRI can provide not only functional data but also give insights into the presence and degree of acute myocardial inflammation, fibrosis, or ischemic injury. Despite the need for sedation during MRI in children, it is increasingly becoming a routine and standard component of both acute and chronic management of cardiomyopathy. With advances in the genetic understanding of the disease, it is likely that genetic medicine may offer rapid and precise diagnoses, improve individual risk stratification, and potentially treat the variety of underlying sarcomeric and metabolic defects. HCM will remain a topic for intense research, where advances in genetic medicine, screening, and population data may combine to prevent unexpected deaths and guide better care for this most common of inherited cardiac conditions.

Intense research is ongoing to improve our understanding of the mechanisms involved with myocardial remodeling and regeneration. Advances in stem-cell biology with the hope of minimizing adverse ventricular remodeling with transplantation or mobilizing stem cells is an area of intense focus. MCS is one of the fastest developing areas in pediatric intensive care and it is very likely that the recent expansion of VAD therapy in children will continue. New continuous-flow pumps are being miniaturized and tested to suit patients of all sizes and to reduce complication rates, particularly in small children. It is likely that as confidence and experience increase, thresholds for VAD use will move toward supporting children who are stable but inotrope dependent, allowing those patients to be discharged home. A focused pediatric database—PediMACS—has been started under the aegis of the Interagency Registry for Mechanically Assisted Circulatory Support (INTERMACS). It is hoped that this worldwide data collection will facilitate research and address knowledge gaps in patient selection, risk factors, and outcomes. To address this common problem of the fragile balance between risk of hemorrhage and risk of thromboembolism, new biocompatible surfaces and anticoagulation strategies are under development. Lastly, the increased number of children on VAD is likely to impact on transplant waiting lists, and with the continuous shortage of donor hearts, alternative therapeutic strategies such as destination therapy or myocardial recovery will become increasingly necessary and attractive.

References

1. Lipshultz SE, Sleeper LA, Towbin JA, et al. The incidence of pediatric cardiomyopathy in two regions of the United States. *N Engl J Med* 2003;348:1647–55.
2. Lipshultz SE. Ventricular dysfunction clinical research in infants, children and adolescents. *Prog Pediatr Cardiol* 2000;12:1–28.
3. Towbin JA, Lowe AM, Colan SD, et al. Incidence, causes, and outcomes of dilated cardiomyopathy in children. *JAMA* 2006;296:1867–76.
4. Kindel SJ, Miller EM, Gupta R, et al. Pediatric cardiomyopathy: Importance of genetic and metabolic evaluation. *J Card Fail* 2012;18:396–403.
5. Cahill TJ, Ashrafian H, Watkins H. Genetic cardiomyopathies causing heart failure. *Circ Res* 2013;113:660–75.
6. Moretti M, Merlo M, Barbati G, et al. Prognostic impact of familial screening in dilated cardiomyopathy. *Eur J Heart Fail* 2010;12:922–7.
7. Cox GF. Diagnostic approaches to pediatric cardiomyopathy of metabolic genetic etiologies and their relation to therapy. *Prog Pediatr Cardiol* 2007;24:15–25.
8. Rusconi PG, Ludwig DA, Ratnasamy C, et al. Serial measurements of serum NT-proBNP as markers of left ventricular systolic function and remodeling in children with heart failure. *Am Heart J* 2010;160:776–83.
9. Maron BJ, Gardin JM, Flack JM, et al. Prevalence of hypertrophic cardiomyopathy in a general population of young adults. Echocardiographic analysis of 4111 subjects in the CARDIA Study. Coronary Artery Risk Development in (Young) Adults. *Circulation* 1995;92:785–9.
10. Gajewski KK, Saul JP. Sudden cardiac death in children and adolescents (excluding Sudden Infant Death Syndrome). *Ann Pediatr Cardiol* 2010;3:107–12.
11. Bos JM, Towbin JA, Ackerman MJ. Diagnostic, prognostic, and therapeutic implications of genetic testing for hypertrophic cardiomyopathy. *J Am Coll Cardiol* 2009;54:201–11.
12. Section on Cardiology and Cardiac Surgery. Pediatric sudden cardiac arrest. *Pediatrics* 2012;129:e1094–e1102.
13. Lipshultz SE, Orav EJ, Wilkinson JD, et al. Risk stratification at diagnosis for children with hypertrophic cardiomyopathy: An

analysis of data from the Pediatric Cardiomyopathy Registry. *Lancet* 2013;382:1889–97.

14. Maron BJ, Spirito P, Ackerman MJ, et al. Prevention of sudden cardiac death with implantable cardioverter-defibrillators in children and adolescents with hypertrophic cardiomyopathy. *J Am Coll Cardiol* 2013;61:1527–35.

15. Maron BJ, Spirito P, Shen W-K, et al. Implantable cardioverter-defibrillators and prevention of sudden cardiac death in hypertrophic cardiomyopathy. *JAMA* 2007;298:405–12.

16. Maron BJ, Chaitman BR, Ackerman MJ, et al.; Working Groups of the American Heart Association Committee on Exercise Cardiac Rehabilitation, and Prevention; Councils on Clinical Cardiology and Cardiovascular Disease in the Young. Recommendations for physical activity and recreational sports participation for young patients with genetic cardiovascular diseases. *Circulation* 2004;109:2807–16.

17. Gersh BJ, Maron BJ, Bonow RO, et al. 2011 ACCF/AHA guideline for the diagnosis and treatment of hypertrophic cardiomyopathy: A report of the American College of Cardiology Foundation/American Heart Association Task Force on Practice Guidelines. *J Thorac Cardiovasc Surg* 2011;142:153–203.

18. Webber SA, Lipshultz SE, Sleeper LA, et al. Outcomes of restrictive cardiomyopathy in childhood and the influence of phenotype: A report from the Pediatric Cardiomyopathy Registry. *Circulation* 2012;126:1237–44.

19. Arimura T, Hayashi T, Kimura A. Molecular etiology of idiopathic cardiomyopathy. *Acta Myol* 2007;26:153–8.

20. Pilmer CM, Kirsh JA, Hildebrandt D, et al. Sudden cardiac death in children and adolescents between 1 and 19 years of age. *Heart Rhythm* 2014;11:239–45.

21. Marcus FI, McKenna WJ, Sherrill D, et al. Diagnosis of arrhythmogenic right ventricular cardiomyopathy/dysplasia: Proposed modification of the Task Force Criteria. *Eur Heart J* 2010;31:806–14.

22. Pignatelli RH, McMahon CJ, Dreyer WJ, et al. Clinical characterization of left ventricular noncompaction in children: A relatively common form of cardiomyopathy. *Circulation* 2003;108:2672–8.

23. Digilio MC, Bernardini L, Gagliardi MG, et al. Syndromic noncompaction of the left ventricle: Associated chromosomal anomalies. *Clin Genet* 2013;84:362–7.

24. Scully RE, Lipshultz SE. Anthracycline cardiotoxicity in long-term survivors of childhood cancer. *Cardiovasc Toxicol* 2007;7:122–8.

25. Lipshultz SE, Adams MJ, Colan SD, et al; American Heart Association Congenital Heart Defects Committee of the Council on Cardiovascular Disease in the Young CoBCSCoC, Stroke Nursing CoCR. Long-term cardiovascular toxicity in children, adolescents, and young adults who receive cancer therapy: pathophysiology, course, monitoring, management, prevention, and research directions: a scientific statement from the American Heart Association. *Circulation* 2013;128:1927–95.

26. Price DI, Stanford LC Jr, Braden DS, et al. Hypocalcemic rickets: An unusual cause of dilated cardiomyopathy. *Pediatr Cardiol* 2003;24:510–2.

27. Maiya S, Sullivan I, Allgrove J, et al. Hypocalcaemia and vitamin D deficiency: An important, but preventable, cause of life-threatening infant heart failure. *Heart* 2008;94:581–4.

28. Cooper LT Jr. Myocarditis. *N Engl J Med* 2009;360:1526–38.

29. Bowles NE, Bowles KR, Towbin JA. Viral genomic detection and outcome in myocarditis. *Heart Failure Clin* 2005;1:407–17.

30. Bowles NE, Ni J, Kearney DL, et al. Detection of viruses in myocardial tissues by polymerase chain reaction. Evidence of adenovirus as a common cause of myocarditis in children and adults. *J Am Coll Cardiol* 2003;42:466–72.

31. Martin AB, Webber S, Fricker FJ, et al. Acute myocarditis. Rapid diagnosis by PCR in children. *Circulation* 1994;90:330–9.

32. Francalanci P, Chance JL, Vatta M, et al. Cardiotropic viruses in the myocardium of children with end-stage heart disease. *J Heart Lung Transplant* 2004;23:1046–52.

33. Tschope C, Bock CT, Kasner M, et al. High prevalence of cardiac parvovirus B19 infection in patients with isolated left ventricular diastolic dysfunction. *Circulation* 2005;111:879–86.

34. Molina KM, Garcia X, Denfield SW, et al. Parvovirus B19 myocarditis causes significant morbidity and mortality in children. *Pediatr Cardiol* 2013;34(2):390–7.

35. Bratincsak A, El-Said HG, Bradley JS, et al. Fulminant myocarditis associated with pandemic H1N1 influenza A virus in children. *J Am Coll Cardiol* 2010;55:928–9.

36. Lindblade CL, Kirkpatrick EC, Ebenroth ES. Eosinophilic myocarditis presenting with pediatric myocardial infarction. *Pediatr Cardiol* 2006;27:162–5.

37. Barton M, Finkelstein Y, Opavsky MA, et al. Eosinophilic myocarditis temporally associated with conjugate meningococcal C and hepatitis B vaccines in children. *Pediatr Infect Dis J* 2008;27:831–5.

38. Chikwava KR, Savell VH Jr, Boyd TK. Fatal cephalosporin-induced acute hypersensitivity myocarditis. *Pediatr Cardiol* 2006;27:777–80.

39. Bhogal N, Grady AM, Ursell PC, et al. Hypersensitivity myocarditis presenting as atrioventricular block and wide complex tachycardia in a toddler. *Congenit Heart Dis* 2008;3:359–64.

40. Cooper LT Jr, Berry GJ, Shabetai R. Idiopathic giant-cell myocarditis—natural history and treatment. Multicenter Giant Cell Myocarditis Study Group Investigators. *N Engl J Med* 1997;336:1860–6.

41. Nugent AW, Daubeney PE, Chondros P, et al. The epidemiology of childhood cardiomyopathy in Australia. *N Engl J Med* 2003;348:1639–46.

42. Basso C, Corrado D, Thiene G. Cardiovascular causes of sudden death in young individuals including athletes. *Cardiol Rev* 1999;7:127–35.

43. Doolan A, Langlois N, Semsarian C. Causes of sudden cardiac death in young Australians. *Med J Aust* 2004;180:110–2.

44. Fabre A, Sheppard MN. Sudden adult death syndrome and other non-ischaemic causes of sudden cardiac death. *Heart* 2006;92:316–20.

45. Noren GR, Staley NA, Bandt CM, et al. Occurrence of myocarditis in sudden death in children. *J Forensic Sci* 1977;22:188–96.

46. Wisten A, Forsberg H, Krantz P, et al. Sudden cardiac death in 15-35-year olds in Sweden during 1992-99. *J Intern Med* 2002;252:529–36.

47. Wren C, O'Sullivan JJ, Wright C. Sudden death in children and adolescents. *Heart* 2000;83:410–3.

48. Weber MA, Ashworth MT, Risdon RA, et al. The role of postmortem investigations in determining the cause of sudden unexpected death in infancy. *Arch Dis Child* 2008;93:1048–53.

49. Dettmeyer R, Baasner A, Schlamann M, et al. Role of virus-induced myocardial affections in sudden infant death syndrome: A prospective postmortem study. *Pediatr Res* 2004;55:947–52.

50. Grangeot-Keros L, Broyer M, Briand E, et al. Enterovirus in sudden unexpected deaths in infants. *Pediatr Infect Dis J* 1996;15:123–8.

51. Noutsias M, Fechner H, de Jonge H, et al. Human coxsackie-adenovirus receptor is colocalized with integrins alpha(v)beta(3) and alpha(v)beta(5) on the cardiomyocyte sarcolemma and upregulated in dilated cardiomyopathy: Implications for cardiotropic viral infections. *Circulation* 2001;104:275–80.

52. Xiong D, Lee GH, Badorff C, et al. Dystrophin deficiency markedly increases enterovirus-induced cardiomyopathy: A genetic predisposition to viral heart disease. *Nat Med* 2002;8:872–7.

53. Badorff C, Lee GH, Lamphear BJ, et al. Enteroviral protease 2A cleaves dystrophin: Evidence of cytoskeletal disruption in an acquired cardiomyopathy. *Nat Med* 1999;5:320–6.

54. Feldman AM, McNamara D. Myocarditis. *N Engl J Med* 2000;343:1388–98.

55. Pankuweit S, Portig I, Lottspeich F, et al. Autoantibodies in sera of patients with myocarditis: Characterization of the corresponding proteins by isoelectric focusing and N-terminal sequence analysis. *J Mol Cell Cardiol* 1997;29:77–84.

56. Kearney MT, Cotton JM, Richardson PJ, et al. Viral myocarditis and dilated cardiomyopathy: Mechanisms, manifestations, and management. *Postgrad Med J* 2001;77:4–10.

57. Aretz HT, Billingham ME, Edwards WD, et al. Myocarditis. A histopathologic definition and classification. *Am J Cardiovasc Pathol* 1987;1:3–14.

58. Bultmann BD, Klingel K, Sotlar K, et al. Fatal parvovirus B19-associated myocarditis clinically mimicking ischemic heart disease: An endothelial cell-mediated disease. *Hum Pathol* 2003;34:92–5.

59. Teele SA, Allan CK, Laussen PC, et al. Management and outcomes in pediatric patients presenting with acute fulminant myocarditis. *J Pediatr* 2011;158:638–43.e631.

60. Lieberman EB, Hutchins GM, Herskowitz A, et al. Clinicopathologic description of myocarditis. *J Am Coll Cardiol* 1991;18:1617–26.

61. McCarthy RE III, Boehmer JP, Hruban RH, et al. Long-term outcome of fulminant myocarditis as compared with acute (nonfulminant) myocarditis. *N Engl J Med* 2000;342:690–5.

62. Freund MW, Kleinveld G, Krediet TG, et al. Prognosis for neonates with enterovirus myocarditis. *Arch Dis Child Fetal Neonatal Ed* 2010;95:F206–F212.

63. Inwald D, Franklin O, Cubitt D, et al. Enterovirus myocarditis as a cause of neonatal collapse. *Arch Dis Child Fetal Neonatal Ed* 2004;89:F461–F462.

64. Drossner DM, Hirsh DA, Sturm JJ, et al. Cardiac disease in pediatric patients presenting to a pediatric ED with chest pain. *Am J Emerg Med* 2011;29:632–8.

65. Durani Y, Egan M, Baffa J, et al. Pediatric myocarditis: Presenting clinical characteristics. *Am J Emerg Med* 2009;27:942–7.

66. Freedman SB, Haladyn JK, Floh A, et al. Pediatric myocarditis: Emergency department clinical findings and diagnostic evaluation. *Pediatrics* 2007;120:1278–85.

67. Ramachandra G, Shields L, Brown K, et al. The challenges of prompt identification and resuscitation in children with acute fulminant myocarditis: Case series and review of the literature. *J Paediatr Child Health* 2010;46:579–82.

68. Felker GM, Boehmer JP, Hruban RH, et al. Echocardiographic findings in fulminant and acute myocarditis. *J Am Coll Cardiol* 2000;36:227–32.

69. Al-Biltagi M, Issa M, Hagar HA, et al. Circulating cardiac troponins levels and cardiac dysfunction in children with acute and fulminant viral myocarditis. *Acta Paediatr* 2010;99:1510–6.

70. Nasser N, Bar-Oz B, Nir A. Natriuretic peptides and heart disease in infants and children. *J Pediatr* 2005;147:248–53.

71. Akhtar N, Ni J, Stromberg D, et al. Tracheal aspirate as a substrate for polymerase chain reaction detection of viral genome in childhood pneumonia and myocarditis. *Circulation* 1999;99:2011–8.

72. Chow LH, Radio SJ, Sears TD, et al. Insensitivity of right ventricular endomyocardial biopsy in the diagnosis of myocarditis. *J Am Coll Cardiol* 1989;14:915–20.

73. Pophal SG, Sigfusson G, Booth KL, et al. Complications of endomyocardial biopsy in children. *J Am Coll Cardiol* 1999;34:2105–110.

74. Schultz JC, Hilliard AA, Cooper LT Jr, et al. Diagnosis and treatment of viral myocarditis. *Mayo Clin Proc* 2009;84:1001–9.

75. Baughman KL. Diagnosis of myocarditis: Death of Dallas criteria. *Circulation* 2006;113:593–5.

76. Gagliardi MG, Bevilacqua M, Di Renzi P, et al. Usefulness of magnetic resonance imaging for diagnosis of acute myocarditis in infants and children, and comparison with endomyocardial biopsy. *Am J Cardiol* 1991;68:1089–91.

77. Price JF, Towbin JA, Dreyer WJ, et al. Outpatient continuous parenteral inotropic therapy as bridge to transplantation in children with advanced heart failure. *J Card Fail* 2006;12:139–43.

78. Hoffman TM, Wernovsky G, Atz AM, et al. Efficacy and safety of milrinone in preventing low cardiac output syndrome in infants and children after corrective surgery for congenital heart disease. *Circulation* 2003;107:996–1002.

79. Namachivayam P, Crossland DS, Butt WW, et al. Early experience with Levosimendan in children with ventricular dysfunction. *Pediatr Crit Care Med* 2006;7:445–8.

80. Lee KJ, McCrindle BW, Bohn DJ, et al. Clinical outcomes of acute myocarditis in childhood. *Heart* 1999;82:226–33.

81. Gagliardi MG, Bevilacqua M, Bassano C, et al. Long term follow up of children with myocarditis treated by immunosuppression and of children with dilated cardiomyopathy. *Heart* 2004;90:1167–71.

82. English RF, Janosky JE, Ettedgui JA, et al. Outcomes for children with acute myocarditis. *Cardiol Young* 2004;14:488–93.

83. Haque A, Bhatti S, Siddiqui FJ. Intravenous immune globulin for severe acute myocarditis in children. *Indian Pediatr* 2009;46:810–11.

84. Drucker NA, Colan SD, Lewis AB, et al. Gamma-globulin treatment of acute myocarditis in the pediatric population. *Circulation* 1994;89:252–7.

85. Klugman D, Berger JT, Sable CA, et al. Pediatric patients hospitalized with myocarditis: A multi-institutional analysis. *Pediatr Cardiol* 2010;31:222–8.

86. Kim HJ, Yoo GH, Kil HR. Clinical outcome of acute myocarditis in children according to treatment modalities. *Korean J Pediatr* 2010;53:745–52.

87. Foerster SR, Canter CE, Cinar A, et al. Ventricular remodeling and survival are more favorable for myocarditis than for idiopathic dilated cardiomyopathy in childhood: An outcomes study from the Pediatric Cardiomyopathy Registry. *Circ Heart Fail* 2010;3:689–97.

88. Aziz KU, Patel N, Sadullah T, et al. Acute viral myocarditis: Role of immunosuppression: A prospective randomised study. *Cardiol Young* 2010;20:509–15.

89. McNamara DM, Holubkov R, Starling RC, et al. Controlled trial of intravenous immune globulin in recent-onset dilated cardiomyopathy. *Circulation* 2001;103:2254–9.

90. Mason JW, O'Connell JB, Herskowitz A, et al. A clinical trial of immunosuppressive therapy for myocarditis. The Myocarditis Treatment Trial Investigators. *N Engl J Med* 1995;333:269–75.

91. Robinson J, Hartling L, Vandermeer B, et al. Intravenous immunoglobulin for presumed viral myocarditis in children and adults. *Cochrane Database Syst Rev* 2005:CD004370.

92. Ahdoot J, Galindo A, Alejos JC, et al. Use of OKT3 for acute myocarditis in infants and children. *J Heart Lung Transplant* 2000;19:1118–21.

93. Abzug MJ, Cloud G, Bradley J, et al. Double blind placebo-controlled trial of pleconaril in infants with enterovirus meningitis. *Pediatr Infect Dis J* 2003;22:335–41.

94. Harmon WG, Sleeper LA, Cuniberti L, et al. Treating children with idiopathic dilated cardiomyopathy (from the Pediatric Cardiomyopathy Registry). *Am J Cardiol* 2009;104:281–6.

95. Kantor PF, Lougheed J, Dancea A, et al; Children's Heart Failure Study Group. Presentation, diagnosis, and medical management of heart failure in children: Canadian Cardiovascular Society guidelines. *Can J Cardiol* 2013;29:1535–52.

96. Frobel AK, Hulpke-Wette M, Schmidt KG, et al. β-blockers for congestive heart failure in children. *Cochrane Database Syst Rev* 2009:CD007037.

97. Duncan BW, Bohn DJ, Atz AM, et al. Mechanical circulatory support for the treatment of children with acute fulminant myocarditis. *J Thorac Cardiovasc Surg* 2001;122:440–8.

98. Paden ML, Conrad SA, Rycus PT, et al. Extracorporeal Life Support Organization Registry Report 2012. *ASAIO J* 2013;59:202–10.

99. Blume ED, Naftel DC, Bastardi HJ, et al. Outcomes of children bridged to heart transplantation with ventricular assist devices: A multi-institutional study. *Circulation* 2006;113:2313–9.

100. Fraser CD Jr, Jaquiss RD, Rosenthal DN, et al. Prospective trial of a pediatric ventricular assist device. *N Engl J Med* 2012;367:532–41.

101. Almond CS, Morales DL, Blackstone EH, et al. Berlin Heart EXCOR pediatric ventricular assist device for bridge to heart transplantation in US children. *Circulation* 2013;127:1702–11.

102. Cassidy J, Dominguez T, Haynes S, et al. A longer waiting game: Bridging children to heart transplant with the Berlin Heart EXCOR device-the United Kingdom experience. *J Heart Lung Transplant* 2013;32:1101–6.

103. Miera O, Potapov EV, Redlin M, et al. First experiences with the heartware ventricular assist system in children. *Ann Thorac Surg* 2011;91:1256–60.

104. Owens WR, Bryant R III, Dreyer WJ, et al. Initial clinical experience with the heartmate II ventricular assist system in a Pediatric Institution: Thoughts and progress. *Artif Organs* 2010;34:600–3.

105. Stiller B, Lemmer J, Merkle F, et al. Consumption of blood products during mechanical circulatory support in children: Comparison between ECMO and a pulsatile ventricular assist device. *Intensive Care Med* 2004;30:1814–20.

106. Thomas HL, Dronavalli VB, Parameshwar J, et al; Steering Group of the UKCTA. Incidence and outcome of Levitronix CentriMag support as rescue therapy for early cardiac allograft failure: A United Kingdom national study. *Eur J Cardiothorac Surg* 2011;40:1348–54.

107. Shuhaiber JH, Jenkins D, Berman M, et al. The Papworth experience with the Levitronix CentriMag ventricular assist device. *J Heart Lung Transplant* 2008;27:158–64.

108. Kouretas PC, Kaza AK, Burch PT, et al. Experience with the levitronix centrimag in the pediatric population as a bridge to decision and recovery. *Artif Organs* 2009;33:1002–4.

109. Maat AP, van Thiel RJ, Dalinghaus M, et al. Connecting the Centrimag Levitronix pump to Berlin Heart Excor cannulae; A new approach to bridge to bridge. *J Heart Lung Transplant* 2008;27:112–5.

110. Kirk R, Dipchand AI, Edwards LB, et al; International Society for Heart and Lung Transplantation. The Registry of the International Society for Heart and Lung Transplantation: Fifteenth pediatric heart transplantation report—2012. *J Heart Lung Transplant* 2012;31:1065–72.

111. Almond CS, Singh TP, Gauvreau K, et al. Extracorporeal membrane oxygenation for bridge to heart transplantation among children in the United States: Analysis of data from the Organ Procurement and Transplant Network and Extracorporeal Life Support Organization Registry. *Circulation* 2011;123:2975–84.

112. Kirklin JK, Naftel DC, Kormos RL, et al. Fifth INTERMACS annual report: Risk factor analysis from more than 6,000 mechanical circulatory support patients. *J Heart Lung Transplant* 2013;32:141–56.

113. Rajagopal SK, Almond CS, Laussen PC, et al. Extracorporeal membrane oxygenation for the support of infants, children, and young adults with acute myocarditis: A review of the Extracorporeal Life Support Organization registry. *Crit Care Med* 2010;38:382–7.

114. Cooper DS, Pretre R. Clinical management of pediatric ventricular assist devices. *Pediatr Crit Care Med* 2013;14:S27–36.

115. Almond CS, Buchholz H, Massicotte P, et al. Berlin Heart EXCOR Pediatric ventricular assist device Investigational Device Exemption study: Study design and rationale. *Am Heart J* 2011;162:425–435.e6.

116. Hetzer R, Potapov EV, Stiller B, et al. Improvement in survival after mechanical circulatory support with pneumatic pulsatile ventricular assist devices in pediatric patients. *Ann Thorac Surg* 2006;82:917–24; discussion 924–5.

117. Ghez O, Liesner R, Karimova A, et al. Subcutaneous low molecular weight heparin for management of anticoagulation in infants on excor ventricular assist device. *ASAIO J* 2006;52:705–7.

118. Rutledge JM, Chakravarti S, Massicotte MP, et al. Antithrombotic strategies in children receiving long-term Berlin Heart EXCOR ventricular assist device therapy. *J Heart Lung Transplant* 2013;32:569–73.

119. Reiss N, El-Banayosy A, Arusoglu L, et al. Acute fulminant myocarditis in children and adolescents: The role of mechanical circulatory assist. *ASAIO J* 2006;52:211–4.

120. Jones CB, Cassidy JV, Kirk R, et al. Successful bridge to recovery with 120 days of mechanical support in an infant with myocarditis. *J Heart Lung Transplant* 2009;28:202–5.

121. Zimmerman H, Covington D, Smith R, et al. Mechanical support and medical therapy reverse heart failure in infants and children. *Artif Organs* 2010;34:885–90.

122. Byrnes JW, Prodhan P, Williams BA, et al. Incremental reduction in the incidence of stroke in children supported with the Berlin EXCOR ventricular assist device. *Ann Thorac Surg* 2013;96:1727–33.

123. Karimova A, Van Doorn C, Brown K, et al. Mechanical bridging to orthotopic heart transplantation in children weighing less than 10 kg: Feasibility and limitations. *Eur J Cardiothorac Surg* 2011;39:304–9.

124. Stein ML, Robbins R, Sabati AA, et al. Interagency Registry for Mechanically Assisted Circulatory Support (INTERMACS)-defined morbidity and mortality associated with pediatric ventricular assist device support at a single US center the Stanford experience. *Circ Heart Fail* 2010;3:682–8.

125. Potapov EV, Stiller B, Hetzer R. Ventricular assist devices in children: Current achievements and future perspectives. *Pediatr Transplant* 2007;11:241–55.

126. Cassidy J, Haynes S, Kirk R, et al. Changing patterns of bridging to heart transplantation in children. *J Heart Lung Transpl* 2009;28:249–54.

127. Aslam S, Hernandez M, Thornby J, et al. Risk factors and outcomes of fungal ventricular-assist device infections. *Clin Infect Dis* 2010;50:664–71.

128. Cabrera AG, Khan MS, Morales DL, et al. Infectious complications and outcomes in children supported with left ventricular assist devices. *J Heart Lung Transplant* 2013;32:518–24.

129. Kuhn B, Shapiro ED, Walls TA, et al. Predictors of outcome of myocarditis. *Pediatr Cardiol* 2004;25:379–84.

130. Why HJ, Meany BT, Richardson PJ, et al. Clinical and prognostic significance of detection of enteroviral RNA in the myocardium of patients with myocarditis or dilated cardiomyopathy. *Circulation* 1994;89:2582–9.

131. Amabile N, Fraisse A, Bouvenot J, et al. Outcome of acute fulminant myocarditis in children. *Heart* 2006;92:1269–73.

132. Daubeney PE, Nugent AW, Chondros P, et al. Clinical features and outcomes of childhood dilated cardiomyopathy: Results from a national population-based study. *Circulation* 2006;114:2671–8.

133. Everitt MD, Sleeper LA, Lu M, et al. Recovery of echocardiographic function in children with idiopathic dilated cardiomyopathy: Results from the pediatric cardiomyopathy registry. *J Am Coll Cardiol* 2014;63:1405–13.

134. Fan Y, Weng YG, Huebler M, et al. Predictors of in-hospital mortality in children after long-term ventricular assist device insertion. *J Am Coll Cardiol* 2011;58:1183–90.

135. Alvarez JA, Orav EJ, Wilkinson JD, et al; Pediatric Cardiomyopathy Registry I. Competing risks for death and cardiac transplantation in children with dilated cardiomyopathy: Results from the pediatric cardiomyopathy registry. *Circulation* 2011;124:814–23.

136. Pahl E, Sleeper LA, Canter CE, et al. Incidence of and risk factors for sudden cardiac death in children with dilated cardiomyopathy: A report from the Pediatric Cardiomyopathy Registry. *J Am Coll Cardiol* 2012;59:607–15.

CHAPTER 74 ■ TREATMENT OF HEART FAILURE: MEDICAL MANAGEMENT

JOSEPH W. ROSSANO, JACK F. PRICE, AND DAVID P. NELSON

KEY POINTS

1 Heart failure is a clinical syndrome characterized by a reduced ability of the heart to fill and/or eject blood to meet the body's metabolic demand. It may occur in the setting of cardiomyopathy, myocarditis, or after cardiac surgery.

2 Angiotensin-converting enzyme inhibitors and β-blockers are the mainstays of chronic management due to their inhibition of the renin–angiotensin–aldosterone system and the sympathetic nervous system. Diuretics are used for control of symptoms.

3 Acute decompensated heart failure is commonly an exacerbation of chronic heart failure.

4 Assessment of perfusion (warm or cold) and congestion (wet or dry) is useful in formulating management plans for patients with acute decompensated heart failure.

5 The primary aim of acute decompensated heart failure therapy is to return the patient to a state of adequate perfusion (warm) and normal or near normal filling pressures (dry).

6 Vasodilators and diuretics are indicated for patients with elevated filling pressures and normal or decreased perfusion.

7 Inotropic agents should be used with caution, as studies from adult patients indicate increased mortality when inotropic agents are used. In patients that fail to respond to inotropic agents, mechanical support may be considered.

8 Low cardiac output syndrome (LCOS) in the early postoperative period is primarily due to transient myocardial dysfunction, compounded by acute changes in myocardial loading conditions, including postoperative increases in systemic and/or pulmonary vascular resistance.

9 At present, direct measure of myocardial performance and/or cardiac output in children is primarily a research tool and not feasible for routine clinical monitoring of patients. Therefore, cardiac output and systemic perfusion

are usually assessed indirectly by monitoring vital signs, peripheral perfusion, urine output, acid–base status and venous oximetry.

10 Blood lactate levels may become elevated only with significant circulatory dysfunction, after the anaerobic threshold has been reached, below the point when oxygen consumption becomes dependent on oxygen delivery.

11 When atrial pressure is low, fluid administration augments end-diastolic volume and increases stroke volume. With successive fluid administration, however, increases in stroke volume become limited due to the nonlinear nature of ventricular diastolic compliance.

12 Use of high-dose catecholamines for inotropic support has disadvantages, as they can increase afterload substantially, promote tachycardia and proarrhythmic effects, increase myocardial oxygen consumption, and depress the myocardial adrenergic response by downregulating β-adrenergic receptors. Phosphodiesterase inhibitors increase cardiac muscle contractility and vascular muscle relaxation without increasing myocardial oxygen consumption or ventricular afterload.

13 In the neonate, the sarcoplasmic reticular system is relatively sparse and undifferentiated, so the neonatal myocardium is more dependent upon extracellular calcium stores for contractile function.

14 Arginine vasopressin has been advocated as a therapeutic option for pediatric patients with refractory hypotension after surgery, to improve systemic arterial blood pressure when conventional therapies fail.

15 Recent data suggest that adrenal dysfunction contributes to morbidity in critically ill adult patients, and low-dose corticosteroid administration has been suggested as an option for patients with refractory LCOS.

Heart failure is a clinical syndrome characterized by a reduced ability of the heart to fill and/or eject blood to meet the body's metabolic demands (1). In children with structural heart disease, this can be the result of pressure or volume overload conditions and resultant ventricular dysfunction, especially in patients with a functionally univentricular heart or systemic morphologic right ventricle. Heart failure is also a common sequela of cardiomyopathies, where abnormal myocardial structure impairs the ability of the heart to contract and/or relax. Among the most common causes of heart failure in infants and children is low cardiac output syndrome (LCOS) after cardiac surgery, which is usually transient and reversible. This chapter discusses the therapeutic options that exist in managing these patients.

MANAGEMENT OF CHRONIC HEART FAILURE

Pharmacological Agents Used for Treatment of Heart Failure

Heart failure is generally a chronic, progressive disorder (2), though certain types of cardiomyopathy such as left ventricular noncompaction can have an undulating phenotype with periods of improvement and/or deterioration in function (3). Another exception is acute myocarditis, especially the fulminant form, in which patients may have a complete recovery of function. Guidelines for the management of chronic heart failure in adults and children have been published by the International Society of Heart and Lung Transplant, the American College of Cardiology, and the American Heart Association (1,4). The primary aim of therapy is to reduce symptoms, preserve long-term ventricular performance, and prolong survival primarily through antagonism of neurohormonal compensatory mechanisms. Since some medications may be detrimental during acute decompensation, the critical care physician should be knowledgeable of the medications and therapeutic goals of chronic heart failure treatment. Furthermore, understanding mechanisms of chronic heart failure may foster improved understanding of the treatment of acute decompensated heart failure.

Diuretics

Treating symptoms of "congestion" is critical to the management of heart failure in both the acute and the chronic setting (1). Diuretics are recommended for patients with symptoms of heart failure and evidence of volume overload. Although these are the most common agents used in the long-term management of heart failure, there is a lack of studies that demonstrate long-term benefits of diuretic treatment. Indeed, data from animal models of cardiomyopathy indicate that furosemide activates the renin–angiotensin–aldosterone system (RAAS) and accelerates the decline of myocardial function (5). Furthermore, a retrospective study of adult heart failure patients identified the use of increased loop diuretic dose as an independent predictor of mortality (6). Loop and thiazide diuretics remain the most commonly used diuretics. In adults, aldosterone antagonists, such as spironolactone, have been shown to improve mortality when added to standard heart failure management (7), though there may be an increase in hyperkalemia (8,9). These agents have not been well studied in children, but pediatric use is expanding, likely secondary to the increased use in adults.

Angiotensin-Converting Enzyme Inhibitors/Angiotensin Receptor Blockers

Angiotensin-converting enzyme (ACE) inhibitors were the first agents to demonstrate improved survival in adults with symptomatic heart failure. These medications decrease the formation of angiotensin II, block the activation of the RAAS, and decrease adrenergic activity (10). Prospective randomized controlled trails of various agents within this class have demonstrated improvement in symptoms with reduced progression of heart failure, decreased hospitalization, and improved survival in adults with chronic heart failure (11–16). The mortality benefit is primarily due to decreased deaths from pump failure. Angiotensin receptor blockers (ARBs), primarily used in adults unable to tolerate ACE inhibitors, have also demonstrated reduction in mortality that is comparable, and possibly superior to the ACE inhibitors (17). The combination of ACE inhibitor and ARB treatment may provide additional benefits to improve left ventricular geometry, ejection fraction, and exercise capacity (18,19).

Although ACE inhibitors have been shown to reduce the Qp:Qs ratio in children with large left-to-right shunt lesions (20), long-term treatment has not been shown to be efficacious. Since heart failure symptoms and ventricular dysfunction are common in infants with single-ventricle hearts, the Pediatric Heart Network conducted a randomized controlled trial of ACE inhibition in this population (21). Administration of enalapril to infants with single-ventricle physiology in the first year of life did not improve somatic growth, ventricular function, or heart failure severity (21). In addition, a trial of ACE inhibition in Fontan patients also failed to demonstrate improvement in resting cardiac index, diastolic function, systemic vascular resistance (SVR), or exercise capacity (22).

Although there have been no large randomized controlled trials of ACE inhibitors in the treatment of children with dilated cardiomyopathy (DCM), there are multiple small studies to suggest efficacy in these patients. In children with DCM, Bengur et al. (23) demonstrated that a single dose of 0.5 mg/kg of captopril increased cardiac index and stroke volume by 22% and decreased SVR without a significant decrease in mean aortic pressure. Stern et al. (24) prospectively studied 12 children with DCM. A 3-month course of captopril (mean dose 1.8 mg/kg/d) was associated with an improvement in left ventricular end-diastolic and end-systolic volumes and reduced aldosterone and plasma atrial natriuretic peptide. Mori et al. (25) reported similar echocardiographic results in a prospective study of patients with aortic and mitral regurgitation treated with ACE inhibitors. A retrospective study of children with DCM reported improved survival with ACE inhibition, although the survival benefit was not statistically significant beyond 1 year of therapy (26). On the basis of the supportive pediatric evidence and abundant adult data, the International Society for Heart and Lung Transplantation (ISHLT) guidelines recommend ACE inhibition for moderate or severe degrees of LV dysfunction in infants and children, and ARB therapy if ACE inhibition is not tolerated.

β-Blockers

As with ACE inhibitors, there is abundant evidence from large randomized controlled trials that β-blockers in adult patients with chronic heart failure demonstrate improvement in symptoms, heart function, frequency of hospitalization, and survival (27–30). Despite negative inotropic properties, the presumed benefit of β-blockade is inhibition of the effects of the sympathetic nervous system (31). Data on β-blocker use in pediatric heart failure are limited and contradictory. Shaddy et al. (32) reviewed the experience of metoprolol in 15 children with DCM at three centers in the United States. Metoprolol was associated with a significant increase in fractional shortening and ejection fraction. Carvedilol use was reviewed in 46 patients with DCM (80%) or palliated congenital heart disease (20%) and was found to be associated with improvement in New York Heart Association (NYHA) functional class and fractional shortening at 3 months (33). A small randomized, placebo-controlled study in 22 children with severe left ventricular dysfunction found that patients given carvedilol had an improvement in ejection fraction and NYHA class over a 3-month period (34). Additionally, 64% of the patients in the carvedilol group improved enough to be taken off the cardiac transplantation list. A large multicenter prospective pediatric study of carvedilol randomized 161 children to placebo, low-dose, or high-dose carvedilol (35). Heart failure outcomes were not different among the treatment groups, but the incidence of heart failure progression was lower than predicted, so the study was thought to be underpowered (35). A prespecified analysis of the interaction effect between ventricular morphology and carvedilol response showed a trend toward improvement in children with DCM and morphologic left ventricles. Although ISHLT guidelines do not recommend β-blockers in infants and children with heart failure (4), β-blockers are often empirically used in children with DCM on the basis of the abundant adult data and the supportive data in children with DCM.

Digoxin

Digoxin, the oldest medication used for treatment of heart failure symptoms, is a cardiac glycoside that improves contractility by inhibiting the Na–K-ATPase pump in the cardiac myocyte membrane. The increase in intracellular sodium is exchanged across the cell membrane by a Na–Ca transporter, which results in increased intracellular calcium and contractility (36).

Although digoxin is effective in alleviating symptoms of heart failure (37), it has not been shown to improve mortality (38), and higher doses are associated with an increase in mortality (39). Based on data from adult studies, the current recommendation of the ISHLT is to use digoxin for symptomatic pediatric patients with the aim of reducing symptoms (4).

Electrophysiological Management of Heart Failure

Arrhythmias are an important consequence and often unrecognized etiology of heart failure in children. Tachycardia-induced cardiomyopathy is uncommon, but reversible. In one series, over 90% of patients presenting with tachycardia-induced cardiomyopathy had resolution of left ventricular dysfunction with medical therapy or radiofrequency ablation (40).

Antiarrhythmic Agents

There is limited evidence for the best choice of an antiarrhythmic agent in children with arrhythmias and heart failure. For arrhythmias where β-blockade is indicated (e.g., re-entrant tachycardia, ectopic focus tachycardia, rate control for atrial fibrillation), metoprolol may be a good choice based on its dual efficacy for heart failure and antiarrhythmic agent. Although its antiarrhythmic efficacy is not as well established, Carvedilol decreases atrial and ventricular arrhythmias in adults after myocardial infarction (41). Amiodarone is an effective antiarrhythmic medication for a variety of arrhythmias. Although amiodarone decreases ventricular arrhythmias in adults with heart failure, effects on survival are contradictory. Some studies suggest a decrease in survival in patients treated with amiodarone (42–44). Patients with ventricular arrhythmias and depressed left ventricular function are at increased risk for sudden death, and an implantable cardioverter-defibrillator (ICD) should be considered (see below).

Cardiac Resynchronization Therapy

Disturbances in the normal electrical conduction of the heart are common in chronic heart failure, and often lead to dyssynchronous contraction. In adults, this is often due to left bundle branch block, which is uncommon in children. Restoration of ventricular synchrony with synchronized biventricular pacing is termed cardiac resynchronization therapy (CRT). In appropriately selected adults, CRT results in reverse remodeling and improved symptoms of heart failure (45). When combined with an ICD, CRT may improve mortality (46). There are limited data on CRT use in children, but initial short-term results demonstrate improved ventricular function with CRT (47). CRT may prove useful for pediatric and adult patients with congenital heart disease with an intraventricular conduction delay, as often seen in patients with tetralogy of Fallot or functionally univentricular hearts (48).

Implantable Cardioverter-Defibrillator

Ventricular arrhythmias and sudden cardiac death (SCD) are common in adults with heart failure. There are limited data on the frequency of sudden death in children with heart failure, but available evidence suggests the incidence is lower than in adult patients (49). The use of an ICD as primary prevention of SCD is well established for adults with both ischemic and nonischemic cardiomyopathy (50). On the basis of existing data, the AHA/ACC/HRS 2008 guidelines for device-based therapy of cardiac rhythm abnormalities recommend the consideration of prophylactic ICD placement for adult patients with an ejection fraction ≤35% with mild to moderate heart

failure symptoms (51). The most recent ISHLT guidelines also include recommendations for children with heart failure. ICD placement is recommended in children with congenital heart disease with documented cardiac arrest or sustained ventricular tachycardia. ICD placement should also be considered for children with cardiomyopathy and recurrent syncope. Because of the apparent reduced frequency of SCD in children with cardiomyopathy and the increased frequency of inappropriate ICD shocks in children, ICD placement is not indicated for children with isolated ventricular dysfunction (51).

MANAGEMENT OF ACUTE DECOMPENSATED HEART FAILURE

Etiology and Pathophysiology

There is no universally accepted definition for acute decompensated heart failure; however, it generally encompasses patients hospitalized for treatment of heart failure (52). There is an estimated one million hospitalizations annually for acute decompensated heart failure in adults (53), and it is the most common reason for hospital admission in patients over 65 years of age. The burden of disease in the pediatric population is not known, but as in adults, most admissions in children are for acute exacerbations of chronic heart failure. In contrast to adult patients, ischemic cardiomyopathy is rare in children and idiopathic DCM is more common. Other important causes of acute decompensated heart failure in children include tachycardia-mediated cardiomyopathy, acute myocarditis, DCM secondary to other etiologies (e.g., anthracycline toxicity, anomalous coronary artery, inborn errors of metabolism), and "high-output" cardiac failure (from arteriovenous malformation, thyrotoxicosis or anemia).

Irrespective of etiology, heart failure is thought to occur after an index event produces an initial decline in heart function (**Fig. 74.1**). This leads to compensatory mechanisms including

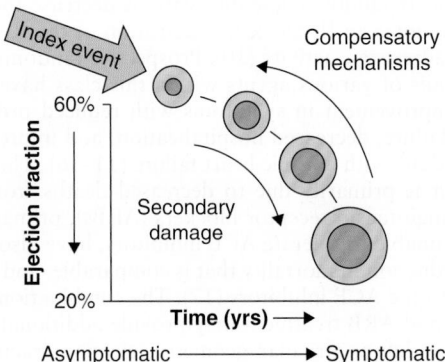

FIGURE 74.1. Pathogenesis of heart failure. Heart failure begins after an index event produces an initial decline in pumping capacity of the heart. Following this initial decline, a variety of compensatory mechanisms are activated, including the adrenergic nervous system, renin–angiotensin system, and cytokine system. In the short term, these systems are able to restore cardiovascular function to a normal homeostasis, so the patient remains asymptomatic. However, with time, the sustained activation of these systems can lead to secondary myocardial injury with pathologic LV remodeling and subsequent cardiac decompensation. The progressive LV remodeling and cardiac decompensation will ultimately lead to a transition from asymptomatic to symptomatic heart failure. (Reproduced with permission pending from Mann DL, Bristow MR. Mechanisms and models in heart failure. *Circulation* 2005;111:2837–49.)

activation of the sympathetic nervous system, salt and water preservation with activation of the RAAS system, and production of inflammatory cytokines (e.g., tissue necrosis factor, interleukin 1). The compensatory mechanisms often delay the onset of symptoms for months or even years. However, the compensatory mechanisms are generally counterproductive over time and contribute to progressive myocardial damage, left ventricular remodeling, and eventual cardiac decompensation. The intensivist must be cognizant that symptoms of heart failure progress independently of the patient's hemodynamic status (54), so heart failure therapy should *not* be titrated on the basis of echocardiographic and/or catheterization results.

Diagnosis and Assessment of Acute Decompensated Heart Failure

The first signs of acute decompensated heart failure are typically respiratory symptoms such as dyspnea, tachypnea, and increased work of breathing. In children, gastrointestinal symptoms such as abdominal pain, vomiting, or diarrhea are also common (55). An increased index of suspicion is required, especially in patients with no prior history of heart failure, as symptoms may overlap with more common clinical entities such as pneumonia or acute gastroenteritis. The cardiac examination may reveal jugular venous distention in older patients, a displaced point of maximal cardiac impulse, a gallop rhythm, or murmur of mitral regurgitation. The liver may be displaced inferiorly, and peripheral edema may be present in older children and adults. The severity of symptoms varies widely from minimal discomfort to cardiogenic shock. The initial physical assessment is critical to guide initial management. A chest radiograph is commonly used to evaluate cardiac size and the degree of pulmonary congestion.

The serum level of B-type natriuretic peptide (BNP) is a sensitive screening tool to help differentiate cardiac dyspnea from other forms of dyspnea in adult patients in the emergency department (56). BNP is a cardiac neurohormone secreted in response to ventricular volume expansion and pressure overload. Serum BNP levels have also been shown to be elevated in pediatric patients with ventricular dysfunction in both the acute and the chronic setting (57). Although BNP assessment in children may aid in making the diagnosis of acute decompensated heart failure, there are no data that the values at the time of admission are predictive of outcome. Other useful laboratory data include assessment of renal function and serum electrolytes, as patients are frequently on chronic diuretics.

Although, quantification of cardiac function is important, the severity of a patient's symptoms *cannot* be predicted by the degree of ventricular systolic dysfunction. Some patients may be chronically stable with ejection fractions of less than 20%, whereas other patients may be quite symptomatic with only mild to moderate dysfunction. Two-dimensional and M-mode echocardiography provide the standard assessment of function with an easily calculated ejection fraction and shortening fraction, but these measures are preload and afterload dependent. Other tools, such as myocardial performance index and Doppler tissue imaging, provide a more quantitative assessment of systolic and diastolic functions that are less dependent on loading conditions of the heart (58).

Preload, an important determinant of cardiac output, is defined as the stretch of the myocardium at end diastole. The stretch on myocytes is determined by the end-diastolic volume (EDV), which correlates with atrial filling pressure. Because of ventricular diastolic stiffness, increases in stroke volume with increasing preload become limited at higher EDVs (Fig. 74.2). Filling pressures that are elevated above normal levels coincide with symptoms in patients with decompensated heart failure, and restoration of filling pressures normal or near normal is

an important endpoint of initial therapy (59). Elevated filling pressures can be estimated clinically with elevated jugular venous pulsations, hepatomegaly, and presence of pulmonary congestion. Measurement of filling pressures can be obtained with central venous catheters. Studies from adults suggest that left ventricular filling pressures can be estimated with moderate sensitivity and specificity with measurement of central venous or pulmonary artery pressure (60). It is unclear whether invasive measurement of filling pressure improves outcome over clinical assessment. A prospective, randomized study in adults with decompensated heart failure found that use of pulmonary artery catheters did not improve outcome, but did increase the occurrence of adverse events (61). Since a central venous catheter is safer and provides comparable information, pulmonary artery catheters are rarely used for hemodynamic assessment of pediatric heart failure patients.

Although most patients with acute decompensated heart failure have elevated filling pressures with adequate tissue perfusion, some patients present with cardiogenic shock. Direct or indirect assessment of cardiac output is thus an important aspect of the initial and the ongoing assessment of patients in heart failure. Indirect measures of cardiac output include mental status, heart rate, extremity temperature, capillary refill time, and urine output. Laboratory assessment of cardiac output includes measurements of acid–base status, lactic acid, and venous oxygen saturation.

In the absence of intracardiac shunting, superior vena cava oxygen saturation correlates well to true mixed-venous oxygen saturation (62). A central line placed into the superior vena cava can thus be used as a surrogate for mixed-venous saturation in patients with and without intracardiac shunting. Data from postoperative patients with congenital heart disease suggest assessment of cardiac output with venous oximetry can improve outcome (63,64). Additionally, regional oxygen saturation via near-infrared spectroscopy can provide a noninvasive surrogate for superior vena cava saturation (65).

Direct measurement of cardiac output can be obtained invasively with pulmonary artery catheters via thermodilution technique. Cardiac output can also be directly calculated by the Fick equation, but this requires measurement of systemic oxygen consumption. A variety of noninvasive techniques for estimation of cardiac output have been developed, including aortic Doppler measurements, carbon dioxide rebreathing, and arterial waveform contour. Validation of these techniques in pediatric patients is limited (66), especially in children with heart failure. Whether routine quantification of cardiac output in pediatric patients with heart failure will improve outcome awaits further inquiry.

Algorithm for Rapid Assessment and Management of Heart Failure

A simple and useful tool to help guide management of the patient with acute decompensated heart failure is the rapid assessment algorithm proposed by Grady et al. (67). As shown in Figure 74.3, patients are classified according to the signs of elevated filling pressures (wet or dry) and adequacy of perfusion (warm or cold). The goal of heart failure treatment is to transition a patient to the "warm and dry" category. Patients who present as "warm and wet" or "cold and wet," generally respond well to medical management. The "cold and dry" state is typically a dire condition, which may require aggressive treatment, such as mechanical support. It should be noted that this conceptual framework was designed for adults with heart failure. Although the benefit of this characterization for children with heart failure has not been validated, it is a useful conceptual framework to approach patient management.

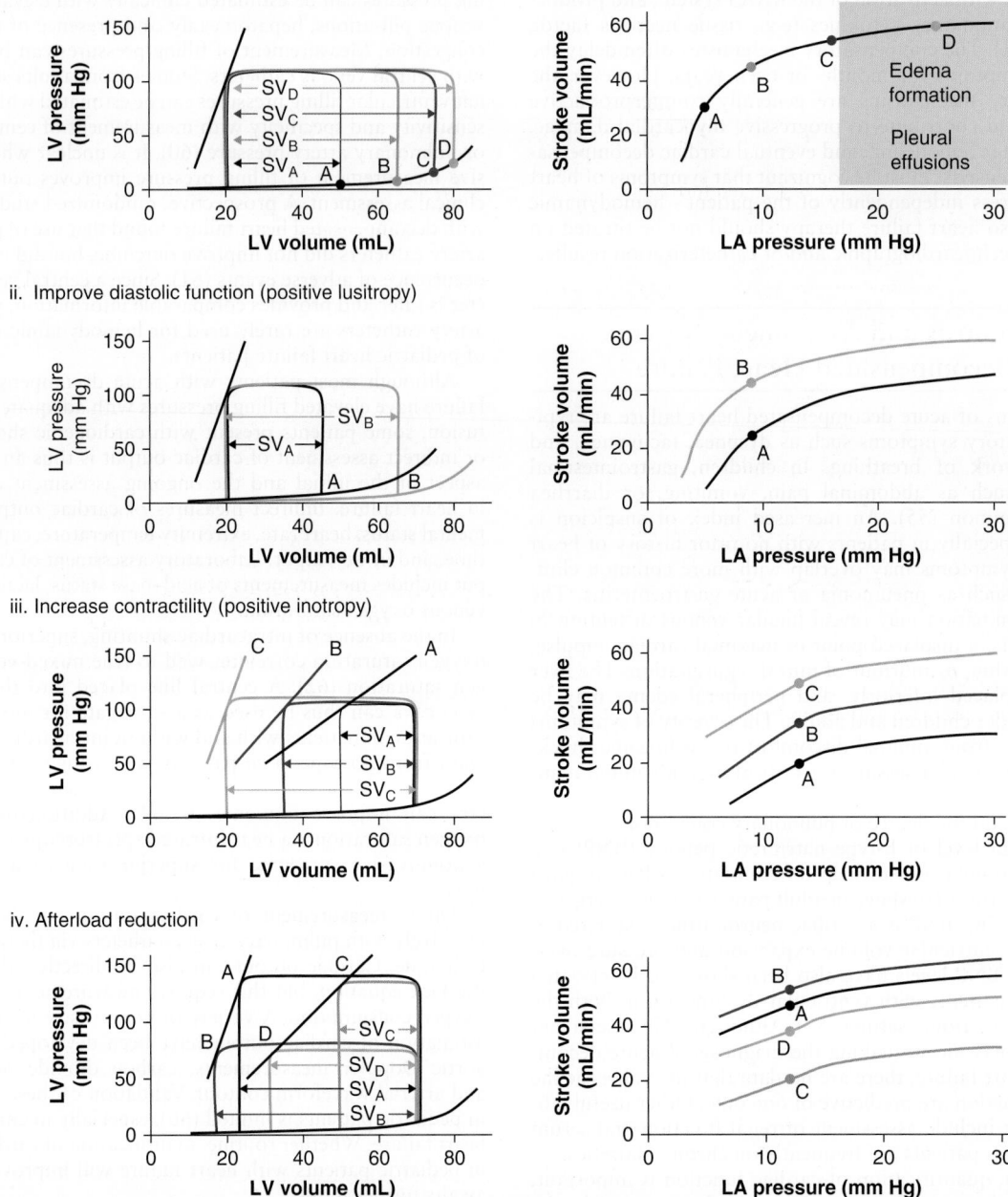

FIGURE 74.2. Paired changes in pressure–volume and Starling relationships with isolated manipulations in preload (i), lusitropy (ii), contractility (iii), and afterload (iv). End-diastolic point A and stroke volume A (SV$_A$) for each pair of graphs represent the initial baseline hemodynamic condition. **Panel i** demonstrates the effect of preload recruitment on the pressure–volume and Starling relationships. Fluid volume administration augments EDV from points A to B, with the increase in stroke volume shown as the difference between SV$_A$ and SV$_B$. Since diastolic compliance is nonlinear, increases in stroke volume are progressively less with further fluid administration (SV$_C$ and SV$_D$). EDVs A, B, C, and D define the diastolic compliance relationship. Preload augmentation is limited by elevations in left ventricular end-diastolic pressure (EDP), which can lead to impaired myocardial perfusion and elevations in atrial pressure, with resultant transcapillary leak and edema formation. **Panel ii** demonstrates beneficial effects of positive lusitropy on the pressure–volume and Starling relationships. Enhanced ventricular compliance corresponds to an increased EDV for the same EDP, thereby augmenting stroke volume without increasing atrial pressure. Enhanced lusitropy results in a greater stroke volume for a comparable atrial pressure. **Panel iii** demonstrates beneficial effects of positive inotropy on the pressure–volume and Starling relationships. Increases in contractility are shown as enhancement of the end-systolic pressure–volume relationship (ESPVR), demonstrated by increases in slopes of lines A to B to C on the left-hand graph. At constant preload, increased contractility enhances ejection during isovolumic contraction, decreasing the end-systolic volume and increasing stroke volume (from SV$_A$ to SV$_B$ to SV$_C$). Enhanced contractility results in a greater stroke volume for a comparable preload. **Panel iv** demonstrates beneficial effects of afterload reduction on the pressure–volume and Starling relationships. From baseline conditions A or C, afterload reduction allows the heart to eject to a lower systolic pressure and volume (points B and D), enhancing ejection and augmenting stroke volume (SV$_A$ to SV$_B$ and SV$_C$ to SV$_D$). At normal contractility (slope AB), the ventricle responds to altered afterload with only a small change in stroke volume (SV$_A$ to SV$_B$). On the other hand, neonatal and failing hearts are particularly sensitive to alterations in afterload. Benefits of afterload reduction are therefore more pronounced in neonatal hearts and in the setting of poor contractility. With reduced contractility (as shown by the reduced slope of ESPVR CD), the increase in stroke volume is greater for a comparable change in afterload. Afterload reduction results in a greater stroke volume for a comparable preload.

	No Congestion	Congestion
Adequate perfusion	"Warm and Dry" A Optimal profile: focus on prevention of disease progression and decompensation	"Wet and Warm" B Diuresis with continuation of standard therapy
Critical hypoperfusion	"Cold and Dry" L Limited further options for therapy	"Wet and Cold" C Diuresis and redesign of regimen with other standard therapies

FIGURE 74.3. Profile of resting hemodynamics. Patients frequently progress from profile A to profile B or profile C. Profile "L" refers to patient's presenting with severely low cardiac output. The letter L was chosen rather than the letter D to avoid the implication that this profile necessarily follows profile C. (Reproduced with permission pending from Grady KL, Dracup K, Kennedy G, et al. Team management of patients with heart failure: A statement for healthcare professionals from The Cardiovascular Nursing Council of the American Heart Association. *Circulation* 2000;102:2443–56.)

Adequate Perfusion with Elevated Filling Pressures; "Warm and Wet"

The patient with congestion but adequate perfusion is the most common presentation of acute decompensated heart failure, and typically responds well to medical therapy. Diuresis is a critical component of the initial management of the patient with elevated filling pressures and may be the only therapy needed in the patient with adequate perfusion. In studies from adult patients, diuretics were found to increase stroke volume, decrease pulmonary capillary wedge pressure, and decrease SVR (68). Diuretics combined with vasodilators have also been shown to decrease mitral regurgitation and increase forward ejection fraction (69). Over-diuresis should be avoided, as volume depletion and renal insufficiency may result. This process in which combined cardiac and renal dysfunction amplifies progression of end-organ damage has been termed the cardiorenal syndrome.

Assessment of systemic perfusion is essential in determining whether to continue chronic therapy for heart failure during acute exacerbations. If perfusion is adequate, β-blockers and ACE inhibitors can generally be continued during hospitalization, while negative inotropic effects of β-blockers may necessitate discontinuation or dose reduction if perfusion is marginal. Some patients may not tolerate acute withdrawal from β-blockade. In adults, continuance of chronic β-blocker therapy during hospitalization is associated with a decreased risk of death or re-hospitalization (70). Initiation of a β-blocker is usually contraindicated while the patient is in decompensated heart failure. Delaying initiation of a β-blocker until the patient has been transitioned back to the "warm and dry" state is generally advised.

Poor Perfusion with Elevated Filling Pressures: "Cold and Wet"

Patients with congestion and poor perfusion typically require intensive care. In one series of adult patients, 20% of patients admitted for heart failure were in this group, and there was a higher risk of death or need for urgent heart transplant in these patients compared with patients with adequate perfusion (71). The initial approach to these patients will depend upon the degree of circulatory compromise. The cornerstone of therapy for these patients is afterload reduction, as this is the most effective way to increase cardiac output in the failing heart (rather than "whipping" it with inotropic agents). Vasodilators and diuretics alone may be adequate therapy for many patients. Avoiding inotropic agents when possible appears to be beneficial. A review of over 15,000 adults hospitalized for heart failure observed a higher in-hospital mortality in patients treated with dobutamine or milrinone compared with patients treated with nitroglycerin or nesiritide (72). This is consistent with prior studies demonstrating adult patients have increased mortality and more adverse events when treated with milrinone (73). Since it is unclear whether the adult data translate to children with heart failure, milrinone tends to be first-line therapy for children with decompensated heart failure in the "cold and wet" state. In children with decompensated heart failure, we try to avoid use of β-adrenergic agonists, especially at higher doses.

There are no pediatric data to support the use of a specific vasodilator for acute decompensated heart failure. Nitroprusside is an effective agent for treatment of heart failure, which has been used in adults for decades (74). The drug has a rapid half-life and can be quickly uptitrated to effect. Blood pressure must be monitored as hypotension can develop. Cyanide toxicity is an important potential side effect, especially with chronic use or renal impairment. There is limited pediatric experience with other vasodilators such as nitroglycerin for heart failure treatment. Nesiritide, human recombinant BNP, has been shown to have positive lusitropic properties, promote vasodilation, improve natriuresis, and inhibit renin and aldosterone. It rapidly improves symptoms in adults with acute decompensated heart failure. There are limited long-term data, and there have been some concerns regarding renal toxicity and the effect on long-term survival (75,76).

Inotropes. Inotropic agents may be required to improve perfusion or treat hypotension in "wet and cold" patients. The decision to use inotropic agents should be based on clinical assessment of end-organ perfusion, and *not* on echocardiographic results. Many patients with significant ventricular dysfunction will remain compensated and may be harmed by inotropes. Traditional inotropic agents used for decompensated heart failure include dobutamine, dopamine, milrinone, and calcium chloride.

Dobutamine. Dobutamine is a β-adrenergic agonist, which stimulates both β_1- and β_2-receptors. β_1-Receptor stimulation increases intracellular cyclic adenosine monophosphate (cAMP), increasing contractility by release of calcium from the sarcoplasmic reticulum. β_2-Receptor activation results in peripheral vasodilation and decreased SVR. The decrease in SVR may cause a reflex tachycardia, although rarely. An increase in heart rate and contractility may result in an undesired increase in myocardial oxygen consumption (77). Although short-term infusions of dobutamine improve symptoms, decrease filling pressures, increase ejection fraction, and improve exercise tolerance (78,79), tachycardia and arrhythmias are common side effects (**Table 74.1**). As noted, dobutamine use has been associated with increased mortality in adult heart failure patients, compared with nesiritide or nitroglycerin.

TABLE 74.1

COMMONLY USED INFUSIONS FOR THE TREATMENT OF HEART FAILURE

■ INOTROPIC AGENT	■ LOADING DOSE	■ INFUSION DOSE RANGE
Dopamine	None	3–10 μg/kg/min
Dobutamine	None	3–20 μg/kg/min
Milrinone	50–100 μg/kg over 60 min	0.25–1 μg/kg/min
Calcium chloride	None	5–20 mg/kg/h
Epinephrine	None	0.03–0.2 μg/kg/min
Arginine vasopressin	None	0.01–0.05 U/kg/h
Hydrocortisone	None	50 mg/m^2/d ÷ Q6 h
Triiodothyronine	None	0.05–0.1 μg/kg/h

This was also the finding of the CASINO (CAlcium Sensitizer or Inotrope or NOne in Low-Output HF Study) trial (80), which compared dobutamine with levosimendan or placebo. In this study, dobutamine use was associated with increased 6-month mortality compared with levosimendan or placebo. For the above reasons, routine use of dobutamine for heart failure has fallen out of favor. It seems likely that other inotropes may have similar detrimental effects for treatment of decompensated heart failure, but they have not been studied extensively. As stated previously, afterload reduction is the cornerstone of treatment rather than inotropic support. *No trial of long-term therapy with a positive inotropic agent has demonstrated improved outcomes in patients with heart failure. Most trials have found increased mortality with positive inotropic agents.*

Dopamine. Dopamine is an endogenous catecholamine. At low doses (2–5 μg/kg/min), there is stimulation of dopamine receptors in the renal, cerebral, coronary, mesenteric, and pulmonary vasculature. Higher doses of dopamine stimulate β-adrenergic receptors, increasing contractility, and heart rate. At higher doses (≥10 μg/kg/min), there is also significant α-adrenergic stimulation, resulting in vasoconstriction and increased systemic and pulmonary vascular resistance (81). There is no evidence to support the use of "renal dose" dopamine. The side-effect profile is similar to dobutamine, including the propensity for tachycardia, arrhythmias, and increased myocardial oxygen consumption. Although there are no clinical trials of dopamine use for treatment of acute decompensated heart failure, a trial of ibopamine, an oral dopaminergic drug, was prematurely stopped because of the increased mortality in the ibopamine-treated patients (82).

Milrinone. The most commonly used agent for acute decompensated heart failure in children is milrinone, a phosphodiesterase (PDE) inhibitor with both vasodilatory and inotropic properties. Milrinone inhibits the breakdown of cAMP by the PDE III isozyme (83). By blocking breakdown of intracellular cAMP, calcium transport into the cell is enhanced and myocyte contractility improved. In addition, reuptake of calcium is a cAMP-dependent process, so these agents may enhance diastolic relaxation of the myocardium by increasing the rate of calcium reuptake after systole. PDE inhibitors increase cardiac muscle contractility, vascular smooth muscle relaxation, and cardiac output without increasing myocardial oxygen consumption or ventricular afterload (84). Although milrinone improves symptoms and decreases filling pressures in adult patients, (85,86), milrinone may not improve long-term survival in patients with heart failure. In a study, of almost 1000 patients, evaluating short-term use of milrinone versus placebo, there was no difference in mortality, hospital length of stay, or hospital readmission (73), but there was an increased incidence of hypotension and arrhythmias

in milrinone-treated patients. Other studies have also failed to demonstrate the long-term benefit of milrinone in adults. A prospective study of oral milrinone for chronic heart failure found that milrinone-treated patients had increased hospitalization, overall mortality, and cardiovascular mortality (87). There are no trials of milrinone in children with acute decompensated heart failure. In a randomized, multicenter trial, milrinone was found to decrease LCOS in children after congenital heart surgery (88). Further investigation is needed to assess the overall efficacy of milrinone in children with acute decompensated heart failure.

Calcium. Calcium chloride has been shown to increase myocardial contractility in the post-arrest setting (89). In the adult heart, calcium released from the sarcoplasmic reticulum accounts for the majority of the calcium that binds to troponin C. In the neonate, the sarcoplasmic reticulum is relatively sparse and undifferentiated, so the neonatal myocardium is more dependent upon extracellular calcium stores for contractile function (90). Contractility is proportional to the level of ionized calcium in the blood (91). In contrast to catecholamines, calcium chloride does not induce tachycardia or arrhythmias. In adult patients, calcium chloride infusions have been discouraged owing to studies implicating calcium with increased myocardial necrosis and worsening diastolic dysfunction (92,93) (Table 74.1). There are no studies in children evaluating the use of chronic calcium chloride for decompensated heart failure, but it has been used extensively in perioperative patients with congenital heart disease. The use of calcium chloride can acutely improve myocardial contractility and cardiac output without excessive tachycardia, especially in younger patients. The long-term safety and efficacy of calcium infusions in children has not been determined.

Levosimendan. Levosimendan is a promising agent in a new class of medications known as calcium sensitizers. As noted in a previous chapter, calcium regulation in the failing myocardium is abnormal with prolonged intracellular calcium transients and a decreased ability to restore low calcium levels in diastole (94). There is a reduced expression of calcium channels in the sarcoplasmic reticulum, and myocardial contraction and relaxation depend primarily on calcium fluxes between the cytosol and extracellular fluid (95). Traditional inotropic agents that increase intracellular calcium are associated with increased oxygen consumption, impaired myocardial relaxation, and arrhythmias (96). Levosimendan is novel since it increases both inotropy and vasodilation without increasing calcium levels or myocardial oxygen demand (97). The enhancement of contractility occurs by binding to troponin C and increasing myofilament sensitivity to calcium. Levosimendan causes vasodilatation via opening of potassium-dependent adenosine triphosphate channels. The unique property of improving cardiac function without increasing intracellular calcium or myocardial oxygen consumption may prove to be a major breakthrough in the treatment of acute and chronic heart failure. Levosimendan has been used safely and effectively in adults with heart failure, with recent studies demonstrating improved mortality. There are isolated case reports of its use in children with severe heart failure postoperatively and in the setting of a DCM (98,99). The drug is not yet available in the United States.

Poor Perfusion with Normal Filling Pressures: "Cold and Dry"

Patients with inadequate perfusion and normal filling pressures represent a tenuous population. Vasodilators may worsen perfusion in patients with marginal blood pressure. In the setting of significantly compromised perfusion or cardiogenic shock, multiple inotropic agents may become necessary, including potent vasoconstrictor agents such as epinephrine or vasopressin. Titration of vasodilation therapy may become feasible if inotropic therapy improves perfusion in these patients, but inotropic agents rarely return these patients to an asymptomatic state. Furthermore, although these agents may be acutely life-saving, they may decrease long-term ventricular function and increase mortality. If there is an inadequate response to vasodilator therapy and increasing inotropic requirements are needed to maintain adequate perfusion, mechanical circulatory support should be considered.

Epinephrine. Epinephrine has dose-dependent actions on α- and β-adrenergic receptors. At low doses, the β-adrenergic receptor response predominates, resulting in vasodilation, increased heart rate, and contractility. At higher doses, α-receptor stimulation mediates vasoconstriction and increased SVR. Although, the increased SVR and contractility may acutely improve perfusion, this may occur at the expense of increased myocardial oxygen consumption and myocardial work. High-dose catecholamines often promote tachycardia and proarrhythmic effects, increase myocardial oxygen consumption, and depress the myocardial adrenergic response by downregulating β-adrenergic receptors. Furthermore, prolonged use of high-dose catecholamines may further amplify cardiomyocyte and sarcomeric injury, thus aggravating diastolic and systolic ventricular dysfunctions (100). Long periods of epinephrine infusion are poorly tolerated by the failing myocardium.

Vasopressin. The use of arginine vasopressin during and postcardiac arrest has been shown to improve return of spontaneous circulation and survival (101). Endogenous vasopressin levels are elevated in children with heart failure (102), but reduced in patients after cardiopulmonary bypass. Vasopressin acts directly upon vascular smooth muscle to increase SVR, but does not have the associated tachycardia found with catecholamines. Vasopressin also acts directly on the myocardium by increasing cytosolic calcium via V1 receptors (103). The use of vasopressin in children to improve low cardiac output in postoperative catecholamine resistant shock has been demonstrated (104). Studies of vasopressin in shock showed an improvement in stroke volume for all different types of shock, suggesting a direct inotropic effect upon the heart. Even if vasopressin has direct myocardial effects, the increased afterload with vasopressin is unlikely to be well tolerated in the failing myocardium for long periods.

Mechanical Support. In the setting of increasing inotrope requirements for the failing myocardium, the situation is dire. Medical therapy is unlikely to return the patient to an asymptomatic state, and continuation of therapy will likely increase the stress on an already failing myocardium. At this point, mechanical support should be considered to "rest the myocardium." In children, mechanical support has generally been used as a bridge to cardiac transplantation. In the setting of a potentially reversible process, such as myocarditis, mechanical support has been used as a bridge for recovery. Mechanical support can reduce the stress on a failing heart to reverse some of the pathologic molecular changes characteristics of heart failure. For example, mechanical support has been associated with reversal of cytoskeletal abnormalities like dystrophin proteolytic cleavage (105). When used in adults with severe heart failure as destination therapy or bridge to possible recovery of function, mechanical support is associated with increased survival and increased quality of life compared to medical therapy (106). A more detailed description of mechanical support is discussed in Chapter 75, but options include short-term support with total cardiopulmonary support from extracorporeal membrane oxygenation (ECMO), medium-term support with centrifugal pump devices, and long-term support with left ventricular assist devices or a total artificial heart. Since heroic efforts such as mechanical support may not be available or desirable in some patients, palliative care may be appropriate.

MANAGEMENT OF LOW CARDIAC OUTPUT SYNDROME AFTER CARDIAC SURGERY

Morbidity and mortality associated with LCOS following cardiac surgery are substantial. During earlier days of infant cardiac surgery, surgical mortality approached 20% (107). Although LCOS is associated with lower mortality in the current era, it results in increased hospital stay, resource utilization, and possible long-term cognitive dysfunction (108). Prompt recognition, diagnosis, and management of LCOS are fundamental to effective cardiac intensive care and essential for optimal patient outcome.

Causes of Low Cardiac Output after Surgery

Low cardiac output after congenital heart surgery is typically multifactorial. Although defects in myocardial systolic or diastolic contractile function usually accompany LCOS, other potential causes of low cardiac output such as altered ventricular loading and residual cardiac lesions should be considered. Changes in ventricular loading are integral to myocardial performance after congenital heart surgery. Ventricular preload is often inadequate, due to blood loss, perioperative fluid shifts, changes in diastolic compliance or physiologic changes resulting from the surgical procedure (e.g., Fontan or shunted single-ventricle physiology) (109). Increases in intrathoracic pressure resulting from tamponade or pneumothorax will limit venous return and impede ventricular filling. Ventricular afterload is often increased after bypass procedures, resulting from bypass-mediated vascular injury and resultant altered vascular reactivity (**Fig. 74.4**). Cardiopulmonary bypass induces both systemic and pulmonary endothelial dysfunctions, presumably due to ischemia–reperfusion injury to the endothelium (110–114). An acute pulmonary hypertension episode causes an acute rise in right ventricular (RV) afterload, which can shift the interventricular septum into the systemic ventricle and decrease the preload of the systemic ventricle. The acute increase in RV afterload and decrease in LV preload can diminish cardiac output dramatically. A pulmonary hypertensive crisis most often presents with acute systemic hypotension and diminished perfusion. Arterial oxygen saturation will decrease only if right-to-left intracardiac shunting can occur.

Residual anatomic or electrophysiologic abnormalities are likely to diminish cardiac output after congenital heart surgery. Uncorrected anatomic defects such as outflow

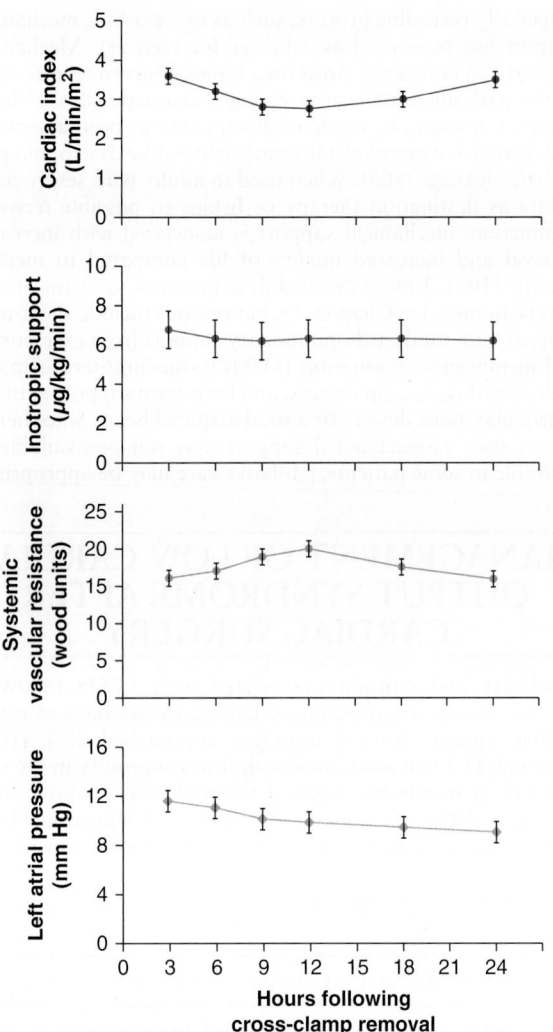

FIGURE 74.4. Serial measurements of cardiac index, inotropic support, SVR, and left atrial pressure after arterial switch procedure. With stable inotropic support, cardiac index falls during the first 12 hours after surgery, returning to normal at 24 hours post-op. During this period, SVR rises, returning to baseline at 24 hours. (Reproduced with permission pending from Wernovsky G, et al. Postoperative course and hemodynamic profile after the arterial switch operation in neonates and infants. *Circulation* 1995;92:2226–35.)

obstruction or valvar insufficiency reduce the effective stroke volume, increasing myocardial demands. Similarly, persistence of a left-to-right intracardiac shunt will yield excessive pulmonary blood flow and diminish systemic blood flow. Low cardiac output could be exacerbated by arrhythmias, which limit ventricular filling and/or compromise atrioventricular synchrony. Careful evaluation for arrhythmias or residual cardiac abnormalities is indicated in any patient with low cardiac output, especially when patients do not follow their expected postoperative course after heart surgery.

Treatment of Low Cardiac Output after Surgery

Management of postoperative LCOS includes optimization of preload and afterload; prompt diagnosis of residual cardiac lesions; prevention of hypoxia, anemia, and acidosis; and administration of pharmacologic agents to improve myocardial contractile function (115). In addition, in low cardiac output associated with right heart failure, some children may benefit from pulmonary vasodilator therapy and/or the presence of an atrial level shunt to allow right-to-left shunting to augment LV preload.

Minimize Oxygen Requirements

Reduced cardiac output and increased systemic oxygen consumption can alter systemic oxygen balance adversely after cardiopulmonary bypass. One study of children aged 2 months to 15 years demonstrated a significant increase in oxygen consumption following cardiopulmonary bypass (116). Peak oxygen consumption correlates significantly with central temperature, so pyrexia in the setting of LCOS should be treated aggressively. A cooling blanket may be useful, but shivering should be avoided since it will increase oxygen consumption. Total oxygen consumption can be decreased by induction of heavy sedation, paralysis, or mild hypothermia to reduce metabolism (117). Case reports of moderate hypothermia for patients with refractory LCOS suggest this as a potential therapy for LCOS (118,119).

Ensure Adequate Preload

Inadequate preload is common in postoperative cardiac surgical patients. Potential causes of hypovolemia include bleeding, excessive ultrafiltration, diastolic dysfunction, and vasodilation from rewarming or afterload reduction (109). Cardiac tamponade or pneumothorax, which impair preload, should always be considered. Myocardial swelling, which may limit myocardial filling and prevent adequate output, may necessitate sternal reopening.

Although true ventricular preload is the end-diastolic ventricular volume, preload assessment can be estimated from atrial pressure. Continual reassessment of the optimal preload is essential, as ventricular compliance and subsequent preload needs often change postoperatively. **Figure 74.2, panel i** shows how preload determination is predominantly a "trial and error" process. When atrial pressure is low, fluid administration augments EDV and increases stroke volume. With successive fluid administration, increases in stroke volume become limited due to the nonlinear nature of ventricular compliance. Preload augmentation is also limited by elevations in left ventricular end-diastolic pressure, which lead to edema formation and potential impairment of myocardial perfusion. Interpretation of hemodynamic pressure monitoring data should always be made with an understanding of the patient's underlying physiology. A stiff ventricle, such as with RV dysfunction after tetralogy of Fallot repair, would be expected to have higher end-diastolic and right atrial pressures than a normal heart and may require higher filling pressures to generate adequate output. These patients may also benefit from lusitropic therapy intended to improve diastolic ventricular filling. **Figure 74.2, panel ii** illustrates how a change in ventricular diastolic compliance affects atrial pressure. Enhanced lusitropy should result in a greater stroke volume for a comparable atrial pressure.

Prompt Recognition of Arrhythmias

Early recognition of postoperative arrhythmias is imperative; therefore, a baseline postoperative surface electrocardiogram should always be obtained for comparison with preoperative and subsequent postoperative tracings. Continuous electrocardiographic monitoring during the postoperative period is also essential. Since sinus bradycardia, bundle branch block, and atrioventricular block can occur after many cardiac surgical procedures, temporary atrial and ventricular pacing wires are typically placed to facilitate pacing, if necessary. Arrhythmias occur frequently in postoperative cardiac surgical patients, and may require overdrive pacing, cardioversion, or pharmacologic intervention (120). Hoffman et al. reviewed the incidence of arrhythmias in postoperative cardiac surgical patients, and observed that nonsustained ventricular and supraventricular tachycardia were most common with incidences of 22% and 12%. Incidence of sustained ventricular, junctional, and supraventricular arrhythmias were 6%, 5%, and 4%, respectively (120). Loss in atrioventricular synchrony can compromise preload, increase pulmonary congestion, and significantly diminish cardiac output; thus, maintenance of atrioventricular synchrony is essential (via pacing, if necessary).

Junctional ectopic tachycardia (JET) is a common tachyarrhythmia that usually occurs in the first 48 hours following surgery, especially after procedures involving closure of a ventricular septal defect and in younger patients (121). It is generally poorly tolerated, especially in patients with unstable hemodynamics. Early recognition of JET and other arrhythmias may be aided by careful surveillance of atrial pressure waveforms; loss of the distinct a and v waves is often the first indication of arrhythmia and/or atrioventricular dyssynchrony. Hypomagnesemia may contribute to the onset of JET, and administration of intravenous magnesium in the early postoperative period may reduce the incidence of JET (122). Once diagnosed, treatment of JET focuses upon reestablishment of atrioventricular synchrony. If the hemodynamics allow, an effort should be made to reduce or discontinue adrenergic agents, which may exacerbate JET (121). Restoration of atrial contribution with pacing, either atrial or dual chamber atrioventricular sequential, is the initial therapy of choice. If the junctional rate is too fast to allow pacing, the goal of pharmacological therapy is to provide rate control to allow institution of pacing. While intravenous amiodarone is generally considered the drug of choice (123), induction of hypothermia and procainamide administration has also been shown to be effective (124). Since the risk of JET increases in the presence of low output ("low cardiac output begets JET"), the diagnosis of JET should prompt the cardiac intensivist to search for other causes of LCOS, including other residual cardiac lesions.

Prompt Diagnosis of Residual Cardiac Lesions

Residual cardiac lesions in the postoperative patient can lead to LCOS and result in increased morbidity and mortality. In patients with LCOS following cardiopulmonary bypass, data from invasive lines and echocardiography should be used to rule out residual structural lesions. Catheterization should be considered if LCOS persists and the etiology remains elusive. Careful evaluation for residual cardiac abnormalities is indicated, especially when patients do not follow their expected postoperative course after heart surgery. Prompt diagnosis of residual structural lesions can help direct medical management optimally, or may prompt surgical or catheter-based intervention.

Treatment of Depressed Myocardial Contractility

Since low cardiac output after pediatric heart surgery is often associated with some level of contractile dysfunction, inotropic support in the early postoperative period is usually necessary. **Figure 74.2, panel iii** demonstrates the beneficial effects of positive inotropy on the pressure–volume and Starling relationships. At constant preload, increased contractility should enhance ejection during systole to increase stroke volume. Since inotropic agents have unwanted side effects, it is important to assess efficacy of these agents following initiation or dosage adjustment. **Figure 74.2** illustrates the potential utility of Starling curves to assess efficacy of most hemodynamic

interventions. The Starling relationship specifies the therapeutic goal of all inotropic agents; enhanced contractility should result in a greater stroke volume for a comparable preload. Since measurement of stroke volume is not routine in postoperative patients, an alternative to the true Starling relationship is illustrated in **Figure 74.5**. Since stroke volume is not easily monitored, indirect measures of cardiac output such as superior vena cava (SVC) oximetry or measures of end-organ perfusion such as urine output may be plotted against atrial pressure to attain a "modified" Starling relationship. Points A–C of **Figure 74.5** illustrate how preload recruitment is used to increase SVC saturation or urine output. Since preload recruitment is limited, inotropic agents are used to improve SVC saturation or urine output by shifting the Starling relationship leftward (point D). Using the modified Starling relationship, the therapeutic goal of enhanced contractility is improvement in systemic blood flow for a comparable preload (reflected as improved SVC saturation and enhanced organ perfusion).

Inotropic agents and vasodilators are routinely used in pediatric cardiac surgical patients to help reestablish adequate myocardial function during and after surgery. Support is often initiated with milrinone and a low-dose infusion of epinephrine. The infusion rate is titrated to produce the desired systemic blood pressure. Since high-dose epinephrine (>0.1 μg/kg/min) frequently results in tachycardia and systemic vasoconstriction, it is often used in combination with intravenous vasodilators such as milrinone or sodium nitroprusside to treat ventricular dysfunction and decrease systemic afterload (or at least attenuate the α_1-effects of epinephrine).

The use of PDE inhibitors, which do not demonstrate many of the shortcomings common to catecholamine therapy, has increased considerably over the past few years. PDE inhibitors improve cardiac index by enhancing both systolic and diastolic functions, and by reducing systemic and pulmonary vascular resistance. The ability to achieve a rapid hemodynamic response upon initiation of milrinone is extremely important after separation from cardiopulmonary bypass, when uncompensated LCOS can quickly result in the deterioration

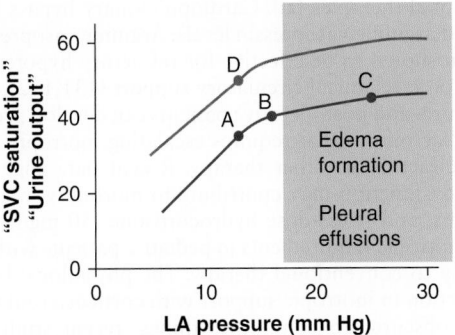

FIGURE 74.5. Modified Starling relationship. Since stroke volume is not easily monitored, indirect measures of cardiac output such as SVC saturation or end-organ perfusion such as urine output may be plotted against atrial pressure to create a "modified" Starling relationship. Fluid administration augments preload and leads to improvement in SVC saturation and end-organ perfusion (point A to point B). Preload augmentation is limited, however; progressive fluid administration ultimately leads to excessive atrial pressures, with resultant edema formation (point C). Alternate ways to improve SVC saturation or urine output include afterload reduction, lusitropic improvement, or inotropic augmentation, which all shift the Starling relationship upward and leftward (point D). The therapeutic goal of enhanced lusitropy, increased contractility, or afterload reduction is improvement in systemic blood flow for a comparable preload (reflected as improved SVC saturation and enhanced organ perfusion).

of hemodynamic status and subsequent secondary organ dysfunction. For patients at high risk for LCOS, some centers prefer to load with milrinone during bypass to avoid potential hypotension. The multicenter prophylactic intravenous use of milrinone after cardiac operation in pediatrics (PRIMACORP) study demonstrated that the use of milrinone in children early after congenital heart surgery reduces the incidence of LCOS. Since renal dysfunction results in delayed clearance of milrinone, patients with renal insufficiency are at risk for toxicity (125,126), so the dose should be adjusted based on creatinine clearance to avoid excessive vasodilation, especially in neonates.

Calcium supplementation and calcium-sensitizing agents also warrant discussion. Cardiac contraction and relaxation are mediated by cyclic fluctuations in cytoplasmic calcium concentration. Hypocalcemia may occur in the postoperative period, especially in patients with 22q11 deletion syndrome or neonates with transient hypoparathyroidism. Transfusion of citrate-treated blood (which chelates calcium) and administration of loop diuretics may exacerbate hypocalcemia. Ionized calcium, the physiologically active form of calcium, should be monitored frequently in the postoperative period and normal or supernormal levels maintained with supplementation. Many centers use calcium infusions routinely in neonates after cardiopulmonary bypass to augment and stabilize extracellular ionized calcium (Table 74.1). Calcium-sensitizing agents, such as levosimendan, have many potential advantages over traditional inotropic agents.

Although the mechanism remains unclear, investigators have advocated thyroid hormone therapy as a potential treatment for LCOS (127–129). During cardiopulmonary bypass, circulating levels of the thyroid hormones triiodothyronine (T_3) and thyroxine (T_4) are reduced; these deficiencies can persist for several days and may play a role in postoperative myocardial depression (127). Administration of T_3 to children after congenital heart surgery results in hemodynamic improvement, although it is unclear if this improves clinical outcomes (127–130).

Arginine vasopressin has been advocated as a therapeutic option for pediatric patients with refractory hypotension after surgery, to improve systemic arterial blood pressure when conventional therapies fail. Cardiopulmonary bypass leads to decreased arginine vasopressin levels. Arginine vasopressin has also been shown to be effective for refractory hypotension in patients on mechanical circulatory support (131,132).

Both pre- and postoperative patients can develop prolonged low cardiac output that requires escalating inotropic support and is refractory to other therapy. Recent data suggest that adrenal dysfunction may contribute to morbidity in critically ill patients, and stress-dose hydrocortisone (50 mg/m²/d) can reduce inotropic requirements in pediatric patients with LCOS refractory to conventional therapy. The physiologic basis for the reduction in inotropic support with corticosteroid therapy remains obscure. To complicate things, recent studies have raised questions about what levels of cortisol truly represent adrenal dysfunction (133).

Afterload Reduction for Systemic Ventricular Failure

Elevated afterload is particularly detrimental to the neonatal heart, especially when compounded by postoperative myocardial dysfunction. Afterload reduction is often beneficial in postoperative patients showing signs of LCOS. Furthermore, if high-dose catecholamines cannot be avoided, afterload reduction/vasodilator therapy should be considered to counter catecholamine vasoconstrictor effects. Figure 74.2, panel iv demonstrates the beneficial effects of afterload reduction on pressure–volume and Starling relationships. This panel also demonstrates an important principle: Benefits of afterload

reduction are pronounced in neonatal hearts and in the setting of poor contractility. With neonatal hearts or impaired contractility, afterload reduction is useful particularly to augment stroke volume and overall cardiac output. As with inotropic agents, it is important to assess efficacy of these agents following initiation or dosage adjustment since vasodilator agents also have unwanted side effects. As shown in Figure 74.2, the therapeutic goal of afterload reduction should be a greater stroke volume for a comparable preload. As noted previously, however, since measurement of stroke volume is not routine in postoperative patients, the modified Starling relationship can be used to assess efficacy of most hemodynamic interventions, including afterload reduction. As shown in Figure 74.5, the therapeutic goal of afterload reduction is improvement in systemic blood flow for a comparable preload (reflected as improved SVC saturation and enhanced organ perfusion).

Some centers advocate use of the potent vasodilator phenoxybenzamine, an α-adrenergic blocking agent, in selected pediatric patients after cardiac surgery (134). Since phenoxybenzamine is a potent vasodilator with a very long half-life (>24 hours), its use may be complicated by severe hypotension. For this reason, many centers prefer to use sodium nitroprusside for afterload reduction and vasodilator therapy in patients with congenital heart disease. Although it is a less potent vasodilator, the therapeutic effects of nitroprusside are easier to titrate due to its very short half-life and rapid onset of action. PDE inhibitors are also commonly used for afterload reduction in pediatric patients with congenital heart disease. These agents are useful particularly in the postoperative pediatric cardiac surgical patients because enhanced inotropic and lusitropic effects are combined with systemic and pulmonary vasodilation. In patients who require high doses of adrenergic agents, it may be necessary to use one or more vasodilator agents simultaneously. Sodium nitroprusside has also been advocated in patients with excessive pulmonary blood flow after Norwood palliation (135). In such patients, the dual effects of nitroprusside include afterload reduction to improve myocardial performance and reduction of SVR to improve the balance of pulmonary and systemic blood flow.

Management of Right Ventricular Failure

Right heart failure is a common complication of congenital heart surgery and, thus, a common cause of LCOS. Factors contributing to postoperative RV dysfunction include difficulties with right heart myocardial protection and right ventriculotomy, which is required for the surgical correction of many congenital heart lesions. Patients undergoing right heart procedures, including tetralogy of Fallot and Fontan procedures, often demonstrate restrictive physiology (diastolic RV dysfunction), characterized by antegrade diastolic pulmonary arterial flow coinciding with atrial systole (136,137).

Children with acute RV restrictive physiology have a decreased cardiac index because the stiff right ventricle has impaired diastolic filling (138). These patients typically have a slower postoperative recovery and a prolonged stay in the ICU with longer periods of inotropic and ventilatory support. Alterations in LV filling may also occur, due to the hypertensive RV. Alterations in ventricular compliance make patients with RV failure particularly sensitive to alterations in venous return caused by intrathoracic pressure changes. As discussed below, these patients benefit from ventilation strategies that minimize intrathoracic pressure (136,137,139,140). Patients with RV failure may benefit from manipulation of pulmonary vascular resistance (PVR) to minimize RV afterload. PDE inhibitors are particularly beneficial in these patients, due to the combined lusitropic and pulmonary vasodilatory effects.

The ability to maintain a right-to-left shunt at the atrial level is beneficial in patients with RV dysfunction. In patients undergoing the modified Fontan procedure, fenestration between the Fontan pathway and atrium is associated with reduced pleural effusion and significantly shorter hospital stays (141). In patients who undergo tetralogy of Fallot repair, a right-to-left atrial shunt can be similarly facilitated by maintaining the patency of the foramen ovale or by creating a small fenestration in the atrial septum.

Ventilation Strategies after Pediatric Cardiac Surgery

Cardiopulmonary Interactions

Since the cardiorespiratory system functions as a unit, ventilation (both spontaneous and mechanical) can have a profound effect on hemodynamics. Since these effects may be particularly pronounced in children following cardiac surgery, an understanding of the interactions between the cardiovascular and respiratory systems is crucial to management of these patients. Alterations in intrathoracic pressure and lung volume affect dynamic and loading conditions of the right and left ventricle differently, often having opposing effects. A transient increase in intrathoracic pressure decreases RV preload and LV afterload, whereas spontaneous inspiration or a decrease in intrathoracic pressure increases RV preload and LV afterload. Effects of ventilation on RV afterload/PVR depend primarily upon lung volume, with PVR being lowest at functional residual capacity. Since effects of intrathoracic pressure changes are opposite for the right and left ventricles, the ventilation strategy depends upon whether right or left ventricular dysfunction predominates. In patients with systemic ventricular contractile dysfunction, positive intrathoracic pressure may be beneficial because the predominant effect is to reduce LV afterload. On the other hand, venous return effects of positive intrathoracic pressure are amplified in lesions with no right ventricle (Glenn and Fontan procedures) or in patients with RV failure, especially patients with restrictive physiology after tetralogy of Fallot repair (136,137,140). These effects highlight the central role of ventilator management in management of patients with low cardiac output.

Lung Recruitment in Patients with Congenital Heart Disease

Although lung recruitment is recognized to be an important principle for ventilation of patients with respiratory failure, lung volume is also key to management of patients with congenital heart disease. In addition to the lung volume effects on PVR, adequate lung volume ensures optimal lung compliance and pulmonary gas exchange. Ventilation strategies for patients with congenital heart disease should strive to maintain an "open lung," striving for a normal functional residual capacity.

Effects of Positive-Pressure Ventilation in LV Failure

Positive intrathoracic pressure is often beneficial in patients with systemic ventricular dysfunction due to diminished LV afterload. In addition to optimal lung recruitment, higher levels of positive end-expiratory pressure may thus be hemodynamically beneficial in these patients. Tidal volumes should be maintained in the range of 6–10 mL/kg to avoid overdistension, which could increase PVR and RV afterload (142). Furthermore, there is evidence that shorter inspiratory times may augment systemic ventricle filling in patients with systemic ventricular dysfunction (143). Since alterations in thoracic pressure may have opposing hemodynamic effects, the hemodynamic effects of all ventilatory maneuvers should be carefully assessed.

Effects of Positive-Pressure Ventilation in RV Failure

Alterations in RV compliance make patients with RV failure particularly sensitive to changes in systemic venous return caused by changes in intrathoracic pressure. Spontaneous inspiration enhances diastolic flow and, overall cardiac output in these patients, so early extubation may be beneficial. Because of the detrimental effects of positive-pressure ventilation on RV dynamics, alternative modes of ventilation have been advocated, including negative-pressure and high-frequency jet ventilation (HFJV). Since HFJV reduces mean airway pressure and PVR while maintaining a similar $Paco_2$, it may be ideally suited to patients with RV dysfunction and/or pulmonary hypertension. In postoperative Fontan patients, HFJV decreased mean airway pressure, reduced PVR, and increased cardiac index (144). Similarly, negative-pressure ventilation has been shown to augment cardiac output in patients with restrictive RV physiology (136,137,140) and Fontan physiology (139). Although technical challenges associated with negative-pressure ventilation in postoperative cardiac surgery patients have prevented its widespread use, ventilation strategies used for patients with RV failure should aim to minimize mean airway pressure while maintaining lung volume at functional residual capacity, where lung function and gas exchange are optimal.

MEDICAL MANAGEMENT OF MYOCARDITIS

Care of a patient presenting with a clinical picture and history suggestive of myocarditis varies depending on the severity of myocardial involvement (145). Many patients present with relatively mild disease, with minimal respiratory compromise and only mild congestive heart failure. These patients require close monitoring to watch for disease progression. Experimental animal studies suggest that bed rest may prevent an increase in intramyocardial viral replication in the acute stage (146); thus, it appears prudent to limit activity at time of diagnosis. General supportive care is provided such as preventing hypoxemia, maintaining cardiac output at levels that supply adequate tissue perfusion and prevent metabolic disturbances, using diuretics for removal of excess extracellular fluid volume, and using anticoagulation (aspirin, warfarin, and/or heparin) to reduce the likelihood of a thrombotic/embolic phenomenon.

Afterload Reduction

Since it is more effective to reduce the work on the heart than to "whip a failing heart," afterload reduction is the cornerstone of therapy for patients with myocarditis and clinically significant contractile dysfunction. Sodium nitroprusside is often used alone or in conjunction with other inotropic agents (see below), especially if the patient requires an agent with vasoconstrictor properties. More recently, PDE inhibitors such as intravenous milrinone have been used to provide both inotropy and afterload reduction. In some circumstances, nesiritide may be beneficial (147). When chronic oral therapy is tolerated, ACE inhibition and diuretics are typically prescribed (148). Addition of a β-blocker such as carvedilol or metoprolol may also be beneficial (149–151).

Circulatory Support

Since catecholamines generally aggravate myocardial injury, their use should be carefully assessed and their doses should be minimized. Low-dose dopamine or dobutamine (<5 μg/kg/min) may provide some assistance in the presence of decreased ventricular function. Higher doses of catecholamines should prompt consideration for mechanical support, especially if more potent catecholamines are needed, such as epinephrine or norepinephrine. Although low-dose epinephrine may be temporarily necessary to maintain blood pressure and/or systemic perfusion, it is our practice to consider mechanical circulatory support if prolonged high-dose epinephrine (> 0.1 μg/kg/min) is necessary. These patients are at high risk for progressive shock or cardiac arrest. Since all inotropic agents have some detrimental effects, we strongly advocate goal-oriented therapy with SVC saturation monitoring to guide inotrope and vasodilator therapy.

For patients unresponsive to medical therapy, mechanical support is indicated (see Chapter 75). Transplantation becomes necessary in patients who do not acutely recover despite medical and mechanical support of the failed myocardium.

Antiarrhythmic Agents

Arrhythmias in these patients should be vigorously treated when they do occur (152). Antiarrhythmic therapy for supraventricular tachyarrhythmias may include β-blockers, procainamide, or digoxin, although digoxin is usually avoided in patients with suspected myocarditis. Ventricular arrhythmias may respond to lidocaine. Intravenous amiodarone may be preferable for refractory arrhythmias or if ventricular function is depressed. Despite aggressive treatment of these arrhythmias, rapid deterioration to ventricular fibrillation may occur, especially in the very young. Complete atrioventricular block requires immediate temporary pacing with possible need for a permanent pacing system. Chronic arrhythmias may persist long after the acute disease has subsided (152), so children who recover from myocarditis should be followed long term.

Immune Modulation

The use of immunosuppressive agents in suspected or proven viral myocarditis is controversial (153–156). Some animal studies have suggested an exacerbation of virus-induced cytotoxicity in the presence of immunosuppressive drugs, possibly due to interference with interferon production. The Myocarditis Treatment Trial analyzed the use of immunosuppressive and steroid therapy (157) in adult patients. There was no improvement among patients treated with azathioprine versus cyclosporine along with prednisone and conventional medical therapy. Although immunosuppressive therapy has not been shown to be beneficial in most patients with histologically confirmed myocarditis, we advocate combined treatment with intravenous immunoglobulin (IVIG) and pulse-dose steroids for patients with the fulminant necrotic myocarditis phenotype of myocarditis. Because of anecdotal reports of benefit, patients with suspected fulminant necrotic myocarditis are treated with intravenous methylprednisolone (10 mg/kg every 8 hours for three total doses).

A frequently used but unproven therapeutic option for children with myocarditis is the use of IVIG. This is based on the observational, nonrandomized study of Drucker et al. (158), who investigated its use in 21 of 46 children with myocarditis. Patients receiving IVIG had better left ventricular function at follow-up, and 1-year survival tended to be higher although the data did not reach statistical significance because of the small number of patients in the study. At most centers, patients with myocarditis are typically treated with one to two doses of 1 g/kg of IVIG.

MEDICAL MANAGEMENT OF CARDIOMYOPATHIES

Treatment Strategies for Dilated Cardiomyopathy

Acute management of a child newly diagnosed with DCM should include an effort to rule out myocarditis or surgically correctable causes (i.e., anomalous left coronary artery arising from the pulmonary artery, aortic arch obstruction). Supportive care of heart failure symptoms should be provided and risk of complications minimized (such as thromboembolic events or arrhythmias). If an intramural thrombus is detected by echocardiography, systemic anticoagulation is indicated. Arrhythmias are a potential cause of sudden death in DCM patients, so newly diagnosed patients should have inpatient telemetry and Holter monitoring performed. If supraventricular or ventricular arrhythmias are identified, they should be treated to preserve cardiac output. Electrolyte imbalances should be identified and corrected. Choice of an antiarrhythmic agent should be balanced against its potential to further depress ventricular function. Short-term management of patients with heart failure arising from DCM should consist of the same supportive care used in management of heart failure stemming from other conditions (see above). Typically, this includes IV diuretics for symptomatic relief from venous congestion, and intravenous vasodilators or inotropes to augment cardiac output. Once the acute decompensation has been controlled, the treatment strategy should transition to oral afterload reduction and neurohormonal inhibition, with a regimen of ACE inhibitors, β-blockers, and diuretics. The overall goal of management of patients with DCM is symptomatic treatment and optimization of long-term outcome.

Treatment Strategies for Hypertrophic Cardiomyopathy

Therapy of hypertrophic cardiomyopathy (HCM) is directed at reduction of symptoms, prevention of untoward complications, and prevention of SCD. When identified, patients should have risk assessment for SCD. Risk stratification is challenging in children, but it is important to identify patients at high risk for SCD who might benefit from ICD placement. An ICD is recommended for patients who survive an SCD episode or who experience one or more episodes of sustained ventricular tachycardia. These patients are considered high risk (51), but represent only a small percentage of the total population of patients with HCM. Electrophysiologic testing is thought to have a low prognostic value in evaluation of children with HCM, so it is not considered useful for risk stratification (37). Medical therapy with β-blockers or non-dihydropyridine calcium channel blockers (e.g., verapamil) is the first-line approach to patients with HCM. Both groups of drugs reduce heart rate, which improves ventricular filling by prolonging diastole. β-Blockers and verapamil may also reduce severe LV outflow obstruction. Disopyramide, a type I antiarrhythmic drug, has also been used to reduce symptoms and outflow tract obstruction. Although they may alleviate symptoms in some patients, diuretics should be used with caution as a reduction in preload may increase the outflow obstruction. Likewise, use of ACE inhibitors could alter loading conditions and worsen the outflow gradient. A subset of patients will progress to end-stage HCM characterized by decreased LV systolic function, thinning of the walls secondary to fibrosis and LV dilation. These patients should be managed for heart failure with standard accepted medical and/or surgical therapy. Management of arrhythmias may also be necessary with medical and/or invasive strategies. Not all arrhythmias are ventricular in nature; up to 20% of adult patients with HCM develop atrial fibrillation, which may require antiarrhythmic therapy and anticoagulation. Nonmedical therapies include surgical myomectomy, pacemaker therapy, and alcohol septal ablation, to relieve outflow tract obstruction with varying degrees of success. Regardless of the intervention, procedures to reduce outflow tract obstruction do not reduce the risk of SCD secondary to ventricular arrhythmias. Infective endocarditis is a relatively rare complication and occurs mainly in patients with severe outflow tract obstruction, typically in the region of the thickened anterior leaflet of the mitral valve.

Therapeutic Strategies for Restrictive Cardiomyopathy

There has been no consistent approach to therapy of restrictive cardiomyopathy RCM in pediatric patients. A variety of medications have been administered in combinations, including digoxin, afterload reducing agents, calcium channel blockers, and β-blockers. Owing to the lack of uniformity of treatment and the small number of patients in each study, the benefits or risks of these therapies cannot be determined. Risks and benefits of ACE inhibition in pediatric RCM remain to be determined. In four pediatric patients with RCM, Bengur reported that captopril lowered aortic pressure by 24% without an increase in cardiac output, when administered during cardiac catheterization (4). Although they suggest that captopril should not be used in patients with RCM, acute decompensation was not reported in other studies, but neither was therapeutic benefit of ACE inhibitors established. Modulation of neurohormonal activation by ACE inhibitors may affect fibroblast activity, interstitial fibrosis, intracellular calcium handling, and myocardial stiffness. In adults with diastolic heart failure, the use of ACE inhibitors has been suggested, but data are limited. In adults with diastolic dysfunction, tachycardia is poorly tolerated; therefore, β-blockers or calcium channel blockers have been suggested as part of the treatment regimen. Rivenes reported that β-blocker therapy blunted rapid heart rates in patients in whom significant ST segment depression occurred with tachycardia (46). At present, medical therapy remains supportive and should be initiated during an inpatient hospitalization. Diuretics may be useful in patients with signs and symptoms of venous congestion, but over-diuresis should be avoided. Because of the high incidence of thromboembolic events, antiplatelet therapy or anticoagulants should be administered. Since development of pulmonary hypertension is common, mortality is high, and current medical therapy appears to be ineffective, cardiac transplantation is the therapy of choice. When comparing survival of RCM patients with and without cardiac transplantation, it is evident that transplantation results in longer survival (55). Most patients should be evaluated and listed for transplantation at the time of presentation. While listed for transplantation, patients should have Holter monitoring performed every 6 months or as symptoms dictate, to evaluate for signs of ischemia, ventricular arrhythmias, or conduction disturbances. Implantable defibrillators should be considered for patients with evidence of ischemia and/or ventricular arrhythmias. Strenuous physical activity should be avoided.

Therapeutic Strategies for Arrhythmogenic Right Ventricular Dysplasia

Management of patients with arrhythmogenic RV dysplasia consists of antiarrhythmic agents, but the only therapy with survival benefit appears to be ICD placement. In addition, therapies for heart failure may be instituted as the disease progresses toward a pattern similar to DCM. Cardiac transplantation is required in some cases.

Therapeutic Strategies for Left Ventricular Noncompaction

Treatment of left ventricular noncompaction cardiomyopathy (LVNC) is dependent on associated comorbidities. Patients with the hypertrophic phenotype with or without depressed systolic function or the dilated phenotype should be treated as outlined above. Aggressive anticoagulant therapy should be considered in cases of thrombus or systemic embolic events. In patients with associated mitochondrial myopathy, a combination of riboflavin, thiamine, coenzyme Q10, and carnitine may be considered. Serial Holter monitoring of patients with LVNC should be considered as there is an increased risk of arrhythmias. Ventricular arrhythmias have been associated with this condition and may prompt ICD placement. Patients that are refractory to adequate medical therapy may require consideration for cardiac transplantation.

CONCLUSIONS AND FUTURE DIRECTIONS

Heart failure is common in the care of critically ill children. Advances made in the treatment of heart failure over the last several decades have improved the course of patients, even with severe ventricular dysfunction. Blockade of neurohormonal activation is the cornerstone of heart failure management. There remains a paucity of data on the treatment of acute decompensated heart failure in pediatric patients. Although severe ventricular dysfunction and postoperative LCOS can often be managed with medical therapy, mechanical support is increasingly utilized in patients with marginal perfusion despite aggressive medial therapy.

The future directions for heart failure treatment for pediatric patients will likely include further investigation of long-term treatment of single and/or systemic right ventricles as there is a burgeoning population of patients surviving with palliated congenital heart disease. All of these patients will likely develop significant heart failure with time. As it does not appear that the supply of donor organs will increase significantly, alternatives to long-term management of refractory heart failure are needed. The increased use of mechanical support and the expansion of mechanical support to include destination therapy for pediatric or congenial heart disease may be considered.

References

1. Hunt SA, Abraham WT, Chin MH, et al. ACC/AHA 2005 Guideline Update for the Diagnosis and Management of Chronic Heart Failure in the Adult: A report of the American College of Cardiology/American Heart Association Task Force on Practice Guidelines (Writing Committee to Update the 2001 Guidelines for the Evaluation and Management of Heart Failure): Developed in collaboration with the American College of Chest

Physicians and the International Society for Heart and Lung Transplantation: Endorsed by the Heart Rhythm Society. *Circulation* 2005;112(12):e154–235.

2. Mann DL. Mechanisms and models in heart failure: A combinatorial approach. *Circulation* 1999;100(9):999–1008.

3. Pignatelli RH, McMahon CJ, Dreyer WJ, et al. Clinical characterization of left ventricular noncompaction in children: A relatively common form of cardiomyopathy. *Circulation* 2003;108(21): 2672–8.

4. Rosenthal D, Chrisant MR, Edens E, et al. International Society for Heart and Lung Transplantation: Practice guidelines for management of heart failure in children. *J Heart Lung Transplant* 2004;23(12):1313–33.

5. McCurley JM, Hanlon SU, Wei SK, et al. Furosemide and the progression of left ventricular dysfunction in experimental heart failure. *J Am Coll Cardiol* 2004;44(6):1301–7.

6. Eshaghian S, Horwich TB, Fonarow GC. Relation of loop diuretic dose to mortality in advanced heart failure. *Am J Cardiol* 2006;97(12):1759–64.

7. Pitt B, Zannad F, Remme WJ, et al. The effect of spironolactone on morbidity and mortality in patients with severe heart failure. Randomized Aldactone Evaluation Study Investigators. *N Engl J Med* 1999;341(10):709–17.

8. Pitt B, Williams G, Remme W, et al. The EPHESUS trial: Eplerenone in patients with heart failure due to systolic dysfunction complicating acute myocardial infarction. Eplerenone Post-AMI Heart Failure Efficacy and Survival Study. *Cardiovasc Drugs Ther* 2001;15(1):79–87.

9. Svensson M, Gustafsson F, Galatius S, et al. How prevalent is hyperkalemia and renal dysfunction during treatment with spironolactone in patients with congestive heart failure? *J Card Fail* 2004;10(4):297–303.

10. Brunner-La Rocca HP, Vaddadi G, Esler MD. Recent insight into therapy of congestive heart failure: Focus on ACE inhibition and angiotensin-II antagonism. *J Am Coll Cardiol* 1999;33(5):1163–73.

11. The CONSENSUS Trial Study Group. Effects of enalapril on mortality in severe congestive heart failure. Results of the Cooperative North Scandinavian Enalapril Survival Study (CONSENSUS). *N Engl J Med* 1987;316(23):1429–35.

12. Cohn JN, Johnson G, Ziesche S, et al. A comparison of enalapril with hydralazine-isosorbide dinitrate in the treatment of chronic congestive heart failure. *N Engl J Med* 1991;325(5):303–10.

13. The SOLVD Investigators. Effect of enalapril on survival in patients with reduced left ventricular ejection fractions and congestive heart failure. *N Engl J Med* 1991;325(5):293–302.

14. Pfeffer MA, Braunwald E, Moye LA, et al; The SAVE Investigators. Effect of captopril on mortality and morbidity in patients with left ventricular dysfunction after myocardial infarction. Results of the survival and ventricular enlargement trial. *N Engl J Med* 1992;327(10):669–77.

15. Packer M, Poole-Wilson PA, Armstrong PW, et al; ATLAS Study Group. Comparative effects of low and high doses of the angiotensin-converting enzyme inhibitor, lisinopril, on morbidity and mortality in chronic heart failure. *Circulation* 1999;100(23):2312–8.

16. The SOLVD Investigators. Effect of enalapril on mortality and the development of heart failure in asymptomatic patients with reduced left ventricular ejection fractions. *N Engl J Med* 1992;327(10):685–91.

17. Sharma D, Buyse M, Pitt B, et al; Losartan Heart Failure Mortality Meta-analysis Study Group. Meta-analysis of observed mortality data from all-controlled, double-blind, multiple-dose studies of losartan in heart failure. *Am J Cardiol* 2000;85(2):187–92.

18. Hamroff G, Katz SD, Mancini D, et al. Addition of angiotensin II receptor blockade to maximal angiotensin-converting enzyme inhibition improves exercise capacity in patients with severe congestive heart failure. *Circulation* 1999;99(8):990–2.

19. Wong M, Staszewsky L, Latini R, et al. Valsartan benefits left ventricular structure and function in heart failure: Val-HeFT echocardiographic study. *J Am Coll Cardiol* 2002;40(5):970–5.

20. Webster MW, Neutze JM, Calder AL. Acute hemodynamic effects of converting enzyme inhibition in children with intracardiac shunts. *Pediatr Cardiol* 1992;13(3):129–35.

21. Hsu DT, Zak V, Mahony L, et al. Enalapril in infants with single ventricle: Results of a multicenter randomized trial. *Circulation* 2010;122(4):333–40.

22. Kouatli AA, Garcia JA, Zellers TM, et al. Enalapril does not enhance exercise capacity in patients after Fontan procedure. *Circulation* 1997;96(5):1507–12.

23. Bengur AR, Beekman RH, Rocchini AP, et al. Acute hemodynamic effects of captopril in children with a congestive or restrictive cardiomyopathy. *Circulation* 1991;83(2):523–7.

24. Stern H, Weil J, Genz T, et al. Captopril in children with dilated cardiomyopathy: Acute and long-term effects in a prospective study of hemodynamic and hormonal effects. *Pediatr Cardiol* 1990;11(1):22–8.

25. Mori Y, Nakazawa M, Tomimatsu H, et al. Long-term effect of angiotensin-converting enzyme inhibitor in volume overloaded heart during growth: A controlled pilot study. *J Am Coll Cardiol* 2000;36(1):270–5.

26. Lewis AB, Chabot M. The effect of treatment with angiotensin-converting enzyme inhibitors on survival of pediatric patients with dilated cardiomyopathy. *Pediatr Cardiol* 1993;14(1):9–12.

27. CIBIS-II Investigators and Committees. The Cardiac Insufficiency Bisoprolol Study II (CIBIS-II): A randomised trial. *Lancet* 1999;353(9146):9–13.

28. Hjalmarson A, Goldstein S, Fagerberg B, et al; MERIT-HF Study Group. Effects of controlled-release metoprolol on total mortality, hospitalizations, and well-being in patients with heart failure: The Metoprolol CR/XL Randomized Intervention Trial in congestive heart failure (MERIT-HF). *JAMA* 2000;283(10): 1295–302.

29. Packer M, Coats AJ, Fowler MB, et al. Effect of carvedilol on survival in severe chronic heart failure. *N Engl J Med* 2001;344(22):1651–8.

30. Poole-Wilson PA, Swedberg K, Cleland JG, et al. Comparison of carvedilol and metoprolol on clinical outcomes in patients with chronic heart failure in the Carvedilol or Metoprolol European Trial (COMET): Randomised controlled trial. *Lancet* 2003;362(9377):7–13.

31. Packer M. Current role of beta-adrenergic blockers in the management of chronic heart failure. *Am J Med* 2001;110(suppl 7A):81S–94S.

32. Shaddy RE, Tani LY, Gidding SS, et al. Beta-blocker treatment of dilated cardiomyopathy with congestive heart failure in children: A multi-institutional experience. *J Heart Lung Transplant* 1999;18(3):269–74.

33. Bruns LA, Chrisant MK, Lamour JM, et al. Carvedilol as therapy in pediatric heart failure: An initial multicenter experience. *J Pediatr* 2001;138(4):505–11.

34. Azeka E, Franchini Ramires JA, Valler C, et al. Delisting of infants and children from the heart transplantation waiting list after carvedilol treatment. *J Am Coll Cardiol* 2002;40(11): 2034–8.

35. Shaddy RE, Boucek MM, Hsu DT, et al. Carvedilol for children and adolescents with heart failure: A randomized controlled trial. *JAMA* 2007;298(10):1171–9.

36. Gheorghiade M, Adams KF Jr, Colucci WS. Digoxin in the management of cardiovascular disorders. *Circulation* 2004; 109(24):2959–64.

37. Lee DC, Johnson RA, Bingham JB, et al. Heart failure in outpatients: A randomized trial of digoxin versus placebo. *N Engl J Med* 1982;306(12):699–705.

38. The Digitalis Investigation Group. The effect of digoxin on mortality and morbidity in patients with heart failure. *N Engl J Med* 1997;336(8):525–33.

39. Rathore SS, Curtis JP, Wang Y, et al. Association of serum digoxin concentration and outcomes in patients with heart failure. *JAMA* 2003;289(7):871–8.

40. Arora G, Cannon BC, Kim JJ, et al. Tachycardia-induced left ventricular dysfunction in infants and children (abstract). *Pediatr Cardiol* 2005;26:501.

41. McMurray J, Kober L, Robertson M, et al. Antiarrhythmic effect of carvedilol after acute myocardial infarction: Results of the Carvedilol Post-Infarct Survival Control in Left Ventricular Dysfunction (CAPRICORN) trial. *J Am Coll Cardiol* 2005;45(4): 525–30.

42. Bardy GH, Lee KL, Mark DB, et al. Amiodarone or an implantable cardioverter-defibrillator for congestive heart failure. *N Engl J Med* 2005;352(3):225–37.

43. Singh SN, Fletcher RD, Fisher SG, et al. Amiodarone in patients with congestive heart failure and asymptomatic ventricular arrhythmia. Survival Trial of Antiarrhythmic Therapy in Congestive Heart Failure. *N Engl J Med* 1995;333(2):77–82.

44. Doval HC, Nul DR, Grancelli HO, et al. Randomised trial of low-dose amiodarone in severe congestive heart failure. Grupo de Estudio de la Sobrevida en la Insuficiencia Cardiaca en Argentina (GESICA). *Lancet* 1994;344(8921):493–8.

45. Abraham WT, Fisher WG, Smith AL, et al. Cardiac resynchronization in chronic heart failure. *N Engl J Med* 2002;346 (24):1845–53.

46. Bristow MR, Saxon LA, Boehmer J, et al. Cardiac-resynchronization therapy with or without an implantable defibrillator in advanced chronic heart failure. *N Engl J Med* 2004;350 (21):2140–50.

47. Dubin AM, Janousek J, Rhee E, et al. Resynchronization therapy in pediatric and congenital heart disease patients: An international multicenter study. *J Am Coll Cardiol* 2005;46(12):2277–83.

48. Cecchin F, Frangini PA, Brown DW, et al. Cardiac resynchronization therapy (and multisite pacing) in pediatrics and congenital heart disease: Five years experience in a single institution. *J Cardiovasc Electrophysiol* 2009;20(1):58–65.

49. Dimas VV, Denfield SW, Cannon BC, et al. Arrhythmias and sudden cardiac death in children with dilated cardiomyopathy (abstract). *Circulation* 2004;110:III–761.

50. Goldberger Z, Lampert R. Implantable cardioverter-defibrillators: Expanding indications and technologies. *JAMA* 2006;295 (7):809–18.

51. Epstein AE, DiMarco JP, Ellenbogen KA, et al. ACC/AHA/HRS 2008 Guidelines for Device-Based Therapy of Cardiac Rhythm Abnormalities: A report of the American College of Cardiology/American Heart Association Task Force on Practice Guidelines (Writing Committee to Revise the ACC/AHA/NASPE 2002 Guideline Update for Implantation of Cardiac Pacemakers and Antiarrhythmia Devices): Developed in collaboration with the American Association for Thoracic Surgery and Society of Thoracic Surgeons. *Circulation* 2008;117(21):e350–408.

52. Adams KF Jr, Fonarow GC, Emerman CL, et al. Characteristics and outcomes of patients hospitalized for heart failure in the United States: Rationale, design, and preliminary observations from the first 100,000 cases in the Acute Decompensated Heart Failure National Registry (ADHERE). *Am Heart J* 2005;149(2):209–16.

53. Thom T, Haase N, Rosamond W, et al. Heart disease and stroke statistics—2006 update: A report from the American Heart Association Statistics Committee and Stroke Statistics Subcommittee. *Circulation* 2006;113(6):e85–151.

54. Mann DL. Heart failure as a progressive disorder. In: Mann DL, ed. *Heart Failure: A Companion to Braunwald's Heart Disease.* 1st ed. Philadelphia, PA: Saunders, 2004:123–8.

55. Towbin JA. Myocarditis. In: Allen HD, Gutgesell HP, Clark EB, et al, eds. *Moss and Adams' Heart Disease in Infants, Children, and Adolescents, Including the Fetus and Young Adult.* 6th ed. Philadelphia, PA: Lippincott Williams & Wilkins, 2001:1197–215.

56. Maisel AS, Krishnaswamy P, Nowak RM, et al. Rapid measurement of B-type natriuretic peptide in the emergency diagnosis of heart failure. *N Engl J Med* 2002;347(3):161–7.

57. Koulouri S, Acherman RJ, Wong PC, et al. Utility of B-type natriuretic peptide in differentiating congestive heart failure from lung disease in pediatric patients with respiratory distress. *Pediatr Cardiol* 2004;25(4):341–6.

58. McMahon CJ, Nagueh SF, Eapen RS, et al. Echocardiographic predictors of adverse clinical events in children with dilated cardiomyopathy: A prospective clinical study. *Heart* 2004;90(8): 908–15.

59. Stevenson LW, Massie BM, Francis GS. Optimizing therapy for complex or refractory heart failure: A management algorithm. *Am Heart J* 1998;135(6 pt 2 suppl):S293–309.

60. Drazner MH, Hamilton MA, Fonarow G, et al. Relationship between right and left-sided filling pressures in 1000 patients with advanced heart failure. *J Heart Lung Transplant* 1999;18(11):1126–32.

61. Binanay C, Califf RM, Hasselblad V, et al. Evaluation study of congestive heart failure and pulmonary artery catheterization effectiveness: The ESCAPE trial. *JAMA* 2005;294(13): 1625–33.

62. Freed MD, Miettinen OS, Nadas AS. Oximetric detection of intracardiac left-to-right shunts. *Br Heart J* 1979;42(6):690–4.

63. Tweddell JS, Hoffman GM, Mussatto KA, et al. Improved survival of patients undergoing palliation of hypoplastic left heart syndrome: Lessons learned from 115 consecutive patients. *Circulation* 2002;106(12 suppl 1):I82–9.

64. Taeed R, Schwartz SM, Pearl JM, et al. Unrecognized pulmonary venous desaturation early after Norwood palliation confounds Qp:Qs assessment and compromises oxygen delivery. *Circulation* 2001;103(22):2699–704.

65. Tortoriello TA, Stayer SA, Mott AR, et al. A noninvasive estimation of mixed venous oxygen saturation using near-infrared spectroscopy by cerebral oximetry in pediatric cardiac surgery patients. *Paediatr Anaesth* 2005;15(6):495–503.

66. Kim JJ, Dreyer WJ, Chang AC, et al. Arterial waveform analysis: An accurate means of determining cardiac index in children (abstract). *Pediatr Cardiol* 2005;26:505.

67. Grady KL, Dracup K, Kennedy G, et al. Team management of patients with heart failure: A statement for healthcare professionals from The Cardiovascular Nursing Council of the American Heart Association. *Circulation* 2000;102(19):2443–56.

68. Wilson JR, Reichek N, Dunkman WB, et al. Effect of diuresis on the performance of the failing left ventricle in man. *Am J Med* 1981;70(2):234–9.

69. Stevenson LW, Brunken RC, Belil D, et al. Afterload reduction with vasodilators and diuretics decreases mitral regurgitation during upright exercise in advanced heart failure. *J Am Coll Cardiol* 1990;15(1):174–80.

70. Butler J, Young JB, Abraham WT, et al. Beta-blocker use and outcomes among hospitalized heart failure patients. *J Am Coll Cardiol* 2006;47(12):2462–9.

71. Nohria A, Tsang SW, Fang JC, et al. Clinical assessment identifies hemodynamic profiles that predict outcomes in patients admitted with heart failure. *J Am Coll Cardiol* 2003;41(10): 1797–804.

72. Abraham WT, Adams KF, Fonarow GC, et al. In-hospital mortality in patients with acute decompensated heart failure requiring intravenous vasoactive medications: An analysis from the Acute Decompensated Heart Failure National Registry (ADHERE). *J Am Coll Cardiol* 2005;46(1):57–64.

73. Cuffe MS, Califf RM, Adams KF Jr, et al. Short-term intravenous milrinone for acute exacerbation of chronic heart failure: A randomized controlled trial. *JAMA* 2002;287(12):1541–7.

74. Guiha NH, Cohn JN, Mikulic E, et al. Treatment of refractory heart failure with infusion of nitroprusside. *N Engl J Med* 1974;291(12):587–92.

75. Sackner-Bernstein JD, Kowalski M, Fox M, et al. Short-term risk of death after treatment with nesiritide for decompensated heart failure: A pooled analysis of randomized controlled trials. *JAMA* 2005;293(15):1900–5.

76. Sackner-Bernstein JD, Skopicki HA, Aaronson KD. Risk of worsening renal function with nesiritide in patients with acutely decompensated heart failure. *Circulation* 2005;111(12):1487–91.

77. Schulz R, Rose J, Martin C, et al. Development of short-term myocardial hibernation. Its limitation by the severity of ischemia and inotropic stimulation. *Circulation* 1993;88(2):684–95.

78. Biddle TL, Benotti JR, Creager MA, et al. Comparison of intravenous milrinone and dobutamine for congestive heart failure secondary to either ischemic or dilated cardiomyopathy. *Am J Cardiol* 1987;59(15):1345–50.

79. Adamopoulos S, Piepoli M, Qiang F, et al. Effects of pulsed beta-stimulant therapy on beta-adrenoceptors and chronotropic responsiveness in chronic heart failure. *Lancet* 1995;345(8946):344–9.

80. Aairis MN, Apostolatos C, Anastassiadis F, et al. Comparison of the effect of levosimendan, or dobutamine or placebo in chronic low output decompensated heart failure. Calcium Sensitizer or Inotrope or None in low output heart failure (CASINO) study (abstract). In: Program and abstracts of the European Society of Cardiology, Heart failure Update 2004.

81. Shekerdemian LS, Redington A. Cardiovascular pharmacology. In: Chang AC, Hanley FL, Wernovsky G, et al. eds. *Pediatric Cardiac Intensive Care*. 1st ed. Baltimore, MD: Lippincott Williams & Wilkins, 1998:45–65.

82. Hampton JR, van Veldhuisen DJ, Kleber FX, et al. Randomised study of effect of ibopamine on survival in patients with advanced severe heart failure. Second Prospective Randomised Study of Ibopamine on Mortality and Efficacy (PRIME II) Investigators. *Lancet* 1997;349(9057):971–7.

83. Bailey JM, Miller BE, Kanter KR, et al. A comparison of the hemodynamic effects of amrinone and sodium nitroprusside in infants after cardiac surgery. *Anesth Analg* 1997;84(2):294–8.

84. Chang AC, Atz AM, Wernovsky G, et al. Milrinone: Systemic and pulmonary hemodynamic effects in neonates after cardiac surgery. *Crit Care Med* 1995;23(11):1907–14.

85. Anderson JL. Hemodynamic and clinical benefits with intravenous milrinone in severe chronic heart failure: Results of a multicenter study in the United States. *Am Heart J* 1991;121(6 pt 2):1956–64.

86. Seino Y, Momomura S, Takano T, et al; Japan Intravenous Milrinone Investigators. Multicenter, double-blind study of intravenous milrinone for patients with acute heart failure in Japan. *Crit Care Med* 1996;24(9):1490–7.

87. Packer M, Carver JR, Rodeheffer RJ, et al; The PROMISE Study Research Group. Effect of oral milrinone on mortality in severe chronic heart failure. *N Engl J Med*. 1991;325(21):1468–75.

88. Hoffman TM, Wernovsky G, Atz AM, et al. Efficacy and safety of milrinone in preventing low cardiac output syndrome in infants and children after corrective surgery for congenital heart disease. *Circulation* 2003;107(7):996–1002.

89. Kay JH, Blalock A. The use of calcium chloride in the treatment of cardiac arrest in patients. *Surg Gynecol Obstet* 1951;93(1):97–102.

90. Schwartz SM, Duffy JY, Pearl JM, et al. Cellular and molecular aspects of myocardial dysfunction. *Crit Care Med* 2001;29(10 suppl):S214–9.

91. Lang RM, Fellner SK, Neumann A, et al. Left ventricular contractility varies directly with blood ionized calcium. *Ann Intern Med* 1988;108(4):524–9.

92. Katz AM. Biochemical "defect" in the hypertrophied and failing heart: Deleterious or compensatory? *Circulation* 1973;47(5):1076–9.

93. Katz AM. Potential deleterious effects of inotropic agents in the therapy of chronic heart failure. *Circulation* 1986;73(3 pt 2):III184–90.

94. Gwathmey JK, Copelas L, MacKinnon R, et al. Abnormal intracellular calcium handling in myocardium from patients with end-stage heart failure. *Circ Res* 1987;61(1):70–6.

95. Katz AM, Lorell BH. Regulation of cardiac contraction and relaxation. *Circulation* 2000;102(20 suppl 4):IV69–74.

96. Felker GM, O'Connor CM. Inotropic therapy for heart failure: An evidence-based approach. *Am Heart J* 2001;142(3):393–401.

97. Ukkonen H, Saraste M, Akkila J, et al. Myocardial efficiency during levosimendan infusion in congestive heart failure. *Clin Pharmacol Ther* 2000;68(5):522–31.

98. Braun JP, Schneider M, Dohmen P, et al. Successful treatment of dilative cardiomyopathy in a 12-year-old girl using the calcium sensitizer levosimendan after weaning from mechanical biventricular assist support. *J Cardiothorac Vasc Anesth* 2004;18(6):772–4.

99. Braun JP, Schneider M, Kastrup M, et al. Treatment of acute heart failure in an infant after cardiac surgery using levosimendan. *Eur J Cardiothorac Surg* 2004;26(1):228–30.

100. Singh K, Communal C, Sawyer DB, et al. Adrenergic regulation of myocardial apoptosis. *Cardiovasc Res* 2000;45(3):713–9.

101. Wenzel V, Krismer AC, Arntz HR, et al. A comparison of vasopressin and epinephrine for out-of-hospital cardiopulmonary resuscitation. *N Engl J Med* 2004;350(2):105–13.

102. Price JF, Towbin JA, Denfield SW, et al. Arginine vasopressin levels are elevated and correlate with functional status in infants and children with congestive heart failure. *Circulation* 2004;109(21):2550–3.

103. Xu YJ, Gopalakrishnan V. Vasopressin increases cytosolic free [Ca2+] in the neonatal rat cardiomyocyte. Evidence for V1 subtype receptors. *Circ Res* 1991;69(1):239–45.

104. Rosenzweig EB, Starc TJ, Chen JM, et al. Intravenous arginine-vasopressin in children with vasodilatory shock after cardiac surgery. *Circulation* 1999;100(19 suppl):II182–6.

105. Vatta M, Stetson SJ, Perez-Verdia A, et al. Molecular remodelling of dystrophin in patients with end-stage cardiomyopathies and reversal in patients on assistance-device therapy. *Lancet* 2002;359(9310):936–41.

106. Rose EA, Gelijns AC, Moskowitz AJ, et al. Long-term mechanical left ventricular assistance for end-stage heart failure. *N Engl J Med* 2001;345(20):1435–43.

107. Parr GV, Blackstone EH, Kirklin JW. Cardiac performance and mortality early after intracardiac surgery in infants and young children. *Circulation* 1975;51(5):867–74.

108. Bellinger DC, Wypij D, Kuban KC, et al. Developmental and neurological status of children at 4 years of age after heart surgery with hypothermic circulatory arrest or low-flow cardiopulmonary bypass. *Circulation* 1999;100(5):526–32.

109. Burrows FA, Williams WG, Teoh KH, et al. Myocardial performance after repair of congenital cardiac defects in infants and children. Response to volume loading. *J Thorac Cardiovasc Surg* 1988;96(4):548–56.

110. Schermerhorn ML, Tofukuji M, Khoury PR, et al. Sialyl lewis oligosaccharide preserves cardiopulmonary and endothelial function after hypothermic circulatory arrest in lambs. *J Thorac Cardiovasc Surg* 2000;120(2):230–7.

111. Schermerhorn ML, Nelson DP, Blume ED, et al. Sialyl Lewis oligosaccharide preserves myocardial and endothelial function during cardioplegic ischemia. *Ann Thorac Surg* 2000;70(3):890–4.

112. Sellke FW, Tofukuji M, Stamler A, et al. Beta-adrenergic regulation of the cerebral microcirculation after hypothermic cardiopulmonary bypass. *Circulation* 1997;96(9 suppl):II-304–10.

113. Stamler A, Wang SY, Aguirre DE, et al. Cardiopulmonary bypass alters vasomotor regulation of the skeletal muscle microcirculation. *Ann Thorac Surg* 1997;64(2):460–5.

114. Wessel DL, Adatia I, Giglia TM, et al. Use of inhaled nitric oxide and acetylcholine in the evaluation of pulmonary hypertension and endothelial function after cardiopulmonary bypass. *Circulation* 1993;88(5 pt 1):2128–38.

115. Lowes BD, Simon MA, Tsvetkova TO, et al. Inotropes in the beta-blocker era. *Clin Cardiol* 2000;23(3 suppl):III11–6.

116. Li J, Schulze-Neick I, Lincoln C, et al. Oxygen consumption after cardiopulmonary bypass surgery in children: Determinants and implications. *J Thorac Cardiovasc Surg* 2000;119(3):525–33.

117. Moat NE, Lamb RK, Edwards JC, et al. Induced hypothermia in the management of refractory low cardiac output states following cardiac surgery in infants and children. *Eur J Cardiothorac Surg* 1992;6(11):579–84; discussion 85.

118. Dalrymple-Hay MJ, Deakin CD, Knight H, et al. Induced hypothermia as salvage treatment for refractory cardiac failure following paediatric cardiac surgery. *Eur J Cardiothorac Surg* 1999;15(4):515–8.

119. Deakin CD, Knight H, Edwards JC, et al. Induced hypothermia in the postoperative management of refractory cardiac failure following paediatric cardiac surgery. *Anaesthesia* 1998;53(9):848–53.

120. Hoffman TM, Wernovsky G, Wieand TS, et al. The incidence of arrhythmias in a pediatric cardiac intensive care unit. *Pediatr Cardiol* 2002;23(6):598–604.

121. Hoffman TM, Bush DM, Wernovsky G, et al. Postoperative junctional ectopic tachycardia in children: Incidence, risk factors, and treatment. *Ann Thorac Surg* 2002;74(5):1607–11.

122. Dorman BH, Sade RM, Burnette JS, et al. Magnesium supplementation in the prevention of arrhythmias in pediatric patients undergoing surgery for congenital heart defects. *Am Heart J* 2000;139(3):522–8.

123. Raja P, Hawker RE, Chaikitpinyo A, et al. Amiodarone management of junctional ectopic tachycardia after cardiac surgery in children. *Br Heart J* 1994;72(3):261–5.

124. Walsh EP, Saul JP, Sholler GF, et al. Evaluation of a staged treatment protocol for rapid automatic junctional tachycardia after operation for congenital heart disease. *J Am Coll Cardiol* 1997;29(5):1046–53.

125. Lindsay CA, Barton P, Lawless S, et al. Pharmacokinetics and pharmacodynamics of milrinone lactate in pediatric patients with septic shock. *J Pediatr* 1998;132(2):329–34.

126. Lebovitz DJ, Lawless ST, Weise KL. Fatal amrinone overdose in a pediatric patient. *Crit Care Med* 1995;23(5):977–80.

127. Portman MA, Fearneyhough C, Ning XH, et al. Triiodothyronine repletion in infants during cardiopulmonary bypass for congenital heart disease. *J Thorac Cardiovasc Surg* 2000;120(3):604–8.

128. Carrel T, Eckstein F, Englberger L, et al. Thyronin treatment in adult and pediatric heart surgery: Clinical experience and review of the literature. *Eur J Heart Fail* 2002;4(5):577–82.

129. Bettendorf M, Schmidt KG, Grulich-Henn J, et al. Tri-iodothyronine treatment in children after cardiac surgery: A double-blind, randomised, placebo-controlled study. *Lancet* 2000;356(9229):529–34.

130. Portman MA, Slee A, Olson AK, et al. Triiodothyronine Supplementation in Infants and Children Undergoing Cardiopulmonary Bypass (TRICC): A multicenter placebo-controlled randomized trial: Age analysis. *Circulation* 2010;122(11 suppl):S224–33.

131. Argenziano M, Choudhri AF, Oz MC, et al. A prospective randomized trial of arginine vasopressin in the treatment of vasodilatory shock after left ventricular assist device placement. *Circulation* 1997;96(9 suppl):II-286–90.

132. Morales DL, Gregg D, Helman DN, et al. Arginine vasopressin in the treatment of 50 patients with postcardiotomy vasodilatory shock. *Ann Thorac Surg* 2000;69(1):102–6.

133. Wald EL, Preze E, Eickhoff JC, et al. The effect of cardiopulmonary bypass on the hypothalamic-pituitary-adrenal axis in children. *Pediatr Crit Care Med* 2011;12(2):190–6.

134. Tweddell JS, Hoffman GM, Fedderly RT, et al. Phenoxybenzamine improves systemic oxygen delivery after the Norwood procedure. *Ann Thorac Surg* 1999;67(1):161–7; discussion 7–8.

135. Rossi AF, Sommer RJ, Lotvin A, et al. Usefulness of intermittent monitoring of mixed venous oxygen saturation after stage I palliation for hypoplastic left heart syndrome. *Am J Cardiol* 1994;73(15):1118–23.

136. Shekerdemian LS, Schulze-Neick I, Redington AN, et al. Negative pressure ventilation as haemodynamic rescue following surgery for congenital heart disease. *Intensive Care Med* 2000;26(1):93–6.

137. Shekerdemian LS, Bush A, Shore DF, et al. Cardiorespiratory responses to negative pressure ventilation after tetralogy of fallot repair: A hemodynamic tool for patients with a low-output state. *J Am Coll Cardiol* 1999;33(2):549–55.

138. Chaturvedi RR, Shore DF, Lincoln C, et al. Acute right ventricular restrictive physiology after repair of tetralogy of Fallot: Association with myocardial injury and oxidative stress. *Circulation* 1999;100(14):1540–7.

139. Shekerdemian LS, Bush A, Shore DF, et al. Cardiopulmonary interactions after Fontan operations: Augmentation of cardiac output using negative pressure ventilation. *Circulation* 1997;96(11):3934–42.

140. Shekerdemian LS, Shore DF, Lincoln C, et al. Negative-pressure ventilation improves cardiac output after right heart surgery. *Circulation* 1996;94(9 suppl):II49–55.

141. Bridges ND, Mayer JE Jr, Lock JE, et al. Effect of baffle fenestration on outcome of the modified Fontan operation. *Circulation* 1992;86(6):1762–9.

142. Cheifetz IM, Craig DM, Quick G, et al. Increasing tidal volumes and pulmonary overdistention adversely affect pulmonary vascular mechanics and cardiac output in a pediatric swine model. *Crit Care Med* 1998;26(4):710–6.

143. Meliones J, Kocis K, Bengur AR, et al. Diastolic function in neonates after the arterial switch operation: Effects of positive pressure ventilation and inspiratory time. *Intensive Care Med* 2000;26(7):950–5.

144. Meliones JN, Bove EL, Dekeon MK, et al. High-frequency jet ventilation improves cardiac function after the Fontan procedure. *Circulation* 1991;84(5 suppl):III364–8.

145. Parrillo JE. Myocarditis: How should we treat in 1998? *J Heart Lung Transplant* 1998;17(10):941–4.

146. Gauntt C, Huber S. Coxsackievirus experimental heart diseases. *Front Biosci* 2003;8:e23–35.

147. Jefferies JL, Denfield SW, Price JF, et al. A prospective evaluation of nesiritide in the treatment of pediatric heart failure. *Pediatr Cardiol* 2006;27(4):402–7.

148. Rezkalla S, Kloner RA, Khatib G, et al. Beneficial effects of captopril in acute coxsackievirus B3 murine myocarditis. *Circulation* 1990;81(3):1039–46.

149. Blume ED, Canter CE, Spicer R, et al. Prospective single-arm protocol of carvedilol in children with ventricular dysfunction. *Pediatr Cardiol* 2006;27(3):336–42.

150. Shaddy RE. Beta-adrenergic receptor blockers as therapy in pediatric chronic heart failure. *Minerva Pediatr* 2001;53(4):297–304.

151. Williams RV, Tani LY, Shaddy RE. Intermediate effects of treatment with metoprolol or carvedilol in children with left ventricular systolic dysfunction. *J Heart Lung Transplant* 2002;21(8):906–9.

152. Friedman RA, Kearney DL, Moak JP, et al. Persistence of ventricular arrhythmia after resolution of occult myocarditis in children and young adults. *J Am Coll Cardiol* 1994;24(3):780–3.

153. Chan KY, Iwahara M, Benson LN, et al. Immunosuppressive therapy in the management of acute myocarditis in children: A clinical trial. *J Am Coll Cardiol* 1991;17(2):458–60.

154. Frustaci A, Chimenti C, Calabrese F, et al. Immunosuppressive therapy for active lymphocytic myocarditis: Virological and immunologic profile of responders versus nonresponders. *Circulation* 2003;107(6):857–63.

155. Weller AH, Hall M, Huber SA. Polyclonal immunoglobulin therapy protects against cardiac damage in experimental coxsackievirus-induced myocarditis. *Eur Heart J* 1992;13(1):115–9.

156. Parrillo JE. Inflammatory cardiomyopathy (myocarditis): Which patients should be treated with anti-inflammatory therapy? *Circulation* 2001;104(1):4–6.

157. Mason JW, O'Connell JB, Herskowitz A, et al; The Myocarditis Treatment Trial Investigators. A clinical trial of immunosuppressive therapy for myocarditis. *N Engl J Med* 1995;333(5):269–75.

158. Drucker NA, Colan SD, Lewis AB, et al. Gamma-globulin treatment of acute myocarditis in the pediatric population. *Circulation* 1994;89(1):252–7.

CHAPTER 75 ■ TREATMENT OF HEART FAILURE: MECHANICAL SUPPORT

IKI ADACHI, LARA SHEKERDEMIAN, PAUL A. CHECCHIA, AND CHARLES D. FRASER Jr.

KEY POINTS

❶ The number of children with heart failure has been increasing, resulting in growing demand for mechanical circulatory support (MCS) in the pediatric population.

❷ Because of an oxygenator, extracorporeal membrane oxygenation (ECMO) should be considered a device for "cardiac *and* pulmonary" support.

❸ Short-term ventricular assist devices (VADs) provide better decompression of a failing ventricle than do ECMO, and hence is the device of choice when the etiology of heart failure is deemed acute process.

❹ Long-term VADs offer the opportunity to rehabilitate the patients while waiting for heart transplantation, making them better surgical candidates.

❺ There are certain situations, such as posttransplant chronic graft failure, where VAD support is not an ideal solution. Total artificial heart can be a superior option in such settings although currently total artificial heart is a realistic option only for older adolescents due to device size.

The history of mechanical circulatory support (MCS) development spans more than 50 years. The first clinical ventricular assist device (VAD) implantation was performed by DeBakey in 1963 (1), which was 4 years earlier than the first orthotopic heart transplantation by Barnard in South Africa (2). In 1969, a total artificial heart was used in human for the first time by Cooley (3). Interestingly, both of these "firsts" in MCS occurred even before the first clinical use of extracorporeal membrane oxygenation (ECMO) in 1971 by Hill (4). Thanks to continuing improvements in device technology and a growing spectrum of MCS devices available, adults with end-stage heart failure are now treated with devices that can be tailored to their individual needs. In contrast, MCS for children has significantly lagged behind their adult counterpart (5). Indeed, ECMO has long been the mainstay or even the only modality for MCS in children. This frustrating situation has, however, started to change. Following the Berlin Heart Investigational Device Exemption trial (6), the U.S. Food and Drug Administration (FDA) granted Humanitarian Device Exemption approval of the Berlin Heart EXCOR in late 2011. The EXCOR has become the first pediatric-specific VAD that has gained widespread acceptance worldwide, with the potential to transform the outlook for children with end-stage heart failure who are awaiting transplantation. As pediatric patients are so divergent in terms of size and cardiac physiology, appropriate device selection and good understanding of each device are keys to success. In this chapter, we will discuss several types of MCS devices available for children, particularly focusing on VADs.

HEART FAILURE IN CHILDREN

❶ The number of children with heart failure has been increasing, resulting in growing demand for MCS in the pediatric population. A recent analysis (2009) of 15 million pediatric hospitalizations using the Healthcare Cost and Utilization Project Kids Inpatient Database revealed an increasing number of pediatric hospital admissions for heart failure (a 30% increase over 3 years) (7). Possible explanations include better recognition of pediatric cardiomyopathy with earlier intervention with medical therapy and advancements in surgery and perioperative care for children with congenital heart disease (CHD), leading to increased long-term survival of this patient population. One of the inevitable consequences of improved survival of these patient groups will be an increased incidence of end-stage heart failure in children, adolescents, and young adults. Typical examples of end-stage heart failure in the setting of operated CHD involve children whose morphological right ventricle is sustaining the systemic circulation and who progress to failure of that systemic ventricle. While cardiac transplantation remains the treatment of choice for end-stage heart failure, it is unlikely that this growing need can be addressed by transplantation only due to the static number of donor organs available. Indeed, numbers of heart transplantation procedures worldwide has been stagnant for over a decade (8).

While pediatric MCS is in rapid evolution, there has been significant refinement of MCS therapy in adults over the last decade. The most significant change to have an impact on patient management strategy was the emergence of durable intracorporeal (implantable) devices such as the HeartMate II (Thoratec, Corp., Pleasanton, CA). Owing to the impressive efficiency of these devices with relatively low morbidity profiles, the indications for device placement have changed, making the early institution of the device a reasonable option in preference to escalating medical management and to improve outcome (9). In adults, VADs are used as a bridge to transplant, as a bridge to recovery (10), or as destination therapy (for patients who opt against transplantation or for whom transplantation is not an option) (11).

The scope of the use of the HeartMate II and other intracorporeal devices in the pediatric population is limited by body size, and they can therefore only be used to provide MCS in larger children and adolescents. Although miniaturized intracorporeal devices for smaller children are on the horizon, the Berlin EXCOR, a paracorporeal pulsatile device, is the only currently available option for this group of patients. When comparing the data of the Berlin Heart Investigational Device Exemption (IDE) trial (6) to that of initial European experience (12), it is likely that higher success rates (~90% in IDE trial vs. 70% in Europe) can be achieved with very careful patient selection and management at higher volume centers (5). However, the Berlin Heart EXCOR is associated with significant morbidity profiles (stroke in ~30%, bleeding in 40%–50%, and infection in 50%–60%). The incidence of complications in children with pulsatile VADs is greater than in adults with intracorporeal devices. This significant complication rate in children suggests the need for careful assessments of the risks and benefits when considering device placement.

PATIENT SELECTION

MCS for any patient is indicated when the benefits of MCS are deemed to outweigh the risks. Since each patient and each device has unique risk profiles, the appropriateness of MCS and the timing of this need to be determined on a case-by-case basis, by the multidisciplinary team, the family, and where appropriate the patient. Special consideration should be given to not only medical, but also social aspects (i.e., family situation and support, prior compliance with medication, etc.). MCS selection should also be influenced by the institutional experience. As with all interventions, one's threshold to provide a therapy changes as the confidence in that therapy to produce beneficial and consistent outcomes for patients increases.

There are other confounding issues that must be considered in providing MCS in children and when choosing the most appropriate device for a given child. Children with CHD may have anatomic variations that pose significant difficulty in cannulation for MCS (e.g., abnormal size and location of the aorta, unusual location or shape of the ventricle). Previous surgical procedures may jeopardize the application of MCS with derangement of anatomy and of circulatory physiology. These include systemic-pulmonary artery shunts or disconnected caval veins or pulmonary artery after Glenn or Fontan operations. In addition to careful attention to the anatomy and circulatory physiology, a thorough understanding of the unique pathophysiological features of pediatric heart failure is an absolute prerequisite to a successful outcome with MCS.

At present, long-term VAD support in children requires candidacy for heart transplantation. When considering contraindications to MCS in children, extreme prematurity, very low body weight (<2.0 kg), significant preexisting neurologic injury, a constellation of congenital anomalies with poor prognosis (unlikely survival beyond childhood), and major chromosomal aberrations are generally accepted contraindications for MCS. Multisystem organ failure may be a relative contraindication, but does not necessarily exclude patients from MCS if reversal of organ function is predicted once hemodynamic improvement is achieved. Indeed, it has been well documented that liver and renal dysfunction improve after restoration of hemodynamic stability with MCS (13,14).

DEVICE SELECTION

Device selection for initial MCS in children with heart failure is ideally limited to cardiac support with VADs, which support the left ventricle (LVAD), right ventricle (RVAD), or both (BiVAD). However, some children with acute decompensated heart failure also have significant pulmonary dysfunction, which is most often reversible and may require cardiopulmonary support; in such case temporary support with ECMO

may be indicated. Moreover, if the patient is in cardiopulmonary arrest with ongoing cardiopulmonary resuscitation, then ECMO is the initial support of choice as this can be rapidly initiated (peripherally) and will provide support to both right and left heart as well as the lungs. Our own institutional Pediatric MCS guideline is depicted in **Figure 75.1**.

EXTRACORPOREAL MEMBRANE OXYGENATION

We will not discuss ECMO in detail since ECMO is separately covered in Chapter 40. Instead, we briefly describe the role of veno-arterial (VA) ECMO in heart failure management, particularly focusing on its difference from that of VAD.

ECMO is a temporary device and should be confined to short-term support for heart failure. Although it has previously been used for this purpose, ECMO has little or no real role in bridging children to heart transplantation. The fact that ECMO is not suitable to provide long-term support for bridge-to-transplant is clearly shown by the Berlin Heart trial (6). There is a significant survival benefit of long-term VAD support over ECMO support for patients waiting for heart transplantation. This is of increased importance because of longer waiting duration on the transplant list in the recent era. The negative effects of ECMO are evident even after patients are bridged to cardiac transplant. Mortality rate posttransplant is higher in patients supported with ECMO compared with those who had VAD support, irrespective of diagnosis (15).

Controversy exists, however, regarding the best mode of MCS if anticipated support duration is short (<2 weeks). Many pediatric heart centers utilize ECMO irrespective of the etiologies of heart failure. ECMO should not be a device for pure circulatory support in our opinion. Because it contains an oxygenator, ECMO should be considered a device for "cardiac *and* pulmonary" support. A fundamental question regarding device selection would be if the patient needs pulmonary support. Because of disadvantages inherently associated with an oxygenator, we believe it is preferable that ECMO be reserved for situations when there is a clear need to support the lungs. A clear example would be extracorporeal cardiopulmonary resuscitation, as discussed earlier. Other potential applications of ECMO for circulatory support would include the presence of significant pulmonary hypertension, hemodynamic instability due to septic shock, or severe pulmonary edema resulting from ventricular dysfunction (16,17). A very specific situation in which ECMO should be considered in the setting of isolated ventricular failure would be as temporary support for patients after stage 1 palliation of hypoplastic left heart syndrome. Even in this setting, however, a conversion to a short-term VAD might be an option provided that pulmonary function is preserved.

The advantages of short-term VADs compared with ECMO include the simplicity of the circuit and, more importantly, better decompression of the failing ventricle. The lack of an oxygenator and the simpler circuit configuration invoke less inflammation, which results in a lower level of anticoagulation requirement (18). Better ventricular decompression is critical in patients with acute heart failure in whom there is a reasonable chance of cardiac recovery (e.g., acute myocarditis). Short-term VAD support with a centrifugal pump provides excellent decompression of the left heart (or systemic ventricle), with immediate impact on left atrial pressure, pulmonary venous hypertension, pulmonary edema, and lung function. It is clear that short-term VADs that directly drain the left heart provide better decompression of a failing left ventricle than do ECMO that has only indirect effect on the left heart. **Figure 75.2** illustrates this principle, where inflow to the venous cannula of a VA ECMO circuit in the right atrium (RA) only drains the left heart if there is a patent

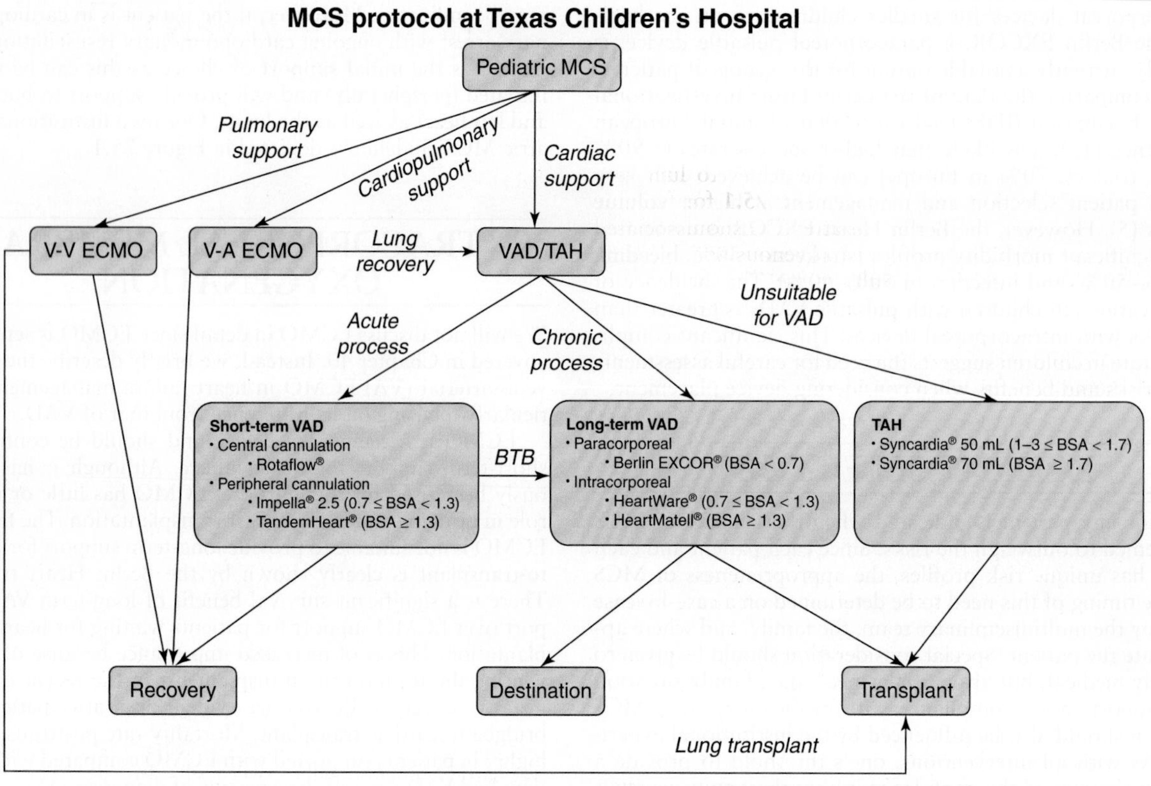

MCS protocol at Texas Children's Hospital

FIGURE 75.1. Mechanical circulatory support protocol from Texas Children's Hospital. Type of MCS support is determined by considering the following factors: (a) which organ(s) to support (e.g., heart only, lungs only, or both heart and lungs), (b) anticipated duration of MCS support based on the etiologies of heart failure, (c) patient's body size, (d) the goal of MCS support (e.g., recovery, destination, or transplant). MCS, mechanical circulatory support; V-V ECMO, veno-venous extracorporeal membrane oxygenation; V-A ECMO, veno-arterial extracorporeal membrane oxygenation; VAD, ventricular assist device; TAH, total artificial heart; BSA, body surface area.

foramen ovale. Conversely, inflow to the LVAD comes from a cannula placed directly on the left side of the heart in the left atrium. Hence, short-term VAD support may provide a better chance of recovery than do ECMO support based on anecdotal

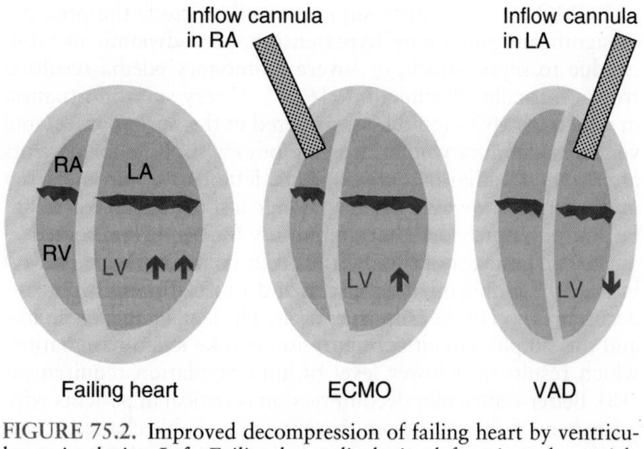

FIGURE 75.2. Improved decompression of failing heart by ventricular assist device. **Left:** Failing heart displaying left atria and ventricle volume distension. **Center:** Moderate improvement of left atria and ventricle volume distension by placing veno-arterial extracorporeal membrane oxygenator inflow (blood return to device) cannula in right atria (indirect decompression). **Right:** Marked improvement of left atria and ventricle volume distension by placing left ventricular assist device inflow (blood return to device) cannula in left atria (direct decompression). RA, right atria; RV, right ventricle; LA, left atria; LV, left ventricle; ECMO, extracorporeal membrane oxygenator; VAD, ventricular assist device.

experience in MCS that suggests that better decompression is associated with a better chance of cardiac recovery.

There are, however, certain situations where ECMO support may be preferable to VAD in the setting of acute heart failure or shock with preserved oxygenation. ECMO is preferred when the right heart is unable to provide "adequate" flow in order to fill the left heart (and therefore the systemic circulation). Suboptimal right heart output can be due either to inherent right ventricular dysfunction (e.g., severe cardiac allograft rejection), intractable ventricular arrhythmias, or pulmonary hypertension. Inadequacy of the right heart can also occur when the demand for total cardiac output is extraordinarily increased beyond what even a healthy ventricle can provide, for example, in the setting of septic shock. MCS for septic shock is very different in a sense that the flow requirement can be exceedingly high (e.g., 150%–200% flow). Such a high cardiac output cannot be achieved with LVAD support alone since the right heart cannot cope with such high demands. Another example of a situation where ECMO would be the modality of choice is when pulmonary blood flow is supplied by a ventricle to pulmonary artery conduit (e.g., stage 1 palliation for hypoplastic left heart syndrome with a right ventricle to pulmonary artery conduit). In this setting, VA ECMO support is necessary as pulmonary blood flow and oxygenation would not be adequate once the systemic ventricle were decompressed on VAD.

Management

Following initiation of VA ECMO, systemic vascular resistance is typically elevated. This can be due to a combination of the low cardiac output with an elevated afterload, as well as the need for high doses of vasoconstrictors prior to ECMO support. Once ECMO support is established, inotropic agents (particularly vasoconstrictors) should ideally be discontinued and systemic vasodilators should be considered in order to optimize flows and perfusion to the organ beds. Ventilator settings are typically weaned to lung protective mode. Once "full-flow" (see **Table 75.1** for full-flow calculation) support is established, attention should be paid to the cardiac filling pressures (central venous and left atrial pressures, where available). Ideally, these should be low in keeping with the goal of unloading the heart when support is initiated. Furthermore the waveform of the arterial line can provide valuable insights into the adequacy of decompression of the systemic ventricle. If the heart is decompressed well, there should be minimal ejection from the patient's own heart, as evidenced by completely or nearly flat waveform, rather than a continued pulsatile waveform, which can be associated with increased myocardial work, left atrial hypertension, pulmonary edema, and a delay in cardiac recovery. Potential causes of inadequate decompression with "full-flow" support would typically include volume overload during resuscitation process, systemic vasoconstriction, inadequate size or suboptimal location of an inflow cannula, and aortic insufficiency. This can also be seen in the setting of significant systemic-to-pulmonary collaterals.

If the chest x-ray shows significant pulmonary venous congestion and particularly if the patient displays pulmonary edema, a decision has to be made promptly regarding how to improve decompression of the systemic ventricle. There has been controversy regarding how often left atrial decompression is necessary during VA ECMO support in children with severe heart failure. While some investigators estimated the frequency that pediatric patients would require left atrial decompression on ECMO to be ~22% (19), others reported that half the patients in their clinical series developed lung edema, thereby benefitting from left atrial decompression (20).

There are several options for left atrial decompression in patients placed on VA ECMO support for acute heart failure. Balloon atrial septostomy, or blade septectomy followed by balloon septostomy using the transcatheter technique is a widely used approach that has the appeal of being minimally invasive (21,22). The procedure can be done using fluoroscopy or even at the bedside with echocardiographic guidance (23). If ECMO has been established with central cannulation, addition of a left atrial cannula is also an option (20). Be aware that a potential complication with this approach is thrombosis within the cannula due to the limited flow. Percutaneous left atrial vent placement is also an option during ECMO support (24,25), but this technique can be challenging, especially in small children.

TABLE 75.1

CALCULATIONS USED TO DETERMINE "FULL FLOW" FOR MECHANICAL CIRCULATORY SUPPORT

A. Patient's body weight <10 kg
  $0.15 \times$ (weight in kg) [L/min]
B. Patient's body weight $\geq$ 10 kg: based on patient's age
  Age $\leq$2 years old: $3.0 \times$ body surface area [L/min]
  Age $\leq$4 years old: $2.8 \times$ body surface area [L/min]
  Age $\leq$6 years old: $2.6 \times$ body surface area [L/min]
  Age $\leq$10 years old: $2.5 \times$ body surface area [L/min]
  Age >10 years old: $2.4 \times$ body surface area [L/min]

SHORT-TERM VENTRICULAR ASSIST DEVICE IN PATIENTS WITH HEART FAILURE

Indication

As already mentioned, in many centers, ECMO still remains the mainstay of MCS regardless of the etiology or the likely clinical course of heart failure. However, we would suggest an approach where, if expertise and experience allow, VAD be the modality of choice and ECMO be reserved for when there are clear clinical advantages of this over VAD such as in the presence of severe pulmonary dysfunction, following ECPR or in the presence of other factors already discussed. Aside from the advantage of a smaller circuit volume, smaller circuit area, and the need for less systemic anticoagulation, the most significant difference between the two modes of support is the degree of decompression of the left (systemic) ventricle.

Short-term VAD may be used in children with heart failure secondary to (a) acute processes (e.g., acute myocarditis and acute rejection of a cardiac allograft), (b) acute exaggeration of chronic heart failure (e.g., acute worsening of dilated cardiomyopathy due to superimposed infection), or (c) postoperative ventricular dysfunction (e.g., following reimplantation of anomalous left coronary artery arising from the pulmonary artery and late arterial switch operation with deconditioning of the left ventricle). If the etiologies are acute processes, it is highly likely that the cardiac function will recover with adequate decompression.

VAD Cannulation and Management

The most typical approach for the short-term VAD support for the left ventricle is left atrial to ascending aortic cannulation via sternotomy. Obviously, the necessity of sternotomy is the big downside of this mode of MCS. The inflow cannula is inserted into the left atrium in the area between the Waterston's groove and right-sided pulmonary veins. If the patient has a history of recent surgery that involves a suture line in the left atrium close to the groove, an alternative option for inflow cannula insertion is via the left atrial appendage. Peripheral cannulation of the left atrium through the atrial septum may be considered (26), but this technique is limited to older adolescents (26).

Once the desired VAD flow has been established, inotropic support should be reduced appropriately but not discontinued. Similarly, inhaled nitric oxide should not be automatically discontinued. This is because, unlike ECMO support, the right ventricle typically requires ongoing pharmacologic support when the left heart is mechanically supported. Almost always, however, initiation of vasodilator drugs is necessary to achieve optimal mean arterial pressures since systemic vascular resistance is substantially elevated in most cases. Once full-flow perfusion is achieved with the target mean arterial pressure, adequacy of systemic perfusion is confirmed by physical examination, urine output, clearance of lactate, reversal of acidosis, near-infrared spectroscopy saturations, mixed venous oxygen saturation, end-organ function, etc. Ventilation settings in patients on LVAD should be optimized to maintain a low pulmonary vascular resistance to maximize cardiac output from the native right ventricle and thus provide better filling of the LVAD pump. Unlike an ECMO circuit, the short-term VAD circuit does not contain a heat exchanger. Therefore, desired temperature, usually normothermia, may not be always achievable, especially when the chest is left open in small children. In this setting, alternative strategies to maintain normothermia may be needed, such as overhead radiant infant heater or an external convective warmer.

The decision regarding when to discontinue or transition to other type of support warrants clinical judgment and varies considerably between individuals. As discussed earlier, most patients with acute etiologies of heart failure are expected to recover within a short period of time (typically <2 weeks), sufficiently short for the MCS to be discontinued. Nonetheless, this recovery process should not be confused with reverse-remodeling that denotes favorable alterations in myocardial structure observed in patients with chronic heart failure (i.e., dilated cardiomyopathy) supported with long-term VADs, although some investigators (27) have described functional recovery of the heart in the setting of acute heart failure as "rapid reverse-remodeling." However, short-term VAD use may be too short for the favorable structural changes to occur. Instead, the main purpose of short-term VAD use for acute heart failure is to support the circulation while protecting the lungs until the inflammatory storm subsides and other end-organs recover, aiming toward bridge to recovery.

In our experience with the use of short-term VADs (28), the majority of patients with acute etiologies (17 out of 20, 85%) were successfully bridged to recovery. In particular, 100% recovery was achieved in patients with acute myocarditis (n = 11). Previous reports on ECMO support for acute myocarditis noted survival rates of 63% by the Extracorporeal Life Support Organization registry (29) and 70%–80% at large pediatric centers in North America (27,30). Most patients with acute myocarditis can be supported reasonably well with either mode of MCS (ECMO or short-term VAD). The difference in left heart decompression, however, could make a difference in the severest end of the spectrum, albeit small proportion of the entire patient population, where there is virtually no cardiac contractility. We believe the superior outcome with our approach using the short-term VAD support is

owing to the capability of saving these sickest children who would not have survived without perfect decompression of the left heart.

In contrast, the goal of short-term VAD support in the setting of chronic heart failure is different from that for acute heart failure. Chronic heart failure implies that cardiac recovery is unlikely. These patients will need a more chronic and durable form of heart failure treatment, such as long-term VADs or heart transplantation. Therefore, the major role of the short-term VAD support in the setting of chronic heart failure is initial salvage when the patient acutely deteriorates with an evidence of ongoing end-organ injury (i.e., INTERMACS 1 profile). (The Interagency Registry for Mechanically Assisted Circulatory Support scale is used to classify advanced heart failure patients according to hemodynamic status. Profile/level 1 is worst, 7 is best, see **Table 75.2.**) It has been well shown that preoperative INTERMACS 1 profile is a significant predictor of early mortality after long-term VAD implantation. By stabilizing the hemodynamics, it would be possible to minimize and ideally reverse pulmonary venous hypertension, to improve lung function, and to provide good systemic oxygen delivery to the tissues and organs, making the patient a better candidate for more invasive operation with a long-term VAD.

LONG-TERM VAD

Indication

4 When the etiology of heart failure is chronic in nature and the patient is relatively stable with respect to secondary organ function and functional status (INTERMACS profile 2 or 3),

TABLE 75.2

INTERAGENCY REGISTRY FOR MECHANICALLY ASSISTED CIRCULATORY SUPPORT (INTERMACS) LEVELS

Profile 1	Critical cardiogenic shock	Patient with life-threatening hypotension despite rapidly escalating inotropic support and critical organ hypoperfusion, often confirmed by worsening acidosis and/or lactate levels.
Profile 2	Progressive decline	Patient with declining function despite intravenous inotropic support, which may be manifest by worsening renal function, nutritional depletion, and inability to restore volume balance.
Profile 3	Stable but inotrope-dependent	Patient with stable blood pressure, organ function, nutrition, and symptoms on continuous intravenous inotropic support (or a temporary circulatory support device or both), but demonstrating repeated failure to wean from support due to recurrent symptomatic hypotension or renal dysfunction.
Profile 4	Resting symptoms	Patient can be stabilized close to normal volume status but experiences daily symptoms of congestion at rest or during activities of daily living (ADL). Doses of diuretics generally fluctuate at very high levels. More intensive management and surveillance strategies should be considered, which may in some cases reveal poor compliance that would compromise outcomes with any therapy. Some patients may shuttle between Profiles 4 and 5.
Profile 5	Exertion intolerant	Comfortable at rest and with ADL but unable to engage in any other activity, living predominantly within the house. Patients are comfortable at rest without congestive symptoms, but may have underlying refractory elevated volume status, often with renal dysfunction. If underlying nutritional status and organ function are marginal, patient may be more at risk than INTERMACS Profile 4 and require definitive intervention.
Profile 6	Exertion limited	Patient without evidence of fluid overload is comfortable at rest, and with ADL and minor activities outside the home but fatigues after the first few minutes of any meaningful activity. Attribution to cardiac limitation requires careful measurement of peak oxygen consumption, in some cases with hemodynamic monitoring to confirm severity of cardiac impairment.
Profile 7	Advanced NYHA III	A placeholder for more precise specification in the future, this level includes patients who are without current or recent episodes of unstable fluid balance, living comfortably with meaningful activity limited to mild physical exertion.

From Boyle AJ, Ascheim DD, Russo MJ, et al. Clinical outcomes for continuous-flow left ventricular assist device patients stratified by pre-operative INTERMACS classification. *J Heart Lung Transplant* 2011;30:402–7.

then long-term VADs are the devices of choice. The selection of device is mainly determined by the size of a patient. Currently, the only pediatric long-term VAD that has widespread acceptance worldwide is the Berlin Heart EXCOR (Berlin Heart, Inc. The Woodlands, TX). In older children, adult-sized intracorporeal devices such as HeartMate II (Thoratec Corp. Pleasanton, CA) or HVAD (HeartWare Inc. Framingham, MA) is an additional option. At our heart center, the Berlin EXCOR is used in patients with a body surface area (BSA) of 0.7 m² or smaller whereas the HeartMate II (Thoratec Corp.; Pleasanton, CA) is used in patients with a BSA of 1.3 m² or larger. The HVAD can be used for intermediate range of patients (0.7 < BSA < 1.3 m²) (31).

Prior to making the decision regarding VAD implantation, it is essential to assess carefully the function of the right ventricle as this will directly impact on the device strategy (i.e., LVAD vs. BiVAD). It is not always easy to accurately assess the RV function in the setting of severe LV dysfunction, and some degree of RV dysfunction is almost inevitable in patients with chronic heart failure. To this end, some centers advocate routine use of BiVAD for all patient. However, global experience would suggest that LVAD can provide adequate circulatory support for most children with severe heart failure in whom RV failure is typically secondary to LV failure. Since previous studies have consistently shown clinical outcome with BiVAD is worse than that of LVAD, it would be beneficial to adopt the approach that LVAD alone should be used if possible, with the exception of certain scenarios when RV function is inherently compromised. Examples of compromised RV function include arrhythmogenic right ventricular dysplasia, posttransplant chronic graft dysfunction, and infarction of the right coronary artery territory. One specific population to consider BiVAD support rather than LVAD alone is in patients with restrictive cardiomyopathy, which is typically associated with biventricular dysfunction as well as elevated pulmonary vascular resistance (32).

Management of LVAD

If LVAD support is chosen, an important focus of postoperative care is directed at optimizing the right heart's cardiac output. Since most of these patients supported with an isolated LVAD have at least some degree of RV failure, right heart management is a key to success. The basic principles of preventing right heart failure on LVAD include optimizing cardiopulmonary interactions, minimizing pulmonary vascular resistance, and maintaining right heart cardiac output with the lowest possible central venous pressure. Inotropes are usually required during the early postoperative period, and many centers would advocate the relatively routine use of inhaled nitric oxide. A clinically important question would be then how to assess right heart cardiac output. Echocardiography is a very useful tool in this regard. In fact, many physicians primarily rely on echocardiography. An advantage of a pneumatic paracorporeal device over an intracorporeal device is the fact that the filling status of a pump can be assessed under a direct vision. This is the most direct indicator of right heart cardiac output, provided that there is no significant aortic insufficiency or intracardiac shunting.

SPECIAL CONSIDERATIONS
Bridge to Recovery

As discussed earlier, most "recoverable" hearts have acute, temporary etiologies of heart failure, which is best supported by a short-term VAD. This is because cardiac function usually recovers within a short period of time (often after an acute insult such as acute inflammation secondary to infection, myocarditis, or cardiac surgery). There is, however, a small subset of patients whose heart undergoes myocardial recovery in a more gradual fashion. In these rare instances, patients may benefit from support with a long-term VAD without the ultimate need for transplantation. Recovery from chronic heart failure with the use of a long-term VAD is not well described in pediatric population and largely relates to anecdotal experience (33,34).

VAD as Destination Therapy

In adults, it is becoming more common to employ long-term VAD support for patients who have been deemed not to be transplant candidates and whose cardiac function is unlikely to recover. This strategy, termed "bridge-to-destination" or alternatively "chronic VAD therapy," is currently not a widely accepted option for the pediatric population. We expect, nonetheless, that in the near future, chronic VAD therapy will gain a more important role in the management of pediatric heart failure. Children who might benefit from this therapy include those with certain systemic diseases that preclude transplant candidacy (e.g., Duchenne or Becker muscular dystrophy; patients with malignancy) in whom improvement of quality of life may be offered with VAD support (35,36).

Functionally Univentricular Physiology

As discussed earlier, advancements in congenital heart surgery over the past few decades have resulted in a growing population of survivors, particularly those with a Fontan circulation, who develop circulatory failure late after surgery—typically in adolescence or early adulthood. Although Fontan failure can be multifactorial, VAD support for a single systemic ventricle can improve the failing circulation when the primary etiology of circulatory failure is systolic ventricular dysfunction. This mode of usage is termed "systemic VAD (SVAD)." In our institution, we implanted the HeartMate II in a 15-year-old boy with failing Fontan circulation manifest by protein-losing enteropathy (37). The patient had severely depressed function of his systemic right ventricle, with severe atrioventricular valve regurgitation, and an end-diastolic pressure in the systemic ventricle of more than 20 mm Hg. The hemodynamics were significantly improved with the HeartMate II. He was successfully bridged to transplantation after 72 days of support. Since patients in this category have unique anatomic and physiological features, SVAD treatment must be optimized individually. The location of the systemic ventricle and its apex is critical for device selection; for example—in the presence of dextrocardia, an L-looped arrangement of the ventricles, it may be difficult to implant the HeartMate II as these devices are essentially designed to fit hearts with an apex on the left (levocardia). In patients with a functionally univentricular heart and Fontan circulation, the absence of a subpulmonary ventricle may result in suboptimal filling of an SVAD. Therefore, it is important to ensure almost complete systemic ventricular decompression with a higher VAD setting and optimal cardiopulmonary interactions to encourage passive flow into the pulmonary arteries.

If the primary reason for Fontan failure is pulmonary in origin (i.e., increased transpulmonary gradient), then the placement of a VAD at a subpulmonary position may be an option (38). When the problems are at multiple levels that would preclude the successful application of VAD use, an alternative option may be a total artificial heart (TAH), which will be discussed in the next section.

Total Artificial Heart

5 There are certain situations where VAD support is not an ideal solution. An example would include chronic graft failure after heart transplantation (e.g., chronic rejection, transplant coronary artery disease, etc.). The necessity of immunosuppression for the cardiac graft poses a significant risk for infectious complications when VAD support is provided. In this scenario, the total artificial heart (Syncardia Inc., Tucson, AZ) may make postoperative care much simpler since it eliminates the need of immunosuppressive therapy. The TAH may also be considered if VAD support requires multiple and complex concomitant procedures (e.g., repair or replacement of aortic and/or atrioventricular valves), in the presence of severe aortic regurgitation or if a VAD cannot be placed for anatomic reasons, most typically cardiac position. We implanted a TAH in a 17-year-old boy with a history of congenitally corrected transposition of the great arteries who developed profound biventricular dysfunction, severe aortic insufficiency, and obstruction of the previously placed left ventricle to pulmonary arterial conduit (39). While awaiting cardiac transplantation, he suffered an acute cardiopulmonary collapse resulting in multisystem organ failure. The presence of severe aortic insufficiency precluded any type of temporary support by peripheral cannulation. VAD support would have required BiVAD implantation in addition to aortic valve replacement (or closure) and conduit exchange in the setting of abnormally located ventricles and great arteries (*l*-looped ventricles and *l*-malposed vessels). Given the complexity of the operation, the TAH was chosen as a preferable device to address all anatomical issues. The patient was successfully bridged to heart transplantation following 6 months of support. The TAH should be considered in a minority of patients with end-stage heart failure awaiting transplantation and who cannot be supported with more conventional VAD devices. The use of the TAH in children is technically challenging. The small thorax size in children poses a major limitation in patient selection, with the current system's 70-cc pump size. Soon a smaller system (with a 50-cc pump) will become commercially available and expand the pediatric application of the TAH (40).

CONCLUSION

The rapidly increasing population of pediatric heart failure patients, on a background of a widespread use of MCS in adults, has resulted in a huge growth in the application of MCS in children. There are several types of devices available for pediatric MCS: ECMO, short-term VADs, long-term VADs, and the TAH. A thorough understanding of the unique pathologic features of pediatric heart failure and selection of an optimal device are absolute prerequisites to a successful outcome with MCS for children.

References

1. Hall CW. When did artificial heart implants begin? *JAMA* 1988;259:1650.
2. Barnard CN. Human cardiac transplantation. An evaluation of the first two operations performed at the Groote Schuur Hospital, Cape Town. *Am J Cardiol* 1968;22(4):584–96.
3. Cooley DA, Liotta D, Hallman GL, et al. Orthotopic cardiac prosthesis for two-staged cardiac replacement. *Am J Cardiol* 1969;24(5):723–30.
4. Bartlett RH. Artificial organs: Basic science meets critical care. *J Am Coll Surg* 2003;196:171–9.
5. Adachi I, Fraser CD Jr. Mechanical circulatory support for infants and small children. *Semin Thorac Cardiovasc Surg Pediatr Card Surg Annu* 2011;14:38–44.
6. Fraser CD Jr, Jaquiss RD, Rosenthal DN, et al; Berlin Heart Study Investigators. Prospective trial of a pediatric ventricular assist device. *N Engl J Med* 2012;367:532–41.
7. Rossano JW, Zafar F, Graves DE, et al. Prevalence of heart failure related hospitalizations and risk factors for mortality in pediatric patients: An analysis of a nationwide sampling of hospital discharges. *Circulation* 2009;120:S586.
8. Colvin-Adams M, Smith JM, Heubner BM, et al. OPTN/SRTR 2011 annual data report: Heart. *Am J Transplant* 2013;13(suppl 1):119–48.
9. Kirklin JK, Naftel DC, Kormos RL, et al. Fifth INTERMACS annual report: Risk factor analysis from more than 6,000 mechanical circulatory support patients. *J Heart Lung Transplant* 2013;32(2):141–56.
10. Hetzer R, Muller J, Weng Y, et al. Cardiac recovery in dilated cardiomyopathy by unloading with a left ventricular assist device. *Ann Thorac Surg* 1999;68:742–9.
11. Kirklin JK, Naftel DC, Kormos RL, et al. Third INTERMACS annual report: The evolution of destination therapy in the United States. *J Heart Lung Transplant* 2011;30:115–23.
12. Hetzer R, Potapov EV, Alexi-Meskishvili V, et al. Single-center experience with treatment of cardiogenic shock in children by pediatric ventricular assist devices. *J Thorac Cardiovasc Surg* 2011;141:616–23.
13. Helman DN, Addonizio LJ, Morales DL, et al. Implantable left ventricular assist devices can successfully bridge adolescent patients to transplant. *J Heart Lung Transplant* 2000;19:121–6.
14. Rose EA, Moskowitz AJ, Packer M, et al. The REMATCH trial: Rationale, design, and end points. Randomized evaluation of mechanical assistance for the treatment of congestive heart failure. *Ann Thorac Surg* 1999;67:723–30.
15. Karimova A, Goldman A. Paediatric cardiac mechanical support. In: Stark J, Leval M, Tsang V, eds. *Surgery for Congenital Heart Defects*. 3rd ed. England: John Wiley & Sons Ltd, 2006:229–37.
16. Davies RR, Russo MJ, Hong KN, et al. The use of mechanical circulatory support as a bridge to transplantation in pediatric patients: An analysis of the United Network for Organ Sharing database. *J Thorac Cardiovasc Surg* 2008;135:421–7.
17. Horton S, d'Udekem Y, Shann F, et al. Extracorporeal membrane oxygenation via sternotomy for circulatory shock. *J Thorac Cardiovasc Surg* 2010;139(2):e12–3.
18. MacLaren G, Butt W, Best D, et al. Central extracorporeal membrane oxygenation for refractory pediatric septic shock. *Pediatr Crit Care Med* 2011;12(2):133–6.
19. Hanna BD. Left atrial decompression: Is there a standard during extracorporeal support of the failing heart? *Crit Care Med* 2006;34(10):2688–9.
20. Kotani Y, Chetan D, Rodrigues W, et al. Left atrial decompression during venoarterial extracorporeal membrane oxygenation for left ventricular failure in children: Current strategy and clinical outcomes. *Artif Organs* 2013;37(1):29–36.
21. Rashkind WJ, Miller WW. Creation of an atrial septal defect without thoracotomy. A palliative approach to complete transposition of the great arteries. *JAMA* 1966;196:991–2.
22. Seib PM, Faulkner SC, Erickson CC, et al. Blade and balloon atrial septostomy for left heart decompression in patients with severe ventricular dysfunction on extracorporeal membrane oxygenation. *Catheter Cardiovasc Interv* 1999;46:179–86.
23. Johnston TA, Jaggers J, McGovern JJ, et al. Bedside transseptal balloon dilation atrial septostomy for decompression of the left heart during extracorporeal membrane oxygenation. *Catheter Cardiovasc Interv* 1999;46:179–99.
24. Ward KE, Tuggle DW, Gessouroun MR, et al. Transseptal decompression of the heat heart during ECMO for severe myocarditis. *Ann Thorac Surg* 1995;59:749–51.
25. Aiyagari RM, Rocchini AP, Remenapp RT, et al. Decompression of the left atrium during extracorporeal membrane oxygenation using a transseptal cannula incorporated into the circuit. *Crit Care Med* 2006;34:2603–6.

26. Pavie A, Léger P, Nzomvuama A, et al. Left centrifugal pump cardiac assist with transseptal percutaneous left atrial cannula. *Artif Organs* 1998;22:502–7.
27. Duncan BW, Bohn DJ, Atz AM, et al. Mechanical circulatory support for the treatment of children with acute fulminant myocarditis. *J Thorac Cardiovasc Surg* 2001;122:440–8.
28. Adachi I, Heinle JS, McKenzie ED, et al. The use of short-term ventricular assist devices in children. *J Heart Lung Transplant* 2012;31:S119.
29. Haines NM, Rycus PT, Zwischenberger JB, et al. Extracorporeal life support registry report 2008: Neonatal and pediatric cardiac cases. *ASAIO J* 2009;55(1):111–6.
30. Teele SA, Allan CK, Laussen PC, et al. Management and outcomes in pediatric patients presenting with acute fulminant myocarditis. *J Pediatr* 2011;158:638–43.
31. Stiller B, Adachi I, Fraser CD Jr. Pediatric ventricular assist devices. *Pediatr Crit Care Med* 2013;14(5 suppl 1):S20–6.
32. Kimberling MT, Balzer DT, Hirsch R, et al. Cardiac transplantation for pediatric restrictive cardiomyopathy: Presentation, evaluation, and short-term outcome. *J Heart Lung Transplant* 2002;21(4):455–9.
33. Hoashi T, Matsumiya G, Sakata Y, et al. A novel system of assessing myocardial recovery during left ventricular support: Report of a case. *Surg Today* 2008;38(2):154–6.
34. Lowry AW, Adachi I, Gregoric ID, et al. The potential to avoid heart transplantation in children: Outpatient bridge to recovery with an intracorporeal continuous-flow left ventricular assist device in a 14-year-old. *Congenit Heart Dis* 2012;7(6):E91–6.
35. Jefferies JL, Eidem BW, Belmont JW, et al. Genetic predictors and remodeling of dilated cardiomyopathy in muscular dystrophy. *Circulation* 2005;112:2799–804.
36. Leprince P, Heloire F, Eymard B, et al. Successful bridge to transplantation in a patient with Becker muscular dystrophy-associated cardiomyopathy. *J Heart Lung Transplant* 2002;21:822–4.
37. Morales DL, Adachi I, Heinle JS, et al. A new era: Use of an intracorporeal systemic ventricular assist device to support a patient with a failing Fontan circulation. *J Thorac Cardiovasc Surg* 2011;142(3):e138–40.
38. Prêtre R, Häussler A, Bettex D, et al. Right-sided univentricular cardiac assistance in a failing Fontan circulation. *Ann Thorac Surg* 2008;86(3):1018–20.
39. Morales DL, Khan MS, Gottlieb EA, et al. Implantation of total artificial heart in congenital heart disease. *Semin Thorac Cardiovasc Surg* 2012;24(2):142–3.
40. Syncardia Inc. http://www.syncardia.com/2013-press-releases/syncardias-50cc-total-artificial-heart-receives-two-hud-designations-from-the-fda-for-destination-therapy-and-pediatric-bridge-to-transplant.html. Accessed February 19, 2014.

CHAPTER 76 ■ THORACIC TRANSPLANTATION

STEVEN A. WEBBER, LAURA A. LOFTIS, AARTI BAVARE, RENEE M. POTERA, AND NIKOLETA S. KOLOVOS

KEY POINTS

Cardiac Transplantation

1. There have been significant improvements in survival over the last two decades, almost entirely related to improvements in early outcome.

2. There is increasing use of ventricular assist device support for bridge-to-transplant indications with excellent short-term outcomes.

3. A wide array of immunosuppressive regimens is used in children, but no large, randomized, controlled trials have been performed.

4. Primary graft failure, infection, and acute rejection are the principal causes of death in the first year after transplantation.

5. Rejection with severe hemodynamic compromise is associated with high mortality and requires early diagnosis and aggressive intervention, including mechanical circulatory support when necessary.

6. Graft coronary artery disease is the principal cause of late graft loss.

7. Retransplantation is associated with poor results if performed early after primary transplantation, or during acute rejection events, but is associated with better results when performed for late indications.

8. The ultimate goal of transplantation is the development of donor-specific graft tolerance.

Lung Transplantation

9. End-stage lung disease secondary to cystic fibrosis remains the primary indication for pediatric lung transplantation, although many complex disease states may benefit from transplantation.

10. Advances in extracorporeal technology may provide benefit to patients awaiting transplantation, although further study in children is warranted.

11. High levels of immunosuppression are required for the lung transplant recipient; the risk of opportunistic infection as well as colonization is a major challenge in the posttransplant period.

12. Lung transplant recipients face some of the worst survival statistics among the solid-organ transplants; the development of bronchiolitis obliterans significantly impacts survival.

CARDIAC TRANSPLANTATION

Transplantation offers the only hope for survival and improved quality of life for selected children with end-stage heart disease that is due to either acquired or congenital cardiac defects. Kantrowitz and associates performed the first pediatric transplant in December 1967, only a few days after Dr. Christian Barnard's pioneering operation in an adult. Interest in transplantation of the heart declined throughout the 1970s due to the high mortality that resulted primarily from lack of effective immunosuppressive medications. A resurgence of clinical activity developed in the early 1980s with the introduction of cyclosporine, the first oral immunosuppressive agent with relative specificity for inhibition of

1. T lymphocytes, the primary mediators of allograft rejection. This therapy resulted in dramatic improvements in survival of all transplanted organs. With improvements in candidate and donor selection, preoperative management, surgical technique, and early postoperative care, ~95% of heart transplant recipients are able to leave the hospital alive and in good health after transplantation (1). Furthermore, pretransplant mortality has fallen. This section provides an overview of the current state of the art of pediatric heart transplantation,

focusing on issues of key interest to those who work in the pediatric intensive care unit (PICU).

Indications for Cardiac Transplantation

Transplantation of the heart is generally considered to be indicated when expected survival is under 2 years and/or when the patient has an unacceptable quality of life. Cardiomyopathy (predominantly dilated forms) and complex congenital heart defects remain the primary indications and together account for ~90% of transplantations undertaken in children (2). Worldwide, transplant activity remains relatively constant and reflects a finite donor pool. Diagnoses that lead to transplantation are age-dependent, with congenital heart disease accounting for two-thirds of transplants in the infant age group and cardiomyopathy accounting for a similar proportion among adolescents (2).

The indications for heart transplantation in children were summarized in a 1999 report from the Pediatric Committee of the American Society of Transplantation and in a more recent report from 2007 (3,4). Perhaps the most controversial indication for heart transplantation is hypoplastic left heart syndrome and related pathologies in the newborn. Survival rates in excess of 80% at 1 year may be achieved at experienced centers, with either Norwood reconstruction or primary transplantation for this condition. Median waiting times for newborn heart transplant candidates are ~2 months in the United States (and longer in many US regions and in some other countries), resulting in very high costs of care prior to transplantation, significant pretransplant morbidities, and wait-list mortality as high as 25%. In light of these observations, most centers have moved away from transplantation and toward staged reconstruction for neonates with hypoplastic left heart syndrome. This strategy increases availability of organs for other infants with cardiac disease unsuitable for surgical palliation.

Relative and/or absolute contraindications include chronic infection with either hepatitis B or C, or HIV; prior nonadherence with medical therapy; recent or current treatment of malignancy with inadequate follow-up to ensure likely cure; active acute viral, fungal, or bacterial infections; elevated and *fixed* pulmonary vascular resistance (PVR), inadequate intraparenchymal pulmonary vascular bed; diffuse pulmonary vein stenosis; and major extracardiac disease felt to be nonreversible with heart transplantation (e.g., severe systemic myopathy). Inevitably, some centers consider specific contraindications absolute, whereas others may feel that they are relative. Decision-making is based on consensus discussion among all team members, including intensive care staff.

Evaluation of the Cardiac Transplant Candidate

A vast number of children who undergo heart transplantation evaluation are hospitalized in the PICU. For many, the transplant will occur during the first hospital admission. Thus, the intensivist will be deeply involved in the transplant evaluation, which should include an assessment of expected survival without transplantation, the patient's current quality of life, the potential for alternate surgical or medical therapies, and the inherent risks of the transplant surgery itself. A typical evaluation protocol is shown in **Table 76.1**.

Anatomic and Hemodynamic Considerations

Children with the most complex cardiac anatomy may receive a cardiac transplant, provided the lung vasculature is

adequately developed and PVR is acceptable. The anatomic points of most interest to the surgeon include abnormalities of cardiac and visceral situs (especially anomalies of the systemic and pulmonary venous return) and the size and anatomy of the main and branch pulmonary arteries (including the presence of stenoses, distortions, and nonconfluence). Intracardiac anatomy is less important, as the bulk of the cardiac mass will be explanted. Abnormalities in the relation of the great arteries usually pose few problems. Extreme care on entry to the sternum must be taken when a right ventricular-pulmonary artery conduit or enlarged right atria (after Fontan procedure) is present. Cardiac catheterization is usually indicated pretransplant to assess PVR. Excessive fixed resistance will result in acute donor right ventricular failure. This situation would necessitate the need for a right ventricular assist device in the immediate postoperative period.

In general, children with indexed PVR (PVRI) ≤6 indexed units (IU) are considered low risk for acute donor right heart failure. If resistance is between 6 and 10 IU, the risks are higher, but transplantation is still generally not contraindicated (5). A PVRI in excess of 10 IU is usually considered a contraindication to isolated heart transplantation, unless a major fall is achieved (to well below 10 IU) with pulmonary vasodilator therapy (100% oxygen and/or nitric oxide). In borderline cases, restudy of hemodynamics after several days of inotropic and vasodilator therapy may be necessary. It should be noted, however, that a rapid fall in pulmonary resistance can lead to acute elevation in left atrial pressure in patients with very poor left ventricular function, even precipitating pulmonary edema. Recent data suggest that elevated PVR may be less of a risk than previously believed in patients undergoing transplantation for indications other than CHD (6). Also of recent interest is the observation that VADs can be used to lower PVR in selected wait-list candidates with unacceptable PVR, allowing for successful bridge-to-transplant without posttransplant acute right ventricular failure (7). More experience with this strategy is anticipated in the future.

Laboratory Investigations

The laboratory tests that should be conducted in a transplant candidate are summarized in **Table 76.1**. Blood typing is necessary to ensure ABO compatibility with the transplanted organ, although infants and young children with absent or low anti-A and anti-B isohemagglutinin titers may be safely transplanted

---

TABLE 76.1

EVALUATION OF CANDIDATES FOR HEART TRANSPLANTATION

History and physical examination
Required consultations
Pediatric cardiologist, congenital cardiovascular surgeon, cardiac anesthesiologist, infectious disease specialist, psychiatrist or psychologist, transplant coordinator, social worker
Additional consultations (as required)
Neonatology, genetics, neurology, dental, oncology, immunology, nephrology, nutritional services, physical/occupational therapy, developmental pediatrics, hospital finance
Cardiac diagnostic studies
Chest radiograph, electrocardiogram, echocardiogram, cardiac catheterization
In selected patients: exercise test, ventilation–perfusion scan, chest CT or MRI, pulmonary function tests
Blood type (ABO), anti-HLA antibody screen, complete blood count and white cell differential, platelet count, coagulation screen, blood urea nitrogen, serum creatinine, glucose, electrolytes, calcium, magnesium, liver function tests, lipid profile, brain natriuretic peptide
Serologic screening for antibodies to the following pathogens: cytomegalovirus; Epstein–Barr; herpes simplex virus; varicella-zoster virus; HIV; hepatitis A, B, C, D, and measles; antibodies to *Toxoplasma gondii*
PPD/Mantoux tuberculosis test placement
Update immunizations including hepatitis B, pneumococcal, and influenza (in season)

HIV, human immunodeficiency virus; PPD, purified protein derivative.

across traditional ABO barriers. This strategy was introduced by West et al. (8) in Toronto and is based on the principle that isohemagglutinins against blood group antigens do not normally develop until the latter part of infancy. Transplantation across blood group barriers prior to the development of naturally occurring anti-A and anti-B isohemagglutinins appears to result in outcomes comparable to ABO-compatible transplants (8–10). Furthermore, many of the transplanted infants do not form antibodies against donor blood group antigens during long-term follow-up, possibly due to the development of B-cell tolerance (9,11). This strategy has profound implications for PICU care, as use of blood products pre- and posttransplant must be carefully planned to avoid transfusion of blood products that contain inappropriate anti-A and anti-B antibodies. The strategy of listing for ABO-incompatible organs may increase likelihood of undergoing transplantation, especially for infants of blood type O, potentially decreasing wait-list mortality.

Evaluation for the presence of preformed anti–human leukocyte antigen (HLA) antibodies ("sensitized") is now most commonly performed using the newer, highly sensitive, solid-phase assays (Luminex). Infectious disease evaluation includes serologic testing for cytomegalovirus (CMV), Epstein–Barr virus (EBV), varicella, herpes simplex virus, *Toxoplasma gondii*, HIV, measles, and hepatitis viruses A, B, C, and D. Serologic status for these agents may guide prophylaxis as well as the diagnostic evaluation of posttransplantation fever. The infectious disease evaluation should also include review of immunization history. Those candidates in whom transplantation is not likely to be imminent should undergo an update of appropriate immunizations at the time of the pretransplant evaluation.

Consultations

A multidisciplinary team that includes the transplant cardiologist and surgeon, social worker, transplant coordinator, and infectious disease expert evaluates each candidate. A screening psychiatric/psychological examination of the patient and the family is also very important. The primary purpose of this evaluation is to identify patients and families at high risk for poor psychosocial outcome while waiting for transplantation and after transplantation. Evaluation of past history of nonadherence to medical therapy is critical. Additional consultations may be required from specialist services such as hematology-oncology (when the patient has past history of malignancy), child development, genetics, neurology, and feeding/nutritional specialists. Patients with Fontan circulation require evaluation of the liver for evidence of cirrhosis, and may require formal hepatology consultation.

Evaluation of the Cardiac Donor

Although the intensivist is not usually involved in the donor evaluation process (**Table 76.2**), it is important for the PICU team to know about key aspects of the potential donor. Evaluation of the donor heart begins with a careful review of the history, including donor age and gender, body size, cause of death, presence of any chest trauma, need for cardiopulmonary resuscitation, length of resuscitation, and evaluation of the hemodynamic status of the donor (including blood pressure, heart rate, and central venous pressure, if available). The amount of inotropic support and trends in usage over time are also noted. A history of cardiopulmonary resuscitation is not, in itself, a contraindication to cardiac donation (12,13). It must be recognized that brain death results in dramatic physiologic disturbances in the donor, including temperature instability with hypothermia, circulatory volume changes (most commonly depletion), and neuroendocrine dysfunction, in addition to depletion of circulating thyroxine, cortisol, insulin, glucagon, and antidiuretic hormone.

TABLE 76.2

EVALUATION OF THE CARDIAC DONOR

History
Donor age, height, weight, and gender
Cause of brain death
History of cardiac arrest and length of resuscitation
Evidence of chest trauma
History of IV drug usage
Past history of cardiovascular disease
Distance from transplant center
History of malignancy
Cardiovascular status
Heart rate, blood pressure, central venous pressure
Fluid balance
Blood gas
Types and doses of IV inotropes
Inotropic support increasing or decreasing
Cardiovascular testing
Electrocardiogram
Chest radiograph
Echocardiogram
Cardiac enzymes
Other testing
Infectious disease screen: CMV, EBV, *Toxoplasma gondii*, HIV-1, HIV-2, HTLV-1, HTLV-2, RPR, hepatitis B and C
All culture results since admission to ICU

IV, intravenous; CMV, cytomegalovirus; EBV, Epstein–Barr virus; HIV, human immunodeficiency virus; HTLV, human T-lymphotropic virus; RPR, rapid plasma reagin.

To rule out structural abnormalities and to evaluate cardiac function, a complete echocardiogram should be performed. Most centers avoid the use of donor hearts whose systolic function is more than mildly impaired after treatment with inotropic agents or thyroid hormone (e.g., shortening fraction <26%, ejection fraction <50%). Some degree of atrioventricular valvar regurgitation is common after brain death and mild degrees do not constitute a contraindication to organ donation. Pericardial effusion may be indicative of myocardial contusion. A 12-lead electrocardiogram should be performed. Mild, nonspecific ST- and T-wave changes are commonly present and usually reflect central nervous system effects, electrolyte disturbances, or hypothermia; these do not contraindicate organ donation. Interpretation of cardiac enzymes may be difficult in the setting of generalized trauma. However, the elevation in cardiac troponin I levels in donor serum appears to be a useful predictor for acute graft failure after infant heart transplantation. Use of older donors (e.g., >35 years of age) for pediatric recipients is associated with high risk of posttransplant coronary disease and poor long-term survival (14). Furthermore, the negative impact of prolonged graft ischemic time (13,15,16) is further adversely influenced by increasing donor age (13).

Size matching is a critical issue in the selection of potential donors. Most centers avoid undersizing the donor below 75%–80% of recipient weight. Below this, cardiac output of the donor may be insufficient to meet the needs of the recipient. Nevertheless, a recent report suggests that grafts from donors as small as 60% of recipient body weight may be safely used in children (17). These observations require validation in separate cohorts of patients. Use of oversized donors is common. Most candidates will have marked cardiomegaly, leaving ample room within the chest for an oversized donor heart. Use of donor-to-recipient weight ratios of 2.5:1 is common in pediatric practice, and ratios of 3:1 to 4:1 have been successfully used, especially in newborn and infant candidates. Marked oversizing often results in delayed sternal closure. In infant recipients, oversizing has been associated with a more prolonged ventilator course and increased risk of primary graft failure (18). Oversized donor hearts may also give rise to a postoperative syndrome characterized by a high-output state associated with systemic hypertension, raised intracranial pressure, and even mental status changes.

It has been suggested that oversizing of donors may improve outcome when the recipient has significant preoperative pulmonary hypertension. Certainly, significant undersizing should be avoided in the presence of recipient pulmonary hypertension. In adults, it has been shown that use of female donors is associated with higher perioperative mortality when recipient PVR is elevated.

All donors should be screened for CMV, EBV, HIV-1, HIV-2, human T-lymphotropic viruses 1 and 2 (HTLV-1, HTLV-2), and hepatitis viruses A, B, and C. Donors are also screened for syphilis and for antibodies to *T. gondii*. The presence of antibodies to CMV, EBV, or *T. gondii* does not constitute contraindication to transplantation but helps to guide post-transplantation therapy and surveillance. Evidence of donor retroviral infection (HIV or HTLV) is considered an absolute contraindication to heart transplantation. The presence of donor hepatitis B surface antigen is also usually considered an absolute contraindication to heart donation. The usage of hepatitis C-positive donors remains controversial. Donors must also be avoided when there is evidence of other important donor-transmissible infections such as West Nile Virus.

Surgical Techniques of Graft Implantation

Detailed reviews of surgical techniques are outside the scope of this text and have been reviewed by Pigula and Webber (19). The *biatrial anastomosis* for cardiac transplantation has been applied to thousands of patients of all ages with excellent results (**Fig. 76.1**). Despite the great success of this technique, the result is a nonanatomically correct one, with large atrial cavities. The resulting abnormal atrial geometry is thought to contribute to tricuspid valve dysfunction and sinus node dysfunction. For these reasons, many centers now perform *bicaval anastomosis* in children of all ages who undergo orthotopic heart transplantation (**Fig. 76.1**). Some specific forms of congenital heart disease lend themselves particularly well to the bicaval technique, for example, in patients who have had previous Mustard or Senning operations or Glenn anastomoses. The bicaval technique may be associated with superior caval vein stenosis, especially in infants (20).

Transplantation for congenital heart disease is often performed after multiple palliative procedures and may present formidable surgical challenges. The anatomic substrate can be broadly classified as abnormalities of the systemic venous return, abnormalities of the pulmonary venous return, and abnormalities of the great vessels, including hypoplastic left heart syndrome. Surgical modifications of the two basic techniques are required for transplantation of these anatomic variants. Abnormalities of systemic venous return are among the most challenging anatomic variants to transplant. Fashioning unobstructed connections in a patient undergoing heart transplantation with left-sided cavae (e.g., in dextrocardia with situs inversus or in heterotaxy syndromes) requires special consideration and planning. Of key importance is procurement of generous sections of donor caval veins, including the innominate vein.

Increasing numbers of children come to heart transplantation after multiple palliative operations have been performed. Often, these operations have involved the pulmonary arteries in the form of systemic-to-pulmonary shunts, cavopulmonary anastomoses, or other procedures. In all cases, as much donor pulmonary artery as possible should be harvested. Most commonly, as

is the case in bidirectional Glenn or Fontan operations, the cavopulmonary anastomosis is taken down, the pulmonary arteries are patched, and bicaval anastomoses are performed. Patch material may take the form of bovine pericardium, homograft, or donor or recipient discard. Repair is best accomplished after recipient cardiectomy and before organ implantation. In the case of discontinuous pulmonary arteries, the donor organ should be procured with the pulmonary bifurcation and pulmonary arteries intact. Direct left and right pulmonary artery anastomoses are then performed. Alternatively, excess donor aorta can be used to connect the right and left pulmonary arteries prior to implantation. Transplantation to a single lung is feasible when there is unilateral absence or severe hypoplasia of a pulmonary artery (21) and should only be performed when the dominant pulmonary artery is well developed and has low PVR.

Few centers currently perform primary transplantation for hypoplastic left heart syndrome. Because of the extensive arch hypoplasia, the donor organ must include the entire transverse and proximal descending aorta en bloc. While most centers perform transplantation of hypoplastic left heart syndrome under circulatory arrest, several techniques have been developed to minimize circulatory arrest time. Regional low-flow perfusion can eliminate the need for circulatory arrest. This technique employs a Gore-Tex tube graft (3.5 mm) anastomosed to the innominate artery, fashioned prior to bypass. Vascular isolation of the brachiocephalic vessels and the descending aorta allows continued perfusion of the brain during cardiectomy as well as graft implantation. This technique provides physiologic cerebral circulatory support and significant somatic circulatory support, such that circulatory arrest can be avoided completely (19).

Postoperative Management and Early Complications

Many of the fundamental principles of early postoperative management after heart transplantation are similar to those for pediatric patients who undergo other procedures with cardiopulmonary bypass (see Chapter 79). Aspects of care that are specific to the transplant recipient are discussed here.

Cardiovascular Considerations

Inotropic Agents. Abnormalities in cardiac function are inevitable due to the obligatory hypoxic–ischemic insult that the donor heart endures. Recovery of systolic function is usually rapid. However, abnormalities in diastolic function may persist for many weeks. Most heart transplant recipients will benefit from low-dose inotropic support in the immediate postoperative period, although often this is only required for 2–3 days. The choice of inotrope will reflect both physician preference and hemodynamic factors such as heart rate, PVR, and blood pressure. Low-dose dobutamine is often used for the first few days. The addition of a combined vasodilator/inotropic agent such as milrinone is logical in the presence of low cardiac output and evidence of high systemic vascular resistance.

Systemic Hypertension. In contrast to the nontransplant cardiac surgical patient, systemic hypertension is common. Many factors contribute to this, including vigorous function of an oversized donor organ and use of high-dose corticosteroids. It is not unusual to observe quite severe systolic hypertension within 24 hours of a successful transplant procedure. Treatment with a variety of IV vasodilators, and sometimes even β blockers, may be necessary. Epicardial pacing wires should be working appropriately if β blockers are to be used, since the freshly transplanted heart is already at risk for transient sinoatrial disease (see below).

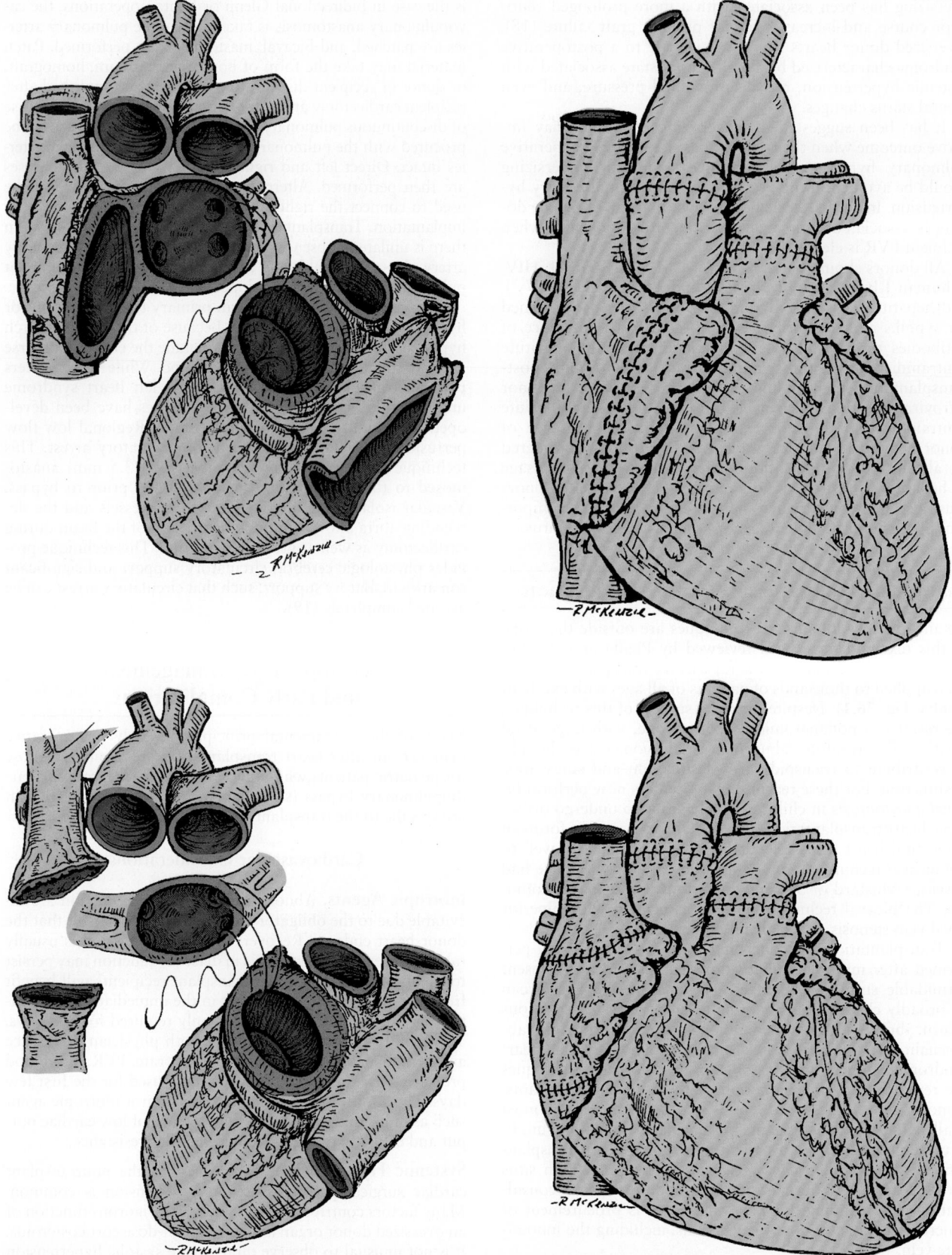

FIGURE 76.1. Orthotopic heart transplantation using the original biatrial technique of lower and Shumway. **A:** The recipient ventricular mass has been excised, and left atrial anastomosis commences after proper graft alignment. **B: Completion. C** and **D:** Heart transplantation using the bicaval technique currently used in many centers. **C:** Generous cavoatrial cuffs remain. The left atrial cuff is trimmed and implantation proceeds from left atrium to IVC, SVC, aorta, and pulmonary artery. **D:** Completion. IVC, inferior vena cava; SVC, superior vena cava.

Pulmonary Vascular Resistance. The importance of PVR as a risk factor for acute donor right ventricular failure was discussed previously. Nitric oxide is begun in the operating room and is used to wean from cardiopulmonary bypass. Acidosis must be avoided, and high levels of inspired oxygen are provided. Generous sedation is provided in the early postoperative period. If necessary, prostaglandin E_1 (PGE_1) can also be used. The right heart may require significant inotropic support, and sometimes epinephrine may be required in addition to milrinone and dobutamine. If right ventricular dysfunction persists with poor cardiac output despite this level of support, then mechanical assistance should be provided.

Cardiac Rate and Rhythm. Postoperative tachyarrhythmias and bradyarrhythmias have been observed in children following heart transplantation. The most common rhythm abnormality (other than sinus tachycardia) is sinus bradycardia, with or without an atrial or junctional escape rhythm. The denervated sinus node generally responds appropriately to exogenous chronotropic agents. A simpler approach is atrial pacing, and all transplant recipients should have temporary pacing wires placed in the operating room. Ventricular ectopy and nonsustained ventricular tachycardia may occur in the first week or two after transplantation but rarely requires treatment. The fresh cardiac allograft has limited ability to increase stroke volume; therefore, establishing an adequate heart rate is important for maintaining cardiac output. It is our practice to target a heart rate of 140–150 beats/min in an infant, while a teenager should have a heart rate of 100 beats/min. Atrial pacing is most commonly used to control the heart rate.

Primary Graft Failure. Both failure to wean from cardiopulmonary bypass and early postoperative graft failure are associated with high mortality. The term *primary graft failure* is often reserved for the finding of acute left ventricular or biventricular failure not due to elevated PVR. Poor donor selection, prolonged ischemic time, poor preservation technique, and hyperacute rejection should all be considered. The latter is extremely rare with routine recipient pretransplant screening for anti-HLA antibodies. When primary graft failure occurs, recovery is frequently possible if the circulation can be supported, which is usually achieved with extracorporeal membrane oxygenation (ECMO) (22). However, recent data suggest that only approximately half of the children supported in this manner for primary graft failure will survive to hospital discharge (23–25). Retransplantation for early graft failure is generally associated with very poor outcomes (26), and many consider this a contraindication to retransplantation.

Respiratory Support. The principles of respiratory support do not differ from those of other pediatric open heart procedures. Early extubation should be the goal. The patient who has required prolonged preoperative mechanical ventilation will usually need more prolonged ventilatory support postoperatively, as retraining of respiratory muscles will be required. Infants with long-standing cardiomegaly will often have significant tracheobronchomalacia, and persistent or recurrent pulmonary atelectasis is not unusual.

Renal Function. The combination of chronic heart failure, cardiopulmonary bypass, and use of cyclosporine or tacrolimus all contribute to postoperative renal dysfunction, which is exacerbated by a postoperative low–cardiac output state. Oliguria is common. Fortunately, acute renal failure is rare in children, and dialysis is seldom required. Persistent oliguria is managed with loop diuretics and low-dose dopamine (e.g., 3–5 mcg/kg/min). Low cardiac output is managed with inotropic agents, as discussed previously. Administration of a continuous furosemide infusion (up to 6 mg/kg/d, maximum of 600 mg/24 hours) may be helpful. These maneuvers are usually successful in stimulating an adequate urine output (>1 mL/kg/h). In some cases, particularly in neonates and infants, IV PGE_1 may also provide a diuretic effect. The primary immunosuppressive agents tacrolimus and cyclosporine are highly nephrotoxic, both acutely and with long-term usage. When urine output remains low, it may be necessary to decrease dosage or hold calcineurin inhibitors in the immediate perioperative period. This is best facilitated by the use of potent T lymphocyte–depleting agents (intravenous "induction therapy"), which provides effective immunosuppression in the first few days after transplantation allowing for more gradual introduction of calcineurin inhibitors.

Gastrointestinal Complications. Gastrointestinal complications are quite common early after pediatric heart transplantation (27). All patients should receive intravenous and, subsequently, oral H_2 antagonists to decrease the risk of stress ulcers in the early postoperative period. These are usually continued until corticosteroids have been weaned to low doses or discontinued. The nasogastric tube is removed as soon as the patient is extubated and able to take oral feeds and medications. Attention is paid to providing optimal calories without use of excessive volumes, as most patients will tend to retain fluid in the early postoperative period. Pancreatitis is not uncommon following transplantation and should be sought in the presence of abdominal pain or unexplained feeding intolerance. Immunosuppressive regimens that avoid the use of azathioprine and corticosteroids may reduce this complication. Symptoms of gastrointestinal perforation may be subtle in small children on immunosuppressive medications, especially if corticosteroids are being used. Many children with chronic heart failure have gastroesophageal reflux disease; this should be aggressively managed but with the knowledge that many drug interactions occur between immunosuppressant medications and drugs used for gastroesophageal reflux disease, including antacids, antihistamines, and prokinetic agents.

Infectious Precautions. Infections are a leading cause of death and morbidity in the first year following heart transplantation. Most severe infections occur during the initial hospitalization. During the first week after transplantation, invasive lines and drains are removed as soon as possible. A short course of antibiotics, typically 72 hours, is given as prophylaxis against mediastinal and wound infection. Usually, a first-generation cephalosporin will suffice. Broader staphylococcal coverage, such as vancomycin, should be considered if the patient has had a prolonged intensive care unit (ICU) stay and has long-standing vascular catheters in place. Such lines are usually replaced in the operating room. Patients colonized with methicillin-resistant *Staphylococcus aureus* are also covered with vancomycin. Oral nystatin is started in the ICU to prevent Candida infections, as well as ganciclovir to prevent early CMV infection if the recipient or donor is seropositive for CMV. Patients at high risk for yeast infections (e.g., patients on pretransplant ECMO) are frequently given prophylaxis with fluconazole. However, it should be noted that all "azole" antifungals have a profound effect on calcineurin-inhibitor metabolism (via the cytochrome P450 system). A marked reduction in tacrolimus or cyclosporine dosing (50%–90% reduction) is required during concomitant use of an azole antifungal agent. Initiation of prophylaxis against *Pneumocystis jiroveci* can follow closer to the time of hospital discharge (28).

Immunosuppression and Early Acute Rejection. High-dose IV methylprednisolone (e.g., 15–20 mg/kg) is given in the operating room. A tapering course of corticosteroids is usually given over the next 1–2 weeks, with the majority of centers historically discharging patients on maintenance corticosteroid therapy (2). However, steroid-free immunosuppressive regimens are increasingly being used in pediatric practice (2,29,30).

TABLE 76.3

POTENTIAL COMBINATIONS OF MAINTENANCE IMMUNOSUPPRESSIVE DRUGS USED IN PEDIATRIC
HEART TRANSPLANTATION

■ NUMBER OF AGENTS	■ POTENTIAL COMBINATIONS	■ COMMENTS
Monotherapy	Tacrolimus or cyclosporine	Monotherapy rarely used with cyclosporine
Dual therapy	Tacrolimus or cyclosporine *with* azathioprine OR mycophenolate mofetil OR sirolimus/everolimus OR corticosteroids	Little experience with the mTOR (target of rapamycin) inhibitors sirolimus and everolimus in children Steroid avoidance increasingly common in pediatric heart transplantation
Triple therapy	Tacrolimus or cyclosporine *with* corticosteroids *with* azathioprine OR mycophenolate mofetil OR sirolimus/everolimus	In triple therapy regimens, mycophenolate mofetil is being used with increasing frequency in lieu of azathioprine

Cyclosporine or tacrolimus is commenced generally within 24–48 hours of surgery once good urine output has been established. Both agents can be given intravenously or enterally. If anti–T-cell induction therapy is used (most commonly, polyclonal rabbit antithymocyte globulin (ATG); less often with an interleukin-2 receptor (IL-2R) antagonist), then there is less urgency to introduce a calcineurin inhibitor in the immediate (first 1–5 days) posttransplant period. Cyclosporine or tacrolimus can then be commenced by the oral route rather than intravenously. Delay in commencement of these agents for several days (under coverage of induction therapy) may be particularly useful when urine output is low or renal function is deteriorating.

3 Numerous strategies are available for maintaining immunosuppression (31,32). All centers currently use a calcineurin inhibitor as the primary immunosuppressive agent, with ~80% of children currently receiving tacrolimus at the time of initial discharge posttransplantation (2). Most centers also use a second, adjunctive agent most commonly mycophenolate mofetil (MMF)/mycophenolic acid (2). More centers are using steroid avoidance regimens or early steroid weaning in children. The principles of maintenance therapy are summarized in **Table 76.3**. In general, agents of similar classes are not given together, as they tend to enhance toxicities. Combination therapies use two or three agents of different classes with different mechanisms of action.

Careful daily assessment looking for signs of rejection is required, although severe rejection before 7–10 days is rare (except in the sensitized patient). Rejection is generally delayed with use of induction therapy. Infants and young children experience less acute rejection than do adolescents. Pallor, increasing tachycardia, abdominal pain, gallop rhythm, and oliguria all are suggestive of severe rejection. Ideally, rejection is identified by echocardiography and/or surveillance biopsy before such signs develop. The electrocardiogram may show reduced precordial voltages. The tempo of rejection can be quite abrupt in the early posttransplant period, and any deterioration in the patient's condition after initial recovery from surgery must be taken very seriously. If evidence of new graft dysfunction is unequivocal, empiric treatment of bolus intravenous corticosteroids is given. Endocardial muscle biopsy generally shows lymphocytic infiltrates (predominantly T cells) with varying degrees of edema and myocyte damage or necrosis. Endomyocardial biopsies are graded according to an internationally agreed classification system developed by the International Society for

Heart and Lung Transplantation (ISHLT) (33). With increasing evidence for the importance of donor-specific anti-HLA antibodies as mediators of acute and chronic graft dysfunction and failure (34–37), the ISHLT also now recommends a standardized approach to the grading of antibody-mediated rejection (AMR) (38), and acute cellular rejection and AMR may require different forms of therapy (32,39).

Medium-term and Late Complications

A detailed discussion of all complications of heart transplantation beyond the immediate postoperative period is outside the scope of this text, and readers are referred to other reviews (33,40). This section focuses on those complications that the intensive care team will be required to manage.

Immunosuppressive therapy aims to prevent or minimize the immune response of the host to donor antigens, while avoiding complications of therapeutic immunosuppression. Immunologic complications of transplantation fall into two main groups—allograft rejection/graft dysfunction (both acute and chronic), reflecting inadequate or ineffective immunosuppression, and manifestations of nonspecific immunosuppression, including infections and malignancy. Finally, nonimmune side effects of immunosuppressive therapy (i.e., tissue and organ toxicities) are an important cause of morbidity, and occasionally mortality, after heart transplantation in children.

Acute Rejection

Patients remain at risk for acute rejection indefinitely. No evidence exists that suggests that heart transplant recipients become truly tolerant to their allograft. The importance of acute rejection episodes becomes evident when causes of death after heart transplant are examined. **4** Data from the ISHLT show that acute rejection/acute graft failure is the most common cause of death between 30 days and 3 years after heart transplantation, accounting for approximately a third of all deaths (2). The peak hazard, or instantaneous risk, for first rejection is between 1 and 3 months after transplantation. By 3 years after transplantation, approximately half of the pediatric heart recipients are free of acute rejection (41). Late acute rejection episodes (occurring beyond the first year after transplantation) appear to carry a particularly poor long-term prognosis (42), especially if associated with graft dysfunction.

When any degree of systolic dysfunction is associated with acute rejection, rapid deterioration is common, even when the patient appears well. Thus, it is prudent to admit all patients with acute graft failure to the ICU for initiation of therapy. If systolic failure is more than mild, IV milrinone should be initiated, and the patient should be monitored for dysrhythmias. Unless graft failure is known to be due to coronary artery disease, treatment for acute rejection/graft dysfunction should be initiated with IV methylprednisolone (10–15 mg/kg, maximum 1 g) daily for 3–5 days. It is optimal to obtain an endomyocardial biopsy if the patient is sufficiently stable, as acute graft dysfunction may be associated with AMR secondary to circulating donor-specific anti-HLA antibodies. Additional therapies may then be required, including plasmapheresis and anti–B-cell/plasma cell agents (39). It should be emphasized that treatment of severe acute rejection should not be delayed while awaiting endomyocardial biopsy or biopsy results. Acute rejection with hemodynamic compromise can be rapidly fatal. Unless specific contraindications exist, such patients should receive full hemodynamic support, including use of mechanical support, as the condition is often reversible in nature. Of interest, recent studies show a fall in the incidence of first year (43) and late (44) acute rejection episodes in the recent era. However, the negative impact of late rejection episodes on the risks of death and development of coronary artery disease (see below) has not changed over time. Furthermore, although the incidences of rejection with preserved graft function and rejection with mild hemodynamic compromise have fallen over time, the incidence of the severest form of rejection (rejection with hemodynamic compromise requiring inotropic support) has not (45), and neither has the death rate for rejection with severe hemodynamic compromise (43). This emphasizes the need for improved recognition and management of the most severe forms of rejection.

Chronic Rejection and Posttransplant Coronary Arterial Disease

The terms *chronic rejection* and *posttransplant arterial disease* are generally used synonymously. Coronary disease subsequent to transplantation is an accelerated vasculopathy that is the leading cause of death among late survivors of pediatric heart transplantation (2,41,46,47). The pathology differs somewhat from that of ischemic heart disease in the normal adult population. Typical allograft coronary arterial disease consists of myointimal proliferation that is generally concentric and involves the entire length of the vessel, including intramyocardial branches. Eventually, luminal occlusion occurs, often with associated inflammation. Both immune and nonimmune mechanisms likely contribute to the development of graft vasculopathy, although immune mechanisms are probably of central importance in young children. Intriguing data have recently been published that show that persistence of viral genome of various viruses (especially adenovirus) detected in the myocardium of heart biopsy samples by polymerase chain reaction (PCR) predicts the development of coronary disease and late graft loss in children (48,49). Use of older donors, donor cigarette usage, late acute rejection episodes, older recipient age, retransplantation, and black race are some of the risk factors reported for the development of posttransplant coronary arterial disease (14,46). CMV infection may also contribute to the development of graft vascular disease (50).

Symptoms of ischemia are often absent, though some children experience episodes of abdominal pain and/or chest pain despite operative denervation of the heart (47). Syncope and sudden death are also common presentations of graft coronary disease in children. In the current era, the diagnosis is most often made during surveillance-selective coronary angiography. Intravascular ultrasound has much greater sensitivity for this diagnosis, though experience in children is much more limited than in adults.

Unfortunately, no curative treatment exists for established coronary arterial disease. Diastolic dysfunction tends to develop early and may be observed even with little evidence of epicardial coronary artery narrowing (51), which may be a reflection of diffuse small-vessel disease in many patients. Once overt systolic failure ensues, survival is poor, and consideration should be given to retransplantation. These patients sometimes require admission to the ICU for heart failure management. As with patients with ischemic myopathy, inotropic agents should be used with great caution. Patients with ischemia-induced syncope should receive automatic implantable cardioverter defibrillators if they are to be discharged from the hospital. However, it may be more prudent to keep such patients in hospital until retransplantation can be performed. β Blockers may be given for their anti-ischemic benefits if heart failure is not advanced and β agonists are not required. Percutaneous coronary interventions may have a role in select patients but are limited by the diffuse and small-vessel nature of the disease (52). Early outcomes for late retransplantation (performed more than 6 months after primary transplant) are similar to those for primary transplantation (26). However, recent data suggest that late outcomes after retransplantation are inferior with decreased long-term survival and increase in transplant-related morbidities, such as chronic renal dysfunction (53). There is little experience with a third transplant, though some success has been achieved (54).

Infections

An increased prevalence of all forms of infection is seen in patients after heart transplantation, compared to the general population of children. Most infections are caused by pathogens that also cause infection in the nonimmunocompromised host. Common examples include respiratory viruses, *Streptococcus pneumoniae*, and varicella virus. All infections that occur in nonimmunocompromised patients can cause greater disease severity in the recipient of a transplanted heart. Of particular note in this respect are infections due to CMV and EBV, which only rarely cause severe disease in the immunocompetent host. Rarely, opportunistic infections are seen due to *P. jiroveci* (28). Although most infections are well tolerated, infection is second only to graft failure as a major cause of death in the first 30 days after transplantation and second only to acute rejection as the main cause of death during the remainder of the first posttransplant year (2). On rare occasion, transplant recipients with severe infection require admission to the ICU. The principles of treatment are broadly the same as for severe infection/septic shock in the nonimmunocompromised host. Severe infection is often associated with immune paralysis; in general, if the child is sick enough to warrant admission to the ICU, maintenance immunosuppression should be temporarily withheld. However, corticosteroids should not be discontinued if they are being used chronically, and stress dosing may be indicated.

Broad-spectrum antibiotic coverage is required in any septic transplant recipient until an organism has been identified. *Streptococcus pneumoniae* infections occur with increased frequency, and antibiotics must be administered to cover this agent. When there is clinical and radiographic evidence of pneumonia and deteriorating clinical status, the clinician should maintain a low threshold for performing bronchoalveolar lavage to obtain deep cultures for viruses, fungi, and bacteria. *P. jiroveci* should be ruled out when hypoxia occurs and characteristic chest x-ray film changes are seen. Respiratory viral pathogens (e.g., respiratory syncytial virus (RSV), influenza, parainfluenza, adenovirus) should be sought when evidence of severe respiratory infection is seen in a heart transplant recipient. While viral respiratory disorders tend to be well tolerated in older children, and when further out from transplantation, acquisition of one of these respiratory viruses in the first few weeks after transplant can cause devastating disease, especially in infants.

Primary CMV infection is less problematic in heart transplant patients than in lung transplant recipients. In the former, pneumonitis is rare, whereas it is a common site of disease in lung and heart–lung recipients who develop primary infection posttransplantation. In heart recipients, gastroenteritis, hepatitis, and bone marrow suppression are relatively common findings. Diagnosis is facilitated by evaluation of peripheral blood by PCR or for antigen (pp65) testing. Diagnosis of CMV *disease* remains a tissue diagnosis. When the diagnosis is made early, treatment with IV ganciclovir and/or oral valganciclovir is usually very effective.

EBV infection in the immunocompromised host can be asymptomatic or cause a nonspecific viral syndrome, mononucleosis, fulminant "viral sepsis," or posttransplant lymphoproliferative disorder (PTLD). The strongest risk factor for the development of PTLD is the development of primary EBV infection posttransplantation, although children who are seropositive for EBV at the time of transplant are not completely protected (55). An analysis of the Pediatric Heart Transplant Study (PHTS) database provides the most comprehensive analysis of PTLD in the pediatric heart population. This study identified 56 cases among 1184 primary transplants (4.7%) at 19 North American centers (56). EBV drove almost 90%, and all but one was of B-cell origin. Most patients were treated with reduced immunosuppression, which resulted in complete remission in 75% of cases. However, relapse occurred in 19%, and the probability of survival after diagnosis was only 75%, 68%, and 67% at 1, 3, and 5 years, respectively. Therapeutic strategies include reduction, or temporary cessation, of immunosuppression and the administration of antiviral agents (without proven benefit), monoclonal antibodies against B-cell antigens (e.g., rituximab, a human/mouse chimeric monoclonal antibody directed against the CD20 antigen), chemotherapy, and, rarely, cellular (adoptive) immunotherapy. With the latter, patients are given infusions of autologous cytotoxic T lymphocytes (cultured *ex vivo*) directed against EBV-specific antigens. This experimental approach is under investigation in children at a small number of centers. Children with fulminant EBV sepsis and some with severe PTLD require admission to the ICU. The major role of the intensivist is general supportive care, recognition and treatment of comorbid infections, and monitoring of graft function that may be compromised at presentation or following therapeutic reduction in immunosuppression. Coordination of care among multiple specialists is an important aspect of the management of these sick patients in the ICU.

Nonimmune Complications

In addition to the consequences of over- or under-immunosuppression, transplant recipients experience a wide array of nonimmune toxicities of immunosuppressive therapies. These include systemic hypertension, hyperlipidemia, glucose intolerance, decreased bone mineral density, and bone marrow suppression (40). One complication worthy of particular attention is that of progressive renal dysfunction due to calcineurin inhibitor renal toxicity, which is becoming increasingly problematic as larger numbers of children survive long term after heart transplantation. Some have already developed end-stage renal failure, requiring renal transplantation (57,58). It is important to carefully monitor renal function in all transplant recipients admitted to the ICU and to make appropriate dose adjustments to relevant medications based on estimates of creatinine clearance. It should be noted that estimates and direct measures of creatinine clearance overestimate glomerular filtration rate in this population and that the severity of renal disease is generally greater than perceived (57). Use of nephrotoxic drugs should be minimized when possible.

Survival

Parents and patients are interested in the chances of survival once a decision has been made to proceed with listing for cardiac transplantation. Despite this, emphasis is rarely given to pretransplant mortality and the optimal timing of transplantation (59). Premature transplantation results in exposure of the recipient to the hazards of transplantation and long-term immunosuppression. Excessive delay may result in death without transplantation or the development of comorbidities that may increase operative risk. These comorbidities include progressive end-organ dysfunction (especially renal), malnutrition associated with advanced heart failure, and progressive rise in PVR. These observations emphasize the importance of studying outcomes after listing the patient for transplantation—and not just after transplantation.

Data from the US Scientific Registry of Transplant Recipients reveal that children in all age groups have substantially shorter waiting times for heart transplants than do adults, but they have a greater risk of death while waiting (http://srtr.transplant.hrsa.gov/). The highest death rate is among infants <1 year of age. The use of ABO-incompatible heart transplants may decrease wait-list mortality in infant heart transplant candidates (60). Several analyses of the PHTS database have focused on understanding risk factors for survival after listing for transplantation and for defining the optimal timing of transplantation (41). It has recently been shown that children awaiting transplant at the lowest urgency status (United Network for Organ Sharing [UNOS] status 2 in the United States) have a very low risk of sudden death while waiting if the underlying etiology is dilated cardiomyopathy. This statistic contrasts with the high risk of sudden death in adults with ischemic etiology who are on the transplant waiting list. These data suggest that routine use of automatic implantable cardioverter defibrillators in all children awaiting transplant is not indicated, though certain subpopulations may benefit.

Data from the registries of the ISHLT (2), the US Scientific Registry of Transplant Recipients (http://srtr.transplant.hrsa.gov/), and the PHTS (41) all demonstrate important trends in posttransplant survival over the last two decades. Importantly, significant improvements in outcome have occurred in recent years (Fig. 76.2), with improved survival being most evident in the infant age group and at smaller volume centers. Most of the improvement appears to be due to reduction in early mortality. One-year survival is now ~90% at many centers, with only a relatively small drop over the following 3–4 years. The PHTS and the ISHLT databases continue to show a slightly higher perioperative and early mortality for infant recipients, but interestingly, these youngest recipients have the greatest conditional graft half-life based on analysis of 1-year survivors (2). It is likely that this reflects a lower incidence of posttransplant coronary artery disease in these very young recipients and a degree of immune privilege. The results of transplantation for congenital heart disease still lag behind those of transplantation for cardiomyopathy; this difference is due to slightly higher perioperative mortality. Importantly, evidence of reduced late survival has been noted among African American pediatric recipients compared to Caucasians (61). The reasons for this discrepancy are under active evaluation.

Very long-term survival beyond two decades does occur for a significant minority of patients undergoing transplantation in childhood (62). Adult survivors of childhood transplantation generally report a good quality of life and demonstrate the ability to obtain an education and to work and live independently (63).

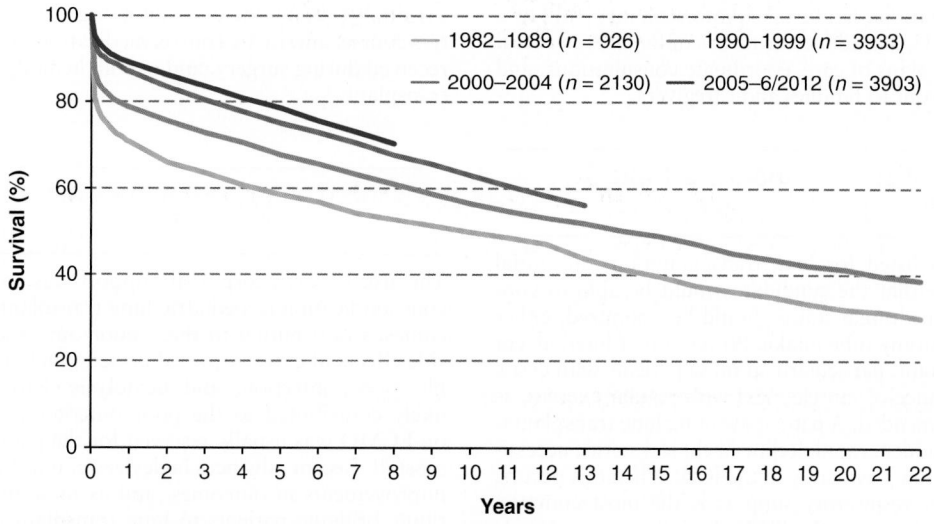

FIGURE 76.2. Pediatric heart transplantation survival by era. Results from the International Society for Heart and Lung Transplantation Registry Report, 2014.

Conclusions and Future Directions

Despite advances in medical and surgical care from the pretransplant through posttransplant periods, heart transplantation remains palliative, and all recipients are at risk for the adverse effects of nonspecific immunosuppression. Current immunosuppressive agents have narrow therapeutic windows and exhibit a wide array of organ toxicities, particularly in young patients. New immunosuppressive regimens have lowered the rates of acute rejection but appear to have had relatively little impact on the incidence of chronic rejection, the principal cause of late graft loss. The ultimate goal is to induce a state of donor-specific tolerance, wherein the recipient will accept the allograft indefinitely without the need for long-term immunosuppression. This quest is currently being realized in animal models of solid-organ transplantation and offers great hope for children undergoing heart transplantation in the future.

LUNG TRANSPLANTATION

Historical Background

Lung transplantation has a rich, albeit somewhat torrid, history. Vladimir Demikhov (64), who also modeled procedures for other solid-organ transplants, performed the first lung transplant on a canine. His findings were presented in May 1947 during Moscow's first All-Union Conference on Thoracic Surgery. Over the next several years, the technique was refined and the first human lung transplant was performed on June 11, 1963, on John Richard Russell, a 58-year-old convicted murderer for the treatment of lung cancer. Pardoned by the governor, he died 18 days later secondary to complications related to rejection and renal failure (65,66). The first pediatric lung transplant was performed in 1987 in a 16-year-old male with familial pulmonary fibrosis (67).

In 2003, Jesica Santillan made world headlines when she inadvertently received an ABO-mismatched donor heart and lungs following an error in compatibility checking. The error was discovered near the end of the case; she was retransplanted 13 days later but sustained a severe brain injury and died several days later.

In May 2005, The UNOS ruled to eliminate the historical measure of having pediatric patients accrue time on a waiting list prior to lung transplantation. UNOS devised a "Lung allocation score" for adults and assigned "Priority Scores" for children. Pediatric candidates were classified as either "Priority 1" or "Priority 2." Children in Priority 1 status had either respiratory failure or pulmonary hypertension with severe associated illness. Additionally, the UNOS ruling directed pediatric organs to children, which was considered a major step forward for children and families who had agonized over the prior allocation scheme.

In 2013, the family of Sarah Murnaghan petitioned a federal judge to order Health and Human Services Secretary Kathleen Sebelius to hold the "Under 12" rule for 10 days such that their 10-year-old daughter with end-stage lung disease would be considered eligible for adult lungs (68). A second family followed suit several days later. Sarah Murnaghan underwent lung transplantation with adult lungs on June 12, 2013; the lungs failed and received a second set of adult donor lungs after a period of time on extracorporeal support. At the time of submission, she had undergone a tracheotomy and required mechanical ventilation for part of the day at home. The fate of the second child could not be ascertained via conventional searches.

Indications for Transplantation

In children, the most common diagnosis for lung transplantation is end-stage lung disease secondary to cystic fibrosis, accounting for over than 50% of lung transplant referrals. The second most common diagnosis is pulmonary hypertension; children may develop this condition primarily or owing to a host of other preexisting conditions, such as complex congenital heart disease, pulmonary hypoplasia secondary to congenital diaphragmatic hernia, or alveolar capillary dysplasia. Additionally, disorders of surfactant protein synthesis may result in end-stage lung disease prompting referral for lung transplantation (69).

Evaluation of the Transplant Candidate

Careful selection and timing of listing of patients is essential to optimize outcomes. At our institution, patients are presented at a multidisciplinary conference such that results of laboratory testing, review of pulmonary function parameters, and anatomic considerations can be taken into account (70). For a patient in the PICU, attendance at these conferences is useful to devise ongoing plans of care, coordinate consultations, and present a united front to families and caregivers.

Care of the Preoperative Lung Transplant Candidate

Once a patient is listed for lung transplantation, the initial strategy would be that the candidate would be able to convalesce. Ideally, nutritional status should be optimized, either via oral or gastrostomy tube intake. Prevention of intercurrent infection is important, particularly in those patients with cystic fibrosis. Maintenance of muscle mass with regular exercise as tolerated is recommended. A patient awaiting lung transplantation may have a sudden, rapid decline in clinical status, necessitating hospitalization, frequently to the ICU. When this occurs, increased need for respiratory support is the most common indication for admission to the PICU. Initially, some patients can be managed with noninvasive mechanical ventilator support; however, many patients will need to be intubated prior to transplantation. Attention to fluid status, renal function, infection, and neurologic functioning become paramount once a patient is hospitalized. Application of noninvasive mechanical ventilatory support such as biphasic level positive airway pressure (BiPAP) may reduce work of breathing with end-stage lung disease. Patients are usually anxious, and initiation of BiPAP may be difficult. Use of low-dose sedatives may be helpful, but care must be taken to avoid excess somnolence. Application of noninvasive support is best initiated and titrated in the ICU setting. Use of transcutaneous carbon dioxide monitoring may be useful in assessing response; any new agitation, somnolence, or hypoxemia should be treated as a failure of therapy.

Intubating a patient with impending respiratory failure secondary to end-stage lung disease, particularly those who have been maintained on noninvasive support, can be challenging. The patient's functional residual capacity is decreased, and the patient maintained on BiPAP may not tolerate its removal. To create ideal intubating conditions, the patient should be placed in 100% oxygen and prior levels of noninvasive support maintained. An experienced airway expert should perform the procedure, and prolonged desaturation should be anticipated. Additionally, these patients frequently have impaired venous return, so compromised cardiac output immediately following the procedure should also be anticipated. Following intubation, patients with obstructive lung disease should be placed on ventilator settings that will allow for a prolonged expiratory phase. Deep sedation and, frequently, neuromuscular blockade are required to facilitate interaction with the ventilator.

Evaluation of the Lung Donor

A comprehensive review of lung donor criteria and allocation is out of scope of this chapter. For the pediatric intensivist, it is important to know that donor factors such as trauma, hemodynamic derangements, and edema may result in the development of reperfusion injury and primary graft dysfunction. For a complete review, the reader is referred to a publication of the American Thoracic Society devoted to this topic (71).

Surgical Techniques of Graft Implantation

For those wishing to review the technical details of lung transplantation, the reader is referred to a review by Boasquevisque et al. (72). For the pediatric intensivist, surgical details that are

essential to know include donor organ ischemic time, operative course, anesthetic course, medications and blood products received during surgery, and overall hemodynamics during the transplant.

Extracorporeal Support as Bridge to Lung Transplantation

The use of extracorporeal support has historically been a contraindication to pediatric lung transplant due to poor outcomes. Contributing to these poor outcomes are the known side effects of extracorporeal devices, including bleeding complications, infection, and hemolysis. Patient selection also likely contributed to the poor outcomes, in that placement on ECMO was usually reserved for the patients that were the most ill. Recent advances in devices and techniques have led to improvements in outcomes, and as these improvements continue, bridging patients to lung transplant using extracorporeal support may become a more viable option.

Early studies in adults reported the perioperative mortality in patients requiring ECMO support as high as 60% (73). More recent studies in adults, however, demonstrate 1-year survival rates posttransplant in patients bridged with ECMO of 60%–75% (74–76). Although this represents an overall improvement when compared to early studies, survival still remains lower than patients not requiring ECMO support. Outcomes in pediatric patients are more difficult to determine given the small amount of data available. In the largest retrospective study, pediatric patients requiring ECMO support in the period prior to transplant have poor outcomes (77). Of 344 patients receiving lung transplants, 15 required ECMO support preoperatively (14 veno-arterial and 1 veno-venous ECMO support). The median duration of ECMO support in these patients was 9.75 days, and all patients survived to transplant. Six patients (40%) were weaned from ECMO prior to transplant, and four of these patients survived to hospital discharge (66%). Of the nine patients that were still on ECMO at the time of transplant, only two (22%) survived to hospital discharge. The 1-year survival in the ECMO group was 33% versus 80.2% in patients not requiring pretransplant ECMO (77). Due to these results, the use of veno-arterial ECMO is considered a contraindication for pediatric lung transplant in many centers. Results of patients bridged to transplant using veno-venous ECMO (VV ECMO) have been encouraging in adults (78,79). Recently, Schmidt and colleagues (80) published a case series of three pediatric patients who were placed on VV ECMO as a bridge to lung transplantation. Two of the three patients, both with a diagnosis of cystic fibrosis, were successfully bridged to transplant and survived to hospital discharge. Importantly, all three of these patients were able to be extubated for a period of time and participate in physical therapy. As in the adult patients in whom this technique has been applied (74,81,82), the ability to awaken and extubate these patients helps to minimize complications related to long-term ventilation and sedation (infection, muscle fatigue, and organ dysfunction) (83,84). The use of VV ECMO is not without risk, however, as one of the patients in this report dislocated the cannula during physical therapy, resulting in desaturation and requiring reintubation and urgent repositioning (80). While the outcomes from small case series employing VV ECMO in pediatric patients are encouraging, larger studies are still needed to determine the feasibility of this technique.

Due to the high mortality in patients requiring ECMO support prior to lung transplant, alternative extracorporeal devices have been attempted to bridge these patients to transplant. One of these devices is the Novalung®. The Novalung®

is primarily designed for patients with hypercarbic respiratory failure. It has been used successfully to bridge adult patients to lung transplant (85,86). In a study of 12 adult patients awaiting lung transplant, 10 were successfully bridged to lung transplant after a mean duration of support on the Novalung® of 15 ± 8 days (87). In this study, eight (80%) of the patients were still alive 1-year posttransplant.

Although the results with the Novalung® are hopeful, it is not currently approved for pediatric use. Because of this, other devices have been used in a similar manner. A recent case report describes the use of a paracorporeal lung assist device in a neonate with alveolar capillary dysplasia (88). This device utilizes the membrane oxygenator from a pediatric ECMO circuit, the Quadrox iD, with cannulation of the pulmonary artery and left atrium. The infant described was supported with this device for a total of 54 days, unfortunately dying from bilateral intracranial hemorrhages (88). This is a promising approach for infants awaiting lung transplant, but further studies are clearly needed.

With continued advances in extracorporeal devices, successful bridging of pediatric patients to lung transplantation may become more feasible. Earlier deployment of these devices, prior to the development of organ dysfunction, may lead to improved long-term survival in this subset of patients.

Postoperative Management and Early Complications

Complete and accurate communication about preoperative recipient and donor status is crucial for the planning of optimal postoperative management strategies of a lung transplant recipient. Donor-related factors that impact postoperative management include donor weight, clinical condition, cause of death, premorbid conditions (related or unrelated to the cause of death), and donor immunologic status against CMV. Donor weight is an important piece of information that helps plan ventilation for the recipient. The severity of illness, clinical condition of the donor prior to death, the cause of death, and other donor premorbidities are known to affect the postoperative function of the transplanted lungs (89). Donor CMV status will determine if the recipient will require pharmacologic prophylaxis. As the waiting list of recipients increases and so do deaths while awaiting transplant, there is increasing acceptance of lungs from suboptimal donors (e.g., low donor PaO_2, or pulmonary infiltrates). This may impact the recipient's postoperative recovery and required management (90). With respect to the transplant recipient, it is essential to understand the reason for transplant, clinical condition pretransplant (ventilation or other respiratory support, cardiac support, colonization/infection pretransplant and drug resistance patterns, nutritional status, and social support system). This information allows for planning of care needed by the patient posttransplant in the ICU, general hospital wards, and also long term for discharge planning.

Acute Complications

Reperfusion Injury/Graft Failure

Reperfusion injury can occur from restoring blood supply to the ischemic donor lungs during and after transplant. Reperfusion injury is characterized by infiltrates on CXR and poor gas exchange that can be self-limited or progress to early graft failure. About 20%–30% of transplant recipients experience some degree of reperfusion damage. Treatment options include inhaled nitric oxide (iNO), PGE_1, positive pressure ventilation, and extracorporeal support. Acute graft failure is a major cause of death in the first 30 days (91).

Acute Rejection

Acute rejection of the donor organ by the recipient's immunologic system can present with poor gas exchange, increasing chest tube drainage, frothy sputum, and worsening gas exchange. Pathologically, acute rejection is seen as infiltrates in the perivascular and interstitial regions with associated airway inflammation (92). Acute rejection is treated with intravenous methylprednisolone, 10 mg/kg/d for 3 days. Rejection refractory to methylprednisolone is treated with ATG for 7–10 days. Recurrent rejection warrants consideration of change in the immunosuppression regimen.

Systemic Inflammatory Response Syndrome

Recipients may demonstrate varying degree of systemic inflammatory response syndrome from immunologic or infectious phenomena in the immediate posttransplant period. Treatment includes supportive care to provide adequate assistance to hemodynamics and organ function.

Bleeding

Postoperative bleeding is not uncommon and can arise from vascular anastomotic sites, surgical planes of dissection, or airways. Factors that increase risk of bleeding include preoperative infections, duration of surgery, and organ function.

Nerve Injury

Phrenic nerve injury is not uncommon especially after bilateral lung transplantation and can complicate postoperative respiratory recovery (93).

Posttransplant Surveillance: Bronchoscopy, Computerized Tomography, Radiographs, Pulmonary Function Testing

Routine postoperative surveillance includes daily chest radiographs while chest tubes are in place. Radiographs allow the provider to follow lung parenchymal changes, assess lung volumes, check catheter and tube position, and to detect evolving effusions. Bronchoscopy is usually performed at 24 hours posttransplant to check for mucosal and anastomotic integrity, graft perfusion, and to facilitate clearance of bronchial secretions/blood. Bronchoscopies are repeated posttransplant, usually at 2, 4, 8, and 12 weeks, then every 3 months thereafter. Transbronchial biopsies are performed at the time of bronchoscopy (94). Chest computerized tomography (CT), ventilation perfusion scans, and pulmonary function tests are performed quarterly for first year after transplant and then semiannually for routine surveillance (95,96). Additional chest radiography, CTs, and bronchoscopies are also performed as needed whenever clinical concern arises with new respiratory symptoms or worsening pulmonary function. CT scans have also been shown to be a useful tool to assess growth of transplanted lungs in infants and young children (97).

Subacute Complications

Anastomotic complications such as airway/vascular dehiscence or stenosis may complicate both the immediate and posttransplant time periods. Airway dehiscence was a common complication in early transplant recipients; this improved after the practice of wrapping omentum around the anastomotic site (designed to restore some bronchial circulation) (98). Omental wrapping is no longer used but donor and recipient peribronchial tissue is approximated near the anastomotic site (99). Bronchial stenosis can affect as many as 10% of lung transplant cases and can be effectively treated with bronchoscopic dilation (100). Transplanted airways grow with somatic growth and bronchial stenosis is not affected by age or size of the recipient (97).

Cardiovascular Considerations

Inotropic Agents and Cardiopulmonary Interactions

The immediate posttransplant lung recipient arrives to the ICU, still intubated, ventilated, and on pressors (e.g., epinephrine, vasopressin) as warranted by the hemodynamics. PGE_1 is routinely administered postoperatively for about 48 hours. It is believed that PGE_1 infusion during and after the ischemic period has the potential to reduce reperfusion injury of the donor lungs. This allows for improved oxygenation and compliance while on the ventilator (101). Recipients are also placed on iNO postoperatively until extubation. Nitric oxide has been described to improve the Pao_2/Fio_2 ratio and decreases pulmonary arterial pressure in postoperative patients with severe graft dysfunction (Pao_2/Fio_2 <150) (102).

Dysrhythmias

Atrial flutter or fibrillation has been reported in nearly 10% of lung transplant cases and is thought to be generated by the electrical aberrance produced by the suture lines for pulmonary venous anastomosis (103,104).

Systemic Hypertension

Hypertension is common in the immediate posttransplant period and is likely multifactorial in etiology. Immunosuppression with high-dose steroids, calcineurin inhibitors, and acute kidney dysfunction (from post-cardiopulmonary bypass and nephrotoxic medications) are common contributors. Severe systemic hypertension may result in surgical site bleeding or derangement in neurologic function. Treatment usually includes short-term antihypertensive agents such as calcium-channel blockers in order to allow for rapid titration of effect.

Respiratory Support

Transplant recipients usually have four chest tubes, two on each side, to drain any surgical bleeding, collections, and pleural effusions. The amount of drainage is expected to decrease over first few days after transplant in the absence of any significant bleeding issues and reperfusion injury to the transplanted lungs. Management goals include achievement of optimal gas exchange, overall negative fluid balance to facilitate improved compliance, and liberation of the patient from sedation and positive pressure ventilation.

Control of Ventilation

Lung transplant recipients are frequently noted to have a specific pattern of breathing characterized by deep and infrequent breaths, due to the denervated donor organs generating a pattern of hyperpneic/hypopneic breathing that may lead to patient–ventilator dyssynchrony, significant discomfort, and agitation. Allowing the patient to dictate the ventilation needs and providing ventilator support that suits the pattern of breathing may facilitate separation from mechanical ventilator support.

Criteria for Extubation

The treatment goal is to be able to extubate as soon as possible to allow weaning of sedatives and to facilitate pulmonary toilet. The requisites for extubation are adequate gas exchange, good mucosal perfusion and integrity on bronchoscopy, and hemodynamic stability. The functional status of the neurologic and renal systems, fluid status, and presence of infection should be taken into consideration prior to extubation.

Gastrointestinal Complications

Gastrointestinal complications are common in the post–lung transplant recipient, especially gastroesophageal reflux disease. Postoperative ileus is also common and requires aggressive preventive and therapeutic strategies to facilitate gut motility (94).

Endocrine Considerations

Hyperglycemia is common and may result from preexisting pancreatic insufficiency in cystic fibrosis patients or from high-dose steroids administered as part of the immunosuppressive regimen. Insulin infusions are the mainstay of therapy and easily titrated.

Renal Function

Acute kidney injury (AKI) is common due to exposure to cardiopulmonary bypass, fluid shifts, and nephrotoxic medications such as immunosuppressive agents (calcineurin inhibitors) and antibiotics (aminoglycosides). Vigilant monitoring to detect early changes in renal function parameters and crucial fluid management are necessary to avoid graft dysfunction while balancing AKI.

Infectious Precautions

Lung transplant recipients are more susceptible than other solid-organ recipients to develop infections because of colonization of recipient and donor airways with organisms. In the early posttransplant period, infections with bacteria and certain viruses, such as adenovirus, influenza, parainfluenza, and RSV, are common. Agents causing late infections include CMV, EBV, and fungal organisms. Infections delay recovery, affect transplanted and other organ function, can hamper immunosuppressive regimens, and are a major cause of morbidity and mortality. Cystic fibrosis patients have increased risk of infections and are specifically prone to infections from colonization with resistant organisms prior to transplant. Aggressive systemic and/or aerosolized antibiotics, antiviral or antifungal therapies, and modification of immunosuppression along with supportive care are warranted to treat infections adequately (105–107).

Immunosuppression

The depth and breadth of knowledge surrounding transplant immunology is expanding rapidly and is out of scope for this chapter; a full review has been published by Heeger and Dinavahi (108). Activation of both the innate and the adaptive responses following transplantation occurs and is the main component of long-term graft survival. The innate nonspecific rapid response activating compliment and toll-like receptor signaling is triggered by the ischemia and healing, potentially adding to the posttransplant injury (109,110). The adaptive immune response is composed of antibody-producing B cells and T cells, and develops slower than innate immune response but is more specific and result in memory (111). This specificity and memory, although essential for controlling and preventing infections, is detrimental to the transplanted organ.

Current immunosuppressive regimens target relatively specific steps in the stimulation or activation of T cells or eliminating alloreactive B cells. Costimulation is required for T-cell activation and the US Food and Drug Administration approved one agent, belatacept, that blocks the interaction between T-cell–expressed CD28 and antigen-presenting cell–expressed CD80, in 2011 (112). Although a number of other potential costimulatory targets are under review, none are currently approved for lung transplantation recipients (113). If both a signal through the T-cell receptor and a second co-stimulatory signal occur, then a number of intracellular activation steps are required for full T-cell activation, including the calcium flux, which in turn activates calmodulin allowing it to bind to calcineurin. This calcium-binding protein is the target of the immunosuppressant drugs cyclosporine A and tacrolimus (108). Following T-cell activation, there is an up-regulation and expression of the high-affinity α chain of the IL-2R (CD25) on the surface of the T cell, which is the target of anti-CD25 monoclonal antibodies basiliximab and daclizumab. Signaling through the IL-2R also mediates progression of the cell cycle, from G1 to S, resulting in proliferation of the T cell. This cascade requires the protein mammalian target of rapamycin, which is the target of sirolimus. The cell-cycle inhibitors, azathioprine and mycophenolic acid, are inhibitors of DNA synthesis and thus inhibit T-cell activation at this stage (108). Corticosteroids inhibit the expression and transcription of several cytokine genes including IL-2, thereby blocking T-cell proliferation and T-cell–dependent immunity (114).

Prior to transplant an alloreactive T-cell repertoire of memory cells against a variety of HLAs may be present as a result of pregnancy, blood transfusion, previous transplant, or chance cross-reactivity with environmental antigens (115–117). These alloreactive memory cells have lower, different costimulatory requirements than naïve cells, are resistant to most immunosuppressant medications, and can rapidly engage effector machinery without a differentiation step and measurements of donor reactive memory cells performed prior to transplant strongly and directly correlate with worse posttransplant outcomes (118–121).

Attempts have been made to reduce these high panel-reactive antibody titers with an induction schema using either intravenous immunoglobulin or plasmapheresis, although there is no currently accepted standard of practice. Another therapeutic strategy to limit antibody-mediated injury is to eliminate alloreactive B cells using therapeutic agents such as rituximab, an antibody specific for CD20 that is capable of depleting B cells (122).

A recent report from the Registry of the ISHLT reviewed data on immunosuppressive regimes for patients receiving lung transplants between January 2001 and June 2011. Induction therapy was used in more than 60% of pediatric recipients, with ~50% of those receiving an IL-2R antagonist and some 15% receiving antilymphocyte globulin or ATG. The number of children receiving IL-2R antagonist induction has been on the rise although this has not been shown to confer a survival benefit. The most common maintenance immunosuppressant drug combination at 1-year posttransplant consisted of a calcineurin inhibitor (tacrolimus was used in 80% and cyclosporine in less than 20%), a cell-cycle inhibitor (MMF was used in 66%), and prednisone. Five years after transplantation, almost all patients remained on prednisone and the use of sirolimus/everolimus had increased (123).

The Washington University group has published on their large cohort of pediatric patients and suggests a combination of cyclosporine, azathioprine, and steroids. For the first-year posttransplant, the target trough cyclosporine blood level is 300–400 ng/mL; following this, levels are maintained at 200–300 ng/mL. The initial steroid dose is 0.5 mg/kg daily of prednisone, which is progressively tapered over time but never stopped entirely. An azathioprine dose of 1.5 mg/kg daily is administered as long as the patient's white blood cell count exceeds 4000 cells/mm^3 (124).

Immunoprophylaxis

⑪ Infectious complications are a leading cause for morbidity and mortality in pediatric lung transplantation, accounting for more than 40% of deaths in the first 12 postoperative months (125). Prophylaxis includes a wide range of antimicrobial agents but there are no well-established protocols. Children who are at high risk for CMV infection (defined as positive recipient or donor serology) receive CMV prophylaxis for 3–6 months, although there is no consensus regarding the length of prophylaxis needed. Pulmonary fungal infections are not uncommon, up to 10% in a recent retrospective, multicenter study and are independently associated with a decreased 12-month posttransplantation survival (126). *P. jiroveci* pneumonia (previously *Pneumocystis carinii*) is another common clinical problem following lung transplantation. The authors of a retrospective study suggested that 12 months of treatment is probably sufficient once immunosuppressive therapy is stable (127).

Vaccine-preventable diseases should not be forgotten as children undergoing lung transplantation are at high risk of infections from these agents. National vaccination guidelines should be followed in pediatric transplant candidates and recipients. Vaccine responses may be decreased after transplantation, and live virus vaccines are not routinely recommended. Vaccinations should also include household contacts (128,129).

Outcomes

⑫ Overall, survival of children after lung transplantation is worse than following any other solid-organ transplant but is not significantly different than that reported in adults. In the first year following transplantation, non-CMV infection and graft failure are the leading causes of death. Beyond 3 years after transplantation, chronic rejection in the form of bronchiolitis obliterans syndrome (BOS) is significant, accounting for ~42% of deaths (125). Benden and colleagues, in reviewing the ISHLT Registry, calculated that the half-life (the estimated time at which 50% of recipients died) for patients who received transplants between January 1990 and June 2010 was just over 6 years for infants and children up to 11 years of age and only 4.3 years for older children and adolescents. Survival in the cohort transplanted between 2002 and June 2010 had a 5-year survival of 54% compared with 46% for children who received allografts between 1995 and 2001 (123). Although detailed information regarding quality of life data is not captured in the ISHLT Registry, functional status of pediatric survivors after lung transplantation was reported to be very good, with no activity limitation in 82% of recipients at 5 years after transplantation (123).

Late-Term Complications

There are numerous comorbidities following lung transplantation. AKI is a common complication immediately following transplantation and is associated with increased risk of chronic kidney disease and all-cause mortality on long-term follow-up (130). Hypertension is the most common comorbidity at 47% at 1 and 5 years after transplantation in surviving recipients who received transplants between April 1994 and June 2011 (123). BOS is also common and increases in prevalence over time (123). Several interventions have impacted the deterioration in lung function seen in BOS, such as azithromycin, altered immunosuppression, photopheresis, and prevention or treatment of gastroesophageal reflux disease (131,132); however, BOS remains a leading cause of chronic graft rejection. Posttransplant lymphoproliferative disease (PTLD) in association with a primary EBV infection is another significant comorbidity, found in 13% of patients in one large cohort. These patients were treated initially with reduction in immunosuppression therapy and those not responding were treated with chemotherapy (124).

According to the ISHLT Registry, in the interval from January 1994 to June 2010, 105 retransplant procedures were reported. Retransplantation was performed for obliterative bronchiolitis in approximately half of the patients and most of the retransplantations occurred in recipients aged less than 12 years (125). For pediatric retransplant procedures performed in this interval, survival was 63% at 1 year, 50% at 3 years, and 38% at 5 years. The justice and equity concerns regarding organ allocation and retransplantation are beyond the scope of this work.

Conclusions and Future Directions

Advances continue in the care of the patient undergoing lung transplantation. Despite improvements, long-term graft survival poses continuing challenges to the patient and management of immunosuppressive regimens and prevention of comorbidity is a mainstay of improved outcome. Patients with end-stage lung disease and progressive critical illness are being considered for transplantation more with increasing frequency and involvement of the pediatric intensivist in the preoperative setting is evolving. The use of paracorporeal technology and improved preoperative donor and recipient management may improve outcomes. Ultimately, preventing or delaying the development of bronchiolitis obliterans will impact survival.

References

1. Webber SA, McCurry K, Zeevi A. Seminar: Heart and lung transplantation in children. *Lancet* 2006;368:53–69.
2. Boucek MM, Edwards LB, Keck BM, et al. Registry of the International Society for Heart and Lung Transplantation: Eighth official pediatric report–2005. *J Heart Lung Transplant* 2005;24:968–82.
3. Canter C, Shaddy R, Bernstein D, et al. Indications for transplantation in pediatric heart disease. *Circulation* 2007;115(5):658–76.
4. Fricker FJ, Addonizio L, Bernstein D, et al. Heart transplantation in children: Indications. *Pediatr Transplant* 1999;3:333–42.
5. Chiu P, Russo MJ, Davies RR, et al. What is high risk? Redefining elevated pulmonary vascular resistance index in pediatric heart transplantation. *J Heart Lung Transplant* 2012;31:61–6.
6. Richmond ME, Law YM, Das BB, et al; Pediatric Heart Transplant Study Investigators. Elevated pre-transplant pulmonary vascular resistance is not associated with mortality in children without congenital heart disease: A multicenter study [published online ahead of print May 9, 2014]. *J Heart Lung Transplant.* doi:10.1016/j.healun.2014.04.021
7. Gandhi SK, Grady RM, Huddleston CB, et al. Beyond Berlin: Heart transplantation in the "untransplantable". *J Thorac Cardiovasc Surg* 2008;136(2):529–31.
8. West LJ, Pollock-Barziv SM, Dipchand AI, et al. ABO-incompatible heart transplant in infants. *N Engl J Med* 2001;344:793–800.
9. Urschel S, Larsen IM, Kirk R, et al. ABO-incompatible heart transplantation in early childhood: An international multicenter study of clinical experiences and limits. *J Heart Lung Transplant* 2013;32(3):285–92.
10. Henderson HT, Canter CE, Mahle WT, et al. ABO-incompatible heart transplantation: Analysis of the Pediatric Heart Transplant Study (PHTS) database. *J Heart Lung Transplant* 2012;31(2):173–9.
11. Conway J, Manlhiot C, Allain-Rooney T, et al. Development of donor-specific isohemagglutinins following pediatric ABO-incompatible heart transplantation. *Am J Transplant* 2012;12(4):888–95.
12. L'Ecuyer T, Sloan K, Tang L. Impact of donor cardiopulmonary resuscitation on pediatric heart transplant outcome. *Pediatr Transplant* 2011;15(7):742–5.
13. Conway J, Chin C, Kemna M, et al; Pediatric Heart Transplant Study Investigators. Donors' characteristics and impact on outcomes in pediatric heart transplant recipients. *Pediatr Transplant* 2013;17(8):774–81.
14. Pahl E, Naftel DC, Kuhn MA, et al. The impact and outcome of transplant coronary artery disease in a pediatric population: A 9-year multi-institutional study. *J Heart Lung Transplant* 2005;24:645–51.
15. Ford MA, Almond CS, Gauvreau K, et al. Association of graft ischemic time with survival after heart transplant among children in the United States. *J Heart Lung Transplant* 2011;30(11):1244–9.
16. Rodrigues W, Carr M, Ridout D, et al. Total donor ischemic time: Relationship to early hemodynamics and intensive care morbidity in pediatric cardiac transplant recipients. *Pediatr Crit Care Med* 2011;12(6):660–6.
17. Tang L, Du W, Delius RE, et al. Low donor-to-recipient weight ratio does not negatively impact survival of pediatric heart transplant patients. *Pediatr Transplant* 2010;14(6):741–5.
18. Huang J, Trinkaus K, Huddleston CB, et al. Risk factors for primary graft failure after pediatric cardiac transplantation: Importance of recipient and donor characteristics. *J Heart Lung Transplant* 2004;23:716–22.
19. Pigula FA, Webber SA. Donor evaluation, surgical technique and perioperative management. Chapter 33. In: Fine R, Webber SA, Harmon W, et al., eds. *Pediatric Solid Organ Transplantation.* Oxford, England: Blackwell Publishing, 2007.
20. Sachdeva R, Seib PM, Burns SA, et al. Stenting for superior vena cava obstruction in pediatric heart transplant recipients. *Catheter Cardiovasc Interv* 2007;70(6):888–92.
21. Lamour JM, Hsu DT, Quaegebeur JM, et al. Heart transplantation to a physiologic single lung in patients with congenital heart disease. *J Heart Lung Transplant* 2004;23:948–53.
22. Fenton KN, Webber SA, Danford DA, et al. Long-term survival after pediatric cardiac transplantation and postoperative ECMO support. *Ann Thorac Surg* 2003;76:843–6.
23. Su JA, Kelly RB, Grogan T, et al. Extracorporeal membrane oxygenation support after pediatric orthotopic heart transplantation [published online ahead of print October 27, 2014]. *Pediatr Transplant.* doi:10.1111/petr.12382
24. Kaushal S, Matthews KL, Garcia X, et al. A multicenter study of primary graft failure after infant heart transplantation: Impact of extracorporeal membrane oxygenation on outcomes. *Pediatr Transplant* 2014;18(1):72–8.
25. Tissot C, Buckvold S, Phelps CM, et al. Outcome of extracorporeal membrane oxygenation for early primary graft failure after pediatric heart transplantation. *J Am Coll Cardiol* 2009;54(8):730–7.
26. Chin C, Naftel D, Pahl E, et al. Cardiac retransplantation in pediatrics: A multi-institutional study. *J Heart Lung Transplant* 2006;25:1420–4.
27. Rakhit A, Nurko S, Gauvreau K, et al. Gastrointestinal complications after pediatric cardiac transplantation. *J Heart Lung Transplant* 2002;21:751–9.
28. Ng B, Dipchand A, Naftel D, et al. Outcomes of *Pneumocystis jiroveci* pneumonia infections in pediatric heart transplant recipients. *Pediatr Transplant* 2011;15(8):844–8.
29. Singh TP, Faber C, Blume ED, et al. Safety and early outcomes using a corticosteroid-avoidance immunosuppression protocol in pediatric heart transplant recipients. *J Heart Lung Transplant* 2010;29(5):517–22.

30. Auerbach SR, Gralla J, Campbell DN, et al. Steroid avoidance in pediatric heart transplantation results in excellent graft survival. *Transplantation* 2014;97(4):474–80.

31. Russo L, Webber SA. Pediatric heart transplantation: Immunosuppression and its complications. *Curr Opin Cardiol* 2004;19:104–9.

32. Irving CA, Webber SA. Immunosuppression therapy for pediatric heart transplantation. *Curr Treat Options Cardiovasc Med* 2010;12(5):489–502.

33. Stewart S, Winters GL, Fishbein MC, et al. Revision of the 1990 working formulation for the standardization of nomenclature in the diagnosis of heart rejection. *J Heart Lung Transplant* 2005;24:1710–20.

34. Feingold B, Park SY, Comer DM, et al. Outcomes after listing with a requirement for a prospective crossmatch in pediatric heart transplantation. *J Heart Lung Transplant* 2013;32(1):56–62.

35. Mahle WT, Tresler MA, Edens RE, et al; Pediatric Heart Transplant Study Group. Allosensitization and outcomes in pediatric heart transplantation. *J Heart Lung Transplant* 2011;30(11):1221–7.

36. Irving C, Carter V, Parry G, et al. Donor-specific HLA antibodies in paediatric cardiac transplant recipients are associated with poor graft survival. *Pediatr Transplant* 2011;15(2):193–7.

37. Rossano JW, Morales DL, Zafar F, et al. Impact of antibodies against human leukocyte antigens on long-term outcome in pediatric heart transplant patients: An analysis of the United Network for Organ Sharing database. *J Thorac Cardiovasc Surg* 2010;140(3):694–9, 699.e1–699.e2.

38. Berry GJ, Burke MM, Andersen C, et al. The 2013 International Society for Heart and Lung Transplantation Working Formulation for the standardization of nomenclature in the pathologic diagnosis of antibody-mediated rejection in heart transplantation. *J Heart Lung Transplant* 2013;32(12):1147–62.

39. Morrow WR, Frazier EA, Mahle WT, et al. Rapid reduction in donor-specific anti-human leukocyte antigen antibodies and reversal of antibody-mediated rejection with bortezomib in pediatric heart transplant patients. *Transplantation* 2012;93(3):319–24.

40. Smith JM, Nemeth TL, McDonald RA. Current immunosuppressive agents: Efficacy, side effects, and utilization. *Pediatr Clin North Am* 2003;50:1283–300.

41. Dipchand AI, Kirk R, Mahle WT, et al. Ten yr of pediatric heart transplantation: A report from the Pediatric Heart Transplant Study. *Pediatr Transplant* 2013;17(2):99–111.

42. Webber SA, Naftel DC, Parker J, et al. Late rejection episodes greater than 1 year after pediatric heart transplantation: Risk factors and outcomes. *J Heart Lung Transplant* 2003;22:869–75.

43. Gossett JG, Canter CE, Zheng J, et al; Pediatric Heart Transplant Study Investigators. Decline in rejection in the first year after pediatric cardiac transplantation: A multi-institutional study. *J Heart Lung Transplant* 2010;29(6):625–32.

44. Ameduri RK, Zheng J, Schechtman KB, et al. Has late rejection decreased in pediatric heart transplantation in the current era? A multi-institutional study. *J Heart Lung Transplant* 2012;31(9):980–6.

45. Everitt MD, Pahl E, Schechtman KB, et al; Pediatric Heart Transplant Study Investigators. Rejection with hemodynamic compromise in the current era of pediatric heart transplantation: A multi-institutional study. *J Heart Lung Transplant* 2011;30(3):282–8.

46. Kobayashi D, Du W, L'ecuyer TJ. Predictors of cardiac allograft vasculopathy in pediatric heart transplant recipients. *Pediatr Transplant* 2013;17(5):436–40.

47. Jeewa A, Dreyer WJ, Kearney DL, et al. The presentation and diagnosis of coronary allograft vasculopathy in pediatric heart transplant recipients. *Congenit Heart Dis* 2012;7(4):302–11.

48. Shirali GS, Ni J, Chinnock RE, et al. Association of viral genome with graft loss in children after cardiac transplantation. *N Engl J Med* 2001;344:1498–503.

49. Moulik M, Breinholt JP, Dreyer WJ, et al. Viral endomyocardial infection is an independent predictor and potentially treatable risk factor for graft loss and coronary vasculopathy in pediatric cardiac transplant recipients. *J Am Coll Cardiol* 2010;56(7):582–92.

50. Webber SA. Cytomegalovirus infection and cardiac allograft vasculopathy in children. *Circulation* 2007;115(13):1701–2.

51. Law Y, Boyle G, Miller S, et al. Restrictive hemodynamics are present at the time of diagnosis of allograft coronary artery disease in children. *Pediatr Transplant* 2006;10:948–52.

52. Lee MS, Sachdeva R, Kim MH, et al. Long-term outcomes of percutaneous coronary intervention in transplant coronary artery disease in pediatric heart transplant recipients. *J Invasive Cardiol* 2012;24(6):278–81.

53. Conway J, Manlhiot C, Kirk R, et al. Mortality and morbidity after retransplantation after primary heart transplant in childhood: An analysis from the registry of the International Society for Heart and Lung Transplantation. *J Heart Lung Transplant* 2014;33(3):241–51.

54. Friedland-Little JM, Gajarski RJ, Yu S, et al. Outcomes of third heart transplants in pediatric and young adult patients: analysis of the United Network for Organ Sharing database. *J Heart Lung Transplant* 2014;33(9):917–23.

55. Chinnock R, Webber SA, Dipchand AI, et al; Pediatric Heart Transplant Study. A 16-year multi-institutional study of the role of age and EBV status on PTLD incidence among pediatric heart transplant recipients. *Am J Transplant* 2012;12(11):3061–8.

56. Webber SA, Naftel D, Fricker FJ, et al. Lymphoproliferative disorders after pediatric heart transplantation: A multi-institutional study. *Lancet* 2006;367:233–9.

57. English RF, Pophal SA, Bacanu S, et al. Long-term comparison of tacrolimus and cyclosporine induced nephrotoxicity in pediatric heart transplant recipients. *Am J Transplant* 2002;2:769–73.

58. Feingold B, Zheng J, Law YM, et al; Pediatric Heart Transplant Study Investigators. Risk factors for late renal dysfunction after pediatric heart transplantation: a multi-institutional study. *Pediatr Transplant* 2011;15(7):699–705.

59. Singh TP, Almond CS, Piercey G, et al. Risk stratification and transplant benefit in children listed for heart transplant in the United States. *Circ Heart Fail* 2013;6(4):800–8.

60. West LJ, Karamlou T, Dipchand AI, et al. Impact on outcomes after listing and transplantation, of a strategy to accept ABO blood group-incompatible donor hearts for neonates and infants. *J Thorac Cardiovasc Surg* 2006;131:455–61.

61. Singh TP, Almond C, Givertz MM, et al. Improved survival in heart transplant recipients in the United States: Racial differences in era effect. *Circ Heart Fail* 2011;4(2):153–60.

62. Copeland H, Razzouk A, Chinnock R, et al. Pediatric recipient survival beyond 15 post-heart transplant years: A single-center experience. *Ann Thorac Surg* 2014;98(6):2145–51.

63. Hollander SA, Chen S, Luikart H, et al. Quality of life and metrics of achievement in long-term adult survivors of pediatric heart transplant [published online ahead of print November 12, 2014]. *Pediatr Transplant*. doi:10.1111/petr.12384

64. Demikhov VP. The homoplastic transplantation of organs. In: *Experimental Transplantation of Vital Organs*. Authorized translation from the Russian by Basil Haigh. New York, NY: Consultants Bureau, 1962:129–35.

65. Transplanting of Lung Apparently Successful. *Tucson Daily Citizen* June 13, 1963:1.

66. Barnett to Free Killer Who Had Lung Transplant. *Miami News* June 26, 1963:3A.

67. Mendeloff EN. The history of pediatric heart and lung transplantation. *Pediatr Transplant* 2002;6:270–9.

68. Judge Rules Temporarily for Pa Girl Who Needs Lungs. *The Philadelphia Inquirer* June 7, 2013.

69. Sweet SC. Pediatric lung transplantation. *Proc Am Thorac Soc* 2009;6:122–7.

70. Kreider M, Kotloff RM. Selection of candidates for lung transplantation. *Proc Am Thorac Soc* 2009;6:20–7.

71. Van Raemdonck D, Neyrinck A, Verleden GM, et al. Lung donor selection and management. *Proc Am Thorac Soc* 2009;6:28–38.

72. Boasquevisque CHR, Yildirim E, Waddel TK, et al. Surgical techniques: Lung transplant and lung volume reduction. *Proc Am Thorac Soc* 2009;6:66–78.

73. Fischer S, Strueber M, Haverich A, et al. Current status of clinical lung transplantation: Patients, indications, techniques and outcome. *Med Klin* 2002;97:137–43.

74. Olsson KM, Simon A, Strueber M, et al. Extracorporeal membrane oxygenation in nonintubated patients as bridge to lung transplantation. *Am J Transplant* 2010;10:2173–8.

75. Hammainen P, Schersten H, Lemstrom K, et al. Usefulness of extracorporeal membrane oxygenation as a bridge to lung transplantation: A descriptive study. *J Heart Lung Transplant* 2011;30:103–7.

76. Toyoda Y, Bhama JK, Shigemura N, et al. Efficacy of extracorporeal membrane oxygenation as a bridge to lung transplantation. *J Thorac Cardiovasc Surg* 2013;145:1065–71.

77. Puri V, Epstein D, Raithel SC, et al. Extracorporeal membrane oxygenation in pediatric lung transplantation. *J Thorac Cardiovasc Surg* 2010;140:427–32.

78. Jackson A, Cropper J, Pye R, et al. Use of extracorporeal membrane oxygenation as a bridge to primary lung transplant: 3 consecutive, successful cases and a review of the literature. *J Heart Lung Transplant* 2008;27:348–52.

79. Nosotti M, Rosso L, Palleschi A, et al. Bridge to lung transplantation by venovenous extracorporeal membrane oxygenation: A lesson learned on the first four cases. *Transplant Proc* 2010;42:1259–61.

80. Schmidt F, Sasse M, Boehne M, et al. Concept of "awake venovenous extracorporeal membrane oxygenation" in pediatric patients awaiting lung transplantation. *Pediatr Transplant* 2013;17:224–30.

81. Turner DA, Cheifetz IM, Rehder KJ, et al. Active rehabilitation and physical therapy during extracorporeal membrane oxygenation while awaiting lung transplantation: A practical approach. *Crit Care Med* 2011;39:2593–8.

82. Hayes D Jr, Kukreja J, Tobias JD, et al. Ambulatory venovenous extracorporeal respiratory support as a bridge for cystic fibrosis patients to emergent lung transplantation. *J Cyst Fibros* 2012;11:40–5.

83. Smits JM, Mertens BJ, Van Houwelingen HC, et al. Predictors of lung transplant survival in EuroTransplant. *Am J Transplant* 2003;3:1400–6.

84. Imai Y, Parodo J, Kajikawa O, et al. Injurious mechanical ventilation and end-organ epithelial cell apoptosis and organ dysfunction in an experimental model of acute respiratory distress syndrome. *JAMA* 2003;289:2104–12.

85. Strueber M, Hoeper MM, Fischer S, et al. Bridge to thoracic organ transplantation in patients with pulmonary arterial hypertension using a pumpless lung assist device. *Am J Transplant* 2009;9:853–7.

86. Cypel M, Waddell TK, de Perrot M, et al. Safety and efficacy of the Novalung Interventional Lung Assist (iLA) Device as a bridge to lung transplantation. *J Heart Lung Transplant* 2010;29(suppl 2):S88.

87. Fischer S, Simon AR, Welte T, et al. Bridge to lung transplantation with the novel pumpless interventional lung assist device NovaLung. *J Thorac Cardiovasc Surg* 2006;131:719–23.

88. Hoganson DM, Gazit AZ, Sweet SC, et al. Neonatal paracorporeal lung assist device for respiratory failure. *Ann Thorac Surg* 2013;95:692–4.

89. Puri V, Scavuzzo M, Guthrie T, et al. Lung transplantation and donation after cardiac death: A single center experience. *Ann Thorac Surg* 2009;88:1609–14.

90. Sundaresan S, Semenkovich J, Ochoa L, et al. Successful outcome of lung transplantation is not compromised by the use of marginal donor lungs. *J Thorac Cardiovasc Surg* 1995;109:1075–9.

91. King RC, Binns OAR, Rodriguz F, et al. Reperfusion injury significantly impacts clinical outcome after pulmonary transplantation. *Ann Thorac Surg* 2000;69:1681–5.

92. Yousem SA, Berry GJ, Cagle PT, et al; Lung Rejection Study Group. Revision of the 1990 working formulation for the classification of pulmonary allograft rejection. *J Heart Lung Transplant* 1996;15 (1, pt 1):1–15.

93. Sheridan PH, Cheriyan A, Doud J, et al. Incidence of phrenic neuropathy after isolated lung transplantation. *J Heart Lung Transplant* 1995;14:684–91.

94. Huddleston CB, Sweet SC, Mallory GB, et al. Lung transplantation in very young infants. *J Thorac Cardiovasc Surg* 1999;118(5):796–804.

95. Elizur A, Faro A, Huddleston CB, et al. Lung transplantation in infants and toddlers from 1990 to 2004 at St. Louis Children's Hospital. *Am J Transplant* 2009;9(4):719–26.

96. Cooper JD, Pearson FG, Patterson GA, et al. Technique of successful lung transplantation in humans. *J Thorac Cardiovasc Surg* 1987;93:173–81.

97. Ro PS, Bush DM, Kramer SS, et al. Airway growth after pediatric lung transplantation. *J Heart Lung Transplant* 2001;20:619–24.

98. Cooper JD, Pearson FG, Patterson GA, et al. Technique of successful lung transplantation in humans. *J Thorac Cardiovasc Surg* 1987;93:173–81.

99. Ramirez J, Patterson GA. Airway complications after lung transplantation. *Semin Thorac Cardiovasc Surg* 1992;4:147–53.

100. Choong CK, Sweet SC, Zoole JB, et al. Bronchial airway anastomotic complications after pediatric lung transplantation: Incidence, cause, management, and outcome. *J Thorac Cardiovasc Surg* 2006;131(1):198–203.

101. Matsuzaki Y, Waddell TK, Puskas JD, et al. Amelioration of postischemic lung reperfusion injury by prostaglandin E1. *Am Rev Respir Dis* 1993;148:882–9.

102. Date H, Triantafillou AN, Trulock EP, et al. Inhaled nitric oxide reduces human lung allograft dysfunction. *J Thorac Cardiovasc Surg* 1996;111:913–9.

103. Gandhi SK, Bromberg BI, Schuessler RB, et al. Left sided atrial flutter—characterization of a novel complication of pediatric lung transplantation in an acute canine model. *J Thorac Cardiovasc Surg* 1996;112:992–1001.

104. Gandhi SK, Bromberg BI, Mallory GB, et al. Atrial flutter—a newly recognized complication of pediatric lung transplantation. *J Thorac Cardiovasc Surg* 1996;112:984–91.

105. Bridges ND, Spray TL, Collins MH, et al. Adenovirus infection in the lung results in graft failure after lung transplantation. *J Thorac Cardiovasc Surg* 1998;116:617–23.

106. Metras D, Viard L, Kreitmann B, et al. Lung infections in pediatric lung transplantation: Experience in 49 cases. *Eur J Cardiothorac Surg* 1999;15:490–4.

107. Apalsch AM, Green M, Ledesma-Medina J, et al. Parainfluenza and influenza virus infections in pediatric organ transplant recipients. *Clin Infect Dis* 1995;20:394–9.

108. Heeger PS, Dinavahi R. Transplant immunology for non-immunologist. *Mt Sinai J Med* 2012;79:376–87.

109. Delves PJ, Roitt IM. The immune system: First of two parts. *N Engl J Med* 2000;343:37–49.

110. Delves PJ, Roitt IM. The immune system: Second of two parts. *N Engl J Med* 2000;343:108–17.

111. McKay DB. The role of innate immunity in donor organ procurement. *Semin Immunopathol* 2011;33:169–84.

112. Vincenti F, Larsen C, Durrbach A, et al; Belatacept Study Group. Costimulation blockade with belatacept in renal transplantation. *N Engl J Med* 2005;353:770–81.

113. Clarkson MR, Sayegh MH. T-cell costimulatory pathways in allograft rejection and tolerance. *Transplantation* 2005;80:555–63.

114. Arya SK, Wong-Staal F, Gallo RC. Dexamethasone mediated inhibition of human T cell growth factor and gamma interferon messenger RNA. *J Immunol* 1984;133:273–6.

115. Pihlgren M, Dubois PM, Tomkowiak M, et al. Resting memory CD8$^+$ T cells are hyperreactive to antigenic challenge in vitro. *J Exp Med* 1996;184:2141–51.

116. Viola A, Lanzavecchia A. T cell activation determined by T cell receptor number and tunable thresholds. *Science* 1996;273:104–6.

117. Welsh RM, Selin LK. No one is naive: The significance of heterologous T-cell immunity. *Nat Rev Immunol* 2002;2:417–26.

118. Pearl JP, Parris J, Hale DA, et al. Immunocompetent Tcells with a memory-like phenotype are the dominant cell type

following antibody-mediated T-cell depletion. *Am J Transplant* 2005;5:465–74.

119. Heeger PS, Greenspan NS, Kuhlenschmidt S, et al. Pretransplant frequency of donor-specific, IFNgamma-producing lymphocytes is a manifestation of immunologic memory and correlates with the risk of posttransplant rejection episodes. *J Immunol* 1999;163:2267–75.

120. Hricik DE, Knauss TC, Bodziak KA, et al. Withdrawal of steroid therapy in African American kidney transplant recipients receiving sirolimus and tacrolimus. *Transplantation* 2003;76:938–42.

121. Nickel P, Presber F, Bold G, et al. Enzyme-linked immunosorbent spot assay for donor-reactive interferon-gamma-producing cells identifies T-cell presensitization and correlates with graft function at 6 and 12 months in renal-transplant recipients. *Transplantation* 2004;78:1640–6.

122. Lefaucheur C, Nochy D, Andrade J, et al. Comparison of combination plasmapheresis/IVIg/anti-CD20 versus high-dose IVIg in the treatment of antibody-mediated rejection. *Am J Transplant* 2009;9:1099–107.

123. Benden C, Ewards LB, Kucheryavaya AY, et al. The registry of the International Society for Heart and Lung Transplantation: Fifteenth pediatric lung and heart-lung transplantation report– 2012. *J Heart Lung Transplant* 2012;31:1087–95.

124. Huddleston CB, Bloch JB, Sweet, SC, et al. Lung transplantation in children. *Ann Surg* 2002;236(3):270–6.

125. Benden C, Aurora P, Edwards LB, et al. The Registry of the International Society for Heart and Lung Transplantation: Fourteenth Pediatric Lung and Heart-Lung Transplantation Report—2011. *J Heart Lung Transplant* 2011;30:1123–32.

126. Danziger-Isakov LA, Worley S, Arrigain S, et al. Increased mortality after pulmonary fungal infection within the first year after pediatric lung transplantation. *J Heart Lung Transplant* 2008;27:655–61.

127. Kramer MR, Stoehr C, Lewiston NJ, et al. Trimethoprim-sulfamethoxazole prophylaxis for *Pneumocystis carinii* infections in heart-lung and lung transplantation—how effective and for how long? *Transplantation* 1992;53(3):586–9.

128. Urschel S, Rieck BD, Birnbaum J, et al. Impaired cellular immune response to diphtheria and tetanus vaccines in children after thoracic transplantation. *Pediatr Transplant* 2011;15:272–80.

129. Benden C, Danziger-Isakov LA, Astor T, et al. Variability in immunization guidelines in children before and after lung transplantation. *Pediatr Transplant* 2007;11:882–7.

130. Wehbe E, Brock R, Budev M, et al. Short-term and long-term outcomes of acute kidney injury after lung transplantation. *J Heart Lung Transplant* 2012;31:244–51.

131. Hayes D Jr. A review of bronchiolitis obliterans syndrome and therapeutic strategies. *J Cardiothorac Surg* 2011;6:92.

132. Abbassi-Ghadi N, Kumar S, Cheung B, et al. Anti-reflux surgery for lung transplant recipients in the presence of impedance-detected duodenogastroesophageal reflux and bronchiolitis obliterans syndrome: A study of efficacy and safety. *J Heart Lung Transplant* 2013;32:588–95.

CHAPTER 77 ■ CARDIAC CONDUCTION, DYSRHYTHMIAS, AND PACING

RICHARD J. CZOSEK, DAVID S. SPAR, JEFFREY B. ANDERSON, TIMOTHY K. KNILANS, AND BRADLEY S. MARINO

KEY POINTS

1. The possible mechanisms of tachyarrhythmias are reentry, increased automaticity, and triggered activity.

2. Until otherwise proven, a wide complex tachycardia should be considered ventricular tachycardia (VT).

3. The most common dysrhythmia in children is supraventricular tachycardia (SVT), specifically atrioventricular reciprocating tachycardia (AVRT) and AV nodal reentrant tachycardia (AVNRT).

4. The presenting symptoms of SVT are age dependent. Infants present with irritability, poor feeding, and, possibly, signs of heart failure, while children present with complaints of palpitations, chest pain, nausea, and dizziness.

5. Acute therapy for SVT includes conversion with adenosine and/or synchronized cardioversion if clinically unstable.

6. IV calcium-channel blockers should be avoided in young patients, particularly infants less than 12 months of age.

7. Long-term treatment for SVT includes medical antiarrhythmic therapy or catheter ablation.

8. Patients with Wolff–Parkinson–White (WPW) syndrome should never be chronically treated with digoxin or a calcium-channel blocker because these medicines enhance conduction through the accessory pathway.

9. The general indications for pacemaker implantation in children include sinus node disease and atrioventricular (AV) block (congenital or acquired). Acquired AV block is typically secondary to mechanical damage during surgical repair of congenital heart disease.

10. Adenosine should not be administered to patients with preexcited atrial fibrillation as this may enhance accessory pathway conduction to the ventricle and induce ventricular fibrillation.

A wide variety of cardiac arrhythmias are seen in the intensive care unit and range from those that are immediately life-threatening to those of little or no consequence. When a cardiac arrhythmia is suspected in the intensive care unit, the first step may not be to specifically diagnose the rhythm mechanism but rather to determine the effects of the rhythm, some of which may need immediate intervention, perhaps without a specific diagnosis. At the other end of the spectrum are rhythms that may initially appear to be benign, but may exert subclinical effects before resulting in hemodynamic collapse. Other arrhythmias may never result in collapse, but their effects may prolong the duration of intensive care admission or mechanical ventilation. Thus, even rhythm abnormalities that do not initially appear to be of hemodynamic significance should be completely investigated.

Most patients in modern intensive care units are on continuous electrocardiographic monitoring with full disclosure review. In addition to surface electrocardiographic recordings, other parameters are frequently helpful in rhythm diagnosis and assessment. Atrial electrical activity may be directly recorded in patients with recent cardiac surgery with use of temporary epicardial wires or in other patients from the esophagus via a bipolar catheter. Atrial or central venous pressure waveforms may also be helpful in arrhythmia diagnosis. Arterial pressure waveforms or pulse oximetry deflections may be important, especially when artifact is present in the electrocardiographic recording.

GUIDE TO INTERPRETATION OF ELECTROCARDIOGRAPHIC RECORDINGS

The electrocardiogram remains the primary modality for diagnosis of cardiac rhythm abnormalities. If full disclosure review is available, the points of initiation and termination and any spontaneous perturbations of the arrhythmia should be identified and reviewed in as many recorded leads as possible.

Identification of atrial activity is often the most helpful first step in the arrhythmia analysis. Printing the ECG on paper may aid in the analysis of the heart rhythm, and marking the location of visible P waves with a pen on paper can help in the identification of the pattern of atrial activity. Measuring calipers can also be quite useful. The atrial mechanism is often regular, and if it is dissociated from ventricular activity, caliper measurements can identify the probable timing of P waves that are concealed by QRS complexes or T waves. Augmented atrial recording with use of the epicardial or esophageal wires can easily identify previously concealed atrial activity. Once all atrial activity has been identified and marked, the atrial rate can be determined. If the atrial rate is the same as the ventricular rate, there is likely to be atrioventricular conduction, ventriculoatrial conduction, or both. If the atrial rate exceeds the ventricular rate, there is AV block of higher than first-degree or nonconducted atrial ectopy. If the ventricular rate exceeds the atrial rate, there is an abnormal ventricular mechanism, which, depending on the ventricular rate, may be due to an inappropriately slow atrial rate (ventricular escape) or to an abnormally fast ventricular rate (VT) with some degree of ventriculoatrial block.

The P-wave axis and morphology and the QRS axis, duration, and morphology should be inspected and, if possible, compared with the P waves during sinus rhythm, and QRS complexes conducted from atrial activity from previous electrocardiographic recordings on the same patient, if they are available. The performance of a multilead electrogram on all patients immediately before interventions anticipated to result in potential intraprocedural or postprocedural arrhythmia is strongly advised for this purpose. P waves with a morphology and axis identical to sinus rhythm seen during tachycardia suggest sinus tachycardia or sinus node reentrant tachycardia, but some automatic atrial tachycardias may have very similar P waves, and careful review and all leads, especially leads V1 and V2, should be undertaken. P waves that are upright in the inferior leads during tachycardia are inconsistent with AVNRT and unlikely to be seen in accessory pathway–mediated tachycardia such as orthodromic AV reentrant tachycardia. Narrow QRS complexes during tachycardia most often indicate a supraventricular mechanism, but VT in young children may have QRS complexes with durations of less than the upper limits of normal for age. If the QRS complexes during a tachycardia are identical in morphology and duration to that seen during sinus rhythm, then the tachycardia has a supraventricular mechanism. Care must be taken to review the QRS morphology in several leads as it may appear similar or even identical in some leads, but quite different in others.

Supraventricular tachycardia may occur with a wide QRS morphology caused by aberrant conduction or ventricular preexcitation. Aberrant conduction may be caused by preexisting conduction system abnormality or block in the conduction system related to a rate faster than the refractory period of a portion of the His–Purkinje system, so-called rate-dependent aberrant conduction. Ventricular preexcitation may be caused by conduction over an accessory AV connection or, less commonly, a connection between the atrium and a fascicle of the conduction system or the ventricular myocardium. Conduction with aberration can usually be distinguished from preexcited conduction by the presence of sharp high-frequency depolarization during the first 40 ms of the QRS complex. This represents normal activation of the ventricle over the functional portion of the conduction system, while the terminal portion of the QRS complexes is delayed. Preexcited conduction will generally show a low-frequency slurred pattern at the beginning of the QRS complex because of activation of ventricular myocardium by the accessory pathway. This pattern may not be present if the accessory pathway inserts into a fascicle of the conduction system, thereby resulting in rapid depolarization of ventricular myocardium by specialist conduction fibers. If aberrant conduction or ventricular preexcitation is seen in previous electrocardiograms from the same patient during sinus rhythm, the pattern may be extremely helpful in the diagnosis of the tachycardia. Again, the availability of multiple leads for comparison may be critical.

THE CARDIAC CONDUCTION SYSTEM

The cardiac conduction system is composed of specialized myocardial cells that can create and propagate electrical depolarizations. The sinus node is the site of normal impulse formation in the heart. Propagation of the impulse occurs through the atrial myocardium to the atrioventricular (AV) node (1).

Refractoriness of AV node cells is both voltage and time dependent. These characteristics result in slowing of conduction between the atrium and ventricle, and potential filtering of rapid or closely coupled beats. From the AV node arises the bundle of His, which penetrates the interventricular septum and divides into right and left bundle branches (fascicles), and the left bundle further divides into an anterior and posterior fascicle. The fascicles propagate the depolarizing wave to the penetrating Purkinje fibers, which carry the electrical depolarization to the ventricular myocardium.

TACHYARRHYTHMIAS

Tachyarrhythmia (an abnormal mechanism of tachycardia) can be classified into three basic electrophysiologic mechanisms: (a) reentry, (b) abnormal automaticity, and (c) triggered activity.

In pediatrics, reentry is most often seen in SVT, but can also be seen in VT (e.g., postoperative congenital cardiac patients). Reentry describes the phenomenon of an electrical wave front "reentering" cardiac tissue. The three essential elements required for the existence of a reentrant circuit include two distinct conducting pathways, slow conduction in one of the pathways, and unidirectional block in one pathway that relies upon the different refractory properties of the two pathways, (Fig. 77.1). An electrical impulse will enter the circuit and begin to pass down the two pathways. If that impulse arrives in one limb of the pathway at such a time that the pathway with the longer refractory period has not recovered from the previous impulse, block will occur in that pathway. If the second pathway has recovered (shorter refractory period), the impulse will propagate down that second pathway. Propagation down that pathway may be slow enough to allow for the recovery of the first pathway, thus allowing the electrical impulse to travel in a retrograde fashion up the first pathway, thereby returning it to the original entry site into the circuit and establishing a reentry circuit. Reentrant arrhythmias typically have a regular rate with a sudden onset and termination. In addition, this type of dysrhythmia can be provoked by an electrical stimulus, such as a premature atrial or ventricular contraction or by pacing maneuvers, and can be terminated by a variety of means, including pacing and direct current cardioversion. Reentrant circuits often involve fixed obstacles, but can also

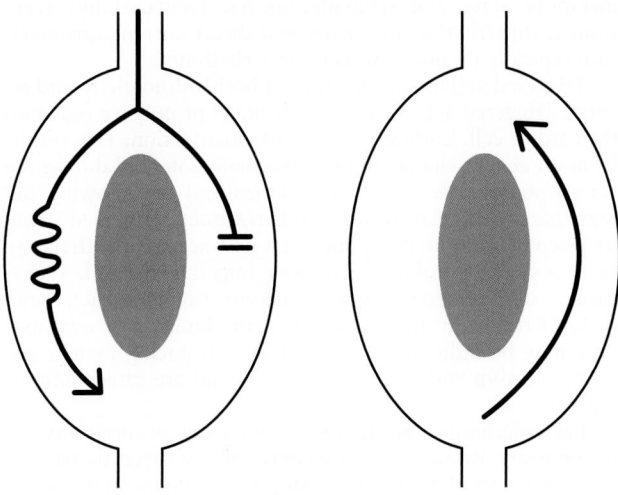

FIGURE 77.1. Schematic diagram representing a reentrant circuit. Requirements for reentry include two pathways, unidirectional block in one pathway (=) and slow conduction in the other pathway (~).

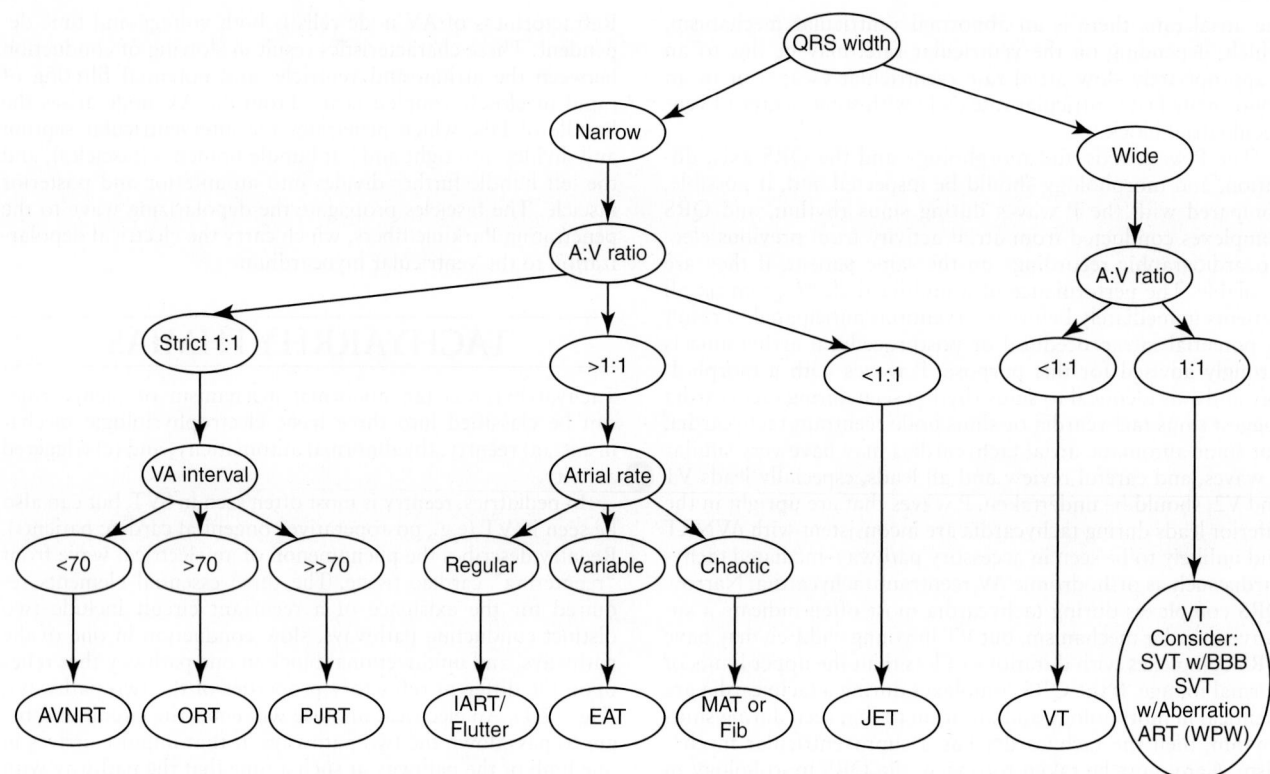

FIGURE 77.2. Diagnostic approach for determining tachycardia mechanism. VA interval (RP interval in text) is measured in milliseconds. ART, antidromic reciprocating tachycardia; AV, atrioventricular; AVNRT, atrioventricular nodal reentrant tachycardia; BBB, bundle-branch block; EAT, ectopic atrial tachycardia; IART, intra-atrial reentrant tachycardia; JET, junctional ectopic tachycardia; MAT, multifocal atrial tachycardia; ORT, orthodromic reciprocating tachycardia; PJRT, permanent junctional reciprocating tachycardia; SVT, supraventricular tachycardia; VA, ventriculoatrial; VT, ventricular tachycardia; WPW, Wolff–Parkinson–White. (From Walsh EP. Clinical approach to diagnosis and acute management of tachycardias in children. In: Walsh EP, Saul JP, Triedman JK, eds. *Cardiac Arrhythmias in Children and Young Adults with Congenital Heart Disease*. Philadelphia, PA: Lippincott Williams & Wilkins, 2001, with permission.)

revolve around "functional obstacles," especially in hearts with previous surgical intervention and scar.

Automaticity refers to the ability of a cell or group of cells to spontaneously depolarize. An abnormal automatic focus can occur in the atria, AV junction, or the ventricles. Automatic tachycardias typically have an irregular rate with a warm-up and cool-down phase. They are sensitive to the adrenergic and metabolic state, and sympathomimetic agents. Unlike reentrant tachyarrhythmias, pacing and direct current cardioversion typically do not convert these arrhythmias.

Triggered activity has features of both automaticity and reentry. Triggered activity involves leakage of positive ions into the cardiac cell, leading to an afterdepolarization. This results from an abrupt change in the membrane potential during the action potential (early afterdepolarization) or following full repolarization (delayed afterdepolarization). Triggered activity resembles automaticity such that new action potentials can be generated by leakage of positive ions into the cell. Tachycardias derived from triggered activity share characteristics of both reentrant and automatic arrhythmias. For example, they may be induced or terminated with pacing maneuvers, have warm-up and cool-down phases, and are catecholamine sensitive.

Each mechanism of tachyarrhythmia may occur at any site in the heart. Reentrant circuits may involve atrial tissue, giving rise to atrial flutter. In postoperative congenital cardiac patients, reentrant pathways around surgical scars have been termed *intra-atrial reentrant tachycardia* (IART). Reentry may also involve pathways within or leading to the AV node, resulting in AVNRT. Reentry that results in VT usually involves

circuits around areas of infarction, surgical scars, or anatomic obstacles. The most common reentrant tachycardias in the pediatric population are those that involve an *accessory pathway*, (2) which is an anomalous electrical connection between atrial and ventricular myocardium across the AV groove. Wolff–Parkinson–White (WPW) syndrome involves an accessory pathway that conducts anterograde (from the atrium to the ventricle) with ventricular preexcitation on surface ECG and participates in AV reciprocating tachycardia. These accessory pathways may support both anterograde and retrograde conduction, while concealed accessory pathways can only support retrograde conduction.

Automatic tachycardias may also originate in any of the cardiac anatomical sites. Multifocal atrial tachycardia (MAT), or chaotic atrial rhythm, is derived from the firing of multiple atrial foci. Increased automaticity near the AV node gives rise to junctional ectopic tachycardia (JET). Finally, some types of VT may arise from isolated foci within the ventricle.

Diagnostic Approach to Tachyarrhythmias

A systematic approach is needed to appropriately diagnose complex tachyarrhythmias (**Fig. 77.2**). A 12-lead electrocardiogram (ECG), telemetry recording, Holter monitor, or event monitor is necessary to determine the arrhythmia mechanism. In postoperative patients, the use of postoperative atrial pacing wires can also be utilized to augment electrical activity on electrocardiogram. Narrow QRS complex tachycardia implies there is conduction through the His–Purkinje system and is

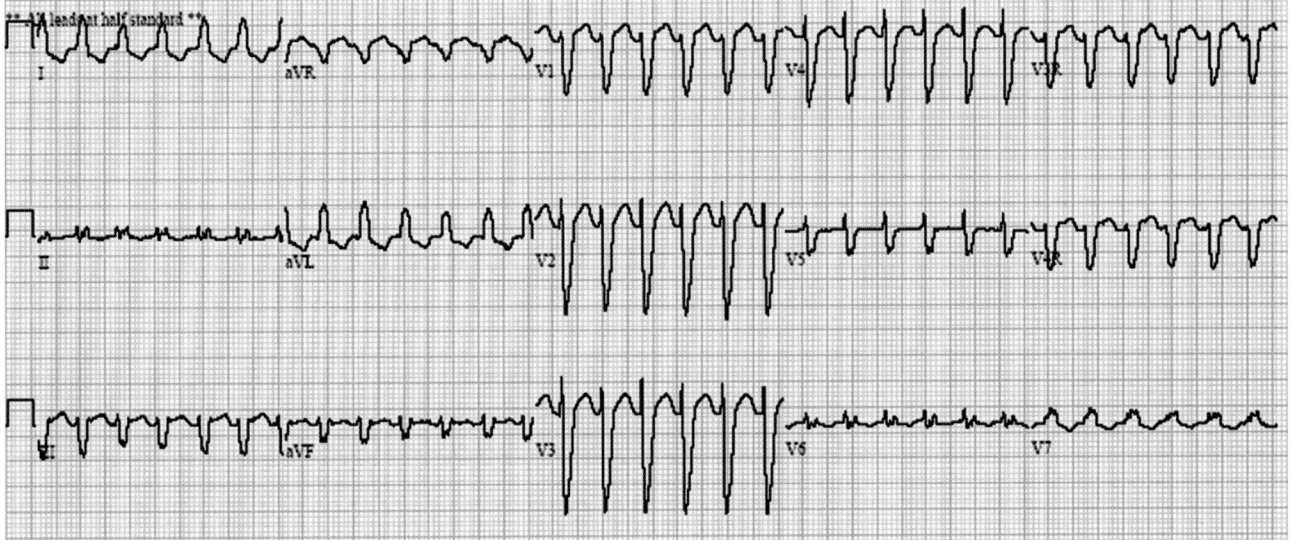

FIGURE 77.3. ECG showing supraventricular tachycardia conducted with aberrancy in a newborn.

therefore supraventricular in origin. A wide QRS complex tachycardia should be assumed to be ventricular in origin but may also be due to a SVT with fixed or rate-dependent aberrancy, or ventricular preexcitation. Reentrant tachycardia that involve an accessory pathway with a narrow QRS complex, anterograde (atria to ventricles) conduction through the AV node, and retrograde (ventricles to atria) conduction through the accessory pathway are called *orthodromic reciprocating tachycardia*. When anterograde conduction occurs down the accessory pathway with retrograde conduction through the AV node, a wide QRS complex tachycardia, called *antidromic reciprocating tachycardia*, results.

The relationship of atrial to ventricular complexes is important to the determination of the tachycardia mechanism. First it should be determined if there is a one-to-one ratio of P waves to QRS complexes, then the relationship between the QRS complex and the P wave should be examined. If the RP interval (VA interval on figure) is <70 ms, typical AVNRT is likely, secondary to near simultaneous depolarization of the atrium and ventricles. If the RP interval is >70 ms, atrioventricular reciprocating tachycardia (AVRT) is the probable etiology, although atypical AVNRT or atrial tachycardia may also be present. Sinus tachycardia may be differentiated from AVNRT or AVRT by a frontal plane P-wave axis of 0 to +90 degrees in a normal situs solitus heart. An A:V ratio >1:1 is typically diagnostic of a primary atrial tachycardia, though AVNRT with 2:1 conduction to the ventricle can be seen. Atrial tachycardia can also occur with 1:1 AV conduction. If the atrial rate is regular, atrial flutter (or IART) is likely. An irregular atrial rate that has a single P-wave morphology, different from the sinus P-wave morphology, and the axis of which is outside of the 0 to +90-degree range suggests ectopic atrial tachycardia (EAT). Finally, an irregular atrial rate with three or more P-wave morphologies suggests MAT. JET may have 1:1 VA conduction or VA dissociation with occasional sinus capture beats and a ventricular rate greater than the atrial rate.

Wide QRS complex tachycardias should be assumed to be ventricular, until proven otherwise. A wide QRS complex tachycardia with AV dissociation (i.e., no relationship between P waves and QRS complexes) and a ventricular rate greater than the atrial rate is diagnostic of VT. A wide QRS complex tachycardia with an A:V ratio of 1 can be VT with retrograde conduction, SVT with aberrancy (**Fig. 77.3**) or preexcited tachycardia.

Specific Diagnosis

Supraventricular Arrhythmias

The most common arrhythmia in the pediatric population is SVT, with a reported incidence of 1 in 250 to 1000 (3). SVT may result from either reentry or abnormal automaticity, with reentry being more common.

Atrioventricular Reciprocating Tachycardia. The most common type of reentrant SVT in children is AVRT, which requires participation of both the atrium and ventricle in the reentrant circuit (2). AVRT utilizes an accessory AV connection and includes orthodromic reciprocating tachycardia and antidromic reciprocating tachycardia (**Fig. 77.4**). In orthodromic AV reciprocating tachycardia, the accessory pathway may only have retrograde conduction, described as a unidirectional retrograde accessory pathway (URAP). SVT may present in the fetus or at any age. Accessory pathway–mediated tachycardias are more common in the fetus, infants, and young children, while AVNRT is more common in adolescents and young adults. Infants frequently will present with symptoms of irritability and poor feeding. If SVT goes undetected, the patient may develop congestive heart failure, manifested as tachypnea, diaphoresis, pallor, and lethargy. Older children may complain of symptoms such as palpitations, chest pain, abdominal pain, or dizziness. Rarely, syncope may occur if the tachycardia rate is sufficiently fast to impair diastolic filling, resulting in hypotension and cerebral hypoperfusion.

Wolff–Parkinson–White Syndrome. WPW syndrome is characterized by a short PR interval and delta wave (which represents ventricular preexcitation prior to normal activation of the AV node and His–Purkinje system) and episodes of tachycardia (**Fig. 77.5**) (4). The incidence of WPW is between 0.1% and 0.3% of the general population and more prevalent in males (5). Congenital heart disease occurs in association with WPW in ~20% of patients. Ebstein's anomaly and L-transposition of the great arteries are the most common associated congenital anomalies (6). WPW syndrome involves an accessory pathway that usually has both antegrade and retrograde conduction, though on occasion the accessory pathway conduction may only be anterograde. SVT may be either orthodromic AV reciprocating tachycardia (down the AV node and up the accessory pathway) or antidromic AV reciprocating

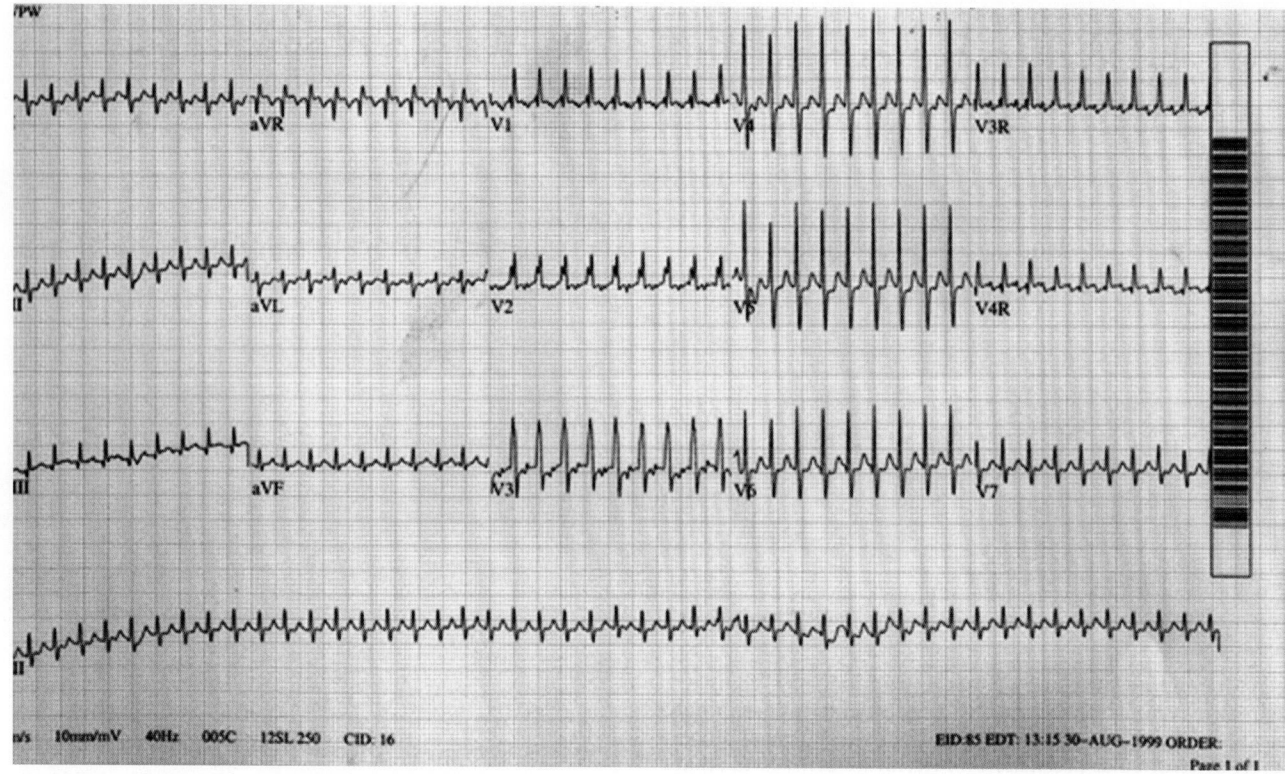

FIGURE 77.4. ECG showing AV reciprocating tachycardia.

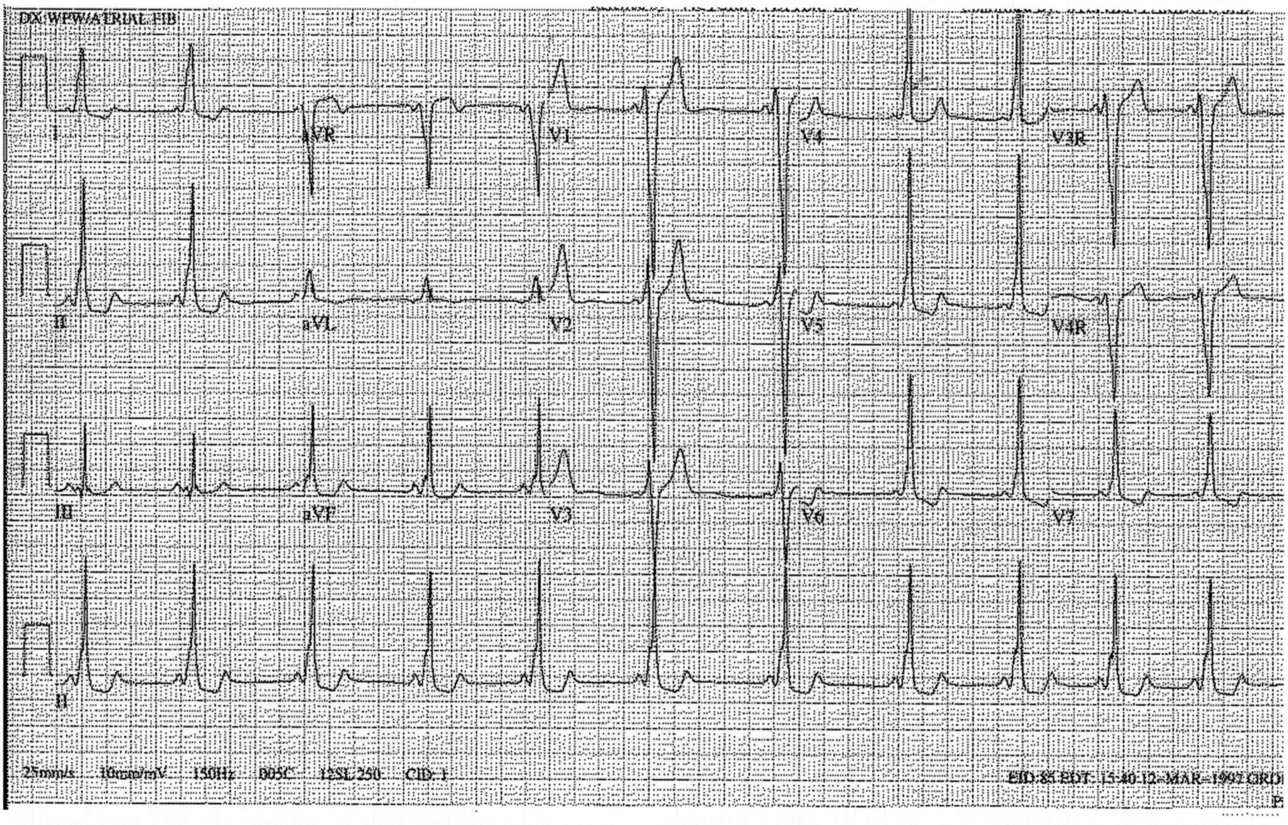

FIGURE 77.5. ECG from a child with Wolff–Parkinson–White syndrome. Note the short PR interval and delta wave.

tachycardia (down the accessory pathway and up the AV node). Orthodromic AV reciprocating tachycardia is more common. Patients with WPW are at an increased risk of atrial fibrillation. If during atrial fibrillation the accessory pathway supports rapid anterograde conduction, hemodynamic instability and sudden death may result. In patients with WPW, the risk of sudden death is low (0.0015 per patient year) (7).

The incidence of WPW in childhood is ~1 in 1000. Of patients who present during infancy, one-third of the patients continue to experience episodes of SVT after 1 year of age (8). Conversely, older patients have a greater chance for SVT recurrence. Some patients with ventricular preexcitation are asymptomatic, and the diagnosis is made incidentally. Risk stratification of the accessory pathway in patients that are asymptomatic is recommended since the first clinical presentation may be sudden cardiac death. Noninvasive testing with an exercise stress test can be used for stratifying patients. Sudden loss of ventricular preexcitation with PR prolongation during exercise suggests a low-risk accessory pathway. The best predictor for patients at risk for sudden death is the measurement of the shortest ventricular preexcited RR interval (SPRR) during atrial fibrillation. Atrial fibrillation can be induced with rapid atrial pacing either via a transesophageal pacing study or a transvenous pacing study. A ventricular preexcited RR interval during atrial fibrillation of <250 ms is considered high risk for rapid conduction through the accessory pathway during atrial fibrillation, which can lead to ventricular fibrillation (9). These patients are candidates for a catheter-ablation procedure. A stepwise approach with (a) exercise stress test, (b) esophageal electrophysiology study, and (c) invasive electrophysiology study/ablation has been proven to be both cost effective and a less invasive method for risk stratifying these patients (10). In 2012, the Heart Rhythm Society in collaboration with the Pediatric and Congenital Electrophysiology Society published guidelines on the management of asymptomatic patients with ventricular preexcitation (11).

Concealed Bypass Tract. Concealed bypass tracts only support retrograde conduction and orthodromic AV reciprocating tachycardia. In view of their inability to propagate extremely rapid atrial rates directly into the ventricle, concealed bypass tracts are highly unlikely to cause hemodynamic instability or sudden death. Orthodromic AV reciprocating tachycardia in patients with WPW and those with concealed bypass tracts are indistinguishable during an episode of tachycardia. Differentiation is possible by evaluating the ECG in sinus rhythm, when the patient with a concealed bypass tract will have a normal PR interval without a delta wave and the patient with WPW will have a short PR interval and delta wave. This difference has important implications for treatment. Patients with a concealed bypass tract present with SVT at any age from infancy through adolescence. An unusual type of SVT that involves a slowly conducting concealed bypass tract is the permanent form of junctional reciprocating tachycardia (PJRT), which has a very long RP interval during the tachycardia. The accessory pathway location in PJRT is typically in the right posterior septum, but has been identified around both the tricuspid and mitral valve annuli. The ECG pattern typically has negative retrograde P waves in leads II, III, and aVF. PJRT is frequently refractory to medical management.

Atrioventricular Nodal Reentrant Tachycardia. The two pathways used as the substrate for the reentrant circuit in AVNRT are electrical approaches to the AV node located in the atrium. The "slow" pathway has slower conduction, often a shorter refractory period, and is anatomically located in the midseptal to posteroseptal region of the AV groove. The "fast" pathway has faster conduction, a longer refractory period, and is located in the anterior aspect of the atrial septum. When these two pathways are present, the patient is

described as having dual AV nodal physiology. Typical AVNRT involves conduction anterograde down the slow pathway and retrograde up the fast pathway. Atypical AVNRT involves conduction anterograde down the fast pathway and retrograde though the slow pathway. The incidence of AVNRT increases with age and represents the most common type of reentrant SVT in adults. In the pediatric population, it is most commonly seen during adolescence. A possible explanation for this is that the AV node undergoes electrophysiologic alterations with age. In one study, dual AV node physiology was found in 15% of children <13 years of age and in 44% of children >13 years of age (1).

Treatment for Atrioventricular Reciprocating Tachycardia. The goal of acute therapy is to terminate the reentrant circuit and restore sinus rhythm. In a patient who presents in shock, attention should be paid to the patient's airway and breathing. If vascular access cannot readily be obtained and/or the patient is in extremis secondary to hemodynamic instability, then direct current cardioversion is indicated. Synchronized cardioversion should be performed with an energy dose of 0.5–1 J/kg.

In the hemodynamically stable patient with AVRT, vagal maneuvers should be attempted. In infants, a bag of ice on the infant's face frequently terminates the SVT by eliciting the diving reflex. First-line medical therapy is adenosine (0.1 mg/kg). Adenosine causes block in the AV node, thereby interrupting the reentrant circuit. Due to its short half-life, adenosine should be administered through a large-bore intravascular catheter placed as close to the heart as possible. The adenosine should be given rapidly and followed with an IV push of saline. Another therapeutic modality is transesophageal pacing, but the placement of an esophageal pacing catheter may be uncomfortable in the conscious patient.

In refractory cases, pharmacologic therapies used in the acute setting include β-blockers (e.g., esmolol), procainamide, calcium-channel blockers (e.g., diltiazem), and amiodarone. For SVT refractory to first-line therapy of adenosine or cardioversion, the Pediatric Advanced Life Support algorithm recommends amiodarone or procainamide. These medications should be used with caution and with the guidance of an electrophysiologist. While IV calcium-channel blockers are an important therapy for SVT in adults, they are contraindicated in young children, especially in those children <1 year of age. Hemodynamic collapse and sudden death have been reported in infants treated with calcium-channel blockers (12).

Chronic therapy attempts to prevent recurrences of SVT and depends upon the type of SVT. Digoxin and β-blockers are first-line oral therapy for chronic prevention. Infants must be monitored for hypoglycemia and hypotension when β-blockers are started. Digoxin is contraindicated in patients with WPW because they may enhance anterograde conduction down the accessory pathway and allow for a more rapid ventricular response during atrial fibrillation (13). For SVT refractory to first-line oral therapy, other agents such as flecainide, sotalol, amiodarone, and verapamil can also be considered with the expert guidance of an electrophysiologist.

Atrial fibrillation in a patient with WPW is an important arrhythmia to recognize. The characteristic ECG finding of atrial fibrillation with WPW is an irregularly irregular wide complex tachycardia. Synchronized cardioversion should be performed in patients with hemodynamic compromise. In the stable patient, specific antiarrhythmic medications that primarily affect the conduction of the accessory pathway should be utilized (e.g., procainamide/amiodarone).

An increasingly popular therapeutic modality for recurrent SVT is catheter ablation, using either radiofrequency energy or cryothermal energy. Catheter ablation involves application of radiofrequency or cryothermal energy via a catheter to the

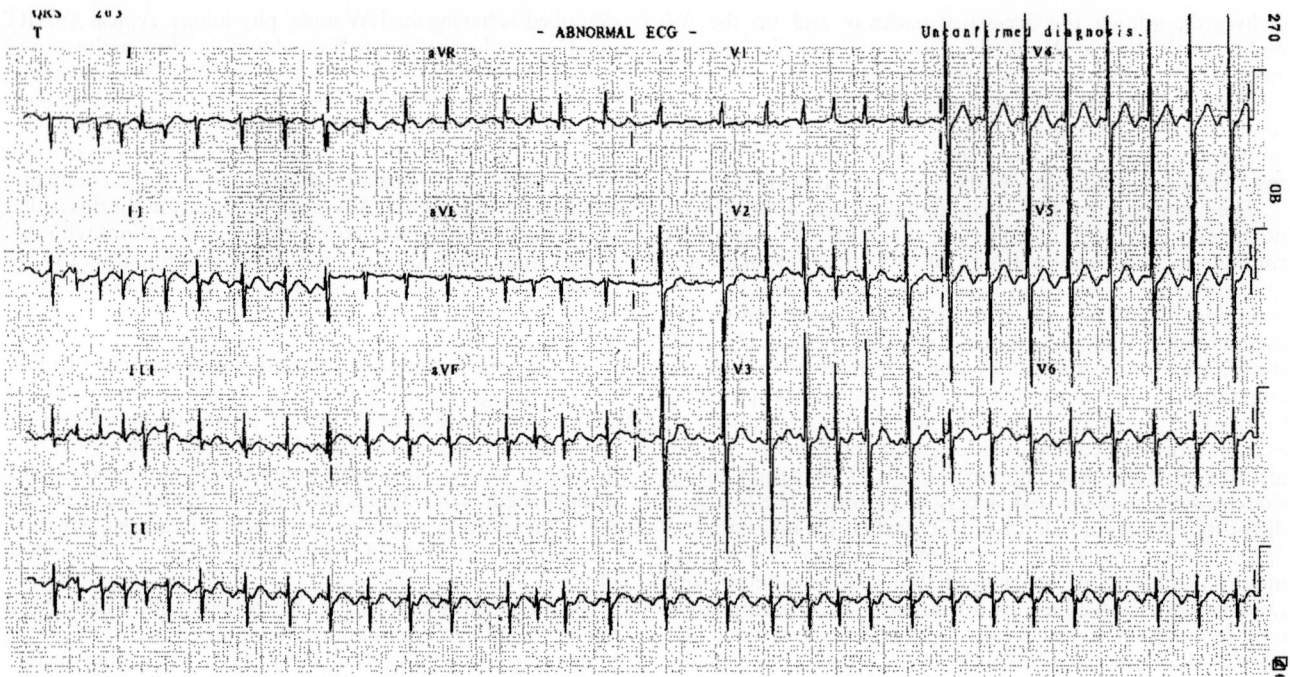

FIGURE 77.6. ECG showing atrial flutter with 2:1 conduction in a newborn. Note the typical flutter waves and "saw-tooth pattern" in leads II, III, and aVF.

arrhythmia substrate (i.e., accessory pathway or AV nodal slow pathway). Catheter ablation has been used successfully to cure various types of arrhythmias in pediatric patients. The success rate for AVRT has been reported between 86% and 97%, depending upon the location of the accessory pathway, and >95% for AVNRT (14,15).

Complication rates are low, with the most common serious complications being AV block, catheter perforation of the myocardium, and thromboembolism. Common indications for catheter ablation of SVT include life-threatening dysrhythmias, medically resistant tachycardias, adverse drug reactions, tachycardia-induced cardiomyopathy, impending cardiac surgery, and patient choice. Cryoablation has been introduced as an alternative means of destroying or altering the arrhythmia substrate. The theoretic advantage of cryoablation is that its effects can potentially be reversed, allowing for its safer use near the AV node (e.g., para-Hisian accessory pathways and slow pathway modifications).

Atrial Flutter/Intra-Atrial Reentrant Tachycardia. Atrial flutter is observed in two distinct groups in the pediatric population: in newborns and in patients with congenital heart disease, especially following atrial surgery for congenital heart defects.

Atrial Flutter. Atrial flutter of infancy is rare but may present in utero or during the newborn period. While uncommon, congenital heart defects may coexist with the dysrhythmia, and echocardiography is recommended to exclude most commonly atrial septal defect, aneurysm of atrial septum, or Ebstein anomaly. The reentrant circuit of atrial flutter of infancy is generally confined to the right atrium. Similar to typical adult atrial flutter, it may utilize the isthmus between the tricuspid valve and the inferior vena cava as the area of slow conduction. Characteristic saw-toothed flutter waves are usually present in leads II, III, and aVF. Atrial rates may reach 600 bpm. There is typically variable conduction to the ventricles, resulting in a ventricular response rate of ≥200 bpm (**Fig. 77.6**).

Atrial flutter in the newborn is converted to sinus rhythm with cardioversion, transesophageal pacing, or medications. Direct current synchronized cardioversion with 0.5–1.0 J/kg is the primary treatment modality given high success and low recurrence rates. Typically, the atrial flutter will not recur and, if there is no other arrhythmia present, the patient does not require long-term antiarrhythmic medications. Medication options include digoxin, procainamide, amiodarone, and sotalol. Procainamide should be used in conjunction with digoxin, as procainamide may slow the flutter rate, resulting in more rapid AV conduction. Digoxin is used to increase the degree of AV block in this setting. Unfortunately, cardioversion with antiarrhythmic medication is not as effective as electrical cardioversion; therefore, they are used as second-line agents. Once atrial flutter in the newborn period is converted to sinus rhythm, recurrence is uncommon (16).

Intra-Atrial Reentrant Tachycardia. Reentrant atrial tachycardia in patients who have undergone surgery for congenital heart disease is referred to as IART (**Fig. 77.7**). The surgical procedures that predispose patients to IART involve surgery in the atria, including atrial septal defect repair, atrial baffling procedures (Senning or Mustard operation) for D-transposition of the great arteries, and the Fontan operation for the univentricular heart. The reentrant circuit may occur anywhere within the atria and frequently incorporates an anatomic barrier or surgical scar. During electrophysiology testing, more than one reentrant circuit may be defined. The typical saw-tooth flutter waves may not be apparent; therefore, the clinician must have a high index of suspicion for the diagnosis. The incidence of IART following congenital heart surgery increases with age. Predisposing factors include surgical scars within the atrium, elevated atrial pressure, abnormal atrial anatomy associated with the primary lesion, and sinus node dysfunction (SND). Atrial rates in IART vary considerably with variable conduction to the ventricle. Symptomatology is related to the ventricular response rate and myocardial function. A fast ventricular response may result in palpitations, syncope, or sudden death. A slower ventricular response rate may result

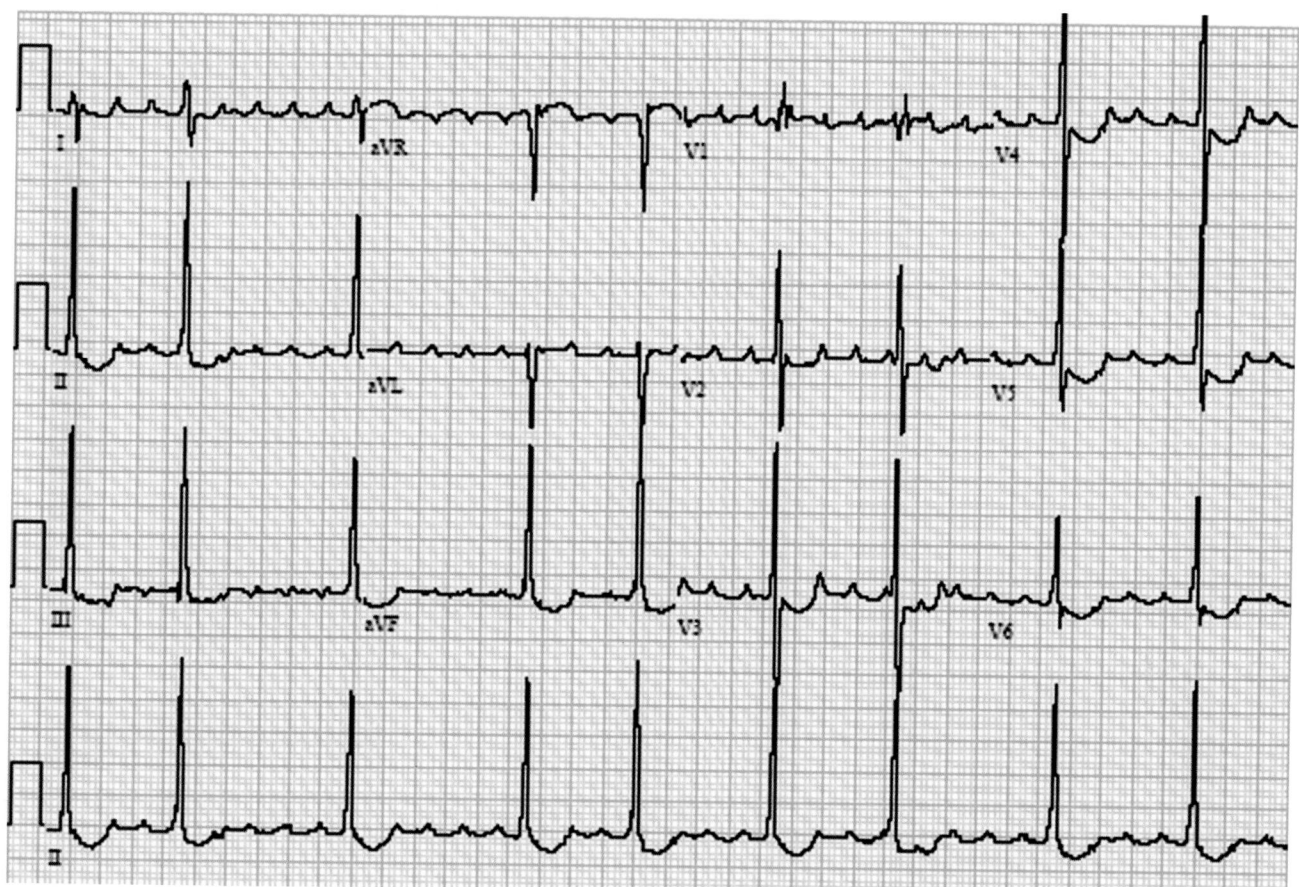

FIGURE 77.7. ECG showing intra-atrial reentrant tachycardia with variable conduction in a child with hypoplastic left heart syndrome status post-Fontan operation.

in gradual fatigue or exercise intolerance, especially in the Fontan patient, as AV synchrony may be crucial for adequate cardiac output. If the ventricular response rate is slow enough, patients may be asymptomatic. Long-standing IART may result in sluggish blood flow in the atria or Fontan pathway and increase the risk for thrombus and thromboembolic events.

Prior to any attempts at converting IART to sinus rhythm, the presence of an atrial thrombus must be ruled out with transesophageal echocardiography unless the patient is known to be in the rhythm <24 hours. Acute therapy typically includes synchronized cardioversion or transesophageal pacing. Antiarrhythmic medications such as propafenone, amiodarone, and sotalol are used in refractory cases. Postcardioversion, the patient remains at a higher risk for thrombus formation secondary to "atrial stunning," and anticoagulation is recommended either with warfarin or with antithrombotic agents (e.g., dabigitran) for one-month postcardioversion (17).

Chronic therapy for IART is often difficult, and may necessitate multiple medications and modalities. Digoxin may be used for rate control but generally has little direct effect on the arrhythmia substrate. Typically, rhythm control is most desirable in patients with congenital heart disease such as the univentricular heart with Fontan palliation or d-TGA with a systemic right ventricle postatrial baffle with cardiac dysfunction. Typical medications for IART include flecainide, propafenone, amiodarone, and sotalol. Other therapeutic modalities include pacemaker placement with antitachycardia pacing and catheter ablation (18). Catheter ablation has been used to interrupt the reentrant circuit. Owing to the presence of multiple reentrant circuits, complex atrial anatomy, and thick atrial muscle, success rates have been in the range of 70%–80%,

with recurrence rates as high as 50% (19). New technologies, such as improved mapping systems and irrigated catheter tips, may help to improve success rates and decrease recurrence.

Automatic Supraventricular Tachycardia. Atrial automatic tachycardias tend to present in children <6 years of age but also occur in older children and adolescents. The heart rate is inappropriately high for the patient's level of activity and appears to be sensitive to the adrenergic state. During sleep or under the influence of sedation, the rate will be slower, or the tachycardia may even be suppressed by normal sinus node activity. These tachycardias tend to be chronic and incessant. At slower rates, they are often not perceived by the patient. Persistence of the tachycardia may eventually lead to a tachycardia-mediated cardiomyopathy. Presentation for many patients includes signs and symptoms of congestive heart failure.

Ectopic Atrial Tachycardia. Ectopic atrial tachycardia (EAT), or *automatic atrial tachycardia,* represents between 4% and 6% of the SVT seen in the pediatric population. EAT arises from a single focus of increased automaticity located within the atria. The firing rate of the ectopic focus is faster than that of the sinus node and overrides the normal sinus node activity. Heart rates can range from 130 to 210 bpm in children and adolescents, but can reach 300 bpm in infants (**Fig. 77.8**). The location of the ectopic focus is most commonly the atrial appendage or the orifices of the pulmonary veins in either atrium, with the right more common than the left. AV block may occur during the tachycardia, but will not interrupt the atrial tachycardia. EAT is associated with conditions that result in atrial dilation, such as AV valve regurgitation and postoperative atrial surgery. In addition, the arrhythmia

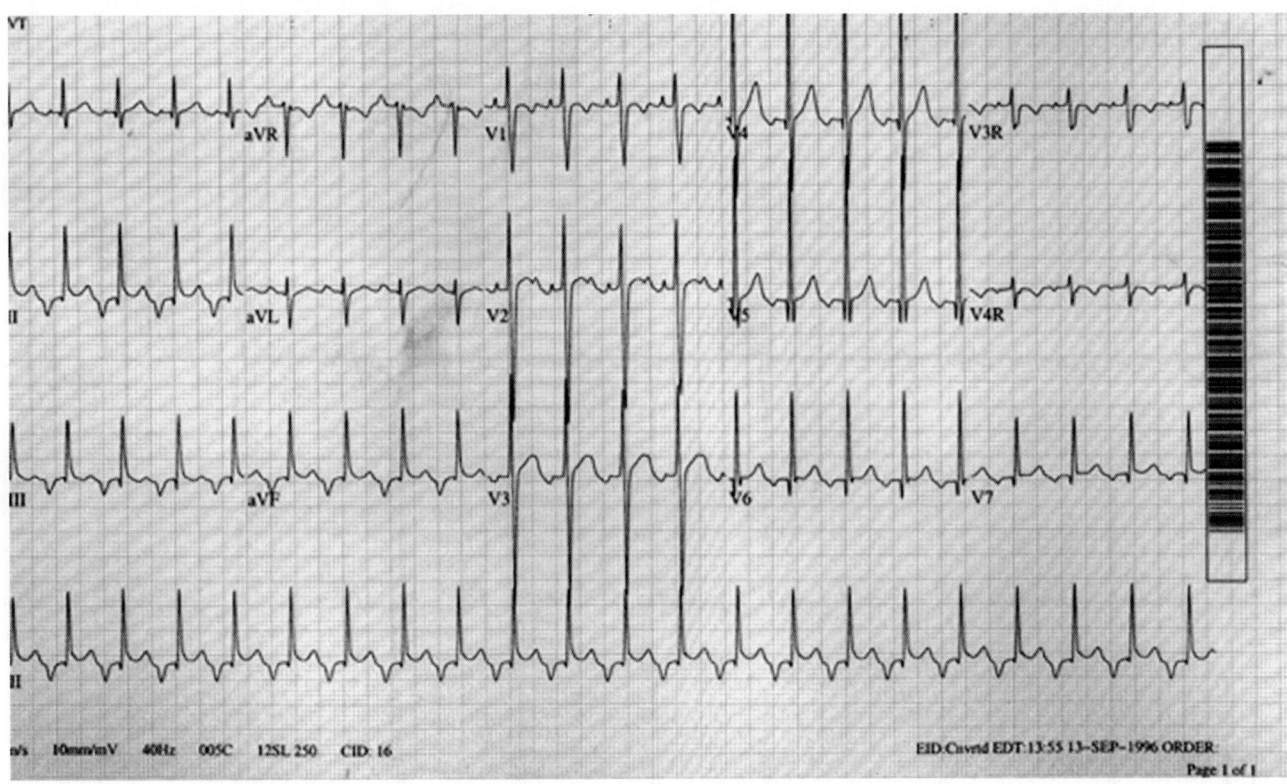

FIGURE 77.8. ECG showing ectopic atrial tachycardia. Note that the P wave is negative in leads II and aVF. Note that this ECG could also represent AV reentrant type with a long RP interval or PJRT with inverted P waves in II, III, and aVF.

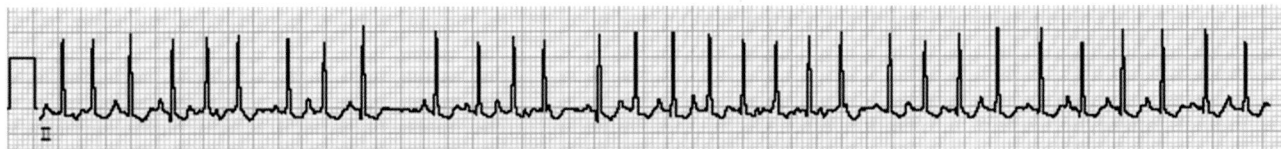

FIGURE 77.9. ECG from an infant with multifocal atrial tachycardia. Note the multiple P-wave morphologies.

has been associated with chronic cardiomyopathy and myocarditis. While some cases of EAT spontaneously resolve, most patients require chronic therapy.

Multifocal Atrial Tachycardia. MAT, or chaotic atrial rhythm, is rare and arises from multiple foci of increased automaticity located within the atria. The tachycardia is defined by the presence of three or more P-wave morphologies. MAT may be confused with atrial fibrillation because of the irregular rhythm and the variable P-wave morphologies (**Fig. 77.9**). The most common presentation is during the newborn period, with up to 50% of patients having an associated cardiac defect or other medical condition. Frequently, this type of tachycardia will spontaneously resolve during the first year of life (20).

Treatment of Ectopic Atrial Tachycardia/Multifocal Atrial Tachycardia. Initial treatment of an automatic SVT involves decreasing the ventricular response rate by slowing AV conduction and decreasing the automaticity of the abnormal focus or foci. Digoxin and calcium-channel blockers can slow conduction through the AV node. Calcium-channel blockers should not be used in children <1 year of age. *β*-blockers, which oppose adrenergic stimulation of the focus, may help suppress the tachycardia. Class IA agents, such as procainamide, and class IC agents, such as flecainide and

propafenone, act by decreasing automaticity and prolonging refractoriness. Class III agents, such as amiodarone and sotalol, can slow conduction throughout the myocardium, including the abnormal focus. Spontaneous resolution of EAT in older patients is unlikely, and catheter ablation tends to be first-line therapy, whereas in younger patients, resolution of EAT is common with low recurrence rates. Catheter ablation of the ectopic focus has become an effective means of curing EAT and is the treatment of choice for medically refractory dysrhythmia. Technical difficulties may arise, as the dysrhythmia is catecholamine sensitive and may be suppressed by sedation. Of note, adenosine, overdrive pacing, and cardioversion will not be successful in converting automatic tachycardias to sinus rhythm.

Junctional Ectopic Tachycardia. JET occurs as a result of enhanced automaticity in the region within or adjacent to the AV junction. JET is characterized by a narrow complex tachycardia with AV dissociation and a ventricular rate faster than the atrial rate (**Fig. 77.10**), though there can be one-to-one VA conduction, or VA Wenckebach. In the pediatric population, JET may be familial and congenital. Patients present during infancy, with some cases detected in utero. Congestive heart failure is frequently the presenting sign and is associated with higher heart rates. Younger patients <6 months old are more likely to have incessant JET. Medical therapy may be weaned

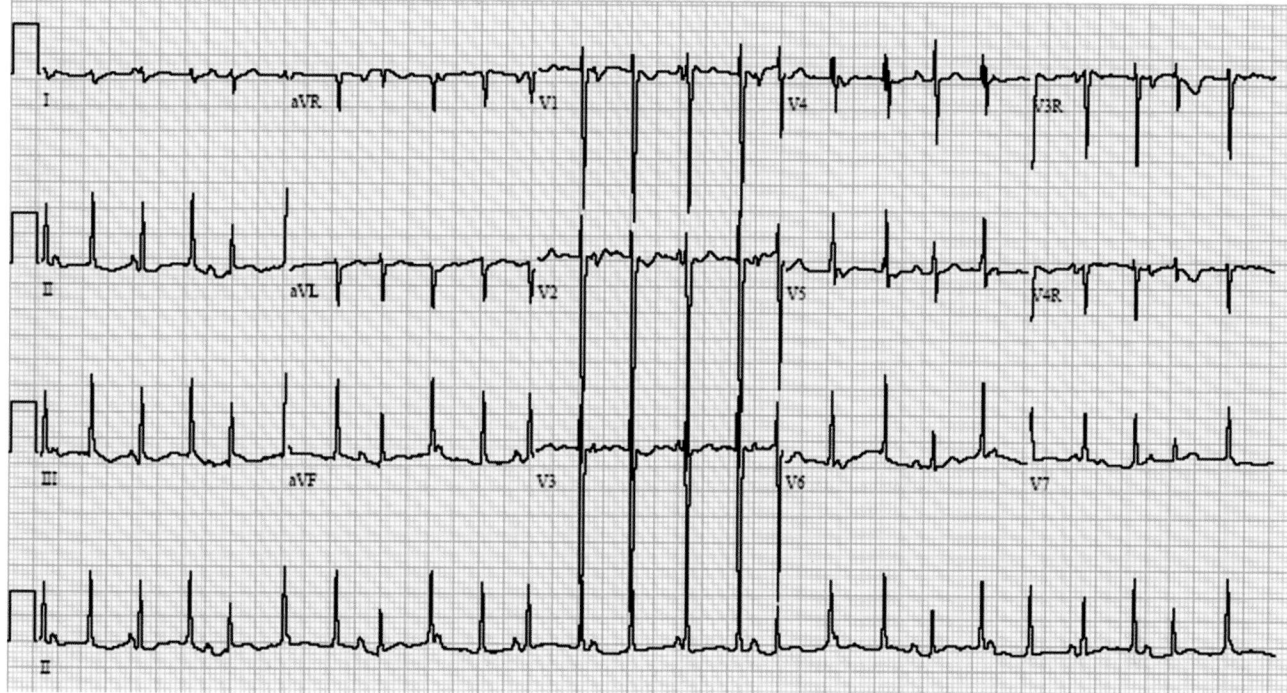

FIGURE 77.10. ECG showing congenital junctional ectopic tachycardia in a newborn. Note the narrow QRS complex with AV dissociation and a ventricular rate that is faster than the atrial rate. There are occasional sinus capture beats seen.

after several months to years in some patients. In one follow-up study, patients who were weaned from their medications were either entirely in sinus rhythm or had intermittent episodes of a slow junctional ectopic rhythm. Sudden death has been reported in this population (21,22).

JET also occurs in the immediate postoperative period following surgery for congenital heart disease. Postoperative JET is usually transient, usually lasting up to 72 hours. Despite its self-limited nature, postoperative JET can cause significant hemodynamic instability. The combination of depressed postoperative myocardial function, tachycardia rates as high as 250 bpm, and loss of AV synchrony may significantly impair cardiac output. With aggressive treatment, the ventricular rate can be slowed, and the patient can be supported until the dysrhythmia resolves. Postoperative JET is most commonly seen following repairs that are near the AV node such as ventricular septal defect closure, tetralogy of Fallot (TOF), and AV canal repairs.

Treatment of Junctional Ectopic Tachycardia. For the congenital form of JET, antiarrhythmic medications are the first line of therapy, with amiodarone being the most successful. Antiarrhythmic therapy may result in enough SND to necessitate the use of a pacemaker (22). Ablation therapy is reserved for the most resistant cases of JET because of the high risk of the development of AV block, though the use of cryotherapy has been shown to be effective without the complication of AV block. Postoperative JET can be treated pharmacologically with amiodarone and/or procainamide. Other nonpharmacologic measures include controlling fever, hypothermia with core temperatures reduced to 35°C, sedation, and avoiding sympathomimetic medications such as epinephrine. Atrial pacing faster than the junctional tachycardia rate can allow for AV synchrony and significantly improve hemodynamics.

Ventricular Arrhythmias

Ventricular Tachycardia. Ventricular arrhythmias in the pediatric population are observed in a variety of patients and

circumstances. VT is defined as three or more ventricular ectopic beats in a row at a rapid rate. In comparison, an accelerated ventricular rhythm occurs at a slower rate (less than 10% above the underlying sinus rate). The differential of any wide QRS complex rhythm should include VT. Following many pediatric cardiac surgical procedures, a prolonged QRS duration can result, usually with a right-bundle-branch block pattern, making the diagnosis of a wide QRS complex tachycardia more difficult after congenital heart disease surgery.

During assessment of a wide QRS complex tachycardia, two important principles should be considered. The QRS complex should have a prolonged duration in VT, but this may be subtle in very young children, as normal measurements of the QRS duration vary with age (**Fig. 77.11**). In addition, VT typically has dissociation of the P waves and QRS complexes, with the QRS complexes occurring at a faster rate. However, children may have retrograde AV node conduction during VT, resulting in retrograde P waves with a 1:1 VA relationship. If it is not possible to determine the P-wave-to-QRS relationship by the surface ECG, recording the atrial activity with a transesophageal electrode catheter or temporary epicardial pacing wires placed at the time of cardiac surgery may be helpful. Finally, symptoms and methods of terminating arrhythmias cannot definitively differentiate between SVT and VT since they are not specific. For example, some types of VT can be sensitive to treatment with adenosine. The possible mechanisms of a wide QRS complex tachycardia are listed in **Table 77.1**.

The patient with a ventricular arrhythmia may be asymptomatic or may present with a cardiomyopathy or cardiac arrest. The patient may have a history of heart disease, but VT may occur in a structurally normal heart. Ischemic heart disease, which is the basis for many of the ventricular arrhythmias noted in the adult population, is rare in pediatric patients. VT in pediatric patients may be associated with a prior surgical repair, myocarditis, cardiomyopathy of any cause, or primary electrical disease. Some wide QRS complex rhythms may occur as a result of marked metabolic or pharmacologic effects

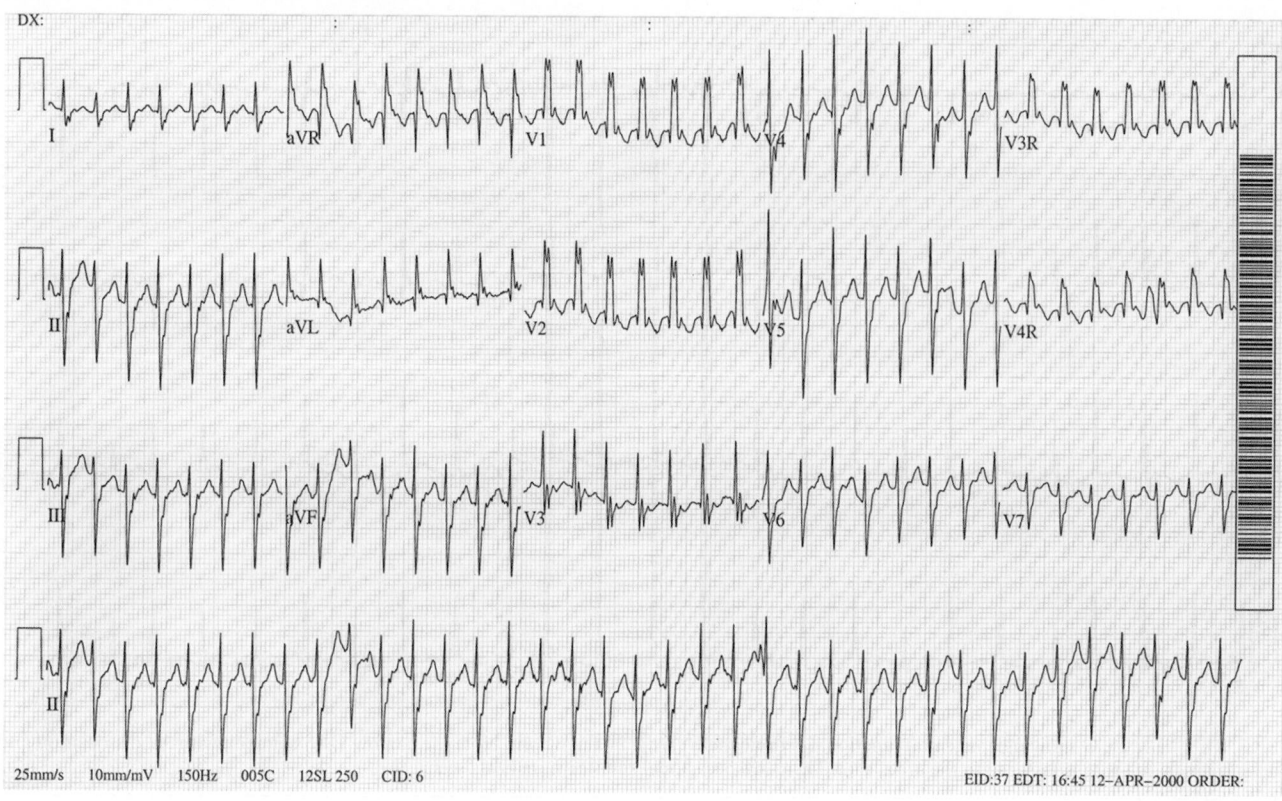

FIGURE 77.11. ECG from an infant with ventricular tachycardia.

on the normal conduction system. Although it is appropriate to manage a wide QRS complex rhythm as a ventricular arrhythmia, other noncardiac etiologies (i.e., hypoxia) should not be overlooked.

The mechanisms by which ventricular arrhythmias occur are the same as those that result in supraventricular arrhythmias: reentry, automaticity, and triggered automaticity. The patient should always be first evaluated clinically for signs of adequate perfusion and hemodynamic stability. If the situation allows, an ECG should be performed. ECG findings that should be noted during the evaluation of a wide QRS complex tachycardia are rate, variability of the R-R interval, QRS duration, QRS complex frontal plane axis, and QRS morphology (monomorphic versus polymorphic). The identification of characteristic features of certain types of VT may allow for more specific and directed therapy.

Isolated premature ventricular complexes are not uncommon in children and are usually benign in the patient with a structurally normal heart, including patients who have ventricular ectopy in a pattern of bigeminy or trigeminy. Although uncommon, frequent premature contractions can lead to

decreased ventricular function (23). On the other hand, in the patient with complex congenital heart disease or a significant cardiomyopathy, premature, ventricular complexes may be a harbinger of more serious arrhythmias. The frequency, timing, and complexity of ventricular ectopy may help to predict the risk of future cardiac events in patients with underlying electrical or myocardial disease (e.g., hypertrophic cardiomyopathy). Ventricular couplets may occur on rare occasion, but nonsustained or sustained runs of VT are generally pathologic and require further investigation.

Ventricular arrhythmias in the child or adolescent with a structurally and functionally normal heart can be well tolerated. When a wide QRS complex tachycardia is irregular, occurs with a gradual onset and termination, and does not respond to cardioversion, an automatic mechanism should be suspected. The most common type of automatic ventricular arrhythmia in the structurally normal heart is that which arises from the outflow tract, typically the right ventricle, which may occur as single, premature ventricular complexes, couplets, or runs of VT. The typical ECG pattern is that of a left-bundle-branch block morphology and inferior frontal plane axis. With a uniform QRS morphology and slower rate, the arrhythmia is frequently asymptomatic and is considered benign with respect to the risk of sudden cardiac events. The arrhythmia appears to arise from the ventricular conal septum, but a specific etiology has not been identified. If other cardiac disease and cardiomyopathy can be excluded with certainty, the prognosis is excellent. Patients with a more incessant form of the arrhythmia that results in an elevated mean daily heart rate may be at risk for the development of a tachycardia-mediated cardiomyopathy (24,25). However, if the rate of the ventricular arrhythmia is <10% faster than the sinus rhythm rate, the rhythm is described as an accelerated ventricular rhythm (Fig. 77.12) (24,26,27). This rhythm is recognized in the newborn with a benign prognosis and usually results in spontaneous resolution of the arrhythmia

TABLE 77.1

MECHANISMS OF A WIDE QRS COMPLEX TACHYCARDIA

Orthodromic atrioventricular reciprocating tachycardia with aberration or bundle-branch block

Antidromic atrioventricular reciprocating tachycardia

Atrial tachycardia with bystander accessory pathway, allowing antegrade conduction (WPW)

Atrioventricular reciprocating tachycardia involving a Mahaim fiber

Ventricular tachycardia

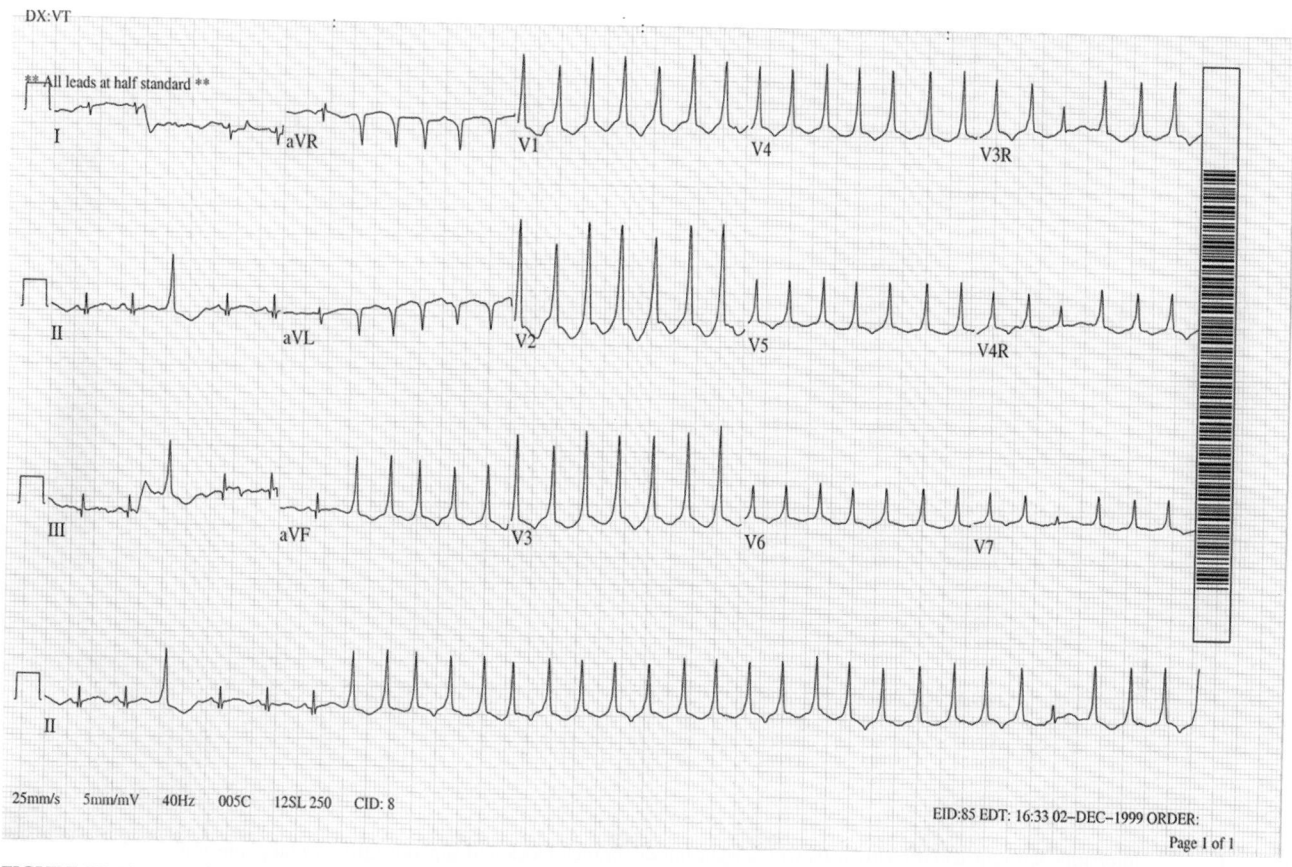

FIGURE 77.12. ECG from a newborn with accelerated ventricular rhythm.

substrate within the first year of life. Although automatic ventricular arrhythmias in the apparently structurally normal heart are generally benign, follow-up is indicated, as isolated instances of significant cardiac events have been reported that probably represent a failure to identify underlying myocardial disease or other risk factors for sudden death.

Patients with an automatic VT may be treated with either medical therapy to suppress the focus or curative catheter-ablation therapy (26,28). The goal of medical therapy is to suppress the active focus or control the rate of the tachycardia. β-blockers and verapamil (verapamil should be avoided in patients <1 year of age) may be effective and have the benefit of being associated with a lower side-effect profile. In infancy and childhood, the majority of patients that require antiarrhythmic therapy will be able to discontinue therapy without relapse of VT. Of those that require medical therapy, the success rates are highest with amiodarone (89%), with sotalol being the most widely used single agent (success rates 62%). Typical indications for catheter ablation include severity of symptoms, failure of drug therapy, incessant VT, and left ventricular dysfunction (25,29). Successful catheter-ablation therapy is performed with the arrhythmia focus usually located within the right ventricular septum, which sometimes must be approached from the left ventricular side. However, indications for catheter ablation are not universal, especially in younger children, because many idiopathic ventricular arrhythmias in the structurally normal heart resolve spontaneously (25,26).

Patients with a structurally normal heart can also develop a reentrant VT. Belhassen described an idiopathic left VT with a right-bundle-branch block pattern and typically a superior frontal plane QRS axis (Fig. 77.13) (30,31). Belhassen (also described as Idiopathic Fascicular or Verapamil sensitive) VT is thought to be maintained by a reentry circuit involving one of the two fascicles of the left bundle. The VT is particularly sensitive to treatment with verapamil or adenosine. This form of VT has been observed in children of all ages and is generally associated with an excellent long-term prognosis (28). If it does not resolve spontaneously or is refractory to medical therapy, the arrhythmia is amenable to catheter-ablation therapy (25,32,33).

In patients who have had prior surgical repair of congenital heart disease, a reentrant mechanism of VT is most commonly identified. The circuit typically occurs in those who have had a ventriculotomy as part of their surgical repair, but any anatomic scar or electrically abnormal area of myocardium may serve as a substrate (34). Surgical incisions and scar serve as a barrier around which the reentry circuit can travel (the large right ventricular outflow tract incision and patch-repair of the ventricular septal defect made in TOF repair). An automatic mechanism can also occur at any ventricular site with enhanced excitability. Thus, the surgical procedures performed, in combination with long-term hemodynamic consequences, create a complex substrate for the development of arrhythmias.

The incidence of VT after repair of TOF ranges from 4.2% to 14.6%, and late sudden death has been reported to be ~6%, ranging between 2% and 9% (35–38). Extensive efforts have been made to identify patients with repaired TOF who are at greatest risk for the development of VT and sudden death in follow-up. A number of demographic (prior palliative shunt, older age at repair, right ventriculotomy), hemodynamic (Higher NYHA class status, LV end diastolic pressure >12 mm Hg), and electrophysiologic variables (QRS duration >180 ms, QRS rate of change) have been proposed as risk factors (Table 77.2), but the risk stratification of individual patients is still suboptimal (39). Programmed ventricular stimulation during an invasive electrophysiologic study has been used to

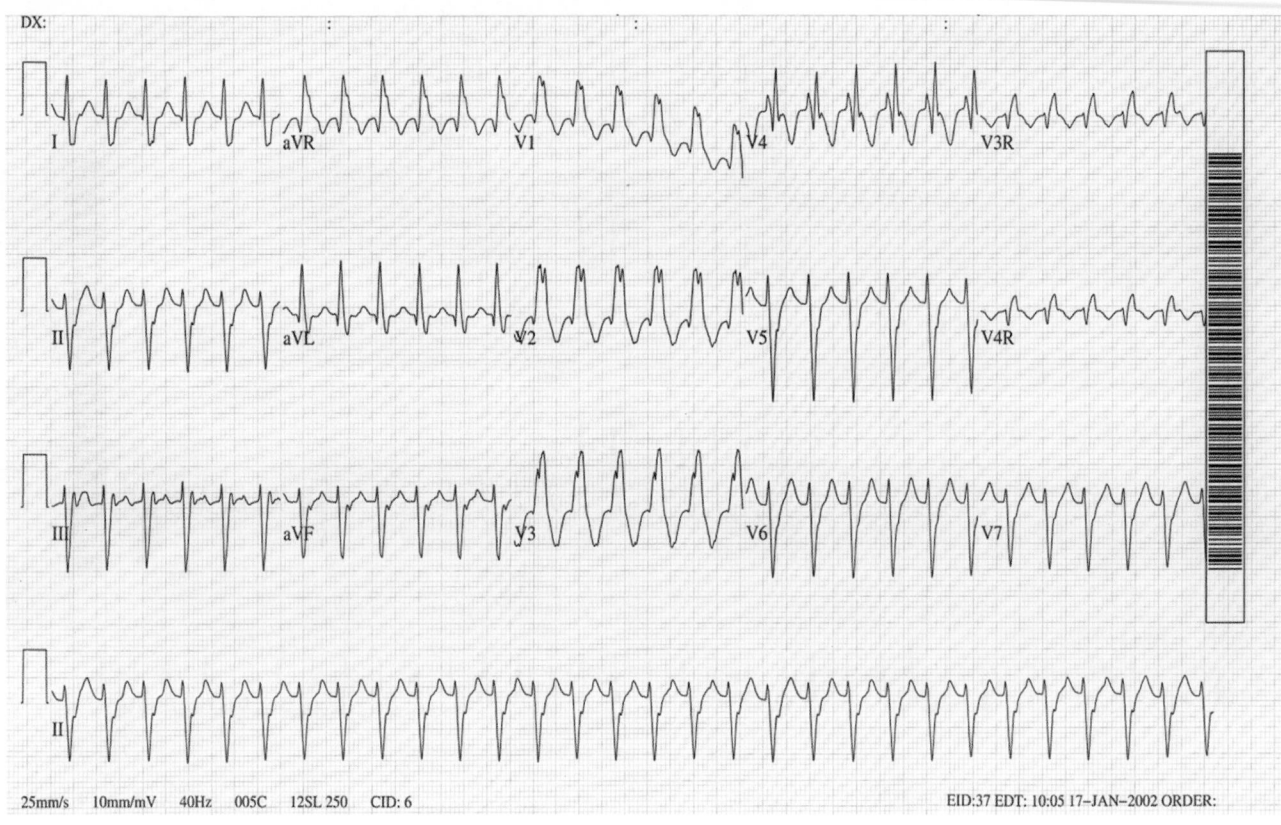

DX:

25mm/s   10mm/mV   40Hz   005C   12SL 250   CID: 6   EID:37 EDT: 10:05 17–JAN–2002 ORDER:

FIGURE 77.13.   Idiopathic left ventricular tachycardia with a right-bundle-branch block and superior QRS frontal plane axis.

help with risk stratification, although the prevalence of inducible, sustained, monomorphic VT is high (36,40). This invasive tool appears to be of some diagnostic and prognostic value, but false-negative studies also occur at a relatively high rate. These electrophysiology studies may contribute to risk-stratification algorithms designed to guide therapy to prevent clinical VT and sudden cardiac death. Although much of the assessment for sudden death in postoperative TOF patients is focused on the cardiac rhythm, it is important to remember that electrophysiologic abnormalities are closely coupled to hemodynamic derangements. Therefore, anatomic and hemodynamic interventions may be as important as antiarrhythmic medications and devices in caring for these patients (41). In patients that have developed pulmonary regurgitation, pulmonary valve replacement reduced the incidence of sustained monomorphic VT, from 22% to 9%. Intracardiac electrophysiologic mapping

TABLE 77.2

PROPOSED RISK FACTORS FOR VENTRICULAR TACHYCARDIA AND SUDDEN DEATH AFTER REPAIR OF TETRALOGY OF FALLOT

Late repair/older age at repair
Older age at follow-up/earlier surgical era
Prior systemic-to-pulmonary artery shunt
Transannular right ventricular outflow tract patch
Right ventricular pressure and/or volume overload
LV end diastolic pressure >12 mm Hg
Residual ventricular septal defect
Ventricular arrhythmias
Atrial arrhythmias
Complete heart block
QRS duration >180 ms

of monomorphic VT in patients with repaired TOF usually demonstrates a macroreentrant circuit around the outflow tract incision/patch, VSD patch, or conal septum, which may be treated with catheter-ablation therapy. Implantable Cardioverter Defibrillators (ICDs) have been used in patients with TOF for both primary and secondary prevention (39). Primary prevention indications such as syncope, QRS duration >180 ms, nonsustained VT, LV ejection fraction <35%, and inducible VT during EP study have been used. Annual rates of shocks are similar for primary and secondary prevention (7%–9%), with a higher LV EDP and nonsustained VT being predictors for ICD shocks in primary prevention.

Patients with other cardiac lesions may also be at risk for ventricular arrhythmias (42,43). Patients enrolled in the Second Natural History study (>15-year follow-up of congenital heart disease that included those with aortic stenosis, pulmonary stenosis, and ventricular septal defect) had a higher frequency of premature ventricular complexes and higher-grade ventricular ectopy than the general population (43,44). Patients with aortic stenosis seem to be the highest risk group, with an increased mortality risk in patients with greater outflow tract gradients. Thus, there are certain groups of patients with repaired and unrepaired congenital heart disease that should be considered at increased risk for ventricular arrhythmias and associated symptoms, including sudden death.

Hypertrophic Cardiomyopathy. Patients with *hypertrophic cardiomyopathy* (HCM) comprise a group with myocardial disease that is prone to ventricular arrhythmias. Hypertrophic cardiomyopathy is a common cardiomyopathy occurring in 1 in 500 adults. Left ventricular outflow tract obstruction may result in ventricular arrhythmias due to coronary artery insufficiency and myocardial ischemia. The histologic findings of the myocardium include disorganization of the cardiac muscle cells, which is also thought to carry an

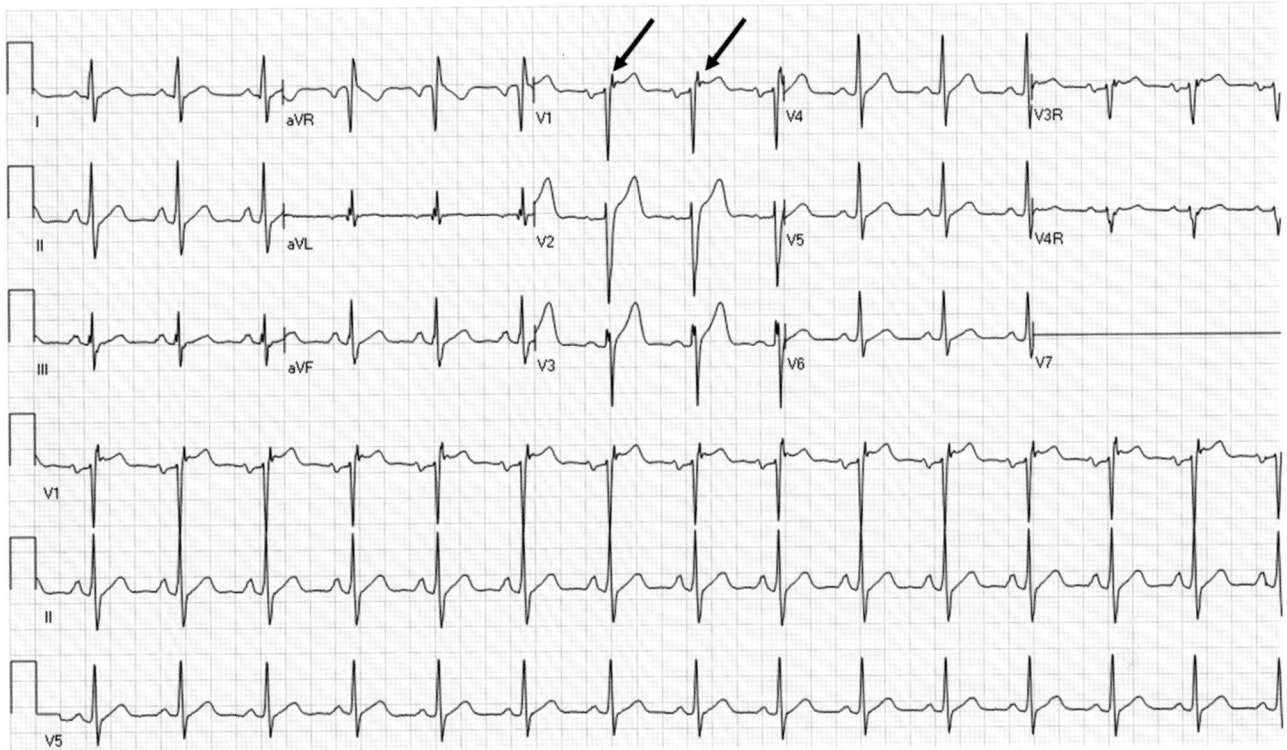

FIGURE 77.14. An ECG demonstrating the Epsilon wave seen in some patients with arrhythmogenic right ventricular cardiomyopathy. *Black arrows* denote the Epsilon waves.

increased potential for arrhythmias. In fact, this microscopic finding seems to put patients at risk regardless of the degree of outflow tract obstruction. Known risk factors for sudden cardiac death (SCD) in adults with HCM include nonsustained VT, family history of sudden death, unexplained syncope, LV thickness >30 mm, and abnormal blood pressure response during exercise (45). ICD implantation is recommended for prevention of SCD in patients with one or more of these major risk factors in adults, but data are limited in the pediatric population if the same risk factors apply (44,45). In a recent study in children with HCM and ICD's, 19% of patients had an appropriate discharge (3% per year for primary prevention). In those patients in which an ICD was placed for primary prevention, there was no difference in ICD discharge rate for those who had 1, 2, or >3 risk factors (14%).

Arrhythmogenic Right Ventricular Cardiomyopathy (ARVC). It is another, less common, cause of VT in, apparently healthy, young people that can cause SCD (46). The pathologic findings may be subtle, and the patient frequently has a normal echocardiogram. The associated VT typically has the morphology of a left-bundle-branch block, as the arrhythmia generally arises from the right ventricular outflow tract. The baseline ECG may reveal T-wave inversion in the right precordial leads (frequently a normal finding in pediatric patients). The QRS complex may be prolonged, and characteristic low-voltage potentials (ε waves) may occur following the QRS complex (Fig. 77.14). The cardiomyopathy involves aneurysmal dilatation and dyskinesis of the right ventricular outflow tract. Histologically, localized replacement or infiltration with fibrous and adipose tissue is seen. Cardiac MRI has become the primary method of identifying the anatomic abnormalities (Fig. 77.15). The diagnosis may be familial or sporadic, with molecular genetic studies showing that it is a disease of the cardiac desmosomes (responsible for cell-to-cell binding) resulting from defective cell adhesion

proteins. There are revised Task Force Criteria from 2010, and the diagnosis is fulfilled by the presence of major and minor criteria including global or regional dysfunction, tissue characterization, repolarization and depolarization abnormalities, arrhythmias, and family history. ICD therapy is recommended in patients with one or more risk factors for SCD, which include early and severe RV dysfunction or advanced disease with biventricular dysfunction, family history of SCD, and symptomatic VT.

Cardiac Tumors These umors, although rare, are another source of ventricular arrhythmias (47). Rhabdomyomas are the

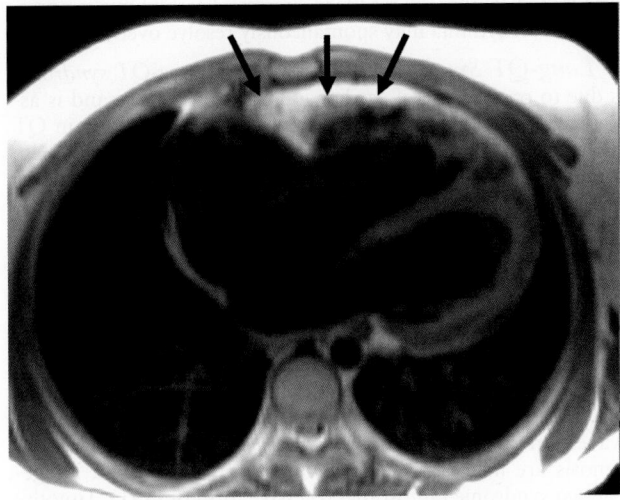

FIGURE 77.15. MRI demonstrating fibrofatty replacement of myocardial tissue. Black arrows denote the fibrofatty replacement.

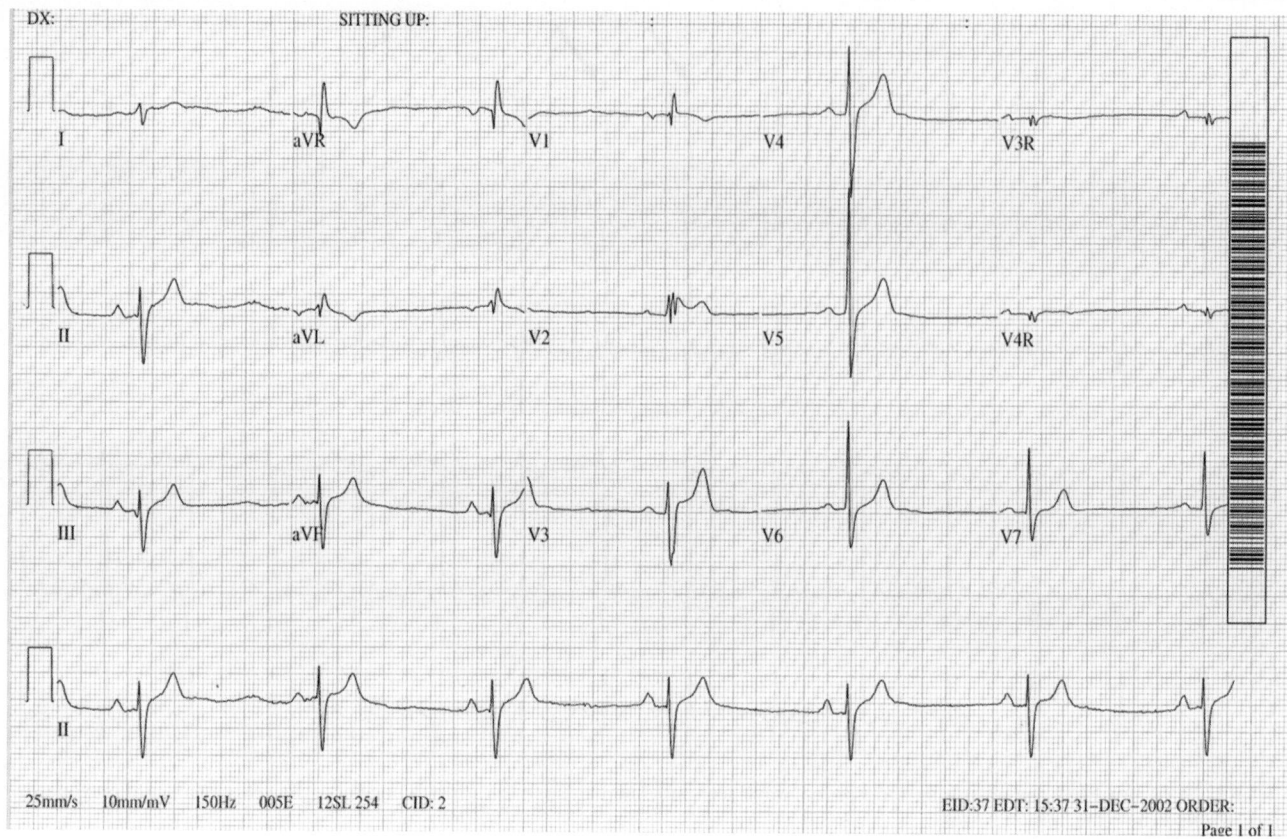

FIGURE 77.16. An ECG pattern observed in patients with Brugada syndrome. Note the right ventricular conduction delay and anterior precordial lead ST segment elevation.

most common cardiac tumor in pediatric patients and are usually found in children with tuberous sclerosis. The tumors are usually multiple and located in the ventricle and interventricular septum. Although many rhabdomyomas regress over time, young patients with rhabdomyomas have been reported to die suddenly or develop congestive heart failure. Treatment of arrhythmias may include medications, catheter ablation, or surgical resection. Fibromas are usually single, large tumors of the ventricle that can be treated successfully with surgical resection. Hamartomas have been described as being associated with incessant VT in infants and have been treated with surgical resection and cryoablation in those refractory to medical therapy. However, if medical therapy results in successful arrhythmia suppression, the arrhythmia may spontaneously resolve over time.

Long-QT Syndrome. The congenital *long-QT syndrome* is due to one of several cardiac ion channelopathies and is associated with abnormal cardiac repolarization resulting in QT prolongation, syncope, cardiac arrest, and sudden death. These symptoms are due to the polymorphic VT (torsades de pointes [TdP]) that occurs as a result of a prolonged duration of the ventricular action potential and early afterdepolarizations that can be propagated to neighboring cells secondary to differences in refractory periods. The electrical abnormality can occur as an inherited congenital problem, an acquired metabolic disturbance, or medication exposure. As the presenting symptom can be a seizure, all patients with a presumed seizure disorder should have a screening ECG. Other ECG findings include bradycardia, 2:1 AV block, abnormal T-wave morphology, prominent U waves, and T-wave alternans. Other associations with the diagnosis are neurosensory hearing loss in Jervelle and Lange-Nielsen syndrome (autosomal recessive form of LQT), Timothy syndrome (LQT8), and Andersen–Tawil syndrome (LQT7). Although several genetic mutations have been recognized to cause

long-QT syndrome, the most common being LQT1 (KCNQ1), LQT2 (KCNH2), and LQT3 (SCN5A), therapy continues to focus on the treatment and prevention of TdP and SCD. Patients at highest risk for SCD include a QTc >500 ms, history of TdP leading to syncope, prepubertal boys and postpubertal girls, and events occurring in the first year of life. Effective therapies include pacing (for bradycardia and pause-dependent episodes of ventricular arrhythmia), magnesium, and β-blockers (e.g., esmolol). Long-term medical therapy for patients with LQT1 and LQT2 are β-blockers (e.g., nadolol/propranolol). Guidelines for ICD therapy include aborted cardiac arrest, breakthrough cardiac events despite adequate medical therapy, and prior LQT triggered events with a QTc >550 ms. It is equally important to avoid cardiac stimulants and medications that are known to prolong the QT interval (some antiarrhythmics, psychotropic medications, erythromycin, and many antifungal agents). There is a complete list of drugs to be avoided at (www.qtdrugs.org). It is important to screen family members, as the presenting symptom of long-QT syndrome may be a life-threatening arrhythmia.

Brugada Syndrome. It is a familial, primary, electrical abnormality with ECG findings that consist of a right ventricular conduction delay and ST segment elevation ("coved" and "saddle" shape elevations) in the anterior precordial leads (V1–V3) (**Fig. 77.16**). Clinically, patients are typically young male adults and present with syncope, ventricular arrhythmias, and sudden death. Several identified mutations affect the SCN5A gene (20%–30% of Brugada patients), which encodes for the cardiac sodium channel. Some families do not have mutations in this gene, indicating that other genetic defects will be found, and that this is a genetically heterogeneous disease. Diagnostic testing includes a provocative drug challenge with a class I antiarrhythmic medication (e.g., procainamide), which may reveal or enhance the characteristic type I Brugada ECG

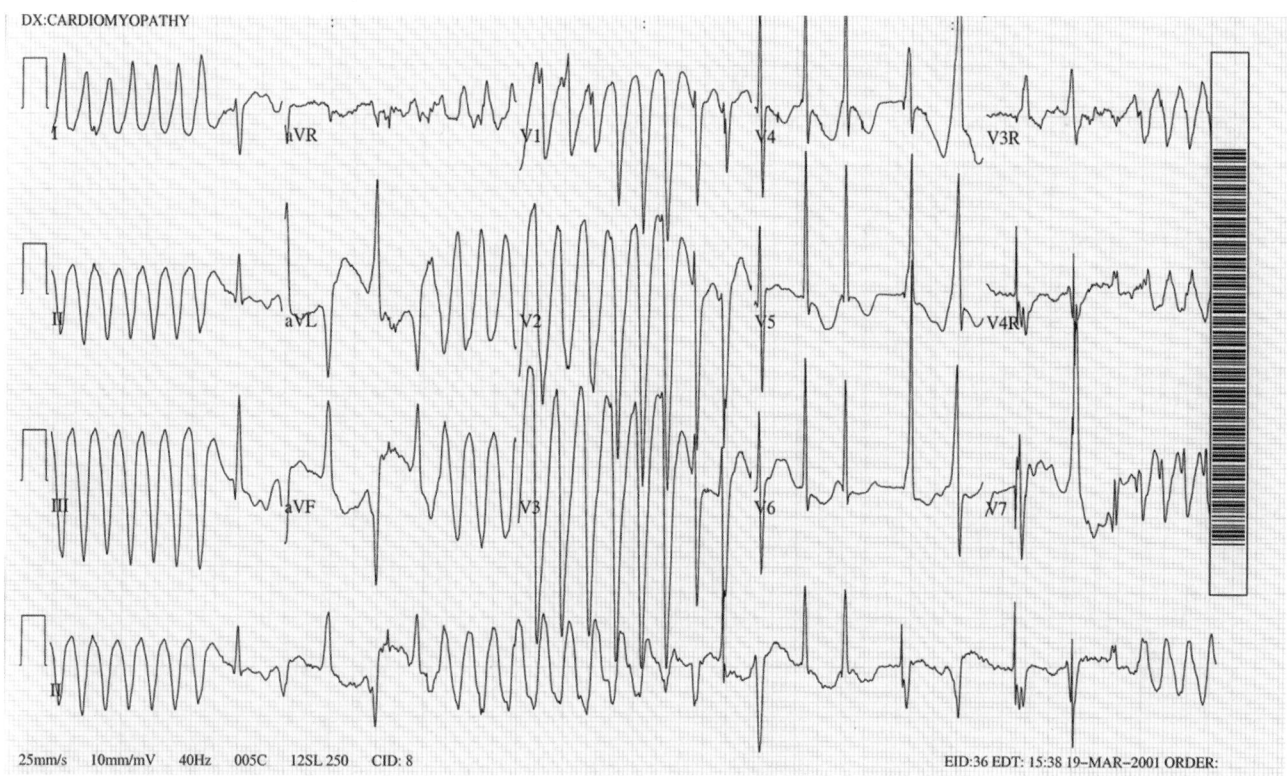

DX:CARDIOMYOPATHY

25mm/s   10mm/mV   40Hz   005C   12SL 250   CID: 8   EID:36 EDT: 15:38 19–MAR–2001 ORDER:

FIGURE 77.17. ECG showing torsades de pointes in a patient with long-QT syndrome.

pattern. The only effective treatment for Brugada syndrome is an implantable defibrillator.

Catecholaminergic Polymorphic VT (CPVT). It has been associated with abnormalities in the cardiac ryanodine receptor (RYR2), which is responsible for the release of calcium from the sarcoplasmic reticulum and calsequestrin-2 (CASQ2), which is a calcium buffering protein of the sarcoplasmic reticulum. It is thought that the increased calcium release is responsible for the development of arrhythmias. Patients develop polymorphic VT or bidirectional VT during exercise and other increased adrenergic states. β-blockers, flecainide, and implantable defibrillators are the mainstay of therapy.

Polymorphic VT should be differentiated from monomorphic VT and is generally poorly tolerated. TdP (**Fig. 77.17**) is recognized by its characteristic pattern of positive and negative oscillations of the QRS complex around the isoelectric baseline, or "twisting of the spikes" (48). It is a pause-dependent arrhythmia that is typically initiated by a premature ventricular complex that occurs during the vulnerable period of ventricular repolarization ("R-on-T phenomenon"). The arrhythmia is highly suggestive of the diagnosis of congenital or acquired long-QT syndrome. Causes of acquired long-QT syndrome should be considered, especially QT-interval-prolonging drugs. TdP should initially be treated with the withdrawal of any aggravating medications and correction of any metabolic abnormalities. Medical therapy should include magnesium supplementation, β-blockers, and lidocaine. Although seemingly counterintuitive, isoproterenol may be beneficial by directly shortening myocardial repolarization times and increasing the heart rate in order to avoid pause-dependent arrhythmias. Patients who experience sustained polymorphic VT with significant hemodynamic compromise despite maximal medical therapy may be candidates for circulatory support with extracorporeal membrane oxygenation or ventricular assist devices. The arrhythmia must be reasonably controlled

before the patient can be considered for an implantable defibrillator, as repeated therapies from a device could escalate arrhythmia activity. *Bidirectional ventricular tachycardia*, another type of polymorphic VT, is characterized by a beat-to-beat alternation of the QRS axis. Bidirectional VT should raise concern for digitalis toxicity or CPVT (**Fig. 77.18**).

Ventricular arrhythmias may arise in several other specific and nonspecific situations. Any condition that can be associated with myocardial inflammation, ischemia, or infarction may result in an increased likelihood of ventricular arrhythmias.

Wide QRS complex rhythms and ventricular arrhythmias are caused by an assortment of systemic causes (**Table 77.3**). Metabolic abnormalities can result in a wide QRS complex tachycardia. Hypoxia and metabolic acidosis can result in sinus tachycardia with delayed conduction through the His–Purkinje system. In addition, electrolyte abnormalities may have direct cellular effects on the myocardium that result in lengthening of the cardiac intervals. For example, hyperkalemia results in prolongation of the PR interval, QRS widening, and lengthening of the QT interval, with a terminal ECG that resembles a sinusoidal waveform (**Fig. 77.19**). Thus, for any critical care patient, the content of IV fluids, parenteral nutrition, and serum electrolytes should be carefully examined if ECG changes suggest an electrolyte abnormality. Physiologic causes of hyperkalemia include metabolic acidosis, such as in diabetic ketoacidosis or cellular death (as with bowel ischemia). The ECG changes seen with hyperkalemia respond promptly to immediate treatment with hyperventilation, calcium, sodium bicarbonate, or glucose/insulin. Finally, drug overdoses (i.e., tricyclic antidepressants) may result in a wide QRS complex rhythm, some of which cause QRS complex prolongation in association with tachycardia.

Management of acute ventricular arrhythmias is dependent on the etiology and hemodynamic stability of the patient. A defibrillator should always be readily available in the event that

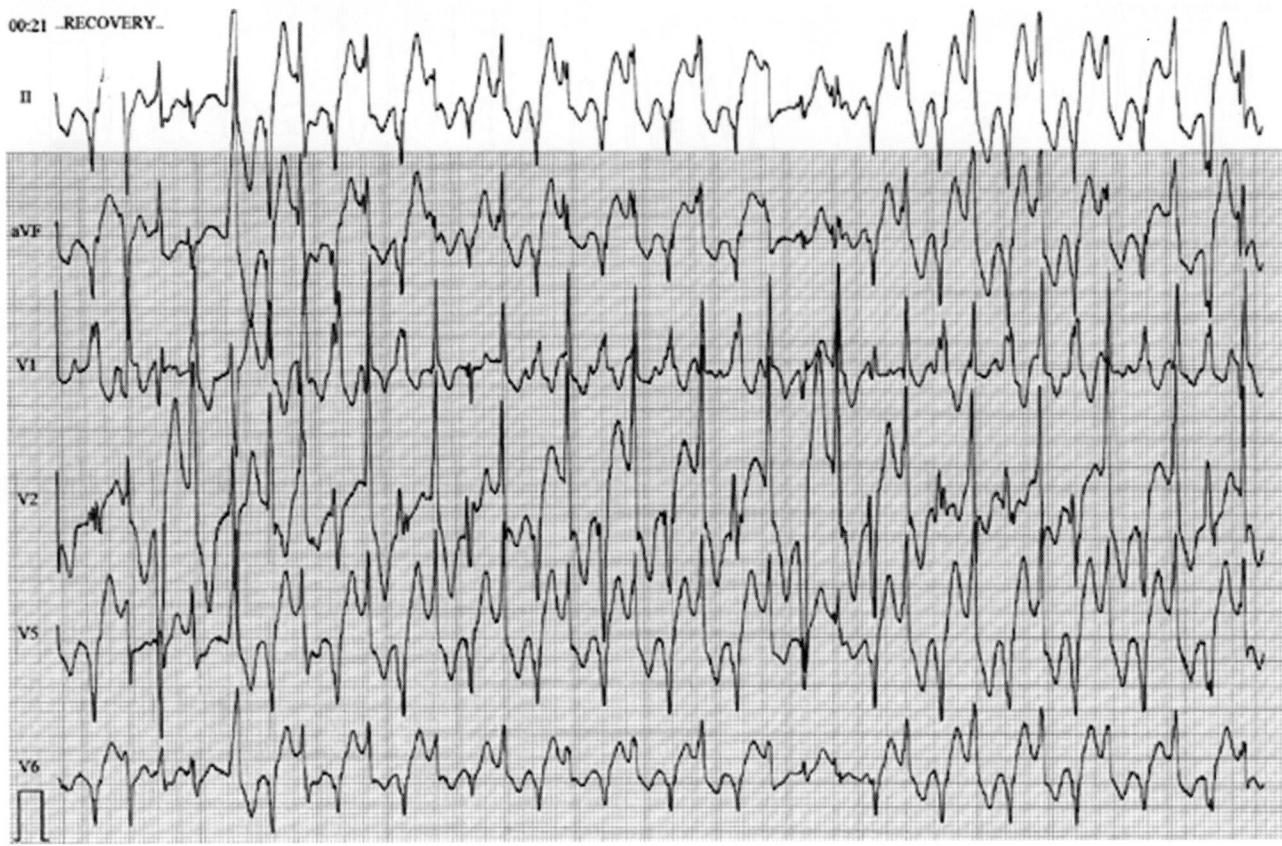

FIGURE 77.18. ECG demonstrating bidirectional ventricular tachycardia. (Courtesy of Dr. Timothy Slesnick.)

TABLE 77.3

SYSTEMIC CAUSES OF VENTRICULAR ARRHYTHMIA

Metabolic	Hyperkalemia
	Hypokalemia
	Hypomagnesemia
	Hypocalcemia
	Hypoxia
	Acidosis
Ischemia	Kawasaki disease
Infectious	Systemic viral infections causing myocarditis
	Systemic bacterial infections causing endocarditis
Toxic	Cocaine/catecholamine infusions/stimulants
	Antiarrhythmic medications
	Digitalis toxicity
	Psychotropic medications
Traumatic	Commotio cordis
	Mechanical irritation/central catheters

the rhythm spontaneously deteriorates, the patient is hemodynamically unstable or develops altered mental status. Medical management or synchronized direct current cardioversion (2 J/kg) may be used to treat a perfusing ventricular arrhythmia or a wide QRS complex arrhythmia with an organized electrical pattern. Expert consultation with an electrophysiologist should be arranged when starting antiarrhythmics (e.g., amiodarone) for a patient in stable VT (49,50). If the rhythm is pulseless or disorganized to the point that the defibrillator cannot recognize distinct QRS complexes, asynchronous defibrillation must be delivered immediately. Chronic therapy is warranted for most patients with spontaneous and sustained VT, unless a reversible and treatable cause is identified. The long-term medical treatment of VT generally involves careful follow-up and the suppression of any recurrences. The ultimate goal is to prevent potentially life-threatening events. Invasive electrophysiologic testing to exclude inducibility may be warranted in some patients. However, sometimes the end point of therapy is not easily determined, as aggressive treatment with some antiarrhythmic agents may result in more morbidity and mortality than the arrhythmia itself. ICD therapy has become more commonly applied in children and is often necessary when symptoms are particularly concerning, significant risk factors exist, or the efficacy of medical therapy is in doubt. The current class I recommendations for ICD's in pediatric patients include (a) survivor of cardiac arrest after evaluation to define the cause of the event and to exclude any reversible causes and (b) patients with symptomatic sustained VT in association with congenital heart disease who have undergone hemodynamic and electrophysiologic evaluation. Catheter ablation or surgical repair may offer possible alternatives in carefully selected patients. The ACC/AHA/HRS 2008 Guidelines for Device-Based Therapy of Cardiac Rhythm Abnormalities include all the ICD recommendations for both adults and pediatric patients (51).

In summary, ventricular arrhythmias are not uncommon in the PICU population and are more likely to be symptomatic if the tachycardia rate is very fast or if myocardial dysfunction is present. If the patient is relatively stable, medical attempts may be made to restore sinus rhythm after an ECG has been performed. Antiarrhythmic medications that affect the sodium and potassium channels of the ventricular myocardium, such as amiodarone and lidocaine, may be most appropriate. Those patients that are hemodynamically unstable should be treated

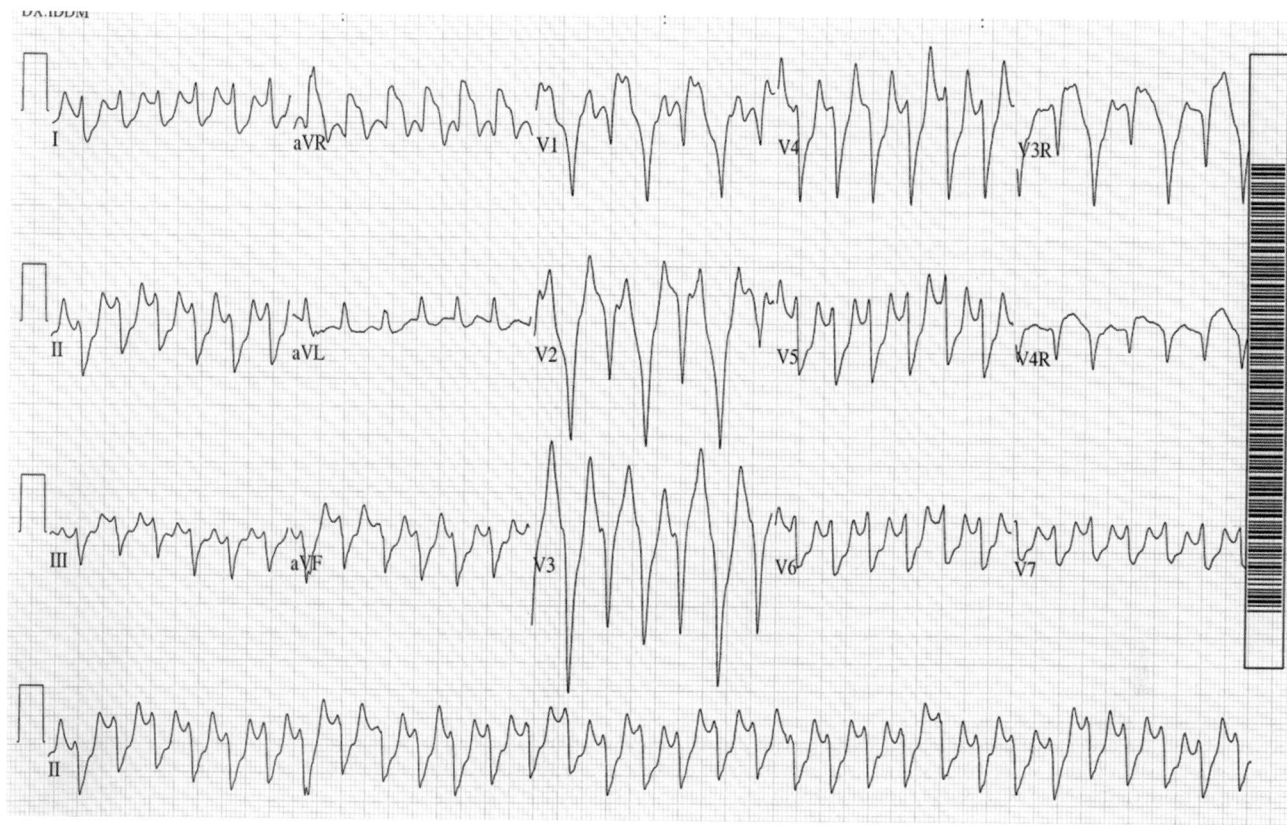

FIGURE 77.19. ECG findings observed with hyperkalemia.

with cardioversion or defibrillation. Automatic and reentrant VT in both patients with and without congenital heart disease are amenable to treatment with catheter-ablation techniques. Finally, if patients are thought to be at significant risk for the development of life-threatening symptoms from VT, placement of an implantable defibrillator should be considered.

BRADYARRHYTHMIAS

In pediatrics, bradycardia is defined as a heart rate that is below the defined age-based range limit. There are multiple mechanistic drivers that can result in bradyarrhythmias including abnormalities in impulse generation or propagation, abnormalities of the central conduction system (including the AV node and/or the distal His–Purkinje system), or the presence of premature atrial complexes that fail to conduct to the ventricle and can result in functional bradycardia. Bradyarrhythmia can be the result of a primary electrical problem, but in intensive care settings, it is often the clinical manifestation of concomitant respiratory, medication or metabolic derived issues.

Diagnostic Approach to Bradyarrhythmias

The differentiation between underlying bradycardia mechanisms is imperative for the proper treatment and clinical management of hemodynamically significant bradycardia. Most etiologies can be elucidated from a combination of standard 12-lead electrocardiogram (ECG) and monitored telemetry when available. The rate and relationship between atrial and ventricular activity on ECG is typically diagnostic of both the site and mechanism causing bradycardia. Determination of the atrial mechanism and rate is the most helpful initial step

when diagnosing the etiology for bradycardia. Close attention should be given to determining when atrial activity is occurring on ECG or telemetry, particularly looking for potential atrial activity that may be partially or completely obscured by QRS and/or T-wave electrical activity. Nonconducted premature atrial complexes, often occur during T-wave activity and can be easily overlooked as the underlying explanation for bradycardia (Fig. 77.20).

After identifying atrial activity, determining whether and how the atrial activity is related to the ventricular activity is the next objective. If the ratio between atrial and ventricular complexes is 1:1 and there is a normal PR interval, the rhythm is most likely sinus bradycardia or ectopic atrial bradycardia. If bradycardia occurs suddenly, it may be the result of an acute increase in vagal tone from an endotracheal tube, sedation, or other vagally mediated medication, or a mechanical cause. If bradycardia is constant and long standing, it may be the result of high vagal tone, medications, sedation, or sinus node disease. Other potential mechanisms for sinus bradycardia include hypoxia, ischemia, central nervous system (CNS) disorders with increased intracranial pressure, hypothyroidism, hypothermia, and medication (digoxin, β-blockers, and calcium-channel blockers).

If the PR interval is prolonged for age but each atrial beat is conducted to the ventricle, then first-degree AV block is present. If there is a relationship between atrial and ventricular activity but the relationship is not 1:1 and there are more atrial complexes than ventricular complexes, there is likely some degree of second-degree AV block. The patterning of the atrial-to-ventricular relationship can delineate the type of second-degree AV block and probable location of central conduction system involvement. If there is no relationship between the atrial and ventricular activity and the atrial rate is faster than the ventricular rate, the patient has complete or high-grade AV block.

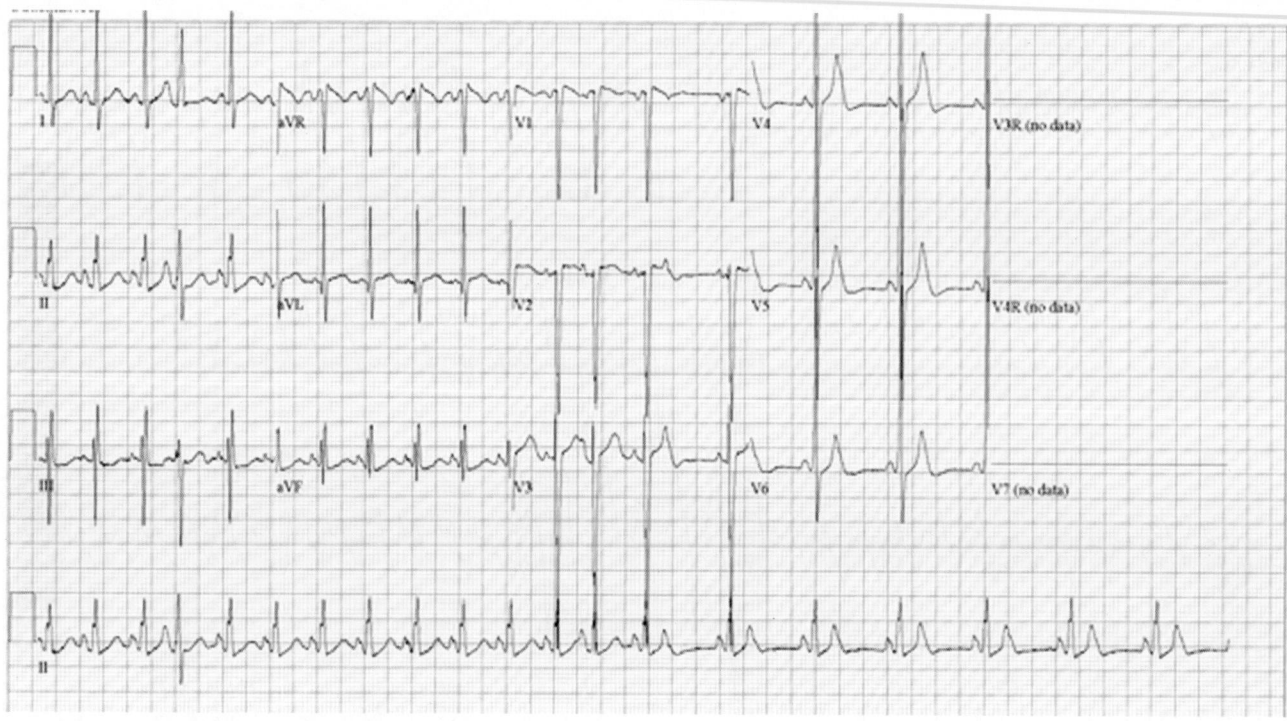

FIGURE 77.20. ECG demonstrating nonconducted premature atrial complexes (PACs) leading to bradycardia. At the beginning of the tracing, there is sinus rhythm with a single PAC. Midway through the tracing, there are frequent PACs in a pattern of bigeminy that are not conducted, resulting in bradycardia. Note the P waves superimposed in the T wave during PAC activity.

If the ventricular rhythm is faster than that of the atrial mechanism and the atrial rhythm is at a bradycardic rate for age, then the underlying rhythm is likely an escape rhythm emanating from either the junction or the ventricle. If the QRS complex is narrow or similar to that seen on previous ECGs, the rhythm is mostly likely a junctional escape rhythm. If there is an acute change in QRS morphology, especially a widening of the QRS complex with initiation of the escape rhythm, the location of the escape mechanism is likely ventricular. Both junctional and ventricular escape mechanisms may have retrograde conduction to the atrium or may have retrograde VA block. When retrograde conduction is present, the atrial activity may be seen following the QRS complex or may occur within the QRS complex itself and be obscured.

Bradyarrhythmia Etiologies

Sinus Node Dysfunction

SND in patients with congenital heart disease is typically the result of surgical scar or suture lines on or around sinoatrial (SA) nodal tissue (52). In the ambulatory setting, clinical manifestations of SND consist of pronounced sinus bradycardia, exercise-induced chronotropic incompetence, and sinus pauses. In the intensive care setting, SND typically presents with an atrial rate that is slower than appropriate for the patient's hemodynamic and clinical scenario, and may manifest with an escape rhythm from the atrium, junction, or ventricle. While most SND is tolerated from a hemodynamic standpoint, the inability to appropriately augment heart rate during concomitant disease processes may lead to hypotension and require treatment.

Patients following cardiac transplantation often have SND secondary to cardiac denervation or direct surgical SA nodal damage. In younger patients, the donor heart may not include the superior vena cava and, potentially, a portion of the right atrium. As the SA node is anatomically located in this area, it may be damaged or not included in the transplanted organ. If the SA node is not included or damaged, there will be SND. If an atrial rate is present, it will be reliant on an atrial escape mechanism from outside the SA node. A similar etiology for SND results from mechanical damage during surgery for congenital heart disease, especially those repairs involving suture and scar lines in the atrium. Common operations that may involve mechanical trauma to the SA node include the atrial-switch operation, Fontan procedure, and repair of atrial septal defects, particularly sinus venosus defects. The outpatient assessment of sinus node function may involve an exercise stress test, ambulatory Holter monitor, pharmacologic challenge, or invasive electrophysiology testing. Although medications have been used, the only reliable means by which to treat symptomatic SND long term is placement of an atrial pacemaker. In the intensive care arena, treatment for SND is often unnecessary, although if clinically significant, medications such as isoproterenol, epinephrine, and atropine may augment the underlying sinus or escape mechanism, but their use must be tempered with potential medication side effects (**Table 77.4**). Patients following surgical cardiac repair often have temporary epicardial wires that may be used for atrial pacing and augmentation of heart rate in the acute setting.

Abnormalities of Atrioventricular Conduction

Abnormalities of the AV conduction system are typically classified on the basis of the relationship between the atrial and ventricular activity. The site of the block within the specialized conduction system may occur in AV nodal tissue or within the more distal His–Purkinje system. Importantly, the type of heart block is often informative to the site of central conduction system involvement as well as prognosis. When the PR interval is prolonged for age, but each atrial beat is conducted to the ventricle, first-degree AV block is present. First-degree AV

TABLE 77.4

TREATMENT FOR HEMODYNAMICALLY SIGNIFICANT BRADYCARDIA

Trendelenburg position (supine with the head lower than the level of the pelvis and feet)

Volume expansion

Pharmacologic interventions

  Anticholinergic agents

    Atropine 0.02–0.04 mg/kg (maximum 1–2 mg) IV/IO

  β-adrenergic agonists and activators of adenylate cyclase

    Isoproterenol infusion: 0.01–2.0 μg/kg/min

    Epinephrine IV bolus: 0.05–0.01 mg/kg; infusion: 0.1–0.5 μg/kg/min

    Glucagon (for β-blocker overdose) 0.03–0.15 mg/kg IV

Digoxin-specific antibody Fab fragments for digoxin toxicity

Temporary transcutaneous or transvenous pacing

Treat reversible causes:

  6 H's: hypoxia, hypovolemia, hydrogen ion (acidosis), hypoglycemia, hypo/hyperkalemia, and hypothermia.

  5 T's: toxins, tamponade, tension pneumothorax, thrombosis (pulmonary), thrombosis (coronary)

block typically results from delayed conduction through the AV node, resulting in an increased PR interval on ECG (**Fig. 77.21**). In patients with congenital heart disease and extensive atrial scaring or myocardial damage, PR prolongation can be the result of slow conduction through the atrial tissue with an increased transit time from the sinus node to the AV node similarly presenting with PR prolongation on the ECG. There are multiple etiologies for first-degree AV block including: increased vagal tone, digoxin or β-blocker administration, viral myocarditis, Lyme disease, hypothermia, electrolyte abnormalities, congenital heart disease, rheumatic fever, or associated cardiomyopathy.

If the atrial and ventricular relationship is not 1:1, there is more atrial activity than ventricular activity, and the patient is not in an atrial tachycardia, then some degree of AV conduction disease is present. When "grouped beating" (the appearance of a repeating pattern of clustered ventricular beats) is present, one should evaluate for potential Mobitz type I second-degree AV block (Wenckebach pattern block). Wenckebach pattern block typically demonstrates progressive PR interval prolongation during the grouped beating, culminating in a nonconducted P wave followed by resetting of the grouped beating pattern (**Fig. 77.22**). The sudden loss of AV conduction without preceding PR interval prolongation is indicative of Mobitz type II second-degree AV block. The distinction between types of second-degree AV block is important as they are usually indicative of different sites of central conduction system involvement. Mobitz type I is typically associated with AV nodal involvement, while Mobitz type II typically involves disease below the AV node in the His–Purkinje system. In the case of progression to complete heart block, patients with complete heart block from AV nodal disease will typically have an escape mechanism from the junction, while patients with disease in the His–Purkinje system that develop complete heart block may have no escape rhythm or one that is sufficiently low that may result in SCD or profound hypotension. Because of this, Mobitz type II heart block is a more concerning pattern and an important distinction in terms of long-term prognosis and management.

Complete heart block, or third-degree AV block, results in complete AV dissociation with the atrial rate faster than the ventricular rate (**Fig. 77.23**). If the ventricular rate is faster than the atrial rate, the patient is likely in an underlying junctional or ventricular rhythm and may or may not have associated heart block. In patients with complete heart block, the QRS morphology can help identify the location of the escape mechanism. Especially in patients with congenital heart disease, it is helpful to compare the rhythm with previous ECGs performed during periods of sinus rhythm. When the escape rhythm arises from the junction (junctional rhythm), the QRS complex should be narrow with a normal QRS axis, although in patients with

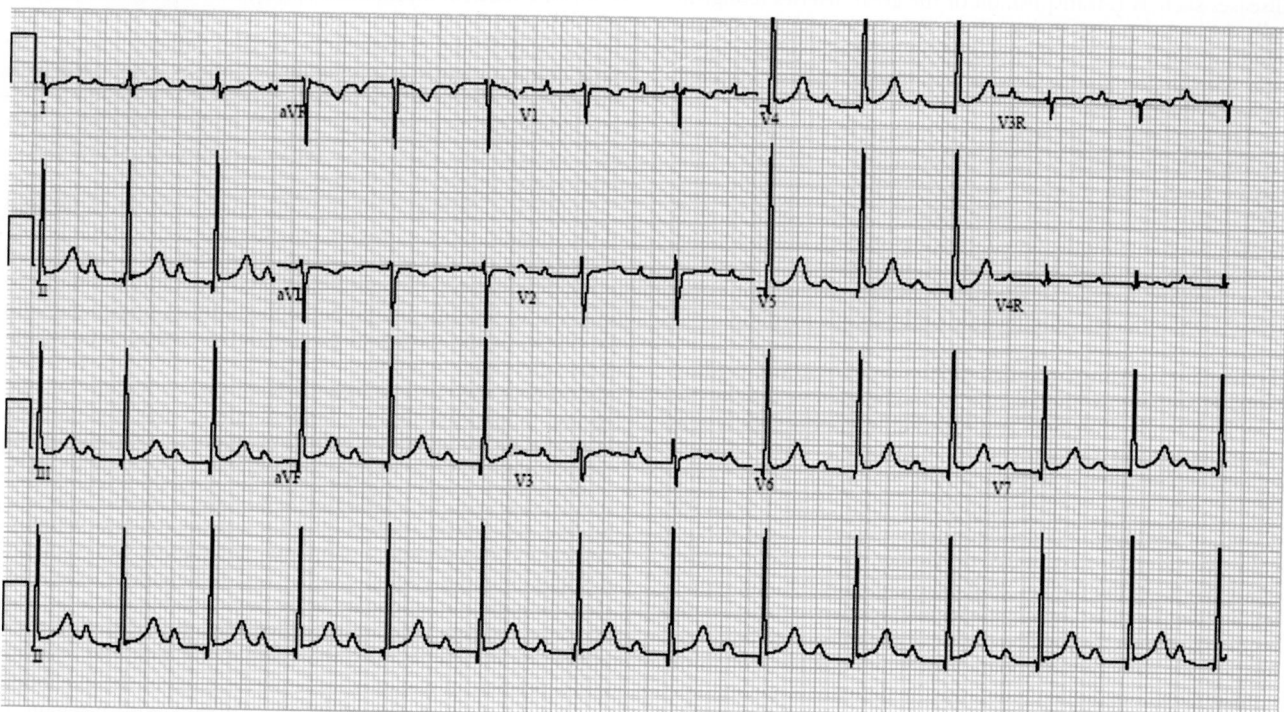

FIGURE 77.21. ECG showing first-degree AV block.

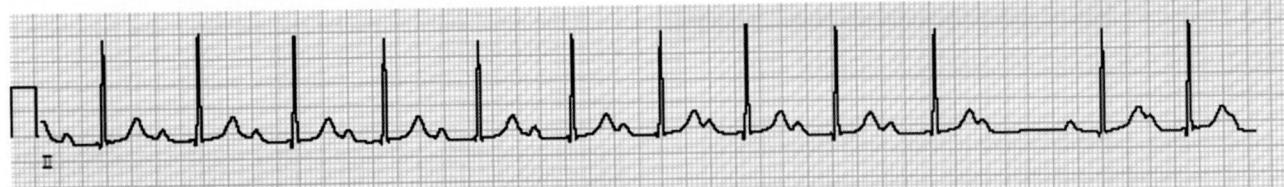

FIGURE 77.22. ECG showing second-degree AV block, Mobitz type I, in a child. Note the progressive prolongation of the PR interval before the blocked P wave.

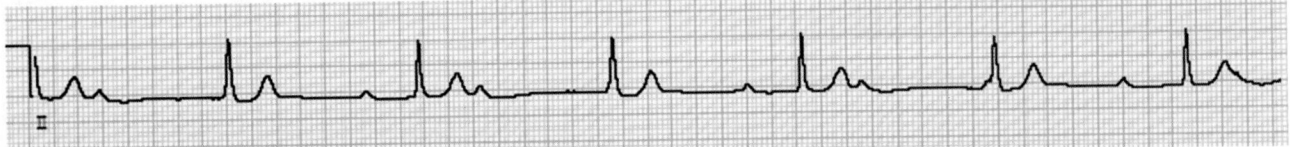

FIGURE 77.23. ECG showing complete heart block in an adolescent. Note the dissociation of the P waves and QRS complexes.

congenital heart disease, there may be baseline abnormalities including abnormal axis and differing levels of conduction system disease, including right-bundle-branch block, and comparison with previous QRS morphology is mandatory for proper diagnosis. If the escape mechanism has a wide QRS morphology and differs from previous QRS morphology documented in sinus rhythm, the escape mechanism is likely ventricular in origin. It should be noted that ventricular rhythms can demonstrate narrow QRS morphology, especially in infants and children with small cardiac mass and in ventricular mechanisms, which penetrate into the distal conduction system. As before, comparison of the QRS morphology with the previous baseline QRS morphology should be done when possible.

Complete heart block may be congenital or acquired (53). The incidence of congenital complete heart block has been estimated to be ~1 in 20,000 live births. Congenital complete heart block can be associated with forms of congenital heart diseases such as L-transposition of the great arteries (congenitally corrected transposition of the great arteries), heterotaxy syndrome (left atrial isomerism), AV canal defect or in association with maternal autoimmune syndromes such as systemic lupus erythematosus.

The fetus with congenital complete heart block may develop hydrops fetalis, which is typically dependent on the rate of the escape mechanism in utero. Postnatally, newborns with complete heart block may be asymptomatic or may present with symptoms related to the reduced cardiac output. In the absence of associated congenital heart disease, management is based on hemodynamic status, the site of the escape mechanism (junctional vs. ventricular), and the rate of the escape rhythm.

Treatment of Abnormalities of Atrioventricular Conduction. Treatment of bradycardia from conduction system disease is dependent on type and location of conduction system involvement and the patient's hemodynamic status. Except in rare circumstances when patients are significantly hemodynamically compromised from concomitant illness or in the setting of postoperative cardiac surgery, no treatment is typically necessary for first-degree or Mobitz type I second-degree heart block. In the patient with asymptomatic Mobitz type II second-degree heart block, acute intervention is usually not required, though the long-term risk of progression to complete heart block with an inadequate ventricular escape mechanism typically dictates intervention with a permanent pacing system. Depending on the clinical scenario, a catheter-based electrophysiology study may be helpful to confirm the location of conduction system disease prior to device implantation.

In newborns with congenital heart block, management is based on clinical hemodynamics and the mechanism and rate of the escape rhythm. In newborns, indications for permanent pacing prior to discharge include average heart rate below 55 bpm, wide complex escape mechanism and hemodynamic instability secondary to bradycardia (51). In asymptomatic neonates and infants with heart rates above 55 bpm and a narrow complex escape rhythm that are otherwise clinically stable, close follow-up with an electrophysiologist as an outpatient is appropriate. In the presence of associated congenital heart disease, permanent pacing is indicated for almost all infants secondary to a significant incidence of death in this group reported to be as high as 29%.

The treatment of acquired complete heart block is dependent on patient stability and the underlying clinical scenario that lead to heart block. The most common scenario for acquired complete heart block in the intensive care setting is the result of collateral mechanical damage during open heart surgery but may occur from traumatic conduction system injury during central line placement or cardiac catheterization. The most common cardiac surgical interventions associated with postoperative heart block include repairs that necessitate manipulation and suturing near the AV node or bundle of His such as atrioventricular canal repairs, ventricular septal defect repairs, and repair of TOF (53).

Immediate management of heart block consists of reversal of the inciting agent whenever possible and stabilization of any hemodynamic compromise. Central lines with distal tips located in the heart should be pulled back, and medications should be reviewed to identify any potential medications associated with AV block. In the setting of postoperative cardiac surgery, patients often have temporary epicardial pacing wires that can used to pace the heart to increase heart rate or restore AV synchrony. In patients without postoperative wires, medications that enhance AV nodal conduction or the rate of the underlying escape mechanism such as epinephrine and isoproterenol can be used to augment the underlying heart rate. If heart block cannot be immediately rectified and the patient remains hemodynamically compromised, a temporary pacing wire can be placed or transcutaneous pacing can be used in emergent situations. After obtaining an adequate heart rate, a stable mode of pacing, or in patients that are hemodynamically stable with their underlying escape rhythm, the decision on long-term pacing with a permanent device is made on the basis of the likelihood of normalization of AV conduction. Patients with mechanical or surgically acquired complete heart block are typically monitored for 7–14 days to allow return of AV conduction. While

AV conduction has been documented to return long after this time period, placement of a permanent pacing system is usually recommended after this one- to two-week wait period.

PRINCIPLES OF TEMPORARY PACING

Temporary pacing wires (usually postsurgical) can be used for pacing patients with SND or AV block, recording atrial electrograms for diagnostic purposes, and overdrive pacing for termination of reentrant arrhythmias. In emergent settings, transcutaneous pacing can be performed, but successful cardiac capture can be difficult to determine clinically, and echocardiogram assistance is often needed for documentation.

Placement of temporary atrial and ventricular pacing wires is standard practice with most cardiothoracic surgical procedures that involve cardiopulmonary bypass. The postoperative wires are attached directly to the epicardial surface of myocardial tissue, and the wires pass through the chest wall and can be attached to an external pacemaker. Depending on surgeon and institution preferences, wires may be placed on the atrium, the ventricle, or both the atrium and the ventricle. Atrial wires can be used to pace the atrium in patients with SND or in patients where a faster heart rate may be beneficial. Atrial pacing is dependent on normal AV nodal conduction for augmentation of the ventricular rate and is not useful in isolation for patients with complete heart block. If ventricular wires are present, pacing of the ventricles can be performed to augment ventricular activity. If only ventricular wires are present, ventricular pacing cannot be synchronized to atrial activity, but in urgent settings, asynchronous ventricular pacing can be lifesaving. If both atrial and ventricular wires are present, pacing can be configured to restore atrial and ventricular synchrony by either tracking atrial activity and pacing the ventricle or pacing both the atrium and the ventricle sequentially.

Temporary pacemakers can be configured for either single or dual chamber pacing. Single chamber pacing denotes pacing and sensing of either the atrium or the ventricle, but not both simultaneously. Dual chamber pacing refers to the pacing and/or sensing of both the atrium and the ventricle. Standard nomenclature published by the North American Society of Pacing and Electrophysiology (NASPE) and the British Pacing and Electrophysiology Group (BPEG) is used to describe pacemaker function and programming. Denotation of pacemaker programming is given as three "positions" displayed as a three-letter code. The first letter or position of the program refers to the chamber, or chambers, which can be paced. The second letter refers to the chamber, or chambers, that can be sensed, and the third letter denotes the response of the device to a sensed event (**Table 77.5**). The fourth and fifth letters refer to advanced programming options that are related to permanent implantable pacemakers with rate-responsive and antitachycardia features but are not typically present in most temporary pacing systems.

Three basic types of temporary pacemaker programming are available based on the goals and needs of transient pacing.

- *Asynchronous or fixed-rate pacing* (AOO, VOO, DOO) describes pacing of the atrium, ventricle, or both atrium and ventricles at a set rate without the ability to sense intrinsic cardiac activity. The device will pace at a preset rate regardless of the patient's underlying rhythm.
- *Single chamber synchronous or demand pacing* (AAI, VVI) describes pacing and sensing of either the atrium or the ventricle. In this mode, the atrium or ventricle will be paced at the programmed lower rate limit unless there is sensed activity from the native heart. If there is native cardiac activity, the device will inhibit subsequent pacing until the rate drops below the lower rate limit.
- *Dual chamber AV sequential pacing* (DDD) refers to a pacing mode that utilizes both atrial and ventricular wires to sense and potentially pace both the atrium and the ventricle in a synchronous manor. If the native atrial rate drops below the lower limit set on the device, atrial pacing will be delivered. If the underlying atrial rate is higher than the lower limit, atrial pacing will be inhibited. Similarly, if the device senses ventricular activity after paced or sensed atrial activity, ventricular pacing will be inhibited or withheld. If there is no sensed ventricular activity, ventricular pacing will be triggered and ventricular pacing is delivered.

Temporary pacing devices have several important programmable features that allow physicians to tailor pacing to the patient's needs and clinical situation and avoid potential issues with pacing. Careful attention is needed to this complex programming, especially in younger aged patients, to avoid potential complications and provide optimal pacing. The lower rate limit refers to the lowest heart rate the device will allow prior to instituting pacing, and should be programmed on the basis of patient age and hemodynamic demands. The upper rate limit refers to the fastest sensed atrial rate at which the

TABLE 77.5

PACEMAKER CODES FROM THE NORTH AMERICAN SOCIETY OF PACING AND ELECTROPHYSIOLOGY AND BRITISH PACING AND ELECTROPHYSIOLOGY GROUP

■ POSITION 1	■ POSITION 2	■ POSITION 3
Chamber paced	Chamber sensed	Response to sensed event
O = none	O = none	O = none
A = atrium	A = atrium	I = inhibited
V = ventricle	V = ventricle	T = triggered
D = dual (A + V)	D = dual (A + V)	D = dual (T + I)

The first two positions of this code are chamber paced and chamber sensed. The third position is described as follows:
D—(dual): In DDD pacemakers, atrial pacing is in the inhibited mode (the pacing device will emit an atrial pulse if the atrium does not contract). In DDD and VDD pacemakers, once an atrial event has occurred (whether paced or native), the device will ensure that an atrial event follows.
I—(inhibited): The device will pulse to the appropriate chamber, unless it detects intrinsic electrical activity. In the DDI program, AV synchrony is provided only when the atrial chamber is paced. On the other hand, if intrinsic atrial activity is present, no AV synchrony is provided by the pacemaker.
T—(triggered): Triggered mode is used only when the device is being tested. The pacing device will emit a pulse only in response to a sensed event.
Adapted from Miller RD. *Miller's Anesthesia.* 6th ed. Philadelphia, PA: Elsevier, 2005.

DDD pacemaker will still deliver ventricular pacing. If the native atrial rate is higher than the programmed upper rate limit, "upper rate phenomenon" will occur, and ventricular pacing will be delivered at a rate below the sensed atrial rate.

Because temporary pacing wires lose the ability to properly sense and pace the heart over time, the capture threshold (the minimum amount of energy delivered per unit of time that is required to depolarize the respective chamber of the heart) and sensitivity should be checked on a daily basis. In most temporary pacemakers, the amount of current delivered can be adjusted, whereas the time that the energy is delivered (pulse width) is fixed. Because of this, the capture threshold is usually denoted as the lowest amount of current that is needed to consistently capture the myocardium. Typically, the programmed pacemaker output is set two to three times the capture threshold value. If there is acute or progressive elevation in the capture threshold or worsening in the ability of the system to sense cardiac activity, intervention with new epicardial wires or an alternate method of chronic pacing may be required if the patient continues to require pacing for hemodynamic stability.

ANTIARRHYTHMIC DRUGS

The choice to initiate antiarrhythmic drugs should be made with the understanding of the potential adverse effects that many of these medications have. Many of the drugs that affect the cardiac conduction system have a narrow therapeutic range and have proarrhythmic properties that can potentially be associated with dangerous or even fatal arrhythmias. When the decision has been made to initiate these medications, it is often necessary to closely monitor patients until a steady drug state has been achieved.

Antiarrhythmic drugs are distinguished by their effects on the two types of action potentials found in the cardiac tissues and on the autonomic nervous system. The fast-response action potential is rich with sodium channels and is found in atrial and ventricular myocytes, as well as in Purkinje fibers. The slow-response action potential is primarily mediated by calcium channels and is present predominantly in sinus node and AV nodal tissues.

The action potential of cardiac myocytes has five distinct temporal phases (Fig. 77.24). During the initial phase (phase 0) of the fast-response action potential, there is rapid depolarization resulting from the change in conformation of sodium channels in the cell membrane and influx of sodium ions. The slope of phase 0 depolarization influences the conduction velocity of cardiac tissue. Repolarization is the return of the action potential to the resting membrane potential and corresponds to phases 1 through 3, the width of the action potential. Repolarization results from inactivation of the inward sodium current and activation of the specialized potassium

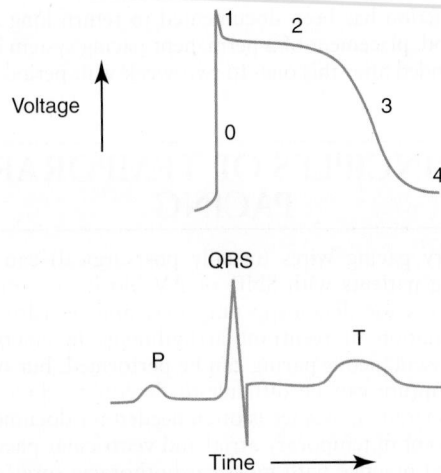

FIGURE 77.24. Fast-response cardiac-action potential and simultaneous correlation with surface ECG events. (From Tanel RE, Levin MD. Pharmacologic treatment of heart disease. In: Bell LM, Vetter VI, eds. *The Requisites in Pediatrics: Pediatric Cardiology*. Philadelphia, PA: Elsevier Mosby, 2006:259, with permission.)

and calcium channels that direct current out of the cell. The period of repolarization determines the refractory period of the cardiac tissue. During phase 4 of the action potential, there is spontaneous depolarization until the cellular threshold membrane potential is reached, triggering the influx of sodium ions characterizing phase 0.

The Vaughan Williams classification of antiarrhythmic drugs, described in 1970, classifies antiarrhythmic drugs by common electrophysiologic properties emphasizing the connection between basic electrophysiologic actions and antiarrhythmic effects. This classification categorizes antiarrhythmic medications into four major groups, although many current medications have multiple (class) actions (**Table 77.6**).

Class I

The class I antiarrhythmic agents include a diverse group of medications that block the rapid sodium channel and delay the upstroke of the action potential, which primarily results in lengthening of the QRS interval. During initiation of these medications, serial surface electrocardiograms must be obtained to monitor for changes in the QRS duration as well as resultant prolongation of the QT interval. Because of the varying effects on the action potential of sodium-channel blockade, the medications are further subclassified into subgroups IA, IB, and IC.

TABLE 77.6

VAUGHN WILLIAMS CLASSIFICATION OF ANTIARRHYTHMIC DRUGS

■ CLASS	■ EFFECT	■ DRUGS
I	Sodium-channel blockade	
Subclass IA		Procainamide, disopyramide, quinidine
Subclass IB		Lidocaine, mexiletine, phenytoin
Subclass IC		Flecainide, propafenone, encainide
II	β-adrenergic receptor blockade	Propranolol, esmolol, atenolol, nadolol, carvedilol
III	Potassium-channel blockade	Amiodarone, sotalol, bretylium
IV	Slow, inward, calcium-channel blockade	Verapamil, diltiazem, nifedipine
Other		Digoxin, adenosine

Class IA

Class IA agents include procainamide, disopyramide, and quinidine. Medications in this group delay repolarization, resulting in action potential lengthening and longer refractory periods. The class IA drugs are unique in their significant effects on the autonomic nervous system. Anticholinergic effects result in increased sinus node activity and more rapid AV node conduction. ECG changes that occur with this class of medications include widening of the QRS complex and prolongation of the QT interval. These medications are useful in treating atrial, ventricular, and AV reentrant tachycardia. The class IA agents all carry a risk of proarrhythmia, with the aggravation of existing arrhythmias or the development of new atrial and ventricular arrhythmias, including TdP. As a result, some hesitate to use these drugs to treat arrhythmias in patients with structural heart disease or congestive heart failure.

Class IB

Medications in the class IB group include lidocaine, mexiletine, and phenytoin. These medications shorten the duration of the action potential. They are primarily used for the treatment of ventricular arrhythmias. Lidocaine has historically been used for the treatment of complex ventricular ectopy, VT, and ventricular fibrillation. It may also be useful for the emergent treatment of arrhythmias that occur in association with prolonged QT syndrome (TdP). Lidocaine has no significant effect on the autonomic nervous system, and proarrhythmia is a rare adverse effect. Mexiletine is an oral medication that is used for chronic outpatient therapy in patients who are responsive to lidocaine.

Class IC

Class IC agents include flecainide, propafenone, and encainide. As with the class IA and class IB agents, these medications inhibit sodium channels in fast-response cells and have a profound depressant effect on conduction velocity, with little effect on the autonomic nervous system. As a whole, the group is used clinically to depress abnormal automaticity and prevent the induction of atrial muscle, ventricular muscle, and accessory pathway reentry circuits. The class IC agents have a relatively high potential for proarrhythmia. Proarrhythmia may lead to cardiac arrest and death, predominantly among patients with underlying heart disease (54,55). When an atrial arrhythmia is treated with a class IC medication, it is important to also use an AV nodal slowing agent, such as a β-blocker or digoxin. This is because the IC medication may slow the atrial tachycardia enough to allow for 1:1 AV conduction in a tachycardia that was previously conducted with some degree of AV block. The resulting ventricular rate, therefore, may be higher after initiating a IC medication, possibly leading to hemodynamic compromise.

Class II

Class II is designated for the β-blockers, which include propranolol, esmolol, atenolol, nadolol, and carvedilol. These medications work by several mechanisms, primarily through competitive inhibition of the cardiac β-adrenergic receptor. Class II medications block endogenous catecholamines and decrease autonomic sympathetic tone. These effects result in slowing of spontaneous discharge from the sinus node, automaticity from other cardiac tissues, and slowing of conduction through the AV node. β-blockers are used to treat all arrhythmias of abnormal automaticity, especially those that are catecholamine driven. In addition, they may be used to treat reentry tachycardias by preventing the premature beats that act as initiating events or by affecting AV nodal conduction when that

structure is part of the arrhythmia circuit. β-blockers are also an important part of the management of long-QT syndrome.

β-blockers can be further classified by their relative cardiac β-receptor activity and their effects on other tissue types. Atenolol has more cardiac β-receptor selectivity, less CNS penetration, and a longer half-life than other β-blockers. Nadolol has less penetration to the brain than other β-blockers, making the incidence of CNS side effects low. Carvedilol and metoprolol have been approved in the United States for the management of congestive heart failure in the adult population, but experience in pediatrics is limited. Patients with chronic congestive heart failure have increased sympathetic nervous system activity that is thought to be related to their clinical deterioration, and β-blocker therapy is thought to interfere with this debilitating neurohormonal pathway.

Class III

The class III agents include amiodarone, sotalol, and bretylium. By definition, class III antiarrhythmic agents prolong the action-potential duration through their actions primarily on potassium channels. These medications work primarily by prolonging the refractory period of myocardial tissue. Amiodarone and sotalol have additional effects on action-potential propagation and variable effects on the autonomic nervous system. Amiodarone is a potent antiarrhythmic agent that is usually reserved for the treatment of potentially life-threatening arrhythmias or arrhythmias that are refractory to other therapies. Amiodarone has been incorporated in advanced cardiac life support treatment algorithms after defibrillation and epinephrine for unstable VT or ventricular fibrillation (49,50). It is also the principal antiarrhythmic agent for JET. Sotalol is used in situations similar to those for amiodarone, but it has the advantage of a faster onset of action and a shorter duration of activity.

Amiodarone and sotalol are used commonly in pediatric practice, while bretylium has been removed from ACLS algorithms because of a high incidence of adverse events, the availability of safer agents, and its limited supply. Amiodarone has a number of serious noncardiac side effects that limit its long-term utility (e.g., nausea and emesis; photosensitivity; optic neuropathy and/or lens cataracts; hypothyroidism; pneumonitis; liver toxicity; neuropathy and neuro-coordination issues, such as tremor and involuntary movements; poor coordination and gait abnormalities; and peripheral neuropathy). Many of these adverse effects are dose related, and may occur with greater frequency when there has been a higher total cumulative dose or longer duration of therapy. Cardiovascular side effects of amiodarone include diminished myocardial function, bradycardia, and, in rare cases, proarrhythmia. Side effects of sotalol include proarrhythmia, including TdP, in 2%–4% of adult patients. Bretylium results in a biphasic norepinephrine response that can be associated with an initial worsening of arrhythmias.

Class IV

Class IV antiarrhythmic drugs are calcium-channel blockers, specifically verapamil, diltiazem, and nifedipine. Of these, verapamil is used most frequently in pediatric practice for the treatment of arrhythmias. Verapamil and the other calcium-channel blockers block the slow, inward calcium current within the sinus node and AV node. This cellular activity decreases sinus node automaticity, slows AV node conduction, and prolongs refractoriness, resulting in sinus bradycardia and prolongation of the PR interval.

Calcium-channel blocking medications are useful in several different tachycardias. Verapamil is most valuable for the treatment of reentrant SVT that involves the AV node. It terminates the tachycardia by interrupting the reentrant circuit in the AV node. Verapamil should be avoided in children <1 year of age. Infants have underdeveloped sarcoplasmic reticulum, and previous reports have described young infants who have responded to IV verapamil with cardiovascular collapse (56). Patients with WPW syndrome should not be treated with calcium-channel blocking medications, as accessory pathway conduction may be enhanced whereas AV nodal conduction may be slowed, particularly during atrial tachycardias. Diltiazem is frequently used for control of the ventricular rate during atrial tachycardia or atrial fibrillation by slowing conduction through the AV node. Calcium-channel blockers are widely used for long-term therapy of pulmonary hypertension, and nifedipine is preferred in those patients, as it has little effect on the sinus node, AV node, and cardiac contractility. In view of its potential for peripheral vasodilation, nifedipine is used for the acute management of hypertension.

Nonclassified Antiarrhythmic Medications

Digoxin

Digoxin is a cardiac glycoside that is useful for the treatment of both arrhythmias and congestive heart failure. Digoxin has slowing effects on the AV node and also reduces automaticity. Specifically, it is used in treating AV reentrant tachycardia by slowing conduction through the AV node and interrupting the circuit. It is also used to achieve control of ventricular rate during an atrial tachycardia by slowing the response of the AV node to the atrial arrhythmia. In view of its ability to decrease automaticity, digoxin may be used for atrial tachycardia, atrial fibrillation, premature atrial complexes, and blocked premature atrial complexes. The mechanism of action is mediated by an increase in vagus nerve tone and decrease in sympathetic efferent activity. Cellular effects are due to binding of digoxin to sodium–potassium adenosine triphosphatase, which inhibits the sodium pump and ultimately increases intracellular calcium. Digoxin should not be used in patients with WPW syndrome owing to its ability to block the AV node, shorten the accessory-pathway effective refractory period, and potentially enhance antegrade conduction across the accessory connection during an atrial tachycardia. Toxic concentrations can result in increased automaticity and triggered arrhythmias.

Digoxin toxicity can result in almost any type of arrhythmia, but the development of arrhythmias is generally a late indicator of toxicity. The ECG signs of digoxin toxicity are different in children as compared with adults. Infants more frequently present with sinus bradycardia and AV block. Older children also have bradyarrhythmias, but can also have atrial and junctional tachyarrhythmias. Pediatric patients, unlike adult patients, rarely develop ventricular tachyarrhythmias. For toxicity, the medication should be discontinued. Serum electrolyte abnormalities should be corrected, while atrial and ventricular arrhythmias can be treated with phenytoin or lidocaine. Atropine or a temporary pacemaker can be used to treat bradycardia or AV block. Digoxin-immune, antigen-binding Fab fragments are specific antibodies that may be used to bind digoxin and may be especially helpful in cases of potentially life-threatening toxicity.

Adenosine

Adenosine is an endogenous purine nucleoside that is useful for terminating AV reentrant tachycardia that utilizes the AV node as a limb of the reentrant circuit. As adenosine blocks AV node conduction, it can be used to help differentiate between an AV reentrant tachycardia and an automatic, ectopic, or reentrant atrial arrhythmia. It will terminate the reentrant circuit by abruptly blocking the AV node, but the atrial tachycardia will persist with block at the AV node, resulting in a ventricular response to the atrial arrhythmia of less than 1:1. When adenosine is administered to terminate or diagnose the etiology of a tachycardia, a 12-lead surface electrocardiogram should be recorded for the duration of the administration to aid with diagnosis of the tachycardia. The effects of adenosine are brief, as the drug is rapidly metabolized with a half-life of <10 seconds. Caffeine and the methylxanthines cause competitive and reversible antagonism via the specific adenosine receptor, requiring higher doses of adenosine for clinical effect. Adenosine should not be administered to patients with preexcited atrial fibrillation as this may enhance accessory pathway conduction to the ventricle and induce ventricular fibrillation. Patients with orthotopic heart transplant have a denervation-induced supersensitivity to adenosine, so this medication should be avoided in this population if possible.

CONCLUSION

Proper recognition and treatment of cardiac arrhythmias can reduce morbidity and mortality in the intensive care unit, reduce admission days, and improve patient comfort and satisfaction. Modern monitoring methods allow for identification of rhythm mechanisms, which in the recent past would have been challenging or impossible. Treatment options including a wide range of antiarrhythmic medications, cardiac pacing from endocardial, epicardial, and cutaneous means, and electrical cardioversion and defibrillation provide great support for the modern intensivist. Acquiring and maintaining the knowledge and skills required, and developing and maintaining collaborative relationships with cardiac electrophysiologists will be a challenge for the future.

References

1. Cohen MI, Wieand TS, Rhodes LA, et al. Electrophysiologic properties of the atrioventricular node in pediatric patients. *J Am Coll Cardiol* 1997;29:403–7.
2. Ko JK, Deal BJ, Strasburger JF, et al. Supraventricular tachycardia mechanisms and their age distribution in pediatric patients. *Am J Cardiol* 1992;69:1028–32.
3. Garson A Jr, Gillette PC. Electrophysiologic studies of supraventricular tachycardia in children. II. Prediction of specific mechanism by noninvasive features. *Am Heart J* 1981;102:383–8.
4. Wolff L, Parkinson J, White PD. Bundle-branch block with short P-R interval in healthy young people prone to paroxysmal tachycardia. *Ann Noninvasive Electrocardiol* 2006;11:340–53.
5. De Bacquer D, De Backer G, Kornitzer M. Prevalences of ECG findings in large population based samples of men and women. *Heart* 2000;84:625–33.
6. Lu CW, Wu MH, Chen HC, et al. Epidemiological profile of Wolff-Parkinson-White syndrome in a general population younger than 50 years of age in an era of radiofrequency catheter ablation. *Int J Cardiol* 2014;174:530–4.
7. Munger TM, Packer DL, Hammill SC, et al. A population study of the natural history of Wolff-Parkinson-White syndrome in Olmsted county, Minnesota, 1953-1989. *Circulation* 1993;87:866–73.
8. Perry JC, Garson A Jr. Supraventricular tachycardia due to Wolff-Parkinson-White syndrome in children: Early disappearance and late recurrence. *J Am Coll Cardiol* 1990;16:1215–20.
9. Klein GJ, Bashore TM, Sellers TD, et al. Ventricular fibrillation in the Wolff-Parkinson-White syndrome. *N Engl J Med* 1979;301:1080–5.

10. Czosek RJ, Anderson J, Cassedy A, et al. Cost-effectiveness of various risk stratification methods for asymptomatic ventricular pre-excitation. *Am J Cardiol* 2013;112:245–50.

11. Pediatric and Congenital Electrophysiology Society (PACES); Heart Rhythm Society (HRS); American College of Cardiology Foundation (ACCF); American Heart Association (AHA); American Academy of Pediatrics (AAP); Canadian Heart Rhythm Society (CHRS); Cohen MI, Triedman JK, Cannon BC, et al. PACES/HRS expert consensus statement on the management of the asymptomatic young patient with a Wolff-Parkinson-White (WPW, ventricular preexcitation) electrocardiographic pattern: Developed in partnership between the Pediatric And Congenital Electrophysiology Society (PACES) and the Heart Rhythm Society (HRS). Endorsed by the governing bodies of PACES, HRS, the American College of Cardiology Foundation (ACCF), the American Heart Association (AHA), the American Academy of Pediatrics (AAP), and the Canadian Heart Rhythm Society (CHRS). *Heart Rhythm* 2012;9:1006–24.

12. Abinader E, Borochowitz Z, Berger A. A hemodynamic complication of verapamil therapy in a neonate. *Helv Paediatr Acta* 1981;36:451–5.

13. Pfammatter JP, Bauersfeld U. Safety issues in the treatment of paediatric supraventricular tachycardias. *Drug Saf* 1998;18: 345–56.

14. Czosek RJ, Anderson J, Marino BS, et al. Linear lesion cryoablation for the treatment of atrioventricular nodal re-entry tachycardia in pediatrics and young adults. *Pacing Clin Electrophysiol* 2010;33:1304–11.

15. Drago F, Placidi S, Righi D, et al. Cryoablation of AVNRT in children and adolescents: Early intervention leads to a better outcome. *J Cardiovasc Electrophysiol* 2014;25:398–403.

16. Texter KM, Kertesz NJ, Friedman RA, et al. Atrial flutter in infants. *J Am Coll Cardiol* 2006;48:1040–6.

17. January CT, Wann LS, Alpert JS, et al. 2014 AHA/ACC/HRS guideline for the management of patients with atrial fibrillation: Executive summary: A report of the American College Of Cardiology/American Heart Association Task Force on practice guidelines and the Heart Rhythm Society. *Circulation* 2014;130(23):2071–104.

18. Stephenson EA, Casavant D, Tuzi J, et al.; ATTEST Investigators. Efficacy of atrial antitachycardia pacing using the Medtronic AT500 pacemaker in patients with congenital heart disease. *Am J Cardiol* 2003;92:871–6.

19. Yap SC, Harris L, Silversides CK, et al. Outcome of intra-atrial re-entrant tachycardia catheter ablation in adults with congenital heart disease: Negative impact of age and complex atrial surgery. *J Am Coll Cardiol* 2010;56:1589–96.

20. Bradley DJ, Fischbach PS, Law IH, et al. The clinical course of multifocal atrial tachycardia in infants and children. *J Am Coll Cardiol* 2001;38:401–8.

21. Villain E, Vetter VL, Garcia JM, et al. Evolving concepts in the management of congenital junctional ectopic tachycardia. A multicenter study. *Circulation* 1990;81:1544–9.

22. Collins KK, Van Hare GF, Kertesz NJ, et al. Pediatric nonpostoperative junctional ectopic tachycardia medical management and interventional therapies. *J Am Coll Cardiol* 2009;53:690–7.

23. Kakavand B, Ballard HO, Disessa TG. Frequent ventricular premature beats in children with a structurally normal heart: A cause for reversible left ventricular dysfunction? *Pediatr Cardiol* 2010;31:986–90.

24. Garson A. Incessant ventricular-tachycardia in infants. *Int Congr Ser* 1990;906:245–8.

25. Crosson JE, Callans DJ, Bradley DJ, et al. PACES/HRS expert consensus statement on the evaluation and management of ventricular arrhythmias in the child with a structurally normal heart. *Heart Rhythm* 2014;11:e55–e78.

26. Pfammatter JP, Paul T. Idiopathic ventricular tachycardia in infancy and childhood—A multicenter study on clinical profile and outcome. *J Am Coll Cardiol* 1999;33:2067–72.

27. Vanhare GF, Stanger P. Ventricular-tachycardia and accelerated ventricular rhythm presenting in the 1st month of life. *Am J Cardiol* 1991;67:42–5.

28. Zeigler VL, Gillette PC, Crawford FA Jr, et al. New approaches to treatment of incessant ventricular tachycardia in the very young. *J Am Coll Cardiol* 1990;16:681–5.

29. Lee GK, Klarich KW, Grogan M, et al. Premature ventricular contraction-induced cardiomyopathy: A treatable condition. *Circulation* 2012;5:229–36.

30. Belhassen B, Shapira I, Pelleg A, et al. Idiopathic recurrent sustained ventricular tachycardia responsive to verapamil: An ECG-electrophysiologic entity. *Am Heart J* 1984;108:1034–7.

31. Thakur RK, Klein GJ, Sivaram CA, et al. Anatomic substrate for idiopathic left ventricular tachycardia. *Circulation* 1996;93:497–501.

32. Smeets JL, Rodriguez LM, Timmermans C, et al. Radiofrequency catheter ablation of idiopathic ventricular tachycardias in children. *Pacing Clin Electrophysiol* 1997;20:2068–71.

33. Timmermans C, Rodriguez LM, Medeiros A, et al. Radiofrequency catheter ablation of idiopathic ventricular tachycardia originating in the main stem of the pulmonary artery. *J Cardiovasc Electrophysiol* 2002;13:281–4.

34. Zeppenfeld K, Schalij MJ, Bartelings MM, et al. Catheter ablation of ventricular tachycardia after repair of congenital heart disease: Electroanatomic identification of the critical right ventricular isthmus. *Circulation* 2007;116:2241–52.

35. Gatzoulis MA, Balaji S, Webber SA, et al. Risk factors for arrhythmia and sudden cardiac death late after repair of tetralogy of Fallot: A multicentre study. *Lancet* 2000;356:975–81.

36. Khairy P, Landzberg MJ, Gatzoulis MA, et al. Value of programmed ventricular stimulation after tetralogy of Fallot repair: A multicenter study. *Circulation* 2004;109:1994–2000.

37. Murphy JG, Gersh BJ, Mair DD, et al. Long-term outcome in patients undergoing surgical repair of tetralogy of Fallot. *N Engl J Med* 1993;329:593–9.

38. Khairy P, Aboulhosn J, Gurvitz MZ, et al.; Alliance for Adult Research in Congenital Cardiology (AARCC). Arrhythmia burden in adults with surgically repaired tetralogy of Fallot: A multi-institutional study. *Circulation* 2010;122:868–75.

39. Khairy P, Harris L, Landzberg MJ, et al. Implantable cardioverter-defibrillators in tetralogy of Fallot. *Circulation* 2008;117:363–70.

40. Alexander ME, Walsh EP, Saul JP, et al. Value of programmed ventricular stimulation in patients with congenital heart disease. *J Cardiovasc Electrophysiol* 1999;10:1033–44.

41. Therrien J, Siu SC, Harris L, et al. Impact of pulmonary valve replacement on arrhythmia propensity late after repair of tetralogy of Fallot. *Circulation* 2001;103:2489–94.

42. Czosek RJ, Anderson J, Khoury PR, et al. Utility of ambulatory monitoring in patients with congenital heart disease. *Am J Cardiol* 2013;111:723–30.

43. Wolfe RR, Driscoll DJ, Gersony WM, et al. Arrhythmias in patients with valvar aortic stenosis, valvar pulmonary stenosis, and ventricular septal defect. Results of 24-hour ECG monitoring. *Circulation* 1993;87:I89–I101.

44. Maron BJ, Spirito P, Ackerman MJ, et al. Prevention of sudden cardiac death with implantable cardioverter-defibrillators in children and adolescents with hypertrophic cardiomyopathy. *J Am Coll Cardiol* 2013;61:1527–35.

45. Maron BJ, Spirito P, Shen WK, et al. Implantable cardioverter-defibrillators and prevention of sudden cardiac death in hypertrophic cardiomyopathy. *JAMA* 2007;298:405–12.

46. Marcus FI, McKenna WJ, Sherrill D, et al. Diagnosis of arrhythmogenic right ventricular cardiomyopathy/dysplasia: Proposed modification of the Task Force Criteria. *Circulation* 2010;121:1533–41.

47. Miyake CY, Del Nido PJ, Alexander ME, et al. Cardiac tumors and associated arrhythmias in pediatric patients, with observations on surgical therapy for ventricular tachycardia. *J Am Coll Cardiol* 2011;58:1903–9.

48. George CH, Higgs GV, Lai FA. Ryanodine receptor mutations associated with stress-induced ventricular tachycardia mediate increased calcium release in stimulated cardiomyocytes. *Circ Res* 2003;93:531–40.

49. Kudenchuk PJ, Cobb LA, Copass MK, et al. Amiodarone for resuscitation after out-of-hospital cardiac arrest due to ventricular fibrillation. *N Engl J Med* 1999;341:871–78.

50. Dorian P, Cass D, Schwartz B, et al. Amiodarone as compared with lidocaine for shock-resistant ventricular fibrillation. *N Engl J Med* 2002;346:884–90.

51. Epstein AE, Dimarco JP, Ellenbogen KA, et al.; American College of Cardiology/American Heart Association Task Force on Practice, American Association for Thoracic Surgery, Society of Thoracic Surgeons. ACC/AHA/HRS 2008 guidelines for device-based therapy of cardiac rhythm abnormalities: Executive summary. *Heart Rhythm* 2008;5:934–55.

52. Triedman JK. Arrhythmias in adults with congenital heart disease. *Heart* 2002;87:383–9.

53. Anderson JB, Czosek RJ, Knilans TK, et al. Postoperative heart block in children with common forms of congenital heart disease: Results from the kid database. *J Cardiovasc Electrophysiol* 2012;23:1349–54.

54. Fish FA, Gillette PC, Benson DW Jr. Proarrhythmia, cardiac arrest and death in young patients receiving encainide and flecainide. The Pediatric Electrophysiology Group. *J Am Coll Cardiol* 1991;18:356–65.

55. Perry JC, Garson A Jr. Flecainide acetate for treatment of tachyarrhythmias in children: Review of world literature on efficacy, safety, and dosing. *Am Heart J* 1992;124:1614–21.

56. Epstein ML, Kiel EA, Victorica BE. Cardiac decompensation following verapamil therapy in infants with supraventricular tachycardia. *Pediatrics* 1985;75:737–40.

CHAPTER 78 ■ PREOPERATIVE CARE OF THE PEDIATRIC CARDIAC SURGICAL PATIENT

JENNIFER J. SCHUETTE, ALAIN FRAISSE, AND DAVID L. WESSEL

KEY POINTS

1 Pediatric cardiac intensive care continues to establish itself as an important and necessary subspecialty.

2 The complexity of heart disease and the expertise necessary to treat these patients require multidisciplinary training and collaborative, integrated care.

3 Expertise is required for care of premature and full-term newborns, infants, and children, as well as the rapidly growing numbers of adults with long-term survival and continuing need for care of their congenital heart disease (CHD).

4 Preoperative neurodevelopmental evaluation in patients with CHD should be standard practice, not only to identify those with impairments but also to identify risk factors and strategies to optimize outcome.

5 Reparative surgery in the newborn is the objective of advanced cardiovascular programs whenever feasible.

6 Diagnosis is usually based in echocardiography and physical examination, with catheterization reserved for complex cases or interventional procedures.

7 Adequate resuscitation of preoperative patients is essential to good outcomes.

8 Balancing single-ventricle physiology and maintaining adequate cardiac output are crucial to achieve preoperative stabilization.

9 Risk stratification and identification of biologic markers are maturing as useful tool sets to guide therapy and to provide benchmarks for outcomes.

10 Therapies for the future will target genetic factors and tailor treatments to the polymorphisms and individual inherited profiles of patients.

11 Fetal diagnosis will increasingly provide advanced knowledge, opportunities for counseling and therapeutic planning, and eventually eliminate unanticipated postnatal circulatory collapse.

Congenital heart disease (CHD) occurs in many different forms. When considered as a single group, it is one of the most common congenital malformations encountered in the newborn population, occurring with an estimated frequency of 1 in 100 live births (1,2). This corresponds to 1.35 million new cases of CHD worldwide each year (3). CHD accounts for 29% of deaths attributed to birth defects, and 5.7% of overall infant mortality; of particular note, 57% of infant mortality attributable to CHD occurs during the neonatal period (4). Significant strides have been made in the past several decades in the preoperative, surgical, postoperative, and long-term care of these patients, resulting in a decline in mortality of between 24% and 39%, depending on the specific defect (5–7). Many factors have been responsible for these gains, including improvements in surgical procedures and techniques, modifications in cardiopulmonary bypass (CPB), and advancements in diagnostic and interventional cardiology. Equally important

1 has been the development of specialized pediatric cardiac intensive care units (CICUs) for the pre- and postoperative management of complex and challenging patients who range in age from preterm neonates to adults. Optimal care of these patients requires an understanding of the subtleties of complex congenital cardiac anomalies, respiratory mechanics and physiology, the transitional circulation of the neonate, pharmacologic and mechanical support of the circulation, airway management, mechanical ventilation, treatment of multiorgan system failure, and the effects of CPB on the heart, lungs, brain,

and abdominal organs. Optimal preoperative care involves (a) initial stabilization, airway management, and establishment of vascular access; (b) a complete and thorough non- or minimally invasive delineation of the anatomic defect(s); (c) resuscitation with evaluation and treatment of secondary organ dysfunction, particularly the brain, kidneys, and liver; (d) cardiac catheterization if necessary—typically for physiologic assessment, interventional procedures such as balloon atrial septostomy or valvotomy, or anatomic definition not discernible by echocardiography (e.g., coronary artery distribution in pulmonary atresia with intact ventricular septum or delineation of aorticopulmonary collaterals in tetralogy of Fallot with pulmonary atresia); and (e) surgical management when cardiac, pulmonary, renal, and central nervous systems are opti-

2 mized. Crucial in this process is the continued communication among medical, surgical, and nursing disciplines.

PATIENT DEMOGRAPHICS

3 With increasing emphasis over the past several decades on early primary repair for many congenital cardiac defects in order to correct cyanosis and reverse pressure and volume loads on the myocardium, the demographic makeup of patients in the ICU has changed substantially. Previously, palliation and deferred definitive repair were the rule for many complex lesions. More recently, interventions on even prematurely born neonates have become more commonplace with encouraging results with respect to morbidity and mortality (8). Although these patients represent a small percentage of admissions to the CICU, they account for long ICU stays and significant resource utilization. Thus, a thorough appreciation of the limited cardiorespiratory reserve and immature organ systems, along with the pathophysiology of CHD, response to surgery, and complications related to CPB in neonates, is essential (9).

Many congenital cardiac defects are either palliated or corrected but not cured. Thus, patients who were operated on 10–20 years ago re-present for additional surgical procedures. They may have residual defects or may have developed progressive pathology associated with the disease itself or with the repair. An increasing number of patients with CHD are surviving into adulthood, so that the span of patients populating the pediatric CICU now ranges from infants under 1000 g with issues of prematurity to middle-aged adults with adult comorbidities. The availability of consultation with multiple disciplines beyond critical care, including neonatology and adult congenital cardiology, has become essential.

NEWBORN CONSIDERATIONS

Care of the critically ill neonate requires an appreciation of the special structural and functional features of immature organs, the interactions of the "transitional" neonatal circulation, and the secondary effects of the congenital heart lesion on other organ systems (9–12). The neonate appears to respond more quickly and profoundly to physiologically stressful circumstances, which may be expressed in terms of rapid changes in pH, lactic acid, glucose, and temperature. Neonates have diminished fat and carbohydrate reserves. The higher metabolic rate and oxygen consumption of the neonate account for the rapid appearance of hypoxia when these patients become apneic. Immaturity of the liver and kidney may be associated with reduced protein synthesis and glomerular filtration, such that drug metabolism is altered and hepatic synthetic function is reduced. These issues may be compounded by the normally increased total body water of the neonate compared to the older patient, along with the propensity of the capillary system of the neonate to leak fluid from the intravascular space. This condition is especially prominent in the lung of the neonate, where the pulmonary vascular bed is nearly fully recruited at rest, and the lymphatic recruitment required to handle increased mean capillary pressures associated with increases in pulmonary blood flow may be unavailable (13,14). The neonatal myocardium is less compliant, less tolerant of increases in afterload, and less responsive to increases in preload than that of the older child. Younger age also predisposes the myocardium to the adverse effects of CPB and hypothermic ischemia implicit in surgical support techniques utilized for reparative operations. These factors do not preclude intervention in the neonate but simply dictate that extraordinary vigilance be applied to the care of these children and that intensive care management plans emerge to account for the immature physiology.

The observed benefits of neonatal reparative operations in patients with two ventricles are numerous (**Table 78.1**). They dictate that care of the newborn with complex CHD before and after CPB is a central feature of cardiac intensive care. Elimination of cyanosis and congestive heart failure early in life will optimize conditions for normal growth and development. Palliative procedures such as pulmonary artery bands and systemic-to-pulmonary artery shunts may not fully address cyanosis or congestive heart failure and may introduce their own set of physiologic and anatomic complications. Some examples of improved outcomes with a single reparative operation rather than staged palliation in a newborn are well known, supported by published literature, and evoke little

TABLE 78.1

ADVANTAGES OF NEONATAL REPAIR

Early elimination of cyanosis
Early elimination of congestive heart failure
Optimal circulation for growth and development
Reduced anatomic distortion from palliative procedures
Reduced hospital admissions while awaiting repair
Reduced parental anxiety while awaiting repair

controversy. Approaches that have been abandoned include banding the pulmonary arteries in truncus arteriosus (15–17), staged repair of type B interrupted aortic arch (18), and staged repair rather than single-session complete repair of transposition of the great arteries with interrupted aortic arch (19,20). In other conditions (such as the severely cyanotic newborn with tetralogy of Fallot), the risk and benefit of neonatal repair versus a palliative shunt are still debated (21,22).

Whereas the neonate may be more labile than the older child, many examples also exist of the enhanced neonatal resilience to metabolic or ischemic injury. In fact, the neonate may be particularly capable of coping with some forms of stress. Tolerance of hypoxia in the neonate is characteristic of many species (23), and the plasticity of the neurologic system in the neonate is well described (24). In neonates with transposition of the great arteries, severe hypoxemia that is sometimes associated with hemodynamic instability prior to balloon atrial septostomy may result in brain injury that is clinically unsuspected; clinically silent strokes in these patients at one time were theorized to be related to the septostomy itself, but subsequent data have cast doubt on this association (25,26). Neonates with obstructive left heart lesions often present with profound metabolic acidosis but can be effectively resuscitated without persistent organ system impairment or sequelae as the rule rather than the exception. The pliability and mobility of vascular structures in the neonate improve the technical aspects of surgery. Reparative operations in neonates take best advantage of normal postnatal changes, allowing more normal growth and development in crucial areas such as myocardial muscle, pulmonary parenchyma, and coronary and pulmonary angiogenesis. Neonatal repair may obviate irreversible secondary organ damage arising from unrepaired or palliative approaches. Postoperative pulmonary hypertensive events are less common in the newborn and more common in the infant who has been exposed to weeks or months of high pulmonary pressure and flow, which seems especially true for such lesions as truncus arteriosus, complete atrioventricular canal defects, and transposition of the great arteries with ventricular septal defects (27,28). Finally, cognitive and psychomotor abnormalities associated with months of hypoxemia or abnormal hemodynamics may be diminished or eliminated by early repair. However, if early reparative surgery results in more exposures to CPB (e.g., repeated conduit changes), which may be associated with cognitive impairment or subtle adverse effects on motor function, then the risk–benefit assessment of early repair must be modified accordingly.

At most centers, the approach to neonates with CHD has been toward complete surgical correction rather than palliation in order to avoid the pathophysiologic consequences and limits on neonatal growth (29). This concept has been extended to include premature newborns who are now commonly admitted to the CICU prior to surgical correction. One in 10 newborns is premature. Despite improvements in ventilation, widespread use of surfactant, and prenatal administration of glucocorticoids, infants who are <30 weeks of gestation carry a significant risk of developing bronchopulmonary dysplasia. The coexistence of CHD and bronchopulmonary dysplasia may worsen the clinical course as a result of elevated pulmonary vascular resistance (PVR). Hence, palliative medical or surgical interventions were often preferred management options in premature infants with CHD. However, current experience with increased mortality after palliative surgery supports the notion that early biventricular repair can be achieved with low mortality (30).

As a group, children with CHD on average fall into the normal range for IQ; however, they are at increased risk for developmental delay and disabilities. This risk is fairly pervasive across the spectrum of CHD, including patients with both cyanotic and acyanotic lesions, those who require neonatal interventions and those who do not, and those who have additional comorbidities: prematurity, genetic anomalies or syndromes, history of mechanical support, need for cardiopulmonary resuscitation at any point, and prolonged hospitalization (31). In patients with complex CHD, neurobehavioral abnormalities such as hypo- and hypertonia, jitteriness, motor asymmetry, and absent suck are reported in more than 50% of newborns; up to 38% of infants have disabilities that include hypotonia, head preference, lethargy, restlessness, agitation, motor asymmetry, and feeding difficulties (32).

Evidence of central nervous system pathology has been demonstrated preoperatively, including in those infants who have not suffered periods of hemodynamic compromise or severe hypoxia postnatally. Preoperative electroencephalograms are frequently abnormal, with epileptiform activity in one fifth of infants and moderate-to-diffuse disturbances in background activity in a third (33). Although cranial ultrasound has been used at some centers and abnormalities have been found in anywhere from 30%–60% of patients, preoperative MRI has a lower false-positive rate and is now considered the gold-standard brain imaging modality in this patient population (34). Abnormalities on MRI are noted in 30%–50% of patients, and include infarction, hemorrhage, white matter injury, and periventricular leukomalacia (35). Preoperative neurodevelopmental evaluation and long-term follow-up should be standard practice to identify those with impairments and to develop individualized strategies to optimize outcome.

PREOPERATIVE MANAGEMENT AND CARE

Successful critical care management of patients with CHD is based on complete, accurate preoperative assessment and adequate preoperative patient preparation. The clinical and laboratory information routinely available preoperatively should be frequently reassessed and integrated with information from continuous monitoring during surgery and the immediate recovery phase. The perioperative team must be cognizant of the physical and laboratory findings that are of particular importance for CHD. Involvement by the intensivist in the preoperative preparation and early postoperative management provides a perspective on the pathophysiology that improves perioperative care.

Physical Examination and Laboratory Data

A complete history and physical examination are required, and when such information is obtained, attention should be directed to the extent of cardiopulmonary impairment, airway abnormalities, and associated extracardiac congenital anomalies. Upper and lower airway problems in patients with Down syndrome, calcium and immunologic deficiencies in patients with aortic arch abnormalities, and renal abnormalities in patients with esophageal atresia and CHD are a few of the associated congenital abnormalities with which the intraoperative

TABLE 78.2

TEN INTENSIVE CARE STRATEGIES TO DIAGNOSE AND SUPPORT LOW CARDIAC OUTPUT STATES

1. Know the cardiac anatomy in detail and its physiologic consequences
2. Understand the specialized considerations of the newborn and implications of reparative rather than palliative surgery
3. Diversify personnel to include expertise in neonatal and adult congenital heart disease
4. Monitor, measure, and image the heart to rule out residual disease as a cause of postoperative hemodynamic instability or low cardiac output
5. Maintain aortic perfusion and improve the contractile state
6. Optimize preload (including atrial shunting)
7. Reduce afterload
8. Control heart rate, rhythm, and synchrony
9. Optimize heart–lung interactions
10. Provide mechanical support when needed

team should be familiar. Intercurrent pulmonary infection is a common and significant finding in chronically overcirculated lungs. The presence, degree, and duration of hypoxemia are important details that, in the absence of iron deficiency, are reflected in a raised hematocrit. The nadir of physiologic anemia during infancy may contribute to left-to-right shunting by decreasing the relative PVR (36). Ten key features required to identify and treat low–cardiac output states in the perioperative period are described in **Table 78.2**.

Chest radiography shows heart size, pulmonary vascular congestion, airway compression, and areas of consolidation or atelectasis. The electrocardiogram may reveal rhythm disturbances and demonstrate ventricular strain patterns (ST- and T-wave changes) characteristic of pathologic pressure or volume burdens on the ventricles. Electrolyte abnormalities caused by congestive heart failure and forced diuresis must also be evaluated preoperatively. Severe hypochloremic metabolic alkalosis may occur in some patients. It may be important to discontinue digoxin preoperatively and to avoid hyperventilation and administration of calcium during induction of anesthesia and preparation for the operating room. The alkalotic, hypokalemic, hypercalcemic, hypotensive, dilated, digoxin-bound myocardium fibrillates with ease.

Echocardiographic and Doppler Assessment

Advances in echocardiographic imaging have had an enormous impact on the diagnosis of CHD. Accurate anatomic diagnosis is now routine in children, without the need for cardiac catheterization. Echocardiography is the preferred imaging modality for assessment of intracardiac anatomic features in young children. However, the intensivist should be aware of the current limitations of echocardiographic and Doppler techniques so that alternative diagnoses can be considered when intraoperative or postoperative findings are inconsistent with the working echocardiographic diagnosis.

Skilled echocardiographers accurately interpret the alignment of cardiac chambers and great vessels but cannot always visualize an atrial septal defect or ventricular septal defect, although color flow-mapping techniques have vastly improved diagnostic capabilities. An atrial septal defect can be indirectly inferred from right ventricular volume overload and interventricular septal shift. Distal pulmonary artery architecture and conduits between a ventricle and a great artery are poorly imaged by echocardiography, and pressure gradients in these areas are not always measurable with Doppler techniques. Evaluation of atrioventricular valve regurgitation may be subjective and nonquantitative. Accuracy of echocardiographic diagnosis is limited by potentially inadequate windows for imaging in the obese patient, the older child, and some postoperative patients. Techniques for three-dimensional (3D) echocardiography are available that may improve diagnostic capabilities, such as defining the mechanism of valve regurgitation (37).

Doppler measurements add greatly to noninvasive diagnostic capabilities. Measurements of pressure gradients across semilunar valves and other obstructions are frequently accurate but may not always correlate with peak systolic ejection gradients measured at catheterization. As good as echocardiographic diagnosis of anatomic defects and Doppler measurements of pressure gradients and valve function have become, the standard for assessment of physiology when other clinical information is ambiguous or contradictory remains cardiac catheterization.

Evaluation of left and right ventricular function in children with CHD is an essential component of the preoperative assessment. Quantitative assessment for left ventricular ejection fraction and shortening fraction is usually made by geometric modeling of the left ventricle, using the Simpson rule. However, the assumptions inherent in this mathematical calculation can lead to markedly inaccurate estimations of ventricular volumes and dynamics. Moreover, the complex geometry of the right ventricle makes this a challenging task and necessitates the use of alternative methods. Developments in echocardiographic techniques, which use 2D echocardiography, Doppler echocardiography, tissue Doppler imaging, and strain rate imaging, have enhanced our ability to accurately assess ventricular function. Doppler techniques offer unique advantages for left and right ventricular function, in that they are independent of geometry and relatively independent of loading conditions (38,39).

An additional modality, transesophageal echocardiography (TEE), may be able to provide additional anatomic information, especially in older or obese patients who have poor transthoracic windows. TEE can be used to confirm preoperative diagnoses, assist in formulating surgical plans, identify residual defects, and guide surgical revisions. Technological advances have expanded the potential uses of TEE, including the recent development of smaller probe sizes, which allow for the safe use of TEE in patients weighing as little as 3.5 kg or less, as well as 3D technology, which optimizes the evaluation of valve anatomy to more clearly identify the site of valve regurgitation (40).

Cardiac Catheterization

When echocardiographic analysis with Doppler measurements and color flow mapping is complete and unambiguous, preoperative assessment may no longer require cardiac catheterization. Catheterization is not typically performed before infant or neonatal operations for ventricular septal defects, complete atrioventricular canal defects, tetralogy of Fallot, interrupted aortic arch, hypoplastic left heart syndrome (HLHS), or coarctation of the aorta. However, in older patients with complex anatomy (e.g., a single ventricle), physiologic data from catheterization may be essential. This technique allows description of the direction, magnitude, and approximate location of intracardiac shunts. Intracardiac and intravascular pressures are measured to determine the presence of obstructions and whether shunt orifices are restrictive or nonrestrictive. Pressure gradients across sites of obstruction must be considered in light of simultaneous blood flow; a small pressure gradient measured at a time of low cardiac output is misleading.

Normally, oxygen saturation does not significantly change from vena cava to pulmonary artery. In the child with CHD, the superior vena cava gives the best indication of true mixed venous oxygen saturation; an increase ("step-up") in saturation

BOX 78-1: CALCULATION OF Q_p:Q_s

Fick equation for Q_s and Q_p:

$$Q_s = \text{Vo}_2/(\text{Cao}_2 - \text{Cmvo}_2)$$
$$Q_p = \text{Vo}_2/(\text{Cpvo}_2 - \text{Cpao}_2)$$

By substituting the equations for oxygen content into the equations for Q_s and Q_p, one can derive a simplified Fick equation for Q_p/Q_s:

$$Q_p/Q_s = (\text{Sao}_2 - \text{Smvo}_2)/(\text{Spvo}_2 - \text{Spao}_2)$$

where Q_s = systemic blood flow, Q_p = pulmonary blood flow, Vo_2 = oxygen consumption, Cao_2 = arterial oxygen content, Cmvo_2 = mixed venous oxygen content, Cpvo_2 = pulmonary vein oxygen content, Cpao_2 = pulmonary artery oxygen content, Sao_2 = arterial oxygen saturation, Smvo_2 = mixed venous oxygen saturation, Spvo_2 = pulmonary venous saturation, and Spao_2 = pulmonary artery saturation

of ≥5% downstream from the superior vena cava suggests the presence of a left-to-right shunt (41), which would occur at the level of the right atrium with an atrial septal defect, in the right ventricle with a ventricular septal defect, and in the pulmonary artery with a patent ductus arteriosus. The magnitude of the left-to-right shunt can be calculated from the Fick equation (see Chapter 71). The oxygen consumption of the patient is usually measured by direct calorimetry, as are the saturation values, but subsequent flow and resistance calculations can be in error. The frequently used term Q_p/Q_s (pulmonary-to-systemic blood flow ratio) can be derived simply from the measured oxygen saturation values (Box 78.1).

The patient whose aortic blood is fully saturated can be safely assumed to have no significant right-to-left shunting. However, when a right-to-left shunt is present, aortic blood is hypoxemic. Blood samples should also be obtained from the pulmonary veins, left atrium, and left ventricle for oxygen saturation determination and ascertainment of the source of desaturated blood. Pulmonary venous desaturation implies a pulmonary source of venous admixture (e.g., pneumonia, atelectasis, or other pulmonary disease). Intrapulmonary shunting may substantially alter the perioperative plan and the postoperative ventilatory requirements of the patient.

In the presence of a left-to-right shunt and elevated PVR, pressure and saturation measurements are often repeated, with the patient breathing 100% oxygen and/or inhaled nitric oxide to assess both the reactivity of the pulmonary vascular bed and any contribution of ventilation–perfusion abnormalities to hypoxemia. If breathing 100% oxygen increases pulmonary blood flow and dramatically increases Q_p/Q_s (with a fall in PVR), potentially reversible processes such as hypoxic pulmonary vasoconstriction are probably contributing to the elevated PVR. The patient with a high, unresponsive PVR and a small left-to-right shunt despite a large shunt orifice may have extensive pulmonary vascular damage from irreversible obstructive pulmonary vascular disease. If so, surgical repair is usually contraindicated (28).

During cardiac catheterization, anatomic abnormalities are identified angiographically. Special, angled views provide specific information about the location and extent of congenital defects (42,43). Ventricular function is assessed angiographically and physiologically (e.g., by pressure measurements). The calculated size of a cardiac chamber may have an important bearing on its ability to support the circulation of a child with hypoplastic ventricles.

Preoperative interventional catheterization may be indicated to optimize conditions for surgical repair. In addition to the classic example of balloon atrial septostomy in neonates with transposition of the great arteries to allow adequate mixing between the parallel circulations (44), preoperative catheter-based procedures can also include device closure of muscular ventricular septal defects in tetralogy of Fallot (45), occlusion of aortopulmonary collaterals prior to Fontan completion (46), and rehabilitation of the pulmonary arteries (47).

One cautionary note should be mentioned to temper the enthusiasm for performing preoperative balloon atrial septostomies in the newborn with single-ventricle physiology. In these patients with mitral stenosis or atresia who may have excess pulmonary blood flow, the large quantity of blood returning to the undersized left atrium may indeed see flow "restricted" across a patent, even stretched open foramen. But the determinant of need for atrial septostomy should be the systemic oxygen saturation levels not the magnitude of the Doppler-measured pressure gradient across the atrial septum. A newborn with HLHS and a Doppler-measured pressure gradient across the atrial septum calculated at 8 mm Hg who has an arterial oxygen saturation level of 82% will not likely benefit from an atrial septostomy and may deteriorate after the procedure since pulmonary blood flow further increases after removal of the flow-related restriction at atrial level. This is in marked contrast to the newborn with HLHS and a 12 mm Hg gradient across the atrial septum who has a widely patent ductus arteriosus and an arterial oxygen saturation of 50%. In this case an atrial septostomy can be life saving and must be done urgently.

Magnetic Resonance Imaging and Angiography

Cardiac magnetic resonance imaging (CMR) has emerged as an important diagnostic modality to complement echocardiographic assessment. CMR provides excellent segmental and anatomic analysis, particularly of the pulmonary veins and thoracic aorta through the use of CMR 3D angiography. Ventricular mass, volume, and function can also be assessed using steady-state free-precession sequences (48,49). Phase-contrast flow-velocity mapping may provide adequate hemodynamic data in some circumstances, obviating the need for diagnostic cardiac catheterization. However, in younger children, temporal and spatial resolution is still technically challenging; moreover, when breath holding is required to avoid respiratory motion artifacts, general anesthesia is often required. Advances continue to be made, and recent CMR imaging sequences allow good anatomic and functional assessment in spontaneously breathing patients, though with less spatial and temporal resolution and at the expense of longer image acquisition times (50).

Contraindications to CMR include pacemakers that are not MR compatible and recently implanted endovascular or intracardiac devices. Computed tomography (CT) is often a reasonable alternative, and can also be of benefit when shorter acquisition times are essential or the risks of general anesthesia are too high to allow for CMR in smaller children. CT angiography generally provides better resolution than CMR, which may be necessary to clearly delineate smaller structures such as pulmonary veins, coronary arteries, and collateral vessels. CT is also the modality of choice to assess the airway and the vascular structures that may surround it. Unlike CMR, CT results in exposure to ionizing radiation, but low-dose scanning protocols are decreasing this risk (51,52).

Assessment of Patient Status and Predominant Pathophysiology

7 Frequently, congenital heart defects are complex and can be difficult to categorize or conceptualize. Rather than trying to determine the management for each individual anatomic defect, a physiologic approach can be taken. The following questions should be asked:

1. How does the systemic venous return reach the systemic arterial circulation to maintain cardiac output? What intracardiac mixing, shunting, or outflow obstruction exist?
2. Is the circulation in series or parallel? Are the defects amenable to a two-ventricle or single-ventricle repair?
3. Is pulmonary blood flow increased or decreased?
4. Is there a volume load or a pressure load on the ventricles?

Appropriate organization of preoperative patient data, preparation of the patient, and decisions about monitoring, anesthetic agents, postoperative care, sedation, and ventilation are best accomplished by focusing on a few major pathophysiologic problems, beginning with whether the patient is cyanotic, in congestive heart failure, or both. Most pathophysiologic mechanisms in the patient's disease that are pertinent to the perioperative plan and to optimal preparation of the patient will focus on one of the following major problems: severe hypoxemia, excessive pulmonary blood flow, congestive heart failure, obstruction of blood flow from the left heart, or poor ventricular function. Although some patients with CHD present with only one problem, many have multiple, interrelated problems.

Severe Hypoxemia

Many of the cyanotic forms of CHD present in the ICU with severe hypoxemia ($PaO_2 < 50$ mm Hg) during the first few days of life, but without respiratory distress. Infusion of prostaglandin E_1 (PGE_1) in patients with decreased pulmonary blood flow maintains or reestablishes pulmonary flow through the ductus arteriosus, which may also improve mixing of venous and arterial blood at the atrial level in patients with transposition of the great arteries (53,54). Consequently, neonates rarely require surgery while they are severely hypoxemic. (One exception is the newborn with obstructed total anomalous pulmonary venous connection, who will present severely hypoxemic with congested lungs and significant distress; these infants do not benefit from PGE_1, and such a diagnosis necessitates emergency surgery and thus must be ruled out by echocardiography). During preoperative preparation with PGE_1, neurologic examination and blood chemistry analysis of renal, hepatic, and hematologic function are necessary to assess the effects of severe hypoxemia during or after birth on end-organ function.

Cyanotic patients who present for surgery after infancy require adequate preoperative and postoperative hydration to prevent the thrombotic problems caused by their elevated hematocrits. The perioperative team should prepare for significant coagulopathy in the cyanotic patient. Premedication must be given cautiously to avoid causing hypoventilation in these patients.

PGE_1 dilates the ductus arteriosus of the neonate with life-threatening ductus-dependent cardiac lesions and improves the patient's condition before surgery. PGE_1 can reopen a functionally closed ductus arteriosus for several days after birth, or it can maintain patency of the ductus arteriosus for an extended period (55,56). The common side effects of PGE_1 infusion (apnea, hypotension, fever, excitation of the central nervous system) are easily managed in the neonate when normal therapeutic doses of the drug (0.01–0.05 μg/kg/min) are used (57,58). However, as PGE_1 is a potent vasodilator, intravascular volume frequently requires augmentation. Patients with intermittent apnea resulting from administration of PGE_1 may require noninvasive positive-pressure ventilation or intubation preoperatively.

PGE_1 usually improves the arterial oxygenation of hypoxemic neonates who have poor pulmonary perfusion due to obstructed pulmonary flow (critical pulmonic stenosis or pulmonary atresia). By providing pulmonary blood flow from the aorta via the ductus arteriosus, an infusion of PGE_1 improves oxygenation and stabilizes the condition of neonates with these lesions. The improved oxygenation reverses the lactic acidosis that may have developed during episodes of severe hypoxia. PGE$_1$ administration for 24 hours usually markedly improves the condition of a severely hypoxemic neonate with restricted pulmonary blood flow (59,60).

Neonates with transposition of the great arteries must have adequate mixing of oxygenated and deoxygenated blood at the atrial level to achieve appropriate oxygen delivery. To accomplish this, balloon atrial septostomy has been applied for over 40 years to create or enlarge an atrial septal defect (44), using echocardiographic guidance in most patients. Hence, balloon atrial septostomy is often performed at the patient's bedside rather than in the catheterization laboratory. It may also be of considerable value in creating an atrial septal defect in any neonate with left atrial hypertension such as HLHS with intact atrial septum. For such patients, fenestration of the atrial septum with an intra-atrial stent is sometimes necessary to maintain patency (61).

Excessive Pulmonary Blood Flow

Excessive pulmonary blood flow is frequently the primary physiologic problem in patients with CHD. The intensivist must carefully evaluate the hemodynamic and respiratory impact of a left-to-right shunt and the extent to which it contributes to the perioperative course in the ICU. Children with left-to-right shunts may have chronic low-grade pulmonary infection and congestion that cannot be eliminated despite optimal preoperative preparation. If so, surgery should not be postponed further; not correcting the defect leaves the patient at risk for recurrent infections, which increases both cardiovascular morbidity and long-term pulmonary sequelae (62). Infections with respiratory syncytial virus (RSV), human metapneumovirus, parainfluenza, and influenza are particularly prevalent in this population, but improvements in intensive care have markedly improved outcomes (63). Additionally, the use of palivizumab for RSV infection prophylaxis has decreased hospitalization rates in CHD patients with RSV by 48% (62).

Aside from the respiratory impairment caused by increased pulmonary blood flow, the left heart must dilate to accept pulmonary venous return that is several times normal. If the body requires more systemic blood flow, the heart responds inefficiently. Most of the increment in cardiac output is recirculated to the lungs. Eventually, symptoms of congestive heart failure appear.

Children with failing hearts increase endogenous catecholamine production and redistribute cardiac output to favored organs by their increased heart rate and decreased extremity perfusion (64). In the most severe cases, the evaluation reveals a child whose body weight is below the third percentile for age and who is tachypneic, tachycardic, and dusky in room air. The child may have intercostal and substernal retractions and skin that is cool to the touch. Capillary refill may be prolonged. Expiratory wheezes are usually audible. Medical management with digoxin, vasodilators, and diuretics may improve the patient's condition, but the diuretics may induce a profound hypochloremic alkalosis and potassium depletion, which may persist after surgery.

These clinical signs and symptoms suggest that profound pathophysiologic alterations have occurred. This information, combined with the anatomic description from the 2D echocardiogram and the physiologic data from cardiac catheterization, permits accurate assessment of the severity of the illness and formulation of an anesthetic plan, a surgical or catheter-based intervention, and a predictable postoperative course.

Obstruction of Left Heart Outflow

Patients who require surgery to relieve obstruction to outflow from the left heart are among the most critically ill children for whom the intensivist must care. These lesions include interruption of the aortic arch, coarctation of the aorta, aortic stenosis, and mitral stenosis or atresia as part of the HLHS (see later discussion). These neonates present with inadequate systemic perfusion and profound metabolic acidosis. The initial pH may be below 7.0 despite a low Paco$_2$. Systemic blood flow is largely or completely dependent on blood flow into the aorta from the ductus arteriosus.

Ductal closure in the neonate with these problems causes dramatic worsening of the patient's condition. The patient becomes critically ill or even moribund and requires PGE$_1$ infusion (see above) for survival. PGE$_1$ allows blood flow into the aorta from the pulmonary artery by maintaining the patency of the ductus arteriosus (59,65), thus creating a systemic circulation in the neonate that depends on right ventricular contractile function and ductal patency. Acidosis, metabolic derangements, and renal failure arise if systemic perfusion is inadequate. PGE$_1$ infusion restores perfusion and aerobic metabolism such that surgery can be deferred until the patient's condition improves. In addition to PGE$_1$ infusion, other supportive measures include ventilatory and inotropic support, as well as correction of metabolic acidosis, hypoglycemia, hypocalcemia, and other electrolyte abnormalities. The stabilization period also allows assessment of the magnitude of end-organ dysfunction caused by the preceding period of inadequate systemic perfusion. Adequacy of resuscitation, rather than severity of illness at presentation, appears to influence postoperative outcome (66,67).

Ventricular Dysfunction

Ideally, the intensivist should participate in the presentation of all preoperative patients who have a planned admission to the ICU, thereby providing an opportunity to understand the extent of ventricular dysfunction preoperatively and providing considerable insight into intraoperative and postoperative events. Although patients with large shunts may have complete mixing of systemic and venous blood and only mild-to-moderate hypoxemia as a result of their excessive pulmonary blood flow, the price paid for near-normal arterial oxygen saturation is chronic ventricular dilation and dysfunction as well as pulmonary vascular obstructive disease. Consequently, decreasing the shunt or a staged approach to single-ventricle repair may be indicated before any other elective surgery can be undertaken. Older patients with CHD and poor ventricular function due to chronic ventricular volume overload (aortic or mitral valve regurgitation or long-standing pulmonary-to-systemic arterial shunts) present a different problem, which may be amenable to afterload reduction to some extent. However, in all of these circumstances, when the heart is dilated and volume overloaded, a propensity for ventricular fibrillation during sedation, anesthesia, and/or intubation of the airway is seen.

Assessment should include an estimation of the patient's functional limitation as an indicator of myocardial performance and reserve, quantification of the degree of hypoxia and the amount of pulmonary blood flow, and evaluation of PVR. For patients with increased Q_p/Q_s, systemic blood flow should be optimized prior to and during induction of anesthesia but without further augmenting pulmonary blood flow. However, during maintenance and emergence from anesthesia, retraction of the lung, positional changes, and abdominal distension may increase the hypoxemia and compromise the function of a dilated, poorly contractile ventricle. If this sequence occurs during surgery, the management must be altered to improve pulmonary blood flow.

In addition, systolic function of the ventricle may be impaired by intrinsic myopathic abnormalities related to drug toxicity (e.g., Adriamycin), inborn enzyme deficiencies, or acquired inflammatory or infectious disease. Patients with such dilated cardiomyopathies require optimization of ventricular performance, with emphasis on inotropic support and afterload reduction. At many centers, these patients are admitted to the ICU for inotropic support and optimization of hemodynamic state prior to a planned surgical intervention. The evidence supporting this practice is not well established in children.

PREOPERATIVE MANAGEMENT OF PATIENTS WITH A SINGLE VENTRICLE

Single-Ventricle Anatomy and Physiology

For a variety of anatomic lesions, the systemic and pulmonary circulations are in parallel, with a single-ventricle effectively supplying both systemic and pulmonary blood flow. The relative proportion of the ventricular output to either the pulmonary or systemic vascular bed is determined by the relative resistance to flow in the two circuits. The pulmonary artery and aortic oxygen saturations are equal, with mixing of the systemic and pulmonary venous return within a "common" atrium. Assuming adequate mixing with normal cardiac output and normal pulmonary venous oxygen saturation, a systemic oxygen saturation (SaO_2) of 80%–85% with a systemic venous saturation (SvO_2) of 60%–65% indicates a Q_p/Q_s of ~1 and hence a balance between systemic and pulmonary flows. Although "balanced," the single ventricle is still required to receive and eject twice the normal amount of blood: one part to the pulmonary circulation and one part to the systemic circulation. A Q_p/Q_s of >1 implies an intolerable volume burden on the heart. While each of the defects associated with single-ventricle physiology involves specific management issues, they all share common management considerations in balancing flow and augmenting systemic perfusion.

Preoperative Management

Changes in PVR have a significant impact on systemic perfusion and circulatory stability, especially preoperatively, when the ductus arteriosus is widely patent. In preparation for surgery, it is important that systemic and pulmonary blood flow be as well balanced as possible to prevent excessive volume overload and ventricular dysfunction that reduces systemic and end-organ perfusion. For example, a newborn with HLHS who has an arterial oxygen saturation of greater than 90%, tachypnea, oliguria, cool extremities, hepatomegaly, and metabolic acidosis has severely limited systemic blood flow. Even though ventricular output is increased, the blood flow that is inefficiently partitioned back to the lungs is unavailable to the other vital organs. Immediate interventions are necessary to prevent imminent circulatory collapse and end-organ injury. In this "over circulated" state, PVR is falling as it should in the normal postnatal state, and the ductus arteriosus is maintained widely patent with prostaglandin infusion to permit unrestricted blood flow from the single right ventricle across the ductus to the systemic vascular bed. Blood flow manipulation through mechanical ventilation and inotrope support may temporarily stabilize the patient (see later discussion), but surgery should not be delayed. Often, the newborn's spontaneous, unassisted ventilatory pattern provides a more stable cardiorespiratory condition than the injudicious use of positive-pressure ventilation and excessive use of vasoactive agents.

Similarly, in a patient with pulmonary atresia and an intact ventricular septum, for example, pulmonary blood flow depends on left ventricular contractile function and ductal patency. As PVR falls, pulmonary blood flow will be excessive

and will eventually steal from the systemic circulation. Preoperative management should focus on an assessment of the balance between pulmonary (Q_p) and systemic flow (Q_s), which is best achieved by a thorough and continuous reevaluation of the clinical examination for adequacy of systemic cardiac output, an evaluation of the chest radiograph for cardiac size and pulmonary congestion, imaging with echocardiography to assess ventricular function and atrioventricular valve competence, and a review of laboratory data for alterations in gas exchange, acid–base status, and end-organ function. A central venous line positioned in the proximal superior vena cava may be useful to monitor volume status and sample for mixed venous oxygen saturation as a surrogate of cardiac output and oxygen delivery. Central venous lines are not necessary in all circumstances; they may have significant complications in small newborns and do not substitute for clinical examination.

Initial resuscitation involves maintaining patency of the ductus arteriosus with a PGE_1 infusion at a rate of 0.01–0.05 μg/kg/min. Intubation and mechanical ventilation are not necessary in all patients. Patients are usually tachypneic, but provided the work of breathing is not excessive and systemic perfusion is maintained without a metabolic acidosis, spontaneous ventilation is often preferable to achieve an adequate systemic perfusion and balance of Q_p and Q_s. A mild metabolic acidosis and low bicarbonate level may be present, but this may not specifically indicate poor perfusion and lactic acidosis. If the presentation involved circulatory collapse and end-organ dysfunction, then a period of days may be required to establish stability and return of vital organ function prior to surgery.

Patients may require intubation and mechanical ventilation due to apnea secondary to PGE_1, to provide additional support in a low–cardiac output state, or for manipulation of gas exchange to assist in balancing the pulmonary and systemic flows. An SaO_2 of >90% indicates pulmonary overcirculation, i.e., Q_p/Q_s > 1.0. PVR can be increased with controlled mechanical hypoventilation to induce a respiratory acidosis, often necessitating sedation and neuromuscular blockade. Ventilation in room air is indicated. While these maneuvers are often successful in increasing PVR and reducing pulmonary blood flow, it is important to remember that these patients have limited oxygen reserve and may desaturate suddenly and precipitously. Controlled hypoventilation in effect reduces the functional residual capacity and, therefore, oxygen reserve, which would be further reduced by the use of a hypoxic inspired gas mixture. An alternate strategy is to add carbon dioxide to the inspiratory limb of the breathing circuit, which will also increase PVR. The limited data available suggest that while either a hypoxic inspired gas mixture or a hypercapnic strategy will decrease Q_p/Q_s to 1, the hypercapnic strategy is more likely to increase cerebral and systemic oxygen delivery (68,69,70). In practice, manipulating inspired gas concentrations is rarely needed in the current era. Patients who have continued pulmonary overcirculation with high SaO_2 and reduced systemic perfusion despite these maneuvers require early surgical intervention to control pulmonary blood flow. At the time of surgery, a snare may be placed around either branch pulmonary artery after the chest is open to effectively limit pulmonary blood flow while the newborn is being prepared for CPB. The rapid improvement in hemodynamics observed with this maneuver has led some to advocate a short period (days) of banding the branch pulmonary arteries in the preoperative newborn with severe congestive heart failure and excessive pulmonary blood flow. This preparatory period may facilitate end-organ recovery prior to more extensive reconstructive surgery such as the first phase of palliation for HLHS.

Decreased pulmonary blood flow in preoperative patients with a parallel circulation is reflected by hypoxemia with an SaO_2 of less than 75%. Preoperatively this may be due to restricted flow across a small ductus arteriosus, increased PVR secondary to parenchymal lung disease, or increased pulmonary venous pressure secondary to obstructed pulmonary venous drainage or a restrictive atrial septal defect. Sedation, paralysis, and manipulation of mechanical ventilation to maintain mild alkalosis may be effective if PVR is elevated. Nitric oxide may also be used in this situation as a specific pulmonary vasodilator. Systemic oxygen delivery is maintained by improving cardiac output with inotropes and maintaining the hematocrit greater than 40%. Among some newborns with HLHS, pulmonary blood flow may be insufficient because the mitral valve hypoplasia in combination with the occasional finding of a restrictive or nearly intact atrial septum severely restricts pulmonary venous return to the heart. The newborn is intensely cyanotic and has a pulmonary venous congestion pattern on chest x-ray. Urgent interventional cardiac catheterization with balloon septostomy or dilation (or stent placement) of a restrictive atrial septal defect may be necessary (71,72). Immediate surgical intervention and palliation may be preferred at some centers.

Systemic perfusion is maintained with the use of volume and vasoactive agents. Inotropic support is often necessary because of ventricular dysfunction secondary to shock states associated with a closing ductus arteriosus at the time of presentation. Systemic afterload reduction with agents such as phosphodiesterase inhibitors (e.g., milrinone) may improve systemic perfusion and reduce atrioventricular valve regurgitation in volume-loaded hearts. However, milrinone may also decrease PVR and thus not fully address the imbalance of pulmonary and systemic flows. Oliguria and a rising serum creatinine level may reflect renal insufficiency from a low cardiac output. Necrotizing enterocolitis is a risk secondary to splanchnic hypoperfusion, and many practitioners prefer not to enterally feed newborns with a wide pulse width and low diastolic pressure (usually <30 mm Hg) prior to surgery. Historically, enteral feeding has been avoided preoperatively in single-ventricle patients awaiting the first stage of palliation, but that practice is now more varied among centers (73). It is important to evaluate end-organ perfusion and function, and optimize the patient's condition prior to surgery.

Prenatal diagnosis of single-ventricle CHD (specifically HLHS) has increased from 37% in the 1990s to 75% for a multiinstitutional cohort of 921 patients with HLHS born between 2005 and 2009 (74,75). Prenatal diagnosis allows for family counseling and the development of a multidisciplinary care plan, genetic testing, and evaluation for associated syndromes and extracardiac anomalies that affect prognosis, identification of complicating conditions (for example, restrictive atrial septum), and possibly fetal intervention (75–78). Interestingly, although preoperative morbidity seems to be improved by prenatal diagnosis, the data are conflicting regarding the effect of prenatal diagnosis on long-term outcomes and survival (74,79–82).

RISK STRATIFICATION IN PEDIATRIC CARDIAC SURGERY

Reliable tools and methods for preoperative risk stratification in pediatric cardiac surgery are essential to fully inform patients and their families, to compare institutions fairly, and to improve postoperative care in pediatric CICUs. Because the field of congenital heart surgery encompasses ~200 diagnoses and 150 procedures, risk assessment is difficult and requires collaboration between experienced clinicians and statisticians. Several scoring systems have been developed for predicting outcome and guiding perioperative therapy in this unique patient population, including the Risk Adjustment in Cardiac Heart Surgery score (RACHS-1) and the Aristotle Comprehensive

Complexity score (83,84). These scoring systems are limited in that they primarily focus on the specific surgical procedure undertaken with sparse additional clinical data. More recently, the Society of Thoracic Surgeons and the European Association of Cardiothoracic Surgery (STS-EACTS) established morbidity and mortality scores and categories, which include a broader array of pre-, intra-, and postoperative clinical data (85,86). Additionally, the Pediatric Cardiac Critical Care Consortium (PC^4) was established in 2009 and has created a multiinstitution clinical database, which provides real-time analysis across centers on numerous quality and outcome metrics for medical and surgical pediatric CICU patients (87). The goal of these efforts is to facilitate comparison of outcomes across cohorts with differing case mixes and to support clinical advances that result in high-quality, cost-effective care for patients with CHD.

Besides methods and scoring that evaluate risk as well as quality of care, a valuable addition to the preoperative evaluation would be a blood marker capable of acutely predicting postoperative morbidity and mortality after congenital heart surgery. Though intra- and postoperative lactate trends have been useful in detecting low–cardiac output syndrome and predicting outcome after CHD repair (88,89), preoperative values do not correlate with postoperative outcomes (90). Preoperative brain natriuretic peptide (BNP) and N-terminal pro-BNP (NTpro-BNP) plasma levels may provide a novel advance in estimating the risk of open-heart surgery in children with CHD. Natriuretic peptides, in particular BNP, are cardiac hormones that are released by ventricular myocytes in response to ventricular dysfunction and wall stress. Specifically, proBNP is released from the myocyte and then cleaved into active BNP and inactive NT-proBNP in the peripheral circulation. Both are measurable in plasma, and it is unclear which will prove to be the more reliable biomarker. Age-specific normative values have been established (91), demonstrating vastly increased circulating BNP in the first postnatal week, which falls dramatically in the first month of life. Increased preoperative plasma levels of NT-proBNP are associated with prolonged postoperative inotropic drug therapy and duration of mechanical ventilation in children who undergo low-risk open-heart surgery (92). Increased preoperative to postoperative BNP ratios may be useful in predicting length of stay, duration of mechanical ventilation, and mortality, but the data are conflicting thus far (93,94). More recent data have shown that pre- and postoperative BNP levels may be lesion and physiology specific, suggesting that additional study in well-defined anatomical populations is needed (95).

CONCLUSIONS AND FUTURE DIRECTIONS

The CICU has become the epicenter of activity in large cardiovascular programs. Nowhere are collaborative practices and multidisciplinary skills more valued or necessary. A curriculum in cardiac intensive care is now formally incorporated into pediatric cardiology training (96). Specialists in this field must have in-depth training in cardiology and critical care and must be well versed in diagnosis and management of multiorgan system dysfunction; this is vital to the discipline of pediatric cardiac intensive care. There has been a dramatic fall in deaths related to CHD, including a decrease of nearly 25% from 1999 to 2006 in the United States (5); while this reduction has been gratifying and is attributable to many factors, achieving 100% survival with minimal morbidity remains the elusive goal, which continues to challenge practitioners.

In the future, new imaging modalities will give us better anatomic and physiologic information. More sophisticated and less-invasive monitoring devices will continue to be developed and refined, aiding in the preoperative care of this fragile patient population. The ways in which the genetic makeup of patients influences outcome will be a focus of future research, along with a clearer understanding of polymorphisms as they relate to risks of CPB. Sophisticated pharmacogenetics will guide drug therapies in the ICU. Increasing clinical trial data will likely guide future patient assessment, and increasing pharmacokinetic data will inform dosage and duration of drug therapies. Discovery and innovation in the basic sciences will lead to new therapies, as it has with treatment of pulmonary hypertension and new inotropic support of the heart. Mechanical support devices suitable for pediatric patients are now available, and will almost certainly be better developed in the future; this will provide options to support patients for longer or even indefinite periods of time, either as bridges to transplantation or even destination therapy. Undoubtedly, clinical teams will continue to become more highly specialized and propel the specialty of pediatric cardiac intensive care to even higher standards, greater patient safety, and better outcomes.

References

1. Botto LD, Correa A, Erickson JD. Racial and temporal variations in the prevalence of heart defects. *Pediatrics* 2001;107(3):E32.
2. Hoffman JI, Kaplan S. The incidence of congenital heart disease. *J Am Coll Cardiol* 2002;39(12):1890–900.
3. van der Linde D, Konings EE, Slager MA, et al. Birth prevalence of congenital heart disease worldwide: A systematic review and meta-analysis. *J Am Coll Cardiol* 2011;58(21):2241–7.
4. Schultz AH, Localio AR, Clark BJ, et al. Epidemiologic features of the presentation of critical congenital heart disease: Implications for screening. *Pediatrics* 2008;121(4):751–7.
5. Gilboa SM, Salemi JL, Nembhard WN, et al. Mortality resulting from congenital heart disease among children and adults in the united states, 1999 to 2006. *Circulation* 2010;122(22):2254–63.
6. Khairy P, Ionescu-Ittu R, Mackie AS, et al. Changing mortality in congenital heart disease. *J Am Coll Cardiol* 2010;56(14):1149–57.
7. Boneva RS, Botto LD, Moore CA, et al. Mortality associated with congenital heart defects in the united states: Trends and racial disparities, 1979-1997. *Circulation* 2001;103(19):2376–81.
8. Reddy VM. Low birth weight and very low birth weight neonates with congenital heart disease: Timing of surgery, reasons for delaying or not delaying surgery. *Semin Thorac Cardiovasc Surg Pediatr Card Surg Annu* 2013;16(1):13–20.
9. Krishnamurthy G, Ratner V, Bacha E. Neonatal cardiac care, a perspective. *Semin Thorac Cardiovasc Surg Pediatr Card Surg Annu* 2013;16(1):21–31.
10. Friedman WF. The intrinsic physiologic properties of the developing heart. *Prog Cardiovasc Dis* 1972;15(1):87–111.
11. Friedman WF, George BL. Treatment of congestive heart failure by altering loading conditions of the heart. *J Pediatr* 1985;106(5):697–706.
12. Romero TE, Friedman WF. Limited left ventricular response to volume overload in the neonatal period: A comparative study with the adult animal. *Pediatr Res* 1979;13(8):910–5.
13. Feltes TF, Hansen TN. Effects of an aorticopulmonary shunt on lung fluid balance in the young lamb. *Pediatr Res* 1989;26(2):94–7.
14. Mills AN, Haworth SG. Greater permeability of the neonatal lung. Postnatal changes in surface charge and biochemistry of porcine pulmonary capillary endothelium. *J Thorac Cardiovasc Surg* 1991;101(5):909–16.
15. Bove EL, Lupinetti FM, Pridjian AK, et al. Results of a policy of primary repair of truncus arteriosus in the neonate. *J Thorac Cardiovasc Surg* 1993;105(6):1057–65; discussion 1065–6.
16. Hanley FL, Heinemann MK, Jonas RA, et al. Repair of truncus arteriosus in the neonate. *J Thorac Cardiovasc Surg* 1993;105(6):1047–56.

17. Chai PJ, Jacobs JP, Quintessenza JA. Surgery for common arterial trunk. *Cardiol Young* 2012;22(6):691–5.
18. McCrindle BW, Tchervenkov CI, Konstantinov IE, et al. Risk factors associated with mortality and interventions in 472 neonates with interrupted aortic arch: A congenital heart surgeons society study. *J Thorac Cardiovasc Surg* 2005;129(2):343–50.
19. Fricke TA, Brizard C, d'Udekem Y, et al. Arterial switch operation in children with interrupted aortic arch: Long-term outcomes. *J Thorac Cardiovasc Surg* 2011;141(6):1547–8.
20. Planche C, Serraf A, Comas JV, et al. Anatomic repair of transposition of great arteries with ventricular septal defect and aortic arch obstruction. One-stage versus two-stage procedure. *J Thorac Cardiovasc Surg* 1993;105(5):925–33.
21. Gladman G, McCrindle BW, Williams WG, et al. The modified blalock-taussig shunt: Clinical impact and morbidity in fallot's tetralogy in the current era. *J Thorac Cardiovasc Surg* 1997;114(1):25–30.
22. Van Arsdell GS, Maharaj GS, Tom J, et al. What is the optimal age for repair of tetralogy of fallot? *Circulation* 2000;102(19 suppl 3):III123–III129.
23. Fisher DJ, Heymann MA, Rudolph AM. Fetal myocardial oxygen and carbohydrate consumption during acutely induced hypoxemia. *Am J Physiol* 1982;242(4):H657–H661.
24. Johnston MV. Plasticity in the developing brain: Implications for rehabilitation. *Dev Disabil Res Rev* 2009;15(2):94–101.
25. McQuillen PS, Hamrick SE, Perez MJ, et al. Balloon atrial septostomy is associated with preoperative stroke in neonates with transposition of the great arteries. *Circulation* 2006;113(2):280–5.
26. Beca J, Gunn J, Coleman L, et al. Pre-operative brain injury in newborn infants with transposition of the great arteries occurs at rates similar to other complex congenital heart disease and is not related to balloon atrial septostomy. *J Am Coll Cardiol* 2009;53(19):1807–11.
27. Taylor MB, Laussen PC. Fundamentals of management of acute postoperative pulmonary hypertension. *Pediatr Crit Care Med* 2010;11(2 suppl):S27–S29.
28. Giglia TM, Humpl T. Preoperative pulmonary hemodynamics and assessment of operability: Is there a pulmonary vascular resistance that precludes cardiac operation? *Pediatr Crit Care Med* 2010;11(2 suppl):S57–S69.
29. Castaneda AR, Mayer JEJ, Jonas RA, et al. The neonate with critical congenital heart disease: Repair—a surgical challenge. *J Thorac Cardiovasc Surg* 1989;98(5, pt 2):869.
30. McMahon CJ, Penny DJ, Nelson DP, et al. Preterm infants with congenital heart disease and bronchopulmonary dysplasia: Postoperative course and outcome after cardiac surgery. *Pediatrics* 2005;116(2):423–30.
31. Marino BS, Lipkin PH, Newburger JW, et al. Neurodevelopmental outcomes in children with congenital heart disease: Evaluation and management: A scientific statement from the american heart association. *Circulation* 2012;126(9):1143–72.
32. Limperopoulos C, Majnemer A, Shevell MI, et al. Neurodevelopmental status of newborns and infants with congenital heart defects before and after open heart surgery. *J Pediatr* 2000;137(5):638–45.
33. Limperopoulos C, Majnemer A, Rosenblatt B, et al. Association between electroencephalographic findings and neurologic status in infants with congenital heart defects. *J Child Neurol* 2001;16(7):471–6.
34. Rios DR, Welty SE, Gunn JK, et al. Usefulness of routine head ultrasound scans before surgery for congenital heart disease. *Pediatrics* 2013;131(6):e1765–e170.
35. Donofrio MT, Duplessis AJ, Limperopoulos C. Impact of congenital heart disease on fetal brain development and injury. *Curr Opin Pediatr* 2011;23(5):502–11.
36. Lister G, Hellenbrand WE, Kleinman CS, et al. Physiologic effects of increasing hemoglobin concentration in left-to-right shunting in infants with ventricular septal defects. *N Engl J Med* 1982;306(9):502–6.

37. Mertens L, Friedberg MK. The gold standard for noninvasive imaging in congenital heart disease: Echocardiography. *Curr Opin Cardiol* 2009;24(2):119–24.

38. Friedberg MK, Rosenthal DN. New developments in echocardiographic methods to assess right ventricular function in congenital heart disease. *Curr Opin Cardiol* 2005;20(2):84–8.

39. Weidemann F, Eyskens B, Sutherland GR. New ultrasound methods to quantify regional myocardial function in children with heart disease. *Pediatr Cardiol* 2002;23(3):292–306.

40. Kamra K, Russell I, Miller-Hance WC. Role of transesophageal echocardiography in the management of pediatric patients with congenital heart disease. *Paediatr Anaesth* 2011;21(5):479–93.

41. Freed MD, Miettinen OS, Nadas AS. Oximetric detection of intracardiac left-to-right shunts. *Br Heart J* 1979;42(6):690–4.

42. Bargeron LM Jr, Elliott LP, Soto B, et al. Axial cineangiography in congenital heart disease. Section I: Concept, technical and anatomic considerations. *Circulation* 1977;56(6):1075–83.

43. Fellows KE, Keane JF, Freed MD. Angled views in cineangiocardiography of congenital heart disease. *Circulation* 1977;56(3):485–90.

44. Rashkind WJ, Miller WW. Creation of an atrial septal defect without thoracotomy. A palliative approach to complete transposition of the great arteries. *JAMA* 1966;196(11):991–2.

45. Bridges ND, Perry SB, Keane JF, et al. Preoperative transcatheter closure of congenital muscular ventricular septal defects. *N Engl J Med* 1991;324(19):1312–7.

46. Banka P, Sleeper LA, Atz AM, et al. Practice variability and outcomes of coil embolization of aortopulmonary collaterals before fontan completion: A report from the pediatric heart network fontan cross-sectional study. *Am Heart J* 2011;162(1):125–30.

47. Dragulescu A, Kammache I, Fouilloux V, et al. Long-term results of pulmonary artery rehabilitation in patients with pulmonary atresia, ventricular septal defect, pulmonary artery hypoplasia, and major aortopulmonary collaterals. *J Thorac Cardiovasc Surg* 2011;142(6):1374–80.

48. Geva T. Introduction: Magnetic resonance imaging. *Pediatr Cardiol* 2000;21(1):3–4.

49. Chung T. Assessment of cardiovascular anatomy in patients with congenital heart disease by magnetic resonance imaging. *Pediatr Cardiol* 2000;21(1):18–26.

50. Seeger A, Fenchel MC, Greil GF, et al. Three-dimensional cine MRI in free-breathing infants and children with congenital heart disease. *Pediatr Radiol* 2009;39(12):1333–42.

51. Bailliard F, Hughes ML, Taylor AM. Introduction to cardiac imaging in infants and children: Techniques, potential, and role in the imaging work-up of various cardiac malformations and other pediatric heart conditions. *Eur J Radiol* 2008;68(2):191–8.

52. Lambert V, Sigal-Cinqualbre A, Belli E, et al. Preoperative and postoperative evaluation of airways compression in pediatric patients with 3-dimensional multislice computed tomographic scanning: Effect on surgical management. *J Thorac Cardiovasc Surg* 2005;129(5):1111–8.

53. Freed MD, Heymann MA, Lewis AB, et al. Prostaglandin E1 infants with ductus arteriosus-dependent congenital heart disease. *Circulation* 1981;64(5):899–905.

54. Butts RJ, Ellis AR, Bradley SM, et al. Effect of prostaglandin duration on outcomes in transposition of the great arteries with intact ventricular septum. *Congenit Heart Dis* 2012;7(4):387–91.

55. Barker CL, Yates RW, Kelsall AW. Prolonged treatment with prostaglandin in an infant born with extremely low weight. *Cardiol Young* 2005;15(4):425–6.

56. Brodlie M, Chaudhari M, Hasan A. Prostaglandin therapy for ductal patency: How long is too long? *Acta Paediatr* 2008;97(9):1303–4.

57. Lewis AB, Freed MD, Heymann MA, et al. Side effects of therapy with prostaglandin E1 in infants with critical congenital heart disease. *Circulation* 1981;64(5):893–8.

58. Browning Carmo KA, Barr P, West M, et al. Transporting newborn infants with suspected duct dependent congenital heart disease on low-dose prostaglandin E1 without routine mechanical ventilation. *Arch Dis Child Fetal Neonatal Ed* 2007;92(2):F117–F119.

59. Donahoo JS, Roland JM, Ken J. Prostaglandin E1 as an adjunct to emergency cardiac operation in neonates. *J Thorac Cardiovasc Surg* 1981;81(2):227.

60. Reddy SC, Saxena A. Prostaglandin E1: First stage palliation in neonates with congenital cardiac defects. *Indian J Pediatr* 1998;65(2):211–6.

61. Gossett JG, Rocchini AP, Lloyd TR, et al. Catheter-based decompression of the left atrium in patients with hypoplastic left heart syndrome and restrictive atrial septum is safe and effective. *Catheter Cardiovasc Interv* 2006;67(4):619–24.

62. Feltes TF, Cabalka AK, Meissner HC, et al; Cardiac Synagis Study Group. Palivizumab prophylaxis reduces hospitalization due to respiratory syncytial virus in young children with hemodynamically significant congenital heart disease. *J Pediatr* 2003;143(4):532–40.

63. Klein MI, Coviello S, Bauer G, et al. The impact of infection with human metapneumovirus and other respiratory viruses in young infants and children at high risk for severe pulmonary disease. *J Infect Dis* 2006;193(11):1544–51.

64. Epstein D, Wetzel RC. Cardiovascular physiology and shock. In: Nichols DG, Ungerleider RM, Spevak PJ, et al., eds. *Critical Heart Disease in Infants and Children*. 2nd ed. Philadelphia, PA: Mosby Elsevier, 2006.

65. Jonas RA, Lang P, Mayer JE, et al. The importance of prostaglandin E1 in resuscitation of the neonate with critical aortic stenosis. *J Thorac Cardiovasc Surg* 1985;89(2):314–5.

66. Jonas RA, Hansen DD, Cook N, et al. Anatomic subtype and survival after reconstructive operation for hypoplastic left heart syndrome. *J Thorac Cardiovasc Surg* 1994;107(4):1121–7; discussion 1127–8.

67. Shamszad P, Gospin TA, Hong BJ, et al. Impact of preoperative risk factors on outcomes after norwood palliation for hypoplastic left heart syndrome. *J Thorac Cardiovasc Surg* 2014;147(3):897–901.

68. Tabbutt S, Ramamoorthy C, Montenegro LM, et al. Impact of inspired gas mixtures on preoperative infants with hypoplastic left heart syndrome during controlled ventilation. *Circulation* 2001;104(12 suppl 1):I159–I164.

69. Ramamoorthy C, Tabbutt S, Kurth CD, et al. Effects of inspired hypoxic and hypercapnic gas mixtures on cerebral oxygen saturation in neonates with univentricular heart defects. *Anesthesiology* 2002;96(2):283–8.

70. Gentile MA. Inhaled medical gases: More to breathe than oxygen. *Respir Care* 2011;56(9):1341–57; discussion 1357–9.

71. Atz AM, Feinstein JA, Jonas RA, et al. Preoperative management of pulmonary venous hypertension in hypoplastic left heart syndrome with restrictive atrial septal defect. *Am J Cardiol* 1999;83(8):1224–8.

72. Vlahos AP, Lock JE, McElhinney DB, et al. Hypoplastic left heart syndrome with intact or highly restrictive atrial septum: Outcome after neonatal transcatheter atrial septostomy. *Circulation* 2004;109(19):2326–30.

73. Pasquali SK, Ohye RG, Lu M, et al. Variation in perioperative care across centers for infants undergoing the norwood procedure. *J Thorac Cardiovasc Surg* 2012;144(4):915–21.

74. Atz AM, Travison TG, Williams IA, et al. Prenatal diagnosis and risk factors for preoperative death in neonates with single right ventricle and systemic outflow obstruction: Screening data from the pediatric heart network single ventricle reconstruction trial. *J Thorac Cardiovasc Surg* 2010;140(6):1245–50.

75. Lowry AW. Resuscitation and perioperative management of the high-risk single ventricle patient: First-stage palliation. *Congenit Heart Dis* 2012;7(5):466–78.

76. Stasik CN, Gelehrter S, Goldberg CS, et al. Current outcomes and risk factors for the norwood procedure. *J Thorac Cardiovasc Surg* 2006;131(2):412–7.

77. Gardiner HM. The case for fetal cardiac intervention. *Heart* 2009;95(20):1648–52.

78. Simpson JM. Fetal cardiac interventions: Worth it? *Heart* 2009;95(20):1653–5.

79. Tworetzky W, McElhinney DB, Reddy VM, et al. Improved surgical outcome after fetal diagnosis of hypoplastic left heart syndrome. *Circulation* 2001;103(9):1269–73.

80. Sivarajan V, Penny DJ, Filan P, et al. Impact of antenatal diagnosis of hypoplastic left heart syndrome on the clinical presentation and surgical outcomes: The australian experience. *J Paediatr Child Health* 2009;45(3):112–7.

81. Satomi G, Yasukochi S, Shimizu T, et al. Has fetal echocardiography improved the prognosis of congenital heart disease? Comparison of patients with hypoplastic left heart syndrome with and without prenatal diagnosis. *Pediatr Int* 1999;41(6):728–32.

82. Verheijen PM, Lisowski LA, Stoutenbeek P, et al. Prenatal diagnosis of congenital heart disease affects preoperative acidosis in the newborn patient. *J Thorac Cardiovasc Surg* 2001;121(4):798–803.

83. Jenkins KJ. Risk adjustment for congenital heart surgery: The RACHS-1 method. *Semin Thorac Cardiovasc Surg Pediatr Card Surg Annu* 2004;7:180–4.

84. Lacour-Gayet F, Clarke D, Jacobs J, et al. The aristotle score: A complexity-adjusted method to evaluate surgical results. *Eur J Cardiothorac Surg* 2004;25(6):911–24.

85. O'Brien SM, Clarke DR, Jacobs JP, et al. An empirically based tool for analyzing mortality associated with congenital heart surgery. *J Thorac Cardiovasc Surg* 2009;138(5):1139–53.

86. Jacobs ML, O'Brien SM, Jacobs JP, et al. An empirically based tool for analyzing morbidity associated with operations for congenital heart disease. *J Thorac Cardiovasc Surg* 2013;145(4):1046, 1057.e1.

87. Gaies M, Pasquali SK, Scheurer MA. Follow the leaders. *World J Pediatr Congenit Heart Surg* 2014;5(1):135–7.

88. Charpie JR, Dekeon MK, Goldberg CS, et al. Serial blood lactate measurements predict early outcome after neonatal repair or palliation for complex congenital heart disease. *J Thorac Cardiovasc Surg* 2000;120(1):73–80.

89. Munoz R, Laussen PC, Palacio G, et al. Changes in whole blood lactate levels during cardiopulmonary bypass for surgery for congenital cardiac disease: An early indicator of morbidity and mortality. *J Thorac Cardiovasc Surg* 2000;119(1):155–62.

90. Rossi AF, Lopez L, Dobrolet N, et al. Hyperlactatemia in neonates admitted to the cardiac intensive care unit with critical heart disease. *Neonatology* 2010;98(2):212–6.

91. Koch A, Singer H. Normal values of B type natriuretic peptide in infants, children, and adolescents. *Heart* 2003;89(8):875–8.

92. Gessler P, Knirsch W, Schmitt B, et al. Prognostic value of plasma N-terminal pro-brain natriuretic peptide in children with congenital heart defects and open-heart surgery. *J Pediatr* 2006;148(3):372–6.

93. Hsu JH, Keller RL, Chikovani O, et al. B-type natriuretic peptide levels predict outcome after neonatal cardiac surgery. *J Thorac Cardiovasc Surg* 2007;134(4):939–45.

94. Mir TS, Haun C, Lilje C, et al. Utility of N-terminal brain natriuretic peptide plasma concentrations in comparison to lactate and troponin in children with congenital heart disease following open-heart surgery. *Pediatr Cardiol* 2006;27(2):209–16.

95. Amirnovin R, Keller RL, Herrera C, et al. B-type natriuretic peptide levels predict outcomes in infants undergoing cardiac surgery in a lesion-dependent fashion. *J Thorac Cardiovasc Surg* 2013;145(5):1279–87.

96. Kulik T, Giglia TM, Kocis KC, et al. American College of Cardiology Foundation, American Heart Association, American College of Physicians Task Force on Clinical Competence (ACC/AHA/AAP Writing Committee to Develop Training Recommendations for Pediatric Cardiology). ACCF/AHA/AAP recommendations for training in pediatric cardiology. Task force 5: Requirements for pediatric cardiac critical care. *J Am Coll Cardiol* 2005;46(7):1396–9.

CHAPTER 79 ■ POSTOPERATIVE CARE OF THE PEDIATRIC CARDIAC SURGICAL PATIENT

RONALD A. BRONICKI, JOHN M. COSTELLO, AND KATE L. BROWN

KEY POINTS

1 Comprehensive postoperative care begins upon admission to the intensive care unit (ICU) with a detailed hand-off from the cardiac surgeon and anesthesiologist, which includes a thorough review of the preoperative history and intraoperative course.

2 Although major advances have occurred in recent years in the conduct of cardiopulmonary bypass, its sequelae continue to impact the recovery of many children following surgery. A thorough understanding of the impact of intraoperative circulatory support techniques on postoperative end-organ function, particularly the cardiovascular, pulmonary, renal, and neurologic systems, is essential.

3 A careful assessment for residual anatomical lesions is warranted upon admission to the ICU after cardiac surgery, and for any patient whose postoperative course deviates from the expected recovery.

4 Given the diverse cardiovascular physiology encountered in the early postoperative period, monitoring and treatment strategies must be tailored for each patient.

5 As the age spectrum and associated noncardiac comorbidities present in patients recovering from congenital heart surgery is quite broad, ranging from premature neonates to middle-age adults, a multidisciplinary team of clinicians is needed to optimize outcomes.

1 The management of the pediatric patient following cardiac surgery is predicated on the clinician having a thorough understanding of a broad fund of knowledge, with an emphasis on pulmonary function, cardiovascular function, and the interaction between these two systems. An appreciation of the patient's preoperative history and intraoperative course, including a deliberate review of all studies, enables the clinician to synthesize a comprehensive plan that is tailored to the needs of a given patient. Postoperative management begins with the physical examination, a survey of respiratory and hemodynamic parameters, as well as radiographs and basic laboratory studies. Based on the integration of all data, a determination of the severity of illness and an initial management strategy is established. At its core, the assessment should attempt to identify residual cardiac lesions and other potential clinical pitfalls. Monitoring strategies are used to provide acute and accurate surveillance, as it is much more advantageous to manage patients in an anticipatory rather than reactionary fashion. Over time, the clinical course is reassessed, assuring that the patient's clinical trajectory is proceeding as expected. The goal of this chapter is to provide the underpinnings necessary for completing these tasks.

GENERAL POSTOPERATIVE CONSIDERATIONS

Respiratory Dysfunction

There are several factors that may contribute to postoperative respiratory dysfunction. Infants in particular are at greater risk for developing respiratory insufficiency following surgery,

as this population has much less respiratory reserve than older children. The functional residual capacity is the lung volume at end-expiration and is set passively by the balance between the inward recoil of the lung and outward recoil of the chest wall. Because the infant has a relatively high chest-wall-to-lung-compliance ratio, the end-expiratory lung volume is reduced, which predisposes the infant to developing atelectasis and pulmonary venous admixture (1). In addition, the infant is less able to defend tidal volume when faced with an increased respiratory load. The highly compliant chest wall is at a mechanical disadvantage, as a significant portion of the energy generated by the respiratory pump is wasted in distorting the rib cage (retractions), rather than in exchanging tidal volume (2). Further compromising ventilatory reserve, the infant diaphragm has less contractile reserve because it contains fewer fatigue-resistant–type muscle fibers and immature sarcoplasmic reticulum (3). Finally, the cross section of the subglottic region is decreased compared with older children, predisposing the infant to the development of upper airway obstruction. Respiratory function evolves over the first year of life, as the chest wall ossifies and respiratory muscles mature (4).

Congenital heart disease and cardiac surgery impact respiratory mechanics (5). Cardiopulmonary bypass (CPB) invariably, but to varying degrees, impairs respiratory function (6). The bioincompatible bypass circuit and pulmonary ischemia–reperfusion injury induce inflammation-mediated structural changes to the pulmonary microvasculature, increasing vascular permeability and extravascular lung water, leading to interstitial edema (7). Further, injury to alveolar epithelium leads to alveolar edema and decreased surfactant bioavailability. Injury to the type II alveolar pneumocyte leads to a decrease in surfactant production while extravasated plasma proteases inactivate surfactant (8). Structural heart lesions that transmit systemic pressure to the pulmonary vasculature while allowing for excessive pulmonary blood flow, such as a large nonrestrictive ventricular septal defect (VSD), also increase extravascular lung water formation and contribute to a decrease in lung compliance. Left-sided heart defects, such as mitral stenosis and left ventricular dysfunction, produce pulmonary venous hypertension and contribute to interstitial pulmonary edema formation. In addition to pulmonary edema and an increase in alveolar surface tension forces, chest wall edema, pleural fluid, and ascites may also contribute to an increase in lung recoil and the propensity for atelectasis.

Airway resistance may be elevated due to several factors. Upper airway obstruction may result from postextubation croup, particularly in the infant. Excessive sedation and analgesia following extubation decrease oropharyngeal muscle tone and compromise upper airway patency. Neurologic lesions such as *recurrent laryngeal nerve injury* and resulting *vocal cord dysfunction* may cause upper airway dysfunction. Lower airway obstruction may result from any cardiac lesion that produces interstitial edema and results from compression of small airways within the bronchovascular sheath. In severe cases of lower airway obstruction, lung volumes are significantly increased, leading to flattened diaphragms and reduced ventilatory capacity, as diaphragmatic preload is decreased (4).

An inefficiency in oxygenation results from a pathophysiologic process that primarily affects alveoli and is characterized by an alveolar to arterial oxygen gradient. Supportive care for parenchymal lung disease includes supplemental oxygen, strategies for reducing extravascular lung water, and the recruitment of atelectatic lung units with end-expiratory pressure. Specific therapies are directed at the underlying condition. Other causes of arterial hypoxemia that are unresponsive to these measures include intracardiac shunting and collaterals with physiologic right-to-left shunting.

Chylothorax is a complication of thoracic surgery due to injury of the thoracic duct or associated lymphatic channels that presents with respiratory distress, worsening oxygenation, or persistent drainage from the postoperative chest tube. Identification of a pleural effusion by postoperative chest x-ray suggests the diagnosis of chylothorax. If the infant has been fed, the pleural effusion appears creamy and the diagnosis is established by triglyceride level >1.2 mmol/liter and a total cell count >1000 cells/microliter (predominantly of lymphocytes). However, the typical postoperative cardiac patient has been fasting, making analysis of pleural fluid often inconclusive. The diagnosis is then established retrospectively when a diet of medium-chain triglycerides (i.e., dietary elimination of long-chain triglycerides) or total parenteral nutrition and other measures directed at chylothorax result in resolution of the pleural effusion.

There are several factors that may impair ventilatory function following cardiac surgery. Ventilatory function is the result of the interplay between neuromuscular competency, which includes the central and peripheral nervous system and respiratory musculature; respiratory muscle energetics, or the relationship between respiratory muscle oxygen delivery and oxygen demand; and respiratory load, which is affected by lung compliance, airway resistance, and ventilatory demand or minute ventilation. Neuromuscular competence may be compromised as a result of central nervous system depression; *diaphragmatic paresis* or *diaphragmatic paralysis*, which has a significant impact in infants due to their diminished respiratory reserve; and disuse atrophy of the respiratory musculature, which may be compounded by malnutrition, the use of muscle relaxants, and glucocorticoid administration. Diaphragm paresis is usually secondary to *phrenic nerve injury* (left more commonly injured), which may be caused by topical application of ice to the area, reoperation and difficult dissection, as well as operation in area of the pulmonary arteries, arch, or superior vena cava (SVC), or from attempts

at central venous access. Diaphragm paresis is most often detected during failed weaning of infants from mechanical ventilatory support. It usually presents as difficulty weaning with CO_2 retention, increased work of breathing, and elevated hemi-diaphragm on chest x-ray. Confirmation often requires ultrasonography or fluoroscopy of the hemi-diaphragms during spontaneous breathing without positive-pressure support.

Respiratory muscle energetics may be compromised due to several factors commonly encountered in the cardiac intensive care setting. Under normal conditions, the arterial–venous oxygen content difference for the diaphragm is high, necessitating an increase in respiratory muscle perfusion when the respiratory load is increased (9). Thus, when cardiac output is limited, ventilatory capacity is reduced (10). An increased respiratory load coupled with a limited cardiac output state, a common convergence of issues in patients with cardiovascular disease, increases the propensity to develop ventilatory failure (11).

Whether ventilatory failure results from neuromuscular incompetence, an excess load, and/or impaired respiratory energetics, it is manifested by hypercapnia with a normal arterial to end-tidal carbon dioxide gradient (<2 mm Hg). The extent to which oxygenation is impaired, which is minimal and readily restored with supplemental oxygen, may be calculated from the alveolar air equation. Management of ventilatory failure involves treating the underlying cause(s) and providing invasive or noninvasive ventilatory support.

Hypercapnia may also result from wasted or deadspace ventilation and is characterized by an elevated arterial to end-tidal carbon dioxide gradient. Any lesion that produces large ventilation-to-perfusion ratios, primarily conditions where pulmonary perfusion is limited, creates inefficiencies in carbon dioxide removal. Often, the amount of deadspace increases with positive-pressure ventilation, as it tends to reduce pulmonary perfusion due to decreases in venous return and increases in right ventricular afterload (see Chapter 70). An understanding of the processes, which impact pulmonary function in patients following cardiac surgery as well as a fundamental understanding of gas exchange, is essential for managing these patients postoperatively. Often, there are several factors, which at any given time impact respiratory function, making the assessment challenging and dynamic.

Cardiovascular Dysfunction

Cardiac function may be impaired for several reasons following surgery. There is invariably some degree of *postoperative systolic dysfunction*, which is in part due to CPB-induced inflammation where mediators such as tumor necrosis factor-α have been shown to impair cardiomyocyte shortening (12,13). Inflammation also produces functional and structural changes to the endothelium, leading to interstitial edema and a decrease in myocardial compliance (14,15). However, the primary mechanism responsible for myocardial dysfunction following surgery is an intraoperative period of ischemia (cardioplegic arrest) compounded by reperfusion injury (see section on cardiopulmonary bypass) (16–18). Other factors that may impact postoperative cardiac function include the surgical approach and preexisting ventricular dysfunction, which may have been due in part to a volume and/or pressure load (see cardiac lesions) (19). Exacerbation of underlying (or the development of new) arrhythmias (e.g., junctional ectopic tachycardia [JET] or heart block) impacts cardiac function and may lead to inadequate cardiac output (see Chapter 77). The pathophysiology and treatment of arrhythmias are covered extensively elsewhere in this section.

The adverse affects of CPB have a disproportionately greater impact on the myocardium of infants, as they have less myocardial reserve than children and adults. The infant cardiomyocyte possesses relatively few and poorly organized contractile proteins, as a majority of the myocyte is composed of noncontractile elements (20). Calcium handling also differs between immature and mature myocardium. Infant myocardium has reduced intracellular stores of calcium and a less-organized sarcoplasmic reticulum compared with mature myocardium (21). As a result, the infant myocardium is less compliant and less responsive to fluid and inotropes and is more susceptible to increases in ventricular afterload than the myocardium of a child or adult (22). The limitations of cardiopulmonary physiology in infants noted above are compounded by the fact that they have a much greater demand on respiratory and circulatory systems. Oxygen consumption per unit mass is much greater than in older children, necessitating a relatively greater cardiac output and minute ventilation.

Vascular function may also be impaired following CPB. As with bypass-induced lung and cardiac injury, the inflammatory response to bypass impacts pulmonary and systemic arterial endothelial function, contributing to heightened pulmonary vascular reactivity and alterations in systemic vascular resistance (see sections on pulmonary hypertension and cardiopulmonary bypass).

Pericardial tamponade may lead to hypotension and cardiac arrest. Tamponade is defined as rapid accumulation of fluid, blood, or air in the pericardial space that increases pericardial pressure and decreases venous return to the heart as the right atrium and ventricle are compressed. Accumulation of blood in the pericardium or mediastinum usually accounts for tamponade in the first 24–48 hours after cardiac surgery. Tachycardia, poor peripheral perfusion, and rising central venous pressure are initial signs of impending tamponade. Pulsus paradoxus, a >10 mm Hg decrease in systolic pressure during inspiration, is the most sensitive sign of tamponade in the postoperative cardiac patient. Echocardiography reveals right atrial and right ventricular compression during diastole. Treatment in the immediate postoperative period involves emergency opening of the sternotomy wound in the pediatric intensive care unit (PICU) and drainage of pericardial fluid. The nonoperative patient with tamponade requires emergency pericardiocentesis.

Cardiopulmonary Interactions

The interactions between respiratory and cardiovascular systems play a prominent role in the pathophysiology of critically ill patients, and the pathophysiology of congenital and acquired cardiovascular disease, and have a significant impact on postoperative cardiovascular function. This subject is covered in detail elsewhere in this textbook (Chapter 70).

Pulmonary Hypertension

Pulmonary arterial hypertension following cardiac surgery arises in relation to cardiac defects associated with long-standing increased pulmonary pressure and blood flow, such as large, nonrestrictive VSDs. Patients with pulmonary venous hypertension resulting from left ventricular dysfunction or obstruction to pulmonary venous return are also at risk. Over time, these hemodynamic conditions contribute to endothelial dysfunction and heightened vascular reactivity, and pulmonary vascular remodeling that consists of progressive smooth muscle hypertrophy and hyperplasia and intimal proliferation. Shear stresses within the pulmonary arterial bed, related to abnormal patterns of blood flow, contribute to pathological changes. Vasoconstriction may be triggered by reduced endogenous nitric oxide production, impaired endothelium-dependent pulmonary artery relaxation, and alterations to the endothelin-1 pathway (23). The "Heath and Edwards Classification" grades 1–6 describe the severity, histological changes, and reversibility of pulmonary arterial disease.

CPB produces a systemic inflammatory response and causes pulmonary ischemia-reperfusion injury. Both components contribute to pulmonary vasoconstriction via further endothelial dysfunction and reduced availability of endogenous nitric oxide (24). Preexisting adverse flow conditions and the concomitant effects of corrective surgery, CPB, and reperfusion injury occasionally result in the evolution of a severe pulmonary hypertensive crises manifested by right ventricular failure and low cardiac output.

Table 79.1 delineates therapeutic measures to alleviate acute pulmonary hypertensive episodes. Intravenous vasodilators are relatively nonselective and may generate systemic hypotension, making them less attractive in the management of acute postoperative pulmonary hypertension. Conversely, inhaled nitric oxide is a selective pulmonary vasodilator delivered as a gas via the ventilator circuit directly into the alveolus. Once there, it rapidly diffuses into adjacent vascular smooth muscle cells where it activates soluble guanylyl cyclase, leading to activation of a cGMP-dependent protein kinase and a signal cascade that ends in smooth muscle relaxation and pulmonary vasodilation. Nitric oxide is quickly deactivated by heme in red blood cells, and thus has no systemic hemodynamic effects. Inhaled nitric oxide has been demonstrated to be efficacious in children with postoperative pulmonary hypertension, in whom it ameliorates pulmonary vasoconstriction (25). Weaning from inhaled nitric oxide may be facilitated by pretreatment with the phosphodiesterase inhibitor sildenafil, which inhibits the inactivation of cGMP within smooth muscle cells (26). Overall, improved outcomes of pulmonary hypertension

TABLE 79.1

CRITICAL CARE STRATEGIES FOR POSTOPERATIVE TREATMENT OF PULMONARY HYPERTENSION

■ ENCOURAGE	■ AVOID
1. Anatomic investigation	1. Residual anatomic disease
2. Opportunities for right-to-left shunt as "pop off"	2. Intact atrial septum in right heart failure
3. Sedation/anesthesia	3. Agitation/pain
4. Moderate hyperventilation	4. Respiratory acidosis
5. Moderate alkalosis	5. Metabolic acidosis
6. Adequate inspired oxygen	6. Alveolar hypoxia
7. Normal lung volumes	7. Atelectasis or overdistension
8. Optimal hematocrit	8. Excessive hematocrit
9. Inotropic support	9. Low output and coronary perfusion
10. Vasodilators	10. Vasoconstrictors/increased afterload

following cardiac surgery in the current era reflect the success of a synergistic approach, which makes use of the full range of therapies and maneuvers available to tackle this problem.

Assessment of Hemodynamics and Oxygen Transport Balance

4 There are several monitoring modalities available to guide the clinician in what is the primary task following surgery, to ensure adequate tissue oxygenation. Although an extensive review of this topic is provided in a separate chapter (Chapter 71), certain aspects of cardiovascular monitoring merit discussion here as well. The conventional approach to hemodynamic monitoring following cardiac surgery is based on the physical examination and the monitoring of routine hemodynamic parameters, such as heart rate, arterial blood pressure, central venous pressure, and urine output. However, studies in adults and children have failed to demonstrate a correlation between estimations of cardiovascular function based on the standard approach and those based on direct measurements (27,28).

Studies in children have demonstrated a poor correlation between estimations of systemic vascular resistance and cardiac output based on the assessment of peripheral pulses, capillary refill time and peripheral to core temperature gradients, and measurements of these hemodynamic parameters (28,29). The central venous pressure gives some indication of ventricular filling; however, studies have demonstrated a poor correlation between this parameter and right ventricular volume (30). The determinants of ventricular filling are the diastolic transmural pressure (the difference in ventricular diastolic and pericardial pressures) and ventricular compliance. Furthermore, in the presence of cardiopulmonary disease, there is no correlation between central venous and left atrial pressures (31,32). Heart rate is affected by many factors, including vasoactive agents, fever, and agitation, and blood pressure is a poor correlate of cardiac output. So, while the clinical estimation of circulatory function and tissue oxygenation begins with an interpretation of these conventional monitoring modalities, the use of additional objective indicators of cardiac function, cardiac output, and oxygen transport balance is needed to establish a timely and accurate assessment of the severity of illness and the responses to interventions.

Measurement of central venous oximetry allows for assessment of the relationship between oxygen demand and delivery (oxygen transport balance). While serum lactate levels assess global oxygen transport balance as well, oxygen extraction increases and becomes critical well before lactate production exceeds its clearance and begins to rise. Cerebral oximetry is used as a surrogate for cerebral venous oxygen saturations and as such is used primarily to assess cerebral oxygen transport balance. Cerebral oximetry is also used as an indicator of global oxygen transport balance. It is important to recall, however, that when cardiac output is limited, blood flow is redistributed away from less vital organs to maintain vital organ perfusion. Thus, cerebral oximetry is a relatively late indicator of a falling cardiac output. Postoperative echocardiograms are essential for creating a comprehensive picture of cardiac function. Pulmonary arterial catheters are seldom used but provide information not obtained elsewhere, including a measurement of cardiac output as well as a direct measurement of pulmonary arterial and left-sided filling pressures.

Maintenance of Tissue Oxygenation

Shock may be defined as inadequate oxygen delivery relative to oxygen demand or impaired oxygen transport balance. This construct provides a comprehensive framework by which to guide therapies for critically ill patients. Several factors are responsible for increasing oxygen demand, including the systemic inflammatory response to bypass, fever, endogenous and exogenous catecholamines, the stress response to surgery, wakefulness, and spontaneous breathing. For those in or at risk for developing shock, therapy begins with minimizing metabolic demand. Mechanical ventilation and unloading of the respiratory pump, sedation and analgesia, and avoiding hyperthermia all serve to decrease oxygen demand and thus favorably impact oxygen transport balance.

Oxygen transport balance may be compromised as a result of impaired oxygen delivery. Impaired oxygenation, anemia, and low cardiac output all may be contributory. Low cardiac output may result from inadequate venous return, ventricular dysfunction, excessive afterload, or arrhythmias. Exacerbation of underlying (or the development of new) arrhythmias impacts cardiac function and may compromise cardiac output. The pathophysiology and treatment of arrhythmias are covered extensively in a separate chapter (Chapter 77). Inadequate preload most often results from an aggressive strategy to decrease total body water, which begins with ultrafiltration performed during CPB and extends into the postoperative period with diuretic therapies. The systemic inflammatory response to bypass may lead to a vascular leak syndrome, decreasing intravascular volume and ventricular preload. A relatively inadequate preload may be due to diastolic dysfunction, where an elevated ventricular filling pressure is needed to maintain an adequate stroke volume, emphasizing the importance of determining the optimal ventricular filling pressure. In either case, volume administration results in a prompt improvement in cardiac output. The lack of improvement suggests that preload reserve is exhausted and either inotropic and/or afterload-reducing therapies are indicated to improve stroke volume. Another cause of inadequate preload is a pericardial effusion and the development of cardiac tamponade, which is characterized by a collapse of the right atrium and cessation of right ventricular filling. The diagnosis begins with an index of suspicion when hypotension fails to respond to volume administration while right atrial pressure and heart rate are rising.

The development of excessive afterload that outpaces compensatory ventricular hypertrophy will cause cardiac output to fall despite what is intrinsically normal myocardium. This most commonly occurs in the setting of pulmonary hypertension, coarctation of the aorta, and malignant hypertension. Acute therapy involves optimizing ventricular filling, inotropic support, vasodilatory agents, and if applicable an intervention to relieve the obstructive lesion.

Low cardiac output following surgery may result from diastolic and/or systolic dysfunction. *Diastolic function* is the ability of the ventricle to receive blood under low pressure and is determined by the process of active relaxation and the passive elastic properties of the heart. Ventricular relaxation is an energy-dependent process involving the reuptake of calcium from the cytosol by the sarcoplasmic reticulum and the extrusion of calcium from the cell. Reduced calcium in the cytosol leads to the unbinding of calcium from the troponin subunit, conformational changes in troponin and tropomyosin, and ultimately the uncoupling of actin–myosin cross bridges. The passive elastic properties of the heart are influenced by the composition of the cardiac interstitium and the myocytes themselves. *Diastolic dysfunction* refers to an abnormality of diastolic distensibility, filling, or relaxation of the ventricle. Thus, the time course of ventricular filling is altered and the resulting pressure is elevated. In diastolic heart failure, an adequate stroke volume is not maintained and, in contrast to systolic failure, the ejection fraction is not depressed and the low-output state results from inadequate ventricular filling. The most common causes of diastolic dysfunction and failure are ischemic myocardium and preexisting conditions that lead to compensatory ventricular hypertrophy such as hypertension or an obstructive lesion.

Therapy for diastolic dysfunction involves volume administration, optimization of heart rate and rhythm (ensuring atrial ventricular synchrony and adequate time for ventricular filling), and minimizing intrathoracic pressure (see cardiopulmonary interaction). Inotropic and afterload-reducing agents are of little benefit, as systolic function is intact. Further, vasoactive agents that induce venodilation decrease ventricular filling pressures and thus reduce systemic and pulmonary venous pressures; however, because the ventricle resides on or near the linear portion of pressure stroke volume curve, a decrease in venous return may cause stroke volume to decrease as well.

Systolic function or contractility is the intrinsic ability of heart muscle to shorten and generate force independent of changes in loading conditions. With a decrease in contractile function, the rate of tension development, and the velocity and extent of fiber shortening decrease. In *systolic dysfunction*, however, the ejection fraction and stroke volume are reduced and the ventricular end-diastolic pressure and volume are elevated. In contrast to the left ventricle, the highly compliant, thin-walled right ventricle has much less contractile reserve. In fact, a significant portion of right ventricular developed pressure and volume outflow is produced by left ventricular contraction, a phenomenon known as systolic ventricular interdependence. With either ventricle, systolic dysfunction renders the ventricle less responsive to volume and more sensitive to increases in ventricular afterload.

Therapy for systolic dysfunction begins with optimizing ventricular loading conditions. Reducing ventricular preload and afterload decreases ventricular wall stress and myocardial oxygen demand while decreasing systemic and pulmonary venous pressures. Ventricular diastolic volume and pressure may be reduced by increasing venous capacitance with venodilators or decreasing intravascular volume with diuretics. As long as an adequate, albeit elevated, ventricular pressure is maintained, stroke volume and cardiac output are unaffected. Reducing afterload also enhances ventricular ejection and may be accomplished pharmacologically or mechanically, the latter resulting from the use of positive-pressure ventilation (see Chapter 70). The ideal inotropic agent increases stroke volume and cardiac output while having minimal effects on heart rate and myocardial oxygen demand.

Vasoactive Therapy

The rationale for selecting vasoactive agents to treat cardiovascular dysfunction is based on right and left ventricular diastolic and systolic function as well as the function of venous capacitance and pulmonary and systemic arterial resistance vessels. There are several vasoactive agents to choose from with varying pharmacokinetic and pharmacodynamic properties. Vasoactive agents that selectively induce venodilation decrease systemic venous return and therefore ventricular diastolic volume and pressure but have no effect on ventricular afterload. Thus, stroke volume and cardiac output do not increase (33). If, however, the ventricle is operating on the ascending portion of its pressure stroke volume curve, venodilation will cause stroke volume to decrease. Vasoactive agents that selectively dilate arterial resistance vessels enhance ventricular ejection; since venous capacitance is unaffected, ventricular diastolic volume and pressure remain largely unchanged (34,35). Inotropic agents increase cardiac output as a result of an increase in ejection fraction and stroke volume and to varying degrees as a result of an increase in heart rate. Ventricular filling pressures remain largely unchanged unless venous capacitance is increased. Myocardial oxygen consumption invariably increases as a result of an enhanced contractile

function and perhaps elevated heart rate. Finally, several vasoactive agents improve diastolic function by improving myocardial oxygen transport balance, and by their direct effects on the myocardium (36).

Catecholamines

The hemodynamic effects of catecholamines are dose-dependent, and are mediated by a variety of adrenergic receptors that use the cAMP-dependent signaling cascade. As intracellular cAMP increases, intracellular calcium metabolism and cellular function are altered. Activation of β-2 receptors leads to vascular smooth muscle relaxation and vasodilation, while activation of β-1 receptors leads to enhanced contractility and, to a lesser extent, increased heart rate. Activation of α-1 receptors leads to vascular smooth muscle contraction and vasoconstriction. β-adrenergic receptors experience agonist-mediated receptor desensitization in which an attenuated physiologic response to β agonists occurs with prolonged exposure to elevated levels of endogenous and exogenous catecholamines. Catecholamines are primarily metabolized by two enzyme systems: catechol O-methyltransferase and monoamine oxidase. All catecholamines have a very short half-life, allowing for easy titration with no need for a loading dose. All catecholamines increase myocardial oxygen demand as a result of their chronotropic and inotropic effects. The agents most commonly associated with induction of dysrhythmias are isoproterenol and epinephrine and, to a lesser extent, dopamine and dobutamine.

Dopamine

Dopamine is the immediate precursor of norepinephrine in the endogenous catecholamine biosynthesis pathway. Approximately half of the dopamine-induced response results from dopamine-induced release of norepinephrine from sympathetic nerve terminals. Dopamine directly stimulates α, β, and dopaminergic receptors. Moderate doses (5–10 mcg/kg/min) have chronotropic and inotropic effects. In adults with congestive heart failure, dopamine significantly increases cardiac output by increasing stroke volume and, to a lesser extent, heart rate. The left ventricular filling pressure either remains unchanged or increases due to vasoconstriction of venous capacitance vessels (37). Data in children are limited but demonstrate similar results (38). At high doses (>10 mcg/kg/min), α-adrenergic effects predominate and systemic vascular resistance begins to increase.

Dobutamine

Dobutamine is a synthetic catecholamine, which provides inotropic support. In adults with ventricular dysfunction, dobutamine significantly increases cardiac output by increasing stroke volume and, to a lesser extent, by increasing heart rate and reducing systemic vascular resistance. In contrast to dopamine, dobutamine consistently decreases ventricular filling pressures (37). Data in children are limited but demonstrate similar results (39).

Epinephrine

Epinephrine is an endogenous catecholamine formed from norepinephrine through N-methylation. It is largely produced by the adrenal medulla in response to stress. Epinephrine provides unparalleled inotropic support, and in low doses (<0.1 mcg/kg/min) decreases systemic and pulmonary vascular resistance and diastolic blood pressure through stimulation of β-2 receptors (40–42). At high doses, activation of α-1 receptors leads to vasoconstriction of venous capacitance and arterial resistance vessels.

Norepinephrine

Norepinephrine is the neurotransmitter of the sympathetic nervous system. It is released from terminal nerve endings and acts locally. Norepinephrine primarily causes vasoconstriction of venous capacitance and arterial resistance vessels by activating α-1 receptors, while providing minor inotropic support. The primary use of norepinephrine is to restore an adequate perfusion pressure in the setting of vasodilatory shock.

Milrinone

Milrinone does not act via adrenergic receptors, and is thus unaffected by adrenergic receptor desensitization, but rather through selective inhibition of phosphodiesterase III. This leads to a reduction of cAMP degradation, causing vasodilation of venous capacitance and pulmonary and systemic arterial resistance vessels while providing modest inotropic support. Studies in children have demonstrated a significant improvement in cardiac output as a result of its inotropic and afterload-reducing properties with little effect on heart rate (43). Because it increases venous capacitance, ventricular filling pressures are decreased (44).

The PRIMACORP study investigated the efficacy and safety of prophylactic milrinone after cardiac surgery in children (45). The multicentered, double-blinded, placebo-controlled study randomized 238 patients to either low- or high-dose milrinone or placebo. The prophylactic use of high-dose milrinone significantly reduced the risk of death or the development of a low–cardiac output syndrome relative to placebo with a relative risk reduction of 55% ($p = 0.023$) in the treated patients. The half-life of milrinone is age-dependent and ranges from <1 hour in children to >3 hours in infants. Milrinone is predominantly cleared via renal excretion; therefore, dosing may need to be adjusted in patients with renal insufficiency.

Nitroprusside

Nitroprusside spontaneously releases nitric oxide, which activates the soluble form of guanylate cyclase producing increased levels of cGMP. Nitroprusside causes dose-dependent dilation of systemic and pulmonary arterial resistance and venous capacitance vessels. In patients with congestive heart failure, nitroprusside increases stroke volume and cardiac output and reduces ventricular filling pressures (46). Nitroprusside decomposes nonenzymatically in the blood, releasing cyanide, which undergoes transsulfuration to form thiocyanate. Cyanide toxicity is a concern when using nitroprusside at high doses for long durations, especially in the presence of hepatic dysfunction, and should be anticipated and monitored. One advantage of nitroprusside is its short half-life of 2 minutes.

Nitroglycerin

Nitroglycerin undergoes biotransformation to yield nitric oxide. Nitroglycerin produces dose-dependent dilation of systemic and pulmonary arterial and venous capacitance vessels and is thus useful in the treatment of congestive heart failure. In low to modest doses (<3 mcg/kg/min), nitroglycerin mainly increases venous capacitance; thus, ventricular filling pressures are reduced without significant changes in stroke volume (47). In higher doses, nitroglycerin reduces systemic and pulmonary vascular resistance and stroke volume and cardiac output increase (48). Nitroglycerin has a short half-life of 2 minutes, allowing for easy titration. In contrast to nitroprusside, tolerance develops rapidly to nitroglycerin due to impaired biotransformation.

Vasopressin

Vasopressin is a hormone that is essential for osmotic and cardiovascular homeostasis (49). In addition to its antidiuretic effect, physiological levels of vasopressin are required for normal vascular tone. Vasopressin interacts with vasopressin-specific receptors with the primary action of stimulating smooth muscle cells to vasoconstrict. Based on these properties, vasopressin may have utility in cardiac arrest and vasodilatory shock. Large prospective randomized controlled trials have not demonstrated improved outcomes with the use of vasopressin in adults with vasodilatory shock (50,51). There has been one prospective randomized controlled trial of vasopressin in pediatric vasodilatory shock, which also failed to demonstrate benefit in those patients receiving vasopressin (52). There have been a few small, retrospective studies on the use of vasopressin following adult and pediatric cardiac surgery that have demonstrated improved fluid balance and reduced need for other vasoactive agents (53–56).

Neurological Issues

The great improvements in mortality following pediatric cardiac surgery in recent years, the concurrent shift toward more complex surgeries at younger ages, and the widespread use of extracorporeal life support (ECLS) technologies have led to an increasing awareness and recognition of neurological issues (57). There is a complex interrelationship between intrinsic patient factors, crucial events leading up to surgery, techniques applied in the operating room, and the postoperative management, all of which contribute to neurological outcomes.

Preoperative Factors

Patients with cardiac disease may have congenital brain abnormalities linked to genetic or syndromic diagnoses. In fetuses with left heart obstructive lesions or transposition physiology, cerebral development may be impaired as a consequence of diminished cerebral blood flow and oxygenation (58). Nearly 20% of full-term neonates with congenital heart disease display evidence of periventricular leukomalacia on preoperative brain magnetic resonance imaging (MRI) (59). Preoperative management strategies are important in determining neurologic outcomes. This is evidenced by the observation that delayed diagnosis of critical neonatal heart disease potentially contributes to cardiovascular collapse and end-organ dysfunction including stroke (60).

The type of congenital heart disease, which determines the choice of operative strategy, may itself be linked to neurodevelopmental outcomes. Operative management, which is a function of the complexity of the underlying defect, has various components, with more prolonged operations being linked to worse outcome. Both CPB and deep hypothermic circulatory arrest (DHCA) contribute to impairments in cerebral pressure autoregulation. CPB techniques applying a pH-stat versus alpha-stat approach and a higher versus lower hematocrit goal appear advantageous, based on various indicators of neurological well-being (61). A detailed study of CPB versus DHCA in patients with transposition of the great vessels initially suggested worse neurological outcomes in the DHCA group at early time points in childhood (62); however, these differences became less discernable as the study subjects grew older, with little evidence that shorter durations of DHCA make a difference (63). A randomized trial comparing low-flow regional cerebral perfusion and DHCA in neonates with hypoplastic left heart syndrome (HLHS) undergoing a stage 1 Norwood operation did not demonstrate differences in neurological outcome between treatment groups (64).

A series of recent studies have assessed cerebral oxygenation measured with near-infrared spectroscopy (NIRS) during and immediately following surgery. Correlations have been identified between lower NIRS values and postprocedural neurological events, including seizures and cerebral

MRI abnormalities (65). Abnormal electroencephalography background and less commonly seizures have been reported postoperatively, and while a high proportion of these resolve, those at the more severe end of the spectrum are linked to poorer developmental outcomes (66). More prolonged periods of DHCA have been linked to the evolution of seizures, and seizures to adverse scores on developmental tests (63).

Low cerebral and mixed venous oxygen saturations have been linked to greater rates of adverse events, such as cardiac arrest, in the intensive care unit (ICU). Cardiac arrest occurs in 1%–3.5% of admissions to the ICU and more frequently in complex patients and has a significant deleterious effect on developmental scores of children with heart disease, after accounting for other important patient-related factors such as prematurity and socioeconomic status (67). Centers have advocated the use of routine postoperative NIRS monitoring alongside treatment protocols aimed at averting or curtailing adverse trends and therefore ultimately improving neurological outcomes. Cardiac arrest and low–cardiac output states are scenarios that may necessitate initiation of ECLS. Approximately 50% of children who survive ECLS and undergo formal neurodevelopmental evaluation are found to have a range of disabilities (68).

Metabolic perturbations of hyperthermia and hyperglycemia may arise following CPB. Hyperthermia can exacerbate brain injury and therapeutic cooling has been shown to be beneficial in neonatal asphyxia (69). While there is no direct evidence that temperature control following cardiac surgery impacts developmental outcome, observational data support active treatment of hyperthermia. There are no data to support the hypothesis that treatment of hyperglycemia benefits neurological outcome, and conversely hypoglycemia (which may arise as a complication of insulin administration) is harmful to the developing brain.

All postoperative cardiac patients require analgesia. Patients who require mechanical ventilation receive sedative agents and the critically ill patient may require neuromuscular blockade. The disadvantages of opiates and sedatives include tolerance and dependence, respiratory depression, and potentially, prolonged mechanical ventilation. The disadvantages of muscle paralysis include impaired neurological assessment and residual weakness. Neuromuscular blockade should be suspended at regular intervals to assess the level and the ability of the patient to move or assessed with use of a twitch monitor. The length of ICU stay is a composite measure that reflects the overall complexity of a postoperative course, including all the issues discussed in this section. Not surprisingly those patients with longer ICU stays have worse developmental outcomes, and any measures that can be taken to minimize the length of stay may have a beneficial impact on neurodevelopmental outcomes (70).

Finally, there is a considerable amount of evidence based on studies in animals that sedatives and analgesics that act by altering synaptic transmission at γ-aminobutyrate type A (benzodiazepines, propofol, and chloral hydrate) and N-methyl-D-aspartate glutamate (ketamine) receptors interfere with normal brain development. Opioids while acting through different receptors have also been shown to have a detrimental effect on the developing brain and neurodevelopmental outcomes. The extent to which these findings can be extrapolated to the clinical setting remains to be determined (71).

Endocrine Disease

Transient postoperative hyperglycemia is an adaptive neuroendocrine response to stress and is very common in critically ill children with cardiac disease. It results from accelerated glucose production, which may be exacerbated by glucocorticoids given during CPB and the development of acute relative resistance to insulin. While the natural physiologic response to stress is a programmed adaptive process, it has been observed that prolonged stress-induced hyperglycemia is linked to various adverse outcomes, including hepatic and renal dysfunction, infection, prolonged ICU stay, and death (72). These data are observational and cannot be used to infer a causal link between hyperglycemia and adverse outcomes.

Conventionally, only children with sustained and more severe hyperglycemia (above 180–270 mg/dL) are managed with insulin therapy following cardiac surgery, unless the child is diabetic. The majority of nondiabetic children do not require insulin, since following cardiac surgery the observed hyperglycemia rapidly resolves. Current evidence does not support the use of insulin therapy to achieve *"tight glycemic control"* (glucose levels of less than 120–140 mg/dL) following pediatric cardiac surgery. A randomized trial of critically ill children, the majority of whom were recovering from cardiac surgery, found that those assigned to receive tight glycemic control had reduced markers of inflammation and ICU length of stay, but 25% of patients experienced severe hypoglycemia (73). A study from the same research group indicated that tight glycemic control led to lower levels of cardiac troponin and reduced inotrope doses after neonatal cardiac surgery (74). A recent randomized trial of 980 children recovering from cardiac surgery found no benefit of tight glycemic control (75).

Adrenal insufficiency leads to hypotension that is resistant to fluid resuscitation and inotropic therapy. A subset of pediatric cardiac surgery patients is affected by transient adrenal insufficiency, manifested by failure to generate an increase in serum cortisol in response to administration of exogenous adrenocorticotrophic hormone (ACTH) or a high ACTH to cortisol ratio (76). Demonstrable improvement with hydrocortisone supplementation has been reported following neonatal cardiac surgery, which has been attributed to the treatment of adrenal insufficiency (76). A prospective evaluation of adrenal function in critically ill pediatric patients found the prevalence of relative adrenal insufficiency to be 19% (77). Occurrence of relative adrenal insufficiency does not appear related to complexity of surgery as manifested by duration of CPB. The supposition is that the etiology of adrenal insufficiency in the PICU is multifactorial as a proportion of children have normal baseline cortisol levels but are nonetheless unable to mount an increment in cortisol in response to ACTH. It is speculated that some patients may have end-organ resistance to cortisol, and the dose of steroid required for an optimal response is unclear. The time course of recovery from adrenal insufficiency is variable and therefore the optimal duration of steroid therapy may be difficult to judge.

The *sick euthyroid syndrome* occurs to a variable degree in all children following pediatric cardiac surgery, regardless of procedure complexity. Transient reductions occur in thyroid-stimulating hormone, total triiodothyronine (T3), free thyroxine (T4), and reverse triiodothyronine (rT3), with an elevation in T3 uptake. These changes in thyroid axis arise in parallel with, but following, surgical intervention, and the degree to which the hormone levels fall mirrors postprocedural clinical indicators such as inotrope scores and organ dysfunction, indicating that they result from, and do not cause, increasing severity of illness. Levels of rT3 return toward normal before T3 levels, which remain low beyond the critical postoperative period, representing an adaptive response to surgical intervention. In light of these observed changes, and mindful that following adult cardiac surgery supplementation with T3 has been noted to improve cardiac contractility, several small studies have evaluated T3 supplementation in infants following cardiac surgery. In summary, the studies are inconclusive and the routine use of T3 supplementation cannot be recommended (78–81).

Gastrointestinal Issues

Poor nutritional states and failure to thrive are common in children with heart disease. Several factors are contributory, including suck–swallow incoordination or gastroesophageal reflux disease leading to poor caloric intake, high energy expenditure, impaired intestinal absorption, and reduced splanchnic blood flow. These factors render patients susceptible to postoperative complications such as infection, necrotizing enterocolitis (NEC), and prolonged recovery from surgery. Fluid restriction for cardiac or renal failure and impediments to enteral feeding such as NEC or severe chylothorax may further compound this cycle. Patients with lower weight for age Z scores are prone to longer ICU stays and have conversely higher-than-normal energy expenditure in the postoperative period (82). Careful attention to a child's nutritional status and gastrointestinal issues is recommended.

The hypermetabolic state generated by CPB is associated with high resting energy expenditure (83). The common use of fluid restriction immediately following surgery contributes to caloric deficit. Complex neonatal patients and those in low–cardiac output states should have parenteral nutrition initiated as soon as possible until the hemodynamic status improves and enteral nutrition is commenced. Feeding algorithms are beneficial in achieving shorter times to achieve full enteral nutrition and reach a better caloric balance during recovery (84).

NEC is an inflammatory bowel condition associated with the use of prostaglandin, low–cardiac output syndrome, and prematurity. NEC is more prevalent in patients with the HLHS and truncus arteriosus although it has been reported in most forms of neonatal heart disease (85). The diagnosis of NEC relies on a combination of clinical, laboratory, and radiological findings of pneumatosis intestinalis with or without additional surgical bowel disease (peritonitis). The treatment consists of intravenous broad-spectrum antibiotics and bowel rest with parenteral nutrition, and surgical intervention if required for bowel necrosis or perforation. *Chylothorax* arises in 1%–5% of children after cardiac surgery. Secondary immune deficiency may develop due to lymphocyte and plasma protein loss in the pleural drainage, and ICU length of stay may be prolonged. The first line of therapy involves feeding with medium-chain triglycerides (which without caloric supplements will lead to a reduction in caloric intake). Refractory cases warrant cessation of enteral feeding and institution of parenteral nutrition.

Congenital gastrointestinal defects may occur in association with conditions linked to congenital heart disease. Examples include malrotation in heterotaxy syndrome, hind gut atresia in VACTER(L) syndrome, esophageal atresia in VACTER(L) or CHARGE syndromes, and a range of malformations in children with chromosomal syndromes (trisomy 21, 8, 5). GERD is commonly associated with infant heart disease and arises even more frequently in syndromic babies. The main stay of treatment is inhibition of acid production from the gastric mucosa and promotion of gastric motility by pharmacologic agents. Patients with symptoms at the severe end of the spectrum may need surgical intervention with placement of a gastric tube and fundoplication in order to achieve adequate weight gain.

Hematological Issues

Immediately following CPB, hypofibrinogenemia, thrombocytopenia, the potential for residual heparinization, and poor clot formation, all exist, which predispose to mediastinal bleeding. The smallest neonates and infants are the most vulnerable, requiring sufficient replacement of the depleted factors such as fibrinogen and platelets, in order to reduce the risk. The use of whole blood is more effective at minimizing bleeding when compared to replacement with separate blood product components (86).

Blood transfusion is frequent following cardiac surgery. A multivariable model to explore the link between red cell transfusion and outcome found that biventricular patients with higher transfusion levels had a greater length of stay, leading the authors to speculate that a modestly restrictive red cell transfusion approach for biventricular patients is reasonable (87). Red cell transfusions may increase oxygen-carrying capacity and thus oxygen delivery; however, the potential adverse effects of transfusion include lung injury, immune modulation, and potential transmission of infection. A recent study of pediatric cardiac surgery patients noted that a restrictive transfusion strategy was safe when compared to a liberal transfusion strategy, supporting this approach in biventricular patients (88). It is hypothesized that single-ventricle patients require a higher hemoglobin level in order to achieve optimal oxygen delivery and this may mitigate some of the potentially harmful effects of transfusion.

In addition to judicious use of blood products, antifibrinolytic agents are beneficial in reducing bleeding in higher-risk patients such as those undergoing reoperations (89). Aminocaproic acid (Amicar) and tranexamic acid are both derivatives of the amino acid lysine, and as enzyme inhibitors they are active against proteins such as plasmin. Aprotinin is a serine protease inhibitor that was linked to postoperative renal failure in adults following cardiac surgery; however, this has not been born out in pediatric studies (90). Activated protein C, which is a component of the clotting cascade, has been used to counter severe bleeding in the cardiac ICU. Activated protein C has been found effective in combating life-threatening hemorrhage in nonrandomized studies; however, the main side effect is the potential for thrombus formation (91).

Lower-flow venous pathways (Fontan) and the use of synthetic material in the circulation (prosthetic heart valves, Gore-Tex shunts) necessitate the use of anticoagulation to prevent thrombosis. Extracorporeal support devices (ventricular assist device and *extracorporeal membrane oxygenation* [ECMO]) require anticoagulation in order to maintain device and cannula patency and integrity, as do intravenous catheters in certain higher-risk patients (for example, where the central veins have been injured by multiple previous interventions). Intravenous unfractionated heparin, an anti-thrombin III inhibitor, is the first-line anticoagulant in the ICU, since it may be titrated to achieve prolonged clotting times in a designated range reflected by the partial thromboplastin time, and can be readily reversed as required, for example, prior to a procedure. A rare complication of heparin is heparin-induced thrombocytopenia. The options for longer-term anticoagulation include (a) Coumadin, which inhibits the synthesis of vitamin K–dependent clotting factors. Coumadin is administered orally once feeds are tolerated and dosing is titrated via the international normalizing ratio. Coumadin has a gradual onset of effect; therefore, an overlap with heparin therapy is required, and is subject to drug interactions when administered in conjunction with hepatic enzyme inhibitors or enhancers. (b) Low-molecular-weight heparin targets anti-factor Xa activity, is administered via subcutaneous injection, and may be titrated to effect against the blood anti-Xa level for use as a long-term anticoagulant in children with a history or predisposition for thrombosis. (c) Antiplatelet agents including aspirin and clopidogrel are orally administered and provide long-term inhibition of platelet aggregation in children at risk of thrombosis in synthetic intravascular material, such as Gore-Tex shunt tubes and the cannulae of ventricular assist devices.

Tissue plasminogen activator (TPA) is a serine protease, which catalyzes the conversion of plasmin to plasminogen, hence lysing blood clots. TPA infusion is a potent means to remove thrombus rather than a measure to prevent its formation (as is the predominant mechanism for the other agents discussed); hence, its major side effect is bleeding.

Infectious Issues

Health-care–associated infections (HAIs) following pediatric cardiac surgery are linked to comorbid medical conditions such as 22q11 deletion that may impair the immune system, preoperative ventilation, greater operative complexity, younger age, blood product exposure, and reoperations (92). Similar patient-related factors are prevalent in cases with prolonged ICU stay, and it is recognized that HAI is inextricably connected to long ICU stays, since patients with greater severity of illness over time have extended dependence on devices, which themselves predispose to HAI (92). Standardized surveillance definitions of specific HAI are issued by the Center for Disease Control and Prevention and are based on a combination of clinical characteristics and laboratory values. Categories include blood stream infections related to central venous lines (CVLs) or vascular access devices (also including arterial lines and ECLS circuits), ventilator-associated pneumonia (VAP), and surgical-site infections (SSI) such as mediastinitis and superficial wound infections. The rate of HAI is reported in terms of the number per 1000 ICU days rather than as a percentage of patients for the purposes of audit and benchmarking. HAI is a measure of ICU morbidity that has rightly been the subject of quality improvement initiatives, given that there is a wealth of evidence that HAI carries an attributed increased risk of mortality, prolongation of ICU stay, and inflation in health-care costs (93). Modifiable risk factors for HAI may be addressed from a range of angles by applying a "bundle approach," whereby all aspects of device insertion, ongoing device handling, and other patient-care issues are actively managed with a focus on each individual issue linked to the risk of infection (94). Examples of components of a bundle approach include removal of a CVL as soon as it is no longer needed, maintenance of patients in a head-up position to reduce the risk of VAP, and optimal timing of pre-procedure antibiotics such that drug levels are optimal at the time of skin incision for the prevention of SSI.

Exposure to broad-spectrum antibiotics, particularly in the presence of intravascular catheters or immune suppression, which may be primary or secondary, predisposes patients to fungal infections. Primary immune deficiency may arise in the context of genetic syndromes such as trisomy 21 and 22q11 deletion, and secondary immune deficiency is induced after transplantation and arises as a result of immunoglobulin leak in chylothorax. Prophylactic antifungal agents are recommended in patients on prolonged broad-spectrum antibiotics and immediately following heart transplantation.

Renal Issues

Renal injury and impairment of kidney function are common problems following cardiac surgery. The pediatric modification of the Risk, Injury, Failure, Loss, and End-Stage Kidney Disease (RIFLE) 2007 (95), or the Acute Kidney Injury Network (AKIN) 2009 (96) graded classifications may be used to describe the level of renal impairment for an individual patient. These validated schemes take into account biochemical parameters such as changes in serum creatinine and duration or severity of oligo-/anuria to objectively categorize renal dysfunction. Prior to such classification schemes being available, renal impairment in postoperative cardiac patients tended to be synonymous with renal support. However, this represents the more severe cases only, and furthermore may incorporate patients with catheters placed to manage fluid accumulation in the peritoneal cavity as a result of high venous pressures (for example, the failing Fontan). Kidney injury affects 40%–50% of cardiac patients following surgery, being more prevalent in younger children, single-ventricle physiology, those with pre-existing renal disease, and following long bypass times (97). Severe forms of renal failure, (AKIN) grade 3, affect 10%–15% of patients, and this group frequently requires renal supportive therapy in the form of peritoneal dialysis, hemodialysis, or hemofiltration.

The etiology of postoperative renal failure is linked to low–cardiac output syndrome and affected patients tend to require higher doses of inotropes and in some cases even mechanical circulatory support. The *"cardiorenal syndrome"* describes the complex interaction of the cardiovascular and renal systems, whereby injury and deterioration in one organ system contribute to dysfunction of the other and vice versa (98). Postoperative renal impairment arises early after surgery and is reversible in the majority of cases (corresponding to type 1 cardiorenal syndrome). The interaction between low cardiac output, poor renal perfusion pressure (high venous pressure with low systemic blood pressure), postbypass inflammation, and nephrotoxic pharmacologic agents contributes to oliguria and increasing fluid overload. It is important to address each component of the cycle in order to support the patient effectively through a crucial postoperative interval, amend all reversible elements of the process, and facilitate recovery.

Renal failure following pediatric cardiac surgery contributes to prolonged mechanical ventilation and extended stays in hospital (99). Reduced clearance of medications such as sedatives and muscle relaxants, and oliguria contribute to pulmonary edema and pleural effusions, which may hinder weaning from mechanical ventilation, predisposing patients to hospital-acquired infections. Mortality rates are higher in patients with postprocedural renal impairment, reflecting their increased complexity and morbidity. The first line of therapy for milder forms of renal impairment (AKIN grade 1) includes fluid restriction, judicious administration of diuretics, optimization of preload and cardiac function, and avoidance of nephrotoxic agents. In a high proportion of patients, the natural time course of low–cardiac output syndrome and the postbypass inflammatory response mean that a diuresis evolves after 24–48 hours, with corresponding recovery of the renal injury. Severe forms of renal impairment (AKIN grades 2 and 3) may lead to fluid overload, acidosis, uremia, or hyperkalemia, and may require renal support.

Peritoneal dialysis is the most common mode of acute renal replacement therapy used in infants. Continuous veno-venous hemofiltration (CVVH) is the recommended approach when peritoneal dialysis fails or is contraindicated because of intra-abdominal pathology. Older children with the acute consequences of renal failure and patients on ECMO may be more effectively supported with CVVH, which is very effective at dialysis and fluid removal. CVVH works by a process of convective ultrafiltration, in which blood is pumped continuously through an extracorporeal hemofilter consisting of a large number of parallel hollow fibers. Plasma fluid containing solutes is removed from the blood by this process and a physiologically balanced solution is infused to the patient in order to maintain fluid and electrolyte balance. CVVH requires the presence of an appropriately sized double-lumen CVL, and anticoagulation with heparin to maintain the integrity of the CVVH circuit. The balancing solution, pump speed, filter size, and anticoagulation management are selected based on local protocols. Once on CVVH, the patient's fluid and caloric intake may be increased liberally, since fluid balance can be titrated easily and effectively via alterations to the rate of the replacement solution.

CARDIOPULMONARY BYPASS

Basic components of a CPB circuit include two venous cannulae that drain systemic venous blood from the superior and inferior vena cava (or one venous cannula from the right atrium), a cardiotomy reservoir, a heat exchanger, a membrane oxygenator, a roller pump, and an arterial filter (**Fig. 79.1**). An arterial cannula returns oxygenated blood to the aorta, although occasionally the innominate, axillary, or femoral artery is used. Occasionally a second arterial cannula is used, such as during repair of an interrupted aortic arch, when one arterial cannula is placed in the ascending aorta and a second in the ductus arteriosus to perfuse the lower body. Tubing connecting these components is minimized in length and diameter in order to decrease priming volumes and exposure of blood to foreign surfaces. Before initiation of CPB, the circuit is "primed" with standardized quantities of crystalloid solution, glucose, buffer (sodium bicarbonate or THAM), heparin, calcium, and either whole blood or packed red blood cells and albumin. As the priming volume of the circuit may exceed the blood volume of a neonate by up to 300%, hemodilution occurs, which not only lowers the hematocrit, but also plasma proteins and clotting factors, leading to decreased oncotic pressure and interstitial edema as well as to a propensity for bleeding. Heparin is administered for the duration of CPB to prevent thrombosis, consumption of clotting factors, and oxygenator dysfunction.

Prior to the onset of CPB, extensive mediastinal dissection is performed and the thymus is subtotally resected for exposure. If present, the ductus arteriosus or any previously placed systemic-to-pulmonary shunts is isolated. Once on full CPB, mechanical ventilation may cease, allowing the lung to collapse. Because infants have a greater rate of oxygen consumption, initial flow rates for infants are higher than adults. By adjusting the heat exchanger, most infants and children are cooled to a variable extent to minimize metabolic needs and oxygen consumption. Hypothermia facilitates surgical exposure by allowing the flow rate to be decreased, which will lessen the amount of blood returning to the heart through aortopulmonary collateral vessels. Hypothermia also allows for greater intervals between cardioplegia applications, and provides protection to the brain and other organs, especially during low-flow states and periods of DHCA. Adverse effects of hypothermia include inflammation and changes in capillary permeability leading to interstitial edema. The degree of hypothermia varies depending on the age of the patient and complexity of the case. For example, mild hypothermia (30°C–34°C) is used for straightforward cases in older children, whereas deep hypothermia (15°C–22°C) is usually reserved for complex repairs, including neonates undergoing aortic arch reconstruction. Because hypothermia causes increased viscosity and red cell rigidity, hemodilution is desirable during moderate to deep hypothermic CPB. The optimal nadir hematocrit to target during CPB is debatable and depends on the degree of hypothermia, pH strategy, and flow rate. In infants, recent clinical trials suggest

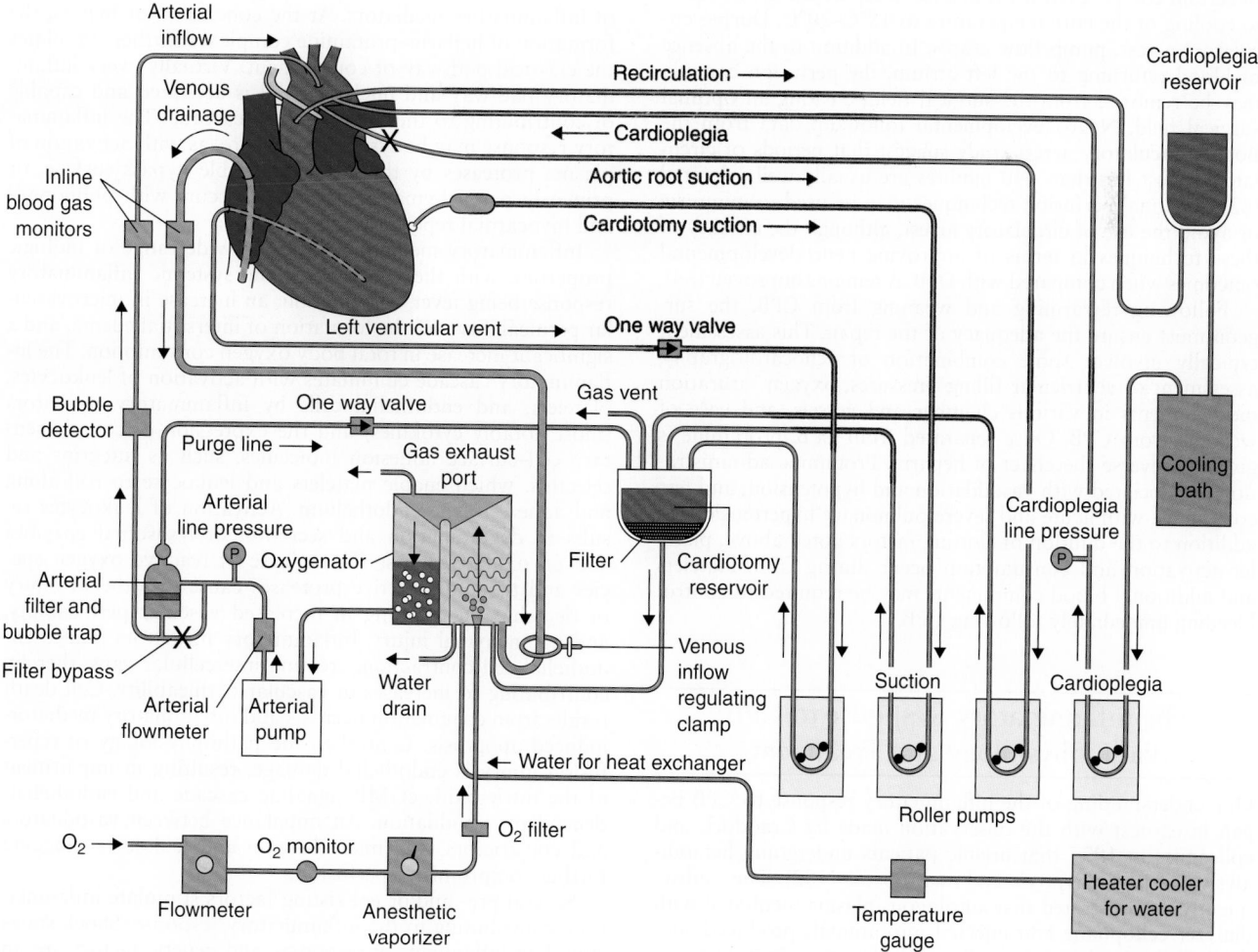

FIGURE 79.1. Extracorporeal cardiopulmonary bypass circuit.

that a nadir hematocrit of 25% is associated with favorable acute and neurodevelopmental outcomes (100).

Temperature has an impact on blood pH. With increasing hypothermia, blood pH becomes progressively alkalotic. Using an alpha-stat strategy, pH is maintained at 7.40 without regard to temperature. With the pH-stat strategy, CO_2 is added to the circuit to maintain a temperature-corrected pH of 7.40. pH management during CPB remains controversial. One clinical trial in infants found that pH stat strategy had modest favorable effects on early outcomes but was not associated with important differences in neurodevelopmental outcomes (61,101).

Selected right heart repairs, such as a pulmonary valve replacement or tricuspid valve surgery, may be performed on CPB with a beating heart provided that no intracardiac communication exists that would allow passage of an air embolus to the systemic circulation. Fibrillatory arrest is another technique that may be used for right heart procedures in the event that an atrial communication exists. To obtain a motionless heart for most other types of intracardiac repairs, the aorta is cross-clamped proximal to the aortic cannula and a cold, potassium-rich cardioplegia solution is delivered via a smaller cannula into the aortic root. Alternatively, cardioplegia may be delivered retrograde through the coronary sinus. Asystole develops once the cardioplegia perfuses the coronary circulation. The combination of cardioplegia and hypothermia provides myocardial protection for several hours. Following placement of the aortic cross clamp, blood from aortopulmonary collaterals will continue to return to the left atrium. DHCA may be used to eliminate left atrial blood return and to facilitate repair of certain complex left heart disease. Deep hypothermia refers to cooling of the core temperature to 18°C–20°C. During circulatory arrest, pump flow ceases. In addition to the absence of blood returning to the left atrium, the perfusion cannula may be removed from the surgical field, creating an optimal surgical field. Neurodevelopmental follow-up data from the Boston circulatory arrest study suggest that periods of circulatory arrest less than ~40 minutes are usually well tolerated (63). Regional perfusion techniques may be used to minimize or avoid the use of circulatory arrest, although the efficacy of these techniques in terms of improving neurodevelopmental outcomes when compared with DHCA remains unproven (64).

Following rewarming and weaning from CPB, the surgeon must ensure the adequacy of the repair. This assessment typically involves some combination of echocardiography, assessment of ventricular filling pressures, oxygen saturation measurements in various chamber and vessels, and ease of weaning from CPB. Once separated from CPB, protamine is given to reverse the effect of heparin. Protamine administration is associated with vasodilation and hypotension, and less commonly, with acute and severe pulmonary hypertension. In addition to the dilution of clotting factors noted above, platelet activation and consumption occur during CPB. Platelets and additional blood components may be required to control bleeding immediately following CPB.

The Inflammatory Response to CPB: Pathophysiology and Treatment

Our understanding of the inflammatory response to CPB began in earnest with the observation made by Craddock and colleagues in 1977 that uremic patients undergoing hemodialysis developed hypoxia and neutropenia (102). They subsequently demonstrated that autologous plasma incubated with dialyzer cellophane and injected into animals produced sudden leukopenia, hypoxia, and a marked increase in pulmonary lymph effluent. Histologic examination demonstrated pulmonary leukosequestration and edema, and the syndrome could

be prevented by inactivation of complement. Subsequently, Kirklin and colleagues demonstrated significant complement activation in adults with the onset of CPB (103). Two years later, Kirklin and colleagues found a positive relationship between complement activation and postoperative morbidity in adults and children undergoing cardiac surgery (104). During the 1980s, additional proinflammatory mediators were discovered and inflammatory mediator assays became readily available. These advances led to a greater understanding of the immunologic response to CPB, as well as other diseases, such as septic shock, trauma, and heart failure.

With exposure of plasma proteases to the non-endothelial lining of the CPB circuit, the contact system and the alternate pathway of complement are activated. The intrinsic and extrinsic coagulation pathways are activated, and ultimately thrombin and plasmin activate the classical pathway of complement. Byproducts of the plasma proteases activate endothelial cells, platelets, leukocytes, macrophages, and parenchymal cells, leading to the production of cellular-derived inflammatory mediators, such as arachidonic acid metabolites, lysosomal enzymes, reactive oxygen species, and cytokines, including interleukins and tumor necrosis factor-α.

Another factor in the pathophysiology of the inflammatory response to bypass is ischemia–reperfusion injury. Myocardial and pulmonary ischemia–reperfusion injury is in large part an inflammatory phenomena (105–107). Following a period of ischemia, reperfusion stimulates the release of additional proinflammatory mediators, particularly reactive oxygen species and cytokines, by parenchymal, endothelial, platelet, and inflammatory cells, contributing to elevated serum levels of inflammatory mediators. At the conclusion of bypass, the formation of heparin–protamine complexes further stimulates the classical pathway of complement. Virtually every inflammatory pathway and nucleated cell is activated and capable of contributing to the inflammatory cascade. The inflammatory response may be systemic in nature, as with activation of plasma proteases by the bioincompatible bypass surface, or primarily parenchymal in nature, as occurs with pulmonary and myocardial reperfusion injury.

Inflammatory mediators possess a wide range of biologic properties, with the hallmark of the systemic inflammatory response being fever, vasodilation, an increase in microvascular permeability and the formation of interstitial edema, and a significant increase in total body oxygen consumption. The inflammatory cascade culminates with activation of leukocytes, platelets, and endothelial cells by inflammatory mediators (most notably cytokines) and the expression of complementary cell–surface adhesion molecules, such as integrins and selectins, which enable platelets and leukocyte to roll along and adhere to the endothelium. Activation of leukocytes results in degranulation and secretion of lysosomal enzymes and an oxidative burst. The release of reactive oxygen species and tissue-destructive proteases cause endothelial injury or detachment, resulting in increased vascular permeability, and parenchymal injury. Inflammatory mediators induce endothelial cell contraction, creating intercellular gaps, thereby contributing to increases in vascular permeability. Cell death results from coagulation necrosis and inflammatory mediator-induced apoptosis. Central to the pathophysiology of reperfusion injury is endothelial damage, resulting in impairment of the nitric-oxide-cGMP signaling cascade and endothelial-dependent vasodilation. An imbalance between vasodilators and constrictors, and microthrombi and leukocyte plugging further compromise reperfusion.

Several pre- and/or coexisting factors stimulate inflammation, contributing to the inflammatory response. Shock states stimulate inflammatory responses and genetic factors are an important determinant of the inflammatory response to a variety of stimuli (108). In hypoxic conditions, hypoxia-inducible factor translocates to the nucleus, where it induces transcription of numerous inflammatory genes (109). Heart failure is characterized by sustained immune activation, reflected in increased circulating levels of inflammatory cytokines and enhanced expression of various inflammatory mediators within the failing myocardium (110). Mechanical cell stress as with a pressure or volume load resulting from structural heart disease stimulates an inflammatory response (111). Inflammatory mediators are not only markers of immune activation but contribute to the pathophysiological process of heart failure by stimulating myocyte apoptosis, myocyte hypertrophy, extracellular matrix alterations, and contractile dysfunction.

With initiation of the proinflammatory cascade, a compensatory anti-inflammatory response ensues, which serves to limit the inflammatory response and extent of tissue injury (112). The discovery of anti-inflammatory mediators followed on the heels of an increasing appreciation of the proinflammatory response and culminated with the coining of the term "Compensatory Anti-inflammatory Response Syndrome" in 1996.

End-Organ Injury and the Inflammatory Response to Cardiopulmonary Bypass

Circulating inflammatory mediators bind to receptors on cerebral vascular and vascular-associated cells, producing an increase in the permeability of the blood–brain barrier and cerebral edema while inducing the central synthesis of intermediate molecules such as prostaglandins and cytokines, which serve as ligands for specific receptors within parenchymal elements of the brain (113). The binding of these intermediate ligands to nuclei within the brain modulates several central functions, such as thermoregulation, behavior (e.g., anorexia, cachexia, and lethargy), the autonomic nervous system, and the hypothalamic–pituitary–adrenal (HPA) axis. Based on animal and clinical studies it does not appear that the bypass-induced systemic inflammatory response causes long-term neurocognitive dysfunction (114,115). The primary mechanism of immune-mediated cerebral injury results from ischemia–reperfusion injury, which may also lead to impaired endothelial-dependent vasodilation and disturbed cerebral pressure autoregulation.

The systemic inflammatory response and pulmonary reperfusion injury impair respiratory function. The importance of reperfusion injury has been demonstrated in several animal and clinical studies (7,105,116,117). Damage to the pulmonary endothelium and alveolar epithelium leads to interstitial and alveolar edema and a decrease in lung compliance. Impaired surfactant production resulting from injury to type II alveolar pneumocytes and the inactivation of surfactant by extravasated plasma proteins further decrease lung compliance. Preexisting lung disease, prolonged duration of CPB and ischemia, and pulmonary venous hypertension contribute to lung injury.

The systemic inflammatory response and pulmonary reperfusion injury also cause pulmonary endothelial dysfunction and increases in pulmonary vascular resistance. As with alveolar injury, animal studies have demonstrated that reperfusion injury plays a major role in the development of pulmonary vascular dysfunction (117,118). Shafique et al. (118) demonstrated that sheep undergoing CPB with pulmonary arterial perfusion maintained vascular function, whereas those animals undergoing total CPB experienced significant alterations in endothelial-dependent vascular responses.

The inflammatory response to bypass and the reperfusion injury that follows cardioplegic arrest lead to myocardial injury and impaired function. Inflammatory mediators, primarily cytokines produced by cardiomyocytes and interstitial cardiac leukocytes, exert a direct effect on the cardiomyocyte,

impairing systolic and diastolic function (12–14). Vaso- and cytogenic edema decrease ventricular compliance, contributing to impaired diastolic function (15). The major insult to the myocardium occurs with reperfusion following cardioplegic arrest (16–18). While calcium overload and myocyte hypercontracture contribute to reperfusion injury, the primary mechanism responsible for myocardial injury is reperfusion-induced inflammation. Cell death results from tissue necrosis and cytokine-mediated apoptosis (18). Because myocardial apoptosis is a part of normal fetal and postnatal maturation, the neonatal myocardium may have an increased vulnerability or susceptibility to apoptosis-related processes following surgery, contributing to postoperative ventricular dysfunction (119). Endothelial dysfunction contributes to the pathophysiological process (120). Decreases in nitric oxide production lead to impaired coronary vasodilatory reserve and because nitric oxide modulates leukocyte–endothelial cell and platelet–endothelial cell interaction, a decrease in nitric oxide bioavailability contributes to the procoagulant and proinflammatory state and microvascular obstruction as a result of thrombosis and leukocyte accumulation (121,122).

The inflammatory response to CPB also affects systemic vascular function. Inflammatory mediators such as histamine, bradykinin, and nitric oxide decrease systemic vasomotor tone. The systemic inflammatory response may also affect vascular function by interfering with the HPA axis, resulting in decreased cortisol production, a relative adrenal insufficiency, and, because cortisol is required for vascular tone, impaired vascular function (123). Some patients may develop vasodilatory shock, a state characterized by systemic hypotension, elevated cardiac output, and decreased arteriolar reactivity that is unresponsive to volume and vasopressors. While a systemic inflammatory response invariably occurs to CPB, why a minority of patients develop vasodilatory shock remains unclear (124,125). Vasoplegia primarily occurs in adults with a reported incidence as high as 20%. Factors identified in adults to be associated with the development of postoperative vasoplegia include a history of long-standing heart failure and the use of certain medications, primarily angiotensin-converting enzyme inhibitors (125). The incidence in children has been demonstrated to be 3% and is much more likely to occur in those children undergoing CPB for heart transplantation or placement of a ventricular assist device (126).

The role of immune-mediated renal injury following bypass has not been extensively studied. Animal models have demonstrated that bypass-induced inflammation results in glomerular and renal tubular damage that is associated with endothelial cell injury and activation and leukocyte sequestration, as well as reduced glomerular filtration rates and creatinine clearance (127,128). Animal models of renal ischemia–reperfusion injury have clearly demonstrated the role of inflammation in producing tubular injury and dysfunction, findings much more dramatic than those reported for CPB-induced inflammation alone (129).

Studies in adults and children have demonstrated that the bypass-induced inflammatory response increases intestinal permeability (130,131). Studies have also demonstrated an inverse relationship between indices of mesenteric perfusion and increases in intestinal permeability during CPB indicating that despite adequate pump flow mesenteric ischemia contributes to intestinal injury (132,133). This may be due in part to nonpulsatile flow stimulating the renin–angiotensin system, leading to increases in mesenteric vascular resistance and contributing to mesenteric ischemia. (134–136). The systemic inflammatory response and reperfusion injury also cause mesenteric endothelial dysfunction and impaired endothelial-dependent vasoreactivity (133). Inflammation and ischemia-related injury compromise the integrity of the mucosa, resulting in bacterial translocation and further stimulation of the inflammatory cascade (137,138). Studies in infants, children, and adults have demonstrated that bacterial translocation during cardiac surgery is common, regardless of whether circulatory arrest is used (138).

Numerous immunomodulatory strategies have been evaluated in animals and clinical trials. The vast majority of pediatric centers in North America and the United Kingdom have incorporated the use of glucocorticoids, modified ultrafiltration (MUF), and heparin-coated circuits into practice (139,140). There have been several relatively small prospective randomized studies in children that have evaluated the role of glucocorticoids in suppressing the inflammatory response to CPB. Initial studies demonstrated an improved postoperative course and evidence of reduced myocardial injury in those patients randomized to glucocorticoids prior to CPB (141–143). Two recently published prospective randomized dose–response studies evaluated whether an additional dose of glucocorticoids was of any benefit (144,145). Patients were randomized to receive a dose of glucocorticoid or placebo 8 hours prior to the intraoperative dose. While each study demonstrated a significant reduction in serum inflammatory mediators in those receiving two doses, neither study demonstrated an improved postoperative course.

MUF is used in the vast majority of pediatric cardiac centers. Ultrafiltration removes water, reverses hemodilution, and eliminates low-molecular-weight substances, including inflammatory mediators. Some studies have shown a significant beneficial effect of MUF on the postoperative course while others have not (146). Heparinization of the contact surface of the circuit was initially done to minimize thrombus formation; subsequently, heparin-bonded circuits have been shown to modify the inflammatory response to bypass, decreasing cytokine release as well as inhibiting the contact system and complement activation (147). Two small prospective randomized studies in children demonstrated significant reductions in serum inflammatory mediator levels and modest improvements in respiratory function and coagulation (148,149).

LESION-SPECIFIC MANAGEMENT

3 A thorough understanding of preoperative anatomy, physiology, diagnostic evaluation, and any prior interventions is essential to provide optimal care in children recovering from cardiac surgery. More detailed information of cardiac embryology, anatomical variants and their physiological correlates, clinical manifestations, and preoperative evaluation is beyond the scope of this textbook, and may be found in a number of excellent pediatric cardiology textbooks. Expected surgical mortality rates for each of the lesions discussed below have been recently published (150).

Patent Ductus Arteriosus

Following ligation of a patent ductus arteriosus (PDA), complications such as a chylothorax (related to thoracic duct injury) and injury of the recurrent laryngeal or phrenic nerves may occur. A subset of premature neonates develops a low–cardiac output state following PDA ligation, likely related to acute alterations in myocardial loading conditions (151). For older infants and children, percutaneous closure of PDAs with coils and other occluding devices may be performed in the cardiac catheterization laboratory. Device embolization, residual shunts, hemolysis, and device-related obstruction of the aorta or the proximal left pulmonary artery are associated complications.

Atrial and Ventricular Septal Defects

Most isolated secundum, primum, or sinus venosus atrial septal defects (ASDs) are electively repaired between 1 and 3 years of age, although some symptomatic patients with prematurity, underlying lung disease, or other comorbidities may benefit from repair in early infancy (152). Patients with large VSDs typically have congestive heart failure and warrant referral for surgical repair in early infancy. Selected infants with large VSDs who are not thought to be candidates for primary repair because of the presence of multiple VSDs with anticipated difficult surgical exposure or noncardiac comorbidities may be palliated with a pulmonary artery band.

Residual defects following isolated ASD repair are uncommon. If the Eustachian valve is mistaken for the lower rim of a secundum ASD, the defect may be closed such that the inferior vena cava is baffled to the left atrium leading to postoperative cyanosis. Obstruction to the SVC or pulmonary veins may occur following sinus venosus ASD repair. Following ASD or VSD closure, most patients do not have low–cardiac output syndrome or other important complications and are candidates for early extubation. Infants with VSDs and significant preoperative congestive heart failure may require a period of diuresis prior to extubation. Various atrial arrhythmias may occur following ASD closure, including transient sinus node dysfunction following repair of sinus venosus defects. JET and heart block may also uncommonly develop following VSD repair. Postpericardiotomy syndrome may develop in the days to weeks following septal defect repair.

Atrioventricular Septal Defects

Most complete atrioventricular septal defects (AVSDs) are referred for surgery between 3 and 6 months of life and use a one-patch, two-patch, or modified single-patch technique. Potential residual lesions include left-sided atrioventricular valve regurgitation, VSD, and pulmonary hypertension. Left atrioventricular valve stenosis is less common, but when present causes elevated left atrial pressures and large atrial waves on the left atrial pressure tracing. Inotropic support and afterload reduction may be indicated to treat left-sided atrioventricular valve regurgitation and pulmonary hypertension. Arrhythmias such as JET and complete heart block may also complicate the postoperative course. Partial AVSDs are usually repaired between 1 and 2 years of age with a patch closure of the ASD and, commonly, suture closure of the cleft in the left-sided atrioventricular valve.

Truncus Arteriosus

As congestive heart failure typically ensues and the risk of inadequate end-organ perfusion increases beyond the first week or two of life, surgical repair of truncus arteriosus is typically undertaken in the newborn period. The operation typically involves VSD closure, removal of the pulmonary arteries from the arterial trunk, and placement of a conduit from the right ventricle to the pulmonary arteries. A subset of patients requires intervention for truncal valve insufficiency and/or an interrupted aortic arch, either of which adds complexity to the operation.

Following repair of truncus arteriosus, potential residual lesions include right ventricular outflow tract obstruction, VSD, and pulmonary hypertension. Truncal valve dysfunction or aortic arch obstruction may be problematic in selected patients. Patients are at risk for developing a variant of right ventricular failure due to restrictive right ventricular physiology (**Table 79.2**). Sternal compression on the right

TABLE 79.2

FACTORS THAT MAY CONTRIBUTE TO RESTRICTIVE RIGHT VENTRICULAR PHYSIOLOGY FOLLOWING NEONATAL RIGHT VENTRICULAR OUTFLOW TRACT RECONSTRUCTION

■ RISK FACTOR	■ ETIOLOGIES
Diastolic dysfunction	Poorly elastic, hypertrophied right ventricle; right ventriculotomy; right ventricular muscle bundle resection; myocardial ischemia-reperfusion injury; noncontractile VSD patch
Deceased right ventricular preload	Tricuspid stenosis
Myocardial ischemia	Injury to conal branch of coronary artery crossing RVOT
	Inadequate coronary perfusion pressure
Volume load	Residual VSD or pulmonary regurgitation
Increased right ventricular afterload	Residual stenosis of the right ventricular infundibulum, pulmonary valve, or pulmonary arteries

RVOT, right ventricular outflow tract; VSD, ventricular septal defect.

ventricular-to-pulmonary artery conduit may further compromise right heart function, and delayed sternal closure or sternal reopening warrants consideration in selected patients. The sequelae of right ventricular failure and pulmonary hypertension may be partially mitigated by leaving a patent foramen ovale at the time of operation, which allows for right-to-left shunting and preservation of left ventricular preload at the expense of mild postoperative cyanosis. Additional treatment options are outlined in **Table 79.3**.

Left ventricular function may be impaired as a result of the volume load imposed on the left ventricle prior to surgery at a time during which diastolic hypotension is present and ventricular perfusion may have been compromised. The severity of the truncal valve pressure gradient is usually decreased postoperatively, as flow across the truncal valve is reduced. However, significant truncal valve regurgitation may compromise coronary blood flow and increase the volume load on the left ventricle. Arrhythmias such as JET, ectopic atrial tachycardia, and complete heart block may occur. A state of low cardiac output may exist related to one or more of the above problems. Given all of these potential issues, supportive care in the immediate postoperative period generally includes vasoactive support, maintenance of atrioventricular synchrony, and standard interventions to mitigate pulmonary hypertension.

Coarctation of the Aorta

Neonates with coarctation of the aorta have a spectrum of presentation, ranging from a well-appearing baby with a murmur and decreased femoral pulses to congestive heart failure and shock. A prostaglandin E1 (PGE$_1$) infusion is indicated once a coarctation is suspected in a neonate, and supportive care for the subset who, present in shock, is provided to allow for resolution of acidosis and recovery of end-organ function prior to surgery. In patients with a coexistent VSD or AVSD, management strategies may be needed to balance the systemic and pulmonary circulations. Older children with an isolated coarctation of the aorta typically have preserved left ventricular function and surgery is undertaken electively.

Several operative techniques are available for coarctation repair, including resection with end-to-end anastomoses, patch aortoplasty, and subclavian flap aortoplasty. Following surgical repair, assessment for residual aortic arch obstruction should occur, which may be due to hypoplasia of the aortic arch or constriction of residual ductal tissue. Neonates who present with a critical coarctation are at risk for significant pulmonary hypertension in the early postoperative period. Beyond the neonatal period, postoperative systemic hypertension is common, due to a combination of pain, baroreceptor

TABLE 79.3

TREATMENT OF RESTRICTIVE RIGHT VENTRICULAR PHYSIOLOGY

■ PHYSIOLOGIC GOALS	■ SPECIFIC TREATMENT STRATEGIES
Optimize ventricular preload	■ Leave patent foramen ovale to preserve left ventricular preload ■ Target right atrial pressure of 10–15 mm Hg ■ Drain significant ascites ■ Maintain atrioventricular synchrony
Inotropic support	■ Judicious use of dopamine, milrinone, and/or epinephrine
Lusitropy	■ Milrinone
Optimize myocardial oxygen supply and demand	■ Maintain coronary perfusion pressure ■ Heart rate control ■ Judicious use of inotropes
Maintain low right ventricular afterload	■ Use lowest possible mean airway pressure to maintain lung volume at functional residual capacity ■ Avoid acidosis ■ Drain pleural effusions, pneumothoraces, or hemothoraces
Minimize systemic oxygen consumption	■ Maintain normothermia ■ Provide adequate sedation and analgesia ■ Consider muscle relaxant

stimulation, and activation of the renin–angiotensin–aldosterone system. Hypertension may contribute to *postcoarctectomy syndrome* (mesenteric arteritis), which is characterized by abdominal pain, fever, ileus, melena, and leukocytosis. As pulsatile flow dramatically increases to vessels beyond the coarctation, thin-walled arterioles may overdistend and rupture, particularly those in the mesentery. Caution is warranted when advancing feeds during the first few postoperative days. Additional early complications include bleeding, chylothorax, phrenic nerve injury, and recurrent laryngeal nerve injury. Spinal cord ischemia leading to paralysis is a rare but important complication following coarctation repair. Older patients with inadequate collateral formation may be at greater risk.

Interrupted Aortic Arch

Neonates with interrupted aortic arch have ductal-dependent systemic blood flow and require a PGE₁ infusion. Corrective surgery involving VSD closure and reconstruction of the aortic arch is typically performed within the first few days of life. Potential residual lesions include a residual VSD, subaortic obstruction, or aortic arch obstruction. Given the extensive suture lines following reconstruction of the aortic arch, bleeding is a postoperative concern and blood pressure should be controlled. Vigilance for pulmonary hypertension is warranted. The most common type of interrupted aortic arch (type B with the interruption between the left subclavian and left carotid arteries) is associated with a 30%–80% incidence of DiGeorge syndrome, making these patients at high risk for hypocalcemia and immune deficiency.

Aortic Stenosis (Valvar, Subvalvar, Supravalvar)

Aortic valve stenosis is the most common type of left ventricular outflow tract obstruction, whereas subvalvar and supravalvar aortic stenosis are encountered less frequently. Neonates with critical aortic valve stenosis may present with severe left ventricular dysfunction and shock and stabilization with PGE₁ may be indicated. Provided that other left-sided structures are adequate for a biventricular repair, treatment options include balloon valvuloplasty or surgical valvotomy. Balloon valvuloplasty is currently the preferred procedure, although evidence that outcomes are superior to surgical valvotomy is lacking.

Following the alleviation of critical aortic valve stenosis, most patients will have a marked improvement in clinical status with recovery of left ventricular function. The residual gradient across the aortic valve may be minimal immediately following intervention, but will often increase as myocardial function and cardiac output improves. Aortic regurgitation may be severe in a minority of cases. Low cardiac output may be present and inotropic support is indicated. The PGE₁ infusion may be continued until the left ventricular function is adequate to support the systemic circulation, as evidenced by predominantly left-to-right ductal flow by lower-extremity pulse oximetry or echocardiography. Pulmonary hypertension may be problematic in the first few days following the intervention. If pulmonary hypertension persists, the adequacy of the intervention and other left-sided heart structures should be reassessed. A minority of neonates will do poorly in the postoperative period due to inadequate size of left heart structures or extensive *endocardial fibroelastosis*. For patients with a poorly functioning aortic valve but otherwise adequate left-sided structures, the aortic valve may be replaced with a homograft or autograft (Ross operation). Those with inadequate left-sided structures may require a Norwood operation.

For older patients recovering from resection of subvalvar aortic stenosis, aortic valve surgery or replacement, or repair of supravalvar stenosis, knowledge of any residual gradient across the left ventricular outflow tract and any aortic regurgitation is important to guide early management. Following aortic root replacement (involving coronary artery reimplantation) or repair of supravalvar stenosis, vigilance should be maintained for signs of coronary ischemia. In most patients, early postoperative care centers on controlling hypertension and monitoring for bleeding in those with extensive aortic suture lines.

Valvar Pulmonary Stenosis

In critical pulmonary valve stenosis, nearly all systemic venous return shunts right to left across a patent foramen ovale or ASD, where mixing occurs with pulmonary venous return. Neonates with critical pulmonary valve stenosis have ductal-dependent pulmonary blood flow, necessitating a PGE₁ infusion. Balloon valvuloplasty is the intervention of choice, and surgical valvotomy is now reserved for those neonates who fail transcatheter intervention. The most common problem encountered following balloon dilation of critical pulmonary valve stenosis is ongoing cyanosis, which may become more significant as the ductus arteriosus constricts several hours following discontinuation of PGE₁ (153). In such patients, right ventricular hypoplasia and poor compliance exist, leading to persistent right-to-left atrial shunting. In this scenario, PGE₁ may be resumed to maintain ductal patency and adequate pulmonary blood flow, thus providing time for right ventricular compliance to improve. Surgical intervention is ultimately required in 15%–25% of neonates with critical pulmonary stenosis, either for technical failure of the balloon valvuloplasty or persistent cyanosis. A systemic-to-pulmonary shunt may be indicated to provide adequate pulmonary blood flow until right ventricle compliance and size improve. If infundibular hypertrophy or residual pulmonary valve stenosis is contributing to the cyanosis, an infundibular patch or pulmonary valvotomy may be required.

Tetralogy of Fallot

The clinical presentation of patients with tetralogy of Fallot is determined to a great extent by the degree of anterior malalignment of the conal septum into the right ventricular outflow tract. Neonates with minimal obstruction to pulmonary blood flow are usually asymptomatic and are well oxygenated soon after birth. These patients may mimic the pathophysiology of an infant with a large VSD and develop congestive heart failure during the first few weeks of life as pulmonary vascular resistance falls. More commonly, however, progressive right ventricular outflow tract obstruction and worsening cyanosis develop. Neonates with tetralogy of Fallot and more severe right ventricular outflow tract obstruction or pulmonary atresia develop excessive cyanosis upon closure of the ductus arteriosus. Such patients may be stabilized with a PGE₁ infusion and referred for early surgical intervention. Indications for surgical intervention for older infants with tetralogy of Fallot include increasing cyanosis or the occurrence of a hypercyanotic episode (i.e., "TET spell").

Complete repair of tetralogy of Fallot includes VSD closure, resection of muscle bundles in the right ventricular outflow tract, a pulmonary valvotomy or leaflet resection, and, if necessary, patch augmentation of the pulmonary valve annulus (i.e., a transannular patch) and proximal pulmonary arteries or placement of a right ventricular-to-pulmonary artery conduit. The repair may be accomplished using a transatrial–transpulmonary approach, thus avoiding the short- and long-term sequelae of a right ventriculotomy.

Some patients manifest restrictive right ventricular physiology following surgery, which is characterized by antegrade flow from the right ventricle into the pulmonary artery during ventricular diastole and results from ventricular diastolic pressure rising above pulmonary arterial diastolic pressure with atrial systole (**Table 79.2**). Patients with restrictive right ventricular physiology have systemic venous hypertension and are thus prone to developing ascites and pleural effusions. Poor right ventricular compliance may lead to inadequate filling and output. Left ventricular filling may also be compromised due to diastolic ventricular interdependence, where right ventricular diastolic hypertension causes the ventricular septum to assume a midline position and in doing so decreases the effective compliance of the left ventricle.

In neonates and young infants at risk for restrictive right ventricular physiology, it may be beneficial for the surgeon to leave a small interatrial communication, allowing for right-to-left shunting and the maintenance of adequate left ventricular filling and cardiac output (**Table 79.3**). Patients may be mildly desaturated initially, but as right ventricular compliance and function improve (usually within a few days), the amount of right-to-left shunting decreases and antegrade pulmonary blood flow and systemic oxygenation increase. If an atrial communication does not exist and severe restrictive right ventricular physiology develops in the early postoperative period, the atrial septum may be opened in the cardiac catheterization laboratory. Additional strategies to improve cardiac output include administering volume and vasoactive agents such as milrinone, which provide *lusitropic* (myocardial relaxation) support. Because biventricular systolic function is most often intact, inotropic and vasodilatory agents are usually of little benefit. Minimizing intrathoracic pressure increases systemic venous return and right ventricular filling, both of which increase right ventricular output (see cardiopulmonary interactions). Loss of atrioventricular synchrony may be poorly tolerated following tetralogy of Fallot repair, particularly in those patients with restrictive right ventricular physiology. JET is the most common arrhythmia seen early following tetralogy of Fallot repair.

Tetralogy of Fallot with Pulmonary Atresia

In a more complicated variant of tetralogy of Fallot with pulmonary atresia, the central pulmonary arteries may be diminutive or absent and one or more *major aortopulmonary collateral vessels* (MAPCAs) are present. The MAPCAs are variable in number and usually arise from the descending aorta, although their origin may be from the ascending aorta, aortic arch, brachiocephalic vessels, or coronary arteries. Pulmonary blood flow may be quite variable depending upon the size and number of MAPCAs and the severity of stenosis within these vessels. Generally such patients do not have ductal-dependent pulmonary blood flow.

Although primary complete repair in early infancy is possible in selected patients, in many cases, a staged series of surgical and transcatheter interventions are required, the timing and conduct of which must be individualized based on underlying anatomy and physiology at presentation (154). If the central pulmonary arteries are small but confluent, the initial operation may involve placement of a systemic-to-pulmonary shunt, an aortopulmonary window, or placement of a right ventricular-to-pulmonary artery conduit to promote growth of these vessels (154,155). Intervention for MAPCAs is customized depending upon their size, the presence or absence of proximal stenosis within the vessel, and a determination as to whether the vessel represents redundant blood supply

to individual lung segments. Redundant MAPCAs can be coil occluded in the cardiac catheterization laboratory or ligated at the time of surgery in order to eliminate left-to-right shunting. If an MAPCA represents the sole source of pulmonary blood flow to a lung segment, the proximal end of the MAPCA is removed from its source and incorporated into the native or newly constructed central pulmonary arteries, such that blood flow to the lung is supplied from a single source (*unifocalization* procedure). Once the pulmonary vascular bed has been optimally recruited, intracardiac repair is completed including VSD closure and (if not previously completed) right ventricular outflow tract reconstruction. A patent foramen ovale or placement of a fenestrated VSD patch may be indicated in those patients with an inadequate pulmonary vascular bed to maintain left ventricular filling (156).

Tetralogy of Fallot Absent Pulmonary Valve Syndrome

In addition to the usual anatomic features of tetralogy of Fallot, patients with absent pulmonary valve syndrome have rudimentary pulmonary valve leaflets. The pulmonary arteries are often severely dilated related to in utero to-and-fro flow (severe regurgitation) across the right ventricular outflow tract. A subset of neonates manifest severe respiratory compromise soon after delivery due to tracheobronchial compression by the aneurismal pulmonary arteries. Prone positioning may be beneficial as gravity may allow the pulmonary arteries to fall off of the airways. Early surgery is indicated, which typically includes plication or replacement of the central pulmonary arteries and placement of a valved right ventricular-to-pulmonary artery conduit. The postoperative course may be complicated by respiratory insufficiency and prolonged mechanical ventilation secondary to distal bronchomalacia and reduced number of alveoli. Those patients without respiratory compromise in the early neonatal period may have their repair delayed until later in infancy.

Pulmonary Atresia with Intact Ventricular Septum

Pulmonary atresia with intact ventricular septum is an uncommon lesion, which is characterized by a membranous or muscular obstruction of the pulmonary valve and varying degrees of right ventricular and tricuspid valve hypoplasia. The left and right pulmonary arteries are usually of normal size. Right ventricle to coronary artery fistulae are present in nearly half of cases, particularly in those with more significant tricuspid valve and right ventricular hypoplasia (157,158). In up to one third of patients with pulmonary atresia and intact ventricular septum, stenosis, interruptions, or ostial occlusions are present in one or more coronary vessels. The myocardium supplied by these coronary arteries is thus dependent on flow from the right ventricle through the coronary fistulae, a condition known as *right ventricular dependent coronary circulation* (RVDCC) (159). In patients with evidence of coronary-cameral fistula by echocardiogram, a cardiac catheterization is required to determine whether RVDCC is present.

All neonates with pulmonary atresia have complete intracardiac mixing and ductal-dependent pulmonary blood flow, and thus PGE_1 is indicated. Provided that the tricuspid valve and right ventricle are of reasonable size and there is no evidence for RVDCC, it is reasonable to reconstruct the right ventricular outflow tract, which allows for regression of right ventricular hypertrophy while promoting right ventricular growth with the anticipation that right-sided heart structures will grow over time enabling a biventricular repair (160). The ASD may be left open to allow for decompression of the right heart and to ensure adequate left ventricular filling. A systemic-to-pulmonary shunt may also be placed, ensuring adequate pulmonary blood flow. Alternatively, the right ventricle may be decompressed in neonates with membranous pulmonary atresia by transcatheter perforation of the pulmonary valve using a stiff wire or radiofrequency ablation catheter followed by balloon valvuloplasty. At best, however, transcatheter intervention avoids the need for early surgical intervention in only approximately one third of patients due to persistent cyanosis, and in this scenario, a systemic-to-pulmonary shunt with or without a right ventricular outflow tract patch is needed. If RVDCC exists, relief of right ventricular outflow obstruction is contraindicated, and the initial operation is a systemic-to-pulmonary artery shunt as the first stage of single-ventricle palliation. Cardiac transplantation may be considered for the unusual infant with severe RVDCC and myocardial dysfunction that precludes single-ventricle palliation.

Residual lesions following intervention in neonates with pulmonary atresia and intact ventricular septum include residual right ventricular outflow tract obstruction and pulmonary regurgitation. Restrictive right ventricular physiology is common following a two-ventricular repair, and management principles are similar to those used following repair of neonatal tetralogy of Fallot or truncus arteriosus (Tables 79.2 and 79.3). In patients palliated with a systemic-to-pulmonary shunt, there exists the potential for pulmonary overcirculation. In patients with coronary-cameral fistulae who have undergone right ventricular decompression, care must be taken to maintain coronary perfusion pressure, and continuous electrocardiogram monitoring for evidence of ischemia is essential.

d-Transposition of the Great Arteries

In d-transposition of the great arteries (d-TGA), the aorta arises from the anatomic right ventricle and the pulmonary artery arises from the anatomic left ventricle. In ~40% of cases, a VSD exists. In this unique parallel circulation, deoxygenated systemic venous blood returns to the right heart and is pumped back to the systemic arterial circulation, and oxygenated pulmonary venous blood passes through the left heart and is pumped back to the lungs. Obligatory intercirculatory mixing may take place at the atrial, ventricular, or great artery level. Neonates with TGA and an intact ventricular septum typically have a patent foramen ovale or ASD that allows for some degree of intercirculatory mixing. A PGE$_1$ infusion may be indicated to maintain ductal patency and increase effective pulmonary blood flow. An emergent balloon septostomy may be indicated to enlarge the atrial communication if severe cyanosis is present (161). High pulmonary vascular resistance may limit effective pulmonary blood flow in some patients, for which measures should be taken to lower pulmonary vascular resistance. An additional benefit of PGE$_1$ is that it is a potent pulmonary vasodilator.

Neonates with TGA and moderate-to-large VSD are generally well oxygenated and do not require a PGE$_1$ infusion provided that the ventricular outflow tracts are unobstructed. With an anterior malalignment VSD, there may be associated right ventricular outflow tract obstruction, aortic valvar stenosis, coarctation of the aorta, or rarely an interrupted aortic arch. Posterior malalignment VSDs are associated with left ventricular outflow tract obstruction, pulmonary stenosis, or atresia. A PGE$_1$ infusion is required for such patients with ductal-dependent systemic or pulmonary blood flow.

In neonates with d-TGA and no significant outflow tract obstruction, the arterial switch operation is performed and septal defects are closed. Using the Lecompte maneuver, the pulmonary artery is typically translocated anterior to the aorta such that its branches drape over the aorta. The coronary arteries are mobilized with a button of periosteal tissue and reimplanted into the neoaorta. If a significant right ventricular outflow tract obstruction is present, a Damus–Kaye–Stansel procedure may be performed as an initial palliation, or as a part of the complete repair including closure of the VSD and placement of a right ventricle-to-pulmonary artery conduit. If significant left ventricular outflow tract obstruction exists, the Rastelli procedure (baffle to close the VSD to the aorta and placement of a right ventricle-to-pulmonary artery conduit) or Nikaidoh operation (aortic root translocation into a surgically enlarged left ventricular outflow tract, VSD closure, and right ventricular outflow tract reconstruction) may be performed (162).

Potential residual lesions following the arterial switch operation include branch pulmonary artery stenosis. Coronary artery stenosis may manifest signs of coronary ischemia and left atrial hypertension. Residual left or right ventricular outflow tract obstruction can be problematic in complex cases. As the morphologic left ventricle adapts to pumping against systemic vascular resistance, inotropic support and afterload reduction may be indicated. The administration of volume should be administered cautiously, as ventricular compliance is impaired. Vigilance for bleeding is required given the extensive aortic suture lines.

Infants with TGA and intact ventricular septum who are referred after 1–2 months of age for the arterial switch operation often require placement of a pulmonary artery band to "prepare" the left ventricle before the arterial switch operation (163). A systemic–to-pulmonary artery shunt is usually required at the time of the pulmonary artery band to ensure adequate pulmonary blood flow. These patients are often critically ill postoperatively with biventricular failure and low cardiac output. Right ventricular function is impaired due to the acute volume load created by the shunt and left ventricular function is impaired as a result of the acute increase in afterload (163,164). Inotropic support and measures to decrease pulmonary overcirculation may be indicated.

Total Anomalous Pulmonary Venous Return

Neonates with isolated obstructed total anomalous pulmonary venous return (TAPVR) typically present with pulmonary venous congestion, cyanosis, and pulmonary hypertension within hours of birth. They require prompt stabilization including mechanical ventilation and inotropic support and emergent surgical intervention. Those with unobstructed TAPVR typically do not present in extremis but rather with a murmur, mild cyanosis, and signs of right ventricular volume overload. Although less urgent, surgical repair is generally performed soon after diagnosis. In infants with supracardiac and infracardiac TAPVR, the pulmonary venous confluence is anastomosed to the back of the left atrium using circulatory arrest, the primitive vertical vein is ligated, and the ASD is closed. If the pulmonary veins drain to the coronary sinus, surgical intervention involves unroofing of the coronary sinus and closure of the ASD.

Patients with obstructed TAPVR are predisposed to pulmonary hypertensive crises following surgery, in part related to abnormal muscularity of the pulmonary arteries and veins, which develops in utero. Pulmonary edema and poor lung compliance are typically present. The left atrium may be small and poorly compliant, and rapid volume infusions may exacerbate pulmonary edema and pulmonary hypertension. The reactive pulmonary hypertension seen in some neonates following repair of TAPVR is exquisitely responsive to inhaled nitric oxide (165).

Single-Ventricle Physiology

Single-ventricle physiology is present when there is complete mixing of systemic and pulmonary venous return and the determinant of pulmonary and systemic blood flow (Q_p and Q_s, respectively) is the relative resistances in the pulmonary and systemic circulations (or the pulmonary vascular resistance–systemic vascular resistance [PVR-to-SVR] ratio). Single ventricle–like physiology may be present in certain neonates with biventricular anatomy, such as those with an interrupted aortic arch and truncus arteriosus, with the caveat being that in some cases there may not be complete mixing of systemic and pulmonary venous return. Ideally, blood flow to the systemic and pulmonary circulations will be relatively balanced, thus minimizing the ventricular volume load while maintaining Q_s. The ratio of systemic and pulmonary blood flow may be calculated by the following modified Fick equation: $Q_p/Q_s = (Sao_2 - Scvo_2)/(Spvo_2 - Spao_2)$, where Sao_2 = aortic saturation (and therefore $Spao_2$ or pulmonary artery oxygen saturation); $Scvo_2$ = central venous saturation (estimated by the SVC oxygen saturation); and $Spvo_2$ = pulmonary venous oxygen saturation. Assuming normal O_2 extraction of 25%–30%, an Sao_2 of ~70%–75% and/or an $Scvo_2$ of ~40%–50% suggest approximately balanced systemic and pulmonary blood flows with $Q_p/Q_s \approx 1$.

It is important to appreciate that if the systemic venous and pulmonary venous oxygen saturations are unknown and normal values are assumed for each when in reality they are decreased, the calculated Q_p-to-Q_s ratio underestimates the degree of pulmonary overcirculation and the propensity to develop inadequate Q_s. Studies have demonstrated that pulmonary venous saturations are not uncommonly depressed following the Norwood procedure, particularly in those patients on room air (166). Clinical parameters such as systemic blood pressure and Sao_2 are not indicators of the Q_p/Q_s ratio or Q_s. And, as discussed under monitoring, estimations of cardiac output based on the physical examination are often discordant from measured values and thus do not necessarily accurately reflect $Scvo_2$ and Q_s. Cerebral NIRS and venous oximetry (Chapter 71) may be used to provide a more robust indication of the $Q_p{:}Q_s$ ratio and more importantly the adequacy of Q_s.

Systemic-to-Pulmonary Artery Shunt

A systemic-to-pulmonary artery shunt may be performed in isolation or as a part of a larger procedure. The most commonly used systemic-to-pulmonary artery shunt is the *modified Blalock–Taussig shunt*. This operation entails placement of a Gore-Tex tube graft between the distal innominate artery or proximal subclavian artery and the pulmonary artery, typically without the use of CPB. An alternative systemic-to-pulmonary artery shunt is a *central shunt*, which involves the placement of a Gore-Tex tube between the ascending aorta and pulmonary artery.

Several postoperative complications may occur following the placement of a systemic-to-pulmonary artery shunt. If the shunt is relatively large, pulmonary blood flow may be excessive and the systemic ventricle will be subjected to volume overload, which may result in inadequate Q_s; conversely, excessive cyanosis may be caused by a relatively small shunt or pulmonary artery stenosis. The absence of a shunt murmur and the abrupt decline or absence of end-tidal carbon dioxide (for intubated patients) suggest acute shunt thrombosis. Observational data suggest that aspirin may have efficacy for minimizing shunt thrombosis risk. Other causes of early postoperative cyanosis are listed in **Table 79.4**. Reported neurological complications following shunt surgery include Horner's syndrome, recurrent laryngeal nerve injury, and phrenic nerve injury (167).

Pulmonary Artery Band

In selected neonates with single ventricular physiology and unobstructed pulmonary and systemic blood flow, a restrictive band is placed on the main pulmonary artery to decrease pulmonary blood flow and thus limit symptoms of congestive heart failure, the adverse effects of volume loading on the ventricle, and the development of pulmonary vascular obstructive disease. Placement of a pulmonary artery band, while conceptually simple, requires substantial surgical judgment. If the band is placed in the setting of high pulmonary vascular resistance, the patient's systemic oxygen saturation in the operating room may indicate a well-balanced circulation. However,

TABLE 79.4

POTENTIAL CAUSES OF EXCESSIVE CYANOSIS FOLLOWING SINGLE-VENTRICLE PALLIATION

	■ STAGE 1 (E.G., NORWOOD, PAB, SP SHUNT)	■ SUPERIOR CAVOPULMONARY ANASTOMOSIS	■ FONTAN
Inadequate pulmonary blood flow	■ Pulmonary hypertension ■ Stenosis of systemic-to-pulmonary shunt ■ Thrombosis of systemic-to-pulmonary shunt ■ Excessive tightness of pulmonary artery band ■ Obstruction to pulmonary venous or left atrial egress	■ Pulmonary hypertension ■ Stenosis of Glenn/hemi-Fontan pathway ■ Thrombosis in Glenn/hemi-Fontan pathway ■ Pulmonary artery stenosis ■ Veno-veno collaterals	■ Pulmonary hypertension ■ Anatomic obstruction to Fontan pathway ■ Thrombosis in Fontan pathway ■ Pulmonary artery stenosis ■ Veno-veno collaterals ■ Pulmonary arteriovenous malformations ■ Baffle leak ■ Oversized fenestration
Pulmonary venous desaturation	■ Atelectasis ■ Pulmonary edema ■ Pleural effusions ■ Pneumonia	■ Atelectasis ■ Pulmonary edema ■ Pleural effusions ■ Pneumonia	■ Atelectasis ■ Pulmonary edema ■ Pleural effusions ■ Pneumonia
Systemic venous desaturation	■ Anemia ■ High Vo_2 ■ Low cardiac output	■ Anemia ■ High Vo_2 ■ Low cardiac output	■ Anemia ■ High Vo_2 ■ Low cardiac output

PAB, pulmonary artery band; SP shunt, systemic pulmonary shunt; Vo_2, oxygen consumption.

as the pulmonary vascular resistance falls over time, pulmonary blood flow may increase, the systemic oxygen saturation level will rise, and signs of congestive heart failure may develop. In contrast, if the pulmonary artery band is relatively tight, the patient may be excessively cyanotic when the anesthetic wears off and oxygen consumption increases in the early postoperative period. If the pulmonary artery band migrates distally on the main pulmonary artery, distortion of the branch pulmonary arteries may develop.

Damus–Kaye–Stansel Procedure

In children with single ventricular physiology and subaortic or aortic stenosis without distal aortic arch obstruction, a Damus–Kaye–Stansel palliation may be performed to provide unobstructed systemic blood flow. This procedure involves anastomosis of the proximal main pulmonary artery and ascending aorta. The distal main pulmonary artery is oversewn and a systemic-to-pulmonary shunt is placed to provide pulmonary blood flow. The postoperative physiology and complications are similar to those seen following the Norwood operation, which are discussed in detail below.

Stage 1 Norwood Procedure

Neonates with HLHS and other single-ventricle heart defects with aortic arch obstruction typically undergo a Norwood operation within the first few days of life. This operation entails anastomosis of the proximal pulmonary artery and the aorta, reconstruction of the aortic arch to allow for unobstructed systemic blood flow, and an atrial septectomy to ensure unobstructed pulmonary venous return. Pulmonary blood flow is provided with either a modified Blalock–Taussig shunt or right ventricular-to-pulmonary artery conduit (Sano shunt). Thus, following the Norwood operation, the single right ventricle pumps blood to the systemic circulation and coronary arteries via the reconstructed aorta ("*neoaorta*"), and to the pulmonary circulation through the systemic-to-pulmonary artery or *Sano shunt*. In a multicenter randomized trial comparing these two shunt types, transplantation-free survival 12 months after randomization was higher with the Sano shunt than with the modified Blalock–Taussig shunt (74% vs. 64%, $p = 0.01$). However, with intermediate-term follow-up, this survival advantage was no longer significant (168).

Several anatomic issues may be present following the Norwood operation. Residual or recurrent aortic arch obstruction may be associated with inadequate perfusion to the lower body and pulmonary overcirculation. The anastomosis of the aorta and pulmonary artery may be narrowed, predisposing to coronary ischemia. Stenosis of the proximal or distal end of a systemic-to-pulmonary artery shunt may contribute to postoperative cyanosis. Sano shunts may be proximally obstructed by right ventricular muscle bundles, and are uncommonly associated with the development of aneurysms at their insertion site into the right ventricle.

Myocardial dysfunction or atrioventricular valve regurgitation may all contribute to inadequate systemic perfusion and a low–cardiac output state. Supportive care includes inotropic support, afterload reduction, and avoidance of both excessive supplemental oxygen and hyperventilation (169). Pulmonary hypertension is uncommon but may occur in patients with a history of a restrictive atrial septum. Other potential causes of hypoxemia are outlined in **Table 79.4**. Delayed sternal closure following the Norwood operation has several potential benefits, including the provision of extra space in patients with myocardial edema and easy access for ECMO cannulation or re-exploration for bleeding.

Superior Cavopulmonary Anastomosis

A superior cavopulmonary anastomosis involves redirection of the SVC blood flow to both pulmonary arteries. Variants include the bidirectional Glenn or hemi-Fontan operation, one of which is commonly performed in infants with single-ventricle physiology before or by approximately six months of age. The bidirectional Glenn operation, also known as the bidirectional cavopulmonary shunt operation, involves an end-to-side anastomosis between the SVC and the pulmonary artery. The hemi-Fontan operation also involves the end-to-side anastomosis between the SVC and the pulmonary artery, but in addition, the proximal SVC is anastomosed to the inferior surface of the pulmonary artery, and a patch is placed at the junction of the SVC and the right atrium. The functional result of this operation is the same as the bidirectional Glenn operation, but it facilitates later completion of the lateral tunnel Fontan operation. Because pulmonary blood flow is passive following a superior cavopulmonary anastomosis, it cannot be performed when pulmonary vascular resistance is elevated. The primary benefit of performing a superior cavopulmonary anastomosis prior to the Fontan procedure is to volume-unload the single ventricle, which leads to ventricular remodeling and reduced morbidity and mortality following the Fontan operation (170–173).

Efforts to maintain a low transpulmonary gradient (i.e., mean pulmonary artery pressure – mean common atrial pressure) in the postoperative period are warranted. Any sizable pneumothoraces, hemothoraces, or pleural effusions should be promptly drained. Cyanosis may be caused by pulmonary venous desaturation, systemic venous desaturation, or inadequate pulmonary blood flow (**Table 79.4**). Ventilatory management following a superior cavopulmonary anastomosis deserves special consideration. As pulmonary blood flow is passive and influenced by intrathoracic pressure, ventilator strategies that minimize airway pressure and maximize exhalation time will enhance pulmonary blood flow, and early extubation is generally desirable. Furthermore, as the upper body and pulmonary vascular beds are in series, pulmonary blood flow is derived in large part from venous return from the brain. Working on the principle that changes in $PaCO_2$ uncouple cerebral blood flow from cerebral metabolism, investigators have demonstrated that, despite concerns of hypoventilation-induced increases in pulmonary vascular resistance, elevated $PaCO_2$ increases pulmonary blood flow and arterial oxygenation (174).

Following a superior cavopulmonary anastomosis, the SVC syndrome may develop, which is characterized by the presence of cerebral and upper extremity venous congestion. SVC syndrome may be caused by a relatively small cross-sectional area of the pulmonary vascular bed, stenosis of the Glenn pathway, or (uncommonly) increased pulmonary vascular resistance (170). Systemic hypertension commonly develops following the superior cavopulmonary anastomosis, likely related to some combination of an intrinsic neurohumoral response to maintain cerebral perfusion pressure in the setting of an acutely elevated cerebral venous pressure, a more efficient circulatory physiology compared with the preoperative state, volume overload, and pain. Chylothorax may complicate the postoperative course in a minority of patients.

Modified Fontan Procedure

The Fontan procedure is generally performed at ~2 years of age. During this operation, the inferior vena cava is connected to the pulmonary arteries, functionally bypassing the heart, and thus separating the systemic and pulmonary circulations and eliminating cyanosis. The lateral tunnel and extracardiac modifications are the Fontan techniques used in the current era. Placement of a 3–4-mm fenestration in the Fontan pathway allows for right-to-left shunting and maintenance of ventricular preload while lowering systemic venous pathway pressures.

Potential residual lesions include obstruction to the Fontan pathway, which may contribute to a low–cardiac output state. A baffle leak in a lateral tunnel Fontan pathway may cause cyanosis. General postoperative strategies are directed at optimizing cardiac output while minimizing the transpulmonary gradient (Table 79.5). Systolic function is generally preserved; however, there is invariably varying degrees of diastolic dysfunction, which is compounded by a reliance on systemic venous pressure to drive blood across the pulmonary circulation. Minimizing airway pressure enhances systemic venous return and ventricular filling. Excessive lung volumes and the resulting increase in pulmonary vascular resistance should be avoided, as they are poorly tolerated in this circulation. Other acute postoperative issues that may be encountered include arrhythmias (e.g., sinus node dysfunction, accelerated junctional rhythm, or JET), and prolonged chest tube drainage. Cyanosis may be caused by pulmonary venous desaturation and right-to-left shunting through collaterals (Table 79.4). Thrombosis may occur in the systemic venous pathway, causing an elevated transpulmonary gradient and low–cardiac output state. Uncertainty exists regarding the efficacy of any anticoagulant or antiplatelet strategy to prevent this complication (175).

Anomalous Origin of the Left Coronary Artery from the Pulmonary Artery

Patients with anomalous origin of the left coronary artery from the pulmonary artery often develop myocardial ischemia as pulmonary vascular resistance and pulmonary artery pressure and thus left coronary artery perfusion pressure decline during infancy. The ensuing congestive heart failure and myocardial dysfunction may be severe, with variable degrees of mitral regurgitation. Some infants will require preoperative mechanical ventilation, inotropic support, and diuresis as temporizing measures while urgent surgery is arranged. The most common surgical approach is transfer of the left coronary artery from the pulmonary artery to the aorta. Alternative options include creation of an intrapulmonary aortocoronary tunnel (Takeuchi repair) or bypass grafting. The primary issue in the postoperative period is management of myocardial dysfunction and

mitral regurgitation, both of which usually gradually improve. ECMO may be required in a small minority of patients.

Ebstein's Anomaly

In Ebstein's anomaly of the tricuspid valve, the septal and posterior leaflets are displaced to some extent into the anatomic right ventricle and are variably adherent to the ventricular septum. The nondisplaced anterior leaflet may be fenestrated and redundant or "sail-like" and cause obstruction of the right ventricular outflow tract. The functional right atrium may be quite enlarged because of tricuspid regurgitation and the fact that the inlet portion of the right ventricle is "atrialized" by the inferiorly displaced tricuspid valve leaflets. ASDs (commonly) and pulmonary valve stenosis or atresia are associated with Ebstein's anomaly. One or more accessory conduction pathways may exist at the tricuspid valve annulus, creating the necessary substrate for atrioventricular reentrant tachycardia.

Right-to-left shunting at the atrial level occurs and may be due to some combination of pulmonary hypertension, pulmonary valve stenosis, or atresia, and right ventricular outflow tract obstruction by the sail-like anterior leaflet of the tricuspid valve. In some neonates, functional pulmonary atresia exists, which develops when the pulmonary artery pressure is greater than the pressure that the Ebsteinoid right ventricle can generate, and the pulmonary valve leaflets fail to open. Severe tricuspid regurgitation and extreme right atrial enlargement may result in pooling of venous return in the compliant right atrium with limited shunting across the ASD to the left atrium. The reduced preload to the left ventricle may contribute to underdevelopment of the left side of the heart and a low–cardiac output state. Neonates with Ebstein's anomaly presenting with significant cyanosis (<75%–80% systemic saturation) should receive PGE_1.

Decision-making for symptomatic neonates with severe Ebstein's anomaly is complex. If pulmonary atresia is present, early consideration must be given to determine whether it is anatomic or functional. If functional atresia is suspected, discontinuation of PGE_1 may lead to ductal constriction and decreased pulmonary artery pressure, which may allow the pulmonary valve leaflets to open (176). Anatomic pulmonary atresia may warrant attempted transcatheter perforation and balloon dilation or surgical placement of a systemic-to-pulmonary shunt. In patients without pulmonary atresia, pulmonary vascular resistance may fall, and systemic-to-pulmonary runoff may occur through the ductus arteriosus, leading to a

TABLE 79.5

ETIOLOGIES OF LOW CARDIAC OUTPUT AFTER THE FONTAN OPERATION

■ RIGHT ATRIAL PRESSURE	■ LEFT ATRIAL PRESSURE	■ ETIOLOGIES
Low	Low	Hypovolemia (bleeding, inadequate preload)
High	Low	Fontan pathway or pulmonary artery obstruction
		Elevated pulmonary vascular resistance
		Clotted fenestration
High	High	Ventricular failure
		Atrioventricular valve stenosis or regurgitation
		Arrhythmia
		Ventricular outflow tract obstruction
		Tamponade

low-output state. Increased pulmonary venous return leads to elevated left atrial pressure, which may inhibit right-to-left atrial shunting and thus contribute to systemic venous hypertension. In this scenario, PGE$_1$ should be discontinued with the aim that subsequent ductal constriction will lead to decreased pulmonary artery pressure, thereby promoting increased antegrade flow across the right ventricular outflow tract and abating symptoms of heart failure. Persistent patency of a large ductus arteriosus may warrant surgical ligation, which may result in dramatic improvement.

For symptomatic neonates who fail medical management as outlined above, there is no single reparative or palliative procedure that has been associated with widespread success. For neonates with both cyanosis and heart failure, one surgical option is to place a systemic-to-pulmonary artery shunt, oversew the tricuspid valve annulus, and perform an atrial septectomy as the first-stage procedure toward Fontan palliation (177). Plication of the right atrium is usually necessary to reduce its volume and promote right-to-left shunting across the atrial septum. Alternatively, a two-ventricle repair may be attempted consisting of a reduction atrioplasty, fenestrated closure of the atrial septum, and tricuspid valvuloplasty (178).

Neonates with Ebstein's anomaly who undergo early surgical intervention are at significant risk for developing a low–cardiac output state, and a number of factors may be contributory. Neonates with a ductus arteriosus or systemic-to-pulmonary shunt and pulmonary and tricuspid regurgitation may develop a circular shunt, which is characterized by the shunting of blood from the aorta through the ductus arteriosus or shunt, retrograde through the pulmonary and tricuspid valves, across the atrial communication and out the left ventricle and aorta (176). In this situation, an emergent reoperation may be required to ligate the ductus arteriosus, limit the shunt size, ligate the main pulmonary artery, or reduce tricuspid regurgitation with a valvuloplasty. Neonates undergoing biventricular repair may have low cardiac output from a combination of residual tricuspid regurgitation and biventricular dysfunction. Interventions to maintain low PVR and SVR are warranted.

CONCLUSIONS AND FUTURE DIRECTIONS

Evidence continues to accumulate that much of the variation in acute and long-term outcomes in children undergoing cardiac surgery is attributable to intrinsic factors, including noncardiac comorbidities and genetic factors. Added to this patient level complexity is the substantial variation that exists in the care of infants and children recovering from cardiac surgery (179). Marked differences also exist in the staffing models used to care for critically ill cardiac patients (180). These facts all highlight the need for additional research in order to determine optimal monitoring and treatment strategies for this patient population. Given growing pressure to reduce healthcare expenditures, more data are urgently needed regarding the cost-effectiveness of the care provided in our ICUs. Finally, as mortality is relatively rare for most surgical procedures in the current era, a greater understanding is needed of the impact of therapies applied in the perioperative period on long-term cardiac function, neurodevelopmental outcomes, and quality of life.

References

1. Fagan DG. Shape changes in static V-P loops from children's lungs related to growth. *Thorax* 1977;32:198–202.

2. Guslits BG, Gaston SE, Bryan MH, et al. Diaphragmatic work of breathing in premature human infants. *J Appl Physiol* 1987;62:1410–5.

3. Keens TG, Bryan AC, Levison H, et al. Developmental pattern of muscle fiber types in human ventilatory muscles. *J Appl Physiol* 1978;44:909–13.

4. Nichols DG. Respiratory muscle performance in infants and children. *J Pediatr* 1991;118:493–502.

5. Lister G, Pitt BR. Cardiopulmonary interactions in the infant with congenital cardiac disease. *Clin Chest Med* 1983;4:219–32.

6. Stayer SA, Diaz LK, East DL, et al. Changes in respiratory mechanics among infants undergoing heart surgery. *Anesth Analg* 2004;98:49–55, table of contents.

7. Anyanwu E, Dittrich H, Gieseking R, et al. Ultrastructural changes in the human lung following cardiopulmonary bypass. *Basic Res Cardiol* 1982;77:309–22.

8. Ochs M, Nenadic I, Fehrenbach A, et al. Ultrastructural alterations in intraalveolar surfactant subtypes after experimental ischemia and reperfusion. *Am J Respir Crit Care Med* 1999;160:718–24.

9. Rochester DF, Briscoe AM. Metabolism of the working diaphragm. *Am Rev Respir Dis* 1979;119:101–6.

10. Aubier M, Trippenbach T, Roussos C. Respiratory muscle fatigue during cardiogenic shock. *J Appl Physiol* 1981;51:499–508.

11. Field S, Kelly SM, Macklem PT. The oxygen cost of breathing in patients with cardiorespiratory disease. *Am Rev Respir Dis* 1982;126:9–13.

12. Gurevitch J, Frolkis I, Yuhas Y, et al. Tumor necrosis factor-alpha is released from the isolated heart undergoing ischemia and reperfusion. *J Am Coll Cardio* 1996;28:247–52.

13. Merx MW, Weber C. Sepsis and the heart. *Circulation* 2007;116:793–802.

14. Blatchford JW III, Barragry TP, Lillehei TJ, et al. Effects of cardioplegic arrest on left ventricular systolic and diastolic function of the intact neonatal heart. *J Thorac Cardiovasc Surg* 1994;107:527–35.

15. Chaturvedi RR, Herron T, Simmons R, et al. Passive stiffness of myocardium from congenital heart disease and implications for diastole. *Circulation* 2010;121:979–88.

16. Hammon JW Jr, Graham TP Jr, Boucek RJ Jr, et al. Myocardial adenosine triphosphate content as a measure of metabolic and functional myocardial protection in children undergoing cardiac operation. *Ann Thorac Surg* 1987;44:467–70.

17. Kronon MT, Allen BS, Halldorsson A, et al. Dose dependency of L-arginine in neonatal myocardial protection: The nitric oxide paradox. *J Thorac Cardiovasc Surg* 1999;118:655–64.

18. Fischer UM, Cox CS Jr, Laine GA, et al. Induction of cardioplegic arrest immediately activates the myocardial apoptosis signal pathway. *Am J Physiol Heart Circ Physiol* 2007;292:H1630–H1633.

19. Graham TP Jr. Ventricular performance in congenital heart disease. *Circulation* 1991;84:2259–74.

20. Legato MJ. Cellular mechanisms of normal growth in the mammalian heart. Part II. A quantitative and qualitative comparison between the right and left ventricular myocytes in the dog from birth to five months of age. *Circ Res* 1979;44:263–79.

21. Chin TK, Friedman WF, Klitzner TS. Developmental changes in cardiac myocyte calcium regulation. *Circ Res* 1990;67:574–9.

22. Romero TE, Friedman WF. Limited left ventricular response to volume overload in the neonatal period: A comparative study with the adult animal. *Pediatr Res* 1979;13:910–5.

23. Celermajer DS, Cullen S, Deanfield JE. Impairment of endothelium-dependent pulmonary artery relaxation in children with congenital heart disease and abnormal pulmonary hemodynamics. *Circulation* 1993;87:440–6.

24. Morita K, Ihnken K, Buckberg GD, et al. Pulmonary vasoconstriction due to impaired nitric oxide production after cardiopulmonary bypass. *Ann Thorac Surg* 1996;61:1775–80.

25. Miller OI, Tang SF, Keech A, et al. Inhaled nitric oxide and prevention of pulmonary hypertension after congenital heart surgery: A randomised double-blind study. *Lancet* 2000;356:1464–9.

26. Namachivayam P, Theilen U, Butt WW, et al. Sildenafil prevents rebound pulmonary hypertension after withdrawal of nitric oxide in children. *Am J Respir Crit Care Med* 2006;174:1042–7.

27. Connors AF Jr, McCaffree DR, Gray BA. Evaluation of right-heart catheterization in the critically ill patient without acute myocardial infarction. *N Engl J Med* 1983;308:263–7.

28. Tibby SM, Hatherill M, Murdoch IA. Capillary refill and core-peripheral temperature gap as indicators of haemodynamic status in paediatric intensive care patients. *Arch Dis Child* 1999;80:163–6.

29. Lobos AT, Lee S, Menon K. Capillary refill time and cardiac output in children undergoing cardiac catheterization. *Pediatr Crit Care Med* 2012;13:136–40.

30. Reuse C, Vincent JL, Pinsky MR. Measurements of right ventricular volumes during fluid challenge. *Chest* 1990;98:1450–4.

31. Toussaint GP, Burgess JH, Hampson LG. Central venous pressure and pulmonary wedge pressure in critical surgical illness. A comparison. *Arch Surg* 1974;109:265–9.

32. Forrester JS, Diamond G, McHugh TJ, et al. Filling pressures in the right and left sides of the heart in acute myocardial infarction. A reappraisal of central-venous-pressure monitoring. *N Engl J Med* 1971;285:190–3.

33. Artman M, Graham TP Jr. Guidelines for vasodilator therapy of congestive heart failure in infants and children. *Am Heart J* 1987;113:994–1005.

34. Nelson GI, Silke B, Forsyth DR, et al. Hemodynamic comparison of primary venous or arteriolar dilatation and the subsequent effect of furosemide in left ventricular failure after acute myocardial infarction. *Am J Cardiol* 1983;52:1036–40.

35. Elkayam U, Weber L, McKay CR, et al. Differences in hemodynamic response to vasodilation due to calcium channel antagonism with nifedipine and direct-acting agonism with hydralazine in chronic refractory congestive heart failure. *Am J Cardiol* 1984;54:126–31.

36. Matter CM, Mandinov L, Kaufmann PA, et al. Effect of NO donors on LV diastolic function in patients with severe pressure-overload hypertrophy. *Circulation* 1999;99:2396–401.

37. Leier CV, Heban PT, Huss P, et al. Comparative systemic and regional hemodynamic effects of dopamine and dobutamine in patients with cardiomyopathic heart failure. *Circulation* 1978;58:466–75.

38. Driscoll DJ, Gillette PC, Duff DF, et al. The hemodynamic effect of dopamine in children. *J Thorac Cardiovasc Surg* 1979;78:765–8.

39. Driscoll DJ, Gillette PC, Duff DF, et al. Hemodynamic effects of dobutamine in children. *Am J Cardiol* 1979;43:581–5.

40. Fitzgerald GA, Barnes P, Hamilton CA, et al. Circulating adrenaline and blood pressure: The metabolic effects and kinetics of infused adrenaline in man. *Eur J Clin Invest* 1980;10:401–6.

41. Allwood MJ, Cobbold AF, Ginsburg J. Peripheral vascular effects of noradrenaline, isopropylnoradrenaline and dopamine. *Br Med Bull* 1963;19:132–6.

42. Barrington K, Chan W. The circulatory effects of epinephrine infusion in the anesthetized piglet. *Pediatr Res* 1993;33:190–4.

43. Chang AC, Atz AM, Wernovsky G, et al. Milrinone: Systemic and pulmonary hemodynamic effects in neonates after cardiac surgery. *Crit Care Med* 1995;23:1907–14.

44. Pagel PS, Hettrick DA, Warltier DC. Influence of levosimendan, pimobendan, and milrinone on the regional distribution of cardiac output in anaesthetized dogs. *Br J Pharmacol* 1996;119:609–15.

45. Hoffman TM, Wernovsky G, Atz AM, et al. Efficacy and safety of milrinone in preventing low cardiac output syndrome in infants and children after corrective surgery for congenital heart disease. *Circulation* 2003;107:996–1002.

46. Appelbaum A, Blackstone EH, Kouchoukos NT, et al. Afterload reduction and cardiac ouptut in infants early after intracardiac surgery. *Am J Cardiol* 1977;39:445–51.

47. Ilbawi MN, Idriss FS, DeLeon SY, et al. Hemodynamic effects of intravenous nitroglycerin in pediatric patients after heart surgery. *Circulation* 1985;72:II101–II107.

48. Miller RR, Vismara LA, Williams DO, et al. Pharmacological mechanisms for left ventricular unloading in clinical congestive heart failure. Differential effects of nitroprusside, phentolamine, and nitroglycerin on cardiac function and peripheral circulation. *Circ Res* 1976;39:127–33.

49. Holmes CL, Patel BM, Russell JA, et al. Physiology of vasopressin relevant to management of septic shock. *Chest* 2001;120:989–1002.

50. Polito A, Parisini E, Ricci Z, et al. Vasopressin for treatment of vasodilatory shock: An ESICM systematic review and meta-analysis. *Intens Care Med* 2012;38:9–19.

51. Russell JA, Walley KR, Singer J, et al. Vasopressin versus norepinephrine infusion in patients with septic shock. *N Engl J Med* 2008;358:877–87.

52. Choong K, Bohn D, Fraser DD, et al. Vasopressin in pediatric vasodilatory shock: A multicenter randomized controlled trial. *Am J Respir Crit Care Med* 2009;180:632–9.

53. Dunser MW, Mayr AJ, Stallinger A, et al. Cardiac performance during vasopressin infusion in postcardiotomy shock. *Intens Care Med* 2002;28:746–51.

54. Alten JA, Borasino S, Toms R, et al. Early initiation of arginine vasopressin infusion in neonates after complex cardiac surgery. *Pediatr Crit Care Med* 2012;13:300–4.

55. Mastropietro CW, Davalos MC, Seshadri S, et al. Clinical response to arginine vasopressin therapy after paediatric cardiac surgery. *Cardiol Young* 2013;23(3):387–93.

56. Rosenzweig EB, Starc TJ, Chen JM, et al. Intravenous arginine-vasopressin in children with vasodilatory shock after cardiac surgery. *Circulation* 1999;100:II182–II186.

57. Goff DA, Luan X, Gerdes M, et al. Younger gestational age is associated with worse neurodevelopmental outcomes after cardiac surgery in infancy. *J Thorac Cardiovasc Surg* 2012;143:535–42.

58. Limperopoulos C, Majnemer A, Shevell MI, et al. Neurologic status of newborns with congenital heart defects before open heart surgery. *Pediatrics* 1999;103:402–8.

59. Mahle WT, Tavani F, Zimmerman RA, et al. An MRI study of neurological injury before and after congenital heart surgery. *Circulation* 2002;106:I109–I114.

60. Brown KL, Ridout DA, Hoskote A, et al. Delayed diagnosis of congenital heart disease worsens preoperative condition and outcome of surgery in neonates. *Heart* 2006;92:1298–302.

61. du Plessis AJ, Jonas RA, Wypij D, et al. Perioperative effects of alpha-stat versus pH-stat strategies for deep hypothermic cardiopulmonary bypass in infants. *J Thorac Cardiovasc Surg* 1997;114:991–1000; discussion 1000–1.

62. Bellinger DC, Jonas RA, Rappaport LA, et al. Developmental and neurologic status of children after heart surgery with hypothermic circulatory arrest or low-flow cardiopulmonary bypass. *N Engl J Med* 1995;332:549–55.

63. Wypij D, Newburger JW, Rappaport LA, et al. The effect of duration of deep hypothermic circulatory arrest in infant heart surgery on late neurodevelopment: The Boston Circulatory Arrest Trial. *J Thorac Cardiovasc Surg* 2003;126:1397–403.

64. Goldberg CS, Bove EL, Devaney EJ, et al. A randomized clinical trial of regional cerebral perfusion versus deep hypothermic circulatory arrest: Outcomes for infants with functional single ventricle. *J Thorac Cardiovasc Surg* 2007;133:880–7.

65. Kussman BD, Wypij D, Laussen PC, et al. Relationship of intraoperative cerebral oxygen saturation to neurodevelopmental outcome and brain magnetic resonance imaging at 1 year of age in infants undergoing biventricular repair. *Circulation* 2010;122:245–54.

66. Gunn JK, Beca J, Penny DJ, et al. Amplitude-integrated electroencephalography and brain injury in infants undergoing Norwood-type operations. *Ann Thorac Surg* 2012;93:170–6.

67. Bloom AA, Wright JA, Morris RD, et al. Additive impact of in-hospital cardiac arrest on the functioning of children with heart disease. *Pediatrics* 1997;99:390–8.

68. Lequier L, Joffe AR, Robertson CM, et al. Two-year survival, mental, and motor outcomes after cardiac extracorporeal life support at less than five years of age. *J Thorac Cardiovasc Surg* 2008;136:976.e3–983.e3.

69. Azzopardi DV, Strohm B, Edwards AD, et al. Moderate hypothermia to treat perinatal asphyxial encephalopathy. *N Engl J Med* 2009;361:1349–58.

70. Newburger JW, Wypij D, Bellinger DC, et al. Length of stay after infant heart surgery is related to cognitive outcome at age 8 years. *J Pediatr* 2003;143:67–73.

71. Loepke AW. Developmental neurotoxicity of sedatives and anesthetics: A concern for neonatal and pediatric critical care medicine? *Pediatr Crit Care Med* 2010;11:217–26.

72. Srinivasan V, Spinella PC, Drott HR, et al. Association of timing, duration, and intensity of hyperglycemia with intensive care unit mortality in critically ill children. *Pediatr Crit Care Med* 2004;5:329–36.

73. Vlasselaers D, Milants I, Desmet L, et al. Intensive insulin therapy for patients in paediatric intensive care: A prospective, randomised controlled study. *Lancet* 2009;373:547–56.

74. Vlasselaers D, Mesotten D, Langouche L, et al. Tight glycemic control protects the myocardium and reduces inflammation in neonatal heart surgery. *Ann Thorac Surg* 2010;90:22–9.

75. Agus MS, Steil GM, Wypij D, et al. Tight glycemic control versus standard care after pediatric cardiac surgery. *N Engl J Med* 2012;367:1208–19.

76. Wald EL, Preze E, Eickhoff JC, et al. The effect of cardiopulmonary bypass on the hypothalamic-pituitary-adrenal axis in children. *Pediatr Crit Care Med* 2011;12:190–6.

77. Menon K, Ward RE, Lawson ML, et al. A prospective multicenter study of adrenal function in critically ill children. *Am J Respir Crit Care Med* 2010;182:246–51.

78. Bettendorf M, Schmidt KG, Grulich-Henn J, et al. Tri-iodothyronine treatment in children after cardiac surgery: A double-blind, randomised, placebo-controlled study. *Lancet* 2000;356:529–34.

79. Chowdhury D, Ojamaa K, Parnell VA, et al. A prospective randomized clinical study of thyroid hormone treatment after operations for complex congenital heart disease. *J Thorac Cardiovasc Surg* 2001;122:1023–5.

80. Mackie AS, Booth KL, Newburger JW, et al. A randomized, double-blind, placebo-controlled pilot trial of triiodothyronine in neonatal heart surgery. *J Thorac Cardiovasc Surg* 2005;130:810–6.

81. Portman MA, Slee A, Olson AK, et al. Triiodothyronine supplementation in infants and children undergoing cardiopulmonary bypass (TRICC): A multicenter placebo-controlled randomized trial: Age analysis. *Circulation* 2010;122:S224–S233.

82. Anderson JB, Beekman RH III, Border WL, et al. Lower weight-for-age z score adversely affects hospital length of stay after the bidirectional Glenn procedure in 100 infants with a single ventricle. *J Thorac Cardiovasc Surg* 2009;138:397.e1–404.e1.

83. De Wit B, Meyer R, Desai A, et al. Challenge of predicting resting energy expenditure in children undergoing surgery for congenital heart disease. *Pediatr Crit Care Med* 2010;11:496–501.

84. Braudis NJ, Curley MA, Beaupre K, et al. Enteral feeding algorithm for infants with hypoplastic left heart syndrome poststage I palliation. *Pediatr Crit Care Med* 2009;10:460–6.

85. McElhinney DB, Hedrick HL, Bush DM, et al. Necrotizing enterocolitis in neonates with congenital heart disease: Risk factors and outcomes. *Pediatrics* 2000;106:1080–7.

86. Manno CS, Hedberg KW, Kim HC, et al. Comparison of the hemostatic effects of fresh whole blood, stored whole blood, and components after open heart surgery in children. *Blood* 1991;77:930–6.

87. Salvin JW, Scheurer MA, Laussen PC, et al. Blood transfusion after pediatric cardiac surgery is associated with prolonged hospital stay. *Ann Thorac Surg* 2011;91:204–10.

88. Willems A, Harrington K, Lacroix J, et al. Comparison of two red-cell transfusion strategies after pediatric cardiac surgery: A subgroup analysis. *Crit Care Med* 2010;38:649–56.

89. Pasquali SK, Li JS, He X, et al. Comparative analysis of antifibrinolytic medications in pediatric heart surgery. *J Thorac Cardiovasc Surg* 2012;143:550–7.

90. Pasquali SK, Hall M, Li JS, et al. Safety of aprotinin in congenital heart operations: Results from a large multicenter database. *Ann Thorac Surg* 2010;90:14–21.

91. Dominguez TE, Mitchell M, Friess SH, et al. Use of recombinant factor VIIa for refractory hemorrhage during extracorporeal membrane oxygenation. *Pediatr Crit Care Med* 2005;6:348–51.

92. Costello JM, Graham DA, Morrow DF, et al. Risk factors for central line-associated bloodstream infection in a pediatric cardiac intensive care unit. *Pediatr Crit Care Med* 2009;10:453–9.

93. Slonim AD, Kurtines HC, Sprague BM, et al. The costs associated with nosocomial bloodstream infections in the pediatric intensive care unit. *Pediatr Crit Care Med* 2001;2:170–4.

94. Costello JM, Morrow DF, Graham DA, et al. Systematic intervention to reduce central line-associated bloodstream infection rates in a pediatric cardiac intensive care unit. *Pediatrics* 2008;121:915–23.

95. Akcan-Arikan A, Zappitelli M, Loftis LL, et al. Modified rifle criteria in critically ill children with acute kidney injury. *Kid Int* 2007;71:1028–35.

96. Mehta RL, Kellum JA, Shah SV, et al. Acute kidney injury network: Report of an initiative to improve outcomes in acute kidney injury. *Crit Care* 2007;11:R31.

97. Li S, Krawczeski CD, Zappitelli M, et al. Incidence, risk factors, and outcomes of acute kidney injury after pediatric cardiac surgery: A prospective multicenter study. *Crit Care Med* 2011;39:1493–9.

98. Ronco C, Haapio M, House AA, et al. Cardiorenal syndrome. *J Am Coll Cardiol* 2008;52:1527–39.

99. Alkandari O, Eddington KA, Hyder A, et al. Acute kidney injury is an independent risk factor for pediatric intensive care unit mortality, longer length of stay and prolonged mechanical ventilation in critically ill children: A two-center retrospective cohort study. *Crit Care* 2011;15:R146.

100. Wypij D, Jonas RA, Bellinger DC, et al. The effect of hematocrit during hypothermic cardiopulmonary bypass in infant heart surgery: Results from the combined Boston hematocrit trials. *J Thorac Cardiovasc Surg* 2008;135:355–60.

101. Bellinger DC, Wypij D, du Plessis AJ, et al. Developmental and neurologic effects of alpha-stat versus pH-stat strategies for deep hypothermic cardiopulmonary bypass in infants. *J Thorac Cardiovasc Surg* 2001;121:374–83.

102. Craddock PR, Fehr J, Brigham KL, et al. Complement and leukocyte-mediated pulmonary dysfunction in hemodialysis. *N Engl J Med* 1977;296:769–74.

103. Chenoweth DE, Cooper SW, Hugli TE, et al. Complement activation during cardiopulmonary bypass: Evidence for generation of C3a and C5a anaphylatoxins. *N Engl J Med* 1981;304:497–503.

104. Kirklin JK, Westaby S, Blackstone EH, et al. Complement and the damaging effects of cardiopulmonary bypass. *J Thorac Cardiovasc Surg* 1983;86:845–57.

105. Kirshbom PM, Jacobs MT, Tsui SS, et al. Effects of cardiopulmonary bypass and circulatory arrest on endothelium-dependent vasodilation in the lung. *J Thorac Cardiovasc Surg* 1996;111:1248–56.

106. Egan JR, Butler TL, Cole AD, et al. Myocardial membrane injury in pediatric cardiac surgery: An animal model. *J Thorac Cardiovasc Surg* 2009;137:1154–62.

107. Buja LM. Myocardial ischemia and reperfusion injury. *Cardiovasc Pathol* 2005;14:170–5.

108. van Deventer SJ. Cytokine and cytokine receptor polymorphisms in infectious disease. *Intens Care Med* 2000;26(suppl 1):S98–S102.

109. Eltzschig HK, Carmeliet P. Hypoxia and inflammation. *N Engl J Med* 2011;364:656–65.

110. Bozkurt B, Mann DL, Deswal A. Biomarkers of inflammation in heart failure. *Heart Fail Rev* 2010;15:331–41.

111. Qing M, Schumacher K, Heise R, et al. Intramyocardial synthesis of pro- and anti-inflammatory cytokines in infants with congenital cardiac defects. *J Am Coll Cardiol* 2003;41:2266–74.

112. Hotchkiss RS, Opal S. Immunotherapy for sepsis—A new approach against an ancient foe. *N Engl J Med* 2010;363:87–9.

113. Rivest S, Lacroix S, Vallieres L, et al. How the blood talks to the brain parenchyma and the paraventricular nucleus of the hypothalamus during systemic inflammatory and infectious stimuli. *Proc Soc Exp Biol Med* 2000;223:22–38.

114. Nussmeier NA, Searles BE. Inflammatory brain injury after cardiopulmonary bypass: Is it real? *Anesth Analg* 2010;110:288–90.

115. Jungwirth B, Kellermann K, Qing M, et al. Cerebral tumor necrosis factor alpha expression and long-term neurocognitive performance after cardiopulmonary bypass in rats. *J Thorac Cardiovasc Surg* 2009;138:1002–7.

116. Lisle TC, Gazoni LM, Fernandez LG, et al. Inflammatory lung injury after cardiopulmonary bypass is attenuated by adenosine A(2A) receptor activation. *J Thorac Cardiovasc Surg* 2008;136:1280–7; discussion 1287–8.

117. Suzuki T, Fukuda T, Ito T, et al. Continuous pulmonary perfusion during cardiopulmonary bypass prevents lung injury in infants. *Ann Thorac Surg* 2000;69:602–6.

118. Shafique T, Johnson RG, Dai HB, et al. Altered pulmonary microvascular reactivity after total cardiopulmonary bypass. *J Thorac Cardiovasc Surg* 1993;106:479–86.

119. Karimi M, Wang LX, Hammel JM, et al. Neonatal vulnerability to ischemia and reperfusion: Cardioplegic arrest causes greater myocardial apoptosis in neonatal lambs than in mature lambs. *J Thorac Cardiovasc Surg* 2004;127:490–7.

120. Lefer AM, Tsao PS, Lefer DJ, et al. Role of endothelial dysfunction in the pathogenesis of reperfusion injury after myocardial ischemia. *FASEB J* 1991;5:2029–34.

121. Gourine AV, Bulhak AA, Gonon AT, et al. Cardioprotective effect induced by brief exposure to nitric oxide before myocardial ischemia-reperfusion in vivo. *Nitric Oxide* 2002;7:210–6.

122. Hataishi R, Rodrigues AC, Neilan TG, et al. Inhaled nitric oxide decreases infarction size and improves left ventricular function in a murine model of myocardial ischemia-reperfusion injury. *Am J Physiol Heart Circ Physiol* 2006;291:H379–H384.

123. Chrousos GP. The hypothalamic-pituitary-adrenal axis and immune-mediated inflammation. *N Engl J Med* 1995;332:1351–62.

124. Checchia PA, Gandhi SK. Defining vasodilatory shock following cardiac surgery in children: When, where, how often? *Pediatr Crit Care Med* 2009;10:409–10.

125. Levin MA, Lin HM, Castillo JG, et al. Early on-cardiopulmonary bypass hypotension and other factors associated with vasoplegic syndrome. *Circulation* 2009;120:1664–71.

126. Killinger JS, Hsu DT, Schleien CL, et al. Children undergoing heart transplant are at increased risk for postoperative vasodilatory shock. *Pediatr Crit Care Med* 2009;10:335–40.

127. Rosner MH, Okusa MD. Acute kidney injury associated with cardiac surgery. *Clin J Am Soc Nephrol* 2006;1:19–32.

128. Bellomo R, Auriemma S, Fabbri A, et al. The pathophysiology of cardiac surgery-associated acute kidney injury (CSA-AKI). *Int J Artif Organs* 2008;31:166–78.

129. Klausner JM, Paterson IS, Goldman G, et al. Postischemic renal injury is mediated by neutrophils and leukotrienes. *Am J Physiol* 1989;256:F794–F802.

130. Braun JP, Schroeder T, Buehner S, et al. Splanchnic oxygen transport, hepatic function and gastrointestinal barrier after normothermic cardiopulmonary bypass. *Acta Anaesthesiol Scand* 2004;48:697–703.

131. Malagon I, Onkenhout W, Klok G, et al. Gut permeability in paediatric cardiac surgery. *Br J Anaesth* 2005;94:181–5.

132. Ohri SK, Velissaris T. Gastrointestinal dysfunction following cardiac surgery. *Perfusion* 2006;21:215–23.

133. Doguet F, Litzler PY, Tamion F, et al. Changes in mesenteric vascular reactivity and inflammatory response after cardiopulmonary bypass in a rat model. *Ann Thorac Surg* 2004;77:2130–7; author reply 2137.

134. Vieira AT, Pinho V, Lepsch LB, et al. Mechanisms of the anti-inflammatory effects of the natural secosteroids physalins in a model of intestinal ischaemia and reperfusion injury. *Br J Pharmacol* 2005;146:244–51.

135. Mallick IH, Winslet MC, Seifalian AM. Ischemic preconditioning of small bowel mitigates the late phase of reperfusion injury: Heme oxygenase mediates cytoprotection. *Am J Surg* 2010;199:223–31.

136. Hart ML, Jacobi B, Schittenhelm J, et al. Cutting edge: A2b adenosine receptor signaling provides potent protection during intestinal ischemia/reperfusion injury. *J Immunol* 2009;182:3965–8.

137. Riddington DW, Venkatesh B, Boivin CM, et al. Intestinal permeability, gastric intramucosal pH, and systemic endotoxemia in patients undergoing cardiopulmonary bypass. *JAMA* 1996;275:1007–12.

138. Lequier LL, Nikaidoh H, Leonard SR, et al. Preoperative and postoperative endotoxemia in children with congenital heart disease. *Chest* 2000;117:1706–12.

139. Allen M, Sundararajan S, Pathan N, et al. Anti-inflammatory modalities: Their current use in pediatric cardiac surgery in the United Kingdom and Ireland. *Pediatr Crit Care Med* 2009;10:341–5.

140. Checchia PA, Bronicki RA, Costello JM, et al. Steroid use before pediatric cardiac operations using cardiopulmonary bypass: An international survey of 36 centers. *Pediatr Crit Care Med* 2005;6:441–4.

141. Bronicki RA, Backer CL, Baden HP, et al. Dexamethasone reduces the inflammatory response to cardiopulmonary bypass in children. *Ann Thorac Surg* 2000;69:1490–5.

142. Schroeder VA, Pearl JM, Schwartz SM, et al. Combined steroid treatment for congenital heart surgery improves oxygen delivery and reduces postbypass inflammatory mediator expression. *Circulation* 2003;107:2823–8.

143. Checchia PA, Backer CL, Bronicki RA, et al. Dexamethasone reduces postoperative troponin levels in children undergoing cardiopulmonary bypass. *Crit Care Med* 2003;31:1742–5.

144. Graham EM, Atz AM, Butts RJ, et al. Standardized preoperative corticosteroid treatment in neonates undergoing cardiac surgery: Results from a randomized trial. *J Thorac Cardiovasc Surg* 2011;142:1523–9.

145. Bronicki RA, Checchia PA, Stuart-Killion RB, et al. The effects of multiple doses of glucocorticois on the inflammatory resposne to cardiopulmonary bypass in children. *World J Pediar Congenit Heart Surg* 2012;3:439–45.

146. Gaynor JW. The effect of modified ultrafiltration on the postoperative course in patients with congenital heart disease. *Semin Thorac Cardiovasc Surg Pediatr Card Surg Annu* 2003;6:128–39.

147. Mangoush O, Purkayastha S, Haj-Yahia S, et al. Heparin-bonded circuits versus nonheparin-bonded circuits: An evaluation of their effect on clinical outcomes. *Eur J Cardiothorac Surg* 2007;31:1058–69.

148. Ozawa T, Yoshihara K, Koyama N, et al. Clinical efficacy of heparin-bonded bypass circuits related to cytokine responses in children. *Ann Thorac Surg* 2000;69:584–90.

149. Grossi EA, Kallenbach K, Chau S, et al. Impact of heparin bonding on pediatric cardiopulmonary bypass: A prospective randomized study. *Ann Thorac Surg* 2000;70:191–6.

150. O'Brien SM, Clarke DR, Jacobs JP, et al. An empirically based tool for analyzing mortality associated with congenital heart surgery. *J Thorac Cardiovasc Surg* 2009;138:1139–53.

151. McNamara PJ, Stewart L, Shivananda SP, et al. Patent ductus arteriosus ligation is associated with impaired left ventricular systolic performance in premature infants weighing less than 1000 g. *J Thorac Cardiovasc Surg* 2010;140:150–7.

152. Lammers A, Hager A, Eicken A, et al. Need for closure of secundum atrial septal defect in infancy. *J Thorac Cardiovasc Surg* 2005;129:1353–7.

153. Fedderly RT, Lloyd TR, Mendelsohn AM, et al. Determinants of successful balloon valvotomy in infants with critical pulmonary stenosis or membranous pulmonary atresia with intact ventricular septum. *J Am Coll Cardiol* 1995;25:460–5.

154. Duncan BW, Mee RB, Prieto LR, et al. Staged repair of tetralogy of Fallot with pulmonary atresia and major aortopulmonary collateral arteries. *J Thorac Cardiovasc Surg* 2003;126:694–702.

155. Rodefeld MD, Reddy VM, Thompson LD, et al. Surgical creation of aortopulmonary window in selected patients with pulmonary atresia with poorly developed aortopulmonary collaterals and hypoplastic pulmonary arteries. *J Thorac Cardiovasc Surg* 2002;123:1147–54.

156. Marshall AC, Love BA, Lang P, et al. Staged repair of tetralogy of Fallot and diminutive pulmonary arteries with a fenestrated ventricular septal defect patch. *J Thorac Cardiovasc Surg* 2003;126:1427–33.

157. Daubeney PE, Delany DJ, Anderson RH, et al. Pulmonary atresia with intact ventricular septum: Range of morphology in a population-based study. *J Am Coll Cardiol* 2002;39:1670–9.

158. Satou GM, Perry SB, Gauvreau K, et al. Echocardiographic predictors of coronary artery pathology in pulmonary atresia with intact ventricular septum. *Am J Cardiol* 2000;85:1319–24.

159. Giglia TM, Mandell VS, Connor AR, et al. Diagnosis and management of right ventricle-dependent coronary circulation in pulmonary atresia with intact ventricular septum. *Circulation* 1992;86:1516–28.

160. Giglia TM, Jenkins KJ, Matitiau A, et al. Influence of right heart size on outcome in pulmonary atresia with intact ventricular septum. *Circulation* 1993;88:2248–56.

161. Rashkind WJ, Miller WW. Creation of an atrial septal defect without thoracotomy. A palliative approach to complete transposition of the great arteries. *JAMA* 1966;196:991–2.

162. Emani SM, Beroukhim R, Zurakowski D, et al. Outcomes after anatomic repair for d-transposition of the great arteries with left ventricular outflow tract obstruction. *Circulation* 2009;120:S53–S58.

163. Boutin C, Jonas RA, Sanders SP, et al. Rapid two-stage arterial switch operation. Acquisition of left ventricular mass after pulmonary artery banding in infants with transposition of the great arteries. *Circulation* 1994;90:1304–9.

164. Wernovsky G, Giglia TM, Jonas RA, et al. Course in the intensive care unit after 'preparatory' pulmonary artery banding and aortopulmonary shunt placement for transposition of the great arteries with low left ventricular pressure. *Circulation* 1992;86:II133–II139.

165. Atz AM, Adatia I, Wessel DL. Rebound pulmonary hypertension after inhalation of nitric oxide. *Ann Thorac Surg* 1996;62:1759–64.

166. Taeed R, Schwartz SM, Pearl JM, et al. Unrecognized pulmonary venous desaturation early after Norwood palliation confounds Gp: Gs assessment and compromises oxygen delivery. *Circulation* 2001;103:2699–704.

167. Odim J, Portzky M, Zurakowski D, et al. Sternotomy approach for the modified Blalock-Taussig shunt. *Circulation* 1995;92:II256–II261.

168. Ohye RG, Sleeper LA, Mahony L, et al. Comparison of shunt types in the Norwood procedure for single-ventricle lesions. *N Engl J Med* 2010;362:1980–92.

169. Tweddell JS, Hoffman GM, Fedderly RT, et al. Phenoxybenzamine improves systemic oxygen delivery after the Norwood procedure. *Ann Thorac Surg* 1999;67:161–7; discussion 167–8.

170. Bradley SM, Mosca RS, Hennein HA, et al. Bidirectional superior cavopulmonary connection in young infants. *Circulation* 1996;94:II5–II11.

171. Tanoue Y, Sese A, Ueno Y, et al. Bidirectional glenn procedure improves the mechanical efficiency of a total cavopulmonary connection in high-risk fontan candidates. *Circulation* 2001;103:2176–80.

172. Fogel MA, Weinberg PM, Chin AJ, et al. Late ventricular geometry and performance changes of functional single ventricle throughout staged Fontan reconstruction assessed by magnetic resonance imaging. *J Am Coll Cardiol* 1996;28:212–21.

173. Penny DJ, Redington AN. Diastolic ventricular function after the fontan operation. *Am J Cardiol* 1992;69:974–5.

174. Bradley SM, Simsic JM, Mulvihill DM. Hypoventilation improves oxygenation after bidirectional superior cavopulmonary connection. *J Thorac Cardiovasc Surg* 2003;126:1033–9.

175. Monagle P, Cochrane A, Roberts R, et al. A multicenter, randomized trial comparing heparin/warfarin and acetylsalicylic acid as primary thromboprophylaxis for 2 years after the Fontan procedure in children. *J Am Coll Cardiol* 2011;58:645–51.

176. Wald RM, Adatia I, Van Arsdell GS, et al LK. Relation of limiting ductal patency to survival in neonatal Ebstein's anomaly. *Am J Cardiol* 2005;96:851–6.

177. Starnes VA, Pitlick PT, Bernstein D, et al. Ebstein's anomaly appearing in the neonate. A new surgical approach. *J Thorac Cardiovasc Surg* 1991;101:1082–7.

178. Knott-Craig CJ, Goldberg SP, Overholt ED, et al. Repair of neonates and young infants with Ebstein's anomaly and related disorders. *Ann Thorac Surg* 2007;84:587–92; discussion 592–83.

179. Wernovsky G, Ghanayem N, Ohye RG, et al. Hypoplastic left heart syndrome: Consensus and controversies in 2007. *Cardiol Young* 2007;17(suppl 2):75–86.

180. Burstein DS, Rossi AF, Jacobs JP, et al. Variation in models of care delivery for children undergoing congenital heart surgery in the United States. *World J Pediatr Congenit Heart Surg* 2010;1:8–14.

CHAPTER 80 ■ PULMONARY HYPERTENSION

JOHN K. MCGUIRE, SILVIA HARTMANN, AND APICHAI KHONGPHATTHANAYOTHIN

KEY POINTS

1 The development of a pediatric pulmonary hypertension (PH) classification systems that incorporates considerations of lung growth and development and the mechanisms specific to children will improve understanding of outcomes and response to therapy in pediatric PH patients.

2 PH is rare in children but remains an important clinical problem in the pediatric ICU as a complication of congenital heart disease, acute lung disease, bronchopulmonary dysplasia, and several other disorders specific to children.

3 Treatment of acute and chronic PH in children is not based on evidence, but rather on extrapolation from adult studies, clinical experience, and consensus expert opinion.

4 Most medications used to treat PH are not approved for that indication in children.

5 The acute pulmonary hypertensive crisis is a medical emergency requiring prompt recognition, reversal of pulmonary vasoconstriction, support for the right ventricle, and treatment of the underlying cause, if possible.

6 Diagnosis, treatment, and long-term follow-up of children with PH require a multidisciplinary team with expertise in the special considerations unique to this special patient population.

Pulmonary hypertension (PH) can be simply defined as an abnormal elevation of the blood pressure in the pulmonary vascular circulation. However, PH has multiple possible etiologies, complex pathophysiology, and a variety of diagnostic and treatment options dependent on individual mechanisms of disease, clinical course, and responses to therapy. This chapter will discuss PH pathophysiology, diagnostic approaches, and treatment considerations of interest to the pediatric intensive care practitioner.

CLASSIFICATION

PH classification has been mainly based on clinical factors, and the most recent scheme is the Dana Point Classification of 2008 established at the 4th World Congress on Pulmonary Hypertension (**Table 80.1**) (1), which included both adult and pediatric patients and used the same *pulmonary arterial hypertension (PAH)* definition for both: mean pulmonary artery pressure ≥25 mm Hg, pulmonary capillary wedge pressure ≤15 mm Hg, and an increased pulmonary vascular resistance (PVR).

In this classification system, Group 1 encompasses etiologies of primary PH and includes idiopathic, familial, and anorexigen medication-induced PH. *Idiopathic pulmonary arterial hypertension* (IPAH) is the most common category in this group and is diagnosed when a patient has no family history of PH, mutations associated with hereditable PAH (HPAH), or identified PAH risk factors. PAH secondary to congenital heart disease and *persistent pulmonary hypertension of the newborn* (PPHN) are also included in Group 1. Groups 2, 3, 4, and 5 comprise what was historically designated as secondary PH. Group 2 describes patients with PH secondary to left-sided heart disease. Patients in this category often initially have pulmonary venous hypertension with elevated pulmonary arterial pressures (PAPs) with normal pulmonary vascular resistive indices (PVRI). Over time, remodeling of the pulmonary vasculature can lead to increased PVRI. An important subgroup

of these patients have PAP elevated out of proportion to the degree of left atrial hypertension and PVRI increase. Group 3 includes patients with PH secondary to lung disease (parenchymal or interstitial) or hypoxia. Hypoxia may be due to chronic upper airway obstruction, such as obstructive sleep apnea, or from low oxygen tension associated with living at high altitude. Group 4 describes patients with chronic thromboembolic PH. Pulmonary arteries are initially obstructed by either thrombus or embolus, and in some patients, there is incomplete resolution of the obstruction, leading to PH. Group 5 is a heterogeneous group of patients with PH from unclear or multifactorial etiologies.

In 2011, a new classification system was proposed that divided pediatric PH patients into 10 categories (**Table 80.2**, modification of Panama Classification) (2). This system attempts to incorporate mechanisms of PH seen more frequently in pediatric patients such as abnormalities of pulmonary development and postnatal pulmonary maladaptation. Notably, the *Panama Classification* uses the term "pulmonary hypertensive vascular disease" rather than "pulmonary hypertension" to specifically exclude children who have PH without increased PVR such as patients with systemic-to-pulmonary shunts. This distinction was made because the treatment of PH secondary to systemic-to-pulmonary shunt is closure of the shunt rather than treatment specifically targeting PAH.

Patients with PH are also classified by measures of the limits the disease places on the individual. This *functional classification*, such as used by the New York Heart Association (NYHA) system (3), has been shown to be a strong predictor of mortality in adult patients and is an important factor in choice of PAH therapy in both adults and children. However, adult classification systems are often less than ideal for use in children with PH, as several of the etiologies seen in children are not adequately considered, nor are developmental factors. Consequently, the Pediatric Task Force meeting in Panama also proposed an extensive functional classification based on age, physical growth, and maturation (4).

TABLE 80.1

WHO CLASSIFICATION OF PULMONARY HYPERTENSION (DANA POINT, 2008)

1.   Pulmonary arterial hypertension
1.1   Idiopathic PAH (IPAH)
1.2   Heritable PAH (HPAH)
1.2.1   Bone morphogenetic protein receptor type 2 (*BMPR2*) mutations
1.2.2   Activin receptor-like kinase (*ALK1*) and endoglin mutations
1.3   Drug- and toxin-induced
1.4   Associated with (APAH)
1.4.1   Connective tissue disease
1.4.2   HIV infection
1.4.3   Portal hypertension
1.4.4   Congenital heart disease
1.4.5   Schistosomiasis
1.4.6   Chronic hemolytic anemia
1.5   Persistent pulmonary hypertension of the newborn (PPHN)
1.6   Pulmonary veno-occlusive disease/pulmonary capillary hemagiomatosis
2.   Pulmonary hypertension due to left heart disease
2.1   Systolic dysfunction
2.2   Diastolic dysfunction
2.3   Valvular disease
3.   Pulmonary hypertension due to lung diseases and/or hypoxia
3.1   Chronic obstructive pulmonary disease
3.2   Interstitial lung disease
3.3   Other pulmonary disease with mixed restrictive and obstructive pattern
3.4   Sleep-disordered breathing
3.5   Alveolar hypoventilation disorders
3.6   Exposure to high altitude
3.7   Developmental abnormalities
4.   Chronic thromboembolic pulmonary hypertension
5.   Pulmonary hypertension with unclear multifactorial mechanisms
5.1   Hematologic disorders: myeloproliferative disorders
5.2   Systemic disorders: sarcoidosis, Langerhans cell histiocytosis, neurofibromatosis type 1, vasculitis
5.3   Metabolic disorders: glycogen storage disease, Gaucher disease, thyroid disorders
5.4   Other: obstruction by tumor mass, chronic renal failure on dialysis

Modified from Ivy D. Advances in pediatric pulmonary arterial hypertension. *Curr Opin Cardiol* 2012;27(2):70–81.

EPIDEMIOLOGY

Several registries describe the pediatric population with PH (5–10). The largest numbers of children with PH are those with transient disease processes, including PPHN and systemic-to-pulmonary shunts, accounting for 82% of patients in a single large registry (9). Most registries exclude patients with transient PH, and in the larger studies, the majority of the remaining patients, approximately 57%–70%, have PAH, either IPAH or HPAH (7,10). The second most common cause of progressive PAH in children is associated with congenital heart disease and comprises 24%–36% of cases, when excluding flow-related PH from systemic-to-pulmonary shunts. Patients with PH due to pulmonary diseases account for 11%–13% of cases, including 5% of patients who have

TABLE 80.2

PROPOSED CATEGORIZATION OF PEDIATRIC HYPERTENSIVE VASCULAR DISEASE

■ GROUP	■ EXAMPLES
1. Prenatal of developmental pulmonary hypertensive disease	■ Associated with oligohydramnios/pulmonary hypoplasia ■ Congenital diaphragmatic hernia ■ Alveolar capillary dysplasia ■ Lymphangiectasia ■ Associated with oligohydramnios/pulmonary hypoplasia
2. Perinatal pulmonary vascular maladaptation	■ Idiopathic PPHN ■ PPHN triggered by another disease process including sepsis or meconium aspiration syndrome ■ Associated with trisomy 21
3. Pediatric cardiovascular disease	■ Associated with systemic-to-pulmonary shunt with increased PVRI ■ Eisenmenger syndrome ■ After repair of TGA, left heart obstruction
4. Bronchopulmonary dysplasia	
5. Isolated pediatric pulmonary hypertensive vascular disease	■ IPAH ■ HPAH ■ Secondary to drug or toxin ■ PVOD/PCH
6. Multifactorial pulmonary hypertensive vascular disease in congenital malformation syndromes	■ Associated with VACTERL syndrome ■ Associated with CHARGE disease ■ Associated with DiGeorge disease ■ Associated with Scimitar complex
7. Pediatric lung disease	■ Associated with cystic fibrosis ■ Associated with sleep-disordered breathing ■ Associated with chest wall and spinal deformities ■ Associated with surfactant protein deficiency
8. Pediatric thromboembolic disease	Secondary to central venous catheters Associated with sickle cell disease Associated with methylmalonic acidemia and homocysteinuria Due to malignancy After splenectomy
9. Pediatric hypobaric hypoxic exposure	
10. Pediatric pulmonary vascular disease associated with other system disorders	■ Associated with portal hypertension ■ Associated with malignancy ■ Due to metabolic disorders ■ Due to autoimmune or autoinflammatory diseases ■ Due to infectious diseases (HIV, schistosomiasis, pulmonary TB) ■ Associated with chronic renal failure

PPHN, persistent pulmonary hypertension of the newborn; PVRI, pulmonary vascular resistance index; TGA, transposition of the great arteries; TOF, tetralogy of Fallot; IPAH, idiopathic pulmonary arterial hypertension; HPAH, heritable pulmonary arterial hypertension; PVOD, pulmonary veno-occlusive disease; PCH, pulmonary capillary hemangiomatosis.
Modified from Ivy D. Advances in pediatric pulmonary arterial hypertension. *Curr Opin Cardiol* 2012;27(2):70–81.

bronchopulmonary dysplasia and 1.4% who have obstructive sleep apnea as the cause of PH (6,10). Etiologies that are uncommon in pediatric patients include PH from connective tissue disease, HIV, drug exposure, and PH associated with portal hypertension.

Overall, chronic PAH is rare in children, with an incidence of approximately 3 cases/million children, especially when compared with the incidence of PPHN, which is approximately tenfold higher at about 30 cases/million children (9). The incidence of IPAH, the most common type of PAH, is 0.48–0.7 cases/million children with a prevalence estimated at 2.2–4.4 cases/million (7,9). A large national registry of more than 3000 pediatric patients with existing PH reported pulmonary hypertensive crises, defined as acute right ventricular failure plus signs of impaired systemic circulation, in 14%–17% of patients, and crises occurred most commonly in the postoperative setting or with upper respiratory infections (9). One study of more than 1000 pediatric patients after surgical repair of congenital heart defects demonstrated a 2% incidence of severe PH defined as systemic or suprasystemic RV pressure (11).

PATHOPHYSIOLOGY OF PH

The Pulmonary Vasculature

In PH, both the function and structure of the pulmonary vasculature are abnormal (Fig. 80.1). Independent of etiology, PH in children is a combination of vasoconstriction, inflammation, structural remodeling of the pulmonary vessels, *in situ* thrombosis, and impaired vascular growth (12,13). Cell types that play key roles in acute and chronic PH include endothelial cells, smooth muscle cells, inflammatory cells, and platelets, and imbalances between the production of endogenous vasodilators and vasoconstrictors contribute to excess pulmonary vasoconstriction (14).

The earliest change is often excessive vasoconstriction of the pulmonary arteriole in the setting of hypoxia. The mechanism is not fully elucidated but likely involves decreased vascular smooth muscle expression and activity of Kv1.5 potassium channels that close in response to hypoxia, leading to depolarization, calcium entry into the pulmonary vascular smooth muscle cell, and vasoconstriction (15). Pulmonary vascular smooth muscle cells in patients with PH may also have increased sensitivity to intracellular calcium from increased activity of Rho A/Rho kinase (ROK) leading to increased vasoconstriction (16).

Histopathological changes in the pulmonary vasculature can involve all layers of the blood vessel wall; however, the vascular wall medial smooth muscle cell is the primary cell type implicated in pathological vascular remodeling (13). In infants with PH, smooth muscle hypertrophy within the vessel media may be the only histological abnormality. Smooth muscle cells may also extend into arterioles that normally do not have a muscular media such as those at the level of the respiratory bronchioles and alveolar ducts. Intimal thickening occurs due to abnormal proliferation of endothelial cells, likely in response to abnormal production of, and altered cellular responses to, growth factors. The endothelial cells in patients with PH produce increased amounts of vasoconstrictors, including endothelin-1 and serotonin (5-HT), while producing decreased amounts of vasodilators, such as nitric oxide and prostacyclin, leading to an imbalance that results in increased PVR (13). In severe disease, endothelial cells may proliferate within the lumen of pulmonary blood vessels to form plexiform lesions that cause vessel obstruction (12).

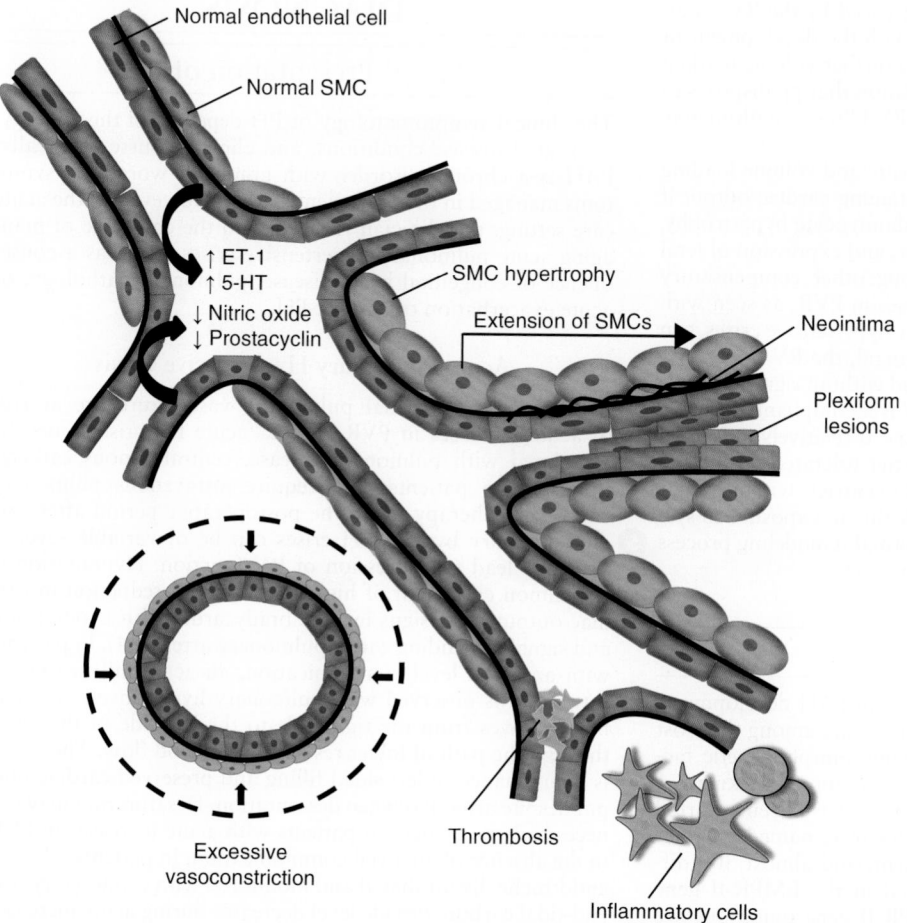

FIGURE 80.1. Pathophysiology of pulmonary hypertension: PH can be due to abnormal function of the pulmonary vasculature with excessive vasoconstriction, increased elaboration of vasoconstricting agents such as endothelin-1 and serotonin as well as decreased production of nitric oxide and prostacyclin from the endothelial cells. Smooth muscle hypertrophy and extension of smooth muscle cells onto arterioles that generally lack musculature also contributes to pulmonary hypertension. In some diseases processes, plexiform lesions, monoclonal expansion of endothelial cells, can obstruct the lumen of pulmonary blood vessels. Chronic thrombosis of pulmonary vasculature and ongoing inflammation of the pulmonary parenchyma can also contribute to increased pulmonary vascular resistance in some instances. SMC, smooth muscle cell; ET-1, endothelin-1; 5-HT, serotonin.

Labels in figure: Normal endothelial cell; Normal SMC; ↑ ET-1 ↑ 5-HT ↓ Nitric oxide ↓ Prostacyclin; SMC hypertrophy; Extension of SMCs; Neointima; Plexiform lesions; Excessive vasoconstriction; Thrombosis; Inflammatory cells

Additional structural changes include increases in fibroblasts and extracellular matrix between the endothelium and the internal elastic lamina, forming a "neointima." Increased adventitial thickness can be seen in patients with PPHN but is unusual in patients with other forms of PH. A reduced cross-sectional area of the vascular bed may be a result of reduced formation of blood vessels due to abnormal angiogenesis or from obstruction of blood vessels by *in situ* thromboses that form in the setting of an abnormal endothelium or in response to inflammatory mediators (13,17). Variable degrees of pulmonary inflammation may contribute to the structural and functional abnormalities in PAH. Cytokines and chemokines may act to promote smooth muscle hypertrophy and increased circulating levels of stromal-derived factor 1 (SDF-1), monocyte chemoattractant protein 1 (MCP-1), and IL-6 have been found in sera of PAH patients (13).

The Right Ventricle in PH

PH increases RV afterload, leading to decreased stroke volume and increased RV end-diastolic blood volume (18). Initial compensatory mechanisms (e.g., Starling response) increase stroke volume in response to cardiomyocyte stretching. However, over time this mechanism is inadequate and to minimize loading of individual cardiomyocytes, the RV hypertrophies. The thickened RV requires a higher filling pressure for the same end-diastolic volume to maintain pulmonary blood flow in the setting of diastolic dysfunction. Neurohormonal mechanisms, including the renin-angiotensin-aldosterone system, are activated to increase circulating blood volume and maintain cardiac output. The increased RV blood volume leads to septal flattening, which not only decreases LV filling and cardiac output by increasing LV end-diastolic pressure, but also decreases the LV assistance in ejecting blood from the RV, thereby exacerbating the volume overload experienced by the RV. Eventual dilation of the RV is associated with the development of tricuspid regurgitation, which leads to further volume loading of the strained RV, and right atrial dilation that predisposes to atrial arrhythmias, which can impair RV filling and ultimately cardiac output (18,19).

Adaptive mechanisms for the pressure and volume loading of the RV are more effective in maintaining cardiac output if PH develops slowly, allowing for cardiomyocyte hypertrophy, increased myocardial connective tissue, and expression of fetal myocardial contractile proteins among other compensatory changes. In comparison, acute increases in PVR, as seen with large pulmonary emboli or pulmonary hypertensive crises, can cause acute RV systolic failure. In general, the RV tolerates a volume load better than a pressure load without significant impairment of cardiac output as the RV is a compliant structure that is able to tolerate increased volume at relatively preserved end-diastolic pressures. PH is also better tolerated during the neonatal period. Neonates have a right ventricle with a similar free wall thickness as the left ventricle due to exposure to systemic pressure *in utero* prior to the normal remodeling process that leads to right ventricular wall thinning.

Genetics

Genetic factors play an important role in PAH development, and TGF-β superfamily protein mutations are among the most important thus far identified (14). Bone morphogenetic factor receptor type-II (BMPR-II), activin receptor-like kinase 1 (ALK-1), and endoglin receptor mutations have been reported (20). The bone morphogenetic proteins were named for their role in bone and cartilage development, and almost 300 different mutations have been identified in the BMPR-II gene found on chromosome 2 (21). BMPR-II gene mutations are the most common identified genetic cause of PAH and have been found in 50%–90% of adults with HPAH. BMPR-II is usually expressed in both pulmonary vascular smooth muscle and endothelial cells, and BMPR-II protein expression is significantly lower in patients with *BMPR2* gene mutations. Reduced BMPR-II function leads to increased pulmonary vascular smooth muscle cell proliferation in response to receptor ligands TGF-β and BMP2, in contrast to people with wild-type BMPR-II proteins who demonstrate inhibition of pulmonary vascular smooth muscle cell proliferation with receptor activation (22). Although mutations in the *BMPR2* gene are inherited in an autosomal-dominant manner, there is incomplete penetrance, ranging from 15%–80%, depending on the specific mutation (20,21). Presence of a BMPR-II mutation is associated with an overall 10%–20% lifetime risk of developing PAH, with other gene interactions or environmental triggers that likely contribute to development of disease.

PH in Acute Lung Disease

PH as a consequence of increased PVR is commonly present in severe lung disease associated with acute lung injury/ARDS, bronchiolitis, pertussis, and other acute pulmonary pathologies, and if associated with RV dysfunction or failure, may be of significant clinical importance. The pathophysiological changes that occur in the pulmonary vasculature in acute lung disease include endothelial dysfunction, pulmonary vascular occlusion, increased vasomotor tone (including hypoxic vasoconstriction), extrinsic pulmonary capillary compression, and, in late stages of lung disease, vascular remodeling (23). A more complete discussion of PH in lung disease is provided in Chapters 47, 49, and 50.

DIAGNOSIS

Clinical Presentation of PH

The clinical symptomatology of PH depends on the etiology, associated disease conditions, and clinical course. Typically, PAH is a chronic disorder with gradually worsening symptoms managed in the outpatient setting. However, in the acute care setting, the clinician is faced with the challenge of managing acute pulmonary hypertensive crises, often as a consequence of congenital heart disease, pulmonary pathology, or acute exacerbation of chronic PH.

Acute Pulmonary Hypertensive Crisis

Patients with abnormal pulmonary vasculature are at risk of acute increases in PVR. These "acute PH crises" may be associated with pulmonary disease, central venous catheter infections in patients who require intravenous pulmonary vasodilator therapy, or in the postoperative period after cardiopulmonary bypass. PH crises can be of variable severity and may lead to depression of RV function. Hypotension is a common early sign of high PVR-induced reduction in cardiac output. Late signs include bradycardia with hypotension and signal impending cardiopulmonary arrest (24). In patients with an atrial level communication, an acute fall in oxygen saturation is observed with pulmonary hypertensive crises as blood moves from the right side to the left side of the heart through the path of lower resistance to blood flow. The result is maintenance of left-sided filling and preserved cardiac output despite arterial oxygen desaturation. Desaturation may not necessarily be evident in patients with acute increases in PVR in the absence of an atrial communication. In patients who are endotracheally intubated and monitored with capnometry, the end-tidal carbon dioxide level decreases during acute increases in PVR as a consequence of reduced pulmonary blood flow. Accordingly, there will be an increase in the arterial to end-tidal carbon dioxide difference as a consequence of increased dead space ventilation. An acute increase in central venous pressure is also expected with acute increases in right ventricular end-diastolic pressure. During a pulmonary hypertensive crisis, increased intensity of a systolic murmur from worsening tricuspid regurgitation and increased hepatomegaly compared with baseline exam may be appreciated.

Chronic PH

Symptoms of chronic PAH are mainly due to the inability to increase cardiac output on exertion. The most common presenting symptom, dyspnea on exertion, has been noted in approximately 65%–75% of patients (7,9,10). Seven percent to 20% of patients have a history of syncope and another 8% have a history of near syncope that reflects cerebral hypoperfusion due to inadequate cardiac output in the setting of exercise. Cyanosis with exercise is reported in 16%–18% of patients and pallor with exertion in 5%. Patients with increasingly severe disease can present with signs of inadequate cardiac output at rest. One study found 11% of patients had dyspnea at rest and 12% had cyanosis at rest (10).

Signs of RV dysfunction may be apparent on physical examination. Auscultation may reveal a loud pulmonic component of the second heart sound (P2) that is associated with high pulmonary artery pressure. Over time, the intensity of P2 may diminish if right ventricular function and right-sided cardiac output worsens. An early systolic or holosystolic murmur may be heard at the left lower sternal border consistent with tricuspid regurgitation as well as an early diastolic murmur indicative of pulmonary insufficiency. Older children may have increased jugular venous pressure noted on inspection of the neck. Abdominal exam can reveal hepatomegaly and ascites, and peripheral edema may be evident on inspection of the extremities.

A comprehensive presentation of the diagnostic approach to children with clinical suspicion of chronic PAH is beyond the scope of this chapter. In general, it is similar to that recommended for adults and is extensively covered in several excellent reviews (1,14). Thus, the discussion here will focus on diagnostic strategies relevant to the pediatric intensive care setting.

PH Diagnostic Evaluation

Electrocardiogram

The electrocardiogram (ECG) may have findings consistent with PH. Almost 80% of patients with IPAH demonstrate right atrial enlargement and 87% demonstrate right ventricular hypertrophy on ECG (6). Additionally, evidence of right ventricular strain may be present.

Echocardiogram

Echocardiography is mandatory in any patient who is suspected to have PH from history and/or physical examination. It is noninvasive, portable, and these features make echocardiography an excellent initial diagnostic tool to assess: (a) presence and severity of PH, (b) RV function, and (c) presence of left heart disease and/or congenital heart disease.

Peak right ventricular systolic pressure (RVSP) can be estimated by the maximal Doppler velocity of the tricuspid valve regurgitation (TR) jet. Using a simplified Bernoulli equation, the RVSP would be equal to $4V^2 + RAP$, where V is the peak velocity of the TR jet and RAP is the mean right atrial pressure (25). Diastolic pulmonary arterial pressure (dPAP) can be estimated by measuring the end-diastolic velocity of pulmonary

regurgitation jet in the same manner. Estimation of the RVSP by TR is problematic when TR is trivial or absent. In a patient with ventricular septal defect (VSD) or patent ductus arteriosus (PDA), RV pressure can be estimated by measuring the peak flow velocity across the VSD or PDA. In absence of these defects, one can gain insight into the pulmonary vascular pressure by visualizing the position of the interventricular septum with the heart in short-axis view (26,27). In the setting of significant PH, the interventricular septum moves leftward, giving the appearance of a D-shaped left ventricle.

Right ventricular size and function can also be assessed by echocardiography. Presence and severity of tricuspid and pulmonary valve regurgitation can be assessed as well as other abnormalities that may be related to PH, such as presence of a pulmonary embolus in the proximal pulmonary artery. Presence of left heart disease must be evaluated in any patient with PH since the treatment and prognosis are very different from PAH. These diseases include various forms of cardiomyopathy, structural heart diseases causing obstruction to left ventricular inflow (e.g., mitral stenosis), cor triatriatum, and pulmonary vein stenosis. The possibility of a congenital heart defect causing left-to-right shunt should also be carefully evaluated.

Cardiac Catheterization

Patients suspected to have group 1 PH (PAH) should undergo cardiac catheterization to define the presence and severity of PH and to rule out anatomic causes of PH that may not be obvious from noninvasive evaluation. Patients with IPAH should also undergo cardiac catheterization for vasoreactivity testing to identify those patients who may benefit from a trial of treatment with calcium channel blockers (CCB) (1,28). To rule out PH from left heart disease (group 2 PH), a left atrial pressure (LAP) or pulmonary arterial wedge pressure (PAWP) should be determined. Any patient with LAP or PAWP exceeding 15 mm Hg would qualify for the diagnosis of PH secondary to left-sided heart disease.

Vasoreactivity Testing

Acute pulmonary vasoreactivity testing is done in the cardiac catheterization laboratory by using a short-acting pulmonary vasodilator such as nitric oxide, epoprostenol, or adenosine. A positive response is defined in adult patients as a reduction in mean PAP at least 10 mm Hg below baseline with a final PAP $\leq$ 40 mm Hg (1,28). In pediatric practice, a conventional definition of a positive response is a fall in mean PAP and PVRI by 20% with and no change or an increase in cardiac output (29). Approximately 40% of children with idiopathic PAH demonstrated pulmonary vasoreactivity as opposed to 10%–26% in adults (30–32). Approximately half of the patients who demonstrated pulmonary vascular reactivity responded well to treatment with long-term CCB therapy (30,32).

Imaging

Plain x-ray films of the chest may show an enlarged cardiac silhouette due to right ventricular hypertrophy in the setting of long-standing PH. The central pulmonary arteries can appear enlarged in the setting of acute or chronic PH. The lung fields can also demonstrate reduced vascularity consistent with decreased pulmonary blood flow. High-resolution computed tomography (CT) scanning of the chest is helpful for excluding pulmonary causes of PH such as interstitial lung disease or emphysema. It can also be used to diagnose pulmonary veno-occlusive disease and pulmonary capillary hemangiomatosis (1). CT pulmonary angiography can be used to diagnose pulmonary thromboembolism (33). Ventilation-perfusion (V/Q) scanning is also useful for evaluating the possibility of pulmonary thromboembolic disease, and a positive V/Q scan should be followed by a method of pulmonary angiography and a coagulopathy evaluation (28). Cardiac magnetic resonance imaging (MRI) may be superior to echocardiography for determining right ventricular volume and contraction and may be used for follow-up of patients with PAH on chronic therapy (34).

Lung Biopsy

In most patients, noninvasive tests and cardiac catheterization are sufficient to determine the etiology and severity of PH. Because of the potential morbidity and mortality associated with the procedure, lung biopsy is generally not required for the initial diagnostic work-up (35). It may be considered in patients who are suspected to have pulmonary veno-occlusive disease, undiagnosed parenchymal lung disease, or in certain patients with congenital heart disease in whom clinical and hemodynamic data are concerning for safety of cardiac surgical repair, as the presence of a severe arteriopathy on lung biopsy may influence the surgical repair strategy (1,36,37). As with any PH patient undergoing general anesthesia or sedation for a procedure, performing lung biopsy in the child with severe PH should be undertaken in a center with specialized expertise (38).

TREATMENT

Because PH is relatively rare in the pediatric age group and diagnosis and treatment require a multidisciplinary approach, the care of these children is usually done in regional tertiary centers with dedicated expertise in pediatric PH. Treatment for patients with an identifiable cause for PH is directed at elimination of the trigger for PH. In those patients in whom the cause is unknown or cannot be eliminated, treatment is targeted at lowering the PAP, supporting RV function, and treating heart failure symptoms such as dyspnea or edema. In adult patients, treatment recommendations are based on evidence (1), whereas in pediatric patients, treatment strategies for acute and chronic pulmonary hypertension have largely been based on extrapolation from adult studies, clinical experience, and consensus of expert opinion (14).

In general, patients with PAH are admitted to the intensive care unit when there is acute decompensation with RV failure and/or syncope. In children with congenital heart disease, PH may be a significant problem in the postoperative period (see Chapter 79). Regardless of cause, cardiovascular decompensation due to an acute pulmonary hypertensive crisis is a medical emergency with the following goals for treatment: (a) recognize that PH is present, (b) prevent or reverse acute pulmonary vasoconstriction (Fig. 80.2), (c) support the failure RV, and (d) treat the underlying cause, if possible. Untreated, an acute pulmonary hypertensive crisis can lead to acute RV failure and complete cardiovascular collapse, and once cardiac arrest ensues, resuscitation outcomes are poor and death is likely (39).

Oxygen and General Supportive Measures

Oxygen has pulmonary vasodilatory effects and should be given to treat hypoxemia or as an adjunct to pulmonary vasodilators. The child should be kept calm to minimize increases in endogenous circulating catecholamines. Noninvasive positive pressure ventilation (NIPPV) may have a role in augmenting oxygenation, treating hypoventilation, providing LV afterload reduction, and reducing work of breathing. However, the benefit of NIPPV must be balanced against its limitations, including increasing patient anxiety and delay of initiation of invasive mechanical ventilation. In the setting of acute right heart failure, inotropic medications such as dobutamine and/or

milrinone can be used to support RV function. Diuretics are used to treat congestive symptoms with careful titration to avoid excessive reduction in intravascular volume, which can decrease preload and further decrease cardiac output and impair renal function.

The decision to intubate a patient is made on an individual patient basis. Invasive mechanical ventilation may offer benefits of providing maximal inspired oxygen concentration, controlling ventilation, facilitating delivery of inhaled nitric oxide, and enabling liberal use of sedation without concern for respiratory depression. However, it must be kept in mind that the intubation and initiation of invasive mechanical ventilation is a high-risk procedure in the patient with acute pulmonary hypertensive decompensation. Anesthetic agents may depress respiration and exacerbate hypoventilation and respiratory acidosis, and vasodilatation may reduce preload and further impair RV output. Thus, close attention must be paid to monitoring hemodynamic status, maintaining preload, and making preparations for institution of resuscitative measures.

Hyperventilation is useful for a severe, acute pulmonary hypertensive crisis in an intubated patient because it can be rapidly performed at the bedside. However, aggressive hyperventilation can cause decreased venous return, alveolar over distention and lung injury, as well as cerebral vasoconstriction; hence, it should be used sparingly and an extreme drop of $Paco_2$ should be avoided (40,41). Hypoxic pulmonary vasoconstriction occurs in atelectatic lung regions and lung over distention can compress alveolar pulmonary blood vessels, further contributing to elevated PVR. Thus, optimal lung volume should be maintained by the use of proper positive endexpiratory pressure (PEEP) and aggressive treatment of the factors that may contribute to lung collapse such as pleural effusion, pneumothorax, or airway obstruction.

Inhaled Nitric Oxide

Nitric oxide (NO) is produced endogenously by vascular endothelium and mediates vasodilatation by causing increased $3'$-$5'$-cyclic guanosine monophosphate (cGMP) within the vascular smooth muscle cells (42). Given by inhalation, NO diffuses through alveolar endothelium of well-ventilated lung regions and causes relaxation of pulmonary vascular smooth muscle. After entering the blood stream, NO is rapidly inactivated by hemoglobin within red blood cells, thus causing minimal systemic side effects. Lack of a significant systemic vasodilatory effect makes inhaled nitric oxide an ideal agent for the critically ill patient with PH. Accumulation of nitrogen dioxide (NO_2) and methemoglobin are the primary potential toxicities associated with its use, though in clinical practice, accumulation of these products is rarely dose limiting.

In an intubated patient, inhaled NO (iNO) is given by a delivery system with automatic adjustment of the gas output based on the concentration of NO measured in the inhaled gas just before entering the endotracheal tube in the inspiratory limb of the ventilator circuit. The range of concentrations used is 1–80 ppm, titrating to the pulmonary vasodilatory effect. The lowest effective dose should be used and the upper limit is usually not more than 20–30 ppm (40,43–46). Abrupt withdrawal or interruption of iNO may aggravate rebound PH; hence, the dose should be gradually decreased to a minimum before discontinuation (43,45,47,48). A system to deliver NO manually should be available for transporting the patient or when there is a technical problem with the ventilator or the delivery system to avoid abrupt termination of iNO administration.

Clinical trials of iNO for treatment of acute PH in children have been done primarily in neonates with PPHN and in children with PH after surgery for congenital heart disease

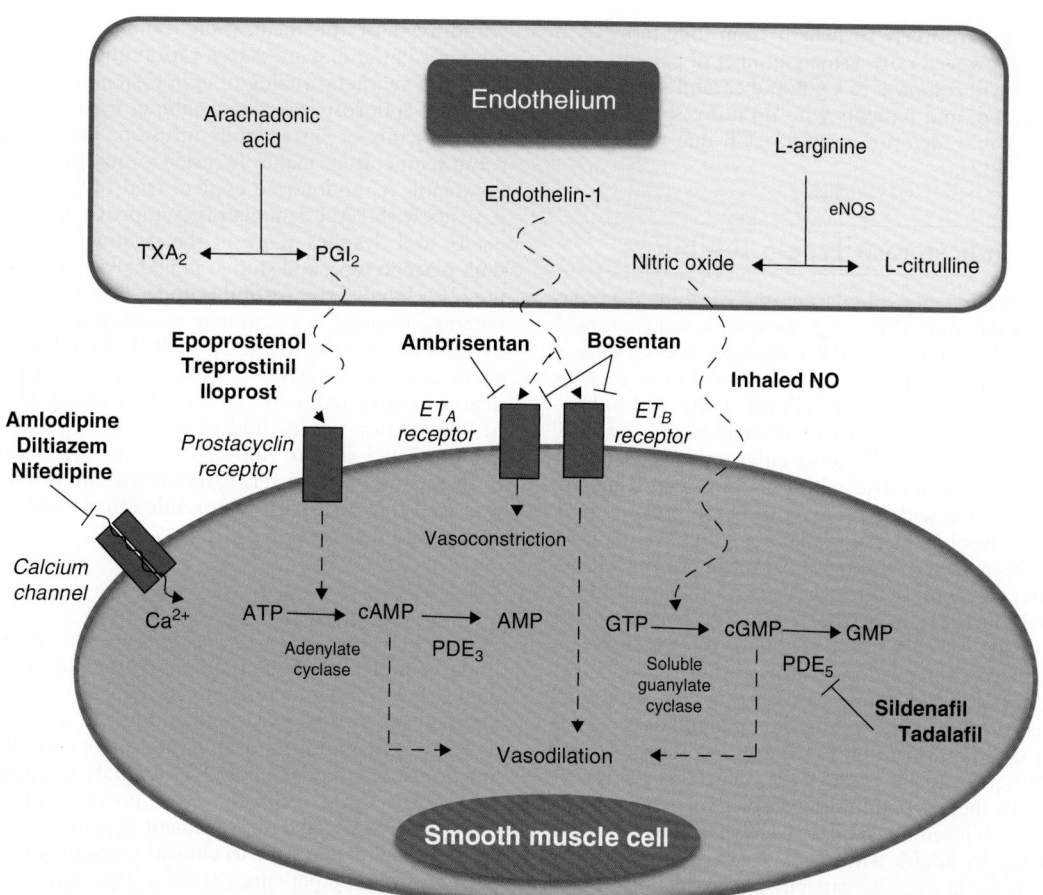

FIGURE 80.2. Pulmonary hypertension pharmacology. Activation of the prostacyclin receptor by endogenous prostacyclin or agonists (epoprostenol, treprostinil, or iloprost) increases the formation of cAMP from adenosine triphosphate (ATP) by enhancing activity of the enzyme adenylate cyclase, which ultimately leads to vasodilation. Endothelial cells also produce endothelin-1, which binds to two types of endothelin receptors on the smooth muscle cell—ETA receptors that lead to smooth muscle cell contraction and ETB receptors that promotes smooth muscle cell relaxation. Bosentan is a nonselective endothelin receptor antagonist and ambrisentan is selective for the ETA receptor and both cause vasodilation by inhibiting the action of endothelin-1. Nitric oxide is elaborated in the endothelial cell and diffuses into the smooth muscle cell where it leads to vasodilation by increasing the production of cGMP through increased activity of soluble guanylate cyclase. Inhaled nitric oxide acts by the same mechanism. Extracellular calcium enters smooth muscle cells through calcium channels and participates in vasoconstriction, which is inhibited by various calcium channel blockers. Sildenafil and Tadalafil inhibit the enzyme PDE5 and thereby increase intracellular cGMP leading to vasodilation. TXA2, thromboxane; PGI2, prostacyclin; eNOS, endothelial nitric oxide synthase; ETA receptor, Endothelin A receptor; ETB receptor, Endothelin B receptor; ATP, adenosine triphosphate; cAMP, cyclic adenosine monophosphate; AMP, adenosine monophosphate; GTP, guanosine triphosphate; cGMP, cyclic guanosine monophosphate; GMP, guanosine monophosphate; PDE3, phosphodiesterase 3; PDE5, phosphodiesterase 5.

(40,44,46,49,50). Nitric oxide has been shown to improve oxygenation and decrease the incidence of ECMO use in term newborns with hypoxic respiratory failure and PPHN, excluding patients with congenital diaphragmatic hernia (44). Given prophylactically in patients deemed at high risk of developing postoperative PH, iNO may decrease the incidence of postoperative PH crises compared with placebo (46). In a study in patients who have already developed postoperative PH, iNO similarly decreased PAP and PVR compared with conventional treatment (hyperventilation) but without the detrimental effects on cardiac preload and cardiac output associated with hyperventilation (40). Whereas iNO appears to have a clinical role in postoperative PH, a Cochrane analysis did not find evidence of effect of iNO on the outcomes reviewed including mortality, number of pulmonary hypertensive crises, or hemodynamic parameters in children after surgery for congenital heart disease (50).

PH associated with acute lung disease is associated with increased mortality (51), and although acute iNO therapy may transiently improve gas exchange and lower PVR, its use has not reduced mortality in large adult studies of lung injury (52,53). Nitric oxide therapy has been shown to be beneficial in PPHN (discussed below) in neonates, but whether iNO should be used in other pediatric patient populations with acute lung disease remains to be determined.

Calcium Channel Blockers

Despite the lack of randomized clinical trials, calcium channel blockers (CCB) such as nifedipine, diltiazem, and amlodipine have been used successfully to treat adults and children with idiopathic PAH for many years (30–32). In general, a positive response on acute pulmonary vasoreactivity testing may predict those who are likely to benefit from long-term CCB therapy (1,30). However, only a small number of patients with idiopathic PAH will response to CCB and careful selection of patients is required, and patients who do not respond to vasodilator testing may deteriorate with CCB due to negative inotropic effects (32).

Phosphodiesterase Type-5 Inhibitors

The cyclic nucleotide phosphodiesterases catalyze degradation of cyclic AMP and GMP, and phosphodiesterase type-5 (PDE5) specifically degrades cGMP in vascular smooth muscle cells. Inhibition of this enzyme by PDE5 inhibitors such as sildenafil results in increased intracellular cGMP and pulmonary vasodilatation. Given orally or intravenously, sildenafil has been shown to reduce PAP and vascular resistance, and the effect is additive to that of nitric oxide (54–56). Acute sildenafil use may be associated with a decrease in blood pressure and/or an increased alveolar-arterial gradient and hypoxemia (54). Sildenafil has been used in the acute PH setting to prevent rebound PH after cessation of nitric oxide (57,58). Sildenafil has also been used to treat term newborn with PPHN in countries where nitric oxide is either not available or too expensive. A recent randomized controlled trial showed that sildenafil improved oxygen index and decreased mortality compared with placebo (59). Another PDE5 inhibitor, tadalafil received US Food and Drug Administration (FDA) approval in the United States in 2009 and can be dosed daily, which may improve compliance with therapy, and initial studies suggest hemodynamic effects in children are similar to sildenafil (60,61).

Sildenafil use in adults with PAH was associated with a significant increase in exercise capacity and reduction of PAP compared with placebo (62,63), and sildenafil is approved by the FDA for use in adult WHO Group 1 PAH patients. A randomized control trial in children with PAH demonstrated improvement in exercise capacity and hemodynamic data in patients taking medium or high doses compared with placebo (64). Although chronic use of sildenafil in children with PAH was generally well tolerated with mild to moderate side effects, such as headache, pyrexia, increased upper respiratory tract infection, vomiting, and diarrhea (64), long-term outcome data showed that high dose sildenafil was associated with higher rates of death, prompting the FDA to issue a warning on prescribing sildenafil to children with PAH. This warning has engendered controversy in the field, as overall mortality rates in the study were lower than historical comparisons. Thus, sildenafil should be used cautiously in children with PH, and particularly for long-term use in children with PAH.

Prostacyclins

Prostacyclin (PGI$_2$) is produced by vascular endothelial cells and exerts vasodilatory effects by increasing 3′-5′-cyclic adenosine monophosphate (cAMP) within vascular smooth muscle cells. Synthetic prostacyclin analogs that have been used to treat PH include epoprostenol, treprostinil, and iloprost. Epoprostenol was the first synthetic prostacyclin approved by the FDA to treat PAH and is currently the drug of choice for IPAH patients with WHO/NYAS functional class IV (1). Because of a short half-life (3–5 minutes), epoprostenol is administered by continuous intravenous infusion. In a randomized controlled trial, epoprostenol improved exercise capacity, quality of life, and survival in patients with idiopathic PAH (65). Side effects are frequent but minor, such as jaw pain, flushing, diarrhea, headache, nausea, and vomiting (65). Long-term side effects are often related to the delivery system such as catheter infection or obstruction and pump malfunction. Abrupt

withdrawal of the medication has been reported to cause rebound PH and acute deterioration and death (29). Treprostinil is a synthetic analog of epoprostenol with a longer half-life than epoprostenol, thus enabling it to be given either by subcutaneous or intravenous infusion. Increased stability at room temperature makes it easier to mix and store than epoprostenol. A randomized control trial of treprostinil in adult patients with PAH demonstrated improvement in exercise capacity and dyspnea score in the treatment group compared with placebo (66), and studies in pediatric patients are promising (29). Inhaled treprostinil is under investigation in pediatric patients. Iloprost is a synthetic prostacyclin analog approved by the FDA for the treatment of PAH by inhalation. In studies of acute use, inhaled iloprost decreased PVR to a similar degree as nitric oxide (67,68). Small randomized control trials of inhaled iloprost in children with PH after cardiac surgery demonstrated similar clinical effects as nitric oxide (69,70). In these studies, short-term administration of inhaled iloprost was well tolerated with minor side effects such as headache, cough, and dizziness.

Endothelin Receptor Antagonists

Endothelin (ET) mediates pulmonary vasoconstriction and also possesses pro-inflammatory effects, which are thought to be the mechanisms by which elevated endothelin activity contributes to PAH. Bosentan is an oral, nonselective endothelin receptor antagonist that binds to both ET$_A$ and ET$_B$ receptors. Randomized control trials of chronic use of bosentan in various forms of PAH demonstrated improvement in hemodynamic data, exercise capacity, and time to clinical worsening compared with placebo in adult patients (71–75). The most significant side effect was dose-dependent elevation of liver transaminases in approximately 10% of patients. These changes were reversible after treatment discontinuation or dose reduction. Other side effects include anemia and peripheral edema. Bosentan has not been approved for use in children with PAH in the United States. However, pediatric studies have suggested safety and efficacy (76), and a pediatric formulation has been approved for use in Europe. Ambrisentan is a selective ET$_A$ receptor that is administered once daily and that shows reduced risk of liver toxicity compared with bosentan; however, data on ambrisentan use in children remain limited (77).

Atrial Septostomy

In patients with severe, refractory PH, creation of a small hole in an atrial septum permits right-to-left atrial shunting at the time when the right ventricle is unable to pump against increased pulmonary pressure. This right-to-left shunt maintains left ventricular preload and output at the expense of increased arterial hypoxemia. Because of the palliative nature and the risks associated with the procedure, it is usually reserved for those with severe heart failure refractory to medical therapy with severe syncopal symptoms and/or while awaiting lung transplantation or when medical therapy such as prostacyclin analog infusion is not available (1,78,79).

Transplantation

Single lung, double lung, or heart–lung transplantation has been used for pediatric patients with PH refractory to other therapies. Between 1990 and 2012, the Registry of the International Society for Heart and Lung Transplantation reported 163 lung transplants performed worldwide for IPAH, the second leading indication for lung transplant in children after cystic fibrosis (80). In children below age 6 years, IPAH was the most common diagnosis for children receiving lung transplant in this time period. The overall 5-year survival was 49% for children receiving lung transplants between 1990 and 2011. Among survivors, functional status was generally good, with 86% of children having no physician-reported activity limitation at 5 years after transplant. Because of the palliative nature of lung transplantation, it is reserved for patients with severe symptoms who are deemed to have poor prognosis despite maximal medical therapy.

PERSISTENT PH OF THE NEWBORN

PPHN occurs mainly in term or late preterm infants and is the result of failure of PVR to fall at birth leading to right-to-left shunting of desaturated blood through a patent foramen ovale and/or ductus arteriosus (81). Mechanisms proposed in idiopathic PPHN include impaired nitric oxide production that occurs in response to the shear stress of lung expansion, failure of arteriolar smooth muscle cell thinning, and the presence of increased extracellular matrix in the pulmonary vasculature that impairs blood vessel distensibility, leading to poor accommodation of the increase in pulmonary blood flow that occurs at birth. Alternatively, PPHN may be associated with primary or secondary lung injury or lung hypoplasia. Treatment of infants with PPHN involves mechanical ventilation with sedation and possibly neuromuscular blockade, inhaled nitric oxide, and high-frequency oscillatory ventilation. Extracorporeal membranous oxygenation (ECMO) has been used successfully to support oxygenation and minimize lung injury in infants refractory to mechanical ventilation until PVR falls. A comprehensive analysis of the ELSO registry reported 81% survival in neonates with PPHN receiving ECMO (82). Sildenafil has been used in resource-limited areas with improved survival of infants with PPHN (59). To date, there have been inadequate quality and quantity of studies to recommend use of magnesium sulfate or milrinone for patients with PPHN (83,84). Patients with PH secondary to irreversible lung dysplasia can present in a manner similar to infants with PPHN. However, these diagnoses are almost universally fatal, and a report from the ECLS Registry reported that a need for initiation of ECLS on or after day 5 of life and duration of ECLS therapy for greater than or equal to 10 days were predictors of the presence of an irreversible lung dysplasia (85).

CONCLUSIONS

In the past two decades, great progress has been made in advancing the understanding of the biology, epidemiology, diagnosis, and treatment of PH in children. The elaboration of a pediatric-specific PH classification system that incorporates considerations of lung growth and development will improve understanding of outcomes and response to therapy in pediatric PH patients. In the pediatric intensive care unit, acute pulmonary hypertensive crises remain a challenging problem. Estimates of 1-year survival after diagnosis of PH are between 86% and 97%, 3-year survival between 80% and 97%, and 5-year survival between 72% and 78% (10). In general, patients with PH associated with congenital heart disease have a better prognosis than those with IPAH. Newer pulmonary vasodilator medications offer the promise of improved survival, reduction in impact of disease, with fewer side effects in both acute and chronic PH. However, despite the increasingly widespread use of pulmonary vasodilator medications, few are approved for use in treating PH in children, and thus long-term studies of these medications in children are urgently needed. A well-coordinated, multidisciplinary approach that incorporates an understanding of patient pathophysiology, rational escalation of therapy, and close follow-up is likely to provide the best opportunity for improved outcomes in individual patients faced with this challenging clinical problem.

References

1. Galie N, Hoeper MM, Humbert M, et al. Guidelines for the diagnosis and treatment of pulmonary hypertension: The Task Force for the Diagnosis and Treatment of Pulmonary Hypertension of the European Society of Cardiology (ESC) and the European Respiratory Society (ERS), endorsed by the International Society of Heart and Lung Transplantation (ISHLT). *Eur Heart J* 2009;30(20):2493–537.

2. Cerro MJ, Abman S, Diaz G, et al. A consensus approach to the classification of pediatric pulmonary hypertensive vascular disease: Report from the PVRI Pediatric Taskforce, Panama 2011. *Pulm Circ* 2011;1(2):286–98.

3. Association CCotNYH. *Nomenclature and Criteria for Diagnosis of Diseases of the Heart and Great Vessels.* 9th ed. Boston, MA: Little, Brown, 1994.

4. Lammers AE, Adatia I, Cerro MJ, et al. Functional classification of pulmonary hypertension in children: Report from the PVRI pediatric taskforce, Panama 2011. *Pulm Circ* 2011;1(2):280–5.

5. Barst RJ, McGoon MD, Elliott CG, et al. Survival in childhood pulmonary arterial hypertension: Insights from the registry to evaluate early and long-term pulmonary arterial hypertension disease management. *Circulation* 2012;125(1):113–22.

6. Fasnacht MS, Tolsa JF, Beghetti M. The Swiss registry for pulmonary arterial hypertension: The paediatric experience. *Swiss Medical Weekly* 2007;137(35–6):510–3.

7. Fraisse A, Jais X, Schleich JM, et al. Characteristics and prospective 2-year follow-up of children with pulmonary arterial hypertension in France. *Arch Cardiovasc Dis* 2010;103(2):66–74.

8. Haworth SG, Hislop AA. Treatment and survival in children with pulmonary arterial hypertension: The UK Pulmonary Hypertension Service for Children 2001–2006. *Heart* 2009;95(4):312–7.

9. van Loon RL, Roofthooft MT, Hillege HL, et al. Pediatric pulmonary hypertension in the Netherlands: Epidemiology and characterization during the period 1991 to 2005. *Circulation* 2011;124(16):1755–64.

10. Berger RM, Beghetti M, Humpl T, et al. Clinical features of paediatric pulmonary hypertension: A registry study. *Lancet* 2012;379(9815):537–46.

11. Lindberg L, Olsson AK, Jogi P, et al. How common is severe pulmonary hypertension after pediatric cardiac surgery? *J Thorac Cardiovasc Surg* 2002;123(6):1155–63.

12. Abman SH, Ivy DD. Recent progress in understanding pediatric pulmonary hypertension. *Curr Opin Pediatr* 2011;23(3):298–304.

13. Rabinovitch M. Molecular pathogenesis of pulmonary arterial hypertension. *J Clin Invest* 2008;118(7):2372–9.

14. Barst RJ, Ertel SI, Beghetti M, et al. Pulmonary arterial hypertension: A comparison between children and adults. *Eur Respir J* 2011;37(3):665–77.

15. Moudgil R, Michelakis ED, Archer SL. The role of k+ channels in determining pulmonary vascular tone, oxygen sensing, cell proliferation, and apoptosis: Implications in hypoxic pulmonary vasoconstriction and pulmonary arterial hypertension. *Microcirculation* 2006;13(8):615–32.

16. Connolly MJ, Aaronson PI. Key role of the RhoA/Rho kinase system in pulmonary hypertension. *Pulm Pharmacol Ther* 2011;24(1):1–14.

17. Rabinovitch M. Pathobiology of pulmonary hypertension. *Annu Rev Pathol* 2007;2:369–99.

18. Haddad F, Doyle R, Murphy DJ, et al. Right ventricular function in cardiovascular disease, part II: Pathophysiology, clinical

importance, and management of right ventricular failure. *Circulation* 2008;117(13):1717–31.

19. Bronicki RA, Baden HP. Pathophysiology of right ventricular failure in pulmonary hypertension. *Pediatr Crit Care Med* 2010;11(suppl 2):S15–22.

20. Newman JH, Trembath RC, Morse JA, et al. Genetic basis of pulmonary arterial hypertension: Current understanding and future directions. *J Am Coll Cardiol* 2004;43(12 suppl S):33S–9S.

21. Machado RD, Eickelberg O, Elliott CG, et al. Genetics and genomics of pulmonary arterial hypertension. *J Am Coll Cardiol* 2009;54(1 suppl):S32–42.

22. Morrell NW. Role of bone morphogenetic protein receptors in the development of pulmonary arterial hypertension. *Adv Exp Med Biol* 2010;661:251–64.

23. Price LC, McAuley DF, Marino PS, et al. Pathophysiology of pulmonary hypertension in acute lung injury. *Am J Physiol Lung Cell Mol Physiol* 2012;302(9):L803–15.

24. Wheller J, George BL, Mulder DG, et al. Diagnosis and management of postoperative pulmonary hypertensive crisis. *Circulation* 1979;60(7):1640–4.

25. Yock PG, Popp RL. Noninvasive estimation of right ventricular systolic pressure by Doppler ultrasound in patients with tricuspid regurgitation. *Circulation* 1984;70(4):657–62.

26. King ME, Braun H, Goldblatt A, et al. Interventricular septal configuration as a predictor of right ventricular systolic hypertension in children: A cross-sectional echocardiographic study. *Circulation* 1983;68(1):68–75.

27. Reisner SA, Azzam Z, Halmann M, et al. Septal/free wall curvature ratio: A noninvasive index of pulmonary arterial pressure. *J Am Soc Echocardiogr* 1994;7(1):27–35.

28. McLaughlin VV, Archer SL, Badesch DB, et al. ACCF/AHA 2009 expert consensus document on pulmonary hypertension a report of the American College of Cardiology Foundation Task Force on Expert Consensus Documents and the American Heart Association developed in collaboration with the American College of Chest Physicians; American Thoracic Society, Inc.; and the Pulmonary Hypertension Association. *J Am Coll Cardiol* 2009;53(17):1573–619.

29. Ivy D. Advances in pediatric pulmonary arterial hypertension. *Curr Opin Cardiol* 2012;27(2):70–81.

30. Barst RJ, Maislin G, Fishman AP. Vasodilator therapy for primary pulmonary hypertension in children. *Circulation* 1999;99(9):1197–208.

31. Rich S, Kaufmann E, Levy PS. The effect of high doses of calcium-channel blockers on survival in primary pulmonary hypertension. *N Engl J Med* 1992;327(2):76–81.

32. Sitbon O, Humbert M, Jais X, et al. Long-term response to calcium channel blockers in idiopathic pulmonary arterial hypertension. *Circulation* 2005;111(23):3105–11.

33. Bergin CJ, Sirlin CB, Hauschildt JP, et al. Chronic thromboembolism: Diagnosis with helical CT and MR imaging with angiographic and surgical correlation. *Radiology* 1997;204(3):695–702.

34. Mullen MP. Diagnostic strategies for acute presentation of pulmonary hypertension in children: Particular focus on use of echocardiography, cardiac catheterization, magnetic resonance imaging, chest computed tomography, and lung biopsy. *Pediatr Crit Care Med* 2010;11(2 suppl):S23–6.

35. Nicod P, Moser KM. Primary pulmonary hypertension. The risk and benefit of lung biopsy. *Circulation* 1989;80(5):1486–8.

36. Rabinovitch M, Keane JF, Norwood WI, et al. Vascular structure in lung tissue obtained at biopsy correlated with pulmonary hemodynamic findings after repair of congenital heart defects. *Circulation* 1984;69(4):655–67.

37. Wilson NJ, Seear MD, Taylor GP, et al. The clinical value and risks of lung biopsy in children with congenital heart disease. *J Thorac Cardiovasc Surg* 1990;99(3):460–8.

38. Galante D. Intraoperative management of pulmonary arterial hypertension in infants and children—Corrected and republished article. *Curr Opin Anaesthesiol* 2011;24(4):468–71.

39. Hoeper MM, Galie N, Murali S, et al. Outcome after cardiopulmonary resuscitation in patients with pulmonary arterial hypertension. *Am J Respir Crit Care Med* 2002;165(3):341–4.

40. Morris K, Beghetti M, Petros A, et al. Comparison of hyperventilation and inhaled nitric oxide for pulmonary hypertension after repair of congenital heart disease. *Crit Care Med* 2000;28(8):2974–8.

41. Umenai T, Shime N, Hashimoto S. Hyperventilation versus standard ventilation for infants in postoperative care for congenital heart defects with pulmonary hypertension. *J Anesth* 2009;23(1):80–6.

42. Atz AM, Wessel DL. Inhaled nitric oxide in the neonate with cardiac disease. *Semin Perinatol* 1997;21(5):441–55.

43. DiBlasi RM, Myers TR, Hess DR. Evidence-based clinical practice guideline: Inhaled nitric oxide for neonates with acute hypoxic respiratory failure. *Respir Care* 2010;55(12):1717–45.

44. Finer NN, Barrington KJ. Nitric oxide for respiratory failure in infants born at or near term. *Cochrane Database Syst Rev* 2006;18(4):CD000399.

45. Macrae DJ, Field D, Mercier JC, et al. Inhaled nitric oxide therapy in neonates and children: Reaching a European consensus. *Intensive Care Med* 2004;30(3):372–80.

46. Miller OI, Tang SF, Keech A, et al. Inhaled nitric oxide and prevention of pulmonary hypertension after congenital heart surgery: A randomised double-blind study. *Lancet* 2000;356(9240):1464–9.

47. Davidson D, Barefield ES, Kattwinkel J, et al. Safety of withdrawing inhaled nitric oxide therapy in persistent pulmonary hypertension of the newborn. *Pediatrics* 1999;104(2 pt 1):231–6.

48. Sokol GM, Fineberg NS, Wright LL, et al. Changes in arterial oxygen tension when weaning neonates from inhaled nitric oxide. *Pediatric Pulm* 2001;32(1):14–9.

49. The Neonatal Inhaled Nitric Oxide Study Group. Inhaled nitric oxide in full-term and nearly full-term infants with hypoxic respiratory failure. *N Engl J Med* 1997;336(9):597–604.

50. Bizzarro M, Gross I. Inhaled nitric oxide for the postoperative management of pulmonary hypertension in infants and children with congenital heart disease. *Cochrane Database Syst Rev* 2005;(4):CD005055.

51. Zapol WM, Snider MT. Pulmonary hypertension in severe acute respiratory failure. *N Engl J Med* 1977;296(9):476–80.

52. Taylor RW, Zimmerman JL, Dellinger RP, et al. Low-dose inhaled nitric oxide in patients with acute lung injury: A randomized controlled trial. *JAMA* 2004;291(13):1603–9.

53. Adhikari NK, Burns KE, Friedrich JO, et al. Effect of nitric oxide on oxygenation and mortality in acute lung injury: Systematic review and meta-analysis. *BMJ* 2007;334(7597):779.

54. Stocker C, Penny DJ, Brizard CP, et al. Intravenous sildenafil and inhaled nitric oxide: A randomised trial in infants after cardiac surgery. *Intensive Care Med* 2003;29(11):1996–2003.

55. Michelakis E, Tymchak W, Lien D, et al. Oral sildenafil is an effective and specific pulmonary vasodilator in patients with pulmonary arterial hypertension: Comparison with inhaled nitric oxide. *Circulation* 2002;105(20):2398–403.

56. Schulze-Neick I, Hartenstein P, Li J, et al. Intravenous sildenafil is a potent pulmonary vasodilator in children with congenital heart disease. *Circulation* 2003;108(suppl 1):II167–73.

57. Atz AM, Wessel DL. Sildenafil ameliorates effects of inhaled nitric oxide withdrawal. *Anesthesiology* 1999;91(1):307–10.

58. Namachivayam P, Theilen U, Butt WW, et al. Sildenafil prevents rebound pulmonary hypertension after withdrawal of nitric oxide in children. *Am J Respir Crit Care Med* 2006;174(9):1042–7.

59. Shah PS, Ohlsson A. Sildenafil for pulmonary hypertension in neonates. *Cochrane Database Syst Rev* 2011;(8):CD005494.

60. Rosenzweig EB. Tadalafil for the treatment of pulmonary arterial hypertension. *Expert Opin Pharmacother* 2010;11(1):127–32.

61. Takatsuki S, Calderbank M, Ivy DD. Initial experience with tadalafil in pediatric pulmonary arterial hypertension. *Pediatr Cardiol* 2012;33(5):683–8.

62. Galie N, Ghofrani HA, Torbicki A, et al. Sildenafil citrate therapy for pulmonary arterial hypertension. *N Engl J Med* 2005;353(20):2148–57.

63. Rubin LJ, Badesch DB, Fleming TR, et al. Long-term treatment with sildenafil citrate in pulmonary arterial hypertension: The SUPER-2 study. *Chest* 2011;140(5):1274–83.

64. Barst RJ, Ivy DD, Gaitan G, et al. A randomized, double-blind, placebo-controlled, dose-ranging study of oral sildenafil citrate in treatment-naive children with pulmonary arterial hypertension. *Circulation* 2012;125(2):324–34.

65. Barst RJ, Rubin LJ, Long WA, et al. A comparison of continuous intravenous epoprostenol (prostacyclin) with conventional therapy for primary pulmonary hypertension. *N Engl J Med* 1996;334(5):296–301.

66. Simonneau G, Barst RJ, Galie N, et al. Continuous subcutaneous infusion of treprostinil, a prostacyclin analogue, in patients with pulmonary arterial hypertension: A double-blind, randomized, placebo-controlled trial. *Am J Respir Crit Care Med* 2002;165(6):800–4.

67. Ivy DD, Doran AK, Smith KJ, et al. Short- and long-term effects of inhaled iloprost therapy in children with pulmonary arterial hypertension. *J Am Coll Cardiol* 2008;51(2):161–9.

68. Rimensberger PC, Spahr-Schopfer I, Berner M, et al. Inhaled nitric oxide versus aerosolized iloprost in secondary pulmonary hypertension in children with congenital heart disease: Vasodilator capacity and cellular mechanisms. *Circulation* 2001;103(4):544–8.

69. Kirbas A, Yalcin Y, Tanrikulu N, et al. Comparison of inhaled nitric oxide and aerosolized iloprost in pulmonary hypertension in children with congenital heart surgery. *Cardiol J* 2012;19(4):387–94.

70. Loukanov T, Bucsenez D, Springer W, et al. Comparison of inhaled nitric oxide with aerosolized iloprost for treatment of pulmonary hypertension in children after cardiopulmonary bypass surgery. *Clin Res Cardiol* 2011;100(7):595–602.

71. Channick RN, Simonneau G, Sitbon O, et al. Effects of the dual endothelin-receptor antagonist bosentan in patients with pulmonary hypertension: A randomised placebo-controlled study. *Lancet* 2001;358(9288):1119–23.

72. Galie N, Beghetti M, Gatzoulis MA, et al. Bosentan therapy in patients with Eisenmenger syndrome: A multicenter, double-blind, randomized, placebo-controlled study. *Circulation* 2006;114(1):48–54.

73. Galie N, Rubin L, Hoeper M, et al. Treatment of patients with mildly symptomatic pulmonary arterial hypertension with bosentan (EARLY study): A double-blind, randomised controlled trial. *Lancet* 2008;371(9630):2093–100.

74. Gatzoulis MA, Beghetti M, Galie N, et al. Longer-term bosentan therapy improves functional capacity in Eisenmenger syndrome: Results of the BREATHE-5 open-label extension study. *Int J Cardiol* 2008;127(1):27–32.

75. Rubin LJ, Badesch DB, Barst RJ, et al. Bosentan therapy for pulmonary arterial hypertension. *N Engl J Med* 2002;346(12):896–903.

76. Ivy DD, Rosenzweig EB, Lemarie JC, et al. Long-term outcomes in children with pulmonary arterial hypertension treated with bosentan in real-world clinical settings. *Am J Cardiol* 2010;106(9):1332–8.

77. Takatsuki S, Rosenzweig EB, Zuckerman W, et al. Clinical safety, pharmacokinetics, and efficacy of ambrisentan therapy in children with pulmonary arterial hypertension. *Pediatr Pulm* 2013;48(1):27–34.

78. Reichenberger F, Pepke-Zaba J, McNeil K, et al. Atrial septostomy in the treatment of severe pulmonary arterial hypertension. *Thorax* 2003;58(9):797–800.

79. Sandoval J, Gaspar J, Pulido T, et al. Graded balloon dilation atrial septostomy in severe primary pulmonary hypertension. A therapeutic alternative for patients nonresponsive to vasodilator treatment. *J Am Coll Cardiol* 1998;32(2):297–304.

80. Benden C, Edwards LB, Kucheryavaya AY, et al. The registry of the international society for heart and lung transplantation: Fifteenth pediatric lung and heart-lung transplantation report—2012. *J Heart Lung Transplant* 2012;31(10):1087–95.

81. Fineman JR, Soifer SJ, Heymann MA. Regulation of pulmonary vascular tone in the perinatal period. *Annu Rev Physiol* 1995;57:115–34.

82. Lazar DA, Cass DL, Olutoye OO, et al. The use of ECMO for persistent pulmonary hypertension of the newborn: A decade of experience. *J Surg Res* 2012;177(2):263–7.

83. Ho JJ, Rasa G. Magnesium sulfate for persistent pulmonary hypertension of the newborn. *Cochrane Database Syst Rev* 2007(3):CD005588.

84. Bassler D, Kreutzer K, McNamara P, et al. Milrinone for persistent pulmonary hypertension of the newborn. *Cochrane Database Syst Rev* 2010(11):CD007802.

85. Lazar DA, Olutoye OO, Cass DL, et al. Outcomes of neonates requiring extracorporeal membrane oxygenation for irreversible pulmonary dysplasia: The Extracorporeal Life Support Registry experience. *Pediatr Crit Care Med* 2012;13(2):188–90.

CHAPTER 81 ■ THE IMMUNE SYSTEM

RACHEL S. AGBEKO, NIGEL J. KLEIN, AND MARK J. PETERS

KEY POINTS

1. The immune system is a phenomenally complex biologic system.
2. Critical illness (both septic and nonseptic) elicits an immune response that is designed to protect the body.
3. An unbalanced immune response may worsen the overall clinical state and exacerbate the level of organ dysfunction.
4. Many examples of congenital immunodeficiency provide the clinician with important insight into infection susceptibility, mechanisms of systemic inflammation, and multiorgan dysfunction.
5. To date, no interventional trial of immune modulation in critically ill children has been of proven benefit, perhaps because of a failure of appropriate targeting.
6. Future clinical trials of immunomodulative agents must evaluate the patient's immunocompetence and inflammatory and infectious status as well as be rigorously tested for *in vivo* efficacy.
7. Therapeutic trials should be appropriately targeted to the immune state of the individual.

The immune system plays a role in every admission to the PICU, either as a component of the initial insult itself or as a consequence of the insult and the supportive care provided. The basic concepts of how host immune mechanisms operate during critical illness are well appreciated. However, less is understood about how these mechanisms contribute to the clinical course seen in the ICU because of the complexity generated by variability in the timing, location, and balance of different parts of the immune response. Interactions between the environment and host genetics are also a huge source of variability that is only now being investigated. This chapter provides a review of the ways in which developments in our understanding of childhood immunologic conditions have shed light on some of the immunologic mechanisms operating in critically ill children.

THE IMMUNE SYSTEM

The immune system is a challenge to understand. To facilitate understanding, dichotomies have been made where a more accurate description might be more nuanced. With evolving understanding, the picture that emerges is of an incredibly complex and interlinking network that incorporates multiple elements: adaptive and innate immunity as well as coagulation, endocrine and nervous systems. The purpose of these interlinking processes is to ward off infectious threats and heal injuries while managing to coexist with benign or beneficial microbes.

A classic paradigm is to distinguish the innate and adaptive immune systems. The *innate* element of the immune system is present at birth. It is the more ancient of the two arms, and provides host defense against a vast array of microbes. The recognition systems employed are targeted against highly conserved structures common to large groups of microorganisms. This targeting is achieved through interactions between host-derived pattern recognition receptors (PRRs) and pathogen-associated molecular patterns (PAMPs) on microbes.

The *adaptive* immune system develops after birth and provides highly specific recognition of both host and foreign antigens, allowing for effective handling of a multitude of microorganisms and for the generation of targeted immunologic memory. While the adaptive and innate systems are often considered as separate entities, the fact that the adaptive immune system has evolved in the presence of the innate system indicates that the two systems are linked, which is exemplified by the shared usage of a number of effector cells and soluble mediators. The key features of the innate versus adaptive immune system are outlined in **Table 81.1**.

TABLE 81.1

CHARACTERISTICS OF THE INNATE VERSUS ADAPTIVE IMMUNE SYSTEM

■ INNATE IMMUNE SYSTEM	■ ADAPTIVE IMMUNE SYSTEM
Older phylogenetically—present in all multicellular organisms	Evolved later—present only in vertebrates
Present from birth	Learned response
Does not require previous exposure	Slower but more definitive
No memory	Memory specific to antigen
Cellular components—phagocytic system (monocytes, macrophages, DCs) and natural killer cells	Cellular components—T and B lymphocytes
Soluble components—cytokines, complement, and acute-phase proteins	Soluble components—immunoglobulins

The perfect immune system would be robust and resilient. It would have the capacity to respond to consecutive or simultaneous infectious and injury threats, have an immediate action, replenish quickly, and contain the response locally without damaging the host. This would require a system to recognize danger quickly and accurately and to contain a threat immediately with minimal collateral damage. It would need to have efficient feedback loops to step up or down responses appropriately. Finally, it would need to dispose of debris effectively. While tremendously effective, human immunity is not so perfect.

The Immune System in Real Life

The initial step in host defense is determination of whether or not matter poses a threat to the host. Initially, this process was thought to be discrimination of "noninfectious self" and "infectious non-self" (1). More recently, the paradigm of discriminating "danger" from "non-danger" (2) has gained favor as the key output from the innate immune system.

This model postulates that the immune system responds to matter that is perceived to pose a threat to the host, that is, antigens that are seen *in a setting of tissue damage*. This model explains phenomena seen in injury (sterile systemic inflammation following trauma or surgery), infection (aggressive responses to some microorganisms while commensals are tolerated), transplantation, and allergy (3). The innate immune system serves as both a sensor and the initial removal apparatus of infection combined with injury.

Some, but not all, of the mechanisms of the host response after tissue damage are understood. Cell and humoral PRRs recognize evolutionarily preserved sequences known as exogenous PAMPs or endogenous danger-associated molecular patterns (DAMPs). Microbes, but not host tissues, express molecular sequences or PAMPs, such as lipopolysaccharide (LPS) or lipoteichoic acid. Examples of host-origin DAMPs are the cytokine high mobility group box 1 (HMGB-1), mitochondria (whole or fractions thereof), and heat shock proteins.

PRRs may be classified according to position and function. They are circulating free receptors (e.g., mannose-binding lectin [MBL]), membrane phagocytic receptors (complement receptor), cytoplasmic signaling receptors, and membrane-bound signaling receptors (e.g., toll-like receptor TLR4).

In response to this PRR ligation, chemotactic substances or "alarmins" are released to draw polymorphonucleated neutrophils, phagocytes as well as antigen-presenting cells, such as dendritic cells (DCs) to the site of concern (4). Here the innate immune system interacts with the more specific adaptive immune system to induce an initially generic but rapidly more specific host response to microbial invasion. This includes the capacity to produce specific antibodies. In addition, the response includes elements to downgrade the response, including anti-inflammatory cytokines and monocyte deactivation.

The innate immune system activates and deactivates many times to return a state of vigilance and response. The term "allostasis" might represent this dynamic process better, rather than the term "homeostasis" given that allostasis incorporates not only feedback loops and set points, but also the complexity of networked interaction and stress responses (5).

IMMUNODEFICIENCY AND INTENSIVE CARE

A number of patients are admitted to the PICU as a result of infectious complications from congenital or acquired immune deficiencies (human immunodeficiency virus [Chapter 84],

TABLE 81.2

SEVERE COMBINED IMMUNODEFICIENCY SYNDROMES

■ DISORDER	■ PHENOTYPE	■ MUTATED GENE	■ MOLECULAR DEFECT
SCID-X1	T − B + NK−	Common g-chain	Absence of receptors for IL-2, IL-4, IL-7, IL-9, IL-15, and IL-21
JAK3 deficiency	T − B + NK−	*JAK3*	Defect of signaling via IL-2, IL-4, IL-7, IL-9, IL-15, and IL-21
IL-7 receptor deficiency	T − B + NK+	IL-7 receptor a	Absence of IL-7 receptor α
RAG-1, RAG-2 deficiency	T − B − NK+	*RAG-1* and *RAG-2*	Defective VDJ recombination
Artemis deficiency	T − B − NK+	Artemis	Defective VDJ recombination; radiation sensitivity
Ligase IV deficiency	T − B − NK+	Ligase IV	Defective VDJ recombination; radiation sensitivity
Cernunnos deficiency	T − B − NK+	Cernunnos	Defective VDJ recombination; radiation sensitivity
Adenosine deaminase deficiency	T − B − NK−	*ADA*	Block in purine salvage metabolism
Purine nucleoside phosphorylase deficiency	T − B + NK+	*PNP*	Block in purine salvage metabolism
T-cell receptor deficiencies	T − B + NK+	CD3ϵ/δ/γ/ζ	Defective T-cell signaling
ZAP70 deficiency	T − B + NK+	*ZAP70*	Defective T-cell signaling
ORAI-1	T + B + NK+	*ORAI-1*	Defective T-cell signaling
CD45 deficiency	T − B + NK+	*CD45*	Defective T- and B-cell signaling
Coronin 1A	T − B + NK+		
P56lck	T − B + NK+		
WHN/Nude SCID	T − B + NK+		
DNA-PKcs	T − B − NK+		
Reticular dysgenesis (adenylate kinase-2 deficiency)	T − B − NK−		
MHC II	T + B + NK+		
CD3 deficiency	T − B + NK+		

VDJ, variable diverse joining.

TABLE 81.3

OTHER CONGENITAL IMMUNODEFICIENCY SYNDROMES

■ DISORDER	■ CHROMOSOME	■ GENE	■ FUNCTION/DEFECT	■ DIAGNOSTIC TESTS
X-linked chronic granulomatous disease	Xp21	gp91phox	Component of phagocyte NADPH	Nitroblue tetrazolium test gp91phox by oxidase-phagocytic respiratory burst immunoblotting; mutation analysis
X-linked agammaglobulinemia	Xq22	Bruton's tyrosine kinase (Btk)	Intracellular signaling pathways essential for pre-B-cell maturation	Btk by immunoblotting or FACS analysis and mutation analysis
X-linked hyper-IgM syndrome (CD40 ligand deficiency)	Xq26 (CD154)	CD40 ligand	Isotype switching, T-cell function	CD154 expression on activated T cells by FACS analysis mutation analysis
Wiskott–Aldrich syndrome	Xp11	WASP	Cytoskeletal architecture formation, immune-cell motility and trafficking	WASP expression by immunoblotting; mutation analysis
X-linked lymphoproliferative syndrome	Xq25	SAP	Regulation of T-cell responses to EBV and other viral infections	Mutation analysis SAP expression—under development
Properdin deficiency	Xp21	Properdin	Terminal complement component	Properdin levels
Type 1 leukocyte adhesion deficiency	21q22	CD11/CD18	Defective leucocyte adhesion and migration	CD11/CD18 expression by FACS analysis; mutation analysis
Chronic granulomatous disease (recessive)	7q11 1q25 16p24	p47phox p67pho p22phox	Defective respiratory burst and phagocytic intracellular killing	p47phox, p67phox, p22phox, expression by immunoblotting; mutation analysis
Chédiak–Higashi syndrome	1q42	LYST	Abnormalities in microtubule-mediated lysosomal protein trafficking	Giant inclusions in granulocytes; mutation analysis
MHC class II deficiency	16p13 19p12	CIITA (MHC2TA) RFXANK	Defective transcriptional regulation of MHC II molecule expression	HLA-DR expression; mutation analysis
RFX5	13q13	RFXAP		
Autoimmune lymphoproliferative syndrome	10q24	APT1 (Fas)	Defective apoptosis of lymphocytes	Fas expression; apoptosis assays; mutation analysis
Ataxia telangiectasia	11q22	ATM	Cell-cycle control and DNA damage responses	DNA radiation sensitivity; mutation analysis
Inherited mycobacterial susceptibility	6q23 5q31 19p13	IFN-γ receptor IL-12 p40 IL-12 receptor b1	Defective IFN-γ production and signaling function	IFN-γ receptor expression; IL-12 expression; IL-12 receptor expression; mutation analysis

WASP, Wiskott–Aldrich syndrome protein; MHC, major histocompatibility complex; FACS, fluorescent activated cell sorting.

severe combined immunodeficiency disease [SCID; Chapter 86], opportunistic infections [Chapter 95], Epstein–Barr virus (EBV) driven lymphoproliferative disease [Chapter 104], tumor lysis syndrome and neutropenic fever [Chapter 115], and idiopathic pneumonitis syndrome, post–bone marrow transplant respiratory failure, and veno-occlusive disease [Chapter 117]). In addition to these severe defects, a number of conditions have been recognized, many originating from single-gene deletions or polymorphisms, that are providing valuable insights into the complex processes of inflammation. Immunodeficiencies are listed in **Tables 81.2** and **81.3**.

The SCID group of primary immune deficiencies is based on profound defects of T lymphocytes (absence or functional) and the presence or absence of B and NK lymphocytes. Other immune deficiencies and immune dysregulation occur in both the adaptive and innate immune system.

Rare primary immunodeficiencies in the innate immune system may offer insight into pathogen recognition pathways and host response. Clinical phenotypes associated with a defective downstream TLR pathway include recurrent pyogenic bacterial infections such as seen in NEMO (NFκB essential modulator) and IRAK-4 (interleukin-1R-associated kinase 4) deficiency.

BALANCE OF SUSCEPTIBILITY VERSUS SEVERITY: CLUES FROM THE IMMUNE SYSTEM

The importance of an intact immune system for protecting children from infection is not in doubt. However, even in patients with profound immunodeficiencies, the frequency, nature, and severity of infectious and inflammatory complications are variable. These factors are, at least in part, determined by the host's remaining functional immune system. Such dysregulated immunity can be seen in a number of scenarios, including in patients with severe combined immunodeficiency early in the process of immune restoration following stem cell transplantation, or in those with *Cryptosporidium* infections and CD40L deficiency. The relationship between infectious susceptibility and severity of the ensuing inflammatory response is complex and frequently determines the clinical course of critically ill patients. A number of defects in the immune system highlight the *balance* between risk of infection and severity of the host response. Five immune networks have been chosen to illustrate this point: complement system, MBL, endotoxin recognition, cytokines and the inflammasome.

Complement System

Complement pathways play a critical role in the destruction of invading microorganisms. Working in concert with the adaptive immune system, activation of the three complement pathways (**Fig. 81.1**) leads to the construction of membrane attack complexes that cause direct lysis and death of the microorganisms (6). During activation, opsonic and chemotactic factors are also generated that facilitate the removal of live and dead organisms from the circulation and from tissues. The importance of these pathways is indicated by the facts that (a) many potentially harmful organisms have mechanisms for avoiding recognition by, or activation of, the complement system, (b) rare complement deficiencies exist in which patients are more vulnerable to infection, and (c) reduced levels of complement proteins in neonates and in the low-protein states of liver disease and nephrotic syndrome may contribute to the susceptibility to infection.

Inherited deficiencies of complement proteins are rare, but affected individuals suffer from an increased risk of bacterial infections. Patients with terminal complement component deficiencies are particularly susceptible to *Neisseria* sp., including *N. meningitidis* (7); however, paradoxically, these episodes of infection are generally less severe than in normal populations. It appears that complement activation, while critical for host

defense against meningococci, leads to more inflammation and clinical deterioration (8). Although the impact of complement deficiencies on the burden of clinical disease in the pediatric population is negligible, such immune defects serve to demonstrate the complex relationship that exists between susceptibility to, and severity from, an infectious insult.

This complex interplay between complement activation, host susceptibility to infection, and inflammatory response is further illustrated by the observation that the complement activation inhibitor Complement Factor H is a susceptibility gene to meningococcal disease (9), but loss of function also predisposes to systemic inflammation (10).

Mannose-Binding Lectin

MBL is a liver-derived plasma protein that recognizes repeating sugar arrays on the surface of many bacteria, fungi, viruses, and parasites. MBL binds to microbes, such as *Staphylococcus aureus* and *N. meningitidis*, and activates complement in an antibody- and C1-complex–independent fashion. In contrast to most complement defects, MBL deficiency is common in the population. Three polymorphisms (codons 52, 54, and 57 in exon 1 of *MBL-2* gene) are associated with a deficiency of circulating functional MBL. Promoter polymorphisms also contribute to levels of the protein. Approximately one-third of the population is deficient in MBL, with 10% having a profound deficiency.

Children with reduced levels of MBL are at an increased risk for many minor infections of childhood and for more frequent and severe infections in the presence of coexisting immunodeficiencies, such as that caused by chemotherapy for the treatment of cancer. Intensive care is an environment in which many of the most basic defenses against infection are compromised: breaches in skin and airway, poor nutrition, gut hypoperfusion, and acquired "immunoparalysis." MBL deficiency appears to

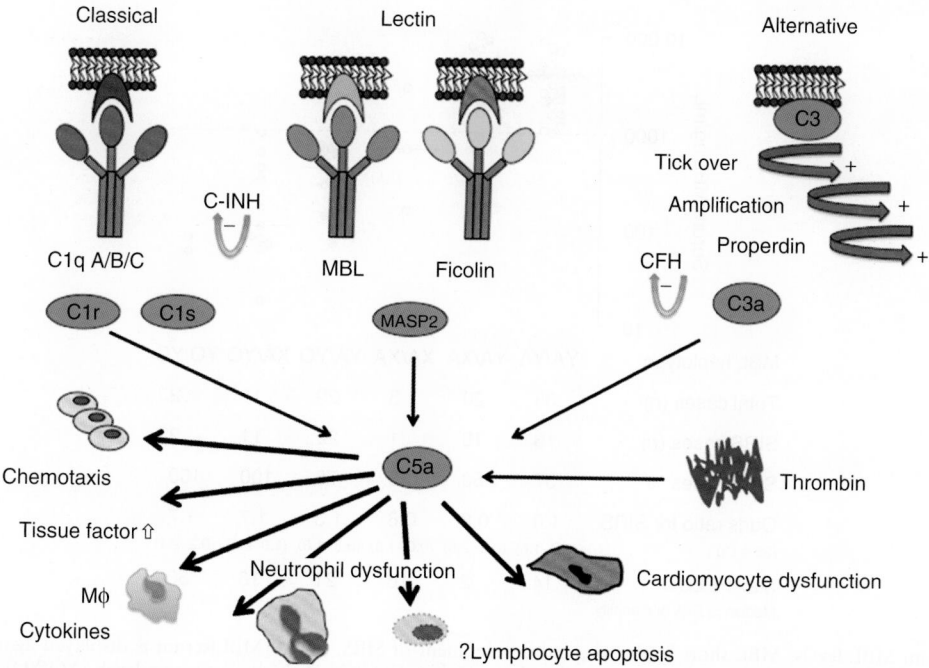

FIGURE 81.1. The complement and lectin pathways. The lectin pathway of complement is activated by MBL and ficolins. On binding to appropriate targets, MBL–MASP-2 complexes cleave C4 and C2 to form C3 convertase (C4bC2a). MBL–MASP-1 complexes may activate C3 directly. Ficolins also work in combination with the MASPs. The classic and alternative pathways also generate C3 convertase enzymes, which cleave C3. The lytic pathway (C5–C9) is common to all three routes of C3 cleavage. MASP, MBL-associated serine proteases; MASP-1, MBL-associated serine protease-1; MASP-2, MBL-associated serine protease 2. C-INH is C1 esterase inhibitor; CFH is Complement Factor H.

be influential in this environment. Children who are admitted to intensive care following infection, trauma, or surgery have a greatly increased risk of developing the systemic inflammatory response syndrome (SIRS) within the first 48 hours of PICU admission if they have MBL deficiency (odds ratio [OR], 7.1; 95% confidence interval [CI], 2.9–19; $p = 0.0001$). This is true for both infectious (OR, 11; 95% CI, 2–57; $p = 0.001$) and noninfectious illness (OR, 5; 95% CI, 1.5–19; $p = 0.018$) (11) (Fig. 81.2). Adults with MBL deficiency and SIRS also have a more severe clinical course and higher risk of death (12,13).

These data suggest that in many cases, residual infection may be contributing to the development of systemic inflammation (14). In order for MBL deficiency to persist despite evolutionary pressure, there must be survival advantages in other situations afforded by these mutations. An advantage of MBL deficiency in some intracellular infections is possible, but recently these genotypes have been shown to attenuate ischemia–reperfusion injury (15). Reduced production of C3a and C5a from this noninfectious stimulus reduces the secondary inflammation. Both mechanisms are active during sepsis, so therapeutic targeting of this pathway would require very detailed understanding of the balance of effects in an individual patient at a particular time point.

Endotoxin Recognition

The archetypal PAMP is the Gram-negative bacterial cell wall component LPS, to which humans are exquisitely sensitive (16). The transmembrane receptor TLR4 complex recognizes the lipid A component of LPS. On binding, the transmembrane receptor TLR4 signals to intracellular components, which, in turn, leads to NFκB-mediated downstream gene expression and cytokine activation. On binding, the transmembrane receptor TLR4 signals to intracellular components, which, in turn, leads to NFκB-mediated downstream gene expression and cytokine activation.

Nonspecific protection against LPS can be provided by circulating humoral factors, for example, LPS-binding protein and antibodies directed against the core of endotoxin (Endo-CAb). All adults have these antibodies, but observed levels vary within populations by more than 80-fold. Higher preoperative levels of IgM EndoCAb are associated with better outcomes following surgery, while higher IgG EndoCAb levels have been linked to survival in sepsis. In one study in children admitted to intensive care after head injury, following surgery, or for other noninfectious reasons, lower levels of IgG EndoCAb were seen in those who went on to develop the SIRS early in their PICU course than in those who did not suffer this complication (17).

Recognition of LPS is complex and involves multiple receptors and mediators. Functional mutations and polymorphisms of proteins involved in LPS recognition and signaling—including TLR4, CD14, MyD88, interleukin receptor-activated kinase (IRAK)-4, and NFκB—have been identified. The pattern of disease susceptibility in relationship to these genetic variants is complex. A number of studies have shown some relationship between reduced responsiveness to LPS and increased susceptibility to bacterial infection and sepsis. However, some benefit may be associated with having a reduced responsiveness to LPS, as such individuals appear to be protected from developing atherosclerosis. The most convincing evidence pertains to rare Mendelian gene defects, rather than common gene variants.

Cytokines

Over the last decade, many studies have found associations between polymorphisms in genes that control levels of immune system cytokines and susceptibility to, and severity of, critical illness. Interpreting results from these studies is not straightforward, partially due to the phase of the condition under investigation. This is exemplified by IL-10, an anti-inflammatory cytokine, the levels of which are critical in the modulation of the proinflammatory/anti-inflammatory balance. Interindividual

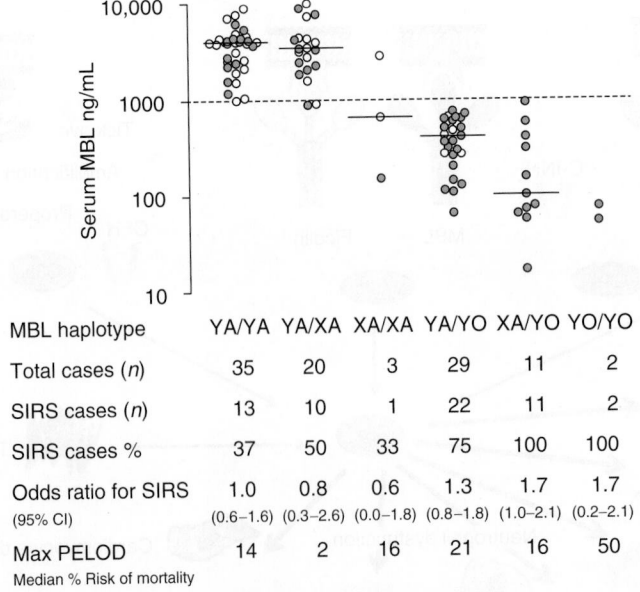

MBL haplotype	YA/YA	YA/XA	XA/XA	YA/YO	XA/YO	YO/YO
Total cases (n)	35	20	3	29	11	2
SIRS cases (n)	13	10	1	22	11	2
SIRS cases %	37	50	33	75	100	100
Odds ratio for SIRS (95% CI)	1.0 (0.6–1.6)	0.8 (0.3–2.6)	0.6 (0.0–1.8)	1.3 (0.8–1.8)	1.7 (1.0–2.1)	1.7 (0.2–2.1)
Max PELOD Median % Risk of mortality	14	2	16	21	16	50

FIGURE 81.2. Serum MBL levels, MBL short haplotype, and development of SIRS. Log10[MBL]serum is displayed against MBL haplotype (exon 1 and promoter polymorphisms) from those associated with the highest (YA/YA) to the lowest serum levels (YO/YO). A clear relationship exists between Log10[MBL]serum and genotype (one-way analysis of variance, p < 0.0001 after correction for multiple comparisons). Filled circles represent cases that developed SIRS; open circles represent cases that did not develop SIRS. The odds ratios (95% CI) for the development of SIRS for each haplotype are shown, as is the risk of mortality derived from the maximum calculated PELOD score. PELOD, pediatric logistic organ dysfunction. (Modified from Dommett RM, Klein N, Turner MW. Mannose-binding lectin in innate immunity: Past, present and future. *Tissue Antigens* 2006;68(3):193–209.)

differences in IL-10 levels are caused, in part, by a number of polymorphisms in the promoter region, found on chromosome 1, including those at positions −1082 (A/G), −819 (C/T), and −592 (C/A). The promoter polymorphism at position −1082 has been most associated with severity of infection (18). A small study showed that patients admitted to ICU with A alleles at this locus had an increased *susceptibility* to sepsis; however, once sepsis was established, the presence of the G allele was associated with higher IL-10 levels and increased mortality (19). Similarly, children with the G allele were more likely to exhibit immunoparalysis and increased complications postcardiac surgery (20).

Functional polymorphisms exist in a number of other genes, the products of which are thought to be important in sepsis, including cytokines such as tumor necrosis factor (TNF), IL-1, and IL-6, and proteins involved in hemostasis and thrombosis, such as plasminogen activator inhibitor 1 and angiotensin-converting enzyme, which has multiple functions, including inflammatory modulation. How, when, and why such genetic variations influence the course and outcome of both infectious and noninfectious conditions are unclear.

The Inflammasome

The inflammasome is an intracellular macromolecular signaling complex that activates caspase-1, which in turn proteolytically activates pro-IL-1β and pro-IL-18 into the potent proinflammatory cytokines IL-1β and IL-18. Assembly of the four known inflammasomes occurs in response to activation of their nucleotide-binding oligomerization domain (NOD) like receptor (NLR) PRR, that is, NLRP1, NLRP3, NLRC4, and AIM2, respectively (21). These complexes respond not only to PAMPs, but also to endogenous DAMPs, and NLRP3 will assemble in response to mitochondrial stress, reactive oxygen species, extracellular ATP, and potassium efflux. This makes the inflammasome a central apparatus in the immune response to infective and sterile insults, as it responds to primary danger matter but

also to danger signals that have been elicited by other parts of the immune system, thus amplifying the inflammatory process.

Given the potential for excessive activation with devastating consequences, the inflammasomes are regulated both at the level of inflammasome sensor molecules and at the level of recruitment of effector components. Our current understanding of the molecular and functional role of inflammasomes is rather rudimentary, and given our previous disappointing experience in therapeutic immunomodulation in critical illness it is prudent to be cautious. Nevertheless, because of a potential central role at different points in the host response, inflammasomes are a promising avenue to explore in modifying systemic inflammation.

It is increasingly apparent that a balance exists between the effective recognition of potentially harmful microbes and the generation of an appropriate host response. A less vigorous inflammatory response might lead to susceptibility to some infections, but may be balanced by a more benign course. Equally, an early vigorous inflammatory response deals with the problem and subsequently shuts off rather than perpetuating ineffective nonresolving inflammation. Between these two states, a state might exist of dynamic homeostasis, also termed allostasis, that is, a zone where the host is still capable of mounting an appropriate response (5).

THE BALANCE BETWEEN PROINFLAMMATION AND ANTI-INFLAMMATION

Systemic Inflammatory Response Syndrome

SIRS can be induced by any major insult that does not result in immediate death. It is typically defined in terms of alterations in simple clinical or laboratory parameters that arise from this insult (22,23) (**Tables 81.4** and **81.5**). In brief, SIRS is defined

---

TABLE 81.4

DEFINITIONS OF SYSTEMIC INFLAMMATORY RESPONSE SYNDROME, INFECTION, SEPSIS, SEVERE SEPSIS, AND SEPTIC SHOCK

SIRS

The presence of at least 2 of the following 4 criteria, one of which must be abnormal temperature or leukocyte count:

Core temperature of ≥38.5°C or ≤36°C.

Tachycardia, defined as a mean heart rate ≥SD above normal for age in the absence of external stimulus, chronic drugs, or painful stimuli;
OR otherwise unexplained persistent elevation over a 0.5 to 4-h time period

OR for children <1 y old: bradycardia, defined as a mean heart rate <10th percentile for age in the absence of external vagal stimulus, β-blocker drugs, or congenital heart disease, or otherwise unexplained persistent depression over a 0.5-h time period

Mean respiratory rate ≥2 SD above normal for age or mechanical ventilation for an acute process not related to underlying neuromuscular disease or the receipt of general anesthesia

Leukocyte count elevated or depressed for age (not secondary to chemotherapy-induced leukopenia) or ≥10% immature neutrophils

Infection

A suspected or proven (by positive culture, tissue stain, or polymerase chain reaction test) infection caused by any pathogen
OR a clinical syndrome associated with a high probability of infection. Evidence of infection includes positive findings on clinical exam, imaging, or laboratory tests (e.g., white blood cells in a normally sterile body fluid, perforated viscus, chest x-ray consistent with pneumonia, petechial or purpuric rash, or purpura fulminans)

Sepsis

SIRS in the presence of, or as a result of, suspected or proven infection

Severe sepsis

Sepsis plus one of the following: cardiovascular organ dysfunction
OR acute respiratory distress syndrome
OR two or more other organ dysfunctions. Organ dysfunctions are defined in **Table 81.5**.

Septic shock

Sepsis and cardiovascular organ dysfunction as defined in **Table 81.5**.

TABLE 81.5

ORGAN DYSFUNCTION CRITERIA

Cardiovascular dysfunction

Despite administration of isotonic IV fluid bolus ≥40 mL/kg in 1 h

Decrease in BP (hypotension) ≤5th percentile for age or systolic BP ≤2 SD below normal for age (**Table 81.6**)

OR Need for vasoactive drug to maintain BP in normal range (dopamine ≥5 mcg/kg/min, or dobutamine, epinephrine, or norepinephrine at any dose)

OR Two of the following:

Unexplained metabolic acidosis: base deficit >5.0 mEq/L

Increased arterial lactate >2 times upper limit of normal

Oliguria: urine output <0.5 mL/kg/h

Prolonged capillary refill: >5 sec

Core to peripheral temperature gap >3°C

Respiratory

Pao_2/Fio_2 <300 in the absence of cyanotic heart disease or preexisting lung disease

OR $Paco_2$ >72 torr or 20 mm Hg over baseline $Paco_2$

OR Proven need for >0.5 Fio_2 to maintain saturation >92%

OR Need for nonelective invasive or noninvasive mechanical ventilation

Neurologic

GCS ≤11 (57)

OR Acute change in mental status with a decrease in GCS ≥3 points from abnormal baseline

Hematologic

Platelet count <80,000/mm³ or a decline of 50% in platelet count from the highest value recorded over the previous 3 days (for chronic hematology/oncology patients)

OR International normalized ratio >2

Renal

Serum creatinine level >2 times upper limit of normal for age or twofold increase in baseline creatinine

Hepatic

Total bilirubin >4 mg/dL (not applicable for newborn)

OR ALT >2 times upper limit of normal for age

BP, blood pressure; GCS, Glasgow Coma Scale; ALT, alanine aminotransferase.

by two or more of the following: (a) hyperthermia or hypothermia, (b) tachycardia or bradycardia, (c) tachypnea, or requirement for ventilatory support, and (d) a pathologic alteration in white cell count. When SIRS is the result of suspected or proven infection, it is termed *sepsis*; however, noninfectious causes, such as burns, trauma, surgery, and pancreatitis, can also cause this clinical picture.

SIRS remains a clinical diagnosis despite advances in the laboratory measurement of hundreds of inflammatory mediators, probably reflecting the complexity of the acute inflammatory response in which multiple mediators have overlapping actions and no single measurement quantifies the inflammatory response effectively. Simple biochemical assessments of end-organ function (platelet count, coagulation times, blood urea nitrogen, creatinine, hepatic enzymes, arterial blood gases, and lactate) form part of the assessment of organ failure that arises from SIRS—but not of SIRS itself (**Table 81.6**).

SIRS and its sequelae represent a continuum of clinical and pathophysiologic severity. Mild-to-moderate SIRS is most likely beneficial; for example, both a raised temperature and

TABLE 81.6

AGE-SPECIFIC VITAL SIGNS AND LABORATORY VARIABLES

■ AGE GROUP	HEART RATE (BEATS/MIN)		■ RESPIRATORY RATE (BREATHS/MIN)	■ LEUKOCYTE COUNT (×10³/MM)	■ SYSTOLIC BLOOD PRESSURE (MM HG)
	■ TACHYCARDIA	■ BRADYCARDIA			
0 days–1 wk	>180	<100	>50	>34	<72
1 wk–1 mo	>180	<100	>40	>19.5 or <5	<75
1 mo–1 y	>180	<90	>34	>17.5 or <5	<100
2–5 y	>140	NA	>22	>15.5 or <5	<94
6–12 y	>130	NA	>18	>13.5 or <4.5	<105
13–<18 y	>110	NA	>14	>11 or <4.5	<117

Lower values correspond to 5th percentile; upper values correspond to 95th percentile.
NA, not applicable.

production of the cytokine TNF facilitate killing of microorganisms. However, a similar response may cause harm, either by being too severe or by spilling over into body compartments where they are not required. Examples include excessive body temperatures raising tissue oxygen demand beyond the available supply and causing rhabdomyolysis, while pathways that involve TNF or IL-6 may contribute to unwelcome myocardial depression (24). After a severe insult, TNF-α peaks very early and decreases quickly, whereas IL-10 may stay elevated over a longer time frame. The circulatory compartment may be hyporeactive to inflammatory stimuli, while simultaneously the tissues might still be in an active inflammatory phase (25).

At a local level, cell–cell interaction lymphocyte apoptosis induces macrophage transforming growth factor beta (TGF-β) production, humoral factors glucocorticoids, and anti-inflammatory cytokines such as IL-10 dampen the immune response. Inherently, these require time for trafficking, gene-regulated production of mediators and transfer of these mediators to the location of interest. In addition, they are ill-fitted to integrate the complex nature of the immune response, nor are they specific in terms of region. This delay in feedback is mitigated by the autonomic system. The vagus nerve has an integrative function with anti-inflammatory properties (26).

Excessive Proinflammation?

Overwhelming sepsis, such as that seen during the acute presentation of meningococcal septicemia, is a powerful reminder to the clinician of the effects of acute immune activation (**Fig. 81.3A** and **B**). The view that sepsis-induced multiorgan failure results exclusively from an excessive, unchecked proinflammatory response typified by mediators such as TNF and IL-1 was widely held through the 1980s and early 1990s. This response overlaps with the predominantly proinflammatory T-helper-1 (Th-1) pattern of immunity associated with cytotoxic T-cell and macrophage activation and suppression of humoral responses. Therefore, initial efforts to find novel therapies for severe sepsis and septic shock focused on blocking elements of this "excessive" proinflammatory response. Important to this concept was the idea of compartmentalization of inflammation: inflammation at the site of infection is critical to infection control, but systemic overflow of inflammation leads to a systemic inflammatory response and secondary organ failure. However, expensive failures of numerous clinical trials of agents designed to block the acute proinflammatory response prompted a reassessment (**Fig. 81.4**) (27). In 1996, Bone (28) suggested that the proinflammatory response does not occur in isolation and that a compensatory anti-inflammatory response syndrome (CARS) is always initiated at the same time. This "arm" of the immune response is typified by such mediators as IL-10, and shares many characteristics with the T-helper-2 (Th-2) response, involving the suppression of macrophage activation and promotion of antibody production.

This important insight raised the concept that wide variability might exist between patients in the nature of the immune response: a predominantly proinflammatory SIRS/Th-1 response in some, and a predominantly anti-inflammatory CARS/Th-2 response in others. These responses may lead to multiorgan failure and death via different routes (**Fig. 81.5**), but the impact of agents that inhibit the proinflammatory processes will be opposite in the two groups. In short, any reduction in early mortality obtained by anti-inflammatory therapies may be negated by increased late deaths in the CARS subgroup of patients. In support of this hypothesis, several studies of anti-inflammatory therapies undertaken in adult septic cohorts demonstrated a reduction in early deaths, which was offset by increased mortality in the subsequent days to weeks. One

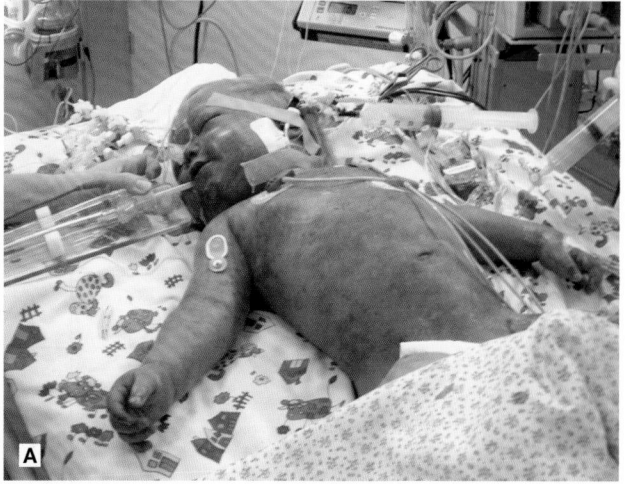

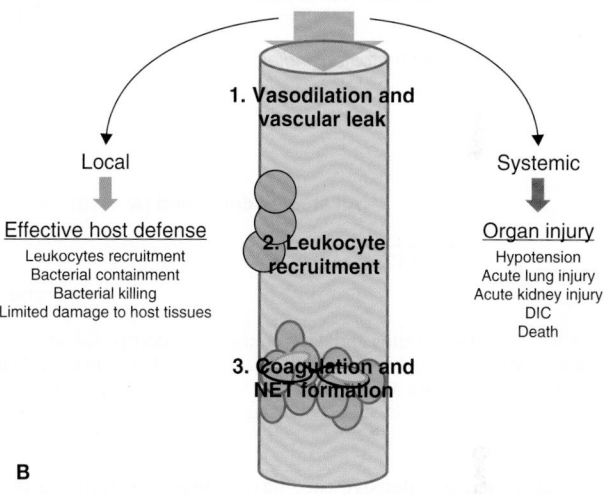

FIGURE 81.3. A: A child with fulminant meningococcal sepsis-induced multiorgan failure. This acute, severe process is an example of an excessive proinflammatory response that may be rapidly fatal. **B:** Fulminant sepsis may, in part, be a reflection of systemic activation of local beneficial host defense mechanisms. NET, neutrophil extracellular trap; DIC, disseminated intravascular coagulation. (From Seeley EJ, Matthay MA, Wolters PJ. Inflection points in sepsis biology: from local defense to systemic organ injury. *Am J Physiol Lung Cell Mol Physiol* 2012;303(5):L355–63, with permission.)

randomized study that attempted to target an anti-inflammatory agent (monoclonal antibody fragment to TNF) showed that a subgroup of patients with high levels of circulating IL-6 (a predominantly proinflammatory cytokine) may have benefited from TNF blockade, whereas the others did not (29).

Balance of Proinflammatory and Anti-inflammatory Response

While clinical studies suggest that the proinflammatory and anti-inflammatory responses probably occur simultaneously following an insult, it is useful to think of the systemic immune response to an insult (septic or nonseptic) as a biphasic response (**Fig. 81.5**). In most cases, the patient's compensatory anti-inflammatory response is proportional to the proinflammatory response, and homeostasis is rapidly restored.

While a small number of children still die of profound cardiovascular collapse early in the course of sepsis, many of

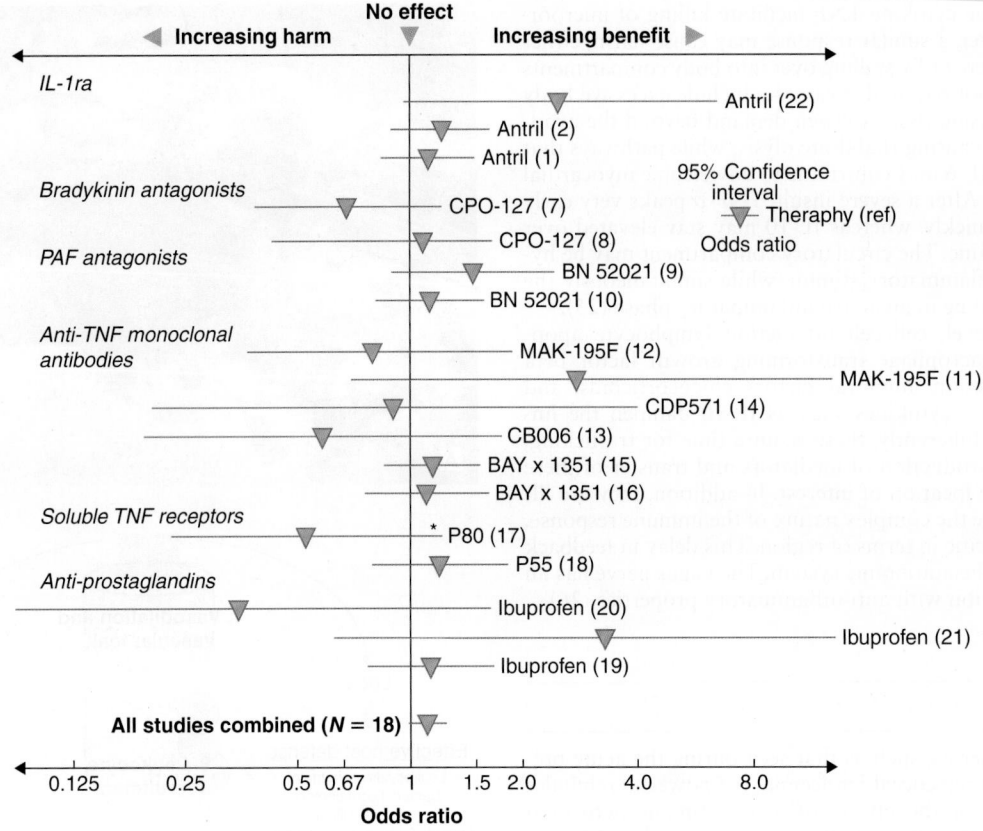

FIGURE 81.4. Odds ratios and 95% confidence intervals for survival in 18 clinical trials of nonglucocorticoid anti-inflammatory agents in adult patients with sepsis and septic shock. (From Zeni F, Freeman B, Natanson C. Anti-inflammatory therapies to treat sepsis and septic shock: A reassessment. *Crit Care Med* 1997;25(7):1095–100, with permission.)

those admitted to intensive care have a brief self-limiting period of SIRS that can be adequately supported using modern intensive care therapy. In patients whose critical condition cannot be reversed with a short intensive care stay, the risk of nosocomial infection influences the morbidity and mortality associated with their stay. Nosocomial infection in PICUs has been estimated to carry an early (4 weeks) relative risk of 3.4 (95% CI, 1.7–6.5). The incidence of nosocomial infection varies according to reports, but in 2011 it was reported that 4% of patients admitted to 183 US hospitals had suffered from

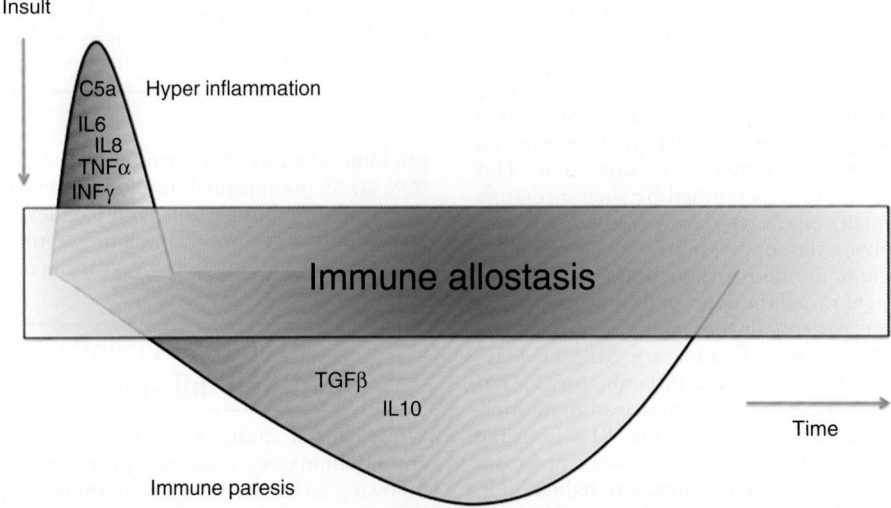

FIGURE 81.5. Immune response in critical illness. Following a primary insult, the patient mounts both a proinflammatory and an anti-inflammatory response. An extreme inflammatory response in either direction will result in cellular and organ injury and death. Within these extremes of what has been termed SIRS and CARS, there lies a "sweat spot" that might be termed "allostasis," where the host is still able to mount an appropriate immune response.

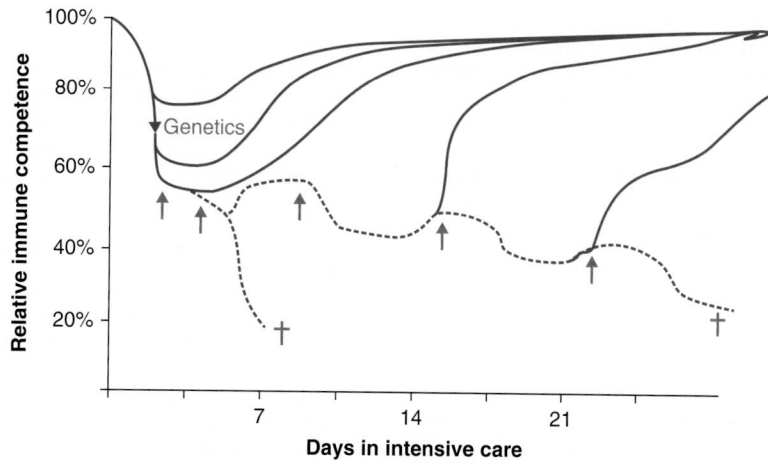

FIGURE 81.6. Possible immune response to primary inflammatory insult and the detrimental effect of secondary insults. Primary insult results in admission to a PICU, which leads to a relative fall in the patient's immune competence. Over the initial week, an attempt is made by the body to restore competency. Genetics (such as cytokine and receptor polymorphisms) may influence the effectiveness by which allostasis is restored. Further insults (↑) to the patient (line sepsis, translocation of bacteria, additional operative procedures) delay recovery of the immune system, prolonging PICU stay and increasing likelihood of a fatal outcome (†).

a healthcare-associated infection. The latest available (2011) National Nosocomial Infection Surveillance report from the Centers for Disease Control in Atlanta demonstrates a continuing reduction in national standardized infection ratio in central line–associated bloodstream infections (CLABSIs) to 0.557 (0.645 in NICUs), in North American PICUs. The crude mean CLABSI rate for adults is 1.1 per 1000 device days (range 0.8 for surgical cardiothoracic and 3.4 for burns units) and 1.4 per 1000 device days for pediatric intensive care admissions. The reason for a continued incidence of nosocomial infection is unclear but does not appear to correlate with patients' initial admitting severity score. It may be that, in an attempt to restore the equilibrium following a proinflammatory SIRS response, some patients generate an excessive anti-inflammatory response, which may explain some of the remaining nosocomial infections.

Excessive Anti-inflammation: "Acquired Immunoparalysis"

An excessive compensatory anti-inflammatory response to the primary insult leaves patients in a state of *acquired immunoparalysis*, in which they are unable to produce an adequate immune response to a new threat, such as a nosocomial infection. In part, this inadequacy is attributable to apoptosis of DCs and lymphocytes in response to the CARS/Th-2 mediators. Further infection during this phase of the patient's illness is likely to progress rapidly, contributing further to organ dysfunction, late multiorgan failure, and death. Failure of clinical trials directed against excessive proinflammation, along with recognition of the biphasic nature of the inflammatory response, has resulted in a general acknowledgment that any future trials should be appropriately targeted to the immune state of the individual patient. Several laboratory tests are being used to classify and monitor the immune status of critically ill patients (30,31). Most studies use two assays to define *acquired immunoparalysis*. One measures the capacity of host monocytes to produce TNF in response to stimulation with endotoxin, while the other measures surface expression of the major histocompatibility complex class II molecule on circulating monocytes (usually the human leukocyte antigen HLA-DR) by flow cytometry. As expression of this molecule is tightly controlled

by a large number of pro- and anti-inflammatory mediators, surface expression levels reflect the balance between pro- and anti-inflammatory responses. Indeed, monocyte HLA-DR expression appears to correlate with in vitro cytokine production in response to bacterial antigens, lymphocyte proliferation in response to recall antigens, and the ability to present new antigens. While clinical studies have shown a contemporaneous relationship between reduced HLA-DR expression and circulating levels of the anti-inflammatory cytokines, to date they have failed to show a direct association between HLA-DR expression and circulating levels of the cytokines TNF-α, IL-10, or TGF-β.

Reduced monocyte surface expression of HLA-DR occurs in critically ill patients over the first few days of ICU admission following surgery, trauma, or sepsis. Although levels between survivors and nonsurvivors do not appear to be significantly different at this stage, lower levels of HLA-DR expression have been found in patients who subsequently develop nosocomial infections. Repeated studies indicate that *persistent* downregulation (>5–7 days) of surface HLA-DR expression on monocytes following an inflammatory insult appears to be associated with late mortality, whereas HLA-DR expression is restored promptly to premorbid levels in survivors following an inflammatory insult.

Ongoing physiologic insults, such as nosocomial infection, endocrine abnormalities, and repeated tissue trauma, propagate a state of immunoparalysis by attenuating recovery of HLA-DR expression, leaving the patient at risk of further infection, late morbidity, and mortality (**Fig. 81.6**).

RESOLUTION VERSUS PERSISTENCE OF THE INFLAMMATORY RESPONSE

The balance between those elements of the immune system determining the susceptibility to infective organisms and the severity of the resultant illness, as well as the pattern of pro- and anti-inflammatory responses in determining the clinical course have been discussed. It may be useful to consider the balance between processes that act to resolve acute inflammation and those that cause it to persist. An overlap obviously exists between this analysis and that discussed previously, with SIRS/Th-1 responses tending to prolong inflammation and CARS/Th-2 responses tending to resolve it, but further elements outside of this axis will be considered.

A key element in resolving the immune response is effective clearance of microorganisms. This requires the presence of activated polymorphonuclear cells (PMNs, or neutrophils) and other phagocytic cells in the appropriate tissue at the appropriate time, with intact cellular processes for killing and disposing of the bacteria. These cells are powerful agents for resolution of the inflammatory response because bacteria that have been recognized, ingested, and killed by PMNs no longer present an inflammatory stimulus. Inability of PMNs to get to the right place at the right time, or to achieve effective killing of bacteria, leads to persistence of the inflammatory response from unresolved infection. Autopsy studies suggest that persistent or unrecognized infections are common in children with sepsis-induced multiorgan failure (32).

Defects in the Removal of Microorganisms

As stated previously, an important function of PMNs is to get to the right place at the right time and to achieve effective killing of bacteria. Conditions in which dysfunctions occur in these steps are associated with severe and often prolonged infections and provide clues as to the value of these processes in resolving infections and restoring homeostasis.

Neutropenia

Chemotherapy-induced neutropenia clearly demonstrates the importance of PMNs. More than 90% of cases of childhood acute leukemia suffer one or more episodes of febrile illness, and infections account for two-thirds of treatment-related deaths in acute myeloid leukemia. Restoration of neutrophil counts is required to clear many infections but (in a paradox similar to the balance of susceptibility versus severity discussed previously) is often associated with a clinical deterioration as the systemic inflammatory response worsens. For example,

worsening of acute lung injury following bone marrow transplantation engraftment is well recognized.

Chemotherapy-associated febrile neutropenic sepsis incidence is reduced by giving recombinant granulocyte colony-stimulating factor (G-CSF), which increases neutrophil counts. This same intervention, however, did not reduce mortality in two trials of pneumonia-associated sepsis.

Leukocyte Adhesion

The mechanisms by which activated leukocytes are recruited into inflamed tissues have been studied in detail (**Fig. 81.7**). This multistep process is modulated by adhesion molecules present on whole cells, such as neutrophils, platelets, and endothelial cells. The importance of these molecules in the inflammatory cascade that may develop into the systemic inflammatory response is supported by animal and human data and by observations in patients who are deficient in elements of this sequence. Several rare conditions exist in which leukocytes do not migrate adequately from the circulation into tissues owing to the absence or dysfunction of these adhesion molecules.

Type 1 leukocyte adhesion deficiency results from a lack of expression of the surface protein CD18, which is necessary for the formation of the β_2 integrin heterodimers that are involved in firm adhesion. Failure of leukocytes to migrate into tissues results in delayed clearance of bacteria. Patients with <1% expression of CD18 present early in life with recurrent bacteremias, progressing to life-threatening infections and requiring bone marrow transplantation for long-term survival. Patients with a moderate phenotype (2.5%–6% of the normal concentrations of protein) have peritonitis, delayed wound healing, and skin infections. Complete absence of CD18 is clearly detrimental in the local control of acute infection and inflammation; therapeutic blockade of CD18 looked promising in animal models (33), but has not translated to human trials. Conversely, anti-CD11a was successful in the chronic inflammatory disease psoriasis (34).

It has been recognized that leukocytes can form complexes either with themselves or with other cell types, including platelets and cell fragments, or "microparticles." These complexes then present a wider array of adhesion molecules than either cell

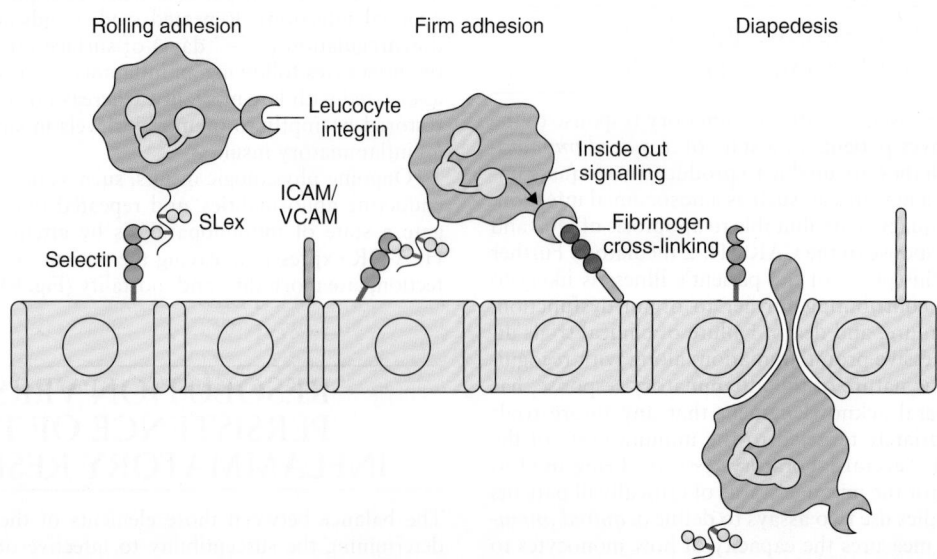

FIGURE 81.7. Mechanism of leukocyte–endothelial interaction. Rolling adhesion mediated by sialyl Lewis^x and other glycosylated structures and selectins. Firm adhesion and diapedesis is mediated by integrins and molecules of the immunoglobulin superfamily (chemokines). ICAM, intercellular cell adhesion molecule; VCAM, vascular cell adhesion molecule.

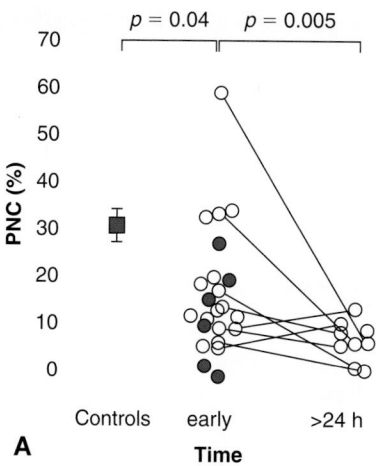

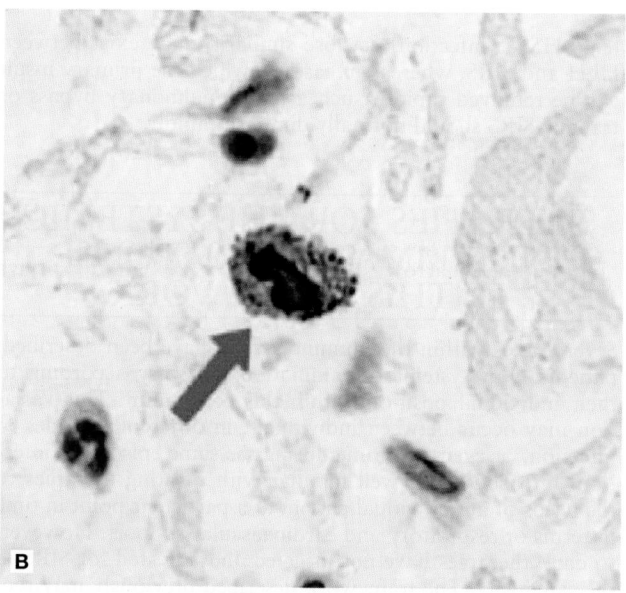

FIGURE 81.8. (A) Platelet neutrophil complexes (PNCs) in 23 cases of acute meningococcal sepsis. Control values for PNC (mean and 95% CIs are shown) were observed in PICU control patients ($n = 20$). Solid circles represent nonsurvivors; open circles represent survivors. The reduced level of PNC on presentation reduced further between 24 and 48 hours. (B) Skin biopsies demonstrated PNC in perivascular infiltrates (CD41 stained).

killing. These patients are deficient in the enzyme NADPH oxidase, which is required for production of the toxic conditions that effect bacterial killing. These patients suffer stubborn infections similar to those seen in patients with leukocyte adhesion deficiency or neutropenia. Interestingly, killing is now thought not to be dependent upon oxidative free radical production but on protease activity and local charge conditions in the vacuole, which cause compensatory ion shifts that disrupt bacterial membranes (37). Granuloma formation probably represents a failure to adequately remove microbial products. These lesions paradoxically may necessitate the use of steroids to reduce the ensuing inappropriate inflammatory response.

Interferon gamma (IFN-γ), an essential cytokine for innate immunity activation, was shown to restore monocyte function in patients with reduced HLA-DR expression. A very small trial of IFN-γ in nine severe sepsis patients showed survival in eight. A larger clinical trial is underway, expected to close in December 2016.

Effective Removal of Prokaryote and Eukaryote Material for Resolution of Infection and the Inflammatory Response

All of the steps just discussed are required for the effective killing of invading microorganisms and the inflammatory response that they generate. However, for the inflammatory response to resolve, an effective removal of cellular (both host and microbial) debris must also occur without further release of proinflammatory elements, such as endotoxin. Importantly, "spent" PMNs undergo apoptosis (programmed cell death) after they have performed these useful functions—and therefore die "silently" without leaving inflammatory cellular debris. Typically, these apoptotic PMNs are, in turn, phagocytosed by tissue macrophages. The processes of apoptosis are significantly altered during systemic inflammation. Several lines of evidence suggest that PMN apoptosis is delayed in sepsis or SIRS. As with all of the systems discussed, this may be beneficial in appropriate circumstances, but harmful in others. Delayed PMN apoptosis may be of benefit by enabling further bacterial clearance, but it may also result in necrotic cell death, which provides a further inflammatory stimulus to the clearing macrophage. The balance between appropriate resolution and harmful persistence of the immune response is, therefore, complex and likely to be very dependent on local factors.

Similarly, apoptosis of lymphocyte subpopulations is differentially affected in both sepsis and SIRS. Insight into the importance of these processes may be gained by considering a condition in which apoptosis is severely abnormal.

Hemophagocytic Lymphohistiocytosis

Hemophagocytic lymphohistiocytosis (HLH) describes a mix of congenital and acquired conditions in which high fever, lymphadenopathy, hepatosplenomegaly, pancytopenia, liver dysfunction, and central nervous system dysfunction are often prominent (**Table 81.7**). Typically, these findings are within the context of an acute infection. Abnormally large and activated cells of myeloid origin (hemophagocytes) are typically found on examination of bone marrow. While these complex conditions are described elsewhere in this text, recent advances in the understanding of the pathogenesis and prevalence of these conditions offer insight into the resolution of the SIRS and sepsis.

Secondary HLH represents a sustained, systemic inflammatory response following a variety of primary insults (viral, bacterial, or fungal) similar to the way in which SIRS represents a nonspecific final pathway after infection, trauma, burns, and

alone. As such, these complexes have a greater capacity to bind to endothelial cells and migrate to tissues. In health, these complexes are constantly forming and dissociating and may act to provide a more activated subpopulation of cells for clearance of bacteria within the circulation or more ready recruitment into tissues. In sepsis, these circulating platelet–neutrophil complexes are reduced, probably due to selective binding to the endothelium and/or migration into the tissues (35) (**Fig. 81.8**). The potential for these primed platelet–neutrophil complexes to cause tissue injury and initiate thrombus formation is considerable and may explain why the combination of low platelets and neutrophils is a good predictor of poor outcome in meningococcal sepsis (36).

Bacterial Killing

Chronic granulomatous disease is a rare condition in which a patient's leukocytes lack the capacity to generate bacterial

TABLE 81.7

CRITERIA FOR THE DIAGNOSIS OF HEMOPHAGOCYTIC LYMPHOHISTIOCYTOSIS

The diagnosis of HLH is established by fulfilling either or both of the following criteria:
1. A molecular diagnosis consistent with HLH (e.g., PRF1, RAB27A, STXBP2, STX11, SH2D1A, UNC13D, or XIAP)
AND/OR
2. Having ≥5 of the following 8 clinical criteria:
   a. Fever
   b. Splenomegaly
   c. Cytopenia affecting 2 cell lineages: hemoglobin <9 g/dL (or 10 g/dL for infants <4 wks of age), platelets <100,000/μL, and neutrophils <1000 μL
   d. Hypertriglyceridemia (>272 mg/dL) and/or hypofibrinogenemia (<150 mg/dL)
   e. Hemophagocytosis in the bone marrow, spleen, or lymph nodes without evidence of malignancy
   f. Low or absent NK cell cytotoxicity (according to local laboratory reference values)
   g. Hyperferritinemia (>500 ng/mL)
   h. Elevated soluble CD25 (IL-2Ra chain >2400 U/mL)

pancreatitis (38). In fact, some reports indicate that HLH and SIRS overlap and coexist in individual cases. An autopsy study of adults who died while in the ICU found evidence of hemophagocytosis on bone marrow examination in 72% of cases; this rose to 83% of cases with sepsis (39). Similarly, children who died of H5N1 influenza virus pneumonia had evidence of hemophagocytosis on lung histology (40). An important distinction is that the outcome for children with active HLH who are in intensive care with multiorgan failure is dismal and much worse than the outcome of those with sepsis-induced multiorgan failure (41,42).

Several cellular mechanisms of congenital predispositions to HLH have been elucidated. Mutations in the genes for perforin are especially important, occurring in 20%–40% of HLH cases. Perforin is a protein found in granules of cytotoxic effector cells, including natural killer cells and activated lymphocytes. Perforin polymerizes in the membranes of target cells to allow entry of the variety of cytotoxic enzymes that cause target cell death via apoptosis. As described previously, apoptosis allows efficient packaging of toxic material (e.g., infected cells) for phagocytosis while causing the minimum amount of inflammatory stimulus. Lack of perforin prevents access of these enzymes, and the inflammatory stimulus of the infected target cell persists. Other defects in this process have been identified, including mutations to the MUNC13-4 and STX 11 genes, which act to prevent the normal release of these same enzymes from cytotoxic T lymphocytes by preventing granule fusion to the plasma membrane. The multiorgan failure seen in HLH, therefore, at least in part, reflects the failure of the normal clearance mechanisms to deal with the toxic debris of microorganisms and infected cells (43).

Macrophage activation syndrome (MAS) may be seen as HLH in the context of rheumatic disease. The overall risk of developing MAS in systemic onset juvenile idiopathic arthritis is 10% with an associated mortality of approximately 20%. Although less common, MAS does occur in other rheumatologic disease, for example, systemic lupus erythematosus, Kawasaki disease, and inflammatory bowel disease. Differentiation of MAS and primary HLH requires a fast turnaround for genetic testing and underscores the overlap in clinical and laboratory parameters.

A possible overlap between HLH and SIRS is that they both reflect extreme examples of powerful proinflammation that have avoided the normal mechanisms for contracting the immune response. Similar failures of toxic substance clearance may occur in sepsis as a result of dysregulated apoptosis. In other words, both prolonged sepsis and HLH conditions can be viewed as relative failures of the host mechanisms to contract the immune response. With a severe or persistent insult

(e.g., H5N1 infection), a close similarity may exist between HLH and SIRS, whereas in cases in which the primary insult can be removed rapidly, such as cardiopulmonary bypass or trauma, SIRS should normally diminish rapidly.

THERAPIES FOR THE SYSTEMIC INFLAMMATORY RESPONSE IN THIS FRAMEWORK

Several axes within the immune system have been described; patients with systemic inflammation will vary according to their individual position within this continuum. This variation may occur between individuals, in different episodes of infection, or even with time during the same episode of infection. Intensivists are well familiar with titrating therapies to the needs of an individual patient at a particular point in time in terms of respiratory and cardiovascular support. However, to date, therapies have not targeted and adjusted for SIRS in the same way. The framework described previously may represent ways of describing individual cases of sepsis/SIRS and targeting therapies to a patient's individual needs. We suggest that existing therapies may yet provide significant advances in the care for such children, if they can be targeted at those individuals with the greatest potential for benefit and the least likelihood of harm.

Therapies That Can Modulate the Balance Between Effective Microbial Killing and the Resultant Inflammatory Response

A proportion of patients who are admitted to the PICU will subsequently be found to have a major defect in their immune system. The vast majority of patients, however, either who are admitted with an infection or who develop an infectious complication while in the PICU, will not have been noted to be at an increased risk for either infection or an excessive inflammatory response prior to admission. The complex nature of how genetic polymorphisms are likely to act in the critical care setting makes therapies targeted at the inflammatory consequences of microbial destruction difficult and potentially dangerous. However, limited data indicate that, in Staphylococcal and Streptococcal toxic shock syndromes, the use of IV immunoglobulin and clindamycin could be beneficial. Both agents act to neutralize the effect of exotoxins—IV immunoglobulin by binding to the exotoxins, and clindamycin by inhibiting the production of exotoxins. Data on how these agents may act in other conditions are limited.

A recombinant version of MBL was developed for therapeutic use and may have provided an opportunity for combining antimicrobial activity with inflammatory modulation. Commercial interests prevailed, and this product is not available as yet. Bactericidal permeability increasing protein (BPI) is an antibacterial molecule with antiendotoxin properties. A recombinant form of this protein, $rBPI_{21}$, may provide a means of killing Gram-negative bacteria, while limiting the potentially harmful inflammatory effects of endotoxin. Clinical studies to date have been disappointing in terms of mortality, even though one study showed a clinically relevant reduction in morbidity with less limb amputations and reduced requirement for platelet transfusions in a randomized trial of $rBPI_{21}$ for meningococcal septic shock (44).

Possible Therapies for Acute Severe Proinflammation

High-Dose Corticosteroids

The effects of exogenous steroids on the immune system are complex and vary according to type, dose, duration, and state of the immune system at the time of administration. Glucocorticoids bind to cytoplasmic glucocorticoid receptors and, via NFκB, act at a transcription level to modulate pro- and anti-inflammatory cytokine levels. Glucocorticoids inhibit production of the proinflammatory cytokines TNF-α, IL-1α, IL-1β, IL-6, IL-8, IL-12, IFN-γ, and granulocyte macrophage CSF (GM-CSF). In addition, glucocorticoids increase transcription of IL-1ra and IL-10, inhibit neutrophil activation, and suppress the synthesis of phospholipase A_2, cyclooxygenase, and inducible nitric oxide synthase. These broad-spectrum anti-inflammatory effects led to their investigation in sepsis.

Large doses of synthetic glucocorticoids (methylprednisolone or dexamethasone) have been investigated in unselected severe sepsis in adults (45). High-dose corticosteroids convey no benefit in septic shock in adults. While some favorable cardiovascular changes were observed, an overall trend toward decreased survival, with high rates of nosocomial infection, was also observed. Within the framework presented in this chapter, steroids might represent an effective intervention against excessive proinflammation that may worsen the risk of excessive anti-inflammation.

The option of high-dose steroids might be reconsidered in pediatric catecholamine-resistant septic shock, in which the risk of early cardiovascular collapse is greater than that of secondary infection. Observational studies suggest that relative adrenal insufficiency may be common and intensive cardiovascular support alone may be insufficient without replacing adequate doses of hydrocortisone (46). If this option is taken forward, any success is likely to be highly dependent on selecting only cases at very high risk of early (proinflammatory) death due to cardiovascular failure. It would also require techniques to limit potentially harmful excessive immunosuppressive effects, including rapid reduction in dosage and great care to reduce the risks of nosocomial sepsis. Moreover, a potential alternative might be venoarterial extracorporeal membrane oxygenation, given the current lower associated morbidity and increasing availability of this modality.

The impact of steroid therapy in a less-than-overwhelming episode of systemic inflammation may be reflected in their use perioperatively in elective cardiac surgery. While the intention was to suppress the post-bypass SIRS response (and indeed a reduction in plasma levels of proinflammatory cytokines has been observed), it remains unclear whether suppression of SIRS is clinically beneficial in these patients. While very little evidence suggests that the use of steroids reduces the morbidity or mortality associated with cardiac surgery, some evidence does suggest that steroids may increase the duration of ventilation and worsen outcome (47–49), perhaps reflecting an excessive immunosuppressive result that leads to an anti-inflammatory state. Indeed, increased IL-10 production has been associated with perioperative steroid use.

Physiologic Doses of Corticosteroids

At physiologic levels, cortisol supports the vascular adrenergic receptor function and inhibits cytokine-induced nitric oxide synthase, thus potentiating vasoconstriction and myocardial contractility. The use of glucocorticoids has been reconsidered with evidence that adrenal failure or *relative adrenal insufficiency* is common in critically ill adults and children. The use of physiologic doses of corticosteroids in adult septic shock remains inconclusive. Two large randomized, controlled trials in septic patients have shown conflicting results in regard to benefit (50,51). Neither is it clear if these steroid doses have significant anti-inflammatory effects. Nonetheless, the most current Surviving Sepsis Campaign guideline for adults recommends the use of physiologic doses of hydrocortisone in patients with poor response to fluid resuscitation and vasopressor therapy (52).

Activated Protein C

Recombinant human activated protein C (rhAPC) possesses anticoagulant, profibrinolytic, and anti-inflammatory properties. Despite early positive trial findings, more recent data did not show benefit and have prompted the manufacturer to remove APC from the market. Whether or not APC may have had benefit in a better-defined subpopulation in sepsis remains unanswered.

Anticytokine Therapies—Monoclonal Antibodies

Effective blockade of TNF is still being assessed in clinical trials. A meta-analysis of 15 randomized placebo controlled trials in severe sepsis in the adult population showed that TNF blockade was safe and had a survival benefit (relative risk 0.93, 95% CI, 0.88–0.98; $p = 0.01$) (53). Given the still reducing mortality in sepsis and the heterogeneity of cytokine profiles in cohorts with a clinical diagnosis of sepsis, we suggest that patients be selected prior to treatment on the basis of some laboratory or clinical parameters that have good positive predictive value for identifying an excessive proinflammatory response. Also, mortality, especially in pediatric sepsis, requires review as the primary endpoint in trials.

HLH poses a hyperinflammatory state in children that might be amenable to anticytokine therapy. A recent retrospective small case series on the use of recombinant IL-1-receptor antagonist (anakinra) in secondary HLH showed clinical improvement after the drug was started (54). Given the nature of the study, it is too early to be able to attribute clinical benefit. The increasing availability of antibodies to other cytokines, such as IL-6, may stimulate further studies to assess a targeted role for cytokine modulation in critical illness.

Possible Therapies for Immunoparalysis

Aggressive Deintensification of Patients

Acquired immunoparalysis will only present a problem if the patient's immune system is challenged beyond the residual capacity to respond. Simple best practices of critical care may reduce this risk dramatically and should not be forgotten during the quest for more innovative solutions. Priority should be given to removal of invasive monitoring lines, endotracheal tubes, and urinary catheters at the earliest possible time to reduce the risk of transient bacteremias in these vulnerable patients.

Stimulating Factors

In one of the landmark studies in sepsis, possible beneficial effects of administration of the proinflammatory cytokine IFN-γ to cases of severe sepsis established the principle that the anti-inflammatory state of acquired immunoparalysis exists and may cause harm following a systemic insult (55). At the time of this writing, a large-scale trial of the targeted use of IFN-γ in patients with acquired immunoparalysis is still underway [ClinicalTrials.gov NCT01649921].

GM-CSF and G-CSF are naturally occurring cytokines that stimulate the number and antimicrobial functions of both neutrophils and monocytes. To date, they have a clear clinical use in the treatment of neutropenia, where their use has been shown to reduce the number of documented infections but not infection-related mortality (56). Interest has extended from their use in accelerating myeloid cell recovery to the potential for benefit from their immune-enhancing properties. In animal models of sepsis, cotreatment with GM-CSF has been shown to enhance pathogen eradication and decrease morbidity and/or mortality (57). However, the outcome in clinical trials has been less clear. Administration of GM-CSF appears to have minimal side effects, to restore monocyte HLA-DR expression and function, and to assist in reducing sepsis episodes, but to date, it has not been shown to affect mortality (58). The effects are even less clear in randomized, controlled, neonatal trials (59). The value of GM-CSF may be greatest if subpopulations with evidence of acquired immunoparalysis are targeted.

A possible role of immunonutrients (arginine, glutamine, eicosapentaenoic acid, Ω-3 fatty acids) as immunomodulating agents has gained attention. Glutamine is an abundant free amino acid in humans, critical for the integrity and function of metabolically active tissues. Under normal conditions, glutamine is a nonessential amino acid. However, in critical illness, glutamine levels in the body decrease, and its endogenous supply cannot match the increased demand. In vivo, circulating glutamine levels have been shown to be significantly reduced in both adults and children following surgery or trauma and to be associated with higher rates of infection (60).

Glutamine has immunomodulatory properties in vitro, with several actions on the immune system, including potentiation of the nonspecific cell-defense mechanisms of heat shock protein (Hsp) production in response to endotoxin and ischemia–reperfusion injury (61). Glutamine infusions enhance Hsp expression in multiple vital organs (heart, lung, and gut) in rat models of intestinal ischemia–reperfusion injury. In models of sepsis and injury, glutamine supplementation has been shown to increase survival, improve immune function, reduce bacteremia, increase gut barrier function, and decrease gastrointestinal mucosal atrophy. In vivo, parenteral supplementation with glutamine in adults has been associated with preservation of monocyte HLA-DR expression, decrease in infectious complications, and shortened hospital stay (62,63).

However, for each study in which glutamine administration to critically ill patients appears to show benefit, a similar study exists with no effect. While this may be attributable to the formulation and dose of glutamine chosen or the route of administration, it may also be that glutamine supplementation is beneficial only when appropriately targeted. A cocktail of glutamine, zinc, selenium, and metoclopramide showed only reduced PICU-acquired nosocomial infection in the subgroup of immune compromised children (64). Similarly, in a randomized trial of parenteral glutamine in surgical infants, the overall incidence of sepsis was not reduced (65).

A mortality benefit has been suggested for enteral feeding with eicosapentaenoic acid, γ-linolenic acid, and antioxidants in adult septic shock cases (66). These observations are perhaps consistent with our framework, despite the lack of patient selection, because these lipids are reported to have both pro- and anti-inflammatory actions (67).

Removal of Inhibitory Plasma Mediators

Addition of IL-10 monoclonal antibodies has been shown to attenuate the inhibitory effect of serum drawn from critically ill patients on control monocyte phenotype and function (68). While IL-10 appears to play an important role in acquired immunoparalysis, it is not the only soluble factor that appears to be acting (68,69). Attempts to eliminate a wide range of different inhibitory factors (as well as possible proinflammatory mediators) have resulted in case reports of hemofiltration, apheresis, and plasmapheresis in critically ill patients. The ability of any of these therapies to change the level of circulating mediators depends on the method used. Conventional plasma exchange does not consistently affect plasma levels of IL-6, IL-6R, TNF-α, TNF-αR, or C-reactive protein. At present, this therapy remains experimental. By comparison, continuous hemofiltration has been shown to minimally reduce inflammatory mediators (complement activation, plasma thromboxane, and proinflammatory cytokines at high-volume filtration) (70,71). Retrospective, single-centered studies suggest that the use of continuous renal hemofiltration in critically ill children improves outcome. The mechanism by which this may be acting is uncertain, and although it may be through an immunomodulating effect, it may also be acting to remove free water, improve fluid balance, and correct acid–base status. A recent meta-analysis on blood purification methods in adult septic shock showed an associated reduced mortality (72). An accompanying editorial discussed potential biases and methodological flaws, but concluded that there was enough scope in blood purification methods to pursue the intervention in adult sepsis at least (73).

CONCLUSIONS AND FUTURE DIRECTIONS

Critical illness (whether infective or noninfective in origin) evokes an immune response that influences the patient's intensive care course. Unlike other vital systems, no accepted physiologic variable or biochemical test exists with which to monitor the complexity and variability of this response. While the immune response has evolved to limit the harmful stimulus, an excessive or unchecked response can result in significant cellular and organ damage.

Biologic systems within the body are designed to both respond to a stressful event and to act to restore physiologic homeostasis. The immune system is no different. For every proinflammatory response, there appears to be a balancing anti-inflammatory response. Under ideal conditions, the inflammatory response is short lived, appropriately sized, and effective during critical illness, and the patient recovers well with limited intensive care support. However, in many clinical scenarios, a balanced immune response is not seen, perhaps due to an inappropriate host immune response (too much or too little) or to the medical management instituted. Broad applications of immunomodulatory agents to patients with critical illness have failed spectacularly, probably because therapies have been administered to patients who vary in their timing, location, and relative balance of immune response.

Future therapeutic trials should target therapy appropriate to the individual inflammatory response of the critically ill patient. To do this, the treating clinician must be able to identify the patient's immunocompetence and inflammatory, as well as infectious, status. Only by understanding the immune response of an individual patient will the clinician be able to more judiciously use antimicrobials and immunomodulating therapies in the setting of critical illness. In addition, the intervention of choice requires robust in vivo efficacy as well as pharmacokinetic/pharmacodynamic data or modeling. Finally, we require an appropriate patient-centered outcome measure with a relevance to the intervention.

References

1. Janeway CA, Jr. The immune system evolved to discriminate infectious nonself from noninfectious self. *Immunol Today* 1992;13(1):11–6.
2. Matzinger P. The danger model: A renewed sense of self. *Science* 2002;296(5566):301–5.
3. Matzinger P. The evolution of the danger theory. Interview by Lauren Constable, Commissioning Editor. *Expert Rev Clin Immunol* 2012;8(4):311–7.
4. Oppenheim JJ, Yang D. Alarmins: Chemotactic activators of immune responses. *Curr Opin Immunol* 2005;17(4):359–65.
5. Brame AL, Singer M. Stressing the obvious? An allostatic look at critical illness. *Crit Care Med* 2010;38(10 suppl):S600–7.
6. Dommett RM, Klein N, Turner MW. Mannose-binding lectin in innate immunity: Past, present and future. *Tissue Antigens* 2006;68(3):193–209.
7. Mathew S, Overturf GD. Complement and properidin deficiencies in meningococcal disease. *Pediatr Infect Dis J* 2006;25(3):255–6.
8. Lehner PJ, Davies KA, Walport MJ, et al. Meningococcal septicaemia in a C6-deficient patient and effects of plasma transfusion on lipopolysaccharide release. *Lancet* 1992;340(8832):1379–81.
9. Davila S, Wright VJ, Khor CC, et al. Genome-wide association study identifies variants in the CFH region associated with host susceptibility to meningococcal disease. *Nat Genet* 2010;42(9):772–6.
10. Agbeko RS, Fidler KJ, Allen ML, et al. Genetic variability in complement activation modulates the systemic inflammatory response syndrome in children. *Pediatr Crit Care Med* 2010;11(5):561–7.
11. Fidler KJ, Wilson P, Davies JC, et al. Increased incidence and severity of the systemic inflammatory response syndrome in patients deficient in mannose-binding lectin. *Intensive Care Med* 2004;30(7):1438–45.
12. Garred P, Strom J, Quist L, et al. Association of mannose-binding lectin polymorphisms with sepsis and fatal outcome, in patients with systemic inflammatory response syndrome. *J Infect Dis* 2003;188(9):1394–403.
13. Gordon AC, Waheed U, Hansen TK, et al. Mannose-binding lectin polymorphisms in severe sepsis: Relationship to levels, incidence, and outcome. *Shock* 2006;25(1):88–93.
14. Felmet KA, Hall MW, Clark RS, et al. Prolonged lymphopenia, lymphoid depletion, and hypoprolactinemia in children with nosocomial sepsis and multiple organ failure. *J Immunol* 2005;174(6):3765–72.
15. Walsh MC, Bourcier T, Takahashi K, et al. Mannose-binding lectin is a regulator of inflammation that accompanies myocardial ischemia and reperfusion injury. *J Immunol* 2005;175(1):541–6.
16. Sauter C, Wolfensberger C. Interferon in human serum after injection of endotoxin. *Lancet* 1980;2(8199):852–3.
17. Stephens RC, Fidler K, Wilson P, et al. Endotoxin immunity and the development of the systemic inflammatory response syndrome in critically ill children. *Intensive Care Med* 2006;32(2):286–94.
18. Schaaf BM, Boehmke F, Esnaashari H, et al. Pneumococcal septic shock is associated with the interleukin-10-1082 gene promoter polymorphism. *Am J Respir Crit Care Med* 2003;168(4):476–80.
19. Stanilova SA, Miteva LD, Karakolev ZT, et al. Interleukin-10-1082 promoter polymorphism in association with cytokine production and sepsis susceptibility. *Intensive Care Med* 2006;32(2):260–66.
20. Allen ML, Hoschtitzky JA, Peters MJ, et al. Interleukin-10 and its role in clinical immunoparalysis following pediatric cardiac surgery. *Crit Care Med* 2006;34(10):2658–65.
21. Latz E, Xiao TS, Stutz A. Activation and regulation of the inflammasomes. *Nat Rev Immunol* 2013;13(6):397–411.
22. Goldstein B, Giroir B, Randolph A. International pediatric sepsis consensus conference: Definitions for sepsis and organ dysfunction in pediatrics. *Pediatr Crit Care Med* 2005;6(1):2–8.
23. Levy MM, Fink MP, Marshall JC, et al. 2001 SCCM/ESICM/ACCP/ATS/SIS International Sepsis Definitions Conference. *Crit Care Med* 2003;31(4):1250–56.
24. Pathan N, Hemingway CA, Alizadeh AA, et al. Role of interleukin 6 in myocardial dysfunction of meningococcal septic shock. *Lancet* 2004;363(9404):203–9.
25. Cavaillon JM, Annane D. Compartmentalization of the inflammatory response in sepsis and SIRS. *J Endotoxin Res* 2006;12(3):151–70.
26. Andersson U, Tracey KJ. Reflex principles of immunological homeostasis. *Annu Rev Immunol* 2012;30:313–35.
27. Zeni F, Freeman B, Natanson C. Anti-inflammatory therapies to treat sepsis and septic shock: A reassessment. *Crit Care Med* 1997;25(7):1095–100.
28. Bone RC. Sir Isaac Newton, sepsis, SIRS, and CARS. *Crit Care Med* 1996;24(7):1125–8.
29. Panacek EA, Marshall JC, Albertson TE, et al. Efficacy and safety of the monoclonal anti-tumor necrosis factor antibody F(ab')2 fragment afelimomab in patients with severe sepsis and elevated interleukin-6 levels. *Crit Care Med* 2004;32(11):2173–82.
30. Cross AS, Opal SM. A new paradigm for the treatment of sepsis: Is it time to consider combination therapy? *Ann Intern Med* 2003;138(6):502–5.
31. Kox WJ, Volk T, Kox SN, et al. Immunomodulatory therapies in sepsis. *Intensive Care Med* 2000;26(suppl 1):S124–8.
32. Amoo-Lamptey A, Dickman P, Carcillo J. Comparative pathology of children with sepsis and MOF, pneumonia without MOF, and MOF without infection. *Pediatr Res* 2001;49:46A.
33. Gardinali M, Borrelli E, Chiara O, et al. Inhibition of CD11-CD18 complex prevents acute lung injury and reduces mortality after peritonitis in rabbits. *Am J Respir Crit Care Med* 2000;161(3, pt 1):1022–9.
34. Leonardi CL, Papp KA, Gordon KB, et al. Extended efalizumab therapy improves chronic plaque psoriasis: Results from a randomized phase III trial. *J Am Acad Dermatol* 2005;52(3, pt 1):425–33.
35. Inwald DP, Faust SN, Lister P, et al. Platelet and soluble CD40L in meningococcal sepsis. *Intensive Care Med* 2006;32(9):1432–7.
36. Peters MJ, Ross-Russell RI, White D, et al. Early severe neutropenia and thrombocytopenia identifies the highest risk cases of severe meningococcal disease. *Pediatr Crit Care Med* 2001;2(3):225–31.
37. Segal AW. How neutrophils kill microbes. *Annu Rev Immunol* 2005;23:197–223.
38. Verbsky JW, Grossman WJ. Hemophagocytic lymphohistiocytosis: Diagnosis, pathophysiology, treatment, and future perspectives. *Ann Med* 2006;38(1):20–31.
39. Strauss R, Neureiter D, Westenburger B, et al. Multifactorial risk analysis of bone marrow histiocytic hyperplasia with hemophagocytosis in critically ill medical patients—A postmortem clinicopathologic analysis. *Crit Care Med* 2004;32(6):1316–21.
40. Henter JI, Chow CB, Leung CW, et al. Cytotoxic therapy for severe avian influenza A (H5N1) infection. *Lancet* 2006;367(9513):870–3.
41. Nahum E, Ben-Ari J, Stain J, et al. Hemophagocytic lymphohistiocytic syndrome: Unrecognized cause of multiple organ failure. *Pediatr Crit Care Med* 2000;1(1):51–4.

42. Ouachee-Chardin M, Elie C, de Saint Basile G, et al. Hematopoietic stem cell transplantation in hemophagocytic lymphohistiocytosis: A single-center report of 48 patients. *Pediatrics* 2006; 117(4):e743–50.

43. zur Stadt U, Schmidt S, Kasper B, et al. Linkage of familial hemophagocytic lymphohistiocytosis (FHL) type-4 to chromosome 6q24 and identification of mutations in syntaxin 11. *Hum Mol Genet* 2005;14(6):827–34.

44. Levin M, Quint PA, Goldstein B, et al. Recombinant bactericidal/permeability-increasing protein (rBPI21) as adjunctive treatment for children with severe meningococcal sepsis: A randomised trial. rBPI21 Meningococcal Sepsis Study Group. *Lancet* 2000; 356(9234):961–7.

45. Sprung CL, Caralis PV, Marcial EH, et al. The effects of high-dose corticosteroids in patients with septic shock. A prospective, controlled study. *N Engl J Med* 1984;311(18):1137–43.

46. Aneja R, Carcillo JA. What is the rationale for hydrocortisone treatment in children with infection-related adrenal insufficiency and septic shock? *Arch Dis Child* 2007;92(2):165–9.

47. Chaney MA. Corticosteroids and cardiopulmonary bypass: A review of clinical investigations. *Chest* 2002;121(3):921–31.

48. Gessler P, Hohl V, Carrel T, et al. Administration of steroids in pediatric cardiac surgery: Impact on clinical outcome and systemic inflammatory response. *Pediatr Cardiol* 2005;26(5):595–600.

49. Morariu AM, Loef BG, Aarts LP, et al. Dexamethasone: Benefit and prejudice for patients undergoing on-pump coronary artery bypass grafting: A study on myocardial, pulmonary, renal, intestinal, and hepatic injury. *Chest* 2005;128(4):2677–87.

50. Annane D, Sebille V, Charpentier C, et al. Effect of treatment with low doses of hydrocortisone and fludrocortisone on mortality in patients with septic shock. *JAMA* 2002;288(7):862–71.

51. Sprung CL, Annane D, Keh D, et al. Hydrocortisone therapy for patients with septic shock. *N Engl J Med* 2008;358(2):111–24.

52. Dellinger RP, Levy MM, Rhodes A, et al. Surviving Sepsis Campaign: International guidelines for management of severe sepsis and septic shock, 2012. *Intensive Care Med* 2013;39(2): 165–228.

53. Qiu P, Cui X, Sun J, et al. Antitumor necrosis factor therapy is associated with improved survival in clinical sepsis trials: A meta-analysis. *Crit Care Med* 2013;41(10):2419–29.

54. Rajasekaran S, Kruse K, Kovey K, et al. Therapeutic role of anakinra, an interleukin-1 receptor antagonist, in the management of secondary hemophagocytic lymphohistiocytosis/sepsis/multiple organ dysfunction/macrophage activating syndrome in critically ill children. *Pediatr Crit Care Med* 2014;15(5):401–8.

55. Docke WD, Randow F, Syrbe U, et al. Monocyte deactivation in septic patients: Restoration by IFN-gamma treatment. *Nat Med* 1997;3(6):678–81.

56. Sung L, Nathan PC, Lange B, et al. Prophylactic granulocyte colony-stimulating factor and granulocyte-macrophage colony-stimulating factor decrease febrile neutropenia after chemotherapy in children with cancer: A meta-analysis of randomized controlled trials. *J Clin Oncol* 2004;22(16):3350–6.

57. Hubel K, Dale DC, Liles WC. Therapeutic use of cytokines to modulate phagocyte function for the treatment of infectious diseases: Current status of granulocyte colony-stimulating factor, granulocyte-macrophage colony-stimulating factor, macrophage colony-stimulating factor, and interferon-gamma. *J Infect Dis* 2002;185(10):1490–501.

58. Bo L, Wang F, Zhu J, et al. Granulocyte-colony stimulating factor (G-CSF) and granulocyte-macrophage colony stimulating factor (GM-CSF) for sepsis: A meta-analysis. *Crit Care* 2011;15(1):R58.

59. Carr R, Modi N, Dore C. G-CSF and GM-CSF for treating or preventing neonatal infections. *Cochr Database Syst Rev* 2003(3):CD003066.

60. Exner R, Tamandl D, Goetzinger P, et al. Perioperative GLY-GLN infusion diminishes the surgery-induced period of immunosuppression: Accelerated restoration of the lipopolysaccharide-stimulated tumor necrosis factor-alpha response. *Ann Surg* 2003;237(1):110–5.

61. Wischmeyer PE, Riehm J, Singleton KD, et al. Glutamine attenuates tumor necrosis factor-alpha release and enhances heat shock protein 72 in human peripheral blood mononuclear cells. *Nutrition* 2003;19(1):1–6.

62. Griffiths RD, Allen KD, Andrews FJ, et al. Infection, multiple organ failure, and survival in the intensive care unit: Influence of glutamine-supplemented parenteral nutrition on acquired infection. *Nutrition* 2002;18(7–8):546–52.

63. Novak F, Heyland DK, Avenell A, et al. Glutamine supplementation in serious illness: A systematic review of the evidence. *Crit Care Med* 2002;30(9):2022–9.

64. Carcillo JA, Dean JM, Holubkov R, et al. The randomized comparative pediatric critical illness stress-induced immune suppression (CRISIS) prevention trial. *Pediatr Crit Care Med* 2012;13(2):165–73.

65. Ong EG, Eaton S, Wade AM, et al. Randomized clinical trial of glutamine-supplemented versus standard parenteral nutrition in infants with surgical gastrointestinal disease. *Br J Surg* 2012;99(7):929–38.

66. Pontes-Arruda A, Aragao AM, Albuquerque JD. Effects of enteral feeding with eicosapentaenoic acid, gamma-linolenic acid, and antioxidants in mechanically ventilated patients with severe sepsis and septic shock. *Crit Care Med* 2006;34(9):2325–33.

67. Mayer K, Gokorsch S, Fegbeutel C, et al. Parenteral nutrition with fish oil modulates cytokine response in patients with sepsis. *Am J Respir Crit Care Med* 2003;167(10):1321–8.

68. Fumeaux T, Pugin J. Role of interleukin-10 in the intracellular sequestration of human leukocyte antigen-DR in monocytes during septic shock. *Am J Respir Crit Care Med* 2002;166(11):1475–82.

69. Mueller A, Kreuzfelder E, Nyadu B, et al. Human leukocyte antigen-DR expression in peripheral blood mononuclear cells from healthy donors influenced by the sera of injured patients prone to severe sepsis. *Intensive Care Med* 2003;29(12):2285–90.

70. Cole L, Bellomo R, Davenport P, et al. Cytokine removal during continuous renal replacement therapy: An ex vivo comparison of convection and diffusion. *Int J Artif Organs* 2004;27(5):388–97.

71. Jiang HL, Xue WJ, Li DQ, et al. Influence of continuous venovenous hemofiltration on the course of acute pancreatitis. *World J Gastroenterol* 2005;11(31):4815–21.

72. Zhou F, Peng Z, Murugan R, et al. Blood purification and mortality in sepsis: A meta-analysis of randomized trials. *Crit Care Med* 2013;41(9):2209–20.

73. Kalil AC, Florescu MC. Blood purification: Can we purify our patients from sepsis? *Crit Care Med* 2013;41(9):2244–5.

CHAPTER 82 ■ NEUROHORMONAL CONTROL IN THE IMMUNE SYSTEM

KATHRYN A. FELMET

KEY POINTS

1. The central nervous system monitors and regulates the immune system in clinically relevant ways.
2. The immunosuppressive effects of the stress response, characterized by catecholamine and glucocorticoid excess, are balanced by the proinflammatory mediators, such as prolactin and vasopressin.
3. In the acute phase of septic shock, inflammation predominates, but during prolonged critical illness, many patients are immune-suppressed.
4. Clinically significant immune suppression may result from failure of the neuroendocrine immune (NEI) system or from the immunosuppressive side effects of NEI mediators used as critical care therapy.
5. Catecholamines, glucocorticoids, somatostatin, and opioids have their immunosuppressive side effects and should be tapered as soon as clinical conditions allow.
6. Future therapies may target the acquired immune suppression of critical illness.
7. Studies of NEI mediators should include an assessment of their impact on immune function.

Through most of the 20th century, scientists considered the immune system to be autonomous and self-regulating despite knowing that well-characterized neural circuits maintain homeostasis in other organ systems. The idea that states of mind, in particular, the stress of urbanization and industrialization, were capable of causing illness gained popularity among physicians and layperson in during the 18th century. During the same era, the power of placebo to mimic subjective outcomes, such as analgesia, was discovered. It was not until the 1960s that the placebo-controlled trial became the standard for testing new medical intervention. Today, we understand that the central nervous system (CNS) guides the mostly autonomous functions of the immune system through both humoral and neural pathways, much as it oversees functions of the heart, digestive, reproductive, and other systems. Although these pathways are not under our conscious control, they exist at the periphery of our experience, are influenced by pain and stress, are subject to suggestion and classical conditioning, and they influence our behavior and subjective experience.

A comprehensive understanding of the feedback loops that allow the CNS to fine-tune the immune response eludes us. Studies in neuroendocrine immune (NEI) interactions have focused on interactions between NEI mediators and individual cell types. While we still cannot hear the whole symphony, what follows is a description of the few notes and melodies that scientists have taught us to recognize.

THE NEUROHORMONAL RESPONSE TO ACUTE STRESS

Outgoing signals from the brain to the immune system were first understood under the paradigm of the stress response. Acute stress causes activation of the sympathetic nervous system (SNS), which leads to epinephrine release; activation of the hypothalamic–pituitary–adrenal (HPA) axis, which leads to cortisol release; and activation of endogenous opioids. Together these systems prepare a body for action by putting growth and housekeeping functions on hold, making fuel substrates available, and supporting blood pressure and intravascular volume. In addition to the immunosuppressive effects of adrenal steroids, endogenous epinephrine and opioids have also been found to have immunosuppressive effects.

The proinflammatory and immune-supportive influence of pituitary peptide hormones on immune function was first recognized in the 1970s. These proinflammatory peptides, such as vasopressin and prolactin, are also released as a part of the stress response. Dozens of molecules produced by the brain or released from nerve terminals have been discovered to have immunomodulatory properties.

Shared Chemical Language of Neuroendocrine and Immune Systems

The neuroendocrine and immune systems share a chemical language. Immune cells express receptors for neurotransmitters and hormones. Endocrine cells, peripheral nerves, and cells of the CNS express receptors for immune-derived cytokines. Immune cells also produce hormones and signaling molecules classically thought of as neurotransmitters. Brain cells produce a wide variety of cytokines (1). Although the complex interplay of all of these signaling molecules remains poorly understood, the profusion of NEI mediators tells us that the brain provides guidance and fine-tuning for the immune response as it does for other organ systems (Fig. 82.1). To do this, the CNS monitors immune function with high acuity, sensing low levels of inflammatory cytokines and very early mediators of inflammation.

Efferent signals   **Afferent signals**

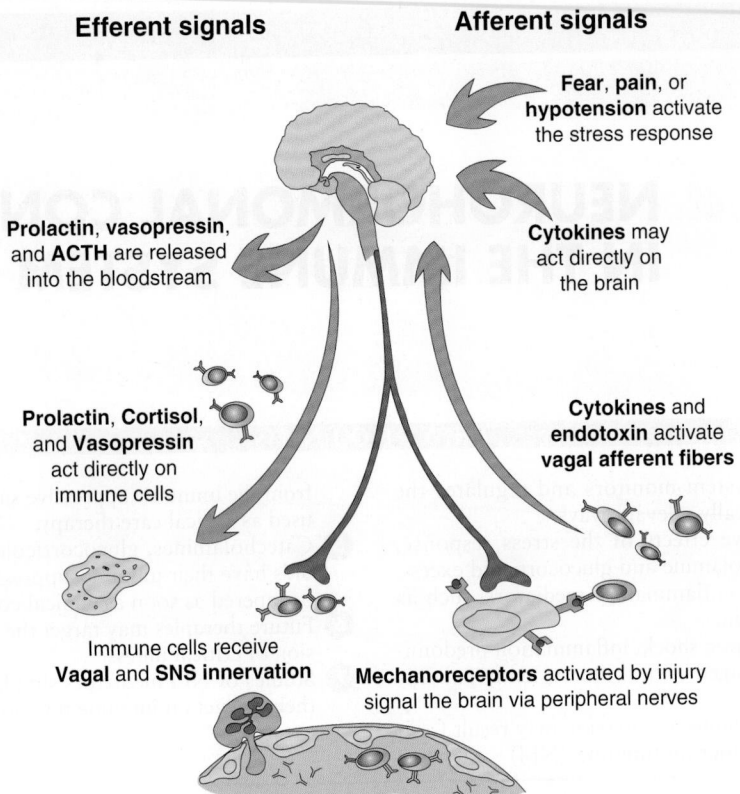

FIGURE 82.1. Bidirectional NEI communication. Stimulation of the acute stress response generates immunosuppressive signals (activation of the HPA axis, the SNS, and endogenous opioids) and immune-supportive signals (release of proinflammatory peptides, such as vasopressin and prolactin). A threat to the homeostatic milieu, in the form of trauma or infection, activates the immune system. Activated immune cells produce cytokines (e.g., TNF-α, IL-1, IL-6), which signal the CNS by stimulating afferent nerves or by circulating directly to the brain. Autonomic nerve activity delivers anti-inflammatory signals in response to immune activation.

The Immune System as a Sensory Organ

This cross talk between cells of the nervous, endocrine, and immune systems is not a static pattern of feedback loops, but a complex, integrated system sensitive to environmental signals perceived by both the brain and the immune system. The immune system can be thought of as a sensory organ that perceives microscopic threats. Day-to-day activities result in wear and tear on epithelial barriers, leading to microbial and other nonself invasion. These peripheral stresses activate immune cells, send signals to the CNS via peripheral or autonomic afferent nerves, and initiate an immunoregulatory response. Centrally mediated immune modulation can be initiated by other sensory input, the simplest example of this being classical conditioning. When an immunosuppressive stimulus (e.g., antilymphocyte serum) is paired with a sensory input (e.g., a flavored drink), the resulting immune suppression can be later reproduced with the flavored drink alone (2).

RECENT NEUROENDOCRINE IMMUNE MEDIATORS APPLIED TO CRITICAL ILLNESS

❶ Although our understanding of NEI interactions is limited, it is still clear that perturbations to any single pathway in this intricate system may have distant reverberations. Because

therapies used in critical care interfere with or mimic many of these pathways, it is incumbent on the intensivist to pay attention to developments in the field of NEI interactions. In the past few years, corticosteroids, growth hormone, and vasopressin—all NEI mediators with immunomodulatory effects—have been proposed as therapeutic agents in the treatment of ICU patients.

Adrenal Replacement Therapy May Have Immunomodulatory Affects

Current recommendations for the use of adrenal replacement therapy in children with sepsis are conservative, calling for their use in patients with fluid refractory, catecholamine-resistant shock and suspected or proven absolute adrenal insufficiency, such as that resulting from chronic steroid exposure or adrenal hemorrhage (3). Corticosteroids are known to have immunosuppressive effects; however, it is unclear whether the small doses used for adrenal replacement will increase patients' susceptibility to nosocomial infection. In the setting of adrenal insufficiency resulting from chronic steroid exposure, the modest doses prescribed to replace adrenal function are unlikely to cause significant additional immune suppression. Recovery from severe sepsis requires a balance between control of inflammation and activation of the specific or adaptive immune response. Studies of adrenal replacement therapy published to date have yet to consider the impact of these drugs on immune function.

Treatment with Growth Hormone Increases Mortality due to Sepsis

The hypercatabolic state seen in critically ill patients has been attributed in part to growth-hormone dysfunction. Trauma, sepsis, and surgery are thought to induce a state of growth-hormone resistance (4,5). The hyperglycemic, catabolic state induced by growth-hormone depletion and resistance is compounded by the normal stress response, the effects of immune-derived cytokines, and inadequate calorie delivery in the ICU (4). Accordingly, exogenous growth hormone was proposed to preserve muscle and improve healing. In small studies, exogenous growth hormone given to postoperative patients and burn patients improved nitrogen balance and protein synthesis, increased muscle strength and lean body mass, and increased the rate of healing (4,6).

Unfortunately, use of exogenous growth hormone in critically ill patients is associated with increased mortality. In two large European studies of growth hormone use in critically ill adults, patients treated with growth hormone had a 1.9- to 2.4-fold relative risk of mortality, mostly because of multiorgan dysfunction syndrome, shock, or uncontrolled infection (7). The reasons behind this unexpected outcome may relate to growth hormone's effect in immune function. At physiologic levels, growth hormone is immunostimulatory, but it has immunosuppressive effects at supraphysiologic levels in vitro (8).

Vasopressin Infusion in Vasodilatory Shock

A large randomized controlled trial comparing norepinephrine to low-dose vasopressin found that vasopressin did not offer a mortality advantage over norepinephrine in adults with septic shock. In a prospectively identified stratum of patients with less severe septic shock, vasopressin was associated with improved survival (9). Because patients treated with vasopressin had greater decreases in a broad array of cytokines, chemokines, and growth factors compared with those treated with norepinephrine, downregulation of the innate immune response has been proposed as a mechanism for this effect (10). As vasopressin has immunosuppressive effects when present in the CNS and immune-supportive effects when present in peripheral tissues (11), it is difficult to predict which effect would predominate during vasopressin infusion in the ICU.

PATHWAYS OF COMMUNICATION

This section summarizes the available data that describe the efferent pathways by which the brain communicates with the immune system, the afferent pathways by which the immune system informs the brain, and the impact of this communication on the function of immune cells. The vast majority of these data have been generated in vitro and in animal models that experimentally impair isolated NEI pathways. From these data, a sense of the overall impact of NEI pathways on the immune system and the critically ill patient as a whole may be synthesized.

Efferent Signals: How the Central Nervous System Communicates with the Immune System

Signals can travel between the brain and immune system on peripheral nerves or in the form of circulating chemical signals, such as hormones or cytokines. Due to the relative ease of experimental modeling, more is known about the humoral control of immune responses than about the signals that travel along nerves. The paucity of data belies the importance of direct innervation in control of immune responses. These pathways are evolutionarily conserved, suggesting a central role to the fine-tuning of the inflammatory response. Neural control has several advantages over humoral control. Humoral control requires molecules to diffuse to and from the site of action. By contrast, direct innervation can carry precise signals that are rapid in onset, discrete in location, and brief in duration.

Autonomic Control of Inflammation: The Cholinergic Anti-inflammatory Pathway

The importance of neural pathways in NEI communication is highlighted by the elegant work of Dr. Kevin Tracey and colleagues, who demonstrated that the vagus nerve is capable of sensing and regulating inflammation using simple and rapid feedback loops. Vagal efferent fibers, distributed throughout the reticuloendothelial system, modulate the immune response to endotoxin through cholinergic signaling (12).

In the presence of endotoxin, macrophages release cytokines that promote inflammation and potentiate activation of the specific immune response (13). Macrophages express nicotinic acetylcholine receptors. The binding of these receptors by an appropriate ligand decreases the release of tumor necrosis factor (TNF)-α and other endotoxin-inducible proinflammatory cytokines (IL-1β, IL-6, and IL-18) without altering release of the anti-inflammatory cytokine IL-10 (12,14) (**Table 82.1**). This acetylcholine-dependent downregulation of inflammation is reproduced by stimulation of the vagus nerve (12,14).

The vagally mediated anti-inflammatory signal seems to impact both local and systemic inflammation. Vagotomized animals release more TNF-α, IL-1, and IL-6 into the circulation during endotoxemia (12). Relative to sham-operated controls, these animals develop more severe local inflammation and are more sensitive to the lethal effects of endotoxin. Stimulation of the vagus nerve or administration of nicotinic acetylcholine receptor agonists reduces inflammatory markers, organ injury, and mortality from sepsis in murine models. Evidence suggests that vagally mediated inhibition of inflammatory responses to antigens routinely encountered in the intestine may protect from autoimmune disease and that some autoimmune disease may be ameliorated by nicotinic acetylcholine receptor agonists (12).

Autonomic Control of Inflammation: The Noradrenergic Pathway

The SNS also innervates the immune system. Postganglionic sympathetic neurons follow vasculature to innervate all primary and secondary lymphoid organs (15). The concentration of noradrenergic fibers in the spleen is concentrated in the white pulp around a central artery. These fibers play a role in controlling blood flow and thus may regulate lymphocyte traffic (16). Noradrenergic fibers also continue into lymphoid tissue without blood vessels. Norepinephrine release from peripheral nerves may impact immune function nonsynaptically by diffusion to the nearby cells of interest (16). The microenvironment around the synapse-like structures at their termination may be bathed in concentrations of norepinephrine as high as 0.3–3 mM on antigenic challenge (15,17). Cells of the bone marrow, thymic epithelial and dendritic cells, monocytes, and macrophages express both α- and β-adrenergic receptors, whereas B and T cells express the β2-adrenergic receptors exclusively (15).

TABLE 82.1

PROINFLAMMATORY AND ANTI-INFLAMMATORY CYTOKINES

	■ PRODUCED BY	■ ACTIONS ON IMMUNE CELLS	■ RELEVANCE IN CRITICAL ILLNESS
Proinflammatory Cytokines			
TNF-α	APCs, NK cells, T cells	Local inflammation, endothelial activation	An early mediator of inflammation and shock
IL-1β	APCs, epithelial cells	T-cell activation, macrophage activation	Causes fever and acute-phase protein production
IL-12	B cells, macrophages	Activates NK cells, induces CD4 T-cell differentiation into Th-1–like cells	Suppresses Th-2
IFN-γ	Th-1 cells, NK cells	Potent macrophage activation, suppresses Th-2 responses	Low levels associated with increased risk of infection
GM-CSF	Macrophages, T cells	Stimulates growth and differentiation of granulocytes and monocytes	Increases HLA-DR expression, may be clinically useful as an immune stimulant
Anti-inflammatory Cytokines			
IL-4	Th-2 cells, mast cells	B-cell activation, suppresses Th-1 cells, IGE switch	Suppresses Th-1 response
IL-10	Th-2 cells, APCs	Potent suppressor of macrophage functions	Suppresses Th-1 response
Other Important Cytokines			
IL-2	T cells	T-cell proliferation, supports Th-1 cells	Most important proliferative factor for T cells
IL-6	T cells, macrophages, endothelial cells	T- and B-cell growth and differentiation	Causes fever, and acute-phase protein production levels are related to severity of systemic inflammation
IL-8	Monocytes, endothelial cells	Chemotactic for neutrophils	Levels are related to severity of systemic inflammation
GCSF	Fibroblasts and monocytes	Stimulates neutrophil growth and differentiation	Exogenous GCSF safely increases neutrophil counts but does not alter mortality

APCs, antigen-presenting cells; HLA-DR, human leukocyte antigen-DR.

In the bone marrow, β-adrenoceptor activation suppresses cell proliferation and differentiation, whereas stimulation of the α-adrenoceptor suppresses myelopoiesis but enhances lymphopoiesis (15). In dendritic cells, monocytes, and macrophages, activation of β-adrenoceptors inhibits the endotoxin-induced release of the proinflammatory cytokines IL-1β, TNF-α, IL-12, and interferon (IFN)-γ and increases the release of the anti-inflammatory cytokines IL-10 and IL-6 in response to endotoxin (15,18). IgG transcription is enhanced by binding to β-adrenergic receptors on B cells (18). In general, catecholamines are believed to favor T helper cell (Th)-2 cytokines and inhibit cellular immunity by suppressing Th-1 cytokine production (16,18). In murine models, activation of the SNS by Lipopolysachharide (LPS) engages an anti-inflammatory reflex that rapidly and dramatically decreases the TNF-α response. It is interesting to note that, in the NEI system, the sympathetic and parasympathetic nervous systems may act synergistically rather than in opposition.

Other Neurotransmitters

Researchers are still discovering new neurotransmitters, hormones, and cytokines, and continue to recognize new NEI roles for well-known molecules. The molecules described here are examples of this interface and add layers of complexity to the NEI system. These substances may function as neurotransmitters in neural pathways or as circulating messengers in humoral pathways.

Opioids. Pain can stimulate the immune response, and both exogenous opioids and endogenous endorphins are known to have immunosuppressive effects. Opioids are thought to induce immune suppression at analgesic doses by binding to classical, naloxone-sensitive opioid receptors in the brain. Immune cells have both classical and nonclassical opioid receptors, but it is unclear to what extent morphine interacts directly with these cells to cause immune suppression in vivo (19,20). Acutely, centrally acting morphine activates the SNS, and most of the observed immunosuppressive effects of morphine may occur via this pathway (21,22). Morphine also activates the HPA axis, which may lead to cortisol-mediated immune suppression, particularly during chronic administration (23).

In vitro, morphine has clear immunosuppressive effects. It decreases B-cell antibody production, reduces the T-cell proliferative response to mitogen, suppresses IL-2 gene expression, increases T-cell apoptosis, and decreases IL-6 levels. It is uncertain to what extent this mechanism is important in vivo (19,24). Acute and chronic exposure to morphine decreases splenic and peripheral natural-killer (NK)-cell activity in animals (20). Treatment with morphine for as little as 36–72 hours impairs macrophage response to monocyte colony-stimulating factor in mice and affects phagocytosis and superoxide production ex vivo (20). In animal models, drugs that potentiate narcotic analgesia, such as clonidine and dexmedetomidine, also have immune suppressive effects (25).

Somatostatin and Somatostatin Receptor Ligands.
Somatostatin analogs (e.g., octreotide) are used in the treatment of gastrointestinal hemorrhage. In addition to decreasing splanchnic blood flow, somatostatin inhibits the release of insulin and decreases secretion and absorption in the gastrointestinal tract (8). Somatostatin has direct immunosuppressive effects in vitro. Somatostatin receptors are expressed on peripheral T and B lymphocytes, on activated monocytes, and in hematopoietic precursors (26,27). In the bone marrow, somatostatin inhibits proliferation, particularly in response to granulocyte colony-stimulating factor (GCSF) (28). Somatostatin strongly inhibits IFN-γ production by T cells, thereby decreasing macrophage activation and antigen presentation (1). The effect of octreotide infusions on immune function in critically ill patients has not been studied.

Other Neuropeptides.
Substance P, a neuropeptide present in afferent nerves in the dorsal horn of the spinal column, was originally discovered to be a mediator of pain sensation. Substance P is powerfully proinflammatory via TNF-α and IL-12 and plays a role in chronic inflammation. In vitro and in vivo, substance P counteracts glucocorticoid-mediated apoptosis (29). Substance P is one of a growing group of neuropeptides that have been shown to have immunoregulatory function. Others include calcitonin gene-related peptide, neuropeptide Y, vasoactive intestinal peptide, pro-opiomelanocortin–related peptides, and β-endorphins (30). Little is known about their function in the normal state or the stress response. Currently, there are no therapeutic agents are known to be directed at them. Further research may prove the importance of these molecules.

Humoral Efferent Pathways

The Hypothalamic–Pituitary–Adrenal Axis

Activation of the HPA axis begins with release of corticotrophin-releasing hormone (CRH) from the hypothalamus in response to cortical signals generated by fear, pain, or hypotension, or in response to immune-derived signal molecules, especially IL-1β, TNF-α, and IL-6 (17). CRH leads to adrenocorticotropic hormone (ACTH) release by the pituitary, which, in turn, causes cortisol release by the adrenal gland. Cortisol inhibits growth and generally increases catabolism while it enhances protein synthesis in the liver, where acute-phase reactants are generated. Cortisol potentiates the vasoconstrictive action of catecholamines and regulates the distribution of total body water (8). In the immune system, corticosteroids reduce circulating numbers of lymphocytes, monocytes, and eosinophils by stimulating apoptosis. Corticosteroids stabilize lysosomal membranes, decrease capillary permeability, impair demargination of white blood cells, impair phagocytosis, and decrease the release of IL-1, preventing fever. Steroids also support a Th-2 (humoral immunity) over a Th-1 (cellular immunity) phenotype (31).

Peptide Hormones: Prolactin and Vasopressin

Prolactin and vasopressin are the immunostimulatory hormones associated with the CNS response to stress. Release of these hormones occurs simultaneously with HPA-axis activation and SNS activation and thus represents an important counterbalance to the immunosuppressive effects of the stress response.

Prolactin, although best known for its role in promoting milk secretion, directly opposes many of the actions of corticosteroids. Prolactin release is stimulated by suckling, IL-1β, IL-2, IL-6, oxytocin, serotonin, and thyrotropin-releasing hormone. Prolactin levels are highest in newborns and lactating mothers but may be suppressed in response to hemorrhage, particularly in the peripartum period (32,33). A prolactin-secretory response to psychological and physical stress is reported (34,35). In the normal state, prolactin secretion is tonically inhibited by hypothalamic dopamine.

In the immune system, prolactin supports circulating lymphocyte numbers as a necessary cofactor for IL-2 and mitogen-stimulated proliferation (34) by opposing glucocorticoid-induced apoptosis (36). Prolactin increases IL-2 production by T cells and is a necessary cofactor for expression of the IL-2 receptor. Prolactin increases antibody production by B cells and increases cytokine-release capacity of macrophages and NK cells (34). The immunosuppressive drug cyclosporine exerts its effect through the prolactin receptor on lymphocytes (37).

Vasopressin is released in response to hypotension and increased serum osmolarity. In children with septic shock, circulating vasopressin levels tend to be elevated (38). Vasopressin has different immunomodulatory effects in the periphery than in the CNS. Circulating or local vasopressin enhances lymphocyte reactions and potentiates primary antibody responses. Peripheral vasopressin favors Th-1 responses (11). Vasopressin can also potentiate the release of prolactin (39). Acting centrally, vasopressin causes release of CRH, but it also has effects on the immune system independent of its effect in stimulating the HPA axis. When given intraventricularly to rats, vasopressin decreases the T-cell response to mitogen, probably via the SNS (40).

Afferent Signals: Alerting the Central Nervous System to a Microbial Threat

The immunoregulatory actions of pituitary hormones, vagal nerve activity, and SNS activation do not occur randomly but in response to information about the current state of immune function that is generated by classical sensory organs and the immune system and synthesized by the brain. The brain is alerted to a microbial threat via both humoral and neural pathways. Cytokines, particularly TNF-α and IL-1β, can act directly, reaching the brain via the bloodstream, or indirectly, by stimulating peripheral afferent nerves (14).

Immune Activation of Afferent Peripheral Nerves

Afferent signals traveling along autonomic and peripheral nerves provide a surveillance system to allow the CNS to monitor immune function. The existence of these neural pathways is supported by the fact that TNF-α and IL-1 released by dendritic cells and macrophages at concentrations too low to reach the brain via the bloodstream can stimulate vagal afferents (12,14). Afferent pathways also collect information about infection and injury independent of immune cells. Both sympathetic and vagal afferents can be directly stimulated by endotoxin, a bacterial product that leads to TNF-α release (12,41). Receptors sensitive to mechanical, thermal, and osmolar changes may also activate vagal sensory fibers, suggesting that the brain can anticipate injury and the resulting inflammation (14). Circulating cytokines can also stimulate sensory nerves.

Inflammation-sensing pathways terminate in the dorsal vagal complex, which consists of the nucleus tractus solitarius (NTS) and the area postrema. The NTS, which receives the main portion of the vagal afferent signal, communicates with the paraventricular nucleus, the site of production of

CRH (14). Inflammation sensed by the vagus nerve increases inflammation-suppressing signals traveling back down the vagus and activates humoral responses via the HPA axis.

Circulating Cytokines

Humoral pathways of immune-to-brain communications revolve around circulating cytokines. Receptors or receptor mRNA in the brain have been found for IL-1α, IL-1β, IL-2, IL-4, IL-6, TNF-α, IFN-γ, macrophage colony-stimulating factor, and stem cell factor (1). Endocrine glands also contain receptors for immune-derived cytokines. Receptors for IL-1α, IL-1β, IL-2, and IL-6 have been described in pituitary, thyroid, pancreas, ovary, and testis (1).

The existence of the blood–brain barrier (BBB) complicates our understanding of humoral pathways of immune-to-brain communication. Proinflammatory cytokines are large lipophobic molecules; therefore, their diffusion into the brain is physically limited (42). Despite this limitation, blockade of brain receptors for proinflammatory cytokines effectively prevents the adaptive behaviors associated with infection, collectively termed the sickness response. When circulating concentrations are high, cytokines are carried across the BBB by saturable transport proteins (43). Circumventricular organs, in which the BBB is weak, are also possible sites of immune-to-brain communication. At these sites, binding of pathogen-associated molecular patterns (PAMPs) to receptors may generate the production of proinflammatory cytokines, which can then enter the brain by volume diffusion (43).

Cytokines may also bind to cell surface receptors on the endothelium of brain capillaries, causing a release of soluble mediators, such as nitric oxide and prostaglandin (43). Soluble mediators may then diffuse into the brain parenchyma and modulate neuron activity. Intracerebral prostaglandins have been proposed as mediators of the febrile response and HPA-axis activation.

Peripheral Responses: The Effects of Neuroimmunomodulation

The brain receives information about potential and ongoing immune responses and sends out signals that modulate these responses. Unfortunately for clinicians, more is understood about pathways of communication than about the nature and effect of the communication itself. What follows here is a review of the immunology central to our current understanding of NEI modulation and a description of the impact of NEI mediators in cases where their effect on functional systems is understood. Because our ability to understand the impact of NEI regulation is limited by our ability to assess the function of the immune system, discussion will be necessarily guided by the scientific methods currently available for evaluation of immune function. At this time, we have tools to assess the impact of NEI mediators on (a) nonspecific immune responses, including behavior and inflammation; (b) on the phenotypes of specific immune responses, particularly Th-1 and Th-2 responses; and (c) on growth and survival of immune cells.

The Sickness Response

The most obvious result of CNS integration of signals from the immune system is a combination of physiologic changes and behaviors associated with recovery, collectively known as the sickness response. In response to illness signaled mainly by TNF-α and IL-1, the CNS initiates physiologic changes, including fever, increased white blood cell count, production of acute-phase proteins in the liver, and increased slow-wave sleep, as well as behavioral changes, including decreased feeding and drinking, and reductions in activity and social interaction (43,42). Alterations in pain sensation are also a part of the sickness response. In the acute phase, the stress response rapidly induces analgesia, presumably by a neural route. Later, inflammatory cytokines induce hyperalgesia, signaling the individual to care for a wound. These changes are not specific to individual pathogens and occur across a wide range of species (42,43).

Inflammation and Phagocytosis

The nonspecific immune response, comprised mainly inflammation and phagocytosis, is even more evolutionarily conserved than the sickness response. Nonspecific immunity is initiated rapidly by microbial invasion or trauma and serves to limit tissue damage and infection to the wound or site of entry. Inflammation and phagocytic cells comprise the first line of defense and recognition. The inflammatory response leads to vasodilation, increased capillary permeability, and an influx of phagocytes, including blood monocytes, neutrophils, and tissue macrophages. Local coagulation limits hematogenous spread of infection. Phagocytic cells recruited by inflammation produce proinflammatory cytokines, primarily IL-1, IL-6, and TNF-α, amplifying the immune response locally (13).

Chemical mediators of the inflammatory response can have systemic effects. The vasodilation, increased capillary permeability, coagulation, and phagocyte diapedesis that prevent local spread of disease can be disastrous globally, causing hypovolemic shock, disseminated intravascular coagulation, and acute respiratory distress syndrome. Consequently, the prevailing paradigm in sepsis research has been that sepsis results from an unbridled hyperinflammatory response. In animal models of sepsis in which large inoculums of bacteria or large doses of lipopolysaccharide are administered, subjects die in the acute phase of their illness from proinflammatory cytokine storm. In these models, anti-inflammatory therapies improve survival.

Corticosteroids, vagal nerve stimulation, SNS activation, circulating catecholamines, and endogenous and exogenous opioids all have anti-inflammatory effects (13,14,44,45). Inflammation is potentiated by prolactin and vasopressin (11,34). Although excessive inflammation can be deadly, anti-inflammatory agents do not improve mortality in human sepsis, in which early death from cytokine storm is usually prevented by medical intervention and the relevant outcome is long-term survival. Recovery from sepsis depends on a balance between proinflammatory and anti-inflammatory signals.

Inflammation recruits phagocytic cells, some of which are responsible for the initiation of the specific immune response. Antigen-presenting cells, such as macrophages and dendritic cells, engulf foreign matter and bacteria, break them down into large molecules, and present these molecules as antigens to T lymphocytes. Antigen presentation is the crucial step in initiating adaptive immunity: impaired antigen presentation is associated with mortality and secondary infection (46). Anti-inflammatory therapies, by virtue of the fact that they mimic pluripotent NEI pathways, tend to have effects beyond simple downregulation of proinflammatory cytokines. Anti-inflammatory therapies can cause immune-cell apoptosis and modulate the specific immune response in ways that may not be favorable for overall survival.

Humoral versus Cellular Immunity

An antigen-specific immune response begins when a T lymphocyte recognizes its specific antigen on the surface of an antigen-presenting cell. The T cell begins to activate and proliferate. Each generation of proliferation takes 8–12 hours; therefore, the generation of a specific immune response takes several days, during which time the organism is dependent on the nonspecific immune response for protection (42). T-cell proliferation is suppressed by catecholamines and supported by prolactin.

The population of T cells that results from this proliferation is not a homogeneous group, as different types of infection require different killing strategies. For instance, as viruses commandeer cellular machinery for their own replication, overcoming a viral infection requires killing of the infected cell. Most viral infections stimulate replication of cytotoxic T cells.

Helper T cells (Th cells) make cytokines that support other cells. The two lines of helper cells, Th-1 and Th-2, are mutually inhibitory and direct different types of immune responses. Th-1 cells are stimulated by pathogens, such as *Mycobacterium tuberculosis*, *Helicobacter pylori*, and *Pneumocystis jirovecii* that accumulate inside the vesicles of macrophages and dendritic cells. A Th-1 or cell-mediated immune response promotes the microbicidal properties of the macrophage and supports the production of immunoglobulin (Ig) G, an opsonizing antibody that facilitates uptake of these pathogens. Cytokines associated with Th-1 responses, IFN-γ, IL-12, and TNF-α are proinflammatory (13). A Th-1 proinflammatory phenotype is associated with autoimmune disease (18).

Extracellular spaces are protected by the Th-2 or humoral immune response. In response to extracellular pathogens (e.g., *Staphylococcus* spp.), Th-2 cells initiate the humoral immune response by activating naïve antigen-specific B cells to produce IgM antibodies. Viruses and intracellular pathogens that travel through these spaces may be neutralized by the binding of specific antibodies. Antibody binding also facilitates uptake of pathogens by phagocytes. The cytokine profile associated with Th-2 humoral immune response is anti-inflammatory, with IL-4 and IL-10 predominating (13). The catecholamine and cortisol excess seen in the stress response favors Th-2 responses (18,31). The impact of vagal nerve activity and other hypothalamic hormones on the Th-1–Th-2 balance is not known.

Septic patients tend to have increased numbers of Th-2 cells relative to the normal Th-1–Th-2 balance and relative to nonseptic, critically ill controls. Whether this finding represents augmentation of humoral immunity or a suppression of cell-mediated immunity is not known. Additionally, this finding has not been correlated with outcomes from sepsis (47). A stress-induced shift to a Th-2 phenotype could be unfavorable in patients infected with a primarily intracellular pathogen.

Apoptosis and Lymphocyte Proliferation

A few days into an episode of sepsis, the catecholamine and cortisol excess of the acute phase suppresses the initial hyperinflammatory state, replacing it with a state of relative immune suppression. Ideally, immune cells are protected by a balance of the proapoptotic forces of adrenal steroids and the antiapoptotic effects of serum prolactin. Once the acute phase of critical illness has passed, the normal pattern of pituitary hormone release and the normal adrenal response to ACTH are disrupted. As a result, cortisol levels often remain elevated (48,49). The balance between proapoptotic and antiapoptotic forces may be further upset in the ICU when patients are treated with prolactin-suppressing dopamine and steroids.

Apoptosis of B and T lymphocytes and dendritic cells has been demonstrated in autopsies of patients who died with sepsis and multiorgan failure (Fig. 82.2). A syndrome of immune paralysis, which consists of lymphoid depletion, deactivation of antigen-presenting cells, and production of anti-inflammatory cytokines, occurring in similar patients has been dubbed the compensatory anti-inflammatory response syndrome (CARS) (46,50). The factors that converge to create the immune paralysis of critical illness are only partly understood, but apoptotic death of immune cells is a causative factor.

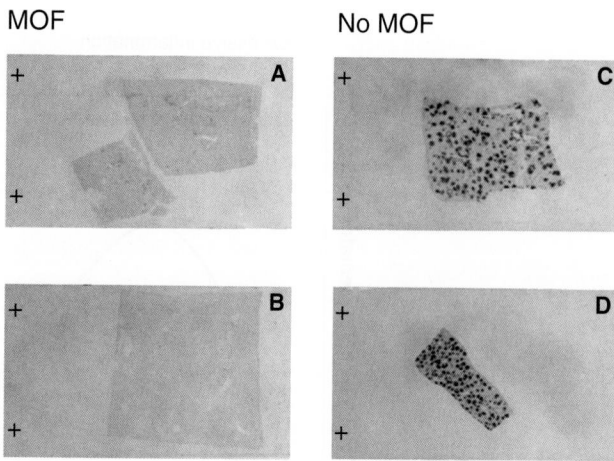

MOF   No MOF

FIGURE 82.2. Depletion of lymphoid elements in patients who died with and without multiorgan failure (MOF). Immunohistochemical staining for B cells in autopsy samples of spleen from patients who died with and without MOF reveals lymphoid depletion that is visible to the naked eye. These are unmagnified images of slides of spleen stained for B cells (CD20). The number and size of lymphoid follicles (dark spots) are dramatically decreased in the patients with MOF. Patients C and D died with normal lymphocyte counts and without MOF; patients A and B died with prolonged lymphopenia (absolute lymphocyte count <1000 for >1 week) and MOF. Staining for DNA changes associated with apoptosis revealed increased apoptosis in patients with lymphoid depletion (not shown).

Immune-cell apoptosis was once thought to be clinically significant only as a marker of immune function; evidence now suggests that apoptosis has functional significance beyond the removal of effector cells (B and T lymphocytes) from the circulation. In vitro, uptake of apoptotic cells by surviving macrophages impairs antigen presentation and potentiates release of the anti-inflammatory cytokine IL-10, while suppressing release of the proinflammatory cytokine IL-12. Adoptive transfer of apoptotic lymphocytes increases mortality from sepsis in animal models, and blocking lymphocyte apoptosis improves survival (51). Clinical trials designed to test inhibitors of apoptosis in sepsis are planned.

IMMUNE COMPETENCE AND FAILURE IN THE PICU

The Acute and Prolonged Phases of Critical Illness

We have alluded to a distinction between the NEI milieu in the first hours or days of critical illness and that seen after several days have elapsed (Fig. 82.3). The acute phase of critical illness is characterized by supranormal release of neuroendocrine mediators from the hypothalamus and pituitary. This secretory activity ensures that short-term goals of blood pressure support and mobilization of fuel substrates are met at the expense of neglecting homeostatic mechanisms, immune function, and cell growth and repair. When a patient's own fight-or-flight response is insufficient to maintain perfusion, shock ensues. During this phase, the anti-inflammatory effect of steroids and catecholamines may be beneficial in many patients. Although clinical trials of anti-inflammatory therapies in sepsis have generally been disappointing, a subset of patients may have a robust inflammatory response that puts them at increased risk of early death from septic shock. During the prolonged

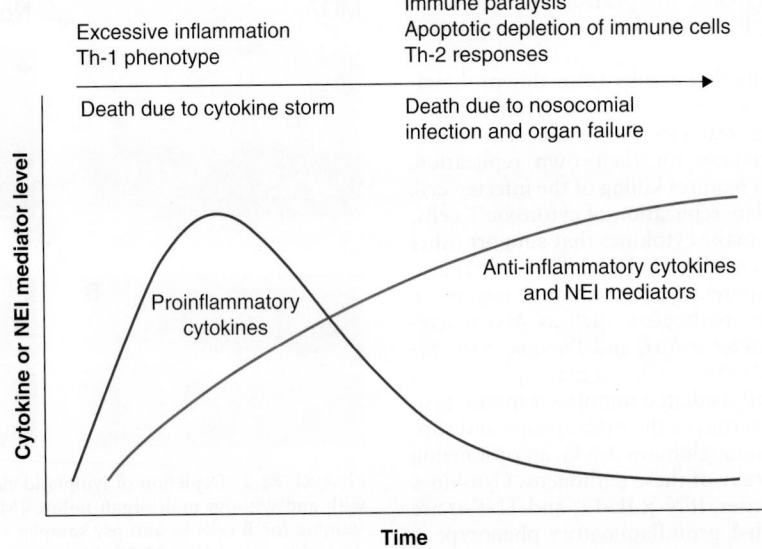

FIGURE 82.3. The acute and prolonged phases of critical illness and sepsis. Early death in sepsis can occur due to overwhelming inflammation with cytokine storm, which causes shock and tissue injury. Therapies directed at decreasing inflammation may be considered during this phase. Resuscitation medications used during this phase, including catecholamines and corticosteroids, are anti-inflammatory. During the prolonged phase of critical illness, patients developed immune paralysis with depletion of lymphoid elements due to apoptosis and decreased antigen-presenting capacity. During this stage, patients are at high risk for secondary infection. Therapies that enhance immune function by activating antigen-presenting cells or by blocking lymphocyte apoptosis may be considered in the future.

phase of critical illness, the effects of fight-or-flight mediators, whether endogenous or exogenous, may be harmful. The body's response to stress has mostly been studied as an acute event that occurs in normal, healthy people. The state of prolonged stress is not well understood, but it is likely that the hormonal milieu associated with survival in the acute phase of resuscitation, that of catecholamine and cortisol excess, may not be appropriate later on. Critically ill patients need a balance between immunosuppressive and immune-supportive signals, between a short-term improvement in blood pressure and long-term cell growth and repair.

Neuroendocrine Immune Failure

Decreased levels of anterior pituitary hormones and loss of the normal pattern of pulsatile release of these hormones characterize the prolonged phase of critical illness (52). ACTH, growth hormone, thyroid-stimulating hormone, prolactin, and luteinizing hormone are all similarly affected. Cortisol levels remain elevated in chronic critical illness despite a fall in ACTH release (46). The metabolic consequence of this neuroendocrine milieu is an impaired ability to use fatty acids as fuel substrates and a tendency to store fat and to waste protein from muscle and organs. The immune consequences are impaired lymphocyte and monocyte function and increased lymphocyte apoptosis. In patients who fail to recover but go on to develop multiorgan dysfunction, the state of catabolism and immune suppression persists even in the absence of exogenous dopamine, glucocorticoids, or other well-known suppressors of the somatotropic axis. Whether the hormonal milieu of prolonged critical illness represents neuroendocrine exhaustion or an adaptive response to chronic stress is unknown. It is also impossible to distinguish NEI failure from iatrogenic effects of the many ICU drugs derived from NEI mediators.

As dysfunction of normal homeostatic mechanisms may occur independently of ICU therapies, it may be tempting to label the neuroendocrine profile of chronically critically ill patients "normal." In fact, prolonged critical illness does not

occur without medical intervention and, in the natural state, these patients would not survive. In the ICU, an appropriate hormone level cannot be judged with reference to norms established in healthy people. Instead, the appropriate hormonal milieu is that associated with the best outcomes, including recovery of organ function, effective wound healing, and freedom from nosocomial infection.

Immunomodulatory Effects of ICU Therapies

Many of the drugs used in the ICU, particularly during resuscitation, owe their potency to native pathways of chemical signaling. Some of these—catecholamines, glucocorticoids, and opioids—have clearly demonstrable immunosuppressive actions. An immunoregulatory role for other drugs (e.g., metoclopramide, octreotide, and vasopressin) is hypothesized based on in vitro data but has not been extensively studied (Fig. 82.4).

Circulating Catecholamines

The effects of catecholamines on the immune system are complex and have mostly been observed in vitro. The extent to which these drugs mimic or suppress the effects of SNS activity on the immune system is not known. In general, catecholamines exert an immunosuppressive effect. Circulating catecholamines have been shown to modulate lymphocyte traffic and circulation in vivo. Within 30 minutes of exogenous administration of catecholamines, lymphocytes and NK cells are mobilized, followed by an increase in circulating granulocytes and relative lymphopenia at 3–4 hours (16). Prolonged infusion of β-agonists may have the opposite effect, reducing numbers and activity of NK cells (16). In vitro, catecholamines inhibit Th-1 and favor Th-2 responses and may inhibit the IL-2–mediated T-cell proliferative response (45).

Catecholamines in pharmacologic doses impact the release of other NEI mediators in vivo. Dopamine at doses as low as 1 μg/kg/min has a powerful inhibitory effect on release of

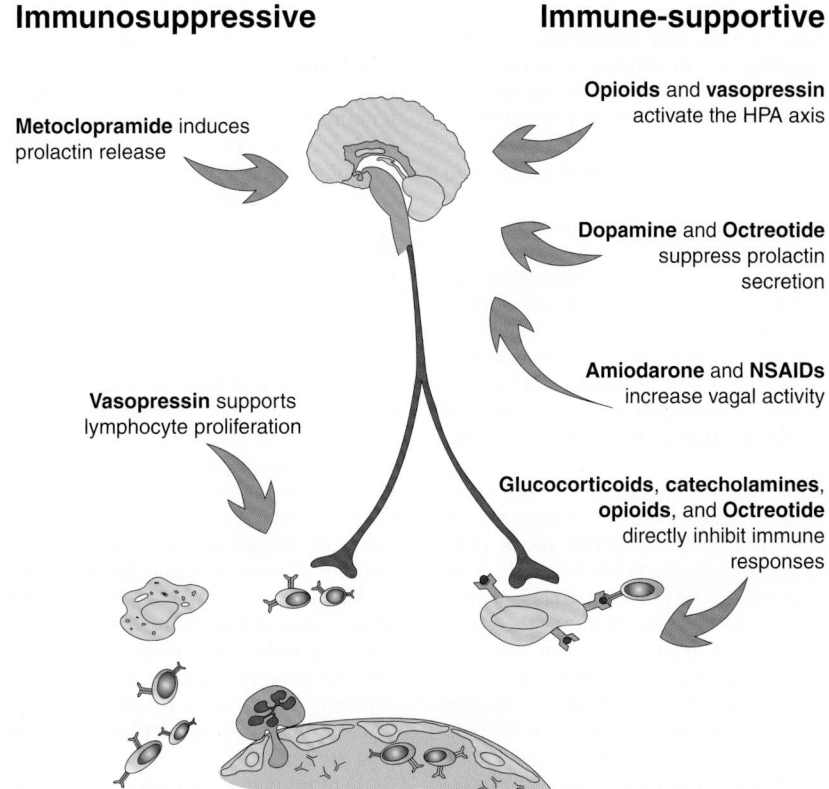

Immunosuppressive

Immune-supportive

Metoclopramide induces prolactin release

Opioids and **vasopressin** activate the HPA axis

Dopamine and **Octreotide** suppress prolactin secretion

Amiodarone and **NSAIDs** increase vagal activity

Vasopressin supports lymphocyte proliferation

Glucocorticoids, catecholamines, opioids, and **Octreotide** directly inhibit immune responses

FIGURE 82.4. Drugs used in the ICU influence immune function. These commonly used ICU drugs can alter neuroendocrine secretory activity and can bind to immune cells directly. Circulating catecholamines and corticosteroids promote Th-2 type immune responses and are broadly anti-inflammatory and immunosuppressive. Opioids and vasopressin activate the HPA axis, leading to cortisol release. Dopamine and octreotide block the release of the immune-supportive hormone prolactin. Opioids and octreotide also have direct effects on immune cells, decreasing lymphocyte proliferation and function of antigen-presenting cells. Amiodarone and nonsteroidal anti-inflammatory drugs (NSAIDs) may increase vagal activity, thus increasing anti-inflammatory signals. The only immune-supportive therapies commonly used in the ICU are vasopressin, which supports lymphocyte function, and metoclopramide, which induces prolactin release.

the proinflammatory mediator prolactin and has been shown to decrease lymphocyte proliferation (48,53). Dopamine-associated hypoprolactinemia has been associated with decreased T-cell response to mitogen ex vivo and with decreased circulating lymphocyte numbers and increased risk of secondary infection in the ICU (53,54). Dopamine inhibits pulsatile release of growth hormone and thus contributes to the catabolic state observed in critical illness (48).

Opioids

Opioid use is ubiquitous in critical care. As discussed previously, opioids have well-documented inhibitory effects on lymphocyte function and survival and on NK cell and macrophage growth and activity. Opioid abusers and their animal-model counterparts have increased susceptibility to infection (55). Studies of the effects of opioids in critically ill patients are limited as in these patients, immune suppression and increased susceptibility to infection is multifactorial.

Glucocorticoids and Adrenal Support

In general, critically ill patients have elevated cortisol, and cortisol levels correspond to the severity of illness. In the acute phase of critical illness, adequate cortisol is necessary for the maintenance of vascular tone and for normal catecholamine responsiveness (56). Even without exogenous steroids, in the face of ongoing stress, cortisol levels in critically ill patients tend to remain elevated despite a decline in ACTH levels (49).

Sustained cortisol production may be due to (a) direct autonomic innervation of steroidogenic cells, (b) paracrine action of the products of the adrenal medulla, or (c) the action of cytokines, which can directly stimulate cortisol production (57,58). Decreased cortisol clearance by the liver may contribute to elevated cortisol levels in prolonged critical illness (49).

In some critically ill patients, the HPA axis seems to have failed. These patients have a cortisol level that is inadequate to their degree of illness or inadequate relative to the ACTH levels measured in their blood. The incidence of relative adrenal insufficiency varies according to author and definition criteria. The incidence has been reported to range from 0% to 75%. Relative adrenal insufficiency is associated with poor outcomes in adults and children (19,59,60). Adrenal replacement therapy has been advocated in patients with catecholamine-resistant shock.

Both endogenous and exogenous steroids suppress fever, promote an anti-inflammatory cytokine profile, cause immune-cell apoptosis, and promote a Th-2/humoral immunity phenotype. The impact of adrenal replacement therapy on immune function and susceptibility to nosocomial infection has not been studied; however, immune suppression almost certainly plays a role in the increased mortality seen in patients with sepsis treated with high-dose glucocorticoids.

The Vagus Nerve

We are only beginning to understand the function of the vagus nerve in modulating the immune system. Little data exist to describe the function of the cholinergic anti-inflammatory pathway in the ICU. Nonsteroidal anti-inflammatory drugs and the antiarrhythmic amiodarone are known to increase vagal activity (14). Vagal tone can be measured using spectral analysis of the oscillation frequencies in heart-rate variability. Beat-to-beat analysis indicates that, among septic patients, nonsurvivors have less variability—thus less vagal tone—than survivors (14).

Patients with vagal nerve stimulators and patients with transplanted organs have disruptions in their cholinergic anti-inflammatory pathways. Vagus nerve stimulators are occasionally used to control intractable seizures. These devices are generally recognized to be safe and have not been associated with increased risk of infection; however, the impact of this therapy on TNF-α synthesis and inflammation has not been investigated. Vagus nerve stimulation has been proposed as a mechanism to treat inflammation in inflammatory bowel dieathe (IBD) (14).

In abdominal-transplant patients, portions of the vagus nerve have been transected. In animal models, vagotomy increases vulnerability to endotoxin-induced septic shock (14). Intestinal transplant patients may be particularly sensitive to this phenomenon, as their graft may have increased permeability to translocated endotoxin and bacteria. Without the effect of the vagus nerve to inhibit TNF-α production in response to endotoxin, these patients may have intermittent elevations in inflammatory cytokines. Elevations in TNF-α, also known as cachexin, may impact the ability of these patients to gain weight. Rejection of an intestinal graft is often accompanied by bacterial translocation from the gut lumen. Sepsis in intestinal transplant patients may evolve more rapidly and may be associated with more profound shock than in other patients.

Assessment and Treatment of Immune Suppression due to Critical Illness

Because good tests for immune function are not available, it is important to maintain vigilance for the immune suppression of critical illness. Strategies to limit exposure to nosocomial infection, such as isolation when appropriate, protocols to minimize catheter-related sepsis, and removal of ICU devices as soon as possible, may be beneficial in all patients. In addition, withdrawal of unnecessary immune suppressants, monitoring of subtle immune dysfunction, and compensation with suppressive antibiotics may minimize the risk for nosocomial infection.

Withdrawal of Unnecessary Immune Suppressants

After the initial period of stabilization, it is important to begin to think about restoring the capacity to grow, heal wounds, build muscle, and fight infection. The intensivist's first step should be to remember the immunosuppressive effects of the drugs that were necessary during resuscitation. Drugs that mimic the acute stress response, such as catecholamines and steroids, should be tapered as soon as hemodynamics or underlying conditions allow. In situations in which catecholamines have no proven benefit, it may be appropriate to consider whether the negative effects on the immune system and on metabolism outweigh the potential benefits of the drug. Intensivists should carefully consider the use of "renal dose" dopamine, which inhibits release of prolactin, one of the very few antagonists to the overwhelmingly immunosuppressive effects of the stress response.

Morphine and other opioids should be used no more than necessary to control a patient's pain. As no analgesic is known to have an efficacy comparable to that of opioids, they remain the analgesic of choice in most situations. Antinociceptive action

is closely linked with opioid-induced immune suppression, and affinity at the μ-receptor correlates with degree of effect on immune function (55). Opioids specific for the χ- or ∂-receptors may induce less immune suppression; therefore, methadone and fentanyl may be slightly less immunosuppressive than morphine (55). Studies of receptor affinity predict that buprenorphine, hydromorphone, oxycodone, oxymorphone, and tramadol are the least immunosuppressive (55). Opioids given locally, as in epidural analgesia, avoid the immunosuppressive complications of systemic administration (55). When the desired effect is anxiolytic, nonopioid alternatives should be considered.

Immune Monitoring and Future Therapies

Once active immune suppressants have been withdrawn to the extent possible, the degree of immune suppression that remains can be assessed. Vascular access, ventilation, surgical wounds, and exposure to antibiotic-resistant organisms place the ICU patient at extremely high risk for infection. The duration of immune suppression correlates strongly with the incidence of related infection so that, over time, even low-grade immune suppression may become clinically significant.

We are not yet able to monitor the state of the stress response activation or interpret the cytokine milieu in these patients, and no NEI mediators are currently available as therapies to support immune function. At this time, the intensivist can only compensate for the immune suppression that exists. The readily clinically available tests to monitor immune function are limited.

Lymphopenia and monocyte deactivation (impaired antigen presentation) have been associated with increased risk of poor outcomes, including nosocomial infection, prolonged hospital stay and mechanical ventilation, multiorgan dysfunction, and death (46,54,61). Lymphopenia can be assessed with a daily complete blood count. When the absolute lymphocyte count is persistently <1000, indicators of T- and B-cell function may be measured. T-cell subsets will help identify patients with low CD4 counts who may benefit from early prophylaxis against fungus or *Pneumocystis jirovecii* pneumonia.

Patients with impaired B-cell function, as evidenced by low immunoglobulin levels, may benefit from IV immunoglobulin. Investigational therapies that target lymphopenia may be available in the near future. Recombinant human prolactin may have therapeutic potential to reverse lymphopenia observed in the ICU and to speed hematopoietic reconstitution after bone marrow transplant (62). Metoclopramide and vasopressin increase pituitary prolactin release (35). Clinical trials of metoclopramide to increase prolactin release in lymphopenic patients are under way.

Monocyte deactivation may be assessed by either flowcytometric evaluation of human leukocyte antigen-DR expression or by ex vivo, endotoxin-stimulated TNF-α production. These tests are still investigational but are being used in clinical trials to assess a patient's immune phenotype for targeted intervention. Patients with persistent infection or documented monocyte deactivation may be candidates for immune stimulants, including GCSF, granulocyte–macrophage colony-stimulating factor (GM-CSF), and IFN-γ. Large clinical trials of GCSF in septic patients were disappointing (63). GM-CSF stimulates cells of monocyte lineage and restores antigen-presenting capacity, the crucial initiating event of the specific immune response (46).

The cholinergic anti-inflammatory pathway may be amenable to pharmacologic intervention. CN1493, a drug currently in phase II trials for the treatment of IBD, may be a prototype for a new class of centrally acting anti-inflammatory agents (14,64). Whether activation of the cholinergic anti-inflammatory pathway could ameliorate symptoms of sepsis and critical illness has yet to be studied.

CONCLUSIONS AND FUTURE DIRECTIONS

The CNS regulates and coordinates immune responses through humoral and neural pathways. Sophisticated manipulation of NEI pathways to ameliorate the hyperinflammatory response of acute sepsis or the acquired immune suppression of critical illness remains out of our reach. NEI pathways have the potential to generate promising drugs for treatment of sepsis. At present, we must be attentive to the immune-modulating consequences of ICU therapies and of the neuroendocrine disarray of prolonged critical illness. We should be vigilant for new therapies aimed at restoring immune function. Perhaps most importantly, we must learn to assess investigational therapies with respect to their potential to impact NEI function. In the evaluation of new drugs, the effects of which derive from their similarity to neurotransmitters or hormone mediators, the possibility of unintended or unrecognized effects on immune function must be considered.

References

1. Besedovsky HO, Del Rey A. Immune-neuroendocrine interactions: Facts and hypotheses. *Endocr Rev* 1996;17(1):64–102.
2. Kusnecov A, Sivyer M, King M, et al. Behaviorally conditioned suppression of the immune response by anti-lymphocyte serum. *J Immunol* 1983;130:2117–20.
3. Dellinger RP, Levy MM, Rhodes A, et al. Surviving sepsis campaign: International guidelines for management of severe sepsis and septic shock: 2012. *Crit Care Med* 2013;41(2):580–637.
4. Carroll P. Treatment with growth Hormone and insulin-like growth factor-1 in critical illness. *Best Pract Res Clin Endocrinol Metab* 2001;15(4):435–51.
5. Noel GL, Suh HK, Stone JG, et al. Human prolactin and growth hormone release during surgery and other conditions of stress. *J Clin Endocrinol Metab* 1972;35:840–51.
6. Gilpin DA, Barrow RE, Rutan RL, et al. Recombinant human growth hormone accelerates wound healing in children with large cutaneous burns. *Ann Surg* 1994;220:19–24.
7. Takala J, Ruokonen E, Webster NR, et al. Increased mortality associated with growth hormone treatment in critically ill adults. *N Engl J Med* 1999;341:785–92.
8. Guyton AC, Hall JH. *Textbook of Medical Physiology.* Philadelphia, PA: WB Saunders, 1996.
9. Russell JA, Walley KR, Singer J, et al. Vasopressin versus norepinephrine infusion in patients with septic shock. *N Engl J Med* 2008;358(9):877–87.
10. Russell JA, Fjell C, Hsu JL, et al. Vasopressin compared with norepinephrine augments the decline of plasma cytokine levels in septic shock. *Am J Respir Crit Care Med* 2013;188(3):356–64.
11. Bell J, Adler MW, Greenstein JI. The effect of arginine vasopressin on autologous mixed lymphocyte reactions. *Int J Immunopharmacol* 1992;14:93–103.
12. Andersson U, Tracey KJ. Reflex principles of immunological homeostasis. *Ann Rev Immunol* 2012;30:313–35.
13. Janeaway CA, Travers P, Walport M, et al. *Immunobiology.* 5th ed. New York, NY: Garland, 2001.
14. Tracey KJ. The inflammatory reflex. *Nature* 2002;420:853–9.
15. Padro CJ, Sanders VM. Neuroendocrine regulation of inflammation [published online ahead of print January 30, 2014]. *Semin Immunol.* doi:10.1016/j.smim.2014.01.003.
16. Elenkov IJ, Wilder RL, Chrousos GP, et al. The sympathetic nerve—an integrative interface between two supersystems: The brain and the immune system. *Pharmacol Rev* 2000;52(4):595–638.
17. Zaloga GP, Marik P. Hypothalamic-pituitary-adrenal insufficiency. *Crit Care Clin* 2001;17(1):25–41.
18. Calcagni E, Elenkov I. Stress system activity, innate and T helper cytokines and susceptibility to immune related diseases. *Ann N Y Acad Sci* 2006;1069:62–76.
19. Joosten KF, de Kleijn ED, Westerterp M, et al. Endocrine and metabolic responses in children with meningococcal sepsis: Striking differences between survivors and non-survivors. *J Clin Endocrinol Metab* 2000;85(10):3746–53.
20. Roy S, Loh HH. Effects of opioids on the immune system. *Neurochem Res* 1996;11:1375–86.
21. Carr DJ, France CP. Immune alterations in chronic morphine treated rhesus monkeys. *Adv Exp Med Biol* 1993;335:35–9.
22. Hall DM, Suo JL, Weber RJ. Opioid-mediated effects on the immune system: Sympathetic nervous system involvement. *J Neuroimmunol* 1998;83(1–2):29–35.
23. Al-Hashimi M, Scott SW, Thompson JP, et al. Opioids and immune modulation: More questions than answers. *Br J Anaesth* 2013l;111(1):80–8.
24. Madden JJ, Whaley WL, Ketelsen D. Opiate binding sites in the cellular immune system: Expression and regulation. *J Neuroimmunol* 1998;83(1–2):57–62.
25. Jang Y, Yeom MY, Kang ES, et al. The antinociceptive effect of dexmedetomidine modulates spleen cell immunity in mice. *Int J Med Sci* 2014;11(3):226–33.
26. Ferone D, Boschetti M, Resmini E, et al. Neuroendocrine-immune interactions: The role of cortistatin/somatostatin system. *Ann N Y Acad Sci* 2006;1069:129–44.
27. Lichtenauer-Kaligis EG, van Hagen PM, Lamberts SW, et al. Somatostatin receptor subtypes in human immune cells. *Eur J Endocrinol* 2000;143:S21–5.
28. Oomen SP, Hofland LJ, van Hagen PM, et al. Somatostatin receptors in the haematopoietic system. *Eur J Endocrinol* 2000;143:S9–14.
29. Dimri R, Sharabi Y, Shoham J. Specific inhibition of glucocorticoid-induced thymocyte apoptosis by substance P. *J Immunol* 2000;164(5):2479–86.
30. Berczi I, Chalmers IM, Nagy E, et al. Immune effects of neuropeptides. *Baillieres Best Pract Res Clin Rheumatol* 1996;10(2):227–59.
31. Greenspan FS, Strewler GJ, eds. *Basic and Clinical Endocrinology.* 2nd ed. Stamford, CT: Appleton and Lange, 1997.
32. Chaudry IH, Ayala A, Ertel W, et al. Hemorrhage and resuscitation: Immunological aspects. *Am J Physiol* 1990;259(4 pt 2):R663–78.
33. Kohm AP, Sanders VM. Norepinephrine and beta 2-adrenergic receptor stimulation regulate CD4+ T and B lymphocyte function in vitro and in vivo. *Pharmacol Rev* 2001;53(4):487–525.
34. Chicanza IC. Prolactin and immunomodulation: In vitro and in vivo observations. *Ann N Y Acad Sci* 1999;876:119–30.
35. Freeman ME, Kanycska B, Lerany A, et al. Prolactin: Structure, function and regulation of secretion. *Physiol Rev* 2000;80(4):1523–631.
36. Fletcher-Chiappini SE, Compton MM, La Voie HA, et al. Glucocorticoid-prolactin interactions in NB2 lymphoma cells: Anti-proliferative versus anticytolytic effects. *Pro Soc Exp Biol Med* 1993;202:345–52.
37. Russell DH, Kibler R, Matrisian L, et al. Prolactin receptors on human T and B lymphocytes: Antagonism of prolactin binding by cyclosporine. *J Immunol* 1985;134(5):3027–31.
38. Lodha R, Vivekanandhan S, Sarthi M, et al. Serial circulating vasopressin levels in children with septic shock. *Pediatr Crit Care Med* 2006;7(3):220–4.
39. Chikanza IC, Petrou P, Chrousos G. Perturbations of arginine vasopressin secretion during inflammatory stress: Pathophysiologic implications. *Ann N Y Acad Sci* 2000;917:825–34.
40. Shibasaki T, Hotta S, Wakabayashi I. Brain vasopressin is involved in the stress induced suppression of immune function in the rat. *Brain Res* 1998;808:84–92.
41. Martelli D, Yao ST, McKinley MJ, et al. Reflex control of inflammation by sympathetic nerves, not the vagus. *J Physiol* 2014;592:1677–86.

42. Maier, SF, Watkins, LR. Cytokines for psychologists: Implications of bi-directional communication for understanding behavior, mood, and cognition. *Psychol Rev* 1998;105:83–107.

43. Dantzer R, O'Connor JC, Freund GG, et al. From inflammation to sickness and depression: When the immune system subjugates the brain. *Nat Rev Neurosci* 2008;9(1):46–56.

44. Levite M. Nerve-driven immunity: The direct effects of neurotransmitters on T-cell function. *Ann N Y Acad Sci* 2000;917:307–21.

45. Oberbeck R, Schmitz D, Wilsenack K, et al. Adrenergic modulation of survival and cellular immune functions during polymicrobial sepsis. *Neuroimmunomodulation* 2004;11(4):214–23.

46. Volk HD, Reinke P, Krausch D, et al. Monocyte deactivation-rationale for a new therapeutic strategy in sepsis. *Intensive Care Med* 1996;22(suppl 4):S474–81.

47. Ferguson NR, Galey HF, Webster NR. T helper cell subset ratios in patients with severe sepsis. *Intensive Care Med* 1999;25:106–9.

48. Van den Berghe G, de Zegher F. Anterior pituitary function during critical illness and dopamine treatment. *Crit Care Med* 1996;24(9):1580–90.

49. Vermes I, Beishuizen A, Hampsink RM, et al. Dissociation of plasma adrenocorticotropin and cortisol levels in critically ill patients: Possible role of endothelin and atrial natriuretic hormone. *J Clin Endocrinol Metab* 1995;80:1238–42.

50. Ward NS, Casserly B, Ayala A. The compensatory anti-inflammatory response syndrome (CARS) in critically ill patients. *Clin Chest Med* 2008;29(4):617–25, viii.

51. Hotchkiss RS, Nicholson DW. Apoptosis and caspases regulate death and inflammation in sepsis. *Nat Rev Immunol* 2006;6:813–22.

52. Van den Berghe G. The neuroendocrine response to stress is a dynamic process. *Best Pract Res Clin Endocrinol Metab* 2001;15(4):405–19.

53. Devins SS, Miller A, Herndon BL, et al. Effects of dopamine on T-lymphocyte proliferative responses and serum prolactin concentration in critically ill patients. *Crit Care Med* 1992;20(12):1644–9.

54. Felmet KA, Hall MW, Clark RS, et al. Prolonged lymphopenia, lymphoid depletion, and hypoprolactinemia in children with nosocomial sepsis and multiple organ failure. *J Immunol* 2005;174(6):3765–72.

55. Budd K. Pain management: Is opioid immunosuppression a clinical problem? *Biomed Pharmacother* 2006;60(7):310–7.

56. Vermes I, Beishuizen A. The hypothalamic-pituitary-adrenal response to critical illness. *Best Pract Res Clin Endocrinol Metab* 2001;15(4):494–507.

57. Ehrhart-Bornstein M, Hinson JP, Bornstein SR, et al. Intra-adrenal interactions in the regulation of adrenocortical steroidogenesis. *Endocr Rev* 1998;19:101–43.

58. Toth IE, Hinson JP. Neuropeptides in the adrenal gland: Distribution, localization of receptors, and effects of steroid hormone synthesis. *Endocr Res* 1995;21:39–51.

59. Annane D, Sebille V, Troche G, et al. A 3 level prognostic classification in septic shock based on cortisol levels and cortisol response to corticotropin. *JAMA* 2000;283(8):1038–45.

60. Beishuizen A, Thijs LG. Relative adrenal failure in intensive care: An identifiable problem requiring treatment? *Best Pract Res Clin Endocrinol Metab* 2001;15(4):513–31.

61. Menges T, Engel J, Welters I, et al. Changes in blood lymphocyte populations after multiple trauma: Association with posttraumatic complications. *Crit Care Med* 1999;27(4):733–40.

62. Richards SM, Murphy WJ. Use of human prolactin as a therapeutic protein to potentiate immunohematopoietic function. *J Neuroimmunol* 2000;109:56–62.

63. Root RK, Lodato RF, Patrick W, et al. Multicenter, double-blind, placebo-controlled study of the use of filgrastim in patients hospitalized with pneumonia and severe sepsis. *Crit Care Med* 2003;31(2):367–73.

64. Matthay MA, Ware LB. Can nicotine treat sepsis? *Nat Med* 2004;10(11):1161–2.

CHAPTER 83 ■ THE POLYMORPHONUCLEAR LEUKOCYTE IN CRITICAL ILLNESS

M. MICHELE MARISCALCO

KEY POINTS

Neutrophil Physiology

1. Neutrophils are uniquely designed to deal with the host's interaction with microbes at mucosal and epithelial surfaces.

2. Neutrophils released from the bone marrow during times of acute infection and injury function differently compared with those released during periods of normal hematopoiesis.

3. Neutrophils released under such conditions are more rigid and more "sticky" and spontaneously produce increased amounts of reactive oxygen species. It is thought that these cells may contribute to organ dysfunction by being trapped in the capillary bed.

Defects in Neutrophil Number and/or Function

4. Neutrophils are critical to host immunocompetence, as is demonstrated by marked recurrent infections in individuals with congenital, developmental, or acquired defects in neutrophil function or number.

Neutrophils and Critical Illness

5. Transfusion-related acute lung injury is more common than previously thought and should be considered in any patient with acute deterioration in lung injury. The effector cell is the neutrophil.

6. The use of granulocyte colony-stimulating factor (G-CSF) decreases hospitalization time of neutropenic patients, whereas its use in the ICU population is far from clear. G-CSF use and recovery from neutropenia may result in lung injury.

7. Granulocyte transfusion and the transfusion of activated neutrophils with blood cell transfusion may contribute to increased organ dysfunction, particularly pulmonary dysfunction. Leukocyte depletion of blood prior to use in extracorporeal membrane oxygenation circuits or use of leukocyte depletion filters in patients in cardiopulmonary bypass may be of use.

Phagocytic leukocytes play a central and critical role in the acute phase of the inflammatory response. They are rapidly mobilized to sites of infection or injury and release an array of cytotoxic molecules to nonspecifically eliminate microbes. Phagocytes are also critical to the normal repair of tissue injury. Individuals with deficits in phagocyte function or number have impairment in wound healing as well as recurring infections. Phagocytes include polymorphonuclear leukocytes (PMNLs), monocytes/macrophages, and dendritic cells. The PMNL system refers to neutrophils, basophils, and eosinophils. PMNLs are grouped together because of their common nuclear morphology and granule content; hence, the name *granulocytes*. This chapter focuses on the neutrophil. Although the neutrophil maintains a central role in the innate immune system, it is also critically involved in many of the pathologic processes that bring patients to the ICU: sepsis, ischemia–reperfusion injury, acute respiratory distress syndrome (ARDS), transfusion-related acute lung injury (ALI), and traumatic injury. A concise review of normal neutrophil physiology and function is provided first. Additional information can be found in several extensive reviews (1,2). Those diseases in which neutrophil function "goes awry" as they relate to the critically ill infant and child, as well as therapies that affect neutrophil function are discussed in the remainder of the chapter.

Leukocytes, other cells of hematopoietic origin, and other cells, such as endothelium and fibroblasts, are often characterized by proteins found on their surface. These proteins often have multiple names, but often they may also be formally identified as human cell differentiation molecules (HCDMs) and given a unique CD (cluster of differentiation) number, nomenclature that was first proposed in 1982. It is thought that the 350 HCDMs now identified are only a small fraction of the possible cell-surface proteins. (The interested reader is referred to the most current list of HCDM at www.hcdm.org, accessed 1/3/2014.)

NEUTROPHIL PHYSIOLOGY

Granulopoiesis, Marrow Release, and Margination

The bone marrow is a large organ (70% larger than the liver) and 50%–60% of its function is dedicated to producing neutrophils. Approximately 100 billion neutrophils leave the bone marrow each day in a healthy adult. The normal ratio of neutrophils to erythroid cells ranges from 2:1 to 3:1. As cells differentiate from hematopoietic stem cells, they undergo

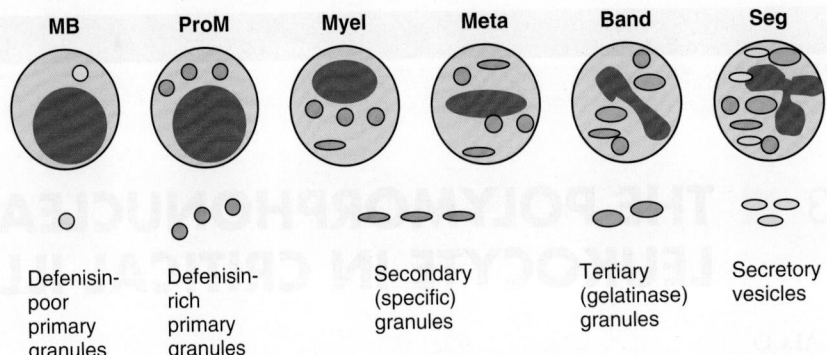

FIGURE 83.1. Neutrophil maturation. Note that granules develop during neutrophil maturation. No further cell division occurs beyond the myelocyte stage. MB, myeloblast; ProM, promyelocyte; Myel, myelocyte; Meta, metamyelocyte; Seg, segmented (mature) neutrophil.

five divisions, from myeloblast to promyelocyte to myelocyte. After the myelocyte stage, they no longer undergo meiosis but remain in the large storage pool (Fig. 83.1). They mature in the storage pool for ~5 days under normal conditions. The nucleus contracts from the large, ovoid shape of the promyelocyte to the "band," and finally to the mature neutrophil with its three- to five-lobed nucleus. Neutrophils circulate for up to 12 hours after their release into the bloodstream.

The elimination of foreign microorganisms through phagocytosis, generation of reactive oxygen metabolites, and release of microbicidal substances is dependent on the mobilization of neutrophilic granules and secretory vesicles. The mature neutrophil contains four granule populations. These granules share common structural features, such as a phospholipid bilayer and an intragranular matrix that contains proteins destined for exocytosis or delivery to the phagosome. Proteins synthesized at the same stage of myeloid cell development localize to the same granule (3). The primary, or azurophil, granule forms during the myeloblast and promyelocyte stage and contains myeloperoxidase and neutrophil elastase (Fig. 83.1 and Table 83.1). Production of myeloperoxidase ceases at the promyelocyte-to-myelocyte stage. Secondary (specific)

TABLE 83.1

NEUTROPHIL GRANULE CONTENTS

■ PROTEIN	■ PRIMARY (AZUROPHIL)	■ SECONDARY (SPECIFIC)	■ TERTIARY (GELATINASE)	■ SECRETORY VESICLE
Membrane proteins				
Cytochrome b_{558}			+	+
CD11b/CD18 (CR3)		+	+	+
fMLF-R		+	+	+
Alkaline phosphatase				+
CD10				+
CD14				+
CD16 (FcγRIIIb)				+
CD35 (CR1)				+
C1qR				+
Matrix proteins				
Myeloperoxidase	+			
Proteinase-3	+			
Leukolysin		+	+	+
Collagenase		+		
Gelatinase		+	+	
Lysozyme	+	+	+	
Defensins	+			
BPI	+			
Cathepsins	+			
Lactoferrin		+		
Elastase	+	+		
Haptoglobin		+		
α_1-Antitrypsin	+			
β_2-Microglobulin		+	+	

CD, cluster of differentiation; CR3, complement receptor 3; BPI, bactericidal/permeability-increasing factor.

granules, which are found in myelocytes and metamyelocytes, contain high concentrations of lactoferrin and low concentrations of gelatinase (matrix metalloproteinase 9, MMP-9). The tertiary granules (gelatinase), found in band cells and segmented neutrophils, are low in lactoferrin and high in gelatinase. The secretory vesicles form in segmented neutrophils. Their membranes contain cytochrome b_{558} (one of the components of the NADPH oxidase system), receptors for complement [CD35 (complement receptor 1, CR1), CD11b/CD18 (Mac-1, CR3)], receptor for complement component 1q (C1qR), and receptors for monovalent and polyvalent immunoglobulin (CD32, CD64, CD16) and for bacterial lipopolysaccharide (CD14). Exocytosis of granules occurs in reverse order, with secretory granules being the easiest to mobilize and the primary granule the least easy, requiring strong phagocytic stimuli.

The primary granule (**Table 83.1**) contains a number of antimicrobial peptides: the four α-defensins (human neutrophil peptide 1 through 4), bactericidal/permeability-increasing protein (BPI), and serprocidins (serine proteases with microbicidal activity: proteinase-3, cathepsin G, and elastase). The α-defensins have microbicidal activity against a broad range of fungi, bacteria, enveloped viruses, and protozoa. They exert their effect through the formation of transmembrane pores. Neutrophil defensins induce chemotaxis of monocytes and lymphocytes. BPI is highly cationic, kills Gram-negative bacteria at nanomolar concentrations, and neutralizes lipopolysaccharide. The serprocidins are cationic polypeptides with proteolytic activity against a variety of extracellular matrix proteins, such as elastin, fibronectin, laminin, type IV collagen, and vitronectin. Unrestrained release of elastase plays a crucial role in the pathogenesis of pulmonary emphysema. The serine proteases have a number of inhibitors: those found in the systemic circulation and in the primary granules (α_1-antitrypsin, also known as α_1-proteinase inhibitor, and α_2-macroglobulin) and those produced by the epithelial and immune cells (secretory leukoproteinase inhibitor and elafin).

The specific and gelatinase granules are formed in the meta-myelocyte stage and continue through maturation until the formation of segmented neutrophils. Specific granules are larger and rich in antibiotic substances. Being more difficult to mobilize than gelatinase granules, they release their contents into the phagolysosome or the exterior of the cell. Gelatinase granules are smaller and more easily exocytosed. They are important primarily as a reservoir of matrix-degrading enzymes and membrane receptors required during neutrophil extravasation. Neutrophils contain three metalloproteinases (MMPs): neutrophil collagenase (MMP-8), gelatinase (MMP-9), and leukolysin (MMP-25) (**Table 83.1**). The MMPs are able to degrade major structural components of the extracellular matrix and are important for the extravasation of neutrophils.

The secretory vesicles are endocytic and constitute a reservoir of membrane-associated receptors required at the earliest phases of neutrophil localization. The secretory vesicles are mobilized in response to a wide variety of inflammatory stimuli. The membranes are rich in CD11b/CD18 (Mac-1, CR3), CD35 (CR1), and receptors for the formylated bacterial peptide [formylmethionyl-leucyl-phenylalanine (fMLF), CD14, and CD16 (FcγRIIIb receptor)].

Maturation of the neutrophil and granule protein synthesis is achieved by the sequential and combined action of transcription factors. More than 40 different growth factors, cytokines, and chemokines regulate PMNL proliferation, differentiation, and cell fate. The most clinically well-known is granulocyte colony-stimulating factor (G-CSF). G-CSF specifically promotes neutrophil proliferation and maturation and enhances neutrophil microbicidal activity when administered in vivo. G-CSF interacts with relatively late hematopoietic progenitors that have already committed to the neutrophil lineage and serves to support their growth and final maturation

into functional neutrophils. Granulocyte–macrophage colony-stimulating factor (GM-CSF) acts on progenitors that are committed to produce either neutrophils or monocytes but can also act on granulocyte precursors directly. As with G-CSF, GM-CSF can enhance neutrophil reactivity when given in vivo.

Neutrophils continuously egress from the sinusoids of the bone marrow. Release is regulated by chemokine receptors expressed on the cells, and their ligand chemokines expressed by stromal cells. Within the circulation, about half of the neutrophils are in the flowing stream; the other half are inaccessible to phlebotomy. This half is called the *marginating pool*. In response to stress, exercise, or IV epinephrine, the neutrophils in the marginating pool are released into the circulating pool. The marginating pool of neutrophils is in the postcapillary venules in major organs and in the capillaries of the lungs. As a result of longer transit times of neutrophils compared with erythrocytes in normal lungs, the concentration of neutrophils within the pulmonary capillary blood is ~40–80 times higher than it is within the blood in large vessels. Neutrophils travel in "hops" through the lung microvasculature, moving quickly through larger capillary segments but stopping and deforming for entry into smaller segments (hence the longer transit times). The neutrophils marginated in the pulmonary bed differ from mature neutrophils, and have increased CXC chemokine receptor 4 (CXCR4). As CXCR4 increases on neutrophils as they age, and the pulmonary vascular endothelial cells express CXC chemokine ligand 12 (CXCL12; stromal derived stem cell factor 1, SDF-1), it is possible that "aging" neutrophils populate the pulmonary reservoir (4).

Neutrophilia occurs after the administration of glucocorticoids. Approximately 60% of the neutrophilia is due to mobilization from the marginated pool, 10% is due to increased bone marrow release, and 30% is due to lengthened half-life in circulation. The administration of G-CSF shortens the transit time of neutrophils through the marrow, particularly in the postmitotic pool. G-CSF has no effect on demargination but delays clearance of neutrophils by inhibiting apoptosis.

In response to inflammatory stimuli or infection, neutrophil production and release significantly increase. Neutrophil release from the bone marrow initially exceeds production, causing a temporary decrease in the bone marrow neutrophil pool. Once the bone marrow neutrophil pool is reestablished, release from the marrow increases and neutrophil count rises. In those individuals with limited neutrophil pool reserves (those with drug-induced neutropenia, those who have received chemotherapy, and in infants) neutrophil count may remain low while the neutrophil pool replenishes.

"Mature" neutrophils released from the bone marrow have altered function after infection, compared with cells produced during the "noninfected" state. They demonstrate decreased chemotaxis, decreased phagocytosis, and an impaired ability to upregulate CD10, a neutral endopeptidase that is present on only mature granulocytes (5,6).

Neutrophil Localization in Infection

The body has a highly coordinated and regulated response to microbes. The first defense is local immunity. The epithelial surface itself functions as a physical barrier. Antimicrobial peptides are released from the epithelium, and secretory IgA is released from submucosal plasma cells. Microbes may be eliminated or controlled at the source; however, if the microbial burden exceeds these processes, then neutrophil recruitment is required to control the infection. Epithelial–bacterial interactions result in the release of cytokines, specifically IL-1 and tumor necrosis factor (TNF)-α, and chemokines, such as IL-8, CXCL8, and G-CSF (7). These cytokines activate the macrophages that reside in submucosa, which in turn amplify the proinflammatory signal with additional release of proinflammatory chemokines and cytokines.

The endothelium of the nearby postcapillary venule, under the immunologic pressure of proinflammatory cytokines, transforms from a nonadhesive surface to one that is proadhesive through the expression of specific ligands on the endothelial surface (**Table 83.2**). Selectins are responsible for the initial capture of the neutrophil from the free-flowing stream and their rolling on the endothelial surface. Selectins are present on both neutrophils (L-selectin, CD62-L) and the endothelial surface (E- and P-selectin, CD62-E and CD62P, respectively) (**Table 83.2**) (8). Members of the immunoglobulin superfamily (IgSF), intercellular adhesion molecule 1 (ICAM-1), and vascular cell adhesion molecule (VCAM) are critical for neutrophil slowing, arrest, and migration on the cell surface (**Fig. 83.2**). The receptors on the neutrophil surface for the IgSF are the β_2 integrins: Mac-1 (CD11b/CD18, CR3), leukocyte functional antigen 1 (LFA-1) (CD11a/CD18), and the β_1-integrin VLA-4 (CD49d/CD29) (**Table 83.2**). The leukocyte integrins are heterodimers comprising α and β subunits. The β subunit may be shared by multiple members of a subfamily, whereas the α subunit confers specificity. The leukocyte integrins are generally functional in an "inactive state" (9). Through a process known as *inside-out signaling*, the integrins change their conformation and become "active," and ligand recognition can occur. The endothelial surface secretes a number of

TABLE 83.2

ADHESION MOLECULES FOR NEUTROPHIL LOCALIZATION TO INFLAMMATORY SITES

■ NAME	■ CD CLASSIFICATION	■ CELL EXPRESSION	■ CONSTITUTIVE/ INDUCIBLE (C/I)	■ LIGAND
Integrin family				
β_1-Integrins				
$\alpha_2\beta_1$ (VLA-2)	CD49b/CD29	Neutrophil	C/I?	Coll I, Coll IV, LN
$\alpha_4\beta_1$ (VLA-4)	CD49d/CD29	Neutrophil	C/I?	FN, VCAM, JAM2
$\alpha_5\beta_1$ (VLA-5)	CD49e/CD29	Neutrophil	C/I?	FN, Tsp
$\alpha_6\beta_1$ (VLA-5)	CD49f/CD29	Neutrophil	C/I?	LN
$\alpha_9\beta_1$		Neutrophil	C/I?	VCAM-1, osteopontin
β_2-Integrins				
$\alpha_L\beta_2$ (LFA-1)	CD11a/CD18	Neutrophil	C	ICAM-1, ICAM-2, ICAM-3, JAM-1
$\alpha_M\beta_2$ (Mac-1, CR3)	CD11b/CD18	Neutrophil	C/I	ICAM-1, C3b, C3bi, Fg, FN, Factor X
$\alpha_X\beta_2$ (p150,95)	CD11c/CD18	Neutrophil	C/I	C3bi, GPIb-IX-V
β_3-Integrins				
$\alpha_V\beta_3$ (vitronectin receptor)	CD51/CD61	Neutrophil	C	vWF, VN, FN, Fg, PECAM-1, Tsp, LN, OSP, Coll I, Coll IV
IgSF and others				
ICAM-1	CD54	T and B cells; Endo; Epi; hepatocytes, pneumocytes, fibroblasts	C/I	LFA-1, Mac-1
VCAM-1	CD102	Endo	I	$\alpha_4\beta_1$, $\alpha_9\beta_1$
JAM-A		Endo, Epi	C	LFA-1, JAM-A
PECAM	CD31	Endo, neutrophil	C	LFA-1, PECAM
CD99	CD99	Endo, neutrophil	C	CD99
Selectins and selectin ligands				
L-selectin	CD62-L	Neutrophil	C	Unknown endo ligand, PSGL-1
P-selectin	CD62-P	Platelet, Endo	C/I	PSGL-1, E-selectin, GPIb-IX-V
E-selectin	CD62-E	Endo	I	PSGL-1
PSGL-1	CD162	Neutrophil	C	P-selectin, E-selectin, L-selectin

This table focuses primarily on adhesion molecules specifically for neutrophil localization to inflammatory sites.

Inducible adhesion molecules: Although ICAM-1 is constitutively expressed on many cell types, its expression can also be induced by the cytokines TNF, IL-1, and IFN-γ after only a brief period (3–4 hours). E-selectin and P-selectin can be induced on endothelial cells by TNF and IL-1 after 3–4 hours of stimulation. VCAM-1 is present on endothelial cells only after cytokine stimulation. Its appearance is delayed compared with the other adhesion molecules. Both endothelial cells (Weibel–Palade bodies) and platelets (α granule) contain an intracellular pool of P-selectin, which can be mobilized to the surface after cell activation. Similarly, Mac-1 and p150,95 are constitutively present on neutrophils, but pools are also present in secretory vesicles that can be easily mobilized.

CD, cluster of differentiation; VLA, very late antigen; Coll I, collagen type I; Coll IV, collagen type IV; LN, laminin; FN, fibronectin; VCAM, vascular cell adhesion molecule; JAM, junctional adhesion molecule; Tsp, thrombospondin; ICAM, intercellular adhesion molecule; IgSF, immunoglobulin gene superfamily; Fg, fibrinogen; GPIb-IX-V, glycoprotein complex present on platelet surface; vWF, von Willebrand factor; VN, vitronectin; PECAM-1, platelet-endothelial cell adhesion molecule 1; OSP, osteopontin; Endo, endothelial cell; Epi, epithelial cells; PSGL-1, P-selectin glycoprotein ligand 1.

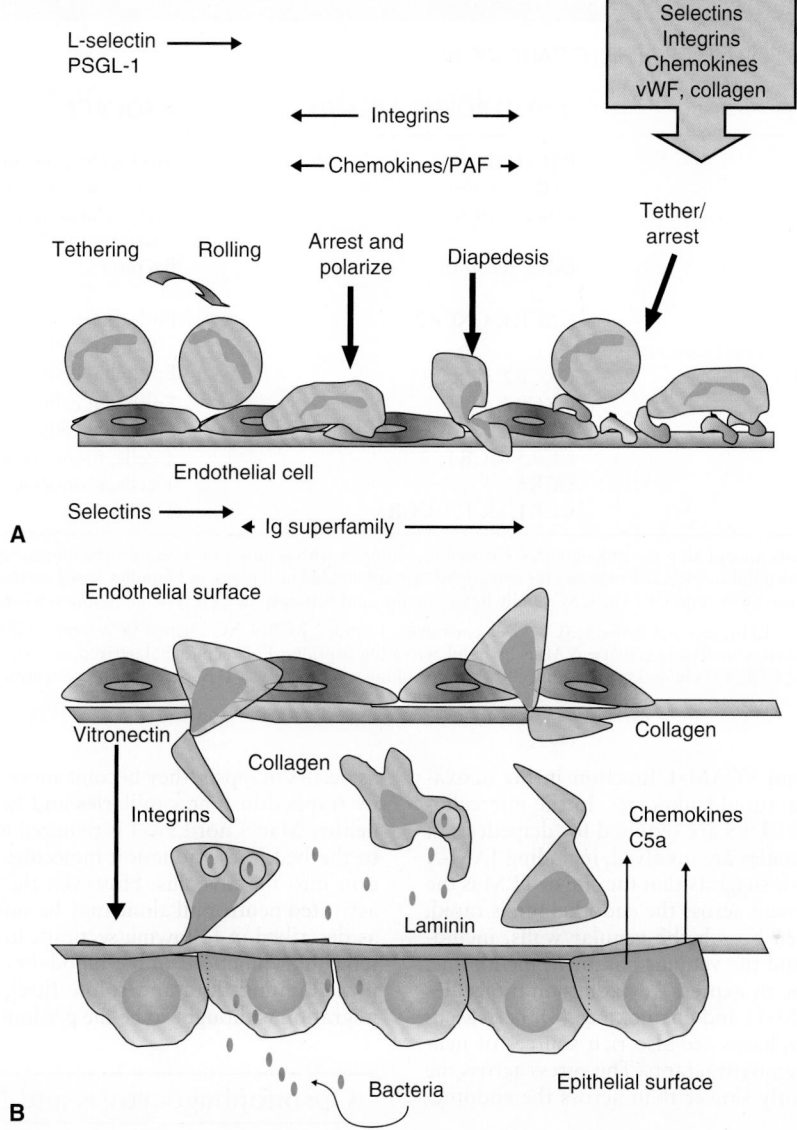

FIGURE 83.2. Neutrophil localization. **A:** In an inflammatory focus, the endothelium, which is normally nonadhesive, becomes proadhesive as a result of activation by cytokines, such as IL-1β and TNF. Neutrophils are tethered from the free-flowing stream and roll on the endothelial lining of the blood vessel, an interaction mediated by all three members of the selectin family. The neutrophils slow, arrest, and change shape (polarize). Integrins and their ligands, the immunoglobulin gene superfamily, mediate the transition from rolling to arrest. This transition is also dependent on the production of activating agents by the endothelial surface, such as PAF and IL-8. The neutrophils then crawl over the surface of the endothelium until they migrate through the endothelial monolayer. There is a hierarchy of molecules needed for transmigration, including PECAM, CD99, and JAM-1, and these specifically occur at the lateral border recycling compartment (LBRC). A neutrophil may be tethered by adherent platelets or another adherent leukocyte. Platelets themselves release chemokines, which activate neutrophils. Platelets may bind directly to von Willebrand factor (vWF) on the endothelial surface or on the basement membrane; alternatively, they may bind to collagen or fibronectin on the exposed basement membrane. In very select vascular beds (the blood–brain barrier for example), neutrophils may migrate directly through the cell body of an endothelial cell. **B:** Neutrophil localization in response to bacterial challenge. Bacteria present on the epithelial surface activate the epithelium to produce neutrophil chemokines NAP-2 (CXCL7) and ENA-78 (CXCL5); complement is activated, and the chemotactic factor C5a is produced. The epithelial surface also produces TNF-α and/or IL-1β, promoting the transition of the adjacent endothelial surface from an antiadhesive to a proadhesive surface. Neutrophils emigrate out of the blood vessel across the endothelial cell lining and crawl through the basement membrane and along the connective tissue. This is mediated by members of the β_1-integrin family and CD11b/CD18 (Mac-1, $\alpha_M\beta_2$). These integrins interact with their specific epitopes in the basement membrane structural proteins (e.g., laminin and vitronectin) and collagen. Neutrophils can continue to emigrate across the epithelial surface. Upon encountering bacteria, neutrophils surround them with plasma membrane, forming a phagolysosome. In the phagolysosome, both oxygen-dependent and oxygen-independent mechanisms are operative, resulting in bacterial killing.

chemokines and lipid-derived products, such as CXCL8 (IL-8) and platelet-activating factor (PAF), which can activate the neutrophil through specific receptors (**Table 83.3**). This step is critical for mediating the transition from rolling to arrest. Once the leukocyte has arrested, it polarizes then "crawls" (also known as diapedesis) through the endothelial lining of

the vessel, either between endothelial cells (transendothelial migration, TEM) or less commonly across the endothelial cell itself (transcellular migration) (10). Most leukocyte TEM occurs in postcapillary venules. Movement of the neutrophil across the endothelium is dependent on a sequential engagement of adhesion molecules. On the apical surface of the

TABLE 83.3

CHEMOTACTIC FACTORS FOR NEUTROPHIL LOCALIZATION

■ ACTIVATING AGENT	■ NEUTROPHIL LIGAND	■ SOURCE
PAF	PAF receptor	Monocytes, endothelial cells
LTB$_4$	LTB$_4$ receptor	Monocytes, neutrophils
C5a	C5a receptor	Anaphylatoxin from complement activation
fMLF	fMLF receptor	Bacteria
CXC and CC chemokines		
IL-8 (CXCL8)	CXCR1, CXCR2	Endothelial cells, monocytes, neutrophils, T cells, epithelial cells
GRO-α, MGSA-α (CXCL1)	CXCR2>CXCR1	Epithelial cells
NAP-2 (CXCL7)	CXCR2	Epithelial cells
ENA-78 (CXCL5)	CXCR2	Epithelial cells
MIP-1α (CCL3)	CCR5, CCR1	T cells, monocytes
MIP-1β (CCL4)	CCR5	T cells, monocytes
RANTES (CCL5)	CCR1, CCR3, CCR5	T cells

Chemokines regulate cell trafficking of all types of leukocytes. Chemokines interact with a subset of seven-transmembrane spanning, G-protein–coupled receptors on the neutrophil surface. Chemokines for neutrophils are subdivided into major subfamilies based on the arrangement of the two amino-terminal cysteine residues CXC and CC. The CXC family has an amino acid between the two cysteine residues, whereas the CC family does not.

PAF, platelet-activating factor; LTB$_4$, leukotriene B$_4$; CXCL, CXC chemokine ligand; CXCR, CXC chemokine receptor; GRO, growth-regulating protein; MGSA, melanocyte growth-stimulating activity; NAP, neutrophil activating peptides; ENA, epithelial derived neutrophil attractant; MIP, macrophage inflammatory peptide; CCL, CC chemokine ligand; CCR, CC chemokine receptor; RANTES, regulated on activation, normal T cell expressed and secreted.

endothelium, ICAM-1 and VCAM-1 function in the activation and adherence of captured leukocytes. In the intercellular borders, PECAM and CD99 are required for diapedesis in vitro. In vivo, other molecules are involved, including JAM-A and ICAM-2. Recent work suggests that the site of TEM is the LBRC (10). While movement across the endothelium is rapid, the neutrophils must then breach the venular walls, including the pericyte sheath and the venular basement membrane. This requires the pericyte to express key adhesion molecules (e.g., ICAM-1 and VCAM-1) and chemokines (8). Perivascular mast cells and macrophages are also rich sources of neutrophil and monocyte chemoattractants. The egress across the venular wall is significantly slower than across the endothelium itself.

Neutrophils migrate toward chemotactic factors released by (a) the bacteria itself (bacterial peptide, fMLF), (b) anaphylatoxins (C5a, C3a) produced after complement activation, and (c) chemokines and arachidonic acid metabolites produced by macrophages and fibroblasts present in the subendothelial matrix (Fig. 83.2). Locomotion through the subendothelial matrix requires additional integrins present on the neutrophils, which recognize matrix proteins, including fibronectin, collagen, vitronectin, and vimentin. Locomotion results in the release of both gelatinase granule and secretory vesicle contents. How neutrophils negotiate the space under basement membrane is still unclear, though given the rapidity of the movement; it is unlikely due to the dissolution of the matrix protein.

In many situations, neutrophil recruitment to the vascular endothelium does not occur in the sequential manner just described. Neutrophils or platelets already recruited to an inflammatory focus can recruit other neutrophils. In vascular beds (such as the liver, kidney, and lung), geometric constraints affect neutrophil localization. In the lung, neutrophil recruitment occurs in the capillary bed; in the liver, it occurs in the sinusoids. Using intravital microscopy, neutrophils appear to "hop" through the capillaries and sinusoids, rather than roll. They spend considerable periods of time in stationary contact with capillary endothelium, and this contact predisposes to adhesive interactions between the neutrophil and the endothelium. As neutrophils are exposed to inflammatory mediators,

as occurs in sepsis, they become more rigid. They are more easily trapped in lung capillaries and hepatic sinusoids. Though neither Mac-1 nor LFA-1 is required for neutrophils to localize to the bed, these adhesion molecules do mediate transmigration into the alveolus. However, the physical trapping of an activated neutrophil alone may be sufficient to result in injury, as described in following sections. In the brain, where the intercellular junctions of the blood–brain barrier are more complex (limiting fluid and solute flux), transcellular neutrophil migration is thought to be the predominate route of TEM (10).

Opsonophagocytosis and Microbial Killing

The ingestion and disposal of microbes is a major aspect of neutrophil function. To facilitate recognition of microbes by neutrophils, these targets are "decorated" with serum opsonins. Opsonins include proteolytic fragments derived from the complement cascade and specific immunoglobulins. Receptors that recognize opsonized bacteria are present on the neutrophil surface (Table 83.4). These receptors include complement receptor 1 (CR1, CD35), CR3 (Mac-1 or CD11b/CD18), and receptors that recognize the Fc portion of immunoglobulin (FcRγ). Three Fcγ receptors recognize either monomeric IgG or complexed IgG. Neutrophils express the low-affinity receptors, FcRγII and FcRγIIIb, CD32 and CD16, respectively. CD16 is present in the gelatinase granules, exocytosis of these granules results in upregulation of CD16. FcγRI (CD64) is a high-affinity Fcγ receptor. Neutrophils express little CD64; however, neutrophils treated with G-CSF or interferon-γ (IFN-γ), or neutrophils obtained from patients with bacterial infection, have dramatically increased amounts of CD64.

Ligation of FCγ and/or complement receptors initiates a cascade of biochemical events that results in the exocytosis of granules, the respiratory burst, and phagocytosis. As neutrophil receptors are activated, the plasma membrane "ruffles" and assumes a bipolar configuration, with the formation of a "head" (or pseudopod) and "tail" (or uropod). The pseudopod surrounds the microbe and fuses at the distal end to form a phagolysosome. The particle is internalized and generally

TABLE 83.4

RECEPTORS FOR PHAGOCYTOSIS ON NEUTROPHILS

■ RECEPTOR	■ CD CLASSIFICATION	■ LIGAND
FcγRI	CD64	Fc portion of IgG (high-affinity receptor)
FcγRIIA	CD32	Fc portion of IgG (low-affinity receptor)
FcγRIIIB	CD16	Fc portion of IgG (low-affinity receptor)
FcαRI		Fc of IgA
CR1	CD35	C3b>C4b>C3bi
CR3 (Mac-1)	CD11b/CD18	C3bi
C1qR		C1q

Complement fragments of C3: C3b, C3bi; complement fragment of C4: C4b; C1q is the q subunit of the complement complex 1. CD, cluster of differentiation.

completely surrounded by plasma membrane. Granules join this newly formed vacuole and discharge their contents within seconds. Release of myeloperoxidase from the primary granule is important for oxygen-dependent killing. Release of other granule contents, such as BPI, lactoferrin, and defensins, is critical for oxygen-independent killing.

The respiratory burst refers to the coordinated consumption of oxygen and production of metabolites that occur when neutrophils are confronted with appropriate stimuli, actions that are the basis of all oxygen-dependent killing by neutrophils and other phagocytes. The NADPH oxidase system is a transmembrane electron system in which NADPH, the primary electron donor on the cytoplasmic side of the membrane, reduces oxygen in the extracellular fluid or within the phagolysosome to form superoxide (O_2^-) (**Fig. 83.3**). In turn, two molecules of O_2^- can spontaneously (or enzymatically through superoxide dismutase) form hydrogen peroxide (H_2O_2). While both H_2O_2 and O_2^- can directly kill bacteria, it is the hydroxyl radical (OH•) and hypohalous acids produced from O_2^- and H_2O_2, respectively, that are the most injurious to microbes (and to healthy tissue/cells, if directly exposed). Myeloperoxidase released from primary granules forms hypochlorous

acid (HOCl) from chloride ion and H_2O_2, which is directly toxic to microbes. Hypochlorous acid can react with amines to form N-chloramines (RNHCl). RNHCl are lipophilic and can readily penetrate cellular membranes. HOCl and RNHCl can inactivate heme proteins, other proteins, and amino acids, and can oxidize DNA. OH• formed in the presence of iron ions (Fe^{3+}) from O_2^- is a strong oxidant. HOCl, H_2O_2, and OH• participate in killing the microbe in the phagocytic vacuole. However, such reactive oxidants also activate latent neutrophilic metalloproteinases, such as collagenase and gelatinase, and inactivate antiproteinases (11).

A central feature of the inflammatory pathology of acute sepsis is accumulation of activated neutrophils within the microcirculation of highly vascular organs such as the liver, leading to immune-mediated tissue damage and organ dysfunction (discussed in more detail later in this chapter). However, recent work suggests that accumulation of neutrophils in the liver enhances clearance of pathogens from the circulation (both viruses and bacteria). This occurs through a process called "NETosis." NETs (neutrophil extracellular traps) are large webs of decondensed chromatin coated with granule proteins that are expelled from activated neutrophils that can

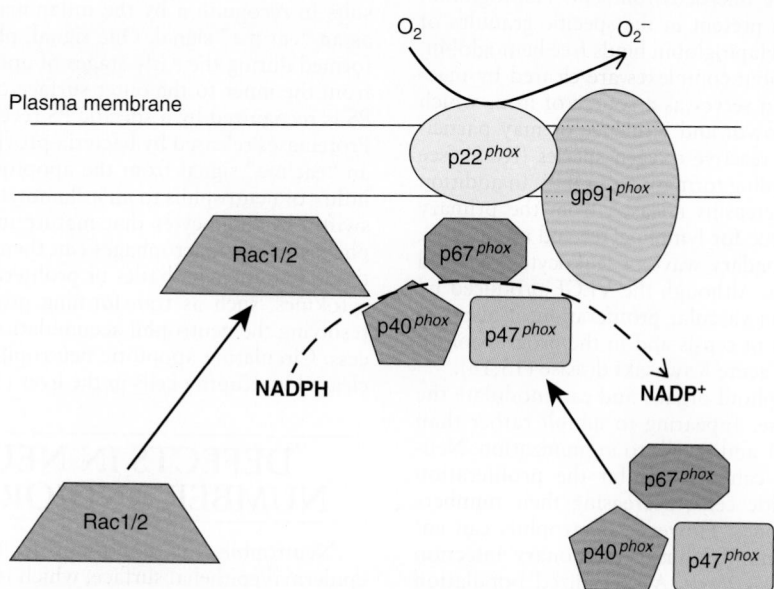

FIGURE 83.3. NADPH oxidase components and activation. On activation of the neutrophil, the three cytosolic components of the NADPH oxidase (p67^{phox}, p47^{phox}, and p40^{phox}) plus either Rac1 or Rac2 are translocated to the membrane of the phagocytic vacuole. The p47^{phox} binds to the membrane component of the NADPH oxidase, cytochrome b_{558} (gp91^{phox} plus p22^{phox}). The NADPH oxidase transfers an electron from NADPH to O_2 to form superoxide (O_2^-). The unstable superoxide is converted to hydrogen peroxide, either spontaneously or by superoxide dismutase.

capture and kill microbes in the extracellular space. This requires interactions with toll-like receptor 4 (TLR4)-activated platelets, and is dependent on neutrophil LFA-1. These intravascular NETs ensnare bacteria and viruses decreasing the circulating pathogen load. However, the intravascular NETs can cause collateral liver damage in both bacterial and viral sepsis modes (12,13).

Modulation of the Immune Response

For many decades, the neutrophil's activity has been presumed limited to "bacterial killing." However, a large body of work demonstrates that the neutrophil has key roles, in both the innate and acquired immune systems, beyond bacterial clearance. Neutrophils have unique pathways that can afford control of gene product at the translational level in response to signals from the environment. Rapid protein synthesis without requirement for new transcription is one of several biologic advantages of "signal-dependent" translation of mRNA that is stored or silent in the basal state. Mature neutrophils can synthesize proinflammatory cytokines (IL-1α and IL-1$\alpha\beta$, IL-6, IL-17, IL-18); anti-inflammatory cytokines (IL-1ra, transforming growth factor β); both CC and CXC chemokines; colony-stimulating factors (G-CSF and macrophage colony-stimulating factor [M-CSF]); angiogenic and fibrogenic factors (vascular endothelial growth factor, VEGF and transforming growth factor alpha) and TNF-superfamily (TNF-α, Fas Ligand, and BAFF or B lymphocyte–activating factor) (14). Production of these proteins occurs under conditions similar to those experienced by an emigrated neutrophil. The amount of protein produced by an individual neutrophil is small compared with a monocyte/macrophage, whereas the amount produced by the large number of emigrated neutrophils is substantially greater. In addition, an emigrated neutrophil may continue to function for many days before it ultimately undergoes apoptosis. Production of cytokines and chemokines by neutrophils are of particular relevance because of their ability to selectively recruit discrete cell populations into sites of injury, therefore regulating leukocyte trafficking (14). Preformed proteins released from granules can also have profound influence on the microenvironment. Haptoglobin, an acute-phase protein, is present in the specific granules of neutrophils (**Table 83.1**). Haptoglobin binds free hemoglobin, and haptoglobin–hemoglobin complexes are cleared by macrophages. Free hemoglobin serves as a source of iron, which may enhance bacterial growth and virulence or may participate in the generation of reactive oxygen species (ROS) (see preceding discussion regarding formation of OH$^\bullet$). In addition to being antimicrobial, defensins released from the primary granule are also chemotactic for lymphocytes and monocytes, thus contributing the secondary wave of leukocytes required for resolution of infection. Although the VEGF produced by neutrophils is important in vascular proliferation, it also has a role in the development of sepsis and in the progression of coronary artery lesions in acute Kawasaki disease (15,16).

Neutrophils enter lymphoid organs and can modulate the adaptive immune response, appearing to inhibit rather than augment the response of T and B cells to immunization. Neutrophil myeloperoxidase can also inhibit the proliferation and activation of dendritic cells, decreasing their numbers in the draining lymph nodes. However, neutrophils can enhance local adaptive immunity during pulmonary infection with *Mycobacterium tuberculosis*. A specialized population of neutrophils reside in the spleen, secrete BAFF, and induce immunoglobulin switching of B cells. Although the bone marrow is not a lymphoid organ, it does contain CD8+ memory T cells and, in very select circumstances, neutrophils may participate more directly in antigen presentation. Neutrophils

also regulate the maturing of the natural killer (NK) cells (patients with severe congenital neutropenia have abnormal NK cell development) (4).

Microvesicles are small intact vesicles ranging in size from 0.1 to 1.0 μm. The extracellular vesicles are observed to bleb off the surface of a number of cell types. Neutrophil-derived microvesicles (NDMVs) are present in small amounts in normal physiologic conditions, but are dramatically elevated in a variety of inflammatory conditions. NDMV composition is dependent on neutrophil state (and stimulating condition). The effect of the NDMV on target cells is absolutely dependent on the proteins/DNA contained within the microvesicle. Thus, NDMV derived from fMLF-stimulated neutrophils can activate endothelial cells to increase the expression of IL-6 and IL-8, and pro-adhesion molecules, and decrease activation of macrophages or neutrophils (reviewed in Refs. 4 and 17).

Clearance of Neutrophils

The half-life of neutrophils is very short, less than 12 hours in the circulation. Circulating neutrophils undergo apoptosis (programmed cell death) and are removed by the reticuloendothelial system of the spleen and bone marrow. In particular, "aging" neutrophils lose CD62-L (L-selectin) on their surface, and upregulation of CXCR4 and CD11b occurs. The ligand for CXCR4 is CXCL12 (SDF-1), which is produced by bone marrow macrophages. Thus, aging neutrophils return to the bone marrow, to be ingested by local macrophages (4).

Neutrophils that migrate to an inflammatory source have a prolonged half-life and increased function. However, these neutrophils do undergo apoptosis and are cleared from the tissue by inflammatory monocytes that have transformed to macrophages. Two apoptotic signal pathways have been characterized: the death receptor and the mitochondrial pathways. Both pathways ultimately result in the activation of caspase 3 and subsequent DNA fragmentation, chromatin condensation, and formation of the apoptotic body. Neutrophils can undergo apoptosis through either mechanism.

The induction of ligands on the apoptotic neutrophil results in recognition by the inflammatory tissue macrophages as an "eat me" signal. One signal, phosphatidylserine (PS), is formed during the early stages of apoptosis, as PS is relocated from the inner to the outer surface of the plasma membrane. PS is recognized by a specific PS receptor on the macrophage. Proteinases released by bacteria provide novel mechanisms for an "eat me" signal from the apoptotic neutrophil. The rapid influx of neutrophils to an inflammatory site must be followed swiftly by monocytes that mature into inflammatory macrophages. These macrophages can then either emigrate from the tissue into the lymphatics or proliferate and secrete reparative cytokines, such as transforming growth factor β_1 (TGF-β_1), resolving the neutrophil accumulation and inflammatory process. Circulating apoptotic neutrophils are almost exclusively cleared by Kupffer cells in the liver (18,19).

DEFECTS IN NEUTROPHIL NUMBER AND/OR FUNCTION

Neutrophils are important to the host defense at the epidermal/epithelial surface, which is continuously exposed to bacteria. Children with neutrophil defects will generally have recurrent bacterial infections of the skin, lung, oropharynx, and perirectal area. New defects in neutrophil function are continuously being identified. The following discussion focuses on several of the more prevalent defects.

Congenital and Developmental

Congenital Neutropenias

Neutropenia can be caused by intrinsic defects in granulocytes or their progenitors. Congenital neutropenias encompass a diverse group; however, all are characterized by low neutrophil count (<500 neutrophils/μL). *Severe congenital neutropenia* appears after birth, with 90% of all children symptomatic within 6 months. Several genetic defects are responsible for this phenotype, the most common have defects in neutrophil elastase, which may also result in cyclic neutropenia. In these children, bone marrow arrest occurs at the promyelocyte or myelocyte stage. Omphalitis is often the presenting sign. These children can also have upper and lower respiratory infections and skin and liver abscesses. In children with *cyclic neutropenia/cyclic hematopoiesis*, a cyclic fluctuation occurs in all hematopoietic lines, though that of the neutrophil line is most marked. Neutrophil counts cycle at an average of 21 days, including periods of severe neutropenia that are 3–10 days in duration. In these children, oral ulcerations, gingivitis, pharyngitis, and tonsillitis are most common. In all of the diseases of severe congenital neutropenia, the use of G-CSF has greatly improved both the life span and the quality of life. Although the long-term use of G-CSF has been lifesaving, children and adults are at risk for developing myelodysplastic syndrome/acute myeloid leukemia.

Other causes of intrinsic defects resulting in neutropenia are Shwachman–Diamond, albinism/neutropenia syndromes (including Chédiak–Higashi Syndrome), bone marrow failure syndromes (acquired and congenital), and neutropenia associated with metabolic abnormalities, which can be a feature of organic acidemias (1).

Defects of Oxidative Metabolism

The most widely recognized and most prevalent defect of neutrophil function is chronic granulomatous disease (CGD), a heterogeneous disease that is characterized by recurrent life-threatening infections with bacteria, fungi, and the formation of abnormal granulomata. The defect is in the NADPH oxidase, the enzyme system responsible for the oxidative burst. The NADPH oxidase is a six-protein complex that has two components—a membrane-bound complex embedded in the walls of the secondary granule (cytochrome b_{558}) and a distinct cytoplasmic component (**Fig. 83.3**). The cytochrome b_{558} is composed of a 91-kDa glycosylated β chain (gp91^{phox}) and a 22-kDa nonglycosylated α chain (p22^{phox}). The cytoplasmic components are p47^{phox}, p67^{phox}, p40^{phox}, and *rac*. The most common genotype of the CGD is the X-linked mutations of gp91^{phox}, accounting for 70% of US cases. Males are affected, and females are carriers. With heavy lionization of the functional gene, an X-linked form of CGD has been reported in females. Defects in p47^{phox} occur in 25% of US cases, and defects in p22^{phox} and p67^{phox} occur in <5%. Clinically, CGD is quite variable and the age at presentation ranges from infancy to late adulthood. Typically, most affected individuals are diagnosed as toddlers and young children. The most frequent sites of infection are lung, lymph nodes, and liver. Of 360 patients in the CGD national registry in 2000, 80% had pneumonia and 68% had an abscess. Osteomyelitis, perianal abscess, and gingivitis are also common (20).

The functional defect is the inability of the NADPH complex to generate superoxide (O_2^-) and the downstream ROS (H_2O_2 and OH$^\bullet$) resulting in defective microbial killing and recurrent infections with catalase-positive bacteria. Organisms that produce their own H_2O_2 but do not degrade it (those that are catalase negative) supply the substrate for the formation of hypohalous acid by the myeloperoxidase released into the phagolysosome by the neutrophil. Note that other granule functions in the CGD neutrophils are intact. The metabolites of superoxide appear to be the mediators of bacterial killing in themselves. However, ROS are required for the activation of the primary granule serine proteases cathepsin G and elastase. Thus, ROS may be involved in other antimicrobicidal pathways in addition to producing a direct microbicidal effect. The overwhelming majority of infections result from *Aspergillus* (40%), *Staphylococcus aureus* (12%), *Burkholderia cepacia* (8%), *Nocardia* (7%), and *Serratia marcescens* (5%) (6). As many as 32% of those with CGD have gastrointestinal involvement, and 38% have urogenital involvement.

The cornerstone of treatment of CGD is trimethoprim/sulfamethoxazole prophylaxis. Since its institution, major infections have been reduced from 1 per year to 1 per 3.5 years; observations include fewer staphylococcal and skin infections and no increases in fungal infections. Itraconazole prophylaxis is routinely recommended in patients with CGD, regardless of age or previous fungal infections. A large, multicentered trial of IFN-γ demonstrated 70% fewer infections, compared with placebo. Long-term follow-up of the prospective trials suggest sustained benefit (21).

Management of infections in these patients is critical to decrease morbidity and reduce mortality. Microbial diagnosis is critical. In severe infections, granulocyte infusions have been used; although they are potentially lifesaving, they may also complicate the ICU course (see later discussion on granulocyte transfusions). As the deletion for X-linked CGD is encoded next to the Kell blood antigen, deletion of the Kell locus may also occur, resulting in CGD with the McLeod phenotype. Hence, a potential transfusion hazard may exist in X-linked CGD patients. If Kell blood antigen-negative individuals are transfused with Kell-positive blood products (or granulocytes), antibodies to Kell antigen may develop. Therefore, all patients with CGD should be screened for Kell antigen. If they are found to be Kell negative, transfusion is best avoided, or Kell-negative erythrocytes or granulocytes should be used.

Defects of Leukocyte Adhesion and Trafficking

Children with recurrent, necrotic bacterial infections, impaired pus formation, and impaired wound healing were first described almost 30 years ago. Leukocyte adhesion deficiency 1 (LAD-1) with defects in the β_2 integrins was identified ~25 years ago.

LAD-1 is an autosomal recessive disorder with mutations in the common chain of the β_2 integrin CD18, which results in a deficiency in number or function of adhesion molecules Mac-1 (CD11b/CD18), LFA-1 (CD11a/CD18), and p150,95 (CD11c/CD18) on the cell surface. Neutrophils cannot adhere and transmigrate to the inflammatory focus. In addition, as Mac-1 is also the complement receptor 3, severely reduced complement-mediated phagocytosis occurs (**Tables 83.2 and 83.4**). Some patients have <1% of expression of these adhesion molecules. With this severe type, children usually present within the first months of life with omphalitis and delayed cord separation. They have severe infections, impaired pus formation, and impaired wound healing. They have neutrophilia at baseline, but with infections, the neutrophil count may rise >100,000/μL. Recurrent infections of the skin, upper and lower airways, bowel, and perirectal area are common and are usually due to *S. aureus* or Gram-negative bacilli. Pathognomonic for neutrophil-adhesion defects, the skin lesions are necrotic, and almost no pus is seen surrounding them. An absence of neutrophil invasion is found on histopathology. In patients with a moderate phenotype, β_2-integrin expression may be up to 30% of normal adult controls. Infections are less ominous, but periodontal disease, leukocytosis, and delayed wound healing are still the rule. In an increasing number of LAD-1 variants, the quantity of β_2-integrin expression is normal, but functional defects occur. Treatment for these children is early and aggressive antibiotics. Bone marrow transplantation is the only definitive treatment for children with LAD-1.

In LAD-2 or congenital disorder of glycosylation IIc (CD-GIIc), defects occur in glycosylation. Selectins must be appropriately glycosylated for full function (**Fig. 83.2A** and **Table 83.2**). In these children, neutrophils cannot be captured from the free-flowing stream; therefore, transition to an arrested cell—a critical step in leukocyte emigration—cannot occur. Although these children do have severe recurrent infections, they also have associated neurodevelopmental defects due to the glycosylation abnormalities.

In LAD-3 (also known as LAD-1/variant), the defect occurs because of the inability of the integrins to be activated. Kindlin proteins are key players in integrin activation. Children with LAD-3 have defects in both neutrophil extravasation and also with platelet aggregation, as kindlin protein III is required for correct integrin activation for both of these cell types. Hematopoietic stem cell transplantation is curative for LAD-1 and LAD-3. Children with LAD-2 also have severe neurologic defects, and stem cell transplantation will not have an effect on the neurologic defects (22).

Developmental Defects in Neutrophil Function

Bacterial infection is a major cause of death and long-term morbidity in preterm neonates. Infection rates among neonates who receive care in the NICU range from 25% to 50%. The large rate of infection is due to immaturity of bactericidal mechanisms. Clinical evidence demonstrates that the neonate's (and, in particular, the preterm infant's) immune incompetence closely patterns that observed in adult patients with profound neutropenia.

Newborn infants, whether born at term or very premature, have peripheral blood counts similar to older children and adults. However, they differ dramatically from adults in their response to sepsis. The profound, sustained neutrophilia with sepsis seen in adults is not found in neonates and premature infants. Instead, neonates and premature infants frequently become neutropenic during infection due to low neutrophil cell mass and an apparent inability to increase the proliferation of the early progenitor pool (23).

Neutrophils isolated from neonatal cord blood have diminished chemotaxis due, in part, to a decreased amount of Mac-1 that is mobilizable from the secretory vesicles and gelatinase granules. They also have diminished L-selectin (CD62-L) and P-selectin glycoprotein ligand-1 (PSGL-1), the ligand for P-selectin. Thus, at least in vitro, neonatal neutrophils have difficulty in being captured from the free-flowing stream, transitioning from a rolling to an arrested cell, and ultimately emigrating across the endothelial cell of the blood vessel. Term infants rapidly establish normal chemotactic function within 1–2 weeks, whereas premature infants, whose chemotactic defect remains for weeks, do not (24).

In contrast, if bacteria are sufficiently opsonized, neonatal neutrophils demonstrate normal phagocytosis, although phagocytosis for *Candida* is decreased compared with adult neutrophils. As is true for term neonates, neutrophils from preterm infants are equally able to phagocytose fully opsonized bacteria (25). Critical is the fact that term or preterm plasma is unable to fully opsonize bacteria. Even adult neutrophils have defective phagocytosis if infant plasma is used for opsonization. Neonatal neutrophils may demonstrate NET formation, and this is paralleled by an unrecognized deficit in extracellular bacterial killing (26).

NEUTROPHILS AND CRITICAL ILLNESS

Neutrophil Function in Critical Illness

Circulating neutrophils from infected or traumatized patients are not the "same" as neutrophils from the same individual in the noninflamed or injured state. In many ways, these neutrophils appear to have already been stimulated. However, they may also be more prepared to fight infections. The high-affinity receptor for immunoglobulin, $Fc\gamma R1$ (CD64), is usually present in low amounts on neutrophils; however, in patients with sepsis, $Fc\gamma R1$ is upregulated dramatically. It is also possible that these differences in neutrophils in patients with sepsis or severe infections may be due to an increased proportion of "aged" cells. Neutrophils have a limited life span in the circulation and, after 12 hours, undergo spontaneous apoptosis. L-selectin (CD62L), which is critical to the initial "tether" of the neutrophil to the inflamed endothelium, decreases as they remain in circulation. L-selectin is markedly diminished as these cells enter into apoptosis. In infection and trauma, circulating neutrophils have decreased markers of apoptosis and decreased L-selectin. Thus, the proportion of aged cells that would normally undergo apoptosis under noninflamed conditions decreases in those individuals with infections. G-CSF and IL-6 increase transit time of neutrophils in the maturational pools and delay apoptosis, and the levels of both are dramatically elevated in sepsis. G-CSF administered to individuals with delayed wound healing demonstrated decreased neutrophil chemotaxis and decreased degranulation. However, respiratory burst and phagocytic activity were increased. Thus, the effects of critical illness on the neutrophil may not be due as much to the "illness" per se, but rather the release of factors which themselves result in a pool of neutrophils with increased inflammatory characteristics.

It has been well recognized for several decades that neutrophils obtained from individuals with infection and trauma have diminished chemotactic function, compared with neutrophils from those same individuals after the infection has resolved. In human sepsis, neutrophil chemotaxis to the bacterial product fMLF and leukotriene B_4 (an arachidonic acid–derived chemotactic factor) is diminished. In patients with sepsis and multiple organ failure, chemotactic response to the chemokine IL-8 is also reduced. Neutrophil Mac-1 (CD11b/CD18) was upregulated in the patients with sepsis and correlated with increased levels of IL-8, compared with normal volunteers. Increased Mac-1, CD64 ($Fc\gamma RI$), and "activation markers" were also found on neutrophils from patients with sepsis and were lower on patients who ultimately died. Neutrophil elastase was found in the serum of patients with severe sepsis and was correlated with disseminated intravascular coagulation. Neutrophil rigidity was increased overall in patients with sepsis. In those patients who recovered, rigidity returned toward normal, whereas in those individuals who did not improve, neutrophils remained rigid. Neutrophils from patients with sepsis have increased spontaneous oxidative burst activity. In traumatized patients, chemotaxis is delayed, spontaneous oxidative burst activity is increased, oxidative activity with stimulation is diminished, and opsonophagocytosis is decreased (reviewed in Ref. 27).

Neutrophils produced and circulating under such conditions contribute to organ injury. Strong evidence exists in animal models that trauma or ischemia results in "activated" neutrophils, and these neutrophils can sequester in remote organs, leading to injury. In adult neutropenic patients with respiratory failure and pneumonia, as many as one-third develop ARDS during their recovery from neutropenia (28). In a cohort of premature infants with respiratory distress who had early-onset neutropenia after birth, those with neutropenia were more likely to require greater inflation pressures on the ventilator and increased inspired oxygen concentration at 12 hours, required mechanical ventilation by 1 week, and more had pulmonary interstitial emphysema, intraventricular hemorrhage, and chronic lung disease compared with the cohort of premature infants with lung disease without neutropenia (29). NETs have been identified in blood smears collected from patients with systemic inflammatory response syndrome (SIRS). In addition, plasma from patients with SIRS is able to induce NET formation by normal neutrophils (30–32). Such examples are compelling evidence that, although neutrophils are critical to the host response, they are also involved in many of the diseases in the ICU.

A compelling theory of damage-associated molecular patterns (DAMPs) may be responsible for the activation of neutrophils in injury and sepsis. DAMPs can include substances that are secreted as a result of cellular activation such as high-mobility group protein B1 (HMGB1), intracellular components such as mitochondrial DNA that are released as result of cellular necrosis, or extracellular matrix components that are released upon tissue damage. DAMPs can active cells of the immune system through germ line–encoded pattern recognition receptors such as TLRs and NOD-like receptors (reviewed in Refs. 27 and 33).

Transfusion-Related Acute Lung Injury

The neutrophil is the effector cell in transfusion-related ALI (TRALI). TRALI is caused by activation of pulmonary neutrophils by activating substances in transfused blood products. The animal models and human studies suggest that, for TRALI to develop, multiple "hits" must occur (34). The first hit results in activation of the endothelium, and a normal antiadhesive surface becomes proadhesive for neutrophils. Neutrophils become activated and sequestered in the lung. This first hit can occur from sepsis, trauma, or massive blood transfusion. The second hit is the infusion of specific antibodies directed against antigens on the neutrophil surface and/or biologic modifiers in the stored blood component, which activate the adherent or trapped neutrophils in the lung, causing neutrophil–endothelial injury, capillary leak, and ALI. Differentiating TRALI from transfusion-associated circulatory overload (hydrostatic pulmonary edema) may be difficult and may require more invasive studies, such as measurement of the left atrial pressure. Blood component and donor management strategies appear to prevent some of TRALI, including the avoidance of blood products from individuals with known leukocyte antibodies, leukoreduction of blood components, shortening the storage time of cellular components to reduce accumulation of cytokines and other biologic response modifiers, and washing cellular components prior to transfusion. This type of injury is being ameliorated by preventing plasma-rich blood products from alloimmunized or all exposed donors from entering the blood supply. However, these efforts have no effect on the "multiple hits" that can lead to TRALI for patients in the ICU (34).

Neutropenia and the ICU

Neutropenia clearly disposes patients to bacteremia, fungemia, and sepsis, but its effect on outcome in patients in the ICU is not completely clear. In adult critically ill patients with cancer, neutropenia does not affect the outcome, even in those individuals with sepsis (35). In a recent Cochrane Review, the use of colony-stimulating factors in patients with febrile neutropenia due to cancer chemotherapy reduced the amount of time spent in the hospital and time for neutrophil recovery,

but no clear survival benefit was seen (36). Well-controlled trials of either G-CSF or GM-CSF in neutropenic patients in the ICU have not been conducted. In small, noncontrolled cohorts of neutropenic patients in the ICU, use of colony-stimulating factors did not reduce the duration of neutropenia, the length of ICU stay, or survival.

In adult critically ill cancer patients, one-third experienced ARDS during neutrophil recovery. These patients were more likely to have leukemia/lymphoma, pneumonia, and prolonged neutropenia (>10 days duration) (28). In adult patients with neutropenia, respiratory status deterioration is associated with G-CSF administration, in particular if individuals have pulmonary infiltrates during neutropenia. Even healthy adults can experience transient respiratory disturbances if they receive G-CSF for granulocyte mobilization for blood progenitor cell transplantation.

The effect of neutropenia on children in the ICU is even less clear. In a large, multicentered study in a cohort of 359 ICU pediatric oncology patients, neutropenia was not associated with increased mortality, though fungal infections and higher Pediatric Risk of Mortality scores were associated with increased mortality (37). In another multicentered study of pediatric oncology patients, those with bacteremia and neutropenia had increased mortality (15%), compared with those who did not have neutropenia (4%, $p < 0.05$) (38). As with adult patients, fungal infections in children with cancer are particularly problematic. Aggressive antineoplastic treatment, severe and long-lasting neutropenia, and/or lymphocytopenia are associated with fungal infections, but mortality is lower in children, compared with adults. In children, risk of death was almost fourfold higher if the patients were already receiving antifungals at the time of diagnosis (39). To date, no studies have been conducted in children to examine changes in lung function with the use of G-CSF. Therefore, recommendations regarding the use of G-CSF in neutropenic, critically ill patients must be individualized. In those neutropenic children with proven or suspected fungal infections in whom mortality is high, G-CSF appears prudent. If neutropenic patients have sepsis (bacteremia and organ failure) again, G-CSF would be indicated. However, those who have pneumonia or another pulmonary process and neutropenia may be at risk for developing worsening respiratory status with the use of G-CSF. Therefore, withholding G-CSF or alternatively administering G-CSF via continuous infusion could be considered.

In a meta-analysis that examined all studies in neonates who received either G-CSF or GM-CSF in addition to antibiotics as treatment for serious infection, no survival benefit was seen at 14 days (40). A single blind, multicenter randomized controlled trial was designed to examine prophylactic administration of GM-CSF in premature infants less than 32 weeks gestation. Although GM-CSF corrected neutropenia, it did not reduce sepsis or improve survival (41). Follow-up of patients at 2 years continued to show no effect of GM-CSF on neurodevelopmental or health outcomes (42).

Use of Colony-Stimulating Factors in Non-neutropenic ICU Patients

Even though a number of studies have been conducted in both neonates (discussed previously) and adults, there is no conclusive evidence that either G-CSF or GM-CSF improves outcome in the non-neutropenic patient. In a meta-analysis of six studies that enrolled ~2000 non-neutropenic adults with pneumonia, G-CSF did not improve outcome (43). However, it is also clear that no excessive morbidity or mortality was associated with G-CSF in this high-risk population. A randomized, double-blind, placebo-controlled trial of G-CSF in non-pediatric patients with septic shock did not demonstrate a survival benefit with the use of G-CSF, and the use of G-CSF was associated with a higher rate of new organ failure (44). It is also important to highlight that G-CSF and GM-CSF cannot be used interchangeably. G-CSF differs from GM-CSF in its specificity of action on developing and mature neutrophils, its effects on neutrophil kinetics, and its toxicity profile. GM-CSF results in priming of monocytes/macrophages and release of inflammatory cytokines. G-CSF also results in production of anti-inflammatory factors. G-CSF or GM-CSF in the non-neutropenic ICU patient should be used only in the context of therapeutic trials.

Use of Granulocyte Transfusion

In light of the previous descriptions of the use of G-CSF to mobilize granulocytes for transfusion, it is hardly surprising that the use of granulocyte transfusions all but disappeared during the 1980s and 1990s. Little therapeutic benefit was observed, and reports surfaced regarding adverse pulmonary responses with granulocyte transfusions. A review of 10 trials for the prophylactic use of granulocyte transfusion demonstrated potentially modest benefit, but all the trials were performed decades ago, and standards of supportive care have changed considerably (45). A review of eight parallel randomized controlled trials, which included 310 patient episodes, examined the use of granulocyte transfusions for treating infections in patients with neutropenia (46). Currently there is inconclusive evidence from these studies to support or refute the generalized use of granulocyte transfusions in adults with neutropenias and infections.

In a meta-analysis of trials in neonates with confirmed or suspected sepsis and neutropenia, no benefit of granulocyte transfusion compared with placebo was observed. In one trial of granulocyte transfusion compared with IV immunoglobulin, a borderline reduction in mortality was associated with granulocyte transfusion (47). All the trials were limited by the number of subjects enrolled (total neonates 105).

Critical Care Therapies and Neutrophil Function

Mechanical Ventilation

Since the early 1990s, studies have demonstrated that "mechanical stretch" of the lung results in lung injury. Mechanical stretch of the alveolar epithelium can lead to the production of proinflammatory cytokines, in particular chemokines for neutrophils. If neutrophils are depleted, ventilator-induced lung injury in animal models can be abrogated. However, in animal models, neutrophil activation occurs early in ventilator-induced lung injury, and injurious ventilation (high tidal volume) results in pulmonary neutrophil sequestration, decreased neutrophil deformability, but no change in adhesion molecule expression. In humans with ALI, the use of conventional ventilation strategy (compared with a protective ventilation strategy) for as little as 36 hours results in increased production of plasma IL-6 and bronchoalveolar fluid, which activated donor neutrophils. In premature infants, the use of mechanical ventilation resulted in activation of circulating neutrophils and monocytes, as measured by increased CD11b/CD18 compared with infants treated with nasal CPAP (48).

Hypothermia

Mild hypothermia (32–34°C) is advocated in adult patients after cardiac arrest and for neonates with hypoxic encephalopathy. However, several lines of evidence suggest that hypothermia increases mortality in patients with sepsis and trauma and that hypothermia favors wound infections. Hypothermia

decreases neutrophil motility, respiratory burst, and phagocytosis, thus potentially decreasing secondary inflammatory injury at the cost of increasing infection risk. Therapeutic hypothermia delays C-reactive protein response and suppresses white blood cell and platelet count in infants with neonatal encephalopathy compared with neonates who received standard care (49). In a separate group of neonates, the hypothermia group had a lower circulating leukocyte count, and with rewarming, only the absolute neutrophil count rebounded. Chemokines, plasma levels of monocyte-chemotactic protein 1 and IL-8, were negatively correlated with their target leukocytes in the hypothermia group suggesting active chemokine and leukocyte modulation by hypothermia (50). Nonetheless, culture-positive sepsis is rare in neonatal encephalopathy (49). In a meta-analysis of randomized controlled trials of therapeutic hypothermia for neonatal encephalopathy, cooling resulted in decreased risk for sepsis (RR 0.87, 95% confidence interval [CI] 0.6–1.26), despite an increased risk of leukopenia (RR 2.40, 95% CI 0.85–6/79) (51).

In a meta-analysis of trials of adult patients who suffered a cardiac arrest, mild hypothermia resulted in a better neurologic outcome compared with normothermia (RR 1.55, 95% CI 1.22–1.97), and there was no difference in the development of pneumonia or sepsis between either treatment (52). Thus, although there are measurable effects on neutrophils and leukocytes of hypothermia, there are no/little data that these result in poor clinical outcomes.

Cardiopulmonary Bypass

In cardiopulmonary bypass (CPB), interaction of the blood elements with the oxygenator membrane and the mechanical stress of the circuit on the cells result in an acute inflammatory process that involves complement activation, production of PAF and other arachidonic intermediates, and activation of the kallikrein system. Neutrophils are activated with increased oxidative burst, and myeloperoxidase, elastase, and lactoferrin are found in the plasma. This inflammatory process is also seen in extracorporeal membrane oxygenation (ECMO). Blood neutrophils from neonates who are being treated with ECMO are activated, and increased neutrophil elastase is found in the plasma, compared with those same neonates before ECMO is initiated. In addition, lung injury worsened once they were placed on ECMO. Leukocyte filtration systems for cardiopulmonary bypass or leukocyte depletion of blood used in ECMO circuits have been used. However, use of the filter itself results in leukocyte activation. Studies to date are heterogeneous, enrolling few patients, with outcomes of modest interest; thus, leukocyte depletion cannot be recommended for ECMO or cardiopulmonary bypass.

Drug Effects

Barbiturates and Anesthetics. Barbiturates, midazolam, and propofol all have profound effects on neutrophils. All inhibit respiratory burst, and barbiturates inhibit chemotaxis, opsonophagocytosis, and intracellular killing. While anesthesia-relevant concentrations may have minimal effects, the considerably higher concentrations used in the ICU place patients potentially at risk for increased infections.

Pentoxifylline and Cyclic AMP Modulators. Pentoxifylline, a xanthine derivative, is a phosphodiesterase inhibitor used in adult patients for treatment of claudication. With the discovery that it also decreases *TNF* gene transcription in sepsis, pentoxifylline has attracted fresh attention as an anti-inflammatory agent. It has numerous functions, including preventing the development of necrotizing enterocolitis in neonates by preserving small-vessel function, preventing endothelial dysfunction in sepsis, enhancing prostacyclin release, and attenuating the release of thromboxane. Pentoxifylline increases erythrocyte and leukocyte deformability, presumably by increasing cyclic AMP levels. In a meta-analysis of four randomized placebo-controlled trials of pentoxifylline in neonatal sepsis as an adjunct to antibiotics, all-cause mortality was reduced with the use of pentoxifylline, and no adverse events were found (53). Given the few patients studied, no recommendation for pentoxifylline use in neonates can be made; however, given the signal for a beneficial effect, larger trials should be developed.

The elevation of intracellular cyclic AMP results in decreased neutrophil adhesion, demonstrated with type IV phosphodiesterase inhibitors (rolipram) and the β_2 agonist isoproterenol, but not with type III phosphodiesterase inhibitors (milrinone). Neutrophils, monocytes, eosinophils, and mast cells have β_2-adrenergic receptors. Activation of neutrophil β_2-adrenergic receptors results in decreased IL-8-induced chemotaxis. Catecholamines, including epinephrine, norepinephrine, dobutamine, and dopamine, depress neutrophil phagocytic ability and production of ROS. Thus, many of the agents used commonly in the ICU can have direct suppressive effects on neutrophil function at the pharmacologic doses achieved.

Corticosteroids. The main anti-inflammatory effects of corticosteroids result from changes in the function of macrophages, monocytes, and granulocytes, including the decreased production of anti-inflammatory cytokines, inhibition of arachidonic acid metabolism, and decreased granulocyte adherence and migration. Lymphocyte number and function are also markedly affected by corticosteroids.

Modulating Neutrophil Function

Anti-integrin Therapy

With the critical role of neutrophils in pathophysiologic diseases, such as shock, ARDS, and ischemia–reperfusion injury, a number of therapies to block neutrophil adhesive function have been proposed and produced. Numerous animal studies have demonstrated that antiadhesive strategies are, in fact, successful. At least in theory, such strategies should also be beneficial in critically ill humans. Initial enthusiasm with this paradigm has given way to a number of negative human studies and a cautious reappraisal of the concept. Studies in traumatic shock, stroke, burns, myocardial infarction, and transplant have demonstrated no benefit of β_2-integrin, LFA-1, or ICAM-1 blockade in humans (54). Use of anti-α_4 or anti-$\alpha_4\beta_7$ therapy in inflammatory bowel disease has had particular success (55,56). Anti-integrin therapy has also been of great use in oncology (57).

Neutrophil Elastase Inhibition

When neutrophils have reduced deformability, such as occurs in sepsis, severe trauma, and ALI, they are potentially trapped in capillaries. These neutrophils may then secrete neutrophil elastase, reactive oxygen products, and other soluble mediators of tissue injury. A selective inhibitor of neutrophil elastase, sivelestat, attenuates leukocyte adhesion in pulmonary capillaries and also attenuates the decreased neutrophil deformability in animal models of sepsis. In humans with ALI, sivelestat infusion for 5 days also attenuated diminished neutrophil deformability. Sivelestat is widely used in Japan for the treatment of ALI. A systematic review and meta-analysis of eight trials (total of 953 subjects) demonstrated no effect of sivelestat on survival at 30 or 180 days in subjects with ALI or ARDS (58). In an exploratory study 13 pediatric patients

who underwent cardiopulmonary bypass received sivelestat prior to the initiation of CPB, and for 24 hours after, control patients received standard care (59). Children who received sivelestat demonstrated less inflammation post-CPB as measured by neutrophil and leukocyte count and C-reactive protein levels.

Leukocyte Depletion

As outlined previously, neutrophils from patients with sepsis are primed by inflammatory factors, they are more rigid, and are more easily trapped in the microcirculation; they readily mobilize secretory granules, ROS and proteolytic enzymes. Leukopheresis has been promulgated for Crohn disease, ulcerative colitis, and systemic lupus erythematosus. Filters used for leukopheresis selectively adsorb neutrophils expressing CD64 and complement receptors, which are abnormally elevated in patients with inflammatory and autoimmune disorders. In small series of patients who have received leukoreduction, there is a clear evidence that these filters appear to select for the neutrophils that are the most activated. Although trials for sepsis and after cardiopulmonary bypass are of interest, they are not of sufficient strength to make a recommendation (27,60). Recent observations in animal studies support the concept of "eliminating" or controlling the hyperactivated neutrophil. In a mouse model, neutrophils crawling toward an agarose bead "studded" with methicillin-resistant *Staphylococcus aureus*, "plugged" the capillaries, and impaired capillary perfusion. This led to parenchymal cell death though the neutrophils were unable to emigrate from the capillaries. This crawling was mediated by β_2- and α_4-integrins, and blocking these integrins postinfection eliminated neutrophil crawling, improved capillary perfusion, and reduced cell death. If the blocking antibodies were used prior to infection, there was increased injury to the tissue (61).

CONCLUSIONS AND FUTURE DIRECTIONS

Many questions remain regarding the manipulation of neutrophil number and function in the PICU population. The neutrophil is at the foundation of the innate immune system. It is absolutely required for maintenance of the organism during the ongoing onslaught by environmental microbes and, in general, is sufficient to control invasion. However, neutrophil function can be compromised in the PICU in a number of circumstances, either by a limitation in number, as occurs with medication or genetic defect, or by limitation in function. Some questions that should be addressed for the care of critically ill children are follows: (a) As neutrophils are activated in transfused blood, should all transfused blood be leukocyte-depleted for patients with ALI or those who are at risk for lung injury? (b) As pentoxifylline is a useful adjunct in neonates with sepsis, will it be useful in the older infant and child? Why has pentoxifylline not had increased use in the septic neonate? (c) Should G-CSF be used in all critically ill neutropenic children or only in those without evidence of lung injury? Should G-CSF be used in the subpopulation of patients who undergo therapies known to induce neutrophil dysfunction, that is, barbiturate infusion and hypothermia? (d) Is the incidence of TRALI in children equal to that in adults? (e) Would pharmacologic manipulation of neutrophils (through the use of neutrophil elastase inhibitors) or the removal of activated neutrophils (through leukodepletion) improve the outcome in those patients who have evidence of activation such as occurs with septic shock or on ECMO?

References

1. Dinauer MC, Newburger PE, Borregarrd N. Phagocyte system and disorders of granulopoiesis and granulocyte function. In: Orkin SH, Nathan DG, Look AT, et al., eds. *Nathan and Oski's Hematology and Oncology of Infancy and Childhood*. Philadelphia, PA: Elsevier Saunders, 2015:773.e729–874.e729.

2. Khanna-Gupta A, Nancy B. Granulocytopoiesis and monocytopoiesis. In: Hoffman RB, Leslie ES Jr, Helen H, et al., eds. *Hematology: Basic Principles and Practice*. 6th ed. Philadelphia, PA: Elsevier, 2013.

3. Faurschou M, Borregaard N. Neutrophil granules and secretory vesicles in inflammation. *Microbes Infect* 2003;5(14):1317–27.

4. Nauseef WM, Borregaard N. Neutrophils at work. *Nat Immunol* 2014;15(7):602–11.

5. Orr Y, Taylor JM, Bannon PG, et al. Circulating CD10-/CD16 low neutrophils provide a quantitative index of active bone marrow neutrophil release. *Br J Haematol* 2005;131(4):508–19.

6. Suwa T, Hogg JC, Klut ME, et al. Interleukin-6 changes deformability of neutrophils and induces their sequestration in the lung. *Am J Respir Crit Care Med* 2001;163(4):970–6.

7. Prince AS, Mizgerd JP, Wiener-Kronish J, et al. Cell signaling underlying the pathophysiology of pneumonia. *Am J Physiol Lung Cell Mol Physiol* 2006;291(3):L297–L300.

8. Nourshargh S, Alon R. Leukocyte migration into inflamed tissues. *Immunity* 2014;41(5):694–707.

9. Herter J, Zarbock A. Integrin regulation during leukocyte recruitment. *J Immunol* 2013;190(9):4451–7.

10. Sullivan DP, Muller WA. Neutrophil and monocyte recruitment by PECAM, CD99, and other molecules via the LBRC. *Semin Immunopathol* 2014;36(2):193–209.

11. Nunes P, Demaurex N, Dinauer MC. Regulation of the NADPH oxidase and associated ion fluxes during phagocytosis. *Traffic* 2013;14(11):1118–31.

12. Jenne CN, Wong CH, Zemp FJ, et al. Neutrophils recruited to sites of infection protect from virus challenge by releasing neutrophil extracellular traps. *Cell Host Microbe* 2013;13(2):169–80.

13. McDonald B, Urrutia R, Yipp BG, et al. Intravascular neutrophil extracellular traps capture bacteria from the bloodstream during sepsis. *Cell Host Microbe* 2012;12(3):324–33.

14. Tecchio C, Micheletti A, Cassatella MA. Neutrophil-derived cytokines: Facts beyond expression. *Front Immunol* 2014;5:508.

15. Hamamichi Y, Ichida F, Yu X, et al. Neutrophils and mononuclear cells express vascular endothelial growth factor in acute Kawasaki disease: Its possible role in progression of coronary artery lesions. *Pediatr Res* 2001;49(1):74–80.

16. Yano K, Liaw PC, Mullington JM, et al. Vascular endothelial growth factor is an important determinant of sepsis morbidity and mortality. *J Exp Med* 2006;203(6):1447–58.

17. Johnson BL III, Kuethe JW, Caldwell CC. Neutrophil derived microvesicles: Emerging role of a key mediator to the immune response. *Endocr Metab Immune Disord Drug Targets* 2014;14(3):210–7.

18. Guzik K, Bzowska M, Smagur J, et al. A new insight into phagocytosis of apoptotic cells: Proteolytic enzymes divert the recognition and clearance of polymorphonuclear leukocytes by macrophages. *Cell Death Differ* 2007;14(1):171–82.

19. Summers C, Rankin SM, Condliffe AM, et al. Neutrophil kinetics in health and disease. *Trends Immunol* 2010;31(8):318–24.

20. Winkelstein JA, Marino MC, Johnston RB Jr, et al. Chronic granulomatous disease. Report on a national registry of 368 patients. *Medicine* 2000;79(3):155–69.

21. Holland SM. Chronic granulomatous disease. *Hematol Oncol Clin North Am* 2013;27(1):89–99, viii.

22. van de Vijver E, van den Berg TK, Kuijpers TW. Leukocyte adhesion deficiencies. *Hematol Oncol Clin North Am* 2013;27(1):101–116, viii.

23. Maheshwari A. Neutropenia in the newborn. *Curr Opin Hematol* 2014;21(1):43–9.

24. Nussbaum C, Gloning A, Pruenster M, et al. Neutrophil and endothelial adhesive function during human fetal ontogeny. *J Leukoc Biol* 2013;93(2):175–84.

25. Prosser A, Hibbert J, Strunk T, et al. Phagocytosis of neonatal pathogens by peripheral blood neutrophils and monocytes from newborn preterm and term infants. *Pediatr Res* 2013;74(5):503–10.

26. Yost CC, Cody MJ, Harris ES, et al. Impaired neutrophil extracellular trap (NET) formation: A novel innate immune deficiency of human neonates. *Blood* 2009;113(25):6419–27.

27. Hazeldine J, Hampson P, Lord JM. The impact of trauma on neutrophil function. *Injury* 2014;45(12):1824–33.

28. Azoulay E, Attalah H, Yang K, et al. Exacerbation by granulocyte colony-stimulating factor of prior acute lung injury: Implication of neutrophils. *Crit Care Med* 2002;30(9):2115–22.

29. Ferreira PJ, Bunch TJ, Albertine KH, et al. Circulating neutrophil concentration and respiratory distress in premature infants. *J Pediatr* 2000;136(4):466–72.

30. Hamaguchi S, Hirose T, Akeda Y, et al. Identification of neutrophil extracellular traps in the blood of patients with systemic inflammatory response syndrome. *J Int Med Res* 2013;41(1):162–8.

31. Hirose T, Hamaguchi S, Matsumoto N, et al. Presence of neutrophil extracellular traps and citrullinated histone H3 in the bloodstream of critically ill patients. *PLoS One* 2014;9(11):e111755.

32. Keshari RS, Jyoti A, Dubey M, et al. Cytokines induced neutrophil extracellular traps formation: Implication for the inflammatory disease condition. *PLoS One* 2012;7(10):e48111.

33. Gunzer M. Traps and hyper inflammation—New ways that neutrophils promote or hinder survival. *Br J Haematol* 2014;164(2):189–99.

34. Middelburg RA, van der Bom JG. Transfusion-related acute lung injury not a two-hit, but a multicausal model [published online ahead of print December 15, 2014]. *Transfusion*. doi:10.1111/trf.12966.

35. Regazzoni CJ, Irrazabal C, Luna CM, et al. Cancer patients with septic shock: Mortality predictors and neutropenia. *Support Care Cancer* 2004;12(12):833–9.

36. Mhaskar R, Clark OA, Lyman G, et al. Colony-stimulating factors for chemotherapy-induced febrile neutropenia. *Cochrane Database Syst Rev* 2014;10:CD003039.

37. Fiser RT, West NK, Bush AJ, et al. Outcome of severe sepsis in pediatric oncology patients. *Pediatr Crit Care Med* 2005;6(5):531–6.

38. Viscoli C, Castagnola E, Giacchino M, et al. Bloodstream infections in children with cancer: A multicentre surveillance study of the Italian Association of Paediatric Haematology and Oncology. Supportive Therapy Group-Infectious Diseases Section. *Eur J Cancer* 1999;35(5):770–4.

39. Castagnola E, Cesaro S, Giacchino M, et al. Fungal infections in children with cancer: A prospective, multicenter surveillance study. *Pediatr Infect Dis J* 2006;25(7):634–9.

40. Carr R, Modi N, Doré C. G-CSF and GM-CSF for treating or preventing neonatal infections. *Cochrane Database Syst Rev* 2003;(3):CD003066.

41. Carr R, Brocklehurst P, Dore CJ, et al. Granulocyte-macrophage colony stimulating factor administered as prophylaxis for reduction of sepsis in extremely preterm, small for gestational age neonates (the PROGRAMS trial): A single-blind, multicentre, randomised controlled trial. *Lancet* 2009;373(9659):226–33.

42. Marlow N, Morris T, Brocklehurst P, et al. A randomised trial of granulocyte-macrophage colony-stimulating factor for neonatal sepsis: Outcomes at 2 years. *Arch Dis Child* 2013;98(1):F46–F53.

43. Cheng AC, Stephens DP, Currie BJ. Granulocyte-colony stimulating factor (G-CSF) as an adjunct to antibiotics in the treatment of pneumonia in adults. *Cochrane Database Syst Rev* 2007;(2):CD004400.

44. Stephens DP, Thomas JH, Higgins A, et al. Randomized, double-blind, placebo-controlled trial of granulocyte colony-stimulating factor in patients with septic shock. *Crit Care Med* 2008;36(2):448–54.

45. Massey E, Paulus U, Doree C, et al. Granulocyte transfusions for preventing infections in patients with neutropenia or neutrophil dysfunction. *Cochrane Database Syst Rev* 2009;(1):CD005341.

46. Stanworth SJ, Massey E, Hyde C, et al. Granulocyte transfusions for treating infections in patients with neutropenia or neutrophil dysfunction. *Cochrane Database Syst Rev* 2005;(3):CD005339.

47. Pammi M, Brocklehurst P. Granulocyte transfusions for neonates with confirmed or suspected sepsis and neutropenia. *Cochrane Database Syst Rev* 2011;(10):CD003956.

48. Turunen R, Nupponen I, Siitonen S, et al. Onset of mechanical ventilation is associated with rapid activation of circulating phagocytes in preterm infants. *Pediatrics* 2006;117(2):448–54.

49. Chakkarapani E, Davis J, Thoresen M. Therapeutic hypothermia delays the C-reactive protein response and suppresses white blood cell and platelet count in infants with neonatal encephalopathy. *Arch Dis Child* 2014;99(6):F458–F463.

50. Jenkins DD, Lee T, Chiuzan C, et al. Altered circulating leukocytes and their chemokines in a clinical trial of therapeutic hypothermia for neonatal hypoxic ischemic encephalopathy. *Pediatr Crit Care Med* 2013;14(8):786–95.

51. Jacobs SE, Berg M, Hunt R, et al. Cooling for newborns with hypoxic ischaemic encephalopathy. *Cochrane Database Syst Rev* 2013;1:CD003311.

52. Arrich J, Holzer M, Havel C, et al. Hypothermia for neuroprotection in adults after cardiopulmonary resuscitation. *Cochrane Database Syst Rev* 2012;9:CD004128.

53. Haque KN, Pammi M. Pentoxifylline for treatment of sepsis and necrotizing enterocolitis in neonates. *Cochrane Database Syst Rev* 2011;(10):CD004205.

54. Yonekawa K, Harlan JM. Targeting leukocyte integrins in human diseases. *J Leukoc Biol* 2005;77(2):129–40.

55. Bickston SJ, Behm BW, Tsoulis DJ, et al. Vedolizumab for induction and maintenance of remission in ulcerative colitis. *Cochrane Database Syst Rev* 2014;8:CD007571.

56. MacDonald JK, McDonald JW. Natalizumab for induction of remission in Crohn's disease. *Cochrane Database Syst Rev* 2007;(1):CD006097.

57. Goodman SL, Picard M. Integrins as therapeutic targets. *Trends Pharmacol Sci* 2012;33(7):405–12.

58. Iwata K, Doi A, Ohji G, et al. Effect of neutrophil elastase inhibitor (sivelestat sodium) in the treatment of acute lung injury (ALI) and acute respiratory distress syndrome (ARDS): A systematic review and meta-analysis. *Intern Med* 2010;49(22):2423–32.

59. Inoue N, Oka N, Kitamura T, et al. Neutrophil elastase inhibitor sivelestat attenuates perioperative inflammatory response in pediatric heart surgery with cardiopulmonary bypass. *Int Heart J* 2013;54(3):149–53.

60. Lewis SM, Khan N, Beale R, et al. Depletion of blood neutrophils from patients with sepsis: Treatment for the future? *Int Immunopharmacol* 2013;17(4):1226–32.

61. Harding MG, Zhang K, Conly J, et al. Neutrophil crawling in capillaries; A novel immune response to *Staphylococcus aureus*. *PLoS Pathog* 2014;10(10):e1004379.

CHAPTER 84 ■ THE IMMUNE SYSTEM AND VIRAL ILLNESS

LESLEY DOUGHTY

KEY POINTS

1. Viral infections can alter host immune function and contribute to bacterial superinfection, asthma exacerbations, autoimmune disease exacerbations, and reactivation of latent viruses during critical illness.

2. Viral and bacterial coinfection occurs frequently in children and may have a role in complications of the viral or bacterial disease.

3. Viral infection can result in increased bacterial adherence to protective mucosal/epithelial barriers.

4. Viral infection can alter many aspects of the innate and acquired immune response leading to vulnerability to bacterial superinfection.

5. Asthmatics are more susceptible to viral infections and have heightened morbidity from exacerbations caused by viral infection.

6. Autoimmune disease exacerbations have been linked to several viral infections—some acute and some reactivated viruses.

This chapter will focus on the impact of common viral infections on immune function. Viral infections, such as human immunodeficiency virus (HIV), deplete lymphocyte subsets and thereby create vulnerability to opportunistic pathogens. As such, HIV represents the most extreme example of immunomodulation induced by viral infection. The impact of HIV viral infection on immune function is well understood; however, the impact of common viral infections, such as influenza A and B, respiratory syncytial virus (RSV), rhinovirus (RV), parainfluenza, adenovirus, enterovirus, and cytomegalovirus (CMV), on host immunity is less well appreciated and will be discussed in this chapter.

One example of immunomodulation by viral infection is seen in bacterial coinfection with influenza. Viral replication and destruction of protective epithelial barriers "open the door" for bacterial infection, additionally the ongoing antiviral immune response alters our ability to mount an appropriate antibacterial immune response. In this way, as depicted in **Figure 84.1**, there is a complex interaction between viral infection, the host antiviral immune response, and bacterial infection that impacts the delicate balance between bacterial eradication and further tissue injury (1).

In addition to increasing the risk of bacterial infection, viruses have been implicated in exacerbations of, and morbidity from, diseases such as asthma and a variety of autoimmune diseases. The data here suggest that viral infection may alter immune function, which sets the stage for disease exacerbation that often leads to critical illness. Acute primary and reactivated latent viral infections (such as CMV in the immunosuppressed population) can be life threatening and aggressive, and prophylaxis and/or treatment is routinely used in transplant recipients at times of peak immunosuppression. Reactivation of such viruses also occurs in critical illness, and the impact of this on critical illness and immune function is not clear. The impact of the immune response to viral infection on a number of disease states will be discussed in further depth in this chapter to introduce the concept that viral infection can have more far-reaching effects on the host than simply acute infection-related symptoms. Given the frequency of infection and the duration of the immune response to common respiratory and gastrointestinal viruses in infancy/childhood, it is possible that these pathogens contribute significantly to vulnerability to, and morbidity from, critical illness in the pediatric population.

APPLICATION TO PEDIATRIC CRITICAL CARE

The frequency of viral infections in the pediatric population warrants consideration of the impact of viral infection on immunity in this population. For the most part, the viral illness is thought to impact on critical illness because of primary infection (bronchiolitis, croup, and influenza); however, these common infections can set the stage for bacterial coinfection that carries the risk of severe morbidity and significant mortality. Data from the recent influenza A H1N1 season highlight this association with coinfection, being not only common but also associated with more severe outcomes. Many data show that significant immune compromise can occur during critical illness of several etiologies (most notably septic shock, acute lung injury, and trauma patients not receiving immunosuppressive medications). During this time, latent viruses, such as CMV, can reactivate and potentially contribute to the severity and survival from critical illness from other etiologies.

Children suffering from asthma exacerbations are a constant presence in the PICU, and the impact of viral infection on asthma exacerbations is considerable. The impact of antiviral immunity on viral control in asthmatics has not been studied in the critically ill asthmatic; however, a routine aspect of care for asthma exacerbations is glucocorticoid therapy. As will be discussed later in the chapter, there is a possibility that immune augmentation may benefit virus-infected asthmatics. An aspect of this disease that is unexplored is the potential use of immune strategies (other than glucocorticoids) to reduce

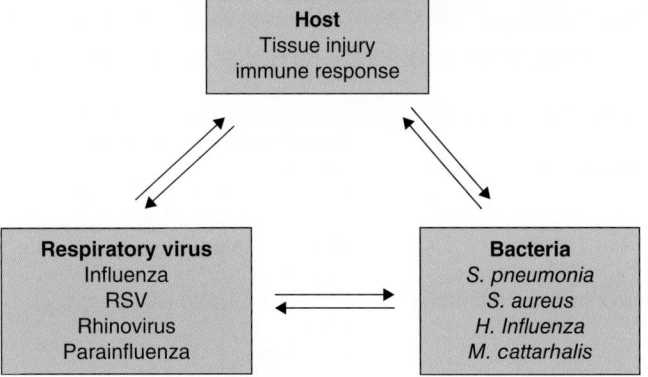

FIGURE 84.1. The interrelationship between viral infections, host immune responses, and bacteria in coinfection. Respiratory viral infection causes airway epithelial cell injury and incites an evolving immune response aimed early at eradicating virus and then tissue repair. The net effect of these responses is an anti-inflammatory milieu leaving the host vulnerable to bacterial coinfection (or subsequent infection) (1).

the impact of viral infection on bronchospastic symptoms in the most severe cases.

Autoimmune disease leading to critical illness is not a common problem in children; however, when it does occur, it can be life threatening and difficult to manage. For the most part, the role of viral infection in this setting has not been examined in children (except in new onset type 1 diabetes mellitus). Like asthma, a thorough knowledge of the association between viral infections and autoimmune disease exacerbation (and in some cases etiology) may provide potential targets for interrupting the influence of viral infection in these settings.

The discussion what follows will present what is known epidemiologically and mechanistically about the impact of viral infection on immune function and its consequences. Given the frequency of viral infection preceding critical illness, these data are pertinent to pediatric critical care.

SCIENTIFIC FOUNDATIONS

Immune Response to Viral Infection

Mucous membrane surfaces, respiratory epithelium, and skin are portals of entry for many viruses. Since viral infections depend on host cellular machinery for survival and replication, entry into cells is a critical early step. This is accomplished by a variety of mechanisms, some of which are common to many viruses and others are virus specific. Examples of mechanisms shared by multiple viruses are fusion with cell membrane (enveloped viruses) and/or endocytosis after binding to cell-surface molecules. Many cell-surface molecules are exploited by viruses to gain entry into cells to facilitate viral replication. Expression of such molecules is cell-type specific and can determine tissue tropism for certain viruses. Examples of exploited host cell-surface molecules include CD4, CCR5, and CXCR4 for HIV; sialic acid residues for influenza and other respiratory viruses; heparan sulfate and proteoglycans for herpesviruses; and coxsackie adenovirus receptor (CAR), and B cell receptors CD21 and C3d for Epstein Barr Virus (2). Once in contact with cells, viral replication and the host antiviral immune response begins. Replication of lytic viruses can directly injure mucosal and epithelial protective barriers by causing cell lysis upon release of viral particles (Table 84.1). Via killing of virus-infected cells, expression of inflammatory mediators, and leukocyte infiltration, the antiviral immune response can cause further tissue injury releasing damage-associated molecules (DAMPs) that

further activate the immune system (3). The immune response to microbial pathogens consists of several phases. The earliest and least specific is the innate immune response followed by a pathogen-specific adaptive immune response leading to immunologic memory. These phases of immune responses include activation of diverse cellular and humoral mediators—many of which are common to many types of infections. The immune response to viral infection involves mechanisms similar to those induced by bacterial infections as well as unique mechanisms. Recognition of viruses by the innate immune system begins by the host recognition of viral pathogen-associated molecular patterns (PAMPs) expressed during viral replication through their interaction with pattern recognition receptors (PRRs), such as the Toll-like receptors (TLRs). Viral PAMPs include virion proteins, hemagglutinin (HA), double-stranded RNA produced during replication of many viruses, F protein from RSV, single-stranded RNA, and viral DNA (4,5). TLR 2, 3, 4, 7, 8, and 9 have been implicated in responses to viral PAMPs. In fact, the initial cellular reactions to viral PAMPs are very similar to those initiated by bacterial PAMPs and are depicted in **Figure 84.2** (4). The innate response is critical for recruitment of effector cells, containment of viral particles, and the initiation of adaptive or antigen-specific immune response necessary for viral eradication and immunologic memory. Binding to TLRs initiates intracellular signal transduction leading to production of proinflammatory cytokines, including type I interferons α and β (IFN-α/β), type III interferons (IFN-λ subtypes), TNF-α, IL-1β, IL-6, and chemokines, such as CCL2, CCL20, and CCR7, which facilitate trafficking of alveolar macrophages, dendritic cells (DCs), and neutrophils to sites of viral invasion (6). Anti-inflammatory cytokines, such as IL-10, soluble TNF-α receptor, and IL-1 receptor antagonist, are also induced. TLR-independent mechanisms for cytoplasmic viral detection also exist including activation of nucleotide-binding and oligomerization domain-like receptors (NLRs) and helicases including retinoic acid–inducible protein (RIG-1). NLRs are a family of multimeric cytosolic structures ultimately capable of converting pro-caspase 1 to its functional form leading to conversion of proforms of IL-1β and IL-18 to their active forms (7). A role for NLRP3 in influenza and RSV has been demonstrated, and more data are emerging to implicate other types of NLRs. The precise activators of NLRP3 are being elucidated; however, it appears that they include conventional PAMPs (dsRNA) as well as reactive oxide species and potassium (K) flux induced during viral replication (7–9). In contrast, RIG-1 is activated by intracellular viral dsRNA produced

TABLE 84.1

MECHANISMS OF BACTERIAL ADHERENCE TO HOST CELLS DURING VIRAL INFECTION

Respiratory epithelial disruption	Loss of mucociliary function
	Basement membrane exposure
Bacterial features	Fimbriae
	Capsule
Expression of viral glycoproteins	Neuraminidase (influenza/parainfluenza)
	Hemagglutinin (influenza/parainfluenza)
	Glycoproteins F and G (RSV)
Upregulation of host cell receptors	CD14, CD15, and CD18
	PAFR
	Complement protein C3
	Fimbriae-associated receptors
	IgA translocating receptor
	Pentameric IgM
Proteins from injured ECM	Fibrinogen
Other	Coupling bacteria to epithelium by RSV
	Altered bacterial adhesins

ECM, extracellular matrix.
Adapted from Mashayekhi A, Shields CL, Shields JA. Transient increased exudation after photodynamic therapy of intraocular tumors. *Middle East Afr J Ophthalmol* 2013;20(1):83–6.

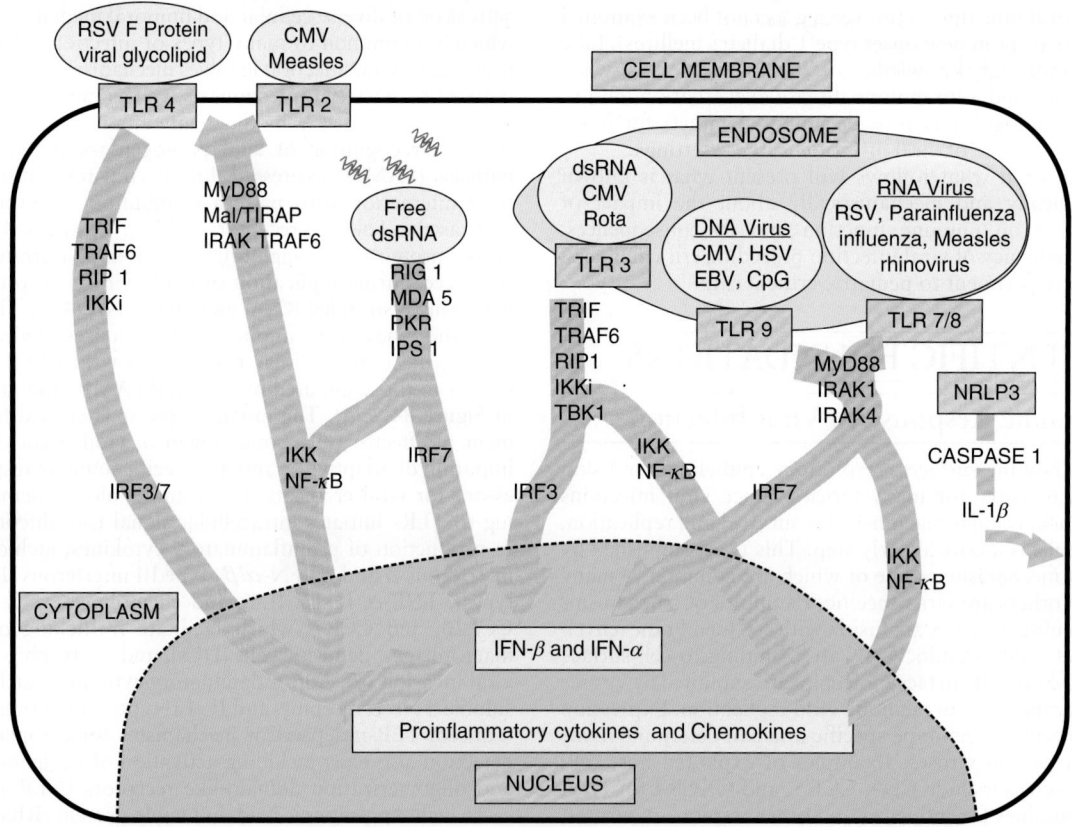

FIGURE 84.2. Early signaling initiated by viral PAMPs. Many viruses are recognized by TLRs. Viral PAMPs also include the fusion protein (F protein) of RSV, dsRNA, DNA, HA protein, and envelope proteins. The PAMPs associated with many viruses capable of signaling through TLRs have not been identified. Intracellularly, many of the adaptor molecules and kinases activated by TLRs are shared and, as with bacteria, ultimately initiate similar inflammatory cascades via NF-κB- and IFN-β-mediated signaling. Both of these pathways are important in containment of viral infections. Since many aspects of the signaling pathways activated by both viral and bacterial PAMPs are shared, the impact of sequential signaling (e.g., viral followed by bacterial) has not been well characterized (4). Rota, rotavirus; CpG, cytosine-phosphate-guanine sites.

during the replication of many viruses. Activation of IRF3 and IRF7 are critical for induction of type 1 interferons (IFN-α/β) that are essential antiviral cytokines (10). These pleiotropic cytokines can affect viral replication by reducing "viral receptor" molecule expression on the host cell surface, inhibition of transcription and translation of viral proteins through IFN-α/β-stimulated genes such as MxA protein, 2'5'-oligoadenylsynthase, double-stranded RNA kinase (PKR), and eukaryotic initiation factor α (eIF-2α), thereby inhibiting viral replication (5,6). In addition to viral proteins, RNA/DNA-mediated activation of the above pathways and DAMPs released from injured tissue including lysed epithelial cell contents can activate innate immune pathways via their respective TLR, RLR, or inflammasomes (10).

IFN-α/β can activate NK cells and macrophages, induce maturation of DCs, and upregulate proteins important in antigen presentation to T cells. Activated CD8 cells differentiate into cytotoxic T cells (CTLs) that contribute to lysis of virus-infected cells and to viral clearance. Macrophages and DCs can bind de novo synthesized intracellular viral peptides via the major histocompatibility complex I (MHC I) and extracellular viral peptides via MHC II. Once activated by viruses, DCs mature as they migrate to draining lymph nodes where they present viral antigens to CD4 T cells via MHC I and CD8 cells via MHC II (5,6). Antigen-activated CD4 cells differentiate to Th1 (proinflammatory), Th2 (anti-inflammatory), regulatory T cells (Tregs), or Th17 (produces the family of IL-17 proteins [IL-17A-D, IL-17E (IL-25), IL-17F], as well as IL-21 and IL-23) depending on the inflammatory milieu (3). Cytotoxic CD8 T cells can eliminate virus by further induction of another essential antiviral cytokine, IFN-γ, by lysis of virus-infected cells via the release of perforin (a membrane pore-forming protein important for cytotoxicity), and by induction of apoptosis through Fas ligand with Fas (CD95) on the virus-infected cells (3,6,11). A result of this immune cascade ideally is eradication of the virus, production of antibodies specific for multiple viral peptides, and creation of memory T cells and B cells important in protection against subsequent infection with the same virus.

IFN-α/β is a critical antiviral cytokine and in the absence of its signaling viral replication is unchecked, and overwhelming viral infection occurs. In chronic viral infection, a lower but sustained IFN-α/β response continues, and despite this, the virus persists. Very cutting edge data have revealed a paradox in IFN-α/β function regarding the role of IFN-α/β in chronic viral infection (12). Lymphocytic choriomeningitis virus (LCMV) typically causes a self-limited mild illness (aseptic meningitis); however, some strains cause chronic viral infection in mice. Blockade of IFN-α/β after the onset of chronic LCMV infection reversed findings seen in chronic viral infection, such as a hyperimmune state, lymphoid tissue destruction resulting in CD4, and IFN-γ-mediated clearance of virus (12–14). Although this is an animal model, its relevance to human disease may be very significant because evidence of IFN-α/β pathway activation in hepatitis C is associated with disease progression and poor response to IFN therapy. Similar findings occur in HIV and latent tuberculosis (12). If these findings hold true in the clinical setting, the use of IFN-α in chronic viral infection may need to be reexamined.

Typically, homeostasis in the lung is maintained by a number of mechanisms, and this homeostasis is important to lung protection as the respiratory tract is continually being challenged by inhaled particulate matter. Immunosuppressive Tregs express the master control transcription factor Forkhead box P3 (FOXP3+) and are critical to this process (10). In RSV and influenza, Tregs are activated and secrete excessive IL-10, thereby dampening Th1 proinflammatory responses. Deletion of these cells in experimental models leads to exaggerated pulmonary inflammation and lung injury (6,10,15). Other cell types that contribute to dampening of the inflammatory

response incited during viral infections include some plasmacytoid DCs, neutrophils by facilitating viral clearance, and airway epithelial cells (AECs) via expression of CD200. CD200 receptors are highly upregulated on airway macrophages during influenza, and ligation leads to suppression of alveolar macrophage response to influenza. Latent TGF-β that is constitutively produced by AECs can be activated by influenza neuraminidase (NA), also resulting in dampening of pulmonary inflammatory responses to viral infection (6,15–17). When the virus is eradicated and the proinflammatory response is resolving, an anti-inflammatory environment evolves to promote healing. Th2 cytokines IL-4 and IL-13 are important mediators and IL-13 is critical to changing the phenotype of macrophages to "alternatively activated macrophages" (M2) that are anti-inflammatory and important to tissue repair (10).

In summary, in addition to the primary proinflammatory responses to respiratory viral infections, negative regulatory mechanisms are activated to limit immune-mediated tissue injury. In simple viral infection, these mechanisms are key to tissue repair; however, they create vulnerability to bacterial infection because of their immune-dampening effects.

IMPACT OF VIRAL INFECTION ON ANTIBACTERIAL DEFENSE

Secondary bacterial infections are associated with several respiratory viral infections. Many reports show that the immune response to respiratory viral infection can compromise antibacterial function contributing to creation of a permissive state for bacterial superinfection (Table 84.2). Many changes have been described that are associated with decreased bacterial killing, and these include phenotype changes of macrophages, diminished recruitment and activation of macrophages and neutrophils, augmented neutrophil apoptosis, and diminished phagocytic function and antigen presentation. In addition, altered differentiation of T cells, suppressed DC, CD4 proliferation, and CD8 T cell cytotoxicity are seen as well. In contrast, there is enhancement of suppressive Tregs (CD4+CD25+) (Table 84.2) (18–21). Th17-derived cytokines are important for neutrophil activation, production of bactericidal proteins, and tissue remodeling that result in antibacterial protection. Unfortunately, IFN-α/β produced during viral infection can suppress differentiation to Th17 cells and diminish the presence of these important antibacterial defenses (3,22). Although these effects may be very important to viral containment and to resolution of the robust antiviral immune response, the cumulative effect of these changes is a permissive environment for bacterial infection, compromised bacterial killing, and skewed antibacterial immune responses.

Respiratory Viruses

Elegant data have demonstrated that during respiratory viral infection there is disruption of protective epithelial barriers as a result of diversion of cell machinery to intracellular viral replication often with direct lysis of infected epithelial cells (18). When protective epithelial barriers are disrupted, mucociliary dysfunction can occur as well as exaggerated bacterial colonization by adherence to exposed basement membrane elements permitting penetration into deeper tissues (see Table 84.1). This concept was demonstrated in experimental human inoculation with influenza followed by the development of detectable airway colonization with Streptococcus pneumoniae 6 days after inoculation with influenza (23). In addition, several studies have demonstrated significantly increased nasopharyngeal colonization with commensal organisms during other respiratory

TABLE 84.2

IMMUNOMODULATORY EFFECTS OF VIRAL INFECTIONS

■ CELL TYPE	■ DECREASED	■ INCREASED
Macrophages	MHC expression	Inflammatory cytokines
	Activation and recruitment	
	Phagocytosis	
	Bacterial killing	
	Antigen presentation	
Neutrophils	Bacterial killing	TLR 2 expression
		Apoptosis
Dendritic cells	Altered IFN-α/β production	Apoptosis
	Altered IFN-γ signaling	
	MHC expression	
	Antigen presentation	
NK cells	Activation	
T cells	CD4 proliferation	Th1 cytokines
	CD8 cytotoxicity	Apoptosis
	Th2 cytokines	
	Treg activation	
	DTH response	
Other	Bone marrow suppression	
	Complement activation	

viral infections (parainfluenza, RSV, and adenovirus) when compared to baseline colonization in the same children (23). Specifically, bacterial adherence is enhanced in areas where epithelium has been denuded. This has been seen in many experimental settings with cell culture and in vivo animal models. In addition, during the 1957 influenza epidemic at autopsy, direct visualization of *Staphylococcus aureus* in the lungs adherent to areas of denuded tracheobronchial epithelium was seen (18,24,25).

Mechanisms of bacterial adherence to infected/disrupted epithelium can be nonspecific as exemplified by bacteria binding to fibrinogen- and fibronectin-binding protein of the exposed extracellular matrix as seen with group A β-hemolytic streptococcus (GAβHS) in influenza A infection models (24). Some mechanisms for increased bacterial adherence during viral infection can be specific for bacterial features. For example, in models of RSV and influenza, enhanced fimbriae- and capsule-mediated binding of nontypable *Haemophilus influenzae*, GAβHS, and *Neisseria meningitidis* to alveolar epithelial cells can occur. These data indicate that viral infection can alter host cell membranes to favor binding to specific bacterial cell wall elements (20,26,27).

Native host cell-surface protein/receptor expression can be upregulated during many viral infections including platelet-activating factor receptor (PAFR), CD14, CD15, and CD18. PAFR, CD14, CD15, complement protein C3, and the polymeric receptor responsible for translocating dimeric IgA or pentameric IgM have been associated with increased adherence of *N. meningitidis* and *Streptococcus pneumoniae* to virus-infected epithelial cells. In some reports, these host proteins facilitate translocation of bacteria across nasopharyngeal mucosa (18).

In addition to altering expression of native host cell proteins/receptors, viral infection can result in the host cell expression of viral glycoproteins. The best-characterized glycoproteins are HA and NA that are expressed on the host cell surface during influenza infections. HA binds to terminal sialic acid residues of host cell surface permitting internalization of virus and fusion of viral envelope with cell membrane leading to penetration into host cells. NA is critical for replication of influenza and parainfluenza because it cleaves sialic acid

residues from host glycoproteins during viral budding from infected cells facilitating release of newly synthesized virus (25,28–32). These sialic acid residues on host proteins provide protection against bacterial adherence and once cleaved by NA, bacteria can adhere and invade. Different strains of influenza possess NA of varying potency, and the NA activity is thought to be a key determinant of the virulence of a given strain and therefore a determinant of the severity of an epidemic. Anti-HA antibodies prevented bacterial superinfection in influenza experimental animal models, and the presumed mechanism was prevention of virus binding to host cells to initiate replication. In an influenza–pneumococcal pneumonia, mouse model increased lethality compared to single infection, and NA inhibitors (NIs) were shown to be protective. In this model, oseltamivir prevented secondary bacterial infection by preventing NA-mediated desialylation of the airway epithelium, thereby decreasing bacterial adherence with a significant reduction in mortality (32–34). These data support an important role for these virus-induced glycoproteins in the susceptibility to bacterial superinfection in the setting of influenza that is highly dependent on HA and NA for successful infection.

Because sialic acid is a binding site for influenza and parainfluenza, another approach is being studied. That approach involves intended desialylation of airway epithelium to prevent viral binding, entry, and replication within the epithelial cell. The drug is called DAS 181, and it consists of a fusion molecule containing a bacterial sialidase conjugated with a part of the amphiregulin molecule that in its native state typically binds to the epidermal growth factor receptor on respiratory epithelium. In DAS 181, the part of amphiregulin that is employed has high affinity for glycosaminoglycans present on the respiratory epithelium and anchors the sialidase in the epithelium (31). It is now in phase II development for treatment of influenza. In contrast to data presented above regarding NIs, studies using this molecule experimentally showed no increase in bacterial adherence and protection from secondary pneumonia (35,36). Clearly these data are discrepant. One hypothesis for the difference in bacterial adherence and infection in these two settings is that during influenza there is tissue damage with other changes in the airway, including exposed basement membrane in addition to desialylation. DAS 181 only causes desialylation without tissue injury (31,36). This drug is also being investigated for use in parainfluenza infection because it too uses sialic acid as a binding receptor for replication (37).

Other viral glycoproteins implicated in susceptibility to bacterial superinfection include glycoproteins F and G that are inserted into the host cell membrane during RSV infection. Expression of glycoprotein G was shown to be involved in exaggerated binding of *N. meningitidis* to RSV-infected epithelial cells experimentally (38–40). In addition, RSV virions bind pneumococci to form complexes that exhibited enhanced adherence to uninfected epithelial cell layers. In this way, RSV directly acted as a coupling agent between bacteria and host cells. In an in vivo model, sequential infection with RSV followed by pneumococcus yielded significantly higher bacteremia compared to pneumococcal infection alone suggesting that by the mechanisms above, RSV may facilitate the penetration of bacteria from the mucosa to the bloodstream (38–40). **Table 84.1** lists many factors induced during viral infection that promote bacterial adherence and facilitate invasion.

Other Viruses

The immunomodulatory effects of viral infection have been elucidated using several viral infection models, including RSV, influenza, hepatitis B, CMV, Epstein–Barr virus (EBV), HIV, and measles virus (MV). Some induced immune defects are shared, and some are unique to specific virus infections. In addition, the duration of these defects is variable, and though typically transient, some are long lasting as with uncontrolled/untreated HIV infection. In some cases, the virus can be cleared as in MV infection; however, in others, many mechanisms of viral-induced immune suppression are thought to contribute to immune evasion and in some, the ability to establish latency rather than being eradicated.

MV infection suppresses many aspects of the immune response leading to profound vulnerability of the host to secondary infections. This immune modulation begins early during viral replication and can persist for many weeks after resolution of the acute MV infection and presence of the virus (41). The clinical importance of this is demonstrated by the frequency of secondary infections occurring after MV infection. The mechanisms reported include depressed delayed-type hypersensitivity (DTH) reactions, poor antigen presentation and poor lymphocyte proliferative response to mitogens, accelerated apoptosis of DCs and lymphocytes, bone marrow suppression, altered IFN-α/β production and signaling, and diminished DC IL-12p70 production with a long-lasting shift toward a Th2 response with sustained elevated levels of IL-4 (42,43). As with other viral infection, triggers for these effects include expression of MV proteins, including HA, fusion proteins H and F, MV nucleoprotein, and the nonstructural proteins C and V. MV can also initiate signaling through host cell receptors, such as CD46 and CD150 both of which are important in regulating complement activation, T cell and macrophage activation, as well as sustaining the Th2 cytokine profile (42). The consequence of these factors is prolonged immunosuppression from a transient viral infection resulting in a high frequency of secondary infections.

Human CMV is an important pathogen and is endemic throughout the world. In addition to its direct pathology, it is a virus capable of modulating the immune response permitting its persistence in a latent state. It is likely that strategies important to its ability to evade the immune system and establish latency are also responsible for the generalized state of immune suppression seen during and transiently after acute CMV infection (44,45). Multiple studies have described

numerous alterations in host immune function, including loss of DTH response to recall antigens, reduced lymphoproliferative responses, and NK cell activity, and suppressed bone marrow myelopoiesis compared to noninfected immunosuppressed individuals (44–46). CMV can infect DCs directly and in doing so modulate the function of this critical aspect of host defense contributing to viral persistence and subsequent immunosuppression. Diminished MHC expression on CMV-infected DCs reduces antigen presentation and T cell proliferation and increases DC-mediated apoptosis of activated T cells experimentally (45,47).

CLINICAL CONSEQUENCES OF VIRAL AND BACTERIAL COINFECTION

Influenza

The association between viral infection and bacterial infection has been repeatedly described for respiratory viruses, such as influenza, RSV, human metapneumovirus, and parainfluenza and secondary bacterial pneumonia. In many reports, antecedent and/or concurrent viral and bacterial infection has been strongly associated with severe morbidity and high mortality (38). Clinically, inflammatory cytokine production in influenza-infected children is altered, and exaggerated immune dysfunction is associated with coinfection and poor outcome (48). Very compelling data to support this association derive from the association of bacterial infection (*Streptococcus pneumoniae* and *Staphylococcus aureus* predominantly) and lethality during influenza pandemics prior to H1N1 in 2009 (49). During the recent H1N1 pandemic, the incidence of bacterial coinfection varied widely; however, in a recent case control examination of 265 children in the New Zealand with confirmed H1N1, ~26% had secondary bacterial infection (50), and in a review of multiple studies the incidence varied between 14% and 39% (51). In a large cohort of H1N1-infected critically ill children in the United States, 33% had a clinical diagnosis of pneumonia or other evidence of bacterial infection within 72 hours of presentation (52,53). Of those infections, *Streptococcus pneumoniae* was the most common, but early methicillin-resistant *Staphylococcus aureus* infection was a risk factor for mortality in children with comorbidities as well as previously healthy children (52,53). From the data prior to H1N1 in 2009, several groups reported increasing incidence of coinfection with higher ICU admissions, ARDS, and mortality in this group compared with influenza alone (52,54,55).

During the 2009 H1N1 pandemic, many studies confirmed this in both adults and children showing that not only was bacterial coinfection associated with more severe disease but was also present in ~30% of fatalities (56,57). Studies comparing pediatric fatalities during the 2009 H1N1 pandemic data to seasonal influenza from other years show that H1N1 did not reveal a higher rate of bacterial coinfection (28% H1N1 vs. 38% seasonal) (58).

Many other studies support this association also demonstrating a 3%–45% incidence of coincident viral and bacterial pneumonia (59,60). In fact, some authors speculate that the seasonal fluctuation of invasive pneumococcal disease peaking in the winter months may be related to winter virus exposure, including influenza and RSV (61). In addition, a possible role for antecedent viral infections including influenza in severe community-acquired methicillin-resistant *Staphylococcus aureus* pneumonia is emerging (62). It has also been noted that the incidence of severe GAβHS also occurs coincident with influenza epidemics (27).

Respiratory Syncytial Virus

Studies have shown a low incidence overall of bacterial coinfection in large cohorts of RSV-infected infants and children. In contrast, studies examining mechanically ventilated infants with severe RSV revealed a high incidence (38%–44%) of bacterial coinfection. The incidence of coinfection may even be higher but not identifiable owing to significant numbers of infants in these studies, who were pretreated with antibiotics or in whom tracheal aspirates were not sent. In these reports, ventilator days were higher in the coinfected group compared with those with RSV alone (63,64). Although the incidence of respiratory viral and bacterial coinfection in infants admitted to the ICU was relatively common (compared to those not requiring ICU care), very few cases of sepsis/septic shock, bacteremia, or meningitis were seen in infants with severe RSV (63,64). Another study showed that 10% (42 of 464) of the infants hospitalized with RSV were preterm infants. There was a higher incidence of bacterial coinfection in preterm infants (average age 2 months) compared to term infants admitted to the ICU (9% vs. 3%), and the length of stay was longer in the coinfected preterm infants (65). Coinfection of RSV with other viral pathogens occurs especially with RV and metapneumovirus. In some cases, disease severity was higher in viral-to-viral coinfection (66,67).

Cytomegalovirus

Typically in immunocompetent people, CMV causes asymptomatic or very mild illness; in some it causes a mononucleosis-like syndrome, whereas in immunosuppressed individuals it can cause severe/fatal disease, involving liver, lung, GI tract, and CNS. Overall, CMV occurs in childhood with 30%–40% incidence within the first year of life increasing thereafter to upwards of 60%–70% in adults (68). CMV infection results in a dormant latent infection status after the acute phase and typically remains in this state. Canonically, immunosuppressed individuals are at significant risk for primary infection (if seronegative), and reactivation is commonly seen (69). With active CMV disease, there is increased risk for secondary infections, malignancies such as posttransplant lymphoproliferative disease, and cardiovascular disease, and overall in this setting active CMV disease is associated with increased mortality. A causal relationship between active CMV and these complications is inferred by reductions in such complications in similar populations that received antiviral prophylaxis (70,71).

Over the last decade, a strong association between critical illness in previously immunocompetent patients and CMV reactivation has been revealed (46,72–75). One such study showed that 33% of critically ill patients developed detectable CMV (multiple methods) by an average of 12 days in the ICU. Over time, not only did CMV become detectable in more patients but the viral load also increased. In this cohort, CMV reactivation was independently associated with death or continued hospitalization at 30 days (75). In a more recent study, in adults with severe sepsis and latent CMV infection, reactivation of CMV occurred in 40%. Although CMV reactivation did not reach statistical significance for mortality, it was associated with increased ICU and hospital length-of-stay as well as increased days of mechanical ventilation suggesting that active CMV infection may complicate recovery from severe sepsis (73). In addition to these important findings, there is an increased incidence of nosocomial infection in the presence of reactivated CMV (46,76). An experimental model suggested that reactivation of this virus caused an increase in circulating inflammatory cytokines and chemokines as well as enhanced pulmonary fibrosis coincident with reactivation 2 weeks after

the onset of polymicrobial sepsis. Ganciclovir prevented these changes. Although this is an animal model, it does suggest that reactivation of CMV could contribute to the overall inflammatory state as well as lung dysfunction (77). This relationship has not yet been studied in children but may be warranted as mounting data demonstrate a potentially significant role for CMV reactivation in adults.

Other Viruses

Numerous reports have demonstrated serious bacterial superinfection as a complication of varicella. Case reports, case series, and epidemiologic studies cite many types of bacterial complications, including necrotizing fasciitis, toxic shock syndrome, septic shock, bacteremia, epiglottitis, spinal epidural abscess, pyogenic arthritis, osteomyelitis, meningitis, orbital cellulitis, and subdural empyema. The primary bacterial culprits are GAβHS and *Staphylococcus aureus* (78–80). In a recent report of severe varicella complications, 46% of 188 patients had secondary bacterial infection (81).

Measles continues to contribute significantly to childhood morbidity and mortality globally, and its complications have been implicated in >1 million deaths annually (32,43). Profound immunosuppression during MV infection has been long appreciated and is a significant cause of measles-related mortality (42,82). This immunosuppression is seen during, and for several weeks following, MV infection, and during this time patients are highly vulnerable to bacterial, other viral infections, parasitic, and other opportunistic pathogens. In some studies, most MV-related deaths are due to pneumonia and/or diarrhea caused by other pathogens during the course of measles.

The above data support the concept that common viral infections likely play an important causal role and may contribute to the severity of serious bacterial illness. The recent H1N1 pandemic demonstrated this relationship in critically ill individuals. The mechanisms for this have not been completely elucidated; however, many potential mechanisms have been demonstrated experimentally. Knowledge of the immune response to viral infections is important in understanding how aspects of viral infection and the host antiviral response impact on the quality of antibacterial defenses. In this regard, it is important to be vigilant for the presence of coinfection in the critically ill with viral infections.

VIRAL INFECTIONS AND ASTHMATIC EXACERBATIONS

Viral infections especially RSV and RV early in life are associated with the development of asthma over time. Respiratory viral infections can precipitate up to 60%–85% of acute asthma exacerbations in children. This association has become significantly stronger since the use of polymerase chain reaction (PCR) virus detection has become more common and the ability to detect RV and metapneumovirus has been developed (83). Multiple respiratory viruses have been implicated in asthma exacerbations; however, in pediatrics, RSV and RV are the most common. One prospective long-term study looked at a cohort of 259 high-risk children (with parental asthma) from birth to 6 years of age and identified viral illness in 90% of wheezing illnesses (84). RV, specifically, has been identified as a major destabilizer of asthma, and in some reports it is found in up to 50%–70% of all asthma exacerbations (85–87).

Experimental RV infections in asthmatic human volunteers have been extensively studied to examine its role in asthma exacerbation. Although RV infection has not typically been identified in the lower airways, this may not be correct in asthmatics. Increased severity of RV infection, a longer duration of airway symptoms, and a greater decline in lung function were reported in asthmatics compared to controls. These data demonstrate that at least in the asthmatic, RV can extend beyond the upper respiratory tract and persist longer (83,88).

A number of findings show that the antiviral response is weakened in asthmatics compared to nonasthmatic controls even when studies have controlled for the use of inhaled corticosteroids and included mild asthmatics (no use of inhaled corticosteroids) (86,88,89). Asthmatics are more susceptible to RV infections, and viral replication in bronchial epithelial cells (BECs) obtained from asthmatics is increased. Greater than 40% of a cohort of 50 asthmatic children had RNA evidence of RV persisting up to 6 weeks after viral infection, which was much longer in stable asthmatics. Asthma exacerbations were more severe in the children with persistence of viral RNA suggesting that the severity of asthma exacerbations may be linked to prolonged RV infection (90).

BECs but not peripheral blood mononuclear cells (PBMCs) from asthmatics have defective production of IFN-β and IFN-λ (type III interferons) during RV infection, indicating that an important antiviral and immunomodulating cytokine is defective in the respiratory compartment when it is needed most (87). IFN-β and -λ are important inducers of apoptosis of RV-infected cells. In another study, cultured BECs from asthmatics infected with RV showed low IFN-β and -λ levels, delayed apoptosis

of infected BECs, and higher viral titers. After treatment with exogenous IFN-β, these findings reversed providing further evidence for an aberrant type I and III interferon response in asthmatics with RV infection (88). Interestingly, in BECs from stable asthmatics the production of IFN-α/β and -λ was comparable to BECs from nonasthmatics indicating that inherently, the ability to produce these interferons is intact but during viral infection it is altered (91). The induction of other proinflammatory cytokines was similar in asthmatic versus healthy BECs, suggesting that all antiviral pathways were not deficient. Other studies have demonstrated a reduced IFN-γ response to RV in PBMCs from asthmatics, suggesting another defect in a critical antiviral mediator (92). It has been suggested that in the presence of an impaired interferon response, a more vigorous inflammatory response (other mediators) may be necessary for virus eradication and in this way may contribute to asthma exacerbation (88).

The asthmatic airway is characterized by the presence of eosinophils and T cells expressing Th2 cytokines, including IL-4, IL-5, and IL-13. It is hypothesized that this environment may also contribute to ineffective antiviral responses. **Figure 84.3** depicts this hypothesis (89). Recently, a therapeutic trial using IFN-β in asthma has been done, and results are pending (93). It will be interesting to see if exogenous IFN-β can provide better control of viral infection in the asthmatic and perhaps diminish the severity of asthma exacerbations.

A Normal host

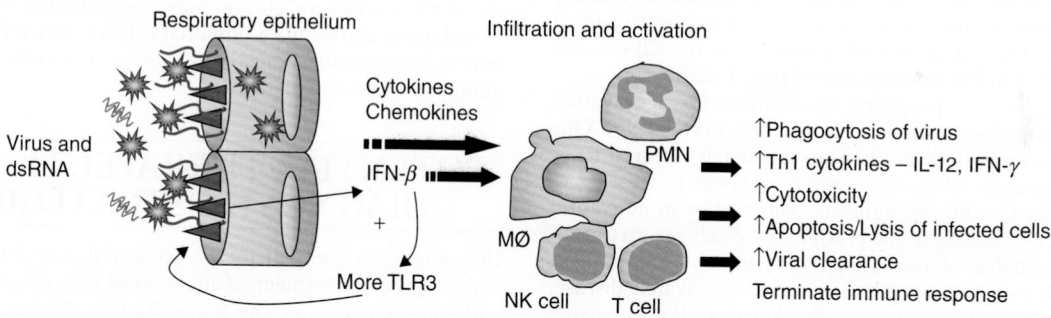

B Asthmatic host

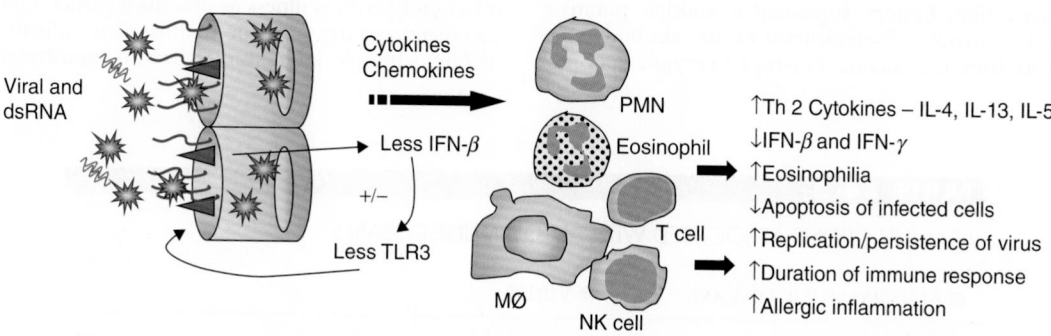

FIGURE 84.3. The antiviral immune response in asthma. Viruses infect respiratory epithelium and dsRNA (released during replication of most viruses) signals through TLR 3, which is constitutively expressed on epithelial cells. Both lead to production of a multitude of cytokines and chemokines, including IFN-β by epithelial cells. IFN-β upregulates TLR 3 leading to further induction of IFN-β. IFN-β induces IFN-α, both of which are pleiotropic cytokines activating a multitude of inflammatory cells, kinases, and regulatory proteins critical for viral containment. **A:** Under normal circumstances, activation and infiltration of inflammatory cells leads to a proinflammatory response including Th1 cytokines that are also important for viral clearance. Effective killing/apoptosis of infected cells occurs promoting viral clearance and resolution of inflammation. **B:** Respiratory epithelial cells from asthmatics produce less IFN-β and TLR 3. Inflammatory cell stimulation is different with infiltration of eosinophils, a Th2 response with less IFN-γ, longer survival of infected cells, and delayed viral clearance (104).

6

VIRAL INFECTIONS AND AUTOIMMUNE DISEASE EXACERBATIONS

Viral infection has been thought to be among the triggers for exacerbation of autoimmune disease as well as a potential etiology and has been extensively investigated. The viruses most closely associated with autoimmune phenomenon include CMV, HSV, EBV, human herpesvirus (HHV) 6 and 7, hepatitis C, parvovirus B19, and MV (68,94). **Table 84.3** lists the viruses implicated in autoimmune diseases. The association has been identified by detection of viral DNA by PCR, detection of virus-specific proteins in serum or affected tissues (such as synovium, skin, neurons, and bowel mucosa), or positive IgM serology, indicating very recent infection at the time of exacerbation or presentation of autoimmune disease (68,95). Many of these viruses can remain in the host in a latent fashion and can become activated during stress or systemic inflammation by proinflammatory cytokines or during immunosuppressed states. It is unclear whether reactivation of these viruses from their latent state is a product of the inflammatory response activated during an autoimmune exacerbation or if viral reactivation is provocative for autoimmune exacerbations. Most of the existing evidence is correlative rather than causal in that evidence of these viruses can be found during exacerbations or at the onset of the diseases (96,97). Another association for which there is considerable data is between coxsackie B4 (CB4) and type 1 diabetes mellitus. This association may be causal because more newly diagnosed type 1 diabetics have increased anti-CB4 antibodies and enteroviral RNA in PBMCs compared to controls (98). In addition, "diabetogenic strains" of CB4 have been identified from new onset diabetics that are capable of transferring pancreatic β cell destruction to animal models (98). These data present a strong case for CB4 as one etiologic factor in the development of type 1 diabetes.

There are several proposed mechanisms for aggravation of autoimmune diseases by the above viruses (96,97,99). One frequently hypothesized mechanism is what is referred to as molecular mimicry where the immune response to viral infection cross-reacts with self-antigens. This results in activation of T and B cells leading to the production of self-reactive autoantibodies capable of mediating tissue injury. Alternatively, viruses such as CMV, during primary or reactivated disease, can activate antigen-presenting cells (APCs) and/or virus-specific T cells resulting in activation of preexisting autoreactive T cells in susceptible individuals. This phenomenon is called bystander activation. Epitope spreading is another putative mechanism that involves diversification of autoantibody epitope specificity from the dominant epitope to cryptic epitopes that may be revealed during virus-mediated tissue injury. Exposure of cryptic epitopes can result in anti-self-immune responses to proteins that prior to damage are not considered foreign (68,96,99).

A key antiviral cytokine produced during the immune response to most viruses is IFN-α. There is a great deal of data implicating IFN-α in the development of autoimmune diseases, such as systemic lupus erythematosus (SLE), thyroid disease, and type 1 diabetes. SLE patients have high circulating IFN-α levels and evidence of activation of IFN-α-regulated genes. In addition, there are many reports of patients receiving therapeutic IFN-α for diseases, such as hepatitis C, who develop autoimmune phenomenon, such as SLE, type 1 diabetes, psoriasis, inflammatory arthritis, or Sjögren syndrome and autoimmune thyroid diseases (100,101). IFN-α is known to potentiate immune responses through differentiation of monocytes to macrophages, augmented capacity for antigen presentation, and increased T cell stimulation and survival. These effects may promote survival of autoreactive T cells and B cells leading to autoantibody-mediated tissue damage. Since viral infections also potently induce IFN-α, it is possible that the presence of IFN-α (administered exogenously or produced endogenously) is responsible for the association of viral infections with autoimmune exacerbations (100).

There are implications to critical illness caused by autoimmune disease if viral infection can precipitate exacerbations. Generally, the therapy for autoimmune exacerbations includes pulse steroids and adjustment of other anti-inflammatory regimens. Viral infections, either primary or reactivated, are known to be significant pathogens in the context of immunosuppressed states (hematopoietic stem cell and solid organ transplants). As with these states, it may be prudent to evaluate the host fully for new or reactivated viral infection by serum PCR when an autoimmune exacerbation occurs. This would guide and define a potential role for antiviral treatment during autoimmune exacerbations requiring augmentation of immunosuppressive regimens.

POTENTIAL THERAPEUTIC AND DIAGNOSTIC STRATEGIES

Unfortunately, the paucity of successful antiviral therapies makes specific treatment of many viral infections impossible with the exception of the herpes family viruses. Data have emerged over the last several years to support the use of some indirect antivirals that may impact on the contribution of viral infection to critical illness as described earlier. One important therapeutic strategy for the treatment of influenza is the use of NIs. Multiple large studies have demonstrated reduction

---

TABLE 84.3

VIRAL INFECTIONS ASSOCIATED WITH AUTOIMMUNE DISEASES

■ AUTOIMMUNE DISEASE	■ VIRUS
Type 1 diabetes mellitus	Coxsackie B4, enteroviruses, rotavirus
Multiple sclerosis	Measles, EBV, HHV-6
Rheumatoid arthritis	CMV, parvovirus B19
Sjögren syndrome	EBV, CMV, HHV-6, hepatitis C
Systemic lupus erythematosus	CMV, EBV, hepatitis C, parvovirus B19
Inflammatory bowel disease	CMV, EBV, measles

Adapted from Osawa R, Singh N. Cytomegalovirus infection in critically ill patients: A systematic review [Review]. *Crit Care* 2009;13(3):R68.

in length of illness by 1–4 days if a NI is begun within the first several hours of influenza symptoms. In addition, prophylactic use has also been effective for high-risk populations and recently exposed individuals. What has also become clear from these studies is that NI treatment has reduced the incidence of otitis media by 44%, lower respiratory tract complications requiring antibiotics by 55%, and hospitalizations for any cause by 59% (102). These clinical data confirm mouse data showing that treatment with a NI improved survival in a model of secondary pneumococcal pneumonia created 7 days after influenza infection. Improvement was seen even when the NI was administered as late as 5 days after the onset of influenza. NI treatment did not reduce viral titers but did reduce bacterial adherence. These data suggest that inhibition of NA decreases NA-mediated changes in respiratory epithelium permissive for bacterial colonization and establishment of pneumonia (30,33). **Figure 84.4** depicts a schematic diagram of hypothetical impact of NI on bacterial adherence/infection. These data support the use of NI agents not only to reduce the morbidity from influenza but also to reduce secondary bacterial infection in high-risk children. Since these drugs are not FDA approved for use in infants <1 year, further work must be done to establish the safety and efficacy in that age group. Conversely, DAS 181, an inhaled conjugated sialidase molecule, is also in trials for influenza (31). Experimental data do not show enhanced bacterial adherence or infection as the data for NA inhibitions would predict.

Given current data demonstrating multifaceted immune compromise during viral infection, constant vigilance for the presence of coinfection at the time of presentation or superinfection later during the viral illness is prudent. Lower respiratory bacterial coinfection is common in influenza, RSV, and parainfluenza infections in immunocompetent children at presentation (103). No data exist describing the incidence of superinfection developing during or after admission to the ICU for critical illness or in high-risk infants and children related to these viruses. One could surmise that the incidence of either coinfection or superinfection developing later in a viral course in high-risk children, critically ill presentations, or stalled clinical improvement situations might be even higher than that in immunocompetent children. Perhaps it is prudent to consider that viral infection in such settings may not be the unifying and sole diagnosis and that further workup may be warranted at presentation and if needed later during the course of the viral infection. Certainly this question deserves further study in children to effectively answer this question and appropriately guide care in the most vulnerable infants and children.

Many data show increased incidence of adverse bronchospastic complications of respiratory viral infections in asthmatics (40,86,90,92,104). Given the interesting data showing innate immune defects in asthmatics, strategies to augment innate and acquired immune function need to be explored as well to alter the exaggerated immune vulnerability to complicated viral infection (104). Results from a study using IFN-β in asthma exacerbations during viral infections are pending (93).

Recent data indicate that human herpesvirus of many types (CMV, EBV, HSV, HHV) reactivation can occur with fairly high prevalence in critically ill patients who have been traditionally

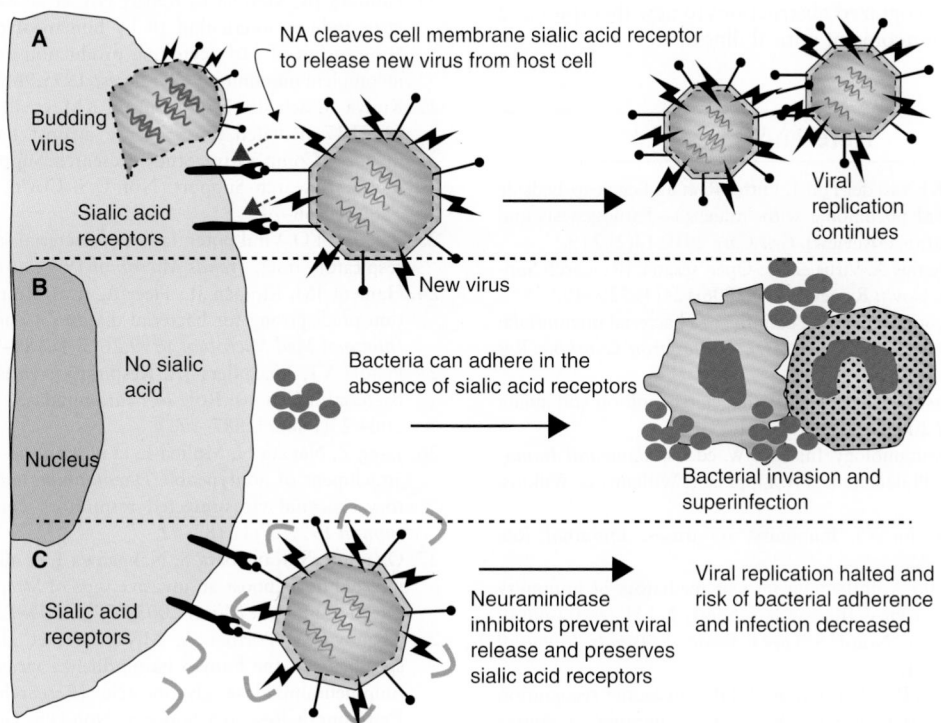

FIGURE 84.4. Mechanism of action of neuraminidase inhibitors. **A:** New virus is released from the cell surface by neuraminidase cleavage of hemagglutinin bound to sialic acid cell receptors. New virus continues to replicate leading to destruction of infected tissue clinical symptomatology. **B:** Bacteria such as pneumococcus can adhere to cell surfaces in the absence of sialic acid residues leading to bacterial superinfection. **C:** Neuraminidase inhibitors block the release of new viruses limiting viral replication and spread to other cells. Also by limiting neuraminidase activity, protective sialic acid residues are preserved decreasing bacterial adherence and invasion (102). Neuraminidase (✗); hemagglutinin (↑); neuraminidase inhibitor (⌒); neuraminidase activity (= =▶).

considered "immunocompetent" as well as the immunosuppressed populations. Life-threatening complications from reactivation of some of these viruses are well documented in the immunosuppressed, and therefore, aggressive monitoring, prophylaxis, and/or treatment with ganciclovir, high titer anti-CMV IgG, or acyclovir for HSV are commonly used at times of maximal immunosuppression. The contribution of reactivation of various herpes family viruses in the critically ill has not been fully defined; however, with new data showing an association with poor outcomes from severe sepsis, it is possible that there may be a role for anti-CMV therapy in this setting and certainly it warrants further investigation.

CONCLUSIONS AND FUTURE DIRECTIONS

Viral infection is a constant nemesis in children. Data have emerged over the last 10 years to support the concept that viral infections may have a more pronounced and far-reaching effect on the host than previously understood. The data presented here are meant to introduce the consequences of some common viral infections on host immunity, including viral infections not previously thought to contribute to host defense alteration, such as RV and influenza. Better mechanistic understanding of the impact of viral infection and the immune response may lead to better strategies for prophylaxis against viral infection and prevention of superinfection. In addition, better understanding of the contribution of viral infection to exacerbations of asthma and autoimmune diseases may provide insight into critical immune interactions and pathways to target in order to maintain the diseases described above in a stable uncomplicated state. In the case of viral reactivation in critical illness, prevention and/or treatment of these pathogens may eliminate unrecognized obstructions to new therapies and may improve the outcome of critical illness.

References

1. van der Sluijs KF, van der Poll T, Lutter R, et al. Bench-to-bedside review: Bacterial pneumonia with influenza—Pathogenesis and clinical implications [Review]. *Crit Care* 2010;14(2):219.
2. Marsh M, Helenius A. Virus entry: Open sesame [Research Support, Non-U.S. Gov't; Review]. *Cell* 2006;124(4):729–40.
3. Ballinger MN, Standiford TJ. Postinfluenza bacterial pneumonia: Host defenses gone awry [Review]. *J Interferon Cytokine Res* 2010;30(9):643–52.
4. Akira S, Uematsu S, Takeuchi O. Pathogen recognition and innate immunity. *Cell* 2006;124(4):783–801.
5. Ertl H. Viral immunology. In: Paul W, ed. *Fundamental Immunology*. 5th ed. Philadelphia, PA: Lippincott Williams & Wilkins, 2003:120–28.
6. Braciale TJ, Hahn YS. Immunity to viruses. *Immunol Rev* 2013;255(1):5–12.
7. Pang IK, Iwasaki A. Inflammasomes as mediators of immunity against influenza virus [Research Support, N.I.H., Extramural; Research Support, Non-U.S. Gov't; Review]. *Trends Immunol* 2011;32(1):34–41.
8. Ichinohe T, Lee HK, Ogura Y, et al. Inflammasome recognition of influenza virus is essential for adaptive immune responses [Research Support, N.I.H., Extramural; Research Support, Non-U.S. Gov't]. *J Exp Med* 2009;206(1):79–87.
9. Lupfer C, Kanneganti TD. The expanding role of NLRs in antiviral immunity. *Immunol Rev* 2013;255(1):13–24.
10. Yoo JK, Kim TS, Hufford MM, et al. Viral infection of the lung: Host response and sequelae. *J Allergy Clin Immunol* 2013;132(6):1263–76.
11. van de Sandt CE, Kreijtz JH, Rimmelzwaan GF. Evasion of influenza A viruses from innate and adaptive immune responses [Review]. *Viruses* 2012;4(9):1438–76.
12. Odorizzi PM, Wherry EJ. Immunology: An interferon paradox [Comment]. *Science* 2013;340(6129):155–6.
13. Wilson EB, Yamada DH, Elsaesser H, et al. Blockade of chronic type I interferon signaling to control persistent LCMV infection [Research Support, N.I.H., Extramural]. *Science* 2013; 340(6129):202–7.
14. Mashayekhi A, Shields CL, Shields JA. Transient increased exudation after photodynamic therapy of intraocular tumors. *Middle East Afr J Ophthalmol* 2013;20(1):83–6.
15. Snelgrove RJ, Goulding J, Didierlaurent AM, et al. A critical function for CD200 in lung immune homeostasis and the severity of influenza infection. *Nat Immunol* 2008;9(9):1074–83.
16. Carlson CM, Turpin EA, Moser LA, et al. Transforming growth factor-beta: Activation by neuraminidase and role in highly pathogenic H5N1 influenza pathogenesis [Research Support, N.I.H., Extramural; Research Support, Non-U.S. Gov't]. *PLoS Pathog* 2010;6(10):e1001136.
17. Schultz-Cherry S, Hinshaw VS. Influenza virus neuraminidase activates latent transforming growth factor beta [Research Support, Non-U.S. Gov't; Research Support, U.S. Gov't, P.H.S.]. *J Virol* 1996;70(12):8624–9.
18. Hussell T, Williams A. Menage a trois of bacterial and viral pulmonary pathogens delivers coup de grace to the lung. *Clin Exp Immunol* 2004;137(1):8–11.
19. Mobbs KJ, Smyth RL, O'Hea U, et al. Cytokines in severe respiratory syncytial virus bronchiolitis. *Pediatr Pulmonol* 2002;33(6):449–52.
20. Okamoto S, Kawabata S, Terao Y, et al. The *Streptococcus* pyogenes capsule is required for adhesion of bacteria to virus-infected alveolar epithelial cells and lethal bacterial-viral superinfection. *Infect Immun* 2004;72(10):6068–75.
21. Panuska JR, Merolla R, Rebert NA, et al. Respiratory syncytial virus induces interleukin-10 by human alveolar macrophages. Suppression of early cytokine production and implications for incomplete immunity. *J Clin Invest* 1995;96(5):2445–53.
22. Kudva A, Scheller EV, Robinson KM, et al. Influenza A inhibits Th17-mediated host defense against bacterial pneumonia in mice [Comparative Study Research Support, N.I.H., Extramural; Research Support, Non-U.S. Gov't]. *J Immunol* 2011; 186(3):1666–74.
23. Bakaletz LO. Viral potentiation of bacterial superinfection of the respiratory tract. *Trends Microbiol* 1995;3(3):110–4.
24. Hament JM, Kimpen JL, Fleer A, et al. Respiratory viral infection predisposing for bacterial disease: A concise review. *FEMS Immunol Med Microbiol* 1999;26(3–4):189–95.
25. Peltola VT, McCullers JA. Respiratory viruses predisposing to bacterial infections: Role of neuraminidase. *Pediatr Infect Dis J* 2004;23(1 suppl):S87–97.
26. Jiang Z, Nagata N, Molina E, et al. Fimbria-mediated enhanced attachment of nontypeable *Haemophilus influenzae* to respiratory syncytial virus-infected respiratory epithelial cells. *Infect Immun* 1999;67(1):187–92.
27. Okamoto S, Kawabata S, Nakagawa I, et al. Influenza A virus-infected hosts boost an invasive type of *Streptococcus* pyogenes infection in mice. *J Virol* 2003;77(7):4104–12.
28. Alymova IV, Portner A, Mishin VP, et al. Receptor-binding specificity of the human parainfluenza virus type 1 hemagglutinin-neuraminidase glycoprotein [Research Support, N.I.H., Extramural; Research Support, Non-U.S. Gov't]. *Glycobiology* 2012;22(2):174–80.
29. Gubareva LV, Kaiser L, Hayden FG. Influenza virus neuraminidase inhibitors. *Lancet* 2000;355(9206):827–35.
30. McCullers JA. Insights into the interaction between influenza virus and pneumococcus. *Clin Microbiol Rev* 2006;19(3):571–82.
31. Nicholls JM, Moss RB, Haslam SM. The use of sialidase therapy for respiratory viral infections. *Antiviral Res* 2013;98(3):401–9.

32. Peltola VT, Murti KG, McCullers JA. Influenza virus neuraminidase contributes to secondary bacterial pneumonia [Research Support, N.I.H., Extramural; Research Support, Non-U.S. Gov't; Research Support, U.S. Gov't, P.H.S.]. *J Infect Dis* 2005;192(2):249–57.

33. McCullers JA, Bartmess KC. Role of neuraminidase in lethal synergism between influenza virus and *Streptococcus pneumoniae* [Comparative Study; Research Support, Non-U.S. Gov't; Research Support, U.S. Gov't, P.H.S.]. *J Infect Dis* 2003;187(6):1000–9.

34. McCullers JA. Effect of antiviral treatment on the outcome of secondary bacterial pneumonia after influenza [Research Support, Non-U.S. Gov't; Research Support, U.S. Gov't, P.H.S.]. *J Infect Dis* 2004;190(3):519–26.

35. Hedlund M, Aschenbrenner LM, Jensen K, et al. Sialidase-based anti-influenza virus therapy protects against secondary pneumococcal infection [Research Support, N.I.H., Extramural]. *J Infect Dis* 2010;201(7):1007–15.

36. Nicholls JM, Aschenbrenner LM, Paulson JC, et al. Comment on: Concerns of using sialidase fusion protein as an experimental drug to combat seasonal and pandemic influenza [Comment Letter]. *J Antimicrob Chemother* 2008;62(2):426–8; author reply 8–9.

37. Moscona A, Porotto M, Palmer S, et al. A recombinant sialidase fusion protein effectively inhibits human parainfluenza viral infection in vitro and in vivo [Research Support, N.I.H., Extramural; Research Support, Non-U.S. Gov't]. *J Infect Dis* 2010;202(2):234–41.

38. Borchers AT, Chang C, Gershwin ME, et al. Respiratory syncytial virus—A comprehensive review. *Clin Rev Allergy Immunol* 2013;45(3):331–79.

39. Hament JM, Aerts PC, Fleer A, et al. Direct binding of respiratory syncytial virus to pneumococci: A phenomenon that enhances both pneumococcal adherence to human epithelial cells and pneumococcal invasiveness in a murine model. *Pediatr Res* 2005;58(6):1198–203.

40. Lotz MT, Peebles RS Jr. Mechanisms of respiratory syncytial virus modulation of airway immune responses [Research Support, N.I.H., Extramural; Research Support, U.S. Gov't, Non-P.H.S.; Review]. *Curr Allergy Asthma Rep* 2012;12(5):380–7.

41. Naniche D, Oldstone MB. Generalized immunosuppression: How viruses undermine the immune response. *Cell Mol Life Sci* 2000;57(10):1399–407.

42. Griffin DE. Measles virus-induced suppression of immune responses [Research Support, N.I.H., Extramural; Review]. *Immunol Rev* 2010;236:176–89.

43. Moss WJ, Griffin DE. Measles [Research Support, N.I.H., Extramural; Research Support, Non-U.S. Gov't; Review]. *Lancet* 2012;379(9811):153–64.

44. Frascaroli G, Varani S, Mastroianni A, et al. Dendritic cell function in cytomegalovirus-infected patients with mononucleosis. *J Leukoc Biol* 2006;79(5):932–40.

45. Osawa R, Singh N. Cytomegalovirus infection in critically ill patients: A systematic review [Review]. *Crit Care* 2009;13(3):R68.

46. Jaber S, Chanques G, Borry J, et al. Cytomegalovirus infection in critically ill patients: Associated factors and consequences. *Chest* 2005;127(1):233–41.

47. Raftery MJ, Schwab M, Eibert SM, et al. Targeting the function of mature dendritic cells by human cytomegalovirus: A multilayered viral defense strategy. *Immunity* 2001;15(6):997–1009.

48. Hall MW, Geyer SM, Guo CY, et al. Innate immune function and mortality in critically ill children with influenza: A multicenter study [Multicenter Study; Research Support, N.I.H., Extramural; Research Support, Non-U.S. Gov't; Research Support, U.S. Gov't, P.H.S.]. *Crit Care Med* 2013;41(1):224–36.

49. Iverson AR, Boyd KL, McAuley JL, et al. Influenza virus primes mice for pneumonia from *Staphylococcus aureus* [Research Support, N.I.H., Extramural; Research Support, Non-U.S. Gov't]. *J Infect Dis* 2011;203(6):880–8.

50. Dalziel SR, Thompson JM, Macias CG, et al. Predictors of severe H1N1 infection in children presenting within Pediatric Emergency Research Networks (PERN): Retrospective case-control study. *BMJ* 2013;347:f4836.

51. Jaber S, Conseil M, Coisel Y, et al. ARDS and influenza A (H1N1): Patients' characteristics and management in intensive care unit. A literature review [Review]. *Ann Fr Anesth Reanim.* 2010;29(2):117–25.

52. Eriksson CO, Graham DA, Uyeki TM, et al. Risk factors for mechanical ventilation in U.S. children hospitalized with seasonal influenza and 2009 pandemic influenza A* [Research Support, N.I.H., Extramural; Research Support, Non-U.S. Gov't]. *Pediatr Crit Care Med* 2012;13(6):625–31.

53. Rice TW, Rubinson L, Uyeki TM, et al. Critical illness from 2009 pandemic influenza A virus and bacterial coinfection in the United States [Multicenter Study; Research Support, N.I.H., Extramural]. *Crit Care Med* 2012;40(5):1487–98.

54. Reed C, Kallen AJ, Patton M, et al. Infection with community-onset *Staphylococcus aureus* and influenza virus in hospitalized children. *Pediatr Infect Dis J* 2009;28(7):572–6.

55. Finelli L, Fiore A, Dhara R, et al. Influenza-associated pediatric mortality in the United States: Increase of *Staphylococcus aureus* coinfection [Comparative Study Multicenter Study]. *Pediatrics* 2008;122(4):805–11.

56. Lucas S. Predictive clinicopathological features derived from systematic autopsy examination of patients who died with A/H1N1 influenza infection in the UK 2009–10 pandemic. *Health Technol Assess* 2010;14(55):83–114.

57. Lee EH, Wu C, Lee EU, et al. Fatalities associated with the 2009 H1N1 influenza A virus in New York city. *Clin Infect Dis* 2010;50(11):1498–504.

58. Cox CM, Blanton L, Dhara R, et al. 2009 pandemic influenza A (H1N1) deaths among children—United States, 2009–2010. *Clin Infect Dis* 2011;52(suppl 1):S69–74.

59. O'Brien KL, Walters MI, Sellman J, et al. Severe pneumococcal pneumonia in previously healthy children: The role of preceding influenza infection. *Clin Infect Dis* 2000;30(5):784–9.

60. Tsolia MN, Psarras S, Bossios A, et al. Etiology of community-acquired pneumonia in hospitalized school-age children: Evidence for high prevalence of viral infections. *Clin Infect Dis* 2004;39(5):681–6.

61. Talbot TR, Poehling KA, Hartert TV, et al. Seasonality of invasive pneumococcal disease: Temporal relation to documented influenza and respiratory syncytial viral circulation. *Am J Med* 2005;118(3):285–91.

62. Gonzalez BE, Hulten KG, Dishop MK, et al. Pulmonary manifestations in children with invasive community-acquired *Staphylococcus aureus* infection. *Clin Infect Dis* 2005;41(5):583–90.

63. Kneyber MC, Blusse van Oud-Alblas H, van Vliet M, et al. Concurrent bacterial infection and prolonged mechanical ventilation in infants with respiratory syncytial virus lower respiratory tract disease. *Intensive Care Med* 2005;31(5):680–5.

64. Thorburn K, Harigopal S, Reddy V, et al. High incidence of pulmonary bacterial co-infection in children with severe respiratory syncytial virus (RSV) bronchiolitis. *Thorax* 2006;61(7):611–5.

65. Resch B, Gusenleitner W, Mueller WD. Risk of concurrent bacterial infection in preterm infants hospitalized due to respiratory syncytial virus infection. *Acta paediatr* 2007;96(4):495–8.

66. Midulla F, Scagnolari C, Bonci E, et al. Respiratory syncytial virus, human bocavirus and rhinovirus bronchiolitis in infants [Research Support, Non-U.S. Gov't]. *Arch Dis Childhood* 2010;95(1):35–41.

67. Semple MG, Cowell A, Dove W, et al. Dual infection of infants by human metapneumovirus and human respiratory syncytial virus is strongly associated with severe bronchiolitis [Research Support, Non-U.S. Gov't]. *J Infect Dis* 2005;191(3):382–6.

68. Soderberg-Naucler C. Does cytomegalovirus play a causative role in the development of various inflammatory diseases and cancer? *J Intern Med* 2006;259(3):219–46.

69. Russell MY, Palmer A, Michaels MG. Cytomegalovirus infection in pediatric immunocompromised hosts [Review]. *Infect Disord Drug Targets* 2011;11(5):437–48.

70. Munoz-Price LS, Slifkin M, Ruthazer R, et al. The clinical impact of ganciclovir prophylaxis on the occurrence of bacteremia in orthotopic liver transplant recipients. *Clin Infect Dis* 2004;39(9):1293–9.

71. Kalil AC, Levitsky J, Lyden E, et al. Meta-analysis: The efficacy of strategies to prevent organ disease by cytomegalovirus in solid organ transplant recipients [Meta-Analysis]. *Ann Intern Med* 2005;143(12):870–80.

72. Chiche L, Forel JM, Roch A, et al. Active cytomegalovirus infection is common in mechanically ventilated medical intensive care unit patients. *Crit Care Med* 2009;37(6):1850–7.

73. Heininger A, Haeberle H, Fischer I, et al. Cytomegalovirus reactivation and associated outcome of critically ill patients with severe sepsis [Research Support, Non-U.S. Gov't]. *Crit Care* 2011;15(2):R77.

74. Heininger A, Jahn G, Engel C, et al. Human cytomegalovirus infections in nonimmunosuppressed critically ill patients. *Crit Care Med* 2001;29(3):541–7.

75. Limaye AP, Kirby KA, Rubenfeld GD, et al. Cytomegalovirus reactivation in critically ill immunocompetent patients [Research Support, N.I.H., Extramural; Research Support, Non-U.S. Gov't]. *JAMA* 2008;300(4):413–22.

76. Jain M, Duggal S, Chugh TD. Cytomegalovirus infection in non-immunosuppressed critically ill patients [Review]. *J Infect Dev Ctries* 2011;5(8):571–9.

77. Cook CH, Zhang Y, Sedmak DD, et al. Pulmonary cytomegalovirus reactivation causes pathology in immunocompetent mice [Evaluation Studies; Research Support, N.I.H., Extramural]. *Crit Care Med* 2006;34(3):842–9.

78. Chuang YY, Huang YC, Lin TY. Toxic shock syndrome in children: Epidemiology, pathogenesis, and management. *Paediatr Drugs* 2005;7(1):11–25.

79. Laupland KB, Davies HD, Low DE, et al. Invasive group A streptococcal disease in children and association with varicella-zoster virus infection. Ontario Group A Streptococcal Study Group. *Pediatrics* 2000;105(5):E60.

80. Moss RL, Musemeche CA, Kosloske AM. Necrotizing fasciitis in children: Prompt recognition and aggressive therapy improve survival. *J Pediatr Surg* 1996;31(8):1142–6.

81. Cameron JC, Allan G, Johnston F, et al. Severe complications of chickenpox in hospitalised children in the UK and Ireland [Multicenter Study; Research Support, Non-U.S. Gov't]. *Arch Dis Child* 2007;92(12):1062–6.

82. Kerdiles YM, Sellin CI, Druelle J, et al. Immunosuppression caused by measles virus: Role of viral proteins [Research Support, Non-U.S. Gov't; Review]. *Rev Med Virol* 2006;16(1):49–63.

83. Johnston SL. Overview of virus-induced airway disease. *Proc Am Thorac Soc* 2005;2(2):150–6.

84. Jackson DJ, Gangnon RE, Evans MD, et al. Wheezing rhinovirus illnesses in early life predict asthma development in high-risk children [Research Support, N.I.H., Extramural]. *Am J Respir Crit Care Med.* 2008;178(7):667–72.

85. Kennedy JL, Turner RB, Braciale T, et al. Pathogenesis of rhinovirus infection [Research Support, N.I.H., Extramural; Research Support, Non-U.S. Gov't; Review]. *Curr Opin Virol* 2012;2(3):287–93.

86. Heymann PW, Kennedy JL. Rhinovirus-induced asthma exacerbations during childhood: The importance of understanding the atopic status of the host [Comment Editorial; Research Support, N.I.H., Extramural; Research Support, Non-U.S. Gov't]. *J Allergy Clin Immunol* 2012;130(6):1315–6.

87. Sykes A, Edwards MR, Macintyre J, et al. Rhinovirus 16-induced IFN-alpha and IFN-beta are deficient in bronchoalveolar lavage cells in asthmatic patients [Research Support, Non-U.S. Gov't]. *J Allergy Clin Immunol* 2012;129(6):1506–14.e6.

88. Wark PA, Johnston SL, Bucchieri F, et al. Asthmatic bronchial epithelial cells have a deficient innate immune response to infection with rhinovirus. *J Exp Med* 2005;201(6):937–47.

89. Heymann PW, Platts-Mills TA, Johnston SL. Role of viral infections, atopy and antiviral immunity in the etiology of wheezing exacerbations among children and young adults. *Pediatr Infect Dis J* 2005;24(11 suppl):S217–22; discussion S20–1.

90. Kling S, Donninger H, Williams Z, et al. Persistence of rhinovirus RNA after asthma exacerbation in children. *Clin Exp Allergy* 2005;35(5):672–8.

91. Sykes A, Edwards MR, Macintyre J, et al. TLR3, TLR4 and TLRs7–9 induced interferons are not impaired in airway and blood cells in well controlled asthma. *PLoS One* 2013;8(6):e65921.

92. Martin JG, Siddiqui S, Hassan M. Immune responses to viral infections: Relevance for asthma. *Paediatr Respir Rev* 2006;7(suppl 1):S125–7.

93. Hansel TT, Johnston SL, Openshaw PJ. Microbes and mucosal immune responses in asthma [Research Support, Non-U.S. Gov't; Review]. *Lancet* 2013;381(9869):861–73.

94. Lossius A, Johansen JN, Torkildsen O, et al. Epstein-Barr virus in systemic lupus erythematosus, rheumatoid arthritis and multiple sclerosis-association and causation [Review]. *Viruses* 2012;4(12):3701–30.

95. Pakpoor J, Giovannoni G, Ramagopalan SV. Epstein-Barr virus and multiple sclerosis: Association or causation? [Research Support, Non-U.S. Gov't; Review]. *Expert Rev Neurother* 2013;13(3):287–97.

96. Getts DR, Chastain EM, Terry RL, et al. Virus infection, antiviral immunity, and autoimmunity. *Immunol Rev* 2013; 255(1):197–209.

97. Munz C, Lunemann JD, Getts MT, et al. Antiviral immune responses: Triggers of or triggered by autoimmunity? [Research Support, N.I.H., Extramural; Research Support, Non-U.S. Gov't; Review]. *Nat Rev Immunol* 2009;9(4):246–58.

98. Devendra D, Eisenbarth GS. Interferon alpha—A potential link in the pathogenesis of viral-induced type 1 diabetes and autoimmunity. *Clin Immunol* 2004;111(3):225–33.

99. Kivity S, Agmon-Levin N, Blank M, et al. Infections and autoimmunity—Friends or foes? [Review]. *Trends Immunol* 2009;30(8):409–14.

100. Crow MK, Kirou KA. Interferon-alpha in systemic lupus erythematosus. *Curr Opin Rheumatol* 2004;16(5):541–7.

101. Hasham A, Zhang W, Lotay V, et al. Genetic analysis of interferon induced thyroiditis (IIT): Evidence for a key role for MHC and apoptosis related genes and pathways. *J Autoimmun* 2013;44:61–70.

102. Moscona A. Neuraminidase inhibitors for influenza. *N Engl J Med* 2005;353(13):1363–73.

103. Michelow IC, Olsen K, Lozano J, et al. Epidemiology and clinical characteristics of community-acquired pneumonia in hospitalized children. *Pediatrics* 2004;113(4):701–7.

104. Message SD, Johnston SL. The immunology of virus infection in asthma. *Eur Respir J* 2001;18(6):1013–25.

CHAPTER 85 ■ IMMUNE MODULATION AND IMMUNOTHERAPY IN CRITICAL ILLNESS

MARK W. HALL AND JENNIFER A. MUSZYNSKI

KEY POINTS

1. Abnormal regulation of the immune response—overactivity *or* underactivity of the immune system—is the cause of adverse outcomes in many forms of critical illness.

2. Therapies aimed at reducing levels of proinflammatory mediators in human sepsis by specifically targeting lipo-polysaccharide (LPS), tumor necrosis factor (TNF)-α, IL-1β, and others have been overwhelmingly unsuccessful in improving outcomes.

3. The role of methylprednisolone in the treatment of acute respiratory distress syndrome (ARDS) continues to be controversial, with recent evidence suggesting that its use beyond the second week of ARDS may be harmful.

4. Innate immune function is dynamic following a proinflammatory insult, such as trauma or sepsis. A subsequent or concurrent compensatory downregulation of innate immune function can be expected and, when severe, is termed *immunoparalysis*.

5. Immunoparalysis can be quantified through measurement of HLA-DR expression on circulating monocytes, with increased risks of adverse outcomes if <30% of mono-cytes are HLA-DR$^+$. Another important measure of innate immune function is the capacity of whole blood to produce TNF-α when stimulated ex vivo. Severe reduction in the ex vivo TNF-α response is similarly associated with adverse outcomes.

6. Immunoparalysis can be reversed through the use of immunostimulatory agents, including interferon (IFN)-γ or granulocyte–macrophage colony-stimulating factor (GM-CSF), or by withholding exogenous immunosuppres-sion, likely with beneficial effects of outcome.

7. Critically ill patients with persistent neutropenia should be treated with granulocyte colony-stimulating factor, and consideration should be given to the use of prophy-lactic therapy for pneumocystis pneumonia and fungal infections.

8. Adaptive immune dysfunction, including lymphopenia, anergy, and skewing toward anti-inflammatory T cells, is associated with increased risk of death in sepsis and multi-organ dysfunction syndrome. Use of appropriate prophy-laxis against pneumocystis pneumonia and fungal infec-tions, avoidance of lymphotoxic drugs, and treatment of hypogammaglobulinemia with IV immunoglobulin (IVIG) are important aspects of care for the critically ill lympho-penic patient.

9. To date, immunonutrition with n-3 polyunsaturated fatty acids or arginine has no role in the PICU.

10. Critical illnesses themselves and most of the therapies used to treat critically ill children have effects on the immune response. The development of routine immune monitor-ing protocols, including measurement of cell counts *and* immune function (e.g., HLA-DR expression or ex vivo TNF-α response), will be crucial to the identification of patients with overactive or underactive immune systems so that individualized treatment plans can be implemented.

The immune response and its regulation by the host is critical for the mounting of a successful defense against invading patho-gens and for facilitating healing and repair of injured tissues. Much of the morbidity seen in the ICU, however, is a direct con-sequence of abnormal regulation of this immune response. The classic example of this maladaptive scenario is the case of sep-tic shock, whereby an overly robust proinflammatory response causes far more tissue damage than the original infection that initiated it. At the same time, it is important to appreciate that pathology also occurs when the pendulum swings in the other direction. It is intuitive that children with underactive immune systems as the result of chemotherapy or treatment with immu-nosuppressive medications are at high risk for the development of infectious complications. Perhaps less intuitive is the notion that an overactive endogenous compensatory anti-inflammatory immune response can follow or accompany a proinflammatory insult and can result in significant morbidity and mortality *without* the influence of exogenous immunosuppressants. The restoration and maintenance of a responsive immune system with a homeostatic balance between proinflammatory and anti-inflammatory forces should be a goal of modern critical care medicine and has, thus far, proven difficult to achieve.

Historically, attempts at immunomodulation in the ICU have been largely focused on the abrogation of the proinflam-matory response in such conditions as sepsis and acute respira-tory distress syndrome (ARDS). It should be remembered that a great many patients suffer from iatrogenic immunosuppres-sion as the result of treatment for malignancy, transplantation, or autoimmune disease. The history and role of immunomodu-lation and special considerations for the management of im-munocompromised patients will be reviewed in this chapter.

TARGETING PROINFLAMMATION

A detailed review of the immunology of inflammation can be found elsewhere in this text. To briefly review, the cyto-kines tumor necrosis factor (TNF)-α, IL-1β, and interferon

(IFN)-γ are proinflammatory cytokines released by innate immune cells (TNF-α, IL-1β) and lymphocytes (IFN-γ) in response to an inflammatory stimulus. The signaling pathways associated with the production of proinflammatory cytokines in immune cells include the mitogen-activated protein kinase and nuclear factor-κB (NF-κB) pathways. The cytokine that has been most reliably associated with adverse outcomes in the setting of proinflammatory disease is IL-6, likely because IL-6 is released in response to more potent proinflammatory cytokines and, therefore, serves as a *marker* for inflammation. IL-6, while an inducer of the acute phase response, has significant anti-inflammatory properties of its own. More potent anti-inflammatory cytokines, produced by both innate and adaptive immune cells, include IL-10 and transforming growth factor (TGF)-β. Innate immune cells include neutrophils, monocytes, macrophages, and dendritic cells, while adaptive immune cells include T and B lymphocytes.

Severe Sepsis and Septic Shock

The classic signs and symptoms of severe septic disease, including fever, altered vascular tone, and increased capillary permeability, are largely the result of the effects of proinflammatory cytokines rather than the offending pathogen itself. It is not difficult to understand, therefore, why a great deal of time and energy was spent in the 1980s and 1990s developing and testing regimens to target proinflammatory mediators in severe sepsis and septic shock.

Anti-endotoxin Strategies

The first studies performed in this area focused on gram-negative lipopolysaccharide (LPS). First using pooled anti-sera rich in anti-LPS activity (1,2), then using monoclonal anti-LPS antibodies (3,4), investigators tried in vain to consistently demonstrate a survival benefit in septic adults. One phase III trial was stopped after interim analysis demonstrated a trend toward *higher* mortality in treated patients (5). Recombinant bactericidal/permeability-increasing protein (BPI), an endogenous antimicrobial peptide capable of neutralizing endotoxin, was evaluated in a phase III trial in children with meningococcemia. While recombinant BPI conferred no improvement in survival, functional outcome was better in the treated group (6).

Anti-cytokine Strategies

Recombinant IL-1 receptor antagonist (IL-1ra), a naturally occurring IL-1β antagonist, underwent two large phase III trials, both of which failed to show improvement in adult sepsis survival (7,8). TNF-α has been similarly targeted with neutralizing monoclonal antibody therapy. Four major anti-TNF antibody studies have been performed in septic adults to date, including the NORASEPT I and II and INTERSEPT trials (9–11), which demonstrated no improvement in 28-day survival in the treatment arms. The subsequent MONARCS trial showed a slight but statistically significant reduction in 28-day mortality in the

subgroup of patients with plasma IL-6 levels of >1000 pg/mL (12), suggesting that the most profoundly inflamed patients may benefit from TNF-α depletion. Antagonists of bradykinin (deltibant) and platelet-activating factor (lexipafant) have also failed to show survival benefit in adults (13,14).

Activated Protein C

It should be noted that significant overlap exists between the inflammatory and hemostatic pathways. Activated protein C (APC) is an endogenous protein with anti-thrombotic, profibrinolytic, and anti-inflammatory properties that has been studied in septic adults and children. Despite initially encouraging results in the subset of adults with the most severe illness (APACHE II scores $\geq$25 or $\geq$2 organ failure *and* an absence of risk factors for severe bleeding, including recent surgery) (15), the pediatric phase III trial that followed was stopped at its planned interim analysis for lack of efficacy (16). Recombinant human APC has subsequently been removed from the market for safety concerns, largely related to bleeding risk.

Corticosteroids

The role of corticosteroids in adult and pediatric critical illness remains controversial. It was once thought that methylprednisolone or dexamethasone would, by virtue of their anti-inflammatory properties, have beneficial effects in the setting of the proinflammatory storm of sepsis. Two meta-analyses published in the mid-1990s concluded that the use of these drugs was associated with an *increased* risk of mortality from sepsis in adults (17,18). Two more recent meta-analyses demonstrated a survival *benefit* associated with the use of a 5- to 7-day course of low-dose hydrocortisone (200–300 mg/day) in adults with severe sepsis or septic shock (19,20). This difference may be explained by the fact that hydrocortisone has far less glucocorticoid (immunosuppressive) activity and far more mineralocorticoid (hemodynamic supporting) activity than either methylprednisolone or dexamethasone (**Table 85.1**). It should be noted that, while subsequent studies have demonstrated faster shock resolution with hydrocortisone use in sepsis, the mortality benefit has not been consistently seen (21). Hydrocortisone use for hemodynamic support in septic children has yet to be studied in a randomized, controlled trial.

Extracorporeal Therapies

Another approach to the restoration of immunologic homeostasis is the bulk removal of inflammatory mediators through hemofiltration, membrane adsorption, plasmapheresis, or plasma exchange [reviewed in (22)]. An advantage of most of these techniques is that no single mediator is targeted; rather, large concentrations of cytokines can be removed at once. Disadvantages include the need for dedicated large-bore IV access, exposure to blood products (plasma exchange), and the likely need for relatively long-term therapy. In fact, most prospective studies of extracorporeal therapies in sepsis have been small, involved short-term treatment (1–2 days), and have been largely unsuccessful

TABLE 85.1

RELATIVE POTENCIES OF CORTICOSTEROIDS

■ DRUG	■ ANTI-INFLAMMATORY (IMMUNOSUPPRESSIVE)	■ MINERALOCORTICOID
Dexamethasone	30	0
Methylprednisolone	5	1
Hydrocortisone	1	5

in demonstrating improved outcomes. Of these therapies, plasmapheresis and plasma exchange have shown the most promise in prospective trials, perhaps because plasma exchange involves the replacement of patient plasma with donor plasma, thereby both removing unwanted mediators and replacing potentially deficient ones (23–25). In particular, restoration of plasma activity of von Willebrand factor–cleaving protease, ADAMTS13, via plasma exchange has been reported to improve outcomes in the setting of pediatric thrombocytopenia-associated multiple organ failure (TAMOF) (26).

Acute Respiratory Distress Syndrome

The immunomodulators that have been studied most extensively in the setting of ARDS are the glucocorticoids. Reduction of inflammation and inhibition of the fibroproliferative phase of ARDS seem to be reasonable therapeutic goals in the management of this syndrome. In 1998, improved pulmonary function, reduction in organ failure, and improved survival were demonstrated in adults with unresolving ARDS at 7 days who received a prolonged course of methylprednisolone (27). Subsequent studies have questioned these findings, including a prospective study of 180 adults that failed to show a survival benefit and, in fact, showed *increased* mortality rates in patients whose methylprednisolone was started >14 days after the onset of ARDS (28). Yet another adult ARDS study, this time using lower doses and earlier initiation of methylprednisolone, demonstrated improvements in morbidity and mortality (29). To date, no studies have been performed to address this question in the pediatric population.

Cardiopulmonary Bypass

Exposure of leukocytes and complement to the tubing and membranes associated with extracorporeal procedures, including cardiopulmonary bypass (CPB), is known to induce a potent proinflammatory response. While significant advances have been made in the development of less bioreactive coatings for these devices, many practitioners continue to rely on systemic anti-inflammatory agents to attenuate this response [reviewed in (30)]. The administration of glucocorticoids to the patient and/or bypass pump has been shown to reduce neutrophil activation and proinflammatory cytokine release. Attempts to effect bulk removal of proinflammatory cytokines through modified ultrafiltration during CPB have yielded variable results. It should be noted that the impact of these strategies aimed at reducing the proinflammatory response to CPB on patient outcomes is far from clear. Multiple pediatric studies now suggest that a prolonged, severe anti-inflammatory response following pediatric CPB may, in fact, be harmful (31–33).

IMMUNOPARALYSIS

The recurrent failure of treatments targeting the proinflammatory response is coincident with burgeoning experimental and clinical evidence that an overactive *anti-inflammatory* response frequently predominates in the ICU, is often occult, and can be highly pathologic. For many years it has been known that a major inflammatory insult typically results in a compensatory anti-inflammatory response syndrome characterized by reduction in cell-surface marker expression on innate immune cells and increased production of anti-inflammatory cytokines, including IL-10 (34,35). In the 1990s, investigators began associating severe depression of innate immune function with adverse outcomes following trauma, sepsis, and transplantation (36–38). This phenomenon, termed *immunoparalysis*, has

been quantified in two major ways. First, surface expression of the class II major histocompatibility complex molecule HLA-DR, important in antigen presentation, has been shown to be reduced in circulating monocytes from patients with compensatory anti-inflammatory response syndrome. Severe reduction in HLA-DR expression, such that <30% of circulating monocytes are strongly HLA-DR$^+$ by flow cytometry, is characteristic of immunoparalysis. A more functional measure of innate immune capability is the ex vivo LPS-induced TNF-α production assay. In this test, an aliquot of whole blood is incubated with a standard concentration of LPS, and TNF-α production is measured in the supernatant. Patients with immunoparalysis will demonstrate a severe reduction in their ability to make TNF-α ex vivo. Specific cutoffs for the definition of immunoparalysis by this method will vary, depending on the type and dose of LPS used, the volume of blood tested, and the duration of incubation.

While the specific causes of immunoparalysis are poorly understood, it is becoming clear that medications, ICU therapies such as transfusions, and genetic and epigenetic factors all are likely to play a role (33,39,40). Patients with this syndrome exhibit skewing toward a T_H2-like immune phenotype with high levels of circulating IL-10. In fact, anti–IL-10 neutralizing antibodies have been shown to partially reverse experimental immunoparalysis induced by incubation of healthy monocytes with plasma from septic adults (41).

The adaptive arm of the immune system is also involved in the compensatory anti-inflammatory response syndrome. Lymphocyte depletion, in the form of widespread apoptosis in lymphoid organs as well as circulating lymphopenia, has been associated with mortality and secondary infection in critically ill adults and children (42,43). Further, highly immunosuppressive regulatory T cells are thought to be resistant to this wave of apoptosis, and their persistence may perpetuate the immunoparalyzed phenotype (44–46). Lymphocytes from septic patients have also been shown to demonstrate reduced cytokine production capacity, as well as upregulation of the inhibitory cell-surface molecule PD-1 (programmed cell death-1 protein) (47). The net result of these effects can be combined innate and adaptive immune suppression in the critically ill patient, though the timing of these changes is somewhat controversial.

Lymphocyte-mediated responses are thought to take place over a longer time frame than innate immune responses, largely due to the typical lymphocyte requirement for antigen presentation and clonal expansion. Numerous investigators, however, have demonstrated downregulation of lymphocyte signaling pathways very early in the course of critical illness in adults and children (48–51). These mRNA studies have shown high levels of transcripts for proinflammatory innate immune mediators in circulating leukocytes alongside reduced levels of adaptive gene expression. This observation has led to the development of two models of innate immune suppression in the ICU (**Fig. 85.1**). In the serial model, a proinflammatory surge is followed by a compensatory anti-inflammatory phenotype, which, if persistent, is associated with adverse outcomes. Of note, patients may already be in the anti-inflammatory phase of their illness at the time of ICU presentation. In the simultaneous model, both proinflammatory and anti-inflammatory responses are upregulated at the same time, in line with the aforementioned transcriptome studies. It is likely that both models have merit, though suppression of *functional* measures of immunity (cell-surface marker expression, cytokine production capacity), both early and late have been associated with adverse outcomes.

Significance

The laboratory measures of immunoparalysis described earlier represent evidence that some patients' compensatory

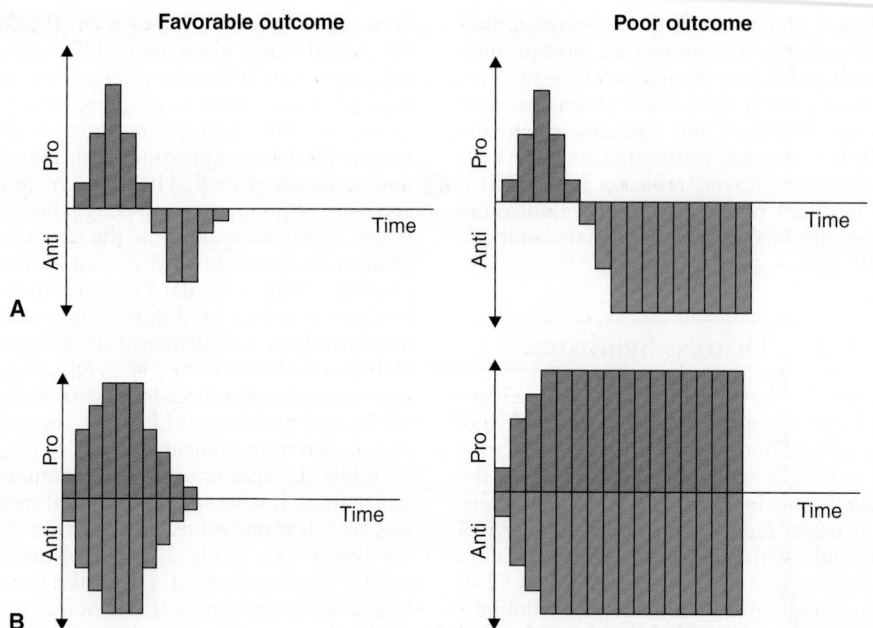

FIGURE 85.1. Models of critical illness–associated immune suppression. In the serial model (A), a proinflammatory surge is temporally followed by a compensatory anti-inflammatory state. If severe and prolonged, this is associated with adverse outcomes. In the simultaneous model (B), a mixed response occurs, with both proinflammatory and anti-inflammatory systems being activated concurrently. Restoration of homeostasis is associated with good outcomes in both models.

anti-inflammatory response, while initially an adaptive attempt to restore immunologic homeostasis, can progress to a maladaptive state, which can be thought of as a type of secondary immunodeficiency. While some reports suggest that critical illness–induced immune suppression is only clinically relevant if present for more than a few days (38,52,53), more recent data indicate that *early,* severe reductions in innate immune function can predict morbidity and mortality in critically ill children (33,54,55).

Mounting evidence suggests that immunoparalysis is reversible, with beneficial effects on clinical outcomes, through the use of immunostimulatory agents or through the tapering of exogenous immunosuppression. Dramatic improvement has been demonstrated in monocyte function and survival rates in adult transplant patients with sepsis and immunoparalysis when immunosuppression was tapered (with no coincident increase in graft rejection) (38). The drugs IFN-γ, granulocyte–macrophage colony-stimulating factor (GM-CSF), and flt3-ligand (56) have been shown to reverse experimental immunoparalysis. Two small, uncontrolled case series have demonstrated reversal of immunoparalysis and suggested improved survival in adult septic patients following in vivo treatment with IFN-γ and GM-CSF, respectively (57,58). In 2005, improved monocyte function and enhanced clearance of infection were demonstrated in a prospective, randomized, controlled trial of GM-CSF in septic adults (59). More recently, immunophenotype-driven trials, in which GM-CSF was given only to subjects whose immune function testing demonstrated immunoparalysis, have shown prompt reversal of immunoparalysis and improved outcomes in critically ill adults (60) and children (53).

Indeed, across-the-board administration of immunostimulating agents to critically ill patients is unlikely to yield improvements in outcomes. For example, a recent Cochrane Database meta-analysis suggested that, while safe, drugs like GM-CSF have no proven benefit in the treatment or prevention of systemic infections in the NICU (14). The disadvantage of the majority of interventional studies on this subject to date is that most were performed with no a priori knowledge of the

patient's immune state. It is therefore critically important that standardized assays of innate immune function be employed to survey for immunoparalysis and target patients who may benefit from inclusion in prospective trials of immunostimulatory agents. The feasibility of highly standardized, multicenter immune function testing has recently been demonstrated in critically ill children with influenza (54).

PATIENTS WITH OVERT IMMUNOSUPPRESSION

Impairment of immune function in the ICU is frequently the result of overt iatrogenic or endogenous inhibition of the immune response. Immunosuppressive medications continue to be the mainstay of treatment for children with cancer, transplantation, autoimmunity, and other chronic inflammatory diseases (**Table 85.2**). Newer antibody-based or recombinant therapies target highly specific aspects of immune function, but are nonetheless immunosuppressive (**Table 85.3**). Accordingly, these patients are known to be at high risk for morbidity and mortality due to infection complications. Similarly, children with primary (congenital) and secondarily acquired (e.g., HIV) immunodeficiencies pose a management challenge for the ICU practitioner. An overarching principle in the care of children with overt immunodeficiency is to remove the offending immunosuppressive agent whenever possible and/or to administer the appropriate immunologic supplementation to the deficient child. Obvious examples of this principle include the withholding of chemotherapy from a child with sepsis and the administration of IV immunoglobulin (IVIG) to a hypogammaglobulinemic child. It is sometimes the case, however, that the clinical situation precludes these options (chemotherapy has already been given, transplant rejection is a concern, or no specific immunologic supplementation is available). Three common scenarios in which overt immunosuppression is a concern are discussed in what follows.

TABLE 85.2

COMMONLY USED NON–ANTIBODY-BASED IMMUNOSUPPRESSIVE AGENTS

■ CLASS	■ DRUG	■ TARGET	■ NONIMMUNE TOXICITIES
Glucocorticoids	Methylprednisolone Dexamethasone Prednisone	Inhibition of proinflammatory and cell-proliferation gene transcription in lymphocytes and other immune cells	Hypertension, hyperglycemia, impaired wound healing, neuromuscular weakness, growth impairment
Calcineurin inhibitors	Tacrolimus (FK506) Cyclosporine A (CsA)	Inhibition of T cell signaling pathways	Nephrotoxicity, CNS toxicity (including seizures), tremor, hypertension, hyperglycemia (FK506), hirsutism (CsA)
TOR protein kinase inhibitor	Sirolimus	Inhibition of T and B cell proliferation	Hyperlipidemia, hypertension, thrombocytopenia, rash
Antimetabolite	Azathioprine Mycophenolate mofetil	Purine synthesis inhibition	Bone marrow suppression, diarrhea, cholestasis

CNS, central nervous system; TOR, target of rapamycin.

The Neutropenic Patient

Severe, prolonged neutropenia most commonly results from the administration of myelosuppressive chemotherapy in the context of cancer treatment, but can also be seen with infection-induced marrow failure and as an unintended side effect of numerous drugs, including antibiotics. It has been understood for decades that an absolute neutrophil count (ANC) of <500 cells/mm^3 is associated with increased incidence of sepsis and death in patients with malignancy. Prophylaxis against pneumocystis pneumonia and candidal infections with trimethoprim/sulfamethoxazole and fluconazole, respectively, should be considered in this population when patients are critically ill. Use of the drug granulocyte colony-stimulating factor (GCSF) has become the standard of care in the treatment of cancer patients with fever and neutropenia. Administration of GCSF results in increased myelopoiesis and neutrophil maturation. The National Comprehensive Cancer Network now advocates the use of a colony-stimulating factor in patients with a 20% risk of developing febrile neutropenia (61). Another therapeutic option for the treatment of severely neutropenic children with life-threatening infection is the administration of donor leukocytes via granulocyte transfusion. This approach requires an element of planning, as a suitable donor is typically pretreated with GCSF for a period of time prior to leukapheresis. Further complicating this approach is the fact that donor leukocytes can induce a potent proinflammatory response following infusion. A 2005 Cochrane Database meta-analysis concluded that evidence to support or contraindicate the use of granulocyte transfusion therapy is inconclusive, but subgroup analysis suggested that patients who received >1 × 10^{10} cells per dose fared better than those receiving lower doses (62). In sum, while neutropenia may not be avoidable, safe and effective approaches can reduce its effect on morbidity and mortality.

The Lymphopenic Patient

Lymphopenia frequently accompanies critical illness and has been associated with increased risk of death and secondary infection. It is especially important to note that the definition of lymphopenia varies by age, with infants and toddlers requiring more robust lymphocyte numbers to remain immunocompetent (Table 85.4). However, some authors have chosen an absolute lymphocyte count (ALC) <1000 cells/mm^3 as diagnostic of clinically relevant lymphopenia across all age groups (42). Causes of lymphopenia in the PICU include drug-related marrow failure (including chemotherapy), infection-induced bone marrow suppression, HIV infection, and lymphocyte loss via chylothorax drainage.

The HIV pandemic has taught numerous lessons about the importance of lymphocyte function in protecting against infection. Chief among them is the importance of appropriate antimicrobial prophylaxis in the setting of prolonged lymphopenia. CDC recommendations currently include the administration of trimethoprim/sulfamethoxazole, dapsone, or pentamidine for pneumocystis pneumonia prophylaxis in children with severe reductions in CD4$^+$ T cell count.

One potential consequence of lymphocyte depletion is a lack of antibody production by B cells. Assessment of quantitative immunoglobulin levels can identify patients with

TABLE 85.3

ANTIBODY-BASED AND RECOMBINANT IMMUNOSUPPRESSIVE AGENTS

■ THERAPY	■ EXAMPLE	■ POTENTIAL USES
Anti-TNF-α	Infliximab, Etanercept	IBD, autoimmune arthritis
Anti-CD20	Rituximab	B cell leukemia/lymphoma, multiple sclerosis, autoimmune arthritis
Anti-IL-2Rα	Basiliximab, Daclizumab	Transplant rejection
Anti-T cell (polyclonal)	Anti-thymocyte globulin	Transplant rejection
Anti-IL-6R	Toclizumab	Autoimmune arthritis
Recombinant IL-1ra	Anakinra	Autoimmune arthritis, NOMID

RA, receptor antagonist; IBD, inflammatory bowel disease; NOMID, neonatal onset multisystem inflammatory disease.

TABLE 85.4

CENTERS FOR DISEASE CONTROL DEFINITIONS OF SEVERE REDUCTIONS IN CD4$^+$ COUNT IN CHILDREN

■ AGE (YEARS)	■ CD4$^+$ COUNT (CELLS/MM^3)
<1	<750
1–5	<500
6–12	<200

Adapted from National Pediatric and Family HIV Resource Center; National Center for Infectious Diseases; Centers for Disease Control and Prevention. 1995 revised guidelines for prophylaxis against *Pneumocystis carinii* pneumonia for children infected with or perinatally exposed to human immunodeficiency virus. *MMWR Recomm Rep* 1995;44(RR-4):1–11.

hypogammaglobulinemia who may benefit from replacement with IVIG. While the role of IVIG in the empiric management of critical illness in the *absence* of low IgG levels is somewhat controversial, as detailed below, the use of IVIG in the treatment of hypogammaglobulinemia in the ICU is not.

It is noteworthy that many therapies commonly used in the practice of critical care medicine may themselves promote or exacerbate lymphopenia. Glucocorticoids, for example, are potent inducers of lymphocyte apoptosis. Dopamine use has similarly been associated with the development of lymphopenia, presumably through its inhibitory effect on the neuroendocrine axes, most notably prolactin, which is known to be a necessary growth factor for lymphocytes. Currently, no lymphocyte-specific colony-stimulating factors are available that can be used to bolster lymphocyte numbers, though several agents (e.g., anti-PD-1 and rhIL-7) have shown promise (63); however, elimination of lymphopenia-inducing agents, when possible, should be strongly considered, especially when suitable alternatives exist (e.g., another catecholamine or fenoldopam in place of dopamine).

The Transplant Patient

Patients who have undergone transplantation are placed in the double bind of taking medicines that place them at high risk for the development of infection, without which they are likely to reject their allograft. Multidrug regimens, including calcineurin inhibitors, corticosteroids, and other immunosuppressives (e.g., mycophenolate or azathioprine), are frequently employed to shut down the adaptive immune response against the transplanted organ, often with significant systemic toxicities. The suppressive effects of these regimens are not limited to the adaptive immune response, but inhibit the innate response as well with reductions in monocyte function associated directly or indirectly with calcineurin inhibition. Lastly, most transplant regimens rely on plasma drug levels and end-organ toxicity to drive dose titration rather than on direct measures of immune function.

Several strategies can be employed to promote improved outcomes in the transplant patient with critical illness. First, antimicrobial prophylaxis is crucial for the prevention of secondary infection. Perhaps the most comprehensive set of recommendations in this regard comes from the Centers for Disease Control Guidelines for Preventing Opportunistic Infection in Hematopoietic Stem Cell Transplant Recipients (64) (Table 85.5). While not necessarily generalizable to all transplant populations, they highlight the scope of the problem and identify a rational approach to prophylaxis. Second, the use of antibody-based immunosuppressive regimens, including anti–IL-2 receptor antibodies, has been shown to be an effective antirejection strategy without the systemic toxicity profiles of drugs, such as cyclosporine and tacrolimus (65). Lastly, the ICU practitioner can rapidly taper the exogenous immunosuppression to allow for a more robust immune response in the setting of suspected or proven infection. The impressive effect of this strategy was displayed by Volk et al., (37) who, in the mid-1990s, demonstrated 90% patient survival (with 98% graft survival in that group) in immunoparalyzed adult transplant

TABLE 85.5

ROUTINE PREVENTIVE REGIMENS FOR PEDIATRIC HEMATOPOIETIC STEM CELL TRANSPLANT RECIPIENTS

■ INFECTION	■ INDICATION	■ FIRST-LINE DRUG
Bacterial infections	Severe hypogammaglobulinemia (serum IgG level <400 mg/dL) at <100 d after transplant	IVIG 400 mg/kg/mo (or as needed to keep IgG level >400 mg/dL)
Candida species	Allogeneic recipients or high-risk autologous recipients from transplant to engraftment or until 7 d after ANC >1000 cells/mm^3	Fluconazole 3–6 mg/kg/d PO or IV (6 mo – 13 y); or 400 mg PO or IV daily (>13 y). Max dose 600 mg/d
Cytomegalovirus	All patients from engraftment through day 100	Ganciclovir 5 mg/kg/dose IV every 12 h for 5–7 d, followed by 5 mg/kg/dose IV daily for 5 d/wk
Pneumocystis jirovecii pneumonia	Allogeneic recipients or high-risk autologous recipients until 6 mo posttransplant (longer if immunosuppression continued or GVHD)	Trimethoprim/sulfamethoxazole (TMP/SMX; 150 mg TMP/750 mg SMX) PO twice daily 3 times weekly [Alternative regimens available; see *MMWR Recomm. Rep* 2000;49(RR-10):1–128]
Herpes simplex virus	Seropositive patients from the beginning of conditioning therapy until engraftment	Acyclovir 250 mg/m^2/dose IV every 8 h or 125 mg/m^2/dose IV every 6 h
Varicella-zoster virus	Postexposure prophylaxis in actively immunosuppressed patients	Varicella-zoster immunoglobulin 125 units/10 kg body weight IM (max dose 625 units)
Methicillin-resistant *Staphylococcus aureus*	Known MRSA carriers	Mupirocin calcium ointment 2% to nares twice daily for 5 d or to wounds daily for 2 wk

Recommendations include vaccination against influenza, respiratory syncytial virus, *Streptococcus pneumoniae*, and *Haemophilus influenzae* type b.
GVHD, graft-versus-host disease; IM, intramuscularly; MRSA, methicillin-resistant *Staphylococcus aureus*.
Adapted from Centers for Disease Control and Prevention; Infectious Disease Society of America; American Society of Blood and Marrow Transplantation. Guidelines for preventing opportunistic infections among hematopoietic stem cell transplant recipients. *MMWR Recomm Rep.* 2000;49(RR-10):1–128.

patients with sepsis when they underwent rapid tapering of immunosuppression. Immunoparalyzed patients who did not undergo rapid tapering experienced an 8% survival rate (37).

A major impediment to the optimal titration of immuno-suppressive therapy in transplant patients is the reliance on drug levels as the primary indicator of immunosuppression. While plasma tacrolimus levels of <10 ng/mL and cyclosporine A levels of <200 ng/mL can be generally thought of as mildly-to-moderately immunosuppressive, functional assays of the immune response, such as ex vivo LPS-induced TNF-α production capacity, have the potential to serve as more relevant targets for titration of these potent drugs.

INTRAVENOUS IMMUNOGLOBULIN

Polyclonal IVIG has been administered to adults and children *without* preexisting hypogammaglobulinemia in the context of sepsis, with mixed results. A recent meta-analysis of IVIG use for the treatment of suspected or proven infection in critically ill neonates showed no effect on mortality with empiric use. It did show, however, that mortality risk was lowered when IVIG was used in the setting of proven infection (66). A 2004 meta-analysis of high-quality adult studies failed to show a reduction mortality risk when IVIG was empirically used in the treatment of sepsis (67). However, in a 2005, prospective, randomized, controlled trial in children <2 years of age with sepsis, 3 days of polyclonal IVIG treatment resulted in improved survival to discharge and in shorter durations of PICU stay (68). Interestingly, it appears that IVIG may be of particular benefit in the setting of severe invasive group A strep infection (69).

A subset of IVIG trials has employed a product that is enriched in the IgM fraction of immunoglobulin. Evidence suggests that IgM-enriched IVIG may be beneficial in postoperative sepsis in adult patients, though a multicentered, randomized, controlled trial failed to show benefit in the setting of chemotherapy-induced neutropenic sepsis (70,71).

IMMUNONUTRITION

Another approach that has been taken to effect immunomodulation in the ICU is through immunonutrition. With this strategy, patients are provided with nutritional supplementation that, in the course of metabolism, has an effect on the immune response. The two substrates that have been the focus of the most investigation are the n-3 polyunsaturated fatty acids (PUFA) and the amino acid arginine.

The n-3 PUFAs, including docosahexaenoic, eicosapentaenoic, and α-linoleic acid, are thought to promote an anti-inflammatory immune state through at least two mechanisms. By incorporating into the cell's phospholipid membrane, n-3 PUFAs compete with arachidonic acid precursors, resulting in lower arachidonic acid production. The n-3 PUFAs are themselves less favorable substrates for eicosanoid formation. In addition, n-3 PUFAs directly inhibit nuclear receptors, including peroxisome proliferator-activated receptor (PPAR-γ), which results in impairment of the propagation of the inflammatory response. Administration of n-3 PUFAs has been shown in vitro and in vivo to be associated with T_H2 polarization, reduced innate and adaptive immune function, and reduced plasma concentrations of proinflammatory cytokines, though no mortality benefit has been definitively shown (72).

Arginine, by contrast, is thought to promote a more vigorous immune response through augmentation of intracellular killing and lymphocyte function. A 2001 meta-analysis of 22 studies in critically ill adults concluded that arginine

supplementation resulted in *higher* mortality in treated patients, though its use was associated with a lower overall infection rate (73). More recent studies have explored the use of combined formulas, including n-3 PUFAs, arginine, and other supplements, in critically ill adults and children (74). While subtle differences in cytokine profiles have resulted, a significant impact on clinical outcomes has yet to be reliably demonstrated. Though it is important to note that these studies did not employ a priori measures of immune function to screen for such conditions as immunoparalysis, routine use of immunonutrition cannot currently be recommended.

THE IMPACT OF CRITICAL ILLNESS ON INFLAMMATION

In addition to overt immunosuppression with drugs (e.g., tacrolimus) and endogenous phenomena (e.g., immunoparalysis), the ICU practitioner must be aware of the profound immunologic effects of many of the therapies routinely used in the ICU. Catecholamines, for example, can enhance (α receptors) or inhibit (β receptors) the immune response. Bactericidal antibiotics can transiently exacerbate the inflammatory response due to release of bacterial components at the time of cell death. Conversely, β-lactams can lead to immunodeficiency through bone marrow suppression, while macrolides are known to impair proinflammatory cytokine production. Opioids are inducers of lymphocyte and macrophage apoptosis and can induce the anti-inflammatory cytokine TGF-β. Insulin is thought to have significant anti-inflammatory properties both through reduction of hyperglycemia-induced proinflammatory cytokine production and through direct inhibition of the NF-κB pathway. Even furosemide is thought to be immunologically active, resulting in attenuation of the inflammatory response in mononuclear cells. Red blood cell transfusion, another staple of ICU management, is now thought to be immunosuppressive as well, particularly in relation to long RBC storage times (39).

Concomitant organ failure and other conditions associated with critical illness further complicate the picture. Hepatic failure, with its associated impairment of cytokine clearance, is frequently associated with a proinflammatory state. Uremic plasma from patients with renal failure has been shown to induce apoptosis in innate and adaptive immune cells. As noted earlier, extracorporeal therapies, including hemodialysis and continuous venovenous hemofiltration, can promote the inflammatory state through immune reactions to plastic tubing and membranes. Hyperglycemia, the control of which is now the target of prospective clinical trials in the PICU, has been clearly shown to be a potent activator of the NF-κB pathway in innate immune cells. Conversely, the endogenous stress-induced cortisol response, though less immunosuppressive than some exogenous glucocorticoids, inhibits proinflammatory cytokine production in leukocytes. These examples illustrate that the effects of these competing forces in a critically ill child can be confusing at best, but they also illustrate the need for assessment of the overall immune phenotype of the patient in determining the proper course of therapy (Fig. 85.2).

CONCLUSIONS AND FUTURE DIRECTIONS

From the proinflammatory storm of sepsis to the anti-inflammatory dominance of immunoparalysis, it is clear that ICU patients span a spectrum of immune activity. It is naïve to assume that one type of immunotherapy will be suitable for all patients with a given condition. As such, the success or

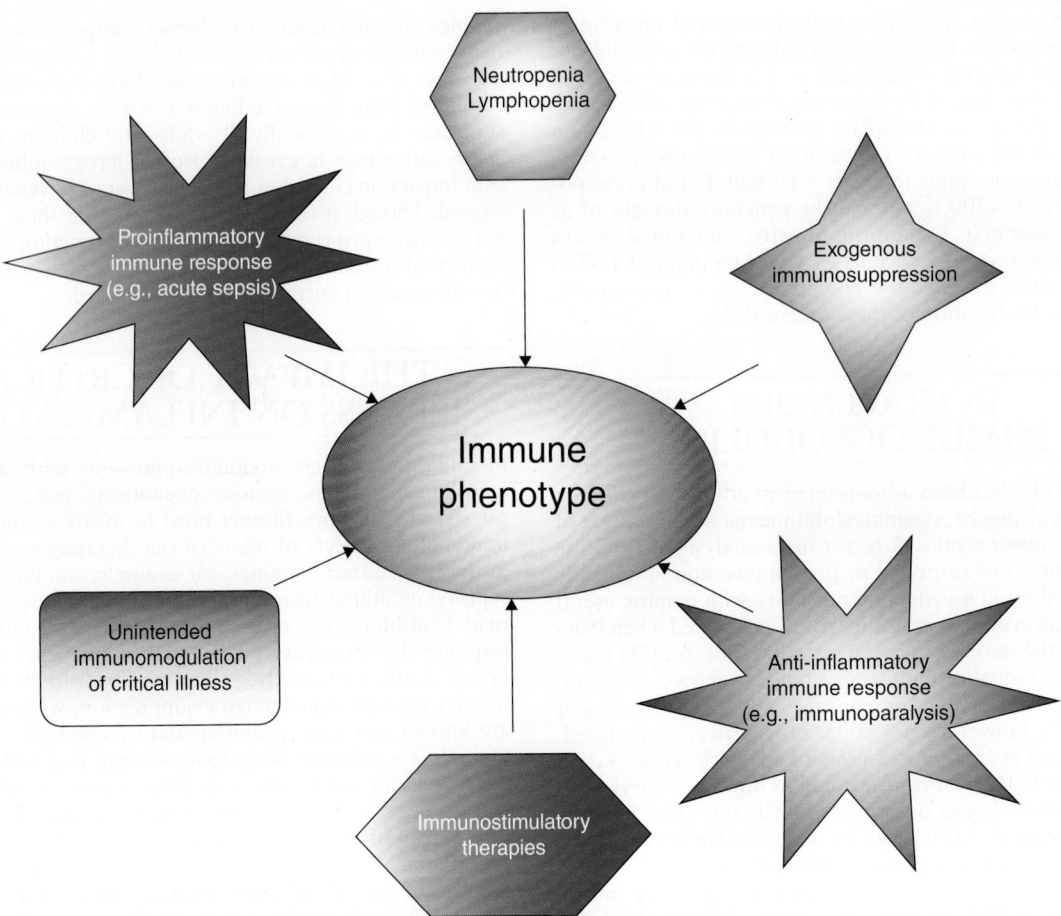

FIGURE 85.2. The ICU immunophenotype. The patient's overall immune phenotype is determined by the net effects of proinflammatory and anti-inflammatory forces acting to influence the inflammatory balance. Many of these forces are occult, necessitating immune monitoring.

failure of any therapy directed at the restoration of immuno-logic homeostasis is likely to be dependent on the right patient receiving the right therapies at the right time. To that end, a program of immune monitoring is essential for directing treatments to patients who are most likely to benefit from them. Innate immune monitoring, through quantification of monocyte HLA-DR expression or ex vivo TNF-α production capacity, is relatively easy to accomplish, but is in need of standardization across the critical care community. Similarly, standardized adaptive immune monitoring regimens, including lymphocyte cell counts, ex vivo lymphocyte stimulation assays, and lymphocyte cell-surface marker quantitation, can and should be developed. Immune function–specific clinical trials targeting innate and/or adaptive immune failure in critical illness are, thankfully, in various stages of development and execution. Along with this type of monitoring and modulation, the practitioner should continue to be vigilant in instituting appropriate prophylactic therapy when indicated, and wisely titrating medications that have immunologic effects, both overt and subtle.

Perhaps the most important method of immunomodulation is that achieved through immunization. Prevention of disease, rather than its treatment, should continue to be the highest goal of the medical community. We should therefore continue to advocate for routine immunization against organisms such as *Haemophilus influenzae*, *Streptococcus pneumoniae*, and *Neisseria meningitis*. Similarly, high-risk children should receive prophylaxis against respiratory syncytial virus and influenza. The development of new vaccine programs, including immunization against *Pseudomonas* species in high-risk populations, holds promise to further extend this umbrella of protection.

Lastly, as is apparent from the above discussion, the vast majority of data that describe the relationships between immune function and critical illness continue to come from adult studies. Significant developmental influences, most of which remain unknown, very likely immunologically differentiate infants from older children and adolescents. Multicentered descriptive and interventional studies remain necessary to address this major gap in the literature and promote immunologic homeostasis in the PICU.

References

1. The Intravenous Immunoglobulin Collaborative Study Group. Prophylactic intravenous administration of standard immune globulin as compared with core-lipopolysaccharide immune globulin in patients at high risk of postsurgical infection. *N Engl J Med* 1992;327(4):234–40.
2. Calandra T, Glauser MP, Schellekens J, et al. Treatment of gram-negative septic shock with human IgG antibody to *Escherichia coli* J5: A prospective, double-blind, randomized trial. *J Infect Dis* 1988;158(2):312–9.
3. Bone RC, Balk RA, Fein AM, et al.; The E5 Sepsis Study Group. A second large controlled clinical study of E5, a monoclonal antibody to endotoxin: Results of a prospective, multicenter, randomized, controlled trial. *Crit Care Med* 1995;23(6):994–1006.
4. Greenman RL, Schein RM, Martin MA, et al.; The XOMA Sepsis Study Group. A controlled clinical trial of E5 murine monoclonal IgM antibody to endotoxin in the treatment of gram-negative sepsis. *JAMA* 1991;266(8):1097–102.

5. McCloskey RV, Straube RC, Sanders C, et al.; CHESS Trial Study Group. Treatment of septic shock with human monoclonal antibody HA-1A: A randomized, double-blind, placebo-controlled trial. *Ann Intern Med* 1994;121(1):1–5.

6. Levin M, Quint PA, Goldstein B, et al.; rBPI21 Meningococcal Sepsis Study Group. Recombinant bactericidal/permeability-increasing protein (rBPI21) as adjunctive treatment for children with severe meningococcal sepsis: A randomised trial. *Lancet* 2000;356(9234):961–7.

7. Fisher CJ Jr, Dhainaut JF, Opal SM, et al.; Phase III rhIL-1ra Sepsis Syndrome Study Group. Recombinant human interleukin 1 receptor antagonist in the treatment of patients with sepsis syndrome: Results from a randomized, double-blind, placebo-controlled trial. *JAMA* 1994;271(23):1836–43.

8. Opal SM, Fisher CJ Jr, Dhainaut JF, et al.; The Interleukin-1 Receptor Antagonist Sepsis Investigator Group. Confirmatory interleukin-1 receptor antagonist trial in severe sepsis: A phase III, randomized, double-blind, placebo-controlled, multicenter trial. *Crit Care Med* 1997;25(7):1115–24.

9. Abraham E, Anzueto A, Gutierrez G, et al.; NORASEPT II Study Group. Double-blind randomised controlled trial of monoclonal antibody to human tumour necrosis factor in treatment of septic shock. *Lancet* 1998;351(9107):929–33.

10. Abraham E, Wunderink R, Silverman H, et al.; TNF-alpha MAb Sepsis Study Group. Efficacy and safety of monoclonal antibody to human tumor necrosis factor alpha in patients with sepsis syndrome: A randomized, controlled, double-blind, multicenter clinical trial. *JAMA* 1995;273(12):934–41.

11. Cohen J, Carlet J; International Sepsis Trial Study Group. INTERSEPT: An international, multicenter, placebo-controlled trial of monoclonal antibody to human tumor necrosis factor-alpha in patients with sepsis. *Crit Care Med* 1996;24(9):1431–40.

12. Panacek EA, Marshall J, Fischkoff S. Neutralization of TNF by a monoclonal antibody improves survival and reduces organ dysfunction in human sepsis: Results of the MONARCS trial. *Chest* 2000;2000(118S):88S.

13. Fein AM, Bernard GR, Criner GJ, et al.; CP-0127 SIRS and Sepsis Study Group. Treatment of severe systemic inflammatory response syndrome and sepsis with a novel bradykinin antagonist, deltibant (CP-0127): Results of a randomized, double-blind, placebo-controlled trial. *JAMA* 1997;277(6):482–7.

14. Suputtamongkol Y, Intaranongpai S, Smith MD, et al. A double-blind placebo-controlled study of an infusion of lexipafant (platelet-activating factor receptor antagonist) in patients with severe sepsis. *Antimicrob Agents Chemother* 2000;44(3):693–6.

15. Dhainaut JF, Laterre PF, Janes JM, et al. Drotrecogin alfa (activated) in the treatment of severe sepsis patients with multiple-organ dysfunction: Data from the PROWESS trial. *Intensive Care Med* 2003;29(6):894–903.

16. Goldstein B, Nadel S, Peters M, et al. ENHANCE: Results of a global open-label trial of drotrecogin alfa (activated) in children with severe sepsis. *Pediatr Crit Care Med* 2006;7(3):200–11.

17. Cronin L, Cook DJ, Carlet J, et al. Corticosteroid treatment for sepsis: A critical appraisal and meta-analysis of the literature. *Crit Care Med* 1995;23(8):1430–9.

18. Lefering R, Neugebauer EA. Steroid controversy in sepsis and septic shock: A meta-analysis. *Crit Care Med* 1995;23(7):1294–303.

19. Annane D, Bellissant E, Bollaert PE, et al. Corticosteroids for severe sepsis and septic shock: A systematic review and meta-analysis. *BMJ* 2004;329(7464):480.

20. Minneci PC, Deans KJ, Banks SM, et al. Meta-analysis: The effect of steroids on survival and shock during sepsis depends on the dose. *Ann Intern Med* 2004;141(1):47–56.

21. Sprung CL, Annane D, Keh D, et al. Hydrocortisone therapy for patients with septic shock [published online ahead of print January 11, 2008]. *N Engl J Med* 2008;358(2):111–24.

22. McMaster P, Shann F. The use of extracorporeal techniques to remove humoral factors in sepsis. *Pediatr Crit Care Med* 2003;4(1):2–7.

23. Busund R, Koukline V, Utrobin U, et al. Plasmapheresis in severe sepsis and septic shock: A prospective, randomised, controlled trial. *Intensive Care Med* 2002;28(10):1434–9.

24. van Deuren M, Santman FW, van Dalen R, et al. Plasma and whole blood exchange in meningococcal sepsis. *Clin Infect Dis* 1992;15(3):424–30.

25. Westendorp RG, Brand A, Haanen J, et al. Leukaplasmapheresis in meningococcal septic shock. *Am J Med* 1992;92(5):577–8.

26. Nguyen TC, Han YY, Kiss JE, et al. Intensive plasma exchange increases ADAMTS-13 activity and reverses organ dysfunction in children with thrombocytopenia-associated multiple organ failure. *Crit Care Med* 2008;36(10):2878–87.

27. Meduri GU, Headley AS, Golden E, et al. Effect of prolonged methylprednisolone therapy in unresolving acute respiratory distress syndrome: A randomized controlled trial. *JAMA* 1998;280(2):159–65.

28. Steinberg KP, Hudson LD, Goodman RB, et al. Efficacy and safety of corticosteroids for persistent acute respiratory distress syndrome. *N Engl J Med* 2006;354(16):1671–84.

29. Meduri GU, Golden E, Freire AX, et al. Methylprednisolone infusion in early severe ARDS: Results of a randomized controlled trial [published online ahead of print April 12, 2007]. *Chest* 2007;131(4):954–63.

30. Rubens FD, Mesana T. The inflammatory response to cardiopulmonary bypass: A therapeutic overview. *Perfusion* 2004;19(suppl 1):S5–12.

31. Allen ML, Peters MJ, Goldman A, et al. Early postoperative monocyte deactivation predicts systemic inflammation and prolonged stay in pediatric cardiac intensive care. *Crit Care Med* 2002;30(5):1140–5.

32. Allen ML, Hoschtitzky JA, Peters MJ, et al. Interleukin-10 and its role in clinical immunoparalysis following pediatric cardiac surgery. *Crit Care Med* 2006;34(10):2658–65.

33. Cornell TT, Sun L, Hall MW, et al. Clinical implications and molecular mechanisms of immunoparalysis after cardiopulmonary bypass. *J Thorac Cardiovasc Surg* 2011;143(5):1160–6.

34. Volk HD, Reinke P, Docke WD. Clinical aspects: From systemic inflammation to 'immunoparalysis'. *Chem Immunol* 2000;74:162–77.

35. Bone RC. Immunologic dissonance: A continuing evolution in our understanding of the systemic inflammatory response syndrome (SIRS) and the multiple organ dysfunction syndrome (MODS). *Ann Intern Med* 1996;125(8):680–7.

36. Doughty L, Carcillo JA, Kaplan S, et al. The compensatory anti-inflammatory cytokine interleukin 10 response in pediatric sepsis-induced multiple organ failure. *Chest* 1998;113(6):1625–31.

37. Reinke P, Volk HD. Diagnostic and predictive value of an immune monitoring program for complications after kidney transplantation. *Urol Int* 1992;49(2):69–75.

38. Volk HD, Reinke P, Krausch D, et al. Monocyte deactivation—Rationale for a new therapeutic strategy in sepsis. *Intensive Care Med* 1996;22(suppl 4):S474–81.

39. Muszynski J, Nateri J, Nicol K, et al. Immunosuppressive effects of red blood cells on monocytes are related to both storage time and storage solution [published online ahead of print October 11, 2011]. *Transfusion* 2012;52(4):794–802.

40. Westendorp RG, Langermans JA, Huizinga TW, et al. Genetic influence on cytokine production in meningococcal disease. *Lancet* 1997;349(9069):1912–3.

41. Fumeaux T, Pugin J. Role of interleukin-10 in the intracellular sequestration of human leukocyte antigen-DR in monocytes during septic shock. *Am J Respir Crit Care Med* 2002;166(11):1475–82.

42. Felmet KA, Hall MW, Clark RS, et al. Prolonged lymphopenia, lymphoid depletion, and hypoprolactinemia in children with nosocomial sepsis and multiple organ failure. *J Immunol* 2005;174(6):3765–72.

43. Hotchkiss RS, Tinsley KW, Swanson PE, et al. Sepsis-induced apoptosis causes progressive profound depletion of B and CD4[+] T lymphocytes in humans. *J Immunol* 2001;166(11):6952–63.

44. Venet F, Pachot A, Debard AL, et al. Increased percentage of CD4+CD25+ regulatory T cells during septic shock is due to the decrease of CD4+CD25− lymphocytes. *Crit Care Med* 2004;32(11):2329–31.

45. Venet F, Chung CS, Kherouf H, et al. Increased circulating regulatory T cells (CD4(+)CD25(+)CD127(−)) contribute to lymphocyte anergy in septic shock patients. *Intensive Care Med* 2009;35(4):678–86.

46. Monneret G, Debard AL, Venet F, et al. Marked elevation of human circulating CD4+CD25+ regulatory T cells in sepsis-induced immunoparalysis. *Crit Care Med* 2003;31(7):2068–71.

47. Boomer JS, To K, Chang KC, et al. Immunosuppression in patients who die of sepsis and multiple organ failure [published online ahead of print December 22, 2011]. *JAMA* 2011;306(23):2594–605.

48. Wong HR, Freishtat RJ, Monaco M, et al. Leukocyte subset-derived genomewide expression profiles in pediatric septic shock [published online ahead of print December 17, 2009]. *Pediatr Crit Care Med* 2010;11(3):349–55.

49. Tang BM, McLean AS, Dawes IW, et al. The use of gene-expression profiling to identify candidate genes in human sepsis. *Am J Respir Crit Care Med* 2007;176(7):676–84.

50. Tang BM, Huang SJ, McLean AS. Genome-wide transcription profiling of human sepsis: A systematic review [published online ahead of print December 31, 2010]. *Crit Care* 2010;14(6):R237.

51. Xiao W, Mindrinos MN, Seok J, et al. A genomic storm in critically injured humans [published online ahead of print November 24, 2011]. *J Exp Med* 2011;208(13):2581–90.

52. Monneret G, Lepape A, Voirin N, et al. Persisting low monocyte human leukocyte antigen-DR expression predicts mortality in septic shock. *Intensive Care Med* 2006;32(8):1175–83.

53. Hall MW, Knatz NL, Vetterly C, et al. Immunoparalysis and nosocomial infection in children with multiple organ dysfunction syndrome. *Intensive Care Med* 2011;37(3):525–32.

54. Hall MW, Geyer SM, Guo CY, et al. Innate immune function and mortality in critically ill children with influenza: A multicenter study [published online ahead of print December 12, 2012]. *Crit Care Med* 2013;41(1):224–36.

55. Mella C, Suarez-Arrabal MC, Lopez S, et al. Innate immune dysfunction is associated with enhanced disease severity in infants with severe respiratory syncytial virus bronchiolitis [published online ahead of print December 04, 2012]. *J Infect Dis* 2013;207(4):564–73.

56. Wysocka M, Montaner LJ, Karp CL. Flt3 ligand treatment reverses endotoxin tolerance-related immunoparalysis. *J Immunol* 2005;174(11):7398–402.

57. Docke WD, Randow F, Syrbe U, et al. Monocyte deactivation in septic patients: Restoration by IFN-gamma treatment. *Nat Med* 1997;3(6):678–81.

58. Nierhaus A, Montag B, Timmler N, et al. Reversal of immunoparalysis by recombinant human granulocyte-macrophage colony-stimulating factor in patients with severe sepsis. *Intensive Care Med* 2003;29(4):646–51.

59. Rosenbloom AJ, Linden PK, Dorrance A, et al. Effect of granulocyte-monocyte colony-stimulating factor therapy on leukocyte function and clearance of serious infection in nonneutropenic patients. *Chest* 2005;127(6):2139–50.

60. Meisel C, Schefold JC, Pschowski R, et al. Granulocyte-macrophage colony-stimulating factor to reverse sepsis-associated immunosuppression: A double-blind randomized placebo-controlled multicenter trial. *Am J Respir Crit Care Med* 2009;180(7):640–8.

61. McNeil C. NCCN guidelines advocate wider use of colony-stimulating factor. *J Natl Cancer Inst* 2005;97(10):710–1.

62. Stanworth SJ, Massey E, Hyde C, et al. Granulocyte transfusions for treating infections in patients with neutropenia or neutrophil dysfunction. *Cochrane Database Syst Rev* 2005;(3):CD005339.

63. Hotchkiss RS, Monneret G, Payen D. Immunosuppression in sepsis: A novel understanding of the disorder and a new therapeutic approach [published online ahead of print February 23, 2013]. *Lancet Infect Dis* 2013;13(3):260–8.

64. Dykewicz CA. Summary of the guidelines for preventing opportunistic infections among hematopoietic stem cell transplant recipients. *Clin Infect Dis* 2001;33:139–44.

65. Di Filippo S. Anti-IL-2 receptor antibody vs. polyclonal anti-lymphocyte antibody as induction therapy in pediatric transplantation. *Pediatr Transplant* 2005;9:373–80.

66. Ohlsson A, Lacy JB. Intravenous immunoglobulin for suspected or subsequently proven infection in neonates. *Cochrane Database Syst Rev* 2004:CD001239.

67. Pildal J, Gotzsche PC. Polyclonal immunoglobulin for treatment of bacterial sepsis: A systematic review. *Clin Infect Dis* 2004;39:38–46.

68. El-Nawawy A, El-Kinany H, Hamdy El-Sayed M, et al. Intravenous polyclonal immunoglobulin administration to sepsis syndrome patients: a prospective study in a pediatric intensive care unit. *J Trop Pediatr* 2005;51:271–8.

69. Norrby-Teglund A, Ihendyane N, Darenberg J. Intravenous immunoglobulin adjunctive therapy in sepsis, with special emphasis on severe invasive group A streptococcal infections. *Scand J Infect Dis* 2003;35:683–9.

70. Hentrich M, Fehnle K, Ostermann H, et al. IgMA-enriched immunoglobulin in neutropenic patients with sepsis syndrome and septic shock: a randomized, controlled, multiple-center trial. *Crit Care Med* 2006;34:1319–25.

71. Rodriguez A, Rello J, Neira J, et al. Effects of high-dose of intravenous immunoglobulin and antibiotics on survival for severe sepsis undergoing surgery. *Shock* 2005;23:298–304.

72. Mayer K, Gokorsch S, Fegbeutel C, et al. Parenteral nutrition with fish oil modulates cytokine response in patients with sepsis. *Am J Respir Crit Care Med* 2003;167:1321–8.

73. Heyland DK, Novak F, Drover JW, et al. Should immunonutrition become routine in critically ill patients? A systematic review of the evidence. *JAMA* 2001;286:944–53.

74. Briassoulis G, Filippou O, Kanariou M, et al. Temporal nutritional and inflammatory changes in children with severe head injury fed a regular or an immune-enhancing diet: A randomized, controlled trial. *Pediatr Crit Care Med* 2006;7:56–62.

CHAPTER 86 ■ IMMUNE DEFICIENCY DISORDERS

TRACY B. FAUSNIGHT, E. SCOTT HALSTEAD, SACHIN S. JOGAL, AND JENNIFER A. MCARTHUR

KEY POINTS

1. Primary immunodeficiency disease, once thought to be a rare occurrence, is more common than originally thought. The pediatric critical care provider needs a sound working knowledge of primary immunodeficiency, as prompt identification and diagnosis of these disorders allows for early institution of appropriate therapy and, potentially, improved outcomes among these high-risk patients.
2. The intensivist should recognize a child presenting with a second invasive bacterial infection, an opportunistic infection, and/or an infection slow to respond to conventional therapy as a patient in need of an immunologic workup.

Disorders Predominantly Affecting Immunoglobulins

3. Antibody defects are the most prevalent primary immune deficiency; thus, laboratory evaluation should generally first focus on the possibility of humoral deficiency.
4. Antibody defects most commonly predispose patients to sinopulmonary infections with encapsulated organisms.
5. An early clue to an immunoglobulin deficiency is the finding of a low total protein level in the presence of a normal albumin level on routine blood analysis.
6. Immunoglobulin replacement may be helpful in the control and clearance of severe infections in patients with known immunodeficiency, and IV administration at physiologic replacement doses of 400–500 mg/kg is most appropriate.

Disorders Predominantly Affecting Cellular Function

7. Although less common than antibody defects, predominantly cellular immune defects may also be encountered by the pediatric intensivist. The cardinal clinical features of T-cell dysfunction are fungal infections, chronic viral infections, opportunistic infections, autoimmune disorders, and malignancies.
8. Dysgammaglobulinemia is a frequent consequence of T-cell dysfunction, given the necessary role of T-cell signaling for immunoglobulin class switching and affinity maturation.
9. Infants with DiGeorge syndrome (DGS) and velocardiofacial syndrome have a characteristic 22q11.2 deletion and frequently manifest T-cell deficiency. The 22q11.2 deletion syndrome is the most common cellular immune defect that is likely to present to the pediatric intensivist as a result of congenital heart disease and/or hypocalcemia.

Immunodeficiency with Cytotoxic Defects

10. Hemophagocytic lymphohistiocytosis (HLH) and macrophage activation syndrome (MAS) are both characterized by uncontrolled inflammation.
11. MAS is typically seen in patients with autoimmune disease and often resolves with aggressive treatment of the underlying autoimmune disorder.
12. HLH can be either familial or acquired and often requires much more aggressive therapy than MAS, including hematopoietic stem cell transplantation (HSCT).

Immunodeficiency with Combined Antibody and Cellular Defects

13. Combined antibody and cellular immune deficiencies are generally characterized by the early onset of viral and fungal infections, usually resulting in growth failure.
14. The intensive care of an infant suspected or known to have severe combined immunodeficiency (SCID) should include strict isolation and the use of only irradiated, CMV-negative, and leukocyte-depleted blood products.
15. The infant with SCID may benefit from aggressive antiviral therapies in addition to antibiotics and intravenous immunoglobulin (IVIG). An immunologist or hematologist should be involved early in the care of these infants to facilitate arrangements for HSCT, the most successful therapy for SCID.
16. Early recognition of a combined immunodeficiency is extremely important not only for treating the infections but in directing care, as there is no uniform approach to treating these disorders.

Disorders Affecting Phagocyte Function

17. Primary neutrophil disorders may also be encountered by the intensivist and may be divided into two broad categories: diseases associated with decreased numbers of neutrophils (neutropenia) and those with impaired neutrophil function.
18. Granulocyte colony-stimulating factor (GCSF) therapy may play a role in the treatment of neutropenic disorders. Prophylactic antibiotics, IVIG, and IFN-γ may be useful in the treatment of some functional neutrophil disorders.

Complement Deficiency

19 Complement deficiencies are likely to present to the intensivist in the form of invasive infections (most notably meningococcal disease), hereditary angioedema (HAE), or rheumatologic disorders, especially systemic lupus erythematosus (SLE).

20 In addition to deficits in the classical complement pathway, deficiencies in mannan-binding lectin (MBL) may also contribute to disease states relevant to the pediatric critical care provider, including sepsis, Kawasaki disease, and autoimmune disorders.

21 C1 esterase inhibitor concentrate infusion therapy can be lifesaving for children with acute upper airway obstruction or severe gastrointestinal symptoms secondary to HAE.

Innate Immune Signaling Defects

22 Primary immunodeficiencies associated with impaired toll-like receptor (TLR) signaling have been described; infections can range from mild to severe, including herpes encephalitis.

Immunodeficiency and Cancer Predisposition

23 Several primary immune deficiencies, including Wiskott–Aldrich syndrome (WAS), ataxia telangiectasia, SCID, Kostmann syndrome, and X-linked lymphoproliferative disease (XLP) are associated with an increased risk of cancer.

24 The mechanisms contributing to this association are not completely understood and are likely multifactorial in origin.

Immunologic Effects of Cancer and Its Treatment

25 Most cancer patients are immunocompromised as a result of their underlying disease and/or their antineoplastic therapy.

26 Several cancer treatment–related factors, including neutropenia, loss of mucosal integrity, and T-cell dysfunction, contribute to this immunocompromised state.

Immune Dysfunction Associated with Hematopoietic Stem Cell Transplant

27 Immune suppression is most severe among those patients who receive an allogeneic HSCT. The replacement of the functional lymphohematopoietic system of the host with that of a donor requires intense immunosuppression, often in a patient whose underlying disease has rendered him or her immunocompromised.

28 HSCT patients remain profoundly immunocompromised until effective immune reconstitution occurs, which is a complex and prolonged process that requires months to years.

29 Immune reconstitution following HSCT is influenced by patient-, disease-, and transplant-related factors. Importantly, cellular reconstitution does not necessarily correlate with functional recovery.

30 The occurrence of graft-versus-host disease (GVHD) in the HSCT patient will significantly impede the recovery of normal immune function.

PRIMARY OR CONGENITAL IMMUNE DEFICIENCY DISORDERS

The pediatric intensivist is frequently confronted with severe and life-threatening infections. While the majority of these infections can be attributed to environmental risk factors and invasive monitoring, immune deficiency is a consideration in **1** select cases. The incidence of congenital immune deficiency is estimated to be from 1 in 10,000 to 1 in 2000 live births (1), but these children are overrepresented at tertiary care centers where expert immunologic care is available. The intensivist should recognize a child presenting with a second invasive bacterial infection, an opportunistic infection or an infection slow to respond to conventional therapy as a patient in need of an immunologic **2** workup. With antibody defects being the most prevalent type of immune deficiency, laboratory evaluation should generally focus first on the possibility of humoral defects. Specific pathogens and characteristic host responses, however, may indicate the likelihood of a cellular, phagocytic, or innate immune defect. A summary of the diseases addressed in this chapter can be found in **Table 86.1**. Excellent reviews of primary immune deficiency are readily available and have been published previously (2,3).

DISORDERS PREDOMINANTLY AFFECTING IMMUNOGLOBULINS

Defects predominantly affecting antibody production and function comprise 65% of the congenital immunodeficient **3** population (4). Included within this category are defects of questionable clinical significance, such as isolated IgM deficiency, isolated IgA deficiency, and IgG subclass deficiencies. Only the disorders involving quantitative total IgG deficiency and predictable immunologic consequences are discussed here. Antibody defects predispose patients to sino-**4** pulmonary infections with encapsulated organisms, such as *Streptococcus pneumoniae* and *Haemophilus influenzae*. The patient presenting with severe pneumonia, which has been poorly responsive to antibiotic therapy, deserves quantitative assessment of immunoglobulin (IG) levels. Bacterial sepsis would be a less common presentation of an antibody defect, but poor responsiveness to therapy might again raise this concern.

X-linked Agammaglobulinemia

Since the original description of X-linked agammaglobulinemia (XLA) in 1952 by Colonel Ogden Bruton (5), significant advances have facilitated the accurate diagnosis and effective therapy of XLA. This defect occurs at an estimated incidence of 1 in 190,000 live male births based on birth rate data from a recent US XLA registry (6). Due to the persistence of maternal immunoglobulin, most XLA patients are not diagnosed until after the first 6 months of life. Surprisingly, adults with some residual IgG production have also been reported within this spectrum of disease. While most patients develop symptoms between ages 6 and 12 months, some may have a delayed presentation. The majority present between 2 and 5 years (6). A presentation with recurrent and refractory sinopulmonary infections is the rule, usually involving extracellular

TABLE 86.1

SUMMARY OF PRIMARY IMMUNE DEFICIENCY DISORDERS

CATEGORY	NAME	TYPE OF DEFICIENCY	GENE	PRIMARY ORGANISMS	USUAL SITES	TREATMENT	ASSOCIATED FINDINGS
Humoral	1. X-linked agammaglobulinemia	Absent or low levels of all immunoglobulins	BTK	Encapsulated bacteria, enteroviruses	Sinopulmonary, GI	IVIG/SCIG, antibiotics as needed	Respiratory failure, bronchiectasis, sepsis, diarrhea
	2. Common variable immunodeficiency	Low levels of IgG, ± low IgA, IgM	ICOS, TACI	Encapsulated bacteria	Sinopulmonary, GI	IVIG, antibiotics as needed	T-cell dysfunction, autoimmunity
	3. Transient hypogammaglobulinemia	Low levels of immunoglobulins until age 4 years	Unknown	Encapsulated bacteria	Sinopulmonary	None	None
	4. Hyper-IgM syndrome	Low levels of IgG and IgA, neutropenia	CD154, CD40, AICDA, UNG, NEMO	Encapsulated bacteria, PJP, *Cryptosporidium*	Sinopulmonary, lymph nodes, GI, liver	IVIG, antibiotics as needed, TMP-SMX	PJP, autoimmunity, chronic liver disease, cancer
Cellular	1. 22q11.2 deletion syndrome (DGS/velocardiofacial syndrome)	Thymic hypoplasia, absence of mature T cells	TBX 1	*Candida*, viruses, PJP	MM, skin, lung	Antifungals as needed, TMP-SMX, thymic transplant/HSCT?	Congenital heart disease, hypoparathyroidism, hypocalcemia
	2. IFN-γ-IL-12 axis	Decreased or absent IFN-γ receptor	IFNGR1, IFNGR2, IL12RB1	Mycobacteria, *Salmonella*, *Listeria*	Pulmonary, bone, lymph nodes	SC IFN-γ antibiotics as needed, HSCT	None
Cytotoxic defects	1. Hemophagocytic lymphohistiocytosis	NK-cell and cytotoxic T-cell dysfunction	IL12B, PFR, MLNC13-4, STX 11	EBV, protozoa, bacteria	Blood/bonemarrow, liver, CNS	Corticosteroids, cyclosporine A, etoposide, HSCT?	Fever, ↑triglycerides, ↓fibrinogen, ferritin
	2. Macrophage activation syndrome	IL-1 dysregulation?	MUNC13-4?	Nonspecific viruses or bacteria	Blood, liver, CNS	Corticosteroids, cyclosporine A, FFP	Juvenile idiopathic arthritis, systemic lupus erythematosus
Combined disorders	1. Severe combined immunodeficiency	Dysplastic thymus, low or absent levels of immunoglobulins, lymphopenia	IL2R gamma, JAK3, RAG1/2, ZAP-70, PNP, ADA, IL-7	Encapsulated bacteria, *Candida*, viruses, PJP	Sinopulmonary, MM, skin, liver, GI, blood	IVIG, TMP-SMX, antibiotics, antivirals, antifungals, HSCT, gene therapy?	Fatal without HSCT, enzyme replacement, or gene therapy
	2. Bare lymphocyte syndrome	Partial or complete absence of MHC class I or MHC class II on T cells	MHC Class I: unknown; MHC Class II: RFX-ANK, MHC2TA, RFX5, RFXAP	Encapsulated bacteria, *Candida*, viruses	Sinopulmonary, skin, GI	Antibiotics, HSCT?	Eczema, autoimmunity, lymphadenopathy
	3. Autoimmune lymphoproliferative syndrome	Elevated $\alpha\beta$ double negative T cells	FAS, FASLG, CASPIO	None	Lymph nodes	Mycophenolate, sirolimus	Autoimmunity, malignancy
	4. Immune deficiency, polyendocrinopathy, X-linked	T-regulatory cell dysfunction	FoxP3	*Staphylococcus*, gram-negative bacteria, PJP, *Candida*, CMV	Sinopulmonary, MM, skin, GI	Steroids, sirolimus, antibiotics as needed, HSCT?	Growth failure, IDDM, eczema, rash, autoimmunity
	5. Autoimmune polyendocrinopathy–candidiasis–ectodermal dystrophy	T-cell anergy to candida antigen stimulation, variable B-cell defects	AIRE	*Candida*	MM, skin	Antifungals	Autoimmunity, hypoparathyroidism, Addison disease

(continued)

TABLE 86.1 (continued)

SUMMARY OF PRIMARY IMMUNE DEFICIENCY DISORDERS

CATEGORY	NAME	TYPE OF DEFICIENCY	GENE	PRIMARY ORGANISMS	USUAL SITES	TREATMENT	ASSOCIATED FINDINGS
	6. Wiskott–Aldrich syndrome	Low levels of IgM, elevated IgA, B- and T-cell dysfunction	WASP	Encapsulated bacteria, PJP, *Candida*, viruses	Sinopulmonary, MM, skin	IVIG, antibiotics as needed, HSCT	Eczema, bleeding, thrombocytopenia, HSM, malignancy, autoimmunity
	7. X-linked lymphoproliferative disorder	T- and B-cell dysfunction, low immunoglobulins	SH2D1A	EBV	Sinopulmonary, lymph nodes, liver	Rituximab or etoposide, acutely IVIG, HSCT	Lymphadenopathy, hepatic necrosis, HLH, malignancy
	8. Ataxia telangiectasia	Low levels of IgA and IgG$_2$, cutaneous anergy	ATM	Encapsulated bacteria	Sinopulmonary	IVIG, antibiotics as needed	Muscle weakness, ataxia, malignancy, telangiectasias
	9. Dedicator of cytokinesis 8 deficiency	Dysfunctional T-cell expansion, lymphopenia, B-cell dysfunction, elevated IgE	DOCK 8	*Staphylococcus aureus*, viruses (esp. herpes, HPV, molluscum)	Sinopulmonary, skin	Antibiotics, HSCT?	Eczema, severe allergies, asthma, malignancy
Neutropenia	1. Severe congenital neutropenia	Neutrophil maturation defect	ELANE?HAX1	Pyogenic bacteria	Skin, MM, lymph node, blood	GCSF	Agranulocytosis, MDS/AML
	2. Cyclic neutropenia	Neutrophil maturation defect	ELANE?	Pyogenic bacteria	Skin, MM, lymph node	GCSF	Periodic fevers, aphthous ulcers
	3. Primary autoimmune neutropenia	Antibody directed against neutrophil	Unknown	Pyogenic bacteria	Sinopulmonary, skin	Antibiotics, TMP–SMX, GCSF	URI, may resolve by age 3
	4. Shwachman–Diamond syndrome	Neutropenia, T-, B-, and NK-cell abnormalities	SBDS	Pyogenic bacteria	Sinopulmonary	GCSF, antibiotics as needed	Pancreatic insufficiency, leukemia, skeletal anomalies, pancytopenia, MDS
Neutrophil dysfunction	1. Neutrophil adhesion defects, LAD-1/LAD-2/LAD-3	Abnormal neutrophil migration	CD18/Sialyl-Lewis X, FERMT3	*Staphylococcus* species, gram-negative bacteria, fungi	Skin, lymph node, MM, liver, bone	Antimicrobials, HSCT, oral fucose—LAD-2	Gingivitis, impaired wound healing, UC separation delayed
	2. Hyper-IgE syndrome	Impaired chemotaxis, T- and B-cell dysfunction	Unknown	*Staphylococcus* species, *Streptococcus* species	Skin, lung (abscesses with pneumatoceles)	*Staphylococcus* prophylaxis, antibiotics as needed, IVIG?	Skeletal/connective tissue abnormalities, eczema, ↑eosinophils
	3. Chronic granulomatous disease	Oxidative burst and bactericidal activity impaired	gp91^{phox}, p22^{phox}, p47^{phox}	*Staphylococcus* species, catalase-positive bacteria, fungi	Sinopulmonary, lung, bone, liver, GI, skin, MM	Antifungal prophylaxis, TMP–SMX, IFN-γ, HSCT	Intestinal and bladder obstruction, osteomyelitis, liver abscesses
	4. Chediak–Higashi syndrome	Abnormal degranulation	LYST	Pyogenic bacteria	Sinopulmonary, Skin	Ascorbic acid, folate, antibiotics as needed	Bleeding, albinism, HLH, peripheral neuropathy

	Defect	Gene/component	Organisms	Site	Treatment	Clinical features
Complement						
1. C1, C2, C3, C4	Low component levels	C1, C2, C3, C4	Encapsulated organisms	Skin, blood	Antibiotics as needed	Lupus-like syndrome
2. C5–9	Absent membrane attack complex	C5–9	Meningococci	Blood, meninges	Vaccination, early antibiotic therapy	Recurrent meningitis
3. Properdin deficiency	Unstable C3 and C5 convertases	PFC	Meningococci	Blood, meninges	Vaccination, early antibiotic therapy	Recurrent meningitis
4. Mannon-binding lectin deficiency	Impaired MASP-activation	MBL	Various bacteria	Sinopulmonary, meninges, blood	Antibiotics as needed	Autoimmunity, ↑SIRS/severity, Kawasaki disease?
5. Mannan-binding lectin–associated serine protease 2 deficiency	Decreased MASP-2 levels	MASP-2	Various bacteria	Sinopulmonary, meninges, blood	Antibiotics as needed	↑Risk febrile neutropenia in cancer patients
6. Hereditary angioedema	Low C4 and C1-INH	C1-INH	None	GI, upper respiratory tract, extremities	C1-INH replacement, kinin-pathway modulators, FFP	Abdominal crises, airway obstruction
Toll-like receptors						
MYD88 serineprotease deficiency, IRAK-4 deficiency	Impaired TLR signaling	NEMO, IRAK-4	Gram-positive bacteria	Sinopulmonary, Blood	Antibiotics as needed	Recurrent sepsis

GI, gastrointestinal; SC, subcutaneous; NEMO, nuclear factor-κB essential modulator; PJP, *Pneumocystis jirovecii* pneumonia; MM, mucous membrane; TMP–SMX, trimethoprim–sulfamethoxazole; FFP, fresh frozen plasma; PNP, polynucleotide phosphorylase; HSM, hepatosplenomegaly; IDDM, insulin-dependent diabetes mellitus; SBDS, Shwachman–Bodian–Diamond syndrome; URI, upper respiratory infections; UC, umbilical cord.

pyogenic bacteria, such as pneumococci, streptococci, meningococci, *H. influenzae*, and *Pseudomonas aeruginosa*. Infections with fungal pathogens and even *Pneumocystis jirovecii* are occasionally reported (7). In addition, there is a unique susceptibility to enteroviral infections in patients with XLA; poliomyelitis was a significant risk for these children in the era of oral polio vaccine. Neutropenia is present in up to 25% of XLA patients at the time of diagnosis (8,9). Recognition of hypoplastic lymphoid tissue in the setting of invasive infection should heighten suspicion of a disorder, such as XLA, in which mature B cells are absent from both lymphoid tissues and the circulation. Mature B cells, which comprise the bulk of tonsilar and lymphoid follicular tissue, are virtually absent from the circulation (<1% of circulating lymphocytes). Plasma cells and immunoglobulins are consequently also lacking, such that immunoglobulin levels are <10% of normal, and antigen-specific responses cannot be demonstrated. An early clue to immunoglobulin deficiency is the finding of a low total protein level in the presence of a normal albumin level on routine blood analysis (since gammaglobulin comprises the largest fraction of the total protein measurement). The genetic defects of XLA are mutations in the Bruton tyrosine kinase (*BTK*) gene at Xq22. A diagnosis can be supported by genotyping, but the absence of mature B cells in the peripheral blood demonstrated by flow cytometry analysis of B-cell surface markers (CD19 and/or CD20) in the presence of normal T-cell numbers is virtually diagnostic of XLA in a male (10).

The mainstay of therapy is immunoglobulin replacement. In the intensive care setting, immunoglobulin replacement therapy can be helpful in the control and clearance of severe infections, and IV administration at physiologic replacement doses of 400–500 mg/kg is most appropriate. Children with a known diagnosis of IgG deficiency may benefit from intravenous immunoglobulin (IVIG) at the time of infections (11). In spite of consistent IgG replacement therapy, a significant proportion of XLA patients progress to bronchiectasis, and chronic antibiotic therapy is recommended for this subset of patients (12). With currently available treatment, most patients lead productive and relatively infection free lives.

Common Variable Immunodeficiency

Common variable immunodeficiency (CVID) describes a group of primary immunodeficiencies that usually present during the second or third decades of life, although ~20% will present during the pediatric years. Total IgG levels in CVID are less than two standard deviations below the mean for age, but generally not as low as those found in XLA. Usually IgA levels are low, and many will have reduced IgM levels (13). The incidence of CVID is estimated to be between 1 in 25,000 and 1 in 50,000 individuals. Patients present in a fashion similar to XLA with recurrent sinopulmonary disease related to encapsulated organisms. Sarcoidosis-like pulmonary granulomas and lymphoid hyperplasia may complicate the interpretation of pulmonary infections. Malabsorptive symptoms should prompt a workup to rule out *Giardia lamblia* infection and autoimmune enteritis similar to celiac enteropathy and/or inflammatory bowel disease. Autoimmune cytopenias are found in 10% of CVID patients, and multiple other autoimmune disease manifestations are reported. Nearly half of these patients manifest mild cellular immune deficiency characterized by chronic viral and fungal infections. Impaired cellular immunity probably underlies the 8- to 13-fold increase in total malignancies in this population and the 438-fold increase in lymphomas among females with CVID (14). Again, immunoglobulin levels are not typically as low as those in XLA, and mature B cells are detected by flow cytometry, but most patients have decreased memory B cells

(13). Impaired vaccine responses, in particular to diphtheria and tetanus toxoid antigens, are most helpful in defining this disorder. Treatment involves intravenous or subcutaneous antibody replacement, being careful to use IgA-depleted products in IgA-deficient patients because of the potential risk of anaphylaxis in those patients who may have anti-IgA antibodies (15). Patients with granulomatous disease have been treated with corticosteroids, and more recently, with etanercept after careful consideration of malignant and infectious etiologies (16). The +448A polymorphism of the TNF-α gene has been associated with granuloma formation in CVID patients (17). There is significant genetic heterogeneity in the CVID population. The largest subgroup (10%) identified thus far relates to mutations in the transmembrane activator and calcium modulator and cyclophilin ligand interactor (*TACI*) gene (18). A smaller subgroup has been found to have mutations in the inducible T-cell costimulator gene (*ICOS*). Occasionally, patients with mutations in genes associated with more classical immunodeficiencies, such as BTK and SH2D1A (mutated in X-linked lymphoproliferative disease [XLP]), have been described (2).

Transient Hypogammaglobulinemia of Infancy

A number of premature, and occasionally, term infants develop an exaggerated hypogammaglobulinemia at the natural nadir of maternal immunoglobulin between 6 and 9 months of age. While immunoglobulin values in these infants overlap with those of immunodeficient infants, normal antigen responses can eventually be demonstrated and most of these infants mature to have normal immunologic function. Normalization of IgG levels can be expected between 2 and 4 years of age. Upper respiratory infections are common in these infants, and only rarely can IVIG use be justified to treat more invasive infections. The occurrence of invasive infections and the need for IVIG therapy should prompt reconsideration of a mild XLA phenotype, early onset CVID, or a CID.

Hyper-IgM Syndrome

The occurrence of hypogammaglobulinemia with normal to high IgM levels was first recognized in males. It is now clear that both an X-linked defect in the CD40 ligand (CD154) and autosomal defects in CD40 (CD40 AR), activation-induced cytidine deaminase (AICDA) deficiency, AICDA C-terminal domain defects, uracil DNA glycosylase (UNG), and nuclear factor (NF)-κB signaling (NEMO) lead to the hyper-IgM (HIGM) phenotype (19). The resultant immunologic dysfunction with these mutations is defective CD40 signaling by B cells affecting class-switch recombination and sometimes somatic hypermutation. The X-linked form accounts for 65%–70% of all cases. These males generally present in infancy with upper and lower respiratory tract infections, and up to 40% will present with interstitial pneumonitis from *P. jirovecii* infection. Diarrhea is another common presenting symptom, often associated with *cryptosporidium* infection. Cytopenias, lymphoid hyperplasia, inflammatory bowel disease, and seronegative arthritis are not infrequent manifestations of autoimmune disease in HIGM patients, reflecting T-cell dysfunction. The patients with CD40 AR will also have a similar, combined immunodeficiency (CID) presentation. Significant early mortality from chronic liver disease and malignancy has justified trials of stem cell transplantation for these patients. The other HIGM presentations appear as pure humoral defects (19).

DISORDERS PREDOMINANTLY AFFECTING CELLULAR FUNCTION

7 Defects localized within the T-cell compartment affecting either maturation of T cells or specific T-cell functions are considered here. Dysgammaglobulinemia, as in the HIGM syndrome, is a frequent consequence of T-cell dysfunction, given the necessary role of T-cell signaling for immunoglobulin class switching and affinity maturation. Thus, some degree **8** of antibody deficiency will accompany most cellular defects. The cardinal clinical features of T-cell dysfunction are fungal infections, chronic viral infections, opportunistic infections, autoimmune disorders, and malignancies.

22q11.2 Deletion Syndrome

Infants with *DiGeorge syndrome* (DGS) and velocardiofacial syndrome have a characteristic 22q11.2 deletion and **9** frequently manifest T-cell deficiency due to lack of normal thymic development. The frequency of these deletion syndromes is ~1 in 4000 persons. Genes within the characteristic deletion on chromosome 22 direct neural crest migration into the third and fourth pharyngeal arches, and the absence of these genes results in conotruncal cardiac defects, parathyroid hypoplasia, and thymic hypoplasia. The most common cardiac anomalies in DGS, in order of prevalence, are interrupted aortic arch type B (IAA type B), persistent truncus arteriosus, tetralogy of Fallot, right aortic arch, ventricular septal defect, and patent ductus arteriosus. Of all patients with IAA type B, up to 80% have DGS. Of all patients with persistent truncus arteriosus and tetralogy of Fallot, 35% and 10%, respectively, have DGS (20,21).

The characteristic deletion can be demonstrated by FISH probe in 90% of infants with the DiGeorge phenotype and a smaller percentage of infants with the velocardiofacial phenotype (4). Most DGS infants are recognized during the neonatal period due to congenital heart defects and/or hypocalcemia symptoms, such as tetany or seizures. There is a poor correlation, however, between genotype and phenotype, particularly with regards to thymic hypoplasia. Even in the presence of the characteristic 22q11.2 deletion clinical syndrome of cardiac defects, hypocalcemia, and facial dysmorphology, complete thymic absence (complete DiGeorge) occurs in no more than 5% of affected infants. The remainder has variable degrees of thymic hypoplasia, altered T-cell kinetics, and occasional increased susceptibility to infection. In one series of 195 patients defined by the 22q11.2 deletion, only minimal difficulties with bacterial infections were noted, while a significant incidence of autoimmune disease, such as juvenile rheumatoid arthritis and immune thrombocytopenic purpura, was reported (22).

In the immediate postnatal period, absolute CD3 counts <50 predict poor T-cell function and the potential need for immune reconstitution with either a thymic or hematopoietic stem cell transplant (HSCT) (23). Spontaneous improvement in T-cell numbers and function has been documented, and serial T-cell counts are needed to distinguish complete DGS from delayed T-cell maturation. Infants with absolute CD3 counts below 1500 at birth should receive *P. jirovecii* prophylaxis. In addition, only cytomegalovirus (CMV)-negative and irradiated blood products should be transfused to avoid risks of infection and graft-versus-host disease (GVHD). Perioperative corticosteroid treatment may confound the immunologic workup in those infants requiring immediate cardiac surgery, and thus, repeat flow cytometry studies should be considered at ~1 month of age.

Defects in the IFN-γ-IL-12 Axis

Other predominantly cellular defects include defects in the IFN-γ-IL-12 axis, chronic mucocutaneous candidiasis, idiopathic CD4 lymphopenia, and natural killer (NK) cell dysfunction (2). The IFN-γ-IL-12 axis is an important component of the defense against intracellular organisms, such as mycobacteria, *Salmonella*, and *Listeria*. Systemic infections with atypical mycobacteria and fatalities after bacille Calmette–Guerin (BCG) immunizations have been described in patients with abnormalities of this axis. Defects causing increased susceptibility to mycobacterial infections have been described in various portions of the IFN-γ receptor, the IL-12 receptor, and IL-12. This group of disorders has been referred to as mendelian susceptibility to mycobacterial disease (24). The severity of infections and response to IFN-γ therapy depends on the location and severity of the defect. Patients who have the most severe form of the disease, complete IFN-γ receptor 1 deficiency, may be candidates for HSCT. Unlike the other disorders within this group, these patients will have no response to IFN-γ therapy because they have a complete deficiency of the IFN-γ receptor (25).

IMMUNODEFICIENCY WITH CYTOTOXIC DEFECTS

Hemophagocytic Lymphohistiocytosis and Macrophage Activation Syndrome

10 Hemophagocytic lymphohistiocytosis (HLH) and macrophage activation syndrome (MAS) comprise a spectrum of disorders related to defective NK cells or cytotoxic T cells. Both disorders share the same diagnostic criteria and the pathophysiology of **11** both disorders is characterized by uncontrolled inflammation. However, MAS is typically seen in patients with autoimmune **12** disease and often resolves with aggressive treatment of the underlying autoimmune disorder. HLH requires much more aggressive therapy, often including HSCT.

HLH is often divided into familial HLH and acquired HLH. Clinically, the different types are often indistinguishable with the exception that the familial forms present at <1 year of age in 70%–80% of the cases, while the acquired forms may present at any age. Familial forms of HLH may also be associated with an immunodeficiency, most notably Chediak–Higashi syndrome, Griscelli syndrome type 2, and XLP. HLH is a frequent, but not absolute component of these disorders. Although acquired HLH is usually associated with infections, it may also occur with malignancy, inborn errors of metabolism, and after HSCT (26).

Several genetic mutations have been discovered in familial HLH. Between 20% and 50% of families have a defect in the perforin gene (*PRF*). This defect results in the production of a nonfunctional (defective) perforin protein. Perforin is secreted by cytotoxic T cells and NK cells. Perforin protein functions to perforate the cell membrane of target cells, thereby enabling the entry of granzymes into the target cell. This process ultimately results in apoptosis of the target cell (27). A mutation in the *MUNC13-4* gene accounts for up to 20% of patients with familial HLH. Patients with this defect are unable to release granules from cytotoxic T cells in a normal manner (28). A third genetic locus, which involves the syntaxin 11 (*STX11*) gene, has been described in familial HLH patients. Syntaxin 11 is a protein believed to be important in intracellular trafficking. Patients with mutations involving this gene may have a slightly milder phenotype than the other forms of familial HLH. However, they may also be at more risk for myelodysplastic syndrome (MDS), acute myelocytic leukemia (AML), and developmental delay (29).

Patients with the underlying immunodeficiencies that frequently develop HLH (Chediak–Higashi syndrome, Griscelli syndrome, and XLP) have also been found to have genetic mutations associated with impaired cytotoxic abilities. Patients with Chediak–Higashi syndrome have been found to have mutations in the *CHSI/LYST* gene. The LYST protein is involved in fusing granules to cell membranes. Griscelli syndrome patients who develop HLH have been noted to have mutations in the *RAB27A* gene. RAB27A plays a role in vesicle movement. Patients with these defects have been found to have poor cytotoxic function. XLP is associated with defects in the *SAP/SH2D1A* gene. The protein encoded by this gene is important for the recruitment of signaling molecules involved in cytotoxic immunity (28).

The pathophysiology involved in HLH and MAS is incompletely understood. However, it is known that it involves a severe, uncontrolled inflammatory response. Patients who develop HLH have ongoing stimulation of NK cells and cytotoxic T-lymphocytes. These cells continue to produce high levels of inflammatory cytokines, which, in turn, activate histiocytes. These activated cells infiltrate tissues and cause the clinical picture seen in HLH (30).

Patients with HLH typically present with high and prolonged fevers associated with hepatosplenomegaly. Neurologic symptoms, a rash, and lymphadenopathy may also occur. An infectious source may or may not be found. The infections typically associated with HLH are viruses, especially Epstein–Barr virus (EBV), but bacteria and protozoa have also been described as triggering agents (26). At first presentation, these patients may not appear to be critically ill. However, their condition may rapidly deteriorate into a life-threatening illness if HLH is not diagnosed and appropriate treatment is not initiated promptly. The Histiocyte Society has devised diagnostic guidelines to account for variability of presentation (Table 86.2).

Patients must meet five of eight clinical criteria, as shown in Table 86.2, to make the diagnosis. As other critical illnesses (e.g., sepsis, systemic inflammatory response syndrome (SIRS), and multiorgan dysfunction) may often meet these criteria (31) and therapy for HLH is not benign, clinical judgment is important in deciding whether or not to give a critically ill patient what may be potentially toxic or lifesaving therapy. There are a handful of case reports of patients not felt to have the more

severe familial HLH who were treated conservatively with observation alone (32) or a combination of methylprednisolone, IVIG, and plasmapheresis (33) who had reasonable outcomes.

Improvements in the ability to quickly determine whether or not a patient has the more severe familial form of HLH versus a secondary form that may respond to a more conservative approach will be very helpful in the future. A new assay that evaluates NK-cell degranulation may be promising to help differentiate the familial from the secondary form of HLH (34).

Patients who do not receive timely therapy develop a severe SIRS characterized by end-organ damage. Although it is disconcerting for an intensivist to administer chemotherapy to critically ill children with SIRS, patients with the most severe forms of HLH will not improve until appropriate treatment is initiated and time is of the essence. Prompt initiation of therapy is crucial to successful treatment.

Prior to the Histiocyte Society developing their first treatment protocol for HLH, HLH-94, the mortality rate for HLH was close to 100%. However, with the institution of HLH-94, survival improved to 66% for those able to be treated with HSCT. Patients with familial HLH had a 50% survival rate overall. However, there were no survivors of familial HLH without HSCT (35). The Histiocyte Society revised HLH-94 based on their outcome data, and patients are now being treated on the revised protocol, HLH-2004. The protocol is quite similar but patients are being treated earlier with cyclosporine and there are slight changes in the treatment of patients with central nervous system (CNS) disease (27). Treatment for HLH initially involves controlling the exuberant inflammatory response and treating any underlying infection or malignancy. Corticosteroids are used to help decrease cytokine and chemokine production. Dexamethasone was chosen by the Histiocyte Society for HLH-2004, as it crosses the blood–brain barrier and patients with HLH may have CNS involvement. Cyclosporine A is used for its ability to inhibit activation of T-lymphocytes. Etoposide is used for its toxicity to monocytes and histiocytes (26). These three medications are the mainstay of therapy in the HLH-2004 protocol. Intrathecal therapy is also utilized for patients with CNS disease. Once patients are in remission, those with a known familial disease or genetic mutation, those with severe persistent disease, or those with reactivation of their disease go on to HSCT when an appropriate donor is identified. For patients who achieve

TABLE 86.2

DIAGNOSTIC GUIDELINES FOR HEMOPHAGOCYTIC LYMPHOHISTIOCYTOSIS

The diagnosis of HLH can be made by one of the following:
1. Molecular diagnosis consistent with HLH (*PRF* mutation, *MUNC13-4* mutation, etc.)
OR
2. Having 5 of the following 8 criteria:
 a. Fever
 b. Splenomegaly
 c. Cytopenias affecting ≥ 2 cell lines
  Hemoglobin < 9 g/dL (≤10g/dL for infants <4 weeks of age)
  Platelet count < 100,000/μL
  Neutrophils < 1000/μL
 d. Hypertriglyceridemia (≥265 mg/dL) and/or hypofibrinoginemia (≤150 mg/dL)
 e. Hemophagocytosis in bone marrow, spleen, or lymph nodes without evidence of malignancy
 f. Low or absent NK-cell activity
 g. Hyperferritinemia (≥500 μg/L)
 h. Elevated soluble CD25 (IL-2Rα chain) ≥ 2400 U/mL

Adapted from Henter JI, Horne A, Arico M, et al. HLH-2004: Diagnostic and therapeutic guidelines for hemophagocytic lymphohistiocytosis. *Pediatr Blood Cancer* 2007;48:124–31.

remission and do not have genetic disease, therapy is discontinued in order to avoid the need for HSCT if possible (27). MAS has the same clinical presentation as HLH, but MAS is more responsive to immunosuppressive therapies. While most reports of MAS in the literature involve systemic onset juvenile idiopathic arthritis (SOJIA) patients, there are case reports of MAS in the context of several other connective tissue and autoinflammatory diseases (36). In addition, one of the authors has personal experience with three children on hyperalimentation for short gut syndrome who developed MAS. In this setting, MAS resolved once intralipid infusions were reduced to the minimum fatty acid requirements.

Management of MAS involves withdrawal of potentially hepatotoxic medications, including nonsteroidal anti-inflammatory medications, administration of high–dose pulse corticosteroids (Solumedrol 30 mg/kg, maximum 1 g/day), and additional treatment with cyclosporine A for rapidly progressive and refractory cases (37). Criteria for early identification of MAS have been proposed. A decrease in platelet count, combined with a DIC-like coagulopathy and hepatic dysfunction, is a very sensitive and specific triad of the diagnosis of MAS. Clinical criteria, which are less specific, include CNS dysfunction, evidence of hemorrhage, and hepatomegaly. The demonstration of hemophagocytosis is not required for diagnosis, but hemophagocytosis in a bone marrow aspirate from a patient with SOJIA is virtually diagnostic of MAS (38). Perforin mutations are found in only a small minority of SOJIA patients who experience MAS. NK-cell function also tends to be normal in these patients. The excessive activation and proliferation of T cells and macrophages, which results in unrestricted release of inflammatory cytokines, is clearly the result of an aberrant inflammatory response. Recent laboratory and therapeutic experiences indicate that IL-1 dysregulation may be at the heart of MAS occurring in the context of SOJIA (39).

IMMUNODEFICIENCY WITH COMBINED ANTIBODY AND CELLULAR DEFECTS

Patients affected by CIDs, in general, manifest failure to thrive and recurrent infections with opportunistic pathogens, such as CMV, *Candida albicans* (thrush), and *P. jirovecii* pneumonia. It is important to note that *P. jirovecii* infection in an infant nearly always indicates a CID. Other common findings include chronic diarrhea, recurrent bacterial infections, and failure to clear adequately treated infections. Maternal–fetal or transfusion-acquired GVHD from "donor" lymphocytes is another prominent feature in infants with CID. The CIDs represent a spectrum of disease, the more severe being severe combined immunodeficiency (SCID).

Severe Combined Immunodeficiency

SCID represents a genetically heterogenous group of condition that as a whole is the prototype of CIDs. The incidence of SCID is estimated to be from 1 in 100,000 to 1 in 150,000 individuals. These infants usually present in the first month of life with refractory oral candidiasis and persistent viral infections. *P. jirovecii* is a frequent cause of morbidity and mortality in this group of infants. Absolute lymphopenia <2000 cells/mm^3 is a common laboratory finding, even on cord blood specimens (40). Flow cytometry will generally indicate very low absolute CD3 or T-cell numbers. Maternal T-cell engraftment, however, may dramatically affect the fetal T-cell population, and thus, clinical suspicion of SCID can justify lymphocyte proliferation assays regardless of lymphocyte counts. B and NK cells may be present or absent, depending on the specific defect (**Table 86.3**).

T-cell–deficient, B-cell–present (T−B+) SCID is the largest subtype of SCID and is most commonly related to mutations in the IL-2 receptor (*IL2R*) gene on the X chromosome, which encodes the cytokine receptor gamma chain (γ_c) common to multiple cytokine receptors. Janus kinase 3 (JAK3) mediates γ_c signal transduction, therefore, JAK3 mutations result in a similar phenotype, although the pattern of inheritance is autosomal recessive (AR). Approximately 50% of both T- and B-cell–deficient (T−B−) SCID is related to mutations in the genes (RAG1/2) that regulate the somatic recombination of immunoglobulin and T-cell receptor genes during B- and T-cell development. Partial function of RAG1 or RAG2 is one cause of *Omenn syndrome*, which is characterized by erythroderma, eosinophilia, lymphoid hyperplasia, and hypogammaglobulinemia (41). Circulating lymphocytes in RAG1/2-deficient patients are primarily NK cells. Metabolic defects in the purine salvage pathway do not spare NK cells, and thus, patients who present with adenosine deaminase (ADA) deficiency often have the most profound lymphopenia. Multiple skeletal abnormalities, including dysplasia of vertebral bodies and flaring of the costochondral junctions, may be seen in up to 50% of these infants. In addition to ADA deficiency, several other immune-osseous syndromes combine skeletal abnormalities with variable degrees of CID, including short-limbed dwarfism with and without ectodermal dysplasia, cartilage hair hypoplasia, CID with metaphyseal dysplasia, and Schimke immune-osseous dysplasia. The intensive care of an infant suspected or known to have SCID should include strict isolation and the use of only irradiated, CMV-negative, and leukocyte-depleted blood products. The intensivist should maintain a high index of suspicion for *P. jirovecii* infection, and both respiratory secretions and stool should be tested for a variety of pathogens. The infant with SCID may benefit from aggressive antiviral therapies in addition to antibiotics and IVIG. An immunologist or hematologist should be involved early in the care of

TABLE 86.3

LYMPHOCYTE PHENOTYPES CHARACTERISTICALLY ASSOCIATED WITH THE FORMS OF SEVERE COMBINED IMMUNODEFICIENCY DISEASE (53,91)

| ■ FORM OF SCID | T CELLS | | | ■ B CELLS | ■ NK CELLS |
	■ CD3	■ CD4	■ CD8		
X-linked, Jak3, IL-2R, IL-7R	↓	↓	↓	Normal	↓
RAG1/2	↓	↓	↓	↓	Normal
ADA	↓	↓	↓	↓	↓
MHC II	Normal	↓	Normal	Normal	Normal
ZAP-70, MHC I	Normal	Normal	↓	Normal	Normal

these infants to facilitate arrangements for HSCT, which remains the most successful therapy for SCID. Survival rates of
>90% can be accomplished with HLA-matched sibling donor
transplants, and even haploidentical transplants from a parent
are reported to be successful in at least 75% of cases (42).

Combined Immunodeficiency Disease

Combined immunodeficiency disease (CID) is at the less severe
end of the spectrum and involves variable degrees of T- and
B-cell dysfunction. With the growing number of identified
CIDs, we have tried to classify the syndromes by the underlying pathway affected with the knowledge that the pathways
exhibit a high degree of overlap and that any classification
schema is ultimately flawed.

Deficiencies in Antigen Presentation Pathways

Bare Lymphocyte Syndrome

Crucial to the adaptive immune system is the capture, processing, and presentation of peptide antigens to both CD4$^+$ and
CD8$^+$ T cells. Fortunately, genetic mutations that interrupt
this system are rare. Bare lymphocyte syndrome (BLS) is a rare
disorder characterized by partial or complete disappearance
of major histocompatibility complex (MHC) molecules from
the surface of cells and can be characterized by the surface
MHC expression (43). Patients with type I BLS have a reduction or absence of MHC class I molecules. Their susceptibility
to infection seems to be inversely proportional to the number
of MHC class I molecules as patients with total absence suffer from frequent infection and have low levels of antibodies.
Patients with transporter-associated antigen-processing protein (TAP) deficiencies are categorized as having type I BLS.
Patients with type II BLS have a deficiency in MHC class II
molecules, which, fortunately, is rare with ~100 unrelated
patients reported worldwide. These patients present with the
same constellation of symptoms of other CIDs with frequent
recurrence of bacterial, viral, and fungal infections, but are
more severe than type I BLS, and have a life expectancy of only
a few years. HSCT is the only known treatment of MHC class
II deficiency, yet these patients have a higher incidence GVHD
than other recipients (44).

Deficiencies in Apoptosis and Tolerance

Autoimmune Lymphoproliferative Syndrome

Autoimmune lymphoproliferative syndrome (ALPS) is characterized by abnormal lymphoproliferation (with patients having lymphadenopathy, splenomegaly, and hepatomegaly) that
develops at a young age (median 11.5 months). Autoimmunity
is common and often manifested as immune-mediated cytopenias. ALPS is due to defects in the Fas/FasL apoptotic pathway
that the immune system uses to downregulate normal immune
responses. Most patients have mutations in the *FAS* gene, and
are inherited in an autosomal dominant (AD) pattern as FAS
defects are dominant negative, heterozygous, missense mutations in the intracellular death domain. FAS mutations often
have variable penetrance with family members showing a wide
spectrum from severe to absent phenotypes. ALPS patients
have an increased incidence of secondary malignancies. This
leads to a diagnostic dilemma as ALPS is difficult to distinguish from lymphomas. Diagnostic criteria include chronic
lymphoproliferation, increased peripheral frequency of double
negative (CD4$^-$ CD8$^-$) T cells, and defective in vitro Fas-
mediated apoptosis. Whereas rituximab and splenectomy are

the mainstay of treatment for refractory autoimmune cytopenias, these treatments are relatively contraindicated in ALPS;
antiproliferative agents, such as mycophenolate and sirolimus,
have shown more success (45).

Immune Deficiency, Polyendocrinopathy, X-linked Syndrome

The defining clinical characteristics of immune deficiency,
polyendocrinopathy, X-linked (IPEX) syndrome are enteropathy, eczematoid rash, and early endocrinopathy, most often,
diabetes mellitus. Up to 50% of patients will present prior to
diagnosis with a serious infection, usually *Staphylococcus*,
Candida, or CMV. Autoimmune cytopenias and splenomegaly
are also frequently noted at presentation. Therapy with sirolimus may be more effective than other forms of immunosuppression for the autoimmune manifestations of this disorder
(46). Immunologic studies are surprisingly normal in most
patients because the responsible *FoxP3* gene mutations on
Xp11.23 impair the normal function of CD4$^+$CD25$^+$ regulatory T cells without otherwise impairing T- or B-cell function.
Survival beyond age 2 is unusual, although milder phenotypes
have been reported. The value of HSCT for this disorder remains unclear.

Autoimmune Polyendocrinopathy Candidiasis Ectodermal Dystrophy

Autoimmune polyendocrinopathy candidiasis ectodermal
dystrophy (APECED) patients usually present with chronic
mucocutaneous candidiasis in infancy, followed by hypoparathyroidism (4–5 years), and then Addison disease (later in
childhood). The complete triad presents itself in two-thirds of
patients. APECED patients have mutations in the autoimmune
regulator (*AIRE*) gene, which functions in thymic medullary
epithelial cells to present multiple self-proteins, and thereby induces self-tolerance (47). Absence/loss of function of the protein leads to a failure of tolerance and autoimmunity. Patients
often have autoantibodies to IFN-α and IFN-ω, providing a
means of diagnosis. Treatment consists of management of the
underlying symptoms and included antifungal, mineralocorticoids, and thyroid replacement therapies.

Deficiencies in Activation and Differentiation

Wiskott–Aldrich Syndrome

Wiskott–Aldrich syndrome (WAS) is an X-linked disorder
often presents with the classic triad of eczema, thrombocytopenia, and immunodeficiency. Boys present with bleeding
within the first year of life, often in the nursery, with bloody
diarrhea or prolonged oozing from a circumcision. Platelets
in WAS patients are abnormally small and defective as compared to the relatively large and functionally normal platelets
seen in immune thrombocytopenic purpura. The intensivist
caring for a WAS patient must be cognizant of both the bleeding and infection risks. Infections often involve encapsulated
organisms related to the inability to produce antibodies in
response to polysaccharide antigens. IgM levels are typically
low as reflected by low isohemagglutinin (blood group) antibodies. B-cell dysfunction is apparent early while T-cell
dysfunction is progressive over time. The mutated WAS protein (WASP) connects T-cell signaling to critical cytoskeletal
regulatory mechanisms necessary for T-cell activation (41).
Minor dysfunction of WASP may be associated with X-linked
thrombocytopenia in some families, and a single case of a
WASP mutation in a patient with X-linked neutropenia has
been reported (2). Autoimmune phenomena are common
manifestations of T-cell dysfunction in WAS. Although IVIG

therapy and splenectomy may help maintain platelet counts and minimize infections, an HLA-matched HSCT from a sibling or from a cord blood bank offers the best chance of long-term survival.

X-linked Lymphoproliferative Disease

The often life-threatening presentation of XLP, or Duncan disease, represents an abnormal immune response to EBV infection. In most cases, it is related to mutations in the *SH2D1A* gene, which encodes the signaling lymphocyte activation molecule–associated protein (SAP) (48). The frequency of XLP is undoubtedly underestimated because of the variability of clinical presentations, due to differing SAP mutations. Classically, patients present with massive lymphadenopathy, hepatic necrosis, and bone marrow failure, much like posttransplant lymphoproliferative disease. This acute presentation of XLP is responsible for the reported 70% mortality by age 10. The remaining 30% may present late, with varying degrees of immune deficiency, ranging from mild hypogammaglobulinemia to CID. As many as one-third of long-term survivors will eventually develop a lymphoreticular malignancy; a 200-fold increased risk of lymphomas is seen in XLP. The diagnosis of XLP is facilitated by positive EBV serology and, more specifically, blood or tissue polymerase chain reaction assays. Bone marrow examination will often indicate hemophagocytosis. Rapid diagnosis is now available by flow cytometry, which documents the absence of intracellular SH2D1A staining in CD8$^+$ T cells (49). Etoposide and rituximab have proven useful in the therapy of acute lymphoproliferation in patients diagnosed prior to EBV exposure (50).

Ataxia Telangiectasia

Patients with ataxia telangiectasia present with delayed ambulation and speech followed by deterioration of gross and fine motor skills. Cerebellar ataxia and oculocutaneous telangiectasias become evident around ~7 years of age. Frequent pulmonary infections may be related to subtle antibody defects or swallowing dysfunction and aspiration. Deficiencies in both humoral and cellular immunity have been reported. Median survival in the Ataxia Telangiectasia Clinical Center at the Johns Hopkins Hospital has recently been reported to be 25 years, with mortality frequently attributed to malignancy. Mutations in the *ATM* gene increase sensitivity to ionizing radiation and lead to a lack of DNA double-strand break recognition and repair. The 10%–30% lifetime prevalence of malignancies is attributable to this defective DNA repair mechanism.

Dedicator of Cytokinesis 8 Deficiency

The constellation of eczema, pneumonia, recurrent skin abscesses, and elevated serum IgE is the usual clinical finding in hyper-IgE syndrome (HIES), which has an AD pattern of inheritance. However, some patients also have increased cutaneous viral illnesses, severe allergies (both food and environmental), and asthma in addition to these symptoms, with an AR pattern of inheritance. These patients have been found to have a deficiency in the *DOCK8* (dedicator of cytokinesis 8) gene. In laboratory models, absence of DOCK8 expression limits T-cell expansion and secondary antibody response to specific antigens; patients with DOCK8 deficiency have a CID. This disease has a high morbidity and mortality rate, with 7 deaths (ages 6–21 years) in a case series of 32, the largest reported series known. Long-term recommendations are unclear, HSCT has been successful in 2 patients, but 2 patients with milder disease have survived without HSCT and are currently in their 40s (51).

DISORDERS AFFECTING PHAGOCYTE FUNCTION

Neutrophil Disorders

Disorders of polymorphonuclear leukocytes, neutrophils, are also relatively uncommon. Patients with these disorders are at increased risk of serious infections that may result in the need for critical care services. It is important for the intensivist to be familiar with these disorders as prompt identification and referral to a hematologist or clinical immunologist may facilitate early diagnosis and institution of appropriate adjunctive therapy. Early recognition and therapy may result in improved outcomes for these high-risk patients.

In order for neutrophils to combat invading pathogens, they must be able to perform a number of complex functions. First and foremost, they must be able to proliferate and mature in the bone marrow. During their maturation, neutrophils form granules that contain bactericidal and hydrolytic proteins important for killing pathogens. Once mature, they must emigrate from the bone marrow into the systemic circulation. There, they must undergo several complex processes. The first is *rolling*, a process in which the neutrophil rolls loosely along the endothelial surface. Once it approximates its target, it binds tightly to the endothelial surface and becomes flattened through a process termed *adhesion*. Finally, the neutrophil must migrate across the endothelium via a process termed *diapedesis*. In order for rolling, adhesion and diapedesis to occur, the neutrophil must communicate with the endothelial surface through the use of cell surface proteins, including selectins, integrin, intercellular adhesion molecule (ICAM)-1, and platelet endothelial cell adhesion molecule (PECAM)-1. Once through the endothelial membrane, the neutrophil is attracted to the invading pathogen by chemotactic factors, including lipopolysaccharide (LPS), IL-1, TNF-α, and IFN-γ via a process called *chemotaxis*. Upon reaching the appropriate site, the neutrophil digests the offending pathogen through *opsonization* and *phagocytosis*. Opsonization is the process where opsonins (such as IgG or C3b) are bound to the pathogen. These opsonins then bind to their receptors on the neutrophil (Fc receptors and complement receptors) allowing the neutrophil to phagocytose (digest) the pathogen (4). These various complex interactions between neutrophils, endothelial cells, and other components of the immune system provide many opportunities where neutrophil function can be impaired. In general, neutrophil disorders can be divided into two broad categories: diseases associated with decreased numbers of neutrophils (neutropenia) and those with impaired neutrophil function.

The group from Meir Medical Center, Israel's main center for neutrophil function studies, reviewed data on 998 pediatric and adult patients over 21 years referred for workup of neutrophil dysfunction (52). Through their retrospective review of these patients, they identified patients at highest risk for an identifiable neutrophil disorder. Patient characteristics most likely to have an identifiable neutrophil disorder included those with (a) positive family history, (b) young age, (c) deep-seated infections, (d) multiorgan involvement, (e) opportunistic infections, and (f) tissue granulomas of unknown etiology. The authors concluded that patients with any of these characteristics should be considered for investigation of a neutrophil disorder.

Disorders Associated with Primary Neutropenia

Severe Congenital Neutropenia and Cyclic Neutropenia

In addition to the more common acquired forms of neutropenia, such as that secondary to cancer and its therapy, there are also congenital causes of neutropenia that must be considered. Severe congenital neutropenia (SCN) and cyclic neutropenia are examples of inherited neutropenic disorders. Both of these conditions have been associated with mutations in the gene encoding neutrophil elastase, ELA2, or ELANE. Several heterozygous mutations of ELANE have been described in nearly all patients with cyclic neutropenia, and in most patients with SCN (53). However, the role that these ELANE mutations play in the pathophysiology of these disorders has not been well established (54). There is growing evidence that there are modifying genes involved in the pathogenesis of these ELANE-related disorders as patients with the same ELANE mutation may have very different phenotypes. One patient may have cyclic neutropenia while the other has SCN (55).

Mutations involving other genes have also been described in patients with SCN. Mutations in the WAS gene have been described in patients with X-linked SCN. HAX1 mutations have recently been discovered in the AR form of SCN known as *Kostmann syndrome*. Extremely rare mutation in GF11 and G6PC3 causing SCN have also been described (56).

Myeloid precursor cells from patients with these conditions demonstrate an abnormal response to hematopoietic growth factors. However, they commonly respond to treatment with granulocyte colony-stimulating factor (GCSF). This response to GCSF decreases the degree of neutropenia, and therefore, the rate of serious infection (57). Patients with SCN have profound neutropenia (an absolute neutrophil count (ANC) <500 neutrophils/m³), and they experience recurrent bacterial infections beginning in the first year of life. Infections are commonly caused by *Staphylococcus aureus* and *P. aeruginosa*. Pathophysiologically, this disease is characterized by a maturational failure of promyelocytes to myelocytes (57). Clinically, these children have a risk of death from sepsis of 0.9% per year as well as a significant risk of malignant transformation to MDS/AML. The risk of development of MDS/AML increases with time ranging from 2.9% per year during the first 6 years of therapy with GCSF up to 8.0% per year after 12 years of treatment (58). In a recent study from Sweden, the risk of developing MDS/leukemia for patients with SCN was as high as 31% (59). In patients at high risk of malignant transformation, such as those receiving high-dose GCSF or who possess the Gly185Arg mutation of the ELANE gene, HSCT should be given strong consideration (60).

Cyclic neutropenia is a rare AD disorder. Patients with cyclic neutropenia experience recurrent episodes of severe neutropenia lasting 3–6 days and occurring in cycles of every 14–36 days. Although these patients may be asymptomatic, during neutropenic cycles they may develop aphthous ulcers, gingivitis, stomatitis, and cellulitis and are at increased risk of mortality from serious infection (57). In contrast to patients with severe SCN, these patients do not appear to be at increased risk for the development of MDS/AML (54).

Autoimmune Neutropenia

Autoimmune neutropenia must also be considered in the differential diagnosis of neutropenia. This type of neutropenia may be either primary or secondary. Secondary autoimmune neutropenias are associated with inflammatory diseases, such as rheumatoid arthritis (i.e., Felty syndrome) and systemic lupus erythematosus (SLE). Often, these patients will have additional hematologic abnormalities, such as thrombocytopenia and/or hemolytic anemia. Successful treatment and control of the underlying disease is the most effective therapy for the neutropenia.

Primary autoimmune neutropenia most commonly begins in the newborn period and is frequently diagnosed within the first several months of life. These patients have significant neutropenia at presentation, with an ANC often <500–1000 neutrophils/m³. However, severe infections, such as pneumonia,

sepsis, and meningitis, are relatively uncommon, occurring in only about 10% of these children. Most patients present with relatively benign infections, such as otitis media, upper respiratory infections, and dermatitis, and the disease commonly resolves spontaneously by 2–3 years of age. Autoimmune neutropenia, as its name implies, is caused by antibodies directed against the neutrophil. These antibodies are frequently directed against the HNA-1a and HNA-1b antigens, although antibodies to the CD11/CD18 complex, CD35, and FcγRIIb have been described. Testing for these antibodies is often falsely negative, and thus, repeat testing is indicated if the diagnosis is strongly suspected. In patients with a serious clinical course, a maturational arrest in the myelocyte/metamyelocyte stage may be detected upon examination of the bone marrow. This is thought to occur because the antibodies directed toward the mature neutrophils also attack their precursors in the bone marrow. The treatment for patients with a benign form of autoimmune neutropenia may simply be antibiotics as needed to treat infections or antibiotic prophylaxis with agents, such as trimethoprim–sulfamethoxazole. For patients with serious infections, GCSF has been found to be beneficial and is considered first-line therapy. Although corticosteroids and IVIG have been utilized, they do not appear to be as beneficial as GCSF (4,61). A new test for autoimmune neutropenia, which is a direct granulocyte immunofluorescence test (D-GIFT), has recently been reported to be more sensitive than previous methods. This may decrease the need for the repeated testing frequently required to diagnose primary autoimmune neutropenia (62).

Shwachman–Diamond Syndrome

Shwachman–Diamond syndrome is a rare autosomal disorder associated with neutropenia, exocrine pancreatic insufficiency, skeletal abnormalities, recurrent infections, and occasionally, pancytopenia. It is caused by a mutation in the gene encoding the Shwachman–Bodian–Diamond syndrome protein. The neutropenia associated with this disorder may be persistent or cyclic. Moreover, in addition to neutropenia, these patients may also have abnormalities of T cell, B cell, and NK lymphocytes (4). GCSF therapy is useful in this condition to reduce the risk of serious infection. These children are at increased risk of myelodysplasia and leukemia independent of the use of GCSF (57).

Disorders of Neutrophil Function

Defects of Neutrophil Adhesion

In addition to disorders associated with an absolute decrease in the number of neutrophils, several conditions have been identified in which neutrophil function is compromised. For example, in leukocyte adhesion disorders, neutrophils are unable to bind appropriately to the endothelial surface, complete diapedesis, and migrate to the site of infection. First described in the 1980s, leukocyte adhesion deficiency type 1 (LAD-1) is an AR disorder caused by genetic mutations encoding CD18, the γ subunit of the neutrophil adhesion molecule LFA-1. The neutrophils of patients with this disorder are unable to adhere appropriately to the endothelial surface, and therefore, are unable to migrate toward the site of infections. Patients often present with recurrent, severe infections and may have a history of delayed umbilical cord separation. The most frequent pathogens are enteric gram-negative bacteria, *S. aureus*, *Candida*, and *Aspergillus* species. These patients also exhibit impaired wound healing and have elevated neutrophil counts in the peripheral blood because their neutrophils are not able to marginate (57). Although rare, other types of leukocyte adhesion disorders have been described. LAD type 2 patients have impaired fucose metabolism that can affect the expression of fucosylated receptors on the neutrophil, which are important for leukocyte rolling along the vessel wall. Patients with this disorder are characterized by immunologic deficiencies as well as mental retardation, short stature, and distinctive facies. These patients may benefit from oral fucose therapy (4). A mutation involving RAC2, a neutrophil GTPase important for the function of the neutrophil actin cytoskeleton, has also been described. This patient had a similar phenotype to patients with LAD-1 and was treated successfully with a matched related HSCT (4). Recently LAD III has been described. These patients have impaired activation of β-integrins 1, 2, and 3 due to a genetic defect of the *FERMT3* gene. This defect causes abnormalities in kindlin-3 protein expression. Patients with LAD III have severe recurrent infections, bleeding tendency, and leukocytosis. Some patients have been described as having bony defects similar to osteopetrosis. Treatment for these patients includes prophylactic antibiotics and blood transfusions, and HSCT has also been used with success (63).

Hyper-IgE Syndrome (Job Syndrome)

HIES (or Job syndrome) is an immunodeficiency first described by Buckley et al. in 1972. The classic form of the disease is characterized by recurrent staphylococcal infections, eczema, recurrent respiratory infections with persistent pneumatoceles, elevated IgE levels, eosinophilia, abnormal cytokine and chemokine expression, and T-cell dysfunction. Neutrophil chemotaxis may be impaired in some patients. Patients have been described as having coarse facial features, joint hyperextensibility, osteopenia, and prolonged retention of primary teeth, but the features may be quite variable (4).

Sporadic, AD, and AR forms have been described with the sporadic and AD forms fitting the classical description. Mutations in the *STAT3* gene have been recently discovered in patients with the AD form of HIES. The stat3 molecule plays an important role in signal transduction of multiple cytokines. Patients with mutations in the *STAT3* gene have problems with maturation of Th17 CD4 cells. This likely is the cause of the increased susceptibility to infection in patients with AD HIES (64). The only treatment known to be of clear benefit is antibiotic prophylaxis against staphylococcal infections, although IVIG may be of benefit in individual patients (65).

Defects of Phagocytosis

Impaired phagocytic function has also been identified as a condition associated with increased risk of infection. Neutrophils have Fcγ receptors on their surface that bind IgG and signal the cell to phagocytose invading pathogens. A number of genetic polymorphisms have been described within the different classes of Fcγ receptors that influence this function. In vitro studies have demonstrated impaired phagocytosis in individuals with a particular genotype of the FcγRII receptor. This same genotype has been detected with increased frequency in patients with severe meningococcal disease when compared to healthy controls (66). This finding may have potential implications for genetic screening and prophylactic immunization of family members of patients with severe meningococcal disease.

Defects of Intracellular Killing

Chronic granulomatous disease (CGD) is caused by a mutation in any of the four structural genes (gp91^{phox}, p22^{phox}, p47^{phox}, and p67^{phox}) of the NADPH oxidase apparatus. The majority of cases are inherited in an X-linked recessive manner (gp91^{phox}), while the others are AR. The disease is characterized by recurrent infections of the skin, lungs, and liver as well as by excessive granuloma formation that can obstruct the gastrointestinal or genitourinary tract. Most infections are caused by *S. aureus*, *Burkholderia cepacia*, *Aspergillus* species, *Nocardia* species and *Serratia marcescens*. *S. aureus* liver abcesses are highly suspicious for the diagnosis of CGD. Patients with CGD are most susceptible to catalase-positive microorganisms.

This diagnosis can be made by laboratory tests, which analyze superoxide formation, such as the nitroblue tetrazolium test or by flow cytometry with dihydrorhodamine dye (57). The defect in NADPH oxidase causes an inability of the neutrophil to produce superoxide and its metabolites, thereby impairing the ability of the neutrophil to kill ingested microorganisms. Patients with CGD are commonly treated with the prophylactic antimicrobials trimethoprim–sulfamethoxazole and itraconazole to prevent bacterial and fungal infections, respectively. IFN-γ therapy has also been found to be effective for these patients reducing infection rates by 70% when compared to placebo. HSCT has been curative in this patient population; however, transplant-related complications require careful consideration before this procedure is undertaken (67). Alternatively, a recent study looking at quality-of-life indicators as measured by the Pediatric Quality of Life Inventory (PedsQL) compared children with CGD treated conservatively to those treated with HSCT. This study found that children who received HSCT scored comparable to that of healthy children on the PedsQL. However, children treated conservatively scored significantly lower than healthy children. This information may be helpful to parents faced with deciding whether or not to have their child undergo HSCT (68). Two additional disorders to consider in the differential of CGD include severe glucose-6-phosphate dehydrogenase deficiency and myeloperoxidase deficiency, both of which present with a milder phenotype.

Disorders of Neutrophil Granules

Immunodeficiencies may also result from defective formation of neutrophil granules. Chediak–Higashi syndrome, an AR disorder, is the best characterized of these disorders. The genetic mutation causing Chediak–Higashi syndrome involves the *LYST* gene. This gene encodes a protein involved with the formation and function of vacuoles. The severity of the phenotype varies with the type of mutation (69). Neutrophils from these patients have impaired chemotaxis, and they are characterized by large perinuclear granules. In addition, elastase and cathepsin G may be absent from their neutrophil granules.

Patients with Chediak–Higashi disease have abnormalities in both the hematologic and the neurologic systems. Clinical features include recurrent bacterial infections, peripheral nerve disorders, mental retardation, autonomic dysfunction, partial albinism, silvery colored hair, and platelet dysfunction. Patients often die in the first decade of life of a lymphoproliferative process termed the accelerated phase. This process is similar to HLH. If patients survive into the second or third decade of life, they often develop a debilitating peripheral neuropathy and eventually die of infection. Although HSCT appears to prevent the accelerated phase, it does not prevent the neurologic sequelae (69).

Neutrophil-specific granular deficiency is a rare autosomal disorder that is characterized by the absence of neutrophil granules. Patients with this disease may have recurrent severe infections, particularly with *Staphylococcus aureus*, *Staphylococcus epidermidis*, and enteric bacteria. The neutrophils of these patients are not able to migrate properly. Similar to patients with severe neutropenia, the severity of these infections may be underestimated by clinical exam because their neutrophils are unable to migrate properly to the site of infection to create visible suppuration and inflammation. Therefore, aggressive treatment with antibiotics and early consideration of surgical management are indicated (67). A recent case of an infant with neutrophil-specific granule deficiency causing intractable diarrhea was described. Due to the severity of her disease causing feeding intolerance and failure to thrive, the infant underwent HSCT. The child is doing well 1 year after HSCT, able to tolerate full enteral feedings, and has resolution of her recurrent infections (70).

Unknown Etiology of Neutrophil Dysfunction

Patients with severe glutathione deficiency have been found to have recurrent bacterial infections. This is felt to be due to defective granulocyte function. However, the exact mechanism is unknown. These patients also have chronic metabolic acidosis, hemolytic anemia, and progressive neurologic symptoms, including mental retardation, seizures, spasticity, ataxia, and intention tremor. Patients with glutathione synthetase deficiency have low levels of glutathione. Patients are treated with vitamin C and E supplementation to help protect cells from oxidative stress and bicarbonate to correct the acidosis. N-acetyl-cysteine is not recommended due to the risk of accumulation of intracellular cysteine (71).

COMPLEMENT DEFICIENCY

Normal Function

The complement system is a key component of innate immunity, acting to protect the host from microorganisms (72). The complement system may be activated via three distinct pathways, all of which require activation of the complement protein C3 (**Fig. 86.1**) (73). The classical pathway is activated by antigen–antibody complexes derived from acquired immunity. The alternative pathway is triggered by the recognition of pathogen-associated molecular patterns (PAMPs) on the surface of bacteria by C3 activated by spontaneous hydrolysis. Finally, complement may be activated by the lectin pathway beginning with the detection of bacterial surface carbohydrates (i.e., mannose) by mannan-binding lectin (MBL) protein. This results in the induction of MBL-activated serine proteases (MASPs) and activation of the complement cascade. A clear understanding of the complement cascade and the biologic functions of the individual components provides insight into the clinical manifestations of complement deficiencies.

Complement C1, a complex macromolecule, initiates activation of the classical pathway and plays a significant role in host defense against pathogens (72). C1 is composed of a recognition protein, C1q, in association with a tetramer composed of two proteases, C1r and C1s. The C1q recognition protein mediates the binding of C1 to a target cell or molecule. The binding of C1 results in the subsequent activation of C4, C2, and ultimately C3. Of note, all three pathways of complement activation converge at C3 and lead to the formation of C3a and C5a and the terminal membrane attack complex, C5b–C9. Activated C3 is critical to opsonization. Activated C5 has numerous effects important in the pathogenesis of sepsis with C5b initiating the formation of the terminal membrane attack complex (72,73). The terminal membrane attack complex functions to lyse the cell membrane of the target cell. The classical pathway may be initiated without antigen–antibody complexes by the direct binding of bacteria, viruses, and apoptotic cells to C1q and subsequent activation of the cascade.

The alternative complement pathway is critical to innate immunity and also serves to activate complement in the absence of antibody. C3 is again the pivotal component. Under normal physiologic conditions, C3 in the plasma is activated via slow hydrolysis and interaction with alternative pathway proteins. Once C3 is activated, the pathway progresses identical to the classical pathway (**Fig. 86.1**). Of note, the alternative pathway C3 convertase is highly unstable and requires properdin for stability.

MBL is the initiating protein for the lectin pathway of complement activation. MBL recognizes specific carbohydrate sequences on the surface of microbes. Once bound to these surfaces, MBL activates two proteases, MASP-1 and MASP-2, which share structural homology with C1r and C1s. MASP-2 triggers the complement cascade by activating C4 while MASP-1 is believed to activate C3 directly.

Complement Regulation

The complement system is critical to the host defense system as it damages invading organisms and produces tissue inflammation. However, strict control of the complement system is essential to prevent complement-mediated destruction of host tissues. Many regulatory proteins exist that function in this role. For example, C1 esterase inhibitor (C1-INH) is a glycoprotein that recognizes and inactivates activated C1r and C1s. Because it is consumed during the process of inactivation, high levels of C1 inhibitor must be produced requiring the activation of two gene sites (73). In fact, deficiency of C1-INH results in hereditary angioedema (HAE) (described later).

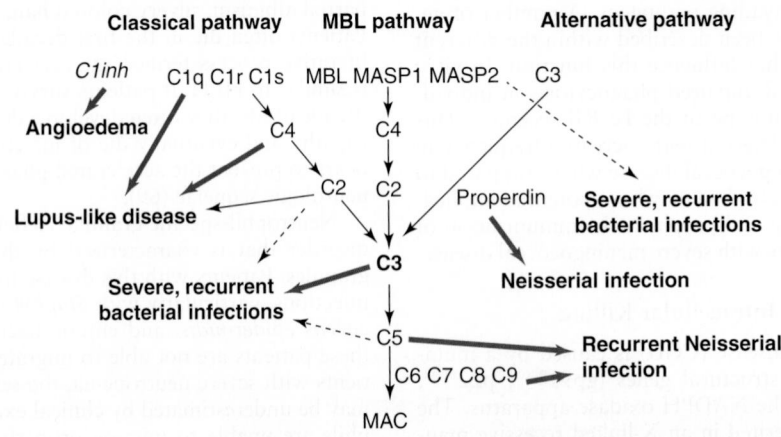

FIGURE 86.1. The figure depicts the complement components involved in activation of the three pathways of the complement cascade and consequences of specific deficiencies. MAC, membrane attack complex. (From Paul WE, ed. *Fundamental Immunology.* 7th ed. Philadelphia, PA: Lippincott Williams & Wilkins, 2013.)

Several other regulatory proteins function at different points of the complement cascade to help minimize destruction of host tissues. It is believed that this occurs as a result of protected sites on microorganisms. When C3b binds to the membrane of microbes, it is positioned in such a way that regulatory proteins (factors H and I) cannot reach it, and therefore, cannot inactivate it. On the other hand, when C3b binds host tissues, it is not protected from factors H and I, and therefore, it can be quickly degraded (73).

Deficiencies and Disease

The association of complement deficiencies with disease states is not well established because of difficulties in estimating the prevalence of complement deficiencies (74). However, there are disorders in which an association with a defect in the complement system has clearly been demonstrated. Rheumatologic disorders (especially *systemic lupus erythematosus*), increased susceptibility to invasive infections (notably *recurrent meningococcal disease*), and *hereditary angioedema* represent the most common pediatric clinical settings in which complement deficiency is suspected (74).

Classic and Alternative Pathway Deficiencies

An increased susceptibility to invasive infection is a prominent feature of many patients with inherited complement deficiencies (4,74,75). Although complement protects against a variety of pathogens, patients with complement deficiency are most susceptible to bacterial infections (4,74,75). Moreover, the specific type of infection tends to be associated with the component of the complement cascade that is deficient. For example, children deficient in C3, important for opsonization, are at increased risk for infections from encapsulated organisms where opsonization is the critical component of host defense. Eighty percent of C3-deficient individuals have significant infections, as compared to 42% of C1-deficient, 33% of C4-deficient, and 50% of C2-deficient individuals (4,75). The lower incidence of infections in the three latter groups would appear to be related to their intact alternative pathway and the ability to activate C3 through this alternative mechanism. In fact, alternative pathway deficiencies are quite rare.

The terminal components of the complement cascade, C5 through C9, form the membrane attack complex, which is responsible for bacterial lysis and death (4). However, because C3 is not deficient, opsonization remains intact, and these patients are not excessively susceptible to encapsulated bacteria. Instead, these patients with deficiencies in terminal components of the complement cascade display increased susceptibility to *Neisseria* infections, in which bactericidal activity is critical to host defense. *Neisseria meningitides* is also the most common pathogen among patients with X-linked properdin deficiency (74), the most common complement deficiency of the alternative pathway.

In addition to an increased incidence of meningococcal infections among patients with a terminal membrane attack complex complement deficiency, these children may also present with unusual patterns of infection. For example, types of meningococci commonly considered avirulent may cause fulminant sepsis or meningitis in these children (4). Infections from *Neisseria* serogroups W-135 and Y have been reported with increased frequency among patients deficient in the terminal components of the complement cascade (74). Interestingly, a few studies suggest that meningococcal disease may have less morbidity and lower mortality in complement-deficient patients (75).

Vaccination against meningococcal disease may be important for these patients (74). Not only do these patients appear to mount normal antibody responses to the administration of the tetravalent meningococcal vaccine, but because the median age for meningococcal disease in terminal complex deficiency and properdin deficiency is late adolescence, there is usually time for effective vaccination (74,75). Vaccination with the tetravalent meningococcal vaccine may be particularly important for properdin deficiency patients (74).

Lectin Pathway Deficiencies

In addition to deficits in the classical complement pathway, deficiencies in MBL and MASPs may also contribute to disease states relevant to the pediatric critical care provider. MBL is a soluble pathogen-recognizing molecule capable of binding to microbes and activating complement via MASPs. Low levels of MBL have been reported in children deficient in opsonizing activity and with increased susceptibility to infection (76,77). Moreover, low levels appear to predispose to febrile neutropenia and infection among cancer patients undergoing chemotherapy (77) In fact, among cancer patients undergoing gastrointestinal surgery, MBL levels were significantly lower in patients who developed sepsis, SIRS, or pneumonia (78,79). This association has not been found in all studies and is less apparent in patients undergoing intensive chemotherapy, such as treatment for AML and/or conditioning for allogeneic HSCT, in which phagocytic function is strongly suppressed (77). In addition, MASP-2 deficiency is also implicated in the increased risk of febrile neutropenia in pediatric cancer patients (80). It is also associated with increased risk of recurrent infections in children with allergic disorders (81).

Among critically ill patients, MBL deficiency not only appears to increase susceptibility to sepsis and septic shock but also may be associated with worse outcomes. In a post hoc analysis of Van den Berghe's landmark study of intensive insulin therapy in critically ill patients, conventionally treated nonsurvivors had significantly lower MBL levels on admission, at day 5, and at conclusion of the study than conventionally treated survivors (82). Moreover, among the subset of these patients with bacteremia, lower MBL levels were again detected among nonsurvivors. In another report, MBL genotype variant alleles were associated with a greater risk of sepsis, severe sepsis, septic shock, and mortality among 272 critically ill adults (83). In that study, serum MBL concentrations were inversely related to the severity of the sepsis. However, in a similar study, genotypes resulting in low MBL levels were associated with an increased risk of bacterial infections, but not with an increased rate of sepsis, septic shock, or mortality in adults admitted to an ICU (84).

In a pediatric study, Fidler et al. (85) evaluated both MBL genotypes and MBL levels in 100 consecutive admissions to a tertiary care PICU. Children with an MBL variant allele had an eightfold increased risk of developing SIRS, as compared to those with a wild-type genotype, after adjusting for age, sex, and ethnicity. In that study, an association was also noted between the severity of the systemic response to infection and MBL variant alleles. MBL serum levels closely correlated with the MBL genotype, and thus, low MBL levels (<1000 ng/mL) identified children at increased risk of SIRS. In contrast, in a study of very low birth weight infants, MBL genotypes were not associated with an increased risk of sepsis (86).

In addition to sepsis, there is data suggesting that low MBL levels, as well as MBL variant genotypes, may be related to a number of other disorders. For example, autoimmune disorders, such as SLE, rheumatoid arthritis, celiac disease, and inflammatory bowel diseases have all been associated with low levels of MBL although the data is far from conclusive (77). There is also data suggesting that low levels of MBL may be associated with the occurrence and the disease pattern of Kawasaki disease. In a Dutch study, children with Kawasaki disease were more likely to exhibit MBL variant genotypes as compared to controls (87). In fact, among children <1 year of age, MBL variant genotypes were associated with a higher incidence of coronary artery involvement (87). In a study of Chinese patients with Kawasaki disease, MBL genotypes were found to modulate arterial stiffness, which is an important cardiovascular risk factor in children with Kawasaki disease (88). In that study, however, MBL genotype distributions did not differ between patients and controls, or between patients with and without coronary artery aneurysms (88). MBL deficiency has also been associated with a number of other conditions, including rejection among heart transplant recipients, atherosclerosis, myocardial infarction, recurrent spontaneous abortions, and other obstetric and gynecologic complications (77).

Treatment for MBL deficiency is currently being investigated (77). The safety of infusing MBL, purified from donor plasma as well as clinical grade recombinant MBL, has been established in phase I trials. Clinical trials testing the potential benefits of MBL reconstitution in deficient individuals remain to be performed.

Hereditary Angioedema

HAE is a rare AD disorder with an estimated frequency of 1 in 10,000 to 1 in 50,000 individuals (89,90). Almost half of all patients will have symptoms before puberty. Affected children can have involvement of skin, abdomen, or upper airway (89,90). This edema can cause limb swelling, painful abdominal crises, and life-threatening airway obstruction. Airway edema may take several hours to develop, although there is one report of a child dying from asphyxiation within 20 minutes of the onset of symptoms (91). The edema may persist for up to 4 days. Approximately 50% of HAE patients will have throat swelling at some point in their lifetime (89); however, for most patients, the edema tends to involve the intestines more frequently than the larynx.

HAE is primarily the result of a deficiency in the C1 esterase inhibitor protein (C1-INH) caused by a deletion, duplication, or mutation in the C1 esterase inhibitor gene (89,90). Two primary forms of HAE represent almost all patients; HAE type I is characterized by a reduced concentration of C1-INH and HAE type II is characterized by a dysfunctional C1-INH. Both also have a very low C4 level. Type I accounts for 80%–85% of patients. There is also a rare form, HAE type 3, which has the same clinical presentation but there are no abnormalities in C4 and C1-INH level or function (89,90).

Without effective treatment, the disease has a high mortality, and diagnosis may be delayed in the absence of a family history. A high index of suspicion must be maintained by the intensive care practitioner because distinguishing HAE from acquired angioedema facilitates treatment (92). A C4 level is the appropriate screening test for this disorder. Analysis of both C1-INH level and function is most commonly used to establish the diagnosis.

The scenario in which the critical care provider is most likely to encounter HAE is in the setting of acute laryngeal edema causing upper airway obstruction or with intestinal obstruction. In both instances, rapid resolution of symptoms is vital. Treatment options include plasma derived C1-INH concentrate, kinin-pathway modulators, and fresh frozen plasma, if C1-INH is not available (90). C1-INH concentrate infusion is the treatment of choice for acute upper airway obstruction or severe gastrointestinal symptoms secondary to HAE. In children with suspected HAE, *any* upper airway symptom merits treatment with C1-INH concentrate, if available (90). Moreover, in treating intestinal obstruction from HAE, failure of clinical improvement following C1-INH infusion warrants consideration of alternative diagnoses for the abdominal symptomatology (92).

Rheumatologic Disorders

In addition to an increased susceptibility to infections, complement-deficient patients are at increased risk for rheumatologic disorders, most notably, SLE. The association between SLE and inherited C2 deficiency was recognized over 30 years ago. C2-deficient SLE is quite similar to genuine SLE, although antinuclear and dsDNA antibody levels are low or undetectable (74,93,94). Also, SLE may be even more common among patients with a complete deficiency of C1 or C4 than those with a C2 deficiency (93,94).

INNATE IMMUNE SIGNALING DEFECTS

The innate immune system uses pattern recognition receptors (PRRs), such as toll-like receptors (TLRs), to detect the presence microbial pathogens. TLRs are cell surface and intracellular pattern recognition receptors critical to the identification of invading microbes by recognizing the PAMPs of the microorganisms. The TLR–PAMP interaction triggers a complex signaling cascade that ultimately results in the activation of NF-κB and activated protein-1 (AP-1). These two factors regulate the transcription of a multitude of genes encoding proinflammatory cytokines critical to the innate host defense. Ten TLR members have been identified, and many of their inflammatory pathways overlap with 10 identified IL-1 receptor (IL-1R) family members. Many of the TLRs and IL-1Rs contain intracellular domain known as the Toll-IL-1R domain (TIR). This TIR domain recruits adaptors proteins, including MyD88 and TRIF proteins, which recruit cytosolic kinases, such as IL-1R–associated kinases (IRAKs). The canonical TIR pathway depends on MyD88. The IRAKs form a complex and activate both NF-κB and mitogen-activated protein kinases (MAPKs). NF-κB is a transcription factor sequestered in the cytoplasm of resting cells through association with the inhibitor of NF-κB (IκB) proteins. Upon cell stimulation, IκBs are phosphorylated at two conserved critical amino-terminal serine residues by the IκB kinase (IKK) complex of which NEMO is a component, leading to the ubiquitination of the IκBs and their subsequent degradation. Immunodeficiencies of the noncanonical TIR or alternative pathway have been described. Patients with genetic mutations of TLR3, UNC93B, and TRAF3 have an increased susceptibility to herpes simplex encephalitis (95). Four primary immunodeficiencies associated with the canonical TIR MyD88-dependent pathway have been described to date.

Two separate AR immunodeficiencies are caused by mutations in the *IRAK4* (44) and *MyD88* (96) genes, which lead to aberrant upstream innate signaling. Interestingly, patients with IRAK4 and MyD88 deficiencies present with nearly identical immune phenotypes. Neither mutation leads to any developmental abnormalities, and these children have increased susceptibility to infection, but primarily only to pyogenic, encapsulated, gram-positive bacteria (e.g., *Streptococcus pneumoniae* and *Staphylococcus aureus*). Their infections occur early in life, and the condition appears to improve with age, presumably because with age adaptive immunity maturation compensates for the innate immunodeficiency.

X-linked anhidrotic ectodermal dysplasia with immunodeficiency is caused by mutations in the *NEMO* gene (97), which as described earlier, acts downstream of IRAK4 and MyD88. These patients may present with absent or conical teeth, dry skin due to absence or decreased number of eccrine sweat glands, and hypohidrosis with sparse scalp, and eyebrow hair due to abnormal development of ectoderm-derived structures. In addition, these children experience an increased susceptibility to a wide variety of severe infections. Their overall prognosis is poor, with approximately half dying of overwhelming infection during childhood. The presence of conical incisors in a male with unusual infections suggests the need to assess for NEMO mutations.

An AD form of anhidrotic ectodermal dysplasia with immunodeficiency has also been reported (98) and is caused by mutation of the gene encoding IκBα. This condition, phenotypically similar to the X-linked form, is characterized by abnormal development of ectoderm-derived structures and associated with multiple severe infections. The clinical features of the autosomal form, however, appear more severe and include severe T-cell dysfunction. HSCT has recently been used to successfully treat the immunodeficiency of AD anhidrotic ectodermal dysplasia; however, HSCT did not prevent the abnormalities of ectodermal dysplasia.

IMMUNODEFICIENCY AND CANCER PREDISPOSITION

As described previously, several inherited immunodeficiency disorders have an increased risk of cancer, including WAS, ataxia telangiectasia, SCID, Kostmann syndrome, and XLP. In addition, patients with acquired immunodeficiencies, such as the acquired immunodeficiency syndrome, and those receiving immunosuppressive therapy following organ transplantation also have an increased susceptibility to cancer. This association of immunodeficiency with a predisposition to cancer suggests that an intact immune system provides a surveillance mechanism to eliminate transformed cancer cells from the body. This theory of immune surveillance against malignant cells is supported by laboratory studies in which mice deficient in the IFN-γ receptor developed tumors more frequently, and more rapidly, upon exposure to carcinogens than control mice, and this may be a reflection of the lack of NK cells in these mice. More recent evidence supports that NK cells play a significant role in immune surveillance as mice deficient for the inhibitory NK receptor, NKG2D, have an increased susceptibility to epithelial and lymphoid malignancies that express the ligand for NKG2D on their surface (98).

On the other hand, the hypothesis for immune surveillance against cancer would appear to only partially explain the association between immunodeficiency and malignancy. For example, patients with severe immunodeficiencies are at increased risk for developing only specific types of cancers, mainly lymphoid malignancies (leukemias and lymphomas). The lack of increased risk for most other forms of cancer suggests that other factors must contribute to the development of malignancy. Moreover, in some immunodeficient conditions, cells have an increased susceptibility to genetic disruption and survive to be transformed into a malignant phenotype. For example, in patients with ataxia telangiectasia, disruption of the *ATM* gene increases the risk for DNA damage from radiation, and therefore, predisposes cells to become malignant independent of the immunodeficient state of this disease. In addition, immunodeficiency states are also associated with an increased risk for infections that may contribute to the malignant transformation of cells. EBV infection, which has been linked to the evolution of lymphomas or lymphoproliferative disorders in posttransplant patients, represents one such example.

In summary, although the association between immunodeficiency states and a predisposition to cancer has been established, the mechanisms contributing to this association are not completely understood and are likely multifactorial in origin.

IMMUNOLOGIC EFFECTS OF CANCER AND ITS TREATMENT

Predisposition to Immunodeficiency Associated with Cancer

In addition to immunodeficiency states predisposing to cancer, conversely, it is widely accepted that most cancer patients are immunocompromised as a result of their underlying disease and/or their antineoplastic therapy. Many of these patients present with some degree of immunocompromise even prior to receiving cytotoxic therapy (99). For example, patients with acute leukemia are often pancytopenic at the time of diagnosis, and leukemia and lymphoma patients have long been known to have impaired neutrophil function. Additionally, both sarcoma and lymphoma patients have been found to present with reduced peripheral blood B- and T-cell populations (99,100). Further, functional impairments from intracranial and other solid tumors may predispose cancer patients to infection prior to therapy for a variety of reasons. Thus, oncology patients are likely to be immunocompromised prior to any cytotoxic cancer treatment.

However, in addition to this underlying predisposition, antineoplastic therapy further compromises the immune function of these patients and places them at increased risk of severe infection. Several treatment-related factors, including neutropenia, loss of mucosal integrity, and T-cell dysfunction contribute to an increased susceptibility of invasive infections in pediatric cancer patients.

Dating back to Bodey's landmark study of 1966, treatment-induced neutropenia has been established as one of the most significant risk factors for severe infection among cancer patients. In fact, the more severe the neutropenia, both in terms of absolute number and duration, the greater the risk of infection. In terms of absolute number, most bacteremias and bacterial pneumonias occur when the ANC is <100 cells/mm^3 (99). In terms of duration, treatment-induced neutropenia that persists for more than a week is associated with increasing risk of infection (99). In fact, the prompt return of neutrophils following cytotoxic therapy portends a favorable outcome even in the setting of a documented infection (99).

Although neutropenia clearly predisposes oncology patients to bacteremia and sepsis, its impact on outcome is less well established. Fiser et al. (101) reported that among pediatric cancer patients with severe sepsis who required both mechanical ventilation and inotropic support, there was no difference among survivors and nonsurvivors in the percentage of patients with neutropenia (ANC <500 cells/mm^3) (68% and 72% respectively, $p = 0.824$). In contrast, Viscoli et al. (102) noted a difference in mortality based on the presence or absence of neutropenia (ANC <1000 cells/mm^3) among children with cancer and a documented bloodstream infection (15% and 4% respectively, $p = 0.03$). Wisplinghoff et al. (103) reported that the crude mortality rate for neutropenic patients was 36% as compared to 31% for those without neutropenia among 2340 adult patients with cancer and a nosocomial bloodstream infection ($p = 0.053$).

In addition to neutropenia, the impact of antineoplastic therapy on other effector cell lines of the immune system further impedes normal immune function. The impact of T-cell dysfunction is particularly detrimental and is the subject of much recent study. As with other hematopoietic cell subtypes, T cells are depleted following cytotoxic cancer therapy. The regeneration of T cells, however, is often prolonged and incomplete. In light of this, cancer patients are susceptible to viral, fungal, and parasitic infections long after the end of their therapy and neutrophil recovery. In fact, CD4$^+$ T-cell subpopulations are more severely depleted in relation to their CD8$^+$ counterparts in patients receiving intensive chemotherapy regimens rendering these patients even more susceptible to opportunistic infection (99,100). In addition to the viral, fungal, and parasitic infections, these patients may also have an increased susceptibility to some bacterial infections, including *Legionella*, *Listeria*, *Salmonella*, *Mycobacterium tuberculosis*, and atypical mycobacteria (104). Moreover, T-cell dysfunction has been attributed to an increased risk of EBV-associated lymphoproliferative disorder and posttransfusion GVHD. Patients who have received protracted intensive chemotherapy and/or who have undergone allogeneic HSCT are at highest risk of complications related to T-cell deficiency states.

In addition to the impact on essential cell lines of the immune system, anticancer therapy also increases the risk of infection in pediatric cancer patients in a number of other ways. For example, the gastrointestinal tract has many rapidly dividing cells placing it at risk for significant toxicity from antineoplastic therapy. This toxicity includes disruption of the mucosal barrier fostering the systemic spread of pathogens. Severe oral mucositis exemplifies this toxicity and has been associated with a significantly increased risk of α-hemolytic streptococcal bacteremia in oncology patients and HSCT recipients (105). Moreover, the pain and discomfort of mucositis often interferes with normal nutrition resulting in an increased risk of malnutrition and the need for parental alimentation. Both of these conditions have been associated with an increased risk of infection and/or impaired immune function. In addition, disruptions of the integumentary barrier including the placement of indwelling catheters and the inherent risk of infection associated with these lines further predispose these children to sepsis. Functional impairments induced by antineoplastic therapy (e.g., generalized weakness, swallowing difficulties, skin breakdown) may also increase susceptibility to infectious pathogens.

IMMUNE DYSFUNCTION ASSOCIATED WITH HEMATOPOIETIC STEM CELL TRANSPLANT

As described previously, immunosuppression is common with most antineoplastic therapy; however, it appears to be most severe in the setting of allogeneic HSCT. This is due primarily to the fact that the process requires the near complete replacement of the host lymphohematopoietic system. For this to successfully occur, intense immunosuppression of the host is required; a host that is likely already immunocompromised as a result of underlying disease and previous therapy. Thus, HSCT patients will be profoundly immunocompromised until effective immune reconstitution occurs. Immune reconstitution, however, is a complex and prolonged process. In fact, although neutrophil engraftment may occur early in the posttransplant period, complete immune reconstitution requires months to years.

In terms of immune reconstitution, children differ from adults in two potentially important ways (3). First, the presence of a thymus greatly enhances both the kinetic and functional recovery of adaptive immunity in the pediatric transplant patient. This results in several beneficial effects, including improved recovery of naïve T cells. Faster recovery of CD4$^+$ T-cell levels has been associated with a decreased risk of opportunistic infection following HSCT engraftment (3,106). Second, there appears to be a lower incidence of GVHD in children when compared to adults. The presence of GVHD contributes significantly to immunosuppression by both impeding immune restoration and requiring further immunosuppressive therapy (3,107).

Immune reconstitution following HSCT is influenced by patient-, disease-, and transplant-related factors. These factors include patient age, underlying disease, disease status, transplant type (autologous vs. allogeneic), preparative regimen, the presence of infection, HLA compatibility, GVHD, and the stem cell source, mobilization, and manipulation techniques. In addition, it is important to note that cellular reconstitution does not necessarily correlate with functional recovery, and innate immunity reconstitution precedes that of adaptive immunity (3).

Innate Immunity Recovery

Natural Killer Cells

NK cells are one of the initial lymphoid cells to recover following HSCT. As such, they play crucial roles in direct cytotoxicity and antibody-dependent cytotoxicity of infected as well as tumor cells. Their role has been implicated in protection against viral infections (particularly CMV) and GVHD, as well as increasing the graft versus leukemia (GVL) effect in certain transplant settings (83). The reconstitution of NK cells has been extensively evaluated in the posttransplant period. NK-cell levels appear to return to normal within 1–2 months following HSCT, seemingly independent of transplant type, stem cell source, patient age, and GVHD (3). Also, it appears as though functional recovery occurs simultaneously with the return of NK cellularity. This is potentially very important to the recipient, given the antimicrobial and antitumor effects of these cells.

Neutrophils, Macrophages, and Monocytes

Granulocytes and monocytes also recover early in the posttransplant period with neutrophil recovery preceding that of monocytes and tissue macrophages (3). However, recovery of these cells differs from that of NK cells in two important ways. First, their recovery is influenced by transplant-related factors, such as stem cell source and GVHD. For example, an unmanipulated matched sibling stem cell graft will have more differentiated precursors allowing quicker recovery of these subsets of cells than a graft composed entirely of the more primitive CD34+ stem cell. Second, in both animal and human studies, recovery in cellularity does not necessarily correspond with functional recovery (3). For example, reconstituted phagocytes have impaired bactericidal activity for at least 2 months following allogeneic HSCT placing the child at increased risk of pyogenic infection and infection-related mortality (3).

Dendritic Cells

Although, the exact mechanisms are still in question, dendritic cells play an important part in immune function after allogeneic bone marrow transplantation. Dendritic cell recovery also occurs relatively early in the post-HSCT setting (3). Although these cells reconstitute to pretransplant levels within 2 months of transplant, it takes up to 1 year to recover to levels of healthy individuals (108). In addition, much like neutrophil recovery, manipulations in the stem cell source appear to influence the speed of dendritic cell recovery (3). Although the relationship between cellular and functional recovery of these cells has not been well established, there is data suggesting that early dendritic cell recovery may serve to protect the transplant recipient against infection (109). Low levels of dendritic cells during the periengraftment period have also been associated with an increased risk of relapse, acute GVHD, and death (110).

Adaptive Immunity Recovery

Reconstitution of Humoral Immunity

In the early post-HSCT period, it is primarily the host plasma cells, which have survived the preparative regimen, that produce IgG (107). Progenitor cells contained in the allograft only begin to give rise to naïve B cells producing IgM 4–6 months after the transplant. Isotype switching, resulting in production of IgG, and subsequently IgA, can only occur with CD4+ T-helper cells, and thus, occurs much later (3,107). In fact, IgG levels may remain abnormal for up to 1 year following transplant and IgA levels for as long as 2 years (3,107). Even when normal levels of IgG are achieved, an oligoclonal pattern may be present limiting their utility (107). The presence of severe acute GVHD or chronic extensive GVHD has been associated with reduced numbers of B cells and diminished availability of CD4$^+$ T-helper cells, thereby further impeding reconstitution of humoral immunity (107). In general, B-cell recovery tends to occur before T-cell reconstitution (3). The type of transplant, however, may impart different reconstitution of cells. Lymphocyte subset populations (especially CD4 T cells) tend to be higher after allogeneic peripheral blood stem cell transplant (PBSCT), as opposed to bone marrow transplant. This is associated with decreased risk of severe infections (especially fungal) in patients receiving PBSCT (111).

T-cell Recovery

T-cell reconstitution is critical for immune competency and is believed to occur via two pathways. The first is a thymic-independent pathway termed homeostatic peripheral expansion (HPE), which merely involves the expansion of mature T cells that survived the preparative regimen, that were contained within the allograft, and/or that were given via donor lymphocyte infusions (107). These T cells are both quantitatively and qualitatively deficient. Also, HPE results in a T-cell pool limited to cells activated by the antigenic milieu of the host, with negligible number of cells having activity for antigens absent at the time of expansion (112). This limited repertoire significantly impedes the ability to generate effective clonal T-cell responses against microbes and tumor cells (3).

Recovery of thymic function, therefore, provides the optimal pathway for T-cell reconstitution. Unfortunately, thymic recovery does not generally occur for several months following allogeneic HSCT (3,107). Thymic recovery is hampered by age-related decrements in thymic function, as well as by cytotoxic-, radiation-, and/or GVHD-induced thymic injury (107). In light of this, recovery of normal T-cell number and function often does not occur within the first year following HSCT (3,107).

GVHD is particularly detrimental to immune reconstitution (107). First, the process is directly toxic to the thymic microenvironment. GVHD may also impair negative selection of T cells that react to host antigens. This combination not only results in decreased thymic function and recovery, but fosters further GVHD. In addition, by causing widespread apoptosis, GVHD limits the effectiveness of HPE, thereby hindering thymic-independent immune restoration (113). Finally, the immunosuppressants needed to treat GVHD further diminish both thymic function and HPE. Thus, both the pathophysiology of GHVD and the immunosuppression required to treat this condition prolong the course of immune reconstitution following HSCT.

FUTURE DIRECTIONS

As described in this chapter, several specific genetic mutations have recently been identified as the cause of most of the well-defined immunodeficiency conditions. For several disorders, notably CVID, several different mutations may lead to the same phenotype. The genetic basis of more subtle cytokine signaling defects and molecular pattern recognition deficits await clarification. Polymorphisms in cytokine signaling pathways may clarify minor variations in immune function that are presently unexplained. Therapeutic advances in the future are likely to include even more convenient and effective methods of HAE treatment. Enhancement of cellular immune function may be feasible with available cytokine therapies. For children with severe defects justifying HSCT, strategies for enhancing

immune tolerance should allow for chimerism following stem cell "mini" transplants, thereby lessening the risks of postablation infection and GVHD. The ultimate therapeutic goal for single gene defects, however, is gene replacement therapy. Gene therapy for SCID continues to improve; although the first trial demonstrated the successful replacement of the γ_c gene in 20 patients with X-linked SCID with 17 patients cured, 5 patients developed leukemia. Forty patients with ADA-SCID have undergone gene therapy, with the majority receiving clinical benefit and 29 patients off ADA replacement. Since 2000, no malignancies have been reported (114). The new generation of self-inactivated lentiviral or retroviral vectors is thought to play a role in this improved outcome.

References

1. Matamoros FN, Mila LJ, Espanol BT, et al. Primary immunodeficiency in Spain: First report of the National Registry in Children and Adults. *J Clin Immunol* 1997;17:333–9.
2. Bonilla FA, Geha RS. Update on primary immunodeficiency diseases. *J Allergy Clin Immunol* 2006;117:S435–441.
3. Auletta JJ, Lazarus HM. Immune restoration following hematopoietic stem cell transplantation: An evolving target. *Bone Marrow Transplant* 2005;35:835–57.
4. Stiehm ER, Ochs HD, Winklestein JA, eds. *Immunologic Disorders in Infants and Children*. 5th ed. Philadelphia, PA: Elsevier Saunders, 2004.
5. Bruton OC. Agammaglobulinemia. *Pediatrics* 1952;9:722–8.
6. Winklestein JA, Marino MC, Lederman HM, et al. X-linked agammaglobulinemia. *Medicine* 2006;85:193–202.
7. Buckley RH. Immunodeficiency diseases. *JAMA* 1992;268:2797–806.
8. Aghamohammadi A, Cheraghi T, Rezaei N, et al. Neutropenia associated with X-linked agammaglobulinemia in an Iranian referral center. *Iran J Allergy Asthma Immunol* 2009;8:43–7.
9. Kanegane H, Taneichi H, Nomura K, et al. Severe neutropenia in Japanese patients with X-linked agammaglobulinemia. *J Clin Immunol* 2005;25:491–5.
10. Bonilla FA, Bernstein IL, Khan DA, et al. Practice parameter for the diagnosis and management of primary immunodeficiency. *Ann Allergy Asthma Immunol* 2005;94:S1–63.
11. Orange JS. Congenital immunodeficiencies and sepsis. *Pediatr Crit Care Med* 2005;6:S99–107.
12. Plebani A, Soresina A, Rondelli R, et al. Clinical, immunological, and molecular analysis in a large cohort of patients with X-linked agammaglobulinemia: An Italian multicenter study. *Clin Immunol* 2002;104:221–30.
13. Cunningham-Rundles C. The many faces of common variable immunodeficiency. *Hematology Am Soc Hematol Educ Program* 2012;2012:301–5.
14. Cunningham-Rundles C, Siegal FP, Cunningham-Rundles S, et al. Incidence of cancer in 98 patients with common varied immunodeficiency. *J Clin Immunol* 1987;7:294–9.
15. Burks AW, Sampson HA, Buckley RH. Anaphylactic reactions after gamma globulin administration in patients with hypogammaglobulinemia. Detection of IgE antibodies to IgA. *N Engl J Med* 1986;314:560–4.
16. Lin JH, Liebhaber M, Roberts RL, et al. Etanercept treatment of cutaneous granulomas in common variable immunodeficiency. *J Allergy Clin Immunol* 2006;117:878–82.
17. Mullighan CG, Fanning GC, Chapel HM, et al. TNF and lymphotoxin-alpha polymorphisms associated with common variable immunodeficiency: Role in the pathogenesis of granulomatous disease. *J Immunol* 1997;159:6236–41.
18. Castigli E, Wilson SA, Garibyan L, et al. TACI is mutant in common variable immunodeficiency and IgA deficiency. *Nat Genet* 2005;37:829–34.

19. Davies EG, Thrasher AJ. Update on the hyper immunoglobulin M syndromes. *Br J Haematol* 2010;149:167–80.

20. Sullivan KE. DiGeorge syndrome/velocardiofacial syndrome: The chromosome 22q11.2 deletion syndrome. *Adv Exp Med Biol* 2007;601:37–49.

21. Carotti A, Digilio MC, Piacentini G, et al. Cardiac defects and results of cardiac surgery in 22q11.2 deletion syndrome. *Dev Disabil Res Rev* 2008;14:35–42.

22. Jawad AF, McDonald-Mcginn DM, Zackai E, et al. Immunologic features of chromosome 22q11.2 deletion syndrome (DiGeorge syndrome/velocardiofacial syndrome). *J Pediatr* 2001;139:715–23.

23. Gennery AR. Immunological aspects of 22q11.2 deletion syndrome. *Cell Mol Life Sci* 2011;69:17–27.

24. Cottle L. Mendelian susceptibility to mycobacterial disease. *Clin Genet* 2010;79:17–22.

25. Roesler J, Horwitz ME, Picard C, et al. Hematopoietic stem cell transplantation for complete IFN-gamma receptor 1 deficiency: A multi-institutional survey. *J Pediatr* 2004;145:806–12.

26. Janka GE. Familial and acquired hemophagocytic lymphohistiocytosis. *Eur J Pediatr* 2007;166:95–109.

27. Henter JI, Horne A, Arico M, et al. HLH-2004: Diagnostic and therapeutic guidelines for hemophagocytic lymphohistiocytosis. *Pediatr Blood Cancer* 2007;48:124–31.

28. Verbsky JW, Grossman WJ. Hemophagocytic lymphohistiocytosis: Diagnosis, pathophysiology, treatment, and future perspectives. *Ann Med* 2006;38:20–31.

29. Rudd E, Goransdotter Ericson K, Zheng C, et al. Spectrum and clinical implications of syntaxin 11 gene mutations in familial haemophagocytic lymphohistiocytosis: Association with disease-free remissions and haematopoietic malignancies. *J Med Genet* 2006;43:e14.

30. Weitzman S. Approach to hemophagocytic syndromes. *Hematology Am Soc Hematol Educ Program* 2011;2011:178–83.

31. Castillo L, Carcillo J. Secondary hemophagocytic lymphohistiocytosis and severe sepsis/systemic inflammatory response syndrome/multiorgan dysfunction syndrome/macrophage activation syndrome share common intermediate phenotypes on a spectrum of inflammation. *Pediatr Crit Care Med* 2009;10:387–92.

32. Belyea B, Hinson A, Moran C, et al. Spontaneous resolution of Epstein-Barr virus-associated hemophagocytic lymphohistiocytosis. *Pediatr Blood Cancer* 2010;55:754–6.

33. Demirkol D, Yildizdas D, Bayrakci B, et al. Hyperferritinemia in the critically ill child with secondary hemophagocytic lymphohistiocytosis/sepsis/multiple organ dysfunction syndrome/macrophage activation syndrome: What is the treatment? *Crit Care* 2012;16:R52.

34. Bryceson YT, Pende D, Maul-Pavicic A, et al. A prospective evaluation of degranulation assays in the rapid diagnosis of familial hemophagocytic syndromes. *Blood* 2012;119:2754–63.

35. Trottestam H, Horne A, Arico M, et al. Chemoimmunotherapy for hemophagocytic lymphohistiocytosis: Long-term results of the HLH-94 treatment protocol. *Blood* 2011;118:4577–84.

36. Rigante D, Capoluongo E, Bertoni B, et al. First report of macrophage activation syndrome in hyperimmunoglobulinemia D with periodic fever syndrome. *Arthritis Rheum* 2007;56:658–61.

37. Mouy R, Stephan JL, Pillet P, et al. Efficacy of cyclosporine A in the treatment of macrophage activation syndrome in juvenile arthritis: Report of five cases. *J Pediatr* 1996;129:750–4.

38. Ravelli A, Magni-Manzoni S, Pistorio A, et al. Preliminary diagnostic guidelines for macrophage activation syndrome complicating systemic juvenile idiopathic arthritis. *J Pediatr* 2005;146:598–604.

39. Pascual V, Allantaz F, Arce E, et al. Role of interleukin-1 (IL-1) in the pathogenesis of systemic onset juvenile idiopathic arthritis and clinical response to IL-1 blockade. *J Exp Med* 2005;201:1479–86.

40. Buckley R. The long quest for neonatal screening for severe combined immunodeficiency. *J Allergy Clin Immunol* 2012;129:597–604.

41. Villa A, Santagata S, Bozzi F, et al. Partial V(D)J recombination activity leads to Omenn syndrome. *Cell* 1998;93:885–96.

42. Buckley RH, Schiff SE, Schiff RI, et al. Hematopoietic stem-cell transplantation for the treatment of severe combined immunodeficiency. *N Engl J Med* 1999;340:508–16.

43. Shrestha D, Szollosi J, Jenei A. Bare lymphocyte syndrome: An opportunity to discover our immune system. *Immunol Lett* 2012;141:147–57.

44. Picard C, Puel A, Bonnet M, et al. Pyogenic bacterial infections in humans with IRAK-4 deficiency. *Science* 2003;299:2076–9.

45. Teachey DT. New advances in the diagnosis and treatment of autoimmune lymphoproliferative syndrome. *Curr Opin Pediatr* 2011;24:1–8.

46. Torgerson TR, Ochs HD. Immune dysregulation, polyendocrinopathy, enteropathy, X-linked: Forkhead box protein 3 mutations and lack of regulatory T cells. *J Allergy Clin Immunol* 2007;120:744–50; quiz 751–42.

47. Kisand K, Peterson P. Autoimmune polyendocrinopathy candidiasis ectodermal dystrophy: Known and novel aspects of the syndrome. *Ann N Y Acad Sci* 2012;1246:77–91.

48. Filipovich AH, Zhang K, Snow AL, et al. X-linked lymphoproliferative syndromes: Brothers or distant cousins? *Blood* 2010;116:3398–408.

49. Tabata Y, Villanueva J, Lee SM, et al. Rapid detection of intracellular SH2D1A protein in cytotoxic lymphocytes from patients with X-linked lymphoproliferative disease and their family members. *Blood* 2005;105:3066–71.

50. Milone MC, Tsai DE, Hodinka RL, et al. Treatment of primary Epstein-Barr virus infection in patients with X-linked lymphoproliferative disease using B-cell-directed therapy. *Blood* 2005;105:994–6.

51. Su HC. Dedicator of cytokinesis 8 (DOCK8) deficiency. *Curr Opin Allergy Clin Immunol* 2010;10:515–20.

52. Wolach B, Gavrieli R, Roos D, et al. Lessons learned from phagocytic function studies in a large cohort of patients with recurrent infections. *J Clin Immunol* 2011;32:454–66.

53. Ancliff PJ, Gale RE, Liesner R, et al. Mutations in the ELA2 gene encoding neutrophil elastase are present in most patients with sporadic severe congenital neutropenia but only in some patients with the familial form of the disease. *Blood* 2001;98:2645–50.

54. Sera Y, Kawaguchi H, Nakamura K, et al. A comparison of the defective granulopoiesis in childhood cyclic neutropenia and in severe congenital neutropenia. *Haematologica* 2005;90:1032–41.

55. Newburger PE, Pindyck TN, Zhu Z, et al. Cyclic neutropenia and severe congenital neutropenia in patients with a shared ELANE mutation and paternal haplotype: Evidence for phenotype determination by modifying genes. *Pediatr Blood Cancer* 2010;55:314–7.

56. Vandenberghe P, Beel K. Severe congenital neutropenia, a genetically heterogeneous disease group with an increased risk of AML/MDS. *Pediatr Rep* 2011;3(suppl 2):e9.

57. Lekstrom-Himes JA, Gallin JI. Immunodeficiency diseases caused by defects in phagocytes. *N Engl J Med* 2000;343:1703–14.

58. Rosenberg PS, Alter BP, Bolyard AA, et al. The incidence of leukemia and mortality from sepsis in patients with severe congenital neutropenia receiving long-term G-CSF therapy. *Blood* 2006;107:4628–35.

59. Carlsson G, Fasth A, Berglof E, et al. Incidence of severe congenital neutropenia in Sweden and risk of evolution to myelodysplastic syndrome/leukaemia. *Br J Haematol* 2012;158:363–9.

60. Connelly JA, Choi SW, Levine JE. Hematopoietic stem cell transplantation for severe congenital neutropenia. *Curr Opin Hematol* 2012;19:44–51.

61. Capsoni F, Sarzi-Puttini P, Zanella A. Primary and secondary autoimmune neutropenia. *Arthritis Res Ther* 2005;7:208–14.

62. Ito T, Taniuchi S, Tsuji S, et al. Diagnosis of autoimmune neutropenia by neutrophil-bound IgG and IgM antibodies. *J Pediatr Hematol Oncol* 2011;33:552–5.

63. Hanna S, Etzioni A. Leukocyte adhesion deficiencies. *Ann N Y Acad Sci* 2012;1250:50–5.

64. Mogensen TH, Jakobsen MA, Larsen CS. Identification of a novel STAT3 mutation in a patient with hyper-IgE syndrome. *Scand J Infect Dis* 2013;45(3):235–8.

65. Bilora F, Petrobelli F, Boccioletti V, et al. Moderate-dose intravenous immunoglobulin treatment of Job's syndrome. Case report. *Minerva Med* 2000;91:113–6.

66. Dahmer MK, Randolph A, Vitali S, et al. Genetic polymorphisms in sepsis. *Pediatr Crit Care Med* 2005;6:S61–73.

67. Rosenzweig SD, Holland SM. Phagocyte immunodeficiencies and their infections. *J Allergy Clin Immunol* 2004;113:620–6.

68. Cole T, McKendrick F, Titman P, et al. Health related quality of life and emotional health in children with chronic granulomatous disease: A comparison of those managed conservatively with those that have undergone haematopoietic stem cell transplant. *J Clin Immunol* 2013;33(1):8–13.

69. Zarzour W, Kleta R, Frangoul H, et al. Two novel CHS1 (LYST) mutations: Clinical correlations in an infant with Chediak-Higashi syndrome. *Mol Genet Metab* 2005;85:125–32.

70. Wynn RF, Sood M, Theilgaard-Monch K, et al. Intractable diarrhoea of infancy caused by neutrophil specific granule deficiency and cured by stem cell transplantation. *Gut* 2006;55:292–3.

71. Ristoff E, Larsson A. Inborn errors in the metabolism of glutathione. *Orphanet J Rare Dis* 2007;2:16.

72. Goldfarb RD, Parrillo JE. Complement. *Crit Care Med* 2005;33:S482–4.

73. Cunnion KM, Wagner E, Frank MM. Complement and kinin. In: Parslow TG, Stites DP, Terr AL, et al., eds. *Medical Immunology*. 10th ed. New York, NY: McGraw-Hill, 2001:175–88.

74. Sjoholm AG, Jonsson G, Braconier JH, et al. Complement deficiency and disease: An update. *Mol Immunol* 2006;43:78–85.

75. Figueroa JE, Densen P. Infectious diseases associated with complement deficiencies. *Clin Microbiol Rev* 1991;4:359–95.

76. Super M, Thiel S, Lu J, et al. Association of low levels of mannan-binding protein with a common defect of opsonisation. *Lancet* 1989;2:1236–9.

77. Thiel S, Frederiksen PD, Jensenius JC. Clinical manifestations of mannan-binding lectin deficiency. *Mol Immunol* 2006;43:86–96.

78. Siassi M, Hohenberger W, Riese J. Mannan-binding lectin (MBL) serum levels and post-operative infections. *Biochem Soc Trans* 2003;31:774–5.

79. Ytting H, Christensen IJ, Jensenius JC, et al. Preoperative mannan-binding lectin pathway and prognosis in colorectal cancer. *Cancer Immunol Immunother* 2005;54:265–72.

80. Schlapbach LJ, Aebi C, Otth M, et al. Deficiency of mannose-binding lectin-associated serine protease-2 associated with increased risk of fever and neutropenia in pediatric cancer patients. *Pediatr Infect Dis J* 2007;26:989–94.

81. Cedzynski M, Atkinson AP, St Swierzko A, et al. L-ficolin (ficolin-2) insufficiency is associated with combined allergic and infectious respiratory disease in children. *Mol Immunol* 2009;47:415–9.

82. Hansen TK, Thiel S, Wouters PJ, et al. Intensive insulin therapy exerts antiinflammatory effects in critically ill patients and counteracts the adverse effect of low mannose-binding lectin levels. *J Clin Endocrinol Metab* 2003;88:1082–8.

83. Garred P, Storm JJ, Quist L, et al. Association of mannose-binding lectin polymorphisms with sepsis and fatal outcome, in patients with systemic inflammatory response syndrome. *J Infect Dis* 2003;188:1394–403.

84. Sutherland AM, Walley KR, Russell JA. Polymorphisms in CD14, mannose-binding lectin, and Toll-like receptor-2 are associated with increased prevalence of infection in critically ill adults. *Crit Care Med* 2005;33:638–44.

85. Fidler KJ, Wilson P, Davies JC, et al. Increased incidence and severity of the systemic inflammatory response syndrome in patients deficient in mannose-binding lectin. *Intensive Care Med* 2004;30:1438–45.

86. Ahrens P, Kattner E, Kohler B, et al. Mutations of genes involved in the innate immune system as predictors of sepsis in very low birth weight infants. *Pediatr Res* 2004;55:652–6.

87. Biezeveld MH, Kuipers IM, Geissler J, et al. Association of mannose-binding lectin genotype with cardiovascular abnormalities in Kawasaki disease. *Lancet* 2003;361:1268–70.

88. Cheung YF, Ho MH, Ip WK, et al. Modulating effects of mannose binding lectin genotype on arterial stiffness in children after Kawasaki disease. *Pediatr Res* 2004;56:591–6.

89. Bernstein JA. Update on angioedema: Evaluation, diagnosis, and treatment. *Allergy Asthma Proc* 2012;32:408–12.

90. Sardana N, Craig TJ. Recent advances in management and treatment of hereditary angioedema. *Pediatrics* 2011;128:1173–80.

91. Bork K, Siedlecki K, Bosch S, et al. Asphyxiation by laryngeal edema in patients with hereditary angioedema. *Mayo Clin Proc* 2000;75:349–54.

92. Boyle RJ, Nikpour M, Tang ML. Hereditary angio-oedema in children: A management guideline. *Pediatr Allergy Immunol* 2005;16:288–94.

93. Jonsson G, Truedsson L, Sturfelt G, et al. Hereditary C2 deficiency in Sweden: Frequent occurrence of invasive infection, atherosclerosis, and rheumatic disease. *Medicine (Baltimore)* 2005;84:23–34.

94. Pickering MC, Botto M, Taylor PR, et al. Systemic lupus erythematosus, complement deficiency, and apoptosis. *Adv Immunol* 2000;76:227–324.

95. Picard C, Casanova JL, Puel A. Infectious diseases in patients with IRAK-4, MyD88, NEMO, or IkappaBalpha deficiency. *Clin Microbiol Rev* 2011;24:490–7.

96. von Bernuth H, Picard C, Jin Z, et al. Pyogenic bacterial infections in humans with MyD88 deficiency. *Science* 2008;321:691–6.

97. Doffinger R, Smahi A, Bessia C, et al. X-linked anhidrotic ectodermal dysplasia with immunodeficiency is caused by impaired NF-kappaB signaling. *Nat Genet* 2001;27:277–85.

98. Courtois G, Smahi A, Reichenbach J, et al. A hypermorphic IkappaBalpha mutation is associated with autosomal dominant anhidrotic ectodermal dysplasia and T cell immunodeficiency. *J Clin Invest* 2003;112:1108–15.

99. Pizzo PA, Poplack DG. *Principles and Practice of Pediatric Oncology*. 4th ed. Philadelphia, PA: Lippincott Williams and Wilkins, 2002.

100. Mackall CL, Fleisher TA, Brown MR, et al. Lymphocyte depletion during treatment with intensive chemotherapy for cancer. *Blood* 1994;84:2221–8.

101. Fiser RT, West NK, Bush AJ, et al. Outcome of severe sepsis in pediatric oncology patients. *Pediatr Crit Care Med* 2005;6:531–6.

102. Viscoli C, Castagnola E, Giacchino M, et al.; Supportive Therapy Group—Infectious Diseases Section of the Italian Association of Paediatric Haematology and Oncology. Bloodstream infections in children with cancer: A multicentre surveillance study of the Italian Association of Paediatric Haematology and Oncology. *Eur J Cancer* 1999;35:770–4.

103. Wisplinghoff H, Seifert H, Wenzel RP, et al. Current trends in the epidemiology of nosocomial bloodstream infections in patients with hematological malignancies and solid neoplasms in hospitals in the United States. *Clin Infect Dis* 2003;36:1103–10.

104. Mackall CL. T-cell immunodeficiency following cytotoxic antineoplastic therapy: A review. *Stem Cells* 2000;18:10–8.

105. Ruescher TJ, Sodeifi A, Scrivani SJ, et al. The impact of mucositis on alpha-hemolytic streptococcal infection in patients undergoing autologous bone marrow transplantation for hematologic malignancies. *Cancer* 1998;82:2275–81.

106. Small TN, Avigan D, Dupont B, et al. Immune reconstitution following T-cell depleted bone marrow transplantation: Effect of age and posttransplant graft rejection prophylaxis. *Biol Blood Marrow Transplant* 1997;3:65–75.

107. Fry TJ, Mackall CL. Immune reconstitution following hematopoietic progenitor cell transplantation: Challenges for the future. *Bone Marrow Transplant* 2005;35(suppl 1):S53–7.

108. Porta MD, Rigolin GM, Alessandrino EP, et al. Dendritic cell recovery after allogeneic stem-cell transplantation in acute

leukemia: Correlations with clinical and transplant characteristics. *Eur J Haematol* 2004;72:18–25.

109. Damiani D, Stocchi R, Masolini P, et al. Dendritic cell recovery after autologous stem cell transplantation. *Bone Marrow Transplant* 2002;30:261–6.

110. Reddy V, Iturraspe JA, Tzolas AC, et al. Low dendritic cell count after allogeneic hematopoietic stem cell transplantation predicts relapse, death, and acute graft-versus-host disease. *Blood* 2004;103:4330–5.

111. Storek J, Dawson MA, Storer B, et al. Immune reconstitution after allogeneic marrow transplantation compared with blood stem cell transplantation. *Blood* 2001;97:3380–9.

112. Mackall CL, Bare CV, Granger LA, et al. Thymic-independent T cell regeneration occurs via antigen-driven expansion of peripheral T cells resulting in a repertoire that is limited in diversity and prone to skewing. *J Immunol* 1996;156:4609–16.

113. Brochu S, Rioux-Masse B, Roy J, et al. Massive activation-induced cell death of alloreactive T cells with apoptosis of bystander postthymic T cells prevents immune reconstitution in mice with graft-versus-host disease. *Blood* 1999;94:390–400.

114. Cavazzana-Calvo M, Fischer A, Hacein-Bey-Abina S, et al. Gene therapy for primary immunodeficiencies: Part 1. *Curr Opin Immunol* 2012;24:580–4.

CHAPTER 87 ■ **BACTERIAL SEPSIS**

NEAL J. THOMAS, ROBERT F. TAMBURRO, SURENDER RAJASEKARAN, JULIE C. FITZGERALD, SCOTT L. WEISS, AND MARK W. HALL

KEY POINTS

1. The International Consensus Conference on Pediatric Sepsis and Organ Dysfunction was convened to develop pediatric-specific definitions for systemic inflammatory response syndrome, sepsis, severe sepsis, and septic shock. These definitions provide the framework for the evaluation and analysis of sepsis across patient and study populations.

2. This overall prevalence of pediatric sepsis is 0.89 per 1000 children, with a national estimate of prevalence of severe sepsis of >75,000 cases. The greatest prevalence is in newborns (9.70 per 1000) and decreases to a low of 0.23 per 1000 in children 10–14 years of age.

3. While many viruses may cause the sepsis syndrome in isolation, the presence of bacterial coinfections, particularly methicillin-resistant *Staphylococcus aureus*, should be suspected in patients with a viral syndrome and severe sepsis.

4. An ever-growing body of literature suggests that the genetic composition of an individual influences the risk of developing sepsis and the outcome from that septic process. In fact, data suggest that death from infection has a stronger heritable component than death from cancer or cardiovascular disease.

5. The presence of a comorbid condition predisposes significantly to both the incidence and outcome of pediatric sepsis.

6. Any device that breaches the skin barrier and remains in place creates the potential for contamination of the device and subsequent bacteremia. Most endemic transmission follows the route of nose to hand to device from either the patient or the healthcare worker. Healthcare-associated infections are a large source of morbidity and have a high cost, making them a prime target for quality improvement initiatives.

7. Septic shock is commonly a combination of distributive, hypovolemic, and cardiogenic shock. Septic shock requires manifestations of decreased organ perfusion by definition.

8. Sepsis in children is much different than in adults. While some children, especially those in whom sepsis is recognized early in the course of infection, can present with the classic adult picture of "warm," vasodilated shock signified by an increase in cardiac output and a decrease in systemic vascular resistance, most children will present with "cold" shock, with an increase in systemic vascular resistance and a decrease in cardiac output, requiring inotropic support as opposed to a vasopressor. Children often change sep-

sis phenotype during their course, and therapies that may have been appropriate on one day may not be beneficial, or may even be harmful, on another.

9. A critical part of the evaluation of the patient with suspected sepsis is the identification of an infectious source. Current guidelines recommend obtaining cultures and administering empiric broad-spectrum antibiotics within 1 hour of presentation.

10. The first hours following the diagnosis of severe sepsis represent an important opportunity for intervention to reverse shock and prevent or attenuate organ dysfunction.

11. The American College of Critical Care Medicine revised their clinical practice parameters for hemodynamic support of pediatric and neonatal patients in septic shock in 2009 (1). These parameters were also briefly reviewed in 2012 in a revision of the adult sepsis guidelines (2). These important documents were based upon review of the medical evidence and consensus expert opinion and fulfill an essential role in the standardization of pediatric sepsis treatment.

12. Goals of therapy for the initial management of pediatric septic shock include prompt recognition of decreased perfusion based on the clinical exam, administration of up to 60 mL/kg of crystalloid or colloid, initiation of antibiotics within 15 minutes of recognition of decreased perfusion, and initiation of inotropic agents for fluid-refractory shock within 60 minutes of shock recognition.

13. In bacterial sepsis, early diagnosis and intervention will result in improved outcomes. Compromised systemic perfusion can often be diagnosed clinically by poor skin perfusion and signs of decreased organ function. The use of hemodynamic monitoring may complement the clinical detection of compromised perfusion as well as assist in clinical decision making.

14. Healthcare-associated infections (HAIs) contribute significantly to hospital-associated morbidity, mortality, and costs. Critically ill children have an increased risk of sepsis related to HAIs due to a high rate of comorbid conditions, depressed immune function, and the presence of indwelling catheters and tubes.

15. The case-fatality rate from pediatric sepsis in 2005 was 8.9%, not significantly changed from 2000, but decreased from 1995. In the United States, there were 75,255 pediatric hospitalizations in 2005 involving severe sepsis, with an associated cost of $4.8 billion.

INTRODUCTION AND DEFINITION

Brief Overview

Bacterial sepsis is a major cause of morbidity and mortality in children and a common reason for children to require pediatric intensive care unit (PICU) resources. Worldwide, sepsis is the most common cause of deaths in infants, as it can occur secondary to pneumonia, diarrhea, malaria, and other invasive bacterial diseases. Conversely, in developed countries, great progress has been made in the treatment of this heterogeneous, infectious condition, with the vast majority of children surviving sepsis. This chapter will serve to identify the epidemiology, etiology, pathophysiology, clinical presentation, clinical management, quality indicators, outcomes, and future directions of bacterial sepsis in children.

Definitions

The sepsis syndrome represents the systemic inflammatory response to suspected or proven infection. The associated signs and symptoms can include fever, tachycardia, tachypnea, abnormal peripheral white blood cell count, and evidence of organ dysfunction, but a practical framework for diagnostic criteria was lacking until the 2001 International Sepsis Definitions Conference (3). The definitions that resulted, including systemic inflammatory response syndrome (SIRS), sepsis, severe sepsis, and septic shock, were specific to adults. Thus,

an International Consensus Conference on Pediatric Sepsis and Organ Dysfunction was convened to develop pediatric-specific definitions for SIRS, sepsis, severe sepsis, and septic shock, which were published in 2005 (4,5) (**Table 87.1**). To date, these definitions provide the framework for the evaluation and analysis of sepsis in children.

The definition of SIRS requires the presence of at least two of four criteria, one of which is an abnormal temperature or leukocyte count. Upper and lower limits of these four SIRS criteria for the six specific age groups were established by consensus opinion (**Table 87.2**). Sepsis is defined as SIRS in the presence of, or as a result of, a suspected or proven infection. Severe sepsis and septic shock are defined as sepsis plus the presence of organ dysfunction. Recently, emphasis has been placed on the distinction between *definitions* and *thresholds* (2). Definitions are simply parameters used to identify the presence of one of these conditions; in contrast, thresholds are therapeutic targets. For example, in the recently published International Guidelines for Management of Severe Sepsis and Septic Shock in adults, sepsis-induced hypotension is defined as a mean arterial pressure <70 mm Hg, but the therapeutic target is a mean arterial pressure ≥65 mm Hg (2).

Although these definitions for SIRS, sepsis, severe sepsis, and septic shock have become well entrenched in pediatric practice and research, problems still exist. For example, a recent, single-center study screened over 1700 patients for the presence of severe sepsis or septic shock and found only a moderate level of agreement between the consensus conference definitions (as described above) and a clinical diagnosis as offered by a member of the medical team in the electronic medical record, or an administrative diagnosis as ascertained from International Classification of Diseases discharge diagnoses (6). Moreover, a

---

TABLE 87.1

DEFINITIONS OF SYSTEMIC INFLAMMATORY RESPONSE SYNDROME, INFECTION, SEPSIS, SEVERE SEPSIS, AND SEPTIC SHOCK IN CHILDREN

SIRS

The presence of at least two of the following four criteria, one of which must be abnormal temperature or leukocyte count:
Core temperature of >38.5°C or <36°C
Tachycardia, defined as a mean heart rate >2 SD above normal for age in the absence of external stimulus, chronic drugs, or painful stimuli
OR otherwise unexplained persistent elevation over a 0.5- to 4-h period
OR for children <1 y old: bradycardia, defined as a mean heart rate <10th percentile for age in the absence of external vagal stimulus, β-blocker drugs, or congenital heart disease or otherwise unexplained persistent depression over a 0.5-h period
- Mean respiratory rate >2 SD above normal for age or mechanical ventilation for an acute process not related to underlying neuromuscular disease or the receipt of general anesthesia
- Leukocyte count elevated or depressed for age (not secondary to chemotherapy-induced leukopenia) or >10% immature neutrophils

Infection

A suspected or proven (by positive culture, tissue stain, or polymerase chain reaction test) infection caused by any pathogen OR a clinical syndrome associated with a high probability of infection. Evidence of infection includes positive findings on clinical exam, imaging, or laboratory tests (e.g., white blood cells in a normally sterile body fluid, perforated viscus, chest x-ray consistent with pneumonia, petechial or purpuric rash, or purpura fulminans)

Sepsis

SIRS in the presence of, or as a result of, suspected or proven infection

Severe Sepsis

Sepsis plus one of the following: cardiovascular organ dysfunction OR acute respiratory distress syndrome OR two or more other organ dysfunctions

Septic Shock

Sepsis and cardiovascular organ dysfunction

From Goldstein B, Giroir B, Randolph A; International Consensus Conference on Pediatric Sepsis. International pediatric sepsis consensus conference: Definitions for sepsis and organ dysfunction in pediatrics. *Pediatr Crit Care Med* 2005;6:2–8, with permission.

TABLE 87.2

AGE-SPECIFIC VITAL SIGNS AND LABORATORY VARIABLES (LOWER VALUES FOR HEART RATE, LEUKOCYTE COUNT, AND SYSTOLIC BLOOD PRESSURE ARE FOR THE 5TH AND UPPER VALUES FOR HEART RATE, RESPIRATION RATE, OR LEUKOCYTE COUNT FOR THE 95TH PERCENTILE)

■ AGE GROUP	HEART RATE (beats/min)		■ RESPIRATORY RATE (breaths/min)	■ LEUKOCYTE COUNT, LEUKOCYTES ($\times 10^3$/mm)	■ SYSTOLIC BLOOD PRESSURE (mm hg)
	■ TACHYCARDIA	■ BRADYCARDIA			
0 d–1 wk	>180	<100	>50	>34	<59
1 wk–1 mo	>180	<100	>40	>19.5 or <5	<79
1 mo–1 y	>180	<90	>34	>17.5 or <5	<75
2–5 y	>140	NA	>22	>15.5 or <6	<74
6–12 y	>130	NA	>18	>13.5 or <4.5	<83
13 to <18 y	>110	NA	>14	>11 or <4.5	<90

From Goldstein B, Giroir B, Randolph A; International Consensus Conference on Pediatric Sepsis. International pediatric sepsis consensus conference: Definitions for sepsis and organ dysfunction in pediatrics. *Pediatr Crit Care Med* 2005;6:2–8, with permission.

precise characterization and staging of patients with sepsis is still lacking. A conceptual framework for analyzing sepsis was proposed as part of the 2001 International Sepsis Definitions Conference (3). Known by the acronym "PIRO," this classification scheme for sepsis stratifies patients on the basis of their *P*redisposing conditions, the nature and extent of the *I*nsult (in the case of sepsis, infection), the nature and magnitude of the host *R*esponse, and the degree of concomitant *O*rgan dysfunction. The value of PIRO-based scoring systems in pediatric sepsis merits further study.

Epidemiology

Bacterial sepsis is a worldwide problem that is confounded by its multiple etiologies and myriad risk factors. The most comprehensive study to examine the epidemiology of severe sepsis in the US reported that, in 1995, >42,000 cases of severe sepsis occurred in children who were ≤19 years of age, with an incidence of 0.56 cases per 1000 population annually (7). This study was duplicated in 2013, demonstrating an increase in the prevalence of severe sepsis, mainly due to an increase in the prevalence of severe sepsis in newborns (8). This overall prevalence had increased to 0.89 per 1000 children, with a national estimate of prevalence of severe sepsis of >75,000 cases. The greatest prevalence was in newborns (9.70 per 1000) and decreased to a low of 0.23 per 1000 in children 10–14 years of age (Table 87.3). It is important to recognize that the highest rate of severe sepsis in this youngest age group was due to the inclusion of very-low-birth-weight infants, where the prevalence of severe sepsis markedly increased in the recent cohort. Despite this wide disparity in incidence across age groups, mortality was fairly consistent at ~6%–10% for all age groups.

Etiology

The most common sites of infection in children are respiratory, blood, genitourinary, abdominal, device-related, soft tissue, and central nervous system (Fig. 87.1). The bacterial pathogens

TABLE 87.3

PREVALENCE OF PEDIATRIC SEVERE SEPSIS: 1995, 2000, AND 2005

■ VARIABLE	■ 1995	■ 2000	■ 2005
Seven state pediatric population	17,146,000	18,332,173	18,846,000
Percent of U.S. pediatric population	22.7	22.8	23.1
Pediatric hospitalizations, *n*	1,586,253	1,569,329	1,563,597
Severe sepsis case, *n*	9675	12,089	17,542
National estimate, *n*	42,370	53,410	75,255
Prevalence (per 1,000 population)[a]	0.56	0.63	0.89
Incidence by age group			
Newborns	4.50	5.37	9.70
Normal birth weight	2.40	2.40	2.50
Low birth weight	2.40	2.00	1.80
Very low birth weight	1.80	2.80	4.60
Nonnewborn infants	1.85	2.21	2.25
1–4 y	0.49	0.44	0.52
5–9 y	0.22	0.19	0.23
10–14 y	0.20	0.21	0.23
15–19 y	0.37	0.40	0.48

[a]Prevalence for newborns is expressed per 1,000 live births in the five states, where birth weight data were available (Massachusetts, Maryland, New Jersey, New York, Virginia).
From Hartman ME, Linde-Zwirble WT, Angus DC, et al. Trends in the epidemiology of pediatric severe sepsis. *Pediatr Crit Care Med* 2013;14(7):686–93.

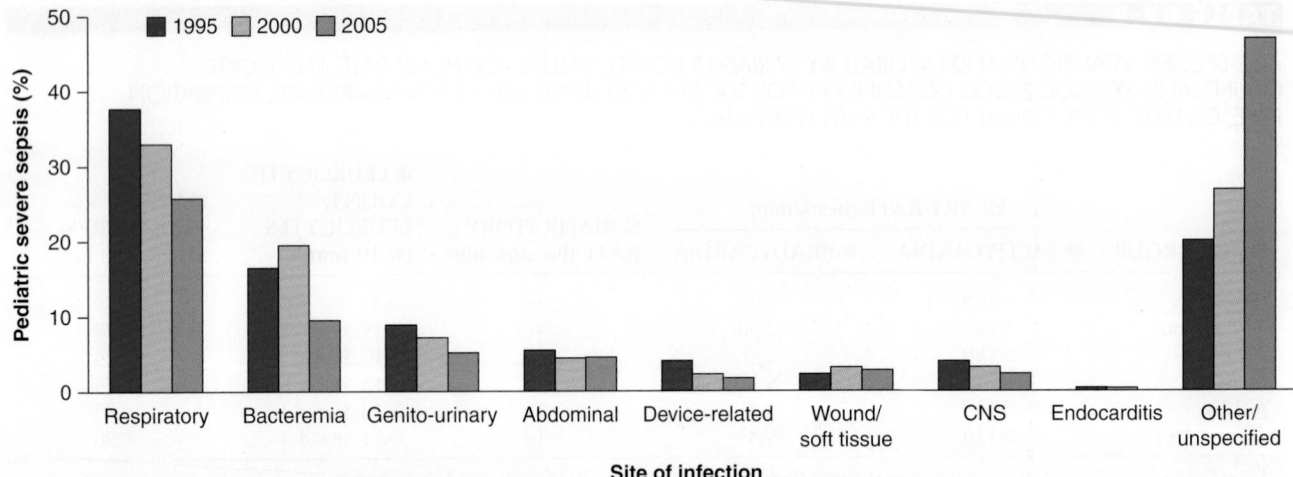

FIGURE 87.1. Site of infection associated with pediatric severe sepsis: 1995 *(blue bar)*, 2000 *(tan bar)*, and 2005 *(green bar)*. Of those cases where site of infection was known, respiratory and bacteremia were the most common sites of infection in all years. There was a significant increase in the proportion of wound and soft-tissue infections over time ($p < 0.0001$). The proportion of severe sepsis cases without documented site of infection or causative organism increased over time, from only 20% of cases in 1995 to 46% of cases in 2005. (From Hartman ME, Linde-Zwirble WT, Angus DC, et al. Trends in the epidemiology of pediatric severe sepsis. *Pediatr Crit Care Med* 2013;14(7):686–93.)

that cause severe sepsis vary by age, institution, and presence of underlying risk factors including immunocompromising condition, indwelling vascular catheter, and immunization status. Gram-positive bacteria, mainly *Staphylococcus* and *Streptococcus* species, remain the most prevalent organisms isolated (9). However, gram-negative organisms, including *Escherichia coli*, *Klebsiella* species, and *Pseudomonas aeruginosa*, are also frequently identified, especially in neonates, patients with neutropenia, and hospital-acquired sepsis (10). Overall, the most common bacterial pathogens isolated from children with severe sepsis are listed in **Table 87.4**. Although less common, meningococcal infections, especially in unimmunized populations, and the toxic shock syndrome caused by toxin-producing strains of *Staphylococcus aureus* and *Streptococcus pyogenes* remain important additional causes of sepsis in children, and can result in significant morbidity and mortality. Notably, a microbial pathogen may not be isolated in up to 75% of children with sepsis (6,11). This "culture-negative" sepsis may indicate a host response to bacterial components, such as endotoxin, released into the circulatory system, insufficient sensitivity of

current diagnostic testing, or result from antibiotic treatment before obtaining bacterial cultures.

Streptococcus agalactiae (group B streptococcus) was the predominant organism associated with neonatal sepsis in the first 3 days of life until the widespread adoption of intrapartum chemoprophylaxis in the early 1990s. The rate of other bacteria that cause early-onset sepsis, including *Escherichia coli*, *Listeria monocytogenes*, enterococcus, non–group D α-hemolytic streptococci, and nontypable *Haemophilus influenzae*, has remained constant (12). Presently, *Staphylococcus* is the most common infecting organism among neonates, causing about a quarter of all cases of neonatal sepsis (9) and reflecting the impact of nosocomial infections in this age group. Approximately 90% of these episodes are due to coagulase-negative staphylococcus, with *S. aureus* implicated in the other 10%. *P. aeruginosa*, gram-negative enteric bacteria, and environmental bacilli are also significant causes of hospital-acquired sepsis. Low birth weight remains a significant risk factor for severe sepsis, and respiratory and cardiovascular diseases are commonly observed underlying conditions in newborn sepsis.

TABLE 87.4

CAUSATIVE ORGANISMS FOR PEDIATRIC SEVERE SEPSIS: 1995, 2000, AND 2005

	CASES (%)			CASE FATALITY (%)		
ORGANISM	■ 1995	■ 2000	■ 2005	■ 1995	■ 2000	■ 2005
Meningococcus	1.2	0.7	0.4	12.4	10.8	10.6
Haemophilus influenzae	0.8	0.5	0.4	4.2	5.0	1.6
Pseudomonas	3.3	3.0	2.4	10.4	8.1	6.4
Echerichia coli	4.6	4.0	2.5	9.7	10.3	6.6
Staphylococcus (all types)	15.8	12.9	6.8	9.7	8.5	7.1
Staphylococcus aureus	2.6	4.9	3.6	2.6	8.1	6.4
Streptococcus (all types)	7.8	5.8	3.3	11.4	8.1	8.2
Pneumococcus	0.9	1.0	0.4	21.5	11.3	5.1
Group B *streptococcus*	1.3	0.4	0.4	8.9	2.2	6.4
Virus	5.6	3.1	2.9	7.3	6.6	4.0
Fungus	6.4	9.5	5.3	11.7	10.1	8.6

Includes data for only those cases where the causative organism was identified (37.6% of all cases, *n* = 14,433).
From Hartman ME, Linde-Zwirble WT, Angus DC, et al. Trends in the epidemiology of pediatric severe sepsis. *Pediatr Crit Care Med* 2013;14(7):686–93.

In older children, the gram-positive organisms *S. aureus* and *Streptococcus* species are most common, often arising from a respiratory or skin/soft tissue source (13,14). Sepsis associated with a thrombophlebitis should raise the suspicion of *Fusobacterium necrophorum*. Primary bacteremia without a focal source is less common in older children compared to infants (7). The prevalence of septicemia due to *H. influenzae* type b (Hib), *Streptococcus pneumoniae*, and *Neisseria meningitidis* has significantly decreased over the past two decades in developed countries due to the advent of conjugated vaccines for these bacteria. Invasive disease in a healthy, immunized population due to Hib, especially, is now virtually nonexistent. The rates of invasive pneumococcal disease have also declined dramatically in both immunized and unimmunized children since the introduction of the 7-valent pneumococcal conjugate vaccine in 2000 (15). Rickettsial infections can also manifest as sepsis. In endemic areas of the US, *Rickettsia rickettsiae* causes Rocky Mountain spotted fever and may present similarly to meningococcemia with fever, shock, and petechial rash. Human ehrlichioses (human monocytic ehrlichiosis due to *Ehrlichia chaffeensis*, human granulocytic anaplasmosis due to *Anaplasma phagocytophila*, and granulocytic ehrlichiosis due to *Ehrlichia ewingii*) can be mistaken for Rocky Mountain spotted fever (16). Human monocytic ehrlichiosis is more likely to present with a rash, and skin manifestations are unusual in human granulocytic anaplasmosis.

Comorbidities that depress host immunity, such as malignancies, renal failure, hepatic failure, HIV/AIDS, and immunosuppressant medications, are common among patients with severe sepsis or septic shock. Certain conditions predispose to sepsis with certain bacteria (Table 87.5). For example, in patients with febrile neutropenia and other immunocompromising conditions, typical gram-positive and gram-negative organisms remain common but more unusual pathogens, including *Streptococcus viridians*, *P. aeruginosa*, *Enterobacter*, *Citrobacter*, and *Acinetobacter* species, and *Stenotrophomonas maltophilia*, are important sources of sepsis in this population (17). In children with sickle cell disease and other causes of functional asplenia, gram-positive bacteria (especially *S. pneumoniae*) predominate, but other encapsulated bacteria, including *Salmonella*, are also commonly identified. In hospital-acquired bacterial sepsis, such as catheter-associated

TABLE 87.6

ENVIRONMENTAL CONDITIONS THAT PREDISPOSE THE HOST TO SPECIFIC BACTERIA

■ ORGANISM	■ ENVIRONMENTAL SOURCE
Listeria monocytogenes	Food, especially dairy and pork products
Enterococcus faecium	Commercial chicken and meat products
Clostridium perfringens	Soil
Salmonella	Poultry, pork, beef, egg, and dairy products
Yersinia	Pork, chitterlings (pork intestines), and dairy products
Vibrio vulnificus	Seawater and undercooked seafood (clams, oysters, and mussels)

bloodstream infections, coagulase-negative *Staphylococcus* is most commonly isolated, followed by gram-negative organisms, including *P. aeruginosa*, *E. coli*, *Klebsiella* species, and *Enterobacter* (10,18). Lastly, certain foods are linked with pathogens (Table 87.6). Children with inherent or acquired predisposition to sepsis are discussed later in this chapter.

While many viruses (e.g., influenza, adenovirus, dengue) may cause the sepsis syndrome in isolation, the presence of bacterial coinfections, particularly methicillin-resistant *Staphylococcus aureus* (MRSA), should be suspected in patients with a viral syndrome and severe sepsis. In a recent study of 838 children with the 2009 pandemic influenza A (H1N1) virus, early (within 72 hours) *S. aureus* respiratory coinfection occurred in 9% of patients of which 48% were MRSA (19). MRSA coinfection was identified as an independent risk factor for mortality. Secondary bacterial pneumonia due to *S. aureus*, *S. pneumoniae*, nontypable *H. influenzae*, and *Moraxella catarrhalis* following primary infection with RSV or other common respiratory viruses is also a common problem in the critically ill child (20).

The prevalence of bacterial strains exhibiting antibiotic resistance is increasing in both community and hospital-acquired sepsis (21,22). Multidrug-resistant organisms include MRSA, β-lactam-resistant and multidrug-resistant *pneumococci*, vancomycin-resistant *enterococci*, extended-spectrum β-lactamase-producing gram-negative enteric pathogens, and carbapenem-resistant *Pseudomonas*. Local resistance patterns need to be considered when selecting empiric antibiotic therapy.

MECHANISM OF DISEASE: CORE PATHOPHYSIOLOGY

Host Risk Factors

Genetic Predisposition

An ever-growing body of literature suggests that the genetic composition of an individual influences the risk of developing sepsis and the outcome from that septic process. In fact, data suggest that death from infection has a stronger heritable component than death from cancer or cardiovascular disease (23). Recently, much work has focused on identifying genetic polymorphisms that code for inflammatory molecules essential for host defense and studying their association with the

TABLE 87.5

CLINICAL CONDITIONS THAT PREDISPOSE THE HOST TO SPECIFIC BACTERIA

■ CONDITION	■ BACTERIA
Asplenia	*Streptococcus pneumoniae*
Polysplenia	*Salmonella*
Sickle cell disease	*Streptococcus pneumoniae*
	Salmonella
Nephrotic syndrome	*Streptococcus pneumoniae*
HIV/AIDS	*Streptococcus pneumoniae*
	Haemophilus influenzae type b
	Staphylococcus aureus
	Pseudomonas aeruginosa
Complement deficiencies	*Neisseria meningitidis*
C5, C6, C7, C8, C9	*Neisseria gonorrhoeae*
Iron overload	*Yersinia enterocolitica*
	Listeria monocytogenes
	Vibrio vulnificus
Neutropenia	*Streptococcus viridans*

HIV, human immunodeficiency virus; AIDS, acquired immune deficiency syndrome.

occurrence and severity of infection. For example, expression of tumor necrosis factor (TNF)-α, a key component of the inflammatory cascade of sepsis, has been associated with polymorphisms in the gene's promoter region (24). An adenine substitution at the −308 base pair, the TNF2 allele, is associated with increased production of TNFα (25). Moreover, the TNF2 allele has been associated with the development of sepsis, sepsis severity, and mortality from sepsis in some, but not all, reports (26).

Additionally, a polymorphism at the platelet activator inhibitor (PAI)-1 promoter site has been identified and has been found to be associated with outcomes from sepsis. Children homozygous for the 4G/4G allele with meningococcemia have been found to have higher plasma concentrations of PAI-1 and worse outcomes as compared to other genotypes (27).

Polymorphisms in the coding region for toll-like receptors (TLRs) have also been found to influence the susceptibility and response to infectious challenges. For example, the coding region for TLR-2 contains a polymorphism at the 753 site involving the replacement of glutamine with arginine. This polymorphism may result in a less vigorous response to gram-positive infection, and has been associated with the risk of recurrent infection (28) and urinary tract infection (29). Polymorphisms in the TLR-4 coding region have been associated with decreased responsiveness to lipopolysaccharide in humans (30) and increased risk of gram-negative infections in murine models (31).

In addition to these examples, polymorphisms in the genes that code for other components of the inflammatory response, including Fc-γ receptors, mannose-binding lectin, interleukin (IL)-1, (IL-1RA), IL-6, IL-10, protein C, bacterial permeability increasing protein, and heat shock proteins, have also been identified. The effects of these polymorphisms on sepsis outcomes in children remain unclear. Genes related to the sepsis process also appear to be influenced by epigenetic changes (32). These changes may impede the immune response long after the initial infection. In children with septic shock, suppression of genes associated with the adaptive immune response appears to occur in conjunction with epigenetic changes (33).

The effects of polymorphisms and epigenetic changes on the inflammatory response to infection are complex and multifactorial. Despite the recent surge in this field of research, translating these findings into clinically relevant information remains a challenge. Functional phenotypic assessment of candidate polymorphisms remains controversial because the same variant may have very different effects in different populations (34). Moreover, the traditional approach of case–control designs is limited by the potential for confounding or spurious associations (34). Any conclusions regarding relationships between disease state and polymorphic alleles must be tempered until confirmed in additional populations by independent investigators. Despite these limitations, large-scale studies may be critical in developing a clear understanding of the genetic determinants of sepsis so that truly personalized sepsis treatments can be developed.

Race/Ethnicity/Gender/Age Differences

Other factors, such as race, ethnicity, gender, and age, may influence the incidence and outcomes from sepsis. Several large epidemiologic adult studies have demonstrated that African-Americans are more likely to be hospitalized for severe sepsis than are Caucasians, though racial influences on mortality are less clear. One such study included over 300,000 trauma patients and found that African-American race was independently associated with a higher likelihood of developing posttraumatic sepsis (35). In another analysis, the racial differences in severe sepsis were notable for a higher infection rate and a higher risk of acute organ dysfunction in African-Americans (36). Unfortunately, less is known about this in pediatrics. Among newborns, data suggest worse sepsis outcomes among African-American children. A recently published longitudinal study of severe sepsis in children suggested that non-White Hispanics are accounting for a higher proportion of cases of severe sepsis than previously reported (8); however, that study does not account for potential changes in the population demographics over time.

In contrast, the effect of gender on sepsis has been more thoroughly investigated. Several studies have demonstrated a significantly higher incidence of severe sepsis in males than in females. The aforementioned epidemiological study of severe sepsis in children reported an increased incidence of severe sepsis among males from 1995 to 2005 (8). In another large epidemiologic study of pediatric sepsis, there were no differences between prepubertal males and females with sepsis in terms of mortality or initial severity of illness (37). However, among postpubertal children with sepsis, males had a significantly higher mortality rate than females. This difference in mortality, however, was no longer significant after controlling for the initial severity of illness and the hospital center, suggesting that the difference in mortality may be due to the initial higher severity of illness in males. These results also suggest that the response of males and females to therapies directed against sepsis is similar. Several potential explanations for these differences in postpubertal males and females have been offered including differences in hormones, comorbidities, the infectious etiology, and health-related behaviors including the time to seek medical care. Differences in the incidence and outcomes among the sexes may also be secondary to differences in the immune response. Both humoral and cell-mediated immune responses to antigen challenge are enhanced in females as compared to males. Numerous studies also support the view that hormones of the endocrine system, including different concentrations of sex steroids, contribute to the difference in immunologic response between the genders.

In addition to gender, it has been long established that age influences the incidence and outcome of sepsis, even among pediatric subgroups (9,38,39). More recent data support this contention and suggest that the prevalence of severe sepsis is increasing among all age groups, but most notably among newborns (8) (Table 87.3). This appears to be due, in large part, to a 2.5-fold increase among very low-birth-weight infants, though the prevalence among older adolescents (15–19 years) has also increased significantly. In terms of mortality, infants less than 1 year of age demonstrate higher sepsis-related mortality than any other age group, with children less than 1 year of age having a case-fatality rate that approximates twice that of children over 1 year (8). Very-low-birth-weight infants have the highest sepsis-related case-fatality rate of all age groups (Fig. 87.2).

Comorbidities

The presence of a comorbid condition predisposes significantly to both the incidence and outcome of pediatric sepsis (8,38). Although the proportion of septic children with a comorbid condition appears to be decreasing, an underlying comorbidity is still reported in approximately 40% of septic children; if prematurity is included as a comorbidity, that number exceeds 60%. The most common comorbidities vary by age, but include neuromuscular, cardiovascular, and respiratory disorders. In infants less than 1 year of age, chronic lung disease and congenital heart disease are the most commonly reported comorbidities, with neuromuscular disorders and neoplasms being the most common in children over 1 year of age. Not surprisingly, case-fatality rates among septic children with a comorbid condition have remained higher than those of children with sepsis who do not have such a coexisting condition.

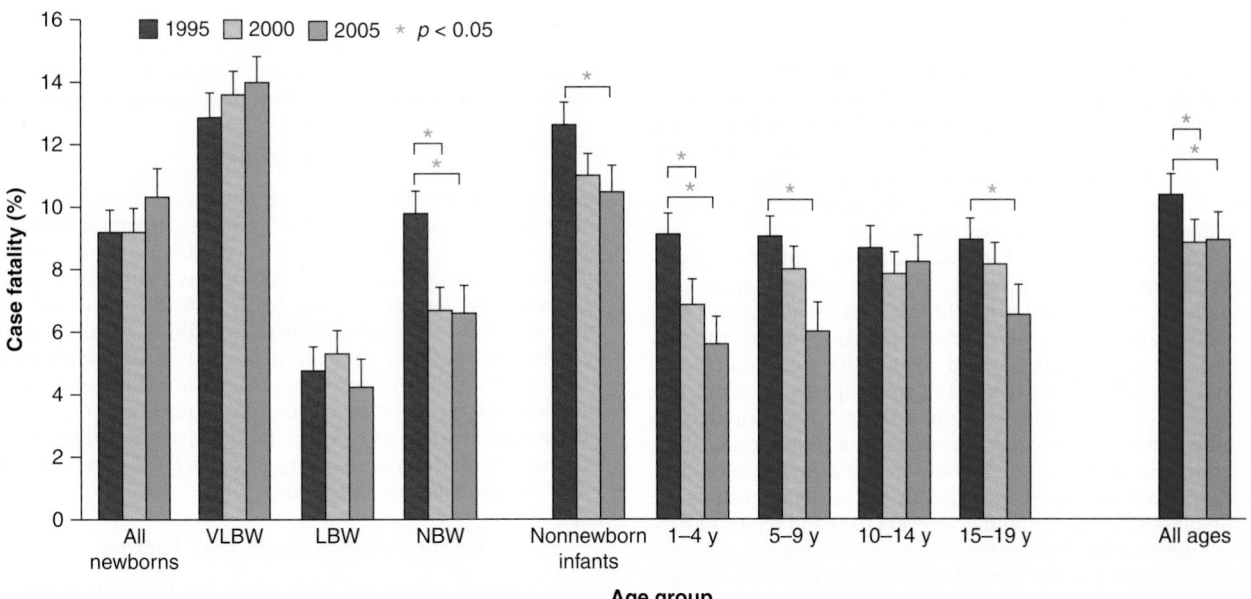

FIGURE 87.2. Mortality related to pediatric severe sepsis: 1995 *(blue bar)*, 2000 *(tan bar)*, and 2005 *(green bar)*. Case fatality from pediatric severe sepsis decreased in every age group over time except in newborns. In this group, fatality for infants with normal birth weight *(NBW)* or low birth weight *(LBW)* dropped but fatality for infants with very low birth weight *(VLBW)* increased by 7.8%. *p value less than 0.05. (From Hartman ME, Linde-Zwirble WT, Angus DC, et al. Trends in the epidemiology of pediatric severe sepsis. *Pediatr Crit Care Med* 2013;14(7):686–93.)

This is true in every age group in children with comorbidities (9) (**Fig. 87.3**) and mortality from sepsis is increased in children when sepsis occurs after surgical procedures.

Environmental Risk Factors

Sepsis can result from infections related to bacterial exposures from the environment as well as those from medical devices and procedures. Any device that breaches the skin barrier and remains in place creates the potential for contamination of the device and subsequent bacteremia. Most such transmission follows the route of nose to hand to device from either the patient or the healthcare worker. Healthcare-associated infections (HAIs) are a large source of morbidity and have a high cost, making them a prime target for quality improvement initiatives.

Central Venous Lines

The use of indwelling central venous catheters in the PICU creates the opportunity for nosocomial bloodstream infections. Gram-positive bacteria, largely *Staphylococcus*, are usually present on the patient's skin before placement of the device.

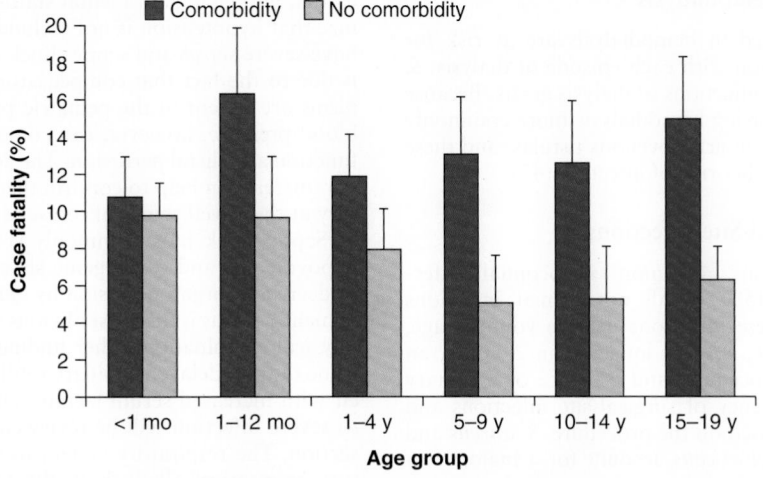

FIGURE 87.3. Case fatality of children with severe sepsis by age and comorbidity. Case fatality was highest in children 1–12 months old and was significantly higher among children with any underlying disease. Results for children who were <1 month old and 1–12 months old are from the five states (Massachusetts, Maryland, New Jersey, New York, and Virginia) in which neonates could be identified (*n* = 6349, or 66% of the entire 7-state cohort). Results for children >1 year of age are from the entire 7-state cohort (*n* = 9675); 95% confidence intervals are shown by *error bars*. (From Watson RS, Carcillo JA, Linde-Zwirble WT, et al. The epidemiology of severe sepsis in children in the United States. *Am J Respir Crit Care Med* 2003;167:695–701, with permission.)

In contrast, healthcare workers may introduce gram-negative organisms present on their hands during manipulation of IV devices. Central line-associated blood stream infections (CLABSIs) are now viewed as preventable rather than inevitable. In fact, the estimated number of CLABSIs in ICUs in the United States fell from 43,000 in 2001 to 18,000 in 2009, with the largest reductions in those infections caused by *S. aureus* (40). Approximately half of all catheter-related infections are now due to coagulase-negative *Staphylococcus* and *Enterococcus* species, followed by *Candida*, *S. aureus*, and then gram-negative organisms (*K. pneumoniae*, *Enterobacter* species, *P. aeruginosa*, *E. coli*, and others) (41). Factors associated with an increased risk for catheter-related infection include the very young, the chronically ill, and those with poor nutritional status, loss of skin integrity, and neutropenia. Specific risk factors for CLABSI identified in pediatric ICU populations include parenteral nutrition, presence of a gastrostomy tube, and duration of ICU central venous access (42), as well as certain practices associated with care of the catheter, such as use of alteplase in malfunctioning catheters (43) and repair of broken catheters (44). Use of bundles or guidelines for insertion and maintenance of the central venous catheter, including use of chlorhexidine skin baths, antibiotic-impregnated catheters, regular assessment of the need for the catheter, and audits of compliance can help decrease the rate of CLABSI (41).

Urosepsis

Although pyelonephritis and secondary sepsis can result from bacteriuria and urinary tract infections, isolated episodes of cystitis are far more common. Longer duration of urinary catheterization is the largest risk factor for urinary tract infection in the critically ill child (45). Virtually all closed-system urinary catheters are colonized within 30 days of placement, and open systems are colonized much sooner. The catheter bypasses the natural defenses against urinary tract infection, such as urine flow and substances secreted by the mucosa that inhibit adhesion of bacteria. Higher rates of infection are associated with diarrhea, low urine flow, and urinary stasis. An important modifiable risk factor is duration of catheterization. The most common bacteria associated with infection are *E. coli*, other gram-negative bacilli, *Enterococcus*, and *Candida* (46).

Hemodialysis

Arteriovenous fistulas used in hemodialysis are at risk for contamination and infection with each episode of dialysis. *S. aureus* causes most of the infections of dialysis grafts. Because of their size, children receiving hemodialysis more commonly have tunneled catheters than arteriovenous fistulas, and these catheters carry an even higher risk of infection (47).

Surgical-Site Infections

Surgical-site infections are common nosocomial infections, accounting for ~15% of all nosocomial infections (48). Risk factors for these infections include younger age, a contaminated procedure, surgery longer than 2 hours, an abdominal or thoracic procedure, and presence of a urinary catheter. The exact frequency of surgical-site infections and the microbiology differ based on the procedure. *S. aureus* and coagulase-negative *Staphylococcus* account for a majority of pediatric surgical-site infections, but gram-negative organisms are becoming more prominent (49).

Osteomyelitis

Nonhematogenous osteomyelitis is uncommon in children but can be associated with open fractures, fascial infections, implanted devices, and chronic open ulcers. *S. aureus* is the typical pathogen, but enteric gram-negative organisms and anaerobic bacteria can infect exposed bone. Osteomyelitis is a rare complication of intraosseous line use. Bone biopsy with culture is the definitive method for diagnosis of osteomyelitis.

Endocarditis

Right-sided endocarditis is being diagnosed more often with the increased use of indwelling venous catheters; however, preexisting congenital heart disease remains the most common risk factor for endocarditis. Endocarditis that occurs within 2 months of cardiac surgery (early postoperative endocarditis) develops as a consequence of thrombi forming at the surgical site(s). These sites can become infected with bacteria introduced via the bypass pump, from a surgical wound infection, secondary to a catheter-associated infection, or from an exposed pacemaker wire. *S. aureus* and viridans *Streptococcus* are responsible for the majority of cases (50). Fungi are also becoming increasingly important.

Other Environmental Risk Factors

Some bacteria associated with sepsis are linked to exposure to specific environmental sources (**Table 87.6**). Identifying a source can be difficult but is important in preventing other cases.

CLINICAL PRESENTATION AND DIFFERENTIAL DIAGNOSIS

Clinical Presentation

To effectively treat sepsis, it must be rapidly recognized by healthcare providers. A very high index of suspicion is required from the onset of symptoms, as the diagnosis of severe sepsis is a clinical one, made by signs of decreased tissue and organ perfusion on physical examination. The clinical presentation can vary widely depending on many factors including the timing of the infection, the organism responsible for the shock state, and the patient's previous state of health. The classic constellation of clinical signs of sepsis includes change in temperature (either hyperthermia or hypothermia), tachypnea and tachycardia, and change in mental status. It is important to recognize that hypotension is not included in this list. Children can have severe sepsis and septic shock without hypotension. This is due to the fact that compensatory vasoconstrictive mechanisms are potent in the pediatric population. Preservation of blood pressure, however, can come at the expense of cardiac function and distal perfusion. The addition of basic laboratory parameters can help to confirm the diagnosis but are unnecessary at the initial stages of resuscitation.

Septic shock, most commonly a combination of distributive, hypovolemic, and cardiogenic shock, requires manifestations of decreased organ perfusion by definition. Whereas a change in mental status is the most obvious symptom to note on a brief physical examination, other findings could include decreased urine output, delayed capillary refill, or an increased base deficit with increased serum lactate. The cardiovascular response to severe infection will be reviewed in detail in the following section. The respiratory system usually exhibits a compensatory respiratory alkalosis in the face of metabolic acidosis. However, pulmonary edema, pneumonia, and/or pediatric acute respiratory distress syndrome may lead to an impairment of this compensatory mechanism. The central nervous system may demonstrate changes in mental status (including somnolence or agitation) and, if the decrease in cerebral perfusion is severe, seizures. Both the renal and hepatic systems may also be injured by decreased organ perfusion, necessitating the monitoring of urine output as well as renal and hepatic function testing. Hematologic failure can occur in the form of DIC, thrombocytopenia (which may cause purpura or petechiae), or bone marrow failure.

Hemodynamic Data

Since normal hemodynamic parameters vary across the pediatric age spectrum, abnormal vital signs must be defined by the age of the child. Definitions published by the International Consensus Conference on Pediatric Sepsis stratified children into the age groups listed in **Table 87.2** (5). The heart rate response to sepsis is most commonly tachycardia, and maintained variability in heart rate can be an encouraging sign. Bradycardia may signify severe infection, particularly in the neonatal period; bradycardia in older children usually signifies a near-terminal event. Hypotension is not required for the diagnosis of sepsis or septic shock and may not be present due to the fact that the children can maintain their blood pressure until the point of decompensation. Definitions of systemic hypotension, based on systolic blood pressure, are also outlined in **Table 87.2**.

It is clear that sepsis in children is much different than in adults. Some children, especially those in whom sepsis is recognized early in the course of infection, can present with the classic adult picture of "warm," vasodilated shock characterized by an increase in cardiac output and a decrease in systemic vascular resistance. Most children, however, will present with "cold" shock with an increase in systemic vascular resistance and a decrease in cardiac output, requiring inotropic support as opposed to a vasopressor. Accordingly, prolonged capillary refill and instantaneous capillary refill can both represent signs of sepsis in children. Moreover, children often change from one phenotype to the other during their course of sepsis, and therapies that may have been appropriate on one day of sepsis may not be beneficial, or may even be harmful, on another (51). Therefore, obtaining serial hemodynamic data may be important in pediatric sepsis due to its dynamic nature.

Laboratory Abnormalities

Pro- and anti-inflammatory cytokines, direct cellular injury, mitochondrial dysfunction, and endothelial damage account for many of the characteristic laboratory findings of sepsis. Leukocytosis often occurs due to demargination of polymorphonuclear cells (PMNs) and increased production and release of immature PMNs from the bone marrow. Neutropenia can develop in the setting of bone marrow failure or if the PMNs are consumed peripherally as they attach to endothelial cells and become ensnared in capillaries. Platelet count is likely to decrease early due to increased peripheral consumption and increase later as a result of reactive thrombocytosis.

Acute-phase reactants are synthesized in the liver, including C-reactive protein, amyloid, α_1-acid glycoprotein, haptoglobin, fibrinogen, ceruloplasmin, and α_1-antitrypsin, in response to IL-1 and IL-6 stimulation. Serum levels of albumin, prealbumin, transferrin, and retinol-binding protein may fall, as a result of decreased production or capillary leak. Serum iron and zinc levels often fall due to uptake by liver cells and inflammatory cells, while copper levels increase in response to higher concentrations of ceruloplasmin. Anemia can be seen in septic children due to underproduction of red blood cells, hemolysis from endothelial damage and microcirculatory changes, and resuscitation-related hemodilution.

Sepsis places considerable metabolic stress on the host. Accelerated use of energy sources can lead to an increase in free fatty acids, hyperglycemia, and protein catabolism. An elevated lactate indicates cellular injury or transition to anaerobic metabolism. The central venous oxyhemoglobin saturation ($ScvO_2$) may be low due to decreased cardiac output and increased metabolic demands, leading to increased oxygen extraction. Alternatively, $ScvO_2$ can be high as a result of mitochondrial dysfunction (tissue dysoxia) and decreased oxygen consumption.

Coagulation abnormalities are common. Fibrinogen, factor V, factor VIII, protein C, and antithrombin levels are often decreased, while tissue factor is increased. Prothrombin time and partial thromboplastin time are prolonged in the majority of patients with DIC. Fibrin degradation products are also present in most septic patients with DIC. D-Dimer is elevated in 90% of patients and is more specific for DIC than fibrin degradation products (52). The peripheral smear will demonstrate microangiopathic changes.

Differential Diagnosis

Other Infectious Diseases

Candidemia is common in premature infants but is unusual in otherwise healthy infants. Other risk factors for fungal sepsis are immunocompromised status, receipt of parenteral nutrition, presence of central venous catheter, and exposure to broad-spectrum antibiotics. Viruses can also present in a fashion indistinguishable from a bacterial process in young infants, especially herpes simplex. In certain circumstances, a TORCH complex (toxoplasma, rubella, cytomegalovirus, and herpes simplex virus) agent should be considered. Varicella, primary herpes simplex, adenovirus, and respiratory syncytial virus can cause serious, life-threatening infections in pediatric patients, and can be particularly severe in immunocompromised patients and patients with history of extreme prematurity. Influenza infection can present with fever, respiratory failure, and shock. Rabies virus must be considered, especially if the patient had contact with a bat or raccoon. Bioterrorism has resurrected the threat of smallpox and anthrax.

Other Noninfectious Diseases

Severe Kawasaki disease, Stevens–Johnson syndrome, drug reactions, juvenile rheumatoid arthritis, pancreatitis, hemophagocytic lymphohistiocytosis, myocarditis, and systemic lupus erythematosus can all masquerade as sepsis. Many of these diseases can also be complicated by superimposed bacterial sepsis. Other causes of SIRS include trauma, burns, and autoimmune disorders. Children with neutropenia can manifest symptoms consistent with SIRS without being infected. Children can also present with SIRS and shock after certain antibody and cytokine therapies for treatment of malignancies. A thorough history and complete physical exam are essential when looking for noninfectious causes of SIRS. Past problems and procedures, recent medications, travel, and potential exposures can all aid in the diagnosis.

Diagnosis

A critical part of the evaluation of the patient with suspected sepsis is the identification of an infectious source. This includes procurement of bacterial cultures from blood as well as sterile specimens from other potential sites of infection that could include cerebrospinal fluid (CSF), urine, respiratory secretions, pleural fluid, skin lesions, vaginal specimens, synovial fluid, or peritoneal fluid. Blood cultures should be obtained from all lumens of indwelling central venous catheters (unless the device was inserted <48 hours prior), as well as at least one culture drawn percutaneously (1). When feasible, it is preferable to obtain specimens before the administration of antimicrobial agents but it is never appropriate to delay treatment of a critically ill child while waiting to obtain cultures. Current guidelines recommend obtaining cultures and administering empiric broad-spectrum antibiotics within 1 hour of presentation. It is important to use sterile techniques to collect specimens, as contamination is a major cause of false-positive cultures. It is essential to recognize that blood cultures are not 100% sensitive in detecting bacteremia. Bacteremia may be transient or intermittent, there may be a low bacterial burden, or the inciting organism may be slow growing. In addition, the sensitivity of blood cultures is partially dependent upon the volume of blood collected. An inappropriately low blood inoculant volume will increase the risk of false-negative culture results. In adults, each additional milliliter of blood cultured increases microbial recovery by up to 3%, though in general the relatively higher bacterial burden in blood found in infants and children with sepsis does allow for smaller blood sampling in younger patients (53). The recommended amount of blood per culture for different age groups is 1–2 mL in neonates, 2–3 mL in infants, 3–5 mL in children, and 10–20 mL in adolescents.

For some infections—particularly nonbacterial pathogens—other diagnostic testing (e.g., viral culture, polymerase chain reaction [PCR], rapid immunoassay antigen test, or direct immunofluorescent antibody staining) may be helpful to establish the source of infection. Viral cultures can yield diagnostic information if obtained with the appropriate method and materials. Sites suitable for sampling include conjunctiva, nasopharynx, urethra, vagina, and vesicles or ulcers on skin and mucous membranes. Blood and CSF can also be sent for viral culture, but specific PCR assays are more sensitive. PCR-based tests are particularly useful to detect herpes simplex, enteroviruses, Ebstein–Barr, cytomegalovirus, and respiratory viruses (e.g., influenza, RSV, adenovirus, parainfluenza, human metapneumovirus). For detection of fungemia, ordinary blood cultures are often sufficient with the advent of modern laboratory detection systems, though it is recommended to alert your microbiology laboratory for concerns of a potential fungal infection as special media or incubation conditions can improve pathogen recovery. Adjunctive tests for fungal disease include galactomannan and β-D-glucan. Galactomannan is recommended when concern for invasive aspergillosis is high, but insufficient data about β-D-glucan precludes its use in pediatrics (54). Large pediatric studies ongoing in the United States and Europe should help to inform the utility of β-D-glucan in children.

The introduction of rapid, non–culture-based diagnostic methods, including DNA amplification by PCR, mass spectroscopy, and microarrays, has the potential to improve the overall rate of, and time to, pathogen identification. These methodologies could be particularly useful for difficult-to-culture pathogens or in clinical situations where empiric antimicrobial agents have been administered before culture samples were obtained (55). In addition, as our understanding of the determinants of antimicrobial resistance continues to improve, these techniques may also be able to identify antibiotic-resistant strains faster than culture-based approaches.

The role of biomarkers to differentiate bacterial sepsis from other noninfectious causes of inflammation remains controversial. White blood cell count, including the presence of immature PMNs ("bands"), and C-reactive protein may be informative but are neither sensitive nor specific for bacterial sepsis. A myriad of novel biomarkers have been studied in adult and pediatric sepsis (56). The most promising is procalcitonin, a precursor to calcitonin, which is upregulated in the presence of bacterial and fungal disease to a greater degree than in viral or noninfectious inflammatory states (57). However, the diagnostic utility of procalcitonin for bacterial sepsis in pediatric patients

is yet to be established. Biomarkers could also help to guide safe discontinuation of antimicrobial therapy when infection is unlikely. For example, multiple studies in sepsis show that procalcitonin levels fall quickly as appropriate antibiotic therapy is initiated, and low procalcitonin levels have successfully reduced the duration of antimicrobial therapy without adverse effects in hospitalized patients when an infectious source could not be identified (58). Finally, biomarkers may improve risk stratification of patients for clinical decision making and enrollment into clinical trials. For example, serum interleukin-8 levels of 220 pg/mL or less, measured within 24 hours of admission to the PICU, had a negative predictive value of 95% for 28-day mortality in pediatric septic shock (59). It is likely that combinations of biomarkers will prove more useful than any single assay. Wong et al. recently used genome-wide expression profiling to derive and test a panel of 12 protein biomarkers to predict outcome and reported a 99% (95% CI: 96%, 100%) negative predictive value for mortality (60).

CLINICAL MANAGEMENT/ TREATMENT

Importance of Early Intervention

Early diagnosis and intervention in the treatment of bacterial sepsis is crucial to achieve optimal outcomes, particularly in high-risk patients who may not be able to mount an effective immune response. This population includes children with primary immunodeficiency, transplantation, malignancy, chemotherapy-induced leukopenia, and other secondary immunodeficiencies. While not necessarily immunosuppressed, children with other comorbidities, including chronic lung disease or congenital heart disease, may not be able to tolerate the cardiorespiratory derangements associated with sepsis. Accordingly, these special populations deserve close monitoring and consideration for early referral to a tertiary care center.

The first hours following the diagnosis of severe sepsis represent an important opportunity for intervention to reverse shock and prevent or attenuate organ dysfunction. Perhaps the best illustration of this principle is the study that showed that fluid resuscitation with >40 mL/kg (average 60 mL/kg) in the first hour of treatment conferred a dramatic survival advantage to children with septic shock, compared to those who received less fluid in the same time frame (61). This notion of early and aggressive resuscitation was replicated in adult patients in whom goal-directed therapy on outcomes from severe sepsis and septic shock was examined (62). While a recent study of African children suggested increased mortality associated with rapid fluid resuscitation, it should be noted that many subjects had severe anemia related to malarial infection (63). The generalizability of these results to the general sepsis population is likely to be low.

Another example of the timeliness of a therapy being related to its efficacy can be found in the use of antibiotics. While the administration of antibiotics should not take precedence over resuscitation, shorter time to the receipt of correct empiric antibiotics has been associated with improved outcomes in the settings of adult sepsis and pediatric severe community-acquired pneumonia (64,65). It is now generally recommended that a de-escalating approach to the use of empiric antimicrobial agents be adopted, with broad-spectrum agents being transitioned to the narrowest possible spectrum drugs once culture and susceptibility data are known. Empiric antibiotic therapy must be tailored to provide coverage for community-acquired or nosocomial pathogens (for children who have been hospitalized for >48 hours or who are at high risk for developing nosocomial infection), taking into account regional, hospital, and unit-specific resistance patterns.

Guidelines for Early Clinical Management

⓫ The American College of Critical Care Medicine (ACCM) revised their clinical practice parameters for hemodynamic support of pediatric and neonatal patients in septic shock in 2009 (1). These parameters were also briefly reviewed in 2012 in a revision of the adult sepsis guidelines (2). These important documents were based upon review of the medical evidence and consensus expert opinion, and this section will serve as a review of these guidelines. The ACCM clinical practice parameters define shock by clinical parameters (hypothermia *or* hyperthermia, altered mental status, and abnormal peripheral vasodilation *or* vasoconstriction), hemodynamic variables (inadequate organ perfusion pressure), and oxygen-use measures such as central venous saturation (Scvo$_2$). A detailed algorithm is provided (**Fig. 87.4**) that is notable for its rigorous time line. Within the first 5 minutes of the diagnosis of shock, the child's airway and breathing should be maintained and IV access established. Continuous pulse oximetry, cardiorespiratory monitoring, urine output ⓬ measurement, and frequent vital sign assessment are necessary. Isotonic fluid boluses (normal saline or colloid) should be administered IV in 20 mL/kg aliquots up to and over 60 mL/kg in the next *15 minutes*, while the patient is monitored for hypoglycemia and hypocalcemia if the shock state is not reversed. If shock persists despite the administration of 60 mL/kg of IV fluid, the authors recommend establishing arterial and central venous access and initiating therapy with a dopamine infusion. It should be noted that the ACCM guidelines recommend the initiation of inotropic support via peripheral IV access until central venous access is obtained. If the shock state is not reversed with a dopamine dose of 10 μg/kg/min, it is recommended to transition to an epinephrine infusion in the setting of vasoconstrictive (cold) shock or central norepinephrine for vasodilatory (warm) shock. The former is characterized by poor peripheral pulses, prolonged capillary refill, and diminished peripheral pulses compared to central pulses. Patients with warm shock demonstrate bounding peripheral pulses, erythematous skin, and instantaneous capillary refill. Children with septic shock, in contrast to adults, frequently present in cold shock with low cardiac output and high systemic vascular resistance, and children who present in warm shock often transition to cold shock over the first 48 hours of illness (51). Thus, titration of inotropic or vasopressor support should be based upon frequent reassessment of the child's hemodynamic state.

Should either type of shock state be persistent despite adequate intravascular volume status and an appropriate inotrope or vasopressor regimen, the authors recommend consideration of the use of hydrocortisone for empiric treatment of adrenal insufficiency. A great deal of evidence suggests that a state of adrenal insufficiency can develop in the context of a severe inflammatory insult. It is postulated that this is due to inhibitory effects of high levels of proinflammatory cytokines at the hypothalamic, pituitary, adrenal, and target tissue levels. The topic of corticosteroid treatment in sepsis continues to be a source of controversy. Use of highly potent glucocorticoids was associated with increased mortality in the setting of adult sepsis, but subsequent work suggested that a short course of low-dose hydrocortisone may be associated with improved mortality and more rapid shock reversal in adult severe sepsis and septic shock (66). This may be due to the fact that hydrocortisone has less glucocorticoid effect and more mineralocorticoid effect than drugs such as methylprednisolone or dexamethasone. More recent work has confirmed beneficial effects on shock reversal, but has called into question the mortality benefit (67). Pediatric data are sorely lacking in this area. Risk factors that favor the use of hydrocortisone include prior corticosteroid use, purpura fulminans, HIV infection, and chronic pituitary or adrenal abnormalities. Specific definitions for the diagnosis and management of relative adrenal insufficiency continue to be debated. In addition to the risk factors for adrenal insufficiency noted above, the 2009 update of the ACCM guidelines indicate that a basal cortisol level of <18 μg/dL, a peak ACTH-stimulated cortisol concentration of <18 μg/dL, or catecholamine-resistant shock are indications for hydrocortisone replacement. A loading dose of 2 mg/kg is followed by maintenance dosing, either every 6 hours or as a continuous infusion, with a total daily dose of 2 mg/kg. The guidelines indicate that this point in the algorithm should be reached *within 60 minutes* of the diagnosis of shock if it is not reversed with fluid and catecholamine therapy. It is noteworthy that the adult 2013 Surviving Sepsis guidelines no longer recommend using ACTH stimulation testing to drive hydrocortisone replacement (2).

Should shock continue to be present in the second hour of resuscitation, the ACCM guidelines recommend therapies based upon the patient's clinical, hemodynamic, and oxygen-use phenotype. Patients with normal blood pressure who demonstrate cold shock and Svo$_2$ <70% should be treated with afterload reduction with careful attention to preservation of preload. Children who demonstrate low blood pressure, cold shock, and Svo$_2$ <70% should be treated with titration of epinephrine and ongoing optimization of volume status. Children with refractory shock despite volume loading and titration of first-line cardiovascular medications may require the addition of a second-line agent. These include milrinone in the volume-loaded cold shock patient, and vasopressin in the warm shock patient. While not FDA-approved in the US, the calcium potentiator levosimendan and the type III phosphodiesterase inhibitor enoximone represent potential advanced therapeutic options elsewhere.

Should these maneuvers fail to reverse shock, the authors recommend advanced cardiovascular monitoring to direct ongoing therapy to maintain normal perfusion pressure and maintain the cardiac index between 3.3 and 6 L/min/m². Such forms of monitoring, discussed below, include the use of a pulmonary artery catheter (PAC), a pulse index contour cardiac output (PiCCO) catheter, a femoral artery thermodilution catheter, or Doppler echocardiography. For children with refractory shock, a final recommendation is to consider the use of extracorporeal membrane oxygenation (ECMO) as a rescue therapy for life-threatening septic shock (Chapter 40). Survival rates with ECMO in the treatment of refractory pediatric septic shock have been reported to be as high as 74% (68).

Evaluation and management of airway and breathing should also accompany hemodynamic resuscitation in the setting of sepsis. The provision of supplemental oxygen will assist in reversal of oxygen supply/demand mismatch. Further, in the septic patient, as much as 20%–25% of cardiac output may be diverted to muscles of respiration to fuel respiratory compensation for metabolic acidosis. Mechanical ventilatory support can offload work of breathing and allow for redirection of cardiac output to vital organs. While invasive mechanical ventilation has historically played this role in sepsis resuscitation, noninvasive ventilatory support is increasingly used for this purpose, despite a lack of evidence demonstrating efficacy.

Although endotracheal intubation may be helpful, it may be associated with negative consequences. First, the provision of positive intrathoracic pressure is likely to result in a decrease in venous return. In a hypovolemic septic patient, this reduction in venous return can result in clinically significant decreases in cardiac output and blood pressure. Accordingly, additional isotonic IV fluid should be readily available and/or given as a bolus around the time of intubation to assure adequate preload. Second, the choice of sedative/analgesic for

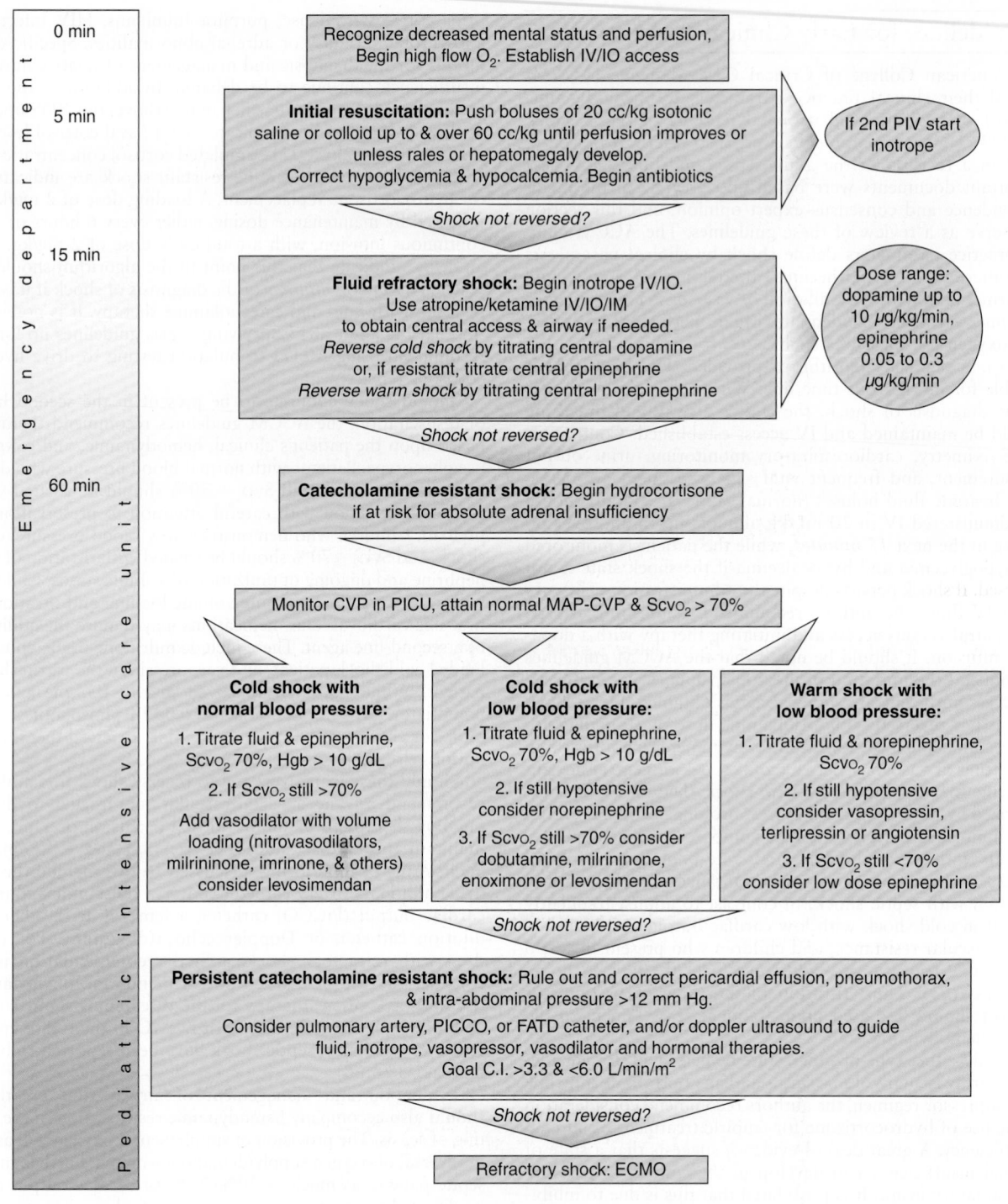

FIGURE 87.4. Algorithm for time-sensitive, goal-directed stepwise management of hemodynamic support in infants and children. (Reproduced from Brierley J, Carcillo J, Choong K, et al. Clinical practice parameters for hemodynamic support of pediatric and neonatal septic shock: 2007 update from the American College of Critical Care Medicine. *Crit Care Med* 2009;37:666–88.)

intubation is important. Etomidate, once popular for its acute blood pressure-sparing properties, is also known to impair adrenal cortisol production. Studies have now associated a single intubating dose of etomidate with increased mortality risk in septic adults and children (69). As a result, etomidate should typically be avoided in this setting in favor of ketamine for sedation for invasive procedures in the setting of sepsis.

Subacute Management

Multiorgan Dysfunction

Although the progression of sepsis to multiple organ dysfunction syndrome (MODS) is poorly understood, it is highly likely that poor perfusion, hypoxia, hyperglycemia, and acidosis all contribute to the process. Detailed attention to organ system support is essential because the cumulative burden of organ system failure increases the likelihood of mortality, with the risk of mortality increasing with each additional organ system failure. Lung dysfunction, which commonly accompanies sepsis, tends to occur early and persist, in contrast to shock, which also occurs early but tends to either rapidly resolve or progress to death. Serious abnormalities of liver function, coagulation, and CNS function tend to occur hours to days after the onset of sepsis and tend to persist. In addition to the number of organ failures, the severity of each failure affects the prognosis.

Ventilation Strategies

Nearly 50% of all adult patients with severe sepsis will develop ARDS, and the prevalence in children is likely similar. The response to sepsis often requires a high minute ventilation in the face of decreased compliance of the respiratory system, increased airway resistance, decreased diffusion, and impaired muscle efficiency (70). Based on the data from adult patients, lung-protective ventilation should be considered. Multiple trials in adults have now demonstrated the benefit of a high positive end-expiratory pressure and low-tidal-volume approach. The goal of mechanical ventilation is to maintain a reasonable level of oxygenation while keeping the fraction of oxygen in inspired gas (FiO_2) below 0.6, allowing for some hypercapnia with the buffered pH >7.25. Nonconventional modes of ventilation, such as airway-pressure-release ventilation or high-frequency oscillatory ventilation, may be required to support oxygenation and minimize lung toxicity.

Renal Replacement Therapy

Acute kidney injury frequently accompanies severe sepsis and portends a poor prognosis, with increased mortality in children. For patients with acute kidney injury who require continuous renal replacement therapy (CRRT), the presence of sepsis, MODS, and fluid overload greater than 20% at the time of CRRT initiation are significantly associated with higher mortality (71).

Hemofiltration can clear some mediators of inflammation and, combined with the benefit of treating fluid overload, may be beneficial in sepsis even in the absence of acute kidney injury. In high-cutoff hemofiltration, a high-flux hemofilter with an *in vivo* cutoff point of ~60 kDa is used, which allows for clearance of molecules up to that size. The ACCM guidelines recommend consideration of CRRT for fluid removal after shock resuscitation for sepsis patients who are >10% fluid overloaded and unable to achieve the desired fluid balance with urine output. In septic shock, with its attendant hemodynamic instability, continuous venovenous hemofiltration is better tolerated than intermittent hemodialysis. Once CRRT is commenced in patients with sepsis, it is important to reassess dosing of antibiotics and measure therapeutic levels wherever practical.

Cardiac Monitoring

Compromised systemic perfusion can often be diagnosed clinically by poor skin perfusion and signs of decreased organ function. However, this can be challenging given the dynamic nature of pediatric sepsis. The goal of treating septic shock is to maintain the perfusion pressure above the critical point below which blood flow to organs is compromised. For example, maintenance of mean arterial pressure with norepinephrine has been shown to improve urine output and creatinine clearance in hyperdynamic sepsis. Several monitoring modalities can be helpful in sepsis resuscitation.

Monitoring of the central venous pressure (CVP) allows for the assessment of the adequacy of fluid resuscitation. Fluid-refractory shock is defined as the persistence of signs of shock after the administration of sufficient fluids to achieve a CVP of 8–12 mm Hg. CVP is best measured from a catheter in the internal jugular or subclavian vein, though useful data can be trended from femoral venous catheters. In addition, the monitoring of $ScvO_2$ may provide insight as to the adequacy of oxygen delivery. Decreased $ScvO_2$ may reflect a cardiac output that is insufficient to meet the metabolic demands of the tissues. A difference of >30% points between systemic saturations and $ScvO_2$ suggests inadequate cardiac output. Alternatively, sepsis can be associated with abnormalities in oxygen extraction or utilization, resulting in an abnormally high $ScvO_2$. A randomized clinical trial of early goal-directed therapy for pediatric septic shock found that the group in which $ScvO_2$ was maintained at 70% for the first 72 hours of pediatric ICU admission had improved survival and better organ function (72). $ScvO_2$ measurement and trending can be accomplished either continuously, using a central venous catheter that contains an oximeter, or intermittently, using laboratory co-oximetry from specimens obtained near the right atrium.

In the setting of refractory, catecholamine-resistant septic shock, the ACCM guidelines recommend the use of advanced hemodynamic monitoring to target a goal cardiac index of 3.3–6.0 L/min/m^2 (**Fig. 87.4**). Historically this measurement was accomplished using a PAC, but the routine use of these catheters is falling out of favor with pediatric and adult intensivists alike. A study of over 3000 adults, including patients with sepsis, demonstrated no statistical difference in mortality or morbidity with PAC use when controlling for severity of illness (73). Alternative approaches for the quantitation of cardiac index and other hemodynamic variables include the use of a PiCCO or femoral artery thermodilution catheter. These devices are often easier and potentially safer to place than a pediatric PAC and can provide intermittent or continuous hemodynamic monitoring. Echocardiography can be helpful in the estimation of cardiac output as well. More recently, inferior vena cava diameter and inferior vena cava collapsibility measured by ultrasound have been used to assess the adequacy of fluid resuscitation in adults with sepsis (74). For circumstances in which the knowledge of pulmonary artery pressures is crucial, however (e.g., a septic patient who may have pulmonary hypertension), a PAC is still the monitoring device of choice.

Transfusion

It would seem intuitive that optimizing hemoglobin levels would improve outcomes from sepsis by augmenting oxygen delivery. In fact, transfusion of red blood cells in the setting of anemia and low $ScvO_2$ is an element of early goal-directed sepsis therapy in adults. However, the efficacy of blood transfusion in sepsis is controversial. One recent study of adults using propensity-matched modeling analysis suggested that blood transfusion was independently associated with a lower risk of 7- and 28-day mortalities (75). Previous work, however, suggested that liberal red blood cell transfusion practices in adults may be associated with higher mortality (76,77). A randomized, controlled trial in stable, critically ill children found that a restrictive transfusion threshold of hemoglobin 7 g/dL did not increase adverse outcomes compared to the more liberal threshold of hemoglobin 9 g/dL (78). A subgroup analysis of the children with sepsis in that trial showed no differences in the incidence of MODS, duration of mechanical ventilation, oxygenation indices, and ICU days between groups (79). The results of these and other trials call into question the current ACCM guideline, which recommends transfusion if the hemoglobin is <10 mg/dL and the patient is in septic shock.

Monitoring of ScvO$_2$ might be one way to weigh the necessity of transfusions and clinically assess their value in resuscitating patients with sepsis.

Nutrition

Sepsis may promote a catabolic state and negative nitrogen balance, and this effect may be accentuated by exogenous steroids. Prolonged bed rest and inactivity also produce a negative nitrogen balance in healthy individuals. Thus, a hypermetabolic state such as sepsis, in concert with bed rest and inactivity, may result in malnutrition. Following the initial resuscitation of the critically ill patient, the nutritional status should be assessed and a plan of nutritional management developed. It is best to utilize the enteral route if possible. Enteral nutrition has been advocated as a means of reducing villous atrophy with its inherent increased intestinal permeability, thereby reducing the incidence of gut translocation and septic complications.

Recently, a large multicenter cohort study of mechanically ventilated children in the PICU demonstrated that a higher percentage of goal energy intake was reached via the enteral route with significantly lower 60-day mortality compared to those receiving parenteral nutrition (80). Patients admitted to units that utilized a feeding protocol had a lower prevalence of acquired infections and this association was independent of the amount of energy or protein intake.

In addition, studies suggest that early enteral feeding of critically ill children on vasoactive drugs and mechanical ventilation is feasible and may be well tolerated. Patients with sepsis who require vasopressors and narcotics often have a degree of gastroparesis and thus may benefit from transpyloric feeding, which may be associated with a shorter time interval to full-strength feeds and a decreased incidence of nosocomial pneumonia. The European Society of Parenteral and Enteral Nutrition recommends that if critically ill patients are not expected to be feeding by mouth within 3 days, enteral nutrition should be commenced. Enteral feedings have additional theoretical advantages, including gastric pH buffering, avoidance of the use of parenteral-nutrition catheters, a more physiologic pattern of enteric hormone secretion, the ability to administer a complete nutritional mixture that includes fiber, and lower costs (70). It is important to note that enteral immunonutrition with L-arginine, ω-3 fatty acids, zinc, and selenium has not been shown to be beneficial in severe sepsis.

Glycemic Control

Hyperglycemia with insulin resistance is common in critically ill children. This may be related to hypoinsulinemia and/or insulin resistance in the setting of sepsis. Tight glycemic control is thought to lead to improvements in white blood cell function and phagocytosis and suppression of the hepatic acute-phase response. There is an association between mortality and longer duration of hyperglycemia and higher peak serum glucose levels in pediatric critical illness (81). The clinical utility of tight glycemic control, however, is unclear in septic children. Children are generally more prone to hypoglycemia when treated with insulin; therefore, insulin therapy should be used cautiously. There are ongoing randomized clinical trials in critically ill children to continue to investigate the optimal blood glucose levels to target and methods to safely achieve glycemic control.

Source Control of Infection

Source control predominantly includes the drainage of infected fluid collections, debridement of infected tissue, and removal of infected devices or foreign bodies. Obvious sources of infection, such as surgical wounds and indwelling foreign bodies

(central venous catheters, ventriculoperitoneal shunts, urinary catheters, etc.), should be carefully scrutinized. If the patient has a central line, for example, both peripheral blood and blood drawn from the catheter should be cultured. The length of time to bacterial growth and the colony count often determine if the catheter is the infectious source. A colony count that is 5–10 times greater from the catheter compared to the peripheral blood is indicative of an infected device. A quantitative culture that yields at least 100 CFU/μL is diagnostic of a central venous catheter infection. If bacteremia persists with appropriate antibiotics, the catheter should be removed. Deep abscesses can be drained with help from the surgical or interventional radiology services, and thus could provide both diagnosis and therapy. Complex fluid collections may require advanced imaging for diagnosis. The prompt identification of necrotizing soft-tissue infections requires immediate surgical debridement.

Other Therapies for Acute Management of Sepsis

A number of treatments aimed at attenuating the inflammatory response during sepsis have been the subject of prospective research in humans as adjunctive therapy. Activated protein C (APC) is an endogenous molecule with antithrombotic, profibrinolytic, and anti-inflammatory properties. The use of recombinant human APC was associated with a significant reduction in mortality in a specific subset of adults with severe sepsis in a large prospective, randomized, double-blinded, placebo-controlled study (82). However, a pediatric phase III follow-up study aimed at promoting resolution of organ dysfunction was stopped at its planned interim analysis due to lack of efficacy (83). Subsequent concerns over safety have resulted in the withdrawal of APC from the market.

Another example of a failed approach to adjunctive treatments in sepsis is that of anti-cytokine therapy. In an effort to reduce the proinflammatory burden in the acute phase of sepsis, numerous adult trials were performed targeting reduction or inactivation of lipopolysaccharide, interleukin-1β, TNF-α, and other mediators. These trials were uniformly unsuccessful. The reasons underlying the failure of these trials were likely multifactorial including the heterogeneity of the septic population, variability in the timing between disease onset and drug administration, the redundancy of proinflammatory cytokine pathways, and unintended immune suppression associated with anti-cytokine therapy.

Extracorporeal therapies such as hemofiltration, plasmapheresis, and plasma exchange represent another approach to the acute restoration of inflammatory homeostasis in sepsis. These treatments are predicated upon bulk removal of inflammatory mediators through diffusion, convection, or membrane adsorption. Plasma exchange offers the additional advantage of replacement of plasma proteins that may become depleted in sepsis, e.g., von Willebrand factor-cleaving protease inhibitor. Data from large, randomized, controlled trials are lacking. However, several small, controlled trials suggest a survival benefit associated with prolonged treatment with plasmapheresis or plasma exchange, particularly in the setting of thrombocytopenia-associated multiple organ failure (84).

The IV administration of polyclonal IV immunoglobulin (IVIG) has also been studied in the context of sepsis in both children and adults with conflicting results. A meta-analysis of IVIG use for the treatment of neonatal infection showed no effect on mortality with empiric use but did show a reduction in mortality risk when used in the context of proven infection (85). These data were supported when a meta-analysis of IVIG use in adult sepsis failed to show a reduction in mortality risk (86), though some investigators have shown improvement in outcomes with IVIG use in the setting of streptococcal toxic shock syndrome (87). A subset of IVIG trials has used a product that is enriched in the IgM fraction of immunoglobulin. Both retrospective and prospective evidence suggests that IgM-enriched IVIG may be beneficial in adults with severe sepsis (88). At present, the benefit of IVIG in pediatric sepsis is still unclear, and it is not currently a part of the ACCM guidelines for pediatric sepsis treatment, with the exception of toxic shock syndrome.

PREVENTION OF SEPSIS

Healthcare-Associated Infections

Given that up to two-thirds of children who develop sepsis have an underlying comorbidity and will likely require frequent hospitalization, successful prevention of sepsis may be highly dependent on eliminating HAIs (6,9,38). HAI are those that occur during a hospitalization when no evidence for that infection was present at the time of admission. HAIs include bloodstream infections (e.g., central line–associated bloodstream infections [CLABSI]), pneumonia and tracheitis (e.g., ventilator-associated pneumonia and tracheitis [VAP and VAT, respectively]), urinary tract infections (e.g., catheter-associated urinary tract infections [CAUTI]), and surgical-site infections. HAIs contribute significantly to hospital-associated morbidity, mortality, and costs. Critically ill children have an increased risk of sepsis related to HAIs due to a high rate of comorbid conditions, depressed immune function, and the presence of indwelling catheters and tubes. Durations of invasive mechanical ventilation and reintubation are commonly reported risk factors for VAP (89). The presence of a central venous catheter for ≥7 days and a bladder catheter for ≥3 days are risk factors for CLABSI and CAUTI, respectively (45,90). In light of this, much attention has been directed to decreasing the incidence of HAIs. Implementation of protocolized insertion and maintenance care practices in 29 PICUs reduced the CLABSI rate from 5.2 to 2.3 per 1000 catheter-days between 2006 and 2009 (91). The Pediatric SCRUB trial, a cluster-randomized, crossover trial in 10 PICUs, showed a decreased rate of bacteremia with daily chlorhexidine bathing in a per-protocol analysis (92). In 2002, the Society of Critical Care Medicine, in collaboration with other organizations, published guidelines intended to provide evidence-based recommendations for preventing catheter-related infections. These guidelines emphasized the following areas: (a) educating and training healthcare providers who insert and maintain catheters; (b) using maximal sterile barrier precautions during central venous catheter insertion; (c) using a 2% chlorhexidine preparation for skin antisepsis; (d) avoiding routine replacement of central venous catheters as a strategy to prevent infection; (e) using antiseptic/antibiotic-impregnated, short-term central venous catheters if the rate of infection is high despite adherence to other strategies; and (f) removing the catheter as soon as possible (93).

High-Risk Patient Populations

Along with decreasing nosocomial infections, another important strategy is the early identification of high-risk patient populations who may be at increased risk for sepsis.

Burns

Improved resuscitation and respiratory support of burn victims has resulted in reduced rates of early death from shock in this patient population but a concomitant increase in late mortality from infection. Infection rates in children hospitalized for burns, including CLABSI, CAUTI, and VAP/VAT, appear to be higher than in critically ill nonburn patients and are similar to rates of other immunocompromised groups (94). Burn patients are predisposed to sepsis for a number of reasons: (a) a global decrease in cellular immune function is associated with burns; (b) neutropenia is common, neutrophil function is depressed, and T-cell transcription is altered; (c) these patients are at risk for increased gut permeability; and (d) bacteremia may occur with wound manipulations.

Trauma

Trauma is another significant risk factor for sepsis. Traumatically injured children are at risk for both injury-related and nosocomial infections. Injury-related infections are primarily wound, intra-abdominal, and CNS infections, while HAIs include respiratory, bloodstream, and urinary tract infections (95). HAIs are most common among mechanically ventilated trauma victims, head-injured patients, and those who require prolonged immobilization or hospitalization (96).

Human Immunodeficiency Virus

HIV-infected children are also at increased risk of viral, bacterial, and fungal sepsis, and the case-fatality rate for nonopportunistic infections may be greater for them than in non–HIV-infected children. Functional abnormalities and apoptosis of CD4$^+$ T lymphocytes, with defective IL-2 and IF-γ production, render patients particularly susceptible to viral and intracellular organisms (97). In addition, associated defects of B-lymphocyte function, natural killer cell activity, neutrophil bactericidal activity, and defective antigen-specific immunoglobulin production (despite an increase in total globulin fraction) predispose children to bacterial sepsis. The use of highly active antiretroviral therapy (HAART) has markedly decreased the rate of progression to acquired immune deficiency syndrome and the prevalence of complications related to HIV, including sepsis and overall mortality (98). The impact of the initiation of HAART on morbidity during acute episodes of sepsis has not been established.

Asplenia

Children born without a spleen or who have impaired splenic function secondary to disease (e.g., sickle cell disease) or splenectomy are at significantly increased risk of life-threatening bacterial sepsis, particularly due to encapsulated organisms. Guidelines for vaccination and prophylactic antibiotics to prevent pneumococcal, meningococcal, and Hib disease have been established for these children (99). Antibiotic prophylaxis is recommended for all children <5 years of age and for at least 1–2 years after splenectomy, though some guidelines propose a longer duration (100).

Cancer and Hematopoietic Stem-Cell Transplantation

Children with neoplasia account for nearly 13% of all cases of severe sepsis in children who are 1–9 years of age and ~17% of cases in children who are 10–19 years of age (9). However, oncology patients should not be considered a homogeneous group, as significant differences exist in their predisposition to sepsis. Leukemia/lymphoma patients have diseased bone marrow and tend to receive more intensive myeloablative therapy than solid tumors, resulting in disruption of normal immune function. As a result of these factors, neutropenic bacteremia appears to occur more frequently among leukemia patients. In addition to the type of cancer, the state of the disease and its treatment may influence the predisposition to sepsis. Not surprisingly, infection rates are significantly higher in patients who receive more intensive protocols. Moreover, hematologic parameters, particularly neutropenia (absolute neutrophil count <500 cells/mm^3), have long been used to identify oncology patients at risk for sepsis, with a well-established relationship between decreased leukocyte numbers and an increased risk of infection. It has been shown that temperature >39.0°C in neutropenic cancer patients increases the likelihood that the patient is bacteremic. Oncology patients who have undergone bone marrow transplantation are at highest risk of death from sepsis (101).

Selective Decontamination

Selective decontamination, aimed at minimizing the risk of nosocomial infection, involves the use of oral nonabsorbable and systemic antibiotics to eliminate potentially pathogenic enteric bacteria while causing minimal effect on endogenous anaerobic flora. Although its efficacy remains controversial, meta-analyses have demonstrated a decrease in nosocomial respiratory infections after *selective oral decontamination* with topical agents and a small decrease in bacteremia and mortality after *selective digestive decontamination* (SDD) that includes intravenous antibiotics (102). Although concern for promoting antimicrobial resistance has been raised, this was not evident in a meta-analysis of 64 studies (103). Limited data from critically ill children suggest that selective decontamination may lead to fewer nosocomial infections. Oral chlorhexidine gluconate is currently recommended by the Surviving Sepsis Campaign because it is relatively easy to administer, decreases the risk of nosocomial infection, and reduces the potential concern over promotion of antimicrobial resistance by other SDD regimens (2).

Prophylaxis

Antimicrobial agents are commonly prescribed to prevent infections in children despite the fact that the efficacy of this practice is unsubstantiated for most conditions. The use of prophylactic antibiotics has been categorized into three major indications: (a) postexposure, (b) periprocedure, and (c) prevention in high-risk populations. Antibiotics are recommended following exposure to specific pathogens, such as *N. meningitidis*, to reduce the risk of developing disease. Second, antibiotics can reduce the likelihood of infection following a procedure when the period of risk is defined and brief, the expected pathogens have predictable antimicrobial susceptibilities, and the site is accessible to antimicrobial agents. The periprocedure use of antibiotics to prevent bacterial endocarditis in children with specific cardiac lesions is a well-established example of this form of prophylaxis. The importance of this practice is emphasized by the fact that endocarditis is associated with the highest case-fatality rate of all forms of pediatric sepsis (9). The third category of prophylactic antibiotic use is to prevent infections in specific high-risk patient populations, as in the asplenic child.

QUALITY INDICATORS

Acute Management Benchmarks

The ACCM practice parameters for pediatric septic shock outline guidelines for quality care in pediatric sepsis (1,2). Goals of therapy for the initial management of pediatric septic shock include prompt recognition of decreased perfusion based on the clinical exam, administration of up to 60 mL/kg of crystalloid or colloid and initiation of antibiotics within 15 minutes of recognition of decreased perfusion, and initiation of vasoactive agents for fluid-refractory shock within 60 minutes of shock recognition. The practice parameters also recommend

the evaluation of blood glucose and calcium levels within the first minutes of sepsis management, and evaluation of lactate during the initial period of pediatric ICU stabilization. While there are few data in pediatrics to support all of the practice guidelines, treatment of pediatric septic shock in accordance with the first edition of the ACCM practice parameters for pediatric septic shock has been associated with significantly improved survival (104). These types of data, along with the strength of the adult studies demonstrating improvement in outcome using "bundles" of recommendations, have led to the current trend of using multifaceted recommendations for sepsis care and for quality benchmarking of this care.

Sepsis Bundle Development

The surviving sepsis campaign was started in 2002 with a plan to create international guidelines for the management of sepsis. The goals of the campaign are to increase awareness, improve diagnosis, to educate practitioners, and to create standard treatment guidelines and methods for sepsis management. The first guidelines were published in 2004 and were updated in 2012 (2). This campaign has proven effective, with decreases in mortality paralleling increases in compliance with bundle guidelines (105). In 2011, the world federation of pediatric intensive care and critical care societies announced the pediatric global sepsis initiative. This initiative is analogous to the surviving sepsis campaign, except that it provides pediatric-specific education, treatment bundle recommendations, and checklists. This initiative also stratifies the bundled recommendations based on the level of industrialization and local resources. Additionally, the initiative provides a voluntary database to track compliance and outcomes. Early data provide further support that compliance with the bundled sepsis care decreases mortality (106). Many hospitals have initiated local sepsis treatment bundles, often focusing on improving acute care delivery in the ED setting. These programs have demonstrated that compliance with bundles can improve time to antibiotic and fluid bolus administration. Compliance with bundled care has also been associated with shorter hospital length of stay, but improvement in other outcomes has not yet been described (107,108).

OUTCOMES

Estimates of the precise number of childhood deaths that are attributable to sepsis are greatly limited by the inexact information that is available. In the largest study performed to examine the scope of pediatric sepsis and outcomes from this disease process in the United States, the case-fatality rate in 2005 was 8.9%, not significantly changed from 2000, but decreased from 1995 (8) (**Fig. 87.2**). The most common infecting organisms in all three epochs were *Staphylococcus* species. Case fatality associated with *Staphylococcus aureus* increased, whereas fatality associated with *Staphylococcus pneumoniae* decreased by 75%. Nationally, there were 75,255 pediatric hospitalizations in 2005 involving severe sepsis, with an associated cost of $4.8 billion (109).

Worldwide, severe sepsis is an even more daunting issue. According to the latest World Health Organization Report, approximately 6.6 million children die each year before reaching their fifth birthday, and almost two-thirds of deaths each year occur as a result of infectious diseases, such as severe infections, acute respiratory infections, and diarrheal diseases (110) (**Fig. 87.5**). One of the goals of the World Health Organization is to move sepsis treatment knowledge to developing countries worldwide in order to decrease these preventable deaths.

Mortality from sepsis appears to be linked to the severity of MODS, given the collective increase in the risk of death

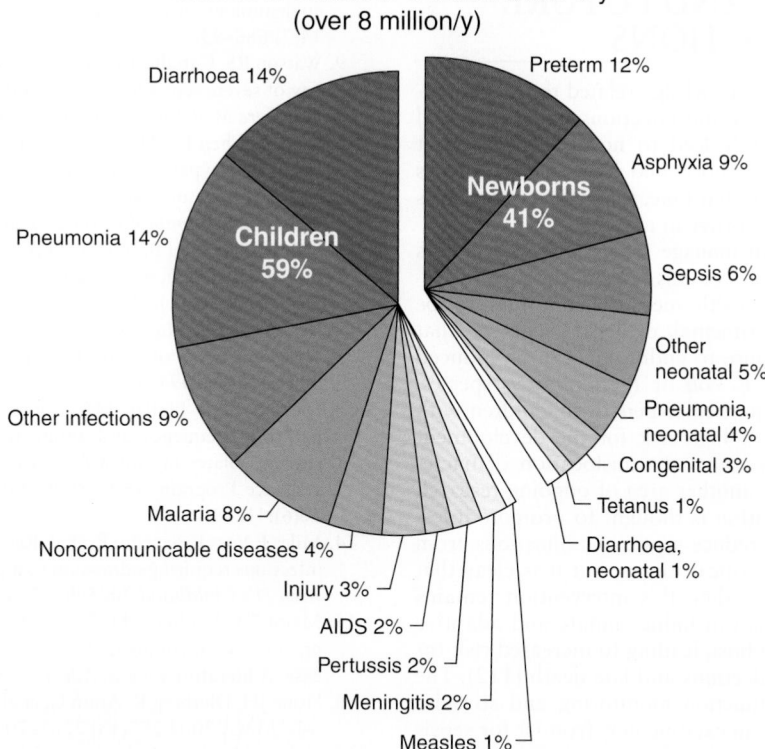

Causes fo deaths in children under 5 y
(over 8 million/y)

FIGURE 87.5. The causes of death in children <5 years of age worldwide. (Source: Unicef 2013 IGME child mortality report.) http://www.childinfo.org/files/Child_Mortality_Report_2013.pdf)

associated with increasing severity of organ dysfunction when a scaled and weighted pediatric MODS score is used. Each unit increase in the pediatric logistic organ dysfunction score is associated with a sharp rise in mortality (111) (Fig. 87.6). A similar trend was seen in a separate cohort of children in whom mortality increased from 7% in those with single-organ failure to 53% in those with four or more organs failing (9).

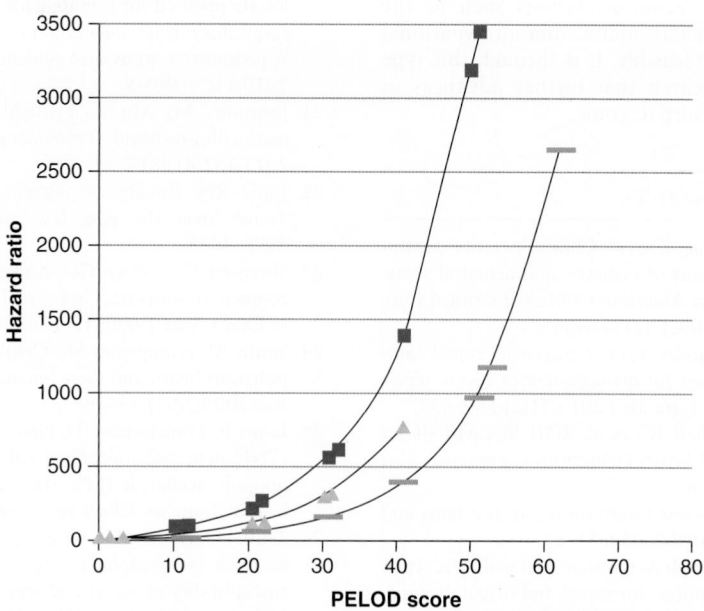

FIGURE 87.6. Observed cumulative hazard ratios (HR) of death of the pediatric logistic organ dysfunction (PELOD) score (which may range from 0 to 71) and the diagnostic category of septic state in the study population (593 children); HR of death is calculated by multiplying HR of the PELOD score (1.096PELOD score) by HR of diagnostic category, i.e., no systemic inflammatory response syndrome (SIRS) (*diamond*); SIRS, sepsis (*dash*); severe sepsis (*triangle*); and septic shock (*square*). (From Leclerc F, Leteurtre S, Duhamel A, et al. Cumulative influence of organ dysfunctions and septic state on mortality of critically ill children. *Am J Respir Crit Care Med* 2005;171: 348–53, with permission.)

SUMMARY AND FUTURE DIRECTIONS

We continue to expand our knowledge related to the interaction between the human host and infectious pathogens, and this knowledge will hopefully lead to novel therapies that have a beneficial impact on short- and long-term outcomes in children with sepsis. Until that time, the mainstay of sepsis therapy continues to be supportive in nature.

Perhaps the best way to manage sepsis is to prevent its occurrence in the first place. For this reason, the most effective sepsis-related public health measure continues to be routine vaccination. Experimental evidence suggests that a protective immune response to endotoxin can be induced from vaccines made from *E. coli* or *Pseudomonas* species. Such vaccines could be of particular benefit to children with chronic illnesses who are at high risk for the development of nosocomial sepsis. Prevention of translocation of bacteria through the intestine is another area of ongoing research interest. Early enteral nutrition is thought to promote intestinal barrier function and reduce septic complications from burns and other forms of critical illness, but it is clear that much more knowledge regarding this intervention remains to be learned. Lastly, sepsis can induce innate and adaptive immune suppression in the host, leading to increased risk for the development of new infections and late death (112). The development of immune function monitoring and stimulation approaches represents an exciting new frontier for sepsis management in children.

The vast majority of large-scale prospective, randomized, controlled trials of sepsis therapies have been performed in adults. The relative infrequency of severe sepsis and septic shock in children and the relatively low pediatric mortality compared to adults make the design and implementation of these studies difficult. In fact, investigators will likely need to target outcomes other than mortality (e.g., length of stay, morbidity) when conducting clinical trials in septic children. As care becomes more standardized across PICUs, with the assistance of evidence-based recommendations such as the ACCM clinical practice parameters, multicenter interventional research should become more feasible. It is through this type of rigorous collaborative research that further advances in pediatric sepsis treatment are sure to come.

References

1. Brierley J, Carcillo JA, Choong K, et al. Clinical practice parameters for hemodynamic support of pediatric and neonatal septic shock: 2007 Update from the American College of Critical Care Medicine. *Crit Care Med* 2009;37(2):666–88.
2. Dellinger RP, Levy MM, Rhodes A, et al. Surviving sepsis campaign: International guidelines for management of severe sepsis and septic shock: 2012. *Crit Care Med* 2013;41(2):580–637.
3. Levy MM, Fink MP, Marshall JC, et al. 2001 SCCM/ESICM/ACCP/ATS/SIS International Sepsis Definitions Conference. *Crit Care Med* 2003;31(4):1250–6.
4. Randolph A. International sepsis forum on sepsis in infants and children. *Pediatr Crit Care Med* 2005;6:S1–64.
5. Goldstein B, Giroir B, Randolph A. International pediatric sepsis consensus conference: Definitions for sepsis and organ dysfunction in pediatrics. *Pediatr Crit Care Med* 2005;6(1):2–8.
6. Weiss SL, Parker B, Bullock ME, et al. Defining pediatric sepsis by different criteria: Discrepancies in populations and implications for clinical practice. *Pediatr Crit Care Med* 2012;13(4):e219–26.
7. Watson RS, Carcillo JA. Scope and epidemiology of pediatric sepsis. *Pediatr Crit Care Med* 2005;6(3 suppl):S3–5.
8. Hartman ME, Linde-Zwirble WT, Angus DC, et al. Trends in the epidemiology of pediatric severe sepsis*. *Pediatr Crit Care Med* 14(7):686–93.
9. Watson RS, Carcillo JA, Linde-Zwirble WT, et al. The epidemiology of severe sepsis in children in the United States. *Am J Respir Crit Care Med* 2003;167(5):695–701.
10. Lee CY, Chen PY, Huang FL, et al. Microbiologic spectrum and susceptibility pattern of clinical isolates from the pediatric intensive care unit in a single medical center—6 years' experience. *J Microbiol Immunol Infect* 2009;42(2):160–5.
11. Gaines NN, Patel B, Williams EA, et al. Etiologies of septic shock in a pediatric emergency department population. *Pediatr Infect Dis J* 2012;31(11):1203–5.
12. Baltimore RS, Huie SM, Meek JI, et al. Early-onset neonatal sepsis in the era of group B streptococcal prevention. *Pediatrics* 2001;108(5):1094–8.
13. Diekema DJ, Pfaller MA, Jones RN. Age-related trends in pathogen frequency and antimicrobial susceptibility of bloodstream isolates in North America: SENTRY Antimicrobial Surveillance Program, 1997–2000. *Int J Antimicrob Agents* 2002;20(6):412–8.
14. Miles F, Voss L, Segedin E, et al. Review of Staphylococcus aureus infections requiring admission to a paediatric intensive care unit. *Arch Dis Childhood* 2005;90(12):1274–8.
15. Myint TT, Madhava H, Balmer P, et al. The impact of 7-valent pneumococcal conjugate vaccine on invasive pneumococcal disease: A literature review. *Adv Ther* 30(2):127–51.
16. Stone JH, Dierberg K, Aram G, et al. Human monocytic ehrlichiosis. *JAMA* 2004;292(18):2263–70.
17. Hakim H, Flynn PM, Knapp KM, et al. Etiology and clinical course of febrile neutropenia in children with cancer. *J Pediatr Hematol Oncol* 2009;31(9):623–9.
18. Yogaraj JS, Elward AM, Fraser VJ. Rate, risk factors, and outcomes of nosocomial primary bloodstream infection in pediatric intensive care unit patients. *Pediatrics* 2002;110(3):481–5.
19. Randolph AG, Vaughn F, Sullivan R, et al. Critically ill children during the 2009–2010 influenza pandemic in the United States. *Pediatrics* 2011;128(6):e1450–8.
20. Levin D, Tribuzio M, Green-Wrzesinki T, et al. Empiric antibiotics are justified for infants with respiratory syncytial virus lower respiratory tract infection presenting with respiratory failure: A prospective study and evidence review. *Pediatr Crit Care Med* 2010;11(3):390–5.
21. Iwamoto M, Mu Y, Lynfield R, et al. Trends in invasive methicillin-resistant *Staphylococcus aureus* infections. *Pediatrics* 2013;132(4):e817–24.
22. Jones RN. Resistance patterns among nosocomial pathogens: Trends over the past few years. *Chest* 2001;119(2 suppl):397S–404S.
23. Sorensen TI, Nielsen GG, Andersen PK, et al. Genetic and environmental influences on premature death in adult adoptees. *N Engl J Med* 1988;318(12):727–32.
24. Smith AJ, Humphries SE. Cytokine and cytokine receptor gene polymorphisms and their functionality. *Cytokine Growth Factor Rev* 2009;20(1):43–59.
25. Louis E, Franchimont D, Piron A, et al. Tumour necrosis factor (TNF) gene polymorphism influences TNF-alpha production in lipopolysaccharide (LPS)-stimulated whole blood cell culture in healthy humans. *Clin Exp Immunol* 1998;113(3):401–6.
26. Teuffel O, Ethier MC, Beyene J, et al. Association between tumor necrosis factor-alpha promoter −308 A/G polymorphism and susceptibility to sepsis and sepsis mortality: A systematic review and meta-analysis. *Crit Care Med* 2009;38(1):276–82.
27. Brouwer MC, Read RC, van de Beek D. Host genetics and outcome in meningococcal disease: A systematic review and meta-analysis. *Lancet Infect Dis* 2012;10(4):262–74.
28. Kutukculer N, Yeniay BS, Aksu G, et al. Arg753Gln polymorphism of the human toll-like receptor-2 gene in children with recurrent febrile infections. *Biochem Genet* 2007;45(7–8):507–14.

29. Tabel Y, Berdeli A, Mir S. Association of TLR2 gene Arg753Gln polymorphism with urinary tract infection in children. *Int J Immunogenet* 2007;34(6):399–405.

30. Michel O, LeVan TD, Stern D, et al. Systemic responsiveness to lipopolysaccharide and polymorphisms in the toll-like receptor 4 gene in human beings. *J Allergy Clin Immunol* 2003;112(5):923–29.

31. Poltorak A, He X, Smirnova I, et al. Defective LPS signaling in C3H/HeJ and C57BL/10ScCr mice: Mutations in Tlr4 gene. *Science* 1998;282(5396):2085–8.

32. Carson WF, Cavassani KA, Dou Y, et al. Epigenetic regulation of immune cell functions during post-septic immunosuppression. *Epigenetics* 2011;6(3):273–83.

33. Wong HR, Freishtat RJ, Monaco M, et al. Leukocyte subset-derived genomewide expression profiles in pediatric septic shock. *Pediatr Crit Care Med* 2010;11(3):349–55.

34. Lin MT, Albertson TE. Genomic polymorphisms in sepsis. *Crit Care Med* 2004;32(2):569–79.

35. Kisat M, Villegas CV, Onguti S, et al. Predictors of sepsis in moderately severely injured patients: An analysis of the National Trauma Data Bank. *Surg Infect (Larchmt)* 2013;14(1):62–8.

36. Mayr FB, Yende S, Linde-Zwirble WT, et al. Infection rate and acute organ dysfunction risk as explanations for racial differences in severe sepsis. *JAMA* 2010;303(24):2495–503.

37. Ghuman AK, Newth CJ, Khemani RG. Impact of gender on sepsis mortality and severity of illness for prepubertal and postpubertal children. *J Pediatr* 2013;163(3):835–40.e1.

38. Odetola FO, Gebremariam A, Freed GL. Patient and hospital correlates of clinical outcomes and resource utilization in severe pediatric sepsis. *Pediatrics* 2007;119(3):487–94.

39. Wynn J, Cornell TT, Wong HR, et al. The host response to sepsis and developmental impact. *Pediatrics* 2010;125(5):1031–41.

40. Centers for Disease Control and Prevention. Vital signs: Central line-associated blood stream infections—United States, 2001, 2008, and 2009. *MMWR Morb Mortal Wkly Rep* 2011;60(8):243–8.

41. Weber DJ, Rutala WA. Central line-associated bloodstream infections: Prevention and management. *Infect Dis Clin North Am* 2011;25(1):77–102.

42. Wylie MC, Graham DA, Potter-Bynoe G, et al. Risk factors for central line-associated bloodstream infection in pediatric intensive care units. *Infect Control Hosp Epidemiol* 31(10):1049–56.

43. Rowan CM, Miller KE, Beardsley AL, et al. Alteplase use for malfunctioning central venous catheters correlates with catheter-associated bloodstream infections. *Pediatr Crit Care Med* 14(3):306–9.

44. Lundgren IS, Zhou C, Malone FR, et al. Central venous catheter repair is associated with an increased risk of bacteremia and central line-associated bloodstream infection in pediatric patients. *Pediatr Infect Dis J* 2012;31(4):337–40.

45. Matlow AG, Wray RD, Cox PN. Nosocomial urinary tract infections in children in a pediatric intensive care unit: A follow-up after 10 years. *Pediatr Crit Care Med* 2003;4(1):74–7.

46. Langley JM. Defining urinary tract infection in the critically ill child. *Pediatr Crit Care Med* 2005;6(3 suppl):S25–9.

47. Fadrowski JJ, Hwang W, Frankenfield DL, et al. Clinical course associated with vascular access type in a national cohort of adolescents who receive hemodialysis: Findings from the Clinical Performance Measures and US Renal Data System projects. *Clin J Am Society Nephrol* 2006;1(5):987–92.

48. Bratzler DW, Hunt DR. The surgical infection prevention and surgical care improvement projects: National initiatives to improve outcomes for patients having surgery. *Clin Infect Dis* 2006;43(3):322–30.

49. Bucher BT, Guth RM, Elward AM, et al. Risk factors and outcomes of surgical site infection in children. *J Am Coll Surg* 2011;212(6):1033–8.e1.

50. Day MD, Gauvreau K, Shulman S, et al. Characteristics of children hospitalized with infective endocarditis. *Circulation* 2009;119(6):865–70.

51. Ceneviva G, Paschall JA, Maffei F, et al. Hemodynamic support in fluid-refractory pediatric septic shock. *Pediatrics* 1998;102(2):e19.

52. Bick RL. Disseminated intravascular coagulation current concepts of etiology, pathophysiology, diagnosis, and treatment. *Hematol Oncol Clin North Am* 2003;17(1):149–76.

53. Reimer LG, Wilson ML, Weinstein MP. Update on detection of bacteremia and fungemia. *Clin Microbiol Rev* 1997;10(3):444–65.

54. Fisher CE, Stevens AM, Leisenring W, et al. The serum galactomannan index predicts mortality in hematopoietic stem cell transplant recipients with invasive aspergillosis. *Clin Infect Dis* 2013;57(7):1001–4.

55. Klouche M, Schroder U. Rapid methods for diagnosis of bloodstream infections. *Clin Chem Lab Med* 2008;46(7):888–908.

56. Standage SW, Wong HR. Biomarkers for pediatric sepsis and septic shock. *Expert Rev Anti Infect Ther* 2011;9(1):71–9.

57. Becker KL, Snider R, Nylen ES. Procalcitonin assay in systemic inflammation, infection, and sepsis: Clinical utility and limitations. *Crit Care Med* 2008;36(3):941–52.

58. Schuetz P, Albrich W, Mueller B. Procalcitonin for diagnosis of infection and guide to antibiotic decisions: Past, present and future. *BMC Med* 2011;9:107.

59. Wong HR, Cvijanovich N, Wheeler DS, et al. Interleukin-8 as a stratification tool for interventional trials involving pediatric septic shock. *Am J Respir Crit Care Med* 2008;178(3):276–82.

60. Wong HR, Salisbury S, Xiao Q, et al. The pediatric sepsis biomarker risk model. *Crit Care* 2012;16(5):R174.

61. Carcillo JA, Davis AL, Zaritsky A. Role of early fluid resuscitation in pediatric septic shock. *JAMA* 1991;266(9):1242–5.

62. Rivers E, Nguyen B, Havstad S, et al. Early goal-directed therapy in the treatment of severe sepsis and septic shock. *N Engl J Med* 2001;345(19):1368–77.

63. Maitland K, Kiguli S, Opoka RO, et al. Mortality after fluid bolus in African children with severe infection. *N Engl J Med* 2011;364(26):2483–95.

64. Muszynski JA, Knatz NL, Sargel CL, et al. Timing of correct parenteral antibiotic initiation and outcomes from severe bacterial community-acquired pneumonia in children. *Pediatr Infect Dis J* 2011;30(4):295–301.

65. Kumar A, Roberts D, Wood KE, et al. Duration of hypotension before initiation of effective antimicrobial therapy is the critical determinant of survival in human septic shock. *Crit Care Med* 2006;34(6):1589–96.

66. Annane D, Bellissant E, Bollaert PE, et al. Corticosteroids for severe sepsis and septic shock: A systematic review and meta-analysis. *BMJ* 2004;329(7464):480.

67. Sprung CL, Annane D, Keh D, et al. Hydrocortisone therapy for patients with septic shock. *N Engl J Med* 2008;358(2):111–24.

68. MacLaren G, Butt W, Best D, et al. Central extracorporeal membrane oxygenation for refractory pediatric septic shock. *Pediatr Crit Care Med* 2011;12(2):133–6.

69. Chan CM, Mitchell AL, Shorr AF. Etomidate is associated with mortality and adrenal insufficiency in sepsis: A meta-analysis*. *Crit Care Med* 2012;40(11):2945–53.

70. Wheeler AP, Bernard GR. Treating patients with severe sepsis. *N Engl J Med* 1999;340(3):207–14.

71. Hayes LW, Oster RA, Tofil NM, et al. Outcomes of critically ill children requiring continuous renal replacement therapy. *J Crit Care* 2009;24(3):394–400.

72. de Oliveira CF, de Oliveira DS, Gottschald AF, et al. ACCM/PALS haemodynamic support guidelines for paediatric septic shock: An outcomes comparison with and without monitoring central venous oxygen saturation. *Intens Care Med* 2008;34(6):1065–75.

73. Sakr Y, Vincent JL, Reinhart K, et al. Use of the pulmonary artery catheter is not associated with worse outcome in the ICU. *Chest* 2005;128(4):2722–31.

74. Haydar SA, Moore ET, Higgins GL III, et al. Effect of bedside ultrasonography on the certainty of physician clinical decision-making for septic patients in the emergency department. *Ann Emerg Med* 2012;60(3):346–58 e4.

75. Park DW, Chun BC, Kwon SS, et al. Red blood cell transfusions are associated with lower mortality in patients with severe sepsis and septic shock: A propensity-matched analysis*. *Crit Care Med* 2012;40(12):3140–5.

76. Hebert PC, Wells G, Blajchman MA, et al. A multicenter, randomized, controlled clinical trial of transfusion requirements in critical care. Transfusion Requirements in Critical Care Investigators, Canadian Critical Care Trials Group. *N Engl J Med* 1999;340(6):409–17.

77. Vincent JL, Baron JF, Reinhart K, et al. Anemia and blood transfusion in critically ill patients. *JAMA* 2002;288(12):1499–507.

78. Lacroix J, Hebert PC, Hutchison JS, et al. Transfusion strategies for patients in pediatric intensive care units. *N Engl J Med* 2007;356(16):1609–19.

79. Karam O, Tucci M, Ducruet T, et al. Red blood cell transfusion thresholds in pediatric patients with sepsis. *Pediatr Crit Care Med* 2011;12(5):512–8.

80. Mehta NM, Bechard LJ, Cahill N, et al. Nutritional practices and their relationship to clinical outcomes in critically ill children—an international multicenter cohort study*. *Crit Care Med* 40(7):2204–11.

81. Srinivasan V, Spinella PC, Drott HR, et al. Association of timing, duration, and intensity of hyperglycemia with intensive care unit mortality in critically ill children. *Pediatr Crit Care Med* 2004;5(4):329–36.

82. Dhainaut JF, Laterre PF, Janes JM, et al. Drotrecogin alfa (activated) in the treatment of severe sepsis patients with multiple-organ dysfunction: Data from the PROWESS trial. *Intens Care Med* 2003;29(6):894–903.

83. Goldstein B, Nadel S, Peters M, et al. ENHANCE: Results of a global open-label trial of drotrecogin alfa (activated) in children with severe sepsis. *Pediatr Crit Care Med* 2006;7(3):200–11.

84. Nguyen TC, Han YY, Kiss JE, et al. Intensive plasma exchange increases a disintegrin and metalloprotease with thrombospondin motifs-13 activity and reverses organ dysfunction in children with thrombocytopenia-associated multiple organ failure. *Crit Care Med* 2008;36(10):2878–87.

85. Ohlsson A, Lacy JB. Intravenous immunoglobulin for suspected or subsequently proven infection in neonates. *Cochrane Database Syst Rev* 2004(1):CD001239.

86. Pildal J, Gotzsche PC. Polyclonal immunoglobulin for treatment of bacterial sepsis: A systematic review. *Clin Infect Dis* 2004;39(1):38–46.

87. Norrby-Teglund A, Ihendyane N, Darenberg J. Intravenous immunoglobulin adjunctive therapy in sepsis, with special emphasis on severe invasive group A streptococcal infections. *Scand J Infect Dis* 2003;35(9):683–9.

88. Yavuz L, Aynali G, Aynali A, et al. The effects of adjuvant immunoglobulin M-enriched immunoglobulin therapy on mortality rate and renal function in sepsis-induced multiple organ dysfunction syndrome: Retrospective analysis of intensive care unit patients. *J Int Med Res* 2012;40(3):1166–74.

89. Elward AM, Warren DK, Fraser VJ. Ventilator-associated pneumonia in pediatric intensive care unit patients: Risk factors and outcomes. *Pediatrics* 2002;109(5):758–64.

90. Niedner MF, Huskins WC, Colantuoni E, et al. Epidemiology of central line-associated bloodstream infections in the pediatric intensive care unit. *Infect Control Hosp Epidemiol* 2011;32(12):1200–8.

91. Miller MR, Niedner MF, Huskins WC, et al. Reducing PICU central line-associated bloodstream infections: 3-year results. *Pediatrics* 2011;128(5):e1077–83.

92. Milstone AM, Elward A, Song X, et al. Daily chlorhexidine bathing to reduce bacteraemia in critically ill children: A multicentre, cluster-randomised, crossover trial. *Lancet* 381(9872):1099–106.

93. O'Grady NP, Alexander M, Dellinger EP, et al. Guidelines for the prevention of intravascular catheter-related infections. *Infect Control Hosp Epidemiol* 2002;23(12):759–69.

94. Gastmeier P, Weigt O, Sohr D, et al. Comparison of hospital-acquired infection rates in paediatric burn patients. *J Hosp Infect* 2002;52(3):161–5.

95. Patel JC, Mollitt DL, Pieper P, et al. Nosocomial pneumonia in the pediatric trauma patient: A single center's experience. *Crit Care Med* 2000;28(10):3530–3.

96. White JR, Dalton HJ. Pediatric trauma: Postinjury care in the pediatric intensive care unit. *Crit Care Med* 2002;30(11 suppl):S478–88.

97. Hogan CM, Hammer SM. Host determinants in HIV infection and disease. Part 1: Cellular and humoral immune responses. *Ann Intern Med* 2001;134(9, pt 1):761–76.

98. Hatherill M. Sepsis predisposition in children with human immunodeficiency virus. *Pediatr Crit Care Med* 2005;6(3 suppl):S92–8.

99. Price VE, Dutta S, Blanchette VS, et al. The prevention and treatment of bacterial infections in children with asplenia or hyposplenia: Practice considerations at the Hospital for Sick Children, Toronto. *Pediatr Blood Cancer* 2006;46(5):597–603.

100. Davies JM, Lewis MP, Wimperis J, et al. Review of guidelines for the prevention and treatment of infection in patients with an absent or dysfunctional spleen: Prepared on behalf of the British Committee for Standards in Haematology by a working party of the Haemato-Oncology task force. *Br J Haematol* 2011;155(3):308–17.

101. Kutko MC, Calarco MP, Flaherty MB, et al. Mortality rates in pediatric septic shock with and without multiple organ system failure. *Pediatr Crit Care Med* 2003;4(3):333–7.

102. Liberati A, D'Amico R, Pifferi S, et al. Antibiotic prophylaxis to reduce respiratory tract infections and mortality in adults receiving intensive care. *Cochrane Database Syst Rev* 2009(4):CD000022.

103. Daneman N, Sarwar S, Fowler RA, et al. Effect of selective decontamination on antimicrobial resistance in intensive care units: A systematic review and meta-analysis. *Lancet Infect Dis* 2013;13(4):328–41.

104. Han YY, Carcillo JA, Dragotta MA, et al. Early reversal of pediatric-neonatal septic shock by community physicians is associated with improved outcome. *Pediatrics* 2003;112(4):793–9.

105. Levy MM, Dellinger RP, Townsend SR, et al. The surviving sepsis campaign: Results of an international guideline-based performance improvement program targeting severe sepsis. *Crit Care Med* 2010;38(2):367–74.

106. Kissoon N, Carcillo JA, Espinosa V, et al. World federation of pediatric intensive care and critical care societies: Global sepsis initiative. *Pediatr Crit Care Med* 2011;12(5):494–503.

107. Larsen GY, Mecham N, Greenberg R. An emergency department septic shock protocol and care guideline for children initiated at triage. *Pediatrics* 2011;127(6):e1585–92.

108. Paul R, Neuman MI, Monuteaux MC, et al. Adherence to PALS sepsis guidelines and hospital length of stay. *Pediatrics* 2012;130(2):e273–80.

109. Hall MJ, Williams SN, DeFrances CJ, et al. Inpatient care for septicemia or sepsis: A challenge for patients and hospitals. *NCHS Data Brief* 2011;(62):1–8.

110. Report UIcm.

111. Leclerc F, Leteurtre S, Duhamel A, et al. Cumulative influence of organ dysfunctions and septic state on mortality of critically ill children. *Am J Respir Crit Care Med* 2005;171(4):348–53.

112. Frazier WJ, Hall MW. Immunoparalysis and adverse outcomes from critical illness. *Pediatr Clin North Am* 2008;55(3):647–68, xi.

CHAPTER 88 ■ PRINCIPLES OF ANTIMICROBIAL THERAPY

CHERYL L. SARGEL, TODD KARSIES, LULU JIN, AND KEVIN SPICER

KEY POINTS

1. Antibiotic decisions are often more complex in the ICU than in other settings because of an increased risk for unusual infections, a need for consideration of organ failure and extracorporeal devices/drains, as well as a higher risk of poor outcomes, including death, if an incorrect treatment course is chosen.

2. The need for appropriate cultures cannot be overemphasized. Every attempt should be made to obtain blood cultures prior to initiation of antimicrobial therapy, as well as preantibiotic specimens from other possibly infected sites (e.g., cerebrospinal fluid, urine, lower respiratory tract, pleural fluid). Viral studies and fungal antigen testing should be considered in the appropriate patient.

3. Many adult, and some pediatric, studies have found an association between inappropriate initial empiric antibiotics and increased mortality, increased length of stay, and delayed recovery in sepsis.

4. Understanding which organisms are prevalent locally and which antibiotics are most effective against these organisms can enhance antibiotic decisions even after patients' risk for particular organisms has been determined. Knowledge of local unit and community microbiology can be useful in developing a unit-based ICU empiric antibiotic strategy.

5. In critically ill children with viral respiratory infections, coinfection with bacterial pathogens may occur in 40%–50% of children with respiratory syncytial virus (RSV) bronchiolitis requiring mechanical ventilation. For this reason, cultures, including lower respiratory cultures, are justified from all children requiring intubation and mechanical ventilation for bronchiolitis, along with empiric antibiotic coverage for at least 48–72 hours until culture results return.

6. In general, unless there are compelling reasons to do otherwise, once the pathogen and susceptibilities are known, antimicrobials should be targeted with a spectrum as narrow as possible. Appropriate and improved use of antimicrobials is first and foremost an issue of patient safety and quality.

7. Administering large volumes of fluids, use of extracorporeal support devices, drains, plasmapheresis, and renal replacement therapies can all significantly impact a patient's volume status and drug distribution. Changes in end-organ function, such as liver, renal, and cardiovascular dysfunction and recovery, can affect drug metabolism and elimination.

8. The use of therapeutic drug monitoring should be considered in all drugs in which this is an option.

9. Effective antibiotic treatment requires more than simply matching a drug with a microorganism. The key is integration of the drug's unique disposition characteristics in the individual patient (i.e., pharmacokinetics [PK]) with an understanding of the drug's clinical activity (i.e., pharmacodynamics [PD]).

INTRODUCTION

Infections and antibiotic administration are extremely common in critically ill children admitted to the PICU. Antibiotic decisions are often more complex in the ICU than in other settings because of an increased risk for unusual infections, a need for consideration of organ failure, the presence of extracorporeal devices, and a higher risk of poor outcomes if an incorrect treatment course is chosen.

General Approach to Antibiotics in the PICU

Patients will commonly present with symptoms suspected to stem from an infectious etiology and will require empiric antibiotic therapy while awaiting results of cultures and other testing. Empiric antibiotic selection can be accomplished using an escalation or a de-escalation strategy. In an *escalation* strategy, relatively narrow-spectrum antibiotics are initially prescribed. Antibiotic coverage is later expanded to cover a broader range of pathogens based on culture results or if there is no clinical improvement. *De-escalation* strategies initially prescribe very broad–spectrum antibiotics to provide empiric coverage for a wider range of organisms. Antibiotics are then narrowed based on culture and susceptibility results and clinical improvement, or discontinued if another cause for critical illness is found. In either strategy, once culture results are obtained, antibiotics are tailored to provide adequate coverage of the pathogen and the narrowest possible spectrum.

The need for appropriate cultures cannot be overemphasized. Every attempt should be made to obtain blood cultures prior to initiation of antimicrobial therapy (1), as well as preantibiotic specimens from other possibly infected sites (e.g., cerebrospinal fluid [CSF], urine, lower respiratory tract, pleural fluid). Viral studies and fungal antigen testing should be considered in the appropriate patient. While a respiratory viral diagnosis may not prompt additional therapy, identification could allow for antibiotic de-escalation depending on the clinical context (2,3); however, for critically ill children diagnosed with a viral respiratory infection who do not have airway cultures, the possibility of a secondary bacterial infection should be considered as coinfection is not uncommon (4).

Pitfalls of Antibiotic Overuse

Although aggressive antibiotic use in the PICU can often be justified, it is not without potential negative consequences involving both the individual patient and the larger community. Antimicrobials account for the more commonly seen drug-associated adverse events, ranging in severity from rash to anaphylaxis and including organ injury (renal or hepatic impairment) and drug–drug interactions. Overuse can also lead to antibiotic-associated diarrhea/colitis and superinfection with drug-resistant bacteria and fungi. Additionally, perturbation of resident flora within the individual's microbiome may impact susceptibility to later infections (5). On the larger community level, there is concern for increasing antimicrobial resistance, which has been associated with antimicrobial exposure (6,7).

EMPIRIC ANTIBIOTIC THERAPY IN THE PICU

There is growing evidence that initial appropriate empiric antibiotics are essential in critically ill patients with infection. The term "appropriate empiric antibiotics" refers to antibiotics administered at, or near, the time of culture to which the cultured organism(s) ultimately prove susceptible. Many adult ❸ studies have found an association between inappropriate initial empiric antibiotics and increased mortality, increased length of stay, and delayed recovery in sepsis. These findings have been seen in global sepsis (8), healthcare-associated MRSA sepsis (9), gram-negative sepsis (10), ventilator-associated pneumonia (VAP) (11), and healthcare-associated pneumonia (HCAP) (12). The HCAP study importantly noted that antibiotic escalation *after* culture results were obtained still lead to an increased risk of death as compared with those who were prescribed initially appropriate antibiotics. A recent meta-analysis demonstrated significant mortality benefit in sepsis when providing initial appropriate empiric antibiotics, with a number needed to treat (NNT) of 10 patients to prevent 1 death (13). Studies on initial antibiotic appropriateness in critically ill children are lacking, although increased mortality has been associated with inappropriate empiric antibiotics for children with bacteremia in all settings (14) and increased resource utilization in severe community-acquired pneumonia (15).

Along with appropriate antibiotic choice, it is also vital to begin the correct antibiotics as quickly as possible. The importance of this is highlighted in consensus guidelines for both adult and pediatric septic shock (1,16). Studies have demonstrated increased mortality associated with delay in initiation of antibiotics in adults with septic shock. In fact, mortality was increased by >7% for each hour antibiotics were delayed after the onset of hypotension (17). Puskarich et al. (18) also found increased mortality for each hour delay in appropriate antibiotic administration after shock recognition in patients receiving early goal-directed therapy. A similar effect has been reported in adults with respiratory infections (11) and in children with severe community-acquired pneumonia (15).

Overview of Empiric Antibiotics and Antibiotic Resistance

The rise of antibiotic-resistant bacteria has made empiric antibiotic selection more challenging. Organisms once only seen in nosocomial infections are now being acquired outside of the

hospital and even without contact with the healthcare system. Community-acquired methicillin-resistant *Staphylococcus aureus* (CA-MRSA) is an increasing problem and is presenting as increasingly invasive infections. Gram-negative bacilli also pose a treatment challenge, particularly those with potential antibiotic resistance, such as *Pseudomonas aeruginosa* and extended-spectrum β-lactamase–producing species. In adults, there is awareness of these healthcare-associated infections, but there is much less appreciation for this type of infection in children, and indeed the pediatric literature discussing healthcare-associated infections often evaluates only hospital-acquired infections (19–21).

Given the importance of early appropriate empiric antibiotics, there are several approaches that have been proposed to ensure coverage even for antibiotic-resistant pathogens. First, one could prescribe very broad–spectrum antimicrobials to all children admitted to the PICU with suspected infection (22). This approach would make it highly likely that the empiric coverage would, indeed, cover the vast majority of pathogens that might be cultured. This would, however, expose many patients to the toxicities of broad-spectrum antibiotics and may increase drug costs. A second approach would be to stratify children based on their risk for potentially resistant pathogens, similar to what is recommended in adult guidelines. Those with minimal risk could be treated with narrower-spectrum agents targeting community-acquired/commonly susceptible organisms, and children felt to have increased risk for potentially resistant organisms could be empirically treated with broader-spectrum antibiotics. Commonly used risk factors for potentially resistant pathogens include:

- recent hospitalization,
- recent antibiotic exposure,
- immunosuppression due to disease or medications, and
- chronic structural lung disease.

A regimen for these patients might include MRSA coverage as well as coverage for gram-negative pathogens, including *P. aeruginosa*. For adults, there are published consensus guidelines that can aid risk assessment and antibiotic decisions (**Table 88.1**) (23–25). Unfortunately, no guidelines currently exist for children, and it is unknown whether application of adult guidelines is appropriate for the pediatric population.

Empiric antiviral or antifungal coverage will likely not be necessary for most PICU patients. However, patients with recent exposure to antibacterials, indwelling central venous catheters, or immune compromise may be at higher risk for fungal disease (26,27). Empiric antiviral therapy should be considered for critically ill patient with suspected influenza (28,29) and may also be appropriate in cases of encephalitis or after solid-organ or hematopoietic stem cell transplant (HSCT), or in the critically ill newborn where herpes simplex infection is suspected.

Empiric Management Strategies for Antibiotic-Resistant Infections

One of the most important tools intensivists have to aid empiric antibiotic selection is a local, unit-specific antibiogram summarizing the antibiotic susceptibilities of all pathogenic ❹ bacteria identified in their PICU (**Fig. 88.1**). Understanding which organisms are prevalent locally and which antibiotics are most effective against these organisms can enhance antibiotic decisions even after a patient's risk for particular organisms has been determined. Knowledge of local unit and community microbiology can be useful in developing a unit-based ICU empiric antibiotic strategy. For example, units with high rates of *Stenotrophomonas maltophilia* may wish

TABLE 88.1

RISK FACTORS FOR INFECTION DUE TO HEALTHCARE-ASSOCIATED ORGANISMS IN ADULTS

- Recent antimicrobial therapy (7+ days within the past 30–90 days)
- Hospitalization ≥5 days
- Recent hospitalization (at least 2 days in past month)
- Resident in chronic care facility
- Systemic corticosteroid therapy (>10 mg prednisone equivalent daily)
- Chronic dialysis
- Home infusion or wound care
- Known exposure to resistant pathogen (household or community)
- Immunosuppressive disease or medications
- Malnutrition
- Structural lung disease

Adapted from Mandell LA, Wunderink RG, Anzueto A, et al. Infectious Diseases Society of America/American Thoracic Society consensus guidelines on the management of community-acquired pneumonia in adults. *Clin Infect Dis* 2007;44(suppl 2):S27–72; Malone DC, Shaban HM. Adherence to ATS guidelines for hospitalized patients with community-acquired pneumonia [published online ahead of print October 26, 2001]. *Ann Pharmacother* 2001;35(10):1180–5; American Thoracic Society; Infectious Diseases Society of America. Guidelines for the management of adults with hospital-acquired, ventilator-associated, and healthcare-associated pneumonia [published online ahead of print February 09, 2005]. *Am J Respir Crit Care Med* 2005;171(4):388–416.

to include coverage of this organism for all patients at risk for healthcare-associated infections.

To further address the issue of resistant bacteria, combination antibiotic therapy is a strategy that has emerged. This approach has been shown to improve mortality in critically ill adults with community-acquired pneumonia (6, 23,30). There are guidelines and evidence to support combination empiric therapy in HCAP, VAP, sepsis, and septic shock (31–37). The best approach to ensure coverage of resistant gram-negative organisms appears to be an antipseudomonal β-lactam or carbapenem combined with an aminoglycoside (AG) rather than fluoroquinolone (38). Importantly, once a pathogen is identified, de-escalation to monotherapy appears to be safe and preferred, provided there is clinical improvement (31,39,40). Another strategy that may be helpful to address antibiotic-resistant bacteria in an empiric antibiotic protocol is antibiotic heterogeneity (e.g., cycling) (41,42). In this approach, antibiotics for specific organisms (e.g., gram-negative bacilli) are rotated such that there are time periods where a particular antimicrobial is the preferred agent for all patients and other periods where that drug is restricted and another is preferred. Cycling does not improve antibiotic appropriateness but rather attempts to decrease the development of resistance. Antibiotic cycling has been proposed as a potential component of an antimicrobial stewardship program (43) and has mixed evidence as to its benefits in both gram-positive and gram-negative infections (44–48). At this time, recommendations cannot be made for or against cycling.

A final approach to resistant bacteria focuses on discontinuation. Specifically, it is important to consider the use of shorter antibiotic courses for infections in the ICU. Studies in adults suggest that shorter antibiotic courses, perhaps ≤7 days, may be as effective as longer courses while theoretically decreasing pressure for the development of antibiotic resistance, particularly in the setting of gram-negative infections (33). There is currently active ongoing research examining the use of biomarkers to safely shorten treatment courses without negatively impacting outcomes.

Another special situation that deserves mention is the infant or child admitted to the PICU with a viral respiratory infection. While a respiratory viral diagnosis may not prompt additional therapy, identification could allow for antibiotic de-escalation depending on the clinical context (2,3); however, consideration of bacterial coinfection in critically ill children with viral respiratory infections is crucial. Serious bacterial infections in infants with bronchiolitis are quite uncommon outside of the ICU, and a recent Cochrane Review found no evidence to support antibiotic therapy for children with bronchiolitis across the board (49). However, in critically ill children with respiratory syncytial virus (RSV) bronchiolitis requiring mechanical ventilation, coinfection with bacterial pathogens may occur in 40%–50% of cases (4,50,51). Additionally, bacterial coinfections, particularly with *S. aureus*, are frequently seen in patients with influenza requiring ICU admission (52,53). For these reasons, cultures, including lower respiratory cultures, are justified from all children requiring intubation and mechanical ventilation for viral lower respiratory infections, along with empiric antibiotic coverage until culture results are known (54).

DE-ESCALATION AND STEWARDSHIP

In general, unless there are compelling reasons to do otherwise, once the pathogen and susceptibilities are known, antimicrobials should be targeted with a spectrum as narrow as possible (55,56).

If cultures were obtained and remain negative at 48–72 hours, then the clinician faces an important decision. Depending on the patient's clinical course, the patient who has improved could have therapy de-escalated or discontinued, with subsequent clinical observation and reculturing and reinitiation of therapy with clinical worsening. Rapid improvement in inflammatory markers (e.g., procalcitonin, C-reactive protein [CRP]), as well as clinical improvement, is reassuring and lends more weight toward de-escalation. A short duration of therapy (e.g., no more than 5 days) may be sufficient in such a clinical scenario, although for sepsis and septic shock, duration of 7–10 days may be more appropriate based on current adult guidelines (1).

The culture-negative patient whose condition is unchanged is more problematic. Without positive cultures or other data strongly supportive of infection, the need for ongoing antimicrobial therapy is unclear. One should consider possible de-escalation in a stepwise approach and limiting the duration of therapy. There is no evidence that prolonged empiric antibiotic coverage in the absence of an identified organism results in improved clinical outcome and such continuing therapy may

FIGURE 88.1. An excerpt from a PICU-specific antibiogram showing susceptibilities of commonly-isolated organisms to frequently-used antibiotics within one institution. Cipro, ciprofloxacin; Unasyn, ampicillin and sulbactam; Zosyn, piperacillin and tazobactam; LFGNR, lactose-fermenting gram-negative rods; NLFGNR, non-lactose-fermenting gram-negative rods; CONS, coagulase-negative staphylococci.

ORGANISM	#isolate	Penicillins			Cephalosporins					Aminoglycosides			Others				Levofloxacin
		Ampicillin	Unasyn	Zosyn	Cefazolin	Cefuroxime	Ceftriaxone	Ceftazidime	Cefepime	Gentamicin	Tobramycin	Amikacin	Aztreonam	Meropenem	Sulfatrim	Cipro	
LFGNR																	
E. cloacae	28	0		79	0		79	79	96	100	100	100		100	93	100	100
E. coli	40	48	82	94	83		88	90	88	85	88	91		100	88	98	91
K. oxytoca	17	0	60	88	19		50	63	60	56	56	69		100	63	100	100
K. pneumoniae	31	0	100	90	73		83	83	85	83	80	96		100	80	90	100
S. marcescens	14	0		93	0		93	93	100	86	79	100		100	100	100	100
NLFGNR																	
A. baumanii	11	0	50	20	0		0	25	25	25	25	20	0	22	25	25	0
A. xylosoxidans	8			88				100					20	38	88	0	
Mucoidal P.	10			40				30	20	50	60	50		30	0	70	
aeruginosa	167			90				81	89	79	85	91	68	80	0	90	92
P. aeruginosa																	
S. maltophilia	33			64(Tim)				41						0	91		79
Staphylococcus																	
CONS	41	0			10					49					46		
S. aureus	140	6			56					86					95		
Streptococcus																	
E. faecium	6	0															
Enterococcus sp. (not faecium)	18	100								100							
S. pneumoniae	16					44	69								50		

in fact be harmful (57,58). Consideration of noninfectious etiologies should also occur.

In the patient showing clinical deterioration, thought should be given to repeating cultures, expanding laboratory or radiographic work-up, engaging consultants, and reviewing trends of inflammatory markers. Additionally, one may need to consider escalation of antimicrobial therapy (e.g., broadening from β-lactam/β-lactamase to a carbapenem) or starting empiric antifungal therapy for the culture-positive patient who deteriorates while on antimicrobial therapy that is appropriate for the initial infection. It is vital to not only suspect new nosocomial infection but also remember the importance of source control (e.g., a drainable abscess), and to ensure appropriate dosing is being utilized.

Biomarkers of Infection

Specific laboratory markers of infection would be helpful as decisions are made regarding antimicrobial therapy. Identifying markers that are sufficiently specific for bacterial infection in the individual critically ill patient has been challenging. Markers, such as CRP and procalcitonin, have shown promise, but current knowledge is insufficient for such data to provide clear direction with treatment decisions (59,60). CRP values show significant overlap in bacterial, viral, and fungal infections. Absolute values may be less helpful than trends over time (61,62). Decreasing CRP levels may allow for more confidence in therapeutic decisions, such as discontinuation of antimicrobial therapy. Procalcitonin may be elevated not only in relation to bacterial infection but also in noninfectious conditions (63). Procalcitonin levels have been used as part of an antimicrobial stewardship program, and its use has been shown to reduce antibiotic use without increasing patient morbidity/mortality (64).

Antibiotic Stewardship

Concerns about increasing bacterial resistance and decreasing availability of new antimicrobials have resulted in the development of antimicrobial stewardship programs in many healthcare facilities. The primary goal of these programs is "to optimize clinical outcomes while minimizing unintended consequences of antimicrobial use, including toxicity, the selection of pathogenic organisms (such as *Clostridium difficile*), and the emergence of resistance" (43). A traditional approach to antimicrobial stewardship is to restrict access to targeted antibiotics or classes, perhaps by requiring preauthorization for use of specific antimicrobials. The prescriber must then justify the use of specific antibiotic either prior to or within a short period of time after its initiation. Although such an approach has been shown to decrease use of specific antibiotics, it is not always clear that overall antibiotic use is reduced. Additionally, there are concerns with prescriber autonomy and the development of an adversarial relationship between prescribers and the antimicrobial stewardship team.

More recently, the focus of antimicrobial stewardship programs has shifted to a process known as "prospective audit and feedback." In this approach, the prescriber initiates therapy, and review of the antimicrobial is made at 48–72 hours allowing for culture results, initial work-up, and evaluation of the early clinical course to be considered. Decisions are then made regarding de-escalation, escalation, continuation, or discontinuation of the specific therapy. This approach allows for initial prescriber autonomy and may promote a less adversarial relationship between prescriber and antimicrobial stewardship staff, but requires sufficient resources to be able to identify patients and provide adequate clinical review. Prospective

audit with feedback has been demonstrated to reduce antibiotic use in a tertiary care pediatric facility (65).

Additional strategies of antimicrobial stewardship include clinical guidelines, education for prescribers, and the use of strategies for antibiotic heterogeneity (e.g., antibiotic cycling), although the clinical impact of these strategies remains unclear. Regardless of the presence of a formal antimicrobial stewardship program, consideration should be given to involving the pediatric infectious diseases consultant under many circumstances commonly found in the PICU. The consultant can provide a perspective focused on the infectious disease issues, which may be especially important in patients who are immunocompromised, when there are mixed pathogens, or the identified pathogen is rare or unusual.

PHYSIOLOGIC CHANGES IN CRITICALLY ILL PATIENTS— IMPACT ON DOSING

There are many physiologic changes that occur during periods of critical illness than can affect drug dosing. Administration of large volumes of fluids, use of extracorporeal support devices, drains, plasmapheresis, and renal replacement therapies can all significantly impact a patient's volume status and drug distribution. Changes in end-organ function, such as liver, renal, and cardiovascular dysfunction and recovery, can affect drug metabolism and elimination. Along with these changes, epidemiologic changes in the pediatric population include an increasing prevalence of pediatric obesity and improved survival of severely impaired pediatric patients who may remain pediatric-sized into adulthood.

Volume Status

Changes in volume of distribution (Vd) and clearance (CL) of antibiotics may alter the plasma concentration of antimicrobials at the target site. Capillary leak syndrome is commonly seen in critically ill patients presenting with sepsis or septic shock. Vd of hydrophilic drugs (e.g., AGs, β-lactams, glycopeptides, lipopeptides, echinocandins, fluconazole, acyclovir, ganciclovir) in these patients is increased leading to lower-than-expected plasma concentrations and risk of treatment failure. Other interventions in the ICU, such as the presence of extracorporeal circuits, may further change the Vd of hydrophilic drugs.

Drains and Drug Loss

Postsurgical drains are placed in critically ill patients to assist with the removal of fluids from affected body cavities. The rate of drainage may significantly differ depending on the type and setup of the drainage system. The amount of antimicrobial loss may be related to the amount of output from the drainage system as well as the degree of hydrophilicity of the antimicrobial. Overall, patients may require higher doses to maintain a therapeutic plasma drug concentration.

There are currently no guidelines on empiric dosing adjustment in patients with postsurgical drains. However, using the highest recommended dose or frequent monitoring of drug levels in patients with postsurgical drains may be beneficial to account for potential drug loss.

Extracorporeal Membrane Oxygenation

A review of the Extracorporeal Life Support Organization (ELSO) registry has shown that 12% of extracorporeal membrane oxygenation (ECMO) cases have been complicated by infection (66). The effects of the ECMO circuit on drug delivery present a special challenge in managing antibiotics. Common mechanisms for altered pharmacokinetics include circuit binding, increased Vd, and decreased drug elimination. Lipophilic and/or highly protein-bound drugs (e.g., voriconazole, fluoroquinolones) are likely to be sequestered in the circuit, whereas hydrophilic drugs (e.g., β-lactams, AGs) are influenced by hemodilution. Information on drug disposition during ECMO, particularly with current circuit technology, is often insufficient to make meaningful recommendations for adjusting antimicrobial drug dosing. The use of therapeutic drug monitoring should be considered in all drugs in which this is an option.

Plasmapheresis

The amount of a particular drug that is removed during plasmapheresis is determined by factors related to the apheresis procedure and pharmacokinetic parameters of the drug. Drugs that are present in the plasma, and are not sequestered within blood cells or tissues, will be effectively removed during the procedure. Factors influencing the amount of drug removed include the duration of the procedure, the volume of plasma removed, and the frequency of plasmapheresis. In general, drugs with a low Vd (<0.2 L/kg) and/or a high degree of protein binding (>80%) are more likely to be removed by plasmapheresis. Antimicrobials known to be removed during plasmapheresis are ampicillin, ceftriaxone (variable), AGs, vancomycin (variable), and teicoplanin. The number of published, controlled studies evaluating removal of antimicrobials during plasmapheresis is very limited.

End-Organ Function

Renal function, hepatic function, and cardiovascular function will all have a significant impact on the elimination and metabolism of drug within the body. These assessments need to occur on a daily basis as a patient may have progressive organ decline or recovery. Improper dosing during these phases of organ dysfunction places the patient at risk for potential overdosing and adverse effects, or underdosing and a suboptimal response. The optimal assessment of end-organ function has not been established, contributing to variability in practice.

Renal Function

The approach to renal function assessment can occur as both indirect and direct measurements, and identification of those at risk can be done by using the pRIFLE criteria (67). Glomerular filtration rate (GFR) is an important parameter used to indicate renal function. Indirect measurement of GFR using serum creatinine values is relatively easy to do with readily available data. Patients with lower-than-expected muscle mass for age or size may, however, be at higher risk for overestimation of GFR using creatinine-based calculations. In these instances, an alternative measurement of GFR may be required.

Use of cystatin C may be superior to creatinine in that the production appears to be independent of sex, body size, or age; however, there are limitations. Laboratory assays have not been standardized and may result in great variability, nor are they widely available. Equations that use both serum creatinine and cystatin C for GFR estimates appear to be more accurate than use of either indicator alone (68).

Direct measurement of GFR can be accomplished by administering a known quantity of a marker whose elimination is dependent on being freely filtered by the kidney, and then obtaining levels at specific time points to calculate the elimination rate. Radioisotopes and AG serum drug concentrations can be used for this purpose, as an estimated GFR can be calculated, for example, from the AG elimination rate. As GFR is inversely proportional to serum creatinine, one can then make daily adjustments to the GFR using subsequent creatinine values and proportionality of the calculated AG clearance. See **Table 88.2** for equations to estimate GFR.

For patients requiring renal replacement therapy (RRT), additional considerations need to be made. First, it should be determined if the patient has any residual kidney function, which may be contributing to drug clearance. Serum creatinine is unsuitable for use as a marker for renal function as it will undergo clearance via the RRT. The mode of RRT should also be taken into consideration as each mode of RRT will have a different effect on drug distribution and clearance. Circuits that malfunction and/or require replacement may lead to short-term loss or accumulation of drug if dosing strategies are not simultaneously adjusted. Patients who are on intermittent hemodialysis (IHD) should have drug doses timed to be administered at the end of their IHD sessions. If this is unable to be accomplished, a supplemental dose to be given after IHD may be indicated. For those patients on (PD), changes in dwell time, number of cycles per day, and dextrose concentration may all affect the efficiency of the dialysis, and therefore drug removal rate. Patients who are being treated for peritonitis and who are on peritoneal dialysis could have the additional consideration of adding anti-infective drugs to the dialysate as a mode of anti-infective delivery.

If the patient is on a medication that can be monitored, such as an AG or vancomycin, frequent drug levels may be helpful in determining the net effect of the RRT with or without any residual renal function. In the case where drug levels cannot be obtained, there is very little guidance in the way of optimizing dosing. Reference manuals as well as primary

TABLE 88.2

EQUATIONS TO ESTIMATE RENAL FUNCTION VIA GLOMERULAR FILTRATION RATE

■ METHOD	■ AGE	■ EQUATION
Bedside Schwartz	1–16 y	GFR (mL/min/1.73 m²) = (0.413 × height in cm) / S_{cr}
(IDMS)-traceable Modification of Diet in Renal Disease (MDRD)	Adult	GFR (mL/min/1.73 m²) = $175 \times (S_{cr})^{-1.154} \times (age)^{-0.203}$ (× 0.742 if female) (× 1.212 if African American) (conventional units)
Cockcroft–Gault (CG)	Adult	GFR (mL/min) = [((140–age) × weight)/(72 × S_{cr})] (× 0.85 if female)
Creatinine–cystatin C equation	Adult	GFR (mL/min/1.73 m²) = $177.6 \times S_{cr} -0.65$ x $(-0.105 + 1.13 \times S_{cys}) -0.57$ × age in y–0.20 (× 0.82 if female) (× 1.11 if African American)

S_{cr}, serum creatinine in mg/dL; S_{cys}, serum cystatin C in mg/L; IDMS, isotope dilution mass spectrometry.

literature searches may offer some guidance on the need for dose adjustment for specific drugs.

Liver Function

As many as 70% of drugs currently on the market undergo some form of hepatic metabolism, and antibiotics remain one of the most common classes of medications leading to drug-induced liver injury in the United States and Europe (69). Critically ill patients, particularly those with septic shock, are at high risk of liver injury, which can lead to poor hepatic drug metabolism. Patients may also have chronic liver failure and may experience additional insults of acute on chronic liver dysfunction.

Patients who are on potentially hepatotoxic medications should have routine liver function test (LFT) screening. Abnormalities in these laboratory tests can indicate the presence of a problem, but not the extent. Most patients will make a complete to near-complete recovery with no other intervention on discontinuation of the offending agent.

It is important to understand the consequences of liver dysfunction on drug dosing and physiologic effects. Vd can be affected for many highly protein-bound drugs as hepatic protein synthesis is diminished. Bilirubin has a high binding affinity for albumin and may displace other highly protein-bound drugs, such as ceftriaxone, if levels are elevated. This will lead to higher free (active) fractions of drug and an increased risk of toxicity. Ascites and third-spacing fluids will increase the Vd for water-soluble drugs, such as AGs. Dose adjustments that account for increased fluid or drainage of this fluid is likely to be necessary, along with frequent drug level monitoring. While changes in drug metabolism can be difficult to predict, general rules can be applied. The more severe the liver injury, the more it can be assumed that drug metabolism will be affected. Phase I reactions (oxidation [i.e., P450 reactions], reduction, hydrolysis) will be affected more than phase II reactions (glucuronidation, sulfation, gluta-thione conjugation, acetylation, methylation). Determining proper drug dosing in the setting of liver dysfunction should include an analysis of the degree of liver damage suspected, the dependence of a drug on hepatic metabolism, the type of metabolism (flow or enzyme dependent, type of enzymatic metabolism), the degree of protein binding, Vd, and whether or not any suitable alternatives are available, which may offer an improved safety profile.

Obesity

Obesity is defined as a body mass index (BMI) at or above the 95th percentile for children of the same age and gender. Physiologic changes in obesity can alter both the Vd and clearance of many commonly used antimicrobials. Antimicrobial dosing in obese children is challenging because of a lack of data in this population. In adult patients, the absorption of drugs does not appear to be significantly modified in the presence of obesity. Drug distribution into tissue, however, is dependent on body composition, blood flow, drug lipophilicity, and plasma protein binding. For most weight-based antimicrobials, the maximum dose used in pediatric patients should not exceed maximum adult dosing, though dosing of vancomycin and daptomycin are based on total body weight. Acyclovir dosing in obese pediatric patients is based on a patient's ideal body weight (IBW). AGs are dosed based on an adjusted body weight in patients weighing >120% of their IBW or >95% BMI for pediatrics (70). For amphotericin products, animal models suggest that liposomal amphotericin may distribute into fat more readily than the deoxycholate, colloidal

dispersion, or lipid complex formulations. It has therefore been suggested to dose liposomal amphotericin using IBW with a correction for increased blood volume. For drugs that can be monitored through serum drug levels, adjusting doses based on serum levels may be the most optimal way to ensure that obese patients are dosed appropriately.

APPLICATION OF PHARMACOKINETICS–PHARMACODYNAMICS TO ANTIBIOTIC THERAPEUTICS

Effective antibiotic treatment requires more than simply matching a drug with a microorganism (71). The key is integration of the drug's unique disposition characteristics in the individual patient (i.e., pharmacokinetics [PK]) with an understanding of the drug's clinical activity (i.e., pharmacodynamics [PD]). There are several crucial pharmacodynamic variables that are linked to microbiologic effect: time-dependent versus concentration-dependent; and bacteriostatic versus bactericidal activities of different antibiotics (Fig. 88.2A).

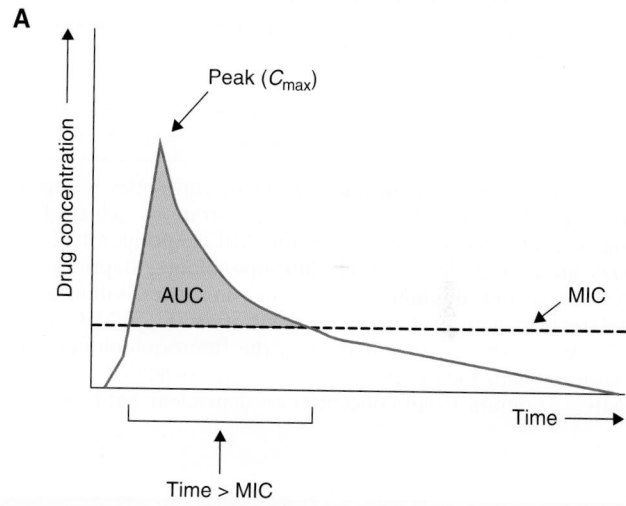

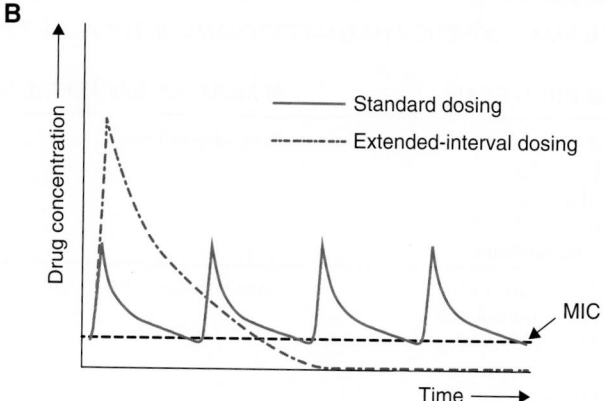

FIGURE 88.2. Pharmacokinetic/pharmacodynamics factors affecting antibiotic potency. **A:** Bacterial killing may be time-dependent (time with drug concentration > MIC), concentration-dependent (C_{max}/MIC), or both (AUC/MIC). **B:** Extended-interval dosing can be used with some antibiotics, though prolonged periods of time without detectable drug levels (>8 hours) should be avoided.

Time Dependency

The activity of time-dependent antibiotics is driven by the relationship between the concentrations achieved at the site of the infection relative to the minimum inhibitory concentration (MIC) of the microbe. The MIC is defined as the lowest concentration of an antibiotic that is needed to hinder the growth of bacteria. Time-dependent antibiotics can be divided into two groups for PK/PD targets: those that lack a postantibiotic effect (PAE) and those that display a moderate PAE. The PAE is a property that prevents bacterial growth for short duration of time even when antibiotic concentrations fall below the MIC. In the first group (time dependent with no PAE), the target PK/PD parameter is maximizing time > MIC. Antibiotics in this group include penicillins, carbapenems, cephalosporins, erythromycin, and linezolid. Increases in drug concentration beyond the MIC do not result in greater killing, however, maximizing the duration of time in which antibiotic concentrations are above the MIC will. This pharmacodynamic principle is exploited in continuous or extended infusion administration. For time-dependent drugs with a moderate PAE, the target PK/PD goal is to maximize the daily area under the curve (AUC)/MIC. This represents the ratio of the integral of the drug concentration over time above MIC to the organism's MIC. A larger AUC can be achieved with an increased peak concentration (C_{max}) and/or longer time spent above MIC. Antibiotics in this group include azithromycin, clindamycin, vancomycin, and tetracyclines (**Table 88.3**).

Concentration Dependency

The activity of concentration-dependent antibiotics is driven by the relationship between the concentrations achieved at the site of infection relative to the MIC. Antimicrobials in this group include the AGs, fluoroquinolones, daptomycin, ketolides, and amphotericin. In some instances, killing correlates best with peak serum concentration (C_{max})/MIC (e.g., the AGs), whereas in others (e.g., the fluoroquinolones and azithromycin) the effect is more strongly correlated to AUC/MIC. Common to all concentration-dependent antibiotics is

that they are relatively slowly bactericidal and demonstrate a PAE (**Table 88.3**).

Bacteriostatic/Bactericidal Properties

Antibiotics are defined as bactericidal if they kill the susceptible bacteria, or bacteriostatic if they slow the growth or reproduction of susceptible bacteria. These definitions apply only to the particular organism (or strain) against which it has been tested under the particular test conditions used, and not necessarily as a blanket statement for the antimicrobial itself. At high concentrations, bacteriostatic agents are often bactericidal against some susceptible organisms. Similarly, antibacterial agents that are considered to be bactericidal as a broad class may only exhibit bacteriostatic activity at low concentrations (72).

Continuous Infusion versus Standard/Bolus Dosing

Continuous infusion of antibiotics is based on the time-dependent killing properties of antibiotics, such as β-lactams and glycopeptides, allows for consistent steady-state concentrations, and maximizes time > MIC. Overall, evidence supporting continuous infusion of antibiotics is lacking in pediatric patients, however, several reports have been published. These include studies of ceftazidime in pediatric patients with cystic fibrosis (CF) and pediatric cancer patients with febrile neutropenia, which have described improved target attainment as well as tolerability of the continuous infusion regimens (73,74). The disadvantages of this method of administration should not be overlooked, however. Some β-lactams may not be stable at room conditions for long enough to allow for extended infusion, and additional dedicated lines may be needed, given incompatibilities with other drugs.

In a recent meta-analysis, it was concluded that there was no clinical advantage observed for prolonged infusion of β-lactams, though a large multicenter RCT is needed (75). If continuous infusion is used, the use of bolus dosing prior to

TABLE 88.3

PHARMACOKINETIC–PHARMACODYNAMIC INTERFACE (CONCENTRATION- VS. TIME-DEPENDENT TARGETS)

■ DRUG CLASS	■ MODE OF BACTERIAL KILLING	■ PHARMACODYNAMIC DETERMINANT
β-Lactams Linezolid Macrolides (not azithromycin) Lincosamides	Time-dependent	Time > MIC
Aminoglycosides Fluoroquinolones Metronidazole Telithromycin Daptomycin Quinupristin/dalfopristin	Concentration-dependent	C_{max}/MIC
Tetracyclines Azithromycin Clindamycin Glycopeptides	Time/concentration-dependent	AUC/MIC and C_{max}/MIC

the start of the infusion may be vital in ensuring that the target drug concentrations are achieved early.

Extended-Interval Aminoglycoside Dosing

AGs display concentration-dependent killing and a reliable PAE and are commonly used in combination with β-lactams for the treatment of serious gram-negative infections. Giving a larger dose will increase the C_{max} optimizing the C_{max}/MIC ratio and the AGs bactericidal activity (**Fig. 88.2B**). Providing longer intervals between doses allows for a greater time for drug elimination and decreases the risk for drug accumulation and toxicity (associated with elevated trough concentrations). Extended-interval aminoglycoside dosing (EIAD) has been evaluated as a method of improving the efficacy and safety of AGs. EIAD generally involves administering the total daily dose every 24 hours. In a prospective randomized trial of adult patients, EIAD achieved lower trough serum concentrations and resulted in a significantly lower incidence of nephrotoxicity, when compared with traditional dosing (76). However, a meta-analysis of pediatric patients did not show any significant difference between EIAD and traditional dosing in incidence of nephrotoxicity, though this occurrence is generally lower in children when compared with adults at baseline (77). This meta-analysis also did not find any significant difference in the clinical or microbiological failure between EIAD and traditional dosing arms. One concern in employing an EIAD strategy in children is that faster clearance will lead to a significant portion of a 24-hour dosing interval with undetectable drug levels, which may exceed the duration of the PAE. It is generally recommended to not exceed an 8-hour duration without detectable drug levels when using EIAD.

Overall, there is a lack of consensus on target population, appropriate dosing, ideal interval, and therapeutic drug monitoring with the use of EIAD in the pediatric population. EIAD has, however, been used in selected pediatric patient populations (CF patients, neutropenic patients). Pediatric patients, owing to their larger Vd, may require a higher daily mg/kg dose than adult patients when using the EIAD strategy.

As EIAD has not been evaluated in patients with impaired renal function, or in certain patient populations (e.g., those with extensive burns, obesity, or ascites) in which the Vd for AGs is significantly altered, it is not recommended to use EIAD in these patients. There are also certain infections, including meningitis, osteomyelitis, persistent bacteremia, and *Enterococcus* spp. endocarditis where EIAD is not the most appropriate approach to dosing AGs.

ANTIBACTERIAL AGENTS

β-Lactams

The β-lactams are comprised of several classes of drugs (penicillins, cephalosporins, monobactams, and carbapenems) based on their similarity of structure and mechanism of action. All have some variation of a β-lactam ring, and their mechanism of action results in inhibition of synthesis of the bacterial peptidoglycan cell wall by binding to a penicillin-binding protein (PBP). PBPs are only expressed during cell division, so β-lactams are only effective in bacteria that are actively dividing. There are three mechanisms of resistance that have emerged against β-lactams: development of β-lactamases, alterations in PBPs, and changes in cell membrane permeability.

Two important groups of β-lactamases have emerged and are expressed in both gram-positive and gram-negative bacteria. Group 1 β-lactamases (also referred to as "AmpC" β-lactamases) hydrolyze virtually all β-lactams except carbapenems and are resistant to inhibition by clavulanate. These enzymes are chromosomally encoded on a sequence labeled *ampC* in *P. aeruginosa*, *Enterobacter cloacae*, *Serratia marcescens*, *Citrobacter freundii*, and *Morganella morganii*. Group 2 β-lactamases include a wide variety of enzymes primarily encoded on plasmids, which commonly contain resistance determinants to other antibiotic classes. Group 2 β-lactamases include extended-spectrum β-lactamases (ESBLs) and are especially prevalent in *Klebsiella* and *E. coli*. Both group 1 and 2 β-lactamases are promoted by, and resistant to, the third-generation cephalosporins, and organisms expressing them are most reliably treated with a carbapenem (78).

β-Lactam resistance based on the alteration of PBPs are found on penicillin-resistant *Streptococcus pneumoniae*, MRSA, and most hospital-acquired coagulase-negative staphylococci. In penicillin-resistant pneumococcus, mildly resistant strains can achieve cure with high doses of β-lactam, plus vancomycin (in the case of meningitis). The β-lactam resistance in MRSA and coagulase-negative staphylococci is high grade and must be treated with an alternative class of drug.

Transport across the outer membrane in gram-negative bacteria is necessary for β-lactams to reach their target PBP and occurs through channels created by porins. A change in these porin channels infers β-lactam resistance, as observed in *Pseudomonas* spp.

In general, β-lactams have an excellent record for safety and have a broad range of antimicrobial activity, often making them the first choice for empiric therapy of both hospital- and community-acquired infections. β-Lactams are bactericidal in dividing cells (except against *Enterococcus* spp., in which they are bacteriostatic) and display time-dependent killing (PK/PD target is T > MIC). Most drugs within this class undergo little drug metabolism and are primarily excreted through the kidneys (with the exception of oxacillin and nafcillin). Dose adjustment in renal insufficiency and during dialysis is likely to be needed if using this drug class. Routine drug level monitoring is not available, making individualized drug dosing/optimization nearly impossible.

Penicillins

All penicillins contain a β-lactam ring and a thiazolidine ring (6-aminopenicillanic acid nucleus) to which various side chains are attached. Alterations in these side chains provide the differences seen in antimicrobial spectrum and pharmacologic variances.

Mechanism of Action and Resistance. The penicillins bind to PBP on the bacterial cell wall, resulting in inhibition of synthesis of the bacterial peptidoglycan, cell wall breakdown, and cell death. The emergence of penicillin resistance among *S. aureus* is due to β-lactamase production (a penicillinase). This stimulated the development of the penicillinase-resistant penicillins (e.g., nafcillin).

Spectrum of Activity. Penicillin G has a relatively narrow spectrum, including coverage against most *Streptococcus* spp. (**Table 88.4**) (79). Drug modifications have led to the development of aminopenicillins with enhanced gram-negative coverage (e.g., ampicillin), antistaphylococcal penicillins (e.g., nafcillin), and antipseudomonal penicillins (e.g., ticarcillin, piperacillin). The combination of these drugs with a β-lactamase inhibitor, such as sulbactam or clavulanate, allows for enhanced coverage of anaerobes and some staphylococci.

TABLE 88.4

SPECTRUM OF ACTIVITY FOR SELECTED PENICILLINS

	Natural Pcns	Antistaphylococcal Pcns	Amino Penicillins		Antipseudomonal Penicillins			
	PCN G	METHACILLIN OXACILLIN NAFCILLIN	AMPICILLIN	AMPICILLIN-SULBACTAM	TICARCILLIN	TICAR-CLAV	PIPERCILLIN	PIP-TAZO
Gram (+)								
S. pneumoniae	+	+	+	+	+	+	+	+
S. viridans	+/−	+/−	+/−	+/−	+/−	+/−	+/−	+/−
E. faecalis	+	0	+	+	+/−	+/−	+	+
E. faecium	+/−	0	+/−	+	+/−	+/−	+/−	+/−
S. aureus	0	+	0	0	0	0	0	+
S. aureus MRSA	0	0	0	0	0	0	0	0
Gram (−)								
N. meningitidis	+	0	+	+	0	+	+	+
M. catarrhalis	0	0	0	+	0	+	+/−	+
H. influenzae	0	0	+/−	+	+/−	+	+/−	+/−
E. coli	0	0	+/−	+	+/−	+	+	+
Klebsiella sp.	0	0	0	0	0	+	+	+
Enterobacter sp.	0	0	0	0	+	+	+	+
Serratia sp.	0	0	0	0	0	+	+	+
P. aeruginosa	0	0	0	0	+	+	+	+

It should be noted that penicillins lack atypical coverage and have only modest anaerobic coverage. The latter is improved with addition of a β-lactamase inhibitor.
PCN, penicillin; Ticar, ticarcillin; Clav, clavulanate; Pip, piperacillin; Tazo, tazobactam.
Adapted from Gilbert DN, Moellering RC Jr, Eliopoulos GM, et al. *Sanford Guide to Antimicrobial Therapy.* 43rd ed. 2013.

TABLE 88.5

PHARMACOKINETIC PROPERTIES OF SELECTED PENICILLINS

■ NAME	■ HALF-LIFE (HOUR)	■ VD (L/KG)	■ PROTEIN BINDING (%)	■ ROUTE OF ELIMINATION	■ DOSE ADJUSTMENT CONSIDERATION	■ DIALYZABLE
Penicillin G	0.5–1.2	0.53–0.67	65	Renal	Renal	Yes
Ampicillin	1–1.8	19.5–27	10–18	Renal	Renal	Yes
Oxacillin	0.5–1.8	0.39–0.43	94	Hepatic, renal	Renal	No
Nafcillin	0.75–1.9	0.85–1.5	90	Hepatic, renal	Renal + hepatic	No
Ticarcillin-clav	1–1.2	0.22	45–65	Renal	Renal + hepatic	Yes
Piperacillin-tazo	0.7–1.4	0.24	26–33	Renal	Renal	Yes

clav, clavulanate; tazo, tazobactam.

Metabolism and Distribution. The penicillins vary markedly in biodisposition from drug to drug (Table 88.5). Many are not well absorbed from the gastrointestinal tract and are therefore administered parenterally. Protein binding varies markedly from a low of ~17% for ampicillin to >90% for nafcillin. Few of these drugs undergo any significant metabolism, although some display hepatic elimination. Most excretion is renal, employing both glomerular filtration and tubular secretion. Significant developmental changes occur in elimination half-life during the first year of life, and doses may need to be adjusted according to the patient's age or renal function. Virtually all of the parenteral penicillins penetrate into the CSF in concentrations that are adequate to treat meningitis when meningeal inflammation is present. In the absence of inflammation, very little penetration occurs.

Adverse Effects. Adverse events occur rarely and can be extremely varied in their presentation. The major toxic effects are allergic reactions. In approximate order of decreasing frequency, manifestations of allergy to penicillins include maculopapular rash, urticarial rash, fever, bronchospasm, vasculitis, serum sickness, exfoliative dermatitis, Stevens–Johnson syndrome, and anaphylaxis (80,81). It is possible to substitute other β-lactam agents for a penicillin with a low risk of cross-reactivity. If potentially severe or life-threatening allergy is present or microbial susceptibility patterns do not permit substitution, desensitization can be performed. Other adverse events are rare and can include hematologic changes, such as thrombocytopenia, eosinophilia, and a positive Coombs reaction. Inhibition of platelet aggregation through binding on platelet adenosine diphosphate receptors can occur, although clinically significant bleeding is rare. Additional adverse effects may include: interstitial nephritis, noted especially with the penicillinase-resistant penicillins; electrolyte abnormalities (especially with sodium and potassium); and bone marrow suppression, particularly neutropenia, observed with prolonged use of virtually all of the penicillins. Seizures are a possibility in the case of massive overdoses or if accumulation due to renal insufficiency occurs. Changes in GI flora leading to diarrhea, possibly pseudomembranous colitis and C. *difficile* infections, are also possible.

Drug Interactions. Few drug–drug interactions of clinical significance are reported with the penicillins. Of note is the fact that probenecid, which competes with the penicillins for renal tubular secretion, prolongs the elimination half-life of penicillin or ampicillin. Antipseudomonal penicillins and extended-spectrum penicillins have been shown to interact in vitro with AGs, causing AG degradation (resulting in falsely low appearing drug levels). Theoretically, concomitant use with bacteriostatic agents may reduce the

bactericidal effects of penicillins by slowing the rate of bacterial growth.

Cephalosporins

Mechanism of Action and Resistance. The cephalosporins, like penicillins, bind to PBP on the bacterial cell wall, resulting in inhibition of synthesis of the bacterial peptidoglycan, cell wall breakdown, and cell death. Cephalosporins contain modifications that make the β-lactam ring more resistant to hydrolysis by penicillinases, create modified pharmacokinetic properties, and alter antimicrobial activity. Bacterial resistance to cephalosporins has been described by three mechanisms: production of β-lactamases, alteration of the PBPs, and alteration of bacterial permeability.

Spectrum of Activity. Cephalosporins are classified into generations and as generations increase, their stability in the presence of various β-lactamases also increases. Lower generations retain better gram-positive coverage, with improving gram-negative coverage and loss of some gram-positive coverage as generations escalate (Table 88.6). Cefepime (fourth generation) is important as it provides excellent gram-negative coverage, antipseudomonal coverage, and regains much of the gram-positive coverage that was lost in the third generation. Ceftaroline (fifth generation) further extends the coverage provided by cefepime, by also including MRSA and *Enterococcus* spp. into its spectrum. It is important to remember that currently available cephalosporins do not have reliable activity against enterococci, coagulase-negative staphylococci and MRSA (with the exception of ceftaroline for the three proceeding organisms), *Listeria monocytogenes*, and S. *maltophilia*.

Metabolism and Distribution. The cephalosporins vary markedly in biodisposition with patient age and agent (Table 88.7). Dosage must be adjusted on the basis of both patient age and renal function. Of the five generations of cephalosporins, only the drugs in the third and fourth generations penetrate into the CSF reliably enough to be used to treat bacterial meningitis. Ceftriaxone is not recommended in neonates (up to 28 days) owing to the high degree of protein binding and related concerns about bilirubin displacement. Cefotaxime should be substituted, if indicated, during the neonatal period.

Few of the cephalosporins undergo any significant metabolism. Several of those in the third generation have sufficient biliary excretion to make them useful in the treatment of hepatobiliary infections (e.g., cefoperazone and ceftriaxone). Most excretion, however, is renal via glomerular filtration, necessitating dosing modifications with age-related and disease-related changes in renal function.

TABLE 88.6

SPECTRUM OF ACTIVITY FOR SELECTED CEPHALOSPORINS

	1st Gen.	2nd Gen.	3rd Gen.		4th Gen.	5th Gen.
	■ CEFAZOLIN	■ CEFOTETAN CEFOXITIN CEFUROXIME	■ CEFOTAXIME CEFTRIAXONE	■ CEFTAZIDIME	■ CEFEPIME	■ CEFTAROLINE
Gram (+)						
S. pneumoniae	+	+	+	+	+	+
S. viridans	+	+	+	+/−	+	+
E. faecalis	0	0	0	0	0	+
S. aureus	+	+	+/−	+/−	+	+
S. aureus MRSA	0	0	0	0	0	+
Gram (−)						
N. meningitidis	0	+/−	+	+/−	+	+
M. catarrhalis	+/−	+	+	+	+	+
H. influenzae	+	+	+	+	+	+
E. coli	+	+	+	+	+	+
Klebsiella sp.	+	+	+	+	+	+
Enterobacter sp.	0	0	+	+	+	+
Serratia sp.	0	0	+	+	+	+
P. aeruginosa	0	0	0	+	+	+/−

It should be noted that cephalosporins lack atypical coverage and have only modest anaerobic coverage (with the exception of cefoxitin).
Adapted from Gilbert DN, Moellering RC Jr, Eliopoulos GM, et al. *Sanford Guide to Antimicrobial Therapy.* 43rd ed. 2013.

Adverse Effects. Gastrointestinal side effects are most common. Allergic reactions also occur in 1%–3% of patients, but are not as frequent as those seen with the penicillins. The cross-reactivity of cephalosporins in patients with documented penicillin allergy is somewhat higher than in the general population, but is likely to be safe. When cephalosporins were given to patients in whom penicillin allergy was documented by skin testing; only 1 of 99 developed a clinically significant reaction.

More rare adverse reactions include positive Coombs reactions, hemolytic anemia, bone marrow suppression, thrombocytosis, acute tubular necrosis, inhibition of platelet aggregation, and mild transaminase elevations. Ceftriaxone has been associated with the formation of biliary sludge in the gallbladder, which, in some critically ill patients, may lead to

signs and symptoms of cholecystitis. In 2007, the FDA released a safety alert warning against concomitant ceftriaxone and intravenous calcium administration owing to the formation of precipitates and patient deaths, and in 2009 this was revised to include only neonates. Risk of new onset seizures has been described when using cefepime, particularly in patients with renal impairment who have not had proper dose adjustment performed (82).

Clinical Indications. First-generation cephalosporins are used primarily for skin and skin structure infections (SSSIs) as well as perioperative prophylaxis against SSSI, given the excellent gram-positive activity. In the newborn period, ampicillin plus cefotaxime has become a standard regimen for the

TABLE 88.7

PHARMACOKINETIC PROPERTIES OF SELECTED CEPHALOSPORINS

	■ NAME	■ HALF-LIFE (HOUR)	■ VD (L/KG)	■ PROTEIN BINDING (%)	■ ROUTE OF ELIMINATION	■ DOSE ADJUSTMENT CONSIDERATION	■ DIALYZABLE
1st. Gen.	Cefazolin	1.5–5	~0.2	74–86	Renal	Renal	Yes
2nd Gen.	Cefuroxime	1–6	—	33–50	Renal	Renal	Yes
	Cefoxitin	0.75–1.5	0.2	65–79	Renal	Renal	Yes
	Cefotetan	3.5	8–14 (L)	76–91	Renal, biliary	Renal	No
3rd Gen.	Cefotaxime	1–4.6	0.15–0.55	31–50	Renal	Renal	Yes
	Ceftriaxone	4.1–16	0.3–0.55	85–95	Renal, biliary	None	No
	Ceftazidime	1.9–4.7	0.28–0.4	<10%	Renal	Renal	Yes
4th Gen.	Cefepime	1.7–5	0.3–0.51	20	Renal	Renal	Yes
5th Gen.	Ceftaroline fosamil	2.4	18.3–21.6 (L)	20	Renal, biliary	Renal	—

treatment of infants with suspected sepsis and/or meningitis. Ceftriaxone has become the standard therapeutic intervention for such children admitted to the hospital beyond the first month of life. Ceftazidime and cefepime have become standard agents for empiric therapy in critically ill children, those with fever and neutropenia, and those with nosocomial infections in the ICU. It should be noted that additional empiric gram-positive coverage, sufficient to cover MRSA or penicillin-resistant pneumococcus, may be indicated in the critically ill child with suspected infection.

Aztreonam

Aztreonam is a bactericidal monobactam whose spectrum is limited to aerobic gram-negative bacteria, such as members of the Enterobacteriaceae family and *P. aeruginosa*. It is devoid of gram-positive or anaerobic activity. Aztreonam can act synergistically with AGs when treating susceptible infections. Aztreonam is well distributed into most body fluids and tissues, including CSF. Approximately 30%–50% of the drug is bound to plasma proteins. It is eliminated from the body by primarily via the kidney (via filtration and active tubular secretion) and also by hepatic mechanisms. Aztreonam is removed by dialysis.

Aztreonam is not considered first-line therapy for any infections in pediatric patients and should not be used as empiric monotherapy, given its limited spectrum of activity. It can be useful, however, in patients who have a documented β-lactam allergy or in situations in which nephrotoxicity is a concern. Aztreonam can also be administered via inhalation, and carries an FDA-approved indication for this route in the treatment of *P. aeruginosa* infections in patients with CF.

Carbapenems

Carbapenems share the basic β-lactam structure with penicillins and cephalosporins; however, a structural alteration confers additional stability in the presence of many β-lactamases.

Mechanism of Action and Resistance. Carbapenems bind to all of the PBPs having the greatest affinity for PBP1 and PBP2, and are bactericidal. The carbapenems are highly resistant to β-lactamases, although bacteria expressing carbapenemases called New Delhi metallo-β-lactamase have emerged and are a global threat (83). *Pseudomonas* spp., in particular, may acquire resistance to the carbapenems through multiple outer membrane mutations or development of an efflux pump after sustained exposure to the drug. *Stenotrophomonas* isolates usually are intrinsically resistant.

Spectrum of Activity. Carbapenems possess a broad spectrum of antibacterial activity against aerobic and anaerobic gram-positive and gram-negative pathogens, and are among the broadest antibacterials currently available (**Table 88.8**). The ability to exert a PAE varies by bacterial isolate.

Metabolism and Distribution. Carbapenems are not absorbed after oral administration, and are only available for parenteral administration. Meropenem, imipenem/cilastatin, and doripenem are well distributed in most body fluids and tissues, including the CNS (**Table 88.9**). Protein binding tends to be low with the above-mentioned drugs. Ertapenem is an exception in that it is highly protein bound and should not be used in the treatment of pediatric meningitis owing to insufficient CNS penetration. Excretion of unchanged drug is principally via renal glomerular filtration, and age-related and renal dosing adjustment is necessary. Imipenem is degraded by a proximal tubular brush border enzyme, dehydropeptidase I, resulting in ineffective urinary concentrations in treating serious urinary tract infections. Thus, for clinical use, imipenem is administered along with a competitive inhibitor of dehydropeptidase I, cilastatin.

Adverse Effects. The adverse effect profile of carbapenems is similar to other β-lactams. Additionally, seizures have been reported in some patients with reduced renal function who are receiving high-dose therapy with imipenem. Patients with an underlying seizure disorder should receive carbapenems with

TABLE 88.8

SPECTRUM OF ACTIVITY FOR SELECTED CARBAPENEMS

	Carbapenems			
	■ DORIPENEM	■ ERTAPENEM	■ IMIPENEM	■ MEROPENEM
Gram (+)				
S. pneumoniae	+	+	+	+
S. viridans	+	+	+	+
E. faecalis	+/−	0	+	+/−
E. faecium	0	0	+/−	0
S. aureus	+	+	+	+
S. aureus MRSA	0	0	0	0
Gram (−)				
N. meningitidis	+	+	+	+
M. catarrhalis	+	+	+	+
H. influenzae	+	+	+	+
E. coli	+	+	+	+
Klebseilla sp.	+	+	+	+
Enterobacter sp.	+	+	+	+
Serratia sp.	+	+	+	+
P. aeruginosa	+	0	+	+

It should be noted that carbapenems lack atypical coverage but have excellent anaerobic coverage.
Adapted from Gilbert DN, Moellering RC Jr, Eliopoulos GM, et al. *Sanford Guide to Antimicrobial Therapy*. 43rd ed. 2013.

TABLE 88.9

PHARMACOKINETIC PROPERTIES OF SELECTED CARBAPENEMS

■ NAME	■ HALF-LIFE (HOUR)	■ VD (L/KG)	■ PROTEIN BINDING (%)	■ ROUTE OF ELIMINATION	■ DOSE ADJUSTMENT CONSIDERATION	■ DIALYZABLE
Doripenem	1	16.8 (L)	8–9	Renal	Renal	Yes
Ertapenem	2.5–4	0.12–0.2	85–95	Renal	Renal	Yes
Imipenem/ cilastatin	1–3	0.14–0.23	13–21	Renal	Renal	Yes
Meropenem	1–2.7	0.3–0.47	2	Renal	Renal	Yes

caution. The overall incidence of these adverse effects with meropenem is somewhat lower than that seen with imipenem/cilastatin. Seizures have been rarely reported with ertapenem.

Drug Interactions. There are few serious drug interactions reported with the carbapenems. A notable exception is a very serious drug interaction that occurs between carbapenems and valproic acid, resulting in subtherapeutic valproic acid levels. This interaction can be prolonged and can persist even after the carbapenem has been discontinued. This tends to be resistant to increases in valproic acid dosing. Accordingly, this drug combination should be avoided (84). Probenecid reduces renal clearance of carbapenems, resulting in increased concentrations within the body.

Clinical Indications. The carbapenems are very broad–spectrum agents that provide rational and effective empiric antimicrobial coverage in the treatment of serious infections, particularly nosocomial/healthcare-acquired infections or infections in the immunocompromised patient, noting the lack of antipseudomonal coverage by ertapenem. Caution against overuse and concerns of development of resistance make de-escalation strategies paramount with empiric use. Ertapenem should not be used for pediatric meningitis owing to poor CNS penetration.

Aminoglycosides

Mechanism of Action and Resistance

AG antibiotics inhibit bacterial protein synthesis by irreversibly binding to the 30S ribosomal subunit and are bactericidal. Resistance is commonly derived from enzymes that inactivate AGs, from decreased transport into the cell, or from mutations affecting proteins in the bacterial ribosome. The genes encoding these enzymes are transferred on plasmids; thus, there can be cross-resistance between members of the class. Amikacin is the most stable AG against these enzymes and can often be used in cases of gentamicin or tobramycin resistance.

Spectrum of Activity

AGs are used to treat aerobic gram-negative bacteria. Cellular uptake of an AG is an oxygen-dependent, active transport process; thus, anaerobic bacteria are universally resistant. While not clinically useful when used alone against gram-positive bacteria, AGs exhibit synergistic activity with other antimicrobial agents against staphylococci, streptococci, and enterococci.

Metabolism and Distribution

AGs are poorly absorbed from the GI tract; thus, for the treatment of systemic infections, these drugs must be administered parenterally. The AGs are not metabolized and are excreted completely unchanged via renal glomerular filtration. AG clearance can therefore be used as a direct and accurate measurement of GFR. Hepatic disease does not interfere with AG elimination. AGs are large, hydrophilic, cationic molecules that do not cross the blood–brain barrier well. Concentrations in the CSF are low and variable, and therefore, they should not be used as single agents to treat meningitis.

Adverse Effects

The most commonly recognized adverse effects are ototoxicity and nephrotoxicity, which limit the clinical use of AGs. Ototoxicity can be either vestibulotoxicity, occurring in up to 15% of patients, or cochleotoxicity, occurring in 2%–25% of patients. Ototoxicity is bilateral, symmetrical, nonreversible, and may be delayed or immediate. Complaints of tinnitus should be taken seriously. AG-associated nephrotoxicity has been reported to occur in ~8%–26% of patients. Nephrotoxicity can be reversible, resulting from proximal tubular necrosis and likely due to elevated trough levels. Close monitoring of renal function is vital during AG.

Allergic reactions, including rash, fever, and eosinophilia, are uncommon and occur in ~1%–3% of patients. AG-associated neuromuscular weakness can occur, though it is uncommon. The exact mechanism is unknown, but may be due to competitive antagonism of acetylcholine activity at the neuromuscular junction. Patients at particular risk to experience AG-induced neuromuscular weakness include those with myasthenia gravis, severe hypocalcemia, infantile botulism, or those who have recently received neuromuscular-blocking agents and/or steroids.

Therapeutic Drug Monitoring

AGs are distributed throughout extracellular water and are sensitive to changes in extracellular body water composition. The commonly accepted Vd of AGs varies by age, and age-specific dosing algorithms should be followed. AG pharmacokinetics is known to be altered in patients with renal dysfunction, CF, burns, meningitis, and an abnormal body habitus. Doses should be individualized by obtaining drug levels early in the course of therapy in high-risk populations.

Serum drug levels are suggested as objective parameters to direct AG dosing in addition to interpretation of clinical status and culture data (Table 88.10). Peak serum concentrations are related to drug efficacy, while trough concentrations are associated with drug toxicity. Guidelines are lacking for when drug level monitoring should occur, although volume overload, unstable renal function, and prolonged courses should all warrant close monitoring. Patients utilizing extracorporeal circuits should have therapeutic drug monitoring performed with changes in devices or fluid removal strategy.

TABLE 88.10

THERAPEUTIC DRUG CONCENTRATION TARGETS OF COMMONLY USED IV AMINOGLYCOSIDES

■ NAME	■ TARGET PEAK—TRADITIONAL	■ TARGET TROUGH—TRADITIONAL	■ TARGET PEAK—HDEI	■ TARGET TROUGH—HDEI	■ TARGET AUC_{0-24}
Gentamicin	8–10	<2	>20	≤1	70–120
Tobramycin	8–10	<2	>20	≤1	70–120
Amikacin	25–30	<8	>60	≤3	210–360

HDEI, high-dose extended-interval.

Drug Interactions

Medications, such as nonsteroidal anti-inflammatory medications, IV contrast, amphotericin, diuretics, and others, that can induce ototoxicity or nephrotoxicity may lead to increased risk of developing these side effects, and concomitant use should be judicious. Some penicillins have been shown to interact in vitro with AGs, causing degradation of the latter. For patients on very high–dose β-lactams or with renal insufficiency, there is concern that this interaction may also occur in vivo. Lastly, as noted above, concomitant use of an AG with corticosteroids and/or neuromuscular-blocking agents has been associated with prolonged neuromuscular weakness.

Clinical Indications

AGs exhibit concentration-dependent killing, a pronounced PAE, with PK/PD targets for maximizing peak/MIC and AUC/MIC ratios. AGs are used initially as empiric combination therapy for serious aerobic gram-negative infections. The 2005 IDSA/ATS guidelines for treatment of HCAP pneumonias recommend 5 days of initial double coverage (25). Antimicrobial synergy between antipseudomonal β-lactams and AGs has been theorized, with clinical evidence for this best described with infections due to *P. aeruginosa*, *Serratia*, *Acinetobacter*, *Citrobacter*, and *Enterobacter* spp. Data in the immunocompromised host with pseudomonal infections show a better survival and cure rate in patients who are treated with this combination, but may not be beneficial for all febrile neutropenic patients (85). Another argument for combination therapy is to increase the likelihood receiving an initially appropriate antibiotic. Combination therapy may also reduce the induction of resistance within a treatment course, but may increase the incidence of adverse effects, such as nephrotoxicity. Evidence exists that both supports and refutes the strategy of double coverage (86).

AGs also are indicated in the treatment of serious enterococcal infections, as susceptible enterococci are killed synergistically when given with penicillin or ampicillin. The levels of AG necessary to produce gram-positive synergy are lower than those required for gram-negative infections, and dosing is proportionally much lower. Synergy between AGs and β-lactams or glycopeptides can also be exploited in the treatment of serious infections due to other gram-positive organisms, including viridans streptococci, group B streptococci, *S. aureus*, and coagulase-negative staphylococci.

Glycopeptides

Mechanism of Action and Resistance

The glycopeptides (e.g., vancomycin) inhibit cell wall synthesis in replicating bacteria by binding to cell wall precursor units, inhibiting transpeptidation reactions. The alarming rise of vancomycin-resistant enterococci (VRE) is due to evolution of a readily transferable plasmid, which results in profoundly reduced affinity for vancomycin. There are also increasing reports of intermediate and resistant *S. aureus* and *Staphylococcus epidermidis* isolates, related to thickened cell walls (*S. aureus*) and production of biofilm (*S. epidermidis*). *S. aureus* MIC > 2 should prompt evaluation of alternative antibiotic therapy (87).

Spectrum of Activity

These drugs are bactericidal against most gram-positive bacteria, with the exception of the enterococci, against which it is bacteriostatic. Vancomycin cannot pass across the membrane of gram-negative bacteria to reach the cell wall, and therefore, has no utility in the treatment of gram-negative infections.

Metabolism and Distribution

The glycopeptides are not absorbed enterally. Vancomycin is irritating and erratically absorbed when given intramuscularly, and must be given intravenously for systemic use. Teicoplanin may be given intramuscularly or intravenously. Approximately 55% of vancomycin and 90% of teicoplanin is bound to plasma protein. The Vd varies based on age and ranges from 0.5 L/kg for premature neonates to 0.75 L/kg for adults. Vancomycin distributes to most body fluids and tissues, but because of its large molecular size, penetration into some infected spaces, such as devitalized wounds, is poor. Vancomycin does not penetrate well into the CNS unless the meninges are inflamed. The glycopeptides are not metabolized. Most drug elimination occurs as unchanged drug via renal glomerular filtration (80%–90%). Renal function should be closely monitored for patients on vancomycin, with dosing intervals extended to allow for adequate clearance of drug. Most pediatric patients will require dosing intervals of every 6 hours, whereas many adult patients will need intervals of every 8–12 hours. Vancomycin dosing should begin at 15 mg/kg/dose based on actual body weight, even for obese patients.

Adverse Effects

A large number of adverse effects have been reduced by removing the impurities found in earlier formulations. "Red man syndrome," characterized by flushing, pruritus, tachycardia, and an erythematous rash, is associated with the rapid IV administration of vancomycin. This is due to vancomycin-induced histamine release. Pretreatment with an antihistamine and slowing the vancomycin infusion rate reduce the frequency and severity of this reaction. This reaction is generally not observed with teicoplanin.

Current estimates suggest that the incidence of vancomycin-associated ototoxicity and nephrotoxicity approximates 2% and 5%, respectively, and their occurrences are dependent on the presence of other confounding variables, such as concurrent administration of known ototoxic and nephrotoxic drugs, patient age, and severity of disease. Nephrotoxicity tends to be reversible, whereas little is known about true vancomycin-induced ototoxicity.

Therapeutic Drug Monitoring

Vancomycin exhibits time-dependent killing, and an AUC/MIC ratio of ≥ 400 has been established as a pharmacodynamic target. Trough serum concentrations should always be maintained >10 mg/L to minimize development of resistance. Trough serum vancomycin concentrations of 15–20 mg/L are recommended for treatment of serious or complicated infections, such as bacteremia, endocarditis, osteomyelitis, meningitis, and hospital-acquired pneumonia caused by S. aureus. Peak vancomycin concentrations are unlikely to be helpful. Initial doses of >2000 mg/dose may warrant drug level monitoring early in the treatment course to ensure safe and effective dosing. Patients with unstable renal function, changes in volume status, or changes in extracorporeal therapies should prompt frequent drug levels.

Drug Interactions

Concomitant use of drugs known to cause ototoxicity and nephrotoxicity with vancomycin may result in additive effects. There is also a potential to increase the neuromuscular-blocking effects of neuromuscular blockers.

Clinical Indications

Therapy is indicated for the empiric or definitive treatment of infections caused by, or suspected to be, MRSA or other resistant gram-positive organism, or as an alternative to β-lactam therapy in children with an allergy. β-Lactams have superior penetration into most body spaces compared to vancomycin, making β-lactams the preferred agent if the organism is susceptible. The empiric use of vancomycin in the treatment of immunocompromised or critically ill patients remains controversial. Local resistance patterns establishing prevalence of MRSA should be utilized to determine if empiric vancomycin is warranted.

Telavancin is a newer semisynthetic derivative of vancomycin, indicated for the treatment of adults with complicated SSSIs. The rate of nephrotoxicity has been reported to be higher with telavancin compared to vancomycin (88). Telavancin is confirmed to prolong the QT interval and is a risk factor for developing torsade de pointes.

Oxazolidinones (Linezolid)

Linezolid binds to the P site of the 50S ribosomal subunit, preventing formation of a complex that initiates protein synthesis. Linezolid is active against gram-positive organisms, including staphylococci, streptococci, enterococci, gram-positive anaerobic cocci, and gram-positive bacilli, such as *Corynebacterium* spp. and *L. monocytogenes*, and devoid of activity against gram-negative bacteria. It is bacteriostatic against enterococci and staphylococci, and bactericidal against streptococci. Linezolid is available in both parenteral and oral preparations, the latter allowing convenient, effective home therapy once clinical stability has been established. Linezolid is not nephrotoxic and does not require adjustment in renal dysfunction, but does undergo hepatic metabolism via oxidation. One of the more common adverse effects noted with linezolid is myelosuppression and elevations in hepatic function tests. Therapy for >8 weeks has been associated with peripheral neuropathy, optic neuritis, and lactic acidosis. Drug interactions are rare, but linezolid does have a weak MAO-I–like structure, and combination with other serotonergic agents and/or a high tyramine diet may result in a serotonin syndrome.

Lipopeptides

Daptomycin is a concentration-dependent, bactericidal, parenteral agent that binds to bacterial cell membranes leading to depolarization, loss of membrane potential, and cell death. Daptomycin has activity against virtually all isolates of S. aureus, coagulase-negative staphylococci, and enterococci (including VRE), but published experience describing its use in children is limited. Resistance is rare, but reports are beginning to emerge. The most significant toxicity is musculoskeletal damage and elevation in creatine kinase. Daptomycin is indicated for treatment of complicated skin and soft-tissue infections, complicated bacteremia, and right-sided endocarditis; however, it cannot be used for the treatment of pneumonia owing to inactivation by pulmonary surfactant.

Quinupristin/Dalfopristin

Quinupristin/dalfopristin (Q/D) inhibits protein synthesis by binding to the 50S ribosomal subunit, similar to macrolides. Q/D is active against gram-positive cocci, including *S. pneumoniae*, *Enterococcus faecium* (but not *Enterococcus faecalis*), and coagulase-positive and coagulase-negative staphylococci. Q/D is also active against *Mycoplasma pneumoniae*, *Legionella* spp., and *Chlamydia pneumoniae*, and gram-negative organisms *Moraxella catarrhalis* and *Neisseria* spp. The combination is bactericidal against streptococci and many strains of staphylococci but bacteriostatic against *E. faecium*. Resistance has been described by changes on the binding site, production of inactivating enzymes, and development of efflux pumps. Q/D should be reserved for treatment of serious infections caused by multiple-drug-resistant gram-positive organisms, such as VRE. Adverse effects are rare and consist mostly of myalgias. Drug interactions are possible, as Q/D inhibits CYP3A4.

Clindamycin

Clindamycin binds exclusively to the 50S subunit of bacterial ribosomes suppressing protein synthesis. Clindamycin is active against susceptible strains of pneumococci, *Streptococcus pyogenes*, and viridans streptococci, methicillin-sensitive S. aureus (MSSA) (and some strains of MRSA), and most anaerobic gram-positive bacteria. Largely all aerobic gram-negative bacilli are resistant. Susceptibility to atypical organisms is variable. Clindamycin is widely distributed in many fluids and tissues, including bone, but not in the CSF, even when the meninges are inflamed. In the critical care field, clindamycin may prove most useful for treatment of abscesses, anaerobic infections, as a narrow-spectrum alternative for susceptible MRSA infections, or as an adjunct in toxic shock syndromes. Clindamycin has been shown to inhibit toxin production by both S. aureus and S. pyogenes (89). It should be noted that clindamycin use, among other antibiotics, has been associated with the development of C. difficile colitis.

Fluoroquinolones

Concern for arthropathy and tendon injury initially seen in juvenile animals during preclinical testing has led to limited use of fluoroquinolones in pediatric patients. Nevertheless, their broad spectrum of activity and enteral availability have given way to a great deal of off-label use in pediatric patients. More recently, pediatric indications have been added for systemic ciprofloxacin and levofloxacin.

Mechanism of Action and Resistance

Fluoroquinolones are bactericidal, inhibiting bacterial DNA-topoisomerase (gram-positive organisms)/DNA-gyrase (gram-negative organisms), which are necessary for bacterial DNA replication and some aspects of transcription and repair. Quinolones do not interact with mammalian DNA-gyrase at concentrations achieved after routine dosing. Resistance to fluoroquinolones is most commonly a result of mutations that alter drug binding to DNA-topoisomerase/gyrase or the result of expression of multidrug efflux pumps that extrude the antibiotic from the bacterial cell. Resistance is more often a class effect, but not necessarily to other antibiotic drug classes.

Spectrum of Activity

Fluoroquinolones are effective against many gram-negative pathogens, including *P. aeruginosa*. Newer agents (levofloxacin, gatifloxacin, and moxifloxacin) also have improved pneumococcus coverage (**Table 88.11**). They also have activity against atypical respiratory pathogens (*M. pneumoniae*, *C. pneumoniae*, and *Legionella*). This renders them excellent choices for both community- and hospital-acquired respiratory infections.

Metabolism and Distribution

Limited data are available regarding pharmacokinetics of fluoroquinolones in infants and children. The fluoroquinolones are available in both IV and enteral formulations. Oral bioavailability approaches 100%, offering the clinician an enteral option in the patient who lacks IV access, but food–drug interactions, particularly with ciprofloxacin, need to be adequately addressed to ensure proper drug delivery. These drugs undergo primary hepatic metabolism, and dosage adjustments may be necessary for most patients with liver disease. Dose adjustments are generally not required in mild-to-moderate renal dysfunction, but are necessary if severe renal disease is present.

Adverse Effects

Nausea, diarrhea, headache, and dizziness are the most common adverse events in adults. Less common adverse effects have included skin rash, photosensitivity reactions, CNS manifestations (headache, confusion, and dizziness), and hepatotoxicity. Some quinolones may cause prolongation of the QT interval. Reports of joint complaints in teenage patients with CF receiving ciprofloxacin have appeared, but the incidence of true quinolone-associated arthropathy in young children is unknown (90).

Drug Interactions

Enteral administration of fluoroquinolones with divalent and trivalent cation-containing antacids, sucralfate, iron, as well as food or tube feeds containing these elements results in chelation and substantially reduces the absorption.

Concomitant use of systemic corticosteroids may increase the risk of arthropathy and tendon rupture. The risk of QTc prolongation increases when fluoroquinolones, particularly moxifloxacin, are used in combination with other medications, which can also prolong the QTc interval (e.g., methadone, ondansetron, and haloperidol). Ciprofloxacin in combination with theophylline derivatives may decrease the metabolism of theophylline derivatives, resulting in toxicity. Several quinolones (ciprofloxacin, norfloxacin, and ofloxacin) are strong inhibitors of CYP1A2 and weak-to-moderate

TABLE 88.11

SPECTRUM OF ACTIVITY FOR FLUROQUINOLONES

	Fluroquinolones			
	■ CIPROFLOXACIN	■ LEVOFLOXACIN	■ MOXIFLOXACIN	■ GATIFLOXACIN
Gram (+)				
S. pneumoniae	+/−	+	+	+
S. viridans	0	+	+	+
E. faecalis	0	+	+	+
E. faecium	0	0	+/−	+/−
S. aureus	+	+	+	+
S. aureus MRSA	0	0	+/−	+/−
L. monocytogenes	+	+	+	+
Gram (−)				
N. meningitidis	+	+	+	+
M. catarrhalis	+	+	+	+
H. influenzae	+	+	+	+
E. coli	+	+	+	+
Klebseilla sp.	+	+	+	+
Enterobacter sp.	+	+	+	+
Serratia sp.	+	+	+	+
P. aeruginosa	+	+/−	+/−	+/−

It shozuld be noted that fluroquinolones have excellent atypical coverage and generally poor anaerobic coverage.
Adapted from Gilbert DN, Moellering RC Jr, Eliopoulos GM, et al. *Sanford Guide to Antimicrobial Therapy*. 43rd ed. 2013.

inhibitors of CYP3A4. Caution and appropriate adjustment may be necessary when using other agents that utilize these enzyme pathways.

Clinical Indications

Fluoroquinolones have a broad spectrum of activity and good penetration into many body compartments. The American Academy of Pediatrics has released a guideline statement on the use of fluoroquinolones in pediatrics, stating that use may be justified in special circumstances in which infection is caused by a multidrug-resistant pathogen for which there is no safe and effective alternative (91). The newer agents, with enhanced *S. pneumoniae* coverage, have proven to provide excellent monotherapy in the treatment of adult CAP and HCAP, although they are not recommended for first-line therapy in children. Fluoroquinolone-containing regimens may also prove to be useful as part of combination therapy with an antipseudomonal β-lactam to spare the nephrotoxic effects of an AG for those patients at higher risk of nephrotoxicity.

Macrolides and Related Drugs

Mechanism of Action and Resistance

Macrolides are bacteriostatic compounds that competitively bind to the 50S ribosomal subunit, antagonizing bacterial protein synthesis by interfering with translocation of tRNA and peptide bond formation. Resistance to macrolides has been characterized by three mechanisms: changes to the 23S ribosomal subunit, an efflux pump, and enzymatic inactivation.

Spectrum of Activity

Macrolides are active against atypical pathogens, such as *Mycoplasma*, *Legionella*, and *Chlamydia*, as well as many community-acquired pathogens, such as pneumococcus, MSSA, and *S. pyogenes*. They have less activity against *Haemophilus influenzae*, although the newer macrolides are superior to erythromycin in this regard. They are the drugs of choice for eradication of *Bordetella pertussis*.

Metabolism and Distribution

Erythromycin is degraded by the acidic environment of the stomach, resulting in reduced bioavailability and emergence of various preparations to overcome this problem. Clarithromycin and telithromycin undergo significant first-pass metabolism (bioavailability 50%–60%). Once in the bloodstream, macrolides are widely distributed throughout the body, with the exception of CNS. Serum protein binding is modest and variable. Macrolides have significant intracellular concentrations (e.g., ~95% of azithromycin), leaving relatively low extracellular concentrations, and thus, they are not always clinically effective against extracellular organisms (e.g., *H. influenzae*) and have enhanced effectiveness against intracellular pathogens, such as *Chlamydia* and *Legionella*.

Elimination of macrolide antibiotics, with the exception of azithromycin, is mainly through hepatic metabolism via CYP3A4 and biliary excretion. Dose adjustment is not necessary in renal or hepatic impairment, with the exception of clarithromycin and telithromycin where dose reduction is recommended in severe renal impairment.

Adverse Effects

The most common adverse effects associated with erythromycin are abdominal pain and diarrhea. More serious adverse effects associated with erythromycin administration include hepatic toxicity, ototoxicity, and cardiac toxicity. Hepatotoxicity resembles a hypersensitivity reaction, which may be delayed up to 14 days after discontinuation. Ototoxicity is reversible. Prolongation of the QT interval and ventricular tachyarrhythmias are the most common manifestations of cardiac toxicity (erythromycin > clarithromycin > azithromycin), and caution should be utilized when combining other medications known to prolong the QT interval.

Telithromycin is contraindicated in patients with myasthenia gravis due to reports of disease exacerbations, leading to the development of respiratory failure. Development of hepatotoxicity has also limited its use.

Drug Interactions

A number of important drug–drug interactions have been reported to occur in patients who receive macrolides. Many drug interactions exist via the CYP3A4 enzyme. Macrolides are enzymatic substrates as well as strong inhibitors. Any other drug that interacts with CYP3A4 will likely have an impact on serum macrolide levels or vice versa. Drugs that are reported to result in clinically important drug interactions with macrolides include carbamazepine, corticosteroids, cyclosporine, warfarin, digoxin, benzodiazepines, and theophylline. A case of sudden cardiac death has been described in an adult taking concomitant methadone (92).

Pharmacodynamically, the binding site on the 50S ribosome subunit is the same target bound by other antibiotics, most notably clindamycin and Q/D, potentially resulting in antibacterial antagonism if these medications are coadministered.

Clinical Indications

Use of both oral and parenteral erythromycin has been largely replaced by use of azithromycin, which is most commonly used as part of a combination regimen for the treatment of community-acquired infections of the respiratory tract, and importantly *B. pertussis*.

Tetracyclines and Related Drugs

Mechanism of Action and Resistance

Tetracyclines are bacteriostatic antibiotics that inhibit protein synthesis by binding reversibly to the 30S subunit of the bacterial ribosome. Drug entry into cells is via both active transport and passive diffusion. Resistance to tetracyclines has been described by three mechanisms: (1) impaired intracellular concentration (lack of entry into or efflux pump out of the cell), (2) impaired binding to the ribosome, and (3) enzymatic inactivation. Resistance is primarily plasmid mediated and often inducible, and cross-resistance within the class depends on which mechanism is active. Tigecycline, a glycylcycline, has a reduced affinity for most efflux pumps, thus retaining activity against many organisms that have developed tetracycline resistance via this mechanism (93).

Spectrum of Activity

Tetracyclines have a broad range of activity, including many aerobic and anaerobic gram-positive and gram-negative bacteria, as well microorganisms that are resistant to cell wall–active agents, such as *Rickettsia*, *Coxiella burnetii*, *M. pneumoniae*, *Chlamydia* spp., *Legionella* spp., *Ureaplasma*, and *Plasmodium* spp. Tetracyclines are active against many spirochetes, such as *Borrelia burgdorferi* (Lyme disease) and some nontuberculosis strains of mycobacteria (e.g., *Mycobacterium marinum*). Tigecycline is generally considered bacteriostatic;

however, bactericidal activity has been demonstrated against isolates of *S. pneumoniae* and *Legionella pneumophila*, and remains active against methicillin-resistant staphylococci. Importantly, tetracyclines are not active against *Pseudomonas*, *Proteus*, and *Providencia* spp.

Metabolism and Distribution

Tetracyclines are widely distributed throughout the body, including low levels within the CSF. They accumulate in reticuloendothelial cells of the liver, spleen, and bone marrow, and in bone, dentine, and enamel of unerupted teeth. Tetracyclines are excreted mainly in bile and urine, and undergo enterohepatic circulation. Adjustment in renal impairment may be necessary, with exception for doxycycline and tigecycline as they are eliminated by nonrenal mechanisms.

Adverse Effects

Children may develop permanent brown discoloration of the teeth, with the highest risk if it is given before the first dentition; however, pigmentation of permanent teeth may develop during calcification if administration between the ages of 2 months and 5 years occurs. Thrombophlebitis frequently follows intravenous administration. This irritant effect is used therapeutically during pleurodesis when drug is instilled into the pleural space.

Other adverse reactions commonly encountered are nausea, vomiting, diarrhea, and photosensitivity. Hepatotoxicity, pancreatitis, and azotemia are serious but uncommon reactions. Pseudotumor cerebri may develop in young infants, even when given in the usual therapeutic doses, and is reversible on discontinuation of the drug.

Drug Interactions

Tetracyclines form chelation complexes, which lead to incomplete absorption when given in conjunction with other di- and trivalent cations, and therefore should not be administered enterally with dairy products, antacids, multivitamins, or iron supplements (tigecycline is only available IV). The anticoagulant effects of warfarin may be enhanced by some tetracyclines. Carbamazepine, (fos)phenytoin, and barbiturates may increase metabolism of some tetracyclines, leading to lower antibiotic levels.

Clinical Indications

Given their broad antimicrobial spectrum, tetracyclines can be used in the treatment of many infections. However, extensive use in animal farming has led to increased resistance among gram-positive and gram-negative organisms, and availability of other better tolerated, easier to administer, and effective antimicrobials has made tetracyclines most often reserved for use in the treatment of rickettsial diseases, and *Mycoplasma* and *Chlamydia* infections.

ANTIFUNGAL DRUGS

Most serious fungal infections occur in immunocompromised patients. A general lack of pediatric studies with newer antifungal agents and decreased predictability of in vitro susceptibility testing for antifungal drugs complicates these treatments. However, substantial advances have been made with the introduction of newer classes of antifungals.

Drug targets for fungi are different than that for bacteria, given that they are eukaryotes with unique cell wall structures (**Fig. 88.3**). A summary of pharmacokinetic properties of selected antifungal drugs is provided in **Table 88.12** (94).

Polyenes

Amphotericin B has traditionally been the gold standard treatment for most critical fungal infections. There are four formulations of amphotericin B: conventional amphotericin B (C-AMB), liposomal amphotericin B (L-AMB), amphotericin B lipid complex (ABLC), and amphotericin B colloidal dispersion (ABCD). Conventional amphotericin B is highly toxic, which led to the development of the latter three formulations.

Mechanism of Action and Resistance

Amphotericin B binds to ergosterol, the principal sterol component of the fungal cell membrane, leading to cell death. Furthermore, oxidative species are generated that damage fungal mitochondria. It is rare for resistance to develop during treatment of infection.

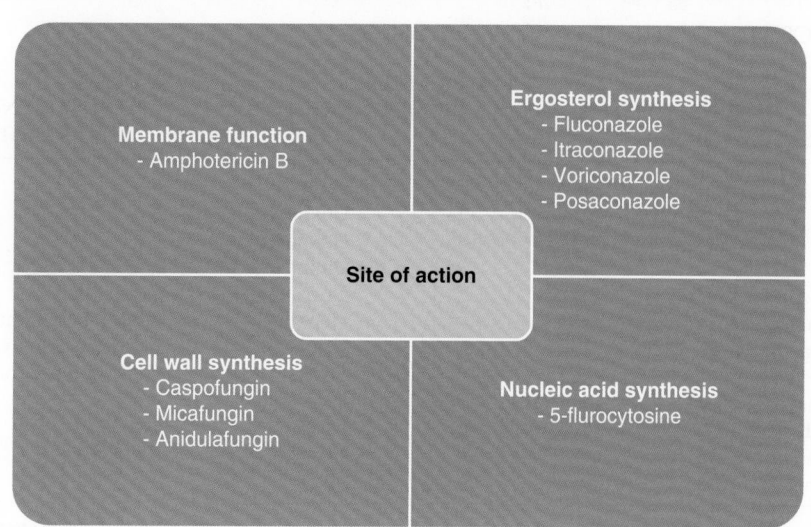

FIGURE 88.3. Sites of action for antifungal drugs.

Spectrum of Activity

Experimentally, amphotericin has concentration-dependent killing, with a prolonged PAE. Susceptible pathogens include *Candida, Aspergillus*, non-*Aspergillus* molds, *Cryptococcus*, the endemic fungal pathogens, such as *Histoplasma, Blastomyces, Coccidioides*, and *Sporothrix*, and the agents of mucormycosis. Some fungal organisms, such as *Candida lusitaniae* and the molds *Aspergillus terreus, Fusarium*, and *Pseudallescheria boydii*, display intrinsic amphotericin B resistance.

Metabolism and Distribution

Amphotericin B is not absorbed enterally and must be given intravenously. The drug is distributed widely in tissues, with liver, kidney, and lung being the organs with the highest concentrations, and bronchial secretions and CNS with the lowest. Nevertheless, amphotericin B has been used successfully for selected CNS infections, particularly *Cryptococcus* and *Coccidioides*, although intraventricular administration may also be required. The mechanisms of elimination are unknown. Blood levels are not influenced by renal or hepatic insufficiency; however, weight may play an important role in pediatric patients. Pharmacokinetic studies suggest that pediatric patients weighing <20 kg may require higher dosing of liposomal products than heavier children.

Adverse Effects

Amphotericin B use is associated with significant toxicities, although it is generally better tolerated in children than in adults. Toxicity can be infusion related (fever, chills, rigors, nausea and vomiting, arthralgias, myalgias, respiratory distress, and hypotension) or dose related (nephrotoxicity, hypokalemia, hypomagnesemia, bicarbonate wasting, and anemia). Use of antipyretics, meperidine, and hydrocortisone are thought to reduce infusion-related symptoms. Dose-related toxicities correlate with cumulative exposure. Use of an every-other-day dosing regimen after the patient has stabilized, or providing a sodium load may decrease the incidence and severity of nephrotoxicity. The lipid-complexed amphotericins demonstrate decreased toxicity, primarily dose-related toxicities, when compared with C-AMB.

Drug Interactions

Concomitant nephrotoxic medications can increase the risk of nephrotoxicity. Corticosteroids may enhance the hypokalemia associated with amphotericin use. Antifungal agents also decrease the effectiveness of many of the available "probiotic" agents, such as *Saccharomyces boulardii*. There is a theoretical concern of therapeutic antagonism of amphotericin if used in combination with the azole class, owing to azoles' inhibition of ergosterol synthesis.

Clinical Indications

Use is FDA-approved for patients with systemic mycoses, primary invasive aspergillosis, and for empiric therapy for febrile neutropenic patients who have not responded to antibacterial therapy, the later use having decreased owing to the development of newer, less-toxic antifungals.

Azoles

Azoles are divided into two classes: imidazoles and triazoles. Triazoles have less effect on human sterol synthesis and may be better tolerated, thus drug development has focused more on triazoles.

Mechanism of Action and Resistance

All of the azoles inhibit the enzyme lanosterol 14α-demethylase, necessary for the synthesis of ergosterol, found in the fungal cell membrane, resulting in inhibition of cell growth and death.

Azole resistance has been documented, particularly in *Candida* spp. The mechanisms include multidrug efflux pumps, alterations of enzymes in the synthetic pathway for ergosterol, upregulation of the target enzymes (resulting in overwhelming the drugs' mechanism of action), and replacement of ergosterol. Multiple resistance mechanisms may be present. Resistance to one azole does not necessarily imply resistance to others, for example, fluconazole-resistant *Candida* spp. usually remain susceptible to voriconazole and posaconazole.

TABLE 88.12

PHARMACOKINETIC PROPERTIES OF SELECTED ANTIFUNGAL DRUGS

	■ NAME	■ HALF-LIFE (HOUR)	■ VD (L/KG)	■ PROTEIN BINDING (%)	■ ROUTE OF ELIMINATION	■ DOSE ADJUSTMENT CONSIDERATION	■ DIALYZABLE
Polyenes	C-AMB	50	4	>95	Feces	No	No
	L-AMB	100–153	0.1–0.16	>95	Unknown	No	No
	ABLC	173	131	>95	Unknown	No	No
	ABCD	30	4.3	>95	Unknown	No	No
Azoles	Fluconazole	15–30	0.65	12	Urine	Renal, dialysis	Yes
	Itraconazole	36	10	99	Hepatic	GFR <10 mL/min	No
	Voriconazole	6–9	4.6	58	Urine	Ethnicity, age, liver, GFR <50 mL/min	No
	Posaconazole	20–66	1774 (L)	>98	Feces, renal	No	No
Echinocandins	Anidulafungin	43–52	30–50 (L)	84	Feces	No	No
	Caspofungin	8–13	—	97	Urine, feces	Renal	No
	Micafungin	12–15	0.39	99	Feces	No	No

Adapted from Lepak AJ, Andes DR. Antifungal PK/PD considerations in fungal pulmonary infections [published online ahead of print December 15, 2011]. *Semin Respir Crit Care Med* 2011;32(6):783–94.

Spectrum of Activity

Azoles are active against many *Candida* spp., *Cryptococcus neoformans*, *Blastomyces dermatitidis*, *Histoplasma capsulatum*, *Coccidioides* spp., and *Paracoccidioides brasiliensis*. Fungi with variable susceptibility include *Aspergillus* spp. and *Fusarium*. *Candida krusei* and the agents of mucormycosis are intrinsically resistant. Posaconazole has slightly improved activity in vitro against the agents of mucormycosis.

Metabolism and Distribution

Itraconazole, voriconazole, and posaconazole are cleared almost exclusively by the liver, and no dose adjustment is required for renal insufficiency. However, use of enteral voriconazole is preferred if GFR is <50 mL/min as the IV vehicle accumulates, the consequences of which are unknown. Fluconazole has a wide distribution with excellent CNS penetration, is cleared by the kidneys, and dose adjustment in renal failure/dialysis is necessary. Itraconazole, ketoconazole, and posaconazole are highly protein bound. Consequently, they are neither dialyzed nor reliable for the treatment of CNS infections. Voriconazole is metabolized via CYP2C19, a polymorphic enzyme, and exhibits nonlinear pharmacokinetics. As many as 20% of non-Indian Asians may achieve voriconazole levels fourfold higher than other patients because of genetic polymorphisms (95), and therapeutic drug monitoring may be warranted.

Clinical Indications

Fluconazole is the first-line agent for suspected *Candida albicans* infections without septic shock, in the treatment and secondary prophylaxis of cryptococcal meningitis, as well as prophylactic use in severely immunosuppressed patients. Resistance to selected *Candida* spp. has become more frequent, giving increasing concern for the prophylactic use of this agent. *C. krusei* and some isolates of *Candida glabrata* are intrinsically resistant to fluconazole, and the incidence of these infections has increased. Fluconazole has no clinically relevant activity against *Aspergillus* or other molds.

Itraconazole is the azole of choice for infections due to the dimorphic fungi *Histoplasma*, *Blastomyces*, and *Sporothrix*. Itraconazole possesses in vitro activity against most *Aspergillus* spp., but is not the azole of choice. Effectiveness and use can be limited by poor bioavailability, drug–drug interactions, and lack of CNS penetration.

Voriconazole has excellent activity against *Candida* spp. (including fluconazole-resistant species, such as *C. krusei*) and the dimorphic fungi, and is the treatment of choice for invasive aspergillosis. Treatment of CNS disease has not been well studied, but several reports suggest that it may be useful for susceptible CNS infections. Voriconazole is not active against Zygomycetes. Therapeutic drug monitoring (trough levels) are available for voriconazole and should be considered for long-term therapy, patients at risk for genetic polymorphism of CYP2C19, pediatric patients, and those with abnormal body habitus or hepatic function.

Posaconazole possesses the broadest activity of the class, including virtually all *Candida* spp., *Cryptococcus*, nearly all *Aspergillus* spp., and non-*Aspergillus* molds, including many *Fusarium* spp. and *P. boydii*. It is also the only azole to date active against Zygomycetes, including *Rhizopus* and *Mucor*. Posaconazole is only available enterally, and absorption is significantly enhanced when given with high-fat meals and in the presence of an acidic environment, thus absorption may be inadequate for patients who are not being enterally fed or who are on medications to increase gastric pH.

Adverse Effects

The most common adverse effects are mild and include nausea, abdominal pain, headache, and mild elevations of hepatic transaminases. Significant transaminase elevations are infrequent, and fulminant hepatitis with the newer azoles, while reported, is rare. Voriconazole has several distinct side effects not noted with other azoles. Temporary visual disturbance (blurred vision, photophobia, and optic neuritis) occurs in up to one-third of patients, often during the first week of therapy. Hallucinations and rash, sometimes severe, are also rarely reported.

Drug Interactions

Drug–drug interactions with other agents metabolized via CYP 450 enzymes are common to all of the azoles, though to varying degrees. Clinically significant interactions include benzodiazepines, barbiturates, phenytoin, carbamazepine, tacrolimus, sirolimus, cyclosporine, warfarin, rifampin, omeprazole, and calcium-channel blockers. Full review of the patient's medication profile for drug–drug interactions, medication adjustments, and monitoring requirements is essential on initiation or discontinuation of an azole.

Echinocandins

Echinocandins, the most recently developed class, share a notably favorable safety profile with lack of significant drug–drug interactions. Presently, three echinocandins have been licensed by the FDA: caspofungin, micafungin, and anidulafungin.

Mechanism of Action and Resistance

Echinocandins inhibit 1,3-β-d-glucan synthase, the enzyme responsible for the production of the polysaccharide 1,3-β-d-glucan, a component of the fungal cell wall. This causes the formation of a defective cell wall, cellular instability and lysis in yeasts, and aberrant hyphal growth in molds. Echinocandins are fungicidal against *Candida* spp., but fungistatic against *Aspergillus*. Mutations in the gene encoding for elements of the 1,3-β-d-glucan synthase complex have been associated with *Candida* resistance to echinocandins.

Spectrum of Activity

The echinocandin spectrum is limited to all isolates within *Candida* and *Aspergillus* spp., including *C. krusei*, *C. glabrata*, and *C. lusitaniae*. Echinocandins have no activity against *Cryptococcus*, Zygomycetes, *Fusarium*, and *Pseudallescheria* and its asexual form *Scedosporium*, or *Trichosporon*. Presently, resistance to the echinocandins among *Candida* and *Aspergillus* is very rare.

Metabolism and Distribution

All echinocandins must be administered IV. They are highly protein bound, have poor penetration into the CNS, and do not undergo any renal clearance. Caspofungin and micafungin are both metabolized in the liver. Dosage adjustment is suggested for moderate-to-severe hepatic insufficiency, but not for renal insufficiency. Anidulafungin is slowly degraded in human plasma, and dose adjustments are not necessary in either renal or hepatic insufficiency.

In general, children tend to have lower drug levels than adults when given comparable doses, and as such, larger doses are given to pediatric patients on an mg/kg or mg/m^2 basis.

Clinical Indications

Echinocandins are rational choices for patients with suspected or proven disease caused by *Candida* or *Aspergillus*, especially those who are failing more conventional therapy, or who have sepsis or septic shock. They are noninferior to L-AMB as antifungal therapy in febrile neutropenia. Most of the experience in the treatment of invasive aspergillosis has been collected in open-label studies directed toward patients who are unresponsive to or intolerant of other agents. Clinical response in this context, either when used alone or with voriconazole, is ~50%.

Adverse Effects

The most frequent adverse effects are pain and phlebitis at the injection site. Occasional small increases in liver transaminases and histamine-like reaction during infusion may occur.

Drug Interactions

Cyclosporine has been shown to increase caspofungin levels by ~35%, and tacrolimus levels have been reported to be reduced by ~20% during caspofungin administration.

Combination Antifungal Therapy

Despite recent advances in antifungal therapy, outcomes still remain poor. Combination antifungal therapy utilizing different classes may be considered for some patients who are failing to respond to single-agent therapy; however, this strategy remains poorly investigated. Combination therapy has been shown successful in the treatment of cryptococcal meningitis (98); however, other animal and in vitro models have shown reduced efficacy with combination therapy, in particular combination therapy with azoles and polyenes. Efforts to further investigate combination therapy have more heavily focused on

combinations with echinocandins and triazoles; however, the ideal combinations of agents for a given pathogen have not been determined.

ANTIVIRAL AGENTS (NON-HIV)

Medication Summary

Viruses are obligate intracellular organisms, dependent on host cells for replication. Antiviral agents must either block viral entry or exit from the cell or be active inside the host cell. Antiviral drugs are static, not cidal, against replicating (not latent) viruses. There are no standardized in vitro susceptibility tests for antiviral agents. Antiviral therapy is currently available for herpesviruses, hepatitis C virus (HCV), hepatitis B virus (HBV), papillomavirus, influenza, and HIV; however, we will focus specifically on antiviral agents likely to be encountered by the pediatric intensivist (**Table 88.13**). These include acyclovir, ganciclovir, cidofovir, foscarnet, and antivirals used to treat influenza infections. Less likely to be utilized, but still of significance, is the antiviral ribavirin, which may be used for the treatment of severe RSV, or experimentally in the treatment of other viral infections.

Mechanisms of Action

The mechanisms of action of the noninfluenza antivirals all share a common final pathway in that they inhibit viral DNA synthesis. Acyclovir, ganciclovir, cidofovir, and ribavirin are nucleoside/nucleotide analog derivatives, which are preferentially incorporated into the viral DNA resulting in chain termination. Foscarnet inhibits viral nucleic acid synthesis by interacting directly with herpesvirus DNA polymerase or HIV reverse transcriptase. Ribavirin's mechanism of action is not completely understood, but relates to alteration of cellular nucleotide pools and inhibition of viral messenger RNA synthesis, potentially leading to lethal mutagenesis of the viral genome.

TABLE 88.13

SUMMARY OF ANTIVIRAL DRUGS

■ DRUG	■ PRIMARY ICU INDICATION	■ CNS PENETRATION	■ DOSE LIMITING ADVERSE EFFECT	■ OTHER ADVERSE EFFECTS	■ DRUG INTERACTIONS
Acyclovir	HSV 1, HSV2, VZV	Yes	Nephrotoxicity	CNS toxicity, neutropenia (in neonates)	Nephrotoxic agents, mycophenolate, Zoster vaccination
Ganciclovir	CMV	Yes	Myelosuppression	↑Creatinine	Imipenem, nephrotoxic agents, myelosuppressive agents
Cidofovir	Adenovirus	No	Nephrotoxicity	Proximal tubular dysfunction, ↓intraocular pressure, uveitis	Nephrotoxic agents,[a]
Foscarnet	CMV	Yes	Nephrotoxicity	Electrolyte abnormalities, genital ulcerations	Other QTc prolonging agents
Ribavirin	RSV, HCV	Aerosol: no	Hemolytic anemia, teratogenicity, interference with respiratory equipment	CNS and psychiatric disturbances	Aerosol: none

[a]As probenacid must be administered along with cidofovir, drug interactions with probenacid should also be taken into account (e.g., increased serum concentrations of β-lactams).

Resistance

Resistance to acyclovir and ganciclovir is mainly encountered in immunocompromised patients, resulting from reduced intracellular drug activation or altered viral DNA polymerase. Cidofovir- and foscarnet-resistant viruses are infrequent, but may occur due to mutations in viral DNA polymerase. Cidofovir resistance may be higher in patients with prior prolonged exposure to ganciclovir or with CMV strains displaying high-level resistance to ganciclovir. Resistance to ribavirin has not been reported for RSV infections.

Spectrum of Activity

Acyclovir has in vitro and clinical activity against herpes simplex virus type 1 (HSV-1), HSV type 2 (HSV-2), weaker activity against varicella-zoster virus (VZV), and very weak activity against Epstein–Barr virus (EBV), cytomegalovirus (CMV), and human herpesvirus 6 (HHV-6). Acyclovir has no in vitro or in vivo activity against viruses outside of the herpesvirus group. Ganciclovir has activity against all herpesviruses, but most notably against CMV and HHV-6. Cidofovir has in vitro antiviral activity against all of the HHVs, including most that are resistant to acyclovir, ganciclovir, and foscarnet. Additionally, activity is displayed against adenovirus, human papilloma and polyoma viruses, and poxviruses (e.g., monkeypox, smallpox, and vaccinia). Foscarnet has activity against several HHVs, including HSV-1 and HSV-2, VZV, CMV, and HHV-6, as well as HBV. It also has activity against the HIV-1 reverse transcriptase. Ribavirin has a broad spectrum of antiviral activity against RNA viruses, including RSV, HCV, measles, hantaviruses, and Lassa viruses.

Clinical Practice

Acyclovir

Intensivists will primarily use acyclovir for neonatal herpes, HSV encephalitis, and HSV and VZV infections in immunocompromised patients. Acyclovir is also used prophylactically to suppress reactivation of latent HSV (e.g., HSV-seropositive bone marrow transplant patients).

Ganciclovir

Ganciclovir is the established agent of choice in the treatment of CMV as well as disseminated HHV-6 infections. Reduction of immunosuppressive medications, if applicable, should also be employed as part of the treatment strategy for these diseases. Severe cases of CMV pneumonitis may also benefit from combined therapy with intravenous immunoglobulin or CMV immunoglobulin to reduce mortality. Given the high morbidity and mortality of CMV infection, ganciclovir or valganciclovir is used as prophylaxis in transplant recipients. While effective against HSV-1, HSV-2, and VZV infection in humans, acyclovir remains preferred as the first-line agent as it has a better side effect profile.

Cidofovir

Cidofovir is most likely to be in the treatment of adenovirus infection in immunocompromised patients, particularly HSCT recipients, as dissemination can occur quickly, with high mortality. Cidofovir should also be considered as second-line therapy for any serious herpetic or CMV infections that are resistant to other antiherpetic drugs. Probenecid

and aggressive fluid hydration are given in conjunction with each dose of cidofovir to prevent cidofovir reuptake and nephrotoxicity.

Foscarnet

While foscarnet is active against HHVs, its principal role is its use as a second-line agent in HHV disease that is unresponsive to less-toxic drugs, particularly acyclovir and ganciclovir. Foscarnet may be considered first line in the case of CMV infection in the already neutropenic host (e.g., HSCT recipient awaiting engraftment) in whom the bone marrow suppressive effects of ganciclovir limit its use.

Ribavirin

Aerosolized ribavirin is approved in the United States for treatment of RSV bronchiolitis, but is generally not recommended since treatment has not been consistently shown to improve outcomes. Combination with intravenous immunoglobulin may reduce mortality of RSV infection in HSCT recipients and other immunocompromised patients. Occasionally, ribavirin has been used to treat other infections, such as severe influenza, adenovirus, vaccinia, parainfluenza, measles virus infections, and hemorrhagic fevers. There is insufficient evidence to recommend ribavirin in these instances; however, in the critically ill patient unresponsive to other therapies, ribavirin could be considered. Intravenous ribavirin is investigational in the United States. Pregnant women should not directly care for patients receiving ribavirin aerosol.

ANTIVIRAL AGENTS (INFLUENZA)

During the 2009 influenza A H1N1 pandemic, recommendations were made to give anti-influenza therapy empirically for critically ill children with respiratory symptoms regardless of age or duration of symptoms. The recommended duration of therapy was driven largely by response to treatment. These recommendations have since been incorporated into guidelines for the treatment of influenza disease (96). Children at higher risk for influenza complications who are recommended to receive antiviral treatment for suspected or confirmed influenza include: children aged <2 years; children with chronic pulmonary, cardiovascular, renal, hepatic, hematological, neurologic/neurodevelopmental, and metabolic disorders; immunosuppressed children; children who take long-term aspirin therapy; American Indians/Alaska Natives; morbidly obese children; and children who reside in chronic care facilities.

Two classes of antiviral agents are licensed for use in the United States for treatment of influenza: neuraminidase inhibitors (NIs) (oseltamivir and zanamivir) and the adamantanes (amantadine and rimantadine) (**Table 88.14**). NIs inhibit influenza virus neuraminidase, which is responsible for detachment of virions from the infected cell's membrane and for viral penetration through respiratory secretions. Adamantanes block the uncoating of influenza A virus preventing penetration of virus into host and inhibit assembly of progeny virions. The NIs have activity against influenza A and B viruses, whereas the adamantanes have activity only against influenza A viruses. Accordingly, oseltamivir and zanamivir are recommended first-line empiric agents on the basis of recent viral surveillance and resistance data indicating that >99% of currently circulating influenza virus strains in the United States are sensitive to these medications (96). There are currently two intravenous NIs, peramivir and zanamivir, currently under investigation in ongoing clinical trials.

TABLE 88.14

SUMMARY OF ANTI-INFLUENZA DRUGS

■ DRUG	■ MECHANISM OF ACTION	■ AVAILABILITY	■ AGE APPROVED FOR USE	■ INFLUENZA ACTIVITY BY STRAIN
Oseltamivir	NI	Enteral	≥1 y, can be used <1 y if EUA	A, B
Zanamivir	NI	Powder for oral inhalation	≥7 y	A, B
Zanamivir	NI	IV, investigational	***	A, B
Amantadine	Adamantane	Enteral	≥1 y	A, although high resistance
Rimantadine	Adamantane	Enteral	≥17 y	A, although high resistance
Peramivir	NI	IV, investigational	***	A, B

NI, neuraminidase inhibitor; EUA, Emergency Use Authorization.

***stands for the fact that there is no age for approved use as the medications, at the time of writing this, are still investigational.

ANTI-INFECTIVES FOR *MYCOBACTERIUM* TUBERCULOSIS

Mycobacteria are a difficult group of organisms to treat, owing to their thick lipid dense cell wall that is difficult to penetrate, a high concentration of drug efflux pumps, and a propensity to exist intracellularly within the host. Multidrug regimens must be used to limit selection of resistant strains. Therapy is typically initiated with a four-drug regimen of isoniazid, a rifamycin, and pyrazinamide plus either ethambutol or streptomycin. Isoniazid–rifampin combination therapy will cure the vast majority of susceptible *Mycobacterium tuberculosis* (TB). Adding pyrazinamide to this combination for the first 2 months decreases total duration of therapy from 9 months to 6 months. Ethambutol and streptomycin are added to provide additional coverage in the case of drug resistance, but they do not add to the overall efficacy of isoniazid and rifamycin in susceptible strains. Newer drugs and delivery systems are currently being investigated with the primary purpose of shortening treatment courses.

Isoniazid

The prodrug isoniazid enters the cell by passive diffusion and is then converted to its active form. Synthesis of components of the mycobacterial cell wall is inhibited, resulting in cell death. Resistance to isoniazid is due to one of several mutations, often in the enzyme that activates the drug. Isoniazid is well absorbed from the GI tract and readily distributed into all body fluids and tissues, including the CSF.

Metabolism is via acetylation by liver *N*-acetyltransferase and can vary genetically among individuals, as people may be "slow" acetylators (common among Inuit and Japanese populations) or "fast" acetylators (common among individuals of Scandinavian, Jewish, and North African white descent). Use of daily dosing in fast acetylators is usually acceptable; however, if there is malabsorption or if once weekly dosing is utilized, subtherapeutic levels can result. Slow acetylators may be at higher risk for isoniazid-induced hepatotoxicity. Dose adjustments are not necessary in renal or hepatic insufficiency; however, isoniazid should be discontinued if it is thought to be the cause of new onset hepatitis.

The most common and serious adverse reaction is hepatitis. Ten to twenty percent of patients will experience mild increases in liver aminotransferases and remain otherwise asymptomatic. One percent of patients will have symptomatic, potentially fatal, hepatitis requiring cessation of drug. CNS side effects are also common, such as peripheral neuropathy, memory loss, and seizures, due to increased excretion of pyridoxine. Administration of pyridoxine can reverse or prevent the CNS side effects. Other reactions include anemia, lupus-like syndrome, tinnitus, and GI upset. The potential for many drug–drug interactions exist as isoniazid inhibits the metabolism of several drugs, including phenytoin, carbamazepine, anticoagulants, benzodiazepines, and vitamin D, and is a weak monoamine oxidase inhibitor.

Rifamycins

Rifamycins (rifampin, rifapentine, and rifabutin) inhibit bacterial RNA synthesis by binding to the β subunit of DNA-dependent RNA polymerase, blocking RNA transcription. Rifampin, the most commonly used within the class, is bactericidal for mycobacteria. Resistance develops when the target binding site is altered. In addition to *Mycobacterium*, rifampin has activity against most gram-positive bacteria, including MRSA, and some gram-negative microorganisms, such as *Neisseria meningitidis* and *H. influenzae*.

Rifampin is available as enteral and IV forms, but when given enterally, it should be given on an empty stomach to improve absorption. Rifampin is highly lipophilic and widely distributed into body tissues and fluids, often staining them orange. CSF penetration is poor if meninges are not inflamed. Drug metabolism occurs in the liver to an active metabolite, and then excretion in the bile (60%–70%) and urine (~30%). Importantly, rifampin is a substrate of P-glycoprotein, and strong inducer of CYP1A2, CYP2A6, CYP2B6, CYP2C19, CYP2C8, CYP2C9, CYP3A4, and P-glycoprotein.

There are numerous drug–drug interactions of which the intensivist must be aware, some of which affect sedation (benzodiazepines), other antimicrobials (use with voriconazole is contraindicated), and many others. Concomitant drug therapy review must occur during initiation and discontinuation of rifampin, and frequently changes are necessary. The most common adverse reactions are rash, fever, and nausea and vomiting. For patients with preexisting liver disease or on other hepatotoxic medications, hepatitis and liver failure can occur.

Pyrazinamide

Pyrazinamide is activated within an acidic environment (pH of 5.5) and is converted to active pyrazinoic acid by mycobacterial pyrazinamidase. The specific mechanism of action is unknown, but likely involves disruption of the cell membrane and alterations in transport. Resistance may be due to impaired uptake of pyrazinamide or mutations in the gene that encodes for conversion of pyrazinamide to its active form.

Pyrazinamide is well absorbed, widely distributed throughout the body, including the CSF, and concentrates in the epithelial fluid of the lungs. Drug metabolism occurs in the liver via microsomal deamidase (not P450 mediated), with metabolites being excreted by the kidney. Drug clearance and Vd increase with patient mass, resulting in variations in half-life and AUC. Dosing should be reduced if patients have a GFR <30 mL/min. Hemodialysis removes pyrazinamide, and doses should be administered after dialysis.

Pyrazinamide may increase the risk of rifampin induced liver injury, and may increase cyclosporine levels. Major adverse effects of pyrazinamide include hepatotoxicity (in 1%–5% of patients), nausea, vomiting, drug fever, and hyperuricemia (inhibits excretion of urate). This happens in nearly all patients, and is not a reason to discontinue therapy.

Streptomycin

Streptomycin is an AG antibiotic that shares the same mechanism of action and resistance as other drugs within this class. Streptomycin is mostly active against extracellular TB, as it has poor intracellular penetration.

Ethambutol

Ethambutol inhibits an essential polymerization component of the mycobacterial cell wall. Resistance typically arises due to a mutation in the target enzyme or by enhanced efflux pumps. Ethambutol has activity against most mycobacteria.

Ethambutol has ~80% absorption from the GI tract. Children have reduced absorption so that good peak concentrations of drug are often not achieved with standard dosing. Distribution is extensive with high concentrations in kidneys, lungs, saliva, and red blood cells, but low in the CSF. About 20% of drug is metabolized in the liver by alcohol and aldehyde dehydrogenase, and ~50% of drug is eliminated unchanged by the kidneys, therefore dose adjustments must be made in patients with GFR <50 mL/min. If patients are receiving hemodialysis, doses should be administered after dialysis as 5%–20% of drug is removed.

Ethambutol is generally well tolerated by most patients. Around 50% of patients will experience hyperuricemia, with many fewer experiencing effects, such as paresthesias, GI upset, increase in liver aminotransferases, and drug fever/rash. Reversible, dose-related visual disturbances, such as loss of red/green differentiation and optic neuritis, are the most serious adverse effects and may necessitate drug discontinuation.

ANTIMALARIAL DRUGS

Most cases of malaria are considered to be uncomplicated and can be treated with oral therapy. Patients with severe disease must be aggressively treated (see chapter on international infections for more details). Recommendations in the United States given by the CDC for the treatment of pediatric severe malaria from all regions include treatment with quinidine gluconate plus one of the following: doxycycline, tetracycline, or clindamycin. An alternative regimen that remains investigational in the United States, but available through the CDC, is artesunate followed by one of the following: atovaquone–proguanil, clindamycin,

or mefloquine. The WHO recommends artesunate as first-line therapy for treatment of severe malaria in African children, as a result of the AQUAMAT (artesunate vs. quinine in the treatment of severe falciparum malaria in African children) trial, which demonstrated a significant mortality reduction in the artesunate group compared to the quinine group (97), and concluded that those data, together with a meta-analysis of all trials comparing artesunate and quinine, strongly suggest that parenteral artesunate should replace quinine as the treatment of choice for severe falciparum malaria worldwide. A summary of antimalarial drugs is provided in **Table 88.15**.

Quinidine

Quinidine gluconate is the only readily available first-line agent for the treatment of severe malaria in the United States. Quinidine is a class IA antiarrhythmic, but in patients with malaria, quinidine acts primarily as an intraerythrocytic schizonticide, with little effect on sporozoites. Quinidine is cidal to *Plasmodium vivax* and *Plasmodium malariae*, but not to *Plasmodium falciparum*. Resistance to quinidine among malaria strains from Southeast Asia and Southern America is increasing, and use of artemisinin derivatives should be highly considered if disease is contracted within a highly resistant region.

Quinidine should be administered IV for the treatment of severe malaria, but can be given IM if IV access cannot be established. Quinidine is metabolized in the liver to inactive substances, is a substrate of CYP2C9, CYP2E1, CYP3A4, P-glycoprotein, and is an inhibitor of CYP2C9, CYP2D6, CYP3A4, P-glycoprotein, leading to many drug–drug interactions. Renal excretion is minimal, but dose adjustments should be made if GFR is <10 mL/min or if the patient is on hemodialysis. Patients with severe liver disease have a larger Vd and impaired clearance, therefore, larger loading doses and reduced maintenance doses are indicated.

Quinine is associated with a triad of dose-related toxicities: cinchonism (tinnitus, high-tone deafness, visual disturbances, headache, dysphoria, nausea, vomiting, and postural hypotension), hypoglycemia (due to hyperinsulinemia), and hypotension. Cinchonism occurs frequently and is reversible on drug discontinuation. Hypotension is rare and most often is associated with excessively rapid infusions. Electrocardiographic monitoring is recommended during IV quinidine administration as QTc prolongation and arrhythmias have been reported. Rarely, severe hematologic effects as a result of a hypersensitivity reaction may occur. "Blackwater fever" is described by massive hemolysis, hemoglobinemia, and hemoglobinuria that leads to anuria, renal failure, and in some instances death, and should result in immediate discontinuation of quinidine. In people with Glucose-6-Phosphate Dehydrogenase deficiency, hemolysis is also a concern, but this tends to be milder reaction.

Artesunate

Artesunate is one of a number of artemisinin derivatives, which also include artemether, artemotil, and dihydroartemisinin (DHA). Artesunate is not FDA-approved in the United States but is commonly used elsewhere in the world. The mechanisms of action of artemisinins are not fully understood. Resistance is limited, but is emerging in Cambodia and Thailand. Artemisinins have a rapid action against all of the erythrocytic stages of the parasite (including transmissible gametocytes) resulting in a rapid clinical benefit and decreased transmission of malaria. Artemisinins have short half-lives and recurrence of infecting parasites and illness can occur if these drugs are not used in combination with a longer-acting agent.

TABLE 88.15

SUMMARY OF ANTIMALARIAL DRUGS

■ DRUG	■ USE
Chloroquine	Treatment and chemoprophylaxis of infection with sensitive parasites
Amodiaquine[a]	Treatment of infection with some chloroquine-resistant *P. falciparum* strains and in fixed combination with artesunate
Piperaquine[a]	Treatment of *P. falciparum* infection in fixed combination with dihydroartemisinin
Quinine	Oral and intravenous[a] treatment of *P. falciparum* infections
Quinidine	Intravenous therapy of severe infections with *P. falciparum*
Mefloquine	Chemoprophylaxis and treatment of infections with *P. falciparum*
Primaquine	Radical cure and terminal prophylaxis of infections with *P. vivax* and *P. ovale*; alternative chemoprophylaxis for all species
Sulfadoxine–pyrimethamine (Fansidar)	Treatment of infections with some chloroquine-resistant *P. falciparum*, including combination with artesunate; intermittent preventive therapy in endemic areas
Atovaquone–proguanil (Malarone)	Treatment and chemoprophylaxis of *P. falciparum* infection
Doxycycline	Treatment (with quinine) of infections with *P. falciparum*; chemoprophylaxis
Halofantrine[a]	Treatment of *P. falciparum* infections
Lumefantrine[b]	Treatment of *P. falciparum* malaria in fixed combination with artemether (Coartem)
Artemisinins (artesunate, artemether,[b] dihydroartemisinin[a])	Treatment of *P. falciparum* infections; oral combination therapies for uncomplicated disease; intravenous artesunate for severe disease

[a]Not available in the United States.
[b]Available in the United States only as the fixed combination Coartem.

Artesunate should be administered IV (preferred) or IM for the treatment of severe malaria; however, rectal administration is also effective and may be of value in settings with limited resources. In patients with renal or hepatic failure, artesunate dosages do not need to be adjusted. Artesunate is a prodrug that is rapidly hydrolyzed to an active metabolite, dihydroartemisinin. Dihydroartemisinin undergoes hepatic metabolism via CYP2B6, CYP2C19, and CYP3A4 to inactive metabolites. Despite interaction with CYP 450 system, there are no known interactions between artesunate and other drugs. The most common adverse reactions are nausea, vomiting, anorexia, and dizziness. More serious adverse effects include neutropenia, anemia, hemolysis, and elevated levels of liver enzymes, neurotoxicity, and embryotoxicity.

References

1. Dellinger RP, Levy MM, Carlet JM, et al. Surviving Sepsis Campaign: International guidelines for management of severe sepsis and septic shock: 2008 [published online ahead of print December 26, 2007]. *Crit Care Med* 2008;36(1):296–327.

2. Barenfanger J, Drake C, Leon N, et al. Clinical and financial benefits of rapid detection of respiratory viruses: An outcomes study [published online ahead of print August 02, 2000]. *J Clin Microbiol* 2000;38(8):2824–8.

3. Oosterheert JJ, van Loon AM, Schuurman R, et al. Impact of rapid detection of viral and atypical bacterial pathogens by real-time polymerase chain reaction for patients with lower respiratory tract infection [published online ahead of print October 19, 2005]. *Clin Infect Dis* 2005;41(10):1438–44.

4. Woods CR, Bryant KA. Viral infections in children with community-acquired pneumonia [published online ahead of print February 02, 2013]. *Curr Infect Dis Rep* 2013;15(2):177–83.

5. Blaser MJ, Falkow S. What are the consequences of the disappearing human microbiota? [published online ahead of print November 10, 2009]. *Nat Rev Microbiol* 2009;7(12):887–94.

6. Shorr AF, Owens RC Jr. Guidelines and quality for community-acquired pneumonia: Measures from the Joint Commission and the Centers for Medicare and Medicaid Services [published online ahead of print June 16, 2009]. *Am J Health Syst Pharm* 2009;66(12 suppl 4):S2–7.

7. Doyle JS, Buising KL, Thursky KA, et al. Epidemiology of infections acquired in intensive care units [published online ahead of print April 21, 2011]. *Semin Respir Crit Care Med* 2011;32(2):115–38.

8. Garnacho-Montero J, Garcia-Garmendia JL, Barrero-Almodovar A, et al. Impact of adequate empirical antibiotic therapy on the outcome of patients admitted to the intensive care unit with sepsis [published online ahead of print December 12, 2003]. *Crit Care Med* 2003;31(12):2742–51.

9. Rodriguez-Bano J, Millan AB, Dominguez MA, et al. Impact of inappropriate empirical therapy for sepsis due to health care-associated methicillin-resistant *Staphylococcus aureus* [published online ahead of print February 13, 2009]. *J Infect* 2009;58(2):131–7.

10. Shorr AF, Micek ST, Welch EC, et al. Inappropriate antibiotic therapy in Gram-negative sepsis increases hospital length of stay [published online ahead of print October 05, 2010]. *Crit Care Med* 2011;39(1):46–51.

11. Luna CM, Aruj P, Niederman MS, et al. Appropriateness and delay to initiate therapy in ventilator-associated pneumonia [published online ahead of print January 03, 2006]. *Eur Respir J* 2006;27(1):158–64.

12. Zilberberg MD, Shorr AF, Micek ST, et al. Antimicrobial therapy escalation and hospital mortality among patients with health-care-associated pneumonia: A single-center experience [published online ahead of print July 22, 2008]. *Chest* 2008;134(5):963–8.

13. Paul M, Shani V, Muchtar E, et al. Systematic review and meta-analysis of the efficacy of appropriate empiric antibiotic therapy for sepsis [published online ahead of print August 25, 2010]. *Antimicrob Agents Chemother* 2010;54(11):4851–63.

14. Ashkenazi S, Samra Z, Konisberger H, et al. Factors associated with increased risk in inappropriate empiric antibiotic treatment

of childhood bacteraemia [published online ahead of print July 01, 1996]. *Eur J Pediatr* 1996;155(7):545–50.

15. Muszynski JA, Knatz NL, Sargel CL, et al. Timing of correct parenteral antibiotic initiation and outcomes from severe bacterial community-acquired pneumonia in children [published online ahead of print October 30, 2010]. *Pediatr Infect Dis J* 2011;30(4):295–301.

16. Brierley J, Carcillo JA, Choong K, et al. Clinical practice parameters for hemodynamic support of pediatric and neonatal septic shock: 2007 update from the American College of Critical Care Medicine [published online ahead of print March 28, 2009]. *Crit Care Med* 2009;37(2):666–88.

17. Kumar A, Roberts D, Wood KE, et al. Duration of hypotension before initiation of effective antimicrobial therapy is the critical determinant of survival in human septic shock [published online ahead of print April 21, 2006]. *Crit Care Med* 2006;34(6):1589–96.

18. Puskarich MA, Trzeciak S, Shapiro NI, et al. Association between timing of antibiotic administration and mortality from septic shock in patients treated with a quantitative resuscitation protocol [published online ahead of print May 17, 2011]. *Crit Care Med* 2011;39(9):2066–71.

19. Casado RJ, de Mello MJ, de Aragao RC, et al. Incidence and risk factors for health care-associated pneumonia in a pediatric intensive care unit [published online ahead of print April 19, 2011]. *Crit Care Med* 2011;39(8):1968–73.

20. Cunningham DJ, Brilli RJ. Risk of healthcare-associated pneumonia in the pediatric intensive care unit: Opportunity lost/new frontier established [published online ahead of print July 20, 2011]. *Crit Care Med* 2011;39(8):2013–4.

21. de Mello MJ, de Albuquerque Mde F, Lacerda HR, et al. Risk factors for healthcare-associated infection in a pediatric intensive care unit [published online ahead of print October 02, 2009]. *Pediatr Crit Care Med* 2010;11(2):246–52.

22. Toltzis P, Dul M, O'Riordan MA, et al. Meropenem use and colonization by antibiotic-resistant Gram-negative bacilli in a pediatric intensive care unit [published online ahead of print December 06, 2008]. *Pediatr Crit Care Med* 2009;10(1):49–54.

23. Mandell LA, Wunderink RG, Anzueto A, et al. Infectious Diseases Society of America/American Thoracic Society consensus guidelines on the management of community-acquired pneumonia in adults. *Clin Infect Dis* 2007;44(suppl 2):S27–72.

24. Malone DC, Shaban HM. Adherence to ATS guidelines for hospitalized patients with community-acquired pneumonia [published online ahead of print October 26, 2001]. *Ann Pharmacother* 2001;35(10):1180–5.

25. American Thoracic Society; Infectious Diseases Society of America. Guidelines for the management of adults with hospital-acquired, ventilator-associated, and healthcare-associated pneumonia [published online ahead of print February 09, 2005]. *Am J Respir Crit Care Med* 2005;171(4):388–416.

26. Ostrosky-Zeichner L, Sable C, Sobel J, et al. Multicenter retrospective development and validation of a clinical prediction rule for nosocomial invasive candidiasis in the intensive care setting [published online ahead of print March 03, 2007]. *Eur J Clin Microbiol Infect Dis* 2007;26(4):271–6.

27. Hermsen ED, Zapapas MK, Maiefski M, et al. Validation and comparison of clinical prediction rules for invasive candidiasis in intensive care unit patients: A matched case-control study [published online ahead of print August 19, 2011]. *Crit Care* 2011;15(4):R198.

28. Smith SM, Gums JG. Antivirals for influenza: Strategies for use in pediatrics [published online ahead of print August 31, 2010]. *Paediatr Drugs* 2010;12(5):285–99.

29. Yu H, Liao Q, Yuan Y, et al. Effectiveness of oseltamivir on disease progression and viral RNA shedding in patients with mild pandemic 2009 influenza A H1N1: Opportunistic retrospective study of medical charts in China [published online ahead of print September 30, 2010]. *BMJ* 2010;341:c4779.

30. Frei CR, Attridge RT, Mortensen EM, et al. Guideline-concordant antibiotic use and survival among patients with community-acquired pneumonia admitted to the intensive care unit [published online ahead of print March 09, 2010]. *Clin Ther* 2010;32(2):293–9.

31. Garnacho-Montero J, Sa-Borges M, Sole-Violan J, et al. Optimal management therapy for *Pseudomonas aeruginosa* ventilator-associated pneumonia: An observational, multicenter study comparing monotherapy with combination antibiotic therapy [published online ahead of print June 22, 2007]. *Crit Care Med* 2007;35(8):1888–95.

32. Wilke M, Grube RF, Bodmann KF. Guideline-adherent initial intravenous antibiotic therapy for hospital-acquired/ventilator-associated pneumonia is clinically superior, saves lives and is cheaper than non guideline adherent therapy [published online ahead of print August 05, 2011]. *Eur J Med Res* 2011;16(7):315–23.

33. Kollef MH, Golan Y, Micek ST, et al. Appraising contemporary strategies to combat multidrug resistant gram-negative bacterial infections—Proceedings and data from the Gram-Negative Resistance Summit [published online ahead of print September 01, 2011]. *Clin Infect Dis* 2011;53(suppl 2):S33–55; quiz S6–8.

34. Vogelaers D, De Bels D, Foret F, et al. Patterns of antimicrobial therapy in severe nosocomial infections: Empiric choices, proportion of appropriate therapy, and adaptation rates—A multicentre, observational survey in critically ill patients [published online ahead of print February 04, 2010]. *Int J Antimicrob Agents* 2010;35(4):375–81.

35. Micek ST, Welch EC, Khan J, et al. Empiric combination antibiotic therapy is associated with improved outcome against sepsis due to Gram-negative bacteria: A retrospective analysis [published online ahead of print February 18, 2010]. *Antimicrob Agents Chemother* 2010;54(5):1742–8.

36. Kumar A, Zarychanski R, Light B, et al. Early combination antibiotic therapy yields improved survival compared with monotherapy in septic shock: A propensity-matched analysis [published online ahead of print July 20, 2010]. *Crit Care Med* 2010;38(9):1773–85.

37. Heyland DK, Dodek P, Muscedere J, et al. Randomized trial of combination versus monotherapy for the empiric treatment of suspected ventilator-associated pneumonia [published online ahead of print December 20, 2007]. *Crit Care Med* 2008;36(3):737–44.

38. Christoff J, Tolentino J, Mawdsley E, et al. Optimizing empirical antimicrobial therapy for infection due to gram-negative pathogens in the intensive care unit: Utility of a combination antibiogram [published online ahead of print January 09, 2010]. *Infect Control Hosp Epidemiol* 2010;31(3):256–61.

39. Eachempati SR, Hydo LJ, Shou J, et al. Does de-escalation of antibiotic therapy for ventilator-associated pneumonia affect the likelihood of recurrent pneumonia or mortality in critically ill surgical patients? [published online ahead of print May 12, 2009]. *J Trauma* 2009;66(5):1343–8.

40. Heenen S, Jacobs F, Vincent JL. Antibiotic strategies in severe nosocomial sepsis: Why do we not de-escalate more often? [published online ahead of print March 21, 2012]. *Crit Care Med* 2012;40(5):1404–9.

41. Masterton RG. Antibiotic heterogeneity [published online ahead of print December 07, 2010]. *Int J Antimicrob Agents* 2010;36(suppl 3):S15–8.

42. Takesue Y, Nakajima K, Ichiki K, et al. Impact of a hospital-wide programme of heterogeneous antibiotic use on the development of antibiotic-resistant Gram-negative bacteria [published online ahead of print March 30, 2010]. *J Hosp Infect* 2010;75(1):28–32.

43. Dellit TH, Owens RC, McGowan JE Jr, et al. Infectious Diseases Society of America and the Society for Healthcare Epidemiology of America guidelines for developing an institutional program

to enhance antimicrobial stewardship [published online ahead of print December 19, 2006]. *Clin Infect Dis* 2007;44(2):159–77.

44. Sandiumenge A, Lisboa T, Gomez F, et al. Effect of antibiotic diversity on ventilator-associated pneumonia caused by ESKAPE Organisms [published online ahead of print June 11, 2011]. *Chest* 2011;140(3):643–51.

45. Merz LR, Warren DK, Kollef MH, et al. The impact of an antibiotic cycling program on empirical therapy for gram-negative infections [published online ahead of print December 15, 2006]. *Chest* 2006;130(6):1672–8.

46. Cadena J, Taboada CA, Burgess DS, et al. Antibiotic cycling to decrease bacterial antibiotic resistance: A 5-year experience on a bone marrow transplant unit [published online ahead of print May 29, 2007]. *Bone Marrow Transplant* 2007;40(2):151–5.

47. Smith RL, Evans HL, Chong TW, et al. Reduction in rates of methicillin-resistant *Staphylococcus aureus* infection after introduction of quarterly linezolid-vancomycin cycling in a surgical intensive care unit [published online ahead of print September 02, 2008]. *Surg Infect (Larchmt)* 2008;9(4):423–31.

48. Sarraf-Yazdi S, Sharpe M, Bennett KM, et al. A 9-year retrospective review of antibiotic cycling in a surgical intensive care unit [published online ahead of print March 27, 2012]. *J Surg Res* 2012;176(2):e73–8.

49. Spurling GK, Doust J, Del Mar CB, et al. Antibiotics for bronchiolitis in children [published online ahead of print June 17, 2011]. *Cochrane Database Syst Rev* 2011;(6):CD005189.

50. Thorburn K, Harigopal S, Reddy V, et al. High incidence of pulmonary bacterial co-infection in children with severe respiratory syncytial virus (RSV) bronchiolitis [published online ahead of print March 16, 2006]. *Thorax* 2006;61(7):611–5.

51. Duttweiler L, Nadal D, Frey B. Pulmonary and systemic bacterial co-infections in severe RSV bronchiolitis [published online ahead of print November 24, 2004]. *Arch Dis Child* 2004;89(12):1155–7.

52. Blyth CC, Webb SA, Kok J, et al. The impact of bacterial and viral co-infection in severe influenza [published online ahead of print April 11, 2012]. *Influenza Other Respi Viruses* 2013;7(2):168–76.

53. Rice TW, Rubinson L, Uyeki TM, et al. Critical illness from 2009 pandemic influenza A virus and bacterial coinfection in the United States [published online ahead of print April 19, 2012]. *Crit Care Med* 2012;40(5):1487–98.

54. Levin D, Tribuzio M, Green-Wrzesinki T, et al. Empiric antibiotics are justified for infants with respiratory syncytial virus lower respiratory tract infection presenting with respiratory failure: A prospective study and evidence review. *Pediatr Crit Care Med* 2010;11(3):390–5.

55. Rea MC, Dobson A, O'Sullivan O, et al. Effect of broad- and narrow-spectrum antimicrobials on *Clostridium difficile* and microbial diversity in a model of the distal colon [published online ahead of print July 10, 2010]. *Proc Natl Acad Sci U S A* 2011;108(suppl 1):4639–44.

56. Stewardson AJ, Huttner B, Harbarth S. At least it won't hurt: The personal risks of antibiotic exposure [published online ahead of print July 22, 2011]. *Curr Opin Pharmacol* 2011;11(5):446–52.

57. Aarts MA, Brun-Buisson C, Cook DJ, et al. Antibiotic management of suspected nosocomial ICU-acquired infection: Does prolonged empiric therapy improve outcome? [published online ahead of print June 15,2007]. *Intensive Care Med* 2007;33(8):1369–78.

58. Chastre J, Luyt CE, Combes A, et al. Use of quantitative cultures and reduced duration of antibiotic regimens for patients with ventilator-associated pneumonia to decrease resistance in the intensive care unit [published online ahead of print August 09, 2006]. *Clin Infect Dis* 2006;43(suppl 2):S75–81.

59. Reinhart K, Meisner M. Biomarkers in the critically ill patient: Procalcitonin [published online ahead of print March 29, 2011]. *Crit Care Clin* 2011;27(2):253–63.

60. Vincent JL, Donadello K, Schmit X. Biomarkers in the critically ill patient: C-reactive protein [published online ahead of print March 29, 2011]. *Crit Care Clin* 2011;27(2):241–51.

61. Vincent JL. Clinical sepsis and septic shock—Definition, diagnosis and management principles [published online ahead of print June 28, 2008]. *Langenbeck Arch Surg* 2008;393(6):817–24.

62. Silvestre J, Povoa P, Coelho L, et al. Is C-reactive protein a good prognostic marker in septic patients? [published online ahead of print January 27, 2009]. *Intensive Care Med* 2009;35(5):909–13.

63. Ciaccio M, Fugardi G, Titone L, et al. Procalcitonin levels in plasma in oncohaematologic patients with and without bacterial infections [published online ahead of print January 22, 2004]. *Clin Chim Acta* 2004;340(1–2):149–52.

64. Albrich WC, Dusemund F, Bucher B, et al. Effectiveness and safety of procalcitonin-guided antibiotic therapy in lower respiratory tract infections in "real life": An international, multicenter poststudy survey (ProREAL) [published online ahead of print July 12, 2012]. *Arch Int Med* 2012;172(9):715–22.

65. Newland JG, Banerjee R, Gerber JS, et al. Antimicrobial stewardship in pediatric care: Strategies and future directions [published online ahead of print January 12, 2013]. *Pharmacotherapy* 2012;32(8):735–43.

66. Bizzarro MJ, Conrad SA, Kaufman DA, et al. Infections acquired during extracorporeal membrane oxygenation in neonates, children, and adults [published online ahead of print May 25, 2010]. *Pediatr Crit Care Med* 2011;12(3):277–81.

67. Akcan-Arikan A, Zappitelli M, Loftis LL, et al. Modified RIFLE criteria in critically ill children with acute kidney injury [published online ahead of print March 31, 2007]. *Kidney Int* 2007;71(10):1028–35.

68. Ferguson MA, Waikar SS. Established and emerging markers of kidney function [published online ahead of print February 09, 2012]. *Clin Chem* 2012;58(4):680–9.

69. Grant LM, Rockey DC. Drug-induced liver injury [published online ahead of print March 28, 2012]. *Curr Opin Gastroenterol* 2012;28(3):198–202.

70. Choi JJ, Moffett BS, McDade EJ, et al. Altered gentamicin serum concentrations in obese pediatric patients [published online ahead of print October 29, 2010]. *Pediatr Infect Dis J* 2011;30(4):347–9.

71. Roberts JA, Lipman J. Antibacterial dosing in intensive care: Pharmacokinetics, degree of disease and pharmacodynamics of sepsis [published online ahead of print August 04, 2006]. *Clin Pharmacokinet* 2006;45(8):755–73.

72. Pankey GA, Sabath LD. Clinical relevance of bacteriostatic versus bactericidal mechanisms of action in the treatment of Gram-positive bacterial infections [published online ahead of print March 05, 2004]. *Clin Infect Dis* 2004;38(6):864–70.

73. Rappaz I, Decosterd LA, Bille J, et al. Continuous infusion of ceftazidime with a portable pump is as effective as thrice-a-day bolus in cystic fibrosis children [published online ahead of print December 29, 2000]. *Eur J Pediatr* 2000;159(12):919–25.

74. Dalle JH, Gnansounou M, Husson MO, et al. Continuous infusion of ceftazidime in the empiric treatment of febrile neutropenic children with cancer [published online ahead of print December 07, 2002]. *J Pediatr Hematol Oncol* 2002;24(9):714–6.

75. Tamma PD, Putcha N, Suh YD, et al. Does prolonged beta-lactam infusions improve clinical outcomes compared to intermittent infusions? A meta-analysis and systematic review of randomized, controlled trials [published online ahead of print June 24, 2011]. *BMC Infect Dis* 2011;11:181.

76. Rybak MJ, Abate BJ, Kang SL, et al. Prospective evaluation of the effect of an aminoglycoside dosing regimen on rates of observed nephrotoxicity and ototoxicity. [published online ahead of print July 02, 1999]. *Antimicrob Agents Chemother* 1999;43(7):1549–55.

77. Contopoulos-Ioannidis DG, Giotis ND, Baliatsa DV, et al. Extended-interval aminoglycoside administration for children: A

meta-analysis [published online ahead of print July 03, 2004]. *Pediatrics* 2004;114(1):e111–8.

78. Vardakas KZ, Tansarli GS, Rafailidis PI, et al. Carbapenems versus alternative antibiotics for the treatment of bacteraemia due to Enterobacteriaceae producing extended-spectrum beta-lactamases: A systematic review and meta-analysis [published online ahead of print August 24, 2012]. *J Antimicrob Chemother* 2012;67(12):2793–803.

79. Gilbert DN, Moellering RC Jr, Eliopoulos GM, et al. (Eds.) The Sanford Guide to Antimicrobial Therapy 2013. 43rd ed. Antimicrobial Therapy, Inc, Sperryville, VA; 2013.

80. Weiss ME, Adkinson NF. Immediate hypersensitivity reactions to penicillin and related antibiotics [published online ahead of print November 01, 1988]. *Clin Allergy* 1988;18(6):515–40.

81. Lagace-Wiens P, Rubinstein E. Adverse reactions to beta-lactam antimicrobials [published online ahead of print January 10, 2012]. *Exp Opin Drug Saf* 2012;11(3):381–99.

82. Chatellier D, Jourdain M, Mangalaboyi J, et al. Cefepime-induced neurotoxicity: An underestimated complication of antibiotherapy in patients with acute renal failure [published online ahead of print March 22, 2002]. *Intensive Care Med* 2002;28(2):214–7.

83. Johnson AP, Woodford N. Global spread of antibiotic resistance: The example of New Delhi metallo-beta-lactamase (NDM)-mediated carbapenem resistance [published online ahead of print January 19, 2013]. *J Med Microbiol* 2013;62(pt 4):499–513.

84. Miller AD, Ball AM, Bookstaver PB, et al. Epileptogenic potential of carbapenem agents: Mechanism of action, seizure rates, and clinical considerations [published online ahead of print April 01, 2011]. *Pharmacotherapy* 2011;31(4):408–23.

85. Paul M, Dickstein Y, Schlesinger A, et al. Beta-lactam versus beta-lactam-aminoglycoside combination therapy in cancer patients with neutropenia [published online ahead of print July 03, 2013]. *Cochrane Database Syst Rev* 2013;6:CD003038.

86. Marcus R, Paul M, Elphick H, et al. Clinical implications of beta-lactam-aminoglycoside synergism: Systematic review of randomised trials [published online ahead of print February 05, 2011]. *Int J Antimicrob Agents* 2011;37(6):491–503.

87. Jacob JT, DiazGranados CA. High vancomycin minimum inhibitory concentration and clinical outcomes in adults with methicillin-resistant *Staphylococcus aureus* infections: A meta-analysis [published online ahead of print October 24, 2012]. *Int J Infect Dis* 2013;17(2):e93–100.

88. Nannini EC, Corey GR, Stryjewski ME. Telavancin for the treatment of hospital-acquired pneumonia: Findings from the ATTAIN studies [published online ahead of print October 04, 2012]. *Exp Rev Anti Infect Ther* 2012;10(8):847–54.

89. Tanaka M, Hasegawa T, Okamoto A, et al. Effect of antibiotics on group A Streptococcus exoprotein production analyzed by two-dimensional gel electrophoresis [published online ahead of print December 24, 2004]. *Antimicrob Agents Chemother* 2005;49(1):88–96.

90. Adefurin A, Sammons H, Jacqz-Aigrain E, et al. Ciprofloxacin safety in paediatrics: A systematic review [published online ahead of print July 26, 2011]. *Arch Dis Child* 2011;96(9):874–80.

91. Bradley JS, Jackson MA. The use of systemic and topical fluoroquinolones [published online ahead of print September 29, 2011]. *Pediatrics* 2011;128(4):e1034–45.

92. Winton JC, Twilla JD. Sudden cardiac arrest in a patient on chronic methadone after the addition of azithromycin [published online ahead of print October 30, 2012]. *Am J Med Sci* 2013;345(2):160–2.

93. Gales AC, Sader HS, Fritsche TR. Tigecycline activity tested against 11808 bacterial pathogens recently collected from US medical centers [published online ahead of print December 11, 2007]. *Diagnost Microbiol Infect Dis* 2008;60(4):421–7.

94. Lepak AJ, Andes DR. Antifungal PK/PD considerations in fungal pulmonary infections [published online ahead of print December 15, 2011]. *Semin Respir Crit Care Med* 2011;32(6):783–94.

95. Kuo IF, Ensom MH. Role of therapeutic drug monitoring of voriconazole in the treatment of invasive fungal infections [published online ahead of print November 01, 2009]. *Can J Hosp Pharm* 2009;62(6):469–82.

96. Fiore AE, Fry A, Shay D, et al. Antiviral agents for the treatment and chemoprophylaxis of influenza—Recommendations of the Advisory Committee on Immunization Practices (ACIP) [published online ahead of print January 21, 2011]. *MMWR Recomm Rep* 2011;60(1):1–24.

97. Dondorp AM, Fanello CI, Hendriksen IC, et al. Artesunate versus quinine in the treatment of severe falciparum malaria in African children (AQUAMAT): An open-label, randomised trial [published online ahead of print November 11, 2010]. *Lancet* 2010;376(9753):1647–57.

98. Perfect JR, Dismukes WE, Dromer F, et al. Clinical practice guidelines for the management of cryptococcal disease: 2010 update by the infectious diseases society of America. *Clin Infect Dis* 2010;50(3):291–322.

CHAPTER 89 ■ DENGUE AND OTHER HEMORRHAGIC VIRAL INFECTIONS

SIRIPEN KALAYANAROOJ AND RAKESH LODHA

KEY POINTS

Dengue Hemorrhagic Fever and Dengue Shock Syndrome

1. Dengue infection is now endemic in more than 100 countries. It is caused by dengue virus (four serotypes) that belongs to Flaviviridae family.

2. The clinical manifestations of dengue virus infection vary from asymptomatic to severe, life-threatening dengue hemorrhagic fever (DHF) and dengue shock syndrome (DSS) that require intensive care.

3. DHF and DSS are characterized by profound capillary leak and thrombocytopenia.

4. Suggested pathogenic mechanisms include increased replication of a serotype of dengue virus enhanced by the presence of nonneutralizing antibodies, complement activation, and increased cytokine levels.

5. Laboratory findings include hemoconcentration and thrombocytopenia.

6. The diagnosis is confirmed by viral culture (initial 5 days of illness), detection of NS1 antigen or demonstration of specific IgM antibodies (after first 5 days of illness).

7. Supportive care and proper fluid therapy are the cornerstones of management. Fluid therapy is guided by clinical response and monitoring of hematocrit.

8. No specific antiviral drugs for dengue infection are available.

9. Early detection and proper fluid therapy can reduce case fatality rates in DHF/DSS to <1%.

Viral Hemorrhagic Fevers

10. VHF, caused by various viruses belonging to the Flaviviridae family (Kyasanur forest disease, Omsk, dengue, and yellow fever viruses), the Bunyaviridae family (Congo, Hantaan, and Rift Valley fever viruses), the Arenaviridae family (Junin, Machupo, Guanarito, and Lassa viruses), and the Filoviridae family (Ebola and Marburg viruses) are characterized by hemorrhagic manifestations.

11. Ebola, Marburg, Lassa, and Crimean-Congo hemorrhagic fever viruses can spread from person to person.

12. The clinical manifestations of these syndromes are quite similar. The severity in variable and the case fatality rates may be up to 90%. The diagnosis can be confirmed by viral isolation or serologic tests.

13. The principle involved in management of all of these diseases, especially hemorrhagic fever with renal syndrome (HFRS), is the reversal of dehydration, hemoconcentration, renal failure, and protein, electrolyte, or blood losses.

14. IV ribavirin may be effective in reducing mortality in Lassa fever and HFRS.

DENGUE INFECTIONS

Background

Dengue viral infections can present with a wide spectrum of clinical illnesses from the common *dengue fever (DF)* to the more severe presentations of *dengue hemorrhagic fever (DHF)* and *dengue shock syndrome (DSS)* (1). Increasing reports of unusual presentations of dengue have caused the World Health Organization (WHO) Southeast Asian Region Office (SEARO) to add a classification of *expanded dengue syndrome (EDS)* (or unusual manifestation of dengue, UD), which includes severe CNS, liver, myocardial, or abdominal dysfunction (2). More than half of the EDS or UD cases are due to prolonged shock and delay in diagnosis of DSS, the remaining cases are due to dengue infections in hosts with comorbidities or co-infections. Although uncommon, there are reports of dengue with neurological involvement (3–7) and one report of confirmed dengue viral encephalitis from Brazil (8).

Epidemiology

1. Dengue infections were reported more than 370 years ago in tropical, subtropical, and temperate areas. Early reports (1953–1979) of DHF as a distinct entity originated from Southeast Asia and Western Pacific Regions and the majority of cases were children below 15 years of age. Since the 1980s, the incidence of dengue has increased dramatically and become a major world health problem. Both adults and children, male and female are susceptible hosts to dengue infections. The WHO and the Pediatric Dengue Vaccine Initiative (PDVI) have estimated that about 2.5–3.6 billion people (approximately half of the world population in tropical and subtropical countries) are at risk of dengue infection. An estimated 50–400 million dengue infections with 100 million symptomatic cases occur worldwide every year (2,9). About 500,000 DHF patients require hospitalization and approximately 12,500 of those die each year (case fatality rate [CFR] of 2.5%) (2). In 1993, the 46th World Health Assembly

adopted a resolution on dengue prevention and control, which urged that strengthening national and local programs for the prevention and control of dengue be among the foremost health priorities of countries where the disease is endemic. Currently more than 130 countries from Asia, Australia, Central and South Americas, Eastern Mediterranean, and Africa have reported dengue infections. Without early diagnosis and proper management, the CFR may be as high as 10%–30%. With WHO SEARO (1,2) guidelines for dengue management and modern intensive supportive therapy, such rates can be reduced to less than 1%. The dengue CFR in Southeast Asia (Bangladesh, Bhutan, India, Indonesia, Maldives, Myanmar, Nepal, Sri Lanka, Thailand, and Timor Leste) was reported as 0.79% (ranged from 0% to 2.2%) in 2009 (2).

Virus

DF, DHF, DSS, and EDS are caused by infection with any of the four dengue virus (DENV) serotypes, DENV-1, DENV-2, DENV-3, or DENV-4. These four dengue viruses are small (50 nm), single-stranded RNA viruses, belonging to the genus *Flavivirus* and family Flaviviridae based on antigenic and biologic characteristics. A fifth serotype, the first in 50 years, has been recently reported (10). The Dengue virion consists of a nucleocapsid with cubic symmetry enclosed in a lipoprotein envelope. The dengue virus genome codes for three structural proteins (capsid protein [C], membrane-associated protein [M], and envelope protein [E]) and seven nonstructural proteins (NS1, NS2a, NS2b, NS3, NS4a, NS4b, NS5). NS1 (45 kDa) is of diagnostic and pathological importance. Infection with any one serotype confers lifelong immunity to that serotype and temporary cross-protection (months) to *secondary infection* with one of the other serotypes. All four dengue viruses have been associated with epidemics of DF with a varying degree of severity (with or without DHF) (2). Infection with DENV-2 is more likely to cause shock than other serotypes, whereas DENV-3 is associated with more liver involvement (11–13).

Transmission

Aedes aegypti and *Aedes albopictus* mosquitoes are the two most important vectors of dengue viruses for human transmission. Dengue virus can also be transmitted through blood transfusion and by vertical transmission. The transmission of dengue depends on biotic (virus and host) and abiotic factors (temperature, humidity, and rainfall). The extrinsic incubation period in mosquito is 8–12 days before the mosquito can transmit the viruses and thereafter, remains infected for the rest of its life (4–6 weeks). The typical incubation period after a mosquito bite to a human (intrinsic incubation period) is 4–6 days (range 3–14 days) (2). Knowledge of the incubation period allows the physician to rule out dengue when symptoms arise in a traveler >14 days after return from an endemic area.

PATHOGENESIS AND PATHOPHYSIOLOGY

Dengue viruses are inoculated by an *Aedes* mosquito bite and then spread to regional lymph nodes and reticulo-endothelial organs, where they multiply and ultimately enter the blood stream. The association between the occurrences of DHF/DSS with secondary infections implicates immuno-pathogenesis. Both innate immunity (NK cells and complement system) and adaptive immunity (humoral and cell-mediated immunity)

play role in this pathogenesis of DHF/DSS (14,15). Enhancement of immune activation during secondary dengue infection leads to an exaggerated cytokine response resulting in increased vascular permeability (16). The leakage in DHF/DSS is unique because of selective leakage of plasma in the pleural and peritoneal spaces and because of the short duration of leakage, 24–48 hours. The potential for a rapid recovery and the absence of vascular inflammation indicate functional changes in vascular integrity rather than structural damage of the endothelium (2,17–19).

The dendritic cells (DCs) are antigen-presenting cells of the immune system and reside in tissues that are in contact with the external environment (skin, nose, stomach, intestine, and lungs). The DCs in the tissues internalize the virus, where it resides in cystic vacuoles, vesicles, and endoplasmic reticulum. After the phagocytosis and antigen processing, the DCs release a number of cytokines, including tumor necrosis factor (TNF)-α and interferon (IFN)-α, which lead to activation of other virus-infected and virus-uninfected DCs in a paracrine manner. IFN-γ is an important second signal for secretion of bioactive IL-12 from DCs in addition to its effect on the expression of molecules that are involved in stimulating an antigen-specific T-cell response. During a secondary dengue infection, memory T cells produce early IFN-γ and CD40L in the DC microenvironment, leading to greater DC activation, T-cell stimulation, and cytokine release (especially IL-12). The viremia may be cleared, but the cascade of events initiated by the early, poorly controlled type 1 cytokine response (a strong cellular immune response—usually involving IL-2, IFN-γ, IL-12, and TNF-β) contributes to the pathogenesis of DHF/DSS. Increased levels of TNF-α, soluble TNF-α receptor, and IFN-γ levels are present in patients with DHF/DSS as compared with those with DF (14–16).

The mechanism of antibody-dependent enhancement has been proposed (16,20). It has been observed that sequential infection with any two of the four serotypes of dengue virus results in DHF/DSS in an endemic area. Serotype cross-reactive antibodies generated from previous primary infection with a particular dengue viral serotype are not highly specific for the other serotypes involved in secondary infections. These cross-reactive antibodies bind to the virions but are unable to neutralize them. There is an enhanced uptake of antibody-coated virions, which results in greater antigen presentation by the infected dendritic cells to the T cells and more rapid activation and proliferation of memory T cells. The cytokines produced by the activated T cells have an important role in the pathogenesis of the DHF/DSS (14,15).

Cytokines are implicated in the pathogenesis of vascular compromise and hemorrhage in dengue virus infection. Dengue viral infection causes the release of both inflammatory and inhibitory cytokines, and the net outcome will depend on the balance of cytokine actions. The levels of T-cell activation markers (soluble IL-2 receptor, soluble CD4 and CD8, IL-2, IFN-γ), monokines (TNFα, IFN-β), and granulocyte-macrophage colony-stimulating factor (GM-CSF) are increased with even higher levels present in patients who develop DHF/DSS. Elevated IL-6 levels are associated with a higher incidence of both shock and ascites. Similarly, high levels of IL-8 can be recovered from serum and pleural fluid of patients with DSS (16).

Complement activation mediated by nonstructural viral protein NS1 leads to local and systemic generation of anaphylatoxins and terminal complement complex (SC5b-9), which may contribute to the pathogenesis of the vascular leakage that occurs in patients with DHF/DSS (16).

Endothelial cells also undergo apoptosis, which causes disruption of the endothelial cell barrier and the syndrome of generalized vascular leakage. The mast cells may play a role in the initiation of chemokine-dependent host responses to dengue virus infection. Assessment of microvascular leakage using strain-gauge plethysmography in children with DHF and DSS found that, although the coefficient of microvascular permeability (K_f) was higher in children with either DHF or DSS as opposed to that in healthy controls, no significant difference existed between the two groups (DHF, DSS), suggesting a similar pathogenic mechanism (21).

Dengue viral infection is commonly associated with *thrombocytopenia*; one postulated mechanism is molecular mimicry. Antibodies against dengue virus proteins, especially NS1, cross-react with platelet surface proteins and cause thrombocytopenia. These antibodies cause both platelet lysis via complement activation and the inhibition of adenosine diphosphate-induced platelet aggregation. Like the markers of inflammation, the titers of these immunoglobulin M (IgM) antibodies are increased in patients with DHF/DSS compared with DF (15). Dengue virus infection can also activate blood clotting and fibrinolytic pathways. Mild disseminated intravascular coagulation (DIC) (22), liver injury, and thrombocytopenia together contribute to hemorrhagic tendency.

Central nervous system (CNS) involvement also has been identified (3,4,6,7,23) and has been attributed to direct neurotropic effect of dengue virus (8).

The degree of viral load correlates with severity of DHF/DSS (24,25).

The risk factors for DHF/DSS are (16,19):

■ Virus strain—DENV-2 > DENV-3, DENV-4 > DENV-1
■ Preexisting antidengue antibody
■ Age of host—younger children are at increased risk
■ Secondary infection
■ Genetic predisposition (26,27)
■ Hyperendemicity—two or more virus serotypes circulating simultaneously at high level.

Pathology

Most fatalities in DHF/DSS occur within 24 hours after shock. The following are the autopsy finding from hundreds of DHF/DSS death in Thailand in the year 1960 (17). Gross findings reveal some degree of hemorrhage in the skin and subcutaneous tissue. Hemorrhage may appear as hemorrhagic rash, petechiae, or ecchymosis, especially around needle puncture marks. Frank hemorrhage may appear in patches in the subcutaneous tissue. The heart typically shows flame-shaped subendocardial hemorrhage in the left ventricular septum and occasionally over the papillary muscles. Hemorrhage may be present in nasal mucosa, gums, gastrointestinal tract, and the liver (subcapsular). While hemorrhage may be striking, especially in cases with prolonged shock, the amount of hemorrhage is not excessive and frank bleeding in serous cavities is rare. Adrenal cortical tissue hemorrhage was found in only two cases. The meninges and brain show only petechial hemorrhage. Massive bleeding into the brain and spinal tissue have not been reported. Serous effusion with high protein content (>1 g/dL) is common in the pleural, abdominal, and occasionally in the pericardial space. The amount of effusion results in a significant fluid loss in the 24-hour period before death. Analysis of the effusion shows a high protein content, mostly albumin and low-molecular-weight globulin, thus rendering it an exudate rather than a transudate, even though there is only small number of leukocytes in the fluid. Analysis of the plasma in the blood reveals corresponding low levels of protein, especially albumin. The most striking findings at autopsy are the negative findings—no gross pathologic damage to major organs in rapidly fatal DHF/DSS nor evidence of suprainfections (bacterial pneumonia, cystitis, or pyelonephritis).

The pathology of DHF/DSS in fatal cases generally reveals no gross or microscopic evidence of severe organ pathology to explain the cause of death. In cases with prolonged shock, consequences of shock on organs, intravascular clotting, and hemorrhage are seen. Despite some display of neurological symptoms (encephalopathy) there is no convincing evidence of encephalitis (neuronal damage due to dengue virus) but there has been one report of dengue encephalitis from Brazil (8). Dengue encephalitis/encephalopathy has been reported with serological or virological confirmation but no pathological confirmation.

Bone marrow biopsy reveals hypocellularity early (in the febrile phase) which may contribute to hemorrhage, while at the time of shock and in most fatal cases, the bone marrow appears normocellular or even hypercellular. Young megakaryocytes proliferate and enter the circulation in high numbers.

The kidneys show immune complex glomerulonephritis with deposition of immunoglobulin and complement on the glomerular capillaries.

Classification

❷ Dengue classifications have been controversial. **Figure 89.1** shows the 1997 WHO classification of dengue, which has been criticized because it does not include all dengue cases, especially those with severe or unusual manifestations (28–32). DHF can be subdivided into grades I–IV on the basis of severity. The WHO SEARO modified the 1997 WHO classification slightly to recognize the following dengue infection syndromes: *viral-like illness, dengue fever (DF), dengue hemorrhagic fever (DHF), dengue shock syndrome (DSS),* and *expanded (atypical or unusual) dengue syndrome (EDS)* (2). **Figure 89.2** shows the 2009 WHO classification, which divides dengue into *uncomplicated* and *severe* cases. In practice, many clinicians in endemic areas prefer the WHO SEARO classification.

DHF (DHF grades I and II), DSS (DHF grades III and IV), and EDS are considered *severe* in the 2009 WHO classification because they may lead to complications and death without proper management. DHF grades I and II are non-shock cases: a grade of II requires that the patient has spontaneous bleeding while a grade of I requires only a positive tourniquet test (see below). DHF grades III and IV are shock cases; a grade of IV requires that the patients have prolonged and profound shock with no blood pressure or no palpable pulse. The majority of dengue presentations (up to 80%–90% of symptomatic cases) are DF, which is mostly a mild illness and rarely leads to death.

DHF and DSS patients differ from DF patients because of plasma leakage during the critical phase. Minor bleeding manifestations, petechiae, epistaxis, and gum bleeding are usually found in all dengue infected patients, but significant bleeding mostly occurs in DHF/DSS and EDS patients. EDS was not described in the first three decades of DHF outbreaks (between 1950s and 1980s). While EDS is still uncommon, there are now increasing reports of EDS especially in countries with new outbreaks and especially in adult patients. The majority of EDS cases are the result of prolonged shock with manifestations of multiple organs failure, comorbidities, and co-infections in dengue-infected hosts. EDS can be found in both DF and DHF/DSS cases (i.e., with or without plasma leakage) (1,33). The percentage of DHF/DSS/EDS patients is minimal compared with viral-like illness and DF patients, but it is very important that clinicians detect and properly manage severe dengue early in order to prevent shock, complications, and death. During the first few days of fever, it may be difficult to differentiate DF from DHF/DSS patients (18,19,34–39).

results in 5–10 minutes, but is still expensive in most dengue endemic countries. This NS1 Ag has a good specificity (>95%) but low sensitivity (40%–70%) so it is to be used with extreme caution, that is, a negative test does not rule out dengue (2,45).

Commonly used serologic tests to detect antibodies include IgM antibody-capture enzyme-linked immunosorbent assay (MAC-ELISA) test and IgG antibody-capture enzyme-linked immunosorbent assay (GAC-ELISA) test. The MAC-ELISA and GAC-ELISA tests measure dengue-specific IgM and IgG antibodies that can differentiate dengue from Japanese encephalitis virus infection and also differentiate primary and secondary dengue infections (46). A commercially available strip test for IgM and IgG antibodies requires only a drop of serum and gives results within a few minutes. The hemagglutination inhibition (HI) test measures IgG antibodies, is sensitive and reproducible test, but is rather complicated and requires paired sera collected at an interval of 1–2 weeks; hence it is not done in most endemic countries. A combined kit for NS1 Ag and IgM/IgG antibodies is available for dengue confirmation (47).

MANAGEMENT

7 **8** Management of suspected dengue is mainly supportive and symptomatic treatment. There are no specific antiviral or anti-plasma leakage drugs. The management depends on the phase of their clinical illness: febrile, critical (leakage), and convalescence (2,34,37,39,48).

Febrile Phase

Management in the febrile phase is mostly symptomatic with supportive treatment. Only paracetamol is recommended to reduce the height of fever, both in children and in adults. Aspirin and NSAID are contraindicated because they may cause gastritis (and massive bleeding) or Reye's syndrome. In addition, aspirin causes platelet dysfunction. Tepid sponge baths should be added if high fever persists to decrease the risk of paracetamol overdose and hepatotoxicity. A warm shower may be recommended for adults and older children. An antiemetic may be given for nausea/vomiting. Other supportive and symptomatic medicines may be given according to the clinical signs and symptoms (e.g., anticonvulsants, antihypertensive drugs, H2-blocker or proton pump inhibitors). Antibiotics are not indicated if there are no associated bacterial infections. *Steroids have no benefit in DHF/DSS* (24,49,50).

Most children with dengue can tolerate a soft diet, fruit juice, or milk. An oral electrolyte solution is used in cases of severe anorexia, nausea, or vomiting. Red, black, or brown foods are avoided so that stool discoloration is not misinterpreted as blood. Some patients with moderate to severe dehydration may need to be observed or admitted to the hospital for IV fluids to correct dehydration. The rate of IV fluid administration is reduced as soon as possible to prevent later fluid overload during the reabsorption phase after plasma leakage (see below).

Uncomplicated DF is usually managed at home, but parents should be advised to bring the child back to hospital without delay for the following indications (which may indicate early shock):

- No clinical improvement during resolution of the fever
- Severe abdominal pain
- Vomiting
- Significant bleeding
- Mental status change (drowsiness, stupor, restlessness, behavior changes)
- Cold-clammy sweating
- Anuria for 4–6 hours.

Indications for Observation/Admission

Observation is indicated for suspected dengue patients who have moderate to severe dehydration during the febrile phase and for those who still appear ill after fever has resolved (may indicate an impending critical phase). Specific admission guidelines include the following:

1. Shock or impending shock
   1.1. Narrow pulse pressure (≤20 mm Hg) is commonly observed in children and is usually due to plasma leakage.
   1.2. Hypotension is commonly observed in adults and patients with significant bleeding. Older children and adults may present with postural hypotension.
   1.3. Some patients may present with clinical signs of shock, that is, rapid and weak pulse, delayed capillary refill time (>2 seconds), cold-clammy skin, or skin mottling with normal blood pressure. Note that shock in dengue patients may not be due to plasma leakage, but rather to other conditions, such as hypoglycemia or excessive vomiting.
2. Rising Hct ≥ 20% and thrombocytopenia
3. Clinical deterioration *during defervescence*
4. Leukopenia and/or thrombocytopenia with poor clinical condition, poor appetite, or other warning signs
5. Significant bleeding.

Some patients may be observed or admitted to the hospital earlier than the usual on the basis of the following indications:

1. *High risk patients: Prolonged shock, obesity, infants, the elderly, pregnancy, bleeding, comorbidities, altered mental status, or behavioral change*
2. No care-takers at home
3. Unreliable follow-up.

Critical Phase (Leakage Phase)

Detection of early plasma leakage (rising Hct, CXR, ultrasonography, or hypoalbuminemia) is important to make the diagnosis of DHF. Leukopenia and/or thrombocytopenia usually precede plasma leakage and hence may serve as an indicator of impending plasma leakage. Such patients are then monitored for the critical period, especially those with poor appetite or other warning signs.

Hospitalized dengue patients are admitted to a unit with a mosquito-free environment for close monitoring and to prevent nosocomial dengue transmission. Individual bed nets are not practical for both patients and healthcare team. The absence of fever for >1 day indicates resolution of viremia, at which time there is no further risk of viral dissemination from mosquito bites. Most of the DHF/DSS cases do not need to be managed in intensive care unit (ICU), but do need close monitoring.

Monitoring

The monitoring protocol depends on the clinical condition.

- Febrile, but otherwise well appearing patients: record temperature, appetite, intake and output, vomiting, abdominal pain, bleeding.
- DHF patients: Vital signs q 4 h, Hct q 4–6 h and urine output q 6–8 hours for 24–48 hours of the critical phase.
- Shock patients: Hourly urine output (0.5 mL/kg/h is the optimum amount of urine in children with dengue) and

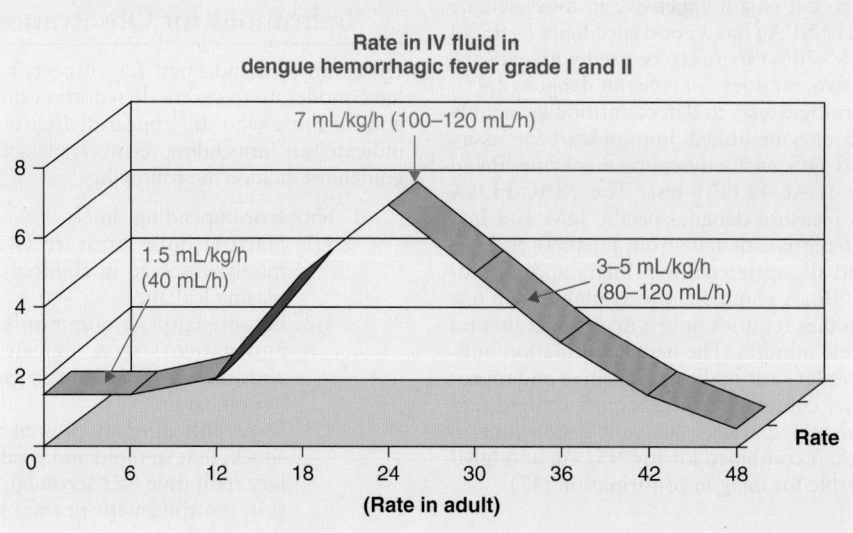

FIGURE 89.6. Rate of IV fluid administration for children and adults with nonshock DHF (grades I and II).

vital signs q 15 min until stable, then q 1–2 h × 4 hours, then q 2–3 h.
- Temperature is recorded q 6 h for all DHF/DSS patients (more frequently is those with high fever).

VOLUME REPLACEMENT

General Principles

The principle of volume replacement in DHF/DSS patients is to give the *minimal amount required to maintain effective circulatory* volume. The IV fluid should be isotonic and similar to electrolyte concentrations lost into the pleural and peritoneal spaces, e.g., normal saline solution (NSS), lactate Ringer's solution (LR), or acetate Ringer's solution (AR). Randomized controlled trials have failed to reveal an advantage of colloid solutions over crystalloid solutions (51).

The *total volume replacement during the critical period is maintenance (M) + 5% deficit (D)* (about 4.6 L in adult) and *the estimated total duration for IV fluid administration is about 36–60 hours.* Complications often occur if the total volume or duration of IV fluid exceeds this estimation. Inadequate fluid resuscitation risks prolonged shock whereas overzealous fluid administration risks fluid overload, respiratory failure, and multiple organs failure. IV fluid with addition of 5% dextrose is preferred because these DHF/DSS patients usually have poor appetite and marginal levels of blood sugar.

IV fluid is to be given only in those patients who enter the critical period and cannot tolerate adequate oral intake. There is no need to administer IV fluid for those patients with good appetite and no vomiting. *The total volume given to DHF/DSS patients includes both oral (fruit juices, milk, or electrolyte solutions only) and IV fluid.* Plain water without electrolytes is avoided because it may aggravate hyponatremia and contribute to more plasma leakage or convulsions.

Fluid Administration for Nonshock Patients (DHF Grades I and II)

IV fluid administration in DHF grades I and II patients should be started at the minimum rate needed to maintain intravascular volume and gradually increased according to the rate of plasma leakage and then decreased after plasma leakage subsides (Fig. 89.6). Table 89.1 shows the recommended IV fluid rate based on the percentage rise in Hct. If the patient is just entering the critical period (i.e., platelet count <100,000 cells/mm³, Hct rising 5%–10%), start IV fluids at half maintenance rate (1.5 mL/kg/h or 40 mL/h for adult). If Hct has risen by 10%–20%, start IV fluids at the maintenance rate (3 mL/kg/h or 80 mL/h for adult) or maintenance +5% deficit rate (5 mL/kg/h or 100–120 mL/h for adult). If Hct has risen >20%, start IV fluid at the rate of 7–10 mL/kg/h for children or 150–200 mL/h for adults. Table 89.2 compares the administration in children and adults. The total duration of IV fluid should not be more than 60–72 hours.

TABLE 89.1

RATE OF IV FLUID ADMINISTRATION BASED ON ELEVATION OF HEMATOCRIT FOR CHILDREN AND ADULTS WITH DHF GRADES I AND II

■ PERCENTAGE RISE IN HCT	■ RATE OF IV IN CHILDREN (mL/kg/h)	■ RATE IN ADULT (mL/h)
5–10	1.5	40
10–20	3–5	80–120
>20	7–10	150–200

Hct elevation based on the standard for age, sex, and population or a known baseline Hct; Hct, hematocrit.

TABLE 89.2

RATE OF IV FLUID ADMINISTRATION BASED ON ESTIMATES OF MAINTENANCE NEEDS AND EXISTING DEFICITS FOR CHILDREN AND ADULTS WITH DHF GRADES I AND II

■ TOTAL VOLUME REPLACEMENT	■ CHILDREN (mL/kg/h)	■ ADULT (mL/h)
M/2	1.5	40
M	3	80
M + 5% D	5	100–120
M + 7% D	7	150–200
M + 10% D	10	300–500

M, Maintenance Fluid Administration; D, Deficit Fluid Administration.

Fluid Administration for Shock Patients (Grade III)

The amount and rate of IV fluid resuscitation for DSS (DHF grade III) is much less compared with other kinds of shock (septic shock, anaphylactic shock, or hypovolemic shock). **Figures 89.7** and **89.8** display the fluid management protocol for grade III patients (compensated shock), who should receive Ringer's lactate or normal saline at a rate of 10 mL/kg/h for children (or 500 mL/h in the adult) for 1–2 hours. Fluid administration is reduced to 7 mL/kg/h for the child (or 250 mL/h in the adult) for another 1–2 hours and then reduced further to 5 mL/kg/h (child) or 100–120 mL/h (adult) for 4–6 hours. After 12 hours of shock, IV fluid should be at maintenance rates for 4–6 hours before reducing to rates designed simply to keep the vein open (KVO) (**Fig. 89.7**). The total duration of IV fluid should not exceed 24–36 hours.

DSS is usually differentiated from other kinds of shock by demonstrating an elevated Hct and a low platelet count. The

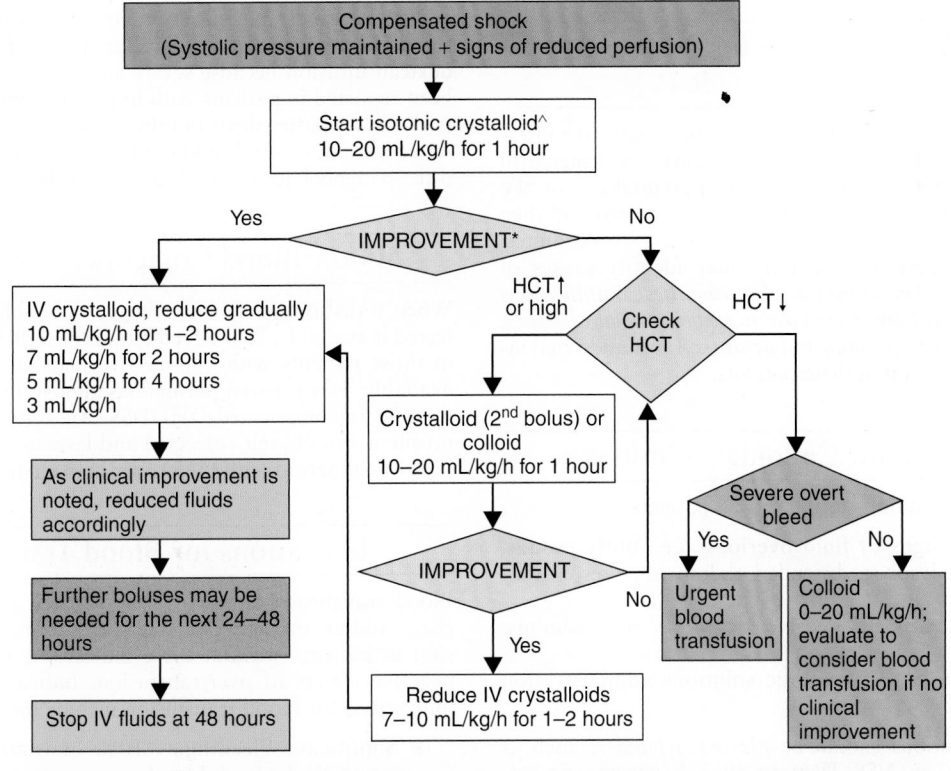

FIGURE 89.7. Algorithm for fluid management in dengue-compensated shock (grade III). (Reproduced with permission from: World Health Organization. *Handbook for Clinical Management of Dengue.* Geneva, Switzerland: WHO, 2012. http://apps.who.int/iris/bitstream/10665/76887/1/9789241504713_eng.pdf)

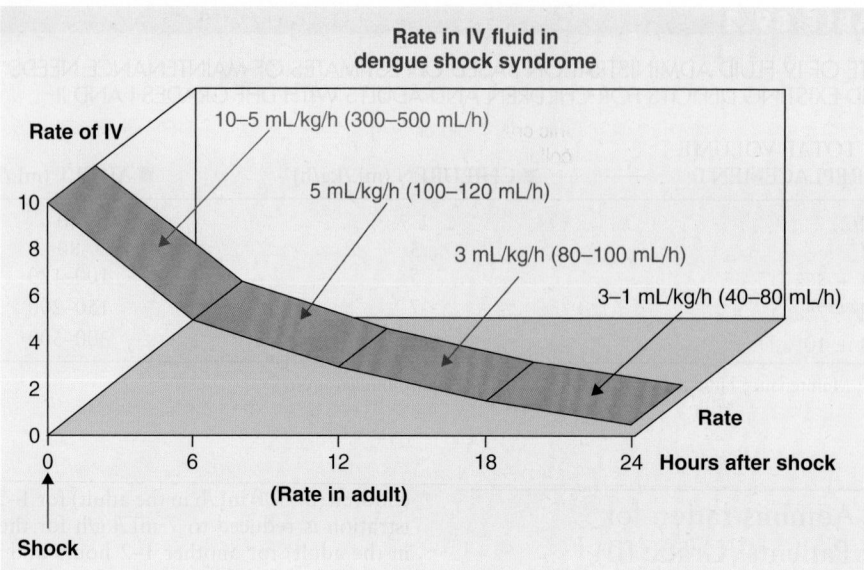

FIGURE 89.8. Rate of IV fluid administration in children and adults with dengue shock syndrome.

elevated Hct alone (usually hemoconcentration >25%–30% of the baseline Hct) can be used to diagnose DSS in uncomplicated cases without internal bleeding.

Fluid Administration for Profound Shock Patients (Grade IV)

As expected, grade IV patients require more aggressive intravenous hydration than do grade III patients. As depicted in **Figure 89.9**, isotonic crystalloid is given at 20 mL/kg/h (or "IV push") until the blood pressure (BP) can be restored and then reduced. If the BP cannot be restored within 15–30 minutes, additional laboratory investigations may identify causes of prolonged shock. *The common abnormalities/complications associated with prolonged DSS are massive internal bleeding, hypoglycemia, hypocalcemia, and acidosis.* Liver and renal injuries are also common in these patients.

Indication for Colloidal Solutions

We use colloidal solutions for DHF/DSS patients

- with overt signs of fluid overload (i.e., puffy eyelids, tachypnea, dyspnea, distended abdomen, or respiratory distress)
- with persistently elevated Hct despite IV fluid administration
- with a history of hypotonic solutions administration before shock.

Colloidal solutions should be *plasma expanders* such as *10% Dextran-40 in NSS*. Dextran-40 is hyper-oncotic (osmolarity = 400 mOsm), has high osmolarity compared with plasma (280–300 mOsm), and is designed to draw interstitial fluid into vascular space. Other colloids (plasma substitutes) are not recommended in the treatment of DHF/DSS because their osmolarity is equal to that of plasma. Six percent hetastarch (Voluven) may be used if dextran-40 is not available; however, it is considered less effective in dextran 40 in lowering the Hct and maintaining intra-vascular volume (52).

Dextran-40 is infused at 10 mL/kg/h (or 500 mL/h for adults) and will lower the Hct by 10% points. An Hct reduction >10%, after hydration with dextran-40 may indicate bleeding. The total recommended dose is 30 mL/kg/day. In severe cases, additional doses of dextran-40 may be considered. Patients should be monitored closely during the first few minutes of the dextran infusion because severe anaphylactoid reactions have been reported in patients with hypersensitivity. Fluid overload with oliguria after dextran infusion may be treated with furosemide. Dextran-40 should not be used for initial resuscitation if the patients had not received IV fluid before.

Blood/Blood Component Transfusion

When transfusing for hemorrhage, whole blood (WB) is preferred if available. Packed red blood cells (PRBC) are indicated in those patients with volume overload or when WB is not available. Fresh frozen plasma has almost no role in the treatment of uncomplicated DHF/DSS. An abnormal coagulation profile is usually self-corrected and lasts only a few days during critical period with the proper management.

Indications for Blood Transfusion

Blood transfusion is usually reserved for significant hemorrhage and anemia complicating shock management. Transfusion in patients without these indications may result in the negative effects of overtransfusion. Indications and relative indications for blood transfusion include the following:

- Significant bleeding (>10% of total blood volume; >6–8 mL/kg in children).
- No significant rise of Hct in DSS patients (by definition have shock). DSS patients usually have a rise of Hct >25%–30% from baseline at the time of shock.
- Fall in Hct without clinical or vital signs improvement.
- Patients with refractory shock despite IV fluid hydration (e.g., women with hypermenorrhea/abnormal vaginal bleeding, patients with severe abdominal pain [peptic ulcer] and those with hemoglobinuria).

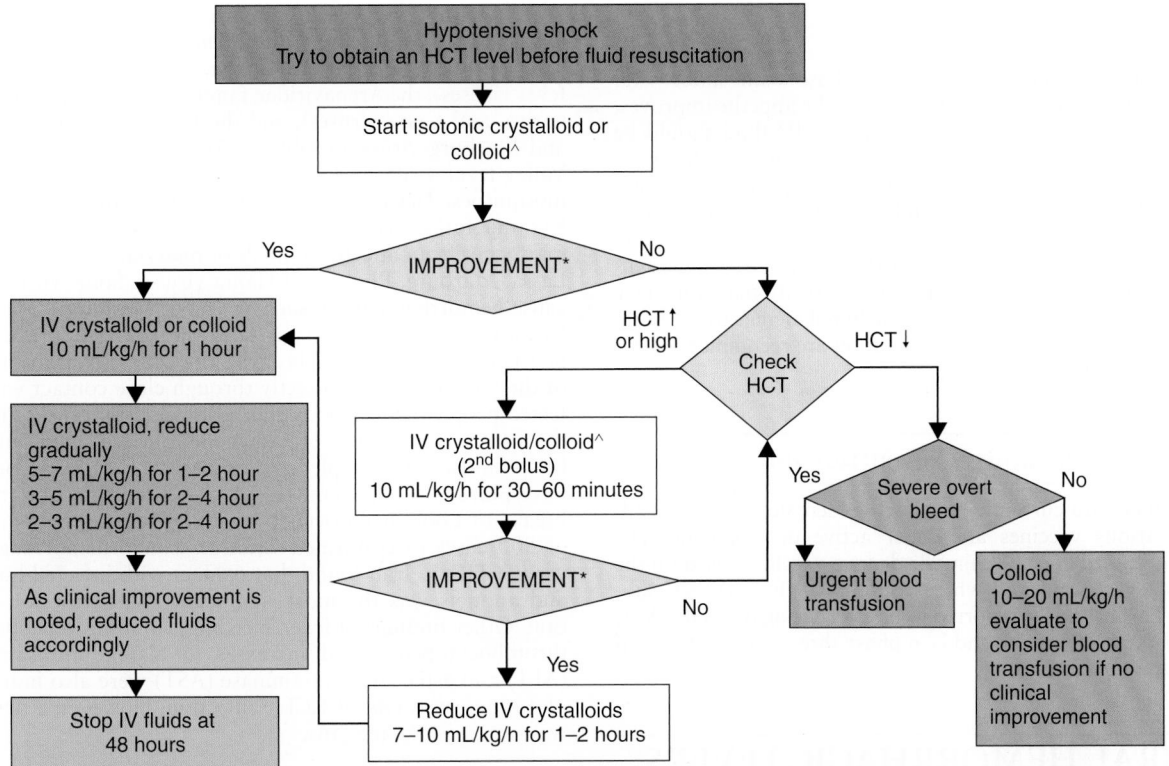

FIGURE 89.9. Algorithm for fluid management in hypotensive shock (grade IV). (Reproduced with permission from: World Health Organization. *Handbook for Clinical Management of Dengue*. Geneva, Switzerland: WHO, 2012. http://apps.who.int/iris/bitstream/10665/76887/1/9789241504713_eng.pdf.)

Amount of Blood to Transfuse

- Transfuse amount equivalent to estimated losses.
- If internal (concealed) bleeding or estimation is not possible, transfuse WB 10 mL/kg or PRBC 5 mL/kg.

Measurements of the Hct before and after blood transfusion are very important to assess the degree of bleeding and develop a subsequent management plan.

Transfusion Rate

- Blood is usually transfused at the rate of 5 mL/kg/h. If DHF/DSS patients have signs of fluid overload, a slower rate is recommended and in some cases diuretic administration (furosemide 1 mg/kg/dose IV) is recommended before, during, or after blood transfusion, depending on the phase of the DHF/DSS patients.
- If the child is in shock, blood can be given as IV push to restore the BP as soon as possible; the rate is then reduced once the BP is restored.

Platelet Transfusion

Platelet transfusion is only considered in patients with significant bleeding and thrombocytopenia. Prophylactic platelet transfusion in the absence of clinical bleeding is not used regardless of the degree of thrombocytopenia unless the patient had previously received antiplatelet or anticoagulant medications because of comorbidities (53). Patients with fluid overload should not receive platelet transfusions even if there is clinical bleeding because of the risk of the pulmonary edema or heart failure.

Special Investigations and Management in DHF/DSS Patients Who Do Not Response Well to the Conventional IV Fluid Management

An urgent, directed laboratory investigation is indicated in high-risk DHF/DSS, especially in the presence of refractory or recurrent shock, fluid overload, massive bleeding, liver failure, or other organ involvement (including EDS patients). The following laboratory studies should be checked and corrected immediately if there are abnormalities:

- **A—Acidosis:** Venous or capillary blood gas, to check for acidosis
- **B—Bleeding:** Hct, to check for bleeding (or hemoconcentration). Blood type and cross-match, for possible transfusion
- **C—Calcium and electrolyte:** Hypocalcemia or other electrolyte imbalances may contribute to shock
- **S—Blood sugar:** Hypoglycemia is common because of malnutrition, poor intake, and liver failure.

Convalescence Phase

When patients enter convalescence phase with stable vital signs, the Hct returns to baseline values, the appetite improves, and urine output increases. At his point, IV fluid should be stopped especially when reabsorption of plasma into the circulation has started. In some patients with large pleural effusion and ascites, transient high blood pressure with strong pulse may be observed together with diuresis. Furosemide IV may be necessary to treat fluid overload manifested by hypertension, dyspnea, and tachypnea. Some patients may still have poor appetite due to bowel ileus or hypokalemia from diuresis. Fruits or fruit juices or KCl solution are recommended for these patients.

Future Directions: Prevention and Vaccines

While there are currently no effective dengue vaccines available, various vaccines are under active development. The most advanced one is a chimeric dengue vaccine, based on the yellow fever strain and which contains all four DENV subtypes. This vaccine is reported to be effective against DENV-1, DENV-3, and DENV-4 and is in phase three trials in Asia and Latin America (54,55).

VIRAL HEMORRHAGIC FEVERS

Viral hemorrhagic fevers (VHF) compose a group of clinical syndromes that are characterized by hemorrhagic manifestations. Disseminated intravascular coagulopathy appears to be the common pathogenetic feature of these illnesses.

The pathogenic viruses are from the Flaviviridae family (Kyasanur forest disease, Omsk, dengue, and yellow fever viruses), Bunyaviridae family (Congo, Hantaan, and Rift Valley fever viruses), the Arenaviridae family (Junin, Machupo, Guanarito, and Lassa viruses), and the Filoviridae family (Ebola and Marburg viruses) (Table 89.3). The dengue viruses, Rift Valley fever virus, and yellow fever virus are transmitted by mosquitoes. Ticks are responsible for transmission of Omsk, Kysanur forest disease, and Congo viruses. Human infection may occur from infected animals or materials in case of Junin, Lassa, Marburg, Ebola, and Hanta viruses. Some viruses that cause hemorrhagic fever, such as Ebola, Marburg, Lassa, and Crimean-Congo hemorrhagic fever viruses, can spread from one person to another. This type of secondary transmission of the virus can occur directly through close contact with infected people or their body fluids. It can also occur indirectly through contact with objects contaminated with infected body fluids. For example, contaminated syringes and needles have played an important role in spreading infection in outbreaks of Ebola hemorrhagic fever and Lassa fever. A report of 800 cases of confirmed Crimean-Congo hemorrhagic fever (CCHF) in Iran found that contact with infected humans and animals was the most significant risk factor for infection. Other findings of fever, bleeding, vomiting, leucopoenia, thrombocytopenia, and increases in alanine transaminase (ALT) and aspartate transaminase (AST) were also indicative of an increased risk of CCHF infection. However, a tick bite was not a risk factor (56).

Clinical Features

The clinical features of different types of viral hemorrhagic fevers are summarized in **Table 89.4** (5,57).

TABLE 89.3

VARIOUS VIRAL HEMORRHAGIC FEVERS

■ DISEASE	■ VIRUS	■ VECTOR	■ GEOGRAPHIC AREAS
Crimean-Congo hemorrhagic fever	Congo virus	Ixodid ticks (*Hyalomma*)	Bulgaria, western Crimea, Rostov-on-Don and Astrakhan regions, Pakistan, Afghanistan, Arabian Peninsula, South Africa, Oman, southern Russia
Kyasanur forest disease	Kysanur forest disease virus	Ticks	Mysore State, India
Omsk hemorrhagic fever	Omsk virus	Ticks	South central Russia, northern Romania
Rift Valley fever	Rift Valley fever virus	Mosquitoes	North, Central, East, and South Africa; Saudi Arabia; Yemen
Argentine hemorrhagic fever	Junin virus	Rodent	Argentina
Bolivian hemorrhagic fever	Machupo virus	Rodent	Amazonian Bolivia
Lassa fever	Lassa virus	Rodent (*Mastomys*)	Nigeria, Sierra Leone, Liberia
Marburg disease	Marburg virus	Unknown	Congo Republic, Germany, Yugoslavia, Zimbabwe, Kenya, South Africa
Ebola hemorrhagic fever	Ebola virus	Unknown	Northern Zaire, southern Sudan, Uganda, Central and West Africa
Hemorrhagic fever with renal syndrome	Hanta virus	Rodents (*Apodemus agrarius, Clethrionomys glareolus, Apodemus flavicollis*)	Japan, Korea, Far Eastern Siberia, north and central China, European and Asian Russia, Scandinavia, Czechoslovakia, Romania, Bulgaria, Yugoslavia, Greece
Yellow fever	Yellow fever virus	Mosquitoes (*Aedes* and *Haemogogus*)	Tropical areas of Africa and the Americas

TABLE 89.4

CLINICAL FEATURES OF VIRAL HEMORRHAGIC FEVERS

■ DISEASE	■ INCUBATION PERIOD (D)	■ CLINICAL FEATURES	■ CASE FATALITY
Crimean-Congo hemorrhagic fever	3–12	Fever, severe headache, myalgia, abdominal pain, anorexia, nausea, and vomiting; erythematous facial or truncal flush and injected conjunctivae; hemorrhagic enanthem on the soft palate and a fine petechial rash on the chest and abdomen. Large areas of purpura and bleeding from gums, nose, intestine, lungs, or uterus may be seen. Hepatomegaly in absence of icterus. In severe illnesses, CNS symptoms and signs may be seen	2%–50%
Kyasanur forest disease	3–8	Severe myalgia, prostration, and bronchiolar involvement. Often presents without hemorrhage but occasionally with severe gastrointestinal bleeding, bronchopneumonia, acute renal failure, and focal liver damage, meningoencephalitis	3%–10%
Omsk hemorrhagic fever	3–8	Moderate epistaxis, hematemesis, and a hemorrhagic enanthem but no profuse hemorrhage, bronchopneumonia	1%–10%
Rift Valley fever	3–6	Fever, headache, prostration, myalgia, anorexia, nausea, vomiting, conjunctivitis, and lymphadenopathy, purpura, epistaxis, hematemesis, and melena	~1%
Argentine, Venezuelan, and Bolivian hemorrhagic fever and Lassa fever	~7–14	Fever, headache, diffuse myalgia, anorexia, sore throat, dysphagia, cough, oropharyngeal ulcers, nausea, vomiting, diarrhea, pains in chest, abdomen, pleuritic chest pain; tourniquet test may be positive. Hypovolemic shock may be accompanied by pleural effusion and renal failure; respiratory distress (airway obstruction, pleural effusion, or congestive heart failure); neurologic symptoms, seizures	10%–40%
Marburg disease and Ebola hemorrhagic fever	4–7	Headache, malaise, drowsiness, lumbar myalgia, vomiting, nausea, and diarrhea. Maculopapular eruption, often hemorrhagic, dark red enanthem on the hard palate, conjunctivitis, and scrotal or labial edema. Gastrointestinal hemorrhage in severe illness. Hypotension and coma in severe cases. DIC and thrombocytopenia are seen in most patients	Marburg disease: 25% Ebola hemorrhagic fever: 50%–90%
Hemorrhagic fever with renal syndrome (Hanta, Puumala)	9–35	Fever, petechiae, mild hemorrhagic phenomena, mild proteinuria. Thrombocytopenia, petechiae, proteinuria. Hypotension may follow defervescence. Hemoconcentration, ecchymoses, oliguria. Confusion, extreme restlessness. Fatal cases may manifest retroperitoneal edema and marked hemorrhagic necrosis of the renal medulla	5%–10%
Yellow fever	3–6	Abrupt onset. Fever, headache, severe myalgias, diarrhea, vomiting, severe prostration, conjunctival suffusion, photophobia, cervical and axillary adenopathy, and more rarely, splenomegaly or hepatosplenomegaly. Papulovesicular lesions involving the soft palate and pulmonary manifestations are frequent during the first stage of the illness. The second stage of the illness is associated with neurologic involvement. Hemorrhagic manifestations are similar to those observed with other viral hemorrhagic fevers	<10%

Diagnosis

Healthcare providers must have a high index of suspicion for VHF in endemic areas. In nonendemic areas, histories of recent travel, recent laboratory exposure, or exposure to an earlier case should evoke suspicion of a viral hemorrhagic fever. In all VHF, the virus can be recovered during the early febrile stage. Bunyaviruses can be recovered from acute-phase serum by inoculation into tissue culture or living mosquitoes. Argentine, Bolivian, and Venezuelan hemorrhagic fever viruses can be isolated from acute-phase blood or throat washings by inoculation intracerebrally into guinea pigs, infant hamsters, or infant mice. Lassa virus may be isolated from acute-phase blood or throat washings by inoculation into tissue cultures.

For Marburg disease and Ebola hemorrhagic fever, acute-phase throat washings, blood, and urine may be inoculated into tissue culture, guinea pigs, or monkeys. The viruses are readily identified by electron microscopy, with a filamentous structure that differentiates them from all other known agents.

Specific complement-fixing and immunefluorescent antibodies appear during convalescence. The viruses of hemorrhagic fever with renal syndrome (HFRS) can be recovered from acute-phase serum or urine by inoculation into tissue culture. A variety of antibody tests using viral subunits are becoming available.

Serologic diagnosis depends on demonstrating seroconversion—a fourfold or greater increase in immunoglobulin G antibody titer in acute and convalescent serum samples taken 3–4 weeks apart. Viral RNA may also be detected in blood or tissues, using reverse-transcriptase PCRs.

Handling blood and other biologic specimens is hazardous and must be performed by specially trained personnel. For those hemorrhagic fever viruses that can be transmitted from person to person (Ebola, Marburg, Lassa, and Crimean-Congo hemorrhagic fever viruses), avoiding close physical contact with infected people and their body fluids is the most effective way of controlling the spread of disease. Infection-control techniques include barrier nursing, isolating infected individuals, and wearing protective clothing. Other infection-control recommendations include proper use, disinfection, and disposal of instruments and equipment (needles, thermometers, etc.) used in treating or caring for patients with VHF.

VHF isolation precautions include the following:

- Isolating the patient (universal, contact, droplet)
- Wearing protective clothing in the isolation area, in the cleaning and laundry areas, and in the laboratory; protective gear should include a scrub suit, gown, apron, two pairs of gloves, mask, head cover, eyewear, and rubber boots
- Cleaning and disinfecting spills, waste, and reusable equipment safely
- Cleaning and disinfecting soiled linens and laundry safely
- Using safe disposal methods for nonreusable supplies and infectious waste
- Providing information about the risk of VHF transmission to health facility staff
- Reinforcing use of VHF isolation precautions with all health facility staff

Differential Diagnosis

Mild cases of hemorrhagic fever are similar to many self-limited systemic bacterial or viral infections. In severe cases, the differential diagnoses include typhoid fever, typhus, leptospirosis, or a rickettsial spotted fever.

Treatment

Ribavirin administered IV is effective in reducing mortality in Lassa fever and HFRS (58). The principle involved in management of all of these diseases, especially HFRS, is the reversal of dehydration, hemoconcentration, renal failure, and protein, electrolyte, or blood losses. The management of hemorrhage should be individualized. Transfusions of fresh blood and platelets are frequently given. Good results have been reported in a few patients after the administration of clotting factor concentrates. The efficacy of other modalities, such as corticosteroids, ε-aminocaproic acid, pressor amines, or α-adrenergic blocking agents has not been established. Sedatives should be selected with regard to the possibility of kidney or liver damage. The successful management of HFRS may require renal dialysis. Although extensive study of vaccines for VHF is ongoing, and some vaccines are in advanced stages of development, no vaccines are currently available for most of these diseases (57). Several Ebola vaccines appear efficacious in nonhuman primates suggesting that a vaccination against Ebola virus is feasible (59).

There is a recent report of a novel synthetic adenosine analogue, BCX4430, which has been shown to inhibit infection of distinct filoviruses in human cells (60). Postexposure administration of BCX4430 protects against Ebola virus and Marburg virus disease in rodent models and completely protects macaques from Marburg virus infection when administered up to 48 hours after infection. BCX4430 also has broad-spectrum activity against bunyaviruses, arenaviruses, paramyxoviruses, coronaviruses, and flaviviruses.

Prognosis and Prognostic Factors

The case fatality rates are shown in **Table 89.4**. Filoviruses (Ebola, Marburg) are responsible for case fatality rates that are among the highest reported for any human pathogen, exceeding 90%. The presence of significant volume depletion, coupled with hemodynamic instability, is a poor prognostic sign in patients with VHF infection. In the largest case study of Ebola-Zaire infection, terminally ill patients typically presented with signs of severe volume loss, including obtundation, anuria, and shock (61). In these patients, tachypnea was the most significant criterion that differentiated between fatal and nonfatal outcomes. Tachypnea was associated with bleeding from mucosa and puncture sites, anuria, and hiccups; tachypnea preceded death by only a few days. Impaired consciousness and splenomegaly have been reported as independent predictors of mortality in Crimean-Congo hemorrhagic fever.

CONCLUSIONS AND FUTURE DIRECTIONS

VHF can be caused by a variety of viruses, which could be used for bioterrorism. Better understanding of the pathogenesis and evaluation of antiviral drugs and other therapeutic modalities is necessary to improve outcomes.

References

1. WHO. *Dengue Hemorrhagic Fever: Diagnosis, Treatment and Control.* Geneva, Switzerland: WHO, 1997.
2. WHO SEARO. *Comprehensive Guidelines for the Prevention and Control of Dengue and Dengue Hemorrhagic Fever.* Revised and expanded ed. Geneva, Switzerland: WHO, 2011.
3. Lum LC, Lam SK, Choy YS, et al. Dengue encephalitis: A true entity? *Am J Trop Med Hyg* 1996;54(3):256–9.
4. Misra UK, Kalita J, Syam UK, et al. Neurological manifestations of dengue virus infection. *J Neurol Sci* 2006;244:117.
5. Piggot DC. Hemorrhagic fever viruses. *Crit Care Clin* 2005; 21:765–83.
6. Solomon T, Dung NM, Vaughn DW, et al. Neurological manifestations occurring during dengue fever infections. *Am J Trop Med Hyg* 1993;48:793.
7. Solomon T, Dung NM, Vaughn DW, et al. Neurological manifestations of dengue infections. *Lancet* 2000;355:1053.
8. Araujo FM, Araujo MS, Nogueira RM, et al. Central nervous system involvement in dengue: A study in fatal cases from a dengue endemic area. *Neurology* 2012;78(10):736–42.
9. Beatty ME, Leston GW, Margolis HS. Estimating the global burden of dengue. *Am J Trop Med Hyg* 2009;81:231.
10. Normile D. Surprising new dengue virus throws a spanner in disease control efforts. *Science* 2013;342:415.
11. Kalayanarooj S, Nimmannitya S. Clinical and laboratory presentations of dengue patients with different serotypes. *Dengue Bull* 2000;24: 53–9.
12. Pongritsakda V, Chunharas A. Hepatic failure in DHF patients [Thai]. *Ramathibodi Hosp J* 1986;1:11–8.
13. Vaughn DW, Green S, Kalayanarooj S, et al. Dengue viremia titer, antibody response pattern, and virus serotype correlate with disease severity. *J Infect Dis* 2000;181(1):2–9.
14. Kurane I, Matsutani T, Rothman AL, et al. T-cell responses to dengue virus in humans. *Trop Med Health* 2011;39(suppl 4):45–51.
15. Mathew A, Srikiatkhachorn A, West K, et al. B-cell responses during primary and secondary dengue virus infections in humans. *J Infect Dis* 2011;204(10):1514–22.
16. Halstead SB. Pathophysiology and pathogenesis of dengue hemorrhagic fever. In: Thongcharoen P, ed. *Monograph on Dengue/*

Dengue Hemorrhagic Fever. New Delhi, India: WHO regional Office for South-East Asia, 1993:80–103.

17. Bhamarapravati N. Pathology of dengue hemorrhagic fever. In: Thongcharoen P, ed. *Monograph on Dengue/Dengue Haemorrhagic Fever.* New Delhi, India: WHO SEARO, 1993:72–9.

18. Nimmannitya S. Clinical manifestations and management of dengue/dengue hemorrhagic fever. In: Thongcharoen P, ed. *Monograph on Dengue/Dengue Hemorrhagic Fever.* New Delhi, India: WHO regional Office for South-East Asia, 1993:48–54, 55–61.

19. Nimmannitya S. Dengue hemorrhagic fever: Diagnosis. In: Gubler DJ, Kuno G, eds. *Dengue and Dengue Hemorrhagic Fever.* Wallingford, England: CAB International, 1997:133–45.

20. Halstead SB. Pathogenesis of dengue: Challenges to molecular biology. *Science* 1988;239:476–81.

21. Bethell DB, Gamble J, Loc PP, et al. Noninvasive measurement of microvascular leakage in patients with dengue hemorrhagic fever. *Clin Infect Dis* 2001;32:243–53.

22. Krishnamurti C, Kalayanarooj S, Cutting MA, et al. Mechanisms of hemorrhage in dengue without circulatory collapse. *Am J Trop Med Hyg* 2001;65(6):840–7.

23. Patey O, Ollivaud L, Breuil J, et al. Unusual neurologic manifestations occurring during dengue fever infection. *Am J Trop Med Hyg* 1993;48:793.

24. Tassaniyom S, Vasanawathana S, Chirawatkul A, et al. Failure of high dose methylprednisolone in established dengue shock syndrome: A placebo-controlled, double-blinded study. *Pediatrics* 1993;92(1):111–5.

25. Teeraratkul A, Limpakanchanarat K, Nisalak A, et al. Predictive value of clinical and laboratory findings for early diagnosis of dengue hemorrhagic fever. *Southeast Asian J Trop Med Pub Health* 1990;21:686–97.

26. Sakuntabhai A, Turpaiboon C, Casademont I, et al. A variant in CD209 promoter is associated with severity of dengue disease. *Nat Genet* 2005;37:507–13.

27. Stephens HAF, Klaythong R, Sirikong M, et al. HLA-A and -B allele associations with secondary dengue virus infections correlate with disease severity and the infecting viral serotype in ethnic Thais. *Tissue Antigens* 2002;60(4):309–18.

28. Chhour YM, Ruble G, Hong R, et al. Hospital-based diagnosis of hemorrhagic fever encephalitis, and hepatitis in Cambodian children. *Emerg Infect Dis* 2002;8:485.

29. Cao XT, Ngo TN, Wills B, et al. Evaluations of the WHO standard tourniquet test and a modified tourniquet test in the diagnosis of dengue infection in Vietnam. *Trop Med Int Health* 2002;7:125.

30. Deen JL, Harris E, Wills B, et al. The WHO dengue classification and case definitions: Time for reassessment. *Lancet* 2006;368:170.

31. Phuong CX, Nhan NT, Kneen R, et al. Clinical diagnosis and assessment of severity of confirmed dengue infections in Vietnamese children: Is the WHO classification system helpful? *Am J Trop Med Hyg* 2004;70:172.

32. Srikiatkhachorn A, Rothman AL, Gibbons RV, et al. Dengue—How best to classify it. *Clin Infec Dis* 2011;53(6):563–7.

33. Nimmannitya S, Thisyakorn U, Hemsrichart V. Dengue hemorrhagic fever with unusual manifestations. *Southeast Asian J Trop Med Pub Health* 1987;18(3):392–7.

34. Kalayanarooj S, Nimmannitya S. *Guidelines for Dengue Hemorrhagic Fever Case Management.* Bangkok, Thailand: Bangkok Medical, 2004.

35. Kalayanarooj S, Vaughn DW, Nimmannitya S, et al. *Early Diagnostic Indicators in Dengue* (Thai) [Research paper]. Bangkok, Thailand: Thai Ministry of Public Health, 1996.

36. Kalayanarooj S, Vaughn DW, Nimmannitya S, et al. Early clinical and laboratory indicators of acute dengue illness. *J Infect Dis* 1997;176:313–21.

37. Kalayanarooj S. Standardized clinical management: Evidence of reduction of dengue hemorrhagic fever case-fatality rate in Thailand. *Dengue Bull* 1999;23:10–16.

38. Nimmannitya S. Clinical manifestations of dengue/dengue hemorrhagic fever. In: *Monograph on Dengue/Dengue Hemorrhagic Fever.* New Delhi, India: WHO, 1993;48–54.

39. Nimmannitya S. Dengue fever/dengue hemorrhagic fever: Case management. *Trop Med (Nagasaki)* 1994;36:249–56.

40. Srikiathchachorn A, Srikiatkhachorn A, Krautrachue A, et al. Natural history of plasma leakage in dengue hemorrhagic fever: A serial ultrasonographic study. *Pediatr Infect Dis J* 2007;26(4):283–90.

41. Kalayanarooj S, Chansiriwongs V, Nimmannitya S. Dengue patients at the Children's Hospital, Bangkok: A 5-year review. *Dengue Bull* 2002;26:33–43.

42. Kalayanarooj S, Nimmannitya S, Suntayakorn S, et al. Can doctors make an accurate diagnosis of dengue? *Dengue Bull* 1999;23:1–9.

43. Vaughn DW, Green S, Kalayanarooj S, et al. Dengue in early febrile phase: Viremia and antibody response. *J Infect Dis* 1997;176:322–30.

44. Kalayanarooj S. A study of erythrocyte sedimentation rate in dengue hemorrhagic fever. *Southeast Asian J Trop Med Pub Health* 1989;20(3):325–30.

45. DeOliveira Poersch C, Pavoni DP, Queiroz MH, et al. Dengue virus infections: Comparison of methods for diagnosing the acute disease. *J Clin Virol* 2005;32:272.

46. Innis BL, Nisalak A, Nimmannitya S, et al. An enzyme-linked immunosorbent assay to characterize dengue infections where dengue and Japanese encephalitis co-circulate. *Am J Trop Med Hyg* 1989;40(4):418–27.

47. Blacksell SD, Mammen MP, Thongpaseuth S, et al. Evaluation of the Panbio dengue nonstructural 1 antigen detection and immunoglobulin M antibody enzyme-linked immunosorbent assays for the diagnosis of acute dengue infections in Lao. *Diagn Microbiol Infect Dis* 2008;60:43.

48. Kalayanarooj S. Clinical Manifestations and Management of Dengue/DHF/DSS. *Trop Med Health* 2011;39(suppl 4):83–7.

49. Panpanich R, Sornchai P, Kanjanaratanakorn K. Corticosteroids for treating dengue shock syndrome. *Cochrane Database Syst Rev* 2006;CD003488.

50. Sumarmo, Talago W, Asrin A, et al. Failure of hydrocortisone to affect dengue shock syndrome. *Pediatrics* 1982;69(1):45–9.

51. Wills BA, Nguyen MD, Ha TL, et al. Comparison of three fluid solutions for resuscitation in dengue shock syndrome. *N Engl J Med* 2005;353:877.

52. Kalayanarooj S. Choice of colloidal solution in dengue hemorrhagic fever patients. *J Med Assoc Thai* 2008;91(suppl 3):S97–103.

53. Wongpiromsarn T. Effect of platelet transfusion in dengue shock syndrome patients. *Thai J Pediatr* 1991;1:71–6.

54. Durbin AP, Whitehead SS. Dengue vaccine candidates in development. *Curr Top Microbiol Immunol* 2010;338:129.

55. Sabchareon A, Wallace D, Sirivichayakul C, et al. Protective efficacy of the recombinant, live-attenuated, CYD tetravalent dengue vaccine in Thai schoolchildren: A randomised, controlled phase 2b trial. *Lancet* 2012;380(9853):1559–67.

56. Mostafavi E, Pourhossein B, Chinikar S. Clinical symptoms and laboratory findings supporting early diagnosis of Crimean-Congo hemorrhagic fever in Iran. *J Med Virol* 2014;86(7):1188–92.

57. Bossi P, Tegnell A, Baka A, et al. Bichat guidelines for the clinical management of haemorrhagic fever viruses and bioterrorism-related haemorrhagic fever viruses. *Eurosurveillance* 2004;9:E1–8.

58. McCormick JB, King IJ, Webb PA, et al. Lassa fever. Effective therapy with ribavirin. *N Engl J Med* 1986;314:20–6.

59. Marzi A, Feldmann H. Ebola virus vaccines: An overview of current approaches. *Expert Rev Vaccines* 2014;13(4):521–31.

60. Warren TK, Wells J, Panchal RG, et al. Protection against filovirus diseases by a novel broad-spectrum nucleoside analogue BCX4430. *Nature* 2014 [epub ahead of print].

61. Bwaka MA, Bonnet MJ, Calain P, et al. Ebola hemorrhagic fever in Kikwit, Democratic Republic of the Congo: Clinical observations in 103 patients. *J Infect Dis* 1999;179(suppl 1):S1–7.

CHAPTER 90 ■ CRITICAL VIRAL INFECTIONS

RAKESH LODHA, SUNIT C. SINGHI, AND JAMES D. CAMPBELL

KEY POINTS

Influenza

1. Influenza infections occur commonly, have a well-defined seasonality, and most infections are mild.
2. Recent pandemic with H1N1 strain caused widespread panic. It highlighted the potential for worldwide spread of new strains.
3. Most of the cases of influenza in children are managed on an ambulatory basis. Of the children needing hospitalization, ~15% need ICU care.
4. It has been hypothesized that cytokine storm plays an important and essential role in causing significant tissue injury and mortality following influenza virus infection.
5. Pneumonia associated with influenza virus infections may result from primary viral infection, bacterial superinfection, or combined bacterial–viral infection.
6. In severe cases, multiple organ systems are involved as manifested by focal and diffuse myocarditis, mediastinal lymph node enlargement and necrosis, and cerebral edema.
7. In addition to the supportive care required for management of critically ill children with influenza, specific antiviral therapy is indicated. The antiviral drugs include M2 protein inhibitors (amantadine and rimantadine) and neuraminidase (NA) inhibitors (oseltamivir and zanamivir).
8. Recent studies have reported a poorer prognosis in children with underlying chronic diseases.

HIV Infection

9. HIV infection has become an important contributor to childhood morbidity and mortality, especially in many developing countries.
10. Children with HIV infection may need admission to PICUs because of respiratory infections and respiratory failure, septic shock, and central nervous system (CNS) disorders.
11. Severe complications of therapy may also become indications for admission into the PICU.
12. The PICU staff should be aware of postexposure prophylaxis.

Measles

13. Measles, a vaccine-preventable infection, is an important cause of death among young children.

14. The conditions associated with measles that may require intensive care include pneumonia, laryngotracheobronchitis, and CNS infections.
15. Vitamin A may be helpful in reducing the morbidity and mortality due to measles.
16. No proven antiviral drugs for measles are available.

Nonpolio Enteroviruses

17. Nonpolio enteroviruses are responsible for a variety of illnesses.
18. Some of the respiratory, myocardial, and CNS infections may be severe enough to require intensive care.
19. The mainstay of care is supportive treatment.

Severe Varicella Infections

20. Varicella (chickenpox), a common and usually self-limited exanthematous illness, may result in severe manifestations, such as pneumonia, hepatitis, encephalitis, and disseminated intravascular coagulation (DIC).
21. The diagnosis can usually be made on the basis of clinical features and can be confirmed by virologic studies.
22. Acyclovir is the drug of choice; valacyclovir, famciclovir, and foscarnet are newer alternatives.
23. Recommendations have been made for routine varicella vaccination for all healthy children between 12 and 18 months and to all susceptible children before their 13th birthday, in addition to catch-up vaccination in older children and those who are at high risk of transmission and exposure.

Severe Herpes Simplex Virus Infections

24. Herpes simplex virus (HSV) infections of the lungs and brain can be severe, having high morbidity and mortality.
25. Immunocompromised children and neonates are at a higher risk of severe infections.
26. Acyclovir is the mainstay of therapy.

Various viral infections pose a challenge to the pediatric intensivists throughout the world. Dengue hemorrhagic fever (DHF) and viral hemorrhagic fevers are discussed in Chapter 89, and respiratory syncytial virus (RSV), metapneumovirus, and rhinovirus are discussed in Chapter 48. Influenza has been a major respiratory infection for decades. The recent influenza pandemic has again brought this infection in the forefront. Significant advances in the prevention of mother-to-child HIV transmission has brought down the numbers of new infections but HIV infection continues to have a significant impact on childe health in many developing countries. Measles infection is still a major problem in many developing countries. Herpes viruses are still responsible for serious illnesses that require intensive care. This chapter discusses these infections, with emphasis on the more severe infections.

SEVERE INFLUENZA INFECTIONS

Background

Influenza, though usually a mild and self-contained illness, has the potential to cause significant morbidity as it spreads extensively in the community. While in the last few years, the world was contemplating if the avian influenza virus (H5N1) would adapt for human spread, the recent outbreak of the swine origin virus (H1N1) has surprised many. It continues to be an important cause of mortality.

Epidemiology

Influenza A outbreaks occur almost every year, although their extent and severity vary widely. In the last century, influenza virus caused three pandemics: the Spanish flu in 1918, the Asian flu in 1957, and the Hong Kong flu in 1968. These outbreaks have differed in the extent of spread, the severity of the illness as well as the responsible pathogen (1). The 1918 pandemic, which has often been cited as the most widespread and severe among these, was caused by the H1N1 strain and affected nearly a third of the world's population. It left in its wake nearly 40 million deaths and probably even contributed to the end of the First World War (2). After the control of this outbreak the virus went back to its usual pattern of causing smaller epidemics until in 1957, an antigenically distinct form of the virus again emerged globally in immunologically naïve population. This strain was the H2N2 strain. However, only 11 years after it was first detected, this virus strain was replaced by the H3N2 strain. Until recently this was the major form of influenza in humans (1). The novel H1N1 strain, which is responsible for the current outbreak of swine origin influenza, was first recognized at the border between Mexico and United States in April 2009, and during a short span of 2 months became the first pandemic of the 21st century (3). Prior to this, the same triple-reassorted virus had been isolated in swine as early as 1998 with sporadic infections in humans as well. This outbreak has been a pandemic in the true sense of the term, involving >170 countries and spread over all the continents.

Influenza infections generally have well-defined seasonality. Epidemics usually occur in winter months in the temperate zones. The circulation of the virus in the winters in the Southern Hemisphere sustains influenza viruses when the Northern Hemisphere has summer.

Virus

The influenza virus is a negative-sense RNA virus of the family Orthomyxoviridae with three genera: influenza A, B, and C (4). Influenza A and B viruses are the most important in human disease and, therefore, have been studied more extensively than have influenza C viruses. These viruses have the property of hemagglutination, and influenza A and B also possess the enzyme neuraminidase (NA). These properties reside on a pair of surface glycoproteins, hemagglutinin (HA) and NA for types A and B; however, influenza C has a single glycoprotein with HA, esterase, and fusion activity.

Influenza A is further subtyped into 16 distinct H types and 9 distinct N types based on the HA and NA antigens on the surface of the virus (5). Every year new strains of the virus emerge as its genes undergo continuous point mutations leading to an "antigenic drift." This helps the virus evade host defenses (6). Another characteristic of type A influenza, which is not shared by type B influenza, is that the virus has a segmented genome with eight single-stranded RNA segments. Thus, when the host cell is infected with more than one influenza virus, which is often the case, these genes have the opportunity to get reassorted and produce a very different strain altogether. This "antigenic shift" is responsible for pandemics of influenza, which have been observed in the past (4). The currently circulating strain of swine origin influenza virus of the H1N1 strain has undergone triple reassortment and contains genes from the avian, swine, and human viruses (7). It is believed to be a legacy of the influenza pandemic of the 1918–1919 virus, having adapted over the last nine decades and has now acquired the ability to not only infect but also spread within the human host (5).

Transmission

The most common mode of natural influenza transmission is by inhalation of airborne particles produced by coughing and sneezing (microdroplet method). It can also be spread by direct contact and large-particle aerosols. Unlike other type A influenza virus, which are transmitted by small droplet nuclei, the swine origin influenza virus is transmitted by large-particle respiratory droplets and hence requires a <6-feet distance between the source and the susceptible individual to be present for effective spread.

Importance to Intensivist

Most of the cases of influenza in children are managed on an ambulatory basis. Of the children needing hospitalization, ~15% need ICU care (8). The mortality in hospitalized children is ~0.5%. In addition to the respiratory illness, influenza may also present as encephalopathy, myocarditis, myositis, or with bacterial (particularly *Staphylococcus aureus*) coinfection.

Pathophysiology

Influenza virus predominantly infects the ciliated columnar epithelial cells in the respiratory tract. The receptor on the viral HA attaches to a sialic acid moiety on the cell membrane, following which the virus is endocytosed. Creation of an acid environment by the ion channel activity of the M2 protein and the fusion activity of the HA leads to fusion of the lipid coat with the cell membrane and the entry of the viral RNA into the cytoplasm.

The infection causes necrosis of the ciliated epithelial cells, which is evident early in the clinical course. The virus has cytopathic effects. Usually the immunocompetent hosts are able to control influenza infection by innate and adaptive immune responses; this limits the clinical effects to mild illness. Some of the reassorted influenza viruses are able to replicate more efficiently and can evade the immune responses and may be able to infect lung causing pneumonia.

Many of the symptoms of influenza may be due to the cytokines released in response to the infection. It has been hypothesized that cytokine storm plays an important and essential role in causing significant tissue injury and mortality following influenza virus infection (9,10). Arankalle et al. (11) analyzed viral load in lungs of critically ill patients who died and those who recovered. Both groups showed roughly equivalent titers of virus. In contrast, mortality correlated directly with cytokine storm. Thus, the patients who died had higher cytokine/chemokine levels but equivalent viral titers in pulmonary samples when compared to patients having a milder infection course and recovering. Oldstone et al. (10) have shown that blockade of cytokine storm provided greater protection than antiviral therapy to inhibit virus replication and does so without compromising the host's ability to control and terminate influenza virus infection. They have suggested a protective role for sphingosine-1-phosphate receptors on the pulmonary endothelial cells in the pathogenesis. Some of the reassorted influenza viruses have the ability to infect the lung tissue and also induce an exaggerated immune response that lead to very severe and often fatal pneumonia (9).

Pneumonia associated with influenza virus infections may result from primary viral infection, bacterial superinfection, or combined bacterial–viral infection. Severe influenza pneumonia is characterized by diffuse hemorrhagic alveolar exudates, necrosis of bronchiolar epithelium, peribronchial lymphocytic infiltration, and marked lymphocytic infiltration of the alveolar walls and interstitial lung tissue (12). In severe cases, other organ systems are also affected as manifested by focal and diffuse myocarditis, mediastinal lymph node enlargement and necrosis, and cerebral edema. Reye syndrome is associated with influenza, particularly type B, and with the use of salicylates in children with influenza infection.

Encephalopathy and encephalitis associated with influenza have been reported in children. This complication is being increasingly recognized (13,14). The pathogenesis of influenza-related encephalopathy is still not clear; it is hypothesized that viral invasion of the central nervous system (CNS), proinflammatory cytokines, metabolic disorders, or genetic susceptibility may have a role (13).

Clinical Features

Clinical features of mild influenza infection are similar to many other viral respiratory tract infections. Some clinical features have been seen more commonly in children: —sudden onset symptoms, anorexia, abdominal pain, vomiting, nausea, cervical adenopathy, and temperature >38.9°C. Influenza C viruses cause less severe disease and the duration of the symptoms is shorter. Influenza B may cause an epidemic in which children have typical symptoms of influenza with fever, but many adults in the population will have only mild upper respiratory tract symptoms without significant fever. This is because antigenic changes in influenza B viruses are less frequent; adults are more likely to have protective immunity. In contrast to adults, greater proportion of children is likely to have gastrointestinal manifestations. Some of the younger children may present with febrile seizures.

In uncomplicated illness, the fever usually persists for 2–3 days. A biphasic temperature pattern may occur. Respiratory tract symptoms become more prominent by the second to the fourth day as systemic complaints begin to subside. Dry and hacking cough usually persists for 4–7 days. Nasal and eye complaints are more prominent in influenza B virus infections, and as compared to influenza A infections, systemic complaints like dizziness and prostration are less common.

Recently, many investigators have reported on the clinical features of children hospitalized with pandemic H1N1 influenza infection (15). Randolph et al. (15) described the clinical features of children with confirmed or probable pH1N1 admitted to 35 US PICUs from April 15, 2009 to April 15, 2010 (15). Commonly reported influenza-related signs and symptoms included fever (79%), cough (73%), shortness of breath (54%), vomiting (30%), diarrhea (12%), and seizures (10%) with the median onset 3 days (interquartile range [IQR]: 1–5) ($n = 694$) before PICU admission. At presentation, nearly 10% received vasopressors for shock, 1.3% were in cardiac arrest, and 3.5% had suspected CNS complications. Most patients (64%) presented with evidence of acute lower respiratory disease; 57.5% received assisted breathing on the day of PICU admission (excluding 27 patients on chronic mechanical ventilation) and 8.9% died. Independent risk factors for mortality were female gender, presence of a chronic neurologic condition or immune compromise, diagnosis of acute myocarditis or encephalitis, and early presumed methicillin-resistant *S. aureus* (MRSA) coinfection of the lung. For the 30% of children who were previously healthy, only early presumed MRSA coinfection of the lung, which increased the relative risk (RR) of death eightfold, was strongly associated with mortality.

Risk Factors

Children under 2 years of age, especially infants under 6 months of age, constitute the highest risk group. Any comorbidity appears to increase the risk of severe influenza, but chronic lung diseases (e.g., asthma), neurologic or neuromuscular disorders (cerebral palsy), immunosuppression, diabetes mellitus, and morbid obesity stand out some of the more prevalent comorbid conditions that increase risk of severe disease (16).

Differential Diagnosis

In an intensive care setting, diagnosis of influenza should be considered in children admitted with lower respiratory tract infections. The differential diagnoses include pneumonias due to other pathogens including bacteria and viruses. Though uncommon, influenza could be the causative organism for myocarditis and encephalopathy.

Diagnosis

The definite diagnosis of influenza can be made by the detection of antigen or isolation of virus from respiratory tract secretions or by demonstrating a significant rise in serum antibody during convalescence. *Reverse transcription polymerase chain reaction (RT-PCR)* has been an important advance in the diagnosis of influenza. This has >90% sensitivity versus a 60%–70% sensitivity of the antigen-detecting techniques that use *fluorescent antibodies*. RT-PCR test results require a 2-day turnaround time such that initial therapeutic decision making must often proceed based on clinical criteria alone. Now various multiplex quantitative RT-PCR are available that allow identification of all the important respiratory viruses of children: influenza, parainfluenza, RSV, metapneumovirus, and adenovirus. The sensitivity of the *rapid antigen* test is much lower than RT-PCR and highly variable depending on virus types, sampling techniques, patient age, and duration of illness. Even though this test result is available within 10–30 minutes, a negative rapid antigen test does not rule out influenza.

Management

In addition to the supportive care required for management of critically ill children with influenza, specific antiviral therapy is indicated. The antiviral drugs include M2 protein inhibitors (amantadine and rimantadine) and NA inhibitors (oseltamivir and zanamivir). The inhaled inhibitor zanamivir is approved for use in children 5 years of age and older. Oseltamivir is available for children >2 weeks of age. Oseltamivir and zanamivir appear to have modest benefit in reducing duration of illness in children with influenza (17). Amantadine–rimantadine resistance of influenza A virus results from point mutations of the M2 protein and is being increasingly reported. Hence, Centers for Disease Control and Prevention (CDC) does not currently recommend amantadine and rimantadine (http://www.cdc.gov/flu/professionals/). New and possibly more effective antiviral drugs such as peramivir, laninamivir, and favipiravir have been developed but have not yet been approved for use in United States.

The CDC recommends influenza antiviral treatment for (http://www.cdc.gov/flu/professionals/antivirals/antiviral-use-influenza.htm#indications):

■ Suspected or confirmed influenza infection in children at high risk for complications (see risk factors discussed earlier)
■ Any child hospitalized with suspected influenza regardless of immunization status
■ Children with suspected influenza experiencing or severe complicated course

Treatment should not be delayed while waiting confirmatory tests. Providers should exercise discretion in the use of antiviral therapy for otherwise healthy children, because indiscriminate use may promote viral resistance and deplete available drug supplies.

Prognosis

The prognosis of uncomplicated influenza is usually good. Complications of influenza such as primary influenza pneumonia, staphylococcal pneumonia, encephalitis, and Reye syndrome have a guarded prognosis. Recent studies have reported a poorer prognosis in children with underlying chronic diseases.

HIV INFECTION IN THE CRITICALLY ILL CHILD

HIV infection continues to be an important contributor to childhood morbidity and mortality, especially in many developing countries. The pandemic has undone many of the significant gains in child health. Increasing numbers of infants and children with HIV infection/AIDS are being admitted to PICUs, particularly in certain geographic areas, and a significant proportion of these patients may be first diagnosed during their PICU stay. Most patients are admitted because of respiratory infections and respiratory failure, septic shock, and CNS disorders (18,19). As the number of children receiving antiretroviral therapy increases, severe complications of therapy may also become indications for PICU admission (20). In addition to patient-specific issues, the unique stresses on medical and nursing staff members who care for HIV-infected children require attention and management. Specific infection control, nutritional, and medicolegal strategies will facilitate safe, effective delivery of care to HIV-infected infants and children in the PICU.

Epidemiology

The WHO estimated that, at the end of 2011, nearly 34 million persons worldwide were living with HIV infection; 3.3

million of these were children under 15 years of age (21). In 2011 alone, 1.7 million people were estimated to have died owing to AIDS, including 230,000 children. In 2011, an estimated 330,000 children were newly infected with HIV. More than 90% of HIV-infected individuals live in developing nations. Sub-Saharan Africa accounts for nearly 90% of the world's total population of HIV-infected children. India and Thailand dominate the epidemic in Southeast Asia, with more recent expansion into Vietnam, China, and Cambodia. Worldwide, it is estimated that in 2011, only 28% of children 0–14 years old who were eligible were receiving the life-saving medicines. Without access to antiretroviral therapy, 20% of children who are infected by their mothers (i.e., vertically infected) will progress to AIDS or death during their first year of life, and more than half of HIV-infected children will die before their fifth birthday.

In the United States, virtually all HIV infections in children who are under 13 years of age are the result of vertical transmission from an HIV-infected mother. A minority of children (2%) were infected through receipt of contaminated blood products and/or clotting factors. Vertical transmission is also the major mode of transmission in other parts of the world, but blood, blood products, and unsafe injections contribute to pediatric HIV infection, as well.

HIV-1 and HIV-2

HIV-1 and HIV-2 are members of the Retroviridae family and belong to the *Lentivirus* genus. The HIV-1 genome is single-stranded RNA that is 9.2 kb in size. Long terminal repeats at both ends contain the regulation and expression genes of HIV. The genome has three major sections: the gag region, which encodes the viral core proteins (p24, p17, p9, p6, all derived from the precursor p55); the pol region, which encodes the viral enzymes (reverse transcriptase [p51], protease [p10], and integrase [p32]); and the env region, which encodes the viral envelope proteins (gp120 and gp41, both derived from the precursor gp160). The other products of the genome are regulatory proteins such as tat (pl4), rev (p19), nef (p27), vpr (p15), and vif (p23) (22).

The major external viral protein of HIV-1 is a heavily glycosylated gp120 protein that is associated with the transmembrane glycoprotein gp41. The gp120 contains the binding site for the CD4 molecule, the most common T lymphocyte surface receptor for HIV. Several chemokines serve as coreceptors for the envelope glycoproteins, permitting membrane fusion and entry into the cell. Most HIV strains have a specific tropism for one of the chemokines: the fusion-inducing molecule CXCR4, which has been shown to act as a coreceptor for HIV attachment to lymphocytes, and CCR5, a β-chemokine receptor that facilitates HIV entry into macrophages. Other mechanisms of attachment of HIV to cells are nonneutralizing antiviral antibodies and complement receptors. Following viral attachment, gp120 and the CD4 molecule undergo conformational changes, allowing gp41 to interact with the fusion receptor on the cell surface. Viral fusion with the cell membrane allows entry of viral RNA into the cell cytoplasm. Viral DNA copies are then transcribed from the virion RNA through viral reverse transcriptase enzyme activity, and duplication of the DNA copies produces double-stranded circular DNA. Because the HIV-1 reverse transcriptase is error-prone, many mutations arise, creating wide genetic variation in HIV-1 isolates, even within an individual patient. The circular DNA is transported into the cell nucleus, where it is integrated into chromosomal DNA; this is called the *provirus*. The provirus can remain dormant for extended periods.

HIV-1 transcription is followed by translation. A capsid polyprotein is cleaved to produce, among other products, the virus-specific protease (p10). This enzyme is critical for HIV-1 assembly. The RNA genome is then incorporated into the newly formed viral capsid. As the new virus is formed, it buds through the cell membrane and is released.

HIV diversity, leading to multiple viral groups (groups M [main], O [outlier], N [non-M, non-O]), probably originated from multiple zoonotic infections found in primates in different geographic regions. Group M then diversified to several subtypes (or clades A–H). In each region of the world, certain clades predominate. For example, clade B is found in South America, clade E in Thailand, and clade C in South Africa. Clades are mixed in some patients because of HIV recombination, and some crossing between groups (i.e., M and O) has been reported.

HIV-2 is a rare cause of infection in children. It is most prevalent in Western and Southern Africa. If HIV-2 is suspected, a specific test that detects antibody to HIV-2 peptides should be used.

Transmission

Transmission of HIV-1 occurs via sexual contact, parenteral exposure to blood, or vertical transmission from mother to child. The primary route of infection in the pediatric population is vertical transmission, accounting for virtually all new cases in developed countries. Most large studies in the Unites States and Europe have documented mother-to-child transmission rates in untreated women to be between 12% and 30%. In contrast, transmission rates in Africa and Asia are higher, up to 50%. Perinatal treatment of HIV-infected mothers with antiretroviral drugs has dramatically decreased these rates (23,24).

Vertical transmission of HIV can occur during the intrauterine or intrapartum periods or through breast-feeding. Up to 30% of infected newborns are infected in utero. The highest percentages of HIV-infected children acquire the virus intrapartum. Breast-feeding is an important route of transmission, especially in developing countries. A meta-analysis of prospective studies found that the additional risk of transmission through breast-feeding in women with HIV infection before pregnancy was 14%, compared with a 29% increase in breast-feeding women who acquired HIV postnatally (25). The risk factors for vertical transmission include preterm delivery (<34 weeks gestation), a low maternal antenatal CD4 count, use of illicit drugs during pregnancy, >4 hour duration of ruptured membranes, and birth weight <2500 g (24).

Transfusions of infected blood or blood products have accounted for a variable proportion of all pediatric AIDS cases. Heat treatment of factor VIII concentrate and HIV antibody screening of donors have virtually eliminated HIV transmission to children with hemophilia. Blood donor screening has dramatically reduced, but not eliminated, the risk of transfusion-associated HIV infection. In many developing countries, where screening of blood donors is not uniform, the risk of transmitting HIV infection via transfusion is still significant.

Although HIV can be isolated rarely from saliva, it is in very low titers (<1 infectious particle/mL) and has not been implicated as a transmission vehicle. In younger children, sexual transmission is infrequent, but a small number of cases that resulted from sexual abuse have been reported. In contrast, sexual contact is a major route of transmission in the adolescent population, accounting for most cases.

Pathogenesis

When the mucosa is the portal of entry for HIV, the first cells to be infected are the dendritic cells, which process the antigens introduced and transport them to the lymphoid tissue.

In the lymph node, HIV selectively binds to cells expressing CD4 molecules on their surface, primarily helper T lymphocytes (CD4 cells), and cells of the monocyte–macrophage lineage. Other cells bearing CD4, such as microglia, astrocytes, oligodendroglia, and placental tissue containing villous Hofbauer cells, may also be infected by HIV. CD4 lymphocytes migrate to the lymph nodes that house-infected cells, where they become activated and proliferate, making them highly susceptible to HIV infection. This antigen-driven migration and accumulation of CD4 cells within the lymphoid tissue may contribute to the generalized lymphadenopathy characteristic of the acute retroviral syndrome in adults and adolescents. HIV preferentially infects the very cells that respond to it (i.e., HIV-specific memory CD4 cells), which accounts for the progressive loss of response by these cells and the subsequent loss of control of HIV replication. Usually within 3–6 weeks from the time of infection, a burst of plasma viremia occurs. With establishment of a cellular and humoral immune response within the following 2–4 months, the viral load in the blood declines substantially, and patients enter a phase that is characterized by a lack of symptoms and a return of CD4 cells to only moderately decreased levels (22). Unlike in adults, early HIV-1 replication in children has no apparent clinical manifestations. The viral load increases by 1–4 months, and almost all HIV-infected infants have detectable HIV-1 in peripheral blood by 4 months of age.

In adults and teenagers, the long period of clinical latency (often up to 8–12 years) is not indicative of viral latency. In fact, a very high turnover of virus and CD4 lymphocytes (>1 billion cells/day) occurs, which gradually causes deterioration of the immune system, evidenced particularly by depletion of CD4 cells. These cells may be destroyed by multiple mechanisms: HIV-mediated single-cell killing, formation of multinucleated giant cells of infected and uninfected CD4 cells (syncytia formation), virus-specific immune responses, superantigen-mediated activation of T cells (rendering them more susceptible to infection with HIV), and programmed cell death (apoptosis). The viral burden in the lymphoid organs is greater than that in the peripheral blood during the asymptomatic period. Cell-mediated and humoral responses occur early in the infection. The CD8 T cells play an important role in containing the infection. HIV-specific cytotoxic T lymphocytes (CTLs) develop against both the structural (i.e., env, pol, gag) and regulatory (e.g., tat) viral proteins. The CTL cells control the infection by killing HIV-infected cells before new viruses are produced and by secreting potent antiviral factors that compete with the virus for its receptors (e.g., CCR5). Neutralizing antibodies appear later during the infection and seem to help in the continued suppression of viral replication during clinical latency (22).

Before highly active antiretroviral therapy (HAART) was available, three distinct patterns of disease were described in children. Approximately 10%–20% of HIV-infected newborns in developed countries presented with a rapid disease course, with onset of AIDS and symptoms during the first few months of life and, if untreated, death from AIDS-related complications by 4 years of age (26). In resource-poor countries, >85% of the HIV-infected newborns may have such a rapidly progressing disease.

It has been suggested that if intrauterine infection coincides with the period of rapid expansion of CD4 cells in the fetus, it could effectively infect the majority of the body's immunocompetent cells. Most children in this group have a positive HIV-1 culture and/or detectable virus in the plasma within the first 48 hours of life. This early evidence of viral presence suggests that the newborn was infected in utero. In contrast to the viral load in adults, the viral load in infants remains high for at least the first 2 years of life.

The majority of perinatally infected newborns (60%–80%) present with a second pattern—a much slower progression of disease with a median survival time of 6 years. Many patients in this group have a negative viral culture or PCR in the first week of life and are therefore considered to be infected intrapartum. In a typical patient, the viral load rapidly increases by 2–3 months of age (median, 100,000 copies/mL) and then slowly declines over a period of 24 months. This observation can be explained partially by the immaturity of the immune system in newborns and infants. The third pattern of disease (i.e., long-term survivors) occurs in a small percentage (<5%) of perinatally infected children who have minimal or no progression of disease with relatively normal CD4 counts and very low viral loads for longer than 8 years.

HIV-infected children have changes in the immune system that are similar to those in HIV-infected adults. CD4 cell depletion may be less dramatic because infants normally have a relative lymphocytosis. Therefore, for example, a value of 750 CD4 cells/mm^3 in children <1 year of age is indicative of severe CD4 depletion and is comparable to <200 CD4 cells/mm^3 in adults. Lymphopenia is relatively rare in perinatally infected children and is usually only seen in older children or those with end-stage disease.

B-cell activation occurs in most children early in the infection, as evidenced by hypergammaglobulinemia associated with high levels of anti-HIV-1 antibody. This response may reflect both dysregulation of T-cell suppression of B-cell antibody synthesis and active CD4 enhancement of B lymphocyte humoral responses. CD4 depletion and inadequate antibody responses lead to increased susceptibility to various infections, and the clinical manifestations vary with the severity of immunodeficiency.

Clinical Manifestations

The clinical manifestations of HIV infection vary widely among infants, children, and adolescents. In most infants, physical examination at birth is normal. Initial signs and symptoms may be subtle and nonspecific, such as lymphadenopathy, hepatosplenomegaly, failure to thrive, chronic or recurrent diarrhea, interstitial pneumonia, or oral thrush, and they may be distinguishable from other causes only by their persistence. Whereas systemic and pulmonary findings are common in the Unite States and Europe, chronic diarrhea, wasting, and severe malnutrition predominate in Africa. Symptoms found more commonly in children than in adults include recurrent bacterial infections, chronic parotid swelling, lymphoid interstitial pneumonitis (LIP), and early onset of progressive neurologic deterioration. The HIV classification system is used to categorize the stage of pediatric disease via two parameters: clinical status (**Table 90.1**) and degree of immunologic impairment (**Table 90.2**).

The Spectrum of Diseases in the PICU

The reasons for PICU admission among HIV-infected children may or may not be related to their HIV infection. The causes of PICU admission unrelated to the HIV infection are usually similar to those found in non–HIV-infected children of comparable age. Many children with clinically unsuspected HIV infection are treated in PICUs. In the early stages of the illness, when the immunosuppression is not severe, the children are likely to respond to standard management. In patients with significant immunosuppression, the prognosis is determined by its severity.

The most common HIV-related diseases that lead to PICU admission are respiratory infections and respiratory failure, septic shock, and disorders of the CNS (18,19). Acute respiratory failure secondary to *Pneumocystis jirovecii* or bacterial

infections is the most important cause of PICU admission. Pneumocystis pneumonia is common in HIV-infected children with severe immunodeficiency, and if untreated, is universally fatal.

Respiratory Diseases Complicating HIV Infection

While acute respiratory failure secondary to pneumocystis pneumonia remains one of the most frequent causes of PICU admission among HIV-infected children, the initial diagnostic evaluation of HIV-infected children with respiratory distress should always consider the other causes of infectious pneumonitis: bacterial, fungal, mycobacterial, and viral infections.

Pneumocystis jirovecii Pneumonia. Pneumocystis pneumonia (PCP) is the opportunistic infection that led to the initial description of AIDS. PCP is one of the commonest AIDS-defining illnesses in children in the United States and Europe. However, data regarding the incidence of PCP in children in other parts of the world are scarce. The majority of the cases occur at between 3 and 6 months of life (27). For further details, refer to Chapter 95.

Even if a child develops PCP while on prophylaxis, therapy may be started with trimethoprim/sulfamethoxazole, as the prophylaxis may have failed because of poor compliance or unusual pharmacokinetics. Drug resistance may also be the cause, in which case the use of one of the alternative drugs is recommended. Untreated, PCP is universally fatal. With the use of appropriate therapy, the mortality decreases to <10%. The risk factors for mortality are the severity of the episode and the severity of the immunosuppression.

Recurrent Bacterial Infections. Both cell-mediated and humoral immunity fail as HIV infection progresses. Despite hypergammaglobulinemia, HIV-infected children are at risk for severe and recurrent bacterial infections. Delay in clearing infections may also be caused by the usual pathogens. In various studies from developing countries, up to 90% of HIV-infected children had history of recurrent pneumonias. Initial episodes of pneumonia often occur before the development of significant immunosuppression. As the immunosuppression increases, the frequency increases. The common pathogens for community-acquired pneumonia in these children are *Streptococcus pneumoniae*, *Haemophilus influenzae*, and *Staphylococcus aureus*. However, in children with severe immunosuppression and in hospital-acquired infections, gram-negative organisms, such as *Pseudomonas aeruginosa*, gain importance. The clinical features of pneumonia in HIV-infected children are similar to those in uninfected children. However, in severely immunocompromised children, the signs may be subtle. Often, the response to therapy is slow, and the relapse rates are high. Bacteremia may be more common, seen in up to 50%.

While attempts should be made to isolate the causative organism, such efforts should not delay empirical therapy. Sick children with pneumonia should be treated with parenteral antibiotics. Choices of appropriate antibiotics are often made based on local patterns of etiologies and susceptibilities. In many settings, an appropriate choice would be a combination of a broad-spectrum cephalosporin and an aminoglycoside. In areas where a large proportion of *S. aureus* isolates are resistant to antistaphylococcal antibiotics (MRSA), the empiric inclusion of vancomycin, clindamycin, linezolid, or other drugs to which community-acquired MRSA is usually susceptible should be considered. Children with nonsevere pneumonia can be managed as out-patients with a second- or a third-generation cephalosporin or a combination, such as amoxicillin–clavulanic acid. As *P. jirovecii* pneumonia cannot be excluded at the outset in most HIV-infected children with severe respiratory infections, co-trimoxazole should be added unless another diagnosis has been definitively made.

TABLE·90.1

CLINICAL CATEGORIES OF HUMAN IMMUNODEFICIENCY VIRUS INFECTION

Clinical Category N
    Children who have no signs or symptoms considered to be the result of HIV infection or who have only one of the conditions
        listed in Category A
Clinical Category A
    Children with two or more of the conditions listed below but none of the conditions listed in Categories B and C
    Lymphadenopathy (≥0.5 cm at >2 sites; bilateral = 1 site)
    Hepatomegaly
    Splenomegaly
    Dermatitis
    Parotitis
    Recurrent or persistent upper respiratory infection, sinusitis, or otitis media
Clinical Category B
    Children who have symptomatic conditions other than those listed for Category A or C that are attributed to HIV infection.
        Examples of conditions in clinical Category B include but are not limited to:
    Anemia (<8 g/dL), neutropenia (<1000/mm^3), or thrombocytopenia (<100,000/mm^3) persisting for at least 30 d
    Bacterial meningitis, pneumonia, or sepsis (single episode)
    Candidiasis, oropharyngeal (thrush), persisting for >2 mo in children >6 mo of age
    Cardiomyopathy
    Cytomegalovirus infection, with onset before 1 mo of age
    Diarrhea, recurrent or chronic
    Hepatitis
    HSV stomatitis, recurrent (more than two episodes within 1 y)
    HSV bronchitis, pneumonitis, or esophagitis, with onset before 1 mo of age
    Herpes zoster (shingles) involving at least two distinct episodes or >1 dermatome
    Leiomyosarcoma
    Lymphoid interstitial pneumonia
    Nephropathy
    Nocardiosis
    Persistent fever (lasting >1 mo)
    Toxoplasmosis, onset before 1 mo of age
    Varicella, disseminated
Clinical Category C
    Serious bacterial infections, multiple or recurrent (i.e., any combination of at least two culture-confirmed infections within a
        2-year period), of the following types: septicemia, pneumonia, meningitis, bone or joint infection, or abscess of an internal organ
        or body cavity (excluding otitis media, superficial skin or mucosal abscesses, and indwelling catheter-related infections)
    Candidiasis, esophageal or pulmonary (bronchi, trachea, lungs)
    Coccidioidomycosis, disseminated (at site other than, or in addition to, lungs or cervical or hilar lymph nodes)
    Cryptococcosis, extrapulmonary
    Cryptosporidiosis or isosporiasis with diarrhea persisting >1 mo
    Cytomegalovirus disease, with onset of symptoms at age >1 mo (at a site other than liver, spleen, or lymph nodes)
    Encephalopathy (at least one of the following progressive findings present for at least 2 mo in the absence of a concurrent illness
        other than HIV infection that could explain the findings):
        (a) failure to attain or loss of developmental milestones, or loss of intellectual ability, verified by standard developmental scale or
        neuropsychological tests
        (b) impaired brain growth or acquired microcephaly demonstrated by head circumference measurements or brain atrophy dem-
        onstrated by CT or MRI (serial imaging is required for children <2 y of age)
        (c) acquired symmetric motor deficit manifested by two or more of the following: paresis, pathologic reflexes, ataxia, or gait
        disturbance
    HSV infection causing a mucocutaneous ulcer that persists for >1 mo; or bronchitis, pneumonitis, or esophagitis for any duration
        affecting a child >1 mo of age
    Histoplasmosis, disseminated (at a site other than, or in addition to, lungs or cervical or hilar lymph nodes)
    Kaposi sarcoma
    Lymphoma, primary, in brain
    Lymphoma, small, noncleaved cell (Burkitt syndrome), or immunoblastic or large cell lymphoma of B-cell or unknown
        immunologic phenotype
    Mycobacterium TB, disseminated or extrapulmonary
    Mycobacterium, other species or unidentified species, disseminated (at a site other than, or in addition to, lungs, skin, or cervical
        or hilar lymph nodes)
    Mycobacterium avium complex or *M. kansasii*, disseminated (at site other than, or in addition to, lungs, skin, or cervical or hilar
        lymph nodes)
    Pneumocystis jirovecii pneumonia
    Progressive multifocal leukoencephalopathy
    Salmonella (nontyphoid) septicemia, recurrent

Toxoplasmosis of the brain with onset at >1 mo of age
Wasting syndrome in the absence of a concurrent illness other than HIV infection that could explain the following findings:
  (a) persistent weight loss >10% of baseline, *OR*
  (b) downward crossing of at least two of the following percentile lines on the weight-for-age chart (e.g., 95th, 75th, 50th, 25th, 5th) in a child at least 1 y of age, *OR*
  (c) <5th percentile on weight-for-height chart on two consecutive measurements at least 30 d apart, *PLUS*
     (i) chronic diarrhea (i.e., at least two loose stools per day for >30 d), OR
     (ii) documented fever (for at least 30 d, intermittent or constant)

HIV, human immunodeficiency virus; HSV, herpes simplex virus; TB, tuberculosis.
From Centers for Disease Control and Prevention. 1994 revised classification system for human immunodeficiency virus infection in children less than 13 years of age. *MMWR* 1994;43:6–8.

The principles of supportive care of HIV-infected children admitted to PICU with severe pneumonia are similar to those in non–HIV-infected children.

Tuberculosis. With the spread of the HIV infection, a resurgence in tuberculosis (TB) has occurred. Coexistent TB and HIV infections accelerate the progression of both diseases. HIV-infected children are more likely to have extrapulmonary and disseminated TB; the course is also likely to be more rapid. An HIV-infected child with tubercular infection is more likely to develop the disease than a child without HIV infection. The overall risk of active TB in children who are infected with HIV is at least 5- to 10-fold higher than that in uninfected children (28) (see Chapter 95).

All HIV-infected children with active TB should receive long-duration antitubercular therapy; a 9–12-month therapy is preferred. The American Academy of Pediatrics recommends a total duration of 12 months of anti-TB therapy for children infected with HIV, while the American Thoracic Society/Centers for Disease Control recommend a total of 6 months of therapy, regardless of HIV status (29). A close follow-up is essential to diagnose nonresponse/drug resistance early.

Infection with *Mycobacterium avium-intracellulare*. Pulmonary disease with *Mycobacterium avium-intracellulare* is uncommon in children with HIV infection, despite immunosuppression. The common symptoms and signs include persistent fever, failure to thrive, night sweats, lymphadenopathy, organomegaly, and refractory anemia. The pulmonary lesions are usually limited to lymphadenopathy and localized parenchymal lesions. The diagnosis of disseminated disease primarily depends on isolation of the organism from blood. Current therapy for disseminated *M. avium-intracellulare* infection involves use of a combination of clarithromycin or azithromycin with ethambutol.

Viral Infections. Infections caused by RSV, influenza, and parainfluenza viruses result in symptomatic disease more often in HIV-infected children, in comparison to noninfected children. Infections with other viruses, such as adenovirus and measles virus, are more likely to lead to serious sequelae than are the previously mentioned viruses. As RSV infection most often occurs in children in the first 2 years of life, during which many may not be severely immunocompromised, the severity of illness may not be different from the non–HIV-infected children. In children with AIDS, disseminated cytomegalovirus is a known opportunistic infection, but pneumonia caused by this virus is rare. The principles of diagnosis and treatment of these infections in HIV-infected children are similar to those in non–HIV-infected children.

Fungal Infections. Pulmonary fungal infections usually present as a part of disseminated disease in immunocompromised children. Primary pulmonary fungal infections are uncommon. Pulmonary candidiasis should be suspected in any HIV-infected child with lower respiratory tract infection that does not respond to the common therapeutic modalities. A positive blood culture supports the diagnosis of invasive candidiasis. For other fungal infections, refer to Chapter 95.

Lymphoid Interstitial Pneumonitis. LIP has been recognized as a distinctive marker for pediatric HIV infection and is included as a Class B condition in the revised CDC criteria for AIDS in children. In the absence of antiretroviral therapy, nearly 20% of HIV-infected children develop LIP. The etiology and pathogenesis of LIP are not well understood. Suggested

TABLE 90.2

IMMUNOLOGIC CATEGORIES BASED ON AGE-SPECIFIC CD4 T LYMPHOCYTE COUNTS IN CHILDREN WITH HIV INFECTION

IMMUNOLOGIC CATEGORIES	Age of Child					
	■ <12 MO		■ 1–5 Y		■ 6–12 Y	
	■ CELLS/MM³	■ %	■ CELLS/MM³	■ %	■ CELLS/MM³	■ %
No evidence of suppression	≥1500	≥25	≥1000	≥25	≥500	≥25
Moderate suppression	750–1499	15–24	500–999	15–24	200–499	15–24
Severe suppression	>750	<15	<500	<15	<200	<15

From Centers for Disease Control and Prevention. 1994 revised classification system for human immunodeficiency virus infection in children less than 13 years of age. *MMWR* 1994;43:6–8.

etiologies include an exaggerated immunologic response to in-haled or circulating antigens and/or primary infection of the lung with HIV, Epstein–Barr virus (EBV), or both. LIP is char-acterized by nodule formation and diffuse infiltration of the alveolar septae by lymphocytes, plasmacytoid lymphocytes, plasma cells, and immunoblasts. No involvement of the blood vessels or destruction of the lung tissue occurs.

LIP is usually diagnosed in children with perinatally ac-quired HIV infection when they are >1 year of age, unlike with PCP. Most children with LIP are asymptomatic. Tachy-pnea, cough, wheezing, and hypoxemia may be seen when children present with more severe manifestations; crepitations are uncommon. Clubbing is often present in advanced disease. These patients can progress to chronic respiratory failure. Long-standing LIP may be associated with chronic bronchi-ectasis. The presence of a reticulonodular pattern, with or without hilar lymphadenopathy, that persists on chest x-ray for 2 months or greater and that is unresponsive to antimicro-bial therapy is considered presumptive evidence of LIP. Care should be taken to exclude other possible etiologies. A de-finitive diagnosis of LIP can only be made by histopathology. Children with LIP have a relatively good prognosis compared to other children who meet the CDC surveillance definition of AIDS. However, children with severe disease are likely to manifest with respiratory failure.

Early disease is managed conservatively. The effect of anti-retrovirals on LIP is probably limited. Steroids are indicated if children with LIP have symptoms and signs of chronic pulmo-nary disease, clubbing, and/or hypoxemia. Treatment usually includes an initial 4–12-week course of prednisolone (2 mg/kg/day), followed by a tapering dose, using oxygen saturation and clinical status as a guide to improvement. This treatment is then followed by chronic low-dose prednisolone.

Gastrointestinal Diseases

The pathologic changes in the gastrointestinal tract of chil-dren with AIDS are variable and can be clinically significant. However, only a few conditions may be indications for admis-sion to a PICU. A variety of microbes can cause gastroin-testinal disease, including bacteria (*Salmonella*, *Campylobacter*, *M. avium-intracellulare* complex), protozoa (*Giardia*, *Crypto-sporidium*, *Isospora*, microsporidia), viruses (cytomegalovirus, herpes simplex virus [HSV], rotavirus), and fungi (*Candida*). The protozoal infections are most severe and can be pro-tracted in children with severe immunosuppression. Children with cryptosporidium infestation can have severe diarrhea that leads to hypovolemic shock, which may merit admission to the PICU. AIDS enteropathy, a syndrome of malabsorption with partial villous atrophy not associated with a specific pathogen, is probably the result of direct HIV infection of the gut.

HIV-infected children with marked failure to thrive who are admitted to the PICU primarily for other indications may require supplemental enteral feedings; in some, placement of a gastrostomy tube for nutritional supplementation may be necessary. Few children may need total parenteral nutrition.

Chronic liver inflammation is relatively common in HIV-infected children. In some, hepatitis caused by cytomega-lovirus, hepatitis B or C viruses, or *Mycobacterium avium* complex (MAC) may lead to liver failure and portal hyperten-sion. It is important to recognize that several of the antiretro-viral drugs (e.g., didanosine and protease inhibitors (PIs) may also cause reversible elevation of transaminases. Pancreatitis is uncommon in HIV-infected children, perhaps the result of drug therapy (e.g., didanosine, lamivudine, nevirapine, or pentamidine). Rarely, opportunistic infections (e.g., MAC or cytomegalovirus) may be responsible for acute pancreatitis. The principles of management of these conditions are similar to those in non–HIV-infected children.

Neurologic Diseases

The incidence of CNS involvement in perinatally infected chil-dren may be >50% in developing countries but lower in de-veloped countries, with a median onset at ~1.5 years of age. The most common presentation is progressive encephalopathy with loss or plateau of developmental milestones, cognitive deterioration, impaired brain growth that results in acquired microcephaly and symmetric motor dysfunction. CNS infec-tions (meningitis due to bacterial pathogens, fungi, such as *Cryptococcus*, and a number of viruses) may be responsible for clinical presentations that are indications for PICU admis-sion. CNS toxoplasmosis is exceedingly rare in young infants but may occur in HIV-infected adolescents; the overwhelm-ing majority of these cases have serum IgG anti-toxoplasma antibodies as a marker of infection. The management of these conditions is similar to that in non–HIV-infected children; the response rates and outcomes may be poorer.

Cardiovascular Involvement

Cardiac abnormalities in HIV-infected children are common, persistent, and often progressive; however, most are subclini-cal. In a study of HIV-infected children, left ventricular (LV) structure and function progressively deteriorated in the first 3 years of life, resulting in subsequent persistent mild LV dysfunction and increased LV mass. Chronic mild depres-sion of LV function and elevated LV mass were associated with higher all-cause mortality (30). Children with encepha-lopathy or other AIDS-defining conditions have the highest rate of adverse cardiac outcomes. Resting sinus tachycardia has been reported in up to nearly two-thirds, and marked sinus arrhythmia in one-fifth, of HIV-infected children. Gal-lop rhythm with tachypnea and hepatosplenomegaly appear to be the best clinical indicators of congestive heart failure in HIV-infected children; anticongestive therapy is generally very effective, especially when initiated early. Electrocardiography and echocardiography are helpful in assessing cardiac function before the onset of clinical symptoms.

Renal Involvement

Nephropathy is an unusual presenting symptom of HIV in-fection, more commonly occurring in older symptomatic chil-dren. Nephrotic syndrome is the most common manifestation of pediatric renal disease, with edema, hypoalbuminemia, pro-teinuria, and azotemia with normal blood pressure. Polyuria, oliguria, and hematuria have also been observed in some pa-tients. Hypertension is unusual in these children.

Diagnosis

All infants born to HIV-infected mothers test antibody positive at birth because of passive transfer of maternal HIV antibody across the placenta. Most uninfected infants lose maternal an-tibody between 6 and 12 months of age. As a small proportion of uninfected infants continues to have maternal HIV antibody in the blood for up to 18 months of age, positive IgG antibody tests cannot be used to make a definitive diagnosis of HIV infection in infants who are younger. In a child >18 months, demonstration of IgG antibody to HIV by a repeatedly reac-tive enzyme immunoassay (EIA) and confirmatory test (e.g., Western blot or immunofluorescence assay) can establish the diagnosis of HIV infection.

Although serologic diagnostic tests were the most com-monly used in the past, tests that allow for earlier definitive diagnosis in children have replaced antibody assays as the tests of choice for the diagnosis of HIV infection in infants. Specific viral diagnostic assays, such as HIV DNA or RNA PCR, HIV culture, or HIV p24 antigen immune dissociated p24 (ICD-p24), are essential for diagnosis of young infants born to HIV-infected mothers. By 6 months of age, the HIV culture and/or PCR identifies all infected infants, who are not having any continued exposure owing to breast-feeding. HIV DNA PCR is the preferred virologic assay in developed countries. Plasma HIV RNA assays may be more sensitive than DNA PCR for early diagnosis, but data are limited. HIV culture has similar sensitivity to HIV DNA PCR; however, it is more technically complex and expensive, and results are often not available for 2–4 weeks, compared to 2–3 days with PCR. The p24 antigen assay is less sensitive than the other virologic tests.

Antiretroviral Therapy

Decisions about antiretroviral therapy for pediatric HIV-infected patients are based on the magnitude of viral replication (i.e., viral load), CD4 lymphocyte count or percentage, and clinical condition. The indications for initiation of HAART are detailed in **Table 90.3**. In the developed world, the decision to initiate HAART is based on clinical, immunologic, and virologic parameters. In contrast, in settings in which access to laboratory tests is limited, the decision to treat may be based only on clinical symptoms.

Availability of antiretroviral therapy has transformed HIV infection from a uniformly fatal condition to a chronic infection, with which children can lead a near-normal life. The currently available therapy does not eradicate the virus and cure the child; it rather suppresses the virus replication for extended periods of time. The three main groups of drugs are nucleoside reverse transcriptase inhibitors (NRTIs), non-NRTIs (NNRTIs), and PIs. HAART is a combination of two NRTIs with a PI or an NNRTI. The details of antiretroviral drugs are shown in **Table 90.4**.

Some complications of antiretroviral therapy, such as lactic acidosis, severe pancreatitis, and Stevens–Johnson syndrome, may require care in the PICU. The therapy for these conditions includes discontinuing the offending drug, when possible, and supportive care similar to the care provided for these problems in non–HIV-infected children.

Outcome

Published literature is limited regarding the outcomes after initiation of antiretroviral treatment in critically ill HIV-infected children. In a report from South Africa, it was observed that the majority of HIV-infected children survived to discharge from the PICU, but only half survived to hospital discharge (31). Limitation of intervention decisions, usually made in the PICU, directly influenced short-term survival and the opportunity to commence HAART. Although few critically ill HIV-infected children in developing countries survived to become established on HAART, the long-term outcome of children on HAART remains encouraging.

Prevention of Transmission in the PICU

The staff in the PICU should always adhere to universal precautions, regardless of the presence or absence of known or suspected HIV infection in their patients. Staff may have a greater likelihood of exposure to HIV-contaminated body fluids in the PICU, as compared to other healthcare settings, because of the increased number of invasive procedures performed in the PICU. In case of exposure, the staff should follow the standard guidelines for postexposure prophylaxis (PEP) (32). The majority of HIV exposures will warrant a two-drug regimen, using two NRTIs (zidovudine and lamivudine or emtricitabine [FTC]) or one nucleotide reverse transcriptase inhibitor and one NRTI (tenofovir and lamivudine or emtricitabine). The US Public Health Service now recommends that expanded PEP regimens be PI based. The PI preferred for use in expanded PEP regimens is lopinavir/ritonavir (LPV/RTV). Other PIs acceptable for use in expanded PEP regimens include atazanavir, fosamprenavir, ritonavir-boosted indinavir, ritonavir-boosted saquinavir, and nelfinavir. Although side effects are common

TABLE 90.3

INDICATIONS FOR INITIATION OF HIGHLY ACTIVE ANTIRETROVIRAL THERAPY IN HIV-INFECTED CHILDREN

1. Antiretroviral therapy (ART) should be initiated in all children with AIDS or significant symptoms (clinical Category C or most clinical Category B conditions)
2. ART should be initiated in HIV-infected infants <12 mo of age regardless of clinical status, CD4 percentage, or viral load
3. ART *should be initiated* in HIV-infected children ≥1 y who are asymptomatic or have mild symptoms with the following CD4 values:
   - Age 1 to <3 y
     with CD4 T lymphocyte (CD4 cell) count <1000 cells/mm^3 or CD4 percentage <25%
   - Age 3 to <5 y
     with CD4 cell count <750 cells/mm^3 or CD4 percentage <25%
   - Age ≥ 5 y
     with CD4 cell count <350 cells/ mm^3
     with CD4 cell count 350–500 cells/mm^3
4. ART *should be considered* for HIV-infected children ≥1 y who are asymptomatic or have mild symptoms with the following CD4 values:
   - Age 1 to <3 y
     with CD4 cell count ≥1000 cells/mm^3 or CD4 percentage ≥25%
   - Age 3 to <5 y
     with CD4 cell count ≥750 cells/mm^3 or CD4 percentage ≥25%
   - Age ≥5 y
     with CD4 cell count >500 cells/mm^3
5. Plasma HIV RNA levels >100,000 copies/mL provide stronger evidence for initiation of treatment

From Panel on Antiretroviral Therapy and Medical Management of HIV-Infected Children. *Guidelines for the Use of Antiretroviral Agents in Pediatric HIV Infection.* November 2012. http://aidsinfo.nih.gov/contentfiles/lvguidelines/pediatricguidelines.pdf. Accessed December 10, 2012.

TABLE 90.4

ANTIRETROVIRAL DRUGS COMMONLY USED IN CHILDREN

■ DRUG	■ DOSE	■ SIDE EFFECTS
Nucleoside Reverse Transcriptase Inhibitors		
Abacavir	3 mo to 13 y: 8 mg/kg/dose q 12 h >13 y: 300 mg/dose q 12 h (max: 300 mg/dose)	Hypersensitivity
Didanosine	0–3 mo: 50 mg/m²/dose q 12 h 3 mo to 13 y: 90–150 mg/m² q 12 h (max: 200 mg/dose) >13 y: <60 kg: 125 mg tablets q 12 h >13 y: >60 kg: 200 mg tablet q 12 h (higher dose for powder preparations)	Peripheral neuropathy, pancreatitis, abdominal pain, diarrhea
Emtricitabine	Neonate/infant dose (aged 0 to <3 mo): ■ Oral solution: 3 mg/kg once daily Pediatric dose (aged ≥3 mo to 17 y): ■ Oral solution: 6 mg/kg (maximum dose 240 mg) once daily ■ Capsules (for children who weigh >33 kg): 200 mg once daily Adolescent (aged ≥18 y)/adult dose: ■ Oral solution: 240 mg (24 mL) once daily ■ Capsules: 200 mg once daily	Minimal toxicity
Lamivudine (3TC)	1 mo to 13 y: 4 mg/kg q 12 h >13 y: <50 kg: 4 mg/kg/dose q 12 h >13 y: >50 kg: 150 mg/kg/dose q 12 h	Pancreatitis, neuropathy, neutropenia
Stavudine (d4T)	1 mo to 13 y: 1 mg/kg q 12 h >13 y: 30–60 kg: 30 mg q 12 h >13 y: >60 kg: 40 mg q 12 h	Mitochondrial toxicity, headache, gastrointestinal upset, neuropathy
Tenofovir disoproxil fumarate (TDF)	Neonate/infant dose: not FDA approved or recommended for use in neonates/infants aged <2 y Pediatric dose (aged ≥2 y to <12 y)[a]: ■ 8 mg/kg/dose once daily Adolescent (aged ≥12 y and weight ≥35 kg)[a] and adult dose: ■ 300 mg once daily	Renal insufficiency, proximal renal tubular dysfunction that may include Fanconi syndrome; decreased bone mineral density (BMD)
Zidovudine	Neonates: 2 mg/kg q 6 h 3 mo to 13 y: 90–180 mg/m² q 6–8 h >13 y: 200 mg q 8 h or 300 mg q 12 h	Anemia, myopathy
Nonnucleoside Reverse Transcriptase Inhibitors		
Efavirenz	>3 y: 10 to <15 kg: 200 mg q 24 h 15 to <20 kg: 250 mg q 24 h 20 to <25 kg: 300 mg q 24 h 25 to <32.5 kg: 350 mg q 24 h 32.5 to <40 kg: 400 mg q 24 h >40 kg: 600 mg q 24 h	Skin rash, central nervous system symptoms, increased transaminase levels
Etravirine (ETR)	Not approved for use in neonates/infants, and in children aged <6 y Antiretroviral-experienced children and adolescents aged 6–18 y (and weighing at least 16 kg): ■ 16 kg to <20 kg: 100 mg twice daily ■ 20 kg to <25 kg: 125 mg twice daily ■ 25 kg to <30 kg: 150 mg twice daily ■ ≥30 kg: 200 mg twice daily Adult dose (antiretroviral-experienced patients): ■ 200 mg twice daily following a meal	Rash, including Stevens–Johnson syndrome Hypersensitivity reactions
Nevirapine (NVP)	2 mo to 13 y: 120 mg/m² (max 200 mg) q 24 h for 14 d, followed by 120–200 mg/m² q 12 h *OR* <8 y: 7 mg/kg q 12 h >8 y: 4 mg/kg q 12 h >13 y: 200 mg q 24 h for 14 d; then increase to 200 mg q 12 h if no rash or other side effects	Skin rash, Stevens–Johnson syndrome
Rilpivirine (RPV)	Not approved for use in neonates/infants and children Adolescent (>18 y of age)/adult dose (antiretroviral [ARV]-naive patients only): ■ 25 mg once daily	Depression, mood changes, insomnia, headache, rash

■ DRUG	■ DOSE	■ SIDE EFFECTS
Protease Inhibitors		
Atazanavir (ATV)	Not approved for use in neonates/infants and children <6 y Dose for children ≥6 y: both atazanavir and ritonavir (RTV) given once daily with food ■ 15 to <20 kg: ATV 150 mg + RTV 100 mg ■ 20 to <32 kg: ATV 200 mg + RTV 100 mg ■ 32 to <40 kg: ATV 250 mg + RTV 100 mg ■ ≥40 kg: ATV 300 mg + RTV 100 mg	Prolonged ECG PR interval, first-degree symptomatic atrio-ventricular block in some patients Hyperglycemia Fat maldistribution Nephrolithiasis
Darunavir (DRV)	Not approved for use in neonates/infants and children <3 y 3 to <18 y of age and weighing ≥10 kg ■ 10 to <11 kg: DRV 200 mg + RTV 32 mg ■ 11 to <12 kg: DRV 220 mg + RTV 32 mg ■ 12 to <13 kg: DRV 240 mg + RTV 40 mg ■ 13 to <14 kg: DRV 260 mg + RTV 40 mg ■ 14 to <15 kg: DRV 280 mg + RTV 48 mg ■ 15 to <30 kg: DRV 375 mg + RTV 50 mg ■ 30 to <40 kg: DRV 450 mg + RTV 60 mg ■ ≥40 kg: DRV 600 mg + RTV 100 mg	Skin rash, including Stevens–Johnson syndrome and erythema multiforme Hepatotoxicity
Fosamprenavir (FPV)	Aged ≥6 mo to 18 y: twice-daily dosage regimens <11 kg: FPV 45 mg/kg + RTV 7 mg/kg 11 kg to <15 kg: FPV 30 mg/kg + RTV 3 mg/kg 15 kg to <20 kg: FPV 23 mg/kg + RTV 3 mg/kg ≥20 kg FPV: 18 mg/kg + RTV 3 mg/kg	Diarrhea, nausea, vomiting Skin rash (FPV has a sulfonamide moiety. Stevens–Johnson syndrome and erythema multiforme have been reported)
Indinavir (IDV)	Not approved for use in neonates/infants and children Adolescent/adult dose: ■ 800 mg IDV + 100 or 200 mg RTV every 12 h	Hyperbilirubinemia, nephrolithiasis
Lopinavir/ritonavir (LPV/r)	Infant dose (14 d to 12 mo): ■ Once-daily dosing is not recommended ■ 300 mg/75 mg LPV/r/m² of body surface area twice daily Pediatric dose (>12 mo to 18 y): ■ Once-daily dosing is not recommended ■ 300 mg/75 mg LPV/r/m² of body surface area per dose twice daily	Diarrhea, fatigue, headache, nausea, and increased cholesterol and triglycerides
Nelfinavir (NFV)	NFV should not be used for treatment in children aged <2 y <13 y: 45–55 mg/ kg q 12 h >13 y: 1250 mg q 12 h (max 2000 mg)	Diarrhea, abdominal pain
Ritonavir (RTV)	<13 y: 350–400 mg/m² q 12 h (starting dose: 250 mg/m²) >13 y: 600 mg q 12 h (starting with 300 mg)	Bad taste, vomiting, nausea, diarrhea, rarely, hepatitis, toxic epidermal necrolysis and Stevens–Johnson syndrome
Saquinavir	50 mg/kg q 8 h >13 y: soft gel capsules, 1200 mg twice daily	Diarrhea, headache, skin rash
Tipranavir (TPV)	**Pediatric dose (aged <2 y):** Not approved for use in children aged <2 y **Pediatric dose (2–18 y of age):** Not recommended for treatment-naive patients Body surface area dosing: ■ TPV 375 mg/m² + RTV 150 mg/m², both twice daily (maximum dose: TPV 500 mg + RTV 200 mg, both twice daily)	Rare cases of fatal and nonfatal intracranial hemorrhage, skin rash

[a]There are concerns about decreased BMD, especially in pre-pubertal patients and those in early puberty (Tanner Stages 1 and 2).
From Panel on Antiretroviral Therapy and Medical Management of HIV-Infected Children. *Guidelines for the Use of Antiretroviral Agents in Pediatric HIV Infection*. November 2012. http://aidsinfo.nih.gov/contentfiles/lvguidelines/pediatricguidelines.pdf. Accessed 10, December 2012.

with NNRTIs, efavirenz may be considered for expanded PEP regimens, especially when resistance to PIs in the source person's virus is known or suspected. Caution is advised when efavirenz is used in women of childbearing age because of the risk of teratogenicity. PEP should be initiated as soon as possible, preferably within hours rather than days of exposure. If a question exists concerning which antiretroviral drugs to use or whether to use a basic or expanded regimen, the basic regimen should be started immediately rather than delaying PEP administration. PEP should be administered for 4 weeks, if tolerated.

Conclusions and Future Directions

HIV infection in children is a serious problem in many developing countries. The severe manifestations of HIV infection, conditions resulting from severe immunosuppression, and drug toxicities may require intensive care. Development of a vaccine to prevent HIV infection is a high priority. More efficacious antiretroviral drugs that have fewer adverse effects are also necessary. Making available antiretroviral therapy at an affordable cost remains a considerable challenge. In the short term, finding effective ways to control vertical transmission from mother to child may help in substantial reduction in childhood HIV infection load.

MEASLES

13 Measles (rubeola) remains an important cause of death among young children, despite the availability of a safe and effective vaccine for nearly four decades. Unlike in industrialized countries, measles remains a common illness in many developing countries, where >95% of measles deaths occur. More than 30 million people are affected each year by measles. In 2010, an estimated 139,300 measles deaths occurred globally, most of them in children (33). In countries where measles has been largely eliminated, cases imported from other countries are now the most important source of infection. Unimmunized children, even in prosperous countries, remain at risk of acquiring the infection and when infected can suffer a severe course (34). Severe measles is particularly likely in poorly nourished young children, especially those who do not receive sufficient vitamin A or whose immune systems have been weakened by HIV/AIDS or other diseases.

Description of Organism

Measles virus is a large, pleomorphic RNA virus (100–300 nm in diameter) belonging to the Paramyxoviridae family. The virus genome is a linear strand of RNA that contains ~15,900 nucleotides (molecular weight: 4.5×10^6 D). The virus can easily be inactivated by heat, ultraviolet light, lipid solvents, and extremes of pH. All measles strains are antigenically homogeneous.

Transmission

The measles virus is spread from an infected individual to a new host by the respiratory route via aerosolized droplets of respiratory secretions. Close person-to-person contact can facilitate transfer of nasal secretions of a patient to the nose of the host. There is no known animal reservoir, and asymptomatic carriers are unknown.

Pathogenesis and Pathophysiology

The primary site of initial infection is the respiratory epithelium of the nasopharynx. The virus multiplies locally and then spreads to the regional lymphoid tissue. A primary viremia follows (day 2–3 after infection), leading to seeding of the reticuloendothelial system and extensive replication. Between the days 8 and 10 of infection, an extensive secondary viremia occurs and infection in the skin, conjunctivae, and the respiratory tract is established; the clinical syndrome of measles becomes evident at this time. The viral burden reaches its maximum height between the days 11 and 14 and, thereafter, rapidly

declines. Immunologically compromised patients may have defective clearing of the virus and increased severity of organ involvement. Malnourished children often experience more severe measles infections than do well-nourished children. The mortality rate for measles infection is increased (25%–50%) in infants and young children in Africa with edematous malnutrition (35).

Widespread distribution of multinucleated giant cells is the characteristic pathologic feature of measles. Of the various organ systems involved, the most prominent are the lungs and the brain. In fatal cases, a striking proliferation of the respiratory epithelia, with formation of peribronchiolar fibroepithelial nodules and cystic transformation of tracheobronchial glands, has been demonstrated. The lung tissues may show marked interstitial pneumonitis with diffuse endothelial cell and pneumocyte degeneration. The brain sections show a paucicellular inflammatory infiltrate with diffuse neuronal damage. However, these findings are found in severe cases and cannot be considered representative of the pathology in all cases of measles.

Clinical Features

14 The incubation period of measles is ~8–12 days. The first sign of infection is usually high fever, which begins ~8–12 days after exposure and lasts 1–7 days. During this initial stage, the child may develop cough, coryza (runny nose), conjunctivitis (the 3 Cs), and an enanthem—small white (appear as grains of salt on a reddened wet background) *Koplik spots* usually found on the buccal mucosa near the molars. Children are usually very irritable. After several days of fever, a rash develops, usually beginning on the face (often in the hairline) and upper neck. The rash is initially erythematous and maculopapular; typical of measles rash is the coexistence of discrete and confluent red maculopapules. Microvesicles may be seen on the top of the erythematous base. Over a period of ~3 days, the rash proceeds downward, eventually reaching the hands and feet. The rash lasts for 5–6 days and then fades. The rash occurs, on average, at day 14 after exposure to the virus, with a range of 7–18 days. Pharyngitis, cervical lymphadenopathy, diarrhea, vomiting, laryngitis, and croup may also occur during the illness.

Atypical measles, a clearly defined clinical syndrome that occurred in previously vaccinated individuals (specifically those who received a killed measles vaccine that is no longer available) after exposure to natural measles, is no longer seen. This illness was characterized by high fever, petechial rash, and pneumonitis and was caused by immune complex deposition. It had a different progression of the rash (cephalad from the extremities).

Some children infected with measles develop complications and can present with a rapidly progressive illness.

Pneumonia

Primary viral involvement of the lungs is common with measles infections. It is characterized by hyperinflation and fluffy perihilar infiltrates. Unilateral, segmental involvement has also been observed. Infants with measles-associated lower respiratory tract infections may present with features suggestive of bronchiolitis. Extensive infection may lead to significant hypoxemia. Children with defects in cell-mediated immunity are particularly prone to develop severe pneumonia. Although measles virus itself can lead to severe pulmonary disease, secondary bacterial pneumonias are also responsible for some measles-related complications and deaths. Children with measles infections have an increased susceptibility to bacterial infections. This propensity may be due to multiple causes: disruption of the respiratory tract epithelium, non-specific suppression of immune responses by measles infection, and vitamin A deficiency. The bacterial pneumonias are usually due to common respiratory pathogens: *H. influenzae*, *Streptococcus pneumoniae*, and *Staphylococcus aureus*. In some studies, coinfection with viruses (parainfluenza and adenovirus) has been reported. Depending on the setting, ~5%–10% of children hospitalized with measles will require intensive care. One study reported that 15 of 237 children hospitalized with measles required intensive care (36); severe respiratory distress that required mechanical ventilation was the reason for the PICU admission in all cases in this series. Acute respiratory distress syndrome and air leaks are examples of complications among the children in this series (36).

Other respiratory complications include otitis media, mastoiditis, laryngitis, and laryngotracheobronchitis, including severe laryngotracheobronchitis. In developing countries, where latent TB infection is common, immune suppression during measles infection may lead to development of reactivation disease.

Neurologic Involvement

Neurologic involvement of measles occurs in children with the reported incidence of encephalitis being ~0.5–1.0 per 1000 measles cases. Measles virus can result in three different forms of CNS infections (37): acute progressive infectious encephalitis, acute postinfectious encephalitis, and subacute sclerosing panencephalitis (SSPE). The acute progressive form of brain disease, also referred to as inclusion body encephalitis, reflects a direct attack by the virus under conditions of yielding cell-mediated immunity. The postinfectious acute disease is interpreted to reflect an autoimmune reaction. Symptoms of encephalitis usually develop in the second week of illness. Some children have rapid deterioration, and increased intracranial pressure and herniation may occur. Cerebellar ataxia, myelitis, and motor deficits have been reported. Survivors may have sequelae, such as seizures, deafness, and motor deficits. SSPE is a rare CNS disease with progressive degenerative loss of intelligence, behavioral difficulties, and seizures.

Other *unusual complications* of measles include myocarditis and pericarditis; clinical consequences of such involvement are rare. Some children infected with measles virus may have bleeding manifestations related to thrombocytopenia. Severe disease may lead to DIC.

Differential Diagnosis

The differential diagnosis of measles includes all illnesses in which erythematous maculopapular rash occurs, such as rubella, erythema infectiosum, roseola infantum, enteroviral infections, infectious mononucleosis, *Mycoplasma pneumoniae* infections, and drug reactions. The typical course and pattern of rash usually allow the diagnosis to be made clinically.

Diagnosis

In endemic areas, the diagnosis is usually clinical. For confirmation, demonstration of specific antimeasles IgM antibody in serum is the most commonly used modality. Other means of making the diagnosis include rise in IgG antibodies to measles (acute and convalescent sera) and isolation of the virus from urine, blood, throat, or nasopharyngeal secretions. Measles is highly contagious with a 90% infection rate in unimmunized domestic contacts. The identification of prodromal signs (Koplik spots, 3 Cs) may help with earlier isolation of infectious individuals.

Treatment

The treatment for mild infections is supportive. A systematic review suggests a possible beneficial effect of antibiotics in preventing complications such as pneumonia, purulent otitis media, and tonsillitis in children with measles; however, methodologic problems preclude a definitive recommendation for antibiotics in measles unless there is a bacterial superinfection (38). Children who require hospitalization must be managed for the complications. Randomized clinical trials have demonstrated reduction in morbidity and mortality in severe measles with use of vitamin A (39). These findings led to the recommendation to treat all children who require hospitalization with a dose of 200,000 IU of vitamin A. The WHO and UNICEF recommend vitamin A for all children with measles in regions where vitamin A deficiency is a problem or the case fatality ratio for measles is 1% or more. The dose should be repeated after 24 hours.

In a systematic review, no significant reduction in the risk of mortality in the vitamin A group was seen when all of the studies were pooled, using the random-effects model (RR, 0.70; 95% confidence interval [CI], 0.42–1.15) (40). However, using megadoses of vitamin A (200,000 IU) on 2 consecutive days was associated with a reduction in the risk of mortality in children <2 years of age (RR, 0.18; 95% CI, 0.03–0.61) and a reduction in the risk of pneumonia-specific mortality (RR, 0.33; 95% CI, 0.08–0.92). The literature includes a few reports of successful use of inhaled and IV ribavirin in severe infections (41), but no controlled trials have been conducted. The associated bacterial infections should be managed with appropriate antimicrobials. Supportive care and monitoring are important in severe infections, as multiple organ systems may be affected.

Prognosis

The complication rates are higher in malnourished children, immunocompromised children, and in those with vitamin A deficiency. Patients with measles who require intensive care have a high risk for death or long-term complications, even when treated in a modern PICU (36). One study reported 26% mortality in 15 children with measles who were admitted to the PICU (36). Acute respiratory distress syndrome, air leaks, and bacteremia were the most severe complications in these patients.

Conclusions and Future Directions

Measles, a vaccine-preventable infection, is an important cause of death among young children in developing countries. The conditions that may require intensive care include pneumonia, laryngotracheobronchitis, and CNS infections. Vitamin A may be helpful in reducing the morbidity and mortality due to measles. No proven antiviral drugs for measles are available. Improving the availability of vaccine and ensuring adequate immunization of susceptible children are the most important challenges in the prevention of measles-associated mortality. Development and evaluation of antiviral agents that are effective against measles virus are required. In the short term, identification of children who may benefit the most from early intensive care is essential and will aid in early institution of intensive care and in prioritizing the available resources.

NONPOLIO ENTEROVIRAL INFECTIONS

Enteroviruses are nonenveloped, single-stranded RNA viruses in the Picornaviridae family; the subgroups are polioviruses, coxsackieviruses, and echoviruses. Newer enteroviruses are classified by numbering. Although >60 different serotypes have been identified, 11 account for the majority of disease. Enteroviruses are ~30-nm particles that consist of a naked, protein capsid and dense central core of RNA. Enterovirus capsids are composed of four proteins: VP1, VP2, VP3, and VP4; the first three are surface proteins, and the last lies on the inner surface. These proteins are the determinants of host range and tissue tropism. The genetic material of the enteroviruses is a single-stranded, positive-sense RNA molecule. Cleavage of a long polyprotein that is translated from the genome leads to formation of four capsid proteins and seven nonstructural proteins.

In the United States, enteroviruses have been found to be responsible for 33%–65% of acute febrile illnesses and 55%–65% of hospitalizations for suspected sepsis in infants during the summer and fall, and 25% year-round. In tropical and semitropical areas, enteroviruses frequently circulate year-round. Large outbreaks of enterovirus infections can occur. Outbreaks of hand-foot-mouth disease associated with severe CNS and/or cardiopulmonary disease due to enterovirus 71 have occurred in recent years in Australia, Japan, Malaysia, and Taiwan, and community outbreaks of enterovirus meningitis have been reported (42). Factors associated with increased incidence and/or severity of enterovirus infection include young age, male sex, poor hygiene, overcrowding, and low socioeconomic status; >25% of symptomatic enterovirus infections occur in infants. Breast-feeding reduces the risk of infection in infants.

Pathogenesis

After the initial contact of the virus with oral or respiratory mucosa, implantation occurs in the pharynx and the gastrointestinal tract. Within 24 hours, the infection spreads to regional lymphoid tissue. Minor viremia occurs thereafter, usually on day 3, leading to infection of many secondary sites; this phase coincides with onset of clinical symptoms. Multiplication of the virus at secondary infection sites leads to major viremia, which often lasts until day 7 of infection. CNS infection may occur, along with infection of secondary sites or during the phase of major viremia. With the appearance of antibody in the blood, viremia ceases and the viral load in the secondary infection sites decreases. However, virus may continue to replicate in the gastrointestinal tract for many weeks.

Clinical Features

Enteroviral infections vary from mild to fatal illnesses. The spectrum of mild illnesses includes nonspecific febrile illness, common cold, pharyngitis, herpangina, stomatitis, and parotitis. Croup may be caused by coxsackie and echovirus infections; however, this illness is milder when compared to croup caused by influenza and parainfluenza viruses. The respiratory tract infection may result in bronchitis, bronchiolitis, or pneumonia caused by coxsackie and echovirus infections. Some of these infections may be severe, and the child may require intensive care. Pleurodynia, characterized by fever and spasmodic chest and upper abdominal muscular pain, is rarely diagnosed now. The major etiologic agents in epidemic pleurodynia were coxsackie B3 and B5. Gastrointestinal manifestations occur commonly in coxsackie and echoviral infections; manifestations other than diarrhea and vomiting include peritonitis, mesenteric adenitis, appendicitis, hepatitis, and pancreatitis.

Various serotypes of coxsackie and echoviruses have been implicated in causation of pericarditis and myocarditis. These are often associated with involvement of other organ systems.

Neurologic illness is a frequent manifestation of infection with enteroviruses; the most common illness is aseptic meningitis. Encephalitis, paralytic disease due to infection of anterior horn cell infection, Guillain–Barré syndrome, transverse myelitis, and cerebellar ataxia may occur. The genitourinary manifestations include nephritis, orchitis, and epididymitis. Arthritis and myositis may be caused by coxsackie virus infections. Skin rashes are common with enterovirus infections and may be maculopapular, morbilliform, petechial, or small vesicles. A common distribution is on the palms, soles, and oral mucosa, leading to the so-called hand-foot-mouth syndrome.

Laboratory Diagnosis

As highlighted in the previous section, enteroviral illnesses have a wide range of manifestations, and, therefore, one must have a high index of suspicion to make the diagnosis. The clinical presentation may be mistaken for bacterial infections or other viruses that cause similar illnesses. The diagnosis of enterovirus infection can be confirmed by virus isolation and detection. The samples may be collected from the nasopharynx, throat, stool, rectal swab, blood, urine, and cerebrospinal fluid (CSF). Viral isolation in culture usually takes less than a week. The virus may be detected in the body fluids by nucleic acid techniques: cDNA and RNA probes and PCR. Serology is usually not used for diagnosis.

Treatment

The mainstay of care is supportive treatment. IV immunoglobulin has been used in neonates with severe disseminated infection and is used for children with persistent CNS infection due to immune deficiencies that cause hypogammaglobulinemia. The antiviral drug pleconaril may have limited benefit for treatment of severe enteroviral infections, particularly neurologic infections, myocarditis, and infections in immunodeficient patients (43). It is not approved for use in the United States, but may be obtained under investigational new drug (IND) application. In absence of any evidence indicating any benefit, corticosteroids should be avoided in severe illnesses. Children with enteroviral infections require universal and contact precautions when admitted to healthcare facilities.

Conclusions and Future Directions

Nonpolio enteroviruses are responsible for variety of illnesses. Some of the respiratory, myocardial, and CNS infections may be severe enough to require intensive care. The mainstay of care is supportive treatment. The challenges that impact control of nonpolio enteroviruses include development and evaluation of simpler and rapid diagnostic methods, antiviral drugs, and cost-effective supportive care.

SEVERE VARICELLA INFECTIONS

Varicella (chickenpox) is a common and usually self-limited exanthematous illness of childhood. The varicella vaccine program in the United States, begun in 1995, has led to a dramatic reduction in varicella cases including children hospitalized with severe varicella (44). However, primary varicella can result in severe manifestations, such as pneumonia, hepatitis, encephalitis, and DIC, particularly in certain groups: neonates, pregnant women, adolescents, adults, and the immunocompromised. Varicella–zoster virus (VZV) establishes lifelong latency in the dorsal root ganglia after the primary infection. Reactivation of virus leads to zoster (shingles), which is usually characterized by a pruritic vesicular rash in a dermatomal pattern in immunocompetent patients. Zoster may manifest as a more severe illness in immunocompromised patients and can involve multiple dermatomes and viscera. Up to 3.5% of children with chickenpox may have a complicated course (45). Deaths are uncommon, with the reported figure <2 deaths per 100,000 in children between 1 and 14 years of age (46).

Description of Virus

VZV is a member of the Herpesviridae family and consists of viral DNA inside an icosahedral nucleocapsid surrounded by lipid envelope. Primary infection with VZV presents as varicella (chickenpox), while reactivation presents as localized cutaneous infection, called zoster (shingles). VZV produces cytopathic effects in cells that are indistinguishable from those produced by HSVs.

Clinical Features

Transmission of varicella occurs by either airborne droplets or contact with secretions or infected vesicular fluid. The incubation period is typically 2 weeks, with a range of 10–21 days. Chickenpox is characterized by a rash, low-grade fever, and malaise. Patients may have prodromal constitutional symptoms 1–2 days before the onset of rash. The rash, which evolves from maculopapules to pruritic vesicles to crusts, often initially appears on the trunk or face and spreads over days to involve the entire body. Groups, or crops, of skin lesions, which number on average 250–500 in the unvaccinated child, progress from macules to vesicles to crusts. Simultaneously having lesions in various stages of evolution is a clinical hallmark of chickenpox. Most patients with varicella make an uneventful recovery after ~1 week. However, some patients may develop the complications described in the next sections.

Bacterial Superinfection

Secondary bacterial complications can occur in skin, soft tissues, and other sites and is often caused by group A *Streptococcus* (GAS) and *Staphylococcus aureus*. Varicella is a particularly important risk factor for severe invasive GAS infections in previously healthy children, and an increasing proportion of these cases in the United States have been associated with varicella. A GAS infection should be considered in any child with varicella who also has localized skin findings of erythema, warmth, swelling, or induration, and in any child with varicella who becomes febrile after having been afebrile, who has a temperature of >39°C beyond day 3 of illness, or who has any fever beyond day 4 of illness. When present, GAS infections are usually painful, and initially, the amount of pain is frequently out of proportion to the clinical findings (47).

Pneumonia

VZV pneumonia is the most serious complication of disseminated VZV infection, with mortality rates of 9%–50%. Reported prevalence of VZV pneumonia has varied from <5% to 50% of all varicella infections in adults (48). Most cases of VZV pneumonia have been reported in immunocompromised adults and in those with chronic lung disease.

Varicella pneumonia usually presents 1–6 days after the onset of the rash and is associated with tachypnea, chest tightness, cough, dyspnea, fever, and occasionally, with pleuritic chest pain and hemoptysis. Chest symptoms may start before the appearance of the skin rash. Physical findings are often minimal, and chest x-rays typically reveal nodular or interstitial pneumonitis. Findings of VZV pneumonia on chest x-ray consist of multiple 5- to 10-mm, ill-defined nodules that may be confluent and fleeting. Hilar lymphadenopathy and pleural effusion are unusual. The small, round nodules usually resolve within a week after the disappearance of the skin lesions but may persist for months. Usually resolving in 3–5 days in milder disease, the small nodules may persist for several weeks in widespread disease. The lesions calcify and can persist as numerous, well-defined, randomly scattered, 2- to 3-mm dense calcifications (49).

High-resolution CT of the chest in patients with varicella pneumonitis usually shows 1- to 10-mm, well-defined and ill-defined nodules that are diffuse throughout both lungs. Nodules with a surrounding halo of ground-glass opacity, patchy ground-glass opacity, and coalescence of nodules are also seen. These findings disappear concurrently with healing of skin lesions after antiviral chemotherapy (49).

Encephalitis

Encephalitis is another serious complication of varicella infection. See Chapters 91 and 95 for more details.

Disseminated Varicella and Zoster

Disseminated varicella and zoster with multivisceral involvement is classically described in immunocompromised patients, particularly those with deficient cell-mediated immunity, bone marrow and renal transplant recipients, and AIDS patients. Even with treatment, the disease carries a very high mortality. Less common complications include transverse myelitis, Guillain–Barré syndrome, purpura fulminans, myocarditis, arthritis, and fulminant hepatic failure. Refer to Chapter 95 for diagnosis and management.

Conclusions and Future Directions

Varicella (chickenpox) is a common and, usually, self-limited exanthematous illness. However, primary varicella can result in severe manifestations, such as pneumonia, hepatitis, encephalitis, and DIC. The challenge is to achieve and improve vaccine availability at affordable cost and wider immunization coverage. Identification of the profile of children who may benefit the most from early intensive care may help in early institution of intensive supportive care. The role of corticosteroids in severe varicella pneumonia should be investigated.

SEVERE HERPES SIMPLEX VIRUS INFECTIONS

HSV infection is one of the most common human viral infections and frequently involves the skin, mucous membranes, and the genitalia. CNS and pulmonary involvement, although less frequent, carry high morbidity and mortality. Immunocompetent patients with HSV infection usually have asymptomatic or mild disease, while immunocompromised patients have a higher risk of disseminated disease, with involvement of multiple organ systems. HSV infection in neonates tends to be severe, with high chances of CNS and visceral dissemination and subsequent morbidity and mortality. Neonatal HSV infection, caused by HSV-2 in ~70% of cases, is estimated to occur in ~1 in 4000 newborns in the United States (50). Herpes simplex encephalitis (HSE) is the most commonly identified cause of sporadic viral encephalitis beyond 6 months of age. Estimated frequency varies from 4 per million per year in the United States to 2.5 per million per year in Sweden (51).

Description of the Virus

HSV is an enveloped virus with double-stranded linear DNA genome, which is enclosed in a regular icosahedral protein capsid; the outer envelope is acquired from the nuclear membrane of host cells and contains various viral glycoproteins. Two distinct strains of HSV, which differ by 50% in their DNA structure, are recognized. HSV-1, which causes orolabial, ocular, and CNS infection, is more prevalent than HSV-2, which is the predominant cause of genital infections, neonatal infections, and aseptic meningitis.

Pathogenesis

Primary oropharyngeal HSV-1 infection results in axoplasmic transport of virus to the trigeminal sensory ganglion, where it establishes latency. Latent HSV-1 is detectable in the trigeminal ganglia of virtually all seropositive individuals. The majority of cases of HSE are due to reactivated virus from dorsal root ganglia, but virus can also reach the CNS via olfactory bulbs during viremia of primary infection. Evidence also suggests persistence of HSV genome in the CNS of asymptomatic individuals. Whether this latent virus could reactivate and cause encephalitis is not clear (51). Neonatal infection is most frequently acquired during the intrapartum period, and primary infection in the mother, rupture of membranes >6 hours, and fetal invasive monitoring appear to increase the risk.

Clinical Features

HSV infections commonly involve oral and genital skin and mucosa. Visceral involvement in herpes is not common, but it carries high morbidity and mortality.

Infections of the Central Nervous System

HSE is a life-threatening manifestation of HSV infection of the CNS. Although HSE is rare, mortality rates reach 70% in the absence of therapy, and only a minority returns to normal function (51). This dreaded manifestation of HSV infection can occur within weeks after birth (neonatal HSV disease) or in childhood or adulthood (HSE). Most cases of neonatal HSV disease are caused by HSV-2, whereas virtually all cases of HSE are caused by HSV-1. HSV encephalitis is discussed in detail in Chapter 91.

Pneumonia

HSV pneumonia is classically seen in immunocompromised patients, but a few case reports describe its occurrence in immunocompetent individuals. HSV pneumonia, particularly in immunocompromised patients, carries a high mortality. The diagnosis of this and other infections caused by the herpes virus family are made difficult by the phenomenon of latency. In that these viruses can be found in healthy people previously infected and in that many of these viruses commonly infect humans, distinguishing the presence of latent virus in people with infections due to other causes and infection caused by the virus itself is difficult.

Disseminated Involvement

Extensive cutaneous and visceral dissemination of HSV is seen in certain children with immune deficiencies, such as severely malnourished children, transplant recipients, patients with malignancies or other conditions that require immunosuppression, patients on high-dose steroid therapy, AIDS patients, burns patients, or patients with other immunodeficiencies, particularly those affecting T lymphocytes. Disseminated disease in these patients may manifest as a sepsis-like syndrome with fever or hypothermia, leukopenia, hepatitis, DIC, and shock and often results in death. This form of herpes has a high mortality, even with appropriate therapy.

Neonatal Herpes

Neonatal herpes may manifest in one of three ways. The least severe form is disease limited to skin, eyes, and mucous membranes (SEM disease), which presents usually between days 5 and 19 of life. Disseminated HSV is rapidly progressive and has a high mortality rate. It also usually has onset before the third week of life. Neonatal HSV disease may also be localized to the CNS. Clinicians may fail to make an early diagnosis because children often have no associated cutaneous findings (52). Most surviving infants with CNS or disseminated disease have neurologic sequelae, and the mortality rate in the absence of therapy is very high (80%) for babies in the latter category. Early recognition and treatment may improve outcome (53). As the clinical features may be nonspecific, the diagnosis is often not considered and administration of therapy is delayed.

Diagnosis

Cutaneous HSV infections can be diagnosed rapidly by microscopic examination of stained scrapings from the vesicles for giant cells and intranuclear inclusions (Tzanck smear). This method, when compared to viral culture, has a specificity of ~90% and sensitivity of 80% in males and 50% in females (54). HSV PCR has been found to be as sensitive as viral culture for diagnosis of cutaneous HSV infection and has the advantage of allowing rapid diagnosis (55).

PCR of the CSF is the method of choice for diagnosis of HSE, but CSF PCR results can be negative in the first 72 hours following illness onset. CSF virus culture is of little value in all patients. For details of the role of neuroimaging, see Chapter 91.

Neonatal herpes may occur in the absence of skin lesions; therefore, if the infection is suspected, swabs of the mouth, nasopharynx, conjunctiva, rectum, skin lesions, mucosal lesions, and urine should be promptly taken and submitted for virus culture. Evidence of disseminated or CNS infection should be sought using liver function tests, complete blood cell count, CSF analysis, and chest x-ray, if respiratory abnormalities are present. Microscopic examination, culture, and PCR assay of bronchoalveolar lavage fluid may help in the diagnosis of HSV pneumonia.

Management

Serious HSV infections require treatment with IV acyclovir. The recommended dose for children (neonates require higher doses, see what follows) and adults with HSE is 10 mg/kg every 8 hours for 21 days. It is also recommended that all patients with HSE undergo a CSF PCR for HSV at the end of 14 days to document elimination of replicating virus. Neonatal and disseminated forms of HSV also require treatment with IV acyclovir. The dose recommended for neonatal HSV encephalitis and neonatal disseminated infection is 20 mg/kg every 8 hours for 21 days, while SEM disease requires treatment for 14 days (56). Dosing of acyclovir may need to be adjusted for degree of renal impairment. Emergence of acyclovir-resistant strains has been particularly reported in immunocompromised patients on acyclovir therapy. The drug of choice for acyclovir-resistant HSV strains is IV foscarnet.

Prognosis

With therapy, most infants with SEM HSV infection improve. The mortality rate is significantly higher in the neonates with disseminated infection and encephalitis. The risk of death is increased in neonates who are in or near coma at presentation, have disseminated intravascular coagulopathy, or are premature. In babies with disseminated disease, HSV pneumonitis is also associated with greater mortality. For HSV infection limited to the skin, eyes, or mouth, the presence of ≥3 recurrences of vesicles has been reported to be associated with an increased risk of neurologic impairment, as compared with ≤2 recurrences (53).

Conclusions and Future Directions

HSV infections of the lungs and brain can be severe, having high morbidity and mortality. Immunocompromised children are at a higher risk for severe infections. Neonates are at a greater risk for severe disease. Acyclovir is the mainstay of therapy. However, HSV diagnosis often goes unsuspected. Given the difficulty in making the clinical diagnosis of HSV, the growing worldwide prevalence, and the availability of effective antiviral therapy, the need to develop rapid, accurate laboratory diagnosis of patients with HSV is clear, as is the need to evaluate the benefit of early administration of acyclovir in patients with suspected severe HSV infection without waiting for virologic confirmation. Development of a vaccine to prevent HSV infection should receive high priority for eventual control of HSV infection.

References

1. Kilbourne ED. Influenza pandemics of the 20th century. *Emerging Infect Dis* 2006;12:9–14.
2. Taubenberger JK. The origin and virulence of the 1918 "Spanish" influenza virus. *Proc Am Philos Soc* 2006;150:86–112.
3. Chang LY, Shih SR, Shao PL, et al. Novel swine-origin influenza virus A (H1N1): The first pandemic of the 21st century. *J Formos Med Assoc* 2009;108:526–32.
4. Dolin R. Influenza. In: Kasper DL, Braunwald E, Fauci AS, et al., eds. *Harrison's Principles of Internal Medicine*. New York, NY: McGraw Hill, 2005:1066–70.
5. Morens DM, Taubenberger JK, Fauci AS. The persistent legacy of the 1918 influenza virus. *N Engl J Med* 2009;361:225–9.
6. Glezen WP. Influenza viruses. In: Feigin RD, Cherry JD, Demmler GJ, et al., eds. *Textbook of Pediatric Infectious Diseases*. Philadelphia, PA: Saunders, 2004:2024–40.
7. Newman AP, Reisdorf E, Beinemann J, et al. Swine influenza A (H1N1) triple reassortant virus infection, Wisconsin. *Emerg Infect Dis* 2008;14:1470–2.
8. Tran D, Vaudry W, Moore DL, et al; IMPACT investigators. Comparison of children hospitalized with seasonal versus pandemic influenza A, 2004–2009. *Pediatrics* 2012;130:397–406.
9. Kuiken T, Riteau B, Fouchier RAM, et al. Pathogenesis of influenza virus infections: The good, the bad and the ugly. *Curr Opin Virol* 2012;2:276–86.
10. Oldstone MBA, Teijaro JR, Walsh KB, et al. Dissecting influenza virus pathogenesis uncovers a novel chemical approach to combat the infection. *Virology* 2013;435:92–101.
11. Arankalle VA, Lole KS, Arya RP, et al. Role of host immune response and viral load in the differential outcome of pandemic H1N1(2009) influenza virus infection in Indian patients. *PLoSOne* 2010;5:e13099.
12. Mulder J, Hers JFP. *Influenza*. The Netherlands: Walters-Noordhoff International School Book Service, 1972.
13. Amin R, Ford-Jones E, Richardson S, et al. Acute childhood encephalitis and encephalopathy associated with influenza. A prospective 11 year review. *Pediatr Infect Dis J* 2008;27:390–5.
14. Maricich SM, Neul JL, Lotze TE, et al. Neurologic complications associated with influenza A in children during the 2003–2004 influenza season in Houston, Texas. *Pediatrics* 2004;114:e626–33.
15. Randolph AG, Vaughn F, Sullivan R, et al. Critically ill children during the 2009–2010 influenza pandemic in the United States. *Pediatrics* 2011;128(6):e1450–8.
16. CDC. Prevention and control of seasonal influenza with vaccines. *MMWR Recomm Rep* 2013;62:1.
17. Wang K, Shun-Shin M, Gill P, et al. Neuraminidase inhibitors for preventing and treating influenza in children (published trials only). *Cochrane Database Syst Rev* 2012;4:CD002744.
18. Cooper S, Lyall H, Walters S, et al. Children with human immunodeficiency virus admitted to a paediatric intensive care unit in the United Kingdom over a 10-year period. *Intensive Care Med* 2004;30:113–8.
19. Zar HJ, Apolles P, Argent A, et al. The etiology and outcome of pneumonia in human immunodeficiency virus-infected children admitted to intensive care in a developing country. *Pediatr Crit Care Med* 2001;2:108–12.
20. Rey C, Prieto S, Medina A, et al. Fatal lactic acidosis during antiretroviral therapy. *Pediatr Crit Care Med* 2003;4:485–7.
21. UNAIDS Report on the Global AIDS Epidemic 2012. http://www.unaids.org/en/media/unaids/contentassets/documents/epidemiology/2012/gr2012/20121120_UNAIDS_Global_Report_2012_with_annexes_en.pdf. Accessed March 5, 2013.
22. Luzuriaga K, Sullivan JL. Viral and immunopathogenesis of vertical HIV-1 infection. In: Pizzo PA, Wilfert CM, eds. *Pediatric AIDS*. 3rd ed. Philadelphia, PA: Lippincott Williams & Wilkins, 1998:89–104.
23. Chi BH, Adler MR, Bolu O, et al. Progress, challenges, and new opportunities for the prevention of mother-to-child transmission of HIV under the US President's Emergency Plan for AIDS Relief. *J Acquir Immune Defic Syndr* 2012;60(suppl 3):S78–87.
24. Fowler MG, Simonds RJ, Roongpisuthipong A. Update on perinatal HIV transmission. *Pediatr Clin North Am* 2000;47:21–38.
25. Dunn DT, Newell ML, Ades AE, et al. Risk of human immunodeficiency virus type 1 transmission through breastfeeding. *Lancet* 1992;340:585–8.
26. Luzuriaga K, Sullivan JL. Viral and immunopathogenesis of vertical HIV-1 infection. *Pediatr Clin North Am* 2000;47:65–78.
27. Abrams EJ. Opportunistic infections and other clinical manifestations of HIV disease in children. *Pediatr Clin North Am* 2000;47:79–108.
28. Chan SP, Birnbaum J, Rao M, et al. Clinical manifestations and outcome of tuberculosis in children with acquired immunodeficiency syndrome. *Pediatr Infect Dis J* 1996;15:443–7.
29. American Thoracic Society/Centers for Disease Control and Prevention/Infectious Diseases Society of America. Treatment of tuberculosis. *Am J Respir Crit Care Med* 2003;167:603–62.
30. Fisher SD, Easley KA, Orav EJ, et al. Mild dilated cardiomyopathy and increased left ventricular mass predict mortality: The prospective P2C2 HIV Multicenter Study. *Am Heart J* 2005;150:439–47.
31. Cowburn CA, Hatherill M, Eley B, et al. Short-term mortality and implementation of antiretroviral treatment for critically ill HIV-infected children in a developing country. *Arch Dis Child* 2007;92:234–41.
32. Updated US Public Health Service Guidelines for the Management of Occupational Exposures to HIV and Recommendations for Postexposure Prophylaxis. *MMWR (RR 9)* 2005;54:1–19.
33. World Health Organization. *Measles Fact Sheet*. http://www.who.int/mediacentre/factsheets/fs286/en. Published February 13, 2013. Accessed March 5, 2013.
34. Van Den Hof S, Smit C, Van Steenbergen JE, et al. Hospitalizations during a measles epidemic in the Netherlands, 1999–2000. *Pediatr Infect Dis J* 2002;21:1146–50.

35. Anonymous. Severity of measles in malnutrition. *Nutr Rev* 1982;40:203–5.

36. Abramson O, Dagan R, Tal A, et al. Severe complications of measles requiring intensive care in infants and young children. *Arch Pediatr Adolesc Med* 1995;149:1237–40.

37. Norrby E, Kristensson K. Measles virus in the brain. *Brain Res Bull* 1997;44:213–20.

38. Kabra SK, Lodha R. Antibiotics for preventing complications in children with measles. *Cochrane Database Syst Rev* 2013; 8:CD001477.

39. Hussey GD, Klein MA. Randomized, controlled trial of vitamin A in children with severe measles. *N Engl J Med* 1990;323:160–4.

40. Huiming Y, Chaomin W, Meng M. Vitamin A for treating measles in children. *Cochrane Database Syst Rev* 2005;4:CD001479.

41. Stogner SW, King JW, Black-Payne C, et al. Ribavirin and intravenous immune globulin therapy for measles pneumonia in HIV infection. *South Med J* 1993;86:1415–8.

42. Cardosa MJ, Perera D, Brown BA, et al. Molecular epidemiology of human enterovirus 71 strains and recent outbreaks in the Asia-Pacific region: Comparative analysis of the VP1 and VP4 genes. *Emerg Infect Dis* 2003;9:461–8.

43. Nowak-Wegrzyn A, Phipatanakul W, Winkelstein JA, et al. Successful treatment of enterovirus infection with the use of pleconaril in 2 infants with severe combined immunodeficiency. *Clin Infect Dis* 2001;32:E13–4.

44. Reynolds MA, Watson BM, Plott-Adams KK, et al. Epidemiology of Varicella Hospitalizations in the United States, 1995–2005. *J Infect Dis* 2008;197(suppl 2):S120.

45. Fornaro P. Epidemiology and cost analysis of varicella in Italy: Results of a sentinel study in the pediatric practice. Italian Sentinel Group on Pediatric Infectious Diseases. *Pediatr Infect Dis J* 1999;18:414–9.

46. Fairley CK, Miller E. Varicella-zoster virus epidemiology—A changing scene? *J Infect Dis* 1996;174:S314–19.

47. American Academy of Pediatrics. Tuberculosis. In: Pickering LJ, ed. *Red Book Report of the Committee on Infectious Diseases.* 25th ed. Elk Grove Village, IL: American Academy of Pediatrics, 2000:593–613.

48. Feldman S. Varicella-zoster virus pneumonitis. *Chest* 1994; 106:22–7.

49. Kim EA, Lee KS, Primack SL, et al. Viral pneumonias in adults: Radiologic and pathologic findings. *Radiographics* 2002; 22:S137–49.

50. Committee on Fetus and Newborn, Committee on Infectious diseases, American Academy of Pediatrics. Perinatal herpes simplex virus infections. *Pediatrics* 1980;66:147–9.

51. Tyler KL. Herpes simplex virus infections of the central nervous system: Encephalitis and meningitis, including Mollaret's. *Herpes* 2004;11:57A–64A.

52. Kimberlin DW. Neonatal herpes simplex infection. *Clin Microbiol Rev* 2004;17:1–13.

53. Whitley R, Arvin A, Prober C, et al. Predictors of morbidity and mortality in neonates with herpes simplex virus infections. The National Institute of Allergy and Infectious Diseases Collaborative Antiviral Study Group. *N Engl J Med* 1991;324:450–4.

54. Nahass GT, Goldstein BA, Zhu WY, et al. Comparison of Tzanck smear, viral culture, and DNA diagnostic methods in detection of herpes simplex and varicella-zoster infection. *JAMA* 1992;268:2541–4.

55. Cohen PR. Tests for detecting herpes simplex virus and varicella-zoster virus infections. *Dermatol Clin* 1994;12:51–68.

56. Kimberlin DW, Lin C-Y, Jacobs RF, et al. Natural history of neonatal herpes simplex virus infections in the acyclovir era. *Pediatrics* 2001;108:223–9.

CHAPTER 91 ■ CENTRAL NERVOUS SYSTEM INFECTIONS

PRATIBHA D. SINGHI AND SUNIT C. SINGHI

KEY POINTS

Bacterial Meningitis

1. Meningitis is inflammation of the meninges that presents acutely when bacterial or viral and subacutely when mycobacterial or fungal.
2. Bacterial meningitis is a serious bacterial infection that is often missed clinically, and cerebrospinal fluid (CSF) should be obtained when suspected.
3. CSF in bacterial meningitis has elevated polymorphonuclear neutrophils, low glucose, and high protein.
4. Bacterial meningitis must be treated emergently with a broad-spectrum antibiotic.
5. The top three causes of bacterial meningitis include *Haemophilus influenzae*, *Neisseria meningitidis*, and *Streptococcus pneumoniae*; the incidence of Hib and pneumococcal meningitis has decreased dramatically in countries with universal immunizations against these organisms but not in other countries.

Aseptic Meningitis

6. Aseptic meningitis has high polymorphonuclear leukocytes (PMNs) initially and then high lymphocyte counts.
7. Aseptic meningitis is mainly caused by viruses but is also caused by tuberculosis (TB) and other agents.

Encephalitis and Myelitis

8. Encephalitis is inflammation of brain parenchyma, and myelitis is the inflammation of the spinal cord.
9. Most agents that cause meningitis may spread to the brain and spinal cord.
10. Arboviruses are the most common cause of epidemic encephalitis.
11. Herpes simplex is the most common cause of sporadic encephalitis.
12. Herpes simplex encephalitis (HSE) must be treated promptly with acyclovir.
13. Japanese encephalitis (JE) can be prevented with vaccination.
14. Acute disseminated encephalomyelitis (ADEM) is a postinfectious autoimmune reaction treated with high-dose steroids.

Brain and Spinal Cord Abscess

15. Lumbar puncture is often contraindicated when a brain abscess is suspected.
16. Antimicrobial therapy with drainage is often necessary in treating central nervous system (CNS) abscesses.

Cerebrospinal Fluid Shunt Infection

17. Most shunt infections are due to *Staphylococcus* spp.—*Staphylococcus epidermidis* and *Staphylococcus aureus*.
18. Antibiotics, shunt removal, and external drainage are often required for appropriate management of shunt infections.

Fungal Infections

19. Fungal CNS infections often have an insidious onset.
20. Most fungal CNS infections are due to hematogenous spread from the lung.
21. Mucormycosis occurs via direct spread from sinuses.
22. Amphotericin B remains an appropriate initial empiric antimicrobial for most suspected fungal infections of CNS.
23. Newer and effective antifungal agents are now available.

Parasitic Infections

24. Most parasitic infections of the CNS are subacute, but some can be acute and severe.
25. The most important etiologic clue to parasitic infection is living in or visiting an endemic area.

Infections of the central nervous system (CNS) are among the most devastating infectious diseases, causing death and disability worldwide. They often present as serious medical emergencies, and institution of early, appropriate intensive care is of utmost importance in reducing mortality and morbidity. This chapter is structured to familiarize the intensivist with common CNS infections, to help generate differential diagnoses, and to develop an appropriate treatment plan. It does not attempt to cover all possible infections that may affect the CNS.

A discussion on meningitis—bacterial, aseptic, and tubercular—is followed by sections on encephalitis and myelitis, with special emphasis on herpes, Japanese encephalitis (JE), and acute disseminated encephalomyelitis (ADEM). A section on brain abscess and epidural abscess, with emphasis on aspects relevant to the intensivist, is also included.

ANATOMY AND PHYSIOLOGY

As important aspects of CNS anatomy and physiology are discussed in Chapter 55, specific implications of anatomic and/ or physiologic issues will be identified in this chapter as they pertain to the specific infections under discussion.

PATHOGENESIS

To cause CNS infections, pathogens must gain access either to the subarachnoid space to cause meningitis or to the brain and spinal cord parenchyma to cause encephalitis, myelitis, or a CNS abscess. Most infections spread to the CNS through the bloodstream; however, different pathogens go to different anatomic locations. The organisms that typically cause bacterial meningitis rarely cause brain abscess, and those found in brain abscesses rarely cause meningitis. At times, the CNS may be infected by direct spread of organisms from an infective focus adjacent to the brain (otitis media, sinusitis, dental abscess) or from a cerebrospinal fluid (CSF) shunt or skull fracture.

CLINICAL PRESENTATION

The main features of CNS infections are fever, headache, and altered sensorium. Focal neurologic signs may also be seen. However, these symptoms and signs are nonspecific and can be seen in noninfectious CNS syndromes as well. Hence, a comprehensive evaluation is necessary to narrow the differential diagnosis. Epidemiologic risk factors for CNS infections and physical examination may provide etiologic clues. Broadly, a child with CNS infections may present with any of the following syndromes.

Acute Meningitis Syndrome

Acute meningitis syndrome presents as acute onset over a few hours to a few days of fever, headache, vomiting, photophobia, neck stiffness, and altered sensorium. An acute upper respiratory tract infection may precede the onset of meningitis by a few days. Examples of CNS infections that present with an acute meningitis syndrome include bacterial and viral meningitis.

Subacute or Chronic Meningitis Syndrome

Onset is usually gradual, often without any evident predisposing condition. Fever is often present but tends to be lower than in acute meningitis. Progression is slower over a few weeks. Examples of CNS infections that present with a subacute or chronic meningitis syndrome include tuberculous and fungal meningitis.

Acute Encephalitis Syndrome

Acute encephalitis may be diffuse or focal. In diffuse encephalitis, alteration of sensorium is predominant and occurs earlier in the course of disease than in acute meningitis. Seizures are seen more frequently than with meningitis and often during the initial phase of disease. Focal encephalitis reflects tropism of some viruses for specific locations in the CNS, such as temporal lobe infection by herpes simplex virus (HSV).

Encephalopathy with Systemic Infection

Many systemic infections involve the CNS, and CNS symptoms may be the presenting feature in some cases. For example, shigellosis, typhoid fever, malaria, rickettsial diseases, and infective endocarditis may directly involve the CNS or present as septic encephalopathy. It is therefore important to consider systemic infection as a possible underlying cause in children with encephalopathy.

Postinfectious Syndromes

ADEM, transverse myelitis, optic neuritis, and multiple sclerosis (MS) are disorders of demyelination of the CNS (collectively referred to as *idiopathic inflammatory diseases of the CNS*) that may present global or focal neurologic deficits days to weeks after recovery from an infectious illness, suggesting an autoimmune phenomenon triggered by infection or vaccine.

DIAGNOSIS

A general diagnostic approach to a patient with suspected CNS infection must include a thorough history and physical. Chronicity of signs and symptoms will help to categorize the illness according to one of the just-mentioned syndromes. Significant history, such as ill contacts, trauma, surgery, travel, insect bites, contact with animals, and sexual activity, may help to determine etiology. Premorbid or comorbid conditions, such as prior viral illness, immunodeficiency, presence of CSF shunt, associated diarrhea, respiratory illness, sinusitis, rash, arthritis, and other associated signs and symptoms, are important. Laboratory tests may include general assessment with complete blood count, chemistry panel, C-reactive protein (CRP), liver function tests (LFTs), urine analysis, and other testing to assess systemic illness. Specific testing of blood, including blood culture, thick and thin blood smears, polymerase chain reaction (PCR), antigen testing, and serology, may be indicated. General assessment of the CNS, including CSF opening pressure, white blood cell (WBC) and red blood cell (RBC) counts, protein, and glucose, is most often indicated; the usual CSF characteristics of meningitis are listed in **Table 91.1**. Specialized studies on CSF, including Gram stain with aerobic and anaerobic bacterial culture, fungal stain and fungal culture, and acid-fast bacilli stain and mycobacterial culture, should be considered. CSF inspection for parasites, viral culture, PCR, antigen testing, and serology may also be indicated. Neuroimaging, electroencephalogram (EEG), and other studies may add to the diagnosis. Drainage of abscesses and obtaining CNS tissue for histopathology are occasionally required.

MANAGEMENT

As with any other serious illness, management starts with the primary survey to ensure immediate attention to the basic airway, breathing, and circulation (ABCs) of life support before looking for an etiologic diagnosis. A secondary survey, with particular attention to the neurologic examination, meningeal signs, and assessment of the severity of coma, if present, is then undertaken. The physical examination in a child with meningitis is mainly geared toward excluding focal neurologic pathology, determining whether the child has clinically significant elevation of intracranial pressure (ICP), finding any

TABLE 91.1

CEREBROSPINAL FLUID CHARACTERISTICS IN MENINGITIS

■ CHARACTERISTICS	■ VIRAL	■ BACTERIAL	■ TUBERCULAR
WBC/mm^3	N (<5) or raised to 10–100	Raised 100 to >1000	Raised 100–1000
Predominant cell type	Lymphocytes	Neutrophils	Lymphocytes
Glucose (CSF: serum)	N (~0.6) or decreased (<0.4)	Decreased (<0.4 or much lower)	Decreased (<0.4 or lower)
Protein (mg/dL)	N (<50) or up to 100	Raised 100 to >500	Raised 100–500

N, normal.

source of infection elsewhere in the body (e.g., sinusitis, otitis, pneumonia), and identifying any other etiologic clues, such as rashes or skin lesions.

Children with a Glasgow Coma Scale (GCS) score of <8, pharyngeal hypotonia, poor gag reflex, and loss of swallowing reflex require intubation and supplemental oxygen. Appropriate techniques should be used to minimize potential increases in ICP associated with endotracheal intubation (see Chapter 24). Clinical signs and laboratory data that warrant admission of a child with meningitis to the PICU are listed in **Table 91.2**. Antimicrobial therapy must be administered promptly and, due to limited penetration into the CSF, at high doses. Details of antimicrobial therapy are discussed in later sections in which specific etiologies of CNS infection are described.

Any evidence of shock, such as poor perfusion, hypovolemia, and/or hypotension, requires aggressive treatment with normal saline boluses and inotropes, if necessary, to maintain normal blood pressure. Shock in CNS infection may be septic, neurogenic, hypovolemic, or a combination of these.

With increasing severity of illness and raised ICP, the cerebral blood flow (CBF) decreases, especially in the subcortical white matter. The level of impairment of consciousness correlates well with decreased cerebral perfusion, and mortality and sequelae are inversely related to the cerebral perfusion

TABLE 91.2

CHECKLIST OF CLINICAL SIGNS AND METABOLIC DATA THAT WARRANT ADMISSION OF A CHILD WITH MENINGITIS TO THE PICU

■ CLINICAL SIGNS	■ METABOLIC DATA
Glasgow Coma Scale < 8	Significant metabolic acidosis
Airway instability	Hypoxemia
Poor/irregular respiratory effort	Hypercapnia
Respiratory distress	Hyponatremia
Hyperventilation	Anemia
Poor perfusion/hypotension	Neutropenia
Oliguria/anuria	Other: falciparum parasitemia >5%
Hypertension/bradycardia	
Abnormal posturing	
Impaired pupillary response	
Deranged liver/renal functions	
Abnormal doll's eye movements	
Abnormal motor response	
Focal neurologic deficits	
Cranial nerve palsy	
Seizures	
Purpura/bleeding diathesis	

pressure (CPP) and CBF. ICP, therefore, must be maintained within a narrow range in children with meningitis. Although ICP monitoring is not routinely recommended, it may be considered in those children with CNS infection who have clinical signs of moderate-to-severe increase in ICP. The approach to control of ICP in patients with CNS infection follows the same algorithm as in other etiologies of intracranial hypertension.

Seizures are controlled with IV benzodiazepines, generally diazepam or lorazepam. Approximately half of the patients with seizures progress to refractory status epilepticus (SE). SE associated with intracranial infections is more difficult to treat and has a poor outcome (1). The overall approach to the treatment of SE is discussed in Chapter 63.

Alterations in fluid and electrolyte homeostasis are often seen with CNS infection and may be life-threatening if not corrected in a timely fashion. Accurate recording of fluid intake and output and close monitoring of electrolytes are essential. Fever, diminished intake, and vomiting may lead to significant dehydration and hypovolemia. Capillary leak secondary to sepsis can further add to hypovolemia. Diabetes insipidus (DI) may rapidly lead to hypovolemia and hypernatremia due to urinary free water loss. The syndrome of inappropriate secretion of antidiuretic hormone (SIADH) may lead to free water retention, hypoosmolality, and hyponatremia. These conditions must be recognized early to ensure appropriate management.

Fluid restriction to two-thirds of normal maintenance has historically been practiced with the hope that it reduces cerebral edema, presumably aggravated by the SIADH. However, it has been contended that a raised antidiuretic hormone level is an appropriate response to fluid deficit as it returns to normal on fluid administration. A prospective randomized trial of fluid restriction versus maintenance fluids with a clinical outcome (2) showed that restriction of fluids does not improve the outcome in children with meningitis. The increased fluid volume and mild systemic hypertension in children with meningitis may represent a compensatory mechanism to overcome raised ICP and to maintain adequate CBF and perfusion. Restriction of fluids and, thereby, extracellular volume may adversely affect cerebral perfusion and may worsen the outcome. Empiric fluid restriction in children with CNS infection is therefore not justified. A meta-analysis of fluid therapy trials found evidence to support the use of IV maintenance fluids in preference to restricted fluids in the first 48 hours in settings with high mortality rates and in which patients present late, but it found insufficient evidence to guide practice when children present early and mortality rates are lower (3). Fluid therapy should be aimed at maintaining normovolemia and normal blood pressure, thereby maintaining adequate cerebral perfusion. Careful monitoring of hydration status, intravascular volume, electrolytes, and osmolality should guide fluid management.

Hyponatremia should be identified early and corrected slowly over 36–48 hours with normal saline or, occasionally, with 3% saline, after calculating the sodium deficit. It is important to prevent and/or treat hyponatremic seizures. Children with meningitis are also prone to develop hypokalemia due to gastrointestinal losses, hemodilution, osmotherapy, diuretic therapy, and associated septicemia.

BACTERIAL MENINGITIS

Etiology

Worldwide, three major meningeal pathogens (*Haemophilus influenzae*, *Neisseria meningitidis*, and *Streptococcus pneumoniae*) account for the majority of cases, but the proportion caused by each organism is somewhat variable by region and age.

Haemophilus spp. are small, gram-negative, pleomorphic coccobacilli that are either encapsulated or unencapsulated. Encapsulated strains are classified into six types, designated *a* through *f*. Nearly all invasive *H. influenzae* infections are caused by serotype b (Hib). Hib strains have been further classified according to their outer membrane proteins (OMPs), which are useful for epidemiologic studies. Presently, almost all invasive disease worldwide is caused by nine clones of Hib, although nontypeable *H. influenzae* may rarely cause meningitis.

Neisseria spp. are non–spore-forming, nonmotile, kidney-shaped, gram-negative cocci that often appear in pairs (diplococci). Meningococci are classified by serogroups, which have important epidemiologic and prevention-related implications. Although 13 serogroups are recognized, most meningococcal disease is caused by organisms in serogroups A, B, C, Y, and W135. The virulence of meningococci is determined by their capsular polysaccharide, pili, immunoglobulin (Ig) A protease, lipopolysaccharide (endotoxin), OMPs, and outer membrane vesicles. All isolates from invasive infections are encapsulated (serogroup positive), whereas 20%–90% of those isolated from carriers are unencapsulated (nontypeable).

Pneumococci are non–spore-forming, nonmotile, small, gram-positive streptococci that are generally seen in pairs or chains. They are classified into serotypes on the basis of antigenic differences among capsular polysaccharides, which are essential for pneumococcal virulence. Approximately 90 pneumococcal serotypes have been characterized; however, only some of these cause invasive pneumococcal infections. Capsular types 1, 4, 6, 9, 14, 18, 19, and 23 cause ~85% of serious infections in children, a pattern different from that observed in adults. The serotypes that cause meningitis have a strong correlation with those that cause pneumonia and bacteremia.

Gram-negative bacilli can also be implicated in meningitis. Most cases of neonatal meningitis and sepsis due to gram-negative bacilli are caused by *Escherichia coli* strains that bear the K1 capsular polysaccharide antigen, a marker of neurovirulence. In addition to the K1 capsule, many other potential virulence factors for meningitis have been documented. Gram-negative bacterial meningitis in children beyond the neonatal period is generally nosocomial or may be associated with other conditions, such as gut infections, head trauma, neurosurgical procedures, and immunodeficiency. Other Enterobacteriaceae can cause meningitis, including *Klebsiella*, *Salmonella*, *Enterobacter*, and *Pseudomonas* spp.

Group B streptococci are the most common cause of invasive neonatal disease in many countries. They are classified into six main serotypes; type III is responsible for most cases of neonatal meningitis. A decrease in the incidence of neonatal invasive group B streptococcal disease has been seen in developed countries, secondary to treatment of pregnant women with vaginal colonization at the time of delivery.

Listeria monocytogenes is a gram-positive, non–spore-forming, catalase-positive, aerobic rod. An important cause of neonatal meningitis, its source is generally the genital tract infection of the mother. However, nosocomial infection may also occur, particularly in low–birth-weight babies in long-term intensive care.

Staphylococci are gram-positive organisms that are generally seen in pairs or clusters. *Staphylococcus aureus* is a virulent organism that is coagulase positive and causes pneumonia, sepsis, endocarditis, osteomyelitis, and meningitis. It is generally seen in malnourished children with staphylococcal skin lesions, dermal sinuses, or CSF shunts. Secondary meningitis may also be seen in children with head trauma, neurosurgical procedures, or sinusitis.

Anaerobic meningitis may occur in certain conditions, such as rupture of brain abscess; chronic otitis, mastoiditis, or sinusitis; head trauma; neurosurgical procedures; congenital dural defects; gastrointestinal disease; suppurative pharyngitis; CSF shunts; and immunosuppression. *Bacteroides fragilis*, *Fusobacterium* spp., and *Clostridium* spp. are anaerobic pathogens that may cause meningitis.

Epidemiology

Hib remains the leading cause of bacterial meningitis in countries where Hib vaccine has not been introduced, particularly in children <5 years of age, with an estimated incidence rate of 31 cases per 100,000 (4). Approximately 80% of cases develop in unvaccinated children <2 years of age, and nearly all cases occur in children <5 years. Meningitis caused by Hib in the first 2 months of life is rare, presumably because of placental transfer of protective maternal bactericidal antibodies. Natural immunity develops after 3 years of age, and concentrations of polyribosylribitol phosphate antibodies reach adult values by 7 years of age (5). The two main factors that determine risk for disease are nasopharyngeal carriage and the concentration of circulating anticapsular antibody. High-risk factors for invasive Hib infection include sickle cell anemia, asplenia, CSF fistulas, and chronic pulmonary infections. If children >6 years have Hib meningitis, such underlying conditions as otitis media, sinusitis, CSF leaks, and immunodeficiency states, including splenectomy, should be excluded.

Meningococcal meningitis occurs primarily in children and young adults. A wide geographic variation exists between the serotypes of meningococci that are endemic and those that cause epidemics. In developed countries, most cases are due to serogroups B and C. However, serogroup A is responsible for large-scale epidemics in many developing countries, including Africa, India, Nepal, and Saudi Arabia. Age-specific incidence of meningococcal infection is inversely proportional to the presence of serum bactericidal antibodies against serogroups A, B, and C. More than 50% of infants possess bactericidal antibody at birth as a result of transplacental transfer; hence, meningococcal meningitis is rarely seen in the first 3 months of life. An intact complement system is also an important host defense against invasive meningococcal disease. Recurrent or chronic neisserial infections have been associated with rare isolated deficiencies of late complement components (C5, C6, C7, or C8, and perhaps C9) due to the role of complement in opsonophagocytosis. Deficiency or dysfunction of properdin, which is a stabilizing factor of C3 convertase in the alternate complement pathway, also predisposes to meningococcal infections. The time from nasopharyngeal acquisition to bloodstream invasion is short (usually 10 days). The incubation period may also be short, because "secondary" cases commonly occur within 1–4 days of the index case.

Pneumococcal meningitis occurs in all age groups, but maximum incidence rates are seen at the extremes of age with an estimated incidence rate of 17 cases per 100,000 population in children <5 years of age (6). The common predisposing factors include pneumonia, otitis media, sinusitis, CSF fistulas or leaks, head injury, sickle cell disease, and thalassemia major.

Enterobacteriaceae, group B streptococci, and *Listeria* cause meningitis predominantly in neonates. Enterobacteriaceae are normal gut flora, 25% of women are colonized with group B streptococci in the developed world, and may infect or colonize the female gastrointestinal tract, predominantly in the developing world. Aspiration of contaminated secretions, pneumonia, and hematogenous seeding of the meninges result in early-onset meningitis incidence of ~10 per 100,000 (7).

Vaccines against Hib, *S. pneumoniae*, and *N. meningitidis* have decreased the disease burden by 99%, 94%, and 90%, respectively, in countries where vaccines are available. Due to the lack of vaccine availability worldwide, the global disease burden has been reduced by a mere 2%.

Pathogenesis

The development of childhood bacterial meningitis typically progresses through phases that include nasopharyngeal colonization and vascular invasion, meningeal invasion and multiplication in the subarachnoid space, induction and progression of inflammation in the subarachnoid space with associated pathophysiologic alterations, and damage to the CNS.

Nasopharyngeal Colonization and Vascular Invasion

Most organisms that cause bacterial meningitis are transmitted by the respiratory route. They colonize the nasopharyngeal mucosa by adherence to the mucosal epithelium and evasion of mucosal host defense mechanisms. Adherence is mediated through adhesins on the bacterial surface that help surface binding to epithelial cell receptors and differs in various organisms. In *N. meningitidis*, adherence depends on the binding of fimbriae on the bacterial cell wall, whereas in *S. pneumoniae*, it depends mainly on the cell wall components. Host secretory IgA antibodies inhibit adherence and penetration of pathogens. The organisms secrete highly specific endopeptidases that cleave the heavy chains of secretory IgA and impair specific mucosal immunity, allowing the organisms to colonize.

Infection of the nasopharyngeal cells causes injury to the ciliated epithelial cells of the respiratory tract, resulting in loss of protective ciliary activity. Bacteria penetrate the mucosal barrier through either transepithelial or paraepithelial means. A number of bacterial factors help the process of invasion, including pili and lipo-oligosaccharides on the outer membranes of *N. meningitidis* and *H. influenzae* and the binding of *S. pneumoniae* to the polymeric immunoglobulin receptors on the mucosa. Pneumolysin and hyaluronidase of the pneumococci also facilitate mucosal invasion.

To survive in the bloodstream, the pathogens must overcome the host defense systems of circulating antibodies, complement-mediated bacterial killing, and neutrophil phagocytosis. The bacterial polysaccharide capsule operates against these mechanisms. In the absence of specific anticapsular antibodies, nonspecific activation of the alternative complement pathway is the main host defense against encapsulated bacteria. Persons with impaired alternative complement pathways and asplenia are at particular risk for overwhelming sepsis and meningitis by these encapsulated bacteria.

Meningeal Invasion

The blood–brain barrier (BBB) normally protects against meningeal invasion. Penetration of BBB occurs via microbial interactions with host receptors and depends on various neurotropic and virulence factors, including capsule characteristics,

fimbriae, surface proteins of bacteria, and, perhaps, a critical magnitude of bacteremia.

After penetrating the meninges, the bacteria multiply freely in the CSF, which has diminished host defense mechanisms. The bacterial capsular polysaccharides have high antiphagocytic properties, and the CSF has a very low concentration of specific antibody. The bacteria thus multiply rapidly and spread over the entire surface of the brain and spinal cord along penetrating vessels.

Inflammation of the Subarachnoid Space

The multiplication and autolysis of bacteria in the CSF lead to the release of bacterial components, including fragments of cell wall and lipopolysaccharide that trigger a strong inflammatory response in the subarachnoid space by inducing the production and release of inflammatory cytokines and chemokines. These cytokines can be produced by many brain cells, including astrocytes, glia, endothelial cells, ependymal cells, and macrophages. Early-response cytokines include IL-1β, IL-6, and tumor necrosis factor (TNF), which then trigger a cascade of inflammatory mediators, including other interleukins, chemokines, platelet-activating factor, matrix metalloproteinases, nitric oxide (NO), and free oxygen radicals. The increase in cytokines enhances permeability of the BBB and recruits leukocytes from the blood into CSF, leading to CSF pleocytosis. These mediators also affect CBF and cerebral metabolism and contribute to the development of cerebral edema and neurologic sequelae.

Pathophysiology

Disruption of the Blood–Brain Barrier and Changes in Cerebral Blood Flow

Loss of autoregulation leads to changes in CBF, which increases in the early phase and decreases in the later phase of meningitis. The increase in CBF in early meningitis is secondary to the vasodilatory effect of NO. Later, the CBF progressively declines, most likely as a result of vasospasm. Loss of autoregulation also makes cerebral perfusion dependent on the systemic blood pressure, and the cerebral perfusion pressure drops when blood pressure drops.

In addition to the global cerebral hypoperfusion, focal hypoperfusion can occur due to vasculitis of large and small arteries crossing the inflamed subarachnoid space, which can cause ischemic damage that leads to permanent neurologic sequelae. Occlusion or severe stenosis of the intracranial internal carotid artery or of the middle and anterior cerebral arteries or involvement of the large vessels at the base of the brain can lead to stroke and result in paresis.

Neuropathology

Bacterial meningitis includes inflammation of the subarachnoid space, inflammatory involvement of the cerebral blood vessels, and parenchymal brain damage. Histologic examination reveals loss of neurons, generally focal, particularly in patients who have a late mortality. Cerebral edema in bacterial meningitis may be vasogenic, cytotoxic, or interstitial. Vasogenic cerebral edema occurs as a result of increased BBB permeability, which leads to extravasation of large molecules and serum into the brain parenchyma. Cytotoxic edema occurs because of an increase in intracellular water that is secondary to alterations of the cell membrane permeability and loss of cellular homeostasis, with influx of potassium and calcium into the cell. Interstitial edema occurs due to an increase in CSF volume, which may occur due to increased CSF production secondary to increased blood flow in the choroid plexus. Associated decrease resorption of the CSF may also occur because of increased outflow resistance across the arachnoid villi of the sagittal sinus. Interstitial edema is probably the main cause of obstructive hydrocephalus in meningitis. Severe brain edema can cause herniation of brain tissue and compression of the brainstem due to increased ICP. The ICP may also increase because of excessive intracerebral hypertension, including the development of obstructive hydrocephalus, cerebritis, cerebral infarction and cerebral venous thrombosis, SE, and SIADH. Death from meningitis may occur because of critically elevated ICP, extensive cerebral infarction, disseminated intravascular coagulation (DIC), and/or circulatory failure resulting from septic shock and refractory SE.

Clinical Presentation

The clinical presentation of meningitis is variable and is determined by the age of the child, the infecting organism, host resistance, and length of time between onset of illness and first evaluation by a physician. The onset is usually sudden but may occasionally be insidious.

The presentation in neonates and infants is generally nonspecific with fever, poor feeding, vomiting, lethargy, irritability, high-pitched cry, and seizures. Fever may be absent in very small infants and in severely malnourished babies. On examination, the anterior fontanel is full and often bulging, and separation of sutures may be seen. The typical presentation in older children is with acute onset of fever, headache, vomiting, anorexia, photophobia, and altered sensorium. A history of preceding upper respiratory or gastrointestinal infection is often present. Children who are <3 years of age may not be able to complain of headache and may only present with irritability.

On examination, signs of meningeal irritation (stiffness and pain on flexion of the neck), a positive Kernig sign, and positive Brudzinski sign are seen. Older children may adopt a tripod posture with arms held back and straight on sitting surface. Meningeal signs are usually attenuated or absent in malnourished children, neonates, young infants, and deeply comatose children.

Seizures may be the presenting feature in almost 1 in 6 children with meningitis and may recur. Meningitis is a common cause of convulsive SE with fever, and the classic symptoms and signs of meningitis may be absent in such children. Children with fever and seizures should prompt a high index of suspicion for bacterial meningitis. Raised ICP is common in bacterial meningitis. It often manifests with progressive impairment of sensorium with deepening coma, headache, vomiting, and Cushing triad (hyperventilation, hypertension, and bradycardia). Papilledema is uncommon at presentation; if it is present, a CT scan must be obtained to exclude a mass lesion or a complication.

Focal signs are seen in ~14% cases and may be due to subdural collection, cortical infarction, or cerebritis. The progression of symptoms generally depends on the pathogen. Most cases of H. influenzae and pneumococcal meningitis have an acute or subacute progression. Pneumococcal meningitis may start as nonspecific sepsis and progress to meningitis. A fulminant picture with manifestations of sepsis, shock, and rapid progression to death is characteristic for meningococcemia, a syndrome more distinct from meningococcal meningitis.

Associated findings vary according to the organism; patients with meningococcemia may present with a maculopapular rash, which rapidly progresses into a petechial/purpuric rash. Rashes can occasionally be seen in H. influenzae or pneumococcal meningitis. The presence of a petechial rash is highly suggestive of meningococcemia. A child with meningitis should also be examined for other sites of infections, such as pneumonia, otitis media, endocarditis, sinusitis, pyoderma, or joint infections.

Differential Diagnosis

The clinical differential diagnosis in a child with meningitis depends mainly on the age of the child and the clinical syndrome at presentation. Meningitis in neonates and very young infants may present as nonspecific septicemia, without any symptoms or signs of CNS involvement. Lumbar puncture (LP) should be done in all such cases to exclude meningitis. In older infants, febrile seizures are the most important differential diagnosis. In the absence of meningeal signs, meningitis may be missed in these babies. LP should be done in all infants <6 months of age and in all children who present with febrile seizures, who have irritability and/or lethargy, or who look toxic. In children with acute onset of fever and neck rigidity, the differential diagnosis includes aseptic meningitis, pneumonia, and other infections that may cause meningismus, such as retropharyngeal abscess, typhoid fever, cervical lymphadenitis, and, rarely, spinal epidural abscess. A good physical examination and appropriate studies help in excluding most of these conditions. In children with a subacute onset of fever and neck rigidity, causes of chronic meningitis, such as tubercular, fungal, and parasitic infection, must be excluded. A predominantly encephalopathic presentation must be differentiated from encephalitis, Reye syndrome, metabolic problems, hepatic encephalopathy, intoxications, and other causes of coma. Cerebral malaria is an important differential diagnosis in developing countries, particularly in endemic regions. In children with raised ICP and focal signs, cerebral abscess, focal encephalitis (such as herpes), intracranial bleeds, and other space-occupying lesions must be excluded. Urgent neuroimaging is warranted in such cases.

Diagnosis

Early recognition of bacterial meningitis is important for optimal outcome. However, published data suggests that the diagnosis is often missed on initial evaluation. The World Health Organization (WHO) Integrated Management of Childhood Illness referral criteria for meningitis include lethargy, unconsciousness, inability to feed, stiff neck, and seizures. These were found to have a sensitivity of 98% and a specificity of 72% to predict meningitis.

Laboratory Diagnosis

Definitive diagnosis of meningitis is made by analysis and culture of the CSF. If there is a clinical suspicion of meningitis, an LP should be done at the earliest opportunity. Considerable controversy has arisen regarding the safety of the LP in children with CNS infections because of the risk of cerebral herniation following LP. However, a temporal relationship does not necessarily imply causality, and very sick children with meningitis may have herniation even if an LP is not performed. Delay in performing an LP can delay the diagnosis of meningitis and administration of appropriate therapy. LP both provides confirmatory diagnosis and helps in organism identification, which is invaluable for selection of the most appropriate antibiotics, deciding the duration of therapy, and avoiding empiric antimicrobial therapy that most children with CNS infections would otherwise receive. It is recommended that LP be undertaken in all cases of suspected meningitis unless one of the following contraindications is present: raised ICP (unequal pupils, blood pressure/heart rate changes, abnormal respiratory pattern, deep coma/deteriorating consciousness), focal neurologic symptoms or signs (obtain a CT to exclude space-occupying lesion), shock/cardiorespiratory instability, thrombocytopenia (platelet count <40,000/mm³/coagulation disorder), or local infection at LP site.

Antibiotics should, however, be administered in all cases of suspected meningitis even if the LP is delayed. Delay in the administration of antibiotics is associated with increased mortality and morbidity in adults and children. Early antibiotic administration may decrease the yield on culture and Gram stain but does not significantly alter the cellular and biochemical parameters of the CSF.

Obtaining a CT scan before performing the LP is not routinely recommended. A proper history and clinical examination are sufficient in most cases to decide the safety of performing an LP. A CT scan should be obtained only in select cases in which focal neurologic symptoms or signs, clinical evidence of critically elevated ICP, or papilledema are observed, or when doubt exists regarding the diagnosis and a mass lesion or a complication, such as a brain abscess, is suspected. CT is normal in most cases of bacterial meningitis, including those with subsequent herniation. It must be remembered that a normal CT does not rule out raised ICP.

❸ The characteristic CSF findings in bacterial meningitis are increased opening pressure, polymorphonuclear pleocytosis, decreased glucose, and increased protein concentration. A cloudy CSF under pressure can be considered diagnostic of bacterial meningitis. Normal CSF in children has 0–5 mononuclear cells/mm³ (lymphocyte and monocytes); polymorphonuclear cells are very rarely seen. Presence of a single polymorphonuclear cell in the clinical setting of meningitis should be considered significant. In neonates, the upper limit of normal extends to a WBC count of 20–30 WBC/mm³, although the mean count is generally 5–10 WBC/mm³. The CSF vglucose is <40 mg/dL in 50%–60% cases. A ratio of serum to blood glucose of <0.4 was 80% sensitive and 98% specific for diagnosis of bacterial meningitis in children >2 months of age; in term neonates, a ratio of <0.6 is considered abnormal. The CSF may occasionally be completely normal in early stages of bacterial meningitis; a repeat LP after a few hours may show abnormalities. Antibiotic therapy must therefore be started in all cases with a strong suspicion of bacterial meningitis.

The LP may occasionally be traumatic; a grossly traumatic CSF can be used for culture alone. With less traumatic LPs, the WBC and RBC counts in blood and CSF can be used to predict the absence of culture-positive meningitis. A predicted CSF WBC count is calculated using the formula:

$$\text{CSF WBC (predicted)} = \text{CSF RBC} \times (\text{blood WBC/blood RBC})$$

The observed WBC count divided by the predicted WBC gives the observed-to-predicted ratio. The specificity and positive predictive value of an observed-to-predicted ratio of ≤0.01 and a WBC-to-RBC ratio of ≤0.01 were 100% reliable (95% confidence interval, 74–100 and 91–100, respectively) in predicting the absence of culture-positive meningitis.

The Gram stain is a quick, inexpensive, accurate method for organism identification. The positivity of the Gram stain depends on the number of organisms in the CSF. The lower limit for detection is ~10⁵ colony-forming units/mL of CSF, which corresponds to a positive smear in 70%–80% of cases of untreated bacterial meningitis. In case of a clear CSF, smears for Gram stain should be obtained from centrifuged sediment, whereas the fresh, uncentrifuged specimen can be used if the CSF is cloudy. The likelihood of having a positive Gram stain also depends on the specific bacterial pathogen: 90% of cases caused by *S. pneumoniae*, 86% by *H. influenzae*, 75% by *N. meningitides*, 50% by gram-negative bacilli, and approximately one-third of cases caused by *L. monocytogenes* have positive Gram-stain results. False-positive Gram stain may rarely result from observer misinterpretation, or reagent or skin flora contamination.

Acridine orange stain is a fluorochrome that stains the nucleic acid of some bacteria so that they appear bright red orange when seen under a fluorescent microscope. It stains the intracellular bacteria better than the Gram stain and may be positive even when the Gram stain is negative.

CSF culture is positive in the majority of untreated cases of meningitis. Ideally, freshly obtained CSF should be directly plated, and enriched thioglycolate media should be used. The yield is poor in developing countries because of pretreatment with antibiotics, delayed plating, and inadequate storage and transport. Blood culture, pleural fluid, and aspiration of other sterile sites (e.g., petechiae in suspected meningococcemia) can be helpful.

The presence of a polymorphic response with hypoglycorrhachia in an acutely sick and toxic-looking child favors the diagnosis of bacterial meningitis. Most cases of viral meningitis have a lymphocytic response; in some cases, however, an initial polymorphic response may occur. The CSF sugar is generally normal in viral meningitis; occasionally, it may be low but is rarely below 30 mg/dL. On the other hand, ~10% of cases with bacterial infection have an initial lymphocytic predominance. Other clinical parameters, such as a viral prodrome (with the child not looking very toxic), a rash, lymph node, or parotid gland enlargement, may favor the diagnosis of viral meningitis. Although tubercular meningitis (TBM) may occasionally have an acute presentation, generally the symptoms are more prolonged; evidence of tuberculosis (TB) elsewhere in the body, such as lungs, abdomen, and fundus for choroid tubercles, should be investigated.

It is not always possible in children to differentiate between viral and bacterial meningitis based on clinical symptoms or even after blood or CSF analysis using routine investigations. Rules for clinical decision making that are based on certain clinical and laboratory parameters have been devised for this purpose, and some of them have been found to be 100% sensitive and reasonably specific. However, such rules should only be applied after a complete validation process, on patients with the same characteristics as those used for their derivation and validation and, importantly, should not replace the clinician's skill. Rapid diagnostic tests that detect the pathogen by countercurrent immunoelectrophoresis, enzyme-linked immunosorbent assay (ELISA), and latex agglutination are useful in providing early diagnosis in such cases, as well as in suspected cases of partially treated bacterial meningitis. The latex agglutination test is more sensitive than countercurrent immunoelectrophoresis. The latex agglutination test for *S. pneumoniae* and *N. meningitidis* has a specificity of 96% and 100%, respectively but has a lower sensitivity, varying from 69% to 100% for *S. pneumoniae* and from 37% to 70% for *N. meningitidis*. However, a negative bacterial antigen test result does not exclude infection caused by a specific meningeal pathogen.

PCR assays detect the nucleic acids of the common organisms that cause meningitis and are very specific. A PCR sensitivity and specificity of over 90% has been shown for patients with suspected meningococcal disease. The DNA load in PCR has also been correlated with the incidence of mortality in patients with meningococcal disease. PCR for pneumococcus is sensitive and specific in the CSF; however, in blood, it may be false positive because of nasopharyngeal carriage. Broad-range bacterial PCRs that can rapidly detect a number of viable and nonviable organisms have shown a sensitivity of 100%, a specificity of 98%, a positive predictive value of 98%, and a negative predictive value of 100%. These can therefore be used for screening; a subsequent PCR would be needed to identify the specific bacteria. These tests are expensive and not easily available in most developing countries. They are generally used to differentiate partially treated bacterial meningitis from viral meningitis when the Gram stain is negative. To prove tubercular, herpetic, or cryptococcal infection, special staining techniques/tests may be required.

Serum and CSF CRP levels can help in discriminating between bacterial and viral meningitis with high probability and in making a diagnosis of bacterial meningitis in children with fever without focus. However, diagnostic value of serum CRP was not perfectly discriminant in several studies, and caution is advised when attempting to use CRP for diagnostic purposes. In general, raised serum CRP >50 mg/L is a nonspecific indicator of bacterial infection; it falls to normal after 1–2 days of antibiotic therapy. In the presence of CSF pleocytosis, elevated serum CRP levels of >20 mg/L in children <6 years of age and >50 mg/L in older children may help distinguish bacterial from viral meningitis. A serum CRP level of <40 mg/L may be found in bacterial meningitis; however, in the presence of a normal serum CRP level of <10 mg/L, the diagnosis of bacterial meningitis is highly unlikely. An elevated peripheral WBC count is suggestive of infection but may not be seen in all cases of meningitis and is, therefore, a poorly discriminating criterion for deciding on the need for LP in a sick child. CSF cytokines are highly sensitive and specific markers of bacterial infection. Elevated serum procalcitonin (PCT) (>5 μg/L) reportedly has a better sensitivity (99%), specificity (83%), and predictive value than CRP, leukocyte count, IL-6, and interferon-α (8). However, PCT estimation is still experimental and is not available in most resource-poor countries. Increased CSF levels of lactate, Limulus amebocyte lysate, and various cytokines have been reported in bacterial meningitis but have not been substantiated in multiple studies or standardized; determination of these levels is not routinely done for diagnosis of meningitis.

Complications

Several complications may occur with meningitis, either as an acute, early, often reversible phenomenon or as late events that generally result in permanent sequelae. Common complications are listed in Table 91.3.

Raised ICP is present at the time of admission in most patients hospitalized for bacterial meningitis and must be managed aggressively. In a 2004 study, almost half of the children with meningitis who required PICU care had raised ICP. Signs of raised ICP were seen either at admission or developed within 48 hours of admission (9). The increase in ICP is associated with deepening coma and pupillary, respiratory, and blood pressure changes. Cerebral herniation was seen on autopsy in 30% of children dying of meningitis. Children with GCS score of <7 have high incidence of raised ICP.

Seizures, which often occur in the first 2–3 days and cease within 1–3 days, can be due to cortical irritation secondary to the inflammatory process, fever, or electrolyte disturbances.

TABLE 91.3

COMPLICATIONS OF BACTERIAL MENINGITIS

Raised ICP
Seizures
Subdural empyema
Infarcts
Cerebritis
Hydrocephalous
Cranial nerve involvement
Brain abscess
Sensorineural deafness
Disseminated intravascular coagulation

If an EEG performed at the end of antibiotic therapy is normal, the anticonvulsant therapy can be gradually withdrawn. However, if seizure onset is later in the course of illness and is associated with underlying structural damage (e.g., an infarct), anticonvulsant therapy may be required for a longer period.

Subdural effusions are a common complication of meningitis, particularly in Hib meningitis, and may occur in almost half of cases. They are often benign, resolve spontaneously, and do not require any intervention. However, in a child with subdural effusion and persistent or recurrent fever, associated raised ICP, focal signs, or the presence of subdural empyema (Fig. 91.1), a subdural tap is indicated. Subdural effusion was found in 25% of patients; only 6 of 22 required drainage for raised ICP (9).

Cerebritis and infarction present with new focal features and occur because of involvement of the blood vessels in the inflammatory exudate or direct spread of infection from the subarachnoid space to the brain. Cerebritis and infarction may progress to form a cerebral abscess and are associated with a poor outcome.

Ventriculitis, which may occur, particularly in neonates and infants, presents with persistent fever and is diagnosed by CT and ventricular tap. Prolonged systemic antibiotic therapy is necessary in such cases. Drainage of CSF and/or intraventricular administration of antibiotics may also be required. Cranial nerve involvement may occur directly or secondary to raised ICP; the third, sixth, and eighth nerves are commonly involved. Sensorineural deafness occurs in 5%–30% cases, especially with pneumococcal meningitis, because of bacterial involvement of the cochlea through the internal auditory canal or via hematogenous spread. It may be transient or permanent and is associated with low CSF glucose and use of ototoxic antibiotics. Abnormalities in the brainstem-evoked responses occur within days and generally recover at the end of the first 2 weeks, although major deficits may persist. Hearing (brainstem-evoked responses or audiometry) must be formally assessed at the time of discharge.

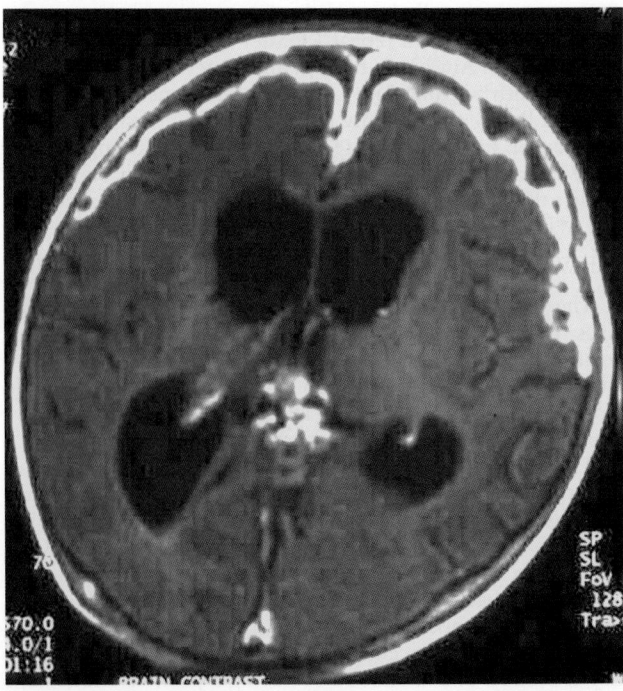

FIGURE 91.1. Contrast MRI showing subdural collections along frontal, parietal convexities and along interhemispheric fissure, with enhancement of dura and parenchymal surface suggestive of subdural empyema.

DIC may occur with fulminant meningococcal and gram-negative infections and requires aggressive therapy. Spread of infection leading to pneumonia, pericarditis, arthritis, and osteomyelitis rarely occurs.

Neuroimaging

The diagnosis of meningitis is made by clinical presentation and CSF analysis. In the early stages of meningitis, a CT scan is often normal. Later, CT may show meningeal enhancement and widening of basal cisterns. However, these findings do not affect therapeutic decisions. A CT scan at presentation is necessary to exclude other pathologies in a child with focal neurologic signs. Later in the illness, CT scan is performed to look for complications if a child does not show clinical improvement or has sudden unexplained deterioration, new-onset seizures, focal neurologic signs, signs of raised ICP, persistent fever, or enlarging head. Routine ultrasound of the head in infants with open fontanel has been found to detect most complications early.

Treatment

If bacterial meningitis is suspected, treatment should be instituted without delay. CSF, blood, and pertinent cultures should ideally be taken before starting antibiotics, but if specimens are difficult to obtain, therapy should be started and specimens obtained later. Most deaths because of bacterial meningitis occur during the first 48 hours of hospitalization. Coma,

raised ICP, seizures, and shock have been identified as significant predictors of death and morbidity. In a study from India, 40% of children with bacterial meningitis required admission to the PICU for one or more indications (9). All children with suspected bacterial meningitis must be kept under vigilant observation and monitoring so that complications (e.g., shock or raised ICP) can be recognized and managed early.

Initial empiric antibiotic therapy should be broad enough to cover all of the likely organisms according to the age of the child and the predisposing condition, and it should be based on sound knowledge of epidemiologic patterns of organisms and resistance patterns. Bactericidal antibiotics are preferred, as they cause more effective sterilization of CSF and improve survival in comparison to bacteriostatic drugs. Targeted antimicrobial therapy is based on organism identification by Gram stain and confirmation on culture. The Infectious Disease Society of America guidelines for empirical and specific antimicrobial therapy and the recommended dosages of the antimicrobials are shown in **Tables 91.4–91.6** (10).

In the United States and other countries where pneumococci resistant to third-generation cephalosporins have emerged, vancomycin is added to the initial empiric regimen. The antimicrobials are given IV; if IV access cannot be secured, intramuscular administration is an acceptable alternative until IV access can be secured. In a study from Africa, the outcome of pneumococcal meningitis was found to be better with the use of continuous infusion of cefotaxime as compared to boluses (11). However, this needs to be studied further. In developing countries, a combination of ampicillin and chloramphenicol may be used if financial constraints prevent the use of cephalosporins (12). However, increasing resistance

---

TABLE 91.4

RECOMMENDATION FOR EMPIRICAL ANTIMICROBIAL THERAPY FOR PURULENT MENINGITIS BASED ON PATIENT AGE AND SPECIFIC PREDISPOSING CONDITION

■ PREDISPOSING FACTOR	■ COMMON BACTERIAL PATHOGENS	■ ANTIMICROBIAL THERAPY
Age		
<1 mo	*Streptococcus agalactiae, E. coli, L. monocytogenes, Klebsiella* spp.	Ampicillin plus cefotaxime or ampicillin plus an aminoglycoside
1–23 mo	*S. pneumoniae, N. meningitidis, S. agalactiae, H. influenzae, E. coli*	Vancomycin plus a third-generation cephalosporin[a,b]
2–50 y	*N. meningitidis, S. pneumoniae*	Vancomycin plus a third-generation cephalosporin[a,b]
>50 y	*S. pneumoniae, N. meningitides, L. monocytogenes;* aerobic gram-negative bacilli	Vancomycin plus ampicillin plus a third-generation cephalosporin[a,b]
Head trauma		
Basilar skull fracture	*S. pneumoniae, H. influenzae,* group A β-hemolytic streptococci	Vancomycin plus a third-generation cephalosporin[a]
Penetrating trauma	*S. aureus,* coagulase-negative staphylococci (especially *S. epidermidis*), aerobic gram-negative bacilli (including *P. aeruginosa*)	Vancomycin plus cefepime, vancomycin plus ceftazidime, or vancomycin plus meropenem
Postneurosurgery	Aerobic gram-negative bacilli (including *P. aeruginosa*), *S. aureus,* coagulase-negative staphylococci (especially *S. epidermidis*)	Vancomycin plus cefepime, vancomycin plus ceftazidime, or vancomycin plus meropenem
CSF shunt	Coagulase-negative staphylococci (especially *S. epidermidis*), *S. aureus,* aerobic gram-negative bacilli (including *P. aeruginosa*), *Propionibacterium acnes*	Vancomycin plus cefepime[c], vancomycin plus ceftazidime[c], or vancomycin plus meropenem[c]

[a]Ceftriaxone or cefotaxime.
[b]Some experts would add rifampin if dexamethasone is also given.
[c]In infants and children, vancomycin alone is reasonable unless Gram stains reveal the presence of gram-negative bacilli.
From Tunkel AR, Hartman BJ, Kaplan SL, et al. Practice guidelines for the management of bacterial meningitis. *Clin Infect Dis* 2004;39:1267–84, with permission.

TABLE 91.5

RECOMMENDATION FOR SPECIFIC ANTIMICROBIAL THERAPY IN BACTERIAL MENINGITIS BASED ON ISOLATED PATHOGEN AND SUSCEPTIBILITY TESTING

■ MICROORGANISM; SUSCEPTIBILITY	■ STANDARD THERAPY	■ ALTERNATIVE THERAPIES
Streptococcus pneumoniae Penicillin MIC	Penicillin G or ampicillin	Third-generation cephalosporin,[a] chloramphenicol
<0.1 μg/mL		
0.1–1.0 μg/mL[b]	Third-generation cephalosporin[a]	Cefepime (B-II), meropenem (B-II)
≥2.0 μg/mL	Vancomycin plus a third-generation cephalosporin[a,c]	Fluoroquinolone[d] (B-II)
Cefotaxime or ceftriaxone MIC ≥ 1.0 μg/mL	Vancomycin plus a third-generation cephalosporin[a,c]	Fluoroquinolone[d] (B-II)
N. meningitis Penicillin MIC	Penicillin G or ampicillin	Third-generation cephalosporin,[a] chloramphenicol
<0.1 μg/mL		
0.1–1.0 μg/mL	Third-generation cephalosporin[a]	Chloramphenicol, fluoroquinolone, meropenem
L. monocytogenes	Ampicillin or penicillin G[e]	Trimethoprim-sulfamethoxazole, meropenem (B-III)
Streptococcus agalactiae	Ampicillin or penicillin G[e]	Third-generation cephalosporin[a] (B-III)
E. coli and other Enterobacteriaceae[g]	Third-generation cephalosporin (A-II)	Aztreonam, fluoroquinolone, meropenem, trimethoprim-sulfamethoxazole, ampicillin
P. aeruginosa[g]	Cefepime[e] or ceftazidime[e] (A-II)	Aztreonam[e] ciprofloxacin[e] meropenem[e]
H. influenzae; β-Lactamase-negative	Ampicillin	Third-generation cephalosporin,[a] cefepime, chloramphenicol, fluoroquinolone
β-Lactamase-positive	Third-generation cephalosporin (A-I)	Cefepime (A-I), chloramphenicol, fluoroquinolone
Staphylococcus aureus		
Methicillin-susceptible	Nafcillin or oxacillin	Vancomycin, meropenem (B-III)
Methicillin-resistant	Vancomycin[f]	Trimethoprim-sulfamethoxazole, linezolid (B-III)
Staphylococcus epidermidis	Vancomycin[f]	Linezolid (B-III)
Enterococcus spp. Ampicillin-susceptible	Ampicillin plus gentamicin	—
Ampicillin-resistant	Vancomycin plus gentamicin	—
Ampicillin- and vancomycin-resistant	Linezolid (B-III)	—

All recommendations are A-III, unless otherwise indicated.
[a]Ceftriaxone or cefotaxime.
[b]Ceftriaxone, cefotaxime-susceptible isolates.
[c]Consider addition of rifampin if the MIC of ceftriaxone is >2 μg/mL.
[d]Gatifloxacin or moxifloxacin.
[e]Addition of an aminoglycoside should be considered.
[f]Consider addition of rifampin.
[g]Choice of a specific antimicrobial agent must be guided by in vitro susceptibility test results.
MIC, minimal inhibitory concentration.
From Tunkel AR, Hartman BJ, Kaplan SL, et al. Practice guidelines for the management of bacterial meningitis. *Clin Infect Dis* 2004;39:1267–84, with permission.

of *H. influenzae* to ampicillin and chloramphenicol, and of pneumococci to penicillin and chloramphenicol, is being reported from Africa and Asia. The mechanism of resistance varies by pathogen; resistance of *H. influenzae* to ampicillin is mediated by a β-lactamase in most cases; therefore, a combination of a β-lactam with a β-lactamase inhibitor may be effective. On the other hand, such a combination would not be effective in pneumococci and meningococci, in which most of the resistance is mediated by change in penicillin-binding proteins.

Meropenem and the newer fluoroquinolones, such as gatifloxacin, moxifloxacin, and trovafloxacin, have been found to be as effective as cephalosporins for treatment of bacterial meningitis; however, they are not included as first choice in standard recommendations. Meropenem has a better CSF penetration as compared to imipenem and may be useful in

patients with meningitis caused by resistant gram-negative bacilli that produce extended-spectrum β-lactamases.

The duration of antibiotic therapy depends on the organism isolated. The standard recommendation has been 7 days for *N. meningitides* and *H. influenzae*, 10–14 days for *S. pneumoniae*, and a minimum of 3 weeks for gram-negative, group B *Streptococcus*, and *Listeria* meningitis. Shorter durations of ceftriaxone have been found effective in children >3 months of age with uncomplicated meningitis. In a multicenter trial in resource-poor countries, the outcome was similar after 5 days versus 10 days of ceftriaxone treatment in children with uncomplicated meningitis due to Hib, *S. pneumoniae* or *N. meningitides* (13). However, short-duration antibiotic therapy is not yet accepted as standard recommendation.

With appropriate antibiotic therapy, the CSF culture and Gram stain become negative within 24–48 hours. The CSF

TABLE 91.6

RECOMMENDED DOSAGES OF ANTIMICROBIAL THERAPY IN PATIENTS WITH BACTERIAL MENINGITIS

TOTAL DAILY DOSE (DOSING INTERVAL IN HOURS)

NEONATES (AGE IN DAYS)

ANTIMICROBIAL AGENT	0–7[a]	8–28[a]	INFANTS AND CHILDREN	ADULTS
Amikacin[b]*	15–20 mg/kg (12–48)	15–30 mg/kg (12–24)	15–30 mg/kg (8)	15 mg/kg (8)
Ampicillin*	100–150 mg/kg (8–12)	150–200 mg/kg (6–8)	200–400 mg/kg (6)	12 g (4)
Aztreonam*	60–90 mg/kg (8–12)	60–120 mg/kg (6–12)	90–120 mg/kg (3–4)	6–8 g (6–8)
Cefepime*	60 mg/kg (12)	60 mg/kg (12)	100–150 mg/kg (8)	4–6 g (8)
Cefotaxime*	100–150 mg/kg (8–12)	150–200 mg/kg (6–8)	200–300 mg/kg (6–8)	8–12 g (4–6)
Ceftazidime*	100–150 mg/kg (8–12)	150 mg/kg (8)	150–300 mg/kg (8)	6 g (8)
Ceftriaxone*	50 mg/kg (24)	50–75 mg/kg (24)	80–100 mg/kg (12–24)	2–4 g (12–24)
Chloramphenicol#	25 mg/kg (24)	25–50 mg/kg (12–24)	75–100 mg/kg (6)	4–6 g (6)[c]
Ciprofloxacin[d]#	—	—	20–30 mg/kg (8–12)	800–1200 mg (8–12)
Gentamicin[b]*	4–5 mg/kg (12–48)	4–7.5 mg/kg (8–24)	7.5 mg/kg (8)	5 mg/kg (8)
Meropenem#	40–60 mg/kg (8–12)	60 mg/kg (8)	120 mg/kg (8)	6 g (8)
Nafcillin*	50–75 mg/kg (8–12)	75–150 mg/kg (6–8)	200 mg/kg (6)	9–12 g (4)
Oxacillin*	50–150 mg/kg (8–12)	75–200 mg/kg (6–8)	200 mg/kg (6)	9–12 g (4)
Penicillin G*	0.1–0.15 mU/kg (8–12)	0.15–0.2 mU/kg (6–8)	0.2–0.4 mU/kg (4–6)	24 mU (4)
Rifampin[e]	—	10–20 mg/kg (12)	10–20 mg/kg (12–24)	600 mg (24)
Tobramycin[b]*	4–5 mg/kg (12–48)	4–7.5 mg/kg (8–24)	7.5 mg/kg (8)	5 mg/kg (8)
TMP-SMZ[f]	—	—	20 mg/kg (6–12)	20 mg/kg (6–12)
Vancomycin[g]#	20–30 mg/kg (12–18)	30–45 mg/kg (6–8)	45–60 mg/kg (6–8)	2–4 g (8–12)

Intravenous dosing is recommended for all antimicrobials for treatment of meningitis; *indicates IV and IM dosing, and #indicates only IV dosing.
[a]Smaller doses and longer intervals of administration may be advisable for very low-birth weight neonates (<2000 g).
[b]Peak and trough serum concentrations must be monitored.
[c]Higher dose recommended for patients with pneumococcal meningitis.
[d]Ciprofloxacin use has been associated with tendon rupture in children <18 years.
[e]Rifampin should only be used as monotherapy for prophylaxis, can be given IV or PO.
[f]Dosage based on trimethoprim component, can be given IV or PO.
[g]Maintain serum, trough concentrations of 15–20 μg/mL.
TMP-SMZ, trimethoprim-sulfamethoxazole.

glucose generally normalizes over 72 hours. The increase in cells and proteins may persist for several days. Fever generally decreases within a week, although it may last for up to 10 days in uncomplicated *H. influenzae* meningitis. Fever that persists for >10 days is considered "persistent," and fever that recurs after 24 hours of an afebrile period is considered "recurrent." Persistent fever may be due to thrombophlebitis, spread of infection (e.g., arthritis), occurrence of complications (e.g., subdural empyema, cerebritis, or ventriculitis), intercurrent viral infections, and, rarely, drug fever. Secondary fever is most often due to nosocomial infections or complications.

A repeat LP during treatment and at the end of therapy is not routinely necessary if the child has improved and is afebrile. Test-of-cure LP is recommended in neonates with gram-negative meningitis.

Indications for repeat LP on appropriate antibiotic therapy are as follows: lack of clinical improvement after 3–4 days, appearance of new symptoms or signs, initial CSF grows resistant/unusual organisms and no clinical improvement occurs within 24–48 hours of specific therapy, and gram-negative meningitis in a neonate.

The inflammatory cascade in patients with bacterial meningitis can lead to tissue damage and worsen the neurologic sequelae. It is believed that antibiotic therapy exaggerates the inflammatory response by causing bacterial lysis and endotoxin release. Steroid therapy has been shown to reduce indices of inflammation, including cerebral edema, elevated ICP, and CSF outflow obstruction in experimental meningitis. A systematic review has shown that dexamethasone, if given prior to or with the first dose of antibiotic therapy, has beneficial effects in

patients with meningitis due to *H. influenzae* and pneumococci (14). The American Academy of Pediatrics recommends the use of dexamethasone in *H. influenzae* meningitis, specifically to reduce the incidence of hearing loss among survivors. A dose of 0.4 mg/kg, 12 hourly for 2 days, has been found to be as effective as 0.15 mg/kg/dose, 6 hourly for 4 days.

However, in developing countries, most children receive antibiotics before a diagnosis of meningitis is made and corticosteroid administration before or with the first dose of antibiotics is rarely possible. Meta-analyses of studies found no beneficial effect of corticosteroid therapy in low-income countries (15–17). The drastic reduction in Hib meningitis in the United States and Europe calls for a relook at the empiric use of dexamethasone. Moreover, dexamethasone may mask the presentation of underlying infections (e.g., brain abscess, TBM, or meningitis due to resistant bacteria), delaying their diagnosis and treatment, hence routine administration of steroids cannot be recommended in developing countries. In developed countries, steroids should be considered prior to or coincident with antibiotic administration in children with suspected Hib meningitis (i.e., children with suspected meningitis who have not been immunized against Hib and/or children with CSF Gram stain showing gram-negative coccobacilli consistent with Hib) in the hope of reducing hearing loss among survivors. The use of steroids for pneumococcal or meningococcal meningitis is controversial in developed countries. Benefit of steroids has not been established in neonatal meningitis.

Oral glycerol for the first 48 hours may reduce neurologic sequelae in children with bacterial meningitis particularly in Hib meningitis. However, a Cochrane analysis concluded that glycerol does not reduce mortality but may reduce hearing loss; currently glycerol is not routinely recommended in bacterial meningitis (18).

Several nonsteroidal anti-inflammatory agents have shown beneficial effects in experimental meningitis. Indomethacin inhibits prostaglandin synthesis by inhibition of cyclooxygenase and has been shown to reduce indices of inflammation and cerebral hyperemia in early phases of meningitis. Pentoxifylline, a methylxanthine phosphodiesterase inhibitor, has several anti-inflammatory properties and has been shown to reduce TNF-α production and indices of CSF inflammation. Platelet-activating factor inhibitors have shown to reduce cerebral edema in experimental pneumococcal meningitis. Recombinant bactericidal/permeability-increasing protein and recombinant protein C may help to reduce severity of sepsis but have poor penetration in CSF and, as such, are unlikely to reduce meningeal inflammation.

The use of human IV immunoglobulin is particularly important for children who have immunoglobulin deficiencies and for neonates who have a limited immunologic response, such as those with group B *Streptococcus* meningitis. Monoclonal antibodies directed at the molecules responsible for leukocyte–endothelial adhesion can be used to reduce CSF leukocytosis and other indices of CSF inflammation.

Prognosis

The mortality rates of meningitis continue to be as high as 15%–20%. Neurologic sequelae are common and include hydrocephalous, spasticity, visual and hearing loss, cognitive deficits, and developmental delay. High serum cortisol levels (420 ng/mL) and high systolic blood pressure were found to be significant predictors of neurologic and hearing sequelae (19). Coma, raised ICP, SE, shock, and respiratory depression are important predictors of morbidity and mortality in children with acute bacterial meningitis (9). Early recognition and prompt management of these factors, preferably in an intensive care setting, are important. Delay in diagnosis is an avoidable adverse prognostic factor.

Prevention

Isolation of children with meningitis caused by *H. influenzae* or *N. meningitidis* until they have received effective antimicrobial therapy for 24 hours is recommended to prevent spread of infection. For *H. influenzae* meningitis, rifampin prophylaxis (20 mg/kg orally, max 600 mg, once daily for 4 days, consider using 10 mg/kg for neonates) is recommended for all household contacts if at least one unvaccinated contact is <4 years old; rifampin prophylaxis for the index case is not needed if ceftriaxone was used but is needed if ampicillin and/or chloramphenicol were used, as they do not eradicate *H. influenzae*.

In treating meningococcal disease, rifampin prophylaxis (10 mg/kg/dose orally, max 600 mg, 12 hourly for 2 days; for neonates: 5 mg/kg/dose) is recommended for household and day care contacts to prevent secondary cases and to reduce nasopharyngeal carriage. A single intramuscular dose of ceftriaxone (125 mg for children <15 years and 250 mg for children ≥15 years and adults) has been found to be better than oral rifampin for eliminating meningococcal group A nasopharyngeal carriage. A single oral dose of 500 mg of ciprofloxacin or 500 mg of azithromycin may be used for adults (>18 years).

Universal immunization against *H. influenzae* has virtually wiped out *H. influenzae* meningitis from developed countries; however, this protocol must still be implemented in many developing countries. Conjugate vaccines for pneumococci and meningococci used for mass immunization in some countries have been shown to reduce disease prevalence dramatically. Until such

time that a similar situation becomes feasible, they could be used in special high-risk situations in developing countries. Universal efforts at introducing mass immunization programs against the common pathogens that cause meningitis in resource-poor countries are the way to prevent this deadly disease.

ASEPTIC MENINGITIS

Aseptic meningitis is a clinical syndrome of meningeal inflammation in which common bacterial agents cannot be identified in the CSF. In general, aseptic meningitis is characterized by a benign clinical course and a lack of long-term sequelae; however, some cases may be associated significant morbidity.

Etiology

Although most cases of aseptic meningitis are caused by viral infections, some may be caused by nonviral pathogens, including fungi, unusual bacteria and mycoplasma, as well as autoimmune diseases, malignancies, and drug reactions. The majority of organisms that can cause meningitis can also penetrate into the brain parenchyma and cause encephalitis (**Table 91.7**). In the past, aseptic meningitis was commonly seen with mumps virus, lymphocytic choriomeningitis virus, and poliovirus. These are uncommon causes in developed countries today but continue to be important causes in many developing countries. Enteroviruses are the most common etiologic agents for aseptic meningitis in both the developing and developed world but will not be discussed in this chapter because of the relatively benign course in an immunocompetent individual. Other viruses, including arboviruses, herpesviruses, paramyxoviruses, and orthomyxoviruses, will be discussed in more detail in the following encephalitis section. Tuberculous meningitis, although grouped under aseptic meningitis by some, actually has an entirely different clinical presentation, pathogenesis, and outcome and will be discussed separately.

TUBERCULAR MENINGITIS

TBM is the most serious complication of TB, especially in children. It is fatal without effective treatment and is associated with significant morbidity even with treatment. CNS TB may take a number of forms, including TBM, tuberculomas, tubercular abscesses, and, rarely, myeloradiculopathy. TBM is the most common.

Etiology

TBM is caused by *Mycobacterium tuberculosis*; meningitis due to *Mycobacterium bovis* or atypical *Mycobacteria*, such as *Mycobacterium avium-intracellulare*, is extremely rare in children.

Epidemiology

A resurgence of TB is being seen both in developing countries and in developed countries due to the association with human immunodeficiency virus (HIV) infection. In addition, multidrug resistance is increasingly common. In 2010, WHO estimated 8.8 million incident cases of TB globally, equivalent to 128 cases per 100,000 population. Most of these occurred in Asia (59%) and Africa (26%) (20). Children, with their relatively compromised cell-mediated immunity, suffer, with a TBM annual incidence rate as high as 32 per 100,000.

TABLE 91.7

COMMON INFECTIOUS CAUSES OF ASEPTIC MENINGOENCEPHALITIS

ORGANISM	DISEASE			DIAGNOSIS		
	INFECTIOUS		POSTINFECTIOUS	CULTURE	PCR	SEROLOGY
	■ PARENCHYMA	■ MENINGES				
Virus						
Adenoviruses	+	+		Y		Y
Arboviruses	++	+				Y
Enteroviruses	+++	++++	+	Y	Y	
Herpesviruses	+++	+	+	Y	Y	Y
Human immunodeficiency viruses	+	+		Y	Y	Y
Influenza A and B viruses	++	+		Y	Y	
Japanese encephalitis virus	++	+	+			Y
Lymphocytic choriomeningitis virus	+	+				Y
Measles	+	+	+	Y		Y
Mumps	++	+	+	Y		Y
Rubella	+	+	+	Y		Y
Rabies	+	+		Y		
Bacteria						
Bartonella henselae	+	+		Y	Y	Y
Bordetella pertussis	+	+		Y	Y	Y
Borrelia burgdorferi (Lyme disease)	++	+		Y		Y
Brucella spp.	+	+		Y		Y
Chlamydia spp.	+	+		Y	Y	Y
Ehrlichia spp.	+	+			Y	Y
Leptospira spp.	++	+		Y	Y	Y
Mycobacteria spp.	++	+		Y	Y	
Mycoplasma spp.	++	+	+	Y	Y	Y
Rickettsia spp.	++	+				Y
Treponema pallidum	++	+			Y	Y
Fungi						
Aspergillus fumigatus	+	+		Y	Y	Y
Blastomyces dermatitidis	+	+		Y		Y
Candida spp.	+	++		Y		
Cryptococcus neoformans	+	+		Y		Y
Coccidioides immitis	+	+		Y		Y
Histoplasma capsulatum	+	+		Y		Y
Others						
Toxoplasma gondii	+	+			Y	Y
Entamoeba histolytica	+		Y		Y	Y
Acanthamoeba	+				Y	
Trichinella	+		Y			
Naegleria	+					

Y, yes; + denotes relative frequency of involvement.

Pathogenesis

Involvement of the CNS mostly occurs during a primary infection in children, whereas in adults, it may occur during reactivation. TBM usually results from the hematogenous spread of bacteria to the CNS from a primary focus elsewhere in the body, usually the lungs. A caseous lesion forms in the cerebral cortex or meninges, increases in size, ruptures, and discharges tubercle bacilli into the subarachnoid space, leading to the formation of a thick gelatinous exudate that infiltrates the corticomeningeal blood vessels, causes inflammation and obstruction of vessels and subsequent infarction of the cerebral cortex. The brainstem and various cranial nerves, particularly nerves III, VI, and VII, are surrounded by the exudates (Fig. 91.2B). The exudate accumulates mostly at the base of the brain and interferes with the normal flow of CSF, leading to hydrocephalus. Vasculitis (Fig. 91.2D), infarction, and hydrocephalus result in severe brain damage. Occasionally, TBM

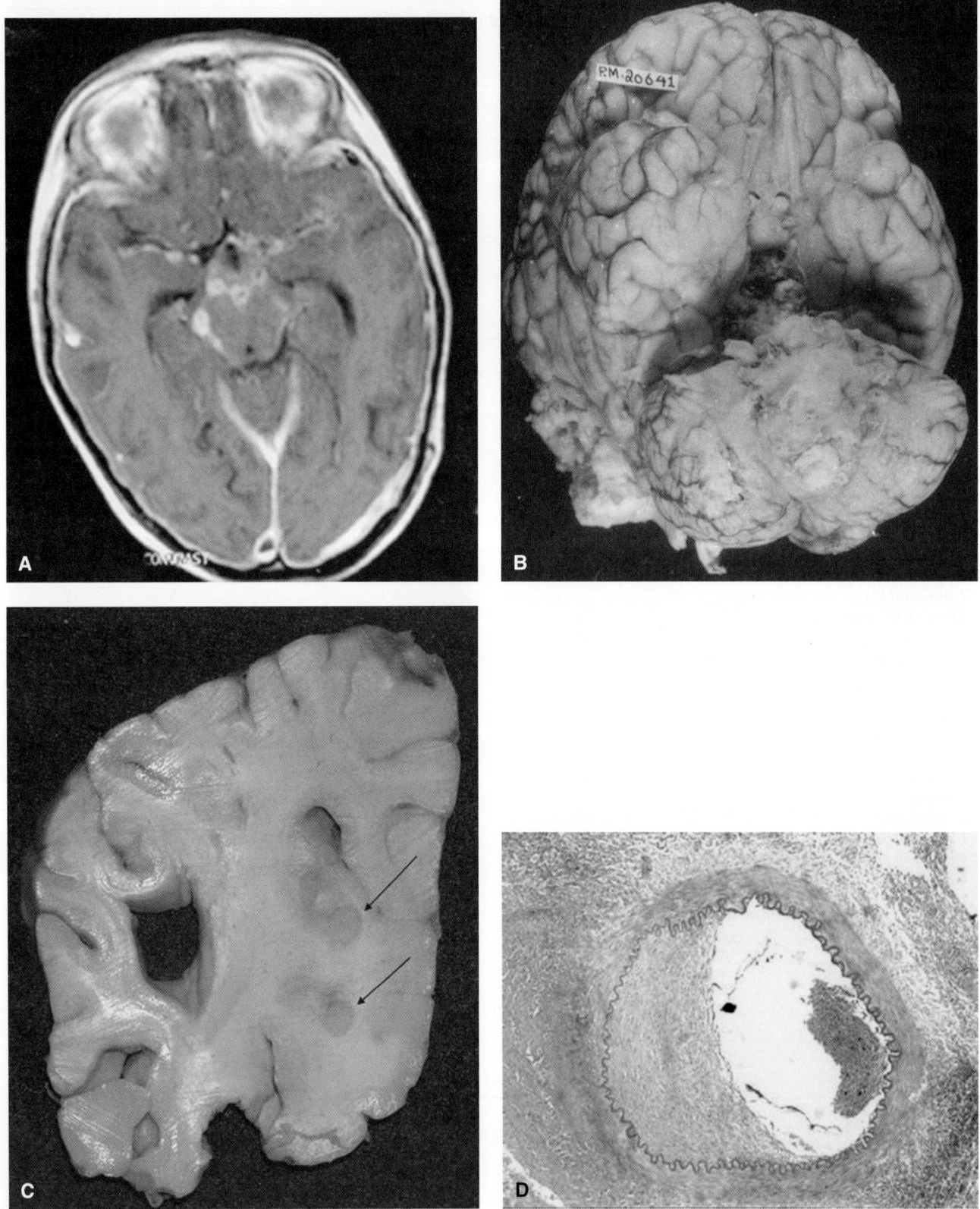

FIGURE 91.2. A: Contrast MRI showing paradoxic development of multiple tuberculomas in a child with TBM shunted for hydrocephalous and on antitubercular therapy. B: On autopsy, the brain showed thick basal exudates encasing the cranial nerves. C: Slices of the brain showing two tuberculomas (*arrows*). D: Histopathology showing intense vasculitis with occlusion of the vessel lumen.

occurs many years after the primary infection when rupture of one or more of the subependymal tubercles discharges tubercle bacilli into the subarachnoid space.

Clinical Presentation

The clinical presentation of TBM is variable. The onset is generally insidious, with low-grade fever, poor feeding, irritability, headache, and vomiting, followed by neck rigidity and altered sensorium. Occasionally, it may be rapid, particularly in infants and young children, who may experience symptoms for only a few days before the onset of acute hydrocephalus, seizures, and cerebral edema. More commonly, the signs and symptoms progress slowly over several weeks and can be divided into three stages (**Table 91.8**). Although the staging system brings objectivity in data comparisons, the progression is not necessarily a smooth continuum in an individual patient. The main presenting clinical symptoms and signs in children include alteration in consciousness (79%), focal neurologic signs (66%), fever (66%), and seizures (53%). Contact with an infected adult can be found in approximately half of cases. No significant difference has been observed in the neurologic findings in HIV-infected and -uninfected children (21).

Diagnosis

The diagnosis of TBM may be difficult because of its nonspecific and variable presentation. In endemic areas, TBM must be considered in the diagnosis of any child with a meningoencephalitic presentation. Differentiation of TBM from partially treated bacterial meningitis is a common problem in developing countries. The CSF is generally clear or straw colored in TBM, with a cell count of 10–500 cells/mm^3, predominantly lymphocytes, although in a few cases polymorphonuclear leukocytes may be present. A "cobweb" formation in the CSF on prolonged standing is highly suggestive of TBM. The CSF glucose is typically <40 mg/dL, and the protein is elevated (generally 150–200 mg/dL but may increase to 1000–2000 mg/dL). Low CSF chloride is no longer considered diagnostic of TBM. Identification or isolation of *Mycobacterium* on smear or culture is the gold standard for diagnosis of TBM. Successful isolation is possible in as many as 80% of cases if multiple samples are processed; however, in general, the yield is much lower. The yield may be increased by using the cobweb or sediment from a large volume of CSF. Radiometric culture (BACTEC) gives early results. CSF PCR, adenosine deaminase

levels, ELISA, and other antigen or antibody detection tests, including detection of interferon-γ from lymphocytes (QuantiFERON and T-SPOT.*TB*), have been reported to be useful with varying degrees of sensitivity and specificity. A combination of CSF adenosine deaminase >10 IU/L and serum >15 IU/L was found to have a specificity of 97% (22). However, none of these tests is diagnostic of TBM. Positive results support, but negative results do not exclude the diagnosis of TBM. The rare "serous" or sterile TBM with a CSF that resembles aseptic meningitis is considered an immunologic reaction to tuberculoprotein. The CSF is often normal in children with tuberculomas.

Neuroimaging

Neuroimaging is extremely valuable in the diagnosis of TBM, particularly because isolation of acid-fast bacilli is not possible in many cases. The CT scan characteristically shows thick basilar enhancement, parenchymal enhancement, hydrocephalus, cerebral edema, early focal ischemia, or infarcts and, sometimes, silent tuberculomas. MRI scan shows similar findings and may detect additional posterior fossa lesions, which may not be detected by CT. Brain involvement has been shown in MRIs of patients with miliary TB without symptoms or signs of CNS involvement. CT or MRI of the brain may, however, be normal during early stages of disease. CT signs of TBM were found to be less prominent in HIV-infected versus HIV-uninfected children (21). Corroborative evidence of TB elsewhere in the body, especially pulmonary involvement on chest x-ray and choroid tubercles on fundoscopy, gastric aspirates for acid-fast bacilli, and family screening for identification of contact, may aid in the diagnosis. The tuberculin skin test is positive in 30%–50% of cases, and a pulmonary focus on chest x-ray is detected in 50%–87% of patients. The diagnosis of TBM depends on a high degree of clinical suspicion, supportive evidence, and specific investigations. Scoring systems have been devised but need further evaluation. Even if the diagnosis is not confirmed, antitubercular therapy should be considered in the presence of meningitis with thick basal exudates.

Treatment

Most children with TBM of insidious onset will not come to the attention of the intensivist; however, some children with an acute, rapidly progressive course and those with serious complications, such as deep coma, stroke, and marked increase in ICP, will need intensive care.

Specific antitubercular therapy should have good BBB penetration and should be directed against both intracellular and extracellular organisms (23). As in other forms of TB, multiple drugs should be used to avoid the emergence of resistance. Initial treatment regimens have varied, using either three or four drugs. All regimens include isoniazid and rifampicin. The third drug used is generally pyrazinamide, but sometimes it is ethambutol or streptomycin. In the four-drug regimen, isoniazid + rifampicin + pyrazinamide + either ethambutol or streptomycin are used. Although clinical trials have shown that the efficacy of streptomycin is approximately equal to that of ethambutol in the initial phase of treatment, the increasing frequency of resistance to streptomycin worldwide has made the drug less useful. Thus, streptomycin is not recommended as being interchangeable with ethambutol unless the organism is known to be susceptible to the drug or the patient is from a population in which streptomycin resistance is unlikely (24). On the other hand, as ethambutol has a poor penetration across the BBB, the WHO recommends that streptomycin be used instead of ethambutol in the initial therapy of cases of TBM (25).

TABLE 91.8

CLINICAL STAGING OF PATIENTS WITH TUBERCULOUS MENINGITIS

Stage I (early) (days to weeks)	Nonspecific symptoms and signs (fever, headache, irritability, malaise)
	Lethargy or alteration in behavior
	No neurologic deficits
	No clouding of consciousness
Stage II (intermediate) (weeks to months)	Meningeal irritation
	Minor neurologic deficits (cranial nerve deficits)
Stage III (late) (months to years)	Abnormal movements
	Convulsions
	Stupor or coma
	Severe neurologic deficits (hemiplegia, paraplegia, decerebration)

The initial regimen is given either daily or twice or thrice weekly for 2 months, followed by a continuation phase generally with two drugs. Pyridoxine is recommended for infants, children, and adolescents who are being treated with isoniazid and who have nutritional deficiencies or symptomatic HIV infection (24). Although different regimens are recommended by various expert groups, in general, certain principles are commonly agreed on for treatment of CNS TB. In the initial phase, four drugs are preferred and a longer duration of continuation phase is advocated. The efficacy of short-course treatment regimens using intermittent supervised therapy has been proven for pulmonary and non-CNS extrapulmonary TB in adults and in children. Although the WHO recommends a 4-month continuation phase for TBM in its Guidelines for National Programmes, current data are inadequate to support short-course regimens for CNS TB.

The regimens recommended by the WHO (25), the American Thoracic Society (24), and the Indian Academy of Pediatrics for CNS TB (26) are listed in Table 91.9. These regimens are used when the organisms are susceptible to standard antituberculous agents. However, resistant strains are being reported from both developed and developing countries, particularly in association with HIV and malnutrition. Resistance to isoniazid or streptomycin is most common; multidrug resistance is seen in 1.4% of cases. Inappropriate or inadequate treatment is the main cause of resistance. Noncompliance is a major issue and is compounded by inappropriate prescribing practices by physicians.

In children, drug resistance in CNS TB is rare and is difficult to establish because of the low rates of organism isolation. It may be suspected if neurologic worsening or absence of clinical or radiologic improvement is seen after adequate therapy for several weeks. In cases where an adult contact has been identified, results of culture susceptibility of specimens obtained from that contact may be used to "confirm" the diagnosis of resistance and to guide the choice of drugs. Most of the data available for resistant TB are from adults. Drug resistance has been reported in some children with TBM. Management of resistant cases is a challenge. Several second-line drugs are available; most of them are expensive. Two or more of these drugs must be introduced simultaneously. The duration of treatment of multidrug-resistant TB is at least 18–24

months. In spite of aggressive treatment, the outcome is not favorable.

Corticosteroids are used with antitubercular therapy, as they reduce the neurologic sequelae of all stages of TBM, especially when they are administered early in the course of disease. Corticosteroids have been found to significantly improve the survival rate and intellectual outcome of children with TBM. Enhanced resolution of basal exudates and tuberculomas has been reported with the use of steroids, although no significant effect on the ICP or the incidence of basal ganglia infarctions was found. In very sick children, dexamethasone is administered IV for the first few days, followed by 1–2 mg/kg/day oral prednisolone, generally given for an initial 6 weeks and tapered off over 2–3 weeks.

Shunt surgery is often necessary in children with TBM who develop hydrocephalous: endoscopic third ventriculostomy has also been tried (27). External ventricular drainage has been used by some as an alternative to shunt surgery. In cases that present with life-threatening ICP secondary to hydrocephalous, an emergency ventricular tap is lifesaving until shunt surgery is done. Shunt surgery in HIV-positive TBM patients has been associated with a poor outcome.

Children with TBM need periodic clinical and radiologic monitoring. Despite adequate antitubercular therapy, improvement in clinical status may take several days, depending on the stage of disease. Some children in deep coma with severe neurologic deficits may take several weeks to improve. Corticosteroid administration is often associated with some clinical improvement within several days. Alleviation of raised ICP after shunt may result in improvement in sensorium within 48–72 hours. A postoperative CT is advised in all cases within 1 week after shunt surgery, or earlier in cases with clinical deterioration or no improvement. The CSF parameters may take months to normalize; CSF glucose returns to normal in 50% cases within 2 months and in the vast majority by 6 months. CSF cellular response and CSF protein levels may take 6 months to normalize.

Paradoxic response, including development of tuberculomas in children (Fig. 91.2A,C), is known even after up to 1 year on standard treatment for TBM (28). The cause and nature of these tuberculomas are poorly understood, but they do not represent failure of drug treatment. This possibility should

TABLE 91.9

RECOMMENDED TREATMENT REGIMENS FOR CENTRAL NERVOUS SYSTEM TUBERCULOSIS

■ THERAPY	■ WHO	■ AMERICAN THORACIC SOCIETY	■ NATIONAL GUIDELINES INDIA
Initial Continuation Phase	2 mo HRZE daily 10 mo HR daily (12 mo total)	2 mo HRZE daily or 2 wk HRZE daily then 6 wk twice weekly[a] 10 mo HR daily or twice weekly	2 mo HRZE daily 7 mo HRE daily (9 mo total, extended to 12 mo in serious cases)

DOSES FOR ANTITUBERCULAR DRUGS FOR CHILDREN[b]

	■ DAILY DOSE mg/kg/24 h	■ TWICE WEEKLY DOSE mg/kg/dose
Isoniazid (max)	10–15 (300 mg)	20–30 (900 mg)
Rifampin (max)	10–20 (600 mg)	10–20 (600 mg)
Pyrazinamide (max)	30–40 (2.0 g)	50–70 (2 g)
Ethambutol (max)	15–25 (1.0 g)	50 (2.5 g)
Streptomycin (max)	20–40 (1.0 g)	25–30 (1.5 g)

[a]All intermittent therapies to be monitored by directly observed therapy (DOT) for the duration of therapy; H, isoniazid; R, rifampicin; Z, pyrazinamide; S, streptomycin; E, ethambutol.
[b]WHO recommendations; WHO does not recommend twice or thrice weekly doses.

be considered whenever a child with tuberculous meningitis deteriorates or develops focal neurologic findings while on treatment. The clinical signs and symptoms may sometimes be severe; corticosteroids are helpful in such cases. Rarely, drug resistance may develop during treatment and is suspected when a patient with TBM shows worsening or cord involvement. Additional antitubercular drugs and steroids are used.

Prognosis

The outcome of TBM correlates most closely with the clinical stage of illness at the time treatment is initiated. The majority of patients in stage 1 have a good outcome, whereas most patients in stage 3 who survive have permanent disabilities, including blindness, deafness, paraplegia, epilepsy, or mental retardation.

ENCEPHALITIS AND MYELITIS

The term *encephalitis* denotes inflammation of brain parenchyma. Encephalitis caused by direct infection of the CNS is called *primary encephalitis*. Clinically, symptoms and signs of cortical or brainstem involvement, such as seizures and altered sensorium, are seen. Pathologically, the brain parenchyma shows (a) inflammation and destruction of neurons, and (b) pathogen detected by direct visualization, tissue staining, immunostaining, or nucleic acid detection. Acute inflammatory demyelination that occurs in temporal association with a systemic viral infection or immunization but without direct viral invasion in the CNS is called *postinfectious encephalitis*. As the spinal cord may also be involved, it is referred to as ADEM. Clinically, symptoms and signs of white matter involvement in addition to gray matter involvement are often seen. Pathologically, demyelination and perivascular aggregation of immune cells in the CNS are noted but not evidence of virus or viral antigen, suggesting an autoimmune etiology. The term *encephalopathy* refers to signs of diffuse cerebral dysfunction and can involve dysfunction that does not have an inflammatory component.

Viral encephalitis may be sporadic or may occur in epidemics. Although epidemic encephalitis has declined in developed countries as a result of improvements in living conditions and mass immunization against many of the childhood exanthems, such as measles, mumps, and rubella, large epidemics of encephalitis, with devastating consequences, continue to occur in many developing countries. Most children with encephalitis are critically ill and require urgent management in the ICU.

Etiology

The most common cause of neonatal encephalitis is HSV, most often HSV type 2 (HSV-2). Other viruses, such as enterovirus or adenovirus, may also cause encephalitis in the neonate. Intrauterine infections, such as cytomegalovirus (CMV), rubella, and toxoplasma, may involve the brain but generally do not present as acute encephalitis.

In childhood, the most common causes of epidemic encephalitis are arthropod-borne viruses (arboviruses) and enteroviruses. Eastern equine encephalitis (EEE) and western equine encephalitis are caused by Alphaviridae. St. Louis encephalitis, West Nile virus encephalitis, and JE are caused by Flaviviridae. Colorado tick fever is caused by an orbivirus, a member of the family Reoviridae. Enteroviruses are viruses that infect primarily the enteric tract and include polio, echo, coxsackie, and other enteroviruses. Adenovirus, Epstein–Barr virus (EBV), measles, mumps, varicella, and the bacterium *Bartonella henselae* also

cause sporadic cases. Subacute sclerosing panencephalitis is a chronic, persistent infection of the measles virus, also quite rare due to the widespread use of measles vaccine. Tick-borne bacterial diseases, such as borreliosis, rickettsial diseases, and ehrlichiosis, may also cause encephalitis. The common etiologies of acute encephalitis are listed in **Table 91.7** and vary by geographic region.

Epidemiology

In a large number of cases of encephalitis, the etiologic agent may not be identified due to lack of investigative facilities. Herpes simplex encephalitis (HSE) is the most common cause of sporadic and severe encephalitis throughout childhood. Two-thirds of the population is infected with HSV type 1 (HSV-1), and one out of four individuals is infected with HSV-2. Approximately, 80% of infections are asymptomatic, and transmission occurs from asymptomatic shedding of virus or via contact with lesions. The majority of encephalitis beyond the neonatal period is caused by HSV-1, although HSV-6 can cause some cases. Most cases of HSV encephalitis are caused by reactivation of latent virus. This topic is discussed in detail later in this chapter.

Arbovirus encephalitis in North America generally occurs in the late summer and fall. St. Louis encephalitis virus and West Nile virus are common vector-transmitted causes of aseptic meningitis and encephalitis throughout America. Birds are the reservoirs, and multiple species of mosquitoes are the principal vectors. Exposure to these mosquitoes may be more likely to occur indoors, as poorly sealed residences appear to be a risk factor. The majority of infections with St. Louis encephalitis and West Nile virus are asymptomatic, but significant neurologic findings, including extrapyramidal signs, optic neuritis, cranial nerve abnormalities, polyradiculitis, myelitis, and seizures may occur. EEE and western equine encephalitis also utilize the bird as reservoir and mosquito as the vector, but horses and humans are dead-end hosts. EEE is the most severe of the four common arboviral encephalitides just discussed, with a fatality rate as high as 50%.

Enteroviruses are endemic in the developed and developing world, with higher transmission rates in summer and fall. Most enteroviral infection is asymptomatic, and meningitis is more common than encephalitis. The only enterovirus against which a vaccine is available is polio, which is slated to follow smallpox in eradication efforts. Target vaccination campaigns address outbreaks in countries where polio transmission occurs, including Nigeria and Pakistan. JE is the leading cause of epidemic encephalitis in many developing countries and will be discussed separately. Rabies, mumps, and measles encephalitis are now rarely seen in developed countries but continue to be seen in many developing countries.

Pathogenesis

Viruses gain access to the CNS by either the hematogenous or the neuronal route. The mechanism of spread to the CNS by either of these routes depends on various viral factors, site of entry, and viral replication in intermediate cells. The host factors that prevent this access include local immune response at the site of entry, systemic immune responses, and protection offered by the BBB. The mechanism of spread to the CNS and the host response influence the clinical manifestations of neurologic disease.

Hematogenous spread is the main pathway of viral spread in human beings. Enteroviruses and arboviruses represent viruses that spread to the CNS through viremia, although their site of entry differs. The virus first replicates at the local site of entry and causes primary viremia. It then infects secondary tissue and undergoes secondary replication, causing an extensive viremia that seeds the CNS. Viral entry into the epithelium is prevented by protective layers of keratin; breaks in this defensive layer can result in increased risk of infection by viral entry into the subepithelial layer or directly into the blood. The conjunctival, respiratory, oral, and nasopharyngeal epithelial layers are nonkeratinized and allow easy entry for viruses that spread through the respiratory route or by large droplets.

After crossing the epithelial barrier and entering a receptive cell, primary replication occurs. The virus can then reach a lymph node and replicate there, or it can bypass the lymph node and enter the bloodstream, causing primary viremia, which leads to seeding of other organs and often marks the onset of clinical illness. In the blood, the virus may circulate freely in the plasma or be attached to or inside cells. Most viruses undergo secondary replication in the liver and spleen, which are highly vascular structures. Secondary viremia follows, and high titers of virus are released in the bloodstream for prolonged periods, leading to the seeding of target organs. As the CNS is protected by the BBB, large numbers of viruses are required to gain access to the brain cells or CSF. The exact mechanisms of viral transport from blood to brain and of viral endothelial cell tropism are not well known. The viruses enter the endothelial cells of arteries, arterioles, and capillaries and cause damage that leads to vasculitis, hemorrhage, and thrombosis. The viruses then enter the CSF and may either involve the meninges alone or enter the brain parenchyma and cause encephalitis.

Viruses can also spread to the CNS via neurons. Viremia and neuronal spread to the CNS can occur concurrently and are not mutually exclusive. Rabies and HSV represent viruses that reach the brain by peripheral neuronal spread, which occurs along peripheral or cranial nerves. Rabies virus classically infects by the myoneural route; however, very rarely, infection can occur from corneal transplantations and via aerosolized route. Following a bite by a rabid animal, rabies virus replicates locally in the soft tissue. It then enters the peripheral nerve and travels by anterograde and retrograde intra-axonal transport to infect neurons in the brainstem and hippocampus and throughout the brain. Cranial nerves, particularly the olfactory nerve, may also provide a pathway for viral access to the CNS. The olfactory neurons are not protected by the BBB and, therefore, provide easy neuronal access to the brain. HSV can infect the brain through the olfactory system and the trigeminal nerve. The inferomedial temporal lobe, which has direct connection with the olfactory bulb, is the initial site of early HSV encephalitis.

After gaining access to the CNS, the virus attaches itself to the host cells. The capsid or envelope proteins bind with receptors of host cells. The mechanism of cell entry varies among enveloped and nonenveloped viruses. Enveloped viruses enter the cell by either direct fusion or receptor-mediated endocytosis. Nonenveloped viruses may undergo structural changes or proteolysis; the capsid protein then fuses with the cell membrane and releases the viral genome into the cytoplasm. Once the viral genome enters the cell, viral replication occurs in the nucleus or the cytoplasm. Positive-stranded viral mRNA is produced, and gene products are subsequently translated. When viral protein synthesis begins, the host protein synthesis decreases, and host cell functions are affected. Within the brain, spread from one cell to another may involve multiple mechanisms.

A number of host and viral factors, including the route of infection, genetic composition of the virus, receptor differences, and so on, may influence neurotropism.

Host factors, such as age, sex, immunity, and genetic differences, also influence the extent, location, and severity of viral CNS disease. Viral infections in very young children are often much more serious, with a higher morbidity and mortality than in older children. Enterovirus infections in children <2 weeks can produce a severe systemic infection, including meningitis or meningoencephalitis, with high morbidity and mortality. In contrast, older children rarely have severe disease or significant morbidity. Physical activity may increase the risk of acquisition or severity of viral infection. Exercise has been associated with increased risk of paralytic poliomyelitis and may result in an increased incidence of enteroviral myocarditis and aseptic meningitis.

The host resists viral infections via both cellular and systemic immune defense mechanisms. Certain enzymatic pathways are activated that destroy viral nucleic acid transcripts and stimulate secretion of interferons. Interferons inhibit viral penetration, replication, translation, and assembly. However, some viruses have developed resistance to interferons, and, occasionally, the inflammatory response itself may cause damage to brain tissue with destruction of the infected neurons. In postinfectious encephalitis, the immune response is misdirected against the brain itself and causes immune-mediated demyelination.

Clinical Manifestations

The clinical manifestations of encephalitis vary according to the site, severity of parenchymal involvement, and a number of host factors. Most viruses that cause encephalitis simultaneously involve the meninges, causing "meningoencephalitis," while some viruses (e.g., rabies) do not have significant meningeal involvement.

In neonates, encephalitis generally presents with nonspecific symptoms and signs of systemic sepsis, including fever, poor feeding, irritability, lethargy, seizures, or apnea. History of maternal fever in the peripartum may be present in some cases of enterovirus or adenovirus infections. History of maternal genital herpes is seen in only 20%–27% of infants with herpes infection. Hence, an absence of parental history of HSV infection does not exclude neonatal HSV infection. Skin lesions in the neonate are seen in some cases of neonatal herpes encephalitis. Focal neurologic signs may be present in some but not in all neonates. As specific signs of encephalitis may not be present, strong consideration should be made to performing HSV PCR in neonates with suspected sepsis from whom CSF is obtained for bacterial culture.

The usual presentation of encephalitis in older children is with acute-onset fever, headache, seizures, behavioral changes, and rapid alteration in sensorium, progressing to coma. A prodromal illness with myalgias, fever, anorexia, and lethargy, reflecting the systemic viremia may be seen in some cases. Alteration in sensorium, the hallmark of encephalitis, generally occurs early and progresses rapidly, as compared to meningitis. Seizures are common and may be generalized or focal. The neurologic symptoms may vary from subtle to severe, and depending on the degree of meningeal involvement, symptoms and signs of meningitis, including photophobia, vomiting, and stiff neck, may be present. Other symptoms and signs depend on the neuroanatomic site of involvement. Cortical involvement may lead to disorientation and confusion, basal ganglia involvement to movement disorders, and brainstem involvement to cranial nerve dysfunction. Associated spinal cord involvement (myelitis) may cause flaccid paraplegia with abnormalities of the deep tendon reflexes.

A careful physical and neurologic examination is essential. A quick neurologic evaluation includes GCS and evaluation for any life-threatening signs of raised ICP. Subsequently, a detailed examination of sensory, motor, and cerebral function can be undertaken to elicit any focal neurologic signs.

Etiologic differentiation of encephalitides may not be possible on the basis of clinical features and usual laboratory tests.

However, certain diagnostic clues can be obtained from the history and examination and from epidemiology. A history of recent travel, exposure to persons with infections, and insects or animal bites should be obtained. A history of focal seizures, personality changes, and aphasia suggests herpes encephalitis. Fever with severe pharyngitis and fatigue may indicate EBV encephalitis. Fever, parotitis, and dysphagia suggest mumps encephalitis. Fever, conjunctivitis, and the characteristic rash of measles indicate measles encephalitis. History of a dog bite or bat exposure with characteristic behavioral changes and predominant bulbar involvement suggests rabies. The furious type of rabies with agitation, characteristic hydrophobia, or hypersalivation is much more common than the "paralytic" or "dumb" type with flaccid ascending paralysis. Exposure to kittens suggests *B. henselae* (cat-scratch) encephalitis. Encephalitis in summer with a suggestive rash is seen with Rocky Mountain spotted fever (petechial), enteroviruses, arboviruses (maculopapular), and Lyme disease (erythema migrans). Epidemics of JE generally occur after the rainy season during mosquito breeding periods; signs and symptoms of basal ganglia involvement are further diagnostic clues.

Differential Diagnosis

Encephalitis must be differentiated from other causes of encephalopathy and coma. Bacterial meningitis may present with encephalopathic components due to the pathophysiology discussed previously, increased ICP, and global CNS dysfunction. Cerebral malaria is an important, eminently treatable condition that must be differentiated urgently in many developing countries. This subject is discussed in Chapter 93. Other febrile encephalopathies, such as those caused by *Salmonella* and *Shigella*, would generally have suggestive symptoms and signs of the primary illness. Fever and the presence of focal signs help in distinguishing encephalitis from encephalopathies secondary to metabolic problems and toxins. Children with Reye syndrome present with afebrile encephalopathy following a prodrome of nausea and vomiting. They have mild hepatomegaly, hypoglycemia, some elevation of liver transaminases with mild hyperbilirubinemia (serum bilirubin < 5 mg/dL), and elevated blood ammonia levels.

A biphasic illness, with antecedent viral illness, rash, or immunization followed by sudden onset meningoencephalitis with multifocal motor deficits indicates ADEM (see later section). Several differential diagnoses that should be considered in a child with an encephalitic presentation are listed in **Table 91.10**.

Diagnosis

Given the more significant outcome of encephalitis, compared to aseptic meningitis, aggressive determination of etiology is often sought. The CSF can be obtained by LP once the child is hemodynamically stable, the ICP is not significantly elevated, and focal lesions have been excluded. In general, CSF findings in encephalitis are nonspecific, and CSF abnormalities seldom correlate with clinical or histologic severity of encephalitis.

CSF analysis is helpful only in a few cases. Generally, the CSF is clear and colorless; the opening pressure may be high in children with raised ICP. CSF cell count and protein are generally slightly elevated or may be normal, and the glucose concentration is often normal. CSF pleocytosis (>5 WBC/mm³) is seen in >95% of cases of acute viral encephalitis and is typically lymphocytic. In the early phase of infection, a mixed pleocytosis that consists of both polymorphonuclear and mononuclear cells and later becomes lymphocytic may

TABLE 91.10

DIFFERENTIAL DIAGNOSIS OF ACUTE ENCEPHALITIS/ MENINGOENCEPHALITIS ACUTE DISSEMINATED ENCEPHALOMYELITIS

Infectious
Bacterial meningitis
Tuberculous meningitis
Cerebral malaria
Cryptococcal meningoencephalitis
Brain abscess

Metabolic
Hepatic coma
Reye syndrome
Uremia
Hypoglycemia
Hypoosmolar or hyperosmolar states
Organic acidemias
Amino acidopathies
Urea cycle defects
Fat oxidation defects
Mitochondrial disorders
Acute intermittent porphyria

Toxic
Shigellosis
Salmonella
Drugs
Lead encephalopathy
Carbon monoxide poisoning
Pertussis

Vasculitic
Systemic lupus erythematosus
Polyarteritis nodosa

Other
Benign raised ICP
Trauma
Nonconvulsive status epilepticus
Neoplasms
Cerebrovascular accidents

be seen. A polymorphonuclear predominance may persist throughout the illness in some types of infection, notably EEE. Atypical lymphocytes in the CSF may occasionally be seen in EBV and CMV encephalitis. Evaluation of the CSF early in the course of acute encephalitis may yield few or no cells. Such a finding does not exclude the diagnosis, and a repeat LP after 1–2 days is often helpful in subsequently demonstrating pleocytosis. CSF pleocytosis >500 WBC/mm³ may be seen in ~10% cases. Vasculitis or tissue necrosis causes extravasation of RBCs into CSF and elicits CSF leukocytosis with increased polymorphonuclear cells. RBCs in the CSF may be seen in late stages of HSV encephalitis. The possibility of a traumatic LP must be excluded. Very rarely, subarachnoid hemorrhage from occult trauma or a vascular malformation may be considered. A very low CSF glucose is unusual in viral encephalitis, and other causes, including bacterial meningitis and TBM, must be considered.

Confirmatory diagnosis is performed by culture, rapid diagnostic tests (including antigen detection and PCR), demonstration of rise in specific antibody titer, and direct visualization of the organism (29). The need for biopsy is less common now than in the past but may be an option of last resort. An etiologic agent is identified in a variable number of cases, but rarely exceeds 60%.

Success of viral culture depends on cells inoculated and is highly dependent on the capabilities of the virology laboratory, the quality of the sample provided, and information provided by the clinician that allows laboratory personnel to perform specific testing. PCR has replaced viral culture for identification of HSV and enteroviruses from the CSF and is available for CMV, EBV, varicella-zoster virus (VZV), human herpesvirus (HHV)-6, HIV, influenza, adenovirus, *Mycoplasma*, *Mycobacteria*, *Rickettsia*, and others. PCR assays are usually highly sensitive and specific. However, false positives may occur because of contamination of laboratory specimens, and false negatives may occur because the infectious encephalitis process may not be near enough to the meninges or CSF or because of the presence of inhibitory factors in the CSF. As the viral genomic material remains in the CSF from weeks to months, its detection helps in confirming the antecedent viral infection in cases of postinfectious encephalitis. Quantitative as well as qualitative DNA amplification techniques may be of value.

Isolation of pathogens from sites other than the CNS may provide a clue to diagnosis. Culture from sites of entry and primary viral replication, such as conjunctivae, nasopharynx, and rectum are useful in identifying enteroviruses and adenoviruses. CMV is readily cultured from urine.

Rapid diagnostic tests provide a diagnosis before diagnosis by culture. PCR and direct fluorescence antibody staining can be performed on cells scraped from the base of lesions (HSV or VZV).

Serology may be helpful if high titers are identified acutely or at least a fourfold rise is noted when measured 3–4 weeks later. An antibody index (measure of specific antibody in CSF compared to the serum) may be useful to determine if infection is localized to the CNS. Serologic tests may lack specificity, and tests for antibodies vary in their quality. Attention should be paid to which antibody detection method has highest sensitivity and specificity (ELISA or other), as well as to the antibody (IgG, IgM, other, or both) being tested. Elevated levels of myelin basic protein in the CSF suggest demyelinating injury as in ADEM. Intrathecal oligoclonal bands are seen occasionally in postinfectious encephalitis, in contrast to MS, in which they are often present.

EEG may be complementary to neuroimaging in the diagnosis of encephalitis and may help in distinguishing generalized from focal encephalitis. In generalized encephalitis, the EEG typically shows diffuse slowing with high-voltage slow waves; occasionally, spikes and spike wave activity may be seen. In focal encephalitis, focal EEG abnormalities, including focal slow waves or spikes, may be seen. The EEG is particularly helpful in HSV encephalitis, wherein characteristic *periodic lateralized epileptiform discharges (PLEDs)* may be seen. However, it must be remembered that PLEDs are not seen in all cases of HSV encephalitis and that the presence of PLEDs is not sine qua non with HSV encephalitis, as PLEDs are also seen in other conditions, including infarcts and other focal lesions.

Before the advent of rapid diagnostic tests, brain biopsy for histologic examination, viral culture, and fluorescent antibody staining was a diagnostic option. This process is now rarely used for the specific diagnosis of encephalitis.

Other tests that may provide diagnostic clues include the peripheral blood smear, which generally shows lymphocytosis. Marked leukocytosis may be seen in EEE. Leukopenia and thrombocytopenia are seen in rickettsial infection, measles, and viral hemorrhagic fever. Characteristic cytoplasmic inclusions in monocytes, known as *morulae*, are seen in ehrlichiosis. Finding of malarial parasites in the smear helps to confirm a diagnosis of cerebral malaria.

Chest x-ray may help in the diagnosis of TB, mycoplasma, or legionella. A full-thickness skin biopsy from the nape of the neck, where numerous hair follicles are located, has a high sensitivity (50%–90%) and a specificity of almost 100% for diagnosis of rabies.

Neuroimaging

Children with suspected encephalitis are often critically ill and have raised ICP; therefore, an LP cannot be performed at presentation in some cases. Neuroimaging is the most important urgent investigation required in such cases.

MRI is a sensitive method of diagnosing encephalitis that detects brain inflammation and edema in the cerebral cortex, the gray–white matter junction, the basal ganglia, or the cerebellum. Specific areas of involvement may suggest the etiology, as with involvement of the inferomedial temporal lobe and frontal lobes in HSV; bilateral thalamic and basal ganglia involvement in JE; hippocampal, cerebellar, and mesencephalic areas in rabies; and disseminated lesions in brainstem and basal ganglia in EEE.

MRI is the diagnostic modality of choice in differentiating acute infectious encephalitis from ADEM. In ADEM, the MRI shows multiple patchy areas of involvement of the white matter and, at times, the deep gray matter of the brain; the spinal cord may also be involved in some cases. Demyelination is best seen in T2-weighted and FLAIR images. Gadolinium contrast enhancement of lesions may be seen in some cases. Lyme disease and MS may also involve diverse areas of brain, brainstem, and spinal cord. Gadolinium also confirms that the multifocal areas of demyelination in ADEM are all of the same stage, in contrast to MS, in which the lesions are of different stages. However, acute presentation of MS that requires management in the PICU is rarely seen in children.

MRI may be insensitive in detecting encephalitis early, especially in neonates with higher brain-water content. The CT scan may help to exclude a bleed or a space-occupying lesion in a suspected case but is not significantly useful for the diagnosis of encephalitis.

Treatment

Acute encephalitis is a neurologic emergency. All children with altered sensorium and a clinical suspicion of encephalitis should be admitted to the PICU for management of life-threatening problems, observation and monitoring of the course of illness, and differentiating from other causes of coma.

CNS infections, particularly meningoencephalitides, are the most common cause of refractory SE in the PICU (1) and must be managed energetically (30). Continuous EEG and cerebral function monitoring is warranted. Specific antimicrobial therapy should be initiated as soon as an etiologic agent is reasonably suspected or identified. Bacterial, fungal, and parasitic etiologies of encephalitis require specific antimicrobial therapy. Antiviral therapy is important for treatment of HSV encephalitis and must be administered promptly in all suspected cases (see later section on Herpes Encephalitis). Acyclovir is not effective for CMV encephalitis, for which ganciclovir or foscarnet must be used (31). Amantadine and rimantadine are effective against influenza A, whereas oseltamivir and zanamivir are effective against both influenza A and B. Highly active antiretroviral therapy (HAART) is available for HIV infection. No specific antiviral therapy is available for enteroviral and arboviral encephalitis. Passive immunity in the form of IV immune globulin may be helpful in immunocompromised individuals who cannot mount an effective immune response. The role of high-dose steroid therapy has not been established in acute viral encephalitis. High-dose dexamethasone was not found to be useful in a study of JE.

Prognosis

The immediate and long-term outcome in encephalitis is determined by several factors, including etiology, host factors (e.g., age and immune status), severity of illness, level of consciousness at presentation, early intensive management, and institution of specific therapy. Most arboviral encephalitides except EEE and JE have a good prognosis in children. The prognosis of HSV encephalitis has improved significantly with use of early acyclovir therapy. Children with severe encephalitis and/or delayed therapy may be left with permanent neurologic deficits.

HERPES ENCEPHALITIS

HSV is the most common cause of fatal sporadic encephalitis in childhood. Human disease can be caused by any of the eight herpes viruses: HSV-1, HSV-2, VZV, CMV, HHV-6 and HHV-7, EBV, and Kaposi sarcoma herpes virus (HHV-8). Also, one simian herpes virus, B virus (cryptotetia-crypta), occasionally causes serious human disease that involves the CNS. All of these viruses have similar biologic characteristics, can remain latent for long periods of time, and can become reactivated. However, most HSE beyond the neonatal period is caused by HSV-1 and, occasionally, HHV-6; most neonatal HSE is caused by HSV-2.

Epidemiology

HSE occurs worldwide, in developed and developing countries. It occurs sporadically at any time of the year and does not occur in epidemic form. Humans are the sole reservoirs of the virus. HSV remains latent in most cases and is transmitted during reactivation. The acquisition of HSV-1 is influenced by geographic location, socioeconomic factors, and age. Primary infection occurs early in children from developing countries and lower socioeconomic strata, whereas it is generally delayed until adolescence in more affluent populations from developed countries.

HSV-2 is generally acquired in adults by sexual contact and may either cause genital infection or be excreted asymptomatically during primary or recurrent infections. Neonates acquire the infection from infected mothers. HSE can occur at any age; both sexes are equally affected. Primary infection often occurs in childhood.

Pathogenesis

HSV is acquired by respiratory droplets or by direct contact with infectious secretions through close contacts with a person excreting HSV. The virus is transported from the abraded skin or mucous membrane by retrograde axonal flow to the dorsal root ganglia, where it replicates. It may cause primary infection with viremia at this time or become latent, as a result of host–virus interaction. The primary infection may disseminate to various organ sites in neonates and children with poor immunity. The latent virus can become spontaneously reactivated at any time. Stress, exercise, fever, immune suppression, and tissue damage are some of the known risk factors for reactivation.

Encephalitis can be caused by both primary and recurrent HSV infection. The route of primary CNS infection is thought to be the olfactory and trigeminal nerves, which explains the neurotropism of HSV to the temporal lobe. Whether reactivation of virus occurs within a previously infected brain tissue or in the olfactory or trigeminal nerves with subsequent passage to the brain is not yet fully understood. The role of host immunity is also poorly defined. Recently specific genetic factors have been associated with the development of HSE in children.

Fetal or neonatal disease is generally acquired from the infected mother, rarely in utero, and more commonly during birth through direct contact with infected secretions in the genitalia. Postnatal contact with HSV accounts for a small number of cases. The disease may present either in a disseminated form, isolated CNS involvement, or with involvement of skin, eyes, and mouth. In the disseminated form, the CNS is most likely infected via the hematogenous route, whereas isolated encephalitis probably occurs through intraneuronal spread.

Clinical Presentation

Neonates

Intrauterine infection may manifest in the neonate with skin vesicles or scarring and involvement of the eyes (e.g., chorioretinitis or optic atrophy) and brain (e.g., microcephaly or encephalomalacia). Clinical presentation of disseminated disease is similar to bacterial sepsis. Symptoms start approximately a week after birth and include poor feeding, lethargy, irritability, and seizures, and may sometimes progress to shock with multiorgan failure. Herpetic lesions of the skin or mucosa are seen in 20%–30% cases and provide a clinical clue to diagnosis. In neonates with isolated encephalitis, the clinical symptomatology of encephalitis is similar to that of encephalitis with disseminated disease; skin lesions are often seen after ~2 weeks of age.

Children

HSE in children generally presents acutely with fever, headache, vomiting, and focal seizures, followed within a few days by alteration in sensorium. Neck stiffness may occur in some cases. At times, preceding nonspecific influenza like symptoms of malaise, lethargy, or mild irritability may be present. Behavioral and personality changes and difficulty with speech may be noted in some children. Focal neurologic abnormalities develop in most cases, generally reflecting involvement of the temporal or frontal lobes. Raised ICP with papilledema, transtentorial herniation, and hemodynamic instability follows. Focal signs and personality changes may provide etiologic clues. HSE has no other specific clinical markers. Presence of herpetic skin lesions has no correlation with concurrent encephalitis. The course of HSE is generally rapid and may be fatal unless specific therapy is started early. Early diagnosis is therefore essential.

Differential Diagnosis

It may not be possible to differentiate HSE from other causes of encephalitis on the basis of clinical features alone. Comparison of positive versus negative findings in brain biopsies revealed that most of the "positive" cases presented with features of focal encephalitis. Presence of focal seizures and frontotemporal signs, including behavioral changes and speech difficulties, are clues but are not specific for HSE.

A number of conditions may mimic HSE, including other viral encephalitis, such as EEE, JE, western equine encephalitis, St. Louis encephalitis, EBV, and other viral infections. The differential diagnosis should also include bacterial and fungal infections (e.g., early brain abscess) and other infections, including tubercular, rickettsial, toxoplasma, and collagen vascular diseases.

Diagnosis

In the absence of skin lesions, making a clinical diagnosis of herpes is problematic (32), particularly in neonates. Swab cultures from conjunctiva, nasopharynx, and rectum may detect early infection. The MRI is not as helpful in neonates as in older children because of diffuse involvement and high brain-water content of the neonatal brain. PLEDs on EEG, if seen, add to the diagnosis but are not specific for herpes.

Laboratory Diagnosis

Identification of HSV in the CSF by PCR is a rapid, highly sensitive (95%) and specific (almost 100%) test that has become the gold standard for diagnosis of HSE. CSF PCR may be negative during the first 3 days of illness and should therefore be repeated in a few days in suspected HSE cases, as the PCR may then become positive. The PCR may also be negative if it is done too late in the illness—after 10–14 days (33). Antibodies to HSV in the CSF take a few days to develop; hence, immunologic tests to detect them are not helpful for early diagnosis of HSE. A fourfold rise in antibody titer over a few weeks may be helpful for a retrospective diagnosis. Antibodies in the CSF are not specific for HSE and, per se, are not helpful in diagnosis. Isolation of the virus from the CSF by culture is possible in less than half of cases with HSE. Identification of virus at sites other than CSF by direct fluorescence antibody, PCR, or culture in the context of clinical symptomatology suggestive of encephalitis is adequate to make the diagnosis of HSE. CSF shows variable pleocytosis predominantly polymorphic in the first 24–48 hours, followed by a lymphocytic response. RBCs may be seen secondary to the necrotizing nature of HSE; at times, the CSF may be xanthochromic. Mild elevation of protein with normal glucose levels is usually seen. As with all other encephalitides, in a small number of cases the CSF may be normal in the early phase of illness.

Characteristic EEG findings in HSE are aforementioned PLEDs, often seen arising from the involved temporal region. With progression of disease, they may spread to the other temporal lobe within a few days. PLEDs and/or focal temporal slowing were seen in 90% of PCR-positive patients at symptom onset, compared with only 30% of the PCR-negative group. Sensitivity of the EEG recordings decreases after 48 hours. However, PLEDs may not be seen in some children and may also be seen in conditions other than HSE, such as other focal encephalitides, infarct, and hypoxic-ischemic injury.

Brain biopsy was once the most important diagnostic test for diagnosis of HSE when PCR and sophisticated neuroimaging facilities were not available. Currently, with a combination of MRI, CSF PCR, and EEG, a diagnosis of HSE can be made with reasonable accuracy.

Neuroimaging

MRI is often the first diagnostic investigation, as LP may be contraindicated in children with raised ICP and focal signs. Involvement of inferofrontal and mediotemporal lobes with gyral swelling and cerebral edema is characteristic (**Fig. 91.3**). However, infants and young children may show a more diffuse and often bilateral involvement. The MRI is much more sensitive than CT and detects changes earlier than CT in cases of HSE. If an MRI facility is not immediately available, a CT scan may be obtained. Low-density areas in a unilateral medial temporal lobe and insular cortex are seen. Small areas of hemorrhage may also be seen in these regions. The CT may appear normal in very early phases of the disease, and abnormalities may be visible only after 4–5 days of illness.

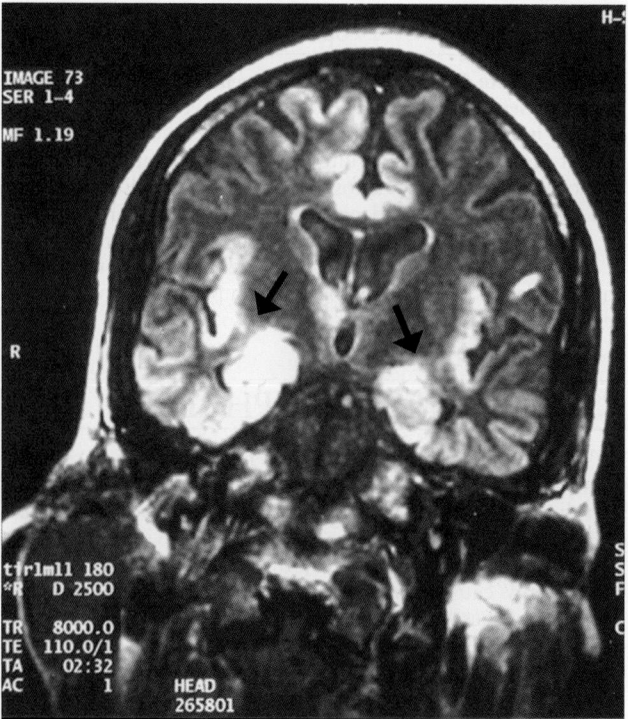

FIGURE 91.3. Coronal FLAIR-MRI showing hyperintense signal involving bilateral temporal lobes and cingulate gyri in a case of herpes encephalitis (*arrows* point between the hyperintense insula laterally and medial temporal lobe inferiorly).

Treatment

A child with suspected HSV should be managed on an urgent basis in the ICU with prompt administration of acyclovir. In children, 30 mg/kg/day IV divided every 8 hours for 14–21 days is the treatment of choice, whereas for neonatal HSE, 60 mg/kg/day IV divided every 8 hours for 21 days is recommended; negative PCR is often obtained prior to discontinuation of therapy. Oral acyclovir or valacyclovir prophylaxis for 3–6 months after neonatal infection has also been advocated by some experts to prevent relapses. Newer antiviral agents, such as famciclovir, ganciclovir, vidarabine, and foscarnet, have also been tried in HSE. No evidence suggests that any of these is better than acyclovir unless resistance is documented. Corticosteroid administration concurrent with acyclovir was a significant predictor of favorable outcome at 3 months after infection in a retrospective study of adults with HSE (34). A multinational, prospective, randomized, controlled study is under progress to determine the effectiveness of corticosteroids in HSE (35).

Prognosis

Early administration of acyclovir has considerably reduced the morbidity and mortality associated with HSE. A delay of ≥48 hours in starting therapy is associated with a poor prognosis. Relapse of HSE has been documented in 12% of acyclovir-treated adult patients and is considered to be secondary to immunologically mediated pathogenicity. Outcome is poor in neonates with disseminated disease, with a 50% mortality rate and 50% of survivors with neurologic sequelae. Mortality is lower (~14%) in neonates with isolated encephalitis.

JAPANESE ENCEPHALITIS

JE is an important arthropod-borne encephalitis endemic in Asia, particularly India, Nepal, Philippines, Thailand, Cambodia, Vietnam, Myanmar, and some parts of China. Approximately 3 billion people live in endemic regions, and ~50,000 cases, with 10,000 deaths, reported annually. JE is the most common form of epidemic and sporadic encephalitis in the tropical region of Asia. The epidemics generally occur after the rainy season in rural areas with rice fields.

Etiology

The JE virus is an enveloped, single-stranded, RNA flavivirus that is antigenically related to St. Louis encephalitis virus, West Nile virus, and Murray Valley virus. It was first isolated in Japan in 1933 and contains several polypeptides encoded by a single, long, open-reading frame. Genomic sequencing of a number of isolates that originate from various geographic regions is known.

JE is a zoonotic disease maintained by a pig–mosquito–pig and bird–mosquito–bird cycle. Pigs and wild birds are the natural hosts of the virus. Pigs serve as amplifier hosts. Bats can also carry the virus for a long time. Humans are incidental dead-end hosts and acquire the disease by the bite of mosquitoes that have fed on infected pigs and birds. The vector mosquitoes are generally *Culex* spp. and breed in rice fields and stagnant water.

Pathophysiology

Following a bite by an infected mosquito, the initial viral replication may occur in regional lymph nodes. The CNS involvement occurs via the hematogenous route. Viremia lasts for 4–5 days. The binding of JE virions to the cells in the CNS is possibly assisted by certain neurotransmitter receptors. Basal ganglia involvement is usually seen.

Clinical Presentation

JE affects mainly children and young adults. The incubation period is 5–15 days, and most infections are either asymptomatic or mildly symptomatic. JE infection that progresses to encephalitis often starts acutely with fever, headache, tiredness, nausea, vomiting, and diarrhea and progresses within a few days to confusion, irritability, and coma. The onset may be abrupt, with high fever, chills, and seizures, with rapid progression to altered sensorium and neurologic deficits. Seizures occur in ~75% of children but are less common in adults. Meningismus and headache are more common in adults than in children. Extrapyramidal signs, including masklike facies, rigidity, tremor, and choreoathetosis, are seen in some cases. Dystonia is more common in children as compared to adults (36). Upper-motor neuron facial palsy occurs in ~10% of cases. In a small number of cases, the illness may start with flaccid paralysis of one or more limbs, generally the legs, with no loss of consciousness. Subsequently, altered sensorium may occur in approximately one-third of cases. Rise in ICP may occur and lead to cerebral herniation.

Differential Diagnosis

The differential diagnosis of JE is similar to that of other encephalitides. During an epidemic, JE should be suspected in any child with sudden onset fever and altered sensorium.

The presence of extrapyramidal symptoms and signs in a child with encephalitis strongly suggests the diagnosis of JE. However, laboratory confirmation is essential.

Diagnosis

The diagnosis of JE is made based on clinical presentation, epidemiologic risk factors, and supporting laboratory data. If CSF can be obtained safely, lymphocytic pleocytosis with moderate elevation of protein and a normal glucose may be seen. The CSF may be acellular or shows polymorphonuclear predominance in early stages. The virus can be isolated from the CSF by inoculating into 2- to 4-day-old mice or by infection of cell cultures. Viral antigens can be detected in the CSF by indirect immunofluorescence assay. Viral antibodies can be detected by rapid serologic assays, such as IgM-capture ELISA (MAC-ELISA) and IgG-ELISA. IgM is more specific early in infection and is positive in nearly all patients at ~7 days, IgG increases later in the course of illness. Monoclonal antibodies (mAbs) have also been used for diagnosis, and real-time PCR for JE is available (37). Virus detection in mosquitoes can also be analyzed by ELISA, and viral isolation can be done by insect bioassay. Diffuse slowing is commonly seen on EEG. Theta and delta coma, burst suppression, and, occasionally, epileptiform activity are suggestive.

Neuroimaging

CT scans show hypodense areas in the thalamus, basal ganglia, midbrain, and brainstem in approximately half of JE cases. MRI scans are more sensitive. Abnormal signals that are hypointense on T1-weighted and hyperintense on T2-weighted images that involve the thalami and basal ganglia bilaterally are characteristic (**Fig. 91.4**). The cerebral hemispheres and cerebellum may also show abnormal signals.

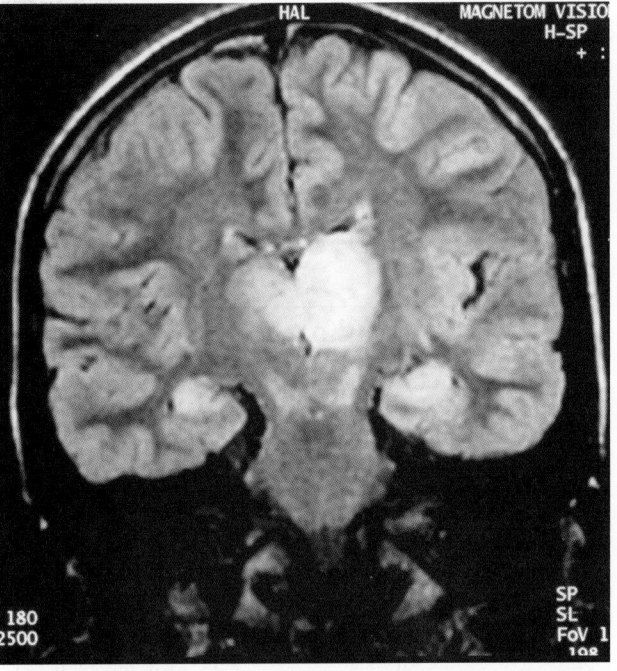

FIGURE 91.4. Coronal FLAIR-MRI showing bilateral hyperintense signal involving the hippocampus, thalamus, and midbrain in a case of JE.

Treatment

Children with symptomatic JE are usually seriously ill and require urgent intensive and supportive care. No specific therapy exists for JE. Use of recombinant interferon is investigational.

Prognosis

Approximately 25%–30% cases are fatal and almost half of those who survive have residual neurologic sequelae. Focal neurologic deficits and altered sensorium at presentation have been correlated with neurologic sequelae.

Prevention and Control

Vaccination against JE is the most effective way of preventing epidemics. Currently, a mouse-brain–derived, inactivated vaccine is being used and is recommended for people living in or traveling to endemic areas for >30 days. Three doses of the vaccine are generally advised; however, two doses have been found to be equally protective. A single dose may provide some protection and may be beneficial for countries with limited resources. A live, attenuated vaccine is also available and found to be effective. Use of vaccine has considerably reduced the number of JE cases in Japan, China, and Korea.

Mosquito control measures that employ larvicidal and adulticidal techniques have been used. Water management systems with alternate drying and wetting in rice fields and the use of neem-based products as fertilizers suppress the breeding of culicine vectors. Personal protective measures to reduce mosquito bites are important.

ACUTE DISSEMINATED ENCEPHALOMYELITIS

ADEM is an inflammatory demyelinating disorder of the CNS that usually follows infections or, less frequently, immunization. It is most frequently seen in children and young adults and is usually a monophasic illness; occasionally, it can be multiphasic, at which time it must be differentiated from MS (38). The common preceding infections are respiratory and gastrointestinal viral illnesses; however, ADEM has been reported following many viral and bacterial infections. Postimmunization encephalomyelitis occurs most commonly after measles, mumps, rubella, and rabies vaccination.

Pathogenesis

The essential feature of ADEM is an inflammatory patchy demyelination with preservation of axon cylinders, perivenular round cell inflammation, and prominence of microglial cells in the inflammatory exudate. The exact mechanism of the demyelination is incompletely understood because most patients with ADEM recover completely. It is mainly extrapolated from experimental allergic encephalomyelitis and is considered to occur secondary to immunodysregulation in susceptible individuals. T-helper cells become sensitized to autoantigens, such as myelin proteins, leading to a complex inflammatory cascade, with release of lymphokines and other mediators of inflammation, as well as disruption of the BBB. Typically, the subcortical white matter is affected; sometimes additional gray matter lesions are seen.

Epidemiology

ADEM is increasingly being reported from both developed (39) and developing countries (40), possibly due to increased availability of MRI; however, an actual increase may also have occurred. ADEM is more common in the winter months. Typical cases of ADEM occur 5–20 days after an infectious illness or, sometimes, immunization. Risk factors are incompletely identified but may include genetic susceptibility, pathogen characteristics, immunization, and other factors. The overall annual incidence of ADEM is ~0.4 per 100,000 (39). The incidence of severe forms of ADEM (e.g., hemorrhagic encephalomyelitis) that may follow measles has diminished in developed countries because of widespread immunization.

Clinical Presentation

ADEM can occur at any age but is generally seen in young children. The mean age at presentation is ~7 years, with a slight male preponderance. Most cases have an acute meningoencephalitic presentation with fever, headache, and irritability, progressing rapidly to altered sensorium and, often, an abrupt multifocal neurologic deficit (40). However, evolution of signs may occur over a few days in a small number of cases. Seizures are seen in ~25%–33% of cases and may be focal or generalized. A history of preceding infectious illness or immunization 1–3 weeks prior to the illness can be elicited in most but not all cases. Although any part of the CNS may be involved, the common sites include the white matter tracts, deep gray matter, spinal cord, and optic nerves. Hemiparesis or quadriparesis may be present. Ataxia is predominant in some cases and extrapyramidal symptoms, such as choreoathetosis or dystonia, may occur in others. In the affected limbs, the muscle tone is generally increased with increased stretch reflexes, upgoing plantar reflexes, and, at times, clonus. Predominant brainstem involvement may occasionally be seen. Simultaneous involvement of the spinal cord may present with a transverse myelitis-like presentation. When optic neuritis occurs, it is usually bilateral; however, involvement of the second eye may follow involvement of the first eye. Other cranial nerve palsies may also occur. Mental or psychiatric disturbances have also been reported. A fulminant presentation with rapid deterioration may occur in a few cases, particularly in children <3 years of age.

Differential Diagnosis

Because of the variability of presentation, a number of conditions may warrant consideration. It is important to exclude infectious meningoencephalitis by CSF examination in suspected cases. Characteristic neuroimaging and exclusion of other diagnoses are necessary to establish the diagnosis.

Diagnosis

A clinical definition of ADEM has recently been put forth by the Brighton collaboration of the Centers for Disease Control and Prevention (https://brightoncollaboration.org/public/what-we-do/setting-standards/case-definitions/available-definitions.html). One of three levels of diagnostic certainty may be established with the presence of encephalopathy or focal/multifocal CNS findings on MRI imaging that are consistent with ADEM. Relapse and alternate diagnoses detract from diagnostic certainty.

CSF may show pleocytosis or may be normal and is not helpful in making a diagnosis of ADEM. RBCs may be seen in cases of hemorrhagic encephalitis. Elevated CSF HSV or Lyme titers do not exclude the possibility of associated ADEM. Oligoclonal bands are positive in ~10% cases. CSF myelin basic protein concentration, reflecting demyelination, may be elevated. The EEG may show focal or generalized slowing and, at times, spikes or sharp waves or rhythmic δ activity. Elevation of WBC, platelet, CRP, and sedimentation rates may be seen occasionally.

Neuroimaging

The CT scan shows low-density abnormalities in approximately half of cases and is far less sensitive than MRI. The MRI scan is the diagnostic modality of choice. The lesions are best visualized on T2-weighted or proton density sequences. Multiple, large confluent centrifugal white matter lesions seen generally at the junction of deep cortical gray and subcortical white matter are characteristic (**Fig. 91.5**). The lesions are generally patchy in distribution but may be fairly symmetric. Lesions may also be seen in deep gray matter, basal ganglia, and thalami in a third of cases. The brainstem, optic nerves, cerebellum, and spinal cord may also be involved. Periventricular and corpus callosum lesions are less common in childhood ADEM, as compared to MS. Gadolinium enhancement, which is typically uniform and usually not very dense, is variably seen. In fulminant cases, areas of hemorrhage may be seen. The lesions of ADEM are typical but not pathognomonic; variations in the character or distribution of lesions may occasionally be seen and necessitate differentiation from other conditions, such as HSV-2

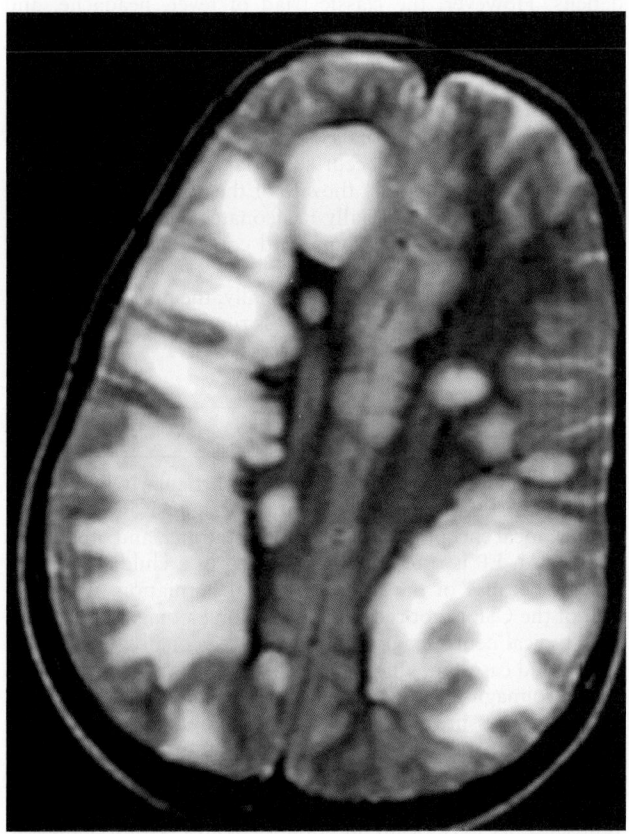

FIGURE 91.5. T2-weighted axial image showing large bilateral asymmetric areas of T2 white matter hyperintensities in ADEM.

encephalitis, Lyme disease, stroke, and MS. Ring enhancement of lesions or mass effect sometimes found in ADEM may suggest abscess, neurocysticercosis (NCC), or tumor. Certain features on MRI, such as large, ill-defined, subcortical white matter lesions, or involvement of deep gray matter sparing of corpus callosum, may help to differentiate the initial presentation of ADEM from MS (41). Rarely, the MRI may be normal on initial presentation and may show lesions characteristic of ADEM if repeated several weeks later, even though patients may be showing clinical improvement, suggesting that a normal initial scan does not necessarily exclude the diagnosis of ADEM and that the appearance of new lesions during recovery from ADEM may not necessarily represent worsening.

Other imaging methods, such as magnetization-transfer MRI, single-photon emission CT scanning, or nuclear MR spectroscopy, have been tried, but none is pathognomonic. Diagnosis of ADEM should be made on clinical grounds in conjunction with neuroimaging.

Treatment

The mainstay of treatment is IV methylprednisolone given in a dose 20–30 mg/kg/day for 3–5 days. Improvement may be observed in some cases within hours but usually occurs over several days. Generally, a taper of oral steroids for 3–6 weeks is used. Concern over treatment with steroids in light of HSE in the differential is occasionally raised. Currently, no evidence is convincing that the use of steroid in the context of HSV infection treated with acyclovir is harmful; clinical judgment regarding the most likely diagnosis must be used.

Plasmapheresis and IV immune globulin 2 g/kg/day for 2–3 days have also been used, especially in cases in which meningoencephalitis cannot be excluded, and it is feared that corticosteroids might worsen the course of infection. To date, no evidence is convincing that treatment with a combination of IV corticosteroids and IV immune globulin is better than either modality alone.

Prognosis

Most children with a mild-to-moderate illness who receive appropriate therapy show good recovery. Acute mortality is rare. Fulminant cases, particularly in children <2 years, are at higher risk. Residual deficits are seen in approximately one-third of cases and include motor, visual, autonomic, and intellectual deficits, as well as epilepsy. Children with transverse myelitis may have residual bladder and bowel dysfunction and motor deficits. MRI lesions resolve slowly over a period of several months, and most disappear by 6 months. A small number of children may have recurrent ADEM during the taper of corticosteroid therapy. This condition usually responds to increasing the corticosteroid dose and prolonging the therapy. Others may have recurrent attacks of ADEM after complete clinical and radiologic recovery. These children often respond to a repeat course of methylprednisolone and oral steroids. Among those who have recurrence, most have a single attack of ADEM; some children may have two or three attacks in a year or two following the initial attack and then do not have further recurrences for several years. A very small number may have repeated recurrences, such that they cannot be weaned off of steroids. Nonsteroidal immunosuppressants have been tried in such cases. These patients do not manifest the immunologic changes of MS, but whether they represent an overlap between the two remains to be determined.

BRAIN AND SPINAL CORD ABSCESS

Abscesses in the brain and spinal cord can occur as a primary event or, occasionally, as a complication of bacterial meningitis. Although uncommon in most developed countries, brain abscesses are not infrequently seen in developing countries. CNS abscesses are important to the intensivists, as they represent an eminently treatable form of serious, potentially fatal, localized CNS infection.

Etiology

The common pathogens include anaerobic bacteria, gram-negative organisms, streptococci, and staphylococci. Many unusual aerobic and anaerobic organisms may also cause brain abscess. Except in neonates, where gram-negative organisms (particularly *Citrobacter diversus*, *Enterobacter sakazakii*, and *Proteus mirabilis*) are the most common pathogens, the specific organism is determined mainly by the underlying cause of the brain abscess. In children with cyanotic heart disease, the most common organisms are the α-hemolytic streptococci. In cases with subacute bacterial endocarditis, streptococci and *S. aureus* are common. In posttraumatic cases, *S. aureus* is the most common pathogen. In children with otitis or sinusitis, anaerobic or aerobic streptococci, *B. fragilis*, *Proteus* spp., *Pseudomonas*, or *H. influenzae* may be isolated. Polymicrobial involvement is seen in approximately a third of cases. In cases secondary to meningitis, the etiologic organisms are those that caused the meningitis.

Pathogenesis

Infection of the brain parenchyma may occur because of hematogenous spread or direct spread from an adjacent infected focus. Hematogenous spread may occur in any child with bacteremia but is common in children with predisposing factors. Cyanotic congenital heart disease, particularly tetralogy of Fallot, is the most common underlying condition. Polycythemia with increased blood viscosity possibly leads to microinfarcts, which make the cerebral parenchyma vulnerable to bacterial seeding. Chronic pulmonary infection, subacute bacterial endocarditis, and immunocompromised status are other predisposing factors. Direct spread of infection may occur from chronic otitis, mastoiditis, a sinusitis, after penetrating trauma, and after neurosurgical procedures. Congenital defects such as dermal sinuses, epidermoid cysts, and encephaloceles, may become infected and rarely may lead to brain abscess or intramedullary abscess of the spinal cord (42). Brain abscess secondary to meningitis is rare if early appropriate therapy is initiated. However, in neonates and in children with gram-negative meningitis, particularly with *Citrobacter*, *Enterobacter*, and *Proteus* infections, brain abscess is not uncommon.

Following hematogenous infection, the pathogens localize, generally at the gray–white matter junction in the brain, and cause cerebritis. Poor vascular supply in the white matter and at the gray–white interface allows organisms to affect these areas. The inflammation and edema progress over a few days to weeks, leading to central necrosis with formation of a surrounding capsule of inflammatory granulation tissue. This progression occurs in four stages. The first stage of "early cerebritis" consists of leukocytic infiltration and focal brain edema, not clearly demarcated from normal brain parenchyma. This stage lasts 1–3 days and is followed by "late cerebritis," in which central liquefaction necrosis is surrounded

by an area of neovascularization and fibroblastic infiltration, forming an ill-defined beginning of a capsule. This phase lasts from day 4 to day 9 and is followed by a phase of early capsule formation. The necrotic center shrinks, and the fibroblastic capsule becomes well formed. The fourth phase is late capsule formation, in which a dense fibrous capsule is surrounded by reactive astrocytes and glial cells, marked edema, and neovascularization. This phase generally occurs after 2 weeks of infection. Progression from the onset of early focal cerebritis to late capsule formation may take from 4 to 6 weeks. In some cases, however, the progression may be rapid and rupture of the abscess may occur into the ventricular system.

Although most often seen in the cerebral hemisphere, brain abscesses may occur in the cerebellum as well as in the brainstem. In the cerebral hemispheres, the distribution of abscess in the frontal, parietal, and temporal lobes is almost equal. The site of abscess is often determined by the etiologic factors. Abscesses secondary to ear infection are located generally in the unilateral temporal lobe or cerebellum, and those following sinusitis are located in the frontal lobe. In children with cyanotic heart disease, abscesses are generally seen in the distribution of the middle carotid artery. Intramedullary abscess of the spinal cord is seen at the site of an anatomic spinal defect in the majority of patients. Hematogenous spread from a urogenital, gastrointestinal, or other source can also occur. The abscess may be solitary or multiple. Multiple abscesses are particularly seen in infections with gram-negative organisms and *S. aureus* and in neonates.

Clinical Presentation

The presentation is generally subacute, with fever, headache, vomiting, altered sensorium, seizures, and focal neurologic deficits. However, the classic triad of fever, headache, and vomiting seen in adults is seen in only half of childhood cases. Seizures may be focal or generalized and are seen in almost half of cases. A bulging fontanelle and increasing head size may be seen in infants, and neck rigidity may be seen in older children. Papilledema, sixth-nerve palsy, and occasionally, cerebral herniation syndromes may occur secondary to raised ICP. Focal deficits are determined by the site of the abscess but may not necessarily be seen, especially in neonates and young infants. Meningismus, pyramidal signs, and cranial nerve palsies are often associated with a brainstem abscess. Hydrocephalus may develop due to mass effect. Occasionally, the presentation may be acute or even abrupt if the abscess ruptures in the ventricles or if hemorrhage occurs in the abscess cavity.

Diagnosis

A high index of suspicion is essential, particularly in children with high-risk factors. The differential diagnosis includes neoplasms, focal encephalitis, subdural hematoma, and other mass lesions. An LP is often contraindicated in a child with brain abscess because of the risk of cerebral herniation. Examination of the CSF is not required for making a diagnosis in cases with typical neuroimaging findings. Occasionally, in carefully considered cases, in which doubt in diagnosis remains even after neuroimaging, an LP may be performed. The CSF is generally under pressure and shows a mild-to-moderate pleocytosis, elevation of protein, and normal glucose. In some cases, it is possible that no cells are seen. Marked pleocytosis (in thousands/mm^3) may be seen if the abscess has ruptured into the ventricles, as may occur in some neonates. Gram stain and culture are generally negative, unless the abscess has ruptured.

Confirmation of the etiologic organism is achieved by aspiration of the abscess and analysis and culture of the aspirated contents. Other sources of organism identification, such as blood culture or aspiration from sinuses or mastoids, should also be considered. The EEG may show focal slowing or, occasionally, spikes over the region of the abscess. Periodic lateralizing discharges or diffuse slowing may also be seen. The EEG may be normal in some cases.

Neuroimaging

A CT scan or MRI with contrast is warranted in all suspected cases. Contrast-enhanced CT scan shows a characteristic ring-enhancing lesion with central hypodensity and surrounding edema in a mature abscess (**Fig. 91.6**). In early cases of cerebritis, the ring enhancement may be incomplete. Mass effect with midline shift may be seen. The MRI is more sensitive than CT in diagnosis of cerebritis. Rarely, a radionuclide ^{99m}TC-pertechnetate scan may be necessary to identify early focal cerebritis. In countries where TB is endemic, a pyogenic abscess must be differentiated from a tubercular abscess. Tubercular abscesses are generally seen at the base of the brain, especially in the cerebellum (**Fig. 91.7**). MR spectroscopy may sometimes be necessary to differentiate an abscess from a neoplasm.

Treatment

Antibiotic therapy with surgical drainage or excision of the abscess is required in most cases. In children, aspiration under CT guidance is used more frequently because of the low mortality and morbidity associated with the procedure. Multiple

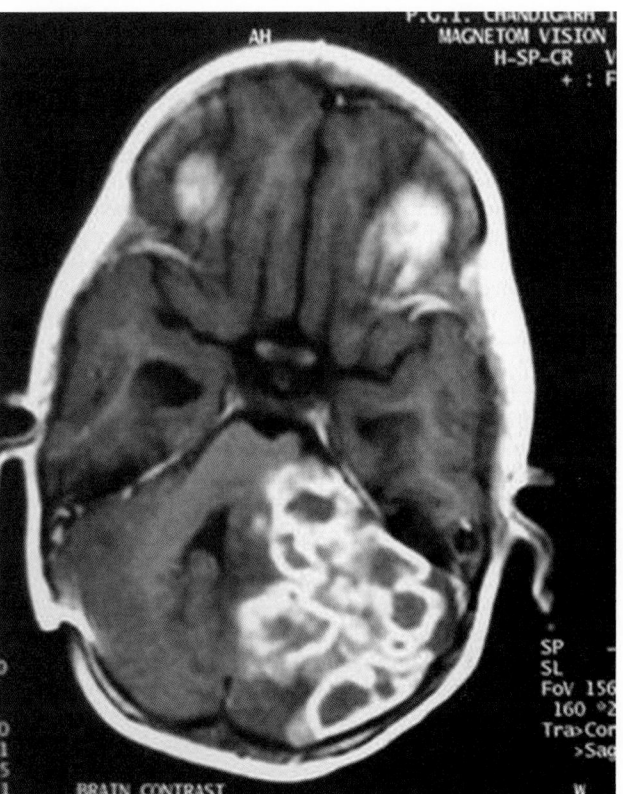

FIGURE 91.7. Contrast MRI showing multiple, conglomerate tubercular abscesses with thick, enhancing, irregular margins and surrounding edema in the cerebellum.

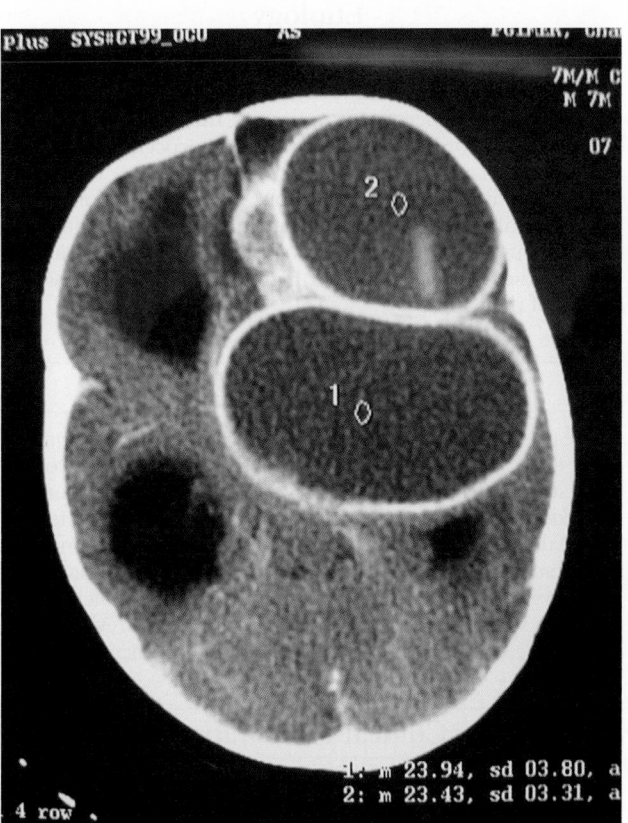

FIGURE 91.6. Contrast-enhanced CT showing multiple staphylococcal brain abscesses with ring enhancement and midline shift.

aspirations are often required. Excision is undertaken if no clinical improvement ensues despite multiple aspirations and antibiotics. Very small abscesses or those in critical areas of the brain may be managed with medical treatment alone. The choice of antibiotics depends on the suspected causative organism. Empiric antibiotic therapy before organism identification typically consists of a broad-spectrum combination of agents to cover anaerobic, gram-negative, and staphylococcal species. Cefotaxime or any other third- or fourth-generation cephalosporin with metronidazole is generally used. If *S. aureus* is suspected or identified, vancomycin should be added. It may be modified according to the underlying predisposing condition and the immune status of the child. Definitive antibiotic therapy is dictated by the organism identified. IV antibiotics in highest doses are required for at least 6 weeks in most cases (43). Corticosteroids given IV at presentation help to reduce cerebral edema and raised ICP. The fear that they may reduce penetration of antibiotics in the abscess cavity has not been substantiated. Follow-up scans are done periodically after surgical drainage/excision to determine the response.

Prognosis

Mortality is high in newborns and young infants and in children with multiple large abscesses and cyanotic heart disease; children with intramedullary abscess of the spinal cord have higher morbidity than children with subdural abscesses, epidural abscesses, or adults. Rupture of brain abscess into the ventricular system can be a life-threatening event unless managed immediately and aggressively. Outcome is poor in cases with low GCS score, gram-negative organisms, and associated sepsis (44). Intramedullary abscess of the spinal cord can result in necrosis of the spinal cord, resulting in permanent neurologic deficit. Brain and spinal cord abscesses, if detected late, are associated with significant neurologic morbidity. The residual deficits depend on the site of the abscess and may include hemiparesis, cranial nerve palsies, cognitive deficits, and epilepsy. Increasing availability of imaging procedures has helped in early identification and better management of brain and spinal cord abscesses and has led to significant decrease in mortality and morbidity. Early decompression is associated with improved outcome.

SUBDURAL EMPYEMA

Subdural empyema is a suppurative collection in the subdural space. It is an important focal intracranial infection that is often a complication of acute bacterial meningitis and may require early intensive management.

Etiology

In children in whom subdural empyema is a complication of meningitis, the organisms are those that cause meningitis. In others, the organisms are similar to those that cause brain abscesses.

Pathogenesis

Spread of infection to the subdural space may occur either as a complication of meningitis or, occasionally, by direct spread from infected sinuses or otitis media, osteomyelitis of skull bones, or head trauma. The emissary veins that traverse the subdural space become infected, and as the subdural space is not limited by attachment, pus collection can be large. Most subdural collections are seen over the cerebral hemispheres, but some may involve the parafalcine region. The majority of subdural empyemas are unilateral; infants may have bilateral involvement. Large collections behave like space-occupying lesions and may cause dangerous elevations of ICP and extensive involvement of brain parenchyma.

Clinical Presentation

The onset is subacute, with fever, headache, vomiting, and, often, seizures. Neck rigidity and focal signs may be present. Infants present with poor feeding, irritability, fever, full fontanelle, and an enlarging head. Persistent or recurrent fever in a child who has bacterial meningitis with focal seizures or other focal neurologic signs suggests a subdural empyema.

Diagnosis

The diagnosis of a subdural empyema is made by neuroimaging. A contrast-enhanced, crescent-shaped, hypodense lesion, at times with loculations, is characteristic. The enhancement is generally linear, along the dura; at times enhancement of underlying brain parenchyma may also be seen (Fig. 91.1). MRI is more sensitive than CT for detecting small collections and for differentiating from cerebritis and thrombosis. The density difference of the collection can distinguish sterile from purulent collections. Purulent collections are hyperintense to the CSF in both T1- and T2-weighted images.

Analysis of the subdural fluid obtained by subdural tap or surgical drainage reveals a purulent fluid with marked leukocytosis. Organism identification can be performed by Gram stain and culture. An LP is often contraindicated. Peripheral blood leukocytosis is not specific.

Treatment

Removal of the purulent collection and IV administration of appropriate antibiotic therapy in high doses for 3–6 weeks are warranted. Antibiotics are chosen according to the suspected source of infection. Surgical removal of an adjacent source of infection, such as chronic otitis media or osteomyelitis, is also necessary. Repeat scans are required periodically to assess the possibility of reaccumulation and to monitor the course. Supportive therapy is provided on the same principles as for meningitis or brain abscess.

Prognosis

The morbidity and mortality associated with subdural empyema has declined significantly with the use of early appropriate medical and surgical intervention. Common residual deficits after large subdural empyemas include hemiparesis and focal seizures.

EPIDURAL ABSCESS

A cranial epidural abscess is a collection of suppurative material between the dura and the cranium. Spinal epidural abscesses also occur, although not commonly in children.

Etiology

The common causative organisms include staphylococci, streptococci, and some anaerobic organisms, such as B. fragilis. In spinal epidural abscesses, S. aureus is the most common organism. Other organisms, such as pneumococci, streptococci, and salmonellae, may be responsible in some cases. The spread of infection is usually hematogenous but may occasionally occur by local spread of an adjacent infection or secondary to spinal trauma. Over half of spinal epidural abscesses are located in the thoracic or lumbar regions, often on the posterior aspect of the cord.

Pathophysiology

In the case of cranial epidural abscess formation, the pathogens enter the extradural space by either direct spread from a contiguous site of infection or secondary to trauma or a neurosurgical procedure. In spinal epidural abscesses, the spread of infection is usually hematogenous. Progression of inflammation leads to spinal cord ischemia and even infarction. Inflammation of blood vessels causes vasculitis and venothrombophlebitis; increase in size of abscess causes spinal compression. A combination of these factors causes ensuing spinal dysfunction.

Clinical Presentation

Children with a cranial epidural abscess present with fever, headache, vomiting, neck rigidity, focal seizures, and focal neurologic deficits, including hemiparesis. Children with spinal epidural abscess present with fever, back pain, and symptoms and signs of spinal cord compression. Localized tender swelling may be found at the site of the pain. Progression may lead to bladder and bowel involvement. A sensory level may be seen in late cases. The rate of progression is variable; generally, an interval of few days passes from the onset of symptoms to complete paraplegia. However, in some cases the child may be paralyzed within hours, resembling acute transverse myelitis. In infants, the initial presentation may be nonspecific and similar to sepsis, resulting in late detection after deficits have already occurred.

Diagnosis

An LP is contraindicated, as it is associated with risk of accidentally spreading infection to the CSF and spinal herniation in cases of complete spinal block. If done, CSF may show leukocytosis, elevated protein, and hypoglycorrhachia. As with subdural abscesses, the diagnosis of epidural abscess is made by neuroimaging. MRI is more sensitive than CT and shows an enhancing lenticular collection between the dura and the cranium or the cord (**Fig. 91.8**). If spinal epidural abscess is suspected, the entire spine should be scanned, as multiple abscesses may be present. Plain radiographs of the spine and contrast myelography have no role in diagnosis.

Treatment

Treatment involves surgical drainage, appropriate antibiotics, and supportive management. As *S. aureus* is a common pathogen, the initial antibiotic therapy consists of a combination of antibiotics to cover staphylococci and gram-negative organisms. Once the abscess is drained and the organism identified, the appropriate antibiotic therapy is administered IV for 4–6 weeks. No scientific evidence supports the use of corticosteroids.

Prognosis

Early appropriate management has led to a significant decrease in mortality and morbidity. The outcome is determined by the severity of neurologic deficits, particularly paralysis, at

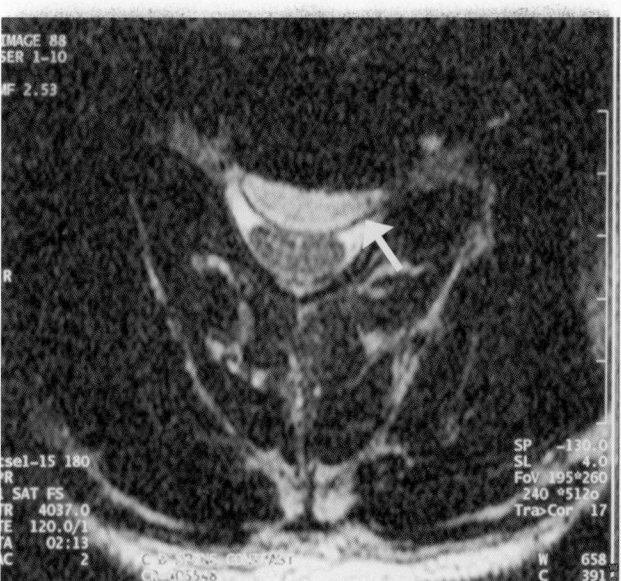

FIGURE 91.8. Contrast MRI at the cervical level showing a well-defined hyperintense extradural collection (*arrow*) in the spinal canal, causing cord compression.

the time of presentation. As with intramedullary and subdural abscesses, the urgency with which decompression is accomplished is critical. Paralysis for >36 hours before intervention is associated with a poor prognosis. Complete recovery may be expected in children who do not have paralysis at presentation.

CEREBROSPINAL FLUID SHUNT INFECTION

CSF shunts are placed by neurosurgeons to relieve pressure from CSF accumulation and brain parenchymal displacement when hydrocephalus is present. CSF shunts may direct CSF from the ventricles to the peritoneum (ventriculoperitoneal), atrium (ventriculoatrial), or to the outside world (externalized). Ventriculoperitoneal shunts are the most common.

Etiology

More than two-thirds of all shunt infections are caused by staphylococcal species. In a number of series, *Staphylococcus epidermidis* has been most frequently isolated (45), whereas in others, *S. aureus* and other coagulase-negative staphylococci have predominated. Gram-negative enteric organisms, usually *E. coli*, *Klebsiella*, *Proteus*, and *Pseudomonas* spp. are responsible for 6%–20% of infections. Streptococcal species are found in 8%–10% of infections. Multiple organisms are cultured in 10%–15% of infections. The traditional meningitic pathogens (*H. influenzae*, *S. pneumoniae*, and *N. meningitidis*) have been described in 5% of shunt infections. Other less common organisms, such as fungi and commensal microbes (e.g., diphtheroids), may rarely be responsible.

Epidemiology

The incidence of shunt infection has declined over the years to <4%. Several factors, including more refined shunt materials, improvement in operating room facilities and surgical techniques, pretreatment of shunt assembly in bacitracin solution, and a reduction in preshunting invasive studies (e.g., pneumoencephalography), are some of the factors responsible. Shunt infections generally occur in a bimodal distribution from the time of last shunt surgery. Almost, 70%–85% of the infections occur within 6 months of surgery. The second peak of infections occurs after 12 months.

Pathogenesis

Shunt devices act as foreign bodies and interfere with natural host defense mechanisms, such as chemotaxis and phagocytosis. Shunt catheters have been shown in vitro to decrease the motility of neutrophils, hindering their ability to phagocytose bacteria in effective numbers. In addition, staphylococci form an extracellular mucoid biofilm called "slime," which increases bacterial adherence to the shunt and decreases susceptibility to antibiotics. Shunt infection is more common in infants <6 months of age at the time of surgery, most likely because of a relatively deficient immune response to bacterial infection or a higher skin bacterial density. Shunts may become infected by several mechanisms: colonization at the time of surgery; breakdown of the surgical wound or of the skin that overlies the shunt, which allows direct access of microbes to the shunt; retrograde infection from the distal end through transluminal passage of bacteria; and hematogenous seeding and infection of CSF shunts, which occurs infrequently.

Clinical Presentation

Most children present with fever, headache, vomiting, lethargy, irritability, and change in mental status. Occasionally, seizures, cranial nerve palsies, visual deficits, and neck rigidity may be seen. The classic symptoms of infection, such as fever and pain, may be absent in some cases. The infected intact surgical wound or cellulitis along the shunt may be associated with local pain and erythema. Infection of the proximal end may result in meningitis or ventriculitis in ~30% cases; however, intracranial empyemas and abscesses are rarely seen. Spread of infection to the distal end may cause peritonitis with abdominal pain and distension.

Diagnosis

A high degree of suspicion for infection helps in early diagnosis. The prerequisites for a diagnostic label of shunt infection are no meningitis/ventriculitis and a sterile CSF culture at the time of shunt placement, shunt in place for at least 24 hours, and a positive CSF culture obtained from the shunt/LP. The gold standard for diagnosis of shunt infection is the isolation of organism from culture of the shunt or of the fluid in contact with it. The risk of infection after a single diagnostic shunt tap appears to be low, and obtained CSF can be evaluated for infection. A high WBC count in the CSF is highly correlated, but sometimes the CSF counts may be normal. CSF glucose may be low or normal; CSF protein levels are typically not raised. Certain patients, even in the absence of infection, may have an elevated CSF white count, generally eosinophilic, probably due to a hypersensitive reaction to the presence of shunt tubing. A positive CSF Gram stain and culture are diagnostic and extremely important in deciding the course of treatment. Culture of CSF obtained from the shunt more often identifies the causative organism, as compared with CSF from the LP or ventricular tap. Antibiotic administration before obtaining CSF decreases the yield. The peripheral WBC count and blood cultures are usually not helpful. Ultrasonography in neonates and young infants may show ventriculitis or a "CSFoma," which strongly suggest infection. A CT scan or MRI is useful if early postoperative scans are available for comparison. An increase in ventricular size because of associated shunt malfunction is often seen. Patients with infection of the distal end may show abdominal pseudocysts around the shunt.

Treatment

Various management regimens have been used, but a combination of antibiotics, shunt removal, and external drainage is perhaps most effective. Some authors recommend shunt removal only if the infection is severe or nonresponsive to antibiotics. Ventriculitis associated with shunt infection appears to clear more quickly with external drainage. The drainage tube should be changed every few days and placed preferably at different sites to avoid repeated discharge of organisms due to colonization of drainage tube lying in the infected ventricle. External drainage provides access to CSF, which can be examined daily to help monitor infection and allows administration of intraventricular antibiotics. The antibiotics used for staphylococcal coverage include cloxacillin or vancomycin, often in conjunction with aminoglycosides. Rifampicin can be added to augment the therapy. Third-generation cephalosporins and aminoglycosides can be used for gram-negative bacteria. Because it is bacteriostatic, chloramphenicol is not recommended in the treatment of shunt infections. Intraventricular therapy with vancomycin and aminoglycosides

(gentamicin, amikacin, and netilmicin) has also been used; whether this is more effective than IV therapy alone is not established. The duration of therapy is dependent on the organism isolated, the extent of infection as determined by cultures obtained after externalization and CSF chemistries, and cell count. Generally, 2–3 weeks of therapy are required; once the CSF is sterile for several consecutive days, a new shunt is inserted.

Prevention

Use of prophylactic antibiotics before and after surgery helps in reducing subsequent shunt infection (46) if infection rates at an institution are >5%. However, centers vary in their practice.

FUNGAL INFECTIONS OF THE CENTRAL NERVOUS SYSTEM

Most patients with a fungal infection of the CNS have some predisposing deficiency in immune response, very often caused by neutropenia, lymphoreticular malignancy, lymphoma, malnutrition, use of immunosuppressive drugs, potent broad-spectrum antibiotic therapy, or acquired immunodeficiency due to HIV infection. Direct inoculation may occur during neurosurgical procedures, such as ventriculoperitoneal shunt placement, or following head injury.

Etiology

The large number of fungi that can infect the CNS can be divided into those that can cause disease in a healthy host (*Cryptococcus, Histoplasma, Blastomyces, Coccidioides immitis, Sporothrix* spp., etc.) and those that cause opportunistic infection in immunocompromised host (*Candida* spp., *Aspergillus* spp., Zygomycetes, and *Trichosporon* spp.), although *Cryptococcus* and *Candida* spp can infect both healthy and immunocompromised hosts.. The fungal infections that may be suspected according to underlying predisposing factors are shown in **Table 91.11**.

TABLE 91.11

FUNGAL INFECTIONS THAT MAY BE SUSPECTED IN PRESENCE OF VARIOUS PREDISPOSING FACTORS

■ PREDISPOSING FACTOR	■ FUNGI MOST LIKELY TO CAUSE INFECTION
Prematurity	*Candida albicans*
Primary immunodeficiency (e.g., CGD, SCID)	*Candida, Cryptococcus, Aspergillus*
Corticosteroids	*Cryptococcus, Candida*
Cytotoxic agents	*Aspergillus, Candida*
Secondary immunodeficiency (e.g., AIDS)	*Cryptococcus, Histoplasma*
Iron chelator therapy	Zygomycetes
Intravenous drug abuse	*Candida,* Zygomycetes
Ketoacidosis, renal acidosis	Zygomycetes (*Mucor*)
Trauma, foreign body	*Candida*

CGD, chronic granulomatous disease; SCID, severe combined immunodeficiency; AIDS, acquired immunodeficiency syndrome.

Epidemiology

In recent times, opportunistic fungal infections in immunologically compromised hosts have increased worldwide. However, the true incidence of fungal CNS infection is unknown. *Candida* and *Aspergillus* spp. are ubiquitous and disseminate from endogenous sources. *Candida neoformans*, an encapsulated yeast, is an environmental fungus and is found in soil and bird droppings. The incidence of cryptococcal meningitis has risen with the increased prevalence of HIV infection, and is currently estimated at ~1 per 100,000. Of the varieties of *C. neoformans*, variety *grubii*, having type A serotype, and variety *neoformans*, having type D serotype, are worldwide in distribution, while variety *gatti* has BC serotypes and is found

in tropical and subtropical regions (Australia, Southeast Asia, central Africa, and California), particularly on flowering eucalyptus trees. *Coccidioides, Histoplasma,* and *Blastomyces* have been reported in different parts of the United States. Zygomycetes and *Trichosporon* also have a ubiquitous distribution (**Table 91.12**).

Pathogenesis

With the exception of mucormycosis, the primary site of infection is usually in the lungs and rarely in skin, from which hematogenous spread occurs to the CNS (**Table 91.12**). Pulmonary infection occurs from inhalation of fungal particles

---

TABLE 91.12

GEOGRAPHIC DISTRIBUTION, PREDISPOSING HOST CHARACTERISTICS, PRIMARY PATHOGENIC MECHANISM, AND PREDOMINANT CLINICAL SYNDROME OF VARIOUS FUNGAL CENTRAL NERVOUS SYSTEM INFECTIONS

■ FUNGUS	■ DISTRIBUTION/ FREQUENCY	■ PRIMARY PATHOGENESIS	■ PREDISPOSING HOST CHARACTERISTICS	■ USUAL CLINICAL SYNDROME
1. *Cryptococcus* variety *neoformans*, variety *gatti*, variety *grubii*	Worldwide/common in Australia, Southeast Asia, Central Africa, California	Pulmonary infection from inhalation of small yeast (basidiospore) Dissemination involves CNS in 30%–50%; often meningitis	Impaired cell-mediated immunity (HIV infection)	Meningitis Meningoencephalitis Cryptococcoma
2. *Coccidioides* (*C. immitis*)	South and Central America, Southern United States/occasional	Pulmonary infection from inhalation of arthroconidia. Dissemination in 0.2%; up to 30% have meningitis; also involves thoracic and lumber spine	Impaired cell-mediated immunity	Meningitis
3. Histoplasma (*H. capsulatum*)	Parts of United States (Midwest)/rare	Inhalation of spores, dissemination rare; of these, 10%–25% have CNS infection, more in patients with AIDS	Impaired cell-mediated immunity	Meningitis
4. *Blastomyces* (*B. dermatitidis*)	Parts of United States (Southeast)/rare	Inhalation of spores from soil leads to primary granulomatous lesion of lung, skin: Dissemination in up to one-third of patients	No prominent risk factor or immune defect	Meningitis Mass lesions
5. *Candida* (*C. albicans, C. tropicalis, C. parapsilosis,* and others)	Normal flora of body/common	Pulmonary or GI primary, hematogenous dissemination, CNS involvement in 50% with dissemination; most often leads to meningitis in infants. Direct inoculation via trauma, VP shunt placement, indwelling catheter	Patients with impaired cell-mediated immunity, neutropenia, phagocytic defects, prematurity, broad-spectrum antibiotics, corticosteroid therapy, hyperalimentation, malignancy, indwelling catheters, diabetes, abdominal surgery, thermal injury	Meningitis Abscess
6. *Aspergillus* (*A. fumigatus, A. flavus, A. terreus*)	Ubiquitous/occasional	Hematogenous spread in immunocompromised host from pulmonary primary. Direct extension from paranasal sinus or following head trauma. Surgery	Immunocompromised host (T-cell defects, phagocytic defects, neutropenia, GVHD)	Abscess Infarct
7. Zygomycosis (*Mucor*)	Ubiquitous/infection only in immunocompromised/occasional	Direct extension to CNS from nasal or paranasal sinuses. Hematogenous, rarely. Angioinvasive, causes cerebrovascular occlusion and infarction	Diabetes, diabetic ketoacidosis, malignancy, immunosuppressive therapy, IV drug users, deferoxamine chelation therapy, renal acidosis	Rhino-orbital-cerebral syndrome Venous thrombosis Infarct Abscess

AIDS, acquired immune deficiency syndrome; VP, ventriculoperitoneal; GVHD, graft-versus-host disease.

(yeast or basidiospores of cryptococci, arthroconidia of *Coccidioides*, and spores of *Histoplasma* and *Blastomyces*). The pulmonary infection often remains subclinical or asymptomatic. Sometimes, it may cause pneumonia of varying severity, including diffuse interstitial pneumonia in immunocompromised patients. Dissemination from lung is rare in *Coccidioides* and *Histoplasma*. *Blastomyces* causes a granulomatous lung lesion, which may disseminate in up to one-third of patients and involve the CNS. Zygomyces (*Mucor* spp.) spread directly into the CNS from paranasal sinuses through tissue planes and blood vessels; *Aspergillus* may also spread through this route or through the hematogenous route. *Candida* generally colonizes skin and GI mucosa and in immunocompromised patients can invade and spread to the CNS primarily through the hematogenous route. Direct inoculation of *Candida* may occur during head injury or neurosurgical procedure, such as ventriculostomy and ventriculoperitoneal shunt placement. Rarely, direct spread occurs from osteomyelitis of skull or vertebrae.

cranial nerve palsies, and infarction. *Coccidioides immitis* causes widespread basal meningitis. *Candida* causes meningitis mainly in neonates. *Cryptococcus neoformans* and *Candida* cause meningoencephalitis. In cryptococcosis, clusters of organisms spread through the brain, with little or no surrounding inflammatory responses, predominantly involving basal ganglia and cortical gray matter. The typical cystic lesion contains gelatinous polysaccharide, which can be detected in CSF. *Aspergillus*, Zygomycetes, *Blastomyces*, and candidiasis cause focal lesions. Disseminated candidiasis, especially *C. albicans*, and *C. tropicalis*, and disseminated aspergillosis (**Fig. 91.9A,B**) produce microabscesses. *Aspergillus* and mucormycosis infections are characterized by extensive angioinvasion. Damage of and penetration through endothelial cells and extracellular matrix lining the blood vessels contribute to the spread and the resultant vasculitis predisposes to infarction and hemorrhage. *Aspergillus* (all species—*A. fumigatus*, *A. flavus*, *A. terreus*) is the most common cause of CNS focal infections in organ-transplant recipients.

Pathology

CNS fungal involvement can occur as meningitis, meningoencephalitis, focal lesion, infarction or abscess. Fungal meningitis predominantly involves the base of the brain. *Cryptococcus neoformans*, when disseminated, may involve the CNS in up to 90% of cases, causing infection of the subarachnoid space. The basic lesion is a combination of suppurative and granulomatous inflammation. The chronic inflammatory response leads to thickening of meninges, hydrocephalus, arteritis,

Clinical Features

Fungal infections have no pathognomonic signs and symptoms. However, some characteristic clinical features, such as new-onset seizures and insidious onset may help. The literature contains many reports of patients who presented with new-onset seizures and deteriorated or died before a fungal cause was diagnosed. Fungal infection should be included in the differential diagnosis of new-onset seizures, especially in any child with predisposing factors.

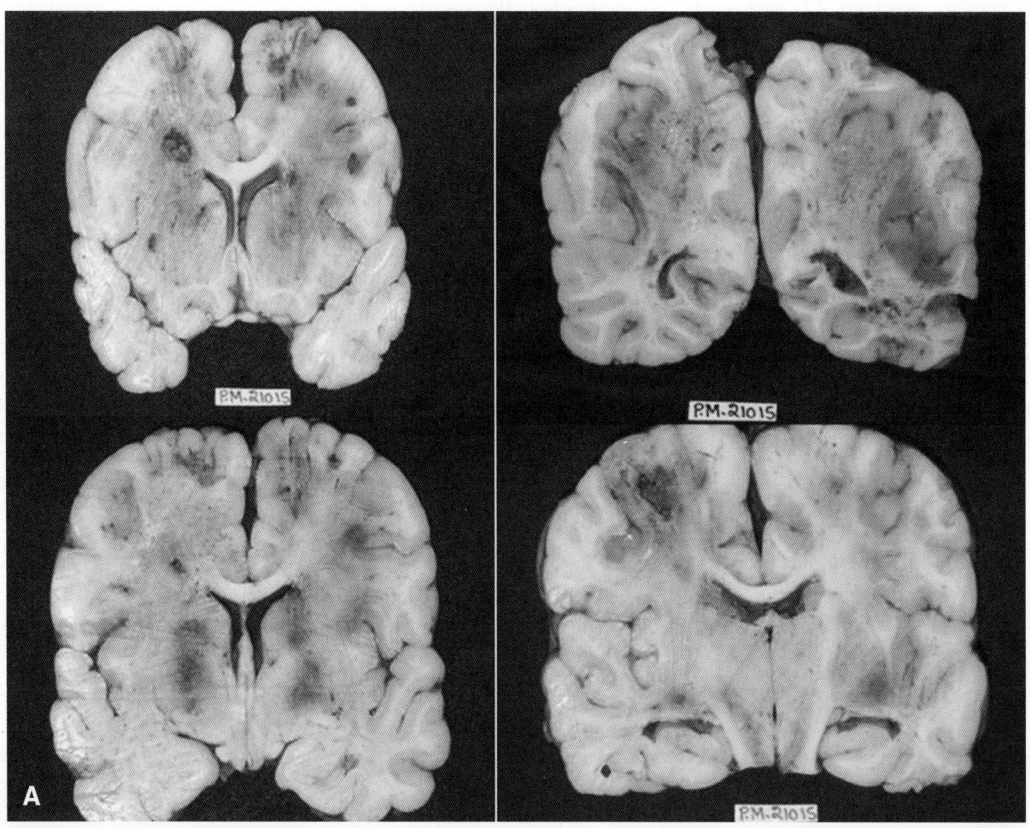

FIGURE 91.9. A: Cut sections of the brain showing multiple necrotic lesions caused by *Aspergillus* in a child with disseminated aspergillosis. **B:** Histopathology showing (*A*) ulcerated bronchial mucosa with many fungal hyphae (GMS stain), (*B*) invasion of vessel wall by fungal hyphae, and centrifugal spread with acute angle dichotomous branching of *Aspergillus hyphae*, as seen with (*C*) PAS stain and (*D*) GMS stain. GMS, Gomori methenamine silver; PAS, periodic acid-Schiff.

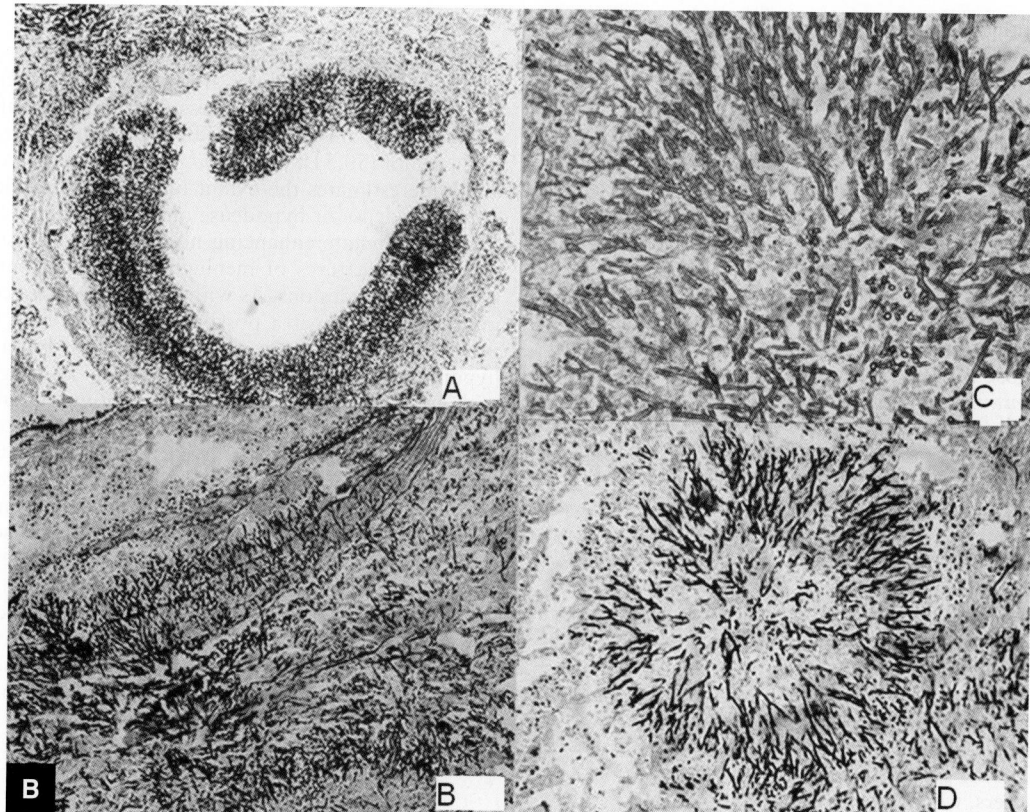

FIGURE 91.9. *(continued)*

FUNGAL MENINGITIS

The common causes are *Cryptococcus neoformans*, *Coccidioides immitis*, *Candida*, and *Aspergillus*. Clinical manifestations of fungal meningitis are less stereotyped than the manifestations of bacterial meningitis. Cryptococcal meningitis is often acute or subacute in HIV-infected children (47) and in those with T-cell suppression. Patients usually present with some combination of fever, headache, lethargy, nausea, vomiting, neck rigidity, impaired mental status, convulsion, and focal neurologic deficits (47). Raised ICP may develop acutely or during progression of the disease. Severe symptoms and signs may develop within days in patients with cryptococcal meningitis who are receiving high-dose corticosteroid therapy or in those with HIV infection. Fungal meningitis should always be a consideration in the differential diagnosis of a patient with a subacute or chronic meningitis syndrome (48).

RHINO-ORBITAL-CEREBRAL MUCORMYCOSIS

Rhino-orbital-cerebral mucormycosis is a major presentation of zygomycosis (*Rhizopus* and *Mucor* spp.), often in patients with poorly controlled diabetes. It presents with orbital pain, nasal discharge, and facial edema. Proptosis and visual loss may occur. Involvement of carotids may cause hemiparesis. Subsequently, trigeminal nerve and adjacent brain may be involved—classically found in mucormycosis, in which blackish necrotic areas are seen in the palate and nasal turbinates. Aspergillosis or mucormycosis may produce sudden onset of neurologic deficit due to vasculitis. Rarely, subarachnoid hemorrhage occurs due to mycotic aneurysmal bleed.

BRAIN ABSCESS

Brain abscess is the most common presenting feature of CNS aspergillosis. 10%–15% of patients with invasive *Aspergillus* infection have CNS involvement, which commonly presents as single or multiple brain abscesses with focal neurologic deficits (49). Fungal brain abscess can occasionally be caused by yeast (*Candida*, *Cryptococcus* spp.) and dimorphic fungi (*Histoplasma*, *Coccidioides*, *Blastomyces* spp.) in immunocompromised patients. Patient presents with focal neurologic signs, raised ICP or seizures, often accompanied by headache. Scedosporiosis of the CNS in near-drowning victims presents mainly as multiple brain abscesses.

SPINAL CORD SYNDROME

Fungal infections of spinal cord are rare. *Aspergillus* spp. may rarely cause aspergilloma, epidural abscess, and spinal arachnoiditis. Arachnoiditis can also occur from cryptococcal infection.

Diagnosis

It is important to suspect fungal infections in a given clinical context. In the presence of a predisposing condition, such as HIV infection, children who present with fever with or without CNS signs should have an LP for CSF analysis and culture. CSF examination usually reveals high proteins, low glucose, and mononuclear leukocytosis ranging between 20 and 500 cells/mm^3. Polymorphonuclear leukocytosis is more likely in *Aspergillus*, Zygomycetes, or

Blastomyces infection. Cell count may be normal or <20 cells/mm³ in patients with HIV infection or those on high-dose corticosteroid therapy.

Direct microscopic examination of CSF mixed with India ink on a slide is helpful in identification of encapsulated cryptococci in >50% cases. In patients with HIV infection, the yield may be up to 80%.

CSF cultures are frequently negative. Sometimes fungi require days to weeks to grow in culture medium. *Candida* takes several days, cryptococci 3–10 days, while *Histoplasma* and *Coccidioides* may take up to 6 weeks. Cisternal CSF may yield organism when lumbar CSF is negative. *C. neoformans* has the best yield on culture; it is positive in up to 90% patients, especially in those with HIV infection. *Blastomyces* and *Histoplasma capsulatum* rarely yield positive culture. In coccidioidal meningitis, culture may be positive in ~50%. Methenamine silver stain of a direct aspirate or biopsy is very helpful in identification of *Aspergillus* and Zygomycetes, which cause tissue invasion and infarction.

Latex agglutination test using CSF is positive (titer 1:8 or more) in up to 90% and is highly specific for cryptococcal meningitis. The test is diagnostic and may be positive early in the infection, even when culture is negative (48). False-negative results are uncommon and repeated negative tests over 1 month exclude the diagnosis (26).

Complement fixating antibody titer of ≥1:32 is found in CSF of 90% of coccidioidomycosis cases. CSF complement fixating antibody titers are diagnostic of meningitis; the test is negative, even in the presence of high serum complement fixating antibody titers, when meningitis is absent.

Diagnosis of *Aspergillus* infection can be made by assaying serum or CSF galactomannan, a polysaccharide marker on *Aspergillus* cell wall. A galactomannan index value of >0.5 in serum has a sensitivity and specificity exceeding 80%. Immunologic tests to detect specific antibodies in CSF are also available for *Histoplasma*, Zygomycetes, and *Sporothrix*, but these are not very specific. Serologic tests available for diagnosis of *Candida* and *Aspergillus* have not been evaluated specifically for CNS infection using CSF. PCR has shown promise in diagnosis of fungal meningitis, but requires further studies.

Neuroimaging

CT and MRI scans findings are generally nonspecific for basal involvement, associated abscess, and areas of infarction and are frequently mistaken for TBM, pyogenic brain abscess, or brain tumor (50,51). In *Candida* CNS infections, CT scan usually underestimates the extent of the disease. Microabscesses appear isodense or hypodense on nonenhanced CT and show multiple punctate enhancing nodules on contrast study. MR scan shows features of meningitis, vasculitis, infarction and ring-enhancing lesions. As with all meningitides, communicating hydrocephalus is a possible complication of fungal meningitis that is apparent at imaging. Fungal brain abscess are hypointense on T1- and hyperintense on T2-weighted images with well-defined contrast enhancement in immunocompetent patients. In immunocompromised patients, abscesses appear patchy, irregular walled T2 hyperintense lesions without contrast enhancement. They also have a high apparent diffusion coefficient (ADC) as compared to a low ADC seen in pyogenic and tubercular abscesses. Cryptococcomas are seen as small enhancing lesions. Clusters of round-to-oval low-density cystic lesions in basal ganglia and thalamic region on CT strongly suggest cryptococcal infection. In rhino-orbital-cerebral mucormycosis, imaging reveals opacification of paranasal sinuses with variable mucosal thickening and bony erosion. Intracranial findings may include thrombosis of cavernous sinus and infarct involving internal carotid artery territory.

Treatment

Optimal treatment includes specific antifungal therapy (Table 91.13), measures to control raised ICP, supportive treatment, surgical intervention, and management of underlying risk factors such as hyperglycemia, acidosis, and reversal of immunosuppression. Amphotericin B (deoxycholate) remains the most used and successful drug for fungal infections of CNS (Table 91.13), although concentrations of the drug in the CSF is generally low or even immeasurable. Lipid formulation of amphotericin B, such as liposomal amphotericin B (AmBisome) 3–5 mg/kg/day IV once daily, may be a better

TABLE 91.13

ANTIFUNGAL THERAPY RECOMMENDED IN COMMON FUNGAL CENTRAL NERVOUS SYSTEM INFECTION

■ FUNGUS	■ ANTIFUNGAL AGENT	■ DOSE	■ ROUTE	■ DURATION
Cryptococcus neoformans	Amphotericin B; +5-FC[a] then Fluconazole	1 mg/kg/d q24h (3–5 mg/kg/d of Lf-AmB) 100 mg/kg/d q6h 6–12 mg/kg/d q6h	IV PO PO	2 wk 2 wk HIV patients: indefinite Non-HIV patients: 6 mo to 1 y
Candida albicans and other	Lf-Amphotericin B ±5-FC then Fluconazole	3–5 mg/kg/d q24h 100 mg/kg/d q6h 10 mg/kg loading, then 6–12 mg/kg/d q24h	IV PO PO/IV	2 wk 4–6 wk Several weeks till clinical, CSF and radiologic resolution
Aspergillus fumigatus	Amphotericin B ±5-FC or Voriconazole	1–1.5 mg/kg/d q24h 100–150 mg/kg/d q6h 6 mg/kg, 2 doses 12 h apart, then 4 mg/kg q12h[b]	IV PO IV/PO	6 mo to 1 y
Coccidioides immitis	Amphotericin B, then fluconazole	0.7–1 mg/kg/d 10 mg/d loading then 5–6 mg/kg/d	IV PO	4 wk Lifelong

[a]5-FC levels should be monitored 2–4 h after oral dose after 3–4 days, with target peak 40–60 μg/mL.
[b]By IV infusion, 5 mg/mL strength, maximum rate 3 mg/kg/h.

alternative to conventional amphotericin B, especially in the setting of renal dysfunction. Some clinicians have used an intrathecal dose (0.025–1.5 mg) twice weekly as a last resort. It may cause vasculitis and arachnoiditis. Common adverse effects of intrathecal amphotericin include nausea, vomiting, and headache.

Flucytosine penetrates well into CSF and achieves concentrations that approach 75% of simultaneous serum concentrations. However, administering flucytosine alone for treatment of CNS fungal infections is associated with a high risk of treatment failure because of development of in vitro and in vivo resistance. When flucytosine is administered in combination with amphotericin B or fluconazole, relapse rate is lower when compared with amphotericin B alone.

Of the azoles, fluconazole is effective against *Cryptococcus* and *Candida*. It crosses the BBB easily and has a long half-life in the CNS. However, CSF sterilization is slower as compared to an amphotericin B–containing regimen. Itraconazole has potent antifungal activity against a broad spectrum of fungi, including *Aspergillus*. Although it has very limited penetration into the CSF, it has been successful in the treatment of cryptococcal meningitis in patients with HIV infection. Voriconazole is a new broad-spectrum triazole with remarkable activity against *Aspergillus*, *Fusarium*, *Scedosporium*, and dematiaceous fungi. Penetration into the CSF and early favorable clinical experience make voriconazole the drug of choice in CNS aspergillosis and scedosporiosis.

Caspofungin, first in the class of echinocandins, works by blocking the synthesis of glucan, a major component of the fungal cell wall. Caspofungin is fungicidal against *Candida* spp. and active against *Aspergillus*. Activity against *Fusarium*, *Rhizopus*, and *Trichosporon* is limited. Micafungin and anidulafungin are second-generation echinocandins with antifungal spectrum and efficacy similar to caspofungin. All echinocandins have low oral bioavailability and distribute well into tissues, but poorly into the CNS and eye. Transaminase monitoring is recommended during treatment. Anidulafungin is unique in that it undergoes elimination by chemical degradation in bile rather than via hepatic metabolism, thus not requiring dose adjustment in hepatic insufficiency (52). Echinocandins alone are infrequently used to treat CNS infections. Caspofungin is effective alone or in combination with polyenes, such as amphotericin, for refractory invasive *Candida* infection and in combination with voriconazole in refractory CNS infection due to *Aspergillus* spp. Micafungin is also approved for use in children, including preterm infants.

In cryptococcal meningitis, amphotericin B plus flucytosine has proven successful. This combination sterilizes CSF within 2 weeks. Amphotericin B alone produces cures in >50% of patients, with a risk of considerable drug-related toxicity. Amphotericin B at a dose of 1 mg/kg/day IV is used with flucytosine 100 mg/kg/day PO divided q6h for at least 2 weeks, followed by fluconazole (12 mg/kg/day) for 8–10 weeks. In patients with HIV infection, a repeat LP should be performed 2 weeks after starting amphotericin to ensure that CSF pressure is normal and CSF is sterile before shifting to maintenance fluconazole, which is continued indefinitely as suppressive therapy to prevent relapses. Intraventricular amphotericin B has been used successfully in cases with a poor prognosis.

Cryptococcomas in the brain parenchyma are much less common than meningeal disease. In small and multiple lesions, antifungal chemotherapy alone is generally successful, although fluconazole may be needed for an extended period of up to 2 years. Large cryptococcomas (>3 cm) located in surgically accessible areas may be considered for surgical removal.

In CNS cryptococcal infection, corticosteroid administration should be discontinued; if it is not possible to do so, the dose must be reduced rapidly and as far as the underlying disease permits. Relapse rate is very high in patients with

underlying HIV infection, well above 50%, and in non-HIV infection patients, it is ~15%–25%. Most relapses occur in the first 3–6 months after cessation of therapy; hence, the need for prolonged suppressive therapy in patients with HIV infection. Unexpected deaths or loss of vision during the first 1–2 weeks of treatment may occur in some patients with HIV infection and cryptococcal meningitis. These patients deteriorate suddenly and may manifest a dramatic increase in ICP. The pathogenesis of such an event is not fully understood. External CSF drainage should be considered in these patients.

In coccidioidal meningitis control of infection is achieved through the use of fluconazole or intrathecal amphotericin B. Oral fluconazole (12 mg/kg/day) is tried first, and intrathecal amphotericin B is used only as an alternative regimen, beginning with 0.1 mg/day, increased as tolerated up to 0.5 mg/day. The need for continuing therapy may be guided by monitoring CSF cells and glucose; the target is 10 cells/mm^3 or less with normal CSF glucose concentrations for at least 1 year. A lowering of the CSF antibody titer is also considered a good prognostic sign.

In *Candida* meningitis, amphotericin B is the primary therapeutic agent, preferably in combination with flucytosine, as it has synergistic activity against *Candida*. It is followed by fluconazole.

Aspergillus infections of the CNS are very difficult to eradicate. High doses of amphotericin B have rarely been successful in arresting the infection. Voriconazole may be considered as a first choice for *Aspergillus* meningitis because it has both IV and oral formulations and early studies suggest that 25% of patients may respond. Aforementioned retrospective data in adults support addition of caspofungin to voriconazole for invasive aspergillosis. In patients with Zygomycetes (*Rhizopus*, *Mucor*) or *Aspergillus* infection with invasion of blood vessels and resultant infarction, in addition to high-dose amphotericin B (1.5 mg/kg/day) or liposomal amphotericin (5–7.5 mg/kg/day), direct surgical removal of infected tissue should be undertaken if lesions are accessible.

The management of fungal brain abscesses is not well standardized. *Blastomyces* and *Histoplasma* abscesses have been successfully removed surgically, with concomitant amphotericin B treatment. Dematiaceous fungi that cause brain abscesses are surgically removed or debulked as primary therapy for cure, along with antifungal agents.

If *Candida* or cryptococcal meningitis develops in a patient with a shunt in place, eradication of infection is best achieved by removing the shunt and treating with antifungal agents.

Prognosis

The most important determinant of the outcome of fungal CNS infections is the causative fungus and the patient's underlying condition. The outcome of cryptococcal CNS infection is usually better than that of other forms of fungal meningitis. In cryptococcal meningitis, convulsions and focal neurologic deficits are independent predictors of in-hospital mortality in HIV-infected children (47). Poor prognostic factors associated with failure of amphotericin B therapy or relapse after therapy include an initial positive CSF India ink test result, high CSF opening pressure, low CSF leukocyte counts (<20 cells/mm^3), cryptococci isolated from extraneural sites, absent anticryptococcal antibody, initial CSF or serum cryptococcal antigen titer of 1:32 or more, posttreatment titers of 1:8 or more, corticosteroid therapy, lymphoreticular malignancy, and a CSF glucose concentration that remains abnormal during 4 weeks or more of therapy (48). Very high CSF antigen titers (≥1:1024), low serum albumin concentration, and low CD4 cell count (<5 cells/mL), and increased ICP in excess of 250 mm H$_2$O predict failure to rapidly sterilize CSF in patients with HIV infection (48).

The mortality with *Candida* meningitis is 10%–20%. Children may be left with permanent neurologic or mental deficits. Poor prognostic factors for patients with *Candida* meningitis include diagnosis made >2 weeks after symptom onset, CSF glucose concentrations <35 mg/dL, and development of intracranial hypertension, and focal neurologic deficits (48).

In childhood, CNS aspergillosis overall mortality in cases reported after 1990 is 40%, which is a tremendous improvement over case fatality rate of 83% in cases reported before 1990. Surgery is independently associated with survival and together with antifungal therapy, it significantly improves outcome (49). However, in patients with disseminated aspergillosis with CNS involvement mortality is 100%.

CNS zygomycosis has a very high mortality. Dissemination and young age (<1 year) are independent risk factors for death in children. As in aspergillosis, antifungal therapy and particularly surgery reduced risk of death by 92% and 84%, respectively (53).

The attributable mortality in *Histoplasma* meningitis is 20%–40%, and relapse rate is as high as 50%. Only 50% patients with coccidioidal meningitis survive initial treatment, and most have extremely high risk of relapse and frequently require lifelong suppressive therapy.

Prevention

A cryptococcal vaccine has been developed but is not yet licensed. Fluconazole therapy for ≥1 year can reduce the number of cryptococcal meningitis cases in HIV-infected patients. Both fluconazole and itraconazole can prevent cryptococcal meningitis cases in HIV-infected adult patients, but survival benefit is seen only in specific patient population. Azole prophylaxis is recommended in children with low CD4 count, living in endemic area and who are not on or are in early stages of highly active antiretroviral therapy. The use of azoles as prophylactic agents to prevent histoplasmosis and coccidioidomycosis in HIV-infected patients is under investigation.

PARASITIC INFECTIONS

Once considered limited to the tropics, parasitic infections are being widely reported across the world. Increasing travel and immigrating populations are responsible for this change. A large number of parasites can affect the CNS. Most of them cause chronic or subacute involvement; however, some may present acutely either with a meningoencephalitic presentation or as a mass lesion with marked cerebral edema and raised ICP. These cases would present to the intensivist. A discussion of all parasitic CNS infections is beyond the scope of this chapter. Some of the parasites that can involve the CNS and their clinical manifestations are listed in **Table 91.14**. Cerebral malaria and NCC are discussed separately.

Etiology

In any case of suspected parasitic infection, the most important etiologic clue is obtained by a detailed history, particularly related to travel to, or immigration from, endemic areas. Some parasitic infections, such as falciparum malaria, manifest clinically within a few days, whereas others, such as NCC, may manifest several months or even years after infection. It is important to inquire about both recent travel and past travel to endemic areas. History of suggestive mode of acquisition, such as blood transfusion for malarial parasite, bathing in a pond for *Naegleria*, exposure to tsetse fly for African trypanosomiasis, or reduviid bug for American trypanosomiasis, is

TABLE 91.14

COMMON PARASITIC CENTRAL NERVOUS SYSTEM INFECTIONS

■ PARASITE	■ CLINICAL MANIFESTATIONS
Protozoa	
Plasmodium falciparum	Cerebral malaria
Ameba	Meningitis/meningoencephalitis
Entamoeba histolytica	Meningitis/meningoencephalitis
Acanthamoeba	Meningoencephalitis
Naegleria	
Trypanosoma	
brucei (*rhodesiense* or	
gambiense)	
cruzi	
Toxoplasma gondii	
Helminths (worms)	
Cestodes (flatworms)	Seizures/meningoencephalitis
Taenia solium	Mass lesion with raised ICP
(neurocysticercosis)	
Echinococcus (hydatid	Solitary/multiple
cyst) (multilocularis/	Seizures
granulosus)	
Nematodes (roundworms)	
Trichinella	Meningoencephalitis
Strongyloides	Meningoencephalitis
Ascaris	Seizures

also important. Underlying immune status of the child, such as HIV-positive status, corticosteroid therapy, and asplenia, may indicate possible specific opportunistic parasitic diseases, such as toxoplasmosis.

Epidemiology

Amebae have a worldwide distribution. *Entamoeba histolytica*, transmitted by the fecal–oral route, is carried by ~0.5 billion individuals worldwide, causing symptoms in 500 million and death in 100,000 each year. Disseminated disease with CNS involvement occurs in a fraction of this subset. Free-living ameba, including *Acanthamoeba* and *Naegleria*, are found in fresh or brackish water, and disease occurs in warm months, when exposure is increased. *Trypanosoma* are transmitted by vectors, including the tsetse fly in Africa and reduviid bug in Central and South America. *Trypanosoma brucei* is the etiologic agent of African trypanosomiasis (also known as African sleeping sickness), with *T. brucei rhodiense* causing East African trypanosomiasis and *T. brucei gambiense* causing West African trypanosomiasis. *Trypanosoma cruzi* is the etiologic agent of American trypanosomiasis (Chagas disease). It is estimated that ~700,000 cases of American trypanosomiasis and 400,000 cases of African trypanosomiasis occur each year. Exact incidence rates of CNS trypanosomiasis are not known but increase with length of illness. *Toxoplasma gondii* is acquired most commonly by ingestion of oocysts present in cat feces or through ingestion of tissue cysts of contaminated meat that is undercooked. Seroprevalence of toxoplasmosis varies from several percentages in countries such as Thailand to 90% in France. The largest disease burden is in neonates born to mothers with primary toxoplasmosis during gestation and in immunocompromised individuals. Echinococcosis is caused by a larval form of the tapeworm *Taenia echinococcus*. Cystic echinococcosis is caused by *Echinococcus granulosus*, found worldwide in association with sheep herding. *Echinococcus multilocularis* involves the CNS less often, is associated with exposure to wild rodents and foxes, and is only found in the northern hemisphere. Nematodes, such as *Trichinella* and *Ascaris*, are found in soil in tropical areas with poor sanitation. *Strongyloides* is also endemic in tropical climes with poor sanitation, but infection occurs by penetration through exposed skin.

Pathogenesis

Infection by the parasite (e.g., *E. histolytica*, *Acanthamoeba*, *Toxoplasma*, *Echinococcus*, and *Ascaris*) typically occurs through the gastrointestinal tract, via a vector (e.g., malaria, trypanosomiasis), or by skin penetration (*Strongyloides*). The parasite typically undergoes a stage of multiplication, followed by hematogenous seeding of the CNS. *Naegleria* penetrates via the nasal mucosa and spreads via olfactory nerves to the CNS.

Clinical Presentation

The clinical presentation of parasitic CNS disease varies considerably based on the causative agent. Symptoms of acute meningitis or meningoencephalitis are most typical, with fever, headache, vomiting, photophobia, neck stiffness, and altered sensorium. New-onset seizures are another common clinical presentation, as in NCC. Cystic echinococcal infection may present insidiously over years with a slowly enlarging cyst, causing headache and progressing toward neurologic deficit and herniation.

Diagnosis

The CSF may be diagnostic in certain cases, such as finding of free-floating amebae in the case of *Naegleria* or Giemsa stain for trypanosomiasis. A positive serology in serum or CSF may suggest NCC; rise in specific IgM titer for toxoplasmosis is highly suggestive. PCR studies are also available for some parasites. Various investigations may be of use in diagnosis, such as blood film for malaria or presence of eosinophilia for helminths.

Neuroimaging

Neuroimaging may reveal characteristic findings, such as a scolex seen within the cyst in NCC. The presence of a round, thin-walled cyst filled with fluid isointense to CSF suggests hydatid due to *Echinococcus* (**Fig. 91.10**), whereas small, ring-enhancing lesions (particularly in deep gray matter) in a child with HIV suggest toxoplasmosis.

Treatment

The supportive management in the ICU is principally similar to other CNS infections. Specific antiparasitic therapy would depend on the etiologic organism. Surgical removal of large cysts is indicated in some cases. Rupture of the cyst should be avoided, as it can induce anaphylactic shock.

NEUROCYSTICERCOSIS

NCC is the most common parasitic infection of the CNS and an important cause of epilepsy in the tropics. The clinical presentations are variable and depend on the stage and location

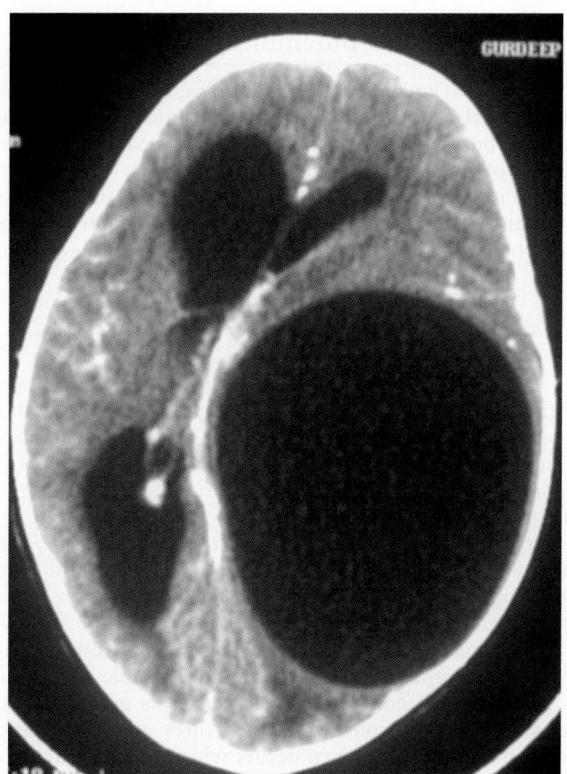

FIGURE 91.10. Contrast-enhanced CT showing a large, rounded cystic lesion with imperceptible walls with midline shift and mass effect, causing ventricular dilatation on the opposite side—hydatid cyst.

of cysts. Most cases present with seizures, and approximately one-third of cases have symptoms and signs of raised ICP. Generally, the presentation is not serious enough to warrant admission to the PICU; however, some cases may present with significant cerebral edema, leading to either an encephalitic presentation or a mass effect.

Etiology

NCC is caused by infestation of the CNS with encysted larvae of *Taenia solium*. Humans acquire intestinal infection (taeniasis, tapeworm) from pigs by ingestion of undercooked pork infected with *T. solium* cysticerci. In the intestine, cysticerci develop into adult worms and release thousands of eggs that are extremely contagious. Open defecation and inadequate sewerage cause contamination of soil with infected stools. The intermediate host is the pig that becomes infected by grazing on soil contaminated with parasitic eggs. The eggs hatch into larvae, invade the intestinal mucosa, and reach the muscles or the brain, where they mature into cysticerci over a period of 3 weeks to 2 months. When humans consume undercooked pork that contains the cysts, the life cycle of the parasite is completed.

Cysticercosis in humans is acquired through the fecal–oral route by ingestion of contaminated raw vegetables or food prepared by carriers of tapeworms; rarely, it is due to auto-ingestion of ova in patients who have intestinal tapeworms. After ingestion of *T. solium* eggs, larvae (oncospheres) form and penetrate the intestinal mucosa, with subsequent migration throughout the body and penetration of the CNS, skeletal muscle, subcutaneous tissue, and the eyes, where mature cysts form.

Epidemiology

Cysticercosis is endemic in Latin America, Mexico, India, sub-Saharan Africa, and China. NCC is not limited to developing countries but is also seen in many developed countries, mainly because of increasing number of immigrants from endemic areas. It is estimated that >1000 new cases of NCC are diagnosed in the United States each year. Approximately 20 million people are infected worldwide, and ~50,000 die from the disease every year.

Pathogenesis

Cysticerci may live within host tissues for years without causing any inflammation or disease, as they have various mechanisms for evading host response, including inhibition of complement activation and suppression of cellular immune response.

The cyst has four stages: The *vesicular (metacestode) stage* marked by is a fluid-filled cyst with a thin wall and an eccentric opaque scolex. This cyst degenerates to the *colloidal stage*, when gelatinous material appears in cyst fluid, followed by the *granular nodular stage* in which the cyst contracts and the walls are replaced by focal lymphoid nodules and necrosis. Finally, in the *nodular calcified stage*, the granulation tissue is replaced by collagenous structures and calcification. Symptomatology most often occurs when the cyst transitions from the living vesicular to the dying colloidal stage, releasing inflammatory mediators. Inflammation and (less commonly) subsequent calcification serve as a nidus for seizure activity.

Clinical Manifestations

The clinical presentation of NCC is variable and depends on the stage and location of the cysts; it is classified into parenchymal and extraparenchymal types.

Parenchymal Neurocysticercosis

The common clinical manifestations include:

■ Seizures in 70%–90% cases, more frequent in children as compared to adults. In a large series of 500 children, seizures were reported in 95% cases (54). Most seizures are complex partial; approximately one-fourth is simple partial. Generalized seizures are less common. Seizures are generally brief; SE has been reported in 2%–32% cases.
■ Elevated ICP with headache and vomiting in almost one-third of cases. Papilledema has been reported in 2.3%–6.6% of children.
■ Focal neurologic deficits in 4% of children are determined by the location of the cysts.
■ Encephalitis: Children and adolescents with numerous cysts and marked diffuse cerebral edema may occasionally present with severe acute raised ICP and an encephalitic picture. They are difficult to treat and have a poor prognosis.

Extraparenchymal Neurocysticercosis

Extraparenchymal involvement is rare in children and includes (a) ventricular involvement, presenting as obstructive hydrocephalous or chronic meningitis; (b) subarachnoid involvement, presenting as basilar arachnoiditis or chronic meningitis; cysts may enlarge, become racemose, and cause mass effects; (c) spinal involvement, with cysts that may be located in the leptomeningeal space or within the cord; radicular pain, paresthesias, and spinal cord compression may occur; intramedullary cysts may present as transverse myelitis with paraplegia and sphincteric disturbances; and (d) ophthalmic involvement, which may affect the subretinal space, vitreous humor, subconjunctiva, or anterior chamber, and may cause visual deficits, sudden blindness, and similar symptoms.

Other presentations of NCC include hydrocephalous, vasculitis, and stroke. Stroke is due to vasculitis secondary to cysticercus arachnoiditis at the base of the brain. The infarcts are generally small, and lacunar; occasionally, large infarcts due to occlusion of middle cerebral or internal carotid artery may occur. Numerous unusual presentations, including dorsal midbrain syndrome, papillitis, ptosis, and cerebral hemorrhage, may also be seen. Fever is unusual in NCC.

Diagnosis

The gold standard for diagnosis of NCC is pathologic confirmation through biopsy or autopsy. Practically, the diagnosis rests mainly on neuroimaging. Immunologic tests have not proven to be very sensitive or specific for diagnosis of NCC, particularly for single lesions. Low positivity from 17% to 25% has been reported in children with NCC (55). ELISA of CSF and serum shows high false-positive and false-negative reactions. Enzyme-linked immunoelectrotransfer blot assay using purified glycoprotein antigens from *T. solium* cysticerci was reported to be highly specific and nearly 100% sensitive for patients with either multiple active parenchymal cysts or extraparenchymal NCC. However, sensitivity is less for patients with either single cysts or calcifications. A crude soluble extract ELISA was found to be more sensitive and specific than dot blot assay. Peripheral eosinophilia is variably reported. CSF is normal in parenchymal NCC; in NCC meningitis, it may show mild pleocytosis with some elevation of protein and hypoglycorrhachia. The cellular response may be polymorphonuclear or lymphocytic. Diagnostic criteria for human cysticercosis and NCC were revised to make them specific for the diagnosis of NCC. In clinical practice, it may not be feasible to apply these diagnostic criteria. In view of the pleomorphism of the disease, NCC should be kept in the differential diagnosis of a wide variety of neurologic disorders, particularly seizures, and appropriate neuroimaging studies should be undertaken to confirm the diagnosis.

Neuroimaging

The characteristic CT picture consists of small, low-density, ring- or disc-enhancing lesions, with perilesional edema. The scolex appears as a bright, high-density, eccentric nodule in these cysts and is pathognomonic of NCC. Enhancing lesions represent degenerating (colloidal vesicular) cysticerci. In most cases, the lesions (termed *single, small, enhancing CT lesions*) are single and <20 mm in size (**Fig. 91.11A**). Some may have multiple lesions; NCC with numerous cysts produces the "starry-sky" appearance typical of NCC. Calcifications are few millimeters in size and may be single or multiple. Vesicular cysts appear as small, round, nonenhancing lesions with CSF-density cystic fluid; the wall is isodense to the brain parenchyma.

In subarachnoid NCC, the CT findings include hydrocephalous, tentorial enhancement, and occasionally, infarcts. Cystic hypodense lesions, representing racemose cysts, may rarely be seen in the sylvian fissure or cerebellopontine angle. Intraventricular NCC manifests as hydrocephalous; rarely, intraventricular cysts may be identified.

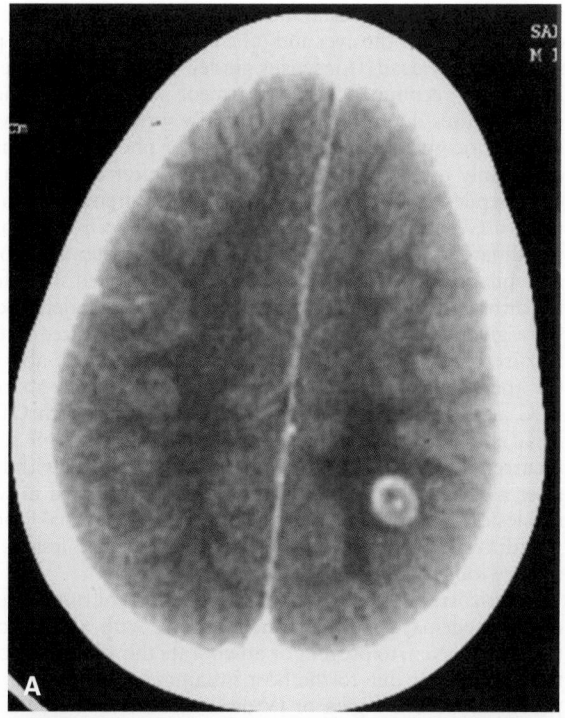

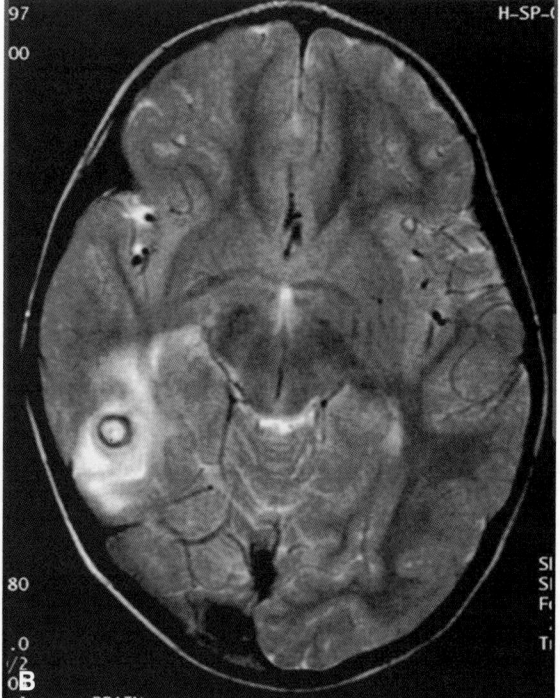

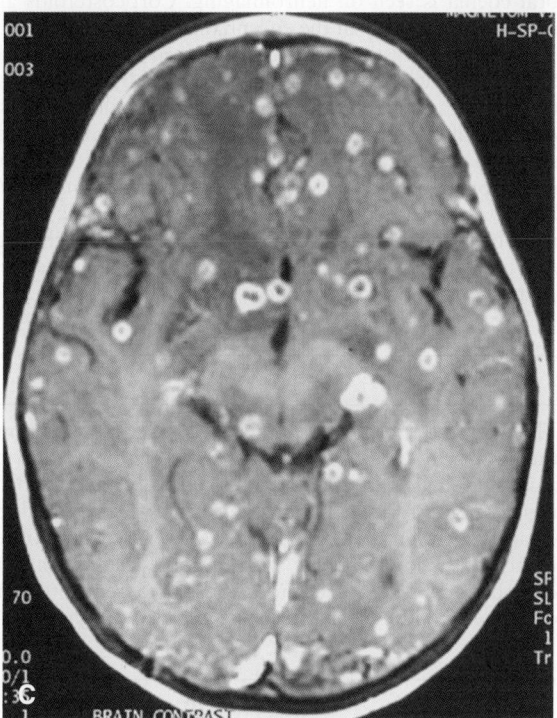

FIGURE 91.11. Neurocysticercosis (NCC). **A:** Contrast-enhanced CT showing a single, small, ring-enhancing lesion (SSECTL) with a well-defined eccentric scolex, and perilesional edema. **B:** T2-weighted MRI showing a single NCC lesion with a scolex and bright perilesional edema. **C:** Contrast MRI showing multiple, ring-enhancing NCC lesions in a small, multiple NCC.

MRI is more sensitive than CT for visualization of extraparenchymal cysts and identification of scolex. On T1-weighted images, live cysts are seen as round lesions, either isointense or slightly hyperintense to the CSF, with a scolex that is hyperintense or isointense to white matter. On T2-weighted images, the cysts are isointense to CSF and the perilesional edema appears bright (**Fig. 91.11B**). The scolex may not be seen because of the high intensity cystic fluid. The scolex is better seen on proton density–weighted images. Gadolinium-enhanced MRI shows ring enhancement of lesion (**Fig. 91.11C**). Calcified lesions appear hypointense on all MR imaging sequences and may at times be missed.

Proton MR spectroscopy is under investigation for evaluation of inflammatory granulomas. Presence of a lipid peak reportedly indicates a tuberculoma; low levels of metabolites with a poor signal-to-noise ratio could indicate NCC. MR spectroscopy may also help in differentiating NCC from a neoplasm.

Other Imaging

Radiographs of skeletal muscles to look for calcified cysts and stool examination for tapeworms are rarely positive. If a subcutaneous nodule is detected in a child with suspected NCC, it should be biopsied to corroborate the diagnosis.

Differential Diagnoses

Parenchymal Neurocysticercosis

In a child with a single, small, enhancing CT lesion, if the scolex is not visualized, the differential diagnoses include:

- Tuberculoma, particularly in developing countries. Raised ICP, progressive focal neurologic deficit, size of CT lesion >20 mm, lobulated irregular shape, and marked edema, causing midline shift favor the diagnosis of tuberculoma but are not absolute criteria. Tests for exclusion of TB (e.g., Mantoux skin test and chest x-ray) should be done in all cases.
- Other parasitic granulomas, such as toxoplasmosis and, rarely, schistosomiasis, sparganosis, and paragonimiasis
- Neoplasms, such as low-grade astrocytoma or cystic cerebral metastasis
- Microabscess
- Fungal lesion, particularly cryptococcosis, and rarely, histoplasmosis or sarcoidosis
- Most of these are rare in children.

Extraparenchymal Neurocysticercosis

Hydrocephalous with racemose NCC in the subarachnoid space may simulate a low-density tumor. Meningitis due to NCC must be differentiated from other causes of meningitis, particularly tubercular and fungal meningitis.

Treatment

A child with an encephalitic presentation requires intensive care management similar to any other encephalitis. IV steroids are used to reduce the cerebral edema, and anticonvulsants to control the seizures. Cysticidal therapy is not used in the acute phase, as it may provoke a further inflammatory response and worsen the edema. It may be considered later in select cases once the edema subsides and the child is stable. Praziquantel and albendazole are the two drugs that have been found effective against *T. solium* cysticerci. Albendazole has been found to be more efficacious, less expensive, and better tolerated than praziquantel. It has better penetration into the subarachnoid space, its bioavailability increases with coadministration of steroids, and it is currently the drug of choice for treatment of NCC. Oral albendazole has been used in a dose of 15 mg/kg/day in two to three divided doses for 28 days. Shorter durations of 14 days to 8 days have also been used. In a placebo-controlled trial of 1 week versus 4 weeks of albendazole therapy in children with one to three enhancing lesions, both regimens were found to be equally effective (56). Oral praziquantel is used in a dose of 50–100 mg/kg/day divided into three doses for a period of 15 days. However, a single-day praziquantel therapy (25 mg/kg/dose every 2 hours × three doses) has been reported to be effective and comparable to 7-day treatment with albendazole. Combination therapy with praziquantel and albendazole has also been used (57). Evidence-based guidelines of the American Academy of Neurology recommend the use of cysticidal therapy (with albendazole and steroid) in most cases of parenchymal NCC (58).

Cysticidal therapy should not be used in the following cases: (a) markedly raised ICP, particularly in disseminated NCC, as sudden elevations of ICP may occur secondary to the host inflammatory response; such cases should be treated with steroids alone; (b) ophthalmic NCC, as the host response may cause damage to the eye; and (c) calcified lesions, as the parasite is already dead. Consensus guidelines for the treatment of NCC (59) recommend that treatment should be individualized. Seizures due to NCC are usually well controlled with a single anticonvulsant. Carbamazepine or phenylhydantoin are commonly used. Recurrence of seizures after discontinuation of antiepileptic drugs is less (10.5%) in children than in adults (50%). Generally, antiepileptic drugs have been used for approximately a 2-year seizure-free interval. Shorter durations of antiepileptic drugs may be sufficient. A controlled study found no difference in seizure recurrence when antiepileptic drugs were given for a 1-year versus a 2-year seizure-free interval. Seizure recurrence correlated significantly with an abnormal CT (persistence or calcification of lesion) and an abnormal EEG at the time of withdrawal. Children with both CT and EEG abnormalities had a significantly higher risk of seizure recurrence. Thus, anticonvulsant therapy may be withdrawn after a 1-year seizure-free interval in those children in whom the lesion has disappeared and the EEG is normal prior to withdrawal. Children with persistent or calcified lesions may require longer therapy.

Corticosteroids are used for short periods of time to reduce cerebral edema, generally concomitantly with anticysticercal therapy, if given, to prevent or ameliorate the adverse reactions that may occur due to the host inflammatory response. Oral prednisolone 1–2 mg/kg or IV dexamethasone is used if cerebral edema is seen on neuroimaging. Corticosteroids are the mainstay of therapy in the encephalitic form of NCC.

Surgery for cyst removal has been used in ophthalmic NCC. Shunt placement is necessary in cases with hydrocephalus; use of steroids and albendazole reduces shunt failure. Endoscopic removal of cysts from the ventricles may obviate the need for shunt placement. Successful medical treatment of subarachnoid, spinal, and other forms of extraparenchymal NCC has led to a decrease in the role of surgery in NCC. Follow-up must be individualized. A repeat CT after 3–6 months is generally indicated to determine whether the lesions have resolved partially or completely, are persisting, or have calcified.

Prognosis

The outcome depends on the type of NCC, cyst location, and the number of cysts. Patients with NCC who present with seizures and single parenchymal cysts generally have a good prognosis; seizures are well controlled in most cases, and lesions disappear within 6 months in over 60% cases. Risk of seizure recurrence is low. Patients with multiple lesions, particularly disseminated NCC and calcifications, have frequent seizure recurrences. NCC encephalitis has a guarded prognosis.

Prevention

Proper animal husbandry, hygiene, and sanitation can eradicate transmission of *T. solium* from pigs to humans. Mass treatment of the population with praziquantel did not show lasting benefits.

CONCLUSIONS AND FUTURE DIRECTIONS

In summary, CNS infections have varied etiology, clinical presentation, treatment course, and prognosis. It is important that the intensivist is familiar with the clinical syndromes and the epidemiology, so that an appropriate differential diagnosis may be generated, diagnostic tests obtained, and empiric and specific treatment initiated. Future directions in the understanding, diagnosis, and management of CNS infection will undoubtedly include improved molecular diagnostic techniques, including PCR and multiplex PCR, for a larger number of etiologic agents, which will enhance the understanding of the epidemiology of CNS infections, as well as their etiology. Advances in molecular microbiology and immunology will also enhance the understanding of pathogenesis and allow for the development of improved therapeutic and preventive measures.

ACKNOWLEDGMENT

Some of the figures are courtesy of Prof. N. Khandelwal and Prof. R.K. Vasishta from the Departments of Radiodiagnosis & Imaging and Histopathology, PGIMER, Chandigarh.

References

1. Singhi S, Murthy A, Singhi P, et al. Continuous midazolam versus diazepam infusion for refractory status epilepticus. *J Child Neurol* 2002;17:106–10.

2. Singhi S, Singhi P, Srinivas B, et al. Fluid restriction does not improve the outcome of acute meningitis. *Pediatr Infect Dis J* 1995;14:495–503.

3. Oates-Whitehead RM, Maconochie I, Baumer H, et al. Fluid therapy for acute bacterial meningitis. *Cochrane Database Syst Rev* 2005;3:CD004786.

4. Watt JP, Wolfson LJ, O'Brien KL, et al. Burden of disease caused by *Haemophilus influenzae* type b in children younger than 5 years: Global estimates [published online ahead of print September 15, 2009]. *Lancet* 2009;374(9693):903–11.

5. Saez-Lorens X, McCracken GH. Bacterial meningitis in children. *Lancet* 2003;361:2139–48.

6. O'Brien KL, Wolfson LJ, Watt JP, et al. Burden of disease caused by *Streptococcus pneumoniae* in children younger than 5 years: Global estimates [published online ahead of print September 15, 2009]. *Lancet* 2009;374(9693):893–902.

7. May M, Daley AJ, Donath S, et al.; for Australasian Study Group for Neonatal Infections. Early onset neonatal meningitis in Australia and New Zealand, 1992–2002. *Arch Dis Child Fetal Neonatal Ed* 2005;24:533–7.

8. Alkholi UM, Abd Al-Monem N, Abd El-Azim AA, et al. Serum procalcitonin in viral and bacterial meningitis. *J Glob Infect Dis* 2011;3:14–8.

9. Singhi S, Khetarpal R, Baranwal AK, et al. Intensive care needs of children with acute bacterial meningitis: A developing country perspective. *Ann Trop Pediatr* 2004;24:133–40.

10. Tunkel AR, Hartman BJ, Kaplan SL, et al. Practice guidelines for the management of bacterial meningitis. *Clin Infect Dis* 2004;39:1267–84.

11. Pelkonen T, Roine I, Cruzeiro ML, et al. Slow initial β-lactam infusion and oral paracetamol to treat childhood bacterial meningitis: A randomised, controlled trial. *Lancet Infect Dis* 2011;11:613–21.

12. Prasad K, Singhal T, Jain N, et al. Third-generation cephalosporins versus conventional antibiotics for treating acute bacterial meningitis. *Cochrane Database Syst Rev* 2004;2:CD001832.

13. Molyneux E, Nizami SQ, Saha S, et al.; CSF 5 Study Group. 5 versus 10 days of treatment with ceftriaxone for bacterial meningitis in children: A double-blind randomised equivalence study. *Lancet* 2011;28(377):1837–45.

14. Van de Beek D, de Gans J, McIntyre P, et al. Corticosteroids for acute bacterial meningitis. *Cochrane Database Syst Rev* 2003;3:CD004405.

15. Sankar J, Singhi P, Bansal A, et al. Role of dexamethasone and oral glycerol in reducing hearing and neurological sequelae in children with bacterial meningitis. *Indian Pediatr* 2007;44:649–56.

16. Brouwer MC, McIntyre P, de Gans J, et al. Corticosteroids for acute bacterial meningitis. *Cochrane Database Syst Rev* 2010;(9):CD004405.

17. Van de Beek D, Farrar JJ, de Gans J, et al. Adjunctive dexamethasone in bacterial meningitis: A meta-analysis of individual patient data. *Lancet Neurol* 2010;9:254–63.

18. Wall EC, Ajdukiewicz KM, Heyderman RS, et al. Osmotic therapies added to antibiotics for acute bacterial meningitis. *Cochrane Database Syst Rev* 2013;3:CD008806. doi:10.1002/14651858. CD008806.

19. Singhi SC, Bansal A. Serum cortisol levels in children with acute bacterial and aseptic meningitis. *Pediatr Crit Care Med* 2006;7:74–8.

20. WHO Report. Global tuberculosis control. http://apps.who.int/iris/bitstream/10665/44728/1/9789241564380_eng.pdf?ua=1, accessed 3rd Nov 2014.

21. Van der Weert EM, Hartgers NM, Schaff HS, et al. Comparison of diagnostic criteria of tuberculous meningitis in human immunodeficiency virus-infected and uninfected children. *Pediatr Infect Dis J* 2006;25:65–9.

22. Cho BH, Kim BC, Yoon GJ, et al. Adenosine deaminase activity in cerebrospinal fluid and serum for the diagnosis of tuberculous meningitis. *Clin Neurol Neurosurg* 2013;115(9):1831–6.

23. Singhi P, Singhi S. Central nervous system tuberculosis. *Curr Treat Options Infect Dis* 2001;3:481–92.

24. Blumberg HM, Burman WJ, Chaisson RE, et al.; American Thoracic Society; Centers for Disease Control and Prevention; Infectious Disease Society of America. Treatment of tuberculosis. *Am J Respir Crit Care Med* 2003;167:603–62.

25. WHO Rapid Advice – Treatment of tuberculosis in children. http://whqlibdoc.who.int/publications/2010/9789241500449_eng.pdf. accessed 3rd Nov 2014.

26. Kumar A, Gupta D, Nagaraja SB, et al. Updated national guidelines for pediatric tuberculosis in India. *Indian Pediatr* 2013;50(3):301–6.

27. Tandon V, Mahapatra AK. Management of post-tubercular hydrocephalus [published online ahead of print September 17, 2011]. *Childs Nerv Syst* 2011;27(10):1699–707. doi:10.1007/s00381-011-1482-1.

28. Kumar R, Prakash M, Jha S. Paradoxical response to chemotherapy in neurotuberculosis. *Pediatr Neurosurg* 2006;42:214–22.

29. Cunha BA. The clinical and laboratory diagnosis of acute meningitis and acute encephalitis [published online ahead of print May 30, 2013]. *Expert Opin Med Diagn* 2013;7(4):343–64. doi:10.1517/17530059.2013.804508.

30. Kneen R, Michael BD, Menson E, et al. National Encephalitis Guidelines Development and Stakeholder Groups. Management of suspected viral encephalitis in children—Association of British Neurologists and British Paediatric Allergy, Immunology and Infection Group national guidelines [published online ahead of print November 18, 2011]. *J Infect* 2012;64(5):449–77. doi:10.1016/j.jinf.2011.11.013.

31. Steiner I, Budka H, Chaudhuri A, et al. Viral meningoencephalitis: A review of diagnostic methods and guidelines for management [published online ahead of print March 03, 2010]. *Eur J Neurol* 2010;17(8):999–e57. doi:10.1111/j.1468-1331.2010.02970.x.

32. De Tiege X, Rozenberg F, Burlort K, et al. Herpes simplex encephalitis: Diagnostic problems and late relapse. *Dev Med Child Neurol* 2006;48:60–3.

33. Kennedy PG, Steiner I. Recent issues in herpes simplex encephalitis. *J Neurovirol* 2013;19(4):346–50.

34. Kamei S, Sekizawa T, Shiota H, et al. Evaluation of combination therapy using acyclovir and corticosteroid in adult patients with herpes simplex virus encephalitis. *J Neurol Neurosurg Psychiatry* 2005;76:1544–9.

35. Martinez-Torres F, Menon S, Pritsch M, et al.; GACHE Investigators. Protocol for German trial of acyclovir and corticosteroids in herpes-simplex-virus-encephalitis (GACHE): A multicenter, multinational, randomized, double-blind, placebo-controlled German,

Austrian and Dutch trial [ISRCTN45122933]. *BMC Neurol* 2008;29(8):40. doi:10.1186/1471-2377-8-40.

36. Kalita J, Misra UK, Pandey S, et al. A comparison of clinical and radiological findings in adults and children with Japanese encephalitis. *Arch Neurol* 2003;60:1760–4.

37. Saxena V, Mishra VK, Dhole TN. Evaluation of reverse-transcriptase PCR as a diagnostic tool to confirm Japanese encephalitis virus infection [published online ahead of print February 26, 2009]. *Trans R Soc Trop Med Hyg* 2009;103(4):403–6. doi:10.1016/j.trstmh.2009.01.021.

38. Krupp LB, Banwell B, Tenembaum S. Consensus definitions proposed for pediatric multiple sclerosis and related disorders. *Neurology* 2007;68(16 suppl 2):S7–12.

39. Leake JA, Albani S, Kao AS, et al. Acute disseminated encephalomyelitis in childhood: Epidemiologic, clinical, and laboratory features. *Pediatr Infect Dis J* 2004;23:756–64.

40. Singhi P, Ray M, Singhi S, et al. Acute disseminated encephalomyelitis in North Indian Children. *J Child Neurol* 2006;21:851–7.

41. Dale RC, Branson JA. Acute disseminated encephalomyelitis or multiple sclerosis: Can the initial presentation help in establishing a correct diagnosis? *Arch Dis Child* 2005;90:636–9.

42. Simon JK, Lazareff JA, Diament MJ, et al. Intramedullary abscess of the spinal cord in children: A case report and review of the literature. *Pediatr Infect Dis J* 2003;22:186–92.

43. Arlotti M, Grossi P, Pea F, et al.; GISIG (Gruppo Italiano di Studio sulle Infezioni Gravi) Working Group on Brain Abscesses. Consensus document on controversial issues for the treatment of infections of the central nervous system: Bacterial brain abscesses. *Int J Infect Dis* 2010;14(suppl 4):S79–92.

44. Nathoo N, Nadvi SS, Narotam PK, et al. Brain abscess: Management and outcome analysis of a computed tomography era experience with 973 patients. *World Neurosurg* 2011;75:716–26.

45. Lee JK, Seok JY, Lee JH, et al. Incidence and risk factors of ventriculoperitoneal shunt infections in children: A study of 333 consecutive shunts in 6 years. *J Korean Med Sci* 2012;27(12):1563–8.

46. Kestle JR, Riva-Cambrin J, Wellons JC 3rd, et al. A standardized protocol to reduce cerebrospinal fluid shunt infection: The Hydrocephalus Clinical Research Network Quality Improvement Initiative. *J Neurosurg Pediatr* 2011;8:22–9.

47. Gumbo T, Kadzirange G, Mielke J, et al. *Cryptococcus neoformans* meningoencephalitis in African children with acquired immunodeficiency syndrome. *Pediatr Infect Dis J* 2002;21:54–6.

48. Perfect JR. Fungal meningitis. In: Scheld WM, Whitley RJ, Marra CM, eds. *Infections of the Central Nervous System.* 3rd ed. Philadelphia, PA: Lippincott Williams and Wilkins, 2004:691–712.

49. Dotis J, Iosifidis E, Roilides E. Central nervous system aspergillosis in children: A systematic review of reported cases. *Int J Infect Dis* 2007;11(5):381–93.

50. Khandelwal N, Gupta V, Singh P. Central nervous system fungal infections in tropics. *Neuroimaging Clin N Am* 2011; 21(4):859–66.

51. Mathur M, Johnson CE, Sze G. Fungal infections of the central nervous system. *Neuroimaging Clin N Am* 2012;22(4):609–32.

52. Chen SC, Slavin MA, Sorrell TC. Echinocandin antifungal drugs in fungal infections: A comparison. *Drugs* 2011;71(1):11–41.

53. Zaoutis TE, Roilides E, Chiou CC, et al. Zygomycosis in children: A systematic review and analysis of reported cases. *Pediatr Infect Dis J* 2007;26(8):723–7.

54. Singhi PD, Ray M, Singhi SC, et al. Clinical spectrum of 500 children with neurocysticercosis and response to albendazole therapy. *J Child Neurol* 2000;15:207–13.

55. Singhi P, Singhi S. Neurocysticercosis in children. *J Child Neurol* 2004;19:482–92.

56. Singhi P, Devi D, Khandelwal N. One week versus four weeks of albendazole therapy for neurocysticercosis in children: A randomized, placebo-controlled, double-blind trial. *Pediatr Infect Dis J* 2003;22:268–72.

57. Kaur S, Singhi P, Singhi S, et al. Combination therapy of praziquantal and albandazole versus albandazole alone in children with single lesion NCC—A randomized placebo controlled double blind trial. *Pediatr Infect Dis J* 2009;28:403–6.

58. Baird RA, Wiebe S, Zunt JR, et al. Evidence-based guideline: Treatment of parenchymal neurocysticercosis: Report of the guideline development subcommittee of the American Academy of Neurology. *Neurology* 2013;80(15):1424–9.

59. Garcia HH, Evans CAW, Nash TE, et al. Current consensus guidelines for treatment of neurocysticercosis. *Clin Microbiol Rev* 2002;15:747–56.

CHAPTER 92 ■ NOSOCOMIAL INFECTIONS IN THE PICU

JASON W. CUSTER, JILL SIEGRIST THOMAS, AND JOHN P. STRAUMANIS

KEY POINTS

1 Adherence to infection-control practices, including hand hygiene, is still one of the most beneficial and unfortunately overlooked methods to prevent nosocomial infections.

2 Isolation precautions are critical to the prevention of transmission of infections within the hospital and need to be put in place at the time of admission based on the likely pathogenic organisms or disease process.

3 Surveillance cultures at the time of admission can decrease nosocomial spread of resistant organisms and should be considered if the infection rate or carrier state in the community is high.

4 Prevention of catheter-related bloodstream infections (CRBSIs) begins at the time of placement with adherence to sterile technique. Care of the catheter site and use of antiseptic- or antibiotic-impregnated catheters can further decrease the risk of infection.

5 Routine removal or rotation of central venous catheters does not reduce the risk of CRBSIs.

6 Prevention of ventilator-associated pneumonia is facilitated by the use of a bundled protocol which includes elevation of the head of the bed and daily readiness-for-extubation assessments.

Since the beginning of medical practice, there have been nosocomial infections—the transmission of infection from medical practitioner or hospital environment to patient. It was not until medical procedures became increasingly invasive and the expectation that infections are curable with antibiotics that the topic of nosocomial infections became an area of interest in the medical field. Well before this, even before Louis Pasteur's germ theory, Ignaz Semmelweis made an important clinical observation and correlation in terms of preventing nosocomial infections in 1847. He realized that his close friend and colleague died of symptoms identical to puerperal fever after his finger was cut during an autopsy on a woman who died of puerperal fever. Semmelweis further noted that a midwife-run obstetric ward had a rate for puerperal fever of only 2%. This was in stark contrast to his ward run by physicians, which had an infection rate of over 12%. The physicians performed autopsies in the morning on women who had died of puerperal fever before examining their patients on the obstetric ward. Semmelweis instituted the practice of making the students wash their hands with a chlorinated lime solution prior to examining their patients. As a result, the infection rate dropped to <2% in the following year. To this day, hand washing remains one of the most important safeguards in preventing nosocomial infection (1).

Nosocomial infections are important to consider, treat, and, most importantly, prevent in any hospital setting, especially in the ICU. Hospital-acquired infections can lead to significant morbidity and mortality. Infection-control measures can greatly impact this effect. It is equally important to prevent the infection of hospital personnel to diminish the risk of spreading infection to other patients and prevent missed days of work, which could impact the ability to staff the PICU. There are additional financial costs associated with nosocomial infections, including hospital costs, loss of productivity of healthcare personnel, and loss of income to families from missing time at work. State, Federal, and private payers have recently instituted financial penalties on hospitals when potentially preventable complications such as nosocomial infections occur during the hospital admission.

DEFINITIONS

1 In discussing nosocomial infections, it is important to have an understanding of several definitions. A *nosocomial infection* is any infection a patient acquires within the hospital setting, which is not present at admission. Even if symptoms develop after discharge, such infections should be considered nosocomial. *Community-acquired infections* are those present at the time of admission even if they do not necessarily cause symptoms at the time of admission. The differentiation between community-acquired and nosocomial infections may take some investigation and is dependent on incubation times as well as ancillary testing such as sensitivities and genetic typing of the organism. *Surgical site infections* are associated with the surgical procedure itself, including the wound and the direct surgical field exposed during the procedure. Other infections at distant sites, even though the surgical procedure or anesthesia for the procedure put the patient at risk for such an infection, are considered nosocomial but not surgical site infections. *Colonization* is the growth or presence of potentially infectious organisms in a cavity, on a surface, in tissue, in body fluids, or even associated with a medical device without causing a host reaction, a clinically adverse event, or disease.

There is a wide variation in how nosocomial infection rates are reported. It may be noted as a percentage of patients, number of infections per 100 patients, or number of infections per 1000 device days. The latter method is used by the Centers for Disease Control and Prevention's (CDC) National Health & Safety Network (NHSN). The NHSN system does report surgical site infections in terms of number of infections per 100 procedures. The surgical site infections are further classified as superficial, incisional and deep, or involving the organ space involved in the operation. Where possible, this chapter will report rates using these standards.

OVERVIEW AND EPIDEMIOLOGY

The CDC estimates that in the United States there are 2 million nosocomial infections annually leading to increased mortality with a conservative estimate of an additional $5.7–$6.8 billion (US dollars) in healthcare costs as a result (2). Although it may not be possible to eliminate all nosocomial infections, one-third or more could be prevented with implementation of organized infection-control programs. Given the incidence, mortality, morbidity, and cost of nosocomial infections, those which could be prevented but were not may be considered a source of medical error. Despite even the best infection-control program, there will always be the risk of nosocomial infection in the ICU due to the unique nature of the critically ill or injured patient. However, many adult and pediatric ICUs across the country have achieved zero nosocomial infections for prolonged periods of time.

The risk of nosocomial infection depends on a variety of factors. The location within the hospital plays an important role with the highest rates typically occurring in the ICU. Even the type of ICU influences the nosocomial infection rate with different rates seen in medical, surgical, trauma, burn, neurological/neurosurgical, and cardiac ICUs. The PICU is unique in that it typically cares for many or all of these subsets of patients over the pediatric age range. Another unique factor in the PICU is that different aged patients will have different incidence patterns of the various types of hospital-acquired infections. For children <5 years of age, the top three nosocomial infections are bloodstream infections (BSIs), pneumonia, and urinary tract infections (UTIs). In children between 5 and 12 years of age, the top three acquired infections are pneumonia, BSIs, and UTIs. In the adolescent population, BSIs

are followed by UTIs and then pneumonia in incidence. The location of the hospital plays a role as well with an increased risk of nosocomial infection being noted in developing nations. All types of nosocomial infections when standardized to device days were increased in the ICUs of developing nations in a study by Rosenthal et al. The device utilization rates were noted to be similar in the developed and developing nation ICUs, making the increased infection rate more likely to be secondary to factors within the ICUs, hospitals, or national healthcare systems (3,4) (**Table 92.1**).

General Risk Factors

In addition to the location within the hospital and the type of ICU, there are general risk factors that are independent of the type of nosocomial infection. Although these risk factors can influence the likelihood of contracting a nosocomial infection, only a few can be realistically altered to impact nosocomial infection rates.

The age of the patient can affect the risk of nosocomial infection. Younger children, particularly neonates, have the highest risk in the pediatric population. The relative immaturity of the immune system at this point of life coupled with common ICU interventions, which bypass the physical barriers to infections such as skin and mucosal surfaces, is responsible for the increased risk. The use of parenteral nutrition with high glucose concentrations and lipids is an additional risk factor for infection. Premature infants are impacted the most by these factors, which explain why neonatal ICUs (NICUs) have higher nosocomial infection rates than PICUs. Patients who are immunosuppressed from chemotherapy, human immunodeficiency virus infection, or steroid use are similarly at an increased risk for developing a nosocomial infection.

Severity of illness as predicted by the Pediatric Risk of Mortality (PRISM) score has been correlated to risk of nosocomial infections. In a study by Arantes et al., a PRISM score above

TABLE 92.1

COMPARISON OF DEVICE USE AND RATES OF DEVICE-ASSOCIATED INFECTION IN THE ICUS OF THE US NATIONAL NOSOCOMIAL INFECTION SURVEILLANCE SYSTEM AND THE INTERNATIONAL NOSOCOMIAL INFECTION CONTROL CONSORTIUM (INICC)

■ VARIABLE	■ US NNIS ICUs 1992–2004	■ INICC ICUs 2002–2005
Rate of device use[a]		
Mechanical ventilators	0.43 (0.23–0.62)	0.38 (0.19–0.64)
CVCs	0.57 (0.36–0.74)	0.54 (0.22–0.97)
Urinary catheters	0.78 (0.65–0.90)	0.73 (0.48–0.94)
Rate per 1000 device days[a]		
VAP	5.4 (1.2–7.2)	24.1 (10.0–52.7)
CVC-associated bloodstream infection	4.0 (1.7–7.6)	12.5 (7.8–18.5)
Catheter-associated UTI	3.9 (1.3–7.5)	8.9 (1.7–12.8)
Proportion of device-associated infections with resistance, %[b]		
MRSA	59	84
Ceftriaxone-resistant *Enterobacteriaceae*	19	55
Ciprofloxacin-resistant *P. aeruginosa*	29	59
VRE	29	5

[a]Overall (pooled) and 10th to 90th percentile range for US NNIS teaching hospitals; overall (pooled) and range of individual countries for the INICC hospitals.
[b]Overall (pooled) data from NNIS, 1992–2004 (300 hospitals) and from INICC, 2002–2005.
NNIS, National Nosocomial Infection Surveillance System; INICC, International Nosocomial Infection Control Consortium; UTI, urinary tract infection.
From Rosenthal VD, Maki DG, Salomao R, et al. Device-associated nosocomial infections in 55 intensive care units of 8 developing countries. *Ann Intern Med* 2006;145(8):582–91, with permission.
Data from National Nosocomial Infections Surveillance (NNIS) System Report, data summary from January 1992 through June 2004, issued October 2004. *Am J Infect Control* 2004;32:470–85.

13 predicted nosocomial infection in a Brazilian PICU with 78.9% sensitivity, 64.4% specificity, 21.8% positive predictive value, and 96.1% negative predictive value. Independent risk factors of developing a nosocomial infection were length of stay, prior antimicrobial therapy, and device utilization ratios, with the latter two being the best predictors of nosocomial infection risk (5).

Understaffing is an independent risk factor for acquiring nosocomial infections. This is most likely owing to the fact that adherence to good hand hygiene has been shown to be inversely correlated to workload. This has been noted for BSIs and ventilator-associated pneumonia (VAP). Understaffing increases workload and therefore nosocomial infection risk. In a study of US NICUs, understaffing by 0.11 of a nurse per infant increased the risk of infection from 9% to 14%. Understaffing by 0.22 nurses per infant increased the risk to 21% (**Fig. 92.1**). Simply increasing staffing with temporary staff does not reverse this trend. This is likely due to disruption of the normal communication within the interdisciplinary team and familiarity with best practices (6–8).

Red blood cell transfusions have been found to be an independent risk factor for the development of nosocomial infections in critically ill adult ICU patients. In a single-center prospective, observational study, the incidence of nosocomial infection was 14.3% in transfused patients and 5.8% in nontransfused patients. Each unit of packed red blood cells administered increased the risk of developing a nosocomial infection by 9.7%. Increasing severity of illness did not affect the risk of developing a nosocomial infection. However, within each quartile of probability of survival, the transfused group had a higher rate of nosocomial infection, which was significant in all but the most severely ill patients with a probability of survival <25%. Those patients with >25% probability of survival had higher mortality rates, longer ICU stays, and longer hospitalizations compared to nontransfused patients. A pediatric study also found the increased risk of nosocomial infection associated with transfusion. However, a dose response was not seen with increasing number of units transfused, but mortality was greater in those receiving three or more units (9,10) (**Fig. 92.2**).

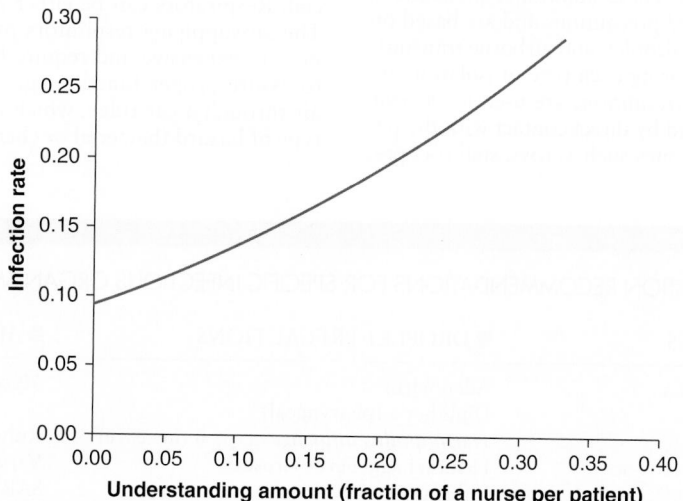

FIGURE 92.1. Predicted risk-adjusted infection by nursing unit understaffing amount. (Modified from Rogowski JA, Staiger D, Patrick T, et al. Nurse staffing and NICU infection rates. *JAMA Pediatr* 2013;167(5):444–50.)

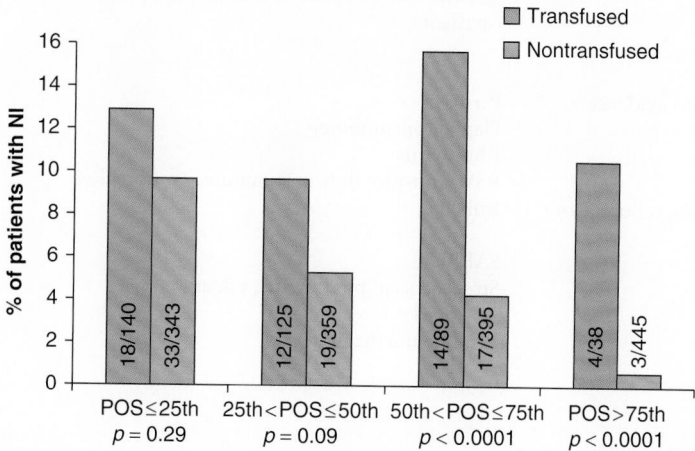

FIGURE 92.2. Nosocomial infection (NI) rates adjusted for probability of survival (POS). The overall rate of NI in transfused patients was significantly higher than in nontransfused patients ($p < 0.0001$; Cochran–Mantel–Haenszel test). Numbers within the bars indicate the number of patients with NI/total in each group. The *p* values beneath each bar refer to the significance level of the within-group comparisons (Student's *t*-tests). (From Taylor RW, O'Brien J, Trottier SJ, et al. Red blood cell transfusions and nosocomial infections in critically ill patients. *Crit Care Med* 2006;34(9):2302–8, with permission.)

Isolation Precautions

Prevention of nosocomial illness can be, in large part, facilitated through the use of isolation precautions. These precautions can be divided into two categories: standard and transmission-based precautions. *Standard precautions* should be used at all times and are designed to prevent the practitioner from coming in contact with potentially infectious bodily fluids. The most important standard precaution is hand hygiene. Soap and water hand washing is considered the gold standard. Use of waterless antiseptic agents is appropriate unless there is the presence of visible dirt, proteinaceous bodily fluids such as blood, or when contamination with spores is likely. Soap and water are necessary under these circumstances. Hand hygiene must be done both before and after patient contact even if gloves are worn. Barriers such as gloves, masks, eye protection, and nonsterile gowns should be worn when contact with bodily fluids or secretions are likely.

Transmission-based precautions are aimed at protection against transmission of infectious organisms from patients with documented or suspected infection as well as those colonized with specific organisms. These additional precautions are over and above the standard precautions and are based on route of transmission: contact, droplet, and airborne transmission. Common organisms requiring each type of isolation are listed in **Table 92.2**. *Contact precautions* are used for a wide variety of organisms that spread by direct contact with the patient or indirect contact via fomites such as toys, stethoscopes, and unwashed hands. Contact isolation should include single-patient rooms or cohorting, gowns, and gloves in addition to standard precautions. *Droplet precautions* are used for organisms that spread short distances, <3 feet away, from the patient via coughing or sneezing. Droplet isolation includes single-patient rooms or cohorting of patients with the same organism. Healthcare providers should wear a mask with an eye shield in addition to following standard precautions. Some organisms such as adenovirus and influenza require both contact and droplet precautions. *Airborne precautions* include additional safeguards to be taken for organisms transmitted by air currents such as tuberculosis, measles, and varicella. Patients should be in private rooms with negative air flow. For measles and varicella isolation, susceptible healthcare providers should avoid contact if possible. For other organisms requiring airborne precautions, a fitted respirator should be worn while in the patient's room. Isolation should be based on the clinical symptoms or conditions present at admission and should always begin even before the organism is isolated (11) (**Table 92.3**).

For protection against airborne infections, the selection of the correct type of respirator and having a proper fit are crucial. Respirators can be either air-supplying or air-purifying. The air-supplying respirators provide the greatest protection but are expensive and require high amounts of maintenance to assure proper functioning. Air-purifying respirators filter air through a cartridge, which must be selected based on the type of hazard (bacterial or chemical) to be exposed to. These

---

TABLE 92.2

TRANSMISSION-BASED ISOLATION RECOMMENDATIONS FOR SPECIFIC INFECTIOUS ORGANISMS AND ILLNESSES

■ CONTACT PRECAUTIONS	■ DROPLET PRECAUTIONS	■ AIRBORNE PRECAUTIONS
Colonization or infection with a multidrug-resistant bacteria	Adenovirus	*Mycobacterium tuberculosis*
Clostridium difficile	Diphtheria (pharyngeal)	
Conjunctivitis, viral and hemorrhagic	*Haemophilus influenzae* type B (invasive)	Rubeola virus (measles)
Diphtheria (cutaneous)	Hemorrhagic Fever viruses	Varicella-Zoster virus
Enteroviruses	Influenza	SARS
Escherichia coli O157:H7 and other Shiga toxin-producing *E. coli*	Mumps	Viral hemorrhagic fevers
Hepatitis A virus	*Mycoplasma pneumoniae*	
	N. meningitidis (invasive)	
	Parvovirus B19 during the phase of illness before onset of rash in immunocompetent patients	
Herpes simplex (neonatal, mucocutaneous or cutaneous)		
Herpes zoster (localized with no evidence of dissemination)	Pertussis	
Human meta-pneumovirus	Plague (pneumonic)	
Impetigo	Rhinovirus	
Major (noncontained) abscesses, cellulitis, or decubitus ulcer	RSV (consider during community outbreaks)	
Parainfluenza virus	Rubella	
Pediculosis (lice)		
RSV	SARS	
Rotavirus	Streptococcal pharyngitis, pneumonia, or scarlet fever	
Salmonella species	Viral hemorrhagic fevers	
Scabies		
Shigella species		
S. aureus (cutaneous or draining wounds)		
Viral hemorrhagic fevers (Ebola, Lassa, or Marburg)		

Some organisms may include more than one type of isolation. This list is not all inclusive. Data from American Academy of Pediatrics. Infection Control for Hospitalized Children. *Red Book: 2012 Report of the Committee on Infectious Diseases*. Pickering LK, ed. 29th ed. Elk Grove Village, IL: American Academy of Pediatrics, 2012.

TABLE 92.3

CLINICAL SYNDROMES OR CONDITIONS WARRANTING PRECAUTIONS IN ADDITION TO STANDARD PRECAUTIONS TO PREVENT TRANSMISSION OF EPIDEMIOLOGICALLY IMPORTANT PATHOGENS PENDING CONFIRMATION OF DIAGNOSIS[a]

■ CLINICAL SYNDROME OR CONDITION[b]	■ POTENTIAL PATHOGENS[c]	■ EMPIRIC PRECAUTIONS[d]
Diarrhea		
Acute diarrhea with a likely infectious cause	Enteric pathogens[e]	Contact
Diarrhea in patient with a history of recent antimicrobial use	*Clostridium difficile*	Contact; use soap and water for handwashing
Meningitis	*N. meningitidis*	Droplet
	Enteroviruses	Contact
Rash or exanthems, generalized, cause unknown		
Petechial or ecchymotic with fever	*N. meningitidis*	Droplet
	Hemorrhagic fever viruses	Add contact plus face/eye protection
Vesicular	Varicella-zoster virus	Airborne and contact
Maculopapular with coryza and fever	Measles virus	Airborne
Respiratory tract infections		
Pulmonary cavitary disease	*Mycobacterium tuberculosis*	Airborne
Paroxysmal or severe persistent cough during periods of pertussis activity in the community	*Bordetella pertussis*	Droplet
Viral infections, particularly bronchiolitis and croup, in infants and young children	Respiratory viral pathogens	Contact and droplet until adenovirus, rhinovirus, and influenza virus excluded
Risk of multidrug-resistant microorganisms[f]		
History of infection or colonization with multidrug-resistant organisms	Resistant bacteria	Contact
Skin, wound, or UTI in a patient with a recent stay in a hospital or chronic care facility	Resistant bacteria	Contact until resistant organism is excluded by cultures
Skin or wound infection		
Abscess or draining wound that cannot be covered	*S. aureus*, group A	Contact

[a]Infection-control professionals are encouraged to modify or adapt this table according to local conditions. To ensure that appropriate empiric precautions are implemented, hospitals must have systems in place to evaluate patients routinely according to these criteria as part of their preadmission and admission care.

[b]Patients with the syndromes or conditions listed may have atypical signs or symptoms (eg, pertussis in neonates may present with apnea, paroxysmal or severe cough may be absent in pertussis in adults). The clinician's index of suspicion should be guided by the prevalence of specific conditions in the community and clinical judgment.

[c]The organisms listed in this column are not intended to represent the complete or even most likely diagnoses but, rather, possible causative agents that require additional precautions beyond **StandardPrecautions** until a causative agent can be excluded.

[d]Duration of isolation varies by agent and the antimicrobial treatment administered.

[e]These pathogens include Shiga toxin-producing *Escherichia coli* including *E coli* O157:H7, *Shigella*organisms, *Salmonella* organisms, *Campylobacter* organisms, hepatitis A virus, enteric viruses including rotavirus, *Cryptosporidium* organisms, and *Giardia* organisms. Use masks when cleaning vomitus or stool during norovirus outbreak.

[f]Resistant bacteria judged by the infection control program on the basis of current state, regional, or national recommendations to be of special clinical or epidemiologic significance.

respirators are protective but not to the same degree as the air-supplying devices. Disposable respirators are air-purifying or filtering devices. The N95 respirators are the most commonly used ones in healthcare settings. The letter designates the mask's reaction to oil. N means not oil proof. If exposed to oil, the filtering efficiency of the mask may not be maintained. There are also oil-resistant masks and oil-proof masks, designated R and P, respectively. The number indicates the filtering efficiency of the mask with an adequate seal. The number 95 identifies the mask as having the ability to filter at least 95% of particles with a median diameter of 0.3 μm or greater. Most respirators have limitations when used by individuals with facial hair, and specialized devices may be necessary (12).

The personal protective equipment which should be worn is determined by the organism being isolated. To assure the maximal effect of the protective equipment, it must be donned and removed in the proper order. After performing hand hygiene, the gown should be donned first, followed by the mask or respirator assuring proper fit. The goggles or face shield is placed on after the mask and then finally the gloves. When removing the protective items, the following sequence should be followed to prevent self-inoculation or exposure to infectious particles. First remove the gloves. Pull them off away from the body, and consider the outer surface of the glove as being contaminated. With one gloved hand, remove the other glove by pulling on the outer surface. Keep the removed glove in the gloved hand, and then place the ungloved fingers under the cuff of the remaining glove pulling it off inside out with the first glove inside the second. Discard of the gloves properly. Remove the goggles or face shield by touching only the sides or headband since the outer, forward facing surface is potentially contaminated; discard or store for cleaning appropriately. Remove the gown by pulling down and away from the body touching only the inside of the gown because the front and sleeves are contaminated. Roll into a bundle with the inner surface of the gown on the outside of the bundle and discard. Finally remove the mask without touching the front surface by pulling on the straps or ties from behind, discard. Perform hand hygiene (13).

Hand Hygiene Compliance

Despite 150 years passing since Semmelweis nearly eradicated the transmission of nosocomial infections on his obstetric ward, present-day practitioners wash their hands less than half of the time. The best practice is to wash with soap and water before and after patient contact. Even with the use of alcohol-based hand sanitizers placed near patient care areas, the compliance rate remains low. Observational studies put the usage rate of any hand hygiene at 14%–48%. Pittet et al. noted an improvement from 48% to 66% in hand hygiene compliance with the initiation of an educational program. Over the course of the program, the nosocomial infection rates decreased from 16.9% to 9.9%. There are differences in the compliance rate among various practitioners. Interestingly, those with less medical training have better compliance rates. Healthcare assistants were 64% compliant followed by nurses and nursing students (49%); ancillary personnel including dieticians, therapists, and phlebotomists (46%); and with physicians and medical students performing the worst with only a 26% hand hygiene compliance rate. Factors that can impact hand hygiene include workload, staffing shortages, and the availability of sinks. The use of alcohol-based solutions can improve the latter in that it does not depend on the presence of sinks or running water. Additional factors that may help improve compliance are that the alcohol-based preparations tend to cause less irritation and drying of the hands as well as saving practitioner time compared with soap and water. Studies have proven that the alcohol-based solutions are effective against infection, including viruses, as long as hands are not visibly soiled. For visible soilage or when *Clostridium* spores are potentially present, soap and water must be used (6,14–17).

The presence of an active infection-control program and surveillance program can lower nosocomial infection rates by as much as one-third compared with hospitals without such programs. Surveillance programs enable hospitals to monitor trends and allow for interventions when indicated (18).

Surveillance Cultures

3 The increasing incidence of resistant organisms colonizing and infecting people in the community impacts the risk of developing a nosocomial infection in the hospital. As the incidence rises in the community, there is an increased risk of falsely identifying a community-acquired infection as nosocomial and of transmitting these community infections to other patients, thus causing a true nosocomial infection. In areas where there is a high level of resistant organisms in the community, it may be worth screening for these infections at admission. This approach has most notably been used with screening for methicillin-resistant *Staphylococcus aureus* (MRSA). The first step in screening is to identify those patients at high risk for MRSA both to prevent false positives when evaluating for nosocomial infection and to control cost. Patients considered having an increased risk of MRSA colonization or infection include (a) patients with a prior MRSA infection or identified colonization; (b) patients who have been frequently hospitalized, particularly if there has been an admission in the prior 6 months; (c) interhospital transfers from high-incidence regions; (d) residents of chronic care facilities; and (e) patients with chronic skin lesions. All patients with a high risk of carriage of MRSA should be screened at admission and/or admitted to isolation. The admission screening is most commonly performed by culturing the anterior nares, but other sites such as wounds or skin lesions, catheter sites, tracheostomies, and the umbilicus in neonates can be used.

Following admission screening, surveillance screening is done to identify new, hospital-acquired infections. The frequency of such screening varies from weekly to monthly depending on the local prevalence of MRSA. Discussions with infection-control personnel can aid in determining the frequency of screening needed as well as which areas or patients in the hospital warrant such monitoring. Screening in the ICU is beneficial due to the high incidence of patients at risk for MRSA colonization; the high frequency of use of invasive devices, which can increase the risk of nosocomial transmission; and the ability to prevent spread to a population who can ill afford an additional infection. The use of routine screening in other areas of the hospital should be determined based on the recommendations of the local infection-control officer. The routine screening of medical staff is not currently recommended. It may be considered in difficult-to-control outbreaks. Once a patient is identified as being colonized with MRSA, they should be isolated, informed of their colonization status, and considered for treatment to clear the colonization (19). This approach has been used for MRSA colonization and infections but could be used for a variety of organisms if the frequency in the community or hospital warrants such an approach and when adequately specific and sensitive screening tests are available.

Once screening or other surveillance measures have been used to identify patients with organisms that are likely to be spread by nosocomial transmission, cohorting of patients with the same organism and the staff caring for them may be beneficial. The theory is that after contact with one infected patient, the next contact of the healthcare worker would be a patient with the same organism and thus diminish the spread of the infection to a naïve patient. Standard precautions still need to be used to prevent infection or colonization of the healthcare workers and minimize the risk of spreading infection. This approach has proven successful for MRSA and vancomycin-resistant enterococci (VRE) in a variety of settings. The Dutch have used such a strategy for 20 years in patients known to have MRSA to decrease the prevalence of MRSA infections to <2% despite a high prevalence in the surrounding countries. Similar techniques have been used for MRSA in Finnish nursing homes and statewide surveillance in Rhode Island as well as for VRE using a regional approach in the United States (6).

CATHETER-RELATED BLOODSTREAM INFECTIONS

Intravascular catheters are essential in the critical care setting to provide stable and secure access for caloric dense nutrition, medications, fluids, and blood products. They also have many diagnostic uses that include a means to monitor laboratory values, to assess treatments and to measure vital pressures, as well as aid in goal-directed therapies. Although these lines offer great benefit in the critically ill patients, they are not without risk and can act as a conduit for infection if not inserted and cared for properly. It is estimated that 15 million central venous catheter (CVC) days occur in ICUs each year (20). Approximately 80,000 catheter-related infections occur in ICU patients and have been shown in multiple analyses to dramatically increase morbidity and healthcare costs (21). Various adult and pediatric studies from individual units have placed the additional cost to the hospital admission of a nosocomial BSI to be in the range of $34,000–$56,000 (US dollars) (18,22). Catheter-related bloodstream infection (CRBSI) has come to the forefront as a preventable complication with the goal of eliminating this complication from the healthcare landscape.

DEFINITIONS

Terminology for catheter-related infections can be confusing. Published guidelines from the CDC have set criteria for diagnosing BSIs involving intravascular catheters (21). A catheter-**related** bloodstream infection (CRBSI) is a clinical definition that requires more extensive testing to pinpoint the central line as the source of the infection. CRBSI is either a bacteremia or a fungemia documented with at least one peripherally obtained blood culture obtained from a vein and not a catheter. Clinical evidence of an infection, including a host response, must be present that cannot be attributed to any source other than the catheter. The growth of an organism in the bloodstream must be documented by (a) a positive semiquantitative or quantitative culture of a catheter segment with an organism identical in species and antibiogram as isolated from a peripheral blood culture; (b) simultaneously drawn peripheral and line quantitative blood cultures with greater than a 5:1 ratio in catheter blood versus peripheral blood colony counts; or (c) a differential in timing of culture positivity of >2 hours between the catheter and peripheral blood culture where the catheter culture is positive first. CRBSI may be difficult to establish and is often not used for surveillance (23). A catheter-**associated** bloodstream infection (CABSI) has less rigorous criteria and requires the presence of central line being in place during the 48 hours prior to the drawing of the positive culture and compelling evidence that the infection is related to the line. This definition is helpful for surveillance but can overestimate the true incidence of bloodstream infections (21).

EPIDEMIOLOGY

Coagulase-negative staphylococci are the most common cause of pediatric nosocomial BSIs, accounting for 20% to nearly 50% of isolates. Gram-negative bacteria account for 25% of PICU nosocomial BSIs. S. aureus and Candida species are responsible for $10% each throughout the pediatric age range. Other organisms causing nosocomial BSIs are dependent upon the age of the child and other clinical factors. Beta-hemolytic streptococci are more prevalent in the neonatal population, causing 8.5% of the hospital-acquired infections in this age group. There is a bimodal peak for enterococcal infections seen in infants and patients 13–65 years of age, with 9.4% and 8.5% of isolates, respectively. Klebsiella species are the third most common isolates at 7.3% behind coagulase-negative staphylococci and S. aureus in the pediatric oncology population (21,24–26).

Diagnosis and Treatment of Catheter-Related Infections

Definitive diagnosis of a catheter-related infection can be difficult, which certainly complicates management decisions as far as catheter removal. Most symptoms such as fever, chills, and rigors have poor specificity and as a result CVCs should not be removed for fever alone. Site inflammation with or without purulence and positive bloodstream cultures have better specificity but low sensitivity. As a result, surveillance cultures are not recommended, and cultures should only be obtained when a CRBSI is suspected. Use of clinical judgment is important, and if the patient has fever with only mild to moderate symptoms, the catheter should not be routinely removed. Cultures positive for common nosocomial BSIs such as coagulase-negative staphylococci, S. aureus, and Candida species without an identified source of infection and in the presence of a CVC should raise suspicion for the possibility of a CRBSI (20).

Two blood cultures should be obtained when a catheter-related infection is suspected and at least one of them, if not both, should be drawn percutaneously. When paired central and peripheral cultures are sent, it is recommended that they either be quantitative cultures or be qualitative cultures with continuously monitored differential time to positivity to aid in the diagnosis of a CRBSI. A differential time to positivity at least 2 hours earlier for the central-line culture compared with the peripheral culture is indicative of a central venous line infection, with a sensitivity of 91% and a specificity of 94%. This method is simpler for most hospital laboratories and is at least as accurate as quantitative cultures. Once the decision has been made to remove the line, the catheter tip should be sent for quantitative or semiquantitative cultures; qualitative broth cultures are not recommended (**Fig. 92.3**). The skin should be prepped prior to removal, then the catheter removed with sterile forceps, the distal portion cut, and sent for culture. For pulmonary artery catheters (PACs), the most likely positive portion of the apparatus is the tip of the sheath introducer rather than the PAC tip. Exchanging the catheter over a guidewire avoids the risks associated with needle puncture at a new site; however, it does not lower the risk of infection. For those patients with suspected line infections and mild to moderate symptoms (in addition to fever), a change over a guidewire may be an alternative while awaiting blood and catheter tip cultures. The previously exchanged line should be removed and replaced at a different site if a CRBSI is verified and:

- Clinical symptoms are not improving with antibiotics.
- A virulent pathogen (e.g., fungus, Pseudomonas aeruginosa, S. aureus) has been identified.
- The identified organism is difficult to eradicate (e.g., Propionibacteria).

Nontunneled catheters may be replaced once appropriate antibiotic therapy has been instituted. The catheter may not need to be removed in patients without evidence of persistent BSI or if there is a culture positive, coagulase-negative staphylococcal infection in the absence of local or metastatic infectious complications. For both conditions, appropriate antibiotic therapy is indicated (**Fig. 92.4**). Persistent bacteremia or lack of clinical improvement after removal of the colonized catheter with the patient on antimicrobial therapy should prompt a thorough evaluation for infective endocarditis, septic thrombosis, and other distant sites of infectious seeding, especially if symptoms are present more than 3 days after catheter removal (20,22,27,28).

In children, placing a new line may be difficult compared with adults, and some authors have reported successful treatment of central-line infections without removal of the device. Such management should include close observation of the clinical condition with prompt removal if clinical deterioration occurs. Initial therapy should be broad spectrum and based on the likely organisms causing the infection based on typical isolates for the hospital as well as predominant sensitivity patterns. Typical empiric coverage should include Gram-positive and Gram-negative coverage. It is important to cover for methicillin-resistant staphylococci with its increasing presence in both the hospital and the community. Initial therapy is usually vancomycin along with a third-generation cephalosporin or aminoglycoside, though extended-spectrum Gram-negative coverage (e.g., drugs with anti-pseudomonal activity) may be appropriate depending on the clinical situation. For severe infections in patients who are immunosuppressed or if yeast species are isolated or highly suspected, the addition of antifungal coverage is appropriate. Once an isolate's sensitivities are known, the antibiotic regimen should be appropriately adjusted to prevent the selection of resistant organisms. Success rates in treating infections with

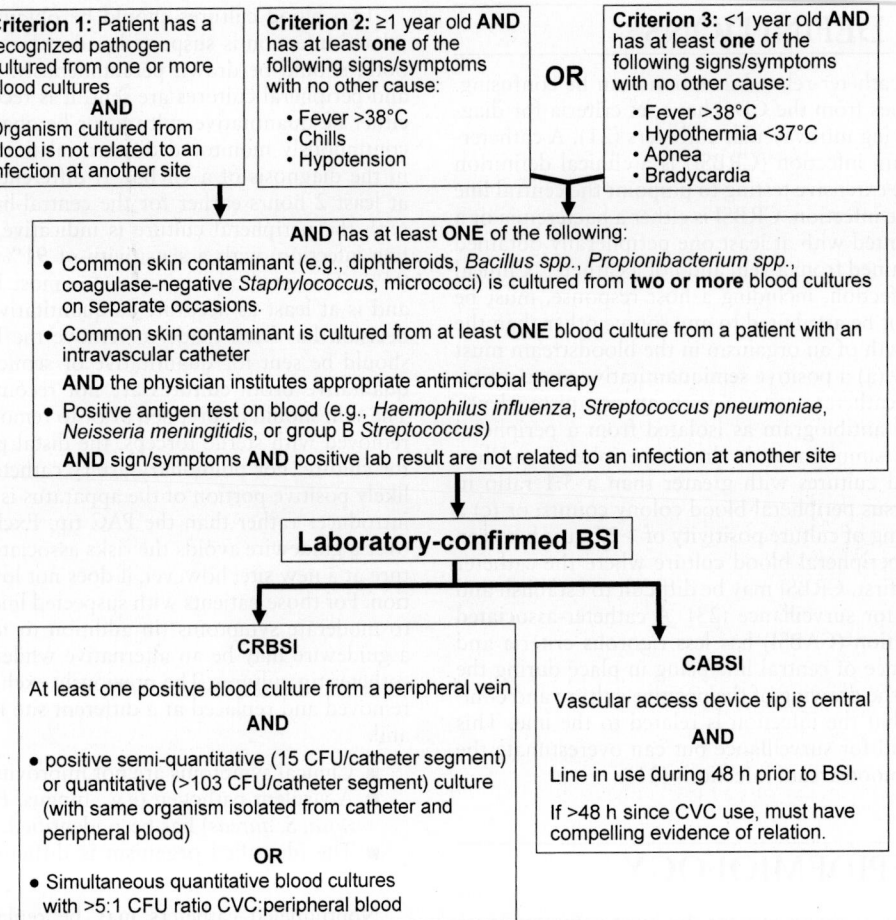

Criterion 1: Patient has a recognized pathogen cultured from one or more blood cultures **AND** Organism cultured from blood is not related to an infection at another site

Criterion 2: ≥1 year old **AND** has at least **one** of the following signs/symptoms with no other cause:
• Fever >38°C
• Chills
• Hypotension

OR

Criterion 3: <1 year old **AND** has at least **one** of the following signs/symptoms with no other cause:
• Fever >38°C
• Hypothermia <37°C
• Apnea
• Bradycardia

AND has at least ONE of the following:
• Common skin contaminant (e.g., diphtheroids, *Bacillus spp.*, *Propionibacterium spp.*, coagulase-negative *Staphylococcus*, micrococci) is cultured from **two or more** blood cultures on separate occasions.
• Common skin contaminant is cultured from at least **ONE** blood culture from a patient with an intravascular catheter
  AND the physician institutes appropriate antimicrobial therapy
• Positive antigen test on blood (e.g., *Haemophilus influenza, Streptococcus pneumoniae, Neisseria meningitidis,* or group B *Streptococcus*)
  AND sign/symptoms **AND** positive lab result are not related to an infection at another site

Laboratory-confirmed BSI

CRBSI
At least one positive blood culture from a peripheral vein
AND
• positive semi-quantitative (15 CFU/catheter segment) or quantitative (>103 CFU/catheter segment) culture (with same organism isolated from catheter and peripheral blood)
OR
• Simultaneous quantitative blood cultures with >5:1 CFU ratio CVC:peripheral blood

CABSI
Vascular access device tip is central
AND
Line in use during 48 h prior to BSI.
If >48 h since CVC use, must have compelling evidence of relation.

FIGURE 92.3. BSI diagnostic flow diagram. A CRBSI can also be confirmed with at least one positive blood culture from a peripheral vein and a differential time to positivity at least 2 hours earlier for a central-line culture. CFU, colony-forming units. (From Stockwell JA. Nosocomial infections in the pediatric intensive care unit: Affecting the impact on safety and outcome. *Pediatr Crit Care Med* 2007;8(suppl 2):S21–37, with permission.)

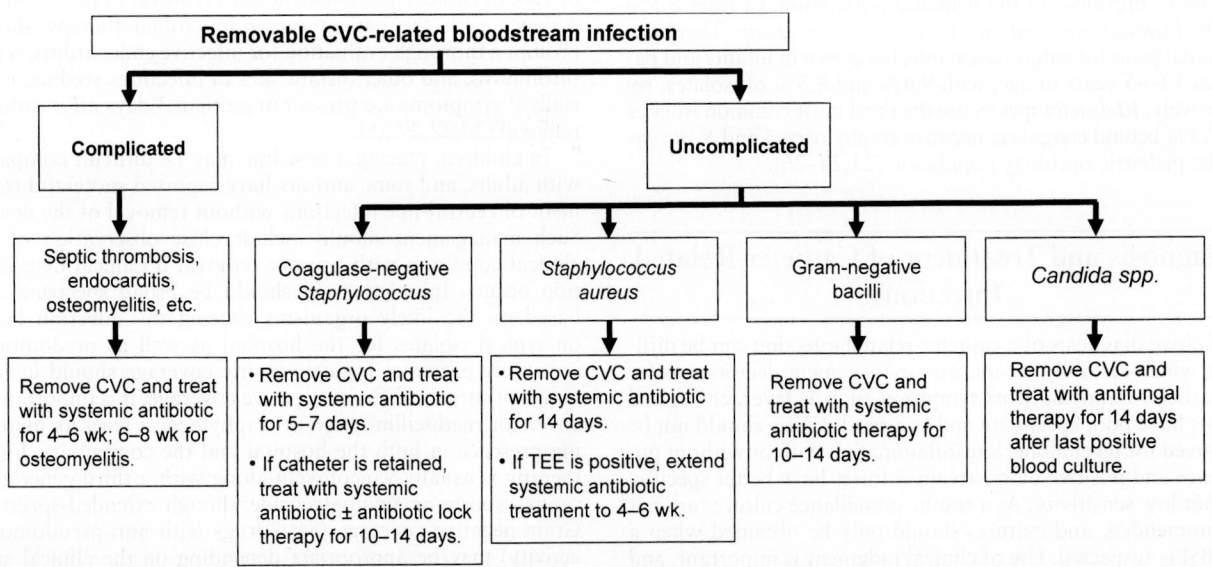

Removable CVC-related bloodstream infection

Complicated

Uncomplicated

Septic thrombosis, endocarditis, osteomyelitis, etc.

Coagulase-negative *Staphylococcus*

Staphylococcus aureus

Gram-negative bacilli

Candida spp.

Remove CVC and treat with systemic antibiotic for 4–6 wk; 6–8 wk for osteomyelitis.

• Remove CVC and treat with systemic antibiotic for 5–7 days.
• If catheter is retained, treat with systemic antibiotic ± antibiotic lock therapy for 10–14 days.

• Remove CVC and treat with systemic antibiotic for 14 days.
• If TEE is positive, extend systemic antibiotic treatment to 4–6 wk.

Remove CVC and treat with systemic antibiotic therapy for 10–14 days.

Remove CVC and treat with antifungal therapy for 14 days after last positive blood culture.

FIGURE 92.4. Approach to the management of patients with nontunneled CVC-related bloodstream infection. Duration of treatment will depend on whether the infection is complicated or uncomplicated. The catheter should be removed, and systemic antimicrobial therapy should be initiated, except in some cases of uncomplicated catheter-related infection due to coagulase-negative staphylococci. For infections due to *S. aureus*, transesophageal echocardiography (TEE) may reveal the presence of endocarditis and help to determine the duration of treatment. (From Mermel LA, Farr BM, Sherertz RJ, et al. Guidelines for the management of intravascular catheter-related infections. *Clin Infect Dis* 2001;32(9):1249–72, with permission.)

the offending line in place are successful in up to 90% of coagulase-negative infections using a minimum of 10–14 days of treatment. Infections caused by fungi or Gram-negative organisms are extremely resistant to treatment if the catheter is left in place, so all central lines should be removed under these circumstances and treatment should be a minimum of 14 days. Removal of the catheter in coagulase-negative staphylococci infections requires only a 5–7-day course of therapy. Regardless of the culture results, if the child does not respond or worsens within the first 3 days of antibiotic therapy, the line should be removed (20,27).

Prevention of Catheter-Related Infections

The cause of central venous line infection can be from many sources, which depend on the conditions under which the line was placed, emergently versus in a controlled situation, experience of the operator, site selection, ongoing line care, and other extrinsic factors. The most common route of infection for percutaneous lines in the ICU is migration of skin organisms down the external surface of the catheter to the bloodstream. This can be greatly influenced by catheter care as well as the patient's own bacterial flora. Other sources of line-associated infection can be grouped into the following categories: (a) hematogenous spread from distant sites with increased risk due to biofilm and clot formation on the catheter surface and is influenced by type of catheter material as well as the presence of antiseptic or antibiotic coatings; (b) infection via contaminated infusate, which is rare in the United States but may be more prominent in developing nations; (c) colonization of the catheter hub, especially with long-term catheters; (d) transducer or intravenous tubing contamination; or (e) contamination of the catheter prior to insertion, which can occur in the manufacturing process, due to the use of expired catheters, or by contamination at the time of insertion through operator error or improper site preparation (20,22,27) (**Fig. 92.5**).

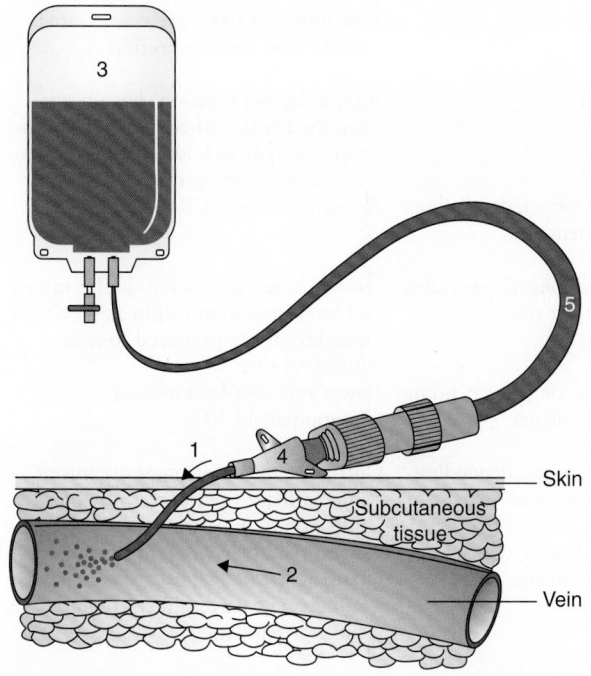

FIGURE 92.5. Mechanisms of nosocomial bloodstream infection. (1) Migration of skin bacteria down external surface of catheter; (2) Hematogenous spread from distal sites; (3) Contaminated infusate; (4) Colonization of catheter hub; (5) Contamination of transducer or IV tubing.

Prevention strategies begin with education and training of the critical care staff on the placement and maintenance of central lines. It has been shown that mandatory education of physicians and nurses as well as the establishment of a unit-based infection-control nurse position can reduce the rate of CRBSI (29). Incorporated into the education was real-time feedback to the staff about rates of infection to raise awareness. The program also incorporated a daily discussion of the need for central access to aid in timely line removal. Recent CDC guidelines for the prevention of CRBSI highlight the importance of a multilayered approach.

Hand Washing: Strong emphasis should be placed on thorough hand washing prior to insertion, which is basic clinical practice. Aseptic technique should be maintained throughout insertion (21).

Skin Preparation: Skin preparation should be performed with a 2% aqueous chlorhexidine gluconate solution. Chlorhexidine has been proven to lower catheter-related infections compared with both 10% povidone–iodine and 70% alcohol. Where a 2% solution of chlorhexidine is not available or contraindicated, povidone–iodine or 70% alcohol should be used. Chlorhexidine preparations should not be used on infants younger than 2 months of age due to possible absorption through the immature skin.

Maximal Barrier Precautions: After adequate skin preparation, full barrier precautions, which include a large sterile or full-body drape, long-sleeved sterile gown, cap, mask, and sterile gloves, should be taken. Use of full barrier precautions reduces the risk of infection compared with standard precautions consisting of a small drape and sterile gloves.

Catheter Site Dressing: Once the line is secured, a dressing should be applied. The use of transparent, semipermeable polyurethane dressings further secures the device and allows for visual inspection of the catheter and insertion site. Proper dressings can allow for bathing, reduce skin irritation and through less frequent dressing changes, can save personnel time and reduce the risk of introducing infection. These points favor use even though studies have yet to find improvement in catheter infection rates compared with standard gauze and tape dressings. If the insertion site is bleeding or oozing, a gauze dressing should be utilized until this is resolved. Regardless of the type of dressing utilized, it should be replaced when damp, soiled, loosened, or visual inspection of the site is needed. The insertion site should be monitored, and if tenderness occurs the dressing should be removed and a thorough examination should be performed (21).

Examination of the use of chlorhexidine-impregnated sponge dressings at the site of catheter insertion revealed, through a meta-analysis, a reduction in bacterial colonization and showed a trend toward the prevention of catheter-related infections (30). A randomized control trial in critically ill adults showed a significant reduction in catheter-related infections with the use of a chlorhexidine-impregnated sponge dressing even when background rates were low. The chlorhexidine-impregnated sponge is effective only in preventing extraluminal surface infections and not the intraluminal infections, which are more common in long-term indwelling catheters (31). One minor risk is a local dermatitis, which is more common in neonates, making its use not yet warranted in this population. Antibiotic ointments should not be used at the insertion site because there is a potential risk of developing resistance as well as an increase in the risk of colonization with *Candida* species. A catheter hub containing 3% iodinated alcohol in an antiseptic chamber is available in Europe. Studies have shown a fourfold reduction in the incidence of catheter infections. Currently available devices have been modified to prevent small amounts of iodinated alcohol from entering the bloodstream occurred in earlier models. The use of antibiotic lock prophylaxis and systemic antibiotic prophylaxis with vancomycin and other antibiotics is not recommended owing to the risk of creating antibiotic resistance (18,22,27,28,32,33).

Central-Line Choice and Antimicrobial/ Antiseptic-Impregnated Catheters

One of the most underrated means of reducing catheter-related infections is prompt removal of the catheter once it is no longer needed. Additionally, placing a line with only the number of lumens required for care decreases the risk of developing a catheter-related infection. A higher number of lumens increases infection risk. In children requiring multiple lumen catheters in the PICU, the lines are typically manipulated frequently, which increases the risk of developing an infection (27).

In adult studies, there is a significantly lower infection risk of the subclavian site compared with the internal jugular site. However, this must be balanced by the increased risk of complications as well as operator experience and expertise. Observational studies on dialysis lines have found internal jugular lines to have a lower infection rate. There is a higher colonization rate at the femoral site with an increased risk of catheter infection in the adult population. This has not been found in studies of pediatric patients, where femoral sites were associated with fewer mechanical complications and had an equivalent infection rate compared with catheters at other sites. When selecting a catheter site for the pediatric patient, the infectious risks, the risks of insertion, and the skills of the operator should be weighed.

In the pediatric population, the femoral site is a viable option as long as nonfemoral sites are considered and utilized in the older pediatric patients because they likely have similar infection risks compared with adults (18,22,27). The type of line inserted must be determined by the patient's needs and the infectious risks associated with the line (Table 92.4). Polyvinyl chloride and polyethylene catheters are less likely to impede bacterial adherence to the catheter and as a result are not usually available from manufactures in the United States. Teflon and polyurethane catheters are associated with fewer line-related infections.

Infection risk can be further reduced by coating or impregnating CVCs with antiseptics or antibiotics. Various catheters are approved by the Food and Drug Administration for use in children over 3 kg. Chlorhexidine and silver sulfadiazine–coated catheters have been shown to reduce infection risk compared with standard catheters. These studies have only examined catheters with the coating on the external catheter surface. The literature supports that a reduction in infection rate when antibiotic-impregnated catheters are incorporated into a multilayer approach to the reduction of central line–associated infections showed a significant decrease in infection rates (34). These catheters also significantly increase the time to central-line infection from an average of 5–18 days (35). The beneficial infection-control aspects of the catheter should be realized over the first 14 days. Despite treated catheters being more expensive than nontreated catheters, a cost savings of $68–$391 (US dollars) per catheter was found in one study, provided there is a high infection rate despite first implementing other more economical interventions (36).

TABLE 92.4

DESCRIPTION OF VASCULAR ACCESS DEVICES AND RISK OF INFECTION

■ CATHETER TYPE	■ ENTRY SITE	■ LENGTH	■ COMMENTS
Peripheral venous catheters (short)	Usually inserted in veins of forearm or hand	<8 cm	Phlebitis with prolonged use; rarely associated with bloodstream infection
Peripheral arterial catheters	Usually inserted in radial artery; can be placed in femoral, axillary, brachial, posterior tibial arteries	<8 cm	Low infection risk; rarely associated with bloodstream infection
Midline catheters	Inserted via the antecubital fossa into the proximal basilic or cephalic veins; does not enter central veins	8–20 cm	Anaphylactoid reactions have been reported with catheters made of elastomeric hydrogel; lower rates of phlebitis than short peripheral catheters
Nontunneled CVCs	Percutaneously inserted into central veins (subclavian, internal jugular, or femoral)	8 cm or longer, depending on patient size	Account for most CRBSIs
PACs	Inserted through a Teflon introducer in a central vein (subclavian, internal jugular, or femoral)	30 cm or longer, depending on patient size	Usually heparin-bonded; similar rates of bloodstream infection as CVC; subclavian site preferred to reduce infection risk
PICCs	Inserted into basilic, cephalic, or brachial veins and enter the superior vena cava	20 cm or longer, depending on patient size	Lower rate of infection than nontunneled CVCs
Tunneled CVCs	Implanted into subclavian, internal jugular, or femoral veins	8 cm or longer, depending on patient size	Cuff inhibits migration of organisms into catheter tract, lower rate of infection than nontunneled CVC
Totally implantable	Tunneled beneath skin and have devices that are subcutaneous port accessed with a needle; implanted in subclavian or internal jugular vein	8 cm or longer, depending on patient size	Lowest risk for CRBSI; improved patient self-image; no need for local catheter site care; surgery required for catheter removal
Umbilical catheters	Inserted into either umbilical vein or umbilical artery	6 cm or less, depending on patient size	Risk for CRBSI similar to catheters placed in umbilical vein versus artery

PICCs, peripherally inserted central catheters.
From O'Grady NP, Alexander M, Dellinger EP, et al. Guidelines for the prevention of intravascular catheter-related infections. The Hospital Infection Control Practices Advisory Committee, Center for Disease Control and Prevention, US. *Pediatrics* 2002;110(5):e51, with permission.

An infection rate over 3.3 per 1000 catheter days may favor the added cost in adults, where the average NNIS BSI rate ranges from 2.9 to 5.9 infections per 1000 catheter days. With the average NNIS pediatric BSI rate of 7.6 per 1000 catheter days in the United States, there may be benefit in the pediatric population as well. Recently, catheters with antiseptic coating on both the external and the luminal surfaces have been introduced. Preliminary studies have found improved anti-infective activity with these catheters. Resistance to chlorhexidine has been seen in vitro but not noted in clinical use. There have been rare reports of anaphylaxis to chlorhexidine/sulfadiazine catheters, nearly all of which have been in Japan, and as a result the catheters are not available commercially there (22,33). Catheters impregnated internally and externally with the antibiotics minocycline and rifampin have been shown lower infection rates compared with externally coated chlorhexidine/sulfadiazine catheters in a randomized multicenter trial. The half-life of antimicrobial activity against *Staphylococcus epidermidis* is 25 days, and the catheters begin showing beneficial effects after 6 days of use. As with the antiseptic catheters, bacterial resistance is possible and has been seen in vitro; however, minocycline- or rifampin-resistant organisms have yet to be reported in clinical use. The decision to implement antiseptic- or antibiotic-impregnated catheters should be based on the rate of infection after a careful implementation of standard precautions with education, maximal sterile barrier precautions, and the use of optimal skin cleansing (21).

Central-Line Replacement

Literature from adult studies initially suggested the need for central-line replacement every few days due to the higher cumulative risk of catheter infection over time. More recent data have disproved these earlier studies through randomized controlled studies. Replacement at a new site carries all the risks associated with insertion and does not lower the cumulative risk of infection. A meta-analysis of 12 studies investigating the replacement of central lines over guidewires failed to show any benefit in reducing infection (37).

The pediatric literature is quite different from adult literature on this topic. For peripheral venous catheters, there is no increase in phlebitis risk with increased duration of catheter use as long as it was placed under aseptic conditions. Peripheral arterial catheters, which include femoral and axillary arterial lines, have increased risk of infection the longer the catheter is in place and if the system permits backflow into the pressure tubing. However, the risk of infection is constant at 6.2% from day 2 to day 20 following insertion. Therefore, routine replacement of arterial lines is not recommended. The routine replacement of CVCs is not recommended owing, in part, to the limited number of vascular sites in children. This is substantiated by one large study (*n* = 397 catheters), where no relation to the time of catheter use and the daily probability of infection was found.

Routine replacement of tubing and infusion sets has been proven to decrease the risk of catheter infection. Tubing for peripheral and central lines should be changed no more frequently than every 72 hours for routine fluids. Infusion sets used for blood, blood products, and lipid infusions should be changed within 24 hours of starting the infusion. For arterial lines, the tubing and the transducer should be changed at 96-hour intervals. Stopcocks used in-line with the tubing and catheter are commonly contaminated up to 50% of the time. The impact of stopcock microbial growth on catheter infections is unknown, and there is no recommendation for frequency of replacement. It is recommended that a 15-second friction scrub with either 70% alcohol or 3/15% chlorhexidine/70% alcohol be used to sterilize entry ports every time they are accessed.

Common sense would dictate changing stopcocks with tubing changes and when soiled or potentially contaminated (22,27).

Other Interventions

As central-line infections continue to be a significant cause of nosocomial morbidity and mortality, there has been an effort to look at other interventions that may contribute to lower rates. Recently, a group investigated the effect of tight glycemic control in postoperative pediatric cardiac surgery patients on healthcare-associated infections. This study failed to show a reduction in healthcare-associated infections, including central line–associated bloodstream infections (38). More large studies are needed to investigate other interventions that can potentially reduce the burden of these infections.

Performance Improvement

With the cause of central line–related infections being multifactorial, it is often a multifactorial approach that is best when attempting the reduction rates. Instituting and enforcing care and maintenance "bundles" along with continuing education has shown to reduce infection rates in multiple populations and in multiple settings (39). Assigning a multidisciplinary team including physicians, nurses, and infection-control personnel can aid in maintaining vigilance and increasing awareness.

Extracorporeal Membrane Oxygenation

The risk factors identified for nosocomial infections associated with extracorporeal membrane oxygenation (ECMO) are prolonged ECMO support, support for cardiac disease, undergoing a major surgical procedure immediately prior to or while on ECMO, and having an open chest while on ECMO. The reported nosocomial infection rate for children on ECMO is 11% for all patients requiring support with subgroup infection rates of 8% for neonates and 13.5% for patients on ECMO for cardiac diagnoses. The nosocomial infections associated with ECMO include wound infections of the neck and chest, BSIs, UTIs, and respiratory infections. Potential reasons for the increased risk of infection while on ECMO include loss of the skin barrier to infection, especially for those patients requiring an open chest, alteration of lymphocyte subsets, a decrease in peripheral natural killer cells, and decreased total B cell counts. Yeast infections are noted as well and are believed to be due to the use of broad-spectrum antibiotics (40).

NOSOCOMIAL RESPIRATORY INFECTIONS

If infections of eye, ear, nose, and throat in addition to pneumonia are included, respiratory tract is the most common site of nosocomial infections for nearly all ages of patients in the PICU (3). Much attention has been placed on VAP as a common and preventable nosocomial infection. Other hospital-acquired respiratory infections include sinusitis, otitis media, and tracheitis. Respiratory syncytial virus (RSV) can be an important pathogen in nosocomial infections due to its annual outbreaks in the community and the number of children hospitalized as a result. However, practitioners must be cognizant of the possibility of other organisms with similar signs and symptoms entering the PICU and being a potential nosocomial infection, such as severe acute respiratory syndrome (SARS) and influenza.

The sources of nosocomial respiratory infections in the PICU are multiple and may come from the hospital environment, therapeutic and diagnostic equipment, hospital staff, family members, and even other patients. Environmental sources include fomites such as toys and cribs improperly cleaned between patient use, and contamination of hospital water sources with organisms such as *Legionella*. Contamination of the patient's respiratory tract can occur from devices in direct contact with the patient, including laryngoscopes blades, endotracheal tubes (ETTs), nasoenteric tubes, suction catheters, and bronchoscopes, as well as those with indirect contact, including mechanical ventilators, ventilator tubing, nebulizers, and oxygen delivery devices. Cross-contamination between devices such as rigid laryngoscope blades and handles can occur, highlighting the need for standardized decontamination, sterilization, and maintenance of respiratory equipment. Inadequate reprocessing of laryngoscopes has been linked to nosocomial infections and subsequent patient deaths in an NICU (41). The human vector most likely to transmit infection to the patient is the hospital staff. Poor hand hygiene and improper isolation practices are the most common risk factors. Family members and other patients can also transmit an infection to the PICU patient. All of these factors must be considered and controlled to minimize nosocomial respiratory tract infections.

Ventilator-Associated Pneumonia

Nosocomial pneumonia is one of the most common hospital-acquired infections in both adults and children, causing significant morbidity, mortality, increased utilization of healthcare resources, and excess cost. Nosocomial pneumonia can occur in any patient but is more common in infants, young children, and patients over 65 years of age. Those at highest risk for acquiring pneumonia in the PICU are patients who require intubation and mechanical ventilation. The increased risk is due to the bypassing and alteration of the host defenses. Inoculation of the formerly sterile lower respiratory tract can occur in part because the vocal cords are stented open by the ETT, increasing the risk of secretion aspiration and colonization of the aerodigestive tract. The risk of nosocomial pneumonia is increased 6–20-fold in patients who require mechanical ventilation compared with those patients not ventilated. Duration of mechanical ventilation is considered to be the greatest risk factor for the development of VAP, with the highest risk within the first 2 weeks of intubation. Independent risk factors for the development of VAP in children are immunodeficiency, immunosuppression, and neuromuscular blockade. Additional risk factors include genetic syndromes with neuromuscular weakness, burns, steroid administration, and use of total parenteral nutrition. As in adults, children are at higher risk for VAP with prior antibiotic use, longer ICU lengths of stay, use of indwelling catheters due to hematogenous spread, use of H_2-antagonist therapy, tracheal reintubation, and transport out of the ICU while intubated. The presence of a nasoenteric tube increases risk because it provides a direct route from the upper gastrointestinal tract to the oropharynx. Other associated therapies that affect risk of nosocomial pneumonia include in-line nebulizers and frequent manipulation of ventilator circuits. Recent studies estimate that the national VAP rate in children accounts for 15%–23% of nosocomial infections. The pooled mean PICU VAP rates reported by the NHSN are 0.6–2.3 episodes per 1000 ventilator days and vary based on ICU type with the highest rates reported in pediatric medical ICUs. The reported NICU VAP rate is inversely related to the patient's birth-weight category. The highest NICU VAP rates were reported in patients weighting ≤750 g with the incidence decreasing as birth weight increases (42). VAP is associated with an increased duration in mechanical ventilation, increasing the length of ventilation by as much as 5–11 days. It is also linked to an increased PICU length of stay, increasing the duration by as much as 20–34 days. Nosocomial pneumonia has the highest mortality rate of all pediatric nosocomial infections, with attributable rates ranging from 19% to 70%. Underlying illness, preterm age, time of onset of VAP, and causative organism may be important determinants of morbidity (17,43,44).

The pathogenesis of VAP begins with colonization of the lower respiratory tract from bacteria that enter the airway through or around the ETT. The type of pathogen and the pattern of antimicrobial resistance depend on the local prevalence and susceptibility patterns. In contrast with nonventilated patients, bacterial organisms identified most often in VAP are Gram-negative, with *Pseudomonas aeruginosa* being the most common species identified in PICUs. Other important organisms in this group are *Escherichia coli*, *Klebsiella pneumoniae*, and *Enterobacter* spp., which are being reported with an increased frequency in PICUs in the United States. The second most common bacterial etiology of pediatric nosocomial pneumonia is the Gram-positive organisms. Frequently isolated bacteria are *S. aureus* and coagulase-negative staphylococci. The mortality rate is less than that seen with the Gram-negative organisms. *S. aureus* and *S. epidermidis* are common causes of nosocomial pneumonia in the NICU population and are typically the result of hematogenous spread. Anaerobic nosocomial pneumonia is rare in the pediatric population but accounts for 23% of nosocomial pneumonias in adults, perhaps in part due to the difficulty in isolating the organisms and the inability to obtain protected brush specimens in children. Viruses, predominantly RSV, are the most common cause of nosocomial respiratory infections. Fungal infections are exceedingly rare but may occur in children who are immunosuppressed, especially if they frequently receive broad-spectrum antibiotics. The incidence of polymicrobial infections is high and has been reported at 38% in the PICU and 58% in the NICU (17,44).

Diagnosis of Ventilator-Associated Pneumonia

VAP in children is defined by the Center for Disease Control (CDC) as new onset of pneumonia in a patient after 48 hours of mechanical ventilation. Updated CDC guidelines for adults have introduced the ventilator-associated events (VAEs) surveillance definition algorithm in an attempt to provide more objective definitions of pulmonary infectious events in mechanically ventilated patients (45). This algorithm uses a stepwise approach before arriving at the diagnosis of possible or probable VAP. A CDC working group is currently examining whether this concept can also be applied to children.

Simplified Ventilator-Associated Event Algorithm

1. Baseline stability on mechanical ventilation ≥2 days
2. Worsening oxygenation
3. *Diagnosis: Ventilator-Associated Condition (VAC)*
4. Onset of fever/hypothermia or leukocytosis/leukopenia AND new administration of antibiotics within 2 days of worsening oxygenation
5. *Diagnosis: Infection-Related Ventilator-Associated Condition (IVAC)*
6. Purulent tracheal secretions and positive (semi-)quantitative culture
7. *Diagnosis: Probable Ventilator-Associated Pneumonia (VAP)*

Currently in children, VAP can be classified based on the time onset, with early onset pneumonia occurring within the first 4 days of mechanical ventilation; subsequent diagnoses are classified as late onset pneumonia. The diagnosis of VAP can be problematic as the direct examination and culture of lung tissue is the accepted gold standard. Since lung biopsy incurs attendant risks and autopsy data are increasingly rare, diagnosis is made on clinical, radiologic, and microbiologic grounds. The diagnosis of VAP in infants and children can be made on clinical grounds without microbiologic evidence. The set clinical diagnostic criteria and the alternate criteria, which vary by age, are listed in **Table 92.5**. Although diagnosis can be made

TABLE 92.5

SPECIFIC SITE ALGORITHMS FOR CLINICALLY DEFINED PNEUMONIA (PNU1)

■ RADIOLOGY	■ SIGNS/SYMPTOMS/LABORATORY
Two or more serial chest radiographs with at least **one** of the following[a,b]: ■ New or progressive **and** persistent infiltrate ■ Consolidation ■ Cavitation ■ Pneumatoceles, in infants ≤1 year old NOTE: In patients **without** underlying pulmonary or cardiac disease (e.g., respiratory distress syndrome, bronchopulmonary dysplasia, pulmonary edema, or chronic obstructive pulmonary disease), <u>one definitive</u> chest radiograph is acceptable.[a]	For ANY PATIENT, at least **one** of the following: ■ Fever (>38°C or >100.4°F) ■ Leukopenia (<4000 WBC/mm^3) or leukocytosis (≥12,000 WBC/mm^3) ■ For adults ≥70 years old, altered mental status with no other recognized cause **and** at least **two** of the following: ■ New onset of purulent sputum,[c] or change in character of sputum,[d] or increased respiratory secretions, or increased suctioning requirements ■ New onset or worsening cough, or dyspnea, or tachypnea[e] ■ Rales[f] or bronchial breath sounds ■ Worsening gas exchange (e.g., O$_2$ desaturations (e.g., Pao$_2$/Fio$_2$ ≤240),[g] increased oxygen requirements, or increased ventilator demand) ALTERNATE CRITERIA, for infants ≤1 year old: Worsening gas exchange (e.g., O$_2$ desaturations [e.g., pulse oximetry <94%], increased oxygen requirements, or increased ventilator demand) **and** at least **three** of the following: ■ Temperature instability ■ Leukopenia (<4000 WBC/mm^3) or leukocytosis (≥15,000 WBC/mm^3) and left shift (≥10% band forms) ■ New onset of purulent sputum[c] or change in character of sputum,[d] or increased respiratory secretions or increased suctioning requirements ■ Apnea, tachypnea,[e] nasal flaring with retraction of chest wall or grunting ■ Wheezing, rales,[f] or rhonchi ■ Cough ■ Bradycardia (<100 beats/min) or tachycardia (>170 beats/min) ALTERNATE CRITERIA, for child >1 year old or ≤12 years old, at least **three** of the following: ■ Fever (>38.4°C or >101.1°F) or hypothermia (<36.5°C or <97.7°F) ■ Leukopenia (<4000 WBC/mm^3) or leukocytosis (≥15,000 WBC/mm^3) ■ New onset of purulent sputum^3, or change in character of sputum,[d] or increased respiratory secretions, or increased suctioning requirements ■ New onset or worsening cough, or dyspnea, apnea, or tachypnea.[e] ■ Rales[f] or bronchial breath sounds ■ Worsening gas exchange (e.g., O$_2$ desaturations [e.g., pulse oximetry <94%], increased oxygen requirements, or increased ventilator demand)

Centers for Disease Control. Ventilator-associated pneumonia (VAP) event. Available at http://www.cdc.gov/nhsn/PDFs/pscManual/6pscVAPcurrent.pdf Published January 2014, accessed October 26, 2014.

[a]Occasionally, in non-ventilated patients, the diagnosis of healthcare-associated pneumonia may be quite clear on the basis of symptoms, signs, and a single definitive chest radiograph. However, in patients with pulmonary or cardiac disease (for example, interstitial lung disease or congestive heart failure), the diagnosis of pneumonia may be particularly difficult. Other non-infectious conditions (for example, pulmonary edema from decompensated congestive heart failure) may simulate the presentation of pneumonia. In these more difficult cases, serial chest radiographs must be examined to help separate infectious from non-infectious pulmonary processes. To help confirm difficult cases, it may be useful to review radiographs on the day of diagnosis, 3 days prior to the diagnosis and on days 2 and 7 after the diagnosis. Pneumonia may have rapid onset and progression, but does not resolve quickly. Radiographic changes of pneumonia persist for several weeks. As a result, rapid radiographic resolution suggests that the patient does not have pneumonia, but rather a non-infectious process such as atelectasis or congestive heart failure.

[b]Note that there are many ways of describing the radiographic appearance of pneumonia. Examples include, but are not limited to, "air-space disease", "focal opacification", "patchy areas of increased density". Although perhaps not specifically delineated as pneumonia by the radiologist, in the appropriate clinical setting these alternative descriptive wordings should be seriously considered as potentially positive findings.

[c]Purulent sputum is defined as secretions from the lungs, bronchi, or trachea that contain >25 neutrophils and <10 squamous epithelial cells per low power field (×100). If your laboratory reports these data qualitatively (e.g., "many WBCs" or "few squames"), be sure their descriptors match this definition of purulent sputum. This laboratory confirmation is required since written clinical descriptions of purulence are highly variable.

[d]A single notation of either purulent sputum or change in character of the sputum is not meaningful; repeated notations over a 24-hour period would be more indicative of the onset of an infectious process. Change in character of sputum refers to the color, consistency, odor and quantity.

[e]In adults, tachypnea is defined as respiration rate >25 breaths per minute. Tachypnea is defined as >75 breaths per minute in premature infants born at <37 weeks gestation and until the 40th week; >60 breaths per minute in patients <2 months old; >50 breaths per minute in patients 2-12 months old; and >30 breaths per minute in children >1 year old.

[f]Rales may be described as "crackles".

[g]This measure of arterial oxygenation is defined as the ratio of the arterial tension (Pao$_2$) to the inspiratory fraction of oxygen (Fio$_2$).

on clinical and radiographic grounds, determination of the causative organism is necessary to direct antibiotic therapy. For adults and older children, bronchoalveolar lavage and protected-specimen brush collection have been used with success. Bronchoscopy and protected-specimen brush collection can be difficult to perform in children due to ETT size limitations. Feasibility in critically ill infants and children, safety, and reduced costs favor tracheal aspiration as a method of culturing tracheal secretions, yet this method has low specificity due to colonization of the ETT and upper airway.

Recognized methods to determine the causative organism include positive blood cultures that cannot be attributed to another source, positive cultures from pleural fluid, a positive bronchoalveolar lavage or protected brush specimen quantitative culture, a direct microscopic exam showing $\geq 5\%$ of cells from a bronchoalveolar lavage sample containing intracellular bacteria, a histopathologic exam demonstrating evidence of fungal hyphae, abscess formation in the bronchioles and alveoli or a positive quantitative culture of lung parenchyma, and a positive detection of viral antigen or antibody from respiratory secretions (44,46). Once nosocomial pneumonia is suspected, empiric treatment should be started, covering the most likely organisms with consideration of the hospital's resistance patterns. When a specific causative agent is identified, antibiotic coverage should be adjusted. If the diagnostic workup is negative and a viral etiology is suspected, the discontinuation of antibiotics may be considered.

Prevention of Ventilator-Associated Pneumonia

❻ The prevention of nosocomial pneumonia begins with active surveillance and early recognition of VAP by a multidisciplinary team, including physicians, advanced practice and bedside nurses, and respiratory therapy and infection-control staff. Healthcare personnel who care for patients at risk for developing nosocomial pneumonia should receive education regarding VAP risk factors, evidence-based practice

recommendations, unit-based VAP rates, and patient outcomes. As with any infection prevention regimen, adherence to infection-control practices to prevent the iatrogenic spread of infection is critical. Hand hygiene with either alcohol-based solutions or soap and water, along with the use of universal precautions and appropriate isolation are the most effective and least utilized infection-control practices.

In 2004, the Institute for Healthcare Improvement launched their campaign to save 100,000 lives, which included an evidence-based approach to lower mortality in six different areas, one of which was VAP. To achieve this goal, an evidence-based set of guidelines was developed using the adult literature to aid practitioners in decreasing mortality. The ventilator bundle was revised in 2010 and consists of the following key interventions: (a) elevation of the patient's head of bed between 30 and 45 degrees; (b) daily oral care with chlorhexidine; (c) daily "sedation holidays," a break in the administration of sedatives, and a daily readiness-for-extubation assessment; (4) stress ulcer prophylaxis; and (5) deep vein thrombosis prophylaxis. The first three of the listed interventions directly address VAP. The application of such a bundle can reduce the incidence of VAP by as much as 45%, even though the latter two items do not directly address nosocomial pneumonia but are designed to treat complications commonly seen in sedate, sedentary, adult ICU patients. Many pediatric centers have implemented only the low-risk interventions such as elevating the head of the bed, performing the readiness-to-extubate test, and using stress ulcer prophylaxis as there are minimal data addressing the usage and effectiveness of the adult ventilator bundle elements in infants and children. VAP bundle items frequently utilized in pediatric centers are aimed at addressing specific risk factors (**Table 92.6**) (47).

Implementation of a pediatric-specific VAP bundle in a single-center PICU resulted in a significant reduction in the overall VAP infection rate. The baseline rate and implementation incidence were recorded as 5.6 and 8.8 infections per 1000 ventilator days, respectively. Utilization of the pediatric-specific VAP bundle decreased the unit's incidence to 0.3 infections per 1000 ventilator days with an infection rate of 0.2%. In addition to including elements similar to those found in adult VAP bundles

TABLE 92.6

COMMONLY UTILIZED PEDIATRIC VENTILATOR-ASSOCIATED PNEUMONIA BUNDLE ITEMS

Items to prevent iatrogenic spread of infection
   Adherence to good hand hygiene practices
   Use of universal precautions
   Use of appropriate isolation techniques based on infectious organism (proven or suspected)
Items to prevent aspiration of gastric contents
   Elevate the head of the bed between 30 and 45 degrees
   Monitor/drain gastric contents
Items to improve oral hygiene
   Oral rinsing/cleaning with chlorhexidine (0.12%)
   Use of toothbrush and oral swabs in daily oral care
Items to decrease ETT risk factors
   Use of in-line suction equipment where appropriate and available
   Suction of the hypopharynx prior to endotracheal suctioning and repositioning
Items to avoid contamination of respiratory equipment
   Dedicated oropharyngeal suction equipment
   Prevention of accumulation of respiratory circuit condensates
   Prevention of contamination of ventilation equipment
Items to decrease the duration of mechanical ventilation
   Daily readiness-for-extubation trials
   Neuromuscular blockade holidays

Adapted from Curley MA, Schwalenstocker E, Deshpande JK, et al. Tailoring the Institute for Health Care Improvement 100,000 Lives Campaign to pediatric settings: The example of ventilator-associated pneumonia. *Pediatr Clin North Am* 2006;53(6):1231–51.

such as head of bed elevation and scheduled mouth care, unit-specific elements such as the usage of heated wire ventilator circuits were included with general strategies to reduce VAP (48).

Maintenance of a semirecumbent position with head of bed elevation between 30 and 45 degrees is important. A multivariable analysis of risk factors associated with VAP revealed maintenance of a semirecumbent position during the first 24 hours of mechanical ventilator resulted in up to a 67% reduction in VAP (43). Elevation of the head of the bed prevents aspiration of gastric contents. This risk can be further minimized by gastric decompression with gastric tubes and the routine monitoring of gastric residuals. In adult studies, the use of a 0.12% chlorhexidine oral rinse solution in patients in surgical intensive care was associated with a decreased incidence of VAP. Although frequently included in pediatric VAP bundles, the usage of a 0.12% chlorhexidine oral solution has not been shown to be effective in significantly reducing the incidence of VAP in children, regardless of age stratification. In a Brazilian study of pediatric patients undergoing cardiac surgery, the incidence of VAP was 18.3% and 15% in the chlorhexidine versus the placebo group. Prophylactic postoperative usage of a 0.12% chlorhexidine solution did not impact the length of mechanical ventilation, need for reintubation, duration of antibiotic usage, or time interval between surgery and nosocomial pneumonia diagnosis (49).

Minimizing the length of time that the patient requires mechanical ventilation is important in preventing nosocomial pneumonia. Prompt treatment and reversal of the condition that necessitated mechanical ventilation must occur. A mechanism should be established by which to assess the patient's readiness to be extubated once the underlying condition is resolved. Adult VAP bundles have included sedation holidays to assess patients' respiratory strength and to ensure that patients are not excessively sedated. For most children in the PICU, sedation holidays are impractical, as they could potentially result in unintended extubations, particularly in children who are too young to cooperate or comprehend the necessity of the critical care interventions to which they are being subjected. Instead, the use of constant, high-dose sedation should be avoided, and appropriate sedation scales should be used. If neuromuscular blockade is being used, it is reasonable to intermittently hold the muscle-relaxing agents if clinically appropriate. Another potential, albeit unproven, element of a pediatric VAP bundle should be the daily assessment as to whether or not the patient can be extubated (**Fig. 92.6**). This should be done on a daily basis from the day of intubation to the day of successful extubation, unless a clinical contraindication is present. One of the main benefits of the readiness-for-extubation test is that it occurs regardless of whether the patient is thought by the clinicians to be ready for extubation. The method noted in the figure is one example of an extubation-readiness test; individual modifications may be required based on institutional practices (47).

While minimizing the duration of mechanical ventilation is important in preventing VAP, it is the presence of the ETT that imparts the risk of VAP and not the act of positive-pressure ventilation. In a meta-analysis of 12 studies that examined pneumonia rates in adult patients who received noninvasive or invasive ventilation, a benefit was found to noninvasive ventilation in terms of lessening the risk for developing pneumonia [relative risk, 0.31; 95% confidence interval (CI), 0.16–0.57; $p = 0.0002$]. Studies have also found that patients managed with noninvasive ventilation have a shorter ICU length of stay and a decreased mortality rate. When appropriate, noninvasive ventilation should be considered as a potential method by which to decrease VAP risk (50,51).

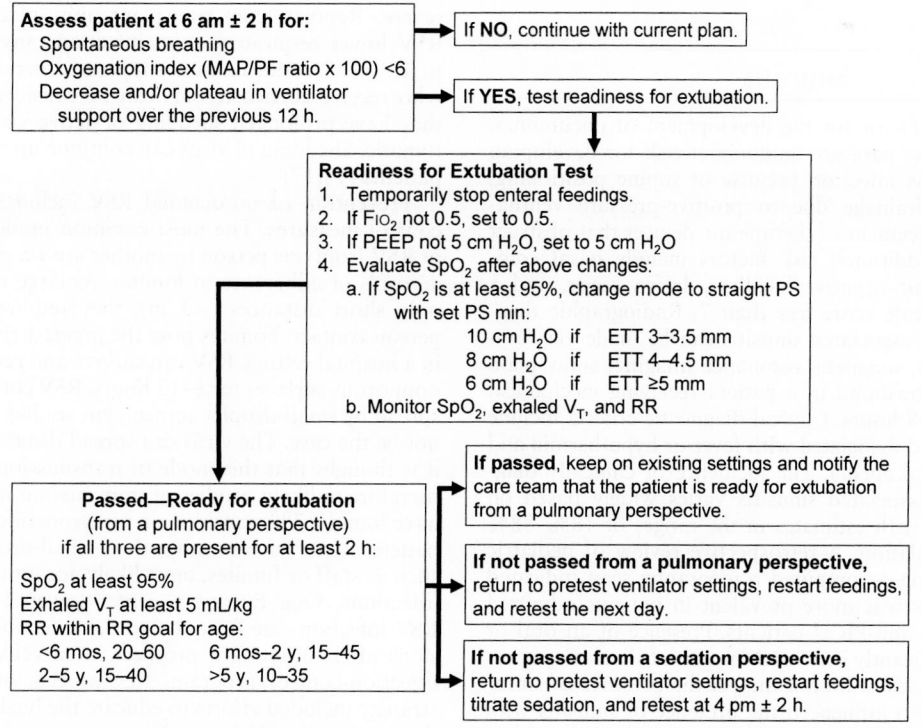

FIGURE 92.6. Daily test for patient readiness for extubation. In this model, prescreening for suitability for extubation is assessed over a 2-hour period. If prescreening criteria are met, feeds are held and the patient is brought to low-ventilation settings for a trial on pressure support ventilator settings for a trial on pressure support ventilation. If the patient does well based on present criteria, extubation is considered. MAP, mean arterial pressure; PF ratio, Pao_2/Fio_2 ratio; PEEP, positive end-expiratory pressure; RR, respiratory rate. (From Curley MAQ, Arnold JH, Thompson JE, et al. Clinical trial design: Effect of prone positioning on clinical outcomes in infants and children with acute respiratory distress syndrome. *J Crit Care* 2006;21:23–32, with permission.)

Additional preventive measures focus on reducing or eliminating aspiration of contaminated oropharyngeal or gastric secretions, colonization of the aerodigestive tract, and the usage of contaminated equipment. In additional to maintaining a semirecumbent position, adult studies provide increasing evidence that subglottic drainage of secretions significantly diminishes the risk of VAP. These specialized ETTs are both expensive and not yet available for the majority of the pediatric population because of size limitations. The findings of these studies led to the practice of suctioning the hypopharynx to clear secretions in pediatric patients. This suctioning should be performed prior to suctioning the ETT to prevent aspiration of hypopharyngeal secretions should the patient cough, prior to the manipulation of the ETT during retaping or repositioning, and prior to moving the patient in bed. If using a cuffed ETT, a cuff pressure of 20 cm H_2O should be maintained to reduce aspiration. The usage of acid suppressive therapy may increase colonization of the aerodigestive tract. Usage of H_2-antagonists and proton pump inhibitors for adult patients who are not at a high risk for developing a stress ulcer or stress gastritis remains controversial. Meta-analyses yield inconsistent results regarding the increased risk of VAP. The risk of developing a stress ulcer or gastritis should be balanced against the risk of developing VAP. The type of heater-humidification or heat and moisture exchangers in ventilator circuits has not been found to influence the incidence of VAP. However, if condensation should occur in the ventilator circuit, it could potentially become contaminated and theoretically cause an infection. Therefore, the condensate should be routinely removed from the circuit through the use of a trap. Ventilatory circuits should be changed when visibly soiled or malfunctioning. Staff should be conscientious and avoid contamination of respiratory equipment such as the end of the ventilator circuit, the resuscitation bag, and suction equipment to further diminish the risk of VAP (43,47,50).

Sinusitis

Sinusitis is a risk factor for the development of pneumonia. Patients in intensive care are uniquely at risk for developing a nosocomial sinus infection because of supine positioning, decreased sinus drainage due to positive-pressure ventilation, and nasal placement of therapeutic devices that obstruct sinus drainage. Additional risk factors include nasal colonization with Gram-negative bacilli, sedative usage, and a Glasgow Coma Scale score less than 7. Radiographic diagnosis of ventilator-associated sinusitis can be made via computed tomography, magnetic resonance imaging, sinus plain radiograph, or ultrasound in a patient receiving mechanical ventilation for >48 hours. Clinical diagnostic criteria include purulent sinus fluid associated with fever or hypothermia and leukocytosis or leukopenia. The incidence of clinically diagnosed ventilator-associated sinusitis varies widely based on study population with estimates in the ranges of 18%–88% in the adult population. A retrospective review of pediatric patients undergoing a computed tomography scan indicated incidental sinusitis was more prevalent in patients admitted to the PICU than non-PICU patients. Presence of an oral or nasal device significantly increased the risk of sinusitis, yet nasal versus oral location did not impact the presence of sinusitis. Patient age also influenced the presence of sinusitis with younger age constituting a specific risk factor for the presence of radiographic sinusitis (52). In adult patients, radiographic evidence of ventilator-associated sinusitis but not confirmed clinical infection is more likely in patients with nasotracheal or nasogastric devices versus patients with orotracheal or orogastric devices. Gram-negative aerobic pathogens account for the majority of ventilator-associated sinusitis followed by

Gram-positive aerobic pathogens. Infection is often polymicrobial with *Pseudomonas* species and *Streptococcus* species isolated most frequently. Sinusitis in intubated patients can evolve into VAP, bacteremia or sepsis. Presence of clinically diagnosed ventilator-associated sinusitis is associated with a higher risk of VAP. Many risk factors of sinusitis can be addressed through the usage of VAP bundles, which include elevation of the head of bed, attention to good oral hygiene, and consideration of daily interruption of sedation (53).

Respiratory Syncytial Virus

RSV is one of the most common etiologies of pediatric nosocomial respiratory tract infections in the PICU and is the most common nosocomial infection overall on pediatric wards. Forty percent of these nosocomial RSV infections occur in the lower respiratory tract. RSV is different from other organisms that cause nosocomial infections in that although those children with underlying cardiopulmonary disease may have more severe infections, healthy children more commonly contract nosocomial RSV infections. The risk factors for contracting an RSV nosocomial infection are young age, especially neonates, underlying chronic illness such as cardiac or pulmonary disease, a long hospitalization, overcrowding or staff shortages, and, most importantly, hospitalization during the RSV endemic season. An additional source of nosocomial RSV infection is healthcare workers. It is estimated that half of the staff on pediatric wards during an RSV season become infected. The symptoms that the staff experiences vary from mild to significant, and up to 20% may have an asymptomatic infection. Reinfection is common, even in the same season, because immunity to RSV is incomplete. Immunocompromised patients deserve special mention for two reasons. First, depending on the degree of immunosuppression, the illness can be quite severe. Reports from transplant units place mortality from RSV lower respiratory tract infections anywhere from 20% to 100%. Second, immunosuppressed neonates and children who receive corticosteroids can be considered in this group; they have prolonged shedding of active virus even if asymptomatic. Shedding of virus can continue up to 3 weeks in these patients (14,17).

Prevention of nosocomial RSV includes simple infection control measures. The most common modes of transmission of RSV from one person to another are via either large-droplet aerosols or adherence to fomites. As large droplets can travel only short distances (<1 m), they require close person-to-person contact. Fomites pose the greatest risk of transmission in a hospital setting. RSV can survive and remain infectious on nonporous surfaces for 6–12 hours. RSV could theoretically be spread by small-droplet aerosol, but studies have found this to not be the case. The virus can spread distances up to 7 m, but it is thought that this mode of transmission is inefficient and therefore unlikely. Studies of transmission in multi-bed rooms have found a 3% transmission rate from infected to uninfected patients (14). Factors other than small-droplet transmission, such as staff or fomites, most likely account for many of these infections. One European center lowered their nosocomial RSV infection rate from 1.1 to 0.1 infections per 100 admissions after initiating a prospective surveillance and targeted infection-control program. Key aspects of the intervention strategy included efforts to educate the healthcare team about the modes of RSV transmission, prospective surveillance for RSV infection, early diagnosis, a strict cohorting and isolation policy, and daily disinfectant of surfaces in the isolation rooms (54). Although some case reports suggest the usage of passive immunization to control nosocomial outbreaks in NICUs, no data are available to support the usage of Palivizumab in controlling nosocomial outbreaks of RSV.

Influenza and Other Respiratory Viruses

Most respiratory viruses can be transmitted and contained using the methods described for RSV. SARS deserves special attention and is discussed in the next section. A very effective method of preventing the nosocomial transmission of influenza is through the annual immunization of healthcare workers.

Severe Acute Respiratory Syndrome

Evaluation of infection control practices during the SARS outbreak in 2003 reveals a great deal about the effectiveness of these practices for SARS and other respiratory pathogens. Personal protective equipment appeared to be quite effective in preventing acquisition of SARS. It was found that consistent wearing of either a simple surgical mask or an N95 respirator was more effective than inconsistent use, with a 13% versus 56% infection rate, respectively. A trend, albeit not statistically significant, of better protection was found with the N95 respirator compared with a surgical mask. However, in Vietnam, at least one hospital with documented SARS cases controlled the spread with only surgical masks during the first 3 weeks of the outbreak. Potential reasons for this equality of protection include the fact that the N95 respirators were not properly fitted and thus no better than surgical masks or that the healthcare workers may not have removed personal protective equipment in the proper order. Additional infection control measures used to prevent large-droplet transmission of infectious agents during the SARS outbreak included "physical space interventions" such as separation of patients, methods to decrease infectious aerosols during at-risk therapies, and environmental decontamination and containment. It was noted that certain procedures seemed to increase the transmission of SARS in instances in which it is postulated that smaller droplets, which can travel further distances, are formed. These procedures included intubation, continuous positive-airway pressure, and nebulization therapy (55).

NOSOCOMIAL URINARY TRACT INFECTIONS

In incidence studies of nosocomial infections, including patients of all ages and in all hospital locations, UTIs are the most frequent behind respiratory and BSIs. The actual rate of catheter-associated UTIs (CAUTIs) in ICUs varies based on the type of unit and ranges from 3.1 to 7.4 per 1000 catheter days. The higher incidences have been described in burn and neurologic units. The NHSN database notes that the PICU nosocomial urinary tract rates to be 4.0–4.4 infections per 1000 catheter days, with the highest incidence in pediatric cardiothoracic ICUs (42). Secondary urosepsis is uncommon in the PICU population. A study of PICU patients with nosocomial UTIs found that 58% were female, the mean age in the infected group was 4.6 years, all patients had urinary catheters in place for at least 3 days, and 26.9% were catheterized for 8 days or longer. The infected group showed a trend toward increased mortality. Multiple regression analysis in this study found having prior cardiac surgery as the only significant risk factor. Additional studies found through multivariate analysis that the nosocomial UTI risks are increased based on duration of catheterization, female sex, absence of systemic antibiotics, and disconnection of the catheter-collecting tube junction. Most infections are caused by a single organism, with 82% identified as Gram-negative bacteria or yeast species. Twenty percent of nosocomial UTIs have antibiotic resistance. In the

PICU, a UTI can be challenging to diagnose, as the patient will not have the typical symptoms (e.g., frequency and dysuria) due to the severity of the critical illness or due to a catheter being in place and masking these symptoms (56).

The acquisition of a CAUTI by critically ill patients is associated with increased morbidity, prolonged hospital length of stay, bacterial resistance, and greater healthcare expenditures. Changes in reimbursement policies have increased attention to the usage of indwelling urinary catheters, their correlation with UTIs, and the prevention of associated nosocomial infections. The effectiveness of a multidisciplinary systematic approach to reducing the CAUTI rates in PICU patients is documented in a prospective surveillance study in 10 PICUs across six developing countries. Before implementation of a multifaceted infection-control bundle, CAUTI rates of 5.9 per 1000 urinary catheter days were recorded. The CAUTI rate was reduced from 57% to 2.6% of cases per 1000 catheter days after implementation of program consisting of outcome surveillance, process surveillance, staff education, a practice bundle of preventive interventions, and feedback on CAUTI rates and performance. A marked increase in hand hygiene compliance was observed, no doubt contributing to the reduction in CAUTIs (57).

Additional core strategies to prevent or decrease nosocomial UTIs include minimizing exposure to urinary catheters by using them only when truly indicated, using a sterile insertion technique, maintaining uninterrupted use of a closed collection system, and removing the device as soon as possible— ideally in <3 days. Automatic urinary catheter reminder and stop orders are effective in reducing the duration of catheterization and associated CAUTIs. Portable ultrasound devices can be used in patients with low urine output to reduce unnecessary catheter insertion. No pediatric studies have been reported, but the usage of antimicrobial/antiseptic-impregnated catheters can be considered if the CAUTI rate is not decreasing after implementation of a comprehensive strategy to decrease nosocomial UTIs (56,58).

NOSOCOMIAL GASTROINTESTINAL INFECTIONS

Nosocomial diarrhea is defined as loose stools occurring >48 hours after admission, a stool frequency of at least two per 12 hours, and no identified noninfectious cause of the loose stools. In general, nosocomial diarrhea accounts for up to 35% of all pediatric hospital-acquired infections. The reported PICU rate is 4%–5%. Outside the PICU, viral etiologies as a group predominate and are usually similar organisms as seen in the community such as rotavirus, adenovirus, and Norwalk virus. The single most common organism isolated in the PICU and on the general ward is *Clostridium difficile*. *C. difficile* is almost exclusively isolated as a cause of diarrhea in children over 1 year of age. It is believed that, although present in the gastrointestinal tract of newborns, *C. difficile* does not typically cause disease in neonates and young infants. The organisms responsible for nosocomial diarrhea are typically spread by the fecal–oral route, which may explain the fact that most children with at least viral etiologies of their diarrhea are incontinent (i.e., diapered). Infection-control techniques are important in preventing and controlling nosocomial diarrhea. Good hand hygiene and contact precautions are paramount to this effort. Soap and water hand cleansing is necessary for *C. difficile* since alcohol-based solutions will not kill the spore. The viruses that cause diarrheal illnesses can survive on fomites and other surfaces for several hours, and the spores of *C. difficile* can survive over a day on such inanimate surfaces. With attention to hydration and electrolyte status, mortality from nosocomial diarrhea is rare, but dehydration is always a concern, especially in young children (3,57).

Necrotizing Enterocolitis

The etiology of necrotizing enterocolitis is multifactorial; however, nosocomial, epidemic outbreaks do occur in NICUs. In a review of epidemics, Boccia et al. found that they last ~8–10 weeks, with an average of 10.5 cases per epidemic, and common organisms were identified in nearly half of the epidemics. The mortality rate of recent cases was <10%. Affected centers used infection-control measures focused on preventing orofecal transmission to limit the epidemic such as strict use of hand washing, the use of gloves, isolation of the infected newborns, cohorting of cases, and the closing of some units. The proposed mechanism is orofecal transmission to susceptible premature infants, increased virulence of the organism, or the synergistic action of two microorganisms. Identified organisms in outbreaks have been *E. coli*, *K. pneumoniae*, *Enterobacter cloacae*, *Clostridium butyricum*, *Clostridium difficile*, *S. epidermidis*, Coronavirus, Rotavirus, and Echovirus. Often the causal organism is not identified. There is a controversy as to whether *Clostridia* species are causative organisms since they may be part of the normal intestinal flora (60).

SURGICAL SITE INFECTIONS

The NHSN tracks surgical site infections for a variety of surgical procedures. These data are broken down by site or when enough data are available by specific operation. The rates are further stratified by risk index category. The risk index is determined by the anesthetic risk on the basis of the American Society of Anesthesiologists preoperative assessment scores, whether or not the surgical field is contaminated, and duration of the operative procedure as benchmarked against a preset standard for each operation. The NHSN surgical site infection rates include data from adult and pediatric patients. Causative organisms of pediatric surgical site infections are most commonly caused by *S. aureus* with 20% of all reported infections although these are more commonly seen in patients 2 months of age and under. Coagulase-negative staphylococci and *P. aeruginosa* account for ~14% each of all pediatric surgical site infections. *P. aeruginosa* is isolated more commonly from surgical site infections in children over 2 months of age (3). Adult studies of chlorhexidine bathing have shown a decrease in surgical site infections. Pediatric studies are lacking, but such bathing may be considered in high-risk patients.

Nosocomial Central Nervous System Infections

Nosocomial central nervous system infections usually involve a surgical site or the presence of a foreign body. The NHSN reported that pooled mean rates for craniotomy are 0.91, 1.72, and 2.41 infections per 100 operations for zero, one, and either two or three risk index categories, respectively. The risk of a surgical site infection from a ventricular shunt with zero risk categories is 4.42 per 100 operations, whereas it is 5.36 per 100 if one or more risk index categories (wound class, duration of operation, and American Society of Anesthesiology score) are present. Other central nervous system operations have a combined surgical site infection rate of 1.53 per 100 operations (61).

A review of children who underwent 281 intracranial surgeries for craniofacial surgery found an incidence of 3.2 surgical site infections per 100 operations. No superficial infections were noted in this retrospective study. Of the nine reported infections, two were deep incisional infections involving the fascial and muscular layers, and seven involved deeper structures such as the bone and dura. Several risk factors for infection were identified in this population and included repairs of syndromic craniosynostosis and an oblique facial cleft. With a more complicated preoperative diagnosis, the infectious risk was increased (OR, 13.0; 95% CI, 2.6–64.4). Additional factors increasing risk of nosocomial infection included an increased duration of surgery (OR, 12.1; 95% CI, 2.4–59.9), closure of the overlying skin under tension (OR, 12.5; 95% CI, 3.0–52.6), and the presence of more than four surgeons during the operative procedure (OR, 6.3; 95% CI, 1.2–32.0). Demographics such as age and gender as well as associated medical conditions and previous surgical procedures including tracheotomy and ventriculoperitoneal shunt were not associated with higher rates of infection (62).

A prospective analysis of 1000 parenchymatously placed monitors at a single center over an 8-year period was performed and included pediatric patients. Two-thirds of the devices were placed in patients with traumatic head injury. Probe tip cultures were obtained in 547 cases, with 91.5% of the cultures negative for bacterial growth. Forty-six (8.5%) of the cultures were positive. *S. epidermidis* grew in nearly half of the positive cultures (47.8%). Other organisms isolated included *E. coli* (19.7%), *Corynebacterium* (10.9%), and *S. aureus* (6.6%). There was no difference in the incidence of positive culture probe tips whether the device was placed in the ICU or operating room. No patients had evidence of infection at the insertion site (63).

Epidural catheters are often used in the ICU to manage pain. The reported infection rates in these catheters range from 0% to 0.7% in published studies. A study of 1458 pediatric patients with postoperative epidural catheters found no epidural abscesses over a 6-year period. Local superficial infections are not frequently reported, but the rate appears similar to those of intravascular lines. The proposed mechanism of infection is similar to intravenous lines as well. Possible sources of epidural catheter infection include skin contamination, introduction of bacteria by the needle or catheter, hematogenous spread, or contamination of the infusate. Risk of infection can be reduced in the same manner as in the placement of intravascular lines. Attention to aseptic technique during placement, adequate skin preparation and disinfection prior to placement, and maintenance of appropriate dressings are important safety measures to prevent infection of the catheter and the epidural space. The duration of catheter use also influences the risk of infection as is seen in intravascular catheters. The longer the catheter is in place, the higher the risk of infection. However, the majority of infections occur within the first 5 days after insertion (64). In a prospective study of 210 children receiving short-term epidural analgesia, no serious systemic infections such as meningitis or epidural abscess were noted. The incidence of dressing contamination, cellulitis, and bacterial colonization was more common in caudally placed catheters compared with lumbar catheters. There was little difference in the incidence of Gram-positive organism positive cultures between the two sites. Caudal catheters were much more likely to be contaminated with Gram-negative organisms, 16% versus 3% (65).

Selected Surgical Site Infections

Adult rates of surgical site infections following cardiovascular surgery are between 1.5 and 2.3 infections per 100 operations. Retrospective studies in pediatrics have put the rate in children at 0.5–5 infections per 100 operations. The low rate of 0.5 may have been an underestimate due to study design. Two more recent, prospective pediatric studies have placed the rate at 2.3–3.4 infections per 100 operations. In these studies, the wound infection rate ranged from 1 to 1.5 per 100 operations, whereas the organ space infection rate (sternal osteomyelitis and mediastinitis) ranged from 0.8 to 2.4 per 100 surgeries. Over half of the infections in children were caused by *S. aureus* followed in frequency by coagulase-negative staphylococci, enterococci, and *Enterobacter* species. These organisms accounted for nearly 90% of the isolated bacteria in the two studies. Debridement when appropriate and intravenous antibiotics were the therapies administered to these patients. Risk factors for surgical site infection have been identified and can be divided pre-, intra-, and postoperative categories. Preoperative risks include younger age at time of surgery, a higher American Society of Anesthesiologists score, a longer preoperative inpatient length of stay, a prior sternotomy, and an elevated leukocyte band count. Intraoperative factors that affect the incidence of surgical site infections are the duration of the surgery, cardiopulmonary bypass, and circulatory arrest. Postoperative factors associated with infection risk include failed primary closure of the chest, low cardiac output, infection at another site, and the duration of use for mechanical ventilation, central venous line, and urinary catheter. In a multivariable analysis, a longer duration of surgery (OR, 1.4, 95% CI 1.2–1.8) and <1 month of age at the time of surgery (OR, 14, 95% CI 3.3–58.4) were independently associated with pediatric cardiovascular surgical site infection. Patients without a surgical site infection had a median surgical time of 150 minutes (range 45–450 minutes), while those children with a wound infection had a median duration of 233 minutes (range 80–600 minutes). Children with sternal osteomyelitis or mediastinitis had a median surgery length of 270 minutes (range 135–450 minutes, $p = 0.0005$ compared with those patients without infection). In another study, the incidence of surgical site infection based on age was 7.6% for <1 month, 3.9% for 1–12 months of age, 3.5% for 1–4 years of age, and 1.6% for children over the age of 4 years of age. Children over the age of 1 year were more likely to be bacteremic with positive blood cultures than younger children (73% vs. 17%, $p = 0.001$) (66,67).

Mediastinitis

Mediastinitis is rare in the PICU population and is defined by purulent discharge in the mediastinal space necessitating surgical debridement, positive cultures from the mediastinal space, or sternal instability in the presence of positive blood cultures. The incidence ranges from 0.04% to 3.9% with most studies placing the rate at ~1% in the postcardiac surgery population despite intravenous perioperative prophylaxis. Gram-positive organisms account for approximately two-thirds of the infections with *S. aureus*, causing the majority of the Gram-positive infections with the remainder nearly all due to coagulase-negative Staphylococcus. A third of the cases are due to Gram-negative bacteria with *P. aeruginosa* responsible for half the infections. Polymicrobial infections are infrequent, and fungal infections are rare. Mediastinitis occurs at a mean of 11 days following sternotomy with Gram-positive infections occurring later than Gram-negative infections, 13 versus 6.5 days, respectively. Concurrent bacteremia is found in 40%–50% of the patients with mediastinitis. Gram-positive mediastinitis has positive blood cultures 67% of the time, and Gram-negative mediastinitis has positive cultures in 18% of cases. In a multivariable analysis, delayed sternal closure was found to be an independent risk factor for the development of Gram-negative mediastinitis (68).

CONCLUSIONS AND FUTURE DIRECTIONS

Nosocomial infections are an important and mostly preventable cause of morbidity and mortality in the PICU. Although not all nosocomial infections may be able to be eliminated in part due to the unique nature of the PICU patient, the incidence can be dramatically reduced through the use of infection-control measures. Simple interventions such as consistent use of hand hygiene, isolation practices, adherence to sterile technique, raising the head of the bed, and judicious use with prompt removal of central lines, urinary catheters, and ETTs can dramatically affect nosocomial infection rates. Use of care bundles and the joining of collaborates can increase effectiveness of these and other measures by standardizing the approach to nosocomial infection prevention. Although all nosocomial infections may not be preventable, our goal as pediatric critical care practitioners should be zero. Consistent use and monitoring the effectiveness of infection-control measures will go a long way toward achieving the goal.

The medical community needs to take action on reducing and preventing nosocomial infections. Future efforts should be directed toward improved differentiation of community-acquired from nosocomial infections; reducing the development of resistant organisms through judicious use of antibiotics via antibiotic stewardship to render nosocomial infections less problematic; designing ICUs to allow proper isolation practices and to facilitate hand hygiene; and developing constraint design or forcing functions to assure compliance with hand hygiene and infection-control bundles. Pay for performance and loss of reimbursement from insurers may be the eventual impetus for change in healthcare systems toward eradicating hospital-acquired infections.

References

1. Tan SY, Brown J. Ignac Philipp Semmelweis (1818–1865): Hand washing saves lives. *Singapore Med J* 2006;47(1):6–7.
2. Scott RD. The Direct Medical Costs of Healthcare-Associated Infections in US Hospitals and the Benefits of Prevention. Centers for Disease Control. http://www.cdc.gov/hai/pdfs/hai/scott_costpaper.pdf. Accessed September 1, 2013.
3. Richards MJ, Edwards JR, Culver DH, et al. Nosocomial infections in pediatric intensive care units in the United States. National Nosocomial Infections Surveillance System. *Pediatrics* 1999;103(4):e39.
4. Rosenthal VD, Maki DG, Salomao R, et al. Device-associated nosocomial infections in 55 intensive care units of 8 developing countries. *Ann Intern Med* 2006;145(8):582–91.
5. Arantes A, Carvalho Eda S, Medeiros EA, et al. Pediatric risk of mortality and hospital infection. *Infect Control Hosp Epidemiol* 2004;25(9):783–5.
6. Bonten MJ. Infection in the intensive care unit: Prevention strategies. *Curr Opin Infect Dis* 2002;15(4):401–5.
7. Rogowski JA, Staiger D, Patrick T, et al. Nurse staffing and NICU infection rates. *JAMA Pediatr* 2013;167(5):444–50.
8. Stone PW, Pogorzelska M, Kunches L, et al. Hospital staffing and health care-associated infections: A systematic review of the literature. *Clin Infect Dis* 2008;47(7):937–44.
9. Taylor RW, O'Brien J, Trottier SJ, et al. Red blood cell transfusions and nosocomial infections in critically ill patients. *Crit Care Med* 2006;34(9):2302–8; quiz 2309.
10. White M, Barron J, Gornbein J, et al. Are red blood cell transfusions associated with nosocomial infections in pediatric intensive care units? *Pediatr Crit Care Med* 2010;11(4):464–8.

11. American Academy of Pediatrics. Infection control for hospitalized children. In: Pickering LK, Baker CJ, Long SS, et al, eds. *Red Book: 2006 Report of the Committee on Infectious Diseases.* 27th ed. Elk Grove Village: American Academy of Pediatrics, 2006:153–64. NOTE: *Used 29th version of Red Book in electronic format – need to check page numbers and reference in printed version*

12. Martyny J, Glazer CS, Newman LS. Respiratory protection. *N Engl J Med* 2002;347(11):824–30.

13. CDC. http://www.cdc.gov/HAI/pdfs/ppe/ppeposter1322.pdf. Accessed September 1, 2013.

14. Hall CB. Nosocomial respiratory syncytial virus infections: The "Cold War" has not ended. *Clin Infect Dis* 2000;31(2):590–6.

15. Pittet D, Hugonnet S, Harbarth S, et al. Effectiveness of a hospital-wide programme to improve compliance with hand hygiene. Infection Control Programme. *Lancet* 2000;356(9238):1307–12.

16. Randle J, Clarke M, Storr J. Hand hygiene compliance in healthcare workers. *J Hosp Infect* 2006;64(3):205–9.

17. Zar HJ, Cotton MF. Nosocomial pneumonia in pediatric patients: Practical problems and rational solutions. *Paediatr Drugs* 2002;4(2):73–83.

18. Farr BM. Preventing vascular catheter-related infections: Current controversies. *Clin Infect Dis* 2001;33(10):1733–8.

19. Coia JE, Duckworth GJ, Edwards DI, et al. Guidelines for the control and prevention of methicillin-resistant Staphylococcus aureus (MRSA) in healthcare facilities. *J Hosp Infect* 2006; 63(suppl 1):S1–44.

20. Mermel LA, Farr BM, Sherertz RJ, et al. Guidelines for the management of intravascular catheter-related infections. *Clin Infect Dis* 2001;32(9):1249–72.

21. O'Grady NP, Alexander M, Burns LA, et al. *Guidelines for the Prevention of Intravascular Catheter-Related Infections, 2011.* Atlanta, GA: CDC Guidelines.

22. O'Grady NP, Alexander M, Dellinger EP, et al. Guidelines for the prevention of intravascular catheter-related infections. The Hospital Infection Control Practices Advisory Committee, Center for Disease Control and Prevention, U.S. *Pediatrics* 2002;110(5):e51.

23. Horan TC, Andrus M, Dudeck MA. CDC/NHSN surveillance definition of health care-associated infection and criteria for specific types of infections in the acute care setting. *Am J Infect Control* 2008;36:309–32.

24. Burton DC, Edwards JR, Horan TC, et al. Methicillin-resistant Staphylococcus aureus central line-associated bloodstream infections in US intensive care units, 1997–2007. *JAMA* 2009;301:727–36.

25. Gaynes R, Edwards JR. Overview of nosocomial infections caused by gram-negative bacilli. *Clin Infect Dis* 2005;41:848–54.

26. Wisplinghoff H, Bischoff T, Tallent SM, et al. Nosocomial bloodstream infections in US hospitals: Analysis of 24,179 cases from a prospective nationwide surveillance study. *Clin Infect Dis* 2004;39(3):309–17.

27. de Jonge RC, Polderman KH, Gemke RJ. Central venous catheter use in the pediatric patient: Mechanical and infectious complications. *Pediatr Crit Care Med* 2005;6(3):329–39.

28. Slaughter SE. Intravascular catheter-related infections. Strategies for combating this common foe. *Postgrad Med* 2004;116(5):59–66.

29. Costello JM, Morrow DF, Graham DA, et al. Systematic intervention to Reduce Central Line–Associated Bloodstream Infection Rates in a Pediatric Cardiac Intensive Care Unit. Pediatrics. *Pediatrics* 2008;121(5):915–23.

30. Ho KM, Litton E. Use of chlorhexidine-impregnated dressing to prevent vascular and epidural catheter colonization and infection: A meta-analysis. *J Antimicrob Chemother* 2006;58(2):281–7.

31. Levi I, Katz J, Solter E, Samra Z, et al. Chlorhexidine-impregnated dressing for prevention of colonization of central venous catheters in infants and children. A randomized control study. *Pediatr Infect Dis J* 2005;24(8):676–9.

32. Coffin SE, Zaoutis TE. Infection control, hospital epidemiology, and patient safety. *Infect Dis Clin North Am* 2005;19(3):647–65.

33. Mermel LA. New technologies to prevent intravascular catheter-related bloodstream infections. *Emerg Infect Dis* 2001;7(2):197–9.

34. Bhutta A, Gilliam C, Honeycutt M, et al. Reduction of bloodstream infections associated with catheters in paediatric intensive care unit: Stepwise approach. *BMJ* 2007;334:362–5.

35. Chelliah A, Heydon KH, Zaoutis TE, et al. Observational trial of antibiotic-coated central venous catheters in critically ill pediatric patients. *Pediatr Infect Dis J* 2007;26:816–20.

36. Veenstra DL, Saint S, Sullivan SD. Cost-effectiveness of antiseptic-impregnated central venous catheters for the prevention of catheter-related bloodstream infection. *JAMA* 1999;282:554–60.

37. Cook D, Randolph A, Kernerman P, et al. Central venous catheter replacement strategies: A systematic review of the literature. *Crit Care Med* 1997;25:1417–24.

38. Agus MS, Steil GM, Wypij D, et al. Tight glycemic control versus standard care after pediatric cardiac surgery. *N Engl J Med* 2012;367(13):1208–19.

39. Rinke ML, Chen AR, Bundy DG, et al. Implementation of Central Line Maintenance care bundle in hospitalized pediatric oncology patients. *Pediatrics* 2012;130(4):e996–1004.

40. O'Neill JM, Schutze GE, Heulitt MJ, et al. Nosocomial infections during extracorporeal membrane oxygenation. *Intensive Care Med* 2001;27(8):1247–53.

41. Muscarella LF. Reassessment of the risk of healthcare-acquired infection during rigid laryngoscopy. *J Hosp Infect* 2008;68(2):101–7.

42. Edwards JR, Peterson KD, Mu Y, et al. National Healthcare Safety Network (NHSN) report: Data summary for 2006 through 2008, issued December 2009. *Am J Infect Control* 2009;37(9):783–805.

43. Coffin SE, Klompas M, Classen D, et al. Strategies to prevent ventilator-associated pneumonia in acute care hospitals. *Infect Control Hosp Epidemiol* 2008;29(suppl 1):S31–40.

44. Venkatachalam V, Hendley JO, Wilson DF. The diagnostic dilemma of ventilator-associated pneumonia in critically ill children. *Pediatr Criti Care Med* 2011;12(3):286–96.

45. Magill SS, Klompas M, Balk R, et al. Developing a new, national approach to surveillance for ventilator-associated events. *Crit Care Med* 2013;41:2467–75.

46. Centers for Disease Control. Ventilator-associated pneumonia (VAP) event. http://www.cdc.gov/nhsn/PDFs/pscManual/6pscVAPcurrent.pdf. Published January 2012. Accessed September 1, 2013.

47. Curley MA, Schwalenstocker E, Deshpande JK, et al. Tailoring the Institute for Health Care Improvement 100,000 Lives Campaign to pediatric settings: The example of ventilator-associated pneumonia. *Pediatr Clin North Am* 2006;53(6):1231–51.

48. Bigham MT, Amato R, Bondurrant P, et al. Ventilator-associated pneumonia in the pediatric intensive care unit: Characterizing the problem and implementing a sustainable solution. *J Pediatr* 2009;154(4):582–7.

49. Jácomo AD, Carmona F, Matsuno AK, et al. Effect of oral hygiene with 0.12% chlorhexidine gluconate on the incidence of nosocomial pneumonia in children undergoing cardiac surgery. *Infect Control Hosp Epidemiol* 2011;32(6):591–6.

50. Flanders SA, Collard HR, Saint S. Nosocomial pneumonia: State of the science. *Am J Infect Control* 2006;34(2):84–93.

51. Hess DR. Noninvasive positive-pressure ventilation and ventilator-associated pneumonia. *Respir Care* 2005;50(7):924–9; discussion 929–31.

52. Moore BM, Blumberg K, Laguna TA, et al. Incidental sinusitis in a pediatric intensive care unit. *Pediatr Crit Care Med* 2012;13(2):e64–7.

53. Agrafiotis M, Vardakas KZ, Gkegkes ID, et al. Ventilator-associated sinusitis in adults: Systemic review and meta-analysis. *Resp Med* 2012;106(8):1082–95.

54. Simon A, Khurana K Wilkesmann A, et al. Nosocomial respiratory syncytial virus infection: Impact of prospective surveillance and targeted infection control. *Int J Hyg Environ Health* 2006;209(4):317–24.

55. Gamage B, Moore D, Copes R, et al. Protecting health care workers from SARS and other respiratory pathogens: A review of the infection control literature. *Am J Infect Control* 2005;33(2):114–21.

56. Matlow AG, Wray RD, Cox PN. Nosocomial urinary tract infections in children in a pediatric intensive care unit: A follow-up after 10 years. *Pediatr Crit Care Med* 2003;4(1):74–7.

57. Rosenthal VD, Ramachandran B, Dueñas L, et al. Findings of the International Nosocomial Infection Control Consortium (IN-ICC), Part 1: Effectiveness of a multidimensional infection control approach on catheter-associated urinary tract infection rates in pediatric intensive care units of 6 developing countries. *Infect Control Hosp Epidemiol* 2012;33(7):696–703.

58. Gould CV, Umscheid CA, Agarwal RK, et al. Guideline for prevention of catheter-associated urinary tract infections 2009. Healthcare Infection Control Practices Advisory Committee, Center for Disease Control and Prevention. *Infect Control Hosp Epidemiol* 2010;31(4)319–26.

59. Langley JM, LeBlanc JC, Hanakowski M, et al. The role of Clostridium difficile and viruses as causes of nosocomial diarrhea in children. *Infect Control Hosp Epidemiol* 2002;23(11):660–4.

60. Boccia D, Stolfi I, Lana S, et al. Nosocomial necrotising enterocolitis outbreaks: Epidemiology and control measures. *Eur J Pediatr* 2001;160(6):385–91.

61. National Nosocomial Infections Surveillance (NNIS). System Report, data summary from January 1992 through June 2004, issued October 2004. *Am J Infect Control* 2004;32(8):470–85.

62. Yeung LC, Cunningham ML, Allpress AL, et al. Surgical site infections after pediatric intracranial surgery for craniofacial malformations: Frequency and risk factors. *Neurosurgery* 2005;56(4):733–9; discussion 733–9.

63. Gelabert-Gonzalez M, Ginesta-Galan V, Sernamito-Garcia R, et al. The Camino intracranial pressure device in clinical practice. Assessment in a 1000 cases. *Acta Neurochir (Wien)* 2006;148(4):435–41.

64. Dawson S. Epidural catheter infections. *J Hosp Infect* 2001;47(1):3–8.

65. Kost-Byerly S, Tobin JR, Greenberg RS, et al. Bacterial colonization and infection rate of continuous epidural catheters in children. *Anesth Analg* 1998;86(4):712–6.

66. Allpress AL, Rosenthal GL, Goodrich KM, et al. Risk factors for surgical site infections after pediatric cardiovascular surgery. *Pediatr Infect Dis J* 2004;23(3):231–4.

67. Nateghian A, Taylor G, Robinson JL. Risk factors for surgical site infections following open-heart surgery in a Canadian pediatric population. *Am J Infect Control* 2004;32(7):397–401.

68. Long CB, Shah SS, Lautenbach E, et al. Postoperative mediastinitis in children: Epidemiology, microbiology and risk factors for Gram-negative pathogens. *Pediatr Infect Dis J* 2005;24(4):315–9.

CHAPTER 93 ■ INTERNATIONAL AND EMERGING INFECTIONS

TROY E. DOMINGUEZ, CHITRA RAVISHANKAR, MIRIAM K. LAUFER, AND MARK W. HALL

International Infections

Malaria

1. Most deaths are in children <5 years of age in sub-Saharan Africa.
2. Most severe infections are caused by *Plasmodium falciparum* transmitted by *Anopheles* mosquito.
3. Some signs of severe malaria include lactic acidosis, severe anemia, respiratory distress, hypoglycemia, impaired consciousness, and prostration.
4. The level of parasitemia may not reflect true parasite burden, but >5% of parasitized red blood cells suggests severe disease in nonimmune individuals.
5. Cerebral malaria carries a high mortality rate and should be treated with parenteral antimalarials.
6. Severe malaria requires intensive care monitoring and antimicrobial treatment with agents active against *P. falciparum*.
7. ECG monitoring is necessary during quinidine or quinine therapy to assess for cardiac toxicity, including widening of the QRS and QT_C prolongation.
8. Attention to glucose level is critical, as hypoglycemia frequently complicates severe malaria and may contribute significantly to morbidity and mortality.

Typhoid Fever

9. Typhoid fever is a bacterial infection spread by the fecal–oral route without any nonhuman reservoirs.
10. Disease is prevalent in most tropical developing countries but highest on the Indian subcontinent.
11. Diarrhea is more common among children but does not occur in most cases.
12. Death occurs in cases of complicated disease: gastrointestinal bleeding, perforation, or typhoid encephalopathy.
13. Diagnosis can be difficult, as blood cultures have a low sensitivity. Bone marrow culture may have a higher yield, especially after the initiation of therapy.
14. Fluoroquinolone-resistant infections are increasing in Asia and make the treatment of the disease more complicated.
15. Empiric therapy should be IV ceftriaxone until susceptibility of the organism is known.
16. Relapse is common.

Chagas Disease

17. Infection with *Trypanosoma cruzi* causes Chagas disease.
18. Acute infection is usually nonspecific, but subclinical cardiac involvement may occur.

19. After acute infection, untreated patients enter an indeterminate phase.
20. Ten to fifteen percent of patients in the indeterminate phase go on to develop the chronic sequelae of infection: cardiomyopathy and megaviscera.
21. Treatment during the acute phase of illness prevents progression to chronic end-organ damage.

Human African Trypanosomiasis

22. Human African Trypanosomiasis is caused by *T. bruceirhodiense* (East) or *T. bruceigambiense* (West) and results in sleeping sickness.
23. In children, developmental delay may be more prominent than somnolence.
24. Acute and late-stage infections are treated differently. The presence of >5 cells/mm^3 in the cerebrospinal fluid defines late-stage infection.
25. The disease is fatal if untreated.

Leptospirosis

26. Infection with *Leptospira* species causes a chronic low-grade infection in animal hosts who subsequently excrete the organisms into the environment, where they can survive for prolonged periods of time.
27. In urban environments, small rodents are important hosts.
28. The majority of leptospirosis infections are asymptomatic or mild.
29. Icteric leptospirosis (Weil disease) is characterized by renal failure, icterus, and hemorrhagic manifestations.
30. Treatment with penicillin, ceftriaxone, or doxycycline is recommended for symptomatic disease, although the role of therapy has not been definitively established.
31. Mortality rates have been reported to be 5%–25% in hospitalized patients.

Hantavirus

32. Hemorrhagic fever with renal syndrome (HFRS) can be seen with other hantaviruses in Europe and Asia.
33. Infection with American hantaviruses can result in hantavirus pulmonary syndrome (HPS).
34. Rodents are the hosts for disease and transmit disease to humans.
35. HFRS is characterized by fever, renal failure, and hemorrhage and is classically associated with Hantaan or Dobrava viruses.

36 HPS in North America is usually manifest by fever and respiratory disease, but renal failure is common in cases of HPS in South America.

37 The overall mortality rate for HPS in North America is 33%. The mortality rate for HFRS is 5%–10%, but varies with infecting serotype.

Polio

38 Polio is an ongoing public health problem with occasional outbreaks occurring in the developing world.

39 Most polio infections are unapparent and paralytic poliomyelitis is seen in only 1% of all infections.

40 Patients with the paralytic form often require mechanical ventilation for prolonged periods and may benefit from tracheostomy.

41 With no known specific antiviral therapy, care is primarily supportive.

42 Patients with mild weakness may have full recovery, although those with flaccid paralysis usually have residual weakness.

Emerging Diseases

West Nile Virus

43 Human infection is found throughout the United States, except in Alaska and Hawaii, with increasing incidence and severity.

44 West Nile virus (WNV) is a mosquito-borne infection transmitted to humans from bird hosts.

45 Most commonly, infection with WNV results in West Nile fever.

46 West Nile neuroinvasive disease (WNND) develops in <1% of those infected.

47 Weakness commonly occurs with WNND, along with meningitis, encephalitis, or meningoencephalitis.

48 The mortality rate is 4%–14%, with a higher mortality rate seen in patients with encephalitis.

Avian Influenza

49 Avian influenza, including the H5N1 and H7N9 strains, is associated with severe respiratory failure in Southeast Asia and China.

50 Avian influenza is commonly associated with exposure to domestic poultry and wild waterfowl.

51 Suspected cases of person-to-person transmission have been reported. A more highly transmissible strain of the virus would be capable of producing a global pandemic.

52 Symptoms include fever, diarrhea, lower respiratory tract symptoms, and respiratory failure.

53 Treatment with oseltamivir is recommended for treatment and prophylaxis.

54 If a suspected case of avian influenza is identified, isolation measures should be taken immediately, and the laboratory that is processing diagnostic specimens should be warned.

55 The overall morality is ~30%–50%.

Novel Coronavirus Infections

56 Severe acute respiratory syndrome (SARS) was first identified in 2003, and no cases have been reported since 2004.

57 SARS is caused by a novel coronavirus (SARS-CoV), which causes a triphasic course of disease.

58 Infection-control practices are effective at preventing transmission, as the disease is not contagious prior to the onset of symptoms.

59 Children are only rarely affected with the severe form of the disease. Only 2 of 47 children reported to have been infected with the SARS virus during the outbreak required mechanical ventilation.

60 The Middle Eastern Respiratory Syndrome coronavirus represents a potentially important emerging pathogen.

Ebola Virus Disease

61 The ebola virus disease (EVD) outbreak of 2014, centered in the West African countries of Sierra Leone, Liberia, and Guinea, was notable for its massive scale and for the spread of EVD to the United States and Europe.

62 EVD is spread through contact with infected bodily fluids and results in a febrile illness after a 2- to 21-day incubation period.

63 Severe vomiting and diarrhea, hemorrhage, and organ failure typically result.

64 Treatment is largely supportive, including massive fluid resuscitation and organ support therapies, though convalescent plasma, chimeric antibodies, and antivirals may have a role.

65 Rigorous isolation and personal protective equipment are essential for containing outbreaks and protecting staff.

66 While the case fatality rate in developing countries is typically very high, mortality rates in the setting of modern critical care are largely unknown.

Infections are the leading cause of death among children worldwide. Some of the most common infections (e.g., pneumonia and gastrointestinal infections) occur in both developing and industrialized countries. Yet, some life-threatening infections are predominantly transmitted in developing countries due to poor sanitation, the absence of adequate public health infrastructure, and a high density of disease-carrying vectors. Several of the "international" infections discussed in this chapter, such as leptospirosis and hantavirus, also occur in North America.

When a child who has been abroad is evaluated for an illness, many infections cannot be distinguished on clinical grounds alone. Most of the illnesses described in this chapter have a protean presentation, including fever and abdominal and/or respiratory complaints. In addition to the standard intensive care unit (ICU) evaluation, a careful travel history along with a detailed account of potential water, food, and animal exposures can help to narrow the differential diagnosis and point toward the appropriate diagnostic assays and empiric therapy (**Table 93.1**). Most studies of illnesses among returned travelers have focused on the adult population. Diarrhea is one of the most common complaints following travel and frequently requires hospitalization among children (1). Among international travelers, gastroenteritis rarely requires intensive care management.

Emerging infections that originated outside the United States will be discussed. West Nile virus (WNV) reached the east coast of the United States in the late 1990s and has subsequently spread throughout the country. Avian influenza, an infection with the potential for a global pandemic, is currently

TABLE 93.1

CAUSES OF SYSTEMIC FEBRILE ILLNESS AMONG RETURNED TRAVELERS

■ DIAGNOSIS	■ CARIBBEAN	■ CENTRAL AMERICA	■ SOUTH AMERICA	■ SUB-SAHARAN AFRICA	■ SOUTH OR CENTRAL ASIA	■ SOUTHEAST ASIA
Malaria	+	++	++	+++	++	++
Dengue	++	++	++	–/+	++	++
Mononucleosis	+	+	+	+	+	+
Rickettsia	–	–	–	+	+/–	+
Typhoid fever	+	+	+	–/+	++	+

Adapted from Freedman DO, Weld LH, Kozarsky PE, et al. Spectrum of disease and relation to place of exposure among ill returned travelers. *N Engl J Med* 2006;354:119–30.

concentrated in Asia but is spreading via migratory birds throughout the world. Lastly, while hemorrhagic fevers are discussed in detail in Chapter 89, a brief overview of the 2014 ebola virus epidemic will also be presented.

INTERNATIONAL INFECTIONS

Malaria

Mechanism of Disease

Epidemiology. Malaria is the most significant parasitic disease in humans. An estimated 215 million infections occur each year, and these result in an estimated 655,000 deaths. Most severe infections and deaths occur in children <5 years of age in Africa. In developed countries, malaria is also the most common cause of febrile illness without localizing signs in returned travelers from developing countries (2). Infection rates appear to be increasing in travelers, with 1700 such cases reported to the Centers for Disease Control and Prevention (CDC) in 2010, the majority of which (65%) originated in Asia (19%) and the Caribbean/Americas (15%) (www.cdc.gov).

Malaria is transmitted by a bite from the female anopheline mosquito. The areas of highest transmission are found in sub-Saharan Africa, although transmission also occurs in many regions of South Asia, Southeast Asia, the South Pacific, and Central and South America (**Fig. 93.1**). Local outbreaks of malaria in the United States occur almost every year due to imported malarial cases infecting local anopheline mosquitoes (3).

Four species of *Plasmodium* cause malaria infections in humans: *P. falciparum, P. vivax, P. malariae,* and *P. ovale.* Worldwide, infection with *P. falciparum* is most common and is exclusively responsible for nearly all life-threatening malaria disease. The second most common species is *P. vivax.*

Repeated exposure to malaria infection, as experienced by individuals who live in malaria-endemic areas, causes a state of "semi-immunity." Patients are still at risk for infection, but their immune systems are able to control the level of parasitemia, and severe disease is extremely rare. In the areas of highest transmission, semi-immunity occurs around the age of 5 years. In areas of lower transmission, it is delayed or absent. Semi-immunity is lost within 6–12 months of leaving an endemic area (4), which is a particular concern for people born in malaria-endemic areas who are living in developed countries. They may return to their country of origin expecting to still be protected from severe disease and fail to take preventive measures, when in fact they are nearly as susceptible as any malaria-naïve traveler.

Hemoglobinopathies commonly found in African and Asian populations are thought to be the result of evolutionary pressure exerted by malaria over time (5). Red blood cell polymorphisms, including hemoglobins S, C, and E, glucose-6-phosphate dehydrogenase deficiency, pyruvate kinase deficiency, and α-thalassemia, are associated with decreased risk of severe malaria disease. The Duffy antigen located on the surface of the red blood cell is necessary for invasion by *P. vivax.* Most Africans lack this antigen, and, as result, *P. vivax* is extremely rare in Africa.

Etiology. All human *Plasmodia* species follow a similar life cycle. The *Anopheles* mosquito injects sporozoites into the human during the process of taking a blood meal. The sporozoites immediately travel to the liver. In the hepatic stage, which lasts 1–2 weeks, the parasites undergo asexual reproduction and become schizonts; no symptoms are associated with this exo-erythrocytic life-cycle stage. When the schizonts in the liver rupture, merozoites emerge into the bloodstream and begin the erythrocytic stage of infection that is associated with clinical disease. Merozoites infect erythrocytes and mature into trophozoites; these become schizonts. Rupture of infected red cells that contain the schizont forms produces more merozoites capable of invading more red blood cells.

The cycle of multiplication, infection, and rupture results in the clinical manifestations of malaria. The burden of malarial parasites multiplies 12- to 15-fold with each erythrocytic cycle. With *P. falciparum*, these cycles of asexual reproduction last ~48 hours. Some merozoites differentiate into male or female gametocytes that can be taken up during a blood meal by an *Anopheles* mosquito and undergo sexual reproduction in the mosquito midgut. The offspring of the sexual reproduction phase enter the mosquito salivary glands as sporozoites, ready to be transferred to a human host.

Severe disease from *P. falciparum* infection is thought to be due to the ability of infected red cells to adhere to the vessel walls in the microvasculature, a process called *sequestration*, which is associated with end-organ damage. Sequestration in the brain microcirculation is associated with the most dreaded complication of infection—cerebral malaria. Sequestration occurs in other organs. In children in endemic areas, sequestration is prominent in the gastrointestinal tract and the skin (6).

Clinical Presentation and Differential Diagnosis

The initial presentation of uncomplicated malaria is a nonlocalizing febrile illness with fever, chills, headache, and diaphoresis. The fevers may be paroxysmal, reflecting the replicating cycle of the parasites, although the pattern of fever cycles is more common among the non-falciparum species. Other common symptoms include nausea, vomiting, diarrhea, malaise, myalgias, dizziness, diarrhea, and dry cough.

Patients without sufficient antimalarial immunity who present with uncomplicated infection can rapidly deteriorate and develop severe disease, or they may initially present with severe disease. The World Health Organization (WHO) has suggested that the following clinical features help to identify patients at high risk of death: prostration, impaired consciousness, acidotic breathing, multiple convulsions, circulatory collapse, pulmonary edema, abnormal bleeding, jaundice, and hemoglobinuria. Laboratory results that are associated with severe disease include severe anemia, hypoglycemia, acidosis, renal impairment, hyperlactatemia, and hyperparasitemia. The definitions for each of these criteria are listed in **Table 93.2**.

The classic syndrome of severe disease among children is cerebral malaria, as discussed in detail in Chapter 91. Briefly, however, cerebral malaria represents a severe complication of infection with *P. falciparum* and is characterized by coma thought to be due to sludging of parasitized red blood cells in the cerebral microcirculation along with central nervous system (CNS) inflammation (7). Cerebral edema, seizures, intracranial hypertension, and cranial nerve abnormalities are typical. Prompt use of parenteral antimalarial drugs, seizure control, and supportive care are essential. Patients with any impairment of consciousness should be treated as if they have cerebral malaria. Cerebral malaria is fatal if untreated, and

mortality rates of 15%–20% are reported with parenteral antimalarial drugs. No effective malaria-specific neuroprotective strategies have thus far been identified. Residual CNS deficits are common in survivors.

An important feature and marker of disease severity in children with severe malaria is the presence of a metabolic acidosis that reflects several metabolic derangements. The acidosis is commonly found in children with cerebral malaria but is also associated with anemia, hypoglycemia, or hypovolemia. An elevated plasma lactate is often seen with the acidosis. Studies in adults have demonstrated increased production of lactate and elevated lactate-to-pyruvate ratios, suggesting impaired tissue substrate delivery. Hypovolemia that leads to tissue hypoperfusion may be a common cause of metabolic acidosis in children, although experts disagree about this. In patients with severe anemia, the low oxygen-carrying capacity may lead to oxygen consumption and delivery mismatch, with anaerobic metabolism and metabolic acidosis.

Hypoglycemia occurs in 10%–30% of children with severe disease. Parasitized red blood cells consume glucose and increase the demand for glucose in the host. Impairment in the gluconeogenic pathway has been observed in adults with severe malaria and may be an important contributor to the pathogenesis of hypoglycemia and lactic acidosis (8). In addition, the hypoglycemia in adults frequently occurs after the initiation of therapy and is associated with hyperinsulinism.

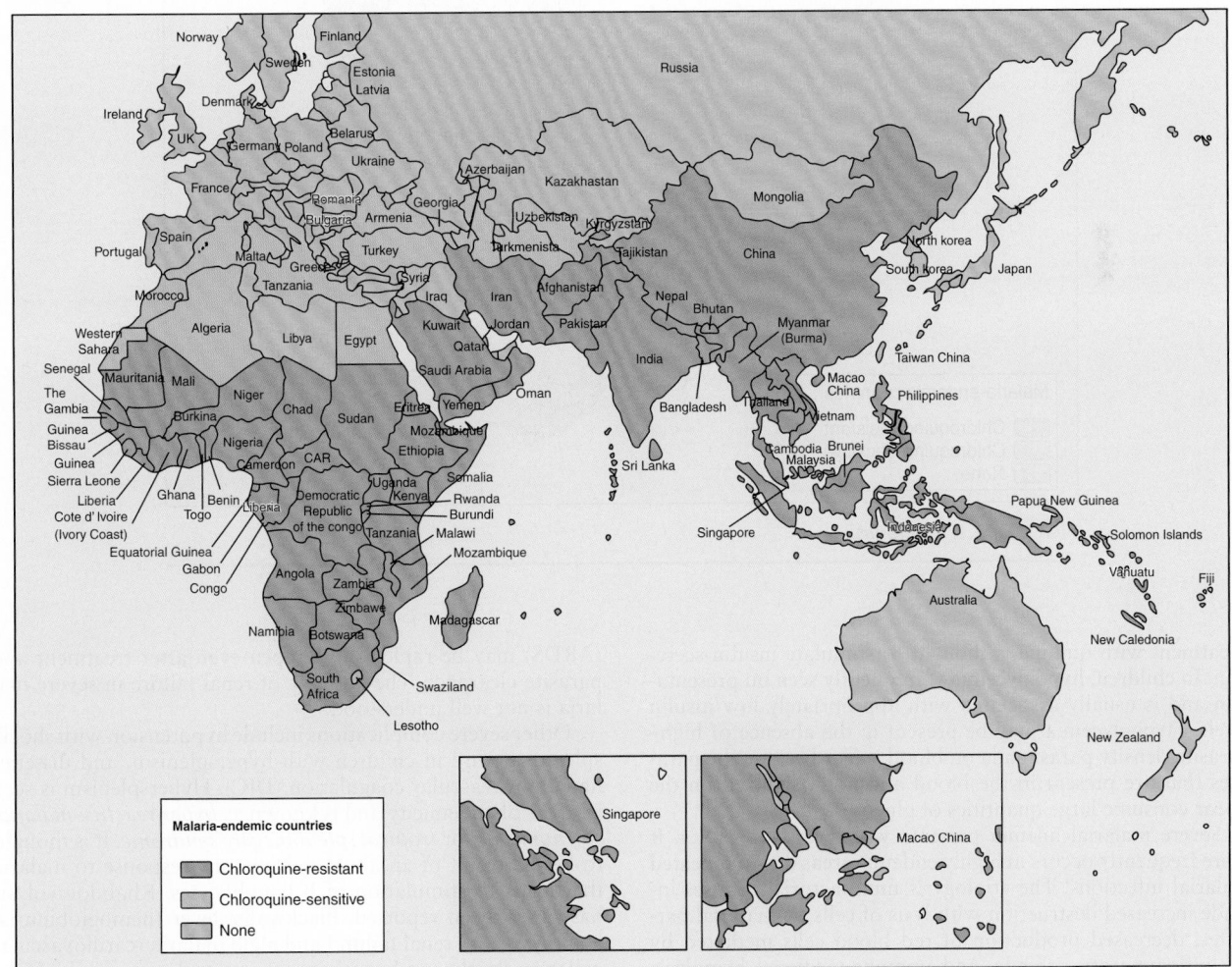

FIGURE 93.1. Distribution of malaria (all species). (From Centers for Disease Control and Prevention. http://wwwn.cdc.gov/travel/yellowBookCh4-Malaria.aspx)

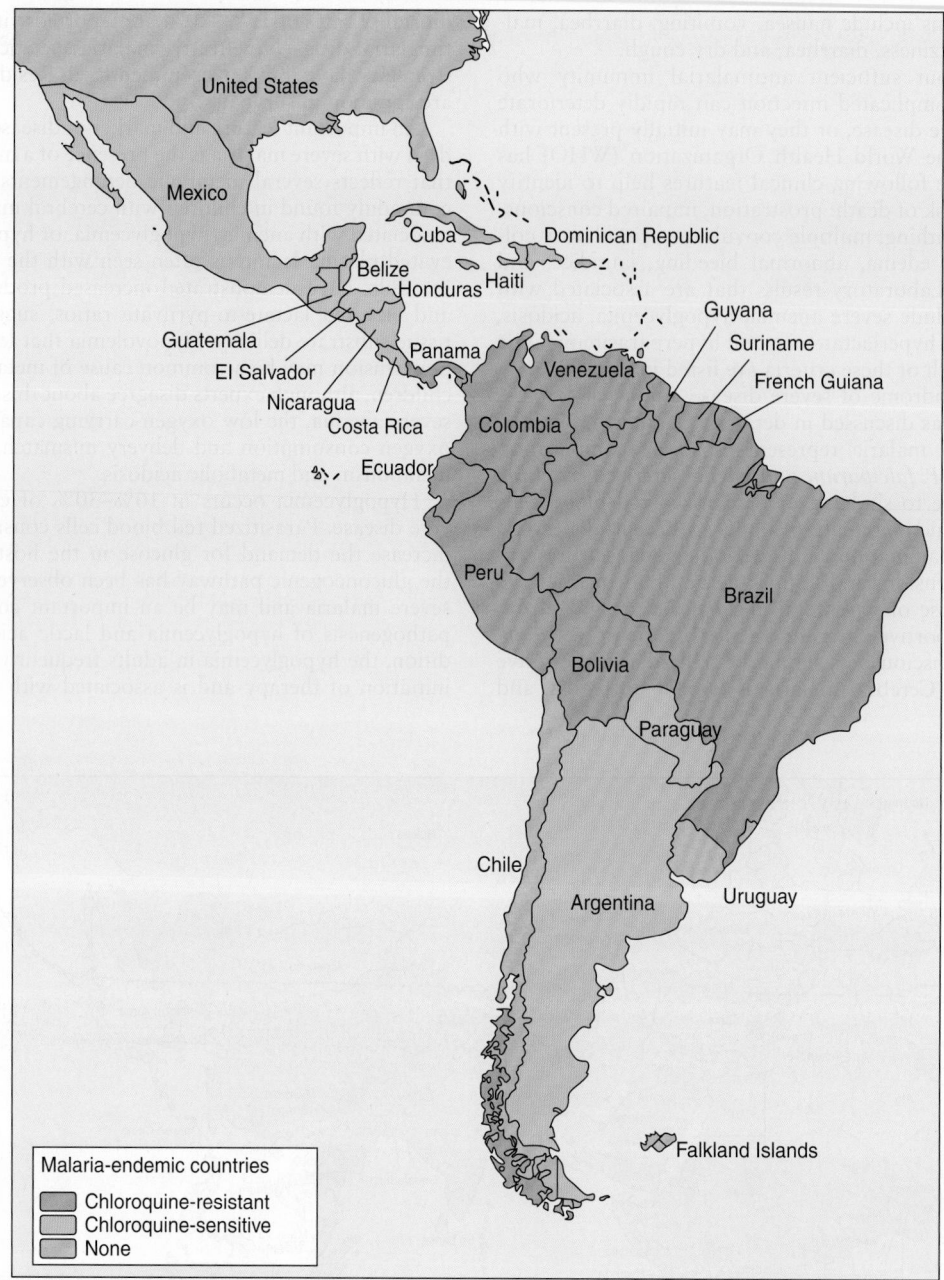

Malaria-endemic countries
- Chloroquine-resistant
- Chloroquine-sensitive
- None

FIGURE 93.1. (*continued*)

Treatment with quinine is thought to stimulate insulin secretion. In children, hypoglycemia is frequently seen on presentation and is usually associated with appropriately low insulin levels. Hypoglycemia may be present in the absence of high–parasite-density parasitemia on blood smear because the parasites that are present in the blood and not visualized on the smear consume large quantities of glucose.

Severe malarial anemia presents with profound pallor. It more frequently occurs in highly endemic areas due to repeated malarial infections. The etiology is multifactorial. Causes include increased destruction with lysis of cells by malarial parasites, decreased production of red blood cells mediated by the inflammatory cascade, and immune-mediated hemolysis of both infected and uninfected cells. Lung and renal disease can be seen in children with severe malaria. The progression to acute lung injury or acute respiratory distress syndrome

(ARDS) may be rapid, and happen even after treatment and parasite clearance. The etiology of renal failure in severe malaria is not well understood.

Other severe complications include hypotension with shock, splenic rupture in children with hypersplenism, and disseminated intravascular coagulation (DIC). Hypersplenism is seen in areas of endemicity and is known as *hyper-reactive malarial splenomegaly* or *tropical splenomegaly syndrome*. It is thought to be the result of an abnormal immune response to malaria that leads to stimulation of B lymphocytes. Rhabdomyolysis has rarely been reported. Blackwater fever (hemoglobinuria, hemolysis, and renal failure) and algid malaria (cardiovascular collapse, shock, and hypothermia) are rarely seen in children.

Laboratory findings in patients with severe malaria include thrombocytopenia, hyperbilirubinemia, anemia, and elevated hepatic transaminases. The white blood cell count can

TABLE 93.2

④ DEFINITION OF POOR PROGNOSTIC SIGNS IN SEVERE MALARIA

Prostration	Inability to sit in a child who was previously able to sit. In infants, can be defined as unable to feed
Impaired consciousness	Coma that lasts at least 30 min after a seizure, with no other cause identified (e.g., meningitis, hypoglycemia). Impairment may be less severe
Respiratory distress (acidotic breathing)	In the absence of abnormalities on auscultation or radiography, normal oxygen saturation
Multiple convulsions	>2 in 24 h
Circulatory collapse	Hypotension with cold, clammy skin
Pulmonary edema	Not due to volume overload
Abnormal bleeding	Spontaneous mucosal bleeding or laboratory evidence of disseminated intravascular coagulopathy
Jaundice	Detected clinically or >3 g/dL (50 μmol/L)
Hemoglobinuria	Macroscopic
Severe anemia	Normocytic anemia with hemoglobin <5 g/dL or hematocrit <15%
Hypoglycemia	<40 g/dL or 2.2 mmol/L
Acidosis	Arterial or capillary pH <7.3 or bicarbonate <15 mmol/L
Renal impairment	Urine output <0.5 mL/kg/h, failure to respond to rehydration, creatinine>3.0 mg/dL
Hyperlactatemia	>5 mmol/L
Hyperparasitemia	>4%–5% in nonimmune children and adults

be normal or low with a left shift. Other nonspecific markers of inflammation such as C-reactive protein and erythrocyte sedimentation rate are usually elevated. Coagulation abnormalities may be present due to DIC. Hypokalemia is seen in ~40% of patients after admission and is thought to be caused by renal potassium loss (9).

In patients returning from an endemic area with a febrile illness, a high suspicion for malarial infection is needed. The initial presentation is often mistaken for influenza. For travelers returning from tropical countries, a variety of nonspecific febrile illnesses might be considered, including typhoid fever, dengue, leptospirosis, and rickettsial diseases. It may be difficult to rule out bacterial sepsis as the etiology of the illness until the blood culture results are available.

Diagnosis. The diagnosis of malaria is established by examining thick and thin blood smears stained with a 3% Giemsa stain. In thick smears, parasites are identified after lysis of the red blood cells. This method is more sensitive than a thin smear (limits of detection, 5–20 parasites/mcL vs. 50–200 parasites/mcL, respectively, for an experienced microscopist). In a thin smear, the parasites are visualized within the erythrocytes (**Fig. 93.2**). This method is useful for determination of species, as the morphology of the parasites and of the infected cells can be appreciated, and for quantification of very high parasitemia if the thick smear is too dense. A single negative set of malaria smears does not rule out the diagnosis of malaria, as parasites move between the bloodstream and sequestration within organs and tissues. Three sets of thick and thin smears 12–24 hours apart have been recommended for establishing a diagnosis in patients with a high likelihood of malaria. Rapid testing with dipstick immunoassays can be used to diagnose malaria or to identify species, though confirmatory microscopy is recommended.

To assess the full extent of the disease, all patients should be assessed for severe disease. Blood glucose, pH, or bicarbonate level, creatinine, and complete blood count must be measured to help classify severity. Blood cultures should also be obtained to evaluate the possibility of a concomitant bacteremia (10,11).

Clinical Management

Specific Antimalarial Therapy. For uncomplicated malaria, the decision for specific antimicrobial therapies depends upon

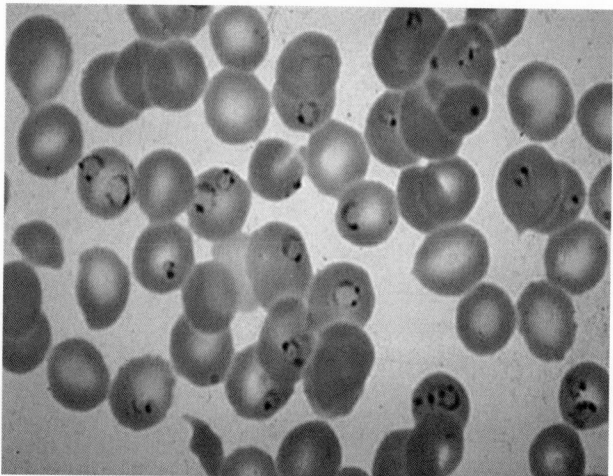

FIGURE 93.2. Malaria thin smear showing parasites within erythrocytes. Courtesy of Dr. Terrie Taylor.

the infecting species and the geographic source of the infection. The appropriate therapies for uncomplicated disease are listed in **Table 93.3**. Although medication can be administered orally, it is recommended that patients remain in the hospital until parasite clearance can be documented, allowing providers to ensure compliance with the medication and monitor for any deterioration in the clinical status.

⑥ Patients with any signs of severe disease should initially be treated with parenteral therapy. Quinine is the mainstay of therapy in endemic areas, although it is not available in the United States. Quinidine is the recommended drug in the United States. As its use as an antiarrhythmic agent is becoming obsolete, pediatric intensive care units (PICUs) should identify a source of quinidine so that they can be prepared for a patient with severe malaria.

The antimalarial treatment regimen for quinidine has not been well studied, and many recommendations are based on recommended dosing of quinine. A loading dose of quinidine is given at the initiation of treatment if the patient did not

TABLE 93.3

TREATMENT OF UNCOMPLICATED AND SEVERE MALARIA

■ DIAGNOSIS	■ THERAPY
Uncomplicated malaria with *P. falciparum* or unknown species: chloroquine sensitive (*only* Central America west of the Panama Canal, Haiti, Dominican Republic)	**Chloroquine phosphate** 10 mg base/kg initial dose, followed by 5 mg base/kg at 6, 24, and 48 h Total dose 25 mg base/kg Maximum adult dose: 1500 mg base
Uncomplicated malaria with *P. falciparum* or unknown species: chloroquine resistant or unknown resistance (all regions except for those mentioned above)	**Atovaquone-proguanil** Adult tabs: 250 mg atovaquone/100 mg proguanil Pediatric tablets: 62.5 mg atovaquone/25 mg proguanil Doses given once per day for 3 days: 5–8 kg: 2 pediatric tabs 9–10 kg: 3 pediatric tabs 11–20 kg: 1 adult tab 21–30 kg: 2 adult tab 31–40 kg: 3 adult tabs >40 kg: 4 adult tabs **Artemether–lumefantrine** 1 tab = 20 mg artemether and 120 mg lumefantrine A total of 6 doses given over 3 days with the second dose following the first by 8 h then 1 dose po bid for the next 2 days 5–<15 kg: 1 tab per dose 15–<25 kg: 2 tabs per dose 25–<35 kg: 3 tabs per dose ≥35 kg: 4 tabs per dose **Quinine sulfate** 8.3 mg base/kg PO TID for 3–7 days Maximum adult dose: 542 mg base/dose *PLUS* one of the following for 7 days **Doxycycline** 2.2 mg/kg PO BID Maximum adult dose: 100 mg/dose **Tetracycline** 25 mg/kg/d divided QID Maximum adult dose 250 mg/dose **Clindamycin** 20 mg/kg/d divided TID **Mefloquine** 15 mg salt/kg PO initial dose, followed by 10 mg salt/kg PO 6–12 h after initial dose Total dose: 25 mg salt/kg Maximum adult dose: 1250 mg salt
Complicated/severe malaria	**Quinidine gluconate** *Continuous infusion*: 6.25 mg base/kg IV over 1–2 h, followed by 0.0125 mg base/kg/min continuous infusion for at least 24 h *Every 8-h dosing*: 15 mg base/kg over 4 h, followed by 7.5 mg base/kg every 8 h Switch to oral therapy when parasite density is <1% Complete 3–7 days of quinidine therapy *PLUS* **doxycycline, tetracycline, or clindamycin** as above. If patient cannot tolerate oral medication, doxycycline or clindamycin may be administered intravenously

Please refer to www.cdc.gov for additional region- or species-specific modifications to this table and/or call the CDC Malaria Hotline at (855) 856-4713, (770) 488-7788, or (770) 488-7100.

receive mefloquine in the previous 12 hours or over 40 mg/kg of quinidine in the previous 48 hours. The treatment regimen is listed in **Table 93.3**. Once the level of parasitemia falls below 1% and the child is able to take oral intake, oral quinidine may be administered at the same dose to complete a total 3- to 7-day course. Clindamycin, tetracycline, or doxycycline is usually administered at the same time as the quinidine. These drugs can be administered orally if the patient can tolerate oral medication and should be continued for 7 days.

Cardiac monitoring is essential during IV quinidine administration due to the risk of prolonged QT, widening of the QRS, and hypotension. An electrocardiogram should be obtained at baseline before beginning the medication. The quinidine infusion should be decreased or stopped if an increase of >50% in the width of the QRS complex, prolongation of the QTc to >0.6 seconds or >25%, or hypotension is seen.

Malaria smears should be repeated every 8 hours when patients have signs or symptoms of severe disease. Quinine and quinidine are slow-acting medications, and it is common for parasites to increase in the blood for the first 24 hours after initiation of therapy. Once the patient has had a good clinical response and has a parasite density <1%, malaria smears can be obtained once or twice daily.

The artemisinin-based therapies are derived from the Chinese medicinal plant, *Artemisia annua*. These drugs are more rapid-acting than most previously developed antimalarial agents and have significantly fewer adverse effects. In addition, resistance to these drugs has not been detected. Artemisinin derivatives are being used to treat severe disease in the United States and abroad. Artemether–lumefantrine was approved by the Food and Drug Administration (FDA) in 2009, and is dosed by weight in children. The parenteral drug artesunate is available upon request on an emergency basis through the CDC to hospitalized patients with severe malaria in the United States who have high levels of parasites in the blood, who cannot take oral medications, or who cannot tolerate (or have failed) quinidine.

Supportive Care. In addition to the specific antimalarial therapy, adequate supportive care is essential to survival. Hypoglycemia is a common complication that leads to increased **8** morbidity and mortality. If hypoglycemia is present, it should be corrected with dextrose infusions. Maintenance fluid administration should include dextrose concentrations sufficient to prevent the development of hypoglycemia in patients with normal glucose levels at presentation.

Fluid and electrolyte management is especially important in children with severe malaria. Metabolic acidosis can often be corrected with volume replacement. In patients with impaired consciousness or any other suspicion of cerebral malaria, volume resuscitation should proceed cautiously, as cerebral edema is common. Indeed, the results of the 2011 Fluid Expansion as Supportive Therapy trial suggested that rapid fluid resuscitation in children with severe malaria-related anemia (hemoglobin <5 g/dL) may be associated with increased mortality regardless of the use of crystalloid or colloid (12). In the absence of intrinsic renal disease, renal output is a good measure of fluid status. Children who remain oliguric after a total of 40 mL/kg bolus infusion of saline should have a central catheter placed to monitor intravascular status (13). Potassium levels may fall during treatment due to an improvement in acid–base status and rise in pH.

The treatment of oliguric renal failure can be accomplished using hemodialysis/hemofiltration or peritoneal dialysis. In a study of adult patients with infection-associated acute renal failure, patients undergoing hemofiltration had a more rapid resolution of acidosis, shorter duration of renal replacement therapy, and lower mortality rate than those treated with peritoneal dialysis (14). The use of dopamine or epinephrine infusions to improve renal blood flow has not been shown to be of benefit (15).

Transfusion. Packed red blood cell transfusions are indicated for patients with symptomatic anemia. The role of exchange transfusion is controversial. No adequate comparative trials have been performed to document a benefit. Anecdotal experience suggests that in cases of high parasite density (>10%), or severe end-organ damage that does not improve with antimalarial therapy, exchange transfusion may be of benefit. The CDC previously recommended considering exchange transfusion if the parasite density is >10% or in the presence of cerebral malaria, non–volume overload pulmonary edema, or renal insufficiency, with the exchanges continuing until the parasitemia falls below 1%. As the result of a 2013 analysis of exchange transfusions for severe malaria, which showed no survival benefit, the CDC no longer recommends the use of exchange transfusions in this setting.

Outcomes

The global mortality rate for patients with severe malaria is 15%–30% with most of the deaths occurring within 24 hours of admission, though reported mortality rates fell by 42% between 2000 and 2012. In malaria-endemic areas, where resources are somewhat limited, impaired consciousness and respiratory distress are strongly associated with death. Among returned travelers who were treated in Europe for *P. falciparum*, the mortality rate was found to be 5%–10% (16). Where malaria is not endemic, increased morbidity and death are often associated with the failure to initially diagnose malaria.

P. falciparum infection has no chronic phase. Once the infection has resolved, it does not emerge again. Recurrence of parasitemia in a patient living in a nonendemic area is due to failed initial therapy. The only long-term sequela of *P. falciparum* infection that has been well described is the neurologic impairment following cerebral malaria.

Future Directions—Malaria

Vaccination against malaria has proven very challenging, though phase I and phase II trials of subunit vaccines are ongoing. Prevention efforts related to mosquito eradication and bite prevention (e.g., insecticide-treated bed netting) have proven effective.

Typhoid

Mechanism of Disease

Epidemiology. Typhoid fever is an enteric fever syndrome caused by *Salmonella enterica* serotype Typhi and occasionally by *S. enterica* serotype Paratyphi. These organisms are only carried by humans, and transmission usually occurs via contaminated food or water. Typhoid fever can be found in many **9** tropical developing countries, as it is a result of poor water sanitation. Over 20 million new cases are reported each year. The highest burden is in Asia, followed by Latin America and Africa (17). Nearly 6000 cases of typhoid fever occur annually in the United States, with over half of returned travelers who develop **10** typhoid fever reporting travel to the Indian subcontinent (18).

The disease afflicts people living in endemic areas as well as travelers to the area due to food- and water-borne exposure. Children <5 years of age are more likely to develop severe forms of the illness and require hospitalization.

Etiology. *S. typhi* is a Gram-negative rod in the family *Enterobacteriaceae*. The organism is ingested, passes through the intestine into the mesenteric lymph nodes, and may travel to the liver and spleen. The organisms replicate in these tissues, usually for 7–14 days, until they enter the bloodstream. The symptoms of typhoid fever begin with the bacteremic phase. The bacteria travel through the blood to cause secondary infections in the liver, spleen, gall bladder, bone marrow, and Peyer patches of the terminal ileum. Although *S. typhi* produces exotoxin, typhoid fever has a remarkably low case fatality rate of <1%. Mortality is a result of unusual complications of the infection.

Clinical Presentation and Differential Diagnosis

The typical presentation of typhoid fever is fever, chills vomiting, anorexia, myalgia, and nonfocal abdominal pain. The fever rises slowly, and as it reaches its peak, it is sustained, unlike the paroxysms of fever typical of malaria. Diarrhea is **11** found in 8%–35% of cases and is more common in children. Although this is a disease that begins with an enteric exposure, constipation may be a presenting complaint.

Physical examination often reveals hepatosplenomegaly and abdominal pain. *Rose spots* are the typical rash of typhoid fever. They are 2–4 mm wide blanching erythematous papules usually found on the trunk. They are frequently transient and may be difficult to see on individuals with dark skin. Relative bradycardia in the face of high fever is typically associated with typhoid fever, although this is not a reliable finding.

CNS manifestations are variable. An "apathetic affect" is common, and intermittent episodes of confusion can occur in the absence of direct infection of the CNS. Altered mental status is a manifestation of typhoid encephalopathy, one of the severe complications of typhoid fever. Seizures may occur in young children.

Laboratory findings are nonspecific. The white blood cell count is often slightly low, although young children may have leukocytosis. Mild increases in liver function tests are common. In severe disease, coagulopathy may be present, with thrombocytopenia and signs of DIC.

Complications of typhoid fever usually occur late in the course of the illness, 1–2 weeks after the onset of symptoms in 10%–15% of patients. Gastrointestinal bleeding is common, but severe bleeding that requires transfusion and possibly surgery is a rare, but life-threatening, form of the disease. Intestinal perforation usually occurs in the ileum, as this is the site of the greatest bacterial replication. Typhoid encephalopathy is usually accompanied by shock and carries a very high mortality rate.

The differential diagnosis depends on the precise travel and exposure history of the patient. Malaria is frequently the leading alternative diagnosis because typhoid and malaria coexist in many regions, and they are among the leading causes of fever without localizing signs in returned travelers. The pattern of fever may distinguish the two diseases: in typhoid, the fever rises gradually and is sustained, while malaria is associated with sudden-onset paroxysms of fever. However, treatment for both infections may be indicated as evaluation is under way. Other diseases to consider include bacterial sepsis of other etiologies, leptospirosis, rickettsial disease, dengue, hepatitis, Epstein–Barr virus, typhus, brucellosis, and tularemia.

Diagnosis. The diagnosis of typhoid fever is challenging. The sensitivity of blood culture has been reported to be as low as 40% but can be as high as 80% when repeat cultures are obtained. The best sensitivity is achieved when large-volume specimens are collected and during the first week of illness. Bone marrow culture is more sensitive than standard blood culture. It remains positive beyond the first week of illness, even after the initiation of antimicrobial therapy.

In endemic areas, the Widal serologic test is used to diagnose typhoid fever. The test is neither reliable nor specific and is therefore not recommended for use in developed countries where other options are available (19,20). Currently, no approved rapid tests exist to diagnose typhoid fever.

Clinical Management

Fluoroquinolones and third-generation cephalosporins are the medications of choice for empiric therapy for typhoid fever. If cultures are positive and the susceptibility patterns are known, treatment may be tailored to the susceptibility pattern of the specific organism. However, the advantage of completing therapy with a fluoroquinolone is that a decreased incidence of chronic intestinal carriage is seen with this class of treatment. For fluoroquinolone-susceptible infections, 5-day duration is sufficient for therapy of uncomplicated disease.

The emergence of fluoroquinolone-resistant *S. typhi* has complicated the treatment of typhoid fever. The problem is most prominent in South Asia and Southeast Asia. Infections with organisms that demonstrate in vitro resistance to the quinolone nalidixic acid and have minimum inhibitory concentrations of fluoroquinolones, such as ciprofloxacin, within the susceptible range, have diminished clinical response to fluoroquinolone therapy. Therefore, organisms that are nalidixic acid-resistant should be managed as fluoroquinolone-resistant infections (21). Treatment of resistant infections requires 10–14 days of therapy with fluoroquinolones at the maximum dose or third-generation cephalosporins. Azithromycin for 5–7 days has shown to be effective against fluoroquinolone-resistant *S. typhi* and successfully eliminates intestinal carriage (22,23). Recommended therapies for typhoid fever are listed in **Table 93.4**.

Hospitalization is required for young children, as they are at higher risk for complication, and for any patients who are suspected of having complicated disease. Persistent vomiting and severe diarrhea are also indications for hospitalization. It may be prudent to hospitalize most patients with typhoid fever for parenteral therapy until the antimicrobial susceptibility is known and an acceptable oral therapy can be selected.

Severe disease requires parenteral therapy for a minimum of 10 days. Controlled clinical trials have demonstrated a benefit of the addition of dexamethasone for treatment of severe typhoid with delirium, obtundation, or shock (3 mg/kg infusion over 1 hour, followed by 1 mg/kg every 6 hours for 8 doses) (24). If dexamethasone is administered, providers should be aware that further intestinal complications may be masked. Severe intestinal bleeding or perforation requires hemodynamic stabilization and surgery. In cases of perforation, the intestine should be explored for additional sites of perforation.

TABLE 93.4

TREATMENT OF TYPHOID FEVER

	■ DRUG	■ DOSE (mg/kg/d)	■ DURATION (d)
Empiric	Ceftriaxone	60	7–14
Fully susceptible	Ciprofloxacin or ofloxacin	15	5–7
	Amoxicillin (second line)	75–100	14
	Trimethoprim/sulfamethoxazole (second line)	8/40	14
Multidrug resistant	Ceftriaxone	60	10–14
	Azithromycin	8–10	7
	Ciprofloxacin or ofloxacin (nalidixic acid–*susceptible* infection)	15	5–7
	Ciprofloxacin or ofloxacin (nalidixic acid–*resistant* infection)	20	10–14

Outcomes

16 Relapse occurs in 5%–10% of appropriately treated infections. The organism is generally identical to the initial infection, although the symptoms are milder. The same treatment can be repeated. Relapse is more common with fluoroquinolone-resistant infections.

Excretion of *S. typhi* can persist beyond the clinical illness. Chronic carriage is defined as excretion for greater than 3 months. This is a rare occurrence among children. If it occurs, prolonged treatment with ciprofloxacin or the combination of amoxicillin and probenecid is recommended for eradication.

Future Directions—Typhoid

The fact that *S. paratyphi* is becoming an increasingly important cause of typhoid fever is of concern because the current typhoid fever vaccines have no activity against *S. paratyphi*.

Chagas Disease

Mechanism of Disease

Trypanosoma cruzi, the etiologic agent of Chagas disease, is
17 one of the most common parasitic infections in humans. The WHO estimates that >100 million people are at risk for the infection and that 7–8 million people are infected throughout Mexico, Central America, and South America. The triatomine type of reduviid bug (kissing bug) is responsible for transmitting the disease to human via feces contamination after a bite or through feces contamination of conjunctiva or mucosa. Housing conditions are important for disease transmission, as the reduviid bugs usually live in the cracks within the walls of mud and straw houses found in rural and poor urban areas. Transfusion-associated *T. cruzi* is another important mode of disease transmission in countries (e.g., Brazil) with a high prevalence of disease. Screening of the blood supply has been established in many endemic areas. The FDA has recently approved an enzyme-linked immunosorbent assay (ELISA) to screen blood, organ, and tissue donations. Screening has been adopted by the American Red Cross and other organizations in the United States (25).

Clinical Presentation and Differential Diagnosis

The initial symptoms of infection with *T. cruzi* are nonspecific and often unrecognized. Beginning 6–10 days after exposure and lasting up to 2 months, patients may develop general malaise. Other associated physical findings may include hepatosplenomegaly, lymphadenopathy, rash, and edema. The reduviid bug has a predilection for biting on exposed areas during sleep, so that the bite occurs in the periorbital or perioral areas and can produce a characteristic swelling of the eyelid and face called *Romaña sign*. Romaña sign may be present in half of the patients with clinically apparent acute disease.

Abnormalities in the heart can develop during the acute illness, and abnormalities on electrocardiogram and chest radiography are common although they generally do not produce
18 symptomatic disease. The changes are due to the inflammatory response to parasites that have a tropism for the cardiac muscle. Life-threatening illness is extremely rare during the acute phase of the infection, although meningitis and myocarditis have been reported.

After acute infection, most patients enter a prolonged asymptomatic period, known as the *indeterminate phase,* and
19 remain in this phase for the rest of their lives. Approximately 15%–30% of patients with indeterminate infection will eventually develop end-organ damage, typically decades after the

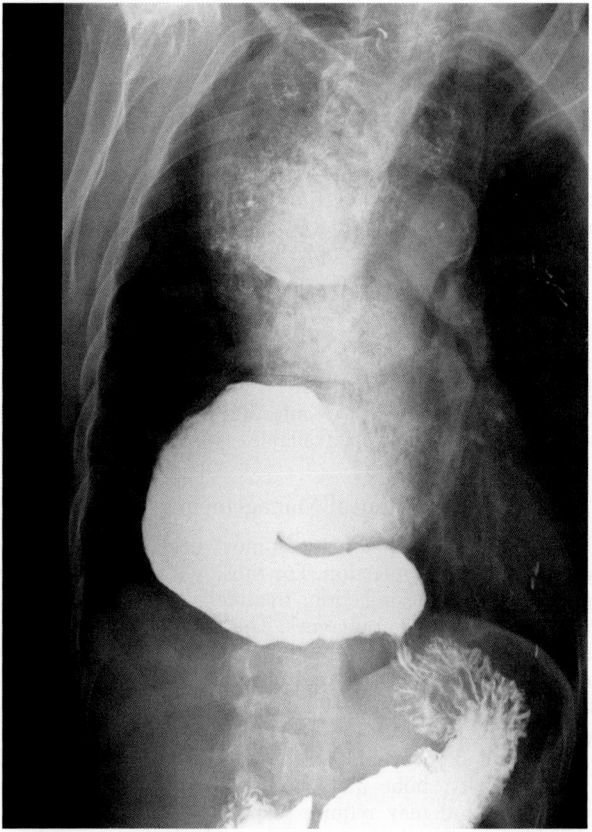

FIGURE 93.3. Megaesophagus due to chronic Chagas disease. Courtesy of Dr. Igor Laufer.

20 initial infection. In normal hosts, chronic infection can occur in the myocardium or the esophagus and colon.

Chagas cardiomyopathy is consistent with a diffuse process. Patients present with chest pain, dizziness, and peripheral edema. Chest x-rays show cardiomegaly in all chambers of the heart. The typical electrocardiographic finding is a right-bundle-branch block. Other conduction abnormalities may also be seen.

Megaviscera syndrome, due to neuronal loss in the gastrointestinal tract, leads to megaesophagus and megacolon. The presenting symptom of megaesophagus is dysphagia, although this occurs late in the disease. The finding on upper gastrointestinal contrast studies is diagnostic (**Fig. 93.3**). Megacolon is associated with constipation and the palpation of a fecaloma on examination. Barium enema can be used to confirm the diagnosis.

Reactivation of *T. cruzi* infection can occur in immunocompromised patients, including those with human immunodeficiency virus (HIV) infection or those receiving immunosuppressive therapy, and in children who are infected before 2 years of age (26). The CNS is the most common site of reactivation. Trypanosome invasion of the brain forms chagoma masses, causing patients to present with headache, fever, cognitive changes, focal neurologic impairment, and seizures. The second site most commonly affected during reactivation is the heart. Cardiac reactivation manifests as acute myocarditis or cardiomyopathy. In patients who already have cardiac damage due to chronic infection, reactivation can lead to new, acute inflammation or worsening congestive heart failure. Reactivation of cardiac disease may occur with or without neurologic disease.

Diagnosis. During the acute phase, parasitemia can be detected in the bloodstream on stained smears or microscopic examination of anticoagulated blood or buffy coat. Organisms may also be visualized in infected organs, including lymph nodes, bone marrow, and pericardial fluid. Xenodiagnosis and blood culture in specific liquid medium may be more sensitive than direct visualization, but the facilities are rarely available and the tests require 2–8 weeks to achieve a diagnosis.

During the indeterminate, chronic phase, the diagnosis can be made by serology. A positive IgM does not differentiate acute from chronic infections, as intermittent rises in IgM are common in chronic infections. A serologic diagnosis can be made using an anti-*T. cruzi* IgG ELISA test, complement fixation, hemagglutination, or indirect immunofluorescence. Because of the poor specificity of these tests, experts generally recommend obtaining two serologic tests to confirm the diagnosis. Clinical diagnostic tests are available through the CDC. Polymerase chain reaction (PCR) is a very sensitive method by which to detect the low-level infection present during chronic infection but is not widely available.

Clinical Management

Treatment of Chagas disease is most beneficial during the acute phase of the infection. For those with end-organ damage due to chronic infection, treatment has not been demonstrated to improve outcomes. The two effective treatment regimens are nifurtimox (15–20 mg/kg/d, divided three times per day) for 90–120 days or benznidazole (5–10 mg/kg/d in two divided doses) for 30–90 days. Patients who weigh <40 kg require higher doses—up to 12 mg/kg/d of nifurtimox and 7.5 mg/kg/d of benznidazole. Common side effects include hypersensitivity, bone marrow suppression, and peripheral neuropathy and may require suspension of treatment with benznidazole. Weight loss, gastrointestinal distress, and psychiatric disturbance may result from treatment with nifurtimox (27). Availability of these drugs varies by country. Only nifurtimox, produced by Bayer in Germany, is available in the United States through the Drug Service of the CDC. Treatment is considered to be successful when both parasitemia is cleared and serology is negative.

During the acute illness, patients may require intensive care for treatment of pancarditis that can result with *T. cruzi* infection. Patients are managed according to the requirement of their cardiomyopathy. Thromboembolism is common, and some suggest the use of anticoagulants for individuals in atrial fibrillation or other thrombogenic arrhythmias. Clinically significant pericardial effusions can occur. Chronic sequelae of Chagas disease, such as cardiomyopathy, megaesophagus, and megacolon, are rare among children. Symptomatic management is required.

For patients with *T. cruzi* reactivation, specific antitrypanosomal treatment is indicated, although survival is uniformly poor. The restoration of the immune system, such as the institution of highly active antiretroviral therapy in patients immunocompromised due to HIV, is important to control the infection.

Outcomes

Patients who are treated during the acute phase achieve a "cure," defined as the disappearance of IgG, in 30%–80% of cases. For those with severe cardiac disease, heart transplant may be an effective long-term solution of Chagas cardiomyopathy, despite the risk of reactivation of chronic infection due to transplant-associated immunosuppression. Sudden death occurs in 38% of patients with Chagas cardiomyopathy, often without a recognized change in cardiac status. Risk factors for death include New York Heart Association stage III or IV heart failure, cardiomegaly on chest x-ray, and left ventricular dysfunction on echocardiogram (28). Immunocompromised individuals with reactivation CNS infection rarely survive beyond 3 months.

Human African Trypanosomiasis

Mechanism of Disease

While recent eradication efforts have met with great success (the WHO estimates that <10,000 people are infected with *Trypanosoma brucei* each year since 2009), human African trypanosomiasis (HAT) remains an important regional health problem. Within Africa, two forms of HAT exist: West African sleeping sickness and East African sleeping sickness, which are caused by infection with *T. brucei gambiense* and *T. brucei rhodesiense*, respectively. Areas with high infection rates include The Congo and Uganda. Outbreaks have been reported in areas of conflict because control activities are abandoned. East African HAT is endemic at a very low rate in Kenya, Mozambique, Zambia, Tanzania, and Malawi. HAT is extremely rare in travelers.

The transmission to humans occurs after a bite from the tsetse fly that results in wound contamination by infected saliva. The habitat and species of tsetse fly are also different for the two regions, with a habitat of forested rivers and shores in western and central Africa and the savannah being the habitat in eastern and southern Africa. Other mechanisms of disease transmission in both areas include blood transfusions, contaminated needles, or congenital transmission.

Trypanosoma are parasitic protozoa that are single-celled flagellates transmitted by biting insect vectors. The life cycle involves both the vector stage and the mammalian host stage when the infective trypomastigote is injected into the bloodstream and is able to reach the CNS.

Clinical Presentation and Differential Diagnosis

In general, the presentation of HAT can be divided into an early, or hemolymphatic, stage and a late, or encephalitic, stage. The difference between the two stages is the presence of CNS involvement. In West African HAT (caused by *T. b. gambiense*), a prolonged asymptomatic period may occur, followed by a febrile stage, in which trypanosomes can be found in the blood and lymphatic systems. During this time, patients develop a nonspecific illness characterized by intermittent fever, myalgia, malaise, and fatigue. Most patients have lymphadenopathy. Pruritus and transient facial edema are rare but may be clues to the diagnosis when present. The late-stage West African HAT occurs after several months of the early febrile illness, although progression to CNS disease is more rapid in children. Headaches and somnolence with night-time insomnia can occur. Developmental delay is more common than somnolence in children. Extrapyramidal signs, cerebellar ataxia, and hemiparesis may occur.

Eastern African HAT (caused by *T. b. rhodiense*) has a more acute presentation. A chancre at the site of inoculation can occur 5–15 days after the bite, with surrounding cellulitis or regional adenopathy. Disease can progress rapidly. Myocarditis is rare, but patients may die due to dysrhythmia or cardiac failure before the neurologic disease becomes clinically apparent.

Lumbar puncture demonstrates an increased number of monocytes and an elevated protein level. A white blood cell count >5 cells/mm^3 is considered positive for CNS disease. Occasionally foamy plasma cells, the pathognomonic Mott morula cells, are found in the cerebrospinal fluid (CSF). CSF total IgM levels may be beneficial in establishing a diagnosis, as they have been found to be elevated in patients with sleeping sickness.

Brain imaging may show basal ganglia involvement such as that seen in Parkinson disease, ventriculomegaly, and asymmetric white matter abnormalities. Electroencephalography in encephalopathic patients may be abnormal, but findings are not pathognomonic. The differential diagnosis includes malaria, tuberculosis, HIV, leishmaniasis, toxoplasmosis, typhoid, and viral encephalitis.

Diagnosis. Definitive diagnosis is made by visualizing trypomastigotes in the blood or tissue. Aspiration of enlarged lymph nodes has a high yield. Thick and thin blood smears are prepared with Giemsa stains, similar to malaria smear preparation. If parasitemia is low, repeated specimens should be examined over different days to increase the sensitivity of diagnosis. Serological testing (for *T. b. gambiense* only) can be helpful. In advanced cases, trypanosomes may be easier to visualize in the CSF than in the peripheral blood. To maximize the utility of the CSF direct examination, 6–8 mL of CSF should be double-centrifuged and the sediment examined.

Clinical Management

Treatment regimens vary based on the infecting organism and stage of illness. *T. b. gambiense* can usually be distinguished from *T. brucei rhodesiense* based on the patient's travel or exposure history. Any patient with evidence of trypanosomiasis and a CSF white blood cell count >5 cells/mm^3 is considered to have late disease, regardless of clinical neurologic status. First-line treatment of the hemolymphatic stage is parenteral pentamidine for *T. brucei gambiense* and IV suramin for *T. brucei rhodesiense*. As use of suramin carries a risk of anaphylactic shock, a test dose must be given first. Eflornithine is only useful for late *T. brucei gambiense* disease; however, convulsions may occur in 6%–7% of treated patients, and bone marrow toxicity is common. For CNS disease, IV melarsoprol is effective for both varieties of HAT. The treatment is highly effective but extremely toxic, with death rates of 4%–6%. Encephalopathy, generalized seizures, coma, and neurogenic pulmonary edema can complicate therapy. Prednisone can be used to decrease these adverse effects without impairment of the treatment efficacy. Polyneuropathy may lead to permanent weakness unless thiamine is administered, and treatment is suspended until symptoms resolve. Combination treatment with nifurtimox and eflornithine has been reported to be effective in the treatment of severe disease due to *T. brucei gambiense*, but not *T. brucei rhodesiense*.

Outcomes

HAT is fatal if untreated. Patients are usually followed up to 2 years after treatment, with periodic lumbar punctures performed to evaluate recurrence of CNS disease. Recurrences require different treatment regimens or higher doses. Long-term prognosis depends on the stage of disease when treatment is initiated and the recurrence of disease, as significant injury to the CNS can occur with disease progression. Significant CNS disease can lead to demyelination, cortical and subcortical atrophy, and multifocal deep white matter lesions. Additionally, hypoxic–ischemic injury may occur as a result of seizures.

Future Directions—Human African Trypanosomiasis

Much of the research on HAT has focused on identification of appropriate targets for drug development. Vector control has been a key factor in the control of this disease in recent years.

Leptospirosis

Mechanism of Disease

Leptospirosis is a bacterial disease caused by the spirochete, *Leptospira interrogans*. Infections can range from being asymptomatic, to causing an influenza-like illness, to causing hemorrhage, renal failure, and death. Leptospires are carried by a variety of wild and domestic animals, including rodents, dogs, and livestock. In most cases, these animals have chronic renal infection with *Leptospira* without any symptoms, and they shed the organisms in their urine. Once excreted, the leptospires survive for months in moist, warm conditions. Transmission frequently occurs due to contact with infected water or moist soil. The most common scenario is flooding of urban areas or fields, leading to the spread of infected excreta and exposure of the human population. Leptospirosis can occur in urban and rural areas of developing countries, as well as through exposures in poor, urban settings in developed countries, recreational and sporting exposures, and through adventurous travel.

The precise burden of the disease is difficult to assess due to frequent under-reporting from developing countries. The clinical presentation mimics other diseases, and cases of leptospirosis are often attributed to other causes. For example, in Southeast Asia, leptospirosis is responsible for up to 13% of nonmalarial fever (29), and it is frequently the etiology of illnesses suspected to be dengue (30,31).

Leptospires are coiled, thin, and flagellated in appearance microscopically and are obligate, slow-growing anaerobes. The bacterial cell wall has a double-membrane architecture and shares features of both Gram-positive and Gram-negative organisms. Cell wall lipopolysaccharide contains antigens to which natural immunity is targeted and is the basis for serovar grouping.

Once gaining entry into the bloodstream, *Leptospira* cause disease through direct infection and through the host immune response. The organisms are highly motile and are able to penetrate and infect a wide variety of organs, including the liver, kidney, lungs, brain, and eyes. A disseminated vasculitis occurs with endothelial damage and inflammatory infiltrates in these end organs.

Clinical Presentation and Differential Diagnosis

Most infections caused by *Leptospira* result in an asymptomatic or mild infection, which is unlikely to come to the attention of a critical care specialist. Severe disease, however, is life-threatening. The clinical course of leptospirosis has been described as being biphasic consisting of an acute (septicemic) phase that usually lasts 1 week, followed by an immune phase. The biphasic nature may not be detected clinically, as patients often come to medical attention after the first phase or may have overlapping syndromes. During the acute phase, the most common symptom is fever, often with chills, and other common symptoms include headache, conjunctival suffusion, myalgia, nausea, and vomiting. Myalgias can be severe. Mild changes in mental status may occur without meningitis. A pretibial papular rash may develop. Jaundice occurs in less than half the identified cases of leptospirosis during the acute phase.

The immune phase is associated with the resolution of these acute symptoms, with an increase in antibody production and excretion of the leptospires in the urine. Typical manifestations of the immune phase are aseptic meningitis and anterior uveitis. CSF analysis reveals a lymphocytic pleocytosis and a high opening pressure. Focal neurologic findings are rare.

The severe icteric form of the disease, Weil disease, may develop as a progression from the initial febrile episode or as a distinct separate phase from the first. It is characterized by jaundice, renal failure, and hemorrhage. Serum bilirubin levels are elevated out of proportion to transaminase levels. Renal failure usually occurs during the second week of the illness. Pulmonary symptoms occur irregularly and may take the form of dyspnea or cough or may be severe with hemorrhage and

ARDS. Thrombocytopenia is common but is not usually associated with DIC.

Hemorrhagic complications can occur in severe disease that is either icteric or anicteric. Purpura, petechiae, epistaxis, and mild hemoptysis are the most frequent manifestations. The pathognomonic sign of leptospirosis, conjunctival suffusion, is due to conjunctival hemorrhage and scleral icterus. Pulmonary hemorrhage can also occur.

In anicteric disease, the white blood cell count may be low, normal, or elevated. Neutrophil predominance is typical. In contrast, lymphocytosis is a hallmark of Weil disease. Elevations in the serum level of muscle enzymes occur in most cases.

Patchy infiltrates seen on chest x-ray are thought to represent areas of intra-alveolar and interstitial hemorrhage. The areas involved are usually at the lung bases and periphery, with bilateral involvement. Histologically, these findings represent endothelial damage and hemorrhage, not inflammatory exudate. Disease can progress to diffuse alveolar infiltrates and radiographic evidence of ARDS.

The differential diagnosis includes other viral infections that are prevalent in the area where the patient resides and/or has traveled and may include common infections in the United States, such as influenza, Ebstein–Barr virus, hepatitis viruses, and community-acquired pneumonia. Other vector-borne infections should be considered based on the appropriate epidemiology and include malaria, dengue, hantavirus, typhoid fever, rickettsial infections, and arbovirus disease. Toxic shock syndrome may also mimic leptospirosis.

Diagnosis. The gold standard diagnostic method is serology using the microscopic agglutination test. The patient's serum agglutinates with *Leptospira* antigen suspensions of known serovars to determine titers. A fourfold increase in antibody titers or conversion from seronegative to a titer >1:100 is considered diagnostic.

Diagnosis of leptospirosis can be made through direct visualization of the organism or by serologic evaluation. Culture of the organism from the CSF or blood during the first week of illness or from the urine during the immune phase is not a dependable method for diagnosis, as it has poor sensitivity and requires 6–8 weeks for growth. Real-time PCR can detect *Leptospira* from clinical samples and may be a rapid, reliable strategy where the assay is available. The added advantage of the real-time PCR is that it offers a quantitative assessment of the bacterial load, which may be associated with prognosis (32).

Clinical Management

The benefit of antibiotic therapy on the outcome of leptospirosis has not been definitively demonstrated. However, some reports suggest that treatment decreases the duration of illness and, in children, it has been observed that antibiotics reduce the duration of thrombocytopenia and extent of renal failure (33). Treatment of severe disease is recommended. Antimicrobials with demonstrated in vivo efficacy against leptospirosis are penicillin, doxycycline, ceftriaxone, and cefotaxime. Doxycycline has typically been reserved for mild or moderate disease. However, in areas endemic for both leptospirosis and rickettsiosis, cephalosporin or doxycycline therapy may be preferable to penicillin therapy because of their activity against coinfecting rickettsia (34). For children in developed countries, initial empiric therapy with an IV cephalosporin should be initiated while the investigation of the etiology is under way. As the Jarisch–Herxheimer reaction (release of endotoxin from large-scale death of bacteria that can follow administration of an antimicrobial in certain diseases) can occur with the initiation of β-lactam therapy, patients should be closely monitored during the first doses.

Aside from antibiotic therapy, management of severe leptospirosis is supportive. Acutely, patients should have prompt treatment of hypovolemia and/or shock and should be assessed for pulmonary involvement and the need for respiratory support. Electrolyte disturbances may also need to be corrected.

Patients with prerenal azotemia should respond well to fluid hydration and electrolyte correction. Most often, the oliguria seen with leptospirosis responds to fluid treatment. In patients with acute, intrinsic renal failure, prompt treatment with renal replacement therapy has been suggested to reduce mortality. Peritoneal dialysis has been demonstrated to be inferior to veno-venous hemofiltration in treating patients with infection associated with renal failure (14). Improvement in mean arterial blood pressure, lowering of heart rate, and normalization of systemic vascular resistance were seen in a small series of patients who underwent hemofiltration for renal failure associated with severe leptospirosis (35).

In patients in whom mechanical ventilation is necessary, lung-protective strategies based upon low tidal volumes (4–6 mL/kg) and high positive end-expiratory pressure to maximize lung recruitment improve outcomes. Inotropic support may be necessary in many of these patients. To evaluate heart function in adult cases of ARDS and circulatory failure, pulmonary artery catheterization has been performed. A common finding is an elevated cardiac output with low systemic vascular resistance, as seen in early septic shock. Furthermore, red blood cell transfusion and correction of thrombocytopenia and coagulopathy with platelet and fresh frozen plasma transfusion may be necessary. Extracorporeal membrane oxygenation (ECMO) has been successful in some severe cases.

Outcomes

Case fatality rates for severe disease range from 5% to 40%. Death has usually been caused by acute renal failure due to acute tubular necrosis and pulmonary hemorrhage. However, mortality rates have been noted to decline in some areas where the use of hemodialysis has become more common.

Among survivors, normalization of glomerular filtration rate occurred by 6 months, although some had a mild persistent defect in urinary concentrating ability. Hepatic function usually returns to normal, although elevated bilirubin levels may persist for weeks. Chronic visual disturbances may persist after other organ system recovery, and anterior uveitis may present several weeks or longer after the acute stage (36).

Future Directions—Leptospirosis

Vaccines are under development for human leptospirosis, though none is currently available. Animal immunization with killed vaccine is widely used, but immunity is short lived and the formulations have high rates of adverse side effects. The mechanism of protection from infection is not yet well enough understood to develop a subunit vaccine.

Hantavirus

Mechanism of Disease

Over 20 types of hantaviruses, part of the Bunyavirus family have been identified in many different rodent populations throughout the world. These infections are associated with two major groups of diseases: the "Old World" viruses in Europe and Asia, which cause hemorrhagic fever with renal syndrome (HFRS), and "New World" viruses found in the Americas, characterized by cardiopulmonary disease and called hantavirus pulmonary syndrome (HPS). Each virus has a specific rodent reservoir. The host rodent develops asymptomatic infection and can excrete infectious virus in urine, feces, and saliva.

Excretion can continue even after the resolution of viremia. Transmission is thought to occur through inhalation of hantavirus aerosols found in rodent feces, although infection may occur through exposure to urine and saliva. No arthropod vectors are necessary.

Human disease begins with inhalation of infected particles that reach the bronchioles or alveoli. Viremia develops with damage to the characteristic endothelial surfaces. On histologic examination, no direct cytopathic effect is seen. The cellular damage of the lung and kidney capillary endothelium, as well as the myocardial depression, is thought to be due to the cytokine response.

Hantavirus was first recognized in the United States in the "Four Corners" region in the southwest in 1993, with a cluster of deaths associated with pulmonary edema presenting with hypotension (37). When the viral strain responsible for this outbreak was identified, it was called the *Sin Nombre Hantavirus*. It is carried by a deer mouse. The infection is rare, with fewer than 500 cases reported in the United States since 1993, and children account for <10% of cases nationwide (38). The states with the highest incidence rates are New Mexico, Montana, Utah, Nevada, Arizona, and Colorado, but cases have been reported from Canada to Mexico.

After identification of the Sin Nombre virus in the United States, cases of HPS due to hantaviruses were identified throughout South America. The most common species in South America HPS is the Andes virus. In Chile, ~500 cases have been reported (39). The seroprevalence of antibodies against the Latin American hantaviruses shows extensive geographic diversity. For example, the seropositive rates in Venezuela, Brazil, and Paraguay are 1.7%, 14.3%, and 42.7%, respectively (40), suggesting that nonvirulent strains frequently circulate in the same region or that the development of disease requires both the virus and an additional factor that is likely environmental.

In Latin America, disease frequently occurs in family clusters and children are often infected. Transmission from person to person is rare but has been reported with the Andes virus in Argentina (41).

The most severe forms of HFRS are cases of the Hantaan virus on the Korean peninsula and the Dobrava virus in the Balkans. A milder disease is caused by the Seoul virus in Southeast Asia. The Puumala virus, found in Scandinavia, Western Europe, and Russia, can cause a benign illness called *nephropathia epidemica* that causes an interstitial nephritis but has also been associated with HFRS.

Clinical Presentation and Differential Diagnosis

Hemorrhagic Fever with Renal Syndrome. HFRS is characterized by fever, renal failure, and hemorrhage. Symptoms usually begin 2–3 weeks after exposure, but incubation may be from 2 days to 6 weeks. The disease has been described to have five phases:

- *Febrile.* The onset of fever may be sudden and accompanied by headache, back and abdominal pain, vomiting, myalgias, weakness, and chills. Flushing and dermatographism may be prominent. This phase lasts an average of 5 days.
- *Hypotensive.* Shock develops. Hemorrhage, capillary leak, proteinuria, leukocytosis, thrombocytopenia, and hypotension may occur. On examination, petechiae and hemorrhage may be noted. Other common findings include hepatosplenomegaly, conjunctivitis, and change in vision.
- *Oliguric.* The oliguric phase usually begins with the return of blood pressure to normal or even hypertension and

may last 3–7 days before improvement in urine output. This is the period with the highest risk of death because patients with fatal disease develop severe hemorrhagic manifestations. Milder cases are associated with nausea and vomiting.
- *Diuretic.* The diuretic phase follows and may last several weeks.
- *Convalescent.* Convalescence may be asymptomatic or associated with some renal abnormalities such as polyuria or hyposthenuria. Permanent renal damage may be a long-term sequela.

Laboratory results show worsening thrombocytopenia and leukocytosis in the febrile and hypotensive phases. Toward the end of this phase, proteinuria can develop, followed by renal insufficiency and electrolyte imbalance during the oliguric phase. Most clinically ill patients have enlarged kidneys on ultrasound, and some have ascites or pleural effusion.

The differential diagnosis is broad and depends on the exposure history of the patient. For patients who have traveled to Asia, rickettsial disease, Dengue virus, and leptospirosis are possible infectious causes. The mild noninfectious etiologies, including renal disease and renal vein thrombosis, might not be easy to differentiate from mild common viral illnesses.

Hantavirus Pulmonary Syndrome

The incubation period for HPS due to the Sin Nombre virus is usually 1–2 weeks but may be much shorter or longer after exposure to infected excreta (39). HPS consists of three phases: a prodromal phase that lasts 3–6 days, a cardiorespiratory phase that lasts 7–10 days, and a convalescent phase. In the prodromal phase, patients usually have nonspecific symptoms of fever, myalgia, and headache. Abdominal pain and diarrhea may also be present. Sore throat is common in children. Patients frequently seek medical care during this time, but the lack of severe disease does not warrant hospitalization. During the cardiopulmonary phase, hospitalization and intensive care are often required. This phase develops rapidly, with most patients having cough, shortness of breath, tachypnea, and tachycardia. Initially, auscultation of the lungs may reveal only mild abnormalities. As the disease progresses, hypotension and hypoxemia develop. Renal insufficiency and bleeding/petechiae have not been seen in children in the United States but are commonly seen in children in South America with Andes virus infection (42).

The most consistent laboratory evaluation abnormality is thrombocytopenia. Other abnormalities include leukocytosis, hemoconcentration (more common in the South American form), myelocytosis, lack of granulation of neutrophils, and >10% lymphocyte with immunoblast appearance (43). DIC may develop. Renal impairment is common in South American HPS and may require dialysis (39).

The initial chest x-ray most commonly demonstrates interstitial edema, and many also have airspace disease. Pleural effusion is common and may help to differentiate HPS from other causes of ARDS (44).

The differential diagnosis includes community-acquired bacterial and viral pneumonias, septic shock with ARDS, initially acute gastroenteritis, leptospirosis, septicemic plague, Colorado tick fever, tularemia, relapsing fever, Rocky Mountain fever ("spotless"), Legionnaire disease, ehrlichiosis, Q fever, coccidioidomycosis, and histoplasmosis. Cardiac shock with high peripheral vascular resistance points toward a viral hemorrhagic fever rather than septic shock (45). Rash with HPS has not been reported in North American children, although petechial rash can be seen in South American infections. A history of peridomestic and/or recreational contact with rodent-infested structures is present in most cases. Severe HFRS may be confused with hemolytic uremic syndrome, but the former lacks a microangiopathic, hemolytic anemia.

Diagnosis

The diagnosis of any hantavirus infection is based on the presence of antibody in a region of the nucleocapsid that is conserved among all species. IgM is almost always present at the time of clinical symptoms, and IgG levels rise early and peak during the first week of illness. A fourfold rise in IgG can distinguish previous exposure from acute infection. An ELISA is available to state health departments through the CDC. In patients from regions where baseline seroprevalence is high, a reverse-transcriptase PCR (RT-PCR) may be required for acute diagnosis. Viral isolation is rarely successful.

Clinical Management

For all serious hantaviral disease, most treatment is supportive. Patients with severe HFRS or HPS require intensive care monitoring and resuscitation to reverse shock and treat circulatory failure, mechanical ventilation for respiratory failure, and the use of renal replacement therapies in some circumstances. The patients require management of increased capillary permeability, myocardial dysfunction, and elevated systemic vascular resistance. The use of ionotropic support with dobutamine has been recommended in the ICU (46). In both children and adults, ECMO has been used in severe cases, and experts recommend the following criteria: cardiac index <2.3 L/min/mm^2, Pao_2/Fio_2 <50 or unresponsive to conventional support. However, these clinicians often begin ECMO before achieving these criteria because decompensation can be so rapid (39).

Although ribavirin is active against hantaviruses in vitro, a small blinded, controlled trial did not demonstrate any benefit of ribavirin in the treatment of HPS (47). Administration of ribavirin within 4 days of onset of illness reduced the incidence of renal failure in HFRS in China. Although end-organ damage is mediated by the host inflammatory response, the use of steroids to mitigate the extent of the damage has not been studied in severe disease.

Outcomes

In patients with HFRS, the outcome depends on the type of infecting virus. Dobrava and Hantaan viruses are associated with more severe disease and have reported mortality rates between 5% and 10%, whereas Seoul virus and Puumala virus have reported mortality rates of 1%–2% and <0.2%, respectively. In severe cases, 15%–20% of the children require renal replacement therapy. Renal insufficiency resolves in most cases.

The overall case fatality for HPS in the United States was 35% in 510 cases from 1993 to 2009 (48). For children in this population, the overall mortality rate has been reported to be similar at 33%, and an elevated prothrombin time was associated with mortality (49,50). Reported mortality rates are higher with Andes virus infection (47%) and may be related to the occurrence of hemorrhage or renal insufficiency (42). Most deaths with HPS are the result of hypoxemia, ventricular dysfunction with hypotension, and arrhythmias (46).

Poliomyelitis

Epidemiology

Poliomyelitis was the first enteroviral disease to be recognized, and a clinical description of the disease was first given in the late 18th century by a London pediatrician. The peak incidence of the disease was during the 1950s, with over 20,000 cases/year occurring in the United States and a large epidemic occurring in Denmark. With vaccination programs, the incidence of disease declined markedly. In the United States, no cases of wild-type poliovirus have been reported since 1986, and vaccine-associated poliomyelitis has not been acquired in the United States since 1999. Endemic cases worldwide have more recently been confined to Africa (western, central, and horn), India, Pakistan, and Afghanistan, with two-thirds of the cases occurring in Nigeria and one-quarter in India (51). Reestablishment of wild-type polio has occurred between 2008 and 2011 in regions affected by instability (Angola, Chad, and the Democratic Republic of the Congo) and importation (Africa, Eastern Europe, Asia).

The peak incidence of poliovirus infections occurs in the summer and fall in temperate climates, with infections occurring year-round in tropical climates. Most infections occur in children <5 years of age. However, in areas of recurrent epidemics, the age distribution shifts to older children and younger adults.

Four types of infection with poliovirus occur: inapparent infection, abortive infection, nonparalytic infection, and paralytic poliomyelitis. Most infections are inapparent and account for 90%–95% of infections. Abortive infections are seen in 4%–8% and result in a mild, nonspecific illness. Aseptic meningitis without evidence of paralysis is seen in 1%–2% of cases. Finally, paralytic poliomyelitis is seen in <1% of infections (52).

Risk factors for paralytic disease with poliovirus infection include older age, pregnancy, recent diphtheria/pertussis/tetanus vaccination, physical exercise at the time of infection, trauma at the time of infection, and tonsillectomy. In areas of endemicity, children <5 years of age account for the vast majority of cases of paralytic polio, as they have most of the infections. Tonsillectomy is a risk factor for the development of the bulbar form of poliomyelitis. Older children and adults, as well as immunodeficient individuals, are at higher risk for vaccine-associated paralytic poliomyelitis. An additional risk factor for vaccine-associated paralytic poliomyelitis is recent intramuscular injection after oral poliovirus vaccination (51,52).

Etiology

Polioviruses are in the enterovirus subgroup of the family *Picornaviridae*. Other enteroviruses include coxsackievirus and echovirus. The viruses are small, single-stranded, positive-sense, RNA viruses with three serotypes. Immunity to one serotype does not confer immunity to the others. The viral genome encodes for four capsid proteins and seven nonstructural proteins. Neutralizing antibodies are made to the capsid proteins. Humans are the only known hosts of poliovirus, although other animals are known to be hosts for other enteroviruses. After infection, viral components and virions are formed intracellularly (51,52).

Infection is spread primarily via the fecal–oral route, although transmission by oral–oral contact may occur as well. In uninfected individuals, the virus enters the mucosa of the pharynx and upper alimentary tract and replicates (alimentary phase). The infection then spreads to lymph tissue (tonsils, lymph nodes, and Peyer patches), where the virus undergoes further multiplication, leading to a minor viremia and seeding of other organs over the next few days (lymphatic phase). By days 3–7, replication in secondary infection sites produces a major viremia with possible CNS infection (viremic phase). By 1 week, specific antibody formation clears the viremia although the virus continues to be shed from the lower intestinal tract for several weeks (51,52).

Replication of poliovirus in the CNS may damage the anterior and dorsal horn cells of the spinal cord and medulla (cranial nerve nuclei and reticular formation), producing the manifestations of paralytic polio. Other affected areas potentially include the midbrain, portions of the hypothalamus and thalamus, and the vermis and midline nuclei of the cerebellum. The white matter of the cerebral cortex and spinal cord are usually spared. The CNS lesions can be more widespread than the clinical manifestations of disease suggest and may be partially reversible (51,52).

Presentation and Differential Diagnosis

Nonparalytic cases of poliomyelitis have evidence of CNS injury without paralysis, including meningismus, muscle spasms, and CSF, which suggests aseptic meningitis. In general, these patients should not require intensive care. Paralytic poliomyelitis is life-threatening in children in the event that respiratory insufficiency develops during the disease course. The incubation period is ~3–5 days for minor illness and 1–2 weeks for CNS involvement. However, the incubation time for paralysis may extend up to 1 month. In children, the disease often progresses in two phases: a minor phase with prodromal symptoms, followed by CNS disease. These symptoms are nonspecific and consist of sore throat, fever, nausea, vomiting, abdominal discomfort, rash, constipation, and flu-like symptoms (51,52).

The paralytic symptoms may not begin for several days after the prodrome. Signs such as toxicity, irritability, higher fever, anxiousness, and the presence of diminished superficial reflexes may herald the onset of paralysis. Weakness may progress over a period of 3–5 days to flaccid paralysis with loss of deep tendon reflexes. The time course can also be of rapid onset with progression over several hours. Transient fasciculations may be observed during disease progression. In general, the lower extremities are more commonly affected than the upper. Muscle spasm may be present prior to the onset of paralysis. As weakness progresses, the patient may have a weak cough, weak cry, and nasal flaring. With severe disease, quadriplegia and respiratory failure occur. In patients with brainstem disease, bulbar symptoms may be present. These signs include pharyngeal hypotonia, hoarseness, deviation of the soft palate, diminished swallowing, increased secretions, aphonia, and "rope" sign (hypotonia of hyoid muscles). Neuronal damage in the brainstem can cause autonomic dysfunction manifest by paralytic ileus, bladder paralysis, cardiac arrhythmias, and systemic hypertension (51,52).

Patients with paralytic poliomyelitis are classified into three clinical groups. Those children with pure spinal poliomyelitis do not have cranial nerve involvement but have muscular weakness and/or paralysis. Respiratory failure, when present, is due to weakness or paralysis of thoracic muscles and diaphragm. This form is most commonly seen and represents 79% of the cases. The second group includes individuals with pure bulbar poliomyelitis that have weakness or paralysis of cranial nerves IX, X, and/or XII primarily. These patients may show signs of agitation or delirium and may have evidence of cardiac dysrhythmias or hypertension, hypothermia, and disordered control of breathing. The respiratory failure in this group of patients is due to extrathoracic airway obstruction and lack of airway clearance of secretions that can lead to aspiration. Pure bulbar poliomyelitis is uncommon and represents 2% of the cases. Those patients with bulbospinal disease account for the remaining 19% of the cases and demonstrate a combination of features. Rarely do patients present with encephalitic poliomyelitis manifest by high fever, mental status changes, spasticity, seizures, and bulbar signs (51,52).

The diagnosis of poliomyelitis is confirmed by poliovirus recovery from the stool and/or oropharynx. The virus may also be isolated from the CSF in some circumstances. Further typing is then performed to rule out a vaccine strain. Serology for the three poliovirus serotypes is problematic in that high titers of neutralizing antibody may be present at the time of presentation. However, the presence of IgM antibodies suggests acute infection (51,52).

The differential diagnosis includes Guillain–Barré syndrome, other enterovirus infections, acute disseminating encephalomyelitis, rabies, botulism, WNV, Ebstein–Barr virus, and other causes of aseptic meningitis or encephalitis (51,52). The presence of flaccid paralysis and lack of significant sensory changes is helpful in ruling out other diseases.

Treatment

Treatment of children with paralytic poliomyelitis is primarily supportive. The focus in the ICU is on the monitoring and management of associated respiratory failure. In patients with bulbar or bulbospinal poliomyelitis, maintenance of airway patency with suctioning and positioning is of importance to ensure adequate ventilation and prevent aspiration of secretions and pneumonia. Close assessment of adequacy of gas exchange by arterial blood gases and noninvasive monitors can help to prevent hypoxia and the consequences of hypoventilation. With airway obstruction or high risk of aspiration, tracheal intubation and mechanical ventilation are necessary. Patients with spinal poliomyelitis who have significant weakness or paralysis of the muscles of respiration may require mechanical ventilation as well. Respiratory failure occurs more frequently in those patients with bulbar poliomyelitis. Given the prolonged time to recovery or residual paralysis that occurs in some patients, tracheostomy may be necessary to provide a stable airway and long-term mechanical ventilation.

No known specific antiviral therapy effectively treats poliovirus infection. Pleconaril is a new oral antiviral agent that has been used to treat enterovirus infections. Use of pleconaril to treat poliomyelitis patients has been reported, but the efficacy is unknown (53). The drug is thought to diminish viral replication by inhibiting viral capsid uncoating.

Analgesia may be necessary in those patients with significant myalgia or headaches. Constipation can also be problematic and require the use of laxatives (51,52). Physical and occupational therapists and physiatrists should be involved to assist with proper positioning, splinting, and therapies to facilitate recovery and prevent contractures. In addition, neurologists, pulmonologists, and infectious disease experts may be of benefit in the evaluation and treatment of severe cases.

Outcomes

Patients with mild weakness may have a complete recovery, although those patients with flaccid paralysis will likely have persistent weakness. If recovery occurs, on average, 60% recovery will occur by 3 months and 80% by 6 months. The time period for improvement does not usually extend beyond 18 months, so that any residual deficits that exist at that time are likely permanent. The mortality rate in paralytic poliomyelitis may be as low as 4% but is higher in adults and in those patients with bulbar disease. The mortality rates in bulbar disease may be as high as 25%–75%. Post-poliomyelitis syndrome occurs in ~25%–40% of patients with a history of paralytic poliomyelitis after a 30- to 40-year time period from infection. These patients have an exacerbation of existing or new weakness and muscle pain (51,52).

Future Directions—Poliomyelitis

With appropriate immunization programs, polio can be eradicated worldwide. Travelers to regions where infection remains endemic should be certain that they are fully immunized prior to arrival.

EMERGING INFECTIONS

West Nile Virus

Mechanism of Disease

The first recognized case of WNV infection occurred in 1937 in a febrile woman in the West Nile province of Uganda and was isolated from children in Egypt during acute febrile illnesses in the 1950s. WNV infections were subsequently associated with outbreaks in Israel, France, South Africa, and India, most commonly causing febrile illness and, rarely, encephalitis or meningitis. In the late 1990s, several outbreaks of encephalitis and meningitis were seen in Russia, Israel, and Romania. The first outbreak in the western hemisphere occurred in 1999 in New York City. Since that time, WNV has rapidly spread in the United States, with over 4000 cases of WNV infection in 2002 and 45 states reporting WNV infections in 2003.

The basis for the increasing incidence and severity of WNV infections is unclear but is potentially related to increasing virulence, changes in host factors, or predisposing chronic disease. Based upon statistics from the New York epidemic, ~1 in 5 patients develop a febrile illness, and 1 in 150 patients develop severe neurologic disease. Most infections with WNV occur during late August to September, with the peak transmission time being between mid-July and December.

The strongest risk factor for the development of West Nile neuroinvasive disease (WNND) and death is advanced age (age >70 years) (54). WNND is also associated with disruption of the blood–brain barrier and immunosuppression and occurs less frequently in children than in adults. Although children may have less exposure to mosquitoes that transmit the disease, it is thought that children likely have more asymptomatic infections or milder disease.

With the increasing prevalence of the WNV, other modes of viral transmission have been identified, including blood transfusion, breast-feeding, organ transplantation, and transplacental infection. No adverse effects of viral transmission to infants have been documented (55,56). At this writing, screening for WNV is being performed on blood components in the United States, using WNV nucleic acid amplification tests to reduce this risk.

WNV is a single-stranded RNA virus from the *Flavivirus* family. WNV is similar to other *Flaviviruses* in the Japanese encephalitis virus complex, including St. Louis encephalitis virus and Japanese encephalitis virus, among others. WNV is sustained through an enzootic cycle between birds and mosquitoes. Mosquitoes of the order *Culex* are important vectors for transmitting WNV infections. Perching birds (sparrows, blue jays, crows, and magpies) are thought to be important hosts for WNV, as they develop a high level of viremia. Viral amplification occurs through bird–mosquito–bird infection cycles, which increases the likelihood of transmission of infection to humans when they are bitten by infected mosquitoes. Humans are believed to be "dead-end" hosts because they develop an insufficient viremia to infect feeding mosquitoes. After human inoculation by feeding mosquitoes infected with WNV, the virus replicates in dendritic cells and ascends to regional lymph nodes, with dissemination to the bloodstream and other organs.

Clinical Presentation and Differential Diagnosis

The incubation period is usually 2–6 days (range, 2–14 days), with prolonged incubations of up to 3 weeks seen in some immunocompromised patients. WNV has been isolated in the blood of immunocompetent individuals 2 days before the onset of symptoms, with clearing of the viremia after ~4 days. In immunocompromised hosts, the viremia can be prolonged and extend up to 1 month after onset. Symptomatic infection associated with WNV has been categorized as West Nile fever and WNND.

In West Nile fever, an abrupt onset of fever occurs, with symptoms that may include headache, myalgia, nausea, vomiting, abdominal pain, or diarrhea. Additionally, sore throat, cough, and maculopapular rash have been described. Most cases have resolution of symptoms within 1 week, but milder symptoms of malaise and fatigue may persist for several weeks.

WNND develops in less than 1% of those infected. In reported cases of pediatric patients in California with WNND, ~50% had meningitis and most commonly presented with headache, nuchal rigidity, and fever. Also, ~50% of the patients had a rash, and one-third had muscle weakness. In those cases with encephalitis, most patients had fever, headache, nuchal rigidity, and alteration in consciousness. Muscle weakness is a prominent part of the clinical manifestation of WNV encephalitis and was seen in ~80% of these patients. Of note, none of these patients had a rash. Patients with encephalitis may have bulbar findings and hyperreflexia as well. Several of the children with encephalitis were also noted to be immunocompromised. All patients with encephalitis were admitted to the PICU (55). Rare extraneurologic complications include myocarditis, pancreatitis, and hepatitis.

Laboratory evaluation may reveal a mild leukopenia or leukocytosis. Hyponatremia can occur in patients with WNND. In patients with WNND, CSF findings can include a mild pleocytosis with lymphocytes, mild-to-moderate protein level elevation, and normal glucose levels. CT and MRI imaging of the brain may initially be normal or show only mild leptomeningeal enhancement despite significant neurologic findings. Follow-up neuroimaging with MRI later in the disease course may show gray matter abnormalities. When performed, electromyography and nerve conduction studies may be consistent with a motor axonal polyneuropathy and demonstrate evidence of anterior horn cell injury.

In patients with WNND, other causes of aseptic meningitis should be considered, including infections with enterovirus and other viruses in the *Flavivirus* family. The presentation with acute muscle weakness may suggest a diagnosis of Guillain–Barré syndrome. Other treatable infections, including herpesvirus infection or bacterial meningoencephalitic, should be considered as well.

Diagnosis. The presence of WNV nucleic acid can be detected using reverse-transcriptase PCR and provides strong evidence of infection. However, WNV nucleic acid often cannot be detected after the viremia has resolved, 3–5 days after the symptoms appear. An IgM ELISA can be performed on the serum or CSF. IgM is detectable 3–5 days into illness. WNV IgM is cross-reactive with other *Flaviviruses*. Therefore, further testing may be required to improve the specificity of the diagnosis. IgM antibody has been known to be detectable in patients up to 1 year after WNV infection.

Clinical Management

Treatment is mainly supportive. Endotracheal intubation may be necessary for airway protection in severe cases of encephalitis. Although rare, seizures may occur, and must be treated aggressively. WNV replication and cytopathogenicity are inhibited by ribavirin and interferon-α in vitro; however, clear benefit has not been demonstrated in patients with WNND, and no controlled trials have been performed.

Outcomes

Overall case mortality in patients with WNV meningoencephalitis has been recently reported to range between 4% and 14%, with virtually all deaths occurring in patients with encephalitis. Children appear to be spared the most severe outcomes: the youngest fatality was in a 19-year-old (56,57).

In adults, half of the patients have reported that they have not recovered physically, functionally, or cognitively at 12 months post-illness. Clinical details regarding the course of pediatric patients with WNV encephalitis are less well studied, given the infrequency of the disease in children. Prolonged neurologic recovery has been reported, with some children having neurologic symptoms for >6 months (55,56).

Future Directions—West Nile Virus

Studies are ongoing to investigate potential therapies for WNV infection (58). Of particular interest is the use of pooled high-titer anti-WNV antibody. A clinical trial of interferon-α is also underway.

Avian Influenza

Mechanism of Disease

Influenza pandemics have swept the world in the past, most notably the "Spanish flu" of 1918–1919 that killed 20–40 million people. Given the pandemic potential, concern about new influenza viruses giving rise to devastating worldwide infection is always there. In 1997, an avian influenza virus strain H5N1 spread from chickens to humans in Hong Kong. It was only controlled after culling every chicken on the island (59). In 2003, an outbreak of H5N1 infection spread throughout Southeast Asia. The infection has spread beyond its origin in Southeast Asia, to central Asia, Africa, and Eastern Europe, likely via the migration of wild birds. Spread to domestic poultry in Eastern Europe has occurred rarely. More recently, an outbreak of H7N9 virus occurred in China in 2013 as the result of exposure to infected poultry, with an ~30% case fatality rate in humans.

The outbreak that began in 2003 is important for several reasons. It was an extremely virulent strain of the virus, causing very high rates of death in both wild and domestic birds. Whereas previously identified avian influenza strains were not found to be spread efficiently by migrating birds, these wild birds are now clearly linked to the spread of infection. This strain of virus has been extremely difficult to control. It has persisted and even spread despite having killed of 150 million infected or exposed birds. Humans have primarily been infected by contact with poultry, although several cases are thought to have occurred through contact with dead wild birds. By the end of 2006, 258 human cases were reported, with 154 deaths. Countries where human cases of avian influenza have occurred include Azerbaijan, Cambodia, China, Djibouti, Egypt, Indonesia, Iraq, Laos, Nigeria, Thailand, Turkey, and Vietnam (60). The activities that have been associated with human cases of avian influenza include handling of diseased birds, playing with infected poultry (especially ducks), and consumption of uncooked poultry (61). Human-to-human transmission has been suspected in several cases (62–64); however, sustained human-to-human transmission has not been documented. In addition, nosocomial transmission to health-care workers has not occurred (65).

Influenza A viruses belong to the family of *Orthomyxoviridae*. Antigenic subtypes are defined by two major surface glycoproteins: hemagglutinin and neuraminidase (NA). *Antigenic drift*, defined as changes within the same viral subtype, is responsible for the annual occurrence of influenza epidemic, whereas *antigenic shift*, with the circulation of a new subtype, has led to pandemics. The reservoir for influenza type A viruses is wild waterfowl. In these birds, influenza A viruses usually cause asymptomatic infection in the gastrointestinal tract, and the virus is transmitted through the fecal–oral route.

Several factors limit the spread of avian influenza to humans. Host-specific infection is mediated by binding to receptors on cells, a necessary step to allow for replication and propagation of infection. Avian viruses tend to bind to α-2,3-Gal-terminated saccharides found on avian intestinal epithelium, and human viruses bind to α-2,6-Gal-terminated saccharides on human respiratory epithelium. Some 2,3-Gal-terminated saccharides are found in the lower respiratory tract and may account for the small number of human cases (66). However, even if infection occurs in a human, it is poorly transmitted because upper respiratory shedding is the most conducive to transmission (67).

Clinical Presentation and Differential Diagnosis

The presenting signs and symptoms may vary, depending on the specific type of avian influenza viral infection. For the avian influenza viruses, the incubation period ranges from 2 to 8 days. The earliest symptoms are high fever and an influenza-like illness with lower respiratory involvement. Upper respiratory symptoms only occur occasionally. Gastrointestinal symptoms, including diarrhea (with or without blood), vomiting, and abdominal pain, are common and may precede the respiratory illness, although the degree of gastrointestinal involvement may vary by clade. Patients usually reach medical attention at the time of the respiratory illness. Almost all patients have signs and symptoms of pneumonia, including dyspnea, increased respiratory rate, and crackles on auscultation. In a comparison of cases of mild versus severe disease, hypoxia never occurred in mild cases, whereas supplemental oxygen was required for all patients with severe disease, either at initial presentation or during the course of the illness (63). As the disease progresses, patients develop ARDS and multiorgan failure, including cardiac dysfunction. Other complications that have been reported include pulmonary hemorrhage, pancytopenia, and systemic inflammatory response syndrome without documented bacteremia.

Low white blood cell count, especially lymphopenia, leukopenia, and thrombocytopenia, is a common laboratory finding. Elevated aminotransferases and creatinine can also occur. The chest x-rays are abnormal and may show a variety of patterns. The most common in the Vietnam epidemic was multifocal consolidation. As respiratory failure and ARDS developed, the x-ray took on a diffuse, ground-glass appearance (68).

As the signs and symptoms of avian influenza viral infection are nonspecific, the most important trigger for consideration of the diagnosis is the potential for exposure, including travel to an area where infection is endemic and contact with poultry, ill birds, or another individual with avian influenza. The WHO tracks cases of human and bird infections and their geographic distribution (http://www.who.int/csr/disease/avian_influenza/en/). Additional diagnoses to consider include causes for influenza-like illnesses, ARDS, and severe community-acquired pneumonia. For individuals with severe pneumonia with a history of travel to Southeast Asia, additional infections should be considered, including leptospirosis and melioidosis. For children who are from medically underserved communities, vaccine-preventable infections such as measles and *Haemophilus influenzae* B may occur.

Diagnosis. The preferred method for diagnosis includes oropharyngeal swab specimens and lower respiratory tract specimens for strain-specific, reverse-transcriptase PCR testing. Throat swabs have higher yield than nasal swabs (63). Specimens should be placed in viral transport medium. Viral antigen testing may also be conducted. The commonly available kits to identify influenza A may detect the presence of avian strains in a minority of cases (63,68). Antigen testing and PCR only require biosafety level (BSL)-2 facilities (69).

Viral isolation of specimens from patients who are suspected of having avian influenza should only be processed in a BSL-3+ facility. If avian influenza is suspected, the laboratory must be informed that a specimen is being submitted.

Clinical Management

The H5N1 and H7N9 viruses are sensitive to the NA inhibitors oseltamivir and zanamivir (70,71). In animal models, the optimal timing of the medication to improve survival is within the first 48 hours. In a series of cases from Thailand, patients who survived received oseltamivir treatment earlier (mean, 4.5 days) than those who did not (mean, 9 days) (72). The standard dose of oseltamivir is given for 5 days: 30 mg twice per day for children ≤15 kg, 45 mg twice a day for those >15–23 kg, 60 mg twice a day for those >23–40 kg, and 75 mg twice a day for those >40 kg. Common adverse effects are nausea and vomiting. Anaphylaxis and severe dermatologic reactions have rarely been reported. In mild cases, the standard approved dose can be administered for 5 days. In cases of severe disease, some experts recommend doubling the standard dose. The increased dose has been shown to have improved efficacy in animal models (73) and is well tolerated in adults but does not have superior efficacy against seasonal influenza (74). Oseltamivir prophylaxis is recommended for 7–10 days after the last exposure in cases of high- to moderate-risk exposures.

Although the avian influenza viruses are susceptible to the NA inhibitors, one case of oseltamivir-resistant H5N1 was isolated from a patient in Vietnam who developed clinical illness after receiving oseltamivir postexposure prophylaxis (75), thus raising the concern that if postexposure prophylaxis were initiated on a wide scale during a threatened epidemic, drug-resistant strains would be selected and propagated.

Oseltamivir is preferred over zanamivir because it is easier to administer. Zanamivir is administered by oral inhalation of a dry powder, making drug delivery difficult in intubated patients and potentially less effective if distributed unevenly in the respiratory system, as can occur in patients with significant lung disease who may not achieve high enough levels in the blood to treat systemic disease. Zanamivir may be preferable for prophylaxis or for less severely ill patients. Other antivirals, such as the amantadane derivatives and ribavirin, have in vitro activity against H5N1 or H7N9. They are not currently recommended for use against avian influenza but may be considered as components of combination therapy, although this strategy has not been well studied. Both NA inhibitor drug dosages must be adjusted for renal failure, as they are renally excreted. Oseltamivir also undergoes significant hepatic metabolism.

Intensive care management is essential for all cases of severe disease. Respiratory failure requiring intubation occurs in most hospitalized patients. Renal dysfunction occurs commonly, although the etiology is unknown. Inotropic support may also be necessary.

Infection control should be addressed immediately if avian influenza infection is suspected. The appropriate infection-control measures (standard, contact, airborne, and eye) should be instituted. In previous outbreaks, hospital staff did not demonstrate serologic evidence of exposure to the virus (76). However, as a widespread pandemic would likely be caused by a more highly transmissible form of the virus, strict infection control should be instituted immediately.

Outcomes

The case fatality rate for hospitalized patients with H5N1 infection is high, with an overall mortality rate reported by the WHO of over 50% of confirmed cases (30% for H7N9). This illness is more severe than the Hong Kong outbreak in 1997 with a very similar virus, in which the case fatality rate was 33%. Death usually occurs due to progressive respiratory failure and multiple organ dysfunction an average of 9–10 days after onset of illness.

Future Directions—Avian Influenza

The key to preventing an avian influenza pandemic is adequate supply of effective vaccine should a highly transmissible strain emerge. The vaccination production strategies that have been studied thus far are similar to the seasonal influenza vaccinations: inactivated virus and live attenuated virus. Using the current technology, the production of these vaccines requires many months of preparation and may pose a safety risk for those involved in production. Newer technology, including recombinant proteins, DNA vaccines, and vector-based delivery, are being developed and tested as vaccines that would be easily produced, safely, on a large scale, and in a timely fashion.

Novel Coronavirus Infections (SARS and MERS)

The last decade has seen the emergence of two novel coronaviruses causing human respiratory disease. These viruses have been shown to be the cause of severe acute respiratory syndrome (SARS) and Middle East respiratory syndrome (MERS). The nomenclature for the viruses themselves is SARS-CoV and Middle Eastern respiratory syndrome coronavirus (MERS-CoV), respectively. While the SARS outbreak of 2003–2004 has not recurred, and the global significance of MERS-CoV is not yet fully known, these viruses merit discussion here given their relatively high case fatality rates and as case studies of the impact of novel viruses.

Epidemiology

The first documented case of SARS occurred in February 2003 in Hong Kong. The index case was a medical physician who traveled from Guangdong province and stayed in a hotel in Hong Kong and infected 12 guests or visitors. By the time this outbreak ended in the summer of 2003, over 8000 people were infected in multiple countries, including Southeast Asia, Canada, the United States, and several European countries, with a significantly high mortality rate in adult cases. New cases of SARS were identified in 2004 but were apparently related to laboratory exposure (77,78). At this writing, no cases have been reported to the CDC or the WHO since 2004. Nonetheless, this section is presented for historic interest and as an example of the rapidity with which an emerging infection can travel worldwide. SARS highlights the potentially disastrous consequences of emerging infections in today's global society.

The disease appears to be transmitted through droplet or fomite contact of the mucous membranes of the respiratory system. The large number of nosocomial cases is thought to be caused by contact with infective droplets generated by the use of respiratory equipment and nebulized medications that would amplify transmission (79). Spread to community occurred through hospital visitors or other health-care workers, representing the primary mode of transmission. Disease in children during the outbreak occurred through sick household contacts or hospital contacts, with no major spread through schools. Two cases of transmission from children to adults were reported, and no instances of child–child transmission were reported. All children and up to 90% of adults in the 2003 outbreak had a positive contact history (80). Implementation of infection-control procedures has been shown to effectively control the spread of SARS. Quarantine measures have been effective, as no instances of transmission have been reported prior to the onset of symptoms. In some outbreaks, some individuals appear to be "super-spreaders," where a few cases result in a disproportionate number of transmissions. Other factors have been identified to be important contributors to the rapid spread of SARS as well. These factors include long incubation period (4–7 days on average, but up to 14 days), insidious onset of symptoms, and infectivity that appears to increase as symptoms progress (77,78,81,82).

Etiology

The etiology of SARS has now been established to be a novel coronavirus (SARS-CoV). The family of coronaviruses includes enveloped, single-stranded RNA viruses that had previously been known only to cause cold symptoms. SARS-CoV is unrelated to known human or animal coronaviruses but is thought to have arisen from interspecies transmission and adaptation. Specifically, interspecies transmission is thought to have potentially occurred in the game markets in southern China, as coronaviruses similar to SARS-CoV have been isolated in civet cats and other wild animals in that region. Recent epidemiologic evidence suggests that Chinese horseshoe bats may be the natural reservoir for SARS-like coronaviruses. Some cases of SARS have had other coinfections, including human metapneumovirus and *Chlamydia* infections, but it is unclear how these coinfections affect the severity or transmissibility of SARS (77,78).

Presentation and Differential Diagnosis

The disease course in SARS has been described as triphasic. Patients with SARS initially present with myalgia, fever, malaise, and chills/rigors after an incubation period of ~4–7 days (phase I). Upper respiratory tract symptoms such as rhinorrhea and sore throat occur less commonly. This phase is associated with viral replication and is transient, with resolution in approximately one-third of cases. The remaining cases develop persistent fever and may have coughing, oxygen desaturation, chest pain, tachypnea, and dyspnea as they develop bronchopneumonia (phase II). This phase has been characterized as an immunopathologic phase and has been thought to be related to an exaggerated host immunologic response. The viral load has been noted to be decreasing during this period. Some patients have also developed a watery diarrhea at this time. The median time from onset of symptoms to hospital admission is 3–5 days (77,78,83–85).

During the course of illness, laboratory data may reveal lymphopenia (56%–90%), thrombocytopenia (13%–41%), and elevated transaminases. Chest radiography demonstrates abnormalities in 60%–100% of cases. Findings include a ground-glass appearance or focal consolidation in the lung bases, peripheral, and/or subpleural areas. In those patients with normal chest x-rays, CT scanning demonstrates abnormalities 67% of the time. Also reported is the development of pneumomediastinum without previous positive-pressure ventilation or intubation, but this occurs later in the disease course (86). Some patients may progress to ARDS with diffuse alveolar damage and pulmonary fibrosis (phase III). Most children have relatively mild disease, with the more severe cases in pediatrics being in the adolescent age group (80,85,86).

Others have noted that establishing a diagnosis of SARS during an outbreak can be problematic if using WHO case definitions, as the symptoms of SARS are similar to other frequently encountered respiratory illnesses in children (87). This finding led to a modification of the definition for probable pediatric cases to include a positive test for SARS-CoV. RT-PCR analyses of nasopharyngeal or stool specimens have been reported to have 50% sensitivity in pediatric patients. A higher sensitivity and fast turnaround time have been found using one-step, real-time RT-PCR to detect viral RNA in plasma. Paired acute and convalescent serology for SARS-CoV is useful for confirmation of infection but not for triage. In addition to specific testing for SARS-CoV, testing for other viral and/or bacterial etiologies for the patient's signs and symptoms should be performed, as coinfection could be present and initial presenting signs may not be reliable to differentiate SARS from non-SARS cases (80,85,86).

Treatment

A key component of treatment is the use of infection-control procedures to control spread of disease through droplets, aerosolization, and fomites. Effective control also involves successful triage of patients based upon definitions of probable and suspected cases. Antimicrobial therapy should be administered for other bacterial etiologies for the patients' signs and symptoms or atypical pneumonia. This therapy might consist of a third-generation cephalosporin and a macrolide in cases of pneumonia and fever. A temporal relationship has been seen between the administration of corticosteroids and clinical improvement in seriously ill pediatric patients. Immunomodulation during this phase of illness (phase II) is thought to have theoretic benefit. Additionally, ribavirin was administered to patients during the outbreak, but SARS-CoV has not been found to be sensitive to this agent in vitro (77).

Terminal events in adult patients have been associated with progressive respiratory failure, multiple organ dysfunction, or intercurrent illness such as myocardial infarction (78,81,84,88).

Outcomes

Approximately 30% of adult patients with SARS-CoV infection require ICU admission, and the mortality rate has been reported to be as high as 50% in older patients. Fewer than 10% of the reported SARS cases have been in children (77,78,83,89). It has been suggested that children <12 years of age have a less severe course of disease, and, to date, no deaths in young children or adolescents have been reported. Approximately 5% of these cases have required PICU admission, and 1% have required mechanical ventilation. In pediatric patients with severe disease, abnormalities in biochemical markers and lymphopenia persist longer. Sore throat and peak neutrophil count have been identified to predict more severe disease in pediatric patients. Most of the pediatric patients treated with steroids have been adolescent patients. In a follow-up study of 47 children (ages 9.8–16 years) 6 months after SARS diagnosis, no child had symptomatic lung disease, and mild lung abnormalities were identified in 34% of patients by high-resolution CT (90). These findings most commonly included residual ground-glass changes and/or air trapping. Two of the 47 children required mechanical ventilation. The need for supplemental oxygen and lymphopenia were identified as risk factors for the noted CT findings. Of 38 patients who underwent pulmonary function testing, only four had abnormal findings, all of which were mild. The findings on high-resolution CT also correlated with diminished aerobic capacity (89).

SARS and MERS

SARS taught us major lessons concerning the control of nosocomial outbreaks of respiratory pathogens. Clinicians must be ever-cognizant of the potential for a new, heretofore undescribed viral infection. Participation in reporting systems and cooperation with public health officials are essential to identify and prevent the spread of emerging diseases. This was highlighted in 2012 when a novel coronavirus was reported to cause acute respiratory failure in Saudi Arabia. This outbreak of what is now referred to as MERS has thus far only been linked to countries in and around the Arabian Peninsula. Human-to-human transmission through close contact has been reported, though large-scale community spread has not been seen. Two cases were imported to the United States through international travel in 2014. Infection with this virus (MERS-CoV), while uncommon, has been associated with a 30% case fatality rate, making it a current target of CDC and WHO investigation.

Ebola Virus Disease

Epidemiology

While hemorrhagic fevers are reviewed in detail in Chapter 89, the scale and global impact of the 2014 ebola virus outbreak merit discussion in this chapter as well. In 2014, there were more than 10,000 cases of laboratory-confirmed ebola virus disease (EVD) in West Africa, with the vast majority of cases occurring in Sierra Leone, Liberia, and Guinea, with sporadic cases reported in Senegal, Nigeria, and Mali. The number of total cases is estimated to be at least twice that, with nearly 6000 deaths officially attributed to EVD in 2014 (www.cdc.gov). This outbreak was notable for its scale and for the spread of EVD out of Africa via infected international travelers or infected international health workers, with such cases reported in Spain and the United States. In both of those countries, subsequent occupational transmission of EVD was documented with at least one health-care worker in Spain and two in the United States becoming infected.

Etiology and Clinical Presentation

EVD is caused by exposure to bodily fluids including blood, urine, vomit, feces, sweat, tears, breast milk, or semen from individuals infected with the ebola virus. Infection with ebola virus, a member of the Filoviridae family, causes fever and nonspecific flu-like symptoms after an incubation period of 2–21 days. Humans are not infectious until they develop symptoms. Patients with EVD usually have vomiting, diarrhea, and rash: some will experience clinically significant internal and external bleeding.

Diagnosis

It is important to distinguish EVD from other, more common sources of fever in West African travelers including malaria and typhoid fever. Blood tests such as antigen-capture ELISA, IgM ELISA, PCR, and viral culture can be diagnostic within a few days of the onset of symptoms. IgM and IgG titers can be helpful in later stages of disease or recovery. Blood testing for EVD is typically conducted at state departments of health and/or the CDC.

Treatment and Outcomes

Treatment for EVD patients includes aggressive hydration including the replacement of massive volumes of gastrointestinal fluid output (up to 10 L a day in adults) (91,92). The remainder of treatment is largely supportive, potentially including mechanical ventilatory support, continuous renal replacement therapy, and management of secondary infections. Patients have also been successfully treated with convalescent plasma from ebola survivors and chimeric monoclonal antibodies against ebola. The experimental antiviral drug brincidofovir has activity against ebola virus, but efficacy in this setting is currently unclear.

Appropriate isolation and use of personal protective equipment (PPE) are essential in the management of patients with, or suspected to have, EVD. While EVD is thought to not be transmissible through the air, the CDC currently recommends airborne infection isolation (including negative pressure rooms) given the possibility of the generation of aerosols in the course of caring for patients. Detailed PPE recommendations are provided on the CDC website.

The global case fatality rate for EVD in 2014 was ~50%, though rates ranging from 25% to 90% have been reported in past outbreaks. It is important to note, however, that a great many nonsurvivors of EVD received little medical care, much less modern intensive care support. With early and aggressive supportive care, it is quite likely that the mortality rate from EVD is much lower, as evidenced by good outcomes from EVD that was occupationally acquired in the United States.

Future Directions

There are many unknowns that confront intensivists who could potentially care for children with EVD. Among these unknowns, it will be important to verify the perceived benefit of transporting children with EVD or suspected EVD to regional specialized centers. It will be essential to determine the best practice for disposal of the large volume of infected waste that EVD patients generate in the ICU. Finally, there are a large number of EVD vaccines and treatments in development and their safety and effectiveness will need to be evaluated.

References

1. West NS, Riordan FAI. Fever in returned travelers: A prospective review of hospital admissions for a 21/2 year period. *Arch Dis Child* 2003;88:432–4.
2. Freedman DO, Weld LH, Kozarsky PE, et al. Spectrum of disease and relation to place of exposure among ill returned travelers. *N Engl J Med* 2006;354:119–30.
3. Eliades MJ, Shah S, Nguyen-Dinh P, et al. Malaria surveillance—United States, 2003. *MMWR Surveill Summ* 2005;54:25–40.
4. Carter R, Mendis KN. Evolutionary and historical aspects of the burden of malaria. *Clin Microbiol Rev* 2002;15:564–94.
5. Williams TN. Red blood cell defects and malaria. *Mol Biochem Parasitol* 2006;149:121–7.
6. Seydel KB, Milner DA Jr, Kamiza SB, et al. The distribution and intensity of parasite sequestration in comatose Malawian children. *J Infect Dis* 2006;194:208–5.
7. Idro R, Marsh K, John CC, et al. Cerebral malaria; Mechanisms of brain injury and strategies for improved neuro-cognitive outcome. *Pediatr Res* 2010;68:267–74.
8. Planche T, Krishna S. The relevance of malaria pathophysiology to strategies of clinical management. *Curr Opin Infect Dis* 2005;18:369–75.
9. Maitland K, Pamba A, Newton CR, et al. Hypokalemia in children with severe falciparum malaria. *Pediatr Crit Care Med* 2004;5:81–5.
10. Berkley J, Mwarumba S, Bramham K, et al. Bacteraemia complicating severe malaria in children. *Trans R Soc Trop Med Hyg* 1999;93:283–6.
11. Bronzan RN, Taylor TE, Mwenechanya J, et al. Bacteremia in Malawian children with severe malaria: Prevalence, etiology, HIV coinfection, and outcome. *J Infect Dis* 2007;195:895–904.
12. Maitland K, Kiguli S, Opoka RO, et al. Mortality after fluid bolus in African children with severe infection. *N Engl J Med* 2011;364:2483–95.
13. Maitland K, Nadel S, Pollard AJ, et al. Management of severe malaria in children: Proposed guidelines for the United Kingdom. *BMJ* 2005;331:337–43.

14. Phu NH, Hien TT, Mai NT, et al. Hemofiltration and peritoneal dialysis in infection-associated acute renal failure in Vietnam. *N Engl J Med* 2002;347:895–902.

15. Day NP, Phu NH, Mai NT, et al. Effects of dopamine and epinephrine infusions on renal hemodynamics in severe malaria and severe sepsis. *Crit Care Med* 2000;28:1353–62.

16. Bruneel F, Hocqueloux L, Alberti C, et al. The clinical spectrum of severe imported falciparum malaria in the intensive care unit: Report of 188 cases in adults. *Am J Respir Crit Care Med* 2001;167:684–9.

17. Crump JA, Luby SP, Mintz ED. The global burden of typhoid fever. *Bull World Health Organ* 2004;82:346–53.

18. Basnyat B. Typhoid and paratyphoid fever. *Lancet* 2005;366:1603.

19. Chart H, Cheesbrough JS, Waghorn DJ. The serodiagnosis of infection with *Salmonella typhi*. *J Clin Pathol* 2000;53:851–3.

20. Olsen SJ, Pruckler J, Bibb W, et al. Evaluation of rapid diagnostic tests for typhoid fever. *J Clin Microbiol* 2004;42:1885–9.

21. Kadhiravan T, Wig N, Kapil A, et al. Clinical outcomes in typhoid fever: Adverse impact of infection with nalidixic acid-resistant *Salmonella typhi*. *BMC Infect Dis* 2005;5:37.

22. Chinh NT, Parry CM, Ly NT, et al. A randomized controlled comparison of azithromycin and ofloxacin for treatment of multidrug-resistant or nalidixic acid-resistant enteric fever. *Antimicrob Agents Chemother* 2000;44:1855–9.

23. Parry CM, Ho VA, Phuong T, et al. Randomized controlled comparison of ofloxacin, azithromycin, and an ofloxacin-azithromycin combination for treatment of multidrug-resistant and nalidixic acid-resistant typhoid fever. *Antimicrob Agents Chemother* 2007;51:819–25.

24. Hoffman SL, Punjabi NH, Kumala S, et al. Reduction of mortality in chloramphenicol-treated severe typhoid fever by high-dose dexamethasone. *N Engl J Med* 1984;310:82–8.

25. Centers for Disease Control and Prevention (CDC). Blood donor screening for Chagas disease—United States, 2006–2007. *MMWR Morb Mortal Wkly Rep* 2007;56:141–3.

26. Ferreira MS, Nishioka SA, Silvestre MT, et al. Reactivation of Chagas disease in patients with AIDS: Report of three new cases and review of the literature. *Clin Infect Dis* 1997;25:1397–400.

27. Rodrigues CJ, de Castro SL. A critical review on Chagas disease chemotherapy. *Mem Inst Oswaldo Cruz* 2002;97:3–24.

28. Rassi A Jr, Rassi A, Little WC, et al. Development and validation of a risk score for predicting death in Chagas' heart disease. *N Engl J Med* 2006;355:799–808.

29. Laras K, Cao BV, Bounlu K, et al. The importance of leptospirosis in Southeast Asia. *Am J Trop Med Hyg* 2002;67:278–86.

30. Bruce MG, Sanders EJ, Leake JA, et al. Leptospirosis among patients presenting with dengue-like illness in Puerto Rico. *Acta Trop* 2005;96:36–46.

31. LaRocque RC, Breiman RF, Ari MD, et al. Leptospirosis during dengue outbreak, Bangladesh. *Emerg Infect Dis* 2005;11:766–9.

32. Truccolo J, Serais O, Merien F, et al. Following the course of human leptospirosis: Evidence of a critical threshold for the vital prognosis using a quantitative PCR assay. *FEMS Microbiol Lett* 2001;204:317–21.

33. Marotto PC, Marotto MS, Santos DL, et al. Outcome of leptospirosis in children. *Am J Trop Med Hyg* 1997;56:307–10.

34. Suputtamongkol Y, Niwattayakul K, Suttinont C, et al. An open, randomized, controlled trial of penicillin, doxycycline, and cefotaxime for patients with severe leptospirosis. *Clin Infect Dis* 2004;39:1417–24.

35. Siriwanij T, Suttinont C, Tantawichien T, et al. Haemodynamics in leptospirosis: Effects of plasmapheresis and continuous venovenous haemofiltration. *Nephrology* 2005;10:1–6.

36. Levett PN. Leptospirosis. *Clin Microbiol Rev* 2001;14:296–326.

37. Duchin JS, Koster FT, Peters CJ, et al. Hantavirus pulmonary syndrome: A clinical description of 17 patients with a newly recognized disease. The Hantavirus Study Group. *N Engl J Med* 1994;330:949–55.

38. Centers for Disease Control. Hantavirus pulmonary syndrome cases by state of residence. http://www.cdc.gov/ncidod/diseases/hanta/hps/noframes/casemap.htm. 2006. Accessed October 7, 2007.

39. Mertz GJ, Hjelle B, Crowley M, et al. Diagnosis and treatment of new world hantavirus infections. *Curr Opin Infect Dis* 2006;19:437–42.

40. Pini N. Hantavirus pulmonary syndrome in Latin America. *Curr Opin Infect Dis* 2004;17:427–31.

41. Martinez VP, Bellomo C, San JJ, et al. Person-to-person transmission of Andes virus. *Emerg Infect Dis* 2005;11:1848–53.

42. Pini NC, Resa A, del Jesús LG, et al. Hantavirus infection in children in Argentina. *Emerg Infect Dis* 1998;4:85–7.

43. Ferres M, Vial P. Hantavirus infection in children. *Curr Opin Pediatr* 2004;16:70–5.

44. Ketai LH, Kelsey CA, Jordan K, et al. Distinguishing hantavirus pulmonary syndrome from acute respiratory distress syndrome by chest radiography: Are there different radiographic manifestations of increased alveolar permeability? *J Thorac Imaging* 1998;13:172–7.

45. Peters CJ, Khan AS. Hantavirus pulmonary syndrome: The new American hemorrhagic fever. *Clin Infect Dis* 2002;34:1224–31.

46. Hallin GW, Simpson SQ, Crowell RE, et al. Cardiopulmonary manifestations of hantavirus pulmonary syndrome. *Crit Care Med* 1996;24:252–8.

47. Mertz GJ, Miedzinski L, Goade D, et al. Placebo-controlled, double-blind trial of intravenous ribavirin for the treatment of hantavirus cardiopulmonary syndrome in North America. *Clin Infect Dis* 2004;39:1307–13.

48. MacNeil A, Ksiazek TG, Rollin PE. Hantavirus pulmonary syndrome, United States, 1993–2009. *Emerg Infect Dis* 2011;17:1195–201.

49. Overturf GD. Clinical sin nombre hantaviral infections in children. *Pediatr Infect Dis J* 2005;24:373–4.

50. Ramos MM, Overturf GD, Crowley MR, et al. Infection with Sin Nombre Hantavirus: Clinical presentation and outcome in children and adolescents. *Pediatrics* 2001;108:E27.

51. Cherry JD. Enteroviruses and parechoviruses. In: Feigin RD, Cherry JD, Demmler GJ, et al., eds. *Textbook of Pediatric Infectious Diseases*. Philadelphia, PA: Saunders, 2004:1984–2034.

52. Centers for Disease Control. Poliomyelitis. http://www.cdc.gov/vaccines/pubs/pinkbook/downloads/polio.pdf. Accessed October 7, 2007.

53. MacLennan C, Dunn G, Huissoon AP, et al. Failure to clear persistent vaccine-derived neurovirulent poliovirus infection in an immunodeficient man. *Lancet* 1908;363:1509–13.

54. Gea-Banacloche J, Johnson RT, Bagic A, et al. West Nile virus: Pathogenesis and therapeutic options. *Ann Intern Med* 2004;140:545–53.

55. Francisco AM, Glaser C, Frykman E, et al. 2004 California pediatric West Nile virus case series. *Pediatr Infect Dis J* 2006;25:81–4.

56. Hayes EB, O'Leary DR. West Nile virus infection: A pediatric perspective. *Pediatrics* 2004;113:1375–81.

57. O'Leary DR, Marfin AA, Montgomery SP, et al. The epidemic of West Nile virus in the United States, 2002. *Vector Borne Zoonotic Dis* 2004;4(1):61–70.

58. Clinical trials for treating West Nile virus disease. http://www.cdc.gov/ncidod/dvbid/westnile/clinicalTrials.htm. Accessed October 7, 2007.

59. Chan PK. Outbreak of avian influenza A(H5N1) virus infection in Hong Kong in 1997. *Clin Infect Dis* 2002;34(suppl 2):S58–S64.

60. World Health Organization. http://www.who.int/influenza/human_animal_interface/influenza_h7n9/Data_Reports/en/. Accessed October 7, 2007.

61. Writing Committee of the World Health Organization Consultation on Human Influenza. Avian influenza A (H5N1) infection in Humans. *N Engl J Med* 2005;353:1374–85.

62. Beigel JH, Farrar J, Han AM, et al. Avian influenza A (H5N1) infection in humans. *N Engl J Med* 1929;353:1374–85.

63. Kandun IN, Wibisono H, Sedyaningsih ER, et al. Three Indonesian clusters of H5N1 virus infection in 2005. *N Engl J Med* 2006;355:2186–94.

64. Ungchusak K, Auewarakul P, Dowell SF, et al. Probable person-to-person transmission of avian influenza A (H5N1). *N Engl J Med* 2005;352:333–40.

65. Apisarnthanarak A, Erb S, Stephenson I, et al. Seroprevalence of anti-H5 antibody among Thai health care workers after exposure to avian influenza (H5N1) in a tertiary care center. *Clin Infect Dis* 2005;40:e16–e18.

66. van Riel D, Munster VJ, de Wit E, et al. H5N1 Virus attachment to lower respiratory tract. *Science* 2006;312:399.

67. Shinya K, Ebina M, Yamada S, et al. Avian flu: Influenza virus receptors in the human airway. *Nature* 2006;440:435–6.

68. Hien TT, Liem NT, Dung NT, et al. Avian influenza A (H5N1) in 10 Patients in Vietnam. *N Engl J Med* 2004;350:1179–88.

69. Outbreaks of avian influenza A (H5N1) in Asia and interim recommendations for evaluation and reporting of suspected cases—United States, 2004. *MMWR Morb Mortal Wkly Rep* 2004;53:97–100.

70. Leneva IA, Goloubeva O, Fenton RJ, et al. Efficacy of zanamivir against avian influenza A viruses that possess genes encoding H5N1 internal proteins and are pathogenic in mammals. *Antimicrob Agents Chemother* 2001;45:1216–24.

71. Leneva IA, Roberts N, Govorkova EA, et al. The neuraminidase inhibitor GS4104 (oseltamivir phosphate) is efficacious against A/Hong Kong/156/97 (H5N1) and A/Hong Kong/1074/99 (H9N2) influenza viruses. *Antiviral Res* 2000;48:101–15.

72. Chotpitayasunondh T, Ungchusak K, Hanshaoworakul W, et al. Human disease from influenza A (H5N1), Thailand, 2004. *Emerg Infect Dis* 2005;11:201–9.

73. Yen HL, Monto AS, Webster RG, et al. Virulence may determine the necessary duration and dosage of oseltamivir treatment for highly pathogenic A/Vietnam/1203/04 influenza virus in mice. *J Infect Dis* 2005;192:665–72.

74. Treanor JJ, Hayden FG, Vrooman PS, et al. Efficacy and safety of the oral neuraminidase inhibitor oseltamivir in treating acute influenza: A randomized controlled trial. US Oral Neuraminidase Study Group. *JAMA* 2000;283:1016–24.

75. Le QM, Kiso M, Someya K, et al. Avian flu: Isolation of drug-resistant H5N1 virus. *Nature* 2005;437:1108.

76. Liem NT, Lim W. Lack of H5N1 avian influenza transmission to hospital employees, Hanoi, 2004. *Emerg Infect Dis* 2005;11:210–5.

77. Chan PK, Tang JW, Hui DS. SARS: Clinical presentation, transmission, pathogenesis and treatment options. *Clin Sci* 2006;110:193–204.

78. Peiris JS, Yuen KY, Osterhaus AD, et al. The severe acute respiratory syndrome. *N Engl J Med* 1918;349:2431–41.

79. Varia M, Wilson S, Sarwal S, et al. Investigation of a nosocomial outbreak of severe acute respiratory syndrome (SARS) in Toronto, Canada. *CMAJ* 2003;169:285–92.

80. Bitnun A, Allen U, Heurter H, et al. Children hospitalized with severe acute respiratory syndrome-related illness in Toronto. *Pediatrics* 2003;112:e261.

81. Booth CM, Stewart TE. Severe acute respiratory syndrome and critical care medicine: The Toronto experience. *Crit Care Med* 2005;33:S53–S60.

82. Hui DS, Chan MC, Wu AK, et al. Severe acute respiratory syndrome (SARS): Epidemiology and clinical features. *Postgrad Med J* 2004;80:373–81.

83. Li AM, Ng PC. Severe acute respiratory syndrome (SARS) in neonates and children. *Arch Dis Child Fetal Neonatal Ed* 2005;90:F461–F465.

84. Manocha S, Walley KR, Russell JA. Severe acute respiratory distress syndrome (SARS): A critical care perspective. *Crit Care Med* 2003;31:2684–92.

85. Wong GW, Li AM, Ng PC, et al. Severe acute respiratory syndrome in children. *Pediatr Pulmonol* 2003;36:261–6.

86. Babyn PS, Chu WC, Tsou IY, et al. Severe acute respiratory syndrome (SARS): Chest radiographic features in children. *Pediatr Radiol* 2004;34:47–58.

87. Li AM, Hon KL, Cheng WT, et al. Severe acute respiratory syndrome: "SARS" or "not SARS." *J Paediatr Child Health* 2004;40:63–5.

88. Brun-Buisson C. SARS: The challenge of emerging pathogens to the intensivist. *Intensive Care Med* 2003;29:861–2.

89. Yu CC, Li AM, So RC, et al. Longer term follow up of aerobic capacity in children affected by severe acute respiratory syndrome (SARS). *Thorax* 2006;61:240–6.

90. Li AM, So HK, Chu W, et al. Radiological and pulmonary function outcomes of children with SARS. *Pediatr Pulmonol* 2004;38:427–33.

91. Schieffelin JA, Shaffer JG, Goba A, et al. Clinical illness and outcomes in patients with ebola in Sierra Leone. *N Engl J Med* 2014;371:2092–100.

92. Lyon GM, Mehta AK, Varkey JB, et al. Clinical care of two patients with ebola virus disease in the United States published. *N Engl J Med* 2014;371:2402–9.

CHAPTER 94 ■ **TOXIN-RELATED DISEASES**

SUNIT C. SINGHI, M. JAYASHREE, JOHN P. STRAUMANIS, AND KAREN L. KOTLOFF

KEY POINTS

Tetanus

1. Tetanus is caused by infection with *Clostridium tetani*, which elaborates a toxin-designated tetanospasmin, which blocks the release of inhibitory neurotransmitters, and causes uninhibited sustained muscle contraction.
2. Worldwide, between 500,000 and 1 million cases occur per year.
3. Trismus and risus sardonicus are the most common initial symptoms, progressing gradually to generalized rigidity and muscle spasms. Mental status is not affected. Cranial nerve palsies occur in cephalic tetanus. Signs of autonomic dysfunction, such as hypertension and tachyarrhythmias, occur 5–7 days after the onset of generalized spasms.
4. Diagnosis is made on clinical grounds alone: No laboratory test is needed.
5. Treatment in the ICU is focused on neutralization of circulating toxin with human tetanus immunoglobulin (500 IU); early intubation/tracheostomy if frequent generalized, pharyngeal or laryngeal spasms occur; penicillin or metronidazole administration; control of muscle spasms with IV benzodiazepines or with neuromuscular blockade in severe cases; and control of hypertension and tachycardia with morphine and either propranolol or labetalol.
6. All survivors must be vaccinated.

Diphtheria

7. Diphtheria is a severe, widespread infectious disease that has the potential to reach epidemic proportions (as seen in Eastern Europe and the former Soviet Union in the 1990s cases and 2500 deaths worldwide in 2011).
8. Most infections are localized at a mucocutaneous site and can result in severe disease if produced by a toxigenic strain of *C. diphtheriae*, manifested by tonsillopharyngitis (90% cases) and pseudomembrane formation.
9. The toxin can cause serious systemic toxic effects, including myocarditis and polyneuritis.
10. The diagnosis is confirmed by the isolation of *C. diphtheriae* from a clinical specimen or a fourfold or greater rise in serum antibody titers.
11. Management consists of immediate administration of diphtheria antitoxin and antibiotics (penicillin or erythromycin), airway management, monitoring of cardiac function (heart rate, blood pressure, and electrocardiogram), and room isolation.
12. The airway should be secured early, as rapid progression of the membrane may preclude a later opportunity.
13. Overall case fatality is 5-10%; increases to 60-70% with complicating myocarditis

14. All survivors must be immunized. All close contacts should be cultured, observed daily for signs of diphtheria for 7 days, and given antibiotic regardless of immunization status (oral erythromycin for 7–10 days or one dose of intramuscular benzathine penicillin).
15. Immunized household contacts should receive a booster dose of toxoid, and unimmunized household contacts should receive primary immunization.
16. Primary control of disease can be achieved with high population immunity (>90%).

Human Botulism

17. Botulism is caused by neurotoxin(s) produced by *Clostridium botulinum*.
18. Neurologic symptoms start with autonomic changes and oculobulbar muscle weakness, followed by symmetric descending weakness of limbs. Sensory system and mentation are usually spared.
19. Diagnosis is based on clinical symptoms to avoid delay in treatment. Detection of toxin in patient's serum, stool, or suspected food confirms the diagnosis.
20. Human botulism immune globulin is reserved for infants. Older children should receive equine botulinum toxin.
21. Supportive treatment should include support of airway and respiratory status. Elective intubation should be considered.
22. An association exists between infant botulism and sudden infant death syndrome.

Toxic Shock Syndrome

23. Toxic shock syndrome (TSS) is an acute, toxin-mediated, multisystem febrile illness mainly caused by *Staphylococcus aureus* and group A Streptococcal infections.
24. TSS is characterized by an abrupt onset of high fever, vomiting, and erythematous rash with rapid deterioration to hypotension and variable degrees of multiorgan failure.
25. The bacterial toxins that cause the disease have been labeled as "superantigens."
26. Staphylococcal TSS has two forms: menstrual (associated with tampon use) and nonmenstrual. TSST-1 is found in nearly all cases of menstrual TSS and in 50% of nonmenstrual TSS, while enterotoxins are found in the other 50% of nonmenstrual TSS.
27. Streptococcal TSS is characterized by early shock and multiorgan failure and often accompanies invasive infections (e.g., rapidly progressive necrotizing fasciitis), sometimes in previously healthy patients.

The goals of management are removal of the source of toxin, appropriate antibiotic therapy, surgical debridement of necrotic tissues, neutralization of toxin with intravenous immunoglobulin therapy (1 g/kg for 2 days), and aggressive supportive therapy for shock (fluids and vasopressors) and multiorgan failure. Clindamycin is recommended for streptococcal TSS and in combination with a β-lactamase-resistant antistaphylococcal antibiotic (cloxacillin, oxacillin, or nafcillin) for staphylococcal TSS.

Most patients require tracheal intubation and mechanical ventilation for shock and for complicating lung disease. Prognosis of streptococcal TSS is worse than staphylococcal TSS.

Several bacterial infections cause illness, not because of direct tissue invasion, but because of the toxin(s) they release. In most of these diseases, toxin(s) often cause a localized disease, which may become a life-threatening systemic disease that requires admission to the PICU. Examples of such diseases include food poisoning and scalded skin syndrome caused by *Staphylococcus aureus*; diarrhea caused by enterotoxigenic *Escherichia coli*, Shiga toxin–producing *E. coli*, *Shigella dysenteriae* type 1, and *Bacteroides fragilis*; anthrax; cholera; gas gangrene; and others. In addition to localized effects, other toxin-mediated diseases cause systemic life-threatening illness that requires intensive care. These diseases are often associated with localized bacterial infection or merely colonization. The toxin is produced at the site of infection or colonization but spreads systemically. In some instances, infection and/or colonization do not occur. For instance, in botulism, ingestion of toxin present in contaminated food causes the disease. Important toxin-producing bacteria and the life-threatening systemic diseases caused by them are listed in **Table 94.1**. Those toxin-related infections that generally require treatment in an ICU are discussed in this chapter.

TETANUS

Tetanus is a potentially fatal disease characterized by hypertonia, muscle spasms, and autonomic instability. Tetanus is caused by the action of tetanospasmin (commonly called *tetanus toxin*), a potent neurotoxin elaborated by the organism *Clostridium tetani* (*C. tetani*).

Tetanus was known to Egyptians over 3000 years ago. Hippocrates gave the first detailed description of the disease in 400 BC, Arthur Nicolaier discovered the tetanus bacterium in 1884, and in 1889 Shibasaburo Kitasato at Koch's Institute obtained the first pure culture of tetanus bacilli. German bacteriologist Emil Von Behring developed a toxin–antitoxin mixture that was an effective vaccine against tetanus. In 1893, Emile Roux, assistant to Louis Pasteur, improved procedures for using serum antitoxin to prevent and to treat tetanus. Tetanus antitoxin was first used during World War I, dramatically reducing the incidence of the disease.

Epidemiology

Tetanus remains a major world health problem despite the availability of active and passive immunization. The World Health Organization (WHO) estimated in 2011 that the number of tetanus-related deaths globally in children <5 years of age was 72,600, of which 61,000 were attributable to neonatal tetanus (1). Worldwide, tetanus affects all age groups, particularly newborns (who account for half of all cases) and children. Lack of seroprotective immunity against tetanus is common among children. Only 45% of children attending an emergency unit of a tertiary care hospital in Africa had seroprotection (2). Tetanus rarely occurs among children who have received the primary series of tetanus toxoid vaccine. In industrialized nations such as the United States, tetanus is a disease of the elderly; a population that was either born before immunization programs were implemented or have an age-related decline in antitoxin levels. Fewer than 75% of adults were immune or partially immune to tetanus in a serosurvey in Australia in 2005 (3).

The Pathogen

Tetanus is caused by *C. tetani*, a drumstick-shaped, anaerobic, Gram-positive bacillus that forms endospores on maturation. The spores are widely distributed (soil, house and operating room dust, freshwater, and saltwater) and may survive for years. They are also present in the feces of a number of animals (sheep, cattle, dogs, cats, chickens, and horses) and in the intestinal tract of as many as 40% of humans. Soil rich in organic matter or treated with animal manure can be highly infective. The spores are resistant to extremes of temperature, moisture, various disinfectants (ethanol, phenol, and, formalin), and to boiling for 20 minutes.

Pathogenesis

Disease is initiated when *C. tetani* spores enter a breach in the skin or mucosa. It typically occurs after acute injury to soft tissue, particularly deep penetrating or puncture wounds and lacerations, in which anaerobic bacterial growth is facilitated. The common portals of infection are wounds on the lower limbs, nonsterile intramuscular (IM) injections, and compound fractures. Tetanus can also occur as a result of animal bites, drug injection with dirty needles, dental abscesses, body piercing, drug abuse (notably skin popping), burns, surgical procedures, and in patients with chronic infections, such as otitis media or decubitus ulcers. The portal of entry is not apparent in approximately one-third of patients.

Inside the wound, in an anaerobic environment, the spores transform into vegetative forms and proliferate. The process is facilitated by the presence of a foreign body, necrotic tissue, or suppuration in the wound. Replicating bacteria do not cause inflammation, and the wound appears benign. The vegetative forms produce two toxins under plasmid control: tetanospasmin and tetanolysin. Tetanolysin damages the viable tissue around the infected wound, lowers the redox potential in the wound, and further facilitates the growth of anaerobic organisms. Tetanospasmin causes the clinical manifestations of tetanus.

Tetanospasmin is a single, 1315-amino-acid polypeptide that acts as a zinc-dependent peptidase. The molecule becomes

TABLE 94.1

COMMON TOXIN-PRODUCING BACTERIA AND THE LIFE-THREATENING SYSTEMIC DISEASES THEY CAUSE

Corynebacterium diphtheria	Diphtheria
C. tetani	Tetanus
C. botulinum	Botulism
Clostridium perfringens	Gas gangrene, food poisoning
Clostridium difficile	Antibiotic-associated colitis
S. aureus	TSS
S. pyogenes (group A streptococcus)	TSS

toxic after being cleaved at serine 458 by a bacterial protease into a heterodimer of a 100-kDa heavy chain and a 50-kDa light chain connected by a disulfide bridge. The heavy chain is further cleaved by pepsin into B and C fragments. The resulting toxin thus comprises the amino-terminal end of a heavy chain (fragment B) linked with a light chain (fragment A) by a di-sulfide bridge (fragment A–B) and a heavier carboxyl-terminal polypeptide (fragment C). Fragment C is responsible for attach-ment to the neuronal cell surface receptors and internalization of toxin, while fragment A–B produces the presynaptic inhibi-tion of neurotransmitter release that results in clinical tetanus.

After entering the body, tetanospasmin spreads via lym-phatics and blood vessels to enter the nervous system at the neuromuscular junction of the lower motor neurons. Although its greatest affinity is for inhibitory systems, a small amount of toxin may also enter sensory and autonomic neurons. The receptor to which toxin binds is thought to be membrane gan-gliosides, but this remains controversial. The toxin spreads through the central nervous system (CNS) by retrograde axo-nal transport to the cell body and transsynaptically to other neurons, particularly the presynaptic inhibitory neurons. The proteins synaptotagmin, syntaxin, and synaptobrevin are in-volved in docking of synaptic vesicles to presynaptic mem-brane and release of the contents of synaptic vesicles into the synaptic clefts. Tetanospasmin cleaves peptide bonds of syn-aptobrevin and inhibits the release of neurotransmitters, pre-dominantly glycine, in the spinal cord and γ-aminobutyric acid (GABA) in the brainstem. The loss of inhibition of α-motor neurons and dysfunction of polysynaptic reflexes result in inhibition of antagonists, causing sustained, uninhibited con-traction of muscles (tetany). Excitatory transmission is also disrupted, causing weakness of muscles.

Blood-borne spread of toxin occurs from the site of entry to the brain at the area postrema of the floor of the fourth ventricle, where the blood–brain barrier (BBB) is nonexistent. This possibly explains the early manifestations of tetanus, such as trismus and nuchal rigidity.

The autonomic dysfunction in tetanus is caused by sev-eral mechanisms, which include the effect of tetanolysin on brainstem and autonomic interneurons, and a direct effect of the toxin on the myocardium and adrenal inhibition. The loss of glycine inhibition by tetanospasmin affects pregan-glionic sympathetic neurons in spinal cord and causes in-creased sympathetic activity and increased catecholamine levels. Tetanospasmin may interfere with the release of ace-tylcholine in peripheral somatic and autonomic nerves, re-sulting in a progressive interference with the inhibition of neuronal transmission. Also, tetanospasmin probably has an angiotensin-converting enzyme–like effect that contributes to hypertension; inhibition by captopril of the effect of tetano-spasmin on synaptobrevin supports this view.

Clinical Features

The incubation period—the time interval between spore inoc-ulation and symptom onset—may vary from 2 days to months (average 2 weeks). In severe forms, the incubation period is shorter, and the period of onset is <48 hours. Tetanus typi-cally evolves as one of four clinical forms, generalized, local-ized, neonatal, or cephalic.

Generalized Tetanus

The most common form of tetanus is generalized teta-nus, which manifests with classical trismus or "lockjaw" (Fig. 94.1), followed by *risus sardonicus* (a facial grimace that results from hypertonia of the orbicularis oris), general-ized muscle rigidity, hyper-reflexia, dysphagia, opisthotonos, and spasms. The body assumes an opisthotonic position that

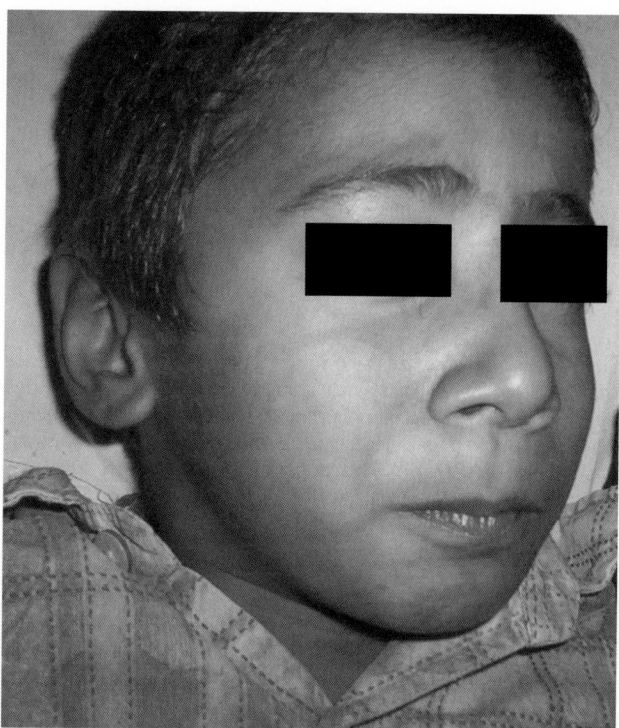

FIGURE 94.1. Typical risus sardonicus in a 9-year-old child with tetanus. (Photo used with permission.)

resembles decorticate posturing (without loss of consciousness) with flexion of the arms and extension of the legs. The muscle spasms are caused by a sudden burst of tonic contraction in muscles and are very painful. Pharyngeal spasms lead to severe dysphagia. If prolonged, spasms may lead to rhabdomyolysis (and its complications), laryngeal obstruction, acute respira-tory failure, and cardiac arrest. Spasms are more prominent in the first 2 weeks, and their severity may increase during this period. Rigidity may last beyond the occurrence of spasms and autonomic disturbances, which usually occur some days after the spasms and reach a peak during the second week of the disease (4). Sympathetic overactivity, associated with ele-vated plasma norepinephrine and epinephrine concentrations, causes fluctuating heart rate, peripheral pallor, labile hyper-tension, and fever with profound sweating. Fluctuations in blood pressure and heart rate appear to be related to changes in systemic vascular resistance rather than cardiac output or left-ventricular filling pressure. These may be accompanied by hypotension and cardiac arrhythmias (paroxysmal supra-ventricular tachycardia, runs of ventricular tachycardia, and ventricular or atrial premature beats). Parasympathetic in-volvement may manifest as excessive salivation and increased bronchial secretions as well as bradycardia and sudden cardiac arrest in severe tetanus. Recovery usually begins after 3 weeks and takes about 4 weeks. However, the clinical course is often unpredictable.

Localized Tetanus

Occasionally, muscle rigidity, often in association with muscle weakness, may remain localized at the site of spore inoculation. Symptoms may be mild, self-limited, and persistent (in par-tially immune hosts), or may progress to generalized tetanus.

Neonatal Tetanus

Neonatal tetanus is a generalized form of tetanus that devel-ops through contamination of the umbilical stump in infants born to inadequately immunized mothers. The contamination may be caused by the use of unsterile instruments to cut the cord or by unhygienic cord care practices (e.g., applying soil or cow dung dressing to the stump) that are prevalent in certain populations. The first signs are poor sucking and excessive crying, followed by variable degrees of trismus, risus sardonicus, and repeated generalized muscle spasms. Apnea may result from spasm of respiratory muscles. The baby cannot be nursed and, unless appropriate treatment is available, is at high risk for death. If the baby survives, spasms subside by the late second or early third week, and swallowing returns by the end of 4 weeks.

Cephalic Tetanus

Cephalic tetanus is an uncommon localized form of disease that is often associated with otitis media and head injuries and affects the cranial nerves. Facial paresis is usually present. A coexisting aerobic infection, often caused by *S. aureus*, may be present. Rarely, extraocular movements are affected, causing "ophthalmologic tetanus."

Diagnosis and Differential Diagnosis

The diagnosis of tetanus is made entirely on clinical grounds (**Table 94.2**). Recent history of injury, bites, or a known portal of entry (such as otitis media, dental abscess, and infected wounds) supports the diagnosis. In patients with trismus or neck stiffness, diagnosis may be difficult in the early phase of disease in the absence of clear evidence of injury. A bedside "spatula test" developed by Apte and Karnad (94% sensitivity and 100% specificity) can be helpful. On insertion of a spatula (or tongue blade) that touches the posterior pharyngeal wall, if the patient gags and expels the spatula, the test is negative, whereas if the patient bites the spatula because of reflex masseter spasms, the test is positive for tetanus (5).

There is no serologic test to determine the presence of toxin in serum or cerebrospinal fluid (CSF). A confirmed history of full active immunization almost excludes tetanus; the failure rate after a full course of tetanus toxoid in immunocompetent population is 4 per 100 million. Culture of *C. tetani* from a suspicious wound is not useful.

The differential diagnoses are few. Trismus caused by peritonsillar and odontogenic abscesses and abdominal rigidity caused by local trauma or peritonitis can be excluded by history and examination. Dystonic reactions to dopamine blockade usually cause torticollis and oculogyric crises but not spasms. Benztropine or diphenhydramine can be administered to rule out such a reaction. Meningitis, meningoencephalitis, and tuberculous meningitis, which cause generalized hypertonia, neck rigidity, and tonic seizures, may sometimes mimic tetanus but can be differentiated by the presence of impaired mental status. Hypocalcemic tetany involves limb muscles more than the trunk and is associated with positive Chvostek and Trousseau signs. Poisoning with strychnine, a direct

antagonist of glycine receptors, closely resembles generalized tetanus. Trismus is absent and abdominal muscles are less rigid in strychnine poisoning. Stiff-person syndrome (a rare neurologic disorder of uncertain etiology) has an insidious onset; hypertonia involves face and jaw muscles minimally and improves during sleep.

Entities that cause diffuse muscle spasms, such as toxidromes and encephalopathies, are accompanied by changes in mental status. The authors described a child with Guillain–Barré syndrome who initially had characteristic stimulation-induced opisthotonos and arching, mimicking tetanus (6). Cephalic tetanus without trismus can be easily mistaken for Bell palsy.

Complications of Tetanus

Hypoxemia that leads to respiratory failure is a major cause of death. Cardiovascular consequences of autonomic instability, including cardiac arrhythmias and cardiomyopathy, sometimes occur and may be less amenable to secondary prevention.

Patients who are treated in the ICU are particularly prone to respiratory complications related to the use of mechanical ventilation (pneumothorax, atelectasis, ventilator-associated pneumonia), nosocomial infection, urinary tract infection related to indwelling catheters, wound sepsis, and gastrointestinal hemorrhage. The most common bacteria-causing infections are those that are Gram negative and *S. aureus*.

Rhabdomyolysis may occur in severe generalized tetanus and may lead to acute renal failure. If the serum creatine kinase level is high or myoglobin is detected in the urine, hydration with normal saline and urinary alkalinization with sodium bicarbonate should be considered. Phrenic and laryngeal neuropathies and other mononeuropathies can occur as a consequence of tetanus. Compression of the common peroneal nerve at the fibular head may produce foot drop.

Management

Tetanus at any age is a medical emergency and is best managed in a referral hospital. Availability of intensive care and critical care protocols has made a significant impact on survival of patients with tetanus (7). Grading of tetanus severity on the basis of Ablett criteria (**Table 94.3**) may help in selecting patients who might most benefit from intensive monitoring and care. Management goals and a proposed protocol for management of severe grades of tetanus appear in **Table 94.4** and include:

1. Neutralization of the unbound toxin
2. Removal of the source of toxin
3. Control of rigidity and muscle spasms
4. Control of autonomic dysfunction
5. Supportive care—airway and ventilation

Neutralization of the Unbound Toxin

Passive immunization to neutralize circulating (unbound) toxin by using antitoxin shortens the course and reduces the severity of tetanus. Human tetanus immunoglobulin (HTIG) is the preparation of choice. It consists of immunoglobulin G and has a half-life of 25 days. The dose of HTIG is 500 IU given IM or IV, although doses as high as 3000–6000 IU have been used. Where HTIG is unavailable, equine anti-tetanus serum may be used after testing for hypersensitivity. Equine anti-tetanus serum has a higher risk of anaphylactic reactions and a short half-life of 2 days but is less expensive. The usual dose of anti-tetanus serum is 500–1000 U/kg; half of the dose is given IM, and half IV. Although HTIG and anti-tetanus serum have effect only on the unbound toxin (which is present in serum samples of only 10% of cases), either one of them

---

TABLE 94.2

CLINICAL CRITERIA FOR DIAGNOSIS OF TETANUS

1. An illness characterized by the acute onset of hypertonia and/or painful muscle contractions (usually of the jaw and neck) and generalized muscle spasms without other apparent causes, such as drug reactions, other CNS disorders, hysteria
2. No history of contact with strychnine
3. Subsequent disease course consistent with tetanus

Adapted from Centers for Disease Control and Prevention. Epidemiologic notes and reports tetanus—Kansas, 1993. *MMWR* 1994;43:309–11.

TABLE 94.3

ABLETT CRITERIA FOR CLASSIFICATION OF SEVERITY OF TETANUS

Grade I	Mild or no respiratory involvement and dysphagia
Grade II	Moderate respiratory involvement and trismus
Grade IIIA	Severe respiratory involvement, generalized rigidity, and major spasms, with no autonomic involvement
Grade IIIB	Severe manifestations as above with autonomic dysfunction

Adapted from Ablett JJL. Analysis and main experience in 82 patients treated in the Leeds tetanus unit. In Ellis M, ed. *Symposium on Tetanus in Great Britain.* Boston Spa, UK: National Lending Library, 1967.

should be administered as soon as possible in all cases, irrespective of the duration or severity of the disease. Whether antitoxin should also be infiltrated locally at the portal of entry is unclear and needs scrutiny.

Intrathecal Administration of Antitoxin. Antitoxin can be administered intrathecally with the assumption that high concentrations of antitoxin in CSF and around the nerve roots will neutralize the toxin bound to neurons in CNS and act on the inhibitory interneurons preventing the release of GABA. Some studies have found it effective, whereas others have not. A randomized trial from Brazil found shorter duration of

occurrence of spasm, hospital stay, and respiratory assistance in adult patients treated with 1000 IU of intrathecal HTIG (8). A meta-analysis of 12 randomized studies that included 484 patients in the intrathecal group and 458 in the IM group concluded that intrathecal therapy was superior to IM therapy (9). The superiority of intrathecal therapy also emerged when the analysis was performed separately for adults and neonates and for high and low doses. Intrathecal anti-TIG (250 IU intrathecal, after removal of equal volume of CSF) in addition to the standard treatment improved the outcome of neonatal tetanus in terms of mortality and hospital stay (10).

Removal of the Source of Toxin

Toxin production may continue in suppurated wounds, wounds with retained foreign bodies, persistent otitis, untreated dental abscess, etc. The portal of entry should, therefore, be identified and treated appropriately with IV antibiotics and extensive wound debridement under local anesthesia after spasms are controlled. After debridement, the wound should be kept clean through regular wound care and aseptic dressing changes.

Antibiotic Therapy

Antibiotic therapy should be given to eradicate toxin-producing *C. tetani*. Although in vitro *C. tetani* is sensitive to metronidazole, penicillin, cephalosporins, carbapenems, and macrolides, crystalline penicillin and metronidazole are generally preferred (**Table 94.5**). Some prefer metronidazole to penicillin because the structure of penicillin is similar to GABA, which is the principal inhibitory neurotransmitter in the CNS. It is

TABLE 94.4

SUGGESTED PROTOCOL FOR TETANUS MANAGEMENT (STEPS IN MANAGEMENT)

A. Stabilization in Emergency Room
1. Assess airway and ventilation, and prepare for endotracheal intubation using rapid-sequence intubation technique, if generalized rigidity or spasm.
2. Establish IV access and obtain samples for electrolytes, blood urea, creatinine, creatine kinase, and urinary myoglobin. If clinically indicated, perform neuroimaging and a lumbar puncture to rule out other diagnosis.
3. Determine and record the portal of entry, incubation period, period of onset, immunization history, and severity grade.
4. Administer diazepam IV, starting with 0.2 mg/kg to control spasms and decrease rigidity. If this causes respiratory depression, intubate using rapid-sequence induction technique.
5. Transfer the patient to a dark isolated room in the ICU.

B. Early management in PICU; first week
1. Administer human tetanus immune globulin (HTIG; 500 units), IM; and tetanus toxoid (0.5 mL) IM, at different sites.
2. Consider intrathecal administration of HTIG (250–1000 IU).
3. Start crystalline penicillin (100,000 IU/kg/d, q 6 h, IV) for 10–14 d or metronidazole (40 mg/kg/d, q 6 h, IV) for 7–10 d.
4. Initiate airway management: endotracheal intubation. Perform a tracheostomy if spasms produce any degree of airway compromise or difficulty in managing secretions.
5. Debride the wound under local anesthesia.
6. Establish a nasogastric tube for feeding.
7. Start continuous monitoring of heart rate, blood pressure, and cardiac rhythm.
8. Continue benzodiazepine infusion (in incremental doses as needed) to control spasms and achieve sedation. If adequate control of spasm is not achieved, administer magnesium IV to achieve a serum magnesium concentration of 4–8 mEq/L (2–4 mmol/L).
9. Initiate neuromuscular junction blockade with IV vecuronium 0.1 mg/kg/h if spasms continue. Continue benzodiazepine for sedation.

C. Continuing management in PICU: next 2–3 wk
1. Control sympathetic hyperactivity with IV propranolol or labetalol. Administer fluids, dopamine, or norepinephrine as and when needed to maintain hemodynamic stability. Avoid diuretics and blood.
2. With sustained bradycardia, atropine is useful; a pacemaker may be needed.
3. Use water or air mattress, to prevent skin breakdown.
4. Maintain benzodiazepines until needed to control spasm/hypertonia. Taper the dose over 14–21 d.
5. Maintain serum magnesium, if used, until spasms are no longer present.

D. Convalescent stage
1. Start physical therapy and supportive psychotherapy
2. Administer a dose of tetanus toxoid.

TABLE 94.5

PHARMACOLOGIC TREATMENT OF TETANUS

■ DRUG	■ DOSE	■ MAJOR SIDE EFFECTS	■ CONTRAINDICATION	■ DURATION
ANTIBIOTICS				
Penicillin G	100,000–200,000 IU/kg/d IV in four divided doses	Local pain, inflammation at injection site, and hypersensitivity may potentiate effects of tetanus toxin due to its GABA agonist effect.	Documented hypersensitivity	10–14 d
Metronidazole	30–40 mg/kg/d IV every 6 h; max, 4 g/d	Neurotoxicity in the form of dizziness, vertigo; rarely, convulsions	Documented hypersensitivity	7–10 d
CONTROL OF SPASMS				
Benzodiazepines				
Diazepam	0.2 mg/kg initial dose through IV infusion, stepped up rapidly in increments until spasms are controlled; usually, 1 mg/kg/h. Change to enteral route in four to six divided doses through nasogastric tube; max 2 mg/kg/h	Respiratory depression, hypotension secondary to vasodilation and myocardial depression. Glycols and benzyl alcohol used as preservatives in IV preparation are toxic when very high doses of diazepam are used.	Shock, respiratory depression	Full doses for 2–3 wk; then, gradually tapered off over 2 wk
Midazolam	0.1–0.3 mg/kg/h as IV infusion	Respiratory depression, hypotension	Shock	
Lorazepam	0.15 mg/kg loading dose, followed by 0.05–0.1 mg/kg/h IV	Respiratory depression, hypotension, toxic glycols, or benzyl alcohol used as preservatives	Hypotension, shock	
Neuromuscular Blocking Agents				
Pancuronium	Initial dose 0.08–0.1 mg/kg; then as IV infusion 0.1 mg/kg/h	Tachycardia, hypertension, and increased cardiac output due to intrinsic sympathomimetic activity. Delayed recovery from paralysis and need for prolonged ventilation	Known hypersensitivity and lack of access to mechanical ventilation	Shortest possible
Vecuronium	Initial dose 0.08–0.1 mg/kg; then as IV infusion 0.1 mg/kg/h	Minimal cardiovascular side effects; the drug is considered "cardiovascularly clean." Complications related to prolonged use are similar to pancuronium.	Used cautiously in the presence of hepatic or renal disease	Shortest possible
Atracurium	Initial dose 0.5 mg/kg; then as IV infusion of 0.5 mg/kg/h	Increases in bronchial secretions, and itching and wheezing due to histamine release	Safe in hepatic and renal disease unlike vecuronium and baclofen	Shortest possible
Intrathecal baclofen	No definite guidelines. Bolus dose of 40-200mcg, followed by 2-20mcg /hour infusion till maximum of 1–2 mg (Santos 2004 paper). Infusion through an epidural catheter placed in the L3–L4 space for prolonged therapy.	Drowsiness, sedation coma, respiratory depression, hypersensitivity. Side effects increase with repeated boluses. Reversible on stopping therapy.	Known hypersensitivity. Used with caution in the presence of respiratory depression and altered sensorium.	7–14 d
CONTROL OF AUTONOMIC INSTABILITY				
Labetalol	IV 0.2–0.5 mg/kg/dose, titrated to effect, max 20 mg/dose. Oral 4 mg/kg/d in two divided doses, max 20 mg/kg/d	Bradycardia, hypotension, congestive heart failure, bronchospasm, rash, dizziness, reversible myopathy (very rarely)	Known hypersensitivity, asthma, cardiogenic shock, bradycardia, pulmonary edema	6–8 wk

■ DRUG	■ DOSE	■ MAJOR SIDE EFFECTS	■ CONTRAINDICATION	■ DURATION
Morphine	0.02–0.1 mg/kg/h as IV infusion or 0.1 mg/kg IV every 4–6 h	Respiratory depression, hence caution in patients with respiratory compromise. Bronchoconstriction, vomiting, and hypotension	Used with caution in advanced liver and renal disease and in known asthmatic.	7–10 d
Magnesium sulfate	25–50 mg/kg/dose IV as an hourly infusion, max dose −2 g/dose, repeated every 6 h, depending on the clinical response and serum magnesium	Hypocalcemia, weakness, sedation, paralysis, hypotension, and bradyarrhythmias (heart block). Serum magnesium levels must be monitored closely, as clinical signs may be missed in a sedated and paralyzed patient.	Oliguria, Compromised renal function	Maintain serum magnesium at ~4–8 mEq/L
Clonidine	Initial 5–10 μg/kg/d in divided doses every 8–12 h PO. Increase to 5–25 μg/kg/d every 6 h gradually	Hypotension, bradycardia, headache, dizziness, fatigue, respiratory depression, Raynaud phenomenon		

believed that, in high doses, penicillin may cause competitive antagonism to GABA and act synergistically with tetanospasmin to worsen the spasms. A randomized, controlled study suggests that benzyl penicillin, benzathine penicillin (single IM injection), and metronidazole are equally effective (11). In the authors' experience clinical outcome is similar with either of the antibiotics in severe, generalized tetanus treated in the PICU (12).

Control of Rigidity and Spasms

Even slight external stimuli, such as noise or touch, can trigger muscle spasms. It is therefore essential to keep the patient's external surroundings as quiet and dark as possible. No one drug or group of drugs has been consistently effective in controlling rigidity and spasms in severe tetanus.

Benzodiazepines. Benzodiazepines (diazepam, midazolam, and lorazepam) are commonly used for control of rigidity and spasms, as they are GABA$_A$ agonists and antagonize the effect of toxin on inhibitory receptors. They control spasms by blocking the polysynaptic reflexes, and work peripherally, without depressing the cortical centers.

Diazepam is a sedative, anticonvulsant, and a muscle relaxant long used as a therapy for tetanus. It has a wide margin of safety and a rapid onset of action and can be given orally, rectally, or intravenously. A meta-analysis of in-hospital deaths caused by tetanus indicated that children treated with diazepam alone had a better chance of survival than those treated with a combination of phenobarbitone and chlorpromazine (13). The dose of diazepam required for control of spasms may vary greatly. At higher doses, diazepam (due to its vehicle propylene glycol) can cause respiratory and myocardial depression, and hyperosmolarity can increase the risk of hemolysis and myoglobinuria. Initial control is achieved with IV diazepam infusion; enteral administration through a feeding tube may be started once spasms are under control (12). After 2–3 weeks of the full dose, the drug is gradually tapered over 2 weeks. Alternatively infusion of midazolam (0.1–0.3 mg/kg/h IV) or lorazepam (0.15 mg/kg IV loading dose, followed by 0.05–0.1 mg/kg/h IV) can be used. Midazolam does not require glycols for solubility and is gaining acceptance as the drug of choice.

Neuromuscular Blockade. Neuromuscular blockade is required when sedatives are not fully effective in controlling rigidity and spasms. Pancuronium (through vagal blockade and inhibition of norepinephrine re-uptake by adrenergic nerves) may cause tachycardia and hypertension and worsen the autonomic instability. Therefore, vecuronium and atracurium are neuromuscular blocking agents of choice in ventilated tetanus patients. Vecuronium is "cardiovascularly clean" and induces minimum autonomic instability but is relatively short-acting and requires continuous infusion. During the period of use of neuromuscular blockade, adequate sedation must be ensured.

Other Drugs. Continuous and intermittent intrathecal administration of baclofen (a GABA$_B$ agonist) has been reported to be useful. It reduced the need for sedation and ventilatory support in adult patients (14). The technique is invasive and expensive, and facilities for ventilation must be available. IV infusion of dantrolene (1–2 mg/kg q 4 hour), a direct-acting muscle relaxant, may be useful in select cases. The sedative agent propofol has been used for its muscle-relaxing properties, but it should not be used alone, as it does not have any GABA activity or analgesic effect. The concentrations of propofol required to control spasms are very high—closer to anesthetic rather than sedative doses. Continuous propofol administration in children raises the concern for propofol infusion syndrome.

Control of Autonomic Dysfunction

Continuous hemodynamic and electrocardiogram monitoring is essential for timely detection of autonomic dysfunction. As with control of spasms, no one class of drugs or combination is known to be consistently effective for management of autonomic dysfunction.

Propranolol, a β-adrenergic blocking agent, is one of the most commonly used drugs for quick control of sympathetic dysfunction, namely tachycardia, hypertension, and supraventricular tachycardia. It should be used in small doses, as it may produce serious side effects. Enteral administration may be dangerous as absorption and response may be erratic because of altered gastrointestinal motility. Labetalol has been used for combined α- and β-adrenergic effect and is currently preferred over other drugs. Esmolol (short-acting β-blocker) reduces catecholamine release and may have advantage over other pure β-blockers.

Morphine acts centrally to reduce sympathetic tone to the heart and vascular system and reduces heart rate and blood pressure. It also has a sedative effect, which is an added advantage.

Magnesium, a presynaptic neuromuscular blocker, inhibits the release of humoral and neuronal catecholamines, and reduces the sensitivity of α-adrenergic receptors. Magnesium infusion is adjusted to maintain a serum magnesium level between 4 and 8 mEq/L, which reduces extreme variability of heart rate and blood pressure and the need for neuromuscular blocking agents and sedatives in adult patients (15). Successful use of magnesium sulfate infusion for control of muscle rigidity and spasm refractory to moderate sedation has been reported in a 12-year-old child. The patient did not require deep sedation, neuromuscular blockade, or mechanical ventilation (16). In the absence of facility to monitor magnesium levels, abolition of patellar reflex may be used as an endpoint (it roughly corresponds to 3.5–4 mmol/L = 7–8 mEq/L) and positive Chvostek's and Trousseau's signs as evidence of hypocalcemia. Magnesium is contraindicated in the presence of renal failure. A meta-analysis of three published studies with 275 participants, however, did not reveal any beneficial effect of magnesium on mortality and ICU needs (17).

Clonidine is a selective partial agonist for α_2-adrenergic receptors in the CNS. It inhibits sympathetic outflow and potentiates parasympathetic activity, produces marked sedation and anxiolysis, and decreases spontaneous motor activity. Further investigation of clonidine as a treatment modality for autonomic dysfunction in tetanus should be conducted.

Other drugs that have anecdotal evidence of potential benefit in tetanus include atropine for parasympathetic autonomic dysfunction, sodium valproate for sedation, angiotensin-converting enzyme inhibitors for hypertension, and adenosine for arrhythmias. To date, their use in tetanus has been largely experimental. The role of pyridoxine is controversial, and corticosteroids are not advised. A nonrandomized trial from Bangladesh has suggested a possible role of vitamin C (1 g/day) as a treatment for tetanus. This study conducted on 117 patients, including 61 children 1–12 years old reported a considerable reduction in mortality with vitamin C (18). Doses and salient features of various drugs commonly used in tetanus are listed in **Table 94.5**.

Supportive Treatment

Supportive treatment in a patient with tetanus should include maintenance of airway and ventilation, proper gastrointestinal function and nutritional support, skin integrity, and prevention of complications of respiratory dysfunction, such as atelectasis and pneumonia.

Airway Management and Ventilatory Support. Patients with tetanus are at risk for hypoxic insult from frequent spasms of laryngeal, diaphragmatic, or respiratory muscles or from drug-induced respiratory failure. Endotracheal intubation should be performed in all patients who have generalized rigidity on arrival, even in the absence of frequent spasms, as the disease is likely to progress in severity for 10–14 days after onset. Children with frequent spasms or who require high-dose IV diazepam or neuromuscular blockade for untill controlled spasms must be intubated. An endotracheal tube should be inserted under sedation and neuromuscular blockade using the rapid-sequence induction technique. A nasogastric tube should be inserted concurrently. No consensus exists regarding the role of early tracheostomy. It is required in patients who have uncontrolled laryngospasm or who receive prolonged ventilation.

Ventilatory support is needed when neuromuscular blockade or high doses of diazepam are used for poorly controlled rigidity and spasms. Controlled ventilation is used initially, till the spasms and rigidity are controlled and not likely to progress (usually by the end of the second week of illness). Gradual weaning from ventilator support is accomplished using modes that allow a graded return to spontaneous respiratory effort.

Strict asepsis, meticulous mouth care, chest physiotherapy, and regular endotracheal tube care are essential to prevent atelectasis, lobar collapse, and pneumonia. Suctioning should be done only when necessary. Adequate sedation is mandatory when all of these interventions are performed to minimize the risk of uncontrolled spasms. Continuous pulse oximetry, respiratory monitoring, and periodic measurements of respiratory dynamics should be undertaken to assess pulmonary functions.

Gastrointestinal and Metabolic Considerations. Energy demand is high in patients with tetanus because of muscular spasms, excessive sweating, and associated sepsis. Therefore, adequate caloric intake should be ensured as early as possible. Enteral feeding, with head elevated to 30–45 degrees, is preferred. Gastrointestinal hypomotility or paralytic ileus may develop as a result of immobility and treatment with morphine. If patients cannot tolerate enteral feedings, parenteral nutrition becomes necessary.

The complications of immobility caused by heavy sedation and paralysis must be minimized. Special water or air mattresses to allow turning the patient with minimal stimulation and to prevent the development of pressure ulcers are preferred. Passive range-of-motion exercises must be instituted early to maintain muscle strength, prevent deformities, and stimulate circulation.

Psychosocial Considerations. Psychosocial care is important for paralyzed patients. It is essential to keep them comfortable and anticipate their needs. Patients' family members should be allowed to participate in care.

Outcome and Prognosis

Mortality rates are <10% in mild generalized disease but are as high as 50% in severe disease with frequent spasms, and are up to 90% in neonates. Death results from various complications, such as respiratory failure, pneumonia, septicemia, and cardiovascular instability. Spasm of the glottis can cause immediate death. Availability of intensive care and mechanical ventilation has helped in reducing early deaths caused by acute respiratory failure and uncontrolled spasms. Autonomic disturbances that appear later in the course of the illness and intensive care-related complications (ventilator-associated pneumonia, gastrointestinal hemorrhage) are now major causes of death.

The prognosis is determined by clinical severity at presentation, incubation period, progression of disease (as determined from "period of onset"—the time interval between first symptoms of tetanus and first generalized spasm), patient's age, portal of entry, and autonomic instability. Generally, the longer the incubation period, the milder the illness and better the prognosis. An incubation period of <1 week tends to be associated with more severe progression of the disease. Tetanus following burns, IM injections, especially quinine, or compound fractures has a poor outcome.

Poor prognostic factors in neonatal tetanus include age <7 days, symptom duration <5 days, fever, and *risus sardonicus*. Respiratory signs at or within 24 hours of admission, respiratory failure that requires mechanical ventilation, fever, and tachycardia are poor prognostic signs. Autonomic dysfunction (presence of labile or persistent hypertension or hypotension, sinus tachycardia or tachyarrhythmia, or bradycardia on electrocardiogram) predicted a poor outcome in adult patients, irrespective of severity of tetanus (19).

Sequelae include enuresis, mild mental retardation, and growth delay. Psychologic after-effects, including a perception of permanent worsening of health, have been reported in adults. Data on this aspect in children are not available.

Prevention

Tetanus is preventable with proper use of tetanus toxoid and HTIG. Active immunization of all survivors of tetanus with tetanus toxoid is imperative to prevent reinfection and further illness. The total amount of toxin produced during disease is inadequate to mount an immune response; therefore, patients with newly diagnosed tetanus must be actively immunized. A serum antibody titer of >0.01 U/mL is considered protective.

Recommendations for primary immunization depend on the age of the patient. A total of five doses of combined diphtheria–pertussis–tetanus (DPT or DTaP) vaccine at ages 2, 4, 6, 15–18 months, and 5 years is recommended. The vaccine may be given simultaneously with hepatitis B and *Haemophilus influenzae* type b (Hib) vaccines. The vaccine confers protective antibody levels in 81%–95% of previously unimmunized people after two doses and in 100% after three doses. A booster dose of tetanus toxoid is recommended every 10 years. Protective antibodies develop rapidly after a booster dose. All pregnant women (including previously immunized women) should receive a booster dose of combined DPT vaccine in the form Tdap, which contains a reduced diphtheria toxoid and acellular pertussis vaccine. The booster dose is given between the 27th and 36th week of pregnancy to confer neonatal immunity via transplacental transfer of antibodies. Pregnant women with unknown or incomplete vaccination histories should receive the series of three tetanus immunizations at times 0, 4, and 6–12 weeks, consisting of two Td doses and one Tdap dose, ideally between the 27th and 36th week of pregnancy (http://www.cdc.gov/vaccines/pubs/preg-guide.htm#tdap).

Postinjury Prophylaxis

Postinjury prophylaxis is not required in people who have received a tetanus toxoid booster dose within the previous 5 years. Children who have received partial immunization need only the remaining doses from the schedule, rather than to restart from the first dose. Although any wound can contain tetanus spores, some wounds are considered to be "tetanus-prone." These include wounds that are contaminated with dirt, saliva, or feces, and puncture wounds (including unsterile injections, missile injuries, burns, frostbite, avulsions, and crush injuries). A semiquantitative bedside test, Tetanus Quick Stick (TQS), can be used to check seroprotection against tetanus in patients with "tetanus-prone" wounds and no clear history of vaccination. It can detect up to 0.1 U of TIG in serum, with 86% sensitivity and 97.6% specificity (20), and can help in avoiding redundant vaccination. If the test is not available, individual with a tetanus-prone wound and an uncertain history of vaccination or the last dose of tetanus toxoid more than 5 years before injury should receive one dose of HTIG and one dose of tetanus toxoid *at separate sites with separate syringes*. HTIG should also be given to immunodeficient patients with a tetanus-prone wound. If doubt exists, a wound should be considered "tetanus-prone." In children, the dose of HTIG should be 500 units IM or IV to achieve adequate antibody concentration (0.1 IU/mL).

Conclusions and Future Directions

Severe tetanus remains a clinical challenge. Drugs that can control spasms and rigidity without causing respiratory depression must be evaluated. Failure to identify ideal drug(s) and limited availability of intensive care and ventilation in developing countries are some of the challenges. A bigger challenge is to find ways to achieve universal immunization of the susceptible population for this fully vaccine-preventable disease.

DIPHTHERIA

Diphtheria is an acute localized infection of skin or respiratory mucous membranes caused by toxin-producing strains of *Corynebacterium diphtheriae*. It is characterized by a pseudomembrane in the throat and a systemic illness that results from absorption of toxin. Edwin Klebs and Fredrick Loeffler, both pupils of Robert Koch, discovered the diphtheria bacillus in 1884. Four years later, Emile Roux discovered the diphtheria toxin secreted by *C. diphtheria*. In 1890, Emil Adolf von Behring at Koch's Institute paved the way for the use of serum therapy, and in 1891, Behring injected the newly prepared protective serum, named "antitoxin," to a severely ill, 8-year-old boy with diphtheria. The boy made a full recovery and became the first human to be cured with specific immunotherapy. The first Nobel Prize in Physiology or Medicine was awarded to Emil Adolf von Behring in 1901 for developing serum therapy for diphtheria.

Epidemiology

The incidence of diphtheria steadily declined in the developed nations following effective immunization programs introduced in the 1920s. However, in the mid-1990s, large epidemics of diphtheria occurred in Eastern Europe and the former Soviet Union. Resurgence of the disease in these countries was largely attributed to waning vaccine immunity in adults and importation of cases from the endemic developing world (21). Surveillance data from the Diphtheria Surveillance Network Countries and WHO European Region for 2000–2009 reported the highest 10-year incidence of 23.8 cases per 1 million person years from Latvia (22).

Diphtheria remains endemic in resource-poor countries. In 2011, diphtheria caused 5000 cases and 2500 deaths globally (23). The annual number of globally reported cases has remained almost unchanged since 2007. An immunization level of 70%–80% in the community is necessary to prevent epidemic spread. The DPT-3 coverage in Southeast Asia and Africa in 2012 was 75% and 72%, respectively, compared to more than 90% coverage in the European, Western Pacific, and American regions (24). Poor socioeconomic standards, overcrowding, delayed reporting to hospital, and nonavailability of or delay in antitoxin administration further contribute to the high mortality in developing countries.

The Pathogen

Clinical diphtheria is caused by toxin-producing corynebacteria—three species (*C. diphtheria*, *C. ulcerans*, and *C. pseudotuberculosis*) of which can produce the diphtheritic toxin. Of these, *C. diphtheriae* is the most common of the potentially toxigenic species associated with epidemic diphtheria and person-to-person spread. It is an aerobic pleomorphic,

Gram-positive, non–acid-fast, nonmotile bacillus that appears slightly curved or club-shaped. It has four subspecies: mitis, gravis, intermedius, and belfanti; each can cause the disease. The only known reservoir for *C. diphtheriae* is man. Transmission of the organism occurs by exposure to respiratory secretions or exudates from the skin lesions. Carriers can transmit the disease, but patients with active infection are more likely to do so. *C. diphtheriae* has been known to survive for weeks in floor dust, suggesting the potential for indirect transmission of infections. In tropical countries, cutaneous diphtheria is the principal source of infection. It may serve as an important reservoir of infection in epidemics of faucial diphtheria. *C. ulcerans* is historically associated with cattle or raw dairy products, and although it is rarely reported, its incidence has slightly increased in Western Europe and the United States in recent years. Currently, however, no direct evidence has been found of person-to-person spread of *C. ulcerans* and *C. pseudotuberculosis*.

Pathogenesis

Both toxigenic and nontoxigenic strains can cause localized mucocutaneous infection, bacteremia, and seeding of distant sites. However, the strains of *C. diphtheriae* that are lysogenized with bacteriophages that contain the structural genes encoding for production of the exotoxin (tox$^+$ strains) produce diphtheria toxin. The toxin is the major virulence factor responsible for severe local and systemic effects.

Diphtheria exotoxin is a 62-kDa polypeptide that includes two segments: the active moiety (A) and the binding segment (B). The latter binds to specific receptors on susceptible cells and allows fragment A to enter into the cell. Fragment A then inhibits protein synthesis by inactivation of elongation factor 2 (EF-2). All human cells are potentially susceptible to the effects of diphtheria toxin because they have receptors for the toxin and contain its substrate, EF-2. The differential effects on various tissues, with predilection for myocardium, peripheral nerves, and kidneys, are poorly explained.

The toxin also causes local destruction of the respiratory mucosa at the site of infection, facilitating formation of a dense coagulum of organism, necrotic epithelial cells, fibrin, and pus cells over the mucosa, the so-called *pseudomembrane*. Formation of pseudomembrane further promotes replication and person–person transmission of diphtheria bacillus. In addition to the toxin, cell wall components such as O and K antigens also contribute to the disease, of which the latter is important for mucosal attachment.

Age and the immunization status of the individual are host factors that are major determinants of disease severity and transmission. Although immunization does not prevent carriage or infection with toxigenic *C. diphtheriae*, antitoxic immunity decreases local tissue spread and necrosis (and therefore ameliorates the incidence and severity of disease). Immunization inhibits replication and transmission of the organism, thus providing herd immunity. It is estimated that 70%–80% of a population must be immunized to prevent epidemic spread. Nonetheless, even populations with very high immunization rates remain vulnerable to diphtheria outbreaks if travelers or immigrants introduce toxigenic strains of *C. diphtheriae*, particularly in crowded conditions with intense exposure (25).

The protective level of serum antitoxin is 0.01 IU/mL. These levels may decline with increasing age and increased vulnerability to the infection. In an Australian study among persons aged ≥50 years, fewer than 60% were immune or partially immune to diphtheria (3). Booster doses may succeed in maintaining sustained antitoxin levels and preventing infections.

Clinical Manifestations

Onset of symptoms may be insidious or abrupt following an incubation period of 2–5 days. Both sore throat and fever are almost universal. Cough and stridor may be presenting features in 65%–70% of unimmunized children with an acute fulminant course. Hoarseness of voice and dysphagia may be evident in 30%–40% of patients (26) (**Table 94.6**). Cervical lymphadenopathy with a brawny edema of the cervical region, described as "bull-neck," is common in severe cases. Unilateral, purulent to blood-tinged nasal discharge is characteristic of nasal diphtheria and is seen in 3%–4% of patients. Nonspecific symptoms, such as nausea, vomiting, malaise, and headache, may precede or coexist with onset of the disease.

The hallmark of respiratory diphtheria is the presence of the characteristic thick adherent fibrinous pseudomembrane on the respiratory epithelium. The membrane looks dull and grayish and bleeds easily on touch. It may be found on the palate, pharynx, tonsils, epiglottis, and larynx, or may extend to the tracheobronchial tree (**Fig. 94.2**). Among patients admitted to the PICU, faucial diphtheria (i.e., involvement of the posterior mouth and the proximal pharynx) is most common (~70%), followed by pharyngolaryngeal (25%), laryngeal (2%–3%), and combined faucial and nasal (4.2%) (27). Laryngeal diphtheria is usually secondary to an extension of faucial diphtheria. Isolated laryngeal membrane, nasal diphtheria, or tracheal membrane without pharyngeal involvement is rare.

Other forms of diphtheria may be seen less commonly. Cutaneous diphtheria infection typically presents as a chronic non-healing ulcer with a gray membrane. Etiologic agents of impetigo (*Streptococcus pyogenes* and *S. aureus*) can often be isolated from the same lesion. Infection is most often found in the tropics and in hosts subjected to inadequate hygiene. Clusters of invasive disease, for example, endocarditis, septic arthritis, and osteomyelitis, have been reported in similar populations.

Complications

Extensive membrane in an unimmunized child who presents within the first 5–6 days of onset of illness with a high leukocyte count should be considered as "severe disease." Delay in initiating treatment in patients with severe disease increases the risk of toxin spread and systemic complications.

Airway Obstruction

Upper airway obstruction is seen in nearly three-fourths of patients with "severe disease." Extension of diphtheritic

TABLE 94.6

SALIENT CLINICAL FEATURES OF DIPHTHERIA

Pseudomembrane	100%
Fever	92.4%
Upper respiratory tract infection	91.6%
Upper airway obstruction	42.3%
Hoarseness	36.7%
Bull-neck	11.3%

$n = 381$.
Data from Pancharoen C, Mekmullica J, Thisyakorn U, et al. Clinical features of diphtheria in Thai children: A historical perspective. *Southeast Asian J Trop Med Public Health* 2002;33:352–4.

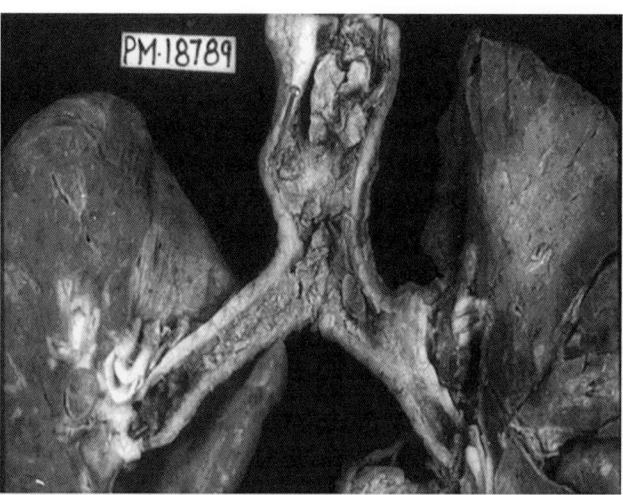

FIGURE 94.2. Gross photograph showing thick diphtheritic membrane on the mucosal aspect of trachea and bronchi. (Courtesy Dr. Ashim Dass, Professor, Department of Histopathology, *PGIMER*, Chandigarh.)

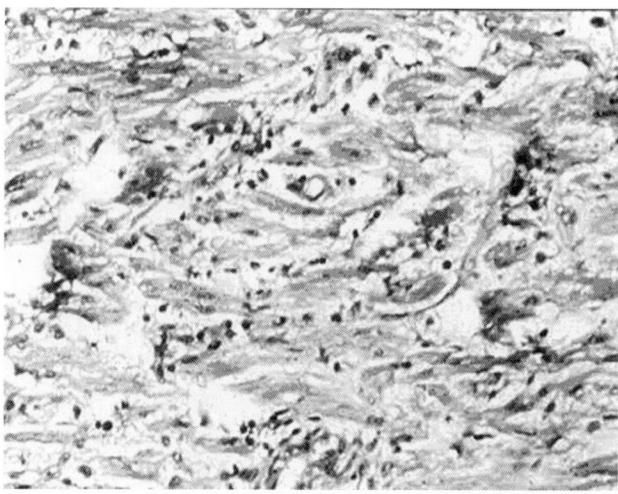

FIGURE 94.3. Microscopy with hematoxylin and eosin (H&E) staining of heart showing foci of necrotic cardiac myocytes with lymphocytic infiltrates in a child with toxic myocarditis caused by diphtheria. (Courtesy Dr. Ashim Dass, Professor, Department of Histopathology, *PGIMER*, Chandigarh.)

membrane into the larynx and tracheobronchial tree is the main cause of airway obstruction. Other contributing factors are soft-tissue edema and necrosis, dislodgement of pharyngeal membrane, and bleeding into the airway. Stridor, hoarseness, aphonia or dysphonia, and respiratory distress are manifestations of an obstructed airway. Ongoing assessment is essential, and the airway should be secured early, as rapid progression of the membrane may preclude a later opportunity. Timely intubation or tracheostomy in patients with airway complications carries a good prognosis. In both children and adults, pulmonary aspiration of the membrane, causing complete airway obstruction, is a common cause of death.

Myocarditis

Myocarditis is one of the most serious complications of diphtheria. Electrocardiographic changes have been reported in 68% of cases (28); symptomatic myocarditis occurs in 10%–25% of patients. In a series from the Kyrgyz Republic in 1995, among 676 patients with respiratory diphtheria, myocarditis occurred in 151 patients (21%) (29). The incidence of myocarditis is much higher (66%) in patients with severe and fulminant disease requiring intensive care (27). On histologic examination, myocardium shows hyaline degeneration and myonecrosis associated with active inflammation in the interstitial spaces and numerous lipid droplets within myofibrils (30) (Fig. 94.3).

Independent predictors of development of myocarditis include shared accommodation, extensive respiratory tract infection with subcutaneous edema (bull-neck), a pseudomembrane score of >2 (0, no membrane; 1, only nose or incomplete tonsillar coverage; 2, confluent coverage of tonsils; 3, as in 2 plus palate and/or pharyngeal wall; 4, as in 3 plus nose and/or larynx), and an elevated aspartate aminotransferase level (31). Subclinical cardiac damage may be identified by the presence of troponin T (32). Adequate immunization and early administration of antitoxin may have some role in preventing myocarditis.

Typically, myocarditis is seen at the end of the second week of illness but may be seen as early as 5 days following the onset of upper respiratory disease in unimmunized patients (27,31). Most of the times, only mild electrocardiographic changes, such as T wave inversion, inappropriate sinus tachycardia, ST

depression, ectopic beats and sinus bradycardia, may be indicative of myocarditis. Symptomatic myocarditis may have varied presentations, including muffled heart sounds, new or altered murmurs, ectopic beats, cardiac enlargement, arrhythmias, cardiogenic shock, or syncope. Diphtheria toxin has a high affinity for the conduction system of the heart, and prolonged PR interval is frequent. Bradyarrhythmias in the form of bundle-branch blocks progressing to complete heart blocks are more common than tachyarrhythmias (Fig. 94.4).

Neuropathy

Diphtheritic polyneuropathy usually occurs 3–16 weeks after the onset of acute diphtheria. Neuropathy has been variably reported to occur in 3%–43% of patients in different case series. A recent large series from India reported neuropathy in 15% of patients (28). The frequency is directly proportional to the severity of diphtheria and timely antitoxin therapy (33). Polyneuropathy could occur, but was attenuated in patients who were vaccinated according to schedule and had received antitoxin within 2–3 days of the onset of acute respiratory symptoms (34).

The neuropathy involves the motor cranial nerves (III, IV, VI, VII, IX, and XII) and the peripheral nerves and is predominantly motor in character. In severe cases, respiratory and abdominal muscles may be involved. Weakness usually begins proximally and spreads distally. Typically, palatal paralysis (nasal twang, dysphonia, and regurgitation of fluids) occurs in the second week, ocular palsies (loss of accommodation, squint, and diplopia) in the third week, and generalized motor weakness after 3–6 weeks of illness. Autonomic disturbances such as tachycardia, hypotension or hypertension, and hyperhidrosis may be seen. CSF may show pleocytosis and elevated protein levels. Complete recovery of neurologic function occurs in most survivors. Resolution usually occurs by 5–6 months, but may take as long as 12 months.

Renal Failure

Renal tubular cells are potentially susceptible to the effects of the exotoxin. Renal failure in diphtheria is generally secondary to acute tubular necrosis but may also be a consequence of decreased cardiac output secondary to myocarditis and cardiogenic shock.

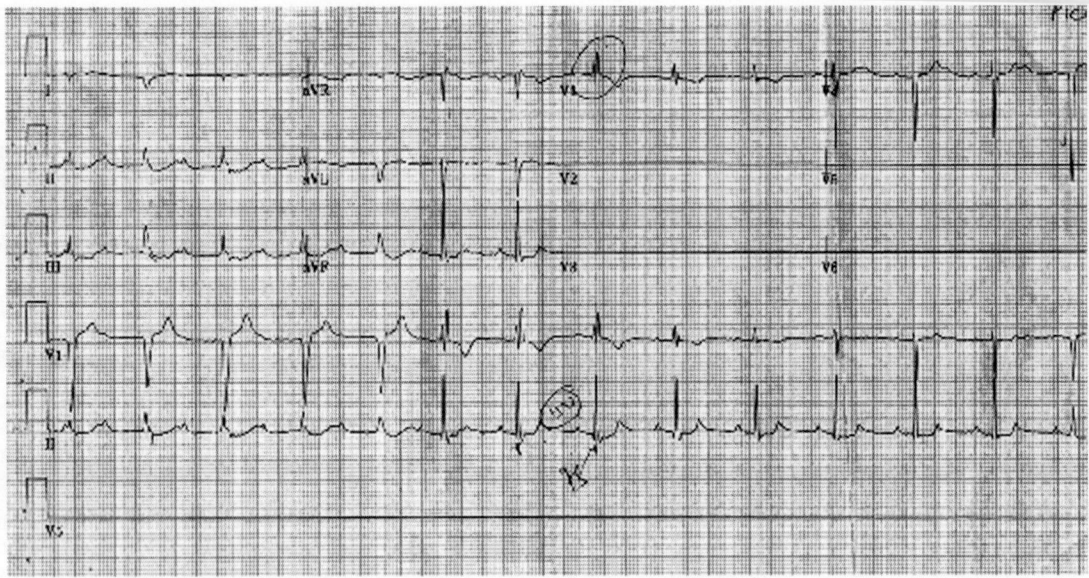

FIGURE 94.4. Electrocardiogram in a patient with diphtheritic myocarditis, showing right bundle-branch block and atrioventricular dissociation.

Thrombocytopenia

Thrombocytopenia and bleeding are considered rare manifestations. However, these have been described in nearly one-third of patients with severe and complicated diphtheria (27).

Diagnosis and Differential Diagnosis

The diagnosis of diphtheria and indication for initiating antitoxin therapy should be based on clinical grounds. The definition recommended by the WHO for a probable clinical case is "an illness characterized by laryngitis or pharyngitis or tonsillitis, and an adherent membrane of the tonsils, pharynx, and/or nose." "A confirmed case is a probable case that is laboratory confirmed or linked epidemiologically to a laboratory confirmed case."

Diphtheria should be suspected in any patient with membranous tonsillopharyngitis, especially if it extends to the uvula and soft palate, or if bull-neck, hoarseness, stridor, unilateral bloody nasal discharge, or palatal palsy is observed. Other conditions that can give rise to a membranous tonsillopharyngitis should be considered in the differential diagnosis. These include acute streptococcal pharyngitis, candidiasis, Vincent angina, infectious mononucleosis, and agranulocytosis (mucositis). At the beginning of the illness, diphtheria can look like any type of tonsillitis, with only a small spot of membrane on the tonsil. Marked edema of the tonsils, uvula, and pharyngeal wall helps distinguish diphtheria from other entities that present as membranous tonsillopharyngitis. Pharyngeal coinfection with group A streptococci (GAS) is common in diphtheria; therefore, identification of streptococcal infection does not exclude diphtheria (35).

Laboratory Diagnosis

Presumptive rapid diagnosis is usually obtained with methylene blue and Gram stain of pharyngeal smear. *C. diphtheriae* is seen as club-shaped, Gram-positive, pleomorphic bacillus with terminal swellings, arranged in a Chinese letter pattern. Diphtheroids that are normal commensals in the throat may give rise to a false-positive test. Isolation of *C. diphtheriae*

from a clinical specimen or fourfold or greater rise in serum antibody is necessary for confirmation of diagnosis.

Successful isolation of *C. diphtheriae* depends on proper collection of swabs and transport to the laboratory. The laboratory must be alerted to the suspicion of diphtheria, as routine cultures are not likely to identify the organism. In cases of respiratory diphtheria, culturing of both nasal and pharyngeal sites improves the rate of isolation. Cultures should be obtained from samples of membrane or a submembrane swab, if possible. In cutaneous disease, samples should be obtained from any wound or skin lesions. Swabs should be immediately streaked on to proper media, including a selective tellurite-containing medium like blood agar, and a Loeffler slant, and then incubated at 35°C–37°C. If a delay in plating is unavoidable, the swab should be transported dry and then incubated overnight in broth that contains plasma or blood before plating. Prior antibiotic use may substantially reduce the yield of culture. Because most microbiology labs in the United States lack the expertise and materials to reliably identify diphtheria, practitioners in the United States should contact their local health department or the Centers for Disease Control and Prevention (CDC) for guidance on correct handling of specimens.

Test for Toxigenicity

Toxigenicity is demonstrated by in vivo and in vitro tests. In vivo tests using guinea pigs are usually slow. In vitro tests are done by immunodiffusion, in which antitoxin-impregnated filter paper is laid over pure growth on solid blood agar culture media (Elek test). Polymerase chain reaction (PCR) detection of sequences from the toxin A subunit and enzyme immunoassay for toxin have also been developed. The results of an Elek test are usually available within 24–36 hours. Use of an immunochromatographic strip test correlates well with the Elek test and may speed identification (36). The PCR test for the presence of tox+ is the fastest, simplest, and most accurate test for toxigenicity. Because both toxigenic and nontoxigenic organisms may coexist in the same patient, at least 10 colonies from a primary culture plate should be tested for toxigenicity.

Additional tests are often performed to evaluate the extent of multisystem involvement. Cultures of blood or other affected sites should be performed as appropriate. Serial electrocardiograms can detect early changes of myocarditis and monitor conduction abnormalities. Cardiac enzymes may be measured to detect myocarditis; elevations in serum aspartate transaminase closely parallel the severity of myocarditis. A chest x-ray and echocardiography should be obtained to assess the cardiac size and contractility, respectively. Platelet counts to detect thrombocytopenia, serum electrolytes, and blood urea nitrogen are obtained to assess renal injury.

Management

Emergency Room Management

Attention must first be given to the airway, breathing, and circulation (ABCs). Once these are stabilized, antitoxin therapy must be initiated immediately after taking appropriate specimens for culture. Airway problems must be anticipated in children who present with extensive disease and bull-neck. Airway should be secured early, as rapid progression of membrane may preclude a later opportunity. Use of accessory muscles of respiration is an indication for immediate airway management. Tracheostomy may serve as a better form of airway (27). Endotracheal intubation is difficult because of a friable upper airway and carries a high risk of dislodgement of the membrane. In patients with severe disease, hemodynamic monitoring should be established to detect early signs of myocarditis.

Indication for Transfer to the ICU

Patients with signs of airway obstruction or myocarditis should be transferred to the ICU immediately. Others who should be transferred to the ICU on priority include unimmunized patients, patients with delayed presentation to hospital (>5 days), delayed antitoxin therapy, or severe pharyngotonsillar disease. These patients are at high risk for systemic complications.

Isolation Policy

Patients with respiratory tract diphtheria should be placed in strict isolation, which should be maintained until therapy has been completed, and two cultures obtained at least 24 hours apart after completion of antibiotic therapy are both negative. Patients, whose initial cultures are negative due to prior antibiotic therapy, should be isolated until completion of antibiotic therapy.

Specific Management

The goals of specific therapy are neutralization of the circulating toxin, eradication of residual bacteria to halt further toxin production, and establishment of active immunity to diphtheria toxin.

Antitoxin. Diphtheria equine antitoxin acts by neutralizing the unbound toxin and prevents its binding to the cell membrane surface receptor cells. The dose of the antitoxin varies from 20,000 to 120,000 units, depending on the site of primary infection, the extent of pseudomembrane, and the delay between onset and seeking of medical advice. After a test dose (see below), the usual recommended dose is 20,000–40,000 units for faucial diphtheria of <48-hour duration, 40,000–80,000 units for faucial diphtheria of >48-hour duration or laryngeal infection, and 60,000–120,000 units for severe toxic state with bull-neck. Therapy is usually given IV over 30–60 minutes. Extensive late or complicated disease should always be treated with doses at the higher end of the range. As antitoxin is a horse serum preparation, it may provoke severe hypersensitivity reactions. A test dose of 50–100 units is recommended 30 minutes prior to giving the therapeutic dose. If any untoward reaction is observed, desensitization must be accomplished before the full dose is given.

Immediate initiation of treatment with antitoxin at the onset of respiratory illness has been shown to decrease mortality by ≥80% compared with case fatality rates in those who receive antitoxin a week after onset (37). It may also prevent spread to susceptible contacts.

Antibiotics. In tox$^+$ infections, antimicrobial therapy eradicates organism, limits toxin production, and prevents locally invasive disease. However, antibiotics are adjuncts and not a substitute for antitoxin. Although *C. diphtheriae* is susceptible to a variety of antibiotics in vitro, only penicillin and erythromycin are currently recommended by the WHO. The standard regimen is as follows:

- Crystalline penicillin 40,000 IU/kg 4–6 hourly IM/IV till toxicity subsides, then procaine penicillin 25–50,000 IU/kg IM once daily for a total of 10–14 days.
- Oral erythromycin 40–50 mg/kg/day (max dose 2 g/day) in four divided doses for 10–14 days if child is sensitive to penicillin.

In an open-label randomized trial in Vietnamese children with diphtheria, penicillin therapy (intramuscular benzyl penicillin 50,000 U/kg/day for 5 days followed by oral penicillin 50 mg/kg/day for 5 days) compared with erythromycin therapy (50 mg/kg/day for 10 days) resulted in early clearance of fever (27 vs. 46 hours; $p = 0.0004$) (38). Erythromycin is the most effective drug for elimination of the carrier state. Antibiotic treatment usually renders patients noninfectious within 24 hours. Untreated patients are infectious for 2–3 weeks. Elimination of the organism should be documented at a minimum of 2 weeks after completion of therapy with two negative cultures of nose, throat, and skin (as appropriate) 24 hours apart. A course of erythromycin is given if end-of-treatment cultures remain positive.

Supportive Therapy

Once specific therapy has been started, monitoring and support of ABCs should continue. Complications should be anticipated and treated accordingly.

Of the treatment options available for diphtheritic myocarditis, neither carnitine nor pacing has been conclusively proven to be of any benefit. Carnitine is a cofactor for the transport of fatty acids into the mitochondria of cardiac cells. Carnitine depletion and fatty acid accumulation in the cytoplasm of cardiac cells have been observed in patients with diphtheria as a consequence of ribosomal damage. Significant reduction in incidence of myocarditis and mortality following DL-carnitine therapy (100 mg/kg/day in two divided doses orally for 4 days) was observed in a large, case-controlled study of 625 patients (39). However, the literature contains no conclusive report regarding its role in prevention of myocarditis.

The severe systolic dysfunction that accompanies bundle-branch blocks and complete heart blocks remains refractory to pharmacologic stimulation and inotropes. Benefit of ventricular pacing for advanced atrioventricular block remains doubtful, and mechanical response to electrical stimulation of the ventricle with pacing may be insufficient in patients with atrioventricular blocks. However, a prospective study from Vietnam suggests that temporary insertion of a pacemaker may improve the outcome in children with diphtheritic myocarditis with severe conduction defects (40).

Outcome and Prognosis

Overall, care fatality rate is 5%–10%. Mortality rates are higher at extremes of age, in severe form of disease, in unimmunized patients, and if antitoxin administration is delayed. Airway complications alone carry a good prognosis if managed in time (27). Mortality in diphtheritic myocarditis may be as high as 60%–70%. The need for inotropic support after pacemaker insertion is a poor prognostic sign (40). The risk of death is increased with thrombocytopenic bleeding or renal failure. Generally, patients who survive diphtheria make a complete recovery. Persistent or progressive cardiac conduction defects have been reported years after the original episode. Some patients die suddenly and unexpectedly weeks after a full recovery. These deaths have been attributed to cardiac arrhythmias secondary to persistent subclinical myocarditis.

Prevention and Treatment for Contacts and Carriers

Clinical diphtheria does not confer natural immunity. Patients who recover from diphtheria should begin or complete active immunization with diphtheria toxoid during convalescence. Persons who have had close contact with diphtheria should have cultures obtained from nose, throat, and skin lesions and receive daily check for development of signs of diphtheria for 7 days. Contacts, regardless of immunization status, and carriers should receive oral erythromycin (40–50 mg/kg/day, maximum 2 g/day) in four divided doses for 7–10 days or IM benzathine penicillin (one dose of 0.6 mega units for patients <5 years of age and 1.2 mega units for those >5 years). The immunization status of the carriers and contacts should be assessed, and booster doses or primary series should be administered as needed. A total of five doses of combined DPT vaccine at ages 2, 4, 6, 15–18 months, and 5 years is recommended during primary immunization. The pediatric formulations of diphtheria toxoid (DTaP and DT) for use among infants and children <7 years of age contain 6.7–25 Lf units of diphtheria toxoid per 0.5 mL dose. However, the concentration of diphtheria toxoid (Td) for use among individuals >7 years of age is reduced to 2 Lf per dose as this not only produces an adequate response but also reduces risk of adverse reactions. In populations where a majority of individuals have protective antitoxin titers, the carrier rate for strains of C. diphtheriae decreases and the overall risk of diphtheria among susceptible individuals is reduced.

Carriers should be placed in strict isolation (for respiratory tract colonization) or contact isolation (for cutaneous colonization) until at least two cultures taken 24 hours apart at least 2 weeks after cessation of therapy are negative for C. diphtheriae. If cultures remain positive, a course of erythromycin should be repeated.

Conclusions and Future Directions

Early diagnosis, prompt administration of antitoxin and antibiotics, and chemoprophylaxis of close contacts and carriers remain the cornerstone of effective prevention and treatment of diphtheria. The primary focus in the developing world should be to ensure age-appropriate immunization universally. Effective therapy of myocarditis and polyneuropathy remains elusive. The future challenges are to find more effective modalities to prevent and treat these serious complications and to find simpler ways to immunize each and every susceptible host.

BOTULISM

Human botulism is caused by the neurotoxin produced by *Clostridium botulinum* and, rarely, by *C. baratii*, *C. butyricum*, *C. novyi*, and *C. bifermentans*. These organisms are ubiquitous, anaerobic, spore-forming, Gram-positive bacilli. The organism and its spores are found in all types of soil; in aquatic sediment from streams, lakes, and coastal waters; in the digestive system of fish and mammals; and in the viscera of shellfish and crabs. Once the spores are in a suitable environment, they germinate, begin to multiply, and produce toxin. Seven heat-labile, antigenic toxin subtypes of *C. botulinum* have been identified and are designated by the letters A through G. Types A, B, E, and, rarely, F cause human botulism. Toxin types C and D cause disease in animals. Type G has been isolated in soil but has not been implicated in human disease (41). Purified botulinum toxin type A is commercially available and is used for cosmetic indications, hyperhidrosis, cervical dystonia, spasticity, and strabismus. Five specific forms of the disease are seen in humans, three of which are infant botulism, food-borne botulism, and wound botulism. The fourth form is thought to be due to intestinal sources and is observed only in patients >12 months of age with symptoms of botulism without a food or wound source of exposure. A fifth form is rarely seen and is a complication of therapeutic use. Each form has its own epidemiology, pathogenesis, prognosis, and treatment. Inhalational botulism does not occur naturally but could potentially result from a biologic warfare application.

Toxin Mechanism

All of the toxin types have the same mechanism of action, which is blocking the release of acetylcholine from nerve endings. The toxin does not cross the BBB but does affect the neuromuscular junction, parasympathetic nerve endings, autonomic ganglia, and acetylcholine sympathetic nerve endings. The toxin enters the body through a wound or mucosal surface. Absorption of the toxin is rapid from the gastrointestinal tract. Toxin type E must first be activated by pancreatic enzymes to cause symptoms. Once in the bloodstream, the toxin enters the neuromuscular junction—specifically, the nerve terminus.

The light chain of the botulinum toxin cleaves one of the soluble *N*-ethylmaleimide-sensitive factor attachment protein receptor (SNARE) proteins. The SNARE proteins form a synaptic fusion complex and allow the acetylcholine-containing synaptic vesicle to fuse with the nerve terminus membrane. Which SNARE protein is cleaved depends upon the toxin type. Toxin types B, D, F, and G cleave synaptobrevin; types A, C, and E cleave SNAP-2; type C cleaves syntaxin. The disruption of any of the SNARE proteins prevents assembly of the synaptic fusion complex. Without this complex, the presynaptic acetylcholine vesicles cannot bind and subsequently release acetylcholine into the synaptic cleft, causing paralysis (**Fig. 94.5**). The nerve cell itself is uninjured by the toxin. Although recovery of synaptic function does occur, it may take months and is achieved through sprouting of new presynaptic axons by the nerve cell with the formation of an entirely new neuromuscular junction (41).

Infant Botulism

Infant botulism is due to ingestion of *C. botulinum* spores. Once in the digestive tract, the spores germinate and the bacteria multiply to colonize the intestines. Toxin is then produced and readily absorbed to cause disease. The colonization occurs in infants because the infant digestive tract lacks the normal intestinal flora to compete with and prevent the growth of *C. botulinum*. Older children and adults routinely ingest *C. botulinum* spores without developing disease due to competition from the normal intestinal flora (42). The transition from infant to adult

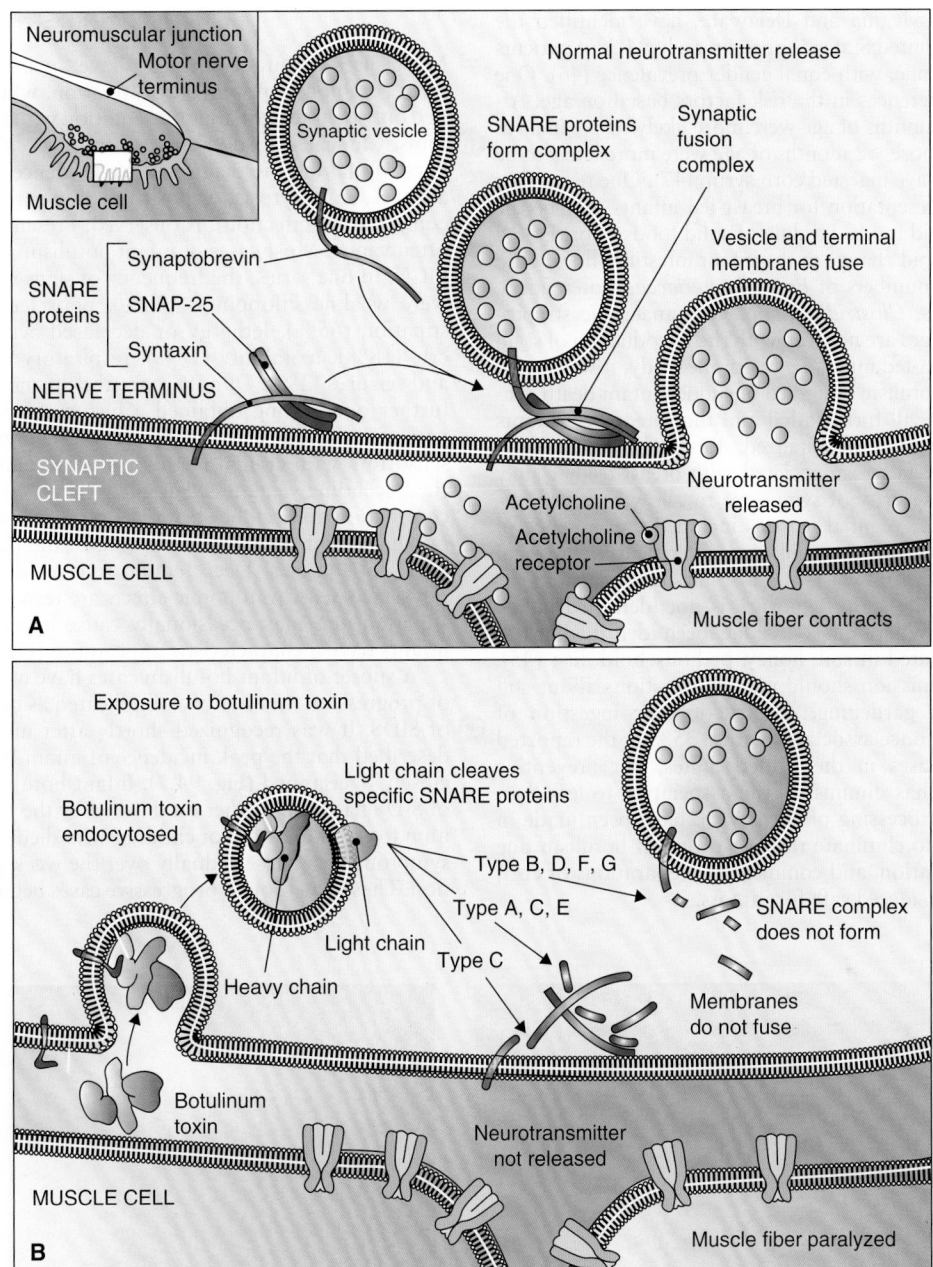

FIGURE 94.5. Mechanism of action of botulinum toxin. **A:** Release of acetylcholine at the neuromuscular junction is mediated by the assembly of a synaptic fusion complex that allows the membrane of the synaptic vesicle that contains acetylcholine to fuse with the neuronal cell membrane. The synaptic fusion complex is a set of SNARE proteins, which include synaptobrevin, SNAP-25, and syntaxin. After membrane fusion, acetylcholine is released into the synaptic cleft and bound by receptors on the muscle cell. **B:** Botulinum toxin binds to the neuronal cell membrane at the nerve terminus and enters the neuron by endocytosis. The light chain of botulinum toxin cleaves specific sites on the SNARE proteins, preventing complete assembly of the synaptic fusion complex, thereby blocking acetylcholine release. Botulinum toxin types B, D, F, and G cleave synaptobrevin; types A, C, and E cleave SNAP-25; and type C cleaves syntaxin. Without acetylcholine release, the muscle is unable to contract. SNARE, soluble NSF-attachment protein receptor; NSF, *N*-ethylmaleimide-sensitive fusion protein; SNAP-25, synaptosomal-associated protein of 25 kDa. (From Arnon SS, Schechter R, Inglesby TV, et al. Botulinum toxin as a biologic weapon: Medical and public health management. *JAMA* 2001;285:1059–70, with permission.)

intestinal flora usually occurs at between 6 and 12 months of age with the introduction of foods. For this reason, infant botulism is rarely, if ever, seen after the age of 1 year.

Epidemiology

Infant botulism is the most common form of disease caused by *C. botulinum* and its toxins, with an annual average of 2.1 reported cases per 100,000 live births in the United States. Cases

of infant botulism have been reported worldwide in all major racial and ethnic groups, with the exception of Africa (43). Given the prevalence of *C. botulinum* in the environment, the global incidence is likely higher than reported. Almost all cases in the United States are caused by either toxin A or B, with a distinctive geographic distribution. Type A is more common from the West Coast to the Rocky Mountains, and type B is more common from the Mississippi River to the East Coast (44,45). California and Utah, along with the Mid-Atlantic states, particularly southeastern Pennsylvania and Delaware, have identified the most cases in the United States. Approximately 94% of patients are <6 months of age, with equal gender prevalence (46). One study revealed differences in the risk factors based on age. Affected infants <2 months of age were more likely to live in a rural area, whereas those ≥2 months of age were more likely to be breast-fed and to have ingested corn syrup (47). One reason for the older age at presentation for breast-fed infants may be the introduction of solid foods. Feeding of solid foods to breast-fed infants causes a rapid change in the infant intestinal flora, with an increase in the numbers of *Enterobacteriaceae*, enterococci, *Bacteroides* species, *Clostridium* spp., and anaerobic streptococci. Similar changes are not seen with the introduction of solid food to the formula-fed infant's diet. In one study, it was found that infants with botulism who died of sudden infant death syndrome (SIDS) were all formula-fed and that breast-fed infants were disproportionately hospitalized. Researchers postulated that breast milk or factors associated with breast-feeding may have lessened the severity of symptoms to allow time to present to the hospital. Potential reasons included the presence of secretory antibodies in breast milk and differences in intestinal microbial flora between breast- and formula-fed infants.

The source of the spore exposure is not identified in the majority of cases. Where the source has been identified, it has typically been isolated in soil, honey, or household dust (45). The history at admission should include questions about soil exposure through gardening, construction, or ingestion of honey. Honey was once associated with ~35% of the reported infant botulism cases in the United States, but preventive health counseling has diminished the association to less than 5%. Changes in processing of corn syrup have been made in the United States to eliminate the risk of infant botulism due to spore contamination, and commercial preparations of corn syrup are now considered safe for infants.

Clinical Features

Most cases of infant botulism have an insidious onset. The most common symptom is constipation, which may be identified only in hindsight after presentation with more severe symptoms. Clinical suspicion and careful physical examination are keys to making the diagnosis. No evidence of infection, such as fever, leukocytosis, or positive cultures (in the absence of a complicating infection), is observed. Presenting symptoms are often vague. Most cases of infant botulism are admitted to the PICU. In one series, the frequency of signs noted at admission were weakness/floppiness (88%), poor feeding (79%), constipation (65%), lethargy or decreased activity (60%), poor cry, (18%), irritability (18%), respiratory difficulties (11%), and seizures (2%). Of note, once the diagnosis was suspected, further questioning obtained a history of constipation in all patients (48). The classic presentation is an infant with normal sensorium with cranial nerve palsies associated with symmetric descending weakness. Fatigue is noted on repetitive muscle contraction and can be elicited by repeated examination of the pupillary light reflex, with slowing of the pupil's constriction over 2–3 minutes. Deep tendon reflexes diminish as the paralysis worsens. Autonomic effects are responsible for the constipation and may occasionally cause hypertension. Affected infants have a characteristic appearance (**Fig. 94.6**).

A subset of infant botulism cases have a more rapid course of progression that has been implicated as one potential cause of SIDS. It was recognized shortly after infant botulism was described that the peak incidence of infant botulism and SIDS closely overlapped (**Fig. 94.7**). Infant botulism as an etiology of SIDS has been further established by the isolation of botulinum toxin in the stool of children who died of SIDS. Typically, symptoms progress gradually over the week prior to presentation. These few rapidly progressive cases begin quickly and can

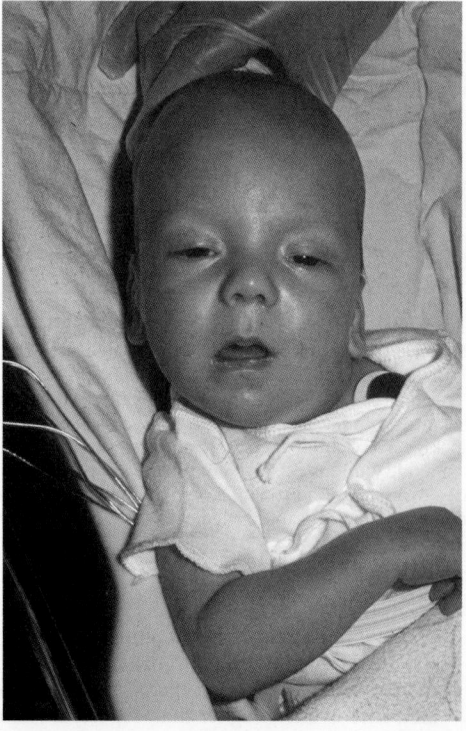
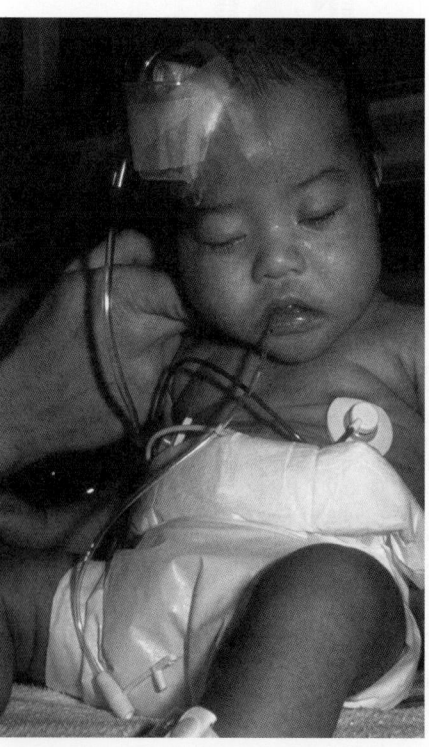

FIGURE 94.6. Photographs showing characteristic appearance of infants affected with botulism. Note the floppy appearance, poor head control, expressionless faces, and ptosis. (Left photo is courtesy of Johnson RO, Clay SA, Arnon SS. Diagnosis and management of infant botulism. *Am J Dis Child* 1979;133:586–93. Right photo is courtesy of Infant Botulism Treatment and Prevention Program, California Department of Public Health.)

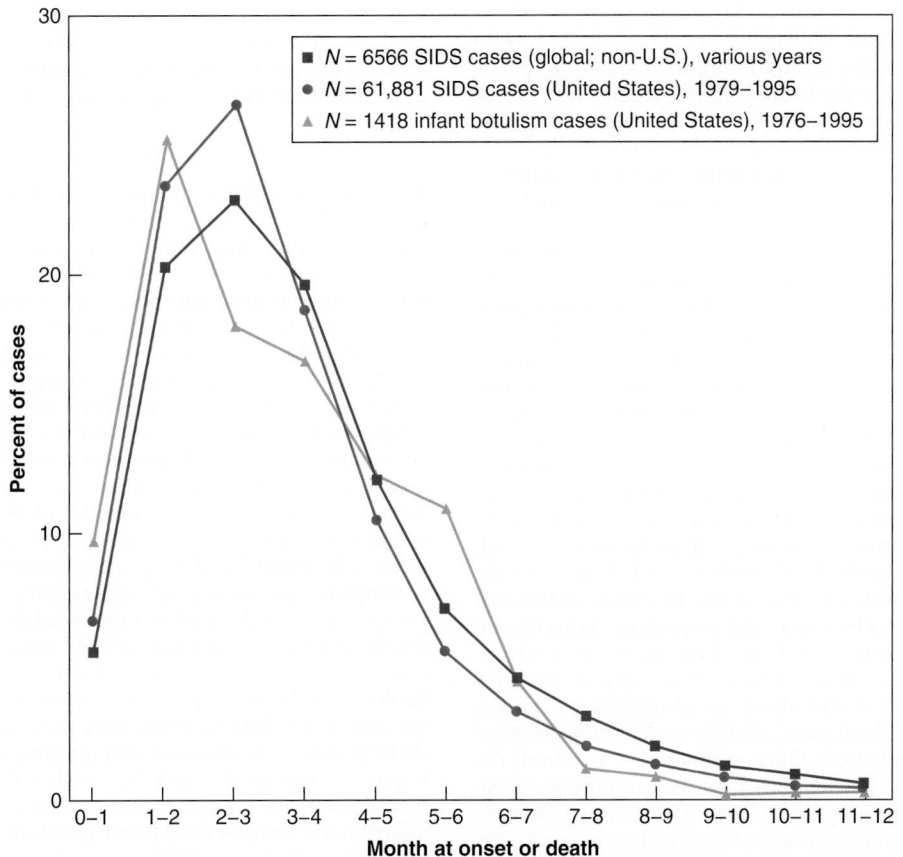

FIGURE 94.7. Epidemiologic data showing closely overlapped peak incidence of infant botulism and SIDS. (From Arnon SS. Infant botulism. In Feigin RD, Cherry J, eds. *Textbook of Pediatric Infectious Diseases.* 5th ed. Philadelphia, PA: WB Saunders, 2003, with permission.)

progress over hours rather than days, with ensuing respiratory or cardiac arrest. The diagnosis of infant botulism may be delayed or even prevented due to this atypical presentation (49).

Diagnosis and Differential Diagnosis

Diagnosis leading to treatment must be made on clinical grounds to avoid delays in potential disease-shortening therapies. Electromyography (EMG) may be helpful in confirming the diagnosis. EMG findings consistent with botulism are small amplitude and overly abundant motor endplate potentials. During repetitive nerve stimulation at 20- and 50-Hz stimulation, a staircase phenomenon is seen. EMG results will usually become positive during the course of the disease but may be equivocal or even negative at presentation. Therefore, a negative EMG study should not prevent treatment if the clinical signs and symptoms are compatible with botulism. In most but not all patients, the stool samples will have an assay positive for toxin or a culture positive for *C. botulinum* (48).

With the appearance of lethargy due to hypotonia, sepsis is a common admitting diagnosis. Infectious causes, such as sepsis, pneumonia, meningitis, and encephalitis, can be ruled out quickly owing to the lack of fever, leukocytosis, or signs of inflammation. CSF studies will be normal to aid in ruling out meningitis, encephalitis, Guillain–Barré syndrome, and poliomyelitis. The weakness in polio is usually asymmetric, which further differentiates it from infant botulism. Myasthenia gravis should not be considered without a history of maternal disease. Encephalopathy, as seen in heavy-metal poisoning or metabolic diseases, is not associated with a normal

electroencephalogram, as would be expected in botulism. Normal electrolytes, acid–base status, ammonia, and liver transaminases eliminate electrolyte abnormalities, hepatic dysfunction, and metabolic disease from the differential diagnosis. Thyroid function testing will be normal, ruling out hypothyroidism. Spinal muscular atrophy has a very similar presentation but can be differentiated by the EMG findings, the presence of tongue fasciculation, and definitively, by positive genetic testing.

Treatment

Once the diagnosis of infant botulism is clinically made, specific therapy should be given as soon as possible, without delaying for confirmatory testing. Human botulism immune globulin as a single dose of 50 mg/kg IV is reserved for the treatment of infant botulism. Observations that most infants with botulism have detectable toxin in their serum prompted a placebo-controlled study to evaluate the efficacy of IV human botulism immune globulin derived from pooled plasma of immunized adult volunteers. The study showed that the immune globulin binds to botulinum toxin and prevents action at the neuromuscular junction. No effect was seen on toxin already bound at the neuromuscular junction making early administration crucial. This study demonstrated significant decreases in hospital length of stay and hospitalization costs when therapy was given within the first 3 days of hospitalization. Late administration has less dramatic effects. In the United States, information on how to obtain botulism immune globulin can be obtained from the California Department of

Health Services' Infant Botulism Treatment and Prevention Program at www.infantbotulism.org or calling 510-231-7600 (available around the clock) (50). Botulism immune globulin is licensed for use only in the United States. Arrangements must be made in individual countries in accordance with regulations for acquisition and use of unlicensed medications. Equine botulinum antitoxin has been used outside the United States as a second-line treatment when botulism immune globulin was not available. A series of patients in Argentina were treated with equine antitoxin and had a decreased hospital and ICU length of stay, shorter duration of mechanical ventilation, and were orally fed sooner compared with those receiving supportive care alone. Minimal adverse effects were noted (51).

Whether or not the child is treated with botulism immune globulin, the prognosis will be greatly affected by providing meticulous intensive care and preventing potential complications. The overall goal of supportive treatment is to prevent hospital-acquired infections, skin breakdown, malnutrition, and airway complications until recovery of the neuromuscular junction is complete. Antibiotics are not indicated unless a complicating infection is involved. If antibiotics are used, aminoglycosides in particular should be avoided owing to the risk of worsening the degree of weakness by effects on the neuromuscular junction. The airway and respiratory status should be closely monitored in an ICU until significant signs of improvement are noted. Monitoring of vital capacity, negative inspiratory force, the child's ability to adequately protect the airway, and arterial blood gases will help to determine the need for mechanical ventilation. Once intubation is required, the risks and benefits of tracheotomy must be carefully weighed. Most children can be managed without tracheotomy. Because of weakness, accidental extubation is rare; when it does occur, it is typically when the patient is being bathed, repositioned, etc. Tracheotomy is associated with a greater duration of the ICU stay. Nutrition should be given enterally via nasojejunal or nasogastric feeding tubes, as indicated (48).

Prognosis

In the United States, the case fatality ratio of infants with botulism who are admitted to the hospital is approaching zero. In areas that do not have PICU facilities, this is not the case. The true mortality rate of infant botulism is unknown and is dependent upon the number of SIDS cases that are due to botulinum intoxication. Children hospitalized with access to intensive care have an excellent prognosis for full recovery, as long as complications do not occur. The risk of such complications can be further minimized by decreasing the length of hospitalization with the use of botulism immune globulin. Use of intravenous human botulism immune globulin within the first 3 days of hospitalization, compared to treatment during hospital days 4 through 7, and no treatment results in significantly shorter hospital admissions (2 vs. 2.9 vs. 5.7 weeks, respectively) (50).

Food-Borne Botulism

Epidemiology

Unlike infant botulism, food-borne botulism is caused by the ingestion of food contaminated with preformed botulinum toxin. The conditions for germination and growth of C. botulinum in food are fairly strict. Anaerobic conditions must exist, with a pH of >4.5, a low sugar and salt content, and a temperature between 4°C and 121°C (42). In the United States, 9.4–9.7 outbreaks occur annually that average ~2.5 cases per outbreak (44). Toxin types A, B, and E predominate in these cases, with a distinct epidemiologic distribution. Large outbreaks are usually associated with restaurants, whereas small outbreaks or single cases are usually related to home-prepared foods, such as home-canned vegetables, fruits, and fish products. Toxin type E is the most common in Alaska (52). The pH of the implicated products is usually >4.6.

Clinical Features

The initial symptoms of food-borne botulism are gastrointestinal. Abdominal pain, nausea, vomiting, and diarrhea occur shortly after ingestion of toxin but are usually not severe enough to cause the victim to seek medical care. Constipation is not seen until after the onset of neurologic symptoms, which occur 1–5 days after consumption of the toxin but usually within 18–36 hours. Onset of neurologic symptoms can vary from person to person, even within the same outbreak. However, they do have a typical order of appearance. The first symptoms to occur are dry mouth due to autonomic nervous system involvement, diplopia from cranial nerve paralysis, and dilated pupils. These bulbar palsies progress to involve the facial muscles and then the muscles of the oropharynx, with symptoms of ptosis, facial droop, depressed gag reflex, dysphagia, dysarthria, and dysphonia. Cranial nerve involvement is complete once the neck muscles become involved. The paralysis continues to descend in a proximal-to-distal pattern, with diaphragmatic involvement typically prior to that of the lower extremities (42,53). The cranial nerve palsies will result in difficulty or inability to speak or swallow, the diaphragmatic involvement will lead to respiratory distress or failure, and the skeletal muscle involvement will interfere with movement. An important feature to recognize is that CNS and/or sensory function are not impaired. As in infant botulism, no signs of infection are seen, as food-borne botulism is intoxication.

Diagnosis

The diagnosis of botulism is based on the recognition of the clinical syndrome. An isolated case, as would be seen with the index case or if affected individuals presented to different hospitals, has a limited differential diagnosis. Once a cluster of cases present with pathognomonic symptoms, as in an outbreak of food-borne botulism, the diagnosis should be straightforward because the diseases in the differential diagnosis of a single case do not cause outbreaks. Common diagnoses entertained in botulism cases are Guillain–Barré syndrome, cerebrovascular accident, myasthenia gravis, tick paralysis, and other intoxications, such as carbon monoxide, organophosphates, and mushrooms. The evaluation of these illnesses with CSF studies, cranial imaging, and Tensilon test will be negative in cases of botulism. EMG may be helpful in making the diagnosis of botulism. Important topics to cover when obtaining the patient's history include the presence of gastrointestinal symptoms and a careful food history of the preceding week, paying particularly close attention to use of home-canned foods, situations in which susceptible foods may have been inadequately stored, and ingestion of marine animals. Confirmatory testing is warranted but should not delay treatment with antitoxin. In food-borne botulism, 10 mL of serum, stool samples, suspect foods in their original containers, and vomitus or gastric secretions (especially if symptoms have recently started) should be tested (42,44,53).

Treatment

Antitoxin (equine cleaved immunoglobulin) is the most important treatment modality. As the binding of the toxin at the neuromuscular junction is irreversible, the goal is to treat the patient with the antitoxin before respiratory symptoms become severe enough to require prolonged ventilation. Late administration of antitoxin does little to shorten the hospital stay and may be of no benefit. Since 2010, a heptavalent botulinum antitoxin with activity against all known botulinum toxins (A–G) has been available in the United States under an investigational new drug protocol through the CDC. This preparation undergoes a process to minimize the presence of immunogenic equine immunoglobulin fragments, which decreases the risk of anaphylaxis or serum sickness significantly. As a result, skin testing with horse serum is no longer indicated (54).

In addition to prompt treatment with antitoxin, patients require close monitoring in an ICU setting. The respiratory status should be closely monitored for deterioration, even after administration of the antitoxin. Vital capacity must be monitored, and mechanical ventilation may be necessary. The paralysis associated with botulism can be lengthy; therefore, tracheotomy may be considered for severely affected individuals. Regardless, careful attention must be paid to preventing complications, such as hospital-acquired infections, skin breakdown, and neuromuscular injury from disuse, which are associated with prolong intensive care admissions.

Prognosis

Prior to the development of critical care as a medical subspecialty, the case fatality rate was >60%, even when high-dose equine antitoxin was used. Between 1950 and 1996, the case fatality rate dropped to 15.5%, and the most recent fatality rates reported are 3%–5%. Disease caused by type A toxin tends to have more severe symptoms and, as a result, has a higher fatality rate than types B and E (42,44,53).

Wound Botulism

Wound botulism is an extremely rare disease, but it has been reported in children. The classic at-risk wound is a crush injury, puncture wound, or gross trauma to an extremity. Toxin is released from bacteria in the wound into the bloodstream, producing neurologic symptoms as described for food-borne botulism. Inflammation, fever, and leukocytosis are often absent in wound botulism, making the diagnosis potentially more difficult. The diagnosis should be considered in a patient who presents with classic symptoms and an at-risk wound. Even wounds that do not appear to be infected should be explored with swabs, and wound exudates and tissue samples should be sent for anaerobic cultures and serum toxin levels. Prompt treatment with antitoxin, as described for food-borne botulism, is indicated, even before laboratory results are available. The case fatality rate is estimated to be 15% (42,44).

Adult (Intestinal) Botulism

Intestinal botulism has a pathophysiology similar to infant botulism and a similar presentation. It is very rare and only occurs in patients with severe alteration of their intestinal bacterial flora, which favors the germination and growth of ingested spores. As a result, the onset of symptoms is more insidious than that seen in infant botulism. The diagnosis should be considered in immunosuppressed patients with the classic neuromuscular findings. Treatment is with botulinum antitoxin, as described in the Food-Borne Botulism section. Confirmatory testing should include stool and serum for toxin, obtained prior to antitoxin administration, as well as stool cultures.

TOXIC SHOCK SYNDROME

Toxic shock syndrome (TSS) is an acute toxin-mediated, multisystem febrile illness caused by *S. aureus* and *S. pyogenes* (group A β-hemolytic streptococcus). It is characterized by high fever, hypotension, vomiting, and erythematous rash

that rapidly progress to variable degree of multiorgan system failure with serious morbidity and mortality. The bacterial toxins that cause the disease have been labeled as "superantigens" (SAgs) due to their ability to bypass usual steps in the antigen-mediated immune response and activate the immune system directly. They bind directly to the major histocompatibility complex (Class II) to trigger a massive activation and expansion of T cells displaying T-cell receptor-specific β-chain variable regions. Superantigens can stimulate over 20% of all T cells; in contrast, conventional antigen stimulates only 1 in 10,000 T cells. The TSS caused by the toxins of these two species of bacteria share certain features, but major differences are apparent in clinical signs, symptoms, morbidity, and mortality. Rarely, other streptococci, including groups B, C, and G, β-hemolytic streptococci, and *S. viridans* (usually in immunocompromised individuals) and *S. suis* (from China) have been reported to cause TSS. *Clostridium sordellii* has been reported as a cause of infection of the female genital tract and fatal TSS (55).

Staphylococcal Toxic Shock Syndrome

Staphylococcal TSS has two forms: menstrual and nonmenstrual. More than 99% cases of menstrual TSS are associated with tampon use. Until early 1980s, menstrual TSS accounted for a vast majority of reported cases; however, by 1990, nonmenstrual TSS exceeded menstrual TSS cases, possibly related to increased awareness and better reporting. Nonmenstrual TSS has been described in nonmenstruating women, children, and men, and is associated with *S. aureus* colonization of nasal packing or focal infection such as wound infection, soft-tissue infections, lymphadenitis, sinusitis, tracheitis, empyema, abscesses, infection following burn, abortion, animal and insect bites, and osteomyelitis.

The incidence of menstrual TSS in the United States is estimated to be ~1 per 100,000 menstruating persons per year with a case fatality rate of 3.3%. Lately, an increase in the incidence of menstrual TSS has been recorded, with the incidence lower in children than in adults (56). Menstrual TSS is caused by TSS toxin 1 (TSST-1) producing strains of *S. aureus*, which colonizes the vagina. Nonmenstrual TSS is caused by toxin-producing *S. aureus* that colonizes skin or mucosa and cause focal sites of staphylococcal infection. Most patients are merely colonized with the offending strain, though some have evidence of *S. aureus* bacteremia or deep tissue infection. The major toxins responsible for all the manifestation of the disease are TSST-1 and enterotoxins A, B, and C (57). TSST-1 is found in nearly all cases of menstrual TSS and in 50% of nonmenstrual TSS, while enterotoxins are found in the other 50% of nonmenstrual TSS. The toxins act together as superantigens that stimulate the release of various cytokines, prostaglandins, and leukotrienes, and are integral in the pathogenesis of the illness. The cytokines cause capillary leak, massive vasodilatation with extravasations of fluids and serum, and consequently severe hypotension and multiple-organ dysfunction. TSST-1 suppresses neutrophil chemotaxis, induces T-suppressor function, and blocks the reticuloendothelial system. Staphylococcal enterotoxins are pyrogenic and enhance susceptibility to lethal shock. Direct toxin-mediated organ injuries to kidney, liver, or myocardium cannot be excluded.

Though the association of tampon use and TSS is very strong, the exact role of tampons in the pathogenesis of TSS remains unclear. Epidemiologic and *in vitro* studies suggest that these toxins are selectively produced in a clinical environment consisting of a neutral pH, a high P_{CO_2}, and an "aerobic" P_{O_2}. Similar conditions are found in the vagina with tampon use during menstruation.

TSST-1 produces an antibody response *in vivo* that is believed to be protective. A survey of 3012 menstruating women between 13 and 40 years shows that 81% of teenagers had protective antibody titers (≥1:32) (58). Patients with TSS lack this protective response. A nonimmune host colonized with a toxin-producing organism that is exposed to growth conditions that induce toxin production is at risk for symptomatic disease.

Clinical Features

Menstrual TSS occurs during or within 2 days of onset or termination of menses. Nonmenstrual TSS is encountered in association with focal staphylococcal infections. The onset is abrupt, with high fever (≥39°C), headache, vomiting, diarrhea, and myalgia, rapidly progressing to hypotension and shock. A diffuse erythematous rash that resembles sunburn appears within 24 hours and may be associated with hyperemia of pharyngeal, conjunctival, and vaginal mucous membranes. Impairment of consciousness can result in somnolence, agitation, disorientation, and obtundation. Gastrointestinal involvement is often pronounced with diffuse abdominal pain. Diarrhea is watery without blood or fecal leukocytes. Renal involvement manifests with pyuria, hematuria, oliguria, and in extreme cases with acute renal failure often in combination with profound hypotension. Recovery from TSS starts within 7–10 days. It is associated with desquamation particularly of palms and soles; hair and nail loss may occur after 1–2 months. Clinicians must remember that desquamation is a feature of convalescence and hence its initial absence does not exclude the diagnosis.

Complications of TSS include acute renal failure, acute respiratory distress syndrome (ARDS), disseminated intravascular coagulation, electrolyte imbalance (hypocalcemia, hypophosphatemia, and hypomagnesemia), rhabdomyolysis, cardiomyopathy, and encephalopathy. Nonmenstrual TSS is more likely to cause renal and CNS complications.

Laboratory Investigations

Nonspecific laboratory abnormalities are found in more than 85% of affected patients. Leukocytosis and moderate thrombocytopenia are common, as are mildly elevated serum transaminase levels. Pyuria, proteinuria, and elevated blood urea nitrogen and creatinine may be seen. These urinary changes are not related to direct infection of the urinary tract by the staphylococci. About 40% of patients may have elevated serum creatine phosphokinase levels more than twice the normal range; a few patients may also have myoglobinuria. Symptomatic hypocalcemia has been observed in a few patients.

Diagnosis and Differential Diagnosis

The diagnosis of TSS is based on clinical signs, and no rapid definitive diagnostic test exists. The CDC has established a set of diagnostic criteria on the basis of clinical and laboratory findings (Table 94.7). When the illness lacks one of the defining criteria, the term "probable TSS" is used.

The differential diagnosis of TSS is broad (Table 94.8). Fever, vomiting, and diarrhea may mimic gastroenteritis. High fever, headache, myalgias, vomiting, and rash may mimic any acute viral infection. Progression to impaired consciousness that results in somnolence, agitation, disorientation, or obtundation may necessitate a lumbar tap to exclude a diagnosis of bacterial meningitis. When headache, disorientation, and thrombocytopenia dominate the clinical picture, the condition may resemble meningococcemia. In its milder forms, TSS may resemble Kawasaki disease because of fever, rash, and desquamation. Hypotension and renal failure are not characteristic of Kawasaki disease. Conversely, lymphadenopathy, a major

---

TABLE 94.7

CENTERS FOR DISEASE CONTROL AND PREVENTION: CASE DEFINITION OF STAPHYLOCOCCAL TOXIC SHOCK SYNDROME 2010

Clinical criteria: An illness with the following clinical manifestations:
1. Fever—temperature ≥38.9°C (102°F)
2. Rash—diffuse macular erythroderma
3. Desquamation—1–2 wk after onset of illness, particularly palms and soles
4. Hypotension—systolic blood pressure ≤90 mm Hg for adults or less than fifth percentile by age for children <16 years of age; orthostatic drop in diastolic blood pressure ≥15 mm Hg from lying to sitting, orthostatic syncope, or orthostatic dizziness
5. Multisystem involvement—three or more of the following:

Gastrointestinal: vomiting or diarrhea at onset of illness

Muscular: severe myalgia or creatine phosphokinase level at least twice the upper limit of normal for laboratory

Mucous membrane: vaginal, oropharyngeal, or conjunctival hyperemia

Renal: blood urea nitrogen or creatinine at least twice the upper limit of normal for laboratory or urinary sediment with pyuria (≥5 leukocytes per high-power field) in the absence of urinary tract infection

Hepatic: total bilirubin, serum alanine aminotransferase (ALT), or serum aspartate aminotransferase (AST), at least twice the upper limit of normal for laboratory

Hematologic: platelets <100,000/mm³

CNS: disorientation or alterations in consciousness without focal neurologic signs when fever and hypotension are absent

Laboratory criteria

Negative results on the following tests, if obtained:
1. Blood, throat, or CSF cultures (blood culture may be positive for *S. aureus*)
2. Rise in titer to Rocky Mountain spotted fever, leptospirosis, or measles

Case classification

Probable: A case which meets laboratory criteria and four of five clinical criteria

Confirmed: A case which meets laboratory criteria and all five clinical criteria described above, including desquamation, unless the patient dies before desquamation occurs

Adapted from Centers for Disease Control and Prevention. CSTE position statement 10-ID-14 (page last reviewed and updated on January 17, 2014).

TABLE 94.8

DIFFERENTIAL DIAGNOSIS IN TOXIC SHOCK SYNDROME

■ INFECTIOUS	■ NONINFECTIOUS
Acute viral syndrome	Kawasaki disease
Acute gastroenteritis	Acute rheumatic fever
Acute pyelonephritis	Systemic lupus erythematosus
Legionnaire disease	Thrombophlebitis
Leptospirosis	Tumor
Lyme disease	Hematoma
Meningococcemia/	Hemolytic uremic syndrome
meningococcal meningitis	
Typhus	
Streptococcal scarlet fever	
Rocky Mountain	
spotted fever	
Septic shock	

Adapted from Herzer CM. Toxic shock syndrome: Broadening the differential diagnosis. *J Am Board Fam Pract* 2001;14:131–6.

criterion for diagnosis of Kawasaki disease, is usually absent in TSS. The other diagnosis most commonly entertained in cases of TSS is scarlet fever. The typical epidemiological setting and the absence of pharyngeal GAS are the most important differential features. The characteristic rash of TSS allows differentiation from all other entities.

Treatment

Immediate and aggressive management of shock forms the cornerstone of management. To ensure adequate perfusion of vital organs, volume replacement with appropriate crystalloids and colloids is a must. Vasoactive therapy may be required to normalize blood pressure and to improve perfusion once volume repletion is accomplished. Hypoproteinemia may worsen peripheral edema, but colloids should be used with extreme caution in a setting of leaky capillaries. Children are more likely to require respiratory support.

All possible sites of staphylococcal infection must be examined to remove preformed toxin and to stop further toxin production. Infected wounds and necrotizing skin lesions should be debrided immediately. All packings and foreign objects, including retained tampons, should be removed. Abscesses should be drained and irrigated.

Parenteral administration of a β-lactamase-resistant antistaphylococcal antibiotic is recommended after appropriate cultures have been taken. Cloxacillin, oxacillin, or nafcillin in combination with aminoglycosides are the first-line agents. Clindamycin and vancomycin can be used in patients who are allergic to penicillin or if methicillin-resistant *S. aureus* (MRSA) is suspected. The newer agents such as daptomycin or tigecycline can be considered if resistance to glycopeptides is suspected. Addition of clindamycin in severe cases will halt toxin production. Therefore, clindamycin should be used in combination with a β-lactamase-resistant antistaphylococcal antibiotic for the first few days to decrease the synthesis of TSST-1. No prospective study on antibiotic use in treating TSS has been reported.

Antibiotics do not shorten the duration of acute illness but are useful in decreasing the organism load, the risk of bacteremia, and the rate of relapse. Treatment of an acute episode of TSS with a β-lactamase-resistant antibiotic is believed to decrease the likelihood of recurrent TSS. Eradication of toxigenic strains of *S. aureus* may require prolonged antibiotic administration (59). Some studies have recommended a 2-week

course of antistaphylococcal antibiotic wherein elimination of carriage is important. Use of combination therapy with rifampicin, mupirocin, or both might decrease the risk of recurrence by eliminating carriage. Further studies should be conducted.

Intravenous immunoglobulin (IVIG), 1 g/kg for 2 days, is suggested for severe cases in which conventional therapies fail to control symptoms in 6 hours, although its efficacy has not been confirmed. As the disease occurs in patients who are seronegative to the implicated staphylococcal toxins, IVIG probably provides the needed antibodies to neutralize the antitoxin. *In vitro* studies suggest that staphylococcal superantigens are not inhibited as efficiently as streptococcal superantigens by IVIG; hence, a higher dose of IVIG may be required for therapy of staphylococcal TSS (60). Plasma exchange has been found to reduce circulating toxins and mediators of TSS. Corticosteroids are not effective.

Outcome and Prognosis

The overall fatality rate from TSS in children has been reported to be 3%–5% (56). Sequelae include prolonged muscle weakness, abnormal renal function, behavioral changes, and memory impairment.

One of the striking features of TSS is its propensity to recur. Several reports of recurrent menstrual and nonmenstrual TSS can be found in the literature. Failure to eradicate colonization with *S. aureus* predisposes the patient to recurrent nonmenstrual TSS. Women with recurrent menstrual TSS have persistent colonization with a toxigenic strain of *S. aureus* and persistent absence of neutralizing antibody. For women who have recurrent menstrual TSS, tampon use should be discontinued, and oral antistaphylococcal antibiotics should be administered before and during each menstrual period until anti-TSST-1 titers rise. Patient education about proper use of tampons and recognition of early signs of disease are important.

Streptococcal Toxic Shock Syndrome

Streptococcal TSS (STSS) is a severe, potentially fatal form of infection caused by invasive GAS. It is characterized, by early shock and multiorgan failure. Although staphylococcal TSS is often associated with colonization, GAS TSS most often accompanies invasive GAS infection. Population-based studies in Canada and the United States have documented an annual incidence of invasive GAS infection of 1.5–5.2 cases/10,000 population, with higher incidence at the extremes of age. The rates of invasive GAS are several fold higher in the developing countries (>10 per 100,000), and a review of global data in 2005 estimated that 97% of cases and deaths due to invasive GAS occur in developing countries (61). Approximately 8%–14% of patients with invasive GAS infection have associated STSS (62), and its presence increases case fatality. In a recently published data from Europe, incidence of streptococcal TSS was 13% among all streptococcal infections and 7-day case fatality was 44% (63).

The Pathogen and Pathogenesis

GAS is a Gram-positive organism. It is classified by the presence of surface proteins, primarily M and T antigens. The strains that are encapsulated and rich in M protein are more virulent. Most of the strains responsible for STSS have M protein types 1 and 3. Extracellular products of GAS include the hemolysins; streptolysins O and S; and pyrogenic exotoxins A, B, C, and F. The streptococcal exotoxins possess superantigenic properties and trigger massive T-cell proliferation and cytokine release in the same way as staphylococcal superantigens. A strong association between infection with strains that produce pyrogenic exotoxin A gene and STSS has been reported (64). The factors that determine the severity of infection are not fully understood. Protective antibody levels to specific M protein and streptococcal superantigens were lower in patients with invasive streptococcal infection and STSS compared with healthy controls (65).

Clinical Features

In children, STSS commonly occurs following varicella or during the use of nonsteroidal anti-inflammatories (66); in others, the focus could be pharyngitis (66). Onset is abrupt with pain, fever, vomiting, diarrhea, and early shock (just as with staphylococcal TSS). In STSS with necrotizing fasciitis, pain is the most common initial symptom; it is severe and out of proportion to physical findings and usually involves an extremity or the abdomen. Influenza-like syndrome consisting of fever, nausea, vomiting, and diarrhea may occur in 20% of patients. Hypotension may be a presenting sign or develop shortly after presentation. Hypothermia may occur in patients with shock. Confusion is present in more than half of the patients. Erythematous rash as seen in staphylococcal TSS is seen only in 10% cases of STSS. Eight percent of patients have clinical signs of soft-tissue infection, such as localized swelling and erythema, which often progress to necrotizing fasciitis and myositis and require surgical debridement, fasciotomy, or amputation. In 20% of patients without soft-tissue infection, clinical symptoms may suggest endophthalmitis, myositis, perihepatitis, peritonitis, myocarditis, or overwhelming sepsis.

The systolic blood pressure normalizes within 4–8 hours with antibiotics, fluids, and vasoactive agents only in 10% of patients. In most cases, the shock persists and organ dysfunction may progress. Multiple-organ dysfunction may precede shock. Renal failure progresses within 48–72 hours, and many patients require dialysis. ARDS is seen in nearly half of the patients; with the majority requiring mechanical ventilation. Coagulopathy with disseminated intravascular coagulation is frequently present on admission. Rarely severe thrombotic disseminated intravascular coagulation in the form of purpura fulminans has been reported.

Diagnosis

The criteria for definition of STSS have been defined (**Table 94.9**). In a child with fever, diarrhea, vomiting, and abdominal pain, rapid onset of septic shock should raise the possibility of STSS. A search for site of infection and early multiorgan dysfunction should be made.

Laboratory Investigation

Renal involvement is indicated by the presence of hemoglobinuria and by serum creatinine values that are usually >2.5 times normal; creatine kinase level is useful in detecting deeper soft-tissue infections. Mild leukocytosis may be seen as in any other infection, but what is more striking is the shift to left. The percentage of immature neutrophils (band forms, metamyelocytes and myelocytes) can reach 40%–50%.

Hypocalcemia, hypoalbuminemia and elevated liver transaminases are commonly found at the time of admission. Bacteremia is common in STSS; blood culture is positive in 60% (56). Cultures from sites of infection, including tissue taken at surgery, CSF, pleural fluid, and synovial fluid can yield organism in up to 95% of cases.

Treatment

The goals of management are removal of source of toxin (appropriate antibiotic therapy and surgical debridement of necrotic tissues), neutralization of toxin (IVIG therapy), and aggressive supportive therapy for shock (fluids and vasopressors) and multiorgan failure.

TABLE 94.9

CENTERS FOR DISEASE CONTROL AND PREVENTION: CASE DEFINITION OF STREPTOCOCCAL TOXIC SHOCK SYNDROME 2010

Clinical Criteria
An illness with the following clinical manifestations:
- Hypotension: A systolic blood pressure less than the fifth percentile by age for children aged less than 16 tears.
- Multiorgan involvement characterized by two or more of the following:
  - Renal impairment: Creatinine greater than or equal to twice the upper limit or normal for age. In patients with preexisting renal diseases, a greater than twofold elevation over the baseline level.
  - Coagulopathy: Platelets $\leq100,000$/mm^3 ($\leq100 \times 10^6$/L) or disseminated intravascular coagulation, defined by prolonged clotting times, low fibrinogen level, and the presence of fibrin degradation products.
  - Liver involvement: Elevated alanine aminotransferase, aspartate aminotransferase, or total bilirubin levels greater than or equal to twice the upper limit of normal for the age. In patients with preexisting liver disease, a greater than twofold increases over the baseline.
  - ARDS: defined by acute onset of diffuse pulmonary infiltrates and hypoxemia in the absence of cardiac failure or by evidence of diffuse capillary leak manifested by acute onset of generalized edema, or pleural or peritoneal effusion with hypoalbuminemia.
  - A generalized erythematous muscular rash that may desquamate.
  - Soft-tissue necrosis, including necrotizing fasciitis or myositis, or gangrene.

Laboratory Criteria for Diagnosis
Isolation of group A streptococcus

Case Classification
Probable: A case that meets the clinical case definition in the absence of another identified etiology for the illness and with isolation of group A streptococcus from a nonsterile site.
Confirmed: A case that meets the clinical case definition and with isolation of group A streptococcus from a normally sterile site (e.g., blood or CSF, or less commonly, joint, pleural, or pericardial fluid).

Adapted from Centers for Disease Control and Prevention. CSTE Position statement 09-1D-60 (page last reviewed and updated on January 17, 2014).

GAS remain sensitive to penicillin, but aggressive GAS infection responds less well to penicillin. It has been suggested that failure of penicillin is these situations is because of the Eagle effect wherein a high inoculum of organisms reaches a stationary phase of growth more quickly, making penicillin less effective (penicillin and other β-lactams are more efficacious against rapidly growing bacteria).

Clindamycin is more efficacious as it is both a potent suppressor of bacterial toxin production and not affected by the size of the inoculum or stage of growth. It facilitates phagocytosis of streptococcus by inhibiting M protein synthesis. Clindamycin possesses a longer postantibiotic effect than β-lactams and also causes suppression of lipopolysaccharide-induced monocyte synthesis of tumor necrosis factor. Studies have demonstrated a lower fatality rate with clindamycin use in GAS necrotizing fasciitis. Therefore, an antibiotic combination of high-dose penicillin and clindamycin should be given when concomitant invasive GAS infection is suspected. In cases of β-lactam intolerance, macrolides and clindamycin can be used. In resistant cases, Linezolid, daptomycin, or tigecycline can be used (67). Depending on the clinical presentation, particularly if it includes necrotizing fasciitis, empirical simultaneous coverage for Gram negatives, anaerobes and possibly *S. aureus* (including MRSA) should be considered until a specific organism is identified.

The presence of necrotizing fasciitis or myositis mandates immediate surgical debridement and constitutes a surgical emergency. The rapidity with which the infection spreads often outpaces the rate of surgical debridement. Most patients may require a second debridement procedure to ensure that all necrotic, infected, and devitalized tissues are removed.

Neutralization of circulating toxin is desirable, and it is in this context that role of IVIG in TSS has emerged. IVIG has been shown to inhibit the activation of T cell by superantigens and to down regulate the production of tumor necrosis factor-α. Commercial IVIG contains neutralizing antibodies to streptococcal exotoxin. Although inconclusive, evidence suggests that IVIG in STSS confers a survival benefit in adults (68). American Academy of Pediatrics committee on infectious disease recommends IVIG for STSS based on the above cited study in patients refractory to several hours of aggressive therapy. IVIG is usually given in a dose of 1 g/kg for 2 days at the slightest suspicion of STSS. A more recent study in children, however, did not find improved outcomes with use of IVIG (69). Perhaps this was due to overall low mortality in IVIG untreated patients rather than lack of efficacy of IVIG.

Supportive management of shock and multiorgan failure form the main thrust therapy. Volume deficits are massive due to external and interstitial loss, combined with peripheral vasodilatation and peripheral pooling. Vasopressors are required after adequate volume replenishment as in any septic shock. Frequent monitoring of hemodynamic status, urine output, acid–base status, and lactate levels should be performed to assess organ perfusion. Patients should also be monitored for development and progression of multiple-organ dysfunction.

Most patients with STSS require tracheal intubation and mechanical ventilation for septic shock and for complicating ARDS. The role of hyperbaric oxygen in STSS remains uncertain.

Prognosis

Prognosis of STSS is worse than staphylococcal TSS. Mortality associated with STSS in children is 5%–10%; much lower than that in the adults (30%–70%) (56). Beneficial effects of prophylactic antibiotics for prevention of STSS in burn patients have been suggested, but there is no consensus regarding their use (70).

CONCLUSION AND FUTURE DIRECTION

Early diagnosis on the basis of "defined" clinical criteria, antibiotics, supportive fluid, and vasoactive drug therapy remains the mainstay of management of TSS. IVIG is the most successful adjunctive therapy.

A better understanding of the molecular mechanism, pathogenesis, and host characteristics may help in developing more definite rapid diagnostic and therapeutic options for this potentially fatal condition. Development of specific antitoxin(s) that can neutralize the toxins that mediate TSS is necessary. Other priorities include evaluating antibiotic options and defining more precisely the role of IVIG.

References

1. World Health Organization. Immunization Vaccines and Biologicals. Monitoring and Surveillance: Tetanus. http://www.who.int/immunization/monitoring_surveillance/burden/vpd/surveillance_type/passive/tetanus/en/. Accessed March 8, 2013.
2. Orimadegun AE, Orimadegun BE, Adepoju AA. Immunity against tetanus infection, risk factors for non-protection, and validation of a rapid immunotest kit among hospitalized children in Nigeria. *Front Neurol* 2013;4:142.
3. Gidding HF, Backhouse JL, Burgers MA, et al. Immunity to diphtheria and tetanus in Australia: A national serosurvey. *Med J Aust* 2005;183:301–4.
4. Mazzei de Davila CA, Davila DF, Donis JH, et al. Autonomic nervous system dysfunction in children with severe tetanus: Dissociation of cardiac and vascular sympathetic control. *Braz J Med Biol Res* 2003;36:815–9.
5. Apte NM, Karnad DR. Short report: The spatula test: A simple bedside test to diagnose tetanus. *Am J Trop Med Hyg* 1995;53:386–7.
6. Baranwal AK, Singhi SC. Hyperextension of spine: Unusual presentation of Guillain Barré syndrome. *Arch Dis Child* 2002;87:359.
7. Brauner JS, Vieira SR, Bleck TP. Changes in severe accidental tetanus mortality in the ICU during two decades in Brazil. *Intens Care Med* 2002;28:930–5.
8. Miranda-Filho DB, Ximenes RA, Barone AA, et al. Randomized controlled trial of tetanus treatment with antitetanus immunoglobulin by the intrathecal or intramuscular route. *BMJ* 2004;328:615–7.
9. Kabura L, Ilibagiza D, Menten J, et al. Intrathecal vs. intramuscular administration of human antitetanus immunoglobulin or equine tetanus antitoxin in the treatment of tetanus: A meta-analysis. *Trop Med Int Health* 2006;11:1075–81.
10. Ahmad A, Qaisar I, Naeem M, et al. Intrathecal anti-tetanus human immunoglobulin in the treatment of neonatal tetanus. *J Coll Physicians Surg Pak* 2011;21:539–41.
11. Ganesh Kumar AV, Kothari VM, Krishnan A, et al. Benzathine penicillin, metronidazole and benzyl penicillin in the treatment of tetanus: A randomized controlled trial. *Ann Trop Med Parasitol* 2004;98:59–63.
12. Singhi S, Jain V, Subramanian C. Postneonatal tetanus: Issues in intensive care management. *Indian J Pediatr* 2001;68:267–72.
13. Okoromah CN, Lesi FE. Diazepam for treating tetanus. *Cochrane Database Syst Rev* 2004;(1):CD003954.
14. Santos ML, Mota-Miranda A, Alves-Pereira A, et al. Intrathecal baclofen for treatment of tetanus. *Clin Infect Dis* 2004;38:321–8.
15. Attygalle D, Rodrigo N. Magnesium as first line therapy in the management of tetanus: A prospective study of 40 patients. *Anaesthesia* 2002;57:811–17.
16. Geneviva GD, Thomas NJ, Kees-Folts D. Magnesium sulfate for control of muscle rigidity and spasms and avoidance of

mechanical ventilation in pediatric tetanus. *Pediatr Crit Care Med* 2003;4:480–4.

17. Rodrigo C, Samarakoon L, Fernando SD, et al. A meta analysis of magnesium for tetanus. *Anaesthesia* 2012;67:1370–4.

18. Hemila H, Koivula TT. Vitamin C for preventing and treating tetanus. *Cochrane Database Sys Rev* 2013;11:CD006665

19. Wasay M, Khealani BA, Talati N, et al. Autonomic nervous system dysfunction predicts poor prognosis in patients with mild-to-moderate tetanus. *BMC Neurol* 2005;5:2.

20. Hatamabadi HR, Abdalvand A, Safari S, et al. Tetanus Quick Stick as an applicable and cost-effective test in assessment of immunity status. *Am J Emerg Med* 2011;29:717–20.

21. Galazka A. The changing epidemiology of diphtheria in the vaccine era. *J Infect Dis* 2000;181:S2–9.

22. Wagner KS, White JM, Lucenko I, et al. Diphtheria in the postepidemic period, Europe 2000–2009. *Emerging Infect Dis* 2012;18:217–25.

23. World Health Organization. Immunization Vaccines and Biologicals. Monitoring and Surveillance: Diphtheria. http://www.who.int/immunization/monitoring_surveillance/burden/vpd/surveillance_type/passive/diphtheria/en/. Accessed March 8, 2013.

24. Centers for Disease Control and Prevention. Global routine vaccination coverage 2012. *MMWR* 2013;62:858–61.

25. Ohuabunwo C, Perevoscikovs J, Griskevica A, et al. Respiratory diphtheria among highly vaccinated military trainees in Latvia: Improved protection from DT compared with Td booster vaccination. *Scand J Infect Dis* 2005;37:813–20.

26. Pancharoen C, Mekmullica J, Thisyakorn U, et al. Clinical features of diphtheria in Thai children: A historical perspective. *Southeast Asian J Trop Med Public Health* 2002;33:352–4.

27. Jayashree M, Shruthi N, Singhi S. Predictors of outcome in patients with diphtheria receiving intensive care. *Indian Pediatr* 2006;43:155–60.

28. Kole AK, Roy R, Kar SS, et al. Outcomes of respiratory diphtheria in a tertiary referral infectious disease hospital. *Indian J Med Sci* 2010;64:373–77.

29. Kadirova R, Kartoglu HU, Strebel PM. Clinical characteristics and management of 676 hospitalized diphtheria cases, Kyrgyz Republic 1995. *J Infect Dis* 2000;181:S110–5.

30. Hadfield TL, McEnvoy P, Polotsky Y, et al. The pathology of diphtheria. *J Infect Dis* 2000;181:S116–20.

31. Lumio JT, Groundstroem KW, Huhtala H, et al. Electrocardiographic abnormalities in patients with diphtheria: A prospective study. *Am J Med* 2004;116:78–83.

32. Kneen R, Nguyen MD, Solomon T, et al. Clinical features and predictors of diphtheritic cardiomyopathy in Vietnamese children. *Clin Infect Dis* 2004;39:1591–8.

33. Piradov MA, Pirogov VN, Popova LM, et al. Diphtheritic polyneuropathy. Clinical analysis of severe forms. *Arch Neurol* 2001;58:1438–42.

34. Krumina A, Logina I, Donaghy M, et al. Diphtheria with polyneuropathy in a closed community despite receiving recent booster vaccination. *J Neurol Neurosurg Psychiatr* 2005;76:1555–7.

35. Quick ML, Sutter RW, Kobaidze K, et al. Risk factors for diphtheria: A prospective case control study in the Republic of Georgia, 1995–1996. *J Infect Dis* 2000;181:S121–9.

36. Engler KH, Efstratiou A, Norn D, et al. Immunochromatographic strip test for rapid detection of diphtheria toxin: Description and multicenter evaluation in areas of low and high prevalence of diphtheria. *J Clin Microbiol* 2002;40:80–3.

37. Singh J, Harit AK, Jain DC, et al. Diphtheria is declining but continues to kill many children: Analysis of data from a sentinel centre in Delhi, 1997. *Epidemiol Infect* 1999;123:209–15.

38. Kneen R, Pham NG, Solomon T, et al. Penicillin vs. erythromycin in the treatment of diphtheria. *Clin Infect Dis* 1998;27:845–50.

39. Ramos A, Barrucand L, Elias PRP, et al. Carnitine supplementation in diphtheria. *Indian Pediatr* 1992;29:1501–5.

40. Dung NM, Kneen R, Kiem N, et al. Treatment of severe diphtheritic myocarditis by temporary insertion of a cardiac pacemaker. *Clin Infect Dis* 2002;35:1425–9.

41. Arnon SS, Schechter R, Inglesby TV, et al. Botulinum toxin as a biological weapon: Medical and public health management. *JAMA* 2001;285:1059–70.

42. Sobel J. Botulism. *Clin Infect Dis* 2005;41:1167–73.

43. Koepke R, Sobel J, Arnon SS. Global occurrence of infant botulism, 1976–2006. *Pediatrics* 2008;122:e73–82.

44. *Handbook for Epidemiologists, Clinicians, and Laboratory Workers*. Atlanta, GA: Centers for Disease Control and Prevention, 1998.

45. Midura TF. Update: Infant botulism. *Clin Microbiol Rev* 1996;9:119–25.

46. Arnon SS. Infant botulism: Anticipating the second decade. *J Infect Dis* 1986;154:201–6.

47. Spika JS, Shaffer N, Hargrett-Bean N, et al. Risk factors for infant botulism in the United States. *Am J Dis Child* 1989;143:828–32.

48. Schreiner MS, Field E, Ruddy R. Infant botulism: A review of 12 years' experience at the Children's Hospital of Philadelphia. *Pediatrics* 1991;87:159–65.

49. Mitchell WG, Tseng-Ong L. Catastrophic presentation of infant botulism may obscure or delay diagnosis. *Pediatrics* 2005;116:e436–8.

50. Arnon SS, Schechter R, Maslanka SE, et al. Human botulism immune globulin for the treatment of infant botulism. *N Engl J Med* 2006;354:462–71.

51. Vanella de Cuetos EE, Fernandez RA, Bianco MI, et al. Equine botulinum antitoxin for the treatment of infant botulism. *Clin Vaccine Immunol* 2011;18:1845–9.

52. Sobel J, Tucker N, Sulka A, et al. Foodborne botulism in the United States, 1990–2000. *Emerg Infect Dis* 2004;10:1606–11.

53. Shapiro RL, Hatheway C, Swerdlow DL. Botulism in the United States: A clinical and epidemiologic review. *Ann Intern Med* 1998;129:221–8.

54. Hill SE, Iqbal R, Cadiz CL, et al. Foodborne botulism treated with heptavalent botulism antitoxin. *Ann Pharmacother* 2013;47:e12.

55. Fischer M, Bhatnagar J, Guarner J, et al. Fatal toxic shock syndrome associated with Clostridium sordellii after medical abortion. *N Engl J Med* 2005;353:2352–60.

56. Chuang YY, Huang YC, Lin TY. Toxic shock syndrome in children: Epidemiology, pathogenesis, and management. *Paediatr Drugs* 2005;7:11–25.

57. Dinges MM, Orwin PM, Schievert PM. Exotoxins of *Staphylococcus aureus*. *Clin Microbiol Rev* 2000;13:16–34.

58. Personnel J, Hansmann MA, Delaney ML, et al. Prevalence of toxic shock syndrome toxin 1-producing Staphylococcus aureus and the presence of antibodies to this superantigen in menstruating women. *J Clin Microbiol* 2005;43:4628–34.

59. Andrews MM, Parent EM, Barry M, et al. Recurrent nonmenstrual toxic shock syndrome: Clinical manifestations, diagnosis and treatment. *Clin Infect Dis* 2001;32:1470–9.

60. Darenberg J, Soderquist B, Normark BH, et al. Differences in potency of intravenous polyspecific immunoglobulin G against streptococcal and staphylococcal superantigens: Implications for therapy of toxic shock syndrome. *Clin Infect Dis* 2004;38:836–42.

61. Donald EL. Toxic shock syndrome. Major advances in pathogenesis, but not treatment. *Crit Care Clin* 2013;29:651–75.

62. Baxter F, McChesney J. Severe group A streptococcal infection and streptococcal toxic shock syndrome. *Can J Anesth* 2000;47:1129–40.

63. Lamagni TL, Darenberg J, Luca-Harari B, et al. Epidemiology of severe Streptococcus pyogenes disease in Europe. *J Clin Microbiol* 2008;46:2359–67.

64. Eriksson BKG, Andersson J, Holm SE, et al. Invasive group A streptococcal infections: TIMI isolates expressing pyrogenic exotoxins A and B in combination with selective lack of toxin-neutralising antibodies are associated with increased risk of streptococcal toxic shock syndrome. *J Infect Dis* 1999;180:410–8.

65. Basma H, Norrby-Teglund A, Guedez Y, et al. Risk factors in the pathogenesis of invasive group A streptococcal infections: Role of protective humoral immunity. *Inf Immun* 1999;67:1871–7.

66. Chiang MC, Jaing TH, Wu CT, et al. Streptococcal toxic shock syndrome in children without skin and soft tissue infection: Report of four cases. *Acta Paediatr* 2005;94:763–5.

67. Lappin E, Ferguson AJ. Gram-positive toxic shock syndromes. *Lancet Infect Dis* 2009;9:281–90.

68. Darenberg J, Ihendyane N, Sjolin J, et al. Intravenous immunoglobulin G therapy for streptococcal toxic shock syndrome: A European randomized double blind placebo controlled trial. *Clin Infect Dis* 2003;37:333–40.

69. Shah SS, Hall M, Srivastava R, et al. Intravenous immunoglobulin in children with streptococcal toxic shock syndrome. *Clin Infect Dis* 2009;49:1369–76.

70. Rashid A, Brown AP, Khan K. On the use of prophylactic antibiotics in prevention of toxic shock syndrome. *Burns* 2005;31:981–5.

CHAPTER 95 ■ OPPORTUNISTIC INFECTIONS

SUSHIL K. KABRA AND MATTHEW B. LAURENS

KEY POINTS

Cytomegalovirus (CMV) Infection

1. CMV is a virus in the herpes group and a common cause of infection in patients with primary immune deficiency, HIV infection, an organ transplant, or who require cancer chemotherapy.
2. CMV can involve all organ systems; the organism is transmitted congenitally through an infected birth canal and postnatally by breast milk, saliva, and blood (via infected white cells).
3. CMV pneumonia is a major cause of morbidity and mortality.
4. Diagnosis can be established by serology, polymerase chain reaction (PCR), antigenemia, and viral culture.
5. Administration of antiviral drugs (ganciclovir, foscarnet) in immunocompromised hosts improves outcome.

Varicella Zoster Virus (VZV) Infection

6. VZV is a DNA virus that typically causes benign infections of the skin and mucous membranes.
7. VZV can lead to visceral dissemination and pneumonia in children with cancer, AIDS, congenital defects of cell-mediated immunity, or those who have received organ transplantation.
8. Varicella can be diagnosed on the basis of physical findings, vesicle scrapings using direct fluorescent antibody, serology, or PCR.
9. The high-risk group, of susceptible individuals, exposed to varicella should be given immune globulin (either VZIG or IVIG up to 96 hours after exposure).
10. Immunocompromised patients should receive IV acyclovir.
11. Experience with efficacy of famciclovir and valacyclovir in children is limited.

Human Herpes Virus Type 6 (HHV-6)

12. HHV-6 is the most widespread among the human herpes viruses and causes exanthem subitum in immunocompetent children. HHV-6 is an emerging pathogen in immunocompromised hosts and experience is limited concerning clinical manifestations, diagnosis, and treatment.
13. HHV-6 has been associated with clinical disease (pneumonia, encephalopathy) in patients with HIV infection and who have received a hematopoietic stem cell or solid organ transplant.
14. Diagnostic tests for HHV-6 includes serology, culture, immunohistochemistry, and nucleic acid assays.
15. Treatment is not well established; antiviral drugs that can be used are ganciclovir, valganciclovir, acyclovir, valacyclovir, cidofovir, and foscarnet.

Candida Infections

16. *Candida* species are recognized as a leading contributor to morbidity and mortality in patients with oncohematologic malignancies, HIV infection, primary immunodeficiencies, prolonged neutropenia, diabetes, corticosteroid administration, broad-spectrum antibiotic treatment, IV hyperalimentation, or indwelling central venous lines.
17. The portals of entry are usually lesions of the gastrointestinal tract, oral mucosa, or skin puncture sites, and organisms can disseminate by the hematogenous route to one or more organs.
18. Common sites of infection in patients with disseminated candidiasis include lungs, kidneys, liver, spleen, and brain.
19. Diagnosis of *Candida* infections is based on clinical findings, examination of tissue, and body fluid culture.
20. First-line therapy includes amphotericin B, fluconazole, and voriconazole.
21. Caspofungin and Micafungin are indicated as a first-line treatment in adults and may be considered in pediatric patients.

Pneumocystis jiroveci

22. *P. jiroveci* (earlier known as *P. carinii*) is now classified as a fungus based on ribosomal RNA and other microbiologic characteristics.
23. Patients at higher risk for pneumocystis pneumonia (PCP) include infants with severe malnutrition, children with primary immunodeficiencies, hematologic malignancies, HIV infection, and recipients of solid organ or hematopoietic stem cell transplants.
24. PCP is diagnosed through direct identification of organisms from lung tissue or induced sputum specimens.
25. The first-line treatment for PCP is with TMP-SMZ, given either intravenously or orally, regardless of previous prophylactic regimen.
26. No randomized, controlled trials have been conducted to evaluate trimethoprim/dapsone combination, pyrimethamine/sulfadoxine combination, clindamycin, primaquine, or atovaquone in children.

Invasive Aspergillosis

27. *Aspergillus* is a group of ubiquitous fungal organisms found in soil and other settings that include the hospital environment. *Aspergillus* organisms enter the body via the respiratory route.
28. Susceptible hosts include recipients of lung, hematopoietic stem cell, and liver transplants; those who received treatment for malignancy, chronic granulomatous disease, or

HIV infection; and those on immunosuppressive chemotherapy.

29 Invasive pulmonary aspergillosis is manifested most commonly as necrotizing bronchopneumonia.

30 Diagnosis is established by demonstration of organisms on body fluids or tissue.

31 Voriconazole is the treatment of choice for invasive aspergillosis.

32 Diagnosis is difficult, as imaging findings are nonspecific and noninvasive tests (galactomannan assay) are difficult to interpret in children.

Mucormycosis

33 Infections by members of the mucormycosis class of fungi occur in children with hematopoietic malignancies, organ transplantation, and diabetes.

34 Mucormycosis may involve lungs, brain, sinuses, kidneys, and skin.

35 The organism invades blood vessels and may disseminate to other sites. Sudden death may occur due to massive pulmonary hemorrhage, mediastinitis, or airway obstruction.

36 Isolation of fungi is difficult; diagnosis is established by histopathology and tissue culture.

37 Treatment consists of prompt management of the underlying medical condition, reduction of immunosuppression, antifungal therapy (lipid formulation amphotericin B), and surgical debridement.

38 A noninvasive method for diagnosis is not available.

Cryptococcus

39 *C. neoformans*, a yeast-like encapsulated fungus, causes disease in immunocompromised patients.

40 The disease primarily presents as subacute or chronic meningitis and may involve all organ systems in disseminated disease.

41 Diagnosis of cryptococcal pulmonary infection is suggested by characteristic clinical and radiographic findings, sputum culture, serologic assays for IgG and IgM, and serologic testing for cryptococcal polysaccharide antigen by latex agglutination.

42 Treatment consists of combination of amphotericin B and flucytosine.

Histoplasmosis

43 Histoplasmosis is a systemic disease caused by the dimorphic fungus *H. capsulatum*.

44 Histoplasmosis occurs more commonly in children with HIV infection.

45 Clinical manifestations include acute, progressive, life-threatening infection that presents as unexplained fever, weight loss, respiratory complaints, abdominal pain, and diarrhea.

46 Diagnosis is made via culture, fungal stain, antigen detection, and serologic tests for antibodies.

47 Amphotericin B is the standard therapy for serious infections, followed by itraconazole for long-term suppressive therapy.

Nontuberculous Mycobacteria

48 Nontuberculous mycobacteria pathogens frequently cause opportunistic infections associated with AIDS and primary immune deficiency disorders.

49 Clinical manifestations of disseminated disease include lymphadenopathy and gastrointestinal tract involvement.

50 Diagnosis is based on culture and PCR.

51 Treatment depends on the organism involved and site of infection. Commonly used drugs for pulmonary disease are clarithromycin and ethambutol, with other antituberculosis drugs used in disseminated disease.

52 Epidemiology, clinical features, and management protocols have not been well established.

Mycobacterium tuberculosis

53 HIV and tuberculosis (TB) form a lethal combination because each increases the other's progress.

54 TB can occur in HIV-infected individuals at any CD4 count.

55 TB in HIV-infected children may be more severe, progresses very fast, and causes more extrapulmonary manifestations.

56 Diagnosis of TB in children is very difficult. No simple test exists for confirmation of diagnosis. Diagnosis is based on demonstration of acid-fast bacilli (AFB) in sputum or other body fluid. In the absence of AFB, a diagnosis of probable TB can be made on the basis of a history of contact with adults with TB, a positive tuberculin skin test, and compatible radiologic findings.

57 A newer test, the automated nucleic acid amplification test, performed on sputum or on gastric aspirates may give results within 2 hours for the presence of *Mycobacterium tuberculosis* and of its resistance to rifampicin.

58 Treatment for TB depends on the clinical syndrome and consists of anti-TB drugs for 6–12 months.

Toxoplasmosis

59 Disseminated *T. gondii* infection in immunocompromised patients has emerged as a potentially fatal pathogen.

60 Common presentations include fever, encephalitis, pneumonia, myocarditis, and bone marrow suppression.

61 Confirmation of the diagnosis is either through serologic methods (reserved for immunocompetent hosts) or molecular methods, such as PCR.

62 Treatment consists of administration of pyrimethamine, sulfadiazine, and folinic acid.

Cryptosporidium Infection

63 *Cryptosporidium* spp. causes severe diarrheal in children with HIV infection, primary immunodeficiencies, or acute leukemia on chemotherapy.

64 Diagnosis of cryptosporidium infection is made by examination of stool.

65 Treatment is not satisfactory. The current therapy includes supportive care with administration of nitazoxanide.

Opportunistic infections typically do not cause disease in a person with a healthy immune system but generally affect people with a poorly functioning or suppressed immune system because of immunodeficiency or immunosuppression.

These infections can be severe to fatal, but early recognition and treatment may improve outcomes. The diagnosis of infections in immunocompromised pediatric patients remains a difficult challenge as presenting clinical signs and symptoms may be atypical and serologic testing may be unreliable. Immunocompromised children include those with congenital defects of host defense and defects in cell-mediated or humoral immunity, but the major expansion of this population has occurred with increased hematopoietic stem cell and solid organ transplantation, successful treatment of childhood malignancies, and the use of immunomodulatory agents for chronic diseases such as Crohn disease and rheumatoid arthritis. These developments have significantly increased the population of children at risk for opportunistic infections, and the list of organisms that lead to infections in these groups has become extensive and continues to grow. Pediatric intensivists are likely to see increasing numbers of children survive with primary immunodeficiencies or receive immunosuppressive therapy for treatment of malignancies, autoimmune disorders, or transplantation. For this reason, it is critical that all practitioners are able to recognize signs and symptoms of infections in these patients.

Conditions that predispose to opportunistic infections, common opportunistic infections, their diagnostic approach, and management of these infections are reviewed in this chapter.

DEFECTS IN THE IMMUNE SYSTEM AND OPPORTUNISTIC PATHOGENS

Defects in the immune system may occur due to primary or secondary immune deficiency disorders. Other causes include irradiation, removal of thymus, and administration of biological agents (various antibodies). Immune deficiency disorders impair immune responses to microbial agents, and thus defects may predispose to infections due to particular microbial agents. For example, B-cell defects leads to hypogammaglobulinemia and predisposes to bacterial infections while children with chronic granulomatous diseases are more prone for development of infections due to *Staphylococcus* and *Aspergillus*. Various immune defects and risk for development of infections due to microbial agents are given in **Table 95.1**.

TABLE 95.1

CONDITIONS PREDISPOSING AN INDIVIDUAL TO OPPORTUNISTIC INFECTIONS

■ MAJOR DEFECTS IN IMMUNE SYSTEM	■ CLINICAL CONDITIONS	■ INFECTIONS/CLINICAL MANIFESTATIONS
B-cell defects (humoral deficiencies)	Agammaglobulinemia, hypogamma-globulinemia, selective IgA deficiency, IgG subclass deficiencies, common variable immune deficiency, hyper-IgM syndrome	Infections with *S. aureus*; encapsulated organisms, such as *S. pneumoniae, H. influenzae*; and gram-negative organisms, such as *Pseudomonas* species Arthritis due to echoviruses, coxsackieviruses, adenoviruses, and *U. urealyticum* Infections due to *P. jiroveci* (*P. carinii*) pneumonitis, and *Cryptosporidium*
T-cell defects (cell-mediated immunity)	Thymic dysplasia (DiGeorge syndrome), defective T-cell receptor, defective cytokine production, T-cell activation defects, CD8 lymphocytopenia	Disseminated viral infections due to herpes simplex, varicella zoster, and CMV Progressive pneumonia caused by parainfluenza, respiratory syncytial virus, cytomegalovirus, varicella, and *P. jiroveci* Superficial and systemic fungal infections and parasitic infections. Severe mucocutaneous candidiasis; disseminated BCG disease after BCG vaccination
Combined B- and T-cell defects	Severe combined immunodeficiency, Omenn syndrome, Wiskott-Aldrich syndrome, ataxia telangiectasia, hyper-IgE syndrome	Infections caused by bacteria, fungi, or viruses Chronic diarrhea, mucocutaneous or systemic candidiasis, *P. jiroveci* pneumonitis, and CMV early in life Infections with *S. pneumoniae* or *H. influenzae* type b, *P. jiroveci* Late-onset recurrent sinopulmonary infections from bacteria and respiratory viruses Recurrent episodes of *S. aureus* abscesses of the skin, lungs, and musculoskeletal system
Abnormalities in phagocytic system	Inadequate numbers (congenital or acquired), Chronic granulomatous disease, leukocyte adhesion deficiency, Chédiak-Higashi syndrome	Recurrent pyogenic and fungal infections due to *Pseudomonas, S. marcescens*, and *S. aureus*, and fungi such as *Aspergillus* and *Candida* present as cellulitis, perirectal abscesses, or stomatitis Pulmonary infection, suppurative adenitis, subcutaneous abscess, liver abscess, osteomyelitis, and sepsis due to fungi or bacteria (*Staphylococcus*) Gastric outlet obstruction, urinary tract obstruction, and enteritis or colitis History of delayed cord separation and recurrent infections of the skin, oral mucosa, and genital tract, Predisposed to development of ecthyma gangrenosum and pyoderma gangrenosum

■ MAJOR DEFECTS IN IMMUNE SYSTEM	■ CLINICAL CONDITIONS	■ INFECTIONS/CLINICAL MANIFESTATIONS
Disorders of the complement system	Disorders involving any one of the complement components, asplenia, splenic dysfunction due to hemoglobinopathies, splenectomy	Infections due to *Salmonella* spp. and encapsulated bacteria including *S. pneumoniae* and *H. influenzae*. These agents can cause sepsis, pneumonia, meningitis, and osteomyelitis
Infections occurring with acquired immunodeficiencies	HIV and other virus infections, cancer chemotherapy, immunosuppressive therapy after organ transplant, diabetes mellitus, sickle cell disease, severe malnutrition	Similar to cell-mediated immune deficiency Neutropenic patients: infections due to gram-positive cocci and gram-negative organisms, such as *P. aeruginosa*, *E. coli*, and *Klebsiella* Fungal infections due to *Candida* and *Aspergillus* in prolonged neutropenia

CMV, cytomegalovirus; BCG, Bacille Calmette-Guérin.

APPROACH TO THE PATIENT WITH SUSPECTED OPPORTUNISTIC INFECTION

The approach to patients with suspected opportunistic infections will depend on underlying illness, site of infection, and severity of illness. A stepwise approach may improve outcome of opportunistic infection:

1. Ascertain predisposing factors (immune deficiency; severe malnutrition; exposure to chemotherapy, biological agents, or chronic steroids; implanted devices; nephrotic syndrome; etc.).
2. Identify underlying disease (primary or secondary immune deficiency).
3. Determine the site of infection (chest, gastrointestinal tract, genitourinary tract, blood stream, etc.).
4. Assess for likely etiological agents (bacteria, fungus, virus, mycobacterium, etc.).
5. Consider recent infections and antimicrobial resistance profiles that may persist in the host.
6. Assess severity of illness.
7. Start antibiotics to cover likely etiological agents.

OPPORTUNISTIC INFECTIONS IN PEDIATRIC INTENSIVE CARE SETTINGS

Patients with opportunistic infections frequently present to the PICU for treatment of fulminant infections, such as respiratory infections, sepsis, infections of the central nervous system (CNS), or multiorgan dysfunction. In patients with underlying immunodeficiency, the clinical course is potentially fulminant and case fatality remains high. Clinical signs and symptoms may provide important clues of immunodeficiency, as well as the possible etiologic agent of the infection, knowledge which is of paramount importance in instituting appropriate treatment.

OPPORTUNISTIC INFECTIONS DUE TO VIRUSES

Cytomegalovirus Infection

Cytomegalovirus (CMV) is in the herpes virus group and is a common infection in all children but can have devastating

❶ effects in the immunocompromised. The organism can be transmitted congenitally through an infected birth canal and postnatally by breast milk, saliva, urine, and blood transfusion (via infected white cells). Both humoral and cellular immune mechanisms are important in protection against CMV. Individuals not exposed to CMV before acquired immunosuppression (due to organ or hematopoietic stem cell transplantation [HSCT]), as evidenced by negative anti-CMV testing, and who subsequently acquire the virus by transfusion or other means are particularly at risk for severe CMV disease. Individuals previously exposed to CMV who subsequently receive immunosuppressive therapy are at significant risk for "reactivation" pneumonia. Approximately 50% of patients with aplastic anemia or hematologic malignancy treated by allogeneic marrow transplantation develop CMV infection. CMV may also be a copathogen with other opportunistic organisms, including *Pneumocystis jiroveci* and *Aspergillus* spp., especially in AIDS patients and patients following HSCT. The incidence has decreased significantly since the introduction of active antiretroviral treatment in patients infected with HIV (1).

Clinical Manifestations

Congenital CMV infection is a well-known clinical entity beyond the scope of this chapter. CMV as an opportunistic infection presents with varying clinical manifestations as it can **❷** infect almost all organ systems of the body (**Table 95.2**).

❸ Pulmonary involvement associated with CMV infection is a major cause of serious, often fatal, interstitial pneumonia in children with congenital immunodeficiency, AIDS, organ or HSCT, or malignancy on chemotherapy. It is a known complication of pediatric heart and lung transplantations. CMV pneumonitis usually occurs 1–3 months following transplantation and begins with symptoms of fever and a dry, nonproductive cough and progressive dyspnea that may require ventilatory support. It may occur as the only disease manifestation or be part of a disseminated CMV infection. Coinfection with other pathogens, especially gram-negative enteric bacteria and fungal pathogens in transplant recipients and *P. jiroveci* in patients with AIDS, can occur. The differential diagnosis of CMV pneumonitis in immunocompromised patients includes bacterial pneumonia (*Chlamydia*, *Mycoplasma*), infection with protozoa (*Toxoplasma gondii*), and fungal pneumonia (*Candida*, *Aspergillus*, or *P. jiroveci*). Noninfectious causes of pneumonitis, such as pulmonary hemorrhage, aspiration pneumonia, immune reconstitution inflammatory syndrome (related to causes other than CMV), and pulmonary damage from chemotherapeutic agents, should also be considered in the differential diagnosis of CMV pneumonia.

TABLE 95.2

CLINICAL MANIFESTATIONS OF CYTOMEGALOVIRUS INFECTION

■ ORGAN INVOLVED	■ SUSCEPTIBLE HOSTS	■ CLINICAL FEATURES
Mononucleosis syndrome	Immunocompetent and immunosuppressed persons; reactivation infection in immunosuppressed	Fever, severe malaise, headache, myalgia, abdominal pain with diarrhea Less common features: interstitial pneumonitis, myocarditis and pericarditis, arthralgias and arthritis, maculopapular rashes, adrenal insufficiency, splenic infarction, ulcerative colitis, and proctitis, Guillain-Barré syndrome, and meningoencephalitis
Respiratory system	Congenital immunodeficiency, AIDS, organ or marrow transplantation, or malignancy	Fever, dry/nonproductive cough, dyspnea, retractions, wheezing, and hypoxia, which require ventilatory support Coinfection with other pathogens, especially gram-negative enteric bacteria and fungal pathogens in transplant recipients and *P. jiroveci* in patients with AIDS
Eyes	Severe immunosuppression, especially in HSCT recipients and patients with AIDS	Rapidly progressive retinitis with white perivascular infiltrates, hemorrhage, with a necrosis Peripheral retinitis Conjunctivitis, corneal epithelial keratitis and disk neovascularization
Liver and hepatobiliary system	Recipients of hematopoietic stem cell, liver, heart, and lung transplant and patients with cancer or AIDS	Fever, thrombocytopenia, and lymphopenia or lymphocytosis with mild hepatomegaly Occasionally granulomatous hepatitis Jaundice and hyperbilirubinemia usually do not occur
Gastrointestinal system	Patients with AIDS and those with organ transplant	Esophagitis, gastritis, gastroenteritis, pyloric and small bowel obstruction, duodenitis, colitis, proctitis, pancreatitis, hemorrhage, and acalculous cholecystitis
Central nervous system syndrome	Patients with AIDS and those with organ transplant	Meningoencephalitis headache, photophobia, nuchal rigidity, memory deficits, and inability to concentrate Ascending paralysis caused by myelitis, with or without vasculitis or necrosis Polyradiculopathy in patients with AIDS
Other organs systems	Renal and heart transplant patients AIDS patients	Myocarditis: heart failure, cardiomegaly, electrocardiographic abnormalities, and poor left ventricular function on echocardiography Endocrinopathy: Addison's disease

A clinical condition called *mononucleosis syndrome* may occur due to CMV infection. In children, it is relatively less common as compared with adolescents and young adults. It may occur in immunocompetent as well as immunosuppressed patients. After initial infection, it will be reactivated with immunosuppression. Clinical course is subacute and includes fever, malaise, headache, myalgia, abdominal pain, and loose stools. There may be enlargement of liver, spleen, and peripheral lymph nodes. Investigations may show peripheral lymphocytosis with atypical lymphocytes and mildly elevated liver enzymes (**Table 95.2**). Similar clinical picture may be present in infections due to Epstein-Barr virus (EBV), hepatitis A or B virus, and HIV.

Over the last two to three decades, CMV retinitis has emerged as a common manifestation of CMV disease in patients with severe immunosuppression, especially in HSCT recipients and patients with AIDS. Children receiving chemotherapy for acute lymphoblastic leukemia and suffering from common variable immune deficiency have been reported to have CMV-related retinitis (2). CMV produces characteristic white perivascular infiltrates and hemorrhage, with a necrotic, rapidly progressive retinitis. Peripheral retinitis can be asymptomatic, or the complaints may be minimal and nonspecific; it is especially difficult to detect in infants and young children. At an advanced stage, it can cause blurred vision, decreased visual acuity, visual field defects, and blindness. Early diagnosis using visual field testing and/or ophthalmologic evaluation

facilitates prompt institution of antiviral therapy, which may be sight saving. CMV may also produce conjunctivitis, corneal epithelial keratitis, and disk neovascularization. The differential diagnosis of CMV retinitis includes other causes of retinal lesions, such as ocular toxoplasmosis, candidal infection of the retina, syphilis, herpes simplex virus (HSV), lymphocytic choriomeningitis virus infection, and varicella.

CMV hepatitis may occur in recipients of hematopoietic stem cell, liver, heart, or lung transplantation and in patients with cancer on chemotherapy or AIDS (3). It manifests as fever, thrombocytopenia, and lymphopenia or lymphocytosis with mild hepatomegaly. Hepatitis due to CMV infection may occur in liver transplant patients and is difficult to differentiate from acute rejection. The clinical manifestations are nonspecific and include prolonged pyrexia, leukopenia, thrombocytopenia, elevated transaminase and bilirubin levels, and hepatic failure. Other hepatic manifestations include vanishing bile duct syndrome, cholangitis, and chronic rejection (in liver transplant recipients). The differential diagnosis of CMV hepatitis includes other causes of viral hepatitis (EBV, HSV, enterovirus, adenovirus, and hepatitis A, B, and C), toxoplasmosis, bacterial hepatitis (including ascending cholangitis), and noninfectious causes (ischemic injury, vascular thrombosis, hemolysis, rejection, and drug- or toxin-induced hepatitis).

Gastrointestinal manifestations of CMV infection in immunocompromised patients (especially those with AIDS and those who have undergone hematopoietic stem cell, kidney, intestinal, or liver transplantation) include esophagitis, gastritis, gastroenteritis, pyloric and small bowel obstruction, duodenitis, colitis, proctitis, pancreatitis, hemorrhage, and acalculous cholecystitis. The differential diagnosis of CMV gastroenteritis/colitis includes infection with bacteria such as *Salmonella*, *Shigella*, *Clostridium difficile*, *Campylobacter*, *Yersinia*, and *Mycobacterium avium-intracellulare*. Viruses like HSV and adenovirus may also cause gastroenteritis mimicking CMV infection. Parasitic infection with *Cryptosporidium*, *Giardia*, and amebae should also be considered in differential diagnosis of CMV-related gastroenteritis. The differential diagnosis of CMV esophagitis and gastritis includes reflux esophagitis, acid peptic disease, HSV, *Candida* esophagitis, histoplasmosis, and TB.

Postnatal CMV meningoencephalitis is relatively uncommon. It is characterized by photophobia, nuchal rigidity, and altered sensorium. Clinical manifestation mimicking Guillain-Barré syndrome may occur in immunocompromised children. CMV polyradiculopathy characterized by leg pains, parasthesias, and flaccid paralysis is more common in adults, but may occur in older children as well (4).

CMV myocarditis has been documented in children who have undergone renal and heart transplant. These patients may manifest as congestive cardiac failure, may show cardiomegaly on x-ray film, ST segment and/or T wave changes on electrocardiogram (ECG), and poor left ventricular ejection fraction on echocardiography. Diagnosis can be confirmed by documenting CMV inclusion bodies on biopsy and demonstration of CMV DNA in tissue.

Immunosuppressed patients, especially those with AIDS, may manifest clinical endocrinopathies caused by CMV infection, such as adrenal insufficiency and adrenal necrosis. Involvement of skin due to CMV may manifest as localized cutaneous ulcers or a widespread maculopapular rashes.

Diagnosis

CMV is diagnosed by serology, polymerase chain reaction (PCR), antigenemia, and viral culture. For suspected CNS infections, PCR of cerebrospinal fluid (CSF) for CMV is the most sensitive diagnostic method (5).

Immunocompetent Hosts. Serology is used primarily in healthy patients to distinguish primary infection from reactivation. Acute serum IgG and IgM titers are obtained at the onset of illness. The presence of CMV IgG titer indicates that the patient has been infected with CMV in the past. Interpretation of CMV IgM antibody requires more careful evaluation, considering other processes that might produce cross-reacting antibody or polyclonal responses (e.g., rheumatoid factor). The presence of CMV IgM indicates current or recent CMV infection. CMV IgM antibody persists for 6 weeks in healthy adults and may be present for 3–6 months after primary infection. CMV IgG avidity index may be helpful to diagnose primary infection though avidity assays are not available commercially. Low avidity index (30%) suggests recent primary infection, within the past 2–4 months, and high avidity index (>60%) suggests a past or recurrent CMV infection (6). Primary infection is diagnosed if the patient is CMV IgG negative on acute presentation and becomes positive when convalescent titers are drawn. CMV IgM titers may be low or slightly elevated in the face of acute infection that is primary or reactivated. For previously healthy individuals, serum PCR testing for CMV may not be positive in patients with acute mononucleosis due to CMV (7).

Immunocompromised Hosts. CMV isolated from immunocompromised patients does not equate with CMV disease, but documentation of primary infection (that usually causes disease) by seroconversion or viremia in a previously seronegative

patient is important. In transplant recipients, primary CMV infection usually occurs 4–12 weeks after transplant. In immunocompromised children, reactivated CMV cannot reliably be diagnosed in spite of viral shedding in urine, saliva, or respiratory secretions. Among recipients of solid organ transplant, isolation from buffy coat or antigenemia correlates with CMV disease. Both serologic PCR and pp65 antigenemia testing for CMV in these patients appear to be sensitive (>90%) for diagnosis; however, neither are very specific (around 60%) to differentiate active or recurrent disease from latent infection (8). When followed longitudinally, these quantitative measures are useful as a signal of recurrence and may indicate a need for treatment (9). Either quantitative serologic PCR or pp65 antigenemia may be used to monitor viral loads during antiviral therapy, but are not interchangeable. More recently, quantification of CMV DNA by fully automated real-time PCR has been described as promising advance for early diagnosis and monitoring of treatment of CMV infection in immunocompromised hosts (10,11). For HSCT recipients and patients with AIDS, plasma detection of CMV DNA by PCR tends to correlate with clinical severity of disease. Among immunocompromised patients, quantitative PCR assays also correlate viral load with risk of CMV disease. However, it must be stated that the quantity of CMV DNA in blood that is predictive of disease varies with the method of measurement, type of sample, and the clinical setting. Among recipients of solid organ transplant, 2000–5000 genome copies/mL of plasma is identified as a useful cutoff value to determine significant risk of CMV disease.

Management

In the immunocompetent host, no treatment is indicated. It is suggested only in severe or life-threatening disease.

Among the immunocompromised, 85% of patients with AIDS and CMV retinitis improve or show stabilization of lesions after induction therapy with ganciclovir, valganciclovir, foscarnet, or cidofovir. Induction followed by continuous maintenance therapy to prevent relapse during continued immunosuppression is indicated in immunocompromised hosts with acquired CMV retinitis. At diagnosis, oral valganciclovir or intravenous ganciclovir is given daily for 2–3 weeks, followed by maintenance treatment 5–7 times a week. For single-agent induction therapy, foscarnet demonstrated a survival advantage over ganciclovir. Combination therapy with ganciclovir and foscarnet is associated with longer time to recurrence, compared with monotherapy. Oral ganciclovir may be considered for patients who are CMV seropositive and have CD4 <50/mm^3.

For solid organ transplant recipients, different regimens of antiviral agents, immunoglobulins, and combinations are used at different centers for prevention and treatment of CMV. Most include prophylaxis for CMV disease with immunoglobulin (IG) therapies including intravenous immune globulin (IVIG) or CMV-specific IVIG, antiviral agents, or some combination before and during the period of highest risk. One of the protocols of combining antiviral agent with IVIG includes the administration, for the first 20 days, of IV ganciclovir, 2.5 mg/kg three times daily plus IVIG, 500 mg/kg every other day (10 doses). This is followed by IV ganciclovir, 5 mg/kg three to five times per week for 20 more doses, and IVIG, 500 mg/kg twice a week for eight more doses. Dosages should be adjusted in patients with renal failure.

Preemptive therapy is an alternative in allogeneic HSCT recipients, for whom regular lab screening with antigenemia or PCR determines the need for initiation of antiviral therapy. This strategy is associated with a survival advantage. However, autologous and stem cell HSCT recipients have lower risk of CMV disease and might not warrant prophylaxis. For those who do acquire CMV pneumonia post–hematopoietic stem cell transplant, combined therapy with intravenous ganciclovir and IVIG or CMV-IVIG is indicated.

In recipients of renal transplant, prophylactic antiviral therapy is recommended (a) when the donor or recipient is seropositive and antilymphocyte treatment is part of the immunosuppressive regimen and (b) for seronegative recipients of grafts from seropositive donors. Furthermore, preemptive therapy with valganciclovir may reduce potential complications of interstitial fibrosis and tubular atrophy.

Prevention

Prevention of CMV disease is achieved through reducing risks associated with blood transfusion, including screening of donors, freezing red cells prior to infusion, removing the buffy coat, and the use of transfusion filters. For infants who consume breast milk, pasteurization or freezing milk prior to consumption reduces the risk of transmission. In the hospital setting, standard precautions are sufficient to block transmission. In the community, CMV prevention includes consideration of day care and school avoidance and good hygienic habits.

Varicella Zoster Virus Infection

Varicella zoster virus (VZV) is a DNA virus that typically causes benign infections of the skin and mucous membranes. It may cause both varicella and zoster in the normal host. However, in certain groups (neonates, children with cancer, HSCT, AIDS, congenital defects of cell-mediated immunity, and organ transplant) VZV can lead to visceral dissemination and pneumonia. HIV-infected children who develop varicella in the setting of severe immunodeficiency are at high risk to develop zoster. Patients undergoing HSCT for a malignant disorder are at higher risk for developing zoster than those with nonmalignant disorders (12). Elderly individuals with lesser induration or erythema when skin tested with VZV antigens were at more risk of developing herpes zoster (13).

Clinical Features

VZV infection may be confined to skin or may be disseminated. In immunocompromised hosts, VZV infection is severe and disseminated, the febrile phase may last longer, and fresh vesicles may continue to appear for a longer period. Skin lesions are more intense on trunk, bigger in size, and may be hemorrhagic. Mucosal surfaces of the entire gastrointestinal tract may be involved, and disease manifests as dysphagia, chest pain, abdominal pain, and bleeding (14). The most serious manifestation of VZV infection in an immunocompromised host is primary varicella pneumonia. The clinical presentation of varicella pneumonia is nonspecific and includes fever, cough, dyspnea, chest pain, cyanosis, and hemoptysis. The chest x-ray typically reveals a diffuse nodular or miliary pattern, most pronounced in the perihilar region (15). Varicella pneumonia may be complicated by acute respiratory distress syndrome, rhabdomyolysis, acute hepatitis, and disseminated intravascular coagulation (16).

CNS complications of VZV include cerebellar ataxia and encephalitis. Patients with varicella may develop ischemic strokes and radiologic and histopathologic evidence of CNS vasculitis. Ocular manifestations of VZV infection include conjunctivitis, keratitis, iridocyclitis, panuveitis, and acute retinal necrosis. Sudden loss of vision due to retrobulbar optic neuritis and retinitis following varicella in a vaccinated child with acute lymphoblastic leukemia has also been reported (17). Other uncommon but important manifestations of varicella infection in immunocompromised hosts include fulminant hepatic failure, myocarditis, arrhythmias, and progression to dilated cardiomyopathy and endocarditis (18).

Diagnosis

Herpes zoster can be diagnosed on the basis of physical findings, vesicle scrapings, serology, or PCR. Physical findings are characteristic and diagnostic. In immunocompromised hosts, vesicles are more common on the trunk; they are bigger in size, umbilicated, and more frequently hemorrhagic. Laboratory confirmation includes scraping of vesicles in the first few days following their appearance may help in identification of the virus. After unroofing a vesicle, the fluid can be sent for viral culture as well as direct fluorescent antibody testing. The direct fluorescent antibody test is advantageous, as the results are more rapidly obtained and can differentiate HSV from VZV. The *Tzanck smear* of vesicle scrapings will show multinucleated giant cells but is not specific for VZV. Vesicular fluid and skin scraping subjected to viral culture and supplemented with PCR may improve diagnosis.

Specific IgM suggests recent infection with VZV. Acute and convalescent titers of serum IgG for varicella zoster will show a rise in antibody titer in immunocompetent persons but not in the immunocompromised. Most serum antibody testing methods are not sensitive enough to identify vaccine-induced immunity. Other investigations include fluorescent antibody to membrane antigen method, latex agglutination, and enzyme-linked immunosorbent assay. PCR testing for VZV is very sensitive and can be performed on body fluids including blood spot samples or tissue specimens.

Management

Management of VZV Exposure. Susceptible persons exposed to varicella should be given immune globulin (either varicella zoster immune globulin [VZIG] or IVIG up to 96 hours after exposure). The VZIG IM dose is 1.25 mL (125 IU) for every 10 kg of body weight, with a maximum IM dose of 6 mL (625 IU). To maximize benefit, immune globulin should be given as soon as possible after exposure. Those who are susceptible include

- immunocompromised children without history of varicella or varicella immunization;
- children with cellular immune deficiencies or other immune system problems;
- pregnant women without evidence of immunity;
- newborn infants whose mothers had onset of chickenpox within 5 days before delivery or within 48 hours after delivery;
- hospitalized premature infants ≥28 weeks' gestation whose mothers lack a history of chickenpox or serologic evidence of protection;
- hospitalized premature infants <28 weeks' gestation or ≤1000 g birth weight, regardless of maternal history or serologic status.

Significant exposures include

- residents of the same household;
- face-to-face indoor playmates;
- for varicella, hospital exposure in the same multibed room or adjacent beds in a large ward, face-to-face contact with an infectious staff member or patient, or visit by a person deemed contagious;
- for zoster, intimate contact (touching or hugging) with a contagious person;
- for newborns, onset of maternal chickenpox ≤5 days before delivery or within 48 hours after delivery; immune globulin is not indicated if the mother has zoster.

Exposure to varicella merits airborne and contact precautions from 8 until 21 days after the onset of rash in the index case, and for 28 days after exposure to the index case in those treated with VZIG or IVIG. For those who have received high-dose immune globulin (400 mg/kg or greater) within 3 weeks before exposure, a second dose is not indicated.

Management of VZV Disease. Treatment of varicella in immunocompetent children is not recommended. However, those with increased risk for moderate-to-severe varicella should be considered candidates for oral therapy with acyclovir or valacyclovir in pediatric patients aged 2 or more. Those at increased risk include people >12 years of age, those with chronic cutaneous or pulmonary disorders, those receiving long-term salicylate therapy, and those receiving short, intermittent, or aerosolized courses of corticosteroids. Therapy should be started within 24 hours of the rash appearance. Pregnant women should not be routinely treated with acyclovir for varicella, as the risks to the fetus are unknown. However, IV acyclovir is indicated for pregnant women with serious complications of varicella. Salicylates should be avoided in children with varicella, as they increase the risk of Reye syndrome.

Immunocompromised patients should receive IV acyclovir. The IV dose of acyclovir for children is 1500 mg/m^2/day (30 mg/kg/day for adolescents) in three divided doses. Oral, high-dose acyclovir (80 mg/kg/day in four divided doses) can be considered in patients who are mildly immunosuppressed and at lower risk for developing severe varicella. The use of VZIG is indicated for immunocompromised persons who are exposed and has not shown benefit in those who have established disease. Experience with efficacy of famciclovir and valaciclovir in children is limited. (11)

Airborne and contact precautions should be maintained in patients with varicella for 5 days after appearance of the rash and while vesicular lesions are present. For those with disseminated varicella, airborne and contact precautions should be maintained for the duration of the illness. Children with varicella may return to school when their lesions have crusted over.

Management of Herpes Zoster Disease. In immunocompromised patients, intravenous acyclovir is the therapy of choice for acute herpes zoster. Treatment should be initiated as soon as vesicles are recognized to prevent progression to disseminated disease. After the initial infection is controlled, a switch to oral therapy can be considered. For patients who do not respond clinically to acyclovir, drug susceptibility testing should be pursued and alternative therapy with intravenous foscarnet or cidofovir considered.

Prevention

The mainstay of prevention of varicella includes a combination of vaccination of the general population, proper isolation of suspected and known cases, administration of VZIG within 96 hours of exposure to immunocompromised hosts, and isolation of susceptible contacts. Hospitalized patients with varicella should be placed in negative air flow rooms and cared for by staff with evidence of immunity. Immunocompromised children should also be placed on acyclovir therapy immediately after exposure and continued for 1–2 weeks. For pediatric solid organ transplant recipients, pretransplant vaccination of these patients and their household contacts should be prioritized. For hematopoietic stem cell transplant recipients, acyclovir prophylaxis reduces VZV infection posttransplant (19).

Immunocompetent patients with localized herpes zoster should be placed on standard precautions with their lesions covered. For immunocompromised patients and immunocompetent patients with disseminated herpes zoster lesions, airborne and contact precautions should be instituted until all lesions are dry and crusted over. Immunocompromised patients

with localized herpes zoster should also be placed on airborne and contact precautions until disseminated disease is excluded.

Herpes Virus Type 6

Human herpes virus 6 (HHV-6) is a DNA virus that is the etiologic agent for most cases of roseola and is among the most widespread of the human herpesviruses. The virus remains latent in the body after primary infection and reactivates in immunocompromised patients. HHV-6 infection occurs in nearly 50% of all recipients of HSCT and in 20%–30% of recipients of solid organ transplant 2–3 weeks following the procedure and is associated with higher morbidity and mortality.

Clinical Features

In immunocompetent children, HHV-6 causes exanthem subitum, febrile episodes without skin rash, and non-EBV and non-CMV infectious mononucleosis. The clinical features in immunocompromised children are nonspecific. It has been suggested that the viral infection and activation result in clinical symptoms, including fever, skin rash, pneumonia, bone marrow suppression, encephalitis, and rejection (20). Most cases of HHV-6–associated pneumonia involve immunocompromised patients, especially those who have received a hematopoietic stem cell transplant or who have been infected by HIV. Encephalitis may also manifest in persons living with HIV and reactivated HHV-6.

Diagnosis

Testing for HHV-6 includes serology, culture, immunohistochemistry, and nucleic acid assays. Serology testing is usually reserved for the immunocompetent and is not useful in posttransplant patients. PCR testing on tissue samples is a commonly used test for HHV-6. The disadvantage of this method is that it does not differentiate between active and latent infection. Other methods include serum plasma PCR and reverse transcriptase (RT) PCR, which detect virus that is circulating and are thought to be indicative of active infection. However, the best method for detection of active HHV-6 is quantitative RT-PCR analysis of body secretions. This method is sensitive and efficient and allows direct determination of viral burden in the host (21).

Management

While treatment is not indicated in healthy children, those who are immunocompromised may experience severe disease. Antiviral therapies have not been evaluated in randomized clinical trials. Drugs commonly used when indicated are the same as those used for treatment of CMV, including ganciclovir cidofovir, and foscarnet. In vitro studies indicate that ganciclovir is superior to acyclovir in treating HHV-6, and several case reports support treatment with ganciclovir, particularly in HHV-6 encephalitis. Foscarnet is another alternative that shows in vitro activity against HHV-6. Cidofovir shows good activity in vitro, but its use is limited by associated nephrotoxicity and limited experience (22). In addition to these therapies, patients may benefit from a reduction in immunosuppression. Adoptive T-cell immunotherapy is currently being explored as a potential adjunctive therapy.

Prevention

Routine prophylaxis or preemptive therapy to prevent HHV-6 infection is not indicated. However, prophylaxis with ganciclovir has proven efficacious in preventing HHV-6 reactivation in HSCT patients (23). A potential pitfall is that prophylaxis has been shown to promote resistance of CMV to ganciclovir.

FUNGAL INFECTIONS

Candidiasis

Candida spp. are recognized as a leading contributor to morbidity and mortality in patients with oncohematologic malignancies, HIV infection, primary immunodeficiencies, prolonged neutropenia, diabetes, corticosteroid administration, broad-spectrum antibiotic treatment, IV hyperalimentation, and presence of central venous lines. Invasive fungal infections are increasing. Data on invasive candidiasis are limited. Available data suggest that over the last two decades the epidemiology of invasive candidal infection has changed and now more infections due to non–*Candida albicans* species infections have been noticed (24). The frequency of *Candida* species in 64 patients from a PICU was *C. tropicalis* (48.4%), *C. albicans* (29.7%), *C. guilliermondii* (14.1%), *C. krusei* (6.3%), and *C. glabrata* (1.6%) (25). In the pediatric intensive care setting, the risk factors for increased incidence of candidal infection include the presence of a central venous catheter and the receipt of either vancomycin or other antimicrobials with activity against anaerobic organisms for >3 days.

Intrinsic differences may exist between different populations sampled. For instance, malnutrition may favor the presence of yeast species other than *C. albicans* (26). Neutropenic children colonized with *C. tropicalis* are at higher risk for dissemination compared with those colonized with *C. albicans* (27).

Clinical Features

Acute disseminated candidiasis occurs in immunocompromised hosts. Disseminated candidiasis may affect different organ system including lungs, kidneys, liver, spleen, and brain. The portals of entry are usually lesions of the gastrointestinal tract, oral mucosa, or skin (puncture sites). Organisms may disseminate via the hematogenous route to the tissues of one or more organs. The clinical manifestations depend on extent and the site of involvement. The clinical features are nonspecific in infants and children and are similar to those with sepsis caused by other organisms. Presence of the ocular lesions of endophthalmitis and maculopapular rash in an immunocompromised state suggest a possibility of candidal sepsis. The skin lesions consist of generalized rashes or discrete, firm, erythematous papules that measure 0.5–1 cm in diameter. A nodular center is often surrounded by an erythematous halo. Candidiasis may involve bones, joints, heart, and CNS. Osteomyelitis of bones may develop in young infants and children. Cardiac involvement may be in the form of endocarditis, myocarditis, or arrhythmia. CNS involvement may occur in disseminated candidiasis and is more common in preterm infants and young children.

Oral candidiasis can be an early sign of illness or of disease progression in HIV/AIDS. The sites commonly involved are buccal mucosa and dorsal and lateral surfaces of tongue. Submucosal edema and bleeding may occur while plaques are removed. Esophageal candidiasis is one of the important clinical manifestations of candidal infection in immunocompromised hosts. Patients may have concurrent oropharyngeal candidiasis, odynophagia, retrosternal pain, fever, nausea/vomiting, drooling, dehydration, hoarseness, and upper gastrointestinal bleeding. *Candida* infection may also manifest as epiglottitis.

Gastrointestinal candidiasis may occur in children with immune deficiency disorders and cancer and after surgery. It may involve the stomach, intestine, or hepatobiliary system. Peritonitis due to *Candida* spp. may occur secondary to bowel perforation, peritoneal dialysis, or intestinal surgery. Clinical manifestations are nonspecific and include abdominal distention, fever, vomiting, and abdominal pain.

The airway, from pharynx to bronchi, may be involved. A child may present with hoarseness of voice, low-grade fever, tachypnea, or nonspecific physical examination findings. Pulmonary infection may be complicated by development of abscess and empyema.

Renal involvement in children with candidemia is relatively common and includes renal microabscesses, papillary necrosis, calyceal distortion, and obstruction due to fungal ball or perinephric abscesses.

C. albicans may be associated with vaginitis in immunocompetent as well as immunocompromised hosts. Clinical features include swelling and erythema of vaginal mucosa with creamy white discharge and involvement of perineal skin.

Diagnosis

Diagnosis of *Candida* infections is based on clinical findings and tissue and body fluid culture. Mucocutaneous candidiasis is diagnosed clinically and can be confirmed with demonstration of budding yeast from scrapings of skin or mucosal lesions. Species identification can be done by culture.

Diagnosis of invasive candida infection can be made by demonstration of fungal element beyond stratum corneum in skin biopsy. Endoscopy is useful for diagnosis of esophageal candidiasis. Tissue samples can be stained and cultured, and the addition of potassium hydroxide to specimens may help to identify yeast and pseudohyphae. For retinal candidal infections, ophthalmologic examination identifies characteristic findings.

Candidal infections in solid organs may be seen on CT or ultrasound studies, but characteristic findings typically occur late in the course of the disease. Four ultrasound patterns of hepatosplenic candidiasis have been described. The first pattern, described as having a "wheel-within-a-wheel" appearance, consists of a central hypoechoic area of necrosis that contains fungi surrounded by an echogenic zone of inflammatory cells. A hypoechoic rim is noted at the periphery. The second pattern is a "bull's-eye" configuration, consisting of a central echogenic nidus surrounded by a hypoechoic rim. In general, this second pattern occurs in patients with active fungal infection and a relatively normal white blood cell count. The third pattern consists of a uniformly hypoechoic nodule and is the most common pattern seen on ultrasound; however, it is the least specific appearance of candidiasis and may simulate metastatic disease or lymphoma. The fourth pattern consists of echogenic foci, with variable degrees of posterior acoustic shadowing. This pattern occurs in later stages of infection and generally indicates early resolution. In contrast-enhanced CT, fungal microabscesses usually appear as multiple, round, discrete areas of low attenuation, generally ranging from 2 to 20 mm. Diagnosis of disseminated candidiasis is difficult as sensitivity of blood culture is 50%–70%. Diagnosis can be established with clinical features and demonstration of candida species from otherwise sterile body fluid like spinal fluid, blood, or bone marrow.

The advancement of in situ hybridization techniques has permitted rapid detection of *Candida* spp. in a matter of hours. Serologic techniques to detect candidal antigens are being perfected to improve diagnostic methods. Specifically, the $(1\rightarrow3)$ β-D-glucan assay has shown high sensitivity and specificity as an adjunct for diagnosis of invasive fungal infections (28).

Management

Evidence-based guidelines for the treatment of candidiasis are published by the Infectious Disease Society of America (29,30). Oropharyngeal candidiasis is treated with topical therapy using clotrimazole cloches or oral nystatin or amphotericin B suspensions; however, systemic therapy with fluconazole is also effective (ketoconazole or itraconazole are alternatives). Esophageal disease should be treated with systemic therapy with oral or intravenous fluconazole or oral itraconazole for 2–3 weeks. For invasive candidiasis in neonates, conventional amphotericin B is the drug of choice, and combination therapy with flucytosine may benefit those with CNS disease. For immunocompromised patients with suspected systemic candidemia, first-line therapies include lipid formulation amphotericin B, caspofungin, or voriconazole. Safety and efficacy of voriconazole has been established in children >12 years of age. For yeast specimens identified as *C. albicans* and for isolates that are susceptible, fluconazole therapy should be used. The length of antifungal therapy for candidemia is 14 days, starting from the first negative blood culture. For disseminated disease, patients are treated until clinical, radiologic, or microbiologic resolution is achieved (30).

Another mainstay in the treatment of invasive candidiasis is the removal of infected vascular lines and hardware, which improves morbidity and mortality in this patient population. Special consideration should be given to patients with tunneled catheters, as these are unlikely to be sources of infection, and to febrile neutropenic patients who are more likely to become candidemic due to gut translocation than via central catheter infection. All candidemic patients should have a dilated eye examination by an ophthalmologist to look for signs of invasive ocular disease, as this would require prolonged antifungal therapy (31).

Prevention

Prevention of invasive candidiasis and associated sequelae involves prophylactic therapy. Studies in the adult ICU setting have demonstrated that invasive candidiasis can be prevented by fluconazole prophylaxis, but decreased mortality was not observed. These studies also report no increase in fluconazole-resistant *Candida* species during the study period. Patients who may benefit from antifungal prophylaxis with fluconazole include neonates whose birth weight is <1000 g, solid organ transplant recipients, patients hospitalized in an intensive care unit with high rates of invasive candidiasis, patients with chemotherapy-induced neutropenia, and HSCT recipients with neutropenia (29). Postoperative prophylaxis for 1–2 weeks with fluconazole or liposomal amphotericin B is indicated after liver, pancreas, and small bowel transplant. For chemotherapy-induced neutropenia, prevention with fluconazole, posaconazole, itraconazole, or caspofungin is indicated during induction and for the duration of neutropenia.

Pneumocystis jiroveci

P. jiroveci, earlier known as *P. carinii*, is a eukaryotic microorganism of uncertain taxonomy that can infect numerous mammalian hosts. Developing from a small, unicellular "trophozoite" into a "cyst" that contains eight "sporozoites," its life cycle superficially resembles those seen in both the protozoa and fungi. Morphologic and ultrastructural observations have led some investigators to conclude that the organism is a protozoan, while others feel that it more closely resembles a fungus. Phylogenetic analysis of *Pneumocystis* 16S-like rRNA demonstrates it to be a member of the fungi family.

Patients at higher risk for *P. jiroveci* pneumonia include infants with severe malnutrition and children with primary immunodeficiencies (combined immune deficiency and hyper-IgM syndrome), hematologic malignancies, HIV infection, and recipients of solid organ or hematopoietic stem cell transplants. Patients with solid tumors (especially who receive high-dose

corticosteroids for brain neoplasms) and patients with inflammatory or collagen-vascular disorders (especially who receive immunosuppressive therapy for systemic lupus, juvenile idiopathic arthritis, and Wegener granulomatosis) have been identified as subgroups at increased risk for *P. jiroveci* pneumonia. Other factors associated with *P. jiroveci* pneumonia include the intensity of the immunosuppressive regimen and tapering doses of corticosteroids (32).

Clinical Features

Clinical manifestations and outcome of children infected with *P. jiroveci* is variable and is determined by underlying disease and extent of immune suppression. The onset of illness may be fulminant or insidious.

The clinical manifestations of *P. jiroveci* pneumonia in HIV-infected and non–HIV-infected children differ. Patients with AIDS typically have a longer duration of symptoms and a more insidious presentation. Hypoxemia may be less intense. Organisms appear to be abundant in AIDS patients and can usually be identified in sputum/induced sputum, bronchoalveolar lavage (BAL) fluid, or even gastric lavage samples. Physical findings may reveal respiratory distress as indicated by tachypnea, nasal flaring, and intercostal, subcostal, or supracostal retractions. In fulminant infection, cyanosis may be present. Initially, auscultation of chest may be normal despite hypoxia and tachypnea. In advanced stage of illness, scattered crackles and rhonchi/wheezing may be detected. Infants with HIV infection or pulmonary alveolar proteinosis may have polymicrobial infections, especially with *P. jiroveci* and CMV, and the manifestations are severe in these patients and are more likely to require ventilatory support.

Though the carriage rates of *P. jiroveci* in immunosupressed children without AIDS is low, their clinical illness due to pneumocystis pneumonia (PCP) may be particularly abrupt in onset and more rapidly progressive. Even within these patients, the course varies widely. In children, fever is generally present and of high grade. It often precedes the onset of nonproductive cough, tachypnea, and severe dyspnea. The time of onset of clinical disease in non-AIDS, high-risk patients is unpredictable, but disease often occurs after discontinuance or a reduction in the dose of corticosteroid therapy (32). Though pneumocystis infection predominantly causes pneumonia, cases of extrapulmonary or disseminated infection of pneumocystis have been described. Extrapulmonary pneumocystosis represents <1% of all cases of infection with *P. jiroveci*. Extrapulmonary spread of *P. jiroveci* infection occurs via both lymphatic and hematogenous routes. Several organs or tissues may be involved, but the most common sites are lymph nodes, spleen, liver, and bone marrow. While all patients with disseminated forms of this infection die rapidly, survival for patients with AIDS is possible if systemic treatment is provided, if a single extrapulmonary site is involved, and if no concomitant pneumonia is present.

Diagnosis

PCP is diagnosed through direct identification of organisms from lung tissue or induced sputum specimens. While identification of organisms from lung biopsy specimens is the gold standard for diagnosis, other methods of identification may be adequate. A meta-analysis of diagnostic procedures to identify PCP found that sputum induction in patients with HIV infection is adequate for diagnosis, compared with BAL specimens. The yield was increased with immunofluorescence testing versus cytochemical staining (33). Additionally, PCR testing for PCP using induced sputum or BAL fluid can increase the diagnostic yield for HIV patients with suspected PCP. The results of PCR testing in immunocompetent patients should be interpreted cautiously as it may indicate colonization (34).

Management

Pneumocystis disease can progress quickly, and the success of treatment depends largely on the stage of disease at the time of treatment initiation. Therefore, prompt diagnosis and treatment are essential. The first-line treatment for PCP is intravenous (IV) trimethoprim-sulfamethoxazole (TMP-SMZ), regardless of previous prophylactic regimen. The initial IV dosage is 15–20 mg/kg/day of the trimethoprim component, divided every 6–8 hours. With good clinical response, this can be transitioned to oral therapy to complete a 21-day course. Second-line treatments include IV pentamidine isethionate, oral dapsone with oral or IV TMP-SMZ, or oral atovaquone.

For patients who present with moderate-to-severe disease (PO_2 <70 mm Hg or PaO_2-to-PaO_2 gradient >35 mm Hg), early corticosteroid administration is also indicated and should be started within the first 72 hours of therapy. The recommended regimen is oral prednisone, 40 mg (1 mg/kg if < 40 kg) twice daily for days 1–5, then 40 mg daily for days 6–10, and 20 (0.5 mg/kg if < 40 kg) mg daily for days 11–20. Alternatively, IV methylprednisolone can be given at 75% of the recommended prednisone dose if indicated (35). Patients may deteriorate after the first 3–5 days of treatment due to the inflammatory response generated (35). Treatment failure is diagnosed if no clinical improvement occurs despite 4–8 days of appropriate therapy. There are no controlled trials to inform the management of treatment failures in children. However, we recommend switching to IV therapy if the patient had been receiving oral therapy. If IV therapy with the same antibiotic is unsuccessful, the patient may be switched to a different antibiotic. Patients who have not tolerated or responded to TMP-SMZ may be treated with pentamidine, 4 mg/kg/day by IV route once daily. Other drugs include trimethoprim/dapsone combination, pyrimethamine/sulfadoxine combination, clindamycin, primaquine, and atovaquone.

Prevention

Prevention of PCP includes appropriate prophylaxis. For HIV-positive patients with CD4 counts of <200/mm^3, daily prophylaxis with TMP-SMZ is indicated. If this therapy cannot be tolerated, second-line therapies should be used, including dapsone, dapsone and pyrimethamine, atovaquone, or aerosolized pentamidine. Prophylaxis should continue until the CD4 count is >200/mm^3 for 3 months. Those with extrapulmonary disease should not be given future prophylaxis with aerosolized pentamidine due to the possibility of recurrence of extrapulmonary infection. For patients who experience PCP, prophylaxis should continue indefinitely (36).

Invasive Aspergillosis

Aspergillus is a group of ubiquitous fungal organisms found in soil and other settings, including the hospital environment. The pathogenic species include *A. fumigatus, A. niger*, and *A. flavus. A. fumigatus* is the most common species responsible for pneumonia in immunocompromised hosts. In tissue, the organisms form septate hyphae with regular 45-degree dichotomous branching, best seen with methenamine-silver staining. The organisms enter the body via the respiratory route. Aspergillosis of the lung is often preceded or accompanied by invasion of the nose and paranasal sinuses in susceptible hosts.

Clinical Features

Susceptible hosts include children with hematologic malignancies (either primary or relapse), allogeneic HSCT, granulocytopenia, corticosteroid usage (for malignancy or autoimmune disease), immunosuppressive therapies, immunodeficiencies (chronic granulomatous disease), severe combined immunodeficiency, and organ transplantation (heart–lung transplantation) (37). Invasiveness appears to depend on the genetic and immune status of the host and on the extent and duration of exposure to spores. Disseminated aspergillosis, defined as infection of two or more noncontiguous organs, is the most severe form of clinical aspergillosis. Patients usually have pulmonic disease and widespread organ involvement (**Table 95.3**).

TABLE 95.3

CLINICAL MANIFESTATIONS OF INVASIVE ASPERGILLOSIS

■ ORGAN SYSTEM	■ PATIENTS PREDISPOSED	■ CLINICAL MANIFESTATIONS
Respiratory system	Organ transplant patients, chronic granulomatous disease, HIV infection, and immunosuppressive chemotherapy	Necrotizing bronchopneumonia or hemorrhagic infarction, single or multiple abscesses, granulomata, or lobar infiltrates. Patients may present with fever, dyspnea, nonproductive cough, mild hemoptysis, and pleuritic chest pain, necrotizing bronchitis with pseudomembrane formation, invasive tracheitis, tracheoesophageal fistula, and pleural aspergillosis In CGD: direct extension from the lungs to the chest wall
Paranasal sinuses	Profound neutropenia associated with chemotherapy or recipient of organ transplant	Sinusitis: direct extension to the orbit, early bone destruction, fever, cough, epistaxis, headache, sinus pain, periorbital swelling, and nasal congestion; duskiness or necrosis of the nasal septum or inferior turbinates
Eyes	Organ transplant patients, chronic granulomatous disease, HIV infection, and immunosuppressive chemotherapy	Fungal endophthalmitis: pain, photophobia, and diminished visual acuity Retinal hemorrhage, infarction, focal retinitis, and vitreitis Fungal keratitis and episcleritis Orbital cellulites: diplopia, periorbital edema, proptosis, and pain on lateral gaze
Central nervous system	Immunosuppressed patients	Brain abscess: single or multiple in cerebrum or cerebellum Present with neurologic deficits, hemiparesis, cranial nerve palsies, or seizures Meningeal signs may be absent

■ ORGAN SYSTEM	■ PATIENTS PREDISPOSED	■ CLINICAL MANIFESTATIONS
Bones and joints	Immunosuppressed patients, CGD	Vertebral and rib osteomyelitis: cord compression due to epidural abscess secondary to vertebral osteomyelitis
Heart	Patients with open-heart surgery	Endocarditis: persistent fever, evidence of embolic phenomena, and disseminated intravascular coagulopathy
		Pericarditis: cardiac tamponade
Genitourinary system	Immunosuppressed patients	Urinary tract infection: fever, chills, and microhematuria
		Unilateral flank pain may occur with ascending infection
Other organ systems		Abscesses: liver, thyroid, testis, spleen, and adrenals

HIV, human immunodeficiency virus; CGD, chronic granulomatous disease.

Invasive pulmonary aspergillosis is manifested most commonly as necrotizing bronchopneumonia or hemorrhagic infarction, although single or multiple abscesses, granulomata, or lobar infiltrates are occasionally present. Positive-surveillance nasal cultures for *Aspergillus* frequently precede the development of invasive pulmonary aspergillosis. Patients may present with fever, dyspnea, nonproductive cough, mild hemoptysis, and pleuritic chest pain (especially prominent in patients with hemorrhagic pulmonary infarction). Coexisting sinusitis is a common finding in neutropenic children. In children with chronic granulomatous disease, direct extension from the lungs to the chest wall may occur. Unusual clinical manifestations in children include necrotizing bronchitis with pseudomembrane formation, invasive tracheitis, tracheoesophageal fistula, and pleural aspergillosis (38). Acute, invasive sinusitis is rare in children and occurs almost exclusively in patients with profound neutropenia associated with chemotherapy or following organ transplant. In the setting of profound immunosuppression, the course may be fulminant, with early bone destruction, direct extension to the orbit and anterior cranial fossa, widespread dissemination, and a high mortality rate. Fever, cough, epistaxis, headache, sinus pain, periorbital swelling, and nasal congestion are the most common clinical signs. Examination typically shows nasal crusting with rhinorrhea, sinus tenderness, nasal or oral ulceration, and duskiness or necrosis of the nasal septum or inferior turbinates. Multiple sinus involvement with opacification or air-fluid levels can be demonstrated radiographically or by CT. Biopsy and culture of the nasal or sinus mucosa demonstrate large numbers of hyphae, and fungal cultures typically yield *A. fumigatus*, *A. flavus*, or, less often, *Rhizopus* or *Candida*.

Otomycosis may occur in immunosuppressed children due to *A. niger* or *A. fumigatus*. Occasionally, otitis externa and mastoiditis may occur in malnourished children.

Cutaneous aspergillosis is a common manifestation of invasive disease in immunocompromised children secondary to hematogenous dissemination or local spread. Local spread may result either from direct inoculation of the skin at sites of local trauma (IV catheter sites, burn wounds, or diaper dermatitis). Cutaneous lesions progress from erythematous or violaceous papules or plaques through a hemorrhagic bullous stage to a purpuric ulcer with central necrosis and eschar formation, called *ecthyma gangrenosum*.

In disseminated *Aspergillus* infection, fungal endophthalmitis may be an important finding. Patients may have pain, photophobia, and diminished visual acuity. Examination of the retina shows retinal hemorrhage, focal retinitis, and vitreitis. Unusual ocular manifestations include bilateral retinal infarction secondary to disseminated disease and fungal keratosis due to direct inoculation of spores into the eye and episcleritis.

Orbital cellulitis may occur even in immunocompetent patients secondary to invasive sinusitis. Infection spreads locally through destroyed orbital walls and may involve the retro-orbital space. Patients may present with diplopia, periorbital edema, proptosis, and pain on lateral gaze (39). Aspergillosis of the CNS may result from direct spread from the paranasal sinuses or, more commonly, from widespread dissemination in immunosuppressed patients. CNS aspergillosis is rare but has very high fatality rates. The disease may be associated with single or multiple abscesses in the cerebrum or cerebellum. Patients may present with neurologic deficits, hemiparesis, cranial nerve palsies, or seizures. Meningeal signs may be absent.

Involvement of bones due to *Aspergillus* infection is uncommon. It may follow direct extension of infection from lungs, overlying skin, a surgical or traumatic wound, or hematogenous spread. Vertebra and ribs are the commonly involved bones. Invasive aspergillosis may present as cord compression due to epidural abscess secondary to vertebral osteomyelitis in children with chronic granulomatous disease.

Aspergillus endocarditis may occur during open-heart surgery or as part of disseminated disease. Clinical features include persistent fever, evidence of embolic phenomena, and disseminated intravascular coagulopathy after cardiac surgery. Echocardiography may be useful for the detection of mycotic aneurysms, intracardiac vegetations, or intra-aortic vegetations (40). Pericarditis due to spread from contiguous pleural foci may occur, and these patients may develop cardiac tamponade.

Infection of the genitourinary tract with *Aspergillus* may result from hematogenous spread or ascending infection. Clinical manifestations include fever, chills, and microhematuria. Unilateral flank pain may occur with ascending infection.

Abscesses due to *Aspergillus* species may develop in immunocompromised children in the liver, thyroid, testis, spleen, and adrenal glands. The infection may spread either as part of hematogenous infection or as local extension.

Diagnosis

Chest x-ray findings are nonspecific. CT of the chest may give a clearer view with characteristic halo sign or air-crescent sign, though this is not diagnostic. The diagnosis can be established by doing CT chest followed by BAL, transthoracic percutaneous needle aspiration, or video-assisted thoracoscopic biopsy as standard procedures (41). Older children and adults are more likely to show the classic cavitation and air-crescent formation than do young children (Fig. 95.1). A diagnostic adjunct is the galactomannan assay, commonly used in adults. This assay is difficult to interpret in children because of the differences in pediatric and adult values. Pediatric studies have shown a false-positive rate of 40% using the serum galactomannan assay, as compared with a false-positive rate of 1% in adults. Potential reasons for the age-related difference are (a) pediatric gut flora may contain cross-reactive antigens to the assay and (b) the antigen may be found in

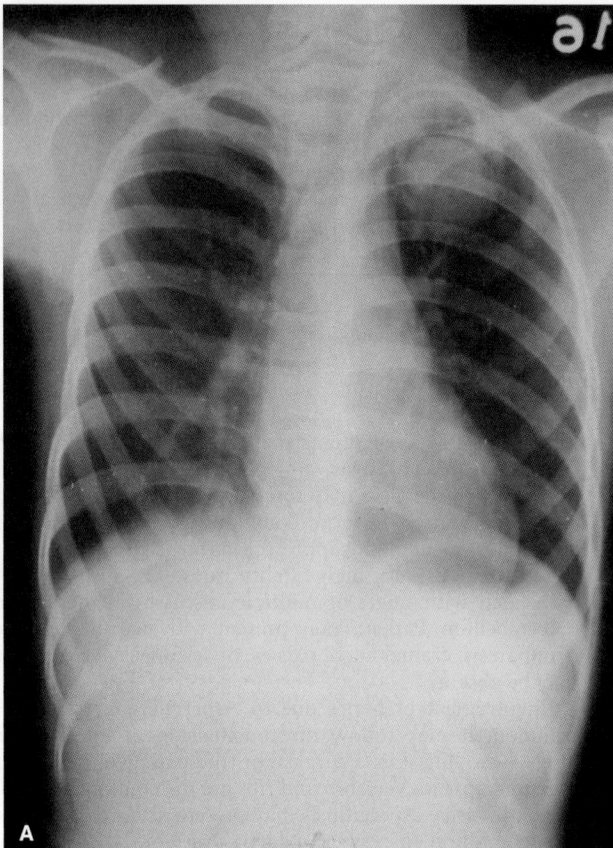
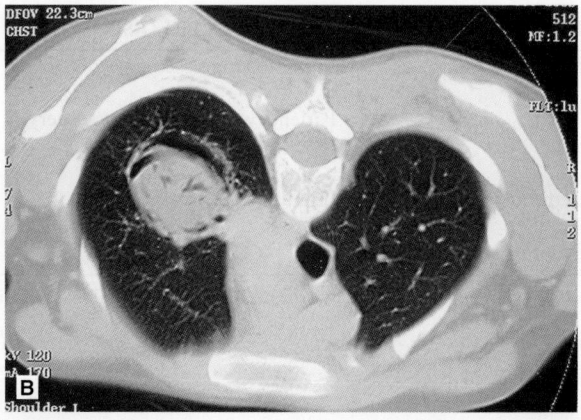
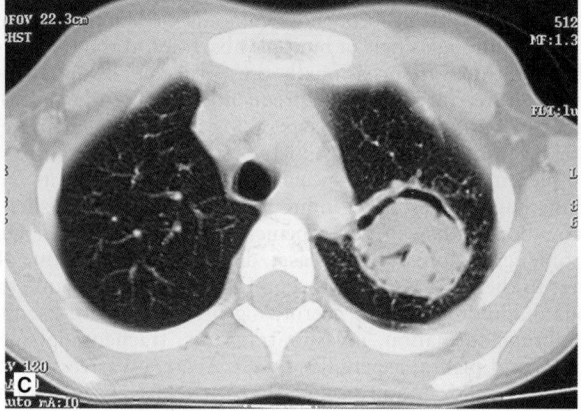

FIGURE 95.1. X-ray and chest CT films of 8-year-old girl suffering from pulmonary aspergillosis. **A:** X-ray of chest, showing homogenous round shadow in left upper zone. **B (prone) and C (supine):** CT scan of chest, showing a fungal ball in left upper lobe; note shift in mass within capsule with change in patients' position. This patient underwent lobectomy of left upper lobe. Histopathology and culture showed *Aspergillus fumigatus*.

infant formula. Furthermore, patients with chronic granulomatous disease who have positive lung biopsy specimens for aspergillosis have been shown to be galactomannan negative. Therefore, this test should not be used alone to diagnose invasive aspergillosis in children, but may be a useful adjunct to inform treatment decisions (41).

In the laboratory, wet preparations of BAL fluid or tissue specimens can be examined using potassium hydroxide or Gomori methenamine-silver nitrate stain to look for the typical morphologic features of *Aspergillus*. Galactomannan testing of BAL fluid has been reported to be useful for diagnosis of invasive pulmonary aspergillosis (42). Identification from tissue culture renders a definitive diagnosis and is isolated readily from lung, sinus, and skin biopsy specimens on Sabouraud dextrose agar or brain–heart infusion media. Blood culture specimens rarely yield positive results.

If allergic aspergillosis is suspected clinically, results of *Aspergillus*-specific IgE serology, eosinophilia, and a positive skin test can provide evidence for the diagnosis. As with invasive candidiasis, a potential adjunct for the diagnosis of invasive fungal disease that has been used successfully in adults is the β-D-glucan detection assay (43). This assay has not yet been standardized for the pediatric population.

The utility of PCR for the diagnosis of invasive aspergillosis is limited. Assays are not standardized, nor are they commercially available. A positive result from a BAL specimen may indicate colonization with a low positive predictive value. A negative result may be helpful to exclude aspergillosis. A recent study using Pan-AC real-time PCR assay has suggested its utility in children suffering from acute leukemia who were suspected to have fungal infection (45).

Management

Voriconazole is the treatment of choice for invasive aspergillosis. The Red Book (2011) recommends voriconazole dosing in children (2–12 years of age) of 9 mg/kg/dose IV/PO every 12 hours for 2 loading doses, followed by 9 mg/kg/dose IV/PO daily. For invasive fungal infections, the IV route is preferred for initial therapy, which can be converted to oral therapy after clinical improvement. Children may metabolize voriconazole at greater rates than do adults and show significant intra- and interindividual pharmacokinetic variation (44). Because clinical outcomes depend on attaining therapeutic drug levels, serum trough concentrations should be monitored after the third dose. Voriconazole dosing is then adjusted to maintain trough concentration >1 mcg/ml and <5.5 mcg/ml. The duration of therapy is at least 12 weeks and depends on the clinical response. Conventional or lipid formulations of amphotericin B should be considered for second-line therapy. For children who do not respond to either voriconazole or amphotericin, IV caspofungin at 70 mg/m² loading dose followed by 50 mg/m² once daily is an alternative therapy. Caution should be exercised when using voriconazole to treat invasive aspergillosis as, unlike amphotericin, it does not have activity against zygomycosis. Breakthrough infections with zygomycosis have been reported while treating invasive aspergillosis with voriconazole. Infections of the eye should be treated with intraocular amphotericin B and vitrectomy.

Prevention

Outbreaks of *Aspergillus* infection have been reported among immunosuppressed patients at hospitals that are undergoing renovation or construction. Measures to reduce the risk of aspergillosis in this population include the use of containment systems for construction/remodeling of facilities, routine cleaning of water spigots and air systems (including air filters), excluding plants and flowers from rooms, avoiding nuts and spices that are often contaminated, and minimizing the use of nonsterile biomedical devices and adhesive tape. The use of high-efficiency particulate air filters and laminar flow in patient's rooms also decreases risk. Though prophylactic regimens exist for prevention of invasive aspergillosis in adults using amphotericin B, itraconazole, caspofungin, and voriconazole, none of these strategies has been tested in children. For patients with leukemia or other immunosuppression who have invasive aspergillosis, continued use of antifungal therapy during future immunosuppression is advised as a preventive measure.

Mucormycosis

Mucormycosis is an acute and often fatal infection caused by a fungus of the Mucorales order of the Zygomycetes class. Infections by members of the mucormycosis class of fungi typically arise in patients with substantial underlying immunosuppression, such as critically ill premature newborns and older children with underlying hematopoietic malignancies, organ transplantation, and diabetes. The route of infection is by **(33)** inhalation of spores that often colonize paranasal sinuses (46).

Clinical Features

The organisms that cause mucormycosis may involve lungs, brain, sinuses, kidneys, and skin. Pulmonary involvement **(34)** may present with persistent fever, chest pain, hemoptysis, and weight loss. Cavitation may occur. The organism invades blood vessels and may disseminate to the brain and other sites. Sudden death may occur due to massive pulmonary hemorrhage, mediastinitis, or airway obstruction.

(35) Rhinocerebral mucormycosis, though relatively uncommon, may cause fatal infection. Sinusitis may occur in children with underlying diseases such as malignancies. It may progress to involve orbits and brain. Multiple abscesses in brain may manifest as headache, vomiting, fever, focal deficits, loss of vision, and occasionally seizures.

Primary cutaneous mucormycosis is an uncommon, deep, and aggressive fungal infection that occurs mainly in immunosuppressed or diabetic patients. Skin involvement may begin as a vascular, hemorrhagic, erythematous plaque and rapidly progress to a dark, necrotic, painful ulcer with erythematous border on the extremities or other parts of body. Gangrenous cellulitis may be one of the serious manifestations in critically ill, premature newborns and older children with underlying hematopoietic malignancies and/or following HSCT.

Diagnosis

Diagnosis of zygomycosis is achieved through a high level of suspicion and aggressive pursuit of tissue culture. Often, mucormycosis is not suspected among hematology patients, as most patients are presumed to have aspergillosis. The direct morphologic classification of tissue culture specimens remains the standard for diagnosis. While wet mounts of sputum, sinus secretions, or BAL fluid are often negative, positivity denotes invasive zygomycosis that should be treated. Cultures of blood or urine are also rarely positive. Invasive testing procedures, including fine-needle aspirates of lesions in deep tissue, transbronchial biopsies of pulmonary lesions, sinus tissue samples, scrapings of mucocutaneous lesions, or samples of deep tissue **(36)** lesions, yield higher results (47).

Various methods can be used to detect Mucorales, including wet mount treated with potassium hydroxide, Gomori's methenamine-silver staining, hematoxylin and eosin staining, and periodic acid-Schiff staining. Histopathologic specimens show evidence of vascular invasion. CT of the chest may identify infiltrates suggestive of Mucorales that are not seen on chest x-ray. A real-time, quantitative PCR (qPCR) assays, targeting the 28S ribosomal RNA gene, for the diagnosis of zygomycosis caused by *Rhizopus*, *Mucor*, *Rhizomucor*, and *Cunninghamella* species has shown good sensitivity and specificity (47).

Management

The mainstays of treatment include a combination of early diagnosis, treatment of the underlying medical condition, reduction of immunosuppression, antifungal therapy, and surgical debridement. After the patient is diagnosed, predisposing **(37)** factors such as hyperglycemia and metabolic acidosis should be corrected to increase survival. Immunosuppressive therapy should be decreased or postponed until the mucormycosis is under control. Improvement of outcomes is related to neutrophil recovery, and antifungal therapy has been ineffective in patients with persistent neutropenia. Granulocyte colony-stimulating factor and granulocyte-macrophage colony-stimulating factor should be considered as adjunct therapy to enhance neutrophil activity against zygomycoses. Lipid formulation of amphotericin B is the antimicrobial therapy of choice for the treatment of mucormycosis (48) although higher doses are necessary due to resistance. After the infection is controlled or in case of intolerance, daily oral posaconazole can be used with caution as it may be less effective than amphotericin and may interact with immunosuppressants in transplant patients. Another option in refractory cases is the concomitant use of a lipid formulation of amphotericin B and an echinocandin. Evidence exists for the effectiveness of hyperbaric oxygen therapy against zygomycosis, and it should be considered where available. Lastly, surgical debridement of mucormycosis lesions results in increased survival compared with patients who are treated medically (47).

Prevention

Prophylactic amphotericin is not indicated for prevention of mucormycosis, but future periods of immunosuppression should also include antifungal therapy in those with a history of disease. Other prevention strategies include control of underlying predisposing factors, such as diabetes, and judicious use of deferoxamine and corticosteroids (47).

Cryptococcosis

Cryptococcosis is a serious fungal disease of humans and animals caused by *Cryptococcus neoformans*, a yeast-like encapsulated fungus. Infection is acquired by inhalation of fungus **(39)** into the lungs. It may remain silent or may develop serious CNS infection. Immunosuppression, such as HIV infection, malignancies, organ transplantation, primary immune deficiencies, and corticosteroid therapy are risk factors for cryptococcosis. Of the two varieties, *C. neoformans* var. *neoformans* is more common and mainly infects immunocompromised hosts, whereas in immunocompetents, the infection is exclusively caused by var. *gatti*.

Clinical Manifestations

The disease primarily presents as subacute or chronic meningitis, although involvement of other organs such as liver, spleen, skin, lymph node, eye, bones, adrenals, and ears may also be

involved. Cryptococcal meningitis more frequently occurs
in patients with severe immunosuppression including AIDS.
These patients commonly present with headache and fever.
Clinical manifestations are that of raised intracranial pressure
in the form of headache, vomiting, alteration of consciousness,
papilledema, and seizures. Other manifestations of cryptococcal meningitis include neck stiffness, impaired mental function, cranial nerve lesions, visual deficits, seizures, diplopia,
focal neurologic deficits, photophobia, and abnormal cerebellar signs.

Pulmonary illness is relatively rare in children. Disseminated
cryptococcosis may present with cough or chest pain, weight
loss, fever, hemoptysis, hepatosplenomegaly, and cutaneous
findings (e.g., ulcers, nodules, vesicles, abscesses, papules, and
cellulitis). Occasional cases of cryptococcosis presenting as
acute abdomen or mimicking pulmonary metastasis in Wilms
tumor have been reported (49).

Diagnosis

Diagnosis is based on demonstration of organisms in body fluids (CSF, urine, BAL, sputum, fluid from skin lesion) using
India ink stain. The diagnosis of cryptococcal pulmonary infection is suggested by characteristic clinical and radiographic
findings, sputum culture, serologic assays for IgG and IgM,
and serologic testing for cryptococcal polysaccharide antigen
by latex agglutination. High titers of antigen (≥1:1024) are
associated with high burden of organisms and a poor host
immune response. High titers are associated with poor therapeutic response. The titers decrease with fungal clearance by
smear. However, antigen may remain in tissue/fluid in low titers for prolonged period (50). Even in asymptomatic patients,
chest x-ray findings of diffuse infiltrations with hilar adenopathy may be seen. Sputum culture results are more likely to be
positive in patients with AIDS than in those without severely
depressed T-cell function. Furthermore, sputum culture and
cryptococcal-specific antibody testing are difficult to interpret,
as they may indicate colonization. Latex agglutination studies
for cryptococcal antigen in serum are thought to reflect disseminated infection, but may be negative in those with isolated
pulmonary disease. The definitive diagnosis of *Cryptococcus*
is via biopsy or fine-needle aspiration. The organism is slow-
growing in culture, requiring a week to proliferate, making
tissue culture slow and difficult. To improve yield and turnaround time, tissue specimens should be tested for cryptococcal antigenemia via in situ hybridization.

Cryptococcal meningitis is suggested by increased intracranial pressure and/or visualization of encapsulated yeast cells in
CSF using India ink stain. Serum blood culture may yield the
organism if the lysis-centrifugation technique is used. Cryptococcal polysaccharide antigen studies on CSF or serum yield
results in 90% of patients infected.

Management

Immunocompetent patients with isolated pulmonary disease
usually clear the organism without antifungal agents. For immunocompromised patients with isolated pulmonary disease,
CSF and serum should be evaluated for evidence of disseminated disease. HIV-infected patients with disseminated disease
(including meningitis) should be treated with a combination
of amphotericin B deoxycholate and flucytosine for at least
2 weeks or until CSF testing is negative, then continue with
fluconazole for a minimum of 8 additional weeks of therapy.
Patients who are immunosuppressed should be treated with a
longer course of therapy. Patients who initially test positive for
CNS disease should undergo repeat lumbar puncture testing
after 2 weeks to document negative CNS culture results and
improvement in intracranial pressure. Refractory cases can be

treated with amphotericin B therapy (including liposomal formulations) with flucytosine. A third-line regimen of high-dose
fluconazole and flucytosine may also be considered. While
CSF cryptococcal antigenemia likely correlates with clinical
outcomes, routine testing is not currently recommended for
monitoring response.

Prevention

The mainstay of prevention is chronic suppressive therapy
for HIV-positive children with fluconazole who have had
Cryptococcus in the past and continuation of this therapy according to clinical judgment. After 6 months of chronic suppressive therapy and a CD4 count of at least 200 cells/mm^3,
discontinuation of prophylaxis may be considered as long as
the CD4 count is sustained. Those who have cellular immunodeficiency, AIDS (especially with CD4 count <100/mm^3),
or are on high-dose corticosteroids should avoid contact with
birds.

Histoplasmosis

Histoplasmosis is a systemic disease caused by the dimorphic
fungus *Histoplasma capsulatum*, which exists as a soil sapro-
phyte. Histoplasmosis occurs throughout the world including
tropical, subtropical, and temperate regions.

Clinical Features

Histoplasmosis occurs in immunocompetent as well as immunocompromised children. Disseminated histoplasmosis
generally occurs in immunocompromised children. Clinical
manifestations of disseminated histoplasmosis include prolonged, unexplained fever, cough, respiratory difficulty abdominal pain, weight loss, and diarrhea. Liver, spleen, and
lymph nodes may be enlarged. Skin may show mucocutaneous
lesions, maculopapular rash, papules, nodules, pustules, and
ulcerative lesions. Children may present with meningitis or
encephalitis and focal brain lesions (51).

Diagnosis

The diagnosis of histoplasmosis is made via culture, fungal
stain, antigen detection, and serologic tests for antibodies.
Cultures of lung tissue or BAL specimens are positive in 85%
of those with acute pulmonary disease, but much less in those
with more limited pulmonary histoplasmosis. Blood cultures
are more likely to yield organism if the lysis-centrifugation
technique is utilized. The organism requires weeks to grow
in culture, and this method, while the gold standard for identification, is often used to confirm antigen testing results.
Rapid results of antigen testing of pulmonary, CSF, urine, and
blood are fairly sensitive for disseminated disease (sensitivity is
higher in urine than blood). The only drawback is that cross-
reactivity can occur with penicilliosis, paracoccidioidomyco-
sis, blastomycosis, and African histoplasmosis. Furthermore,
antigen levels can be followed as therapy is initiated to determine the success of treatment. Fungal silver or Wright stain
can be used on peripheral blood or tissue culture to diagnose
histoplasmosis. Serologic tests for *Histoplasma* antibodies typically yield 80%–90% positivity for those with disseminated
or acute pulmonary disease, but they may not be useful due to
lack of production early in the disease course and in immunosuppressed patients.

Imaging findings are nonspecific. X-ray film of chest (CXR)
may show enlarged hilar nodes (multiple nodular shadows in
lung parenchyma). CT scan of chest may show nodular shadows that may not be seen on CXR.

Management

No treatment is indicated for immunocompetent children with primary pulmonary histoplasmosis, as the disease usually follows a self-limited course. For complicated disease in children, including those who are immunocompromised, the treatment of histoplasmosis generally follows treatment guidelines for adults. Amphotericin B deoxycholate is the standard therapy for acute primary pulmonary histoplasmosis and other serious infections, followed by itraconazole for long-term suppressive therapy, which should last for 12 months in those with severe immunosuppression. Those with mild to moderate progressive disseminated histoplasmosis can be treated with itraconazole oral therapy for 12 months after an initial loading dose. Second-line therapies include voriconazole and posaconazole. For isolated pericarditis, drainage of pericardial fluid and nonsteroidal anti-inflammatory drugs are the mainstays of therapy—no antifungals are indicated.

Prevention

To prevent histoplasmosis in immunocompromised patients, encourage them to avoid traveling to endemic areas and walking inside caves where bird droppings may aerosolize readily. It is also important to know the serologic status of patients diagnosed with immunodeficiency or in whom transplantation is considered, especially if they spent time in endemic areas (no recommendations exist for prophylaxis). For children who have completed 1 year of itraconazole therapy after treatment of initial infection, continuation of itraconazole therapy may be considered in cases of severe immunosuppression or relapse.

MYCOBACTERIAL INFECTIONS

Mycobacterial infections are frequent, opportunistic pathogens associated with AIDS. With the onset of the AIDS epidemic, disease due to both *Mycobacterium tuberculosis* and atypical strains such as *M. avium-intracellulare* have been increasingly recognized in both AIDS and non-AIDS immunodeficient populations. Those infected with the HIV are particularly susceptible to TB, either by the reactivation of latent infection or by a primary infection with rapid progression to active disease (52).

Nontuberculous Mycobacteria

Nontuberculous mycobacteria, ubiquitous organisms in the environment, historically have not caused invasive disease in immunocompetent hosts. However, increasing numbers of case reports document the spectrum of disease caused by these bacteria in otherwise healthy individuals in the past three decades (53).

Clinical Features

Lymphadenitis is the most common manifestation of infection due to nontuberculous mycobacteria. The majority of patients present with an enlarged palpable mass and preceding constitutional symptoms. The lymph node involvement may be multiple, with the most common site being the cervical region. Cases of disseminated *M. avium* complex with gastrointestinal tract involvement have been reported in HIV-infected children, HSCT recipients, and patients with interferon (IFN)-γ receptor-1 deficiency. Common clinical findings include prolonged fever, weight loss, lymphadenopathy, hepatosplenomegaly, diarrhea, anemia, and leucopenia (54).

Diagnosis

Diagnostic testing for atypical mycobacteria depends on the involved site of infection. Diagnosis can be established by cultures from body fluids on radiometric or continuously monitored automated blood culture systems. Possibility of contamination from environment is a major challenge in interpretation of culture results of sputum. In disseminated infection in HIV-infected patients, blood culture has a sensitivity of 90%–95%. Culture may be positive in 7–10 days for *M. avium* complex. Differentiation from *M. tuberculosis* and identification of species can be achieved by DNA probes or DNA sequencing. A presumptive diagnosis can be made by demonstration of histiocytes containing numerous acid-fast bacilli (AFB) in bone marrow or other tissue including lymph node.

For suspected pulmonary disease, three sputum specimens obtained on three different days should be sent for AFB smear and culture. PCR testing is becoming the gold standard for detection of atypical mycobacterial infection and should be performed on at least one sputum specimen and any AFB smear-positive specimen.

Susceptibility testing for atypical mycobacterium is useful for appropriate management of disease, but these results might not correlate with clinical efficacy. In addition to general susceptibility testing, some organism-specific testing recommendations are important to consider. For *M. avium-intracellulare*, susceptibility to clarithromycin should be tested if the patient was previously on macrolide therapy, is currently failing therapy, or is intolerant to current therapy. *M. kansasii* isolates should be tested for susceptibility to rifampin, as resistance does not develop during the course of therapy. Susceptibility testing is recommended only for *M. marinum* if patients fail to respond to initial therapy.

Management

Therapy for atypical mycobacterial infections depends on the organism and the site of involvement. For lymphadenitis due to *M. avium-intracellulare* or other atypical mycobacteria, surgical excision, if complete, is sufficient without antimicrobial therapy. If excision is not possible or incomplete, therapy with clarithromycin or azithromycin should be considered. The appropriate length of therapy, however, is not established (55).

For pulmonary disease due to *M. avium* complex, the treatment of choice includes clarithromycin and ethambutol, with rifabutin added for severe disease. Alternative therapies include azithromycin, ciprofloxacin, levofloxacin, or amikacin. This therapy should be continued until the patient is culture negative for 12 months.

Prevention

Atypical mycobacterial infection is difficult to prevent, as these organisms are ubiquitous in the environment, and immunocompromised populations are particularly susceptible. In patients who are HIV positive, prophylaxis with azithromycin or clarithromycin is indicated for those aged <2, aged 2–5 years with a CD4 count of <200/mm^3, and aged ≥6 years with a CD4 count of <100/mm^3. This prophylaxis should continue for patients who are on antiretroviral therapy until their CD4 count is above the threshold for their age for at least 6 months and having completed at least 6 months of antiretroviral therapy.

Mycobacterium tuberculosis

The majority of children with TB are managed on an ambulatory basis or hospitalized in wards. A small proportion may require admission to PICUs, including those with disseminated disease (severe combined immune deficiency, HIV infection), CNS TB, hemoptysis, and respiratory failure due to acute endobronchial spread in the setting of immune suppression.

Clinical Features

TB can occur in HIV-infected individuals at any CD4 count, which is in contrast to other opportunistic infections that generally occur when CD4 counts significantly decline. When children who are infected with HIV develop TB, the clinical picture is similar to TB in the immunocompetent child, although the disease tends to progress more rapidly and the clinical manifestations are more severe. An increased tendency for extrapulmonary disease and dissemination may be seen, as well as involvement of unusual sites and atypical chest x-ray findings. Extrapulmonary involvement occurs in more than 70% of patients with TB and preexisting AIDS (56). Children with disseminated TB may have fever, respiratory difficulty, lymphadenopathy, hepatosplenomegaly, and occasionally skin lesions.

Diagnosis

The diagnosis of TB in an immunocompromised patient requires a heightened suspicion and diagnostic modalities beyond the traditional purified protein derivative (PPD) skin test. If PPD testing is utilized, a positive test for those who are immunosuppressed is defined as induration of >5 mm in diameter. A positive PPD test without evidence of clinical disease (e.g., absence of pulmonary symptoms or chest x-ray findings) indicates latent TB infection while the addition of x-ray findings and pulmonary symptoms are consistent with active TB disease.

Evaluation for pulmonary TB should include a chest x-ray, although some experts would argue that lymphadenopathy characteristic of TB infection is best visualized on CT scan. In addition, sputum or gastric aspirate samples should be sent for AFB smear and culture for patients with pulmonary symptoms. For children and adolescents with suspected TB, the best test is the early-morning gastric aspirate, obtained on awakening via a nasogastric tube on two separate days, or induced sputum using hypertonic saline inhalation by nebulizer. If a sample returns positive for AFB, confirmation via culture or PCR is required, as other mycobacteria can give positive results for this test. Evaluation for nonpulmonary TB includes AFB smear and culture of suspected sterile body sites, including CSF and lymph node or other biopsy specimens. PCR testing for TB can also be performed on these specimens to improve diagnostic yield. For patients with suspected disseminated disease, mycobacterial blood cultures can be obtained for diagnosis. Positive cultures for TB should be evaluated for drug sensitivity testing (35).

Automated nucleic acid amplification test on sputum/gastric aspirates may give results within 2 hours for presence of *Mycobacterium tuberculosis* and its sensitivity to rifampicin. A systematic review suggests a sensitivity of 90% and specificity of 98% for pulmonary TB and sensitivity of 80% and specificity of 86% for extrapulmonary TB. The sensitivity of pulmonary TB in children was lower (74%) in children than that of 90% in adult patients (57).

Management

Latent TB infection is managed with a single drug regimen (depending on the resistance pattern in particular geographic regions or the index case). For isoniazid-susceptible latent TB, the child is treated with isoniazid once daily for 6–9 months. In cases with isoniazid resistance, rifampin may be given once daily for 6 months. A combination of three drugs, including pyrazinamide, was associated with high rates of hepatotoxicity in some studies.

The recommended treatment for TB disease in patients who are HIV positive should be considered in other immunosuppressed pediatric populations and includes an intensive phase of 8 weeks followed by a continuation phase of 9–12 months. The regimen for an initial intensive phase includes isoniazid, rifampin, pyrazinamide, and ethambutol. The continuation phase can be given as a daily regimen of isoniazid plus rifampin or an intermittent regimen of isoniazid and rifampin thrice weekly. The length of the continuation phase is 9 months for pulmonary TB and 12 months for extrapulmonary TB (58). Caution is advised for HIV patients on antiretroviral therapy, as many of these drugs have overlapping toxicities and additive side effects. Substantial pharmacokinetic interactions occur between the rifamycin component of anti-TB treatment and antiretroviral drugs, especially protease inhibitors and nonnucleoside reverse transcriptase inhibitors. The key therapeutic principles that underlie the treatment of HIV–TB are (a) treatment of TB always takes precedence over the treatment of HIV infection; (b) in patients who are already on highly active antiretroviral therapy (HAART), it must be continued with appropriate modifications in both HAART and anti-TB treatment; and (c) in patients who are not receiving HAART, the need for, and timing of, initiation of HAART should be decided on an individual basis after assessing the short-term risk of disease progression and death, based on CD4$^+$ count and type of TB.

Treatment of TB should be based on drug resistance in the index case, in the local geographic area, or in the country of origin for imported cases. The local health department maintains data on local patterns of TB resistance and can advise if a three- or four-drug regimen should be used. Local health departments should also be notified of any new case of TB so that investigation and testing of contacts can begin. Directly observed therapy is offered in many countries through local health departments/facilities. The World Health Organization has recommended category-based treatment for children in high-endemic areas (58) (**Table 95.4**).

Management of extrapulmonary TB includes chemotherapy and consideration of other therapies. No evidence suggests that surgery in addition to chemotherapy provides added benefit for spinal TB (59). For pericarditis associated with TB, adjunctive corticosteroids should be considered, but not routinely given for treatment, as no advantage has been proven.

Monitoring for treatment success is essential for treatment of TB. For patients with evidence of pulmonary TB, sputum specimens should be obtained monthly until two consecutive specimens are negative. Patients should be followed clinically and radiographically for evidence of treatment success. Routine laboratory testing is not indicated to monitor for adverse medication effects unless elevated transaminase levels are noted at baseline (35).

Prevention

A successful approach to prevention of TB comprises many strategies, including hospital infection control measures, case-finding and managing contacts, pharmacotherapy for contacts, and consideration for Bacille Calmette-Guérin vaccine in select populations. Though most children with TB are not contagious (except those with cavitary lesions, positive sputum AFB smears, laryngeal involvement, pulmonary infection, or suspected congenital infection), they are often exposed by a visiting family member who is infectious. For this reason, many hospitals attempt to place these children in a negative-pressure room, with caregivers using particulate respirators. The local health department should be immediately informed when a child tests positive for TB. The health department will direct testing of contacts to identify others who have been exposed and, potentially, the index case. Those who test positive

TABLE 95.4

WORLD HEALTH ORGANIZATION STANDARDIZED TUBERCULOSIS TREATMENT REGIMENS FOR CHILDREN

■ EPIDEMIOLOGIC SETTING	■ CLINICAL SYNDROME	■ SUGGESTED REGIMENS
High HIV prevalence or high Isoniazid resistance	Suspected or confirmed pulmonary TB or peripheral lymphadenitis	2 HRZE 4 HR
Low HIV prevalence or low isoniazid resistance	Extensive pulmonary disease, suspected or confirmed pulmonary TB or peripheral lymphadenitis	2 HRZE 4 HR
All	Tuberculous meningitis; Suspected or confirmed osteoarticular TB	2 HRZE 10 HR
MDR TB	Proven or suspected pulmonary TB or tuberculous meningitis	Regimen should include fluoroquinolone

TB, tuberculosis; H, isoniazid; R, rifampicin; Z, pyrazinamide; E, ethambutol; S, Streptomycin; 2 HRZE 4 HR, 2 months of 4 drugs (HRZE) followed by 4 months of 2 drugs (HR); 2 HRZ 4 HR, 2 months of 3 drugs (HRZ) followed by 4 months of 2 drugs (HR); 2 HRZE 10 HR: 2 months of 4 drugs (HRZE), followed by 10 months of 2 drugs (HR).
From World Health Organization. 2010. *Rapid Advice: Treatment of Tuberculosis in Children*. Geneva, Switzerland: World Health Organization. WHO/HTM/TB/2010.13. http://whqlibdoc.who.int/publications/2010/9789241500449_eng.pdf.

should be given appropriate therapy on the basis of their diagnosis of latent infection or TB disease. Bacille Calmette-Guérin vaccination should be considered for children who live in an environment in which they are exposed to TB that is either not being treated or is resistant to isoniazid and rifampin, and from which the child cannot be removed. In countries with universal Bacille Calmette-Guérin vaccination programs, immunocompromised children who are in contact with adults whose sputum smear is positive for TB should be treated with isoniazid prophylaxis for 6–9 months. If the index case has documented isoniazid resistance, the child may be treated with rifampicin for 6 months. If the index case has documented resistance to isoniazid and rifampicin, the child may be treated with two drugs (e.g., ethambutol and fluoroquinolones) for 9–12 months.

PARASITIC INFECTIONS

Toxoplasmosis

59 Toxoplasmosis is a parasitic infection. *Toxoplasma gondii* infects cats and other animals and secondarily infects human, causing congenital toxoplasmosis during intrauterine infection.

Clinical Features

60 Patients with AIDS, agammaglobulinemia, or marrow or stem cell transplant may develop disseminated *T. gondii*—a potentially fatal condition. Common presentations include fever, encephalitis, pneumonia, myocarditis, and bone marrow suppression. It may manifest similar to mononucleosis syndrome.

Diagnosis

The diagnosis of infection due to toxoplasma is made on the basis of clinical presentation with confirmation either by demonstration of trophozoites (in body fluids or tissues), by serologic methods (reserved for immunocompetent hosts), or by molecular methods (PCR). In infants and other immunocompromised patients (i.e., HIV patients) with a suspected diagnosis of toxoplasma, sera should be sent for PCR testing.

61 In immunocompetent patients, toxoplasma-specific IgG will peak in serum 1–2 months after infection and may remain positive for life. A fourfold rise in serum IgG is consistent with infection. A positive IgM titer for *T. gondii* indicates recent or acute infection. IgM titers may not be positive until 1 month after onset of infection and may take up to 2 years to fall.

HIV-1–infected patients with suspected toxoplasma encephalitis should undergo serologic testing, CSF analysis including PCR testing, and serum PCR testing. They are usually positive for serum toxoplasma IgG. Definitive testing for toxoplasma encephalitis involves a brain biopsy, with organisms seen on hematoxylin and eosin stains. CSF testing for toxoplasma via PCR is highly specific (96%–100%) but is associated with a low sensitivity (50%) (35).

Management

HIV-positive and other immunosuppressed patients with *T. gondii* encephalitis or other systemic manifestations should be treated with sulfadiazine, pyrimethamine, and folinic acid (leucovorin). Clindamycin can be substituted for sulfadiazine. Pyrimethamine penetrates the brain parenchyma, while folinic acid prevents hematologic toxicities associated with its use. **62** TMP-SMZ is reported to be effective and better tolerated but has less in vitro activity, and practitioners have less experience with its use in the setting of toxoplasma encephalitis. Therapy should be given for at least 6 weeks, with longer courses for extensive disease or evidence of incomplete response. Corticosteroids should be considered for CNS disease when CSF protein is highly elevated >1000 mg/dL or when a mass effect associated with focal lesions is seen. Patients should be monitored for clinical and radiologic improvement. Leucovorin dosage can be increased if bone marrow suppression develops. Brain biopsy and change in treatment regimen should be considered in patients who deteriorate within the first 2 weeks of therapy (35).

Prevention

HIV-positive pregnant women with a history of toxoplasma infection and CD4 count of <200/mm³ should be placed on prophylaxis with TMP-SMZ to prevent reactivation and neonatal infection. HIV-positive patients and other immunosuppressed persons who have been treated for toxoplasma encephalitis should be placed on lifelong prophylaxis with sulfadiazine, pyrimethamine, and folinic acid. Prophylaxis may be discontinued if immune reconstitution occurs as evidenced by a sustained CD4 count of >200/mm³ for 6 months (35).

CRYPTOSPORIDIUM INFECTION

Cryptosporidium spp. is a major cause of diarrheal disease in both immunocompetent and immunodeficient individuals. The most severe disease is seen in individuals with defects in the T-cell response. Children with HIV infection, primary immunodeficiencies (most notably severe combined immunodeficiency syndrome), and acute leukemia seem to be most at risk from cryptosporidiosis.

Clinical Features

Immunocompromised patients, including children with severe malnutrition, suffer from severe and prolonged watery diarrhea. Disease may be fatal. In addition, body systems other than the gastrointestinal tract may be affected. Cryptosporidium may cause cholangitis (particularly sclerosing cholangitis), pancreatitis, and respiratory symptoms. Cryptosporidium may also cause respiratory symptoms. In most patients with respiratory symptoms, coinfection with typical or atypical mycobacterium occurs.

Diagnosis

Diagnosis of cryptosporidium is made by examination of stool, which can be performed using a modified acid-fast stain to look for oocysts. However, due to increased sensitivity and specificity, immunofluorescence microscopy and enzyme-linked immunoassays are now the methods of choice for identifying cryptosporidium in stool. Molecular methods for diagnosis are currently being used primarily for research purposes and are not available for clinical use.

Management

Infection in immunocompetent persons is self-limiting and does not require treatment. However, in the immunocompromised, treatment is indicated. The current therapy for immunocompromised children with cryptosporidiosis, in addition to electrolyte management and replacement of fluids, is nitazoxanide. However, the effect of nitazoxanide on the course of cryptosporidiosis has been reported as marginal, with little significant benefit (60). Immunocompromised patients require a different dosing regimen than immunocompetent patients for nitazoxanide (61). The suggested administration of nitazoxanide is 500 mg doses orally twice daily for 3 days in adults and adolescents, 200 mg doses twice daily for 3 days in children aged 4–11 years, and 100-mg doses twice daily for 3 days in children aged 1–3 years. Therapy may be given for up to 14 days in an attempt to clear infection.

Prevention

Immune reconstitution is essential to preventing cryptosporidiosis in immunocompromised patients living with HIV (61). Those with diarrhea should not use public recreational waters until 2 weeks after diarrhea is resolved. In areas where drinking water is contaminated, it should be boiled before consumption. Handwashing and other personal hygiene measures will help to limit exposure and to prevent infection both within and outside the healthcare system.

CONCLUSIONS AND FUTURE DIRECTIONS

Opportunistic infections are common causes of morbidity and mortality in children admitted in PICUs. The predisposing conditions include primary or secondary immune deficiencies.

The common conditions include primary immune deficiency of T cells and B cells, complement deficiency, or phagocytic defects. Acquired immune deficiencies include children with HIV infections, children on immunosuppressant therapy for organ or hematopoietic stem cell transplant, and children with autoimmune illness including collagen-vascular diseases and the like.

Patients with opportunistic infections present to PICUs with respiratory infections, sepsis, infections of the CNS, or multiorgan dysfunction. Due to underlying immune deficiency, the clinical course is fulminant and the case fatality is high. Clinical signs and symptoms may provide important clues of the immune deficiency and the possible etiologic agent of infection. Children with humoral immune deficiency conditions contract infections due to *S. aureus*, encapsulated organisms such as *S. pneumoniae* and *H. influenzae*, and with gram-negative organisms such as *Pseudomonas* spp. These patients may develop arthritis due to echoviruses, Coxsackie viruses, adenoviruses, and *Ureaplasma urealyticum*. Some of these patients may develop infections due to *P. jiroveci* (*P. carinii*) pneumonitis, and *Cryptosporidium*. Children with T-cell deficiency disorders are more prone to disseminated viral infections due to HSV, VZV, and CMV and may develop progressive pneumonia caused by parainfluenza, respiratory syncytial virus, cytomegalovirus, varicella, and *P. jiroveci*. They may also develop superficial and systemic fungal infections, parasitic infections, and disseminated bacilli Calmette-Guérin disease after vaccination for that disease. Children with phagocytic disorders are more prone for recurrent pyogenic and fungal infections due to *Pseudomonas*, *Serratia marcescens*, and *S. aureus*, and fungi such as *Aspergillus* and *Candida*. Patients may present with cellulitis, perirectal abscesses, stomatitis, pulmonary infection, suppurative adenitis, subcutaneous abscess, liver abscess, osteomyelitis, and sepsis. Early recognition of diagnosis of immune deficiency disorders and etiologic agents with appropriate laboratory tests may help in institution of appropriate treatment.

To make rational use of antibiotics in critically sick children, it is important that PICUs have a surveillance system for etiologic agents and their sensitivity in opportunistic infections. The first-line empirical therapy may be decided on the basis of surveillance data.

Cultures are not a very efficient method by which to diagnose viruses, fungi, and mycobacterial species. Therefore, continued development of noninvasive and rapid diagnostic methods for these infections in children would greatly improve accurate and rapid diagnosis and facilitate targeted treatment strategies.

References

1. Guibert G, Warszawski J, Le Chenadec J, et al; French Perinatal Cohort. Decreased risk of congenital cytomegalovirus infection in children born to HIV-1-infected mothers in the era of highly active antiretroviral therapy. *Clin Infect Dis* 2009;48:1516–25.
2. Singh R, Singh R, Trehan A, et al. Cytomegalovirus Retinitis in an ALL child on exclusive chemotherapy treated successfully with intravitreal ganciclovir alone. *J Pediatr Hematol Oncol* 2013;35(3):e118–9.
3. Zekri AR, Mohamed WS, Samra MA, et al. Risk factors for cytomegalovirus, hepatitis B and C virus reactivation after bone marrow transplantation. *Transpl Immunol* 2004;13:305–11.
4. Zaucha-Prazmo A, Wojcik B, Drabko K, et al. Neurological manifestation of CMV disease after allogeneic haematopoietic stem cells transplantation–A case report. *Ann Univ Mariae Curie Sklodowska [Med]* 2004;59:198–200.
5. Boivin G. Diagnosis of herpes virus infections of the central nervous system. *Herpes* 2004;11(suppl 2):4A–56A.

6. Grangeot-Keros L, Mayaux JF, Lebon P, et al. Value of cyto-megalovirus (CMV) IgG avidity index for the diagnosis of primary CMV infection in pregnant women. *J Infect Dis* 1997; 175:944–50.

7. Navalpotro D, Gimeno C, Navarro D. PCR detection of viral DNA in serum as an ancillary analysis for the diagnosis of acute mononucleosis-like syndrome due to human cytomegalovirus (HCMV) in immunocompetent patients. *J Clin Virol* 2006; 35:193–6.

8. Hernando S, Folgueira L, Lumbreras C, et al. Comparison of cytomegalovirus viral load measure by real-time PCR with pp65 antigenemia for the diagnosis of cytomegalovirus disease in solid organ transplant patients. *Transplant Proc* 2005;37:4094–6.

9. Kumar A, Kumar D, Boivin G, et al. Cytomegalovirus (CMV) virus load kinetics to predict recurrent disease in solid organ transplant patient with CMV disease. *J Infec Dis* 2002;186:829.

10. Boaretti M, Sorrentino A, Zantedeschi C, et al. Quantification of cytomegalovirus DNA by a fully automated real-time PCR for early diagnosis and monitoring of active viral infection in solid organ transplant recipients. *J Clin Virol* 2013;56:124–8.

11. Bravo D, Clari MÁ, Costa E, et al. Comparative evaluation of three automated systems for DNA extraction in conjunction with three commercially available real-time PCR assays for quantitation of plasma Cytomegalovirus DNAemia in allogeneic stem cell transplant recipients. *J Clin Microbiol* 2011;49:2899–904.

12. Aytaç S, Yalçin SS, Küçükbayrak O, et al. Dynamics in children and adolescents who experience varicella zoster virus infections after haematopoietic stem cell transplantation: A case-control study. *Epidemiol Infect* 2011;139:1701–9.

13. Okuno Y, Takao Y, Miyazaki Y, et al. Assessment of skin test with varicella-zoster virus antigen for predicting the risk of herpes zoster. *Epidemiol Infect* 2013;141(4):706–13.

14. Takatoku M, Muroi K, Kawano-Yamamoto C, et al. Involvement of the esophagus and stomach as a first manifestation of varicella zoster virus infection after allogeneic bone marrow transplantation. *Intern Med* 2004;43:861–4.

15. Welgama U, Wickramasinghe C, Perera J. Varicella-zoster virus infection in the Infectious Diseases Hospital, Sri Lanka. *Ceylon Med J* 2003;48:119–21.

16. Mantadakis E, Anagnostatou N, Danilatou V, et al. Fulminant hepatitis due to varicella zoster virus in a girl with acute lymphoblastic leukemia in remission: Report of a case and review. *J Pediatr Hematol Oncol* 2005;27:551–3.

17. Yoshida M, Hayasaka S, Yamada T, et al. Ocular findings in Japanese patients with varicella-zoster virus infection. *Ophthalmologica* 2005;219:272–5.

18. Abrams D, Derrick G, Penny DJ, et al. Cardiac complications in children following infection with varicella zoster virus. *Cardiol Young* 2001;11:647–52.

19. Kim DH, Kumar D, Messner HA, et al. Clinical efficacy of prophylactic strategy of long-term low-dose acyclovir for varicella-zoster virus infection after allogeneic peripheral blood stem cell transplantation. *Clin Transplant* 2008;22:770–9.

20. Yoshikawa T. Human herpesvirus-6 and -7 infections in transplantation. *Pediatr Transplant* 2003;7:11–7.

21. Ihira M, Enomoto Y, Kawamura Y, et al. Development of quantitative RT-PCR assays for detection of three classes of HHV-6B gene transcripts. *J Med Virol* 2012;84:1388–95.

22. De Bolle L, Naesens L, Clercq ED. Update on human herpesvirus 6 biology, clinical features, and therapy. *Clin Microbiol Rev* 2005;18:217–45.

23. Rapaport D, Engelhard D, Tagger G, et al. Antiviral prophylaxis may prevent human herpesvirus-6 reactivation in bone marrow transplant recipients. *Transplant Infect Dis* 2002;4:10–6.

24. Cugno C, Cesaro S. Epidemiology, risk factors and therapy of candidemia in pediatric hematological patients. *Pediatr Rep* 2012;4:e9.

25. Singhi SC, Reddy TC, Chakrabarti A. Candidemia in a pediatric intensive care unit. *Pediatr Crit Care Med* 2004;5:369–74.

26. Jabra-Rizk MA, Falkler WA Jr, Enwonwu CO, et al. Prevalence of yeast among children in Nigeria and the United States. *Oral Microbiol Immunol* 2001;16:383–5.

27. Kumar CP, Sundararajan T, Menon T, et al. Candidosis in children with onco-hematological diseases in Chennai, south India. *Jpn J Infect Dis* 2005;58:218–21.

28. Mularoni A, Furfaro E, Faraci M, et al. High levels of beta-D-glucan in immunocompromised children with proven invasive fungal disease. *Clin Vaccine Immunol* 2010;17:882–3.

29. Pappas PG, Kauffman CA, Andes D, et al. Infectious Diseases Society of America. Clinical practice guidelines for the management of candidiasis: 2009 update by the Infectious Diseases Society of America. *Clin Infect Dis* 2009;48:503–35.

30. Pappas PG, Rex JH, Sobel JD, et al. Guidelines for treatment of candidiasis. *Clin Infect Dis* 2004;38:161–89.

31. Ostrosky-Zeichner L, Pappas PG. Invasive candidiasis in the intensive care unit. *Crit Care Med* 2006;34:857–63.

32. Russian DA, Levine SJ. Pneumocystis carinii pneumonia in patients without HIV infection. *Am J Med Sci* 2001;321:56–65.

33. Cruciani M, Marcati P, Malena M, et al. Meta-analysis of diagnostic procedures for Pneumocystis carinii pneumonia in HIV-1-infected patients. *Eur Respir J* 2002;20:982–9.

34. Turner D, Schwarz Y, Yust I. Induced sputum for diagnosing Pneumocystis carinii pneumonia in HIV patients: New data, new issues. *Eur Resp J* 2003;21:204–8.

35. Benson CA, Kaplan JE, Masur H, et al. Treating opportunistic infections among HIV-infected adults and adolescents. *MMWR* 2004;53(RR15):1–112.

36. P Nesheim S, Read JS, Serchuck L, et al. Guidelines for the prevention and treatment of opportunistic Infections among HIV-exposed and HIV-infected children: Recommendations from CDC, the National Institutes of Health, the HIV Medicine Association of the Infectious Diseases Society of America, the Pediatric Infectious Diseases Society, and the American Academy of Pediatrics. *MMWR Recomm Rep* 2009;58(RR-11):1–166.

37. Brissaud O, Guichoux J, Harambat J, et al. Invasive fungal disease in PICU: Epidemiology and risk factors. *Ann Intensive Care* 2012;2:6.

38. Miyake F, Yoshikawa T, Fujita A, et al. Pneumonia with marked pleural effusion caused by Aspergillus infection. *Pediatr Infect Dis J* 2006;25:186–7.

39. Gupta AK, Ghosh S, Gupta AK. Sinonasal aspergillosis in immunocompetent Indian children: An eight-year experience. *Mycoses* 2003;46:455–61.

40. Rao K, Saha V. Medical management of *Aspergillus flavus* endocarditis. *Pediatr Hematol Oncol* 2000;17:425–7.

41. de Mol M, de Jongste JC, van Westreenen M, et al. Diagnosis of invasive pulmonary aspergillosis in children with bronchoalveolar lavage galactomannan. *Pediatr Pulmonol* 2013;48(8): 789–796. doi:10.1002/ppul.22670.

42. Hsu LY, Ding Y, Phua J, et al. Galactomannan testing of bronchoalveolar lavage fluid is useful for diagnosis of invasive pulmonary aspergillosis in hematology patients. *BMC Infect Dis* 2010;10:44.

43. Odabasi Z, Mattiuzzi G, Estey E, et al. Beta-D-glucan as a diagnostic adjunct for invasive fungal infections: Validation, cutoff development, and performance in patients with acute myelogenous leukemia and myelodysplastic syndrome. *Clin Infect Dis* 2004;39:199–205.

44. Michael C, Bierbach U, Frenzel K, Lange T, Basara N, Niederwieser D, Mauz-Körholz C, Preiss R. Voriconazole pharmacokinetics and safety in immunocompromised children compared to adult patients. *Antimicrob Agents Chemother* 2010;54:3225–32.

45. Mandhaniya S, Iqbal S, Sharawat SK, et al. Diagnosis of invasive fungal infections using real-time PCR assay in paediatric acute leukaemia induction. *Mycoses* 2012;55:372–9.

46. Lanternier F, Sun HY, Ribaud P, et al. Mucormycosis in organ and stem cell transplant recipients. *Clin Infect Dis* 2012;54: 1629–36.

47. Gonzalez CE, Rinaldi MG, Sugar AM. Zygomycosis. *Infect Dis Clin N Am* 2002;16:895–914.

48. Walsh TJ, Gamaletsou MN, McGinnis MR, et al. Early clinical and laboratory diagnosis of invasive pulmonary, extrapulmonary, and disseminated mucormycosis (zygomycosis). *Clin Infect Dis* 2012;54(suppl 1):S55–60.

49. Chaudhary MW, Sardana K, Kumar P, et al. Disseminated infection with *Cryptococcus neoformans* var neoformans in an 8 years immunocompetent girl. *Indian J Pediatr* 2005;72:85.

50. Lu H, Zhou Y, Yin Y, et al. Cryptococcal antigen test revisited: Significance for cryptococcal meningitis therapy monitoring in a tertiary Chinese hospital. *J Clin Microbiol* 2005;43:2989–90.

51. Fischer GB, Mocelin H, Severo CB, et al. Histoplasmosis in children. *Paediatr Respir Rev* 2009;10:172–7.

52. Tran DQ. Susceptibility to mycobacterial infections due to interferon-gamma and interleukin-12 pathway defects. *Allergy Asthma Proc* 2005;26:418–21.

53. Wentworth AB, Drage LA, Wengenack NL, et al. Increased incidence of cutaneous nontuberculous mycobacterial infection, 1980 to 2009: A population-based study. *Mayo Clin Proc* 2013;88(1):38–45.

54. Ding LW, Lai CC, Lee LN, et al. Lymphadenitis caused by nontuberculous mycobacteria in a university hospital of Taiwan: Predominance of rapidly growing mycobacteria and high recurrence rates. *J Formos Med Assoc* 2005;104:897–904.

55. Mandell DL, Wald ER, Michaels MG, et al. Management of nontuberculous mycobacterial cervical lymphadenitis. *Arch Otolaryngol Head Neck Surg* 2003;129:341–4.

56. Chan SP, Birnbaum J, Rao M. Clinical manifestation and outcome of tuberculosis in children with AIDS. *Pediatr Infect Dis J* 1996;15:443–7.

57. Chang K, Lu W, Wang J, et al. Rapid and effective diagnosis of tuberculosis and rifampicin resistance with Xpert MTB/RIF assay: A meta-analysis. *J Infect* 2012;64:580–8.

58. World Health Organization. 2010. *Rapid Advice: Treatment of Tuberculosis in Children*. Geneva, Switzerland: World Health Organization. WHO/HTM/TB/2010.13. http://whqlibdoc.who.int/publications/2010/9789241500449_eng.pdf.

59. Swanson AN, Pappou IP, Cammisa FP, et al. Chronic infections of the spine: Surgical indications and treatments. *Clin Orthop* 2006;444:100–6.

60. Zardi EM, Picardi A, Afeltra A. Treatment of cryptosporidiosis in immunocompromised hosts. *Chemotherapy* 2005;51:193–6.

61. Smith HV, Corcoran GD. New drugs and treatment for cryptosporidiosis. *Curr Opin Infect Dis* 2004;7:557–64.

CHAPTER 96 ■ PRINCIPLES OF GASTROINTESTINAL PHYSIOLOGY, NUTRITION, AND METABOLISM

PATRICK O'NEAL MAYNORD AND Z. LEAH HARRIS

KEY POINTS

Gastrointestinal Tract Anatomy and Physiology

1 The gastrointestinal (GI) tract serves distinct roles in metabolism, immunity, cell signaling, and hormonal modulation.

2 Water homeostasis and water recirculation occur throughout the GI tract in the form of secretion and reabsorption.

3 Bacterial colonization, fermentation, and energy balance are intimately linked.

4 Neuroendocrine control of the GI tract and metabolism are critical and hormones secreted from the GI tract play an important role in the regulation of appetite, metabolism, motility, and immune function.

The Gut as an Immune System

5 The gut microbiome is a major determinant of nutritional bioavailability.

6 Susceptibility to infectious complications is directly related to a patient's nutritional status.

7 An appreciation of the benefits of immune-enhanced diets for specific patient populations is necessary but it is premature to institute immunonutrition for all critically ill patients.

8 Probiotic use needs to be studied in greater detail but offers an intriguing mechanism to control gut flora and maintain an individual's gut integrity.

Energy Expenditure and Metabolism

9 Energy expenditure refers to the amount of energy used by an individual to complete the daily metabolic functions.

10 Total energy expenditure = basal energy expenditure (resting energy expenditure or basal metabolic rate) + activity energy expenditure (all daily activities).

11 Indirect calorimetry is essential to measure the true energy requirement of a patient.

12 Careful attention to macronutrient requirements will help prevent unintended cumulative excesses or deficits of energy and protein in critically ill children.

13 Both overfeeding and underfeeding are prevalent in the PICU, and their impact on outcomes needs to be studied further in this population.

Key Nutrients

14 Adequate and appropriate nutrition, implemented early, is critical in treating malnutrition in the ICU.

15 Malnutrition is associated with increased morbidity and mortality in the ICU.

16 Determination of macronutrient (protein, fat, carbohydrate) composition of the diet is an important aspect in nutrition prescription.

17 Micronutrients—trace elements, vitamins, electrolytes—are essential and deficiencies may result in clinical deterioration.

Body Composition

18 Malnutrition is associated with worse outcomes from critical illness. The prevalence of malnutrition has remained steady over the past decades.

19 Body composition is used as a surrogate for nutritional state.

20 Body mass index has become a proxy for body fat percentage.

21 Methods of measuring body composition are varied, offer limited agreement, and need to be further studied.

22 Future studies must examine the association between childhood obesity and clinical outcome in critically ill children and provide optimal nutritional strategies.

Enteral versus Parenteral Nutrition

23 Enteral feeding during critical illness maintains intestinal tropism, stimulates the immune system, reduces bacterial translocation, and is associated with decreased cost.

24 Further studies are needed to determine optimal timing, site, volume, and composition of feeds in critically ill children. Until then, a uniform consensus-based approach may help achieve nutrition delivery goals in the PICU.

Issues with nutrition in the management of critically ill children range from how much to feed (i.e., what is the resting energy expenditure [REE] of a critically ill child?), to what to feed (macronutrient and micronutrient composition), and even how to feed (e.g., route of delivery). Implementation of an evidence-based nutritional management protocol increases the likelihood that critically ill patients receive enteral feeds and is associated with shortened duration of mechanical ventilation (1). However, a comprehensive understanding of the nutritional needs of critically ill children and nutrient delivery goals continue to elude us. Mounting evidence reveals that clinical outcome in the ICU is influenced by genetic variability in energy metabolism, stress response, and inflammation, but the extent of this effect is poorly understood.

Controlling for nutrient intake and distinguishing among the effects of various nutrients and vitamins ingested from food complicate the design and interpretation of studies aimed at assessing nutrient-dependent outcomes in both healthy and critically ill populations. Individual nutrient bioavailability adds a further complexity to interpretation of studies of nutrient supplementation. The identification of single-nucleotide polymorphisms within populations has led to the concept of "personalized designer medicine" (2). The notion that diets can be customized based on individual genetic profiles to decrease the risk of disease underscores two new areas of nutritional research: *nutrigenomics* and *nutrigenetics*. The future of nutraceuticals may depend upon translating gene-based differences into health outcome differences.

Currently, $34 billion dollars per year are spent by American adults on alternative medicines, the large bulk of this being multivitamins and dietary supplements (including fish oils). The evidence to support or advise against the use of multivitamin and mineral supplements for the prevention of chronic disease in the general population is insufficient (3). The lack of randomized, controlled trials makes it difficult for those who work in the field of nutrition to form evidence-based recommendations. Potential clearly exists for adverse effects from the consumption of multivitamin supplements. The World Health Organization and UNICEF have recognized that "although the benefits of iron supplementation have generally been considered to outweigh the putative risks, there is some evidence to suggest that supplementation at levels recommended for otherwise healthy children carries the risk of increased severity of infectious disease in the presence of malaria and/or undernutrition" (4).

The goals of this chapter are to introduce the relevance of nutrition in disease as it relates to energy and metabolism to critical illness, review macronutrients and micronutrients and their significance in health, discuss the role of immunonutrition in the management of critically ill children, and present a review of gastrointestinal (GI) physiology. In presenting the principles of nutrition and metabolism in critically ill children, it is hoped that nutrition will be viewed as adjuvant therapy in combating disease states and that, like pharmaceuticals, nutrition will one day be "personalized" for individualized care and support. Likely we will learn that implementing caloric restriction may benefit outcomes for some diseases (5), the benefits of a ketogenic diet may well have more to do with mitochondrial health (6), the nutrition of the parents and grandparents are more predictive of our patients' health (7), and that continuous feeding puts demands on the cell that need to be carefully balanced (8).

GI TRACT ANATOMY AND PHYSIOLOGY

The Stomach

The GI tract represents the portal of entry for multiple nutrients and also the largest surface area exposed to the external world. In fact the GI tract has a surface area equivalent to a tennis court. The stomach can be thought of as a muscular bag lined with a complex epithelium designed to secrete acid that begins the breakdown of foodstuffs and maintains a sterile entry point into the intestinal tract. Anatomically a food bolus passes through the gastroesophageal junction and enters the fundus of the stomach. The fundus and corpus of the stomach harbor the gastric acid–secreting parietal cells and pepsinogen-secreting chief cells, which initiate the digestive process and the production of the chyme, the semiliquid, partially digested food. Next, chyme is escorted into the gastric antrum where the surface epithelium secretes alkaline fluid to buffer the chyme prior to entry into the duodenum. The gatekeeper to the small intestine is the pylorus, which consists of the pyloric antrum and the pyloric sphincter, a circular muscular ring that acts as a sieve between the antrum and the duodenum.

The stomach has three layers of smooth muscle that are collectively known as the muscularis. There is an inner circular layer, middle longitudinal layer, and an incomplete oblique layer on the outside. When food enters the esophagus, the fundus undergoes receptive relaxation to allow room for the incoming bolus. Adaptive relaxation occurs when food enters the fundus allowing a larger pool of liquids to be stored while propelling the solids toward the pylorus. In the corpus of the stomach are pacemaker neurons that coordinate forward motility of luminal contents down to the pylorus. The pylorus allows small particles to pass but large particle movement is restricted thereby allowing mechanical disruption and digestion of food. In addition, this allows time for enzymatic degradation to occur with gastric acid and pepsinogen (9).

Acid Secretion

The stomach is lined by a complex epithelium with numerous tubular gastric glands that reach deep into the muscularis mucosa. Within these gastric glands are parietal cells that secrete acid, chief cells that secrete pepsinogen, and enteroendocrine cells that include enteric-chromaffin–like (ECL) cells and somatostatin-secreting D cells. In the neck of the gland, pluripotent stem cells migrate up or down the neck differentiating into the various cell lines. Parietal cells are responsible for gastric acid secretion by means of the hydrogen-potassium ATPase pump. The pump transports hydrogen cations into the gastric lumen and potassium from the gastric lumen into the cell. In the resting phase, parietal cells store the proton tubular vesicles within the cell. Following stimulation these vesicles are transported to the apical membrane. There are three stimulatory receptors on the parietal cell: the muscarinic receptor (M_3), the Type B cholecystokinin receptor (CCKb), and the H_2 histamine receptor, all located on the basolateral membrane. Parasympathetic vagal nerve fibers release acetylcholine that stimulates the M_3 receptor allowing intracellular calcium flux and stimulating the proton pump. Histamine produced by the ECL cells stimulates histamine receptors, activating adenylyl cyclases that increase cyclic AMP levels and lead to activation of the proton pump. Gastrin is the third stimulatory molecule that binds the CCKb receptors. CCKb activation increases intracellular calcium, activating the proton pump. Gastrin is produced in the G-cell of the basal membrane in the antrum. Vagal stimulation triggers the release of gastrin-releasing peptide (GRP) from cells of the gastric fundal mucosa. GRP binds G-cells triggering gastrin secretion. Gastrin binds the CCKb to the receptor but also increases histamine release from ECL cells. Protein is the major stimulant for gastrin release. Recently it has been discovered that gastrin serves other functions in the mucosa that include guiding maturation of parietal cells and migration of immature cells within the gland.

Acid secretion can be described in terms of three phases: the cephalic, gastric, and intestinal. The cephalic phase of acid secretion is stimulated by discussion, sight, or smell of food. The gastric phase of acid secretion is stimulated by gastric distention and chemical factors such as protein, amino acids, and alcohol. During the intestinal phase, acid secretion occurs in response to intestinal distention and protein digestion. The development of the stomach is completed at 14–15 weeks of gestation. In fact, premature infants at 24 weeks' gestation are able to maintain gastric pH below 4 from the first day of life. The control factor in the production of gastric acid is the parietal cell mass. Maximal acid output is ~0.2 mEq/kg beginning in infancy and continuing through adulthood.

Postprandial acid hypersecretion is prevented by negative feedback loop involving somatostatin. When the pH in the stomach falls below 3, somatostatin is released suppressing the release of gastrin and histamine via a paracrine mechanism. Somatostatin also directly inhibits acid secretion from parietal cells. Pepsinogen is secreted via the chief cells. In the presence of acid, pepsinogen is cleaved into pepsin, a protease, which begins the digestion of protein. The maintenance of an acidic environment without injuring the stomach is a complex process only now being understood. The surface mucous cells and mucous neck cells secrete mucus via exocytosis. Mucus contains water, small amounts of electrolytes, glycoproteins, and bicarbonate. Stimuli for mucus production include acetylcholine and prostaglandins. Mucus acts by slowing the effusion of acid from the gastric lumen to the mucosa and also lubricating the stomach during the mechanical stress of digestion. Mucus cannot be broken down by gastric acid but is damaged by bile salts, ethanol, and nonsteroidal anti-inflammatory drugs, thus leading to injury.

H^+ cannot pass through the apical membrane of the mucosa; however, it can diffuse between cell junctions and reach the basolateral surface. In elevated concentrations this can cause mucosal injury. The bicarbonate $[HCO_3^-]$ concentration of the mucosa prevents injury. The mucosal parietal cells possessing a bicarbonate/chloride anti-porter, such that every proton transferred out of the cell secretes bicarbonate to the basolateral membrane. This helps neutralize the acid that reaches the basolateral membrane. The bicarbonate/chloride anti-porter is activated by prostaglandins. In addition, an Na^+/H^+ anti-porter also drives sodium into the cell and hydrogen into the lumen. In the critical care setting, the protection of gastric mucosa and prevention of stress ulceration is of foremost concern particularly in the setting of hypoperfusion. The use of H_2 blockers, such as ranitidine, or proton-pump inhibitors, such as omeprazole, seeks to limit gastric acid secretion to promote mucosal healing (10,11).

Nutrient Absorption and Osmoregulation

In addition to chyme preparation, the stomach also aids in nutrient absorption. Parietal cells secrete intrinsic factor (IF), an essential cofactor in absorption of vitamin B_{12}. In addition, gastric acid promotes processes that improve Ca^{2+} and Fe^{2+} absorption in the duodenum.

The stomach is also the first regulator of osmolarity in the gut. Water homeostasis and water recirculation occur throughout the GI tract in the form of secretion and reabsorption. The stomach has an amazing capacity to handle extremely hypotonic fluid as well as extremely hypertonic solids and deliver an isosmotic chyme to the duodenum for absorption. The apical membrane of the gastric epithelium is impermeable to water and small molecules. This impermeability protects the epithelium from osmotic swings that occur during digestion. Large quantities of water move through the epithelium and via a paracellular route accompany gastric acid in order to balance the osmolarity. One mechanism of water movement, via aquaporin (AQP) channels in the secretory glands of the stomach, basolateral membrane, and microcapillary bed, allows rapid flux of water from capillary vessels through the basement membrane and into the secretory gland to address changing osmolarity into the stomach antrum. Of note, AQP

channels (types 1–10) have varying expression throughout the GI tract. In the stomach, types 1, 3, and 4 are highly expressed and changes in their expression pattern have been associated with atrophic gastritis in the antrum of the stomach. During critical illness, decreased gastric motility has led to the use of transpyloric feeds to achieve adequate enteral nutrition (EN). The loss of osmoregulation during transpyloric feeds particularly during advancement of caloric density can lead to malabsorption, diarrhea, and electrolyte derangements (9,10,12).

The Small Intestine

The small intestine's primary function is toward further breakdown of the chyme into micronutrients for absorption. This task is accomplished by an integrated system of specialized epithelium, commensal bacteria, immune tissue, and a system for handling pancreatic and biliary secretions. In addition, gut motility is highly coordinated by the enteric nervous system (ENS), the "gut brain," to provide proper mixing and propulsion of chyme to maximize absorption. Breakdown in any of the systems can lead to multiple complications in the critically ill patient, so much so that some authors have termed the gut as the "motor" of critical illness (13). The duodenum represents the entry point into the small intestine. Here acidic chyme mixes with pancreatic secretions containing chymotrypsin and trypsinogen. Chymotrypsin and trypsinogen are activated by enterokinase on the surface of epithelial cells to the active proteolytic enzymes trypsin and chymotrypsin that digest proteins into peptides. Bile salts are secreted into the duodenum, which emulsifies fats and exposes them to pancreatic lipases to initiate triglyceride breakdown to monoglycerides and free fatty acids (FAs). The duodenum also receives pancreatic amylase initiating breakdown of starch into maltose, dextrins, and maltotriose. In addition, pancreatic secretions are rich in bicarbonate to buffer the acidic chyme received from the stomach. As luminal contents progress, further digestion is accomplished via brush border enzymes on the surface of the epithelium as well as digestion via commensal bacteria. This efficient system has remarkable absorptive capacity and less than 5% of dietary fat is found in the feces (14).

Intestinal Epithelial Anatomy

The anatomy of the small intestine is such that surface area contact with lumen substrate is maximized. In fact, 95% of nutrient absorption occurs in the small intestine. Kerckring's folds (mucosal folds), villi, and microvilli increase the surface area 600-fold compared to a pipe of the same length and diameter. The microvillus border is sometimes referred to as a brush border. The epithelium of the intestine contains a single layer of columnar cells. Three of the cell lines (absorptive enterocytes, goblet cells, and enteroendocrine cells) are produced from multipotent stem cells originating in the crypts. The fourth cell line, Paneth cells, migrates down the villi and resides in the crypts. Enterocytes are the functional cells involved in the absorption of macronutrients (carbohydrate, fat, and protein). Goblet cells are columnar epithelial cells that secrete mucins and trefoil factors. Mucins are polysaccharide- and glycoprotein-containing secretions that form the glycocalyx mucous barrier on the epithelium and limit luminal bacterial contact with the gut epithelium. Trefoil stimulates epithelial regrowth and repair. There are 10 different enteroendocrine cell lines making up 1% of the epithelium. They function to secrete various peptides and hormones in response to the luminal environment that acts locally on neighboring cells (paracrine function), local neural networks (neuronal function), or into the lamina propria (endocrine function). They provide input into maintaining appropriate motility, glucose homeostasis, pancreatic exocrine function, epithelial integrity, gall bladder contractility, hunger, and satiety. Enterocytes, goblet cells, and enteroendocrine cells all migrate from crypt to the distal villi where they undergo spontaneous apoptosis and are shed into the lumen. The epithelium is turned over every 4–5 days. Paneth cells migrate into the deepest portion of the crypt where they secrete antimicrobial peptides into the lumen and are interspersed with the stem cells. Paneth cells also secrete trophic factors that play a role in stem-cell maintenance and growth (15,16).

The enterocytes of the epithelium are joined together laterally by junctional complexes consisting of tight junctions, adherens junctions, desmosomes, and gap junctions. Tight junctions are located apically at the intercellular space. Adherens junctions are located beneath the tight junction and they function together with adjacent cells as a "fence" to limit paracellular movements of molecules into the lamina propria (the layer beneath the epithelium). Desmosomes are focal adhesions between cells that are connected to the cytoskeleton. Gap junctions are protein tubes that function as intercellular channels linking the interior of adjacent cells for the movement of small ions and molecules. This global barrier system allows for the generation of the different osmotic environments of the lumen, epithelium, and capillary systems and the preservation of electrical polarity for the diffusion of ions. The lamina propria is a layer beneath the epithelium consisting of cells of the innate and acquired immune system, the ENS, endocrine system, myofibroblasts, and cell matrix (17).

Pathways Across the Epithelium

Solutes may take five paths across the intestinal epithelium. The transcellular pathway is reserved for small lipophilic and hydrophilic molecules utilizing passive diffusion. AQP proteins located in the crypts and surface villi allow for passive flux of water, sodium, and chloride. The paracellular route allows medium-sized hydrophilic compounds to pass via the tight junctions. This route is impermeable to proteins and bacterial antigens. Large molecules, like proteins and bacterial antigens, can be taken up by endocytosis followed by transcytosis in small vesicles across the cell toward the basal membrane. Active carrier-mediated absorption is responsible for most nutrient absorption, including carbohydrates, fat, many proteins, and vitamins. Dysfunction involving any of these pathways can lead to barrier dysfunction. Intestinal barrier dysfunction is linked to many clinical diseases including intestinal hypersensitivity, irritable bowel syndrome, and the elevated intestinal permeability that has been implicated in critical illness as a mechanism of multiple organ dysfunction syndrome (18).

Ion Transport

The secretion and absorption of electrolytes and fluids are essential functions of the small intestine epithelium. A healthy adult GI tract can secrete 8–10 L of fluid per day in addition to 1.5–2 L of oral input. However, the net flow across the ileocecal junction is 2 L/day. The net movement of water and solute is dependent on the establishment of an electrochemical gradient generated by the active transport of Na^+, Cl^-, and HCO_3^- within the enterocyte. The basolateral membrane is lined with Na^+/K^+ exchange pumps. These pumps, when activated by ATP, exchange $3Na^+$ from the enterocyte into the basolateral and paracellular space in exchange for $2K^+$. This efflux of sodium maintains an intracellular Na^+ content of ~50 mEq/L. The luminal environment has a sodium content of roughly 150 mEq/L. As sodium is pumped into the interstitial space between enterocytes, an increased sodium concentration is formed and water from the lumen can then diffuse down an osmotic gradient across the tight junctions into the paracellular space. The apical membrane of the enterocyte is lined with

Na^+/H^+ exchangers. Sodium enters the enterocyte from the lumen in exchange for H^+ secretion into the lumen. Sodium cotransport with glucose and amino acids is also an important mechanism of sodium absorption into the enterocyte. Thus, a gradient for sodium is created from the lumen into the enterocyte. Once these have diffused into the interstitial space of the villi they are rapidly absorbed by the capillary network. Thus, water absorption occurs against an osmotic gradient. Globally speaking, the proximal duodenum absorbs water primarily in an osmotic fashion, whereas the distal jejunum and colon absorb water against an osmotic gradient. Cl^-/HCO_3^- exchangers on the apical membrane facilitate secretion of HCO_3^- into the lumen while Cl^- moves into the enterocyte. Metabolism in the enterocyte generates CO_2, which combines with H_2O and then, via carbonic anhydrase, forms the H^+ and HCO_3^- that drive these exchanger pumps. Duodenal bicarbonate secretion regulates the pH of chyme entering from the stomach.

Secretion of Cl^- requires the coordination of basolateral $Na^+K^+/2Cl^-$ cotransporters (NKCC) and the cystic fibrosis transmembrane conductance regulator (CFTR) in the apical membrane. In the crypts, $2Cl^-$ move into the enterocyte from the interstitium, along with Na^+ and K^+. The apical CFTR transporter then pumps Cl^- across the apical membrane into the crypt via a cAMP-dependent activation. The result is an increase in Cl^- ions in the crypts. As Cl^- increase in the local lumen at the crypts creating an electronegative gradient, that then allows Na^+ to move into the lumen via the tight junctions. As NaCl moves into the crypts, water follows via osmosis. The circulation of secretion from the crypts to the apex provides an ample bath of fluid to support digestion at the epithelial level. The control of Na^+H^+ transporters, apical Cl^- channels, NKCC, and sodium/glucose cotransporters or linked transporters (SGLT) is handled via intracellular second messenger production including cAMP, cGMP, threonine, calcium, inositol phosphates, and phospholipids. The tight control over secretion and absorption of water and electrolytes is exhibited by the impact of pathogens that deregulate the system. The pathogen *Vibrio cholera* stimulates cellular cAMP production via permanent activation of adenylyl cyclase and activates CFTR-mediated Cl^- secretion resulting in massive fluid secretion and diarrhea. Water also moves into the lumen based on the lumen osmolarity. As chyme enters the duodenum it is initially isosmotic, but during digestion the breakdown of macromolecules into micromolecules increases the luminal osmolarity. The hyperosmolar luminal environment draws water into the lumen via osmosis. Nutrient absorption including fat, protein, and carbohydrate will be covered in a separate section (19,20).

The Large Intestine

- The colon, in its essence, is an organ dedicated to nutritional salvage. The endpoint of colonic transit is the recovery of electrolytes, water, and energy. In the normal adult, ~10 L a day of fluid enter the small intestine, and 7.5 L are absorbed in the small intestine with another 1.5 L absorbed in the colon. Partially absorbed sugars and dietary fiber entering the colon are fermented by commensal bacteria into short-chain FAs, which are then absorbed for energy utilization. To accomplish this task, the colon has a specialized epithelium with similar cell lines as the intestine but designed for a different geography. Bacteria also make their presence known through a variety of effects including energy scavenging, host–biofilm interactions, and crowding out of invasive species.

The epithelial layer of the colon consists of a single sheet of columnar epithelial cells dotted with crypts. Crypts are finger-like invaginations of epithelial cells into the lamina propria that form the basic unit of colonic function. There are three cell types within the colon: columnar, goblet, and enterochromaffin. Notably absent are the Paneth cells found in the small intestine. Columnar cells (the functional enterocyte of the large intestine) and goblets cells make up 95% of the total cell mass, with the remaining 5% attributed to the enterochromaffin community. Much like the small intestine, cells originate in the deepest crypt as a multipotent stem cell and differentiate as they rise to the surface. Columnar cells function to secrete and absorb liquids and electrolytes. Goblet cells secrete mucus to provide lubrication to the forming feces in response to mechanical stimuli and parasympathetic input.

Absorption and secretion in the colon was once thought to be a segregated function in the sense that the crypts secreted fluid and the surface epithelial was responsible for absorption. Recent discoveries have clarified that secretion and absorption can occur in either location. Water and ion transport within the large intestine functions in a manner analogous to the small intestine. Basolateral Na^+/K^+ ATPase pumps establish low intracellular sodium content. Apical Na^+/H^+ exchange pumps bring sodium into the cell and H^+ out. Cl^-/HCO_3^- exchangers bring Cl^- in and secrete HCO_3^-. Thus, net absorption of NaCl from the luminal environment is similar to the small intestine. The Na^+/H^+ and Cl^-/HCO_3^- are tightly coupled to allow electroneutral absorption of NaCl. Water absorption in response to the net movement of NaCl can occur via the transcellular pathway or paracellular pathway. Recently AQP channels have been identified in the apical and basolateral membranes to facilitate water absorption. These mechanisms are found throughout the entirety of the colon. The distal colon has in addition an electrogenic pathway for the absorption of Na^+. Epithelial Na^+ channel (ENaC) found on the apical membrane of distal colonic epithelial cells absorbs Na^+ down the electrogenic gradient created by Na/K ATPase. Cl^- then enters cell via the apical Cl^- channels or via paracellular route. Aldosterone increases the absorptive activity of both the proximal intestine Na^+H^+ and the distal colon ENaC.

Secretion occurs in the healthy colon to maintain the transport of mucus out of the crypts and into the lumen. The maintenance of apical secretion of Cl^- and HCO_3^- requires the same cellular components previously described in the small intestine. Namely, apical Cl^- channels (including CFTR) and apical K^+ channels are responsible for active secretion. Basolateral NKCC channels and Na^+K^+ ATPase channels ensure adequate ion influx into the intracellular space, maintaining a stable net cell ion concentration. Paracellular pathway allows for the efflux of water in response to shifts in the osmolarity (21,22).

Bacterial Colonization, Fermentation, and Energy Balance

In the newborn, bacterial colonization occurs during the birth process. The vaginal flora shifts at the end of pregnancy such that *Lactobacillus* and *Prevotella* predominate and are responsible for early colonization. Neonates born via C-section tend to be colonized by skin flora namely *Staphylococcus*, *Corynebacterium*, and *Propionibacterium*. Throughout life the bacterial content changes in response to diet. These changes in flora have been implicated in inflammatory bowel disease, obesity, and development of the innate immune system. Bacterial counts rise from the proximal to the distal end of the gut. The stomach contains very few aciduric, Gram-positive bacteria such as lactobacilli and streptococci. As one enters the small intestine, aerobic bacteria appear and gradually transition to anaerobes in the large intestine. Bacterial counts in the terminal ileum are 10^7 organisms/mL but once across the ileocecal valve the number increases to 10^{12} organisms/mL.

The colonic bacteria function in energy harvest by fermenting starch, unabsorbed sugars, and cellulosic and noncellulosic polysaccharides into short-chain fatty acids (SCFAs) and gases. The most important SCFAs are acetate, propionate, and butyrate. Absorbed SCFAs are used directly as an energy source by enterocytes and additionally are transported out of the colon into peripheral tissue. Propionate serves as a substrate for gluconeogenesis in the liver as well as regulation of cholesterol synthesis. SCFAs contribute ~6%–10% of the entire energy requirement in humans. This contribution can be increased in the setting of higher dietary fiber ingestion. SCFAs also act on energy balance by functioning as intracellular signaling molecules interacting with G-protein-coupled receptors to stimulate leptin and peptide YY (PYY) secretion. Acetate has an anti-inflammatory activity via reduction of lipopolysaccharide-stimulated tumor necrosis factor (TNF)-α release from neutrophils and increasing peripheral blood antibody production. Other anti-inflammatory properties of SCFAs include regulation of the intestinal epithelial function, but are beyond the scope of this chapter. In addition to SCFAs, microbes in the gut are responsible for the production of the major source of vitamin K in the diet. This is most evident by the vitamin K deficiency at birth when the GI tract is sterile (13,23,24).

The Physiology of Absorption

Absorption of nutrients is the primary function of the intestinal tract. The transformation of foodstuff into useable energy is a complex process that requires specialized epithelial machinery, careful control of transit, and an integrated system to accomplish this task in an efficient and safe manner. As previously discussed, the morphologic characteristics of the intestine are suited to maximize surface area for absorption.

Carbohydrates represent the majority of the energy supply in the human diet, accounting for >50% of calories in the western diet. Oligo- and polysaccharides represent the majority of these starches and they cannot be absorbed to any appreciable amount by the small intestine directly. Two enzymatic steps that take place in the brush border are required. Starch, primarily in the form of amylopectin and amylose, is cleaved initially by α-amylase in the duodenum. Amylose is hydrolyzed into maltose and maltotriose, while amylopectin into dextrins. Maltose, maltotriose, and dextrin interact with brush border disaccharidases anchored in the apical membrane of enterocytes. These disaccharidases (maltase, glucoamylase, isomaltase, sucrase, and lactase) in turn produce D-glucose, D-fructose, and D-galactose. The SGLT in the intestine is associated with these enzymes and utilizes the luminal to intracellular sodium gradient to transport glucose into the enterocyte. Glucose can also move via osmosis in and out of the cell. Galactose can also use the SGLT. Factors affecting carbohydrate absorption include gastric emptying, small intestine contact time, pancreatic amylase function, and the thickness and contents of the unstirred layer above the epithelium. In general, slowed motility in the small intestine facilitates nutrient absorption. The mechanisms of motility will be addressed in neural control (14,25).

The absorption of protein is one of the central tasks of the intestine. There are three phases: the luminal phase, the brush border phase, and the cytoplasmic phase. The luminal phase begins to a minor extent in the stomach with acidic degradation and pepsin digestion that release a small amount of free amino acids. Functional breakdown begins in the duodenum with the influx of pancreatic proteases that begin the cleavage of polypeptides. Inactive peptidases, including trypsinogen, chymotrypsinogen, procarboxypeptidases, and proelastases, are secreted into the duodenal lumen as chyme enters. Enterokinase in the small intestinal surface cleaves trypsinogen into trypsin.

Trypsin then activates the other precursors into their active forms. The action of these peptidases cleaves large polypeptides into peptides 2–8 amino acids (aa) in length and a minor number of free amino acids. In the upper jejunum (and to a lesser extent in the proximal ileum) the bulk of protein is absorbed via the brush border mechanism. Amino-oligopeptidases cleave the polypeptides into free amino acids and peptides 2–3 aa in length. Specific amino acid transporters exist on the surface of the epithelial. Na^+/aa cotransport occurs via use of the sodium gradient developed by Na^+K^+ ATPase pump. Transport is also driven by the proton-motive force. Specific transporters exist for specific groups: (a) neutral amino acids; (b) cationic amino acids and cysteine; (c) proline, hydroxyproline, and glycine; (d) anionic amino acid transport; and (e) taurine and β-amino acids. A review of the specific transporters for each of these and specific disease states from their deficiencies is beyond the scope of this chapter. Peptide carriers also exist on the surface and transport dipeptides and tripeptides into the cytoplasm of enterocytes, where the tripeptidases and dipeptidases hydrolyze them into separate amino acids. The basolateral membrane also has specific Na^+- and non-Na^+-coupled transporters that move amino acids into the lamina propria, where they are absorbed into the veins of the villi for transport to the portal vein.

In addition to absorption of protein, enterocytes also use amino acids scavenged from the lumen for their own energy source. In fact, the gut is a high energy-expending organ accounting for the 12% of energy use in the body yet only making up 5% of the total body mass. Enterocytes preferentially utilize certain amino acids as an energy source. The utilization rate changes as one transitions from a high-growth phase during neonatal life to adult patterns after growth is completed. Luminal glutamine, glutamate, and aspartate are major enterocyte fuel sources in addition to glucose. Lysine and threonine are additionally important in neonates during rapid growth. The oxidation of these acids is increased during enteral feeding when energy demand is higher. Specific amino acids are also channeled into specific pathways to maintain enterocyte health. Threonine is used for mucin production. Glutamate is used preferentially in mucosal glutathione synthesis. The function of glutamine as a fuel source and precursor for nucleotides forms the physiologic basis for its use in immunonutrition (14,25,26).

Fat absorption is an important source of energy, particularly in the growing newborn. Approximately 90% of fat ingested with a meal consists of triglycerides, with the remainder being phospholipids, cholesterol FAs, and fat-soluble vitamins. In addition to energy, fat in infant formula and human milk provide essential FAs of the n-6 and n-3 series [linoleic and α-linolenic acid (ALA), respectively]. Long-chain polyunsaturated FAs derived from linoleic acid and ALA are also found in human milk. Absorption of these nutrients is essential for grey matter health as well as retinal development.

Triglyceride digestion is initiated in the stomach by gastric lipase (HGL). Emulsification takes place in the stomach without requiring bile salts. HGL is secreted in response to ingestion of a meal. HGL acts on the surface of milk globules to start their breakdown. As fat particles enter the duodenum, pancreatic colipase-dependent triglyceride lipase (PTL) is secreted as well as bile salts to begin the hydrolysis and emulsification of fat, respectively. The acidic contents of the stomach trigger the release of secretin, which in turn stimulates the pancreas to secrete bicarbonate and water. The increase in pH aids in lipase function and also draws the FAs to the surface of the lipid droplet. The key enzyme in phospholipid breakdown, pancreatic phospholipase A2 (PLA2), hydrolyzes phospholipids. Of note both PTL and PLA2 are relatively deficient in preterm and newborn infants. Instead in this population, there are two nonspecific lipases, pancreatic lipase-related protein-2 (PLRP2) and bile salt-stimulated lipase (BSSL), which are the

dominant lipases. Of interest, BSSL is also a product of the lactating mammary gland. These lipases are nonspecific and particularly well suited to the digestion of milk fat.

As bile and pancreatic lipase mix with fat globules, simple and mixed bile salt micelles and unilamellar vesicles of bile form via the following process. Bile lipids and enzymes adsorb to the oil–water interface. Here the lipases can be activated by colipase and bile salt lipases hydrolyze the lipids into FAs, monoglycerides, cholesterol, and lysophospholipids. Large multilamellar droplets are formed, which are then emulsified further by bile salts to the mixed micelle. Mixed micelles and unilamellar vesicles both coexist together in the duodenum as an aqueous suspension. Both of these particles can then be absorbed from the intestinal lumen.

FA absorption occurs via a carrier-mediated transport utilizing the transmembrane sodium gradient. Monoglyceride absorption occurs via passive diffusion. Absorption begins in the distal duodenum and is finished in the distal jejunum. Bile salts are reabsorbed in the terminal ileum where they undergo enterohepatic circulation. Functionally, micelles bump into the brush border where the local acidic environment allows the FAs to disassociate from the bile salts.

After penetration through the membrane, long-chain FAs are formed into chylomicrons for transport to the lymphatic system where, as medium-chain FAs, they are transported into the liver via the portal vein. Chylomicron formation requires several steps. Long-chain FAs are bound by cytosolic proteins and then carried to the endoplasmic reticulum (ER) where they undergo conversion to triacylglycerol (TAG). Microsomal triacylglycerol transport protein transports TAG to an enlarging lipid droplet. The TAG then binds to one of the apolipoproteins in the ER and moves to the Golgi apparatus. Vesicles carrying TAG bud off the Golgi apparatus and bind to the basolateral membrane of the enterocyte where the TAG is excreted into the lymphatics as chylomicrons. Ultimately they make their way into the venous system via the thoracic duct (27).

Neural Control of the GI Tract

Neural control of the gut is essential to fulfill the GI tract's physiologic purpose. All steps in regulation of food acquisition, appetite, motility, absorption, immune function, perfusion, and repair mechanism are to some extent under neural regulation. The ENS functions as the "gut brain." In fact if the gut is isolated from the rest of the body the gut can continue to function remarkably well. The ENS integrates with local reflexes triggered by muscle, chemosensory, and mucosal level information. Containing 100 million nerve cells it is the second largest group of nerve cells after the brain. There are two major plexuses within the ENS; the myenteric plexus regulating muscle activity and the submucosal plexus regulating mucosal level function. These two plexuses interact with each other via hardwire reflexes. Higher levels of integration occur with the spinal cord and brain. The prevertebral sympathetic ganglia are the site of integration of peripheral reflex pathways and preganglionic sympathetic fibers from the spinal cord. Brain centers supply descending sympathetic and parasympathetic outflow to the gut via the fibers travelling with autonomic nervous system. The gut itself sends up sympathetic and parasympathetic outflow to the central nervous system (28,29).

Motility

The muscle structure of the gut is arranged in three layers: an outer longitudinal layer, the muscularis externa, and an inner circular layer, the muscularis interna. There is also a small submucosal layer, the muscularis mucosa. In the stomach the neural control is predominantly mediated by vasovagal reflexes, responsible for both passive relaxation, to allow a food bolus to enter, as well as for regulation of the lower esophageal sphincter tone, to prevent reflux. However, beginning in the stomach and continuing into the small and large intestine, the muscle layers exhibit rhythmic, phasic contractions. The pacemaker activity controlling these activities is generated through the activity of the interstitial cells of Cajal (ICC) within the myenteric layers separating the longitudinal muscle and the circular muscle. This allows the muscle layers to share a common pacemaker activity. The ICC's function is dependent on the influx and efflux of Ca^+ within the cells. The propagation occurs via gap junctions that electrically couple the cells. The rhythmic waves that knead and propel stomach contents into the intestine are generated in the ICC. The ICC form the link between the myenteric plexus and the smooth muscle cells of the inner and outer layers of muscle There are multiple patterns of movements within the intestine all governed by the ENS and its interaction with higher CNS centers.

Peristalsis involves the rapid orthograde movement of contents toward the anus. Segmentation is mixing movements that improve absorption and expose intestinal contents to additional surface area. The migrating myoelectric complex (MMC) is a slow orthograde propulsive movement occurring every 90 minutes in the fasted state. The MMC moves residual contents 1–4 cm/minute. This aids in prevention of bacterial overgrowth in the small intestine by sweeping contents back into the colon. Retropulsion is the expulsion of noxious substances from the small intestine back into the stomach followed by vomiting. The conversion from one type of movement to another is tightly coordinated depending on current luminal conditions. Intrinsic sensory neurons in the lumen respond to luminal chemistry, mechanical distortion of the mucosa, and direct mechanical distortion of their processes in the lumen. These neurons send action potentials to various local motor neurons to appropriately coordinate motility in response to the luminal environment. For example, FAs sensed in the lumen lead to the conversion of propulsive movements to mixing movements. Nociceptors detect pathogens and cause retropulsion in the small intestine and stomach and propulsion and fluid secretion in the large intestine.

Fluid movement is also tightly controlled by interaction of the ENS with the sympathetic pathways, the vasoconstrictor pathways, and the secretomotor pathways. Blood volume and blood pressure receptors in the circulation change the activity of these pathways such that fluid shifts promote fluid retention or secretion in response to whole-body fluid balance. Enteric neural reflexes control the shift of water and electrolytes in either the lumen-to-capillary direction or capillary-to-lumen direction. Enteroendocrine cells also interact with the ENS. Enteroendocrine cell receptors detect luminal contents and secrete second messengers that interact with the local neurons as well as vagal and spinal sensory neurons (28–30).

Neural Control of Inflammation

Nerve fibers from sympathetic nervous system innervated the gut lymphoid tissue where they function to maintain control over both inflammatory and anti-inflammatory functions in response to the local or whole-body inflammatory state. The autonomic nervous system plays an important role in regulating the communication between the brain and the gut immune system. In response to stimuli (i.e., shock or injury), intestinal macrophage activation occurs as well as cytokine release. These inflammatory signals stimulate vagal afferent nerves, which feed into brain nuclei. The brain sends efferent signals back to the gut via the vagus nerve. The release of acetylcholine by the vagus nerve deactivates and inhibits local macrophage activity and cytokine release. In an animal model of inflammation, stimulation of the vagus nerve results

in cholinergic activity and downregulation of inflammation; this is referred to as the "cholinergic anti-inflammatory pathway." The cholinergic anti-inflammatory pathway serves as a physiologic monitor to keep inflammation under tight control. Notably, the anti-inflammatory cytokines IL-10 and transforming growth factor-10 are activated by this cholinergic pathway. This is essential to maintain the beneficial interaction between normal bacterial flora, the gut epithelium, and its immune function (31,32).

GI Perfusion

Arterial blood flow comes to the gut from the superior mesenteric artery, the celiac artery, and the inferior mesenteric artery. The celiac and superior mesenteric arteries feed the small intestine and the liver, which are the most metabolically active organs of the body. As the arteries branch, the smaller branches distribute throughout the mesentery, meeting on end, and forming a functional circle of arteries around the bowel. Smaller branches enter the bowel wall and vascular plexuses are formed in the serosa and submucosa. Arterioles of the submucosa branch into the intestinal villi and form a counter current system within the villus. The anatomy is such that arteriolar oxygen entering the base of the villi can diffuse directly into the lamina and the venules. This system functionally renders the distal tip of the villi with a lower oxygen tension than the base. The degree of diffusion is flow rated such that as flow increases, more oxygen is delivered to the distal villi. During fasted conditions, 20%–25% of the total cardiac output is allocated to the hepatosplanchnic circulation. Following a meal, this percentage doubles.

In the normal physiologic state, splanchnic blood flow is tightly regulated at the local level by chemical mediators, ENS responses, and sympathetic nervous system responses and at the global level via circulating vasoactive substances, systemic perfusion, and systemic sympathetic responses. Local mechanisms of perfusion control include pressure/flow autoregulation, reactive hyperemia, and hypoxic vasodilatation. A balance between vasoconstriction and vasodilation maintains appropriate flow (33–35).

Perfusion Control: The Balance of Vasoconstriction and Vasodilation

Alpha agonists, predominantly norepinephrine, produce vasoconstriction in the gut. In addition, angiotensin II and endothelin-1 (ET-1) are powerful local vasoconstrictors. The predominant local vasoconstrictor during shock is ET-1. The endothelial cells of the splanchnic vasculature contain endothelin-converting enzyme, which produces ET-1 where it functions as a paracrine hormone. There are two subtypes of ET-1 receptors: ET-1$_A$ and ET-1$_B$. ET-1$_A$ receptors are found on vascular smooth muscle in the muscularis, submucosa, and mucosa bowel wall and their stimulation leads to vasoconstriction of vessels early in circulatory shock from hypovolemia. This action is part of a global splanchnic response during shock that mobilizes stored fluid and blood from the small vasculature of the splanchnic beds to increase circulating volume. This phenomenon has been termed the "circulatory sink" and is seen during the mobilization of fluid during exercise. ET-1$_B$ has two subtypes ET-1$_{B1}$ and ET-1$_{B2}$. ET-1$_{B2}$ is expressed on vascular smooth muscle and stimulation results in vasoconstriction. ET-1$_{B1}$ is actually vasodilatory in nature and is most likely responsible for clearing ET-1 but the mechanism is not well understood. In addition, vasopressin and angiotensin are local potent intestinal vasoconstrictors. During low-flow states, the vasoconstrictive response is mediated by the renin–angiotensin system, the endothelin system, the sympathetic nervous system, and vasopressin. Sympathetic discharges from the CNS lead to vasoconstriction via increased adrenal catecholamine secretion as well as local vasoconstriction mediated by splanchnic level neuronal discharges increasing local norepinephrine production.

The main local vasodilators are prostacyclin (PGI$_2$), endothelial derived hyperpolarizing factor, and low levels of nitrous oxide (NO). Prostaglandins are locally produced and act as vasodilators during low-flow states and after mucosal injury. NO is produced at a consistent low level by the endothelium to maintain perfusion through vasodilatation. The low-level NO production can become unregulated during circulatory shock resulting in severe shunting of blood through the vascular bed without adequate time for local oxygen extraction. Systemically produced catecholamines can also induce local vasodilation via β_2 and dopamine receptors (33–35).

Intestinal Response to Feeding, Impaired Splanchnic Blood Flow, and Reperfusion

During enteral feeding the splanchnic blood flow increases by as much as 40%–60%, a phenomenon referred to as intestinal hyperemia. The degree of hyperemia is specific to the nutritional content of the meal with fat inducing the highest increase in blood flow. The hyperemic response is key in linking oxygen delivery to the gut during its most metabolically active time, i.e., digestion. The necessary linkage between adequate local blood flow and luminal nutrient content is best demonstrated during tissue hypoxia. During circulatory shock the splanchnic vasoconstrictive response occurs to preserve global cardiac output. The gut epithelium can become oxygen starved, allowing for several enzymes to convert from dehydrogenases to oxidases. Local NO production is markedly increased. Once adequate blood flow is restored to the system, these enzyme systems generate free oxygen radicals resulting in local damage, termed the *intestinal reperfusion injury*. Luminal nutrients during this oxygen-depleted time can overwhelm the ATP-dependent absorption system resulting in local cellular ischemia. Enteral feeding during hypotension can lead to oxygen demand/supply mismatching causing increased mucosal permeability. However, the mismatch can be partially balanced by the intestinal hyperemic response to enteral feeding. Of note, the mesenteric vasoconstrictive response that occurs during hypovolemic and circulatory shock can persist well beyond the time that other hemodynamic parameters have normalized including heart rate, blood pressure, and acidosis (33–35).

Neuroendocrine Control of the GI Tract and Metabolism

Hormones secreted from the GI tract play an important role in the regulation of appetite, metabolism, motility, and immune function. During critical illness or convalescence, these functions may become deregulated and lead to disordered function of motility and catabolism.

Ghrelin is a 28-aa peptide secreted from the stomach and proximal intestine. In health, ghrelin levels steadily increase during fasting and peak just before normal meal times. Ghrelin functions as a strong appetite stimulant. In addition, it increases stomach acid secretion, and gastric and small intestine motility, and potentiates the normal release of growth hormone (GH). In fact, ghrelin was discovered as an endogenous ligand for the GH secretagogue receptor. Ghrelin stimulates the organism to eat, prepares the GI tract for the arrival of food, and prepares the body metabolically to utilize nutrients. In one study, low ghrelin levels were associated with delayed gastric emptying and decreased appetite. Ghrelin's role in motility has made it a drug target for investigations in postoperative ileus and

diabetic gastroparesis. Ghrelin also has implications outside the GI tract, and fasting ghrelin levels were markedly elevated in adults with sepsis compared to fasted healthy controls (36). In addition, high ghrelin levels were associated with survival in sepsis. This coincides with previous animal work that showed ghrelin-preserved cardiac contractility, improved endothelium-dependent vascular relaxation, and had a survival benefit in laboratory animals (37–39).

During cachexia of chronic illness (e.g., COPD, chronic heart failure, or renal failure), ghrelin levels are significantly elevated. The same observations hold true for children with heart failure and renal failure (40,41). In fact, a ghrelin-resistant state has been proposed, as the appetite-promoting effects of ghrelin seem to be blunted in these populations of patients. Recently, ghrelin has been used in small trials as a means of improving appetite, weight gain, and in one small study a means of improving cardiac function. Ghrelin infusions induced a positive energy balance, stimulated food intake, induced adiposity, improved cardiovascular function, and decreased levels of proinflammatory cytokines IL-1β, IL-6, and TNF-α while increasing levels of the anti-inflammatory cytokine IL-10 (42–44). Ghrelin's overall role in critical illness, recovery from critical illness, and cachexia will undoubtedly represent a prominent role in research during the coming years (36,45).

Motilin is related to ghrelin and has receptors throughout the GI tract. As its name implies, motilin primarily functions to promote motility in the interdigestive phase. Of note, erythromycin binds motilin receptors and is used to promote motility in patients during critical illness. One should note that tachyphylaxis occurs in 60% of patients after 7 days, due to downregulation of the motilin receptors (36).

Cholecystokinin is stored in the proximal small intestine and is secreted following stimulation by luminal fat and protein. Secretion of CCK leads to gallbladder contraction, an increase in pancreatic fluid secretion, slowed gastric emptying, and accelerated small intestine transit. Overall, its actions promote absorption of fat and protein. During critical illness, CCK levels are elevated and associated with delayed gastric emptying (46).

PYY can be thought of as the opposite of ghrelin, inhibiting motility and promoting satiety. PYY is predominantly secreted by the colon, and to a lesser degree the small intestine and stomach. Fat and protein are the greatest stimulus of its release. Short-chain FAs produced by commensal bacteria in the stomach also stimulate PYY release, slowing local motility allowing more time for energy harvesting. PYY levels are elevated in critical illness and correlate with poor motility and early satiety (23,36).

Glucagon-like peptide-1 (GLP-1) and *glucagon-like peptide-2* (GLP-2) are hormones secreted from the L-cells of the small intestine and colon in response to luminal nutrients. GLP-1 serves to slow gastric emptying and blunt the hyperglycemic response to glucose via increasing insulin secretion and decreasing glucagon secretion. Of note, the changes in insulin and glucagon occur only in the presence of glucose. Given this profile, GLP-1 has been studied as a means of preventing hyperglycemia in critically ill patients. GLP-2 does not regulate gastric emptying or hyperglycemia but has been demonstrated to stimulate intestinal growth, absorptive function, and promote intestinal mesenteric perfusion (36).

THE GUT AS AN IMMUNE SYSTEM

It is likely that diet is one of the most modifiable determinants of human health. We now know that indeed "we are what we eat" and that our individual nutrition patterns not only affect our body composition but also dramatically impact our gut microbiome. The nutritional value of our food is not merely the food itself but how well the microbial community that lives in our gut is able to extract and digest the individual nutrients. Studies in humanized gnotobiotic mice reveal that switching diets resulted in an entirely new gut microbiome within a single day (47). The implications that this has on how quickly our microbiome changes in the face of illness are profound, especially when we consider the addition of antibiotics and starvation into the equation. Both the bacteria that make up the microbiome and their spatial organization within the gut environment are important. The human microbiome is enriched with genes involved in multiple metabolic processes essential for human energy expenditure and growth: thiamine and pyridoxine biosynthesis, amino acid metabolism, and dietary polysaccharides to name a few (48).

Immunonutrition

The notions that (a) nutrition is beneficial to critically ill patients, and (b) EN is preferred to parenteral nutrition in the critically ill have been well studied. A systematic review of the literature revealed that, indeed, EN resulted in a decrease in infectious complications in critically ill adults and reduced hospital costs (49). In a review of 13 studies in which multiple small clinical studies were pooled to allow a more precise estimation of treatment effect, no difference in length of ICU stay, number of ventilator days, or mortality was shown, but EN was associated with fewer infectious complications. For many, this single observation is frequently heralded as proof that providing EN to the critically ill maintains a normal immunity. Further, the hyperglycemia that occurs more frequently with parenteral than with EN is suggested to increase the likelihood for a bacterial bloodstream complication. Thus, nutrition provided to the gut offers both a protective effect on maintaining the mucosal barrier and delivers nutrients critical for normal immune function.

The concept of immunonutrition was born out of the observation that nutritional deficiencies are associated with immunodeficiencies. Protein calorie malnutrition is associated with leukotriene reduction and impaired microbial ingestion and killing. Cellular immunity is much more sensitive to protein calorie malnutrition: thymus structure and function deteriorate, and T-cell memory response to antigen is reduced. Studies of the mechanisms of nutrient modulation of the immune response provided critical insight as to how nutrition and immunity are related. However, the corollary to this work has proven controversial, in that some believe that if certain nutrients are required for normal immune functioning, then certainly diets with enhanced specific nutrients must be more immuno-beneficial. However, a better outcome is not necessarily guaranteed with enhanced nutrient supplementation. The identification of certain nutrients as being immunomodulators has generated significant interest and will be discussed in detail in this section.

Three areas of the immune defense system represent targets for specific nutritional manipulation: the mucosal barrier, cellular immunity, and the inflammatory response. The duality of the small-bowel epithelia is remarkable; the mucosa must be both permeable for nutrient uptake and protective against a wide variety of antigens, resident bacteria, and invading microorganisms. The mucosal surface is coated by mucins that are synthesized and secreted by goblet cells and interspersed among the absorptive enterocytes. The mucous coat provides a layer of protection and acts as a filter, allowing smaller nutrients to pass through and keeping larger molecules (antigens, pathogens) out. The cell-surface structure itself acts as a barrier to antigen trafficking: microvilli density, rhythmic movement, and negative charge are combined to repel macromolecules, antigens, and microorganisms. Thus, any disease process

that results in altered charge, decreased microvilli number, or microvilli atrophy makes the host imminently susceptible to disease and infiltration by antigens and microorganisms.

Antigens pass through the mucosal barrier into the enterocyte and are either taken up via endocytosis and rapidly degraded by lysosomes (major pathway), or they pass through the cell untouched and are released into the systemic circulation (minor pathway). The GI tract is composed of a single layer of epithelial cells and antigens/nutrients can pass through the cell via a transcellular trafficking pathway or between the tight junctions that connect these cells via paracellular transport. Transcellular trafficking involves a clathrin-mediated endocytosis in which a ligand bound to its receptor aggregates in high concentration within a clathrin-coated pit that subsequently invaginates to produce a vesicle. These receptor-rich microdomains are not randomly found along the cell surface but rather are static structures called *caveolae* that are cholesterol- and sphingolipid rich. Caveolae represent specialized areas on the cell surface where pit-mediated endocytosis takes place. Certain pathogens have adapted to penetrate the cell at the caveolae; Shiga toxin and cholera toxin (a) can bind to the lipid-enriched "rafts" that bind the sphingolipid-enriched caveolae, and (b) are internalized via clathrin-mediated endocytosis. Vesicles, with nutrients or pathogens, fuse with an endosome within the cell. In the endosome, an acidification process occurs that results in ligand–receptor uncoupling, with trafficking of the ligand across the endosome membrane and recycling of the receptor back to the cell surface. The acidification process both allows for recycling of the receptor (which avoids limiting transportation of ligands and nutrients by the need for de novo synthesis of receptors) and provides another barrier to infection by killing pathogens trapped in the acidified endosome. Nutrients, antigens, macromolecules, and pathogens that successfully transverse the cell are transported to the systemic circulation (50). Paracellular transport through gaps in tight junctions and pores that open between epithelial cells occurs following activation of certain apical membrane-coupled transport systems (Na$^+$-glucose-coupled transport), which signals opening a pore in the tight junction. With an average pore radius of 5 nm, many small molecules and proteins can readily pass through. So too can pathogens and cholera toxins readily induce pore opening and cytoskeleton reorganization, allowing for the trafficking of larger macromolecules.

Processed antigens are further presented to T-lymphocytes within or beneath the enterocyte epithelium by the major histocompatibility complex class I and class II molecules on the enterocyte surface. The role of this antigen presentation in the development of tolerance is critical. Under conditions of infection and inflammation, costimulatory cytokine production in conjunction with antigen presentation by the enterocyte on its cell surface is capable of generating a significant immune response. Ongoing research is directed toward studying how manipulation of the mucosal surface may alter an immune response versus developing tolerance in cases of food allergy, inflammatory bowel disease, and celiac disease.

Glutamine

Glutamine is the most prevalent amino acid in the human body. It serves as a nitrogen donor and is essential for the synthesis of purine, pyrimidines, nucleotides, and glutathione. The high requirement by rapidly proliferating cells for glutamine explains the significant requirement for this amino acid by the intestinal mucosa. In 1991, investigators revealed that glutamine-supplemented enteral or parenteral solutions were associated with increased mucosal thickness, improved integrity of the mucosal barrier, and reduced bacterial translocation across the enterocyte mucosal barrier. Glutamine supplementation has been associated with heat shock protein (hsp70) induction, reduced heat shock-induced cell death, restoration of mucosal immunoglobulin (IgA), enhanced bacterial clearance in peritonitis, and enhanced production of both intestinal and hepatic glutathione stores.

Glutamine supplementation of parenteral nutrition in a double-blinded, randomized, controlled trial did not improve intestinal permeability or nitrogen balance, decrease infection rate, or improve survival in newborn and infant children who underwent digestive-tract surgery (51). These findings are in contrast to those of a prospective, controlled, double-blinded, randomized, multicentered study in critically ill adults from 16 different surgical ICUs, which found that patients who received the glutamine-supplemented parenteral nutrition (0.5 g/kg/day) had fewer bloodstream infections, lower incidence of pneumonia, and a lower rate of requirement for insulin to manage hyperglycemia (52). Whereas no study to date has conclusively confirmed the benefit of glutamine in nutritional supplementation during critical illness, neither risk nor adverse outcome appears to be associated with its delivery either enterally or parenterally.

Arginine

Arginine is a versatile dibasic amino acid that plays many roles in cellular homeostasis. The liver and gut are the two organs that are critical for arginine homeostasis. Hepatic arginase activity rapidly converts the majority of liver arginine to urea. This process is regulated at the level of the intestine, which converts dietary arginine into citrulline, thereby limiting the concentration of arginine presented to the liver. Citrulline is converted back to arginine by argininosuccinate synthetase and argininosuccinate lyase, enzymes that are nearly absent in the enterocyte and liver. Thus, arginine in the form of citrulline passes through the enterocyte, enters the circulation, bypasses the liver, and is captured by the kidneys. Renal citrulline uptake is highly efficient, and the kidney converts 80% of gut citrulline into circulating serum arginine. Thus, arginine, the precursor for multiple proteins and signaling molecules, can enter the body as arginine or as citrulline. Concern for increasing hepatic urea stores by supplementing enteral diets with arginine has been studied, and citrulline successfully increased the arginine pool and restored nitrogen balance in rats that underwent intestinal resection (53).

Arginine is metabolized in the liver and gut via the arginase pathway into urea and ornithine. Ornithine is a critical regulator of cell proliferation and differentiation; critical for the formation of proline and hydroxyproline; a precursor for polyamine, histidine, and nucleic acid synthesis; an essential promoter of thymic growth and development; and stimulator of the release of a plethora of hormones, including insulin, prolactin, glucagon, and GH. More importantly, arginine is a unique substrate for the signaling molecule NO, which is formed by the oxidation of L-arginine by NO synthase. Three separate NO isoenzymes have been characterized: inducible NO (iNO), endothelial NO, and neuronal NO. iNO plays a significant role as an immunomodulator. Early studies documented the effect of enteral arginine on increased lymphocyte and monocyte proliferation and enhanced T-helper cell formation. Multiple studies in wound healing have shown a significant improvement in results with patients on arginine supplementation (25–30 g/dose), such as enhanced protein synthesis, improved wound healing, increased nitrogen balance, increased insulin-like growth factor 1 levels, and enhanced immuno-activity (54).

Although it may appear that arginine would enhance immune function, clinical studies suggest that NO potentiates the systemic inflammatory response in patients with sepsis and is associated with worse outcomes (55). The use of a nonselective NO synthase inhibitor is associated with increased mortality (56).

Early clinical trials that studied the benefit of oral citrulline in reducing pulmonary hypertension in children who underwent cardiopulmonary bypass and who were at risk for the development of pulmonary hypertension showed some promising results. In one study, 40 children were randomized to receive 5 perioperative doses of either oral citrulline or placebo. Postoperative pulmonary hypertension developed in 30% of the placebo group and 15% of the citrulline group. Despite concerns for the study size and design, the conclusion that oral citrulline supplementation may be effective in reducing postoperative pulmonary hypertension is intriguing (57).

Nucleotides

Nucleotides are by definition composed of a heterocyclic base, a sugar, and one or more phosphate groups, and they are the building blocks that compose RNA and DNA. The sugar is usually a five-carbon sugar—either ribose (RNA) or deoxyribose (DNA). The nucleotides/deoxynucleotides can be classified as either purines (adenosine or guanosine) or pyrimidines (thymidine, uridine, cytidine). Nucleotides are also the primary components of coenzyme A (CoA), flavin adenine dinucleotide (FAD), flavin mononucleotide (FMN), nicotinamide adenine dinucleotide (NAD), and nicotinamide adenine dinucleotide phosphate (NADP). During catabolic stress or protein malnutrition, de novo nucleotide biosynthesis is severely impaired. Rapidly dividing cells are the most sensitive to this loss, and immune cells appear to be exceptionally susceptible. T-helper cells are selectively lost, and IL-2 production is impaired with selective dietary loss of urines and pyrimidines (54). In animal models, an association of increased susceptibility to *Staphylococcus aureus* and *Candida albicans* sepsis is seen during nucleotide deficiency (58). No randomized clinical trial has been conducted to explore whether the demand for nucleotides can exceed the endogenous production or to determine the safety of enhancing nucleotides in either parenteral or EN.

Omega-3 Polyunsaturated Fatty Acids

Omega-3 polyunsaturated fatty acids (PUFAs) are metabolized to the 3-series of prostanoids and the 5-series of leukotrienes. As compared to the metabolites of the other subclass of long-chain omega FAs (omega-6), these prostanoids and leukotrienes lack the inflammatory and immunosuppressive characteristics, notably vasoconstriction, induced platelet aggregation, impaired cytokine secretion, defective leukocyte migration, and abnormal macrophage function. In fact, evidence suggests that nutritional intervention with omega-3 PUFAs modulates and downregulates inflammatory eicosanoids and prostaglandin E_1 production. Omega-3 PUFAs are obtained from fish or canola oils and provide an excellent lipid energy source (58). FAs are characterized by the number of carbon atoms, the number of double bonds, and the position of the first double bond. An omega-3 PUFA has the first double bond at position C-3 from the methyl end. Important examples of the omega-3 PUFAs are ALA, eicosapentaenoic acid (EPA), and docosahexaenoic acid (DHA). ALA contains 18 carbon atoms, EPA contains 20, and DHA contains 22. ALA is the precursor to EPA and DHA. Deficiencies of these PUFAs have been associated with delayed growth, skin lesions, decreased visual acuity, delayed learning ability, and neuropathology (54). Diets higher in monounsaturated FAs and PUFAs are believed to decrease risk of heart disease, in particular because they can lower levels of low-density lipoprotein cholesterol and triglycerides. PUFAs are also called *essential FAs* because they are not synthesized by the human body and must be obtained in our diet.

Previous anecdotal studies suggested that omega-3 PUFAs were able to ameliorate the symptoms of multiple inflammatory diseases, such as rheumatoid arthritis, psoriasis, Crohn's disease, and ulcerative colitis. Small, randomized, controlled trials that have studied omega-3 PUFAs and clinical improvement in cystic fibrosis, autism, depression, and asthma have been encouraging. Considerable interest was generated in the possibility that the 3-omega PUFAs acted in reducing proinflammatory cytokines (IL-1 and IL-6), oxidative injury, and lipid peroxidation. One group showed that the administration of omega-3 PUFAs as part of total parenteral nutrition significantly decreased energy requirements, was well tolerated, and did not downregulate lipogenic genes, plasma triglyceride levels, or lipid oxidation, and did not affect glucose metabolism (59). In a single-centered, prospective, randomized, controlled, unblinded study, 100 patients with acute lung injury were randomized to receive a standard enteral diet versus a standard diet supplemented with EPA and γ-linoleic acid (GLA) for 14 days. EPA/GLA-treated patients had shorter lengths of ventilation and improved respiratory mechanics. However, improvements in oxygenation at days 4 and 7 in the EPA/GLA-enriched group were lost by day 14, and length of stay and survival were the same (60).

The safety of PUFAs in children has been established and in fact has been shown to be safe in reversing parenteral nutrition-associated liver failure (61). That said, clinical guidelines and indications for use in critical illness are currently limited and in 2009 the American Society for Parenteral and Enteral Nutrition and the Society for Critical Care Medicine published joint guidelines stating that immunomodulating enteral formulas were appropriate in most critically ill patient populations but should be used cautiously in patients with sepsis (62), while a meta-analysis found that continuous infusion of PUFAs incorporated into a nutritional regimen for patients with acute respiratory distress syndrome reduced organ dysfunction/failure by >80% and adult mortality by 60% (63). Rice et al. (64) reported worsened outcomes and no mortality benefit with fish oil supplementation.

Branch-Chain Amino Acids

The branched-chain amino acids (BCAA) include leucine, isoleucine, and valine and account for 35%–40% of the dietary essential amino acids in the body's protein pool and 14%–18% of the total amino acids found in muscle proteins. Studies in the 1970s suggested that the exogenous supplemented BCAA had anabolic properties. In a review of all known studies that characterize the effect of the BCAAs as anticatabolic agents under conditions of burns, sepsis, or trauma, investigators concluded that leucine alone possesses protein-regulatory properties and is solely responsible for the decreased protein degradation observed (65). Leucine promotes protein synthesis and inhibits protein degradation via a leucine-specific signaling of the mechanistic target for rapamycin. Leucine supplementation was associated with improved muscle recovery following rigorous muscle exercise in healthy volunteers (66). Clearly, the "leucine concept" deserves to be evaluated in a randomized, controlled trial before endorsing its use.

Immunonutrition and the concept of immuno-enhancing diets remain controversial but represent an important shift in our approach to nutrition; dietary manipulation of the immune system adds yet another therapeutic tool to our armamentarium to fight disease states. A systematic review of 22 randomized trials concluded that while immunonutrition may have decreased infectious disease complications, it was not associated with an overall mortality advantage and that the treatment effect was patient-population specific (67). Advances in basic science and clinical trials are increasing clinicians' understanding of which patients and which diseases are most amenable to adjuvant nutritional therapy. Recognizing the specific patient populations that will benefit from immunonutrition will be the task for the next decade. Current consensus reports on immune-enhancing diets recommend that those who should receive early EN with an immuno-enhancing diet are (a) moderately or severely malnourished patients (albumin <3.5 g/dL) who undergo elective GI surgery, (b) severely malnourished patients with albumin <2.8 g/dL who undergo colonic or rectal surgery, and (c) patients who have suffered blunt and penetrating torso trauma (68).

In the first blinded, prospective, randomized, controlled clinical trial to study early enteral administration of immunonutrition in critically ill children, 100 children admitted to a single PICU were randomized within the first 12 hours to receive either an enteral formula supplemented with glutamine, arginine, omega-3 PUFAs, and antioxidants or a control formula. Randomization, prepared formula masking, and energy calculations were performed by a single, blinded individual. Both formulas provided adequate energy protein balance, with the supplemented immuno-enhancing diet providing more favorable effect on nitrogen balance, decreased gastric colonization rates, and a decreasing trend in nosocomial infections. No difference was observed in length of stay or mortality (69). However, a more careful analysis of the data suggests a trend for increased mortality among the immunonutrition-fed group. Concern that these deaths may have been in children who were admitted with sepsis sparked an intense debate (70). A clear position on the effectiveness and safety of immuno-enhanced diets for both children and adults has yet to be determined. This topic warrants well-designed, randomized studies as the field of immunonutrition grows.

Probiotics

The use of *probiotics* (which contain microbes) and *prebiotics* (which promote the growth of microbes) in pediatric practice to modify the intestinal environment increases as we learn more about the changes in gut microbiome, struggled to deal with antibiotic resistance and search for innovative methods to manipulate endogenous defense systems against populations of pathogenic bacteria pre- and postcolonization. By definition, probiotics are live microorganisms, which, when administered in adequate amounts, confer a health benefit by maintaining and/or repopulating a damaged microbiome. The mechanism(s) of this conferred cytoprotection is still being determined. Theories include enhanced intestinal barrier function, improved mucus production, and upregulation of protective cytokines and innate and cellular immune responses. The role of probiotics in the management of allergies, eczema, gastroenteritis (acute and chronic), *Clostridium difficile* infections, and inflammatory bowel disease has been studied with some promise in children (71). An initial randomized placebo-controlled trial of probiotics in PICU was halted prematurely after early analysis revealed a nonsignificant but positive association between the treatment group that received *Lactobacillus rhamnosus* and nosocomial illness as defined as pneumonia, bacteremia, and/or tracheobronchiolitis (72). A study evaluating the effectiveness of probiotics in preventing candida colonization in critically ill children enrolled 150 children that had been on antibiotics for at least 48 hours to be randomized to receive either probiotics or placebo. Probiotics contained *Lactobacillus acidophilus*, *Lactobacillus rhamnosus*, *Bifidobacterium longum*, *Bifidobacterium bifidum*, *Saccharomyces boulardii*, and *Saccharomyces thermophilus*. Rectal candida colonization was assessed over a 14-day study period. While both groups had similar candidal colonization rates on Day 0, by Day 7 and then Day 14, the probiotic group had fewer total colonized patients. The placebo group had a greater incidence of candiduria (37% vs. 17%) as compared to the probiotic group. There were no differences in candidemia although there was a suggestion of protection in the probiotic group (1.6% candidemia rate in the probiotic group and 6.35% in the placebo group, but not statistically significant). The study is an important first step in determining if probiotics can decrease the rate of invasive candidiasis and affect PICU morbidity and mortality (73). The vast majority of studies attempting to delineate a benefit for probiotics for critically ill adults have been underpowered and unrevealing as seen in probiotic use in patients with hepatic encephalopathy and patients with severe necrotizing pancreatitis (74,75). In a meta-analysis reviewing ~1400 patients from multiple studies, all using a *Lactobacillus*-based probiotic, the data suggested that while the administration of probiotics did not significantly reduce ICU or hospital mortality rates, it did reduce the incidence of ICU-acquired pneumonia and ICU length of stay (76). Caution still needs to be exercised with probiotic use in adult critically ill patients who appear to be more at risk for endocarditis, bacteremia, and bowel ischemia. Large-scale, well-designed randomized control trials are needed for both adult and pediatric patients in ICUs to determine the future of probiotic use in critically ill individuals.

ENERGY EXPENDITURE AND METABOLISM

The metabolic response of critically ill individuals, both adult and children, is characterized by an increase in REE. Defined as the amount of calories required by the body during a nonactive, 24-hour period, the REE (calories/day) represents 70%–80% of the calories used by the body. The REE is synonymous to the *resting* metabolic rate, which defines the energy required to maintain normal, basal physiologic functioning. A more sophisticated measurement, the *basal* metabolic rate, represents the amount of energy expended while at rest at a neutral temperature and under fasting conditions (12-hour fast).

The REE is useful in optimizing nutrition management for the patient. While critically ill individuals have a greater REE than healthy controls and have an increased caloric need over their "resting" state, a formula by which to derive REE is useful to prevent the underfeeding or overfeeding of individuals. A common calculation for predicted energy expenditure uses the Harris–Benedict equations, which take into account gender, age, height, and weight.

The Harris–Benedict equations have been found to overestimate the actual energy expenditure measurements calculated

by indirect calorimetry (IC) by 6%–15% (77). The Harris–Benedict equation is likely the most accurate for use in adult critical care units if an activity factor is taken into account when deriving the predicted energy expenditure (78). The Harris–Benedict equations are only two of many equations available to calculate REE. Others include the Food and Agriculture Organization/World Health Organization/United Nations University equation and the Schofield-height/weight (Schofield-HW) equation (Table 96.1). For any of the calculations, a large variation between individuals should be considered when their measured energy expenditure is compared to the calculated amount.

As the large variations in critically ill children can lead to inaccuracy in predictions when using these equations, IC is the only accurate method to determine REE. Energy expenditure can be determined by IC using a metabolic cart that allows gas exchange measurements. The IC device is used to measure volumetric oxygen consumption (Vo_2) and volumetric carbon dioxide production (Vco_2) and the REE is derived using the modified Weir equation; REE = 3.94 (Vo_2) + 1.11 (Vco_2) × 1.44. The ratio of Vco_2 to Vo_2 is the respiratory quotient (RQ), which may indicate the utilization of carbohydrates, fats, and proteins as they are converted to energy substrate.

Respiratory Quotient

In the Krebs cycle, energy is derived from catabolism of macronutrients (fats, carbohydrate, and protein) to acetyl-CoA, which is then oxidized to smaller particles and chemical form of energy (ATP). All of these processes require consumption of oxygen and production of carbon dioxide as a byproduct. The RQ, as measured, does include a contribution for protein-derived energy, but due to the extreme variability in which complex amino acids are metabolized, no single RQ value can be "assigned" to the oxidation of protein. The physiologic range of RQ is 0.67–1.3. An RQ >1.0 indicates a greater oxidation of carbohydrate as compared to fat and a relatively large production of carbon dioxide. A value above 1 might indicate the need to decrease the total calorie intake or decrease the carbohydrate-to-fat ratio. An RQ of <0.81 represents a greater oxidation of fat, which may indicate a need to increase the total calorie intake or increase the carbohydrate-to-fat ratio. However, the sensitivity of RQ to energy adequacy is low, and hence it may not be an accurate indicator of underfeeding

TABLE 96.1

EQUATIONS FOR CALCULATING RESTING ENERGY EXPENDITURE

Harris-Benedict Equations (calories/d)

Male: 66.5 + [13.8 × weight (kg)] + [5.0 × height (cm)] – [6.8 × age (y)]

Female: 655.1 + [9.6 × weight (kg)] + [1.8 × height (cm)] – [4.7 × age (y)]

FAO/WHO/UNU (calories/d)

Male (3–10 y): REE = [22.7 × weight (kg)] + 495

Female (3–10 y): REE = [22.5 × weight (kg)] + 499

Male (10–18 y): REE = [12.2 × weight (kg)] + 746

Female (10–18 y): REE = [17.5 × weight (kg)] + 651

Schofield-HW (calories/d)

Male (3–10 y): REE = [19.6 × weight (kg)] + [1.033 × height (cm)] + 414.9

Female (3–10 y): REE = [16.97 × weight (kg)] + [1.618 × height (cm)] + 371.2

Male (10–18 y): REE = [16.25 × weight (kg)] + [1.372 × height (cm)] + 515.5

Female (10–18 y): REE = [8.365 × weight (kg)] + [4.65 × height (cm)] + 200

REE, resting energy expenditure; FAO, Food and Agriculture Organization; WHO, World Health Organization; UNU, United Nations University; HW, height weight.

or overfeeding and must not be used as such for fine adjustments to the dietary intake (79).

Indirect Calorimetry

IC or metabolic carts are not routinely used in PICUs for a variety of reasons: technical difficulties in performing the technique on mechanically ventilated children, lack of experience in handling expired gases, limitations on its use for patients requiring high-inspired oxygen, and lack of resources. To maximize the results of a metabolic cart and to improve accuracy, (a) infused feeds need to be held constant for at least 12 hours, and intermittent or cyclic feeds held for at least 4 hours; (b) ventilator settings must remain constant for 6 hours; and (c) no procedures (including dialysis) are usually performed for 2 hours before testing. Over the last 5 years there has been a resurgence of interest in the use of IC in the PICU. As intensivists are recognizing the importance of matching energy needs and are wary of both overfeeding and underfeeding, more IC is being studied and in distinct pediatric critical care populations. With the caveats outlined above in place, practitioners are now employing modern metabolic carts to derive the REE with the modified Weir equation. The modified equation converts the volume of oxygen consumed (Vo_2) and the volume of CO_2 (Vco_2) produced per minute into a value for REE expressed (calories). It differs from the standard Weir equation in that the gas concentration measured by the REE machine is reported in L/minute, not mL/minute (80). In a study by Li et al., energy expenditure and caloric and protein intake during the first 72 hours following cardiopulmonary bypass and Norwood procedure were studied. Vo_2, Vco_2, and RQ were determined and the patient's energy expenditure was calculated using the modified Weir equation. The results revealed that these children were hypermetabolic for the first 48 hours following repair. The authors raised the question of effect this underfeeding might have on outcomes (81). More recently, another study evaluated energy expenditure in children following severe traumatic brain injury (TBI) and utilizing a similar methodology (REE calculated from Harris–Benedict equation) determined that the patients studied were not hypermetabolic as had been previously described in the literature and ascribed new neurocritical care neuroprotective measures as possible mediators of metabolism. Both these studies again confirm diet as a previously invisible intervention that we need to be more thoughtful of in our interpretation of outcomes (82). Other studies have similar mixed results with the TICACOS—Tight Caloric Control Study—identifying that mechanically ventilated ICU patients who had their nutritional supplementation guided by IC were in fact more overfed than control patients and while their outcomes trended to reduced mortality they had an increased incidence of infections and a longer length of stay (83–87).

Which method to use to determine REE: the modified Weir or the modified Harris–Benedict? In a study of severely burned children (>40% body surface area), REE was measured by IC and compared with predicted equations when the children were assessed to be their most hypermetabolic. For all children, good agreement was obtained between the three sets of equations used to calculate REE. Unfortunately, the predicted REEs were significantly lower than the measured REEs (mean difference of 635 kcal/day; 95% confidence interval, 525–745 kcal/day; $p < 0.05$). The authors concluded that IC should be used to determine energy expenditure until more accurate equations are developed for this hypermetabolic group of critically ill patients (88). On the other hand, a number of recent studies in children admitted to the PICU after surgery, bone marrow transplantation, or even on extracorporeal membrane oxygenation (ECMO) have REE that are similar to or lower than that seen in healthy children (89–91). In a study

that compared the predictive value of four separate equations to determine REE (as compared to IC) in children with bronchopulmonary dysplasia, the Harris–Benedict equations were the best to predict REE, while the Schofield-HW equations had the best agreement for control children (92). The authors concluded that while all prediction equations underestimated REE in children with a chronic disease (bronchopulmonary dysplasia), the appropriate equation could be a useful tool toward preventing undernutrition and promoting growth.

In critically ill children, the ability to accurately predict energy expenditure is essential. Underfeeding results in nutrient depletion, protein-energy malnutrition, decreased immunocompetence, and increased morbidity and mortality. Overfeeding may induce thermogenesis, hepatic fat deposition, and increased carbon dioxide production. Although it seems intuitive that the severity of illness would affect energy metabolism, this factor was not studied in children until 2000. In a prospective study in critically ill children, investigators hypothesized that measured energy expenditure during critical illness would be lower than predicted energy expenditure and that nutritional and clinical indices would correlate (93). In a group of 37 children (24% with sepsis, 24% with TBI, 13% with respiratory failure, 21% with transplant, and 16% post-cardiac surgery), measured energy expenditure was found to be significantly lower than predicted energy expenditure. Measured energy expenditure did not differ substantially by disease or by administration of muscle relaxation but was different when protein intake, use of vasoactive agents, and sedation were factored in. A study of energy expenditure in children with severe head injury compared four sets of REE prediction equations to measured energy expenditure and found significant variation between predicted and measured for all equations, with more than half of all children having differences of >10% (94). Because the predictive equations may be inaccurate in critically ill children, IC (95–98) is necessary to determine the energy expenditure and guide accurate treatment of the metabolic response during critical illness. A targeted approach to IC in children with the highest risk of metabolic instability has been suggested and might be helpful in resource-limited settings (99).

KEY NUTRIENTS

The goals of nutrition have grown in focus from maintaining lean body mass to include using nutrition as an intervention to modulate the immune response, minimize oxidative stress, normalize gut integrity, and maintain glycemic control. Clinicians need to better understand the components of the nutrition they provide and their contribution as immunomodulators and specific energy sources. As well, it must be determined which patients need active nutritional intervention and which nutrients are optimal to deliver. As a simple, inexpensive indicator of potential morbidity, albumin remains the recommended lab value to obtain for nutritional assessment. In a retrospective cohort study, serum albumin was identified as the single best indicator of outcome in adult surgical patients: a serum albumin <3.25 g/dL was predictive of worse postoperative outcomes (100). With more than 200 enteral formulas available and a growing list of components and their effects, sorting out the macronutrient and micronutrient requirements and deciding upon the optimal nutrient delivery is more complicated than ever before.

Macronutrients

Like adults, infants and children rely on the metabolism of macronutrients (carbohydrates, fats, and protein) to meet their energy demands. Oxidation of carbohydrates usually begins with glycolysis, the conversion of glucose to two molecules of pyruvate. Pyruvate oxidation follows, in which pyruvate is transported to the mitochondria to be converted to acetyl-CoA, followed by the tricarboxylic acid (TCA) cycle, in which acetyl-CoA (from many sources) is converted to energy, carbon dioxide, and water. β-oxidation of FAs produces acetyl-CoA, which again enters into the TCA cycle. The acetyl-CoA produced by fat β-oxidation during periods of decreased glucose intake is converted to ketones in the liver and converted by the brain back to acetyl-CoA for entry into the TCA cycle. Proteins enter either as precursors for acetyl-CoA or as other intermediaries of the TCA cycle.

Energy produced per gram of the substrate metabolized is as follows:

- Carbohydrate   4–5 kcal/g
- Protein   4–5 kcal/g
- Fat   9 kcal/g

The most significant difference between children and adults is in their macronutrient reserves. A review of body composition over age groups (infant, child, and adult) reveals that, whereas carbohydrate as a percentage of total body weight is relatively constant (0.4%), differences in fat reserve/composition (infant, 14%; child, 17%; adult, 19%) and protein (infant, 11%; child, 15%; adult, 18%) are substantial (101). Clearly, children have half of the protein stores and a third of the fat stores of adults, and thus have much less available at times of injury or illness. Therefore, the composition of the macronutrients for infants and children must be specialized. Current recommendations for energy and protein requirements in healthy individuals are (101) (requirements in critically ill children are likely to be quite varied):

- Infants   2.2 g/kg/day protein, 120 kcal/kg/day total cal
- Children   1.0 g/kg/day protein, 70 kcal/kg/day total cal
- Adults   0.8 g/kg/day protein, 35 kcal/kg/day total cal

Glucose

Glucose production in children is critical to meet their energy demands, especially during illness. It is imperative to provide adequate carbohydrate calories so that autocatabolism and further consumption of depleted carbohydrate stores are minimized. Glucose is the preferred energy substrate for the brain, red blood cells, and renal medulla. It is this increased need for glucose in children that drives the breakdown of skeletal muscle to generate glucose in times of nutrient intake deprivation. Without adequate carbohydrate replacement, the catabolism of the diaphragm and intercostal muscles causes additional compromise of respiratory function in an already ill child. Initial attempts at pediatric nutritional support produced regimens that were high in glucose and protein with minimal fat. This unbalanced supplementation caused excess glucose to be converted to fat, with subsequent generation of carbon dioxide, and led to increased respiratory effort. The current goal is to provide a balanced supplementation composed of fat, glucose, and protein. Estimations for carbohydrate requirement in adult patients are available but may be difficult to apply in the critically ill (102).

Fats

Fats are listed in six categories: total fat, saturated FA, monounsaturated FA, polyunsaturated FA, trans-FA, and dietary cholesterol. To provide basal, or resting, metabolic needs, saturated FAs require more energy to burn than do unsaturated FAs. Free FAs, released from glycerol in the hydrolysis of triglycerides, are the primary lipid source for energy. The glycerol released following triglyceride breakdown is converted to pyruvate, which is shuttled into glucose metabolism as a gluconeogenic precursor. Critically ill children who do not receive lipids develop essential FA deficiencies within a week (101). To prevent this condition, incorporation of an appropriate fraction of essential FAs in the prescribed diet, linoleic acid (4.5% total calories), and linolenic acid (0.5% total calories) is recommended. Currently available lipid preparations provide essential free FAs but are associated with a risk of an increased incidence of pneumonia in adult intensive care patients. Free FAs interfere with leukocyte function, and hyperlipidemia is associated with decreased oxygenation in premature infants who receive IV fat infusions. Neonates have a theoretical risk of IV lipid displacing unconjugated bilirubin and causing kernicterus. Restricting the infusion of lipid to 2–3 g/kg/day protects against bilirubin displacement (101).

Proteins

Unlike the storage of fat, the body has no storage depots of protein. Approximately 98% of the amino acids are incorporated in proteins, and protein recycling represents the major pathway for amino acid/protein utilization. Newborns have a protein turnover twice as active as adults: 6.7 g/kg/day versus 3.5 g/kg/day. Burns, trauma, and ECMO cause protein turnover to increase further. A 100% increase in urinary nitrogen excretion is seen with bacterial sepsis in infants, and a 100% increase in protein breakdown is seen if they require ECMO support. Amino acid supplementation has been shown to be successful in restoring negative protein balance, but limited data exist to guide optimal protein delivery. To provide adequate amino acids for wound healing, protein synthesis, and preservation of skeletal muscle mass, the recommended protein requirements during critical illness are as follows (103,104):

- Low-birth-weight infants   3–4 g/kg/day
- Term neonates   2–3 g/kg/day
- Children   1.5 g/kg/day

Protein administration >6 g/kg/day is associated with toxicity to the liver and kidneys and should be avoided. Infants should receive 43% of protein as essential amino acids, and children should receive 36%. While infants should receive a minimum of 30% of their calories from fat, children should receive a maximum of 30% of total calories from fat and no more than 10% of their calories from saturated or unsaturated fats (105).

Micronutrients

Micronutrients are classified as *vitamins* [A (retinol), B_1 (thiamin), B_2 (riboflavin), B_3 (niacin), B_5 (pantothenic acid), B_6 (pyridoxine), B_7 (biotin), B_9 (folate), B_{12} (cobalamin or cyanocobalamin), C, D, E (tocopherol), and K], *trace elements/minerals* (zinc, iron, copper, selenium, fluoride, iodine, chromium, molybdenum, cobalt, and manganese), and *amino acids* (glutamine, arginine, homocysteine). The significance of these micronutrients lies in the unique disease states that result from their deficiency. Divided into fat-soluble (vitamins A, D, E, and K) and water-soluble (vitamins B and C), vitamins are organic compounds required by humans in small amounts from the diet. Minerals are elements that originated in the atmosphere and earth's crust and were likely incorporated into energy metabolism secondary to their abundance in the soil.

Vitamin A (retinol) is a member of the family of compounds known as the *retinoids*. β-carotene and other carotenoids that are converted into retinoids are frequently referred to as *provitamin A carotenoids*. Retinol ($C_{20}H_{30}O$) can be oxidized to either of the metabolically active forms retinal ($C_{20}H_{28}O$)

or retinoic acid (RA) ($C_{20}H_{28}O_2$). RA is integral in regulating gene transcription. Correctly classified as hormones, based on their ability to affect gene expression, RA and its isomers (all-trans RA and 9-cis RA) are transported to the nucleus via cytoplasmic RA-binding proteins and participate in an elaborate cascade of nuclear gene regulation via binding to specific RA receptors (either RA receptor, RAR, or retinoid X receptor, RXR). Once bound, both RAR and RXR are able to form either homodimers or heterodimers and complex to a specific RA response element that is located on the 5' end of a host of genes that are critical for cellular differentiation and regulation of embryonic limb development, cardiac development, ocular and otic development, GH expression, development and differentiation of T-lymphocytes, and stem-cell differentiation into red blood cell precursors. RAR and RXR are also capable of forming heterodimers with several other nuclear receptors including but not limited to thyroid hormone receptors and vitamin D receptors (VDRs).

Retinol also plays a unique and essential role in the formation of the visual pigment rhodopsin. Following transport to the retina, retinol is stored as a retinyl ester in the retinal pigment epithelial cells; 11-cis retinal, derived from the retinyl ester, binds to opsin in the interphotoreceptor matrix of the rod cell to form rhodopsin. Vitamin A deficiency leads to decreased retinal and is the leading cause of blindness in developing nations.

Thiamin (Thiamine, B₁) is a water-soluble B vitamin required for the coenzyme thiamin pyrophosphate, which is a critical component of multiple dehydrogenase enzymes—pyruvate dehydrogenase, α-ketoglutarate dehydrogenase, and branched-chain ketoacid dehydrogenase—all located in the mitochondria and required for ATP generation. In addition, thiamine triphosphate is concentrated in both nerve and muscle cells and is believed to activate ion channels. A deficiency of B_1 results in beriberi, which was first described in Chinese literature in 2600 BC and has three forms: (a) dry beriberi, characterized by peripheral neuropathy; (b) wet beriberi, characterized by neurologic and cardiovascular abnormalities (congestive heart failure); and (c) cerebral beriberi, best characterized by Wernicke disease. Thiamine disease is usually associated with either inadequate intake (malnutrition) or alcoholism. Less common causes include a diet high in thiaminase-rich foods (raw fish, ferns) and/or foods high in antithiamine factors (betel nuts). Thiamine loss can also occur during hemodialysis. Thiamine deficiency is easily remedied with thiamine replacement and fortification in diet. The cardiac disease appears somewhat reversible while the neurologic injury remains fixed.

Riboflavin (B₂) is a water-soluble B vitamin essential for the coenzyme, FAD and FMN. Flavins (coenzymes derived from riboflavin) and flavoproteins (proteins that use a flavin coenzyme) participate in numerous redox pathways, in particular glutathione reductase, glutathione peroxidase, and xanthine oxidase. Methylene tetrahydrofolate reductase is a FAD-dependent enzyme that maintains the folate coenzyme responsible for converting homocysteine to methionine. Cataracts and migraine headaches have been ascribed to decreased levels of riboflavin. Deficiency is usually caused by inadequate intake or, rarely, by impaired absorption.

Niacin (B₃) is an essential ligand for the enzymes NAD and NADP. The transfer of electrons during oxidation–reduction reactions is predominantly NAD/NADP dependent, and more than 200 enzymes require NAD/NADP. Niacin deficiency is usually secondary to inadequate intake. It may also occur with administration of isoniazid, inadequate absorption of tryptophan (Hartnup disease), or inadequate synthesis of niacin from tryptophan (carcinoid syndrome). The late stage of severe niacin deficiency is known as *pellagra*, the symptoms of which are dermatitis, diarrhea, dementia, and, if untreated, death. Niacin

can be synthesized from tryptophan and, as such, severe tryptophan deficiencies may also present clinically as pellagra.

Pantothenic acid, B₅, is found in every living cell in the form of CoA, an enzyme critical for glucose metabolism, fat metabolism, protein homeostasis, cholesterol synthesis, steroid synthesis, neurotransmitter synthesis, and heme synthesis. Its ubiquitous expression is due to the acetate group donated by CoA for all acetylation reactions required for life. With the exception of that experimentally induced, pantothenic acid deficiency is unknown.

Vitamin B₆ exists in multiple forms, but pyridoxine and pyridoxal 5'-phosphate are the two most common. Humans cannot synthesize B_6 and are thus susceptible to disease from abnormalities in this class of B vitamin. Infant seizures are associated with pyridoxine deficiency, in which seizures are the final manifestation. Irritability, depression, and confusion can frequently occur with this disorder. Pyridoxal phosphate is linked to nucleic acid synthesis, steroid hormone synthesis, heme-oxygen–carrying capacity, red blood cell formation, and neurotransmitter synthesis and secretion. Homocysteine, an intermediate in the metabolism of methionine, can be metabolized by either a folate/B_{12} pathway or a B_6 pathway. The risk of cardiovascular disease is significantly increased in patients with elevated homocysteine levels, and trials are underway to examine the risk of cardiovascular disease in relation to B_6 levels. Deficiency can be due to inborn enzyme abnormalities, inadequate intake, or as a complication of administration of either isoniazid or estro-progestational hormones.

Biotin (B₇) (the vitamin formerly known as H) searched for an identity for many decades before being classified as a B-complex vitamin. Biotin is essential for FA metabolism, gluconeogenesis, leucine metabolism, and histone biotinylation/DNA replication and transcription. FA metabolism requires four separate carboxylases to transfer carbon dioxide, using bicarbonate as its one-carbon substrate. Biotin is the cofactor for each of these carboxylase reactions:

- Acetyl-CoA carboxylase catalyzes the formation of malonyl-CoA.
- Methylcrotonyl-CoA carboxylase catalyzes leucine metabolism.
- Propionyl-CoA carboxylase catalyzes cholesterol and FA metabolism.
- Pyruvate carboxylase is critical for gluconeogenesis.

Once the carboxylase reaction has occurred, biotin is recycled and cleaved from the holocarboxylase by a biotinidase. The biotinidases have been determined to be critical for the selective biotinylation of histones involved in gene transcription and DNA packaging. Biotin deficiency may result from either a biotinidase mutation that interrupts effective biotin recycling or severe dietary restriction. Despite being required by all organisms, biotin is synthesized exclusively by bacteria, yeasts, molds, and select plant species. Bacteria in the human intestine are thought to play a role in biotin homeostasis. The signs and symptoms of biotin deficiency include an erythematous, scaly skin eruption distributed around the eyes, nose, mouth, and perineum, as well as alopecia, conjunctivitis, and neurologic abnormalities. "Biotin deficiency facies" is composed of a rash around the eyes, nose, and mouth, along with an unusual distribution of facial fat. In biotin-deficient infants, the neurologic findings are hypotonia, lethargy, and developmental delay. In adults, the neurologic findings are lethargy, depression, hallucinations, and paresthesias of the extremities. Because biotin requirements are low and it is so readily available, deficiency is rare. One cause is prolonged consumption of raw egg whites. Avidin, a protein in egg whites that is inactivated by cooking, scavenges and binds biotin, leading to deficiency. Other causes of biotin deficiency include genetic inborn errors, extended parenteral nutrition, pregnancy, or long-term anticonvulsant therapy.

Folic acid, B₉ and folate coenzymes are uniquely required to mediate one-carbon unit transfers and may act as both donors and acceptors. Folates are required for methionine synthesis, homocysteine regulation, rapidly dividing cell growth, and DNA methylation. Folate deficiency manifests with bone marrow abnormalities, megaloblastic or macrocytic anemia, and hypersegmented neutrophils, and is followed by abnormalities associated with disrupted homocysteine metabolism. The link between rapid cell growth and folates resulted in research that linked neural tube defects with low folate levels. Adequate folate is critical for DNA and RNA synthesis, and the neural tube is most susceptible to injury during the period between gestational days 21 and 27. It is the link with homocysteine metabolism (folate has an effect of lowering elevated homocysteine levels) that suggests that a folate-rich diet is associated with decreased heart disease. Folates also appear to be of benefit in reducing colorectal cancer risk, Alzheimer disease, and cognitive impairment. Folate deficiency can be caused by inadequate intake, malabsorption (celiac disease, alcoholism), pregnancy and lactation, hemodialysis, and medications (methotrexate, phenytoin, primidone, sulfasalazine, triamterene, and trimethoprim-sulfamethoxazole).

Vitamin B₁₂ (cobalamin or cyanocobalamin) is the largest and most complex of the vitamins and is unique in that it contains cobalt. Cyanocobalamin and methylcobalamin are required for the function of the folate-dependent enzyme methionine synthase (also known as tetrahydrofolate-methyltransferase or 5′-tetrahydrofolate-homocysteine methyltransferase), which produces methionine from homocysteine. In the acidity of the stomach, B₁₂ is released from food stuffs and binds to a family of proteins referred to as *R-proteins* or *R-binders*. In the alkaline environment of the duodenum, the R-proteins are degraded by pancreatic enzymes, and B₁₂ is released and binds to the IF.

The B₁₂–IF complex then traffics through the enterocyte coupled to calcium metabolism. Deficiency can cause anemia (usually macrocytic megaloblastic anemia) or demyelination (numbness, tingling, ataxia). Deficiency can be seen with abnormalities of the stomach (intact stomach is needed for acid environment and R-protein), pancreas (releases proteolytic enzymes that cleave R-protein), gastric parietal cells (release IF), and terminal ileum (where cyanocobalamin is absorbed). The most common causes of B₁₂ deficiency are inadequate intake, autoantibodies against gastric parietal cells (pernicious anemia), and malabsorption. It has also been reported with metformin administration.

Vitamin C (L-ascorbate), a potent antioxidant and reductant, must be ingested and obtained from the diet. Vitamin C is required for collagen synthesis, neurotransmitter release, carnitine synthesis, and redox stability. Scurvy, seen in severe vitamin C deficiency, is fatal if left untreated. While many studies reflect on the link between vitamin C and lower rates of heart disease, stroke, and cancer, many of the participants in these studies were also on a weight-loss program that included increased fruits and vegetables in their diet and decreased meats/fat. It is unclear if vitamin C is truly associated with decreased cardiovascular disease and reduced risk of many cancers. Because the body cannot store vitamin C, ascorbic acid deficiency occurs soon after fresh supply becomes inadequate.

Vitamin D is a group of fat-soluble vitamins essential for maintaining calcium homeostasis. Vitamin D₃ (cholecalciferol) is synthesized in the skin after it is consumed in the diet or after exposure to ultraviolet light. It is then transported to the liver, where it is hydroxylated to the form 25-hydroxycholeclaciferol (calcidiol). An additional hydroxylation occurs in the kidneys, producing 1, 25-dihydroxycholecalciferol (calcitriol), which is the active form of the vitamin. The biologic effects of vitamin D are mediated through a nuclear transcription factor, the VDR. Upon binding active vitamin D, the complex enters the nucleus and associates with the RXR. The VDR–RXR complex, in the presence of 1,25-dihydroxyvitamin D, binds to the vitamin D response elements and initiates a cascade that modulates the transcription of numerous genes, including gene expression of transport proteins that are responsible for calcium absorption in the intestine. In addition to its presence in the intestine, the VDR is on bone, kidney, and parathyroid cells. The activation of the VDR on these sites is responsible for maintenance of blood levels of calcium and phosphorus and of bone mineral content. Vitamin D is also involved in immune modulation through VDR activation on the surface of T cells and antigen-presenting cells, leading to cell proliferation and differentiation. Severe vitamin D deficiency is seen in the PICU as rickets, osteopenia, or osteoporosis—all due to failure of the bone to mineralize. The main cause of vitamin D deficiency is inadequate intake; rarely, it is secondary to inadequate exposure to ultraviolet light.

The last 5 years have heralded keen interest in the link between vitamin D levels and critical illness in particular respiratory illness. Studies in adults and children have shown an association of vitamin D deficiency with increased viral respiratory illness and sepsis. Perhaps regulated by the 25(OH)D direct effect on the production of cathelicidin hCAP-18, an antimicrobial peptide (106,107), there is a clear association of low vitamin D levels and pediatric critical illness. Lower 25(OH)D levels were associated with higher PICU illness severity on day of admission although critically ill children admitted for a suspected infectious etiology did not have uniformly lower 25(OH)D levels (108). When comparing vitamin D levels in critically ill children, postoperative cardiac surgery patients had lower vitamin D levels than their counterparts in the PICU although 25(OH)D levels did not correlate with ICU length of stay or mortality. Further, these same postoperative cardiac surgery patients also had a higher inotrope requirement (109). Understanding the link between vitamin D and critical illness in children and the implications of supplementing critically ill children with vitamin D upon admission to the PICU remains to be studied.

Vitamin E is a term that broadly covers eight forms of this fat-soluble antioxidant vitamin: four tocopherols and four tocotrienols. *α*-tocopherol is the most active form of vitamin E and appears to be an antioxidant that prevents lipid peroxidation and cell membrane destruction. Vitamin E deficiency is seen in children with fat malabsorption syndromes (cystic fibrosis, pancreatic insufficiency, gastrectomy, Crohn's disease, and cholestatic liver disease), very low–birth-weight neonates, and abetalipoproteinemia. Vitamin E deficiency presents with ataxia, peripheral neuropathy, myopathy, and a pigmented retinopathy.

Vitamin K represents a group of fat-soluble vitamins that are essential for the normal functioning of a host of clotting factors. This fat-soluble vitamin has a single function: the γ carboxylation of glutamic acid such that calcium binding occurs and a signaling pathway generates a clot. Vitamin K-dependent coagulation factors are synthesized in the liver. Newborn infants are the most susceptible to vitamin K deficiency and hence bleeding; they therefore receive vitamin K injections shortly after birth. Other causes of vitamin K deficiency include inadequate intake, abnormal intestinal absorption, or administration of vitamin K antagonists.

Trace Elements and Minerals

The trace elements and minerals comprise a long list of compounds found in minute quantities in the body. A micronutrient is considered "essential" if the body maintains homeostatic control over its uptake into the bloodstream or tissue and its elimination. The following are considered essential micronutrients: cobalt, copper, chromium, fluorine, iron, iodine, manganese, molybdenum, selenium, and zinc. Nickel, tin, vanadium, silicon, and boron have been classified as important micronutrients. Aluminum, arsenic, barium, bismuth, bromine, cadmium, germanium, gold, lead, lithium, mercury, rubidium, silver, strontium, titanium, and zirconium are all found in plant and animal tissue; however, their importance is still being determined. A systematic review investigated whether supplementing critically ill patients with trace elements and minerals improved survival (110). Trace elements that appeared to support antioxidant function were the most advantageous. Selenium and zinc were examined in 11 eligible studies. Multivitamin supplementation alone was not associated with any benefits.

Selenium is a trace element nutrient that functions as a cofactor for reduction of antioxidant enzymes such as glutathione peroxidases and thioredoxin reductase. Selenium-dependent enzymes are involved in peroxide degradation, cellular redox, transcriptional regulation, cytokine excretion, and thyroid hormone deiodination. Selenoprotein P appears to regulate immune and endothelial cell function. As critically ill patients have been noted to have low glutathione peroxidase activity, it has been hypothesized that low selenium levels are associated with increased mortality. A meta-analysis of critically ill patient outcomes following selenium supplementation revealed a trend toward a reduction in 28-day mortality following sepsis. Further studies are necessary to determine the impact of this trace element in the management of septic patients (111,112).

Many of the trace elements are transition metals with a free electron in their outer valence that can participate as both a reductant and oxidant. The ability of these compounds to participate both as antioxidants and catalysts in oxidative stress injury makes their trafficking and their appropriate cellular compartmentalization essential. In particular, mitochondria are most susceptible to redox injury.

Recent interest has been generated utilizing coenzyme Q_{10} (ubiquinone) in the management of pediatric cardiomyopathy. Coenzyme Q_{10} is a vitamin-like substance present in the mitochondria that is essential for generating ATP. In the role as a substrate to enhance cellular energy production, exogenous coenzyme Q_{10} (idebenone) has been used in adults with promising results with heart failure with or without cardiomyopathy. Studies in six children with idiopathic dilated cardiomyopathy (2 months to 11 years) revealed an increase in fractional shortening and ejection fraction in five out of six cases after 8 months of treatment (113). The topic deserves the design and conduct of a larger trial before a conclusion can be drawn, but the concept is intriguing.

Refeeding Syndrome

For decades the discussion on refeeding syndrome centered on patients with adolescent eating disorders or children being cared for with short gut syndrome. Both patient populations educated us on the principles of slow initiation of enteral feeds, vigilant monitoring of electrolytes and trace elements, and, in particular, for the clinical signs of hypophosphatemia, hypomagnesemia, and hypokalemia. The etiology of these disturbances is secondary to the effects of starvation on insulin synthesis and secretion. Insulin concentrations decrease while glucagon levels increase during starvation resulting in the rapid conversion of glycogen stores to glucose. Many parallel pathways are activated as the body shifts from carbohydrate metabolism to fat metabolism and undergoes catabolism of fat and muscle to provide an energy substrate: (a) gluconeogenesis occurs resulting in glucose synthesis via lipid and protein breakdown products; (b) adipose stores release large

quantities of FAs and glycerol; (c) muscle releases amino acids; and (d) ketone bodies and free FAs replace glucose as the major energy source. During refeeding, insulin secretion resumes, in response to increased carbohydrate intake, resulting in increased glycogen, fat, and protein synthesis. This process requires phosphates, magnesium, and potassium, which are already depleted secondary to the previous starvation state. Formation of phosphorylated carbohydrate compounds further depletes intracellular ATP and 2,3-diphosphoglycerate. Thiamine exists as a pyrophosphate and is an essential cofactor in glycolysis at the step of pyruvate dehydrogenase converting pyruvate to acetyl-CoA for subsequent incorporation into the Krebs cycle. Thus, thiamine deficiency results in cellular oxidative failure, a shunting of pyruvate into an anaerobic path and clinically manifests as a lactic acidosis (114).

We now see refeeding syndrome in the PICU under different contexts: (a) children that have not received adequate nutrition for >10 days as a result of their critical illness; (b) chronically ill children on parenteral nutrition for supplementation that are neither receiving adequate nutrition as a result of poor oral intake and because of hyperalimentation modification in the face of pharmaceutical recalls and additive shortages; (c) athletes practicing starvation for competition; (d) patients with liver failure; (e) patients who present with excessive vomiting or diarrhea that has limited oral intake; and (f) oncology patients (115). In all these cases, recommendations for prevention would include early hypocaloric feeding that is slowly increased coupled with micronutrient supplementation to replete inadequate stores prior to the initiation of a more robust caloric challenge (116).

BODY COMPOSITION

Multiple models have been developed to differentiate body compartments. In the *basic two-compartment model*, the body is divided into a fat compartment and a fat-free mass compartment. While simple, this model has allowed for subtle changes in each compartment to be studied during growth, maturation, illness, and starvation. While total body mass may stay the same, it is changes in these body compartments that have heralded larger physiological changes. As our studies of energy metabolism and nutrition have deepened, so too has the complexity of body compartment models reflecting a greater sophistication in analyzing the whole body at either an *atomic* level, *molecular* level, *cellular* level, or *functional* level. The atomic model breaks down the whole body into oxygen, carbon, hydrogen, and electrolytes. The molecular model differentiates mineral, fat, protein, and water. The cellular model measures cell mass, extracellular fluid, extracellular solids, and fat. The functional model delineates skeletal muscle, adipose tissue, bone, blood, and other. With the exception of the atomic model, body composition is a term used to delineate distinct tissue types by percentage of fat and then everything else: muscle, bone, and water that an individual is made up of. These percentages enable comparisons of compartments during the aforementioned periods of nutrient excess or deficiency. More commonly, body percentage of fat is used as a surrogate for determining physical leanness and is particularly relevant as we have become more aware of the medical comorbidities associated with obesity. Recently, body mass index (BMI) has become a proxy for body fat percentage in many circles and is calculated by dividing weight by height (117).

Routine anthropometry has been an integral component for studying health, weight, and body composition for decades. A simple and inexpensive method, a routine anthropometric assessment includes weight, length, head circumference, abdominal circumferences, and skinfold thickness. In truth these measurements more successfully present body density. Other methods to follow body composition include underwater weighing, whole-body air displacement plethysmography, bioelectric impedance analysis, near-infrared interactance, body average density measurements, and dual-energy X-ray absorptiometry (DXA) scans. Anthropometric measurements may be inaccurate in critically ill patients with fluid shifts and edema as well as being age and disease specific (118,119).

DXA scans offer a new application for an old modality. DXA scans are able to measure three distinct body compartments: bone mineral, lean soft tissue, and adipose tissue. The lean soft tissue compartment is composed of the metabolically active body cell mass and any extracellular fluid and is really a subtraction of fat and bone mineral mass from the total DXA measurement. Previously utilized exclusively for bone mineral density measurements, this technology provides accurate estimates of bone mineral and the two other compartments—the lean soft tissue compartment and adipose tissue compartment. At the 2013 International Society for Clinical Densitometry Position Development Conference on body composition, the reporting section for the society recommended that all DXA body composition reports should contain parameters of BMI, bone mineral density, body mass composition, total mass, total lean mass, total fat mass, and percent fat mass (120).

The impact of obesity on critical illness in children remains an area for further investigation. In the 2010 study by Srinivasan et al. evaluating the impact of childhood obesity on likelihood of survival to hospital discharge following in-hospital pediatric cardiopulmonary resuscitation, the authors concluded that indeed childhood obesity was associated with worse outcomes. Obesity was defined as ≥95th weight-for-length percentile if <2 years old or >95% BMI-for-age percentile if >2 years old. Obesity was more likely to be associated with males, non-cardiac disease, and malignancy, and is inversely related with heart failure and was associated with a lower rate of survival to hospital discharge after in-hospital pediatric cardiopulmonary resuscitation. The same study evaluated underweight patients (defined as ≤5% weight-for-length percentile if <2 years old or <5% BMI-for-age percentile if >2 years old) and discovered that underweight was not associated with worse outcomes (121).

A follow-up study in 2013 by Goh et al. similarly evaluated the effect of obesity on mortality, length of mechanical ventilation, and length of stay for critically ill children. There was a retrospective cohort of children requiring mechanical ventilation and underweight children were excluded from the study. Weight z-score was used to categorize patients. In this study, critically ill overweight, obese, and severely obese children who were mechanically ventilated had similar parameters as compared to normal-weight controls (122). A recent systematic review of the literature looking at the influence of obesity on clinical outcomes in hospitalized children revealed that childhood obesity may be a risk factor for higher mortality in hospitalized children who are critical ill, carry an oncologic diagnoses, or are transplant candidates. The group recommended that further studies were needed to better understand the relationship between obesity and clinical outcomes (123). The definition of obesity is varied in these studies, and a uniform definition would help determine its impact on clinical outcomes.

ENTERAL VERSUS PARENTERAL NUTRITION

The last two decades have heralded a new commitment to enteral feeding accompanied with an aggressive feeding tube-placement strategy. The recognition that even small feed volumes could significantly maintain a normal gut flora, minimize

bacterial overgrowth, decrease the rate of drug-resistant bacteria emergence, and reduce bacterial translocation was accepted by the critical care community, although implementation remains poor. While the importance of calories and maintaining "normal" gut function were recognized, macronutrients and micronutrients were quickly recognized to be essential ligands for the signaling process critical for cellular responses to illness, and macronutrient and micronutrient composition and caloric content became important.

Markers of nutritional sufficiency are lacking. Vitamin levels are variable, and micronutrient pools are rapidly depleted. Macronutrient values appear to provide the most accurate serum markers of nutrition status. Albumin, prealbumin, transferrin, and retinol-binding proteins represent the four proteins most commonly measured to assess protein malnutrition and extrapolated to reflect total body nutrient needs. The serum protein half-lives of these proteins are:

Albumin (3.5–5.5 g/dL)	20 days
Transferrin (200–400 mg/dL)	8 days
Prealbumin (16–35 mg/dL)	2 days
Retinol-binding protein (2.6–7.6 mg/dL)	10 hours

It is clear that early implementation of a nutritional regimen improves clinical outcomes, decreases infection rate, and reduces hospital stay. A review of adult critical care outcome studies confirms that malnutrition, defined as inadequate nutritional support to meet metabolic demand, is associated with increased morbidity and mortality, increased dependency on ventilatory support, increased nosocomial infection rates, and impaired wound healing. The adult ICU literature also reveals that enteral feeds are superior to parenteral feeds. Despite providing caloric and substrate support, parenteral nutrition is associated with increased incidence of central-line and wound infections (124,125). Secondary hepatobiliary dysfunction is associated with parenteral feeds. Parenteral nutrition does not confer the gastric-stimulated gut peristalsis or neutralization of gastric acid that protects from both ulcer development and bacterial translocation that are accomplished with enteral feeds. Hence, EN is the mode of choice for nutrient delivery in the ICU.

Despite all of the benefits of implementing enteral feeding, delays in initiating feeding regimens are commonplace. An adult study was conducted to examine outcomes in critically ill patients in both medical and surgical ICUs before and after implementation of an evidence-based nutritional management protocol. Feeding tubes were placed within 24 hours of admission to the ICU and patients were randomized to a protocolized feeding algorithm by 48 hours. This approach resulted in fewer days to feed (2.9 ±1.7 vs. 3.2 ±2.0) and fewer mechanical ventilation days (11.2 ±19.5 vs. 17.9 ±31.3), with no difference in length of stay or mortality between the groups. Not surprising, patients with better premorbid nutritional status and those who tolerated full enteral feeds early were less likely to die than those with poor premorbid nutritional deficiencies and those who had difficulty tolerating or advancing their enteral diet (1). Repeat studies to address the benefit of early feeding while recognizing the potential harm of overfeeding and potential hyperglycemia have been conducted since then with a trend to continue to support early EN and revealing an association with reduced mortality. In a meta-analysis by Doig et al. (126), six randomized clinical trials in adults were evaluated and confirmed a mortality reduction with the introduction of enteral feeds within the first 24 hours of ICU admission. While undersized, the results were promising. A 2009 ASPEN Clinical Guidelines: Nutrition Support of the Critically Ill Child similarly reviewed all the data on enteral feeding in children and concluded similarly that there was not sufficient data to recommend early enteral feeds nor the site for feeding (gastric versus post-pyloric) and outcome measures in the majority of pediatric studies were evaluating ability to reach full nutrition rather than mortality (127).

Whereas adult ICU feeding protocols start at a rate of 25 mL/hour and target a gastric intraluminal volume of <100 mL to indicate an excessive gastric residual after 4 hours of feeding, pediatric protocols require volume and rate adjustment based on patient size and age. In a retrospective comparison chart review that evaluated the use of a nasogastric feeding protocol in a PICU, time to reach goal feedings was the single most significant difference identified as a result of establishing a protocol. Twenty percent of the patient population was receiving inotropes, and 80% was receiving sedation. While patients enterally fed early had improved tolerance to feeds (less vomiting, less diarrhea, and less constipation), no differences in ICU stay or hospital length of stay were noted (128). While length of stay, days on ventilator, and total hospital days may not differ between the groups, it is interesting to note that surviving children uniformly have prealbumin values on day 5 of feeding that are significantly higher than nonsurvivors (106). Uniform institutional feeding protocols are expected to guide bedside nutrient delivery, and increase the likelihood of achieving nutrient delivery goals in the PICU. The role of feeding protocols in critically ill children needs to be further elaborated. Splanchnic blood flow and the effect of inotropes and/or sepsis on intestinal mucosal oxygenation remain substantially understudied (129). It is interesting that in multiple studies where nasogastric feedings are initiated by protocol in critically ill children (sepsis and TBI, no cardiovascular postoperative patients, or other pediatric surgical patients) have failed to document gut catastrophes associated with intestinal ischemia secondary to feeding (130,131).

The reduction in gastric motility associated with critical illness and an increased risk for pulmonary aspiration appears to be another barrier to early feeding. Transpyloric feeding (placing a tube in the first to fourth segment of the duodenum) was compared with nasogastric feeds in terms of tolerance, complications, and outcomes. Despite the many limitations of the study, the authors were able to conclude that transpyloric feeding was well tolerated, desired calories were reached more rapidly, and the patients required less sedation (132). The major impediment to most pediatric feeding studies is difficult adherence to feeding and a propensity to halt feeds in the face of procedures. In an attempt to determine the size of feeding volume in patients with acute lung injury who were being mechanically ventilated, an adult study—the EDEN Randomized Trial—was conducted. Patients were randomly assigned trophic versus full enteral feeds within 48 hours of developing acute lung injury. One thousand patients were entered into the study and the main outcome measure was number of ventilator-free days to study day 28. While the trophic fed group never attained the caloric goals of the group that was fully fed, there were no differences in outcomes between the two groups in terms of ventilator-free days, 60-day mortality, or infectious complications. Valuable information from this study was confirmation that gastric feeding was well tolerated (85% of all initial feeding regimens were gastric) and 90% of all patients were on feeds by 48 hours of admission (133). Further upon 1-year follow-up, there was no difference in physical function, survival, employment status, quality of life, and cognitive functioning (134). Studies are still needed to determine timing, site, volume, and composition of feeds in critically ill children. Enteral feeding remains the first choice in those patients who can tolerate gut utilization.

CONCLUSIONS AND FUTURE DIRECTIONS

For decades, pediatric intensivists have studied physiology during disease states, developed strategies to improve outcome,

and evaluated the effectiveness of therapeutic interventions. We have committed ourselves to practicing evidence-based medicine as best as possible and continually push the frontier of clinical and translational medicine to seek solutions for the problems our patients present with. Despite this background, questions remain regarding the metabolic response to injury and illness, the ability to estimate macronutrient needs, the way to overcome barriers to nutrient delivery, and the understanding of alterations in substrate handling in critically ill children. Perhaps the most important consideration is the prioritization of nutrition support in the PICU.

Recent studies have shown association between nutrient delivery and outcomes in this population. Despite this, we continue to know very little about the nutritional health of our patients, seldom titrate nutrition to metabolic need, assume that formula composition can be identical regardless of age, weight, or illness, and rarely consider the effect of medications on our gut microbiome or the effect of microbiome changes secondary to illness on absorption and metabolism.

Diet is the most modifiable determinant of human health. The time has come for us to lay the foundation for incorporating nutrition into our armamentarium of care. Do critically ill cells want to be fed or starved? Do mitochondria want to be continuously fed or allowed breaks to replenish oxidative health? Can we identify which patients need early nutrition? Early micro–macronutrient supplementation and what that supplementation looks like? Are anthropometric variables what we should be measuring during critical illness or are there better "biomarkers" to trend? We need results based on investigation that has been carefully stratified by age (or in some instances, gestational age), weight, illness, nutritional status, and gut microbiome. Our patients' outcomes depend on our understanding how to use diet as a treatment modality during specific periods and types of critical illness.

References

1. Barr J, Hecht M, Flavin KE, et al. Outcomes in critically-ill patients before and after implementation of an evidence-based nutritional management protocol. *Chest* 2004;125:1446–57.
2. Subbiah MTR. Nutrigenetics and nutraceuticals: The next wave riding on personalized medicine. *Transl Res* 2007;149:55–61.
3. National Institutes of Health (NIH) State-of-the-Science Panel. National Institutes of Health (NIH) State-of-the-Science Conference Statement: Multivitamin/mineral supplements and chronic disease prevention. *Ann Intern Med* 2006;145:364–71.
4. Sazawal S, Black RE, Ramsan M, et al. Effects of routine prophylactic supplementation with iron and folic acid on admission to hospital and mortality in preschool children in a high malaria transmission setting: Community-based, randomized, placebo-controlled trial. *Lancet* 2006;367:133–43.
5. Casaer MP, Mesotten D, Hermans G, et al. Early versus late parenteral nutrition in critically ill adults. *N Engl J Med* 2011;365:506–17.
6. Wallace DC, Fan W, Procaccio V. Mitochondrial energetics and therapeutics. *Annu Rev Pathol* 2010;5:297–348.
7. Buescher JL, Musselman LP, Wilson CA, et al. Evidence for transgenerational metabolic programming in Drosophila. *Dis Model Mech* 2013;6(5):1123–32.
8. Davies AR, Morrison SS, Bailey MJ, et al; ENTERIC Study Investigators; ANZICS Clinical Trials Group. A multicenter, randomized controlled trial comparing early nasojejunal with nasogastric nutrition in critical illness. *Crit Care Med* 2012;40(8):2342–8.
9. Soybel DI. Anatomy and physiology of the stomach. *Surg Clin N Am* 2005;85:875–94.
10. Ramsay PT, Carr A. Gastric acid and digestive physiology. *Surg Clin N Am* 2011;91:977–82.
11. Dimaline R, Varro A. Attack and defence in the gastric epithelium—A delicate balance. *Exp Physiol* 2007;92(4):591–601.

12. Laforenza U. Water channel proteins in the gastrointestinal tract. *Mol Aspects Med* 2012;33(5–6):642–50.

13. Clark JA, Coopersmith CM. Intestinal crosstalk: A new paradigm for understanding the gut as the "motor" of critical illness. *Shock* 2007;28(4):384–93.

14. Caspary WF. Physiology and pathophysiology of intestinal absorption. *Am J Clin Nutr* 1992;55:299S–308S.

15. Vereecke L, Beyaert R, van Loo G. Enterocyte death and intestinal barrier maintenance in homeostasis and disease. *Trends Mol Med* 2011;7:10.

16. Cheng H, Leblond CP. Origin, differentiation and renewal of the four main epithelial cell types in the mouse small intestine. V. Unitarian theory of the origin of the four epithelial cell types. *Am J Anat* 1974;141:537–61.

17. Fink MP. Intestinal epithelial hyperpermeability: Update on the pathogenesis of gut mucosal barrier dysfunction in critical illness. *Curr Opin Crit Care* 2003;9(2):143–51.

18. Keita AV, Söderholm JD. The intestinal barrier and its regulation by neuroimmune factors. *Neurogastroenterol Motil* 2010;22:718–33.

19. Venkatasubramanian J, Ao M, Rao MC. Ion transport in the small intestine. *Curr Opin Gastroenterol* 2010;26:123–8.

20. Malakooti J, Saksena S, Gill RK, et al. Transcriptional regulation of the intestinal luminal Na^+ and Cl^- transporters. *Biochem J* 2011;435:313–25.

21. Geibel J. Secretion and absorption by colonic crypts. *Annu Rev Physiol* 2005;67:471–90.

22. Milla PJ. Advances in understanding colonic function. *J Pediatr Gastroenterol Nutr* 2009;48 (suppl 2):S43–S45.

23. Krajmalnik-Brown R, Ilhan ZE, Kang DW, et al. Effects of gut microbes on nutrient absorption and energy regulation. *Nutr Clin Pract* 2012;27:201.

24. Macfarlane S, Bahrami B, Macfarlane GT. Mucosal biofilm communities in the human intestinal tract. *Adv Appl Microbiol* 2011;75:111–43.

25. Mourad FH, Saadé NE. Neural regulation of intestinal nutrient absorption. *Progr Neurobiol* 2011;96:149–62.

26. Bröer S. Amino acid transport across mammalian intestinal and renal epithelia. *Physiol Rev* 2008;88:249–86.

27. Lindquist S, Hernell O. Lipid digestion and absorption in early life: an update. *Curr Opin Clin Nutr Metab Care* 2010;13:314–20.

28. Schemann M. Control of gastrointestinal motility by the "Gut Brain"—The enteric nervous system. *J Pediatr Gastroenterol Nutr* 2005;41:S4–S6.

29. Furness J. The enteric nervous system and neurogastroenterology. *Nat Rev Gastroenterol Hepatol* 2012;9:286–94.

30. Lee HT, Hennig GW, Fleming NW, et al. The mechanism and spread of pacemaker activity through myenteric interstitial cells of Cajal in human small intestine. *Gastroenterology* 2007;132:1852–65.

31. De Jonge WJ, The FO, van der Zanden EP, et al. Inflammation and gut motility; Neural control of intestinal immune cell activation. *J Pediatr Gastroenterol Nutr* 2005;41:S10–S11.

32. Maloy KJ, Powrie F. Intestinal homeostasis and its breakdown in inflammatory bowel disease. *Nature* 2011;474(7351):298–306.

33. Jakob SM. Clinical review: Splanchnic ischaemia. *Crit Care* 2002;6(4):306–12.

34. Cresci G, Cúe J. The patient with circulatory shock: To feed or not to feed? *Nutr Clin Pract* 2008;23:501.

35. Ackland G. Understanding gastrointestinal perfusion in critical care: so near, and yet so far. *Crit Care* 2000;4:269–81.

36. Deane A, Chapman MJ, Fraser RJL, et al. Bench-to-bedside review: The gut as an endocrine organ in the critically ill. *Crit Care* 2010;14:228.

37. Wu R, Chaung WW, Dong W, et al. Ghrelin maintains the cardiovascular stability in severe sepsis. *J Surg Res* 2012;178(1):370–7.

38. Nagaya N, Kangawa K. Ghrelin improves left ventricular dysfunction and cardiac cachexia in heart failure. *Curr Opin Pharmacol* 2003;3(2):146–51.

39. Wu R, Zhou M, Cui X, et al. Upregulation of cardiovascular ghrelin receptor occurs in the hyperdynamic phase of sepsis. *Am J Physiol Heart Circ Physiol* 2004;287(3):H1296–H1302.

40. Arbeiter AK, Buscher R, Petersenn S, et al. Ghrelin and other appetite-regulating hormones in paediatric patients with chronic renal failure during dialysis and following kidney transplantation. *Nephrol Dial Transplant* 2009;24(2):643–6.

41. Yilmaz E, Ustundag B, Sen Y, et al. The levels of Ghrelin, TNF-alpha, and IL-6 in children with cyanotic and acyanotic congenital heart disease. *Mediators Inflamm* 2007;2007:32403.

42. Nagaya N, Moriya J, Yasumura Y, et al. Effects of ghrelin administration on left ventricular function, exercise capacity, and muscle wasting in patients with chronic heart failure. *Circulation* 2004;110(24):3674–9.

43. Kodama T, Ashitani J, Matsumoto N, et al. Ghrelin treatment suppresses neutrophil-dominant inflammation in airways of patients with chronic respiratory infection. *Pulm Pharmacol Ther* 2008;21(5):774–9.

44. Waseem T, Duxbury M, Ito H, et al. Exogenous ghrelin modulates release of pro-inflammatory and anti-inflammatory cytokines in LPS-stimulated macrophages through distinct signaling pathways. *Surgery* 2008;143(3):334–42.

45. Akamizu T, Kangawa K. The physiologic significance and potential clinical applications of ghrelin. *Eur J Intern Med* 2012;23:197–202.

46. Nguyen NQ, Fraser RJ, Bryant LK, et al. The relationship between gastric emptying, plasma cholecystokinin, and peptide YY in critically ill patients. *Crit Care* 2007;11(6):R132.

47. Turnbaugh PJ, Ridaura VK, Faith JJ, et al. The effect of diet on the human gut microbiome: A metagenomic analysis in humanized gnotobiotics mice. *Sci Transl Med* 2009;1(6):1–10.

48. Turnbaugh PJ, Gordon JI. An invitation to the marriage of metagenomics and metabolomics. *Cell* 2008;134:708–13.

49. Gramlich L, Kichian K, Pinilla J, et al. Does enteral nutrition compared to parenteral nutrition result in a better outcomes in critically ill adult patients? A systematic review of the literature. *Nutrition* 2004;20:843–8.

50. Snoeck V, Goddeeris B, Cox E. The role of enterocytes in the intestinal barrier function and antigen uptake. *Microbes Infect* 2005;7:997–1004.

51. Albers MJ, Steyerberg EW, Hazebroek FW, et al. Glutamine supplementation of parenteral nutrition does not improve intestinal permeability, nitrogen balance, or outcome in newborns and infants undergoing digestive-tract surgery: Results from a double-blind, randomized, controlled trial. *Ann Surg* 2005;241:599–606.

52. Dechelotte P, Hasselmann M, Cynober L, et al. L-alanyl-L-lutamine dipeptide-supplemented total parenteral nutrition reduces infectious complications and glucose intolerance in critically ill patients: The French controlled, randomized, double-blind, multicenter study. *Crit Care Med* 2006;34:598–604.

53. Osowska S, Moinard C, Neveux N, et al. Citrulline increases arginine pool and restores nitrogen balance after massive intestinal resection. *Gut* 2004;53:1781–6.

54. Suchner U, Kuhn KS, Furst P. The scientific basis of immunonutrition. *Proc Nutr Soc* 2000;59:553–63.

55. Ochoa JB, Makarenkova V, Bansal V. A rational use of immune enhancing diets: When should we use arginine supplementation? *Nutr Clin Pract* 2004;19:216–25.

56. Lopez A, Lorente JA, Steingrub J. Multiple-center, randomized, placebo-controlled, double-blind study of the nitric oxide synthase inhibitor 546C88: Effect on survival in patients with septic shock. *Crit Care Med* 2004;32:21–30.

57. Smith HAB, Canter JA, Christian KG, et al. Nitric oxide precursors and congenital heart surgery: A randomized controlled trial of oral citrulline. *J Thorac Cardiovasc Surg* 2006;132:58–65.

58. Kudsk KA. Immunonutrition in surgery and critical care. *Annu Rev Nutr* 2006;26:463–79.

59. Tappy L, Berger MM, Schwarz JM, et al. Metabolic effects of parenteral nutrition enriched with n-3 polyunsaturated fatty acids in critically ill patients. *Clin Nutr* 2006;25:588–95.

60. Singer P, Theilla M, Fisher H, et al. Benefit of an enteral diet enriched with eicosapentaenoic acid and gamma-linolenic acid in ventilated patients with acute lung injury. *Crit Care Med* 2006;34:1033–8.

61. de Meijer VE, Gura KM, Meisel JA, et al. Fish oil-based emulsions prevent and reverse parenteral nutrition-associated liver disease: The Boston experience. *JPEN J Parenter Enteral Nutr* 2009;33(5):541–7.

62. McClave SA, Martindale RG, Vanek VW, et al. Guidelines for the provision and assessment of nutrition support therapy in the adult critically ill patient: Society of Critical Care Medicine (SCCM) and American Society for Parenteral and Enteral Nutrition (A.S.P.E.N). *JPEN J Parenter Enteral Nutr* 2009;33(3):277–316.

63. Pontes-Arruda A, Demichele S, Seth A, et al. The use of an inflammation-modulating diet in patients with acute lung injury or acute respiratory distress syndrome: A meta-analysis of outcome data. *JPEN J Parenter Enteral Nutr* 2008;32(6):596–605.

64. Rice TW, Wheeler AP, Thompson BT, et al; NIH NHLBI Acute Respiratory Distress Syndrome Network of Investigators. Enteral omega-3 fatty acid, gamma-linolenic acid, and antioxidant supplementation in acute lung injury. *JAMA* 2011;306(14):1574–81.

65. De Bandt JP, Cynober L. Therapeutic use of branched-chain amino acids in burn, trauma and sepsis. *J Nutr* 2006;136:308S–13S.

66. Shimomura Y, Yamaoto Y, Bajotta G, et al. Nutraceutical effects of branched-chain amino acids on skeletal muscle. *J Nutr* 2006;136:529S–532S.

67. Heyland DK, Novak F, Drover JW, et al. Should immunonutrition become routine in critically ill patients? A systematic review of the evidence. *JAMA* 2001;286:944–53.

68. Sacks GS, Genton L, Kudsk KA. Controversy of immunonutrition for surgical critical-illness patients. *Curr Opin Crit Care* 2003;9:300–5.

69. Briassoulis G, Filippou O, Hatzi E, et al. Early enteral administration of immunonutrition in critically ill children: Results of a blinded randomized controlled clinical trial. *Nutrition* 2005;21:799–807.

70. Leite HP, Iglesias SBO. Are immune-enhancing diets safe for critically ill children? *Nutrition* 2006;22:579–80.

71. Crooks NH, Snaith C, Webster D, et al. Clinical review: Probiotics in critical care. *Crit Care* 2012;16(6):237.

72. Honeycutt TC, El Khashab M, Wardrop RM III, et al. Probiotic administration and the incidences of nosocomial infection in pediatric intensive care: A randomized placebo-controlled trial. *Pediatr Crit Care Med* 2007;8(5):452–8.

73. Kumar S, Bansal A, Chakrabarti A, et al. Evaluation of efficacy of probiotics in prevention of candida colonization in a PICU—a randomized controlled trial. *Crit Care Med* 2013;41(2):565–72.

74. McGee RG, Bakens A, Wiley K, et al. Probiotics for patients with hepatic encephalopathy. *Cochrane Database Syst Rev* 2011;(11):CD008716.

75. Gou S, Yang Z, Liu T, et al. Use of probiotics in the treatment of severe acute pancreatitis: A systematic review and meta-analysis of randomized controlled trials. *Crit Care* 2014;18(2):R57.

76. Barraud D, Bollaert PE, Gibot S. Impact of the administration of probiotics on mortality in critically ill adult patients: A meta-analysis of randomized controlled trials. *Chest* 2013;143(3):646–55.

77. Coss-Bu JA, Jefferson LS, Walding D, et al. Resting energy expenditure and nitrogen balance in critically ill pediatric patients on mechanical ventilation. *Nutrition* 1998;14(9):649–52.

78. Alexander E, Susla G, Burstein AH, et al. Retrospective evaluation of commonly used equations to predict energy expenditure in mechanically ventilated, critically ill patients. *Pharmacotherapy* 2004;24:1659–67.

79. McClave SA, Lowen CC, Kleber MJ, et al. Clinical use of the respiratory quotient obtained from indirect calorimetry. *JPEN J Parenter Enteral Nutr* 2003;27(1):21–6.

80. Weir JB. New methods for calculating metabolic rate with special reference to protein metabolism. *J Physiol* 1949;109(1–2):1–9.

81. Li J, Zhang G, Herridge J, et al. Energy expenditure and caloric and protein intake in infants following the Norwood procedure. *Pediatr Crit Care Med* 2008;9(1):55–61.

82. Mtaweh H, Smith R, Kochanek PM, et al. Energy expenditure in children after severe traumatic brain injury. *Pediatr Crit Care Med* 2014;15(3):242–9.

83. Singer P, Anbar R, Cohen J, et al. The tight calorie control study (TICACOS): A prospective, randomized, controlled pilot study of nutritional support in critically ill patients. *Intensive Care Med* 2011;37(4):601–9.

84. Hulst JM, van Goudoever JB, Zimmermann LJ, et al. The effect of cumulative energy and protein deficiency on anthropometric parameters in a pediatric ICU population. *Clin Nutr* 2004;23(6):1381–9.

85. Villet S, Chiolero RL, Bollmann MD, et al. Negative impact of hypocaloric feeding and energy balance on clinical outcome in ICU patients. *Clin Nutr* 2005;24(4):502–9.

86. Mehta NM, Bechard LJ, Cahill N, et al. Nutritional practices and their relationship to clinical outcomes in critically ill children—an international multicenter cohort study. *Crit Care Med* 2012;40(7):2204–11.

87. Mikhailov TA, Kuhn EM, Manzi J, et al. Early enteral nutrition is associated with lower mortality in critically ill children. *JPEN J Parenter Enteral Nutr* 2014;38(4):459–66.

88. Suman OE, Mlcak RP, Chinkes DL, et al. Resting energy expenditure in severely burned children: Analysis of agreement between indirect calorimetry and prediction equations using the Bland-Altman method. *Burns* 2006;32:335–42.

89. Chwals WJ. Overfeeding the critically ill child: Fact or fantasy? *New Horiz* 1994;2(2):147–55.

90. Mehta NM, Bechard LJ, Dolan M, et al. Energy imbalance and the risk of overfeeding in critically ill children. *Pediatr Crit Care Med* 2011;12(4):398–405.

91. Vazquez Martinez JL, Martinez-Romillo PD, Diez Sebastian J, et al. Predicted versus measured energy expenditure by continuous, online indirect calorimetry in ventilated, critically ill children during the early postinjury period. *Pediatr Crit Care Med* 2004;5(1):19–27.

92. Bott L, Béghin L, Marichez C, et al. Comparison of resting energy expenditure in bronchopulmonary dysplasia to predicted equation. *Eur J Clin Nutr* 2006;60(11):1323–9.

93. Briassoulis G, Venkataraman S, Thompson AE. Energy expenditure in critically ill children. *Crit Care Med* 2000;28:1166–72.

94. Havalad S, Quaid MA, Sapiega V. Energy expenditure in children with severe head injury: Lack of agreement between measured and estimated energy expenditure. *Nutr Clin Pract* 2006;2:175–81.

95. Verhoeven JJ, Hazelzet JA, van der Voot E, et al. Comparison of measured and predicted energy expenditure in mechanically ventilated children. *Intensive Care Med* 1998;24(5):464–8.

96. Vazquez Martinez JL, , J, et al. Predicted versus measured energy expenditure by continuous, online indirect calorimetry in ventilated, critically ill children during the early postinjury period. *Pediatr Crit Care Med* 2004;5(1):19–27.

97. White MS, Shepherd RW, McEniery JA, et al. Energy expenditure in 100 ventilated, critically ill children: Improving the accuracy of predictive equations. *Crit Care Med* 2000;28(7):2307–12.

98. Framson CM, LeLeiko NS, Dallal GE, et al. Energy expenditure in critically ill children. *Pediatr Crit Care Med* 2007;8(3):264–7.

99. Mehta NM, Bechard LJ, Leavitt K, et al. Cumulative energy imbalance in the pediatric intensive care unit: Role of targeted indirect calorimetry. *JPEN J Parenter Enteral Nutr* 2009;33(3):336–44.

100. Kudsk KA, Tolley EA, DeWitt RC. Preoperative albumin and surgical site identify surgical risk for major postoperative complications. *JPEN J Parenter Enteral Nutr* 2003;27:1–9.

101. Agus MSD, Jaksic T. Nutritional support of the critically ill child. *Curr Opin Pediatr* 2002;14:470–81.

102. Martindale RG, Maerz LL. Management of perioperative nutrition support. *Curr Opin Crit Care* 2006;12:290–4.

103. Bechard LJ, Parrott JS, Mehta NM, et al. Systematic review of the influence of energy and protein intake on protein balance in critically ill children. *J Pediatr* 2012;161(2):333–9.

104. Botrán M, López-Herce J, Mencía S, et al. Enteral nutrition in the critically ill child: Comparison of standard and protein-enriched diets. *J Pediatr* 2011;159(1):27–32.

105. Briassoulis G, Zavras N, Hatzis T. Malnutrition, nutritional indices and early enteral feeding in critically ill children. *Nutrition* 2001;17:548–57.

106. Liu PT, Stenger S, Li H, et al. Toll-like receptor triggering of a vitamin D-mediated human antimicrobial response. *Science* 2006;311(5768):1770–3.

107. Gombart AF, Borregaard N, Koeffler HP. Human cathelicidin antimicrobial peptide (CAMP) gene is a direct target of the vitamin D receptor and is strongly up-regulated in myeloid cells by 1,25-dihydroxyvitamin D3. *FASEB J* 2005;19(9):1067–77.

108. Madden K, Feldman HA, Smith EM, et al. Vitamin D deficiency in critically ill children. *Pediatrics* 2012;130(3):421–8.

109. Rippel C, South M, Butt WW, et al. Vitamin D status in critically ill children. *Intensive Care Med* 2012;38(12):2055–62.

110. Heyland D, Dhaliwal R, Suchner U, et al. Antioxidant nutrients: A systematic review of trace elements and vitamins in the critically ill patient. *Intensive Care Med* 2005;31:327–37.

111. Angstwurm MW, Engelmann L, Zimmermann T, et al. Selenium in Intensive Care (SIC): Results of a prospective randomized, placebo-controlled, multiple-center study in patients with severe systemic inflammatory response syndrome, sepsis, and septic shock. *Crit Care Med* 2007;35(1):118–26; comment 206–7.

112. Angstwurm MW, Gaertner R. Practicalities of selenium supplementation in critically ill patients. *Curr Opin Clin Nutr Metab Care* 2006;9(3):233–8.

113. Elshershari H, Ozer S, Ozkutlu S, et al. Potential usefulness of coenzyme Q_{10} in the treatment of idiopathic dilated cardiomyopathy in children. *Int J Cardiol* 2003;88:101–2.

114. Manzanares W, Hardy G. Thiamine supplementation in the critically ill. *Curr Opin Clin Nutr Metab Care* 2011;14(6):610–7.

115. Byrnes MC, Stangenes J. Refeeding in the ICU: An adult and pediatric problem. *Curr Opin Clin Nutr Metab Care* 2011;14(2):186–92.

116. Casaer MP, Van den Berghe G. Nutrition in the acute phase of critical illness. *N Engl J Med* 2014;370(13):1227–36.

117. Flegal KM, Ogden CL, Yanovski JA, Freedman DS, Shepherd JA, Graubard BI, and Borrud LG. High adiposity and high body mass index -for-age in US children and adolescents overall and by race-ethnic group. *Am J Clin Nutr.* 2010; 91(4): 1020–1026.

118. Freitas Júnior IF, Rupp de Paiva SA, de Godoy I, et al. Comparative analysis of body composition assessment methods in healthy men and in chronic obstructive pulmonary disease patients: anthropometry, bioelectrical impedance and dual-energy X-ray absorptiometry. *Arch Latinoam Nutr* 2005;55(2):124–31.

119. Kulkarni B, Mamidi RS, Balakrishna N, et al. Body composition assessment in infancy and early childhood: Comparison of anthropometry with dual-energy X-ray absorptiometry in low-income group children from India. *Eur J Clin Nutr* 2014;68(6):658–63.

120. Petak S, Barbu CG, Yu EW, et al. The Official Positions of the International Society for Clinical Densitometry: Body composition analysis reporting. *J Clin Densitom* 2013;16(4):508–19.

121. Srinivasan V, Nadkarni VM, Helfaer MA, et al; American Heart Association National Registry of Cardiopulmonary Resuscitation Investigators. Childhood obesity and survival after in-hospital pediatric cardiopulmonary resuscitation. *Pediatrics* 2010;125(3):e481–e488.

122. Goh VL, Wakeham MK, Brazauskas R, et al. Obesity is not associated with increased mortality and morbidity in critically ill children. *JPEN J Parenter Enteral Nutr* 2013;37(1):102–8.

123. Bechard LJ, Rothpletz-Puglia P, Touger-Decker R, et al. Influence of obesity on clinical outcomes in hospitalized children: A systematic review. *JAMA Pediatr* 2013;167(5):476–82.

124. Mikhailov TA. Early enteral nutrition is associated with lower mortality in critically ill children. *JPEN J Parenter Enteral Nutr* 2014;38(4):459–66.

125. Skillman HE, Mehta NM. Nutrition therapy in the critically ill child. *Curr Opin Crit Care* 2012;18(2):192–8.

126. Doig GS, Heighes PT, Simpson F, et al. Early enteral nutrition, provided within 24 h of injury or intensive care unit admission, significantly reduces mortality in critically ill patients: A meta-analysis of randomized controlled trials. *Intensive Care Med* 2009;35(12):2018–27.

127. Mehta NM, Compher C; A.S.P.E.N. Board of Directors. A.S.P.E.N. Clinical Guidelines: Nutrition support of the critically ill child. *JPEN J Parenter Enteral Nutr* 2009;33(3):260–76.

128. Petrillo-Albarano T, Pettignano R, Asfaw M, et al. Use of feeding protocol to improve nutritional support through early, aggressive enteral nutrition in the pediatric intensive care unit. *Pediatr Crit Care Med* 2006;7:340–4.

129. Sasbon JS, Cardigni G. Nutritional support in the critically ill child: Fast food or haute cuisine. *Pediatr Crit Care Med* 2006;7:395–6.

130. Briassoulis G, Zavras NJ, Hatzis TD. Effectiveness and safety of a protocol for promotion of early intragastric feeding in critically ill children. *Pediatr Crit Care Med* 2001;2:113–21.

131. Briassoulis G, Tsorva A, Zavras N, et al. Influence of an aggressive early enteral nutrition protocol on nitrogen balance in critically ill children. *J Nutr Biochem* 2002;13:560–9.

132. Sanchez C, Lopez-Herce J, Carrillo A, et al. Early transpyloric enteral nutrition in critically ill children. *Nutrition* 2007;23:16–22.

133. National Heart, Lung, and Blood Institute Acute Respiratory Distress Syndrome (ARDS) Clinical Trials Network; Rice TW, Wheeler AP, Thompson BT, et al. Initial trophic vs full enteral feeding in patients with acute lung injury: The EDEN randomized trial. *JAMA* 2012;307(8):795–803.

134. Needham DM, Dinglas VD, Bienvenu OJ, et al. One year outcomes in patients with acute lung injury randomised to initial trophic or full enteral feeding: Prospective follow-up of EDEN randomised trial. *BMJ* 2013;346:f1532.

CHAPTER 97 ■ NUTRITIONAL SUPPORT

WERTHER BRUNOW DE CARVALHO, ARTUR F. DELGADO, AND HEITOR PONS LEITE

KEY POINTS

1 The World Health Organization defines severe undernutrition as a weight–height ratio of more than 3 standard deviations below the median for the population (Z score −3). Similarly, the Waterlow criteria define severe undernutrition as a body weight-for-height that is <70% of the weight-for-height of the population median.

2 Undernutrition constitutes an important risk factor for increased morbidity, mortality, length of hospital stay, and medical costs.

3 Severe undernutrition is associated with decreased cardiac output, renal solute clearance, and intestinal absorption.

4 Undernutrition combined with stress (from a response to trauma, sepsis, or burns) leads to a complex neuro-endocrine-immunologic response marked by hypercatabolism and hyperglycemia.

5 The majority of critically ill children tolerate early enteral nutrition well with the possibility of improved survival if caloric and nutrient goals are met.

NUTRITIONAL ASSESSMENT

It is known that in critically ill patients, anthropometric assessment is difficult to interpret because the measurements may be confounded by fluid retention and swelling. However, the consensus is that this assessment is very important for the nutritional evaluation and monitoring of patients in the PICU (1–4).

HISTORY AND PHYSICAL EXAMINATION

A good history and physical examination are the first steps toward establishing the requirements for nutritional support. The need for specialized nutritional support is often clinically obvious but detailed histories of the illness, of food intake, and of weight loss are important to establish a nutritional therapeutic plan. Nutritional repletion is indicated by weight gain, loss of edema, increased muscle strength, increased work capacity, improvement in appetite, and sense of well being (3–6).

Poor nutritional status has been associated with decreased respiratory function, impaired wound healing, and immune and gastrointestinal dysfunctions. Despite its high prevalence, malnutrition in hospitalized patients is poorly recognized by pediatricians. The classical presentation with signs of kwashiorkor is rare in children and adolescents with chronic diseases but the physical examination may reveal signs of malnutrition such as hair loss or change in texture, skin atrophy, pallor, etc. (7–10).

ANTHROPOMETRIC EXAMINATION

Anthropometric measurements are useful to assess nutritional alterations prior to hospital admission and to document the effects of long-term therapeutic interventions. However, they may not accurately reflect acute nutritional deterioration under conditions of metabolic stress. Despite the limitations in acutely ill children who are admitted to the PICU, anthropometric measurements are vital to allow for an objective assessment, enabling the detection of undernutrition and aiding in the planning and monitoring of nutritional support throughout the hospital stay. Anthropometric markers (measurements) are useful to document the severity of undernutrition upon admission to hospital. The anthropometric data for a population reflect its health, growth, and development status (3,6,8). As opposed to anthropometric markers, many biochemical markers do not have standardized values per age ranges.

There are well-established criteria for the nutritional assessment of a child without associated comorbidities, including those developed by the World Health Organization (WHO), the Center for Diseases Control and Prevention (CDC), and the National Center for Health Statistics (NCHS). All criteria assume a predictable sequence of events during nutritional deprivation beginning with weight loss and followed by linear stunting. Typical measurements use the weight–age ratio, the height–age or length–age ratio, the weight–height or length ratio and the BMI–age ratio, where:

BMI (Body Mass Index) = body weight (kg) ÷ height (m^2)

1 WHO criteria (http://www.who.int/childgrowth/standards/en/) compare the child's weight–length ratio or weight–age ratio against a population median. If the weight–height ratio is more than 2 standard deviations below the population median, the child is considered to be moderately undernourished. This standard deviation difference is defined as a Z score, which expresses how many standard deviations the child's ratio is from the population median. For instance, if the child's ratio was 3 standard deviations below the median, he or she would be considered to have a Z score of −3 indicating severe undernutrition or wasting. The presence of symmetrical edema may be additional sign of severe undernutrition under WHO criteria.

The Waterlow criteria express the child's anthropomorphic ratios as percentage of population medians determined from standard growth charts. Specifically, acute malnourishment ("wasting") is determined by the ratio of the child's *actual* weight as percentage of the *expected* weight for height, where the expected weight for height can be obtained by plotting the child's height on the 50th percentile line of the growth curve to obtain the height-age. The 50th percentile for weight at the height age is defined as the *expected* weight for height. Children whose actual weight is less than 90%, 80%, or 70% of their expected weight for height are considered to have mild, moderate, or severe acute undernutrition, respectively. Similarly, children whose height is less than 95%, 90%, or 85% of their expected height for age have mild, moderate, or severe stunting, respectively, reflecting chronic malnutrition.

Clinical circumstances and comorbidities may confound height and weight measurements. Critically ill children are usually confined to bed, and accurate height or length values may not be available. Fluid and electrolyte imbalance, renal and liver malfunction with edema and/or ascites, or tumor mass may impair the accuracy of weight measurement. This difficulty in measuring weight and height can hinder the diagnosis and management of the nutritional status using the usual ratios.

Critically ill patients may undergo an intense protein catabolic process and have changes in body composition due to loss of muscle mass and rearrangement of total body water. Therefore, measurements that define the body compartments in more detail become more important, even as prognostic indices in the assessment of this patient. In the anthropometric assessment, circumference measurements and skinfolds are simple methods to estimate the body composition, for they reflect both the fat and fat-free components. The WHO recommends the mid-upper arm circumference (MUAC) to estimate the total skeletal muscular protein. A reduced fat-free mass (FFM)/height ratio is an important predictor of increased mortality (3,6). Once again, these measurements may be less reliable in the setting of edema.

NUTRITIONAL STATES

Undernutrition

Undernutrition is common at hospital admission and tends to worsen during hospitalization. In Europe and North America, 40%–50% of hospitalized patients are at risk of malnutrition (3–5). Several studies performed in Brazil and in other countries demonstrated that malnutrition can affect 50% of children and adolescents during hospitalization, although the classical kwashiorkor presentation is rare in critically ill infants, children, and adolescents with chronic diseases such as those in ICUs (9).

In hospital, undernutrition constitutes an important risk factor for increased morbidity, mortality, length of hospital stay, and medical costs (4). Specific associations have been reported between poor nutritional status, decreased respiratory function, impaired wound healing, and immune and gastrointestinal dysfunctions (6,7,11). Hence, proper enteral or parenteral nutritional support should be provided in ill children who are unable to feed normally and who are at risk of undernutrition. To prevent undernutrition-related complications, patients should be assessed for nutritional state and risk of becoming malnourished at the time of hospital admission, and optimal nutrition must be guaranteed in ill children who are unable to feed orally. A nutritional therapeutic plan on admission is essential to ensure adequate nutritional support during the course of illness (12).

Critically ill, undernourished children are less able to handle substrate, liquid, and solute overload. The most common absorptive disturbances involve carbohydrates (particularly lactose) and fats. Reductions in cardiac output, glomerular filtration rate, renal blood flow, or renal solute excretion capacity may arise from undernutrition. Intracellular potassium and sodium pump activity is lowered. In view of these limitations, caution is urged in initial phases of treatment as excessive volume intake of water and nutrients may cause complications or death (7). Well-nourished children who are likely to return to normal feeding within 4–5 days do not generally require artificial nutritional support, whereas undernourished patients with hypermetabolism or hypercatabolism should receive treatment as swiftly as possible (8).

Starvation

Fasting (a reduction or absence of the intake of nutrition) becomes starvation when suffering or the process of perishing occurs. The physiologic changes that occur with severe malnutrition and starvation may be a result of inadequate intake of energy and basic nutrients (simple starvation) or it can be a result of increased energy expenditure (EE) unmatched by adequate intake (stress starvation). Stress starvation can develop more quickly than simple starvation (7,9,13) (**Table 97.1**).

For didactic purposes, the starvation response may be divided into three phases, although the biochemical events overlap and depend on baseline nutritional status, comorbidities, and the extent of the nutrient restriction (complete or partial). During phase I, glucose remains the primary source of energy and is produced by the breakdown of absorbed carbohydrate and glycogen stored in muscle and liver. Phase I begins after the consumed meal has been digested and the body has entered the postabsorptive phase. Glycogen stores are usually exhausted within 24 hours in young children.

During phase II, fats become the primary source of energy after glycogen stores have been depleted. Lipolysis mobilizes fat stores to release free fatty acids, which are oxidized to ketone bodies (aceto-acetate and β-hydroxybutyrate). These ketone bodies serve as an alternative source of energy for the brain in the face of limited glucose supply. Laboratory analysis reveals mild ketoacidosis at this stage. Proteolysis liberates amino acids from muscle to support gluconeogenesis and mitigate the risk of hypoglycemia. Hormonal changes including falling insulin levels and rising glucagon (and other counterregulatory hormone) levels contribute to maintenance of serum glucose levels.

If starvation continues, the fat stores become exhausted and the body enters phase III of starvation. During this phase proteins become the major source of energy. This phase is characterized by further breakdown of muscle (including cardiac muscle) in order to support gluconeogenesis, a process known as "protein wasting."

Adaption to starvation involves reducing EE by suppressing metabolic rate, body temperature, and delaying growth/reproduction (10,13). During stress starvation, the normal adaptative responses of simple starvation, which conserve body protein, are overridden by the neuroendocrine and cytokine

TABLE 97.1

SIMPLE VERSUS STRESS STARVATION

	■ SIMPLE STARVATION (>72 H)	■ STRESS STARVATION
Metabolic rate	↓	↑
Protein catabolism (relatively)	↓	↑
Protein synthesis (relatively)	↓	↑
Protein turnover	↓	↑
Nitrogen balance	↓	↓↓
Gluconeogenesis	↓	↑
Ketosis	↑↑	None
Glucose turnover	↓	↑
Blood glucose	↓	↑
Salt and water retention	?	↑↑↑
Plasma albumin	None	↓↓

effects of injury. Metabolic rate rises rather than falls, ketosis is minimal, protein catabolism accelerates to meet the demands for tissue repair and for gluconeogenesis, and there is hyperglycemia and glucose intolerance. Salt and water retention is exacerbated, and this may result in a kwashiorkor-like state with hypoalbuminaemia and edema.

Refeeding Syndrome

Refeeding syndrome (nutritional recovery syndrome) is a potentially lethal condition that can occur usually within 1–3 days after reinstitution of nutrition following 5–10 days of fasting. Patients at risk include those with severe undernutrition and anorexia nervosa. The major manifestations of refeeding syndrome include the following:

- Hypophosphatemia
- Hypokalemia
- Hypomagnesemia
- Fluid overload
- Thiamine deficiency

The pathophysiology of refeeding syndrome begins with a contraction of intracellular spaces and depletion of major intracellular ions (phosphorus, potassium, and magnesium) during starvation, yet normal serum levels are maintained (14). Refeeding of carbohydrates increases glucose levels, stimulates insulin release and induces protein, glycogen, and fat synthesis. Elevated insulin levels shift phosphorus, potassium, magnesium, and thiamine to the intracellular space. Hence serum levels of these ions may fall rapidly.

Cardiovascular manifestations of refeeding syndrome include heart failure and dysrhythmias. Preexisting cardiac atrophy from starvation exacerbated by thiamine and phosphate deficiency make the patient vulnerable to heart failure and fluid overload. Because most severely undernourished patients are bradycardic, the restoration of a "normal" heart rate may be a sign of impending heart failure.

Pulmonary complications of refeeding syndrome involve respiratory muscle weakness. A weak cough reflex leads to retained airway secretions, atelectasis, and pneumonia. Hypophosphatemia may lead to ventilatory failure.

Neurologic complications may entail seizures, delirium, and frank encephalopathy from thiamine deficiency (Wernicke's encephalopathy).

Prevention is the key to management of refeeding syndrome. Electrolytes abnormalities should be anticipated and corrected when discovered in the severely undernourished child. Nutritional supplementation (especially caloric intake from carbohydrates) should be advanced gradually. Excess fluid and sodium administration are avoided. Observation for cardiac arrhythmias is particularly important, as this is the major cause of fatalities. Vitamin supplementation (especially thiamine) should also be implemented with refeeding and continued for at least 10 days.

Hypercatabolism

A hypercatabolic state occurs in response to many clinical conditions (sepsis, trauma, burns, etc.) and is characterized by an increase in circulating catabolic hormones and inflammatory cytokines as well as insulin resistance. Hyperglycemia, glucose intolerance, and insulin resistance are common features of critically ill patients, especially in patients with sepsis or septic shock.

Nutrition in children with severe infection, trauma, or following major surgery is hampered by the hormonal and metabolic changes associated with the systemic inflammatory response (8,15,16). The systemic inflammatory response activates the sympathetic nervous system and the hypothalamic–pituitary–adrenal axis. These responses are characterized by changes in glucose and lipid metabolism, along with increased protein turnover and breakdown, which results in increased EE, a negative nitrogen balance, and muscle protein loss. Deamination of branched-chain amino acids supplies amino acids for the protein synthesis required for wound healing and the immunologic response (production of immunoglobulins and acute-phase reactants) (15,16). Peripheral resistance to insulin action ensures continued glucose production with hyperglycemia, reduced glucose oxidation, and storage as hepatic glycogen. Increased lipolysis provides free fatty acids for energy and glycerol for gluconeogenesis (16–18). Levels of catecholamines, cortisol, glucagon, growth hormone, aldosterone, and antidiuretic hormone are increased, and insulin is generally elevated but not sufficiently to impede hyperglycemia. Insulin secretion is initially suppressed by the α-adrenergic mechanism and later increased together with glucagon levels. Peripheral resistance to growth hormone action occurs, with a reduction in insulin-like growth factor (IGF)-1 secretion, while hyperglycemia and lipolytic effects remain. Increased counterregulating hormone concentrations induce insulin- and growth hormone-resistant states (a characteristic sign of stress), which results in protein catabolism and the utilization of carbohydrate and fat stores to meet the increased basal metabolic rate. All of these mechanisms constitute the interaction between the nervous, endocrine, and immunologic systems in an effort to mediate stress (19–21).

An additional pathophysiologic process is the synthesis and release of inflammatory and metabolic response mediators by monocytes (primarily Kupffer cells and alveolar macrophages). These mediators include cytokines, products of arachidonic acid metabolism, and platelet activation factors. (Interleukin 6 is an important cytokine that causes an inflammatory response and increases nutritional risk.) Acting locally or distally, they promote changes in cell function and metabolism. Such mediators also act directly on hypothalamic activity, influencing the release of classic stress hormones (9,17). Continued hypermetabolism results from complicating factors, such as hypotension or infection, leading to accelerated malnutrition and lowering of immunologic function (15,17,22).

Obesity

Childhood obesity is a public health crisis of epidemic proportions throughout the world, with an estimated prevalence of 10%–25% (23). Severe childhood obesity is defined as a body mass index (BMI) >35 kg/m². Pseudotumor cerebri, slipped capital femoral epiphysis, steatohepatitis, cholelithiasis, and sleep apnea represent some of the major comorbidities associated with severe obesity (1,24). Obese adults with severe respiratory failure have higher mortality rates (24,25). Recent data also suggest that obesity may be associated with increased mortality in critically ill children (26). Special problems for morbidly obese patients in the PICU include the following:

- Difficult airway
- Risk of gastroesophageal reflux and acid aspiration
- Obstructive sleep apnea and obstructive hypoventilation (requiring caution with use of opioids and sedative medications)
- More rapid desaturation during rapid sequence intubation (decreased functional residual capacity and increased O_2 consumption)
- Drug dosing usually based on lean body weight or ideal body weight rather than total body weight

Insulin resistance is associated with obesity and may be secondary to the presence of adipocytokines. As a result, morbidly obese patients exhibit variable glucose homeostasis including glucose intolerance, overt type II diabetes, or metabolic syndrome. Clinical clues to the presence of insulin resistance include abdominal obesity, acanthosis nigricans, hirsutism, muscle cramps, hypertension, and hypertriglyceridemia, among others.

Nutritional management of the morbidly obese patient takes into account comorbidities, special ICU problems, and insulin resistance. Excess carbohydrate administration may lead to increased CO_2 production and delayed weaning from mechanical ventilation. Insulin resistance may produce hyperglycemia, which has been associated with poor ICU outcomes. Therefore some adult studies have suggested the use of hypocaloric—high protein diets in adults with obesity (27). The goal is to avoid the complications of CO_2 retention, hyperglycemia, and fatty liver, while achieving positive nitrogen balance, which may promote wound healing. There are no randomized controlled trials on this approach in children.

NUTRITIONAL MANAGEMENT

Although some critically ill children present in a hypermetabolic state (major burns, multiple injuries, and prolonged admission), the majority have a lower EE than healthy children, particularly those receiving mechanical ventilation or sedation and muscle relaxation. The aims of nutritional therapy during critical illness are to provide fluids and nutrients in adequate quantities to maintain vital functions and homeostasis, to recover the activity of immune system, to reduce the risks of overfeeding, and to ensure an adequate supply of protein and energy sources necessary to minimize the protein catabolism and nitrogen loss. Implementation of evidence-based recommendations improved the provision of nutritional support and was associated with improved clinical outcomes (8–10,21). Conversely, several reports have shown that inadequate provision of nutrients is associated with increased physiologic instability in critically ill patients (8,22,28).

Component Requirements

An effective nutritional plan requires understanding of the individual components to be provided via the enteral or parenteral route.

Fluid Intake

Fluid requirements depend on a patient's clinical picture. Daily assessment of weight, urinary osmolality, and fluid balance provides a good estimation of hydration state. Fever, increased ambient temperature, hypermetabolism, and liquid loss through diarrhea or digestive juices all imply further water loss and call for increased water intake. A significant weight loss from one

day to the next tends to reflect abnormal liquid loss, and conversely, marked weight gain may be the result of excessive water intake or retention. Fluid losses through diarrhea or ileostomy drainage should be replaced daily. Fluid retention that stems from the changes in endothelial permeability that occurs with the systemic inflammatory response may require fluid restriction. Hypoxia and systemic hypotension may cause renal cortical or tubular necrosis, compromising renal function. In the presence of acute renal insufficiency, the volume required to supply protein-calorie needs should be administered in association with renal replacement therapy to remove excess fluid. Once the systemic inflammatory response has resolved, and if there is no further need to restrict volume, an increase of up to 50% over basal fluid requirements can be made to improve nutrient intake and promote anabolism (11,19,29–31).

Energy Intake

Adequate energy intake in critically ill children is essential to provide sufficient substrates for metabolic functions during the acute phase of the disease process, in addition to providing for growth of the child. However, excessive amounts of energy, particularly in the form of glucose, can be deleterious to the patient and can result in lipogenesis, increased respiratory quotient, increased carbon dioxide production, hepatic steatosis, and liver dysfunction. The caloric requirement for sedated infants in intensive care during acute metabolic stress is limited to that needed to reach basal metabolic rate plus a stress factor, which, depending on the clinical situation, is between 1.1 and 1.2 (18,19,30,32).

The basal metabolic rate in newborns and infants is ~50–55 kcal/kg/day and falls steadily until adolescence to 25 kcal/kg/day. This calculation represents only an estimate of energy needs, considering that the rules tend to overestimate EE and can vary by up 30% over any given 24-hour period (1,8,33).

Electrolyte Intake

In addition to meeting basal requirements, electrolyte intake must also replace abnormal losses that occur in situations associated with alterations in water and electrolytic balance, such as sepsis, malnutrition, and refeeding syndrome. Undernutrition leads to losses in intracellular potassium, magnesium, and phosphorus and increases in sodium and water. Although monitoring of sodium, potassium, and calcium serum levels is integral to routine care, too little attention has been given to phosphorus in patient follow-up. The demand for phosphorus is greater in children because it is needed for the formation of new tissues, a state that puts a critically ill patient with severe malnutrition at higher risk of developing hypophosphatemia (19,28,34,35). The recommended amounts of electrolytes by parenteral route are shown in Table 97.2.

TABLE 97.2

DAILY ELECTROLYTE REQUIREMENTS BY PARENTERAL ROUTE

■ ELECTROLYTE	■ NEONATES (mEq/kg)	■ INFANTS/CHILDREN	■ ADOLESCENTS
Sodium	2–5	2–6 mEq/kg	Individualized
Chloride	1–5	2–5 mEq/kg	Individualized
Potassium	1–4	2–3 mEq/kg	Individualized
Calcium	3–4	1–2.5 mEq/kg	10–20 mEq
Phosphorus	1–2	0.5–1 mmol/kg	10–40 mmol
Magnesium	0.3–0.5	0.3–0.5 mEq/kg	10–30 mEq

Adapted from ASPEN. Board of Directors and The Clinical Guidelines Task Force. Guidelines for the use of parenteral and enteral nutrition in adult and pediatric patients. *JPEN J Parenter Enteral Nutr* 2002;26(1):97SA–128SA.

Carbohydrate

Hydrated glucose, supplies 3.4 kcal/g and as the main source of carbohydrate in parenteral and enteral nutrition, is vital to supply the central nervous system, red blood cells, leukocytes, and renal medulla. The maximum rate of glucose that can be oxidized by adults and adolescents is 5 mg/kg/min (19).

Excessive intake of calories in the form of glucose can give rise to increased metabolic rate, hyperglycemia, and hepatic alterations. Glucose intake that exceeds 18 g/kg/day (equivalent to a 12.5 mg/kg/min infusion rate) in neonates can lead to lowered energy benefit, increased hepatic lipogenesis, and increased CO_2 production.

The glucose infusion rate in full-term newborns required to prevent hypoglycemia is between 3 and 4 mg/kg/min, and these values are generally higher in extremely premature births. Acute stress and corticosteroid therapy are conditions that call for reduced glucose intake. Hyperglycemia may trigger glycosuria (with osmotic diuresis), hamper immunologic function and healing, and may be associated with intracranial hemorrhage and worse neurologic prognosis. Should hyperglycemia occur, the cause must be treated, and the concentration or rate of glucose infusion reduced (2,18,36,37).

The role of a *tight glycemic control* regimen in which insulin administration is used to maintain serum glucose in a specified normal range (e.g., ~70–130 mg/dL) has been the subject of intense debate. Two smaller randomized controlled trials have suggested reduced morbidity or mortality with tight glycemic control compared with conventional glycemic control (e.g., serum glucose 130–200 mg/dL) in critically ill children, especially those with severe burns (38,39). However, a recent large randomized controlled trial involving 13 centers and over 1300 children with cardiac and noncardiac diagnoses failed to show a significant mortality or morbidity benefit from tight glycemic control, although hospital costs were significantly reduced in the noncardiac population undergoing tight glycemic control (40). The tight glycemic control group also experienced an increased incidence of hypoglycemia as has been demonstrated in other studies. Therefore, the current balance of the evidence appears to favor conventional glycemic control with careful monitoring of serum glucose levels to avoid hypoglycemia. The severely burned child appears to be an exception to this recommendation, where tight glycemic control with insulin administration appears to decrease the incidence of infection, sepsis, and organ dysfunction associated with the intense catabolic and inflammatory response to a burn (39).

Lipids

Lipids are the primary energy source for infants and young children. In addition to providing energy, they supply essential fatty acids and lipid-soluble vitamins required for growth and development of tissues, including the brain (30,41). Medium-chain fatty acids are a rapid source of energy. They are spontaneously hydrolyzed in the intestinal lumen, independent of pancreatic lipase and bile salts, for absorption and are not dependent on plasma binding with albumin or carnitine for use in mitochondria (21,42,43).

Fatty acids from the ω-6 and ω-3 families and their derivatives originate from linoleic acids and α-linolenic acids, respectively, and are considered vital. The ω-6 fatty acids are derived chiefly from animal and vegetable fats, while ω-3 fatty acids are found mainly in deep-water fish oil sources. Endogenous production is insufficient to ensure suitable concentrations of polyunsaturated fatty acids (PUFAs). Both ω-6 and ω-3 PUFAs are considered metabolic antagonists. The series 6 PUFA, linoleic acid (18:2 ω-6) forms ω-linoleic acid (18:3 ω-6), which converts to arachidonic acid (20:4 ω-6), which is the precursor of series 2 prostaglandins (PGE_2), thromboxane A_2 (TXA_2), and series 4 leukotrienes (LT4). These molecules are involved in inflammation, modulation of the immune system, regulation of vascular tone, and platelet aggregation. An excess of ω-6 PUFA may elevate the synthesis of proinflammatory eicosanoids, which may depress immune defense and increase the systemic inflammatory response (28,41,44).

The series 3 PUFA, α-linolenic acid (18:3 ω-3) is converted into eicosapentaenoic acid (20:5 ω-3) and docosahexaenoic acid (22:6 ω-3), which are precursors of series 3 prostaglandins (PGE_3), thromboxane A_3 (TXA_3), and series 5 leukotrienes (LT5). Series 3 PUFAs play a key role during pregnancy and in the growth and development of a child in the first years of life. Docosahexaenoic acid, in particular, is incorporated into the brain of the fetus from the first 3 months of pregnancy to the 8th month of postnatal life. As neonates are unable to fully synthesize docosahexaenoic and arachidonic acids from their precursors, these fatty acids must be present in their diet. The ω-3 PUFAs possess few inflammatory properties compared with ω-6 PUFAs, but they inhibit production of inflammatory eicosanoids and decrease production of inflammatory cytokines, providing potential benefit in chronic disease and during the acute stress response (28,41,43,44). Infant diets should supply 30% of energy in lipid form, where 1%–2% of energy intake is derived from linoleic acid and 0.5% is derived from α-linolenic acid (41).

Amino Acids

The hypercatabolic state of injury or sepsis is characterized by a marked negative nitrogen balance. It has been reported that increasing the nitrogen intake in septic adult patients results in an increased nitrogen balance over a wide range of nitrogen intakes. There are limited data with regard to total protein intake in critically ill children, with only a few studies in the literature in the pediatric burn or surgical populations. Higher protein intakes in critically ill children were recommended on the basis of a higher protein turnover in this population when compared with healthy children whose requirements ranged between 1 and 3.5 g/kg/day (1,2,19).

Estimates of protein requirements should be made on an individual basis, as these may differ according to the child's age, clinical condition, intake of energy and other nutrients, and quality of the protein given. Protein needs using the parenteral route are lower than through the enteral route: 2.5–3.0 g/kg/day of parenteral protein promotes nitrogen retention in newborns and in young infants. Emphasis is generally given to growth in planning protein intake, provided the patient is relatively metabolically stable. However, in hypercatabolic patients, the goal of protein administration is to minimize the effects of nitrogen loss, partially offsetting protein catabolism, thereby calling for different amino acid needs. Increased protein intake does not lower catabolism, nor does it reverse the endocrine alterations that caused it; however, a positive nitrogen balance is needed to enable return to anabolism (17,19,28,45).

Parenteral protein needs also vary according to age. Recommended intakes are 2.5–3 g/kg/day for neonates, 2–2.5 g/kg/day for infants, 1–1.2 g/kg/day for older children, and 0.8–1 g/kg/day for adolescents. The proportion of protein as caloric source should represent 8%–15% of total energy intake, attaining 20% or more in hypercatabolic states (19).

Incorporation of protein depends on adequate intake of all essential and nonessential amino acids and intake of nitrogen to synthesize it; it also depends on the minimum quantity of nonprotein energy, equivalent to 25 kcal for every gram of amino acid. To promote anabolism, the nitrogen:nonprotein calorie ratio must lie between 1:150 and 1:250 (between 1:90 and 1:150 in hypercatabolism). One gram of protein provides 4 kcal; 1 g of protein corresponds to 0.16 g of nitrogen, or 1 g nitrogen is contained in 6.25 g of protein (19,46).

Clinical situations associated with hypercatabolism should be monitored for specific amino acid deficits in which patients can benefit from selective administration. Under these conditions, certain amino acids deemed nonessential may be considered *conditionally indispensable*. In this context, L-glutamine is the amino acid which has been most investigated (47,48).

Micronutrient Intake

Micronutrients act as cofactors in metabolic processes and in the elimination of oxygen-free radicals. Besides increasing utilization of micronutrients, critical illness may affect micronutrient metabolism through (a) reduced intestinal absorption; (b) loss of water-soluble micronutrients (diarrhea, tubes, fistula, dialysis) and increased utilization on the extreme end of the scale, resulting in marked losses in zinc, copper, and selenium; and (c) intracellular release and excretion in urine, especially zinc, secondary to increased tissue protein turnover (especially in skeletal muscle), which occurs in the acute-phase response. Scant information is available regarding the needs, bioavailability, and efficacy of micronutrient supplementation during metabolic stress (49). Most recommendations tend to be based on the needs of stable children and do not pertain to disease (**Tables 97.3** and **97.4**).

Plasma zinc concentrations are low in critically ill children. Plasma zinc can be correlated with measures of inflammation

(C-reactive protein and interleukin-6), and low plasma zinc concentrations can be associated with the degree of organ failure. Zinc is a very important micronutrient and more data are necessary with larger studies of shifts in plasma zinc concentrations in critically children to potentially identify patients who might benefit from zinc supplementation (50,51).

Prior malnutrition, drug use, acute and chronic disease, surgery, trauma, and anabolism increase micronutrient requirements. Actual needs of each patient cannot be determined, and although formulas for IV use are generally adequate, some may be lacking in certain nutrients such as zinc and water-soluble vitamins. Additional intake is likely needed during the anabolic period following hypercatabolic states. In the absence of consensus on the supplementary quantities needed during stress, administration at normally recommended levels for IV use is indicated (19,52).

Recent studies have demonstrated that enteral zinc supplementation could have a benefit in immunocompromised, long-stay intensive care patients (age 1–17 years) to prevent sepsis (20 mg/day) or that zinc could be given as adjunct treatment to reduce the risk of antibiotic treatment failure in infants aged 7–120 days with serious bacterial infection (10 mg/day) (50,51).

TABLE 97.3

DAILY TRACE ELEMENT REQUIREMENTS BY PARENTERAL ROUTE

ELEMENT	NEWBORNS (mcg/kg)		<5 Y (mcg/kg)	OLDER CHILDREN AND ADOLESCENTS
	■ PRETERM	■ FULL TERM		
Zinc	400	300	100	2–5 mg
Copper	20	20	20	200–500 mcg
Selenium	2.0	2.0	2–3	30–40 mcg
Chromium	0.20	0.20	0.14–0.2	5–15 mcg
Manganese	1.0	1.0	2–10	50–150 mcg
Iodine	1.0	1.0	1.0	–

Adapted from Greene HL, Hambidge K, Schanler R, et al. Guidelines for the use of vitamins, trace elements, calcium, magnesium and phosphorus in infants and children receiving total parenteral nutrition: Report of the Subcommittee on Clinical Practice Issues of the American Society for Clinical Nutrition. *Am J Clin Nutr* 1988;48:1324–42.

TABLE 97.4

DAILY VITAMIN REQUIREMENTS BY PARENTERAL ROUTE

■ VITAMIN	■ PRETERM INFANTS (kg/body weight)	■ CHILDREN AND FULL-TERM INFANTS (Total Dose)
A (UI)	1640	2300
E (mg)	2.8	7
K (mcg)	80	200
D (UI)	160	400
C (mg)	25	80
Thiamin (mg)	0.35	1.2
Riboflavin (mg)	0.15	1.4
Pyridoxine (mg)	0.18	1.0
Niacin (mg)	6.8	17
Pantothenic acid (mg)	2.0	5
Biotin (mcg)	6.0	20
Folate (mcg)	56	140
B_{12} (mcg)	0.3	1.0
Vitamin K (mcg)	–	200
Carnitine (mg)	20	2–10 mg/kg/d

Adapted from Greene HL, Hambidge K, Schanler R, et al. Guidelines for the use of vitamins, trace elements, calcium, magnesium and phosphorus in infants and children receiving total parenteral nutrition: Report of the Subcommittee on Clinical Practice Issues of the American Society for Clinical Nutrition. *Am J Clin Nutr* 1988;48:1324–42.

NUTRITIONAL THERAPY

Enteral Nutrition

In critically ill children, nutritional treatment must be oriented to deliver substrates that favor the maintenance of organ function and recovery from disease. The enteral route is preferable as it prevents intestinal atrophy and reduces infectious complications when compared with parenteral nutrition. It is also less expensive and provides a corresponding reduction in hospital costs. Most studies have shown that enteral nutrition in critically ill children is well tolerated and presents a minimal risk of complications. A historic cohort study that spanned a 12-year period reported an increase in enteral feeding and a decrease in parenteral nutrition use when promoted by an ongoing education program in nutrition support (chiefly when the nutrition-support team began to assume responsibility for the nutrition support). Those infants who received enteral nutrition for longer periods during hospitalization presented an 83% lower risk of death (5,10,34,53).

Enteral nutrition is indicated in children who have a viable gastrointestinal tract and when oral intake is either not possible or is insufficient to meet the nutritional needs of the patient. In this context, conditions that justify the enteral route include prematurity, mechanical pulmonary ventilation, severe malnutrition, hypermetabolic states, and neurologic diseases. The best point in time at which to begin enteral nutrition is also a question of debate. Critically ill children are particularly vulnerable to the effects of fasting and prolonged stress as they have a lower percentage of muscle and fat and higher basal energy requirements than do adults. The majority of critically ill children tolerate early enteral nutrition well with no increase in complications. Enteral intake of a high percentage of prescribed dietary energy goal was associated with improved 60-day survival (19,34,53–55). It would therefore appear reasonable to recommend that critically ill children not be kept fasting for more than 24–48 hours. However, many critically ill children start nutrition too late and do not receive the prescribed energy delivery, usually because of the need for fluid restriction, interruptions due to procedures, poor tolerance, or mechanical problems (the tube becomes obstructed or dislodged).

Parameters that indicate adequate intestinal function are the presence of bowel sounds, absent abdominal distension or vomiting, and a small quantity of gastric residue. As measurement of blood perfusion from the digestive tract using gastric tonometry is not routinely performed, signs of adequate intestinal perfusion in the critical patient include stabilized vital signs, no continuous requirement for administration of fluid volume or vasoactive drugs, and a normalized acid–base balance and serum lactate. The use of vasopressor agents and neuromuscular blockers are not an obstacle to use enteral nutrition in the majority of the patients in the PICU. Enteral nutrition intolerance can be a sign of intestinal hypoperfusion. However, retrospective data suggest that most (70%) of critically ill children tolerate enteral feeding while receiving cardiovascular drugs for hemodynamic support (56). Those patients who do not tolerate sufficient feeding volume through the enteral route may benefit from a combination of parenteral and enteral nutrition. This kind of treatment increases protein and energy intakes, promotes protein anabolism in critically ill infants in the first days after admission. Since this is an important target of nutritional support, increased protein and energy intakes by a combination of routes can be useful in select patients (22,55,57–59).

Selection of the most suitable diet to meet the patient's needs requires knowledge of the formula composition, as well as of possible alterations in the physiologic processes of digestion and absorption secondary to the disease. The following items should be considered regarding the patient: digestive and absorptive capacity of the gastrointestinal tract; specific nutritional needs, which differ depending on the patient's clinical picture; and the need for fluid or electrolyte restriction (42,60). With regard to the formula, the degree of absorption is determined by the form and concentration of each nutrient (e.g., whole or hydrolyzed protein, lactose, or glucose polymers). Severity and variability of disease dictate the metabolic and nutritional profile of each patient, with each case requiring a specific formulation. A number of diets for special situations have osmolarity levels and concentrations of electrolytes that are formulated for use in adults and are excessive for children due to the risk of diarrhea and hypertonic dehydration (34,42,54,55). The main pediatric enteral feeding formulas with their indications and contraindications are listed in **Table 97.5**.

Another key factor is that high-osmolarity formulas may cause diarrhea when administered through duodenal or jejunal routes. The American Academy of Pediatrics recommends that osmolarity of infant formulas for oral or intragastric administration be <460 mOsm/kg (1,34,42). We suggest the use of formulas with osmolarity of 300–310 mOsm/kg for duodenal or jejunal administration.

Human milk is indicated as the exclusive food source in infants up to 6 months of age. After 6 months, solid foods can be introduced, and breast milk is continued up to at least the age of 12 months or older. Contraindications of breastfeeding are (a) maternal infections caused by microorganisms transmittable through maternal milk, (b) inborn errors of metabolism or other conditions that cause intolerance to the components of human milk (e.g., galactosemia or tyrosinemia), and (c) maternal exposure to foods, drugs, or environmental agents that, when excreted by human milk, can harm the infant. Infant formulas are recommended in situations where human breastmilk is precluded.

Cow's milk-based formulas fulfill the nutrient needs of healthy children when used exclusively up to the age of 4–6 months. (The American Academy of Pediatrics recommends avoiding an unmodified cow's milk diet in infants <12 months of age because of the increased renal solute load and the risk of iron-deficiency anemia.) Their main carbohydrate source, as in maternal milk, is lactose and the caloric density of infant formula is 0.67 kcal/mL (the same as human milk) (1,42). Protein levels in infant formula are generally 1.5 times that of maternal milk but the ratio of whey protein to casein is 60:40 (similar to human milk). The main whey protein in the formulas is β-lactoglobulin, whereas in human milk, it is α-lactalbumin. In the preparation process, cow's milk is substituted with polyunsaturated vegetable fat, which improves digestibility and increases the concentration of essential fatty acids. Some amino acids, such as taurine are added, as well as micronutrients such as iron. Cow's milk formulas can be used as a substitute or supplement for maternal milk in children whose mothers are not breastfeeding (or do not do so exclusively), as a substitute in children for whom breast-feeding is contraindicated, and as a supplement for breast-fed children with insufficient weight gain (1).

Soy-based formulas are indicated for children with cow's-milk protein or lactose intolerance. In term infants, soy formulas promote growth and bone mineralization to the same degree as cow's milk-based formulas. They are milk free and have sucrose and hydrolyzed starch carbohydrates. They contain minerals and vitamins in greater quantities than milk-based formulas to compensate for the presence of possible mineral absorption antagonists such as soy phytates (1).

Protein hydrolysate formulas are processed by enzymatic hydrolysis of different protein sources, such as bovine casein/whey and soy. The hydrolysate consists of free amino acids, dipeptides, and tripeptides that do not require additional digestion. These formulas are lactose free, their carbohydrate source can be tapioca starch, corn syrup, or corn starch. Fats are provided by a blend of medium- and long-chain triglycerides in varying amounts.

TABLE 97.5

ENTERAL FEEDING: FORMULAS, INDICATIONS, AND CONTRAINDICATIONS

■ FORMULA	■ INDICATIONS	■ CONTRAINDICATIONS
Cow's milk-based formulas, iron-fortified	Healthy term infants	Cow's milk protein intolerance; lactose intolerance
Cow's milk-based, lactose-free formulas	Lactase deficiency/lactose intolerance	Cow's milk protein intolerance; galactosemia (enough galactose remains)
Cow's milk-based, low mineral/ electrolyte formula	Hypocalcemia/hyperphosphatemia renal disease	Cow's milk protein intolerance (Note: This is a low-iron formula; iron should be supplied from other sources)
Cow's milk-based, high (86%) medium-chain-triglyceride formula	Severe fat malabsorption, chylothorax	Monitor for signs of essential fatty acid deficiency if used for prolonged periods
Cow's milk-based follow-up formula	Older infants who are eating solid foods	No advantage over breast-feeding or standard infant formula for the first year of life (according to the American Academy of Pediatrics)
Soy-based formula (milk-free, lactose-free)	Galactosemia; hereditary or transient lactase deficiency; documented IgE-mediated allergy to cow's milk; vegetarian-based diet	Birth weight <800 g Prevention of colic or allergy Cow's milk protein-induced enterocolitis or enteropathy
Soy-based formula with fiber	Diarrhea	Constipation
Casein-hydrolysate formulas	Allergies; intact protein sensitivity	Note: Infants with severe cow's milk protein allergies may react to whey protein hydrolysate formula
Amino acid-based	Malabsorption due to gastrointestinal or hepatobiliary disease and not responsive to hydrolyzed protein formulas	
Human milk fortifiers	Preterm/low-birth-weight infants	Fortifiers are low in iron; additional iron should be supplied from other sources
Preterm formulas	Preterm/low-birth-weight infants	
Preterm discharge formulas	Former preterm/low-birth-weight infants from hospital discharge through 9 mo of age	

Adapted from ASPEN. Board of Directors and The Clinical Guidelines Task Force. Guidelines for the use of parenteral and enteral nutrition in adult and pediatric patients. *JPEN J Parenter Enteral Nutr* 2002;26(1):97SA–128SA.

Protein hydrolysates are recommended for children who are intolerant to whole-milk formulas because of decreased intestinal length, absorptive capacity, or pancreatic or hepatobiliary diseases. These formulas might be considered during the systemic inflammatory response, when alterations in permeability and reduction of the absorptive surface of the intestinal epithelium take place (1,31). No pediatric studies are available that compare whole diets (breast milk, cow formula, or soy formula) with partially digested formulas in relation to ICU outcomes. The studies that do exist were conducted in heterogeneous adult groups and show no evidence of major favorable clinical outcome associated with their use. Unfortunately, they do not take into account the nutritional status of the patients, which represents an important factor for increased intestinal permeability (11).

Amino acid–based formulas (elemental formulas) are indicated for patients who have protein hypersensitivity unresponsive to hydrolyzed protein formulas (1,19).

Immune-enhancing formulas. The terms immunonutrition and pharmaconutrition have become widespread in recent years. These terms refer to the concept that nutrition provides not only energy substrates but also substances that are lacking in the critically ill and/or that modify the inflammatory and immune responses. Studies have demonstrated immunostimulating properties of nutrients, such as glutamine, arginine, ω-3 chain fatty acids, probiotics, nucleic acids, and antioxidants, used in conjunction or separately in critically ill patients (61,62). Given the higher cost of these diets, both safety and cost benefits have been considered in a few studies that reveal conflicting results. Although immunonutrition may reduce the rate of infectious complications in trauma and perioperative

adult patients, a clear position on its effectiveness has yet to be established. One pediatric-blinded design study demonstrated a decrease in morbidity associated with immunonutrition but no effect on mortality or length of stay (54). The possibility that immunonutrition may be harmful to some critically ill patients is raised by a randomized trial with higher mortality in adults who received enteral immunonutrition compared with standard nutrition (63). It has been suggested that overstimulation of the inflammatory response by an immune-enhancing diet can be harmful for the critically ill (63). Given the potential risk of harm reported and the fact that these formulas have not been designed according to pediatric standards, their use is not currently recommended in critically ill children (62).

Method of enteral feeding. Gastric feeding is more physiologic than *postpyloric feeding* (duodenal or jejunal) and easier to access, but may be limited by intolerance due to gastric dysfunction and excessive residual volumes. Postpyloric feeding may help to overcome these problems and avoid feeding interruptions and reduce aspiration risks. Routine placement of a nasojejunal tube when a reduced gastric residual volume is evidenced, but is not recommended. Studies have shown that the incidence of pneumonia, hospitalization time, mortality, and energy delivery are similar in patients with gastric or jejunal tube (64). In children and adolescents, even those on mechanical ventilation, it is common to use the gastric route for administration of enteral nutrition (59). Transpyloric (ideally jejunal) continuous feeding may be employed in children who do not tolerate gastric feedings or are at risk for aspiration (65). Careful patient selection, a team specializing in this task, and institutional protocols are recommended (**Fig. 97.1**).

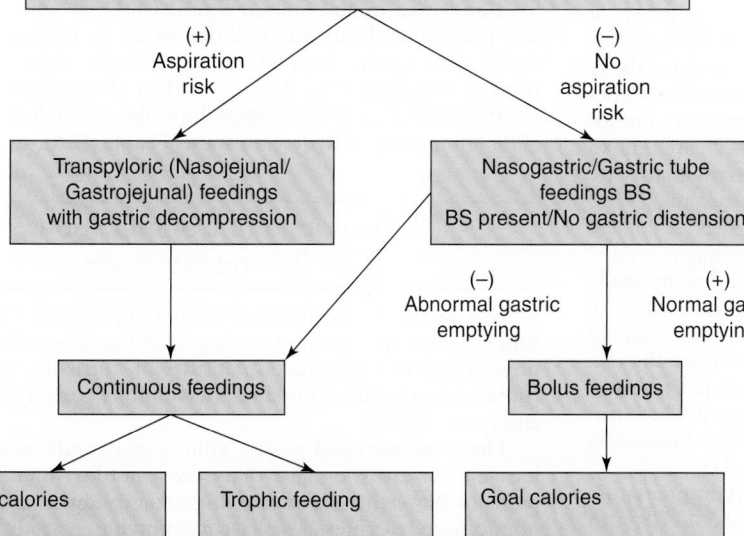

Oral route unavailable
or
unable to protect airway

Nutrition assessment, weight on admission
identify caloric goal[5]

Head of bed elevated 30° unless contraindicated[7]

Evaluate for risk of aspiration[7]
(Depressed gag/cough, altered sensorium, delayed gastric emptying,
GE reflux, severe bronohospasm, history of reflux)

(+)
Aspiration
risk

(−)
No
aspiration
risk

Transpyloric (Nasojejunal/
Gastrojejunal) feedings
with gastric decompression

Nasogastric/Gastric tube
feedings BS
BS present/No gastric distension

(−)
Abnormal gastric
emptying

(+)
Normal gastric
emptying

Continuous feedings

Bolus feedings

Goal calories

Start: 1–2 mL/kg/h
(max 25 mL/h)
(or 0.5 mL/kg/h if risk
of gut ischemia)

Advance:
<1 y: 1–5 mL/h q 4 h
>1 y: 5–20 mL/h q 4 h
until goal reached.

Trophic feeding

1–2 mL/kg/h
or
20 mL/h

Full-strength formula
or breast milk

Goal calories

Start: 1/2 Goal volume
(Full-strength feeding
volume required to reach
caloric goal). Bolus
feedings divided q 3 h
(if < 6 mo) or
q 4 h (if > 6 mo of age).

*If volume intolerant, try
smaller volumes more
frequently or continuous
feedings.*

Advance: Increase
each feeding by 25%
volume until goal
reached.

Constipation

(For age >1 mo/nonneutropenic)
No stool after 48 h of enema

Day#1
Prune juice

Day#2
Glycerin supp.

Docusate
(<3 y: PO 10 mg BID)
(3–6 y: PO 20 mg BID)
(6–12 y: PO 50 mg BID)
(≥12 y: PO 100 mg BID)

Senna (Discontinue after 2 normal
stools)
(1 mo–2 y: PO 2.5 mL BID)
(2–5 y: PO 3.75 mL BID)
(5–12 y: PO 7.5 mL BID)
((≥12 y: PO 1 Tab BID)

Fleet enema (for age > 2 y)
- Pediatric fleets enema: 2–12 y
  (66 mL/bottle)1 enema
- Adult fleet enema: ≥12 y

Diarrhea
(>4 Loose stools/24 h)

Discontinue laxatives (senna) and
stool softeners (docusate)

Discontinue any sorbitol-containing
medication

Review osrnolarity of formula

Consider withdrawal from opiates

Consider change in formula, or hold
tube feedings until diarrhea resolves

Stool viral studies/*Clostridia (C.)
difficile*

Stool *C. difficile* toxin and culture
(if on antimicrobials).

Enteral feeding intolerance
Gastric residual volumes (GRV) recorded prior to each bolus feed or q 4 h in patients on
continuous gastric feedings with abdominal discomfort, distension or emesis.

If GRV > 150 mL; or 5 mL/kg, or > 1/2 volume of previous feeding; or > total 2 hourly infusion
rate in patients on continuous feeding–hold feedings and repeat GRV after 2 h. If repeat GRV
is elevated, hold feedings and monitor GRV of 4 h.

If abdominal distension, (abdominal girth increased for 2 consecutive measurements)
or abdominal discomfort or emesis × 2–hold feedings for 4 h and reassess.

FIGURE 97.1. Enteral nutrition support algorithm. GE, gastroesophageal; BS, bowel sounds; EN, enteral nutrition; PO, per oral; BID, twice daily; q, every. (From Mehta NM. Approach to enteral feeding in the PICU. *Nutr Clin Pract* 2009;24(3):377–87.)

Enteral Nutrition for Premature Newborns

In feeding premature infants, it should be considered that immaturity of digestive function, increased growth rate, and limited energy reserves make this group particularly sensitive to overfeeding. Nutrition through enteral tube feeding using expressed breast milk from the baby's mother has obvious benefits over formula and is associated with a lower risk of necrotizing enteritis and death. The use of supplements to maternal milk has been recommended in very-low-birth-weight (VLBW) premature newborns because increased calcium, phosphorus, proteins, and caloric content allows for greater weight gain (28,66).

Enteral fasting may diminish the functional adaptation of the immature gastrointestinal tract and prolong the need for parenteral nutrition with its attendant infectious and metabolic risks. Early trophic feeding, giving infants very small volumes of milk during the first week after birth, may promote intestinal maturation, enhance feeding tolerance and decrease time to reach full enteral feeding. Growth-restricted preterm infants are at increased risk of developing necrotizing enterocolitis (NEC) and initiation of enteral feeding is frequently delayed. There is no evidence that this delay is beneficial and it might further compromise nutrition and growth (28,34,66). Recent study demonstrated that the early introduction of enteral feeding in growth-restricted, preterm infants results in earlier achievement of full enteral feeding and does not appear to increase the risk of NEC (67). When use of maternal breast milk is not possible, a special formula for preterm newborns may be used. These formulas have added nutrients but lack the digestion facilitators and protective factors present in maternal milk (42).

Low duodenal lipase and biliary acid activity in premature neonates reduce absorption of fats ingested to 65%–70%. In this respect, maternal milk is particularly advantageous because it contains its own lipase, which aids triglyceride digestion. Medium-chain triglycerides (MCTs) are added to formulas for premature infants in an attempt to reverse the tendency of poor fat absorption. To compensate for lower carbohydrate absorption and digestion that result from lactase deficiency, these formulas, in addition to lactose, also contain additional glucose polymer, given that active transport of monosaccharides by intestinal mucous is present in premature infants (28,66).

Premature infants, due to their needs for higher quantities of protein and owing to their limited metabolizing capacity, run the risk of developing uremia, metabolic acidosis, and neurologic disturbances if protein intake exceeds metabolic capacity. Formulas for premature infants contain greater protein levels than do term infant formulas (up to 3 g/100 kcal). These formulas specifically contain higher amounts of cysteine because premature infants are enzymatically immature and poorly convert methionine into cysteine, making this amino acid conditionally essential. Calcium, phosphorus, and vitamin D are also present in greater concentrations in these formulas, allowing for higher bone incorporation and rates of bone mineralization similar to those in intra-uterine life. Due to their raised concentrations of protein and minerals, these formulas exert a higher renal solute load than do formulas for term newborns. Formulas developed for premature infants yield higher calorie (0.81 kcal/mL), protein, vitamin, and mineral levels, along with lower lactose levels than do formulas for term children. Use of these formulas in indicated up to the postnatal age of 9 months (1).

Enteral Nutrition for Children Aged 1–10 Years

With energy density of 1 kcal/mL, formulas for children aged 1–10 years vary in osmolarity from 300 to 650 mOsm/L and are lactose free. Vitamin and trace elements can be met with a total intake of 950–2000 mL. Patients with fluid restriction may require vitamin and trace element supplementation. Isotonic formulas are preferred for pediatric patients because they allow transpyloric tube feeding (1). Formulas for transpyloric administration usually have a osmolarity of 300–310 mOsm/kg.

Enteral Nutrition for Children Older than 10 Years

These patients can be fed adult formulas, formulas not suitable for younger children because of the elevated renal solute load and inadequate vitamin levels. Children whose calorie and protein needs are elevated due to severe trauma or burn injury may receive high-nitrogen and high-calorie formulations (1.5 kcal/mL) (1). Because of their elevated protein and electrolyte levels, the use of these formulas in children requires close monitoring of hydration status (**Table 97.5**).

Difficulties and Complications with Enteral Nutrition

Enteral nutrition can present a number of practical difficulties. Initial delays are common, owing to reduced bowel motility, prescription of inadequate quantities of nutrients, and interruptions as a result of nursing interventions or delayed gastric emptying (57,68).

The total aspirated gastric volume is considered a simple measure for assessing gastrointestinal motility in critically ill patients. Nevertheless, increased gastric residual volume may not accurately express low gastric emptying. A study in adult patients compared data on gastric residual volume with clinical and radiologic evidence of gastroparesis and found no correlation among the variables (59). High residual volume is not necessarily indicative of intolerance; conversely, low residual volume does not indicate tolerance. The main causes and examples of gastrointestinal intolerance are shown in **Table 97.6**.

The general incidence of diarrhea in children in the PICU ranges from 35% to 63%, but in one pediatric study, the incidence was reported as only 5.6%. Diarrhea has been attributed to a series of factors such as food osmolarity, formula type, low serum albumin concentration, and medication interactions (69). Some guidelines for enteral nutrition in hospitalized adults note that simultaneous use of some medications, particularly antibiotics, is often the cause of diarrhea in enteral nutrition (19). These guidelines recommend to reduce the suppression of gastric acidity and provide interruption of feeding, which allows pH to fall and helps to prevent bacterial overgrowth. It has also been suggested that, occasionally, a fiber-containing formula may improve enteral nutrition-related diarrhea. The most frequent mechanical, gastrointestinal, and metabolic complications, along with their probable causes and corresponding treatments are summarized in **Tables 97.7, 97.8, and 97.9**, respectively (34).

Complications may also occur with enteral nutrition and concomitant medication use. Some medications can be incompatible with enteral diets and others may cause tube blockage when given in parallel.

Parenteral Nutrition

Parenteral nutrition aims to restore or maintain nutritional status while promoting growth and is indicated when the gastrointestinal tract is compromised by disease or treatment or when the enteral route alone is unable to meet nutritional needs. Previously well-nourished patients without likelihood of

TABLE 97.6

CAUSES OF GASTROINTESTINAL INTOLERANCE

■ CAUSE	■ EXAMPLES
Site and speed of nutrition delivery	High delivery speed, postpyloric feeding
Diet type	Low fiber content, high-osmolarity
Drug-related	Laxatives, antibiotics, proton pump inhibitors, nonsteroidal anti-inflammatory drugs, medications that contain magnesium, antihypertensives
Infectious	Contaminated food, excessive bacterial growth in the small bowel, *Clostridium difficile*
Lactose deficiency	Primary and secondary
Poor fat absorption	Pancreatic dysfunction, hepatic disease, celiac disease

TABLE 97.7

MECHANICAL COMPLICATIONS OF ENTERAL NUTRITION

■ COMPLICATION	■ PROBABLE CAUSE	■ PREVENTION
Tube blockage	Failure to regularly irrigate tube	Flush tube with water after each diet infusion
	Medication administration via tube	Use medications in liquid form and flush tube with water following administration of medicines
	Fiber-rich diet	Use a 10-caliber tube to infuse fiber-rich diets
Pulmonary aspiration	Reduction in protective reflexes of airways, gastric atonia, ileum, badly placed tube	Choose postpyloric route in patient with reduced level of consciousness or who is on mechanical ventilation. Infuse diet slowly with child in elevated decubitus position; monitor gastric residue
Poor or shifted-tube position	Incorrect insertion technique; coughing or vomiting	Correct tube insertion technique; monitor position daily
Accidental tube withdrawal	Agitated patient; inadequate affixation	Correct tube attachment; monitor constantly, sedate when necessary

TABLE 97.8

GASTROINTESTINAL COMPLICATIONS OF ENTERAL NUTRITION

■ COMPLICATION	■ PROBABLE CAUSE	■ PREVENTION/TREATMENT
Diarrhea	Overly fast infusion	↓ infusion speed
	High-osmolarity diet	↑ dilution or change of formula
	Lactose intolerance	Use lactose-free formula
	Formula with high lipid level	↓ level of fat in the diet
	Food intolerance	Use hydrolyzed protein formula
	Medicines (metoclopramide, aminophylline, erythromycin, sorbitol, xylitol, magnesium, phosphorus)	Do not use antidiuretics; consider vancomycin or metronidazole orally. Avoid medicine administration via tube
	Change in intestinal flora due to antibiotic therapy	Aseptic preparation and administration technique; infusion flask must not remain exposed to ambient temperature for >8 h
	Bacterial and diet contamination	Choose ready diets and closed infusion systems
Abdominal distension	Use of antacids and antibiotics, overly fast infusion; hypertonic formula or with high fat level, narcotic use, ileum	Consider suspending drugs ↓ flow or volume of infusion; consider formula change; review use of drugs causing gastric atonia
Nausea and vomiting	Multifactorial	↓ flow; consider change of formula; exclude infectious process
Intestinal obstipation	Diet poor in residues; dehydration	Consider fiber-rich diet; maintain adequate hydration

receiving effective enteral nutrition in 5–7 days are candidates for parenteral nutrition. It is recommended that commencement of parenteral nutrition not be delayed beyond 48 hours in severely malnourished patients or neonates who are not receiving enteral nutrition, provided they are hemodynamically and metabolically stable. In this context, parenteral nutrition should be used mainly in chronically malnourished patients, in those at risk of malnutrition due to acute disease or postsurgical complications, in those with syndromes of poor intestinal absorption, and in premature neonates (10,19,28,35).

METABOLIC COMPLICATIONS OF ENTERAL NUTRITION

■ COMPLICATION	■ PROBABLE CAUSE	■ PREVENTION/TREATMENT
Hyperglycemia	Metabolic stress	↓ infusion rate; monitor glycosuria and glycemia
Dehydration	High-osmolarity diets, inadequate liquid intake	Monitor electrolytes, urea, hematocrit ↓ protein intake ↑ liquid intake
Hypokalemia	Anabolism and intake shortage; losses through diarrhea, digestive juices, or diuretic use	Frequent monitoring of potassium
Hyperkalemia	Renal insufficiency; metabolic acidosis	↓ potassium intake, treat underlying cause
Hypernatremia	Hypertonic formulas; inadequate liquid intake	Consider formula change ↑ liquid intake
Hypophosphatemia	Refeeding of the severely malnourished; use of antacids	Frequent monitoring of phosphate
Hypercapnia	Hypercaloric diet with high level of carbohydrates in patients with respiratory insufficiency	↑ proportion of lipids as caloric source

Parenteral nutrition is much more costly than enteral nutrition and is subject to complications. Therefore, in addition to considering the cost–benefit ratio, proper implementation should also consider assessment and monitoring of nutritional and metabolic needs, access route, and formulation (5).

Nutritional need is the main factor that determines access route, with preference given to the peripheral venous route when use will be <2 weeks. Usually, peripheral veins can support solutions with glucose concentrations of up to 12.5%. This glucose concentration limit does not take into account solution osmolarity and is valid for solutions that contain glucose and electrolytes in quantities equivalent to basal needs (19,30,48,70).

In parenteral nutrition solutions, amino acids, electrolytes, and glucose contribute to the final osmolarity of the solution. Concentrations of glucose higher than 8% generally have osmolarity of >600 mOsm/L, independent of amino acid concentration. In the case of intermediate concentrations between 6% and 8%, raised osmolarities are found when amino acid concentrations are ≥10%. Notably, even infusions of solutions with osmolarity of ~600 mOsm/L have been associated with thrombophlebitis in peripheral veins (48,71).

Infusion time is another factor to be considered. Data from an experimental study in which parenteral nutrition solutions with increasing osmolarities were given suggest that vein tolerance of increased osmolarity lessens with increased infusion time (71). The tolerated osmolarity by normal-flow peripheral veins was 820 mOsm/kg for 8 hours, 690 mOsm/kg for 12 hours, and 550 mOsm/kg for 24 hours. Superficial peripheral veins, due to their low flow, are prone to sclerosis or phlebitis during hypertonic solution infusion, as well as leakage of solution and consequent injury to the subcutaneous tissue. High-osmolarity solutions should be administrated through a central vein (48,70).

The osmolarity of the parenteral nutrition solution must be known prior to administration, particularly when the solution is suspected to be hypertonic. The formula below has been validated for estimating parenteral nutrition osmolarity in children (72).

$$\text{Osmolarity (mOsm/L)} = (A \times 8) + (G \times 7) + (Na \times 2) + (P \times 0.2) - 50$$

where A = amino acids (mg/L), G = glucose (g/L), Na = sodium (mEq/L), P = phosphorus (mg/L). This formula is useful in cases in which the final glucose concentrations is >7% or when it is <7% and aminoacids are >10%, conditions that do not guarantee a final solution osmolarity of <600 mOsm/L. Those children unable to receive nutrition through the enteral

route for 2 weeks or more and whose needs cannot be met by the peripheral route must receive parenteral nutrition in a central vein. To lower the risk of phlebitis secondary to parenteral nutrition, solutions with osmolarity >600 mOsm/L should be administered in a central vein (48).

IV lipid emulsions are very important and can ensure provision of essential fatty acids and allow caloric intake to be increased without the need or inconvenience of greater glucose intake. Conventional lipid emulsions are essentially composed of soybean oil and phospholipids from egg yolk and are available in 10% and 20% concentrations. They contain excessive quantities of PUFAs (55% linoleic and 9% linolenic acids) and insufficient amounts of α-tocopherol. They also contain long-chain triglycerides (LCTs) or a mixture of these with MCTs in equal ratio, which speeds lipid metabolization. Emulsions of 20% concentrations are more easily cleared in patients receiving high doses of lipids, an advantage over lower-concentration emulsions. Two other types of emulsions have become available: the first is an olive oil– and soy oil–based emulsion, which, by virtue of its predominantly monounsaturated fatty acid makeup (80% olive oil), is less subject to lipid peroxidation; the second contains a soy oil and olive oil mix, with MCTs in fish oil that contains the ω-3 eicosapentaenoic and docosahexaenoic acids, with a lower ω-6/ω-3 ratio. It is enriched with α-tocopherol to inhibit lipid peroxidation in cell membranes due to high levels of long-chain PUFAs. This lipid emulsion, besides being a source of energy and essential fatty acids, also has a beneficial effect in reducing inflammation and modulating the immune system, given its balanced level of ω-6 and ω-3 fatty acids (44). With a lower proportion of PUFAs, the olive oil-based lipid emulsion is well tolerated in premature neonates and may represent a promising alternative to parenteral nutrition in this patient group (41). Nevertheless, the benefit of these new lipid emulsions has yet to be proven in terms of clinical outcome.

Children in metabolic stress states have increased serum levels of triglycerides, fatty acids, and glycerol due to increased lipolysis. Elevated concentrations of plasma triglycerides (>200 mg/dL) saturate the lipoprotein lipase system, resulting in clearance through phagocytosis by the liver's endothelial-reticular system and the lungs and possible depression in immunologic function (41,43,46). The immunosuppressive effect of lipid emulsions has yet to be established; further evidence is needed from *in vivo* studies.

Infusion of lipid emulsions in high doses has been reported to impair respiratory function and hemodynamics, with inflammatory changes, edema, and surfactant alterations in adults with acute lung injury. Adverse effects depend on the mixture of lipid used, with MCT/LCT lipid emulsions causing fewer alterations in respiratory failure than LCT. Given that no studies have been reported in children, it is advisable to closely monitor lipid intake during the acute phase of respiratory failure (12). In newborn infants who cannot receive sufficient enteral feeding, IV lipid emulsions should be started no later than on the third day of life, but may be started on the first day of life. Preterm infants who weigh <1000 g deserve special attention because of their limited tolerance to IV lipids (73). The use of lipid emulsions in newborns—particularly in the premature infants with sepsis, thrombocytopenia, respiratory discomfort, or jaundice—has been the subject of discussion regarding risk of adverse effects, such as impaired oxygenation, reduced immunologic function, and increased levels of free bilirubin. Compared with older children, premature and low-weight newborn patients exhibit slower lipid clearance and lower lipoprotein lipase activity, likely due to immaturity of hepatic function and reduced adipose tissue mass. The upper limit of triglyceride plasma concentration tolerated by the premature is not well known (28,41).

IV lipid infusion can reduce arterial Po_2 through the following mechanisms: (a) through eicosanoid production, which vasodilates vessels around poorly ventilated alveoli causing intrapulmonary shunt and hypoxemia; and (b) the deposition of fat in the capillary-alveoli membrane. This effect is minimized by slowing the infusion of lipid emulsion over 20–24 hours (46,70).

Hyperlipidemia in the premature with jaundice increases the risk of kernicterus with free fatty acid molar:albumin ratio of greater than 6:1 as fatty acids compete with bilirubin for binding sites on albumin. Icteric premature newborns should be started on 0.5 g/kg/day doses, increasing after bilirubin levels fall or on determination of free fatty acid levels. No increase in fatty acid and free bilirubin concentrations have been seen following lipid intake of up to 3 g/kg/day. Liver function tests should be monitored when lipid emulsions are given. If evidence of progressive hepatic dysfunction or cholestasis is seen, a decrease in lipid administration should be considered, especially if other concurrent morbidities (e.g., sepsis, thrombocytopenia) are present. Lipid administration in amounts that supply at least the minimal essential fatty acid requirements are necessary to maintain normal platelet function. In patients with severe thrombocytopenia, lipid administration can activate mechanisms that contribute to platelet aggregation, reduced lifespan, and promote hemophagocytosis. Therefore, in patients with thrombocytopenia, serum triglyceride concentrations should be monitored and a reduction of parenteral lipid dosage considered (19,28,32,74).

Carnitine facilitates the transport of long-chain fatty acids through the mitochondrial membrane for later oxidation and energy production. Given the low serum and tissue levels of carnitine in newborns, its administration has been recommended in the presence of persistent hypertriglyceridemia or in infants who are exclusively on parenteral nutrition for >4 weeks. Nevertheless, no clear evidence exists regarding the benefits of carnitine supplementation in neonates who receive parenteral nutrition (43).

Lipid emulsions should be administered over 24 hours. Infusion of lipid emulsions as 3-in-1 solutions (protein, sugar, lipid in same container) is not recommended, particularly when calcium concentrations exceed 8.5 mEq/L, as the mixture is not complete and the stability of the emulsion may be impaired. Administration in the Y- or 3-route tap connection is also not recommended, as the mixture in low-caliber tubes is also incomplete (48,70). Heparin does not improve utilization of IV lipids and should not be given with lipid infusion on a routine basis, unless indicated for other reasons (48). Lipid emulsions should be protected by validated light-protected tubing during phototherapy to decrease the formation of hydroperoxides (48,70).

Additional Considerations

The supply of at least some nutrition enterally is important, especially in children on TPN for long periods, as small quantities of food have trophic effects on the intestine, reduce bacterial translocation, improve gastric motility, and promote biliary flow (55). It has been suggested that TPN cycling for children on prolonged TPN may reduce continuous, nonphysiologic, hepatic stimulation and assist visceral protein synthesis (75).

Manganese should be included in parenteral nutrition solutions in sufficient quantities to meet daily requirements. Care should be taken with manganese delivery as long-term administration can lead to toxic symptoms from a buildup. Manganese intoxication may provoke parkinsonian-like symptoms, with muscle weakness, stiffness, trembling, ataxia, asthenia, and speech difficulties (76).

Several parenteral component-nutrition solutions (albumin, heparin, calcium, phosphate salts) contain aluminium. Any additional supply of aluminium raises risk of toxicity in children on TPN, owing to the element's tendency to become incorporated into body tissues (48,70).

If prolonged TPN is predicted (>2 weeks), hepatic function tests should be performed, particularly in VLBW neonates, to obtain measurements that might suggest the likelihood of hepatic disease or cholestasis (28). Increased bilirubin and transaminase are late indicators of cholestasis. The earliest indicator, albeit nonspecific, is γ-glutamyl transpeptidase, and its specificity increases when it is used in conjunction with alkaline phosphatase (77). The etiopathogenesis of hepatopathy is multifactorial, and cholestasis-associated risk factors include absence of enteral feeding, immaturity, infection, hypoxia, excessive glucose and caloric intake, and toxicity of amino acids (such as methionine) or trace elements (including copper, chromium, and manganese). TPN light oxidation, medications, and deficit in nutrients such as taurine, choline, fatty acids, and minerals have all been associated with increased incidence of cholestasis (74).

Parenteral Nutrition Combined with Enteral Nutrition

Peripheral parenteral nutrition is an effective method of administering nutritional support to patients with mild to moderate nutritional deficiencies who are unable to receive enteral nutrition or for whom enteral nutrition alone cannot meet energy needs. Adults with this kind of nutrition therapy had improvement in prealbumin and CD4 cell count (78). In other study, early addition of enteral and parenteral nutrition in patients with chronic obstructive pulmonary disease under mechanical ventilation (MV) accelerated weaning from MV and reduced length of hospitalization and cost during treatment (58). More research is needed to determine the effects of combination of enteral and parenteral nutrition on clinical outcomes in critically ill patients who are poorly intolerant to enteral nutrition (78).

Optimizing the increased substrate requirement for the critically ill by initiating timely nutrition support and ensuring tight glycemic control with insulin is now considered central for improved intensive care outcomes. Supplemental parenteral combined with enteral nutrition could be an effective alternative to achieve 100% of energy and protein targets in the beginning of hospitalization (78).

Underfeeding

Fluid and electrolyte complications are also related to inadequate intake. Hyponatremia (sodium <135 mmol/L) occurs with sodium depletion or water intoxication. Hypokalemia may result from insufficient intake or increased losses of potassium (vomiting, diarrhea, digestive fistula, malnutrition). Treatment consists of increased potassium intake. Hypophosphatemia is the result of inadequate phosphorus intake or an increase in phosphorus intracellular shift and uptake during the anabolic protein phase. It represents a frequent complication in malnourished patients during the refeeding process. Treatment consists of increasing phosphorus intake. Hypocalcemia occurs due to insufficient intake or excessive losses of calcium, or poor intestinal absorption, or it is concomitant with hypomagnesemia (chronic diarrhea, digestive fistula, or malnutrition). Osteopenia chiefly results from the inability to supply sufficient amount of calcium and phosphorus to a patient with a limited volume intake through TPN. Osteopenia may occur in 30% of newborns who weigh <1500 g and undergo prolonged TPN without enteral feeding. Other children at risk include those with fluid or protein restrictions treated chronically with diuretics. Routine measurement of levels of calcium, phosphorus, and alkaline phosphatase is useful for detecting signs of metabolic bone disease. Generally, alkaline phosphatase serum levels are high and phosphorus levels are low in children with osteopenia. Calcium levels are typically maintained at the expense of bone reabsorption, although the presence of acute and chronic acid–base disturbances may influence this calcium-level control. Treatment of hypocalcemia consists of increasing calcium intake and correcting associated fluid and electrolyte disturbances: metabolic or respiratory alkalosis, hypomagnesemia, and hyperkalemia, possibly using vitamin D (19,24,35,48).

Hypoglycemia is one of the most serious TPN complications, given its neurologic consequences and the fact that premature newborns are high-risk patients due to their limited glycogen reserves (48,79).

Patients on TPN at risk of iron deficiency include premature newborns, those with low or no enteral intake, and chiefly, those who present with poor absorption or fluid loss. Iron can be administered using oral, intramuscular, or parenteral routes for prophylaxis or treatment. Iron overload is linked to increased risk of sepsis in malnourished children who have low transferrin levels and is associated with increasing requirements for vitamin E (48,70).

Zinc deficiency is seen in patients with severe diarrhea, poor absorption, digestive fistula, and insufficient zinc intake. Children with zinc deficiency present with characteristic cutaneous lesions (enteropathic acrodermatitis) (80). Low selenium can cause cardiomyopathy, whereas excessive intake leads to toxic manifestations, such as alopecia, headache, nausea, and garlic-like breath odor (49).

Overfeeding Syndrome

Overfeeding syndrome occurs when nutrient intake exceeds energy need, resulting in increased fat synthesis (48). Overfeeding is probably underappreciated in the PICU setting (81). Overfeeding is associated with fatty infiltration of the liver, hyperglycemia, hypertriglyceridemia, increased metabolic rate, and electrolyte disturbances (19). Furthermore, increased glucose and caloric intake may result in increased oxygen uptake, increased carbon dioxide (CO_2) production, and CO_2 retention in children with pulmonary or cardiac insufficiency. Hypermetabolic and malnourished patients are more susceptible to these respiratory problems (70). Hyperglycemia is a frequent complication in children who receive TPN and is caused by a drop in the patient's glucose tolerance (resistance to insulin or the presence of the counterregulating hormones during stress: cortisol and glucagon). Hyperglycemia can provoke an osmotic diuresis from glycosuria leading to dehydration, and

more complicated fluid management. Control of hyperglycemia is usually established by reducing glucose concentrations, although adequate supply of calories may be affected. The use of insulin is indicated only in children unresponsive to reduced glucose supply. Another potential complication of overfeeding with glucose is an increase in the risk of infectious complications secondary to hyperglycemia (16,32,37,79,82). If insulin is required, it is vital to perform close monitoring of glucose and acid–base conditions (18).

Intolerance to lipid use may occur in children who are preterm, septic, or malnourished, have hepatic or renal insufficiency, or in those who are receiving steroids (73). The use of some medicines that contain lipids (e.g., propofol and amphotericin B) may contribute to a sufficient quantity of energy in relation to total daily intake and may increase the possibility of hyperlipidemia. Triglyceride levels must be measured 4 hours following commencement of IV fat infusion or 4 hours after any increased infusion rate, given that hypertriglyceridemia tends to occur within this time frame (48). High levels of triglycerides may also be attributed to carnitine deficiency, as premature newborns below 34 weeks have a limited stock of carnitine (43). Interpretation of data concerning IV fat infusion and pulmonary dysfunction is complicated, as adverse effects seem to depend on the dose, administration rate, the presence of peroxides, and the clinical condition of the lungs. On rare occasions, IV fat infusion has been associated with thrombocytopenia (28).

The safety margin for administration of amino acids is wide, having minimal likelihood of causing an impact on blood ammonia levels. However, ammonia levels in children who present with hepatic failure must be carefully monitored and controlled (46,48).

NUTRITIONAL MONITORING

Nutritional Biomarkers

Serum levels of electrolytes, urea, lactate, ammonia, proteins, arterial blood gas, glucose (glycosuria), triglycerides, and nitrogen balance are all parameters for monitoring (9,29,45,83).

Nitrogen balance is the difference between nitrogen intake and nitrogen excreted. It assesses the suitability of protein intake and degree of hypercatabolism. However, it is not an indicator of protein reserves but only signifies metabolism and ingestion over 24 hours. It can be expressed by the following formula:

$$\frac{\text{ingested protein (g/24 h)}}{6.25} - \frac{\text{urinary urea (g/24 h)}}{2.14} + 4^{*}$$

This estimate must be made in the absence of diarrhea or abnormal losses. A 24-hour urinary volume is required. The aim is to obtain a positive nitrogen balance as a reflection of anabolism. If the balance proves negative, it could be due to insufficient protein ingestion or hypercatabolism. Unmeasured losses (burns, renal disease, diarrhea, and protein-losing enteropathy) can contribute to a negative nitrogen balance that is not reflected by the calculation.

It was shown that the amount of protein intake necessary to maintain a nitrogen balance in critically ill patients appears to vary depending on the level of stress, severity of inflammatory response, and the status of organ function (3,8,9,15). Several studies have reported nitrogen balance in critically ill children. Nitrogen excretion is related to the degree of injury

---

*Estimated value of extraurinary nitrogen losses, used in adolescents and adults only (the Wilmore nomogram is used in younger children [28]).

and the metabolic state, with urinary urea nitrogen reported as being between 170 and 254 mg/kg/d in critically ill children (3,6,8,9,21,46).

Serum Proteins

It is not always possible to identify inflammatory response in severely ill children through clinical means. Serial monitoring of proteins such as C-reactive protein and the acute-phase reactants may, by identifying return to anabolism, enable timely increase in nutritional supply and help avoid the risk of overfeeding. A decrease in serum C-reactive protein levels to <2 mg/dL can be interpreted as resolution of stress and return to anabolism, a change which is also reflected by increased serum levels of albumin and prealbumin (20,29). Serum levels of transport proteins can fall in response to metabolic stress or rise upon simple resolution of the process. In the presence of inflammation, their measurement is only valuable in conjunction with that of C-reactive protein, as this provides a reference parameter to assess the course of the inflammatory response (3,9,45,83).

C-reactive protein is an acute-phase reactant normally present in minute quantities in the blood of healthy individuals, increasing in concentration in several inflammatory states, and considered a good indicator of bacterial infection and postsurgical complications. It is synthesized in the liver in response to cytokine stimulation, mainly by IL-6. Serum levels increase 6–8 hours following injury, peaking at 24–48 hours. It has a short half-life (8–12 hours), and, in the absence of complications, serum levels return to basal values within ~4 days (3,9).

Procalcitonin, with its half-life of 24 hours, is advantageous for its greater sensitivity in detecting sepsis and its more rapid elevation than C-reactive protein, although it is associated with a higher cost. Those proteins whose plasma concentrations drop below basal levels in response to inflammatory reaction are known as *acute-phase negative reactants*. Synthesis may be normal or reduced, but both catabolism and flow into extravascular space are increased (3,8).

The principal nutritional proteins are albumin, prealbumin, apolipoprotein A1, retinol-binding protein, transferrin, and fibronectin. Prealbumin, due to its short half-life and the fact that it is affected by malnutrition, is the most relevant protein as a plasma protein pool marker. It is synthesized by the liver and has a half-life of 2 days. Its serum concentration falls rapidly when calorie and protein intake is below normal but rises soon after the initiation of nutritional support; therefore, it is useful in detecting acute malnutrition. Although normally considered an indicator of nutritional state, it has been better employed in monitoring response to nutritional support in critically ill patients. In practice, interpreting its level during illness can prove difficult, as it may fall in response to metabolic stress or rise upon simple resolution of the process. Ideally, it should be assessed together with C-reactive protein to provide a reference parameter for the magnitude of inflammatory response (3).

Serum albumin, given its relatively long half-life and redistribution from the extravascular pool, may not accurately reflect protein-calorie malnutrition. Although malnutrition is an important factor in the regulation of albumin production, serum albumin concentration is influenced by various nonnutritional factors such as inflammation, infection, hepatic failure, and dilution from fluid overload. This variability in serum concentration can impair its validity as a nutritional parameter in patients who have acute-phase response and metabolic stress. The transcapillary flow of plasma proteins secondary to endothelial lesion is the main underlying mechanism to explain hypoalbuminemia in critically ill patients. Its magnitude may be related to the severity of the metabolic response. In the initial stage of the inflammatory process, an increase in permeability of the

microcirculation occurs, allowing greater transcapillary flow of plasma proteins (29). This event may be more important in the postoperative period of cardiac surgery because the contact of blood with the surface of cardiopulmonary bypass tubes may produce an endothelial lesion that, in turn, is a triggering factor of the systemic inflammatory response (45). Data in a pediatric study suggest that concentration of serum albumin may be associated with higher risks of mortality and postsurgical infection and longer periods of hospitalization following cardiac surgery (20,45). Thus, in critically ill patients, hypoalbuminemia is more indicative of the degree of metabolic stress than are alterations in nutritional state.

Other Inflammatory Markers

Interleukin 6 (IL-6), a proinflammatory cytokine, is recognized as an early marker of the systemic inflammatory response syndrome (SIRS) in several disease models. It can be used to determine whether the inflammatory response is present and its intensity (17). Recently, serum concentrations of IL-6 have been associated with the capacity to identify patients with a potential nutritional risk (9,17). Other studies suggest that undernourished patients retain the capacity to produce a positive acute-phase response during infection with an increase in interleukins (9,17).

Plasma Triglyceride Concentrations

Triglyceride levels in serum or plasma should be monitored in patients who receive lipid emulsions, particularly in those with significant risk for hyperlipidemia (e.g., sepsis, trauma, liver or renal diseases, use of steroids, extremely low-birth-weight infants). No data define the triglyceride level at which adverse effects may occur. In children with mild hypertriglyceridemia (175–225 mg/dL), steady increases in infusion rates are recommended. At moderately elevated concentrations (225–275 mg/dL), infusion rates should be reassessed without further increase until levels have normalized. At concentrations that exceed 400 mg/dL, it is recommended that infusion be halted for 12–24 hours and then resumed at 0.02–0.04 g/kg/h (43,48).

Measured EE (Indirect Calorimetry)

Failure to accurately estimate energy requirements may result in underfeeding or overfeeding. Many methods to assess the resting EE in critically ill patients have been described, but all of them have limitations. Indirect calorimetry (IC), although being currently considered to be the "gold standard," has technical limitations such as requiring trained personnel with available time, the need for an inspired oxygen fraction of less than 60%, and requiring equipment of high cost, but this method allows the assessment of EE for adequate energy supply, monitoring of the volume of oxygen consumption during weaning from mechanical ventilation, and measurement of the respiratory quotient. Moreover, with IC, it is possible to determine the required type and amount of macronutrient substrates. However, when applying IC, it is important to be aware of methodologic pitfalls to avoid potential inaccuracies. For example, a recent study demonstrated that there was no relationship between EE and clinical severity evaluated using the PRISM, PIM2, and PELOD scales or with the anthropometric nutritional status or biochemical alterations. Finally, it was concluded that neither nutritional status nor clinical severity is related to EE. Therefore, EE must be measured individually in each critically ill child using IC. Only patients who are hemodynamically stable with an inspired F_{IO_2}

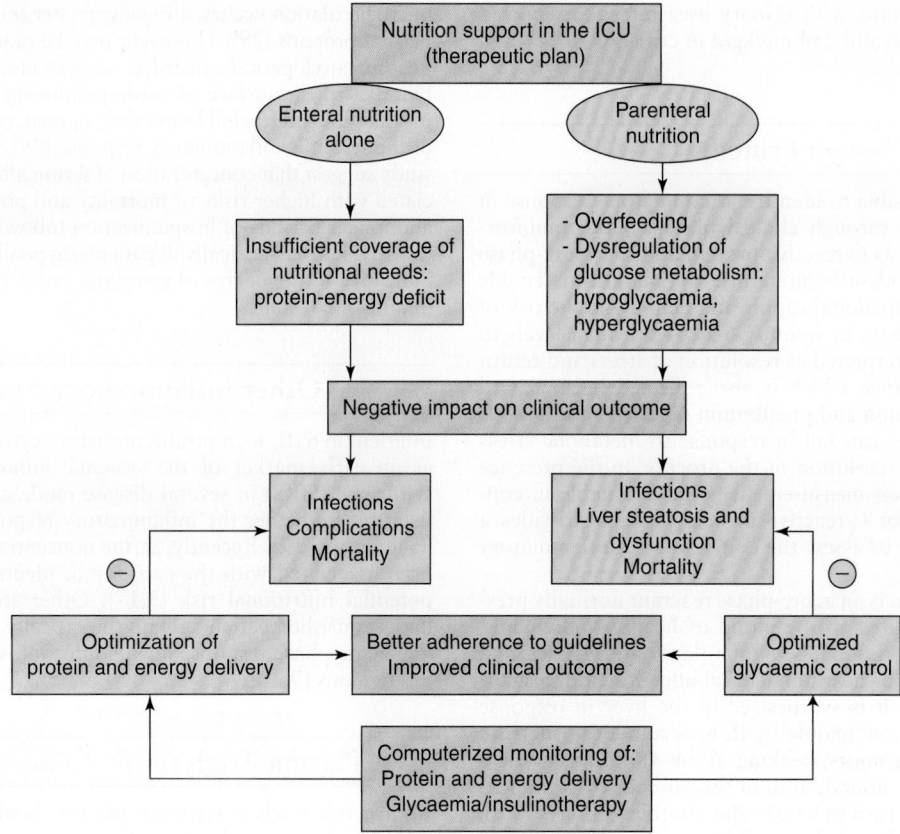

FIGURE 97.2. Flow chart to guide the use of nutrition therapy. (Adapted of guidelines of European Society of Parenteral and Enteral Nutrition.)

of <0.6, no air leaks around the endotracheal tube, adequate sedation, no fever, and no anaerobic metabolism can be reliably tested with IC. In the recovery phase of critical illness, the energy needs can increase to levels above those for normal, healthy children. Another aspect of energy measurement is the time required to measure the EE by IC. In a clinical setting, total daily EE is usually estimated with a 1-to-2-hour measurement, while EE can change throughout the day. When it is not possible to perform IC, EE can be calculated using a predictive formula (see Chapter 96), but a disparity can be observed between equation-estimated EE, measured resting EE, and total energy intake in some studies. This can result in a high incidence of underfeeding or overfeeding. Targeted IC on high-risk patients selected by a dedicated nutrition team may prevent cumulative excesses and deficits in energy balance (8,84–86). **Figure 97.2** summarizes the use and monitoring of nutrition therapy.

CONCLUSIONS AND FUTURE DIRECTIONS

Increased understanding of the pathophysiology of metabolic stress, the application of new concepts in nutrition and metabolism, and the implantation of multidisciplinary nutritional therapy teams within the hospital setting can bring a therapeutic plan and improvement in the quality of nutritional intervention. Furthermore, insights into how the genotype of the individual influences response to nutrients can better enable the application of this knowledge. Nutrigenomics, a science that studies the interface among nutrients and cellular and genetic processes has the potential to make this kind of genotyping a reality. The variability in response to nutrients

determined by genetic polymorphism can influence inflammatory mediator production. A field within enteral nutrition that is open to further investigation is that concerning how genetic polymorphism can affect the efficacy of the so-called immunomodulating diets. In practical terms, nutrigenomics emerges with the perspective that future nutritional support, in addition to taking into account nutritional state and individual needs, considers the standard genotypical response to nutrients, with the goal of preventing or curing diseases. Perfecting this science would likely result in lowering the rates of morbidity and mortality of severely malnourished patients who gain greatest benefit from nutritional intervention.

References

1. Kleinman RE. *Pediatric Nutrition Handbook*. 5th ed. American Academy of Pediatrics, 2003;55–97.
2. Kochanek PM, Carney N, Adelson PD, et al; American Association for the Surgery of Trauma; Child Neurology Society; International Society for Pediatric Neurosurgery, et al. Guidelines for the acute medical management of severe traumatic brain injury in infants, children, and adolescents. *J Trauma* 2003;54 (suppl 6):S235–310.
3. Koletzko B, Goulet O, Hunt J, et al; for the Parenteral Nutrition Guidelines Working Group. Guidelines on paediatric parenteral nutrition of the European Society of Paediatric Gastroenterology, Hepatology and Nutrition (ESPGHAN) and the European Society for Clinical Nutrition and Metabolism (ESPEN), Supported by the European Society Paediatric Research (ESPR). *J Pediatr Gastroenterol Nutr* 2005;41(suppl 2):S19–27.
4. Hiesmayr M. Nutrition risk assessment in the ICU. *Curr Opin Clin Nutr Metab Care* 2012;15(2):174–80.

5. Correia MI, Waitzberg DL. The impact of malnutrition on morbidity, mortality, length of hospital stay and costs evaluated through a multivariate model analysis. *Clin Nutr* 2003;22: 235–9.

6. Zamberlan P, Delgado AF, Leone C, et al. Nutrition therapy in a pediatric intensive care unit: Indications, monitoring, and complications. *JPEN J Parenter Enteral Nutr* 2011;35(4):523–9.

7. Ashworth A. Treatment of severe malnutrition. *J Pediatr Gastroenterol Nutr* 2001;32:516–8.

8. Botrán M, López-Herce J, Mencía S, et al. Relationship between energy expenditure, nutritional status and clinical severity before starting enteral nutrition in critically ill children. *Br J Nutr* 2011;105(5):731–7.

9. Delgado AF, Okay TS, Leone C, et al. Hospital malnutrition and inflammatory response in critically ill children and adolescents admitted to a tertiary intensive care unit. *Clinics (Sao Paulo)* 2008;63(3):357–62.

10. Gurgueira GL, Leite HP, Taddei JA. Outcomes in a pediatric intensive care unit before and after the implementation of a nutrition support team. *JPEN J Parenter Enteral Nutr* 2005;29:176–85.

11. Brewster DR, Manary MJ, Menzies IS, et al. Intestinal permeability in kwashiorkor. *Arch Dis Child* 1997;76:236–41.

12. Skillman HE, Mehta NM. Nutrition therapy in the critically ill child. *Curr Opin Crit Care* 2012;18(2):192–8.

13. Hasan TF, Hasan H. Anorexia nervosa: A unified neurological perspective. *Int J Med Sci* 2011;8(8):679–703.

14. Hearing SD. Refeeding syndrome. *BMJ* 2004;328:908–9.

15. Anand K. The stress response to surgical trauma: From physiological basis to therapeutic implications. *Prog Food Nutr Sci* 1986;10:67–132.

16. Bistrian B. Hyperglycemia and infection: Which is the chicken and which is the egg? *JPEN J Parenter Enteral Nutr* 2001;25(4):180–1.

17. Briassoulis G, Venkataraman S, Thompson A. Cytokines and metabolic patterns in pediatric patients with critical illness. *Clin Dev Immunol* 2010;2010:354047. Published online May 16, 2010.

18. Gore D, Chinkes D, Heggers J. Association of hyperglycemia with increased mortality after severe burn injury. *J Trauma* 2001;51(3):540–4.

19. American Society of Enteral and Parenteral Nutrition Board of Directors: The Clinical Guidelines Task Force. Guidelines for the use of parenteral and enteral nutrition in adult and pediatric patients. *JPEN J Parenter Enteral Nutr* 2002;26 (suppl 1):1SA–138SA.

20. Leite HP, Fisberg M, Vieira JG, et al. The role of insulin-like growth factor I, growth hormone and plasma proteins in surgical outcome of children with congenital heart disease. *Pediatr Crit Care Med* 2001;2(1):29–35.

21. Watters JM, Wilmore DW. The metabolic responses to trauma and sepsis. In: Degroot LJ, Jameson JL. *Endocrinology.* Philadelphia, PA: WB Saunders, 1989;2367–93.

22. Allen JM. Vasoactive substances and their effects on nutrition in the critically ill patient. *Nutr Clin Pract* 2012;20(10):1–5.

23. deOnis M, Blossner M, Borghi E. Global prevalence and trends of overweight and obesity among preschool children. *Am J Clin Nutr* 2010;92(5):1257–64.

24. Port AM, Apovian C. Metabolic support of the obese intensive care unit patient: A current perspective. *Curr Opin Clin Nutr Metab Care* 2010;13(2):184–91.

25. Srinivasan V, Nadkarni VM, Helfaer M, et al. Childhood obesity and survival after in-hospital pediatric cardiopulmonary resuscitation. *Pediatrics* 2010;125(3):e481–8.

26. Bechard LJ, Rothpletz-Puglia P, Touger-Decker R, et al. Influence of obesity on clinical outcomes in hospitalized children: A systematic review. *JAMA Pediatr* 2013;167(5):476–82.

27. Dickerson RN, Boschert KJ, Kudsk KA, et al. Hypocaloric enteral tube feeding in critically ill obese patients. *Nutrition* 2002;18(3):241–6.

28. Deme S, Poindexter B, Leitch C. Nutrition and metabolism in the high-risk neonate. Part 2; Parenteral mutrition. In: Fanaroff

A, Martin R, eds. *Neonatal-Perinatal Medicine.* 7th ed. St. Louis, MO: Mosby, 2002;598–617.

29. Fleck A, Raines G, Hawker F, et al. Increased intravascular permeability: A major cause of hypoalbuminaemia in disease and injury. *Lancet* 1985;1(8432):781–4.

30. Heird WC, Driscoll JM Jr, Schullinger JN, et al. Intravenous alimentation in pediatric patients. *J Pediatr* 1972;80(3):351–72.

31. Johnston JD, Harvey CJ, Mengies IS, et al. Gastrointestinal permeability and absorptive capacity in sepsis. *Crit Care Med* 1996;24:1144–9.

32. Chwals WJ. Overfeeding the critically ill child: Fact or fantasy? *New Horizons* 1994;2(2):147–55.

33. Anderson D. Nutritional assessment and therapeutic interventions for the preterm infant. *Clin Perinatol* 2002;29:313–26.

34. Baker S. Enteral nutrition in pediatrics. In: Rombeau JL, Rollandelli RH, eds. *Enteral and Tube Feeding.* Philadelphia, PA: WB Saunders, 1997;349–67.

35. Greene HL, Hambidge K, Schanler R, et al. Guidelines for the use of vitamins, trace elements, calcium, magnesium and phosphorus in infants and children receiving total parenteral nutrition: Report of the Subcommittee on Clinical Practice Issues of the American Society for Clinical Nutrition. *Am J Clin Nutr* 1988;48:1324–42.

36. Chourdakis M, Kraus MM, Tzellos T, et al. Effect of early compared with delayed enteral nutrition on endocrine function in patients with traumatic brain injury: An open-labeled randomized trial. *JPEN J Parenter Enteral Nutr.* 2012;36(1):108–16.

37. Khaodhiar L, McCowen K, Bistrian B. Perioperative hyperglycemia, infection or risk? *Curr Opin Clin Nutr Metab Care* 1999;2:79–82.

38. Vlasselaers D, Milants I, Desmet L, et al. Intensive insulin therapy for patients in paediatric intensive care: A prospective, randomized controlled study. *Lancet* 2009;373(9663):547–56.

39. Jeschke MG, Kulp GA, Kraft R, et al. Intensive insulin therapy in severely burned pediatric patients: A prospective randomized trial. *Am J Respir Crit Care Med* 2010;182(3):351–9.

40. Macrae D, Grieve R, Allen E, et al. A randomized trial of hyperglycemic control in pediatric intensive care. *N Engl J Med* 2014;370(2):107–18.

41. Koletzko B, Göbel Y, Engelsberger I, et al. Parenteral feeding of preterm infants with fat emulsions based on soybean and olive oils: Effects on plasma phospholipid fatty acids. *Clin Nutr* 1998;17(suppl):25.

42. Fomon SJ. Potential renal solute load: Considerations relating to complementary feedings of breastfed infants pediatrics. *Pediatrics* 2000;106(suppl 5):1284.

43. Magnussum G, Bobert M, Cederblad G, et al. Plasma and tissue of lipids, fatty acids and plasma carnitine in neonates receiving a new fat emulsion. *Acta Paediatr* 1997;86:638–44.

44. Carpentier YA, Simoens C, Siderova V, et al. Recent developments in lipid emulsions: Relevance to intensive care. *Nutrition* 1997;13(suppl 9):S73–8.

45. Leite HP, Fisberg M, Carvalho WB, et al. Serum albumin and clinical outcome in pediatric cardiac surgery. *Nutrition* 2005;21:553–8.

46. Paisley J, Baron KA, Hay WW, et al. Safety and efficacy of low versus high parenteral amino acid intakes in extremely-low-birth-weight neonates (ELBW) immediately after birth. *Pediatr Res* 2000;47:293A.

47. Poindexter BB, Ehrenkranz RA, Stoll BJ, et al. Parenteral glutamine supplementation does not reduce the risk of mortality or late-onset sepsis in extremely low birth weight infants. *Pediatrics* 2004;113(5):1209–15.

48. Shulman RJ, Phillips S. Parenteral nutrition in infants and children. *J Pediatric Gastroenterol Nutr* 2003;36:587–607.

49. Shenkin A, Alwood MC. Trace elements in adult intravenous nutrition. In Rombeau JL, Rolandelli RH, eds. *Clinical Nutrition Vol. II: Parenteral Nutrition.* 3rd ed. Philadelphia, PA: WB Saunders, 2000.

50. Bhatnagar S, Wadhwa N, Aneja S, et al. Zinc as adjunct treatment in infants aged between 7 and 120 days with probable

serious bacterial infection: A randomised, double-blind, placebo-controlled trial. *Lancet* 2012;379:2072–8.

51. Carcillo JA, Dean JM, Holubkov R, et al; Eunice Kennedy Shriver National Institute of Child Health and Human Development (NICHD) Collaborative Pediatric Critical Care Research Network (CPCCRN). The randomized comparative pediatric critical illness stress-induced immune suppression (CRISIS) prevention trial. *Pediatr Crit Care Med.* 2012;13(2):165–73.

52. Cvijanovich N, King J, Flori H, et al. Zinc homeostasis in pediatric critical illness. *Pediatr Crit Care Med* 2009;10(1):29–34.

53. Lucas C, Moreno M, Lopez-Herce J, et al. Transpyloric enteral nutrition reduces the complication rate and cost in the critically ill child. *J Pediatr Gastroenterol Nutr* 2000;30:176–81.

54. Briassoulis G, Filippou O, Hatzi E, et al. Early enteral administration of immunonutrition in critically ill children: Results of a blinded randomized controlled clinical trial. *Nutrition* 2005;21:700–807.

55. Dunn L, Hutman S, Weiner, et al. Beneficial effects of early hypocaloric enteral feeding on neonatal gastrointestinal function: Preliminary report of a randomized trial. *J Pediatric* 1988;112:622–9.

57. Adams S, Batson AS. Study of problems associated with the delivery of enteral feed in critically ill patients in five ICUs in the UK. *Intensive Care Med* 1997;23:261–6.

58. Grigorakos L, Sotiriou E, Markou N, et al. Combined nutritional support in patients with chronic obstructive pulmonary disease (COPD), under mechanical ventilation (MV). *Hepatogastroenterology* 2009;56(96):1612–4.

59. McClave SA, Snider JL, Lowen CC, et al. Use of residual volume as a marker for enteral feeding intolerance: Prospective blinded comparison with physical examination and radiographic findings. *JPEN J Parenter Enteral Nutr* 1992;16:99–105.

60. McClave SA, Sexton L, Spain DA, et al. Enteral tube feeding in the intensive care unit: Factors impeding adequate delivery. *Crit Care Med* 1999;27:1252–6.

61. Heyland DK, Novak F, Drover J, et al. Should immunonutrition become routine in critically ill patients? A systematic review of the evidence. *JAMA* 2001;286:944–53.

62. Leite HP, Iglesias SB. Are immune-enhancing diets safe for critically ill children? *Nutrition* 2006;22:579–80.

63. Bertolini G, Iapichino G, Radrizzani D, et al. Early enteral immunonutrition in patients with severe sepsis: Results of an interim analysis of a randomized multicentre clinical trial. *Intensive Care Med* 2003;2:834–40.

64. Davies AR, Morrison SS, Bailey MJ, et al. A multicenter randomized controlled trial comparing early nasojejunal with nasogastric nutrition in critical illness. *Crit Care Med* 2012;40:2342–8.

65. Mehta NM. Approach to enteral feeding in the PICU. *Nutr Clin Pract* 2009;24(3):377–87.

66. Lavoie PM. Earlier initiation of enteral nutrition is associated with lower risk of late-onset bacteremia only in most mature very low birth weight infants. *J Perinatol* 2009;29(6):448-54.

67. Leaf A, Dorling J, Kempley S, et al. Early or delayed enteral feeding for preterm growth-restricted infants: A randomized trial. *Pediatrics* 2012;129(5):e1260–8.

68. Heyland DK, Cook DJ, Winder B, et al. Enteral nutrition in the critically ill patient: A prospective survey. *Crit Care Med* 1995;23:1055–60.

69. Kelly TW, Patrick MR, Hillman KM. Study of diarrhea in critically ill patients. *Crit Care Med* 1983;11:7–9.

70. Shulman R. New developments in total parenteral nutrition for children. *Curr Gastroenterol Rep* 2000;2:253–8.

71. Takashi T, Asanami S, Kubo S. Experimental infusion phlebitis: Tolerance osmolality of peripheral venous endothelial cells. *Nutrition* 1998;14:496–501.

72. Pereira-da Silva L, Virella D, Henriques G, et al. A simple equation to estimate the osmolarity of neonatal parenteral nutrition solutions. *JPEN J Parenter Enteral Nutr* 2004;28:34–7.

73. Sentipal-Walerius J, Dolberg S, Mimouni F. Effect of pulsed dexamethasone therapy on tolerance of intravenously administered lipids in extremely low birth weight infants. *J Pediatr* 1999;134:229–32.

74. Buchman A, Ament M, Sohel M, et al. Choline deficiency causes reversible hepatic abnormalities in patients receiving parenteral nutrition: Proof of human choline requirement: A placebo-controlled trial. *JPEN J Parenter Enteral Nutr* 2001;25(5):260–8.

75. Maehan J, Georgeston K. Prevention of liver failure in parenteral nutrition-dependent children with short bowel syndrome. *J Paediatr Surg* 1997;32:473–5.

76. Dickerson RN. Manganese intoxication and parenteral nutrition. *Nutrition* 2001;17:689–93.

77. Nanji A, Anderson F. Sensitivity and specificity of liver function tests in detection of parenteral nutrition-associated cholestasis. *JPEN J Parenter Enteral Nutr* 1985;9:307–8.

78. Heidegger CP, Romand JA, Treggiari MM, et al. Is it now time to promote mixed enteral and parenteral nutrition for the critically ill patient? *Intensive Care Med* 2007;33(6):963–9.

79. Jones MO, Pierro A, Hammond P, et al. Glucose utilization in the surgical newborn infant receiving total parenteral nutrition. *J Pediatric Surg* 1993;28:1121–5.

80. Hardy G, Reilly C. Technical aspects of trace element supplementation. *Curr Opin Nutr Metab Care* 1999;2:277–85.

81. Srinivasan V, Spinella PC, Drott HR, et al. Association of timing, duration, and intensity of hyperglycemia with intensive care unit mortality in critically ill children. *Pediatr Crit Care Med* 2004;5:329–36.

82. Mehta NM, Bechard LI, Dolan M, et al. Energy imbalance and risk of underfeeding in the PICU. *Pediatr Crit Care Med* 2011;12(4):398.

83. Kanakoudi F, Drossou V, Tzimouli V. Serum concentration of 10 acute-phase proteins in healthy term and preterm infants from birth to 6 months. *Clin Chem* 1995;41:605–8.

84. Basile-Filho A, Auxiliadora Martins M, Marson F, et al. An easy way to estimate energy expenditure from hemodynamic data in septic patients. *Acta Cir Bras* 2008;23(suppl 1):112–7; discussion 117.

85. Martinez JL, Martinez-Romillo PD, Sebastian JD, et al. Predicted versus measured energy expenditure by continuous, online indirect calorimetry in ventilated, critically ill children during the early post-injury period. *Pediatr Crit Care Med* 2004;5:19–27.

86. Mehta NM, Bechard LI, Leavitt K, et al. Cumulative energy imbalance in the pediatric intensive care unit: Role of targeted indirect calorimetry. *JPEN J Parenter Enteral Nutr* 2009; 33:336–44.

CHAPTER 98 ■ SECRETORY AND MOTILITY ISSUES OF THE GASTROINTESTINAL TRACT

EITAN RUBINSTEIN AND SAMUEL NURKO

KEY POINTS

1. Gastrointestinal complications are common in the intensive care unit (ICU).
2. Multiple causes of diarrhea in the ICU exist. It is often helpful to subdivide between infectious and noninfectious.
3. Replacement of fluids and electrolytes and establishment of hemodynamic stability are the major goals in diarrhea management.
4. Critical illness is associated with a variety of systemic effects that have been implicated in potentially contributing to gastrointestinal hypomotility.
5. Management of hypomotility must focus on eliminating underlying condition (when possible) and supportive care.
6. In the setting of critical illness, gastroesophageal reflux (GER) can be serious and potentially life threatening.

Critically ill children face many challenges on the road to recovery. Gastrointestinal (GI) complications remain one of the most common issues encountered in the intensive care unit (ICU), and the ability to tolerate nutrition and intestinal function have been noted to affect outcomes, morbidity, and mortality (1,2). Whether GI complications are the cause or a marker for poor outcomes remains unclear.

Most of the literature involving GI complications in the ICU involves adults; however, children encounter similar issues. Pérez-Navero et al. (3) reviewed the incidence of GI complications among critically ill children fed via enteral nutrition and found an incidence of vomiting in 17.9%, abdominal distension in 13.2%, diarrhea in 11.3%, excessive gastric residue in 4.7%, aspiration in 1.9%, and GI hemorrhage in 0.9%. This chapter will focus on specific GI problems that result from diarrhea or hypomotility.

DIARRHEA

1. Diarrhea has been reported as the most common GI complication encountered in the ICU (4), with a prevalence ranging from 14% to 78% (5–8). It is an important condition that must be recognized because severe diarrhea leads to dehydration, malnutrition, electrolyte imbalances, skin breakdown, and hemodynamic instability (9). The definition of diarrhea varies. In general terms, it may be thought of as an intestinal alteration that produces more frequent and/or looser stools. In adults, it has been defined as three or more loose or liquid stools per day with stool weight greater than 200–250 g/day (2). In children, a stool output greater than 10 cc/kg/day is consistent with diarrhea.

Etiologies of Diarrhea that Develops in the ICU

Diarrhea in the ICU is usually multifactorial and may be a reflection of the severity of underlying illness and gut dysmotility (10). Several factors have been associated with a higher incidence, or risk, of developing diarrhea in the ICU (**Table 98.1**). Such factors include increased severity of illness, oxygen saturation levels, glucose control, albumin concentration, white blood cell count (5), and the need for mechanical ventilation (11). Other important factors relate to the acquisition of nosocomial infections, like *Clostridium difficile*, and of diarrhea associated with antibiotic use (8,12). In general terms, the causes of diarrhea in the ICU can be classified into one of two major categories: infectious and noninfectious.

Noninfectious causes include diarrhea that is induced by enteral feedings, fecal impaction, the side effects of medications, psychological stress, diagnostic test reagents, certain tumors, endocrine disorders, malabsorption, intestinal ischemia, exacerbation of inflammatory bowel disease, and hypoalbuminemia (9). Diarrhea is a frequently reported complication of enteral feedings, affecting up to 12%–78% of adult patients, even in the absence of GI dysfunction (5,8). Enteral feeding-related diarrhea might be associated with intolerance to enteral nutrients during illness (or after fasting), decreased absorptive capacity of the enteral mucosa, or the effect of osmolar load from the enteral formula. A short period of enteral fasting has been associated with the development of duodenal mucosal atrophy in critically ill patients (13). The role that formula osmolarity plays in the development of diarrhea is not clear. Even though findings are contradictory (11,14), the use of hyperosmolar formulas needs to be approached with caution as higher osmolality may result in excessive intraluminal volume and subsequent diarrhea (15). The delivery site of feedings should also be considered. A randomized controlled study conducted by Davies et al. showed no overall difference in diarrhea when feeds were delivered into the stomach as opposed to postpyloric (16,17). However, the jejunum is more reliant on isosmotic feeds, so hyperosmotic feeds and bolus feeds (bolus feeds cause *dumping syndrome*) into the jejunum have been associated with diarrhea. A decrease in the absorptive ability of the bowel can significantly interfere with nutrient uptake and lead to an *osmotic diarrhea* (fluid is drawn into the intestine by the increase in osmotically active contents).

Hypoalbuminemia has been implicated as a predisposing factor for diarrhea in the critically ill (18–20), and patients with chronic hypoalbuminemia seem to have a higher degree

TABLE 98.1

CAUSES OF DIARRHEA DEVELOPING IN THE PICU

Infectious
  Bacteria—*C. difficile* (±*pseudomembranous colitis in severe cases*)
  Other bacteria (*Salmonella* spp., *Shigella* spp., *Campylobacter jejuni*, *Yersinia enterocolitica*, *Vibrio cholerae*, *Escherichia coli*—
    enteropathogenic, enterotoxigenic, enteroinvasive, enteroaggregative, and enterohemorrhagic)
    Viruses (rotavirus, norovirus, sapovirus, adenovirus, astrovirus)
    Other (*Giardia, Cryptosporidium, Entamoeba*)
Noninfectious
  Enteral nutrition
    Malabsorption
    Prolonged fasting >5 d
    Hyperosmolar formula
  Medication related
    Contrast dye
    Antibiotic use
    Opioid or benzodiazepine withdrawal
  Other
    Intestinal ischemia
    Toxic megacolon (secondary to bacterial infection, Hirschsprung disease, or inflammatory bowel disease)
    Hypoalbuminemia (<2.5 g/dL), especially chronic severe hypoalbuminemia
    Fecal impaction
    Psychological stress
    Tumor (hormone secreting—carcinoid, gastrinoma, VIPoma, mastocytosis)
    Endocrine disorder (adrenal insufficiency, hyperthyroidism)
    Inflammatory bowel disease exacerbation
    Overuse of stool softeners

of diarrhea than those with acute hypoalbuminemia suggesting that chronicity of malnutrition might be more important than disease severity when it comes to diarrhea (8).

Malabsorption of nonabsorbable solutes in the GI tract, such as carbohydrates, causes osmotic diarrhea. In addition, bacterial fermentation of a portion of the nonabsorbed carbohydrate reaching the colon results in the formation of short-chain fatty acids, which further contributes to the osmotic load presented to the colon and limits water reabsorption. In addition, short-chain fatty acids stimulate peristalsis. Bile acid malabsorption has also been associated with diarrhea in the critically ill (21).

Another factor is the use of antibiotics. They can act via direct effects on the GI tract as well as via their association with the development of *C. difficile* (8,12). Diarrhea associated with antibiotic use that is not due to development of *C. difficile* infections is likely due to a direct increase in intestinal motility or to a reduction in bacterial fermentation of carbohydrates. Either of these causes will cease shortly after the antibiotic is discontinued. The risk factors that put ICU patients at risk of *C. difficile* and other infections include antibiotic use, immune compromise, and acid blockade (22). Infectious diarrhea is troublesome due to the risk of spread of the infection from patient to patient. In adults, the most common cause of infectious diarrhea in the ICU is *C. difficile*, but *Salmonella*, rotavirus, and norovirus have also been associated with outbreaks (9). In children, while much of the focus is on *C. difficile*, it is estimated that 91%–94% of hospital-acquired infectious diarrhea is due to virus, especially rotavirus (9).

Recent years have witnessed an increase in the occurrence of *C. difficile*. The antibiotics most frequently implicated in *C. difficile* infection in children are ampicillin, penicillin, cephalosporins, amoxicillin, and clindamycin (23). Although diarrhea is considered the hallmark of *C. difficile*, it can also present with abdominal pain, and a lack of diarrhea could indicate severe ileus (9). Ang et al. (24) noted in his adult population that admission to the ICU carried a moderate risk of

acquiring *C. difficile*. Its acquisition increased mortality from a baseline of 29%–34%. In another study, the 30-day mortality of patients with *C. difficile* infection in the ICU was demonstrated to be close to 40% and a 6% mortality rate was directly attributed to the infection (9). Others, however, have noted that if treated early, ICU-acquired *C. difficile* was not independently associated with increased mortality and only marginally impacted the length of stay in the ICU (6). *C. difficile* is diagnosed by testing the stool for specific toxins, or by new PCR methodologies. If toxin assays are used, it is important to remember that there are two toxins that can be associated with *C. difficile* infections (A and B) and that not all commercially available assays measure both. PCR detection is now being commonly used (25). Rarely, it may be necessary to perform emergency endoscopic procedures to establish the diagnosis. In those cases the typical pseudomembranes are seen (26).

Another type of diarrhea that can develop in the ICU patient is *secretory diarrhea*. This type of diarrhea is voluminous, and unlike osmotic diarrhea does not stop when the patient is fasted. It usually occurs from active intestinal secretion (e.g., secondary to cholera toxin), and it results in major shifts in fluid and electrolytes. It can occur in the setting of critical illness or systemic processes that affect the GI tract. It is often possible to differentiate osmotic from secretory diarrhea, which may help in the management. Osmotic diarrhea typically has less stool volume per day, a lower Na content, a pH of <5, tests positive for reducing/nonreducing sugars, and usually responds to fasting.

Evaluation and Management

A thorough history will help determine if triggers are present, which could be discontinued (like medications) or treated (infections, malabsorption, and underlying inflammatory bowel disease) (2,27). Physical examination will help determine the presence of impaction. Gross stool examination can detect blood, leukocytes, mucus, ova, and parasites. Presence of leukocytes suggests presence of invasive or toxin-producing microorganism in the gut. The pH and presence of reducing substances in the stool may indicate the presence of carbohydrate malabsorption.

The discontinuation of enteral feeds during diarrhea is not always justified (27). Feedings, however, may need to be adjusted to decrease osmolar load via the reduction of infusion rate, repositioning of feeding tube or dilution of nutrition formula (2). If there is evidence of carbohydrate malabsorption (low pH and reducing substances in stool), the formulas may need to be diluted or the infusion rate lowered. It is important to remember that formulas, which contain sucrose (a nonreducing substance), can produce an osmotic diarrhea and test negative for reducing substances. When there is severe osmotic diarrhea from malabsorption, it is likely that there is significant damage to the absorptive surface of the intestine, and it may be necessary to change to more predigested formulas.

The replacement of fluids and electrolytes and the establishment of hemodynamic stability are the major goals in diarrhea management. Fluid and electrolyte management in the ICU are reviewed in other sections.

The role of probiotics in the ICU is controversial. Some authors have demonstrated clinical improvement with their use (1,28,29), but others have not (30,31). Other therapies such as the addition of soluble fiber to feeds have also been suggested to prolong transit time and decrease diarrhea (2).

Specific treatment needs to be administered in the case of infections like C. *difficile*. The most commonly used treatments are oral metronidazole and vancomycin, although recent studies have shown the efficacy of rifaximin. The enteral route is preferred, but anecdotal experience suggests that parenteral metronidazole may also be effective (32).

In the cases of secretory diarrheas, it may be necessary to slow down intestinal secretions with the use of loperamide, or similar agents although they must be used with caution in the critically ill (33). Loperamide is not indicated in children <3 years old or who may suffer overgrowth of invasive infectious organisms associated with dysentery if motility is slowed.

Severe skin breakdown is another complication of significant diarrhea that should be anticipated, prevented when possible, and aggressively treated when it occurs.

INTESTINAL HYPOMOTILITY (ILEUS)

Several conditions resulting in critical illness and admission to ICU are associated with GI motility dysfunction. These include respiratory failure (particularly when mechanical ventilation is used), increased intracranial pressure, sepsis, trauma, postoperative conditions, burns, and cardiac injury (34).

The absence of a uniform definition of GI hypomotility is a major hurdle in establishing its prevalence in the ICU. Some of the common terms used to describe motility dysfunction include feeding intolerance, abdominal distension, and/or the presence or absence of bowel sounds. *Ileus* is often defined as transient impairment of GI motility, which is clinically characterized by delayed passage of stool and flatus, absent bowel sounds, nausea, vomiting, abdominal distension, and accumulation of gas and fluid in the bowel (35,36). Bowel sounds have been used as a marker of intestinal motility but there is little evidence that the absence of bowel sounds indicates that enteral nutrition should be withheld (37) in the critically ill. The drainage of liquid and air from the stomach may reduce the components that create bowel sounds and enteral feeding may provide those components and produce bowel sounds.

Regardless of the definition, hypomotility is a frequent phenomenon encountered in the ICU. Although the incidence of

ileus has been reported in 50%–80% of the critical care population, the absence of a biomarker makes it hard to establish the true prevalence (35). Some authors have noted abdominal distension in 10.6%–46% of patients in the ICU (4). Gastric hypomotility is one of the most frequent encountered complications in critically ill children receiving gastric feeds. Reduced GI motility has been noted in 50% of critically ill children with subsequent delay in gastric emptying (1).

The exact pathophysiology of GI hypomotility in the ICU patient is not well understood. Mechanical ventilation, increased intracranial pressure, infections, sepsis, volume overload with intestinal wall edema, hypotension, vasoactive drugs reducing splanchnic blood flow, direct catecholamine-induced inhibition of intestinal motility, and electrolyte disorders have all been associated with hypomotility (38). In patients with acute respiratory failure, a history of liver disease has been associated with a higher risk of ileus (4). Altered proximal gut motility has been associated with such factors as increased intracranial pressure, intra-abdominal pressure, and metabolic abnormalities (such as hyponatremia, hypernatremia, hypokalemia, hyperkalemia, hypomagnesemia, and hyperglycemia) (39).

Mechanical ventilation is associated with abnormal proximal gastric motor responses to small intestinal nutrients that include less-frequent and lower-amplitude fundic volume waves (40). Dive et al. (41) found that 42% of mechanically ventilated patients exhibited patterns of hypomotility or complete lack of peristalsis. Mechanical ventilation can also contribute to splanchnic hypoperfusion via increased intrathoracic pressure, increased plasma–renin–angiotensin–aldosterone activity and elevated catecholamines in the setting of high levels of positive end-expiratory pressure (8). Cytokine production during mechanical ventilation can also lead to splanchnic hypoperfusion and impaired intestinal smooth muscle function (42–44).

Shock can result in elevated proinflammatory mediators and reduced splanchnic perfusion inducing functional and structural changes in the GI tract, which can alter the tolerance to enteral nutrition (1,8,45). Hypoperfusion and then reperfusion of the splanchnic vascular bed can lead to significant damage to GI epithelium and mucosa as well as altered GI motility (8,46,47). The role of gastric residual volume measurements in the ICU is unclear. Recent literature questions the use of gastric residual volumes as a marker of enteral nutrition tolerance or the risk of aspiration pneumonia (48,49).

The gastric and duodenal reflexes appear to be abnormal in the critically ill. Chapman et al. performed antro-pyloro-duodenal manometry in critically ill patients and noted stimulation of pyloric- and suppression of antral pressure by duodenal nutrients compared to healthy controls; these motor responses contributed to reduced gastric emptying. They suggest that duodenal feedback is pathologically increased in the critically ill and the presence of smaller than usual amounts of nutrients in the duodenum can activate a reflex that inhibits gastric emptying. Hyperglycemia and catecholamine use may contribute to this increased duodenal feedback to the introduction of duodenal nutrients in the critically ill (50). Diminished functional association between proximal and distal gastric motility in the critically ill patient has also been reported (51).

Critical illness is associated with a variety of systemic effects on the body, which have also been implicated as potentially contributing to hypomotility. Elevated levels of proinflammatory cytokines such as IL-2 and IL-6 and tumor necrosis factor lead to increased leukocyte migration and inflammation in the muscularis of the intestinal wall, which can have inhibitory effects on contractility (35). Tachykinins (such as substance P and neurokinin) have been shown to be elevated in critical illness and associated with intestinal hypomotility (52). Elevation of plasma cholecystokinin both in fasting and nutrient-stimulated states in critical illness has been associated with delayed gastric emptying (53). In a canine model

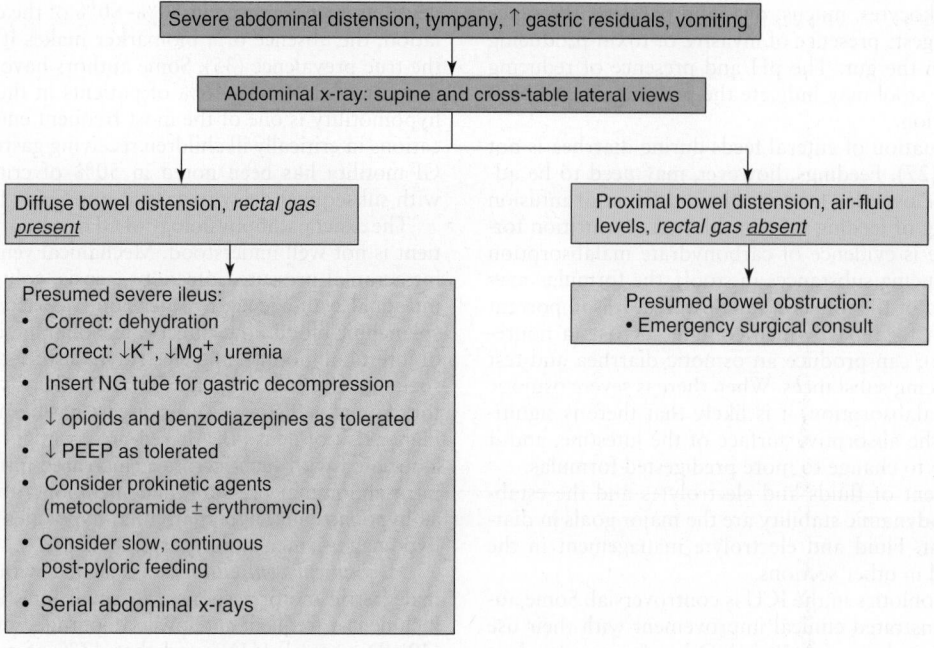

FIGURE 98.1. Management algorithm for severe ileus. ↑, increased; ↓, decreased; NG, nasogastric; K⁺, potassium; Mg⁺, magnesium; PEEP, positive end-expiratory pressure.

of sepsis, nitric oxide (NO) and vasoactive intestinal peptide were elevated and associated with suppression of migrating motor complexes (44).

Corticotrophin-releasing factor, which has been shown to increase in stress, has been noted in animal models to cause a delay in gastric emptying via increased corticosteroid levels (54). Endotoxemia by bacterial lipopolysaccharide via ligation to Toll-like receptor 4 activation was noted to impair GI smooth muscle activity (55). The sympathetic stimulation associated with stress and injury correlated with a decreased motility via a decrease in acetylcholine release in an animal model (35,56).

Postoperative ileus is usually considered an expected occurrence. The stomach and duodenum tend to return to function in the first 24–48 hours and the colon within 72 hours after abdominal surgery (38). Ileus is secondary to disturbances of intestinal motility (in particular of the migrating motor complex, which is the intrinsic motor activity of the small bowel) that result in reduced flushing of luminal contents to the colon. This stagnation of luminal contents can lead to microbial overgrowth and bacterial translocation (38). The most significant complication of ileus might be secondary to increased luminal pressure, which can lead to gut wall ischemia and increased intra-abdominal pressure (39).

Medications used in the ICU for cardiovascular support and pain management (especially opioids) are also likely to contribute to GI dysfunction. Most sedatives (e.g., benzodiazepines, barbiturates) decrease gastric motility and can also interfere with feeding tolerance. There is little evidence regarding the effect of the sedative dexmedetomidine on intestinal motility. It is postulated that the reduction in opioid administration afforded by the use of dexmedetomidine may decrease the likelihood of intestinal hypomotility.

The use of high doses of catecholamines may reduce intestinal perfusion. However, the effect of catecholamine infusions on feeding tolerance is unclear. Some data suggest impaired GI motility and an increase in complications with feeds during catecholamine infusions (e.g., dopamine) (1,57–59). In contrast, other preliminary evidence suggests that some patients

receiving vasoactive medications may tolerate enteral nutrition (60,61). A large randomized controlled trial is needed to resolve this question.

Management

❺ Management needs to focus on eliminating the underlying condition (if possible) and supportive care to minimize the effects of hypomotility and its complications (**Fig. 98.1**). Medications that inhibit GI motility such as catecholamines, sedatives, and opioids should be decreased or withdrawn if possible, and conditions impairing motility such as electrolyte imbalance and hypovolemia should be corrected (2,8,38).

Nutrition is an important factor, which can influence outcome in the critically ill. Hence, most of the focus revolves around ensuring proper nutrition. In adult burn patients, institution of early enteral feeds (in <18 hours after injury) was associated with lower rates of gastroparesis and the need for parenteral nutrition (62). If gastric feeds are not tolerated due to gastroparesis, postpyloric feeds might be a suitable option. Although postpyloric feeds are usually well tolerated, they must be administered with caution in critically ill children (63). The Working Group on Abdominal Problems (WGAP) of the European Society of Intensive Care Medicine (ESICM) recommended that in the setting of gastroparesis, postpyloric feeds be considered when prokinetic therapy is not effective. The hesitation for early institution of postpyloric feeds was due to the risk of severe small bowel dilatation and perforation in rare cases (2). In pediatrics, the use of transpyloric tubes is very common and for the most part tolerated well. Nonetheless, despite their rarity it is important to be mindful of potential complications such as small intestine intussusception (64) and minor GI hemorrhage (16).

Prokinetic agents can be helpful in improving hypomotility. Erythromycin has been noted to increase upper GI tract motility in the critically ill and mechanically ventilated patient (65,66). It activates motilin receptors on smooth muscle cells and enteric neurons to facilitate neurotransmitter release stimulating high-amplitude, antral, migrating myenteric complex III contractions, which propagate across the pylorus into the duodenum (34). Along with an increased amplitude of antral contractions, it can also improve antroduodenal coordination (66–68). While at low doses it exhibits prokinetic effects, higher doses seem to induce strong antral contraction, which could slow duodenal-to-cecal transit (38,69,70). Aside from dose, duration of administration should also be considered as prolonged administration (greater than 3 or 4 days) has been associated with reduced efficacy (71).

Metoclopramide has also been used as a prokinetic agent for the therapy of hypomotility though effects seem limited to the proximal gut. It increases gastric motility and has a moderate stimulant effect on the small bowel (38). It improves antroduodenal coordination and reverses the inhibitory effects of dopamine on GI motility (8,58). It is a dopamine D_2 receptor antagonist, 5-HT_3 receptor antagonist, and 5-HT_4 receptor agonist. It exerts its prokinetic effects by facilitating acetylcholine release from enteric cholinergic neurons (5-HT_4 receptors), dopamine D_2 receptor antagonism in the myenteric plexus, and direct smooth muscle contraction via muscarinic receptor sensitization (34,72). Unfortunately, due to its crossing the blood–brain barrier, its use can lead to side effects in 10%–20% of patients (69). The most significant side effect is irreversible tardive dyskinesia, which has been associated with long-term use or high doses. Due to its side-effect profile, the FDA has placed a black box warning on its use. As with erythromycin, prokinetic effects of the drug also diminish rapidly over time (71).

While both erythromycin and metoclopramide have prokinetic properties separately, using both agents together has been seen to be more successful than erythromycin alone in allowing gastric feed tolerance (73).

Other drugs such as domperidone and cisapride are not routinely available in the US, but have been used in other countries. Domperidone acts as an antagonist at the peripheral dopamine D_2 receptor (38,69). Its antidopamine effects can stimulate gastric motility, resulting in improved emptying of solids and liquids (69). Cisapride is a 5-HT_4 receptor agonist that stimulates antral and duodenal contractions, improves antroduodenal coordination, and accelerates gastric emptying and small bowl transit (38). It acts by stimulating myenteric cholinergic nerves with subsequent increase in acetylcholine release (74,75). However, cisapride has been associated with Q-T prolongation, torsades de pointes, ventricular tachyarrhythmias, and sudden death (69). Due to cisapride's association with cardiac arrhythmias (some resulting in death), it has been withdrawn from the US market.

Octreotide has also been demonstrated to have prokinetic properties. It is a synthetic octapeptide that shares an essential four–amino acid sequence with somatostatin. At low doses it can stimulate motility via induction of migrating motor complexes. However, at higher doses, it has antisecretory effects, which may inhibit motility (69). Octreotide can have inhibitory effects on antral function, so it is often necessary to administer a prokinetic when it is being used (76).

Neostigmine works as a cholinergic agonist by its actions as a cholinesterase inhibitor (69). Its prokinetic effects are more significant in the distal intestinal tract (especially the colon) where it stimulates contractility. It does, however, carry potentially significant side effects due to its cholinergic properties such as increased secretions, bradycardia, abdominal cramping, blurred vision, bladder cramps, increased micturition, and stimulation of acid secretion (69). It can be used in cases of acute colonic pseudoobstruction, like Ogilvie syndrome (acute colonic obstruction and dilation without mechanical blockage).

Opioids, which carry significant unwanted GI side effects such as hypomotility, are frequently used in the critically ill. Opioid antagonists have been developed to counteract the GI motility impairment but preserve the opiate's analgesic function. Methylnaltrexone is a pure mu-opioid antagonist that has peripheral effects. Because of its poor lipid solubility it does not cross the blood–brain barrier and does not interfere with the central analgesic effect of opioids (77). It has been shown to prevent the delayed gut transit time induced by methadone (78). Alvimopan is a different peripherally acting mu-opioid receptor antagonist. It is orally effective and, as with methylnaltrexone, does not cross the blood–brain barrier, so it does not compromise analgesia. Its use has been shown to speed recovery of bowel function (79–81). It is currently approved for management of postoperative ileus after bowel resection in adults. Long-term data for these agents is not yet available. Because of unknown long-term side effects, a consensus statement from the WGAP of the ESICM in 2012 could not recommend their routine use (2).

Laxatives can improve colonic transit and have been recommended to avoid bowel dysfunction (38). Due to delayed onset of action, laxative drugs should be given prophylactically (2). If necessary, rectal administration of laxatives may be an option.

It is important to remember that if patients are still unable to tolerate enteral nutrition despite all efforts, the use of parenteral nutrition should be instituted. Parenteral nutrition, however, carries its own risks such as catheter-related infection, thrombophlebitis, and electrolyte derangements (3).

Prognosis

GI hypomotility has been associated with a worse outcome in the ICU patient. Ileus is identified as a clinical factor that increases the risk for aspiration, nutritional deficiencies, sepsis, and prolonged ventilation (35). Along with feeding difficulty and undernutrition, ileus can affect volume status and circulation, as well as the hepatic, pulmonary, renal, and neurologic systems. Nguyen et al. reported that critically ill patients with impaired gastrointestinal transit (IGT) had longer ICU stays and were less likely to reach nutritional targets than controls. A higher dose of opioids were noted to be a major risk factor for development of IGT (82). Reintam et al. noted that mortality was increased when bowel dysfunction was present. They reported a mortality of 11.3% of those with normal bowel sounds compared to 22.6% and 36% in those with abnormal or absent bowel sounds, respectively (7).

GASTROESOPHAGEAL REFLUX

In children, particularly infants, gastroesophageal reflux (GER) is very common and usually benign. In the setting of critical illness, particularly with intubation and ventilation, the condition can be very serious and potentially life threatening related to aspiration, or in intubated patients to ventilator-associated pneumonia (VAP) (83–87).

Etiologies

Children with chronic lung disease and structural tracheal and esophageal anomalies have a higher prevalence of GER (88). Neurologically impaired infants are especially at high risk for GER. Other factors such as prolonged supine positioning, esophageal dysmotility, increased intra-abdominal pressure (secondary to seizures and hypertonicity), central vomiting, and lower esophageal sphincter immaturity also increase the risk of GER (88).

As discussed in previous sections, critical illness is associated with significant GI dysmotility. GI dysmotility can lead to increased gastric residuals and abdominal distension (89).

Both a decreased propulsive motor activity of the esophagus (90) and gastric emptying delay (91) have been described in the critically ill regardless of underlying cause.

The combination of lower esophageal hypotension, esophageal body dysmotility, and gastroparesis places patients at a very high risk for GER and subsequent aspiration (92). Nind et al. found that in mechanically ventilated, critically ill adults, gastroesophageal reflux disease (GERD) was predominantly due to very low or absent lower esophageal sphincter pressure. They also noted that motor response to reflux (secondary peristalsis) was significantly impaired (93). Along with dysmotility, the presence of nasogastric tube has also been described as contributor to GER (94).

The use of a proton-pump inhibitor (PPI) for stress ulcer prophylaxis in the ICU is common. PPI use has been shown to be associated with an increased risk for the development of respiratory infection in otherwise healthy children that use them chronically (95). The role of acid blockade in the development of VAP is controversial. Some adult studies have shown increased rates of VAP when acid blocking agents are used over the gastroprotective agent sucralfate (which does not alter gastric pH) (96,97). Other studies have failed to demonstrate a similar increase (98). It is also unclear if different acid blocking agents carry different risk. Miano et al. (99) reported that pantoprazole use was associated with VAP in 9.3%, which was significantly higher than the 1.5% in those using ranitidine. Other studies have failed to note different rates of VAPs between acid blocking agents (100). Pediatric data are limited but also have contradicting results. Sharma et al. (101) noted an increased rate of VAP in patients using ranitidine. Other studies noted no difference when comparing patients exposed to acid blocking agents (omeprazole and ranitidine), the gastroprotective agent sucralfate, and those not receiving stress ulcer prophylaxis (102,103).

Management

There are two aspects to the management of GERD: one is to control acidity, improve dysmotility, and gastric emptying, and the other is to avoid complications (aspiration and malnutrition). The medical therapy to improve dysmotility is discussed above. The use of acid inhibition is usually achieved with the administration of PPIs. ICU patients are at increased risk of stress ulcers, and the use of acid inhibition with PPIs has been found to be protective. Therefore, most ICU patients at risk of developing GERD-related complication will be on acid blockade. Acid blockade has also been shown to be very effective for the treatment of GERD. As mentioned, it remains unclear if use of acid blockade increased the risk of VAP but pediatric data for the most part have shown no increase in such risk (102,103).

Feeding is an important aspect of recovery for the critically ill. The presence of GERD may prevent adequate caloric intake because of vomiting and aspiration. Given that parenteral nutrition is associated with risks including infection, thrombophlebitis, and electrolyte derangement (3), enteral feeds need to be used when possible. Enteral feeds are considered more physiologic and can decrease GI mucosal atrophy. Gastric and postpyloric feeding represent the two main methods for enteral nutrition in the critically ill. Given the possible complications associated with gastric feedings, it is very common to use postpyloric feedings in the ICU setting, although there is limited evidence to support its routine use (16).

Some studies have shown a decrease in vomiting and VAP in critically ill adults on postpyloric feedings (104). A pediatric study, however, showed no difference in vomiting or presence of pepsin in tracheal aspiration in children receiving gastric versus small bowel feeds; however, they did find that the gastric group achieved a lower percentage of their daily caloric goals then the small bowel group (105).

Aside from the possible reduction of VAP, Lyons at al. (106) evaluated the role of postpyloric feeds during extubation. No difference was noted in adverse events (defined as GERD, feeding intolerance, and pulmonary aspiration) in groups that had postpyloric feeds during endotracheal extubation compared to those made NPO 4 hours before and 4 hours after. Postpyloric feeds may be useful if gastric feeds have been tried and failed or if significant risk factors for aspiration or history of aspiration exist. Transpyloric tubes may be associated with complications due to malposition and in centers with limited resources may increase interruptions to enteral nutrition (107).

It has been suggested that in critically ill patients, with presence or significant risk for GER (and its complications), a fundoplication may be indicated. Barnes and colleagues (108) evaluated 10 infants in the NICU who were determined to have GER, had suffered life-threatening respiratory episodes, and failed medical management. The infants were deemed ICU dependent due to recurrent life-threatening respiratory episodes. Infants underwent a Nissen fundoplication with eight having a gastrostomy tube inserted at that time. Following surgery, authors reported no further life-threatening episodes specifically attributable to GER and all infants were able to discontinue antireflux medications without demonstrable consequences (100). A more recent review of ventilator-dependent infants who underwent fundoplication to help wean them off ventilation found that while all were successfully weaned from ventilation, 34% had recurrence of symptoms and 38% died within the study period. One patient's death was attributed to operative morbidity (missed tracheoesophageal fistula) and one died after having recurrent pneumonias despite the report the fundoplication was intact. The other eight deaths were not deemed related to recurrence of reflux. It is important to note that all 26 patients had complex comorbidities (88).

CONCLUSIONS AND FUTURE DIRECTIONS

The presence of GI disturbances in the ICU patient may have an important impact on their treatment and prognosis. An effort to establish the etiology needs to be undertaken. The treatment needs to be focused on treated specific etiologies, in providing nutritional support, and in avoiding complications. Given the impact that GI dysfunction has on ICU patients, their nutrition, and their complications, the future will focus on research geared to trying to understand the pathophysiology of gastrointestinal dysfunction in ICU patients, as well as to find better ways to prevent them and treat them.

References

1. Lopez-Herce J. Gastrointestinal complications in critically ill patients: What differs between adults and children? *Curr Opin Clin Nutr Metab Care* 2009;12(2):180–5.
2. Reintam Blaser A, Malbrain ML, Starkopf J, et al. Gastrointestinal function in intensive care patients: Terminology, definitions and management. Recommendations of the ESICM Working Group on Abdominal Problems. *Intensive Care Med* 2012;38(3):384–94.
3. Pérez-Navero JL, Dorao Martínez-Romillo P, López-Herce Cid J, et al. [Artificial nutrition in pediatric intensive care units]. *An Pediatr (Barc)* 2005;62(2):105–12.
4. Dark DS, Pingleton SK. Nonhemorrhagic gastrointestinal complications in acute respiratory failure. *Crit Care Med* 1989;17(8):755–8.

5. Jack L, Coyer F, Courtney M, et al. Diarrhoea risk factors in enterally tube fed critically ill patients: A retrospective audit. *Intensive Crit Care Nurs* 2010;26(6):327–34.

6. Zahar JR, Schwebel C, Adrie C, et al. Outcome of ICU patients with *Clostridium difficile* infection. *Crit Care* 2012;16(6):R215.

7. Reintam A, Parm P, Kitus R, et al. Gastrointestinal symptoms in intensive care patients. *Acta Anaesthesiol Scand* 2009;53(3):318–24.

8. Mutlu GM, Mutlu EA, Factor P. GI complications in patients receiving mechanical ventilation. *Chest* 2001;119(4):1222–41.

9. Bobo LD, Dubberke ER. Recognition and prevention of hospital-associated enteric infections in the intensive care unit. *Crit Care Med* 2010;38(8, suppl):S324–S334.

10. Chang RW, Jacobs S, Lee B. Gastrointestinal dysfunction among intensive care unit patients. *Crit Care Med* 1987;15(10):909–14.

11. Smith CE, Marien L, Brogdon C, et al. Diarrhea associated with tube feeding in mechanically ventilated critically ill patients. *Nurs Res* 1990;39(3):148–52.

12. Marcon AP, Gamba MA, Vianna LA. Nosocomial diarrhea in the intensive care unit. *Braz J Infect Dis* 2006;10(6):384–9.

13. Hernandez G, Velasco N, Wainstein, et al. Gut mucosal atrophy after a short enteral fasting period in critically ill patients. *J Crit Care* 1999;14(2):73–7.

14. Heimburger DC, Sockwell DG, Geels WJ. Diarrhea with enteral feeding: Prospective reappraisal of putative causes. *Nutrition* 1994;10(5):392–6.

15. Barrett JS, Shepherd SJ, Gibson PR. Strategies to manage gastrointestinal symptoms complicating enteral feeding. *JPEN J Parenter Enteral Nutr* 2009;33(1):21–6.

16. Davies AR, Morrison SS, Bailey MJ, et al. A multicenter, randomized controlled trial comparing early nasojejunal with nasogastric nutrition in critical illness. *Crit Care Med* 2012;40(8):2342–8.

17. Lopez-Herce J, Mencia S, Sanchez C, et al. Postpyloric enteral nutrition in the critically ill child with shock: A prospective observational study. *Nutr J* 2008;7:6.

18. Brinson RR, Kolts BE. Hypoalbuminemia as an indicator of diarrheal incidence in critically ill patients. *Crit Care Med* 1987;15(5):506–9.

19. Brinson RR, Kolts BE. Diarrhea associated with severe hypoalbuminemia: A comparison of a peptide-based chemically defined diet and standard enteral alimentation. *Crit Care Med* 1988;16(2):130–6.

20. Hwang TL, Lue MC, Nee YJ, et al. The incidence of diarrhea in patients with hypoalbuminemia due to acute or chronic malnutrition during enteral feeding. *Am J Gastroenterol* 1994;89(3):376–8.

21. DeMeo M, Kolli S, Keshavarzian A, et al. Beneficial effect of a bile acid resin binder on enteral feeding induced diarrhea. *Am J Gastroenterol* 1998;93(6):967–71.

22. Cunningham R, Dial S. Is over-use of proton pump inhibitors fuelling the current epidemic of *Clostridium difficile*-associated diarrhoea? *J Hosp Infect* 2008;70(1):1–6.

23. Brook I. Pseudomembranous colitis in children. *J Gastroenterol Hepatol* 2005;20(2):182–6.

24. Ang CW, Heyes G, Morrison P, et al. The acquisition and outcome of ICU-acquired *Clostridium difficile* infection in a single centre in the UK. *J Infect* 2008;57(6):435–40.

25. Humphries RM, Uslan DZ, Rubin Z. Performance of Clostridium difficile toxin enzyme immunoassay and nucleic acid amplification tests stratified by patient disease severity. *J Clin Microbiol* 2013;51(3):869–73.

26. Gebhard RL, Gerding DN, Olson MM, et al. Clinical and endoscopic findings in patients early in the course of *Clostridium difficile*-associated pseudomembranous colitis. *Am J Med* 1985;78(1):45–8.

27. Wiesen P, Van Gossum A, Preiser JC. Diarrhoea in the critically ill. *Curr Opin Crit Care* 2006;12(2):149–54.

28. Madsen K. Probiotics in critically ill patients. *J Clin Gastroenterol* 2008;42(suppl 3, pt 1):S116–S118.

29. Frohmader TJ, Chaboyer WP, Robertson IK, et al. Decrease in frequency of liquid stool in enterally fed critically ill patients given the multispecies probiotic VSL#3: A pilot trial. *Am J Crit Care* 2010;19(3):e1–e11.

30. Ferrie S, Daley M. Lactobacillus GG as treatment for diarrhea during enteral feeding in critical illness: Randomized controlled trial. *JPEN J Parenter Enteral Nutr* 2011;35(1):43–9.

31. Honeycutt TC, El Khashab M, Wardrop RM III, et al. Probiotic administration and the incidence of nosocomial infection in pediatric intensive care: A randomized placebo-controlled trial. *Pediatr Crit Care Med* 2007;8(5):452–8; quiz 464.

32. Simor AE. Diagnosis, management, and prevention of *Clostridium difficile* infection in long-term care facilities: A review. *J Am Geriatr Soc* 2010;58(8):1556–64.

33. Shah SB, Hanauer SB. Treatment of diarrhea in patients with inflammatory bowel disease: Concepts and cautions. *Rev Gastroenterol Disord* 2007;(7, suppl 3):S3–S10.

34. Fraser RJ, Bryant L. Current and future therapeutic prokinetic therapy to improve enteral feed intolerance in the ICU patient. *Nutr Clin Pract* 2010;25(1):26–31.

35. Caddell KA, Martindale R, McClave SA, et al. Can the intestinal dysmotility of critical illness be differentiated from postoperative ileus? *Curr Gastroenterol Rep* 2011;13(4):358–67.

36. Kehlet H, Holte K. Review of postoperative ileus. *Am J Surg* 2001;182(5, suppl 1):3S–10S.

37. McClave SA, Martindale RG, Vanek VW, et al. Guidelines for the provision and assessment of nutrition support therapy in the adult and critically ill patient. *JPEN J Parenter Enteral Nutr* 2009;33:277–316.

38. Fruhwald S, Holzer P, Metzler H. Gastrointestinal motility in acute illness. *Wien Klin Wochenschr* 2008;120(1-2):6–17.

39. Madl C, Druml W. Gastrointestinal disorders of the critically ill. Systemic consequences of ileus. *Best Pract Res Clin Gastroenterol* 2003;17(3):445–56.

40. Nguyen NQ, Fraser RJ, Chapman M, et al. Proximal gastric response to small intestinal nutrients is abnormal in mechanically ventilated critically ill patients. *World J Gastroenterol* 2006;12(27):4383–8.

41. Dive A, Moulart M, Jonard P, et al. Gastroduodenal motility in mechanically ventilated critically ill patients: A manometric study. *Crit Care Med* 1994;22(3):441–7.

42. Lodato RF, Khan AR, Zembowicz MJ, et al. Roles of IL-1 and TNF in the decreased ileal muscle contractility induced by lipopolysaccharide. *Am J Physiol* 1999;276(6, pt 1):G1356–G1362.

43. Cullen JJ, Caropreso DK, Ephgrave KS, et al. The effect of endotoxin on canine jejunal motility and transit. *J Surg Res* 1997;67(1):54–7.

44. Cullen JJ, Caropreso DK, Hemann LL, et al. Pathophysiology of adynamic ileus. *Dig Dis Sci* 1997;42(4):731–7.

45. Rokyta R Jr, Matějovic M, Krouzecký A, et al. Enteral nutrition and hepatosplanchnic region in critically ill patients—friends or foes? *Physiol Res* 2003;52(1):31–7.

46. Spain DA, Kawabe T, Keelan PC, et al. Decreased alpha-adrenergic response in the intestinal microcirculation after "two-hit" hemorrhage/resuscitation and bacteremia. *J Surg Res* 1999;84(2):180–5.

47. Bassiouny HS. Nonocclusive mesenteric ischemia. *Surg Clin North Am* 1997;77(2):319–26.

48. DeLegge MH. Managing gastric residual volumes in the critically ill patient: An update. *Curr Opin Clin Nutr Metab Care* 2011;14:193–6.

49. Kuppinger DD, Rittler P, Hartl WH, et al. Use of gastric residual volume to guide enteral nutrition in critically ill patients: A brief systematic review of clinical studies. *Nutrition* 2013;29:1075–9.

50. Chapman M, Fraser R, Vozzo R, et al. Antro-pyloro-duodenal motor responses to gastric and duodenal nutrient in critically ill patients. *Gut* 2005;54(10):1384–90.

51. Nguyen NQ, Fraser RJ, Bryant LK, et al. Diminished functional association between proximal and distal gastric motility in critically ill patients. *Intensive Care Med* 2008;34(7):1246–55.

52. Holzer P, Holzer-Petsche U. Tachykinins in the gut. Part I. Expression, release and motor function. *Pharmacol Ther* 1997;73(3):173–217.

53. Nguyen NQ, Fraser RJ, Chapman MJ, et al. Feed intolerance in critical illness is associated with increased basal and nutrient-stimulated plasma cholecystokinin concentrations. *Crit Care Med* 2007;35(1):82–8.

54. Coşkun T, Bozkurt A, Alican I, et al. Pathways mediating CRF-induced inhibition of gastric emptying in rats. *Regul Pept* 1997;69(3):113–20.

55. Scirocco A, Matarrese P, Petitta C, et al. Exposure of Toll-like receptors 4 to bacterial lipopolysaccharide (LPS) impairs human colonic smooth muscle cell function. *J Cell Physiol* 2010;223(2):442–50.

56. Fukuda H, Tsuchida D, Koda K, et al. Inhibition of sympathetic pathways restores postoperative ileus in the upper and lower gastrointestinal tract. *J Gastroenterol Hepatol* 2007;22(8):1293–9.

57. Levein NG, Thörn SE, Lindberg G, et al. Dopamine reduces gastric tone in a dose-related manner. *Acta Anaesthesiol Scand* 1999;43(7):722–5.

58. Levein NG, Thorn SE, Wattwil M. Dopamine delays gastric emptying and prolongs orocaecal transit time in volunteers. *Eur J Anaesthesiol* 1999;16(4):246–50.

59. Tarling MM, Toner CC, Withington PS, et al. A model of gastric emptying using paracetamol absorption in intensive care patients. *Intensive Care Med* 1997;23(3):256–60.

60. King W, Petrillo T, Pettignano R. Enteral nutrition and cardiovascular medications in the pediatric intensive care unit. *JPEN J Parenter Enteral Nutr* 2004;28:334–8.

61. Panchal AK, Manzi J, Connolly S, et al. Safety of enteral feedings in critically ill children receiving vasoactive agents [published online ahead of print August 28, 2014]. *JPEN J Parenter Enteral Nutr.* doi:10.1177/0148607114546533

62. Jacobs DG, Jacobs DO, Kudsk KA, et al. Practice management guidelines for nutritional support of the trauma patient. *J Trauma* 2004;57(3):660–78; discussion 679.

63. López-Herce J, Sánchez C, Carrillo A, et al. Transpyloric enteral nutrition in the critically ill child with renal failure. *Intensive Care Med* 2006;32(10):1599–605.

64. Kincaid MS, Vavilala MS, Faucher L, et al. Feeding intolerance as a result of small-intestine intussusception in a child with major burns. *J Burn Care Rehabil* 2004;25(2):212–4; discussion 211.

65. Deane AM, Wong GL, Horowitz M, et al. Randomized double-blind crossover study to determine the effects of erythromycin on small intestinal nutrient absorption and transit in the critically ill. *Am J Clin Nutr* 2012;95(6):1396–402.

66. Dive A, Miesse C, Galanti L, et al. Effect of erythromycin on gastric motility in mechanically ventilated critically ill patients: A double-blind, randomized, placebo-controlled study. *Crit Care Med* 1995;23(8):1356–62.

67. Annese V, Janssens J, Vantrappen G, et al. Erythromycin accelerates gastric emptying by inducing antral contractions and improved gastroduodenal coordination. *Gastroenterology* 1992;102(3):823–8.

68. Fraser R, Shearer T, Fuller J, et al. Intravenous erythromycin overcomes small intestinal feedback on antral, pyloric, and duodenal motility. *Gastroenterology* 1992;103(1):114–9.

69. Thompson JS, Quigley EM. Prokinetic agents in the surgical patient. *Am J Surg* 1999;177(6):508–14.

70. Coulie B, Tack J, Peeters T, et al. Involvement of two different pathways in the motor effects of erythromycin on the gastric antrum in humans. *Gut* 1998;43(3):395–400.

71. Nguyen NQ, Chapman MJ, Fraser RJ, et al. Erythromycin is more effective than metoclopramide in the treatment of feed intolerance in critical illness. *Crit Care Med* 2007;35(2):483–9.

72. Park MI, Camilleri M. Gastroparesis: Clinical update. *Am J Gastroenterol* 2006;101(5):1129–39.

73. Nguyen NQ, Chapman M, Fraser RJ, et al. Prokinetic therapy for feed intolerance in critical illness: One drug or two? *Crit Care Med* 2007;35(11):2561–7.

74. Heyland DK, Tougas G, Cook DJ, et al. Cisapride improves gastric emptying in mechanically ventilated, critically ill patients. A randomized, double-blind trial. *Am J Respir Crit Care Med* 1996;154(6, pt 1):1678–83.

75. Spapen HD, Duinslaeger L, Diltoer M, et al. Gastric emptying in critically ill patients is accelerated by adding cisapride to a standard enteral feeding protocol: Results of a prospective, randomized, controlled trial. *Crit Care Med* 1995;23(3):481–5.

76. DiLorenzo C, Lucanto C, Flores AF, et al. Effect of sequential erythromycin and octreotide on antroduodenal manometry. *J Pediatr Gastroenterol Nutr* 199;29:293–6.

77. Yuan CS. Methylnaltrexone mechanisms of action and effects on opioid bowel dysfunction and other opioid adverse effects. *Ann Pharmacother* 2007;41(6):984–93.

78. Yuan CS, Foss JF, O'Connor M, et al. Methylnaltrexone for reversal of constipation due to chronic methadone use: A randomized controlled trial. *JAMA* 2000;283(3):367–72.

79. Webster L, Jansen JP, Peppin J, et al. Alvimopan, a peripherally acting mu-opioid receptor (PAM-OR) antagonist for the treatment of opioid-induced bowel dysfunction: results from a randomized, double-blind, placebo-controlled, dose-finding study in subjects taking opioids for chronic non-cancer pain. *Pain* 2008;137(2):428–40.

80. Irving G, Pénzes J, Ramjattan B, et al. A randomized, placebo-controlled phase 3 trial (Study SB-767905/013) of alvimopan for opioid-induced bowel dysfunction in patients with non-cancer pain. *J Pain* 2011;12(2):175–84.

81. Akca O, Doufas AG, Sessler DI. Use of selective opiate receptor inhibitors to prevent postoperative ileus. *Minerva Anestesiol* 2002;68(4):162–5.

82. Nguyen T, Frenette AJ, Johanson C, et al. Impaired gastrointestinal transit and its associated morbidity in the intensive care unit. *J Crit Care* 2013;28(4):537.e11–537.e17.

83. Turton P. Ventilator-associated pneumonia in paediatric intensive care: A literature review. *Nurs Crit Care* 2008;13(5):241–8.

84. Drakulovic MB, Torres A, Bauer TT, et al. Supine body position as a risk factor for nosocomial pneumonia in mechanically ventilated patients: a randomised trial. *Lancet* 1999;354(9193):1851–8.

85. Allen Furr L, Binkley CJ, McCurren, et al. Factors affecting quality of oral care in intensive care units. *J Adv Nurs* 2004;48(5):454–62.

86. Hunter JD. Ventilator associated pneumonia. *Postgrad Med J* 2006;82(965):172–8.

87. Montejo Gonzalez JC, Estebanez Montiel B. [Gastrointestinal complications in critically ill patients]. *Nutr Hosp* 2007;(22, suppl 2):56–62.

88. Macharia EW, Eaton S, de Coppi P, et al. Fundoplication in ventilator-dependent infants with gastro-oesophageal reflux. *Eur J Pediatr Surg* 2012;22(1):91–6.

89. Landzinski J, Kiser TH, Fish DN, et al. Gastric motility function in critically ill patients tolerant vs. intolerant to gastric nutrition. *JPEN J Parenter Enteral Nutr* 2008;32(1):45–50.

90. Kölbel CB, Rippel K, Klar H, et al. Esophageal motility disorders in critically ill patients: A 24-hour manometric study. *Intensive Care Med* 2000;26(10):1421–7.

91. Chapman MJ, Besanko LK, Burgstad CM, et al. Gastric emptying of a liquid nutrient meal in the critically ill: Relationship between scintigraphic and carbon breath test measurement. *Gut* 2011;60(10):1336–43.

92. Quigley EM. Critical care dysmotility: Abnormal foregut motor function in the ICU/ITU patient. *Gut* 2005;54(10):1351–2; discussion 1384–90.

93. Nind G, Chen WH, Protheroe R, et al. Mechanisms of gastroesophageal reflux in critically ill mechanically ventilated patients. *Gastroenterology* 2005;128(3):600–6.

94. Ferrer M, Bauer TT, Torres A, et al. Effect of nasogastric tube size on gastroesophageal reflux and microaspiration in intubated patients. *Ann Intern Med* 1999;130(12):991–4.

95. Canani RB, Cirillo P, Roggero P, et al. Therapy with gastric acidity inhibitors increases the risk of acute gastroenteritis and community-acquired pneumonia in children. *Pediatrics* 2006;117(5):e817–e820.

96. Prod'hom G, Leuenberger P, Koerfer J, et al. Nosocomial pneumonia in mechanically ventilated patients receiving antacid, ranitidine, or sucralfate as prophylaxis for stress ulcer. A randomized controlled trial. *Ann Intern Med* 1994;120(8):653–62.

97. Driks MR, Craven DE, Celli BR, et al. Nosocomial pneumonia in intubated patients given sucralfate as compared with antacids or histamine type 2 blockers. The role of gastric colonization. *N Engl J Med* 1987;317(22):1376–82.

98. Cook D, Guyatt G, Marshall J, et al. A comparison of sucralfate and ranitidine for the prevention of upper gastrointestinal bleeding in patients requiring mechanical ventilation. Canadian Critical Care Trials Group. *N Engl J Med* 1998;338(12):791–7.

99. Miano TA, Reichert MG, Houle TT, et al. Nosocomial pneumonia risk and stress ulcer prophylaxis: A comparison of pantoprazole vs. ranitidine in cardiothoracic surgery patients. *Chest* 2009;136(2):440–7.

100. Barkun AN, Adam V, Martel M, et al. Cost-effectiveness analysis: Stress ulcer bleeding prophylaxis with proton pump inhibitors, H_2 receptor antagonists. *Value Health* 2013;16(1):14–22.

101. Sharma H, Singh D, Pooni P, et al. A study of profile of ventilator-associated pneumonia in children in Punjab. *J Trop Pediatr* 2009;55(6):393–5.

102. Lopriore E, Markhorst DG, Gemke RJ. Ventilator-associated pneumonia and upper airway colonisation with Gram negative bacilli: The role of stress ulcer prophylaxis in children. *Intensive Care Med* 2002;28(6):763–7.

103. Yildizdas D, Yapicioglu H, Yilmaz HL. Occurrence of ventilator-associated pneumonia in mechanically ventilated pediatric intensive care patients during stress ulcer prophylaxis with sucralfate, ranitidine, and omeprazole. *J Crit Care* 2002;17(4):240–5.

104. Hsu CW, Sun SF, Lin SL, et al. Duodenal versus gastric feeding in medical intensive care unit patients: A prospective, randomized, clinical study. *Crit Care Med* 2009;37(6):1866–72.

105. Meert KL, Daphtary KM, Metheny NA. Gastric vs. small-bowel feeding in critically ill children receiving mechanical ventilation: A randomized controlled trial. *Chest* 2004;126(3):872–8.

106. Lyons KA, Brilli RJ, Wieman RA, et al. Continuation of transpyloric feeding during weaning of mechanical ventilation and tracheal extubation in children: a randomized controlled trial. *JPEN J Parenter Enteral Nutr* 2002;26(3):209–13.

107. Martinez EE, Bechard LJ, Mehta NM. Nutrition algorithms and bedside nutrient delivery practices in pediatric intensive care units: An international multicenter cohort study. *Nutr Clin Pract* 2014;29:360–7.

108. Barnes N, Robertson N, Lakhoo K. Anti-reflux surgery for the neonatal intensive care-dependent infant. *Early Hum Dev* 2003;75(1-2):71–8.

CHAPTER 99 ■ GASTROINTESTINAL BLEEDING

SABINA MIR AND DOUGLAS S. FISHMAN

KEY POINTS

1. Patients in a critical care unit are at high risk of gastrointestinal bleeding from stress-related mucosal ulcers and may benefit from prophylactic antisecretory therapy.

2. Initiate broad-spectrum antibiotic coverage and medical reduction of portal hypertension early in the course of acute variceal bleeding.

3. A clear nasogastric aspirate does not exclude a bleeding source proximal to the ligament of Treitz.

4. Investigate infectious etiologies in acute bloody diarrhea: *Escherichia coli* O157:H7, *Shigella*, *Salmonella*, *Yersinia*, *Campylobacter*, and *Clostridium difficile*.

INTRODUCTION AND EPIDEMIOLOGY

Gastrointestinal (GI) bleeding is a common condition in the pediatric age group with a higher incidence in children admitted in the intensive care unit (ICU). The reported incidence of GI bleeding in the pediatric ICU (PICU) is 6%–25% (1–3). Fortunately, the risk of life-threatening bleeding in children admitted in the PICU with upper GI bleeding is only 0.4% (3). Critically ill patients have an increased risk of GI bleeding secondary to multiple comorbidities (high blood pressure, mechanical ventilation (2), disseminated intravascular coagulopathy (DIC), medications, circulatory shock, trauma, and septicemia).

In 2009, 23,383 children aged 11–15 years were admitted in US hospitals with a diagnosis of GI bleeding. The highest mortality rates associated with GI bleeding were in cases with intestinal perforation (8.7%) and esophageal perforation (8.4%). Children with GI bleed had higher rates of comorbidities (12.3% vs. 2.3%; p<.001) (4).

In adult patients, non variceal upper GI bleeding is associated with costs ranging from $3180 to 8890 per admission and a mortality of 3.5% (5). The severity of upper GI bleeding may range from self-resolving benign conditions to progressive and life-threatening bleeding that prompts immediate intervention. This chapter focuses on the initial approach, diagnostic investigation, and management (medical and therapeutic) of GI bleeding in the PICU.

ANATOMICAL LOCATION

GI bleeding is broadly divided into upper and lower GI tract, depending on the anatomical origin. The ligament of Treitz, located at the junction of the end of the duodenum and beginning of the jejunum, provides the division between the upper and lower GI tracts; upper bleeding originates proximal to the ligament, and lower bleeding originates distally. Upper GI bleeding is further characterized into variceal and non-variceal bleeding. It is essential to exclude other, non-GI, sites where bleeding may originate, such as from the nose or lungs, as different management is required.

DEFINITIONS AND CLINICAL PRESENTATION

Hematemesis is vomiting fresh blood and indicates a rapidly bleeding lesion.

Coffee ground emesis is vomit with a dark brown color due to the effects of gastric acid on the blood.

Melena is a dark-, black-, or tar-colored stool, secondary to bleeding from above the ileocecal valve or, if colonic transit time is slow, from proximal large bowel. A small volume of blood in the stomach can cause melena for 3–5 days and may not indicate ongoing bleeding.

Hematochezia is the passage of bright red blood per rectum or maroon-colored stools, resulting from a colonic source or massive upper GI bleeding.

Obscure GI bleeding (OGIB) is blood loss that occurs with a negative upper endoscopy and colonoscopy or obvious source from basic imaging.

ETIOLOGY

There are numerous causes of GI bleeding in the pediatric population, varying with the age of the child. **Tables 99.1–99.3** summarize the etiology of GI bleeding in children (6).

DIAGNOSTIC EVALUATION

A detailed history, including medications that may potentiate GI bleeding (e.g., anti platelet agents and non steroidal anti-inflammatory drugs [NSAIDS]), and physical examination are important in elucidating the cause and source of bleeding. Physical findings characteristic of underlying disease can help establish the diagnosis (**Table 99.4**). There are a number of interventional options available for diagnostic evaluation and intervention; they are described in the following section and the next, and summarized in **Figure 99.1**.

TABLE 99.1

CAUSES OF NON VARICEAL UPPER GASTROINTESTINAL BLEEDING IN CHILDREN

■ NEWBORN	■ INFANT	■ CHILD-ADOLESCENT
Swallowed maternal blood	Esophagitis	Esophagitis
Maternal breast milk irritation	Maternal breast milk irritation	*H. pylori* (gastritis)
Stress gastritis, ulcers	Duodenitis	Salicylates, NSAIDS
Vitamin K deficiency	Peptic ulcer disease	Mallory–Weiss tear
Vascular malformation	Mallory–Weiss tear	Duodenal Crohn
Milk protein sensitivity	Gastric esophageal duplication	Vascular malformation
Necrotizing enterocolitis	Salicylates, NSAIDS	Dieulafoy lesion
Hemophilia	Foreign body	Coagulopathy (DIC, ITP)
Gastric esophageal duplication	Coagulopathy (DIC, ITP)	
Maternal ITP	Vascular malformation	
	Dieulafoy lesion	

DIC, disseminated intravascular coagulopathy; ITP, idiopathic thrombocytopenic purpura; NSAIDS, non steroidal anti-inflammatory drugs.

TABLE 99.2

CAUSES OF VARICEAL GASTROINTESTINAL BLEEDING IN CHILDREN

■ PREHEPATIC	■ POSTHEPATIC	■ INTRAHEPATIC
Portal vein thrombosis	Budd–Chiari syndrome	Biliary atresia
Splenic vein thrombosis	Congestive heart failure	Autoimmune hepatitis
Arteriovenous fistula	Inferior vena cava obstruction	Metabolic liver disease (Wilson disease, hemachromatosis)
	Constrictive pericarditis	Toxins
		Sinusoidal obstruction syndrome (veno-occlusive disease)
		Infectious hepatitis

The Nasogastric Tube

An assessment of active bleeding (and gastric decompression) can be determined by nasogastric (NG) tube placement, although the role of tube placement is controversial. A meta-analysis of adult patients with GI bleeding revealed that blood or coffee ground material in an NG aspirate has a 44% sensitivity, 95% specificity, and positive likelihood ratio of 9.4 for UGI bleeding (7). In a study of 520 patients that underwent NG aspirate prior to endoscopy for UGI bleed, 15% had a clear aspirate but were found to have an upper GI lesion on

endoscopy (8). Hence, a clear NG aspirate does not exclude a bleeding source proximal to the ligament of Treitz. Conversely, the presence of blood in the NG aspirate generally confirms the diagnosis of UGI bleeding in an otherwise consistent clinical context and provided swallowed blood can be ruled out. On balance, we favor the placement of an NG tube in children in the PICU with suspected UGI bleeding to confirm the diagnosis and improve the conditions for endoscopy. Potential

TABLE 99.3

CAUSES OF LOWER GASTROINTESTINAL BLEEDING IN CHILDREN

■ NEONATE	■ INFANT	■ CHILD-ADOLESCENT
Hemorrhagic disease of newborn	Anal fissure	Anal fissure
Coagulopathy	Infectious colitis	Infectious colitis
Milk protein sensitivity	Intussusception	Polyp
Necrotizing enterocolitis	Meckel diverticulum	Vascular malformation
Volvulus	Volvulus	Inflammatory bowel disease
Vascular malformation	Vascular malformation	Vasculitis (Henoch–Schönlein purpura)
Hirschsprung disease enterocolitis	Intestinal duplication	Intestinal duplication

TABLE 99.4

PHYSICAL EXAMINATION

■ SYSTEM	■ SIGN	■ SUSPECTED DIAGNOSIS
Eyes	Jaundice	Cirrhosis
	Iritis	IBD
Skin	Hemangiomas, telangiectasia	Vascular anomalies
	Petechia, bruises	Cirrhosis, DIC
	Jaundice	Cirrhosis
	Purpura	HSP
	Skin tags, anal fissures, erythema nodosum, pyoderma gangrenosum	IBD
Abdomen	Hepatosplenomegaly, ascites	Cirrhosis
	Distension, rebound tenderness	Bowel perforation
Joints	Arthritis	HSP, IBD

DIC, disseminated intravascular coagulopathy; HSP, Henoch–Schönlein purpura; IBD, inflammatory bowel disease.

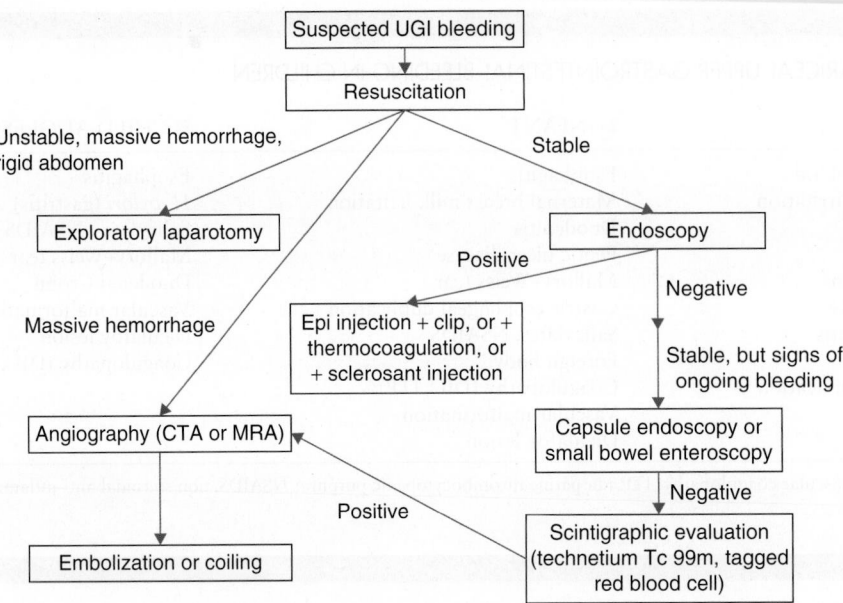

FIGURE 99.1. Diagnostic algorithm for severe upper GI hemorrhage. Epi, epinephrine.

complications of NG tube insertion should be considered in patients with basil skull fracture, severe facial trauma, clotting disorders, esophageal varices, esophageal tumors, or esophageal surgery.

Laboratory Tests

Hemodynamic changes (e.g., tachycardia, hypotension) are signs of hypovolemic shock and require immediate resuscitation measures prior to further evaluation. Initial laboratory investigations (complete blood count and coagulation profile)

should be instituted during resuscitation. Once the child is hemodynamically stable, additional laboratory testing (**Table 99.5**) to investigate the cause and to direct therapy may include liver panel, metabolic panel, erythrocyte sedimentation rate (ESR), C-reactive protein (CRP), and stool cultures (*E. coli* O157:H7, *Shigella*, *Salmonella*, *Yersinia*, *Campylobacter*, and *Clostridium difficile* [*C. diff*] PCR). Fecal and gastric contents can be tested for the presence of hemoglobin using a guaiac-based test to detect occult bleeding. False-positive guaiac reactions occur with intake of red meat, raw fruits or vegetables, and other foods with peroxidase activity. Inflammatory markers (ESR and CRP) are useful when inflammatory bowel disease is considered.

TABLE 99.5

INVESTIGATION

■ INVESTIGATION	■ INDICATION
Laboratory	
Complete blood count	Assess severity of bleeding (anemia and thrombocytopenia)
PT/INR and PTT	Coagulopathy (liver dysfunction, DIC)
BUN/Cr	High ratio (>30) suggestive of UGI bleed (in adults)
Stool culture	Infectious colitis (*Shigella, Salmonella, Yersenia, Campylobacter,* and enteropathic *E. coli*) Stool PCR for *C. diff*
ESR/CRP	Infectious and inflammatory disorders
Guaiac-based tests	Detection of hemoglobin in gastric or fecal content
Imaging	
X-ray	Foreign body, bowel perforation or obstruction
Abdominal ultrasound	Portal hypertension, vascular malformation, intussusception
Radionuclide scanning	TPT (Meckel scan), detection of heterotopic gastric mucosa
CT/MRI abdomen	Mass, vascular malformation, intestinal duplication
Angiography	In massive UGI bleed (bleeding must be at least 0.5 mL/min to be detected
Endoscopy	
Esophagogastroduodenoscopy	For assessing acute UGI bleeding requiring transfusion or unexplained recurrent bleeding
Colonoscopy	Polyps, colitis, vascular malformations
Enteroscopy	Small bowel polyps, ulcers, colitis, vascular malformations
Wireless capsule study	Small bowel polyps, ulcers, colitis, vascular malformations

DIC, disseminated intravascular coagulopathy; UGI, upper gastrointestinal; TPT, technetium 99m pertechnetate.

Radiologic and Nuclear Medicine Imaging

Plain x-ray film may be useful in the setting of suspected GI perforation or intestinal obstruction presenting with bleeding. Ultrasonography with Doppler flow is useful for the evaluation of portal hypertension, liver disease, large vascular anomalies (arteriovenous malformations, hemangiomas), and intussusception. Air contrast or barium contrast enema can be used to confirm the diagnosis and treat colonic intussusception. Regular and angiographic CT and MRI are noninvasive and useful in detecting mass lesions and vascular malformations. These modalities are noninvasive but may require sedation. Technetium 99m pertechnetate (TPT) rapidly binds to gastric mucosa and is useful in detecting ectopic gastric mucosa, particularly Meckel diverticulum. The sensitivity of TPT scintigraphy has been reported to range from 50% to 91% (9,10). Pretreatment with pentagastrin, histamine H_2 blockers, or glucagon is reported to enhance the sensitivity of the Meckel scan (11). The low negative predictive (0.74) limits the clinical utility of a Meckel scan in patients with lower GI bleeding in the presence of anemia (12,13).

Bleeding sites can be visualized by a tagged red blood cell (RBC) scan if the rate of bleeding is greater than 0.5 mL/min. Angiography (interventional or CT) is an alternative in massive bleeding (greater than 0.5 mL/min) or when endoscopic evaluation and therapy are difficult. These modalities provide an approach for both diagnosis and the potential for therapeutic embolization or coiling (13). In a case series of 34 patients aged 7–92 years, with OGIB or lower GI bleed, angiography identified the source of bleed in 31% (14) (**Fig. 99.1**).

Endoscopic Evaluation

GI endoscopy is a highly effective method to identify the source and to treat UGI bleeding. It is indicated in GI bleed requiring blood product transfusions, recurrent bleeding, or if additional diagnostic information is needed. There are no guidelines or indications for early endoscopy in children as compared to adults with GI bleeding. Urgent endoscopy with surgical backup may be required in variceal and non variceal bleeding refractory to medical therapy. Urgent endoscopy performed within 24 hours is recommended in adults with Hb <8 g/dL and hypovolemic shock after initial resuscitation (15). In adults, early upper endoscopy for GI bleed is associated with a decreased need for blood transfusion and a shorter hospital stay without change in mortality (16,17).

The administration of proton pump inhibitors (PPIs) and prokinetic agents in relation to endoscopic evaluation has been studied. Administration of PPIs is commonly used as pharmacologic acid suppression therapy in management of UGI bleeding. They allow platelet aggregation and clot formation by inhibiting gastric acid production. A Cochrane meta-analysis of six randomized control trials of PPI use before endoscopy reported a reduced need for endoscopic intervention for UGI bleeding with the PPI use as compared to placebo, but showed no significant differences in mortality, rebleeding, or need for surgery (18). The use of high-dose intravenous (IV) PPI after endoscopy in patients with bleeding ulcers has shown to reduce the risk of rebleeding as compared to placebo [HR-Heart Rate], 3.9; [95% confidence interval (CI), 1.7–9.0] (19).

The optimal regimen of PPI administration (continuous infusion vs. interval dosing) to achieve a neutral gastric pH is unclear. Investigation of dosing shows that high-dose IV PPI (omeprazole or esomeprazole, 80-mg bolus followed by 8 mg/h for 72 hours) reduced rebleeding ($p = 0.02$) compared to standard dose for adults with bleeding peptic ulcers (20). Choice of PPI depends on availability at individual institutes.

Prokinetics is useful for promoting gastric motility and movement of retained blood for better visualization during endoscopy. In a meta-analysis, a decreased rate of repeat endoscopy in UGI bleed has been reported with administration of IV prokinetic (erythromycin: 3–5 mg/kg to max of 250 mg IV; or metoclopramide: 0.1–0.2 mg/kg to max of 10 mg IV) 20–120 minutes prior to procedure (OR-Odds Ratio, 0.55; 95% CI, 0.32–0.94) (21).

Various modalities are available to provide effective endoscopic hemostasis in patients with GI bleeding. Sclerotherapy with injection of several available sclerosants (e.g., sodium morrhuate, ethanol, ethanolamine, fibrin, and cyanoacrylate glue) is frequently used (22). Hemostasis of bleeding sites may also be achieved endoscopically by using clips, band ligation, and several types of cautery (15). Available cautery devices include mono-, bi-, or multipolar electrocautery, argon plasma coagulation, and heater probes. In a meta-analysis comparing available endoscopic modalities for treating peptic ulcer disease (PUD), a lower risk of further bleeding was seen when therapeutic interventions (sclerosant, thermal therapy, fibrin glue, or clips) were used in combination with epinephrine injection versus using epinephrine injection alone (relative risk (RR), 0.40; 95% CI, 0.23–0.68). There was no significant difference in efficacy of achieving hemostasis with clip placement alone as compared to sclerosant or heater probes thermocoagulation (23).

Newer modalities such as wireless capsule endoscopy and enteroscopy are currently available to evaluate the small bowel and OGIB in children (22). Small bowel visualization for GI bleeding is indicated in suspected Crohn disease (CD), hereditary polyposis syndrome, OGIB, and evaluation of abdominal pain (24–26). In wireless capsule endoscopy, the patient swallows a video capsule made of biocompatible gastric acid-resistant material that allows noninvasive visualization of the entire small bowel by taking multiple pictures (27). This method does not allow mucosal biopsy or therapeutic interventions. Capsule endoscopy has been safely used in children as young as 10 months of age (25); it is safe and feasible with a sensitivity to detect GI bleed (28,29). In 49 adult patients with upper GI bleed, a capsule study detected blood in 83.3% of cases compared to NG aspiration (33.3%) (30). The diagnostic yield of capsule endoscopy has shown to be significantly higher than angiography (53.3% vs. 20%; $p = 0.016$) (31). Enteroscopy allows visualization of the entire small intestine with the benefit of therapeutic interventions (polypectomy, biopsies, and cautery). In a pediatric cohort of 30 patients, enteroscopy was done for suspected small bowel disease. Twenty two had occult GI bleed. In majority of patients, enteroscopy provided information for further treatment (32). However, in a comparison study between capsule endoscopy and enteroscopy in adult patients with OGIB, capsule endoscopy detected a lesion in 44.9% of the cases and enteroscopy in 53.4% ($p = 0.01$) (33).

Colonoscopy allows direct visualization of the entire colon, making it useful for diagnosis and treatment of a variety of lower GI bleeding disorders (colitis, polyps, and vascular malformations). Therapeutic interventions to achieve hemostasis during colonoscopy include epinephrine injection therapy, clipping, electrocoagulation, and argon plasma coagulation (34). To optimize visualization, a proper bowel cleanout is important. Certain conditions (e.g., fulminant colitis, suspicion of toxic megacolon, GI obstruction, and perforation) are relative contraindications for a colonoscopy (35). Colonoscopy can also be performed with a combined gastroenterology and surgical team to decompress the bowel or provide additional diagnostic information at the time of surgical intervention (14).

MANAGEMENT

Immediate management for GI bleeding may require airway protection and insertion of two large bore IV catheters for hemodynamic resuscitation by volume replacement (**Fig. 99.2**). NG tube placement indications and contraindications are discussed above in evaluation. Currently, there are no prospective randomized trials to support the utility of NG lavage in UGI bleed (36). Packed RBCs or whole blood is generally transfused to a goal of Hb 7–8 g/dL (37,38). Overtransfusion in patients with variceal bleeding is particularly hazardous and may exacerbate bleeding. Very rapid blood loss may require blood transfusion for volume resuscitation in the face of seemingly normal serum hemoglobin measurement. Some authors have suggested a goal of >10 g/dL in adults with lower GI bleeding (34). The preceding scenarios illustrate that while Hb 7–8 g/dL is a typical goal for a hemodynamically stable patient, the optimal transfusion plan and goal Hb need to be tailored to the individual patient depending on factors such as decompensated shock, ongoing blood loss, and the presence of underlying disease (e.g., cyanotic heart disease and portal hypertension).

Coagulopathy secondary to liver failure is a complex phenomenon involving decrease in procoagulants and anticoagulants (protein C, protein S, and antithrombin III), vitamin K deficiency from cholestasis (resulting in decreased synthesis of factors II, V, VII, IX, and X in addition to protein C and S), hypofibrinogemia, increased platelet destruction, and impaired platelet function. The INR is unreliable in liver failure patients and does not indicate risk of bleeding.

Underlying coagulopathy from liver disease or DIC may require replacement with platelets, fresh frozen plasma (FFP), and vitamin K. However, it is unrealistic to aim for complete correction of coagulopathy and thrombocytopenia as this may potentially result in volume overload increasing the risk of variceal rebleeding, raised intracranial pressure, and pulmonary edema (39). Administration of vitamin K, cryoprecipitate, FFP, and platelets is recommended in patients with active bleeding and prior to an invasive procedure (40). A platelet count of 50,000/μL is the goal for patients who are actively bleeding and prior to invasive procedures (41). FFP in the absence of bleeding is typically not recommended as it does not appear to reduce the risk of GI bleeding. Recombinant activated factor VII is not recommended for variceal bleeding based on randomized control trials (42).

Acid blockers may have a beneficial role in management of GI bleed. One explanation is that increasing the gastric pH indirectly stabilizes clot formation. Available pharmacological drugs (**Table 99.6**) target acid suppression (intravenous PPI, histamine [H$_2$] blockers). Choice of medication depends on availability. There is insufficient evidence on high- versus low-dose PPI in the presence of GI bleed. Cochrane review that included 13 studies (1716 patients) found no benefit of high-dose over low-dose PPI (43).

Vasoactive medications (vasopressin, somatostatin, and octreotide) are used in acute management of bleeding from portal hypertension. Vasopressin increases splanchnic vascular tone, causing a decrease in arterial splanchnic flow and portal venous pressure (44). Due to the vasoconstriction, side effects include organ ischemic injury. Octreotide and somatostatin decrease azygos blood flow, resulting in decreased variceal flow (45). The largest pediatric series on the efficacy of octreotide in children with portal hypertension was reported by Eroglu et al., who found that 71% of patients stopped bleeding with administration of octreotide (46).

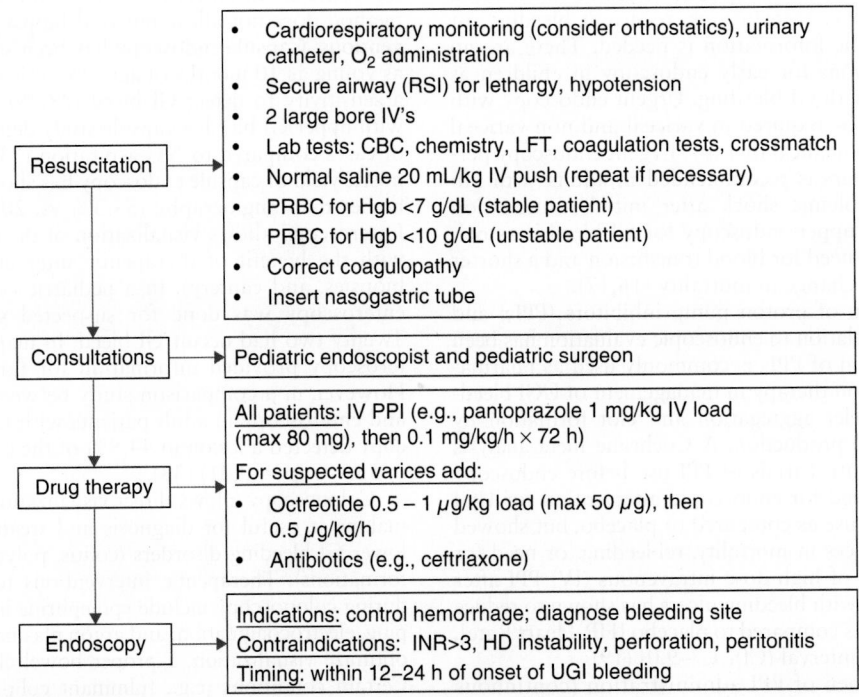

Resuscitation
- Cardiorespiratory monitoring (consider orthostatics), urinary catheter, O$_2$ administration
- Secure airway (RSI) for lethargy, hypotension
- 2 large bore IV's
- Lab tests: CBC, chemistry, LFT, coagulation tests, crossmatch
- Normal saline 20 mL/kg IV push (repeat if necessary)
- PRBC for Hgb <7 g/dL (stable patient)
- PRBC for Hgb <10 g/dL (unstable patient)
- Correct coagulopathy
- Insert nasogastric tube

Consultations
Pediatric endoscopist and pediatric surgeon

Drug therapy
All patients: IV PPI (e.g., pantoprazole 1 mg/kg IV load (max 80 mg), then 0.1 mg/kg/h × 72 h)
For suspected varices add:
- Octreotide 0.5 – 1 μg/kg load (max 50 μg), then 0.5 μg/kg/h
- Antibiotics (e.g., ceftriaxone)

Endoscopy
Indications: control hemorrhage; diagnose bleeding site
Contraindications: INR>3, HD instability, perforation, peritonitis
Timing: within 12–24 h of onset of UGI bleeding

FIGURE 99.2. Emergency management for severe UGI bleeding. A goal-directed approach involving a multidisciplinary team (intensivist, endoscopist, surgeon) is indicated. The management proceeds from resuscitation to emergency consultation, drug therapy, and endoscopy. For esophageal varices alternative management includes balloon tamponade (Sengstaken Blakemore tube), surgical shunt, and transjugular intrahepatic portosystemic shunt (TIPS). CBC, complete blood count; EST, endoscopic sclerotherapy; EVL, endoscopic variceal ligation.

TABLE 99.6

PHARMACOLOGICAL THERAPIES

■ DRUGS	■ DOSE
Vasoconstriction	
(for acute management of bleeding secondary to portal hypertension)	
Vasopressin	0.002–0.005 units/kg/min, maximum 0.01 units/kg/min (continuous IV)
Octreotide	0.5–2 µg/kg bolus (max 100 µg), then 0.5–1 µg/kg/h (continuous IV)
Acid Suppression	
Ranitidine	2–4 mg/kg/day divided 6–8 h, maximum 200 mg/d (IV)
Lansoprazole	0.6–1.8 mg/kg daily (IV)
Omeprazole	40 mg/1.72 m² daily (IV)
Esomeprazole	1 mo–1 y: 0.5 mg/kg daily; 1–17 y (less than 55 kg): 10 mg daily; > 55 kg: 20 mg daily (IV)
Pantoprazole	1 mg/kg/d, maximum 40 mg (IV)
Cytoprotection	
Sucralfate	40–80 mg/kg/d divided 6 h, maximum 1 g/day (oral)
Misoprostol	100–200 µg every 6–8 h (oral)

IV, intravenous.

Octreotide has a longer half-life than somatostatin and is therefore more commonly used.

SPECIFIC CONDITIONS

Neonatal GI Bleeding

Swallowed maternal blood during birth or nursing from cracked nipples can present with hematemesis in neonates within the first few days of life. Hemorrhagic disease of the newborn is a rare entity in the developed world with an estimated incidence of 0.01%–0.44% (47,48). It is a preventable and treatable condition secondary to vitamin K deficiency that responds to administration of vitamin K. Neonatal food allergies to cow's milk or soy protein represent a spectrum of disorders from sensitivity to severe enterocolitis presenting with hematemesis and/or hematochezia. Other causes of neonatal GI bleeding include necrotizing enterocolitis, liver disease, and hemorrhagic gastropathy.

A retrospective study on 100 critically ill neonates during a 5-month period identified mechanical ventilation as the main risk factor for GI bleeding. The cause of bleeding seems to be multifactorial. Neonates on ventilation are sicker to begin with. The added effects of stress-induced mucosal injury, coagulopathy, trauma from NG/endotracheal tubes, and GI complications from multiorgan failure hypotension, and prolonged delivery were additional risk factors for gastric mucosal lesion (49). Preterm infants exposed to indomethacin, dexamethasone, mechanical ventilation, and *nil per os* status may benefit with stress-ulcer prophylaxis (49,50). High-pressure mechanical ventilation is an independent risk factor for UGI bleed in children (2). A decrease in cardiac output from high positive end-expiratory pressure, which compromises splanchnic blood, can contribute to GI complications (51).

Ulcers and Gastritis

Gastroduodenal ulcers are rare in children. The estimated incidence of acid related or PUD (peptic ulcer disease) in the US pediatric population in 2008 ranged from 0.5 to 4.4/100,000 individuals (52). *Helicobacter pylori* (*H. pylori*) is a well-recognized cause of gastric and duodenal ulcers, more prevalent in underdeveloped countries compared to those with higher socioeconomic status (53). It is the primary cause of duodenal ulcers in children (54). There are several pharmacological regimens for eradication of *H. pylori*, mostly using a combination of two antibiotics plus a PPI. The most commonly used regimen is "triple therapy" with amoxicillin, clarithromycin, and a PPI. Metronidazole may be substituted for amoxicillin in patients allergic to penicillin. The duration of therapy is usually 7–14 days. Optimal treatment is based on the antibiotic susceptibility and the resistance pattern in the specific region (55). "Quadruple therapy" should be attempted in geographic regions with known resistance to triple therapy antibiotics or in patients who have recently received triple therapy antibiotics. The quadruple therapy is defined by the addition of bismuth to a PPI and two antibiotics to which helicobacter is sensitive (e.g., metronidazole or tetracycline).

Secondary etiologies of PUD include stress (shock, sepsis, trauma, burns, multiorgan failure, surgery) and medications (typically NSAIDS and steroids) (56). Impaired blood flow to the gut mucosa, dysmotility, loss of mucosal protective layer from impaired prostaglandin production, decreased gastric pH, and ischemia are implicated in the pathogenesis of stress ulcers in critically ill patients. A systematic review of the literature found that prophylactic therapy against stress ulcers and gastritis (including omeprazole, ranitidine, sucralfate, or almagate) in critically ill children was more likely to prevent UGI bleeding compared to no treatment (57). Randomized controlled trials in critically ill adults comparing PPI to histamine H_2 receptor antagonists for preventing UGI bleed demonstrated PPI to be more efficacious (RR, 0.36; 95% CI, 0.19–0.68; $p = 0.002$; $I = 0\%$) (58).

Patients in critical care units are at high risk of GI bleeding from stress-related mucosal ulcers and may benefit from prophylactic antisecretory therapy. Conversely, there was no difference in mortality and pneumonia rates between the treatment and no treatment groups. While there are a number of methodologic problems with meeting inclusion criteria in the few (2–3) randomized controlled trials and more study is needed, it is our practice to offer routine prophylactic acid suppression with a PPI to the critically ill child. The literature for adult patients notes that there is little data but suggests that acid suppression therapy may be discontinued once there is an improvement in mucosal blood flow and the patient is tolerating enteral nutrition (59,60).

Hematopoietic Stem-cell Transplant/ Immunosuppressed Patients

GI complications are a major cause of mortality and morbidity of hematopoietic stem-cell transplantation (HSCT) recipients (61). Etiologies of GI bleeding include infectious enteritis, mainly from cytomegalovirus (CMV) and *C. difficile*. Noninfectious causes include graft-versus-host disease (GVHD), typhlitis, and autoimmune and radiation-induced colitis.

In a retrospective study of 142 pediatric HSCT patients, the occurrence of melena and hematochezia was associated with ICU admission and increased risk of death within 100 post transplant days (61). Another adult retrospective study of 447 HSCT recipients reported that severe hemorrhage from any source doubled the mortality rate. They also found that patients with acute GVHD of skin and GI tract had a 2.9-fold higher risk of hemorrhage from any source (62). High-dose chemotherapy is another factor associated with GI bleeding.

Immunosuppressed individuals (secondary to disease or medications) (63,64) are at a high risk for *C. difficile* infection and require early recognition and treatment. The clinical presentation can include diarrhea, hematochezia, toxic megacolon, and perforation. Fecal enzyme immunoassay for *C. difficile* toxins is a commonly available diagnostic test with a sensitivity of 63%–94% and specificity of 75%–100%. Real-time PCR of toxins A and B has a sensitivity of 90%–95% and specificity 95%–96% (65). Available antibiotics for treatment include metronidazole, oral vancomycin, rifaximin, and fidaxomicin. In a recent phase 3 clinical trial, fidaxomicin was shown to be superior to vancomycin for treatment of *C. difficile* (66). Fecal bacteriotherapy, or fecal transplant, is a strategy for recurrent *C. difficile* infections, but is not widely available (67–69). Patients with fulminant *C. difficile* colitis may benefit from surgical intervention.

CMV enteritis is a less common presentation of CMV infection after HSCT. It is usually observed relatively late in the post engraftment period (2–3 months after transplant). (Please also see Chapters 90 and 117.) The management of the HSCT patient at risk of CMV is complicated by a combination of factors including the high risk of CMV infection, the increased mortality rates associated with CMV infection in the immune-compromised host, and the marrow toxicity of antiviral therapy, especially ganciclovir. Therefore, many centers avoid prophylactic ganciclovir, but start it preemptively (i.e., in the absence of symptoms) as soon as a surveillance test (serology, quantitative PCR, or culture) suggests CMV infection. Histologic examination of intestinal tissue after endoscopy or colonoscopy may aid in making the diagnosis.

Typhlitis (neutropenic enterocolitis) is an inflammation of the colon with or without involvement of the small bowel. It occurs in approximately 5% of patients with chemotherapy-induced neutropenia, with a lower incidence in the pediatric population (70,71). Typhlitis classically presents as abdominal pain, fever, vomiting, and diarrhea, rapidly progressing to hemorrhage and perforation. In neutropenic patients, these classical signs and symptoms may be absent, due to inability to mount an effective inflammatory response. Hence, a high index of suspicion is necessary to provide early imaging for detection of occult typhlitis in this population. Treatment is supportive with bowel rest, parenteral nutrition, and broad-spectrum antibiotic coverage for gram-positive and gram-negative organisms, including *Pseudomonas*, *C. difficile*, and fungus. Surgical management needs to be considered in the setting of persistent GI bleeding, perforation, and obstruction failing supportive therapy with decompression of the bowel. Colonoscopy in this setting carries a very high risk of perforation.

Patients with severe neutropenia have a high risk of bacteremia with GI procedures. The British Society of Gastroenterology guidelines recommend antibiotic prophylaxis prior to GI procedures (variceal sclerotherapy, esophageal dilation, laser therapy, and endoscopic retrograde cholangiopancreatography) in patients with a neutrophil count <500/μL (0.5 × 10⁹/L) (72).

Inflammatory Bowel Disease

Inflammatory bowel disease is broadly categorized as ulcerative colitis (UC) and CD, both of which can manifest with GI bleeding. Although up to 60% of children with CD may present with hematochezia, life-threatening GI hemorrhage is rare. Conversely, severe acute UC is a life-threatening condition with 1%–2% mortality and approximately 20%–25% patients require colectomy within 5 years of disease onset (73,74). UC requires aggressive supportive and medical management with timely involvement of the surgeons in case of failure to medical therapy. IV corticosteroids are the first line of treatment for moderate-to-severe disease, and rescue therapy with tacrolimus, infliximab, or cyclosporine is recommended for failure to respond to steroids in 3–5 days. Uncontrolled lower GI hemorrhage is an indication for colectomy in UC. Other indications for colectomy include failure of rescue therapy by days 6–10, toxic megacolon, or bowel perforation. Detailed management of acute severe UC is beyond the scope of this chapter (75,76).

Variceal Bleeding

Gastroesophageal varices develop secondary to portal hypertension. Causes of portal hypertension (**Table 99.2**) can be prehepatic, hepatic, or extrahepatic. Portal hypertension is defined as an increase in venous pressure greater than 10 mm Hg (normal: 5–10 mm Hg) in the vessels that bring blood from the GI tract and spleen to the liver. Variceal hemorrhage may occur at pressure greater than 12 mm Hg (44). Splanchnic vasodilatation increases portal vein flow and maintains portal hypertension, leading to the formation of porto-systemic collaterals in the esophageal, gastric, and colonic vessels. Approximately two-thirds of children with varices present with hematemesis or melena (77). Hematochezia may indicate anorectal varices or portal colopathy.

With advances in medical management and efficacious therapeutic interventions, the mortality rate from variceal bleeding in adults has been significantly decreased (78). Mortality in children from first bleeding episode is approximately 5%–15% (79). In children, cirrhosis is often secondary to biliary atresia (BA). The risk of death is higher for children with BA presenting with esophageal variceal bleeding (80) and with a higher rate of bleeding within the first year (81). In a Finnish series of 47 children with failed hepatoportoenterostomy for BA, surveillance endoscopy was recommended as young as 6 months of age (82).

After immediate resuscitation (**Fig. 99.2**), the management of portal hypertension in patients with intrahepatic disease (cirrhosis) can be broadly classified into reduction of portal pressure (vasoconstriction and shunts) and obliteration of varices (endoscopic band ligation, sclerotherapy, and glue) (83). Available pharmacological drugs (**Table 99.6**) target acid suppression (intravenous PPI, histamine [H₂] blockers) and portal vasoconstriction (vasopressin, somatostatin, and octreotide, which lower portal pressure by decreasing the splanchnic flow). Cirrhotic patients are prone to bacterial infections as a result of integration of multiple factors causing increased gut permeability. Antibiotic prophylaxis in individuals with cirrhosis and UGI bleed should be considered and has been shown to decrease mortality compared to placebo or no antibiotic (84–86). Treatment involves the initiation of broad-spectrum antibiotic coverage and medical reduction of portal hypertension early in the course of acute variceal bleeding. It is not known if bacterial infections are the cause of an acute variceal bleed or result from a bleeding episode. However, it is associated with rebleeding and possible mortality in patients with severe liver disease (87). The British Society of Gastroenterology guideline suggests fluoroquinolones (88). The American Association for Study of Liver Disease and American College of Gastroenterology guidelines in 2007 suggested IV ceftriaxone as being more effective (89,90).

Several procedural interventions should be considered in the patient with variceal bleeding. In the presence of severe hemorrhage, balloon tamponade (Sengstaken–Blakemore or Linton tubes) may serve as a temporary measure for uncontrolled bleeding from esophageal or gastric varices. The use of these tubes in very young children may be limited by available sizes. To control variceal bleeding, randomized control trials have not shown a benefit of emergency sclerotherapy versus vasoactive drug administration (91). Effective prophylactic sclerotherapy has been reported in infants with BA (mean age: 13 months; mean weight: 8.2 kg) (92). Successful obliteration of varices by sclerotherapy was achieved in 92%–95% of patients. A randomized control trial compared children who underwent endoscopic variceal ligation (EVL) (*n* = 25) to those who had endoscopic sclerotherapy (*n* = 24). Obliteration of varices was higher in the EVL group than the sclerotherapy group (*p* < 0.0001) with no significant difference in the recurrence rate after a 22-month follow-up period (85). A pilot pediatric study with 18 subjects (age < 2 years; weight < 10 kg) reported gastric variceal eradication in all cases after a mean of 1–2 sessions of cyanoacrylate glue (93). A systemic review that included 17 trials of 1817 adults found no benefit of sclerotherapy over vasoactive medications in patients presenting with GI bleeding secondary to cirrhosis (91). Another option of treatment for life-threatening variceal bleeding while waiting for a liver transplant is transjugular intrahepatic portosystemic shunt (TIPS). The TIPS procedure creates a portacaval shunt (stent placement between intrahepatic portal vein and hepatic vein) that results in decreased portal venous pressure. TIPS is reserved for cases that have failed pharmacological and endoscopic interventions to control bleeding (94). Complications of the TIPS procedure include hepatic encephalopathy, shunt stenosis, liver failure, and hepatic perforation during placement.

SUMMARY AND FUTURE DIRECTIONS

Advances in therapeutic endoscopy, imaging modalities, and drug therapy have revolutionized the management of GI hemorrhage. In addition to general measures to achieve hemodynamic stability, specific management of bleeding depends on the etiology. Therefore, a detailed history, physical examination, and a thoughtful diagnostic approach are essential. Considering the multiple comorbidities of children in the ICU and risk of GI bleeding, a multidisciplinary approach to optimize care and prevent GI hemorrhage cannot be overemphasized.

Future directions for improving management of GI bleeding include (a) generating a pediatric scoring system based on clinical signs and symptoms to determine prognostic factors and to categorize those who may benefit from early endoscopic interventions, (b) establishing evidence-based guidelines for stress-ulcer prophylaxis in critically ill children, and (c) identifying factors that may predict response or failure to treatment in variceal bleeding.

References

1. Chaibou M, Tucci M, Dugas MA, et al. Clinically significant upper gastrointestinal bleeding acquired in a pediatric intensive care unit: A prospective study. *Pediatrics* 1998;102(4 pt 1):933–8.
2. Deerojanawong J, Peongsujarit D, Vivatvakin B, et al. Incidence and risk factors of upper gastrointestinal bleeding in mechanically ventilated children. *Pediatr Crit Care Med* 2009;10(1):91–5.
3. Lacroix J, Nadeau D, Laberge S, et al. Frequency of upper gastrointestinal bleeding in a pediatric intensive care unit. *Crit Care Med* 1992;20(1):35–42.
4. Pant C, Sankararaman S, Deshpande A, et al. Gastrointestinal bleeding in hospitalized children in the United States. *Curr Med Res Opin* 2014;30(6):1065–9.
5. Parker DR, Luo X, Jalbert JJ, et al. Impact of upper and lower gastrointestinal blood loss on healthcare utilization and costs: A systematic review. *J Med Econ* 2011;14(3):279–87.
6. Fox VL. Gastrointestinal bleeding in infancy and childhood. *Gastroenterol Clin North Am* 2000;29(1):37–66, v.
7. Srygley FD, Gerardo CJ, Tran T, et al. Does this patient have a severe upper gastrointestinal bleed? *JAMA* 2012;307(10):1072–9.
8. Aljebreen AM, Fallone CA, Barkun AN. Nasogastric aspirate predicts high-risk endoscopic lesions in patients with acute upper-GI bleeding. *Gastrointest Endosc* 2004;59(2):172–8.
9. Fries M, Mortensson W, Robertson B. Technetium pertechnetate scintigraphy to detect ectopic gastric mucosa in Meckel's diverticulum. *Acta Radiologica* 1984;25(5):417–22.
10. Sfakianakis GN, Haase GM. Abdominal scintigraphy for ectopic gastric mucosa: A retrospective analysis of 143 studies. *AJR Am J Roentgenol* 1982;138(1):7–12.
11. Saremi F, Jadvar H, Siegel ME. Pharmacologic interventions in nuclear radiology: Indications, imaging protocols, and clinical results. *Radiographics* 2002;22(3):477–90.
12. Swaniker F, Soldes O, Hirschl RB. The utility of technetium 99m pertechnetate scintigraphy in the evaluation of patients with Meckel's diverticulum. *J Pediatr Surg* 1999;34(5):760–4; discussion 5.
13. Meyerovitz MF, Fellows KE. Angiography in gastrointestinal bleeding in children. *AJR Am J Roentgenol* 1984;143(4):837–40.
14. Kim CY, Suhocki PV, Miller MJ Jr., et al. Provocative mesenteric angiography for lower gastrointestinal hemorrhage: Results from a single-institution study. *J Vasc Interv Radiol* 2010;21(4):477–83.
15. Hwang JH, Fisher DA, Ben-Menachem T, et al. The role of endoscopy in the management of acute non variceal upper GI bleeding. *Gastrointest Endosc* 2012;75(6):1132–8.
16. Barkun AN, Bardou M, Kuipers EJ, et al. International consensus recommendations on the management of patients with nonvariceal upper gastrointestinal bleeding. *Ann Intern Med* 2010;152(2):101–13.
17. Jairath V, Kahan BC, Logan RF, et al. Outcomes following acute nonvariceal upper gastrointestinal bleeding in relation to time to endoscopy: Results from a nationwide study. *Endoscopy* 2012;44(8):723–30.
18. Sreedharan A, Martin J, Leontiadis GI, et al. Proton pump inhibitor treatment initiated prior to endoscopic diagnosis in upper gastrointestinal bleeding. *Cochrane Database Syst Rev* 2010;7:Cd005415.
19. Lau JY, Sung JJ, Lee KK, et al. Effect of intravenous omeprazole on recurrent bleeding after endoscopic treatment of bleeding peptic ulcers. *N Engl J Med* 2000;343(5):310–6.
20. Liu N, Liu L, Zhang H, et al. Effect of intravenous proton pump inhibitor regimens and timing of endoscopy on clinical outcomes of peptic ulcer bleeding. *J Gastroenterol Hepatol* 2012;27(9):1473–9.
21. Barkun AN, Bardou M, Martel M, et al. Prokinetics in acute upper GI bleeding: A meta-analysis. *Gastrointest Endosc* 2010;72(6):1138–45.
22. Fisher L, Lee Krinsky M, Anderson MA, et al. The role of endoscopy in the management of obscure GI bleeding. *Gastrointest Endosc* 2010;72(3):471–9.
23. Laine L, McQuaid KR. Endoscopic therapy for bleeding ulcers: An evidence-based approach based on meta-analyses of randomized controlled trials. *Clin Gastroenterol Hepatol* 2009;7(1):33–47; quiz 1–2.
24. Barth BA. Enteroscopy in children. *Curr Opin Pediatr* 2011;23(5):530–4.
25. Jensen MK, Tipnis NA, Bajorunaite R, et al. Capsule endoscopy performed across the pediatric age range: Indications, incomplete studies, and utility in management of inflammatory bowel disease. *Gastrointest Endosc* 2010;72(1):95–102.
26. Nishimura N, Yamamoto H, Yano T, et al. Safety and efficacy of double-balloon enteroscopy in pediatric patients. *Gastrointest Endosc* 2010;71(2):287–94.
27. Barth BA, Donovan K, Fox VL. Endoscopic placement of the capsule endoscope in children. *Gastrointest Endosc* 2004;60(5):818–21.

28. Meltzer AC, Ali MA, Kresiberg RB, et al. Video capsule endoscopy in the emergency department: A prospective study of acute upper gastrointestinal hemorrhage. *Ann Emerg Med* 2013;61(4):438–43.e1.

29. Nadler M, Eliakim R. The role of capsule endoscopy in acute gastrointestinal bleeding. *Ther Adv Gastroenterol* 2014;7(2):87–92.

30. Gralnek IM, Ching JY, Maza I, et al. Capsule endoscopy in acute upper gastrointestinal hemorrhage: A prospective cohort study. *Endoscopy* 2013;45(1):12–9.

31. Leung WK, Ho SS, Suen BY, et al. Capsule endoscopy or angiography in patients with acute overt obscure gastrointestinal bleeding: A prospective randomized study with long-term follow-up. *Am J Gastroenterol* 2012;107(9):1370–6.

32. Shen R, Sun B, Gong B, et al. Double-balloon enteroscopy in the evaluation of small bowel disorders in pediatric patients. *Dig Endosc* 2012;24(2):87–92.

33. Shishido T, Oka S, Tanaka S, et al. Diagnostic yield of capsule endoscopy vs. double-balloon endoscopy for patients who have undergone total enteroscopy with obscure gastrointestinal bleeding. *Hepatogastroenterology* 2012;59(116):955–9.

34. Wong Kee Song LM, Baron TH. Endoscopic management of acute lower gastrointestinal bleeding. *Am J Gastroenterol* 2008;103(8):1881–7.

35. Leung A, Wong AL. Lower gastrointestinal bleeding in children. *Pediatr Emerg Care* 2002;18(4):319–23.

36. Pallin DJ, Saltzman JR. Is nasogastric tube lavage in patients with acute upper GI bleeding indicated or antiquated? *Gastrointest Endosc.* 2011;74(5):981–4.

37. Bardou M, Benhaberou-Brun D, Le Ray I, et al. Diagnosis and management of nonvariceal upper gastrointestinal bleeding. *Nat Rev Gastroenterol Hepatol* 2012;9(2):97–104.

38. Lacroix J, Hebert PC, Hutchison JS, et al. Transfusion strategies for patients in pediatric intensive care units. *N Engl J Med* 2007;356(16):1609–19.

39. Shneider BL, Bosch J, de Franchis R, et al. Portal hypertension in children: Expert pediatric opinion on the report of the Baveno v consensus workshop on methodology of diagnosis and therapy in portal hypertension. *Pediatr Transplant* 2012;16(5):426–37.

40. Stravitz RT, Kramer AH, Davern T, et al. Intensive care of patients with acute liver failure: Recommendations of the U.S. Acute Liver Failure Study Group. *Crit Care Med* 2007;35(11):2498–508.

41. Drews RE, Weinberger SE. Thrombocytopenic disorders in critically ill patients. *Am J Respir Crit Care Med* 2000;162(2 pt 1):347–51.

42. Bosch J, Thabut D, Albillos A, et al. Recombinant factor VIIa for variceal bleeding in patients with advanced cirrhosis: A randomized, controlled trial. *Hepatology* 2008;47(5):1604–14.

43. Neumann I, Letelier LM, Rada G, et al. Comparison of different regimens of proton pump inhibitors for acute peptic ulcer bleeding. *Cochrane Database Syst Rev* 2013;6:Cd007999.

44. Mileti E, Rosenthal P. Management of portal hypertension in children. *Curr Gastroenterol Rep* 2011;13(1):10–6.

45. Heikenen JB, Pohl JF, Werlin SL, et al. Octreotide in pediatric patients. *J Pediatr Gastroenterol Nutr* 2002;35(5):600–9.

46. Eroglu Y, Emerick KM, Whitingon PF, et al. Octreotide therapy for control of acute gastrointestinal bleeding in children. *J Pediatr Gastroenterol Nutr* 2004;38(1):41–7.

47. Autret-Leca E, Jonville-Bera AP. Vitamin K in neonates: How to administer, when and to whom. *Paediatr Drugs* 2001;3(1):1–8.

48. Van Winckel M, De Bruyne R, Van De Velde S, et al. Vitamin K, an update for the paediatrician. *Eur J Pediatr* 2009;168(2):127–34.

49. Kuusela AL, Maki M, Ruuska T, et al. Stress-induced gastric findings in critically ill newborn infants: Frequency and risk factors. *Intensive Care Med* 2000;26(10):1501–6.

50. Ojala R, Ruuska T, Karikoski R, et al. Gastroesophageal endoscopic findings and gastrointestinal symptoms in preterm neonates with and without perinatal indomethacin exposure. *J Pediatr Gastroenterol Nutr* 2001;32(2):182–8.

51. Mutlu GM, Mutlu EA, Factor P. GI complications in patients receiving mechanical ventilation. *Chest* 2001;119(4):1222–41.

52. Brown K, Lundborg P, Levinson J, et al. Incidence of peptic ulcer bleeding in the US pediatric population. *J Pediatr Gastroenterol Nutr* 2012;54(6):733–6.

53. Perez-Perez GI, Rothenbacher D, Brenner H. Epidemiology of Helicobacter pylori infection. *Helicobacter* 2004;9(suppl 1):1–6.

54. Ertem D. Clinical practice: Helicobacter pylori infection in childhood. *Eur J Pediatr* 2013;172(11):1427–34.

55. Graham DY, Fischbach L. Helicobacter pylori treatment in the era of increasing antibiotic resistance. *Gut* 2010;59(8):1143–53.

56. Beejay U, Wolfe MM. Acute gastrointestinal bleeding in the intensive care unit. The gastroenterologist's perspective. *Gastroenterol C lin North Am* 2000;29(2):309–36.

57. Reveiz L, Guerrero-Lozano R, Camacho A, et al. Stress ulcer, gastritis, and gastrointestinal bleeding prophylaxis in critically ill pediatric patients: A systematic review. *Pediatr Crit Care Med* 2010;11(1):124–32.

58. Alhazzani W, Alenezi F, Jaeschke RZ, et al. Proton pump inhibitors versus histamine 2 receptor antagonists for stress ulcer prophylaxis in critically ill patients: A systematic review and meta-analysis. *Crit Care Med* 2013;41(3):693–705.

59. Hurt RT, Frazier TH, McClave SA, et al. Stress prophylaxis in intensive care unit patients and the role of enteral nutrition. *JPEN J Parenter Enteral Nutr* 2012;36(6):721–31.

60. Marik PE, Vasu T, Hirani A, et al. Stress ulcer prophylaxis in the new millennium: A systematic review and meta-analysis. *Crit Care Med* 2010;38(11):2222–8.

61. Barker CC, Anderson RA, Sauve RS, et al. GI complications in pediatric patients post-BMT. *Bone Marrow Transplant* 2005;36(1):51–8.

62. Pihusch R, Salat C, Schmidt E, et al. Hemostatic complications in bone marrow transplantation: A retrospective analysis of 447 patients. *Transplantation* 2002;74(9):1303–9.

63. Ananthakrishnan AN, Issa M, Binion DG. Clostridium difficile and inflammatory bowel disease. *Gastroenterol Clin North Am* 2009;38(4):711–28.

64. Ananthakrishnan AN, McGinley EL, Binion DG. Excess hospitalisation burden associated with Clostridium difficile in patients with inflammatory bowel disease. *Gut* 2008;57(2):205–10.

65. Crobach MJ, Dekkers OM, Wilcox MH, et al. European Society of Clinical Microbiology and Infectious Diseases (ESCMID): Data review and recommendations for diagnosing Clostridium difficile-infection (CDI). *Clin Microbiol Infect* 2009;15(12):1053–66.

66. Louie TJ, Miller MA, Mullane KM, et al. Fidaxomicin versus vancomycin for Clostridium difficile infection. *N Engl J Med* 2011;364(5):422–31.

67. Brandt LJ, Reddy SS. Fecal microbiota transplantation for recurrent clostridium difficile infection. *J Clin Gastroenterol* 2011;45(suppl):S159–67.

68. Kelly CR, de Leon L, Jasutkar N. Fecal microbiota transplantation for relapsing Clostridium difficile infection in 26 patients: Methodology and results. *J Clin Gastroenterol* 2012;46(2):145–9.

69. Mattila E, Uusitalo-Seppala R, Wuorela M, et al. Fecal transplantation, through colonoscopy, is effective therapy for recurrent Clostridium difficile infection. *Gastroenterology* 2012;142(3):490–6.

70. Fike FB, Mortellaro V, Juang D, et al. Neutropenic colitis in children. *J Surg Res* 2011;170(1):73–6.

71. Gorschluter M, Mey U, Strehl J, et al. Neutropenic enterocolitis in adults: Systematic analysis of evidence quality. *Eur J Haematol* 2005;75(1):1–13.

72. Andreyev HJ, Davidson SE, Gillespie C, et al. Practice guidance on the management of acute and chronic gastrointestinal problems arising as a result of treatment for cancer. *Gut* 2012;61(2):179–92.

73. Gower-Rousseau C, Dauchet L, Vernier-Massouille G, et al. The natural history of pediatric ulcerative colitis: A population-based cohort study. *Am J Gastroenterol* 2009;104(8):2080–8.

74. Hart AL, Ng SC. Review article: The optimal medical management of acute severe ulcerative colitis. *Aliment Pharmacol Ther* 2010;32(5):615–27.

75. Turner D, Travis SP, Griffiths AM, et al. Consensus for managing acute severe ulcerative colitis in children: A systematic review and joint statement from ECCO, ESPGHAN, and the Porto IBD Working Group of ESPGHAN. *Am J Gastroenterol* 2011;106(4):574–88.

76. Van Assche G, Vermeire S, Rutgeerts P. Management of acute severe ulcerative colitis. *Gut* 2011;60(1):130–3.

77. Beppu K, Inokuchi K, Koyanagi N, et al. Prediction of variceal hemorrhage by esophageal endoscopy. *Gastrointest Endosc* 1981;27(4):213–8.

78. Chalasani N, Kahi C, Francois F, et al. Improved patient survival after acute variceal bleeding: A multicenter, cohort study. *Am J Gastroenterol* 2003;98(3):653–9.

79. van Heurn LW, Saing H, Tam PK. Portoenterostomy for biliary atresia: Long-term survival and prognosis after esophageal variceal bleeding. *J Pediatr Surg* 2004;39(1):6–9.

80. Miga D, Sokol RJ, Mackenzie T, et al. Survival after first esophageal variceal hemorrhage in patients with biliary atresia. *J Pediatr* 2001;139(2):291–6.

81. Duche M, Habes D, Roulleau P, et al. Prophylactic endoscopic sclerotherapy of large esophagogastric varices in infants with biliary atresia. *Gastrointest Endosc* 2008;67(4):732–7.

82. Lampela H, Kosola S, Koivusalo A, et al. Endoscopic surveillance and primary prophylaxis sclerotherapy of esophageal varices in biliary atresia. *J Pediatr Gastroenterol Nutr* 2012;55(5):574–9.

83. Garcia-Tsao G, Bosch J. Management of varices and variceal hemorrhage in cirrhosis. *N Engl J Med* 2010;362(9):823–32.

84. Chavez-Tapia NC, Barrientos-Gutierrez T, Tellez-Avila FI, et al. Antibiotic prophylaxis for cirrhotic patients with upper gastrointestinal bleeding. *Cochrane Database Syst Rev* 2010(9):Cd002907.

85. Gines P, Fernandez J, Durand F, et al. Management of critically-ill cirrhotic patients. *J Hepatol* 2012;56(suppl 1):S13–24.

86. Thalheimer U, Triantos CK, Samonakis DN, et al. Infection, coagulation, and variceal bleeding in cirrhosis. *Gut* 2005;54(4):556–63.

87. Lee YY, Tee HP, Mahadeva S. Role of prophylactic antibiotics in cirrhotic patients with variceal bleeding. *World J Gastroenterol* 2014;20(7):1790–6.

88. Jalan R, Hayes PC. UK guidelines on the management of variceal haemorrhage in cirrhotic patients. British Society of Gastroenterology. *Gut* 2000;46(suppl 3–4):Iii1–iii15.

89. Garcia-Tsao G, Sanyal AJ, Grace ND, et al. Prevention and management of gastroesophageal varices and variceal hemorrhage in cirrhosis. *Hepatology* 2007;46(3):922–38.

90. Garcia-Tsao G, Sanyal AJ, Grace ND, et al. Prevention and management of gastroesophageal varices and variceal hemorrhage in cirrhosis. *Am J Gastroenterol* 2007;102(9):2086–102.

91. D'Amico G, Pagliaro L, Pietrosi G, et al. Emergency sclerotherapy versus vasoactive drugs for bleeding oesophageal varices in cirrhotic patients. *Cochrane Database Syst Rev* 2010;3:Cd002233.

92. Hidaka H, Nakazawa T, Wang G, et al. Long-term administration of PPI reduces treatment failures after esophageal variceal band ligation: A randomized, controlled trial. *J Gastroenterol* 2012;47(2):118–26.

93. Rivet C, Robles-Medranda C, Dumortier J, et al. Endoscopic treatment of gastroesophageal varices in young infants with cyanoacrylate glue: A pilot study. *Gastrointest Endosc* 2009;69(6):1034–8.

94. Boyer TD, Haskal ZJ. The role of transjugular intrahepatic portosystemic shunt in the management of portal hypertension. *Hepatology* 2005;41(2):386–400.

CHAPTER 100 ■ ABDOMINAL COMPARTMENT SYNDROME

MUDIT MATHUR AND J. CHIAKA EJIKE

KEY POINTS

1. Intra-abdominal pressure (IAP) can be measured easily using the indirect intravesical method by creating a fluid column through saline instillation into the urinary bladder (1 mL/kg up to 25 mL, or a standard volume of 3 mL irrespective of weight) and recording the pressure across this fluid column.

2. Abdominal perfusion pressure (APP) appears to be a better predictor of outcome from intra-abdominal hypertension (IAH) than mean arterial pressure, IAP, or other traditionally used resuscitation endpoints.

3. IAH and abdominal compartment syndrome can lead to multi–organ system failure and are associated with increased morbidity and mortality in critically ill patients.

4. Clinical examination is not a reliable substitute for measuring IAP.

5. A high index of suspicion should be used in initiating serial IAP monitoring in patient populations at risk for developing IAH and abdominal compartment syndrome.

6. Infants and children with catecholamine refractory shock should have IAP measured to rule out IAH.

7. Principles of medical management include treating the underlying condition, improving abdominal wall compliance, evacuating intraluminal contents, optimization of fluid balance, identification and evacuation of abdominal fluid collections, and optimizing regional and systemic perfusion.

8. Surgical decompression and open abdomen management may be needed if medical management fails.

INTRODUCTION

Increased pressure in a confined anatomical space affects local circulation and threatens the function and viability of the organs contained within. Abdominal compartment syndrome (ACS) results from a sustained pathological increase in intra-abdominal pressure (IAP) leading to organ dysfunction and failure. The term ACS was first coined by Kron et al. (1) in 1984, though the adverse effects of IAP have been known for over one hundred years. Pediatric surgeons have long recognized that staged closure of omphaloceles reduces the risk of excessive intraperitoneal tension and improves outcome of abdominal wall repair in newborns (2). ACS is an increasingly recognized complication in critically ill children with varied underlying medical and surgical pathology. Recent efforts by a multispecialty group of healthcare professionals (The World Society of Abdominal Compartment Syndrome [WSACS]) have led to the development of consensus definitions for the diagnosis and management of ACS in adults and children (3,4).

CONSENSUS DEFINITIONS

The WSACS recently released updated consensus definitions that for the first time include specific definitions applicable to children (5).

IAP is the steady-state pressure concealed within the abdominal cavity. IAP in critically ill children is approximately 4–10 mm Hg.

Intra-abdominal hypertension (IAH) in children is a sustained or repeated pathologic elevation in IAP > 10 mm Hg (>12 mm Hg in adults). IAH can be classified by severity on the basis of the IAP reading: Grade I (12–15 mm Hg), Grade II (16–20 mm Hg), Grade III (IAP 21–25 mm Hg), or Grade IV (IAP > 25 mm Hg) (3). The clinical significance of grading IAH is unclear but may be useful when comparing patient populations between studies.

ACS in children is defined as a sustained elevation in IAP greater than 10 mm Hg associated with new or worsening organ dysfunction that can be attributed to elevated IAP.

ACS may be classified as primary, secondary, or tertiary, depending on its origin and the underlying condition. Primary ACS is associated with an injury or disease in the abdomen or pelvis (e.g., abdominal trauma or peritonitis). Secondary ACS originates from outside the abdomino-pelvic region (e.g., massive fluid resuscitation for septic shock). Tertiary ACS occurs when ACS redevelops after medical or surgical treatment of primary or secondary ACS.

Abdominal perfusion pressure (APP) is the mathematical difference between the mean arterial pressure (MAP) and the IAP (APP = MAP − IAP). This is analogous to the concept of cerebral perfusion pressure (6). Normative data for APP are not available for children. The threshold APP below which organ dysfunction ensues is likely to be lower in children than the 60 mm Hg value used in adults because normal MAP values are lower in children (7,8).

Clinical Interpretation of IAP Values

The consensus definitions serve as the basis for diagnosing various grades of IAP elevation in children. Elevation of IAP above normal constitutes IAH and leads to physiologic changes within the abdominal cavity and beyond. Initial effects include reduction in perfusion to abdominal organs, but can progress to affect multiple extra-abdominal organ systems if untreated. It is important to recognize that there

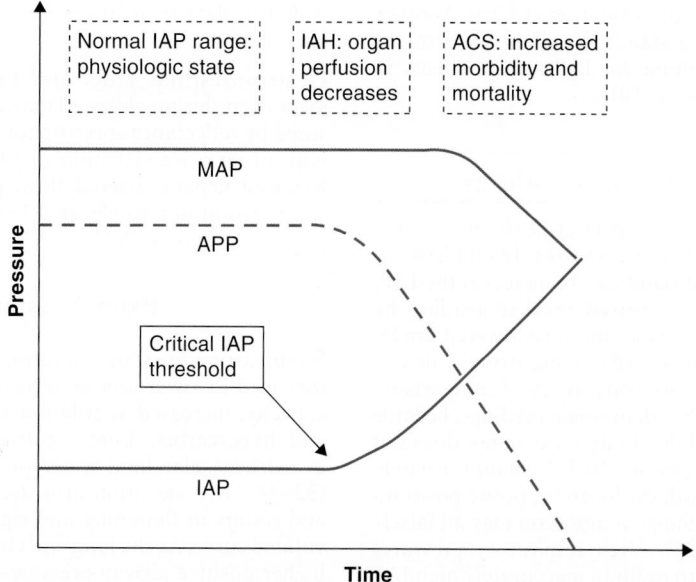

FIGURE 100.1. The intra-abdominal hypertension spectrum: With progression from normal IAP to IAH, APP falls and organ perfusion is compromised. If untreated, IAH may lead to ACS, increasing morbidity, and mortality. MAP, mean arterial pressure; APP, abdominal perfusion pressure; IAP, intra-abdominal pressure; IAH, intra-abdominal hypertension; ACS, abdominal compartment syndrome.

is a spectrum of IAP elevation that culminates in ACS. Early recognition and management of IAH and ACS are important to prevent progression to multisystem organ dysfunction and death (Fig. 100.1). The increase in IAP is exponential beyond a "critical IAP" threshold and leads to reduced APP, decreased organ perfusion, and end-organ injury.

The exact threshold beyond which IAP compromises organ perfusion may vary among patients. It may depend on comorbidities and the stage of progression of the causative pathophysiology. Thus, monitoring APP closely may be more useful than relying on the IAP values alone. Serial IAP monitoring and comprehensive medical and surgical management, using goal-directed optimization of APP, systemic perfusion, and organ function have been shown to improve survival in adults with IAH/ACS (9).

Optimal APP in the pediatric population is unknown, but is likely lower than that in adults, due to lower age-dependent MAP in infants and children (10). In a study of 585 neonates and children undergoing laparoscopy, cardiopulmonary function was affected at IAP as low as 6 mm Hg in newborns and at 12 mm Hg in older children (11). Elevated IAP in the 9–13 mm Hg range has been associated with exacerbation of necrotizing enterocolitis in newborns (12). This supports the updated definition by the WSACS with an IAP threshold for defining IAH and ACS in children that is lower than that used in adults.

TECHNIQUES FOR MEASURING IAP

IAP is measured with the patient supine, in the absence of abdominal muscle contraction, and recorded in mm Hg at end-expiration using a closed, de-bubbled system with the pressure transducer zeroed at the mid-axillary line. The techniques for measuring IAP are broadly classified into two categories.

Indirect Methods

These methods are based on measuring IAP indirectly across the walls of an intra-abdominal organ or structure. The indirect method used most commonly is the intravesical method performed via a urinary catheter. When the bladder is drained or has a minimal volume, the IAP is transmitted through the bladder's compliant wall and is measured by transducing the urinary catheter. A minimum volume of 3 mL or 1 mL/kg up to a maximum of 25 mL saline is instilled into the Foley catheter to establish a continuous fluid column with the pressure transducer, and IAP is recorded (10). IAP may be measured using a fluid column, in which case the reading is in cmH$_2$O and should be converted to mm Hg by dividing by 1.36. Bladder detrusor muscle spasm may occur during saline instillation; thus, allowing time (30 seconds to 1 minute) for equilibration of pressures permits an accurate steady-state IAP to be measured (13). IAP should be expressed in mm Hg and measured at end-expiration in the supine position after ensuring that abdominal muscle contractions are absent and with the transducer zeroed at the level of the mid-axillary line.

Intragastric, intrauterine, venacaval, and intrarectal sites have also been described for indirect measurement of IAP (14–16). The intravesical method is most often used in clinical practice because it is simple, reliable, and easily performed at the bedside. Kimball et al. using a standardized protocol for intravesical measurement demonstrated that intraobserver and interobserver variation in IAP readings is minimal (Pearson's correlation coefficient 0.934 and 0.950, respectively) (17). Indirect intravesical IAP measurement can be performed using a commercially available kit or assembled low-cost components.

Direct Method

This method measures IAP directly from the peritoneal space using a pressure transducer or a fluid column. Direct measurement of IAP involves the placement of a needle or catheter into the peritoneum, making it more invasive, and generally less preferred than indirect measurement. However, if a preexisting catheter (such as a peritoneal dialysis catheter) is in place, the direct method can be used with equal ease (18).

The agreement between direct IAP measurement and indirect intravesical measurement has been studied in children. Two studies have shown that intravesical IAP measurement was most accurate with 1 mL/kg saline instilled into the bladder as compared with larger volumes of instillation (18,19). Another study suggests that instilling a standard volume of 3 mL is as reliable as the 1 mL/kg volume for IAP measurements in children weighing less than 50 kg (10).

Variables Affecting IAP Readings

Many factors commonly encountered in critically ill patients may affect the accuracy of IAP measurements. In children, elevation of the head of the bed significantly increases the IAP. An elevation from 0° to 30° increased the IAP reading by 2 mm Hg (20). If the head of the bed cannot be lowered briefly for IAP measurement, subsequent IAP readings should also be measured at the same elevation for consistency of comparison. In this case, the IAP trend, rather than single readings, become more important. Unlike in adults, body mass index does not appear to affect IAP measurement (20,21). Inappropriately large instillation volume, transducer location, prone positioning, inadequate sedation, coughing, or agitation may all falsely raise measured IAP (13,21–24). High respiratory pressures and obesity have been shown to result in inaccurately high IAP in adults (23). Air bubbles or a "vapor lock" in the transducer tubing may also lead to erroneous measurements (24).

ANATOMY AND PATHOPHYSIOLOGY

Anatomy

The abdomen occupies a central position in the body and contains several major organs. The abdominal contents are encased in a compartment with fairly rigid posterior (spine and back muscles) and inferior (bony pelvis and pelvic floor) walls and relatively more compliant anterolateral (abdominal wall muscles and fascia) and superior (diaphragm) constraints. As a result, increase in IAP may first lead to anterolateral abdominal distension and upward displacement of the diaphragm, but then starts to compromise the perfusion, viability, and function of various intra-abdominal and extra-abdominal organ systems as IAH progresses to ACS (25).

Pathophysiology

Abdominal Contents

Abdominal Vasculature. Even with mild induced IAH in human volunteers (median IAP 12–15 mm Hg, grade I IAH), compression and distortion of the inferior vena cava (IVC) and portal vein can be demonstrated by sonography. Progressive increase in IAP may further affect IVC flow and patency. The resistive index in renal arteries also increases, suggesting direct compression of renal parenchyma and microvasculature (26).

Kidneys. External pressure of 70–80 mm Hg applied to the abdomen with an inflatable bladder underneath a girdle raised the IAP measured in the IVC to 20 mm Hg and decreased renal plasma flow and glomerular filtration rate by 25%. Urine volume declined dramatically while IAP was high and recovered upon release of the girdle (27).

In a prospective study of 123 adults in a mixed medical/surgical ICU, of whom 30% had IAH, IAP of 12 mm Hg was found to be the best cutoff (with a sensitivity of 91%, specificity 67%, and area under receiver operating characteristic curve 0.85) for acute kidney injury (AKI) using the Risk Injury Failure Loss and End-stage renal disease (RIFLE) criteria for acute renal dysfunction. IAH was an independent predictor of AKI with an odds ratio of 2.44 (28). There are no specific pediatric data to help define an IAP threshold predictive of kidney injury.

Gastrointestinal Tract and Liver. Gastric mucosal oxygen saturation during elective laparoscopic surgery in adults measured by reflectance spectrophotometry decreased significantly with progressive elevation of IAP to 8 and 12 mm Hg (29). Reduced hepatic arterial flow, portal venous flow, and IVC compression due to elevated IAP may further exacerbate hepatic congestion (30,31).

Extra-Abdominal Organs

Respiratory System. Elevation of the diaphragm from IAH may lead to lower lobe atelectasis, reduced functional residual capacity, increased ventilation–perfusion mismatch, hypoxia, and hypercarbia. Lung neutrophil activation and increase in extravascular lung water may further worsen lung injury (32–36). IAP elevation also decreases chest wall compliance and results in flattening and rightward shift of the pressure–volume curve. As the lung and chest wall compliance decreases, higher positive airway pressures will be needed to deliver the same tidal volume (35). At an IAP of 16 mm Hg, pulmonary compliance decreases by 50% as was seen in adults undergoing laparoscopic cholecystectomy (37). In ARDS resulting from extrapulmonary pathology, IAP elevation above 16 cmH$_2$O (12 mm Hg) was associated with a significant increase in chest wall elastance (38). Interestingly, this observation coincides with the IAP threshold associated with a decrement in kidney function as discussed above. This supports the concept of a critical IAP threshold above which multiple organ systems are affected.

Cardiovascular System. MAP rises initially as systemic vascular resistance (SVR) increases. Pulmonary vascular resistance and pulmonary artery pressure are also increased. At first, cardiac output is maintained but decreasing venous return soon results in a fall in cardiac output. With progressive IAP elevation, the pulmonary capillary wedge pressure (PCWP) increases and cardiac index decreases further (32). Simple assessment of fluid responsiveness is difficult as both CVP and PCWP readings may be falsely elevated. Acute rises in IAP cause decreased LV compliance and regional wall motion abnormalities due to increased LV afterload. Regional blood flow redistribution leads to further reduction of flow to the abdomen (39).

Central Nervous System. A 15-kg weight placed on the abdomen in moderately ill neurosurgical patients led to increases in intracranial pressure (ICP), jugular venous pressure, CVP, and PCWP. However, MAP transiently increased as well, such that CPP was maintained (40). Based on these physiologic observations, decompressive laparotomy (DL) has been utilized as a management tool for refractory elevation in ICP in patients with "multiple compartment syndrome" (increased ICP, IAP, and intrathoracic pressure after severe brain injury) (41).

Multisystem Organ Failure

IAH affects multiple organ systems and its cascading effects may get amplified by common ICU interventions. Fluid resuscitation aimed at restoring adequate preload and MAP may result in "third-spaced" peritoneal fluid and bowel wall edema, thus contributing to incremental IAP elevation. As IAH progresses, it initiates a vicious cycle with IVC compression reducing venous return, the resulting decrement in cardiac output further compromising organ perfusion and function. Supporting this core principle is the observation that APP appears to be a better predictor of outcome in adults with IAH than do MAP, IAP, or other traditionally used resuscitation endpoints in shock states such as lactate, pH, base deficit, or urinary output (6).

EPIDEMIOLOGY

There are no population-based data or multicenter studies describing the prevalence of IAH in children. In a point prevalence study done in a mixed medical/surgical ICU population, IAH (defined as IAP > 12 mm Hg) was present at admission in 32% of adult patients. ACS (defined in this study as IAP > 20 mm Hg) occurred in 12.9% of patients with IAH and in 4.2% of the overall patient cohort. The occurrence of IAH was a significant independent predictor of mortality (relative risk 1.85) (42).

In retrospective single-center studies, ACS was seen in 0.6%–1% of PICU patients with a 40%–60% associated mortality (43,44). In a prospective study where study consent could be obtained in one-third of mechanically ventilated infants and children admitted to the PICU, IAH was observed in 22% and ACS in 7%. Overall, ACS was seen in 14/294 (4.7%) admissions. Again, the associated mortality was high (50% with ACS vs. only 8.1% without ACS). IAP and ACS were both independent predictors of mortality (odds ratio 1.53 and 9.09, respectively). Both the IAP and a PRISM score greater than 17 were predictive of developing ACS (8). Other conditions that have been associated with a risk for developing ACS mainly reported in adult studies include abdominal surgery, major trauma, burns, high-volume crystalloid resuscitation, polytransfusion, positive fluid balance, oliguria, prone positioning, increased head of bed angle, intra-abdominal infection/abscess, laparoscopy with excessive insufflation pressures, damage-control laparotomy, anemia, acidosis, coagulopathy, hypothermia, bacteremia, increased APACHE-II or SOFA score, and high gastric regional to end-tidal carbon dioxide differences (5,42,45).

COMMON ETIOLOGIES

Though IAH and ACS can occur in any critically ill child, certain PICU patient populations are at greater risk. A list of some medical and surgical conditions where IAH and ACS occurs in children is provided in **Table 100.1**. These conditions can be broadly classified into four categories: reduced abdominal domain/decreased abdominal compliance, increased intraluminal contents, increased intra-abdominal contents, and patients needing massive resuscitation.

CLINICAL PRESENTATION AND RECOGNITION OF IAH AND ACS

IAH can only be determined by objective IAP measurement. It is important to note that clinical palpation is *not* sufficient for estimating IAP or deciding on the presence of IAH. The sensitivity of clinical examination alone in detecting raised IAP has been examined in two studies and found to be quite poor. Clinicians could identify elevated IAP in 40% of patients with the IAP > 10, and in 56% when the IAP was over 15 mm Hg (63). Even with IAP over 18 mm Hg, clinicians are able to detect it by abdominal palpation in only 60% of patients (64). Thus, measuring IAP is the only reliable way to know what the IAP is and to detect IAH early.

When clinical manifestations resulting from sustained IAH become evident, ACS is present. The common features seen in ACS are a distended abdomen associated with hemodynamic instability, oliguria or anuria, metabolic acidosis, and respiratory deterioration (43,65).

IAH can cause and/or result from organ dysfunction in critically ill patients with varying underlying etiologies. Morbidity

TABLE 100.1

PEDIATRIC POPULATIONS AT RISK FOR ACS

Primary ACS
Decreased abdominal compliance/reduced abdominal domain
  Gastroschisis (46)
  Pentalogy of Cantrell (47)
Increased intraluminal contents
  Small intestine intussusception (48)
  Ileus (49)
  Hirschprung disease (50)
Increased abdominal contents
  Intra-abdominal trauma (edematous viscera) (51)
  Intestinal transplantation (52)
  Intra-abdominal bleeding/retroperitoneal bleeding (53)
  Gastrointestinal bleeding (54)
  Extracorporeal life support (54)
  Nonpancreatic pseudocyst (55)
  Abdominal tumors (56,57)
  Burkitt lymphoma (9)
  Pyonephrosis/obstruction megaureter (58)
  Pancreatitis (49)
  Tension pneumoperitoneum/intestinal perforation (59)
  Peritonitis/intra-abdominal infection (8)
  Infectious enterocolitis (50)
  Postsurgical complication (abdominal surgery) (50)
  Bowel obstruction or perforation (49,50)
Secondary ACS
Capillary leak/fluid resuscitation
  Sepsis/septic shock (8,49)
  Toxic shock syndrome (8)
  Dengue shock syndrome (60)
  Trauma shock (61)
  Cardiogenic shock/cardiac arrest (8)
  Burns (49,62)

ACS, abdominal compartment syndrome; IAP, intra-abdominal pressure.
Source: Ejike JC, Mathur M, Moores DC. Abdominal compartment syndrome: Focus on the children. *Am Surg* 2011;77(suppl 1):S72–7.

and mortality related to IAH and ACS can be prevented by using serial IAP measurements performed in at-risk patients (**Table 100.1**) to identify those with progressive IAH and guide early management. Infants and children with catecholamine refractory shock should have IAP measured to rule out IAP > 12 mm Hg as recommended in the latest American College of Critical Care Medicine/Pediatric Advanced Life Support practice parameters for the management of shock in infants and children (66). Overt ACS, with a rigid abdomen and multiple organ failure, is easy to recognize, but is often irreversible and life threatening (67). Evolving physiologic changes such as rising serum lactate, worsening metabolic acidosis, decreasing urine output, worsening pulmonary compliance with elevated peak and plateau pressures, hypercapnia, hypoxemia, and decreasing cardiac output in the setting of IAH may be better triggers for initiating management targeted at lowering IAP.

IAP should be monitored in patients at increased risk for ACS and in patients with IAH or ACS until their risk factors have resolved. The WSACS recommends IAP monitoring when any known risk factor for IAH/ACS is present in a critically ill or injured patient (5).

MEDICAL MANAGEMENT

Medical management is based on the principles of treating the underlying conditions that led to the development of IAH, supporting organ function, and lowering the IAP (**Table 100.2**).

TABLE 100.2

IMPORTANT PRINCIPLES FOR MANAGEMENT
OF ACS IN CHILDREN

Serial IAP measurements
Treat the underlying condition and preexisting comorbidities
Implement IAP lowering interventions
Evacuate intraluminal contents
Evacuate intra-abdominal space occupying lesions
Minimize capillary leak/avoid excessive fluid resuscitation
Improve abdominal wall compliance
Optimize systemic (MAP) and APP
Recognize and support ongoing organ dysfunction
Surgical abdominal decompression
Temporary abdominal closure/open abdomen management
Permanent abdominal closure

ACS, abdominal compartment syndrome; IAP, intra-abdominal pressure; MAP, mean arterial pressure; APP, abdominal perfusion pressure.

There is a range of interventions from simple to increasingly complex that are directed at reduction of IAP and prevention of organ dysfunction (3).

1. Improving abdominal wall compliance: Adequate sedation and neuromuscular blockade (when necessary) may be used to improve abdominal wall compliance. Several studies have demonstrated a prompt drop in IAP (4–12 mm Hg) with the use of neuromuscular blocking agents (20,22). Removal of constrictive abdominal dressings, eschars, or intra-abdominal packing may need to be considered.

2. Evacuation of intraluminal contents: Strategies include using naso-gastric, oro-gastric, and/or rectal tubes; administering enemas or prokinetic agents when appropriate, to help evacuate intestinal contents; and minimizing or stopping enteral feeds to decrease gastric contents. Rectal and colonic decompression using endoscopy may also be useful.

3. Identification and evacuation of space occupying abdominal lesions: Free intraperitoneal fluid or air can be evacuated by paracentesis or percutaneous catheter drainage (55,68). In some cases, placement of drains using ultrasound or CT guidance may avoid the need for laparotomy. Space occupying lesions may need to be removed surgically or embolized using interventional radiology techniques.

4. Optimizing fluid balance: Excessive resuscitation fluids (especially crystalloids) may lead to the development of IAH and ACS with associated increases in mortality and should be avoided (69,70). Clinicians should aim for a net negative or zero fluid balance as soon as possible after achieving hemodynamic stability. Judicious use of diuretics, ultrafiltration via continuous renal replacement therapy, or hemodialysis (if tolerated) may be considered.

5. Optimizing systemic and regional perfusion, and organ function: Development or worsening of multi–organ system dysfunction is an integral part of the definition of ACS. Surveillance through continuous hemodynamic monitoring (with caution interpreting individual CVP or PCWP values in the presence of IAH/ACS), laboratory assessment, and imaging studies can help detect and monitor progression of failing organs that need support. Therapies to achieve an adequate APP should be the overarching goal for effective organ support in the presence of respiratory, cardiovascular, and renal failure. Other organ systems such as the hepatic,

gastrointestinal, and neurologic are also affected but are not as readily recognized in the critically ill patient (30,31,71). The affected organ systems require specific and escalating support while ACS is treated.

Adult recommendations consider surgical decompression for IAP over 25 mm Hg refractory to medical management with onset of new organ dysfunction or failure (3). In children, a more suitable trigger for surgical decompression may be progression of IAH to ACS with early detection of new and progressive organ dysfunction despite medical management, rather than reliance on a specific IAP threshold.

SURGICAL MANAGEMENT

Surgical management options include decompression using paracentesis, a percutaneously or surgically placed catheter/drain, or decompressive laparotomy (DL). The strategy used may be selected on the basis of the underlying condition that led to ACS and the findings on radiologic investigations (e.g., abdominal ultrasound or CT scan). A percutaneously placed catheter can be used to drain free peritoneal fluid and relieve ACS in children receiving ECMO and to minimize the risk of bleeding (68). DL is the specific treatment of choice for patients with ACS refractory to medical management (5). It entails making an incision through all layers of the abdominal wall to provide access to the abdominal cavity (72). Surgical exploration of the abdomen is an essential part of DL to identify occult primary causes of ACS or identify and treat consequences of ACS such as bowel ischemia or necrosis.

The optimal timing for DL remains a subject of debate. Abdominal decompression should be performed before irreversible organ damage occurs, for improved outcomes. There may only be a small window of opportunity for surgical decompression and exploratory laparotomy because of the patient's progressive multiorgan dysfunction, making them less than ideal candidates for anesthesia and surgery. However, prolonged attempts at preoperative stabilization may result in an unnecessary delay in the definitive treatment for ACS, namely DL. Organ dysfunction may become irreversible and the risk for mortality and morbidity higher. Surgical decompression in the ICU at the bedside may help prevent unnecessary delays in trying to secure an operating room (OR) and decrease inherent risks in transporting an unstable patient with ACS to the OR. In a recent case series describing infants and children with ACS, PICU and OR were used in equal proportion as locations for performing DL (67). Patients without primary intra-abdominal pathology who develop secondary ACS may be better candidates for DL in the PICU. Patients with suspected primary intra-abdominal pathology may be best dealt with in the OR where specific surgical resources are more easily accessible if unexpected pathology is discovered. Ultimately, patient stability, hospital resources, and surgeon's preference dictate where DL is performed.

DL is associated with significantly improved patient survival in ACS (9,49). It improves physiologic parameters associated with ACS and mortality in both adults and children (43,50,67,68). Pearson and colleagues studied 26 children with ACS who required emergency laparotomy. Many manifested overt ACS with oliguria, high ventilator settings, vasopressor requirement, and IAP range 12–44 (mean 25 mm Hg). Following DL, there was an improvement in the oxygen index, mean airway pressure, and vasopressor score; urine output, however, continued to be minimal for 12 hours (67). The overall mortality was 58% in this retrospective cohort. Beck et al. retrospectively studied 10 children with 15 episodes of ACS. After DL, the MAP, PaO_2, PaO_2/FIO_2 ratio, $PaCO_2$, peak inspiratory pressures (PIP), positive end-expiratory pressures (PEEP), urinary output, and base deficit all returned to pre-ACS values (43). In another recent study, early DL and open abdomen management using a vicryl mesh in 28 children with ACS (25 primary and 3 secondary ACS) defined as IAP >12 mm Hg and *one* organ dysfunction led to an overall mortality of only 21% (49). These children underwent early DL guided by the use of a therapeutic algorithm that focused on timely decompression. The survival outcome in this cohort appears to be favorable compared with previous studies that have shown survival rates of only 40%–60% (8,43,67). However, the populations included in these studies are quite different and do not lend themselves to direct comparison.

Clinical Consequences of Surgical Decompression

ICU clinicians should be prepared to manage sudden hypovolemia that may occur as venous capacitance is reestablished following surgical decompression for ACS. Acute changes in respiratory dynamics occur as the chest wall compliance dramatically improves, and PEEP and peak inspiratory pressure (or HFOV mean airway pressure) may need to be rapidly weaned. Electrolyte abnormalities resulting from reperfusion of compromised tissues such as hyperkalemia, acidosis, hyperphosphatemia, or hypocalcemia may precipitate an acute decompensation, though the patient should stabilize quickly once these issues are promptly addressed. In one case series, surgical decompression improved oxygenation, ventilation, cardiac output, atrial filling pressures, and urine output within 15 minutes (73).

Open Abdomen Management

This strategy involves electively leaving the abdomen open after laparotomy in patients at risk for developing ACS postoperatively. The fascia and skin are left unopposed following laparotomy, and a temporary abdominal closure (TAC) dressing is applied (6,9,49,67). This may also be necessary after operations in which edematous viscera preclude easy fascial closure, when adult-sized organs are transplanted in small children, or when second-look surgery is anticipated (74,75). This practice has increased survival in patients with abdominal wall defects, trauma, intestinal and liver transplantation, and ACS (52). Options for TAC include spring-loaded silastic silo, vacuum pack, Wittmann patch, and vacuum-assisted closure systems (74). The main goal in management of the open abdomen is to primarily close the abdomen as soon as it is clinically safe to do so and avoid or minimize complications.

CONCLUSIONS

ACS is a relatively uncommon but potentially lethal condition associated with varied medical and surgical diagnoses. Serial IAP monitoring should be done in patients at risk for elevated IAP or those with evolving IAH, and APP should be calculated and addressed. ACS lies at the end of the IAH spectrum and is associated with 21%–60% mortality in children. Identifying IAH and preventing its progression to ACS through early medical and/or surgical management may help alleviate the morbidity and mortality associated with ACS in children.

FUTURE DIRECTIONS

Many of the current consensus-based recommendations for managing IAH and ACS in children are guided by data from adult patients. Consistent application of IAH and ACS

definitions specific to pediatric patients is needed not only for optimal clinical management but also for achieving more uniform research design. Future studies should aim to identify evidence-based management approaches that result in improved outcomes in children. Studies to determine correlation between APP and organ dysfunction are vital in order to define APP thresholds at which organ dysfunction occurs in infants and children. Identifying specific APP thresholds may in turn be helpful in guiding goal-directed therapy in managing IAH and ACS. Application of currently available noninvasive tools such as near-infrared spectroscopy to evaluate tissue oxygenation in intra-abdominal organs might be useful in early detection of organ dysfunction. Identifying early markers for organ dysfunction might help individualize medical therapy and determine the optimum time for surgical decompression before ACS becomes irreversible. Long-term studies should be conducted to evaluate the impact of abdominal decompression techniques and open abdomen management in infants and children.

References

1. Kron IL, Harman PK, Nolan SP. The measurement of intra-abdominal pressure as a criterion for abdominal re-exploration. *Ann Surg* 1984;199(1):28–30.
2. Gross RE. A new method for surgical treatment of large omphaloceles. *Surgery* 1948;24(2):277–92.
3. Cheatham ML, Malbrain ML, Kirkpatrick A, et al. Results from the international conference of experts on intra-abdominal hypertension and abdominal compartment syndrome. II: Recommendations. *Intensive Care Med* 2007;33(6):951–62.
4. Malbrain ML, Cheatham ML, Kirkpatrick A, et al. Results from the international conference of experts on intra-abdominal hypertension and abdominal compartment syndrome. I: Definitions. *Intensive Care Med* 2006;32(11):1722–32.
5. Kirkpatrick AW, Roberts DJ, De Waele J, et al. Intra-abdominal hypertension and the abdominal compartment syndrome: Updated consensus definitions and clinical practice guidelines from the World Society of the Abdominal Compartment Syndrome. *Intensive Care Med* 2013;39(7):1190–206.
6. Cheatham ML, White MW, Sagraves SG, et al. Abdominal perfusion pressure: a superior parameter in the assessment of intra-abdominal hypertension. *J Trauma* 2000;49(4):621–6; discussion 6–7.
7. Ejike JC, Mathur M, Moores DC. Abdominal compartment syndrome: Focus on the children. *Am Surg* 2011;77(suppl 1):S72–7.
8. Ejike JC, Humbert S, Bahjri K, et al. Outcomes of children with abdominal compartment syndrome. *Acta Clin Belg Suppl* 2007(1):141–8.
9. Cheatham ML, Safcsak K. Is the evolving management of intra-abdominal hypertension and abdominal compartment syndrome improving survival? *Crit Care Med* 2010;38(2):402–7.
10. Ejike JC, Bahjri K, Mathur M. What is the normal intra-abdominal pressure in critically ill children and how should we measure it? *Crit Care Med* 2008;36(7):2157–62.
11. Baroncini S, Gentili A, Pigna A, et al. Anaesthesia for laparoscopic surgery in paediatrics. *Minerva Anestesiol* 2002;68(5):406–13.
12. Sukhotnik I, Riskin A, Bader D, et al. Possible importance of increased intra-abdominal pressure for the development of necrotizing enterocolitis. *Eur J Pediatr Surg* 2009;19(5):307–10.
13. Chiumello D, Tallarini F, Chierichetti M, et al. The effect of different volumes and temperatures of saline on the bladder pressure measurement in critically ill patients. *Crit Care* 2007;11(4):R82.
14. Sugrue M, Buist MD, Lee A, et al. Intra-abdominal pressure measurement using a modified nasogastric tube: description and validation of a new technique. *Intensive Care Med* 1994;20(8):588–90.
15. Gudmundsson FF, Viste A, Gislason H, et al. Comparison of different methods for measuring intra-abdominal pressure. *Intensive Care Med* 2002;28(4):509–14.

16. Dowdle M. Evaluating a new intrauterine pressure catheter. *J Reprod Med* 1997;42(8):506–13.

17. Kimball EJ, Mone MC, Wolfe TR, et al. Reproducibility of bladder pressure measurements in critically ill patients. *Intensive Care Med* 2007;33(7):1195–8.

18. Davis PJ, Koottayi S, Taylor A, et al. Comparison of indirect methods of measuring intra-abdominal pressure in children. *Intensive Care Med* 2005;31(3):471–5.

19. Suominen PK, Pakarinen MP, Rautiainen P, et al. Comparison of direct and intravesical measurement of intraabdominal pressure in children. *J Pediatr Surg* 2006;41(8):1381–5.

20. Ejike JC, Kadry J, Bahjri K, et al. Semi-recumbent position and body mass percentiles: Effects on intra-abdominal pressure measurements in critically ill children. *Intensive Care Med* 2010;36(2):329–35.

21. De Waele JJ, De Laet I, De Keulenaer B, et al. The effect of different reference transducer positions on intra-abdominal pressure measurement: A multicenter analysis. *Intensive Care Med* 2008;34(7):1299–303.

22. De Laet I, Hoste E, Verholen E, et al. The effect of neuromuscular blockers in patients with intra-abdominal hypertension. *Intensive Care Med* 2007;33(10):1811–4.

23. De Keulenaer BL, De Waele JJ, Powell B, et al. What is normal intra-abdominal pressure and how is it affected by positioning, body mass and positive end-expiratory pressure? *Intensive Care Med* 2009;35(6):969–76.

24. Malbrain ML, Léonard M, Delmarcelle D. A novel technique of intra-abdominal pressure measurement: validation of two prototypes [abstract]. *Critical Care* 2002;6(suppl 1):P4. doi:10.1186/cc1739, available at http://ccforum.com/content/6/S1/P4.

25. Epelman M, Soudack M, Engel A, et al. Abdominal compartment syndrome in children: CT findings. *Pediatr Radiol* 2002;32(5):319–22.

26. Cavaliere F, Cina A, Biasucci D, et al. Sonographic assessment of abdominal vein dimensional and hemodynamic changes induced in human volunteers by a model of abdominal hypertension. *Crit Care Med* 2011;39(2):344–8.

27. Bradley SE, Bradley GP. The effect of increased intra-abdominal pressure on renal function in man. *J Clin Invest* 1947;26(5):1010–22.

28. Dalfino L, Tullo L, Donadio I, et al. Intra-abdominal hypertension and acute renal failure in critically ill patients. *Intensive Care Med* 2008;34(4):707–13.

29. Schwarte LA, Scheeren TW, Lorenz C, et al. Moderate increase in intraabdominal pressure attenuates gastric mucosal oxygen saturation in patients undergoing laparoscopy. *Anesthesiology*. 2004;100(5):1081–7.

30. Cresswell AB, Wendon JA. Hepatic function and non-invasive hepatosplanchnic monitoring in patients with abdominal hypertension. *Acta Clin Belg Suppl* 2007(1):113–8.

31. Sakka SG. Indocyanine green plasma disappearance rate as an indicator of hepato-splanchnic ischemia during abdominal compartment syndrome. *Anesth Analg* 2007;104(4):1003–4.

32. Ridings PC, Bloomfield GL, Blocher CR, et al. Cardiopulmonary effects of raised intra-abdominal pressure before and after intravascular volume expansion. *J Trauma* 1995;39(6):1071–5.

33. Rezende-Neto JB, Moore EE, Melo de Andrade MV, et al. Systemic inflammatory response secondary to abdominal compartment syndrome: Stage for multiple organ failure. *J Trauma* 2002;53(6):1121–8.

34. Ranieri VM, Brienza N, Santostasi S, et al. Impairment of lung and chest wall mechanics in patients with acute respiratory distress syndrome: Role of abdominal distension. *Am J Respir Crit Care Med* 1997;156(4 pt 1):1082–91.

35. Pelosi P, Quintel M, Malbrain ML. Effect of intra-abdominal pressure on respiratory mechanics. *Acta Clin Belg Suppl* 2007(1):78–88.

36. Quintel M, Pelosi P, Caironi P, et al. An increase of abdominal pressure increases pulmonary edema in oleic acid-induced lung injury. *Am J Respir Crit Care Med* 2004;169(4):534–41.

37. Obeid F, Saba A, Fath J, et al. Increases in intra-abdominal pressure affect pulmonary compliance. *Arch Surg* 1995;130(5):544–7; discussion 7–8.

38. Gattinoni L, Pelosi P, Suter PM, et al. Acute respiratory distress syndrome caused by pulmonary and extrapulmonary disease. Different syndromes? *Am J Respir Crit Care Med* 1998;158(1):3–11.

39. Robotham JL, Wise RA, Bromberger-Barnea B. Effects of changes in abdominal pressure on left ventricular performance and regional blood flow. *Crit Care Med* 1985;13(10):803–9.

40. Citerio G, Vascotto E, Villa F, et al. Induced abdominal compartment syndrome increases intracranial pressure in neurotrauma patients: A prospective study. *Crit Care Med* 2001;29(7):1466–71.

41. Scalea TM, Bochicchio GV, Habashi N, et al. Increased intra-abdominal, intrathoracic, and intracranial pressure after severe brain injury: Multiple compartment syndrome. *J Trauma* 2007;62(3):647–56; discussion 56.

42. Malbrain ML, Chiumello D, Pelosi P, et al. Incidence and prognosis of intraabdominal hypertension in a mixed population of critically ill patients: A multiple-center epidemiological study. *Crit Care Med* 2005;33(2):315–22.

43. Beck R, Halberthal M, Zonis Z, et al. Abdominal compartment syndrome in children. *Pediatr Crit Care Med* 2001;2(1):51–6.

44. Diaz FJ, Fernandez Sein A, Gotay F. Identification and management of Abdominal Compartment Syndrome in the Pediatric Intensive Care Unit. *P R Health Sci J* 2006;25(1):17–22.

45. Balogh Z, McKinley BA, Holcomb JB, et al. Both primary and secondary abdominal compartment syndrome can be predicted early and are harbingers of multiple organ failure. *J Trauma* 2003;54(5):848–59; discussion 59–61.

46. Tsai MH, Huang HR, Chu SM, et al. Clinical features of newborns with gastroschisis and outcomes of different initial interventions: Primary closure versus staged repair. *Pediatr Neonatol* 2010;51(6):320–5.

47. Suehiro K, Okutani R, Ogawa S, et al. Perioperative management of a neonate with Cantrell syndrome. *J Anesth* 2009;23(4):572–5.

48. Kincaid MS, Vavilala MS, Faucher L, et al. Feeding intolerance as a result of small-intestine intussusception in a child with major burns. *J Burn Care Rehabil* 2004;25(2):212–4; discussion 1.

49. Steinau G, Kaussen T, Bolten B, et al. Abdominal compartment syndrome in childhood: diagnostics, therapy and survival rate. *Pediatr Surg Int* 2011;27(4):399–405.

50. Neville HL, Lally KP, Cox CS Jr. Emergent abdominal decompression with patch abdominoplasty in the pediatric patient. *J Pediatr Surg* 2000;35(5):705–8.

51. Perks DH, Grewal H. Abdominal compartment syndrome in the pediatric patient with blunt trauma. *J Trauma Nurs* 2005;12(2):50–4.

52. Grevious MA, Iqbal R, Raofi V, et al. Staged approach for abdominal wound closure following combined liver and intestinal transplantation from living donors in pediatric patients. *Pediatr Transplant* 2009;13(2):177–81.

53. DeCou JM, Abrams RS, Miller RS, Gauderer MW. Abdominal compartment syndrome in children: Experience with three cases. *J Pediatr Surg* 2000;35(6):840–2.

54. Lam MC, Yang PT, Skippen PW, et al. Abdominal compartment syndrome complicating paediatric extracorporeal life support: Diagnostic and therapeutic challenges. *Anaesth Intensive Care* 2008;36(5):726–31.

55. Oray-Schrom P, St Martin D, Bartelloni P, et al. Giant nonpancreatic pseudocyst causing acute anuria. *J Clin Gastroenterol* 2002;34(2):160–3.

56. Roberts S, Creamer K, Shoupe B, et al. Unique management of stage 4S neuroblastoma complicated by massive hepatomegaly: Case report and review of the literature. *J Pediatr Hematol Oncol* 2002;24(2):142–4.

57. Chung PH, Wong KK, Lan LC, et al. Abdominal compartment syndrome after open biopsy in a child with bilateral Wilms' tumour. *Hong Kong Med J* 2009;15(2):136–8.

58. Kavaguti SK, Mackevicius BR, de Andrade MF, et al. Abdominal compartment syndrome caused by massive pyonephrosis in an infant with primary obstructive megaureter. *Case Report Med* 2011; article ID is 174167, p. 1–4.
59. Ng E, Kim HB, Lillehei CW, et al. Life threatening tension pneumoperitoneum from intestinal perforation during air reduction of intussusception. *Paediatr Anaesth* 2002;12(9):798–800.
60. Gala HC, Avasthi BS, Lokeshwar MR. Dengue shock syndrome with two atypical complications. *Indian J Pediatr* 2012;79(3):386–8.
61. Morrell BJ, Vinden C, Singh RN, et al. Secondary abdominal compartment syndrome in a case of pediatric trauma shock resuscitation. *Pediatr Crit Care Med* 2007;8(1):67–70.
62. Jensen AR, Hughes WB, Grewal H. Secondary abdominal compartment syndrome in children with burns and trauma: A potentially lethal complication. *J Burn Care Res* 2006;27(2):242–6.
63. Kirkpatrick AW, Brenneman FD, McLean RF, et al. Is clinical examination an accurate indicator of raised intra-abdominal pressure in critically injured patients? *Can J Surg* 2000;43(3):207–11.
64. Sugrue M, Bauman A, Jones F, et al. Clinical examination is an inaccurate predictor of intraabdominal pressure. *World J Surg* 2002;26(12):1428–31.
65. Schein M, Wittmann DH, Aprahamian CC, et al. The abdominal compartment syndrome: The physiological and clinical consequences of elevated intra-abdominal pressure. *J Am Coll Surg* 1995;180(6):745–53.
66. Brierley J, Carcillo JA, Choong K, et al. Clinical practice parameters for hemodynamic support of pediatric and neonatal septic shock: 2007 update from the American College of Critical Care Medicine. *Crit Care Med* 2009;37(2):666–88.
67. Pearson EG, Rollins MD, Vogler SA, et al. Decompressive laparotomy for abdominal compartment syndrome in children: before it is too late. *J Pediatr Surg* 2010;45(6):1324–9.
68. Prodhan P, Imamura M, Garcia X, et al. Abdominal compartment syndrome in newborns and children supported on extracorporeal membrane oxygenation. *ASAIO J* 2012;58(2):143–7.
69. Daugherty EL, Hongyan L, Taichman D, et al. Abdominal compartment syndrome is common in medical intensive care unit patients receiving large-volume resuscitation. *J Intensive Care Med* 2007;22(5):294–9.
70. Balogh Z, McKinley BA, Cocanour CS, et al. Supranormal trauma resuscitation causes more cases of abdominal compartment syndrome. *Arch Surg* 2003;138(6):637–42; discussion 42–3.
71. De laet I, Citerio G, Malbrain ML. The influence of intraabdominal hypertension on the central nervous system: Current insights and clinical recommendations, is it all in the head? *Acta Clin Belg Suppl* 2007(1):89–97.
72. Anand RJ, Ivatury RR. Surgical management of intra-abdominal hypertension and abdominal compartment syndrome. *Am Surg* 2011;77(suppl 1):42–5.
73. Cullen DJ, Coyle JP, Teplick R, et al. Cardiovascular, pulmonary, and renal effects of massively increased intra-abdominal pressure in critically ill patients. *Crit Care Med* 1989;17(2):118–21.
74. Ejike JC, Mathur M. Abdominal decompression in children. *Crit Care Res Pract* 2012; article ID is 180797, p. 1–11.
75. Karpelowsky JS, Thomas G, Shun A. Definitive abdominal wall closure using a porcine intestinal submucosa biodegradable membrane in pediatric transplantation. *Pediatr Transplant* 2009;13(3):285–9.

CHAPTER 101 ■ THE ACUTE ABDOMEN

EDUARDO J. SCHNITZLER, TOMAS IÖLSTER, AND RICARDO D. RUSSO

KEY POINTS

1 The most frequent cause of acute abdomen in previously healthy children is acute appendicitis.

2 Acute appendicitis in infants and small children may have an unclear initial presentation. It is sometimes associated with diarrhea, and the diagnosis is often delayed until after it progresses to generalized peritonitis.

3 The most frequent cause of intestinal obstruction is acquired adhesions, the management of which may only require decompression and intestinal rest.

4 Timely diagnosis of intussusception is critical to facilitate a quick resolution and avoid progression to intestinal ischemia and obstruction.

5 Midgut volvulus associated with malrotation is a severe condition with rapid development of ischemia; if suspected, it requires an urgent surgical consultation for a decision regarding surgical intervention.

6 During the care of newborns, especially premature infants, necrotizing enterocolitis (NEC) remains prevalent

and carries a high risk of morbidity and mortality in severe cases. The prevention, early diagnosis, and appropriate combined clinical–surgical management of NEC are essential to improve survival and reduce long-term morbidity.

7 Severe acute pancreatitis is less frequent in the pediatric population; however, it can be devastating when accompanied by local and systemic intense inflammatory responses.

8 The most frequent pediatric abdominal complications seen in the pediatric intensive care unit include gastrointestinal hemorrhage, postoperative ileus, acalculous cholecystitis, pseudomembranous colitis, toxic megacolon, and abdominal compartment syndrome.

9 Recognizing the etiology of abdominal pain or of episodes that simulate the acute abdomen in systemic illnesses, such as diabetic ketoacidosis, acute porphyria, sickle cell crisis, Henoch–Schönlein purpura, or Kawasaki disease, is essential for adequate management.

INTRODUCTION

The term *acute abdomen* is a clinical syndrome characterized by rapid onset of signs and symptoms indicating an intra-abdominal pathology that requires prompt decision making and often emergent surgical intervention. Presenting signs might include abdominal pain, signs of inflammation, or other symptoms. A diverse spectrum of diseases may produce similar signs and symptoms that culminate in abdominal pain. Accurate and timely clinical assessment is essential to diagnose the underlying pathology and begin appropriate medical or surgical treatment (1).

EVALUATION OF THE EVIDENCE

Due to the paucity of medical evidence, most of the decisions related to the management of children with acute abdomen in the pediatric intensive care unit (PICU) are based on consensus or expert opinion. Conversely, most of the published controlled clinical trials or prospective series are from the adult population; unfortunately etiology, complications, and clinical scenarios differ considerably from those found in children.

To help evaluate the available literature, we use the following modified quality of evidence grading (2) in this chapter:

1. Grade A—decisions based on systematic reviews, meta-analysis, or at least one randomized, controlled trial applicable to the adult critical patient (A−) or the pediatric critical patient (A+).

2. Grade B—evidence based on at least one cohort study or case–control studies applicable to the adult critical patient (B−) or the pediatric critical patient (B+). Only recommendations based on this type of evidence (A or B) are emphasized.

3. Grade C—evidence based on case series, consensus, or expert opinion.

CLINICAL ASSESSMENT

Causes of acute abdomen are listed in **Table 101.1** and are divided into three diagnostic groups:

- primary abdominal pathology (originating from the gastrointestinal tract);
- abdominal pathology as a consequence of critical illness (secondary); and
- abdominal manifestations in some systemic diseases that may present as acute abdomen.

Four basic processes may provoke signs and symptoms of acute abdomen: infection or inflammation, obstruction, perforation, and ischemia. A fifth process, gastrointestinal hemorrhage, may be associated with acute abdomen, and is described in more detail in Chapter 99. Most patients with primary abdominal pathology do not require admission to the PICU, provided that diagnosis and treatment (usually surgical) are instituted promptly. However, if the child's abdominal pathology progresses to ischemia and perforation, the severity

TABLE 101.1

CAUSES OF ACUTE ABDOMEN

Primary abdominal pathology
- Mechanical obstruction
  - Intussusception, peritoneal adhesion, others
- Acute intestinal ischemia
  - Malrotation, volvulus, others
- Infection/inflammation
  - Peritonitis, intra-abdominal abscess, fistula
  - Enteritis, neutropenic enterocolitis
  - Acute pancreatitis
  - Acute cholecystitis[a]
- Hollow viscera perforation
- Abdominal trauma
- Diseases linked to the reproductive organs

Abdominal pathology of the critical patient
- Gastrointestinal hemorrhage
- Ileus
- Pseudomembranous colitis
- Toxic megacolon
- Abdominal compartment syndrome

Abdominal manifestations of systemic diseases
- Diabetic ketoacidosis
- Acute intermittent porphyria
- Henoch-Schönlein purpura
- Kawasaki disease
- Sickle cell crisis

[a]Cholecystitis can also present as an abdominal pathology of the critical patients.

of this presentation with the risk of multiorgan dysfunction necessitates perioperative care in the PICU.

The critically ill patient may present with complications that compromise the function of the gastrointestinal tract. Intestinal ileus, acute cholecystitis, toxic megacolon, abdominal compartment syndrome, intra-abdominal collections, and tertiary peritonitis are some of the complications of critical illness that may contribute to the patient's morbidity and mortality. These complications may progress to multiorgan failure and subsequent death.

Finally, diverse systemic diseases may cause conditions that generate or simulate an acute surgical abdomen. The history and clinical examination may be suggestive of a systemic disease that presents as an acute abdomen caused by direct or indirect lesions of the gastrointestinal tract. (Please refer to **Table 101.1**.)

The etiology and the rapidity of disease progression dictate the clinical presentation and the condition of the patient. A volvulus-associated bowel ischemia usually progresses rapidly to a life-threatening situation, unless it is promptly recognized and treated. An acute appendicitis, if unrecognized or treated inappropriately, may lead to a critical condition. Any one of the conditions assigned to the diagnostic groups in **Table 101.1** may necessitate admission to the PICU for monitoring and management of multiorgan failure. Timely recognition may be challenging as patients often manifest with multiple organ dysfunction and deterioration of consciousness. Clinical presentations may overlap among the three groups; hence a strict classification or categorization is not intended. Rather, the goal of this chapter is to distinguish scenarios and to outline an approach that allows diagnosis and management in a timely fashion.

INITIAL MANAGEMENT OF THE CHILD WITH AN ACUTE ABDOMEN

Primary Evaluation and Stabilization

One of the most important initial determinations to be made is whether the patient requires an urgent laparotomy or laparoscopy for diagnosis and treatment. The initial approach, as in any other emergency, includes a quick assessment of the severity of the condition and the potential complications (**Fig. 101.1**). If the child is clinically unstable or if an intra-abdominal catastrophe is a possibility, establishing an adequate airway, ensuring gas exchange, and maintaining circulation must be prioritized. Intra-abdominal catastrophe may be suspected based on clinical examination. The presence of severe abdominal distension, board-like rigidity, abdominal ecchymoses, or discoloration may be signs of a severe abdominal condition. Monitoring of pulse oximetry, heart rate, electrocardiogram, and noninvasive blood pressure is essential to guide therapy. Two large-bore peripheral venous catheters for vascular access should be established as quickly as possible, and blood and urine samples should be obtained for complete blood count, coagulation profile, chemistries, blood typing and cross matching, blood cultures, and urine studies. Fluid boluses should be administered rapidly until appropriate perfusion has been established, and empiric broad-spectrum intravenous antibiotic treatment should be initiated whenever an infectious etiology is suspected. Early surgical review and imaging studies, such as abdominal radiography and/or ultrasound, may guide therapeutic decisions.

If perforation, peritonitis, or ischemic bowel compromise is suspected, immediate surgical intervention is necessary. If the diagnosis is not clear, further options include an abdominal computerized tomography (CT) scan, an observation period with serial abdominal examination, or an urgent diagnostic surgery (exploratory laparotomy). When bowel obstruction is suspected, initial management will depend on the probable cause and the presence of clinical signs compatible with ischemia. In these patients, nil per os and placement of a nasogastric (NG) tube for stomach decompression are necessary.

History

As soon as the child is stable and intra-abdominal catastrophe is ruled out, a detailed history of the presenting signs and symptoms and sequence of events should be obtained. The presentation and sequence of such symptoms as fever, vomiting, diarrhea, constipation, urinary symptoms, and pelvic symptoms in female teenagers are important for the diagnosis. When possible, localization and radiation of the pain should be determined. History should include previous medical pathologies, previous surgery, chronic drug therapy, recent trauma, and possibility of accidental ingestion of harmful substances in young children. This process is usually undertaken simultaneously as primary evaluation and stabilization of airway and cardiorespiratory status is ongoing.

Physical Examination

Following initial resuscitation, the clinical examination of the abdomen should be thorough and systematic. Inspection may reveal significant findings, such as distension, masses, hernias, surgical scars, or other alterations in the skin. The presence of petechiae, purpura, or rash may be suggestive of a

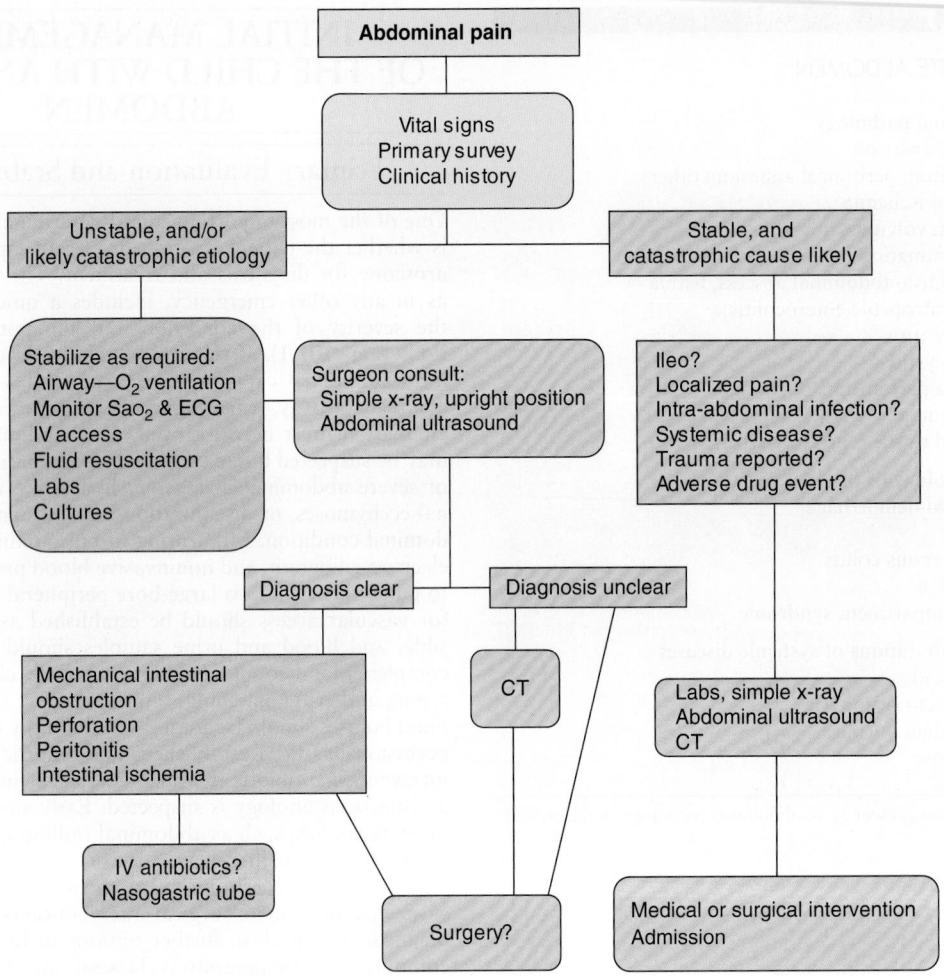

FIGURE 101.1. Initial approach to child with acute abdomen.

systemic disease. Auscultation should precede palpation to avoid modification of the peristalsis by external stimulation. Bowel sounds are typically altered during abdominal pathology. However, sometimes, findings may not be typical; bowel sounds may be absent in mild diseases or may be present even during intra-abdominal catastrophes. Abdominal percussion helps to differentiate between gaseous distension (tympanic) and distension due to masses or ascites (dull). Abdominal palpation should be gentle, and the child's attention should be distracted. Palpation should be systematic, beginning with a superficial examination in the most distant quadrant from the site of maximum pain and moving slowly toward the painful area. The interexaminer reliability in physical examination of children with abdominal pain performed by emergency medicine physicians (residents and attending physicians) and the pediatric surgeon may be variable (3). When comparing residents and attending physicians for the evaluation of the presence or absence of abdominal signs, investigators have reported less-than-moderate chance-adjusted agreement (κ range: −0.04 to 0.38). Because of the lack of reliability of the abdominal examination, abdominal x-ray and/or ultrasound are almost always indicated when abdominal pathology is suspected and the diagnosis is not immediately obvious. Examination of the inguinal and scrotal regions is essential to detect possible hernias or changes of the scrotal appearance. Digital rectal examination should not be performed routinely

in the evaluation of abdominal pain or acute abdomen. It can be useful for the evaluation of occult blood, local masses, and rectal lesions (4). Pelvic examination is only indicated for adolescents in whom the pain is suggestive of gynecologic pathology. Pregnancy tests should be included as part of the laboratory examination for all postpubertal females. In cases of suspected sexual abuse of prepubescent girls, the pelvic examination should be performed by very experienced gynecologists after the patient has been deeply sedated or anesthetized.

Once the cause of the acute abdomen has been established, it is necessary to consider its severity and possible complications. Abdominal emergencies are dynamic and will change within hours. The child should be assessed frequently to rule out evolving complications and to determine the need for timely surgical intervention. The critically ill child who is receiving mechanical ventilation is usually sedated and may be receiving muscle relaxants. In this situation, physical examination may not reflect the abdominal pathology, and a high degree of suspicion is essential. Clinical worsening, persistence of signs of infection or inflammation, increased NG fluid losses, or persistence of ileus should be considered as possible markers of underlying abdominal pathology. Frequent clinical examination and serial imaging studies will indicate the need for more invasive procedures. Children with immunocompromise or low white-cell counts may not be able to mount an appropriate inflammatory response and hence may not manifest the clinical signs of acute abdomen.

Diagnostic Imaging

A discussion of abdominal diagnostic imaging can be found in Chapter 102 (Diagnostic imaging of the abdomen). The plain abdominal x-ray is useful for the diagnosis of bowel obstruction, renal lithiasis, pneumoperitoneum, and pneumatosis intestinalis (**Fig. 101.2**). In bowel obstruction, the distribution of air may show a few localized loops (sentinel loops) of small intestine and/or cecum, distended loops of small bowel in an organized, obstructive pattern, or in the upright view, numerous air-fluid levels. Sometimes, the finding of opacity in the upper abdomen that obscures the caudal border of the liver may help to confirm the diagnosis of intussusception. Conversely, the presence of air or opacities suggestive of feces in the cecum may help to exclude a diagnosis of intestinal pathology, although specificity and sensitivity are low. Abdominal ultrasound and CT scan are the two principal tools for the assessment of the child with abdominal emergencies.

The use of CT scan has been restricted because of the long-term cancer risk related to radiation exposure (5). The double-contrast CT scan helps to determine the size and location of an intra-abdominal mass and its relation to other organs, and it is useful to study the cause of an intestinal obstruction and to evaluate pancreatic, retroperitoneal, and pelvic pathology (6).

Analgesia

One of the common concerns of the pediatric intensivist is the potential masking of important clinical signs during optimal management of analgesia in a child being evaluated for an acute abdomen. The traditional view in adult and pediatric emergency medicine, based on expert opinion, has been to avoid giving analgesia before the surgeon's evaluation. A systematic review that included adult and pediatric patients noted that although opioid administration may alter the physical examination findings, these changes do not result in management errors (7). In adults with acute abdominal pain the use of opioid analgesia does not increase the risk of diagnostic error or the risk of error in making decisions regarding treatment (8). *Recommendation A (−).*

PRIMARY ABDOMINAL PATHOLOGY

Bowel Obstruction

Bowel obstruction is a mechanical blockage to the transit of the intestinal contents that may be either intrinsic (intraluminal or from the bowel wall) or due to extrinsic compression. The former may include obstruction secondary to *Ascaris lumbricoides* (still existent in developing countries) or intussusception, whereas causes of extrinsic compressions may include postsurgical adhesions or incarcerated hernia (**Table 101.2**). Prolonged complete bowel obstruction will usually cause plasma leakage into the extracellular space ("third spacing") and dehydration. It may also lead to intestinal ischemia due to distension, to systemic infections, and finally, to death.

Congenital causes of small bowel obstruction include annular pancreas, malrotation-volvulus, malrotation-Ladd bands, Meckel diverticulum with volvulus or intussusceptions, and inguinal hernia. Other congenital anomalies such as intestinal duplication, remnant omphalomesenteric duct, or mesenteric cyst can originate intestinal obstruction by means of internal hernia or volvulus (9). Duodenal or ileal atresias are congenital causes diagnosed during the newborn period. Congenital obstructions of the colon include Hirschsprung disease, pseudo-obstruction, volvulus, and colonic duplication. In the immediate neonatal period, imperforate anus or colonic atresia may be diagnosed.

The most frequent causes of acquired obstructions are postsurgical adhesions and intussusception. Crohn disease (CD) may also be a cause of small bowel obstruction. In patients

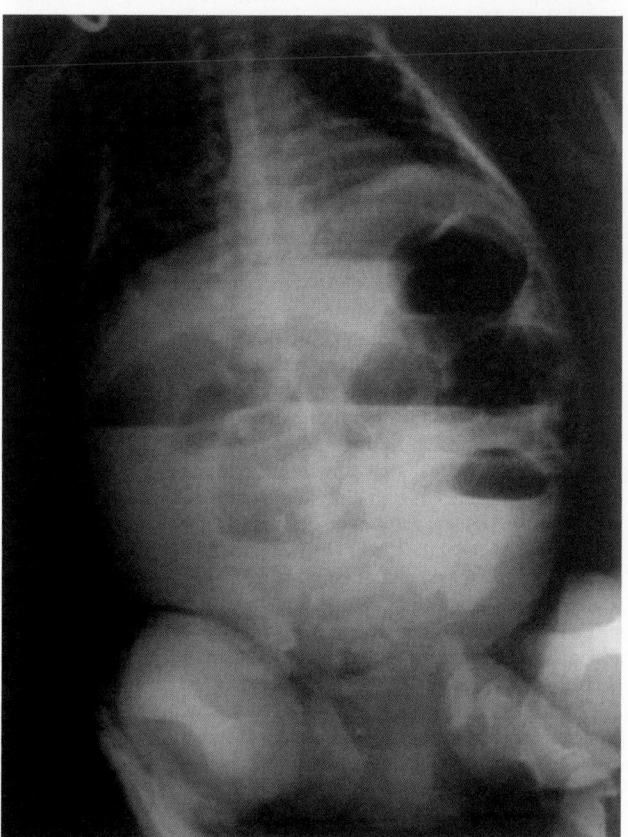

FIGURE 101.2. Paralytic ileus. Enteritis.

TABLE 101.2

MECHANICAL OBSTRUCTION

Obstruction due to adhesions
Intussusception
Incarcerated hernia
Tumoral obstruction
Crohn disease
Duodenal hematoma
Obstruction due to *Ascaris lumbricoides*
Malrotation—midgut volvulus
Meckel diverticulum with volvulus or intussusception
Volvulus or hernia in congenital anomalies (e.g., intestinal duplication cyst)
Annular pancreas
Duodenal or ileal atresia[a]
Hirschsprung disease
Toxic megacolon
Chronic intestinal pseudo-obstruction
Imperforate anus[a]
Colonic atresia[a]

[a]Diagnosis can be made in the immediate neonatal period.

with cystic fibrosis, obstructive syndromes in the distal ileum or in the colon may be present. Less frequent causes include duodenal hematoma and superior mesenteric artery syndrome.

The clinical presentation of bowel obstruction may include cramping abdominal pain, nausea, bilious vomiting, and absence of intestinal transit when the obstruction is complete. Diarrhea, sometimes bloody, may signal the onset of obstruction before intestinal transit ceases. Cramping abdominal pain changes to continuous pain when intestinal ischemia begins. Typically, symptoms are more sudden, intense, and progressive than in ileus, where symptoms are less intense and have a slower progression. The patient with mechanical obstruction presents with severe pain and systemic signs, such as tachycardia, sweating, and, occasionally, shock. Abdominal distension may be generalized when the obstruction is in the distal bowel, or it may be absent in proximal obstruction, such as duodenal or jejunal obstruction due to bowel malrotation. Bowel sounds are usually increased. External examination of the abdominal wall may reveal previous scars, implicating postsurgical adhesions as a possible cause of obstruction. Palpation may reveal the presence of intra-abdominal masses or hernias. Signs of peritoneal irritation, such as rebound tenderness or abdominal rigidity, are suggestive of ischemia and perforation. No clinical or laboratory findings can clearly predict the presence of intestinal ischemia during mechanical obstruction; clinical judgment by an experienced surgeon is essential in deciding the best moment for surgical intervention (**Table 101.3**).

Plain abdominal x-rays may reveal air-fluid levels in the small bowel, dilated small bowel, or colon loops, as well as intestinal wall edema or minimal intestinal gas distal to the obstruction. The upright or lateral position is necessary to visualize air-fluid levels (see **Fig. 101.2**). Abdominal CT scan is the study of choice to identify less clear causes of obstruction or to evaluate the presence of ischemia (10), although most of the evidence is from adult studies. Unnecessary imaging studies should never delay exploratory laparotomy when an urgent indication is clear. Abdominal ultrasound is useful for the diagnosis of intussusception, and the presence of free fluid may suggest a collection secondary to bowel perforation. In the intensive care setting, the diagnosis of mechanical obstruction may be difficult in a child requiring mechanical ventilation and sedation. Increased NG tube output and the absence of stool output or flatus may be key signs for the diagnosis

TABLE 101.3

BOWEL OBSTRUCTION

Clinical presentation
 Sudden, intense, and progressive symptoms
 Cramping abdominal pain
 Nausea and bilious vomiting
 Diarrhea and enterorrhagia (onset)
 Bowel sound increased (onset)
 Absence of intestinal transit (complete obstruction)
 Continuous pain, peritoneal irritation (ischemia or perforation)
 Tachycardia, sweating, hypovolemia, shock
 Abdominal distension (in relation with level of obstruction)
 Increase nasogastric-tube output

Imaging
 Plain abdominal x-ray
 CT scan
 Bedside ultrasound (useful in diagnosis of intussusception)

Management
 Hydration
 Placement of nasogastric tube
 Evaluation of surgical resolution

of bowel obstruction. Presurgical insertion of an NG tube is useful to control vomiting, to measure fluid losses, and to control pain. However, the patient should be fully conscious, with intact airway-protective reflexes before any attempt is made to insert the NG tube. If these criteria cannot be satisfied, the airway should be secured first using a rapid-sequence intubation technique (Chapter 24, Airway Management).

Surgical resolution of complete obstruction is a priority, and any delay will influence the outcome. Postponing surgery for >24 hours in a complete obstruction increases the risk of ischemia and intestinal resection (11). An expeditious surgical intervention in the presence of persistent signs of obstruction or signs of ischemia is recommended. *Recommendation: Grade B (−)*.

Intussusception

Intussusception represents the most common cause of acute abdomen in infants and preschool children and usually presents within the first 2 years of life, with a peak incidence between 5 and 9 months of age. It occurs when one segment of the intestine (proximal) is telescoped into the adjacent segment (distal). In most cases, no lead point can be identified, and these cases are regarded as idiopathic, possibly linked to swollen Peyer patches (lymphoid tissue) in the terminal ileum (>90% of cases). Lead points may be noted in children <3 months but are especially frequent in children >2 years (2%–8% of cases). Meckel diverticulum, mesenteric lymph nodes, intestinal polyps, hemangioma, mucosal hemorrhage, and lymphoma are all causes of lead points. The most frequent form of intussusception involves the ileocolic region, where the terminal ileum is telescoped into the colon. Less frequent types of intussusception are ileoileal, cecocolic, or combinations (e.g., ileoileocolic). Ileoileal intussusception may be present after abdominal surgery, usually within the first 5 days. During intussusception, mesenteric venous drainage of the intussuscepted segment is obstructed, resulting in increased volume of the segment, edema, and mucosal bleeding. The apex of the intussusception may extend and displace itself through the interior of the colon. When intussusception is resolved within the first 24 hours, most cases do not present with ischemic compromise; however, after 24 hours, the risk of severe ischemia and intestinal gangrene increases progressively.

The typical presentation involves a previously healthy infant who presents with severe paroxysmal colicky pain accompanied by drawing up of the legs and intense weeping. Initially, the child recovers between episodes; however, if the diagnosis is delayed, progressive lethargy occurs in most cases. Emesis is usually present, and normal stools may be present during the initial phase. Passage of (red) currant jelly stool or presence of blood on rectal examination may be seen in the first 12 hours but may also occur later. A slightly tender, sausage-shaped mass may be palpable in the subhepatic region of the abdomen (**Table 101.4**). However, the triad of colicky abdominal pain, red currant jelly stools (or hematochezia), and a palpable abdominal mass is present only in 30% of patients. Children with delayed diagnosis or perforation secondary to hydrostatic or pneumatic reduction may develop critical illness with compromised perfusion and sepsis. The initial diagnosis is suspected on clinical examination and may be confirmed by an abdominal ultrasound, which is a very sensitive test, and if a competent ultrasonographer has ruled out intussusception using ultrasound, no further imaging tests should be necessary to search for that diagnosis.

For nonsurgical reduction, the use of pneumatic enema or saline-solution enema under ultrasound guidance has a success rate of 70%–90% when performed within the first 48 hours. Both methods were found to be accurate in the diagnosis and

TABLE 101.4

INTUSSUSCEPTION

Clinical presentation
  Severe paroxysmal colicky pain[a]
  Emesis
  Normal or currant jelly (red) stools[a]
  Sausage-shaped mass palpable[a]
  Progressive lethargy
  Late diagnosis (perforation, shock, sepsis)
Imaging
  Ultrasound
Management
  Nonsurgical reduction (when early diagnosis)—air or saline-
    solution enema with ultrasound or fluoroscopic guidance
  Surgical reduction or resection (when late diagnosis or lead
    point identified)

[a]Classic triad is present only in 30% of cases.

reduction of intussusception (12). *Recommendation A(+).* Perforation rates during pneumatic reduction have been reported to occur in 0.1%–0.2% of cases. Barium enema may cause perforation and chemical peritonitis and is, therefore, contraindicated. Factors predicting successful reduction with enema are proximal colon localization and the experience of the provider, measured by the volume of procedures (13).

Nonsurgical reduction is contraindicated when symptoms have been present for >48 hours or in the presence of shock, peritoneal irritation, perforation, pneumatosis, or ultrasound findings that predict failure of a nonsurgical intervention or are suggestive of the presence of a lead point. When nonsurgical reduction fails or is not possible, urgent laparotomy approach is the rule. The need for surgical reduction or bowel resection and the risk of complications are directly related to the time that elapses between onset of symptoms and laparotomy. Intussusception may recur within the first 6 months and is more frequent during the first day after reduction.

Peritoneal Adhesions

Fibrous adhesions following abdominal surgery are a frequent cause of bowel obstruction, representing as much as 33% of all cases. The reported incidence of bowel obstruction due to adhesions in children after abdominal surgery is 2%–3% and may present as soon as 2 weeks after the procedure. Postsurgical adhesions may produce folding or strangling of the bowel loops or, less frequently, may predispose to intestinal volvulus secondary to loop distension and peritoneal shortening. The presence of fever, leukocytosis, or signs of peritonitis is suggestive of intestinal ischemia. Usual treatment includes NG tube placement, hydration, and presurgical antibiotic therapy effective against gram-negative aerobic and anaerobic bacteria and enterococci. If ischemia is not associated with bowel obstruction from adhesions, spontaneous recovery without the need for surgery is possible. If after 48 hours a patient with uncomplicated adhesive bowel obstruction receiving conservative treatment does not improve, the use of oral contrast study with gastrografin may reduce length of stay and allow earlier feeding initiation when the study shows normal contrast passage (14).

Other Causes of Intestinal Obstruction

Other causes of the intestinal obstruction include incarcerated hernia, intestinal strictures related withCD, Meckel diverticulum, and, rarely, neoplastic pathology such as intestinal lymphoma, Wilms tumor, or neuroblastoma.

Hirschsprung disease, or congenital aganglionic colon, is usually diagnosed during the neonatal period due to the presence of meconium retention, or failure to pass meconium within 24 hours after birth. However, in some cases, this sign may be absent and presentation may occur later with signs of acute enterocolitis, bowel obstruction, or sepsis. Enterocolitis is the principal cause of morbidity and mortality in children with this disease (15). Hirschsprung disease is diagnosed by anorectal manometry and rectal mucosal biopsy. Colonic contrast study shows an area of transition between the colon that is proximal to the obstruction and the distal aganglionic, narrowed segment. Children with chronic intestinal pseudo-obstruction present with symptoms within the first months of life; these include abdominal distension, vomiting, chronic constipation, failure to thrive, diarrheal episodes, and abdominal pain. The diagnosis is usually suspected due to the absence of anatomical causes of obstruction. Diagnosis is confirmed by manometric studies and bowel biopsy, which should reveal muscular fiber involvement or compromise of the enteric nervous system.

Intestinal Ischemia

Bowel ischemia is the final common pathway of many abdominal pathologies and may arise following progression of anatomical malformations, such as malrotation or intestinal volvulus. It may also develop after delayed management of abdominal pathology, such as intussusception, incarcerated hernia, or any other complete mechanical obstruction that has not been promptly resolved. Bowel ischemia during the postoperative period following repair of a coarctation of the aorta, although infrequent, has been clearly reported. Furthermore, intestinal mucosal ischemia may occur during or after cardiac surgery in children. Much less frequently, arterial mesenteric thrombosis and venous occlusive thrombosis are reported as causes of intestinal ischemia or gangrene in the pediatric population. Colonic ischemia may be secondary to vasculitic processes as the hemolytic uremic syndrome (**Table 101.5**).

Patients with severe bowel ischemia progress from mucosal ischemia to transmural necrosis and bowel perforation. Combined sepsis and multiorgan failure are frequently present. In nonintubated, conscious children, the apparent lack of proportion between the severe referred pain and the lack of early clinical findings may be suggestive of the diagnosis. The presence of abdominal distension, severe hypovolemia and hemoconcentration, refractory metabolic acidosis, or hematochezia may lead to the diagnosis. During the initial phase in patients with no obvious surgical pathology, useful diagnostic tests include sigmoidoscopy, colonoscopy, and multidetector CT. When signs of perforation are present, surgery must not be delayed.

Midgut volvulus secondary to malrotation of the bowel may cause one of the most severe forms of bowel ischemia in

TABLE 101.5

INTESTINAL ISCHEMIA

Malrotation—midgut volvulus
Intussusception (late diagnosis)
Incarcerated hernia (late diagnosis)
Complete intestinal obstruction
Surgical repair of coarctation of the aorta
Postoperative period of cardiac surgery
Arterial mesenteric thrombosis
Venous occlusive thrombosis
Hemolytic uremic syndrome

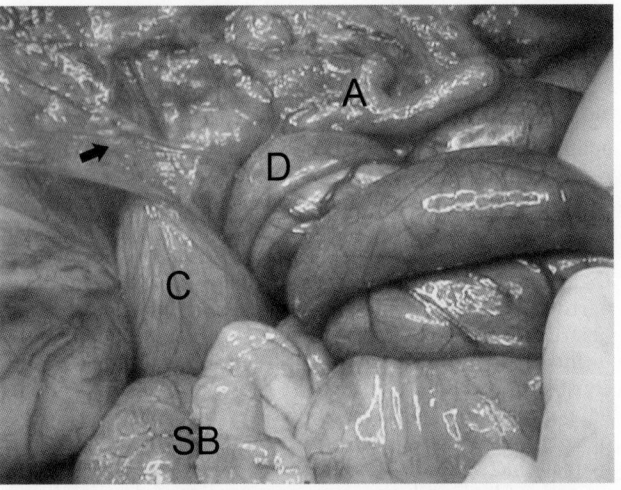

FIGURE 101.3. Operative photograph of midgut volvulus caused by a short mesenteric artery pedicle. *A*, appendix; *D*, duodenum; *C*, colon; *SB*, small bowel; *arrow*, peritoneal bands (Ladd).

children. An abnormal orientation of the intestine in which the ascending colon is not fixed to the right side of the abdomen is associated with a stretching of the base of the intestinal mesentery and allows Ladd′s bands to kink the duodenum predisposing volvulus generation. The mesenteric vessels and bowel are twisted and fixed in the volvulus, which leads to intestinal ischemia and necrosis (**Figs. 101.3 and 101.4**). This diagnosis should be suspected in infants and children with severe abdominal pain and bilious vomiting. A child admitted with intestinal ischemia or necrosis is usually in shock and may or may not present with abdominal distension (depending on the localization of the volvulus), and the abdominal

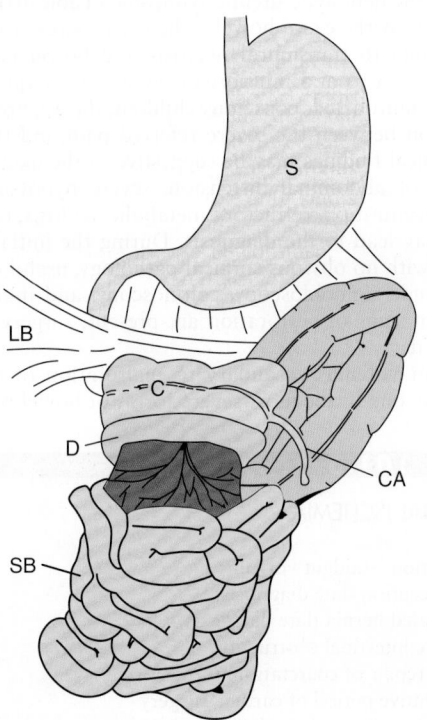

FIGURE 101.4. Volvulus. *S*, stomach; *LB*, Ladd bands; *C*, colon; *CA*, appendix; *D*, duodenum; *SB*, small bowel.

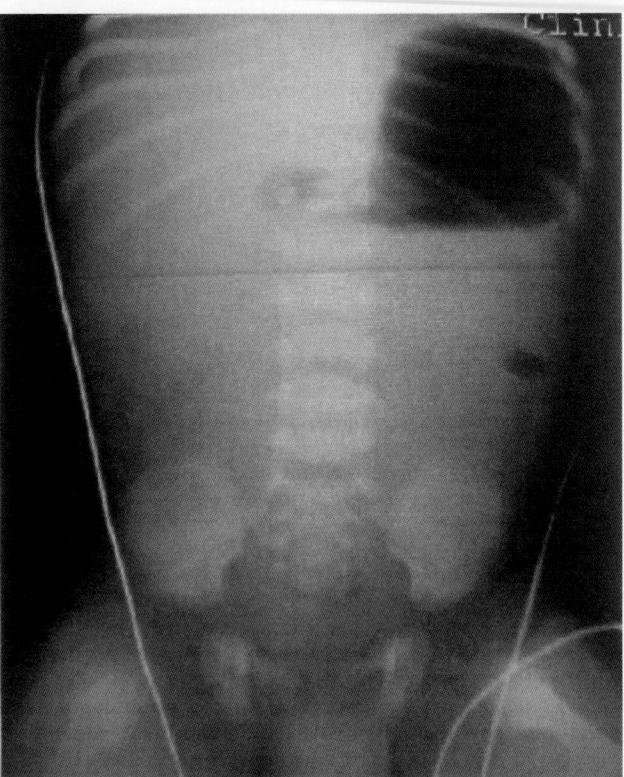

FIGURE 101.5. Abdominal x-ray showing a double-bubble (stomach and duodenum) image.

wall may appear to be blue. Hematochezia is a late sign. The presence of diarrhea does not exclude the diagnosis. Occasionally, the disease may present with less clear signs or even with a normal abdominal x-ray. The classic radiologic findings are the double-bubble sign (**Fig. 101.5**) that shows an abdomen with scarce intestinal air with two air bubbles, one in the stomach and one in the duodenum, air-fluid levels, abnormal position of the cecum, and absence of distal air. Although ultrasound or abdominal CT may yield the diagnosis, contrast studies under fluoroscopic control (upper gastrointestinal series) remain the diagnostic gold standard. Treatment is always surgical (16). When volvulus is present, the whirlpool sign due to the twisted bowel mesentery can be observed in the CT scan. In a study about the risk of intestinal gangrene in patients with small bowel volvulus, nonbilious vomiting, leukocytosis, and elevated C reactive protein were significant findings in multivariate analysis (17).

Peritonitis

Peritonitis is an inflammation of the peritoneal lining of the abdominal cavity that usually results from infectious, chemical, or peritoneal processes. The perforation of the appendix is the most frequent cause. In young children, this diagnosis may be difficult or delayed until diffuse peritonitis is present. Primary peritonitis occurs when the source of infection is outside of the abdomen and reaches the peritoneal cavity via hematogenous or lymphatic dissemination. Secondary peritonitis originates from the rupture or extension of an intra-abdominal viscus or abscess (polymicrobial etiology). Tertiary peritonitis occurs when one or more surgical procedures fail to control an intra-abdominal infectious process. Other intra-abdominal infections are listed in **Table 101.6**.

TABLE 101.6

PERITONITIS AND INTRA-ABDOMINAL INFECTIONS

Peritonitis

Primary peritonitis: no apparent intra-abdominal pathology
   Single organism
   Ascites (cirrhosis, portal hypertension, nephrotic syndrome)
   Associated with peritoneal dialysis
Secondary peritonitis: associated with perforation of intestinal wall secondary to obstructive, ischemic, or inflammatory process
   Polymicrobial organisms
   Appendiceal perforation, bowel ischemia, Crohn disease
   Gangrenous cholecystitis, dehiscence in enteroanastomosis
Tertiary peritonitis: peritonitis following failure of more than one surgical procedure undertaken to control an intra-abdominal focus of infection
   Nosocomial polymicrobial organisms and presence of facilitator material

Other intra-abdominal infections

Intra-abdominal abscess: solid organ, interintestinal, periappendiceal, subhepatic, subphrenic, pelvic, peripancreatic, or retroperitoneal abscess
Acute cholecystitis
Fistulae: lateral or partial and complete or terminal
Congenital infected (Meckel diverticulitis, urachal remnant, etc.)
Pelvic inflammatory disease
Enteritis: invasive or cytotoxin-producing organism
Hemolytic uremic syndrome
Neutropenic enterocolitis or typhlitis

Primary Peritonitis

It is possible to define two types of primary peritonitis: spontaneous bacterial peritonitis (SBP) and peritoneal dialysis-related peritonitis (PDRP). SBP is a rare peritoneal infection with no apparent intra-abdominal pathology, such as perforation, abscesses, or other intra-abdominal sources of infection. Primary peritonitis is usually caused by a single organism, the most frequent being *Streptococcus pneumoniae*, group A streptococci, *Escherichia coli*, or other enteric bacteria. Children who have undergone splenectomy are especially susceptibility to SBP caused by encapsulated organisms.

In children with ascites caused by cirrhosis, portal hypertension, or nephrotic syndrome, the diagnosis of primary peritonitis should be suspected and should be sought in the presence of fever, increased ascites, or a worsening clinical condition. The most frequent causative agents are *Enterococcus*, *Streptococcus*, *Staphylococcus*, or enteric bacteria (e.g., *E. coli* or *Klebsiella pneumoniae*). In children with ascites caused by cirrhosis or nephrotic syndrome, the disease may have an insidious progression without significant clinical findings. At other times, especially in patients with nephrotic syndrome, primary peritonitis may present with severe hypovolemic shock.

In children with ascites, diagnostic paracentesis should be undertaken whenever spontaneous peritonitis is suspected, and the presence of a neutrophil count >250 cells/m^3 in the ascitic fluid confirms the diagnosis. Gram-stain examination of the ascitic fluid has a low sensitivity, and culture may be negative in up to 50% of cases. Initial empiric antibiotic treatment includes ceftriaxone or cefotaxime in combination with aminoglycosides. The results of the culture sensitivity will guide the definitive therapy.

The diagnosis of PDRP should be suspected among patients receiving peritoneal dialysis in the presence of fever, local signs at the entry site of the cannula, or changes in the characteristics of the dialysate. Confirmed (positive culture),

probable (positive gram stain but negative culture), or possible (negative gram stain an culture) diagnosis is defined by the presence of symptoms of peritoneal inflammation and >100 white cells/μL (polymorphonuclear >50%) (18). The empiric antibiotic treatment depends on the predominant infections in each center.

Secondary Peritonitis

Secondary peritonitis occurs when bacteria enter the peritoneal cavity through a perforation or rupture of the intestinal wall or other viscus as a consequence of an obstructive, ischemic, or inflammatory process. The rupture of an abscess into the peritoneal cavity is another mechanism. This process may develop in previously healthy children as a community-acquired infection, with the progression of appendicitis as the most frequent cause. Complicated ischemic processes, including intussusception, midgut volvulus, or incarcerated hernias, may be other causes. In addition, perforation may be the consequence of the progression of inflammatory diseases, such asCD, gangrenous cholecystitis, typhlitis, or peripancreatic abscesses. The dehiscence of sutures during the postoperative period of an enteroanastomosis or complications during the course of a traumatic intra-abdominal injury are the most frequent causes of peritonitis produced by nosocomial bacteria that colonize the gastrointestinal tract of hospitalized patients. In postpubertal females, organisms such as *Neisseria gonorrhoeae* and *Chlamydia trachomatis* may invade the pelvic cavity through the fallopian tubes.

The clinical picture of secondary peritonitis includes high fever, diffuse abdominal pain, and vomiting. The physical findings consist of rebound tenderness, abdominal wall rigidity, and diminished or absent bowel sounds. Most children with peritonitis secondary to appendicular perforation improve with surgical treatment and antibiotic therapy and do not need admission to the PICU. However, some children may develop third-space fluid losses, shock, or acute respiratory distress syndrome. Laboratory tests may show leukocytosis, and the upright abdominal x-ray may show free air in the abdominal cavity, ileus, and signs of obstruction or obliteration of the psoas shadow.

The critically ill child with an abdominal infection is common in the PICU; the seriousness of illness may be the consequence of the progression of inflammatory, infectious, or mechanical processes and, many times, may be exacerbated by diagnostic delays or delays during initial management. These children may develop recurrent sepsis and multiorgan failure, which increases the risk of mortality. Frequent surgical evaluation is essential for determining the need for further diagnostic studies or surgery. As secondary peritonitis is caused by rupture of a hollow viscus, the typical microbiologic finding is polymicrobial flora in the peritoneal fluid. The most frequent pathogens include enteric gram-negative bacteria (*E. coli*, *Klebsiella*, *Enterobacter*, etc.) and anaerobes (*Bacteroides fragilis*, *Clostridium* spp., and others) (19). The site of perforation determines the inoculum and type of bacteria. Most secondary peritonitis incidences are a consequence of appendicular inflammation and are caused by community pathogens. Therefore, these infections are usually sensitive to antibiotics that are effective against gram-negative and anaerobic bacteria. The recovery depends on adequate and timely surgery and the addition of broad-spectrum antibiotic treatment. Ninety percent of children recover adequately and do not require admission to the PICU. In patients with secondary generalized peritonitis, surgery is mandatory.

Tertiary Peritonitis

Tertiary peritonitis is defined by the appearance of peritonitis following the failure of one or more surgical procedures undertaken to control an intra-abdominal focus of infection. It is characterized by the presence of nosocomial polymicrobial flora, such as coagulase-negative *Staphylococcus*, *Candida*, *Enterococcus*, *Pseudomonas*, or *Enterobacter*.

Intra-abdominal Abscesses

Solid-organ abscesses may develop in abdominal viscera, such as liver, spleen, kidneys, pancreas, or uterine adnexa, as well as in the interintestinal, periappendiceal, subhepatic, pelvic, and retroperitoneal spaces. Intra-abdominal abscesses may be caused by community-acquired infections such as those secondary to appendicular infection, or they may be the consequence of complications related to surgical procedures. Pelvic abscesses may present symptoms such as rectal tenesmus and dysuria. A rectal digital examination may be useful when this process is suspected. Physiologic predictors of postoperative abscess in children with perforated appendicitis are age, weight and body mass index (more frequent in older and/or obese children), diarrhea on presentation, and persistence of fever in postoperative period (20). Abdominal ultrasound is useful for the diagnosis and to guide percutaneous drainage of intra-abdominal fluid collections. The CT scan is the best diagnostic tool for intra-abdominal or pelvic infections, and the use of oral and intravenous contrast significantly improves the diagnostic sensitivity during this procedure. A thorough clinical examination of the surgical wounds and drain sites performed by an experienced surgeon, combined with contrast studies through fistulous conduits, may add useful data.

The choice of initial empiric antibiotic therapy depends on the suspicion of a community-acquired or nosocomial infection. No antibiotic scheme has been shown to be superior. A combination of an aminoglycoside (amikacin or gentamicin) or a third- or fourth-generation cephalosporin with an antianaerobic antimicrobial (clindamycin or metronidazole) is the most frequently used regimen for intra-abdominal abscesses (21). Single antibiotic regimens with imipenem, meropenem, or piperacillin-tazobactam have not been shown to be superior and are more expensive. Seven days of treatment are sufficient, provided that an appropriate resolution of the intra-abdominal focus has been achieved.

Adequate source control refers to the surgical removal or drainage of the primary cause. Antibiotic treatment without drainage of the source may be effective only for small abscesses. For a well-circumscribed, accessible abscess that is not loculated, percutaneous drainage is the desired procedure in conjunction with adequate antibiotic treatment. Percutaneous drainage may be the definitive solution, or it may buy time to stabilize the patient before definitive surgery. Interloop abscesses and fluid collections may be recurrent or persistent sources of infections for which antibiotics have poor penetration. These collections are best treated by ultrasound- or CT-guided needle aspiration or with laparotomy. Possible complications related to failure to control the source include local complications, such as abdominal wall infection, suture dehiscence, enteric fistulas, or recurrent or tertiary peritonitis. Systemic complications include recurrent sepsis, septic shock, and multiorgan failure.

Necrotizing Enterocolitis

Necrotizing enterocolitis (NEC) is a common and devastating condition during the neonatal period. The incidence is between 0.3 and 2.4 per 1000 live births in the United States, being more frequent among younger preterm neonates (22). It is characterized by bowel necrosis and multisystem organ failure. NEC usually occurs during the second week of life after the initiation of enteral feeds, and the diagnosis is based on physical examination, laboratory studies, and abdominal radiographies. Over the past four decades, its etiology and physiopathology have been cause of intense investigation and debates (23,24).

Overall, up to 25%–50% of patients with NEC require surgical intervention. Morbidity can be high with many patients needing long-term neurologic and intestinal rehabilitation despite which adverse neurodevelopmental outcomes are frequent (25). Need for significant bowel resection is one of the most severe complications of NEC and is the major cause of short-bowel syndrome in pediatric patients. Mortality is variable and ranges from 20% to 30% among infants that require surgery (26).

Prenatally administered glucocorticoids act as an intestinal maturation factor and can help to prevent NEC. The following risk factors have been associated with NEC: (a) preterm birth, (b) enteral feedings, (c) dysfunctional motility, (d) reduced intestinal blood flow, (e) microbe-induced proinflammatory epithelial signaling, and (f) enteroinvasive microbe infection (27).

A large, multicenter network database from Canada and the United States shows a prevalence of NEC of around 7% among newborns with a birth weight between 500 and 1500 g (28). Despite the advances in knowledge, the rate of cases of NEC has increased during the last decade due to the success of modern neonatal intensive care and the increase in numbers of extremely preterm survivors. NEC is rare in term infants and is usually associated with congenital cardiovascular disease, intestinal atresia (Apple-peel), sepsis, hypotension, premature rupture of membranes, chorioamnionitis, and exchange transfusion. Infants with NEC have a high incidence of nosocomial infections, have a slower growth rate, and have longer intensive care and hospital stays.

There is indirect evidence that inappropriate microbial colonization is a risk factor to develop NEC. There are many reports of institutional and outbreaks; however, the responsible organisms vary between outbreaks. Exposure to antibiotics may not only delay beneficial colonization by normal gastrointestinal flora but also promote development of pathogenic germs. The possible roles of probiotic and prebiotic agents are currently being evaluated without a clear demonstration of their benefit.

The diagnostic suspicion is basically clinical. Pediatric surgeons must be involved as soon as NEC is suspected to participate in the follow-up and decision making. Characteristic clinical signs of NEC are feeding intolerance, abdominal distention, tenderness, and sometimes gross occult blood in stools. The abdominal wall can present with reddish or bluish discoloration and is painful at palpation. The NG tube may retrieve variable volumes of gastric and later bilious residuals. General clinical signs include temperature instability, alterations in the glucose levels, lethargy, apnea, bradycardia, or hypotension.

Once NEC is suspected, radiological and laboratory tests must be done. Anteroposterior and left decubitus x-ray serial exams (every 6 hours) allow assessment of the progress and severity of the disease. Abdominal radiographic views can show irregular gas distribution with intestinal distension, pneumoperitoneum (**Fig. 101.6**), pneumatosis, portal venous gas (**Fig. 101.7**), or a fixed loop. The presence of gas in the portal venous tree is thought to be due to the passage of gas from the bowel wall in patients with pneumatosis and it is considered a bad prognostic data. A fixed-loop pattern in serial x-ray tests plus an erythematous (**Fig. 101.8**) and painful abdominal wall is pathognomonic of gut necrosis. Ultrasonography allows detection of the site of a blocked perforation by the presence of an intestinal mass.

Laboratory studies include examination of the full blood count, acid–base status, lactic acid level, electrolytes, glucose,

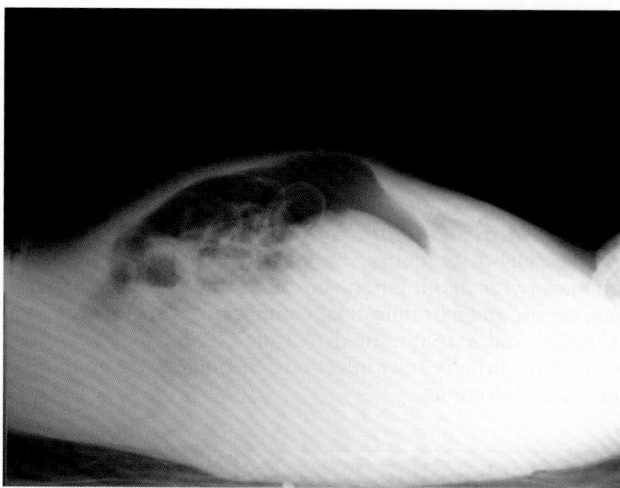

FIGURE 101.6. Pneumoperitoneum.

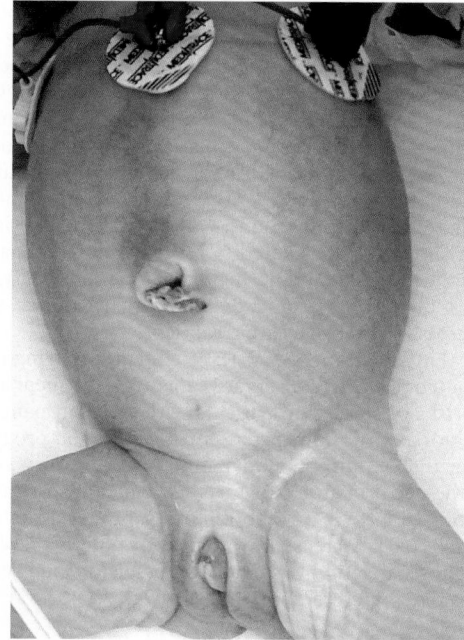

FIGURE 101.8. Abdominal distention and local erythema in a newborn with NEC.

reactive protein C, procalcitonin, and blood cultures. There is no specific laboratory study that confirms NEC diagnosis.

Medical treatment consists of gut rest, antibiotic therapy against enteropathogenic bacteria and clinical stabilization of the septic syndrome including hemodynamic support, respiratory assistance, and correction of hematologic, hydroelectrolytic, and metabolic alterations. Gastric decompression with orogastric tube is mandatory to reduce contents of swallowed air and minimize gut distention. Discontinuation of enteral feeds is usually indicated for ~7–10 days. Total parenteral nutrition should be used until enteral alimentation can deliver adequate amount of calories.

Broad-spectrum antibiotics should be started in all patients; if positive blood cultures are obtained, treatment should be modified according to antibiotic sensibility. Transfusions are often necessary to maintain hemoglobin and platelet counts, which are frequently altered in NEC.

Up to 50% of these patients need surgery. Surgical priorities are control of the sepsis by removal of necrotic bowel and preservation of as much intestine as possible to avoid short-bowel syndrome. Clinical deterioration and/or x-ray data of gut perforation are the most important indications for surgery. In many situations, however, defining the best moment for surgery can be difficult. There has been discussion regarding whether peritoneal drainage is a better option than laparotomy as surgical approach. The most recent evidence suggests that surgery is the best option. A meta-analysis showed a 50% increase in mortality with peritoneal drainage compared to laparotomy. *Recommendation A (+) (29).*

Neutropenic Enterocolitis and Typhlitis

Typhlitis, also known as neutropenic enterocolitis, is an acute life-threatening abdominal condition characterized by transmural necrotizing inflammation of the cecum with possible extension to the terminal portion of the ileum and the ascending colon. It occurs most frequently in children receiving chemotherapy for lymphomas, leukemias, and solid tumors or after conditioning for bone marrow transplantation, but it can also present in children receiving immunosuppressive therapy for solid-organ transplants and children with acquired immunodeficiency syndrome.

The most frequent symptoms are abdominal pain and fever, but other symptoms such as nausea, vomiting, and diarrhea are frequently present. Pain may be localized in the right iliac fossa or may be diffuse with peritoneal reaction appearing between 10 and 14 days after chemotherapy. Presence of abdominal distension or peritoneal reaction is associated with more severe disease. Neutropenia (absolute neutrophil count <500 cells/μL) is found in most of the patients; however, it may not be present in all of the cases (30). The diagnosis is confirmed by an ultrasound or CT scan, which characteristically shows thickening of the walls of the cecum or other involved areas. Other findings may include mucosal edema, fat or mesenteric infiltration, pneumatosis, hepatic portal venous gas, and free cavity fluid.

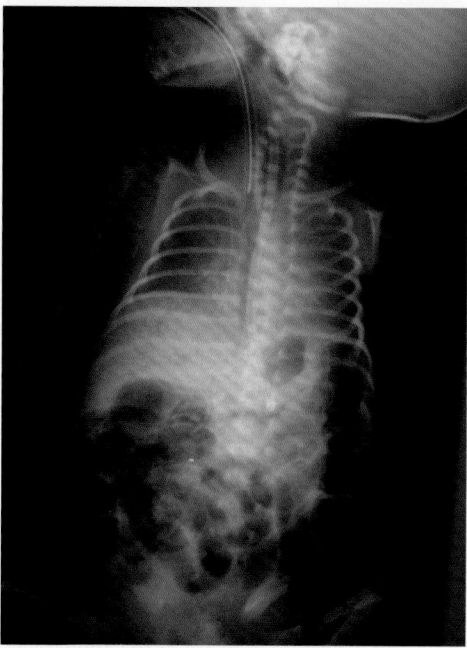

FIGURE 101.7. Portal venous gas in patient with NEC.

Treatment is based on the administration of broad-spectrum antibiotics and intestinal rest while maintaining a close observation. Parenteral nutrition should be given during the acute phase of the disease until enteral feeds can be started. Owing to intestinal paralysis with gastric fluid retention, placement of an NG tube is usually necessary. Platelets and red blood cells should be replaced as needed, and recombinant granulocyte colony-stimulating factor should be administered for normalization of the neutrophil count. Appropriate analgesia with morphine should be considered to relieve abdominal pain. Severe complications, including hemodynamic instability, acute respiratory distress syndrome, or other organ failures, should receive the usual intensive care treatment.

Surgical intervention is now less frequent following reports of good outcomes with conservative medical treatment and the inherent risks of surgery in patients with frequent pancytopenia. Signs of perforation, persistent bleeding, or progressive worsening that require hemodynamic or respiratory support indicate the need of surgery. Mortality, which historically has been high, is improving; some reports show levels as low as of 0%–10% (31). Increased awareness of typhlitis leading to early diagnosis, together with the progress in management, has probably contributed to improved survival.

Fistulae

Fistulae are abnormal epithelialized ducts that connect two hollow viscera or a hollow viscus with the skin. The intestinal wall defects may be partial (lateral fistulae) or complete (terminal fistulae). The presence of a distal obstruction transforms a lateral fistula into a functional terminal fistula. Fistulae may occur in the context of an intestinal operation and in the presence of an inflammatory process. During the development of a fistula and before it finally connects to the skin or to another viscus, the conduit may act as an occult source of infection. Fistulae may develop with an abscess in their tract, or they may develop without intraperitoneal collections. Fistulae tracts must be studied to find their origin, even though the clinical picture and recent history may suggest it. The best way to study the tract is by injecting water-soluble contrast material through a catheter that is introduced into the external opening and obtaining a sinogram (fistulogram). Very short fistulae that have a direct contact between the gastrointestinal tract and the skin are the most difficult to close (32). Abdominal and pelvic CT scans are important diagnostic tools for studying fistulae, especially because they may be associated with intra-abdominal infectious foci.

In high-output fistulae, close measurement and replacement of fluid losses and monitoring of electrolytes are essential to avoid severe derangements. The factors that influence spontaneous closure include the child's nutritional status, the absence of a distal obstruction, and the absence of abscess cavities within the tract. General therapy includes antibiotic treatment until the resolution of the intra-abdominal infection, initial intestinal rest, care of the skin surrounding the external ostium, and parenteral nutritional support. Low-output distal fistulae may be adequately controlled with enteral feeding with elemental diets or partially digested formulae. Fifty percent of enterocutaneous fistulae close spontaneously within the first month. Octreotide or somatostatin can be used to decrease fistula output but its benefit is not clear. When spontaneous closure is not achieved, surgical correction is indicated.

Enteritis

Enteritis is an intestinal infection that may mimic an acute abdomen. Intestinal infections may be caused by a wide variety of enteropathogenic organisms, including bacteria, viruses, and parasites. They often present with fever and gastrointestinal symptoms such as vomiting, bloody diarrhea, severe abdominal pain, and tenesmus. The process may progress to submucosal compromise and complete involvement of the intestinal wall, producing ileus, systemic bacterial migration, and sepsis. The finding of leukocytes in the feces indicates the presence of an invasive or cytotoxin-producing organism, such as *Salmonella*, *Shigella*, *Campylobacter jejuni*, enteroinvasive *E. coli*, *Clostridium difficile*, or *Yersinia enterocolitica*. The specific diagnosis requires culture of the organism and/or immunoassay for toxin. Enteric infections may produce bacteremia, sepsis, and extraintestinal complications such as seizures (*Shigella*) and extraintestinal foci of infection, including osteomyelitis, urinary tract infections, meningitis, peritonitis, or soft tissue infections.

Hemolytic Uremic Syndrome

In previously healthy hosts, the presence of bloody diarrhea caused by the verotoxin-producing *E. coli* 0157 may develop into hemolytic uremic syndrome. In this disease, the classic triad consists of microangiopathic hemolytic anemia, thrombocytopenia, and oliguria and may be associated with severe complications of the gastrointestinal tract (mainly severe ischemic lesions in the colon). This complication frequently raises the dilemma of an acute surgical abdomen, which would complicate the placement of a peritoneal catheter for dialysis in a child with acute renal failure. The ischemic lesions may progress to perforation or total segmentary gangrene. Ischemic colitis as a part of the extrarenal involvement of the diarrhea associated with hemolytic uremic syndrome is a major determinant of morbidity and mortality (33).

Acute Pancreatitis

The International Study Group of Pediatric Pancreatitis defines acute pancreatitis (AP) when two of the following findings are present: (a) abdominal pain compatible with AP, (b) serum amylase and/or lipase values >3 times upper limits of normal, and (c) imaging findings of AP (34).

Inflammation of the pancreas can cause an acute abdomen and life-threatening disease when it is severe or in the presence of local complications, such as necrosis, pseudocyst formation, or pancreatic abscesses. These cases may develop systemic inflammatory manifestations or multiorgan failure. Approximately 30% of pediatric cases have no identifiable cause, and the remainder of cases are either obstructive (e.g., choledochal cysts, pancreatic duct stricture, or stones) or nonobstructive (e.g., trauma, hemorrhage, infection, or medications) in origin. In an important single-center report (35), the identifiable causes of pancreatitis were medication-induced (19.9%), biliary tract disease (12%), trauma (7.6%), transplantation (7.6%), and structural (5.2%). Ma et al. (36) reported the risk factors associated with biliary pancreatitis. They found that Hispanic children had a higher probability to suffer biliary pancreatitis than white or black children. Amylase/lipase values were significantly higher in cases of AP with biliary etiology compared to other causes, and aspartate aminotransferase was an independent predictor.

Hereditary forms of pancreatitis may arise from mutations in the trypsinogen gene and in the cystic fibrosis transmembrane regulator gene. Genetic assays can detect alterations and help to explain some cases of recurrent pancreatitis, previously categorized as idiopathic. Milder inflammations with only abdominal pain and moderate increase of the amylase and lipase level are usually the consequence of viral infections and some systemic diseases.

TABLE 101.7

SEVERE ACUTE PANCREATITIS

Types
  Obstructive (gallstone, choledochal cyst, pancreatic duct
    stricture)
  Nonobstructive (trauma, infection, drugs)
  Hereditary forms or idiopathic

Clinical presentation
  Abdominal pain, vomiting, abdominal distension, and
    guarding
  Systemic inflammatory response syndrome, shock, jaundice,
    ascites, and pleural effusion
  Labs: amylase >300 U/L, lipase >900 U/L

Imaging
  Ultrasound to evaluate obstructive causes and pseudocyst
    control
  CT to confirm diagnosis and evaluation of necrotic areas
  ERCP for suspected or proven lithiasis acute pancreatitis

Treatment
  Fluid resuscitation
  Control of hypocalcemia or hyperglycemia
  Analgesics
  Nasogastric tube
  Nutrition: parenteral (initial) and enteral nutrition (when
    tolerated)
  Evaluation of antibiotic treatment
  Evaluation of percutaneous draining, fine-needle aspiration
    or laparotomy to resolve the complications (pseudocysts,
    necrosis, abscess)

ERCP, endoscopic retrograde cholangiopancreatography.

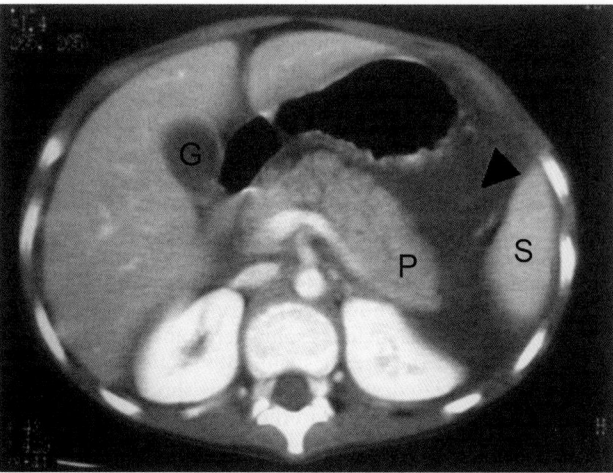

FIGURE 101.9. CT of acute pancreatitis. *P*, inflamed pancreas; *S*, spleen; *G*, gallbladder; *arrow*, free fluid.

Pancreatitis is rare in the previously healthy child. The patient usually presents as acutely ill with nausea, vomiting, and abdominal pain (**Table 101.7**). The pain is usually epigastric and may radiate toward the back. Abdominal distension and muscular guarding are frequent features in children. The child is irritable and may adopt an antalgic position, such as sitting forward with flexed legs or lying in lateral decubitus position. Hemodynamic compromise, fever, jaundice, ascites, hypocalcemia, and pleural effusion may be present. Mortality is high and is linked to the systemic inflammatory response syndrome and multiorgan failure. The diagnosis should be considered in children with acute abdomen and/or systemic inflammatory response syndrome without a clear cause or in the presence of probable etiologic factors (e.g., lithiasic pathology). The diagnosis is confirmed by increased serum amylase and lipase levels of at least three times the normal value (>300 and 900 U/L, respectively). Even though the lipase elevation is sensitive and more specific in adults, this has not been validated in pediatric patients. The enzyme levels diminish progressively after the first days; therefore, the time elapsed since the beginning of symptoms will affect the sensitivity of enzyme concentrations as a diagnostic method. Pancreatic enzymes may also be elevated in other situations, including perforated gastroduodenal ulcers, intestinal perforation or occlusion, peritonitis, acidosis, and renal failure.

Ultrasound and CT scan are the diagnostic studies used to confirm the diagnosis, evaluate the etiology, and search for complications of pancreatitis (**Fig. 101.9**). Ultrasound is helpful in locating gall stones in the pancreatic or common bile ducts. However, as its sensitivity is lower during AP, it is convenient to repeat the ultrasound during the course of the disease. When the pancreas can be visualized, the structural characteristics and the findings in the adjacent tissues contribute to the diagnosis and follow-up. Possible findings include increased size, peripancreatic fluid collections, structural heterogeneity, and abscesses. In 20% of pediatric cases, the initial ultrasound is normal. The plain abdominal x-ray film may reveal indirect signs, such as sentinel loop, ileus, blurring of the psoas, transverse colon dilation, or pancreatic calcification. The CT scan is the most useful study to confirm the diagnosis and to exclude other causes of acute abdomen. The use of contrast allows the identification of necrotic areas. When contrast cannot be used, MRI is an alternative. MR cholangiopancreatography and endoscopic ultrasonography have been incorporated recently as diagnostic tools in pediatric care. Endoscopic retrograde cholangiopancreatography has been accepted as an essential method for the evaluation of patients with recurrent pancreatitis and in selected case of AP or choledocholithiasis (37).

Management includes early fluid resuscitation, hemodynamic stabilization, and oxygen supplementation. An adequate fluid and electrolyte balance should be maintained (38). NG tube insertion is necessary to relieve symptoms, especially in patients with gastric atony. Patients should receive parenteral nutrition while enteral feedings are being withheld. Analgesics are necessary for pain control, but opioids should be used with caution because of possible biliary spasm. Hypocalcemia and hyperglycemia may require treatment with calcium supplementation and insulin infusion, respectively. Gastric acid secretions should be suppressed using antacids.

The data on the use of prophylactic antibiotics are contradictory in adults (39). No clear evidence exists to support prophylactic antibiotic treatment in preventing infection of the necrotic areas. However, infection of these necrotic areas is the most severe local complication and is associated with high mortality. When the area of necrosis exceeds 30% of the parenchyma, the risk of infection is increased. Antibiotic treatment may be considered in this group and continued for 1–2 weeks. *A precise recommendation cannot be made due to the contradictory evidence; however, we favor the use of prophylactic antibiotics in this setting.*

Enteral feeding can be started once the symptoms subside and the levels of pancreatic enzymes decrease; however, ~20% of patients will not tolerate feeding. The effects of feeding should be monitored by clinical examination and serial serum enzyme levels. A meta-analysis that compared parenteral with enteral nutrition in adult patients with AP described a significantly lower risk of infection (relative risk [RR], 0.45; 95% confidence interval [CI], 0.26–0.78), reduced need for surgery to control pancreatitis (RR, 0.48; 95% CI, 0.22–0.1), and reduced length of hospital stay (mean reduction, 2.9 days; 95% CI, 1.6–4.3 days) in the enteral group (40). However, no differences were found in mortality or noninfectious complications. Enteral nutrition should be introduced early and replace parenteral nutrition as soon as the enteral tolerance is adequate. *Recommendation: Grade A (−).*

Endoscopic retrograde cholangiopancreatography should be performed in patients with suspected or proven lithiasic AP, or when AP coexists with cholangitis, jaundice, or dilation of the common bile duct. It is advisable to perform this procedure within the first 72 hours after the onset of symptoms. The endoscopic procedure includes sphincterotomy, the extraction of gallstones, and the use of stents (38). Patients with mild pancreatitis associated with cholelithiasis should have cholecystectomy performed as part of their treatment.

One of the most frequent complications during the course of the disease is the formation of pseudocysts, named for the capsule that is formed by granulation tissue without an epithelial layer. These are diagnosed by ultrasound studies, are usually asymptomatic, and resolve spontaneously. The term *pseudocyst* is used for the collections that persist for >4 weeks after the initiation of the disease. When pseudocysts are associated with persistent or recurrent vomiting, pain, ileus, and elevated enzymes, or they jeopardize adjacent structures, a surgeon should be consulted and percutaneous drainage or laparotomy should be considered. Local infection should be suspected in the presence of fever, leukocytosis, pain, or abdominal guarding. CT scan is useful during follow-up and to guide invasive draining procedures.

In the presence of signs of sepsis and tomographic demonstration of pancreatic or peripancreatic necrosis, a fine-needle aspiration should be performed to obtain material for culture to confirm or exclude the diagnosis of infected necrotic tissue. If the diagnosis is confirmed, surgical drainage or interventional radiology should be considered. If symptoms persist for >7 days, if necrotic area is >30%, or if any necrotic area exists in association with sepsis, cultures should be obtained through guided, fine-needle aspiration. Patients with infected necrosis will require surgical debridement or percutaneous drainage of all of the cavities that contain necrotic material. Surgery is recommended after 2 weeks of disease onset. Patients with noninfected necrosis can usually be managed without surgical treatment (38). The mortality from AP in children is significantly lower than in adults; however, in severe disease, it can be as high as 10%.

Inflammatory Bowel Disease

Inflammatory bowel disease is a chronic condition that includes two important different entities, ulcerative colitis (UC) and CD. Clinical manifestations include abdominal pain, diarrhea, vomiting, lethargy, dehydration, weight loss, anemia, hypoalbuminemia, or signs of systemic toxicity in some cases. Manifestations of severe abdominal disease are acute bloody diarrhea, acute ileitis, and acute abdomen. Fistulas, abscesses, perforations, and intestinal obstruction are possible causes of acute abdomen in CD, whereas UC can present with toxic dilatation of the colon, potentially resulting in toxic megacolon with high risk of perforation or severe bleeding. These complications can happen at different stages of the disease including at initial presentation. Initial management should be aimed at achieving clinical stability. Correction of electrolyte abnormalities, volume replacement, and treatment of septic complications are essential. Imaging studies contribute to making the initial diagnosis or evaluating abdominal complications. Abdominal CT scan and MRI may help to identify transmural lesions and bowel dilations and to exclude strictures. Endoscopy

shows patchy lesions and granulomas and is used for initial diagnosis. Biopsies of the lesions should be obtained to confirm the diagnosis.

Once initial stabilization has been obtained, specific steroid treatment should be started. Alternative immunosuppressive agents can be considered as rescue therapy. Rescue therapies should not delay surgical treatment when needed.

Gastrointestinal hemorrhage can be a severe complication. Although in some cases it can stop spontaneously, in others, persistent or massive hemorrhage needs aggressive management. Intra-abdominal abscesses are usually localized in the terminal ileum and can be diagnosed with abdominal ultrasound or CT scan. Percutaneous drainage in combination with antibiotic treatment is frequently effective. In cases of ineffective drainage, surgical treatment should be used. Bowel obstruction is most frequent in ileal CD. Obstruction is usually not complete and improves with medical treatment that includes enteral rest, gastric drainage, adequate fluid reposition, and frequent radiologic evaluation. If obstruction is complete, surgical treatment is indicated. Toxic megacolon is described below.

Pelvic Inflammatory Disease

Pelvic inflammatory disease (PID) is an infection of the upper genital tract that most frequently involves the endometrium and fallopian tubes. In the pediatric population, it can be the cause of acute lower abdominal pain in sexually active female adolescents. It is secondary to the ascension of microorganisms from the lower genital tract into the upper genital tract. The clinical presentation is variable and the most frequent symptoms in mild disease are dyspareunia (pain during sexual activity), lower abdominal pain, and vaginal discharge. Patients with severe PID are ill-appearing and often have intense pain, fever, or vomiting. Laboratory findings include elevated erythrocyte sedimentation rate and/or leukocytosis. Abdominal complications include tubo-ovarian abscess, ectopic pregnancy, and chronic pain.

As diagnosis of PID can be difficult, the following diagnostic criteria are frequently used: one or more findings of cervical motion tenderness, uterine tenderness, or adnexal tenderness on pelvic examination; and one or more additional findings of oral temperature higher than 38°C, abnormal cervical or vaginal mucopurulent discharge, presence of abundant numbers of white blood cells on saline microscopy of vaginal fluid, or laboratory documentation of cervical infection with *N. gonorrhoeae* or *C. trachomatis* (41). Treatment objectives are elimination of the infection and prevention of long-term sequelae. Parenteral antibiotic recommendations include cefoxitin, 2 g IV every 6 hours, plus doxycycline, 100 mg IV every 12 hours, or clindamycin, 900 mg IV every 8 hours, plus gentamicin, 2 mg/kg/dose IV every 8 hours.

ABDOMINAL PATHOLOGY OF THE CRITICAL PATIENT

A dysfunction of the gastrointestinal tract has severe consequences for the critically ill child due to both its negative effect on nutrition and the complications related to bacterial overgrowth and possible bacterial translocation. The gastrointestinal and abdominal complications that can affect a critically ill child include gastrointestinal hemorrhage, ileus, acute cholecystitis, ischemic colitis, pseudomembranous colitis, and toxic megacolon due to *C. difficile* or other bacterial infections, pancreatitis, and abdominal compartment syndrome (Table 101.1).

Ileus

Ileus is defined as intestinal dysmotility in the absence of a mechanical obstruction. Signs and symptoms include diminished or absent bowel sounds, failure to pass stools or flatus, abdominal distension, vomiting or increased drainage through the NG tube, and increased gastric residual volume during enteral feeds. Severe consequences of ileus can include ischemia, perforation, or compartment syndrome. The three types of ileus are adynamic, spastic, and ischemic. The latter is observed in hemodynamically unstable patients or in patients with nonocclusive mesenteric ischemia. Increased air in the small bowel, intestinal distension, or air-fluid levels are radiographic signs suggestive of ileus, but they do not allow for differentiation of a functional ileus from a mechanical obstruction. The abdominal CT has a high sensitivity and specificity to differentiate ileus from mechanical obstruction (10). The causes of ileus are multiple in the critically ill child, the most frequent being intestinal manipulation during abdominal surgery. The ileus may extend from 3 to 5 days after a major intra-abdominal surgery; the small bowel recovers its motility within the first 24 hours, whereas the stomach and colon take longer. Severe sepsis can cause ileus by means of diminishing visceral muscle contractility.

The presence of ileus predisposes to the following problems: risk of vomiting and aspiration pneumonia, intestinal ischemia, fluid and electrolyte imbalances, sepsis, and difficulty in reestablishing nutrition. Decrease in intestinal transit, which results in intraluminal bacterial multiplication, may be a cause of sepsis that begins a cycle that leads to recurrent and severe sepsis and results in multiorgan failure. Narcotic administration is another contributing factor for ileus. Narcotics act by stimulating μ-opioid receptors that inhibit peristalsis and diminish visceral smooth muscle tone. The decrease in analgesia seen with opioid tolerance does not correlate with decreased gastrointestinal effects; therefore, higher doses worsen constipation. Severe hypokalemia, exogenous catecholamines, general anesthetics, and a diversity of medicines, such as benzodiazepines, calcium-channel blocking agents, and anticholinergics, may be involved in the development of ileus.

The prevention of ileus includes adequate fluid resuscitation, a rational use of vasopressors, timely weaning of opioids, and the institution of early enteral feeding. Nutrients help to maintain intestinal mucosa trophism and motility. The advantages of early nutrition in the critically ill child are well known and the absence of bowel sound is not a contraindication to enteral feeding. In a systematic review of adults that compared early postoperative feeding with initial fasting, a decrease in the length of stay and a reduction in the risk of infection were observed in the former (42). *Recommendation: Grade A.*

The primary treatment for ileus is gastric decompression with an NG tube, which reduces the risk of vomiting and aspiration pneumonia. Data on the pharmacologic management of ileus in children are scarce. The use of promotility drugs should be undertaken with caution and only after ruling out surgical and other causes of an acute abdomen.

Acute Cholecystitis

Acute cholecystitis is less common in children than in adults, but its incidence in the pediatric population appears to be rising, especially among the critically ill. In children, most cholecystitis is acalculous and frequently related to dehydration, certain infections, or systemic diseases, such as leptospirosis or Kawasaki disease (43). Calculous cholecystitis may present in premature infants, hemolytic diseases, or cystic fibrosis, or it may be associated with total parenteral nutrition irrespective of the underlying clinical disease. Calculous or acalculous cholecystitis is a known complication during the postoperative course of diverse surgical procedures, including cardiovascular, orthopedic, or general surgery. It may also be observed in patients who are admitted to the PICU due to multiple trauma or severe burns. It is one of the causes to be ruled out in the septic patient suspected of having an intra-abdominal infection.

The classic clinical presentation of cholecystitis, which consists of right upper-quadrant pain, fever, and jaundice (Charcot triad), has a low sensitivity and specificity in critically ill patients (44). The laboratory findings are nonspecific and may include leukocytosis, as well as elevated serum levels of bilirubin, γ-glutamyl transpeptidase, and other liver enzymes (ALT, AST). Ultrasound is the most useful diagnostic test; compatible findings include thickening of the gallbladder wall and the presence of pericholecystic fluid. Other less frequent signs are the double wall (edema of the gallbladder wall), the halo sign (intramural gas), and the presence of gallbladder distension. The absence of gallstones does not exclude the diagnosis.

Initial treatment of acute cholecystitis consists of supportive care and the administration of antibiotics that are effective against gram-negative strains, enterococcus, and anaerobes. Ultrasound- or CT-guided percutaneous drainage of the gallbladder is the recommended treatment in adults, especially when they are clinically unstable. The obtained material should be cultured for guidance of antibiotic treatment in accordance with bacterial sensitivities. However, in 50% of cases, the culture may be negative. Cholecystectomy is indicated when the process cannot be resolved by means of percutaneous cholecystostomy or when this procedure is contraindicated. Urgent cholecystectomy may be necessary during complications such as acute cholangitis or gallstone pancreatitis.

Pseudomembranous Colitis

C. difficile is a gram-positive, anaerobic, spore-forming rod that can be responsible for the development of colitis. The pathogenic strains produce two major exotoxins: A and B. The spores must germinate in the anaerobic environment of the colon before toxin can be released. The annual incidence of *C. difficile* infection among hospitalized children in the United States has increased from 7.2 cases/10,000 hospitalizations in 1997 to 12.8 cases/10,000 hospitalizations in 2006 (45). Manifestations of disease range from mild diarrhea to pseudomembranous colitis, which occurs in 3%–5% of carriers and less frequently toxic megacolon. Severe *C. difficile* infection can be suspected in the presence of fever, rigors, abdominal pain, leukocytosis (>15,000 cells/μL), increase in serum creatinine, endoscopic findings consistent with pseudomembranous colitis, or evidence of colitis in CT scan. Toxic megacolon is discussed separately.

C. difficile usually affects patients who are receiving or have received antibiotics during the previous 3 weeks. The possibility of infection increases, the longer the child stays in the hospital. The diagnosis is confirmed by means of stool culture that grows *C. difficile* and stool assays for toxins using enzyme-linked immunosorbent assay, the cytotoxin test in tissue cultures (to detect toxin B), or polymerase chain reaction assays. Clinicians must be aware of which test the laboratory is using to identify *C. difficile* toxin, because negative tests do not always exclude the presence of toxin.

Treatment with metronidazole (30 mg/kg/d, maximum 500 mg/dose; IV/PO) three times daily is used for mild-to-moderate cases of *C. difficile* infection. Severe infection is treated with vancomycin (10 mg/kg/dose; maximum 500 mg/dose, PO/NG) every 6 hours. In the presence of systemic compromise, ileus or toxic megacolon, oral vancomycin plus the addition of IV metronidazole (every 8 hours) is recommended. Broad-spectrum antibiotics should be stopped or avoided, if possible, to stimulate the recovery of the endogenous flora. In addition to specific antibiotic therapy and fluid and electrolyte replacement, the patient should be isolated, and caregivers should wear gowns and gloves. Strict hand-washing precautions should be in effect for every patient in the PICU, but are reinforced for patients with C. *difficile*.

Toxic Megacolon

Toxic megacolon represents a severe complication of colonic inflammation. It presents as an acute abdomen characterized by colonic dilation with systemic toxicity in patients with underlying inflammatory or infectious diseases. The most frequent etiologies are inflammatory bowel diseases, especially UC and less frequently CD and C. *difficile* infection; however, *Salmonella, Shigella, Yersinia, C. jejuni, E. coli*, cytomegalovirus, or rotavirus among others infections may also be the cause. Patients with UC can develop toxic megacolon even during the initial presentation. Diverse predisposing factors in these patients include treatment interruption, hypokalemia, the use of antidiarrheals, or colonoscopy.

Diagnosis is suspected by the presence of systemic toxicity and imaging studies showing colonic dilatation. Clinical signs of systemic compromise include fever, tachycardia, leukocytosis, dehydration, or electrolyte imbalances. Altered levels of consciousness and hypotension, which are characteristically described in the adult population, seem to be less frequent in children (46). Examination of the abdomen may show distension, tenderness, and reduced bowel sounds or signs of peritonitis that may indicate colonic perforation. The most severe cases can progress to septic shock and multiorgan failure. Radiologic diagnosis of colonic dilatation is critical for the diagnosis. Plain abdominal x-ray shows dilatation of the colon most frequently in the ascending and transverse portions. Fluid-air levels and alteration of the normal haustration can also be evident. CT scan shows colonic dilation, submucosal edema, areas of wall thickening, or areas of wall thinning, and it is useful to detect intra-abdominal complications. Ultrasound may aid in the diagnosis also by demonstrating the colonic dilatation.

Management of toxic megacolon is based on the treatment of the underlying disease, close monitoring, and supportive care of involved organs with circulatory and ventilatory support when necessary. Electrolyte abnormalities that deteriorate the tone of the colon, especially hypokalemia and dehydration, should be corrected. Severe anemia and hypoglycemia need to be corrected. The use of drugs that inhibit colonic movement should be avoided or discontinued as soon as possible. Bowel rest with parenteral nutrition is necessary during the acute phase; however, NG suction has no effect on colonic dilatation and is usually not necessary. Treatment of the underlying disease varies according to the etiology. For UC, steroid therapy should be started rapidly. For refractory UC, other immunosuppressive therapy can be considered as a rescue therapy but without delaying surgical treatment when needed. If an infectious cause is suspected, appropriate antimicrobial treatment should be started. When the cause is not clear, empiric treatment with metronidazole may be considered. The utilization of enteral probiotics that may act by stimulating the immune response is being evaluated.

If there is not a rapid response to medical treatment, surgical resection usually by subtotal colectomy may be necessary. Absolute indications for surgery include clinical deterioration with progression to organ failure, signs of peritonitis or perforation, and uncontrollable bleeding. Mortality due to toxic megacolon can be high, especially when surgery is delayed.

ACUTE ABDOMINAL MANIFESTATION OF SYSTEMIC DISEASES

Some pediatric patients may present with symptoms of an abdominal surgical emergency in the context of systemic diseases. Recognizing these situations may avoid unnecessary surgical interventions and allow an appropriate treatment without delays (Table 101.1). *Diabetic ketoacidosis* may present with abdominal pain, vomiting, a tense abdomen with guarding, and absent bowel sounds, simulating an acute abdomen.

Porphyrias are both hereditary and acquired diseases in which the activity of the enzymes responsible for the heme biosynthesis pathways is partially or completely deficient. *Acute intermittent porphyria* may present with nausea, vomiting, abdominal pain, diarrhea, constipation, or ileus and may occasionally be confused with an acute surgical abdomen. The presence of other neurologic symptoms, such as hypotonia, peripheral neuropathy, or seizures, is suggestive of this diagnosis. The Watson–Schwartz test, which is used as urinary screening to detect porphobilinogen, has high sensitivity but low specificity, and the diagnosis should be confirmed by means of chromatographic measurement. *Rheumatologic diseases* may cause abdominal complications that include ischemic lesions due to mesenteric vascular compromise. The clinical manifestations depend on the caliber of the affected vessels and the degree of obstruction. The most severe cases may result in infarction or gangrene. Other complications include perforations, intussusception, intestinal volvulus, and colonic strictures. Episodes of AP have also been described. *Henoch–Schönlein purpura* is a vasculitis that affects small vessels and is the most frequent cause of nonthrombocytopenic purpura in children. The association of colicky abdominal pain, arthralgia or arthritis, edema in dependent or distensible areas, palpable nonthrombocytopenic purpura, and proteinuria is the basis of the diagnosis. Severe abdominal pain may be the only symptom, and recognizing the diagnosis can avoid unnecessary surgery. The pain is usually colicky and may be accompanied by fecal occult blood or hematemesis. Occasionally, intestinal manifestations may be severe, and such complications as intussusception or intestinal perforation may be present. *Kawasaki disease* was associated with a 4.6% (10 cases) incidence of severe abdominal symptoms at presentation in a series of 219 children (47). In a majority of this subset, the presentation of acute abdomen was not accompanied by sufficient signs for the diagnosis of Kawasaki disease. Two to four days after admission, the characteristic signs appeared: maculopapular rash, conjunctivitis, mucositis, cervical adenitis, and edema of the feet and hands. The most frequent abdominal signs were acute abdominal pain, distension, emesis, jaundice, and hepatomegaly. *Sickle cell disease* is a hereditary illness that presents with chronic hemolytic anemia and recurrent episodes of pain as cardinal manifestations. The episodes of acute pain, previously called *sickle cell crisis*, are based on the occlusion of the bone marrow vascular bed that leads to bone infarction and release of inflammatory mediators. Severe abdominal pain can be one of the clinical manifestations.

FUTURE DIRECTIONS

Our ability to diagnose abdominal emergencies with precision continues to improve with the use of new imaging technologies. However, early diagnosis depends on the clinical skills of the emergency pediatrician, the intensivist, and the pediatric surgeon. On the other hand, rising healthcare costs prompt us to carefully evaluate the benefits of diagnostic studies in relation to their cost efficiency. Minimally invasive surgical techniques and laparoscopy are being used more frequently; however, standard surgical skills to resolve abdominal emergencies are critical. Most cases of acute abdomen in healthy children can be easily resolved with an appropriate diagnosis and timely intervention. When diagnosis is delayed or management is not optimal, the complications can be severe. An updated review of clinical and diagnostic findings in acute appendicitis and intussusception has been included for this purpose. New clinical challenges are emerging as a consequence of improved survival in very low-birth-weight infants and children who undergo complex surgery or solid-organ, bone marrow, or intestinal transplantation; in those with acquired immunodeficiency syndrome; and in those with previously fatal oncologic pathology. Finally, some systemic diseases that may present as an abdominal emergency should be considered among the diagnostic possibilities.

References

1. Jones S, Claridge J. Acute abdomen. In: Townsend JR, Beauchamp D, Evers BM, et al., eds. *Sabiston Textbook of Surgery.* 17th ed. Philadelphia, PA: WB Saunders; 2004:1219–35.

2. Grade of Recommendation, Assessment, Development, and Evaluation (GRADE) Working Group. Grading quality of evidence and strength of recommendations. *BMJ* 2004;328:1490–94.

3. Yen K, Karpas A, Pinkerton HJ, et al. Interexaminer reliability in physical examination of pediatric patients with abdominal pain. *Arch Pediatr Adolesc Med* 2005;159:373–6.

4. Kessler C, Bauer SJ. Utility of the digital rectal examination in the emergency department: A review. *J Emerg Med.* 2012;43:1196–204.

5. Miglioretti DL, Johnson E, Williams A, Greenlee RT et al. The use of computed tomography in pediatrics and the associated radiation exposure and estimated cancer risk. *JAMA Pediatr.* 2013; 167:700–7.

6. Bogusevicius A, Maleckas A, Pundzius J, et al. Prospective randomized trial of computer-aided diagnosis and contrast radiography in acute small bowel obstruction. *Eur J Surg* 2002;168:78–83.

7. Manterola C, Vial M, Moraga J, et al. Analgesia in patients with acute abdominal pain. *Cochrane Database Syst Rev* 2011;CD005660.

8. Ranji SR, Goldman LE, Simel DL, et al. Do opiates affect the clinical evaluation of patients with acute abdominal pain? *JAMA* 2006;296:1764–74.

9. Saito J. Beyond appendicitis: evaluation and surgical treatment of pediatric acute abdominal pain. *Curr Opin Pediatr* 2012;24:357–64.

10. Scaglione M, Romano S, Pinto F, et al. Helical CT diagnosis of small bowel obstruction in the acute clinical setting. *Eur J Radiol* 2004;50:15–22.

11. Bickell N, Federman A, Aufses A. Influence of time on risk of bowel resection in complete small bowel obstruction. *J Am Coll Surg* 2005;201:847–54.

12. Meyer JS, Dangman BC, Buonomo C, et al. Air and liquid contrast agents in the management of intussusception: A controlled, randomized trial. *Radiology* 1993;188:507–11.

13. Curtis JL, Gutierrez IM, Kirk SR, et al. Failure of enema reduction for ileocolic intussusception at a referring hospital does not preclude repeat attempts at a children's hospital. *J Pediatr Surg* 2010;45:1178–81.

14. Bonnard A, Kohaut J, Sieurin A, et al. Gastrografin for uncomplicated adhesive small bowel obstruction in children. *Pediatr Surg Int* 2011;27:1277–81.

15. Frykman PK, Short SS. Hirschsprung-associated enterocolitis: Prevention and therapy. *Semin Pediatr Surg* 2012; 21:328–35.

16. Millar AJ, Rode H, Cywes S. Malrotation and volvulus in infancy and childhood. *Semin Pediatr Surg* 2003;12:229–36.

17. Lin YP, Lee J, Chao HC, et al. Risk factors for intestinal gangrene in children with small-bowel volvulus. *J Pediatr Gastroenterol Nutr* 2011;53:417–22.

18. Thompson AE, Marshall J, Opal S. Intraabdominal infections in infants and children: Descriptions and definitions. *Pediatr Crit Care Med* 2005;6:S30–5.

19. Roehrborn A, Thomas L, Potreck O, et al. The microbiology of postoperative peritonitis. *Clin Infect Dis* 2001;33:1513–19.

20. Fraser JD, Aguayo P, Sharp SW, et al. Physiologic predictors of postoperative abscess in children with perforated appendicitis: Subset analysis from a prospective randomized trial. *Surgery* 2010;147:729–32.

21. Mazuski JE, Sawyer RG, Nathens AB, et al. The Surgical Infection Society guidelines on antimicrobial therapy for intra-abdominal infections: Evidence for the recommendations. *Surg Infect* 2003;3:175–233.

22. Christensen RD, Gordon PV, Besner GE. Can we cut the incidence of necrotizing enterocolitis in half—Today? *Fetal Pediatr Pathol* 2010;29:185–98.

23. Berman L, Moss RL. Necrotizing enterocolitis: An update. *Semin Fetal Neonatal Med* 2011;16:145–50.

24. Neu J, Walker WA. Necrotizing enterocolitis. *N Engl J Med* 2011;364:255–64.

25. Martin CR, Dammann O, Allred EN, et al. Neurodevelopment of extremely preterm infants who had necrotizing enterocolitis with or without late bacteremia. *J Pediatr* 2010;157:751–6.

26. Fitzgibbons SC, Ching Y, Yu D, et al. Mortality of necrotizing enterocolitis expressed by birth weight categories. *J Pediatr Surg* 2009;44:1072–5.

27. Alexander VN, Northrup V, Bizzarro MJ. Antibiotic exposure in the intensive care unit and the risk of necrotizing enterocolitis. *J Pediatr* 2011;159:392–7.

28. Hollman RC, Stoll BJ, Curs AT, et al. Necrotizing enterocolitis hospitalizations among neonates in the United States. *Paediatr Perinat Epidemiol* 2006;20:498–506.

29. Sola JE, Tepas JJ III, Koniaris LG. Peritoneal drainage versus laparotomy for necrotizing enterocolitis and intestinal perforation: A meta-analysis. *J Surg Res* 2010;161:95–100.

30. Rizzatti M, Brandalise SR, de Azevedo AC, et al. Neutropenic enterocolitis in children and the young adults with cancer: Prognostic value of clinical and image findings. *Pediatr Hemato Oncol* 2010;27:462–70.

31. Sundell N, Boström H, Edenholm M, et al. Management of neutropenic enterocolitis in children with cancer. *Acta Paediatr* 2012;101:308–12.

32. West M. Conservative and operative management of gastrointestinal fistulae in the critically ill patient. *Curr Opin Crit Care* 2000;6:143–7.

33. Gallo E, Gianantonio CA. Extrarenal involvement in diarrhoea-associated haemolytic-uraemic syndrome. *Pediatr Nephrol* 1995;9:117–9.

34. Morinville VD, Husain SZ, Bai H, et al. Definitions of pediatric pancreatitis and survey of present clinical practices. *J Pediatr Gastroenterol Nutr* 2012;55:261–5.

35. Lautz TB, Turkel G, Radhakrishnan J, et al. Utility of the computed tomography severity index (Balthazar score) in children with acute pancreatitis. *J Pediatr Surg* 2012;47:1185–91.

36. Ma MH, Bai HX, Park AJ. Risk factors associated with biliary pancreatitis in children *J Pediatr Gastroenterol Nutr* 2012;54:651–6.

37. Otto AK, Neal MD, Slivka AN, et al. An appraisal of endoscopic retrograde cholangiopancreatography (ERCP) for pancreaticobiliary disease in children: Our institutional experience in 231 cases. *Surg Endosc* 2011;25:2536–40.

38. Athens A, Curtis R, Beale R, et al. Management of the critically ill patient with severe acute pancreatitis. *Crit Care Med* 2004;32:2524–36.

39. Isenmann R, Runzi M, Kron M, et al. Prophylactic antibiotic treatment in patients with predicted severe acute pancreatitis: A placebo-controlled, double-blind trial. *Gastroenterology* 2004;126:997–1004.

40. Marik E, Zaloga G. Meta-analysis of parenteral nutrition versus enteral nutrition in patients with acute pancreatitis. *Br Med J* 2004;328(7453):1407.

41. Banikarim C, Chacko MR. Pelvic Inflammatory Disease in Adolescents. *Semin Pediatr Infect Dis* 2005;16:175–180.

42. Lewis SJ, Andersen HK, Thomas S. Early enteral nutrition within 24 h of intestinal surgery versus later commencement of feeding: A systematic review and meta-analysis *J Gastrointest Surg* 2009;13: 569–75.

43. Lobe TE. Cholelithiasis and cholecystitis in children. *Semin Pediatr Surg* 2000;9:170–6.

44. Trowbridge RL, Rutkowski NK, Shojania KG. Does this patient have acute cholecystitis? *JAMA* 2003;289:80–6.

45. Zilberberg MD, Tillotson GS, McDonald C. *Clostridium difficile* infections among hospitalized children, United States, 1997–2006. *Emerg Infect Dis* 2010;16:604–9.

46. Benchimol EI, Turner D, Mann EH, et al. Toxic megacolon in children with inflammatory bowel disease: Clinical and radiographic characteristics. *Am J Gastroenterol* 2008;103: 1524–153.

47. Zulian F, Falcini F, Zancan L, et al. Acute surgical abdomen as presenting manifestation of Kawasaki disease. *J Pediatr* 2003;142:731–5.

CHAPTER 102 ■ DIAGNOSTIC IMAGING OF THE ABDOMEN

SWAPNIL S. BAGADE AND REBECCA HULETT BOWLING

KEY POINTS

❶ The plain abdominal radiograph is the most common imaging technique in the PICU but exposes the child to ionizing radiation.

❷ The plain abdominal radiograph is used to
   a. confirm proper position of catheters and tubes,
   b. diagnose pneumoperitoneum with gas seen between the liver and the abdominal wall in the left lateral decubitus position, and
   c. diagnose bowel obstruction with dilated proximal bowel loops and absent gas in the distal bowel.

❸ Ultrasound is an excellent imaging tool in children because of the absence of ionizing radiation. However, overlying bowel gas may limit visualization.

❹ Ultrasound is the imaging technique of choice for
   a. intussusception ("target sign"; sensitivity and specificity ~100%),

   b. guiding paracentesis in patients with ascites,
   c. detection of hepatic vascular complications after liver transplantation by using Doppler ultrasound, and
   d. focused abdominal sonography for trauma (FAST) to locate free fluid or hemoperitoneum in the upper quadrants and the pelvis.

❺ Computed tomography (CT) requires ionizing radiation and has been associated with increased cancer risk in children.

❻ CT is the imaging modality of choice for evaluation of abdominal injury after blunt trauma in a hemodynamically stable patient.

❶ Plain radiographs are often the initial radiologic investigation used to evaluate a child with abdominal symptoms in the PICU. Other supplemental imaging techniques used include fluoroscopic gastrointestinal procedures with contrast media, ultrasound (US), and advanced cross-sectional imaging with computed tomography (CT) or magnetic resonance imaging (MRI). This chapter discusses these techniques of imaging the abdomen in children, highlighting the role of plain films, with brief discussions of fluoroscopy, US, and advanced imaging of CT and MRI.

PLAIN RADIOGRAPHS

The plain abdominal radiograph is an indispensable tool for both suspected abdominal pathology and the placement of tubes and catheters in children. Since children are more sensitive to radiation and have a longer life expectancy than adults, it is important to minimize radiation exposure. Dose reduction in diagnostic radiology must be achieved without compromising the diagnostic quality of the image. Low-dose techniques using increased tube potential (kVp) between 60 and 70 and a low milliampere-second (mAs) of 2–4 significantly decrease the dose (1).

Various radiographic views for assessment of the abdomen include supine, decubitus, and cross-table (horizontal) lateral. The left lateral decubitus view is preferred over the right lateral decubitus view for detection of a pneumoperitoneum because it is more sensitive (gas is easily seen between liver and abdominal wall). The bowel gas pattern is part of the radiographic assessment. Gas is usually present in the stomach

within 10–15 minutes of birth and fills the large bowel by 12–14 hours (2). The bowel loops should be symmetric and often have a polygonal pattern ("chicken wire") on the supine image (Fig. 102.1). A decubitus film or, less commonly, a cross-table lateral view also shows the bowel gas pattern in another plane (Figs. 102.2 and 102.3). Both views are evaluated for abdominal masses and calcifications. Free intraperitoneal fluid may be seen on a plain film if the amount is sufficient; it will cause the bowel loops to move centrally, with increased opacity in the flanks (Fig. 102.4). The abdominal radiograph may also reveal a lower lobe pneumonia or pleural effusion as the cause of abdominal symptoms. In addition, abnormalities of the soft tissues and bones can be visualized.

❷ Abnormal plain film findings include the following:

Tubes and catheters: An abdominal radiograph is often ordered to assess the position of tubes and catheters after placement. It is important to determine the position of the tubes and catheters to prevent untoward complications associated with their misplacement, kinking, or break in continuity. Common tubes and catheters seen on an abdominal radiograph include umbilical arterial catheter (UAC), umbilical venous catheter (UVC), peripheral and central venous catheters, enteric tube, gastrostomy tube, ventriculoperitoneal shunt tubing, drainage tubes, pH probes, and temperature probes (Figs. 102.5A–C, 102.6A,B, and 102.7).

Bowel obstruction (images can be seen in later sections according to etiology): The typical clinical presentation in a neonate includes poor feeding, vomiting, abdominal distension, and delayed passage of meconium. An increase in postgastric aspirates may also be present. Differentiation between large and small bowel on plain film in the neonate or very young

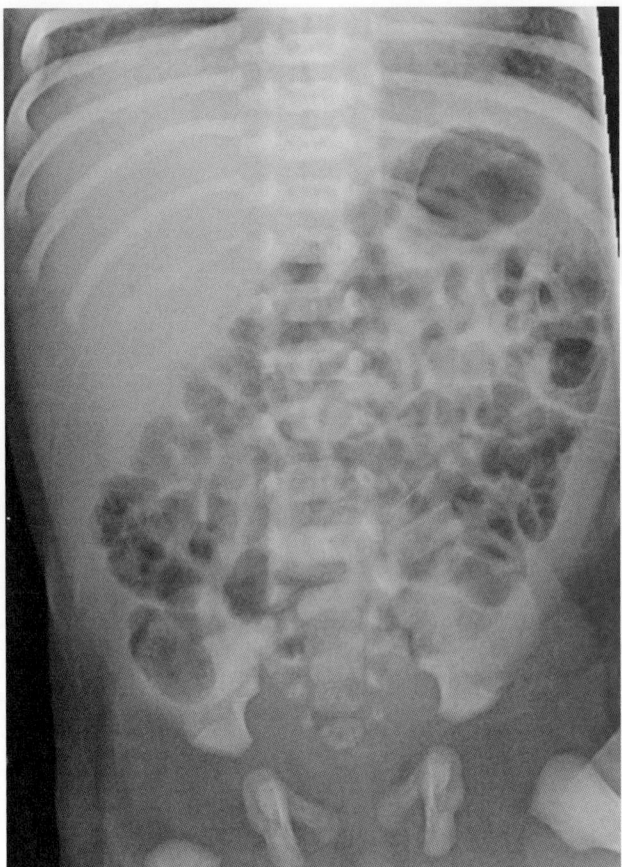

FIGURE 102.1. Normal abdominal bowel gas pattern. Supine AP radiograph of a neonate shows air-filled small-bowel loops in the center and air-filled colon in the periphery of the abdomen. However, in a neonate the differentiation between small and large bowel loops can be difficult. Air-filled stomach is seen in the left upper quadrant. Soft-tissue opacity of the liver occupies the right upper quadrant.

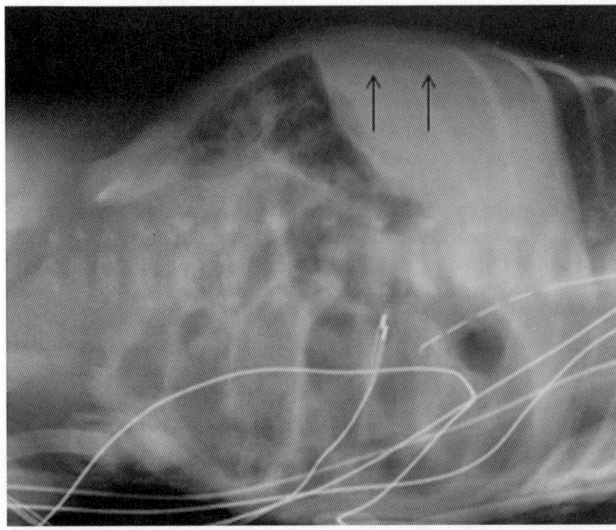

FIGURE 102.2. Left lateral decubitus. Multiple distended loops of bowel are seen. There is minimal free intraperitoneal free air, best seen on the cross-table lateral view as subtle lucency (*arrows*) projecting over the lateral aspect of liver.

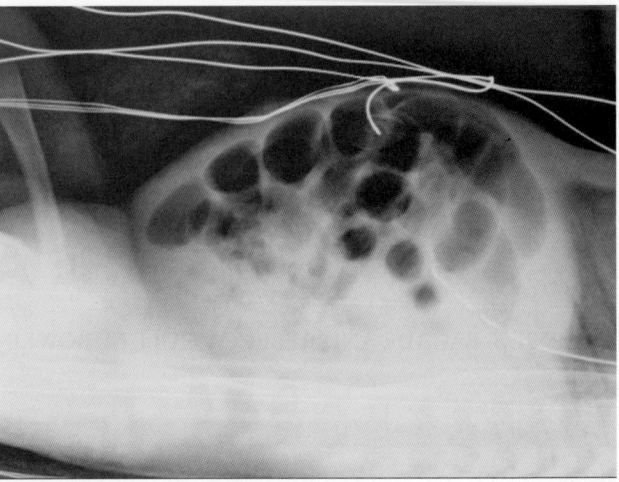

FIGURE 102.3. Supine cross-table lateral (horizontal beam) view. Supine cross-table lateral view in the same patient shows air in the distended bowels. This view is less sensitive for the small amount of free air.

child can be difficult since mucosal landmarks such as valvuli, plicae, and haustra are poorly developed. The radiologic findings in obstruction differ dep ending on the level of pathology. High intestinal obstruction implies obstruction from the stomach to the level of proximal ileum. There may be air

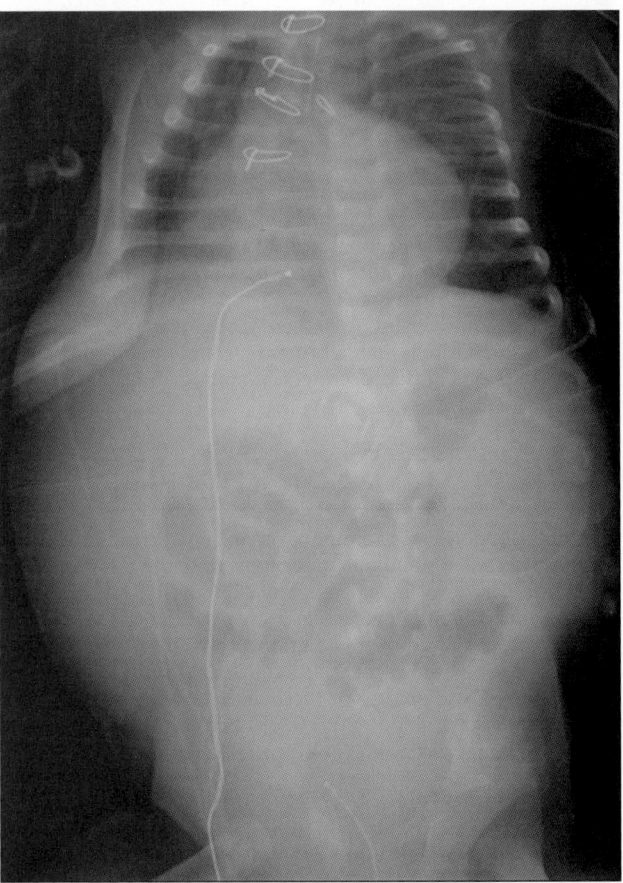

FIGURE 102.4. Ascites. On the abdominal radiograph, there is increased soft-tissue density in the periphery of the abdomen (from the ascitic fluid) with centrally located (floating) bowel loops.

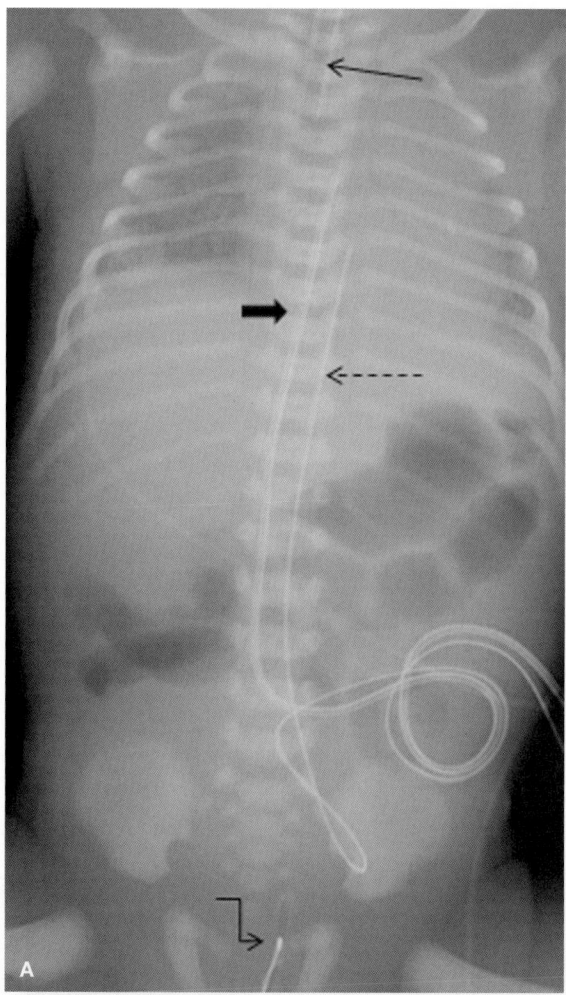

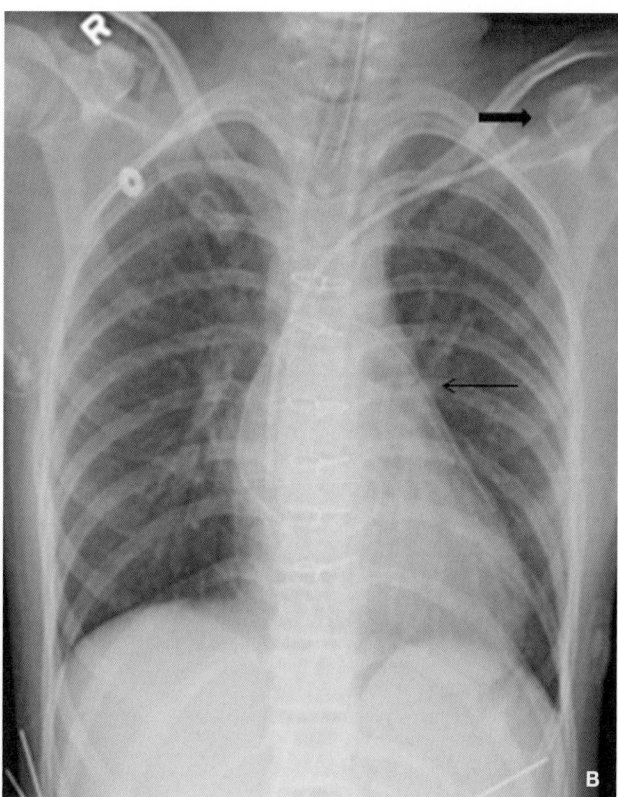

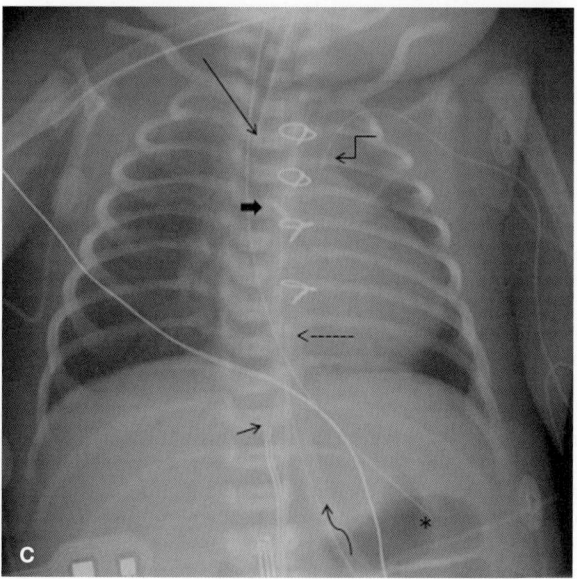

FIGURE 102.5. Positions of tubes and catheters. **A:** UVC terminating in the right atrium (*bold arrow*), while the UAC terminating at the level of T6 (*dotted arrow*). The UVC ideally should be at the level of the diaphragm. The UAC typically turns inferiorly from the umbilicus in the iliac artery and then extends superiorly in the aorta and is expected to terminate at the level varying from T6 to T10. Also seen are the endotracheal tube (*thin arrow*), which should lie at least 1 cm above the carina. A temperature probe is seen in the pelvis (*angled arrow*). **B:** A left-sided subclavian venous catheter (*blocked arrow*) is seen with its tip in the right atrium along with a mediastinal drainage catheter (*thin arrow*). **C:** Frontal view of the chest shows left PICC (peripherally inserted central catheter) line terminating in the left innominate vein region (*angled arrow*), UAC with its tip at the T7–8 level (*dotted arrow*), UVC ending over the left liver lobe (*short arrow*), likely in the ductus venosus. A well-positioned endotracheal tube about 3 cm above the carina (*long arrow*), and a drainage catheter extending in the mediastinum (*curved arrow*), Ductus ligation clip (*blocked arrow*), and the tip of nasogastric tube in the stomach (*asterisk*).

only in the stomach in cases of gastric outlet obstruction such as in pyloric stenosis, antral dyskinesia, or antral web. Two dilated bowel loops (double bubble) are seen with duodenal atresia (DA), annular pancreas, or duodenal web. More dilated bowel loops are present with a jejunal obstruction as in jejunal atresia (3,4). A low bowel obstruction shows multiple loops of dilated bowel in the abdomen. Low intestinal obstruction is seen in conditions involving the ileum, such as meconium ileus and ileal atresia, and pathology of the colon including Hirschsprung disease (HD), meconium plug/small left colon,

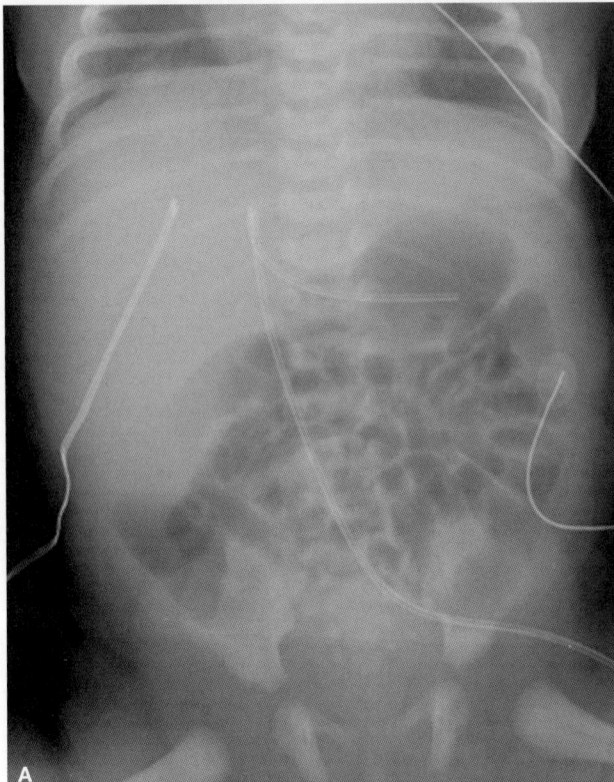 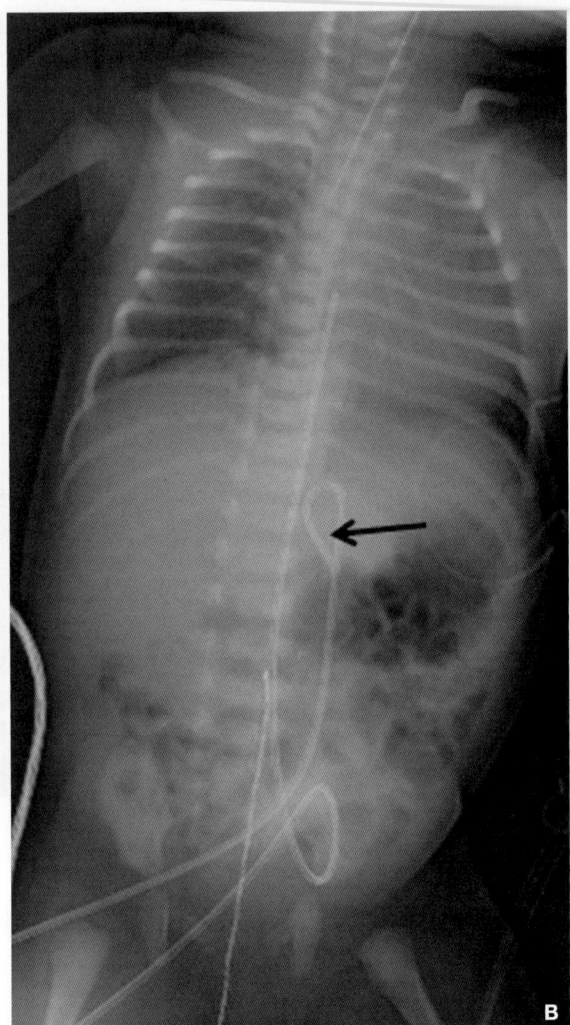

FIGURE 102.6. Malposition of catheter. **A:** The UVC bends to the left to overlie the mid-abdomen and probably extends into the splenic vein. **B:** In another case, the UVC loops near the hepatic hilum, and terminates overlying the left upper quadrant. Ideally, the tip of the UVC is positioned near the inferior cavoatrial junction.

colonic atresia, and imperforate anus. Contrast enemas are helpful in determining whether the colon or distal small bowel is the cause of low intestinal obstruction. In many cases of a high obstruction, the patient is taken to surgery after the plain film is obtained. If there is a concern for malrotation, an upper GI (UGI) study should be performed. In cases of low intestinal obstruction, plain film followed by enema is recommended (5).

Pneumoperitoneum: Causes of pneumoperitoneum in the child include necrotizing enterocolitis (NEC), spontaneous perforation not associated with NEC, ruptured Meckel diverticulum, dissection from pneumomediastinum, gastric perforation (e.g., from a nasogastric tube, mechanical ventilation, indomethacin administration, or child abuse), colonic perforation (possibly secondary to an enema or a rectal thermometer), peritoneal dialysis, paracentesis, recent surgery, and abdominal trauma (6). In older children, perforation in appendicitis, Meckel diverticulitis or ischemic or infective enteritis, and penetrating and blunt abdominal trauma are common causes of pneumoperitoneum (7). Locations of gas in the abdomen include intraluminal, extraluminal, intramural, and intraparenchymal.

Free intraperitoneal air (extraluminal) is seen in nondependent areas (subdiaphragmatic along the liver dome, or along the lateral margin of the liver in a left lateral decubitus view) (**Fig. 102.8A,B**). Portal venous gas can be seen as branching linear lucencies along the periphery of the liver (**Fig. 102.9**). Gas in the biliary tract is more central overlying the liver with a branching tree pattern (8).

Pneumatosis intestinalis: Pneumatosis intestinalis (PI) is when air accumulates within the bowel wall. It is a well-known radiographic finding in cases of NEC, where it portends bowel infarction. Pneumoperitoneum and portal venous gas may be accompanied with PI. PI can also appear in intestinal ischemia, bowel obstruction, graft-versus-host disease, short bowel syndrome, infection with rotavirus, decompensated cardiac disease, and nonischemic colitis (9,10). A more benign occurrence of pneumatosis can be seen in chronic steroid use, immunodeficiency, nutritional deficiencies, bronchopulmonary dysplasia (BPD), or pneumomediastinum. On radiographs, pneumatosis may appear as small linear or bubbly lucencies within the bowel wall (**Fig. 102.10**).

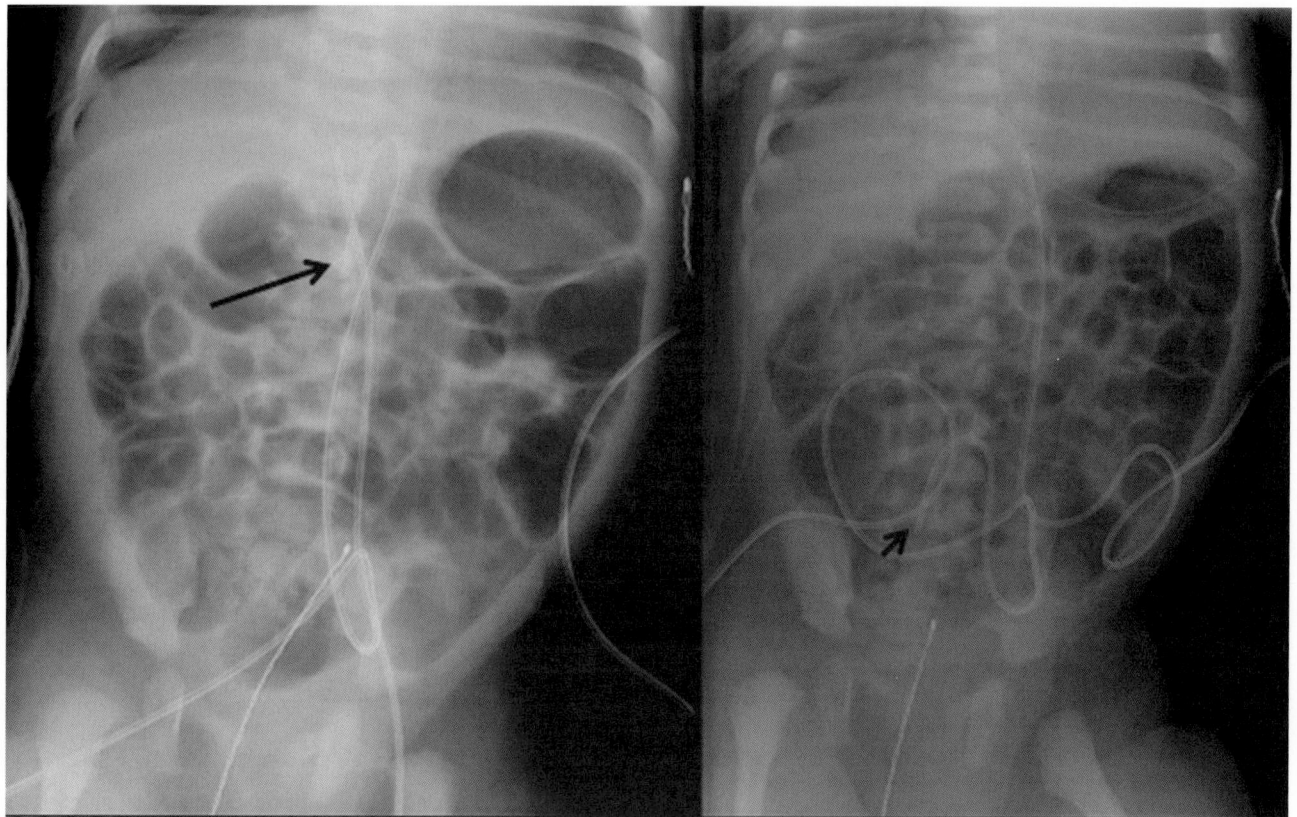

FIGURE 102.7. Neonate with UAC (*arrow*) looped in the aorta overlying the upper abdomen (**left**). Radiograph after attempted repositioning of the UAC (*arrow*) demonstrated the catheter in the right iliac artery (**right**).

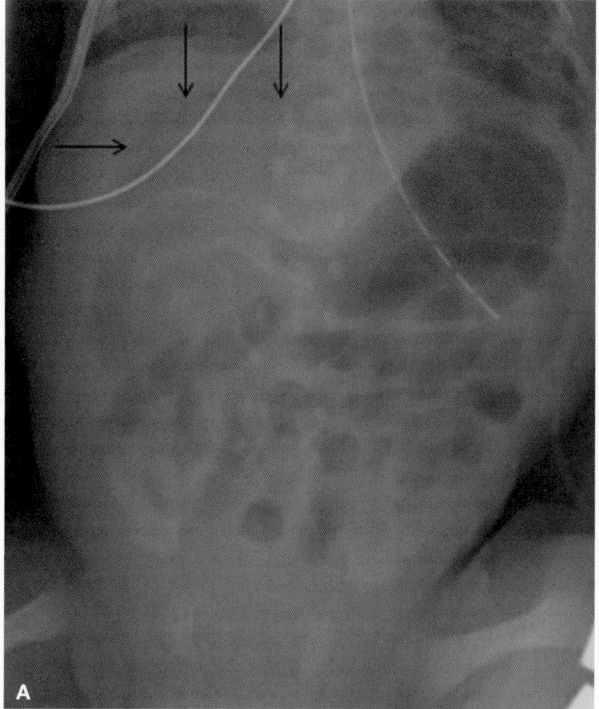

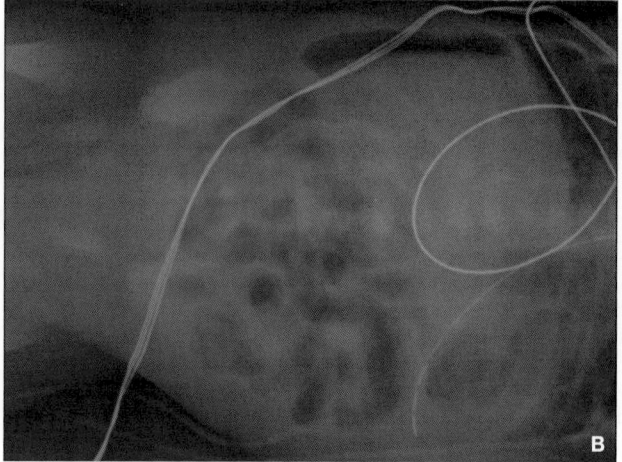

FIGURE 102.8. Pneumoperitoneum. **A:** Large amount of free intra-peritoneal air causing lucency (*arrows*) over upper abdomen and liver. No definite pneumatosis or portal venous gas identified. **B:** Free air is seen bordering the edge of the liver on lateral decubitus view. Patient had bowel perforation.

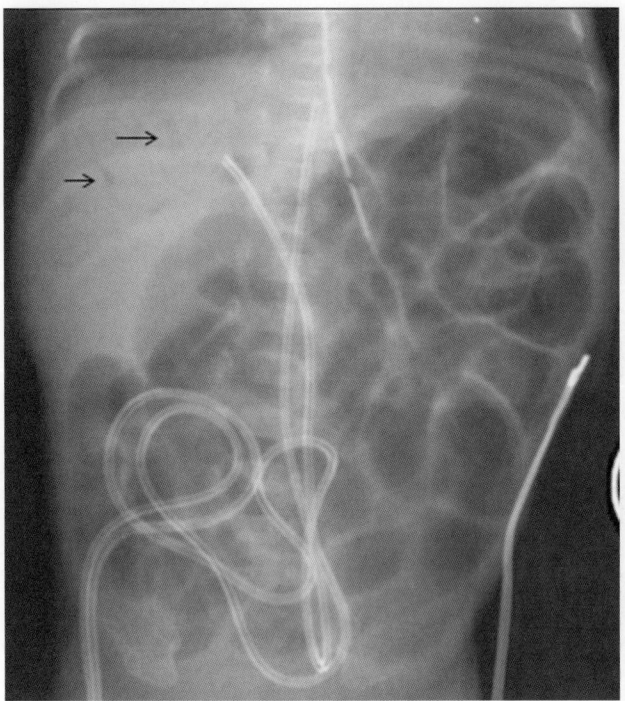

FIGURE 102.9. Portal venous gas. Abdominal radiograph showing branching linear lucencies (*arrows*) along the periphery of the liver owing to portal venous gas.

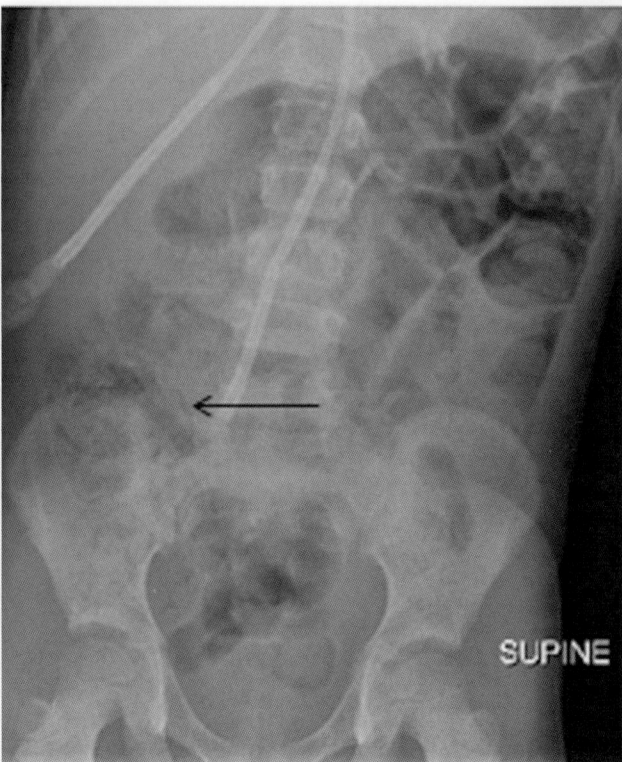

FIGURE 102.10. Pneumatosis intestinalis. Intramural air in the right-sided bowel is seen as streaky lucencies in the right abdomen (*arrow*). This patient was a 7-year-old with inflammation of the ileocecal area who developed PI.

Abdominal masses: The appearance of a soft-tissue opacity or mass is a common finding in a child with abdominal pathology. Plain abdominal radiographs are the initial imaging tests performed in the evaluation of a suspected abdominal mass. The radiographs may help determine the location of the mass, whether there is associated bowel obstruction, and whether calcifications are present. Calcifications are seen in several types of tumors including neuroblastoma and teratoma. Calcifications could also represent stones in the biliary or renal tracts. Sonography is a very useful adjunct study in the workup of abdominal masses.

CONTRAST STUDIES

The UGI series is often modified so that it both answers the clinical question and limits the radiation dose (4,5). An UGI study includes the esophagus, stomach, and duodenum to the duodenojejunal junction and is adequate to assess malrotation. Barium is the most commonly used contrast agent and is excellent for delineating GI tract anatomy. A small-bowel follow-through (SBFT) is used to assess the small bowel beyond the duodenum to the cecum, using serial imaging over several hours (**Fig. 102.11A,B**). Low osmolar, nonionic contrast agents (such as iohexol) are important and have clinical uses, but are much more expensive. These nonionic agents are used when there is concern for possible leak, as in the case of a repaired TE fistula. Hyperosmolar contrast (i.e., gastrografin) can be therapeutic in cases of meconium ileus, meconium plug, and chronic constipation. Water-soluble agents should be used if there is a potential for perforation.

ULTRASOUND

Ultrasonography is a key imaging tool with important applications in diagnosing abdominal pathology in children in the PICU. It is usually the first investigation in a child with a palpable abdominal mass after a plain film. In addition to identifying the solid or cystic nature of the mass, determination of the organ of origin may be assessed. US can be used to evaluate the relationship of the superior mesenteric artery (SMA) with the superior mesenteric vein (SMV) in cases of malrotation (11,12). High-resolution US can be used to evaluate the bowel wall and to detect pneumatosis and portal venous gas. US is the modality of choice to confirm the presence of absence of intussusception. US is also an excellent tool to assess for ascites and can be used to guide paracentesis (**Fig. 102.12**). The lack of ionizing radiation, easy portability, and availability make it an ideal modality for use in children. The disadvantages of US include a potentially limited window in the presence of various catheters, tubes and dressings, interference by overlying bowel gas, as well as operator dependence.

Color and Spectral Doppler

Doppler US is useful in the evaluation of major vessels prior to cardiac shunt surgeries or extracorporeal membrane oxygenation in intensive care patients, and detection of post–liver transplant vascular complications and venous thrombosis. In the case of a post–liver transplant patient, the normal low resistance waveform of the hepatic arterial flow is replaced by a high-resistance waveform with resistive index elevated

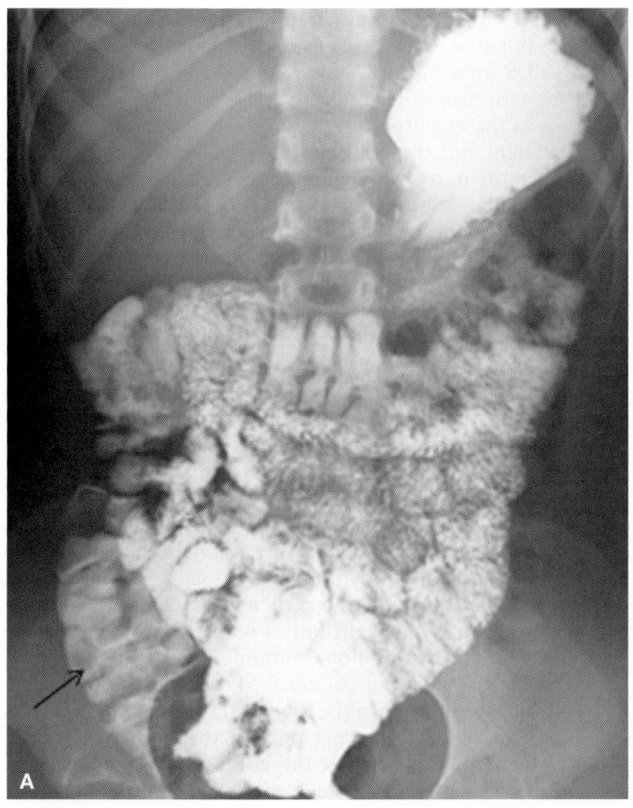

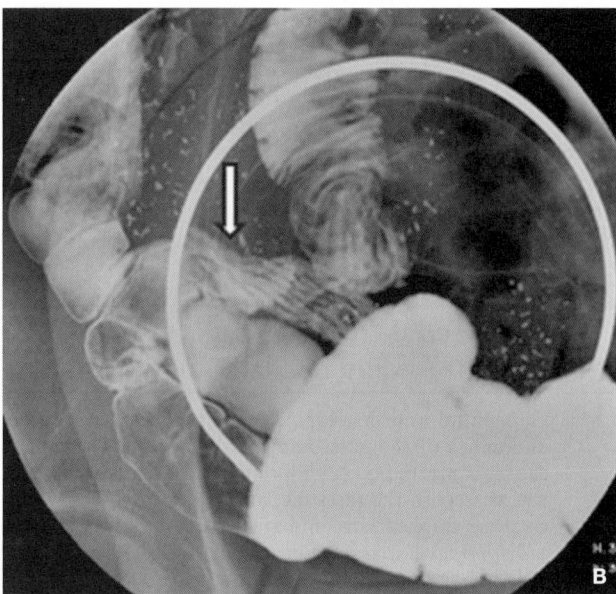

FIGURE 102.11. Small-bowel follow-through study. **A:** Normal appearing bowel loops opacified by barium. An arrow shows the cecum. **B:** Compression views obtained show normal terminal ileum and ileocecal junction (*arrow*).

above 0.8. Hepatic arterial thrombosis is highly suspicious if there is no diastolic and/or systolic hepatic arterial flow. Other vascular complications such as hepatic arterial stenosis, pseudoaneurysm, or venous thrombosis are also detected by Doppler (13). US is the first approach in suspected post–liver transplant complications including hepatic necrosis, perihepatic fluid collections, and biliary obstructions. Doppler also reliably determines the portal vein flow direction and velocity.

COMPUTED TOMOGRAPHY

7 Concern for an increased risk of cancer in children exposed to radiation during CT makes it a less favored imaging modality. CT is performed only when radiographs or US do not diagnose the condition. CT is more useful than US in cases of trauma and to delineate the extent of visceral and intraperitoneal abscesses. The benefits of CT are excellent spatial and contrast resolution; newer scanners are fast enough that the patient may not need sedation. Younger patients receiving IV contrast for the CT often require sedation despite the use of fast scanning techniques because they tend to move when the contrast is administered. When ordering CT imaging, one should consider alternative imaging modalities not involving ionizing radiation such as US or MRI. Research is currently being done to provide CT scanner algorithms that decrease radiation dose while maintaining images of diagnostic quality (14,15). High scanning speed can decrease motion artifacts and at the same time decrease the radiation dose to the patient.

MAGNETIC RESONANCE IMAGING

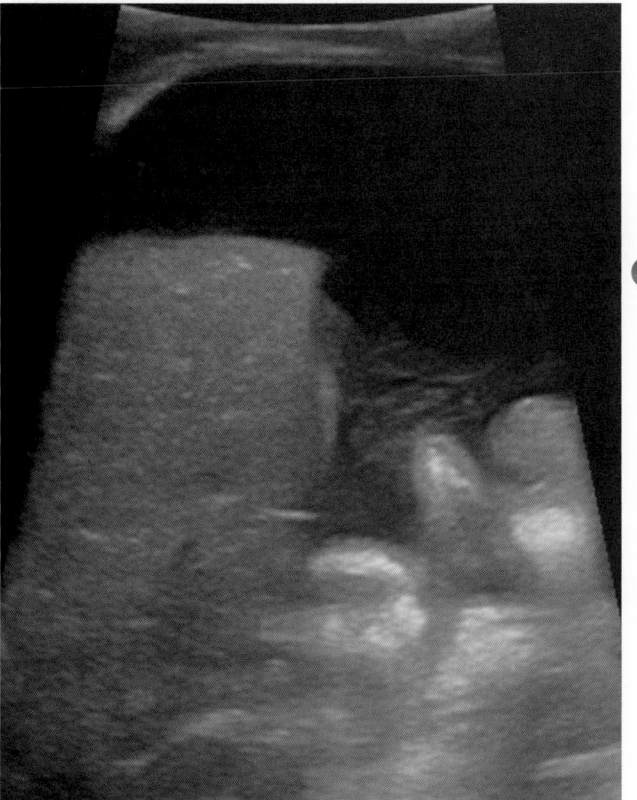

FIGURE 102.12. Ascites. Free abdominal fluid detected on US as anechoic collection under the abdominal wall. Hyperechoic floating bowel loops are seen. Same patient as in **Figure 102.4.**

Improved detail due to better soft-tissue contrast and lack of ionizing radiation make MRI an important problem-solving tool. The limitations for MRI are its cost, availability, and motion artifacts due to long scanning time. Various fast imaging techniques can reduce motion artifact. Techniques such as MR cholangiopancreatography to evaluate biliary and pancreatic abnormalities, MR enterography for gastrointestinal pathologies, and MR urography for evaluation of renal collecting system abnormalities and renal function are available. Diffusion-weighted sequences are used widely for imaging of neoplasms (16).

Differential Diagnosis and Imaging of Abdominal Pathology

1. Congenital and developmental disorders: Congenital anomalies of the gastrointestinal tract are a common cause of morbidity in children. These include obstructive defects in the intestine, anomalies of rotation and fixation, duplications, and anorectal anomalies.
    a. *Esophageal atresia with tracheoesophageal fistula*: Esophageal atresia (EA) is the most common congenital abnormality of the esophagus. It results from failure of division of the primitive foregut (at the fifth gestational week) into two distinct tubes forming the esophagus and the trachea. In almost 90% of cases, EA is associated with a fistula to the posterior wall of the trachea. Proximal EA with distal tracheoesophageal fistula (TEF) is the most common type, seen in 85% of cases. This condition is usually part of the spectrum of **VACTERL** association: Vertebral, (imperforate) Anus, Cardiac, TracheoEsophageal fistula, Renal, and Limb (radial ray). A skeletal survey, cardiac echo, and abdominal US are required investigations in such cases to rule out these associated anomalies. Prenatal US is unlikely to diagnose EA with accuracy; nonspecific findings seen in a few cases are polyhydramnios and nonvisualization of the stomach. A dilated esophageal pouch in the neck with absent abdominal bowel gas may be seen in EA without a distal fistula (**Fig. 102.13A**). The most suggestive finding on the radiograph in a newborn is coiling of the nasogastric tube in the proximal esophagus (**Fig. 102.13B**) (4,5).
    b. *Diaphragmatic (Bochdalek) hernia*: Incomplete closure of the pleuroperitoneal canal results in a posterior lateral diaphragm defect. Newborns with a large hernia beginning early in utero have a poorly developed ipsilateral lung (6). The contralateral lung may also be hypoplastic. Lung volume estimation is performed with serial antenatal USs, and preferably with MRI for prognostic purposes. On the chest radiograph, bowel loops are seen within the thoracic cavity with contralateral mediastinal shift (**Fig. 102.14**). The position of the tip of the nasogastric tube localizes the stomach. The bowel loops ideally are kept deflated in order to decrease intrathoracic pressure until surgical repair is performed.
    c. *Hypertrophic pyloric stenosis*: Hypertrophic pyloric stenosis (HPS) affects 2–3 in 1000 infants and is most common in first-born males. The infant is typically 6 weeks old and presents with vomiting, dehydration, and hypokalemic alkalosis. The caterpillar sign (markedly dilated stomach with exaggerated incisura) may be seen on plain film and represents a distended, peristalsing stomach. US is the imaging gold standard and the method of choice for both diagnosis and exclusion of HPS with a sensitivity and specificity of close to 100% (**Fig. 102.15A,B**)

(17,18). Scanning in the right posterior oblique position is helpful. Prior to vast improvements in US imaging, the UGI was used to evaluate children with projectile vomiting and would show signs such as the mushroom sign, antral shouldering, the string sign, and the double-track sign (redundant mucosa in the narrowed pyloric lumen causing separation of the barium into two channels) (**Fig. 102.15C**). The treatment for HPS is surgical myotomy.
    d. *Congenital gastric/duodenal obstruction*: This includes antral atresia, duodenal atresia, duodenal stenosis (DS), duodenal web (or diaphragm), annular pancreas, and preduodenal portal vein. Duodenal atresia is the most common cause of high intestinal obstruction in a child. Its associations include Down syndrome and congenital heart disease. The diagnostic plain radiograph finding is a double bubble, with air present in the distended stomach and duodenal bulb (**Fig. 102.16A**) (16). The double bubble may also be seen on prenatal US or MRI (**Fig. 102.16B**). The degree of duodenal distension on the radiograph is unreliable in determining the cause of high intestinal obstruction and is therefore unhelpful in ruling out intestinal malrotation with midgut volvulus in an infant with bilious vomiting.
    e. *Malrotation and volvulus*: Malrotation of the intestines results when the intestinal rotation and fixation fails to occur during the 4th through 11th weeks of fetal life. During the course of pregnancy, the bowel rotates to the left of the SMA at the ligament of Treitz. The normal small-bowel mesentery has a broad attachment stretching diagonally from the duodenal-jejunal junction (in the left upper quadrant) to the cecum (in the right lower quadrant). This mesenteric attachment is generally shorter in patients with abnormally rotated bowel, thus creating a high risk of volvulus, which can cause intestinal obstruction and bowel necrosis. Fibrous adhesive (Ladd's) bands are usually present (1,2,4). Plain radiographs often fail to provide convincing evidence of malrotation, but should be obtained as the initial step in order to assess the bowel gas pattern. An upper gastrointestinal contrast series is the gold standard for diagnosis and shows the orientation of the duodenum and position of the duodenal-jejunal junction, which localizes the ligament of Treitz. Radiographic findings of malrotation include displacement of the duodenojejunal junction from its normal left upper quadrant location to the right side and inferiorly with a relative anterior position of the duodenum on the lateral view (**Fig. 102.17A,B**) (5,11). The third part of the duodenum does not cross the midline, and the proximal small bowel is seen on the right side of the abdomen (**Fig. 102.18A,B**). If there is uncertainty about the diagnosis of malrotation on the UGI study, a small-bowel series or enema can be performed to evaluate the position of the cecum. This may demonstrate an abnormally high and medial position of the cecum rather than the normal right lower quadrant location (**Fig. 102.18C**). Manual maneuvers are performed to determine whether the cecum is fixed (normal) or mobile (19). If volvulus occurs, there is spiraling of the small bowel downwards, often to the right of midline (**Fig. 102.18D**). In these cases, demonstration of obstruction of the third or fourth portion of the duodenum is helpful. If bowel necrosis occurs, plain films may show ileus, intestinal pneumatosis, and free intraperitoneal air (in cases of perforation). US is being investigated as a tool for use in

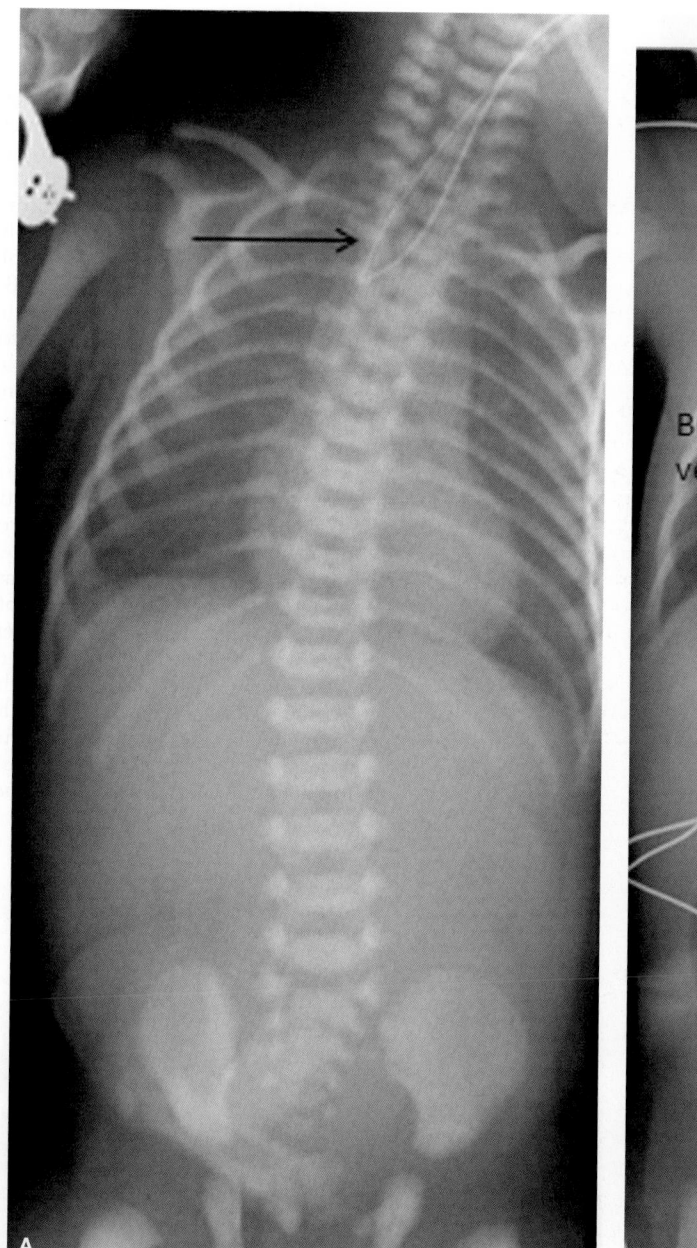
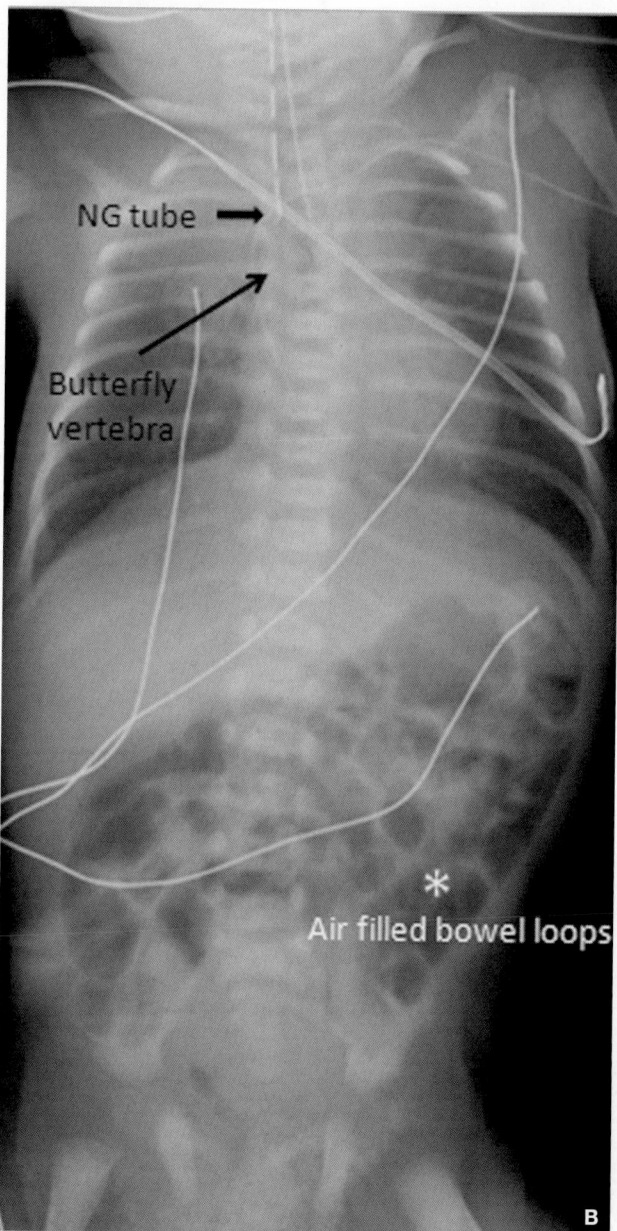

NG tube ➡

Butterfly
vertebra

*
Air filled bowel loops

FIGURE 102.13. Esophageal atresia. **A:** The tip of the nasogastric tube is doubled back on itself in the upper esophagus (*arrow*) and is positioned in the region of the pharynx. Gasless abdomen suggests absence of distal TEF. **B:** Known case of EA with TEF in which the NG tube terminates high in the thorax (*short arrow*). Air-filled bowel loops are seen (*asterisk*). Patient also had 13 ribs with a butterfly T4 vertebra (*long arrow*). EA plus TEF can occur as a part of VACTERL association.

place of the UGI study, but its use for this purpose is currently not widespread and is an area of ongoing research (12). Retroperitoneal position of the third and fourth parts of the duodenum can be confirmed on US. Spiraling of the small bowel around the SMA or twisted vascular pedicle ("whirlpool sign") may be seen on US with or without supplementation by Doppler imaging (12,20).

f. *Jejunal/ileal atresia*: Unlike duodenal atresia, in which there is a failure of recanalization, jejunal/ileal atresia is thought to be due to an intrauterine ischemic event (21,22). The most common presentation of jejunal/ileal atresia is bilious vomiting and abdominal distension. In some cases, failure to pass

meconium is seen. If there is atresia in the proximal small bowel, then meconium is formed by the secretions of the more distal bowel, and the colon is typically normal in caliber. Plain radiographs of the abdomen show several dilated bowel loops, with a paucity of bowel gas distally (**Fig. 102.19A**). In ileal atresia, there is little material entering the colon so that a microcolon (unused colon) is present with or without presence of meconium (**Fig. 102.19B**). Differential diagnosis of ileal atresia includes meconium ileus, small left colon/meconium plug syndrome, or colonic obstruction from HD. Dilated bowel loops can also be seen with high grade stenosis (**Fig.102.19C,D**).

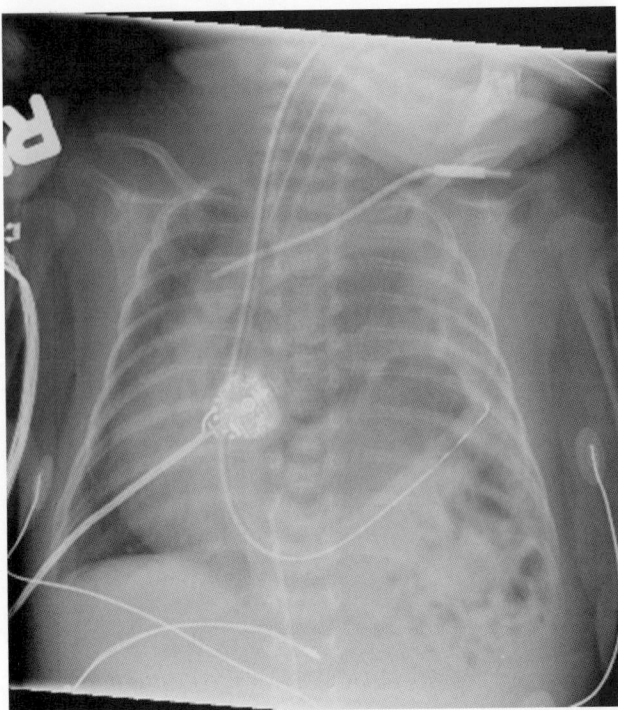

FIGURE 102.14. Diaphragmatic hernia. Newborn with left diaphragmatic hernia with bowel loops in the lower left chest and contralateral mediastinal shift. Tip of the NG tube indicates intrathoracic position of the stomach.

g. *Meconium ileus*: Thick meconium becomes inspissated in the distal ileum and results in a high-grade small-bowel obstruction. This usually occurs in patients with cystic fibrosis as they produce thick, tenacious meconium in utero. On imaging, low intestinal obstruction is noted with a bubbly appearance in the right lower quadrant owing to air mixed with meconium (**Fig. 102.20A**). A water-soluble contrast enema can be diagnostic and therapeutic (21). The enema typically shows a microcolon and multiple filling defects in the terminal ileum (**Fig. 102.20B**). An attempt is made to reflux the contrast into the terminal ileum in order to wash out the thick meconium from the distal small bowel and relieve the obstruction. Serial enemas can be performed as long as the patient remains stable. If the obstruction is not relieved with enemas, surgery is required.

h. *Meconium plug syndrome/small left colon*: This entity is seen more commonly in infants of diabetic mothers. Most patients have delayed passage of meconium and plain films showing multiple dilated loops of bowel throughout the abdomen, indicating a distal obstruction (**Fig. 102.21A**). Multiple filling defects in the distal ileum are seen on hypertonic water-soluble contrast enema. The left side of the colon may be relatively small in caliber, but the remainder of the colon is normal (**Fig. 102.21B**). The enema may be therapeutic in cases of meconium plug causing obstruction and delay in passage of meconium (5). If the patient continues to have obstruc-

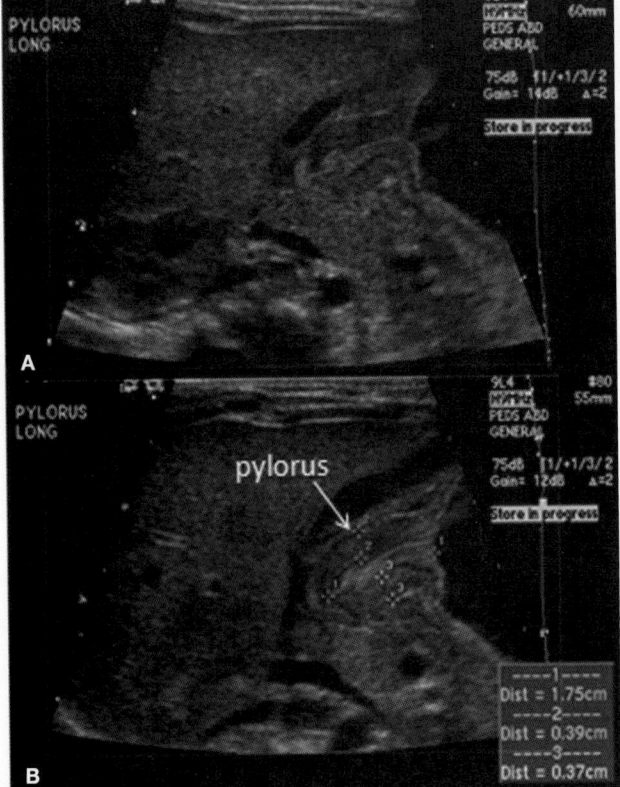

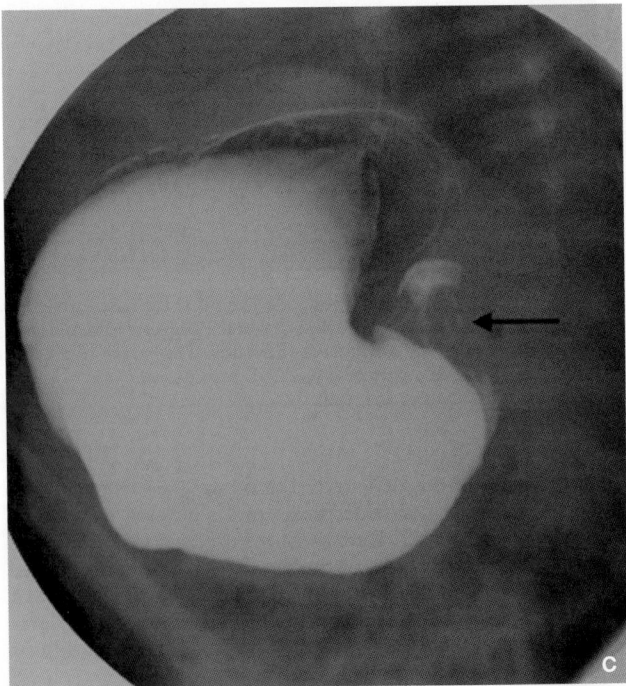

FIGURE 102.15. Pyloric stenosis. **A** and **B:** US shows a hypoechoic mass formed by thickened pyloric muscle with a narrowed and elongated pyloric channel. The length of the pyloric thickening is 1.5 cm, and maximum single-wall thickness of 3 mm is highly suggestive of pyloric stenosis. **C:** UGI barium study on a 10-day-old boy with nonbilious vomiting and distended stomach. The pyloric channel is narrowed and elongated with a double-track appearance (*arrow*) with hypertrophy of the pyloric muscle, consistent with pyloric stenosis.

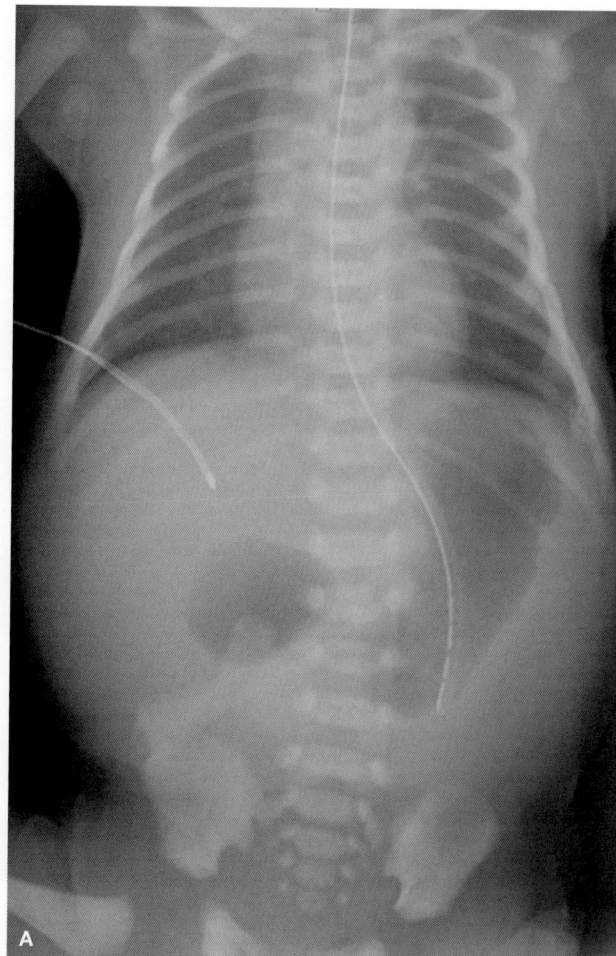

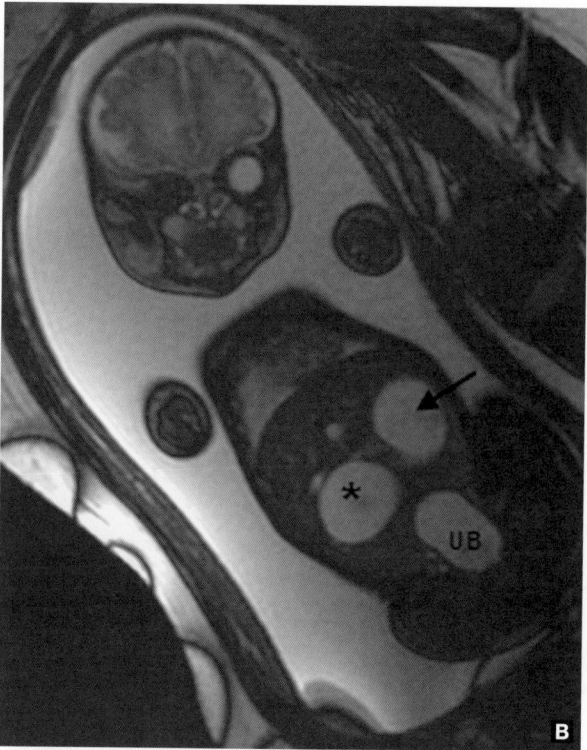

FIGURE 102.16. Duodenal atresia. **A:** Newborn presenting with vomiting. Gas is seen only in the stomach and duodenal bulb, consistent with a double-bubble sign in duodenal atresia. **B:** Prenatal MRI at 33-weeks gestation. There is a double-bubble sign with stomach on the left (*arrow*) and distended proximal duodenum (*asterisk*) of the fetus compatible with duodenal atresia. Urinary bladder (UB) is also seen in the pelvis.

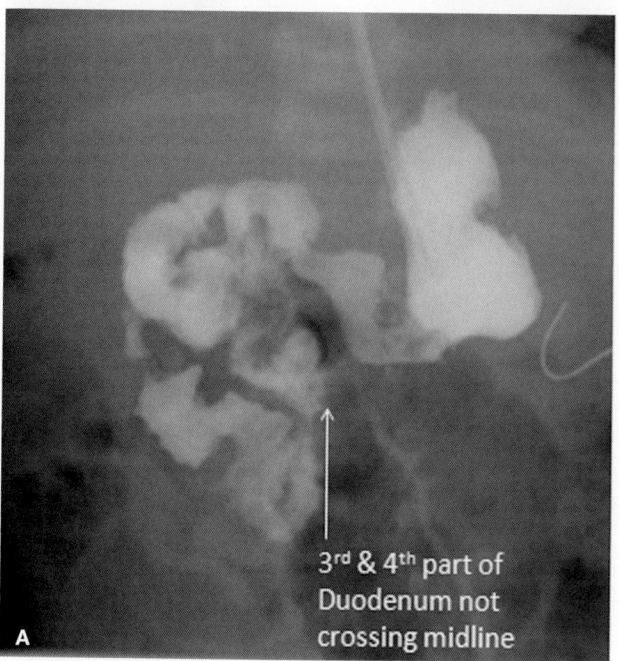

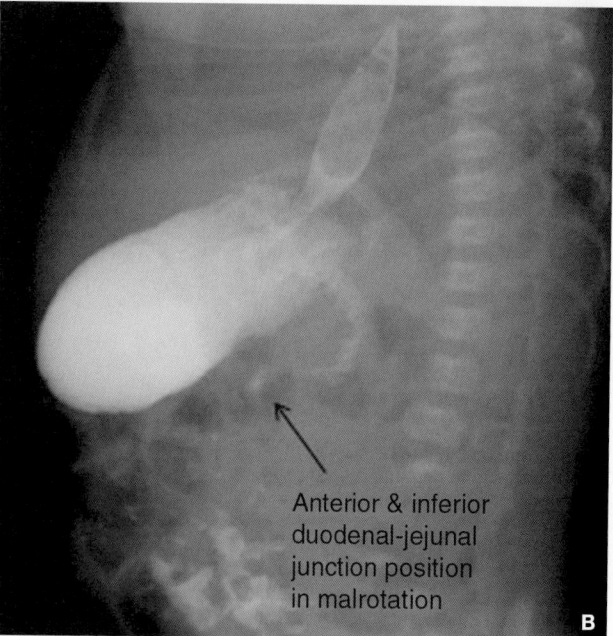

FIGURE 102.17. Malrotation. **A:** Patient presented with bilious vomiting. UGI barium study shows absence of normal configuration of the duodenal C loop with the fourth part staying on the right side of the spine. **B:** The duodenal-jejunal junction is seen displaced inferiorly and anteriorly on the lateral view.

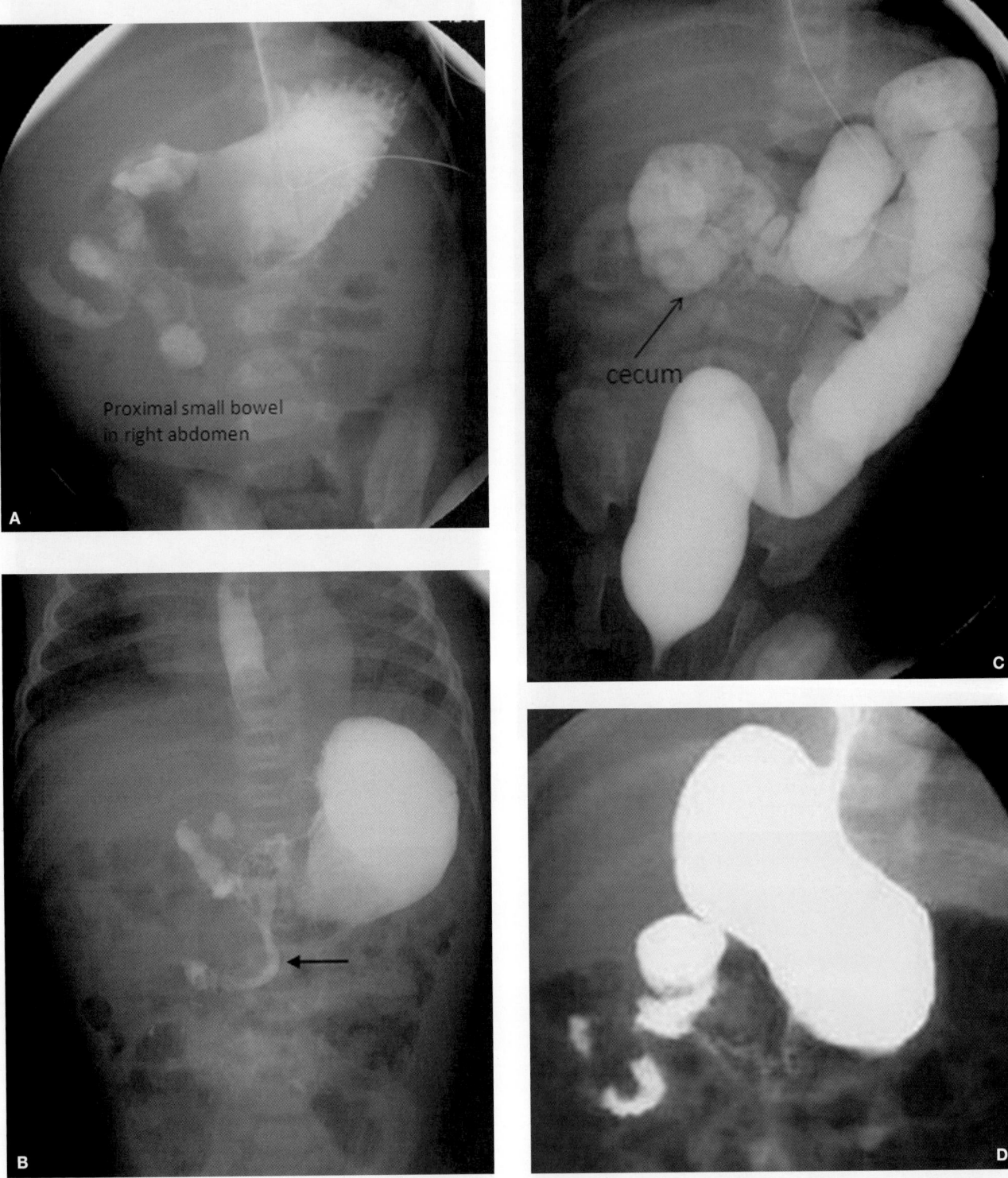

FIGURE 102.18. Malrotation. **A:** 3-week-old with bilious vomiting. UGI study showed that the duodenal sweep does not cross midline. The duodenum and jejunum are positioned within the right hemiabdomen, suggestive of malrotation. **B:** Case of malrotation in which the UGI study shows the third portion of duodenum not crossing the midline and turning inferiorly (*arrow*). **C:** Lower GI study in this patient showed normal filling of the rectum and distal aspect of the colon, with the cecum and terminal ileum appearing freely mobile. The cecum is located abnormally high in the right upper quadrant (*arrow*) of the abdomen. **D:** An example of a case of malrotation in a patient with spiraling of opacified proximal bowel loops in the right upper abdomen with obstruction, suggestive of volvulus.

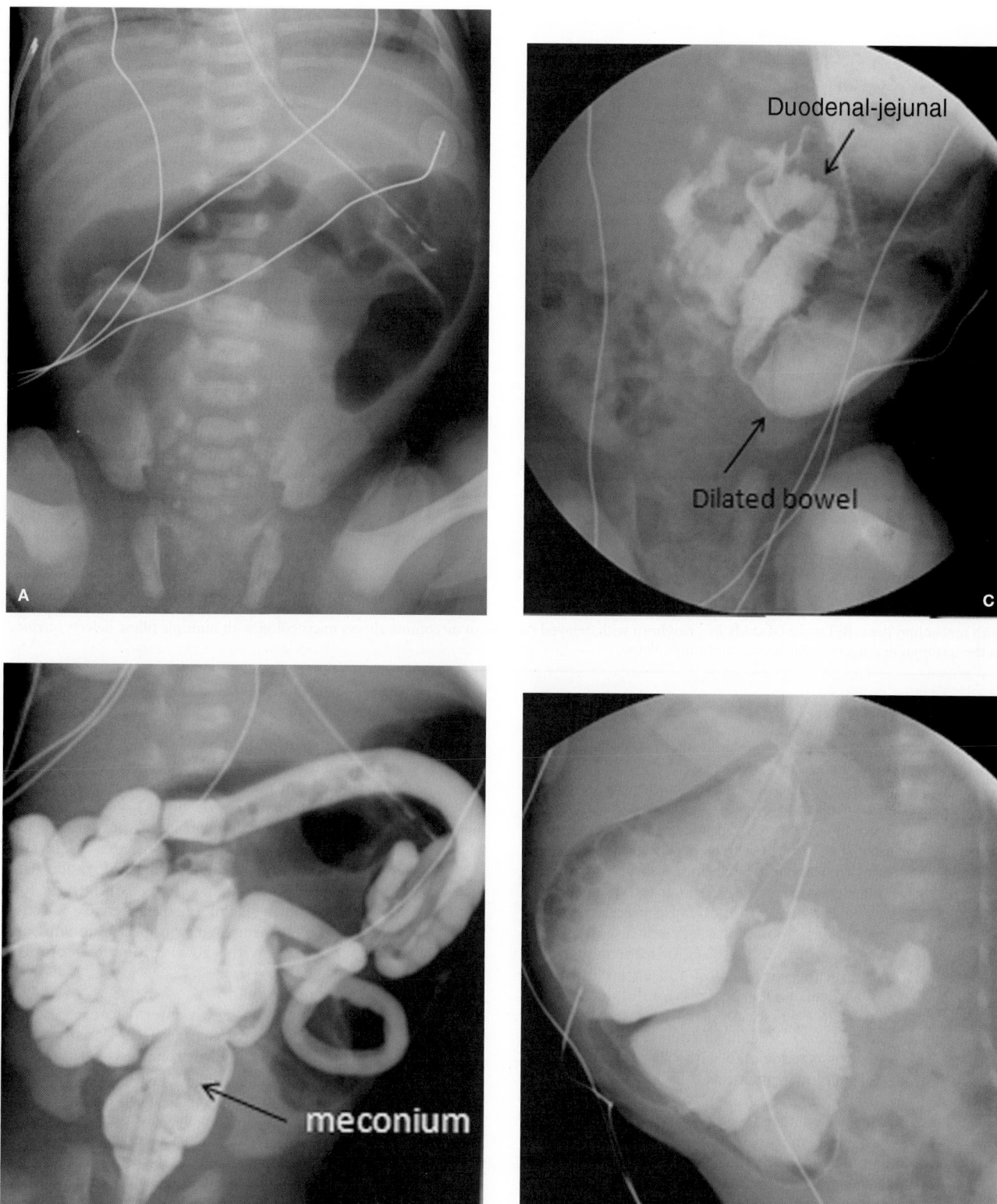

FIGURE 102.19. High intestinal obstruction. A: Jejunal atresia. X-ray abdomen:Few dilated bowel loops in the upper abdomen with paucity of gas distally concerning for UGI obstruction. **B:** Ileal atresia Lower GI study:Contrast enema image demonstrates a normal caliber rectum containing some meconium (*arrow*). Contrast refluxed freely into the terminal and distal ileum. Contrast was not refluxed into the more proximal distended loops of the small bowel. Patient was found to have proximal ileal atresia at surgery. **C:** Jejunal stenosis. Contrast UGI study: The duodenum is normal in caliber, with a normally positioned duodenal-jejunal junction. There is gradual dilatation of jejunum distal to the ligament of Treitz, with a markedly dilated loop at least 7 cm from the ligament of Treitz (*arrow*). **D:** Lateral view demonstrating the same dilated proximal jejunal loop. There was delay in contrast emptying distal to this dilated loop. However, the contrast eventually filled multiple normal caliber small-bowel loops.

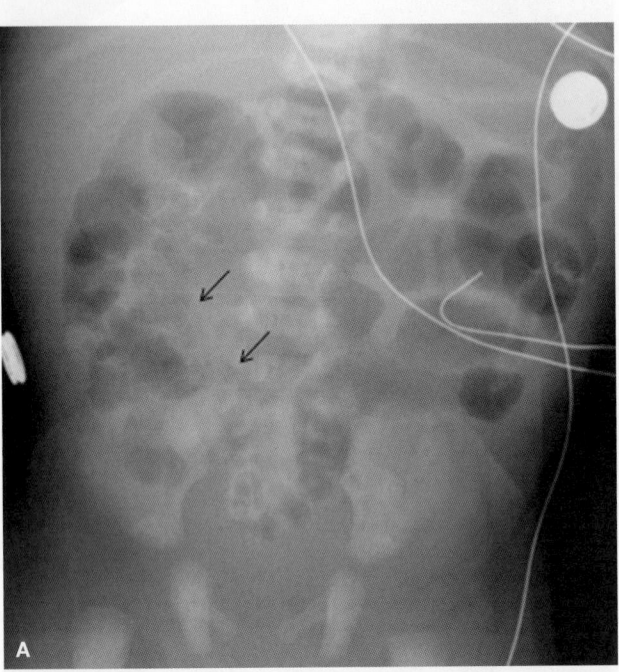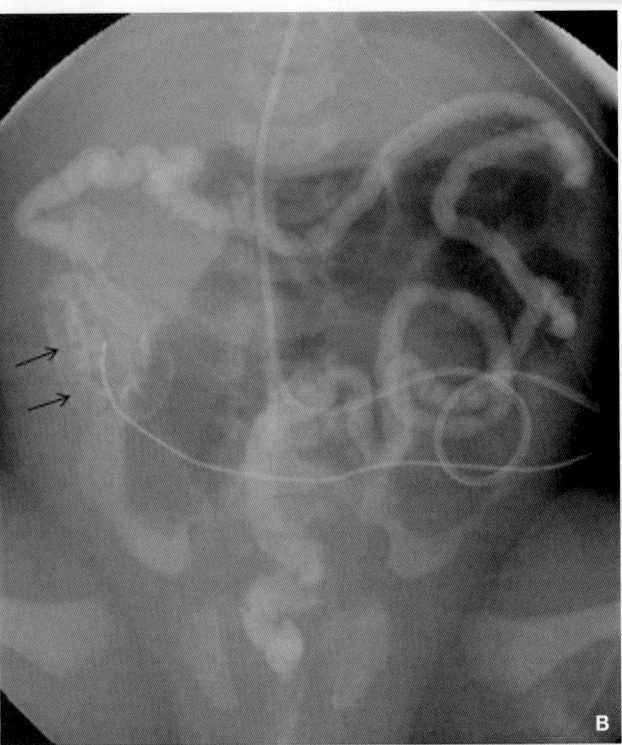

FIGURE 102.20. Newborn with delayed passage of meconium. **A:** Bubbly lucencies are seen within the right lower quadrant (*arrows*) in a patient with meconium ileus. **B:** Lower GI study in a newborn with delayed passage of meconium shows microcolon with multiple filling defects (*arrows*) in the terminal ileum, compatible with meconium ileus.

tive symptoms after repeated enemas, consideration should be given for HD.

i. *Hirschsprung disease*: HD is of unknown etiology with functional low intestinal obstruction resulting from absence of ganglion cells in the myenteric plexus of the distal bowel. Depending on the level of neuronal migration arrest, there may be ultrashort segment disease involving the internal sphincter, short segment disease involving the rectum and a portion of the sigmoid, long segment disease involving a variable portion of colon, or total aganglionosis involving the entire colon and variable portion of small bowel. HD, especially total colonic aganglionosis, can be associated with Down syndrome, cardiac defects, or genitourinary abnormalities. Enterocolitis is associated with HD and can lead to toxic megacolon, which has a higher mortality and morbidity rate (21). On contrast enema, the transition zone is visualized at the site of absent ganglion cells. An abnormal rectosigmoid index is seen with the diameter of the rectum appearing narrower than the diameter of the sigmoid (**Fig. 102.22A,B**). Toxic megacolon appears as mucosal irregularity, colonic dilation, and possibly a colon cut-off sign in the rectosigmoid region with absence of air distally. These patients should not undergo enema, as the risk for perforation is high. Even without an enema, toxic megacolon may lead to perforation, with the finding of pneumoperitoneum (23).

j. *Anorectal malformations*: There are a wide variety of anomalies owing to the failure of the hindgut to cross the puborectalis sling. These include imperforate anus (most common), anorectal atresia, and stenosis. Generally, there is an associated fistula and

a wide range of genital and urinary abnormalities. Plain films demonstrate colonic obstruction. Sacral anomalies can be seen (**Fig. 102.23**). An invertogram (placing the patient upside down) was obtained in the past, but is now not routine. It outlines the distal rectum filled with air and estimates the level of termination of the hindgut and its distance from the skin. However, the specificity is relatively low. Similar information can be obtained by a cross-table prone (rectum up) view. Imperforate anus and a presacral mass with sacral anomalies comprise Currarino triad (5,6).

2. Infectious and inflammatory

a. *Gastroenteritis*: Acute gastroenteritis caused by bacteria, viruses, or parasitic agents is a major cause of morbidity among children across the world (24). Diffuse bowel distension without evidence of focal obstruction is seen on abdominal radiographs (**Fig. 102.24A**). US may be successful in demonstrating thickened bowel wall, particularly in the ileocecal region with or without free peritoneal fluid (**Fig. 102.24B,C**) (25). Management of fluid and nutritional imbalance in these patients precedes further imaging with CT scan, which is reserved for challenging and resistant cases. Bowel wall thickening with enhancement is a nonspecific feature on CT scan in patients with gastroenteritis (26).

b. *Necrotizing enterocolitis*: NEC is a serious gastrointestinal disease of neonates of yet unknown etiology. NEC is characterized by mucosal and transmural necrosis of bowel. Severely ill and premature neonates remain susceptible to NEC. NEC can occur in term infants with polycythemia, hypoxia, complex congenital heart disease, and other illnesses that may

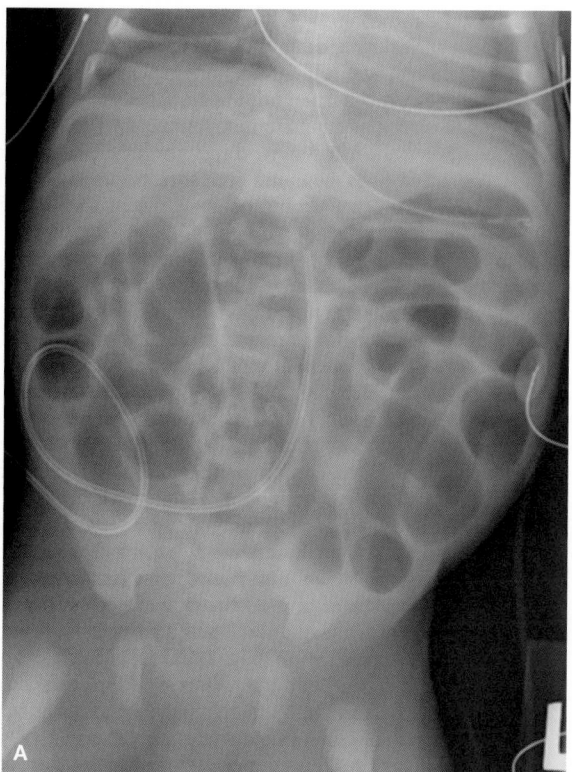
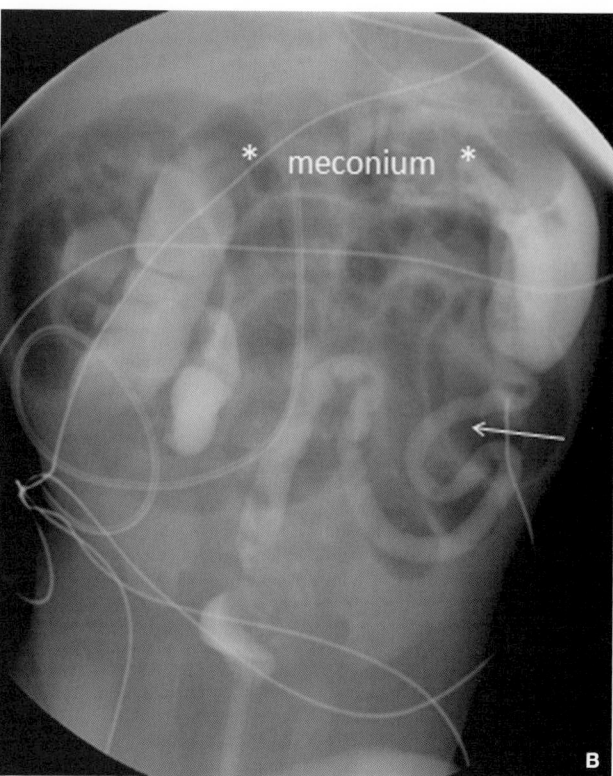

FIGURE 102.21. Meconium plug syndrome. **A:** Newborn with abdominal distension, bile-stained vomiting. Mother has history of magnesium sulfate intake. Multiple mildly dilated loops of bowel are present throughout the abdomen although no air is seen in the rectum. There is no pneumatosis, portal venous gas, or free intraperitoneal air. Findings compatible with distal bowel obstruction from meconium plug/small left colon syndrome. **B:** Lower GI study: Enema was performed with water-soluble iodinated contrast; contrast was run retrograde in the colon. The left colon is small in caliber (*arrow*). The descending colon diameter is 3.6 mm, while that of transverse colon was 15 mm. At a point in the splenic flexure, there is an abrupt caliber change in the bowel, with large meconium plugs seen (*asterisk*) in the transverse colon, suggestive of meconium plug or small left colon.

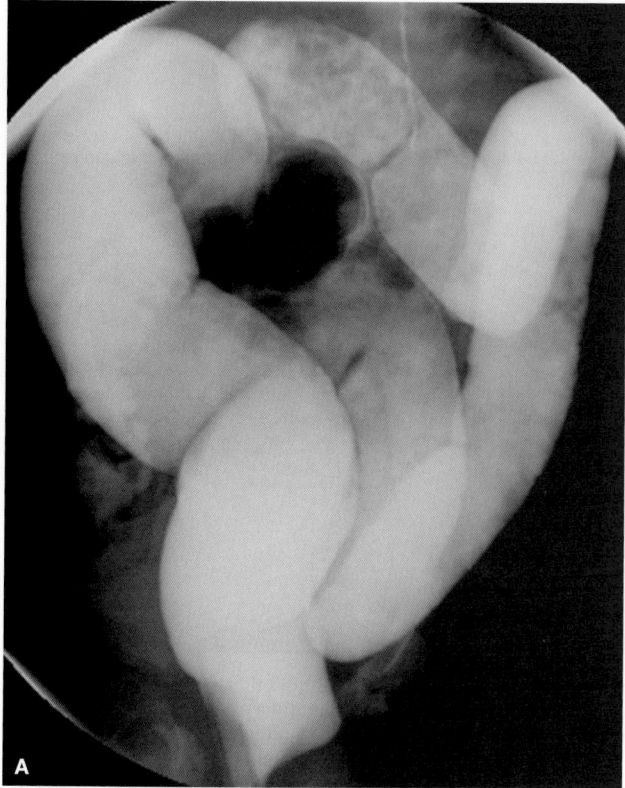
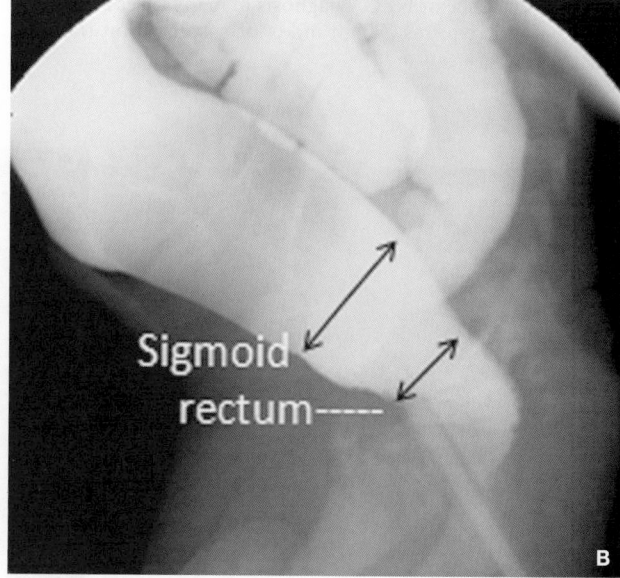

FIGURE 102.22. Hirschsprung disease. **A** and **B:** 4-week-old boy with constipation and poor feeding. Lower GI study with ionic contrast instilled in usual retrograde fashion in the rectum by gravity filling the colon up to the cecum. There is no presacral mass. There is no definite transition zone identified. The diameter of the sigmoid is larger than that of the rectum (rectosigmoid ratio <1, consistent with HD at the rectosigmoid level).

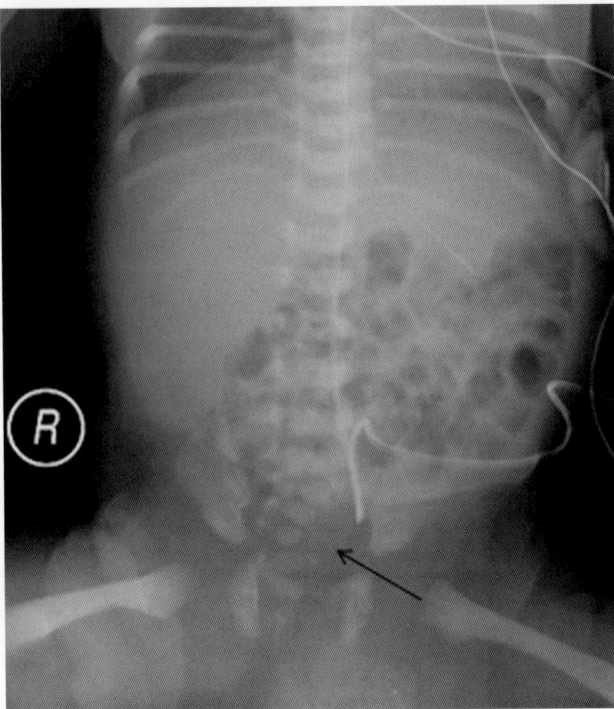

FIGURE 102.23. Sacral dysgenesis. A newborn with known anorectal malformation has a hypogenetic sacrum (*arrow*) seen on the plain film.

predispose the patient to bowel ischemia. Infants of cocaine-abusing mothers are also at risk. If a patient has symptoms concerning for NEC, serial supine and lateral decubitus abdominal radiographs, every 4–6 hours, are performed to monitor for radiographic evidence of NEC. Diagnosis in many cases is difficult and requires a high index of suspicion on the part

of the radiologist (4). Radiographs may demonstrate one or multiple dilated bowel loops that display little or no change in location and appearance with serial studies. Another useful, but nonspecific, sign in NEC is loss of a symmetric distribution of the bowel gas. Other well-known findings include pneumatosis, portal venous gas, and free intraperitoneal air (**Fig. 102.25A–D**). Pneumatosis is present in 50%–75% of patients (8).

c. *Meconium peritonitis*: Meconium when leaked into peritoneum, either by obstruction or by malformation, causes chemical peritonitis. The resulting diffuse peritoneal inflammation results in calcifications scattered throughout the abdomen often seen well on plain films (**Fig. 102.26A**). Calcifications can also be seen in the scrotum as the inflammation spreads via the patent processus vaginalis. US within a few hours of birth can show increased echogenicity of the abdomen (snowstorm pattern). Ascites and bowel wall thickening may also be seen. The inflammation may be localized by fibrosis and form a pseudocyst. Meconium pseudocyst formation can be seen in cases of walled-off bowel perforation. This appears as a cystic mass with a fibrous wall with or without calcification (**Fig. 102.26B**) (2,27).

d. *Hepatitis and hepatic abscess*: Hepatitis can be caused by infections with viruses including hepatitis A, rubella, cytomegalovirus, and herpes, or other organisms such as ameba, toxoplasma, or spirochete, as well as congenital metabolic disorders (alpha-1 antitrypsin deficiency), familial cholestasis, or idiopathic. It usually presents in the first month of age occurring more commonly in boys (28). US shows heterogeneous echogenicity of the liver with or without periportal thickening. The gallbladder and the biliary tree are normal. Often, the US may not show any findings to suggest hepatitis. Hepatobiliary scintigraphy may show delayed clearance of the tracer from the blood pool, with lack of tracer excretion in the common bile duct or bowel, confusing it with biliary atresia. Administration of

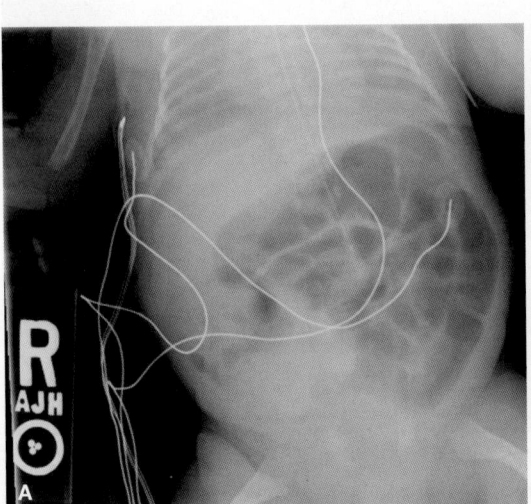
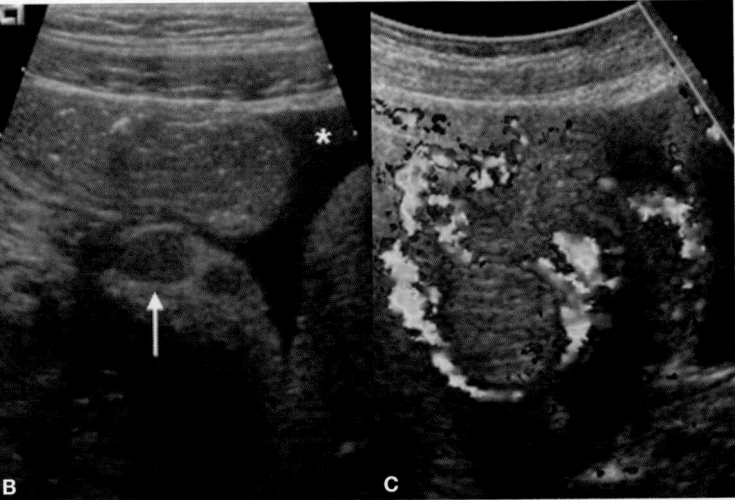

FIGURE 102.24. Gastroenteritis. **A:** 4-week-old boy with abdominal distension and diarrhea. Radiograph shows diffuse bowel dilation with a paucity of bowel gas in the right lower quadrant. **B** and **C:** On US, there is mild bowel thickening in the right lower quadrant with a moderate amount of ascites (*asterisk*) and few mesenteric lymph nodes (*arrow*); Color Doppler shows multiple hyperemic bowel walls consistent with enteritis/colitis.

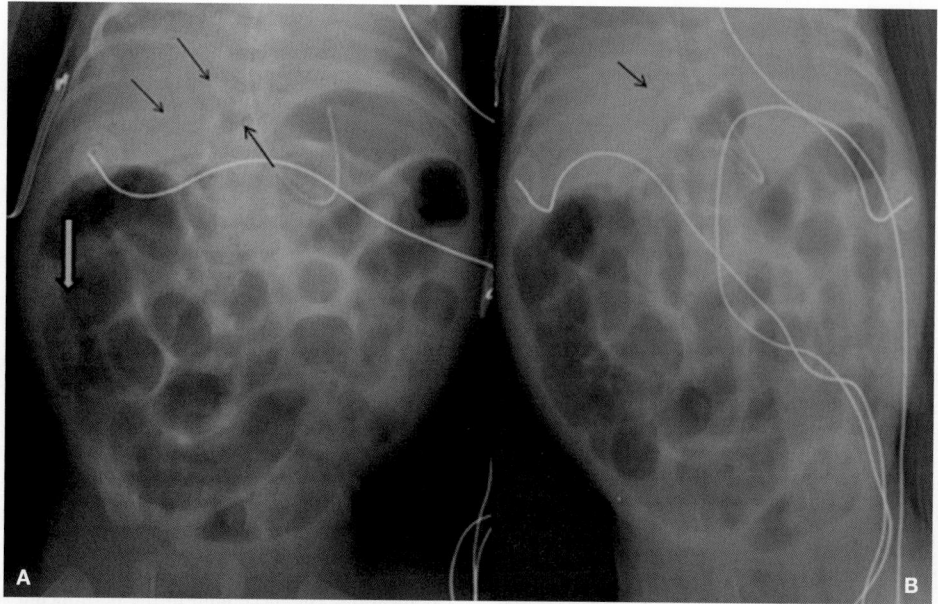

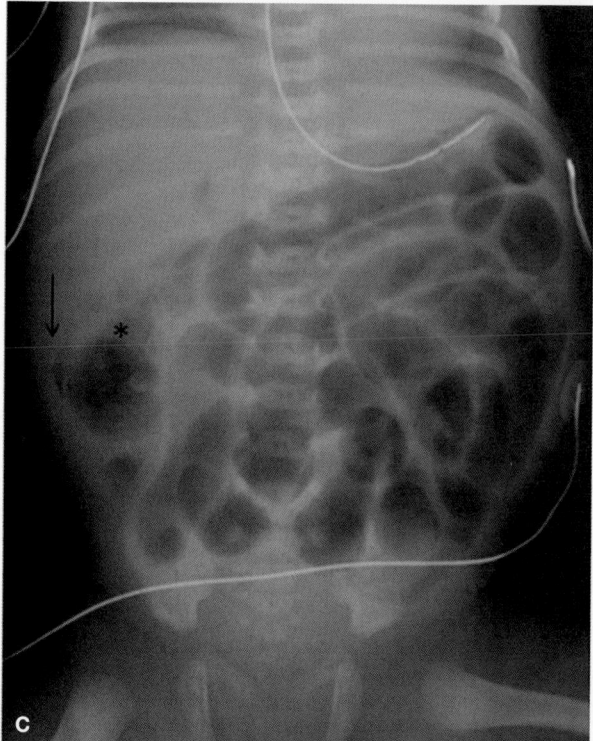

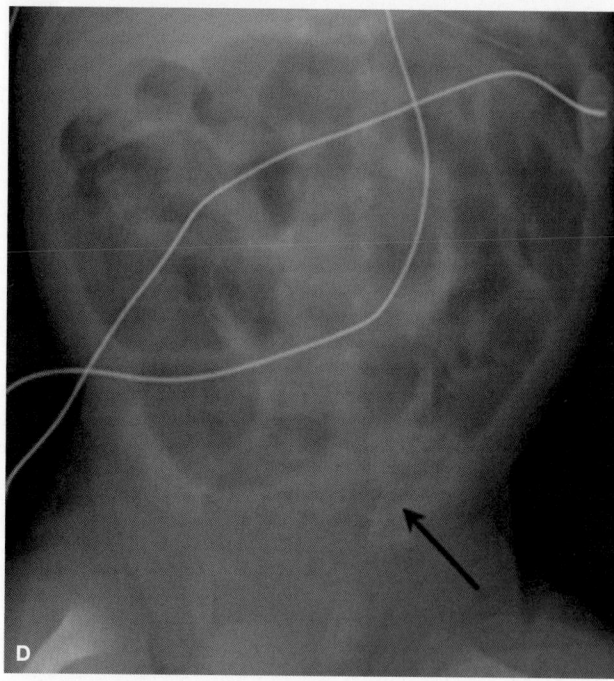

FIGURE 102.25. Necrotizing enterocolitis. **A** and **B:** Dilated bowel loops, bubbly lucencies in the right flank around the bowel loops (blocked *arrow*), suggestive of pneumatosis. There is presence of portal venous gas seen as lucencies in a tree branch pattern radiating from the region of hilum of the liver (*arrows*). No pneumoperitoneum. **C:** NEC with perforation. Mottling (*asterisk*) over the bowel loop in the right abdomen with extraluminal gas (*arrow*). **D:** Mottling due to intramural gas in the left lower quadrant (*arrow*) in a different patient with NEC.

phenobarbital induces the hepatic enzymatic function and shows improved clearance of the radiopharmaceutical and thus differentiates hepatitis from biliary atresia (no biliary excretion of tracer even at 24 hours). Focal hepatic abscesses from pyogenic or fungal infections may occur in children. The most common organism in children with liver abscesses is *Staphylococcus aureus*, while it is *Escherichia coli* in the adult population. These can

occur hematogeneously via (a) the hepatic artery from distant infections, (b) the portal vein from enteritis, (c) the biliary tract, by direct extension from adjacent abdominal process, or (d) secondary to penetrating trauma. US shows a hypoechoic center with irregular margin in a pyogenic abscess. Peripheral heterogenous wall enhancement with a necrotic nonenhancing center on CT is suggestive of abscess in the correct clinical setting. Internal gas

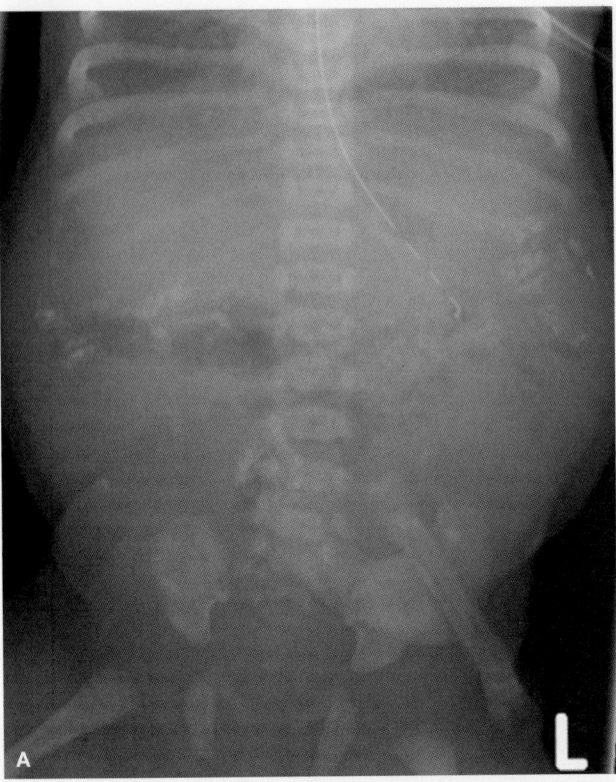

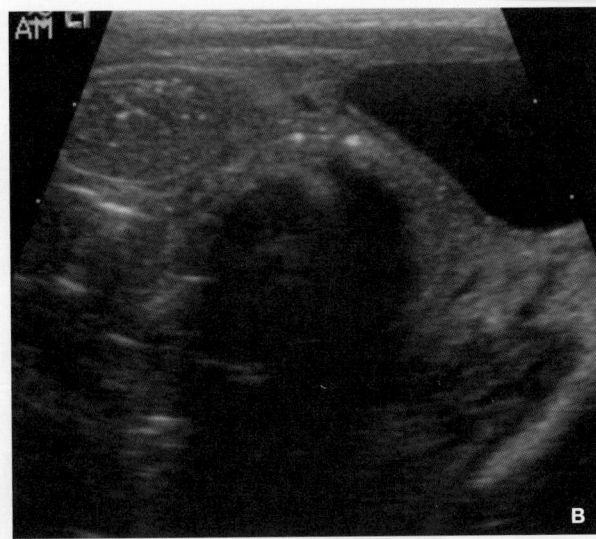

FIGURE 102.26. Meconium peritonitis. **A:** Diffuse coarse abdominal calcification. The meconium in the peritoneum secondary to bowel perforation tends to result in scattered intra-abdominal calcifications. **B:** Meconium pseudocyst: 2-day-old premature girl with abdominal distension and vomiting. US of the lower abdomen shows a collection with an echogenic rim and dirty shadowing that obscures details. Surgery revealed meconium ileus with bowel perforation and cystic meconium collection.

may also be seen (29). Fungal abscesses occur in pediatric patients on chemotherapy, posttransplant, or with neutropenia; they usually are multifocal and small and may not show a necrotic center. Hepatic amebic abscess due to *Entamoeba histolytica* infection secondary to ileocecal involvement are seen less commonly in children and are more common in adults from developing countries. Hepatic echinococcal involvement from *Echinococcus granulosus* gives rise to multiple cysts. Hypoechoic thin-walled lesions on US and hypodense lesions on CT are seen with internal smaller daughter cysts.

e. *Appendicitis*: Acute appendicitis is an important differential in children with acute abdominal pain, and it is the most common cause of a pediatric acute abdomen which leads to surgery (30). While most of the children above 5 years of age have acute abdominal syndrome, patients under 5 years may present with nonspecific symptoms, which may also be seen in conditions such as viral enteritis, intussusception, or mesenteric adenitis (31). US is the first diagnostic study in children for whom an experienced surgeon has determined the findings for appendicitis to be equivocal. If the US is nondiagnostic and urgent diagnosis is indicated, the patient should undergo contrast-enhanced CT (32). The US usually shows a dilated appendix (diameter 7 mm or more) with thickened walls with hyperemia seen on Doppler. Surrounding anechoic fluid and an echogenic appendicolith are other findings sometimes seen on US (**Fig. 102.27A,B**). CT accurately demonstrates the thickened appendix and surrounding inflammatory fat stranding (**Fig. 102.27C,D**). The added advantage of CT lies in detecting peritoneal abscess in case of perforated appendicitis, which might track away at the location other than the right lower quadrant.

Conditions mimicking appendicitis, such as mesenteric adenitis or typhlitis, can also be diagnosed by CT scan with contrast unless there are contraindications. Oral contrast is relatively contraindicated in patients with vomiting. Intravenous contrast is relatively contraindicated in patients with renal insufficiency. Other acute inflammatory conditions involving the right lower quadrant in the pediatric population are typhlitis, Meckel diverticulitis, enteritis, ischemia, and inflammatory bowel disease (33).

f. *Meckel diverticulitis and bleeding*: Meckel diverticulum is the most common embryologic remnant of the omphalomesenteric duct (OMD), seen in 2% of the population. Meckel diverticulum is associated with several complications, including Meckel diverticular bleeding, inflammation with or without perforation, intussusception, bowel obstruction, or neoplasm. Diverticular bleeding is the most common complication seen in younger children. Technetium-99m pertechnetate scintigraphy is the investigation of choice in evaluation of pediatric patients with suspected bleeding from a Meckel diverticulum (**Fig. 102.28**). Similar to appendicitis, diverticulitis results from obstruction of the lumen by an enterolith or foreign body, leading to stasis and bacterial infection. Abdominal plain films would not show any findings than a radiopaque enterolith, if present, or any bowel obstruction secondary to Meckel diverticulitis. The CT scan shows a blind-ending tubular structure in the right lower quadrant or periumbilical region with thickened walls (**Fig. 102.29**), and surrounding fat stranding (34). US has a limited role in imaging of remnants of the OMD. In most cases, the presentation is nonspecific, and it is important to consider the possibility of an OMD remnant as the cause of an acute abdomen in a child.

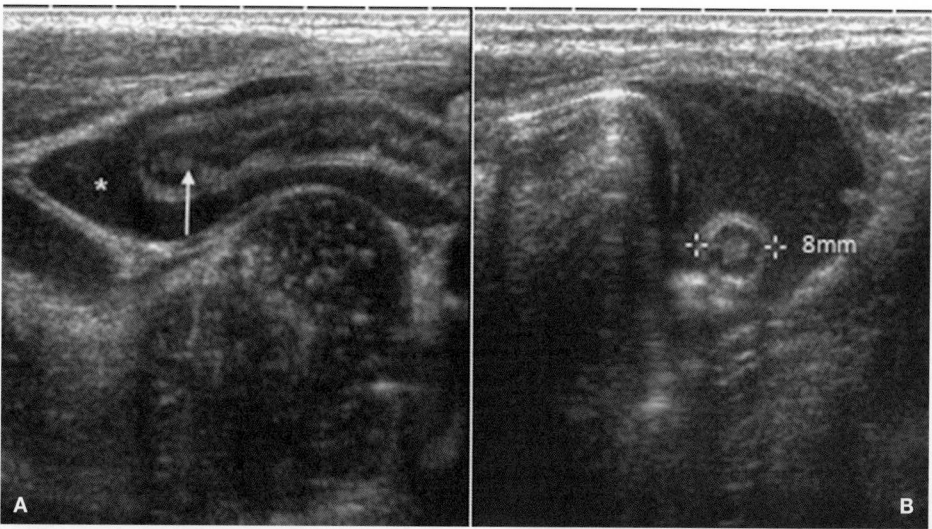

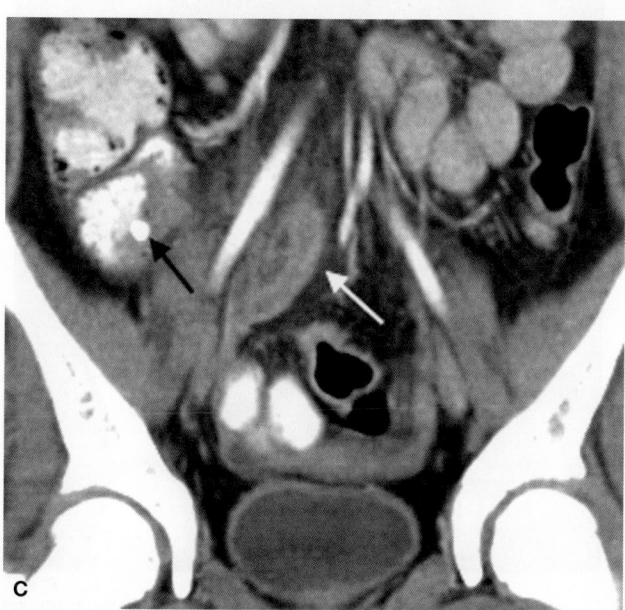

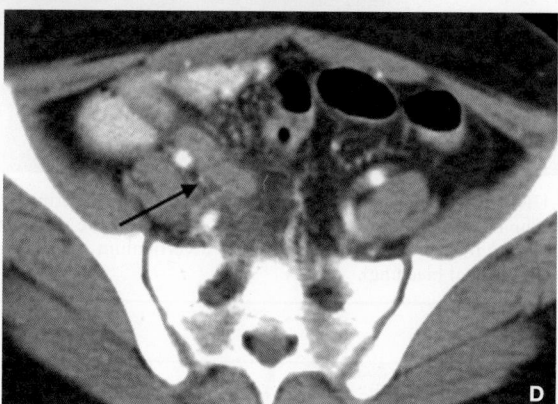

FIGURE 102.27. Appendicitis. **A** and **B:** Longitudinal and transverse US images of an inflamed appendix with a diameter of 8 mm in the right lower quadrant (*arrow*) with surrounding free fluid (*asterisk*). **C:** CT scan with contrast coronal reconstruction shows an inflamed appendix (*white arrow*) in the lower abdomen with thick wall and surrounding fat stranding with a hyperdense appendicolith seen near the cecum (*black arrow*). **D:** Axial images in the same patient showing the inflamed appendix (*arrow*).

g. *Typhlitis or neutropenic colitis:* Typhlitis or neutropenic colitis is inflammation in neutropenic patients involving the cecum, which may also involve the ascending colon or terminal ileum. It is increasingly seen in children undergoing chemotherapy, more commonly in patients with leukemia and lymphoma. Common presentation is with fever, diarrhea, and abdominal pain and may be associated with vomiting and lethargy (35). Bowel wall thickening is the most notable finding on imaging, which is accurately measured by US and correlates with the duration of neutropenia (36). CT scan will show a thickened cecal wall with or without involvement of the terminal ileum (**Fig. 102.30A,B**).

3. Masses

a. *Adrenal:* Adrenal hemorrhage is an important diagnosis for the intensivist and is the most common cause of an adrenal mass in neonates. The hemorrhage can occur prenatally or be due to perinatal stress (birth trauma or hypoxia), particularly in neonates of

diabetic mothers (37). US is the examination of choice for suspected adrenal hematoma. Initial US typically reveals a complex cystic, echogenic mass that may also be seen in cases of neuroblastoma (the most common adrenal mass in older children) (**Figs. 102.31A,B and 102.32**). Another differential is extrapulmonary sequestration of the lung in a subdiaphragmatic location. Sequestration is seen more commonly on the left side, while adrenal hemorrhage is more common on the right. Later, evolution of the hematoma and regression is seen (38). Radiographic findings include later appearance of rim-like calcification around the hemorrhage, whereas stippled calcifications are typical of neuroblastoma (see *renal masses* below).

b. *Liver masses:* MRI is the investigation of choice in patients with liver lesions providing better soft-tissue contrast. US is the initial imaging modality in a child in a hospital setting (39). A precise radiologic diagnosis is sometimes problematic because of nonspecific imaging features. Primary liver tumors are

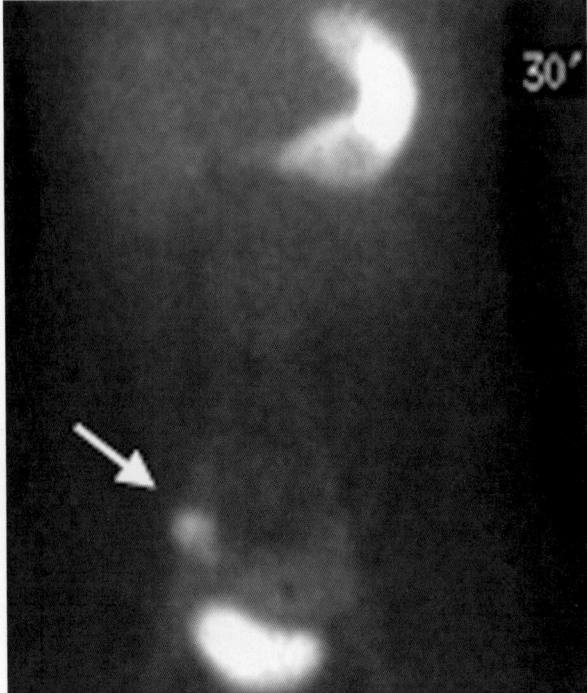

FIGURE 102.28. Meckel diverticular bleeding. Technetium-99m pertechnate scan shows a focus of gastric mucosa in the right lower abdomen (*arrow*), suggestive of Meckel diverticulum (the cause of gastrointestinal bleeding).

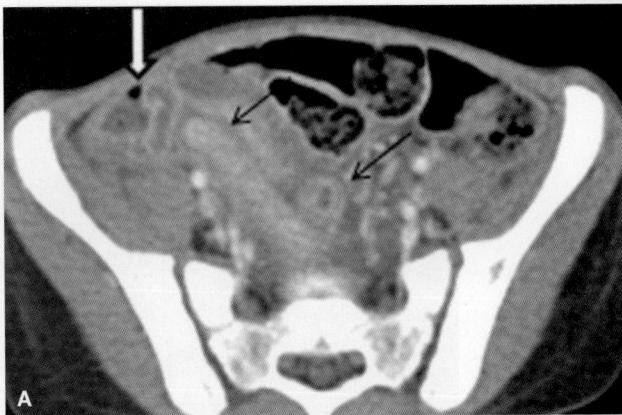

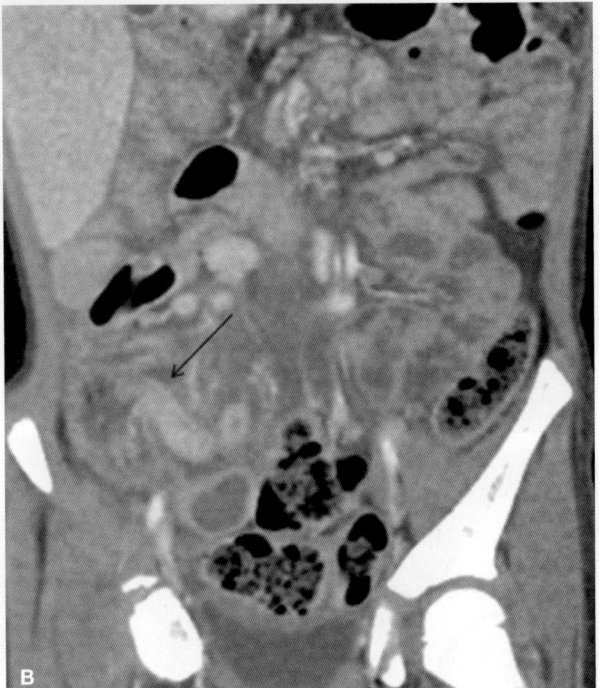

FIGURE 102.30. Bowel inflammation. **A** and **B:** Typhilitis: Images from a CT scan of a 12-year-old patient on chemotherapy presenting with neutropenia, abdominal pain, and diarrhea. Inflamed cecum (*blocked arrow*) and terminal ileum (*black arrows*) with surrounding fluid in the right lower quadrant.

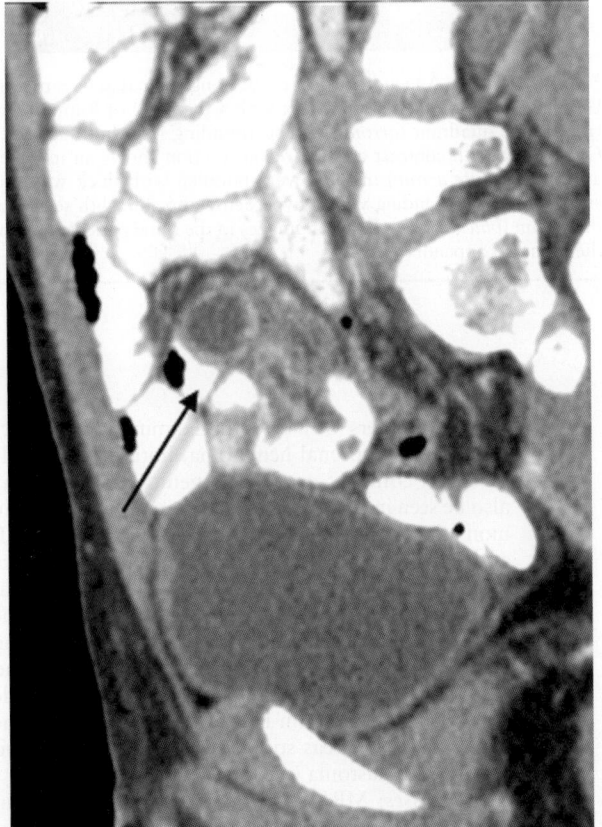

FIGURE 102.29. Meckel diverticulitis. CT scan sagittal image shows a blind-ending loop with thickened wall in the lower abdomen (*arrow*). Surgery showed inflamed Meckel diverticulum.

very rare in the neonatal period; the most frequent are infantile hemangioendothelioma, cavernous hemangioma, mesenchymal hamartoma, hepatoblastoma, and, less commonly, benign or malignant germ cell tumors (40–42). In older children, benign hepatic lesions, including infantile hemangioendothelioma (commonest), hepatic cysts, adenoma, and focal nodular hyperplasia, can occur. Hepatoblastoma is the commonest primary hepatic malignancy in the age group of <5 years, affecting boys twice as often as girls (**Fig. 102.33A,B**). Other malignant tumors in this age group include hepatocellular carcinoma, fibrolamellar carcinoma, angiosarcoma, or lymphoma. Most hepatic masses are metastatic lesions, with the commonest metastases from Wilms tumor and neuroblastoma (29). Lymphoproliferative masses of the liver are now

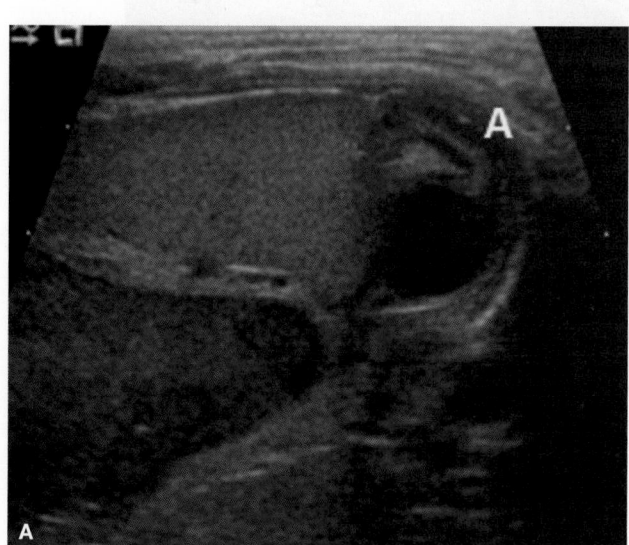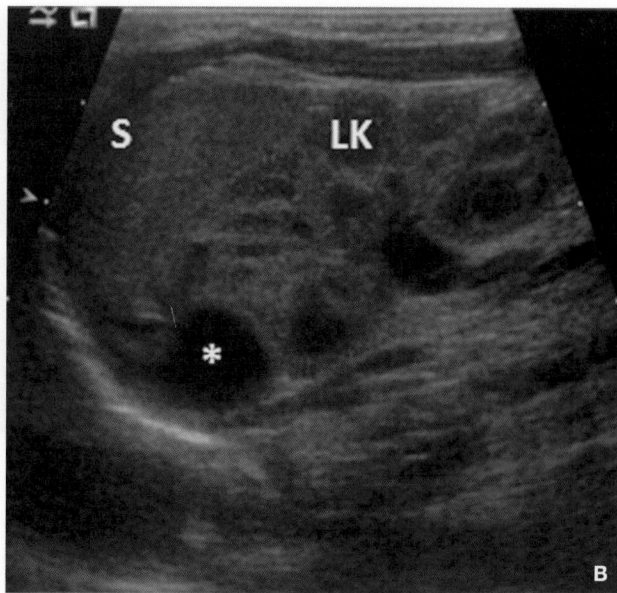

FIGURE 102.31. Adrenal cystic lesion. **A** and **B:** Newborn with incidental finding of a 1.1-cm cystic structure in the left adrenal gland (*asterisk*), likely representing evolving perinatal adrenal hemorrhage. (The adrenal gland [A], spleen [S] and left kidney [LK] are also shown.) A less likely differential consideration is adrenal cystic neuroblastoma. Follow-up US would show gradual evolution in case of hemorrhage.

more commonly seen in children because of increased use of organ transplantation and immunosuppression (39). Choledochal cyst (CC) is a benign congenital anomaly of the biliary tree characterized by cystic dilatation of the extrahepatic and/or intrahepatic bile ducts. US demonstrates a cystic structure in the hepatic hilum. Magnetic resonance cholangiopancreatography (MRCP) is the most accurate preoperative imaging method for characterizing cyst anatomy in detail and

for classifying lesions according to the standard Todani classification (16). Endoscopic retrograde cholangiopancreatography (ERCP) has been used pre- and intra-operatively, can be of diagnostic as well as therapeutic use, but carries a 5% risk of pancreatitis (43,44).

c. *Renal masses*: Hydronephrosis, multicystic dysplastic kidney, and obstructed upper pole of a duplicated collecting system account for the majority of urinary tract masses. Wilms tumor (nephroblastoma) is the

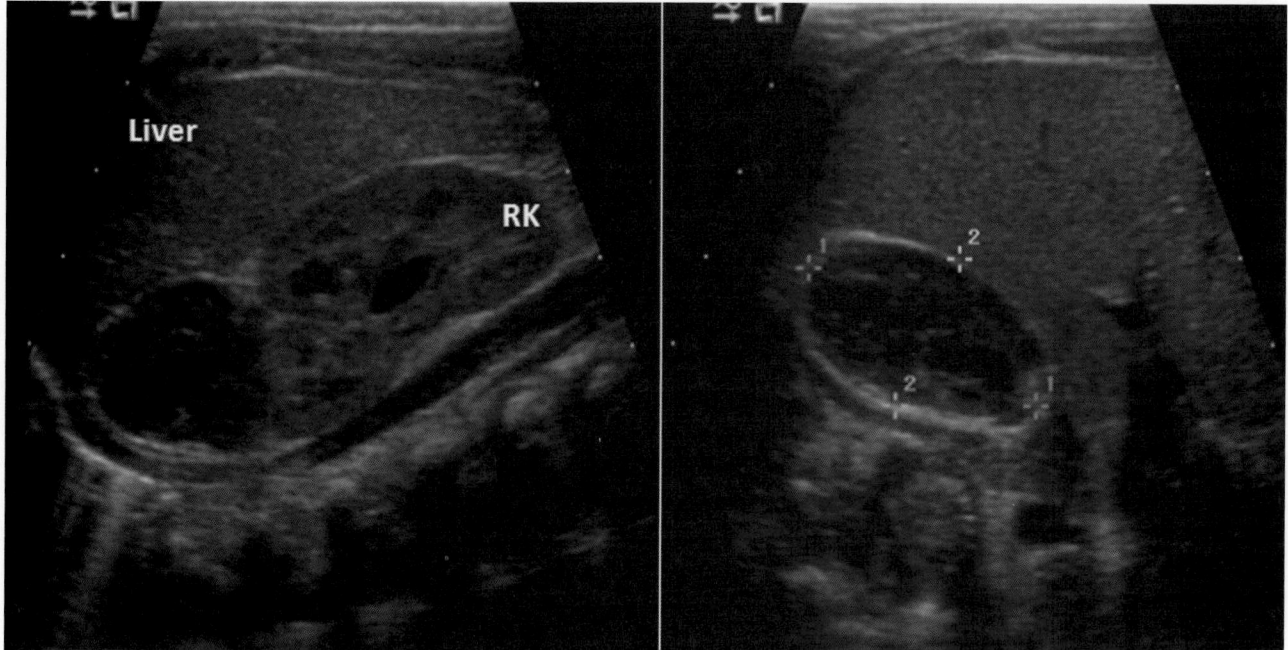

FIGURE 102.32. Adrenal hemorrhage. Transverse and longitudinal US scans through right upper abdomen reveal a heterogeneous hypoechoic 3-cm suprarenal mass; the mass decreased in size on follow-up and most likely represented right adrenal hemorrhage.

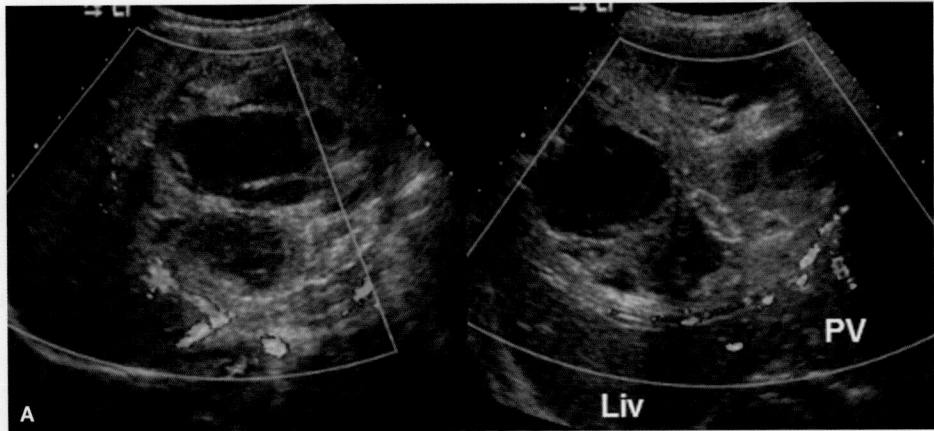

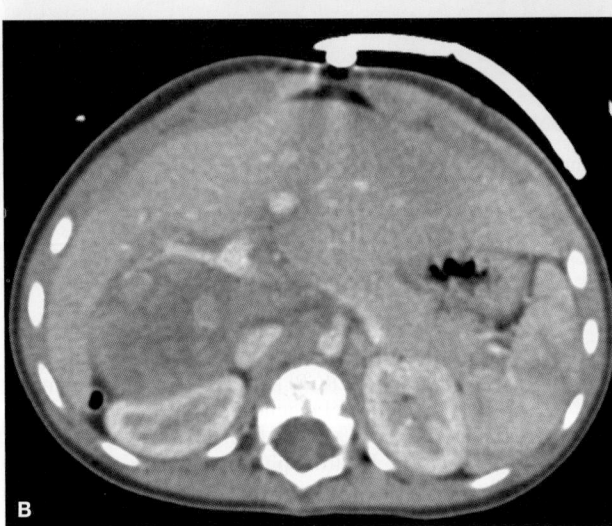

FIGURE 102.33. Hepatoblastoma. A: US in transverse and longitudinal planes demonstrates a solid cystic mass in the right hepatic lobe causing mass effect on the right branch of portal vein. B: CT scan with contrast shows a heterogeneously enhancing lobulated mass in the right hepatic lobe causing mass effect seen on portal vein, right hepatic vein, hepatic artery and inferior vena cava, and compression of the right kidney. Pathology revealed a hepatoblastoma.

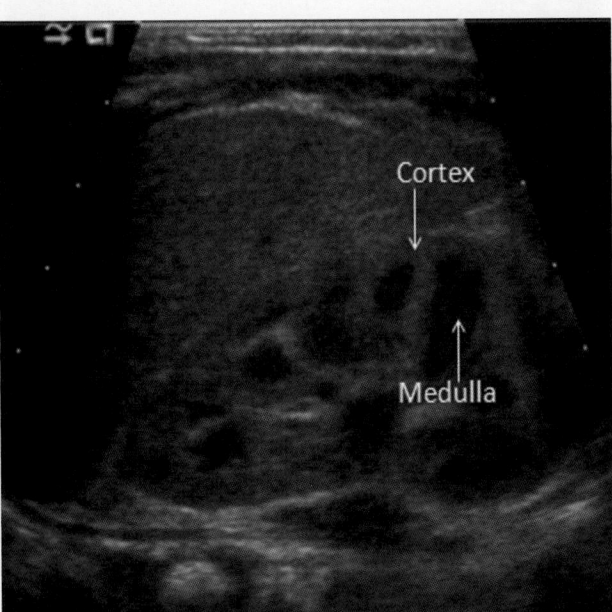

FIGURE 102.34. Neonatal kidney. Normal hyperechoic appearance of the cortex as compared with the medulla. Lobulations may be seen on the renal surface.

most common solid renal mass of childhood, mesoblastic nephroma is the most common solid renal neoplasm in neonates and infants, and renal cell carcinoma is rare before the second decade (3,45). Neuroblastoma is a solid tumor that often arises from the adrenal gland and may be difficult to differentiate from nephroblastoma. Neuroblastoma tends to occur earlier (<2 years vs. 3–4 years), is more invasive, not well marginated, and more likely to contain calcifications. Polycystic kidney, nephroblastomatosis, and renal vein thrombosis are other common renal masses that are detected radiographically. On abdominal radiographs, the soft-tissue renal mass may be seen causing displacement of bowel loops. Calcifications are rare in most of the above-mentioned renal masses. US followed by CT scan and/or MRI is helpful in determining the origin as well as etiology of the masses based on imaging characteristics (**Figs. 102.34** and **102.35A–C**) (46).

d. *Pelvic and genital masses*: The most common genital masses in the newborn are ovarian cystic lesions (47,48). The most common complication of a large ovarian cyst is hemorrhage followed by torsion. The US appearance of an uncomplicated ovarian cyst is an anechoic mass with a thin wall. A hemorrhagic cyst is seen as a cystic structure on US with floating internal echoes. Hydrometrocolpos involves

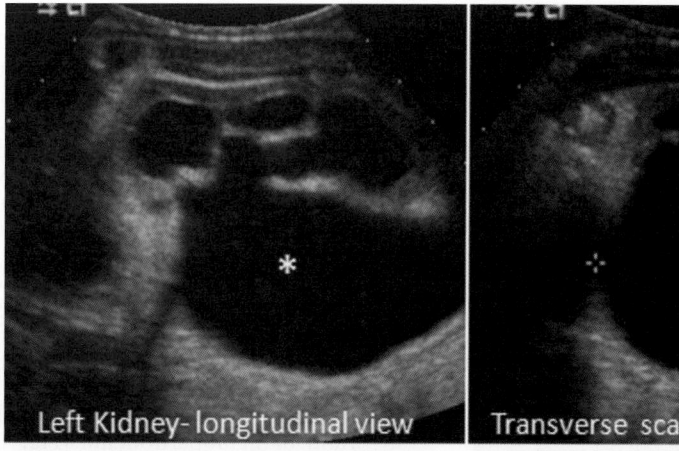

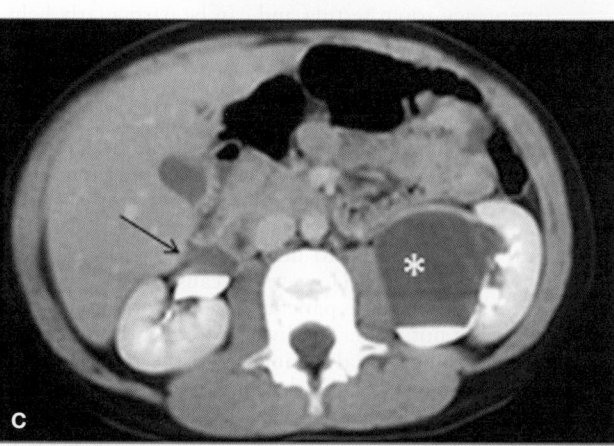

FIGURE 102.35. Hydronephrosis. **A** and **B:** Longitudinal and transverse US images through left kidney demonstrate pelvicalyceal dilation (*asterisk*). The proximal ureter was not dilated (not shown). Ureteropelvic junction obstruction is likely. **C:** Axial CT scan shows left hydronephrosis (*asterisk*) without hydroureter in a pattern consistent with ureteropelvic junction obstruction. The patient also had an extrarenal pelvis (*arrow*) in the right kidney, which is dilated without dilation of the calyces. Contrast is seen layering in the renal pelvis bilaterally.

distension of the uterus and the vagina as the result of fluid accumulation due to an obstruction of the genital tract. US demonstrates a fluid-filled structure posterior to the bladder. Prenatal diagnosis is by MRI, which shows a fetal cystic abdominal mass located in the midline posterior to the bladder (49). Sacrococcygeal teratoma is a germ cell tumor in the presacral location and the most common solid tumor in this location in neonates. Radiography may reveal a soft-tissue mass from the sacrococcygeal region with calcifications. CT or MR with contrast will show the cystic and enhancing solid elements (**Fig. 102.36**) (50).

e. *Gastrointestinal:* The differential diagnoses of an intra-abdominal cystic lesion in the newborn (excluding renal, hepatobiliary, and retroperitoneal origin) include ovarian cyst, enteric duplication cyst, mesenteric cyst (abdominal lymphatic malformations), and meconium pseudocyst. Gastrointestinal masses are second in frequency to masses of genitourinary origin in the neonate, estimated to comprise 15% of neonatal abdominal masses. Most gastrointestinal masses are enteric duplication cysts, occurring more commonly in the ileocecal region. The recognition of the "rim" sign of the cyst wall on US is considered virtually diagnostic of enteric duplication cysts. This comprises the echogenic inner rim of the mucosa and the hypoechoic outer rim of the muscle layer, giving a double layer (**Fig. 102.37A,B**) (51). Peristalsis in the cyst wall is also a helpful sign in the case of a gastrointestinal duplication cyst.

f. *Intussusception:* Intussusception usually occurs in the age group of 3 months to 3 years. The classic clinical triad consists of acute colicky abdominal pain, "currant jelly" or frankly bloody stools, and either a palpable mass or vomiting (4,25). Younger infants with intussusception may be lethargic. A two-view abdominal plain film is recommended as initial imaging. The

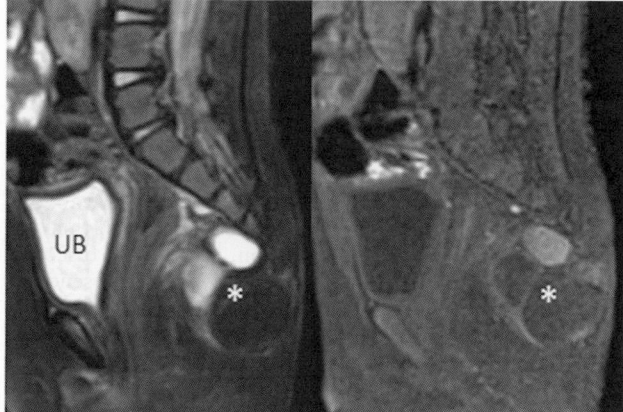

FIGURE 102.36. Sacrococcygeal teratoma. Fat-saturated T2W and postcontrast T1W MRI images show a complex mass arising from the coccyx with T2 bright and T1 hypointense cystic areas. Fatty areas within the mass (*asterisk*) appear dark (UB = urinary bladder).

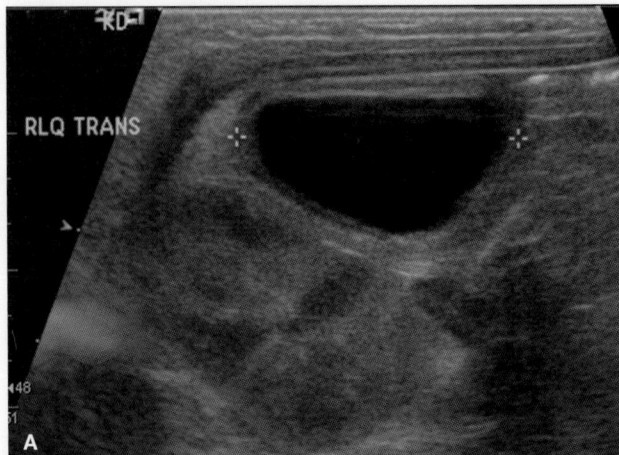

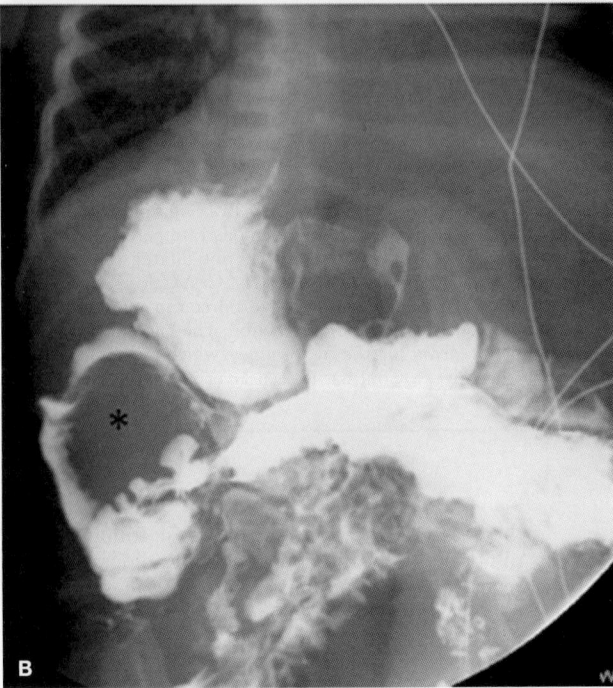

FIGURE 102.37. GI duplication cyst: 6-year-old with abdominal pain. **A:** US revealed a thick-walled anechoic cystic structure within the right mid-abdomen causing mild mass effect on the surrounding bowel. Thick-walled appearance of the cyst is from the bowel lining; this is the gut signature sign. **B:** Barium small-bowel follow-through study shows mass effect from the duplication cyst (*asterisk*) at the ileocecal valve without bowel obstruction.

presence of a curvilinear intraluminal mass in the right upper quadrant is highly specific for intussusception (**Fig. 102.38A**) (52). This finding may not be present, and it is helpful to look for a paucity of bowel gas in the right lower quadrant. Small-bowel obstruction and, in the case of perforation, free intraperitoneal air may be seen. US is a highly sensitive and specific test for intussusception and is the current imaging modality of choice for diagnosis (53). When viewed transversely, the alternating concentric hypoechoic and echogenic layers of an intussusception have an appearance referred to as the "target" or "donut" sign. Longitudinal images are obtained to confirm a bowel-within-bowel appearance; the hypoechoic muscle layer in the outer wall and the echogenic mucosa

on the inside can appear similar to a kidney leading to the pseudokidney sign (**Fig. 102.38B,C**). Reduction of the intussusception can be performed with air or water-soluble contrast enema, and surgical intervention can be avoided in most cases.

4. Trauma

Trauma in neonates is seen mainly in cases of motor vehicle collisions (MVCs) and child abuse. The liver is the most common organ injured following blunt trauma to the neonatal abdomen. In the older child, MVC and sports injuries are common causes of abdominal trauma and commonly result in injuries to the liver, spleen, pancreas, or kidneys. Focused abdominal sonography for trauma (FAST) can be employed, where the right and left upper quadrants and the pelvis are evaluated for the presence of free fluid or hemoperitoneum (**Fig. 102.12**). US is fast and easily available at the bedside in a critical care or emergency room setting and can be particularly helpful in the evaluation of a hemodynamically unstable patient trauma. However, US has technical limitations with variable sensitivity and specificity (54). CT is the imaging modality of choice for evaluation of abdominal injury after blunt trauma in a hemodynamically stable patient (55). CT with intravenous iodinated contrast is useful for evaluating the injured bowel and bladder, as well as vascular injury. Instillation of oral contrast helps to demonstrate small and large bowel injuries (5). However, because of the necessity for evaluating these patients urgently, oral contrast is generally not used. The liver is frequently injured in pediatric abdominal trauma, with the posterior segment of the right lobe the most commonly involved (**Fig. 102.39**) (56). The CT grading system for hepatic trauma by American Association of Surgery in Trauma (AAST) can be employed in older children (**Table 102.1**) (57). The degree of hepatic injury predicts the time required for healing, with mild injuries taking up to 3 months to heal, while severe injuries may take beyond 9 months (58). Splenic injury is usually associated with hemoperitoneum with the blood tracking along the splenorenal ligament into the anterior pararenal space around the pancreas, although 25% cases of splenic injury may not have free blood or fluid in the peritoneum. CT in the venous phase, that is, approximately 70-minute postintravenous contrast, can diagnose splenic lacerations (**Fig. 102.40**). Bowel injury following blunt trauma is rare in a child, but can occur in the form of intramural hematoma or bowel rupture. CT scan without contrast would show a hyperdense mass in the peripancreatic region related to the duodenum with or without mass effect (**Fig. 102.41**). Duodenal hematomas could be diagnosed earlier with UGI studies; however, CT scan can help to detect other associated intra-abdominal injuries (59). In the case of rupture of the bowel wall, one or more findings can be seen, including wall thickening, mesenteric fat infiltration, bowel wall discontinuity, or extraluminal air. However, the presence of a moderate amount of peritoneal fluid not explained by other obvious injuries is also suspicious for bowel injury. Hemoperitoneum on US appears as free fluid with internal echoes. On CT, measurement of density of the peritoneal fluid helps detect the presence of blood, which measures between 30 and 60 HU. Hypotensive patients following blood loss often show hypoperfusion complex, which is a constellation of findings that include abnormally intense contrast enhancement of the bowel wall, mesentery, adre-

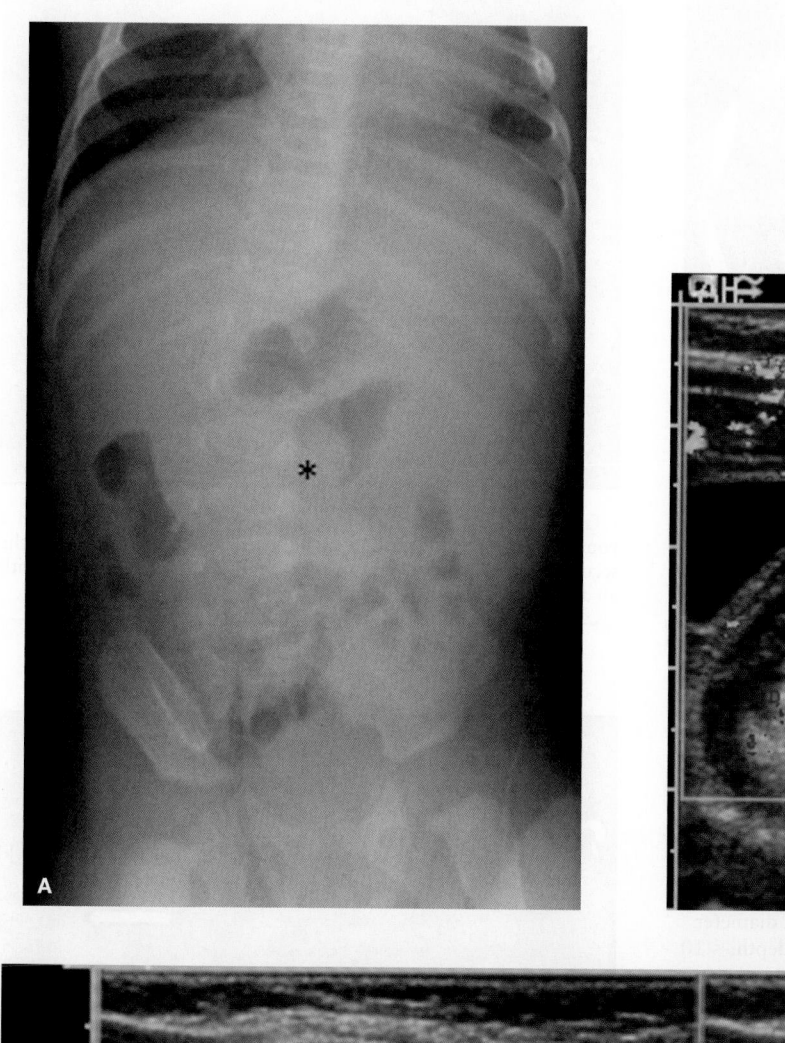

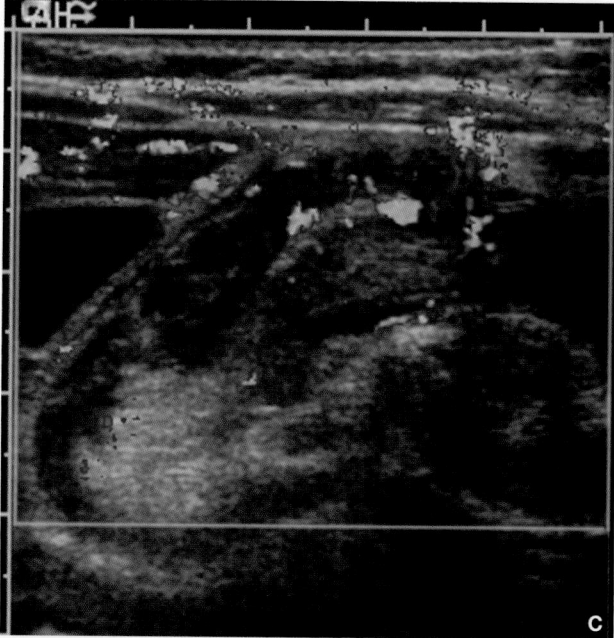

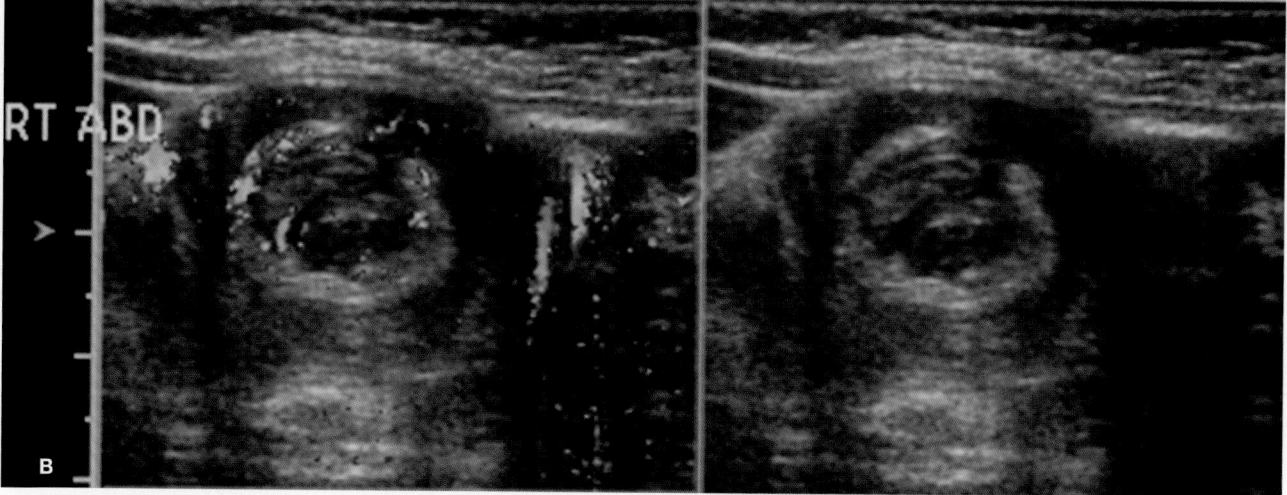

FIGURE 102.38. Intussusception. **A:** 3-month-old female with abdominal pain, vomiting, and lethargy. There is clinical concern for intussusception with an abnormal bowel gas pattern with a soft-tissue mass (*asterisk*) in the center of the abdomen seen on the obstructive series. There was no pneumoperitoneum. **B:** Targeted survey sonogram of the abdomen demonstrates the right upper quadrant ileocolic intussusception. In transverse US images, echogenic serosa of the intussusceptum is seen inside the lumen of intussuscipiens, giving rise to a target sign or donut sign through the intussusception. Color Doppler blood flow is demonstrated within the walls of bowel loops. **C:** Longitudinal image through the intussusception shows a pseudokidney sign. A small amount of free peritoneal fluid is seen.

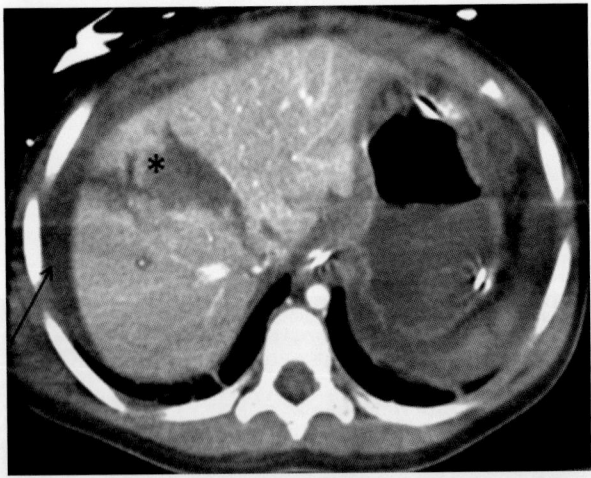

FIGURE 102.39. Liver laceration. Infant with blunt abdominal trauma. CT scan shows irregular hypoattenuation through the right hepatic lobe in keeping with a laceration (*asterisk*). Free abdominal fluid is also noted (*arrow*).

TABLE 102.1

CT GRADING SYSTEM FOR HEPATIC TRAUMA BY AMERICAN ASSOCIATION OF SURGERY IN TRAUMA

■ GRADE	■ DESCRIPTION
I	Hematoma: subcapsular, <10% surface area Laceration: capsular tear, <1 cm in parenchymal depth
II	Hematoma: subcapsular, 10%–50% surface area; intraparenchymal, <10 cm in diameter Laceration: 1–3 cm in parenchymal depth; <10 cm in length
III	Hematoma: subcapsular >50% area ruptured with active bleed; intraparenchymal, >10 cm Laceration: >3 cm in parenchymal depth
IV	Hematoma: ruptured intraparenchymal hematoma with active bleeding Laceration: parenchymal disruption 25%–75% of a hepatic lobe or 1–3 segments in a single lobe
V	Laceration: parenchymal disruption >75% of a hepatic lobe or >3 segments in a single lobe
VI	Vascular: hepatic pedicular avulsion

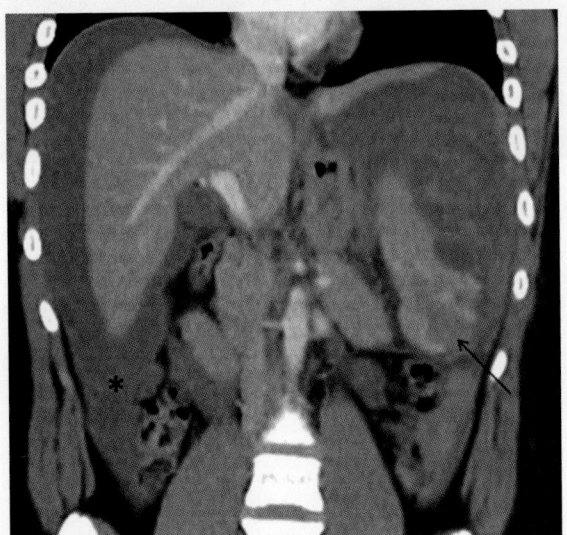

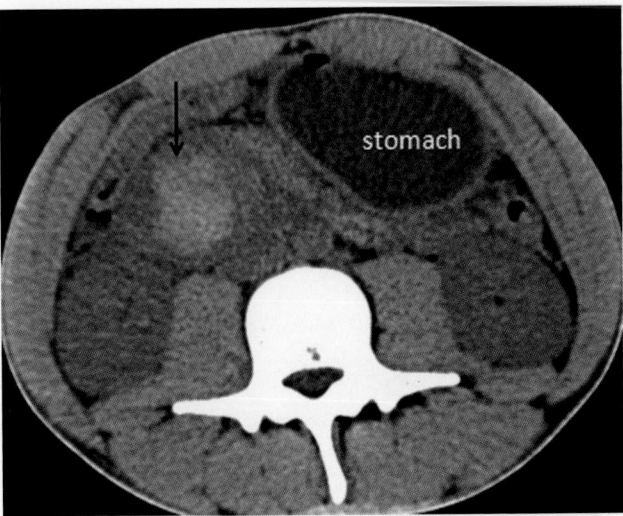

FIGURE 102.41. Duodenal hematoma. Noncontrast CT scan in a young patient in a MVC shows a high-attenuating mass lesion in the second and third portions of the duodenum (*arrow*) compatible with an acute duodenal hematoma.

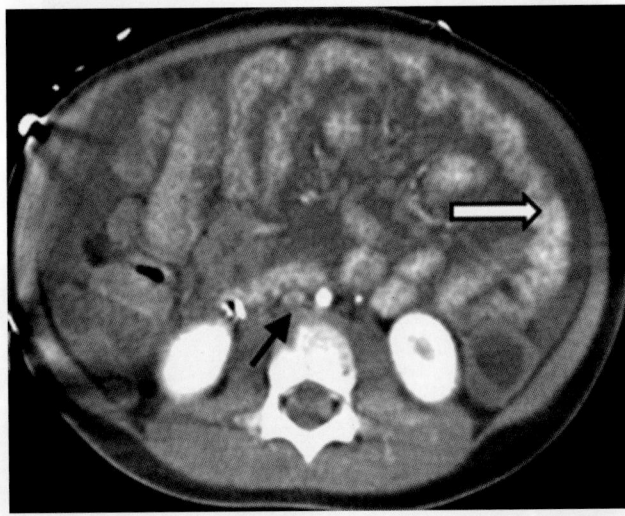

FIGURE 102.42. Hypoperfusion complex. CT scan with contrast of a patient in a setting of blunt abdominal trauma. There is significant enhancement of the bowel mucosa (*blocked arrow*) and kidneys with decreased caliber of the IVC and aorta (*black arrow*), consistent with hypoperfusion complex or shock bowel.

FIGURE 102.40. Splenic injury. CT with contrast of a 17-year-old with blunt abdominal injury following a football game shows splenic lacerations along the inferior pole (*arrow*) with an extensive perisplenic/subcapsular hematoma. CT scan with contrast can also help in detecting areas concerning for active extravasation as described. High-density ascites (*asterisk*) is suggestive of hemoperitoneum.

nals, and kidneys along with decreased caliber of the inferior vena cava (IVC), and aorta (**Fig. 102.42**) (60).

SUMMARY

Diagnostic imaging forms a critical component of management of abdominal conditions in the pediatric patient. Knowledge of applications of various radiologic imaging tests in a child can help the pediatric intensive care provider to request appropriate imaging tests and to provide efficient care. Findings on plain radiographs are helpful for recognition of critical findings in many types of abdominal pathology. The indications and applications of advanced studies including US, CT, and MRI have been provided.

FUTURE DIRECTIONS

In the era of imaging gently, the use of digital radiography with a constant effort to decrease the radiation dose in keeping with ALARA (As Low As Reasonably Achievable) radiation safety guidelines while obtaining diagnostic quality radiographs is necessary. Increased use of modalities without ionizing radiation (US and MRI) and decreased use of CT should be encouraged.

References

1. McParland BJ, Gorka W, Lee R, et al. Radiology in the neonatal intensive care unit: Dose reduction and image quality. *Br J Radiol* 1996;69(826):929–37.
2. Stringer DA. *Pediatric Gastrointestinal Imaging.* St Louis, MO: B.C. Decker, 1989:654.
3. Kirks DR, Rosenberg ER, Johnson DG, et al. Integrated imaging of neonatal renal masses. *Pediatr Radiol* 1985;15(3):147–56.
4. Swischuk LE. *Imaging of the Newborn, Infant, and Young Child.* 4th ed. Baltimore, MD: Williams & Wilkins, 1997:1088.
5. Coley B. Editor in Chief. *Caffey's Pediatric Diagnostic Imaging.* 12th ed. Philadelphia, PA: Mosby, 2013.
6. Kirks DR, Griscom NT. *Practical Pediatric Imaging: Diagnostic Radiology of Infants and Children.* 3rd ed. Philadelphia, PA: Lippincott-Raven, 1998:1226.
7. Bulas DI, Taylor GA, Eichelberger MR. The value of CT in detecting bowel perforation in children after blunt abdominal trauma. *Am J Roentgenol* 1989;153(3):561–4.
8. Coursey CA, Hollingsworth CL, Wriston C, et al. Radiographic predictors of disease severity in neonates and infants with necrotizing enterocolitis. *Am J Roentgenol* 2009;193(5):1408–13.
9. Kurbegov AC, Sondheimer JM. Pneumatosis intestinalis in non-neonatal pediatric patients. *Pediatrics* 2001;108(2):402–6.
10. Shabib SM, Al Mane K, McDonald P. Pneumatosis intestinalis beyond the newborn period. *Saudi J Gastroenterol* 2000;6(1):47–50.
11. Strouse PJ. Disorders of intestinal rotation and fixation ("malrotation"). *Pediatr Radiol* 2004;34(11):837–51.
12. Menten R, Reding R, Godding V, et al. Sonographic assessment of the retroperitoneal position of the third portion of the duodenum: An indicator of normal intestinal rotation. *Pediatr Radiol* 2012;42(8):941–5.
13. Garcia-Criado A, Gilabert R, Berzigotti A, et al. Doppler ultrasound findings in the hepatic artery shortly after liver transplantation. *Am J Roentgenol* 2009;193(1):128–35.
14. Strauss KJ, Goske MJ, Kaste SC, et al. Image gently: Ten steps you can take to optimize image quality and lower CT dose for pediatric patients. *Am J Roentgenol* 2010;194(4):868–73.
15. Yu L, Bruesewitz MR, Thomas KB, et al. Optimal tube potential for radiation dose reduction in pediatric CT: Principles, clinical implementations, and pitfalls. *Radiographics* 2011;31(3):835–48.
16. Darge K, Anupindi SA, Jaramillo D. MR imaging of the abdomen and pelvis in infants, children, and adolescents. *Radiology* 2011;261(1):12–29.
17. Chandler JC, Gauderer MW. The neonate with an abdominal mass. *Pediatr Clin North Am* 2004;51(4):979–97, ix.
18. Hernanz-Schulman M, Sells LL, Ambrosino MM, et al. Hypertrophic pyloric stenosis in the infant without a palpable olive: Accuracy of sonographic diagnosis. *Radiology* 1994;193(3):771–6.
19. Applegate KE, Anderson JM, Klatte EC. Intestinal malrotation in children: A problem-solving approach to the upper gastrointestinal series. *Radiographics* 2006;26(5):1485–500.
20. Karmazyn B. Duodenum between the aorta and the SMA does not exclude malrotation. *Pediatr Radiol* 2013;43(1):121–2.
21. Berrocal T, Lamas M, Gutieerrez J, et al. Congenital anomalies of the small intestine, colon, and rectum. *Radiographics* 1999;19(5):1219–36.
22. Franken EA, Smith WL. *Gastrointestinal Imaging in Pediatrics.* 2nd ed. Philadelphia, PA: Harper & Row, 1982:635.
23. Coran AG, Teitelbaum DH. Recent advances in the management of Hirschsprung's disease. *Am J Surg* 2000;180(5):382–7.
24. Dennehy PH. Acute diarrheal disease in children: Epidemiology, prevention, and treatment. *Infect Dis Clin North Am* 2005;19(3):585–602.
25. Cogley JR, O'Connor SC, Houshyar R, et al. Emergent pediatric US: What every radiologist should know. *Radiographics* 2012;32(3):651–65.
26. d'Almeida M, Jose J, Oneto J, et al. Bowel wall thickening in children: CT findings. *Radiographics* 2008;28(3):727–46.
27. McNamara A, Levine D. Intraabdominal fetal echogenic masses: A practical guide to diagnosis and management. *Radiographics* 2005;25(3):633–45.
28. Gubernick JA, Rosenberg HK, Ilaslan H, et al. US approach to jaundice in infants and children. *Radiographics* 2000;20(1):173–95.
29. Adeyiga AO, Lee EY, Eisenberg RL. Focal hepatic masses in pediatric patients. *Am J Roentgenol* 2012;199(4):W422–40.
30. Sivit CJ, Applegate KE. Imaging of acute appendicitis in children. *Semin Ultrasound CT MR* 2003;24(2):74–82.
31. Rodriguez DP, Vargas S, Callahan MJ, et al. Appendicitis in young children: Imaging experience and clinical outcomes. *Am J Roentgenol* 2006;186(4):1158–64.
32. Kaiser S, Jorulf H, Soderman E, et al. Impact of radiologic imaging on the surgical decision-making process in suspected appendicitis in children. *Acad Radiol* 2004;11(9):971–9.
33. Hoeffel C, Crema MD, Belkacem A, et al. Multi-detector row CT: Spectrum of diseases involving the ileocecal area. *Radiographics* 2006;26(5):1373–90.
34. Levy AD, Hobbs CM. From the archives of the AFIP. Meckel diverticulum: Radiologic features with pathologic Correlation. *Radiographics* 2004;24(2):565–87.
35. Shafey A, Ethier MC, Traubici J, et al. Incidence, risk factors, and outcomes of enteritis, typhlitis, and colitis in children with acute leukemia. *J Pediatr Hematol Oncol* 2013;35(7):514–7.
36. McCarville MB, Adelman CS, Li C, et al. Typhlitis in childhood cancer. *Cancer* 2005;104(2):380–7.
37. Kawashima A, Sandler CM, Ernst RD, et al. Imaging of nontraumatic hemorrhage of the adrenal gland. *Radiographics* 1999;19(4):949–63.
38. Westra SJ, Zaninovic AC, Hall TR, et al. Imaging of the adrenal gland in children. *Radiographics* 1994;14(6):1323–40.
39. Donnelly LF, Bisset GS III. Pediatric hepatic imaging. *Radiol Clin North Am* 1998;36(2):413–27.
40. Isaacs H Jr. Fetal and neonatal hepatic tumors. *J Pediatr Surg* 2007;42(11):1797–803.

41. Chung EM, Cube R, Lewis RB, et al. From the archives of the AFIP: Pediatric liver masses: Radiologic-pathologic correlation. Part 1. Benign tumors. *Radiographics* 2010;30(3):801–26.

42. Chung EM, Lattin GE Jr, Cube R, et al. From the archives of the AFIP: Pediatric liver masses: Radiologic-pathologic correlation. Part 2. Malignant tumors. *Radiographics* 2011;31(2):483–507.

43. De Angelis P, Foschia F, Romeo E, et al. Role of endoscopic retrograde cholangiopancreatography in diagnosis and management of congenital choledochal cysts: 28 pediatric cases. *J Pediatr Surg* 2012;47(5):885–8.

44. Iqbal CW, Baron TH, Moir CR, et al. Post-ERCP pancreatitis in pediatric patients. *J Pediatr Gastroenterol Nutr* 2009;49(4):430–4.

45. Lowe LH, Isuani BH, Heller RM, et al. Pediatric renal masses: Wilms tumor and beyond. *Radiographics* 2000;20(6):1585–603.

46. Hoffer FA. Magnetic resonance imaging of abdominal masses in the pediatric patient. *Semin Ultrasound CT MR* 2005;26(4): 212–23.

47. Ziereisen F, Guissard G, Damry N, et al. Sonographic imaging of the paediatric female pelvis. *Eur Radiol* 2005;15(7):1296–309.

48. Schmahmann S, Haller JO. Neonatal ovarian cysts: Pathogenesis, diagnosis and management. *Pediatr Radiol* 1997;27(2):101–5.

49. Hayashi S, Sago H, Kashima K, et al. Prenatal diagnosis of fetal hydrometrocolpos secondary to a cloacal anomaly by magnetic resonance imaging. *Ultrasound Obstet Gynecol* 2005;26(5):577–9.

50. Kocaoglu M, Frush DP. Pediatric presacral masses. *Radiographics* 2006;26(3):833–57.

51. Khong PL, Cheung SC, Leong LL, et al. Ultrasonography of intra-abdominal cystic lesions in the newborn. *Clin Radiol* 2003;58(6):449–54.

52. del-Pozo G, Albillos JC, Tejedor D, et al. Intussusception in children: Current concepts in diagnosis and enema reduction. *Radiographics* 1999;19(2):299–319.

53. Hryhorczuk AL, Strouse PJ. Validation of US as a first-line diagnostic test for assessment of pediatric ileocolic intussusception. *Pediatr Radiol* 2009;39(10):1075–9.

54. Sivit CJ. Imaging children with abdominal trauma. *Am J Roentgenol* 2009;192(5):1179–89.

55. Browning JG, Wilkinson AG, Beattie T. Imaging paediatric blunt abdominal trauma in the emergency department: Ultrasound versus computed tomography. *Emerg Med J* 2008;25(10):645–8.

56. Stalker HP, Kaufman RA, Towbin R. Patterns of liver injury in childhood: CT analysis. *Am J Roentgenol* 1986;147(6):1199–205.

57. Yoon W, Jeong YY, Kim JK, et al. CT in blunt liver trauma. *Radiographics* 2005;25(1):87–104.

58. Bulas DI, Eichelberger MR, Sivit CJ, et al. Hepatic injury from blunt trauma in children: Follow-up evaluation with CT. *Am J Roentgenol* 1993;160(2):347–51.

59. Berger PE, Kuhn JP. CT of blunt abdominal trauma in childhood. *Am J Roentgenol* 1981;136(1):105–10.

60. Sivit CJ, Eichelberger MR, Taylor GA. CT in children with rupture of the bowel caused by blunt trauma: Diagnostic efficacy and comparison with hypoperfusion complex. *Am J Roentgenol* 1994;163(5):1195–8.

CHAPTER 103 ■ ACUTE LIVER FAILURE AND LIVER TRANSPLANTATION

PIERRE TISSIERES AND DENIS J. DEVICTOR

KEY POINTS

1 Infants and children with acute liver failure (ALF) should be referred to centers with expertise in pediatric liver disease, as determination of an accurate etiologic diagnosis before encephalopathy occurs is critical.

2 Liver support devices may stabilize hemodynamics, improve neurologic status, and give additional time for emergency liver transplantation (LT).

3 Encephalopathy and coagulation parameter (factor V activity, prothrombin time, and international normalized

ratio) kinetics are major ALF severity criteria that aid in deciding whether to perform emergency LT.

4 Care following LT requires a complete understanding of the surgical and medical specificities of hepatic diseases and the management of postoperative complex multiorgan failure.

5 LT has drastically changed prognosis of pediatric ALF and end-stage liver disease.

ACUTE LIVER FAILURE

Acute liver failure (ALF) is a rare disease in most countries but remains endemic in some regions where viral hepatitis is highly prevalent. In the United States, the estimated frequency of ALF is 17 cases per 100,000 per year, inclusive of all age groups. The incidence of ALF in the pediatric population is unknown but accounts for 10%–15% of all pediatric liver transplantations (LTs) (1,2). In neonates and infants, metabolic diseases are the main cause of ALF and many are amenable to medical therapies, which may preclude the need for LT (3,4). In older children, viruses (especially hepatitis A virus), drug-induced hepatotoxicity, and autoimmune hepatitis are the most common identified causes of ALF. The cause of ALF remains undetermined in a large proportion of children (3,5,6). Consensus recommendations regarding management of ALF in adults have been published but these remain scarce for children (7–10). This chapter examines the specificities of ALF in neonates and children with emphasis on definition, emerging causes, clinical presentation, and controversies in management. Available medical therapies for metabolic diseases presenting with ALF in infancy are also discussed.

Definition and Classification of ALF

ALF was originally described, by Trey and Davidson in 1970, as a severe liver injury in a patient with no previous history of liver disease, which progressed to hepatic encephalopathy (HE) within 8 weeks of the initial symptoms (usually onset of jaundice). This definition was inadequate for infants and children who may present with ALF from an asymptomatic metabolic disease with encephalopathy unrelated to ALF or who may not develop encephalopathy in the course of ALF despite an unfavorable outcome. ALF in children is defined as a multisystemic disorder involving severe impairment of liver function, with or without encephalopathy, in the absence of underlying liver disease. Since 1999, the pediatric acute liver failure (PALF) study group, a consortium of 24 active pediatric

hepatology centers, created a database of children with ALF (6). Their criteria for pediatric ALF includes patients from birth through 18 years who meet the following criteria: (a) no evidence of chronic liver disease, (b) biochemical evidence of acute liver injury, and (c) hepatic-based coagulopathy defined as a prothrombin time (PT) ≥15 seconds or an international normalized ratio (INR) ≥1.5 not corrected by vitamin K and the presence of HE, or PT ≥20 seconds or INR ≥2.0 regardless of the presence or absence of clinical HE. In some countries, coagulation factor V <50% is part of the definition of hepatic-based coagulopathy.

Causes of ALF

ALF can be schematically classified into seven categories: metabolic, infective, toxic, autoimmune, malignancy-induced, vascular-induced, or undetermined (18%–47% of cases) (2,3,10–17) (**Table 103.1**). The relationships between these etiologies are highly age-dependent. Early identification of the cause of ALF is of paramount importance for several reasons. In some cases, ALF may be reversed with immediate initiation of specific therapies. This is principally the case in certain metabolic diseases (galactosemia, fructosemia, and hereditary tyrosinemia type 1 [HT-1]), Wilson disease, autoimmune hepatitis, or acetaminophen-induced ALF (4,18). Alternatively, early identification is important when LT is not an option (leukemia and mitochondrial respiratory chain disorders with neurological involvement). These challenges, as well as determining who may recover without LT, highlight the importance **1** of early referral to pediatric liver transplant centers. Finally, some causes require specific therapy to be administered to the patient's family, such as in cases of hepatitis B virus or neonatal herpes infection.

Causes in Neonates and Infants

Among neonates and infants, viral infection and inborn metabolic disorders are the two main causes of ALF.

TABLE 103.1

CAUSES OF ALF IN INFANTS AND CHILDREN ADMITTED AT THE BICÊTRE HOSPITAL PICU (1986–2007) AND COMPARED TO THE PALF STUDY GROUP[a]

CATEGORY	CAUSES	BICÊTRE (1986–2007) MONOCENTER STUDY			PALF[a] (1999–2008) MULTICENTER STUDY[b]		
		<1 Y (*n* = 107)	≥1 Y (*n* = 128)	TOTAL (*n* = 235)	<7 MO (*n* = 149)	≥7 MO (*n* = 554)	TOTAL (*n* = 703)
Metabolic	Galactosemia, tyrosinemia, hemochromatosis, Wilson disease, Reye syndrome, fatty-acid oxidation disorder, mitochondrial respiratory chain disorders	54 (50%)	27 (21%)	81 (34%)	27 (18%)	41 (7%)	68 (10%)
Infectious	HAV, HBV, herpes simplex, HHV6, EBV, enterovirus, adenovirus, parvovirus B19, Dengue fever	19 (18%)	33 (26%)	52 (22%)	20 (13%)	25 (4%)	45 (6%)
Toxic	Acetaminophen, sulfamide, sodium valproate, sulfasalazine, halothane, amanita phalloides, chemotherapy	7 (7%)	25 (19%)	32 (14%)	3 (2%)	108 (19%)	111 (16%)
Autoimmune	Giant cell hepatitis, LKM or LC1 autoimmune hepatitis	8 (7%)	7 (5%)	15 (6%)	0 (0%)	48 (9%)	48 (7%)
Malignancy-induced	Familial lymphohistiocytosis, macrophage activation syndrome, leukemia	7 (7%)	3 (2%)	10 (4%)	-	-	-
Vascular	Veno-occlusive disease, Budd–Chiari syndrome	2 (2%)	1 (1%)	3 (1%)			
Other	Ischemic liver	-	-	-	38 (25%)	64 (12%)	102 (14%)
Undetermined		10 (9%)	32 (25%)	42 (18%)	61 (49%)	268 (48%)	329 (47%)

[a]PALF, Pediatric acute liver failure study group adapted from Ref. 6.
[b]The consortium consists of 24 active pediatric liver transplant centers.HAV, hepatitis A virus; HBV, hepatitis B virus; HHV, human herpes virus; LKM, liver kidney microsome; LC1, liver cytosol 1.
From Devictor D, Tissieres P, Durand P, et al. Acute liver failure in neonates, infants and children. *Expert Rev Gastroenterol Hepatol* 2011;5(6):717–29.

Viral Infections. Enteroviruses, particularly Echovirus, serotype 11, are frequently identified viral causes of ALF in neonates. Severe infection with multiorgan involvement, including the liver, occurs almost exclusively in newborns typically between days 4 and 7 (18,19). Mortality is high, but treatment with a new anti-picornaviral drug, pleconaril, may improve the outcome (20). Neonatal herpes simplex virus (HSV 1 and 2) infection may be transmitted during delivery due to exposure to infected maternal genital secretions or lesions or after birth from infected contacts. Symptoms typically develop after day 5 (18,19,21). Liver failure may occur with disseminated disease (involving the skin, eyes, mucous membranes, brain, and lung) or as the only manifestation. Despite acyclovir therapy, the prognosis is poor. Successful LT has been reported. Although uncommon, primary HSV infections in pregnant women can result in maternal disseminated HSV infection with a mortality reaching 50% (22). Human herpes virus 6 (HHV6), adenovirus, parvovirus B19, and paramyxovirus are other viruses that have also been associated with neonatal acute liver failure.

Inborn Metabolic Disorders. Congenital galactosemia is an autosomal recessive disorder due to a deficiency of the enzyme galactose-1-phosphate uridyltransferase (4,17,23). The onset occurs usually early in the neonatal period. Complete elimination of dietary lactose/galactose results in resolution of liver failure. Galactosemia should be strongly considered in neonates with cataracts and/or *Escherichia coli* sepsis.

Hereditary fructose intolerance (HFI) is an autosomal recessive disorder due to a deficiency of the enzyme fructose-1-phosphate aldolase. Symptoms develop only once fructose is introduced in the diet. Therefore, symptoms do not usually occur in neonates who are fed with fructose-free milk formulas (except for those given medications or rehydration formulas containing fructose, sucrose, or sorbitol). Complete elimination of fructose results in a dramatic improvement within 2 days.

Hereditary tyrosinemia type 1 (HT-1) is an autosomal recessive disorder, caused by a deficiency of fumarylacetoacetate hydrolase, which results in accumulation of toxic metabolites responsible for liver and proximal renal tubular dysfunctions, and porphyria-like crises (24–26). Infants most often present with coagulopathy soon after birth. Clinical signs of liver failure become apparent usually within 1 and 6 months of age. Management includes nitisinone (NTBC [2-(2-nitro-4-trifluoromethylbenzoil)-1,3 cyclohexanedione]) therapy associated with a tyrosine- and phenylalanine-restricted diet, which proves curative in 90% of cases. Infants who do not respond to NTBC are considered for LT.

Mitochondrial respiratory chain disorders (e.g., inborn errors of oxidative phosphorylation) can also cause liver failure (27). Most infants also have extrahepatic features (neurological symptoms, myopathy, proximal renal tubular dysfunction, hypertrophic cardiomyopathy, and hematological and gastrointestinal [GI] disorders), although a few patients are reported with respiratory chain defects isolated to the liver. Prenatal liver disease is present in some cases. A thorough investigation is necessary to exclude significant extrahepatic involvement before LT can be proposed. In some cases, liver dysfunction may precede neurologic involvement for weeks, months, or years.

Inborn errors in bile acid synthesis, such as Δ 4-3-oxosteroid 5β-reductase deficiency, have been recognized as a cause of ALF associated with neonatal cholestasis and normal gamma-glutamyl transferase activity (17,28). Early diagnosis is important because oral administration of chenodeoxycholic acid and/or cholic acid may be curative.

Neonatal hemochromatosis is a rare perinatal disorder of abnormal iron storage associated with intrahepatic and extrahepatic iron accumulation that spares the reticuloendothelial system. The cause of this condition is unclear, but probably due to feto-maternal alloimmunization directed against the fetal liver (29). Liver injury has been identified as early as at 28 weeks of gestation. Oligohydramnios or hydramnios can complicate the pregnancy. Neonates are often premature and/or small for dates. The usual presentation is of acute decompensation of end-stage liver disease (ESLD) in the first few days of life, which leads to death in most cases. Early therapy with high-dose intravenous (IV) immunoglobulin G (IgG) in combination with exchange transfusion has been associated with a 75% survival without LT (29).

Other Causes. Familial hemophagocytic lymphohistiocytosis is a rare disorder involving inappropriate activation of macrophages that can present as ALF (30). Initial management includes chemotherapy, but long-term survival requires a bone marrow transplant. LT is contraindicated due to recurrence in the graft. Five of the following eight criteria need to be present in order to diagnose the condition: fever, cytopenia of two cell lines, hypertriglyceridemia and/or hypofibrinogenemia, hyperferritinemia (>500 μg/L), hemophagocytosis, elevated interleukin-2 (IL-2) receptor (CD25), decreased natural killer cell activity, and splenomegaly (30).

Causes in Children

The most common causes in children ≥1 year of age are drug-induced ALF, autoimmune hepatitis, and viral infections. In the PALF study, drug toxicity represents 19% of causes (mainly acetaminophen overdose). Autoimmune hepatitis and acute viral hepatitis represent 9% and 4% of the causes, respectively (31). In this series, 48% of the causes remained undetermined. In our series, the main causes were viral (infectious) ALF (26%), metabolic (21%), toxic (19%), or undetermined (25%) (18). These large differences could be explained by a center effect (single center's experience vs. a consortium experience) and differences in the exhaustiveness of the laboratory screening as outlined by PALF investigators (6,32).

Drug- or Toxin-Induced ALF. Drug intoxication leads to ALF in a large number of cases, either directly through hepatotoxicity or indirectly through an idiosyncratic reaction. Acetaminophen is the most identifiable cause of ALF in children living in Western countries. Acetaminophen toxicity injures hepatocytes in a dose-dependent fashion. ALF occurs as a result of conversion of acetaminophen to the highly reactive metabolite, N-acetyl-p-benzoquinone imine (NAPQI) through the cytochrome P-450 system. NAPQI is detoxified by glutathione. With depletion of hepatic glutathione stores, NAPQI binds to cysteine groups on protein, forming hepatotoxic protein adducts. There are at least two clinical presentations. The first is an acute, intentional ingestion (mostly teenagers), and the second referred to as a "therapeutic misadventure" relates to the ingestion of multiple doses taken over several days' time with the intent-to-treat clinical symptoms such as pain or fever, frequently in fasting children. If acetaminophen intoxication is suspected, specific therapy with N-acetylcysteine should be started without delay and may still

be useful 48 hours after ingestion (8,33) (see also Chapter 35, Poisoning). Sodium valproate can cause acute hepatic necrosis in 1 in 5000 treated children during the first 4–6 months after initiation of therapy. Such toxicity occurs more frequently in younger children or when associated with other seizure treatments. Sodium valproate-induced ALF has a significant resemblance to Reye syndrome and mitochondrial cytopathy, in which a microvacuolar steatosis associated with centrilobular necrosis is found. In adults, halothane is known to cause ALF in 1 in 35,000 halothane anesthetics, and the frequency increases if two exposures to halothane occur within 6 weeks. However, in children, incidence has been demonstrated to be >1 in 100,000 halothane anesthetics. Its pathogenicity involves an immune reaction with subsequent cellular inflammation and necrosis. Similarly, other volatile anesthetics (enflurane, isoflurane, and sevoflurane) have been documented to cause ALF in children (34). Other drugs, such as carbamazepine, sulfasalazine, antituberculosis drugs, and recreational drugs (ecstasy, cocaine), are involved in drug-induced ALF (35).

Toxin-induced liver injury is uncommon in children. It is mainly related to ingestion of amanita toxin, a known hepatotoxin present in different species of wild mushrooms (*Amanita phalloides*, *Lepiota* species). If the patient presents early with suspected mushroom poisoning, gastric lavage and activated charcoal administration should be performed. Importantly, symptoms (profuse diarrhea, vomiting) and hepatotoxicity are more severe in young children compared to adults, and warrant an early transfer to a pediatric LT center. Penicillin G and silibinin (silymarin) are the accepted antidotes. However, mushroom poisoning continues to have a low rate of transplant-free rate of survival. Phosphorus and carbon tetrachloride intoxication are other potential causes of ALF.

Immune Dysregulation. Autoimmune hepatitis occurs as a result of an immune reaction to liver cell antigens. Patients present with progressive jaundice, encephalopathy, and an uncorrectable coagulopathy over a period of 1–6 weeks. Usually, at least one serum autoimmune marker (e.g., antinuclear antibody, anti-smooth muscle antibody, liver-kidney-microsomal antibody, anti-cytosol type 1, soluble liver antigen) is detected. Diagnosis of autoimmune hepatitis is urgent because treatment with corticosteroids prior to the onset of HE may preclude the need for LT. Macrophage activation syndrome can also be associated with ALF and is frequently secondary to a viral infection (Parvovirus B19, HHV6).

Virus-Induced and Infective ALF. Hepatitis A virus is the most common cause of ALF in endemic areas. It is uncommon in North America or Europe. Hepatitis B-induced ALF is rare in infants, thanks to sero-vaccination (with maternal administration of hepatitis B immunoglobulin during pregnancy) of neonates born to HBsAg-positive mothers. Hepatitis E occurs within endemic areas such as India and Africa. Other virus-induced causes of ALF in children include adenovirus, human herpes virus-6, parvovirus B19, and Epstein–Barr virus (EBV). Bacterial and parasitic infections are usually not associated with ALF, although they may be observed in cases of exotoxin-induced ALF (invasive group A streptococcal infection) or during malignant hyperthermia secondary to malaria. In rare cases, congenital syphilis could cause ALF in infants. Leptospirosis, brucellosis, Q fever, and Dengue fever have been reported to cause ALF.

Metabolic Causes. Fulminant Wilson disease is currently the most common metabolic disease presenting with ALF in children and adolescents and is not observed in children younger than 7 years old (36,37). Biochemical features include evidence of Coombs-negative hemolytic anemia, coagulopathy, modest rises in serum aminotransferase levels, and low alkaline phosphatase in regard to the markedly elevated bilirubin (total bilirubin to alkaline phosphatase <1 μmol/IU). Serum copper and 24-hour urinary excretion of copper are increased and serum ceruloplasmin is decreased (normal in 15% of cases). The diagnosis can be rapidly determined by an ophthalmologist when Kayser–Fleischer rings are seen at slit lamp examination (36,37). Renal function is frequently impaired. Fulminant Wilson disease with HE is considered to be uniformly lethal without transplantation. However, if initiated prior to the onset of HE, chelating agents may preclude the need for an LT. A modified Nazer's Wilson disease score, based on the level of serum bilirubin, aspartate amino transferase, INR, and white blood cells at presentation, may predict the need for transplantation (36). The benefit of albumin dialysis as a bridge to LT has been reported in some anecdotal cases in adults and children (38).

Vascular Causes. In children, as in adults, veno-occlusive disease of the liver (i.e., hepatic vein occlusion following hematopoietic stem cell transplantation or chemotherapy), Budd–Chiari syndrome (i.e., obstruction of the hepatic venous outflow), or "cardiac liver" (congested liver secondary to right heart failure) may present as ALF. A reversible hepatic insufficiency occurs frequently after cardiogenic shock, septic shock, multiorgan failure, or any significant hypoperfusion state.

Diagnosis of ALF

Clinical Manifestations

Clinical symptoms vary according to the cause of ALF and the age of the child (3,5,18,39,40). In the newborn, symptoms are nonspecific, sometimes only related to an altered general condition, failure to thrive, and vomiting, whereas in older children, most have jaundice associated with HE.

In the newborn, the clinical presentation depends on the etiology of ALF. Presentation at birth implies an intrauterine insult such as a congenital infection, neonatal hemochromatosis, or mitochondrial disorders. A later presentation may be related to a bacterial or a viral infection or a metabolic condition unveiled by the introduction of feeding (i.e., galactosemia, HFI, HT-1). A detailed family history, including information on consanguinity, previous miscarriages, neonatal deaths, and liver disease in sibling, is important to record. Early symptoms are nonspecific, sometimes only related to an altered general condition, poor feeding, lethargy, failure to thrive, and vomiting. Jaundice may be absent, especially when inborn metabolic diseases are involved. Encephalopathy can be a late feature and is particularly difficult to diagnose in neonates. Behavioral changes, irritability, and reversal of day/night sleep patterns indicate HE. Convulsions may reflect meningoencephalitic involvement or be related to hypoglycemia. Hepatomegaly is very often present. Splenomegaly and ascites are usually noted in cases of severe disease progressing to cirrhosis. The diagnosis of ALF must be considered in any neonate with coagulopathy. Hypoglycemia and hyperammonemia are common, although these may be related to the underlying disease. High serum transaminases usually result from hepatocyte necrosis associated with acute viral infection, toxin, or ischemic injury. In contrast, there is normal to moderate elevation of transaminases and minimal to moderate jaundice in metabolic liver diseases.

In infants or older children, there is usually a prodromal phase of malaise, nausea, and anorexia. Most often jaundice is a late development. Occasionally, jaundice does not develop (especially when the cause of ALF is a metabolic disease or toxic) and clinical diagnosis of ALF becomes more difficult. Hemorrhage may occur spontaneously, and usually involves the digestive tract. Severe hypoglycemia, which may lead to seizures, is frequently observed (3,5,18,39,40). HE may be absent in

spite of severe liver dysfunction or develop within a few hours to days or weeks from onset of liver failure. In older children, signs and symptoms are similar to those in adults but the classical symptoms of asterixis, tremors, and fetor hepaticus are often absent.

HE is a complex neuropsychiatric syndrome characterized by a reversible chemical and neurophysiologic status that occurs when liver function is altered. HE pathophysiology is complex and multifactorial. Various nonexclusive pathophysiologic mechanisms deserve mention: (a) *the hyperammonemia theory*, in which hyperammonemia is thought to have a "direct" effect on neuronal membranes, enhancement of neuroinhibitory γ-aminobutyric acid (GABA)-mediated transmission by direct activation of GABA receptors, and "indirect" effect on neuronal dysfunction due to disturbance of glutamate neurotransmission and plasma amino acid profile; (b) *the false-neurotransmitter theory*, in which liver failure modifies the plasma amino acid profile (increase in aromatic amino acids, decrease in branched-chain amino acids) that results in alterations to brain metabolism; and (c) *the neuroinhibition, or GABA-benzodiazepine, theory*, which is characterized by increased levels of neuroinhibitory GABA and a synergistic neuroinhibitory effect with benzodiazepine receptor ligands, explaining why, in some cases, use of flumazenil has shown to reverse encephalopathy without affecting outcome; *(d) the liver–brain inflammatory axis:* where systemic and neuroinflammation and microglial activation act synergistically with ammonia on the development of cerebral edema (41). It is essential to recognize the difference between the HE that occurs in chronic liver disease and the acute HE that occurs during ALF, which is often associated with cerebral edema and intracranial hypertension (42,43). HE can occur a few hours to days after jaundice appears. In the newborn, HE is nonspecific and can be reflected only by behavioral changes, agitation, and a high-pitched cry. These signs may precede the development of brisk reflexes, clonus, and appearance of a coma with hypertonia, agitation, and pupillary abnormalities (sluggish, then fixed), followed by a deeper coma with hypotonia and brainstem coning. In older children, signs and symptoms are identical to those in adults. HE is classified into four grades using a modification of the West Haven criteria (Table 103.2) and may demonstrate one of five electroencephalographic (EEG) patterns that correlate with prognosis (see below) (Table 103.3) (3). Status epilepticus may complicate HE, especially in grade IV. HE may be precipitated by disease progression as well as by infection, metabolic abnormalities, GI bleeding, excessive protein load (fresh frozen plasma), and portal vein thrombosis.

A detailed history in suspected cases of ALF might include family members with inheritable disease, birth history, exposure

TABLE 103.2

GRADES OF HEPATIC ENCEPHALOPATHY

I	Changes in behavior, minimal change in level of consciousness, altered sleep (hypersomnia, insomnia, inversed sleep cycle in the newborn)
II	Spatiotemporal disorientation, drowsiness, inappropriate behavior, obvious asterixis
III	Marked confusion, stuporous, respond or not to auditory stimuli, decerebrate posturing to pain, asterixis usually absent
IV	Comatose, unresponsive to pain, decorticate posturing

Adapted from the West Haven criterion; Atterbury CE, Maddrey WC, Conn HO. Neomycin-sorbitol and lactulose in the treatment of acute portal-systemic encephalopathy. A controlled, double-blind clinical trial. *Am J Dig Dis* 1978;23:398–406.

to sick contacts, relevant travel history, potential exposure to toxins, recent medications and dosages, and include symptoms such as onset of fatigue, drowsiness, recent deterioration in neurocognitive functioning, type and color of stool, color of urine, easy bruising, and abdominal pain.

TABLE 103.3

ELECTROENCEPHALOGRAPHIC PATTERN OF ACUTE LIVER FAILURE

Type I	Slow polyrhythmic activity associating 5–6 Hz, 3–4 Hz, 1–2 Hz frequencies with a reactive or inconsistently reactive EEG pattern
Type II	Slow theta-delta (3–4 Hz) activity of 50–100 μV amplitude. Inconsistent or absent EEG reactivity
Type III	Large (100–150 μV) monomorphic delta activity (1–3 Hz). No EEG reactivity
Type IV	Slow, depressed (<1 Hz) pattern, with decreasing amplitude. No EEG reactivity
Type V	Progressive disappearance of EEG activity

Diagnostic Workup

The diagnostic workup of ALF is directed toward establishing a diagnosis and characterizing the severity of liver failure (Table 103.4). Cholestasis is usually present in viral-induced ALF (levels of alkaline phosphatase and gamma-glutamyl transferase are usually elevated), cholestasis may be moderate in toxic ALF, and the absence of hyperbilirubinemia should suggest Reye syndrome. Increases in serum liver enzyme levels are usually proportional to the degree of hepatic necrosis. Marked elevation of liver enzymes (>3000 IU/L) is usually found; however, normal liver enzyme levels may not be favorable and could represent end-stage hepatic necrosis. In this case, decreased liver enzymes are accompanied by increased bilirubin and gamma-glutamyl transferase. Hemostasis abnormalities are closely correlated with severity of ALF. A prolonged PT or INR >2 and a factor V activity <50% are the most potent abnormalities. Additionally, hypofibrinogenemia and altered factor II, VII, and X activities are found. These alterations in hemostasis factors may be associated with a disseminated intravascular coagulopathy. A decreased factor V activity <30% underscores a severe liver injury. Other biochemical abnormalities include hypoglycemia, hyperammonemia, lactic acidosis, and hypoalbuminemia. Respiratory alkalosis secondary to neurogenic hyperventilation is frequently

TABLE 103.4

DIAGNOSTIC WORKUP OF ACUTE LIVER FAILURE

General workup

Na, K, Cl, Mg, Ca, BUN, creatinine, LDH, lactate, ammonia, blood gas, complete blood count, Coombs test, cultures from blood, urine, and CSF, blood group determination, AST, ALT, alkaline phosphatase, gamma-glutamyl transferase, total and conjugated bilirubin, alpha-fetoprotein, prothrombin time, international normalized ratio, partial thrombin time, fibrinogen, factors II, V, VII, IX, X activity, D-dimer.

Metabolic workup

Hereditary tyrosinemia type 1	Urine succinylacetone, wrist x-ray, plasma tyrosine, phenylalanine, methionine
Galactosemia	Red cell galactose-1-phosphate uridyltransferase activity (spot test) and GALT activity
Hereditary fructose intolerance	Mutations by PCR amplification of genomic DNA
Neonatal hemochromatosis	Ferritin level, extrahepatic iron deposition, i.e., salivary gland (biopsy, NMR)
Wilson disease	Serum ceruloplasmin, serum, and urinary copper, Kayser–Fleisher ring
Reye syndrome and fatty-acid oxidation disorders	Urinary and blood organic acid chromatography, carnitine and fatty-acid level
Mitochondrial cytopathy	Blood lactate/pyruvate. 3-OH-butyrate/acetoacetate; organic acids in urine. Mitochondrial DNA, muscle and liver biopsy for quantitative respiratory chain enzyme determination. CSF lactate, creatine kinase, echocardiography
Inborn errors of bile acid synthesis	Serum total bile acids, FAB-MS and GC-MS urine analysis
Urea cycle disorders	Plasma amino acids, urinary orotic acid
Congenital disorder of glycosylation syndrome	Transferrin isoelectric focusing

Infectious workup

Hepatitis A, B; HHV-1, 2, 6; CMV; EBV; VZV; echovirus; adenovirus; enterovirus; parovirus B19; paramyxovirus	Viral serology (mother and infant), keep frozen serum, PCR (blood, CSF), stool culture
Treponema pallidum (syphilis)	VDRL (maternal if newborn)

Other

Familial lymphohistiocytosis and macrophage activating syndrome	Blood triglycerides, cholesterol, ferritin, bone marrow analysis and phenotyping
Autoimmune	Coombs test, autoantibodies, biopsy
Leukemia	Bone marrow study
Neonatal lupus	Maternal autoantibodies
Intoxication	Acetaminophen level, salicylate level, keep frozen urine and blood
Vascular/hypoxic-ischemic	Echocardiography

NMR, nuclear magnetic resonance, OTC, ornithine transcarbamylase; HHV, human herpes virus; VZV, varicella-zoster virus; CSF, cerebrospinal fluid; VDRL, Venereal Disease Research Laboratory test; FAB-MS, fast atom bombardment—mass spectrometry; GC-MS, gas chromatography—mass spectrometry.

observed. Renal failure could indicate hepatorenal syndrome (more frequently observed with viral or toxic ALF). Lactic acidosis may indicate tissue hypoxia and severe liver failure. No optimal tool is available for monitoring time-responsive indicators of liver function. Blood lactate and coagulation parameters may be used, but the response time is slow. Preliminary work using kinetics of the indocyanine green elimination rate measured by pulse-dye densitometry may prove beneficial at the bedside to identify failing or recovery of the liver function (44).

Abdominal sonography allows the assessment of hepatic size, condition of the parenchyma, occurrence of ascites, and an evaluation of the vascular supply. Liver biopsy should be postponed, due to its associated elevated bleeding risk and reduced benefit. However, if required, the transjugular approach should be preferred due to a lower risk of intraperitoneal bleeding after this procedure (45). If mitochondrial respiratory chain defects are suspected, liver and muscle biopsy should be considered.

EEG abnormalities are associated with the various grades of HE. These are characterized by the association of diminished basal activity and the occurrence of characteristic slow triphasic waves that are not found in the youngest child. Five types of EEG pattern can be associated with prognosis (**Table 103.3**). Deceleration of the electric frequency below 2 Hz frequently precedes type IV HE. However, EEG pattern may not discriminate brain death from grade IV HE. Transcranial-Doppler ultrasound, somatosensory-evoked potential, nuclear brain flow, or cerebral angiography may be required to diagnose brain death. Electrical seizures usually indicate grade II or higher HE. Brain computerized tomography (CT) has a limited utility in fulminant liver failure. Although identification of cerebral edema is correlated with poor prognosis, CT scan is not a sensitive modality for detection of cerebral edema (46). Repetitive transcranial-Doppler examination of arterial cerebral flow is emerging as a useful tool with which to identify intracranial hypertension (19,47).

ALF etiologic diagnosis remains undetermined in ~30% of cases. Although most cases are related to an acute etiology, decompensated, previously unrecognized chronic liver disease may appear similar to viral ALF (e.g., fulminant Wilson disease, tyrosinemia, or chronic active autoimmune hepatitis). Decompensated, unrecognized chronic liver disease usually displays nodular and hard hepatomegaly and splenomegaly. The diagnostic workup in infants and children with ALF is summarized in **Table 103.4**.

Complications of ALF

Preoperative and early postoperative complications of FHF are listed in **Table 103.5**.

Cerebral Edema and Intracranial Hypertension

In children, cerebral edema with intracranial hypertension frequently occurs during FHF and is recognized as a major risk for death (1,3,46,48). In the newborn, symptoms include a tense fontanelle, axial hypertonia, oculomotor disturbances, decerebrate posturing, neurovegetative symptoms (apnea, Cushing triad, dysrhythmia), and absence of brainstem reflexes. Death following ALF is attributed to cerebral edema in 40% of cases.

Pathophysiology of intracranial hypertension is complex, involving cytotoxic and vasogenic cerebral edema, increase in blood–brain barrier permeability, increase in cerebral blood flow, loss of vascular cerebral autoregulation, and alteration in cerebral metabolism. Cytotoxic edema may develop in relation to Na^+, K^+-ATPase pump inhibition, ammonium accumulation, and deregulated equilibrium of cerebral osmotic amino acids. Alteration in ammonia metabolism is important in the development of cerebral edema through an effect on the Krebs cycle, an increase in brain lactate, and an increase in extracellular glutamate. It is now shown that cytokines play important synergistic roles in the pathogenesis of increased intracranial pressure (ICP) during ALF through glial activation and ammonia toxicity (41). An association has been demonstrated between cytokines levels (TNF-α, IL-6, and IL-1β) and development of intracranial hypertension in ALF. In addition, a de novo brain production of ammonia during uncontrolled intracranial hypertension was found (49). The nature of the signaling between the failing liver and central neuroinflammation is a current area of research interest (41). On one hand, it is shown that systemic pro- and anti-inflammatory response may initiate the process by direct transfer of cytokines by the way of active transport, interactions with receptors on circumventricular organs lacking blood–brain barrier, or activation of afferent neurons of the vagus nerve. Additionally, evidence suggests that toxins generated by the failing liver (ammonia, glutamate, manganese, neurosteroids) as well as oxidative stress participate, alone or in synergy, in glial activation.

Hemorrhage

In ALF, hemorrhage may occur spontaneously (<10% of patients). Procoagulant proteins (e.g., factors V, VII, X, and fibrinogen) and anticoagulant proteins (e.g., antithrombin, protein C, and protein S) are reduced. This balanced reduction in the pro-and anticoagulant proteins may account for the relative infrequency of clinically important bleeding in the absence of a provocative invasive procedure (vascular access, invasive intracranial monitoring). Use of ultrasound-guided central venous catheter insertion greatly reduces the risk of bleeding due to multiple inadvertent punctures.

TABLE 103.5

PREOPERATIVE AND EARLY POSTOPERATIVE COMPLICATIONS OF ACUTE LIVER FAILURE AND LIVER TRANSPLANTATION

■ PREOPERATIVE	■ POSTOPERATIVE
Cerebral edema, intracranial hypertension, kernicterus	Cerebral edema, intracranial hypertension
Circulatory collapse, dysrhythmia	Hypovolemia, hemorrhage, myocardial dysfunction
Hypoxemia, ARDS	Hypoxemia, ALI-VILI, ARDS
Renal failure, electrolyte disorders (hypoglycemia, hypokalemia, hyponatremia, hypophosphatemia, hypomagnesemia)	Renal failure, electrolyte disorders
Hemostasis disorders, disseminated intravascular coagulopathy, bleeding disorders (gastrointestinal, cerebral)	Anemia, thrombocytopenia, leukopenia, hemostasis disorders, disseminated intravascular coagulopathy
Bacterial sepsis	Bacterial and fungal sepsis
Metabolic disorders, lactic acidosis, hyperammonemia	Abdominal compartment syndrome, acute pancreatitis, hemorrhage (abdominal), primary graft nonfunction, graft vascular anastomosis stenosis/thrombosis, acute graft rejection
Adrenal insufficiency	

ARDS, acute respiratory distress syndrome; ALI, acute lung injury; VILI, ventilator-induced lung injury.

Renal Failure

Renal failure may be secondary to hypovolemia, acute tubular necrosis, or functional renal failure (hepatorenal syndrome). *Hepatorenal syndrome* is defined as a progressive renal insufficiency in patients with liver disease and is characterized by low urine sodium and elevated urinary-to-plasma ratios for creatinine and osmolarity. In patients with ALF, type 1 hepatorenal syndrome is found and defined as a rapid and progressive renal impairment. It is the result of the action of vasoconstrictor systems (i.e., the renin–angiotensin system, the sympathetic nervous system, and arginine vasopressin) on the renal circulation activated as a homeostatic response to improve the extreme underfilling of the splanchnic circulation. As a result, renal perfusion and glomerular filtration rate are greatly reduced but tubular function is preserved. Recognized risk factors are portal hypertension, low mean arterial blood pressure, and dilutional hyponatremia. Hepatorenal syndrome may be precipitated after GI bleeding, septicemia, and dehydration. Nephrotoxic drugs such as aminoglycosides should be avoided. Tubular nephropathy is frequently observed and results in low blood phosphate, magnesium, and potassium. Renal replacement therapy with continuous veno-venous hemofiltration may be necessary in some cases.

Cardiovascular and Pulmonary Complications

Pulmonary edema is an underestimated complication of ALF (up to 35% of patients). Causes may be related to the development of central neurogenic pulmonary edema coupled with fluid overload (syndrome of inappropriate antidiuretic hormone, hyperaldosteronism). In addition, ventilation–perfusion mismatch (loss of hypoxic vasoconstriction due to circulating vasodilatory substances) occurs and results in severe refractory hypoxemia and the hepatopulmonary syndrome of platypnea (shortness of breath when upright) and othrodeoxia (desaturation when upright).

The hemodynamic profile of ALF patients is characterized by cardiac hyperkinesia with elevated cardiac index and low systemic vascular resistances, and in many aspects looks similar to the early phase of septic shock (50). Adrenal insufficiency is frequently found in adults with ALF (up to 68% of cases) and is associated with hemodynamic instability (51). Dysrhythmias, such as sinus tachycardia, ectopic rhythms, and atrioventricular conduction block, are less frequent in children than in adults and are usually associated with electrolyte abnormalities.

Systemic Inflammatory Response Syndrome and Sepsis

A systemic inflammatory response syndrome (SIRS) is observed in 57% of adults with ALF, 68% of whom will develop secondary sepsis (52). Severity of SIRS may be correlated with progression of HE, development of respiratory failure, disseminated intravascular coagulopathy, renal failure, acute pancreatitis, and multiorgan failure. Risk of developing sepsis in the course of ALF is elevated, which may be related to a decreased immune response to pathogens and may be aggravated by invasive procedures inherent in the critically ill condition. Sepsis was shown to aggravate and worsen overall prognosis of patients with ALF and may participate in a quarter of all deaths following ALF. Incriminated pathogens are Gram-negative bacteria, cutaneous bacteria, and fungi (13%–32% of all infections) (53). ALF and septic shock share many phenotypic similarities. In both conditions, overwhelming activation of the immune response occurs, including the production of cytokines, chemokines, and activation of circulating immune cells, such as macrophage, monocytes, NK cells, NK T cells, $\gamma\delta$ T cells, as well as endothelial and Kupffer cells. Role of cytokines and immune response in the pathogenesis of systemic inflammatory response and multiple organ dysfunction syndrome during ALF is increasingly recognized and is thought playing a pivotal role in the initiation, propagation, and resolution of ALF.

Metabolic Complications

Severe hypoglycemia frequently occurs in ALF patients as a result of impaired glycogen storage, decreased gluconeogenesis, hyperinsulinism (decreased insulin degradation and increased insulin resistance), and increased glucose use (anaerobic metabolism) and should be recognized and treated early. The utilization of fat and protein stores leads to breakdown of muscle and adipose tissue. Increased glucagon and growth hormone levels further increase catabolism. Total energy expenditure is increased in ALF. Electrolyte abnormalities, such as hyponatremia, hypokalemia, hypophosphatemia, and hypomagnesemia, can be found in patients with ALF. Kernicterus may precipitate HE and appears if plasma direct bilirubin is >26 mg/dL, especially if blood–brain barrier permeability is increased (acidosis, hypoxemia). Kernicterus typically occurs in cases of fulminant Wilson disease (associated with which hemolytic anemia) (19,54).

Management of ALF

ALF is a challenging medical condition that requires intensive care management to prevent or treat major complications (such as hepatorenal syndrome, encephalopathy, brain edema, intracranial hypertension, bleeding, infections, and multisystem organ dysfunction). Timely and effective treatment may allow liver function to recover or minimize the risk of complications until LT can be performed. Management of ALF is ideally performed in a pediatric ICU (at an LT center) where continuous monitoring and multidisciplinary expertise are available (2,3,5,7,18,55–57).

The child should be admitted to the ICU as soon as signs of clinical or EEG HE develop, factor V activity decreases below 50% of normal, the prothrombin index (PT index = standard PT/observed PT × 100) decreases to below 50%, and/or other organ dysfunction occurs (2,5,18,19,39,57–59).

Because patients with ALF can deteriorate rapidly, transportation within the hospital or between centers must include (a) appropriate staff members who are qualified in advanced airway management, (b) cardiac and respiratory monitoring, and (c) sufficient equipment to initiate new treatment if needed during transfer to manage airway maintenance, circulatory compromise, or cerebral edema. Because the deterioration may be very rapid, families require early support and should be informed of the severity, the prognosis, and therapeutic alternatives (especially LT when appropriate).

Medical Management

General Supportive Care. The mainstay of medical care is to minimize the effect of ALF complications and to limit additional morbidity. Key to manage patients with ALF is avoidance of administering drugs that have no proven beneficial effect (60). It is essential to understand that pharmacodynamic processes and drug kinetics are modified during ALF and therefore toxic effects (neurologic and hemodynamic) could occur. In addition, in some conditions, such as hepatitis A, hepatitis B, and herpes infection, community healthcare measures are required. Anti-infective prophylactic targeted toward Gram-negative bacteria and fungi should be started.

Specific Therapies. Some causes of ALF (e.g., galactosemia, fructosemia, tyrosinemia, hemochromatosis, ornithine transcarbamylase [OTC] defect, Wilson disease, herpetic ALF,

TABLE 103.6

SPECIFIC THERAPIES FOR ACUTE LIVER FAILURE

■ CAUSE	■ TREATMENT	■ QUALITY OF EVIDENCE
Hereditary tyrosinemia	Nitisinone (NTBC or 2-(2-nitro-4-trifluoromethylbenzoyl)-1,3-cyclohexanedione) 1 mg/kg/d orally in 2 doses	II-1
Neonatal hemochromatosis	High-dose intravenous IgG in combination with exchange transfusion	II-1
Herpetic hepatitis (immunocompromised host >1 y of age)	Acyclovir 1500 mg/m^2/d IV	I
Enterovirus hepatitis	Pleconaril[a] 15 mg/kg orally in 3 doses	II-3
Acetaminophen poisoning	Activated charcoal 1 g/kg orally	I
	N-acetylcysteine 150 mg/kg IV over 60 min, then 50 mg/kg over 4 h, followed by 100 mg/kg administered over 16 h	II-1
Mushroom poisoning	Penicillin G 300,000–1 million units/kg/d IV	II-3
	Silymarin 30–40 mg/kg/d IV or orally	

[a]Currently requires investigational drug approval in the United States.
Quality of evidence: I, randomized, controlled trials; II-1, controlled trials without randomization; II-2, cohort or case-controlled analytic study; II-3, multiple time series, dramatic uncontrolled experiments; III, expert opinions.

acetaminophen or mushroom intoxications, and autoimmune FHF) may respond to a specific therapy (Table 103.6).

In the infant, congenital galactosemia and HFI can lead to ALF that is reversible, up to 1 week, if galactose and fructose are removed from the diet. Acute hepatic manifestations of hereditary tyrosinemia can occur early in life and are usually triggered by infection. A low-tyrosine diet does not usually reverse ALF, and the use of nitisinone or NTBC, an inhibitor of the enzyme 4-hydroxyphenylpyruvate dioxygenase, is recommended. NTBC prevents the formation of fumarylacetoacetate (a metabolite toxic to hepatocytes) from tyrosine. Results from an international study showed a dramatic improvement in overall survival for patients with HT-1 (61). Neonatal hemochromatosis treatment is based on prenatal diagnosis, and high-dose IV IgG in combination with exchange transfusion. Implementation of a low-protein diet is the therapy for OTC deficiency and can limit neurologic symptoms. However, in some cases, whole-liver transplantation will be required.

Fulminant Wilson disease is considered to be uniformly lethal without transplantation. Its initial treatment with albumin dialysis, continuous hemofiltration, plasmapheresis, or plasma exchange is directed toward lowering serum copper and limiting further hemolysis. Initiation of treatment with penicillamine (a copper chelator) has risks of hypersensitivity to the drug and worsening of neurologic symptoms in some patients (62).

Although rare, herpetic ALF is devastating and is rapidly lethal unless acyclovir is used. Acyclovir should be started preventively in all newborns with ALF, as delayed initiation could be lethal.

Acetaminophen is a dose-related hepatotoxin, and most cases leading to ALF exceed ingestion of 150 mg/kg lead to ALF. An acetaminophen toxicity nomogram (see Chapter 35, Poisoning) may aid in determining the likelihood of serious liver damage after acute intoxication, but it cannot exclude toxicity due to prolonged administration or in fasting patients. Therefore, if acetaminophen intoxication is suspected, specific therapy should be started without delay. If acetaminophen ingestion is known or suspected to have occurred within a few hours (up to 4 hours), activated charcoal may be useful for GI decontamination. Oral N-acetylcysteine efficiency is not precluded by previous charcoal administration, although the IV route is preferred in patients with ALF and possibly altered mental status or GI bleeding (19,63). N-acetylcysteine should

be given as soon as possible and may still be useful 48 hours after ingestion. N-acetylcysteine in nonacetaminophen ALF is not recommended by the literature, although many expert centers still use it (64).

If early enough, gastric lavage and activated charcoal administration should be performed in cases of suspected mushroom poisoning. Penicillin G and silibinin (silymarin) are the accepted antidotes. Based on a few case reports, N-acetylcysteine is sometimes administered with penicillin G and silibinin. However, mushroom poisoning still has a low transplant-free rate of survival.

Cerebral Edema Management. Cerebral edema and, ultimately, intracranial hypertension should be aggressively treated. Some interventions are supported by more evidence than others, and no uniform protocol has been established. The first line of treatment is to minimize aggravating conditions. Therefore, any precipitating events that can result in hyperammonemia should be avoided. Treatment should include lowering endogenous nitrogen intake (by limiting GI bleeding and infection and preventing slowed intestinal transit) or exogenous nitrogen intake (by keeping protein delivery below 0.5 g/kg/d and avoiding unjustified fresh frozen plasma administration). Administration of oral or rectal lactulose an osmotic cathartic nonabsorbable disaccharide is not recommended anymore as it might increase bowel distension during a subsequent transplant procedure. Neomycin is not recommended and should not be used, as it may precipitate renal failure and has not shown a benefit when combined with lactulose (65). Rifaximin is another agent used in the HE associated with chronic liver failure and whose value has not been proven in ALF. Ornithine aspartate and sodium benzoate have been proposed to decrease serum ammonia, as in Reye syndrome and in urea cycle defects, but hemofiltration remains the main treatment of acute hyperammonemia (66–68). It is important to consider that minimizing neurosensory and painful stimulation (quiet and darkened room, limited nasopharyngeal aspiration) may help control spikes in ICP.

No consensus exists on the use of invasive ICP monitoring. The ultimate goal of this technique is to maintain adequate cerebral perfusion pressure, which may be particularly critical during the anhepatic phase of LT. However, an effect on mortality by this strategy has never been shown. The bleeding risk is higher with subdural or intraparenchymal catheter than with epidural catheter. In the United States, it is estimated that slightly more than half of the adult centers use ICP monitors. Noninvasive methods as transcranial arterial Doppler monitoring are an option and are preferred (19, 47).

In patients with signs (decerebrate posturing, pupillary abnormalities) or measured intracranial hypertension, treatment with mannitol (0.25–0.5 g/kg bolus) is recommended. This dose can be repeated, provided that serum osmolality does not exceed 320 mOsm/L. However, prophylactic use of mannitol is not recommended. Hyperventilation to reduce $PaCO_2$ to 30 mm Hg is known to quickly lower ICP via decreasing cerebral blood flow and concomitant oxygen delivery and, in patients with ALF, to restore loss of cerebral blood flow autoregulation (69). However, in a randomized trial, prophylactic moderate hyperventilation in patients with ALF did not change the outcome (70). While temporary hyperventilation is useful in an attempt to lower ICP in impending herniation, prolonged and prophylactic hyperventilation are not recommended. A controlled trial of hypertonic sodium chloride use in ALF, with a target plasma sodium level of 145–155 mEq/L, was shown to prevent increases in ICP but did not affect mortality. Barbiturate use (thiopental, pentobarbital) may be considered when severe intracranial hypertension does not respond to other therapies; it has been shown to effectively decrease ICP (71). However, systemic hypotension should be anticipated following barbiturate administration and treated with vasopressors (because myocardial depression and vasodilation occur with barbiturate administration, a vasoconstrictor and inotrope may be more effective than a vasoconstrictor alone). Moderate hypothermia (32°C–34°C, 89.6°F–93.2°F) has been shown to prevent the development of brain edema without increasing risk of bleeding and infection (72). Moderate hypothermia prevents increases in ICP during LT for FHF (73). In addition, in a report of 14 adults with FHF and uncontrolled ICP who awaited LT, a moderate hypothermia allowed control of the ICP and successfully bridged 13 patients to LT (74). Corticosteroids and flumazenil are not recommended. Although no controlled data are available, the use of indomethacin and extracorporeal liver-assist devices may soon join the therapeutic arsenal to treat cerebral edema and HE (see below).

Hemorrhage and Digestive Tract Bleeding. In the absence of bleeding or an imminent surgical procedure, *routine* correction of abnormal coagulation values in children with ALF is not indicated because:

- Life-threatening hemorrhage is uncommon probably because ALF decreases both procoagulant and anticoagulant factors.
- The volume load from fresh frozen plasma may worsen ascites.
- The protein load plasma concentrates may worsen encephalopathy.
- Coagulation tests (PTT, INR) can then no longer be used to evaluate liver function.

Vitamin K should be administered intravenously upon admission of the ALF patient to the PICU. Additional doses of vitamin K should be evaluated based on coagulation studies and the response to the initial dose. Profound thrombocytopenia ($<10,000/mm^3$) and hypofibrinogenemia ($<0,5$ g/L) should be corrected if an invasive procedure such as placement of a central venous catheter is planned.

Sucralfate is preferred for prophylaxis against GI hemorrhage. Histamine-2 receptor blockers should be avoided because of their effect on the central nervous system. No study has evaluated proton-pump inhibitors for GI bleeding prophylaxis in ALF patients.

Activated recombinant factor VII administration has been used to treat life-threatening hemorrhage. It induces hemostasis at the site of injury independent of the presence of factor VIII or factor IX by forming complexes with exposed tissue factor. The recommended dosage is 15–30 mcg/kg every 4–6 hours until hemostasis is achieved. A nonrandomized trial of 15 patients with ALF showed an effective temporary correction of coagulopathy when activated recombinant factor VII was used in association with fresh frozen plasma, thereby facilitating the invasive procedure (75). Administration of fresh frozen plasma is hampered by the risk of volume and protein overload and should be thoughtfully evaluated. The use of activated recombinant factor VII has not been shown to alter long-term patient outcomes.

Renal Failure. Acute renal failure is frequent in ALF. Every effort should be made to protect renal function, maintain adequate renal perfusion, and avoid nephrotoxic drugs. If renal failure occurs, dialysis should not be delayed. Continuous, rather than discontinuous, renal replacement therapy is preferred. If dialysis is used, hypophosphatemia and hypomagnesemia may be precipitated. Evidence is limited to support the potential utility of N-acetylcysteine in improving renal function as part of the management of ALF. Use of terlipressin, for type I hepatorenal syndrome, even at a low dose, is not recommended due to the risk of increased cerebral blood flow, hyperemia, and intracranial hypertension (76). Hepatorenal syndrome will reverse in most cases after LT.

Cardiopulmonary Failure. Hypovolemia may be present at admission, but fluid resuscitation should be monitored carefully to avoid volume overload, especially if renal failure occurs. Vasoplegia will generally respond to α-adrenergic agents and they should be used as a first-line therapy for hypotension once intravascular volume has been restored. Adrenal insufficiency can occur in ALF, and hydrocortisone may be beneficial if hemodynamic instability occurs (51). Although myocardial dysfunction is unusual, echocardiographic examination may help to appreciate pulmonary artery pressure, preload condition, and contractility. Respiratory failure, especially severe hypoxemia, may occur and require mechanical ventilation. Patients with grade III or IV encephalopathy may require secured airways. Noninvasive ventilation (bilevel positive airway pressure) is rarely indicated because of the need for airway protection.

Metabolic Disorders. Continuous glucose administration (frequently up to 1 g/kg/h) is necessary and may require a central venous line to deliver high-concentration dextrose in a small fluid volume. Phosphate, magnesium, and potassium supplementation is common. Enteral nutrition (gastric or duodenal) is recommended (stress ulcer prevention) and should be initiated early. Protein intake should be limited to 0.5 g/kg/d. Finally, branched-chain amino acids are not recommended.

Liver Support Devices

Liver support devices have been developed for more than 40 years to circumvent the lack of efficient treatment for ALF (77). The latest generation of liver support techniques can be divided into ex vivo whole-organ perfusion (animal or human), bioartificial liver support using hepatocytes, "detoxification" methods, or a combination of these techniques.

Ex vivo whole-organ perfusion has been used by a number of centers, but no improvement in survival has been found. Results of auxiliary LT for ALF differ significantly between centers, and this procedure is not recommended. Bioartificial liver support incorporates hepatocytes in hollow fibers through which patient blood is filtrated. These systems are either combined with nonbiologic techniques (HepatAssist, MELS) or not (BLSS, Liverx2000, AMC-BAL). Preliminary studies failed to show improved survival. A multicenter, randomized trial that used the HepatAssist device with porcine hepatocytes demonstrated an improvement in patients with FHF of known etiology but not in patients with primary graft dysfunction (78).

Among the nonbiologic detoxification systems, the principal systems involve hemodiafiltration, high-volume plasma exchange, and albumin dialysis. The molecular absorbent recirculating system (MARS) is currently the most widely used nonbiologic liver support system. In MARS, blood is dialyzed against albumin in a three-step process (hemodialysis circuit, activated charcoal, and anion-exchange membrane) aimed at removing albumin-bound toxins, such as fatty acids, bile acids, and bilirubin. MARS was shown to improve liver function and HE in patients with acute decompensation of chronic liver disease and to improve renal function in patients with hepatorenal syndrome (79). Hundreds of patients with ALF have been treated with MARS, with decreases in HE and plasma bilirubin levels. However, the plasma ammonia level is less reduced than with high-performance hemofiltration. Of significant interest is that half of the patients with primary graft dysfunction survived without transplantation, although >80% were placed on the list for retransplantation (80). Two recent adult randomized trials on MARS in ALF and acute-on-chronic liver failure failed to show any impact on survival (81,82). Published experience with MARS and other liver support devices in children is increasing (83–85). A controlled trial conducted to evaluate the hemodynamic consequences of MARS suggested that the vasoplegic hemodynamic status found during ALF could be reversed by albumin dialysis systems (86). Interestingly, during MARS therapy, hemodynamic improvement seems to be related to both increase in stroke volume and systemic vascular resistance, associated with improved levels of renin, aldosterone, and norepinephrine, ❷ strengthening the potential role of circulating factors in ALF pathogenesis (87,88). Currently, hemodynamic stabilization, and prolonged delay between registration and LT while being on assistance are defining the role of extracorporeal liver support devices (37,89). In some major expert centers including the authors', high-flow venovenous hemofiltration has replaced MARS because of convincing results obtained in ammonia detoxification, neurologic improvement, electrolyte homeostasis, and hemodynamic stabilization in all pediatric patients, including newborns (89). It is performed as soon as patients display severe metabolic disturbance (metabolic acidosis, lactic acidosis, hyperammonemia), vasoplegic hemodynamic profile, and HE higher than grade II irrespective of the renal function. Rationale for using continuous venovenous hemofiltration to counteract cytokines-induced vasoplegia during sepsis was based on precept articles showing decrease in plasma cytokines after hemofiltration in adults with sepsis and renal failure (90). Although hemodynamic improvement could not be solely attributable to cytokine clearance, effect of hemofiltration on pro- and anti-inflammatory cytokines is now clearly demonstrated with a net balance in favor of reduced proinflammatory cytokines and decreased immunoparalysis.

None of the 10 controlled trials that evaluated liver support devices showed that liver support devices significantly reduce mortality when compared to standard medical therapy (78,81, 82,91). However, data do suggest that liver support devices may be efficient in other outcomes, such as a bridge to LT, by controlling cerebral edema, stabilizing hemodynamics, thereby providing time to evaluate spontaneous recovery capacity of the failing liver.

Emergency LT for ALF

Emergency LT remains the mainstay of therapy in children with ALF, associated with a long-term survival ranging from 52% in infants to 79% in older children (3,56). The advent of LT in this setting raises several crucial decisions.

The Decision of When to List A Child for Emergency LT.

❸ The decision to list a child for LT depends on the cause and severity of ALF, the potentiality of spontaneous liver regeneration, the availability of a specific therapy that may reverse ALF, and the comorbidities (especially the risk of permanent neurologic damage). Fulminant Wilson disease and undetermined ALF carry the worst prognosis, whereas children with hepatitis A- or acetaminophen-induced ALF have a greater chance of spontaneous recovery without transplantation.

The most common criteria used in adults to assess the need for transplantation are inadequate for children due to a very weak negative-predictive value (39). As in adult studies that showed that the severity of associated organ dysfunction correlated with HE and outcome, the PRISM score reflects the severity of ALF in children (92). Unfortunately, there are no well-defined, universally accepted criteria for LT in children (93).

Although scoring systems may be relevant for epidemiologic purposes, the decision to transplant depends on dynamic clinical and biochemical assessment of the patient's condition (92). Invariably, criteria predicting outcome, either mortality or liver transplant-free survival, include coagulation parameters (PT, INR, factor V), bilirubin, HE, and (in some criteria) age and ALF etiology. Among others, the PALF network refined the King's College criteria to HE grade >2, INR >4, and elevated bilirubin >2 mg/dL (93). Recently, the Liver Injury Units–based score (prothrombin, bilirubin, ammonia) was tested in the PALF cohort and showed better predictive value for transplant-free survival than for death (94). As a synthesis, currently no perfect criteria exist. However, altered coagulation and presence of HE higher than 2 are universally recognized as severity criteria. Emergency LT should be considered if HE greater than grade II is associated with a cofactor V activity below 20% or a prothrombin index below 20% (PT >60 seconds) or INR ≥2 (3). These levels should be adjusted for the age of the child (in infants, encephalopathy may be absent or difficult to diagnose) and the cause of ALF. Other criteria that indicate the need for emergency LT include a rapid decrease in liver size, seizures, ascites, hepatorenal syndrome, a fibrinogen level <1 g/L, bilirubinemia >400 μmol/L, worsening lactic acidosis, and hyperammonemia >150 mmol/L.

The Decision of When Not to List A Child for Emergency LT.

LT may be contraindicated in 11%–20% of cases (3). Diseases not cured with LT such as malignant disease (i.e., leukemia, lymphoproliferative syndrome, and lymphohistiocytosis), Reye syndrome and mitochondrial, respiratory chain, and disorders with neurologic involvement are contraindications to transplantation. As well, findings of uncontrolled intracranial hypertension or uncontrolled multiorgan failure should contraindicate transplantation due to the poor outcome. Children expected to recover spontaneously or under specific therapies should not be listed prematurely for emergency LT.

The Decision About Which Procedure to Do.

A cadaveric whole, split, or reduced-size liver transplant is generally used. The use of split-liver grafts and living-related donors has a favorable impact in decreasing pediatric mortality (47,95,96). Living donor liver transplants for children with ALF remain scarce but are associated with improved survival. Improved outcome for patients receiving a living donor liver transplant is probably related to a lower cold ischemia and waiting time. Auxiliary LT has been used as a bridge to provide necessary time for the native liver to regenerate. It is an ideal option, particularly when the underlying etiology remains undiagnosed and where there is a possibility of native liver regeneration and recovery. Recent clinical studies suggest that hepatocyte transplantation may be useful for bridging patients to LT, for providing metabolic support during liver failure, and for replacing LT in certain metabolic liver diseases (97,98). To date, hepatocyte transplantation has been performed in only a small number of adult patients with ALF with encouraging results (98).

Postoperative Care

Neurologic awakening from coma is the key element in early postoperative evaluation, as it determines the success of overall management. Although the postoperative period is hallmarked by the restoration of liver function and neurologic improvement, postoperative care of patients with ALF is marked by an increased incidence of associated multiorgan failure. Early circulatory resuscitation may be required due to bleeding. It is not unusual to have depressed cardiac outflow associated with inadequate preload. Intra-abdominal pressure (IAP) monitoring is required, especially in small receiver-to-donor weight ratio, because intra-abdominal hypertension and/or abdominal compartment syndrome will precipitate vascular thrombosis, liver hypoperfusion, and graft failure. At our institution, IAP is measured by the means of an intravesical Foley catheter connected through the culture-aspiration port (18-gauge plastic IV infusion catheter) to two three-way stopcocks and a pressure transducer. Before measuring IAP, 1 mL/kg of saline solution is injected into the bladder. Interpretation of IAP measures is based on two important criteria: kinetics of IAP measures and occurrence and/or development of organ failure (oliguria, lactic acidosis, respiratory restrictive syndrome) related to increased IAP (see Chapter 100 for greater detail on intra-abdominal hypertension). Acute pancreatitis can occur after transplantation in patients with ALF and results in a worse prognosis (99). Susceptibility to infection (bacterial, fungal) may lead to sepsis or septic shock. Of significance is posttransplantation generalized edema mainly due to severe capillary leak syndrome that may be secondary to ALF and the perioperative fluid management. High ventilatory pressure may alter respiratory function and gas exchange and decrease abdominal wall compliance, increase IAP and potentially affect graft perfusion. Postoperative hemofiltration may effectively control fluid balance and serve to supplement temporary renal failure. Electrolyte homeostasis is particularly important, as hypophosphatemia may interfere with extubation success.

Outcome

ALF prognosis has significantly improved since the performance of the first emergency LT, shifting from an overall pretransplant survival of 15% to >60% (3,39,100). In a large series of 141 children with ALF from the SPIT registry, the 6-month probability of survival post transplant is 76%. Most post operative death occurs following multiorgan failure, cerebral edema and infection. Pretransplant factors associated with poor postoperative outcome were a grade IV encephalopathy, children younger than 1 year of age, and renal failure requiring dialysis (39).

LIVER TRANSPLANTATION

Pediatric LT is one of the most successful solid organ transplantations (3,101–104). It is a well-established strategy in treating children with ESLD or irreversible ALF. In most centers, the 1-year actuarial survival rate is higher than 90% in elective patients and higher than 70% in children with ALF (40,105). Long-term survival is greater than 80% with excellent health-related quality of life (7,57,106). Advancements in pre-, peri-, and posttransplant management have contributed significantly to improved survival (105). The development of new surgical techniques (reduction hepatectomy, split-LT and living-related LT) have extended the procedure to infants less than 1 year of age and less than 8 kg in weight, which has reduced the waiting list mortality from 25% to 5%. Pediatric LT is being performed in developed countries across the world. Reports of experience from single centers are encouraging, and databases from the Studies in Pediatric Liver Transplantation (SPLIT) group show marked improvements in outcome (11,12,106,107).

Main Indications and Preoperative Evaluation for Pediatric LT

Main Indications for Pediatric LT

The main indications for LT in the pediatric population can be broadly separated in four groups: cholestatic liver diseases, metabolic liver disease, ALF, and liver tumors (**Tables 103.7 and 103.8**) (107). Out of 1187 children transplanted in North America between 1995 and May 2002, 33.5% were ≤12 months old at the time of transplantation, 55.6% had cholestatic disease, and 41.6% had biliary atresia. Of the children transplanted at <1 year of age, 65.6% had biliary atresia (2).

Cholestatic Liver Disease. Biliary atresia is the most common cause of chronic cholestasis in infants and accounts for nearly 50% of the indications for LT in children. Most of these small children have undergone a Kasai procedure (hepatoportoenterostomy) that failed to re-establish effective biliary flow. Consequently, they develop secondary biliary cirrhosis leading to chronic end-stage liver failure. Indications for LT in children with biliary atresia are cholangitis or progressive jaundice (35%), portal hypertension or hepatorenal syndrome (41%), and decreased liver synthetic functions. Intrahepatic cholestasis such as sclerosing cholangitis, Alagille syndrome, nonsyndromic paucity of intrahepatic bile ducts, and progressive familial intrahepatic cholestasis represents ~15% of all transplantations (11).

Metabolic Diseases. Metabolic diseases are the second most common indication for pediatric LT (4,109,108). They include primary hepatic diseases such as Wilson disease, α-1-antitrypsin deficiency, and cystic fibrosis, as well as primarily nonhepatic diseases such as OTC deficiency, Crigler–Najjar syndrome type 1, primary hyperoxaluria type 1, and organic acidemia. In children with primary hyperoxaluria type 1, combined liver and kidney transplantation should be considered when irreversible renal injury from oxalic acid accumulation has developed. However, LT does not correct the enzyme deficiency in other organs except the liver, and patients remain at risk of severe extrahepatic complications. Children transplanted for metabolic diseases generally have excellent outcomes (4,109).

Liver Tumors. Liver tumors are mainly represented by hepatoblastoma. Tumor resection or LT for hepatoblastoma is considered after chemotherapy (110,111). Hepatocellular carcinoma in children is rare and is often secondary to another chronic underlying liver disease. The development of hepatocellular carcinoma has been reported in greater frequency in children with biliary atresia, Alagille syndrome, progressive intrahepatic cholestasis, and tyrosinemia. In children with tyrosinemia, there is a 33% incidence of hepatocellular carcinoma before 2 years of age (105).

Main Contraindications to Pediatric LT

The list of contraindications to LT in children has progressively shortened because surgical techniques and medical management have improved significantly over time (102). Absolute contraindications where LT is futile are (a) unresectable extrahepatic malignant tumor considered incurable by standard oncologic criteria; (b) concomitant end-stage organ failure that cannot be corrected by a combined transplant; (c) multiple organ failure; and (d) irreversible serious neurological damage. Relative contraindications include malignancy that is considered

TABLE 103.7

PEDIATRIC LIVER TRANSPLANTATION, INDICATIONS AND OUTCOMES

	■ DIAGNOSIS	■ BICÊTRE HOSPITAL (1986–2002)	■ PITTSBURGH CHILDREN'S HOSPITAL (1981–1998)	■ SPLIT REGISTRY (1995–2002)
Number of patients		568	808	1092
Number of liver transplantations		648	1113	NA
	Biliary atresia	53%	51%	42%
	Chronic cholestasis	25%	11%	14%
	Metabolic disease	8%	15%	12%
	Fulminant hepatic failure	11%	6%	13%
	Other causes	3%	13%	10%
Liver graft survival		65%[a]	52%[a]	75%[b]
Patient survival		78%[a]	69%[a]	83%[b]

[a]15-year outcome.
[b]3-year outcome.
SPLIT, Studies of pediatric liver transplantation; NA, not available.
From Jain A, Mazariegos G, Kashyap R, et al. Pediatric liver transplantation. A single-center experience spanning 20 years. Transplantation 2002; 73:941–7; Martin SR, Atkison P, Anand R, et al. Studies of pediatric liver transplantation 2002: Patient and graft survival and rejection in pediatric recipients of a first liver transplant in the United States and Canada. Pediatr Transplant 2004;8:273–83.

TABLE 103.8

PATIENT CHARACTERISTICS OF 2982 CHILDREN
WHO UNDERWENT A FIRST LIVER TRANSPLANTATION
(REGISTERED IN SPLIT FROM 1995–2008)

	TOTAL N = 2982	
	■ N	■ %
Age at transplant		
Missing	1	0.0
0–6 mo	260	8.7
6–12 mo	725	24.3
1–5 y	962	32.3
5–13 y	616	20.7
13 + y	418	14.0
Race		
Missing	47	1.6
White	1678	56.3
Black	464	15.6
Hispanic	494	16.6
Other	299	10.0
Sex		
Missing	1	0.0
Male	1407	47.2
Female	1574	52.8
Primary disease		
Biliary atresia	1203	40.3
Other cholestatic or metabolic	837	28.1
Fulminant liver failure	420	14.1
Cirrhosis	196	6.6
Other	326	10.9
Patient status at transplant		
Missing	15	0.5
ICU/intubated	369	12.4
ICU/nonintubated	407	13.6
Hospitalized	514	17.2
Home	1677	56.2

Data from McDiarmid SV, Anand R, Martz BS, et al. A multivariate analysis of pre-, peri-, and post-transplant factors affecting outcome after pediatric liver transplantation. *Ann Surg* 2011;254:145–54.

cured or curable by standard oncologic criteria and treatable infection.

Preoperative Evaluation for LT

Preoperative care includes the consideration of the indications and contraindications for LT, the selection, evaluation, and preparation of the candidates, and their prioritization. The appropriate preoperative evaluation of recipients is crucial to the outcome (102). The first step is to determine whether LT remains the best option and that no other medical therapies, either transitory or definite, could be life sustaining with adequate quality of life. Once the indication is confirmed, the second step is to determine the severity of the disease and assess for any complications or comorbidities. Renal function should be assessed as it may severely impair postoperative care in patients with severe cholestasis (e.g., Alagille syndrome) and patients with hepatorenal syndrome (112). Careful cardiac workup, including echocardiographic exams, should be performed looking at restrictive cardiomyopathy (hyperoxaluria), altered diastolic function and pulmonary hypertension (cholestasis), and pulmonary vein stenosis (Alagille syndrome). In cases in which hepatopulmonary syndrome is suspected, intrapulmonary shunt by scintigraphy may be quantified. In addition, preoperative viral (adenovirus, EBV, cytomegalovirus [CMV], HHV6, HHV8 by quantitative polymerase chain reaction [PCR]) and bacterial (blood and ascites) workup may help in managing postoperative infective complications.

Prioritization of Potential Candidates for LT

In most countries with an established organ transplantation network, graft allocation is based on the concept that organs need to be allocated to the sickest patients. Most systems preferentially allocate pediatric donors to pediatric recipients. However, the policy to allocate organs is undergoing constant modification because of a persistent donor shortage. In the United States, the pediatric end-stage liver disease (PELD) score was introduced in 2002 to stratify the degree of illness in children with similar diseases who are competing for pediatric liver grafts. This score is calculated from a formula based on objective medical criteria including total bilirubin (mg/dL), INR, serum albumin (g/dL), age less than 1 year, and growth failure (height less than 2 standard deviations from the mean for age and gender) (22,102, 113,114). Additional points are awarded for specific risk factors not taken into account in the PELD score, such as hepatopulmonary syndrome, metabolic diseases, and liver tumors. The adoption of the PELD score in the United States has improved the access and accountability of the allocation system. Since the use of the PELD score, fewer children are now dying on the waiting list (102,114). However, the PELD score does not cover all pediatric situations (102). It is currently used only for children up to 12 years old, does not take into account potential complications of ESLD (e.g., hepatopulmonary syndrome), and is not adapted to children with ALF, liver tumors, or metabolic diseases.

Intraoperative Care of Children Undergoing LT

It is not possible to review all the surgical aspects of pediatric LT; however, it is important to have a basic understanding of the processes involved in harvesting the organ from the donor and transplanting it to the recipient. The technical aspects of the arterial reconstruction, the portal vein anastomosis, and the restoration of biliary tract continuity are important to consider as each procedure has its own share of complications. Therefore, the communication between the surgeons, radiologists, and intensivist about the technical aspects is crucial.

The Graft

Donor Selection. Selection of an appropriate liver donor is vitally important to the short- and long-term success of the transplantation. Particular attention is paid to donor's age, cause of brain death, intensive care hospitalization time, infections, hemodynamic stability, and use of vasopressors. No consistent data exist on the effect of donor age on the long-term results of pediatric LT. Up to the early 1980s, the only technical option was to transplant the whole liver of a donor with a weight as close as possible to that of the recipient. However, the shortage of pediatric cadaveric donors resulted in a high mortality rate on the waiting list. The development of techniques that allow surgeons to transplant portion of livers from adult donors has expanded the donor pool and has been a major advancement in reducing the waiting period and improving the survival rates of pediatric LT. Currently, reduced-liver grafts to the left lateral segments and split livers provide the majority of grafts in infants, whereas left or right lobes are used in older recipients (**Table 103.9**).

Whole-Liver Transplantation. To date, whole-organ transplantation is used when a cadaveric donor has an approximate recipient size. When using whole-organ grafts, the donor weight should range 15% above or below that of recipient. Whereas bigger grafts may result in difficulties during abdominal closure and subsequent risk of abdominal compartment syndrome, undersized grafts are associated with significant risk of hemorrhagic necrosis due to excessive portal flow.

Reduced-Size LT. This procedure consists in the procurement of the whole liver from an adult cadaver donor, which is reduced in its size and used in one single recipient. Reduced-size liver graft is most often limited to the left anatomic lobe (segments II, III, IV) or left lateral segment (segments II and III) of the donor liver (**Fig. 103.1**). This technique allows surgeons to overcome differences in size between the donor and the recipient of up to 4 or 5 times. Estimates of donor graft-to-recipient body weight ratio (optimal 1.5%–2%, i.e.,

TABLE 103.9

TRANSPLANT CHARACTERISTICS OF 2982 CHILDREN WHO UNDERWENT A FIRST LIVER TRANSPLANTATION (REGISTERED IN SPLIT FROM 1995–2008)

	TOTAL N = 2982	
	■ N	■ %
Donor organ		
Missing	100	3.4
Live	461	15.5
Whole	1564	52.4
Reduced	482	16.2
Split	375	12.6
Transplant year		
1995–2001	1161	38.9
2002–2008	1821	61.1
Primary immunosuppression		
Missing	128	4.3
Cyclosporine	444	14.9
Tacrolimus	2326	78.0
Other	84	2.8
Donor age		
Missing	213	7.1
0–6 mo	148	5.0
6–12 mo	121	4.1
1–18 y	1482	49.7
18–50 y	932	31.3
≥50 y	86	2.9

Data from McDiarmid SV, Anand R, Martz BS, et al. A multivariate analysis of pre-, peri-, and post-transplant factors affecting outcome after pediatric liver transplantation. *Ann Surg* 2011;254:145–54.

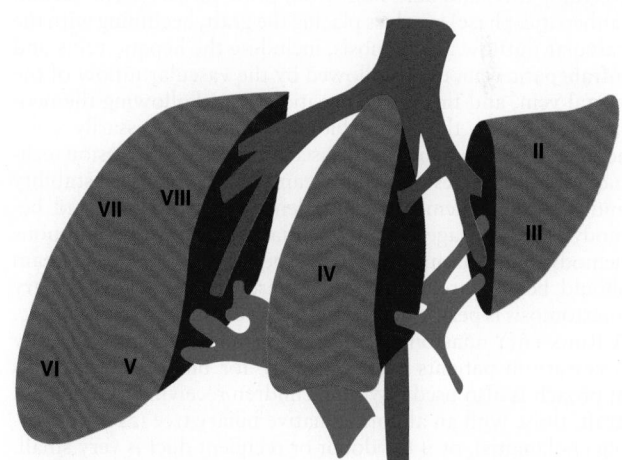

FIGURE 103.1. Couinaud's segmental classification of the liver. Liver segments are determined by portal *(red)* and hepatic veins *(blue)*. (Adapted from Couinaud C. *Le Foie: Études Anatomiques et Chirurgicales.* Paris: Masson, 1957.)

150–200 g, for a recipient who weighs 10 kg) appear to be the most accurate predictor of adequate graft volume. Reduced-size LT shows similar outcomes to whole-liver transplantation (12,13,15,104,115). However, reduced-size LT decreases the pool of livers for adults. Therefore, other options such as split-liver and living-related LT have been developed.

Split-Liver Transplantation. Split-liver transplantation doubles the number of recipients and allows two functional allografts.

The left lateral segment (segments II and III) is transplanted in a child, whereas the right liver is transplanted into an adult. This procedure increases the ischemia time, with an increased risk of primary dysfunction and technical complications. Because split-liver transplantation may require a prolonged ischemic period, selection of donors is crucial (22). The possibility to split the liver in situ (requires a heart beating donor) can reduce the ischemia time. This procedure has shown comparable results to those obtained with conventional techniques.

Living-Related LT. Living-related LT accounts for a substantial amount of the pediatric elective LT performed in many centers across the world and the only possibility for LT in countries where cadaveric organ procurement was not allowed (116,117). The procedure consists in a left lobectomy, during which segments 2 and 3 are separated from the remaining liver. Living-related LT has been widely debated with regard to the ethics of performing major surgery on a healthy person. Donor mortality and morbidity are estimated at ~0.2% and 10%, respectively. Evaluation of the donor and the recipient is crucial. Recipient's size and age are important, because there is evidence that infants and small children do better than older children with living donor transplantation (101). In the majority of cases, living-related transplants register an excellent outcome for pediatric patients, thanks to the possibility of performing the transplant before the child's clinical condition deteriorates. Living-related LT should also be considered in children with ALF when no cadaveric grafts are available.

Graft Implantation

The details of the surgical procedure in the recipient have been described elsewhere (111). In brief, the procedure follows three major phases. The first (hepatectomy phase) begins with the recipient hepatectomy. It is often the most difficult part of the procedure because of complicating features (portal hypertension, coagulopathy, and adhesions from prior surgery). The second (anhepatic, phase) involves placing the graft, beginning with the vascular outflow anastomosis, including the hepatic veins and infrahepatic vena cava, followed by the vascular inflow of the portal vein, and finally the hepatic artery. Following the neo-liver perfusion, the initial blood return is necessarily cold, acidotic, and hyperkalemic (caused by graft cold perfusion techniques) and can result in significant cardiovascular instability and additional hemostatic problems. Optimal fluid and hemodynamic management is essential and requires continuous hemodynamic monitoring. The specialized anesthesia team should be prepared to manage these problems. The biliary anastomosis is performed in the final (postimplantation) phase. A Roux-en-Y anastomosis (hepaticojejunostomy) is obviously necessary in patients undergoing LT for biliary atresia. This approach is also used in young children receiving a segmental graft, those with an abnormal native biliary tree (as in sclerosing cholangitis), or if the donor or recipient duct is very small. A direct choledocho-choledochostomy is possible in other patients with a normal native biliary tract.

The operative procedure is marked by important issues, which may influence postoperative management. Severe portal hypertension may result in critical bleeding during removal of the native liver. Bleeding may occur during dissection of extensive adherences, such as in children with biliary atresia who underwent previous portoenterostomy surgeries. Assessment of the vascular anastomosis is essential (i.e., portal anastomosis in children with biliary atresia may be difficult) as portal vessels are frequently hypoplastic. Arterial anastomosis may preclude important dissection along the infrarenal aorta, with subsequent risk of traumatic lesions to the pancreas. The appearance of the liver graft after unclamping may be informative regarding the quality of the graft. Finally, abdominal closure should be performed in a manner to avoid increased IAP.

❹ Postoperative Care of Children after LT

After LT, children are taken to the PICU for intensive monitoring and management. Management can be divided into two main issues: the general management of a patient after major abdominal surgery and specific considerations regarding LT.

General Postoperative Management

Respiratory. Patients should be weaned from the ventilator and extubated as soon as possible because prolonged mechanical ventilation has been associated with higher mortality and morbidity. In general, children can be extubated within 48 hours after transplantation. However, for some children, a more prolonged course of mechanical ventilation is necessary because of severe fluid overload, increased abdominal pressure, malnutrition, postoperative pain, or other complications such as sepsis, liver dysfunction, refractory ascites, and, in rare cases, right phrenic nerve paresis. Pleural effusions secondary to ascites passing across the diaphragm are common and can be treated with diuretic therapy and pleural puncture. In some cases, a pleural pigtail drainage catheter is required. Continuous monitoring of oxygen saturation, expired carbon dioxide, and frequent assessment of arterial blood gas values should also be performed.

Cardiovascular. Continuous arterial pressure and central venous pressure should be monitored. The abdominal drainage should be assessed hourly for extensive bleeding indicating possible hemorrhage from the vascular anastomosis, or coagulopathy, especially in case of primary nonfunction. Excessive abdominal hemorrhage of more than one blood volume despite correction of postoperative coagulopathy (platelets, clotting factors) may warrant hemostasis laparotomy. Postoperative cardiopulmonary failure is worth mentioning, as restrictive or obstructive cardiomyopathy (hyperoxaluria, chronic cholestasis) and pulmonary hypertension (hepatopulmonary syndrome, pulmonary vein stenosis in Alagille syndrome) may be encountered. Postoperative vasoplegia is frequent and may require vasopressor support. Postoperative monitoring, either invasive or noninvasive (cardiac echocardiography, continuous aortic Doppler), may help in identifying the cause and initiate adequate treatment. Hypertension may be the result of side effects from immunosuppressive agents, volume overload, or pain, but postoperative systemic hypertension may warrant careful neurologic evaluation for raised ICP (cerebral edema in ALF, intracranial hemorrhage).

Gastrointestinal. It is crucial to assess synthetic, metabolic, and excretory function of the graft immediately after transplantation. Absence of intra-abdominal bleeding and rapid correction of coagulation abnormalities are the best indicators of synthetic function. Adequate metabolic function is reflected in normalizing lactate levels and awakening within several hours following the transplant procedure. Clearance of anesthesia is a good indicator of synthetic function. After 48 hours, the total bilirubin, coagulations tests, and transaminases are reliable indicators of liver function. Depending upon the degree of graft injury due to ischemia, the transaminase levels may rise dramatically within 2 days but should be near normal after 7 days.

Renal. Electrolytes and fluid balance should be monitored closely. Massive fluid shifts from ascites or blood loss may result in hypovolemia, hypotension, and metabolic and electrolyte disturbances. With the addition of nephrotoxic drugs, such as tacrolimus and some antibiotics, patients are at higher risk of kidney impairment. Renal replacement therapy may be necessary.

Neurologic. Level of consciousness is an important indicator of graft function. Neurologic evaluation shortly after PICU admission is important. Graft dysfunction is generally indicated by slowness to waken.

Specific Postoperative Considerations

Specific postoperative management of the LT patient includes monitoring for both surgical and medical complications. The incidence of surgical complications has decreased over time, but sepsis and rejection remain significant issues (**Tables 103.5** and **103.10**).

Primary Nonfunction and Subfunction of the Graft. Primary nonfunction of the graft is a rare but catastrophic event. It usually occurs within the first 48 hours following the procedure, and diagnosis is based on absence of neurologic awakening, HE, bleeding, increasing liver enzymes, lactic acidosis, and persisting vasoplegic shock. In cases of split-liver transplant, information regarding the other liver recipient's postoperative course may help in diagnosing primary graft nonfunction. The only therapy is emergency retransplantation. Sub-graft function with persistent coagulopathy is also possible but generally reversible within a few days. Although the cause is unknown, it is likely the result of donor (rather than recipient) factors and is probably related to ischemia/reperfusion injury of the graft, which further emphasizes the critical importance of the donor's selection (cause of cerebral death, hemodynamic stability, normoxia, age, etc.), as previously mentioned.

Vascular Complications. Vascular thrombosis is the main postoperative complication that will cause graft loss. Hepatic artery thrombosis occurs in children (5%–15%) 3 times more frequently than in adults, usually within the first 30 days after transplantation (104,118). This complication is directly related to the size of the vessels and thus is most likely in the smallest pediatric recipients and/or small liver grafts. Prevention of hepatic artery thrombosis in these situations is based on anticoagulation, antiplatelet aggregation therapy, and avoiding hemoconcentration. Hepatic artery thrombosis can occur with various clinical presentations, which may include acute allograft failure, biliary obstruction, or sepsis. Suspected hepatic artery thrombosis requires prompt evaluation with duplex sonography, magnetic resonance angiography, or angiogram. Successful thrombectomy is possible if hepatic artery thrombosis diagnosis is made before graft necrosis occurs. Hepatic artery thrombosis can also occur as a late complication and can manifest as biliary strictures, bilomas, or sepsis. These biliary complications are particularly frequent after hepatic artery thrombosis because

the hepatic artery offers most of the vascularization to the bile duct. In the case of biliary tract necrosis due to hepatic artery thrombosis, the only option is retransplantation. Early portal vein thrombosis usually occurs within the first week (median, 2 days) after transplantation and requires emergency thrombectomy in most cases. It occurs in 5%–10% of recipients. It is more frequent in children transplanted for biliary atresia, because of preexisting portal vein hypoplasia. Refractory ascites may indicate a portal thrombosis or stenosis of suprahepatic veins.

Biliary Complications. Bile duct complications (bile leaks, stenosis, and strictures) are usually a result of technical problems or of ischemic injury of the donor duct (119). Early leaks can be diagnosed by the appearance of bile in the drains. Many leaks resolve with decompression by transhepatic tube drainage. Surgical revision of the anastomosis should be performed for those patients with bile peritonitis and those with persistent leaks. As discussed earlier, bile complications resulting from bile duct ischemia secondary to early hepatic artery thrombosis generally require retransplantation (**Table 103.11**). Biliary strictures can occur later, even years after transplant, presenting as bile duct dilatation on ultrasound or recurrent cholangitis. They can be definitively diagnosed and treated with percutaneous transhepatic cholangiography with stenting and dilatation, but surgical revision may be necessary in some cases.

Infections. Infection is the most common source of morbidity and mortality following LT. Because of immunosuppression,

TABLE 103.11

INDICATIONS FOR RETRANSPLANTATION OF THE LIVER

Primary nonfunction	22%
Chronic allograft rejection	21%
Hepatic artery thrombosis	18%
Portal vein thrombosis	17%
Acute allograft rejection	7%
Atypical acute allograft rejection	6%
Biliary complications	3%
Recurrent or de novo viral diseases	5%
Other	1%

Data from Farmer DG, Venick RS, McDiarmid SV, et al. Predictors of outcomes after pediatric liver transplantation: An analysis of more than 800 cases performed at a single institution. *J Am Coll Surg* 2007;204:914–6.

TABLE 103.10

SPECIFIC POSTOPERATIVE COMPLICATIONS AFTER LIVER TRANSPLANTATION IN CHILDREN

REFERENCES	YEAR	LIVER TRANSPLANTATION	COMPLICATIONS %				
		N	HAT	PVC	SHV	BILIARY	DIGESTIVE
Bourdeaux et al. (125)	2009						
Total		235	7.6	9.4	1.7	21.7	NA
LRDT		100	1	13	0	30	NA
Fouquet et al. (7)[a]	2005	280	17	11	NA	20	11
Diamond et al. (15)[b]	2007						
Total		2192	7.6	5.5	NA	12	9.8
LRDT		360	6.7	7.5	NA		11.1
Ueda et al. (102)[c]	2006	600	3.3	7.5	3.7	14.5	5.7
Heaton et al. (113)[c]	2008	50	6	4	NA	14	

[a]Liver transplantation only for biliary atresia.
[b]Complication occurring within the first month after transplantation.
[c]Living related liver transplantation only.
LRDT, living related donor transplantation; HAT, hepatic artery thrombosis; PVC, portal vein complication (thrombosis or stenosis); SHV, stenosis of the hepatic vein anastomosis.

patients are at risk of developing nosocomial and opportunistic infections. In addition, the patient's preoperative condition may be a risk factor for sepsis. Bacterial sepsis occurs in the immediate posttransplant period and is more frequently due to Gram-negative enteric organisms, *Enterococcus* and *Staphylococcus* species. Fungal sepsis (*Candida* spp., *Aspergillus* spp.) may occur in the early posttransplant period and hold an elevated mortality if severe infection occurs, making monitoring of colonization index and early treatment mandatory. Frequent postoperative prophylactic regimens include acyclovir, an antifungal agent, a β-lactam antibiotic, and trimethoprim-sulfamethoxazole. Although viral and opportunistic infections may occur later after transplantation, EBV, CMV, herpes simplex, and adenovirus can cause early infection that must be recognized. The risk of developing either EBV or CMV infection is influenced by the preoperative serological status of the transplant donor and recipient. Seronegative recipients receiving seropositive donor organs are at greater risk. The development of effective methods of diagnosis, prophylaxis, and treatment of CMV with ganciclovir or valganciclovir means that these diseases are no longer a significant cause of mortality but morbidity remains high. In contrast, the absence of therapy for EBV means that infection rates are high. The development of molecular genetic diagnosis using quantitative PCR for EBV has resulted in the prevention of progressive disease, or posttransplant lymphoproliferative disease (PTLD) by preemptive reduction of immunosuppression in response to rinsing EBV titers. Various prophylactic protocols have been used to decrease the incidence of symptomatic CMV and EBV infection, although seroconversion in naive recipients inevitably occurs.

Acute Rejection. Despite improved immunosuppressive regimens, acute rejection remains a problem and about 20%–50% of patients develop at least one episode of acute rejection in the first weeks after LT (57). It can occur later, and is often associated with immunosuppressant noncompliance. The clinical picture includes fever, ascites, and jaundice. Rejection is generally suspected because of increasing liver enzymes and increase in gamma-glutamyl transferase level. Liver biopsy is the key for diagnosis, and histologic findings of acute rejection are a mixed portal inflammatory infiltrate, predominantly mononuclear cells associated with portal and central vein endothelitis and bile duct damage. The primary treatment is a short course of high-dose methylprednisolone, which is effective in treating rejection in 80% of cases.

Other Complications and Retransplantation. Early second look reoperation is used in several centers for the best diagnosis and treatment of bile leakage, hemorrhage, bowel injury, and sepsis. GI perforation occurs in 20% of children with biliary atresia. Acute pancreatitis occurs in <2% of children who undergo LT but is associated with high mortality (57). Retransplantation is not an uncommon event. Its overall incidence ranges from 10% to 20% and occurs mainly within the first 30 days following initial transplantation (11,120). The majority of retransplantation results from acute allograft damage caused by hepatic artery thrombosis, primary nonfunction, or acute graft rejection (**Table 103.11**).

PTLDs are a heterogeneous group of diseases, ranging from benign lymphatic hyperplasia to lymphomas. It is favored by the intensity of the immunosuppression, an EBV seronegative host, and an EBV seropositive donor. Treatment of PTLDs is based on the clinical aggressiveness of the syndrome and the immunological cell typing. In all cases documented PTLD requires an immediate decrease or withdrawal of immunosuppression. If the tumor expresses the B cell marker CD20, the anti-CD20 monoclonal antibody rituximab is indicated.

In general, recurrence of the primary liver disease in the graft is uncommon in children since liver disease requiring LT is usually congenital biliary atresia and therefore LT is curative.

However, a recurrence is possible if the LT indication is a primary sclerosing cholangitis. De novo autoimmune hepatitis can occur in any graft, regardless of the original disease, and is therefore not considered recurrence of the disease, but a new entity (121). It may be associated with the use of steroid-free regimes and occurs in 2%–3% of children. This form of graft dysfunction is associated with an increasing incidence of nonspecific antibodies (ANA, SMA, and rarely LKM), graft hepatitis, and elevated immunoglobulins and may be related to the progressive development of graft hepatitis with fibrosis. Chronic hepatitis has been recently recognized as a prevalent problem in late allograft dysfunction (58,102). Liver biopsy shows portal inflammation. The treatment of this condition is not clear.

Immunosuppression

The immune system recognizes the liver graft as "non-self" and begins a destructive immune response mediated principally by the T lymphocytes, especially the CD4+ T cell. In addition, IL-2 activates the secretion of cytotoxic T cells, B cells, and macrophages. To avoid destruction of the liver graft, immunosuppressive drugs must be administered. The immunosuppressive agents must interrupt the activation of CD4+ T cells and IL-2 production. The incidence of acute and chronic rejection has declined following the development of newer immunosuppressive drugs, which are more easily absorbed such as cyclosporine microemulsion or more potent such as tacrolimus. The following are the main immunosuppressive drugs used in pediatric LT.

Corticosteroids. Corticosteroids are effective in both the prevention and the treatment of graft rejection. Their mechanisms of action are unclear, but they inhibit IL-2 and reduce the proliferation of T cells (helper and suppressor T cells, cytotoxic T cells) and the migration and activity of neutrophils. However, corticosteroids have important side effects. Their use is associated with increased incidence of infection (bacterial, viral, and fungal), increased risk for malignancy, and detrimental metabolic effects in children. The most common metabolic side effects include bone marrow suppression, hypertension, diabetes mellitus, polyphagia, obesity, gastric ulcers, and sodium and water retention. Long-term use may result in osteoporosis, growth retardation, avascular necrosis of joints, and depression. For these reasons, most pediatric centers have currently adopted steroid-free immunosuppressive protocols, combining calcineurin inhibitors and antibody to the IL-2 receptors of T cells (basiliximab).

Calcineurin Inhibitors. Progress in LT in the last 20 years has been characterized in large part by the introduction of calcineurin inhibitors (*cyclosporine, tacrolimus*) that today represent the keystone of most immunosuppressive protocols. These drugs inhibit T cell response and bind to intracellular proteins called immunophilins. This complex binds to and inhibits the phosphatase activity of calcineurin, which results in a block of the transcription of cytokines, particularly IL-2. The use of calcineurin inhibitors is associated with side effects, which include nephrotoxicity, neurotoxicity, and hypertension. Most of them are reversible after dose reduction or discontinuation of the drug. The introduction of cyclosporine in the 1980s was a major advancement because it led to significant increases in survival rates (patient and graft) and a reduction in the incidence and severity of rejection. Administration of cyclosporine usually begins intravenously, during or after LT, with maintenance doses delivered orally. Absorption is dependent on the presence of bile. Therefore, hepatic dysfunction might limit the absorption of cyclosporine. Microemulsions of cyclosporine are more easily absorbed and allow more stability of the desired blood concentration. However, many drugs interact with cyclosporine. Therefore, serum drug levels should be monitored closely. Cyclosporine is also associated with cosmetic side effects such as hypertrichosis and gingival hyperplasia. For all these reasons, over the last 10 years, the use of tacrolimus has increased, and nowadays it is preferred to cyclosporine. Tacrolimus is 100 times more potent than cyclosporine. Moreover, tacrolimus is associated with less hyperlipidemia and a lower cardiovascular risk than cyclosporine. Comparison between tacrolimus and cyclosporine shows similar 1-year survival (patient and graft) as well as steroid-resistant rejection in children. Tacrolimus can be given as a 24-hour continuous IV infusion or orally. Daily determination of calcineurin inhibitors' blood level is essential because it will help in dosing immunosuppressive therapy, and in balancing between the risk of infection (in case of over dosage) and rejection (in case of under dosage). Desired concentration of calcineurin inhibitors depends upon the time posttransplant. At 0–3 months posttransplant, cyclosporine and tacrolimus target levels are 200–250 and 10–15 mg/L, respectively. At 4–12 months posttransplant, cyclosporine and tacrolimus levels should be at 150–200 and 8–10 mg/L, respectively. After 1 year, the optimal levels are 50–100 mg/L for cyclosporine and 5–8 mg/L for tacrolimus.

IL-2 Receptor Antibodies. T cells involved in acute rejection act by exposing activation markers such as the IL-2 receptors. Anti-IL-2 receptor antibodies (*basiliximab*) combined with calcineurin inhibitors have drastically improved graft survival. Basiliximab is a chimeric (mouse and human) monoclonal antibody. Its safety and tolerability are excellent. As previously mentioned, the combination of these drugs allows steroid-free immunosuppression with no harmful effect on graft acceptance. The patient receives two doses of basiliximab: the first one should be given 6 hours after organ reperfusion, and the second on day 4 after transplantation. This approach reduces hypertension, growth retardation, and the cosmetic effects of steroid therapy.

Other Immunosuppressive Drugs. *Mycophenolate mofetil*, a selective inhibitor of the inosine monophosphate dehydrogenase (necessary for B and T cell growth), has been successfully used as an alternative immunosuppressive agent in patients with chronic rejection, refractory rejection, or severe calcineurin inhibitor toxicity. Large interindividual variations indicate the need for therapeutic drug monitoring and individualized dosing. *Sirolimus* (rapamycin) is a macrolide antibiotic with immunosuppressive properties that acts by blocking T cell activation by way of IL-2R post–receptor signal transduction. It has been used as a rescue treatment in chronic rejection and calcineurin inhibitor toxicity.

5 ## Results and Outcome for Pediatric LT

Although the potential complications are numerous, the overall results of pediatric LT are excellent, especially for long-term outcome, as most indications for pediatric LT do not recur within the transplanted allograft, whereas disease recurrence represents a significant cause of long-term graft loss in adults.

Short-Term Results

Survival rates vary according to the age at transplantation and the underlying diagnosis. Survival for children less than 1 year old has improved dramatically. The univariate predictors of graft loss are age less than 6 months, calculated creatinine clearance less than 90, pre-LT hospitalization, pre-LT mechanical ventilation, repeat LT, and infants transplanted for reasons other than cholestatic liver disease. Neonates represent a special population and their outcomes from LT are worthy of consideration (17,117,122). Although small babies have higher complication rates and longer hospital stays following transplantation, neonatal liver transplant recipients now have similar patient and graft survival compared with older children. The underlying diagnosis at transplantation also has an effect on outcomes. Patients with ALF have worse early and long-term survival rates. Although the patient and graft survival are dependent on surgical techniques and patient care, their influence on survival is limited to the initial perioperative period and does not affect long-term outcome. Early postoperative death is mainly related to sepsis, graft failure, multiorgan failure, and cardiopulmonary and neurologic complications, whereas late mortality is mainly related to sepsis. From the SPLIT database, a total of 42 pre-, peri-, and posttransplant variables were evaluated in 2982 pediatric recipients of a first LT (107). Factors affecting patient and graft outcome at 6 months included reoperation for any cause (increased the risk for both patient and graft loss by 11-fold) and reoperation exclusive of specific complications (by 4-fold). Vascular thrombosis, bowel perforation, septicemia, and retransplantation, each independently increased the risk of patient and graft loss (by three- to fourfold). The only baseline factor with similarly high relative risk for patient and graft loss was if recipients required intensive care unit and were intubated at time of transplant.

Overall survival of children after LT is 70%–80% in the largest series, and 15-year graft survival is between 52% and 65% (Table 103.7). As techniques and patient care improve, actual survival can exceed 85% (39). Ten years after transplant, 79% of children attend normal school and in 69% of them school performance is not delayed (7,123). Clinical factors associated with improved post-LT health-related quality of life 20 years after LT are younger age at LT, allograft longevity, and strong social support. In a recent study, more than 90% of pediatric survivors completed high school. After LT, 34% of pediatric recipients married, and 79% remained married at 20-year follow-up (124). Effective transition strategies from childhood to adulthood are important in adolescents since nonadherence to treatment is common (123). One study has reported the psychological adjustment of 116 pediatric LT recipients reaching adulthood. In this study, 76% considered their quality of life as good or very good. Poor compliance with medications was reported by 45% of them. Anxiety, loneliness, and negative thoughts were expressed by 53%, 84%, and 47% of the patients, respectively. Among them, 11% were being cared for by psychologists or psychiatrists (106).

Long-Term Results and Quality of Life

Despite these encouraging results, late complications are possible. Seventy-three per cent of long-term survivors have abnormal liver histology with centrilobular fibrosis mainly due to chronic rejection (123). Resistant linear growth impairment is also common in the pediatric liver transplant population (125). Renal dysfunction has been noted in more than 30% of long-term survivors. This has modified immunosuppressive practices in at-risk transplant recipients. Current immunosuppressive agents are also associated with an increased risk for diabetes, dyslipidemia, and obesity (59,126). Lifestyle modification and minimization of immune suppressants can be effective in reducing these risks. In summary, LT gives children with a potentially lethal disease an excellent long-term prognosis and quality of life.

CONCLUSIONS AND FUTURE DIRECTIONS

Long-term outcomes for infants and children undergoing LT are excellent and have improved over time. The history of pediatric LT has clearly shown that success is dependent on constant collaboration between pediatricians, hepatologists, surgeons, nurses, transplant coordinators, dieticians, psychologists, and social workers. The incidence of acute and chronic rejection has fallen following the development of newer immunosuppressive drugs and protocols. Appropriate indications for LT and selection of the most appropriate donor and surgical procedure are critical. One major problem remains the lack of donors. In the United States, the total number of pediatric liver donors has decreased in 10 years from 20% to 12% (127). Donation after cardiac death offers a new possibility to increase the pool of potential donors (101,128). In children with ALF, increased interest is centered on the possibility of providing temporary liver support with extracorporeal devices (artificial and bioartificial) or on hepatocyte transplantation and their use either as a bridge to LT or to obviate the need for it. As long-term survival increases, attention has now focused on the quality of life achieved by children undergoing transplantation (106,123,124).

FINANCIAL DISCLOSURES/ ACKNOWLEDGMENT

No sources of funding were used to assist in the preparation of this manuscript. The authors have no conflicts of interest that are directly relevant to the content of this manuscript.

References

1. Jain A, Mazariegos G, Kashyap R, et al. Pediatric liver transplantation. A single-center experience spanning 20 years. *Transplantation* 2002;73:941–7.

2. McDiarmid SV, Anand R, Lindblad AS; SPLIT Research Group. Studies of Pediatric Liver Transplantation: 2002 update. An overview of demographics, indications, timing, and immunosuppressive practices in pediatrics transplantation in the United States and Canada. *Pediatr Transplant* 2004;8:284–94.

3. Devictor D, Desplanques L, Debray D, et al. Emergency liver transplantation for fulminant liver failure in infants and children. *Hepatology* 1992;16:1156–62.

4. Durand P, Debray D, Mandel R, et al. Acute liver failure in infancy: A 14-year experience of a pediatric liver transplantation center. *J Pediatr* 2001;139:871–6.

5. Dhawan A. Etiology and prognosis of acute liver failure in children. *Liver Transpl* 2008;14:S80–S84.

6. Narkewicz MR, Dell Olio D, Karpen SJ, et al. Pattern of diagnosis evaluation for the causes of pediatric acute liver failure: An opportunity for quality improvement. *J Pediatr* 2009;555:801–6.

7. Fouquet V, Alves A, Branchereau S, et al. Long-term outcome of pediatric liver transplantation for biliary atresia: A 10-year follow-up in a single center. *Liver Transpl* 2005;11:152–60.

8. Kortsalioudaki C, Taylor RM, Cheesman P, et al. Safety and efficacy of N-acetylcysteine in children with non-acetaminophen-induced acute liver failure. *Liver Transpl* 2008;14:25–30.

9. Lee WM, Squires RH Jr, Nylberg SL, et al. Acute liver failure: Summary of a workshop. *Hepatology* 2008;47:1401–15.

10. Venick RS, Mc Diarmid SV, Farmer DG, et al. Rejection and steroid dependence: Unique risk factors in the development of pediatric post-transplant de novo auto-immune hepatitis. *Am J Transplant* 2007;7(4):955–63.

11. Ng V, Anand R, Martz K, et al. Liver retransplantation in children: A SPLIT database analysis of outcome and predictive factors for survival. *Am J Transplant* 2008;8(2):386–95.

12. Roberts JP, Hulbert-Shearon TE, Merion RM, et al. Influence of graft type on outcomes after pediatric liver transplantation. *Am J Transplant* 2004;4(3):373–7.

13. Becker NS, Barshes NR, Aloia TA, et al. Analysis of recent pediatric orthotopic liver transplantation outcomes indicates that allograft type is no longer a predictor of survivals. *Liver Transpl* 2008;14(8):1125–32.

14. Black DD. The continuing challenge of "indeterminate" acute liver failure. *J Pediatr* 2009;555:770.

15. Diamond IR, Fecteau A, Millis JM, et al. Impact of graft type on outcome in pediatric liver transplantation: A report from Studies of Pediatric Liver transplantation (SPLIT). *Ann Surg* 2007;246(2):301–10.

16. Sartorelli MR, Comparcola D, Nobili V. Acute liver failure and pediatric ALF: Strategic help for the pediatric hepatologist. *J Pediatr* 2010;156:342.

17. Shanmugam NP, Bansal S, Greenough A, et al. Neonatal liver failure: Aetiologies and management. State of the art. *Eur J Pediatr* 2011;170(5):573–81.

18. Devictor D, Tissieres P, Afanetti M, et al. Acute liver failure in children. *Clin Res Hepatol Gastroenterol* 2011;35:430–7.

19. Polson J, Lee WM. AASLD position paper: The management of acute liver failure. *Hepatology* 2005;41:1179–97.

20. Aradottir E, Alonso EM, Shulman ST. Severe neonatal enteroviral hepatitis treated with pleconaril. *Pediatr Infect Dis J* 2001;20(4):457–9.

21. Kimberlin DW, Lin CY, Jacobs RF, et al. Natural history of neonatal herpes simplex virus infections in the acyclovir era. *Pediatrics* 2001;108:223–9.

22. Sauerbrei A, Wutzler P. Herpes simplex and varicella-zoster virus infections during pregnancy: Current concepts of prevention, diagnosis and therapy. Part 1: Herpes simplex virus infections. *Med Microbiol Immunol* 2007;196:89–94.

23. Segal S, Berry GT. Disorders of galactose metabolism. In: Scriver CR, Beaudet AL, Sly WS, et al., eds. *The Metabolic and Molecular Bases of Inherited Diseases*. 7th ed. New York, NY: McGraw-Hill, 1995:967–1000.

24. Grompe M. The pathophysiology and treatment of hereditary tyrosinemia type 1. *Semin Liver Dis* 2001;21:563–71.

25. Holme E, Lindstedt S. Nontransplant treatment of tyrosinemia. *Clin Liver Dis* 2000;4(4):805–14.

26. McKiernan PJ. Nitisinone in the treatment of hereditary tyrosinaemia type 1. *Drugs* 2006;66(6):743–50.

27. Lee WS, Sokol RJ. Mitochondrial hepatopathies: Advances in genetics and pathogenesis. *Hepatology* 2007;45:1555–65.

28. Gonzales E, Gerhardt MF, Fabre M, et al. Oral cholic acid for hereditary defects of primary bile acid synthesis: A safe and effective long-term therapy. *Gastroenterology* 2009;137(4):1310–20.

29. Rand EB, Karpen SJ, Kelly S, et al. Treatment of neonatal hemochromatosis with exchange transfusion and intravenous immunoglobulin. *J Pediatr* 2009;155:566–71.

30. Henter JI, Horne A, Aricó M, et al. HLH-2004: Diagnostic and therapeutic guidelines for hemophagocytic lymphohistiocytosis. *Pediatr Blood Cancer* 2007;48:124–31.

31. Squires RH, Shneider BL, Bucuvalas J, et al. Acute liver failure in children: The first 348 patients in the pediatric acute liver failure study group. *J Pediatr* 2006;148:652–8.

32. Schwarz KB, Dell Olio D, Lobritto SJ, et al. Analysis of viral testing in nonacetaminophen pediatric acute liver failure. *J Pediatr Gastroenterol Nutr* 2014;59(5):616–23.

33. Schmidt LE, Larsen FS. Prognostic implications of hyperlactatemia, multiple organ failure, and systemic inflammatory response syndrome in patients with acetaminophen-induced acute liver failure. *Crit Care Med* 2006;34:337–43.

34. Subcommittee on the National Halothane Study of the Committee on Anesthesia. Summary of the National Halothane Study. Possible association between halothane anesthesia and postoperative hepatic necrosis. *JAMA* 1966;197(10):775–88.

35. Reube A, Koch DG, Lee WM. Drug-induced acute liver failure: Results of a U.S. multicenter, prospective study. *Hepatology* 2010;52:2065–76.

36. Dhawan A, Taylor RM, Cheeseman P, et al. Wilson's disease in children: A 37-year experience and revised King's score for liver transplantation. *Liver Transpl* 2005;11:441–8.

37. Tissières P, Chevret L, Debray D, et. al. Fulminant Wilson's disease in children: Appraisal of a critical diagnosis. *Pediatr Crit Care Med* 2003;4:338–43.

38. Rustom N, Bost M, Cour-Andlauer F, et al. Effect of molecular adsorbents recirculating system treatment in children with acute liver failure caused by Wilson disease. *J Pediatr Gastroenterol Nutr* 2014;58(2):160–4.

39. Baliga P, Alvarez S, Lindblad A, et al. Post-transplant survival in pediatric fulminant hepatic failure: The SPLIT experience. *Liver Transpl* 2004;10:1364–71.

40. Berg CL, Steffick DE, Edwards EB, et al. Liver and intestine transplantation in the United States 1998-2007. *Am J Transplant* 2009;9 (4, pt 2):907–31.

41. Butterworth RF. The liver-brain axis in liver failure: Neuroinflammation and encephalopathy. *Nat Rev Gastroenterol Hepatol* 2013;10(9):522–8.

42. Blei AT. Medical therapy of brain edema in fulminant hepatic failure. *Hepatology* 2000;32:666–9.

43. Tissieres P, Devictor D. Drug treatment of encephalopathy associated with fulminant liver failure. *CNS Drugs* 1999;11:335–49.

44. Inderbitzin D, Muggli B, Ringger A, et al. Molecular absorbent recirculating system for the treatment of acute liver failure in surgical patients. *J Gastrointest Surg* 2005;9:1155–61; discussion 1161–2.

45. Mammen T, Keshava SN, Eapen CE, et al. Transjugular liver biopsy: A retrospective analysis of 601 cases. *J Vasc Interv Radiol* 2008;19(3):351–8.

46. Alper G, Jarjour IT, Reyes JD, et al. Outcome of children with cerebral edema caused by fulminant hepatic failure. *Pediatr Neurol* 1998;18:299–304.

47. Aggarwal S, Brooks DM, Kang Y, et al. Noninvasive monitoring of cerebral perfusion pressure in patients with acute liver failure using transcranial Doppler ultrasonography. *Liver Transpl* 2008;14:1048–57.

48. Lee WS, McKiernan P, Kelly DA. Etiology, outcome and prognostic indicators of childhood fulminant hepatic failure in the United Kingdom. *J Pediatr Gastroenterol Nutr* 2005;40:575–81.

49. Wright G, Shawcross D, Olde Damink SWM, et al. Brain cytokine flux in acute liver failure and its relationship with intracranial hypertension. *Metab Brain Dis* 2007;22:375–88.

50. Larsen FS, Strauss G, Knudsen GM, et al. Cerebral perfusion, cardiac output, and arterial pressure in patients with fulminant hepatic failure. *Crit Care Med* 2000;28:996–1000.

51. Harry R, Auzinger G, Wendon J. The clinical importance of adrenal insufficiency in acute hepatic dysfunction. *Hepatology* 2002;36:395–402.

52. Rolando N, Wade J, Davalos M, et al. The systemic inflammatory response syndrome in acute liver failure. *Hepatology* 2000;32:734–9.

53. Mekala S, Jagadisan B, Parija SC, et al. Surveillance for infectious complications in pediatric acute liver failure—A prospective study. *Indian J Pediatr* 2015;82(3):260–6.

54. Larsen FS. Optimal management of patients with fulminant hepatic failure: Targeting the brain. *Hepatology* 2004;39:299–301.

55. Cochran JB, Losek JD. Acute liver failure in children. *Pediatr Emerg Care* 2007;23:129–35.

56. Farmer DG, Venick RS, McDiarmid SV, et al. Fulminant hepatic failure in children: Superior and durable outcomes with liver transplantation over 25 years at a single center. *Ann Surg* 2009;250:484–93.

57. Ng VL, Fecteau A, Shepherd R, et al. Outcomes of 5 years survivors of pediatric liver transplantation: Report on 461 children from a North American multicenter registry. *Pediatrics* 2008;122 (6):e1128–e1135.

58. Evans HM, Kelly DA, Mc Kiernan PJ, et al. Progressive histological damage in liver allografts following pediatric liver transplantation. *Hepatology* 2006;43(5):1109–17.

59. Everhart JE, Lombardero M, Lake JR, et al. Weight change and obesity after liver transplantation: Incidence and risk factors. *Liver Transpl Surg* 1998;4(4):285–96.

60. Stravitz RT, Kramer AH, Davern T, et al. [Intensive care of patients with acute liver failure: Recommendations of the U.S. Acute Liver Failure Study Group]. *Crit Care Med* 2007;35:2498–508.

61. Holme E, Lindstedt S. Tyrosinaemia type I and NTBC (2-(2-nitro-4-trifluoromethylbenzoyl)-1,3-cyclohexanedione). *J Inherit Metab Dis* 1998;21:507–17.

62. Roberts EA, Schilsky ML. A practice guideline on Wilson disease. *Hepatology* 2003;37:1475–92.

63. Larson AM, Polson J, Fontana RJ, et al. Acetaminophen-induced acute liver failure: Results of a United States multicenter, prospective study. *Hepatology* 2005;42:1364–72.

64. Squires RH, Dhawan A, Alonso E, et al. Intravenous N-acetylcysteine in pediatric patients with nonacetaminophen acute liver failure: A placebo-controlled clinical trial. *Hepatology* 2013;57(4):1542–9.

65. Curioso WH, Monkemuller KE. Neomycin should not be used to treat hepatic encephalopathy. *BMJ* 2001;323(7306):233.

66. Debray D, Yousef N, Durand P. New management options for end-stage chronic liver disease and acute liver failure: Potential for pediatric patients. *Paediatr Drugs* 2006;8:1–13.

67. Kircheis G, Wettstein M, Dahl S, et al. Clinical efficacy of L-ornithine-L-aspartate in the management of hepatic encephalopathy. *Metab Brain Dis* 2002;17:453–62.

68. Summar M. Current strategies for the management of neonatal urea cycle disorders. *J Pediatr* 2001;138:S30–S39.

69. Strauss G, Hansen BA, Knudsen GM, et al. Hyperventilation restores cerebral blood flow autoregulation in patients with acute liver failure. *J Hepatol* 1998;28:199–203.

70. Ede RJ, Gimson AE, Bihari D, et al. Controlled hyperventilation in the prevention of cerebral oedema in fulminant hepatic failure. *J Hepatol* 1986;2:43–51.

71. Forbes A, Alexander GJ, O'Grady JG, et al. Thiopental infusion in the treatment of intracranial hypertension complicating fulminant hepatic failure. *Hepatology* 1989;10:306–10.

72. Karvellas CJ, Todd Stravitz R, Battenhouse H, et al. Therapeutic hypothermia in acute liver failure: A multicenter retrospective cohort analysis. *Liver Transpl* 2015;21(1):4–12.

73. Jalan R, Olde Damink SW, Deutz NE, et al. Moderate hypothermia prevents cerebral hyperemia and increase in intracranial pressure in patients undergoing liver transplantation for acute liver failure. *Transplantation* 2003;75:2034–9.

74. Jalan R, Olde Damink SWM, Deutz NEP, et al. Moderate hypothermia in patients with acute liver failure and uncontrolled intracranial hypertension. *Gastroenterology* 2004;127:1338–46.

75. Shami VM, Caldwell SH, Hespenheide EE, et al. Recombinant activated factor VII for coagulopathy in fulminant hepatic failure compared with conventional therapy. *Liver Transpl* 2003;9:138–43.

76. Shawcross DL, Davies NA, Mookerjee RP, et al. Worsening of cerebral hyperemia by the administration of terlipressin in acute liver failure with severe encephalopathy. *Hepathology* 2004;39:471–5.

77. Kjaergard L, Liu J, Als-Nielsen B, et al. Artificial and bioartificial support systems for acute and acute on chronic liver failure. *JAMA* 2003;289:217–22.

78. Demetriou AA, Brown RS Jr, Busuttil RW, et al. Prospective, randomized, multicenter, controlled trial of a bioartificial liver in treating acute liver failure. *Ann Surg* 2004;239:660–7; discussion 7–70.

79. Heemann U, Treichel U, Loock J, et al. Albumin dialysis in cirrhosis with superimposed acute liver injury: A prospective, controlled study. *Hepatology* 2002;36:949–58.

80. Steiner C, Mitzner S. Experiences with MARS liver support therapy in liver failure: Analysis of 176 patients of the International MARS Registry. *Liver* 2002;22(suppl 2):20–5.

81. Bañares R, Nevens F, Larsen FS, et al. Extracorporeal albumin dialysis with the molecular adsorbent recirculating system in acute-on-chronic liver failure: the RELIEF trial. *Hepatology* 2013;57(3):1153–62.

82. Saliba F, Camus C, Durand F, et al. Albumin dialysis with a noncell artificial liver support device in patients with acute liver failure: A randomized, controlled trial. *Ann Intern Med* 2013;159(8):522–31.

83. Bourgoin P, Merouani A, Phan V, et al. Molecular Absorbent Recirculating System therapy (MARS) in pediatric acute liver failure: A single center experience. *Pediatr Nephrol* 2014;29(5):901–8.

84. Ringe H, Varnholdt V, Gratopp A, et al. Continuous veno-venous single-pass albumin haemodiafiltration in children with acute liver failure. *Pediatr Crit Care Med* 2011;12:257–64.

85. Singer AL, Olthoff KM, Kim H, et al. Role of plasmapheresis in the management of acute hepatic failure in children. *Ann Surg* 2001;234:418–24.

86. Schmidt LE, Wang LP, Hansen BA, et al. Systemic hemodynamic effects of treatment with the molecular adsorbents recirculating system in patients with hyperacute liver failure: A prospective controlled trial. *Liver Transpl* 2003;9:290–7.

87. Lai WK, Haydon G, Mutimer D, et al. The effect of molecular adsorbent recirculating system on pathophysiological parameters in patients with acute liver failure. *Intensive Care Med* 2005;31:1544–9.

88. Laleman W, Wilmer A, Evenepoel P, et al. Effect of the molecular adsorbent recirculating system and Prometheus devices on systemic haemodynamics and vasoactive agents in patients with acute-on-chronic alcoholic liver failure. *Crit Care* 2006;10:R108.

89. Chevret L, Durand P, Lambert J, et al. High-volume hemofiltration in children with acute liver failure. *Pediatr Crit Care Med* 2014;15(7):e300–e305.

90. Bellomo R, Tipping P, Boyce N. Continuous veno-venous hemofiltration with dialysis removes cytokines from the circulation of septic patients. *Crit Care Med* 1993;21:522–6.

91. Tissières P, Sasbon J, Devictor D. Liver Support for fulminant hepatic failure: Is it time to use the Molecular Absorbents Recycling System in children? *Pediatr Crit Care Med* 2005;6:585–91.

92. Tissieres P, Prontera W, Chevret L, et al. The pediatric risk of mortality score in infants and children with fulminant liver failure. *Pediatr Transplant* 2003;7:64–8.

93. Sundaram V, Shneider BL, Dhawan A, et al. King's College Hospital Criteria for non-acetaminophen induced acute liver failure in an international cohort of children. *J Pediatr* 2013;162(2):319–23.

94. Lu BR, Zhang S, Narkewicz MR, et al. Evaluation of the liver injury unit scoring system to predict survival in a multinational study of pediatric acute liver failure. *J Pediatr* 2013;162(5):1010–6.

95. Faraj W, Dar F, Bartlett A, et al. Auxiliary liver transplantation for children with acute liver failure. *Ann Surg* 2010;251:351–6.

96. Farmer DG, Venick RS, McDiarmid SV, et. al. Fulminant hepatic failure in children: Superior and durable outcomes with liver transplantation over 25 years at a single center. *Ann. Surg.* 2009; 250:484–93.

97. Fox IJ, Chowdhury JR. Hepatocyte transplantation. *Am J Transplant* 2004;4(suppl 6):7–13.

98. Pareja E, Cortes M, Bonora A, et al. New alternatives to the treatment of acute liver failure. *Transplant Proc* 2010;42:2959–61.

99. Tissières P, Simon L, Debray D, et al. Acute pancreatitis after orthotopic liver transplantation in children: Incidence, contributing factors and outcome. *J Pediatr Gastroenterol Nutr* 1998; 26(3):315–20.

100. Moghazy MW, Ogura Y, Mutsuko M, et al. Pediatric living-donor liver transplantation for acute liver failure: Analysis of 57 cases. *Transpl Int* 2010;23:823–30.

101. Abt PL, Fisher CA, Singhal AK. Donation after cardiac death in the US: history and use. *J Am Coll Surg* 2006;203(2):208–25.

102. Kamath BM, Olthoff KM. Liver transplantation in children: Update 2010. *Pediatr Clin North Am* 2010;57:401–14.

103. Kelly DA. Current issues in pediatric transplantation. *Pediatr Transplant* 2006;10(6):712–20.

104. Martin SR, Atkison P, Anand R, et al. Studies of Pediatric Liver Transplantation 2002: patient and graft survival and rejection in pediatric recipients of a first liver transplant in the United States and Canada. *Pediatr Transplant* 2004;8(3):273–83.

105. Ueda M, Oike F, Ogura Y, et al. Long-term outcomes of 600 living donor liver transplantations for pediatric patients at a single center. *Liver Transpl* 2006;12:1326–36.

106. Dommergues JP, Letierce A, Gravereau L, et al. Current lifestyle of young adults after liver transplantation during childhood. *Am J Transplant* 2010;10:1643–51.

107. McDiarmid SV, Anand R, Martz BS, et al. A multivariate analysis of pre-, peri-, and post-transplant factors affecting outcome after pediatric liver transplantation. *Ann Surg* 2011;254:145–54.

108. Florman S, Shneider B. Living-related liver transplantation in inherited metabolic liver disease: Feasibility and cautions. *J Pediatr Gastroenterol Nutr* 2001;33(4):520–1.

109. Kayler LK, Rasmussen CS, Dykstra DM, et al. Liver transplantation in children with metabolic disorders in the United States. *Am J Transplant* 2003;3(3):334–9.

110. Austin MT, Leys CM, Feurer ID, et al. Liver transplantation for childhood hepatic malignancy: A review of the United Network for Organ Sharing (UNOS) database. *J Pediatr Surg* 2006; 41(1):182–6.

111. Avila LF, Luis AL, Hernandez F, et al. Liver transplantation for malignant tumors in children. *Eur J Pediatr Surg* 2006;16(6):411–4.

112. Ginès P, Guevara M, Arroyo V, et al. Hepatorenal syndrome. *Lancet* 2003;362:1819–27.

113. Freeman RB Jr, Wiesner RH, Harper A, et al. The new liver allocation system: Moving toward evidence-based transplantation policy. *Liver Transpl* 2002;8(9):851–8.

114. McDiarmid SV, Merion RM, Dykstra DM, et al. Selection of pediatric candidates under the PELD system. *Liver Transpl* 2004;10(10, suppl 2):S23–S30.

115. Hong JC, Yersiz H, Farmer DG, et al. Long-term outcomes for whole and segmental liver grafts in adult and pediatric liver transplant recipients: A 10-year comparative analysis of 2988 cases. *J Am Coll Surg* 2009;208:682–91.

116. Heaton N, Faraj W, Melendez HV, et al. Living related liver transplantation in children. *Br J Surg* 2008;95:919–24.

117. Wiesner RH, Mc Diarmid SV, Kamath PS, et al. MELD and PELD: Application of survival models to liver allocation. *Liver Transpl* 2001;7(7):567–80.

118. Duffy JP, Hong JC, Farmer DG, et al. Vascular complications of orthotopic liver transplantation: Experience in more than 4,200 patients. *J Am Coll Surg* 2009;208:896–905.

119. Peclet MH, Ryckman FC, Pedersen SH, et al. The spectrum of bile duct complications in pediatric liver transplantation. *J Pediatr Surg* 1994;29(2):214–9.

120. Bourdeaux C, Brunati A, Janssen M, et al. Liver retransplantation in children. A 21-year single-center experience. *Transpl Int* 2009;22(4):416–22.

121. Hubscher S. What does the long-term liver allograft look like for the pediatric recipient? *Liver Transpl* 2009;15 (suppl 2):S19–S24.

122. Grabhorn E, Richter A, Fischer, et al. Emergency liver transplantation in neonates with acute liver failure: Long-term follow-up. *Transplantation* 2008;86(7):932–6.

123. Bell LE, Bartosh SM, Davis CL, et al. Adolescent transition to adult care in solid organ transplantation: A consensus conference report. *Am J Transplant* 2008;8(11):2230–42.

124. Duffy JP, Kao K, Co CY, et al. Long-term patient outcome and quality of life after liver transplantation: Analysis of 20-year survivors. *Ann Surg* 2010;252:652–61.

125. Alonso EM, Shepherd R, Martz KL, et al. Linear growth patterns in prepubertal children following liver transplantation. *Am J Transplant* 2009;9(6):1389–97.

126. Hathout E, Alonso E, Anand R, et al. Post-transplant diabetes mellitus in pediatric liver transplantation. *Pediatr Transplant* 2009;13(5):599–605.

127. Magee JC, Krishnan SM. Benfield MR, et al. Pediatric transplantation in the United States, 1997-2006. *Am J Transplant* 2008;8:935–45.

128. Naim MY, Hoehn KS, Hasz RD, et al. The Children's Hospital of Philadelphia's experience with donation after cardiac death. *Crit Care Med* 2008;36(6):1729–33.

CHAPTER 104 ■ PEDIATRIC INTESTINAL AND MULTIVISCERAL TRANSPLANTATIONS

GEOFFREY J. BOND, KATHRYN A. FELMET, RONALD JAFFE, KYLE A. SOLTYS, JEFFREY A. RUDOLPH, DOLLY MARTIN, RAKESH SINDHI, AND GEORGE V. MAZARIEGOS

KEY POINTS

1 **Causes of irreversible intestinal failure** in children are predominantly due to surgical conditions (mostly short gut syndrome from volvulus, necrotizing enterocolitis, gastroschisis, etc.). In addition, medical conditions can lead to functional intestinal failure, such as motility disorders (e.g., intestinal pseudo-obstruction), and enterocyte dysfunction, such as microvillus inclusion disease.

2 **Indications for intestinal transplantation** include (a) evidence of liver dysfunction or failure, (b) loss of major venous access, (c) frequent central line-related sepsis, and (d) recurrent episodes of severe dehydration despite intravenous fluid management.

3 **Recipient operations should be tailored** to the specific indications for each patient and include isolated intesti-

nal transplantation, combined liver and intestinal transplantation, and multivisceral transplantation including the stomach (with or without the liver).

4 **Immunosuppression for intestinal transplantation** is based on tacrolimus and antibody induction therapy.

5 Current modifications in intestinal transplantation include pretreatment of the recipient with an antilymphocyte antibody such as either antithymocyte antibody or basiliximab to eliminate maintenance steroid use postoperatively.

6 **Sepsis following intestinal transplantation** should prompt a rapid search for technical complications (intra-abdominal abscess, anastomotic dehiscence, etc.) and immunologic causes (rejection may lead to bacterial translocation, over-immunosuppression places the recipient at risk of infection).

Intestine was one of the first organs to be transplanted (1), but early case reports noted a high incidence of graft loss from rejection, infection, and technical complications (2). In 1987, a 3-year-old girl received a multivisceral abdominal graft that included the stomach, duodenum, pancreas, small bowel, colon, and liver and survived with good intestinal graft function for 6 months (3). A modification of this operation was reported in 1989 that involved transplantation of a "cluster" of organs consisting of the liver and the pancreaticoduodenal complex (**Fig. 104.1**) (4). Unfortunately, until 1990, there were only two survivors of isolated cadaveric intestinal grafts (5,6). In 1989, the introduction of the immunosuppressive agent tacrolimus (FK506, Prograf) revolutionized the field by permitting successful transplantation of human intestinal grafts (alone or as part of a multivisceral graft) (7).

INDICATIONS

Diseases associated with loss of intestinal function and the need for transplantation can be divided into surgical and nonsurgical etiologies. Patients with surgical causes generally suffer from loss of bowel length after resections due to ischemia, obstruction, or from strictures and fistulas (as with Crohn disease). With nonsurgical causes of intestinal failure, the anatomic length and gross morphology of the intestine are often normal. Nonsurgical causes of intestinal failure include motility disorders (e.g., intestinal pseudo-obstruction, Hirschsprung disease) (8,9) and disorders of enterocyte function (e.g., microvillus inclusion disease) (10). **Table 104.1** lists the indications

for transplantation in the case experience at the University of Pittsburgh and Children's Hospital of Pittsburgh.

Parenteral nutrition (PN) is the standard of care for patients with intestinal failure who are unable to maintain a normal nutritional, fluid balance and electrolyte state (11,12). The management of intestinal failure should be multidisciplinary and provide a medical focus to optimize nutritional status while minimizing cholestatic liver injury and a surgical focus to consider options (such as stoma closure or bowel lengthening) that reduce the need for total PN (TPN) and, ultimately, transplantation (13,14). A group of patients persist who develop irreversible intestinal failure and suffer from complications of indefinite PN therapy. Transplantation of the intestine either alone or accompanied by other intra-abdominal organs (liver, stomach, duodenum, pancreas) may be lifesaving for these patients (15).

Decisions regarding the best transplant options are based on the anatomic and functional integrity of the remaining gut and abdominal organs as well as their vascular supplies. Liver replacement in intestinal transplant candidates is based on biochemical dysfunction (hyperbilirubinemia, transaminase abnormalities, hypoalbuminemia, thrombocytopenia, and coagulopathy), the presence of bridging fibrosis or cirrhosis on liver biopsy, and the presence of portal hypertension. Hypercoagulable patients deficient in protein S, protein C, and antithrombin III (16) may develop diffuse thromboses within the splanchnic system and undergo transplantation for mesenteric venous hypertension rather than for intestinal failure. Unfortunately, liver transplantation may not be technically feasible because of extensive portomesenteric thrombosis in some patients.

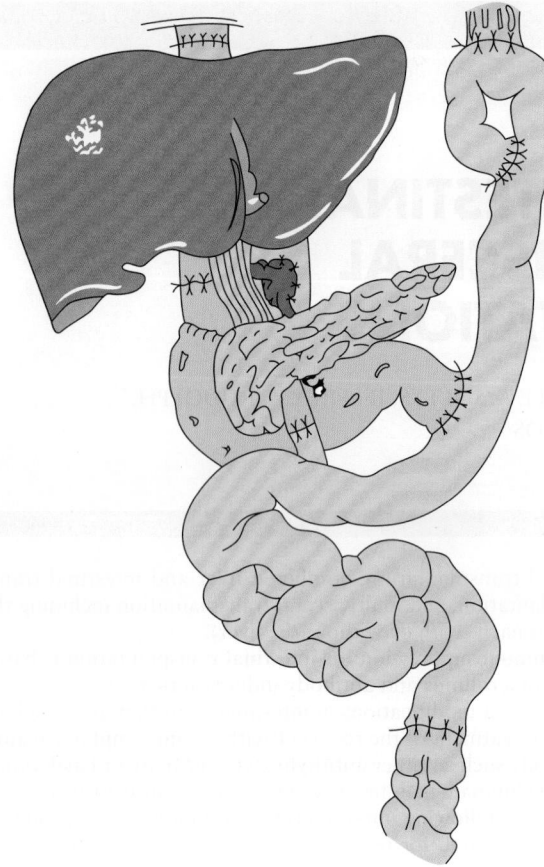

FIGURE 104.1. Cluster allograft (*shaded portion*), including the liver, pancreas, and duodenal segment of small intestine. (From Starzl TE, Todo S, Tzakis A, et al. Abdominal organ cluster transplantation for the treatment of upper abdominal malignancies. *Ann Surg* 1989;210:374–86.)

In October 2000, the Center for Medicare and Medicaid Services (CMS) in the United States approved intestinal, combined liver and intestinal, and multivisceral transplantation (17,18) at centers of excellence as a standard of care for patients with irreversible intestinal failure who could no

TABLE 104.1

INDICATIONS FOR COMPOSITE AND ISOLATED INTESTINAL TRANSPLANTATION

■ PEDIATRIC PATIENTS	■ ADULT PATIENTS
Volvulus	Trauma
Gastroschisis	Superior mesenteric artery thrombosis
Necrotizing enterocolitis	Crohn disease
Intestinal atresia	Desmoid tumor
Pseudo-obstruction	Volvulus
Microvillus inclusion disease	Familial polyposis
Intestinal polyposis	Gastrinoma
Hirschsprung disease	Budd–Chiari disease
Trauma	Intestinal adhesions
	Pseudo-obstruction
	Inflammatory bowel disease
	Radiation enteritis

longer be maintained on PN because of (a) impending liver failure, as manifested by jaundice or elevated liver injury tests, clinical findings (splenomegaly, varices, coagulopathy), history of stomal bleeding, or hepatic cirrhosis on biopsy; (b) loss of major venous access defined as more than two thromboses in the great vessels (subclavian, jugular, and femoral veins); (c) frequent central line-related sepsis consisting of more than two episodes of systemic sepsis per year or one episode of line-related fungemia associated with septic shock or acute respiratory distress syndrome; or (d) recurrent episodes of severe dehydration despite intravenous fluid management.

CLINICAL MANAGEMENT OF THE PRETRANSPLANT CHILD IN THE PICU

Intensive care of children with intestinal or combined intestinal and liver failure presents a unique set of challenges that fall into two categories: (a) PN dependence and the associated vascular access issues, and (b) the development of liver disease. PN dependence and the long-term requirement for central access bring a set of problems (discussed in detail in the next section). Liver disease develops in 40%–60% of infants who require long-term PN for intestinal failure, and although it may not ultimately require liver transplant, it can complicate their management (also discussed in detail in a later section) (19). Both problems are compounded by the long wait times before size-appropriate organs are available (often 6 months to 1 year), and they make it important for potential intestinal transplant candidates to be referred to a transplant service for evaluation as soon as possible. The success of the intestinal or multivisceral transplantation depends in large measure on the health and nutritional status of the transplant recipient. Even if the child does not ultimately require a transplant, early referral to a center experienced in the management of intestinal failure, including surgical and transplantation options, can dramatically impact outcomes.

The goal of critical care is to keep the child in optimal condition to receive a transplant. For this reason, the intensivist should be in close communication with the transplant surgeon both to review the patient's status and to discuss PICU interventions that may interfere with the patient's candidacy.

Parenteral Nutrition Dependence

PN-dependent patients have chronic problems with venous access because of infection and thrombosis. Any patient with a central line has increased susceptibility to infection, but intestinal transplant candidates are unique in several ways. Prevention of infection is particularly important since episodes of sepsis contribute to the deterioration in liver function (20,21). The central lines of patients with short gut syndrome can become infected by external contamination of the line or by translocation of bacteria across a gut with inadequate barrier function (22). Because patients have been repeatedly exposed to broad-spectrum antibiotics, and because intestinal stasis contributes to bacterial overgrowth, infections that result from bowel translocation may be multidrug resistant (23). The risk of fungal infections is also increased in this patient group compared to the general population (22). Enteric feedings may help preserve the intestinal mucosal barrier function and decrease infectious complications (23).

Patients with liver failure have impaired immune responses. The oxidative burst function of neutrophil and Kupffer cells is impaired and complement levels are reduced (22,24).

Additionally, adrenal insufficiency with failure of the stress cortisol response is common in patients with acute and chronic liver disease (25,26). The combination of adrenal insufficiency, relative immune deficiency, and the intestinal transplant candidate's requirement for invasive procedures creates a dangerous susceptibility to severe sepsis and septic shock.

Treatment for septic shock should follow established parameters (27) with a few caveats. The cardiac function of intestinal transplant candidates with liver disease is not normal. Patients with severe liver failure may have a hyperdynamic state at baseline, but a blunted contractile response to stress. Both systolic and diastolic ventricular function may be impaired (28). Clinical experience indicates that children with cirrhotic cardiomyopathy may not tolerate large-volume fluid challenge. Resuscitation should be appropriately aggressive, but with careful attention to signs of intravascular volume overload as well as vigilance for concomitant hepatopulmonary or hepatorenal syndrome. Palpation of the liver may not be a reliable indicator of intravascular volume overload in patients with cirrhosis; instead, clinicians should investigate changes in central venous pressure, development of rales on lung exam, and changes on chest x-ray. Echocardiogram can be used in difficult cases to assess cardiac filling and function. In patients with advanced liver disease, albumin may be preferable to crystalloid as a resuscitation fluid to avoid worsening anasarca. High salt loads (e.g., normal saline) should be avoided in established liver disease.

Inotropic or vasopressor agents should be used if clinical signs suggest the child is intravascularly replete. Low diastolic blood pressures may be present in association with advanced liver disease (28,29). Early septic shock in these children follows a vasodilatory pattern commonly seen in adults and may respond to vasopressor agents. In patients with catecholamine unresponsive septic shock, adrenal function should be evaluated with a cortisol level and/or adrenocorticotropic hormone (ACTH) stimulation test. In some cases, it may be appropriate to treat adrenal insufficiency empirically (hydrocortisone bolus and intermittent dosing or continuous infusion) while results of these tests are pending.

When infections cannot be cleared, it may be necessary to remove and replace lines. As children awaiting intestinal transplant are dependent on central access, meticulous care must be given to prevention of infection and preservation of line sites when possible. Intestinal transplant candidates are at high risk for forming clots around central lines that can become occlusive and persist after line removal. An inadequate synthesis of both coagulation factors and anticoagulating factors (e.g., protein C, protein S, and antithrombin III) is common in patients with liver failure (22). The loss of two or more great vessels to thrombosis is part of the criteria for considering transplantation, but clotting in most or all of the available sites for central venous catheterization can make transplantation technically challenging or impossible. When new lines are being placed, care should be taken not to damage the vessel unduly. Before line placement a careful clot history should be taken, and when appropriate, Doppler ultrasound of great vessels should be used to guide the individual performing the procedure. In some cases, especially older children, venograms of the extremities are performed as part of the pretransplant workup to better delineate vascular patency that is not accurately assessed by ultrasound (30,31).

A full discussion of nutritional requirements of children with intestinal failure is beyond the scope of this chapter, but it is important to note (a) that the ability to heal after a major operation is partly dependent on preoperative nutritional status, and (b) that the development of liver disease may be influenced by nutritional and metabolic parameters (19,32). A nutritional specialist should routinely be involved in the care of all prospective intestinal transplant patient regardless of

location. Whether that care occurs at home or in the hospital, attention should be paid to the provision of PN with adequate calories and an appropriate balance of fats, protein, and carbohydrate calories with an appropriate complement of trace elements and minerals.

Adequate nutrition is crucial, but our clinical experience with preoperative intestinal transplant patients suggests that these patients have a tendency to gain excess adipose tissue. When calculating metabolic requirements of these children in the ICU, it is important to include an estimate of their decreased activity on actual caloric expenditure. When possible, delivery of some enteral calories may preserve intestinal epithelial barrier function, decrease the risk or severity of intestinal failure-associated liver disease, and improve hospital mortality (19,33,34).

Liver Failure

Isolated intestinal transplant candidates may have mild, reversible liver disease. Patients awaiting combined liver and small intestinal or multivisceral transplants may persistently struggle with all of the problems seen in hepatic failure over a waiting period that is long compared to isolated liver candidates. Coagulopathy, portal hypertension with ascites and hepatomegaly, variceal bleeding, hypoalbuminemia, hyperbilirubinemia, hyperammonemia with hepatic encephalopathy, and hepatorenal and hepatopulmonary syndrome may all be seen in this patient population. The effects of a long duration of increased abdominal girth, renal dysfunction, and persistent coagulopathy on patients waiting for combined transplants deserve further discussion.

Intestinal transplant candidates with cirrhosis and liver failure have increased abdominal girth due to organomegaly and ascites. In children, especially infants, the enlarged liver and other abdominal contents may impinge on lung volumes and impede respiration. Although the problem is easily overcome with positive pressure ventilation, mechanical ventilation should be considered a last resort in view of the associated problems of sedation, respiratory muscle deconditioning, and ventilator-associated pneumonia. Due to risk of bleeding and infection, tracheostomy is usually contraindicated and should not be performed without consultation with the transplant surgeon. If ascites predominates over organomegaly as a cause of increased abdominal girth, drainage of ascitic fluid may relieve symptoms. Relief is usually temporary, as the circumstances leading to the fluid collection persist. The indications for peritoneal drainage must be weighed against the risk of infection. Additionally, rapid drainage of large volumes of peritoneal fluid may lead to intravascular hypovolemia and shock.

Patients with combined liver and intestinal or multivisceral transplants often have some degree of renal dysfunction that renders them sensitive to fluid overload. Repeated infections with fungus and gram-negative organisms expose these patients to multiple nephrotoxic agents. Additionally, episodes of septic shock can expose the kidney to low-flow states, causing acute tubular necrosis. Hepatorenal syndrome is a very late finding in liver failure but can contribute to renal insufficiency.

Persistent coagulopathy in combined liver and intestinal transplant candidates is a significant complication. Coagulopathy may be managed with administration of clotting factors. It may be impossible to normalize laboratory indicators of clotting function; instead, clinical evidence of bleeding should guide therapy. Intracranial hemorrhage, though rare, can occur. Correction of disordered coagulation with large volumes of clotting factors can lead to fluid overload. Renal insufficiency associated with exposure to nephrotoxic agents can exacerbate this predisposition to fluid overload. In cases of severe or recurrent bleeding, plasma exchange (plasmapheresis) and judicious use of recombinant factor 7 have been used successfully to correct coagulopathy without fluid overload (35,36). Plasma exchange may also have a role as a liver support therapy (36).

Extracorporeal liver support therapy, though in its infancy, someday may have application in combined liver and intestinal or multivisceral transplant patients. Support systems in use today mimic the liver's detoxifying function relying on diffusion of molecules across a membrane (dialysis with or without albumin-enriched dialysate), absorption (by charcoal, albumin), or dilution (exchange of plasma volumes) (37). Bio-artificial liver systems using animal or immortalized human cells are under development.

The pathophysiology of liver failure that causes brain edema and multiple organ failure is not well understood. Unfortunately, none of the extracorporeal liver support systems designed to prevent or reverse these complications have been rigorously evaluated in children (38). Of the therapies under investigation, MARS (molecular adsorbents recirculating system, a system based on albumin dialysis) and plasma exchange have been most extensively used (36,39). Studies with both systems have documented clinical improvement, but it has been difficult to demonstrate survival benefit. At our institution, it has successfully been used in an adult patient to bridge the time until a suitable multivisceral donor could be localized. Someday these systems may help to keep patients healthy enough to undergo a transplant until appropriate organs become available.

THE TRANSPLANT OPERATION

Abdominal Visceral Procurement

Optimal donor selection is imperative to a successful transplant outcome, especially whenever the intestine is involved. Intestine-containing allografts should be assessed

and procured (40–42) by surgeons intimately involved in the specialty. A further technical factor is size disparity, especially in recipients in whom the abdominal domain is reduced from prior resection. This is particularly pronounced in the very young where size-matched donors are infrequent. Both allograft reductions and efforts to provide increased abdominal domain (e.g., abdominal wall transplant or delayed closure) have been attempted to expand the donor pool.

Recipient Operations

Obtaining vascular access, especially when the liver requires transplantation, can be problematic in patients who have multiple thrombosed veins. Innovative therapies, including reopening venous channels (31) and intra-arterial perfusion (43), may be necessary. Access issues are best determined prior to the patient going to the operating room in view of the time constraints involved in minimizing the cold ischemic time of the allograft. Even so, time is often spent at the beginning of the procedure to establish appropriate access. The recipient operation consists of removal of the failed organs after exposure of the vascular anatomy, followed by allograft implantation, as described in the following sections.

Isolated Small Bowel

In cases of surgical short gut, the recipient's diseased small intestine is removed and the superior mesenteric artery (SMA) of the donor bowel is sewn to the infrarenal aorta (or occasionally the native SMA), and the donor superior mesenteric vein is anastamosed to the recipient superior mesenteric vein or inferior vena cava (Fig. 104.2A). The anastamoses are often facilitated by the use of interposition arterial and venous

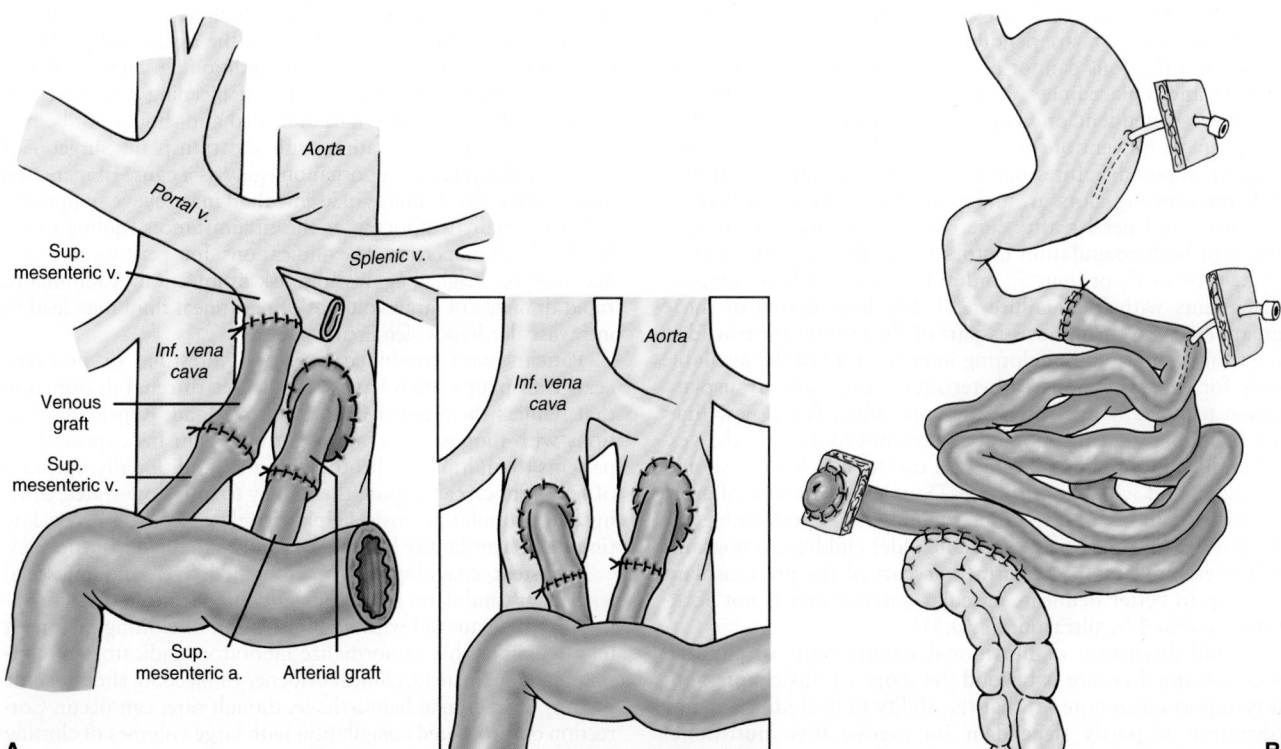

FIGURE 104.2. Arterialization and potential venous drainage options of the isolated small intestine allograft (A). Illustration of an isolated small bowel graft; the distal ileal chimney allows easy access to bowel mucosa (B).

grafts. Intestinal continuity is completed with proximal and distal gastrointestinal anastomoses, and access to the ileum for endoscopic examination is provided by a temporary chimney ileostomy (**Fig. 104.2B**) (44), except in the case of a permanent end ileostomy.

Liver–Small Bowel

The diseased liver is removed, with the retrohepatic vena cava preserved in situ ("piggyback"), and a permanent portacaval shunt draining the native stomach and pancreas is performed (**Fig. 104.3A**). Prior to implantation of the allograft (**Fig. 104.3B**), the double arterial stem of the celiac and superior mesenteric arteries (using the Carrel patch technique) is connected to the infrarenal aorta using a donor aortic conduit homograft. A proximal jejunojejunostomy, ileocolostomy, and a temporary distal ileostomy complete the operation. The allograft duodenum remains in continuity with the allograft biliary system (45).

Multivisceral Transplantation

After removal of the native liver, distal stomach, duodenum, pancreas, and intestine, the retroperitoneal aorta is exposed and the multivisceral graft (**Fig. 104.4A**) is connected to its vascular inflow and outflow. With a full multivisceral transplant (liver included), the suprahepatic venous attachment is completed initially followed by the aorto-aortic anastomosis. No portal vein anastomosis is required in this procedure as the recipient's portal vein and its inflow native organs (gastrointestinal tract, pancreas, and liver) are removed with the enterectomy. Patients with a normal native liver receive a modified multivisceral procedure where allograft portal venous return is directed into the recipient's native portal vein (**Fig. 104.4B**), preserving the native liver.

A gastro-gastric anastomosis, coloenteric anastomosis, and a chimney ileostomy are routinely performed. A pyloroplasty is also necessary owing to vagal denervation to avoid gastric outlet obstruction. In all types of intestinal recipients, the ileostomy is primarily placed to allow for ease of allograft monitoring via ileoscopy and ileal allograft biopsies. Takedown of the ileostomy can be performed once oral nutrition is consistently adequate and a stable immunosuppressant regimen has been achieved with less need for frequent endoscopic surveillance.

POSTTRANSPLANT MANAGEMENT

Immunosuppression

The immunosuppression regimens used at the University of Pittsburgh from 1990 to 2012 are presented in **Table 104.2**. Currently, thymoglobulin is given as a single 5-mg/kg dose preallograft reperfusion. Methylprednisolone is given as a bolus (2 mg/kg IV) as a lymphocyte-depleting premedication to limit the cytokine reaction; subsequent low-dose steroid therapy is weaned over the first 3–6 months posttransplant (46). Recent modifications in intestinal transplantation include pretreatment of the recipient with antilymphocyte antibody such as antithymocyte antibody or basiliximab to eliminate maintenance steroid use postoperatively. Rejection is treated with optimization of tacrolimus levels, supplemental corticosteroids, and monoclonal or polyclonal antibody if necessary. Additional or alternative agents have occasionally been used, including azathioprine, rapamycin, and mycophenolate mofetil, especially in the face of complications such as renal dysfunction and recurrent rejection, although their efficacy appears to be less than that of the standard agent(s).

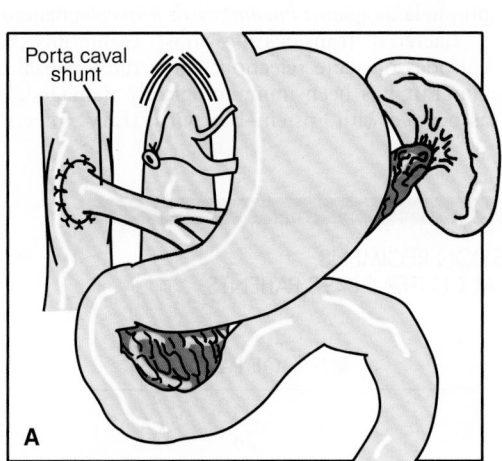

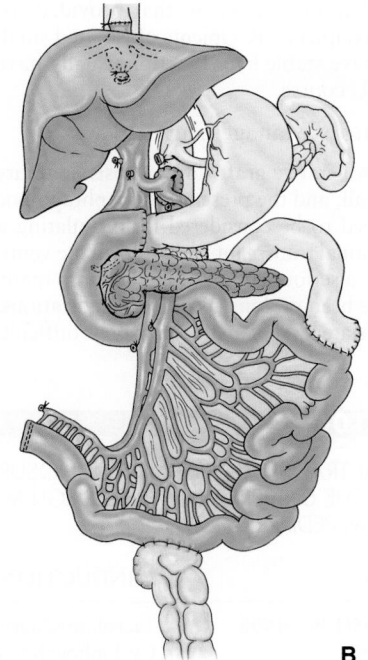

FIGURE 104.3. Combined liver and small intestinal allograft. Systemic portacaval shunt allows venous outflow of retained pancreas and stomach from recipient (**A**). Composite liver and intestine graft with preservation of the duodenum in continuity with the graft jejunum and hepatobiliary system (**B**).

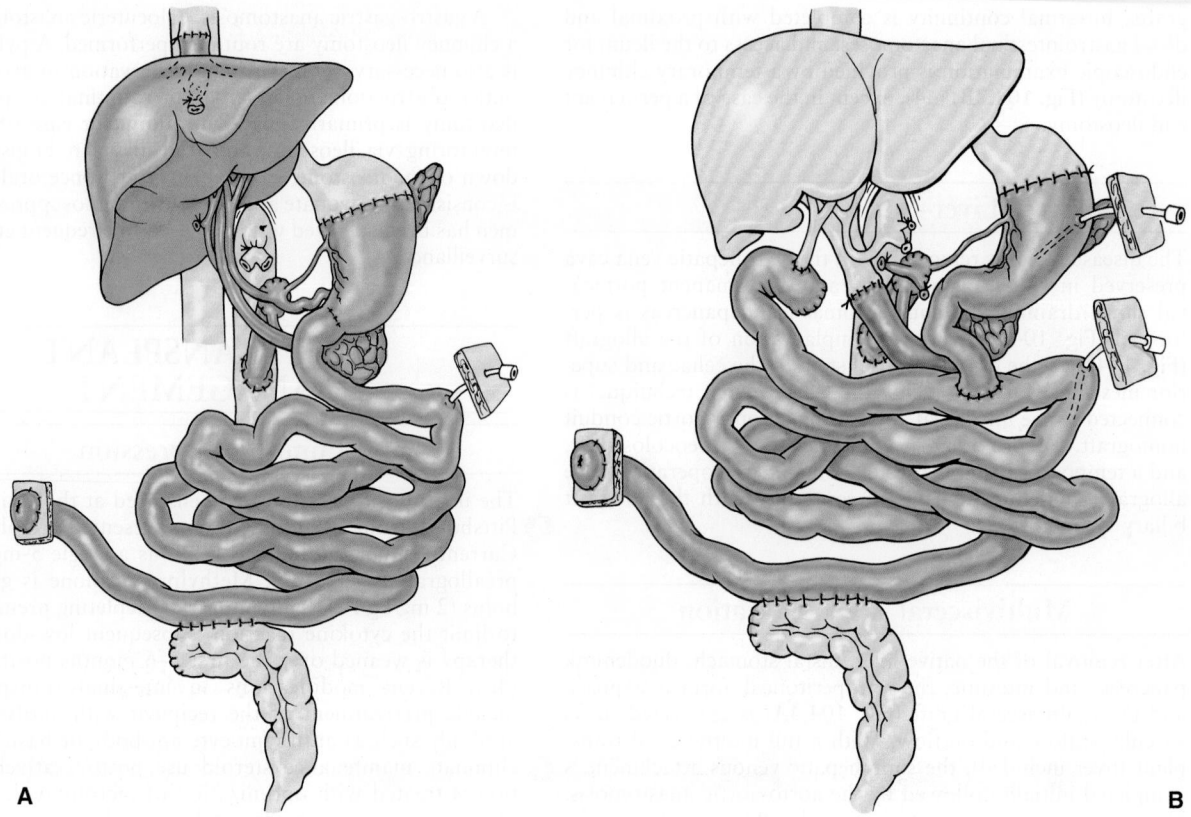

FIGURE 104.4. Diagrams of multivisceral donor organs: complete (**A**), modified multivisceral (**B**).

Postoperative Care

For recipients with pretransplant liver failure, postoperative care is similar (although more intense) to that provided for isolated liver transplant recipients. Recipients of isolated small bowel transplants who have stable liver function usually have a more routine initial ICU course.

Ventilatory Management

Pretransplant status, postoperative graft status, sepsis, inability to close the abdominal wall, and the presence of diaphragmatic weakness or paralysis need to be considered in formulating a plan for weaning the intestinal transplant patient from the ventilator. Pain management is a serious complicating factor as many of the older patients have been on long-term pain medications, and obtaining the appropriate level of analgesia may be difficult.

Infection Control

Recipients of intestinal grafts receive prophylactic, broad-spectrum intravenous antibiotics. Antiviral prophylaxis currently includes a 2-week course of intravenous ganciclovir (5 mg/kg twice daily IV) with concomitant administration of CMV-specific hyperimmune globulin (Cytogam) (150 mg/kg IV at 2, 4, 6, and 8 weeks posttransplant and 100 mg/kg/dose IV at 12 and 16 weeks posttransplant and oral ganciclovir) to CMV-negative recipients who receive an allograft from a CMV-positive donor. Oral administration of trimethoprim–sulfamethoxazole (80 mg po three times weekly) is used for the lifetime of the patient as prophylaxis against *Pneumocystis jirovecii* pneumonia.

Bacterial translocation most commonly occurs during episodes of acute rejection, when the mucosal barrier of the allograft has been immunologically damaged, or in enteritis associated with Epstein–Barr virus (EBV) infection (47).

TABLE 104.2

INTESTINAL TRANSPLANTATION: IMMUNOSUPPRESSION REGIMENS BY ERA AT THE UNIVERSITY OF PITTSBURGH MEDICAL CENTER IN 498 PATIENTS (ADULT, 269; PEDIATRIC, 229)

■ YEARS	■ INDUCTION	■ NO. OF PATIENTS
1990–1995/1997–1998	Tacrolimus/steroids	83
1995–1997	Cyclophosphamide	24
1998–2001	Daclizumab	61
2002–2012	Thymoglobulin/campath preconditioning protocol	330
Total		498

Gastrointestinal Function and Assessment

The normal intestine is pink, nonedematous, and occasionally demonstrates contractions. Postoperative changes in the ileal stoma should be promptly investigated and vascular, technical, or immunologic causes ruled out (48). Dramatic and rapid changes may be seen in recipients of a positive tissue typing crossmatch, especially B-cell, which may herald a vascular humoral type of rejection (49).

Routine endoscopic surveillance is used to assess graft integrity and for the diagnosis of intestinal rejection. Zoom endoscopy has been used in some centers to try to establish a prompt visual tool to diagnose rejection; however, as the changes are not specific, it is yet to receive widespread application.

Normal stomal output is 40–60 mL/kg/day. No reliable serum tests exist for monitoring the function of intestinal grafts. Data on prospective markers, such as citrulline or stool calprotectin, have been inconclusive (50–52).While PN is continued in the early postoperative weeks, enteral nutrition is introduced once integrity of the gastrointestinal tract has been demonstrated by contrast study, usually at 1 week posttransplant.

Management of Complications

Graft Rejection

Intestinal allograft rejection may be clinically asymptomatic or present with fever, abdominal pain, distention, nausea, vomiting, or a sudden change (increase or decrease) in stomal output. The stoma may be normal in appearance or lose its normal velvety appearance and become friable or ulcerated. Histologically (53), the rejection is graded by the degree of epithelial damage. In mild rejection (**Fig. 104.5A**), apoptosis leads to epithelial cell loss within the deep crypts. In moderate rejection (**Fig. 104.5B**), there is more severe crypt damage with focal crypt loss. Severe rejection (**Fig. 104.5C**) leads to denuded mucosa. Regeneration (**Fig. 104.5D**) occurs by reepithelialization over the surface of a lamina propria devoid of crypts.

Chronic rejection is observed in ~15% of isolated small bowel recipients (54). The presentation may include weight loss, chronic diarrhea, intermittent fever, or gastrointestinal bleeding. Histologically, the features are mostly those of chronic ischemia, such as villous blunting, focal ulcerations,

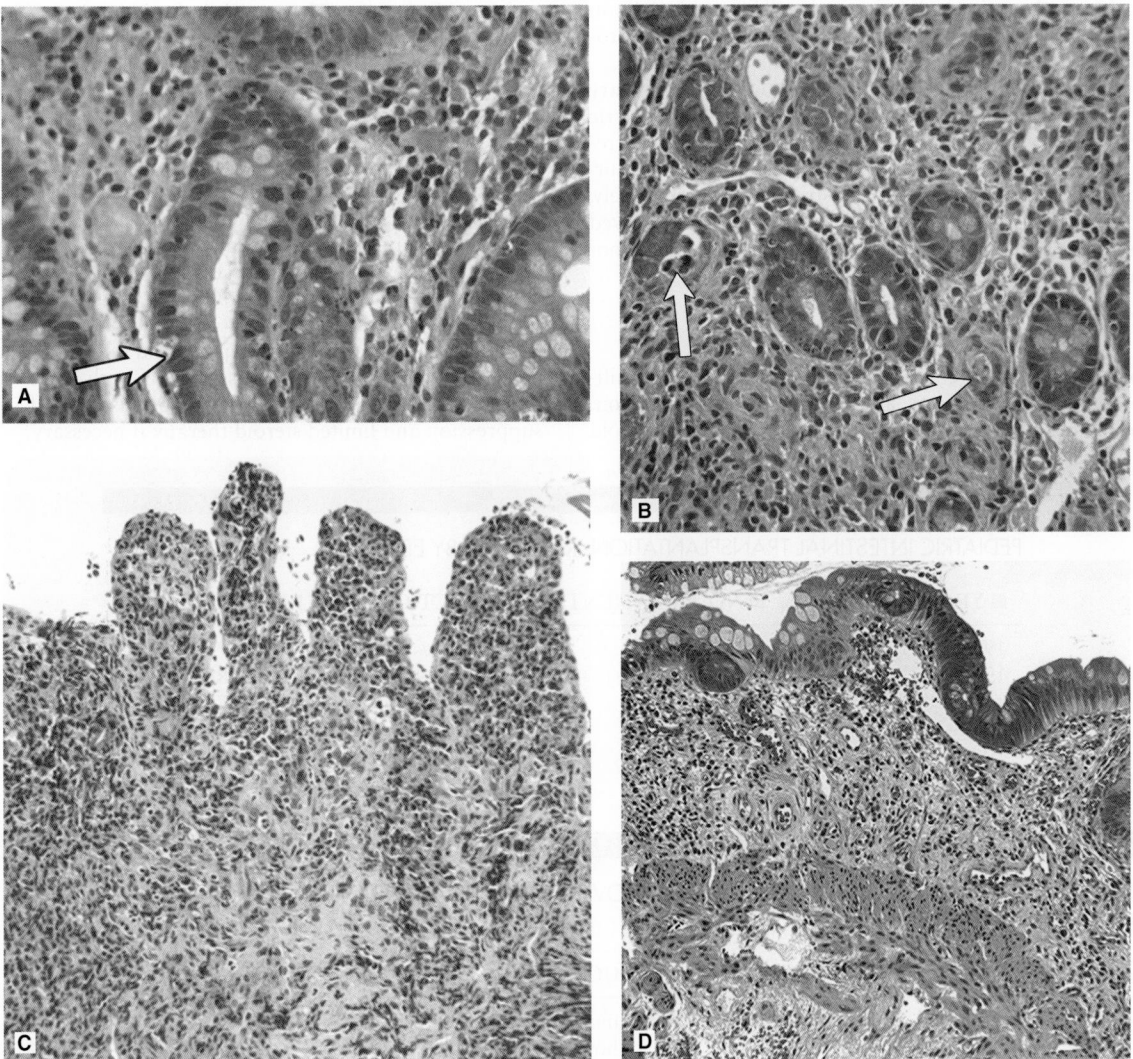

FIGURE 104.5. The rejection is graded by the degree of epithelial damage. In mild rejection (**A**), there is epithelial cell apoptosis *(arrows)* leading to epithelial cell loss within the deep crypts. In moderate rejection (**B**), there is more severe crypt damage *(arrow)* with focal crypt loss. Severe rejection (**C**) leads to denuded mucosa. Regeneration (**D**) occurs by reepithelialization over the surface of a lamina propria devoid of crypts. (Original magnification: ×400, **A** and **B**; ×200, **C** and **D**.)

epithelial metaplasia, and scant cellular infiltrate (55). Full-thickness intestinal biopsies or resections may show obliterative changes of the perforating arteries.

Acute rejection occurs in ~50% of patients with the use of a preconditioning protocol (**Table 104.3**). Reduction in immunosuppression resulted in a concomitant decrease in CMV and EBV disease, especially in pediatric recipients (**Table 104.4**).

Mild graft rejection in most cases responds to intravenous methylprednisolone combined with optimization of tacrolimus levels to 15 ng/mL. Antibody therapy with OKT3 is used when rejection has progressed despite a steroid taper, or as the initial therapeutic agent in cases of severe mucosal injury and crypt damage.

Biliary Complications

The biliary and pancreatic complications from leaks and strictures at anastomoses have been avoided through modification in donor technique to preserve the donor duodenum and the entire pancreas and to maintain the hepato-pancreato-biliary system. A group of patients have been identified who have signs and radiologic evidence of obstruction, perhaps from ampulla of Vater dysfunction. This can occur months to years posttransplantation. These can be managed via percutaneous transhepatic cholangiography (PTC) with balloon dilatation and/or endoscopic retrograde cholangiopancreatogram (ERCP) and stenting or incision of the ampulla (56).

In modified multivisceral grafts, continuity of the biliary axis is surgically reestablished, via either a Roux-en-Y enteric loop or a duct-to-duct in bigger donors and recipients. Correspondingly, these grafts can develop biliary system-related surgical complications (i.e., leaks and obstructions). Alternatively, the native spleen, pancreas, and duodenum may be preserved and gastrointestinal/biliary continuity restored by a duodeno-duodenostomy (57).

Infection

Infectious complications continue to be responsible for significant morbidity and mortality after intestinal transplantation. Sepsis following intestinal transplantation should prompt a rapid search for technical complications (intra-abdominal abscess, anastomotic dehiscence, etc.) and immunologic causes (rejection may lead to bacterial translocation, overimmunosuppression places the recipient at risk of infection). Immunosuppression modifications have decreased the incidence of life-threatening bacterial complications so that fungal and viral infections are the main source of morbidity in current transplant series.

Fungal infections are more common after heavy treatment for rejection, massive antibiotic usage, intestinal leaks, and multiple surgical explorations. The current incidence of cytomegalovirus (CMV) infection is ~13% (**Table 104.4**). Clinical presentation is usually with enteritis (**Fig. 104.6A,B**). Successful clinical management has been accomplished in the majority of episodes using ganciclovir alone or ganciclovir in combination with CMV-specific hyperimmunoglobulin (58). A CMV-positive donor graft transplanted into a CMV-negative recipient is a significant risk factor for CMV disease, but monitoring of CMV PCR with preemptive therapy has allowed the successful use of CMV-mismatched organs.

Posttransplantation lymphoproliferative disease (PTLD) may present as asymptomatic findings at routine endoscopy, EBV enteritis (**Fig. 104.7A**), systemic symptoms, bleeding, lymphadenopathy, or tumors (**Fig. 104.7B**). PTLD has decreased in incidence to 10% (**Table 104.4**) under current immunosuppression. Therapy includes reduction of immunosuppression, antiviral therapy using ganciclovir, acyclovir, and/or hyperimmunoglobulin, rituximab (anti-CD20 monoclonal antibody) and chemotherapy (59).

Graft-versus-Host Disease

Skin changes consistent with graft-versus-host disease (GVHD) were diagnosed by histopathologic criteria in ~5% of cases and confirmed by immunohistochemical studies visualizing donor cell infiltration into the lesions on two occasions or by flow cytometry detecting elevated donor cell chimerism in peripheral blood. Two children died (one with hereditary IgG and IgM deficiency and one from sepsis), and one adult developed a complex chronic GVHD in association with PTLD (60). All other cases have been treated with optimization of immunosuppression and limited steroid therapy if necessary.

TABLE 104.3

PEDIATRIC INTESTINAL TRANSPLANTATION: REJECTION BY ERA

■ YEARS	■ NO. OF PATIENTS	■ INDUCTION	■ REJECTION RATE
1990–1995/1997–1998	48	Tacrolimus/steroids	38 (79%)
1995–1997	16	Cyclophosphamide	14 (88%)
1998–2001	23	Daclizumab	16 (70%)
2002–2012	21	Campath	13 (62%)
2002–2012	121	Thymoglobulin	76 (63%)

TABLE 104.4

PEDIATRIC INTESTINAL TRANSPLANTATION: CYTOMEGALOVIRUS DISEASE AND POSTTRANSPLANTATION LYMPHOPROLIFERATIVE DISEASE BY ERA

■ YEARS	■ NO. OF PATIENTS	■ INDUCTION	■ CMV RATE	■ PTLD RATE
1990–1995/1997–1998	48	Tacrolimus/steroids	11 (23%)	19 (40%)
1995–1997	16	Cyclophosphamide	9 (56%)	3 (19%)
1998–2001	23	Daclizumab	1 (4%)	6 (26%)
2002–2012	21	Campath	3 (14%)	6 (29%)
2002–2012	121	Thymoglobulin	16 (13%)	12 (10%)

CMV, cytomegalovirus; PTLD, posttransplantation lymphoproliferative disease.

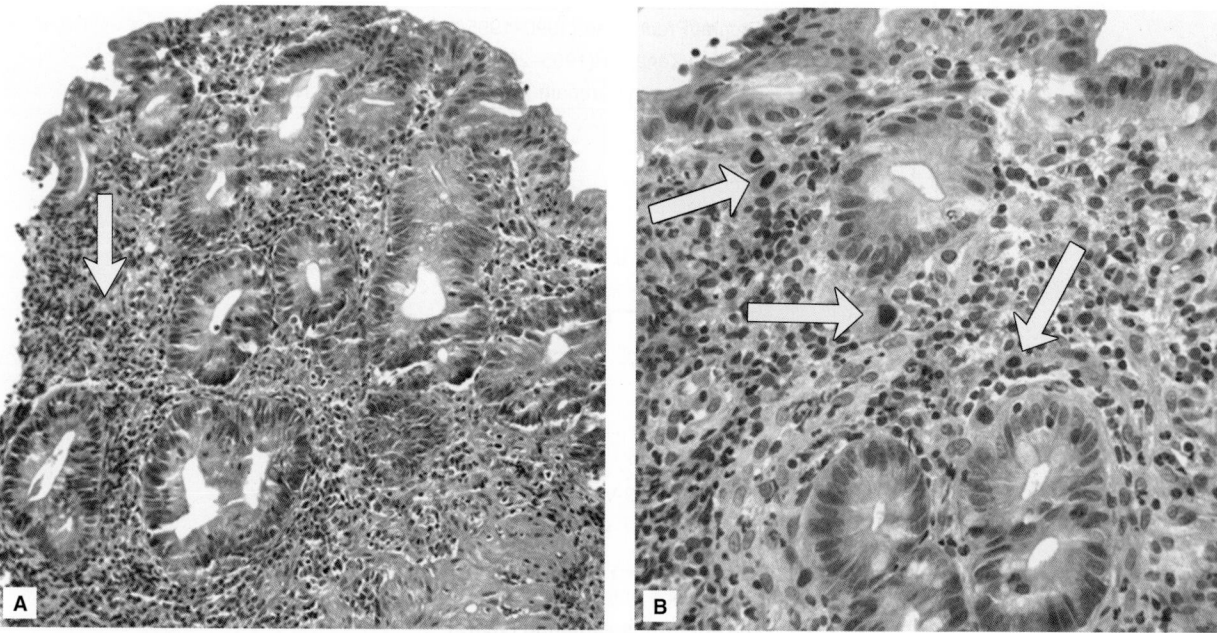

FIGURE 104.6. Cytomegaloviral enteritis is characterized histologically by the presence of characteristic inclusions (×200) *(arrow)* (**A**), by staining for viral antigens *(arrow)* (**B**), or by both. Note the focal neutrophilic inflammation (immunoperoxidase for cytomegalovirus antigens, ×350).

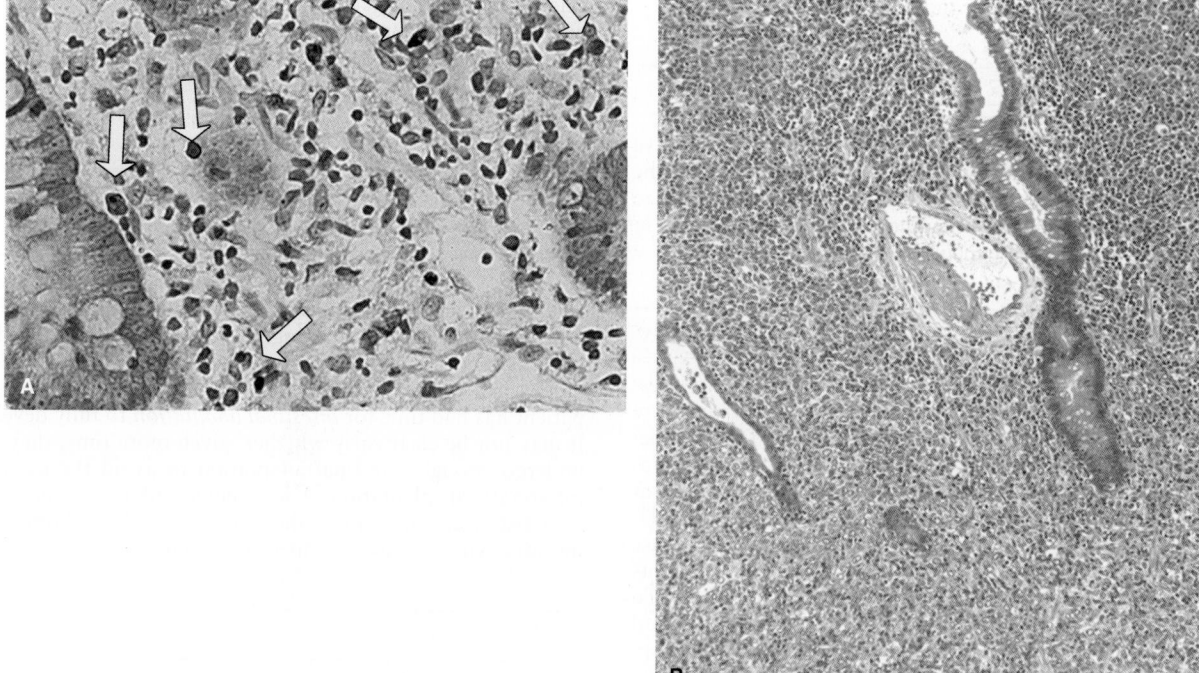

FIGURE 104.7. EBV infection (**A**) is diagnosed when EBER-1 positive nuclei *(arrow)* are seen in an otherwise relatively normal stroma (EBER-1 probe, Vector Red stain, original magnification ×400). Proliferative lymphoid processes (PTLD) distort the local architecture, forming masses (**B**) (H&E, original magnification ×200). EBER (Epstein Barr virus encoded small RNAs).

OUTCOMES

Current overall patient actuarial survival at 1 and 5 years is 90% and 78% (**Fig. 104.8**), respectively, and full nutritional support has been achieved in 91% of surviving patients (61). Optimal donor selection, transplantation of suitable candidates who are free from infection, and attention to detail in the technical performance of the operation are prerequisites for success. However, even under the best of circumstances, the critical care and managing physicians should anticipate potential postoperative difficulties and be prepared to support these patients fully for an extended period of time. Managing the balance between

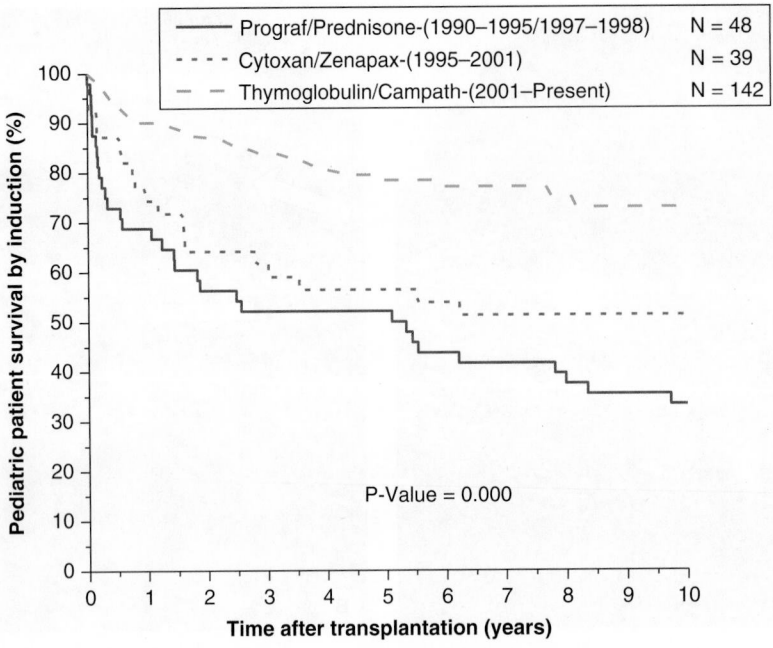

FIGURE 104.8. Patient survival by immunosuppression.

excessive and inadequate immunosuppression in the face of infections or rejection are the most challenging tasks.

FUTURE DIRECTIONS

Although intestinal and multivisceral transplantations have progressed significantly over the last 20 years so that the procedure is more "routine," several issues still challenge the intestinal transplant community and those interested in advancing the field. These include the following.

Allograft Reduction(s) and Organ Availability

The death rate in pediatric recipients awaiting liver and intestinal transplantation is disproportionately higher than those requiring intestinal transplantation alone (62). This is especially the case in the very young patient (<1 year) where obtaining appropriate size-matched donors is difficult. Attempts at increasing the Model for End-Stage Liver Disease (MELD) (used for age ≥12 years)/Pediatric End-Stage Liver Disease (PELD) (used for age <12 years) score to get these patients transplanted earlier have only been marginally successful. To overcome the size disparity, centers at Birmingham (63) and Pittsburgh (64) have undergone a trial of allograft reduction. Although technically successful, the outcomes in some cases have been less than desirable compared to whole transplants, with some recipients remaining dependent on intravenous fluids and line access. Others have adapted poorly after episodes of rejection and required retransplantation.

Live Donor Intestinal and Combined Liver and Intestinal Allografts

Although some of the earliest attempts at intestinal transplantation involved live donors, results were not overly successful, with no long-term survivors, and most suffering from chronic rejection (65). Renewed attempts at this procedure show

early success (66). The need for a live donor-isolated intestinal transplant is unclear because these organs are generally available except for the very young. More interesting is the combined liver and intestinal live donor transplant which may overcome a lack in the appropriate size-matched donor pool for the young infant (67).

Liver Alone Transplantation in Patients with Intestinal Failure

The very young infant with gut dysfunction is more susceptible to PN-associated liver failure. In some infants with short bowel syndrome, the remaining intestine may eventually adapt and become functional enough to become PN-free. Unfortunately, the livers, of some of these infants, may fail before the patient has had time for *intestinal adaptation* to fully develop. It may not be clear early whether, given more time, they will undergo enough intestinal adaptation to avoid the need for intestinal transplantation. A few centers (68,69) have, in this circumstance, transplanted the failing liver alone, hoping the intestine will continue to undergo adaptation.

Utility of the Stomach and Colon

Early experience with the use of donor colon as part of the allograft transplant led to an increased incidence of infectious complications. More recently, the colon has been transplanted in some centers (70) without undue increase in morbidity and mortality. Although technically feasible, it is debatable as to whether this procedure significantly increases fluid resorption compared to pharmacologic manipulation with antidiarrheals to warrant the inherent risks.

Another issue is whether to replace the native stomach in cases of chronic intestinal pseudo-obstruction (CIPO). Our experience is that if there is significant dysmotility in the native stomach, it should be replaced. Failure to do so has frequently led to inability to advance oral feeds. Gastrojejunostomy, although successful in some, has not necessarily been the solution, with some patients still suffering ongoing feeding difficulties. In CIPO, the question has also been raised as to whether a small amount of native rectum can be retained and an ileorectal anastomosis done to avoid committing the patient to a lifelong ileostomy. This procedure has produced adequate functional outcomes in patients who do not have associated urologic involvement or marked rectal abnormalities on manometry.

Optimization of Immunosuppression

Despite progress with outcomes under current strategies, long-term graft function appears to be most limited by chronic rejection and graft loss predicted by the presence of donor-specific antibody (DSA) (71,72). Therapies aimed at antibody-mediated rejection are currently under evaluation (73). Considerable work is needed before we will be able to differentiate patients in whom immunologic activity may allow for drug weaning compared to those at risk of rejection (74,75).

Bioartificial Neointestine

Tissue engineering is an advancing field (76,77) but because the intestine is a complex functional and highly immunologic organ there are significant barriers to bringing this concept to clinical practicality. In theory, a neointestine from autologous human tissue would assist in overcoming immunologic issues, provide prompt access to an organ, and avoid the need for live donation (78).

SUMMARY

There is much hope for continued advancement in the field of intestinal and multivisceral transplantations. Focused multidisciplinary team care is required for this extremely challenging group of patients. Long-term outcomes will improve as immunologic challenges of chronic graft vasculopathy are addressed and immunosuppressant-related complications minimized.

References

1. Starzl TE, Kaupp HA Jr, Brock DR, et al. Homotransplantation of multiple visceral organs. *Am J Surg* 1962;103:219–29.
2. Grant D. Intestinal transplantation: Current status. *Transplant Proc* 1989;21:2869–71.
3. Starzl TE, Rowe M, Todo S, et al. Transplantation of multiple abdominal viscera. *JAMA* 1989;261:1449–57.
4. Starzl TE, Todo S, Tzakis A, et al. Abdominal organ cluster transplantation for the treatment of upper abdominal malignancies. *Ann Surg* 1989;210:374–86.
5. Grant D, Wall W, Mimeault R, et al. Successful small-bowel/liver transplantation. *Lancet* 1990;335:181–4.
6. Goulet OK, Revillon Y, Jan D, et al. Small-bowel transplantation in children. *Transplant Proc* 1990;22:2499.
7. Todo S, Tzakis AG, Abu-Elmagd K, et al. Cadaveric small bowel and small bowel-liver transplantation in humans. *Transplantation* 1992;53:369–76.
8. Bond GJ, Reyes JD. Intestinal transplantation for total/near-total aganglionosis and intestinal pseudo-obstruction. *Sem Ped Surg* 2004;13:286–92.
9. Masetti M, Di Benedetto F, Cautero N, et al. Intestinal transplantation for chronic intestinal pseudo-obstruction in adult patients. *Am J Transplant* 2004;4:826–9.
10. Ruemmele FM, Jan D, Lacaille F, et al. New perspectives for children with microvillous inclusion disease: Early small bowel transplantation. *Transplantation* 2004;77(7):1024–8.
11. Howard L, Ament M, Fleming RC, et al. Current use and clinical outcome of home parenteral and enteral nutrition therapies in the United States. *Gastroenterology* 1995;109:355–65.
12. Pironi L, Joly F, Forbes A, et al. Long-term follow-up of patients on home parenteral nutrition in Europe: Implications for intestinal transplantation. *Gut* 2011;60(1):17–25.
13. Cowles RA, Ventura KA, Martinez M, et al. Reversal of intestinal failure-associated liver disease in infants and children on parenteral nutrition: Experience with 93 patients at a referral center for intestinal rehabilitaton. *J Pediatr Surg* 2010;45(1):84–7; discussion 7–8.
14. Javid PJ, Malone FR, Bittner R, et al. The optimal timing of referral to an intestinal failure program: The relationship between hyperbilirubinemia and morality. *J Pediatr Surg* 2011;46(6):1052–6.
15. Revillion Y, Chardot C. Indications and strategies for intestinal transplantation. *J Pediatr Surg* 2011;46(2):280–3.
16. Casella JF, Lewis JH, Bontempo FA, et al. Successful treatment for homozygous protein C deficiency by hepatic transplantation. *Lancet* 1988;1:435–8.
17. Kaufman SS, Atkinson JB, Bianchi A, et al. Indications for pediatric intestinal transplantation: A position paper of the American Society of Transplantation. *Pediatr Transplant* 2001;5:80–7.
18. American Gastroenterological Association. American Gastroenterological Association medical position statement: Short bowel syndrome and intestinal transplantation. *Gastroenterology* 2003;124:1105–10.
19. Kelly D. Intestinal failure-associated liver disease: What do we know today? *Gastroenterology* 2006;130:s70–7.
20. Kaufmann SS, Loseke CA, Lupo JV, et al. Influence of bacterial overgrowth and intestinal inflammation on duration of PN in children with short bowel syndrome. *J Pediatr* 1997;131:356–61.
21. Sondheimer JM, Asturias E, Cadnapaphornchai M. Infection and cholestasis in neonates with intestinal resection and long-term PN. *J Pediatr Gastroenterol Nutr* 1998;27:131–7.
22. Krasko A, Deshpande K, Bonvino S. Liver failure, transplantation, and critical care. *Crit Care Clin* 2003;19(2):155–83.
23. Pierro A, van Saene HK, Jones MO, et al. Clinical impact of abnormal gut flora in infants receiving parenteral nutrition. *Am Surg* 1998;227:547–52.
24. Panasiuk A, Wysocka J, Maciorkowska E, et al. Phagocytic and oxidative burst activity of neutrophils in the end stage of liver cirrhosis. *World J Gastroenterol* 2005;11(48):7661–5.
25. Marik PE, Gayowski T, Starzl TE; Hepatic Cortisol Research and Adrenal Pathophysiology Study Group. The hepatoadrenal syndrome: A common yet unrecognized clinical condition. *Crit Care Med* 2005;33(6):1254–9.
26. Harry R, Auzinger G, Wendon J. The clinical importance of adrenal insufficiency in acute hepatic dysfunction. *Hepatology* 2002;36(2):395–402.
27. Carcillo JA, Fields AI; American College of Critical Care Medicine Task Force Committee Members. Clinical practice parameters for hemodynamic support of pediatric and neonatal patients in septic shock. *Crit Care Med* 2002;30(6):1365–78.
28. Liu H, Gaskari SA, Lee SS. Cardiac and vascular changes in cirrhosis: Pathogenic mechanisms. *World J Gastroenterol* 2006;12(6):837–42.
29. Moller S, Henriksen JH. Cirrhotic cardiomyopathy: A pathophysiological review of circulatory dysfunction in liver disease. *Heart* 2002;87(1):9–15.
30. Rodrigues AF, van Mourik IDM, Sharif K, et al. Management of end-stage central venous access in children referred for possible small bowel transplantation. *J Pediatr Gastroenterol Nutr* 2006;42:427–33.
31. Lang EV, Reyes J, Faintuch S. Central venous recanalization in patients with short gut syndrome: Restoration of candidacy for intestinal and multivisceral transplantation. *J Vasc Interv Radiol* 2005;16:1203–13.
32. Greer R, Lehnert M, Lewindon P, et al. Body composition and components of energy expenditure in children with end-stage liver disease. *J Pediatr Gastroenterol Nutr* 2003;36(3):358–63.

33. Moore FA, Feliciano DV, Andrassy RJ, et al. Early enteral feeding, compared with parenteral, reduces postoperative septic complications. The results of a meta-analysis. *Ann Surg* 1992;216(2):172–83.

34. Artinian V, Krayem H, DiGiovine B. Effects of early enteral feeding on the outcome of critically ill mechanically ventilated medical patients. *Chest* 2006;129(4):960–7.

35. Brown JB, Emerick KM, Brown DL, et al. Recombinant factor VIIa improves coagulopathy caused by liver failure. *J Pediatr Gastroenterol Nutr* 2003;37(3):268–72.

36. Singer AL, Olthoff KM, Kim H, et al. Role of plasmapheresis in the management of acute hepatic failure in children. *Ann Surg* 2001;234(3):418–24.

37. Chamuleau RA, Poyck PP, van de Kerkhove MP. Bioartificial liver: Its pros and cons. *Ther Apher Dial* 2006;10(2):168–74.

38. Mazariegos G, Chen Y, Squires R. Biological and artificial liver support system in children: A new perspective. *Pediatr Crit Care Med* 2005;6(5):616–17.

39. Tissieres P, Sasbon JS, Devictor D. Liver support for fulminant hepatic failure: Is it time to use the molecular adsorbents recycling system in children? *Pediatr Crit Care Med* 2005;6(5):585–91.

40. Abu-Elmagd K, Bond G, Reyes J, et al. Intestinal transplantation: A coming of age. *Adv Surg* 2002;36:65–101.

41. Abu-Elmagd K, Fung J, Bueno J, et al. Logistics and technique for procurement of intestinal, pancreatic, and hepatic grafts from the same donor. *Ann Surg* 2000;232(5):680–7.

42. Boggi U, Vistoli F, Del Chiaro M, et al. A simplified technique for the en bloc procurement of abdominal organs that is suitable for pancreas and small-bowel transplantation. *J Surg* 2003;10(011):629–41.

43. Bouchek C, Abu-Elmagd K. Alternative route transfusion for transplantation surgery in patients lacking accessible veins. *Anesth Analg* 2006;102:1585–98.

44. Reyes J, Mazariegos GV, Bond GM, et al. Pediatric intestinal transplantation: Historical notes, principles and controversies. *Pediatr Transplant* 2002;6(3):193–207.

45. Bueno J, Abu-Elmagd K, Mazariegos G, et al. Composite liver-small bowel allografts with preservation of donor duodenum and hepatic biliary system in children. *Pediatr Surg* 2000;35(2):291–6.

46. Starzl TE, Murase N, Abu-Elmagd K, et al. Tolerogenic immunosuppression for organ transplantation. *Lancet* 2003;361(9368):1502–10.

47. Sigurdsson L, Green M, Putnam P, et al. Bacteremia frequently accompanies rejection following pediatric small bowel transplantation. *J Pediatr Gastroenterol Nutr* 1995;21(3):356.

48. Bond GJ, Mazariegos GV, Sindhi R, et al. Evolutionary experience with immunosuppression in pediatric intestinal transplantation. *J Pediatr Surg* 2005;40:274–80.

49. Wu T, Abu-Elmagd K, Bond G, et al. A clinicopathologic study of isolated allografts with preformed IgG lymphotoxic antibodies. *Hum Pathol* 2004;35:1332–9.

50. Godolesi G, Kaufman S, Sansaricq C, et al. Defining normal plasma citrulline in intestinal transplant recipients. *Am J Transplant* 2004;4:414–8.

51. Ruiz P, Tryphonopoulos P, Island E, et al. Citrulline evaluation in bowel transplantation. *Transplant Proc* 2010;42(1):54–6.

52. Mercer DF, Vargas L, Sun Y, et al. Stool calprotectin monitoring after small intestine transplantation. *Transplantation* 2011;91(10):1166–71.

53. White FV, Reyes J, Jaffe R, et al. Pathology of intestinal transplantation in children. *Am J Surg Pathol* 1995;19:687–98.

54. Abu-Elmagd KM, Costa G, Bond GJ, et al. Five hundred intestinal and multivisceral transplantations at a single center: Major advances with new challenges. *Ann Surg* 2009;250(4):567–81.

55. Parizhskaya M, Redondo C, Demetris A, et al. Chronic rejection of small bowel grafts: A pediatric and adult study of risk factors and morphologic progression. *Pediatr Dev Pathol* 2003;6:240–50.

56. Papachristou GI, Abu-Elmagd KM, Bond G, et al. Pancreaticobiliary complications after composite visceral transplantation: Incidence, risk, and management strategies. *Gastrointest Endosc* 2011;73(6):1165–73.

57. Cruz RJ Jr, Costa G, Bond G, et al. Modified "liver-sparing" multivisceral transplant with preserved native spleen, pancreas, and duodenum: Technique and long-term outcome. *J Gastrointest Surg* 2010;14(11):1709–21.

58. Manez R, Kusne S, Green M, et al. Incidence and risk factors associated with the development of cytomegalovirus disease after intestinal transplantation. *Transplantation* 1995;59:1110–4.

59. Abu-Elmagd KM, Mazariegos G, Costa G, et al. Lymphoproliferative disorders and de novo malignancies in intestinal and multivisceral recipients: Improved outcomes with new outlooks. *Transplantation* 2009;88(7):926–34.

60. Mazariegos GV, Abu-Elmagd K, Jaffe R, et al. Graft versus host disease in intestinal transplantation. *Am J Transplant* 2004;4(9):1459–65.

61. Reyes J, Mazariegos GV, Abu-Elmagd K, et al. Intestinal transplantation under tacrolimus monotherapy after perioperative lymphoid depletion with rabbit anti-thymocyte globulin (thymoglobulin). *Am J Transplant* 2005;5(6):1430–6.

62. Fryer J, Pellar S, Ormond D, et al. Mortality in candidates waiting for combined liver-intestine transplants exceeds that for other candidates waiting for liver transplants. *Liver Transpl* 2003;9:748–53.

63. de Goyet J, Mitchell A, Mayar AD, et al. En bloc combined reduced-liver and small bowel transplants: From large donors to small children. *Transplantation* 2000;69:555–9.

64. Reyes J, Fishbein T, Bueno J, et al. Reduced-size orthotopic composite liver-intestinal allograft. *Transplantation* 2000;69:555–9.

65. Gruessner RW, Sharp HL. Living-related intestinal transplantation: First report of a standardized surgical technique. *Transplantation* 1997;11:271–4.

66. Benedetti E, Testa G, Holterman M, et al. Application of living donor bowel transplantation to pediatric patients. *Clin Transpl* 2004;13:134.

67. Testa G, Holterman M, John E, et al. Combined living donor liver/small bowel transplantation. *Transplantation* 2005;79(10):1401–4.

68. Botha J, Grant W, Torres C, et al. Isolated liver transplantation in infants with end-stage liver disease due to short bowel syndrome. *Liver Transpl* 2006;12:1062–6.

69. Mazariegos G, Soltys K, Bond G, et al. Isolated liver transplantation in infants with short gut syndrome: Is less better? *Liver Transpl* 2006;12:1040–1.

70. Kato T, Selvaggi G, Gaynor JJ, et al. Inclusion of donor colon and ileocecal valve in intestinal transplantation. *Transplantation* 2008;86(2):293–7.

71. Farmer DG, Venick RS, Colangelo J, et al. Pretransplant predictors of survival after intestinal transplantation: Analysis of a single-center experience of more than 100 transplants. *Transplantation* 2010;90(12):1574–80.

72. Abu-Elmagd KM, Wu G, Costa G, et al. Preformed and de novo donor specific antibodies in visceral transplantation: Long-term outcome with special reference to the liver. *Am J Transplant* 2012;12(11):3047–60. doi:10.1111/j.1600-6143.2012.04237.x.

73. Dick AA, Horslen S. Antibody-mediated rejection after intestinal transplantation. *Curr Opin Organ Transplant* 2012;17(3):250–7.

74. Zeevi A, Britz JA, Bentlejewski CA, et al. Monitoring immune function during tacrolimus tapering in small bowel transplant recipients. *Transpl Immuno* 2005;15:17–24.

75. Kumar AR, Li X, Leblanc JF, et al. Proteomic analysis reveals innate immune activity in intestinal transplant dysfunction. *Transplantation* 2011;92(1):112–9.

76. Chen MK, Beierle EA. Animal models for intestinal tissue engineering. *Biomaterials* 2004;25:1675–81.

77. Duxbury MS, Grikscheit TC, Gardner-Thorpe J, et al. Lymphangiogenesis in tissue-engineered small intestine. *Transplantation* 2004;77(8):1162–6.

78. Levin DE, Grikscheit TC. Tissue-engineering of the gastrointestinal tract. *Curr Opin Pediatr* 2012;24(3):365–70.

CHAPTER 105 ■ **ADRENAL DYSFUNCTION**

ABEER HASSOUN AND SHARON E. OBERFIELD

KEY POINTS

1. Biology of the adrenal function
2. Adrenocortical insufficiency
3. Relative adrenal insufficiency
4. Adrenal hyperfunction
5. Steroid supplementation during critical illness
6. Therapeutic guidelines and steroid preparations

The pathophysiology and management of adrenal disorders that are relevant to the care of children in the ICU are reviewed in this chapter.

BIOLOGY OF ADRENAL FUNCTION

Overview

Four hundred and fifty years ago, Bartholomeo Eustacius (1) described the anatomy of the adrenal gland; shortly thereafter, the zonation of the gland and the distinction of the cortex and medulla were described. The human adrenal glands are located superior to the upper pole of each kidney and can be considered as two unique endocrine organs: the adrenal cortex and the adrenal medulla. Thomas Addison (2) defined the function of the adrenal gland. However, it was really 100 years later, in the 1950s, after performing adrenalectomies in animals, that Brown-S'equard (3) described the adrenal glands as "organs essential for life." Pituitary control of the adrenal function was reported in the 1920s, and this was followed by the isolation of sheep adrenocorticotropic hormone (ACTH) (4). Corticotropin-releasing hormone (CRH) (the hypothalamic releasing factor) was not synthesized until 1981 (5). With respect to the adrenal glomerulosa, primary aldosteronism was described by Conn (6) in the mid1950s, and the regulation of aldosterone by angiotensin II demonstrated afterwards. It is now known that transcription factors are essential for the development of the adrenal gland: SF-1 (steroidogenic factor-1) and DAX1 (dosage-sensitive sex reversal, adrenal hypoplasia congenita, X chromosome) (7).

The adrenal cortex consists of three zones: the outermost, *zona glomerulosa* (15%), from which there is a gradual transition to the middle, *zona fasciculata* (75%), and then a clear transition to the inner most, *zona reticularis* (10%). The *zona glomerulosa* contains relatively small cells with a low cytoplasmic-to-nuclear ratio. It is the primary site of mineralocorticoid synthesis. The *zona fasciculata* has large cells with a high cytoplasmic-to-nuclear ratio and a large number of cytoplasmic lipid vacuoles, which are arranged in columns directed toward the center of the gland (radial cords). This zone is involved in the production of cortisol. The *zona reticularis* contains compact anastomosing cords of cells and an intermediate cytoplasmic-to-nuclear ratio. The *zona reticularis* produces predominantly androgens.

The adrenal medulla should be considered a part of the sympathetic nervous system and is composed of chromaffin cells arranged in nests and cords with sympathetic ganglion cells. In adults, epinephrine is the major catecholamine synthesized and stored in the adrenal medulla. However, this varies with age, for example, at birth norepinephrine is the major catecholamine (8).

In cord blood and in newborns, the concentrations of both cortisol and cortisone are low and about equal, 4–10 μg/100 mL of plasma (9). After 3–4 weeks of life, the cortisol concentration increases in relation to that of cortisone. There is little or no diurnal variation of glucocorticoid concentration until about 4–6 months of age (10). Cortisol secretion rates, corrected for body surface area, remain constant during childhood, puberty, and adulthood, and maintain a diurnal variation. In parallel with cortisol, ACTH peaks between 6 a.m. and 9 a.m, declines to nadir between 11 p.m. and 2 a.m., and then start to rise between 2 a.m. and 3 a.m. (11). Urinary-free cortisol excretion may be higher in perimenarcheal females (12). Aldosterone is secreted at a constant rate during infancy, childhood, and adulthood, albeit the concentrations of aldosterone in infancy tend to be relatively higher than those observed later on in childhood for specific levels of sodium (13). Adrenal androgen secretion is low during childhood. Prior to puberty with onset of adrenarche (physically noted as the onset of pubic hair), there is an increase in the secretion dehydroepiandrosterone (DHEA), dehydroepiandrosterone sulfate (DHEA-S), and androstenedione (9). At the same time, however, there is no change in ACTH concentrations in blood or of the cortisol secretion rate corrected for body size raising the issue as to what stimulates the increase in DHEA/DHEA-S secretion.

Adrenal Cortex

Hormones Produced by the Adrenal Cortex

Three main classes of hormones are produced by the adrenal cortex: *glucocorticoids* (e.g., cortisol), *mineralocorticoids* (e.g., aldosterone), and *sex steroids* (e.g., testosterone, DHEA, and androstenedione).

All steroid hormones are derived from the cyclopentanoperhydrophenanthrene structure that is composed of three cyclohexane rings and a single cyclopentane ring. Although adrenal steroid cells can synthesize cholesterol de novo from acetate,

80% of the cholesterol precursor for adrenal cortex hormone synthesis is provided from circulating plasma lipoproteins. Cholesterol (mainly LDL in circulation) is the precursor for all adrenal steroidogenesis (14).

The biochemical pathways involved in adrenal steroidogenesis are shown in **Figure 105.1**, and the adrenal steroidogenic enzymes and cofactors are illustrated in **Table 105.1**. Conversion of cholesterol to pregnenolone has been described as the rate-limiting step for steroidogenesis, catalyzed by side-chain cleavage enzyme.

However, the true rate-limiting step of adrenal steroidogenesis is the transfer of cholesterol across the inner mitochondrial membrane. This requires the action of the steroidogenic acute regulatory (StAR) protein. At the mitochondrial inner membrane, the side chain of cholesterol is then cleaved to yield pregnenolone, catalyzed by cholesterol side-chain cleavage enzyme (cholesterol desmolase, P450scc, CYP11A1), a cytochrome P450 (CYP) enzyme (15). Pregnenolone then diffuses out of mitochondria and enters the endoplasmic reticulum. The subsequent reactions that occur are zone dependent and are mediated by two groups of enzymes and cofactors (cytochrome P450 enzymes and hydroxysteroid dehydrogenase). These enzymes undergo posttranslational modification with the assistance of electron-donating cofactors. There are two types of P450 enzymes; type 1 P450 enzymes that receive electrons from NADPH via ferredoxin and ferredoxin reductase and type 2 P450 enzymes that receive electron from P450 oxidoreductase (POR) (16). In the *zona glomerulosa*, pregnenolone is converted to progesterone by 3β-hydroxysteroid dehydrogenase (HSD3B2). Progesterone is converted to 11-deoxycorticosterone by steroid 21-hydroxylase (P450c21, CYP21), which is another cytochrome P450 enzyme. In the mitochondria, deoxycorticosterone is then converted to aldosterone by aldosterone synthase (P450aldo, CYP11B2). Aldosterone synthase also performs three successive oxidations: 11β-hydroxylation, 18-hydroxylation, and further oxidation of the 18-methyl carbon to an aldehyde. In the *zona fasciculata*, pregnenolone and progesterone are converted by 17α-hydroxylase (P450c17, CYP17) to 17-hydroxypregnenolone and 17-hydroxyprogesterone, respectively, in the endoplasmic reticulum. This enzyme is not expressed in the zona glomerulosa. 17-Hydroxypregnenolone is converted to 17-hydroxyprogesterone and 11-deoxycortisol by the same 3β-hydroxysteroid and 21-hydroxylase enzymes, respectively, which are active in the zona glomerulosa. 11-Deoxycortisol is converted to cortisol in the mitochondria by steroid 11β-hydroxylase (P450c11, CYP11B1). In the *zona reticularis* and to some extent in the *zona fasciculata*, the 17-hydroxylase (CYP17) enzyme has an additional activity, which is the cleavage of the 17,20-carbon–carbon bond. 17-Hydroxypregnenolone is converted by 3β-hydroxysteroid dehydrogenase to androstenedione.

Regulation of the Adrenal Cortex (Hypothalamic–Pituitary–Adrenal Axis)

The major regulator of glucocorticoid secretion is by ACTH. ACTH is a 39–amino acid peptide that is produced in the anterior pituitary (17), and is synthesized as a part of a large-molecular-weight precursor proopiomelanocortin (POMC).

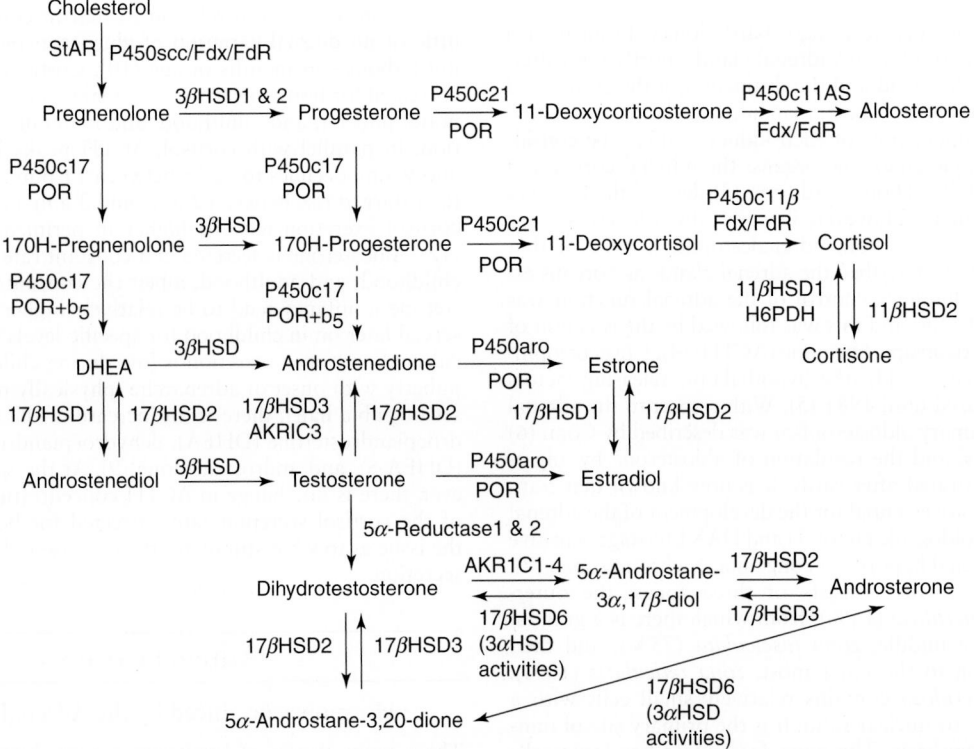

FIGURE 105.1. Major human steroidogenic pathways. Key enzymes and cofactor proteins are shown near *arrows* indicating chemical reactions. P450scc cleaves cholesterol to pregnenolone, the first committed intermediate in steroid biosynthesis. The steroids in the first column are Δ5-steroids, which constitute the preferred pathway to C$_{19}$ steroids in human beings. The *dashed arrow* indicates poor flux from 17α-hydroxyprogesterone to androstenedione via P450c17, and the three *small arrows* below P450c11AS emphasize the three discrete steps with intermediates corticosterone and 18-hydroxycorticosterone. Not all intermediate steroids, pathways, and enzymes are shown. Fdx, ferridoxin; FdR, ferridoxin reductase; HSD, hydroxysteroid dehydrogenase; AKR, aldo–keto reductase. ([© R. J. Auchus] Reprinted with permission from Miller WL, Nichols RJ. The molecular biology, biochemistry, and physiology of human steroidogenesis and its disorders. *Endocr Rev* 2011;32:81–151.)

TABLE 105.1

ADRENAL STEROIDOGENIC ENZYMES AND COFACTORS

■ NAME	■ CELLULAR LOCATION/ACTION	■ CHROMOSOMAL LOCATION
StAR	Cholesterol transport to adrenal and gonadal mitochondria	Active gene: 8 Pseudogene: 13
CYP11A (P450scc)	(Mitochondrial) 20-hydroxylase, 22-hydroxylase, 20,22-desmolase (cholesterol side-chain cleavage)	15q23-q24
3β-HSD 2	(Microsomal) 3β-hydroxysteroid dehydrogenase, Δ4-Δ5-isomerase	1p13.1
CYP17 (P450c17)	(Microsomal) 17α-hydroxylase, 17,20-lyase	10q24-q25
CYP21 CYP21P (P450c21)	(Microsomal) 21-hydroxylase	6p21-active gene and pseudogene
CYP11B1 (P450c11)	(Mitochondrial) 11β-hydroxylase (zona fasciculata/reticularis)	8q22-two homologous CYP11B genes
CYP11B2	(Mitochondrial) 11β-hydroxylase, 18-hydroxylase (CMOI), 18-dehydrogenase (CMOII) (zona glomerulosa)	8q22
P450 Oxidoreductase (64)	Serves as an electron transfer protein to all microsomal P450	7q11.2

Adapted from Kappy M, Allen D, Geffner M. *Pediatric Practice: Endocrinology.* 2nd ed. New York, NY: McGraw-Hill, 2014:366.

ACTH is released in bursts, which vary in amplitude throughout the 24-hour cycle. The normal diurnal rhythm of cortisol secretion is established after infancy. In children and adults, the pulses of ACTH and cortisol are the highest in the early morning hours, become lower in late afternoon, and in the evening reach their nadir 1 or 2 hours after sleep begins. ACTH secretion from the anterior pituitary is stimulated mainly by CRH. This hormone is synthesized by neurons of the parvocellular division of the hypothalamic paraventricular nucleus (17,18). The secretion of ACTH and CRH is predominantly regulated by cortisol through a negative feedback effect. ACTH can also inhibit its own secretion.

Aldosterone secretion is regulated mainly by the renin–angiotensin system and by serum potassium levels (19,20). ACTH plays a very small role in the regulation of its synthesis. Predominantly, in response to decreased intravascular volume, as in dehydration, renin is secreted by the juxtaglomerular apparatus of the kidney. Renin is a proteolytic enzyme that cleaves an α2-globulin produced by the liver called angiotensinogen and results in the formation of angiotensin I, which is cleaved further by angiotensin-converting enzyme (ACE) in the lungs and other tissues yielding the biologically active angiotensin II. Angiotensin II is cleaved further to produce the angiotensin III. Angiotensin II and III are potent stimulators of aldosterone secretion. Angiotensin II occupies a G protein–coupled receptor and activates phospholipase C. Phospholipase C triggers a cascade, which results in a rise in the intracellular calcium and activates protein kinase C and calmodulin-activated (CaM) kinases. CaM kinases increase transcription of aldosterone synthase (CYP11B2), the enzyme needed for aldosterone synthesis (21).

Adrenal Steroid Action

Both cortisol and aldosterone act by binding to intracellular receptors: the glucocorticoid receptor and the mineralocorticoid receptor. These receptors belong to the superfamily of nuclear receptors. They have a common structure that contains a C-terminal ligand-binding domain, a central DNA-binding domain, and an N-terminal hypervariable region. The binding of steroid to its receptor in the cytoplasm results in its dimerization and translocation to the nucleus. In the nucleus, they bind the glucocorticoid response element on the glucocorticoid responsive genes, which results in increased transcription.

Glucocorticoids have regulating effects on carbohydrate, lipid, and protein metabolism. They increase hepatic gluconeogenesis, glycolysis, proteolysis, and lipolysis. Glucocorticoids can result in increased insulin levels, which will inhibit peripheral tissue glucose uptake leading to hyperglycemia. In addition,

glucocorticoids may work in parallel to insulin by stimulating glycogen deposition and production in the liver, which provides protection against starvation. An increase in free fatty acid levels is associated with glucocorticoid administration. This results from glucocorticoid enhancement of lipolysis, decrease of cellular glucose uptake, and decrease in glycerol production. In addition, there is an increase of amino acid substrates that are used in gluconeogenesis due to proteolysis in fat, skeletal muscle, bone, lymphoid, and connective tissues.

Glucocorticoid excess can decrease the levels of free IGF-1 and increase IGFBP-1 resulting in a decrease in free IGF-1. They also exert a direct inhibitory effect on the epiphyses, which results in delayed skeletal maturation and decreased linear growth in children. Although excess glucocorticoids can impair growth, they are also essential for normal growth and development. In the fetus and neonate, they accelerate the differentiation and development of various tissues, such as the development of the hepatic and gastrointestinal systems, as well as the production of surfactant in the fetal lung.

Glucocorticoids also play a major role in immune regulation. They suppress the inflammatory process. Depletion of monocytes, eosinophils, and lymphocytes (T lymphocytes) is observed with the administration of high doses of glucocorticoids. T lymphocytes are reduced more than the B lymphocytes, leading to a predominantly humoral immune response. Glucocorticoids also inhibit immunoglobulin synthesis and stimulation of lymphocyte apoptosis (22). In addition, they block other anti-inflammatory effects, such as histamine and proinflammatory cytokine secretion (e.g., tumor necrosis factor-α, interleukin-1, and interleukin-6).

Glucocorticoids have a positive inotropic effect on the heart that leads to an increase in left ventricular output. They also increase blood pressure by a number of mechanisms that involve the vascular system and the kidneys. In the vascular smooth muscles and the heart, glucocorticoids have a permissive effect on the actions of epinephrine and norepinephrine. They also increase the sensitivity to vasopressor agents, such as catecholamines and angiotensin II, while reducing nitric oxide–mediated endothelial dilatation (23). Hypertension is often observed in patients with glucocorticoid excess; it is thought to be due to the activation of mineralocorticoid receptor.

Glucocorticoids can induce a negative calcium balance by increasing renal calcium excretion and inhibition of calcium absorption by the intestine. Long-term use of glucocorticoid can lead to osteopenia and osteoporosis as they also inhibit the osteoblastic activity. Glucocorticoids also have effects on brain metabolism and mood changes such as emotional liability with irritability, euphoria as well as appetite stimulation and insomnia can occur.

The major role of *mineralocorticoids* is to maintain intravascular volume. This is achieved by sodium retention coupled with the elimination of potassium and hydrogen ions. The main target tissues for the action of mineralocorticoids are the kidney, gut, and salivary and sweat glands. Mineralocorticoids act mainly on the distal convoluted tubules and cortical collecting ducts of the kidney. They stimulate the reabsorption of sodium and the secretion of potassium in the distal convoluted tubules. The mineralocorticoid receptor has a similar affinity for cortisol and aldosterone, yet glucocorticoids have limited mineralocorticoid activity. This is due to the action of 11β-hydroxysteroid dehydrogenase type 2, which converts cortisol to cortisone. Cortisone does not, under normal circumstances, occupy the mineralocorticoid receptor.

The Effects of Stress on Adrenocortical Function

Physical and emotional stress can lead to the increased secretion of ACTH. This involves an immune-endocrine cascade, which results in the activation of the hypothalamic–pituitary–adrenal (HPA) axis. IL-1 is secreted by macrophages in response to immunologic and inflammatory reactions (24). IL-1 triggers a proinflammatory response that will lead to antibody production. At the same time, the CRH–ACTH–cortisol axis is activated (25), leading to increased plasma cortisol concentration, which then results in a negative feedback on the macrophages. IL-6, tumor necrosis factor-α, and IL-1 are other cytokines that have been shown to stimulate CRH release and also to be inhibited by cortisol (26). It has also been observed that the autonomic nervous system can influence interactions of the endocrine immune system (27). A low cortisol level during stress or illness may indicate adrenal insufficiency or depressed and inadequate central nervous system activation of the adrenal axis.

Altered Cortisol Secretion in Systemic Disease

Impaired cortisol metabolism and decreased protein binding can occur in chronic liver disease. It has been suggested that patients may show increased sensitivity to steroid therapy. However, cortisol secretion usually remains normal (28). Renal failure on the other hand results in a reduced excretion of steroid metabolites despite the normal secretion of cortisol.

Altered Aldosterone Secretion in Systemic Disease

It is important to note that aldosterone secretion is increased in hyperkalemia that is associated with renal failure. In patients with heart failure, renin–angiotensin–aldosterone is secreted in response to inadequate systemic perfusion (29). It was also reported that patients with depression can have a significant increase in aldosterone levels during sleep, which was not reported in healthy controls (30).

Adrenal Medulla

The catecholamines, such as dopamine, norepinephrine, and epinephrine, are the main hormones produced by the adrenal medulla. Catecholamine synthesis also occurs in extra-adrenal tissue; the brain, sympathetic nerve endings, and in chromaffin tissue. The biosynthesis of catecholamines is illustrated in **Figure 105.2**. Catecholamine metabolites are excreted in the urine. They include 3-methoxy-4-hydroxymandelic acid (VMA), metanephrine, and normetanephrine. Epinephrine and norepinephrine levels in the adrenal gland vary with age. Norepinephrine is detected in early fetal stages; at birth, it is the principle catecholamine, and in adults (8), it constitutes up to one-third of the pressor amines in the medulla.

In states of stress, high concentration of glucocorticoids has been described in the venous drainage of the adrenal cortex; this exposure is required for the release of epinephrine from the medulla. Loss of basal epinephrine secretion, as well as the response to upright posture, cold pressor, and exercise, has also been reported in patients with glucocorticoid deficiency due to ACTH unresponsiveness (31).

Norepinephrine has no effect on cardiac output. Only epinephrine increases cardiac output. Norepinephrine increases systolic and diastolic blood pressures by increasing peripheral vascular resistance with minimal reduction in the pulse rate. Epinephrine decreases the peripheral vascular resistance with a reduction in the diastolic pressure and an increase in the pulse rate.

❷ ADRENOCORTICAL INSUFFICIENCY

Primary Adrenal Insufficiency

Primary adrenal insufficiency (**Table 105.2**) can result from congenital or acquired lesions of the adrenal cortex, which result in the reduced production of cortisol and occasionally aldosterone. Lesions in the anterior pituitary gland or hypothalamus may cause a deficiency of corticotropin (ACTH) (*secondary adrenal insufficiency*) or CRH (*tertiary adrenal insufficiency*),

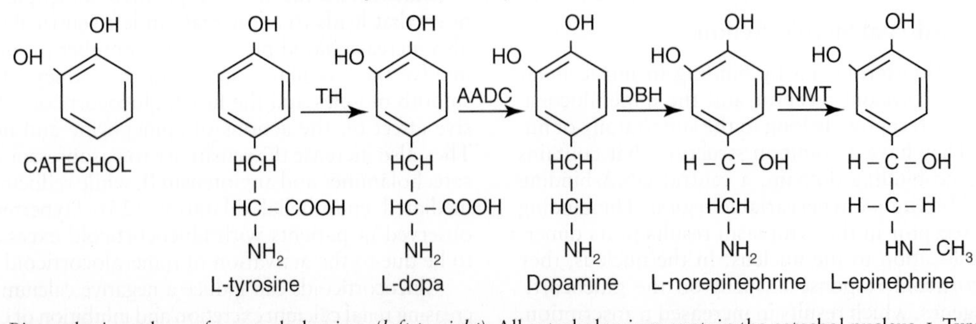

FIGURE 105.2. Biosynthetic pathway for catecholamines (*left to right*). All catecholamines contain the catechol nucleus. L-Tyrosine is converted to L-3,4-dihydroxyphenylalanine (L-dopa) in the rate-limiting step by tyrosine hydroxylase (TH). Aromatic L-amino acid decarboxylase (AADC) converts L-dopa to dopamine. Dopamine is hydroxylated to L-norepinephrine by dopamine β-hydroxylase (DBH). L-Norepinephrine is converted to L-epinephrine by phenylethanolamine-N-methyltransferase (PNMT). (Reprinted with permission from Stewart PM. The adrenal cortex. In: Melmed S, Polonsky KS, Larsen PR, et al., eds. *William's Textbook of Endocrinology.* 12th ed. Philadelphia, PA: Saunders Elsevier, 2011:555.)

TABLE 105.2

ETIOLOGY OF ADRENAL INSUFFICIENCY

1. **Primary Adrenal Insufficiency**
    A. Adrenal hypoplasia or aplasia
        i. X-linked
            a. Duchenne muscular dystrophy and glycerol kinase deficiency (Xp21 deletion)
            b. Hypogonadotropic hypogonadism (*DAX1* mutation)
        ii. Familial glucocorticoid deficiency
            a. Corticotropin-receptor mutations/ACTH unresponsiveness
            b. Alacrima, achalasia, and neurologic disorders (triple A syndrome)
    B. Defects of steroid biosynthesis
        i. Lipoid adrenal hyperplasia (StAR mutation)
        ii. 3β-Hydroxysteroid dehydrogenase deficiency
        iii. 21-Hydroxylase (P450C21) deficiency
        iv. Isolated aldosterone (P450C18) deficiency
        v. P450 Oxidoreductase deficiency
    C. Pseudohypoaldosteronism (aldosterone unresponsiveness)
    D. Adrenoleukodystrophy (peroxisomal membrane protein defect)
    E. Acid lipase deficiency
        i. Wolman disease
    F. Destructive lesions of adrenal cortex
        i. Granulomatous lesions (e.g., tuberculosis)
    G. Autoimmune adrenalitis (idiopathic Addison disease)
        i. Isolated
        ii. Associated with hypoparathyroidism or mucocutaneous candidiasis (type I autoimmune polyglandular syndrome/AIRE gene mutation), or both
        iii. Associated with autoimmune thyroid disease and insulin dependent diabetes (type II autoimmune polyglandular syndrome)
    H. Neonatal hemorrhage
    I. Acute infection (Waterhouse–Friderichsen syndrome)
    J. Mitochondrial disorders
    K. Acquired immunodeficiency syndrome
2. **Secondary Adrenal Insufficiency (ACTH deficiency)**
    A. Isolated
    B. Autosomal recessive
    C. Multiple deficiencies
        i. Pituitary hypoplasia or aplasia
        ii. Destructive lesions (e.g., craniopharyngioma)
        iii. Autoimmune hypophysitis
3. **Tertiary Adrenal Insufficiency**
    A. Isolated
    B. Multiple deficiencies
        i. Congenital defects (e.g., anencephaly, septo-optic dysplasia)
        ii. Destructive lesions (e.g., tumor)
        iii. Idiopathic (e.g., idiopathic hypopituitarism)
4. **Secondary or Tertiary, or Combined Forms of Adrenal Insufficiency**
    A. Iatrogenic
        i. Abrupt cessation of exogenous corticosteroids or corticotropin
        ii. Removal of functioning adrenal tumor
        iii. Adrenalectomy for Cushing disease
        iv. Drug administration: aminoglutethimide, mitotane (o,p′-DDD), metyrapone, ketoconazole
    B. Fetal adrenal suppression—maternal hypercortisolism

and leads to insufficient production of cortisol by the adrenal cortex. The signs and symptoms of adrenocortical insufficiency (**Table 105.3**) vary, determined by the hormones that are deficient and the specific steroids that are oversecreted (as in cases of inborn errors of biosynthesis of cortisol and aldosterone). The clinical features of chronic hypoadrenocorticism may be influenced by additional symptoms resulting from destructive processes that involve the autoimmune system.

Adrenal Crisis Overview

Acute adrenal insufficiency can be life threatening and lead to serious morbidity and mortality. Adrenal crisis may occur in patients with primary adrenal insufficiency and hypopituitarism,

after a stressful insult, such as infection, trauma, dehydration, and abrupt discontinuation of chronic steroid treatment. The patient may complain of abdominal pain, confusion, fever, and fatigue. Hypotension, tachycardia, and dehydration are common signs. Laboratory evaluation shows hyponatremia, hyperkalemia, acidosis, hypoglycemia, and low cortisol level. Treatment includes hydration with normal saline and intravenous **glucocorticoid** administration (32).

Congenital Causes

Congenital Adrenal Hyperplasia. In infancy, the salt-wasting forms of congenital adrenal hyperplasia are the most common cause. These patients most commonly have P450c21

TABLE 105.3

SIGNS AND SYMPTOMS OF ADRENAL INSUFFICIENCY

■ GLUCOCORTICOID DEFICIENCY	■ MINERALOCORTICOID DEFICIENCY	■ ADRENAL ANDROGEN DEFICIENCY
Fasting hypoglycemia	Weight loss	Decreased pubic and axillary hair
Increased insulin sensitivity	Fatigue	Increased β-lipotropin levels
Nausea	Nausea	Hyperpigmentation
Vomiting	Vomiting	
Fatigue	Salt-craving	
Muscle weakness	Hypotension	
	Hyperkalemia, hyponatremia, metabolic acidosis (normal anion gap)	

Adapted from Kappy M, Allen D, Geffner M. *Pediatric Practice: Endocrinology*. 2nd ed. New York, NY: McGraw-Hill, 2014:395.

(21-hydroxylase) deficiency, or deficiency of 3β-hydroxysteroid dehydrogenase. Inability to synthesize cortisol and/or aldosterone can lead to symptoms of salt wasting (shock and vascular collapse) with hyponatremia, hyperkalemia, and acidosis in the newborn period. The patients with salt-wasting crisis usually present in the first week of life. Females with 21-hydroxylase deficiency are easier to diagnose due to virilization of the external genitalia, which results from extra-adrenal androgen production in utero (16). POR deficiency (combined deficiency of P450c17 and P450c21) due to mutation in POR may cause genital ambiguity, is associated with Antley-Bixler syndrome, and hormonal abnormality in the form of cortisol deficiency, virilization in females, and undervirilization in males.

Adrenal Hypoplasia Congenita. Adrenal hypoplasia congenita with adrenal insufficiency also presents with a salt-wasting crisis in the first few weeks of life. However, the presentation can be more delayed into later childhood and adulthood. This disorder is caused by a mutation of the *DAX1* gene. It affects primarily boys who can also present with cryptorchidism and hypogonadotropic hypogonadism, and who do not undergo puberty. This disorder also occurs as part of a syndrome together with Duchenne muscular dystrophy, glycerol kinase deficiency, and mental retardation. The combination of these conditions has been termed a contiguous gene defect (33,34).

Other Congenital Causes of Adrenal Insufficiency. *Familial glucocorticoid* deficiency is another form of inherited adrenal insufficiency. Hypoglycemia, seizures, and increased pigmentation are the presenting symptoms in such patients. These symptoms commonly present in the first decade of life, and patients usually have an isolated deficiency of glucocorticoid, elevated levels of ACTH, and normal aldosterone production. Indeed, salt-wasting symptoms are not common in this type of adrenal insufficiency. The disorder has an autosomal recessive mode of inheritance. Some, but not all, of these patients have been shown to have mutations in the gene for the ACTH receptor.

Triple A syndrome, an autosomal recessive disorder due to mutation in the AAAS, which encodes the protein ALADIN, is an another syndrome of ACTH resistance that occurs in association with achalasia of the gastric cardia and alacrima. Deafness, mental retardation, autonomic dysfunction, and motor neuropathy has been described in these patients (16).

Smith–Lemli–Optiz syndrome (SLOS), an autosomal recessive disorder, results from a defect in the DHCR7 gene that leads to cholesterol biosynthesis defect. Patients present with multiple congenital anomalies and sometimes with adrenal insufficiency (16). Insufficient adrenal cortical function had been described in patients with disorders of cholesterol synthesis or metabolism, such as abetalipoproteinemia and familial hypercholesterolemia. *Wolman disease* is a rare disorder, which results from a mutation in the LIPA gene (16) that results in lysosomal acid lipase defect and intralysosomal accumulation of cholesterol esters in different body organs; this can lead to hepatosplenomegaly, steatorrhea, abdominal distention, bilateral adrenal calcification with adrenal insufficiency, and failure to thrive. Death usually occurs during infancy (35). In *steroid sulfatase deficiency*, patients can present with ichthyosis. This is an X-linked recessive disorder of steroid metabolism. This enzyme deficiency results in accumulation of sulfated 3β-hydroxysteroids in the skin, particularly DHEA-S and cholesterol sulfate (16).

Acquired Causes

Addison disease, historically, was the term applied to primary adrenal insufficiency due mainly to tuberculosis of the adrenal gland. At the present time, the term Addison disease is used to describe primary adrenal insufficiency that is mainly due to autoimmune adrenalitis.

Autoimmune Adrenalitis. Autoimmune adrenalitis is the most common cause (90% of the cases) of acquired adrenal insufficiency (36). Macroscopically, the glands may be too small to be seen, and often only remnants of tissue are found in microscopic sections. The medulla is preserved while the cortex is markedly infiltrated with lymphocytes. Antiadrenal cytoplasmic antibodies and anti-21-hydroxylase (CYP21) are the most frequently reported antibodies. Clinically, Addison disease has also been described in association with two syndromes: type I autoimmune polyendocrinopathy (APS-1), known as the autoimmune polyendocrinopathy/candidiasis/ectodermal dystrophy (APECED) syndrome; and type II autoimmune polyendocrinopathy (APS-2), which consists of Addison disease associated with autoimmune thyroid disease (Schmidt syndrome) or type 1 diabetes (Carpenter syndrome).

Adrenoleukodystrophy. Adrenoleukodystrophy is a potential cause of adrenal insufficiency. Patients have demyelination of the central nervous system due to the accumulation of high levels of very long–chain fatty acids in different tissues, including the adrenal gland, as a result of a mutation in the gene encoding the protein ALDP that leads to impaired β-oxidation in the peroxisomes. Although adrenal insufficiency can be evident in many patients at the time of neurologic presentation, it may also precede the neurologic symptoms by many years. Therefore, the diagnosis should be considered in all patients with Addison disease of unknown etiology and screening for very long fatty acids is advisable (16,37).

Other Acquired Causes. In the last century, *tuberculosis* was considered a common cause of adrenal destruction but is much less prevalent now. *Meningococcemia*, at the present, is the most common infection that causes adrenal insufficiency. It can present as adrenal crisis and is referred to as the Waterhouse–**Friderichsen** syndrome. Although frank adrenal insufficiency is rare, *AIDS* patients may show different subclinical abnormalities in the HPA axis. They may have problems with adrenal hormone production and action, which is often related to the medications that are used in treating this condition.

Adrenal hemorrhage in pediatrics can lead to hypoadrenalism in the neonatal period. It is observed after breech presentation and/or difficult labor. These patients may present with an abdominal mass, anemia, unexplained jaundice, or scrotal hematoma. However, most of the times, the hemorrhage is asymptomatic, limited, and incidental, and identified later by radiographic calcification of the adrenal gland.

Medications, including *rifampin* and *anticonvulsants* (phenytoin, phenobarbital), induce steroid-metabolizing enzymes (cytochrome P450 superfamily) in the liver and reduce the effectiveness and bioavailability of corticosteroid replacement therapy. *Ketoconazole*, by inhibiting adrenal enzymes, can cause adrenal insufficiency. *Mitotane* is cytotoxic to the adrenal cortex. It is used in the treatment of refractory Cushing syndrome and in the treatment of adrenal carcinoma. It may also alter extra-adrenal cortisol metabolism.

Clinical Features of Primary Adrenal Insufficiency

In primary adrenal failure, there is decreased or absent production of one or all three groups of adrenal steroid hormones (38). The signs and symptoms, thus, will vary depending on the hormone that is deficient. Usually the signs and symptoms develop slowly (**Table 105.3**). Most of the patients present with fatigue, muscle pain, and weight loss. Gastrointestinal and orthostatic symptoms are common. Children may present with anorexia, nausea, vomiting, and diarrhea, which can result in growth failure. They may also present with signs of acute adrenal insufficiency precipitated by a febrile illness. Hyperpigmentation is present in >90% of the patients. It may develop over a long period of time, sometimes years. Although this may be difficult to appreciate in individuals with dark complexions, the typical distribution of hyperpigmentation is over the extensor surfaces of the extremities, particularly in sun-exposed areas. The mucous membranes (vaginal mucosa, gingival borders), axillae, and palmar creases are involved, and hyperpigmentation of these areas are the hallmark of Addison disease. Occasionally, the skin pigmentation is generalized. The melanocytes are stimulated by excessively high levels of α-melanocyte–stimulating hormone, which is secreted concomitantly with ACTH (as a response to glucocorticoid deficiency) from the anterior pituitary gland, as both are cleavage products of proopiomelanocortin (39,40).

The clinical presentation of adrenal insufficiency also depends on the age of the patient, and to some extent on the underlying etiology. In early infancy, the most common cause is sepsis, inborn errors of steroid biosynthesis, adrenal hypoplasia congenita, and adrenal hemorrhage. Although infants may present with only a few days of decreased activity with gastrointestinal symptoms, they may deteriorate and become ill very quickly. This is contributed to by the greater requirement for aldosterone in infants than older children; they can deteriorate quickly with rapid occurrence of dehydration and electrolytes abnormalities. In older children with Addison disease, as previously stated, the onset is usually more gradual and is characterized by muscle weakness malaise, anorexia, vomiting, weight loss, and orthostatic hypotension. Hyperpigmentation is often but not necessarily present. Hypoglycemia, hyponatremia, and ketosis are common. Hyperkalemia occurs later in the course of the disease, more in younger than in older children.

Laboratory Findings

Hypoglycemia, hyponatremia, hyperkalemia, and ketosis are common. Hyperkalemia may not manifest in patients who also have significant vomiting and diarrhea, and it can be detected by EKG in critically ill children. The blood urea nitrogen level is elevated if the patient is dehydrated. Cortisol levels may sometimes be at the low end of the normal range but are invariably low when the patient's degree of illness and stress are considered. In primary adrenal insufficiency, ACTH levels are high. Aldosterone level may be within the normal range but inappropriately low in relation to the level of hyponatremia, hyperkalemia, hypovolemia, and elevated levels of plasma renin activity. Hypercalcemia is also associated with Addison disease. Biochemically, adrenal insufficiency is diagnosed by measuring serum cortisol before and 60 minutes after the administration (IV or IM) of cosyntropin (synthetic ACTH). The patient is considered to have a normal response if the 60 minutes cortisol measures ≥ 18 μg/dL (41).

Treatment

Immediate and vigorous treatment of acute adrenal insufficiency is very important. A blood sample should be obtained before therapy for determination of electrolytes, glucose, ACTH, cortisol, aldosterone, and plasma renin activity to establish the etiology of adrenal insufficiency. If it is possible, specifically in infants, 17α-hydroxyprogesterone (steroid precursor) level should be obtained. An ACTH stimulation test can be performed while initial fluid resuscitation is underway. A bolus of 20 mL/kg of 5% dextrose with 0.9% sodium chloride should be given and intravenous fluid can be continued to correct hypoglycemia, hypovolemia, and hyponatremia. Hyperkalemia can be very severe, and this may necessitate the treatment with calcium and/or bicarbonate, potassium-binding resin (sodium polystyrene sulfonate), or intravenous infusion of glucose and insulin. Stress doses of hydrocortisone, preferably a water-soluble form, such as hydrocortisone sodium succinate, should be given intravenously. Acute doses of 10 mg for infants, 25 mg for toddlers, 50 mg for older children, and 100 mg for adolescents should be administered immediately and then every 6 hours for the first 24 hours. These doses may be tapered during the next 24 hours if the patient has a satisfactory progress. Fluids and electrolytes balance is usually achieved by continuous intravenous saline administration, aided by the mineralocorticoid effect of high doses of hydrocortisone. Most of the patients require chronic replacement therapy for their cortisol and aldosterone deficiencies. Hydrocortisone may be given orally in doses of 10 mg/m^2)/day in three divided doses. During stress, such as infection or minor operative procedures, the dose of hydrocortisone should be increased two- to threefold. Major surgery under general anesthesia requires high intravenous doses of hydrocortisone similar to those used for acute adrenal insufficiency. If aldosterone deficiency is present, fludrocortisone (Florinef), a mineralocorticoid, is given orally in doses of 0.05–0.3 mg daily, since there is no intravenous or intramuscular preparation available. Intravenous sodium chloride is administered to help correct sodium levels.

Mineralocorticoid Deficiency

CYP11B2 Deficiencies. Deficiencies in CYP11B2 are associated with two related genetic disorders of aldosterone synthesis. A genetic defect in the CYP11B2 gene impairs the production of mineralocorticoids without compromising glucocorticoid production. It was previously hypothesized that two distinct enzymes carried out 18-hydroxylation and 18-oxidation (now known to be performed by CYP11B2) and two deficiencies were clinically characterized—corticosterone methyloxidase I (CMO I) deficiency and corticosterone methyloxidase II (CMO II) deficiency. More recent analyses have shown definitively that a single protein, encoded by the CYP11B2 gene, catalyzes both of these reactions, as well as the initial 11β-hydroxylation required for aldosterone production (42). Deficiency of CMO I or CMO II causes elevated renin activity and aldosterone deficiency, with the accumulation of steroid precursors prior to the biosynthetic block (DOC and corticosterone in CMO I deficiency; and DOC, corticosterone, and 18-hydroxycorticosterone in CMO II deficiency). These precursors have some mineralocorticoid activity, which compensate partially for the aldosterone deficiency. Thus, partial salt loss is the usual presentation rather than the typical salt-losing crisis of complete mineralocorticoid deficiency. Renal salt wasting and decreased growth velocity develop in these patients, and infants may present only with failure to thrive. The diagnosis is accomplished by laboratory evaluation, which reveals a low aldosterone level and elevated DOC and corticosterone in CMO I deficiency. Laboratory evaluation in CMO II deficiency reveals an increased corticosterone concentration and 18-hydroxycorticosterone, which is accompanied by an increased ratio of 18-hydroxycorticosterone to aldosterone. Treatment consists of giving fludrocortisone (0.05–0.3 mg daily), sodium chloride, or both in order to achieve normal plasma renin activity. With increasing age, due to not fully understood mechanisms, salt-replacement requirements usually improve and drug therapy can often be discontinued. Rarely, there is a third genetic disorder of the CYP11B, in the form of autosomal dominant hypertension caused by a hybrid CYP11B1/CYP11B2 gene.

Pseudohypoaldosteronism. In this condition, the kidneys do not respond to aldosterone. The infant presents with dehydration, hyponatremia, and hyperkalemia despite marked elevation of aldosterone and renin levels. The mutations are either in the gene encoding the mineralocorticoid receptor (autosomal dominant and mild) or in the genes encoding the amiloride-sensitive epithelial sodium channel (autosomal recessive and severe). Treatment with mineralocorticoid is ineffective, and the only effective treatment is with sodium chloride.

Acquired Hypoaldosteronism. As in hyporeninemic hypoaldosteronism, there is damage to the juxtaglomerular apparatus and hence renin deficiency. Patients have hyponatremia, hyperkalemia, and normal or elevated blood pressure with both low aldosterone and plasma renin activity. Patients usually have impaired renal function, as seen in diabetes, SLE, myeloma, amyloid, AIDS, and use of nonsteroidal anti-inflammatory drugs (which is unusual in the pediatric setting). Many patients are asymptomatic, with only mild to moderate hyperkalemia. In the ICU, administration of heparin may exacerbate relative hypoaldosteronism by inhibiting its synthesis and thereby precipitate significant salt wasting and volume loss (43).

Pituitary Disease and ACTH Deficiency (Secondary Adrenal Insufficiency)

By definition, this is due to ACTH deficiency. Pituitary or hypothalamic dysfunction can cause ACTH deficiency, usually associated with deficiencies of other pituitary hormones, such as growth hormone and thyrotropin. Craniopharyngioma and germinoma are the most common causes of corticotropin deficiency. Surgical removal or radiotherapy of tumors in the midbrain can lead, in most of the cases, to damage of the pituitary and/or the hypothalamus with resultant secondary adrenal insufficiency. Very rarely, autoimmune hypophysitis can be the cause of corticotropin deficiency. Congenital lesions

of pituitary alone or with additional midline structure defect may be involved, as in septo-optic dysplasia. More severe developmental anomalies of the brain, such as anencephaly and holoprosencephaly, can also affect the pituitary. Patients with multiple pituitary hormone deficiencies due to mutations in the PROP1 gene have been described with progressive ACTH/cortisol deficiency (44).

Hypothalamic Disease and Corticotropin-Releasing Hormone Deficiency (Tertiary Adrenal Insufficiency)

By definition, this implies a hypothalamic decrease in CRH secretion or production. Most commonly this occurs when the HPA axis is suppressed by prolonged administration of high doses of a potent glucocorticoid and then that agent is withdrawn suddenly or the dose is tapered too rapidly. Patients at risk for this problem are those undergoing treatment for leukemia, asthma, and collagen vascular disease or other autoimmune conditions that require massive doses of potent glucocorticoids and those who have undergone tissue transplants or neurosurgical procedures. The maximum duration and dose of glucocorticoid that can be administered before encountering this problem is not known, but it is assumed that high-dose glucocorticoids (e.g., prednisone 2 mg/kg/day to maximum of 60 mg/day) can be administered for up to about a week without requiring a subsequent slow taper of dose (45). On the other hand, when high doses of dexamethasone are given to children with leukemia, it can take more than a month after therapy is stopped before the return of the integrity of the HPA axis (46,47). These patients, when subsequently subjected to stress, such as severe infections or additional surgical procedures, should be presumed adrenally incompetent for up to 1 year unless documented to have a normal cortisol response to provocative stimulation, for example, ACTH stimulation test. However, even with a normal peak stimulated response to ACTH, any signs of vasomotor instability during surgical procedure warrants immediate glucocorticoid coverage.

Clinical Presentation of Secondary and Tertiary Adrenal Insufficiency

Because the adrenal gland is, by definition, intact in secondary and tertiary adrenal insufficiency, and the renin–angiotensin system is not involved, aldosterone secretion is unaffected. Therefore, the signs and symptoms of secondary and tertiary adrenal insufficiency are hypoglycemia, orthostatic hypotension, or weakness. Electrolytes are usually normal. Hyponatremia may be observed, nevertheless, due to the decreased glomerular filtration rate and decreased free water clearance associated with cortisol deficiency. When secondary adrenal insufficiency is due to an inborn or acquired anatomic defect involving the pituitary, there may be signs of associated deficiencies of other pituitary hormones, such as microphallus and jaundice in infancy or poor growth after the first year of life.

Treatment of Secondary and Tertiary Adrenal Insufficiency

Iatrogenic adrenal insufficiency (caused by chronic glucocorticoid administration) is best avoided by using the smallest effective doses of systemic glucocorticoids for the shortest period of time. When the patient is thought to be at risk, tapering the dose rapidly to a level equivalent to or slightly less than physiologic replacement ($\sim$10 mg/m^2/24 h) and further tapering over several weeks may allow the adrenal cortex to recover without the development of signs of adrenal insufficiency. Patients with anatomic lesions of the pituitary should be treated indefinitely with glucocorticoids. Mineralocorticoid replacement is not required. In cases of a unilateral adrenocortical tumor producing cortisol that, for example, results in Cushing syndrome, the steroid secretion is autonomous and does not require ACTH activation. The high concentration of circulating cortisol will suppress the endogenous CRH/ACTH secretion and result in atrophy of the contralateral adrenal. Following removal of the tumor, the patient is in a condition similar to the cessation of iatrogenic glucocorticoid therapy. It is therefore appropriate to provide exogenous cortisol during the stress of surgery and during postsurgical period. Then therapy can be stopped or tapered depending on the individual's response while under close observation. The patient requires additional steroid coverage at times of intercurrent stress for the next period of 6–12 months.

RELATIVE ADRENAL INSUFFICIENCY DURING A CRITICAL ILLNESS

Critically ill patients may develop glucocorticoid insufficiency at the high point of their illness. The diagnosis can be challenging, due to the variable changes that normally occur as a part of the response of the HPA axis to severe illness. Critical illness can result in an increase in serum cortisol, changes in the circadian rhythm of serum cortisol, decrease in corticosteroid-binding proteins as well as both changes in the number and the sensitivity of tissue glucocorticoid receptors (48). In **Figure 105.3, panel B**, the initial response to stress is illustrated. The early increase in CRH, ACTH, and cortisol levels are usually proportional to the degree of illness. However, due to multiple mechanisms with prolonged illness, there can be impairment of the glucocorticoid rise, which results in acute adrenal insufficiency as seen in **Figure 105.3, panel C**. This phenomenon has been called functional adrenal insufficiency to denote that it is a "functional" and not a "structural" defect that is responsible for the adrenal insufficiency. Another term that describes perturbations of HPA axis during severe illness is "relative" adrenal insufficiency. This term is used by some to describe situations when, although high, absolute cortisol levels are present, they are "relatively" insufficient to overcome the degree of physiologic stress facing patient. Moreover, the patient often cannot mount any additional responses to subsequent stress (49,50). Attempts to define relative adrenal insufficiency may require assessing the response to exogenous administration of ACTH (51). Unfortunately, studies defining relative or functional adrenal insufficiency in children are limited. However, assessment of severely ill children with septic shock have begun to show that both absolute

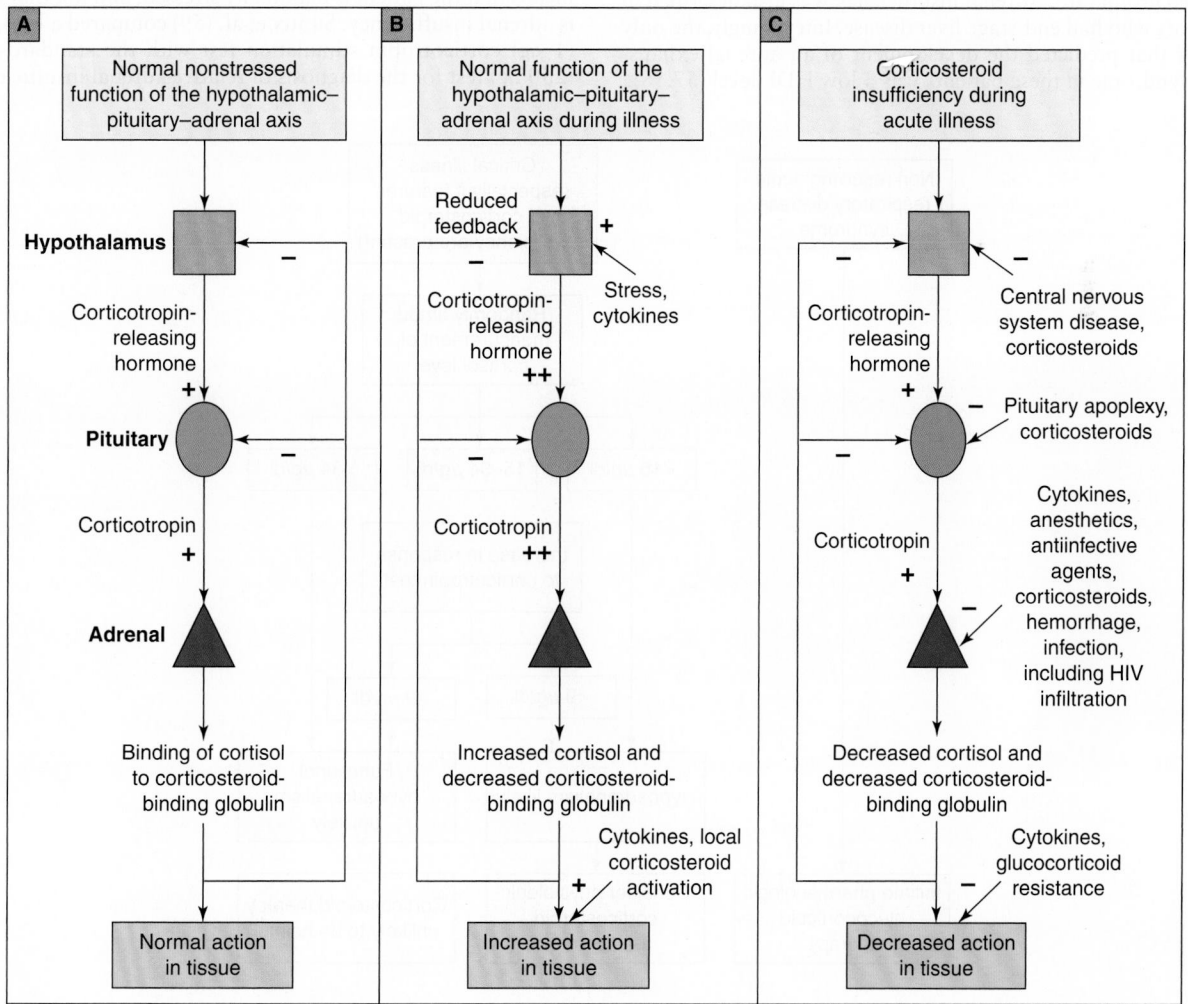

FIGURE 105.3. Activity of the HPA axis under normal conditions (*panel A*), during an appropriate response to stress (*panel B*), and during an inappropriate response to critical illness (*panel C*). A *plus sign* indicates a stimulatory effect, and a *minus sign* an inhibitory effect. (From Cooper M, Stewart P. Corticosteroid insufficiency in acutely ill patients. *N Engl J Med* 2003;348:727–34.)

and relative adrenal insufficiency are common in children with catecholamine-resistant shock and absent in children with fluid-responsive shock (52,53).

Adrenal insufficiency is also common in critical illnesses other than sepsis. Many factors and illnesses in the ICU can contribute to relative adrenal insufficiency, which is seen in trauma, hemorrhagic shock, and following traumatic brain injury (54,55). In a recent study where adrenal insufficiency was reported following traumatic brain injury, patients were considered adrenally insufficient, if, in post-injury, they had an initial cortisol level of <5 μg/dL or two consecutive cortisol levels of ≤15 μg/dL (55). They were also found to have a considerably lower ACTH levels, suggesting secondary adrenal insufficiency, as well. In addition, these patients had higher injury severity scores, hypotension, and etomidate use. The state of adrenal insufficiency was found to be transient, in which most of the survivors showed a normal response to a 1-μg ACTH stimulation test 6 months after injury (55). Other factor that may contribute to relative adrenal insufficiency is being mechanically ventilated. In a recent study of adult ICU patients who required mechanical ventilation for >24 hours, 75% of the patients were found to have adrenal insufficiency. They were considered to have normal adrenal function if they had a plasma cortisol level >25 μg/dL or a 9-μg/dL increment in serum cortisol level than after an ACTH stimulation test. Weaning from mechanical ventilation was significantly higher in the adequate adrenal reserve group than in the hydrocortisone-treated group (56). Adrenal insufficiency was also described in patients who had end-stage liver disease. Interestingly, the only factor that predicted the development of an adrenal exhaustion syndrome in these patients was a low HDL level (57,58).

Clinical Diagnosis of Relative Adrenal Insufficiency in the ICU

Diagnosis of relative adrenal insufficiency can be very difficult. Hemodynamic instability in a critically ill patient, despite adequate fluid resuscitation, can suggest the diagnosis. In addition, an inadequate response to empirical treatment in cases of ongoing inflammation can give clues to the diagnosis. Laboratory tests can be confusing and misleading. In an ICU setting, both high and low cortisol levels can be detected. Many levels have been proposed, under which the patient may be diagnosed with relative adrenal insufficiency. An ACTH stimulation test can be used as a diagnostic tool in an ICU setting (Fig. 105.4). It can be performed the same way as in non–critically ill patients, using 250 μg of synthetic ACTH. The absolute post–ACTH response is yet to be determined, especially in children. The threshold can be the same as in the non–critical patients or may ultimately be found to be higher, to compensate for the level of stress. Annane et al. (51) have studied cortisol levels and cortisol response to corticotropin in patients with septic shock. High-baseline cortisol levels were the most prognostic factor. They also used the absolute cortisol increment of 9 μg/dL above baseline as having prognostic implication. It was reported that <9 μg/dL increment from the baseline, 60 minutes after ACTH administration, is associated with an increased death risk (51). High baseline with low increment probably means that the patient is maximally stressed, and not that there is adrenal insufficiency. Siraux et al. (59) compared a low-dose (1 μg) corticotropin stimulation test with the standard-dose (250 μg) test for the diagnosis of relative adrenal insufficiency.

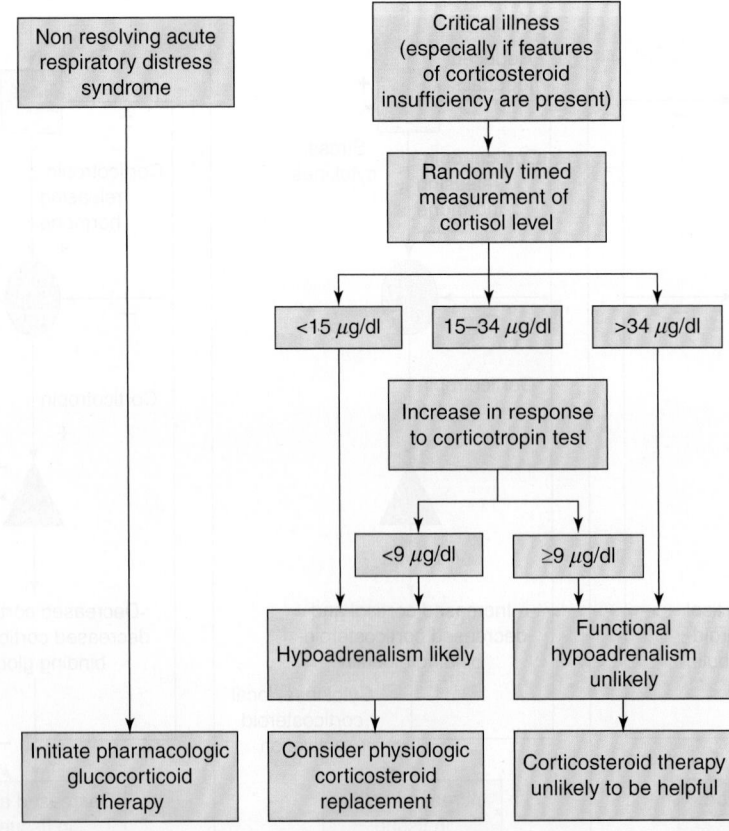

FIGURE 105.4. Investigation of adrenal corticosteroid function in critically ill patients on the basis of cortisol levels and response to the corticotropin stimulation test. The scheme has been evaluated for patients with septic shock. It must be borne in mind, however, that no cutoff value will be entirely reliable. (From Cooper M, Stewart P. Corticosteroid insufficiency in acutely ill patients. N Engl J Med 2003;348:727–34.)

TABLE 105.4

ETIOLOGIES OF DIFFERENT TYPES OF ADRENAL HYPERFUNCTION

■ DISORDER	■ ETIOLOGY
Cushing disease	Pituitary adenoma
Cushing syndrome	Adrenal adenoma
	Bilateral micronodular adrenal hyperplasia (e.g., McCune–Albright syndrome)
	Primary pigmented adrenal hyperplasia (e.g., Carney complex)
	Bilateral macronodular adrenal hyperplasia
	Adrenal carcinoma
	Ectopic ACTH (CRH): nonpituitary ACTH (CRH)-producing tumor
Pseudo-Cushing syndrome	Depression, alcoholism (increased CRH secretion)
Iatrogenic Cushing syndrome	Pharmacologic glucocorticoid therapy

The ACTH stimulation tests were performed consecutively with a minimum of 4 hours space between the low- and the standard-dose tests. Serum cortisol levels were measured at baseline, 30, 60, and 90 minutes post–ACTH administration, an adequate response was an increment in cortisol >9 μg/dL. Nonresponders to the low-dose test had a higher mortality rate than responders to both tests, which suggests that the low-dose test can identify patients in septic shock with inadequate adrenal function (59). These patients had poorer outcomes and would have been missed by the standard-dose test. The authors had suggested that this subgroup may benefit from steroid replacement. Loriaux and Fleseriu (60) have recommended a different approach to diagnose relative adrenal insufficiency in adults. They suggested obtaining two cortisol samples 45 and 60 minutes post–ACTH stimulation test: one for a total cortisol and the second for free cortisol (which will be stored). If the total cortisol value is >20 μg/dL then the patient is considered to have sufficient adrenal response. If the total cortisol level is <10 μg/dL, then the patient has adrenal insufficiency and needs treatment with glucocorticoids. The patients who have values between 10 and 20 μg/dL are categorized in one of two groups, either being critically ill with low protein binding (that may affect the total cortisol value) or having secondary adrenal insufficiency. In either situation, the patient needs to be treated with glucocorticoids while waiting for the free cortisol results. If the free cortisol value is normal then the glucocorticoid treatment can be discontinued (60). In a recent study, Hochwald et al. (61) suggested that a post–ACTH cortisol of <12% from the baseline can be used as a potential marker for relative adrenal insufficiency in low-birth-weight infants.

Studies are warranted in the pediatric age group, to determine the diagnostic criteria of relative AI and whether corticosteroid use in the ICU in these instances benefit the overall outcome in children with suspected relative adrenal insufficiency.

ADRENAL HYPERFUNCTION

Cushing Syndrome

The principal causes of Cushing syndrome in childhood are listed in **Table 105.4**. The most common cause of noniatrogenic Cushing syndrome in children is of adrenal origin. In adolescents who have Cushing disease, a central nervous system lesion, such as an ACTH-secreting adenoma, is more likely the cause of Cushing syndrome.

In the ICU setting, Cushing syndrome in pediatrics is most often iatrogenic and seen in patients who have received exogenous glucocorticoids. The glucocorticoids can be been given for chronic steroid replacement in states of adrenal insufficiency or as a part of high-dose or bolus steroid therapy for renal or rheumatologic disorders. In these instances, the patient may present with physical and biochemical signs of glucocorticoid excess, including cushingoid appearance with moon-like facies, centripetal obesity, short stature, thin extremities with fragile capillaries, hirsutism, and acne. They may also present with delayed puberty and amenorrhea. Hypertension, hyperglycemia or glucose intolerance, and osteopenia are also observed. Patients, who receive chronic treatment with glucocorticoids, should not have abrupt cessation of their glucocorticoid therapy and should receive stress doses of glucocorticoid during the peri-, intra- and postoperative period (see previous discussion under primary adrenal insufficiency).

The diagnosis of Cushing syndrome can be difficult to make in an ICU setting. As previously stated, in the ICU, the circadian rhythm of cortisol secretion is lost and cortisol levels at midnight and 8 a.m. are usually comparable (48). Further, diurnal blood samples from patients under conditions of stress in the ICU may demonstrate high levels of cortisol, making it difficult to differentiate these patients from those with Cushing syndrome. Of course, the diagnosis of Cushing syndrome in the ICU can always be made on clinical grounds using the history and features of physical examination. More specific evaluation can be obtained after the patient is discharged from the ICU to the regular hospital ward.

The treatment of choice for pituitary-related Cushing disease in children is transsphenoidal pituitary microsurgery. Reoperation or pituitary irradiation is performed when relapses occurs. Long-term remission is predicted by low postoperative serum or urinary cortisol concentrations. Patients with benign cortical adenoma can benefit from adrenalectomy. Such adenomas are occasionally bilateral and may require subtotal adrenalectomy. Adrenocortical carcinomas frequently metastasize, especially to the liver and lungs, and the prognosis may be unfavorable despite removal of the primary lesion.

Virilizing Tumors

Virilizing tumors of the adrenal gland are the most common adrenal tumor in childhood. Virilization is the most common presenting symptom and includes accelerated growth velocity, acne, muscular development, precocious development of axillary and pubic hair, and penile enlargement without testicular enlargement in males. In females, signs include hirsutism, masculinization with clitoral enlargement, and the precocious development of axillary and pubic hair with rapid growth. In addition to virilization, 20%–40% of the patients can present with symptoms of cortisol excess. Patients with these tumors have elevated levels of serum DHEA, DHEA-S, androstenedione, and testosterone. Cortisol and aldosterone levels are usually within normal with normal serum electrolytes. Ultrasonography, CT scan, and MRI can be used to diagnose the tumor and metastasis. Histologically, it is often difficult to

TABLE 105.5

PHARMACOLOGIC CHARACTERISTICS OF VARIOUS STEROIDS RELATIVE TO CORTISOL

STEROID	ANTI-INFLAMMATORY GLUCOCORTICOID EFFECT	SALT-RETAINING MINERALOCORTICOID EFFECT	GROWTH-RETARDING GLUCOCORTICOID EFFECT	PLASMA HALF-LIFE (MIN)	BIOLOGIC HALF-LIFE (HOURS)
Cortisone (Hydrocortisone, Cortef)	1.0	1.0	1.0	80–120	8
Cortisone acetate (oral)	0.8	0.8	0.8		
Cortisone acetate (IM)	0.8	0.8	1.3	80–120	8
Prednisone	3.5–4	0.8	5	200	18
Prednisolone (Orapred, Pediapred)	4	0.8		120–300	16–36
Methylprednisolone (Medrol)	5	0.5	7.5		16–36
Dexamethasone	30	0	80	150–300	36–54
9α-Fluorocortisone (Fludrocortisone)		200			
Aldosterone	0.3	200–1000			

Adapted from Sperling M. *Pediatric Endocrinology*. 4th ed. Philadelphia, PA: Saunders, 2008.

differentiate between benign and malignant tumor. Surgery or laparoscopic removal of the tumor is the treatment of choice. Adrenal insufficiency may follow the resection of the adrenal tumor if cortisol excess is a manifestation on presentation.

❺ STEROID SUPPLEMENTATION DURING STRESS OR IN THE PERIOPERATIVE PERIOD

In patients with acute glucocorticoid, or complete adrenal insufficiency, treatment consists of supportive care, treatment of the underlying disease, and hydrocortisone replacement. Supportive care includes administration of fluids, appropriate electrolytes (to treat hyponatremia, hyperkalemia, hypercalcemia, and acidosis), nutritional supplementation, medications, antibiotics, and organ support. It is important to maintain body temperature and glucose levels. Hyperkalemia is a contraindication to the use of succinylcholine. Intubation should be prompt in unstable and obtunded patients. Etomidate, which is a short-acting intravenous anesthetic agent used for the induction of general anesthesia in critically ill patient, has an inhibitory effect on adrenal function. This can result in the depression of the adrenal cortical stress response with reduction of cortisol and aldosterone production (62,63). Etomidate inhibits 11β-hydroxylase, the enzyme required for the conversion of 11-deoxycortisol to cortisol (final step in cortisol synthesis). This side effect is dose dependent and has been shown to increase mortality in septic patients (64). In a recent study of 157 septic intubated patients (110 using etomidate and 47 not using etomidate), clinically significant hypotension was observed in 72% of the patients who received etomidate versus 30% of those who did not ($p < 0.001$). However, the side effect was transient and was not significant to cause long-term effect (65). Another recent study involving 2014 adults with sepsis or septic shock requiring intubation in the ICU looked at 1102 who received etomidate versus 912 who received other induction agents. The etomidate group was more likely to receive steroids after intubation (53% vs. 44%, $p < 0.001$), but there was not a difference in need for vasopressor, duration of mechanical ventilation, length of stay, or mortality (66). Thiopental, propofol, and midazolam do not depress the adrenocortical response to stress, but inhibit steroidogenic enzymes in vitro (67,68). In Cushing syndrome, after surgical resection of the pituitary or adrenal tumor, most patients have transient suppression of the normal CRH/ACTH/adrenal axis, necessitating corticosteroid replacement therapy for several months.

Children who have been exposed to high doses of endogenous (Cushing syndrome or disease) or exogenous steroids are susceptible to osteoporosis and may be at risk of pathologic fractures. Therefore, care should be taken during positioning for procedures in the operating room. These patients may have muscle weakness, so neuromuscular blocking drugs should be used with caution.

Patients with adrenal insufficiency or those who are receiving long-term steroid therapy need appropriate supplemental glucocorticoid therapy in the perioperative period. During general anesthesia, with or without surgery, the cortisol secretion rate in normal subjects increases greatly. Parenteral steroids are needed. Protocols vary; one protocol recommended intramuscular administration of cortisone acetate (that has a biologic activity of 18 hours) at a dose of twice the physiologic daily requirement, 18 hours and then again at 8 hours before the surgical procedure (69). From our experience, the following protocol has been useful: a dose of 25 mg/m^2 of hydrocortisone sodium succinate is given IV stat just prior to anesthesia and is followed by a dose of 50 mg/m^2 as a constant infusion for the period of the surgical procedure; finally, a third dose of ~25–50 mg/m^2 hydrocortisone sodium succinate is given as a constant IV infusion for the rest of the first 24 hours of the surgical day. This is a total of 100–125 mg/m^2 of hydrocortisone sodium succinate over a 24-hour period or ~10 times replacement therapy. This dosing can be followed the next day by three to four times replacement therapy (50 mg/m^2/day) of constant IV infusion of hydrocortisone sodium succinate. Eventually oral therapy is resumed as tolerated.

❻ THERAPEUTIC GUIDELINES/STEROID PREPARATIONS

Various derivatives of steroids are available and can be administered using multiple routes. In order to choose the appropriate product, one must realize that the convention is to describe glucocorticoids according to their anti-inflammatory potency. Further, glucocorticoid preparations vary by their plasma and biologic half-lives and their growth suppressant effects. These actions can differ significantly from the established anti-inflammatory effect. The mineralocorticoid activity of glucocorticoids also varies widely according to the preparation used. In patients who receive phenobarbital or phenytoin, cortisone and prednisolone are cleared rapidly. In hepatic failure, there is a decreased glucocorticoid clearance. In general, the rapidly absorbed steroids are orally administered (they are usually incompletely absorbed) while intramuscularly administered steroids are absorbed slowly but more completely (**Table 105.5**).

In the ICU setting, the most commonly used corticosteroids are those that are intravenously administered. These include intravenous forms of dexamethasone, methylprednisolone, prednisolone, and hydrocortisone. Hydrocortisone has the highest mineralocorticoid activity whereas dexamethasone has none. Thus, in patients with adrenal crisis and hypovolemia, hydrocortisone is the best steroid to use whereas in patients with intracranial tumors or increased intracranial pressure, dexamethasone (which has no mineralocorticoid activity) is the most appropriate steroid to be used.

OUTCOME

Maintenance of normal adrenal function is essential in patients treated in the ICU. In some instances, patients develop relative adrenal insufficiency. Few studies had demonstrated that treatment with steroids can improve outcome in patients with sepsis and septic shock. For patients with respiratory failure, it was demonstrated that early identification of adrenal insufficiency and stress-dose steroid replacement can result in shorter and more successful ventilator weaning (48). Marik et al. (57) have shown in patients with chronic liver failure or post–liver transplant and with adrenal insufficiency in an ICU setting that treatment with a steroid can decrease the requirement for vasopressor therapy. These patients also had a significantly lower mortality rate than those who were not treated (56). Unfortunately, studies of this sort are rare in children.

References

1. Eustachius B. *Tabulae Anatomicae*. Lncisius B, ed. Amsterdam, 1774.
2. Addison T. *On the Constitutional and Local Effects of Disease of the Supra-renal Capsules*. London, England: Highley, 1855.
3. Brown-S'equard CE. Recherches experimentales sur la physiologie et la pathologie des capsules surrenales. *Arch Gen Med* 1856; 5(8):385–401.

4. Li CH, Simpson ME, Evans HM. Adrenocorticotropic hormone. *J Biol Chem* 1943;149:413–24.

5. Vale W, Spiess J, Rivier C, et al. Characterization of a 41-residue ovine hypothalamic peptide that stimulates secretion of corticotropin and β-endorphin. *Science* 1981;213:1394–7.

6. Conn JW. Primary aldosteronism: A new clinical entity. *J Lab Clin Med* 1955;45:3–17.

7. Ikeda Y, Swain A, Weber T, et al. Steroidogenic factor 1 and DAX 1 colocalize in multiple cell lineages: Potential links in endocrine development. *Mol Endocrinol* 1996;10:1261.

8. Kappy M, Allen D, Geffner M. *Pediatric Practice: Endocrinology.* 2nd ed. New York, NY: McGraw-Hill, 2014.

9. Beitins IZ, Bayard F, Anecs IG, et al. The metabolic clearance rate, blood production, interconversion and transplacental passage of cortisol and cortisone in pregnancy near term. *Pediatr Res* 1973;7:509.

10. Onishi S, Miyazawa G, Nishimura Y, et al. Postnatal development of circadian rhythm in serum cortisol levels in children. *Pediatrics* 1983;72:399.

11. Veldhuis JD, Iranmanesh A, Johnson ML, et al. Amplitude, but not frequency, modulation of adrenocorticotropin secretory bursts gives rise to the nyctohemeral rhythm of the corticotropic axis in man. *J Clin Endocrinol Metab* 1990;71(2):452–63.

12. Legro RS, Lin HM, Demers LM, et al. Urinary free cortisol increases in adolescent caucasian females during perimenarche. *J Clin Endocrinol Metab* 2003;88:215.

13. Weldon VV, Kowarski A, Migeon CJ. Aldosterone secretion rates in normal subjects from infancy to adulthood. *Pediatrics* 1967;39:713.

14. Gwynne JT, Strauss JF III. The role of lipoprotein in steroidogenesis and cholesterol metabolism in steroidogenic glands. *Endocr Rev* 1982;3:299–329.

15. Miller WL. Molecular biology of steroid hormone synthesis. *Endocr Rev* 1988;9:295–318.

16. Miller WL, Nichols RJ. The molecular biology, biochemistry, and physiology of human steroidogenesis and its disorders. *Endocr Rev* 2011;32:81–151.

17. Hale AC, Rees LH. ACTH and related peptides. In De Groot LJ, Besser GM, Marshall JC, et al., eds. *Endocrinology.* 2nd ed. Philadelphia, PA: WB Saunders, 1989:363.

18. Saffran M, Schally AV, Benfey BG. Stimulation of the release of corticotropin from the adenohypophysis by neurohypophysical factor. *Endocrinology* 1955;57:439.

19. Laragh JH, Angers M, Kelly WG, et al. Hypotensive agents and pressor substances. The effects of epinephrine, norepinephrine, angiotensin II and others on the secretion of rate of aldosterone in man. *JAMA* 1960;17:234.

20. Kaplan NM. The biosynthesis of adrenal steroids. Effects of angiotensin II, adrenocorticotropin and potassium. *J Clin Invest* 1965;44:2029.

21. Burnay M, Python C, Vallotton M, et al. Role of the capacitative calcium influx in the activation of steroidogenesis by angiotensin-II in adrenal glomerulosa cells. *Endocrinology* 1994;135:751.

22. Cidlowski JA, King KL, Evans-Storms RB, et al. The biochemistry and molecular biology of glucocorticoid-induced apoptosis in the immune system. *Recent Prog Horm Res* 1996;51:457–91.

23. Grunfeld J-P, Eloy L. Glucocorticoids modulates vascular reactivity in the rat. *Hypertension* 1987;10:608–18.

24. Dinarello CA, Mier JW. Current concepts: Lymphookines. *N Engl J Med* 1987;317:940.

25. Sapolsky R, Rivier C, Yamamoto G, et al. Interleukin-1 stimulates the secretion of hypothalamic corticotropin-releasing factor. *Science* 1987;238:522.

26. Chroousos GP, The hypothalamic-pituitary-adrenal axis and immune-mediated inflammation. *N Engl J Med* 1995;332:1351.

27. Besedovsky HO, De Ray A. Immune-neuro-endocrine interactions: Facts and hypotheses. *Endocr Rev* 1996;17:64.

28. McCann V, Fulton T. Cortisol metabolism in chronic liver disease. *J Clin Endocrinol Metab* 1975;40(6):1038–44.

29. Pratt NG. Pathophysiology of heart failure: Neuroendocrine response. *Crit Care Nurs Q* 1995;18(1):22–31.

30. Murck H, Held K, Ziegenbein M, et al. The renin-angiotensin-aldosterone system in patients with depression compared to controls: A sleep endocrine study. *BMC Psychiatry* 2003;3:15.

31. Zuckerman-Levin N, Tiosano D, Eisenhofer G, et al. The importance of adrenocortical glucocorticoids for adrenomedullary and physiological response to stress: A study in isolated glucocorticoid deficiency. *J Clin Endocrinol Metab* 2001;86:5920.

32. Stewart PM. The adrenal cortex. In: Melmed S, Polonsky KS, Larsen PR, et al., eds. *Williams Textbook of Endocrinology.* 12th ed. Philadelphia, PA: Saunders Elsevier, 2011.

33. Patil S, Bartley JA, Murray JC, et al. X-linked glycerol kinase, adrenal hypoplasia, and myopathy maps to X linked glycerol kinase, adrenal hypoplasia, and myopathy maps to Xq21. *Cytogenet Cell Genet* 1985;40:720.

34. Wise Je, Matalon R, Morgan AM, et al. Phenotypic features of patients with congenital adrenal hypoplasia and glycerol kinase deficiency. *Am J Dis Child* 1987;141:744.

35. Assmann G, Seedorf U. Acid Lipase Deficiency: Wolman disease and cholesterol ester storage disease. In: Scriver CR, Beaudet AL, Sly WS, et al., eds. *The Metabolic and Molecular Bases of Inherited Diseases.* New York, NY: McGraw-Hill, 2001:3551–72.

36. Kong M, Jeffcoate W. Eighty-six cases of Addison's disease. *Clin Endocrinol* 1994;41:757.

37. Dubey P, Raymond GV, Moser AB, et al. Adrenal insufficiency in asymptomatic adrenoleukodystrophy patients identified by very long-chain fatty acid screening. *J Pediatr* 2005;146(4):528–32.

38. Nerupt J. Addison syndrome—Clinical studies. A report of 108 cases. *Acta Endocrinol (Copenh)* 1974;76:127.

39. Chang AC, Cochet M, Cohen SN. Structural organization of human genomic DNA encoding the pro-opiomelanocortin peptide. *Proc Natl Acad Sci USA* 1980;77:4890.

40. Li CH. Lipotropin, a new active peptide from pituitary glands. *Nature* 1964;201:924.

41. Speckart PF, Nicoloff JT, Bethune JE. Screening for adrenocortical insufficiency with cosyntropin (synthetic ACTH). *Arch Intern Med* 1971;128(5):761–3.

42. Shizuta Y, Kawamoto T, Mitsuuchi Y, et al. Molecular genetic studies on the biosynthesis of aldosterone in humans. *J Steroid Biochem* 1992;8:981.

43. Oster JR, Singer I, Fishman LM. Heparin induced aldosterone suppression and hyperkalemia. *Am J Med* 1995;98(6):575–86.

44. Reynaud R, Chadli-Chaieb M, Vallette-Kasic S, et al. A familial form of congenital hypopituitarism due to a PROP1 mutation in large kindred: Phenotypic and in vitro functional studies. *J Clin Endocrinol Metab* 2004;89(11):5779–86.

45. Zora JA, Zimmerman TL, Carey EJ, et al. Hypothalamic-pituitary-adrenal axis suppression after short-term, high-dose glucocorticoid therapy in children with asthma. *J Allergy Clin Immunol* 1986;77(1, pt 1):9–13.

46. Kuperman H, Damiani D, Chrousos GP, et al. Evaluation of the hypothalamic-pituitary-adrenal axis in children with leukemia before and after 6 weeks of high-dose glucocorticoid therapy. *J Clin Endocrinol Metab* 2001;86(7):2993–96.

47. Felner EI, Thompson MT, Ratliff AF, et al. Time course of recovery of adrenal function in children treated for leukemia. *J Pediatr* 2000;137(1):21–4.

48. Cooper MS, Stewart PM. Corticosteroid insufficiency in acutely ill patients. *N Engl J Med* 2003;348:727–34.

49. Soni A, Pepper GM, Wyrwinski PM, et al. Adrenal insufficiency occurring during septic shock: Incidence, outcome, and relationship to peripheral cytokine levels. *Am J Med* 1995;98:266–71.

50. Rothwell PM, Udwadia ZF, Lawler PG. Cortisol response to corticotropin and survival in septic shock. *Lancet* 1991;337:582–3.

51. Annane D, Sebille V, Troche G, et al. A 3-level prognostic classification in septic shock based on cortisol levels and cortisol response to corticotropin. *JAMA* 2000;283:1038–45.

52. Den Brinker M, Joosten K, Liem O, et al. Adrenal insufficiency in meningococcal sepsis: Bioavailable cortisol levels and impact of interleukin-6 levels and intubation with etomidate on adrenal function and mortality. *J clin Endocrinol Metab* 2005;90:5110–7.

53. Pizarro C, Troster E, Damiani D, et al. Absolute and relative adrenal insufficiency in children with septic shock. *Crit Care Med* 2005;33:855–9.

54. Hoen S, Asehnoune K, Brailly-Tabard S, et al. Cortisol response to corticotropin stimulation in trauma patients: Influence of hemorrhagic shock. *Anesthesiology* 2002;97(4):807.

55. Cohan P, Wang C, McArthur DL, et al. Acute secondary adrenal insufficiency after traumatic brain injury: A prospective study. *Crit Care Med* 2005;33:2358.

56. Huang CJ, Lin HC. Association between adrenal insufficiency and ventilator weaning. *Am J Respir Crit Care Med* 2006;173(3):276–80.

57. Marik PE, Gayowski T, Starlz TE; for Hepatic Cortisol Research and Adrenal Pathophysiology Study Group. The hepato-adrenal syndrome: A common yet unrecognized clinical condition. *Crit Care Med* 2005;33:1254.

58. Marik PE. Adrenal-exhaustion syndrome in patients with liver disease. *Intensive Care Med* 2006;32:275–80.

59. Siraux V, De Backer D, Yalavatti G, et al. Relative adrenal insufficiency in patients with septic shock: Comparison of low-dose and conventional corticotropin test. *Crit Care Med* 2005;33(11):2479.

60. Loriaux D, Fleseriu M. Relative adrenal insufficiency. *Curr Opin Endocrinol Diabetes Obes* 2009;16:392–400.

61. Hochwald O, Holsti L, Osiovich H. The use of an early ACTH test to identify hypoadrenalism related hypotension in low birth weight infants. *J Perinatol* 2012;32:412–7.

62. Absalom A, Pledger D, Kong A. Adrenocortical function in critically ill patients 24 h after a single dose of etomidate. *Anesthesia* 1999;54:861–7.

63. Wagner RL, White PF. Etomide inhibits adrenocortical function in surgical patients. *Anesthesiology* 1984;61:652.

64. Annane D, Sebille V, Troche G, et al. A 3-level prognostic classification in septic shock based on cortisol levels and on cortisol response to corticotropin. *JAMA* 2000;283:1038–45.

65. Thompson Bastin ML, Baker SN, Weant KA. Effects of etomidate on adrenal suppression: A review of intubated septic patients. *Hosp Pharm* 2014;49(2):177–83.

66. McPhee LC, Badawi O, Fraser GL, et al. Single-dose etomidate is not associated with increased mortality in ICU patients with sepsis: Analysis of a large electronic ICU database. *Crit Care Med* 2013;41:774–83.

67. Crozier TA, Beck D, Schlaeger M, et al. Endocrinological changes following etomidate, midazolam or methohexital for minor surgery. *Anesthesiology* 1987;66:628–35.

68. Robertson WR, Reader SC, Davidson B, et al. On the biopotency and site of action of drugs affecting endocrine tissues with specific reference to the antisteroidogenic effect of anesthetic agents. *Postgrad Med J* 1985;61:145.

69. Sperling M. *Pediatric Endocrinology*. 4th ed. Philadelphia, PA: Saunders, 2008.

CHAPTER 106 ■ DISORDERS OF GLUCOSE HOMEOSTASIS

EDWARD VINCENT S. FAUSTINO, STUART A. WEINZIMER, MICHAEL F. CANARIE, AND CLIFFORD W. BOGUE

KEY POINTS

1 Diabetic ketoacidosis (DKA) is the most frequent cause of diabetes-related death in children, with a mortality rate of 0.2%–0.3%. Over 75%–87% of the mortality in DKA can be attributed to cerebral edema.

2 Correction of dehydration with isotonic fluids and insulin replacement is necessary for optimal management of DKA. Insulin infusion should not be discontinued until DKA resolves. Glucose should be provided to avoid hypoglycemia.

3 Early identification and prompt management of cerebral edema is crucial in improving the outcomes in children with DKA.

4 Hyperglycemic hyperosmolar syndrome (HHS) is underrecognized in children and may be mistaken for DKA.

5 Early and aggressive fluid therapy is critical for effective management of HHS.

6 Mortality in HHS is high, 15% or higher, attributable to circulatory collapse, thrombotic complications, and multisystem organ failure.

7 Hyperglycemia commonly occurs in critically ill nondiabetic children and is associated with increased morbidity and mortality.

8 Neurohormonal factors that accompany stress response lead to insulin resistance, increased glucose production, and hyperglycemia.

9 The optimal management of hyperglycemia in critically ill children is unclear. Controlling blood glucose to a target range of 80–110 mg/dL is likely not beneficial in postoperative cardiac children. The benefit of tight glycemic control in critically ill children with other conditions is uncertain.

10 Except in rare circumstances, hypoglycemia is a defect in fasting adaptation. Understanding the ordered responses to fasting provides the framework for differentiating among the various causes of hypoglycemia and making a prompt diagnosis.

11 Infants, young children, and critically ill children may not present with typical adrenergic symptoms of hypoglycemia. A high index of suspicion should be maintained for these patient populations.

12 Collection of the appropriate blood and urine specimens for determination of alternate fuels and hormones at the time of hypoglycemia provides the most efficient opportunity for determining the etiology of hypoglycemia.

13 Although the outcome of hypoglycemia in a child probably depends on the underlying cause, the clinical significance of insulin-induced hypoglycemia in critically ill children is less clear. Follow-up studies on tight glycemic control trials in children will provide valuable information to answer this question.

DIABETIC KETOACIDOSIS IN CHILDREN

Diabetic ketoacidosis (DKA) is a life-threatening, preventable complication of diabetes mellitus that is characterized by inadequate insulin action, hyperglycemia, dehydration, electrolyte loss, metabolic acidosis, and ketosis. It is the most frequent cause of death in children with type 1 diabetes mellitus. Type 1 diabetes is one of the most common chronic illnesses in children with an incidence of ~3% in young people worldwide (1), and DKA is one of the most common reasons for admission to the PICU (2). DKA occurs in ~15%–70% of children with diabetes at disease onset and in 1%–10% of children with a previous diagnosis of diabetes (3). DKA at diagnosis of type 1 diabetes occurs more commonly in very young children, children without a prior family history of type 1 diabetes, and in families from lower socioeconomic backgrounds. The risk of DKA in children with established type 1 diabetes is associated with infection, intercurrent illness, insulin pump malfunction, purposeful insulin omission,

a history of prior poor metabolic control, concomitant psychiatric disease, peripubertal and adolescent girls, and lower socioeconomic background (3,4).

Definition and Pathophysiology

DKA is defined as a blood glucose concentration >200 mg/dL, with ketonemia/ketonuria, and a venous pH <7.3 or bicarbonate <15 mEq/L (3). The severity of DKA is categorized on the basis of the degree of acidosis (mild: venous pH <7.3 or bicarbonate <15 mEq/L; moderate: pH <7.2 or bicarbonate <10 mEq/L; and severe: pH <7.1 or bicarbonate <5 mEq/L). The primary abnormality is insulin deficiency, which results in hyperglycemia by three mechanisms: increased gluconeogenesis, accelerated glycogenolysis, and impaired peripheral glucose utilization. Early in the progression of type 1 diabetes, the defects in peripheral glucose uptake predominate over the abnormalities in hepatic glucose production, such that postprandial glucose levels are elevated while fasting glucose levels are normal. However, as insulin deficiency becomes progressively more severe and absolute, fasting hyperglycemia occurs. As serum glucose levels exceed the renal threshold of 180 mg/dL, an osmotic diuresis occurs, which results in the loss of extracellular water and electrolytes.

Although insulin deficiency is the primary defect, physiologic stress caused by acidosis and progressive dehydration, as well as coexistent infection or illness, stimulate the release of counter-regulatory hormones (glucagon, catecholamines, and cortisol), which further exacerbate hyperglycemia by increasing hepatic glucose production and further impairing peripheral glucose uptake. Counter-regulatory hormones, particularly epinephrine, also promote lipolysis and free fatty acid release through the activation of adipose tissue hormone-sensitive lipase in adipocytes. Additionally, these hormones activate the hepatic β-oxidation of free fatty acids to ketone bodies, predominantly β-hydroxybutyrate and acetoacetate, which leads to ketoacidosis. Accumulation of ketoacids is the primary cause of the metabolic acidosis in DKA. Although acetone is also formed (causes a fruity odor to the breath), it does not contribute to the acidosis.

The increasing levels of hyperglycemia and acidosis contribute to a vicious cycle. Osmotic diuresis leads to intravascular volume depletion with reduction in renal blood flow and glomerular perfusion, limiting the body's ability to excrete glucose and worsening the hyperglycemia. Likewise, progressive dehydration and acidosis further stimulate the release of counter-regulatory hormones, which accelerates the production of glucose and ketoacids (**Fig. 106.1**). Worsening dehydration then leads to poor peripheral tissue perfusion, with resultant increases in lactic acidosis. Abdominal pain and vomiting are a result of intestinal ileus from ketoacids and dehydration and prevent hydration with oral fluids. The metabolic acidosis leads to potassium transport out of cells into the plasma in exchange for hydrogen and excretion in the urine. Thus, patients with DKA develop a "total-body" deficiency of potassium (intra- and extracellular), which may not correlate with their serum level. Phosphate is affected similarly. A deficiency of 2,3-diphosphoglycerate, a phosphate-containing glycolytic intermediate in red blood cells that facilitates release of oxygen from hemoglobin, may also contribute to the development of lactic acidosis, complicating the ketoacidosis.

As sodium and potassium are excreted in the urine with lactate and ketoacids, hyperchloremia occurs. Electrolyte deficits of up to 5–10 mEq/kg of sodium, 3–5 mEq/kg of potassium, and 0.5–1.5 mmol/kg of phosphate in DKA are not uncommon.

Clinical Presentation and Differential Diagnosis

DKA is not difficult to recognize in a child with known diabetes who is dehydrated, hyperventilating, and obtunded. In the child whose diabetes has not yet been diagnosed, however, it may be confused with gastroenteritis, pneumonia, sepsis, toxic ingestion, or a central nervous system (CNS) lesion. The diagnosis of diabetes (if not already established) is suggested by a history of polyuria, polydipsia, polyphagia, nocturia, or enuresis in a previously toilet-trained child. Weakness and unexplained weight loss may also be presenting features. Abdominal pain, tenderness, and guarding are frequently present in DKA and may be of sufficient intensity to mimic an acute surgical abdomen. Other nonspecific symptoms of DKA, such as mental obtundation, vomiting, and abnormal breathing, are related to the dehydration and acidosis.

DKA in children must be differentiated from such commonly occurring childhood illnesses as urinary tract infection, gastroenteritis, more severe conditions that result in a "surgical abdomen," asthma, and pneumonia. In all of these conditions, symptoms and signs may overlap with diabetes: urinary frequency, polyuria, nocturia, abdominal pain, vomiting, changes in breathing, and dehydration. In particular, extreme hyperglycemia, due to stress hormone excess, and acidosis, due to dehydration and/or fasting, may closely mimic DKA in infants and toddlers with a febrile illness associated with poor oral intake. However, in these children, the absence of polyuria, and polydipsia and the rapid clinical improvement with rehydration alone (without insulin) may differentiate these episodes of stress hyperglycemia from true DKA.

The physical examination findings in DKA are predominantly those of dehydration: tachycardia, delayed capillary refill, dry mucous membranes, and poor skin turgor. Severe acidosis and dehydration may impair cardiac contractility,

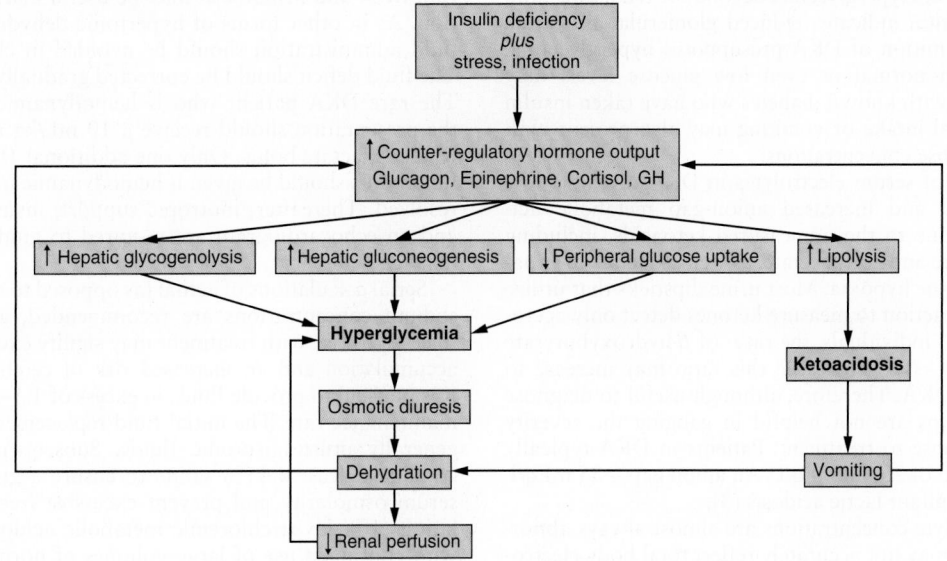

FIGURE 106.1. Pathophysiology of diabetic ketoacidosis. GH, growth hormone.

resulting in hypotension. Respiratory compensation for the metabolic acidosis induces hyperventilation, which may appear as deep sighing respirations (Kussmaul breathing) and may initially suggest a primary respiratory illness. Acetone on the breath yields a fruity odor and may be present but is not reliably detected. Mental status may vary from full alertness to frank coma. Most patients with severe metabolic derangements are lethargic but do not have severe CNS depression and are able to protect their airway.

The primary survey should focus initially on the adequacy of the airway, breathing, a thorough assessment of the circulatory status (heart rate, blood pressure, description of mucous membranes, capillary refill, distal pulses, and warmth of extremities), degree of dehydration (including weight if possible), and mental status. A rough estimation of degree of dehydration should be made to calculate the fluid deficit and facilitate rehydration therapy. A careful examination and written documentation of the neurologic status is critical to serve as a baseline in case of deterioration in neurologic status later in therapy. General physical examination should include respiratory and abdominal examinations, as well as a search for an intercurrent illness that may have served as the precipitating factor for the episode of DKA.

Laboratory Findings

The laboratory evaluation of patients suspected to have DKA includes determination of the blood glucose, plasma or urinary ketones, serum electrolyte concentration, blood urea nitrogen (BUN), creatinine, osmolarity, baseline calcium and phosphorus, and, if infection is suspected, complete blood count and blood culture. Bedside determination of the blood glucose with a glucose-monitoring device and evaluation of the urine for glucose and ketones should be performed as quickly as possible, and treatment should be initiated without waiting for the results of the laboratory assessment to become available. A baseline blood gas measurement should also be made to determine the pH and P_{CO_2}. While venous blood gas measurements suffice in most episodes of DKA, an arterial blood gas measurement should be considered in patients who are suspected to have incomplete respiratory compensation or those with hemodynamic instability.

The initial blood glucose level is characteristically, but not invariably, elevated. Hyperglycemia beyond the renal threshold for glucose filtration indicates reduced glomerular filtration. Although the definition of DKA presupposes hyperglycemia, ketoacidosis with normal or even low glucose levels may occur in patients with known diabetes who have taken insulin recently. Poor oral intake or vomiting may also present with near-normal glucose concentrations.

Measurement of serum electrolytes in DKA reveals a low bicarbonate level and increased anion-gap metabolic acidosis, primarily due to the unmeasured ketoacids, including β-hydroxybutyrate and acetoacetate, as well as lactate in situations of severe tissue hypoxia. Most urine dipsticks that utilize a nitroprusside reaction to measure ketones detect only acetoacetate. In normal individuals, the ratio of β-hydroxybutyrate to acetoacetate is ~1:1. However, this ratio may increase to 10:1 or more in DKA. Therefore, although useful to diagnose ketosis, these strips are not helpful in gauging the severity of DKA or response to treatment. Patients in DKA typically have an anion gap of 20–30 mEq/L. An anion gap >35 mEq/L suggests a concomitant lactic acidosis (3).

Serum electrolyte concentrations are almost always abnormal in DKA and may not accurately reflect total body electrolyte disturbances. Because of the osmotic flux of water from the intracellular space to the extracellular space in the presence of hyperglycemia, serum sodium will be reduced. The actual sodium concentration may be determined by adding 1.6 mEq/L

for each 100 mg/dL rise in glucose concentration >100 mg/dL (5). Furthermore, extreme hypertriglyceridemia may cause the serum sodium concentration to be falsely lowered (dilutional hyponatremia) (6). A normal or elevated sodium level in the setting of severe DKA suggests extreme free water losses. The degree of elevation of the BUN and creatinine, as well as the hematocrit, may also indicate the extent of dehydration (and the possibility of renal damage).

The initial serum potassium may be low, normal, or high, depending on the degree of acidosis and the quantitative urinary losses. However, total body potassium stores are almost always depleted from excessive urinary losses, and normal or low K levels at presentation may be associated with severe hypokalemia once treatment for DKA is initiated. Phosphate, like potassium, is depleted in the setting of DKA, and serum phosphate levels may not accurately reflect total body stores. Serum phosphate level may also decrease during therapy.

Clinical Management

The International Society for Pediatric and Adolescent Diabetes published practice guidelines for the management of DKA in 2009 (3). The guidelines are consistent with those published by the Lawson Wilkins Pediatric Endocrine Society and European Society for Paediatric Endocrinology in 2004 (7). The goals of therapy for DKA are (1) to correct dehydration and electrolyte deficits, (2) to correct acidosis and reverse ketosis, (3) to restore blood glucose to near normal, (4) to avoid complications of therapy, and (5) to identify and treat any precipitating event.

Correction of Dehydration and Electrolyte Deficits

A rough estimation of degree of dehydration should be made to calculate the fluid deficit and facilitate rehydration therapy even though such clinical approximations are subjective and typically inaccurate in estimating the actual degree of dehydration. Furthermore, the dehydration of DKA is hyperosmolar, resulting in a translocation of intracellular water to the extracellular compartment, thus masking the degree of dehydration. Significant total body fluid losses can occur before evidence of changes in vital signs or physical examination. Serum BUN and hematocrit may be useful markers of dehydration. As in other forms of hypertonic dehydration, too rapid fluid administration should be avoided in children in DKA. The fluid deficit should be corrected gradually, over 48 hours. The rare DKA patient who is hemodynamically unstable at the presentation should receive a 10 mL/kg normal saline or Ringer's lactate bolus. Only one additional 10 mL/kg isotonic fluid bolus should be given if hemodynamic instability has not resolved. Thereafter, inotropic support, invasive monitoring, and an echocardiogram are required to guide hemodynamic management.

Serial calculations of actual (as opposed to measured) serum sodium concentrations are recommended, as sodium levels that fail to rise with treatment may signify excessive free water accumulation and an increased risk of cerebral edema (8,9). It is unusual to provide fluids in excess of 1.5–2 times the daily maintenance rate. The initial fluid replacement (first 6 hours) generally utilizes isotonic fluids. Subsequent fluids should contain at least 0.45% saline to ensure a gradual decline in serum osmolarity and prevent excessive free water accumulation (10). Hyperchloremic metabolic acidosis may develop with continued use of large volumes of normal saline. There are no data to support the use of colloids over crystalloids for this patient group (3).

Early potassium replacement is important to correct the deficit. With the initiation of insulin therapy and correction of acidosis, serum potassium levels may drop precipitously as potassium shifts back from the extracellular to the intracellular compartment. In hypokalemic patients, replace potassium at the time of initial volume expansion and prior to starting insulin infusion. Otherwise, potassium should be administered only after adequate renal function is determined, particularly in patients who are hyperkalemic. Electrocardiographic monitoring facilitates early recognition of hyperkalemia (peaked T waves), hypokalemia (flat or inverted T waves), and the development of potentially dangerous cardiac dysrhythmias. Potassium is usually given at a dose of 40 mEq/L of fluid, either as potassium chloride or in combination with potassium phosphate. The latter has the additional advantage of replacing the phosphate deficit. Potassium can also be repleted as potassium acetate, which may theoretically provide buffering equivalents for the metabolic acidosis. The relative risks and benefits of these infusion alternatives in the treatment of DKA in children have not been rigorously studied (3,7). It should be noted that while hypophosphatemia in DKA may predispose to rhabdomyolysis and hemolysis and while low 2,3-diphosphoglycerate levels in DKA may impair tissue delivery of oxygen, complications of hypophosphatemia in DKA are rare, and phosphate replacement may precipitate acute hypocalcemia. Serum calcium should be monitored if phosphate is given. It is recommended to replace phosphate in patients with severe hypophosphatemia and unexplained weakness (3).

Correction of Acidosis and Reversal of Ketosis

Acidosis in DKA reverses with fluid replacement and insulin therapy. Restoration of circulation improves renal perfusion, resulting in acid excretion. Improved tissue perfusion also limits the production of lactic acid in hypoperfused tissues. Insulin administration stops ketoacid production. Acidosis in DKA usually resolves later than hyperglycemia. However, it is important to continue insulin therapy until acidosis resolves while supporting the patient with glucose to prevent hypoglycemia.

Bicarbonate, once considered routine therapy in severe DKA, is no longer thought to be beneficial and is no longer recommended in the treatment of uncomplicated DKA. Most often, dramatic clinical improvement results simply from initial expansion of extracellular fluid volume, reestablishment of adequate peripheral perfusion, and prompt insulin administration. Bicarbonate therapy may lead to paradoxical worsening of CNS acidosis, hypokalemia, sodium overload, late alkalosis, and, theoretically, impaired tissue perfusion due to leftward shift of the oxyhemoglobin dissociation curve. Finally, bicarbonate has been associated, in multivariate analysis, with a higher risk of development of cerebral edema (8). Bicarbonate may still be considered in the setting of severe acidosis with impaired cardiac contractility and vasomotor tone. It may be given in a slow infusion of 1–2 mEq/kg over 60 minutes.

Restoration of Blood Glucose to Near Normal

Insulin therapy, at a dose of 0.05–0.1 U/kg/h, should be initiated immediately after the patient has received initial volume expansion. Because insulin adsorbs to intravenous tubing, 20 mL of the insulin solution should be flushed through the tubing set before connecting to the patient. The insulin infusion can then be started immediately, and there is no need to allow the insulin to "dwell" in the intravenous tubing after the 20-mL flush (11). Intravenous insulin bolus is contraindicated because it may increase the risk of cerebral edema. As with fluid replacement, the aim of therapy is gradual correction of blood glucose (i.e., a reduction of the blood glucose by 50–100 mg/dL/h). However, the serum glucose concentration often falls significantly with initial rehydration alone owing to increased glomerular filtration from improved renal

perfusion. The dose of insulin usually remains at 0.1 U/kg/h until acidosis resolves. Because insulin infusion often results in lowering of the blood glucose concentration before the decrease in ketoacidosis, it is important not to decrease the rate of insulin infusion, but instead to add dextrose to the rehydration fluids to prevent hypoglycemia. Dextrose should be added to the intravenous fluid solution when the serum glucose level falls below 250 mg/dL and should then be titrated to maintain blood glucose at about 200 mg/dL until DKA resolves. This may be accomplished with the simultaneous use of two intravenous solutions that differ only in the dextrose concentration (10% and 0%). Independent manipulation of each infusion allows the dextrose infusion to be varied quickly and efficiently (the so-called "two-bag" system) (12).

Avoidance of Complications of Therapy

Some of the more common complications of DKA therapy are inadequate rehydration, hypoglycemia, hypokalemia, hyperchloremic acidosis, and cerebral edema. Of these, acute cerebral edema is the most serious, and accounts for 75%–87% of the mortality in DKA. Cerebral edema occurs in ~0.5%–1% of episodes of pediatric DKA and carries a mortality rate of over 20% and a rate of permanent neurologic disability of over 25% (13). Cerebral edema is more likely to occur in patients at the time of first diagnosis of diabetes, in younger children, and in those presenting with the most severe degree of dehydration and metabolic derangement. It typically develops within the first 4–12 hours of treatment but may occur as late as 24–48 hours after the start of treatment. Symptoms and signs include headache, confusion, slurred speech, bradycardia, hypertension, and other signs of increased intracranial pressure. A bedside scoring system based on the patient's neurologic status was proposed to diagnose cerebral edema (14). Although a number of causes of acute cerebral edema have been suggested from uncontrolled, retrospective studies, the etiology in many cases is not known. A common proposed mechanism involves a rapid decline in serum osmolality with treatment of DKA. On the basis of this hypothesis, previous recommendations for treatment of DKA advised limiting the rate of rehydration to <4 L/m²/day (15) and avoiding hypotonic fluids (16). Until the precise mechanisms that underlie the development and progression of cerebral edema are elucidated, it appears prudent to correct dehydration evenly over 48 hours (unless the patient is in shock), and monitor neurologic status and laboratory parameters closely.

Treatment of cerebral edema is aimed at lowering intracranial pressure. Reducing the rate of fluid administration by one-third is suggested. Prompt administration of IV mannitol (0.5–1 g/kg over 20 minutes) may be beneficial if given early in the course of cerebral edema. The dose may be repeated in 0.5–2 hours if there is no response to the initial dose. Hypertonic saline (3%), 5–10 mL/kg over 30 minutes, may be used as an alternative or in addition to mannitol. One should keep the patient's head elevated and midline. Tracheal intubation may be needed for impending respiratory failure or airway protection. Although aggressive hyperventilation should be avoided as this decreases cerebral perfusion, care should be taken to match the level of hyperventilation the patient was spontaneously producing as sedating and ventilating the patient at a lower $Paco_2$ than they were producing may worsen acidosis, cause cerebral vasodilation, and increase intracranial pressure if intracranial compliance is limited. Near infrared spectroscopy (NIRS) may be used to assess the ventilatory parameters and resulting $Paco_2$ associated with a favorable cerebral O_2 supply/demand ratio. Intracranial imaging to exclude other pathologies, such as cerebral infarction or thrombosis, should be obtained but not at the expense of timely therapeutic interventions.

Other less common complications of DKA include thrombosis (including cerebral venous sinus thrombosis), a concern in children who require a central venous catheter for access; cardiac dysrhythmias, usually related to electrolyte disturbances; pulmonary edema; renal failure; pancreatitis; rhabdomyolysis; and infection, such as aspiration pneumonia, sepsis, and mucormycosis.

Identification and Treatment of Any Precipitating Event

Infection is a common precipitating event for DKA. Infections should be appropriately worked up and treated. In cases of DKA in children with known diabetes, additional education on insulin omission, or sick day or pump failure management may be needed to prevent another episode of DKA.

Successful management of DKA requires meticulous attention to clinical and laboratory changes. Children with severe DKA or who are at increased risk for cerebral edema should be cared for in the ICU. Clinical monitoring is essential. Vital signs, perfusion, input/output balance, and neurologic status should be documented at least hourly. Cardiac monitoring is recommended owing to the risk of dysrhythmia. Laboratory monitoring should include venous blood glucose concentrations hourly and electrolytes and venous pH every 2–4 hours until normal. BUN and creatinine levels should be followed until they are normal, and calcium should be monitored, particularly if phosphate is administered. Lack of improvement in clinical and biochemical parameters with time suggests an occult infection or inadequate insulin or fluid replacement.

Outcomes

DKA is the most frequent diabetes-related cause of death in children, with a mortality rate of ~0.15%–0.3% across many centers and geographic regions (3,7). With appropriate treatment, complications of DKA, especially cerebral edema, are uncommon.

Conclusions and Future Directions—Diabetic Ketoacidosis

One of the most important areas for further investigation in the management of DKA is in improving prevention strategies. DKA, especially in known diabetics, is preventable. Future research endeavors should also address the basic pathophysiologic mechanisms of cerebral edema, so that treatment algorithms may be optimized to reduce or eliminate this complication of DKA. Differentiation of hyperosmolar coma from DKA and management of DKA in children with type 2 diabetes are areas that require more attention, as increasing numbers of pediatric patients with type 2 diabetes are being recognized. Finally, the use of continuous glucose-monitoring systems that track glucose values and trends in real time to facilitate clinical management of DKA have yet to be fully explored.

HYPERGLYCEMIC HYPEROSMOLAR SYNDROME

Hyperglycemic hyperosmolar syndrome (HHS) is a potentially lethal disorder of decompensated glucose homeostasis. Patients with this syndrome, known formerly as hyperosmolar nonketotic coma or state (HONKC) or hyperglycemic hyperosmolar nonketotic syndrome (HHNS), suffer from the dangerous consequences of marked hyperglycemia and hyperosmolarity. Once thought limited to the adult population, the syndrome is increasingly described in younger patients.

Epidemiology

Cases of extreme hyperglycemia without significant ketosis have been described in adults for more than 100 years (17). Currently, the literature cites the rate of HHS as 17.5 per 100,000 adult patients, with a greater distribution in the elderly and disabled (18). The syndrome affects known diabetics (particularly those with type 2 diabetes) but may also herald its onset. In addition, precipitating factors associated with HHS include infections, coexisting medical problems (e.g., renal failure, pancreatitis), medications (notably, diuretics, steroids, anticonvulsants, and psychotropic drugs), and total parenteral nutrition, as well as other conditions that lead to dehydration, such as burns and heat stroke (18).

HHS was first described in children in 1951, followed by sporadic case reports over the succeeding decades involving patients from infancy through adolescence (19). Often depicted as idiopathic, various triggers akin to those in adults have been ascribed to the syndrome in children. In addition, concerns about an underlying incipient diabetes mellitus ("pseudodiabetes of infancy") or impaired osmoregulatory function have been considered (20). Unfortunately, the lack of data has precluded any reasonable attempt at estimating the syndrome's prevalence in the pediatric population. Nonetheless, a review of published HHS cases in the past decade reveals an increasing number of reports (65 between 2001 and 2008), compared with the roughly 2 dozen reports described in the preceding decade (21–25). In contrast to the various etiologies described in the past, more recent reports noted a near-universal association with diabetic disorders (type 1 and 2 diabetes mellitus). Interestingly, among survivors of HHS, 41% had type 2 diabetes, while 35% had type 1 diabetes. Three-quarters of the patients were obese. Moreover, the risk appears higher in certain ethnic groups, with African Americans representing 70% of pediatric patients (25). This is consistent with the higher risk of type 2 diabetes in African Americans. The epidemic of pediatric obesity and its strong association with altered glucose metabolism, insulin resistance, and, ultimately, type 2 diabetes creates the potential for an increase in the number of cases of HHS in children (26,27).

Pathophysiology

HHS and DKA are often depicted as opposite extremes along the spectrum of decompensated diabetes. In HHS, insulin levels may be sufficient to suppress lipolysis and ketogenesis seen in DKA, but they are inadequate to promote normal anabolic function and inhibit the creation of glucose through gluconeogenesis and glycogenolysis. Thus, HHS may be seen as the presentation of an unrecognized relative insulin deficiency that is triggered by intercurrent illness or medication. The hyperbolic shape of the insulin sensitivity curve may help to explain the seemingly acute decompensation. Regardless of the proximal cause, the resulting surge of counter-regulatory hormones raises glucose levels by both enhanced hepatic glucose generation and worsening insulin resistance. Hyperglycemia itself triggers a heightened inflammatory state, which, in turn, exacerbates glucose dysregulation (28). This maladaptive milieu can precipitate a massive osmotic diuresis and, ultimately, dehydration. The resultant volume contraction reduces the glomerular filtration rate, further elevating glucose levels, and may lead to hyperosmolarity that is prominent in this syndrome. In summary, the disorder "begins" with elevated blood glucose and "progresses with varying degrees of speed toward the development of profound dehydration" (17).

The risks related to the hyperglycemic hyperosmolar state extend beyond the effects of volume contraction and circulatory compromise. The long-term ill effects of hyperglycemia on the microcirculation and macrocirculation have been well described, but evidence shows an association between acute hyperglycemia itself and morbidity and mortality in critically ill patients (29,30). Through a variety of mechanisms, hyperglycemia may cause vascular injury and thrombus formation. It also disrupts the phagocytic and oxidative burst functions of the innate immune system (28,31–34). Finally, hyperglycemia has been shown to disrupt the blood–brain barrier, alter CNS metabolism, and worsen the effects of ischemia on brain tissue (29).

Although HHS and DKA are often placed in the extremes of the continuum of perturbed glucose homeostasis, important distinctions exist from a critical care perspective. For example, in HHS, ketoacidemia is generally neither the underlying nor the most extreme pathophysiologic disturbance. Second, because of the duration of symptoms and the extreme hyperosmolarity of patients with HHS, a much greater degree of volume depletion may be present. It is estimated that DKA patients are 10% dehydrated, whereas HHS patients may typically be 15%–20% dehydrated (35). An early study estimated patients with HHS and coma to be 24% dehydrated (17). Greater electrolyte loss may also be present in HHS as compared with DKA (36). Finally, the existing data suggest that HHS poses a more serious threat to pediatric patients than does DKA, which has a mortality rate of <1%.

Clinical Presentation and Diagnosis

One case series suggests that a failure to consider the diagnosis of HHS greatly contributes to morbidity and mortality (37). Patients with HHS commonly present with a history of weight loss, complaints of polydipsia or polyuria of variable duration, and gastrointestinal distress. Examination reveals that patients are lethargic and often have neurologic impairments that range from a slightly altered sensorium, to focal neurologic deficits, and frank coma (the "nonketotic coma"). These patients are dehydrated and in varying—and often tenuous—states of cardiovascular decompensation. The duration of these symptoms and the ability of the patient to compensate for the prodigious osmotic diuresis dictate the severity of their presentation.

Although the clinical assessment is a crucial aspect of the diagnosis and management of HHS, it can be clouded by a number of factors. First, the onset of symptoms is likely insidious, with an indolent prelude to decompensation and a correspondingly vague history. An altered mental status may further shroud the history (and a workup for mental status changes may not include HHS). Second, the frequent absence of the symptomologic and objective hallmarks of ketoacidemia may obscure the diagnosis. The abdominal discomfort, nausea, and vomiting have been reported to be less severe, and acetone breath and a Kussmaul breathing pattern are not usually present. Finally, assessing the volume status of an obese patient can be difficult, which may obscure both the correct diagnosis and the severity of illness.

Laboratory findings should confirm the presence of marked hyperglycemia (>600 mg/dL) and hyperosmolarity (>330 mOsm/kg). Glucose levels as high as 2580 mg/dL have been reported (23). The traditional diagnostic criteria for HHS also include serum bicarbonate ≥15 mEq/L and a pH ≥7.3 without evidence of significant ketosis (36). Yet most patients recently described had bicarbonate <15 mEq/dL and, in those for whom it was measured, a pH <7.25. Significant ketonuria was also present in more than a quarter of these patients (17,20,27,36,38,39). In fact, DKA/HHS overlap or "mixed" syndromes are not uncommon (40–43). It is important to recognize, moreover, that the level of acidemia in these patients can be influenced by factors other than the degree of ketosis,

such as the severity of shock, the effectiveness of respiratory compensation, and the use of large quantities of normal saline. Laboratory evidence of end-organ injury is typically found, in particular acute kidney injury, as well as rhabdomyolysis and pancreatitis. Finally, patients with this disorder may have significant electrolyte imbalance and, depending on the degree of acidemia, the serum potassium may be initially elevated (35).

Treatment

There have been no clinical trials on the optimal treatment for HHS. However, greater experience with the disorder and a firmer grasp of the pathophysiology has led to more informed recommendations for therapy. Given the potential for life-threatening complications, HHS must be viewed as a matter of medical urgency, if not emergency. As such, it is prudent for patients with HHS to be monitored in an ICU until they are stabilized—even in the absence of profound acidemia. Initial management, as dictated by the degree of hemodynamic compromise and complications on presentation, should emphasize the essentials of ICU care. Accordingly, the early goals of treatment should target airway protection and mechanical ventilation on the basis of Glasgow coma scale and compensatory response as well as the restoration of hemodynamic stability and tissue perfusion. The placement of appropriate cardiovascular monitoring (including arterial and central venous pressure monitoring as indicated) may be required. Electrolytes should be rigorously monitored and repleted on the basis of frequent sampling and hyperglycemia conservatively corrected. Finally, vigilant monitoring for neurologic or other complications, detection and treatment of precipitating causes, and appropriate prophylactic measures should be undertaken.

Given an estimated fluid deficit of ~15%, volume resuscitation is the mainstay of therapy for HHS (35,37,44). Reports from critically ill adults advocate aggressive volume resuscitation (2–3 L of normal saline over the first 2 hours) with replacement of 50% of the deficit in the first 12 hours. Similar recommendations appear in the pediatric and adult emergency medicine literature. Published pediatric guidelines suggest an initial normal saline bolus of 20 mL/kg (repeating as necessary to restore peripheral perfusion), and an appropriate maintenance rate plus replacement of the remaining volume deficit over 24–48 hours (36). Pediatric experts also urge replacement of ongoing urinary losses, which can be exceedingly high in hyperosmolar patients (39,45). As poor outcomes have been associated with failure to recognize and aggressively treat HHS, a timely and appropriate response is essential (35,44,46,47). In areas of ambiguity, central venous monitoring may assist volume status assessment and replacement. Isotonic fluid is generally recommended for the resuscitative phase of treatment, with half-normal saline employed later to complete rehydration.

Although insulin may have salutary, anti-inflammatory benefits, in the absence of significant ketoacidemia, it is felt by many to play a secondary role in the initial management of HHS (44,48). In fact, hyperglycemia can often be partially corrected by reestablishing renal perfusion and glomerular filtration, thereby ensuring a more gradual correction of hyperosmolarity without rapid fluid and electrolyte shifts (48–50). Accordingly, a more guarded approach to insulin therapy is recommended in HHS (0.025–0.05 U/kg/h) with higher doses (0.05–0.1 U/kg/h) suggested for patients with greater acidemia. The blood glucose level should not decline by more than 100 mg/dL/h (39).

Theoretically, the absence of a large ketotic diuresis should lessen the cationic urinary loss. However, the prolonged duration of illness may lead to total body electrolyte depletion. Estimated electrolyte deficit ranges in adults with HHS are

3–7 mmol/kg for phosphate, 4–6 mEq/kg for potassium, and 5–13 mEq/kg for sodium (5). Electrolytes should be monitored carefully and replaced as indicated, with particular attention to potassium shifts with the initiation of insulin therapy. Volume contraction, the use of insulin, and copious amounts of normal saline commonly lead to hypernatremia, which can be addressed with hypotonic fluids, after the initial stage of treatment. Finally, given the risk of rhabdomyolysis, serum creatinine phosphokinase should be closely monitored.

Although current research suggests that hyperglycemia predisposes to thrombogenesis and that HHS in particular predisposes to deep vein thromboses in patients with central venous catheters, the degree of risk of thromboembolism has not been formally assessed. Therefore, current evidence does not support the use of anticoagulation in HHS. Nonetheless, appropriate prophylaxis for deep vein thromboses should be employed.

Outcomes

In the adult population, complications and fatalities associated with HHS are most often due to comorbid conditions (35). In pediatric patients, morbidity includes acute kidney injury, rhabdomyolysis, coma, malignant hyperthermia-type syndrome and significant electrolyte disturbances. Neurologic findings are common in HHS. However, a parallel to the more isolated and devastating intracerebral events (cerebral edema) of DKA has not been established (20,38). In the most recent reports, positive autopsy or CT findings of cerebral edema are rare and described only in the context of multisystem organ failure or sudden cardiac death (21,23,24).

Historically, the adult mortality risk has been cited to be between 15% and 60%, with newer estimates suggesting a risk closer to 15% (36). In children, as the prevalence of the disorder is unknown, only crude approximations of mortality risk are possible. Although a cumulative mortality risk of 23% was calculated from older studies, mortality risk in a more recent cohort was disturbingly high at 37% (25). Deaths in HHS have been attributed to cardiac arrest and refractory dysrhythmias, pulmonary thromboemboli, circulatory collapse, refractory shock, and multisystem organ failure.

Conclusions and Future Directions— Hyperglycemic Hyperosmolar Syndrome

Aside from epidemiologic gaps, a great deal remains to be explained regarding HHS, including (a) clarification of the underlying pathophysiology, with attention to the role of obesity and its relationship with inflammatory mediators, (b) the role of hyperglycemia-induced inflammation in the complications of HHS, (c) a clearer understanding of those patients most at risk for HHS, as well as a method for determining the degree of that risk, and (4) finally and perhaps most importantly, more outcomes data are needed to inform the optimal treatment for this syndrome.

HYPERGLYCEMIA IN CRITICALLY ILL CHILDREN

Hyperglycemia is a significant concern in critically ill children. Although hyperglycemia in the sick, nondiabetic patient was first described in the 19th century by Claude Bernard (28), interest in this metabolic disturbance was not highlighted until the landmark Leuven trial by van den Berghe et al. (51) in 2001. "Stress diabetes," "traumatic diabetes," or "diabetes of

injury," as it was previously called, was thought of as an adaptive response, and the rise in glucose was thought to represent the body's attempt to provide an adequate energy source to combat the stress. Previously, hyperglycemia was considered simply a marker of illness severity that required no significant intervention unless glucosuria occurred. However, in the Leuven trial, controlling blood glucose to normal levels with insulin resulted in a survival benefit among critically ill surgical adults, suggesting a causal relationship between hyperglycemia and worse outcomes (51). With subsequent studies failing to replicate the results of this study, management of hyperglycemia in the nondiabetic critically ill child remains unsettled (52).

Epidemiology of Hyperglycemia

Hyperglycemia is common in critically ill nondiabetic children. However, the exact prevalence is unclear because of the absence of a consensus definition for hyperglycemia. Studies in critically ill adults initially utilized a threshold of ≥110 mg/dL on the basis of the definition used by the World Health Organization and a number of diabetes organizations for impaired fasting glucose (53). A recent clinical practice guideline suggested using a threshold of ≥150 mg/dL for glucose control (54). Surveys of intensivists showed that pediatricians tend to use a higher threshold of 140–160 mg/dL to define hyperglycemia (55,56). Using a threshold of >150 mg/dL, hyperglycemia occurs in 49%–72% of critically ill children (57,58). Certain populations of critically ill children are at a disproportionately increased risk for hyperglycemia. These include children recovering from cardiac surgery, massive burns, traumatic brain injury, and sepsis (58). Patients on mechanical ventilation, vasoactive drug support, and extracorporeal support are also at increased risk for hyperglycemia (59).

Despite the lack of a consensus definition for hyperglycemia, elevated glucose levels have been consistently associated with increased morbidity and mortality in critically ill children. Among all admissions to the PICU, blood glucose >150 mg/dL is associated with a 2.5–10.9-fold increased risk of mortality (57,58). The association holds true for different subsets of critically ill children, including patients who have massive burns, traumatic brain injury, septic shock, and postoperative cardiac patients (58). Nonsurvivors consistently have higher glucose levels compared with survivors (29,60). In addition, hyperglycemia in critically ill children is associated with prolonged ICU stays and higher infection rates (57,61,62). The intensity, timing, and duration of hyperglycemia substantially affect the outcome (58).

Normal Glucose Homeostasis

Maintenance of normoglycemia is a complex process that involves the removal and addition of glucose to the bloodstream. Neurohormonal and autoregulatory mechanisms tightly regulate this process (63).

Noninsulin-mediated uptake of glucose by the CNS accounts for 80% of glucose utilization during basal conditions. Skeletal muscles remove the remaining 20%, half of which is insulin-mediated. After a meal, blood glucose is cleared in nearly equal amounts by the muscle, fat, hepatosplanchnic bed, and noninsulin-requiring tissues, including the CNS. The liver extracts as much as 40% of ingested glucose for conversion to glycogen.

Glut proteins facilitate cellular glucose transport (28,63,64). A number of isoforms have been identified, of which glut1, glut2, and glut4 are thought to play major roles in glucose metabolism. Found in nearly all cells, glut1 is most abundant and is important in basal glucose uptake. Glut2, on the other hand, is found mainly in hepatocytes, where it transports glucose into and out of the hepatocytes. Glut4 facilitates glucose absorption in insulin-responsive cells in the presence of the hormone.

Although nearly all cells are involved in glucose uptake, glucose production occurs only in the liver and the kidneys. Two processes contribute to glucose formation: breakdown of glycogen in the liver and production of new glucose molecules from both the liver and the kidneys. Glycogenolysis provides most of the glucose after an overnight fast. However, with prolonged starvation, glycogen stores are depleted and other sources of energy are utilized.

The balance of uptake and production of glucose is the result of an interaction between a number of hormonal, neural, and hepatic autoregulatory mechanisms. Insulin, glucagon, catecholamines, cortisol, and growth hormone are the major hormones involved in glucose metabolism. Insulin decreases blood glucose levels by enhancing glucose uptake and glycogenesis and conversely inhibiting gluconeogenesis. In contrast, the other hormones, which are also known as counter-regulatory hormones, have the opposite effect of elevating blood glucose by inhibiting glucose uptake and enhancing glycogenolysis and gluconeogenesis.

Different sites within the brain affect glucose control. These centers, which include nuclei in the brainstem and the hypothalamus, affect sympathetic and parasympathetic outflow to the liver, pancreas, and splanchnic circulation to adjust the amount of insulin secreted and the amount of glycogen cleaved into glucose. Peripherally, glucose sensors found in the portal vein and the intestines relay glycemic levels to the brainstem and the hypothalamus. Effectors of these pathways include the pancreas and the adrenal glands, which respond by changing insulin and catecholamine secretion.

The liver also has an intrinsic autoregulatory ability to respond to changing blood glucose levels. The major step in this process is the interconversion of glucose to glucose-6-phosphate, and vice versa, which is mediated by glucokinase and glucose-6-phosphatase. Autoregulation enables the liver to adjust glucose production on the basis of blood glucose levels and availability of the requisite glucose precursors.

Glucose Control during Critical Illness

Hyperglycemia results from the body's systemic response to stress. During stress, the hypothalamic–pituitary–adrenal axis and sympathetic system are activated, leading to increased cortisol and catecholamine secretion (**Fig. 106.1**). Other counter-regulatory hormones and cytokines are secreted as well. The combination of these factors leads to insulin resistance and elevated blood glucose.

Most studies indicate that stress hyperglycemia is a result of glucose overproduction rather than impairment of glucose uptake (63,65,66). The orchestrated rise in the counter-regulatory hormones leads to enhanced hepatic gluconeogenesis and glycogenolysis (**Table 106.1**), which in this abnormal setting are not inhibited by increased blood glucose levels or by increased insulin secretion. Insulin resistance in the liver ensues. Among the counter-regulatory hormones, catecholamines and glucagon are responsible for an initial transient rise in glucose. Epinephrine and norepinephrine promote gluconeogenesis via a cAMP-dependent mechanism. Glucagon, also working through a cAMP-mediated mechanism, increases the activity of hepatic enzymes involved in gluconeogenesis and inhibits the enzymes of glycogenesis. Sustaining hyperglycemia requires the action of cortisol and growth hormone on mRNA transcription. Cytokines such as tumor necrosis factor

TABLE 106.1

MAJOR ACTIONS OF COUNTER-REGULATORY HORMONES AND CYTOKINES IN MEDIATING STRESS HYPERGLYCEMIA

■ HORMONE	■ MECHANISM
Glucagon	Increased gluconeogenesis
	Increased hepatic glycogenolysis
Epinephrine	Skeletal muscle insulin resistance by altering postreceptor signaling
	Increased gluconeogenesis
	Increased skeletal muscle and hepatic glycogenolysis
	Increased lipolysis, increased free fatty acids
	Direct suppression of insulin secretion
Norepinephrine	Increased lipolysis
	Increased gluconeogenesis, but hyperglycemia not marked except at high concentrations
Glucocorticoids	Skeletal muscle insulin resistance
	Increased lipolysis
	Gluconeogenesis increased through provision of substrate
Growth hormone	Skeletal muscle insulin resistance
	Increased lipolysis
	Increased gluconeogenesis
Tumor necrosis factor	Skeletal muscle insulin resistance, altered postreceptor signaling
	Hepatic insulin resistance

Reprinted from McCowen KC, Malhotra A, Bistrian BR. Stress-induced hyperglycemia. *Crit Care Clin* 2001;17(1):107–24.

(TNF)-α, IL-1, and IL-6 worsen hyperglycemia by promoting the secretion of counter-regulatory hormones both centrally and peripherally.

In addition to the effect of increased counter-regulatory hormones on circulating glucose levels, other gluconeogenic precursors, including lactate, alanine, glycerol, and glutamine, are produced during stress (63,65,66). Major sources of lactate are the lungs (in acute lung injury), intestines, and wounds—a reflection of increased rates of glycolysis and possible downregulation of pyruvate dehydrogenase. The liver avidly extracts lactate from the circulation and converts it to glucose. The principal source of alanine is de novo synthesis from pyruvate in skeletal muscle rather than muscle breakdown, whereas glycerol is a by-product of adipocyte lipolysis. Fat mobilization significantly increases during stress. Finally, glutamine provides the primary source of carbon for glucose production in the kidneys.

Glucose uptake during stress is significantly higher than during basal conditions (28,63). Cytokines and hypoxia are some of the factors shown to upregulate glut1 expression and its translocation to the membrane. However, the majority of glucose removal occurs in noninsulin-dependent tissues such as the CNS and red blood cells as a result of the insulin resistance that develops.

Counter-regulatory hormones and cytokines are responsible for the impaired glucose uptake in insulin-dependent tissues (66) (**Table 106.1**). Catecholamines inhibit glucose utilization by increasing glucose-6-phosphate from glycogen in the skeletal muscles. In turn, the phosphorylated form of glucose negatively inhibits hexokinase, the rate-limiting step in glucose catabolism, by decreasing its uptake from the blood. Epinephrine has also been shown to blunt the insulin-induced autophosphorylation of glut4, whereas glucocorticoids and growth hormone attenuate glucose uptake through their effects on glut4 processing. Glucocorticoids prevent the translocation of the protein through the plasma membrane, whereas growth hormone interferes with phosphorylation of the transporter. The latter also inhibits the insulin-signaling cascade. Cytokines are thought to confer peripheral insulin resistance through their interference with the tyrosine phosphorylation and mRNA expression of glut4 (34).

In addition to the direct effects on the glut4 protein, epinephrine, cortisol, growth hormone, and TNF-α stimulate lipase activity in the adipocytes, leading to increased levels of free fatty acids (34,65). Strong evidence suggests that free fatty acids themselves augment insulin resistance through inhibition of the insulin-signaling pathway.

Although insulin resistance seems to be the predominant mechanism leading to hyperglycemia in adults, studies suggest that β-cell dysfunction and decreased insulin production also play a role in increasing blood glucose in critically ill children (67,68).

A number of other factors also contribute to hyperglycemia among critically ill patients (58). Obesity, even in the absence of diabetes, is associated with insulin resistance. Hypothermia and hypoxemia can lead to insulin deficiency, whereas uremia and cirrhosis can increase insulin resistance. Glucocorticoid therapy and exogenous catecholamines produce hyperglycemia through a mechanism similar to their endogenous counterparts. Other underappreciated sources of hyperglycemia in the ICU are hypercaloric nutrition, infusion of dextrose-diluted medications, and the use of high glucose-containing dialysis solutions.

Pathologic Effects of Hyperglycemia

The detrimental effects of hyperglycemia were previously thought to be limited to osmotic diuresis (leading to dehydration and electrolyte imbalance) and HONKC. However, studies show that the effects of elevated glucose levels, even of short duration, are more profound (28). Broadly, the adverse effects of hyperglycemia can be attributed to endothelial dysfunction (28,65,69–71), impaired immune response (28,34,63,65,71,72), and activation of coagulation (73–75).

The data on the deleterious effect of hyperglycemia on the vasculature are derived mainly from adult studies (76,77). Hyperglycemic patients, both diabetic and nondiabetic, have worse outcomes after an acute cardiac or cerebral ischemic event, compared with normoglycemic patients. This finding is attributed to a number of causes, including impaired cardiac contractility, increased frequency of dysrhythmias, disruption of the blood–brain barrier, impaired endothelium-dependent vasorelaxation, and a prothrombotic state. Hyperglycemia, especially when prolonged, leads to nephropathy, neuropathy, and retinopathy.

It is speculated that the effects of hyperglycemia are, at least in part, owing to endothelial dysfunction (28,70). Endothelial cells, such as neurons and red blood cells, do not require insulin for glucose uptake. In the presence of hyperglycemia and upregulated glut1 transporters, the endothelium is confronted with an intracellular glucose load. Normally, when glucose enters the cell, it is diverted to the Krebs cycle to produce ATP. Production of reactive oxygen species, which are easily detoxified by manganese superoxide dismutase, accompanies this process. However, with the high intracellular glucose concentration, superoxide is overproduced and interacts with nitric oxide to form peroxynitrite. The latter compound is capable of nitrating intracellular proteins, including those in the mitochondrial electron transport chain, manganese superoxide dismutase, glyceraldehyde-3-phosphate dehydrogenase,

and voltage-dependent anion channels. Theoretically, nitration of these compounds would suppress electron transport chain activity, impair superoxide detoxification, shuttle glucose into toxic pathways, or induce advanced glycation end-product formation and increased apoptosis. Inhibition of glyceraldehyde-3-phosphate dehydrogenase has been linked to vascular damage in organs and tissues of diabetic patients. Disruption of the mitochondrial respiratory chain activity has been speculated to explain renal injury (78) and critical illness neuropathy (79) in hyperglycemic patients.

High glucose concentrations also alter various components of the immune response (34,71). Normally, in response to injury, vasoactive substances and chemotactic factors from the complement cascade, mast cells, and the kininogen–bradykinin system are released at the site of injury, resulting in increased blood flow and capillary permeability. Neutrophils and, later, macrophages migrate to the area, with resultant phagocytosis and lysis of the offending agent. During hyperglycemia, vasodilation is decreased secondary to impaired endothelial nitric oxide generation, a dysfunctional kininogen–bradykinin system, and reduced mast cell secretion. Hyperglycemia-induced expression of adhesion molecules enhances the interaction between leukocytes and endothelium, preventing the white blood cells from migrating to the area of injury. The interaction is further augmented by activation of nuclear factor-$\kappa\beta$, downregulation of the inhibitory protein I-$\kappa\beta$, and activation of protein kinase C. Concentrations of complement cascade components increase with hyperglycemia. However, complement-mediated functions such as phagocytosis and opsonization are depressed. Chemotaxis, phagocytosis, and generation of reactive oxygen species, which are all functions of neutrophils, are likewise attenuated, with elevated glucose levels impairing clearance of microorganisms. Impairment in the immune response may explain the increased risk of cardiovascular dysfunction (80,81) and infectious complications (71,82) in hyperglycemic patients.

Activation of the coagulation system may also explain some of the deleterious effects of high blood glucose (73–75). Hyperglycemia enhances coagulation by increasing the expression of tissue factor and activating factor VII (75). Multiorgan failure that is commonly associated with hyperglycemia is thought to result from increased coagulation activity leading to microthrombosis.

Management of Hyperglycemia Associated with Critical Illness

The management of hyperglycemia in critically ill patients remains unclear. Historically, insulin therapy was initiated only at the onset of glucosuria because of the belief that osmotic diuresis was the sole adverse effect of high blood glucose. However, with the publication of the Leuven trial, tight glycemic control with insulin infusion became the usual care in adults (51). The excitement with tight glycemic control was later tempered with the results of the Normoglycaemia in Intensive Care Evaluation and Survival Using Glucose Algorithm Regulation (NICE-SUGAR) trial (83). Less is known about the appropriate management of hyperglycemia in critically ill children. A couple of randomized trials have been conducted to elucidate this issue.

In the initial Leuven trial, mechanically ventilated adults admitted to a surgical ICU were randomized to tight glycemic control (with a blood glucose goal of 80–110 mg/dL) or conventional treatment (with a blood glucose goal of 180–200 mg/dL) (51). There was a significant reduction in ICU (risk ratio [RR]: 0.57, 95% confidence interval [CI]: 0.38–0.85) and hospital (RR: 0.66, 95% CI: 0.48–0.92) mortality in the treatment group. The biggest decrease in mortality was seen in patients who stayed in the ICU longer than 5 days and in patients with multiorgan failure and a proven focus of infection. There was also a significant reduction in bloodstream infections, acute kidney injury requiring dialysis or hemofiltration, and critical illness neuropathy in the treatment group. In a follow-up study, critically ill adults who were anticipated to stay in the ICU for at least 3 days were randomized to tight glycemic control or conventional treatment (84). In contrast to the initial trial, there was no significant difference in the mortality between the two groups. However, there was a reduction in acute kidney injury, number of mechanical ventilator days, and duration of ICU and hospital stay in the treatment group.

Subsequent multicenter trials failed to replicate the results of the Leuven trials (52). In fact, the NICE-SUGAR trial showed opposite results (83). In the NICE-SUGAR trial, which is the largest trial on tight glycemic control to date, more than 6000 critically ill adults who were anticipated to stay in the ICU for at least 3 days were randomized to tight glycemic control with a target blood glucose range of 81–108 mg/dL or to conventional glucose control with a target blood glucose range of 180 mg/dL or less. There was a significant increase in 90-day mortality in the treatment group with an RR of 1.10 (95% CI: 1.01–1.20). In addition, there were no significant differences in the risk of acute kidney injury, duration of mechanical ventilation, and duration of ICU and hospital stay. Subsequent meta-analyses of randomized trials on tight glycemic control in critically ill adults showed no overall mortality benefit (52,85,86). However, there may be some benefit in critically ill surgical patients, posttraumatic injury patients, and neurologic injury patients (52,54).

A number of explanations have been put forward to explain the difference in the results of the Leuven and the NICE-SUGAR trials (87). These include differences in comparator groups, glucose measurement technology, feeding strategies, and patient population. On the basis of the available studies, it is currently recommended to maintain blood glucose <180 mg/dL with a range that is more liberal than 80–110 mg/dL in critically ill adults (54,88,89).

Currently, there are two published randomized controlled trials on tight glycemic control in critically ill children (90,91). The first is the pediatric Leuven trial where children admitted to the pediatric ICU were randomized to tight glycemic control with blood glucose target that was normal for age or to the conventional group where insulin was infused to prevent blood glucose from exceeding 214 mg/dL (90). The study was designed to detect a "hypothesized decrease" in C-reactive protein. Approximately 75% of the children enrolled in the study were postoperative cardiac patients. The authors reported a significant reduction in C-reactive protein in the treatment group. In a secondary analysis, there were also significant reductions in mortality (RR: 0.45, 95% CI: 0.21–0.98), duration of ICU stay, days on vasoactive drugs, and risk of secondary infection in the treatment group. However, 25% of children in the treatment group developed hypoglycemia compared with 1% in the control group.

The data from the pediatric Leuven trial suggested that the benefit of tight glycemic control in children came from postoperative cardiac patients. On the basis of these data, Agus et al. (91) randomized children less than 1 year old who underwent repair of congenital heart disease into tight glycemic control versus standard care. There was no significant difference in the primary outcome of rate of health care–associated infections between the two groups. There were also no significant differences in the risk of cardiovascular, respiratory, renal failure, or mortality. The investigators hypothesized that the lack of benefit from tight glycemic control was owing to the limited window of hyperglycemia. Nearly all children in the control group who did not receive insulin had normal glucose within 48 hours after the surgery. With the use of continuous glucose monitoring, only 3% of children in the treatment group developed severe hypoglycemia.

There are currently no formal recommendations to guide the treatment of hyperglycemia in critically ill children (54).

Conclusions and Future Directions—Hyperglycemia

Hyperglycemia in critically ill children continues to be an important management issue. Although hyperglycemia is common in critically ill children and is associated with worse outcomes, it is unclear whether control of blood glucose to normal levels will improve outcomes in critically ill patients. In adults, the data suggest that there may be certain patient populations (i.e., the surgical but not the medically ill patients) who may benefit from tight glycemic control. In children, the data are less clear. It is unlikely that postoperative cardiac patients will benefit from tight glycemic control. We do not have the answer yet for non-postoperative cardiac children. There are three additional trials on tight glycemic control in critically ill children (92–94), with one of the studies enrolling only non-postoperative cardiac patients (93).

HYPOGLYCEMIA IN CHILDREN

Glucose serves as the body's predominant fuel, responsible for at least half of basal energy requirements and almost all of the basal energy needs of the neonate. The brain in particular utilizes glucose at a rate that is 20 times higher than that of the rest of the body, primarily because it cannot use free fatty acids as a fuel source. In neonates, whose brain comprises a relatively greater proportion of body weight, glucose requirements are 5- to 10-fold greater than in older children and adults (8–10 mg/kg/min vs. 1–2 mg/kg/min) (95,96).

The definition of hypoglycemia is controversial. Part of the difficulty in defining hypoglycemia is owing to the use of blood glucose measurement as a surrogate for symptomatic neuroglycopenia (97). Pediatric intensivists tend to use thresholds of 40–80 mg/dL to define hypoglycemia (55). Historically, the parameters for hypoglycemia were based on statistical rather than physiologic grounds. Delayed first feeding of infants commonly resulted in hypoglycemia in the first hours after birth, which may have led physicians to accept lower thresholds of blood glucose as "normal" (97). In the absence of evidence that the infant brain is less sensitive to hypoglycemia than is the brain of an older child or adult, and given that it may actually be more vulnerable to hypoglycemic injury, at least the same rigorous therapeutic standards should be maintained for an infant as those maintained for an adult. Therefore, we recommend that any blood glucose <60 mg/dL deserves treatment (54,98).

The concern for hypoglycemia in critically ill children was highlighted because of the practice of tight glycemic control. With the use of intravenous insulin infusion to maintain a tight blood glucose range, hypoglycemia with blood glucose <60–65 mg/dL may occur in as many as 33% of children receiving this therapy (97). In the absence of insulin, hypoglycemia occurs in 7%–9.7% of children in the ICU.

Pathophysiology

With rare exceptions, hypoglycemia in infants and children is a failure of fasting adaptation. An understanding of normal fasting physiology can provide a framework for diagnosing and treating the various disorders of hypoglycemia.

The elements of fasting include the four alternative fuel pathways: (a) hepatic glycogenolysis, (b) hepatic gluconeogenesis, (c) adipose tissue lipolysis, and (d) hepatic fatty acid oxidation and ketogenesis. These systems are under hormonal control, primarily by insulin, which suppresses the fasting systems, and the counter-regulatory hormones (i.e., glucagon, cortisol, epinephrine and growth hormone), which act to stimulate them.

The first phase of normal fasting occurs 2–3 hours after a meal. Thereafter, circulating glucose that is derived from intestinal absorption of carbohydrates dissipates (Fig. 106.2, pathway A). Insulin secretion is suppressed (X), and counter-regulatory hormones increase (+), allowing glucose to be released from hepatic glycogen stores (B). By 12–16 hours of fasting (and even earlier in sick or premature newborns), glycogen stores are depleted. Muscle and adipose tissue stores are then mobilized during this second phase of fasting. Amino acids derived from muscle breakdown (C) are the primary substrates for the production of new glucose by hepatic gluconeogenesis (D). Fatty acids released from lipolysis of adipose tissue (E) are either utilized directly as a fuel (particularly in muscle) or further oxidized in the liver, generating the energy required for the process of hepatic gluconeogenesis and the formation of ketones (F), an alternate fuel for the brain. Hepatic glycogenolysis is primarily stimulated by glucagon and epinephrine, lipolysis is stimulated by increases in epinephrine and growth hormone, and gluconeogenesis is stimulated by glucagon and cortisol. In the setting of insulin-induced hypoglycemia, lipolysis is inhibited by insulin, resulting in a reduction in ketone production and deprivation of the brain of an alternate energy source (99).

Causes of Hypoglycemia

Multiple factors may cause or contribute to the development of hypoglycemia in critically ill children (54,100,101). Critically ill children may not have adequate glycogen stores as a result of malnutrition, prematurity, or prolonged illness. Renal and hepatic failure may impair gluconeogenesis. Renal failure may also impair insulin metabolism, leading to insulin accumulation and prolonged action of the drug. There may be a relative insufficiency of counter-regulatory hormones that is unable to counteract a drop in blood glucose. Sepsis and asphyxia increase the child's risk of hypoglycemia because of a hyperinsulinemic state from cytokines. Other risk factors

associated with hypoglycemia in critically ill children include age <1 year old, higher severity of illness, and mechanical ventilator and/or vasoactive drug support (101).

One of the most common causes of hypoglycemia in hospitalized children is the acute interruption of high-concentration intravenous dextrose infusion, particularly seen in sick newborns treated with total parenteral nutrition. It is thought that supraphysiologic insulin secretion cannot be downregulated quickly enough when the infusion is abruptly stopped or accidentally blocked or removed (transport off unit for procedures or to the OR for surgery). Inappropriate elevated insulin levels at the time of hypoglycemia, along with suppression of free fatty acids and ketones, are consistent with this phenomenon of transient iatrogenic hyperinsulinism. A similar scenario occurs when continuous renal replacement therapy is abruptly stopped in children receiving insulin infusion. Replacement and dialysate fluids used for continuous renal replacement therapy contain high glucose concentrations such that stopping the therapy without adjusting the insulin infusion dosage results in hypoglycemia.

Medications may induce hypoglycemia; these include insulin, particularly in the setting of diabetic therapy and tight glycemic control (102); sulfonylureas and other antidiabetic drugs, by stimulating insulin release; quinine, pentamidine, and disopyramide, also through augmentation of insulin secretion; β-blockers, by blunting adrenergic response to hypoglycemia; and salicylates and octreotide, whose mechanism is unknown (97). Recreational drugs, such as ecstasy and alcohol intoxication can also cause hypoglycemia. Finally, factitious hypoglycemia due to Munchausen syndrome, in which children or their caregivers surreptitiously administer insulin or an oral secretagogue, may mimic true hyperinsulinism.

Other causes of hypoglycemia that are not specific to critically ill children include inborn errors of metabolism (e.g., glycogen storage disease, disorders of gluconeogenesis and fatty acid oxidation disorders) (Chapter 113), disorders of the hypothalamic–pituitary–adrenal axis (Chapter 105), nesidioblastosis, and genetic syndromes (e.g., Beckwith–Wiedeman syndrome).

Clinical Presentation

Symptoms and signs of hypoglycemia can be divided into those that arise from autonomic responses to hypoglycemia (adrenergic) and those that arise from neurologic dysfunction (neuroglycopenic). Adrenergic symptoms/signs include tremors, diaphoresis, tachycardia, hunger, weakness, and nervousness. Neuroglycopenic symptoms/signs include lethargy; confusion; unusual behavior; and with more severe decrements in blood glucose, seizures, and coma. Autonomic activation usually occurs earlier and at a glucose threshold higher than would cause neuroglycopenia.

Both autonomic and neuroglycopenic symptoms and signs of hypoglycemia are less obvious, or even absent, in infants and young children. Alternative manifestations of hypoglycemia in infants include apnea, pallor, cyanosis, feeding difficulties, tachypnea, respiratory distress, hypothermia, or sepsis-like state. Critically ill children are also less likely to present with the typical signs and symptoms of hypoglycemia because of their ongoing therapy, such as sedative use, or underlying illnesses. Thus, a high index of suspicion must be maintained.

Diagnosis of Hypoglycemic Disorders

A normal child should not become hypoglycemic until all available fuel sources are depleted and counter-regulatory hormone stimulation is maximized, at which time (a) glycogen stores

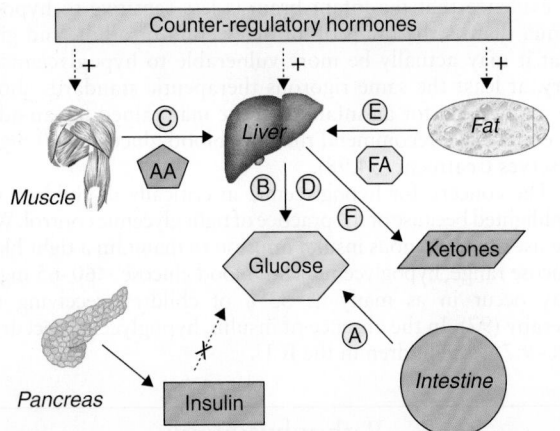

FIGURE 106.2. Pathways of fasting adaptation. See text for details. AA, amino acids; FA, fatty acids. (Adapted from Louis CA, Weinzimer SA. A 12-day-old infant with hypoglycemia: Case report. *Curr Opin Pediatr* 2003;15:333–7.)

will be depleted and no glycemic response to glucagon will occur; (b) lactate will be low, reflecting exhaustion of gluconeogenic stores; (c) free fatty acids and ketones will be elevated; and (d) insulin will be undetectable in the serum. Therefore, in the child with hypoglycemia, in whom at least one control system is defective, analysis of the integrity of all of the control systems at the time of hypoglycemia is required to determine the etiology of the disorder, the so-called "critical sample." The critical sample, which should be obtained prior to treating the hypoglycemia, consists of the primary fuel glucose, alternate fuels (lactate, ketones, and free fatty acids), and controlling hormones (insulin, cortisol and growth hormone). Administration of glucagon, subcutaneously or intramuscularly, at the time of hypoglycemia provides valuable information, as a hyperglycemic response to glucagon signifies persistent hepatic glycogen stores, which is abnormal in the face of hypoglycemia (103). Additional studies to be obtained include electrolytes, ammonia, lactate, acylcarnitine and organic acid profiles, and urinalysis for ketones (Table 106.2).

The duration of fasting tolerance (i.e., time to hypoglycemia from last carbohydrate consumed), amount of glucose required to restore and maintain euglycemia, serum bicarbonate, urinary ketones, and response to glucagon suggest the etiology of the hypoglycemia until the confirmatory critical sample results are known. The presence of acidosis with hypoglycemia indicates an accumulation of either ketones or lactate. Ketoacidosis is a normal response to prolonged fasting, while lactic acidosis generally indicates a block in the gluconeogenic pathway (failure to convert lactate to glucose). However, fasting tolerance of <4–6 hours, significant ketosis, and fatty acid breakdown in a child with hepatomegaly suggest one of the glycogen storage diseases, which are all characterized by the absence of glycemic response to glucagon (<30 mg/dL rise in blood glucose) and normal parenteral glucose requirements to restore and maintain euglycemia. Supraphysiologic glucose requirement, low or absent ketones, and glycemic response to glucagon (>30 mg/dL) are the hallmarks of hyperinsulinism, in which excessive insulin action inhibits glycogenolysis and promotes excessive peripheral glucose uptake. Disorders of fatty acid oxidation are also associated with low or absent ketones, but glucose requirements are normal and glycemic response to glucagon is absent. Hypopituitarism, either simple growth hormone deficiency or multiple pituitary hormone deficiency, is difficult to classify in this framework, as glucose requirements may be supraphysiologic and glycemic response to glucagon inconclusive.

Treatment of Hypoglycemia

In the acute setting, the immediate goal in the treatment of hypoglycemia is to increase the plasma glucose to at least 70 mg/dL. The critical sample should be drawn prior to treatment, if tolerated by the patient. Rapid improvement in blood sugar is normally seen after administration of 10% dextrose, 2 mL/kg by intravenous push, followed by continuous intravenous dextrose at a rate of at least 8 mg/kg/min. When only higher dextrose concentrations are available, doses equivalent to 0.25 g/kg are as follows:

- 2.5 mL/kg of 10% dextrose solution (D10W)
- 1 mL/kg of 25% dextrose solution (D25W)
- 0.5 mL/kg of 50% dextrose solution (D50W)

Glucose levels should be repeated frequently. For continuing hypoglycemia, additional boluses should be given, and the basal glucose infusion should be increased in 10%–15% increments. Some infants with hyperinsulinism require 20 mg/kg/min dextrose to maintain euglycemia.

Definitive treatment of hypoglycemia depends on the underlying condition. Withdrawal of medications that cause hypoglycemia, particularly insulin, usually results in prompt improvement. Likewise, children with hormone deficiencies (e.g., growth hormone deficiency or hypoadrenalism) usually respond well to appropriate hormonal supplementation.

Outcomes

The long-term outcome for children with hypoglycemia depends primarily on the underlying etiology. The primary risk of hypoglycemia in infants and young children relates to

---

TABLE 106.2

CRITICAL SAMPLE FOR EVALUATION OF HYPOGLYCEMIA IN CHILDREN*

■ TEST	■ SAMPLE REQUIREMENTS	■ NORMAL VALUES AT HYPOGLYCEMIA (GLU <55)
Glucose	1 mL serum or plasma	
Electrolytes	1 mL serum	Bicarbonate >18 mEq/L
Lactate	1 mL plasma	<2.5 mmol
Insulin	1 mL serum	<2 mcU/mL
Cortisol	1 mL serum	>20 mcg/dL
Growth hormone	1 mL serum	>7–10 ng/mL
Free fatty acids	1 mL plasma	>1.5 mmol/L
β-Hydroxybutyrate	1 mL plasma	>2 mmol/L
Acetoacetate	1 mL plasma	>2 mmol/L
Ammonia	1 mL plasma	<35 mcmol/L
C-peptide	1 mL EDTA plasma	<0.5 ng/mL
Acylcarnitine profile	1 mL EDTA plasma	
Urine organic acids	5–10 mL urine, frozen stat	
Urine ketones	1–2 mL	Positive

EDTA, ethylenediaminetetraacetic acid.
*Interpretation of a specialist is needed.

neurodevelopmental sequelae. The precise level and duration of hypoglycemia required to cause permanent neurologic dysfunction is unknown. Of the hypoglycemic disorders, children with hyperinsulinism appear to be most vulnerable, with neurodevelopmental complications reported in 26%–44% (104). Younger age at presentation, longer duration of hypoglycemia, and unresponsiveness to medical therapy are associated with greater risk of neurologic sequelae.

In critically ill children, the clinical significance of hypoglycemia is unclear because of the confounding effect of their underlying illnesses. Although hypoglycemia is associated with mortality and worsening organ dysfunction, it is likely that low blood glucose is merely a marker of severity of illness (101). The use of insulin for tight glycemic control has highlighted the intensivists' concern for complications of insulin-induced hypoglycemia (55,56). Insulin impairs ketogenesis and deprives these children's brains of an energy source. Typical neurologic symptoms of hypoglycemia may also be missed owing to their underlying illnesses and treatments they receive. However, because these children are closely monitored in the ICU, they are less likely to be hypoglycemic for prolonged periods of time. In the pediatric Leuven trial, although hypoglycemia occurred in 25% of the children in the treatment group, the presence of hypoglycemia was not independently associated with mortality (90). At follow-up 3–4 years after the study, there was no significant difference in neurocognitive function in those who developed hypoglycemia compared with the rest of the cohort (105). These findings are in contrast to adults where hypoglycemia from tight glycemic control is associated with increased mortality and impaired neurocognitive function (54,106–108).

Conclusions and Future Directions—Hypoglycemia

Hypoglycemia is a significant concern in critically ill children. In the absence of obvious reason for a hypoglycemic episode, children should be worked up for metabolic problems that may explain the low blood glucose. It is likely that the outcomes of hypoglycemia are a reflection of the child's underlying illness. Whether this is also true for insulin-induced hypoglycemia is unclear. Follow-up studies on pediatric trials on tight glycemic control will further inform us of the significance of insulin-induced hypoglycemia in critically ill children.

References

1. Vehik K, Hamman R, Lezotte D, et al. Childhood growth and age at diagnosis with type 1 diabetes in colorado young people. *Diabetic Med* 2009;26:961–7.
2. Sapru A, Gitelman S, Bhatia S, et al. Prevalence and characteristics of type 2 diabetes mellitus in 9–18 year-old children with diabetic ketoacidosis. *J Pediatr Endocrinol Metab* 2005;18:865–72.
3. Wolfsdorf J, Craig ME, Daneman D, et al. Diabetic ketoacidosis in children and adolescents with diabetes. *Pediatr Diabetes* 2009;10(suppl 12):118–33.
4. Rewers A, Chase HP, Mackenzie T, et al. Predictors of acute complications in children with type 1 diabetes. *JAMA* 2002;287:2511–8.
5. Katz MA. Hyperglycemia-induced hyponatremia—calculation of expected serum sodium depression. *N Engl J Med* 1973;289:843–4.
6. Kaminska ES, Pourmotabbed G. Spurious laboratory values in diabetic ketoacidosis and hyperlipidemia. *Am J Emerg Med* 1993;11:77–80.
7. Dunger DB, Sperling MA, Acerini CL, et al. ESPE/LWPES consensus statement on diabetic ketoacidosis in children and adolescents. *Arch Dis Child* 2004;89:188–94.
8. Glaser N, Barnett P, McCaslin I, et al. Risk factors for cerebral edema in children with diabetic ketoacidosis. The Pediatric Emergency Medicine Collaborative Research Committee of the American Academy of Pediatrics. *N Engl J Med* 2001;344:264–9.
9. Harris GD, Fiordalisi I, Harris WL, et al. Minimizing the risk of brain herniation during treatment of diabetic ketoacidemia: A retrospective and prospective study. *J Pediatr* 1990;117:22–31.
10. Harris GD, Lohr JW, Fiordalisi I, et al. Brain osmoregulation during extreme and moderate dehydration in a rat model of severe dka. *Life Sci* 1993;53:185–91.
11. Thompson CD, Vital-Carona J, Faustino EV. The effect of tubing dwell time on insulin adsorption during intravenous insulin infusions. *Diabetes Technol Ther* 2012;14:912–6.
12. Grimberg A, Cerri RW, Satin-Smith M, et al. The "two bag system" for variable intravenous dextrose and fluid administration: Benefits in diabetic ketoacidosis management. *J Pediatr* 1999;134:376–8.
13. Glaser N. Pediatric diabetic ketoacidosis and hyperglycemic hyperosmolar state. *Pediatr Clin North Am* 2005;52:1611–35.
14. Muir AB, Quisling RG, Yang MC, et al. Cerebral edema in childhood diabetic ketoacidosis: Natural history, radiographic findings, and early identification. *Diabetes Care* 2004;27:1541–6.
15. Duck SC, Wyatt DT. Factors associated with brain herniation in the treatment of diabetic ketoacidosis. *J Pediatr* 1988;113:10–4.
16. Harris GD, Fiordalisi I. Physiologic management of diabetic ketoacidemia. A 5-year prospective pediatric experience in 231 episodes. *Arch Pediatr Adolesc Med* 1994;148:1046–52.
17. Arieff AI, Carroll HJ. Nonketotic hyperosmolar coma with hyperglycemia: Clinical features, pathophysiology, renal function, acid-base balance, plasma-cerebrospinal fluid equilibria and the effects of therapy in 37 cases. *Medicine* 1972;51:73–94.
18. Delaney MF, Zisman A, Kettyle WM. Diabetic ketoacidosis and hyperglycemic hyperosmolar nonketotic syndrome. *Endocrinol Metab Clin North Am* 2000;29:683–705, V.
19. Meyer PC, Salt HB. Unusually high blood sugar in a boy. *Br Med J* 1951;1:171–2.
20. Rubin HM, Kramer R, Drash A. Hyperosmolality complicating diabetes mellitus in childhood. *J Pediatr* 1969;74:177–86.
21. Carchman RM, Dechert-Zeger M, Calikoglu AS, et al. A new challenge in pediatric obesity: Pediatric hyperglycemic hyperosmolar syndrome. *Pediatr Crit Care Med* 2005;6:20–4.
22. Fourtner SH, Weinzimer SA, Levitt Katz LE. Hyperglycemic hyperosmolar non-ketotic syndrome in children with type 2 diabetes*. *Pediatr Diabetes* 2005;6:129–35.
23. Hollander AS, Olney RC, Blackett PR, et al. Fatal malignant hyperthermia-like syndrome with rhabdomyolysis complicating the presentation of diabetes mellitus in adolescent males. *Pediatrics* 2003;111:1447–52.
24. Morales AE, Rosenbloom AL. Death caused by hyperglycemic hyperosmolar state at the onset of type 2 diabetes. *J Pediatr* 2004;144:270–3.
25. Rosenbloom AL. Hyperglycemic hyperosmolar state: An emerging pediatric problem. *J Pediatr* 2010;156:180–4.
26. Kaufman FR. Type 2 diabetes in children and youth. *Endocrinol Metab Clin North Am* 2005;34:659–76, ix–x.
27. Bloomgarden ZT. Type 2 diabetes in the young: The evolving epidemic. *Diabetes Care* 2004;27:998–1010.
28. Van den Berghe G. How does blood glucose control with insulin save lives in intensive care? *J Clin Invest* 2004;114:1187–95.
29. Srinivasan V, Spinella PC, Drott HR, et al. Association of timing, duration, and intensity of hyperglycemia with intensive care unit mortality in critically ill children. *Pediatr Crit Care Med* 2004;5:329–36.
30. Van den Berghe G, Wouters PJ, Bouillon R, et al. Outcome benefit of intensive insulin therapy in the critically ill: Insulin dose versus glycemic control. *Crit Care Med* 2003;31:359–66.
31. Carl GF, Hoffman WH, Passmore GG, et al. Diabetic ketoacidosis promotes a prothrombotic state. *Endocr Res* 2003;29:73–82.
32. Edge JA, Jakes RW, Roy Y, et al. The uk case-control study of cerebral oedema complicating diabetic ketoacidosis in children. *Diabetologia* 2006;49:2002–9.

33. Glaser NS, Wootton-Gorges SL, Marcin JP, et al. Mechanism of cerebral edema in children with diabetic ketoacidosis. *J Pediatr* 2004;145:164–71.

34. Turina M, Fry DE, Polk HC. Acute hyperglycemia and the innate immune system: Clinical, cellular, and molecular aspects. *Crit Care Med* 2005;33:1624–33.

35. Magee MF, Bhatt BA. Management of decompensated diabetes. Diabetic ketoacidosis and hyperglycemic hyperosmolar syndrome. *Crit Care Clin* 2001;17:75–106.

36. Kitabchi AE, Umpierrez GE, Murphy MB, et al. Hyperglycemic crises in diabetes. *Diabetes Care* 2004;27(suppl 1):S94–102.

37. Lorber D. Nonketotic hypertonicity in diabetes mellitus. *Med Clin North Am* 1995;79:39–52.

38. Arieff AI. Cerebral edema complicating nonketotic hyperosmolar coma. *Miner Electrolyte Metab* 1986;12:383–9.

39. Zeitler P, Haqq A, Rosenbloom A, et al; Drugs and Therapeutics Committee of the Lawson Wilkins Pediatric Endocrine Society. Hyperglycemic hyperosmolar syndrome in children: Pathophysiological considerations and suggested guidelines for treatment. *J Pediatr* 2011;158:9–14, 14.e1–2.

40. Gerhardt CM, Klingensmith GJ. New-onset diabetes in an obese adolescent: Diagnostic dilemmas. *Nat Clin Pract Endocrinol Metab* 2008;4:578–83.

41. Chumiecki M, Minkina-Pedras M, Chobot A, et al. Nonketotic hyperosmolar syndrome as an acute complication of type 1 diabetes onset in a 20-month-old boy with congenital central nervous system defect. *Pediatr Endocrinol Diabetes Metab* 2012;18:40–4.

42. Umpierrez GE, Smiley D, Kitabchi AE. Narrative review: Ketosis-prone type 2 diabetes mellitus. *Ann Intern Med* 2006;144:350–7.

43. Wachtel TJ, Tetu-Mouradjian LM, Goldman DL, et al. Hyperosmolarity and acidosis in diabetes mellitus: A three-year experience in rhode island. *J Gen Intern Med* 1991;6:495–502.

44. Trence DL, Hirsch IB. Hyperglycemic crises in diabetes mellitus type 2. *Endocrinol Metab Clin North Am* 2001;30:817–31.

45. Krane EJ, Rockoff MA, Wallman JK, et al. Subclinical brain swelling in children during treatment of diabetic ketoacidosis. *N Engl J Med* 1985;312:1147–51.

46. Murthy S, Sharara-Chami R. Aggressive fluid resuscitation in severe pediatric hyperglycemic hyperosmolar syndrome: A case report. *Int J Pediatr Endocrinol* 2010;2010:379063.

47. Canarie MF, Bogue CW, Banasiak KJ, et al. Decompensated hyperglycemic hyperosmolarity without significant ketoacidosis in the adolescent and young adult population. *J Pediatr Endocrinol Metab* 2007;20:1115–24.

48. Gottschalk ME, Ros SP, Zeller WP. The emergency management of hyperglycemic-hyperosmolar nonketotic coma in the pediatric patient. *Pediatr Emerg Care* 1996;12:48–51.

49. Nugent BW. Hyperosmolar hyperglycemic state. *Emerg Med Clin North Am* 2005;23:629–48, vii.

50. West ML, Marsden PA, Singer GG, et al. Quantitative analysis of glucose loss during acute therapy for hyperglycemic hyperosmolar syndrome. *Diabetes Care* 1986;9:465–71.

51. van den Berghe G, Wouters P, Weekers F, et al. Intensive insulin therapy in the critically ill patients. *N Engl J Med* 2001;345:1359–67.

52. Griesdale DE, de Souza RJ, van Dam RM, et al. Intensive insulin therapy and mortality among critically ill patients: A meta-analysis including nice-sugar study data. *CMAJ* 2009;180:821–7.

53. Standards of medical care in diabetes—2012. *Diabetes Care* 2012;35(suppl 1):S11–63.

54. Jacobi J, Bircher N, Krinsley J, et al. Guidelines for the use of an insulin infusion for the management of hyperglycemia in critically ill patients. *Crit Care Med* 2012;40:3251–76.

55. Hirshberg EL, Sward KA, Faustino EV, et al. Clinical equipoise regarding glycemic control: A survey of pediatric intensivist perceptions. *Pediatr Crit Care Med* 2012.

56. Preissig CM, Rigby MR. A disparity between physician attitudes and practice regarding hyperglycemia in pediatric intensive care units in the united states: A survey on actual practice habits. *Crit Care* 2010;14:R11.

57. Faustino EV, Apkon M. Persistent hyperglycemia in critically ill children. *J Pediatr* 2005;146:30–4.

58. Srinivasan V. Stress hyperglycemia in pediatric critical illness: The intensive care unit adds to the stress! *J Diabetes Sci Technol* 2012;6:37–47.

59. Preissig CM, Rigby MR. Pediatric critical illness hyperglycemia: Risk factors associated with development and severity of hyperglycemia in critically ill children. *J Pediatr* 2009;155:734–9.

60. Gore DC, Chinkes D, Heggers J, et al. Association of hyperglycemia with increased mortality after severe burn injury. *J Trauma* 2001;51:540–4.

61. Polito A, Thiagarajan RR, Laussen PC, et al. Association between intraoperative and early postoperative glucose levels and adverse outcomes after complex congenital heart surgery. *Circulation* 2008;118:2235–42.

62. Hirshberg E, Larsen G, Van Duker H. Alterations in glucose homeostasis in the pediatric intensive care unit: Hyperglycemia and glucose variability are associated with increased mortality and morbidity. *Pediatr Crit Care Med* 2008;9:361–6.

63. Mizock BA. Alterations in fuel metabolism in critical illness: Hyperglycaemia. *Best Pract Res Clin Endocrinol Metab* 2001;15:533–51.

64. Ellger B, Debaveye Y, Vanhorebeek I, et al. Survival benefits of intensive insulin therapy in critical illness: Impact of maintaining normoglycemia versus glycemia-independent actions of insulin. *Diabetes* 2006;55:1096–105.

65. McCowen KC, Malhotra A, Bistrian BR. Stress-induced hyperglycemia. *Crit Care Clin* 2001;17:107–24.

66. Taylor JH, Beilman GJ. Hyperglycemia in the intensive care unit: No longer just a marker of illness severity. *Surg Infect* 2005;6:233–45.

67. Preissig CM, Rigby MR. Hyperglycaemia results from beta-cell dysfunction in critically ill children with respiratory and cardiovascular failure: A prospective observational study. *Crit Care* 2009;13:R27.

68. Verhoeven JJ, den Brinker M, Hokken-Koelega AC, et al. Pathophysiological aspects of hyperglycemia in children with meningococcal sepsis and septic shock: A prospective, observational cohort study. *Crit Care* 2011;15:R44.

69. Preiser JC, Devos P, Van den Berghe G. Tight control of glycaemia in critically ill patients. *Curr Opin Clin Nutr Metab Care* 2002;5:533–7.

70. Langouche L, Vanhorebeek I, Vlasselaers D, et al. Intensive insulin therapy protects the endothelium of critically ill patients. *J Clin Invest* 2005;115:2277–86.

71. Losser MR, Damoisel C, Payen D. Bench-to-bedside review: Glucose and stress conditions in the intensive care unit. *Crit Care* 2010;14:231.

72. Stegenga ME, van der Crabben SN, Dessing MC, et al. Effect of acute hyperglycaemia and/or hyperinsulinaemia on proinflammatory gene expression, cytokine production and neutrophil function in humans. *Diabet Med* 2008;25:157–64.

73. Stegenga ME, van der Crabben SN, Blumer RM, et al. Hyperglycemia enhances coagulation and reduces neutrophil degranulation, whereas hyperinsulinemia inhibits fibrinolysis during human endotoxemia. *Blood* 2008;112:82–9.

74. Stegenga ME, van der Crabben SN, Levi M, et al. Hyperglycemia stimulates coagulation, whereas hyperinsulinemia impairs fibrinolysis in healthy humans. *Diabetes* 2006;55:1807–12.

75. Brealey D, Singer M. Hyperglycemia in critical illness: A review. *J Diabetes Sci Technol* 2009;3:1250–60.

76. Mesotten D, Van den Berghe G. Clinical potential of insulin therapy in critically ill patients. *Drugs* 2003;63:625–36.

77. Lacherade JC, Jacqueminet S, Preiser JC. An overview of hypoglycemia in the critically ill. *J Diabetes Sci Technol* 2009;3:1242–9.

78. Vanhorebeek I, Gunst J, Ellger B, et al. Hyperglycemic kidney damage in an animal model of prolonged critical illness. *Kidney Int* 2009;76:512–20.

79. Callahan LA, Supinski GS. Hyperglycemia and acquired weakness in critically ill patients: Potential mechanisms. *Crit Care* 2009;13:125.

80. Hagiwara S, Iwasaka H, Hasegawa A, et al. Hyperglycemia contributes to cardiac dysfunction in a lipopolysaccharide-induced systemic inflammation model. *Crit Care Med* 2009;37:2223–7.

81. Vlasselaers D, Mesotten D, Langouche L, et al. Tight glycemic control protects the myocardium and reduces inflammation in neonatal heart surgery. *Ann Thorac Surg* 2010;90:22–9.

82. Wade C. Hyperglycemia may alter cytokine production and phagocytosis by means other than hyperosmotic stress. *Crit Care* 2008;12:182.

83. Finfer S, Chittock DR, Su SY, et al. Intensive versus conventional glucose control in critically ill patients. *N Engl J Med* 2009;360:1283–97.

84. Van den Berghe G, Wilmer A, Hermans G, et al. Intensive insulin therapy in the medical icu. *N Engl J Med* 2006;354:449–61.

85. Marik PE, Preiser JC. Toward understanding tight glycemic control in the icu: A systematic review and metaanalysis. *Chest* 2010;137:544–51.

86. Wiener RS, Wiener DC, Larson RJ. Benefits and risks of tight glucose control in critically ill adults: A meta-analysis. *JAMA* 2008;300:933–44.

87. Van den Berghe G, Schetz M, Vlasselaers D, et al. Intensive insulin therapy in critically ill patients: NICE-SUGAR or Leuven blood glucose target? *J Clin Endocrinol Metab* 2009;94(9):3163–70.

88. Implement effective glucose control. http://www.ihi.org/knowledge/Pages/Changes/ImplementEffectiveGlucoseControl.aspx. Accessed April 1, 2012.

89. Dellinger RP, Levy MM, Carlet JM, et al. Surviving sepsis campaign: International guidelines for management of severe sepsis and septic shock: 2008. *Crit Care Med* 2008;36:296–327.

90. Vlasselaers D, Milants I, Desmet L, et al. Intensive insulin therapy for patients in paediatric intensive care: A prospective, randomised controlled study. *Lancet* 2009;373:547–56.

91. Agus MS, Steil GM, Wypij D, et al. Tight glycemic control versus standard care after pediatric cardiac surgery. *N Engl J Med* 2012;367:1208–19.

92. Macrae D, Pappachan J, Grieve R, et al. Control of hyperglycaemia in paediatric intensive care (CHIP): Study protocol. *BMC Pediatr* 2010;10:5.

93. Heart and lung failure - pediatric insulin titration trial (half-pint). http://clinicaltrials.gov/ct2/show/NCT01565941. Accessed April 30, 2012.

94. Pediatric intensive care units at Emory Children's Center glycemic control: The PedETrol trial. Accessed April 15, 2012.

95. Bier DM, Leake RD, Haymond MW, et al. Measurement of "true" glucose production rates in infancy and childhood with 6,6-dideuteroglucose. *Diabetes* 1977;26:1016–23.

96. Haymond MW, Sunehag A. Controlling the sugar bowl. Regulation of glucose homeostasis in children. *Endocrinol Metab Clin North Am* 1999;28:663–94.

97. Faustino EV, Hirshberg EL, Bogue CW. Hypoglycemia in critically ill children. *J Diabetes Sci Technol* 2012;6:48–57.

98. Stanley CA, Baker L. The causes of neonatal hypoglycemia. *N Engl J Med* 1999;340:1200–1.

99. Yager JY, Heitjan DF, Towfighi J, et al. Effect of insulin-induced and fasting hypoglycemia on perinatal hypoxic-ischemic brain damage. *Pediatr Res* 1992;31:138–42.

100. Vriesendorp TM, DeVries JH, Hoekstra JB. Hypoglycemia and strict glycemic control in critically ill patients. *Curr Opin Crit Care* 2008;14:397–402.

101. Faustino EV, Bogue CW. Relationship between hypoglycemia and mortality in critically ill children. *Pediatr Crit Care Med* 2010;11:690–8.

102. Faraon-Pogaceanu C, Banasiak KJ, Hirshberg EL, et al. Comparison of the effectiveness and safety of two insulin infusion protocols in the management of hyperglycemia in critically ill children. *Pediatr Crit Care Med* 2010;11:741–9.

103. Finegold DN, Stanley CA, Baker L. Glycemic response to glucagon during fasting hypoglycemia: An aid in the diagnosis of hyperinsulinism. *J Pediatr* 1980;96:257–9.

104. De Leon DD, Stanley CA. Mechanisms of disease: Advances in diagnosis and treatment of hyperinsulinism in neonates. *Nat Clin Pract Endocrinol Metab* 2007;3:57–68.

105. Mesotten D, Gielen M, Sterken C, et al. Neurocognitive development of children 4 years after critical illness and treatment with tight glucose control: A randomized controlled trial. *JAMA* 2012;308:1641–50.

106. Finfer S, Liu B, Chittock DR, et al. Hypoglycemia and risk of death in critically ill patients. *N Engl J Med* 2012;367:1108–18.

107. Hermanides J, Bosman RJ, Vriesendorp TM, et al. Hypoglycemia is associated with intensive care unit mortality. *Crit Care Med* 2010;38:1430–4.

108. Duning T, van den Heuvel I, Dickmann A, et al. Hypoglycemia aggravates critical illness-induced neurocognitive dysfunction. *Diabetes Care* 2010;33:639–44.

CHAPTER 107 ■ DISORDERS OF WATER, SODIUM, AND POTASSIUM HOMEOSTASIS

JAMES SCHNEIDER AND ANDREA KELLY

KEY POINTS

1 Disorders of water, Na^+, and K^+ occur commonly in the pediatric intensive care unit, and these disturbances of fluid and electrolyte homeostasis are generally associated with underlying comorbidities, such as renal dysfunction, diabetic ketoacidosis, diabetes insipidus (DI), chemotherapy, brain tumors, and brain surgery.

2 Evaluation, assessment, and management of fluid and electrolyte disorders require an understanding of the basic factors that regulate homeostasis as well as the differential diagnosis of the underlying conditions that predispose to altering water, Na^+, and K^+ homeostasis.

3 Therapeutic management requires both managing the underlying condition appropriately and being aware that inappropriate therapeutic measures can be an iatrogenic cause of disturbance of fluid and electrolyte homeostasis.

4 In the clinical acute care setting, careful historic information and physical examination are the cornerstone of therapy; however, it must be stressed that physical assessment of the degree of dehydration or hydration is, at best, only an initial estimation; that vital signs, clinical improvement, and biochemical parameters must be monitored closely; and that changes in fluid therapy must be allowed for as necessary.

5 Often, the most complicated disorders of water, Na^+, and K^+ to manage are those in which the basic underlying conditions are changing, such as in syndrome of inappropriate antidiuretic hormone, postoperative craniopharyngioma patients, or patients with known central DI subsequently developing a salt-wasting condition. Frequent laboratory monitoring is exceptionally important in management of these children.

6 Clear potential for morbidity and mortality exists with any disturbance of water, Na^+, and K^+ homeostasis, but perhaps the most common abnormality that results in injury and death is hyponatremia. It must be stressed, however, that prolonged and untreated hypernatremia is also associated with significant injury and death.

7 Recent studies stressed the need to avoid the use of hypotonic fluids during resuscitation, as they are a major cause of iatrogenic hyponatremia. Further, the continued use of hypotonic fluids as maintenance therapy is in question, as critically ill children often have the inability to optimally dilute urine, increasing the risk for the development of hyponatremia.

8 Management of fluid and electrolyte disturbance requires therapeutic flexibility because dogmatic approaches can often lead to undesirable outcomes.

Children in the pediatric intensive care unit (PICU) are frequently admitted with or, even more commonly, develop disorders of water, sodium (Na^+), or potassium (K^+). Water or electrolyte abnormalities may be manifestations of the principle disease process but more often arise from either secondary organ injury or from interventions, such as medications, fluid management, or positive pressure ventilation. The intensivist plays a vital role in recognizing these risks and monitoring for development of these disorders. It is becoming clearer that fluid or electrolyte imbalances have an important influence on the outcome of critically ill children, and, therefore, a thorough understanding of the normal physiology and pathophysiology that leads to these imbalances is fundamental to providing optimal care. Discussions in this chapter focus on the evaluation and management of water, Na^+, and K^+ disorders as they pertain to the critically ill child and will not attempt to be inclusive of all such disorders in less critical settings. Although mentioned in various sections, molecular mechanisms, genetic alterations, animal models, and similar information will not be discussed in detail. Further, sophisticated laboratory studies not generally immediately available to the intensivist will be discussed to only a limited degree. Specifically, discussions will focus on paradigms regarding the clinical evaluation and management of fluid disorders, as appropriate correction of

fluid disturbances in the critically ill child is often paramount for resuscitation and survival.

To provide the foundation for an understanding of the pathophysiologic disturbances, this chapter will include a review of normal physiology and the mechanisms that regulate water, Na^+, and K^+ balance. The disorders of water, Na^+, and K^+ will be discussed as to etiology and most common presentations in the critical care setting. As to the differential diagnosis of the various conditions, the discussions will focus upon the most probable causes that result in admission to a PICU. Fluid management will be discussed, including the differences in initial therapies involving resuscitation, as well as maintenance of hydration and electrolyte control. A review of outcomes related to these electrolyte or fluid disturbances will also be presented as a basis for discussion of potential sources of error.

NORMAL PHYSIOLOGY AND PATHOPHYSIOLOGY

Strict regulation of total body water, Na^+, and K^+ occurs **2** through multiple, often redundant, pathways. Regulation of Na^+ is critical for maintaining extracellular fluid (ECF)

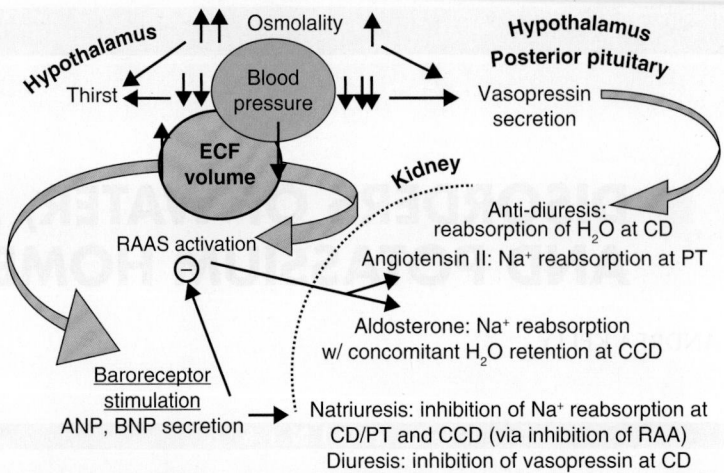

FIGURE 107.1. Regulation of extracellular fluid osmolality and volume. Vasopressin secretion is primarily responsible for preserving plasma osmolality. Secretion of vasopressin by the hypothalamus occurs with as little as a 1% increase in plasma osmolality. Much larger increases in plasma osmolality are required to trigger thirst, the center for which is also located in the hypothalamus. This offsetting likely occurs to avoid simultaneously activating thirst and vasopressin secretion at the lower end of normal plasma osmolality, which would result in overcorrection. Significant decreases in blood pressure/effective extracellular fluid (ECF) volume, communicated to the hypothalamus via cardiovascular baroreceptors, are required to trigger vasopressin secretion. Vasopressin recruits aquaporin-2 water channels in the renal collecting ducts (CD) to promote reabsorption of water and concentration of urine. ECF volume is primarily maintained through Na^+ homeostasis. Decreases in blood pressure/effective ECF volume also activate the renin-angiotensin-aldosterone system (RAAS). Aldosterone promotes reabsorption of Na^+ and water at the renal cortical-collecting duct (CCD), and angiotensin II stimulates Na^+ reabsorption at the proximal tubules (PT). Hypertension/fluid overload activates cardiovascular baroreceptors, leading to A-type natriuretic peptide (ANP) and brain natriuretic peptide (BNP) release. These peptides promote Na^+ and water excretion at the level of the kidney.

volume, while regulation of K^+ is vital for maintaining cellular electrophysiology. Superimposed upon regulation of these electrolytes is water metabolism, which is primarily influenced by changes in serum osmolality and, to a lesser extent, volume status. The kidney is the primary site for regulation of Na^+, K^+, and water, a result of the interplay between multiple hormonal pathways (**Fig. 107.1**).

Renal Handling of Water and Solutes—an Overview

A number of renal factors influence the dilution and concentration of urine. First, the glomerular filtration rate (the amount of renal blood flow that enters the nephron) dictates the maximum amount of fluid that can be delivered to the tubules. The glomerular filtration rate is heavily influenced by renal blood flow through the afferent and efferent arterioles. Vasoconstriction of afferent arterioles decreases glomerular blood flow, thereby decreasing glomerular pressure and filtration, while vasoconstriction of efferent arterioles, to an extent, increases glomerular pressure and filtration. A feedback mechanism, mediated by the macula densa, controls the vasoconstriction and vasodilation of the afferent and efferent arterioles to autoregulate the glomerular filtration rate. When the macula densa "senses" a low glomerular filtration rate, vasodilatation of afferent arterioles (and vasoconstriction of efferent arterioles mediated by angiotensin II) increases glomerular perfusion, thereby increasing the glomerular filtration rate to affect urine output. Conversely, with increased glomerular filtration, the macula densa again provides negative feedback to the afferent and efferent arterioles: vasoconstriction of afferent arterioles (and vasodilatation of efferent arterioles) occurs, decreasing glomerular filtration, slowing fluid transport through the nephron, and allowing increased filtrate

reabsorption and, ultimately, decreased urine output. Afferent and efferent arterioles are regulated by the sympathetic nervous system and angiotensin II, as described later.

Following filtration at the level of the glomerulus, the fluid is delivered to the tubules, where solute absorption varies depending upon the segment. The proximal tubule accounts for 65% of filtrate reabsorption, including that of Na^+, K^+, and water. The descending thin limb of the loop of Henle is permeable to water, urea, and other solutes, while the ascending thin limb is relatively impermeable to water. The thick ascending limb (TAL) and the initial segment of the distal tubule avidly absorb Na^+ and other solutes but are impermeable to water regardless of the status of vasopressin and, hence, are referred to as the *diluting segment* of the kidney. Here, tubular fluid osmolality falls below that of the glomerular filtrate. The late distal tubule and cortical-collecting duct mediate the Na^+-retaining and K^+-wasting effects of aldosterone. In addition, like the collecting duct, they are permeable to water only in the presence of vasopressin.

Na^+ absorption occurs through an active process and facilitates the absorption of many other solutes. Na/K-ATPase, expressed on the basolateral membrane of tubular epithelium, pumps Na^+ into the renal interstitium and ultimately into the peritubular capillaries (**Fig. 107.2**). Activity of this enzyme generates an Na^+ concentration gradient and an electrochemical gradient between the tubule lumen and the tubular cell. These gradients facilitate Na^+ transport from tubular fluid into the tubular epithelium, further supplying Na^+ for the Na/K-ATPase pump. In addition, these gradients drive water reabsorption. Because the cellular concentration of K^+ is already high relative to interstitial fluid, and because the tubular epithelial basolateral membrane is readily permeable to K^+, K^+ driven into the cell by Na/K-ATPase diffuses easily into the interstitium for reabsorption from the filtrate.

From this discussion, it can be concluded that water, Na^+, and K^+ homeostases are not completely independent.

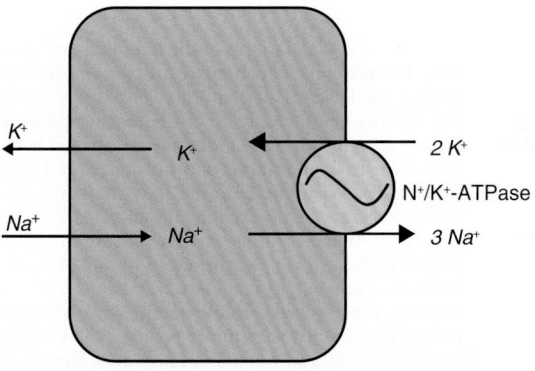

FIGURE 107.2. Na/K-ATPase activity. The Na/K-ATPase is ubiquitously expressed on the plasma cell membrane. Via an ATP-consuming process, this enzyme exchanges three intracellular Na^+ cations for two extracellular K^+ cations to maintain the intracellular-to-extracellular gradients for these two cations. Na^+ can pass down this concentration gradient from the extracellular fluid (ECF) to the intracellular fluid (ICF), whereas K^+ diffuses down its concentration gradient from the ICF to the ECF. The location of these pumps varies depending upon the cell type; they may be distributed evenly along the cell membrane or localized to the basolateral membranes as in renal epithelial cells.

A disorder that primarily affects one of these important body constituents can have a significant impact on another.

Water Homeostasis

The human body is composed of 42%–75% water, with the exact content dependent upon age, gender, and amount of body fat. Approximately two-thirds of the water is located intracellularly. The remaining estimated one-third is located extracellularly and is divided between the interstitium (three-fourths) and plasma (one-fourth) (Fig. 107.3). The solute content of these fluid compartments differs significantly, with K^+ being the primary constituent of intracellular fluid (ICF) and Na^+ being the major electrolyte in ECF. Na/K-ATPase, a plasma membrane enzyme expressed on most cells, is responsible for maintaining this discordant distribution of Na^+ and K^+ in body fluids (Fig. 107.2). It plays a key role in maintaining cellular volume—through its active transport of Na^+ extracellularly; it prevents accumulation of intracellular water that would arise from the significant intracellular concentrations of impermeable proteins and organic compounds. Na/K-ATPase maintains this transcellular gradient through an energy-expending process, exchanging three molecules of intracellular Na^+ for every two molecules of extracellular K^+ (Fig. 107.2).

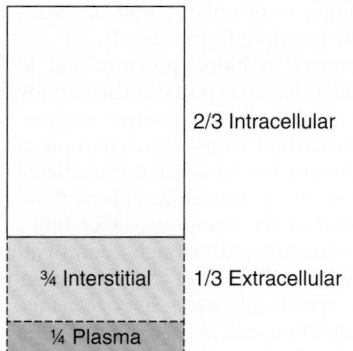

FIGURE 107.3. Approximate body composition of water.

Strict regulation of body water is critical for preserving ECF osmolality within a narrow range. The normal range for blood osmolality is 280–290 mOsm/kg H_2O. Cell membranes are freely water permeable. As a result, when a concentration gradient develops between ECF and ICF, water passively moves from the compartment with the lower to the higher gradient, thus restoring equilibrium. ECF osmolality can be estimated based upon the equation:

$$2 \times Na + [urea\ nitrogen\ (mg/dL)/2.8] + [glucose\ (mg/dL)/18]$$

Urea nitrogen and glucose (in the absence of hyperglycemia/insulin deficiency) freely permeate most cell membranes, with the exception of the blood–brain barrier (BBB), and are considered ineffective osmoles because they do not influence transcellular water flux. Because Na^+ is the prevailing extracellular cation, it and its companion anions largely determine ECF osmolality; that is, plasma Na^+ effectively drives water homeostasis.

Maintenance of body water and, hence, osmolality occurs despite potentially large variations at the sites of regulation: intake and output. Fluid intake is regulated by thirst. Water output is primarily regulated by vasopressin at the level of the kidney. In fact, over 99% of water in the glomerular filtrate is reabsorbed by the renal tubules. However, unregulated (and potentially substantial) water loss can occur through the skin, gastrointestinal tract, and lungs. Normally, insensible loss of water consists of ~300–500 mL/m²/day. In addition, obligate water loss occurs via the kidney in the elimination of solutes. In general, the kidney disposes of 500 mOsm solute/m²/day. The amount of solute to be excreted by the kidney can vary considerably (high-salt diet, normal saline solution), and thus, obligate water losses can vary significantly.

Vasopressin

Arginine vasopressin (AVP), also referred to as antidiuretic hormone (ADH), is a peptide hormone encoded on chromosome 20, and is produced by magnocellular neurons located in the hypothalamus. Their distal axons pass through the pituitary stalk and store AVP until its release into a plexus of capillaries and, together with the terminal axons of oxytocin-producing hypothalamic neurons, constitute the posterior pituitary (Fig. 107.4). The plexuses drain into the systemic circulation through the cavernous sinus and superior vena cava. The posterior pituitary has been reported in animals to store AVP in amounts sufficient for maximal diuresis for a week. As detailed later, AVP production and secretion are regulated by serum osmolality, ECF volume, and blood pressure (Fig. 107.5).

Plasma osmotic pressure is the major determinant of AVP release (Fig. 107.5). Osmotically responsive AVP release is believed to occur through a threshold effect: below a certain osmotic threshold, AVP release is suppressed; above this threshold, AVP release increases in a linear fashion with osmolarity (Fig. 107.6) (1). Individual differences in AVP release exist. In general, the threshold for AVP release is 280–285 mOsm/kg H_2O and for every 1 mOsm/kg H_2O increase in plasma osmolality, plasma AVP increases by 0.4–1 pg/mL to a maximum of 4–5 pg/mL for maximal urinary concentration (2). Individual thresholds for AVP release and AVP responsiveness are at least partly determined by genetics, but these can be altered by nonosmotic inputs such as blood pressure and drugs, as well as by chronic perturbations in plasma osmolality. This fine-tuning of responsiveness is mediated through inhibitory and excitatory inputs that include angiotensin II.

Plasma osmolality is "monitored" via stretch-sensitive channels in osmo-sensitive cells. Changes in plasma osmotic pressure lead to changes in cell volume; stretch-inactivated channels transduce this volume by altering the plasma

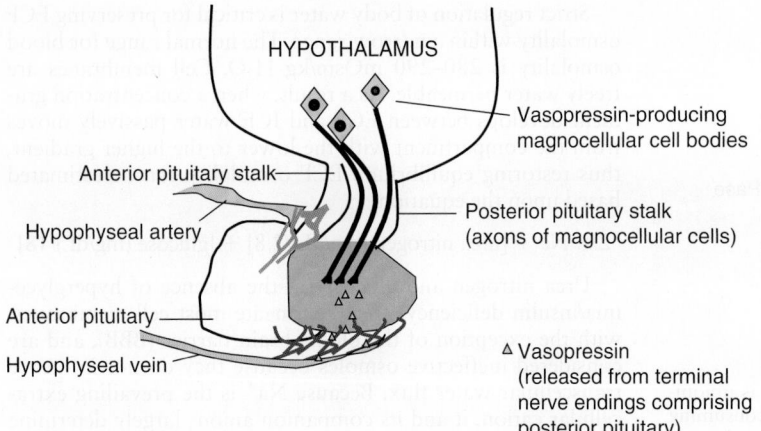

FIGURE 107.4. Anatomy of the hypothalamic-pituitary axis. The pituitary is composed of two embryologically distinct subdivisions. The anterior pituitary is one of several distinct neuroendocrine cell types that produce and secrete growth hormone, adrenocorticotropic hormone, prolactin, thyroid-stimulating hormone, and gonadotropins. It is regulated by the hypothalamus through axons that traverse the anterior pituitary stalk and by the peripheral milieu through the hypophyseal artery. Vasopressin and oxytocin are produced by distinct cell bodies located in the hypothalamus. The axons of these cells compose the posterior pituitary stalk, while the posterior pituitary houses their terminal endings, the storage sites for vasopressin and oxytocin. Hormones from both the anterior and posterior pituitaries are transported to the periphery via the hypophyseal veins.

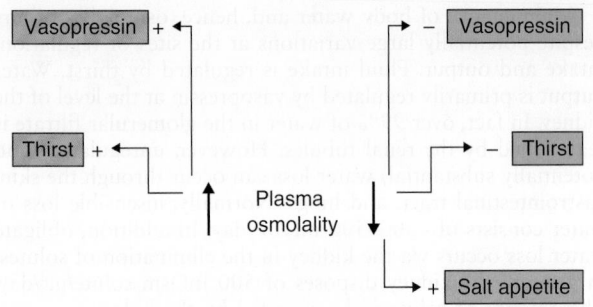

FIGURE 107.5. Responses to changes in plasma osmolality. Slight increases in plasma osmolality stimulate vasopressin secretion; further increases are required to stimulate thirst. Increases in plasma osmolality also suppress salt intake. Decreases in plasma osmolality suppress vasopressin secretion and thirst while activating the salt appetite.

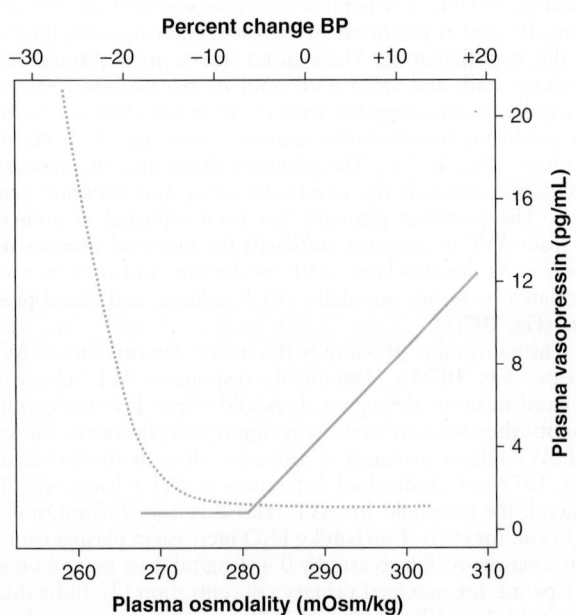

FIGURE 107.6. Plasma concentrations of arginine vasopressin (AVP) in response to plasma osmolality and blood pressure. Note that vasopressin secretion is much less sensitive to small changes in blood pressure (or circulating blood volume) than changes in osmolality. Solid line: Vasopressin response to changes in serum osmolality. *Dotted line:* Vasopressin response to changes in blood pressure. (Adapted from Robertson GL, Athar S. The interaction of blood osmolality and blood volume in regulating plasma vasopressin in man. *J Clin Endocrinol Metab* 1976;42:613–20.)

membrane potential and the likelihood of depolarization. For instance, hyperosmolality leads to cell shrinkage, activation of stretch-inactivated channels, membrane depolarization, and excitation of the neurosecretory cell. This osmotic-sensing capability is intrinsic to vasopressin-producing cells. Local glial cells and neurons in the anterior hypothalamus are also osmosensors and participate in regulating AVP release by magnocellular cells (3). Not all osmotically active solutes stimulate AVP release, highlighting the role of changes in cell volume in transducing the signal for change in plasma osmolality. Na^+ and mannitol are "effective" solutes because they do not freely permeate the cell membrane, leading to an osmotic gradient, shifts in osmosensor water content, and alterations in AVP release. On the other hand, despite their osmotic properties, urea and glucose freely permeate the cell membrane (in the absence of the BBB) and do not generate an osmotic gradient to induce cellular volume changes and AVP release. In the absence of insulin (as occurs in diabetic ketoacidosis, DKA), glucose entry into osmosensing cells is impaired, and glucose becomes a stimulant for AVP release.

Nonosmotic regulation of AVP includes blood pressure and ECF volume (Fig. 107.7), pain, nausea, and hypoglycemia. Normally, pressure receptors tonically inhibit AVP secretion. In contrast to the small increases in osmolality that stimulate AVP release, relatively large decreases in blood pressure (effective ECF volume) are required to mount an AVP response. However, unlike the relationship between osmolality and AVP, which is linear, the relationship between blood pressure (volume) and AVP is exponential: blood pressure decreases of 5%–10% are required to evoke AVP release while decreases of 20%–30% prompt AVP secretion many times above that required for maximal antidiuresis (Fig. 107.6). Smaller changes in blood pressure (ECF volume) modulate AVP responsiveness, with modest decreases in blood pressure sensitizing AVP release to changes in osmolality and increases in blood pressure potentially blunting responses (4).

These responses to blood pressure and ECF volume are mediated through baroreceptors in the cardiovascular system. Activation of neural stretch-sensitive sensors in the cardiac atria, aorta, and carotid arteries leads to tonic inhibition of AVP secretion. Pathways for baroreceptor-mediated AVP secretion are distinct from those of osmoreceptors; these pathways converge at the level of the vasopressin-secreting cells (5). Angiotensin II, both directly and through neural pathways, has also been implicated in AVP release (5). Other nonosmotic stimuli of AVP release, specifically stress, hypoglycemia, nausea, vomiting, and inflammation, can play significant roles as well. In fact, nausea can lead to AVP concentrations 20–40 times that evoked by hyperosmolality. Inflammatory mediators, such as IL-1β and IL-6, have been identified as stimulants of AVP release, and

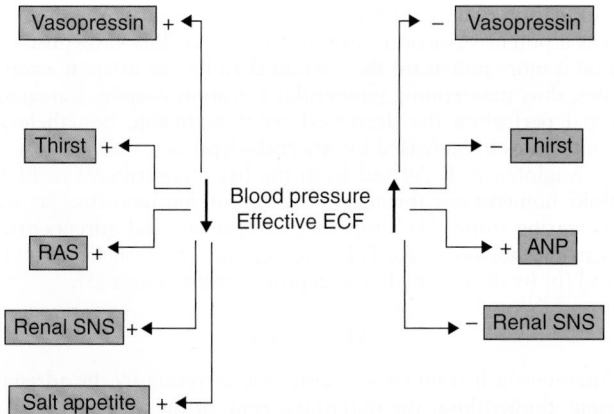

FIGURE 107.7. Responses to changes in blood pressure and effective extracellular fluid (ECF) volume. Detection of increased blood pressure or effective ECF volume by baroreceptors triggers suppression of vasopressin secretion, thirst, and the renal sympathetic nervous system (SNS), while stimulating secretion of A-type natriuretic peptide (ANP). Together, these mechanisms work to lower ECF volume and blood pressure. In contrast, detection of decreased blood pressure or effective ECF volume by baroreceptors triggers secretion of vasopressin, thirst, salt appetite, the renin-angiotensin system (RAS), and the renal sympathetic nervous system to affect water and salt retention and, ultimately, an increase in ECF volume. Discrepancies in blood pressure and effective ECF volume do occur; e.g., an increased ECF volume is ineffective, such as that occurs with congestive heart failure, and causes additional fluid retention.

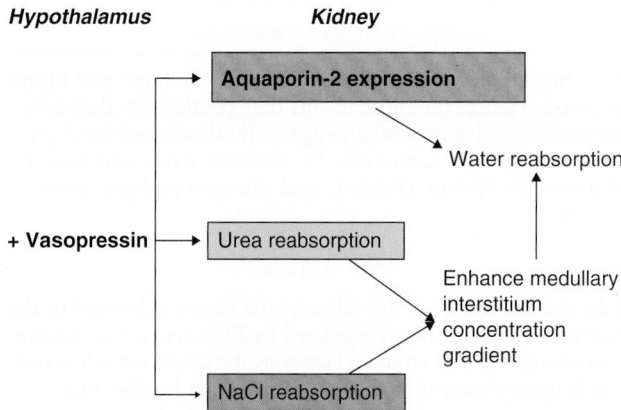

FIGURE 107.8. Effects of vasopressin. Vasopressin secretion by the hypothalamus stimulates fluid retention by increasing aquaporin-2 expression in the renal tubules to promote water absorption from urine. Vasopressin also promotes, to a lesser extent, Na^+ and urea reabsorption in the collecting tubules to help maintain the concentration gradient of the medullary interstitium and the kidney's ability to concentrate urine.

correlate with AVP levels in patients with Kawasaki disease (6). Elevated levels of AVP are common in respiratory illness such as asthma and bronchiolitis (7,8) and have been identified in patients who have undergone spine surgery for scoliosis repair (9–11). Further, high levels of AVP occur early in pediatric sepsis and septic shock (12–14), in contrast to relative deficiency of AVP found in adults with septic shock (15).

Multiple pharmacologic agents can either stimulate (carbamazepine, tricyclic antidepressants, serotonin reuptake inhibitors, nicotine, isoproterenol, vincristine) or inhibit (opioids, ethanol) AVP release. These agents do not appear to have clinical significance in the absence of pathologic conditions.

The primary antidiuretic activity of AVP occurs through recruitment of renal water channels (aquaporin-2) in the collecting duct (4) (**Fig. 107.8**). These collecting ducts traverse the medullary interstitium of the kidney, the site of an increasing concentration gradient, ranging from ~50–60 to 1100–1200 mOsm/kg H_2O. In infants, this range is narrower, 200–600 mOsm/kg H_2O. This concentration gradient is created and maintained primarily by the function of the TAL of the loop of Henle. Specifically, in this diluting segment of the nephron (which also includes the early segment of the distal tubule), the $Na^+/K^+/2Cl^-$ symporter on the luminal surface of the TAL tubular cells increases the interstitial osmolality by pumping these solutes from the lumen of the tubule, while the water remains behind, as this segment of the nephron is impermeable to water. Solutes, such as sodium and urea, subsequently accumulate in the interstitium. In the absence of vasopressin/aquaporin channels, urine is dilute (~50 mOsm/kg H_2O) reflecting the obligate solute losses by the kidney. With the provision of aquaporin channels along the tubular side of the collecting ducts, water is absorbed along the concentration gradient. Urine concentration increases linearly with increasing plasma AVP concentrations until a maximum above which urine can no longer be further concentrated. This maximum, when serum osmolality exceeds 290–295 mOsm/kg, reflects the greatest concentration of the medullary interstitium and

is ~1100–1200 mOsm/kg. This maximum is achieved with plasma AVP concentrations of ~4–5 pg/mL, levels achieved with hyperosmolality but much lower than those attained with hypotension and nausea.

AVP may contribute to this concentration gradient of the corticomedullary interstitium by regulating delivery of urea to the medullary interstitium (16) and increasing sodium chloride channel expression. Chronic polyuria can "wash out" this concentration gradient, preventing maximum concentration of urine despite adequate amounts of AVP. This dilution of the medullary interstitium can occur with excessive fluid intake, such as that occurs with primary polydipsia and diabetes insipidus (DI), and can impact the results of a water deprivation test. AVP is important for transcription of aquaporin-2; chronic deficits could conceivably also impact urine-concentrating ability during water deprivation.

Thirst

Thirst is one of the body's two main mechanisms to protect against the development of hyperosmolality. The thirst center is located in the preoptic medial nucleus in the anterior hypothalamus. As with AVP, thirst is regulated by plasma osmolality and blood pressure/volume status. The osmosensors that activate the preoptic nucleus to trigger the thirst sensation are located in the anterior hypothalamus, specifically the organum vasculosum and subfornical organ, and are outside the BBB (17,18).

Cardiovascular baroreceptors transmit their signals to the thirst center through the vagal and glossopharyngeal nerves via the medulla, while angiotensin II directly stimulates thirst. Hypoosmolality, increased arterial blood pressure, and increased gastric water all inhibit thirst (17,19).

The osmotic threshold for activating thirst may be higher than that for AVP secretion, ~295 mOsm/kg H_2O. This offsetting is hypothesized to occur to prevent simultaneous activation of thirst and AVP secretion, which would obligate frequent water consumption to maintain the set plasma osmolality. In addition, the simultaneous activation of these two mechanisms would predispose to hypoosmolality, as antidiuresis would be occurring with concomitant water intake. Instead, following activation of thirst and consumption of fluids, AVP secretion is suppressed. This suppression occurs prior to decreases in osmolality and is thought to occur to minimize the risk of overcorrection of plasma osmolality.

Sodium Homeostasis

Na^+ plays a key role in maintaining ECF volume and blood pressure. Hence, the mechanisms that regulate its abundance primarily revolve around changes in fluid volume/blood pressure and include natriuretic factors, the renin–angiotensin–aldosterone system (RAAS), and the sympathetic nervous system.

Salt Appetite

Like the thirst center, the salt appetite center is located in the hypothalamus. It, too, is regulated by ECF Na^+ concentration and effective blood volume; however, the desire for salt occurs much more slowly (hours to days) than that for thirst (5).

Renin-Angiotensin System

Two distinct renin-angiotensin systems (RASs) exist: one in the brain and the other in the periphery. The peripheral RAS only has access to the central nervous system (CNS) at sites where the BBB is absent, such as the posterior pituitary and the circumventricular structures (the vascular organ of the laminar terminalis, the subfornical organ, area postrema, median eminence, and neurohypophysis). Both systems play a role in maintaining fluid status, although data are limited in humans with respect to the brain system (5) (**Fig. 107.9**).

Decreases in circulating blood volume/blood pressure detected by baroreceptors in the renal arterioles, extrarenal baroreceptors, and the renal macula densa stimulate renin release from the renal juxtaglomerular cells. Renin release is inhibited by angiotensin II, vasopressin, and atrial natriuretic factor. A proteolytic enzyme, renin, converts hepatically derived angiotensinogen to angiotensin I. Angiotensin-converting enzyme, located throughout the vasculature endothelium (particularly the lung), converts angiotensin I to the active hormone angiotensin II.

Angiotensin II serves a number of roles in maintaining ECF volume. Circulating angiotensin II has access to brain osmoreceptors in the organum vasculosum and subfornical organ. Activation of these receptors stimulates thirst and AVP secretion. Angiotensin II-mediated thirst activation is blunted by increased blood pressure. At the level of the kidney, angiotensin II stimulates Na^+ and water reabsorption (a) directly, by renal proximal tubules, and (b) indirectly, through presynaptic stimulation of intrarenal norepinephrine release and stimulation of adrenal aldosterone secretion (20). Angiotensin II is a potent vasoconstrictor. In the kidney, this vasoconstriction is more potent for the efferent than for the afferent arterioles, thus maintaining glomerular filtration despite decreased renal perfusion; the decreased renal perfusion, nonetheless, contributes to increased filtrate reabsorption.

Angiotensin II derived from the brain contributes to ECF fluid homeostasis through a variety of mechanisms: (a) by increasing thirst, Na^+ appetite, vasopressin and adrenocorticotropic hormone (ACTH) release, and sympathetic output; and (b) by decreasing baroreceptor responsiveness (5).

Aldosterone

Angiotensin II stimulates aldosterone secretion by the adrenal zona glomerulosa, the outermost zone of the adrenal cortex. In addition to angiotensin II, the major regulator for aldosterone secretion, increased plasma K^+ and decreased plasma Na^+ also stimulate aldosterone release.

Like other adrenal steroid hormones, aldosterone is synthesized from cholesterol through the action of a series of enzymes. The mineralocorticoid properties of aldosterone are imparted through its actions on the principal cells of the late distal tubule. Aldosterone binds to a specific mineralocorticoid cell-surface receptor, causing an increase in Na^+ channel expression in the luminal membrane and Na/K-ATPase expression in the basolateral membrane, leading to enhanced Na^+ reabsorption and K^+ excretion (**Fig. 107.10**). Coupled with vasopressin, aldosterone increases ECF: aldosterone-mediated Na^+ reabsorption increases plasma osmolality, triggering vasopressin secretion, and, hence, water reabsorption. In addition, aldosterone increases Na^+/H^+ antiporter activity in renal intercalated cells to enhance hydrogen (H^+) excretion in the urine. Other adrenal hormones, such as cortisol and deoxycorticosterone, also bind the mineralocorticoid receptor to affect salt retention. Despite the many-fold higher plasma concentrations of cortisol over aldosterone, cortisol displays significantly lower levels of mineralocorticoid activity. This specificity is conferred through renal expression of 11-β-hydroxysteroid dehydrogenase type 2, an enzyme that inactivates cortisol to cortisone.

Although only 2%–4% of filtered Na^+ reaches the collecting duct, over a 24-hour period, this amount is substantial. In a 30-kg child (approximate body surface area = 1 m^2) with normal renal function (glomerular filtration rate = 110 mL/min/1.73 m^2), the kidney filters 90 L/day. With a plasma Na^+

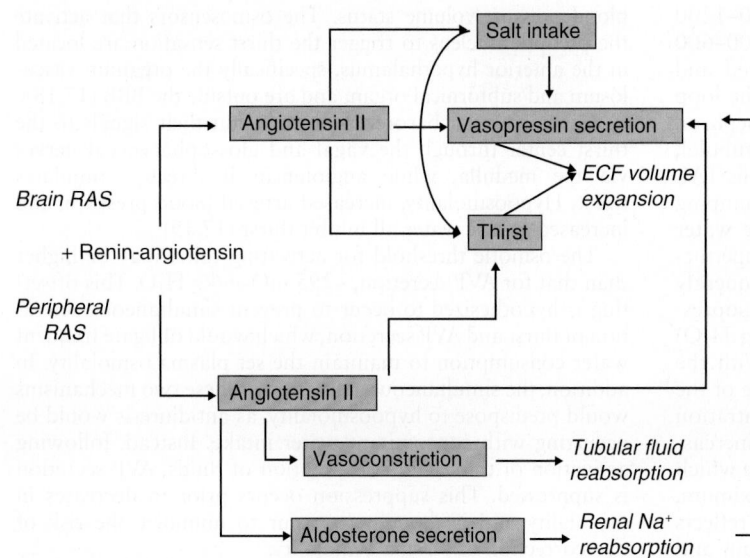

FIGURE 107.9. Effect of the renin-angiotensin system. Both brain and peripheral renin-angiotensin systems (RAS) exist, and both act to preserve extracellular fluid (ECF) volume. Stimulation of both of the systems generates angiotensin II. In the brain, angiotensin II stimulates thirst, salt appetite, and vasopressin secretion. An increase in salt further stimulates thirst and vasopressin secretion. Angiotensin II, generated in the periphery, stimulates thirst, vasopressin secretion, vasoconstriction, which stimulates fluid absorption from the renal tubules, and aldosterone secretion, which promotes renal salt retention. The ultimate result of these intertwined and redundant pathways is an expansion of ECF volume.

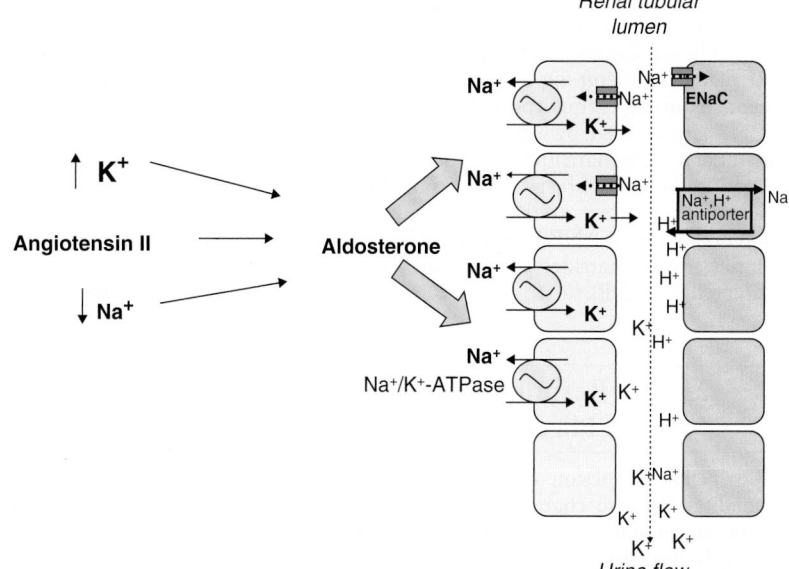

FIGURE 107.10. Stimulants and effects of aldosterone secretion. Hyperkalemia, angiotensin II, and hyponatremia all stimulate aldosterone secretion. Aldosterone then interacts with the mineralocorticoid receptors in the distal tubules to effect Na^+ reabsorption by increasing expression of amiloride-sensitive epithelial Na^+ channels (ENaC) in the apical membrane and Na/K-ATPase activity in the basal membrane. Increased Na^+ reabsorption drives K^+ and hydrogen excretion.

level of 140 mEq/L, ~12,600 mEq of Na^+ will be filtered and 252 mEq (2%) will be delivered to the collecting ducts. The 252 mEq represents ~1.8 L ECF—almost one-third of the total ECF in a 30-kg child. Hence, aldosterone plays a key role in maintaining fluid homeostasis.

Natriuretic Peptides

A number of natriuretic peptides have been identified, the prototype of which is *A-type natriuretic peptide* (ANP); these peptides also include *B-type natriuretic peptide* (BNP), *C-type natriuretic peptide* (CNP) and *urodilatin*. These peptides have a similar 17-amino acid ring structure; their activity spectrum is conferred by their affinity for specific natriuretic receptors. Both CNS and peripheral natriuretic systems exist (**Fig. 107.11**) (5).

ANP, previously referred to as atrial natriuretic peptide, is a 28-amino acid hormone produced both by the hypothalamus and the cardiac atrial myocytes. Atrial myocytes release ANP in response to distention of the cardiac atria, as occurs in the setting of fluid overload. β adrenergic stimulation

also promotes ANP release. ANP lowers circulating volume and, hence, blood pressure through a variety of mechanisms. Through its effects on the renal vasculature, ANP increases the glomerular filtration rate, thereby promoting fluid excretion. It decreases renal Na^+ reabsorption by the distal convoluted tubules and collecting ducts, thereby promoting natriuresis. In addition, it inhibits renin secretion. Given that angiotensin II stimulates ANP secretion, ANP provides negative feedback for the RAS. ANP also directly inhibits aldosterone secretion by the adrenal glomerulosa and relaxes vascular smooth muscle. Hypothalamic ANP may potentiate ANP secretion by the cardiac atria. In addition, ANP participates in water metabolism by inhibiting thirst (5,21).

BNP, formerly referred to as brain natriuretic peptide due to its initial identification in the porcine brain, is a 32-amino acid peptide secreted by the ventricular myocardium in response to excessive stretching (i.e., fluid overload). Its mode of action is similar to that of ANP, although it binds to the natriuretic peptide receptor with much lower affinity. Its half-life is only 22 minutes, allowing it to dynamically reflect the state of the heart. Consequently, plasma BNP concentrations, or

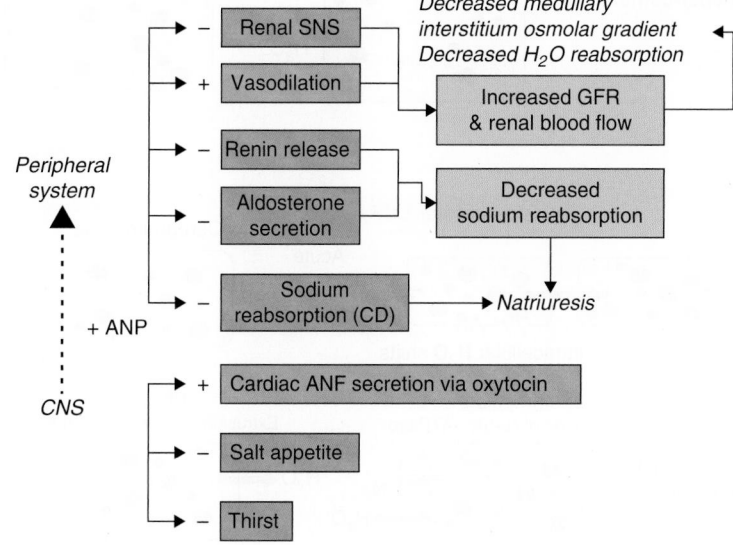

FIGURE 107.11. Activities of A-type natriuretic peptide (ANP). ANP acts both centrally and peripherally to mediate its effects. Centrally, ANP suppresses thirst and salt appetite while promoting additional atrial naturetic factor (ANF) release by the heart. Peripherally, ANP promotes vasodilation and inhibits the renal sympathetic nervous system (SNS) to increase glomerular filtration (GFR) and, ultimately, urine output. In addition, it directly inhibits renin and aldosterone secretion and Na^+ reabsorption at the collecting duct (CD) to promote natriuresis.

the biologically inactive N-terminal fragment (NT-proBNP), are used in the diagnosis and management of congenital or acquired heart disease (22,23) and correlate with outcomes in those patients undergoing congenital heart surgery (24) and in patients requiring extracorporeal membrane oxygenation (25).

CNP is produced by vascular endothelial cells. Although a member of the natriuretic peptide family, CNP does not directly induce natriuresis and is thought to have an autocrine/paracrine effect at the level of the endothelium. This difference between ANP/BNP and CNP arises from selective affinities for the natriuretic receptors (type A for ANP/BNP and type B for CNP).

Cellular Responses to Disturbances in Plasma Osmolality

Proper cellular function depends upon preservation of ICF osmolality. Because changes in ECF osmolality elicit transmembrane cellular shifts in water and solute, the mechanisms previously described are critical for preserving both ECF and ICF homoeostasis. In addition, cellular mechanisms exist to maintain ICF osmolality in the face of chronic perturbations in ECF osmolality. These compensatory mechanisms, however, can predispose to significant disturbances in ICF during therapeutic interventions and, thus, frequently dictate our delivery of fluid and solute to patients.

In response to an increase in plasma osmolality, water is shifted from the ICF to ECF in an attempt to maintain a balance in osmolality (**Fig. 107.12**). A shift of inorganic osmoles, particularly Na^+, is accompanied by a shift of water to the ICF to help prevent cellular dehydration. Additionally, hypothalamic, pituitary, and renal mechanisms are invoked to preserve body water. Significant hyperosmolality occurring abruptly can be accompanied by cellular shrinkage and likely accounts for the abrupt clinical symptomatology that accompanies such perturbations. On the other hand, for many cell types, additional mechanisms operate in response to chronic hyperosmolar states. For instance, in the brain, intracellular idiogenic organic osmoles (taurine, glycine, glutamine, sorbitol, and inositol) accumulate (by increased synthesis and decreased breakdown) over hours to days. These molecules offset increased plasma osmolality and reestablish normal intracellular volume without further increasing intracellular Na^+ and chloride, which can interrupt normal metabolism (26). These "compatible" organic osmoles do not interfere with cellular metabolism. However, the generation of these osmoles presents a therapeutic dilemma for clinicians, as rapid correction of the hyperosmolar state in their presence can lead to accumulation of ICF, leading to cellular swelling (i.e., cerebral edema).

In response to a decrease in plasma osmolality, water is shifted to the intracellular compartment, thereby reestablishing the equilibrium between ECF and ICF (**Fig. 107.13**). The increase in cellular volume that accompanies these shifts

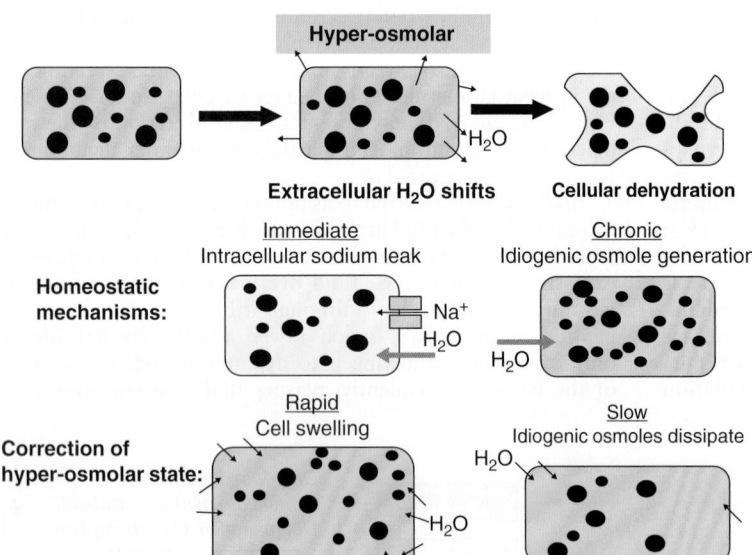

FIGURE 107.12. Cellular responses to hyperosmolality. Hyperosmolar ECF promotes movement of water from the ICF to the ECF and, thus, cell shrinkage. To preserve cell volume, Na^+ leakage into the cell occurs; water accompanies this movement to the intracellular space. The cellular response to chronic hyperosmolality is the generation of "idiogenic osmoles," which shifts water from the ECF to the ICF, preserving cell volume. Rapid correction of the chronic hyperosmolar state causes excessive shifts of water into the ICF because idiogenic osmoles persist intracellularly.

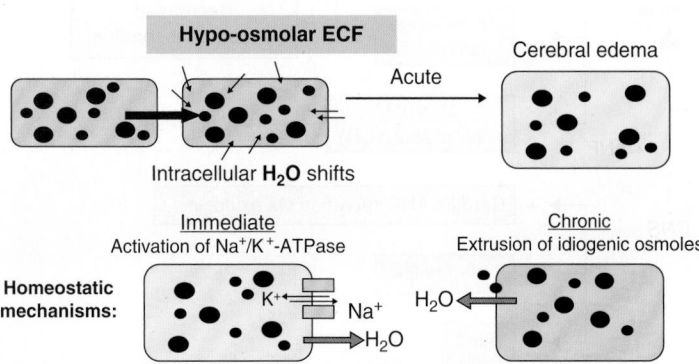

FIGURE 107.13. Cellular responses to hypoosmolality. Hypoosmolar ECF promotes water shifts from the ECF to the ICF. Acutely, large shifts cause cellular edema. To minimize cellular swelling, Na/K-ATPase is activated and water is shunted with Na^+ to the extracellular space. The cell adapts to chronic hypoosmolality by extruding idiogenic osmoles, thus lowering the gradient between the ICF and the ECF.

activates Na/K-ATPase: Na^+ is exported extracellularly and is accompanied by water, minimizing the risk of cellular swelling. To compensate for chronic hypoosmolality, idiogenic osmoles are extruded and normal cell volume preserved (27).

Potassium Homeostasis

K^+ plays a key role in creating the resting membrane potential of the cell and does so because of the significant transcellular concentration gradient maintained through the activity of Na/K-ATPase. The ICF contains nearly 98% of total body (40–50 mEq/kg) K^+ and has a K^+ concentration of 140–150 mEq/L. The concentration of K^+ in the ECF, the site of the remaining 2% of total body K^+, ranges from 3.5 to 5.5 mEq/L. Because K^+ is primarily located intracellularly, plasma K^+ concentration may not accurately reflect changes in total body stores.

As occurs with Na^+ and water, the kidneys play a large role in responding to variable inputs of K^+ to ensure total body K^+ homeostasis. Transport of K^+ with Na^+ occurs in the proximal tubule and TAL and accounts for over 90% of K^+ reabsorbed from glomerular filtrate. The distal tubules and cortical-collecting ducts can then reabsorb the majority of the remaining K^+, if necessary.

Dietary intake frequently exceeds the amount of K^+ available for excretion following the initial reabsorption phase, and secretion of K^+ must occur in the distal tubules and cortical-collecting ducts to prevent a positive K^+ balance. Hence, K^+ regulation largely occurs in the distal tubules and cortical-collecting ducts. With increased plasma K^+ concentration, K^+ directly stimulates its secretion by activating Na/K-ATPase and luminal Na^+ and K^+ channels.

In addition, increases in ECF K^+ stimulate aldosterone secretion, thereby indirectly stimulating K^+ excretion in urine. Aldosterone interacts with the mineralocorticoid receptor in renal principal cells, which comprise the majority of the tubular epithelium in the late distal tubules and cortical-collecting ducts. Stimulation of the mineralocorticoid receptor upregulates Na/K-ATPase activity at the basolateral membrane, resulting in an increase in intracellular K^+ (**Fig. 107.10**). Because the luminal border of the principal cells is highly permeable to K^+ (unlike other renal tubular cells), K^+ can flow down its concentration gradient into the tubular lumen for excretion. Aldosterone also acts upon the colon to stimulate Na^+ reabsorption and K^+ secretion.

Other nonrenal regulators of K^+ include insulin, catecholamines, and acid–base balance. Insulin promotes intracellular K^+ uptake through direct stimulation of Na/K-ATPase; the importance of basal insulin in maintaining plasma K^+ within a normal range is highlighted by insulin-deficient states, which are characterized by hyperkalemia.

The sympathetic nervous system regulates the transcellular K^+ gradient through opposing mechanisms. Stimulation of β_2-adrenergic receptors activates Na/K-ATPase, thereby lowering plasma K^+ concentrations. This activity may prevent excessive ECF K^+ concentrations due to exercise-induced K^+ release by muscles. Stimulation of α-adrenergic receptors triggers movement of K^+ to the ECF.

Metabolic acidosis caused by mineral acids triggers a shift in K^+ to the extracellular space in exchange for hydrogen ions. Respiratory acidosis and metabolic organic acidosis less consistently cause these shifts because blood pH is not the sole determinant of K^+ shifts. Studies suggest that these differences in the setting of metabolic acidoses may arise from the different hormonal responses evoked by organic versus mineral acids, with ketoacids stimulating an insulin response and hydrogen chloride stimulating a glucagon response (28).

CLINICAL PRESENTATION AND DIFFERENTIAL DIAGNOSIS

Many of the disorders resulting in disturbances of Na^+ and K^+ frequently do not cause clinical symptoms unless accompanied by disturbances of hydration. However, children admitted to the PICU frequently have associated respiratory insufficiency, severe muscle weakness, neurologic symptoms (including seizures, coma, tremors, and disorientation), nausea, vomiting, and even cardiac dysrhythmias, all of which could be associated with underlying altered electrolyte levels. Disturbances in Na^+ or K^+ are commonly coincident to other serious comorbidities (such as a child admitted for a head injury and found to have unrelated hyponatremia due to diuretics), or are secondary to iatrogenic causes, such as fluid administration. The etiology of the electrolyte abnormality can often be determined by careful exploration of the information pertaining to the changes that prompted the admission. Determining the rate of onset of the abnormality is vital for understanding the cause as well as risk associated with treatment. A detailed review of systems must be obtained, including onset of mental status changes, gastrointestinal changes (diarrhea or vomiting), appetite or eating alterations, weight loss, changes in skin color or skin tone, and urinary output. Recent medications, including the use of "natural supplements" or laxatives, must be reviewed.

Physical Examination

The physical examination must assess the degree of hydration as judged by vital signs, skin tone, and perfusion. An accurate weight as well as any recent change must be obtained. Careful evaluation of the respiratory system, paying particular attention to respiratory rate, work of breathing, and auscultation might suggest the possibility of pulmonary edema or impending heart failure. Examination should include a search for the possibility of physical abuse, i.e., bruising or burns that might raise the possibility of head trauma (even in those children with a known previous morbidity). Children with chronic illnesses have a well-known increased risk of being victims of nonaccidental trauma (29).

Laboratory and Technical Studies

In addition to a basic metabolic panel, laboratory studies should include ionized calcium, serum magnesium, and studies of acid–base balance. Blood urea nitrogen and creatinine help to evaluate both the potential degree of dehydration and renal function. A spot urinary Na^+ is extremely useful, with urinary Na^+ >20 mmol/L in conditions of hyponatremia indicative of high urinary Na^+ excretion. Direct measurements of plasma and urine osmolalities can be informative in DI and helpful in documenting salt-wasting polyuria. Urine output must be measured and recorded. Dependent upon a number of variables, including age, a urine output >2–3 mL/kg/hour in children (outside of infancy) is excessive.

CT scan of the brain in those patients with potential cerebral edema or brain injury may be indicated. ECG, especially in those patients with disorders of K^+, is necessary for evaluation and for monitoring progress of all patients with water and electrolyte disturbances. Central venous pressure (CVP) is used to assess the degree of dehydration in selected patients. However, due to effects of cardiopulmonary interactions (among other physiologic influences), reliance on a single CVP measurement to assess intravascular volume status may be inappropriate and misleading. Rather, the CVP (as a reliable measure of right atrial pressure) is an accurate assessment of the impedance imposed by the right heart to systemic venous return such that the rise in CVP with fluid accumulation in fact reflects the compliance of the right ventricle.

Disorders of Sodium Balance

Differential Diagnosis of Hypernatremic Conditions

Hypernatremia is defined as the presence of serum Na$^+$ >145 mEq/L. It is estimated that 0.04%–0.2% of hospitalized children are admitted with or develop hypernatremia, the majority developing after hospital admission (30,31). Various factors contributing to the development of hypernatremia are commonly found in ICU patients, such as excess Na$^+$ administration (fluid resuscitation, sodium bicarbonate, and blood product administration), renal concentrating defects, increased insensible water losses (fever, tachypnea, or burns), restricted access to oral fluids, and renal replacement therapy complications. Moritz et al. noted a 22% incidence of hypernatremia (defined as serum Na$^+$ >150 mEq/L) in critically ill patients (31). Most patients who develop hypernatremia are either debilitated by acute or chronic medical conditions or have baseline neurologic impairment prior to the onset of hypernatremia. The disorders that can result in hypernatremic states (as noted in **Table 107.1**) include some that are problems of management in the intensive care setting. The more common disorders are associated with dehydration. Nevertheless, the differential diagnosis of disorders uncommon in the ICU will be included for completeness.

TABLE 107.1

HYPERNATREMIC CONDITIONS

Euvolemia (or mild hypervolemia)
  Hypothalamic hypodipsia
  Congenital central hypoventilation syndrome (CCHS)
  Late-onset congenital hypoventilation syndrome (LOCHS)
  Iatrogenic (excess Na$^+$ administration e.g., hypertonic saline, medicatons, sodium bicarbonate, dialysis)
  Hyperaldosteronism
  Cushing syndrome
Hypovolemia (or mild hypovolemia to euvolemia)
  Water losses
    Renal:
    Diabetes insipidus (central or nephrogenic)
    Diuretics
    Alcohol ingestion
    Recovery after acute kidney injury
    Hyperosmolality (e.g., hyperglycemia)
    Gastrointestinal:
    Gastroenteritis
    Osmotic diarrhea
    Colostomy/ileostomy
    Emesis
    Insensible:
    Burns
    Fever
    High ambient temperature
    Excessive sweating (overheating)
  Decreased fluid intake
    Neurologic impairment
    Restricted access to fluids
    Hypothalamic disorder
    Fluid restriction

Hypernatremic Disorders Generally Associated with Euvolemia. Iatrogenic causes of hypernatremia are generally recognizable because such children are invariably being treated with intravenous (IV) solutions or tube feedings. Administration of sodium bicarbonate for disorders consisting of metabolic acidosis can result in excessive serum Na$^+$ concentrations. The prolonged use of hypertonic saline or even continued use of normal saline (0.9% NaCl) in certain states, such as fluid resuscitation in sepsis or DKA after correction of hyperglycemia and hydration, can result in hypernatremia. Although, more recently, Choong (32), Neville (33), and Montanana (34) have demonstrated the safety of prescribing isotonic saline as maintenance fluids rather than hypotonic saline without any increased incidence of hypernatremia.

Hypothalamic hypodipsia arises from loss of function of the hypothalamic thirst center incurred by brain injury or, less commonly, acquired congenitally. This brain insult may be due to head trauma, brain tumor, or injury sustained during surgery for a CNS abnormality. Affected children often have elevated Na$^+$ levels but remain asymptomatic. Such children are not likely to be admitted to the PICU for hypernatremic dehydration unless a comorbid condition results in critical illness. History of known insufficient fluid intake, brain injury, or developmental delay, lack of polyuria, and previous findings of asymptomatic hypernatremia will distinguish such patients from those with acute hypernatremia. Central hypoventilation syndrome is associated with hypothalamic hypodipsia and can be both congenital and late-onset, although the congenital form is less likely to be associated with hypothalamic problems. The major issues in children with central hypoventilation syndromes are, in fact, due to hypoventilation; therefore, these children might be admitted to the PICU for care because of their need for mechanical respiratory support.

Congenital central hypoventilation syndrome (CCHS) generally presents in the newborn period with periodic apnea and hypoventilation. This condition is often associated with Hirschsprung disease (20% of patients with congenital hypoventilation syndrome) and other autonomic nervous dysfunction, as well as tumors of the neural crest. This condition arises from mutations of the *PHOX 2B* gene that encodes a transcription factor in the developing hindbrain and peripheral nervous system (35). The main issue with children with CCHS is hypoventilation during sleep, which results in hypercapnia and hypoxemia. Affected infants often die with cor pulmonale, respiratory failure, sepsis, and aspiration. However, since identification of mutations in *PHOX 2B* in this syndrome, variable expression of this disorder has been appreciated. In fact, patients with *PHOX 2B* mutations may present later in life, with one such patient identified at 35 years of age following a history of "snoring" throughout life. The genetic pattern of inheritance is autosomal dominant with variable penetrance and expression and with many mutations arising de novo. In general, children with CCHS have normal growth and have intact hypothalamic function, including that of the thirst center (unlike late-onset central hypoventilation syndrome [LOCHS]).

LOCHS overlaps with CCHS because both are associated with neural crest tumors and central hypoventilation during sleep. However, LOCHS is frequently associated with hypothalamic dysfunction, including hypothalamic obesity, variable degrees of hypopituitarism, and hypernatremia secondary to hypodipsia, as well as some degree of vasopressin deficiency (but generally without polyuria) (36). Many children with LOCHS have asymptomatic hypernatremia, with an Na$^+$ concentration of 145–155 mEq/L, but they develop somnolence when Na$^+$ levels exceed these values. *PHOX2B* mutations have not been associated with the majority of LOCHS patients despite the commonality of sleep-associated central hypoventilation and neural crest tumors (as well as Hirschsprung disease). This is especially true of the LOCHS patients with the phenotype of obesity and hypothalamic-pituitary dysfunction.

Primary hyperaldosteronism is largely a disease of adulthood, whereas Cushing syndrome may occur in children (often due to primary adrenal tumors and less commonly due to pituitary adenoma). The more common cause of Cushing syndrome in PICU patients is iatrogenic, due to prolonged use of high-dose glucocorticoids in patients admitted because of worsening of the primary morbidity for which they are receiving glucocorticoid treatment (Chapter 105).

Hypernatremic Conditions Associated with Hypovolemia (or Euvolemia).
Many of the disorders that result in free water loss can be overcome with water intake, and relatively normal Na$^+$ levels and normal hydration can be preserved. However, if the fluid intake in response to free water loss contains significant electrolytes, hypernatremia is the outcome, despite normal hydration. Conversely, loss of free water without replacement will result in dehydration as well as hypernatremia.

DI can arise from vasopressin deficiency (central DI) or vasopressin insensitivity (nephrogenic DI). The various causes of central DI are listed in **Table 107.2**. Children with congenital forms of DI, both central and nephrogenic variants, are rarely admitted to the PICU unless an intercurrent illness interferes with their routine management. The most common reason for children with DI to be admitted to the PICU is for postoperative management of resection of a craniopharyngioma or other midline intracranial tumors such as astrocytoma. These resections are frequently accompanied by reversible injury or edema of the pituitary stalk, although complete and permanent transection can occur. A triphasic response follows severing of the pituitary stalk/injury, beginning with deficiency of vasopressin. This polyuric phase often lasts ~4–5 days. In the second phase, an unregulated release of stored vasopressin from necrotic vasopressin-secreting neurons occurs. This release of vasopressin without any feedback from the normal osmolar or hemodynamic mechanisms is often thought of as syndrome of inappropriate antidiuretic hormone (SIADH). Varying degrees of vasopressin deficiency then ensue, reflecting the extent of retrograde neuronal degeneration of vasopressin-secreting neurons. In general, the higher the injury to the pituitary stalk, the greater the number of vasopressin-secreting axons that will be damaged (as the axons terminate at different levels along the stalk) and the greater the loss of vasopressin-secreting neurons. During this second phase of stored vasopressin release, hyponatremia can occur if fluid management is not curbed and/or vasopressin administration is continued. Following this brief period of vasopressin release, permanent DI is the usual outcome, although loss of over 80%–90% of all vasopressin-secreting neurons must occur for permanent DI to develop. DI can also result from head trauma, which can manifest this "triple phase" as well. Profuse polyuria is evident during the initial phase, but urine output diminishes when stored vasopressin is released. Because the patient is often being managed with aggressive fluid replacement, the intensivist must monitor Na$^+$ often, being cognizant of this second phase that can result in sudden profound hyponatremia. Hypothalamic brain tumors, such as a germinoma or ependymoma, or pituitary stalk lesions, such as histiocytosis, will often present with central DI.

Severe diarrhea or other forms of gastrointestinal loss of water, especially in very young children being treated with oral electrolyte fluid, can result in hypertonic dehydration. The child may be obtunded, with a doughy-like skin that will "tent" when pinched during assessment for degree of dehydration. The history of profuse watery diarrhea and oral electrolyte replacement should alert the admitting physician to administer fluids judiciously.

TABLE 107.2

CAUSES OF DIABETES INSIPIDUS

CENTRAL
Genetic
  Autosomal dominant inheritance
  Autosomal recessive inheritance
  Wolfram syndrome (DIDMOAD syndrome) autosomal recessive
  X-linked recessive inherited (associated with Xq2B)
Anatomic congenital malformation
  Septo-optic dysplasia
  Holoprosencephaly
  Pituitary agenesis
Acquired
  CNS tumors that involve hypothalamus or pituitary stalk (germinoma, craniopharyngioma)
  Trauma—severing pituitary stalk
  Surgery involving pituitary stalk (removal of craniopharyngioma or optic glioma)
  Hypophysitis
  Granulomatous disease—histiocytosis, sarcoid
  Infection—meningitis, encephalitis
  Vascular injury
NEPHROGENIC
Hereditary
  X-linked (AVPR2 gene mutation)
  Aquaporin-2 gene mutation (autosomal recessive, autosomal dominant)
Renal disorders
  Sickle cell disease or trait
  ADPCKD
  Bartter syndrome
  Bardet-Biedl syndrome
  Cystinosis
Acquired
  Hypercalcemia
  Hypokalemia
Drugs
  Lithium
  Cidofovir
  Foscarnet
  Amphotericin B
  Ifosfamide
  Ofloxacin

DIDMOAD—DI, diabetes insipidus; DM, diabetes mellitus; OA, optic atrophy; D, deafness; CNS, central nervous system; AVPR2-arginine vasopressin receptor 2; ADPCKD-autosomal dominant polycystic kidney disease.

The loss of free water due to injury to the skin (as in burns), excessive heat, or fever with profuse sweating is a relatively rare situation in children, except in the well-publicized cases of children locked inside automobiles or enclosed rooms without ventilation during extremely hot weather. The relatively high body surface areas of children predispose them to a higher risk of fluid loss than adults. For each degree elevation of core body temperature above 38°C, basal fluid requirements increase by ~12.5% (37).

Diuretics, such as furosemide, that affect the loop of Henle in the kidney, can result in mild hypernatremia. In addition, the accidental (or intentional) ingestion of alcohol will inhibit vasopressin release and cause excessive loss of free water. In an adolescent, the history of excessive alcohol intake and the clinical findings of vomiting and disturbed mental status with disorientation are indicative of this cause of hypernatremia.

Historical information regarding medications, including diuretics or alcohol ingestion, provides the explanation of the cause of hypernatremia and directs the management as needed. The clinical management of the obtunded adolescent or child due to alcohol exposure is dictated by the dehydration and hypernatremia as well as by the seriousness of alcohol poisoning of brain function.

Differential Diagnosis of Hyponatremic Conditions

The pediatric intensivist must be familiar with the diagnosis and management of hyponatremia, as it occurs in ~25% of hospitalized children, and is even more prevalent in PICU patients (38,39). About 30% of adult ICU patients will develop hyponatremia. In contrast, PICU patients may demonstrate low serum Na^+ levels even more frequently; a prevalence as high as 73% has been reported in children with severe bronchiolitis (39). Furthermore, outcomes are negatively and independently affected by the presence of hyponatremia (39–45). After ensuring true hypoosmolality rather than dilutional hyponatremia (secondary to hyperlipidemia, hyperproteinemia, hyperglycemia, or elevation of some other effective osmole), hyponatremia can be separated into those with clinical euvolemia (or mild hypervolemia) and those with hypovolemia as outlined in **Table 107.3**.

Hyponatremia with Euvolemia. The SIADH, in which the concentration of AVP is pathologically elevated relative to the degree of hypoosmolality, is one of the most common causes of hyponatremia in the PICU. SIADH is seen in a critically ill child with profound hyponatremia in the face of euvolemia (and even hypervolemia) and poor urine output. Due to the excess reabsorption of water, dilute urine cannot be produced, resulting in a urinary Na^+ level that is disproportionately elevated for the degree of hyponatremia. SIADH may arise through multiple mechanisms, but the exact CNS pathophysiologic mechanisms are not completely characterized. Nonphysiologic secretion of AVP is highly prevalent in PICU patients and is associated with a number of conditions, particularly brain injury (CNS surgery or radiation, traumatic brain injury), pulmonary injury, congenital malformations, and positive pressure mechanical ventilation. A number of chemotherapeutic agents used to treat childhood cancer, including vincristine and cyclophosphamide, have also been implicated as causing SIADH. Parenthetically, as discussed later, some of these same chemotherapeutic agents cause renal tubular injury, resulting in salt and water wasting (causing hyponatremia and raising diagnostic and, therefore, management issues). As a result of plasma expansion during SIADH, ANP may be elevated and exacerbate the hyponatremic condition by causing renal salt wasting. This compensatory response has led to

the misdiagnosis of SIADH as cerebral salt wasting (CSW), a hyponatremic condition associated with polyuria and natriuresis, is discussed later. These salt-wasting conditions are part of the major diagnostic dilemmas in managing SIADH, especially in that the primary causes of the conditions overlap.

Hyponatremia due to excessive free water ingestion is extremely uncommon because of the number of endogenous counter-regulatory mechanisms available to prevent such an event from occurring. In critically ill children, in whom the ability to self-regulate fluid intake is often compromised and for whom the renal handling of water is often impaired, free water overload can occur. The use of hypotonic maintenance fluids has been implicated in iatrogenic hyponatremia, prompting many to recommend isotonic solutions for maintenance therapy (33,34,38,46–49). Excessive free water may inadvertently be administered to patients with central DI on vasopressin therapy. In otherwise healthy infants, excessive free water intake due to overdilution of formula or excessive administration of tap/bottled water can also cause hyponatremia. The inability of the infant to handle the free water load has been attributed to immaturity of the kidney, including a low glomerular filtration rate.

In protein-losing disorders, such as in nephrotic syndrome or protein-losing enteropathies (post-Fontan repair), decreased intravascular oncotic pressure leads to interstitial fluid volume expansion, often resulting in symptoms of fluid overload, such as edema or ascites, but also may result in intravascular hypovolemia due to these fluid shifts. Counter-regulatory Na^+-retaining mechanisms are stimulated, resulting in increased total body Na^+ and water but mild hyponatremia. Urinary Na^+ excretion is low.

Decompensated heart failure, with compromised cardiac output, leads to hypervolemia (as evidence by edema) due to increased AVP levels as a result of carotid sinus baroreceptor stimulation. Further, activation of the RAAS results in increased Na^+ uptake in the proximal nephron, which limits free water delivery to the diluting segment. Similar neurohumoral consequences are seen in hepatic failure in which a reduction of effective circulating blood volume results from arterial vasodilatation.

Renal disease, both acute and chronic kidney injury, with reduced glomerular filtration and loss of tubular function, as well as after renal transplant, is a known cause of hyponatremia. Multiple mechanisms exist and involve many of the factors discussed previously in the physiology section, including water retention, unresponsiveness to aldosterone, tubular loss of Na^+, and hyperkalemic metabolic acidosis. This form of hyponatremia is easily recognizable by history, the elevated K^+, elevated phosphorus levels, azotemia, and elevated creatinine levels. The management is more complex and often requires therapeutic measures such as dialysis. The measure of the fractional excretion of sodium (FeNa) can identify the presence of abnormal renal Na^+ loss (if FeNa is greater than 2%) in patients with hyponatremia. FeNa can be calculated as:

$$FeNa = 100 \times (U_{Na} \times S_{Cr})/(S_{Na} \times U_{Cr})$$

where U_{Na} is the urine concentration of Na^+, U_{Cr} the urine concentration of creatinine, S_{Na} the serum concentration of Na^+, and S_{Cr} the serum concentration of creatinine.

Loss of Na^+ through skin can be substantial, especially in patients with cystic fibrosis or adrenal insufficiency during periods of excessive heat, in very febrile patients, or those with significant burns. As mentioned previously, water is also lost during these circumstances, but salt loss is especially concerning in patients with cystic fibrosis, salt-wasting congenital adrenal hyperplasia, and other forms of adrenal insufficiency. Furthermore, hyponatremia can develop if thirst is treated by ingestion of nonelectrolyte fluids during periods of excessive heat and excessive perspiration.

TABLE 107.3

HYPONATREMIC CONDITIONS

Associated with euvolemia (or mild hypervolemia)
SIADH
Iatrogenic—water overload
Protein loss
Renal disease
Skin loss
Central adrenal insufficiency
Hypothyroidism
Associated with hypovolemia
Salt wasting (cerebral, renal tubular)
Primary adrenal insufficiency
Non-ketotic hyperosmolar coma
Drugs (diuretics)

Central adrenal insufficiency (i.e., secondary or tertiary corticotrophin-releasing hormone or ACTH deficiency) results in insufficient glucocorticoid production, especially during stress. Because glucocorticoids (a) have an adjunctive role in aldosterone production, (b) suppress production of nitric oxide (nitric oxide causes vasopressin-independent insertion of aquaporin-2 into renal tubules), and (c) suppress vasopressin production, mild hyponatremia without hyperkalemia can occur with central adrenal insufficiency; this is true as well in the syndromes of ACTH insensitivity. Affected patients do not have the marked water and electrolyte problems of primary adrenal insufficiency because the adrenal zona glomerulosa is regulated by the RAS and not affected by ACTH deficiency. These conditions are discussed in more detail in the chapter concerning adrenal function (Chapter 105).

Hyponatremia Associated with Hypovolemia. This clinical condition occurs as a result of the loss of both water and Na^+. Water is relatively conserved due to hemodynamic (extracellular volume) stimulation of AVP secretion, leading to a decreased serum Na^+ concentration. Salt wasting can occur at the level of the renal tubules either from a primary tubular defect or through medication or a hormone-mediated process. Because salt wasting is associated with simultaneous water loss, it can result in severe hyponatremia and clinical dehydration. Specifically, renal Na^+ and fluid losses can be due to diuretic use, mineralocorticoid deficiency, and CSW.

Prolonged use of diuretics, especially in the presence of concomitant salt restriction, can cause hypovolemic hyponatremia. The loop diuretics, such as furosemide, inhibit Na/K/Cl absorption in the medullary ascending limb of the loop of Henle, causing Na^+ loss but rarely causing hyponatremia. Much more commonly, the use of loop diuretics results in hypernatremia, due to the relative excessive water loss compared to sodium. The thiazide diuretics inhibit the NaCl cotransporter reabsorption at the cortical diluting segments (the early distal convoluted tubule). By impairing urinary dilution, AVP secretion is stimulated through intravascular volume depletion, promoting retention of free water. Therefore, thiazides are associated with greater risk, and studies suggest that hyponatremia is more common and more severe with the thiazides. It is important to note that diuretics are K^+-depleting as well, and correction requires both Na^+ and K^+ replacement.

Primary adrenal crisis, or Addisonian crisis, causes the characteristic findings of hyponatremia and severe hyperkalemia and metabolic acidosis (Chapter 105).

CSW results in Na^+ and water losses from the kidney as a result of a CNS insult, despite normal renal function. The natriuresis resulting from cerebral disease is characterized by

hyponatremia associated with polyuria. The mechanism for CSW remains unclear, with theories pointing to altered RAAS or sympathetic nervous system, as well as natriuretic peptide activity (50). Severe hyponatremia in the setting of persistent urine output raises questions as to whether the patient has (a) SIADH and compensatory ANP production from fluid overload, (b) CSW, or (c) vasopressin insufficiency in the setting of a salt-losing process. The clue to differentiating CSW from SIADH is hydration status. The child with CSW will be dehydrated; the child with SIADH has normal-to-expanded blood volume. The clinical picture becomes more complicated in the child with DI who also develops CSW as a result of underlying CNS pathology, surgery, infection, or radiation therapy. For example, in patients with brain tumor-related DI, chemotherapeutic treatment with salt-wasting agents such as cisplatin can also make management difficult. The finding of a coexisting salt-losing process in the patient with central DI requires vasopressin administration to be withheld; Na^+ concentrations are normalized with salt replacement while intravascular volume is repleted. The clinical and biochemical differences between these often coexisting conditions are listed in **Table 107.4**.

The patient with type 2 diabetes who presents in the nonketotic hyperosmolar state can have significant urinary Na^+ loss from the osmotic diuresis and can have additional salt loss in vomitus. Although the patient is total-body Na^+ depleted, the degree of hyponatremia is more reflective of an osmotic shift in intracellular water, with some degree of dilutional hyponatremia. This cause of hyponatremia and the clinical manifestations of nonketotic hyperosmolar coma are discussed more fully in the section on glucose homeostasis (Chapter 106).

Nonrenal losses of sodium and water can occur in cases of diarrhea, emesis, gastrointestinal drains (i.e., ileostomies) or third-spacing (extravascular volume loss). The kidneys attempt to conserve Na^+, reflected in a urine Na ≤ 20 mmol/L. Close monitoring of a patient's intake and outputs should raise the clinician's awareness of this etiology.

Disorders of Potassium Balance

Differential Diagnosis of Hyperkalemic Disorders

Although the disorders of hyperkalemia are separated into mild, moderate, and severe hyperkalemia in **Table 107.5**, the clinical disturbances might not be reflected by serum concentrations of K^+. In general, mild hyperkalemia refers to plasma K^+ in the 5–6 mEq/L range, moderate hyperkalemia refers to plasma K^+ in the 6–7 mEq/L range, and severe hyperkalemia refers to plasma K^+ levels of >7–8. It is the intracellular content of K^+ that is of major concern. The acid–base

TABLE 107.4

DIFFERENTIATION OF DISORDERS OF WATER AND SODIUM BALANCE SEEN IN CRITICAL CARE

		CLINICAL AND BIOCHEMICAL FINDINGS		
■ DISORDER	■ SERUM SODIUM	■ URINE SODIUM	■ URINE OUTPUT	■ VOLUME STATUS
DI (inadequate treatment)	High	Low	High	Hypovolemic
Excess DDAVP or water excess	Low	Low	Normal or low	Euvolemic/hypervolemic
SIADH	Low	High	Low	Euvolemic/hypervolemic
Salt wasting	Low	High	High	Hypovolemic

DI, diabetes insipidus; DDAVP, 1-deamino(8-D-arginine) vasopressin; SIADH, syndrome of inappropriate antidiuretic hormone.

TABLE 107.5

HYPERKALEMIC CONDITIONS

Mild increase
  Spurious hyperkalemia
  Dietary intake of potassium
  Fasting
Moderate (to severe) increase
  Drugs (ACE-I, ARBs, succinylcholine)
  Cell death (tumor lysis)
  Hyperkalemic periodic paralysis
Severe hyperkalemia
  Chronic and acute renal failure
  Adrenal insufficiency
  Low-renin hyperkalemia

ACE-I, angiotensin-converting enzyme inhibitors; ARBs, angiotensin receptor blockers.

status, serum calcium and Na^+ concentrations, and rate of change in K^+ concentrations all influence the clinical threat of hyperkalemia. Although associated symptoms are rare, complaints vary from fatigue to muscle weakness, disorientation, paresthesias, and palpitations. The major concern is cardiac dysfunction due to the hyperkalemia, as potassium concentrations are intimately responsible for normal cardiomyocyte repolarization, with asystole being the most serious outcome. Initially, a mild elevation in the K^+ level is demonstrated by tall-peaked T waves, moderate elevations by a prolonged P-R interval, and severe elevations by flattened or absent P waves as well as widening QRS intervals (forming the classic sine wave), merging ST waves, and then bradycardia, all of which precede ventricular tachycardia (see **Fig. 107.14**). However, the sensitivity of the ECG to detect hyperkalemia is not reliable. Acker demonstrated that approximately half of the patients with serum potassium levels >6.5 mmol/L did not have ECG changes (51). Further, the progression from a normal ECG to a lethal ventricular dysrhythmia may develop at an unpredictable rate of progression.

Mild Elevations of Potassium Level. Routine serum electrolyte determinations often find mild elevations of K^+ secondary to hemolysis of red blood cells during the blood sampling. Issues related to specimen collection can lead to hemolysis, such as prolonged tourniquet time, inadequate drying time for alcohol skin preparation, collecting blood through the placement of an IV line, and excessive force applied to the syringe

when drawing and transferring the sample. Further, excessive time elapsed between the sample draw and laboratory evaluation, exposure to heat or cold, or mechanical injury to cells with vigorous shaking of the sample during transport will exacerbate the RBC destruction. This form of spurious hyperkalemia (also referred to as *pseudohyperkalemia*) is also likely due to potassium release from activated platelets in the blood sample, and may occur within an hour from the time of the blood specimen collection (52). Although serum K^+ levels may exceed that of the plasma by greater than 0.4 mmol/L, no ECG abnormalities or other clinical consequence result.

Dietary ingestion of high K^+-containing foods or K^+ salt substitutes rarely causes hyperkalemia, but such cases with mild elevation of serum K^+ concentration have been reported. Fasting or chronic starvation, such as that occurs in anorexia nervosa, can result in suppression of insulin production and mild hyperkalemia. The list of drugs that have resulted in mild hyperkalemia is extensive and includes β-blockers, angiotensin-converting enzyme inhibitors, and nonsteroidal anti-inflammatory drugs.

Moderate to Occasionally Severe Elevation of Potassium Levels. A number of drugs, including K^+-sparing diuretics, such as spironolactone, can raise K^+ levels. Other drugs that interfere with the RAS (including angiotensin-converting enzyme inhibitors, angiotensin receptor blockers, and heparin) may cause hyperkalemia. A single dose of the depolarizing neuromuscular blocker succinylcholine will raise serum K^+ levels ~0.5 mEq/L in healthy children. Those with neuromuscular disorders (i.e., muscular dystrophy), burns, and severe crush injuries will have a more profound release of intracellular K^+ and should not receive the drug.

Massive cell death, such as that occurs with tumor lysis or rhabdomyolysis, can cause hyperkalemia. Massive blood transfusion and red cell lysis during mechanical dialysis can similarly cause red cell breakdown and increase serum K^+ levels. Rhabdomyolysis that results in cell death and hyperkalemia can occur secondary to infections (i.e., influenza), crush injury, or catabolism during a fasted state in children with certain inborn errors of metabolism, such as fatty acid oxidation defects. It also has occurred during treatment of DKA because of prolonged use of isotonic saline in the hypernatremic patient after restoration of hydration and fluid volume, as noted by normal glucose levels and normal acid–base balance.

An interesting cause of hyperkalemia is the genetic form of hyperkalemic periodic paralysis. Periodic paralysis includes a group of genetic disorders with mutations in Na^+, calcium, and K^+ channels. Hyperkalemic periodic paralysis presents with attacks of disabling weakness and elevated serum K^+ levels.

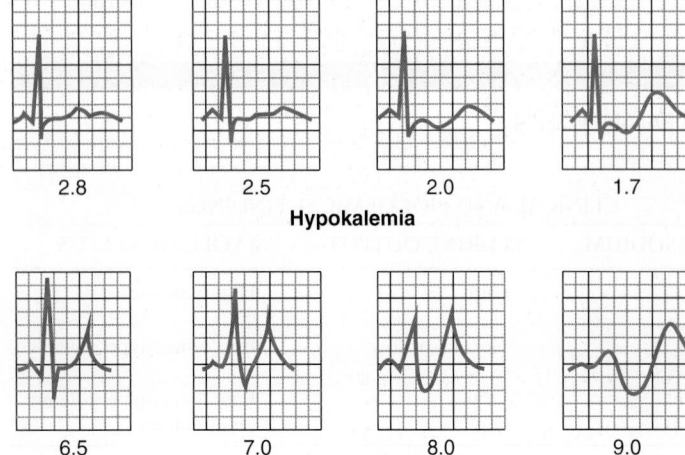

2.8   2.5   2.0   1.7

Hypokalemia

6.5   7.0   8.0   9.0

Hyperkalemia

FIGURE 107.14. Electrocardiographic changes in hypokalemic and hyperkalemic conditions. Serum K^+ in mmol/L. (Lewis JL *Merck Manual online.* www.merckmanuals.com/professional/endocrine_and_metabolic_disorders. Accessed July 21, 2013.)

In a large study of kindreds, mutations of the Na$^+$ channel were found in 64%, and none were found in 36% (53). The onset was young (approximately age 2 years) in those in whom mutations were found and much older (approximately age 14) in those in whom no mutations were found. Attacks were more frequent in those with mutations. The average serum K$^+$ levels ranged between 4.9 and 6.1 mEq/L, with the lower levels in those patients in whom no mutations were found. A number of precipitants for these attacks are known, including cold, exercise, and hunger. Occasionally, cardiac dysrhythmias are found, especially in the form of hyperkalemic periodic paralysis referred to as Andersen–Tawil syndrome (long QT syndrome 7), which arises from mutations in a gene encoding a K$^+$ channel inherited in an autosomal dominant pattern; the phenotype includes cardiac dysrhythmias (as a complication of prolonged QT interval), dysmorphia (including micrognathia, low set ears, clinodactyly, hypertelorism), and periodic paralysis, in the setting of elevated, normal, or low K$^+$.

Potassium Disorders with Marked Elevation of Potassium.

Renal disease, including chronic renal insufficiency, acute kidney injury, and end-stage renal failure, can be associated with significant hyperkalemia. In acute kidney injury, the increase in K$^+$ levels may be rapid and tolerated poorly. In more chronic situations, despite K$^+$ levels of 7–8 mEq/L, cardiac function and ECG findings remain normal. Chronicity of kidney injury often leads to tolerance of even moderately severe hyperkalemia.

Patients with primary adrenal crisis present in shock, dehydration, and often with cardiac dysrhythmias. The biochemical abnormalities include hyponatremia, severe hyperkalemia, and a non-anion gap metabolic acidosis.

Type IV renal tubular acidosis occurs in states of aldosterone deficiency or insensitivity and manifests as persistent hyperkalemia, reduced bicarbonate reabsorption, and potentially mild-to-moderate glomerular insufficiency. One form of type IV renal tubular acidosis is associated with an obstructive uropathy that damages the juxtaglomerular apparatus, leading to hyporeninemia and subsequent hypoaldosteronism. However, in the setting of primary aldosterone deficiency or resistance, renin will be elevated.

Differential Diagnosis of the Hypokalemic Disorders

Hypokalemia, defined as a serum K$^+$ less than 3.5 mEq/L, is one of the most common electrolyte abnormalities faced in the PICU, and is generally less threatening than hyperkalemia. Serum values for K$^+$ can be low due to total body deficiency or, more commonly, due to conditions that result in the intracellular shift of extracellular K$^+$. Nevertheless, low K$^+$ levels can be associated with cardiac dysrhythmias, particularly in the setting of preexisting cardiac dysfunction, or in patients receiving digoxin. ECG changes include flattening or inversion of T waves, ST depression, and development of U waves (see **Fig. 107.14**). Ultimately, automatic dysrhythmias may occur. In general, no symptoms or only mild weakness are present due to decreased skeletal muscle excitability. Certainly, muscular weakness can be associated with ileus or respiratory difficulties. The disorders of hypokalemia are listed in **Table 107.6**.

Drugs are a frequent cause of mild hypokalemia. Loop diuretics (furosemide, bumetanide, ethacrynic acid), particularly if used in conjunction with thiazides, are the most common cause of PICU-associated hypokalemia (54). Other drugs responsible for hypokalemia, especially in the intensive care setting, include glucocorticoids, chemotherapeutic agents, and laxatives used chronically. β-adrenergic agonists (including inhaled β-agonists for bronchodilation as well as systemic sympathomimetics for hemodynamic support) and insulin cause an intracellular shift of K$^+$ from the extracellular space. Gastrointestinal disease

TABLE 107.6

HYPOKALEMIC CONDITIONS

Drugs: diuretics, chemotherapeutic agents (cis-platinum), amphotericin B, penicillin derivatives, β-adrenergic agonists, insulin, aminophylline
Gastrointestinal disease: severe diarrhea, emesis, nasogastric suctioning
Renal losses: metabolic alkalosis, diabetic ketoacidosis, proximal and distal renal tubular acidosis, hypomagnesemia, Bartter syndrome, Gitelman syndrome
Adrenal cortical excess
Primary aldosteronism
Hyporeninemic and Hyperreninemic syndromes
Hypokalemic periodic paralysis

with loss of K$^+$ in stool is also a frequent cause of mild hypokalemia. Children with malignancy are at particular risk for loss of K$^+$ due to gastrointestinal losses, either due to chemotherapy or due to the malignant process.

Primary adrenal cortical disease (adrenal tumors or Cushing disease) occurs frequently in children, and the signs and symptoms are generally quite evident. The incidence and findings are discussed in Chapter 105. Sporadic primary aldosteronism, which includes benign aldosterone-secreting tumors and bilateral adrenal hyperplasia, is unlikely to occur in childhood. However, inherited disorders in the mineralocorticoid pathway are recognized. For instance, recessively inherited defects in 11-β-hydroxysteroid dehydrogenase type 2 cause low-renin hypertension and hypokalemia by interfering with inactivation of cortisol. Failure to inactivate cortisol to cortisone leads to excessive stimulation of the mineralocorticoid receptor by cortisol. In addition, defects in 11-β-hydroxylase cause a form of congenital adrenal hyperplasia that is associated not only with excessive androgen production but accumulation of deoxycorticosterone, a precursor to aldosterone. Deoxycorticosterone has significant mineralocorticoid activity and its accumulation leads to low-renin hypertension and hypokalemia.

Hypokalemic periodic paralysis arises from mutations in either the calcium (more common) or the Na$^+$ channel (53). Attacks are characterized by intermittent muscular weakness (particularly of the shoulders and hips) or generalized paralysis that lasts <24 hours; weakness that compromises breathing and swallowing has also been described. Those with calcium channel defects presented earlier and had more frequent attacks than those with mutations of the Na$^+$ channel.

Bartter syndrome is clinically recognized by failure to thrive, developmental delay, increased renin levels, hypokalemia, and alkalosis. Muscle weakness, muscle cramps, and salt craving may also be present. Hypertension and edema are absent. Hyperplasia of the juxtaglomerular cells, with elevated urinary excretion of prostaglandin E$_2$, is present. Genetic studies have identified four subtypes (55), with the most serious presenting before birth with polyhydramnios and premature delivery, and, immediately after birth, Na$^+$ chloride loss. All subtypes of Bartter syndrome are autosomal recessive in inheritance and are characterized by abnormal NaCl reabsorption in the ascending limb of the loop of Henle.

Gitelman syndrome was considered a variant of Bartter syndrome. Genetic studies now clearly define an autosomal recessive inherited disorder that is distinct from Bartter syndrome. Gitelman syndrome arises from mutations in the thiazide-sensitive Na$^+$ chloride cotransporter. Affected children do not have growth failure or developmental delay. This condition often presents later in childhood with hypokalemia, hypocalciuria, and, frequently, hypomagnesemia. These children characteristically have carpopedal spasm.

MANAGEMENT OF SODIUM AND POTASSIUM DISORDERS

In the pediatric critical care setting, the assessment and management of disorders of Na^+ and K^+ rely on timely clinical evaluations that utilize readily available laboratory tests and other technologies that will provide information rapidly. Genetic studies and the measurement of various hormones, peptides, and urinary metabolites, although important to obtain, often will not be immediately available or useful in the management of the critically ill child. Detailed and complete histories and physical examinations will often provide the information needed to judge the cause of the electrolyte disturbance and initiate resuscitation.

Management

Management of these disorders depends upon the severity of patient compromise and the duration of the water or electrolyte abnormality. The severity of clinical symptoms associated with these electrolyte disturbances depends on the rapidity of development. Management can be divided into resuscitation and maintenance therapies. In addition, management includes addressing the specific electrolyte/water abnormality, while also attending to the underlying cause of the abnormality. In the PICU setting, the intensivist is likely to be confronted with cardiovascular and neurologic compromise as a result of water and electrolyte disorders and be forced to address these issues while minimizing the risk of treatment-incurred complications.

Regardless of the underlying electrolyte abnormality, the dehydrated child requires fluid resuscitation. The initial volume to be administered will depend upon the extent of cardiovascular compromise and generally consists of isotonic solutions, such as 0.9% NaCl or lactated Ringer's solution. While a mildly dehydrated child may only require a 20 mL/kg bolus, repeated boluses may be required for the severely dehydrated child until the cardiovascular status is stabilized. Continued fluid therapy will then depend upon the child's cardiovascular status, remaining fluid deficit, and nature of the electrolyte abnormality. Traditionally, for greater than 50 years, maintenance fluid rates are prescribed based upon the studies of Holliday and Segar, in which fluid therapy is indexed to metabolic rate: 100 mL water/100 kcal/day (56). In general, 1000 mL is required for the first 10 kg, 500 mL for the next 10 kg, and 500 mL for the next 25 kg. Alternatively, maintenance fluids have been determined by providing 300–500 mL/m²/day for insensible fluid losses and an additional 1000 mL/m²/day for normal urine output. This can be adjusted based on the patient's current clinical state. For example, the patient with DI will require 300–500 mL/m²/day and fluid to match the excessive urine output to maintain euvolemia.

Hypernatremia

Hypernatremia with Hypovolemia. Following initial resuscitation with boluses and continuous infusions administered to restore perfusion and correct volume depletion, replacement therapy is required and must address the free water deficit in the child with persistent hypernatremia due to pure water loss or the Na^+ and water deficit, as occurs with hypotonic Na^+ loss. One can calculate the expected change in serum Na^+ with 1 L of a given fluid by the following equation:

Change in serum $[Na^+]$ for each liter of given fluid = (serum $[Na^+]$ – infusate $[Na^+]$)/(liters of total body water +1)

With the use of typical resuscitation fluids (0.9% NaCl), the plasma Na^+ is likely only to decrease slightly [for example,

1 L of 0.9% NaCl in a 30-kg child with total body water of 18 L (30 × 0.6) and plasma Na^+ of 165 will decrease the plasma Na^+ by (165 – 154)/(18 + 1) = 0.6 mEq/L]. Continued use of isotonic saline will not correct the hypernatremia, and a hypotonic solution must be introduced. In the child with known or presumed chronic hypernatremia, the subsequent goal of therapy is to decrease plasma Na^+ by ~0.5 mEq/L every hour (12 mEq/L/24 hours) to reduce the risk of rapid shifts of free water into the intracellular space, causing cerebral edema (57).

For patients with pure water loss (DI), (a) daily water and electrolyte requirements, (b) the free water deficit, and (c) ongoing losses are included in the calculations. For patients with pure water loss, the free water deficit can generally be calculated with the following equation:

$$\text{Free water deficit} = \text{TBWD} \times (\text{actual } [Na^+] - \text{desired } [Na^+])/\text{actual } [Na^+]$$

Or, this can be simplified, by using 140 mEq/L as the desired $[Na^+]$, to:

$$\text{Free water deficit} = \text{TBWD} \times [(\text{actual } [Na^+]/140) - 1]$$

The total body water distribution (TBWD) depends upon the age, gender, and weight of the child and is a product of the weight in kilograms and the water distribution. An extremely obese adolescent may have a water distribution of 0.5; 0.6 is frequently used for the adult male, 0.5 for the adult female, and 0.7 for infants. After the free water deficit is calculated, a desired correction period needs to be determined. The free water deficit can then be used to calculate the rate of free water replacement over the desired correction period. If possible, this free water should be delivered via the gastrointestinal tract, although critically ill children are often unable to safely receive enteral fluids. IV administration will require it to be administered with dextrose or a minimal amount of Na^+; this Na^+ may reflect the daily requirement infused in the water replacement plus the daily water requirement. For acutely acquired hypernatremia (over a few hours), the correction can occur more rapidly, as accumulation of "idiogenic" osmoles has not occurred. Large and rapid shifts occur commonly in the hospitalized child with DI, in whom vasopressin administration, as an infusion of vasopressin or as intermittent doses of vasopressin1-deamino (8-D-arginine) vasopressin (DDAVP), is delayed.

Continued losses must also be addressed. For the child with untreated DI, urine output will essentially reflect free water loss, which can be voluminous unless treated. For the child with central DI, institution of vasopressin by continuous infusion (starting IV infusion dose of 0.5 mU/kg/hour) will curb excessive losses. The continuous vasopressin infusion, with its short half-life of about 10 minutes, allows quick titration and avoids excessive urine output. DDAVP is avoided in the initial management because of its long half-life, preventing fine-tuning of fluid therapy. The use of vasopressin may dictate a recalculation of replacement fluids based upon either (a) normal maintenance fluids of 1500 mL/m²/day or (b) the previously outlined formula by Holliday et al. (56), both of which reflect insensible losses as well as normal urinary losses (not urinary losses under maximally antidiuresed states). In the completely antidiuresed state, maintenance fluid may be less than 50% of normal. For these reasons, calculating the fluid deficit, determining the amount to be replaced over a 24-hour period, establishing the desired positive fluid balance over 6–8-hour intervals, and examining the "ins and outs" and plasma Na^+ over these individual time frames will allow adequate fluid replacement and avoidance of overshooting the goal. For some patients, vasopressin is not an option. In such circumstances, urine output must be replaced with water. One-sixth normal saline (0.15% NaCl) may initially be used to replace hourly urine output. Measurement of urine Na^+ should follow, adjusting the Na$^+$ content of the administered fluid to match the approximate tonicity to maintain stable serum Na$^+$ levels. Again, fluid calculations must consider that usual maintenance fluid (1500 mL/m^2) includes urine output and insensible losses. If all urine output is to be replaced, then the maintenance component of the calculations must reflect insensible water losses only (300–500 mL/m^2/day) and daily electrolyte requirements. Also, additional sources of fluid need to be considered; for instance, antibiotics and other medications can be significant sources of fluid, and should not be ignored.

For the postoperative patient in whom DI is anticipated, urine output and plasma Na$^+$ are closely monitored. As patients frequently receive significant amounts of fluid intraoperatively, initial urine output often represents mobilization of these fluids rather than DI. Additionally, patients commonly receive high-dose glucocorticoids, which can provoke hyperglycemia and diuresis; thus, urine and blood glucose should be monitored. Once the diagnosis of DI is established postoperatively based upon excessive urine output and increasing serum Na$^+$, a continuous infusion of vasopressin can be initiated, as described previously. Again, fluid administration must be tailored to restore insensible fluid losses, replace ongoing urinary losses, and meet daily electrolyte requirements. During correction, frequent measures of serum Na$^+$, as often as every 2 hours, will allow for adjustments to maintain appropriate management. Excessively rapid Na$^+$ correction can lead to cerebral edema and devastating consequences. Patients who develop chronic DI can be managed with intermittent doses of DDAVP. Thiazides may also be used, due to their paradoxical antidiuresis effect (58).

For children with hypotonic Na$^+$ loss (i.e. severe diarrhea, vomitus, nasogastric or drain output), the just-mentioned free water deficit formula may underestimate their losses. The Adrogue–Madias formula calculates the amount that plasma Na$^+$ will drop following infusion of 1 L of fluid of varying components (2):

$$\frac{\text{Infusate [Na}^+\text{]} + \text{plasma [Na}^+\text{]}}{\text{TBWD} + \text{Wt (kg)} + \text{infusate volume (L)}}$$

For a 30-kg child with a TBWD of 0.6 and plasma Na$^+$ of 170 receiving 600 mL (0.6 L) of normal saline solution: (154 – 170)/[(0.6 × 30) + 0.6] = –0.86; the plasma Na$^+$ will decrease by 0.86 mEq/L, whereas use of 600 mL of half-normal saline solution (77 mEq/L) will decrease plasma Na$^+$ by 5 mEq/L. Additional loss must be addressed. For the child with severe diarrhea, vomitus, or nasogastric output, these losses will include water and other electrolytes, and additional fluid supplementation should reflect this fluid composition.

Hypernatremia with Euvolemia or Hypervolemia.
Hypernatremia with normal or overhydration arises from salt loading, as might occur in the child who receives excessive NaCl or sodium bicarbonate during resuscitation. Treatment requires the withdrawal of the Na$^+$ source and the addition of water. For more severely compromised patients with fluid overload, the addition of furosemide to increase Na$^+$ excretion and water may be indicated. The Adrogue–Madias formula, as detailed previously, has its limits but does provide a target for initiating fluid replacement therapy. For patients with renal failure, dialysis may be indicated. Again, close monitoring of serum electrolytes during correction will help prevent iatrogenic hyponatremia.

Hyponatremia

Patients with hyponatremia may present with a variety of total body fluid states, which is the primary physical assessment that is necessary to begin the investigation for the cause. History, including urine output, will often determine the fluid

status, but one cannot overemphasize the utility of the clinical exam. Determination of the hydration status will direct the evaluation as per **Figure 107.15**.

Hyponatremia with Hypovolemia.
With hyponatremic dehydration, the Na$^+$ deficit exceeds the free water deficit. The clinical presentation may largely reflect CNS irritability from hyponatremia or dehydration, and initial management should reflect attention to the clinical situation. CNS findings, such as seizure, frequently reflect an acute decrease in plasma Na$^+$. During an active seizure associated with acute hyponatremia, treatment considerations should include administration of 6 mL/kg of 3% NaCl to raise plasma Na$^+$ by ~5 mEq/L over 20–30 minutes. If no epileptic activity occurs and symptoms primarily reflect dehydration, normal saline solution should be administered; the plasma Na$^+$ will also increase with this step but to a much lesser extent. Again, following initial resuscitation, further correction of the fluid and Na$^+$ deficits must be addressed. Additionally, sources of free water should be discontinued. In general, if a patient has not had a seizure associated with the hyponatremia, it should be assumed that the development of hyponatremia has occurred over an extended period of time and thus should be corrected slowly. Maintenance Na$^+$ and water requirements should be calculated; Na$^+$ and water deficits should be estimated. The total Na$^+$ deficit (in mEq/L) can be calculated as (59):

$$(140 - \text{plasma [Na}^+\text{]}) \times (\text{TBWD} \times \text{Wt in kg})$$

Generally, half of the Na$^+$ deficit is replaced at a rate of 0.5 mEq/hour. Thus, the 30-kg child with a plasma [Na$^+$] of 120 and a distribution of water of 0.6 will have an Na$^+$ deficit of (140 – 120) × (0.6 × 30) = 360 mEq. To begin correcting this child's 20 mEq/L deficit, an initial correction of 10 mEq/L will be replaced at a rate of 0.5 mEq/hour; that is, over 20 hours. If 0.9% NaCl solution is used (154 mEq/L = 0.154 mEq/mL), the infusion rate necessary to correct half of the deficit is (180 mEq/0.154 mEq/mL)/20 hour = 58 mL/hour. Following institution of specific fluid rates and types, the effect of these therapies upon hydration and biochemical parameters must be reviewed every 4–6 hours and, as always, the child's clinical status must be continuously evaluated. Sources of continued salt loss should be investigated. For instance, the child with excessive salt losses from CSW may require additional salt replacement (which can be estimated from the amount of urinary Na$^+$ × the volume of urine). Plasma Na$^+$ in the child with adrenal insufficiency will improve with administration of salt-containing fluids, but initiation of glucocorticoids (which have mineralocorticoid activity at "stress" doses of 100 mg/m^2) and/or mineralocorticoids is also important for stabilization of the patient.

As with the correction of the hypernatremic state, care must be taken to correct the plasma Na$^+$ at the appropriate rate. In an asymptomatic child, the target rate of rise should not exceed 0.5–1 mEq/L per hour to avoid the risk of developing central pontine myelinolysis (CPM). This noninflammatory demyelinating disorder can present with spastic quadriplegia, pseudobulbar palsy, and encephalopathy (60). Hence, if abnormal Na$^+$ losses have abated, the previously healthy child does not require additional IV Na$^+$ replacement once the serum Na$^+$ has reached 130 mmol/L. At that point, normal renal Na$^+$ retention mechanisms are adequate to allow gradual return of serum Na$^+$ to a normal value.

Hyponatremia with Salt-wasting and Known Central DI.
Hyponatremia with salt-wasting and known central DI can be both a diagnostic and a therapeutic challenge. For the child with DI who has been overtreated with vasopressin and water, the salt wasting reflects a normal response to fluid overload, and withholding of fluids and additional vasopressin will permit diuresis and correction of the hyponatremic state. For the

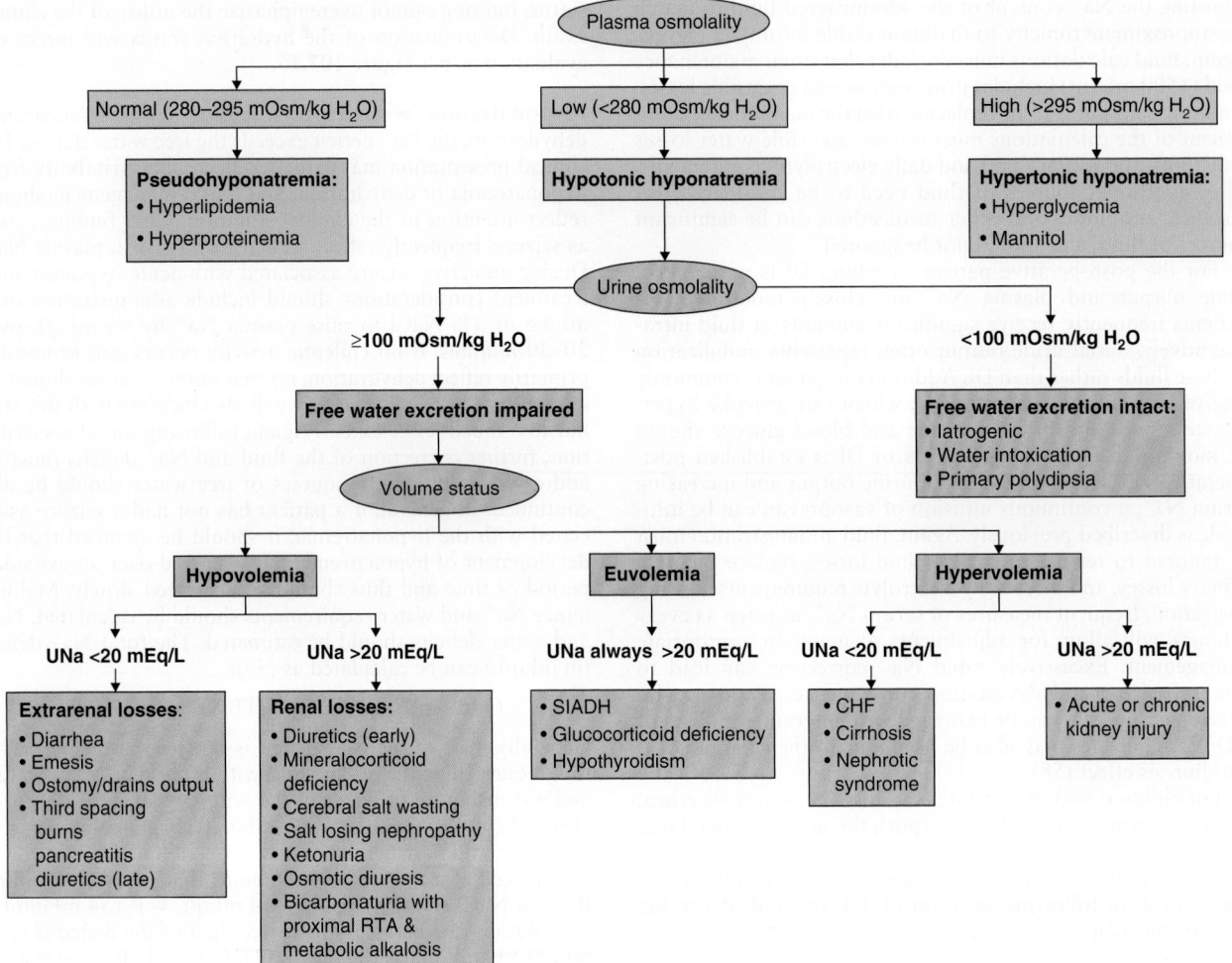

FIGURE 107.15. Diagnostic algorithm and differential diagnosis for hyponatremia (serum Na <135 mEq/L). UNa, urine sodium concentration; RTA, renal tubular acidosis; SIADH, syndrome of inappropriate antidiuretic hormone secretion; CHF, congestive heart failure.

child with DI and either concomitant CSW or natriuresis due to drug toxicity, the approach to hyponatremia can be more problematic. After initial resuscitation, the Na+ deficit should be determined and ongoing urinary Na+ losses should be calculated by measuring urine Na+ and volume. Vasopressin is withheld because it can potentiate hyponatremia. However, a vasopressin drip should be readily available at the bedside, as the waning effect of previously administered vasopressin/DDAVP and resolution of the salt-wasting state may be accompanied by excessive free water losses and rapid increases in plasma Na+. Frequent laboratory evaluations are necessary to avoid radical swings in plasma Na+ levels.

Hyponatremia with Euvolemia or Hypervolemia. This clinical scenario is almost always due to SIADH in critically ill children. It also arises in those with congestive heart failure, liver failure, or those on positive pressure ventilation. Due to changes in intrathoracic pressure and its effect on decreasing systemic venous return to the heart, ANP levels decrease with the use of positive pressure ventilation, leading to the common finding of hypervolemic hyponatremia in mechanically ventilated patients. As with hyponatremic dehydration, initial management depends upon clinical symptoms. Acute decreases in Na+ are associated with lethargy, disorientation, nauseas, vomiting, and muscle cramps. Seizures can develop when there is an acute drop in Na+ levels to less than 120 mEq/L. The

child with symptomatic hyponatremia will require infusion of hypertonic saline. Following initial resuscitation in the symptomatic child, water restriction alone or in combination with hypertonic Na+ chloride and a loop diuretic will increase Na+ without exacerbating the fluid-overloaded state. Those with hypervolemia interfering with adequate respiratory function may require the administration of diuretics. In addition, the underlying cause of the hyponatremia must be addressed. Care must be taken not to attempt to correct a low plasma Na+ level with sodium supplementation alone in the hypervolemic patient, such as with CHF or acute liver failure, as this may worsen the underlying condition, further exacerbate the overhydration, and further impinge upon the patient's stability. Excessive free water intake due to primary polydipsia or to overdiluted infant formula may respond to fluid restriction. However, caution must be taken so that withdrawal of the free water source does not cause over-rapid correction of the plasma Na+. In such cases, it may be necessary to administer hypotonic fluids to control the rate of plasma Na+ rise (59).

Recently, the administration of AVP receptor antagonists (vaptans) has gained attention as a possible therapy for hypervolemic hyponatremia. By blocking the AVP V2 receptor, vaptans enhance free water excretion while minimizing Na+ loss. This new class of medications is FDA-approved for the use in adults with euvolemic or hypervolemic hyponatremia and is most commonly prescribed for inpatient or outpatient treatment of SIADH. Zeltser (61) and Schrier (in the SALT trials) (62) demonstrated efficacy and safety in increasing serum Na^+ levels in adult patients with SIADH. In the "Efficacy of Vasopressin in Heart Failure Outcome Study with Tolvaptan" (EVEREST) trial, the use of tolvaptan safely improved the hyponatremia in adults with congestive heart failure, although no long-term outcome benefit (congestion symptoms, mortality) was identified (63,64). Jones (65) and Sahu (66) report the effective use of conivaptan for correction of severe hyponatremia in young children with congestive heart failure. It has also been reported as an important modality for enabling adequate hydration to prevent tumor lysis syndrome in an oncologic patient with SIADH (67). Although promising, subsequent clinical trials are necessary before routine use of vaptans will be recommended in children with hypervolemic or euvolemic hyponatremia.

Maintenance Fluids and Normal Serum Na^+. The commonly taught Holliday Segar method for the prescription of maintenance fluids in children is based on the daily losses of fluids and electrolytes from urine and insensible losses. However, recently, significant concern has been expressed that this methodology is flawed and inappropriate, as it does not take into consideration the physiologic differences of hospitalized children from the healthy children used to derive the formula. Children with illness requiring hospitalization have multiple nonosmotic factors leading to an excess in secretion of vasopressin, rendering the child unable to dilute urine appropriately. With the administration of hypotonic fluid according to the Holliday Segar formula, most hospitalized children are at significant risk for developing hyponatremia. Importantly, hyponatremia has been identified as an independent risk for increased morbidities, such as permanent brain injury, and mortality in adults (40) and chronically ill or previously healthy children (43,45,68). The use of hypotonic fluids has been shown repeatedly to cause hyponatremia, and is the most important risk factor for the development of hospital-acquired hyponatremia (32,39). In fact, up to 21% of intensive care unit (34) and 41% of postoperative pediatric patients (39,50) have been shown to develop hyponatremia within 24 hours while receiving hypotonic maintenance fluids. Therefore, it has been suggested that these solutions should only be reserved for patients with free water losses (48). Multiple studies have confirmed that the administration of isotonic fluids (i.e., 0.9% NaCl [normal saline]) at maintenance rates prevents the development of hyponatremia (33,34,50). Isotonic maintenance fluids suppress the release of vasopressin and reduce the risk of hyponatremia (69,70). Interestingly, using hypotonic solutions has been identified as the cause of hyponatremia despite normal levels of circulating vasopressin (49). Interestingly, patients on positive pressure mechanical ventilation do not appear to be at increased risk of developing hyponatremia due to free water retention (39,40). The theoretical risks of using isotonic solutions, such as thrombophlebitis, hypertension, or developing hypernatremia, have not been shown to be clinically relevant, supporting the safety of their use as maintenance fluids (32–34).

Hyperkalemia

Hyperkalemia brings the cell membrane potential closer to the threshold for cell membrane depolarization and thus is a significant risk for cardiac conduction abnormalities and muscle weakness/paralysis. When K^+ level is less than 6.5 mEq/L without changes in the ECG, it may only be necessary to discontinue exogenous sources of potassium and medications that limit its excretion, followed by meticulous follow-up. Initial treatment of hyperkalemia in the setting of cardiac conduction abnormalities is two-pronged: stabilize the cell membrane electrical potential and acutely lower the plasma K^+ through redistribution. The former is achieved through administration of 10% (1 g calcium/10 mL) calcium gluconate, 1.0 mL/kg (100 mg/kg) IV over 2–3 minutes (and has been suggested to occur over 20–30 minutes in the setting of digitalis toxicity). Calcium infusion can be repeated in 5 minutes if ECG abnormalities persist. As to the second prong, rapid IV infusion of glucose (0.5–1 g/kg) and regular insulin (0.2 units/g glucose or 0.1–0.2 units/kg) will lower plasma K^+ within 10–20 minutes, with a peak effect between 30 and 60 minutes. IV dextrose should be continued and blood glucose tested to monitor for the development of hypoglycemia or hyperglycemia. Treatment with inhaled β-adrenergic agonists is recommended in adults, and some centers follow this recommendation; however, data are limited in children. A third prong to the treatment of hyperkalemia is the definitive removal of plasma K^+. This can be accomplished with sodium polystyrene sulfonate (Kayexalate), 1 g/kg orally or by rectum in sorbitol solution, if indicated and if not contraindicated by bowel pathology. Loop or thiazide diuretics are useful to increase renal excretion and thus should be considered early in therapy. In the setting of renal failure, dialysis may be required. Data on treatment of hyperkalemia with Na^+ bicarbonate are equivocal, and it is therefore not recommended as monotherapy, although it may have a role in the setting of severe metabolic acidosis or hyperkalemic cardiac arrest (71–73).

Hypokalemia

Management of hypokalemia depends upon the acuity of symptoms and the underlying etiology. The child with hypokalemia-induced paralysis or with hypokalemia-induced ECG changes requires urgent IV treatment (0.5 mEq/kg over 30–60 minutes by continuous IV infusion) and frequent assessments to monitor the response. The child who is on digoxin or has an underlying cardiac defect is at increased risk of dysrhythmias and may require IV treatment at higher doses (1 mEq/kg) and at higher plasma K^+ concentrations. Magnesium replacement may also be necessary to treat hypokalemia.

The child with hypokalemia in the setting of DKA also requires aggressive attention, as glucose and insulin administration will drive K^+ intracellularly and aggravate hypokalemia. In fact, the child in DKA represents a special situation that the intensivist will frequently encounter. K^+ is delivered at higher-than-usual rates (provided that the child is urinating) in the setting of normal plasma K^+ concentrations because, despite significant total body K^+ deficits, the plasma K^+ is normal or elevated as a result of insulin deficiency and the concomitant metabolic acidosis. The K^+ can be administered as a combination of K^+ chloride and K^+ phosphate, as the child with DKA also has a phosphorus deficit. If hypokalemia develops during the course of DKA treatment, and hyperglycemia and acidosis have nearly resolved, lowering the insulin infusion rate will help to address the hypokalemia.

In the PICU setting, mild, asymptomatic deficits are treated slowly with increased IV K^+ supplementation or, if possible, oral replacement. The child on chronic diuretics may need to have these reassessed or have chronic K^+ supplementation initiated.

OUTCOMES: MORBIDITY AND MORTALITY

A discussion of morbidity and mortality is an important exercise as a means by which to determine how clinicians can improve outcome. However, the disorders of water, Na^+, and K^+ do not occur without underlying processes that alter the protective physiologic homeostatic mechanisms meant to prevent dehydration and electrolyte disturbance, and the underlying disease process is often a major contributor to outcome data. Examples of such conditions include DKA, adrenal crisis, acute kidney injury, severe burns, or cystic fibrosis. The outcome in many conditions, therefore, is often related to the homeostatic disturbances of water and electrolytes and to a number of other factors related to the underlying disease. The mortality and morbidity of the various specific conditions that commonly present with disturbed fluid and electrolyte homeostasis are discussed in the chapters pertaining to the respective diseases.

The studies that document outcomes of fluid and electrolyte disturbances generally do not exclude underlying diseases, but they review the outcomes in particular settings, such as intensive care, postoperative care, or inpatient care. Both hypernatremia and hyponatremia have been identified as independently associated with increased mortality and morbidities. Wald identified in greater than 50,000 adult admissions that community-acquired hyponatremia occurred in about 38% and hospital-acquired in about 38%, both of which were independently associated with increased mortality and length of stay (74). This group found a linear increase in mortality with decreases in serum Na^+ levels below 138 mmol/L, although this relationship has not been consistently reported in other literature. The study by Arieff (43) evaluated healthy children admitted for elective surgery to one center over a 6-year period and ascertained that the incidence of hyponatremia was 0.34% (83 of 24,412 consecutively admitted patients), and, of these patients, 7 children (8.4%) died. This study concluded, based upon a prospectively studied group of 16 hyponatremic patients (evaluated by the authors from multiple centers), that the hyponatremia was caused by extrarenal losses and replacement with hypotonic saline. These data indicate that the higher incidence of hyponatremia seen in the hospital setting may reflect the morbidity associated with underlying conditions. A study of 11,702 admissions to one pediatric center over 1 year found that the incidence of hyponatremia (defined as serum Na^+ less than 130 mmol/L) was 1.38%, 57% of which developed while in the hospital; 37 of these 161 cases were otherwise previously healthy children (75). The authors concluded that adverse outcomes, neurologic deficits (3.7%), and death (12%, but many deaths occurred well after correction of hyponatremia) in their study were more closely related to the underlying condition rather than to hyponatremia or its correction. Unfortunately, this study did not provide sufficient information as to the underlying conditions or sufficient data to support the reasoning as to why they suggested that the underlying conditions dictated prognosis. However, multiple studies that have evaluated hyponatremia indicate that hyponatremia in the hospital setting occurs "commonly," a finding no doubt related to the fact that children are admitted to the hospital (and especially the PICU) because of associated severe acute and chronic disease and exposure to drugs, which frequently cause disturbances of water, Na^+, and K^+. Further, as previously discussed, elevated levels of vasopressin are common in critically ill children and lead to the inability to adequately dilute urine, and predispose to hyponatremia. Hasegawa noted that 18% of children admitted to non-intensive care units have hyponatremia on admission; a significant proportion of these children were admitted with a febrile illness (76) and almost all had elevated levels of vasopressin. Moreover, hyponatremia appears to be even more common in critically ill children and is most commonly hospital-acquired. Montanana reported an incidence of hospital-associated hyponatremia of 21% in 121 PICU patients. This hyponatremia was attributed to the provision of hypotonic fluids as maintenance fluid therapy within 24 hours of ICU admission (34). Of 81 postoperative PICU patients with normal baseline serum Na^+, Eulmesekian reported hyponatremia within 24 hours after admission in 31% (39).

Identifying and preventing hyponatremia is of utmost importance as mortality and morbidity increase significantly in hyponatremic patients. Hanna identified a significant incidence of hyponatremia on admission in critically ill children with bronchiolitis, some of whom developed hyponatremic seizures (44). Hyponatremia often develops during hospitalization of bronchiolitic patients, and is associated with prolonged length of PICU stay (39). Halberthal analyzed all children diagnosed with hyponatremia over a 10-year period, and reported that more than half became symptomatic requiring PICU transfer; more alarming was the 20% mortality rate (68). Children with end-stage liver disease awaiting transplant and who remain hyponatremic for at least 7 days have a significantly increased risk of mortality (41). In preterm neonates, hyponatremia seems to be associated with significant deleterious consequences, such as impaired growth, worse neurodevelopment, sensorineural hearing loss, cerebral palsy, and increased mortality (77).

Although less common, hypernatremia is a clinically important metabolic derangement that should not be overlooked. Historically, hypernatremia is more commonly encountered in infants with diarrheal dehydration, but hypernatremia in pediatric inpatients is also commonly associated with inadequate fluid intake in children with chronic medical conditions, particularly those with neurocognitive impairment (31). Hypernatremia (defined as serum Na^+ greater than 150 mEq/L) was identified in 0.22% of 32,000 children admitted to a large tertiary children's hospital; the majority had been admitted for reasons other than hypernatremia. In those in which the hypernatremia was not corrected, mortality was significantly higher. Fifteen percent developed acute or chronic neurologic complications attributed to the hypernatremia (31). Forman identified a 0.04% incidence of hypernatremia in a 10-year study of over 100,000 pediatric admissions; most of the hypernatremia developed during the course of the hospitalization (30). Although mortality was higher in those with hypernatremia, the mortality was not thought to be directly related to the hypernatremia, rather to the underlying morbidity that led to the hypernatremia. Specifically, a high percentage of patients with cerebral palsy composed the cohort of hypernatremic patients. In adult ICU patients, hypernatremia has been associated with increased length of stay and mortality (78,79).

A review of Na^+ disturbances emphasizes that the more common underlying conditions that predispose to hyponatremia during fluid therapy are those with impaired renal water excretion; and, therefore, the use of hypotonic saline solution for resuscitation and maintenance frequently results in hyponatremia (80). The morbidity from hyponatremia is such that >50% (with serum Na^+ <125 mEq/L) will develop encephalopathy. Postoperative patients have a number of factors predisposing to hyponatremia during fluid therapy, including pain, subclinical hypovolemia, and medications that stimulate vasopressin release and, therefore, are susceptible to development of hyponatremia with hypotonic fluid administration. However, although strong proponents of isotonic saline (and even hypertonic saline in certain conditions, such as CSW) for resuscitation and maintenance, the authors also note that hypernatremia is not without neurologic sequelae and death (31,83). The mortality attributed to hypernatremia was 16%, and neurologic complications were noted in 15% of patients (31). This review allows for the use of hypotonic solutions in certain circumstances, especially when fluid volume has been restored and maintained in patients but hypernatremia persists or in the circumstances of ongoing hypotonic fluid losses. The consequences of prolonged hypernatremia include shrinkage of brain volume that can result in cerebral demyelinating lesions, cavernous sinus thrombosis, and rhabdomyolysis. Although demyelinating lesions have generally been associated with hyponatremia, the finding of CPM in severely burned patients who had suffered hyperosmolality, including hypernatremia, suggested that hypernatremia could lead to this neurologic lesion (81). Although uncommon, additional cases of myelinolysis in adults (82,83) and children (29,84–86) in association with hypernatremia make this neurologic insult a real concern in the setting of hypernatremia. Demyelination of brain due to prolonged hypernatremia has been demonstrated in rats and has been attributed to hyperosmolality, although the underlying pathology for this condition remains unclear (87).

Much less pediatric data in terms of incidence, morbidity, and mortality are available for disorders of K^+ in children, as compared with Na^+ disturbances. Hypokalemia has been identified in 3.6% (88) to 14.8% (54) in critically ill children, while hyperkalemia has been reported to occur in 14.4% (88). Potassium abnormalities were associated with both higher mortality and increased length of stay (54,88). Recently, a study of 667 tertiary PICU admissions identified 19% admitted to the PICU with hypokalemia and 12% with hyperkalemia, and the majority of these potassium disorders were mild (89). During the course of PICU hospitalization, 40% of patients developed hypokalemia and 29% hyperkalemia. Severity of hypokalemia was not associated with increased mortality after adjustment for important covariates. Nonetheless, both elevated and low K^+ levels occurring during PICU hospitalization were associated with longer PICU length of stay (89). A study of adult and pediatric patients hospitalized in a university setting found that severe hypokalemia occurred in 2.6% of yearly hospitalizations and that the death rate was 20.4% or 10-fold greater in patients with hypokalemia than that of the entire hospitalized population (89). However, only 11.2% of the patients with hypokalemia were pediatric patients, and the odds ratio for death in children from hypokalemia was 1.00.

It is estimated that the incidence of hyperkalemia in hospitalized patients is 1%–10%, but to what degree spurious hyperkalemia influences the estimate of incidence is not clear. In the Cummings study, 24% of all hyperkalemic samples and almost half of the moderate-to-severe values were due to hemolysis (89). Of these, a significant number were normal values when redrawn. From this data, consideration of retesting when a significant elevation of K^+ is encountered seems appropriate.

The quest to improve outcome by retrospective evaluation of therapy and morbidity and mortality is standard medical practice. In disorders of water and electrolytes, the evaluation therapy in terms of morbidity and mortality is no minor issue. The general consensus is that resuscitation, especially in the dehydrated state, requires careful fluid management and avoidance of the use of hypotonic fluid replacement to prevent iatrogenic hyponatremia. However, a degree of controversy exists as to the appropriate use of hypotonic fluid for maintenance fluid therapy, as originally described by Holliday et al. (56). Montanana (34), Rey (91), and Neville (33) have all shown that the use of isotonic saline rather than hypotonic fluids for maintenance therapy prevents hyponatremia in hospitalized children. Nevertheless, in a recent survey of US pediatric residents, hypotonic maintenance fluids were selected in 78% of the cases (92,93). We cannot ignore, that hypernatremia, especially after fluid volume has been restored, is also life- and brain-threatening (31,83). Holiday et al. would argue that a physiologic approach to maintenance therapy is still appropriate (94). The therapeutic management discussed previously is an attempt to approach resuscitation and maintenance therapy, allowing for some clinical judgment and interventions that are not simply based upon formulas or dogmatic algorithms.

CONCLUSIONS AND FUTURE DIRECTIONS

In conclusion, disorders of water, Na^+, and K^+ homeostasis occur commonly in children in the PICU. Often, these disturbances are associated with underlying conditions that perturb the mechanisms that regulate water and electrolyte homeostasis. At present, the evaluation, management, and therapeutic modalities rely on knowledge of the physiology and potential pathology, with superb clinical judgment and the use of relatively few technical or biochemical modalities. As well, newer pharmacologic therapies based upon even better understanding of mechanisms that regulate water, Na^+, and K^+ homeostasis will allow newer therapeutic strategies.

The new information regarding water, Na^+, and K^+ abnormalities will provide further recognition of the underlying biochemical and genetic disturbances responsible for, or contributing to, these abnormalities. The identification of additional pathways will then provide the foundation for development of diagnostic and therapeutic strategies that may apply to numerous other disease states.

As an example, in congestive heart failure, co-activation of volume overload and volume-depleted response mechanisms occurs: cardiac release of ANP and BNP in response to atrial and ventricular stretch is accompanied by baroreceptor-mediated activation of vasopressin secretion, the sympathetic nervous system, and RAAS. As congestive heart failure progresses, the "volume-depleted" anti-natriuretic and vasoconstrictive responses predominate, and fluid overload ensues. However, traditional treatment of the fluid-overloaded state with diuretics can (a) further activate the sympathetic nervous system and RAAS, and (b) exacerbate hyponatremia. Thus, alternative medications for the treatment are being investigated.

The development of vasopressin-2 receptor antagonists, such as conivaptan and tolvaptan, has a potentially important role in hyponatremia. These agents prevent water reabsorption at the level of the kidney without natriuresis, thus offering removal of excessive water without the hyponatremia that frequently accompanies diuresis. These agents may have a role in the treatment of congestive heart failure and chronic SIADH, but further pediatric investigation is needed.

While much has been learned about the genetics and pathophysiology of disturbances of water, Na^+, and K^+ homeostasis, the challenge remains to understand the development and prevention of their complications.

References

1. Robertson G, Athar S. The interaction of blood osmolality and blood volume in regulating plasma vasopressin in man. *J Clin Endocrinol Metab* 1976;42:613–20.
2. Verbalis JG. Disorders of body water homeostasis. *Best Pract Res Clin Endocrinol Metab* 2003;17:471–503.
3. Voisin DL, Bourque CW. Integration of sodium and osmosensory signals in vasopressin neurons. *Trends Neurosci* 2002;25:199–205.
4. Robertson GL. Antidiuretic hormone. Normal and disordered function. *Endocrinol Metab Clin North Am* 2001;30:671–94, vii.
5. Antunes-Rodrigues J, de Castro M, Elias LL, et al. Neuroendocrine control of body fluid metabolism. *Physiol Rev* 2004;84:169–208.
6. Lim G, Lee M, Kim HS, et al. Hyponatremia and syndrome of inappropriate antidiuretic hormone secretion in kawasaki disease. *Korean Circ J* 2010;40:507–13.
7. van Steensel-Moll H, Hazelzet J, Van der Voort E, et al. Excessive secretion of antidiuretic hormone in infections with respiratory syncytial virus. *Arch Dis Child* 1990;65:1237–39.
8. Rivers R, Forsling ML, Olver RP. Inappropriate secretion of antidiuretic hormone in infants with respiratory infections. *Arch Dis Child* 1981;56:358–63.
9. Lieh-Lai MW, Stanitski DF, Sarnaik AP, et al. Syndrome of inappropriate antidiuretic hormone secretion in children following spinal fusion. *Crit Care Med* 1999;27:622–27.

10. Bell GR, Gurd AR, Orlowski JP, et al. The syndrome of inappropriate antidiuretic-hormone secretion following spinal fusion. *J Bone Joint Surg Am* 1986;68:720–24.

11. Elster AD. Hyponatremia after spinal fusion caused by inappropriate secretion of antidiuretic hormone (SIADH). *Clin Orthop Relat Res* 1985;(194):136–41.

12. Lodha R, Vivekanandhan S, Sarthi M, et al. Serial circulating vasopressin levels in children with septic shock. *Pediatr Crit Care Med* 2006;7:220–24.

13. Leclerc F, Walter-Nicolet E, Leteurtre S, et al. Admission plasma vasopressin levels in children with meningococcal septic shock. *Intensive Care Med* 2003;29:1339–44.

14. Lee JH, Chan YH, Lai OF, et al. Vasopressin and copeptin levels in children with sepsis and septic shock. *Intensive Care Med* 2013;39:747–53.

15. Sharshar T, Blanchard A, Paillard M, et al. Circulating vasopressin levels in septic shock. *Crit Care Med* 2003;31:1752–58.

16. Sands JM. Mammalian urea transporters. *Annu Rev Physiol* 2003;65:543–66.

17. McKinley MJ, Johnson AK. The physiological regulation of thirst and fluid intake. *Physiology* 2004;19:1–6.

18. Stricker EM, Sved AF. Thirst. *Nutrition* 2000;16:821–26.

19. Fitzsimons J. Angiotensin, thirst, and sodium appetite. *Physiol Rev* 1998;78:583–686.

20. DiBona GF. Nervous kidney interaction between renal sympathetic nerves and the renin-angiotensin system in the control of renal function. *Hypertension* 2000;36:1083–88.

21. Suttner SW, Boldt J. Natriuretic peptide system: Physiology and clinical utility. *Curr Opin Crit Care* 2004;10:336–41.

22. Maher KO, Reed H, Cuadrado A, et al. B-type natriuretic peptide in the emergency diagnosis of critical heart disease in children. *Pediatrics* 2008;121:e1484–88.

23. Koulouri S, Acherman R, Wong P, et al. Utility of B-type natriuretic peptide in differentiating congestive heart failure from lung disease in pediatric patients with respiratory distress. *Pediatr Cardiol* 2004;25:341–46.

24. Hsu J, Keller RL, Chikovani O, et al. B-type natriuretic peptide levels predict outcome after neonatal cardiac surgery. *J Thorac Cardiovasc Surg* 2007;134:939–45.

25. Chikovani O, Hsu J, Keller R, et al. B-type natriuretic peptide levels predict outcomes for children on extracorporeal life support after cardiac surgery. *J Thorac Cardiovasc Surg* 2007;134:1179–87.

26. Pasantes-Morales H, Franco R, Torres-Marquez ME, et al. Amino acid osmolytes in regulatory volume decrease and isovolumetric regulation in brain cells: Contribution and mechanisms. *Cell Physiol Biochem* 2001;10:361–70.

27. Ordaz B, Tuz K, Ochoa LD, et al. Osmolytes and mechanisms involved in regulatory volume decrease under conditions of sudden or gradual osmolarity decrease. *Neurochem Res* 2004;29:65–72.

28. Adrogue HJ, Chap Z, Ishida T, et al. Role of the endocrine pancreas in the kalemic response to acute metabolic acidosis in conscious dogs. *J Clin Invest* 1985;75:798.

29. Brown J, Cohen P, Johnson JG, et al. A longitudinal analysis of risk factors for child maltreatment: Findings of a 17-year prospective study of officially recorded and self-reported child abuse and neglect. *Child Abuse Negl* 1998;22(11):1065–78.

30. Forman S, Crofton P, Huang H, et al. The epidemiology of hypernatraemia in hospitalised children in lothian: A 10-year study showing differences between dehydration, osmoregulatory dysfunction and salt poisoning. *Arch Dis Child* 2012;97:502–7.

31. Moritz ML, Ayus JC. The changing pattern of hypernatremia in hospitalized children. *Pediatrics* 1999;104:435–9.

32. Choong K, Kho ME, Menon K, et al. Hypotonic versus isotonic saline in hospitalised children: A systematic review. *Arch Dis Child* 2006;91:828–35.

33. Neville KA, Verge CF, Rosenberg AR, et al. Isotonic is better than hypotonic saline for intravenous rehydration of children with gastroenteritis: A prospective randomised study. *Arch Dis Child* 2006;91:226–32.

34. Montanana PA, i Alapont VM, Ocon AP, et al. The use of isotonic fluid as maintenance therapy prevents iatrogenic hyponatremia in pediatrics: A randomized, controlled open study. *Pediatr Crit Care Med* 2008;9:589–97.

35. Weese-Mayer DE, Berry-Kravis EM, Marazita ML. In pursuit (and discovery) of a genetic basis for congenital central hypoventilation syndrome. *Respir Physiol Neurobiol* 2005;149:73–82.

36. Katz ES, McGrath S, Marcus CL. Late-onset central hypoventilation with hypothalamic dysfunction: A distinct clinical syndrome. *Pediatr Pulmonol* 2000;29:62–8.

37. Winters RW. *The Body Fluids in Pediatrics: Medical, Surgical, and Neonatal Disorders of Acid-Base Status, Hydration, and Oxygenation.* 1st ed. Boston, MA: Little, Brown Medical Division, 1973.

38. Eulmesekian PG, Perez A, Minces PG, et al. Hospital-acquired hyponatremia in postoperative pediatric patients: Prospective observational study. *Pediatr Crit Care Med* 2010;11:479–83.

39. Seifert ME, Welak SR, Carroll CL. Hyponatremia is associated with increased severity of disease in critically ill children with bronchiolitis open access. *Int J Clin Med* 2010;1:37–40.

40. Wald R, Jaber BL, Price LL, et al. Impact of hospital-associated hyponatremia on selected outcomes. *Arch Intern Med* 2010;170:294.

41. Carey RG, Bucuvalas JC, Balistreri WF, et al. Hyponatremia increases mortality in pediatric patients listed for liver transplantation. *Pediatr Transplant* 2010;14:115–20.

42. Kim WR, Biggins SW, Kremers WK, et al. Hyponatremia and mortality among patients on the liver-transplant waiting list. *N Engl J Med* 2008;359:1018–26.

43. Arieff AI, Ayus JC, Fraser CL. Hyponatraemia and death or permanent brain damage in healthy children. *BMJ* 1992;304:1218.

44. Hanna S, Tibby S, Durward A, et al. Incidence of hyponatraemia and hyponatraemic seizures in severe respiratory syncytial virus bronchiolitis. *Acta Paediatr* 2003;92:430–4.

45. Playfor S. Fatal iatrogenic hyponatraemia. *Arch Dis Child* 2003;88:646.

46. Moritz ML, Ayus JC. Prevention of hospital-acquired hyponatremia: A case for using isotonic saline. *Pediatrics* 2003;111:227–30.

47. Hoorn EJ, Geary D, Robb M, et al. Acute hyponatremia related to intravenous fluid administration in hospitalized children: An observational study. *Pediatrics* 2004;113:1279–84.

48. Moritz ML, Ayus JC. Hospital-acquired hyponatremia—Why are hypotonic parenteral fluids still being used? *Nat Clin Pract Nephrol* 2007;3:374–82.

49. Choong K, Arora S, Cheng J, et al. Hypotonic versus isotonic maintenance fluids after surgery for children: A randomized controlled trial. *Pediatrics* 2011;128:857–66.

50. Yee AH, Burns JD, Wijdicks EF. Cerebral salt wasting: Pathophysiology, diagnosis, and treatment. *Neurosurg Clin* 2010;21:339.

51. Acker CG, Johnson JP, Palevsky PM, et al. Hyperkalemia in hospitalized patients: Causes, adequacy of treatment, and results of an attempt to improve physician compliance with published therapy guidelines. *Arch Intern Med* 1998;158:917.

52. Sevastos N, Theodossiades G, Archimandritis AJ. Pseudohyperkalemia in serum: A new insight into an old phenomenon. *Clin Med Res* 2008;6:30–2.

53. Miller T, Da Silva MD, Miller H, et al. Correlating phenotype and genotype in the periodic paralyses. *Neurology* 2004;63:1647–55.

54. Singhi S, Marudkar A. Hypokalemia in a pediatric intensive care unit. *Indian Pediatr* 1996;33:9–14.

55. Proesmans W. Threading through the mizmaze of bartter syndrome. *Pediatr Nephrol* 2006;21:896–902.

56. Holliday MA, Segar WE. The maintenance need for water in parenteral fluid therapy. *Pediatrics* 1957;19:823–832.

57. Adrogué HJ, Madias NE. Hypernatremia. *N Engl J Med* 2000;342:1493–9.

58. Loffing J. Paradoxical antidiuretic effect of thiazides in diabetes insipidus: Another piece in the puzzle. *J Am Soc Nephrol* 2004;15:2948–50.

59. Adrogué HJ, Madias NE. Hyponatremia. *N Engl J Med* 2000;342:1581–89.

60. Pearce J. Central pontine myelinolysis. *Eur Neurol* 2009;61:59–62.

61. Zeltser D, Rosansky S, van Rensburg H, et al. Assessment of the efficacy and safety of intravenous conivaptan in euvolemic and hypervolemic hyponatremia. *Am J Nephrol* 2007;27:447–57.

62. Schrier RW, Gross P, Gheorghiade M, et al. Tolvaptan, a selective oral vasopressin V2-receptor antagonist, for hyponatremia. *N Engl J Med* 2006;355:2099–112.

63. Gheorghiade M, Konstam MA, Burnett JC Jr, et al. Short-term clinical effects of tolvaptan, an oral vasopressin antagonist, in patients hospitalized for heart failure. *JAMA* 2007;297:1332–1343.

64. Konstam MA, Gheorghiade M, Burnett JC Jr, et al. Effects of oral tolvaptan in patients hospitalized for worsening heart failure. *JAMA* 2007;297:1319–1331.

65. Jones RC, Rajasekaran S, PharmD MR, et al. Initial experience with conivaptan use in critically ill infants with cardiac disease. *J Pediatr Pharmacol Ther* 2012;17:78–83.

66. Sahu R, Balaguru D, Thapar V, et al. Conivaptan therapy in an infant with severe hyponatremia and congestive heart failure. *Texas Heart Inst J* 2012;39:724.

67. Rianthavorn P, Cain JP, Turman MA. Use of conivaptan to allow aggressive hydration to prevent tumor lysis syndrome in a pediatric patient with large-cell lymphoma and SIADH. *Pediatr Nephrol* 2008;23:1367–70.

68. Halberthal M, Halperin ML, Bohn D. Lesson of the week: Acute hyponatraemia in children admitted to hospital: Retrospective analysis of factors contributing to its development and resolution. *BMJ* 2001;322:780.

69. Powell KR, Sugarman LI, Eskenazi AE, et al. Normalization of plasma arginine vasopressin concentrations when children with meningitis are given maintenance plus replacement fluid therapy. *J Pediatr* 1990;117:515–22.

70. Brazel PW, McPhee IB. Inappropriate secretion of antidiuretic hormone in postoperative scoliosis patients: The role of fluid management. *Spine* 1996;21:724–27.

71. Mahoney B, Smith W, Lo D, et al. Emergency interventions for hyperkalaemia. *Cochrane Database Syst Rev* 2005;(2):CD003235.

72. Elliott MJ, Ronksley PE, Clase CM, et al. Management of patients with acute hyperkalemia. *Can Med Assoc J* 2010;182:1631–35.

73. Evans KJ, Greenberg A. Hyperkalemia: A review. *J Intensive Care Med* 2005;20:272–90.

74. Wald R, Jaber BL, Price LL, et al. Impact of hospital-associated hyponatremia on selected outcomes. *Arch Intern Med* 2010;170:294.

75. Wattad A, Chiang ML, Hill LL. Hyponatremia in hospitalized children. *Clin Pediatr* 1992;31:153–7.

76. Hasegawa H, Okubo S, Ikezumi Y, et al. Hyponatremia due to an excess of arginine vasopressin is common in children with febrile disease. *Pediatr Nephrol* 2009;24:507–11

77. Moritz ML, Ayus JC. Hyponatremia in preterm neonates: Not a benign condition. *Pediatrics* 2009;124:e1014–16.

78. Waite MD, Fuhrman SA, Badawi O, et al. Intensive care unit–acquired hypernatremia is an independent predictor of increased mortality and length of stay. *J Crit Care* 2013;28:405–12.

79. Stelfox H, Ahmed S, Khandwala F, et al. The epidemiology of intensive care unit-acquired hyponatraemia and hypernatraemia in medical-surgical intensive care units. *Crit Care* 2008;12:R162.

80. Moritz ML, Ayus JC. Preventing neurological complications from dysnatremias in children. *Pediatr Nephrol* 2005;20:1687–700.

81. McKee AC, Winkelman MD, Banker BQ. Central pontine myelinolysis in severely burned patients relationship to serum hyperosmolality. *Neurology* 1988;38:1211–7.

82. Clark W. Diffuse demyelinating lesions of the brain after the rapid development of hypernatremia. *West J Med* 1992;157:571.

83. McComb RD, Pfeiffer RF, Casey JH, et al. Lateral pontine and extrapontine myelinolysis associated with hypernatremia and hyperglycemia. *Clin Neuropathol* 1989;8:284–8.

84. AlOrainy I, O'Gorman A, Decell M. Cerebral bleeding, infarcts, and presumed extrapontine myelinolysis in hypernatraemic dehydration. *Neuroradiology* 1999;41:144–6.

85. Brown WD, Caruso JM. Extrapontine myelinolysis with involvement of the hippocampus in three children with severe hypernatremia. *J Child Neurol* 1999;14:428–33.

86. Shah B, Tobias JD. Osmotic demyelination and hypertonic dehydration in a 9-year-old girl: Changes in cerebrospinal fluid myelin basic protein. *J Intensive Care Med* 2006;21:372–6.

87. Soupart A, Penninckx R, Namias B, et al. Brain myelinolysis following hypernatremia in rats. *J Neuropathol Exp Neurol* 1996;55:106–13.

88. Roa S, Thomas B. Electrolyte abnormalities in children admitted to pediatric intensive care unit. *Indian Pediatr* 2000;37:1348–53.

89. Cummings BM, Macklin EA, Yager PH, et al. Potassium abnormalities in a pediatric intensive care unit frequency and severity. *J Intensive Care Med* 2014;29(5):269–74.

90. Paltiel O, Salakhov E, Ronen I, et al. Management of severe hypokalemia in hospitalized patients: A study of quality of care based on computerized databases. *Arch Intern Med* 2001;161:1089.

94. Rey C, Los-Arcos M, Hernández A, et al. Hypotonic versus isotonic maintenance fluids in critically ill children: A multicenter prospective randomized study. *Acta Paediatr* 2011;100:1138–43.

95. Freeman MA, Ayus JC, Moritz ML. Maintenance intravenous fluid prescribing practices among paediatric residents. *Acta Paediatr* 2012;101:e465–68.

96. Friedman B, Cirulli J. Hyponatremia in critical care patients: Frequency, outcome, characteristics, and treatment with the vasopressin V2 receptor antagonist tolvaptan. *J Crit Care* 2013;28:219.e1–12.

97. Holliday MA, Friedman AL, Segar WE, et al. Acute hospital-induced hyponatremia in children: A physiologic approach. *J Pediatr* 2004;145:584–7.

98. O'Connor C, Starling R, Hernandez A, et al. Effect of nesiritide in patients with acute decompensated heart failure. *N Engl J Med* 2011;365:32–43.

99. Behera SK, Zuccaro JC, Wetzel GT, et al. Nesiritide improves hemodynamics in children with dilated cardiomyopathy: A pilot study. *Pediatr Cardiol* 2009;30:26–34.

100. Domico M, Checchia PA. Biomonitors of cardiac injury and performance: B-type natriuretic peptide and troponin as monitors of hemodynamics and oxygen transport balance. *Pediatr Crit Care Med* 2011;12:S33–42.

101. Reel B, Oishi PE, Hsu J, et al. Early elevations in B-type natriuretic peptide levels are associated with poor clinical outcomes in pediatric acute lung injury. *Pediatr Pulmonol* 2009;44:1118–24.

102. Amirnovin R, Keller RL, Herrera C, et al. B-type natriuretic peptide levels predict outcomes in infants undergoing cardiac surgery in a lesion-dependent fashion. *J Thorac Cardiovasc Surg* 2013;145:1279.

CHAPTER 108 ■ DISORDERS OF CALCIUM, MAGNESIUM, AND PHOSPHATE

KENNETH J. BANASIAK

KEY POINTS

1. Regulation of the serum concentration of calcium is the net sum of the interface between the circulation and three tissues: the intestines, bone, and kidneys.
2. The primary site of regulation of calcium is at the level of the intestine.
3. The primary site of regulation of phosphorus is the kidney.
4. Parathyroid hormone (PTH) and 1,25-dihydroxyvitamin D are the major hormonal regulators of calcium and phosphorus homeostasis.
5. Total serum calcium concentration ranges between 8.8 and 10.8 mg/dL and is 40% protein bound, 50% in a free ionized form, and 5%–10% complexed to small anions.
6. The ionized fraction of calcium is relevant with respect to clinical symptomatology and can be measured directly in the settings of hypoalbuminemia and acid–base disturbances.
7. Hypocalcemia may be manifest by neuromuscular irritability, tetany, seizures, and coma. Symptoms include lethargy, constipation, bone pain, and features of hypercalciuria (hematuria, dysuria, renal stones, and hyposthenuria). In infants, signs of hypocalcemia may be nonspecific, such as poor feeding.
8. Clinical findings of hypocalcemia include Chvostek and Trousseau signs.
9. An important step in assessment of calcium disorders is to determine whether they are PTH-dependent or -independent.
10. Phosphate is ubiquitous in the diet, and hypophosphatemia due to dietary causes is uncommon, except in breast-fed premature infants.
11. Hypophosphatemia is often due to primary renal losses or intracellular–extracellular compartmental shifts.

Calcium, magnesium, and phosphate are critical regulators of cellular and organ function acting as enzyme cofactors and regulators of metabolic function within cells. Magnesium and phosphate are predominantly located within the intracellular space. In contrast, calcium is largely excluded from the intracellular space. However, extracellular calcium is a major determinant of neuromuscular stability. It is important for the clinician to understand the regulation of calcium, magnesium and phosphate, as disruption of the regulation of these ions adversely impacts a variety of physiologic functions.

DISTRIBUTION OF CALCIUM, MAGNESIUM, AND PHOSPHATE

Calcium and magnesium exist in the body as divalent cations (Ca^{2+} and Mg^{2+}). Approximately 99% of the total body calcium resides in the skeleton, whereas the remaining 1% is found in the soft tissues and extracellular spaces. Approximately 40% of plasma calcium is bound to protein, principally albumin, 10% is complexed with anions, and the remaining 50% exists in the unbound, or ionized, form. Ionized calcium is the physiologically important circulating form of calcium within the body.

Approximately 40%–50% of magnesium, which lies within bone, resides in the intracellular space, whereas only 1% is found in the extracellular space. Approximately 20%–30% of plasma magnesium is bound to protein, chiefly albumin (1), whereas the remaining 70%–80% exists in the ionized form or is complexed to citrate, bicarbonate, and phosphate. Similar to calcium, the ionized form of magnesium is the most physiologically significant circulating form of magnesium.

Approximately 85% of total body phosphorus is found in bones and teeth. The remaining total body phosphorus is distributed in the soft tissues (14%) and the extracellular space (1%). Approximately 60% of plasma phosphorous exists in ionized forms of phosphate, hydrogen phosphate (HPO_4^{2-}), and dihydrogen phosphate ($H_2PO_4^-$). The remaining plasma phosphate is complexed to cations, primarily Ca^{2+}, Mg^{2+}, and Na^+, or is bound to plasma proteins.

REGULATION OF CALCIUM, MAGNESIUM, AND PHOSPHATE

The extracellular concentrations of calcium, magnesium, and phosphate are maintained within a normal range through (a) absorption of ingested calcium, magnesium, and phosphate through the intestinal tract; (b) absorption and excretion via the kidney; and (c) mobilization from the bone. All of these processes are regulated by hormonal action.

Intestinal Absorption

Intestinal absorption is the primary site of regulation of total body calcium. Dietary calcium is passively absorbed in a concentration-dependent fashion throughout the small intestine and is actively transported in the duodenum and upper jejunum by mechanisms regulated by 1,25-dihydroxyvitamin D. The efficiency of calcium absorption is increased with reduced dietary intake, rapid growth during childhood, pregnancy, and lactation. Dietary magnesium is principally absorbed in the jejunum and the ileum by both active and passive mechanisms. Magnesium absorption is enhanced during reduced dietary intake. Phosphate is absorbed in the duodenum and jejunum by passive processes and active mechanisms regulated by 1,25-dihydroxyvitamin D. Absorption of phosphate is impeded by the presence of polyvalent cations (e.g., Ca^{2+}, Mg^{2+}, and Al^{3+}) in the intestinal lumen or by deficiency of vitamin D. A small proportion of calcium, magnesium, and phosphate is secreted in digestive juices and excreted via stool.

Renal Handling

Approximately 60%–70% of total plasma calcium, chiefly in its ionized and complexed forms, is filtered by the kidneys, with less than 5% of filtered calcium being excreted in the urine. Most (~70%) of filtered calcium is reabsorbed along with sodium and water in the proximal convoluted tubule (PCT) by a concentration-dependent mechanism. An additional 15%–20% of calcium is reabsorbed in the thick ascending limb of the loop of Henle (TALH). The action of the Na^+–K^+–$2Cl^-$ cotransporter in the thick ascending limb creates a potential difference that favors voltage-dependent absorption of calcium. The remaining 10%–15% of filtered calcium is reabsorbed in the distal convoluted tubule (DCT) by active mechanisms that are poorly understood and that are regulated by parathyroid hormone (PTH) and cyclic AMP.

Approximately 70%–80% of plasma magnesium, in its ionized or complex forms, is filtered in the glomerulus. Approximately 3% of filtered magnesium is excreted in the urine, and 5%–15% is reabsorbed in the PCT by an undefined passive mechanism. The majority of filtered magnesium (60%–70%) is reabsorbed in the TALH as the consequence of a voltage-dependent gradient generated by action of the Na^+–K^+–$2Cl^-$ cotransporter. The remaining 5%–10% of magnesium is reabsorbed in the DCT by an unknown mechanism that is stimulated by PTH (2).

As with calcium and magnesium, the ionized and complexed forms of phosphate are filtered in the glomerulus and accounts for ultrafiltration of 85%–90% of the total plasma phosphate. The amount of phosphate excreted in the urine ranges from 3% to 20% of the filtered load. Nearly 80% of the filtered phosphate is reabsorbed in the PCT through the action of sodium–phosphate (Na–P) cotransporters, which are regulated by PTH. An additional 5% of phosphate is reabsorbed in the DCT by an unknown active mechanism (3). Thus, the kidney is the major site of regulation of total body phosphorous.

Multiple factors can alter renal reabsorption or excretion of calcium, magnesium, and phosphate (1) (**Table 108.1**). Volume expansion, for example with a bolus saline infusion, leads to increased calcium, magnesium, and phosphate excretion primarily due to decreased proximal tubular reabsorption. Hypercalcemia decreases renal blood flow and glomerular filtration rate (GFR) and simultaneously increases excretion of calcium due to decreased reabsorption of calcium in the proximal tubule, loop of Henle, and DCT. The net effect of these two potentially opposing mechanisms is enhanced calcium excretion due to suppression of PTH release by elevated serum calcium levels. The effects of hypercalcemia on phosphate excretion are determined by the duration of the hypercalcemic state. During acute hypercalcemia, reduction in GFR, formation of calcium–phosphate–protein complexes (which prevents ultrafiltration of phosphate), and suppression of PTH release (which prevents phosphate reabsorption in the proximal tubule) contribute to decreased phosphate excretion. In contrast, during chronic hypercalcemia, phosphate excretion increases due to decreased reabsorption via unknown mechanisms. Hypocalcemia induces PTH secretion, which in turn

reduces renal excretion of calcium by enhancing reabsorption in the DCT. Hypocalcemia contributes to reduced excretion of magnesium and phosphate by increasing magnesium absorption in the TALH and by increasing phosphate absorption by an unknown mechanism. Hypermagnesemia has no clear effect on calcium or phosphate excretion but increases magnesium excretion by reducing the fractional reabsorption of magnesium in the proximal tubule and inhibiting reabsorption in the loop of Henle. Conversely, during hypomagnesemia, magnesium excretion is decreased due to increased reabsorption in the loop of Henle by an unclear mechanism. Hyperphosphatemia induces PTH secretion, thereby reducing calcium excretion through increased uptake in the DCT. Hyperphosphatemia has no clear effect on magnesium excretion. Hypophosphatemia increases Na–P cotransporter–mediated reabsorption in the proximal tubule, thereby decreasing phosphate excretion.

Acid–base disturbances have significant effects on renal handling of calcium, magnesium, and phosphate. Both acute and chronic metabolic acidosis induce calciuria by inhibiting epithelial calcium channel type 1 (ECaC1)-mediated uptake of calcium in the distal tubule (4). On the other hand, metabolic alkalosis enhances conductance of calcium through the ECaC1, leading to reduced calcium excretion (4). Metabolic alkalosis reduces renal losses of magnesium by increasing absorption in the loop of Henle. Acute metabolic acidosis does not seem to have any significant effect on phosphate excretion, whereas chronic metabolic acidosis causes phosphaturia by reducing Na–P cotransporter expression at the tubular cell surface, resulting in decreased absorption in the proximal tubule (5). Respiratory acidosis enhances both calcium and phosphate excretion. Respiratory alkalosis decreases renal phosphate excretion but has no effect on calcium excretion. Respiratory acid-base disturbances do not appear to have any significant effect on magnesium excretion.

Multiple medications, in particular diuretics, have a major impact on renal excretion of calcium, magnesium, and phosphate. Thiazide diuretics decrease calcium excretion by enhanced calcium reabsorption in the DCT. In contrast, thiazide diuretics cause a modest increase in magnesium excretion via inhibition of the Na^+–Cl^- cotransporter. Thiazides induce phosphaturia by inhibiting carbonic anhydrase. Loop diuretics augment calcium and magnesium excretion through inhibition of the Na^+–K^+–Cl^- cotransporter in the TALH, which reduces voltage-dependent absorption of both calcium and magnesium. Similar to thiazides, loop diuretics slightly enhance phosphate excretion through inhibition of carbonic anhydrase (6). Other medications such as aminoglycosides, cisplatin, and cyclosporine have been shown to increase magnesium excretion by inhibiting magnesium reabsorption in the loop of Henle (6). These medications generally do not affect calcium or phosphate excretion.

Hormonal Regulation

The plasma concentrations of calcium, phosphate, and, to a lesser degree, magnesium are precisely regulated by several hormones (**Table 108.2**). The key hormones in calcium regulation are PTH, 1,25-dihydroxyvitamin D, and calcitonin.

Parathyroid Hormone

PTH tightly regulates ionized calcium and, to a lesser degree, phosphate levels in the blood and extracellular fluids. PTH is synthesized in the parathyroid gland and is enzymatically cleaved from pre-pro-PTH to pro-PTH and then to PTH prior to its secretion. The signal sequences contained in the pre-prohormone are critical to hormone processing, as

TABLE 108.1

FACTORS AFFECTING RENAL EXCRETION OF CALCIUM, MAGNESIUM, AND PHOSPHATE

FACTORS AFFECTING EXCRETION	CALCIUM — EFFECT ON RENAL EXCRETION	CALCIUM — MECHANISM(S)	MAGNESIUM — EFFECT ON RENAL EXCRETION	MAGNESIUM — MECHANISM(S)	PHOSPHATE — EFFECT ON RENAL EXCRETION	PHOSPHATE — MECHANISM(S)
Volume expansion	↑	↓ reabsorption in PCT	↑	↓ reabsorption in PCT	↑	↓ reabsorption in PCT
Electrolyte disturbances						
Hypercalcemia	↑	↓ reabsorption in PCT, TALH, DCT (↓ PTH)	↑	↓ tubular reabsorption	↓ (acute) ↑ (chronic)	↓ ultrafiltration, ↓ GFR and ↓ PTH (acute); ↓ tubular reabsorption via unknown mechanism (chronic)
Hypocalcemia	↓	↑ reabsorption in DCT due to ↑ PTH	↓	↑ reabsorption TALH	↑ or ↓ (chronic hypocalcemia)	↓ tubular reabsorption secondary to ↑ PTH
Hypermagnesemia	—	—	↑	↓ reabsorption in TALH	—	—
Hypomagnesemia	—	—	↓	↑ reabsorption in TALH	↑	—
Hyperphosphatemia	↓	↑ reabsorption in DCT due to ↑ PTH	—	—	↑	↓ tubular reabsorption due to ↓ Na–P activity
Hypophosphatemia	↑	↓ reabsorption in DCT	↑	↓ reabsorption in TALH	↓	↑ tubular reabsorption due to ↑ Na–P activity
Acid–base disturbances						
Metabolic acidosis	↑	↓ reabsorption in DCT due to ↓ ECaC1 conductance	↑	↓ reabsorption in TALH	↑ (chronic metabolic acidosis)	↓ tubular reabsorption due to ↓ Na–P activity
Metabolic alkalosis	↓	↑ reabsorption in DCT due to ↑ ECaC1 conductance	↓	↑ reabsorption in TALH	↓ ↑	↑ tubular reabsorption due to ↑ Na–P activity
Respiratory acidosis	↑	—	↑	—	↑	—
Respiratory alkalosis	—	—	—	—	—	—
Medications						
Thiazide diuretics	↓	↑ reabsorption in DCT due to inhibition of Na–Cl cotransporter	Minimal ↑	↑ reabsorption in DCT due to inhibition of Na–Cl cotransporter	↑	—
Loop diuretics	↑	↓ reabsorption in DCT due to altered inhibition of Na–K–2Cl cotransporter	↑	↓ reabsorption in DCT due to altered inhibition of Na–K–2Cl cotransporter	↑	Enhancement of phosphate excretion through inhibition of carbonic anhydrase
Aminoglycosides	—	—	↑	↓ reabsorption in TALH	—	—
Cisplatin	—	—	↑	↓ reabsorption in TALH	—	—
Cyclosporine	—	—	↑	↓ reabsorption in TALH	—	—

PCT, proximal convoluted tubule; TALH, thick ascending limb of the loop of Henle; GFR, glomerular filtration rate; ECaC1, epithelial calcium channel type 1.

Modified from Suki WN, Lederer ED, Rouse D. Renal transport of calcium, magnesium, and phosphate. In: Brenner BM, ed. *Brenner and Rector's The Kidney.* 6th ed. Philadelphia, PA: WB Saunders, 2000:520–74.

TABLE 108.2

HORMONAL REGULATION OF CALCIUM AND PHOSPHATE

		EFFECT ON SERUM LEVEL		
■ HORMONE	■ CALCIUM	■ MECHANISM OF ACTION	■ PHOSPHATE	■ MECHANISM OF ACTION
PTH	↑	↑ reabsorption in DCT and TALH	↓	↓ reabsorption in PCT and DCT
Vitamin D	↑	↑ absorption in intestine and reabsorption in DCT	↑	↑ absorption in intestine and reabsorption in DCT
Calcitonin	↓	↓ bone resorption ↓ reabsorption in renal tubules	—	—

TALH, thick ascending limb of the loop of Henle; PCT, proximal convoluted tubule.

mutations at these sites have been seen in hereditary forms of hypoparathyroidism.

PTH binds to cell surface receptors linked to adenylate cyclase within the kidney and bone (7). In the kidney, PTH enhances transcellular reabsorption of calcium in the DCT and paracellular reabsorption in the cortical thick ascending loop of Henle. In contrast, PTH inhibits phosphate reabsorption in the proximal and distal tubules by inducing cellular uptake and proteolytic degradation of the Na–P cotransporters (8). Furthermore, PTH stimulates the conversion of 25-hydroxyvitamin D to $1,25(OH)_2D_3$ in the proximal tubule via induction of transcription of the 25-hydroxyvitamin D 1α-hydroxylase gene (9). PTH enhances release of calcium from bone by increasing expression of the surface protein RANK (receptor activator of nuclear factor κB) ligand, which stimulates osteoclast maturation and activity, leading to bone resorption (10).

PTH secretion is primarily regulated by the blood concentration of ionized calcium. High blood concentrations of ionized calcium decrease PTH secretion, whereas low concentrations of ionized calcium increase PTH secretion. There exists a dose–response relationship of PTH secretion to blood ionized calcium that is sigmoidal in nature. In addition, the greater the rate of fall in blood ionized calcium, the greater the rise in PTH secretion. From the teleological standpoint, these two properties protect against abrupt falls in blood ionized calcium.

When extracellular ionized calcium increases, the ionized calcium binds to G-protein-coupled, calcium-sensing receptors on the parathyroid cell surface, intracellular calcium increases, and PTH secretion decreases. When extracellular ionized calcium falls, binding to the calcium-sensing receptor decreases, intracellular ionized calcium concentration falls, and PTH secretion is increased.

Calcium concentrations can also affect the biosynthesis of PTH. Although the precise mechanism is unknown, hypocalcemia has been shown to enhance PTH gene transcription, enhance PTH mRNA stability, and stimulate PTH mRNA translation. In contrast, hypercalcemia has no effect on production of PTH mRNA.

Phosphate has also been shown to have an effect on PTH synthesis. Elevated blood phosphate indirectly stimulates PTH secretion by reducing blood calcium and 1,25-dihydroxyvitamin D levels (11). PTH secretion can be stimulated directly by markedly elevated levels of phosphate, but the precise mechanism is unknown. 1,25-Dihydroxyvitamin D, although having no direct effect on PTH synthesis, has been shown to inhibit PTH gene transcription.

Vitamin D

Vitamin D is obtained from two primary sources: the skin and dietary supplementation. In the skin, the precursor of vitamin D, 7-dehydrocholesterol, undergoes photochemical cleavage to form previtamin D. Previtamin D then undergoes a temperature-dependent molecular rearrangement to form vitamin D. Vitamin D consumed in the diet is absorbed by the lymphatics and enters the circulation, where it is bound to vitamin D–binding protein and, to a lesser extent, albumin. Vitamin D–binding protein serves to act as a serum reservoir for vitamin D precursors and to modulate serum levels of vitamin D metabolites. In the liver, vitamin D undergoes 25-hydroxylation. Subsequently, the 25-hydroxyvitamin D undergoes 1-hydroxylation by a cytochrome P450 enzyme in the kidney to form the biologically active 1,25-dihydroxyvitamin D (12). 1,25-Dihydroxyvitamin D is metabolized to inactive forms by 24- or 26-hydroxylation side-chain oxidation and cleavage, and is then excreted into bile.

1,25-Dihydroxyvitamin D acts via nuclear receptors to enhance calcium and phosphate absorption primarily in the intestine and, to some extent, in distal renal tubules. 1,25-Dihydroxyvitamin D also functions to promote osteoclast differentiation and bone resorption and to stimulate the synthesis of matrix proteins integral to normal bone mineralization (13). In addition, 1,25-dihydroxyvitamin D has been shown to decrease transcription of PTH. It is unclear whether this effect is critical to PTH regulation under normal conditions, but it has been used as a therapeutic strategy in the treatment of secondary hyperparathyroidism.

Calcitonin

Calcitonin is a 32-amino-acid polypeptide secreted and stored in the C cells of the thyroid gland. Calcitonin has been shown to inhibit renal tubular reabsorption of calcium and osteoclast-mediated bone resorption. The secretion of calcitonin is stimulated by increased blood calcium levels and by glucocorticoids, calcitonin gene-related peptide, glucagon, enteroglucagon, gastrin, pentagastrin, pancreozymin, and β-adrenergic agents. Although calcitonin is known to be important in regulating calcium blood levels in other species, its importance in the human physiologic regulation of calcium is unclear.

DISORDERS OF CALCIUM, MAGNESIUM, AND PHOSPHATE HOMEOSTASIS

Normal Values

Published normal values for total serum calcium range from 8.8 to 10.8 mg/dL (14). Although measurement of total calcium is a well-accepted means of monitoring calcium levels in healthy patients, this measurement may be inaccurate in critically ill patients. Because critically ill patients frequently are

TABLE 108.3

CAUSES OF HYPOCALCEMIA

Inadequate intake or malabsorption
PTH-related
  Impaired parathyroid gland formation
    Congenital agenesis or dysgenesis of the parathyroid glands
      DiGeorge syndrome
      X-linked hypoparathyroidism
  PTH gene mutations
  Parathyroid gland destruction
    Autoimmune polyglandular syndrome type 1
    Inadvertent surgical destruction
    Hemochromatosis
    Thalassemia major
    Wilson disease
  Impaired secretion of PTH
    Hypomagnesemia
    Maternal hypercalcemia
    Calcium-sensing receptor mutations
    Cytokine release
    Respiratory alkalosis
  End-organ resistance to PTH (pseudohypoparathyroidism)
Vitamin D–related
  Inadequate intake or absorption
    Breast-feeding (without vitamin D supplementation)
    Gastrectomy
    Small-bowel surgery
    Celiac disease
    Inflammatory bowel disease
    Cystic fibrosis
  Increased catabolism
    Phenobarbital
    Phenytoin
    Carbamazepine
    Isoniazid
    Rifampin
    Theophylline
  Decreased 25-hydroxylation (hepatic disease)
  Decreased 1-hydroxylation (renal disease)
  Vitamin D resistance
Chelation by anions
  Hyperphosphatemia
  Red blood cell transfusions (citrate)
  Lipid administration
  Pancreatitis (fatty acids)
Other
  Fluoride intoxication
  "Hungry-bone" syndrome
  Critical illness

hypoalbuminemic and because ~40% of calcium is predominantly bound to albumin, it is not infrequent to encounter low total calcium levels in the critically ill. One approach has been to calculate the corrected calcium level based on the serum albumin level using the following equation (3):

$$Ca_{corrected} = Ca_{measured} + [8.0 (4.0 - albumin_{measured} \text{ mg/dL})]$$

However, it may be preferable for the clinician to obtain measurements of ionized calcium in critically ill patients as timely and accurate measurements are readily available via point-of-care testing. Normal values for ionized calcium range between 4.2 and 5.5 mg/dL (1.0–1.4 mmol/dL) (14). Reported normal values of magnesium are 1.5–2.3 mg/dL (14). Normal phosphate levels vary with age, with values ranging from 4.8 to 8.2 mg/dL in newborns and from 2.7 to 4.7 mg/dL in older adolescents (14).

Hypocalcemia

Causes

Hypocalcemia can occur as the consequence of inadequate calcium intake, malabsorption, hormonal imbalance or dysfunction or chelation by anions (**Table 108.3**). PTH-deficient hypocalcemia may be due to impaired synthesis of PTH (either primary dysfunction or hypoplasia or agenesis of the parathyroid glands), inappropriate suppression of PTH secretion, or target organ resistance to PTH. Physiologic deficiency of PTH secretion occurs in neonates ("early neonatal hypocalcemia") during the first 4 days of life. This disorder most commonly occurs in premature infants, low-birth-weight infants, infants of diabetic mothers, and infants born after prolonged, difficult deliveries. Patients recover after several days of nutritional supplementation. Congenital agenesis or dysgenesis of the parathyroid glands has been observed in a number of inherited genetic defects. The most notable are disorders associated with deletions in the chromosome 22q11 region, the locus for DiGeorge syndrome, velocardiofacial syndrome, and conotruncal face syndromes (15). Embryologically, these disorders result as a consequence of maldevelopment of the third and fourth branchial pouches, resulting in thymic aplasia, facial anomalies (hypertelorism, antimongoloid slant of the eyes, short philtrum, low set ears, micrognathia), and aortocardiac anomalies (right-sided aortic arch, tetralogy of Fallot, truncus arteriosus). On occasion, neonatal hypoparathyroidism may be the only presenting symptom of DiGeorge syndrome. Defects in the PTH signal peptide site have been detected in rare cases of congenital hypoparathyroidism (16).

Antibody-mediated destruction of the parathyroid glands has been detected in autoimmune polyglandular syndrome type 1 (APS1), also known as the autoimmune polyendocrinopathy–candidiasis–ectodermal dystrophy (APECED) syndrome, which is caused by mutations in the autoimmune regulator gene (*AIRE*), resulting in hypoparathyroidism, primary adrenal insufficiency, and mucocutaneous candidiasis. The candidiasis is usually the first presenting symptom and is followed by hypoparathyroidism as early as 3 years of age and subsequently adrenal insufficiency.

Postsurgical destruction of the parathyroid glands is the most common cause of hypoparathyroidism and occurs as a complication of thyroidectomy, radical neck dissection for malignancies, or after inadvertent interruption of the blood supply to the parathyroid glands during head and neck surgery. Destruction of the parathyroid glands is a rare complication of radioablative iodine therapy for Graves disease. In addition, parathyroid destruction has rarely occurred as the consequence of (a) deposition of iron in patients with hemochromatosis and (b) thalassemia major and copper deposition in patients with Wilson disease.

Impaired secretion is observed in hypomagnesemia. In the initial stages of hypomagnesemia, PTH secretion is increased. However, as hypomagnesemia persists, intracellular depletion of magnesium develops and impairs PTH secretion. Pronounced suppression of PTH occurs in neonates of mothers with hyperparathyroidism. The resultant maternal hypercalcemia suppresses PTH secretion in the fetus and the responsiveness of the parathyroid glands to hypocalcemia following birth. Autosomal-dominant activating mutations in the gene encoding the calcium-sensing receptor (*CASR*) also cause impaired PTH secretion. With activating mutations, PTH secretion is decreased because the receptor falsely detects low serum calcium concentrations as being normal. Patients with this disorder have mild-to-moderate hypocalcemia and are generally asymptomatic. However, under stress conditions, such as a febrile illness, they can present with seizures or tetany. Disorders that contribute to macrophage-mediated cytokine release, such as Gram-negative sepsis and toxic shock syndrome, have also been found to impair PTH secretion.

End-organ resistance to the action of PTH, or pseudohypoparathyroidism, results from defects in the PTH receptor–adenylate cyclase system (17), specifically in the α-subunit of the GTP (guanosine triphosphate) binding protein G_s. In these disorders, PTH levels are high in the face of hypocalcemia. The disorders are classified by the urinary excretion of cyclic AMP (cAMP) and phosphate in response to PTH administration. In type 1 pseudohypoparathyroidism, decreased urinary excretion of cAMP and phosphate occurs in response to PTH. The type 1 disorders have been divided into three subtypes. In type 1a, an autosomally inherited mutation of the *GNAS1* gene occurs, leading to an inability to activate adenylate cyclase when PTH binds to its receptor. Patients with this defect present with Albright hereditary osteodystrophy, characterized by round facies, short stature, short fourth metacarpal bones, obesity, subcutaneous ossifications, and developmental delay. Patients with type 1b pseudohypoparathyroidism have mutations that affect regulatory elements of *GNAS1* but do not exhibit the Albright phenotype. It is believed that PTH resistance is confined to the kidneys in this disorder. Patients have been described with normal cAMP excretion and decreased phosphate excretion in response to PTH administration (18) and were said to have pseudohypoparathyroidism type 2. This disorder has been seen in some patients with myotonic dystrophy.

Hypocalcemia as the result of low 1,25-dihydroxyvitamin D can occur due to inadequate vitamin D intake or production, increased vitamin D catabolism, decreased 25-hydroxylation in the liver, decreased 1-hydroxylation in the kidney, and vitamin D resistance. Inadequate intake of fatty fishes, milk or other vitamin D–containing foods, exclusive breast-feeding (without vitamin D supplementation), and inadequate sun exposure can lead to vitamin D deficiency and rickets. Inadequate intestinal absorption of vitamin D has been observed in patients with gastrectomy, celiac disease, extensive bowel surgery, inflammatory bowel disease, or pancreatic insufficiency due to cystic fibrosis. Enhanced catabolism of 1,25-dihydroxyvitamin D by activation of the cytochrome P450 system has been reported in patients receiving phenobarbital, phenytoin, carbamazepine, isoniazid, theophylline, rifampin, primidone, and glutethimide. Hepatic 25-hydroxylation of vitamin D is mildly impaired in severe liver disease or dysfunction. Decreased 1-hydroxylation of 25-hydroxyvitamin D occurs in patients with renal disease due to decreased 1-hydroxylase synthesis. Vitamin D resistance occurs as the consequence of mutations that involve the vitamin D receptor gene. These mutations result in impaired signal transduction associated with the vitamin D–receptor interaction producing clinical rickets.

Chelation of ionized calcium by anions is seen in a number of clinical situations. Hyperphosphatemia as a consequence of massive tissue lysis (e.g., tumor lysis syndrome and rhabdomyolysis), or phosphate administration can induce hypocalcemia due to the formation of calcium phosphate precipitates in soft tissues. Hypocalcemia due to complex formation with citrate present in packed red blood cells is typically transient and not clinically significant unless large volumes are transfused rapidly (2 cc/kg/min) or with smaller volumes if liver dysfunction interferes with citrate metabolism. EDTA-containing radiocontrast dyes have been shown to cause hypocalcemia. Administration of lipids or excess release of free fatty acids, as seen in pancreatitis, may also cause hypocalcemia. Other unclassified causes of hypocalcemia include the "hungry-bone syndrome" and fluoride intoxication. The "hungry-bone syndrome" occurs following parathyroidectomy in patients with primary hyperparathyroidism. Persistently high PTH levels result in prolonged bone resorption. Following parathyroid gland resection, the acute drop in PTH leads to pronounced

uptake of calcium, leading to hypocalcemia. Excessive fluoride intake has been shown to inhibit bone resorption.

The hypocalcemia that has been observed in critically ill patients is poorly understood and is likely the consequence of multiple factors (see section "Hypocalcemia in Critical Illness"). Potential mechanisms for hypocalcemia during critical illness include suppression of PTH secretion by cytokines, increased calcium binding to albumin, PTH deficiency, impaired renal hydroxylation of vitamin D, calcium chelation, and hypomagnesemia. Hypocalcemia has been associated with increased mortality in critically ill patients but was found to be a poor independent predictor of mortality (19,20).

Signs and Symptoms

The signs and symptoms of hypocalcemia are most commonly the manifestations of altered function of calcium-dependent excitable tissues such as nerves and skeletal and cardiac muscle (Table 108.4). Patients may report myoclonic jerks and paresthesias of the perioral region, fingers, and toes. In more severe cases, patients may present with seizures, apnea, cyanosis, laryngospasm, tachypnea, tachycardia, and vomiting. On physical examination, percussion of the facial nerve below the zygomatic arch may result in facial muscle contraction (Chvostek sign). Compression of the arm or leg with a blood pressure cuff may result in carpopedal spasm (Trousseau sign). On electrocardiogram, prolongation of the QT interval and nonspecific ST–T wave changes may be observed. Hypocalcemia rarely causes ventricular arrhythmias.

Deficiency of vitamin D due to inadequate intake, 1-α-hydroxylase deficiency (vitamin D dependency type 1), and resistance to vitamin D (vitamin D dependency type 2) result in rickets. Rickets is characterized by abnormal mineralization of bone and growth-plate cartilage, resulting in widening, cupping, and fraying of the bone metaphysis. On clinical examination, skeletal changes include widened wrists, swelling of the costochondral junctions of the ribs (the "rachitic rosary"), and bowing of the legs. In more severe cases of hypocalcemic rickets, symptoms of hypocalcemia may manifest.

Diagnosis and Treatment

Diagnosis of the patient with hypocalcemia should begin with a thorough history of dietary intake (concentrating on sources of calcium and vitamin D). It should also include an investigation of family history of rickets, hypocalcemia, and endocrine disorders. Physical examination should include a close evaluation of the bones and joints.

TABLE 108.4

SIGNS AND SYMPTOMS OF HYPOCALCEMIA

Neuromuscular
  Paresthesias
  Chvostek sign (facial muscle spasm with percussion of nerve)
  Trousseau sign (carpopedal spasm with ischemia)
  Bronchospasm
  Laryngospasm
  Apnea
  Seizures
Cardiac
  Prolonged QT interval
  Nonspecific ST–T wave changes
  Rickets (radiographic findings)
  Epiphyseal widening
  Costochondral widening ("rachitic rosary")
  Genu varum or valgum
  Osteopenia

For most patients, the clinical history may provide a clear etiology, obviating the need for extensive evaluation; this also applies to most critically ill patients in the ICU. For those patients with no clear etiology or suspected rickets, a more extensive evaluation should be performed. Total serum calcium, ionized calcium, and albumin are useful. Other recommended laboratory studies include assessments of blood levels of phosphorus, magnesium, blood urea nitrogen, creatinine, alkaline phosphatase activity, PTH, 1,25-dihydroxyvitamin D, and 25-hydroxyvitamin D. On a random "spot" urine collection, urinary calcium excretion is best interpreted as a calcium/creatinine (mg/mg) ratio.

Urinary phosphorous excretion is very dependent upon diet and body phosphorous status. The ideal assessment is obtained with a fasting 2-hour urine collection, with a concomitant serum sample obtained midway through the urine collection. The tubular reabsorption of phosphate (TRP) is expressed as a percentage of the filtered phosphate load and is calculated by the formula:

$$TRP = 1 - \left[\frac{[P]u \times [Cr]s}{[P]s \times [Cr]u} \right] \times 100\%$$

where [P]u is the concentration of phosphate in urine, [P]s is the concentration of phosphate in serum, [Cr]u is the concentration of creatinine in urine, and [Cr]s is the concentration of creatinine in serum. All units should be identical (e.g., mg/dL)

Serum phosphorus is usually low in patients with vitamin D deficiency and is elevated in renal failure, hypoparathyroidism, and pseudohypoparathyroidism. In vitamin D–dependent rickets type 1, the serum 25-hydroxyvitamin D level is normal and the 1,25-dihydroxyvitamin D is low. Serum alkaline phosphatase activity may be elevated in patients with long-standing vitamin D deficiency but usually not in early disease. A low or normal circulating PTH in the presence of hypocalcemia indicates an inappropriate parathyroid response to hypocalcemia (i.e., functional hypoparathyroidism). Increased PTH secretion is a normal physiologic response to hypocalcemia, so that elevated serum PTH would occur in non-parathyroid–related hypocalcemia, such as in vitamin D deficiency or impaired vitamin D action. Increased PTH levels are usually seen in pseudohypoparathyroidism.

A primary tenet in the treatment of hypocalcemia is to tailor the therapy to the cause of hypocalcemia. Calcium may be given intravenously or orally. For patients who present with acute symptomatic hypocalcemia (i.e., tetany, muscle twitching, carpopedal spasm, laryngospasm, or seizures), a bolus dose of calcium gluconate (100–200 mg/kg or 9–18 mg/kg elemental calcium to a maximum of 1–3 g in adults) should be administered over 10–20 minutes (3,21). A continuous infusion of calcium gluconate may be administered at starting dose of 10–30 mg/kg/h to maintain adequate calcium levels to prevent symptoms. The rate of the infusion can then be titrated based on serial calcium measurements (or ionized calcium if necessary). Much controversy has existed concerning the use of calcium chloride as a better alternative to calcium gluconate for the correction of ionized hypocalcemia. To date, published studies that compare calcium chloride to calcium gluconate show that they have similar bioavailability and are equally effective in correcting ionized hypocalcemia (22,23). We recommend administering IV calcium through a central venous catheter because of a significant risk of tissue necrosis with peripheral administration (24). Calcification of soft tissue may result if extravasation of the infusion occurs (21). All patients receiving IV calcium require close monitoring of total or ionized calcium levels. Cardiac telemetry or electrocardiograms should be used during IV calcium administration to

detect cardiac rhythm disturbances. In hypocalcemic patients with hypomagnesemia, magnesium should be replenished with IV magnesium sulfate or oral magnesium oxide. In patients with concurrent hyperphosphatemia, the elevated phosphate should be corrected with phosphate binders, due to the risk of tissue deposition of calcium phosphate if the calcium–phosphate product exceeds 80 mg^2/dL^2.

$$\text{Calcium–phosphate product} = (Ca)s \times (PO_4)s$$

This calculation is the product of total serum calcium (Ca)s (mg/dL) and the serum phosphorous (PO$_4$)s (mg/dL) levels (for more discussion about calcium–phosphate product and the levels associated with risk of deposition, by age, see section "Hyperphosphatemia").

Once tetany resolves in symptomatic patients receiving IV calcium or in asymptomatic patients who can take enteral calcium, a variety of oral preparations are available, including calcium carbonate (400 mg of elemental calcium/g), calcium glubionate (64 mg of elemental calcium/g), and calcium gluconate (90 mg of elemental calcium/g). A recommended starting dose is 50 mg/kg body weight/24 h of elemental calcium divided into three to four doses. The dose is then titrated based on serum calcium levels (3).

In patients with hypocalcemia secondary to vitamin D deficiency or resistance, vitamin D replacement and adequate dietary calcium intake are the mainstays of therapy. The formulation and dosage of vitamin D required are dependent on the cause of the disorder. Children with deficiency of vitamin D due to poor dietary intake or malabsorption will typically respond to oral vitamin D therapy. Children with nutritional rickets will typically require 1000–5000 IU/d of vitamin D (3). Patients for whom medication compliance is a concern may be treated with a single dose of 600,000 IU of vitamin D. Patients with malabsorption require doses of vitamin D as high as 25,000–50,000 IU/d to correct the deficiency (3). Similarly, patients on phenytoin therapy may require vitamin D supplementation. In patients with renal failure, vitamin D–dependent rickets type 1, hypoparathyroidism, or pseudohypoparathyroidism, reduced 1,25 (OH)$_2$ D synthesis may occur, requiring replacement with 1,25-dihydroxyvitamin D itself (calcitriol; 0.01–0.08 mcg/kg/d in children up to 10 kg; 0.25–1.0 mcg/d in adults) (3,21). Calcium levels should be monitored during the course of therapy.

Hypocalcemia in Critical Illness

Hypocalcemia in critically ill patients has been attributed to alterations in PTH secretion and action, vitamin D deficiency, administration of citrated blood products, and medication administration (13,20,25–27). Ionized hypocalcemia that does not normalize within several days of admission or is <0.8 mmol/L is associated with increased ICU stay and mortality (19,28,29). However, there is no evidence that indicates correction of hypocalcemia in critically ill patients improves outcome (20,21,29). Despite the lack of data supporting improved outcomes, most authors recommend that hypocalcemia should be corrected in critically ill patients with symptomatic hypocalcemia or hemodynamic instability.

Hypercalcemia

Causes

Hypercalcemia generally occurs as the consequence of excessive dietary calcium intake or increased intestinal absorption. These alterations may be related to hormonal imbalance or dysfunction, increased renal reabsorption, or increased bone resorption (**Table 108.5**). One of the earliest descriptions of

TABLE 108.5

CAUSES OF HYPERCALCEMIA

Excessive intake
  "Milk–alkali syndrome"
  Oral calcium supplements
  Parenteral nutrition
PTH-related
  Calcium-sensing receptor mutations
  Multiple endocrine neoplasia type 1
  Multiple endocrine neoplasia type 2a
  Parathyroid adenoma
  Transient neonatal hyperparathyroidism (parathyroid gland
    hyperplasia)
  Chronic lithium toxicity
  Chronic renal failure
  Hyperparathyroidism–jaw tumor syndrome
Humoral hypercalcemia of malignancy (PTHrP-, TNF-, or
  cytokine-mediated)
Vitamin D intoxication
Increased renal reabsorption
  Thiazide diuretics
  Calcium-sensing receptor mutations
Increased bone resorption
  Thyrotoxicosis
  Vitamin A intoxication
  Primary and metastatic tumors
  Cytokine release
  Immobilization
Other
  Williams syndrome
  Subcutaneous fat necrosis

PTHrP, PTH-related peptide; TNF, tumor necrosis factor.

hypercalcemia due to excessive calcium intake is the milk–alkali syndrome, a disorder that was first reported in the early 20th century in patients who ingested excessive amounts of milk and related dairy products and sodium bicarbonate for treatment of peptic ulcer disease. These patients presented with the classic triad of hypercalcemia, metabolic alkalosis, and renal failure. Changes in therapy for peptic ulcer disease led to a significant reduction in the incidence of this disorder, but a resurgence of this disorder has been seen in the past 20 years in patients receiving calcium carbonate as part of their therapy for chronic renal failure. Children who receive oral calcium supplementation for hypocalcemic disorders or as part of their parenteral nutrition are at risk for hypercalcemia.

The most common hormonal imbalance contributing to hypercalcemia is hyperparathyroidism. Primary hyperparathyroidism may occur as the result of mutations in *CASR* or tumors related to defects in the tumor suppressor genes in parathyroid cells (30). Familial hypocalciuric hypercalcemia is the consequence of heterozygous mutations in the *CASR* gene. Parathyroid cells are stimulated and secrete relatively large amounts of PTH in the setting of normal calcium levels (30). When mutations in *CASR* are homozygous, severe neonatal hyperparathyroidism ensues. This rare, autosomal recessive, disorder presents in the neonatal period and can be fatal if diagnosis and treatment are delayed. Parathyroid adenomas that produce excess PTH can be seen as part of multiple endocrine neoplasia type 1 (hyperparathyroidism, tumors of the anterior pituitary and pancreatic islets) and multiple endocrine neoplasia type 2a (hyperparathyroidism, medullary carcinoma of the thyroid, pheochromocytoma) (31). Transient neonatal secondary hyperparathyroidism occurs in infants of mothers

with hypoparathyroidism due to prolonged fetal exposure to hypocalcemia, which stimulates hyperplasia of the parathyroid glands (32). In older children, somatic mutations in parathyroid tumor suppressor genes may lead to the development of pituitary adenomas (30). A mild form of secondary hyperparathyroidism can be seen in patients with chronic lithium toxicity. It is believed that lithium interferes with signaling by the calcium-sensing receptor, leading to excess PTH production. "Tertiary" hyperparathyroidism is seen in children with chronic renal failure. This entity refers to the development of autonomous PTH secretion following chronic "secondary" or physiologic parathyroid gland hyperfunction, for example, due to prolonged hypocalcemia.

A number of childhood malignancies, including rhabdoid tumors of the kidney, congenital mesoblastic nephroma, neuroblastoma, medulloblastoma, leukemia, Burkitt lymphoma, dysgerminoma, and rhabdomyosarcoma, are associated with hypercalcemia of malignancy. Similarly, in adults, squamous cell, breast, renal cell, and bladder cancers may manifest hypercalcemia as a paraneoplastic phenomenon. PTH-related peptide (PTHrP) mediates this hypercalcemia commonly in adults and rarely in children. PTHrP has been shown in vitro and in vivo to stimulate the PTH1 receptor (33). Vitamin D intoxication, typically seen with ingestions of >100,000 units/d of vitamin D, and malignant lymphomas that produce 1,25-dihydroxyvitamin D are uncommon causes of hypercalcemia. Variably elevated circulating levels of $1,25(OH)_2$ have been reported in subcutaneous fat necrosis in infants.

Increased renal absorption of calcium that leads to hypercalcemia can be seen with thiazide therapy and with inactivating mutations of *CASR*. Thiazide diuretics stimulate calcium reabsorption in the DCT.

Hypercalcemia secondary to increased bone resorption may rarely accompany thyrotoxicosis and excess vitamin A ingestion. Tumors that cause bone osteolysis and hypercalcemia (e.g., multiple myeloma and breast cancer) are seen in adults and, rarely, in children. It is believed that tumor necrosis factor β and the interleukins IL-1β and IL-6 released from these tumors stimulate bone resorption. Other causes of hypercalcemia include Williams syndrome and immobilization.

Signs and Symptoms

Signs and symptoms of hypercalcemia are varied, and the severity of the symptoms is correlated with the degree of hypercalcemia (Table 108.6). Severe symptoms are observed in patients with serum calcium levels >15 mg/dL. Patients with a serum level of <15 mg/dL may be asymptomatic. Infants tend to present with gastrointestinal symptoms such as poor feeding, emesis, and failure to thrive. In older children, neurologic symptoms such as altered mental status, psychosis, and hallucinations may be present. Severe hypercalcemia contributes to a hyperpolarization across myocardial membranes, resulting in a shortened QT interval and ventricular dysrhythmias. Hypercalcemia impairs the renal response to antidiuretic hormone (ADH), causing nephrogenic diabetes insipidus and resulting in an inability to concentrate urine and polyuria.

Diagnosis and Treatment

Hypercalcemia in children is uncommon. The diagnosis of the patient with hypercalcemia should begin with a thorough history of dietary intake, medications, vitamin intake, renal function, and familial disorders, including sarcoidosis and other granulomatous diseases, endocrine disorders, and hypercalcemia.

Laboratory investigation should include total serum calcium, serum phosphorus, blood urea nitrogen, creatinine, alkaline phosphatase, urinary calcium, urinary phosphorus,

TABLE 108.6

SIGNS AND SYMPTOMS OF HYPERCALCEMIA

Neuromuscular
  Fatigue
  Weakness
  Lethargy
  Confusion
  Coma
  Hallucinations
  Psychosis
Gastrointestinal
  Poor feeding
  Failure to thrive
  Nausea
  Vomiting
  Constipation
  Pancreatitis (rare)
Cardiac
  Shortened QT interval
  Ventricular dysrhythmias
Renal
  Polyuria
  Hyposthenuria
  Dehydration
  Hypernatremia
  Renal stone formation
  Renal failure

urinary creatinine (for calculation of the calcium/creatinine ratio and the tubular reabsorption of phosphorus), PTH, 1,25-dihydroxyvitamin D, and 25-hydroxyvitamin D. If malignancy is suspected as a cause, a PTHrP level may be useful. An elevated PTH in the presence of hypercalcemia is diagnostic for primary hyperparathyroidism, unless the history and physical examination suggest familial hypocalciuric hypercalcemia, malignancy, or lithium therapy. When distinguishing between primary hyperparathyroidism and familial hypocalciuric hypercalcemia, a urinary calcium:creatinine ratio of <0.01 (mg/mg) raises suspicion for the familial disorder, although the distinction may be difficult to make on clinical grounds (21). A low or normal PTH level should prompt investigation of malignancy-related or other non-PTH-dependent causes of hypercalcemia.

The treatment of hypercalcemia is dependent on its severity. The initial basic tenets of therapy are to restore intravascular volume (as hypercalcemic patients are typically dehydrated) and to enhance renal excretion, which can be accomplished by administration of normal saline at two to three times maintenance fluid rate. If the patient is adequately rehydrated and calcium levels do not decrease, loop diuretics may be administered to enhance renal excretion of calcium but should be done judiciously to avoid intravascular volume depletion. Calcitonin and bisphosphonates, which inhibit bone resorption, are useful adjuncts in severe hypercalcemia (5). Patients with malignancy-related hypercalcemia also have been successfully treated with bisphosphonate. Reasonable success has been achieved with IV administration of pamidronate (a bisphosphonate) in treating selected cases of childhood hypercalcemia. In severe cases in which hydration and medications fail to reduce serum calcium levels, hemodialysis using a low-calcium dialysate can be performed. Glucocorticoids have been useful in treating hypercalcemia secondary to sarcoidosis and vitamin D deficiency (through inhibition of intestinal actions of vitamin D) (21).

Indications for surgery for primary hyperparathyroidism include total calcium level >12 mg/dL, hyperparathyroid crisis (discrete episode of life-threatening hypercalcemia), marked hypercalciuria, nephrolithiasis, impaired renal function, osteitis fibrosa cystica, reduced cortical bone density (measured with dual x-ray absorptiometry or similar technique), bone mass greater than two standard deviations below age-matched controls, classic neuromuscular symptoms, proximal muscle weakness and atrophy, hyperreflexia, gait disturbance, and age <50 years (34).

Hypercalcemia in Critical Illness

Hypercalcemia is uncommon in critically ill pediatric patients. In this setting, malignancy-associated and primary hyperparathyroidism have been found to be the most common causes (35,36). Less common causes include sarcoidosis, prolonged immobilization, and excessive thiazide diuretic use (36,37).

Hypomagnesemia

Causes

Hypomagnesemia generally occurs as the consequence of decreased dietary magnesium intake, malabsorption, decreased renal reabsorption, or redistribution from the extracellular to the intracellular space (Table 108.7). Dietary deficiency of magnesium is exceedingly uncommon due to the presence of magnesium in a wide variety of foods. The three most common scenarios in which nutritional magnesium deficiency can be seen are protein–calorie malnutrition, parenteral nutrition, and alcoholism. In patients with fat malabsorption, free fatty acids in the intestinal lumen chelate magnesium, preventing its absorption. Intestinal malabsorption or syndromes that are characterized by significant diarrhea (e.g., celiac disease, inflammatory bowel disease, and Whipple disease) are associated

TABLE 108.7

CAUSES OF HYPOMAGNESEMIA

Decreased dietary intake or malabsorption
  Protein–calorie malnutrition
  Parenteral nutrition
  Alcoholism
  Diarrhea
  Celiac disease
  Inflammatory bowel disease
Decreased renal reabsorption
  Inherited disorders
  Isolated familial hypomagnesemia
  Primary hypomagnesemia with hypercalciuria
  Primary hypomagnesemia with hypocalcemia
  Bartter syndrome
  Gitelman syndrome
  Medications
  Loop diuretics
  Cisplatin
  Pentamidine
  Cyclosporine
  Aminoglycosides
  Foscarnet
  Amphotericin
Redistribution from the extracellular to the intracellular space
  Insulin therapy
  Hyperinsulinism
  Pancreatitis
  Hyperaldosteronism
  Respiratory alkalosis
  Catecholamines

with increased magnesium loss in the stool. Decreased renal reabsorption of magnesium may occur as the consequence of congenital or acquired renal disorders, medications (loop diuretics, cisplatin, cyclosporine, amphotericin B, and aminoglycosides), or metabolic abnormalities. Inherited disorders associated with renal magnesium wasting include (a) isolated familial hypomagnesemia, (b) familial hypomagnesemia with hypercalciuria [associated with mutations in the paracellin (*PCLN1*) gene], (c) primary hypomagnesemia with hypocalcemia (associated with defects in the TRP gene family), (d) Bartter syndrome [associated with mutations in the genes for the apical sodium–potassium–chloride cotransporter (*BSC1*), the apical inwardly rectifying potassium channel (*ROMK1*), or the basolateral chloride channel (*CLC-Kb*)], and (e) Gitelman syndrome [associated with mutations in the DCT electroneutral thiazide-sensitive sodium–chloride cotransporter (*TSC*)] (38–41).

Patients with isolated familial hypomagnesemia present with hypomagnesemia and hypermagnesuria but no other electrolyte disturbances. Familial hypomagnesemia with hypercalciuria is characterized by hypomagnesemia, hypermagnesuria, and marked hypercalciuria, contributing to hypocalcemia and nephrocalcinosis. Primary hypomagnesemia with hypocalcemia is an autosomal recessive disorder found in Bedouin kindreds; affected patients typically present with hypocalcemia-induced seizures. Bartter syndrome is an autosomal recessive disorder that presents in infancy or early childhood. Patients typically present with sodium wasting, hypokalemic metabolic alkalosis, and hypercalciuria. Gitelman syndrome presents after age 6, and is differentiated from Bartter syndrome by the presence of hypocalciuria. Impaired renal reabsorption of magnesium occurs as a side effect of various medications, including diuretics (most commonly of the loop type), cisplatin, pentamidine, cyclosporine, aminoglycosides, foscarnet, and amphotericin. Typically, renal magnesium wasting resolves within several days of discontinuation of the medication. One exception is cisplatin, with which renal magnesium loss may persist for several months. Intravascular volume expansion, osmotic diuresis (as seen in diabetic ketoacidosis), and polyuria during the recovery phase of acute renal failure have been reported as causes of hypomagnesemia due to renal loss.

The movement of magnesium from the extracellular to the intracellular compartment occurs in a variety of disorders, including insulin therapy for diabetic ketoacidosis and hyperinsulinism associated with the "refeeding syndrome" in chronically malnourished children. Enhanced intracellular uptake of magnesium has also been observed in patients with pancreatitis, hyperaldosteronism, respiratory alkalosis, and elevation in plasma catecholamines. Hypomagnesemia has been observed in patients who undergo cardiopulmonary bypass or require massive transfusion and in those with extensive burn injury or excessive sweating.

Signs and Symptoms

The signs and symptoms of hypomagnesemia do not typically manifest until serum levels fall below 1 mg/dL. The imbalance in serum magnesium typically affects the neuromuscular system and heart. Symptoms are often due to the hypocalcemia from impaired PTH release and hypokalemia, which are also associated with hypomagnesemia. Presenting neurologic signs include muscle weakness and tremors, tetany, Chvostek sign, Trousseau sign, and seizures. Hypokalemia consequent to hypomagnesemia lowers the myocardial action potential threshold, manifesting in nonspecific T-wave changes, U waves, a prolonged QT interval, and ventricular arrhythmias. Hypomagnesemia *per se* can predispose to cardiac dysrhythmias, particularly those of ventricular origin. However, the degree

of risk for dysrhythmias in patients with hypomagnesemia in general and the relative importance of Mg^{2+} deficiency alone versus hypomagnesemia with coexisting hypokalemia or intrinsic cardiac disease in the pathogenesis of the dysrhythmia remain controversial.

Diagnosis and Treatment

The diagnosis of hypomagnesemia can frequently be determined by the clinical history, which should explore dietary intake, gastrointestinal disorders, medications, renal function, and familial disorders. In addition to serum magnesium, serum calcium and potassium levels should be measured. If the cause of hypomagnesemia is unknown, measurement of plasma (P) and urinary (U) magnesium and creatinine concentrations and calculation of the fractional excretion of magnesium (FE_{Mg}) using the equation below can assist in the differentiation between renal and nonrenal causes of hypomagnesemia (3).

$$FE_{Mg} = [(U_{Mg} \times P_{creatinine})/(0.7 \times P_{Mg} \times U_{creatinine})] \times 100$$

Normal values for the fractional excretion of magnesium range from 1% to 8%. In patients with hypomagnesemia due to nonrenal causes, the FE_{Mg} is <2%. In patients with renal magnesium wasting, the FE_{Mg} is >4%. If a renal cause of hypomagnesemia is suspected, an arterial blood gas should be obtained to assess for metabolic alkalosis.

Symptomatic patients or asymptomatic patients with magnesium levels <1 mg/dL require IV replacement with a magnesium salt (3,19). Magnesium sulfate at a dose of 25–50 mg/kg (2.5–5.0 mg/kg of elemental magnesium) given as a slow IV infusion is recommended. Serum magnesium levels should be closely monitored, and the dose should be repeated every 6 hours until levels stabilize. For patients who require long-term therapy or for mild-to-moderate hypomagnesemia, oral supplementation with agents such as magnesium gluconate (5.4 mg elemental magnesium/100 mg), magnesium oxide (60 mg elemental magnesium/100 mg), and magnesium sulfate (10 mg elemental magnesium/100 mg) at doses of 20–40 mg/kg of elemental magnesium per day can be instituted. Patients with hypocalcemia and hypokalemia require replenishment of these minerals.

Hypomagnesemia in Critical Illness

Hypomagnesemia is a relatively common electrolyte abnormality in the ICU setting with rates ranging from 24% to 44% (42–45). Critically ill patients with hypomagnesemia commonly have other coexisting electrolyte abnormalities, including hypocalcemia (most common), hypokalemia, hyponatremia, and hypophosphatemia (42). Common risk factors and causes include sepsis, cardiopulmonary bypass, and drug side effect (most commonly diuretic use) (43,45). Hypomagnesemia has been associated with increased incidence of cardiac arrhythmias following cardiopulmonary bypass (46–49) and increased ICU mortality (42,43). Repletion of magnesium following cardiac surgery has been associated with a decreased incidence of arrhythmias (49). However, there is no current evidence showing that correction of hypomagnesemia is associated with a reduction in ICU mortality. Nonetheless, it is recommended that hypomagnesemia be corrected in critically ill patients.

Hypermagnesemia

Causes

Hypermagnesemia can be the consequence of increased intake or administration of magnesium, decreased renal excretion,

TABLE 108.8

CAUSES OF HYPERMAGNESEMIA

Increased intake
  Laxatives
  Enemas
  Parenteral administration
  Magnesium supplementation
Decreased renal excretion (renal failure)
Cellular release
  Shock
  Trauma
  Burns
Other
  Hypothyroidism
  Hypoaldosteronism

massive cellular release, or other causes (Table 108.8). Hypermagnesemia most commonly occurs in the setting of excess administration of medications that contain magnesium (e.g., cathartics and antacids) or parenteral administration of magnesium to patients with preeclampsia. Patients with renal failure have impaired renal excretion of magnesium, but hypermagnesemia is uncommon unless the patient is receiving magnesium supplementation. Significant cellular lysis with release of intracellular magnesium and consequent hypermagnesemia has been reported in the setting of shock, trauma, and burns. Hypothyroidism and hypoaldosteronism are rare causes of hypermagnesemia.

Signs and Symptoms

The signs and symptoms of hypermagnesemia usually do not manifest until the serum level is >4.0 mg/dL. The manifestations of hypermagnesemia are attributable, in part, to impaired release and binding of acetylcholine at the neuromuscular junction (Table 108.9). Patients may develop muscle weakness, loss of deep tendon reflexes, lethargy, progression to coma, and respiratory failure. Magnesium-induced vasodilatation may cause hypotension. Ileus or decreased gastrointestinal motility may be a presenting sign. Hypermagnesemia also induces significant cardiac effects, including bradycardia, prolongation of the PR and QT intervals, heart block, and cardiac arrest.

Diagnosis and Treatment

The diagnosis of hypermagnesemia may be suggested by the clinical history, which should explore medications and symptoms of renal dysfunction. The basic tenets of therapy

TABLE 108.9

SIGNS AND SYMPTOMS OF HYPERMAGNESEMIA

Neuromuscular
  Muscle weakness
  Muscle paralysis
  Respiratory depression
  Lethargy
  Coma
Cardiac
  Prolonged PR interval
  Prolonged QT interval

for hypermagnesemia are to interrupt magnesium intake and promote magnesium excretion (3,21). Because hypermagnesemia may contribute to hypocalcemia, serum calcium levels should be measured and followed closely during therapy.

Patients with mild, asymptomatic hypermagnesemia and good renal function can be safely treated by stopping the magnesium-containing agent. Patients with significant neuromuscular or cardiac toxicity require measures to enhance magnesium excretion, which can be achieved by hydration with normal saline and administration of a loop diuretic. Alternatively, non-magnesium-containing enemas or a cathartic may be administered. Patients with refractory hypermagnesemia or with renal failure and severe hypermagnesemia may require hemodialysis or peritoneal dialysis to effectively reduce serum magnesium levels. Hypocalcemia should be corrected by calcium replacement. Another scenario involves newborns born to mothers on magnesium for eclampsia who are hypotonic and hypotensive from hypermagnesemia and may require treatment with calcium and normal saline administration to improve blood pressure.

Hypophosphatemia

Causes

Hypophosphatemia occurs as the consequence of (a) decreased dietary phosphate intake or malabsorption, (b) decreased renal reabsorption, (c) increased bone formation, or (d) redistribution of phosphate from the extracellular to the intracellular space (Table 108.10). Hypophosphatemia due to poor intake is uncommon because of the abundance of phosphate in foodstuffs and compensatory ability of the renal tubule to enhance

TABLE 108.10

CAUSES OF HYPOPHOSPHATEMIA

Decreased dietary intake or malabsorption
  Protein–calorie malnutrition
  Disorders of the duodenum and jejunum
  Chronic diarrhea
Decreased renal reabsorption
  PTH-dependent mechanisms
    Hyperparathyroidism
    Tumor release of PTH-related peptide
  PTH-/PTHrP-independent mechanisms
  X-linked hyperphosphatemic rickets and other FGF23-
    related disorders
  Intravascular volume expansion
  Fanconi syndrome
  Vitamin D deficiency
  Medications/toxins
    Acetazolamide
    Glucocorticoids
    Ifosfamide
    Cisplatin
    Pamidronate
    Heavy-metal ingestion
Increased bone formation ("hungry-bone" syndrome)
Redistribution from the extracellular to the intracellular space
  Insulin therapy
  Catecholamine administration
  Theophylline
  Respiratory alkalosis

PTHrP, PTH-related peptide; FGF, fibroblast growth factor.

⑩ reabsorption of phosphate when supply is low. Children with severe protein–calorie malnutrition and premature infants who ingest unsupplemented breast milk (which is low in phosphate content) may develop hypophosphatemia. Critically ill, malnourished patients, in particular those who require mechanical ventilation, may develop hypophosphatemia during refeeding. Administration of carbohydrate in these patients enhances insulin release, which stimulates intracellular uptake ⑪ of phosphate. The combination of phosphate depletion from their baseline poor nutritional state, along with cellular uptake of phosphate, may contribute to symptomatic hypophosphatemia—most commonly muscle weakness—impairing the ability to wean from mechanical ventilation. Malabsorption due to intestinal disorders that affect the duodenum and jejunum (the primary sites for phosphate absorption) and ingestion of phosphate-binding acids are frequently encountered causes of hypophosphatemia.

Increased renal excretion of phosphate may occur by PTH-dependent and PTH-independent mechanisms. Hyperparathyroidism and tumor secretion of PTHrP (discussed previously) decrease the renal TRP. PTH-independent mechanisms of hypophosphatemia include intravascular volume expansion, renal tubular disorders (e.g., X-linked hypophosphatemia and Fanconi syndrome), medications, and toxins. The Fanconi syndrome is a generalized renal tubular wasting of solutes that typically include phosphate, amino acids, glucose, and bicarbonate. Fanconi syndrome may be inherited or acquired and includes renal tubular acidosis and hypophosphatemia (hypokalemia may ensue) as the most clinically significant features. Acetazolamide, glucocorticoids, bicarbonate, ifosfamide, cisplatin, pamidronate, ethanol, and heavy metals also enhance renal excretion of phosphate.

The genetic disorder X-linked hypophosphatemia usually presents as a rachitic disorder in early childhood and is due to mutations in the *PHEX* gene that encodes for an enzyme of the neuropeptidase family (50,51). For reasons that are not clear, elevated serum levels of a novel member of the fibroblast growth factor family, FGF23, are characteristic of X-linked hypophosphatemia and are thought to mediate the renal phosphate wasting. Elevated FGF23 levels are typical of other related causes of hypophosphatemic rickets. These include (a) autosomal-dominant hypophosphatemic rickets (due to specific *FGF23* mutation that prevent its breakdown), (b) autosomal recessive hypophosphatemic rickets (due to mutations in *DMP1*, dentine matrix protein), and (c) oncogenic osteomalacia, in which FGF23 is overproduced by tumors (52).

Other causes of redistribution of phosphate from the extracellular to the intracellular space with resultant hypophosphatemia include increased endogenous insulin production following glucose infusion, insulin therapy for treatment of diabetic ketoacidosis, catecholamine administration, theophylline, and respiratory alkalosis.

Signs and Symptoms

Signs and symptoms of severe hypophosphatemia occur when serum phosphate levels are <1–1.5 mg/dL. The signs and symptoms are believed to be the consequence of intracellular ATP and resultant cellular energy depletion (Table 108.11). The signs and symptoms are variable. Patients may present with hemolysis, leukocyte dysfunction, platelet dysfunction, muscle weakness, paralysis, muscle atrophy, respiratory failure, rhabdomyolysis, and lethargy.

Diagnosis and Treatment

The diagnosis of hypophosphatemia may be suspected from elements of the clinical history, which should explore dietary intake, medications, renal function, and a family history of

TABLE 108.11

SIGNS AND SYMPTOMS OF HYPOPHOSPHATEMIA

Muscle weakness
Paralysis
Coma
Seizures
Respiratory depression
Hemolysis
Leukocyte dysfunction
Platelet dysfunction
Rhabdomyolysis

renal tubular disorders or hyperparathyroidism. Measurement of serum phosphate, total serum calcium, circulating PTH, and vitamin D levels is usually helpful. Patients with serum phosphate levels >2.2 mg/dL do not require aggressive therapy and can be treated with an increased intake of milk (3,21). Patients with serum phosphate levels <1.5 mg/dL and/or symptomatic hypophosphatemia may require treatment with IV phosphate. It has been recommended that patients with asymptomatic severe hypophosphatemia (<1 mg/dL) receive 2.5 mg/kg of elemental phosphorus over 6 hours and that symptomatic patients receive 5 mg/kg of elemental phosphorus also over 6 hours (3,21). When administering intravenous phosphate supplements, patients should be monitored for the development of hypocalcemia, hypomagnesemia, and hypotension.

Hypophosphatemia in Critical Illness

In critically ill patients, hypophosphatemia is most commonly the consequence of phosphate depletion (malnutrition, antacid therapy, diuretic use) or cellular uptake of phosphate (insulin administration, cortisol administration, respiratory alkalosis) (53,54). It occurs commonly following major surgical procedures including cardiac and hepatic surgery (55–58). Patients with severe hypophosphatemia (<1 mg/dL) are at risk for the development of altered mental status, generalized weakness, respiratory insufficiency, myocardial dysfunction, and arrhythmias due to depletion of phosphate energy stores (59–63). Multiple studies have shown an association between hypophosphatemia and increased mortality in critically ill patients. Correction of severe hypophosphatemia is recommended despite the lack of evidence showing a reduction in ICU mortality.

Hyperphosphatemia

Causes

Hyperphosphatemia is the result of increased intake of phosphate, or its decreased renal excretion or redistribution from the extracellular to the intracellular space. Increased intake is an uncommon cause of hyperphosphatemia (Table 108.12), reported in patients with renal failure who are receiving phosphate supplementation and in children receiving phosphate enemas. Acute and chronic renal failure is the most common cause of hyperphosphatemia due to limitations of phosphate excretion, with progressive nephron impairment or loss. Other conditions associated with impaired renal phosphate excretion include acromegaly and tumoral calcinosis, a rare, non-neoplastic disease characterized by hyperphosphatemia, increased 1,25-dihydroxyvitamin D levels, low or normal PTH levels, and periarticular calcium deposition. More common in African Americans, tumoral calcinosis presents with focal hyperostosis and large, lobulated periarticular ectopic calcifications. It may result from loss-of-function mutations in *FGF23*, or *GALNT3*,

TABLE 108.12

CAUSES OF HYPERPHOSPHATEMIA

Increased intake
  Phosphate supplements
  Phosphate-containing enemas
Decreased renal excretion
  Acute and chronic renal failure
  Hypoparathyroidism
  Acromegaly
  Heparin
  Tumoral calcinosis
  Vitamin D intoxication
Redistribution from the extracellular to the intracellular space
  Tumor lysis syndrome
  Rhabdomyolysis
  Hemolysis
  Crush injuries
  Hyperthermia
  Respiratory acidosis
  Metabolic acidosis

a gene encoding an *N*-acetylgalactosaminyltransferase (Gal-NAc-transferase) that is thought to be important in the post-translational modification of FGF23 (64). Respiratory acidosis, metabolic acidosis, tumor lysis syndrome, rhabdomyolysis, hemolysis, crush injuries, and hyperthermia are also associated with hyperphosphatemia.

Signs, Symptoms, Diagnosis, and Treatment

Hyperphosphatemia alone generally does not result in acute physiologic manifestations. Hyperphosphatemia, however, may serve to increase the calcium–phosphate product, which, when >80 mg/dL in infants (>60 in small children and >40 in older children and adults), promotes soft tissue calcification. Acute increases in serum phosphate levels will also result in a hypocalcemic response. Supportive history for the finding of hyperphosphatemia should include a review of dietary intake, medications, and renal function. The basic tenets of treatment are to improve renal filtration and excretion of phosphate through intravascular volume expansion with normal saline and to stop intake of excess phosphate (3,21). Dialysis is effective in decreasing phosphate in renal failure patients with severe hyperphosphatemia.

CONCLUSIONS AND FUTURE DIRECTIONS

Disorders of calcium, magnesium, and phosphate are commonly the result of disruptions in their supply and demand. In addition, hormonal signaling pathways that regulate these minerals may be disrupted. As these pathways and the genetic mutations that affect calcium, magnesium, and phosphate homeostasis are more clearly delineated, tailored therapies directed toward molecular targets within the various biochemical pathways will likely be developed. For example, identification of the calcium-sensing receptor as central to regulation of PTH secretion has resulted in "calcimimetic" medications. These compounds increase the sensitivity of the calcium-sensing receptor to circulating ionized calcium concentrations and have been used to treat selected cases of hyperparathyroidism (65). The use of calcimimetics has included the treatment of increased PTH levels in children with chronic kidney disease (66). The effect of these medications on the calcium-sensing

receptors on the chondrocytes at growth plates in bones and the result of this on growth in children will need to be evaluated.

References

1. Suki WN, Lederer ED, Rouse D. Renal transport of calcium, magnesium, and phosphate. In: Brenner BM, ed. *Brenner and Rector's The Kidney.* 6th ed. Philadelphia, PA: WB Saunders, 2000:520–74.
2. Dai LJ, Ritchie G, Kerstan D, et al. Magnesium transport in the renal distal convoluted tubule. *Physiol Rev* 2001;81:51–84.
3. Greenbaum LA. Pathophysiology of body fluids and fluid therapy. In: Behrman RE, Kliegman RM, Jensen HB, eds. *Nelson Textbook of Pediatrics.* 17th ed. St. Louis, MO: WB Saunders, 2004; MD Consult version.
4. Vennekens R, Prenen J, Hoenderop JG, et al. Modulation of the epithelial Ca^{2+} channel ECaC by extracellular pH. *Pflugers Arch* 2001;442:237–42.
5. Ambuhl PM, Zajicek HK, Wang H, et al. Regulation of renal phosphate transport by acute and chronic metabolic acidosis in the rat. *Kidney Int* 1998;53:1288–98.
6. Topf JM, Murray PT. Hypomagnesemia and hypermagnesemia. *Rev Endocr Metab Disord* 2003;4:195–206.
7. Mannstadt M, Juppner H, Gardella TJ. Receptors for PTH and PTHrP: Their biological importance and functional properties. *Am J Physiol* 1999;277(5, pt 2):F665–F675.
8. Lotscher M, Scarpetta Y, Levi M, et al. Rapid downregulation of rat renal Na/P(i) cotransporter in response to parathyroid hormone involves microtubule rearrangement. *J Clin Invest* 1999;104:483–94.
9. Murayama A, Takeyama K, Kitanaka S, et al. Positive and negative regulations of the renal 25-hydroxyvitamin D_3 1α-hydroxylase gene by parathyroid hormone, calcitonin, and 1α,25(OH)$_2$D$_3$ in intact animals. *Endocrinology* 1999;140:2224–31.
10. Suda T, Takahashi N, Udagawa N, et al. Modulation of osteoclast differentiation and function by the new members of the tumor necrosis factor receptor and ligand families. *Endocr Rev* 1999;20:345–57.
11. Estepa JC, Aguilera-Tejero E, Lopez I, et al. Effect of phosphate on parathyroid hormone secretion in vivo. *J Bone Miner Res* 1999;14:1848–54.
12. Takeyama K, Kitanaka S, Sato T, et al. 25-Hydroxyvitamin D$_3$1α-hydroxylase and vitamin D synthesis. *Science* 1997;277: 1827–30.
13. Zaloga GP, Chernow B. The multifactorial basis for hypocalcemia during sepsis. Studies of the parathyroid hormone-vitamin D axis. *Ann Intern Med* 1987;107:36–41.
14. Price PA. Blood chemistries and body fluids. In: Robertson J, Shilkofski N, eds. *Johns Hopkins: The Harriet Lane Handbook: A Manual for Pediatric House Officers.* 17th ed. St. Louis, MO: Mosby, 2005; MD Consult version.
15. Garabedian M. Hypocalcemia and chromosome 22q11 microdeletion. *Genet Couns* 1999;10:389–94.
16. Sunthornthepvarakul T, Churesigaew S, Ngowngarmratana S. A novel mutation of the signal peptide of the preproparathyroid hormone gene associated with autosomal recessive familial isolated hypoparathyroidism. *J Clin Endocrinol Metab* 1999;84:3792–6.
17. Pearce SH, Williamson C, Kifor O, et al. A familial syndrome of hypocalcemia with hypercalciuria due to mutations in the calcium-sensing receptor. *N Engl J Med* 1996;335:1115–22.
18. Jüppner H, Schipani E, Bastepe M, et al. The gene responsible for pseudohypoparathyroidism type Ib is paternally imprinted and maps in four unrelated kindreds to chromosome 20q13.3. *Proc Natl Acad Sci USA* 1998;95:11798–803.
19. Hastbacka J, Petilla V. Prevalence and predictive value of ionized hypocalcemia among critically ill patients. *Acta Anesthesiol Scand* 2003;47:1264–9.

20. Ward RT, Colton DM, Meade PC, et al. Serum levels of calcium and albumin in survivors after critical injury. *J Crit Care* 2004;19:54–64.

21. Bringhurst FR, Demay MB, Kronenberg HM. Hormones and disorders of mineral metabolism. In: Larsen PR, Kronenberg HM, Melmed S, et al., eds. *Williams Textbook of Endocrinology.* 10th ed. St. Louis, MO: WB Saunders, 2003; MD Consult version.

22. Martin TJ, Kang Y, Robertson KM, et al. Ionization and hemodynamic effects of calcium chloride and calcium gluconate in the absence of hepatic function. *Anesthesiology* 1990;73:62–5.

23. Umpaichitra V, Bastian W, Castells S. Hypocalcemia in children: Pathogenesis and management. *Clin Pediatr* 2001;40:305–12.

24. Ford DC, Leist ER, Algren JR, et al. *Guidelines for Administration of Intravenous Medications to Pediatric Patients.* 2nd ed. Bethesda, MD: American Society of Health-System Pharmacists, 1984.

25. Zaloga GP. Hypocalcemia in critically ill patients. *Crit Care Med* 1992;20:251–62.

26. Buckley MS, Leblanc JM, Cawley MJ. Electrolyte disturbances associated with commonly prescribed medications in the intensive care unit. *Crit Care Med* 2010;38:S253–S264.

27. Lind L, Carlstedt F, Rastad J, et al. Hypocalcemia and parathyroid hormone secretion in critically ill patients. *Crit Care Med* 2000;28:93–9.

28. Egi M, Kim I, Nichol A, et al. Ionized calcium concentration and outcome in critical illness. *Crit Care Med* 2011;39:314–21.

29. Steele T, Kolamunnage-Dona R, Downey C, et al. Assessment and clinical course of hypocalcemia in critical illness. *Crit Care* 2013;17:R106.

30. Beall DP, Henslee HB, Webb HR, et al. Milk alkali syndrome: A historical review and description of the modern version of the syndrome. *Am J Med Sci* 2006;331:233–42.

31. Marx SJ, Agarwal SK, Kester MB, et al. Multiple endocrine neoplasia type 1: Clinical and genetic features of the hereditary endocrine neoplasias. *Recent Prog Horm Res* 1999;54:397–439.

32. Schuffenecker I, Virally-Monod M, Brohet R, et al. Risk and penetrance of primary hyperparathyroidism in multiple endocrine neoplasia type 2A families with mutations at codon 634 of the RET proto-oncogene. *J Clin Endocrinol Metab* 1998;83:487–91.

33. Body JJ. Hypercalcemia of malignancy. *Semin Nephrol* 2004;24:48–54.

34. NIH Conference. Diagnosis and management of asymptomatic primary hyperparathyroidism: Consensus development conference statement. *Ann Intern Med* 1991;114:593–7.

35. Forster J, Querusio L, Burchard KW, et al. Hypercalcemia in critically ill surgical patients. *Ann Surg* 1985;202(4):512–8.

36. Aguilera IM, Vaughan RS. Calcium and the anaesthetist. *Anaesthesia* 2001;55(8):779–90.

37. Lind L, Ljunghall S. Critical care hypercalcemia—A hyperparathyroid state. *Exp Clin Endocrinol* 1992;100(3):148–51.

38. Blostein R, Pu HX, Scanzano R, et al. Structure/function studies of the gamma subunit of the Na,K-ATPase. *Ann N Y Acad Sci* 2003;986:420–7.

39. Konrad M, Schlingmann KP, Gudermann T. Insights into the molecular nature of magnesium homeostasis. *Am J Physiol Renal Physiol* 2004;286:F599–F605.

40. Walder RY, Landau D, Meyer P, et al. Mutation of TRPM6 causes familial hypomagnesemia with secondary hypocalcemia. *Nat Genet* 2002;31:171–174.

41. Wolf MT, Dotsch J, Konrad M, et al. Follow-up of five patients with FHHNC due to mutations in the paracellin-1 gene. *Pediatr Nephrol* 2002;17:602–8.

42. Zafar MSH, Wani JI, Karim R, et al. Significance of serum magnesium levels in critically ill patients. *Int J Appl Basic Med Res* 2014;4:34–7.

43. Saleem AF, Haque A. On admission hypomagnesemia in critically ill children: Risk factors and outcome. *Indian J Pediatr* 2009;76(12):1227–30.

44. Escuela MP, Guerra M, Añón JM, et al. Total and ionized serum magnesium in critically ill patients. *Intensive Care Med* 2005;31:151–7.

45. Dacey MJ. Hypomagnesemic disorders. *Crit Care Clin* 2001;17:155–73, viii.

46. Aglio LS, Stanford GG, Maddi R, et al. Hypomagnesemia is common following cardiac surgery. *J Cardiothorac Vasc Anesth* 1991;5:201–8.

47. Lum G, Marquardt C, Kuri SF. Hypomagnesemia and low alkaline phosphatase activity in patients' serum after cardiac surgery. *Clin Chem* 1989;35:664–7.

48. Prielipp RC, Zaloga GP, Butterworth JF, et al. Magnesium inhibits the hypertensive but not cardiotonic actions of low-dose epinephrine. *Anesthesiology* 1991;74:973–9.

49. Schweigel I, Kopel ME, Finlayson DC. Magnesium reduces the incidence of post-operative dysrhythmias in patients after cardiac surgery. *Anesthesiology* 1989;71:A1163.

50. Liu S, Guo R, Simpson LG, et al. Regulation of fibroblastic growth factor 23 expression but not degradation by PHEX. *J Biol Chem* 2003;278(39):37419–26.

51. Sabbagh Y, Boileau G, Campos M, et al. Structure and function of disease-causing missense mutations in the PHEX gene. *J Clin Endocrinol Metab* 2003;88(5):2213–22.

52. Yu X, White KE. FGF23 and disorders of phosphate homeostasis. *Cytokine Growth Factor Rev* 2005;16(2):221–32.

53. de Menezes FS, Leite HP, Fernandez J, et al. Hypophosphatemia in critically ill children. *Rev Hosp Clin Fac Med Sao Paulo* 2004;59:306–11.

54. Geerse DA, Bindels AJ, Kuiper MA, et al. Treatment of hypophosphatemia in the intensive care unit: A review. *Crit Care* 2010;14:R147.

55. Cohen J, Kogan A, Sahar G, et al. Hypophosphatemia following open heart surgery: Incidence and consequences. *Eur J Cardiothorac Surg* 2004;26:306–10.

56. Zazzo JF, Troche G, Ruel P, et al. High incidence of hypophosphatemia in surgical intensive care patients: Efficacy of phosphorus therapy on myocardial function. *Intensive Care Med* 1995;21:826–31.

57. Goldstein J, Vincent JL, Leclerc JL, et al. Hypophosphatemia after cardiothoracic surgery. *Intensive Care Med* 1985;11:144–8.

58. George R, Shiu MH. Hypophosphatemia after major hepatic resection. *Surgery* 1992;111:281–6.

59. Aubier M, Murciano D, Lecocguic Y, et al. Effect of hypophosphatemia on diaphragmatic contractility in patients with acute respiratory failure. *N Engl J Med* 1985;313:420–4.

60. Fiaccadori E, Coffrini E, Fracchia C, et al. Hypophosphatemia and phosphorus depletion in respiratory and peripheral muscles of patients with respiratory failure due to COPD. *Chest* 1994;105(5):1392–8.

61. Schwartz A, Gurman G, Cohen G, et al. Association between hypophosphatemia and cardiac arrhythmias in the early stages of sepsis. *Eur J Intern Med* 2002;13(7):434–48.

62. Ognibene A, Ciniglio R, Greifenstein A, et al. Ventricular tachycardia in acute myocardial infarction: The role of hypophosphatemia. *South Med J* 1994;87(1):65–9.

63. Bugg NC, Jones JA. Hypophosphatemia pathophysiology, effects and management on the intensive care unit. *Anaesthesia* 1998;53(9):895–902.

64. Topaz O, Shurman DL, Bergman R, et al. Mutations in GALNT3, encoding a protein involved in O-linked glycosylation, cause familial tumoral calcinosis. *Nat Genet* 2004;36(6):579–81.

65. Falchetti A. Calcium agonists in hyperparathyroidism. *Expert Opin Investig Drugs* 2004;14:229–44.

66. Alharthi AA, Kamal NM, Abukhatwah MW, et al. Cinacalcet in pediatric and adolescent chronic kidney disease: A single-center experience. *Medicine* 2015;94:e401.

CHAPTER 109 ■ THYROID DISEASE

ORI EYAL AND SUSAN R. ROSE

KEY POINTS

1 To understand the effects of critical illness on thyroid function, it is necessary to understand the normal physiology of thyroid hormone secretion and action.

2 Most patients in the ICU will exhibit nonthyroidal illness, which probably reflects physiologic adaptation to disease.

3 Currently, treatment of nonthyroidal illness with thyroid hormone therapy is not recommended, nor is thyroid function testing during intercurrent illness. However, if clinical suspicion for hypothyroidism arises, thyroid function tests

should be checked; if hypothyroidism is confirmed, thyroid treatment should be initiated.

4 The two thyroid emergencies, myxedema coma and thyroid storm, are extremely rare in the pediatric population (myxedema coma occurs typically in older patients). However, it is important to recognize the diagnostic features and the precipitating factors and to initiate treatment as soon as possible, as both are life-threatening conditions with high mortality rates if left untreated.

NORMAL PHYSIOLOGY

1 Thyroid hormones play a key role in the regulation of energy expenditure and substrate metabolism and are essential for normal growth and development. A classic feedback control loop exists between the thyroid gland, hypothalamus, and pituitary (**Fig. 109.1**). Thyrotropin-releasing hormone (TRH)

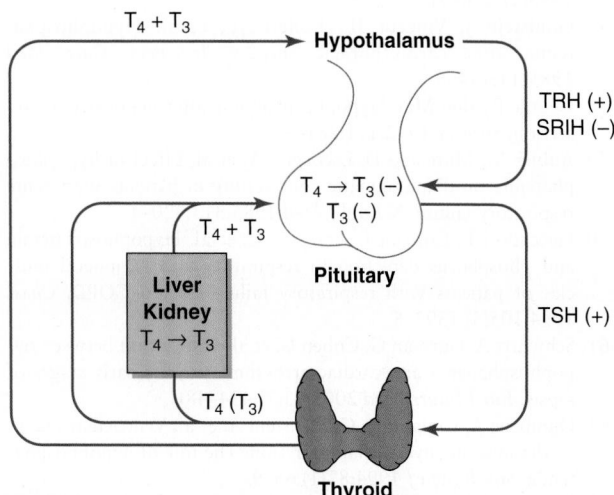

FIGURE 109.1. Basic elements in the regulation of thyroid function. TRH stimulates TSH synthesis and release. TRH synthesis is regulated directly by thyroid hormones. TSH stimulates the thyroid gland to synthesize and secret thyroid hormones. T4 is the predominant secretory product of the thyroid gland, with peripheral deiodination of tetraiodothyronine (T4) to triiodothyronine (T3) in the liver and the kidney, supplying 80% of the circulating T3. Both circulating T3 and T4 inhibit TSH synthesis and release independently; T4 via its rapid conversion to T3. SRIH, somatostatin. (Adapted from www.thyroidmanager.org, permission from Endocrine Education Inc.)

is expressed in the hypothalamus and regulates thyroid-stimulating hormone (TSH) synthesis and secretion by the thyrotroph cells in the pituitary. Serum TSH concentration exhibits a circadian pattern. After it reaches its nadir in the late afternoon, the serum TSH concentration rises to a peak around midnight, remains on a plateau for several hours, and then declines (1). TSH is the major regulator of the morphologic and functional states of the thyroid gland. In addition, an inverse relationship exists between the thyroid organic iodine and the rate of hormone formation.

The substrate for the synthesis of thyroid hormone is circulating iodide. The thyroid gland is able to trap iodide from the circulation by an energy-requiring mechanism. The trapped iodide is oxidized by the enzyme peroxidase. The next step in the synthesis of triiodothyronine (T3) and tetraiodothyronine (T4) is iodination of tyrosine to monoiodotyrosine (MIT) and to diiodotyrosine (DIT). Coupling of two DIT molecules results in the formation of T4. Some T3 is also formed within the thyroid gland by condensation of one molecule of MIT and DIT. The formed T3 and T4 are stored in the thyroid gland in combination with thyroglobulin. Release of T3 and T4 from thyroglobulin in the colloid (fluid that contains thyroglobulin in the lumens of the follicles) occurs by proteolysis and is regulated by TSH (2).

Under normal conditions, 10%–20% of T3 and 100% of T4 in the serum are directly secreted by the thyroid gland. The remaining 80%–90% of T3 is derived from peripheral monodeiodination of T4 by the enzyme 5'-monodeiodinase. Thyroxine (T4) may also be metabolized peripherally by the enzyme 5'-monodeiodinase to reverse T3 (rT3), which is largely metabolically inactive. Three types of monodeiodinase have been described: Type I 5'-monodeiodinase predominantly is expressed in the liver and the kidney and accounts for most circulating T3. Type II 5'-monodeiodinase is located predominantly in the brain, pituitary, and brown adipose tissue, and acts primarily to increase the intracellular levels of T3 in these tissues. Circulating T3 is not active in the brain, and T4 is not active in the brain without this enzyme. Type III 5'-monodeiodinase catalyzes the conversion of T4 to rT3 and of T3 to T2 (diiodothyronine).

In the blood, thyroid hormones are mainly associated with carrier proteins: thyroxine-binding globulin (TBG), prealbumin or transthyretin, and albumin. The prolonged half-life of thyroid hormone is related to its protein binding. The bound form is in equilibrium with free hormones. The most important carrier protein for T4 is TBG. TBG and albumin seem equally important as carrier proteins for T3. The concentrations of free T4 and free T3 approximate 0.03% and 0.30%, respectively, of the total serum thyroid hormone concentration (3). The bound hormone acts merely as a serum reservoir. It is the free hormone that is available to the tissues for intracellular transport and feedback regulation. The free hormones penetrate the cell membrane by carrier-mediated, energy-dependent transport. The carrier-transport system for T3 and T4 is saturable and stereospecific and requires ATP. The two iodothyronines typically do not compete for uptake (4). T4 is monodeiodinated to T3 in the cell cytoplasm.

The cellular cytoplasmic T3 diffuses into the nucleus and initiates its actions by binding to one of two groups of nuclear DNA-bound thyroid hormone receptors (TR), TRα or TRβ. After binding, the T3/TR complex either homodimerizes with a second TR or heterodimerizes to a retinoid x receptor. These complexes directly bind to consensus DNA sequences, resulting in either activation or inhibition of gene transcription (**Fig. 109.2**). The thyroid hormone nuclear receptors are members of the steroid hormone/retinoic acid receptor superfamily and function as DNA transcription factors. The gene for TRα is located on chromosome 17, and the gene for TRβ is on chromosome 3. Each gene is translated to several mRNA species, including TRα1, TRα2, TRβ1, and TRβ2. TRα1 and TRβ1 are the major nuclear receptors present in most tissues. TRα2 is present in developing brain tissue. TRβ2 is present in pituitary and selected brain tissues (3). T3 is the active hormone and has a 15-fold higher binding affinity for the DNA receptor than does T4.

A number of assays have been developed for TSH and free T4 (FT4). One should be aware of the specific assays being used at one's own institution, the normal ranges in these assays, and the possible factors that may interfere with each

assay and cause falsely elevated or falsely decreased results. The ultrasensitive TSH immunoassay uses monoclonal antibodies. With the availability of third- and fourth-generation ultrasensitive assays, TSH can now be measured quickly and with more accuracy than with previous assays. Estimates of the FT4 concentration in serum can be generated by direct and indirect assay. Analog indirect assays for FT4 employ radioimmunoassay. The gold standard for measurement of FT4 uses equilibrium dialysis, which is the most accurate and direct measurement of the concentrations of FT4. FT4 can be measured indirectly by using radiolabeled T4; the proportion that is unbound by protein is determined by dialysis, and the concentration of FT4 can then be calculated as the product of the total hormone concentration and the fraction that is free (4).

❷ CRITICAL NONTHYROIDAL ILLNESS

A decrease in serum T3 and an increase in rT3 levels are characteristic of the fasting state. These are also the most common changes in nonthyroidal illness (NTI) in response to a variety of acute and chronic illnesses, a condition that is referred to as the euthyroid sick syndrome, NTI, or the low-T3 syndrome. The most rapid and consistent findings in NTI are decline in circulating total T3 and free T3 and an increase in the inactivated rT3 concentrations. A major contributing factor to the decrease in the peripheral production of T3 is the decreased conversion of T4 into T3 by type I enzyme 5′-monodeiodinase. The concomitant rise of rT3 appears to be due to impaired rT3 clearance secondary to decreased 5′-monodeiodinase activity during illness, and not so much due to an increase in rT3 production by type III monodeiodinase. The greater the severity of the disease, the greater the decline in serum T3 levels (5,6), greater the rise in rT3, and the greater the reduction in the T3/rT3 ratio (7).

The majority of patients with NTI have a normal or slightly decreased serum FT4 level. Most commonly, serum total and free T3 concentrations are low, whereas serum T4 concentration remains within the normal range. However, with increasing severity of illness, the serum T4 level and that of T3 decrease. In severely ill patients, an additional suppression of the hypothalamic–pituitary hormone release is often observed (6). The concentration of TSH typically remains within the low-to-normal range, but the circadian variation of TSH may be lost, and response of TSH to TRH is blunted. Low TSH level during critical illness is associated with poorer overall prognosis. Various agents, such as dopamine and corticosteroids, may further decrease TSH levels (**Table 109.1**). Patients with prolonged critical illness show diminished TSH pulsatility, as if progressive dysfunction of the hypothalamus is involved, characterized by an absent nocturnal TSH surge and decreased TSH pulse amplitude. The changes in nocturnal TSH secretion in NTI resemble those found in central hypothyroidism, suggesting that hypothalamic changes are involved in this condition. In severe prolonged illness, the changes in thyroid function may be accompanied by a decline in secretion of growth hormone, gonadotropins, and adrenocorticotropic hormone (ACTH) (6–8). During the recovery phase, the TSH level may rise slightly above the normal range. Whether these alterations serve as physiologic adaptation or contribute to further deterioration remains an intriguing question (**Fig. 109.3**). The treatment of NTI is controversial. Multiple studies have addressed this issue in patients with cardiac disease, sepsis, pulmonary disease, burn, and trauma. Brent and Hershman (9) found no difference in mortality between critically ill patients with NTI who were treated with T4 and the control group consisting of critically ill patients with NTI who were

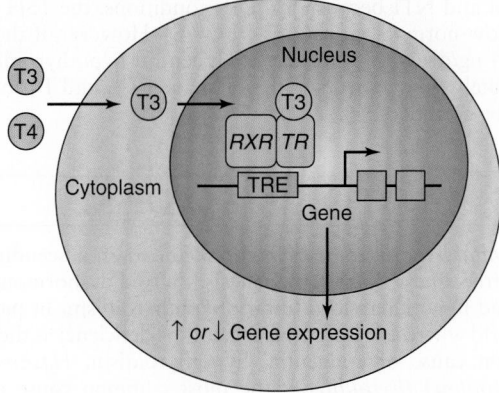

Mechanism of Thyroid Hormone Action

FIGURE 109.2. Thyroid hormones exhibit their action through binding to nuclear receptors. T3 and T4 (the major circulating thyroid hormones) are transported across plasma membranes into peripheral cells, where T4 is monodeiodinated to T3. The cytoplasmic T3 diffuses into the nucleus, where it binds to the thyroid hormone receptors, which in turn, bind to DNA at retinoid x receptor (RXR). The hormone activated receptor binds to thyroid hormone response elements (TRE) and regulates gene transcription and, thus, levels of mRNA. (Adapted from www.thyroidmanager.org, permission from Endocrine Education Inc.)

TABLE 109.1

MEDICATIONS ASSOCIATED WITH HYPOTHYROIDISM

Decreased TSH secretion
  Dopamine
  Glucocorticoids
  Octreotide
Decreased thyroid hormone secretion
  Lithium
  Iodide
  Amiodarone
Decreased T4 absorption
  Cole stipol
  Cholestyramine
  Aluminum hydroxide
  Ferrous sulfate
  Sucralfate
Increased thyroid hormone metabolism
  Phenobarbital
  Rifampin
  Phenytoin
  Carbamazepine

TABLE 109.2

CHANGES IN THYROID FUNCTION TESTS IN HYPOTHYROIDISM AND DURING CRITICAL ILLNESS

	■ TSH	■ T4	■ FT4	■ T3	■ RT3
Primary hypothyroidism	↑↑	↓	↓	↓ or =	↓
Central hypothyroidism	= or ↓	↓ or =	↓ or =	=	↓
NTI, acute phase	=	= or ↑	= or ↑	↓	↑
NTI, prolonged phase	↓	↓	↓	↓↓	↑ or =
Recovery phase	= or ↑	↓ or =	↓ or =	↓ or =	V

V, variable; ↑, increased; ↓, decreased; =, normal range.

NTI from hypothyroidism. However even then, the diagnosis may be difficult because free T4 levels are often unreliable in the face of critical illness.

If the downregulation in NTI is an energy-saving neuroendocrine adaptation to disease, attempts to increase and thereby restore thyroid hormone concentrations may be disadvantageous. At the current time, thyroid hormone therapy should not be initiated in the critical care setting in the absence of clear clinical and laboratory evidence for hypothyroidism (10). However, it is important to distinguish between patients with primary hypothyroidism and patients with NTI (**Table 109.2**). Only those with primary hypothyroidism will benefit from therapy. Patients with primary hypothyroidism almost always have a TSH level above 10 mU/L in parallel with a decreased T4 level. In more severe stages, they also have a decreased T3 level. Although elevated TSH may also occur in NTI upon recovery, it rarely exceeds 10 mU/L. In a situation in which TSH is mildly elevated (TSH 5–20 mU/L) with a low serum concentration of rT3, a low thyroid hormone binding ratio (the ratio between the result of T3 resin uptake for the unknown sample and the result of T3 resin uptake simultaneously obtained in the same assay for standard control sera), and especially a high ratio of serum T3 to FT4 (T3/FT4 >100), the patient is more likely to have hypothyroidism with or without NTI. It is particularly difficult to distinguish between central hypothyroidism and NTI because, in both conditions, the TSH tends to be low-normal, and the FT4 low (8). However, if the FT4 is <0.4 ng/dL with a normal TSH, central hypothyroidism is more likely (few patients with NTI have FT4) and T4 therapy could be considered.

not treated with T4. Treatment with T4 delayed the normalization of thyroid function during recovery. Treatment of critically ill patients with T3 has the potential hazardous effect of increasing metabolic rate, catabolism, and energy expenditure. In view of these considerations, critically ill patients with a low T3 and T4 should *not* be treated with thyroid hormone replacement unless there is also *clinical* evidence of hypothyroidism (8). A full thyroid function panel is needed to distinguish

HYPOTHYROIDISM

Congenital hypothyroidism might be due to (in descending order of frequency) thyroid dysgenesis, thyroid dyshormonogenesis, and hypothalamic–pituitary hypothyroidism. In parts of the world where salt is not iodized, iodine deficiency is the most common cause of congenital hypothyroidism. *Hashimoto's (autoimmune) thyroiditis* is the most common cause of acquired hypothyroidism in children older than 6 years of age in North America. Hashimoto thyroiditis occurs in a genetically predisposed population. A family history of thyroid disease exists in 30%–40% of patients with Hashimoto thyroiditis (3). The disease also has marked predilection for women. Usually, the onset of the disease is insidious, with the thyroid gland enlarged and firm (goiter). Occasionally, the goiter causes local pressure and difficulty in swallowing (**Fig. 109.4**). Most patients have detectable circulating autoantibodies against the thyroid.

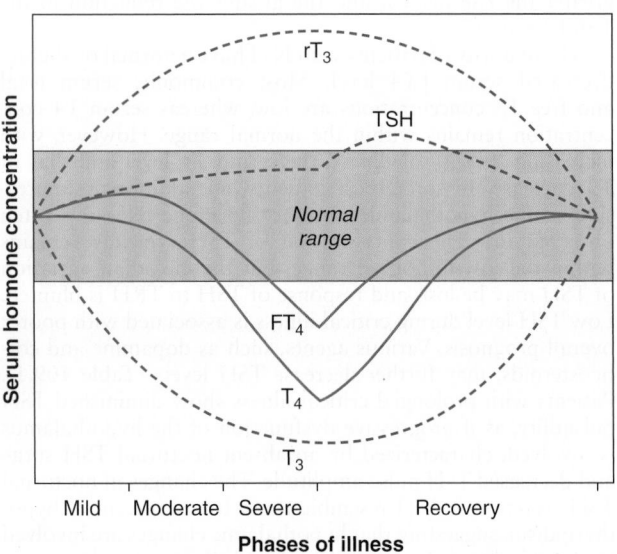

FIGURE 109.3. Changes in thyroid function during critical illness. In the acute phase of illness, the following are observed: reduction in circulating T3; increase in serum rT3; and no change in serum FT4, total T4, or TSH. In phase 2: modest increase in FT4 and further decrease in T3 and increase in rT3. In phase 3: a loss of pulsatile secretion of TSH; decrease in T4, T3, and FT4; and an increase—followed by a decrease—in serum rT3. In the recovery phase: a gradual normalization of parameters; TSH can be elevated in this stage. (From Brent GA, Hershman JM. Effects of nonthyroidal illness on thyroid function tests. In: Van Middlesworth L, ed. *The Thyroid Gland: A Practical Clinical Treatise.* Chicago, IL: Year Book Medical, 1986:83–110, with permission.)

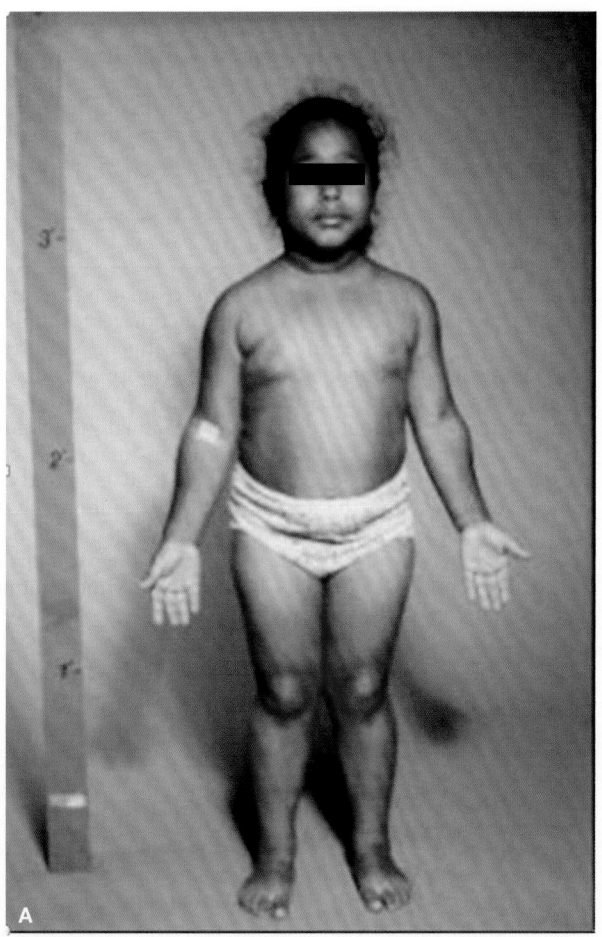

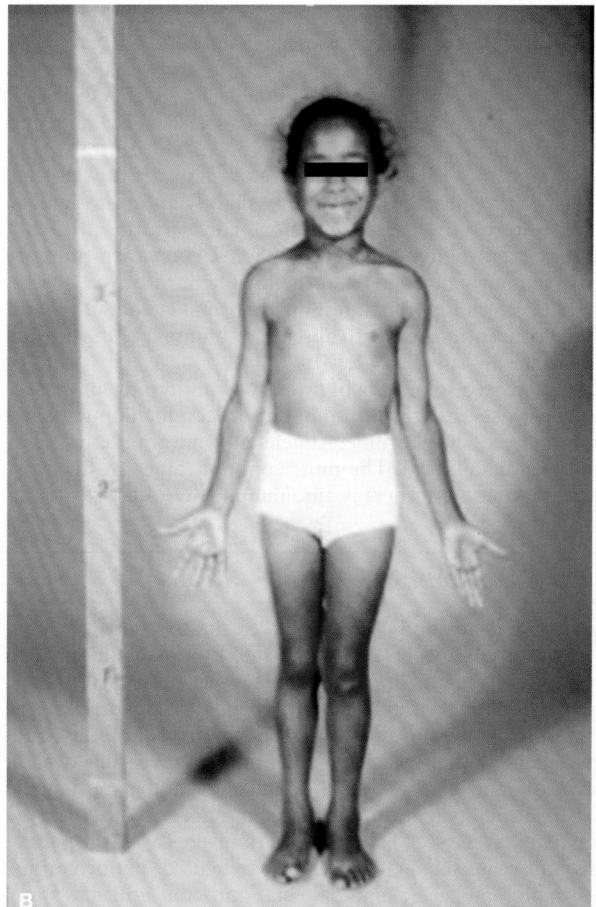

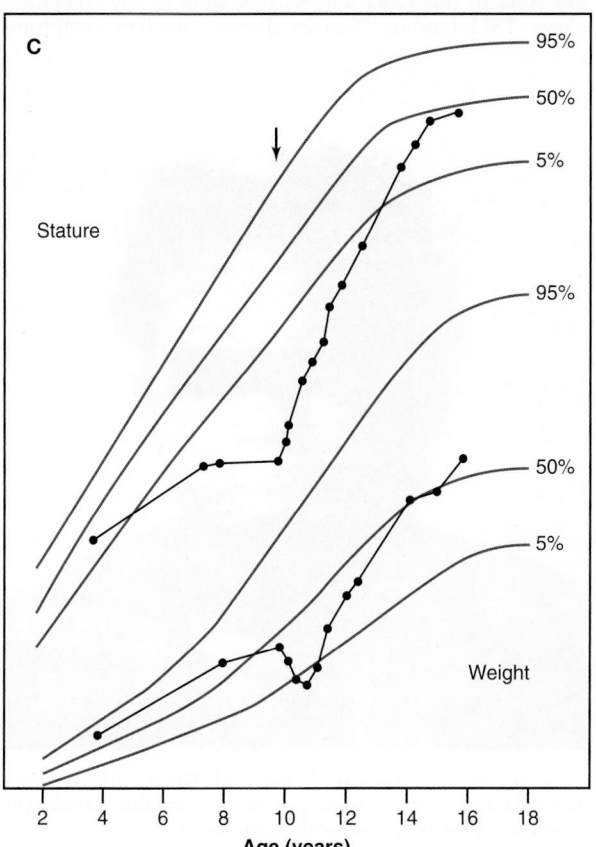

FIGURE 109.4. A 10-year-old girl with severe primary hypothyroidism before (**A**) and after (**B**) treatment. Presenting complaint was poor growth. Note the dull facies, relative obesity, and immature body proportions prior to treatment. At age 10, she had not lost a single deciduous tooth. After treatment was initiated (indicated by the arrow in **C**), she lost six teeth in 10 months and had striking catch-up growth. Bone age was 5 years at a chronologic age of 10. (From www.thyroid-manager.org, with permission from Endocrine Education Inc.)

Hypothalamic or pituitary disorders are frequently associated with TSH deficiency, producing *central hypothyroidism*. All patients with hypothalamic or pituitary disease should have thyroid function tests performed (11). Isolated central hypothyroidism is uncommon and associated with subclinical hypothyroidism and short stature (12). In central hypothyroidism, the TSH is inappropriately low (below normal range, within normal range, or only slightly above normal) in relationship to low thyroid hormone concentrations. In children with central hypothyroidism, the FT4 concentrations are below the normal range or in the lowest third of the normal range. These children manifest an abnormal circadian pattern of TSH concentrations, with absence or blunting of the normal nocturnal TSH surge (1,12,13).

An increased frequency of primary hypothyroidism is associated with several chromosomal disorders, including Turner syndrome, Down syndrome, Klinefelter syndrome, and 18p or 18q deletions (14,15). The most common cause of hypothyroidism in these disorders is autoimmune thyroiditis.

Clinical Manifestations

Hypothyroidism should be considered in any child with subnormal growth and delayed bone age. In most children with hypothyroidism, pubertal development is delayed. Affected girls may present with primary or secondary amenorrhea. The onset of hypothyroidism is usually insidious. Signs and symptoms include lethargy, cold intolerance, bradycardia, weight gain, slow and husky speech, dry coarse skin, spare dry and coarse hair, constipation, muscle pain, anorexia, and delayed deep tendon reflexes (**Table 109.3**). In severe cases, the patient may exhibit myxedematous features (edema of periorbital tissues, hands and feet, macroglossia, and cool and dry skin). Pleural effusion, pericardial effusion, or bowel obstruction may be the first presenting symptom in previously unrecognized longstanding severe hypothyroidism.

Diagnosis

In primary hypothyroidism, serum TSH is usually elevated (>3 mU/mL) (16), and is often the earliest laboratory finding. In secondary or tertiary (central) hypothyroidism, the TSH levels are low, normal, or slightly elevated (<10 mU/L). T4

and FT4 concentrations are low or low-normal (it is not useful to measure T3, as levels are preserved). When the FT4 is in the lowest third of the normal range and the TSH is low or normal, a TSH surge test is needed to confirm the diagnosis of central hypothyroidism. In central hypothyroidism, the TSH surge test shows blunting of the normal nocturnal surge.

Treatment

Most children require therapy with approximately 100 μg/m^2 body surface levothyroxine. Thyroid function tests should be checked 4–6 weeks after initiation of treatment and after a dose change has been made (sooner in newborn and infants), and the dose should be adjusted accordingly. In addition, thyroid function tests should be taken semiannually in children and annually in adolescents (more often in infants). A child with hypothyroidism who is admitted to the ICU should continue thyroid hormone therapy. If the patient cannot take oral medication, T4 should be given intravenously in a dose that is approximately two-thirds of the oral dose (if the patient is unable to take oral intake for only 1 or 2 days, thyroid treatment can be omitted for this short period).

HYPERTHYROIDISM (THYROTOXICOSIS)

The term thyrotoxicosis is often used to describe the hypermetabolic state that results from elevated circulating levels of thyroid hormones. Hyperthyroidism in childhood and adolescence is most commonly the result of *Graves disease*, an autoimmune disorder (**Fig. 109.5**). Autoantibodies against the thyroid gland can be found in the majority of the patients, of which the autoantibodies against the TSH receptor play a key role. In this case, antibody binding to the receptor simulates TSH binding. Graves disease involves symptoms of

TABLE 109.3

MANIFESTATIONS OF HYPOTHYROIDISM

■ SYMPTOMS	■ SIGNS
Fatigue	Thyroid enlargement
Lethargy	Cool, pale skin
Headache	Brittle nails
Weight gain	Bleeding tendencies
Cold intolerance	Alopecia; coarse, spare hair
Somnolence	Macroglossia
Decreased appetite	Bradycardia
Dry skin	Constipation
Hoarseness of voice	Muscle hypertrophy
Constipation	Slowed speech
Menstrual irregularities	Dementia
Myalgias	Slowed reflexes (with delayed relaxation phase)
Paresthesias	Psychosis
Depression	Diminished libido
	Memory defects

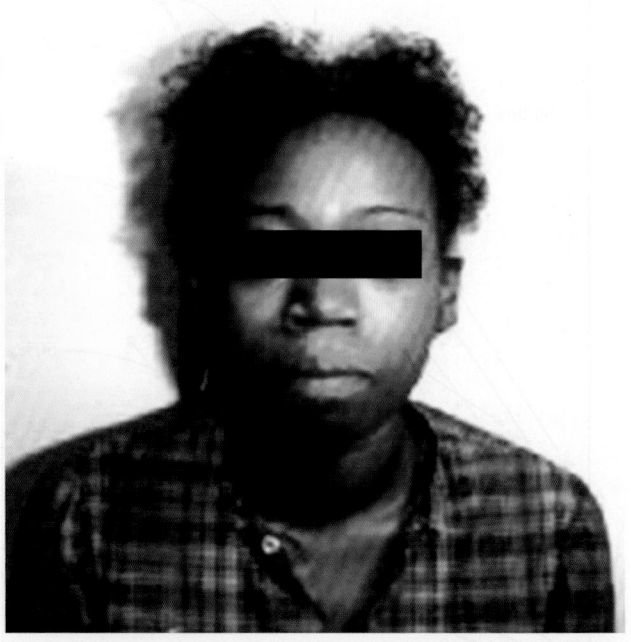

FIGURE 109.5. A 16-year-old girl with Graves disease. Note the exophthalmos, stare, asymmetry of the eyes, and thyroid enlargement. (From www.emedicine.com with permission.)

hyperthyroidism including elevated metabolic rate, eye manifestations, and dermopathy. The disease has a genetic predisposition and is more prevalent in women.

Other causes of hyperthyroidism include toxic multinodular goiter, toxic nodular goiter, exogenous thyroid hormone, iodine-induced thyrotoxicosis, excess release of thyroid hormone, struma ovarii, molar pregnancy, thyroid adenoma, destruction of thyroid tissue with excess hormone release as a result of trauma, subacute thyroiditis, chronic thyroiditis, or post-radiation thyroiditis. In rare cases, hyperthyroidism can be caused by increased TSH secretion as a result of pituitary adenoma (11). There is an association between idiopathic or heritable pulmonary arterial hypertension (PAH) and hyperthyroidism such that PAH patients should be routinely screened for hyperthyroidism. Hyperthyroidism is also part of the differential diagnosis in the sudden cardiorespiratory decompensation of the PAH patient (17).

Generalized *resistance to thyroid hormone* (RTH) involves tissues throughout the body being resistant to the effects of thyroid hormone. In RTH, T4 is high, TSH is normal, and the patients are euthyroid with a small goiter. Pituitary resistance to thyroid hormone (PRTH) is a rare non-neoplastic disorder caused by inherited mutations in the gene for the TRβ1. In this syndrome, T4 is elevated, TSH is unsuppressed, and patients are clinically hyperthyroid. The pituitary gland may be resistant to the feedback inhibitory effects of circulating thyroid hormones, whereas peripheral tissues respond normally, causing patients to experience hyperthyroidism (18). Current thinking suggests that both RTH and PRTH are typically caused by defects in the TRβ1 gene and represent a spectrum of manifestations of the same underlying disorder.

Clinical Manifestations

The onset of thyrotoxicosis is usually insidious, with a period of increasing nervousness, palpitations, increased appetite, and muscle weakness. A cardinal sign is loss of weight despite increased appetite. Other symptoms include fatigue with sleep disturbance, emotional instability, heat intolerance, excessive sweating, tremor, diarrhea, dyspnea, tachycardia, and atrial arrhythmia (**Table 109.4**). On physical examination, findings may include thyroid enlargement; thyroid bruit (continuous murmur directly over the goiter); ophthalmopathy; retraction of the eyelids and lid lag; tremor; hyperactive reflexes; increased precordial activity; tachycardia; atrial fibrillation; warm, smooth, and moist skin; and separation of the end of the fingernail from the nail bed (onycholysis). Proximal muscle weakness is common and may be the dominant manifestation in some individuals (19). Cardiovascular manifestations of thyrotoxicosis are common. The hemodynamic changes of thyrotoxicosis mimic a hyperadrenergic state. These changes are caused by an increase in myocardial β-receptors, which is induced by excessive thyroid hormone. Supraventricular tachyarrhythmias are common. Severe hyperthyroidism may lead to cardiac failure secondary to atrial fibrillation, which causes a decrease in cardiac output in the face of increased circulatory demand. Such cardiac failure usually occurs in patients with underlying heart disease (20). Uncontrolled hyperthyroidism with large goiter secondary to Graves disease may cause edema of the upper airway, a potentially life-threatening situation that requires a high degree of vigilance (21).

Diagnosis

Laboratory findings in patients with hyperthyroidism include increased serum concentrations of T3 and T4 because of

TABLE 109.4
MANIFESTATIONS OF HYPERTHYROIDISM

■ SYMPTOMS	■ SIGNS
Nervousness	Tachycardia
Anxiety	Thyroid enlargement[a]
Heat intolerance	Tremor
Palpitations	Thyroid bruit
Fatigue	Eye signs[b]
Weight loss	Hyperactive reflexes
Tachycardia	Atrial fibrillation
Dyspnea	Hot and moist skin
Weakness	Thin and fine hair
Increased appetite	Onycholysis
Eye complaints[b]	Muscle weakness
Swelling legs	Hyperactive precordial pulse
Hyperdefecation (without diarrhea)	Splenomegaly[c]
Diarrhea	Gynecomastia
Anorexia	Liver palms
Personality change	
Emotional lability	
Impaired concentration	
Insomnia	
Difficulty swallowing	
Menstrual irregularities	

[a]Enlargement of the thyroid may be lacking in fewer than 5% of patients with thyrotoxicosis.
[b]These manifestations are much more common in patients with Graves disease.
[c]Exclusively present in patients with Graves disease.

increased production of these hormones. Occasionally, only the serum T3 concentration is increased (T3 toxicosis). Conversely, it is possible that only the serum T4 concentration is increased (T4 toxicosis). It is more valuable to measure the active thyroid hormone concentrations, free T3 (FT3) and FT4, and to verify that either or both are elevated. The TSH is low and usually undetectable (except in the extremely rare cases of TSH-secreting tumors, TRH-secreting tumors, and selective PRTH). Quantitative human chorionic gonadotropin (hCG), which can cross-react at the TSH receptor level, is elevated in molar pregnancy.

Treatment

Management of hyperthyroidism includes medical treatment, radioactive iodine, or surgery. Previously, children with hyperthyroidism were treated with an antithyroid agent, such as propylthiouracil (PTU), methimazole, or carbimazole (used in Europe). These agents block synthesis of the thyroid hormone by inhibiting oxidation of iodide. In addition, PTU impairs the conversion of T4 to T3 by inhibiting type I 5'-monodeiodinase. However, due to association between PTU and severe liver failure in children and the subsequent black-box warning from the Food and Drug Administration, the use of PTU should be avoided in children (22,23). Methimazole should be the first-choice antithyroid medication, and in countries where it is not available, carbimazole, a drug that is biologically converted to methimazole, may be substituted. An initial dose of methimazole or carbimazole varies from 20 to 40 mg (0.4–0.6 mg/kg) daily PO, divided into two to three doses. In the initial state (before a euthyroid state is achieved), a β-adrenergic blocking agent, such as propranolol, may be added as 10–40 mg/dose

TABLE 109.5

HYPERSENSITIVITY REACTIONS TO ANTITHYROID DRUGS

Rash
Agranulocytosis (accompanied by fever and sore throat)
Arthralgia
Myalgia
Neuritis
Hepatitis (with PTU)
Cholestasis (with methimazole)
Liver necrosis
Thrombocytopenia
Loss of or abnormal pigmentation of the hair
Loss of sensation
Enlargement of lymph nodes or salivary glands
Edema
A lupus-like syndrome
Toxic psychosis
Pruritus
Stevens–Johnson syndrome

TABLE 109.6

COMPLICATIONS OF THYROIDECTOMY

Transient hypocalcemia
Permanent hypocalcemia
Transient recurrent laryngeal nerve palsy
Permanent recurrent laryngeal nerve palsy
Thyroid storm
Hemorrhage

Surgical treatment is used less often than in the past, but it is still an effective treatment option for hyperthyroidism (27). With proper preparation and if performed by an experienced surgeon, the complication rate is relatively low (Table 109.6). Surgery should be considered in patients with a large thyroid gland, severe ophthalmopathy, and a lack of remission with medical treatment. With proper surgical management most patients achieve a rapid remission; some may have recurrence of thyrotoxicosis or may develop hypothyroidism.

(2 mg/kg/day divided q6–12 hours) orally every 6 hours (see Thyroid Storm below). After a euthyroid state is achieved, the methimazole dose should be decreased to maintenance dose (usually 1/3–2/3 of the initial dose given once or twice daily). The doses should be adjusted according to the FT4 concentration, as TSH may remain suppressed for months.

A small percentage of patients develop hypersensitivity reactions to antithyroid drugs; they are usually mild and resolve when the drug is withdrawn, but a severe reaction may occur (Table 109.5). The most common hypersensitivity reaction, occurring in as many as 10% of patients, is a rash that can take many forms, including hives. Among the serious reactions, agranulocytosis is the most common, occurring in fewer than 1% of patients and accompanied by fever and sore throat. Hypersensitivity reaction usually occurs within the first few weeks of treatment. As these medications can affect blood count and liver function tests, it is advisable to perform complete blood count and liver function tests before initiation of an antithyroid drug treatment and to repeat them after the first few weeks of treatment, to help recognize these potential side effects. Suspicion of any serious manifestation should be an indication for discontinuation of antithyroid drug therapy and recourse to surgery or radioactive iodine (20). Usually, it is necessary to continue medical treatment for 2 years before the patient achieves remission.

Patients with hyperthyroidism admitted to the ICU should be monitored carefully for possible development of thyroid storm (see below). Medical treatment should be continued and adjusted according to the thyroid function tests. As no parenteral preparations of antithyroid drugs are available, they must be administered orally or via a nasogastric tube. Rectal administration has also been used.

Radioactive iodine has been used relatively infrequently in childhood owing to the potential risks of leukemia or thyroid cancer in the patient and genetic mutations in their offspring. However, a number of recent reports show that this approach is not associated with an increased risk of these complications and is safe enough to be considered as treatment, particularly in adolescents (24–26). Radioactive iodine is used for treatment of older children and adolescents who fail medical treatment or in whom medical treatment is contraindicated owing to severe side effects. The main complication is primary hypothyroidism. Radioactive iodine may cause thyroid storm.

CRITICAL HYPOTHYROIDISM: "MYXEDEMA COMA"

4 The term myxedema coma is often used to describe clinically severe hypothyroidism. However, this term is a misnomer, because most patients who have severe hypothyroidism do not present with myxedema or in a comatose state. Critical hypothyroidism is characterized by progressive dysfunction of the cardiovascular, respiratory, and central nervous systems. Myxedema is related to organ hypofunction (e.g., cardiac, gastrointestinal [GI], skin, renal) and occurs with prolonged or severe hypothyroidism. If not recognized and treated, the mortality rate is exceedingly high. Myxedema coma is rare in the pediatric population. Typically, patients are older and have known hypothyroidism; however, it can be the initial presentation of hypothyroidism. Myxedema coma occurs most commonly in winter. Common precipitants include infection, trauma, hypothermia, and medications (Table 109.7).

TABLE 109.7

PRECIPITATING FACTORS FOR MYXEDEMA COMA

Infections
  Pneumonia
  Sepsis
  Urinary infections
  Influenza
Surgery
Burns
Trauma
Hypothermia
Drugs
  Sedatives (narcotics, tranquilizers, barbiturates)
  Cardiac medications (amiodarone, β-blockers)
  Lithium
  Phenytoin
  Rifampin
Stroke
GI bleeding
Congestive heart failure

Clinical Manifestations

Cardinal findings include hypothermia and altered mental status. Additional features include bradycardia, hypotension, and hypoventilation. A reduction in hypoxic ventilatory drive results in a lowered respiratory rate, carbon dioxide narcosis and progressive somnolence, which compound the underlying slow mental status of the patient. Respiratory muscle weakness may also occur, further compromising the ability to ventilate. Presence of ascites, pleural effusion, or pericardial effusion may further impede effective ventilation (28). Cardiac contractility is reduced, resulting in a reduction of stroke volume and cardiac output. Cardiac output can be further limited by significant pericardial effusion. If present, myxedema is characterized by decreased metabolic clearance of all substances, reduced intravascular volume with fluid retention in tissues, generalized skin and soft tissue swelling, often with associated periorbital edema, ptosis, macroglossia, and cool, dry skin (Table 109.8).

Diagnosis

The diagnosis of myxedema coma requires low levels of T3 and of T4 (total and free). TSH levels are usually elevated, but may be normal or low in the setting of hypothalamic–pituitary disease or critical illness. Additional laboratory findings include anemia, hyponatremia, hypoglycemia, azotemia, elevated liver enzymes, hypercholesterolemia, and elevated creatinine phosphokinase levels. Hypoxia, hypercapnia, and respiratory acidosis are common.

TABLE 109.8

CLINICAL MANIFESTATIONS OF MYXEDEMA COMA

■ ORGAN SYSTEM	■ CLINICAL FEATURES
Skin and soft tissues	Generalized swelling
	Edema
	Periorbital edema
	Ptosis
	Cool, dry skin
	Coarse, sparse hair
	Macroglossia; hoarseness
Neurologic	Hypothermia
	Lethargy
	Altered mental status
	Psychosis
	Seizures
	Delayed reflex relaxation
Cardiovascular	Bradycardia
	Hypotension
Respiratory	Depressed ventilatory drive
	Hypoventilation
	Hypoxia
	Hypercapnia
GI	Constipation
	Abdominal distention
	Paralytic ileus
	Megacolon
Hematologic	Anemia
	Leukopenia
Renal	Decreased glomerular filtration rate

The occurrence of pericardial effusion in hypothyroidism appears to be dependent on the severity of the disease. Pericardial effusion may be a frequent manifestation in myxedema at an advanced severe stage, but it is rare in hypothyroidism at an early mild stage (29). A chest radiograph may reveal cardiomegaly and pleural effusions. Echocardiography can reveal septal hypertrophy and hypertrophic subaortic stenosis in addition to the pericardial effusion. Electrocardiographic (ECG) findings include sinus bradycardia, decreased voltage with electrical alternans if a pericardial effusion is present, and nonspecific ST and T wave abnormalities. Other ECG abnormalities include prolongation of the QT interval and conduction abnormalities of varying degrees (2).

A lumbar puncture may be indicated to exclude meningitis. An increased opening pressure and elevated protein levels in the cerebral spinal fluid are nonspecific findings associated with myxedema coma (30).

Treatment

The treatment of myxedema coma involves general supportive measures, correction of physiologic derangements, and immediate intravenous replacement of thyroid hormone (30). Patients should be treated in the ICU setting with careful monitoring. In patients who have severe hypotension, vasopressor therapy should be considered. Warm room temperature, blankets, and/or heating pad should be used to correct hypothermia. Rapid correction of hypothermia may cause hypotension and cardiovascular collapse owing to peripheral dilatation. Severe hyponatremia may be treated with hypertonic saline. Hypoglycemia should be treated with continuous dextrose infusion. Precipitating factors should be pursued and treated. Broad-spectrum antibiotics should be considered until infection has been excluded.

The proper initiation of thyroid hormone therapy in myxedema is controversial (30,31). Enteral absorption of T4 may be disrupted by edema of intestinal villi. Most investigators recommend initiating therapy with intravenous T4 alone, with a loading dose of 200–500 μg (4 μg/kg if <50 kg), followed by 50–100 μg/day (1–2 μg/kg if <50 kg). Using T4 alone allows a slow conversion of T4 to T3 in the periphery, thereby reducing the possible adverse cardiac effects that may occur with a large dose of T3, especially in those with preexisting heart disease (2). If combination therapy is begun, a loading dose of 4 μg/kg of T4 and 10 μg of T3 (0.2 μg/kg) may be used, followed by maintenance doses of T4 (50–100 μg daily; 1–2 μg/kg) and T3 (10 μg; 0.2 μg/kg) every 8 hours until oral therapy is initiated. If intravenous T3 alone is used, initial dose should be 10–20 μg (0.2–0.4 μg/kg), followed by 10 μg (0.2 μg/kg) every 4 hours for the first 24 hours, then 10 μg (0.2 μg/kg) every 6 hours for another 1–2 days. Depending on the clinical response, the patient may then be converted to oral T4 therapy. Rapid onset of action of T3 can lead to adverse cardiovascular effects. A study that compared the response of thyroid hormones between intravenous high-dose T4 and oral T4 in affected adults found that with oral administration of 500 μg of T4 on the first day, followed by 100 μg of T4 daily by mouth, plasma T3 and T4 increased slowly, remaining in the hypothyroid range, but clinical response occurred within 24–72 hours (32). The intravenous route involved high peaks of plasma T3 and T4 within 3 hours. IV administration of T4 at the proposed doses causes an abrupt rise in serum T4 to a supraphysiologic level, and then a fall to the normal range in 24 hours. Serum T3 levels rise slightly, and serum TSH levels fall sharply and substantially (31). Whatever the regimen, subsequent thyroid hormone dosing should be guided by frequent measurement of FT4 concentrations. With the IV route, the peak level is reached within 3 hours, with subsequent gradual decline over a few days (32).

Thus, we recommend checking FT4 twice daily when using the IV route to ensure that most levels are within the normal range. When the patient is converted to oral T4, FT4 can be measured once or twice per week.

Cortisol response to stress is blunted during severe hypothyroidism. Most investigators recommend the concurrent administration of "stress dose" corticosteroid therapy, in case of concurrent adrenal insufficiency. Hydrocortisone, 100 mg/m² IV, should be administered initially, followed by 25 mg/m² IV every 6 hours. Cortisol levels should be drawn before initiation of corticosteroid therapy. If the levels are appropriately elevated, the steroid therapy may be safely discontinued. If the cortisol levels are low (<25 μg/dL), steroid therapy should be continued until the critical illness phase is resolved. At a later time, an ACTH stimulation test can be performed to exclude persistence of hypoadrenalism.

6 CRITICAL HYPERTHYROIDISM: "THYROID STORM"

Thyroid storm (or thyrotoxic crisis) is a life-threatening condition caused by the exaggeration of clinical manifestations of thyrotoxicosis. Thyroid storm most commonly occurs in Graves disease. The progression from thyrotoxicosis to life-threatening thyroid storm involves high fever, mental status changes, and evidence of multiorgan dysfunction, including adrenergic crisis (tachycardia, hypertension) and GI hypermotility. Early diagnosis and intervention are crucial to prevent morbidity and mortality. Precipitating factors include thyroid surgery, withdrawal of antithyroid drugs, radioiodine therapy, or the administration of iodinated radiocontrast dyes (**Table 109.9**). In patients who have preexisting thyrotoxicosis, thyroid storm can also be precipitated by systemic insults, including surgery, trauma, severe infection, and diabetic ketoacidosis.

Thyroid storm may be less frequent now than in the past due to the earlier diagnosis and management of hyperthyroidism

TABLE 109.9

PRECIPITATING FACTORS FOR THYROID STORM

Infection
Surgery (thyroidal and nonthyroidal)
Therapy with radioactive iodine
Administration of iodinated contrast dyes or ingestion
  of large stable iodine loads
Withdrawal of antithyroid medication
Amiodarone therapy
Ingestion of excessive amounts of exogenous
  thyroid hormone
Diabetic ketoacidosis
Congestive cardiac failure
Hypoglycemia
Toxemia of pregnancy
Parturition and the immediate postpartum state
Severe emotional stress
Acute manic crisis
Pulmonary embolism
Cerebral vascular accident
Bowel infarction
Acute trauma
Tooth extraction
Vigorous palpation of thyroid gland

(31). If left untreated, the mortality rate ranges between 20% and 30% (33). Thus, prevention, early diagnosis, and aggressive management of thyroid storm are extremely important.

Most studies have not found a significant difference in serum thyroid hormonal levels between uncomplicated hyperthyroidism and thyroid storm (33). Acute and rapid increase in serum levels of thyroid hormones might be the cause of thyroid storm, as evidenced by cases of thyroid storm that present following thyroid surgery, administration of radioactive iodine, and abrupt discontinuation of antithyroid medication. The sympathetic nervous system has been implicated in the pathogenesis of thyroid storm, as many of the manifestations are similar to those seen in conditions of catecholamine excess and administration of β-blockers causes a marked relief of these signs and symptoms. Although the catecholamine levels are within the normal range, thyroid hormones upregulate adrenergic receptor expression and thus affect tissue responsiveness to catecholamines. Another mechanism might be enhancement of the cellular response to thyroid hormones as seen in conditions that precipitate thyroid storm, such as infection, hypoxemia, hypovolemia, and diabetic ketoacidosis.

Clinical Manifestations

Thyroid storm is characterized by four major features: fever, tachycardia, central nervous system dysfunction, and GI symptoms. The fever can progress to frank hyperpyrexia. Sinus tachycardia is usually seen, although a variety of supraventricular arrhythmias may also be present, such as atrial fibrillation. Central nervous system manifestations can range from agitation, restlessness, and emotional lability, to confusion, frank psychosis, and coma. GI symptoms include nausea, vomiting, and diarrhea. A useful scoring system for recognition of thyroid storm is presented in **Table 109.10** (31).

Diagnosis

Laboratory findings include elevated serum total and free thyroid hormonal levels (free T3 and/or free T4), with undetectable TSH. Serum electrolytes are usually normal. Liver function abnormalities, leukocytosis, or leucopenia may also be present.

Treatment

The management of thyroid storm is complicated. Patients with thyroid storm should be monitored and treated in the ICU. The aims of the treatment are to reduce the production and secretion of thyroid hormones, to antagonize the peripheral action of the thyroid hormones, to alleviate signs and symptoms, and to treat the precipitating factor. Supportive therapy includes respiratory support and management of hyperthermia. Phenobarbital may be used for sedation because it stimulates metabolic clearance of thyroid hormone by the liver. Hyperthermia may be treated with cool IV fluids, antipyretics, or cooling blankets.

An early step in the treatment must include complete blockade of new thyroid hormone synthesis using either PTU or methimazole. Methimazole has a better safety profile and is given as a loading dose of 60–100 mg (1.2–2 mg/kg), followed by 20–30 mg (0.4–0.7 mg/kg) every 6–8 hours orally, but it does not provide inhibition of conversion of T4 to T3. PTU had been considered the drug of choice because of its inhibition of peripheral conversion of T4 to T3 in addition to its inhibition of synthesis of thyroid hormone. However, PTU is now known to have more adverse effects, especially hepatotoxicity.

TABLE 109.10

THE PREDICTIVE CLINICAL SCALE FOR THYROID STORM
(BURCH AND WARTOFSKY)

■ PARAMETER TAKEN INTO CONSIDERATION	■ SCORING POINTS
Thermoregulatory dysfunction, temperature (oral; in °F)	
99–99.9	5
100–100.9	10
101–101.9	15
102–102.9	20
103–103.9	25
≥104	30
CNS effects	
Absent	0
Mild (agitation)	10
Moderate (delirium, psychosis, extreme lethargy)	20
Severe (seizures, coma)	30
GI–hepatic dysfunction	
Absent	0
Moderate (diarrhea, nausea/vomiting, abdominal pain)	10
Severe (unexplained jaundice)	20
Tachycardia (beats/min)	
99–109	5
110–119	10
120–129	15
130–139	20
≥140	25
Congestive cardiac failure	
Absent	0
Mild (pedal edema)	5
Moderate (bibasal rales)	10
Severe (pulmonary edema)	15
Atrial fibrillation	
Absent	0
Present	10
Precipitating event	
Absent	0
Present	10

A cumulative score of ≥45 is highly suggestive of thyroid storm, 25–44 is suggestive of "impeding" storm, and <25 is unlikely to represent thyroid storm.
From Rose SR. TSH above 3 is not usually normal. The Endocrinologist 2006; 16: July–Aug.

PTU can be administered as a 600–1000-mg (12–20 mg/kg) loading dose, followed by 200–300 mg (4–6 mg/kg) every 4–6 hours orally. Both PTU and methimazole can be administered rectally, but no parenteral preparation for these drugs is available. As thyrotoxicosis improves, the doses should be gradually lowered to the standard dose ranges (see above: medical treatment of hyperthyroidism).

To block the release of preformed thyroid hormone from the thyroid gland, inorganic iodine should be used. Ideally, iodine therapy should be administered 2 hours after initial thiourea dosing, to allow for initial blockade of iodine organification. Formulations for oral inorganic iodine that can be used include saturated solution of potassium iodide (children, five drops, 250 mg, two to four times per day; infants, two drops, four times per day) and Lugol solution (four to eight drops, three times per day). Iodinated contrast dyes given intravenously, including ipodate and iohexol, are also effective. In addition to blocking thyroid hormone release, these radiocontrast agents interfere with peripheral conversion of T4 to T3 and may antagonize the binding of thyroid hormone to its receptors (30).

Lithium therapy (300 mg or 6 mg/kg every 6 hours) may be used in addition to iodine to block thyroid hormone release. High-dose corticosteroids (hydrocortisone 50–100 mg, IV, every 6–8 hours or 25–50 mg/m² body surface) are also effective in blocking peripheral conversion of T4 to T3. Blocking the action of thyroid hormone is another mainstay of the treatment. In the absence of cardiac failure, a β-adrenergic blocking agent should be added. Beta blockers (e.g., propranolol, 40–80 mg, 0.5 mg/kg, orally, or 1–3 mg/dose IV, every 4–8 hours) are effective in reducing tachycardia, hypertension, and adrenergic symptoms associated with thyrotoxicosis (30). However, a short acting β-blocker such as esmolol given IV may be safer in the critically ill patient by minimizing the risk of cardiovascular collapse and allowing better titration of the medication's effects because of the short half-life (5,20,27). In life-threatening cases in which medical therapy has been proven ineffective, plasmapheresis, plasma exchange, charcoal plasma perfusion, and peritoneal dialysis, have all been used successfully to remove circulating thyroid hormone (34–37).

Following initiation of therapy for thyroid storm, clinical and biochemical improvement should occur within 24 hours, although full recovery may take several days to weeks. In most cases, medical therapy should be used for weeks to months before definitive treatment with radioactive iodine or thyroidectomy. In rare cases, definitive therapy with thyroidectomy may be considered during the acute phase of thyroid storm. Radioactive iodine has no role in the acute management due to therapeutic administration of inorganic iodine, antithyroid drugs, and concerns over excess thyroid hormone release.

CONCLUSIONS AND FUTURE DIRECTIONS

Nonthyroidal illness occurs in most patients admitted to the ICU. At this point, it is not clear whether thyroid hormone administration is beneficial or detrimental. Further large-scale prospective studies are required to determine when such a treatment could be beneficial, on the basis of the clinical presentation, laboratory evaluation, and the primary condition. In addition, these studies should determine the correct treatment (T3 and/or T4) and doses to be used.

Myxedema coma and thyroid storm are extremely rare in the pediatric population. Current treatment has significantly reduced the mortality rate associated with these conditions. However, better understanding of the physiology may enable us to anticipate the development of these complications and prevent them. Improvement in treatment may further decrease the morbidity and mortality. Our recommendations regarding the treatment of these conditions are adopted from studies in adults due to the rarity of these conditions in the pediatric population and may need further adjustments to achieve an optimal outcome.

References

1. Rose SR, Nisula BC. Circadian variation of thyrotropin in childhood. *J Clin Endocrinol Metab* 1989;68:1086–90.
2. Tews MC, Shah SM, Gossain VV. Hypothyroidism: Mimicker of common complaints. *Emerg Med Clin North Am* 2005;23:649–67.

3. Rivkees SA. Thyroid Disorders in Children and Adolescents. In: Sperling MA, ed. Pediatric Endocrinology. 4th ed. Philadelphia, PA: Saunders, 2014; 444–470.

4. Larsen PR, Davies TF, Schlumberger M-J, et al. Thyroid physiology and diagnostic evaluation of patients with thyroid disorders. In: Larsen PR, Kronenberg HM, Melmed SM, et al., eds. *Williams Textbook of Endocrinology.* 10th ed. Philadelphia, PA: Saunders, 2003:331–73.

5. Vanhorebeek I, Van den Berghe G. The neuroendocrine response to critical illness is a dynamic process. *Crit Care Clin* 2006;22:1–15, v.

6. Ligtenberg JJ, Girbes AR, Beentjes JA, et al. Hormones in the critically ill patient: To intervene or not to intervene? *Intensive Care Med* 2001;27:1567–77.

7. Hulst JM, van Goudoever JB, Visser TJ, et al. Hormone levels in children during the first week of ICU-admission: Is there an effect of adequate feeding? *Clin Nutr* 2006;25:154–62.

8. Nylen ES, Muller B. Endocrine changes in critical illness. *J Intensive Care Med* 2004;19:67–82.

9. Brent GA, Hershman JM. Thyroxine therapy in patients with severe nonthyroidal illnesses and low serum thyroxine concentration. *J Clin Endocrinol Metab* 1986;63:1–8.

10. Stathatos N, Levetan C, Burman KD, et al. The controversy of the treatment of critically ill patients with thyroid hormone. *Best Pract Res Clin Endocrinol Metab* 2001;15:465–78.

11. Emerson CH. Central hypothyroidism and hyperthyroidism. *Med Clin North Am* 1985;69:1019–34.

12. Rose SR. Isolated central hypothyroidism in short stature. *Pediatr Res* 1995;38:967–73.

13. Gruñeiro-Papendieck L, Chiesa A, Martínez A, et al. Nocturnal TSH surge and TRH test response in the evaluation of thyroid axis in hypothalamic pituitary disorders in childhood. *Horm Res* 1998;50:252–7.

14. Lomenick JP, Smith WJ, Rose SR. Autoimmune thyroiditis in 18q deletion syndrome. *J Pediatr* 2005;147:541–3.

15. Schaub RL, Hale DE, Rose SR, et al. The spectrum of thyroid abnormalities in individuals with 18q deletions. *J Clin Endocrinol Metab* 2005;90:2259–63.

16. Rose SR. Thyrotropin above 3 is not usually normal. *Endocrinologist* 2006;16:189–90.

17. Trapp CM, Elder RW, Gerken AT, et al. Pediatric pulmonary arterial hypertension and hyperthyroidism: A potentially fatal combination. *J Clin Endocrinol Metab* 2012;97:2217–22.

18. McDermott MT, Ridgway EC. Central hyperthyroidism. *Endocrinol Metab Clin North Am* 1998;27:187–203.

19. Reasner CA, Isley WL. Thyrotoxicosis in the critically ill. *Crit Care Clin* 1991;7:57–74.

20. Davies TF, Larsen PR. Thyrotoxicosis. In: Larsen PR, Kronenberg HM, Melmed SM, et al., eds. *Williams Textbook of Endocrinology.* 10th ed. Philadelphia, PA: Saunders, 2003;374–421.

21. Li Pi Shan W, Hatzakorzian R, Sherman M, et al. Upper airway compromise secondary to edema in Graves' disease. *Can J Anaesth* 2006;53:183–7.

22. Bauer AJ. Approach to the pediatric patient with Graves' disease: When is definitive therapy warranted? *J Clin Endocrinol Metab* 2011;96:580–8.

23. Glinoer D, Cooper DS. The propylthiouracil dilemma. *Curr Opin Endocrinol Diabetes Obes* 2012;19:402–7.

24. Barrio R, López-Capapé M, Martinez-Badás I, et al. Graves' disease in children and adolescents: Response to long-term treatment. *Acta Paediatr* 2005;94:1583–9.

25. Dotsch J, Rascher W, Dorr HG. Graves disease in childhood: A review of the options for diagnosis and treatment. *Paediatr Drugs* 2003;5:95–102.

26. Segni M, Gorman CA. The aftermath of childhood hyperthyroidism. *J Pediatr Endocrinol Metab* 2001;14 (suppl 5):1277–82; discussion 1297–8.

27. Weber KJ, Solorzano CC, Lee JK, et al. Thyroidectomy remains an effective treatment option for Graves' disease. *Am J Surg* 2006;191:400–5.

28. Ringel MD. Management of hypothyroidism and hyperthyroidism in the intensive care unit. *Crit Care Clin* 2001;17:59–74.

29. Kabadi UM, Kumar SP. Pericardial effusion in primary hypothyroidism. *Am Heart J* 1990;120:1393–5.

30. Goldberg PA, Inzucchi SE. Critical issues in endocrinology. *Clin Chest Med* 2003;24:583–606.

31. Sarlis NJ, Gourgiotis L. Thyroid emergencies. *Rev Endocr Metab Disord* 2003;4:129–36.

32. Arlot S, Debussche X, Lalau JD, et al. Myxoedema coma: Response of thyroid hormones with oral and intravenous high-dose L-thyroxine treatment. *Intensive Care Med* 1991;17:16–8.

33. Tietgens ST, Leinung MC. Thyroid storm. *Med Clin North Am* 1995;79:169–84.

34. Ashkar FS, Katims RB, Smoak WM 3rd, et al. Thyroid storm treatment with blood exchange and plasmapheresis. *JAMA* 1970;214:1275–9.

35. Candrina R, Di Stefano O, Spandrio S, et al. Treatment of thyrotoxic storm by charcoal plasmaperfusion. *J Endocrinol Invest* 1989;12:133–4.

36. Herrmann J, Schmidt HJ, Kruskemper HL. Thyroxine elimination by peritoneal dialysis in experimental thyrotoxicosis. *Horm Metab Res* 1973;5:180–3.

37. Tajiri J, Katsuya H, Kiyokawa T, et al. Successful treatment of thyrotoxic crisis with plasma exchange. *Crit Care Med* 1984;12:536–7.

CHAPTER 110 ■ ACUTE KIDNEY INJURY

CHRISTINE B. SETHNA, NATALIYA CHORNY, SMARIKA SAPKOTA, AND JAMES SCHNEIDER

KEY POINTS

1 Acute kidney injury (AKI) is common during critical illness and is associated with significant morbidity and mortality.

2 AKI is defined by the pRIFLE criteria: graded levels of risk assessment (risk, injury, failure) and outcomes (loss and end-stage renal disease).

3 The incidence of AKI is rising primarily because of increased use of intensive care and advanced technologies such as cardiac surgery, bone marrow transplantation, and care of very low-birth-weight premature infants.

4 In the intensive care unit, the most common etiologies of AKI are sepsis, multiple organ dysfunction syndrome, cardiac surgery, and nephrotoxic medication.

5 Biomarkers may aid in early diagnosis and prevention.

6 The etiology of AKI is classified into categories of prerenal, intrinsic, and postrenal.

7 Treatment of AKI is largely supportive and includes optimizing renal perfusion through fluid management and avoidance of nephrotoxins.

Pediatric acute kidney injury (AKI) in the intensive care unit (ICU) is a dynamic process that is multifactorial and complex. Traditionally, AKI is classified into three categories based on the anatomical location of the injury: *prerenal AKI*, *intrinsic renal AKI*, and *postrenal AKI*. Prerenal AKI results from decreased perfusion to the kidney either from volume depletion or decreased circulating volume. Intrinsic AKI is characterized by kidney dysfunction from injury to the glomerular, tubular, or vascular structures of the kidney. Postrenal AKI is caused by obstruction of the lower urinary tract. Despite the growing understanding of the causes and mechanisms of AKI development, very few preventive and therapeutic measures exist.

The clinical landscape of AKI has undergone a dramatic change in recent years. The incidence of pediatric AKI is continuously rising and the etiology of disease has shifted due to the increased use of intensive care and advanced technologies. **1** AKI is a known independent risk factor for increased mortality and morbidity in critically ill children. Therefore, a focus on preventive and therapeutic strategies is paramount. The discovery of early biomarkers is opening up an exciting new era in the diagnosis of AKI. Hopefully, this advance in diagnostic markers will lead to an improvement in prevention and intervention for patients with AKI.

DEFINITION OF AKI

AKI, formerly known as acute renal failure (ARF), is defined as the abrupt onset of renal dysfunction resulting from injurious endogenous or exogenous processes characterized by a decrease in glomerular filtration rate (GFR) and an increase in serum creatinine. This leads to an inability to regulate acid and electrolyte balance as well as failure to excrete waste and fluid. There has been a shift in terminology from "ARF" to "AKI" in order to more accurately describe renal dysfunction as a continuum rather than an absolute failure in kidney function. More than 30 definitions of AKI that appeared in published literature prior to 2004 resulted in variations in the reported incidence and morbidity and mortality rates for AKI (1). To overcome this, standardized definitions for AKI have been proposed. The introduction and subsequent application of standardized definitions into the medical literature has allowed us to gain a better understanding of AKI.

The RIFLE criteria, developed by the Acute Dialysis Quality Initiative group, consists of the acronym for the three graded levels of injury (risk, injury, and failure) based upon either the degree of elevation in serum creatinine or urine output, and two outcome measures (loss and end-stage renal disease) (2). The use of RIFLE criteria in the adult population has been validated and there is a predictive correlation between the different degrees of AKI and mortality (3–5). For **2** pediatric patients, a modified version of RIFLE criteria known as pRIFLE has been proposed (6) (**Table 110.1**). To account for the expected changes in serum creatinine concentration that follow normal pediatric growth, the pRIFLE criteria classifies the severity of AKI based on changes in estimated creatinine clearance and urine output rather than on absolute changes in serum creatinine. pRIFLE staging has been shown in several studies to be independently associated with morbidity and mortality (7,8). Another modified classification of RIFLE, introduced by The Acute Kidney Injury Network (AKIN), takes into account small variations in creatinine and has been validated in adults (9). More recently, the organization Kidney Disease: Improving Global Outcomes (KDIGO) released a definition and staging system for AKI that combines the RIFLE and AKIN criteria and includes pediatric measures (**Table 110.2**) (10,11). However, the criteria have not yet been adequately validated for use in children.

EPIDEMIOLOGY

Much attention is being paid to the importance of AKI in both adults and children. Pediatric AKI is common and on the increase secondary to the increased availability of treatment options for critically ill patients. Advances that have led **3** to a growing population of more susceptible children include stem-cell and solid organ transplantation, the use of immune modulators for various systemic diseases, chronic mechanical ventilation, and improvements in neonatal care.

The understanding of the epidemiology of AKI has changed over recent years. Prior to the standardized definitions of AKI,

TABLE 110.1

PRIFLE CRITERIA

PEDIATRIC-MODIFIED RIFLE (pRIFLE) CRITERIA

	■ ESTIMATED CCI	■ URINE OUTPUT
Risk	eCCI decrease by 25%	<0.5 mL/kg/h for 8 h
Injury	eCCI decrease by 50%	<0.5 mL/kg/h for 16 h
Failure	eCCI decrease by 75% or eCCI <35 mL/min/1073 m²	<0.3 mL/kg/h for 24 h or anuric for 12 h
Loss	Persistent failure >4 weeks	
End	End-stage renal disease	
Stage	Persistent failure >3 months)	

eCCI, estimated creatinine clearance; pRIFLE, pediatric risk, injury, failure, loss, and end-stage renal disease. Akcan-Arikan A, Zappitelli M, Loftis LL, et al. Modified RIFLE criteria in critically ill children with acute kidney injury. *Kidney Int* 2007;71(10):1028–35.

TABLE 110.2

KDIGO CRITERIA

■ STAGE	■ SERUM CREATININE	■ URINE OUTPUT
1	1.5–1.9 times baseline or ≥0.3 mg/dL (≥26.5 μmol/L) increase	<0.5 mL/kg/h for 6–12 h
2	2.0–2.9 times baseline	<0.5 mL/kg/h for ≥12 h
3	3.0 times baseline or increase in serum creatinine to ≥4.0 mg/dL (≥26.5 μmol/L) or initiation of renal replacement therapy or, in patients <18 y, decrease in eGFR to <35 mL/min per 1.73 m²	<0.3 mL/kg/h for ≥24 h or anuria for ≥12 h

Kidney Disease: Improving Global Outcomes (KDIGO) Acute Kidney Injury Work Group. KDIGO clinical practice guideline for acute kidney injury. *Kidney Int Suppl* 2012;2:1–138.

the incidence of AKI in hospitalized children ranged from 0.05% to 1% (12,13) and in critically ill children from 2.5% to 4.5% (14,15). In adults, depending on the definition of AKI used, a single patient population may have an incidence of AKI ranging from 1% to 44% (8). Since the establishment of a standard definition for AKI in 2004, there have been hundreds of studies describing the epidemiology and clinical significance of pediatric AKI. There still exists a significant challenge, though, in understanding the true epidemiology of pediatric AKI due to the variation in use and application of these definitions. Using the pRIFLE definition, Moffett identified an incidence of AKI of 34% in noncritically ill children admitted to Texas Children's Hospital (16), while a study of 2.6 million pediatric admissions in the United States from 4121 hospitals revealed a rate of 3.9/1000 hospitalizations (17). In children admitted to the hospital for acute infections, AKI was found in 13% of patients according to the AKIN criteria (18).

Specifically regarding critically ill children, the incidence of AKI is significantly higher, ranging from 10% to 46% (8,19–22). In the largest study of a heterogeneous population of critically ill children, Schneider demonstrated a 10% incidence of AKI, with more than half having some degree of AKI at the time of PICU admission (8). In another multicenter analysis, AKI was identified in 18% of patients (19). The incidence of AKI is even higher in specialized populations:

- 58%–90% for those requiring mechanical ventilation or victims of trauma (6–8,23)
- 64% for those requiring extracorporeal membrane oxygenation support (24)
- 45% for burn victims (25)

- 30%–56% for children undergoing congenital heart disease surgery (26–28) (with incidence increasing as patients' age decreases)
- 17%–45% for hematopoietic stem-cell transplants (HSCTs) of patients (29,30)

Risk factors associated with development of HSCT-associated AKI are veno-occlusive disease, sepsis, and nephrotoxic medications. Unlike in adults, total body irradiation does not appear to significantly influence the development of AKI (29,30).

Risk factors for AKI differ between developed countries and developing countries. Anochie showed that in a Nigerian cohort of children, acute gastroenteritis was the most common cause, accounting for 29% of patients with AKI (31). In a large multicenter study from Turkey, hypoxic/ischemia injury and sepsis were the most common causes for both neonates and children >30 days of age, although hypoxic/ischemic injury was responsible for a much larger percentage in the neonatal population (43.5% vs. 20.5%) (32). In a recent large U.S. national hospitalization database study of 2.6 million pediatric admissions, AKI was found in 0.39% of all children (17). AKI was identified more commonly in older children, with one third of AKI patients being between 15 and 18 years old. Interestingly, neonates showed the lowest incidence, unlike other smaller studies where neonates seem to develop AKI at a higher rate (16,26). Similar to what has been shown in adults (33), African Americans had the highest rate for a specific race, accounting for 20% of all AKI hospitalizations (17). Further, AKI was associated with the presence of liver disease, respiratory failure, shock, coagulation disorders, mechanical ventilation, blood transfusions, presence of vascular catheters, and delivery of enteral/parenteral nutrition (17).

The epidemiology of AKI has changed over the years as well. In the 1980s, AKI was more commonly due to intrinsic renal disease (acute glomerulonephritis [GN], hemolytic uremic syndrome) and burns (34). More recently, complications from systemic diseases, such as sepsis, multiple organ dysfunction, hematologic and oncologic (stem-cell transplantation) complications, solid organ transplantation, pulmonary failure, congenital heart surgery, complications from neonatal care, and exposure to nephrotoxins, are responsible for the development of AKI (12,32,34). Regarding neonates, similar risk factors have been identified in addition to congenital heart disease with circulatory failure and postoperative complications (17). Longer bypass and cross-clamp times, higher surgical complexity score, higher inotrope score, use of circulatory arrest, and younger age are all associated with the development of AKI after congenital heart surgery (26,35).

ESTIMATION OF GLOMERULAR FILTRATION RATE

GFR Estimation Equations

The gold standard for the measurement of GFR is the urinary clearance of inulin, a solute that is freely filtered at the glomerulus, neither secreted nor reabsorbed by the kidney tubules. This method is expensive and cumbersome. Therefore, assessment of the GFR using creatinine clearance estimation equations is more commonly utilized. The Schwartz equation is the traditional formula used to estimate GFR in children. The Schwartz equation is based on serum creatinine determined by the Jaffe method (36).

Schwartz formula:

$$\text{GFR (mL/min/1.73 m}^2) = k \times \text{height (cm)/serum creatinine (mg/dL)}$$

k = Muscle factor: Premature infant up to 1 year of age = 0.33 (37)
Term infant up to 1 year of age = 0.45 (38)
Child or adolescent girl = 0.55
Adolescent boy = 0.7

The newest and more commonly used enzymatic method for creatinine measurement provides lower values compared with the Jaffe method. Therefore, the original Schwartz equation was adapted to utilize the enzymatically determined serum creatinine. This equation was derived from The Chronic Kidney Disease in Children (CKiD) Study (39). The formula is useful in the GFR range of 15–75 mL/min/1.73 m².

CKiD Schwartz formula:

$$\text{GFR (mL/min/1.73 m}^2) = 0.431 \times \text{height (cm)/serum creatinine (mg/dL)}$$

Children reach adult levels of GFR by the age of 2. The following are reference values for GFR:

>2 years of age 110–120 mL/min/1.73 m²
Premature infants <10 mL/min/1.73 m² (40)
Term infants 10–40 mL/min/1.73 m² (41)

Creatinine

Serum creatinine is the most common laboratory test used to identify reduced GFR, but there are several inherent problems with its measurement. Serum creatinine only accurately reflects GFR in patients with stable kidney function in a steady state.

Therefore, the measurement is inaccurate in those with fluctuating renal function and the rise in creatinine is often delayed. Creatinine is derived from the metabolism of creatine in skeletal muscle and from dietary meat intake. It is freely filtered across the glomerulus and is neither reabsorbed nor metabolized by the kidney. However, ~10%–40% of urinary creatinine is derived from tubular secretion by the organic cation secretory pathways in the proximal tubule, making it a suboptimal marker of estimated GFR. Additionally, serum creatinine is influenced by factors such as diet, hydration status, medications (cimetidine, trimethoprim), and hyperbilirubinemia (42,43).

Normal creatinine values in pediatric patients vary with age and body mass. The following are serum creatinine reference values by age (44):

Newborn – 0.3–1.0 mg/dL (27–88 μmol/L)
Infant – 0.2–0.4 mg/dL (18–35 μmol/L)
Child – 0.3–0.7 mg/dL (27–62 μmol/L)
Adolescent – 0.5–1.0 mg/dL (44–88 μmol/L)

Cystatin C

Cystatin C is a 122-amino-acid low-molecular-weight protein that is a member of the cysteine protease inhibitor family (45). It is produced at a constant rate by all nucleated cells and is freely filtered by the glomerulus, reabsorbed, not secreted, but is catabolized in the tubules (46). Cystatin C blood levels are not significantly affected by age, gender, race, or muscle mass, so it is effective as a marker of glomerular function in cachectic or pediatric patients; or in the case of early AKI, where serum creatinine could underestimate the true renal function (46).

One prospective study in an adult population at risk for AKI showed that a 50% increase of cystatin C level in serum predicted AKI 2 days before the rise in serum creatinine (47). Another study demonstrated that cystatin C had a better correlation with GFR than serum creatinine in critically ill adults (48). Cystatin C levels were also useful for predicting need for renal replacement therapy and correlated with AKI in children suffering from malaria (49). Cystatin C may be superior to creatinine as a marker of GFR, but it should be noted that there are ongoing concerns related to the lack of standardization in cystatin C measurement (42).

Biomarkers

Because of the lag between the timing of renal injury and abnormalities in serum creatinine and urinary output, serum creatinine is a poor marker for early AKI. Significant renal damage has already occurred by the time the diagnosis of AKI has been made. Therefore, there has been a shift in focus to the early detection of AKI by novel biomarkers. There are more than 25 promising candidate biomarkers that are being investigated (50).

Neutrophil Gelatinase-Associated Lipocalin. Neutrophil gelatinase-associated lipocalin (NGAL) is a 25-kDa lipocalin secreted by activated neutrophils and expressed in many cells (e.g., kidney, lungs, stomach, and colon). Plasma NGAL is freely filtered by the glomerulus and is largely reabsorbed in the proximal tubules. After ischemia it is secreted in the thick ascending limb and detected in the urine (51). Urinary excretion of NGAL is likely to occur when concomitant proximal renal tubular injury precludes NGAL reabsorption and/or increases *de novo* NGAL synthesis (52).

In a recent meta-analysis that included more than 4000 adult patients at risk for AKI, NGAL was detected 1–3 days prior to AKI diagnosis (53). In studies of critically ill children, urine and plasma NGAL measurements were shown to predict AKI ~2 days prior to the rise in serum creatinine (54,55).

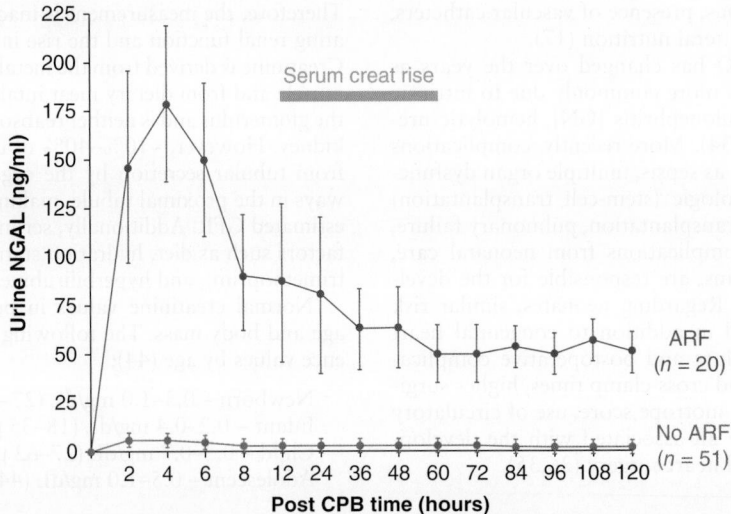

FIGURE 110.1. Neutrophil gelatinase-associated lipocalin (NGAL) preceded the diagnosis of acute kidney injury in children after cardiopulmonary bypass (CPB) surgery. The graph shows urine NGAL (ng/mL) at various times after CPB in patients who subsequently developed AKI (blue) versus those who did not (red). The green bar represents the time when the initial rise in serum creatinine was detected. (Wouters PF, Gehring H, Meyfroidt G, et al. Accuracy of pulse oximeters: The European multi-center trial. *Anesth Analg* 2002;94:13–6.)

NGAL also preceded the diagnosis of AKI in children after cardiopulmonary bypass (CPB) surgery. **Figure 110.1** shows a panel of urine NGAL (ng/mL) at various times after CPB in patients who subsequently developed AKI (blue) versus those who did not (red). The green bar represents the time when the initial rise in serum creatinine was detected. At all post-CPB time points examined, urine NGAL was significantly greater in subjects who developed AKI, as defined by a 50% increase in serum creatinine over baseline (56).

Kidney Injury Molecule-1: Human kidney injury molecule (KIM) is a type 1 transmembrane glycoprotein receptor (with an immunoglobulin and mucin domain) that is not detectable in normal kidney tissue or urine, but is expressed at very high levels in proximal tubule epithelial cells in human and rodent kidneys after ischemic or toxic injury. KIM-1 can be detected in the urine of patients with acute tubular necrosis (ATN) and may serve as a useful biomarker for renal proximal tubular injury allowing early diagnosis of the disease (57).

High urinary KIM-1 expression was evaluated in a cohort prospective study of 201 hospitalized patients with AKI and was associated with adverse clinical outcome (death and need for dialysis) (58). In a case–control study of 20 children after CBP surgery, urinary KIM-1 was found to be elevated 6–12 hours following CBP and remained high up to 48 hours in patients with a greater than 50% increase in serum creatinine, but not in children with normal renal function (59).

Interleukin 18: Interleukin 18 (IL-18) is a pro-inflammatory cytokine that is expressed in the intercalated cell of the late distal convoluted tubule and the collecting duct of the healthy human kidney. These cells have intracellular cysteine protease, which converts the proform of IL-18 to its active form, which then exits the cell and may enter the urine in AKI (60). IL-18 may be used as a marker for proximal tubular injury in ATN. When combined with NGAL, it predicted the duration of AKI in children after cardiac surgery (56).

Liver-type Fatty-Acid-Binding Protein. Liver-type fatty-acid-binding protein (L-FABP) is a protein expressed in the proximal tubule of the kidney. It was found as an early biomarker in urine within 4 hours after surgery in children undergoing CPB who subsequently developed AKI (61). Urinary L-FABP was also found to be significantly higher in patients who did not survive during septic shock and associated AKI, than in the

survivors, with an area under the curve for mortality prediction of 0.99 (62).

N-Acetyl-β-Glucosaminidase. N-acetyl-β-glucosaminidase (NAG) is a newly emerging biomarker of AKI. NAG is a lysosomal enzyme, found predominantly in the proximal convoluted tubules. Increased activity of this enzyme in the urine suggests injury to tubular cells. It has been associated with nephrotoxic medications, contrast nephropathy, and ischemic AKI (63).

Combination of AKI Biomarkers. It is apparent that a combination of biomarkers may achieve the highest diagnostic and prognostic data in early prevention of AKI. One prospective study of 90 adults who underwent cardiac surgery showed that combined analysis of a panel consisting of KIM-1, NAG, and NGAL enhanced the sensitivity of early detection of postoperative AKI (64). Another study evaluating serial measurements of multiple urinary biomarkers after pediatric cardiac surgery revealed a sequential pattern for the appearance of AKI biomarkers, with NGAL and L-FABP being the earliest responders (2–4 hours) and KIM-1 and IL-18 representing the intermediate responders (6–12 hours) (65).

EVALUATION OF ACUTE KIDNEY INJURY

Once the diagnosis of AKI is established, a careful history, review of medications, and physical examination are needed to differentiate between prerenal, intrinsic renal, and postrenal etiologies of AKI if the cause is not immediately apparent. For patients who develop AKI while in the hospital, a precipitating event in the few days prior to the rise in serum creatinine should be sought out (e.g., nephrotoxic exposure, hypotension, or cardiac surgery). The physical examination includes measurement of blood pressure, and evaluation for edema and signs of systemic disease. Initial testing generally includes testing of serum for creatinine, blood urea nitrogen (BUN), electrolytes, including phosphorus, and albumin. Urine should be sent for general analysis, sodium, and creatinine. A complete blood count and renal ultrasound should also be performed (see **Table 110.3**). Additional serologic testing, imaging, and, rarely, renal biopsy may be required to further characterize the etiology of kidney disease.

TABLE 110.3

LABORATORY FINDINGS IN ACUTE KIDNEY INJURY

■ INDICES	■ PRERENAL AKI	■ INTRINSIC AKI: GLOMERULAR	■ INTRINSIC AKI: TUBULO-INTERSTITIAL	■ POSTRENAL AKI
BUN:Creatinine	>20	<10	<10	<10
Urine sodium (mEq/L)				
Children	<10	>20	>20	>20
Neonates	<20–30	>30	>30	>30
FENa(%)				
Children	<1	>2	>2	>2
Neonates	<3	>3	>3	>3
Urine osmolality (mOSm/kg)	>500	<350	<350	<350
Urine specific gravity	>1.020	<1.010	<1.010	<1.010
Urine protein	Usually absent	May be absent or mild to moderate. Not nephrotic range	May be nephrotic range	Variable
Urine sediment	Hyaline casts	Dysmorphic red blood cells, red blood cell casts, lipid casts	Granular casts, muddy brown casts, white blood cell casts, epithelial casts, eosinophils	Variable

AKI, acute kidney injury; BUN, blood urea nitrogen; FENa, fractional excretion of sodium.

Urinalysis. Qualitative urinalysis and microscopic examination of the urine sediment are essential in the evaluation of AKI. A key component of the urinalysis is assessment for proteinuria. The urine dipstick detects albumin and qualitatively measures the protein concentration of 0–2000 mg/dL. The amount of protein can be further quantified by a protein-to-creatinine ratio sent on a random sample; normal is less than 0.2 mg/mg and nephrotic range is greater than 2 mg/mg (66). A first morning urine sample is used to eliminate the confounding variable of benign orthostatic proteinuria. Twenty-four-hour urine collection is generally not recommended as it is often difficult to obtain an accurate urine collection in children. The protein-to-creatinine ratio can be approximated to 24-hour protein by multiplying the ratio by a factor of 0.63; a normal value is less than 4 mg/m^2/h (67). Proteinuria is not typically found in prerenal or postrenal AKI, but can be significant in intrinsic renal disease.

Microscopic evaluation of the urine sediment by an experienced individual is important for identifying an etiology. Urine sediment should be analyzed for the presence of casts, crystals, cellular debris, and red blood cell morphology. The urine dipstick can detect whole blood, hemoglobin, and myoglobin. The presence of red blood cells (RBCs) on microscopy indicates hematuria, while its absence signifies myoglobinuria or hemoglobinuria. The finding of dysmorphic RBCs or RBC casts indicates a glomerular origin of hematuria.

Urine Indices. The urine sodium concentration and fractional excretion of sodium (FENa) are useful tests to help distinguish prerenal from other forms of AKI. In a state of volume depletion, the appropriate renal response is to conserve sodium. Thus, urine sodium is usually less than 20 mEq/L. In ATN, the urine sodium is generally greater than 20 mEq/L due to impaired tubular function (68). However, this does not always hold true because urine sodium concentration may be affected by variations in water reabsorption. FENa is felt to be a more reliable test since it is a measure of sodium handling and is not altered by urine volume. FENa is calculated from a random urine specimen as follows:

$$FENa(\%) = (\text{Urine Sodium} \times \text{Serum Creatinine}/\text{Serum Sodium} \times \text{Urine Creatinine}) \times 100$$

The FENa is expected to be less than 1% in prerenal AKI and greater than 2% in intrinsic and postrenal AKI (68). The ratio is normally higher in neonates due to decreased sodium reabsorption. A limitation of FENa is that it is inaccurate in patients treated with diuretics. The fractional excretion of urea (FE$_{UN}$) is not affected by diuretics and may be used in this scenario. In states of hypovolemia, the FE$_{UN}$ is less than 35%, while, in ATN, it is often greater than 50%.

Urine specific gravity and osmolality may provide useful information as well. The body's normal response to a hypovolemic state is secretion of antidiuretic hormone, which leads to maximal concentration of the urine. Urine osmolality in prerenal AKI is typically greater than 500 mOsm/kg and specific gravity greater than 1.020. In contrast, intrinsic renal disease results in impairment of urine-concentrating ability with urine osmolality usually less than 350 mOsm/kg and specific gravity less than 1.010 (68).

BUN-to-Creatinine Ratio. BUN is preferentially reabsorbed along with sodium in the proximal tubule during hypovolemic states. The proximal tubule is impermeable to creatinine. Thus, a ratio of BUN to creatinine (mg/mg) greater than 20 is suggestive of a prerenal etiology. This should be interpreted with caution as the ratio may also be elevated with gastrointestinal bleeding, steroid use, and decreased muscle mass. A ratio less than 10–15 is common in ATN.

Ultrasound. Ultrasonography of the kidneys and bladder is a valuable tool that provides information about the anatomy of the urinary tract and can assess for the presence of obstruction. Doppler studies allow for the evaluation of the renal vasculature. Ultrasound is the imaging modality of choice in AKI due to the advantages of absence of radiation or iodonized contrast or the need for sedation. The finding of obstruction on ultrasound is diagnostic for postrenal AKI. Ultrasound is usually normal in prerenal AKI. Increased echogenicity of the kidneys may be found in intrinsic AKI.

Prerenal Acute Kidney Injury

Etiology. Prerenal AKI is the end result of decreased blood flow to the renal parenchyma from either volume depletion or decreased effective circulating volume. Hypovolemic states that lead to prerenal AKI include hemorrhage and gastrointestinal, urinary or cutaneous losses. Decreased effective circulating volume may also occur in cases of hypervolemia, such as nephrotic syndrome, cardiac dysfunction, and liver disease. Hypotension as a result of septic or myocardial shock is also a contributor to pre-renal AKI (**Table 110.4**).

Pathophysiology. When cardiac and arterial stretch receptors sense a reduction in mean arterial pressure from decreased cardiac output or systemic vascular resistance, activation of the receptors leads to increased sympathetic tone and release of renin, angiotensin II, aldosterone, and antidiuretic hormone (69). The end result is vasoconstriction of the renal circulation and decreased renal blood flow in order to preserve blood supply to vital organs. Diminished renal blood flow causes a direct reduction in GFR. Nephrons attempt to compensate for this decrease in GFR by releasing prostaglandins and angiotensin II, which preferentially dilate the afferent arterioles and constrict the efferent arterioles, respectively. There is also the myogenic response of the smooth muscle in afferent arterioles that leads to vasodilation when hypoperfusion is detected.

Although there is a decrease in GFR, the glomeruli, interstitium, and tubular structures as well as the renal tubule handling of water and sodium remain intact in pre-renal AKI. Aldosterone avidly reabsorbs sodium while antidiuretic hormone conserves water, leading to decreased urine output. When renal perfusion is restored, the GFR and urine flow return to normal. On the other hand, if diminished renal perfusion persists, pre-renal AKI may convert to intrinsic AKI.

Clinical History and Physical Exam. Children with pre-renal AKI may present with a history of hemorrhage, vomiting, diarrhea, fever, weight loss, or decreased urine output. Signs and symptoms of dehydration or decreased perfusion are present on physical exam. Clinical evidence includes tachycardia, low blood pressure, poor skin turgor, dry mucous membranes, mental status changes, sunken eyes and fontanelle, reduced tears, and capillary refill greater than 2 seconds (70). Cardiac dysfunction, nephrotic syndrome, and liver disease may result in edema.

Diagnostic Evaluation. In pre-renal AKI, the BUN-to-creatinine ratio is greater than 20. The urinalysis usually demonstrates no proteinuria, hematuria, or abnormal urine sediment, although hyaline casts may be present. The specific gravity is elevated with urine osmolality typically greater than 500 mOsm/kg. The urine sodium concentration is expected to be less than 10 mEq/L and the FENa less than 1%, indicative of sodium retention. In neonates, these values are higher (urine sodium less than 20–30 mEq/L and FENa less than 3%).

Management. Management of pre-renal AKI requires treatment of the underlying condition, volume resuscitation, and

maintenance of renal perfusion. Fluid management is discussed in detail later in the chapter. The return of serum creatinine to baseline in response to volume repletion is diagnostic for prerenal AKI.

INTRINSIC RENAL AKI

Intrinsic renal disease may arise from the glomerular, tubulointerstitial or vascular components of the kidney. The most common cause is ATN due to ischemia, although in the ICU intrinsic AKI is frequently multifactorial due to a combination of insults. The causes of intrinsic AKI are listed in **Table 110.5**.

Glomerular Disease

Etiology. GN is a renal disease characterized by inflammation and proliferation of glomeruli with resulting renal dysfunction. The typical presentation of GN is nephritic syndrome, defined as glomerular hematuria, edema, azotemia, and hypertension. IgA nephropathy is the leading cause of GN worldwide, while post-streptococcal glomerulonephritis (PSAGN) is the most common cause in children (71). Rapidly progressive glomerulonephritis (RPGN) is a form of GN that presents with a rapid loss of renal function and is associated with the histological presence of crescents in glomeruli. RPGN may be caused by all forms of GN.

Pathophysiology. Glomerular lesions are a result of immune deposits or in situ formation of immune complexes.

TABLE 110.4

ETIOLOGY OF PRERENAL ACUTE KIDNEY INJURY

Volume depletion
- Gastrointestinal losses (vomiting, diarrhea)
- Hemorrhage
- Skin losses
- Burns
- Diuretics
- Osmotic diuresis (mannitol, glucosuria)

Decreased effective circulating volume
- Septic shock
- Nephrotic syndrome
- Anaphylaxis
- Cardiac dysfunction
- Post–cardiac surgery
- Liver disease

TABLE 110.5

INTRINSIC RENAL CAUSES OF ACUTE KIDNEY INJURY

Glomerular
- IgA nephropathy
- Post–infectious glomerulonephritis
- Henoch–Schonlein Purpura
- Membranoproliferative glomerulonephritis
- Systemic lupus erythematosus
- ANCA-associated vasculitis
- Anti-glomerular basement membrane syndrome

Tubular (acute tubular necrosis)
- Hypoxia/Ischemia
- Sepsis
- Medications
- Toxins
- Pigment nephropathy (rhabdomyolysis, hemolysis)
- Obstruction by crystals (uric acid, tumor lysis syndrome, acyclovir)
- Oxalosis

Interstitial (interstitial nephritis)
- Infectious
- Pyelonephritis
- Infiltration
- Medications

Vascular/Hemodynamic
- Hemolytic uremic syndrome
- Thrombosis
- Polyarteritis nodosa
- Nonsteroidal anti-inflammatory drugs
- ACE inhibitors

ANCA, anti-neutrophil cytoplasmic antibody; ACE, angiotensin-converting enzyme.

Inflammation and proliferation lead to damage of the basement membrane, mesangium, or capillary wall endothelium, which creates a barrier to glomerular filtration. In nephritic syndrome, edema and hypertension are present due to fluid overload and increased hydrostatic pressure.

Clinical History and Physical Examination. Patients with glomerular disease typically present with edema or tea-colored urine. A history of sore throat or skin infection preceding the onset of gross hematuria by 1–3 weeks is suggestive of PSAGN, while an upper respiratory illness at the time of hematuria is indicative of IgA nephropathy. Systemic symptoms such as joint aches, rash, and fever suggest an autoimmune disease or vasculitis. Pulmonary hemorrhage is associated with Goodpastures syndrome and anti-neutrophil cytoplasmic antibody (ANCA) vasculitis. On physical examination, blood pressure measurement is important as hypertension is common with glomerular disease. Edema is most obvious in the morning on awakening located in the periorbital area with a gradual progression to generalized edema with possible ascites and pulmonary edema. Petechiae or purpura may be seen with Henoch–Schonlein Purpura and other vasculitides.

Diagnostic Evaluation. A hallmark of glomerular disease is hematuria and proteinuria on urinalysis. RBC casts and dysmorphic RBCs are indicative of glomerular hematuria. Proteinuria may reach nephrotic range (protein-to-creatinine ratio greater than 2 mg/mg). Urine osmolality is usually less than 350 mOsm/kg. The urine sodium concentration is expected to be greater than 20 mEq/L and the FENa greater than 2%. The BUN-to-creatinine ratio is less than 10. To obtain a specific diagnosis, serum complement levels (C3, C4), anti-streptolysin O antibody, streptozyme, anti-nuclear antibody, double-stranded DNA, anti-glomerular basement membrane antibody, and ANCA may be sent. Hypocomplementemia is suggestive of PSAGN, systemic lupus erythematosus, membranoproliferative glomerulonephritis, shunt nephritis, or bacterial endocarditis. On renal ultrasound, the kidneys may be enlarged and show increased echogenicity compared to the liver. Renal biopsy may aid in the diagnosis of glomerular disease.

Management. Treatment of GN is geared toward the specific disease. PSAGN is a self-limited condition that requires supportive therapy. Immunosuppressive treatments and plasmapheresis may be needed for other forms of GN.

Tubular Disease: Acute Tubular Necrosis

ATN is a process that leads to a decline of renal function due to injury and cell death of the tubular cells of the kidney. ATN is the most common cause of AKI in the ICU. The majority of cases of ATN are due to renal ischemia, sepsis, and nephrotoxins. The pathophysiology, diagnostic evaluation, and management of these are discussed separately.

Ischemic Renal Disease

Etiology. ATN is on a continuum with prerenal disease with progression from the latter when the ischemic insult persists. It frequently occurs in patients with hypotension from sepsis and major surgery. Cardiac surgery with CPB, in particular, is a significant risk factor for AKI (26,35,72).

Pathophysiology. ATN occurs when ischemia persists long enough to induce cell injury and death. ATN generally follows three stages. In the initiation phase, ischemia and reperfusion lead to the release of calcium, reactive oxygen species, and phospholipases in the proximal tubule. Loss of polarity of Na-K-ATPase and integrins in the tubular cells and effacement of the brush border ensue, followed by apoptosis and cell death (73). Obstruction of the tubule lumen by necrosed tubular cells and casts causes an increase in glomerular pressure,

transtubular back leak of glomerular filtrate, and a decline in GFR. In the maintenance phase, there is a sustained reduction in GFR of a variable time period, usually 1–2 weeks. In the recovery phase, the tubule cells regenerate, the obstruction of the tubule lumen resolves, and GFR returns to baseline.

Clinical History and Physical Examination. Patients with ischemic ATN will present with a history of volume depletion similar to those with pre-renal AKI (e.g., vomiting, diarrhea, hemorrhage, or sepsis). ATN may be oliguric or nonoliguric. If the patient is nonoliguric, blood pressure may be normal. Findings on physical exam may suggest dehydration or hypovolemia. Conversely, hypertension and edema may be present in an oliguric patient.

Diagnostic Evaluation. The classic finding on urinalysis in ATN is muddy brown granular casts consisting of sloughed tubular cells. Epithelial cell casts and epithelial cells may also be found. Mild-to-moderate proteinuria may be present, but hematuria is not significant. ATN may often be distinguished from pre-renal AKI by urine indices. Urine osmolality is less than 350 mOsm/kg, urine sodium is greater than 20 mEq/L, and FeNa is greater than 2% in ATN. The BUN-to-creatinine ratio is less than 10. On renal ultrasound, the kidneys may show increased echogenicity compared to the liver.

Management. Most cases of ischemic ATN are reversible if the underlying cause is treated; however, permanent damage with cortical necrosis may occur if the ischemia is severe.

Sepsis

Sepsis is a significant contributor to morbidity and mortality in the pediatric ICU. Sepsis is an independent risk factor for the development of AKI (19,32,74) and sepsis-induced AKI is associated with poor outcomes and increased risk of death in both children and adults (74–76). The pathophysiology of sepsis-induced AKI is not completely understood. The traditional view attributes AKI to ischemia-reperfusion injury secondary to decreased cardiac output and hypotension. However, this idea has been challenged by experimental studies that have shown a variation of renal blood flow in sepsis. Renal blood flow may be normal, decreased, or increased in sepsis (77). Immune-mediated injury, apoptosis, and alterations in intrarenal hemodynamics are thought to play a role in sepsis-induced AKI although the mechanisms are not fully known. Systemic inflammation, release of cytokines, arachidonic acid metabolites, the clotting cascade, and T-cell activation may contribute to kidney injury in sepsis, although it is unclear whether they are true mediators of injury (78). The diagnostic evaluation and management of sepsis-induced AKI are similar to those of ischemic ATN. The underlying cause of sepsis requires treatment.

Nephrotoxins

Drug-induced AKI is a significant preventable cause of AKI. Nephrotoxicity accounts for 16%–25% of AKI in the ICU (79,80). **Table 110.6** lists the most common offenders. The primary mechanisms of nephrotoxicity include direct injury to the tubules, alteration of renal blood flow, and tubular obstruction. *Aminoglycosides* bind to tubular epithelial cells, are taken up by lysosomes, and cause rupture of the lysosomes with resultant necrosis of the tubule cell. The degree of injury is dose and duration dependent; therefore, monitoring of drug levels is essential. *Nonsteroidal anti-inflammatory drugs* (NSAIDs) inhibit prostaglandin synthesis, causing vasoconstriction of the afferent arteriole and reduced blood flow to the glomerulus. NSAIDs may also cause interstitial nephritis and nephrotic syndrome. Similarly, *calcineurin inhibitors* such as tacrolimus and cyclosporine cause vasoconstriction of the afferent arteriole by activating endothelin and

TABLE 110.6

COMMON NEPHROTOXIC MEDICATIONS

- Antimicrobial agents
  - Aminoglycosides
  - Amphotericin B
  - Acyclovir
  - Cidofovir
  - Foscarnet
  - Gancyclovir
  - Pentamidine
  - Quinolones
  - Sulfonamides
  - Vancomycin
- Chemotherapeutic agents
  - Cisplatin
  - Ifosphamide
  - Methotrexate
  - Mitomycin C
  - Streptozocin
- Vasoactive drugs
  - ACE inhibitors
  - Cyclosporine
  - NSAIDS
  - Tacrolimus
  - Rapamycin
- Lithium
- Radiocontrast agents
- Intravenous immune globulin (with sucrose)
- Colloidal agents
  - Dextran 40
  - Hydroxyethyl starch

thromboxane and inhibiting nitric oxide and prostaglandin activity. *Angiotensin-converting enzyme inhibitors* (ACEi) and *angiotensin receptor blockers* (ARBs) block the actions of angiotensin II and cause vasodilation of the efferent arteriole, which reduces glomerular pressure. The nephrotoxic effects of NSAIDs, calcineurin inhibitors, ACEi, and ARBs are potentiated in states of hypovolemia. *Acyclovir* precipitates in the distal tubules and results in tubular obstruction with transtubular back leak of glomerular filtrate. Alkalinization of the urine and adequate hydration may prevent nephrotoxicity from acyclovir (81). *Contrast-induced nephropathy* is caused by the administration of high osmolal ionic radiocontrast agents. The contrast is thought to induce renal vasoconstriction mediated by alterations in nitric oxide, endothelin, and/or adenosine. It is also postulated that ATN is a direct result of the cytotoxic effects of the contrast agents. Preventive measures include use of lower doses of contrast, and avoidance of volume depletion and volume expansion with isotonic intravenous fluids prior to, and continued for several hours after, contrast administration (11). Studies of alkalinization of the urine with sodium bicarbonate (82,83) and N-acetylcysteine (NAC) for the prevention of contrast-induced nephropathy are contradictory (84). NAC is thought to minimize vasoconstriction and oxygen-free radical generation. In general, avoidance of nephrotoxins in patients at risk for or with AKI is the best preventive measure. Drug-induced nephropathy is by and large reversible when the offending agent is removed.

Postrenal Acute Kidney Injury

Etiology. Postrenal AKI ensues when there is bilateral obstruction of the lower urinary tract or obstruction of a solitary kidney. Obstruction may occur anywhere from the level of tubules to the ureters and beyond. The obstructive etiology may be congenital or acquired (see **Table 110.7**).

Pathophysiology. Obstruction to the flow of tubular ultrafiltrate causes an increase in intratubular pressure and hydrostatic pressure in Bowman's space, which is normally negligible as compared with the driving pressure across the glomerular capillary bed. As the pressure in Bowman's space rises, the overall difference in pressure that drives ultrafiltration is reduced and, as a result, GFR is diminished. With unilateral obstruction, the changes in renal function may not be clinically evident due to the compensatory change in the unaffected kidney. However, with bilateral obstruction or obstruction in a solitary kidney, the changes in renal function are significant and may lead to AKI. The severity of obstruction to ultrafiltrate flow on kidney function depends on the site, cause, and the duration of obstruction.

Clinical History and Physical Examination. Many cases of urinary obstruction are diagnosed during the prenatal period with ultrasound. Significant obstruction may lead to oligohydramnios and immature development of the lungs while *in utero*. Other congenitally acquired causes of obstruction may first be discovered during an evaluation for urinary tract infection. Children with postrenal AKI often present with a history of difficult urination, weak urine stream, or anuria. Nephrolithiasis, clots, or masses may present with abdominal or flank pain and/or gross hematuria. Abdominal examination may identify a palpable bladder or abdominal mass.

Diagnostic Evaluation. Renal ultrasound is highly sensitive and specific for the diagnosis of obstruction. A voiding cystourogram may aid further in the diagnosis of posterior urethral valves, ureteropelvic junction obstruction, ureterovesical junction obstruction, and neurogenic bladder. Bladder catheterization can rule out urethral obstruction. The BUN-to-creatinine ratio is typically less than 10. The urinalysis may be variable, but urine indices usually demonstrate urine osmolality less than 350 mOsm/kg, urine sodium greater than 20 mEq/L, and FeNa greater than 1%.

Management. Relief of the obstruction by catheter drainage and/or intervention by pediatric urology is the cornerstone of treatment in postrenal AKI. Patients need to be monitored for post obstructive diuresis, manifested by polyuria and electrolyte abnormalities after the relief of obstruction. The pathophysiology of post obstructive diuresis involves decreased reabsorption of sodium due to altered expression of sodium transporters as well as an accumulation of natriuretic factors during uremia. There is also decreased resorption of bicarbonate, calcium, and chloride, and decreased excretion of potassium and hydrogen ions. The inability to maximally concentrate urine due to a decreased medullary concentrating gradient and decreased response to ADH is also thought to lead to post-obstructive diuresis. Finally, increased production of prostaglandin immediately following the relief of the obstruction may be a contributor.

TABLE 110.7

POSTRENAL CAUSES OF ACUTE KIDNEY INJURY

- Posterior urethral valves
- Bilateral upper tract obstruction (ureteropelvic junction obstruction, ureterovesical junction obstruction)
- Nephrolithiasis (bilateral)
- Clots
- Neoplasm
- Trauma
- Prune belly syndrome
- Neurogenic bladder

Postobstructive diuresis is usually self-limited, lasting 24–36 hours, during which time creatinine clearance will improve rapidly and urinary replacement needs will taper off; rarely, it may last up to months. Management focuses on avoiding severe volume depletion and electrolyte imbalances such as hypokalemia, hyponatremia, hypernatremia, and hypomagnesemia. Volume replacement is appropriate only if there is volume depletion or disturbance of osmolality. As initial urine is isosthenuric, the starting fluid for replacement is 0.45% saline, given at a rate slower than the rate of urine output. Close monitoring of vital signs, volume status, urine output, and electrolyte is important during this period.

PREVENTION AND TREATMENT OF AKI

❼ There is limited evidence in pediatrics regarding effective therapy for AKI. Clinical management is primarily supportive as there are no pharmacologic agents that have been proven to prevent or treat AKI. Early recognition of renal dysfunction and avoidance of nephrotoxins are the best preventive measures. The mainstays of treatment are restoration and maintenance of adequate fluid balance, correction of metabolic and electrolyte derangements, nutritional support, and limitation of further renal injury. When conservative therapy is unsuccessful, renal replacement therapy (RRT) becomes necessary.

Fluid Management

An accurate initial assessment of the patient's intravascular volume status is required to guide initial fluid management. Children with prerenal AKI presenting with signs or symptoms of dehydration, sepsis, or shock require immediate expansion of intravascular volume with the aim of increasing perfusion to vital organs. The initial step in volume resuscitation is intravenous (or intraosseous) repletion of fluids with one or more boluses of 10–20 mL/kg. Isotonic crystalloids (normal saline or Llactated Ringer's) are recommended over colloids (albumin, hydroxyethyl starch, gelatin, and dextran) in patients at risk for AKI or with established AKI, except in cases of hemorrhagic shock (11). Colloids have not been found to be more effective than isotonic crystalloids in reducing the risk of death or need for RRT in critically ill patients (85) and may, in fact, be harmful. Studies have demonstrated that hydroxyethyl starch is associated with increased risk for AKI, need for RRT, and adverse events (86,87). Furthermore, albumin resuscitation has been linked to increased mortality in patients with traumatic brain injury and therefore should be avoided in those cases (88).

After the initial phase of volume expansion, subsequent fluid therapy is based on strict recording of daily inputs, outputs, weight, physical examination, and invasive monitoring as needed. The remaining fluid deficit may be replaced over 24–48 hours while maintaining insensible and ongoing fluid losses. AKI due to prerenal etiologies is usually reversible and responsive to volume resuscitation. Restoration of renal perfusion through volume expansion may be a strategy to prevent progression of prerenal AKI to intrinsic AKI. Current studies evaluating the optimal timing and amount of initial volume resuscitation required to prevent AKI are ongoing. Data from adult patients with septic shock demonstrate that early goal-directed fluid therapy leads to improved mortality and other outcomes (incidence of AKI not reported) (89). Volume expansion has also been successful in patients at risk for AKI in situations such as tumor lysis syndrome, contrast-induced

AKI, and pigment nephropathy. However, once intrinsic AKI is confirmed by continued azotemia, oliguria (<1.0 mL/kg/h in infants, <0.5 mL/kg/h in children), or anuria (<0.2 mL/kg/h) after volume administration, fluid restriction is important in order to prevent volume overload. Studies in adults and children have demonstrated that increased fluid administration and positive fluid balance are associated with increased mortality in AKI (90,91). The RENAL study found that a negative mean daily fluid balance during RRT was associated with decreased risk of death (92). Some strongly suggest consideration of RRT when fluid overload exceeds 10% of body weight and definite initiation of RRT when fluid overload is greater than 15% (90).

The fluid prescription should be tailored to include maintenance needs and replacement of ongoing losses. However, the practice of providing maintenance fluids based on caloric requirements (e.g. Holliday Segar method (93)) is not appropriate in patients with intrinsic AKI. To maintain an even fluid balance, insensible water losses and ongoing losses need to be replaced. Insensible water losses can be estimated as a daily volume of 400 mL/m^2 (~1/3 "maintenance fluid" using Holliday Segar method) given as D5W or D10W at a constant rate (94). Of note, insensible losses are greater in febrile patients and lower in mechanically ventilated patients due to administration of humidified air. Urine losses need to be replaced millimeter for millimeter with 0.45% normal saline. Other ongoing fluid losses (e.g. diarrhea, nasogastric output, etc.) should also be replaced with equivalent volumes. In cases of hypervolemia, a negative fluid balance may be achieved by replacing a fraction of the insensible losses and/or urine output. Strict recording of daily inputs, outputs, and weights is paramount for optimal fluid management in AKI. Bladder catheterization is recommended to confirm oligoanuria and to aid in recording of output.

Diuretics

Oliguric AKI is generally associated with worse outcomes when compared to nonoliguric AKI (95,96); therefore, in theory, there is a strong rationale for the use of diuretics in the prevention of AKI. Diuretics, in particular loop diuretics, may increase urine flow, flush urine debris, reduce glomerular pressure, and increase renal blood flow, preventing tubular obstruction, further ischemic injury, and limiting oxygen consumption (97). Yet, its use to prevent AKI has not been proven, and thus, diuretics are not recommended as a prevention strategy (11).

Diuretics are also not recommended for the treatment of established AKI but can be used to manage volume overload (11). Diuretics may convert oliguric AKI to nonoliguric AKI, which may aid in fluid management. However, the use of diuretics has not been shown to improve outcomes in established AKI. Diuretics do not reduce mortality, need for dialysis, length of RRT, and length of stay or increase recovery of renal function (98,99).

Patients with AKI do not respond normally to diuretics and usually require higher doses (furosemide 2–5 mg/kg/dose) to achieve a response. Nevertheless, multiple doses of furosemide, if not effective, are likely to cause ototoxicity. For that reason, diuretics should be discontinued quickly if there is no improvement. If there is a diuretic response, a continuous infusion of furosemide (0.1–0.3 mg/kg/h) may be started, which may be superior to bolus dosing because overall less drug is needed (100). A study of post–cardiac surgery neonates receiving continuous versus intermittent dosing of furosemide demonstrated similar urine output between groups, but the group on the drip had less drug exposure and more consistent urine output (101).

Vasoactive Agents

The use of vasopressors is recommended in patients with vasomotor shock (not responsive to fluids) to maintain or restore renal perfusion in critically ill patients (11); however, no pharmacologic agents have been proven to prevent or treat AKI.

Dopamine. Low-dose or "renal-dose" dopamine (0.5 to 3–5 μ/kg/min) administered for the prevention of AKI was a wide-spread practice in ICUs that has now been abandoned. Dopamine is thought to increase renal blood flow by promoting vasodilatation and improving urine output by promoting natriuresis. However, adult studies of low-dose dopamine have failed to show benefit and the intervention may even be harmful (102,103). Dopamine has not proven to alter the course of AKI or to convert oliguric to nonoliguric AKI, and has no effect in decreasing the need for dialysis or improving survival in patients with AKI (102,104,105). Complications of dopamine include tachycardia, arrhythmias, myocardial ischemia, and intestinal ischemia. When used as a vasopressor in adult patients with vasomotor shock, dopamine was associated with more adverse events and increased risk of death when compared to norepinephrine. Thus, norepinephrine is recommended as the first-line agent over dopamine for adults in vasomotor shock (106). In contrast, children frequently present with low cardiac output shock and thus vasoactive agents with greater inotropic support such as dopamine, epinephrine, and dobutamine are utilized (107).

Fenoldopam. Fenoldopam is a selective dopamine-1 receptor agonist that increases renal blood flow through systemic vasodilation. Results of adult studies are promising. A meta-analysis of adults after cardiac surgery demonstrated that fenoldopam resulted in reduced need for RRT, shorter hospital stay, and decreased mortality (108). One small clinical trial in neonates after CPB demonstrated no effect on urine output, incidence of AKI, or change in creatinine (109). Additional prospective studies to define the role of fenoldopam in children are warranted.

Theophylline. A potential mechanism of theophylline is blockage of the actions of adenosine, a potent renal vasoconstrictor that is released during ischemia. Given within the first hour of birth, theophylline was associated with improved fluid balance, higher GFR, and lower creatinine in severely asphyxiated newborns (110,111). A single dose of theophylline is recommended to be given to neonates with severe perinatal asphyxia who are at high risk for AKI (11).

Other pharmacologic agents such as nesiritide (synthetic human brain natriuretic peptide), atrial natriuretic peptide, IGF-1, and N-acetylcysteine have not proven to be beneficial and are not recommended for the prevention or treatment of AKI (11,106). An exception to this may be the use of N-acetylcysteine for the prevention of contrast-induced AKI (11).

Electrolyte and Acid–Base Balance

Electrolyte disturbances in AKI are common and are usually asymptomatic; therefore, frequent monitoring of electrolytes is warranted.

Hyperkalemia. Hyperkalemia in AKI results from reduced GFR, decreased secretion of potassium, and extracellular shifts of potassium during acidosis. Hyperkalemia is the most serious electrolyte abnormality associated with AKI with potential for arrhythmia and cardiac death. Electrocardiogram changes in sequence include peaked T waves, prolonged PR interval, flattened P waves, widened QRS complex, sine wave, ventricular tachycardia, and ventricular fibrillation. ECG changes usually do not occur until the plasma potassium concentration is above 6.5 mEq/L.

Patients with AKI should be placed on a potassium-restricted diet and should not receive potassium supplementation unless they are hypokalemic. Mild-to-moderate hyperkalemia (5–6.5 mEq/L) is treated with potassium restriction and medications that remove potassium from the body. Sodium polystyrene sulfonate eliminates potassium via the gastrointestinal tract. The resin exchanges potassium for sodium (1 g/kg lowers potassium 1 mEq/L). It may be given orally or per rectum every 2–6 hours as needed. Adverse reactions include hypernatremia, intestinal obstruction, and gastrointestinal upset. Caution should be used in neonates and premature infants. Loop diuretics may be given to patients who are not anuric to aid in excretion of potassium in the urine.

Treatment of severe hyperkalemia includes calcium gluconate 10% solution (0.5–1.0 mL/kg intravenously over 5–15 minutes) to stabilize the cardiac membrane and the administration of medications that redistribute as well as remove potassium from the body. Albuterol, a β₂ agonist, is readily available in the ICU and works quickly (10–30 minutes) by transporting potassium into cells. Its effect lasts 2–4 hours. Insulin stimulates beta-receptors on the cell membrane and works within 30 minutes (effect lasts 2–4 hours). Insulin is given with glucose to prevent hypoglycemia, which requires large quantities of fluid (0.5–1.0 g of glucose/kg over 30 minutes and 0.1 unit of insulin/kg intravenously). Sodium bicarbonate (1–2 mEq/kg intravenously over 30–60 minutes) also shifts potassium into the cell and works within 30 minutes (lasts 1–2 hours). A drawback of bicarbonate is fluid overload, other electrolyte abnormalities (hypernatremia and hypocalcemia), and risk of cardiac complications. Hyperkalemia refractory to conservative measures may be treated with dialysis.

Metabolic Acidosis. Elevated anion-gap metabolic acidosis is most commonly found in AKI, although the anion gap can be normal. Acidosis is caused by the impaired secretion of titratable and nontitratable acids generated in the body resulting in a consumption of bicarbonate as a buffer and the irregular tubular handling of bicarbonate. In addition, critically ill patients may have higher acid loads due to sepsis or shock. Treatment of acidosis is important to restore normal pH and body metabolism. Supplementation with oral sodium citrate or sodium bicarbonate (oral or intravenous) may be given, although the use of intravenous sodium bicarbonate is controversial due to its adverse side-effect profile.

Hypocalcemia and Hyperphosphatemia. Hyperphosphatemia is attributable to decreased phosphate excretion in the kidney during AKI. As a result, phosphorus binds to calcium resulting in hypocalcemia. Hypocalcemia is exacerbated by the inability of the kidney to generate active vitamin D and parathyroid hormone resistance. The measurement of ionized calcium is important. Restriction of phosphorus in the diet is recommended as well as the use of oral phosphate binders given with meals to bind phosphate in the gastrointestinal tract. Calcium carbonate is the first-line phosphate binder in children. Selvelamer is a non-calcium-containing phosphate binder. Aluminum-containing binders should be avoided in children due to the risk of neurotoxicity due to aluminum accumulation. Severe hypocalcemia can be treated with intravenous calcium preparations.

Glucose. Neuroendocrine axis changes in AKI cause altered carbohydrate metabolism, which may lead to hyperglycemia. KDIGO recommends insulin therapy to target plasma glucose 110–149 in critically ill adults (11). There is evidence that intensive insulin therapy administered to critically ill adult patients is associated with a reduction in the incidence of AKI and improved survival (112). One prospective study of intensive insulin therapy in critically ill children demonstrated improvements in length of stay and inflammatory markers, but no improvement in need for dialysis or peak serum creatinine (113). Studies on insulin therapy in children require further exploration.

Dosing of Medications

Nephrotoxic medications (see **Table 110.6**) should be avoided in patients at risk for AKI or with established AKI as they may worsen renal injury and delay recovery. The use of aminoglycosides for the treatment of infections is not recommended unless there is no suitable alternative (11). For fungal infections, the lipid formulations of amphotericin B are suggested rather than conventional formulations (11). When appropriate, monitoring of drug levels is important as it allows for adjustment of drug dosing. Once AKI is established, medications that are excreted by the kidney require dosage adjustment based on the estimated GFR. Of note, in the early phases of AKI, the GFR is difficult to estimate as a rise in creatinine is known to be delayed.

Hypertension

Hypertension in AKI usually results from volume overload although it may also be renin-mediated. Fluid restriction and avoidance of volume overload may aid in the prevention of hypertension. To prevent sodium and fluid retention, sodium intake should be restricted to 2–3 mEq/kg/d. Hypertension that does not respond to fluid and sodium restriction requires treatment with antihypertensive medications (see **Table 110.8**). Diuretics may be used in patients with nonoliguric AKI and in those with acute GN. Nifedipine, labetalol, hydralazine, and clonidine are medications that work quickly. ACEi and ARBs are contraindicated in AKI because they reduce glomerular pressure and can lead to hyperkalemia. For hypertensive emergency and urgency, continuous infusion with short-acting medications such as nicardipine, labetalol, and sodium nitroprusside are recommended. The aim is to reduce blood pressure slowly, not more than 25% in the first hours of treatment and then gradually to normal over days. RRT may be used to treat hypertension due to volume overload that is not responsive to diuretics.

Nutritional Support

The provision of adequate nutritional and metabolic support is essential in the care of the critically ill child with AKI as they are at increased risk for undernutrition (114). Malnutrition is associated with increased morbidity and mortality in critically ill adult patients with AKI (115,116). Alterations in physiologic metabolism in AKI lead to a state of hypercatabolism, hypoalbuminemia, loss of lean body mass, and increased utilization of fat stores. Hence, optimal nutritional support that provides adequate energy and protein is indicated to sustain anabolism. Patient energy requirements based on measured energy expenditure are estimated to be 0.20–0.26 mJ/kg/d, equal to a caloric intake of 50–60 cals/kg/d (117). In contrast to adults, protein intake is not restricted in children with AKI. Protein requirements are 2–3 g/kg/d for children aged 0–2 years and 1.5 g/kg/d for children and adolescents greater than 2 years (118). Children on RRT require additional protein supplementation (119). Enteral feedings with renal formulas lower in solute load, phosphorus, and potassium are preferred over parenteral nutrition when feasible. The prescription for total parenteral nutrition (TPN) calls for a high concentration of dextrose with less than 20% given as lipids. Additional supplementation of water-soluble vitamins and trace minerals is often necessary, especially while on RRT. The volume of TPN should be concentrated as much as possible to avoid volume overload.

Renal Replacement Therapy

RRT will be covered briefly as it is discussed in further detail in Chapter 41. When AKI cannot be managed by conservative measures, RRT becomes necessary. RRT is a life-supporting therapy that aids in the removal of fluid and solute waste when there is impaired kidney function. There are no specific threshold levels of creatinine, BUN, or electrolytes that are absolute indications to initiate RRT; rather, the broader clinical context is taken into consideration. General indications for RRT are listed in **Table 110.9**.

TABLE 110.8

ANTIHYPERTENSIVE MEDICATIONS

DRUG	CLASS	DOSE	COMMENTS
Furosemide	Loop diuretic	0.5–2 mg/kg oral or IV every 6–12 h Continuous infusion: start 0.05 mg/kg/h	Use only in nonoliguric AKI
Amlodipine	Calcium channel blocker	Oral: 0.05–0.1 mg/kg/d Adult dose: 2.5–5 mg once daily	Avoid use with AV block, neonates, sick sinus
Clonidine	Central α₂ agonist	Oral: 5–25 µg/kg/d PO divided q 6–8 h Transdermal: 0.1–0.3 mg patch	Rebound hypertension with abrupt withdrawal. Start dose at 5–10 µg/kg/d and increase every 5–7 d
Nifedipine	Calcium channel blocker (short acting)	Oral: 0.1–0.25 mg/kg/dose every 4–6 h	Side effects: flushing and tachycardia
Hydralazine	Direct arterial vasodilator (short acting)	Oral: 0.2–2 mg/kg every 6–12 h IV bolus: 0.1–0.5 mg/kg/dose every 3–4 h	Side effects: tachycardia, nausea, lupus-like reactions
Labetalol	α- and β-blocker	Oral: 0.5–1.5 mg/kg every 12 h IV bolus: 0.2–1.0 mg/kg every 10 min PRN Continuous infusion 0.25–3 mg/kg/h IV	Avoid use with bradycardia, AV block, bronchospasm, CHF
Nicardipine	Calcium channel blocker	Continuous infusion 0.5–4 µg/kg/min	May require a large volume infused
Sodium nitroprusside	Arterial and venous vasodilator	Continuous infusion 0.3–10 µg/kg/min IV	Follow for cyanide toxicity. Risk is higher in AKI
Esmolol	β-blocker	Continuous infusion 100–500 µg/kg/min	Avoid use with asthma, IDDM, AV block

From Lexicomp Online, 2013.

TABLE 110.9

INDICATIONS FOR RENAL REPLACEMENT THERAPY

Severe metabolic acidosis unresponsive to bicarbonate therapy
Electrolyte disturbance despite medical therapy
Fluid overload unresponsive to diuretics
Uremic complications, e.g., pericarditis, encephalopathy, coagulopathy
Inborn errors of metabolism: urea cycle defects

RRT modalities include peritoneal dialysis (PD), intermittent hemodialysis (iHD), and continuous renal replacement therapy (CRRT). The choice of modality is influenced by age, size, medical comorbidities of the patient, availability of access placement, and expertise of the treating physicians. For example, PD is preferred in neonates because iHD and CRRT can be technically challenging due to difficult vascular access. Patients who are hemodynamically unstable cannot tolerate high blood-flow rates and rapid fluid removal; therefore, CRRT is the preferred modality. HD and CRRT are used to treat hyperammonemia and inborn errors of metabolism.

Peritoneal Dialysis. PD utilizes the capillaries of the peritoneal membrane as the conduit for dialysis. The surface area of the peritoneal membrane is larger in children relative to adults, which allows for rapid and efficient equilibration of solutes. A single- or double-cuffed Tenckhoff catheter is the recommended access with the exit site orientation preferably downward or lateral facing to reduce the risk of infection. Dialysis solution is instilled and drained manually or via a cycler machine. The dextrose concentration in the solution is chosen based on the amount of ultrafiltration that is desired. A higher dextrose concentration achieves more fluid removal (1.5%, 2.5%, and 4.25% solutions). The dialysis prescription includes exchange volumes of 20–50 mL/kg (10 mg/kg at initiation to reduce risk of leak), dwell times of 25–50 minutes, and drain times of 5–15 minutes. Shorter dwell times result in increased clearance and fluid removal. The advantages of PD are that vascular access is not required and it is a simpler technique. Disadvantages are that PD may be less efficient than HD and CRRT for solute removal and that there is a risk of peritonitis.

Intermittent Hemodialysis. Intermittent HD is an extra-corporeal blood purification treatment that utilizes a counter-current flow of blood and dialysate to allow diffusion of solutes across a semipermeable membrane of the dialyzer. Urea clearance is dictated by the size of dialyzer, blood flow, dialysate flow, and duration of treatment. Fluid removal is achieved by altering hydrostatic pressure within the dialyzer. Vascular access may be either temporary or permanent via the femoral or internal jugular vessels. The subclavian route is discouraged to prevent stenosis in a patient that may require long-term access for RRT. The advantages of intermittent HD are the short treatment times and accurate fluid removal. A disadvantage is that intermittent HD is not tolerated in a hemodynamically unstable patient.

Continuous Renal Replacement Therapy. CRRT is a slow, gentle treatment that is given continuously for 24 hours per day. The principles of CRRT are similar to that of HD with the exception that hemofiltration, through convection, may be used to aid in solute removal. Hemofiltration refers to the use of replacement fluid that is given either pre- or post-filter. There are several available CRRT modalities. Continuous venovenous hemofiltration refers to the use of replacement fluid for convective clearance. Continuous venovenous hemodialysis is similar to the intermittent HD setup using dialysate fluid for diffusion clearance. Continuous venovenous hemodiafiltration uses a combination of dialysate and replacement fluid for effective diffusion and convection clearance of solutes. Used together, there is enhanced solute clearance. The advantages of CRRT are that it can be used in unstable patients, it allows for administration of large daily volumes (nutrition and blood products), and it has accurate fluid removal.

PROGNOSIS

Short-term Outcomes

AKI has consistently been identified as having an independent negative impact on patient outcomes in the PICU. Children, as well as adults, demonstrate a clear increase in mortality, duration of mechanical ventilation, ICU length of stay, and hospital length of stay in the presence of AKI (6,8,19,20,26). Having any degree of AKI at the time of PICU admission is associated with an odds ratio of 5.4 for mortality, which increases to 8.7 if AKI develops during the ICU stay (8). Further, as a validation of the newer standardized definitions, a stepwise increase in mortality and duration of mechanical ventilation occurs with worsening degrees of AKI (6,8,19,20,26). These negative associations with outcomes are consistently reported in general hospitalized populations, PICU populations, as well as all other specialized groups of patients when looked at individually. The paradigm of thinking of the kidney as an innocent bystander of other systemic illness or therapies must change. We now clearly understand that patients do not die with AKI; rather they die *because* of AKI.

Long-term Outcomes

There is limited data on long-term outcomes of children with AKI although there is a suggestion that AKI may increase the risk of developing chronic kidney disease (CKD). In adults, AKI is associated with an acceleration of development of CKD (120). Long-term follow-up of children with known risk for AKI such as childhood cancer survivors, bone marrow transplant recipients, and premature infants have demonstrated increased risk of CKD after long-term follow-up (121–123). One prospective study of children surviving episodes of AKI in the ICU showed that 10% of children developed CKD (defined as albuminuria or GFR <60 mL/min/1.73 m^2) 1–3 years after the AKI episode. In addition, nearly half of the patients were identified as at risk for CKD, defined as having GFR 60–90 mL/min/1.73 m^2, hyperfiltration, or hypertension (124). In another series, 12% (16/129) of children who survived hospitalization after AKI developed end-stage renal disease. In a small group of these children (29 children), 59% had either low GFR, hyperfiltration, microalbuminuria, or hypertension documented 3–5 years after the episode of AKI (125).

CONCLUSIONS

Acute Kidney Injury (AKI) is common in the pediatric intensive care unit and is a known independent risk factor for increased mortality and morbidity in critically ill children. The incidence of AKI has been on the rise due to increased use of intensive care and advanced technologies with the most common etiologies being sepsis, multiple organ dysfunction syndrome, cardiac surgery, and nephrotoxic medication. The development of standardized definitions for AKI has allowed us to improve upon the classification and epidemiology of AKI. Biomarkers such as NGAL may aid in early diagnosis and prevention. However, there are few preventive and therapeutic measures that have been proven to be successful. Treatment of AKI is largely supportive and includes optimizing renal perfusion through fluid management and avoidance of nephrotoxins.

FUTURE DIRECTIONS

With the introduction of standardized definitions of AKI, the true incidence and classification of AKI will be able to be more accurately characterized. Given all that is known about the morbidity and mortality associated with AKI, future research should focus on preventive and therapeutic strategies. The discovery of early biomarkers is opening up an exciting new era in the diagnosis of AKI. Hopefully, this advance in diagnostic markers will lead to an improvement in prevention and intervention for patients with AKI.

References

1. Bellomo R, Kellum J, Ronco C. Acute renal failure: Time for consensus. *Intensive Care Med* 2001;27:1685–8.
2. Bellomo R, Ronco C, Kellum JA, et al. Acute renal failure–Definition, outcome measures, animal models, fluid therapy and information technology needs: The Second International Consensus Conference of the Acute Dialysis Quality Initiative (ADQI) Group. *Crit Care* 2004;8:R204–12.
3. Ricci Z, Cruz D, Ronco C. The RIFLE criteria and mortality in acute kidney injury: A systematic review. *Kidney Int* 2008;73:538–46.
4. Thakar CV, Christianson A, Freyberg R, et al. Incidence and outcomes of acute kidney injury in intensive care units: A Veterans Administration study. *Crit Care Med* 2009;37:2552–8.
5. Uchino S, Bellomo R, Goldsmith D, et al. An assessment of the RIFLE criteria for acute renal failure in hospitalized patients. *Crit Care Med* 2006;34:1913–7.
6. Akcan-Arikan A, Zappitelli M, Loftis LL, et al. Modified RIFLE criteria in critically ill children with acute kidney injury. *Kidney Int* 2007;71:1028–35.
7. Plotz FB, Bouma AB, van Wijk JA, et al. Pediatric acute kidney injury in the ICU: An independent evaluation of pRIFLE criteria. *Intensive Care Med* 2008;34:1713–7.
8. Schneider J, Khemani R, Grushkin C, et al. Serum creatinine as stratified in the RIFLE score for acute kidney injury is associated with mortality and length of stay for children in the pediatric intensive care unit. *Crit Care Med* 2010;38:933–9.
9. Joannidis M, Metnitz B, Bauer P, et al. Acute kidney injury in critically ill patients classified by AKIN versus RIFLE using the SAPS 3 database. *Intensive Care Med* 2009;35:1692–702.
10. Mehta RL, Kellum JA, Shah SV, et al. Acute Kidney Injury Network: Report of an initiative to improve outcomes in acute kidney injury. *Crit Care* 2007;11:R31.
11. KDIGO AKI Work Group. KDIGO clinical practice guidelines for acute kidney injury. *Kidney Int Sup p l* 2012;2:1–138.
12. Vachvanichsanong P, Dissaneewate P, Lim A, et al. Childhood acute renal failure: 22-year experience in a university hospital in southern Thailand. *Pediatrics* 2006;118:e786–91.
13. Devarajan P. Pediatric acute kidney injury: Different from acute renal failure but how and why. *Curr Pediatr Rep* 2013;1:34–40.
14. Bailey D, Phan V, Litalien C, et al. Risk factors of acute renal failure in critically ill children: A prospective descriptive epidemiological study. *Pediatr Crit Care Med* 2007;8:29–35.
15. Medina Villanueva A L-HJ, Lopez Fernandez Y, et al. Acute renal failure in critically-ill children. A preliminary study. *An Pediatr* 2004;61:509–14.
16. Moffett BS, Goldstein SL. Acute kidney injury and increasing nephrotoxic-medication exposure in noncritically-ill children. *Clin J Am Soc Nephrol* 2011;6:856–63.
17. Sutherland SM, Ji J, Sheikhi FH, et al. AKI in hospitalized children: Epidemiology and clinical associations in a national cohort. *Clin J Am Soc Nephrol* 2013;8:1661–9.
18. Imani PD, Odiit A, Hingorani SR, et al. Acute kidney injury and its association with in-hospital mortality among children with acute infections. *Pediatr Nephrol* 2013;28:2199–206.
19. Alkandari O, Eddington KA, Hyder A, et al. Acute kidney injury is an independent risk factor for pediatric intensive care unit mortality, longer length of stay and prolonged mechanical ventilation in critically ill children: A two-center retrospective cohort study. *Crit Care* 2011;15:R146.
20. Bresolin N, Bianchini AP, Haas CA. Pediatric acute kidney injury assessed by pRIFLE as a prognostic factor in the intensive care unit. *Pediatr Nephrol* 2013;28:485–92.
21. Bresolin N, Silva C, Halllal A, et al. Prognosis for children with acute kidney injury in the intensive care unit. *Pediatr Nephrol* 2009;24:537–44.
22. Kavaz A, Ozcakar ZB, Kendirli T, et al. Acute kidney injury in a paediatric intensive care unit: Comparison of the pRIFLE and AKIN criteria. *Acta Paediatr* 2012;101:e126–9.
23. Prodhan P, McCage LS, Stroud MH, et al. Acute kidney injury is associated with increased in-hospital mortality in mechanically ventilated children with trauma. *J Trauma Acute Care Surg* 2012;73:832–7.
24. Zwiers AJ, de Wildt SN, Hop WC, et al. Acute kidney injury is a frequent complication in critically ill neonates receiving extracorporeal membrane oxygenation: A 14-year cohort study. *Crit Care* 2013;17:R151.
25. Palmieri T, Lavrentieva A, Greenhalgh D. An assessment of acute kidney injury with modified RIFLE criteria in pediatric patients with severe burns. *Intensive Care Med* 2009;35:2125–9.
26. Aydin SI, Seiden HS, Blaufox AD, et al. Acute kidney injury after surgery for congenital heart disease. *Ann Thorac Surg* 2012;94:1589–95.
27. Toth R, Breuer T, Cserep Z, et al. Acute kidney injury is associated with higher morbidity and resource utilization in pediatric patients undergoing heart surgery. *Ann Thorac Surg* 2012;93:1984–90.
28. Li S, Krawczeski CD, Zappitelli M, et al. Incidence, risk factors, and outcomes of acute kidney injury after pediatric cardiac surgery: A prospective multicenter study. *Crit Care Med* 2011;39:1493–9.
29. Ricci Z, Di Nardo M, Iacoella C, et al. Pediatric RIFLE for acute kidney injury diagnosis and prognosis for children undergoing cardiac surgery: A single-center prospective observational study. *Pediatr Cardiol* 2013;34:1404–8.
30. Hazar V, Gungor O, Guven AG, et al. Renal function after hematopoietic stem cell transplantation in children. *Pediatr Blood Cancer* 2009;53:197–202.
31. Satwani P, Bavishi S, Jin Z, et al. Risk factors associated with kidney injury and the impact of kidney injury on overall survival in pediatric recipients following allogeneic stem cell transplant. *Biol Blood Marrow Transplant* 2011;17:1472–80.
32. Anochie IC, Eke FU. Acute renal failure in Nigerian children: Port Harcourt experience. *Pediatr Nephrol* 2005;20:1610–4.
33. Duzova A, Bakkaloglu A, Kalyoncu M, et al. Etiology and outcome of acute kidney injury in children. *Pediatr Nephrol* 2010;25:1453–61.
34. Waikar SS, Curhan GC, Ayanian JZ, et al. Race and mortality after acute renal failure. *J Am Soc Nephrol* 2007;18:2740–8.
35. Goldstein SL. Overview of pediatric renal replacement therapy in acute renal failure. *Artif Organs* 2003;27:781–5.
36. Schwartz GJ, Haycock GB, Edelmann CM Jr, et al. A simple estimate of glomerular filtration rate in children derived from body length and plasma creatinine. *Pediatrics* 1976;58:259–63.
37. Brion LP, Fleischman AR, McCarton C, et al. A simple estimate of glomerular filtration rate in low birth weight infants during the first year of life: Noninvasive assessment of body composition and growth. *J Pediatr* 1986;109:698–707.
38. Schwartz GJ, Feld LG, Langford DJ. A simple estimate of glomerular filtration rate in full-term infants during the first year of life. *J Pediatr* 1984;104:849–54.
39. Schwartz GJ, Munoz A, Schneider MF, et al. New equations to estimate GFR in children with CKD. *J Am Soc Nephrol* 2009;20:629–37.

40. Bueva A, Guignard JP. Renal function in preterm neonates. *Pediatr Res* 1994;36:572–7.

41. Chevalier RL. Developmental renal physiology of the low birth weight pre-term newborn. *J Urol* 1996;156:714–9.

42. Ferguson MA, Waikar SS. Established and emerging markers of kidney function. *Clin Chem* 2012;58:680–9.

43. Melnikov VY, Ecder T, Fantuzzi G, et al. Impaired IL-18 processing protects caspase-1-deficient mice from ischemic acute renal failure. *J Clin Invest* 2001;107:1145–52.

44. Hsu CW, Symons JM. Acute kidney injury: Can we improve prognosis? *Pediatr Nephrol* 2010;25:2401–12.

45. *The Harriet Lane Handbook*. 19th ed. St. Louis, MO: Mosby; 2012. By Johns Hopkins Hospital, Kristin Arcara and Megan Tschudy, MD.

46. Laterza OF, Price CP, Scott MG. Cystatin C: An improved estimator of glomerular filtration rate? *Clin Chem* 2002;48:699–707.

47. Urbschat A, Obermuller N, Haferkamp A. Biomarkers of kidney injury. *Biomarkers*;16(suppl 1) 2011;S22–30.

48. Herget-Rosenthal S, Marggraf G, Husing J, et al. Early detection of acute renal failure by serum cystatin C. *Kidney Int* 2004;66:1115–22.

49. Villa P, Jimenez M, Soriano MC, et al. Serum cystatin C concentration as a marker of acute renal dysfunction in critically ill patients. *Crit Care* 2005;9:R139–43.

50. Burchard GD, Ehrhardt S, Mockenhaupt FP, et al. Renal dysfunction in children with uncomplicated, Plasmodium falciparum malaria in Tamale, Ghana. *Ann Trop Med Parasitol* 2003;97:345–50.

51. Vanmassenhove J, Vanholder R, Nagler E, et al. Urinary and serum biomarkers for the diagnosis of acute kidney injury: An in-depth review of the literature. *Nephrol Dial Transplant* 2013;28:254–73.

52. Schmidt-Ott KM, Mori K, Li JY, et al. Dual action of neutrophil gelatinase-associated lipocalin. *J Am Soc Nephrol* 2007;18:407–13.

53. Devarajan P. Neutrophil gelatinase-associated lipocalin (NGAL): A new marker of kidney disease. *Scand J Clin Lab Invest* 2008;241(suppl):89–94.

54. Haase M, Devarajan P, Haase-Fielitz A, et al. The outcome of neutrophil gelatinase-associated lipocalin-positive subclinical acute kidney injury: A multicenter pooled analysis of prospective studies. *J Am Coll Cardiol* 2011;57:1752–61.

55. Zappitelli M, Washburn KK, Arikan AA, et al. Urine neutrophil gelatinase-associated lipocalin is an early marker of acute kidney injury in critically ill children: A prospective cohort study. *Crit Care* 2007;11:R84.

56. Wheeler DS, Devarajan P, Ma Q, et al. Serum neutrophil gelatinase-associated lipocalin (NGAL) as a marker of acute kidney injury in critically ill children with septic shock. *Crit Care Med* 2008;36:1297–303.

57. Mishra J, Ma Q, Prada A, et al. Identification of neutrophil gelatinase-associated lipocalin as a novel early urinary biomarker for ischemic renal injury. *J Am Soc Nephrol* 2003;14:2534–43.

58. Han WK, Bailly V, Abichandani R, et al. Kidney Injury Molecule-1 (KIM-1): A novel biomarker for human renal proximal tubule injury. *Kidney Int* 2002;62:237–44.

59. Liangos O, Perianayagam MC, Vaidya VS, et al. Urinary N-acetyl-beta-(D)-glucosaminidase activity and kidney injury molecule-1 level are associated with adverse outcomes in acute renal failure. *J Am Soc Nephrol* 2007;18:904–12.

60. Han WK, Waikar SS, Johnson A, et al. Urinary biomarkers in the early diagnosis of acute kidney injury. *Kidney Int* 2008;73:863–9.

61. Portilla D, Dent C, Sugaya T, et al. Liver fatty acid-binding protein as a biomarker of acute kidney injury after cardiac surgery. *Kidney Int* 2008;73:465–72.

62. Doi K, Noiri E, Maeda-Mamiya R, et al. Urinary L-type fatty acid-binding protein as a new biomarker of sepsis complicated with acute kidney injury. *Crit Care Med*;38:2037–42.

63. Gibey R, Dupond JL, Alber D, et al. Predictive value of urinary N-acetyl-beta-D-glucosaminidase (NAG), alanine-aminopeptidase (AAP) and beta-2-microglobulin (beta 2M) in evaluating nephrotoxicity of gentamicin. *Clin Chim Acta* 1981;116:25–34.

64. Han WK, Wagener G, Zhu Y, et al. Urinary biomarkers in the early detection of acute kidney injury after cardiac surgery. *Clin J Am Soc Nephrol* 2009;4:873–82.

65. Devarajan P. Neutrophil gelatinase-associated lipocalin: A promising biomarker for human acute kidney injury. *Biomark Med*;4:265–80.

66. Hogg RJ, Portman RJ, Milliner D, et al. Evaluation and management of proteinuria and nephrotic syndrome in children: Recommendations from a pediatric nephrology panel established at the National Kidney Foundation conference on proteinuria, albuminuria, risk, assessment, detection, and elimination (PARADE). *Pediatrics* 2000;105:1242–9.

67. Abitbol C, Zilleruelo G, Freundlich M, et al. Quantitation of proteinuria with urinary protein/creatinine ratios and random testing with dipsticks in nephrotic children. *J Pediatr* 1990;116:243–7.

68. Miller TR, Anderson RJ, Linas SL, et al. Urinary diagnostic indices in acute renal failure: A prospective study. *Ann Intern Med* 1978;89:47–50.

69. Just A. Mechanisms of renal blood flow autoregulation: Dynamics and contributions. *Am J Physiol Regul Integr Comp Physiol* 2007;292:R1–17.

70. Kliegman RM BR, Jenson HB, et al. *Nelson Textbook of Pediatrics*. 18th ed. Philadelphia, PA: WB Saunders; 2007.

71. Rodriguez-Iturbe B, Musser JM. The current state of poststreptococcal glomerulonephritis. *J Am Soc Nephrol* 2008;19:1855–64.

72. Alabbas A, Campbell A, Skippen P, et al. Epidemiology of cardiac surgery-associated acute kidney injury in neonates: A retrospective study. *Pediatr Nephrol* 2013;28:1127–34.

73. Thadhani R, Pascual M, Bonventre JV. Acute renal failure. *N Engl J Med* 1996;334:1448–60.

74. Bellomo R, Wan L, Langenberg C, et al. Septic acute kidney injury: New concepts. *Nephron Exp Nephrol* 2008;109:e95–100.

75. Plotz FB, Hulst HE, Twisk JW, et al. Effect of acute renal failure on outcome in children with severe septic shock. *Pediatr Nephrol* 2005;20:1177–81.

76. Chang JW, Tsai HL, Wang HH, et al. Outcome and risk factors for mortality in children with acute renal failure. *Clin Nephrol* 2008;70:485–9.

77. Langenberg C, Wan L, Egi M, et al. Renal blood flow in experimental septic acute renal failure. *Kidney Int* 2006;69:1996–2002.

78. Gustot T. Multiple organ failure in sepsis: Prognosis and role of systemic inflammatory response. *Curr Opin Crit Care* 2011;17:153–9.

79. Uchino S, Kellum JA, Bellomo R, et al. Acute renal failure in critically ill patients: A multinational, multicenter study. *JAMA* 2005;294:813–8.

80. Hui-Stickle S, Brewer ED, Goldstein SL. Pediatric ARF epidemiology at a tertiary care center from 1999 to 2001. *Am J Kidney Dis* 2005;45:96–101.

81. Guo X, Nzerue C. How to prevent, recognize, and treat drug-induced nephrotoxicity. *Cleve Clin J Med* 2002;69:289–90, 93–4, 96–7; passim.

82. Brar SS, Hiremath S, Dangas G, et al. Sodium bicarbonate for the prevention of contrast induced-acute kidney injury: A systematic review and meta-analysis. *Clin J Am Soc Nephrol* 2009;4:1584–92.

83. Hoste EA, De Waele JJ, Gevaert SA, et al. Sodium bicarbonate for prevention of contrast-induced acute kidney injury: A systematic review and meta-analysis. *Nephrol Dial Transplant*;25:747–58.

84. Fishbane S. N-acetylcysteine in the prevention of contrast-induced nephropathy. *Clin J Am Soc Nephrol* 2008;3:281–7.

85. Perel P, Roberts I, Ker K. Colloids versus crystalloids for fluid resuscitation in critically ill patients. *Cochrane Database Syst Rev* 2013;2:CD000567.

86. Myburgh JA, Finfer S, Bellomo R, et al. Hydroxyethyl starch or saline for fluid resuscitation in intensive care. *N Engl J Med* 2012;367:1901–11.

87. Brunkhorst FM, Engel C, Bloos F, et al. Intensive insulin therapy and pentastarch resuscitation in severe sepsis. *N Engl J Med* 2008;358:125–39.

88. Finfer S, Bellomo R, Boyce N, et al. A comparison of albumin and saline for fluid resuscitation in the intensive care unit. *N Engl J Med* 2004;350:2247–56.

89. Rivers E, Nguyen B, Havstad S, et al. Early goal-directed therapy in the treatment of severe sepsis and septic shock. *N Engl J Med* 2001;345:1368–77.

90. Goldstein SL, Somers MJ, Baum MA, et al. Pediatric patients with multi-organ dysfunction syndrome receiving continuous renal replacement therapy. *Kidney Int* 2005;67:653–8.

91. Payen D, de Pont AC, Sakr Y, et al. A positive fluid balance is associated with a worse outcome in patients with acute renal failure. *Crit Care* 2008;12:R74.

92. Bellomo R, Cass A, Cole L, et al. An observational study fluid balance and patient outcomes in the Randomized Evaluation of Normal vs. Augmented Level of Replacement Therapy trial. *Crit Care Med* 2012;40:1753–60.

93. Holliday MA, Segar WE. The maintenance need for water in parenteral fluid therapy. *Pediatrics* 1957;19:823–32.

94. Hellerstein S. Fluid and electrolytes: Clinical aspects. *Pediatr Rev* 1993;14:103–15.

95. Brivet FG, Kleinknecht DJ, Loirat P, et al. Acute renal failure in intensive care units—causes, outcome, and prognostic factors of hospital mortality; a prospective, multicenter study. French Study Group on Acute Renal Failure. *Crit Care Med* 1996;24:192–8.

96. Frankel MC, Weinstein AM, Stenzel KH. Prognostic patterns in acute renal failure: The New York Hospital, 1981–1982. *Clin Exp Dial Apheresis* 1983;7:145–67.

97. Brater DC. Diuretic therapy. *N Engl J Med* 1998;339:387–95.

98. Cantarovich F, Rangoonwala B, Lorenz H, et al. High-dose furosemide for established ARF: A prospective, randomized, double-blind, placebo-controlled, multicenter trial. *Am J Kidney Dis* 2004;44:402–9.

99. Ho KM, Power BM. Benefits and risks of furosemide in acute kidney injury. *Anaesthesia* 2010;65:283–93.

100. Martin SJ, Danziger LH. Continuous infusion of loop diuretics in the critically ill: A review of the literature. *Crit Care Med* 1994;22:1323–9.

101. Luciani GB, Nichani S, Chang AC, et al. Continuous versus intermittent furosemide infusion in critically ill infants after open heart operations. *Ann Thorac Surg* 1997;64:1133–9.

102. Bellomo R, Chapman M, Finfer S, et al. Low-dose dopamine in patients with early renal dysfunction: A placebo-controlled randomised trial. Australian and New Zealand Intensive Care Society (ANZICS) Clinical Trials Group. *Lancet* 2000;356:2139–43.

103. Lauschke A, Teichgraber UK, Frei U, et al. 'Low-dose' dopamine worsens renal perfusion in patients with acute renal failure. *Kidney Int* 2006;69:1669–74.

104. Friedrich JO, Adhikari N, Herridge MS, et al. Meta-analysis: Low-dose dopamine increases urine output but does not prevent renal dysfunction or death. *Ann Intern Med* 2005;142:510–24.

105. Marik PE. Low-dose dopamine: A systematic review. *Intensive Care Med* 2002;28:877–83.

106. Palevsky PM, Liu KD, Brophy PD, et al. KDOQI US commentary on the 2012 KDIGO clinical practice guideline for acute kidney injury. *Am J Kidney Dis* 2013;61:649–72.

107. Brierley J, Carcillo JA, Choong K, et al. Clinical practice parameters for hemodynamic support of pediatric and neonatal septic shock: 2007 update from the American College of Critical Care Medicine. *Crit Care Med* 2009;37:666–88.

108. Landoni G, Biondi-Zoccai GG, Marino G, et al. Fenoldopam reduces the need for renal replacement therapy and in-hospital death in cardiovascular surgery: A meta-analysis. *J Cardiothorac Vasc Anesth* 2008;22:27–33.

109. Ricci Z, Stazi GV, Di Chiara L, et al. Fenoldopam in newborn patients undergoing cardiopulmonary bypass: Controlled clinical trial. *Interact Cardiovasc Thorac Surg* 2008;7:1049–53.

110. Bakr AF. Prophylactic theophylline to prevent renal dysfunction in newborns exposed to perinatal asphyxia—A study in a developing country. *Pediatr Nephrol* 2005;20:1249–52.

111. Bhat MA, Shah ZA, Makhdoomi MS, et al. Theophylline for renal function in term neonates with perinatal asphyxia: A randomized, placebo-controlled trial. *J Pediatr* 2006;149:180–4.

112. Thomas G, Rojas MC, Epstein SK, et al. Insulin therapy and acute kidney injury in critically ill patients a systematic review. *Nephrol Dial Transplant* 2007;22:2849–55.

113. Vlasselaers D, Milants I, Desmet L, et al. Intensive insulin therapy for patients in paediatric intensive care: A prospective, randomised controlled study. *Lancet* 2009;373:547–56.

114. Kyle UG, Akcan-Arikan A, Orellana RA, et al. Nutrition support among critically ill children with AKI. *Clin J Am Soc Nephrol* 2013;8:568–74.

115. Fiaccadori E, Lombardi M, Leonardi S, et al. Prevalence and clinical outcome associated with preexisting malnutrition in acute renal failure: A prospective cohort study. *J Am Soc Nephrol* 1999;10:581–93.

116. Wooley JA, Btaiche IF, Good KL. Metabolic and nutritional aspects of acute renal failure in critically ill patients requiring continuous renal replacement therapy. *Nutr Clin Pract* 2005;20:176–91.

117. Briassoulis G, Venkataraman S, Thompson AE. Energy expenditure in critically ill children. *Crit Care Med* 2000;28:1166–72.

118. Mehta NM, Compher C. A.S.P.E.N. Clinical Guidelines: Nutrition support of the critically ill child. *JPEN J Parenter Enteral Nutr* 2009;33:260–76.

119. Zappitelli M, Goldstein SL, Symons JM, et al. Protein and calorie prescription for children and young adults receiving continuous renal replacement therapy: A report from the Prospective Pediatric Continuous Renal Replacement Therapy Registry Group. *Crit Care Med* 2008;36:3239–45.

120. Hoste EA, Lameire NH, Vanholder RC, et al. Acute renal failure in patients with sepsis in a surgical ICU: Predictive factors, incidence, comorbidity, and outcome. *J Am Soc Nephrol* 2003;14:1022–30.

121. Hingorani S, Guthrie KA, Schoch G, et al. Chronic kidney disease in long-term survivors of hematopoietic cell transplant. *Bone Marrow Transplant* 2007;39:223–9.

122. Knijnenburg SL, Mulder RL, Schouten-Van Meeteren AY, et al. Early and late renal adverse effects after potentially nephrotoxic treatment for childhood cancer. *Cochrane Database Syst Rev* 2013;10:CD008944.

123. White SL, Perkovic V, Cass A, et al. Is low birth weight an antecedent of CKD in later life? A systematic review of observational studies. *Am J Kidney Dis* 2009;54:248–61.

124. Mammen C, Al Abbas A, Skippen P, et al. Long-term risk of CKD in children surviving episodes of acute kidney injury in the intensive care unit: A prospective cohort study. *Am J Kidney Dis* 2012;59:523–30.

125. Askenazi DJ, Feig DI, Graham NM, et al. 3–5 year longitudinal follow-up of pediatric patients after acute renal failure. *Kidney Int* 2006;69:184–9.

CHAPTER 111 ■ CHRONIC KIDNEY DISEASE, DIALYSIS, AND RENAL TRANSPLANTATION

VINAI MODEM, ROBERT P. WORONIECKI, AND FANGMING LIN

KEY POINTS

1 Chronic kidney disease (CKD) is defined as abnormalities of kidney structure or function, present for >3 months, with implications for health.

2 CKD affects multiple organ systems, and both the kidney and other organ system dysfunction can be more pronounced in critically ill children.

3 Renal replacement therapy is a crucial component of the ICU care for children with end-stage renal disease (ESRD). Treatment of ESRD with dialysis or kidney transplantation requires a collaborative effort between critical care physicians, nephrologist, and surgeons.

Chronic kidney disease (CKD) is a chronic, debilitating condition and has a significant impact on morbidity and mortality (1). The prevalence of and the costs for treating CKD in and out of the pediatric ICU have increased steadily over the past few decades. In this chapter, we will focus on the diagnosis and basic management of CKD for critically ill children in the ICU.

DEFINITION AND RISK FACTORS FOR DEVELOPING CKD

CKD can be diagnosed when there are pathologic abnormalities or markers of kidney damage such as persistent albuminuria (an indicator of ongoing renal injury), or reduced glomerular filtration rate (GFR) <60 mL/min/1.73 m² for ≥3 months (2). Chronic kidney condition is classified into five stages on the basis of the estimated GFR (Table 111.1). End-stage renal disease (ESRD) typically refers to stages IV and V, which require renal replacement therapy (RRT) in the form of either chronic dialysis or renal transplantation. Acute kidney injury (AKI) can become CKD when renal injury and dysfunction persist for >3 months. CKD staging can be used for adults and children at 2 years of age or older.

The prevalence of all stages of CKD has been increasing worldwide (3). In particular, the prevalence of pediatric (0–19 years) ESRD has increased by 32% since 1990. CKD is associated with various comorbidities which could affect ICU outcomes (4). Children with oncologic disease, hematopoietic stem cell transplantation, solid organ transplantation, congenital heart disease, and rheumatologic diseases are at a greater risk for developing CKD. Additional factors contribute to CKD and include repeated insults to the kidney from septic episodes, low cardiac output, and the use of nephrotoxic medications (antibiotics, chemotherapy, and immunosuppressive agents) (5). Patients can also have primary renal disease that progresses to CKD. Common causes of primary renal disease in children include congenital anomalies of the kidney and urinary tract such as aplastic or hypodysplastic

kidneys, obstructive uropathy (e.g., posterior urethral valves), and reflux nephropathy. Tubular disease (e.g., nephronophthisis and polycystic kidney disease), glomerular disease due to focal segmental glomerulosclerosis (FSGS), and vasculitis (e.g., lupus nephritis) also contribute to the development of CKD.

CHRONIC KIDNEY DISEASE IN PATIENTS WITH CRITICAL ILLNESS

2 Renal dysfunction affects multiple organ systems (Fig. 111.1). The extent and severity of involvement depends on the etiology and stage of CKD (6). CKD stages I and II usually show evidence of renal injury and may have clinical manifestations of proteinuria and hypertension. The primary goal of CKD management for these stages is to prevent the progression by reducing proteinuria and controlling hypertension typically with angiotensin-converting enzyme inhibitors (ACEIs) and angiotensin receptor blockers (ARBs), which offer renal protection. As renal function deteriorates to stages III, IV, and V, patients will have multiple manifestations involving various organ systems (Fig. 111.1). In addition to slowing down renal disease progression, it is imperative to address these complications. Management focuses on the treatment of electrolyte and acid–base disturbances, anemia, hyperparathyroidism, malnutrition, and behavioral and psychological disorders.

AKI on CKD

Normal kidneys have a significant functional reserve (Fig. 111.2). This reserve is primarily due to hyperfiltration at the level of individual nephrons. If the number of functional nephrons is reduced, this reserve is decreased. The reduction in the functional reserve is proportional to the severity of CKD (7,8). Chronic hyperfiltration can be associated with

TABLE 111.1

CHRONIC KIDNEY DISEASE STAGING

CKD STAGE	ESTIMATED GFR	CLINICAL IMPACT
Stage I	≥90 mL/min/1.73 m² With evidence of renal injury (albuminuria)	Decreased renal reserve; Risk of CKD progression
Stage II	60–89 mL/min/1.73 m² With evidence of renal injury (albuminuria)	Decreased renal reserve; Risk of CKD progression
Stage III	30–59 mL/min/1.73 m²	Decreased renal reserve; Risk of CKD progression; CKD Complications
Stage IV	15–29 mL/min/1.73 m²	Decreased renal reserve; Risk of CKD progression; CKD Complications; Need for RRT
Stage V	<15 mL/min/1.73 m² (or dialysis)	Decreased renal reserve; Risk of CKD progression; CKD Complications; Need for RRT

hypertension and diabetes and can result in glomerular sclerosis and further loss of nephrons. The CKD kidneys may already be functioning at their maximal capacity. As a result, even mild insults to the kidneys can cause significant deterioration in GFR. Hence, these patients need special attention toward renal protective and supportive care during critical illness (9,10). Frequency and severity of AKI (i.e., need for RRT) increase the risk of CKD progression.

Impact of CKD on the Cardiovascular System

CKD can lead to cardiovascular pathology, including hypertension, vascular wall stiffness, cardiomyopathy, and valvular heart disease (11). These conditions increase the risk of developing congestive heart failure and other cardiac events (dysrhythmias). Vascular complications of hypertension such as posterior-reversible encephalopathy syndrome (PRES) (also called reversible posterior leukoencephalopathy syndrome—RPLS) can occur. In addition to hypertension, uremia, vasculitis, immunosuppressant use, and organ transplant are risk factors for PRES/RPLS that may be seen with CKD or AKI (see also Chapter 64). Rigorous attention to fluid and blood pressure management is essential in children with cardiovascular involvement. Fluid requirements depend on the etiology and severity of CKD. Patients with obstructive uropathy and tubulopathy typically have increased urine output due to concentrating defects. In contrast, patients with hypoplastic/dysplastic kidneys and glomerulopathies are frequently oligoanuric and are at risk for developing fluid overload. Delaying supportive care such as RRTs may adversely affect outcomes in these children.

Vascular access is another important issue that needs a judicious approach in patients with CKD. As the CKD progresses, patients may need an arteriovenous fistula, arteriovenous graft, or dialysis catheter for hemodialysis (HD). Peripherally inserted central catheters (PICCs) have a high rate of venous thrombosis and stenosis limiting the vascular access options (12,13). There is an increased risk of dialysis catheter-related infection as well with prior history of a PICC. Subclavian lines can lead to similar complications such as thrombosis and stenosis, rendering the vasculature on that arm unsuitable for dialysis access.

Hematological and Immune Responses in CKD

Many patients with CKD have anemia, requiring the use of erythropoiesis-stimulating agents (ESAs). During critical illness, there is increased red cell destruction and blood loss. In addition, systemic inflammation increases the resistance to ESAs (14). Therefore, severe anemia may develop in critically ill patients with preexisting CKD. Although blood transfusions may be an easy temporary fix, a conservative approach is warranted. Repeated blood transfusions increase the risk of developing anti-human leukocyte antigen (HLA) antibodies, leading to difficulty in matching with future kidney donors. Every effort should be made to minimize iatrogenic blood loss and blood transfusions.

There are no firm guidelines for the use of ESAs in children with CKD and their use should be individualized. The clinical practice recommendation is to start either recombinant human erythropoietin or darbepoietin alfa plus iron supplementation, if the child's hemoglobin is ≤10 g/dL or the child is symptomatic (e.g., fatigue, cognitive problems, left ventricular hypertrophy) with hemoglobin ≤5th percentile for age. The target hemoglobin range is 11–12 g/dL. Because studies in adults have suggested an increased mortality in CKD patients with hemoglobin >13 g/dL, ESA and iron therapy should be adjusted if hemoglobin >12 g/dL.

Uremia can cause platelet dysfunction, which increases the risk of bleeding. In such patients, desmopressin (dDAVP, usual dose 0.3 μg/kg, intravenously) can be given 30 minutes prior to invasive procedures to promote clotting by stimulating endothelial release of von Willebrand factor multimers. Desmopressin's rapid onset and relative safety make it the preferred approach to lower the bleeding time in uremic patients. Maintaining a normal hemoglobin also lowers the bleeding time, which offers another justification for chronic iron supplementation and ESAs. Prophylactic red cell transfusion simply to lower the bleeding time is discouraged because of the risk of allosensitization, which would complicate a future renal transplantation. Rather, red cell transfusion should be reserved for the patient who is acutely bleeding. Unfortunately, tachyphylaxis usually develops after the second dose of desmopressin. Therefore, alternative therapies to manage platelet dysfunction may be needed, including dialysis, estrogens, or cryoprecipitate.

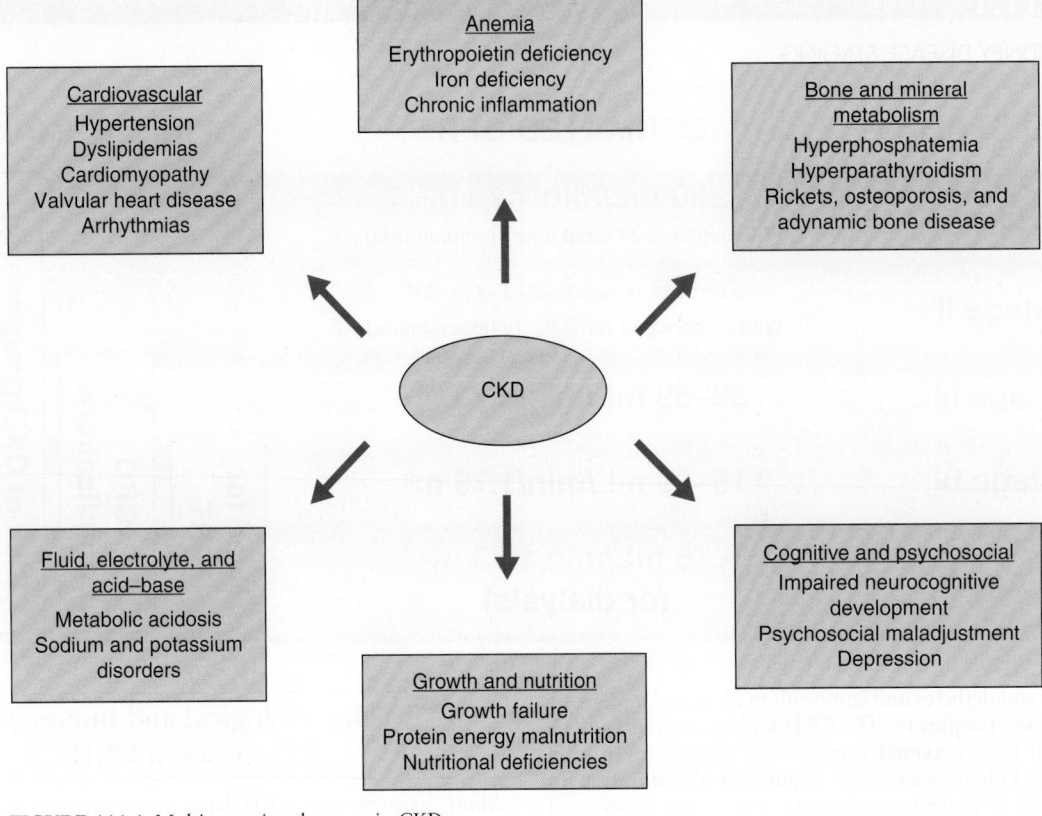

FIGURE 111.1 Multiorgan involvement in CKD.

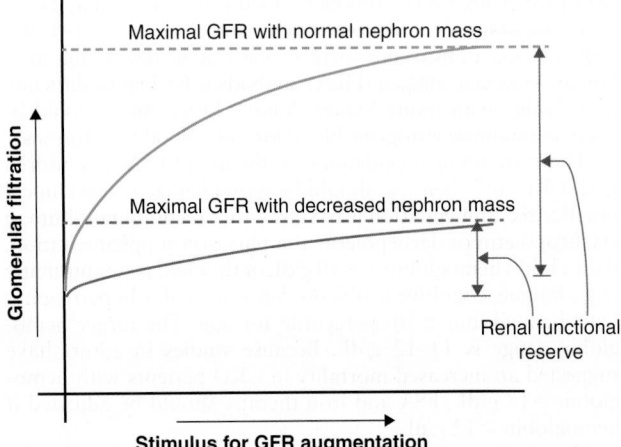

FIGURE 111.2 Renal functional reserve using protein loading as an example. Protein loading, which stimulates hyperfiltration to augment GFR, can be used to assess renal functional reserve. At least a 20% increase in GFR after protein loading is considered normal. The maximal attainable GFR and hence renal reserve decreases in proportion to the reduction in nephron mass. Patients with reduced nephron mass demonstrate lower maximal GFR (*red curve*) compared with subjects with normal nephron mass (*green curve*).

Chronic inflammation and immune dysregulation are frequently seen in CKD (15). The innate immune system is chronically activated, leading to hypercytokinemia and increased levels of acute phase reactants such as C-reactive protein. Markers of chronic inflammation have been linked to complications of CKD and associated with mortality in patients with CKD. On the other hand, adaptive immunity is impaired with poor response to infections. Various factors such as uremic toxins, recurrent endotoxemia, and vitamin D deficiency have all been implicated in the pathogenesis of immune dysregulation in CKD. Both chronic inflammation and impaired adaptive immunity adversely affect the patient's response to critical illness. The presence of indwelling catheters and bacterial and fungal colonization further increases the risk of catheter-related infections.

UNIQUE CHALLENGES IN CHILDREN WITH ESRD

Children with ESRD require chronic dialysis or kidney transplantation. Common reasons for these patients to require ICU care include severe fluid overload, hypertensive crises, severe electrolyte imbalances (hyperkalemia), uremia and its complications, and catheter-related sepsis. Some of the unique challenges in their management are discussed here (16).

Differentiating ESRD from AKI

Previously unrecognized ESRD can present with uremia and its complications. When there is no history of kidney disease, the first step is to distinguish ESRD from AKI. The presence of features of CKD such as anemia, growth failure, and hyperparathyroidism are helpful in this regard. Renal sonogram is very informative in identifying small, echogenic end-stage kidneys and underlying structural abnormalities. In most cases of ESRD, the utility of renal biopsy to identify the underlying causes is limited because end-stage kidneys usually show non-specific changes such as sclerotic glomeruli, atrophic tubules, and fibrotic interstitium. In contrast, an urgent renal biopsy may be essential in some children with AKI, both from diagnostic as well as management perspective.

Fluid Overload

Fluid overload can present as systemic and pulmonary vascular congestion leading to congestive heart failure and hypertension. Very often, the excess of fluid is not obvious during a physical exam but can be detected as weight gain. Patients respond well to aggressive fluid removal. Most patients with chronic dialysis have an estimated "dry weight," and the goal for fluid removal is to reach this weight. However, if they continue to be hypertensive despite reaching the goal, their dry weight needs to be challenged by removing more fluid until symptoms have improved and a new dry weight is established.

Infection of Vascular Access and Peritonitis

Vascular access is the primary site of infection in HD patients. Non-tunneled temporary catheters are at the highest risk for infection followed by tunneled catheters and arteriovenous grafts. Arteriovenous fistulas are the least likely to get infected. Infection could occur at the exit site, in the subcutaneous tunnel, or in the catheter itself. Gram-positive bacteria (e.g., methicillin-resistant *Staphylococcus aureus* [MRSA]) account for the majority of infections. Initial broad-spectrum antibiotic coverage depends on local resistance patterns. Vancomycin for Gram-positive bacteria and aminoglycosides for Gram-negative bacteria are common initial choices. The advantage of these antibiotics is that a single dose will maintain adequate blood concentration through the entire interdialytic period because renal failure limits their excretion. However, one should be mindful about the renal toxicity of aminoglycosides in patients who still have residual renal function. Recurrent infections and multidrug-resistant organisms may require a longer course of antibiotics or even removal of the catheter; however, this measure must be balanced against losing vascular access for dialysis. Catheter-related infections can lead to long-term issues such as vascular stenosis and thrombosis. Some of the preventive approaches to minimizing infections include avoidance of catheters with "Fistula First" initiative; treating MRSA carriers; minimizing access of the catheter for non-dialysis purpose (e.g., blood draws); and using thrombolytics (e.g., tPA), antibiotic, or citrate locks for the catheter.

Similarly, peritoneal dialysis (PD) catheter-related infections occur at the exit site, at the subcutaneous tunnel, or in the catheter itself. These can lead to life-threatening peritonitis and sepsis. Infection with Gram-positive bacteria is the most common. Contamination due to system break during initiation or termination of dialysis is a common source of these bacteria. Peritonitis can be treated with intraperitoneal antibiotics (17). Initial empiric regimen includes both cefazolin for Gram-positive bacteria and ceftazidime for Gram-negative bacteria, including pseudomonas. Other antibiotics that can be used intraperitoneally include vancomycin, aminoglycosides, carbapenems, and fluroquinolones. One needs to be aware of the significant systemic absorption of antibiotics instilled into the peritoneum. Patients with multiple and prolonged antibiotic courses may develop fungal peritonitis due to changes in the microbiome. The risk of fungal peritonitis is particularly high in patients who are malnourished and hypoalbuminemic. Fungal peritonitis, recurrent peritonitis by the same organism, and peritonitis with multidrug-resistant organisms are indications for catheter removal. These patients may need HD for a period of time until the peritoneum is cleared of infection. Repeated episodes of peritonitis can damage the peritoneum and lead to inadequate PD.

DIALYSIS AS A RENAL REPLACEMENT THERAPY

The primary goal of dialysis is to remove metabolic wastes (solute clearance) and fluid. Solute removal is measured in terms of clearance, which is defined as the volume of blood cleared in a unit time. Fluid removal is referred to as ultrafiltration. There are two dialysis modalities, HD and PD, based on the semipermeable membrane used. The choice of using HD versus PD is influenced by multiple factors such as patient condition, family preferences, institutional and family resources, dialysis goals, and the specific advantages or disadvantages of each modality (18).

Hemodialysis

HD uses an artificial semipermeable membrane (holofiber dialysis filter) for solute and water transport and requires an extracorporeal circuit. Blood flows inside the holofibers and dialysate flows outside the holofibers in a countercurrent fashion (see Chapter 41). Solute clearance occurs by diffusion driven by a concentration gradient between the blood and dialysate. The rate of diffusion depends on the size of solute molecules, concentration gradient, and surface area of the filter membrane. Hence, small molecules with larger concentration gradient are cleared faster. Blood flow rate, dialysate flow rate, surface area of the filter, and duration of HD session can be adjusted to achieve the goal clearance. The amount of fluid removed or ultrafiltration is controlled by adjusting the transmembrane pressure gradient across the dialysis membrane. The main advantage of HD is the rapid clearance of solutes and removal of fluid. But the extracorporeal volume and high blood flow rates can potentially cause hemodynamic instability. Infants and unstable patients may need priming of the extracorporeal circuit with blood. Dialysis disequilibrium syndrome, which manifests with neurologic symptoms resulting from cerebral edema, could occur if clearance is rapid, especially on the first dialysis treatment (19). Therefore, it is advised that first dialysis provide no more than 25% urea reduction rate in a uremic patient. In CKD, the large urea (or other organic compound) gradient in the brain may pull fluid in and cause cerebral edema. The needs for vascular access, systemic anticoagulation, specialized equipment, and trained personnel are other considerations in determining whether to proceed with HD.

Thrombus, kinking of the catheter or cracks in the catheter are the common causes of catheter malfunction. Life-threatening blood loss and embolic phenomena are rare but could occur. An x-ray with IV contrast usually helps with identifying some of these problems. Thrombolytic agents (e.g., tPA) usually help with clearing the clots. Occasionally, stripping of the fibrin sheath around and at the tip of the catheter may need to be performed by interventional radiologists. Similarly, thrombotic complications can occur with arteriovenous grafts and fistulas.

Peritoneal Dialysis

The peritoneal membrane is a semipermeable membrane made of mesothelial cells and capillaries of peritoneal cavity, across which water and solute transport occurs in PD. Water clearance occurs with ultrafiltration and is driven by an osmotic gradient. Solute clearance occurs primarily by diffusion and to a much less extent by ultrafiltration (convective clearance) when small molecules move along with the water, called solvent drag. Dwell volume is the amount of dialysate instilled with each cycle and dwell time is the duration for which the dialysate is left in the peritoneal cavity before draining. The rate of solute clearance depends on dwell volume, dwell time, number of cycles, and the characteristics of peritoneal membrane. The rate of water clearance depends on the concentration of the osmotic agent. The PD dialysate fluid typically consists of electrolytes (Na, Mg, Ca, and Cl), buffer (lactate), and an osmotic agent (e.g., dextrose, icodextrin). The concentration of osmotic agent (e.g., 1.5%–4.25% dextrose) can be adjusted to increase or decrease the rate of ultrafiltration. Additives such as heparin (used to prevent fibrin clots, especially in a new PD catheter or during peritonitis), bicarbonate (small amount to adjust the pH of dialysate and provide comfort to the patient), antibiotics, and electrolytes (e.g., potassium) can be added to the dialysate when needed.

PD has a role in acute setting in selected patients (20). One of its major advantages is that it could be performed continuously. In fact it is considered a type of continuous RRT. It is better tolerated than intermittent HD in smaller infants and patients with hemodynamic instability. Technical simplicity, no requirement for systemic anticoagulation and lower cost are other benefits. But, it does require a PD catheter placement and an accessible and functional peritoneum. The dialysis dose will be low with small dwell volumes before the catheter site is completely healed to reduce the risk of leakage and infection.

Inadequate clearance and fluid retention are common problems associated with PD. These can occur in patients with constipation or when the tip of the PD catheter is malpositioned or occluded. An abdominal x-ray is helpful in confirming proper position of the catheter tip as well as evaluating for constipation. In patients with respiratory distress or failure, the abdominal distension from instilling the dialysate can worsen the respiratory symptoms. Also, if the intra-abdominal pressure is greater than 18 cm H_2O, ultrafiltration can occur in the reverse direction with water moving from peritoneal space to intravascular space, resulting in fluid retention (21). Dextrose used as the osmotic agent will be absorbed systemically over time and can lead to hyperglycemia. Hemodynamic instability could occur if there is an excessive fluid loss from dialysis. Therefore, patients need to be monitored for potential complications associated with PD.

RENAL TRANSPLANTATION

Renal transplantation is a form of RRT (22). Patients undergo extensive work-up prior to transplantation. Some patients may require special preparations such as removal of native kidneys (e.g., recurrent UTIs, severe nephrotic syndrome), urologic surgery (e.g., bladder augmentation), and desensitization procedures (e.g., plasmapheresis, immunosuppression). Management around the time of transplant is crucial for kidney graft survival and requires collaboration between transplant surgeons, nephrologists, and critical care physicians.

Surgical and Anesthetic Management

Adequate hydration and stable hemodynamic status of the patient is essential before transplant surgery. In children, a disproportionately large adult donor kidney can take up more than 20% of the cardiac output, necessitating appropriate increase in the patient's cardiac output immediately after the donor kidney is connected. Adequate fluid resuscitation and continued vigilance to maintain effective circulating volume is the key. Some children may require vasopressor support such as dopamine to maintain adequate mean arterial pressure for perfusion of the kidney graft.

Methods for kidney placement largely depend on the size of the patient. Younger children (usually <15 kg) require a transperitoneal approach with a large midline incision and intra-abdominal placement of the kidney graft. Older children (usually >15 kg) could take an extraperitoneal approach in the lower abdomen. Renal vessels are anastomosed with abdominal aorta and inferior vena cava when the kidney is placed intra-abdominally and with iliac vessels when the kidney is placed in the lower abdomen. The donor ureter is implanted into recipient's bladder. With adequate perfusion, the kidney graft will produce urine immediately after vascular anastomosis. The donor kidney undergoes warm and cold ischemia prior to anastomosis with the recipient vessels. Warm ischemia starts when blood supply is interrupted at the time of harvesting to the time the kidney is perfused with cold preservation solution. Cold ischemia time refers to the duration of perfusion with cold preservation solution to anastomosis with recipient vessels. Prolonged warm and cold ischemia times, especially >24 hours, increase the risk of delayed graft function largely due to acute tubular necrosis (ATN). Every effort is made to reduce the ischemic time by the transplant team.

Respiratory Management

The majority of patients are extubated in the recovery room or soon after arriving in the ICU. Fluid overload is one of the main reasons causing delays in extubation. Most of these children have been given a large amount of fluid during the perioperative period while urine output has not increased enough to excrete excess amount of fluid. The patient may develop pulmonary edema with fluid overload. This is especially an issue in patients with underlying cardiopulmonary compromise from CKD.

Hemodynamic and Fluid Management

The primary goal for post-transplant management in the ICU is to ensure adequate perfusion of the new graft. Kidney injury resulting from warm and cold ischemia prior to transplantation as well as lack of intact renal innervation affects autoregulation. As a result, renal blood flow in the graft is blood pressure dependent. Also, as most transplanted kidneys come from adult donors, these require higher mean arterial pressure for perfusion. Hence, blood pressure is monitored very closely during this period. Goal blood pressures vary from patient to patient. Adequate effective circulating volume is essential such that the central venous pressure should be maintained around 8–10 mm Hg. Vasopressors such as dopamine may be needed as well, to maintain adequate blood pressure.

Fluid requirement for the initial 24 hours after transplantation depends on the patient's urine output and hemodynamic status. Typically, patients are placed on a constant rate of dextrose-containing fluids to prevent hypoglycemia and replenish insensible losses. In addition, they receive hourly urine replacement at a 1:1 ratio with 0.45% NaCl. Some patients may have exceedingly high urine output (>500 mL/h), and their urine replacement can be capped off at a maximal rate to prevent fluid overload and stop driving high urine output. After 24–48 hours, if patients continue to have good urine output and show improvement in renal function, urine replacement can be discontinued. The patients can be placed on a constant fluid rate to match the insensible, urinary, and other fluid losses. Electrolytes need to be monitored closely. Patients may develop hypomagnesaemia and hypophosphatemia requiring supplementation. Hypophosphatemia can be a significant problem in patients with very elevated parathyroid hormone levels prior to transplantation. Calcitriol will be helpful to suppress parathyroid function and increase gastrointestinal absorption of phosphate.

Monitoring Renal Function

Urine output and renal clearance are closely monitored. Urine output is a combination of urine produced by the transplanted kidney and patient's native kidneys if present. The transplanted kidney frequently lacks concentrating ability due to ATN, leading to polyuria. Decreased urine output, especially of sudden onset, should be investigated promptly. First, adequate blood pressure and intravascular volume should be ensured. The Foley catheter must be examined for patency since blood clots and debris from the bladder can cause obstruction, which can be cleared by gentle flushing with saline. Some patients have stents placed at the ureterovesical anastomosis, which can potentially dislodge and cause obstruction. Other causes of urinary obstruction include lymphocele and kinking of the ureter. Urinary leak from the anastomotic site or bladder rupture (occurs rarely) can also lead to low urine output. This can result in urinary ascites or urinoma, both of which can be detected by sonogram and require surgical repair. If the patient continues to have poor urine output despite adequate hemodynamic status and lack of urine flow obstruction, an urgent renal sonogram with Doppler flow study is required to assess renal blood flow and vascular anastomoses. Thrombosis of the vascular anastomotic site is a serious complication and can result in graft loss. Small children and those with hypercoagulability (e.g., nephrotic syndrome) are at higher risk for thrombosis. Other important causes of poor urine output and graft dysfunction are acute rejection and recurrence of primary disease (e.g., FSGS, atypical hemolytic uremic syndrome), which might need a renal biopsy to confirm the diagnosis.

Pain Management

Good pain control is an important goal of ICU management. It is usually achieved with an opioid and acetaminophen. However, one needs to be aware of impaired clearance of opioids and accumulation of their active metabolites with renal failure. Before allograft function is established, it is advised to use lower doses at reduced frequency. All patients on opioids should be closely monitored for adverse effects. Patients who receive epidural anesthetic and analgesic infusions for pain control are at risk for vasodilation, especially in the lower extremities, which may lead to hypotension necessitating vasopressor support.

Immunosuppression

Immunosuppression is given to prevent rejection of the transplanted kidney. Induction of immunosuppression is initiated in the operating room. The regimen used depends on the risk profile of the patient and on whether the graft is obtained from a living or deceased donor. Common immunosuppressive agents include lymphocyte-depleting agents (polyclonal and monoclonal antibodies, IL-2 receptor antagonists), calcineurin inhibitors (tacrolimus, cyclosporine A), antiproliferative agents (mycophenolate), and corticosteroids. Acute rejection can occur in the immediate postoperative period. It requires a biopsy for diagnosis and needs to be treated immediately to prevent loss of the graft. Patients with immunosuppression are at risk for infections and need prophylaxis. In the immediate postoperative period, most patients receive antibacterial prophylaxis with cephalosporin. They require cytomegalovirus prophylaxis with ganciclovir, PCP prophylaxis with bactrim, and candida prophylaxis with nystatin or fluconazole for an extended period of time.

Other Postoperative Issues

Anemia, hypertension, and nutrition need to be addressed as well in the postoperative period. The goal with anemia management is to minimize blood transfusions. Repeated transfusions can lead to sensitization to future donors. Some patients may require reinitiation of ESAs. Acute decrease in hemoglobin during the postoperative period can result from hemorrhage, which requires immediate surgical attention. Hypertension can be caused by fluid overload, inadequate pain control, or rebound effect of coming off antihypertensive medications. Depending on the etiology, hypertension can be managed with diuretics (in case of fluid overload), calcium channel blockers, and clonidine. ACEIs and ARBs, which reduce glomerular filtration in the graft, are avoided. Finally, diet is an important aspect of managing a patient with kidney disease. Prior to transplant, patients with ESRD are on Na-, K-, and phosphorus-restricted diet. After transplant, they no longer need these restrictions. Most of them require phosphorus and magnesium supplements. Patients are also at risk for developing glucose intolerance and hyperglycemia from immunosuppressive medications (e.g., tacrolimus, prednisone). It is advised that patients avoid concentrated sweets and reduce carbohydrate intake.

In summary, the prevalence of CKD is increasing in children. CKD presents with unique challenges in ICU management. A multidisciplinary team approach is required to manage the critically ill children with CKD.

References

1. Harambat J, van Stralen KJ, Kim JJ, et al. Epidemiology of chronic kidney disease in children. *Pediatr Nephrol* 2012;27(3):363–73.
2. National Kidney Foundation. K/DOQI clinical practice guidelines for chronic kidney disease: Evaluation, classification, and stratification. *Am J Kidney Dis* 2002;39(2 suppl 1):S1–266.
3. USRDS. Pediatric ESRD. In: NIDDKD, eds. *USRDS 2012 Annual Data Report: Atlas of Chronic Kidney Disease and End-Stage Renal Disease in the United States.* Bethesda, MD: National Institutes of Health, 2012.
4. Wong CJ, Moxey-Mims M, Jerry-Fluker J, et al. CKiD (CKD in children) prospective cohort study: A review of current findings. *Am J Kidney Dis* 2012;60(6):1002–11.
5. Singh N, McNeely J, Parikh S, et al. Kidney complications of hematopoietic stem cell transplantation. *Am J Kidney Dis* 2013;61(5): 809–21.
6. Quigley R. Chronic kidney disease: Highlights for the general pediatrician. *Int J Pediatr* 2012;2012:943904.

7. Bosch JP, Lew S, Glabman S, et al. Renal hemodynamic changes in humans. Response to protein loading in normal and diseased kidneys. *Am J Med* 1986;81(5):809–15.

8. Barai S, Gambhir S, Prasad N, et al. Functional renal reserve capacity in different stages of chronic kidney disease. *Nephrology (Carlton)* 2010;15(3):350–3.

9. Leung KC, Tonelli M, James MT. Chronic kidney disease following acute kidney injury-risk and outcomes. *Nat Rev Nephrol* 2013;9(2):77–85.

10. Yang L, Humphreys BD, Bonventre JV. Pathophysiology of acute kidney injury to chronic kidney disease: Maladaptive repair. *Contrib Nephrol* 2011;174:149–55.

11. Hruska KA, Choi ET, Memon I, et al. Cardiovascular risk in chronic kidney disease (CKD): The CKD-mineral bone disorder (CKD-MBD). *Pediatr Nephrol* 2010;25(4):769–78.

12. Agarwal AK. Central vein stenosis: Current concepts. *Adv Chronic Kidney Dis* 2009;16(5):360–70.

13. Gonsalves CF, Eschelman DJ, Sullivan KL, et al. Incidence of central vein stenosis and occlusion following upper extremity PICC and port placement. *Cardiovasc Intervent Radiol* 2003;26(2):123–7.

14. Prakash D. Anemia in the ICU: Anemia of chronic disease versus anemia of acute illness. *Crit Care Clin* 2012;28(3):333–43, v.

15. Cohen G, Horl WH. Immune dysfunction in uremia—an update. *Toxins (Basel)* 2012;4(11):962–90.

16. Szamosfalvi B, Yee J. Considerations in the critically ill ESRD patient. *Adv Chronic Kidney Dis* 2013;20(1):102–9.

17. Warady BA, et al. Consensus guidelines for the prevention and treatment of catheter-related infections and peritonitis in pediatric patients receiving peritoneal dialysis: 2012 update. *Perit Dial Int* 2012;32(suppl 2):S32–86.

18. Walters S, Porter C, Brophy PD. Dialysis and pediatric acute kidney injury: Choice of renal support modality. *Pediatr Nephrol* 2009;24(1):37–48.

19. Zepeda-Orozco D, Quigley R. Dialysis disequilibrium syndrome. *Pediatr Nephrol* 2012;27(12):2205–11.

20. Warady BA. Paediatrics: Peritoneal dialysis for AKI—Time may be of the essence. *Nat Rev Nephrol* 2012;8(9):498–500.

21. Fischbach M, et al. Measurement of hydrostatic intraperitoneal pressure: A useful tool for the improvement of dialysis dose prescription. *Pediatr Nephrol* 2003;18(10):976–80.

22. Salvatierra O Jr, Millan M, Concepcion W. Pediatric renal transplantation with considerations for successful outcomes. *Semin Pediatr Surg* 2006;15(3):208–17.

CHAPTER 112 ■ HYPERTENSIVE CRISIS

GEORGE OFORI-AMANFO, ARTHUR SMERLING, AND CHARLES SCHLEIEN

KEY POINTS

❶ Hypertensive crisis is characterized by severe hypertension associated with end-organ damage (hypertensive emergency) or impending end-organ damage (hypertensive urgency).

❷ Hypertensive crisis can develop either de novo or as a complication of preexisting essential or secondary hypertension. Any disorder that causes hypertension can give rise to a hypertensive crisis.

❸ Hypertensive crisis is a rapid onset, acute disease and therefore a trigger factor may be implicated in its pathogenesis; these include neurohormonal factors such as the renin–angiotensin system, endothelin, vasopressin, and catecholamines.

❹ The endothelium in resistance vessels plays a central role in blood pressure (BP) homeostasis, as it attempts to compensate for changes in vascular resistance through increased autocrine and paracrine release of vasodilator molecules, such as nitric oxide and prostacyclin.

❺ In sustained severe hypertension, these compensatory endothelium-mediated vasodilator responses are overwhelmed, which leads to endothelial decompensation, endothelial failure, and vasoconstriction.

❻ Clinical manifestations consist of features related to hypertension and those related to target organ injury. The absolute BP is often not as important as the rate of elevation. Acute elevations in BP are less well tolerated and more likely to produce symptoms than are chronic elevations.

❼ Clinical distinction between hypertensive emergency and hypertensive urgency is crucial; however, the principles of treatment are the same.

❽ The principal goals of treatment are tightly controlled BP reduction and prevention of end-organ injury. The recommended aim is to reduce the mean arterial pressure by 20%–25% within a period of 15 minutes to 2 hours. Subsequent rate of reduction of the BP is dictated by clinical status and the rapidity with which the hypertension may have evolved. Too rapid a reduction in BP is to be avoided, as that can worsen end-organ dysfunction *except* in the treatment of hypertensive crisis associated with aortic dissection where appropriate treatment requires rapid reduction of systolic BP to minimize aortic wall stress.

❾ Choice of drugs must take into account organs involved in the disease process and the adverse effect profile.

❿ Although intravenous antihypertensive infusions are preferred in the treatment of hypertensive crisis, oral agents may be used in a select group of patients with hypertensive urgency.

INTRODUCTION AND DEFINITIONS

Blood pressure (BP) generated across a vascular bed is determined by the blood flow and resistance across that bed and is defined by the following equation:

$$\text{Pressure} = \text{flow} \times \text{resistance}$$

Systemic hypertension occurs when there is an increase in blood flow or vascular resistance (or both). The body has intrinsic homeostatic mechanisms that modulate vascular resistance when changes in blood flow occur. Hypertension occurs when these autoregulatory mechanisms fail. The Joint National Committee on Prevention, Detection, Evaluation and Treatment of High Blood Pressure has defined hypertension in children and adolescents as systolic BP and/or diastolic BP ≥95th percentile for age, gender, and height (1). The above formula forms the fundamental basis of treatment of hypertension.

Hypertensive crisis is an acute, life-threatening elevation of BP and represents two processes that are pathophysiologically ❶ distinct: hypertensive emergencies and hypertensive urgencies. *Hypertensive emergency* is defined as sudden, severe hypertension complicated by acute end-organ damage; *hypertensive urgency* is characterized by severely elevated BP without end-organ damage (2). The clinical distinction between these two groups is the *presence* or *absence* of target organ damage—not the absolute level of the BP. The organ systems most frequently involved are those that maintain strict autoregulation to sustain physiologic function, including the central nervous system (CNS), cardiovascular system, and kidneys (Table 112.1). Involvement of these organ systems results in specific clinical syndromes.

Hypertensive Emergency

The hallmark of hypertensive emergency is end-organ injury. Though the brain, eyes, heart, and kidneys could all be involved, among pediatric patients the brain is the most commonly affected and would typically present with signs and symptoms of hypertensive encephalopathy, which may manifest as insidious onset of headache, visual changes, nausea, and vomiting followed by altered mental status, focal neurologic deficits, and coma (3). Ocular involvement may present as retinal hemorrhages, exudates, and papilledema. Cardiac involvement may lead to left ventricular (LV) failure, pulmonary edema, or acute myocardial ischemia. Renal effects may result in hematuria, proteinuria, or azotemia.

TABLE 112.1

MANIFESTATIONS OF HYPERTENSIVE CRISES

■ **HYPERTENSIVE CRISES**
- Hypertensive encephalopathy
- Acute stroke
- Retinopathy
- Acute myocardial ischemia
- Acute LV failure with pulmonary edema
- Dissecting aortic aneurysm
- Acute renal failure
- Microangiopathic hemolytic anemia

Hypertensive Urgency

In hypertensive urgency, there is acute, severe elevation of BP without associated target organ injury (4). Patients experiencing hypertensive urgency may or may not develop symptoms such as severe headache, shortness of breath, epistaxis, or severe anxiety.

PATHOPHYSIOLOGY

Hypertensive crisis can develop either de novo or as a complication of preexisting essential or secondary hypertension (**Table 112.2**). Any disorder that causes hypertension can give rise to hypertensive crisis. The endothelium in resistance vessels plays a central role in BP homeostasis, as it attempts to compensate for changes in vascular resistance through increased autocrine and paracrine release of vasodilator molecules, such as nitric oxide and prostacyclin. With sustained severe hypertension, these compensatory endothelium-mediated vasodilator responses are overwhelmed, which leads to endothelial decompensation, endothelial failure, and vasoconstriction (5). Although the detailed pathophysiology of hypertensive crisis remains to be elucidated, an initial abrupt increase in vascular resistance seems to be a necessary step and is likely related to a sudden surge in humoral vasoconstrictors (6). Activation of the renin–angiotensin system, nitric oxide (NO), endothelin, vasopressin, and catecholamines has been postulated to play important roles in the pathophysiology of hypertensive crises (7–9).

Of these trigger factors, the role of renin–angiotensin system in the pathogenesis of end-organ injury has been the most studied. (For in-depth discussion of renin–angiotensin system, see Chapter 107.) In humans, a rapid elevation of circulating renin levels occurs during transition to malignant hypertension, (10) and in transgenic mice, evidence suggests that the renin–angiotensin system is important for transformation to malignant hypertension and lethality (11). Mice that express the murine renin gene, *Ren-2*, develop severe hypertension compared with controls (12), and rats that are double transgenic for human renin and human angiotensinogen genes develop not only severe hypertension but also an inflammatory vasculopathy similar to that seen in human severe hypertension (13). Angiotensin II has been shown to have direct cytotoxic effects on the vessel wall, some of which seem to be mediated through activation of expression of genes for proinflammatory cytokines (e.g., IL-6) and activation of the transcription factor, NF-$\kappa\beta$ (14,15). Furthermore, inhibition of angiotensin-converting enzyme (ACE) prevents the development of malignant hypertension in transgenic rats that express the murine renin gene (11). Activation of the renin–angiotensin–aldosterone system may be primary or secondary to renal ischemia produced by arteriolar occlusion. The BP elevation may

TABLE 112.2

CAUSES OF HYPERTENSIVE CRISIS

■ DISORDER	■ CAUSE
Essential hypertension	
Primary CNS disease	Spinal cord injury
Renal parenchymal disorders	Reflux nephropathy
	Obstructive uropathy
	Glomerulonephritis
	Interstitial nephritis
	Hemolytic uremic syndrome
	Systemic lupus erythematosis
	Vasculitides
Renovascular disorders	Fibromuscular dysplasia
	Acute renal artery occlusion
	Polyarteritis nodosa
Endocrine disorders	Renin-secreting tumors
	Pheochromocytoma
	Thyroid crisis
	Cushing syndrome
	Conn disease
Ingestions/drugs	Cocaine
	Amphetamines
	Phencyclidine
	Cyclosporine
	Tacrolimus
	Sympathomimetic diet pills
Cardiovascular disorder	Coarctation of the aorta
	Midaortic syndrome
Pre-eclampsia/eclampsia	Pregnancy

induce pressure natriuresis, intravascular volume depletion, and a further increase in renin secretion. Increased angiotensin II causes further renal vasoconstriction and, hence, worsening hypertension.

The ensuing increase in BP generates mechanical stress and injury of the microvasculature, endothelial damage, activation of the renin–angiotensin system, and oxidative stress (4). The endothelial injury results in increased vascular permeability, activation of coagulation cascade, and platelet deposition of fibrin (**Fig. 112.1**). Further progression leads to fibrinoid necrosis of the arterioles with resulting ischemia and the release of additional vasoactive mediators generating a vicious cycle of repeated injury (6,16,17). Activation of the renin–angiotensin system leads to further vasoconstriction and production of proinflammatory cytokines such as interleukin-6 (IL-6) (14,18). The process also triggers an increase in NADPH oxidase activity, which generates the release of reactive oxygen species (ROS) and further tissue injury (19,20).

Nitric oxide (NO) plays a major role in vascular smooth muscle relaxation and vasodilation (nitric oxide is discussed in detail in Chapter 21). NO is predominantly synthesized in the vascular endothelium by the action of endothelial nitric oxide synthase (eNOS) on L-arginine. NO diffuses from the endothelial cells to activate soluble guanylate cyclase and form cGMP in the vascular smooth muscle cells, which causes vascular smooth muscle relaxation, prevention of platelet adhesion, and aggregation, and anti-inflammatory, antiproliferative, and anti-migratory effects on leukocytes, endothelial cells, and vascular smooth muscle cells (21,22). The main characteristic of endothelial dysfunction present in arterial hypertension is the attenuated NO bioavailability (23). Hypertensive patients have increased generation of ROS, which act as potent NO scavengers and reduce NO bioavailability. Additionally, studies in animals have shown that deletion of the eNOS gene as

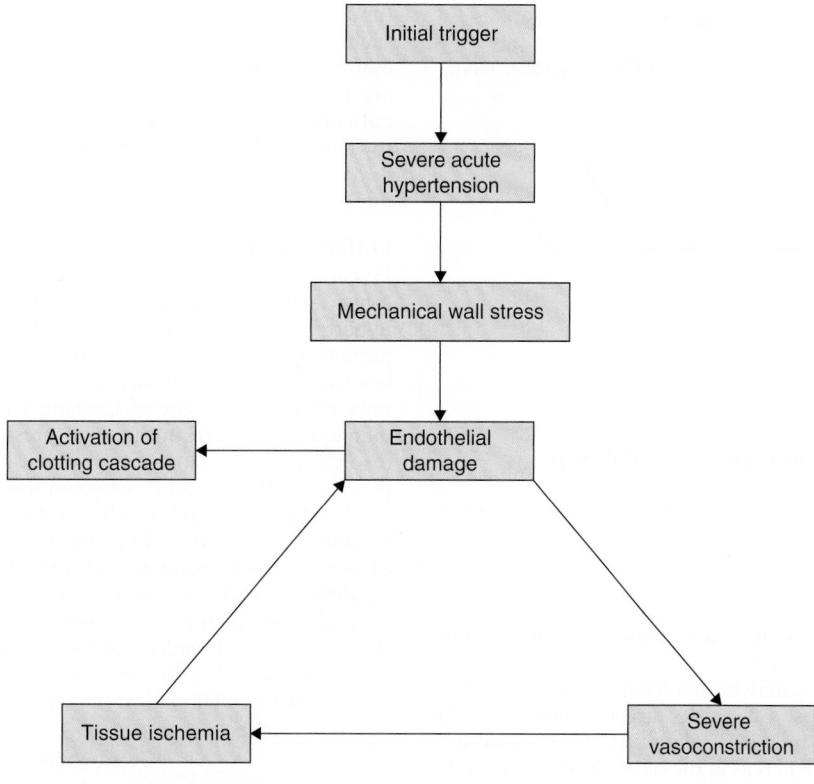

FIGURE 112.1. Pathophysiology of hypertensive crisis.

well as chronic inhibition of NO synthesis with N-nitro-L-arginine methyl ester (L-NAME) leads to development of arterial hypertension (24,25). Studies in both humans and animals show that the restoration of NOS activity by administration of NOS cofactors such as tetrahydrobiopterin (BH_4) or L-arginine result in increased bioavailability of NO, improved endothelial function, and prevention of hypertension (26,27).

Other agents responsible for vasodilation include endothelial-derived hyperpolarizing factor (EDHF) and prostaglandin I_2 (PGI_2). EDHF is potent non-NO, non–prostaglandin-mediated endothelium-dependent vasodilator with a predominant effect on resistance vessels (28). PGI_2 is an eicosanoid of the cyclooxygenase pathway that causes vascular smooth muscle relaxation and inhibits platelet aggregation (29). Endothelin, another endothelium-derived agent, on the other hand, has a potent vasoconstrictor effect and may act alone or in concert with other agents such as thromboxane A_2 (TXA_2), prostaglandin $F_{2\alpha}$ ($PGF_{2\alpha}$), or endothelial-derived constrictor factor (EDCF) to cause vasoconstriction. The relative amounts of the various factors released by the endothelial cell are kept in a tight equilibrium and are dependent on the physiologic circumstance and pathophysiologic status. Disturbance of this equilibrium can result in an acute hypertensive episode.

It is important to note that patients with chronic hypertension may have arterial wall hypertrophy and, therefore, may be relatively protected from the effects of acute BP elevation (26). Conversely, in patients without preexisting chronic hypertension, a hypertensive emergency can develop at a substantially lower BP (5).

Cerebral Autoregulation

The pathophysiologic mechanism of development of hypertensive encephalopathy, though controversial, deserves mention.

Autoregulation of cerebral blood flow (CBF) is governed by the relationship between cerebral perfusion pressure (CPP) and cerebrovascular resistance (CVR).

$$CBF = CPP/CVR$$

CPP can be defined as the difference between the mean arterial pressure (MAP) and the cerebral venous pressure. Under conditions of normal intracranial pressure and central venous pressure, the cerebral venous pressure is negligible; therefore, CBF is directly related to MAP and maintains a reciprocal relationship with CVR. In normotensive adults, CBF is maintained over a wide BP range (MAP between 60 and 150 mm Hg). The range of autoregulation shifts to the right in chronically hypertensive patients (**Fig. 112.2**) (30), a phenomenon that is reversible with long-term BP control (31). This autoregulation is maintained by the appropriate adjustments in CVR. Hypertensive encephalopathy occurs when MAP exceeds the upper limit of autoregulation. Likely mechanisms of hypertensive encephalopathy involve the failure of autoregulation, due to either inappropriate or forced cerebral vasodilation. The abnormal cerebral vasodilation causes excessive CBF, dysfunction of the blood–brain barrier and vascular endothelium, cerebral edema, increased intracranial pressure, and microhemorrhages (5,32). Another suggested mechanism of hypertensive encephalopathy involves decreased CBF from severe cerebral vasoconstriction in response to acute hypertension, but this hypothesis has been heavily disputed (33).

CLINICAL PRESENTATION

The risk of development of hypertensive crisis is greater in patients with secondary hypertension than in patients with essential hypertension. The absolute BP is often not as important as the rate of elevation of the systemic BP. Acute elevations

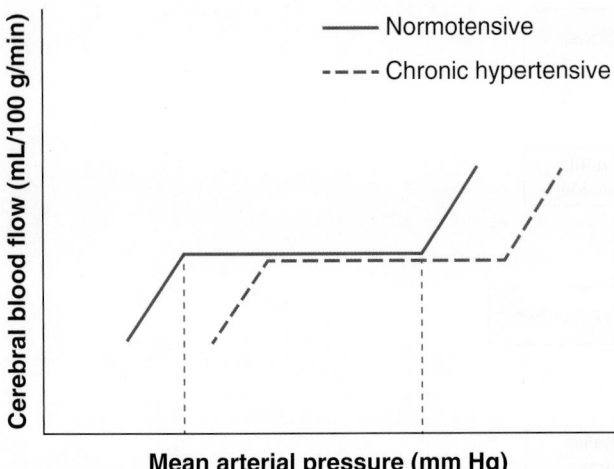

FIGURE 112.2. Cerebral autoregulation and effect of chronic hypertension.

in BP are less well tolerated and more likely to produce symptoms than are chronic elevations.

Clinical manifestations may be divided into features related to hypertension and those related to target organ injury. In the neonate, symptoms and signs related to hypertension are lethargy and irritability, whereas in the older child they include severe headache, dizziness, blurred vision, and epistaxis. Typically, the headache is occipital and more prominent in patients with hypertensive encephalopathy.

Physical examination findings such as altered mental status, papilledema, and pulmonary edema are related to the organs involved (34).

Blood Pressure

It is difficult to apply an absolute BP level to define hypertensive emergencies and urgencies. Normal and abnormal BPs vary very widely with age and body size. Systolic and diastolic BP levels by age and height percentiles are available for children and adolescents (1). Stage II hypertension is defined as systolic or diastolic BP more than 5 mm Hg greater than the 99th percentile for age and height, and this condition requires prompt evaluation and pharmacologic therapy (1).

Neurologic Manifestations

Hypertensive Encephalopathy

Hypertensive encephalopathy is defined as an acute organic brain syndrome, in the setting of severe hypertension, characterized by profound headache, severe nausea and vomiting, blurred vision, and altered mental status. These symptoms may progress to focal or generalized seizures, focal neurologic deficits, and cortical blindness. If not appropriately treated, hypertensive encephalopathy may progress rapidly to cerebral hemorrhage, coma, and death. It occurs as a result of failure of cerebral vascular autoregulation, cerebrovascular endothelial dysfunction, microhemorrhage, blood–brain barrier disruption with cerebral edema, and intracranial hypertension. Hypertensive encephalopathy may be associated with untreated or inadequately treated primary or secondary hypertension. In the pregnant adolescent, it may occur in the setting of preeclampsia and eclampsia. Physical examination findings are consistent with the neurologic symptoms. In some cases,

fundoscopy may reveal evidence of malignant hypertension such as papilledema, retinal hemorrhages, and exudates. These manifestations, a result of failure of cerebral autoregulation, are reversible with BP management. In chronic hypertensive patients, adaptive mechanisms shift cerebral autoregulation to a higher MAP range and provide protection against the development of hypertensive encephalopathy during sudden increases in BP (Fig. 112.2) (35).

Differential Diagnosis of Hypertensive Encephalopathy. Hypertensive encephalopathy must be differentiated from other acute neurologic events that may be associated with hypertension, such as cerebral infarct or hemorrhage. Hypertension in response to cerebral ischemia can be caused by brainstem ischemia or increased intracranial pressure (Cushing's triad). Treatment of Cushing triad must be directed at managing increased intracranial pressure and the underlying disorder and not at lowering systemic BP, which will only compromise CPP and lead to stroke in this setting.

Pseudotumor cerebri, when associated with severe hypertension, may mimic hypertensive encephalopathy. Other causes of hypertension and altered mental status that should be differentiated from a hypertensive crisis include primary renal disease (uremic encephalopathy), hepatorenal syndrome (hepatic encephalopathy), and steroid overdose (altered sensorium). Primary CNS disorders such as stroke and vasculitis may present with similar clinical findings and need to be ruled out.

Acute Stroke

Acute stroke with concomitant severe hypertension poses a diagnostic and management dilemma. The hypertension may be a reflex response to maintain cerebral perfusion, or it may be the cause of the stroke. Careful assessment and management of such patients are imperative. In many patients in whom hypertension is secondary to stroke, the BP tends to resolve spontaneously within 48 hours. The clinical presentation includes acute onset of severe headache, altered mental status, or loss of consciousness associated with focal neurologic findings (e.g., hemiparesis, hemiplegia). The distribution of the focal findings depends on the extent and location of cerebral vascular involvement.

Cardiovascular Manifestations

Myocardial Ischemia

The effects on the left ventricle of the sudden increase in afterload and intracavitary pressure associated with a hypertensive crisis include an increase in oxygen demand and decrease in oxygen supply. Myocardial ischemia results if there is no concurrent increase in coronary blood flow. The sustained increase in myocardial workload leads to LV failure, elevated LV end-diastolic pressure, and pulmonary edema. These pathophysiologic events manifest as acute chest pain, tachypnea, dyspnea, orthopnea, cough, and hemoptysis. Physical examination may reveal rales or gallop on auscultation; chest x-ray may reveal pulmonary edema.

Aortic Dissection

Severe acute hypertension can cause aortic dissection, especially in patients with predisposing syndromes (Marfan, Loeys-Dietz, Ehler-Danlos type 4, Turner and polycystic kidney disease). Severe chest or abdominal pain is the most common symptom of acute aortic dissection. The precise location of the pain depends on the site and the extent of the dissecting process. Syncope, paralysis, and blindness may result from carotid or innominate artery involvement. Dissection of the thoracic aorta may be associated with hemoptysis, orthopnea, and dyspnea, while involvement of the abdominal aorta may cause a variety of gastrointestinal and genitourinary disturbances. The diagnosis of acute aortic dissection should be suspected in a hypertensive patient with abrupt onset of pain, pulse deficits, and signs of end-organ circulatory compromise. Mortality from acute aortic dissection is not from the intimal disruption *per se* but due to the dissecting hematoma, which may rupture or interrupt blood supply to a major organ.

Renal Manifestations

Acute renal dysfunction may be a cause or effect of hypertensive crisis. Among pediatric patients, renal or renovascular disorders are the most common etiologies of severe hypertension. Renal diseases, such as post-streptococcal glomerulonephritis and hemolytic uremic syndrome, are common causes of de novo acute hypertension. Mild proteinuria and elevated serum creatinine can be the result of a primary renal disease or may be secondary manifestations of severe hypertension, and such cases may be difficult to differentiate. In cases where the kidneys are the target organs of severe acute hypertension, the injury may manifest as multiple intraparenchymal hemorrhages with many areas of renal destruction and, eventually, kidney failure, uremia, and death.

CLINICAL EVALUATION

The goal of the initial clinical evaluation is to differentiate hypertensive emergency from urgency. All organ systems at risk of involvement in hypertensive emergencies must be critically assessed. The presence of one organ dysfunction at presentation does not preclude evaluation of others. The history and physical examination must determine the nature, severity, and subsequent management of the hypertensive syndrome. The duration and severity of preexisting hypertension and the presence of previous end-organ damage must be ascertained. History of antihypertensive drug therapy, degree of BP control, and use of any other drugs, including illicit drugs (cocaine, ecstasy, amphetamines, phencyclidine-PCP), must be determined. A focused examination to identify any evidence of end-organ injury is imperative.

BP must be obtained in all four extremities to exclude coarctation of the aorta. Fundoscopic examination is particularly useful because it can distinguish a true hypertensive emergency from hypertensive urgency (the presence of new hemorrhages, exudates, or papilledema, indicates a hypertensive emergency). The cardiovascular assessment should include auscultation for new murmurs of aortic insufficiency (aortic dissection) or mitral insufficiency (myocardial infarction). The presence of parasternal heave or S3 gallop may reflect the presence of heart failure, and crackles in the lung fields may suggest pulmonary edema. Neurologic examination should evaluate level of consciousness, signs of meningeal irritation, visual fields, and focal neurologic deficits.

Initial laboratory investigations include serum electrolytes, urea, creatinine, full blood count with peripheral smear (for evidence of hemolysis), urinalysis, and chest radiograph. An electrocardiograph (ECG) may reveal LV hypertrophy and myocardial ischemia/infarction, and chest radiograph should be obtained and may demonstrate cardiac enlargement, widened mediastinum, or pulmonary edema. Measurement of plasma renin and aldosterone activity may be helpful in making a retrospective diagnosis of hypertension. Once the patient is stabilized, investigations for secondary causes of severe hypertension should be performed, as guided by clinical presentation and laboratory findings (**Table 112.2**). Brain MRI, though not part of the initial work-up, may reveal the characteristic

posterior leukoencephalopathy that predominantly affects the white matter of the parieto-occipital, posterior frontal, and temporal regions of the brain and best appreciated on T$_2$-weighted images (36,37). (Posterior reversible encephalopathy syndrome/reversible posterior leukoencephalopathy syndrome is discussed in Chapter 64.) Pregnancy must be ruled out in female adolescents presenting with hypertensive crisis as this may impact on the approach to treatment and the choice of antihypertensive agents.

TREATMENT

General Principles

While it is important to establish the distinction between hypertensive emergency and hypertensive urgency, the treatment algorithm is the same for either condition. Management requires the immediate assessment of the airway, breathing, and circulation and initiation of appropriate interventions. The patient must be admitted to the PICU and an arterial line placed for continuous, invasive BP monitoring. However, it is imperative that specific antihypertensive therapy is not delayed while these measures are being implemented. The primary goal of therapy is to prevent end-organ injury, not solely to restore BP to normal. Reversible causes must be identified and treated appropriately. A reduction of BP by 25% is believed safe and to still be above the lower limit of CBF autoregulation (38). The recommended initial therapy is to reduce MAP by 20%–25% over a period of 15 minutes to 2 hours. Subsequent rate of reduction of the BP is dictated by clinical status and the rapidity with which the hypertension may have evolved. Too rapid a reduction in BP can worsen end-organ dysfunction and must be avoided. Volume depletion is common in patients with hypertensive crises and may lead to excessive fall in BP during treatment. Careful volume repletion with intravenous crystalloid often restores organ perfusion.

Aortic dissection is the most dramatic and most rapidly fatal complication of severe hypertension. Emergency surgery may be indicated depending on the type and location of the dissection. After insuring airway patency and oxygenation, medical management requires rapid reduction of systolic BP to 100–120 mm Hg or the normal range for age to avoid aortic rupture. Rapid minimization of aortic wall stress is imperative and this can be accomplished by lowering both BP and heart rate and consequently the Dp/Dt (change in BP/change in time) with esmolol. Morphine is indicated for chest pain. If the systolic BP remains above the desired range despite an adequate esmolol infusion, then nitroprusside, nicardipine, or dilitiazem may be added.

Acute postoperative hypertension caused by pain, anxiety, bladder distension, hypothermia, or hypoxemia may present as a hypertensive urgency. A specific underlying cause for postoperative BP elevation should be identified and treated before the implementation of antihypertensive therapy. If the BP remains significantly elevated after appropriate analgesia, bladder drainage, and normalization of O$_2$ saturation and body temperature, then a β-blocker or labetalol (combined α- and β-blocker) may be administered on the assumption the child has experienced an acute catecholamine surge from activation of the sympathetic nervous system.

Postcoarctectomy (paradoxical) hypertension in the first week after relief of coarctation of the aorta can occur after surgical repair or after balloon angioplasty with an incidence of 30%–56% (39,40). Provided the repair is satisfactory, the hypertension usually resolves after several days, though intensive antihypertensive therapy during the early postoperative period is frequently required. Both the sympathetic and renin–angiotensin systems have been implicated in the pathogenesis of paradoxical hypertension (41). Aggressive treatment of the hypertension is crucial if end-organ damage and risk of rupture of surgical suture lines are to be avoided. If an esmolol is insufficient to manage severe paradoxical hypertension after coarctation repair, sodium nitroprusside (SNP) infusion can be added.

Reflex, or rebound, hypertensive crisis is a condition that develops in patients who abruptly discontinue their antihypertensive medications, especially clonidine or β-blockers. The specific therapy is to restart their original medications after an initial BP reduction with labetalol or SNP (4).

Pharmacologic Therapy

Hypertensive urgency can be treated in a non-ICU setting with oral medications over a 24–48-hour period. β-Blockers, diuretics, ACE inhibitors and calcium channel blockers can be used initially in the inpatient setting, and the patient can be discharged with close follow-up after adequate BP control has been attained. However, in the presence of acute end-organ damage, the patient should be admitted to the ICU and treated with intravenous medication.

The aim of drug therapy is to reduce BP in a controlled, predictable, and safe manner, which is best achieved with continuous infusion of pharmacologic agents that have rapid onset, short half-life, and ease of titration. These antihypertensive agents act by inducing vascular smooth muscle relaxation and vasodilation. They enhance organ perfusion and minimize end-organ dysfunction. The choice of drug must take into consideration the patient's risk factors, comorbidities, and the nature and extent of target organ involvement. For example, drugs such as clonidine and methyldopa that significantly affect the central nervous system should be avoided in patients with hypertensive encephalopathy. Also, drugs that act by predominant β-receptor blockade must be avoided in pheochromocytoma crisis, as unopposed α-receptor stimulation may cause a paradoxical worsening of the hypertension. From the wide array of intravenous antihypertensive medications available, the most commonly used in the pediatric population are SNP, fenoldopam, labetalol, and nicardipine, although esmolol has been favored in postcoarctectomy hypertension (**Table 112.3** includes the commonly used antihypertensive infusions). Oral agents have an important place in the management of hypertensive crisis. Those most commonly used are the calcium channel blockers

(e.g., nifedipine), ACE inhibitors (enalapril, captopril), and α_2-agonists (clonidine).

PARENTERAL ANTIHYPERTENSIVE AGENTS

Sodium Nitroprusside

SNP has been used as first-line medication in most cases of hypertensive crisis. It is a nonselective vasodilator with effect on both arterioles and venules. It decreases both systemic and pulmonary vascular resistance. Once infused, SNP interacts with oxyhemoglobin, dissociating immediately to form methemoglobin while releasing free cyanide and nitric oxide. This process is independent of enzyme activity. Nitric oxide activates guanylate cyclase in the vascular smooth muscle, triggering an increase in intracellular cGMP, followed by relaxation of vascular smooth muscle and vasodilation. The free cyanide radical (CN^-) binds to methemoglobin to form cyanomethemoglobin. Each molecule of SNP metabolized results in the release of five cyanide radicals, some of which bind to methemoglobin, with the rest available to be converted to thiocyanate by the rhodanase enzyme in the liver and the kidneys. Any free cyanide that is not rapidly converted to thiocyanate can bind to and inactivate tissue cytochrome oxidase and manifest as tissue hypoxia. Because the conversion of SNP to cyanide is a nonenzymatic process, the amount of CN^- released from SNP depends entirely on the total dose of the drug administered. The subsequent rate at which CN^- is converted to the less toxic thiocyanate by rhodanase enzyme is dependent on the availability of a sulfur donor for the enzyme, usually endogenous thiosulfate derived from the amino acid cysteine. Thiocyanate is cleared by the kidneys with an elimination half-life of 4–7 days. The presence of renal failure or prolonged SNP therapy can cause accumulation of thiocyanate.

SNP has been favored in the management of hypertensive crises because of its rapid onset of action, ease of titration, rapid dissipation of its effects after discontinuation, and almost universal efficacy. It acts within 30 seconds, peak antihypertensive effect occurs within 2 minutes, and its effects persist for 2–4 minutes after cessation of infusion. Most patients respond to a starting dose of 0.3–0.5 μg/kg/min, and the dose may be escalated as needed to rates not exceeding 5 μg/kg/min. Occasionally doses as high as 10 μg/kg/min may be needed for adequate BP response, but this must be administered for

TABLE 112.3

INTRAVENOUS ANTIHYPERTENSIVE DRUGS

■ DRUG	■ STARTING DOSE[a]	■ ONSET OF ACTION	■ PEAK EFFECT	■ HALF-LIFE
Sodium nitroprusside	0.3–0.5 μg/kg/min	30 s	2 min	1–2 min
Fenoldopam	0.1 μg/kg/min	15 min	15–20 min	5 min
Nicardipine	5–10 μg/kg bolus (>1–2 min), then 1–3 μg/kg/min	5–15 min	30 min to 2 h	2–4 h
Labetalol[b]	0.25 mg/kg bolus (>1–2 min), then 0.25 mg/kg/h	2–5 min	5–15 min	6–8 h
Esmolol	300–500 μg/kg bolus (>1–3 min), then 25–200 μg/kg/min	2 min	6–10 min	8 min
Enalaprilat	5–10 μg/kg/dose (>5 min) q8–24 h	10–15 min	1–4 h	11 h

[a]See text for range and max dose.
[b]Labetalol is dosed as mg/kg/h, whereas others are dosed as μg/kg/min.

no longer than 10 minutes to minimize toxicity. Reflex tachycardia usually occurs with SNP therapy and may cause difficulty in obtaining an adequate BP response. In such situations, the addition of a small dose of β-blocker will result in significant improvement in BP control. When used in the treatment of aortic dissection, prior institution of β-blocking agent is imperative as the reflex tachycardia could be extremely deleterious in such patients.

The most common adverse effect of SNP is precipitous hypotension, with or without reflex tachycardia, due to its potent vasodilator effect on both the venous and the arterial beds. This reaction is accentuated in the hypovolemic patient. SNP has been shown to cause increased intracranial pressure raising concern about its use when cerebral compliance is compromised (42).

Cyanide toxicity is a rare, but potentially fatal complication of SNP use. Cyanide toxicity presents as lactic acidosis, tachycardia, seizures, coma, and almond smell on breath. Free cyanide radicals bind and inactivate tissue cytochrome oxidase, leading to tissue anoxia, anaerobic metabolism, and lactic acidosis. Toxic accumulation of cyanide that leads to severe lactic acidosis can occur if SNP is infused at a rate >5 μg/kg/min over a period of several hours, assuming normal rhodanase activity. Patients receiving SNP who demonstrate evidence of tissue hypoxia (metabolic acidosis) must be suspected of having cyanide toxicity. An unexplained increase in venous oxygen saturation may be the first sign of cyanide toxicity. A high-degree suspicion is warranted whenever SNP is used, so that cyanide antidotes can be administered in a timely fashion. A treatment protocol for suspected cyanide toxicity includes the following:

- Discontinuation of SNP infusion
- 100% O_2
- 3% sodium nitrite 4–6 mg/kg IV *slowly*
- Sodium thiosulfate 150–200 mg/kg IV over 15 minutes
- Sodium bicarbonate 1–2 mEq/kg IV to correct metabolic acidosis
- Hydroxocobalamin (vitamin B_{12a}) 70 mg/kg IV $\times$ 1 (controversial)

Methemoglobinemia is another important toxic effect of SNP. Severe methemoglobinemia causes tissue hypoxia and subsequent acidosis. The total SNP required to generate 10% methemoglobinemia exceeds 10 mg/kg (~10 μg/kg/min for more than 16 hours).

Thiocyanate toxicity is the most common clinically observed toxicity of SNP administration and results in nausea, confusion, muscle weakness, psychosis, and seizures. This toxicity occurs predominantly in patients with concomitant renal dysfunction. Thiocyanate levels of 1 mmol/L (60 mg/L) are associated with the onset of neurologic symptoms. Thiocyanate levels should be measured when SNP is used for >48 hours or at doses continuously >4 μg/kg/min. The SNP dose should be titrated to keep thiocyanate levels <0.85 mmol/L (50 mg/L).

In general, cyanide toxicity is more likely to occur if hepatic dysfunction is present, thiocyanate toxicity more likely if there is renal dysfunction or prolonged infusion. Coadministration of SNP with sodium thiosulfate at a ratio of 10:1 (SNP:sodium thiosulfate) has been shown to increase the rate of CN⁻ processing and reduces the risk of cyanide toxicity without altering the efficacy of SNP (43,44). Thiocyanate toxicity may still occur with SNP:sodium thiosulfate coadministration.

Fenoldopam

Fenoldopam is a benzapine derivative of dopamine and a selective dopamine agonist that interacts with DA_1 receptor without significant interaction with DA_2, α_1-adrenergic, or β-adrenergic receptors. Stimulation of the receptor results in vasodilation and, in the kidneys, induces diuresis and natriuresis. During reduction of severely elevated BP, fenoldopam significantly increased creatinine clearance, urinary flow, and sodium and potassium excretion. These unique effects on the kidneys make fenoldopam a particularly attractive drug in the treatment of hypertensive emergencies with renal impairment (45–47).

Peripheral DA_1 receptors are located postsynaptically in the systemic and renal vasculature and at various sites in the nephrons, parathyroid gland, and the gastrointestinal tract (48). DA_1 receptors are also present in the brain, but fenoldopam does not cross the blood–brain barrier. It is not metabolized by the cytochrome P-450 pathway and, therefore, has no significant drug interactions; furthermore, its pharmacokinetics is not altered by hepatic or renal insufficiency. Fenoldopam has a short half-life (5 minutes) and predictable dose response, is easily titrated, and is not associated with precipitous decline in BP. The onset of BP response occurs within 15 minutes of initiation (3 half-lives); therefore, it is recommended that the drug be titrated no more frequently than every 15 minutes. Steady state is reached within 30 minutes, and elimination half-life is about 10 minutes. The recommended starting dose is 0.1 μg/kg/min, titrated to effect to a maximum of 1.6 μg/kg/min (49). In one pediatric case series, doses up to 2.5 μg/kg/min were used successfully without excessive hypotension or clinically significant adverse effects (50). Rebound hypertension after discontinuation is rare with fenoldopam.

The majority of adverse effects associated with fenoldopam are attributable to the vasodilator action of the drug. These include headache, flushing, dizziness, and reflex tachycardia. Most of the adverse effects occur in the first 24 hours of treatment. ECG changes (flattening T waves in anterior and lateral leads) have been reported with fenoldopam, but these have not been shown to have any clinical significance. Elevation of intraocular pressure has been reported (51), but the effect of fenoldopam on intracranial pressure (ICP) has not been well studied (52).

Nicardipine

Nicardipine is a nondihydropyridine derivative calcium channel blocker. It differs from nifedipine by the addition of tertiary amine moiety to the ester side chain pyridine ring and movement of the nitro group to the meta-position of the phenyl ring, making it 100 times more water soluble than nifedipine. Nicardipine acts by blocking calcium influx through voltage-sensitive channels in vascular smooth muscle cells, resulting in smooth muscle relaxation and vasodilation. It can be given as a continuous intravenous infusion and is easily titratable. The pharmacokinetic characteristics of nicardipine include onset of action of 5–15 minutes, peak hypotensive effect at 30 minutes to 2 hours, half-life of 2–4 hours, and a duration of action of 4–6 hours. It is administered as a loading dose of 5–10 μg/kg, given over a minute, followed by a continuous infusion of 1–3 μg/kg/min.

Adverse effects include orthostatic hypotension, tachycardia (reflex), and peripheral edema. Nicardipine undergoes considerable first-pass metabolism in the liver and excretion in the urine, so it requires careful use in patients with hepatic or renal dysfunction. It can be used alone or in conjunction with other antihypertensive agents.

Labetalol

Labetalol is a competitive α_1-adrenergic and β-adrenergic receptor antagonist. The α_1-receptor blockade causes arterial smooth muscle relaxation and vasodilation, and the β-receptor antagonism contributes to the fall in BP by blocking reflex sympathetic stimulation of the heart. In addition, labetalol has intrinsic sympathomimetic activity at β_2 receptors, which may contribute further to the peripheral vasodilation. These actions contribute to the BP lowering effects in patients with hypertension. It is available in oral and intravenous forms, but when taken orally its bioavailability may vary between 20% and 40%. When given intravenously, the β-blocker effect is seven times greater than the α-blocker effect. The hypotensive effect of labetalol begins 2–5 minutes after an IV dose, peaks at 5–15 minutes, and persists for about 2–4 hours (53). The recommended dose in children is an initial dose of 0.25 mg/kg bolus, followed by continuous infusion of 0.25 mg/kg/h, titrated up to 3 mg/kg/h (54). The most common adverse effects associated with labetalol are precipitous hypotension and orthostatic hypotension. Bradycardia, heart block, and bronchospasm (all β-antagonist effects) may also complicate its use.

Esmolol

Esmolol is an intravenous, ultra-short-acting selective β_1-adrenergic antagonist. It has virtually no intrinsic sympathomimetic activity and therefore significant bradycardia can be associated with its administration. Peak hemodynamic effect occurs in 6–10 minutes following an appropriate loading dose. It has a half-life of 8 minutes, and a rapid offset of effect occurs within 15–30 minutes following discontinuation. Esmolol is administered as a bolus of 300–500 μg/kg IV over 1–3 minutes, then 25–200 μg/kg/min. Infusion dose may be titrated by 25–50 μg/kg/min q5–10 minutes for optimal antihypertensive effect to a maximum infusion dose of 1000 μg/kg/min. Adverse effects include bradycardia, hypotension, congestive heart failure, and bronchoconstriction. Esmolol is contraindicated in second- or third-degree heart block and in cardiogenic shock.

Enalaprilat

Enalaprilat is an ACE inhibitor that decreases circulating levels of angiotensin II, reduces serum aldosterone levels, and inhibits the indirect adrenergic effects of angiotensin II. Because angiotensin II stimulates the release of norepinephrine from adrenergic nerve endings and also amplifies the vasoconstrictive effect of α_1-adrenergic stimulation, the antihypertensive effect of enalaprilat is the combined result of decreased vascular smooth muscle tone and its antiadrenergic properties. Enalaprilat reaches peak serum levels rapidly with antihypertensive effects seen within 15 minutes of administration. Because of its potency and rapid onset of action, it must be administered over 5 minutes. Intravenous enalaprilat is started at a dose of 5–10 μg/kg/dose every 8–24 hours to a maximum of 1.25 mg/dose with the dosing frequency based on clinical response. Adverse effects are similar to captopril and rapid drop in BP may occur with intravenous enalaprilat. The Food and Drug Administration has issued a black box warning against the use of enalaprilat in pregnant patients because of the risk of fetal damage or death.

ORAL ANTIHYPERTENSIVE AGENTS

Nifedipine

Nifedipine is a dihydropyridine calcium channel–blocking agent that induces peripheral vasodilation. It is administered either orally or sublingually. Following its administration, nifedipine reduces BP abruptly and therefore has an important role in the management of hypertensive urgencies. The usual dose is 0.25–0.5 mg/kg/dose; however, the lower end of

this range is the preferred starting dose due to the risk of precipitous hypotension. Unfortunately, there is no commercially available pediatric suspension of nifedipine. The smallest commercially available dose is a 10-mg liquid-filled capsule, which can be punctured with a tuberculin syringe to administer either a 2.5-mg dose or a 5-mg dose. The dose may be repeated as needed to a daily maximum of 3 mg/kg. Absorption is nearly complete, but bioavailability is 45%–75% due to first-pass effect. Onset of action is observed within 15–30 minutes and an elimination half-life may be as short as 1.5 hours. Even though its rapid onset of action is viewed as a major advantage, nifedipine must be used with caution since the peripheral vasodilation that follows its administration can trigger an intense reflex adrenergic stimulation with tachycardia as well as activation of the renin–angiotensin system.

Captopril

Captopril, an ACE inhibitor, which works by reducing the levels of circulating angiotensin II represents an important component of the treatment of hypertensive crises. Captopril lowers BP promptly without causing tachycardia and therefore offers distinct hemodynamic advantage over other vasodilator drugs. Captopril is very well absorbed; its antihypertensive effect begins within 15 minutes of administration and can last for up to 2 hours. Elimination half-life is 4–6 hours. The initial dose is 0.3–0.5 mg/kg, and this may be repeated to a maximum daily dose of 6 mg/kg. Patients must be closely monitored after the first dose as an exaggerated hypotensive effect may be observed in patients presenting with acute severe hypertension associated with a high renin state. Adverse effects include cough, hyperkalemia, neutropenia, and, rarely, angioedema. In patients with renovascular hypertension, the glomerular filtration rate is maintained by an increased postglomerular arteriolar resistance caused by angiotensin II. Therefore, in patients with bilateral renal artery stenosis or stenosis in a solitary kidney, captopril and other ACE inhibitors are contraindicated. Autoimmune renal disease with hypertension (e.g., scleroderma) is often associated with high renin states, and ACE inhibitors are to be used with utmost caution. Captopril is also contraindicated in severe renal failure.

Enalapril

Enalapril is an ACE inhibitor. It is a prodrug that is de-esterified in the liver and the kidneys to the active drug, enalaprilat. The initial oral dose of enalapril is 0.08–0.1 mg/kg to a maximum of 5 mg in one to two divided doses per day. When administered orally, it is rapidly absorbed with a bioavailability of 60%, but peak plasma concentration of the active drug, enalaprilat, does not occur until after 4–5 hours. Because of these limitations, enalapril is generally not a preferred drug if an acute drop in BP is necessary.

CONCLUSION AND FUTURE DIRECTIONS

Hypertensive crisis is a serious medical emergency that affects the pediatric population. If untreated, severe end-organ damage can occur. The pathophysiology of hypertensive crisis and the molecular mechanisms that mediate target organ injury are not very well understood. With the elucidation of these molecular mechanisms, translational studies in humans may lead to additional therapeutic options that are directed at both tight BP control and prevention of target organ injury.

References

1. National High Blood Pressure Education Program Working Group on High Blood Pressure in Children and Adolescents. The fourth report on the diagnosis, evaluation, and treatment of high blood pressure in children and adolescents. *Pediatrics* 2004;114(suppl 2):555–76.

2. Singh D, Akingbola O, Yosypiv I, et al. Emergency management of hypertension in children. *Int J Nephrol* 2012;2012:420247.

3. Patel HP, Mitsnefes M. Advances in the pathogenesis and management of hypertensive crisis. *Curr Opin Pediatr* 2005;17(2): 210–14.

4. Aggarwal M, Khan IA. Hypertensive crisis: Hypertensive emergencies and urgencies. *Cardiol Clin* 2006;24(1):135–46.

5. Vaughan CJ, Delanty N. Hypertensive emergencies. *Lancet* 2000;356(9227):411–7.

6. Ault MJ, Ellrodt AG. Pathophysiological events leading to the end-organ effects of acute hypertension. *Am J Emerg Med* 1985;3(6 suppl):10–15.

7. Vilela-Martin JF, Vaz-de-Melo RO, Cosenso-Martin LN, et al. Renin Angiotensin system blockage associates with insertion/deletion polymorphism of angiotensin-converting enzyme in patients with hypertensive emergency. *DNA Cell Biol* 2013;32(9): 541–8.

8. Weismann D, Kleinbrahm K, Hu K, et al. Prevention of hypertensive crises in rats induced by acute and chronic norepinephrine excess. *Horm Metab Res* 2010;42(11):803–8.

9. Vacher E, Richer C, Cazaubon C, et al. Are vasopressin peripheral V1 receptors involved in the development of malignant hypertension and stroke in SHR-SPs? *Fundam Clin Pharmacol* 1995;9(5):469–78.

10. Collidge TA, Lammie GA, Fleming S, et al. The role of the renin-angiotensin system in malignant vascular injury affecting the systemic and cerebral circulations. *Prog Biophys Mol Biol* 2004;84(2–3):301–19.

11. Montgomery HE, Kiernan LA, Whitworth CE, et al. Inhibition of tissue angiotensin converting enzyme activity prevents malignant hypertension in TGR(mREN2)27. *J Hypertens* 1998;16(5):635–43.

12. Mullins JJ, Peters J, Ganten D. Fulminant hypertension in transgenic rats harbouring the mouse Ren-2 gene. *Nature* 1990;344(6266):541–4.

13. Ganten D, Wagner J, Zeh K, et al. Species specificity of renin kinetics in transgenic rats harboring the human renin and angiotensinogen genes. *Proc Natl Acad Sci U S A* 1992;89(16):7806–10.

14. Funakoshi Y, Ichiki T, Ito K, et al. Induction of interleukin-6 expression by angiotensin II in rat vascular smooth muscle cells. *Hypertension* 1999;34(1):118–25.

15. Muller DN, Dechend R, Mervaala EM, et al. NF-kappaB inhibition ameliorates angiotensin II-induced inflammatory damage in rats. *Hypertension* 2000;35(1 Pt 2):193–201.

16. Wallach R, Karp RB, Reves JG, et al. Pathogenesis of paroxysmal hypertension developing during and after coronary bypass surgery: A study of hemodynamic and humoral factors. *Am J Cardiol* 1980;46(4):559–65.

17. van den Born BJ, Lowenberg EC, van der Hoeven NV, et al. Endothelial dysfunction, platelet activation, thrombogenesis and fibrinolysis in patients with hypertensive crisis. *J Hypertens* 2011;29(5):922–7.

18. Han Y, Runge MS, Brasier AR. Angiotensin II induces interleukin-6 transcription in vascular smooth muscle cells through pleiotropic activation of nuclear factor-kappa B transcription factors. *Circ Res* 1999;84(6):695–703.

19. Datla SR, Griendling KK. Reactive oxygen species, NADPH oxidases, and hypertension. *Hypertension* 2010;56(3):325–30.

20. Lassegue B, Griendling KK. NADPH oxidases: Functions and pathologies in the vasculature. *Arterioscler Thromb Vasc Biol* 2010;30(4):653–61.

21. Panza JA, Quyyumi AA, Brush JE Jr, et al. Abnormal endothelium-dependent vascular relaxation in patients with essential hypertension. *N Engl J Med* 1990;323(1):22–7.

22. Hermann M, Flammer A, Luscher TF. Nitric oxide in hypertension. *J Clin Hypertens (Greenwich)* 2006;8(12 suppl 4):17–29.

23. Luscher TF, Vanhoutte PM. Endothelium-dependent contractions to acetylcholine in the aorta of the spontaneously hypertensive rat. *Hypertension* 1986;8(4):344–8.

24. Huang PL, Huang Z, Mashimo H, et al. Hypertension in mice lacking the gene for endothelial nitric oxide synthase. *Nature* 1995;377(6546):239–42.

25. Arnal JF, el Amrani AI, Chatellier G, et al. Cardiac weight in hypertension induced by nitric oxide synthase blockade. *Hypertension* 1993;22(3):380–7.

26. Podjarny E, Hasdan G, Bernheim J, et al. Effect of chronic tetrahydrobiopterin supplementation on blood pressure and proteinuria in 5/6 nephrectomized rats. *Nephrol Dial Transplant* 2004;19(9):2223–7.

27. Fortepiani LA, Reckelhoff JF. Treatment with tetrahydrobiopterin reduces blood pressure in male SHR by reducing testosterone synthesis. *Am J Physiol Regul Integr Comp Physiol* 2005;288(3):R733–6.

28. Ozkor MA, Quyyumi AA. Endothelium-derived hyperpolarizing factor and vascular function. *Cardiol Res Pract* 2011; 2011:156146.

29. Tanaka Y, Yamaki F, Koike K, et al. New insights into the intracellular mechanisms by which PGI2 analogues elicit vascular relaxation: Cyclic AMP-independent, Gs-protein mediated-activation of MaxiK channel. *Curr Med Chem Cardiovasc Hematol Agents* 2004;2(3):257–65.

30. Strandgaard S, Paulson OB. Cerebral blood flow in untreated and treated hypertension. *Neth J Med* 1995;47(4):180–4.

31. Strandgaard S. Autoregulation of cerebral blood flow in hypertensive patients. The modifying influence of prolonged antihypertensive treatment on the tolerance to acute, drug-induced hypotension. *Circulation* 1976;53(4):720–7.

32. MacKenzie ET, Strandgaard S, Graham DI, et al. Effects of acutely induced hypertension in cats on pial arteriolar caliber, local cerebral blood flow, and the blood–brain barrier. *Circ Res* 1976;39(1):33–41.

33. Smeda JS, Payne GW. Alterations in autoregulatory and myogenic function in the cerebrovasculature of Dahl salt-sensitive rats. *Stroke* 2003;34(6):1484–90.

34. Flynn JT, Tullus K. Severe hypertension in children and adolescents: Pathophysiology and treatment. *Pediatr Nephrol* 2009;24(6): 1101–12.

35. Immink RV, van den Born BJ, van Montfrans GA, et al. Impaired cerebral autoregulation in patients with malignant hypertension. *Circulation* 2004;110(15):2241–5.

36. Schneider JP, Krohmer S, Günther A, et al. Cerebral lesions in acute arterial hypertension: The characteristic MRI in hypertensive encephalopathy. *Rofo* 2006;178(6):618–26.

37. McKinney AM, Short J, Truwit CL, et al. Posterior reversible encephalopathy syndrome: Incidence of atypical regions of involvement and imaging findings. *AJR Am J Roentgenol* 2007;189(4):904–12.

38. Strandgaard S, Paulson OB. Cerebral autoregulation. *Stroke* 1984;15(3):413–6.

39. Toro-Salazar OH, Steinberger J, Thomas W, et al. Long-term follow-up of patients after coarctation of the aorta repair. *Am J Cardiol* 2002;89(5):541–7.

40. Fawzy ME, Sivanandam V, Pieters F, et al. Long-term effects of balloon angioplasty on systemic hypertension in adolescent and adult patients with coarctation of the aorta. *Eur Heart J* 1999;20(11):827–32.

41. Leenen FHH, Balfe JA, Pelech AN, et al. Postoperative hypertension after repair of coarctation of aorta in children: Protective effect of propranolol? *Am Heart J* 1987;113(5):1164–73.

42. Hartmann A, Buttinger C, Rommel T, et al. Alteration of intracranial pressure, cerebral blood flow, autoregulation and carbondioxide-reactivity by hypotensive agents in baboons with intracranial hypertension. *Neurochirurgia (Stuttg)* 1989; 32(2):37–43.

43. Hall VA, Guest JM. Sodium nitroprusside-induced cyanide intoxication and prevention with sodium thiosulfate prophylaxis. *Am J Crit Care* 1992;1(2):19–25; quiz 26–17.

44. Schulz LT, Elder EJ Jr, Jones KJ, et al. Stability of sodium nitroprusside and sodium thiosulfate 1:10 intravenous admixture. *Hosp Pharm* 2010;45(10):779–84.

45. Brogden RN, Markham A. Fenoldopam: A review of its pharmacodynamic and pharmacokinetic properties and intravenous clinical potential in the management of hypertensive urgencies and emergencies. *Drugs* 1997;54(4):634–50.

46. Devlin JW, Seta ML, Kanji S, et al. Fenoldopam versus nitroprusside for the treatment of hypertensive emergency. *Ann Pharmacother* 2004;38(5):755–9.

47. Tumlin JA, Dunbar LM, Oparil S, et al. Fenoldopam, a dopamine agonist, for hypertensive emergency: A multicenter randomized trial. Fenoldopam Study Group. *Acad Emerg Med* 2000;7(6):653–62.

48. Oparil S, Aronson S, Deeb GM, et al. Fenoldopam: A new parenteral antihypertensive: Consensus roundtable on the management of perioperative hypertension and hypertensive crises. *Am J Hypertens* 1999;12(7):653–64.

49. Murphy MB, Murray C, Shorten GD. Fenoldopam: A selective peripheral dopamine-receptor agonist for the treatment of severe hypertension. *N Engl J Med* 2001;345(21):1548–57.

50. Tobias JD. Fenoldopam for controlled hypotension during spinal fusion in children and adolescents. *Paediatr Anaesth* 2000;10(3):261–6.

51. Everitt DE, Boike SC, Piltz-Seymour JR, et al. Effect of intravenous fenoldopam on intraocular pressure in ocular hypertension. *J Clin Pharmacol* 1997;37(4):312–20.

52. Hennes HJ, Jantzen JP. Effects of fenoldopam on intracranial pressure and hemodynamic variables at normal and elevated intracranial pressure in anesthetized pigs. *J Neurosurg Anesthesiol* 1994;6(3):175–81.

53. Varon J, Marik PE. Clinical review: The management of hypertensive crises. *Crit Care* 2003;7(5):374–84.

54. Morgenstern BZ. Dosage guidelines for pediatric hypertension. *Mayo Clin Proc* 1995;70(4):406–7.

CHAPTER 113 ■ INBORN ERRORS OF METABOLISM

MICHAEL WILHELM AND WENDY K. CHUNG

General Approach to Inborn Errors of Metabolism

1 Although individually rare, inborn errors of metabolism (IEMs) are collectively common in pediatrics.

2 There should be a high index of suspicion of an IEM in patients with encephalopathy, (cardio) myopathy, hyperammonemia, hypoglycemia, or refractory metabolic acidosis.

3 Prompt initiation of specific therapy can prevent irreversible brain injury.

4 Patients with IEMs may have a number of nonmetabolic complications requiring pediatric intensive care.

Disorders Associated with Lactic Acidosis

5 Primary lactic acidemia should be suspected when a source of tissue hypoperfusion cannot be determined.

6 In disorders of oxidative phosphorylation, lactate levels may fluctuate significantly in the blood, or only be elevated in the cerebrospinal fluid.

7 In diseases of energy metabolism or hypoperfusion, the lactate-adjusted anion gap is normal while it is elevated in the organic acidemias due to the presence of other anions besides lactate.

8 A lactate-to-pyruvate ratio of greater than 25:1 suggests a defect in oxidative phosphorylation.

Metabolic Acidosis without Increased Lactate

9 These disorders should be suspected with intoxication syndromes exhibiting encephalopathy and vomiting associated with marked ketosis.

10 Extracorporeal toxin removal with hemodialysis or hemofiltration may be beneficial with severe presentations that do not respond to conservative therapies.

11 Specific supplemental vitamin/cofactor therapies are indicated in many of these disorders in addition to general management.

12 Liver (and in rare cases renal) transplantation may be beneficial in many of these disorders.

Hypoglycemia

13 Hypoglycemia (<50 mg/dL or <40 mg/dL in neonates) must be promptly treated to prevent permanent brain injury.

14 Critical samples should be obtained at the time of hypoglycemia.

15 The absence of ketones suggests inappropriate hyperinsulinism or a defect in fatty acid oxidation.

16 Hypoglycemia with fasting (often as infants begin sleeping through the night) suggests glycogen storage disorders.

17 C-peptide distinguishes endogenous hyperinsulinism from administered insulin.

Hyperammonemia

18 Hyperammonemia is one of the most critical metabolic conditions as ammonia is extremely toxic to the brain.

19 Prophylactic intubation is indicated with levels >500 μmol/L due to the risk of rapid progression to coma and respiratory depression.

20 Levels >500 μmol/L should be treated with some form of hemodialysis.

21 The more severe cases (>300 μmol/L) are typically due to urea cycle defects.

22 Initial treatment consists of making the patient NPO and making them anabolic with an appropriate glucose and electrolyte infusion.

23 In suspected urea cycle defects, L-arginine, sodium benzoate, and phenylacetate should be added empirically.

Liver Failure

24 Hepatomegaly may help distinguish metabolic causes of liver failure from infectious causes initially.

25 Initial presentation with hepatomegaly, hepatocellular injury, conjugated hyperbilirubinemia, or unconjugated hyperbilirubinemia can suggest the specific metabolic disorder.

26 Associated myopathy and cardiomyopathy suggest a defect of long-chain fatty acid oxidation.

Nonmetabolic Critical Illness in IEMs

27 IEMs can affect hepatic, renal, pulmonary, cardiovascular, and hematologic systems.

28 Certain IEMs are contraindications to specific anesthetic agents.

29 Storage diseases (i.e., the mucopolysaccharidoses) may make endotracheal intubation extremely difficult.

Inborn errors of metabolism (IEMs) result from the deficiency of any one of over 400 enzymes involved in intermediary metabolism. Although individually rare, collectively they are common in pediatrics. Many children with previously diagnosed IEMs will come to the PICU postoperatively following procedures or during an acute metabolic decompensation and will require specialized cardiorespiratory and metabolic management dictated by their underlying IEM. Other children with previously unrecognized IEMs will present in a variety of ways, including change in mental status, shock, metabolic acidosis, vomiting, failure to thrive, developmental delay, intractable seizures, liver failure, and cardiomyopathy. Therefore, pediatric intensivists must have a fundamental understanding of these conditions, including when to suspect an IEM and how to initially manage these patients. This chapter provides a basic framework for approaching the patient with a suspected IEM with particular attention given to management issues that may confront the pediatric intensivist. Because of the large number of IEMs, we present some general concepts initially followed by specific discussions of the more important individual diseases, their presentation, and treatment.

GENERAL APPROACH TO INBORN ERRORS

Pathophysiology of IEMs

Inborn errors often present with nonspecific manifestations that may culminate in critical illness, particularly in young infants or neonates. Because these disorders result from enzyme deficiencies for which 50% of normal activity is usually adequate, they are inherited predominantly in an autosomal recessive fashion. The mitochondrial genome, however, is maternally inherited and thus some mitochondrial disorders are matrilineally transmitted. Furthermore, many mitochondrial diseases depend upon the percentage of the mitochondrial population that carries the mutation (*heteroplasmy*) and therefore manifestations depend on the load of mutant mitochondria in each tissue. Thus, a given mutation may produce varying manifestations in different family members. Specific disorders with X-linked inheritance predominantly affecting males are identified in the appropriate sections.

These diseases manifest as a result of the lack of products of the deficient enzyme, accumulation of upstream metabolites, shunting of accumulated metabolites into other pathways, or some combination of the above. The pathophysiology of IEMs

presenting in the PICU can be categorized into one of the following processes: (a) intoxication from metabolites such as ammonia, amino acid derivatives, or ketoacids, (b) reduced fasting tolerance, (c) derangements of energy metabolism, (d) derangement of neurotransmission, or (e) storage of nonmetabolizable substrates in vital organs or tissues. Table 113.1 lists disorders associated with each of these categories.

Clinical Presentation and Differential Diagnosis

Historical Clues

The history and physical examination may provide clues that a patient has an IEM, though IEMs can masquerade as other causes of critical illness. Commonly, IEMs present with changes in mental status (lethargy, irritability, seizures, and coma) with or without overt cardiorespiratory compromise and can be easily confused with sepsis. Hypothermia may be associated with metabolic decompensation, especially in the urea cycle defects. Furthermore, infection often exacerbates metabolic derangements and precipitates metabolic decompensation owing to increased energy requirements and the frequent association with decreased food intake. Finally, certain IEMs make patients more susceptible to infection (*Escherichia coli* sepsis in galactosemia or neutropenia associated with organic acidurias). Therefore, empiric treatment for suspected sepsis should be initiated after obtaining appropriate cultures.

The child's history may reveal decreased oral intake, due to an intercurrent infection or fasting as an infant begins to sleep through the night. Neonates may present with failure to regain birth weight by the second week of life. The older child may present with recurrent episodes of lethargy and difficulty recovering from minor illnesses. Children of all ages often demonstrate failure to thrive. In rare cases, the specific dietary intake may suggest the diagnosis. Particular foods such as a high-protein meal may induce symptoms, including nausea in urea cycle defects. Ingestion of fruits or sweet foods containing sucrose may trigger decompensation in hereditary fructose intolerance. Children with partial enzymatic deficiencies and milder disorders may even unknowingly alter their diet to avoid foods that make them feel lethargic or ill.

A history of developmental delay, hypotonia, and/or seizures is associated with many of the IEMs. A history of developmental regression is particularly concerning and should prompt a careful search for an IEM, particularly the lysosomal storage and mitochondrial disorders.

TABLE 113.1

CATEGORIES OF INBORN ERRORS OF METABOLISM WITH ACUTE PRESENTATIONS

■ PATHOPHYSIOLOGY	■ LIKELY DISORDERS
Intoxication (encephalopathy)	Urea cycle[a], organic acidemias[a], aminoacidopathies[a]
Reduced fasting tolerance	Glycogen storage disease type I, disorders of gluconeogenesis, fatty acid oxidation defects
Impaired energy production	Mitochondrial disorders, fatty acid oxidation disorders, and disorders of the pyruvate dehydrogenase complex
Altered neurotransmission	Pyridoxine- or folinic acid–dependent epilepsy, nonketotic hyperglycinemia, sulfite oxidase deficiency
Storage disorders/complex macromolecules	MPSs, sphingolipidoses, glycogen storage diseases, peroxisomal biogenesis disorders, congenital disorders of glycosylation

[a]Diseases that may require emergent dialysis.

TABLE 113.2

ODORS ASSOCIATED WITH METABOLIC DISEASES

■ ODOR	■ ASSOCIATED INBORN ERROR(S)
Sweaty feet	Glutaric acidemia (type II), isovaleric acidemia
Maple syrup	MSUD
Mousy	Phenylketonuria
Boiled cabbage	Hypermethioninemia, tyrosinemia type I
Swimming pool	Hawkinsinuria
Rotten fish	Trimethylaminuria, dimethylglycinuria

Features of the family history may suggest a metabolic disease, including parental consanguinity, ethnicity of the patient (hepatorenal tyrosinemia in French Canadians and maple syrup urine disease in Pennsylvania Amish), fetal demise, unexplained deaths or sudden infant death syndrome, developmental delay, seizures, failure to thrive or other unexplained chronic illness. Although the prenatal history is often unremarkable, a history of maternal liver disease or HELLP syndrome may suggest a long-chain fatty acid oxidation disorder. The sex of the patient is relevant in a small number of IEMs that are X linked, such as the urea cycle defect ornithine transcarbamylase deficiency, the carbohydrate defect pyruvate dehydrogenase deficiency E1α, and the defect of the nucleotide salvage pathway Lesch–Nyhan disease.

Physical Examination Findings

On physical examination, the presence of an unusual body or urine odor might suggest a specific organic acidemia (**Table 113.2**), but these odors can be subtle and their absence should not dissuade pursuit of an IEM. Careful attention should be paid to the respiratory pattern (tachypnea may herald sepsis with acute respiratory distress syndrome, Kussmaul respirations occur with metabolic acidosis). It is important to remember, that Kussmaul respirations can be difficult to discern in neonates and other patients with restrictive lung disease.

Progressive hepatosplenomegaly occurs in a number of IEMs as nonmetabolizable substrate accumulates in glycogen storage disorders and lysosomal storage disorders. Dysmorphic features are present at birth in a number of peroxisomal biogenesis disorders, fatty acid oxidation disorders, congenital disorders of glycosylation, and pyruvate dehydrogenase deficiency while they develop progressively over time in the mucopolysaccharidoses (MPSs) as storage material accumulates in the soft tissues and bones. Smith–Lemli–Opitz syndrome, a defect in sterol biosynthesis, may present with ambiguous genitalia and 2/3 toe syndactyly. Ophthalmologic examination may also provide clues to an IEM with cataracts observed in galactosemia and retinal pigmentary changes in Tay Sachs disease and in some of the mitochondrial disorders.

Myopathy demonstrated by hypotonia or cardiomyopathy (hypertrophic or dilated) possibly detected by a heart murmur or signs of heart failure may herald a disorder of fatty acid oxidation, mitochondrial derangement, glycogen storage disorder, or rarely a congenital disorder of glycosylation. IEMs are important causes of cardiomyopathy to exclude in children since these can be treated and in some cases cured such as in the case of Pompe disease.

Laboratory Findings

Routine laboratory test results may suggest an IEM (**Tables 113.3** and **113.4**). A primary respiratory alkalosis may be found with hyperammonemia caused by a urea cycle defect. A metabolic acidosis, particularly with an elevation in anion gap (AG) or in lactate occurs in certain IEMs, though this may also occur in other diseases such as sepsis or hypoperfusion. Children with elevated lactate due to hypoperfusion usually appear quite ill, whereas patients with an IEM may have lactate elevations out of proportion to their degree of illness. The *lactate-adjusted AG* is calculated by subtracting the lactate level (in mmol/L) from the AG and can provide clues to the etiology. In diseases of energy metabolism or hypoperfusion, the lactate-adjusted AG is normal while it is elevated in the organic acidemias due to the presence of other anions besides lactate. The *lactate-to-pyruvate ratio* is also helpful, with normal levels being about 20 when both concentrations are expressed in mmol/L. A consistent ratio <10 suggests a pyruvate dehydrogenase deficiency, which has important therapeutic implications, whereas a consistent ratio >25 occurs in tissue hypoxia, pyruvate carboxylase deficiency, and mitochondrial disorders.

Hypoglycemia may occur in sepsis, liver disease, or any other severe illness (particularly in neonates with limited ability to mobilize glycogen stores). In the setting of other clinical and laboratory findings listed here, hypoglycemia is much more likely to indicate an IEM. The relationship of hypoglycemia to feeding can be helpful in identifying a specific disease. Hypoglycemia that occurs immediately after the ingestion of fructose (fruit or foods containing sucrose) suggests hereditary fructose intolerance and is usually detected when an infant transitions to solid foods. The presence of reducing substance in the urine is further evidence for hereditary fructose intolerance. In most other IEMs, including the glycogen storage diseases, fatty acid oxidation defects, disorders of gluconeogenesis, and some organic acidemias, hypoglycemia occurs with fasting.

The presence or absence of ketones further narrows the differential diagnosis. Normally, in the setting of hypoglycemia, the liver mobilizes ketone bodies as an alternative energy substrate. Therefore, nonketotic hypoglycemia suggests a defect in fatty acid oxidation or ketogenesis. Although normal neonates effectively generate 3-hydroxybutyrate, they have a limited

TABLE 113.3

LABORATORY EVALUATION OF A SUSPECTED INBORN ERROR OF METABOLISM

	■ BLOOD TESTS	■ URINE TESTS	■ CSF TESTS
Initial studies	Blood gas, glucose, electrolytes, basic metabolic panel, ammonia, lactate, pyruvate, β-hydroxybutyrate, transaminases, blood count, coagulation profile, creatinine kinase	Ketones, pH, reducing substances	As indicated
Further workup	Plasma amino acids, plasma acylcarnitine profile, carnitine	Organic acids, amino acids	

TABLE 113.4

RESULTS OF INITIAL LABORATORY TESTS IN INBORN ERRORS OF METABOLISMS

	■ UREA CYCLE DEFECT	■ AMINO ACIDOPATHY	■ ORGANIC ACIDURIA	■ FATTY ACID OXIDATION DISORDER	■ CARBOHYDRATE METABOLISM	■ ELECTRON TRANSPORT CHAIN
Blood pH	↑	↓/–	↓	↓/–	↓	↓
AG	WNL	↑/–	↑	↑/–	↑	↑
Glucose	WNL	+/–	WNL	↓↓	↓↓	+/–
Ammonia	↑↑	WNL	↑	↑	WNL	WNL
Lactate	WNL	WNL	↑/–	WNL	↑	↑↑
Ketones	Neg	↑	↑	↓↓	↑	Neg
LFTs	WNL	WNL	WNL	↑	↑	WNL
Serum amino acids	Abnormal	Abnormal	Abnormal	WNL	WNL	Alanine high
Urine organic acids	Some abnormal	Abnormal	Abnormal	Abnormal	WNL	Lactate in urine
Urine reducing substances	–	–	–	–	+/–	–

WNL, within normal limits; Neg, negative.

capacity to generate acetoacetate. Because urine dipsticks detect only acetoacetate, *serum 3-hydroxybutyrate* levels must be evaluated in the hypoglycemic infant. Conversely, a positive urine dip for ketones in the first month is always abnormal and suggests an organic acidemia or inability to utilize ketone bodies (1). Elevated ketone levels in the nonfasting/nonhypoglycemic patient suggest an organic acidemia or maple syrup urine disease (MSUD).

Evidence of hepatic injury or dysfunction (elevation of transaminases, hyperammonemia, and coagulopathy) provides another clue to a possible IEM. Although hyperammonemia may occur in liver injury owing to sepsis and toxins, levels greater than 400 μmol/L suggest a urea cycle defect and require swift and aggressive intervention to prevent irreversible brain damage. Disorders of mitochondrial metabolism, fatty acid oxidation disorders, and the organic acidemias may all cause secondary hyperammonemia because of interactions between these pathways and the urea cycle within the mitochondria. However, in these disorders, ammonia is elevated to a much lesser degree than the urea cycle defects. In the setting of severe decompensation, a number of IEMs may present with elevated transaminases and coagulopathy. Mitochondrial disorders, neonatal hemochromatosis, Wilson disease, hepatorenal tyrosinemia, galactosemia, Crigler–Najjar syndrome, and Niemann–Pick disease may all present with prominent liver injury.

Although individually each of the above historical, physical, or laboratory findings may occur in a number of disease states, the combination of several of these features increases the likelihood that a given patient has an IEM. In addition to supporting the diagnosis of an IEM, these initial labs help point to specific etiologies (Fig. 113.1). Once an IEM is suspected, specific metabolic tests should be performed, including urine organic acids, plasma amino acids, plasma carnitine levels, and acylcarnitine profile as well as specific tests depending on the suggested diagnoses. The samples for metabolites should be obtained before therapy because pathognomonic metabolites may clear rapidly with resuscitative therapy. Definitive diagnosis beginning with the biochemical signature of the above tests often requires tissue for enzymatic assays and/or molecular

genetic testing and may require several weeks to months for complete evaluation. Molecular genetic testing for panels of genes (mitochondrial disorders, congenital disorders of glycosylation, and glycogen storage disorders) is available to facilitate making the definitive diagnosis.

Clinical Management Principles

As in all cases, initial management begins with provision of adequate respiratory and circulatory support. As will be discussed later in this chapter, securing the airway may require advanced techniques in certain patients with storage diseases such as the MPSs. A number of complications of IEMs may require respiratory support. Encephalopathy may render a patient unable to protect their airway. With profound metabolic acidosis, even with adequate energy production, patients may not maintain an adequate minute ventilation, particularly during infancy. In older children capable of generating large tidal volumes, it may be difficult to maintain an equivalent minute ventilation after administering neuromuscular blockade. Acute worsening of acidosis may necessitate treatment of its complications (i.e., hyperkalemia, worsened cardiovascular function).

Because many of these diseases are associated with emesis and anorexia, patients often present with dehydration. Care must be exerted, however, in volume resuscitation of patients who may have a complicating cardiomyopathy or cerebral edema. Obviously, rapid correction of hypoglycemia requires a bolus of dextrose (2–4 cc/kg of 25% dextrose solution). Furthermore, if an IEM is strongly suspected, all patients should be made NPO and given sufficient intravenous glucose (~10 mg/kg/min or 6 cc/kg/h of a 10% dextrose solution) to prevent catabolism of amino acids and fatty acids, which may increase the production of abnormal metabolic products. Rarely glucose will exacerbate a lactic acidosis, suggesting an error in the pyruvate dehydrogenase complex, in which case changing to a ketogenic diet will improve the metabolic acidosis. The ketogenic diet has even been used successfully in the setting of coincident diabetes and pyruvate dehydrogenase deficiency (2).

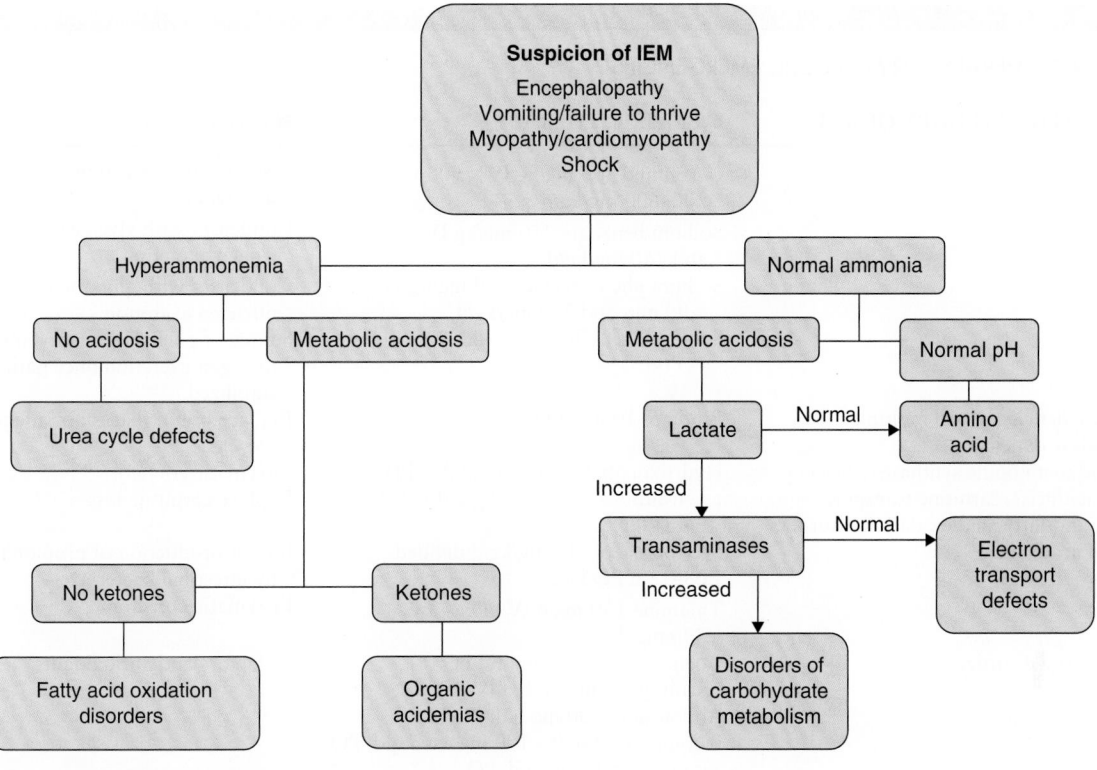

FIGURE 113.1. Categorization of IEMs based on laboratory results.

Older patients with intoxication syndromes may present with cerebral edema and are at greater risk for intracranial hypertension during therapy than neonates since their sutures are closed. Management of the cerebral edema is discussed more extensively in Chapter 61. Intravenous fluids must provide adequate sodium to prevent hyponatremia, which could exacerbate this situation.

Disease-specific therapies must sometimes be initiated empirically prior to obtaining a specific metabolic diagnosis. These will be discussed in the sections pertaining to each category of defect. However, in diseases in which symptoms result from toxic metabolic intermediates (**Table 113.1**), specifically in the setting of hyperammonemia in urea cycle defects or elevated plasma leucine levels in MSUD, direct elimination of these toxins is crucial and must be done quickly to prevent irreversible brain damage. Initial approaches included exchange transfusion with or without peritoneal dialysis (PD), with PD superior to exchange transfusion alone (3,4). Continuous venovenous hemofiltration and dialysis (CVVHD) has become the method of choice when available (5,6). Schaefer et al. (7) showed that CVVHD clears ammonia more rapidly than PD in neonates and is particularly more rapid at clearing elevated leucine levels. Optimal clearance depends on high blood flow rates (and hence catheter size) and dialysis rate (7). In many patients, they were able to achieve clearance rates similar to intermittent hemodialysis without the rebound hyperammonemia seen following that therapy. Importantly, they also showed that rapid elimination of ammonia or leucine correlated with improved neurodevelopmental outcome. Hemofiltration and dialysis have even been used successfully in patients with IEMs requiring ECMO support (8). However, no controlled trials have determined that dialysis improves outcomes and, given the attendant risks, dialysis is typically reserved for patients in coma who do not rapidly respond to

other therapies. Furthermore, dialysis promotes clearance of other amino acids, which can prevent the establishment of an anabolic state in some cases (9).

Another category of diseases that requires brief mention here are those that produce neonatal epileptic encephalopathy. In this setting, a trial of intravenous pyridoxine and folinic acid may produce rapid and dramatic improvement. A number of metabolic diseases require supplementation of specific vitamins or cofactors. Given the low toxicity of these agents, they should be initiated before confirmation of a definitive diagnosis if the specific disease is within the differential diagnosis. General recommendations for empiric therapy on the basis of suspected disease category are given in **Table 113.5**. In all cases, early involvement of a metabolic disease specialist ensures optimal management of these complex patients.

Postmortem Evaluation

Unfortunately some patients with a suspected IEM will die despite aggressive therapy prior to establishing a specific diagnosis. In this setting, making a postmortem diagnosis can have significant implications for the patient's siblings and for genetic counseling of the parents. Therefore, obtaining appropriate specimens for analysis is crucial; 5–10 mL of plasma should be collected in a lithium or sodium heparin tube, separated, and frozen at −70°C. An additional sample of blood should be collected in ethylenediaminetetraacetic acid and stored at room temperature for up to several days for DNA extraction for future genetic analysis. With advances in molecular genetic testing including whole-exome and whole-genome sequencing, samples as a source of DNA have become critical to making a definitive diagnosis.

The earliest sample of urine obtained during the illness should be frozen, as should several milliliters of cerebrospinal

TABLE 113.5

SUPPLEMENTAL THERAPY FOR METABOLIC EMERGENCIES

■ SUSPECTED CATEGORY OF IEM	■ EMPIRIC THERAPY	■ RATIONALE
Urea cycle	L-Arginine 600 mg/kg IV >90 min and 200–600 mg/kg/d	Essential amino acid in all but arginase deficiency
	Sodium benzoate 250 mg/kg IV >90 min and 250 mg/kg/d	Condenses with glycine to enhance nitrogen excretion
	Sodium phenylacetate 250 mg/kg IV >90 min and 250 mg/kg/d	Condenses with glutamine to enhance nitrogen excretion
	Sodium phenylbutyrate 100–200 mg/kg PO tid	Source of phenylacetate to enhance nitrogen excretion once patient is stabilized
Biotinidase deficiency and multiple carboxylase deficiency	Biotin 5–10 mg/d PO	Replace biotin that is not adequately recycled
MMA and methionine synthase deficiency	Hydroxocobalamin 1–5 mg/d IM/IV	Enzymatic cofactor
Organic acidurias, carnitine transport defects, and fatty acid oxidation disorders	L-Carnitine 50–100 mg/kg/d divided bid IV/PO	Replace carnitine losses
Propionic academia	Metronidazole 15 mg/kg/d divided q8–12 h PO/IV	Inhibit production of propionate by intestinal bacteria
MSUD	Thiamine 150 mg/d IV/PO; >3 y 300 mg/d	Enzymatic cofactor
Mitochondrial disorders	Coenzyme Q10 25 mg tid PO Carnitine 50 mg/kg bid IV/PO Alipoic acid 100 mg q.d. PO/IV B complex vitamins 100 mg each q.d. PO Vitamin E 50 units q.d. PO	Cofactors and antioxidants
Ketotic hyperglycinemia	Sodium benzoate 250 mg/kg IV >90 min and 250 mg/kg/d	Condenses with glycine to enhance nitrogen excretion

fluid (CSF). Tissue samples should ideally be obtained as part of a complete autopsy. However, selected tissues can be helpful if the family refuses autopsy. A punch skin biopsy should be obtained pre- or postmortem for a fibroblast culture for enzymatic testing. Postmortem kidney, liver, muscle, and cardiac biopsies should also be performed. Tissues should ideally be obtained as soon as possible after death to preserve enzymatic activity and should be immediately frozen in liquid nitrogen and stored at −70°C. Samples of bile may also provide important information. Again, consultation with a metabolic specialist and careful discussion with the pathologist are extremely important.

Impact of Neonatal Screening

Newborn screening programs have existed in the United States for more than 40 years and are administered on a state level. Although there can be differences in the disorders screened from state to state, since the consensus recommendation of the American College of Medical Genetics all babies born in the United States are screened for the minimum 29 recommended disorders (http://mchb.hrsa.gov/programs/newbornscreening/index.html). A number of online resources will identify the tests currently performed in any given state (http://genes-r-us.uthscsa.edu/). With the widespread use of tandem mass spectrometry, the number of identifiable IEMs has increased dramatically. The results of the child's newborn screening results should be obtained if an IEM is suspected. At the same time, however, a normal neonatal screening test does not exclude the possibility of an IEM in a critically ill patient since not all IEMs can be screened by this methodology, and in some cases deranged metabolism will be periodic with fluctuations in energy requirements.

DISORDERS ASSOCIATED WITH LACTIC ACIDOSIS

Symptoms of lactic acidosis include poor feeding, failure to thrive, lethargy, change in mental status, seizures, hypotonia, ataxia, developmental delay, optic nerve atrophy, deafness, and dysfunction of the most energy-dependent organs (brain, heart, muscle, kidney, and liver). As a general rule, the greater the number of systems involved, the greater the likelihood of a mitochondrial disorder of oxidative phosphorylation. The family history may suggest an IEM when there have been previously affected children within the nuclear family, or similarly but more or less severely affected individuals on the maternal side of the family due to mutations in the maternally transmitted, mitochondrial-encoded genes.

Lactic acidosis results from accumulation of pyruvate, which is converted into lactic acid and alanine. *Primary* lactic acidemia results from defects in either gluconeogenesis or oxidative phosphorylation. Definitive diagnoses of the IEMs causing primary lactic acidosis are often challenging and frequently require tissue biopsies for enzymatic analysis in specialized laboratories and/or genetic testing. Treatment in these cases is often started empirically prior to a definitive diagnosis.

Secondary lactic acidemia results from either anaerobic metabolism or other IEMs that produce less significant degrees of lactic acidosis, often detectable only during an acute metabolic crisis. Secondary lactic acidemia is a consequence of decreased flux through oxidative phosphorylation due to tissue hypoxia or hypoperfusion. Within the intensive care setting, causes of secondary lactic acidemia are much more common than primary etiologies. Many conditions in the PICU promote tissue hypoxia or hypoperfusion sufficient to cause lactic acidosis. In addition, liver injury or malperfusion prevents the normal conversion of lactate into pyruvate. One must, however, be cautious because severe metabolic decompensation due to an IEM can also be associated with cardiopulmonary failure. Therefore, IEMs should always be considered when ⑤ the underlying cause of tissue hypoxia is unknown. The differential diagnosis of IEMs causing secondary lactic acidosis includes many of the organic acidemias (propionic acidemia and methylmalonic acidemia [MMA]), which are associated with accumulation of other acids to a greater extent than lactate and can be readily identified by analyzing urine for organic acids. Definitive diagnoses of the IEMs causing primary lactic acidosis are often challenging and frequently require tissue biopsies for enzymatic analysis in specialized laboratories and/ or molecular genetic testing. Treatment in these cases is often started empirically prior to a definitive diagnosis.

The first step in investigating lactic acidemia is ensuring that the lactic acid is truly elevated. The levels of lactic acid can be artifactually elevated by use of a tourniquet, difficulty obtaining the blood sample, or prolonged time between sample collection and analysis. A primary lactic acidemia is strongly suggested by a significant elevation of lactate (>3–5 mmol/L or greater than twice the normal laboratory level). Arterial or free-flowing venous blood from a catheter should be obtained as venous samples distal to a tourniquet can have falsely elevated lactate levels. Consideration should be given to measuring lactic acid from the CSF if any neurological symptoms are present even without elevated plasma lactate. Fluctuations in levels of lactate with fasting may suggest the underlying etiology. Lactate is most elevated after a prolonged fast in disorders of gluconeogenesis (*fructose bisphosphatase deficiency*), and provocative, carefully monitored fasting studies may be necessary to evaluate these diagnoses. In the setting of a fasting-induced lactic acidosis, measurement of biotinidase can identify readily treatable cases of *biotinidase deficiency*. In other cases of gluconeogenic defects, the patient should be treated by avoiding fasting.

In defects of oxidative phosphorylation, lactate levels may fluctuate significantly in the blood or may only be elevated in ⑥ the CSF. Simultaneous measurement of pyruvate allows determination of the lactate-to-pyruvate ratio. The ratio of lactate to pyruvate reflects the redox potential of the cell and ratios greater than 25 suggest a defect in mitochondrial oxidative ⑧ phosphorylation. Repeated simultaneous measurements of lactate and pyruvate and their relative ratios are often helpful to establish a consistent ratio. Measuring alanine in the blood and CSF also allows for an independent, indirect measurement of defective pyruvate metabolism and is not subject to the same difficulties in measurement as lactate. If a defect in mitochondrial oxidative phosphorylation is suspected, a muscle biopsy should be performed to look for ragged red fibers and to biochemically assess the respiratory chain complexes. In addition, specific genetic testing for conditions such as *MELAS (Mitochondrial Encephalopathy, Lactic Acidosis and Stroke)* and *MERRF (Mitochondrial Encephalopathy with Ragged Red Fibers)* is available. Complete mitochondrial sequencing and deletion analysis as well as sequencing for over 100 nuclear genes involved in oxidative phosphorylation are available; this analysis can be performed on a blood sample and avoid the need for a biopsy. Defects of the *pyruvate dehydrogenase complex* should be treated with a high-fat, low-carbohydrate diet and supplementation with thiamine and lipoic acid. Most of the other mitochondrial defects of oxidative phosphorylation are difficult to treat but can be empirically treated with thiamine, riboflavin, nicotinamide, vitamin E, and coenzyme Q10 while a definitive diagnosis is being established (**Table 113.5**). Sodium bicarbonate can be used to correct the metabolic acidosis, but will not decrease lactic acid production. Experimentally, dichloroacetate (DCA) has been used to treat lactic acidosis and works by activating the pyruvate dehydrogenase

complex (10). In most cases, however, DCA is not appropriate for long-term clinical care outside study protocols because it is still investigational and has been associated with toxic neuropathy.

METABOLIC ACIDOSIS WITHOUT INCREASED LACTATE

Although any metabolic disease may present with modest lactic acidosis during an acute decompensation because of the associated dehydration or hypoperfusion, the organic acidemias and aminoacidopathies typically present with an AG acidosis due to accumulation of the abnormal organic acids or ketoacids, but the AG is *not* predominantly due to elevated lactate. As mentioned above, the lactate-adjusted AG is abnormal in these conditions. Many of these disorders present with significant ketoacidosis, though some (*3-hydroxy-3-methylglutaric aciduria* and *acyl-CoA dehydrogenase deficiency*) do not. Classically the organic acidurias present as massive ketosis and ⑨ metabolic acidosis in a vomiting or lethargic neonate. Making the initial diagnosis of these disorders typically depends upon determination of urine organic acids and serum amino acids, often by mass spectrometry. These disorders are included in the recommended list of IEMs for inclusion in newborn screening programs. In most of these disorders, chronic treatment requires carefully balanced protein intake to provide an adequate supply of essential amino acids while minimizing the load of precursors that cannot be metabolized.

The most common disorders within this category are MSUD, MMA, and propionic acidemia. Most of these disorders present as intoxication syndromes with episodes of encephalopathy and vomiting, particularly during periods of catabolic stress. Thus, they tend to present during the early neonatal period in an infant who initially appears well or during an intercurrent illness. The age-specific differential diagnosis for metabolic acidosis without elevated plasma lactate is given in **Table 113.6**. Because intoxication plays a central role, extracorporeal toxin removal with hemodialysis or hemofiltration may be useful in the acute management of some of these conditions including MSUD when the patient presents with ⑩ neurologic deterioration. Hemodialysis and CVVH/CVVHD have been shown to promote rapid lowering of branched-chain amino acids, particularly when combined with appropriate enteral feeds.

MSUD is a disorder of metabolism of the essential, branched-chain amino acids (BCAAs), valine, leucine, and isoleucine. Normally, the enzyme complex *branched-chain α-ketoacid dehydrogenase*, which requires thiamine pyrophosphate as a coenzyme, decarboxylates all three BCAAs. Infants with the *classic* form present in the first few days of life with

TABLE 113.6

AGE-SPECIFIC DIFFERENTIAL DIAGNOSIS OF METABOLIC ACIDOSIS WITHOUT INCREASED LACTATE

■ AGE AT PRESENTATION	■ METABOLIC DERANGEMENT
Neonate	MSUD, isovaleric acidemia, glutaric acidemia type II, multiple carboxylase deficiency
Infant	MSUD, MMA, propionic acidemia, ketotic hyperglycinemia, biotinidase deficiency
Older children	Biotinidase deficiency, dietary biotin deficiency

vomiting, encephalopathy, and severe metabolic acidosis. The characteristic odor of urine, sweat, and cerumen can provide an important clue to the diagnosis. MSUD has an increased incidence in the Old Order Amish and Mennonites (11) and Ashkenazi Jewish populations (12). Milder forms, with greater residual enzyme activity may present later in life during stress (infection, surgery) in a child with mild developmental delay or failure to thrive. Acute episodes in these nonclassical forms are indistinguishable from those of classic MSUD. Some patients respond dramatically to thiamine supplementation, which should be started empirically in all patients upon presentation.

Isovaleric acidemia results from a deficiency of *isovaleryl CoA dehydrogenase*, which is further down the leucine degradative pathway. The acute form presents much like MSUD, though these patients have a characteristic odor of sweaty socks and may have associated neutropenia.

Propionic acid and *methylmalonic acid* are sequential catabolic products of isoleucine and valine as well as threonine, methionine, cholesterol, and odd-chain fatty acids. Deficiency of the enzymes responsible for their catabolism (*propionyl-CoA carboxylase* and *methylmalonyl CoA mutase*, respectively) results in *ketotic hyperglycinemia*. Because methylmalonyl CoA mutase requires adenosylcobalamin (a metabolite of *vitamin B12*) as a coenzyme, disorders of cobalamin metabolism may also result in secondary MMA. These conditions all present with vomiting, severe ketoacidosis, encephalopathy progressing to coma, and neutropenia. Because of the secondary inhibition of the urea cycle, moderate to severe hyperammonemia may also occur. In addition to supportive care, constipation should be prevented or treated and sterilization of the intestinal tract with metronidazole initiated to minimize production of propionic acid by intestinal bacteria. Carnitine supplementation (50–100 mg/kg/day IV or PO) replaces losses due to propionyl carnitine formation and hastens resolution of metabolic acidosis. Because propionic acidemia may occur as part of *multiple carboxylase deficiency* (see below), biotin (10 mg/day PO) should be provided until a definitive diagnosis is established. Similarly, large doses of cobalamin (1–2 mg/day IV) should be provided to patients with suspected MMA.

Several other IEMs may present primarily with metabolic acidosis, ketosis, and an intoxication syndrome. These include disorders affecting the four *biotin-dependent carboxylases* (acetyl-CoA carboxylase, methylcrotonyl-CoA carboxylase, propionyl-CoA carboxylase, and pyruvate carboxylase). Deficiency of *holocarboxylase synthetase*, which catalyzes the binding of biotin to all the carboxylases, results in the most severe disorder and presents in the first few weeks of life. These patients have rashes that mimic eczema and a tomcat urine odor in addition to the above metabolic derangements. *Biotinidase deficiency* presents similarly in older infants and children, and may be associated with an eczematoid rash. Dietary biotin deficiency may occur in short gut syndrome, inadequate supplementation in parenteral nutrition, prolonged anticonvulsant therapy (13), and significant raw egg consumption. Biotinidase deficiency and acquired biotin deficiency both respond well to biotin supplementation (10 mg/day PO) and can be cured with this simple therapy.

Novel Therapies

Liver transplantation has been performed in more than 50 patients with MSUD (14,15) and provides improved dietary protein tolerance and apparent elimination of episodic decompensations (16). Despite increasing long-term follow-up showing excellent graft and patient survival (15), insufficient data exist to determine whether the risks and costs of this procedure outweigh the benefits. Liver transplantation, including living-donor transplantation (17) (with simultaneous renal

transplant in MMA (18)), has been performed in a small number of patients with other organic acidemias (19). Although initial results suggested an improvement, long-term prognosis remains guarded as, unfortunately, many children develop irreversible neurocognitive deficits prior to transplantation. However, transplantation is increasingly used for patients with recurrent metabolic decompensations inadequately controlled with medical therapies.

HYPOGLYCEMIA

Children with hypoglycemia may present with diaphoresis, pallor, irritability, decreased feeding, jitteriness, temperature instability, lethargy, coma, or seizure. Hypoglycemia must be promptly recognized and treated to prevent damage to the brain. Severe and/or recurrent hypoglycemia can result in permanent brain damage producing a range of injuries, including global mental retardation, behavioral problems and attention deficit disorder, and occipital blindness.

Hypoglycemia is defined as a serum concentration of less than 50 mg/dL or a whole-blood concentration of less than 45 mg/dL. Historically, some neonatologists defined hypoglycemia in a term infant as <35 mg/dL, or less than 25 mg/dL in the preterm infant. However, it is advisable to maintain glucose concentrations greater than at least 40 mg/dL even in a neonate. A patient can appear artifactually hypoglycemic if the blood has been sitting for several hours. Therefore, hypoglycemia should be confirmed with the bedside glucometer reading and a laboratory measurement requested "stat."

Hypoglycemia must be treated promptly and continuously reassessed. Recurrent hypoglycemia is more likely to suggest a serious underlying disorder that will require definitive diagnosis and treatment. Acute treatment in the intensive care setting consists of a bolus of intravenous dextrose, 0.5–1 g/kg given as a 10%–25% solution followed by continuous dextrose infusion to maintain a glucose concentration >70 mg/dL (usually 3–5 mg/kg/min in older children and 5–10 mg/kg/min in neonates). An intravenous line should be in place at all times, and glucose should be monitored at least every 4 hours to ensure normoglycemia.

Although sometimes difficult, it is diagnostically ideal to evaluate the etiology at the time of hypoglycemia (**Fig. 113.2**). **Table 113.7** lists common etiologies of hypoglycemia. It is essential to evaluate the metabolic status by obtaining the "critical sample" as discussed in Chapter 106 during the time of derangement to produce the maximal diagnostic yield. If it is not possible to obtain the critical samples at the time of hypoglycemia, carefully monitored fasting and glucagon challenge studies can be performed later to attempt to replicate the hypoglycemia and obtain critical samples at that time. At the time of hypoglycemia, it is necessary to evaluate the hormonal response, including insulin, growth hormone, and cortisol as well as alternate metabolic substrates, including the appropriate production of ketone bodies. The critical sample should consist of glucose, insulin, growth hormone, cortisol, serum chemistries, liver function tests (LFTs), ammonia, β-hydroxybutyrate, acetoacetate, free fatty acids, and lactate. Insulin measured at the time of hypoglycemia should normally be extremely low or undetectable. Additionally, ketone bodies and free fatty acids should be extremely elevated in the normal physiologic response to hypoglycemia. Failure to appropriately produce ketone bodies during hypoglycemia suggests either inappropriate hyperinsulinemia or a defect in the oxidation of fatty acids or ketone body production. Fatty acid oxidation disorders can then further be evaluated with an acylcarnitine profile, free and total carnitine, urine organic acids, and urine acylglycines.

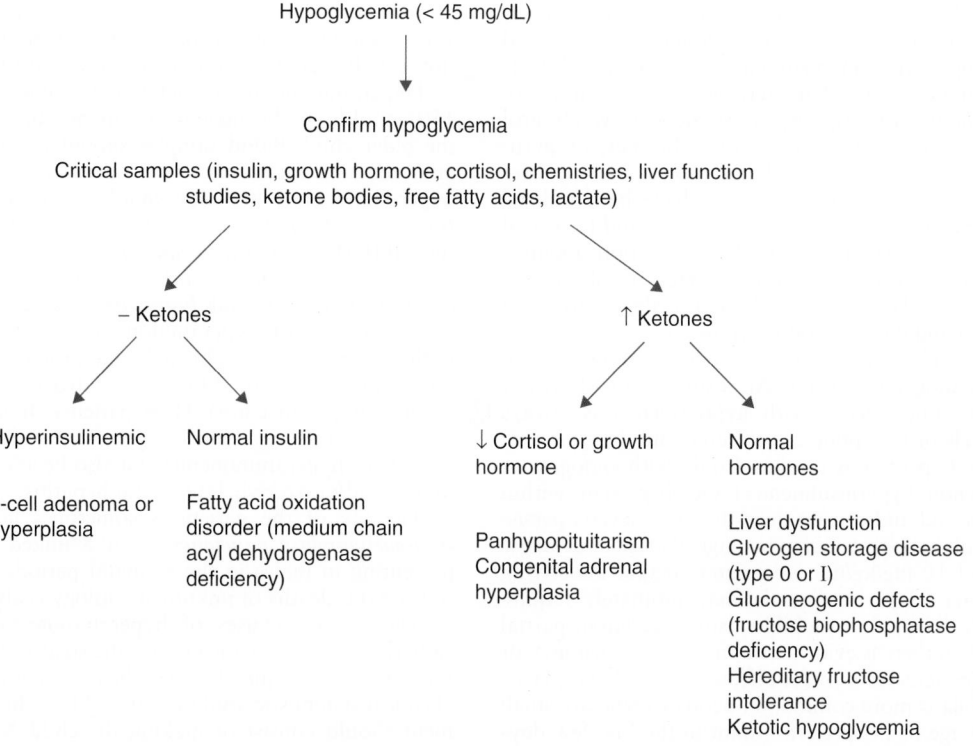

Hypoglycemia (< 45 mg/dL)

↓

Confirm hypoglycemia

Critical samples (insulin, growth hormone, cortisol, chemistries, liver function
studies, ketone bodies, free fatty acids, lactate)

− Ketones   ↑ Ketones

Hyperinsulinemic   Normal insulin   ↓ Cortisol or growth hormone   Normal hormones

β-cell adenoma or hyperplasia   Fatty acid oxidation disorder (medium chain acyl dehydrogenase deficiency)   Panhypopituitarism Congenital adrenal hyperplasia   Liver dysfunction Glycogen storage disease (type 0 or I) Gluconeogenic defects (fructose biophosphatase deficiency) Hereditary fructose intolerance Ketotic hypoglycemia

FIGURE 113.2. Evaluation of hypoglycemia and examples of disorders within each diagnostic category.

The timing of the hypoglycemia in relationship to meals may offer clues to the etiology. Hypoglycemia immediately after a meal suggests provocation by some component of the ingested substance. Infants with *hereditary fructose intolerance* typically present at ~6 months of age when transitioning from breast milk or formula to solid foods, including introduction of fruits and vegetables. Within ~30 minutes of ingesting foods containing fructose or sucrose, they will become acutely hypoglycemic and have transient elevations of transaminases and lactic acid. Treatment for hereditary fructose intolerance consists solely of eliminating fructose and sucrose from the diet and is compatible with normal health, growth, and development. Hypoglycemia associated with a high-protein diet can be provoked by high levels of leucine in disorders such as a deficiency of *glutamate dehydrogenase*, resulting in *hyperinsulinemic hyperammonemia*. Hypoglycemia and liver dysfunction in infancy can also be caused by ingestion of breast milk or cow's milk–based formulas in *galactosemia*, but most cases are now diagnosed by newborn screening and readily treated with a soy-based formula.

Hypoglycemia can also be associated with ingestion of toxins or medications. Oral hypoglycemic agents such as the sulfonylureas can produce acute, rapid hypoglycemia. Other agents such as aspirin, acetaminophen, ethanol, and any hepatotoxic agent can cause hypoglycemia. Generally, the age of the patient and a thorough history will suggest this etiology.

Hypoglycemia associated with fasting for ~8 hours is most characteristic of glycogen storage disorders such as glycogen storage disorder type I (glucose-6-phosphatase deficiency) or glycogen storage disorder type 0 (glycogen synthase deficiency). These disorders frequently present as infants begin to sleep through the night with increased fasting intervals and/or during periods of intercurrent illness associated with anorexia or vomiting. Children with type I glycogen storage

TABLE 113.7

COMMON CATEGORIES AND CAUSES OF HYPOGLYCEMIA

- **Endocrinopathies**
  Growth hormone deficiency
  Cortisol deficiency
  Hyperinsulinism
  - Infants of diabetic mothers
  - Beckwith–Weidemann syndrome
  - Surreptitious insulin
- **Defective hepatic glucose release and/or utilization of available gluconeogenic substrate**
  Ketotic hypoglycemia
  Enzymatic defects
  - Glycogen storage diseases (glycogen synthetase deficiency, glucose-6-phosphatase deficiency)
  - Galactosemia (galactose-1-phosphate uridyltransferase deficiency)
  - Hereditary fructose intolerance (fructose-1-phosphate aldolase)
- **Fatty acid oxidation or ketogenesis disorders**
  Carnitine acyl transferase deficiency
  Long-chain fatty acid acyl-CoA dehydrogenase deficiency
  Medium-chain fatty acid acyl-CoA dehydrogenase deficiency
  Short-chain fatty acid acyl-CoA dehydrogenase deficiency
  Hydroxymethylglutaryl CoA lyase deficiency
- **Toxic**
  Salicylate
  Acetaminophen
  Alcohol
  Oral hypoglycemic agents (biguandies, sulfonylureas)

disease have a biochemical profile of lactic acidosis, hyper-alaninemia, hyperuricemia, and hyperlipidemia associated with their hypoglycemia. Hypoglycemia associated with fasting for ~16 hours is more characteristic of defects in gluconeogenesis (fructose-1,6-bisphosphatase deficiency, glycerol kinase deficiency, pyruvate carboxylase deficiency, or pyruvate kinase deficiency) or fatty acid oxidation disorders. After ~16–24 hours, all the glycogen reserves have been utilized and the body begins to rely on gluconeogenesis and fatty acid oxidation. Definitive diagnosis of all these conditions requires genetic testing or enzyme assays in leukocytes, fibroblasts, or, in some cases, liver. Treatment for these disorders consists of avoiding fasting and dietary modifications.

Hyperinsulinemia causing hypoglycemia can be due to exogenous or endogenous insulin. An insulin value of greater than 10 U/mL simultaneous with hypoglycemia is always abnormal. Levels of C-peptide can differentiate the source of insulin because C-peptide is produced only with *endogenous* insulin. Endogenous hyperinsulinemia typically presents within the neonatal period and can produce the most severe, persistent, and difficult hypoglycemia to manage. Persistent dextrose requirements of 10 mg/kg/min or greater suggest underlying hyperinsulinemia. Hyperinsulinemia may ultimately require treatment with diazoxide to inhibit insulin secretion, partial pancreatectomy if there is evidence of an islet cell adenoma, or near complete pancreatectomy for diffuse islet cell hyperplasia.

Hypoglycemia is more common in neonates who are small for gestational age or the preterm infant in the first few days of life. Additionally maternal diabetes may lead to perinatal hyperinsulinemia and hypoglycemia in the neonate. Hypoglycemia in these situations is always associated with ketosis and usually resolves within the first few days to weeks of life.

Patients with liver disease are also more susceptible to hypoglycemia due to the decreased capacity of the liver to supply glucose through glycogenolysis and gluconeogenesis. This may be a nonspecific manifestation of liver dysfunction and is best treated symptomatically by supplying glucose intravenously.

The physical examination may also provide useful clues as to the etiology of the hypoglycemia. The baby who is large for gestational age and hypoglycemic suggests an infant of a diabetic mother. Macrosomia, hemihypertrophy, macroglossia, umbilical hernia, and ear pits or creases in a neonate suggest *Beckwith–Wiedemann syndrome*. Midline defects with a cleft lip and/or palate or a small penis may suggest panhypopituitarism. Hepatomegaly suggests a glycogen storage disorder or nonspecific liver disease. Inverted nipples and decreased gluteal fat suggest a *congenital disorder of glycosylation* that may be associated with hyperinsulinemia.

A common and relatively benign cause of hypoglycemia is *ketotic hypoglycemia* often seen in toddlers and young children. These children appropriately mobilize fats and have massive ketosis during periods of hypoglycemia. Children with this disorder are most often symptomatic during an intercurrent illness associated with anorexia or a vomiting. This condition can be treated simply by avoiding fasting for more than 12 hours and is usually outgrown by the age of 5–10 years.

HYPERAMMONEMIA

Severe hyperammonemia represents one of the most emergent metabolic conditions. Newborns often present with rapidly progressive decreased feeding, hypothermia, lethargy, apnea, coma, and death within a period of hours in the most severe cases. Elevated concentrations of ammonia are extremely toxic to the brain and cause permanent brain damage even when rapidly corrected. Therefore, it is imperative to suspect and diagnose hyperammonemia early in the clinical course and immediately institute therapy if present. Severe

hyperammonemia can be rapidly progressive and associated with respiratory depression. Therefore, prophylactic intubation is indicated with ammonia levels >500 μmol/L.

Hyperammonemia is defined as ammonia higher than 150 μmol/L in the neonate or higher than 100 μmol/L in the older child. Blood samples should be placed on ice and analyzed immediately to avoid artifactual elevations. Mild hyperammonemia (~< 300 μmol/L) can be associated with *transient hyperammonemia of the newborn* as well as with several IEMs, including *organic acidurias; fatty acid oxidation defects; lysinuric protein intolerance;* and *hyperammonemia, hyperornithinemia,* and *homocitrullinuria syndrome*. More severe degrees of hyperammonemia are typically observed with *urea cycle defects*. In such cases, there is often an associated depression of the blood urea nitrogen (BUN) due to the inability to produce urea. These patients often initially demonstrate a respiratory alkalosis on their arterial blood gas (ABG). Secondary hyperammonemia can also be associated with liver failure and/or overwhelming viral hepatitis.

The sex of the patient is sometimes helpful. *Ornithine transcarbamylase deficiency* is an X-linked disorder usually presenting in males in the neonatal period. A family history of neonatal deaths of unknown etiology is always suspicious.

The various causes of hyperammonemia are metabolically diverse, each requiring specific treatment. Therefore, it is imperative to act quickly to get the results of the necessary biochemical diagnostic studies within 24–48 hours. Initial treatment should consist of making the child NPO and keeping the child anabolic with infusion of only dextrose and electrolytes to meet the age-dependent metabolic demands. Diagnostic laboratory tests should include ABG, serum chemistries, liver function studies, urine organic acids (specifically tested for orotic acid), urinalysis, serum amino acids, acylcarnitine profile, and repeated and frequent measures of ammonia until the rate of rise can be determined. Metabolic acidosis or an increased AG suggests that the diagnosis is not a urea cycle defect. Urinary ketosis with mild hyperammonemia suggests an organic aciduria. *Fatty acid oxidation disorders* should not be associated with urinary ketones, but are often associated with hypoglycemia and elevated creatine phosphokinase (CPK) with *mild* hyperammonemia.

Urea cycle defects are associated with the greatest and most rapid rise in ammonia. Elevations of ammonia rapidly rising beyond 500 μmol/L should be treated with some form of hemodialysis (including CVVHD) if available. PD and exchange transfusion with such severe hyperammonemia are much less efficacious. The specific defect in the urea cycle is important to establish for definitive therapy. However, while awaiting the results of diagnostic studies, in addition to initiation of hemodialysis, patients with suspected urea cycle disorders should be started on intravenous L-arginine to maintain the urea cycle and given loading doses and continuous infusions of sodium benzoate and phenylacetate that can be used to remove ammonia via alternative metabolic pathways utilizing glycine and glutamine to eliminate nitrogen (**Table 113.5**). Sodium benzoate and phenylacetate are Food and Drug Administration approved and can be stocked, but are expensive and rarely used; they may not be available except in tertiary neonatal and pediatric ICUs unless specifically requested. If cerebral edema is suspected, comprehensive management of increased intracranial pressure is indicated, including airway protection and osmotic agents (mannitol or hypertonic saline). Definitive diagnoses of urea cycle defects ultimately depend on biochemical analysis of liver tissue and/or molecular genetic testing. To date, the best long-term treatment for children with urea cycle defects has been liver transplantation (20). However, if significant hyperammonemia has occurred prior to transplant, permanent and irreversible brain damage should be carefully considered by parents prior to pursuing transplantation. For some *urea* *cycle defects* in which enzymes are also active outside the liver, dietary treatment and arginine supplementation in addition to liver transplantation may be necessary. In cases in which the diagnosis was known or suspected prenatally because of a previously affected sibling, neonatal metabolic management and liver transplantation can enable children to avoid neurocognitive damage. Furthermore, neonatal liver transplants have required minimal long-term immunosuppression.

Notably, females heterozygous for the X-linked *ornithine transcarbamylase deficiency* or patients with partial urea cycle defects may demonstrate only periodic metabolic crises with normal intervening metabolic evaluations. In these cases, metabolic crises are associated with ingestion of large amounts of protein and/or a catabolic state induced by an intercurrent illness. Metabolic crises should be managed as outlined above.

LIVER FAILURE

Liver failure associated with elevated transaminases, jaundice, bleeding, edema, and/or hepatomegaly is a common presentation for IEMs. Because the liver is the metabolic center of the body, most processes causing severe hepatic impairment can also cause alterations in metabolic pathways and produce mild hyperammonemia or hypoglycemia. Some inherited disorders cause direct hepatocyte damage, including *hepatorenal tyrosinemia, galactosemia, Wilson disease, α_1-antitrypsin deficiency*, peroxisomal disorders (*Zellweger syndrome* and *Refsum disease*), and defects in cholesterol and bile acid synthesis. Initially, it may be difficult to distinguish these IEMs from infectious causes such as sepsis; hepatitis A, B, or C; cytomegalovirus, Epstein–Barr virus, herpes simplex, and HIV infections; or toxoplasmosis. The size of the liver may aid in differentiation between IEMs and infectious etiologies; hepatomegaly occurs more commonly with IEMs.

Liver function should be assessed with a liver function panel, including albumin, transaminases, direct and indirect bilirubin, alkaline phosphatase, γglutamyltranspeptidase, α-fetoprotein, glucose, ammonia, BUN, prothrombin time, and partial thromboplastin time. If liver disease is suspected, titers and viral cultures of stool and urine should be performed to rule out viral etiologies of hepatitis. Once an inborn error of metabolism is suspected, specialized testing may be necessary including lactate, pyruvate, serum amino acids, urine organic acids (succinylacetone in *hepatorenal tyrosinemia*, dicarboxylic acids in *fatty acid oxidation disorders*, and orotic acid in *urea cycle defects*), bile acids, urinary reducing substances (galactose and fructose), α_1-antitrypsin activity and Pi phenotyping, very long–chain fatty acids for peroxisomal biogenesis disorders, iron and ferritin for hemochromatosis, galactose-1-phosphate uridyl transferase activity for galactosemia, and transferrin isoelectric focusing for congenital disorders of glycosylation. Many hepatic processes will produce a pattern of tyrosyluria and elevated tyrosine and methionine in the serum amino acids. This pattern is usually not diagnostic of hepatorenal tyrosinemia but simply indicates liver dysfunction. A liver biopsy may be necessary to identify storage material within the liver followed by specific enzymatic testing using fibroblasts or liver tissue for definitive diagnosis.

Many children with liver disease present initially with jaundice. As neonates, most babies with inborn errors of hepatic metabolism present with conjugated hyperbilirubinemia. Unconjugated hyperbilirubinemia, in contrast, suggests the diagnosis of *Crigler–Najjar syndrome* or a hemolytic anemia. Crigler–Najjar syndrome is treated with phototherapy and plasmapheresis acutely and ultimately by liver transplantation. α_1-*Antitrypsin deficiency* presents as cholestasis in a minority of infants with the Pi-ZZ phenotype. *Progressive*

familial intrahepatic cholestasis, Dubin–Johnson, and *Rotor syndromes* usually present as conjugated hyperbilirubinemia after 3 months of age. *Hepatorenal tyrosinemia, Niemann–Pick type C*, and *peroxisomal disorders* can also initially present as conjugated hyperbilirubinemia, but all usually progress rapidly to severe liver failure.

Liver failure associated with hepatocellular necrosis can be observed in the neonatal period as well as the older infant. Neonatal liver failure can be caused by infectious etiologies as well as neonatal hemochromatosis, galactosemia, hepatorenal tyrosinemia, urea cycle defects, defects in oxidative phosphorylation, long-chain fatty acid oxidation disorders, and *Niemann–Pick types A and B. Galactosemia* is suggested by reducing substance in the urine if the infant has ingested lactose within the previous 24 hours. Galactosemia may be associated with cataracts and *E. coli* sepsis. Definitive diagnosis is based upon enzymatic testing of blood and is part of newborn screening panels. *Neonatal hemochromatosis* is a rare cause of acute liver dysfunction of largely unknown etiology. Diagnosis is largely by exclusion and demonstration of increased concentrations of serum iron and ferritin and decreased concentrations of transferrin. Abdominal MRI may also be useful to demonstrate increased liver iron stores. *Hepatorenal tyrosinemia* is suggested by rapid hepatic decompensation and greatly elevated α-fetoprotein and is confirmed by demonstration of succinylacetone in the urine. *Defects of long-chain fatty acid oxidation* are suggested by the combination of hepatic necrosis, myopathy, and cardiomyopathy, which may occur in the neonatal period and/or intermittently throughout infancy. Biochemically, these disorders are most specifically associated with elevations in CPK and abnormal acylcarnitine profiles that suggest the specific enzymatic deficiency. *Defects in oxidative phosphorylation* characteristically have multisystem involvement and are associated with increased levels of lactic acid. Definitive diagnosis often rests on a liver biopsy to demonstrate mitochondrial DNA depletion.

In older children, hepatocellular necrosis and encephalopathy suggest a Reye-like syndrome that may be due to an underlying inborn error of metabolism, chronic viral hepatitis, autoimmune disease, or acute intoxication. The differential diagnosis of IEMs presenting with Reye-like syndrome includes *fatty acid oxidation disorders, urea cycle disorders, hepatorenal tyrosinemia, hereditary fructose intolerance, Wilson disease*, and α_1-*antitrypsin deficiency. Wilson disease* is characterized by choreoathetoid movements and dystonia, Kayser–Fleischer rings around the cornea, reduced levels of serum ceruloplasmin, and increased urinary copper. The age of presentation for some of these disorders depends on the degree of the enzymatic deficiency with less severe deficiencies presenting at older ages.

Hepatomegaly is often observed in IEMs, especially those associated with storage of nonmetabolizable large molecules. The combination of splenomegaly with hepatomegaly is more specific for storage disorders. In many of the *lysosomal storage disorders*, liver function is intact although the liver can become extremely enlarged. Lysosomal storage disorders are further suggested by short stature; failure to thrive; or coarse facial features; and developmental delay, hypotonia, or seizures. Many of the *glycogen storage diseases* can also produce hepatomegaly with or without associated hypoglycemia and are often diagnosed by findings of abnormal quantity and/or structure of glycogen on a liver biopsy. *Hemochromatosis* is a rare cause of hepatomegaly resulting from excess storage of iron.

Treatment for many liver diseases caused by IEMs is supportive therapy to treat associated coagulopathies with vitamin K and fresh frozen plasma, edema due to hypoalbuminemia with diuretics and albumin infusion, unconjugated hyperbilirubinemia with phototherapy, and deranged metabolism producing hypoglycemia and hyperammonemia.

Diet should be carefully considered, and in the cases of severe liver dysfunction the child should be made NPO and receive only intravenous dextrose and electrolytes until initial metabolic labs have been evaluated. A growing number of these disorders can ultimately be treated by liver transplant from either a cadaveric liver or a living related donor (21). Disease-specific treatments are available for a few IEMs causing liver dysfunction. A lactose-free, soy-based diet is a simple cure in *galactosemia*. A diet free of fructose and sucrose is curative for *hereditary fructose intolerance*. A low phenylalanine and tyrosine metabolic formula and administration of 2(2-nitro-4-trifluoro-methyl-benzoyl)-1,3-cyclohexanedione (NTBC) have revolutionized treatment for *hepatorenal tyrosinemia* and can allow normalization of hepatic and renal function. *Long-chain fatty acid oxidation disorders* remain problematic to treat, but current treatment relies on a low-fat diet with the majority of fat supplied as medium-chain triglycerides and supplementation with carnitine. Copper chelation is effective treatment for *Wilson disease*, and phlebotomy for *hemochromatosis*.

NONMETABOLIC CRITICAL ILLNESS IN INBORN ERRORS OF METABOLISM

Many IEMs present in the PICU not due to metabolic crisis, but due to the effects on specific vital organ systems. Effects on the hepatic, renal, pulmonary, cardiovascular, and hematologic systems may all have significant implications for the pediatric intensivist. Any disorder producing hepatic or renal insufficiency requires careful dose adjustments of medications cleared by these organs. Because of the rarity of individual IEMs, many recommendations are based on retrospective data, case reports, and anecdotal experience rather than randomized clinical trials. Lactate-containing fluids should not be administered to patients who may not metabolize exogenous lactate (mitochondrial disorders (22) and pyruvate dehydrogenase complex deficiency). Though propofol has been used successfully in mitochondrial disorders (22), it should probably be avoided in fatty acid oxidation defects because of possible predisposition to propofol infusion syndrome (23). Several IEMs place patients at significant risk for *hyperkalemia* and *rhabdomyolysis* leading to myoglobinuria following the use of a depolarizing neuromuscular blocker (succinylcholine), including glycogen storage diseases V (*McArdle disease*) and VII (*Tauri disease*). The absence of acidosis distinguishes this phenomenon from malignant hyperthermia (MH). The mitochondrial disorders, however, may predispose to true MH following the use of a depolarizing agent or volatile anesthetic (24).

IEMs may affect many aspects of the cardiovascular system, including the vessels themselves, the coagulation system, the myocardium, the endocardium, and the pericardium. Extensive reviews of these diseases are outside the scope of this text and can be found elsewhere (25). An increasing number of known abnormalities of proteins involved in the contractile machinery cause *cardiomyopathy*, and these disorders are covered in detail in Chapter 73. Any IEM that impairs energy metabolism, particularly disorders of the mitochondrial respiratory chain and fatty acid oxidation defects may also present with cardiomyopathy, usually dilated rather than hypertrophic. The fatty acid oxidation disorders (including *fatty acyl-CoA dehydrogenase deficiencies* and *glutaric acidemia type II*) may also present with arrhythmias in addition to neonatal cardiomyopathy (26). They are treated primarily with a low-fat diet with minimal amounts of essential fatty acids and supplementation with medium-chain triglycerides and carnitine replacement. *Primary carnitine deficiency*, due to a defect in the carnitine transporter in the heart, liver, and kidneys, presents with cardiomyopathy with or without skeletal myopathy beginning in late infancy or early childhood. *Carnitine-acylcarnitine translocase deficiency* and the severe form of *carnitine palmitoyltransferase-2 deficiency* also present with dilated cardiomyopathy. Treatment with high doses of oral carnitine can be curative for primary carnitine deficiency.

IEMs also affect cardiovascular function in the PICU through their effects on coagulation and microvascular physiology. The *hyperlipoproteinemias* increase cardiovascular risk through atherogenesis. Only type II (*familial hypercholesterolemia*) has consequences in children (27). When hypertriglyceridemia occurs (type IIB), homozygous children can have severe atherosclerotic disease and dilated cardiomyopathy out of proportion to the degree of ischemia. *Homocystinuria* predisposes patients to thromboembolic disease. In the classic form (*cystathionine synthase deficiency*), patients typically present with ectopia lentis after 3 years of age, a Marfanoid habitus and developmental delay. On the other hand, IEMs may promote a bleeding diathesis due to hypersplenism in a number of storage diseases or due to decreased liver synthetic function.

The lysosomal storage diseases often involve both the cardiovascular and respiratory systems, providing a number of challenges for the intensivist and anesthesiologist. Perioperative considerations are reviewed more extensively in other texts (28). Type II glycogen storage disease (*Pompe disease*) results from deficiency of the enzyme *α-1,4-glucosidase* (acid maltase) and causes a hypertrophic cardiomyopathy syndrome with a short P–R interval. These patients also have glycogen storage in other organs causing hypotonia and macroglossia. The X-linked disorder, *Fabry disease (lysosomal α-galactosidase A deficiency)*, causes disseminated glycosphingolipid deposition. Angiokeratomas are characteristic and result from deposition in the skin, typically in a "bathing suit distribution." The cardiovascular manifestations result from deposition causing obstructive vasculopathy, mitral valve thickening, and hypertrophic and eventually dilated cardiomyopathy. Mutations of the γ-subunit of AMP-activated protein kinase (*PRKAG2*) and X-linked lysosome-associated membrane protein (*LAMP2, Danon disease*) result in hypertrophic cardiomyopathy due to glycogen accumulation in the heart and are also associated with ventricular preexcitation (1).

The MPSs can affect both the myocardium and the endocardium (valvular disease). Type I (*Hunter/Scheie*) and Type II (*Hurler*) MPSs result in varying degrees of myocardial and valvular diseases. Although the mucolipidoses, *I-cell disease* and *pseudo-Hurler polydystrophy*, share many features with the MPSs such as valvular disease, reports of cardiomyopathy are rare (29,30). Together with Pompe disease, these lysosomal storage disorders also affect a variety of systems involved in respiratory management in the PICU. The associated dysmorphisms and tracheal narrowing can make endotracheal intubation extremely challenging; a view of the larynx may be unobtainable using direct laryngoscopy. Atlanto-axial instability, particularly in MPS IV (*Morquio syndrome*), must be considered during laryngoscopy as well. These patients are also at high risk for airway obstruction during induction. Therefore, these patients may require fiberoptic intubation or even tracheotomy and should be intubated awake whenever possible. Muscle relaxants are contraindicated before successful intubation unless an easy mask airway can be established.

Novel Therapies

There is increasing long-term experience with *enzyme replacement therapy* for a growing number of lysosomal storage disorders, including Gaucher disease (31), Pompe disease (32–34), Fabry disease (35), MPS I (36,37), and MPS VI (38,39), and this is one question that has actually been addressed by randomized, placebo-controlled trials. Unfortunately, none of these enzymes are able to cross the blood–brain barrier, and therapy is therefore effective only at treating the systemic disease but not the neurological components. Furthermore, though in most cases enzyme replacement therapy effectively prevents further accumulation of material, it may not effectively reverse organ damage already sustained. Therefore, it is not surprising that early therapy appears to offer the greatest benefit (34). Several problems exist with this therapy, including the high cost, need for biweekly intravenous infusions, and, in rare cases, development of neutralizing antibodies (40,41). Anaphylactoid reactions have been reported with infusions of replacement enzymes, which could also bring these patients to the attention of an intensivist. Small molecule inhibitors of substrate accumulation and chaperones to rescue patients' endogenous misfolded proteins are being explored as alternative therapies. Direct intracerebroventricular infusion of enzyme is currently being considered for clinical trials to treat the neurological symptoms. Both these latter approaches have shown promise in animal models.

Hobbs first reported improvement in a patient with Hurler syndrome following *bone marrow transplantation* in 1981 (42). Since then, several other storage disorders, including Krabbe disease (43), metachromatic leukodystrophy (43), and Niemann–Pick type B (44) have been treated with hematopoietic stem cell transplantation (HSCT) with at least partial success. Donor-derived macrophages (or microglia in the central nervous system [CNS]) are able to make and secrete the deficient enzyme, which is taken up by resident, enzyme-deficient host cells, allowing stored material to be cleared, even in the CNS ("cross-correction") (45). However, stabilization or improvement in organ function can occur slowly (CNS) or not at all (bone/heart valves) due to poor penetration of donor macrophages into these tissues. Early treatment (even neonatally) of appropriate patients without severe organ dysfunction dramatically improves outcome and is the justification for adding Krabbe disease to the newborn screening panel in New York. Fortunately, even with obtaining only the modest levels of sustained enzyme production and mixed chimerism, clinical improvement or stabilization has been noted (46). Hurler syndrome remains the most commonly transplanted IEM, and a great deal has been learned about the factors determining disease outcome following transplant in this disorder (45). Increasing experience has also determined which IEMs are most amenable to HSCT and which are not. However, early (neonatal) transplantation may provide benefit in disorders for which transplantation of symptomatic patients has been considered futile (45). Some patients may even benefit from combinations of enzyme replacement therapy, substrate inhibitors, and HSCT either sequentially or simultaneously (47).

CONCLUSIONS AND FUTURE DIRECTIONS

Patients with IEMs frequently present with critical illnesses. Although IEMs are individually rare, collectively they are not infrequent and therefore intensivists are virtually certain to care for such patients. With advances in diagnosis, particularly improved neonatal screening using tandem mass spectroscopy, many patients will be diagnosed before their first metabolic decompensation. However, a normal newborn screening does not rule out all IEMs. A systematic approach to the diagnosis and initial treatment of these disorders is imperative, as is early involvement of a metabolic disease specialist. Early recognition of an IEM and appropriate therapy, including dietary management, cofactor supplementation, and removal of toxic metabolites, improves neurological

outcome for these patients. Additionally, enzyme replacement therapy, substrate inhibitors, and liver transplantation and HSCT are now being used to treat many of these diseases. With improvements in gene delivery, enzyme delivery across the blood–brain barrier, and chaperoning misfolded endogenous proteins, we should be able to improve the treatment for many of these conditions.

References

1. Garganta CL, Smith WE. Metabolic evaluation of the sick neonate. *Semin Perinatol* 2005;29(3):164–72.
2. Henwood MJ, Thornton PS, Preis CM, et al. Reconciling diabetes management and the ketogenic diet in a child with pyruvate dehydrogenase deficiency. *J Child Neurol* 2006;21(5):436–9.
3. Batshaw ML, Brusilow SW. Treatment of hyperammonemic coma caused by inborn errors of urea synthesis. *J Pediatr* 1980;97(6):893–900.
4. Saudubray JM, Ogier H, Charpentier C, et al. Hudson memorial lecture. Neonatal management of organic acidurias. Clinical update. *J Inherit Metab Dis* 1984;7(suppl 1):2–9.
5. de Baulny HO, Benoist JF, Rigal O, et al. Methylmalonic and propionic acidaemias: Management and outcome. *J Inherit Metab Dis* 2005;28(3):415–23.
6. Wong KY, Wong SN, Lam SY, et al. Ammonia clearance by peritoneal dialysis and continuous arteriovenous hemodiafiltration. *Pediatr Nephrol* 1998;12(7):589–91.
7. Schaefer F, Straube E, Oh J, et al. Dialysis in neonates with inborn errors of metabolism. *Nephrol Dial Transplant* 1999;14(4):910–8.
8. Summar M, Pietsch J, Deshpande J, et al. Effective hemodialysis and hemofiltration driven by an extracorporeal membrane oxygenation pump in infants with hyperammonemia. *J Pediatr* 1996;128(3):379–82.
9. Hmiel SP, Martin RA, Landt M, et al. Amino acid clearance during acute metabolic decompensation in maple syrup urine disease treated with continuous venovenous hemodialysis with filtration. *Pediatr Crit Care Med* 2004;5(3):278–81.
10. Stacpoole PW, Nagaraja NV, Hutson AD. Efficacy of dichloroacetate as a lactate-lowering drug. *J Clin Pharmacol* 2003;43(7):683–91.
11. Puffenberger EG. Genetic heritage of the Old Order Mennonites of southeastern Pennsylvania. *Am J Med Genet C Semin Med Genet* 2003;121(1):18–31.
12. Edelmann L, Wasserstein MP, Kornreich R, et al. Maple syrup urine disease: Identification and carrier-frequency determination of a novel founder mutation in the Ashkenazi Jewish population. *Am J Hum Genet* 2001;69(4):863–8.
13. Mock DM, Mock NI, Nelson RP, et al. Disturbances in biotin metabolism in children undergoing long-term anticonvulsant therapy. *J Pediatr Gastroenterol Nutr* 1998;26(3):245–50.
14. Barshop BA, Khanna A. Domino hepatic transplantation in maple syrup urine disease. *N Engl J Med* 2005;353(22):2410–11.
15. Mazariegos GV, Morton DH, Sindhi R, et al. Liver transplantation for classical maple syrup urine disease: Long-term follow-up in 37 patients and comparative united network for organ sharing experience. *J Pediatr* 2012;160(1):116–21.e1.
16. Bodner-Leidecker A, Wendel U, Saudubray JM, et al. Branched-chain L-amino acid metabolism in classical maple syrup urine disease after orthotopic liver transplantation. *J Inherit Metab Dis* 2000;23(8):805–18.
17. Kasahara M, Sakamoto S, Kanazawa H, et al. Living-donor liver transplantation for propionic acidemia. *Pediatr Transpl* 2012;16(3):230–4.
18. Nagarajan S, Enns GM, Millan MT, et al. Management of methylmalonic acidaemia by combined liver-kidney transplantation. *J Inherit Metab Dis* 2005;28(4):517–24.

19. de Baulny HO, Benoist JF, Rigal O, et al. Methylmalonic and propionic acidaemias: Management and outcome. *J Inherit Metab Dis* 2005;28(3):415–23.

20. Morioka D, Kasahara M, Takada Y, et al. Current role of liver transplantation for the treatment of urea cycle disorders: A review of the worldwide English literature and 13 cases at Kyoto University. *Liver Transpl* 2005;11(11):1332–42.

21. Meyburg J, Hoffmann GF. Liver transplantation for inborn errors of etabolism. *Transplantation* 2005;80(1S):S135–7.

22. Vilela H, García-Fernández J, Parodi E, et al. Anesthetic management of a patient with MERRF syndrome. *Paediatr Anaesth* 2005;15(1):77–9.

23. Steiner LA, Studer W, Baumgartner ER, et al. Perioperative management of a child with very-long-chain acyl-coenzyme A dehydrogenase deficiency. *Paediatr Anaesth* 2002;12(2):187–91.

24. Fricker RM, Raffelsberger T, Rauch-Shorny S, et al. Positive malignant hyperthermia susceptibility in vitro test in a patient with mitochondrial myopathy and myoadenylate deaminase deficiency. *Anesthesiology* 2002;97(6):1635–7.

25. Gilbert-Barness E. Cardiovascular involvement in metabolic diseases. *Pediatr Pathol Mol Med* 2002;21(2):93–136.

26. Bonnet D, Martin D, Pascale De L, et al. Arrhythmias and conduction defects as presenting symptoms of fatty acid oxidation disorders in children. *Circulation* 1999;100(22):2248–53.

27. Barness LA. An approach to the diagnosis of metabolic diseases. *Fetal Pediatr Pathol* 2004;23(1):3–10.

28. Katz J, Stewart DJ, eds. *Anesthesia and Uncommon Pediatric Diseases*. 1st ed. Philadelphia, PA: W.B. Saunders, 1987:549.

29. Müller P, Reichenbach H, Möckel A, et al. I-cell disease complicated by unusual dilatative cardiomyopathy. *J Inherit Metab Dis* 2000;23(5):514–6.

30. Steet RA, Hullin R, Kudo M, et al. A splicing mutation in the alpha/beta GlcNAc-1-phosphotransferase gene results in an adult onset form of mucolipidosis III associated with sensory neuropathy and cardiomyopathy. *Am J Med Genet A* 2005;132(4):369–75.

31. Kishnani PS, DiRocco M, Kaplan P, et al. A randomized trial comparing the efficacy and safety of imiglucerase (Cerezyme) infusions every 4 weeks versus every 2 weeks in the maintenance therapy of adult patients with Gaucher disease type 1. *Mol Genet Metab* 2009;96(4):164–70.

32. Klinge L, Straub V, Neudorf U, et al. Enzyme replacement therapy in classical infantile pompe disease: Results of a ten-month follow-up study. *Neuropediatrics* 2005;36(1):6–11.

33. Klinge L, Straub V, Neudorf U, et al. Safety and efficacy of recombinant acid alpha-glucosidase (rhGAA) in patients with classical infantile Pompe disease: Results of a phase II clinical trial. *Neuromuscul Disord* 2005;15(1):24–31.

34. Kishnani PS, Corzo D, Leslie ND, et al. Early treatment with alglucosidase alfa prolongs long-term survival of infants with Pompe disease. *Pediatr Res* 2009;66(3):329–35.

35. Brady RO. Enzyme replacement therapy: Conception, chaos and culmination. *Philos Trans R Soc Lond B Biol Sci* 2003;358(1433):915–9.

36. Wraith JE, Clarke LA, Beck M, et al. Enzyme replacement therapy for mucopolysaccharidosis I: A randomized, double-blinded, placebo-controlled, multinational study of recombinant human alpha-L-iduronidase (laronidase). *J Pediatr* 2004;144(5):581–8.

37. Clarke LA, Wraith JE, Beck M, et al. Long-term efficacy and safety of laronidase in the treatment of mucopolysaccharidosis I. *Pediatrics* 2009;123(1):229–40.

38. Muenzer J, Wraith JE, Beck M, et al. A phase II/III clinical study of enzyme replacement therapy with idursulfase in mucopolysaccharidosis II (Hunter syndrome). *Genet Med* 2006;8(8):465–73.

39. Harmatz P, Yu ZF, Giugliani R, et al. Enzyme replacement therapy for mucopolysaccharidosis VI: Evaluation of long-term pulmonary function in patients treated with recombinant human N-acetylgalactosamine 4-sulfatase. *J Inherit Metab Dis* 2010;33(1):51–60.

40. Kakavanos R, Turner CT, Hopwood JJ, et al. Immune tolerance after long-term enzyme-replacement therapy among patients who have mucopolysaccharidosis I. *Lancet* 2003;361(9369):1608–13.

41. Bénichou B, Goyal S, Sung C, et al. A retrospective analysis of the potential impact of IgG antibodies to agalsidase β on efficacy during enzyme replacement therapy for Fabry disease. *Mol Genet Metab* 2009;96(1):4–12.

42. Hobbs JR, Barrett AJ, Chambers D, et al. Reversal of clinical features of Hurler's disease and biochemical improvement after treatment by bone-marrow transplantation. *Lancet* 1981;2(8249):709–12.

43. Krivit W, Aubourg P, Shapiro E, et al. Bone marrow transplantation for globoid cell leukodystrophy, adrenoleukodystrophy, metachromatic leukodystrophy, and Hurler syndrome. *Curr Opin Hematol* 1999;6(6):377–82.

44. Vellodi A, Hobbs JR, O'Donnell NM, et al. Treatment of Niemann-Pick disease type B by allogeneic bone marrow transplantation. *Br Med J (Clin Res Ed)* 1987;295(6610):1375–6.

45. Wynn R. Stem cell transplantation in inherited metabolic disorders. *ASH Education Program Book* 2011;2011(1):285–91.

46. Conway J, Dyack S, Crooks BNA, et al. Mixed donor chimerism and low level iduronidase expression may be adequate for neurodevelopmental protection in Hurler Syndrome. *J Pediatr* 2005;147(1):106–8.

47. Biswas S, Le Vine SM. Substrate-reduction therapy enhances the benefits of bone marrow transplantation in young mice with globoid cell leukodystrophy. *Pediatr Res* 2002;51(1):40–7.

CHAPTER 114 ■ CANCER THERAPY: MECHANISMS AND TOXICITY

DAVID M. LOEB AND MASANORI HAYASHI

KEY POINTS

1 Modern cancer therapy is often multimodal, including chemotherapy, surgery, and radiotherapy.

2 Chemotherapeutics can be categorized based on structure and function:

2a Alkylating agents, such as nitrogen mustard derivatives and nitrosureas, contain highly reactive alkyl groups that form covalent bonds with DNA, resulting in cross-linking events that lead to cell death by impeding DNA replication.

2b Antimetabolites, such as the antifolate methotrexate and the purine analogs, induce cell death predominantly through interference with DNA synthesis.

2c Topoisomerase inhibitors, such as podophyllotoxins and anthracyclines, induce cell death by interfering with the maintenance of DNA supercoiling.

2d Antimicotubule agents, such as vinca alkaloids and taxanes, interfere with the function of the mitotic spindle.

3 Radiation therapy can be delivered as either photons or protons, and causes cytotoxicity predominantly through the induction of DNA damage.

4 More recently, targeted biologic therapies, such as differentiation therapy using ATRA, immunotherapy for neuroblastoma, small-molecule kinase inhibitors, monoclonal antibodies, and antiangiogenic therapies have started to be used widely in certain diseases.

5 Toxicities of cancer therapies are usually related to interference with the function or survival of normal cell types.

5a Central nervous system toxicities include ifosfamide-induced encephalopathy, araC acute cerebellar syndrome, and methotrexate leukoencephalitis.

5b Anthracyclines cause a cumulative dose-dependent cardiotoxicity, caused by O_2 free radicals and characterized primarily by cardiomyopathy, resulting in congestive heart failure.

5c Bleomycin and radiation therapy are the primary agents that cause pulmonary toxicity. This toxicity is predominantly fibrotic and is worsened by high O_2 tension.

5d Retinoic acid syndrome is a major complication of ATRA treatment for APML, causing respiratory distress, pulmonary infiltrates and pleural effusions.

5e The most common genitourinary toxicities of chemotherapy are the renal tubular dysfunction associated with ifosfamide and cisplatin and the hemorrhagic cystitis caused by cyclophosphamide and ifosfamide.

6 Radiation recall is an inflammatory reaction in a previously irradiated body area. Most commonly, it manifests as an acute dermatitis, but visceral involvement also occurs.

7 Options for the management of chemotherapy overdose are limited. Some agents can be removed by hemodialysis or plasmapheresis. Carboxypeptidase G2, a bacterial enzyme that hydrolyzes methotrexate to inactive metabolites extremely rapidly, is an "antidote" to methotrexate. Methylene blue has been administered to treat ifosfamide overdose.

---

1 Most pediatric malignancies are treated with multimodal therapy, traditionally consisting of chemotherapy, radiation therapy, and surgery. More recently, biologically-based therapies have been developed, including monoclonal antibodies, small-molecule kinase inhibitors, cytokines, differentiation therapies, and antiangiogenic therapies. Some of these treatments have entered the realm of standard of care, while others remain available only in the context of a clinical trial. A clear understanding of the mechanism of action of each of these modalities, along with an understanding of the most common toxicities, is essential to the delivery of optimal critical care to pediatric cancer patients. This chapter will discuss the mechanism of action of the major classes of chemotherapeutic agents, the distinctions between different radiation therapy modalities, and the most common side effects that might be encountered in the critical care setting. A comprehensive discussion of the mechanism of action of each available chemotherapy drug is beyond the scope of this chapter. We will focus on the most commonly used agents in pediatric oncology practice, with an emphasis on discussion of classes of drugs, rather than focusing on individual compounds. The reader is referred to any of several excellent textbooks for a more comprehensive discussion of individual chemotherapy drugs.

MECHANISM OF ACTION OF CHEMOTHERAPEUTICS

Chemotherapy drugs are classified by their mechanism of action. **Table 114.1** lists the commonly used constituents of each major drug class. **Table 114.2** lists some regimens commonly used to treat certain pediatric malignancies. The mechanism of action of each class of drug is discussed in more detail below.

Alkylating Agents

2a The oldest class of chemotherapeutic drugs is the alkylating agents. Mechlorethamine, also known as nitrogen mustard, was the first nonhormonal drug successfully given to a patient

TABLE 114.1

CHEMOTHERAPEUTICS ORGANIZED BY CLASS

■ CLASS	■ DRUGS
Alkylating agents	Cyclophosphamide, ifosfamide, BCNU, CCNU, cisplatin, carboplatin
Antimetabolites	Methotrexate, 6-mercaptopurine, 6-thioguanine, clofarabine
Topoisomerase inhibitors	Etoposide (VP16) and teniposide (VM26) inhibit Topo II Irinotecan and topotecan inhibit Topo I
Anthracyclines	Doxorubicin, daunorubicin, idarubicin, mitoxantrone
Antimicrotubule agents	Vincristine, vinblastine, vinorelbine, paclitaxel, docetaxel

TABLE 114.2

COMMONLY USED CHEMOTHERAPY REGIMENS IN PEDIATRIC ONCOLOGY

■ DIAGNOSIS	■ CHEMOTHERAPY
Acute lymphoblastic leukemia (induction only)	Prednisone or dexamethasone, vincristine, L-asparaginase (and daunorubicin for high-risk patients)
Acute myelogenous leukemia (induction only)	Daunorubicin, cytarabine, etoposide
Osteosarcoma	Methotrexate, cisplatin, doxorubicin (ifosfamide and etoposide added for some patients with poor response to neoadjuvant therapy)
Ewing sarcoma	Vincristine, doxorubicin, cyclophosphamide, alternating with ifosfamide and etoposide
Rhabdomyosarcoma	Vincristine, dactinomycin, cyclophosphamide
Hodgkin disease	**Low risk:** doxorubicin, prednisone, vincristine, cyclophosphamide **Intermediate and high risk:** doxorubicin, bleomycin, vincristine, etoposide, prednisone, cyclophosphamide
Neuroblastoma	**Intermediate risk:** carboplatin, etoposide, cyclophosphamide, doxorubicin **High risk:** cyclophosphamide, topotecan, cisplatin, etoposide, doxorubicin, vincristine
Wilms tumor	**Low risk:** vincristine, dactinomycin **Intermediate risk:** vincristine, dactinomycin, doxorubicin **High risk:** vincristine, doxorubicin, cyclophosphamide, etoposide

for the explicit purpose of treating cancer (1). A number of related agents have subsequently been developed for clinical use. Most alkylating agents commonly used in pediatric oncology are derivatives of nitrogen mustard, including cyclophosphamide and ifosfamide, or derivatives of methylnitrosourea, such as lomustine (CCNU) and carmustine (BCNU). These drugs contain highly reactive alkyl groups that form covalent bonds with DNA and other intracellular macromolecules. Both nitrogen mustard derivatives and nitrosoureas primarily modify the N-7 position of guanine (2); nitrosoureas also alkylate the N-3 position on cytidine (3) or the O-6 position on guanine (4). Following this initial alkylation reaction, the remaining reactive group can interact with a second macromolecule, resulting in either intrastrand or interstrand DNA cross-links. It has been suggested that these cross-links are the events that lead to cytotoxicity, perhaps by impeding DNA replication or by direct mutagenesis (5). While compelling arguments exist to support this hypothesis, direct proof remains lacking.

In addition to the nitrogen mustard and nitrosourea derivatives, platinum-based antitumor compounds also create DNA cross-links. While not true alkylating agents, these compounds have a similar mechanism of action and are therefore sometimes referred to as "nonclassical alkylating agents." The two commonly used platinum-based compounds are cisplatin and carboplatin, which, like the classical alkylating agents, form adducts at the N-7 position of guanine (6). These drugs can form both intrastrand and interstrand cross-links, and these

cross-links are correlated with cytotoxicity (6). As with the classical alkylating agents, the relationship between DNA cross-links and cytotoxicity remains correlative, with definitive proof of causality lacking.

Antimetabolites

Antimetabolites are commonly used by both medical and pediatric oncologists to treat a variety of tumor types. The several classes of antimetabolites are classified based on the metabolic pathways with which they interfere. In pediatric oncology, antifolates and purine antimetabolites are most commonly used; therefore, they will be discussed here to the exclusion of other types of antimetabolites.

Antifolates

In the early 1940s, it was recognized that patients with acute leukemia were folate deficient. This observation prompted a series of investigations culminating in the use of aminopterin by Farber to induce temporary remissions in children with acute lymphoblastic leukemia (ALL). Methotrexate was eventually developed as a clinically useful chemotherapeutic agent because it has a more favorable therapeutic index than aminopterin. Methotrexate acts by competitively inhibiting the enzyme dihydrofolate reductase. Inhibition of this key enzyme for synthesis of thymidine leads to depletion of intracellular thymidine triphosphate and eventually to arrest of DNA synthesis (7). It has also been reported that high doses of methotrexate lead to decreased purine synthesis and ultimately to cell death (8). Another potential mechanism of action of methotrexate is its toxicity to endothelial cells (9). Mounting evidence supports methotrexate as an effective therapy for autoimmune diseases, in part through inhibition of angiogenesis (10)—although the antiangiogenic mechanism is unclear—and this inhibition may play a role in the antineoplastic effects of methotrexate as well.

Purine Antimetabolites

Purine biosynthesis is critical for DNA synthesis and, therefore, for cell replication. The development of drugs that interfere with purine biosynthesis was a major focus in the 1950s, and ultimately led to the awarding of the Nobel Prize to Gertrude Elion and George Hitchings (along with James Black) in 1988 for the development of, among other drugs, 6-mercaptopurine and 6-thioguanine. Clofarabine is the first example of a newer generation of purine antimetabolite (11), and this drug is used mostly to treat relapsed acute leukemias. These drugs are thought to act primarily by being incorporated into growing DNA strands, thereby inhibiting DNA synthesis. Other mechanisms by which these drugs exert their cytotoxicity include inhibition of the activity of enzymes that are necessary for the synthesis of natural purines (adenine and guanine).

Topoisomerase Inhibitors

Topoisomerases are enzymes involved in the maintenance of supercoiling of the DNA double helix (12). They are essential for DNA replication, transcription, and chromosomal segregation—critical processes for cell division and, therefore, for tumor growth. Two classes of topoisomerase inhibitors are type I enzymes, which make single-strand cuts in DNA, and type II enzymes, which make double-stranded cuts. Inhibitors of each type of topoisomerase are in common use in pediatric oncology.

Inhibitors of Topoisomerase II

The two types of topoisomerase II inhibitors are podophyllotoxins and anthracyclines. Etoposide (VP16) is the more commonly used podophyllotoxin, and teniposide (VM26) is rarely used. Etoposide was approved by the FDA in 1983, but it was not clear until 1984 that this drug functioned by inhibiting topoisomerase II. This enzyme modulates DNA topology by passing an intact DNA helix through a transient double-stranded break in the DNA backbone (12). Etoposide poisons topoisomerase II by increasing the steady-state concentration of DNA cleavage complexes (13)—in essence by gluing the enzyme to the broken strand of DNA and preventing repair of the cleaved helix.

In addition to podophyllotoxins, anthracycline antibiotics, such as doxorubicin, daunorubicin, and idarubicin, also inhibit topoisomerase II. First isolated from fermentation products of *Streptomyces peucetius*, anthracycline antibiotics were originally thought to act primarily by virtue of their ability to intercalate between DNA base pairs in the intact double helix. In the 1980s, it was recognized that these compounds are also inhibitors of topoisomerase II (14). Other activities of anthracycline antibiotics include effects on nuclear helicases and the generation of iron free radicals. At present, it is unclear whether the cytotoxicity of these drugs is a result of just one mechanism (inhibition of topoisomerase II), or a combination of all of these activities.

Inhibitors of Topoisomerase I

Inhibitors of topoisomerase I represent a newer class of chemotherapeutic agents. The agents in common use, irinotecan and topotecan, are derivatives of camptothecin, a plant alkaloid obtained from the Camptotheca acuminata tree. These drugs target the DNA–topoisomerase I complex, preventing the reannealing of the nicked DNA strand, which leads to the accumulation of drug-stabilized, nicked DNA strands, causing an arrest of DNA replication and subsequent cell death (15). Other agents in this class are under development.

Antimicrotubule Agents

Vinca Alkaloids

All vinca alkaloids are derived from compounds originally identified in the pink periwinkle plant (older scientific name *Vinca rosea* Linn). Three related compounds are commonly used in the United States: vincristine, vinblastine, and vinorelbine. Vinca alkaloids are thought to produce cytotoxicity through interaction with tubulin, the major protein component of microtubules (16), an interaction that disrupts the structure of the microtubules and leads to dissolution of the mitotic spindle and metaphase arrest of dividing cells. The importance of microtubules in other cellular functions explains the non-cytotoxic effects of these compounds. In particular, neurons require intact microtubules for axonal transport, and disruption of this function causes the well-known peripheral neuropathy associated with vincristine treatment (17).

Taxanes

The original taxane, paclitaxel, was found through a National Cancer Institute program that screened plant extracts for anti-cancer activity (18), and it was initially isolated from the bark of the Pacific yew tree. The major source of taxanes today is a semisynthetic derivative of the needles and other components of more abundant trees, such as the European yew. Docetaxel and paclitaxel are the two most commonly used taxanes, and they act by binding to tubulin at sites distinct from those bound by the vinca alkaloids. Taxanes function by stabilizing microtubules against depolymerization, primarily through an effect on tubulin dissociation rates at both ends of the microtubule (19), affecting dynamic instability of the microtubules, which is critical for normal microtubule dynamics during both mitotic and nonmitotic phases of the cell cycle. Ultimately, this disruption of microtubule dynamics leads to induction of apoptosis. Interestingly, taxanes also inhibit angiogenesis at concentrations below those that are cytotoxic (20). The contribution of this and other effects to the cytotoxicity of taxanes is as yet unclear.

Other Cytotoxic Drugs

Asparaginase

L-Asparaginase hydrolyzes asparagines to aspartic acid and ammonia. In sensitive tumor cells that lack adequate levels of asparagine synthetase, this enzyme depletes the cells of a critical amino acid, thus rapidly inhibiting protein synthesis. DNA and RNA syntheses are eventually also inhibited, and cell death ensues. Asparaginase is particularly used to treat pediatric ALL and, as a single agent, is able to induce complete remission in 50%–60% of patients (21). Interestingly, relapsed patients will achieve a second complete remission with asparaginase alone in 30%–50% of cases. Remissions induced by a single agent are short lived, however; therefore, ALL is always treated with combination chemotherapy.

Cytarabine

Cytarabine (araC) differs from cytidine by the substitution of arabinose for ribose. Uptake into the cell is via the same transport mechanisms that are responsible for uptake of other nucleosides. Once internalized, cytarabine is serially phosphorylated to generate araCTP by deoxycytidine kinase. Cytarabine decreases intracellular concentrations of deoxycytidine by competition for enzymes that are responsible for the activation of cytidine and, thereby, inhibits DNA synthesis. DNA polymerase is also inhibited by incorporation of araCTP into nascent DNA strands, and incorporation of araCTP into DNA correlates with cytotoxicity (22). In addition to these effects, araC also causes cells to synthesize small reduplicated segments of DNA, increasing the possibility of crossovers and recombination (23). Chromosome fragmentation has been observed in cells cultured with araC, possibly reflecting the effects of these small reduplications. The importance of this finding to the cytotoxic effects of the drug remains unclear.

Gemcitabine is another cytidine analog that has recently been introduced into pediatric oncology practice. Like araC, gemcitabine is phosphorylated by nucleoside kinases. Gemcitabine triphosphate competes with dCTP for incorporation into DNA and inhibits DNA polymerase, thus inhibiting DNA synthesis.

THE BASICS OF RADIATION THERAPY

In pediatric oncology, radiation therapy is primarily used in the treatment of solid tumors as a means of local control. For some tumor types, such as Wilms tumor and most central nervous system (CNS) malignancies, radiation is a standard part of therapy. For others, such as Ewing sarcoma, radiation is used to treat patients for whom surgery is not an option or patients who have an inadequate resection. In the past, radiation was used for CNS prophylaxis for all leukemia patients, but due to significant long-term side effects, modern regimens reserve radiation for patients at high risk for CNS involvement. In addition, radiation therapy is sometimes incorporated into bone marrow transplant preparative regimens and in treatment of patients with leukemia who have CNS involvement.

General Principles of Radiation Therapy

Radiation therapy is the delivery of packets of energy to a target tissue with the intention of causing lethal damage to malignant cells while minimizing damage to normal cells. Radiation energy comes in different packets, the most commonly used being photons (for example, from x-rays), although other particles (e.g., protons or electrons) are also used. Different packets of energy possess different properties, including the amount of energy per packet and depth of tissue penetration, and these properties determine the mode of treatment. As the packets deposit their energy, ionization events occur in biologically important molecules, and it is these events that lead to tissue damage and death. These events can occur directly (as when a photon causes the release of an electron from a target biological molecule, and this electron directly damages the molecule) or indirectly (as when a released electron interacts with a neighboring water molecule to generate free radicals, which then damage macromolecules). The dose of energy delivered is measured in Gray (Gy), and 1 Gy = 1 J/kg. An older dose term, *rad*,

is still sometimes used, and 1 rad = 1 cGy = 0.01 Gy. While multiple biological macromolecules can be affected by ionizing radiation, it is thought that induction of double-stranded DNA breaks is the proximate cause of cell death. It is estimated that a 1-Gy dose of x-rays will result in 40 double-stranded DNA breaks per cell (24).

Because double-stranded DNA breaks cause cell death in irradiated tissue, understanding the response to DNA damage is necessary in order to understand the toxicities of radiation. Ionizing radiation initiates a complex cascade of cellular responses that can result in cell-cycle arrest, induction of stress-response genes, induction of apoptosis, or repair of DNA damage. These responses are not mutually exclusive. For example, transient cell-cycle arrest allows time for DNA damage repair prior to mitosis initiation, potentially triggering apoptosis as a result of unrepaired double-strand breaks. The response to DNA damage is a very active field of research, but the details are beyond the scope of this chapter.

Several biologic characteristics of a tumor modify sensitivity to radiation. Oxygenation status of target tissue is a critical factor. It is clear that hypoxic tumors are more resistant to ionizing radiation than are normally oxygenated tumors (25). As cancer cells die within the tumor mass, anoxic regions can "reoxygenate," and cells that had been relatively protected can become more sensitive. Another important determinant of radiosensitivity is position in the cell cycle. Cells in the G2 and M phases of the cell cycle are most sensitive to radiation, while cells in late S phase are relatively resistant (26). This differential sensitivity can lead to a relative synchronization of tumor cells. These factors (oxygenation status and fluxes related to irradiation as well as cell-cycle and tumor synchronization) are taken into account when developing treatment plans.

Types of External-beam Radiation

Typical external-beam radiotherapy is delivered from a Cobalt-60 source and is composed of photons. To minimize dose delivery to normal tissue, perpendicular beams are used to deliver the radiation, with the area of overlap corresponding to the target. Because the beams are rectangular, but most tumors are irregularly shaped, devices known as collimators in the head of the radiation source shape the beam to more closely conform to the shape of the tumor as determined by CT scan. The beam can be further shaped with the use of individually constructed blocks, which shield body regions that are not in the target area. Modern, multileaf collimators provide additional precision to the shape of the beam.

Photons typically deposit energy relatively deep into tissue, with higher-energy photons penetrating deeper than lower-energy photons. Electrons, in contrast, deposit their energy in a relatively shallow range, with a rapid drop-off of energy with increasing depth. Thus, a superficial tumor (such as leukemia cutis) will be more appropriately treated with electron-beam therapy, rather than standard photons.

Like electrons, protons have a very rapid drop-off of energy in the last few millimeters of penetration. Unlike electrons, protons penetrate relatively deep into tissue. Thus, a proton beam can treat a target deeper than an electron beam, but with similar precision in the deposition of energy. Thus, proton-beam radiation is valuable when the target is located deep but adjacent to particularly sensitive normal tissue. Whereas photons and electrons are commonly available, a limited number of centers are capable of delivering proton-beam radiotherapy. Merchant recently reviewed indications for, and results of, proton-beam radiotherapy in pediatric oncology (27).

Targeted Radiation Therapy

Other means of delivering radiation therapy, aside from external beam, are brachytherapy and targeted radiation therapy. Because brachytherapy is unlikely to result in complications requiring critical care, it will not be discussed further. In pediatric oncology, interest is growing in physiologic targeting of radiation. Examples of physiologic targeting include the use of iodine 131 metaiodobenzylguanidine (^{131}I-MIBG) to treat neuroblastoma and samarium-153 ethylene diamine tetramethylene phosphonate ([153]Sm-EDTMP) to treat osteosarcoma. MIBG is a catecholamine precursor that, when labeled with Iodine-123 has been used as a diagnostic imaging tool for neural crest tumors, such as neuroblastoma. Oncologists are exploring the use of ^{131}I-MIBG as a therapeutic tool, based on the concept that neuroblastoma cells concentrate MIBG, allowing the delivery of potentially cytotoxic doses of ^{131}I to the tumor, while sparing normal tissue. The feasibility of this approach in the setting of an autologous peripheral blood stem-cell transplant has recently been demonstrated (28). [153]Sm-EDTMP is a bone-seeking radiopharmaceutical that has been used to treat high-risk osteosarcoma (29). Just as the MIBG targets ^{131}I to neuroblastoma cells, EDTMP targets [153]Sm to osteosarcoma cells, essentially sparing surrounding normal tissue. Like ^{131}I-MIBG, [153]Sm-EDTMP is being delivered in the context of autologous peripheral blood stem-cell support, making it likely that such patients will require critical care.

BIOLOGICAL THERAPY

As our understanding of the biology of pediatric tumors improves, biologically-based therapy is becoming a reality. Biological therapies currently in clinical use include differentiation therapy, immunotherapy, small-molecule kinase inhibitors, and monoclonal antibody therapies. A full review of biologically-based anticancer therapy is beyond the scope of this chapter, but we will discuss examples of each type of biological therapy with an emphasis on agents that have significant enough toxicities that patients run a reasonable risk of needing critical care.

Differentiation Therapy

The best-known example of differentiation therapy is the use of all-trans retinoic acid (ATRA) in the treatment of acute promyelocytic leukemia (APML). APML is well known to the intensivist because of the characteristic profound bleeding diathesis seen at presentation. Prior to the routine use of ATRA, APML was associated with a very poor prognosis, with an overall survival rate of ~20% and 10%–20% of patients dying of hemorrhage during induction therapy. Molecular research into the pathogenesis of this disease revealed that the malignant cells are characterized by the presence of a translocation between chromosomes 15 and 17 that causes the production of a fusion protein that combines the retinoic acid receptor RARα with a nuclear protein called PML. Pharmacologic doses of ATRA overcome the block to differentiation caused by PML-RARα, and the malignant promyelocytes differentiate into granulocytes (30). The advent of ATRA therapy has improved the remission induction rate from 62% to greater than 90% and has significantly decreased the rate of hemorrhagic death.

A second common example of differentiation therapy in pediatric oncology is the use of 13-cis-retinoic acid to treat neuroblastoma. As laboratory work demonstrated that retinoids induce the differentiation of neuroblastoma cells, a large-scale trial was performed that randomized patients with high-risk neuroblastoma to receive either 13-cis-retinoic acid or nothing following a randomization to autologous peripheral blood stem-cell transplant or intensive chemotherapy. Because this study showed a clear survival advantage for patients who were treated with 13-cis-retinoic acid (31), this has become standard of care in the United States.

Immunotherapy

Like differentiation therapy, immunotherapy is gaining acceptance in the treatment of pediatric malignancies. Under the broad category of immunotherapy, are classified such diverse treatments as allogeneic hematopoietic stem-cell transplantation, with or without infusion of donor lymphocytes, and treatment with various recombinant cytokines. Stem-cell transplantation and donor lymphocyte infusions are covered in depth in Chapter 101. Cytokine administration remains a rare event in pediatric oncology, but this approach was pioneered by the National Cancer Institute's efforts at inducing an immune response to metastatic melanoma and to renal cell carcinoma by infusions of interleukin (IL)-2. In neuroblastoma, it has been shown that the disialoganglioside GD2 is uniformly expressed in tumor, but the only normal tissues with significant GD2 expression are normal neurons, skin melanocytes, and peripheral sensory nerve fibers. A chimeric human–murine anti-GD2 monoclonal antibody has been used in early-phase clinical trials, and was shown to be effective, especially when given in combination with GM-CSF and IL-2. Recently, a randomized control study showed clear survival advantage for patients who were treated with a combination therapy of 13-cis-retinoic acid, anti-GD2 antibodies with alternating GM-CSF and IL-2 compared with 13-cis-retinoic acid only (32). This has now become a standard of care in patients with high-risk neuroblastoma following stem-cell transplant. Similar protocols are being explored by the Children's Oncology Group, and over time, manipulation of the immune system via cytokine administration will become a more frequent event.

Small-molecule Kinase Inhibitors

The advent of Gleevec for the treatment of chronic myelogenous leukemia (CML) heralded the era of targeted therapy based on a molecular understanding of tumorigenesis. CML is defined by the presence of a distinctive chromosomal translocation, t(9;22), or the Philadelphia chromosome. This translocation leads to the production of a fusion protein tyrosine kinase called BCR-ABL, and this kinase drives the neoplastic process. Gleevec is a competitive inhibitor of the BCR-ABL tyrosine kinase and causes complete hematologic response as a single agent in 95% of CML patients (33). Many patients with CML achieve long-term remission with Gleevec, and now second-generation tyrosine kinase inhibitors (TKIs) such as Dasatinib and Nilotinib are available for patients with resistant disease. Based on the success of Gleevec, newer TKIs have been developed and are being used in clinical trials for many other diagnoses. Sorafenib, which is a multiple TKI initially used to treat hepatocellular carcinoma and renal cell cancer in adults, is now used increasingly for AML with an internal tandem duplication of FMS-like tyrosine kinase receptor-3 gene (FLT3-ITD). Although the drug commonly causes side effects such as diarrhea and hand–foot skin reaction, this is often manageable by supportive care.

Monoclonal Antibodies

Monoclonal antibody therapy is also finding expanded use in pediatric oncology. Two frequently used monoclonal antibodies target antigens on the surface of lymphocytes. Rituximab is an antibody against CD20, a marker of B lymphocytes, and is seeing increased use in treating non-Hodgkin lymphoma and autoimmune disorders, such as ITP and hemolytic anemia (34). Response to rituximab can be monitored indirectly by measuring CD20-positive cells in the circulation, and they often become undetectable within a day of only one dose of the antibody. Clearance of circulating CD20-positive cells does not necessarily correlate with efficacy, unfortunately, because most CD20-positive cells do not circulate, but are found in spleen and lymph nodes, where they are not easily measured. Another commonly used monoclonal antibody is alemtuzumab, which is anti-CD52. CD52 is a pan-lymphocyte marker, and treatment with alemtuzumab results in a rapid, profound, and long-lasting depletion of circulating T cells, B cells, NK cells, and monocytes. Patients become lymphopenic within 2 weeks and remain lymphopenic for as long as a year after treatment (35). In adult oncology, alemtuzumab is primarily used as therapy for lymphomas, but in pediatric oncology, its primary use is in the context of bone marrow transplantation (BMT)—either as part of an immunoablative preparative regimen or in the prevention or treatment of graft-versus-host disease (GVHD). An appreciation of the profoundly immunosuppressive nature of this drug is critical to appropriately evaluate BMT patients who have received the drug.

Antiangiogenic Therapy

The growth of solid tumors, such as sarcomas, is limited by the availability of oxygen and nutrients, which must be delivered by blood vessels. Aggregates of cancer cells are unable to grow into tumors of greater than 1–2 mm in diameter without an adequate blood supply. The induction of tumor vasculature is referred to as the "angiogenic switch (36)." The major molecular driver of angiogenesis is vascular endothelial growth factor (VEGF). VEGF is overexpressed in multiple malignancies, and targeting of VEGF has been attempted through multiple approaches. One common VEGF-targeted therapy is a monoclonal antibody called bevacizumab. Bevacizumab has been studied in multiple pediatric clinical trials, particularly in CNS tumors and sarcomas, and does provide benefit for patients with some of these tumors, especially glioblastoma multiforme. The drug has been used in combination therapy with more conventional chemotherapeutics such as irinotecan and has been well tolerated, but commonly side effects include poor wound healing, thrombocytopenia, hypertension, proteinuria, and venous thrombosis.

Another antiangiogenic approach is the use of TKIs that target VEGF receptors, including Sunitinib and Cediranib. Sunitinib is an oral multitarget tyrosine kinase receptor inhibitor that inhibits the VEGF receptor as well as other targets such as the platelet-derived growth factor receptors. It has shown effectiveness in renal cell carcinoma and gastrointestinal stromal tumors in adults, and is currently being studied for refractory solid tumors in children. Although this is generally well tolerated, cardiac toxicity has been reported in phase I trials in children. Cediranib, which is also a multitargeted TKI, is known to be a VEGF receptor inhibitor and has been studied in children with refractory solid tumors. Common side effects such as hypertension and prolonged QTc have been reported as dose-limiting toxicities.

TOXICITIES

The management of acute toxicities of cancer therapy often falls to a partnership between the pediatric oncologist and the pediatric intensivist. Understanding the unique toxicities experienced by the pediatric cancer patient is critical to the successful management of the critically ill child with cancer. This section will outline the common therapy-related toxicities that may be experienced by a pediatric cancer patient. Some of these toxicities are covered more extensively in other chapters (e.g., GVHD is covered in the BMT chapter), and the reader is referred to those chapters for more detail. Table 114.3 lists typical toxicities caused by the commonly used chemotherapy drugs. The discussion below is organized by organ system, rather than by individual drug.

Fever in the Neutropenic Patient

The most common side effect of cytotoxic chemotherapy is myelosuppression, which leads to periods of absolute neutropenia. A fever in a neutropenic cancer patient represents

---

TABLE 114.3

TYPICAL TOXICITIES OF COMMONLY USED CHEMOTHERAPY DRUGS

■ DRUG	■ TOXICITIES
Ifosfamide	Renal tubular dysfunction, encephalopathy, hemorrhagic cystitis
Cyclophosphamide	Renal tubular dysfunction, hemorrhagic cystitis, myocardial necrosis
Cytarabine	Cerebellar syndrome, myelopathy, leukoencephalopathy, pulmonary edema, pneumonitis, *Streptococcus viridans* sepsis
Methotrexate	Skin sloughing, nephrotoxicity, encephalopathy, hepatic dysfunction
Anthracyclines	Severe mucositis, congestive heart failure
Bleomycin	Pneumonitis
ATRA	Capillary leak syndrome
L-asparaginase	Pancreatitis
Cisplatin	Renal tubular dysfunction, cardiotoxicity
Vincristine	Peripheral neuropathy, ileus, neuropathic pain
Sorafenib	Hand–foot rash syndrome, thrombocytopenia

Note: Most chemotherapeutic agents cause nausea, vomiting, mucositis, and pancytopenia; therefore, these are not included in this table. This table is *not* intended to be a comprehensive listing of chemotherapy side effects, but rather a list of the most common toxicities that may be encountered by the pediatric intensivist.

a true emergency due to the significant rate of gram-negative bacteremia in such patients, which can rapidly lead to septic shock. Because of the emergent nature of febrile neutropenia, this topic is dealt with in Chapter 99.

Toxicities Related to Bone Marrow Transplantation

Children who have undergone BMT are subject to a number of unique toxicities, including veno-occlusive disease, cytokine storm/engraftment syndrome, and GVHD. BMT patients may also develop fever while they are neutropenic, and many of the immunosuppressive drugs used as prophylaxis or in treatment of GVHD can cause significant, difficult-to-control hypertension. Finally, pneumonitis is a common problem encountered in the post-BMT setting. These topics are covered extensively in other chapters in this text.

Toxicities of the Central Nervous System

5a A number of commonly used chemotherapeutic drugs cause distinct CNS toxicities. The greatest culprit in the pediatric population is ifosfamide. Ifosfamide causes encephalopathy in 10%–30% of patients, with onset of symptoms, which can range from mild (somnolence) to severe (coma or seizure), occurring between 2 and 48 hours after drug administration (37). The mechanism for this toxicity is unclear, although several potential pathophysiologic explanations have been proposed, including accumulation of glutaric acid, which can lead to disturbances in the mitochondrial respiratory chain, ultimately leading to high levels of the ifosfamide metabolite chloracetaldehyde, which is neurotoxic (38). David and Picus investigated risk factors for the development of ifosfamide-induced encephalopathy and found no correlation with renal function or dose of drug. They did, however, find a statistically significant association between encephalopathy and hypoalbuminemia (37). The management of ifosfamide-induced encephalopathy includes discontinuation of the drug and standard supportive measures (discussed in more detail elsewhere in this volume). Several groups have reported of the use of methylene blue for the treatment of ifosfamide-induced encephalopathy, but the lack of any controlled trials (and reports of spontaneous resolution) makes it impossible to determine if this agent is helpful (39). The mechanism by which methylene blue might treat this encephalopathy is also unclear.

Another chemotherapy drug that commonly causes acute CNS toxicity is araC (40). The neurologic toxicities depend on dose and route of administration. Intrathecal araC has been associated with a rapid-onset myelopathy (although this might be related to the use of benzyl alcohol as a diluent) or a slower-onset myelopathy, with symptoms beginning 2 days to 6 months after treatment. On autopsy in many of these patients correlative evidence of demyelination was observed. Other CNS toxicities have also been reported more rarely after intrathecal araC, including seizures and leukoencephalopathy. Seizures have also been described in patients being treated with intravenous high-dose araC. In general, these have been self-limited and do not recur once therapy is stopped. Cerebral dysfunction, usually accompanying cerebellar syndrome, has also been described and usually takes the form of generalized encephalopathy. Cerebral dysfunction also usually resolves spontaneously.

The acute cerebellar syndrome is the most prominent and common neurologic toxicity associated with cytarabine (40). The syndrome is only seen after treatment with high-dose systemic cytarabine and occurs at an incidence of at least 10%. Onset of symptoms is 3–8 days after treatment, and

manifestations include dysarthria, dysdiadochokinesia, dysmetria, and ataxia. The outcome is variable, with complete resolution of symptoms common, but ~30% of adults never regain normal function. Diagnostic evaluation is unrevealing. Risk factors include age (with incidence increasing from 3% in patients under 40 years of age to 30% in patients over 60). Other possible risk factors include renal dysfunction and cumulative exposure to drug, although these are not completely agreed upon. The neuropathology of cerebellar syndrome has been extensively investigated, and findings consistently include the loss of Purkinje cells in the cerebellar hemispheres and vermis with a reactive gliosis. The only effective therapy for this disorder is discontinuation of the drug and institution of supportive care as indicated.

Finally, methotrexate is associated with CNS toxicities when administered intrathecally or at high doses intravenously. Methotrexate can cause an encephalitis after both high-dose systemic administration or after intrathecal administration in up to 5% of patients. Common clinical presentation includes headache, confusion, disorientation, seizures, dysphagia, and weakness, including hemiparesis. The encephalopathy is usually self-limited, resolving over a period of a week. The pathophysiology of this neurotoxicity is unclear. Aminophylline has been used as an adenosine receptor blocker based on the observation that high adenosine levels have been observed in the CSF after methotrexate therapy, leading to intermittent cerebral vasodilation. Although there are reports that administration of aminophylline shortens the duration of encephalopathy, there are no controlled trials, so the use of this agent is of unclear clinical utility.

Cardiac Toxicities

5b The best-known cardiotoxic chemotherapy drugs are the anthracyclines: doxorubicin, daunorubicin, and idarubicin. The mechanism of cardiotoxicity involves the generation of oxygen free radicals, which ultimately lead to irreversible loss of myocardiocytes and the development of cardiomyopathy. Anthracycline cardiotoxicity can be acute or delayed. Acute effects include transient arrhythmias and acute left ventricular failure (41). The acute effects are usually transient and will attenuate after discontinuation of therapy (41). Cardiac injury can also present in a delayed fashion, years or decades after treatment, as new onset congestive heart failure. The most significant risk factor for serious cardiotoxicity is cumulative dose. Many approaches to minimize the risk of cardiotoxicity have been investigated. Other than limiting total exposure, measures that have been investigated include the administration of liposome-encapsulated anthracyclines and the use of cardioprotectants, such as dexrazoxane (Zinecard). Dexrazoxane acts as an iron chelator, prevents the formation of an anthracycline–iron complex that is thought to be a critical mediator of myocardiocyte injury, and thus prevent cardiac damage. Clinical evidence suggests that dexrazoxane does, in fact, reduce cardiotoxicity caused by doxorubicin. Once patients exhibit symptoms of cardiotoxicity, standard treatments should be administered, aimed at decreasing afterload and increasing contractility. Anticoagulation is useful in the setting of severe left ventricular dysfunction and persistent dysrhythmia. Cardiac transplantation remains an option for end-stage cardiomyopathy.

Cyclophosphamide has also been associated with severe cardiotoxicity at high doses, such as are employed in BMT. The estimated incidence in children is 5% in patients treated with marrow ablative doses (41). Risk factors include prior anthracycline chemotherapy and chest irradiation. Clinically, cardiotoxicity presents as congestive heart failure or myocarditis. Severe hemorrhagic cardiac necrosis has been reported as well. Symptoms may be delayed by up to 2 weeks after administration, but can be rapidly fatal, with a 10% mortality rate. With no specific treatment available for cyclophosphamide-induced cardiotoxicity, standard supportive measures are indicated.

Paclitaxel has been associated with asymptomatic bradycardia in up to 29% of treated patients (41). Second- and third-degree heart blocks are also seen, though less frequently. These bradyarrhythmias are reversible. Several cases of acute myocardial infarction after cisplatin therapy have also been reported (42).

Several other drugs have been associated with cardiac toxicities. Amsacrine, an acridine derivative with activity against hematologic malignancies (not commercially available in the United States), can affect cardiac electrophysiology and cause a wide range of EKG changes, including ventricular tachycardia. The arrhythmias can occur within minutes of treatment. More rare are reports of delayed (days after treatment) cardiomyopathy. 5-Fluorouracil has also been reported to induce cardiotoxicity (including arrhythmias, silent ischemia, and even sudden death) in up to 18% of treated patients, occurring mostly in the setting of continuous infusion, rather than bolus dosing. Risk factors include preexisting coronary artery disease and concurrent radiotherapy. The mechanism of this toxicity is unknown.

Pulmonary Toxicities

5c Bleomycin is the chemotherapeutic most frequently thought of in the context of pulmonary toxicity, but other cytotoxic treatments can cause pulmonary fibrosis or edema, including gemcitabine, cytarabine, and radiation therapy. Additionally, a number of drugs (including carmustine, methotrexate, procarbazine, and bleomycin) have been linked with a hypersensitivity pneumonitis syndrome. Also referred to as inflammatory interstitial pneumonitis, this syndrome is characterized by an insidious progression of nonproductive cough, dyspnea, and low-grade fevers. Eosinophilia is noted in the peripheral blood and on lung biopsy, which often also reveals bronchiolitis obliterans with organizing pneumonia. This syndrome resolves with removal of the offending agent, although sometimes oral corticosteroids speed recovery.

Bleomycin toxicity is primarily limited to lungs and skin because these organs lack bleomycin hydrolase. Most commonly, bleomycin causes an interstitial pneumonitis (bleomycin-induced pneumonitis, BIP) and has been reported in up to 46% of patients treated with bleomycin (depending on diagnostic criteria), with mortality seen in 3%. BIP usually begins during therapy and is initially indolent, with a cough and dyspnea on exertion as the primary symptoms. The disorder can progress to dyspnea at rest, tachypnea, and cyanosis. Radiographic findings are nonspecific and may be focal or diffuse, unilateral or bilateral. Interstitial or alveolar infiltrates can be seen on plain film, and CT scan often shows small linear and subpleural nodular lesions in the lung bases. Lung biopsy may show characteristic lesions, such as squamous metaplasia of bronchiolar epithelium, inflammatory cells infiltrating into alveoli and alveolar septa, edema plus focal collagen depositions in these septa, and fibrotic areas. In animal models, the pathogenesis appears to be related to initial endothelial damage, probably mediated through free radical production and release of cytokines, followed by an influx of inflammatory cells, ultimately leading to pulmonary fibrosis. Decrease in diffusion capacity is seen in patients with BIP, although this finding is nonspecific. Decreased vital capacity is also seen and was noted in patients who received combination therapy with bleomycin, etoposide, and cisplatin, but not in patients treated with etoposide and cisplatin alone (43),

suggesting that decreased vital capacity may be a more specific indicator of BIP. High-dose corticosteroids (60–100 mg/day in adults) are frequently used to treat clinically significant BIP, but as yet, no randomized studies demonstrate the efficacy of steroids in this setting. Also of importance to the intensivist is the acute onset of pulmonary edema, often mimicking adult respiratory distress syndrome, in patients previously treated with bleomycin who are exposed to high concentrations of inspired oxygen, as may occur in conjunction with a surgical procedure, even years after chemotherapy is completed. This complication can be minimized by administering the lowest possible concentration of oxygen to patients with a history of treatment with bleomycin.

A vascular leak syndrome, leading to significant, sometimes life-threatening, pulmonary edema, has also been described with infusions of araC or IL-2 (44). The vascular leak is usually reversible with discontinuation of therapy and is treated with diuresis and oxygen. Prostaglandins or cyclooxygenase-2 may attenuate IL-2-induced vascular leak. Vascular leak has also been reported in patients treated with ATRA for APML. The leukemia itself is probably involved in this process, because vascular leak has not been reported in patients treated with ATRA for other disorders. More recently, clofarabine has been associated with a life-threatening capillary leak syndrome (45).

Other chemotherapeutic agents associated with pulmonary toxicity include Mitomycin-C, which causes a delayed-onset interstitial pneumonitis that is symptomatic in ~5% of treated patients, actinomycin D, which acts as a radiation sensitizer, and, rarely, cyclophosphamide or ifosfamide, which can cause pulmonary fibrosis in less than 1% of treated patients.

Radiation therapy can damage capillary endothelial cells and type I pneumocytes, eventually leading to a pneumonitis syndrome. Incidence and severity are primarily related to the amount of lung volume irradiated, total dose delivered, and the fractions into which the total dose is divided. Radiation pneumonitis is rare in patients treated with less than 20 Gy, but is highly likely in patients who receive greater than 60 Gy. Symptoms become evident 2–3 months following completion of therapy, and primarily include complaints of dyspnea and a nonproductive cough. Physical findings are usually minimal. Permanent changes of fibrosis evolve over 6–24 months, but usually stabilize after this time period. No controlled trials of treatment have been conducted for radiation pneumonitis, but objective responses to corticosteroids are seen. Once fibrosis develops, most experts believe that corticosteroids have no further therapeutic role. Clinical symptomatic relief has been reported in patients with pulmonary fibrosis who were treated with pentoxifylline and vitamin E (46).

Retinoic Acid Syndrome

5d The advent of ATRA for the treatment of APML has transformed this disease from one that carried a grave prognosis into one that is frequently curable. The major complication of ATRA treatment is the retinoic acid syndrome, which occurs in as many as 25% of patients with APML who are treated with ATRA. Improvements in recognition and treatment have decreased the mortality of retinoic acid syndrome from 30% to 5%. The diagnosis is established by the presence of at least three of the following signs and/or symptoms in the absence of alternative explanations: fever, weight gain, respiratory distress, pulmonary infiltrates, pleural or pericardial effusions, hypotension, and renal failure (47). The syndrome most commonly manifests approximately 10 days after the start of chemotherapy, but has been reported as rapidly as 2 days into treatment. The pathogenesis is related to tissue infiltration, with newly differentiated granulocytes and cytokine production by these cells. The final pathway is endothelial damage leading to edema, hemorrhage, fibrinous exudates, and respiratory failure. The only specific therapy available for retinoic acid syndrome is dexamethasone. As noted above, improved recognition of the syndrome and prompt institution of steroid therapy have dramatically improved prognosis.

Pancreatitis

It has long been recognized that treatment with L-asparaginase may cause acute pancreatitis. Management of asparaginase-induced pancreatitis is identical to the management of idiopathic pancreatitis, including gut rest. Asparaginase-induced acute pancreatitis can progress to hemorrhagic pancreatitis, and chronic pancreatitis is also seen in some patients.

Urinary Tract Toxicities

Both ifosfamide and cyclophosphamide can cause hemorrhagic cystitis. Ifosfamide is a more potent urotoxin than cyclophosphamide. Both drugs are broken down to produce, among other degradation products, acrolein. Acrolein has been incriminated as the major cause of hemorrhagic cystitis after treatment with these drugs, but the difference between ifosfamide and cyclophosphamide is not accounted for entirely by increased production of acrolein; therefore, other metabolites are probably also involved. Prophylaxis against hemorrhagic cystitis includes aggressive hydration (alkaline intravenous fluids at twice maintenance) and the use of mesna (sodium-2-mercaptoethanesulfonate). Mesna can be administered either orally or intravenously and is rapidly oxidized to dimesna, which is filtered and excreted by the kidneys. Between 30% and 50% of glomerularly filtered dimesna is reduced back to mesna in the renal tubular epithelium by glutathione reductase. Mesna collects in the bladder, where it detoxifies acrolein and other oxazaphosphorine metabolites. Mesna is superior to placebo or to hydration alone in the prevention of hemorrhagic cystitis (48). Uncontrolled hemorrhagic cystitis can be life threatening, and exsanguination can occur. If prophylaxis fails, management includes cystoscopy and clot evacuation, aggressive bladder irrigation, and intravesicle instillation of formalin.

In addition to cystitis, cyclophosphamide and ifosfamide can also cause renal dysfunction, both tubular and glomerular. Ifosfamide is a far more potent nephrotoxin, although nephrotoxicity is seen after very high doses of cyclophosphamide. Proximal tubular dysfunction is the most common form of nephrotoxicity observed and frequently manifests as Fanconi syndrome, with hypophosphatemia, renal tubular acidosis, hypokalemia, hypocalcemia, or hypomagnesemia. Any of these can be quite severe and require aggressive replacement therapy. Distal tubular dysfunction is less common, but nephrogenic diabetes insipidus has been reported. Glomerular toxicity, though more rare, can be severe enough to require dialysis and may become chronic. Hypertension is also seen. The specific mechanism of renal tubular damage caused by these drugs is unknown. Risk factors for ifosfamide nephrotoxicity include age (increased risk in children <5 years old), total dose of ifosfamide (increased risk with total dose >60 g/m²), prior or concurrent treatment with cisplatin (which increases the risk), and preexisting renal impairment (49). A theoretical basis exists for the belief that very high doses of mesna might protect against renal tubular damage caused by ifosfamide, but no clinical studies have been conducted to support this theory. Thus, currently, the only available preventive measures are careful screening of patients and limiting treatment in patients with the risk factors described above.

Cisplatin is also nephrotoxic. Cisplatin accumulates in the proximal tubules, with intracellular concentrations fivefold higher than plasma concentrations (50). Through inhibition of protein synthesis and depletion of glutathione, cisplatin causes the tubular necrosis that underlies its renal toxicity. Cisplatin administration results in a dose-dependent reduction of glomerular filtration rate, hypomagnesemia, hypokalemia, and polyuria. Evidence suggests that aggressive hydration, including the use of mannitol, can attenuate the toxicity of cisplatin. The renal toxicity of cisplatin is usually reversible, but can become chronic and progressive.

Radiation Recall

Radiation recall is an inflammatory reaction in a previously irradiated body area. Most commonly, radiation recall manifests as an acute dermatitis. Reactions can range from a mild maculopapular erythematous skin rash to severe necrosis and occur in a sharply demarcated area corresponding to the prior radiation field. The reaction can occur weeks to years after radiation exposure, and the mechanism of this reaction is unclear. First described in patients treated with actinomycin D, radiation recall has subsequently been described with numerous other antineoplastic drugs and, more recently, even in patients treated with other classes of pharmacologic agents (51). Although skin is the most common organ involved, radiation recall has been reported in lung, esophagus, gut, and the CNS. In visceral organs, it manifests as inflammation of the target organ within a previous radiation field. Numerous hypotheses have been proposed to explain the phenomenon of radiation recall, but none have been proven to explain the process. The most reasonable current explanation is an idiosyncratic drug reaction in a tissue with an altered inflammatory response ratio induced by prior irradiation (51). A dose–response phenomenon is suggested, in that radiation recall is more frequent in areas that receive higher doses of radiation. Also, while numerous drugs have been implicated in radiation recall, nearly 50% of reported cases have been associated with the use of taxanes or anthracyclines. Treatment is straightforward, with the mainstays of therapy being corticosteroids and withdrawal of the offending agent. Topical steroids are appropriate for skin reactions, but clearly systemic steroids are necessary for visceral involvement.

Management of Chemotherapy Overdose

As chemotherapeutic agents can cause life-threatening complications when dosed appropriately, a chemotherapy overdose is certainly an indication for careful evaluation and will likely lead to a need for critical care. The literature contains few reports of the effects of accidental chemotherapy overdose, and even fewer reports of successful, specific treatments. Most reports document the efficacy of aggressive supportive care allowing the patient to recover. Others report specific therapies administered to patients who received an overdose of cisplatin, including plasmapheresis and the administration of sodium thiosulfate. Hemodialysis has not been found to be effective, probably because cisplatin is extensively protein bound and deposits in tissues from which it is unable to be cleared by hemodialysis. Plasmapheresis is expected to be more effective by virtue of removing circulating plasma proteins to which cisplatin is bound. In one patient who was accidentally given a threefold overdose of cisplatin, at the time of overt renal failure, sodium thiosulfate was administered (loading dose of 4 g/m², followed by 2.7 g/m²/day in three divided doses of 0.9 g/m²/dose for 13 days) based on the assumption that this compound would bind the platinum and remove it

TABLE 114.4

USE OF HEMODIALYSIS FOR OVERDOSE OF CHEMOTHERAPY

■ READILY CLEARED BY HEMODIALYSIS	■ NOT CLEARED BY HEMODIALYSIS
Ifosfamide	Etoposide
Methotrexate	Dactinomycin
Cyclophosphamide	Vinca alkaloids
	Anthracyclines

Note: Platinum agents are cleared only if dialysis is initiated rapidly after drug administration. These drugs become protein bound (carboplatin) or distribute into tissue (cisplatin) quickly and are no longer dialyzable. Paclitaxel pharmacokinetics is unaltered in anephric patients undergoing hemodialysis.

from circulation (52). An increase in urinary platinum levels was seen after initiation of this therapy. The other reported specific treatment for cisplatin overdose is the administration of N-acetylcysteine to replenish glutathione and allow the usual detoxification reactions to function (53).

Ifosfamide overdose has been treated with the use of methylene blue. A patient who was accidentally given an overdose of ifosfamide was found to have excessive urinary excretion of glutaric acid and sarcosine, which is compatible with glutaric aciduria type II, a defect in mitochondrial fatty acid oxidation that results from defective electron transfer to flavoproteins (54). This observation led to the administration of 50 mg of methylene blue intravenously, based on the function of methylene blue as an electron acceptor. The severe neurotoxicity experienced by that patient rapidly reversed.

7 Carboxypeptidase G2 (or Glucarpidase) is another recently developed "antidote" to chemotherapy overdose. It is a bacterial enzyme that hydrolyzes methotrexate to its inactive metabolites, 4-deoxy-4-amino-N10-methylpteroic acid and glutamate. Carboxypeptidase G2 has been administered intravenously to patients with delayed methotrexate clearance after they were given appropriate high-dose methotrexate therapy, and more recently, it has been given intrathecally with good results to patients with an accidental intrathecal methotrexate overdose (55). Glucarpidase was recently approved by the FDA for symptomatic, severe methotrexate toxicity.

Hemodialysis is a nonspecific intervention often employed in the treatment of drug overdose. The effects of hemodialysis on the pharmacokinetics of antineoplastic drugs have been recently reviewed (56) and are summarized in **Table 114.4**. Paclitaxel pharmacokinetics is unaltered in anephric patients who are undergoing hemodialysis. Dialysis is effective in clearing cisplatin and carboplatin only within a relatively short time after drug administration due to rapid and stable binding to proteins in serum (carboplatin) or peripheral tissues (cisplatin). Methotrexate and cyclophosphamide are readily dialyzable, with an increased rate of elimination, compared to renal clearance. Ifosfamide is also readily removed by hemodialysis, while etoposide, dactinomycin, vinca alkaloids, and anthracyclines are rapidly and extensively protein bound and not cleared effectively by hemodialysis.

FUTURE DIRECTIONS

The future of pediatric cancer therapy lies not with the development of improved cytotoxic drugs, but rather with the expansion of biologically-based therapies and targeted therapies. The prototype for the potential of these approaches remains the astounding success of ATRA in the treatment of APML. The profound efficacy of Gleevec for the treatment of CML in the absence of significant toxicity further emphasizes the power of biologically-based therapies. The future will

see the expansion of this type of treatment, and hopefully will see the disappearance of highly toxic, highly nonspecific cytotoxic chemotherapy.

References

1. Gilman A. The initial clinical trial of nitrogen mustard. *Am J Surg* 1963;105:574–8.
2. Lawley PD, Brookes P. Acidic dissociation of 7:9-dialkylguanines and its possible relation to mutagenic properties of alkylating agents. *Nature* 1961;192:1081–2.
3. Kohn KW. Interstrand cross-linking of DNA by 1,3-bis (2-chloroethyl)-1-nitrosourea and other 1-(2-haloethyl)-1-nitrosoureas. *Cancer Res* 1977;37(5):1450–4.
4. Pegg AE. Mammalian O6-alkylguanine-DNA alkyltransferase: Regulation and importance in response to alkylating carcinogenic and therapeutic agents. *Cancer Res* 1990;50(19):6119–29.
5. Hall AG, Tilby MJ. Mechanisms of action of, and modes of resistance to, alkylating agents used in the treatment of haematological malignancies. *Blood Rev* 1992;6(3):163–73.
6. Zwelling LA, Kohn KW. Mechanism of action of cis-dichlorodiammineplatinum(II). *Cancer Treat Rep* 1979; 63(9–10):1439–44.
7. Fridland A. Effect of methotrexate on deoxyribonucleotide pools and DNA synthesis in human lymphocytic cells. *Cancer Res* 1974;34(8):1883–8.
8. Hryniuk WM. Purineless death as a link between growth rate and cytotoxicity by methotrexate. *Cancer Res* 1972;32(7):1506–11.
9. Hirata S, Matsubara T, Saura R, et al. Inhibition of in vitro vascular endothelial cell proliferation and in vivo neovascularization by low-dose methotrexate. *Arthritis Rheum* 1989;32(9):1065–73.
10. Billington DC. Angiogenesis and its inhibition: Potential new therapies in oncology and non-neoplastic diseases. *Drug Des Discov* 1991;8(1):3–35.
11. Jeha S, Gandhi V, Chan KW, et al. Clofarabine, a novel nucleoside analog, is active in pediatric patients with advanced leukemia. *Blood* 2004;103(3):784–9.
12. Chen AY, Liu LF. DNA topoisomerases: Essential enzymes and lethal targets. *Annu Rev Pharmacol Toxicol* 1994;34:191–218.
13. Hande KR. Etoposide: Four decades of development of a topoisomerase II inhibitor. *Eur J Cancer* 1998;34(10):1514–21.
14. Tewey KM, Rowe TC, Yang L, et al. Adriamycin-induced DNA damage mediated by mammalian DNA topoisomerase II. *Science* 1984;226(4673):466–8.
15. Pommier Y. Eukaryotic DNA topoisomerase I: Genome gatekeeper and its intruders, camptothecins. *Semin Oncol* 1996; 23(1 suppl 3):3–10.
16. Himes RH. Interactions of the catharanthus (Vinca) alkaloids with tubulin and microtubules. *Pharmacol Ther* 1991;51(2):257–67.
17. Quasthoff S, Hartung HP. Chemotherapy-induced peripheral neuropathy. *J Neurol* 2002;249(1):9–17.

18. Rowinsky EK, Donehower RC. Paclitaxel (taxol). *N Engl J Med* 1995;332(15):1004–14.

19. Schiff PB, Fant J, Horwitz SB. Promotion of microtubule assembly in vitro by taxol. *Nature* 1979;277(5698):665–7.

20. Belotti D, Vergani V, Drudis T, et al. The microtubule-affecting drug paclitaxel has antiangiogenic activity. *Clin Cancer Res* 1996;2(11):1843–9.

21. Capizzi RL, Bertino JR, Handschumacher RE. L-asparaginase. *Annu Rev Med* 1970;21:433–44.

22. Kufe DW, Major PP, Egan EM, et al. Correlation of cytotoxicity with incorporation of ara-C into DNA. *J Biol Chem* 1980;255(19):8900–97.

23. Woodcock DM, Fox RM, Cooper IA. Evidence for a new mechanism of cytotoxicity of 1-beta-D arabinofuranosylcytosine. *Cancer Res* 1979;39(4):1418–24.

24. Radford IR. The level of induced DNA double-strand breakage correlates with cell killing after X-irradiation. *Int J Radiat Biol Relat Stud Phys Chem Med* 1985;48(1):45–54.

25. Belli JA, Dicus GJ, Bonte FJ. Radiation response of mammalian tumor cells. I. Repair of sublethal damage in vivo. *J Natl Cancer Inst* 1967;38(5):673–82.

26. Chaffey JT, Hellman S. Differing responses to radiation of murine bone marrow stem cells in relation to the cell cycle. *Cancer Res* 1971;31(11):1613–5.

27. Merchant TE. Proton beam therapy in pediatric oncology. *Cancer J* 2009;15(4):298–305.

28. Matthay KK, Tan JC, Villablanca JG, et al. Phase I dose escalation of iodine-131-metaiodobenzylguanidine with myeloablative chemotherapy and autologous stem-cell transplantation in refractory neuroblastoma: A new approaches to Neuroblastoma Therapy Consortium Study. *J Clin Oncol* 2006;24(3):500–6.

29. Anderson PM, Wiseman GA, Dispenzieri A, et al. High-dose samarium-153 ethylene diamine tetramethylene phosphonate: Low toxicity of skeletal irradiation in patients with osteosarcoma and bone metastases. *J Clin Oncol* 2002;20(1):189–96.

30. Warrell RP Jr., de The H, Wang ZY, et al. Acute promyelocytic leukemia. *N Engl J Med* 1993;329(3):177–89.

31. Matthay KK, Villablanca JG, Seeger RC, et al. Treatment of high-risk neuroblastoma with intensive chemotherapy, radiotherapy, autologous bone marrow transplantation, and 13-cis-retinoic acid. Children's Cancer Group. *N Engl J Med* 1999;341(16):1165–73.

32. Yu AL, Gilman AL, Ozkaynak MF, et al. Anti-GD2 antibody with GM-CSF, interleukin-2, and isotretinoin for neuroblastoma. *N Engl J Med* 2010;363(14):1324–34.

33. Kantarjian H, Sawyers C, Hochhaus A, et al. Hematologic and cytogenetic responses to imatinib mesylate in chronic myelogenous leukemia. *N Engl J Med* 2002;346(9):645–52.

34. Abdulla NE, Ninan MJ, Markowitz AB. Rituximab: Current status as therapy for malignant and benign hematologic disorders. *BioDrugs* 2012;26(2):71–82.

35. Thursky KA, Worth LJ, Seymour JF, et al. Spectrum of infection, risk and recommendations for prophylaxis and screening among patients with lymphoproliferative disorders treated with alemtuzumab*. *Br J Haematol* 2006;132(1):3–12.

36. Hanahan D, Folkman J. Patterns and emerging mechanisms of the angiogenic switch during tumorigenesis. *Cell* 1996;86(3):353–64.

37. David KA, Picus J. Evaluating risk factors for the development of ifosfamide encephalopathy. *Am J Clin Oncol* 2005;28(3):277–80.

38. Kupfer A, Idle JR. Methylene blue and fatal encephalopathy from ackee fruit poisoning. *Lancet* 1999;353(9164):1622–3.

39. Patel PN. Methylene blue for management of Ifosfamide-induced encephalopathy. *Ann Pharmacother* 2006;40(2):299–303.

40. Baker WJ, Royer GL Jr., Weiss RB. Cytarabine and neurologic toxicity. *J Clin Oncol* 1991;9(4):679–93.

41. Simbre VC, Duffy SA, Dadlani GH, et al. Cardiotoxicity of cancer chemotherapy: Implications for children. *Paediatr Drugs* 2005;7(3):187–202.

42. Schimmel KJ, Richel DJ, van den Brink RB, et al. Cardiotoxicity of cytotoxic drugs. *Cancer Treat Rev* 2004;30(2):181–91.

43. Sleijfer S. Bleomycin-induced pneumonitis. *Chest* 2001;120(2):617–24.

44. Abid SH, Malhotra V, Perry MC. Radiation-induced and chemotherapy-induced pulmonary injury. *Curr Opin Oncol* 2001;13(4):242–8.

45. Curran MP, Perry CM. Clofarabine: In pediatric patients with acute lymphoblastic leukemia. *Paediatr Drugs* 2005;7(4):259–64; discussion 256–65.

46. Delanian S, Balla-Mekias S, Lefaix JL. Striking regression of chronic radiotherapy damage in a clinical trial of combined pentoxifylline and tocopherol. *J Clin Oncol* 1999;17(10):3283–90.

47. Larson RS, Tallman MS. Retinoic acid syndrome: Manifestations, pathogenesis, and treatment. *Best Pract Res Clin Haematol* 2003;16(3):453–61.

48. Siu LL, Moore MJ. Use of mesna to prevent ifosfamide-induced urotoxicity. *Support Care Cancer* 1998;6(2):144–54.

49. Skinner R, Sharkey IM, Pearson AD, et al. Ifosfamide, mesna, and nephrotoxicity in children. *J Clin Oncol* 1993;11(1):173–90.

50. Kuhlmann MK, Burkhardt G, Kohler H. Insights into potential cellular mechanisms of cisplatin nephrotoxicity and their clinical application. *Nephrol Dial Transplant* 1997;12(12):2478–80.

51. Azria D, Magne N, Zouhair A, et al. Radiation recall: A well recognized but neglected phenomenon. *Cancer Treat Rev* 2005;31(7):555–70.

52. Erdlenbruch B, Pekrun A, Schiffmann H, et al. Topical topic: Accidental cisplatin overdose in a child: Reversal of acute renal failure with sodium thiosulfate. *Med Pediatr Oncol* 2002;38(5):349–52.

53. Sheikh-Hamad D, Timmins K, Jalali Z. Cisplatin-induced renal toxicity: Possible reversal by N-acetylcysteine treatment. *J Am Soc Nephrol* 1997;8(10):1640–4.

54. Kupfer A, Aeschlimann C, Wermuth B, et al. Prophylaxis and reversal of ifosfamide encephalopathy with methylene-blue. *Lancet* 1994;343(8900):763–4.

55. Widemann BC, Balis FM, Shalabi A, et al. Treatment of accidental intrathecal methotrexate overdose with intrathecal carboxypeptidase G2. *J Natl Cancer Inst* 2004;96(20):1557–9.

56. Tomita M, Aoki Y, Tanaka K. Effect of haemodialysis on the pharmacokinetics of antineoplastic drugs. *Clin Pharmacokinet* 2004;43(8):515–27.

CHAPTER 115 ■ ONCOLOGIC EMERGENCIES AND COMPLICATIONS

RODRIGO MEJIA, NIDRA J. RODRIGUEZ, JOSE A. CORTES, SANJU S. SAMUEL, FERNANDO F. CORRALES-MEDINA, REGINA OKHUYSEN, RIZA C. MAURICIO, AND WINSTON W. HUH

KEY POINTS

Shock in the Child with Cancer

1 Shock is common *and* of varied etiology in acutely ill pediatric cancer patients such that careful noninvasive and invasive hemodynamic assessment is necessary for optimal management.

2 Critically ill or septic neutropenic patients should undergo resuscitation according to advanced life-support guidelines; cultures should be obtained and broad-spectrum antibiotics should be promptly administered.

Hematologic Emergencies

3 Symptomatic hyperleukocytosis is a medical emergency. The goal of management is to rapidly decrease the white blood cell count, usually through induction chemotherapy or leukopheresis.

4 Hemostatic abnormalities remain a leading cause of morbidity and mortality in childhood cancer.

5 Acute promyelocytic leukemia is a distinct subtype of acute myeloid leukemia that is characterized by severe coagulopathy.

Water, Electrolyte, and Metabolic Emergencies

6 Tumor lysis syndrome is characterized by hyperuricemia, hyperkalemia, hyperphosphatemia, and hypocalcemia.

7 Tumor lysis syndrome may result in renal failure, seizures, and potentially fatal cardiac arrhythmias and is often preventable with appropriate therapy, including hydration and recombinant urate oxidase (rasburicase) administration.

8 Because alkalinization is ineffective when recombinant urate oxidase is used and it has the potential for worsening hypocalcemia, it is no longer recommended as a part of management of tumor lysis syndrome.

Neurologic Emergencies

9 Back pain in a child with known history of malignancy should raise concern for malignant spinal cord compression.

10 MRI is the diagnostic test of choice in suspected posterior reversible encephalopathy, and treatment should include control of hypertension and seizures.

Respiratory Emergencies

11 Patients with anterior mediastinal masses are particularly at high risk of rapid cardiopulmonary collapse when sedated or placed under general anesthesia.

12 The most common cause of massive hemoptysis in the pediatric cancer patient is invasive pulmonary aspergillosis.

Abdominal Emergencies

13 Immunosuppression may blind the typical signs and symptoms of acute abdomen that one expects to find in a healthy child. Clinical vigilance and the use of diagnostic imaging are important for early intervention.

INTRODUCTION

The prognosis and outcome for pediatric cancer patients have gradually improved over the last decades as a result of significant advances in treatment protocols that include newer chemotherapeutic agents, improved radiation techniques, and aggressive supportive care. However, these advanced therapies have been associated with severe and often life-threatening complications that require PICU admission. Especially following hematopoietic stem cell transplantation, these children may have poor outcomes when admitted to the PICU with organ system failure requiring mechanical ventilation and vasopressor support (1). Improved outcomes are seen with early PICU intervention for children with cancer who have low Pediatric Risk of Mortality (PRISM) scores (2) and with aggressive interventions for children with cancer admitted to the intensive care unit with septic shock (3,4). Despite the technological advances and improving outcomes, pediatric hematopoietic stem cell transplant (HSCT) patients remain at high risk for severe sepsis and multiple organ failure. Recent studies have noted improved outcomes and suggest that a more aggressive, individualized therapeutic approach, with earlier application of invasive therapies, may be responsible for improvements in outcome (5–7).

This chapter provides the pediatric intensive care team with information on aspects of care that may be critical to the care of this patient population early in the admission and treatment phase. The special complications encountered by the patient after hematopoietic stem cell transplant are discussed in Chapter 117. Because cancer patients often encounter the same critical illnesses as noncancer patients, the reader will be referred to other chapters in the text where these illnesses are discussed in greater detail.

Based on current knowledge, consideration for admission to the PICU and application of aggressive supportive therapies should occur as *early as possible* in the setting of a deteriorating clinical course. The goals of therapy and the decisions regarding additional therapy should be individualized and continuously reevaluated on the basis of the patient's clinical course to ensure an informed discussion among caregivers, patients, and families concerning the continuation, limitations, or even withdrawal of supportive care.

SHOCK IN THE CHILD WITH CANCER

Children with cancer commonly present to the PICU in shock and are vulnerable to the same insults that cause shock in children without cancer. Hypovolemic shock may complicate chemotherapy-induced diarrhea or surgical bleeding whereas subclinical myocardial dysfunction in children exposed to chemotherapy or radiation may rapidly evolve into critical global myocardial dysfunction with the onset of sepsis (8).

Although overwhelming septic shock may develop very quickly in pediatric oncology patients, most of these children respond well to treatment. In fact, mortality comparable to previously healthy children presenting with community-acquired septic shock has been reported (3,4,6,9). A low threshold for recognizing an evolving critical illness coupled with aggressive treatment are crucial for good outcomes (8). Rapid recognition of tachycardia or deviations from the chronically ill child's baseline vital signs may allow prompt correction of early shock with simple measures such as isotonic crystalloid boluses. A worldwide positive trend in outcomes of pediatric cancer patients admitted to the intensive care unit extends to those presenting with shock and respiratory failure (6).

Septic Shock

The general features of sepsis and septic shock, as well as their management, are discussed at length in Chapters 28 and 87. The development of sepsis or septic shock in the children with cancer presents special challenges because they are immunocompromised. They are commonly profoundly neutropenic, have impaired mucosal barriers, and may have preexisting end-organ dysfunction, making them more vulnerable to multiple organ system failure (MOSF). Their care should be meticulously directed to avoid organ failure, as they have substantially greater mortality from MOSF than do other patients (9). Cardiac function may deteriorate rapidly in these children, who frequently have subclinical myocardial dysfunction (10). Prompt recognition and the institution of goal-directed interventions are of paramount importance to mitigate end-organ injury (**Table 115.1**). Critical interventions include the timely normalization of the heart rate, the cardiac index, the perfusion pressures, and targeting a central venous oxygen saturation ($ScvO_2$) of $\geq 70\%$ (8).

Aggressive fluid resuscitation (traditionally considered to be at least 60 mL/kg in the first hour) with isotonic crystalloid, colloid, or indicated blood products is the cornerstone of septic shock therapy, in the absence of preexisting volume overload or congestive heart failure. Patients with subclinical

TABLE 115.1

EVALUATING A CHILD WITH CANCER AND SEPTIC SHOCK

1. Early admission to the PICU
2. Antimicrobial administration within the first hour
3. Consider resistant bacterial and fungal infections
4. Aggressively search for an infectious source
5. Evaluate for cardiac dysfunction
6. Evaluate for preexisting organ dysfunction
7. Consider the risk of adrenal insufficiency

chemotherapy-induced myocardial dysfunction require extremely close monitoring during fluid resuscitation because congestive heart failure may develop suddenly (see below). Additionally, these patients usually require vasoactive agents to help achieve hemodynamic goals. Serial physical examinations, noninvasive, and in most cases invasive hemodynamic monitoring and echocardiography are useful in determining the status of intravascular volume, cardiac contractility, and systemic vascular resistance. Care should be taken to avoid exacerbating tachycardia that accompanies the systemic inflammatory response. Severe tachycardia may cause coronary insufficiency in children with marginal diastolic pressures, triggering life-threatening dysrhythmias. Careful review and frequent reassessment of clinical and hemodynamic data should be used to guide treatment decisions to optimize myocardial oxygen consumption while improving end-organ perfusion pressures. Brierley and colleagues (10) noted that chronically ill children with chronic venous catheters complicated by septic shock tended to present with a low systemic vascular resistance and high cardiac output, "warm shock," while previously healthy children with community-acquired septic shock displayed more variability in their hemodynamic profiles, with a trend toward higher systemic vascular resistance and lower cardiac output, "cold shock." These findings endorse the need to individualize the use of an inotrope versus a vasoactive agent as a first-line treatment in hypotensive cancer patients. Dopamine or the more potent vasopressor, norepinephrine, are often required in hypotensive children with evidence of decreased systemic vascular resistance unresponsive to fluid administration. Vasopressin may be effective in patients refractory to catecholamines due to its effect through distinct V_1 receptors. Terlipressin, a vasopressin analogue with a longer half-life, is utilized in some countries but is currently not available in the United States.

Calcium administration or infusion may improve refractory cardiomyocyte function in children with ionized hypocalcemia. Children with myocardial dysfunction and evidence of high systemic vascular resistance may respond to afterload reduction with inodilator agents such as milrinone. Milrinone loading doses may be avoided when there are concerns that resultant hypotension may be significant and prolonged. The calcium-sensitizing agent levosimendan is available outside the United States and appears to be useful in the stabilization of children with severe myocardial dysfunction, although its role in the management of pediatric septic shock is unclear.

Ventilator strategies designed to reduce work of breathing, optimize oxygenation, and minimize lung injury are critical. Renal replacement therapies should be applied early if indicated to maintain fluid balance as a means of mitigating injury and breakdown of integument that are associated with fluid overload. Analgesia and sedation may help minimize oxygen consumption and facilitate patient care. Neuromuscular blockade is becoming sparingly used given the concern for prolonged myopathy and neuropathy; the 2008 Surviving Sepsis Campaign recommends they be avoided in adults with sepsis (11).

Corticosteroids are used frequently in pediatric oncology patients as part of their chemotherapy and for control of complications, such as vomiting and graft-versus-host disease (GVHD). The American College of Critical Care Medicine guidelines suggest that the use of corticosteroids should be limited to patients with catecholamine-resistant shock and proven or suspected adrenal insufficiency (8). Other risk factors for adrenal insufficiency in pediatric cancer patients include catastrophic neurologic injury, profound shock with watershed injury to the adrenal glands, and exposure to megestrol acetate or etomidate. The administration of hydrocortisone to children who have absolute or relative adrenal dysfunction may promote rapid improvement in hemodynamic function and decreased requirement for vasoactive agents (12). Corticosteroids, therefore, should be implemented as indicated early and withdrawn as soon as practical. Extracorporeal support techniques and devices may be appropriate for selected patients with underlying malignancies suffering from refractory shock (13,14).

The importance of timely antibiotic administration cannot be overemphasized. Appropriate antibiotic therapy must be implemented within the first hour of contact. This intervention has measurable effects on patient outcome. Most tertiary pediatric cancer centers have protocols in place to ensure that children presenting to the hospital, emergency center, or clinic receive broad-spectrum antibiotics within the first hour of contact. Cultures should be obtained prior to antibiotic administration if possible, with care taken not to delay antibiotic administration. Cultures should be frequently reviewed and antibiotics tailored appropriately to culture results. Source control must be implemented if a focus of infection is identified. Consultation with an infectious disease specialist is often very helpful.

Cardiac Dysfunction

Cardiogenic shock is not uncommon in children with cancer and may be multifactorial. Myocardial dysfunction may evolve very rapidly, regardless of its cause, with corresponding changes in the physical exam. Persistent tachycardia is very common but may be missed, particularly in younger children. A narrow pulse pressure and changes in capillary refill and other indicators of perfusion are important clues. An intermittent or continuous gallop may be noted, along with systemic congestion (anasarca), pulmonary edema, and organ dysfunction. Physicians who care for cancer patients should be mindful that children exposed to chemotherapeutic agents may have acute, transient alterations in cardiac function or may experience a lifelong cardiac disability. Specialized echocardiographic protocols that evaluate diastolic function or provide indicators of myocardial performance under nonload conditions, such as speckle tracking imaging, may be more sensitive than measurements of ejection or shortening fractions (15). Measurement of biomarkers such as troponins and natriuretic peptides may be useful for monitoring children at risk for myocardial dysfunction. Carvedilol and enalapril may be beneficial in the chronic care of such patients. Long-term cardiology follow-up is indicated for these children, given their lifelong increased risk of myocardial dysfunction.

Chemotherapy, particularly anthracyclines may produce subclinical myocardial dysfunction, which may rapidly evolve into florid cardiac failure with stress such as sepsis. Although the anthracyclines (primarily doxorubicin and daunorubicin) are the agents most commonly implicated in myocardial dysfunction, other agents such as cytarabine, cyclophosphamide, 5-fluorouracil, and ifosfamide are capable of causing acute dysrhythmias or cardiac failure, particularly in the presence of electrolyte abnormalities. Clinically significant cardiac dysfunction may also occur in chemotherapy-naïve children. The systemic inflammatory response that accompanies sepsis, other causes of critical illness, or resection of large tumors may precipitate life-threatening, reversible myocardial dysfunction in a pattern reminiscent of takotsubo cardiomyopathy (a transient, stress-related, sympathetic-mediated cardiomyopathy) seen in adults. Although survivors of pediatric cancer have a lifelong risk of cardiovascular dysfunction, much is now understood regarding mitigation of cardiovascular toxicity from anthracyclines and other agents (16).

Cardiac tumors are rare but may cause severe dysfunction in children of all ages. Most of the primary tumors such as rhabdomyomas seen in patients with tuberous sclerosis, while benign in histology, may cause significant hemodynamic compromise or dysrhythmias requiring intervention (17). Other neoplasms may cause severe dysfunction. Catecholamine-secreting tumors such as pheochromocytoma may cause severe cardiomyopathy or fatal tachydysrhythmia with exposure to stress (18). Osteosarcoma and other sarcomas may invade the pericardium causing effusions and tamponade or may cause shock through direct intracavitary extension.

Pericardial Effusions and Cardiac Tamponade

Neoplasms are very common causes of pericardial effusions, accounting for up to 39% of cases in a recent pediatric review. The cancer-related causes of pediatric pericardial effusions in that review included T-cell leukemias, lymphomas, metastatic sarcomas, and complications of acute or chronic graft-versus-host disease (19). Radiation-induced inflammatory changes may cause effusion, which in turn may be exacerbated by thrombocytopenia and coagulopathy. While many pericardial effusions collect gradually, these are well tolerated and can be safely observed. Some effusions consisting of transudates, exudates, purulent material, blood, or air collect rapidly. Intrapericardial pressure eventually exceeds transmural myocardial pressure, compromising diastolic filling and ultimately left ventricular output. Classic signs of cardiac tamponade include tachycardia, jugular venous distension, pulsus paradoxus, Kussmaul sign (respiratory variation of jugular venous distension), muffled heart sounds on auscultation, electrical alternans or generalized low voltages on electrocardiogram, and cardiomegaly with a bottle-shaped heart on a chest radiograph.

Echocardiograms are both sensitive and specific in identifying or excluding a pericardial effusion and are helpful in assessing both the extent of hemodynamic compromise and the efficacy of interventions. Pericardial effusions cannot be conclusively excluded on the basis of a physical examination or a normal chest x-ray. Electrocardiographic changes may be nonspecific, underscoring the importance of echocardiography in this setting.

Relative or functional hypovolemia must be promptly addressed with appropriate fluid therapy as the evaluation progresses. Vasoactive infusions may be necessary but are most effective in the presence of an adequate intravascular volume. Sedation for procedures must be with extreme caution because medications such as morphine, propofol, or benzodiazepines may lower the systemic vascular resistance and lead to severe hypotension or cardiac arrest (20). Agents such as fentanyl or ketamine, which are less likely to precipitate cardiovascular collapse, are safer in this setting. Definitive treatment for tamponade requires the decompression of the pericardium. While image-guided pericardiocentesis with placement of a percutaneous catheter is sufficient for most patients, definitive surgical decompression is necessary in others.

HEMATOLOGIC EMERGENCIES

Febrile Neutropenia

The treatment for most pediatric malignancies is based on aggressive multimodality therapy including systemic antineoplastic agents and radiation therapy. Although this approach has led to impressive improvements in the cure rates for many pediatric malignancies, it has secondary effects on a variety of normal cells including the hematopoietic elements of the bone marrow. The resulting bone marrow suppression produces intermittent periods of leukopenia (especially neutropenia), anemia, and thrombocytopenia of varying severity and duration. The risk of morbidity and mortality because of serious infection during these periods of neutropenia is greatly increased (21). For decades, routine management for patients with cancer presenting with fever and neutropenia (FN) has been emergency hospitalization and empiric broad-spectrum intravenous antimicrobial therapy with or without escalation to include antifungal therapy until resolution of FN and signs of infection (22). This approach has resulted in a lower mortality rate. Nevertheless, complications that require admission to the ICU do exist. Febrile neutropenia risk factors and complications that may require critical care intervention are discussed below.

Fever is defined as a single oral temperature $\geq 38.3°C$ (101°F) or a temperature $\geq 38°C$ (100.4°F) sustained over 1 hour. Axillary temperatures are discouraged and rectal temperatures are contraindicated in neutropenic pediatric patient, as doing so may disrupt the mucosal barrier and create a nidus for infection (22). Neutropenia is defined as an absolute neutrophil count (ANC) of either a single measurement ≤ 500 cells/mm^3 or ≤ 1000 cells/mm^3 with a downward trend of the absolute neutrophil count on two separate peripheral blood counts (23).

Certain patients are at a higher risk for complications due to the intensive nature of their chemotherapy regimens and may require ICU admission during the course of their hospitalization (24). Identification of these patients is important for early implementation of life-saving strategies. The risk of sepsis or invasive bacterial infections increases with the degree and duration of neutropenia. The risk of bacteremia and septicemia increases with an absolute neutrophil count of ≤ 200 cells/mm^3. Neutropenia that lasts longer than 7 days is also a risk factor for a worse outcome. Certain pediatric oncology populations, including those with hematologic malignancies (e.g., relapsed leukemia) and those who have undergone an allogeneic hematopoietic stem cell transplant (HSCT), are at increased risk for prolonged periods of neutropenia due to the intensity and timing of their treatment regimens. Alterations in cytokine production associated with poorly controlled solid malignancies may impair regulation of immune response even in the face of normal neutrophil counts. Treatment with high-dose cytarabine is associated with increased susceptibility to infection and mortality from *Streptococcus viridans* and fungal species (21).

Multiple clinical and laboratory-based criteria for identifying high-risk febrile neutropenic patients have been investigated in various prospective clinical trials (25,26). The clinical and laboratory risk factors that may place a pediatric cancer patient at a higher risk for a serious infection are listed in **Table 115.2**. Furthermore, a presenting temperature $\geq 39.5°C$, capillary refill time ≥ 3 seconds, a low diastolic blood pressure (DBP; defined as DBP which is more than 2 standard deviations below the mean for age), and the presence of oral mucositis were identified retrospectively on multivariate analysis as variables that were significantly associated with the need for critical care therapies in febrile neutropenic children

TABLE 115.2

CLINICAL AND LABORATORY HIGH-RISK FACTORS IN FEBRILE NEUTROPENIA

■ CLINICAL RISK FACTORS	■ LABORATORY-BASED RISK FACTORS
Evidence of shock	Elevated C-reactive protein >10 mg/L
Near-myeloablative chemotherapy (leukemia induction or delayed intensification)	Absolute neutrophil count <200 cells/mm^3
Allogeneic hematopoietic stem cell transplant recipient	Absolute monocyte count <100 cells/mm^3
Relapsed leukemia	Platelet count <50,000/mm^3
Poorly controlled solid malignancies	Gram-negative bacteremia
Pneumonia	
Neutropenic enterocolitis	
Invasive fungal infection	
Severe oropharyngeal mucositis	
Prolonged neutropenia (>7 d)	
High presenting temperature (>39°C)	
High-dose cytosine arabinoside	
Age less than 1 y	

with cancer (27). Research into further laboratory markers of risk, such as interleukin-6 (IL), IL-8, tumor necrosis factor α, interferon γ, and host genetic characteristics associated with infection risk are ongoing.

The human granulocyte colony-stimulating factors (GCSF) filgrastim and pegfilgrastim and the granulocyte-macrophage colony-stimulating factor (GM-CSF) sargramostim are primarily used in patients at high risk for chemotherapy-associated neutropenia. GCSF stimulates the release of neutrophils, whereas GM-CSF enhances the release of both neutrophils and macrophages. Filgrastim is generally given subcutaneously (although it may also be administered using the IV route) in a dose of 5–10 mcg/kg/day; pegfilgrastim's dose is 100 mcg/kg/dose every 14–21 days. GM-CSF, administered subcutaneously, is dosed at 250 mcg/m^2/day. During treatment, white cell count should be monitored daily, and the medication should be continued until neutrophil counts have recovered to more than 1000/mm^3 for 3 consecutive days. The agents may then be discontinued or weaned by half and stopped if no significant drop in neutrophil count is seen for 3 days following the dose reduction. Bone pain, myalgia and a flu-like syndrome are the most commonly reported side effects of these agents; however, increased uric acid and lactate dehydrogenase (LDH) levels have also been noted, and these levels should be monitored in the critically ill patient. Exacerbation of existing inflammatory conditions, such as vasculitis or psoriasis, has also been reported.

Although these medications appear to be safe and effective in the supportive setting, the effect on long-term survival remains unclear. An individualized approach is recommended given the remote risk of serious complications with these agents including allergic reactions, acute lung injury, splenic rupture, precipitation of sickle cell crisis, and secondary leukemia. The human granulocyte-macrophage colony-stimulating factor sargramostim, on the other hand, has been associated with severe capillary leak syndrome, pulmonary edema, pericardial and pleural effusions, and renal and hepatic dysfunction in adult patients.

Very few pediatric clinical trials evaluating the role of filgrastim and pegfilgrastim in the critically ill neutropenic child have been published to date. A large meta-analysis study has been conducted in adult patients with solid tumors and high-risk neutropenia and infections treated with GCSF and antibiotics or antibiotics alone. Findings included significant reductions in duration of neutropenia, length of antibiotic treatment, and number of hospital days (28). Very young premature infants appear to derive a transient benefit in some studies (29–31). *In vivo* and *in vitro* reversal of immunoparalysis has been recently described in a cohort of critically ill pediatric transplant patients, including stem cell recipients. Pegfilgrastim infusions were well tolerated with fewer deaths reported in the children randomized to the intervention. However, further studies are needed (32). In general, the use of GCSF in patients with neutropenia and life-threatening infection has been better studied than has the use of GM-CSF. Given the lack of clear evidence regarding use of GM-CSF in critically ill pediatric cancer patients, consultation with infectious disease specialists should be obtained to evaluate each individualized case, especially if invasive fungal disease is suspected.

Granulocyte transfusions are a consideration in neutropenic children with life-threatening bacterial or fungal infection. A systemic inflammatory response with acute lung injury and fluid overload are common complications in these children (33). Consultation with the child's oncologist may guide optimal use of these measures in children with severe sepsis.

Specific Infectious Complications

Bacteremia. Improved management and antimicrobial prophylaxis have led to a shift in pathogens that complicate the neutropenic state. Fever occurs in approximately 35% (range 10%–60%) of episodes of neutropenia in children and is more common in patients after HSCT or aggressive myeloablative treatment for acute leukemia or lymphoma (34). Overall, documentation of an infectious etiology or focus of infection occurs in only 10%–45% of febrile episodes (34,35). Patients who are not at high risk for a serious infection have an incidence of bacteremia of less than 10% (25). Clinical and laboratory features indicative of a high-risk of infection in febrile neutropenia are listed in **Table 115.2**. Catheter-related infections are the most common source of bacteremia. Other frequently involved sites of bacterial infection include the respiratory tract, the gastrointestinal tract, the skin, and the soft tissues. While the rate of gram-positive infections has increased, the rate of infections caused by gram-negative organisms has remained unchanged. Even though most gram-positive infections are less virulent than gram-negative infections, an exception is α-hemolytic streptococcal species. Certain groups, such as AML patients, are at a higher risk. Mucositis also places these patients at risk for *Streptococcus viridans* infections (36). For this reason, adequate antimicrobial coverage for *Streptococcus viridans* should be instituted for any AML patient or a patient with recent exposure to high-dose cytarabine admitted with fever and neutropenia.

Commonly used antimicrobials for the management of febrile neutropenia are listed in **Table 115.3**. Monotherapy with an antipseudomonal β-lactam agent has been shown to be as effective as combination therapy in patients who are hemodynamically stable without evidence of skin or soft tissue infection, pneumonia, or concern for catheter-related infection (37,38). Current evidence supports the empirical use of piperacillin-tazobactam or cefepime in locations where antimicrobial susceptibility data do not warrant empirical carbapenem (meropenem or imipenem/cilastin) use (39). Ceftazidime is no longer recommended for empiric monotherapy due to its decreasing activity against many gram-negative pathogens (40). Routine initiation of an aminoglycoside in combination with an antipseudomonal β-lactam agent should be avoided because it offers no survival advantage and is associated with increased toxicity and a higher treatment failure rate (37). Even though supportive evidence is lacking, the addition of vancomycin or another agent active against gram-positive pathogens to the initial regimen is a common practice for high-risk patients (41,42). The risk of vancomycin-resistant enterococci (VRE) colonization makes it unwise to add vancomycin to the regimen for uncomplicated febrile neutropenia in low-risk patients. Additional antibiotic agents for suspected or documented bacteremia should be tailored to cover for the most likely organisms, subsequent susceptibility results, as well as resistance patterns in the institution. In summary, an example of empiric antibiotic coverage for the hemodynamically stable patient with uncomplicated febrile neutropenia might be monotherapy with cefepime **or** piperacillin-tazobactam **or** meropenem. If hemodynamic instability or complications are also present, then the following antibiotics should be considered *in addition to* the above monotherapy:

1. Vancomycin (for known MRSA or resistant streptococcal colonization, pneumonia, skin/soft tissue infections, or suspected central line–associated infection)
2. Aminoglycoside (for hypotension, pneumonia, or suspected antibiotic resistance)
3. Metronidazole (for suspected anaerobic infection, abdominal pain, or bloody stools)

Neutropenic Enterocolitis and Typhlitis. Neutropenic enterocolitis is a complication that can involve the distal ileum, cecum, or ascending colon and is seen in patients with prolonged neutropenia. The true incidence of neutropenic enterocolitis is unknown; a review of 145 pooled adult studies found that it developed in 5.3% of patients treated for neoplasias (43). The incidence is reported to be slightly lower in children. One major pediatric cancer center reported 24 cases over a 30-year period (44). The pathogenesis is poorly understood, possibly related to direct cytotoxicity to the intestinal mucosal cells, overgrowth of specific bacterial flora, generalized immunodeficiency with decreased resistance even to normal intestinal bacteria, production of bacterial endotoxins, and many other possible causative agents that have been postulated (45).

TABLE 115.3

SELECT ANTIMICROBIALS FOR MANAGEMENT OF FEBRILE NEUTROPENIA

■ BROAD-SPECTRUM ANTIBIOTICS	■ GRAM-POSITIVE COVERAGE	■ GRAM-NEGATIVE COVERAGE	■ ANAEROBIC COVERAGE
Cefepime	Vancomycin	Aminoglycoside (Gentamicin, Amikacin, Tobramycin)	Metronidazole
Piperacillin-Tazobactam	Ampicillin/Sulbactam	Aztreonam	Clindamycin
Carbapenems (Meropenem, Imipenem)	Linezolid		

Cases involving the cecum are often referred to as *typhlitis*, but the ileum may also be involved. The most common underlying disease in children with typhlitis is leukemia. The classic triad of fever, abdominal pain, and diarrhea may not always be present and is not highly specific, making the clinical diagnosis difficult. Imaging with either ultrasonography or abdominal CT scan with oral and intravenous contrast is essential. CT imaging allows for differentiation from other diagnoses and generally remains the modality of choice. Ultrasonography may also prove useful as a prognostic tool, based on the degree of bowel thickness. It is also easily performed at the bedside of even the most critically ill patients. Bowel wall thickness greater than 4 mm, along with clinical symptoms, confirms the diagnosis. Sepsis and perforation are the most common complications. To date, no prospective, randomized trials have been conducted to study the management of this disease. Current medical approach in patients without perforation consists of bowel rest and decompression, broad-spectrum intravenous antibiotics (including antifungal agents), and sometimes G-CSF. Patients with perforation, obstruction, peritonitis, active gastrointestinal bleeding, or clinical deterioration may require operative intervention including colectomy and diversion. Fortunately, most pediatric patients do not require surgery. Mortality rates currently range from 30% to 50% in adults. Mortality is markedly lower in children at approximately 5%.

Neutropenic colitis is relatively uncommon in children with malignancies. Laparotomy is rarely necessary, and mortality directly from the colitis is low. A precipitous drop in the ANC should raise the level of clinical vigilance/suspicion, particularly if other signs and symptoms are present (46).

Invasive Fungal Infections. Invasive fungal diseases, in particular invasive aspergillosis, are a frequent complication of chemotherapy-induced neutropenia and steroid therapy. Populations at risk include patients with an acute leukemia and those patients who have undergone an allogeneic HSCT. The immunosuppression involved in treating graft-versus-host disease is also another risk factor to be considered. The high mortality rate of disseminated fungal infections results from difficulties in obtaining a reliable and early diagnosis and in establishing a proper treatment (47,48). Historically, *Candida albicans*, *nonalbicans species*, and *Aspergillus fumigatus* have been the most frequently isolated organisms. In recent years, with the advent of fluconazole prophylaxis, the incidence of invasive candidiasis has dropped to less than 5%, with a shift toward nonalbicans species. Another trend seen from the advent of fluconazole prophylaxis is that invasive aspergillosis is slowly becoming the most predominant invasive fungal infection. Due to the nonspecific symptoms, a high index of suspicion for fungal infections is appropriate in any patient with persistent fever and a prolonged neutropenic course. A 2008 international consensus to define invasive fungal infections in cancer patients emphasized the need for early diagnosis and treatment (24). The neutropenic patient with persistent fever for longer than 3–5 days should have empiric coverage expanded to include fungal organisms (26). Amphotericin B, the primary option for antifungal therapy in the past, is well known for adverse effects including fever, chills, hypokalemia, nausea, and vomiting. Newer preparations of amphotericin (AmBisome, Abelcet) as well as the azole group of antifungals (fluconazole, voriconazole, and posaconazole) are associated with fewer side effects. These newer antifungals can be used as initial empiric therapy or treatment for proven mycoses. Voriconazole is considered the drug of choice for treatment of invasive aspergillosis (27). The echinocandin class of antifungals, including caspofungin, micafungin, and anidulafungin, have activity against azole-resistant *Candida* species and *Aspergillus* (49). As with bacterial organisms, therapy should be tailored to specific infection and resistance patterns in the institution so that the most likely fungal organisms are covered. Evidence-based guidelines from the *International Pediatric Fever and Neutropenia Guideline Panel* recommend liposomal amphotericin B or caspofungin as initial empiric antifungal therapy for patients with suspected invasive fungal disease based on neutropenia and prolonged or recurrent fever lasting >96 hours despite appropriate antibacterial therapy (50).

Lower Respiratory Tract Infections. Pneumonia is an uncommon complication of febrile neutropenia. Although routine chest radiography is not warranted, febrile neutropenic patients who present with cough or respiratory distress and hypoxemia require immediate imaging due to the potential for rapid progression of infection. *Pneumocystis (carinii) jiroveci* pneumonia is now rare due to widespread use of trimethoprim-sulfamethoxazole prophylaxis in immunosuppressed patients; however, it should be considered in the differential of any immunocompromised patient who presents with hypoxemia and diffuse patchy infiltrates on chest x-ray. First-line treatment is with intravenous trimethoprim-sulfamethoxazole (with pentamidine as an alternative agent). Corticosteroids should be initiated within 72 hours of initiating therapy for any patient with moderate or severe *Pneumocystis jiroveci* pneumonia ($PaO_2 \leq 70$ mmHg on room air).

Community-acquired infections well known to the general pediatric population (influenza, respiratory syncytial virus, and parainfluenza) can have devastating effects in immunocompromised hosts, especially in transplant patients. Although therapy is available for influenza (neuraminidase and M2 inhibitors), no effective therapy exists for parainfluenza pneumonia. Ribavirin, palivizumab, and respiratory syncytial virus immune globulin have been shown in small, uncontrolled trials to be of some benefit in the management of HSCT patients with respiratory syncytial virus pneumonia.

Mortality from cytomegalovirus (CMV) pneumonitis in HSCT patients is high. Preemptive therapy is the ideal, when a patient has an active (i.e., CMV antigenemia in peripheral blood) but asymptomatic CMV infection. Either intravenous ganciclovir or foscarnet is adequate for preemptive therapy, depending on which prophylactic agent was used prior to detection of CMV antigenemia (51). Although based on uncontrolled studies, current recommended treatment of CMV pneumonia is with a combination of intravenous ganciclovir and immune globulin.

The unique and fragile nature of the pediatric cancer patient requires a truly multidisciplinary approach in the management of infectious complications in the intensive care setting. The intensivist should work in conjunction with the pediatric oncology and infectious disease teams to develop the best management strategy for each patient hospitalized with complications from febrile neutropenia.

Hyperleukocytosis

Definition

Hyperleukocytosis is a laboratory abnormality defined as a peripheral white blood cell (WBC) count greater than 100×10^9/L (100,000/mm³). Leukostasis, which is also known as symptomatic hyperleukocytosis, is considered a medical emergency. It is most commonly seen in patients presenting with acute leukemia.

Etiology

Hyperleukocytosis occurs in 10%–30% of patients with acute lymphoblastic leukemia, 10%–20% patients with acute myeloid leukemia, and the majority of patients with chronic myeloid leukemia (52). Clinically significant hyperleukocytosis can be evident with WBC ≥ 200,000/mm³ in AML and WBC ≥ 300,000/mm³ in ALL and CML. Myeloblasts are larger (350–450 mm³) compared with lymphoblasts (250–350 mm³).

Pathogenesis

The increased morbidity and mortality seen in patients with leukemia presenting as hyperleukocytosis is directly related to its pathogenesis. Hyperleukocytosis is considered an important prognostic factor in certain types of leukemias (53). Factors such as leukostasis, disseminated intravascular coagulation (DIC), and tumor lysis syndrome (TLS) are the major contributors in the pathogenesis of hyperleukocytosis.

Leukostasis. The pathogenesis is not well understood but there are two leading theories. The rheological theory is based on the principle of increased blood viscosity resulting from blasts that are less deformable than mature leukocytes leading to microvascular obstruction and tissue hypoxia (54). The second theory is based on the interaction of blasts with the endothelium and cytokine production (55). The lungs and central nervous system (CNS) are the most common sites of vascular obstruction, although other organs can also be affected. Pulmonary leukostasis can cause respiratory failure likely due to the release of intracellular contents from leukemic cells within the pulmonary vessels causing alveolar damage. CNS involvement is associated with intracranial hemorrhage (**Fig. 115.1**).

DIC. DIC is a pathological syndrome resulting from the formation of thrombin, subsequent activation and consumption of certain coagulant proteins, and production of fibrin thrombi (56). DIC occurs in up to 40% of patients with hyperleukocytosis (52). A leading theory to explain DIC in hyperleukocytosis is based on increased levels of tissue factor that trigger the extrinsic pathway of coagulation via Factor VII activation (57). Hemorrhage in the setting of hyperleukocytosis can result from DIC, although severe thrombocytopenia or other coagulation defects can also be potential causes.

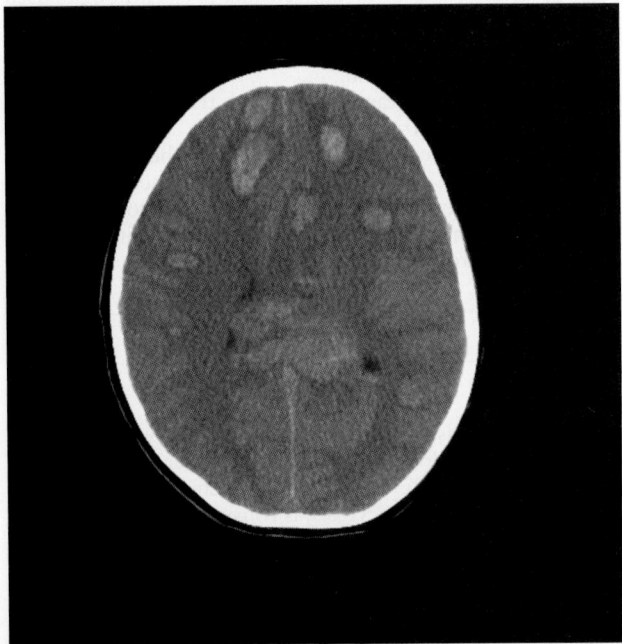

FIGURE 115.1. CT image of stroke secondary to hyperleukocytosis. Multiple, widespread intraparenchymal hemorrhages characteristic of a blast crisis.

TLS. Acute TLS results from the rapid release of intracellular metabolites (potassium, phosphorus, and uric acid). It is present in up to 10% of patients with leukostasis (52). Severe TLS can be seen in hyperleukocytosis due to a high cellular turnover.

Evaluation and Management

The diagnosis of symptomatic hyperleukocytosis is considered a medical emergency as up to 40% of patients die within the first week of presentation (58,59). A diagnosis is established when a leukemic patient with hyperleukocytosis presents with neurologic or respiratory symptoms presumed to be secondary to tissue hypoxia. Clinical signs and symptoms include, but are not limited to tachypnea, dyspnea, hypoxia, visual changes, headache, dizziness, tinnitus, and altered mental status.

The goal of hyperleukocytosis management is to rapidly lower the white blood cell count. Cytoreduction can be achieved with induction chemotherapy, leukopheresis, exchange transfusion, and treatment with hydroxyurea. However, hydroxyurea is primarily reserved for those unable to receive immediate induction chemotherapy (60). Induction chemotherapy is the preferred method of cytoreduction since it not only decreases the WBC count, but also destroys malignant cells. A reduction in the WBC is typically seen within 24 hours. Some centers use low-dose cranial irradiation in patients with hyperleukocytosis and neurologic symptoms. However, there is no convincing evidence to support its routine use (61).

Apheresis refers to the withdrawal of whole blood from the body, separation and retention of one or more components, with the return of the remaining components to the patient (62). For the treatment of hyperleukocytosis, leukapheresis removes the white blood cells while the other components are returned to the patient. A single leukapheresis can reduce the WBC count by 20%–50%. Additional leukapheresis may be performed based on the patient's WBC count response. A goal WBC count ≤100,000/mm³ seems to be acceptable for most practitioners (62). However, leukapheresis should be avoided in patients with acute promyelocytic leukemia (APL) as it can worsen coagulopathy and increase the risk of hemorrhage or thrombosis (63).

Preventing TLS by initiating aggressive hydration and the administration of agents to control uric acid levels such as allopurinol or rasburicase are critical. Supportive care for these patients also includes correction of metabolic abnormalities, respiratory support, correction of coagulopathy, and blood products to maintain a hemoglobin level between 8 and 10 g/dL and a platelet count ≥20,000/mm³. Nevertheless, unnecessary red blood cell transfusions should be avoided until the blast count decreases since this can increase blood viscosity, worsening the symptoms of leukostasis. If red blood cell transfusions are unavoidable prior to a decrease in the blast count, it should be administered slowly and without the use of diuretics. On the other hand, platelet transfusions do not contribute significantly to viscosity. Therefore, aggressive platelet support should be instituted due to a high risk of hemorrhage, particularly intracranial.

Abnormal Hemostasis in Cancer

Hemostatic abnormalities including both thrombosis and hemorrhage remain a leading cause of mortality in patients with cancer. These can be detected clinically, by laboratory testing or by pathologic examination. The degree of hemostatic abnormality is influenced by multiple factors including the type of cancer, extent of disease, treatment-related factors (type of chemotherapy, surgery, radiation therapy, central venous access), inherited thrombophilia, and other acquired risk factors.

The pathogenesis of hemostatic disorders in cancer is complex and reflects the interaction of different mechanisms, including activation of the coagulation and fibrinolytic systems, perturbation of the vascular endothelium, and activation of monocytes and platelets (64). Tumors can produce procoagulant molecules that can activate coagulation either directly or indirectly by initiating an inflammatory response, which further induces the release of more procoagulants (65). Two well-characterized procoagulants in cancer are tissue factor (TF) and cancer procoagulant (CP). In addition, tumor cells also release inflammatory cytokines such as tissue necrosis factor (TNF), interleukin-1 (IL-1), and vascular endothelial growth factor (VEGF) that act on leukocytes and endothelial cells to further enhance the procoagulant activity. Furthermore, these factors play a role in tumor cell growth and metastasis (66). Various laboratory studies in patients with cancer reflect an activation of the coagulation system. These may include mild shortening or prolongation of the prothrombin time (PT) or partial thromboplastin time (PTT), elevated fibrinogen, and mild to moderate thrombocytosis. However, none of these coagulation markers are predictive of thrombosis in patients with cancer nor clinically useful in identifying who may benefit from thromboprophylaxis (67). Cancer treatment may also affect hemostasis, primarily by causing endothelial damage and/or altering the balance of natural anticoagulants in the blood. For example, L-asparaginase is considered prothrombotic due to its effects of decreasing antithrombin III levels resulting in an acquired antithrombin III deficiency.

Hemorrhage in Childhood Cancer

Etiology

Hemorrhage is a potentially serious complication of cancer. The etiology of hemorrhage in children with cancer is commonly multifactorial. Thrombocytopenia is the most common hemostatic abnormality in pediatric cancer. It is typically seen in acute leukemia due to suppression of platelet production by cancer, but it is also seen as a result of chemotherapy in both leukemias and solid tumors. Thrombocytopenia can also be seen in cancer patients with disseminated intravascular coagulation (DIC) due to platelet consumption. In cases of DIC, bleeding can be worsened by the concomitant consumption of coagulation factor proteins. DIC can occur in any type of leukemia or solid tumor. However, it is more commonly associated with acute myeloid leukemia (AML), particularly M3 type of promyelocytic leukemia (APL) (68).

Coagulation disturbances leading to hemorrhage may also be chemotherapy related. For example, agents such as cyclophosphamide, ifosfamide, methotrexate, and doxorubicin are known to cause hemorrhagic cystitis and mucositis. Radiation therapy may also induce local bleeding secondary to blood vessel damage.

Hyperfibrinolysis is another important contributor to hemorrhage in the patient with cancer. It is evident that tumor cells can express proteins on their surface that are important in regulating fibrinolysis and play an important role in the pathogenesis of bleeding. These include urokinase-type (u-PA) and tissue-type plasminogen activators (t-PA) as well as plasminogen activator inhibitors 1 and 2 (PAI-1 and PAI-2) (69). Hemorrhage in patients with cancer can also result from defective hepatic clotting factor synthesis. This can be secondary to liver damage from chemotherapy, primary hepatic malignancy, or metastatic liver disease. In pediatric cancer patients, vitamin K deficiency can also contribute to bleeding complications resulting from decreased vitamin K availability or decreased absorption. Such cases are commonly seen with prolonged antibiotic use, decreased oral intake, and/or diarrhea.

Other etiologies for bleeding in patients with cancer include postsurgical bleeding, presence of acquired inhibitors to clotting factors (e.g., acquired Von Willebrand disease seen in association with Wilms tumor), and direct damage to blood vessels due to tumor growth.

Diagnosis

A thorough clinical evaluation should assess for bruising, petechiae, and/or bleeding. The initial laboratory evaluation should include a complete blood count (CBC), prothrombin time (PT), partial thromboplastin time (PTT), INR, and fibrinogen. A peripheral blood smear should be considered if pseudo-thrombocytopenia is suspected, for example, in a patient with a significantly decreased platelet count but no clinical signs of bleeding. The fibrinogen level is expected to be elevated as an acute phase reactant in patients with cancer but expected to be decreased in DIC.

If PT and/or PTT are prolonged, a mixing study (1:1 mix with normal plasma with repeat PT/PTT immediately and after 1-hour incubation) should be obtained to evaluate for coagulation factor deficiency versus the presence of an inhibitory antibody. If the mixing study corrects the PT and/or PTT, a coagulation factor deficiency must be present. In the setting of cancer, most coagulation factor deficiencies are acquired and not congenital in nature. Specific coagulation factor assays should be ordered for further investigation (factor VII assay if PT is prolonged; factors VIII, IX, XI, and XII if PTT is prolonged). If both PT and PTT are prolonged, evaluate factors II, V, VII, VIII, IX, and X. If the mixing study does not correct either PT or PTT, an inhibitory antibody must be present. Of note, it is important to make sure that the samples are not contaminated with heparin.

Management

Initiate emergency care as indicated, including oxygen administration and intravenous fluids. Specific therapies for management of bleeding in cancer are directed toward forming a stable clot and include local measures such as packing of the nose with or without pressure (70). In addition, topical thrombin or fibrin sealants are useful in mucosal or cutaneous bleeding, but particularly in oral or nasal bleeding (71). Recombinant human thrombin is also now available (72). Surgical control and pressure dressings are recommended in postsurgical bleeding.

In case of bleeding and coagulopathy due to vitamin K deficiency (prolonged PT; decreased factors II, VII, IX, and/or X; normal factors V and VIII), vitamin K can be administered on a daily basis via oral, subcutaneous, or intravenous routes. Response to treatment is monitored by measuring PT.

Antifibrinolytic agents epsilon-aminocaproic acid and tranexamic acid, both lysine derivatives, may be used as adjuvant therapy for bleeding control. These agents inhibit fibrinolysis by inhibiting the proteolytic activity of plasmin. Antifibrinolytics are contraindicated in DIC, thrombosis, and hematuria (increased risk of intrarenal and/or ureteral thrombosis). Both agents are available in the United States in oral and intravenous forms. Since controlled studies of these agents are lacking in childhood cancer, dosage is based on data obtained from noncancer patients. The recommended dose for epsilon-aminocaproic acid is 100 mg/kg/dose every 4–6 hours, whereas for tranexamic acid is 10 mg/kg/dose every 6–8 hours (73).

Recombinant factor VIIa (rFVIIa) is indicated to promote hemostasis in patients with hemophilia A or B with inhibitors. The mechanism of action includes binding of activated factor VII to tissue factor (TF), which activates factor X leading to thrombin generation. rFVIIa also binds the surface of activated platelets independent of TF, activating factor X, and also leading to thrombin generation. The off label use of rFVIIa in childhood cancer has been primarily in the setting of coagulopathy or severe bleeding unresponsive to the use of blood products. The use of 1–2 doses of rFVIIa (60–90 mcg/kg/dose) has been reported in children with leukemia and life-threatening hemorrhages (74). Doses ranging from 75 to 275 mcg/kg (mean 129.6) have been used intraoperatively in pediatric patients with solid tumors as well as during chemotherapy for intra-abdominal tumors (75,76). Nevertheless, since thrombosis has been reported with the use of rFVIIa, it should be used with extreme caution particularly in the setting of DIC and active malignant disease (77). Lower doses of 15–30 mcg/kg, as used in congenital factor VII deficiency, may be safer in regard to its thrombogenic potential. One or two doses of rFVIIa are typically sufficient for bleeding control and subsequent dosing/interval is based on clinical judgment. Unfortunately, there is no validated laboratory test to monitor the efficacy of rFVIIa therapy. Hence, physicians need to use clinical response and cessation of bleeding as the endpoint.

Blood products are certainly indicated to control bleeding and coagulopathy. Packed red blood cells, platelets, and fresh frozen plasma (FFP) should be transfused as clinically indicated. Cryoprecipitate may be preferred for the management of bleeding secondary to DIC due to its greater concentration of fibrinogen compared with FFP. If the patient appears refractory to platelet transfusions due to the presence of alloimmune or autoimmune antibodies, ABO-type specific or HLA-matched platelets are recommended.

Bleeding in Acute Promyelocytic Leukemia

APL is a distinct subtype of acute myeloid leukemia characterized by severe coagulopathy. This propensity is attributed to the release of tissue factor-like procoagulants from the leukemic blasts predisposing to DIC. The coagulopathy seen in APL is complex and consists of classic DIC, systemic fibrinolysis, or hemostatic and vascular defects produced by proteolytic enzymes (68). The risk of bleeding is particularly high during the first 14 days after diagnosis (78). In more than 50% of the cases, APL is associated with DIC. Up to 40% of patients with DIC develop intracerebral or pulmonary hemorrhage during induction chemotherapy or even before the diagnosis is established. Mortality is reported in up to 10% of children with APL who present with DIC. Even higher rates of DIC are reported after chemotherapy is begun. Therefore, supportive measures to correct coagulopathy with transfusion of platelets, FFP, and cryoprecipitate should be aggressively instituted and continued until all clinical and laboratory signs of coagulopathy have disappeared. In addition, invasive procedures including lumbar puncture should be postponed until coagulopathy has resolved. Children with APL treated with all-trans-retinoic acid (ATRA) show earlier normalization of coagulation abnormalities compared with nontreated children (78,79). Hyperfibrinolysis also contributes to bleeding complications in APL. However, antifibrinolytic agents are to be used only in life-threatening bleeding conditions due to the increased risk of thrombosis in the setting of DIC.

Thrombosis in Childhood Cancer

Etiology

A diagnosis of cancer is present in about 20% of thrombosis cases in children (80). Childhood thrombosis is becoming increasingly recognized in part due to improved recognition of symptoms and availability of better imaging. Symptomatic thrombosis has been reported in children with hematologic malignancies as well as solid tumors. However, most thrombotic events with or without a central venous catheter (CVC) occur in children with acute lymphoblastic leukemia (ALL) (81). A prevalence of up to 73% has been reported on the basis of different diagnostic methods and treatment protocols (82). However, symptomatic thrombosis in ALL ranges from 3% to 14% (83). The treatment for CNS and lower extremity embolism is typically 3 months. Treatment for cardiac and pulmonary embolism ranges between 3–6 months of therapy depending on risk factors which may include: active cancer, chemotherapy, presence of a central line, obesity, hormonal treatment (estrogen replacement) inherited or acquired thrombophilia, surgery and immobility (84). The rate of thrombosis in children with solid tumors ranges from 12% to 19% (85). However, children with brain tumors have a lower incidence of thrombosis ranging from 0.6% to 2.8% when compared with children with other solid tumors or leukemia (86). The reported rates of asymptomatic thrombosis in childhood cancer range from 27% to 66% during routine screening with venography (87).

The etiology of thrombosis in childhood cancer is multifactorial. A major risk factor for thrombosis includes the presence of a CVC, but multiple other risk factors also play a role in childhood cancer. These include chemotherapy, radiation, surgery, primary tumor type/size, the presence of metastatic disease, obesity, immobility, total parenteral nutrition, and inherited thrombophilia. Certain chemotherapeutic agents, for example L-asparaginase, are known to increase the risk of thrombosis primarily by reducing antithrombin III levels. Other agents including vincristine, the anthracyclines, and prednisone have also been associated with thrombotic events.

Diagnosis

A thrombus is suspected when the following signs or symptoms are present: pain, swelling, erythema, skin discoloration, increased warmth, collateral veins, unexplained shortness of breath, decreased oxygen saturation, unexplained headache, or changes in the level of consciousness. However, clinical manifestations may vary depending on the characteristics of the thrombus (location and extension) as well as whether it is an acute or a chronic thrombus. Initial laboratory evaluation may reveal an increased D-dimer, which is a marker of clot formation and the resultant fibrinolysis. However, D-dimer is not specific for thrombosis. It is also important to obtain baseline labs to establish the safety of starting anticoagulation therapy (CBC, PT/PTT, and renal function). Screening for inherited thrombophilia is still controversial, and therefore each case should be individualized. Confirmation of thrombosis may be obtained with imaging studies including Doppler ultrasound, venogram (gold standard), computed tomography (CT), magnetic resonance imaging (MRI), or angiogram.

Management

Specific therapies for management of thrombosis include anticoagulation and in selected cases thrombolysis. Since few pediatric clinical trials are available, management is typically extrapolated from the adult data. A few pediatric trials have evaluated anticoagulation prophylaxis in the presence of a CVC and antithrombin III replacement during treatment of ALL. The PROTEKT (PROphylaxis of ThromboEmbolism in Kids) trial, an open-label randomized controlled trial of low-molecular-weight heparin (LMWH) for the prevention of CVC-related thrombosis, failed to show efficacy in children treated with LMWH compared with routine line care (88,89). The PAARKA (Prophylactic Antithrombin replacement in kids with ALL treated with L-asparaginase) trial, a randomized controlled trial evaluating the incidence of thrombosis in children with ALL and a CVC receiving antithrombin III replacement versus no replacement, showed a trend to safety and efficacy with antithrombin

III. However, the trial was not powered to show that antithrombin III replacement was superior to routine care (90).

Anticoagulation should be initiated as soon as possible to minimize thrombus extension or embolization, recurrence, and postthrombotic syndrome. Anticoagulants used commonly in childhood cancer include unfractionated heparin (UFH), LMWH, and vitamin K antagonists. The choice of the agent depends on multiple factors, but LMWH seems to be the most frequently used anticoagulant in childhood cancer. Nevertheless, UFH may be preferred perioperatively or in the intensive care unit due to its shorter half-life and reversibility. The newer anticoagulant agents available for adult use (direct thrombin inhibitors and factor Xa inhibitors) are still not available for use in children (91).

Thrombolysis is considered only in selected cases such as in the presence of extensive thrombosis as seen in major ileofemoral thrombosis, superior or inferior vena cava thrombosis, intracardiac thrombosis, or massive pulmonary embolism with hemodynamic instability. The agent of choice in such cases is tissue plasminogen activator (tPA). Nevertheless, thrombolysis should be used with extreme caution, as it is associated with a significant risk of bleeding. This complication is even more significant and potentially dangerous in the pediatric cancer patient who is already at risk for bleeding complications.

There are limited data on the use of inferior vena cava (IVC) filters to prevent pulmonary embolism in children with cancer. In fact, most of the limited data are reported in children above 5 years of age. The most common indication for IVC filter placement is the presence of a contraindication to anticoagulation, but another reason is anticoagulation failure. Both permanent and retrievable filters have been successfully used in children with leukemia and solid tumors, the majority of which have been Greenfield-type filters (92,93).

WATER, ELECTROLYTE, AND METABOLIC EMERGENCIES

Water, electrolyte, and metabolic disorders are common in pediatric patients with cancer admitted to the PICU. Glomerular and/or tubular disorders may arise from the tumor's direct kidney involvement (Wilms tumor), metastatic infiltration of the renal parenchyma (leukemia, neuroblastoma), urinary tract compression (sarcomas), or as a consequence of the toxic properties of the chemotherapy on the kidney. Water and sodium balance disturbances in particular are frequently found in this patient population. This section will focus on the most significant water, electrolyte, and metabolic emergencies affecting the child with cancer. An in-depth discussion about pathophysiology, diagnosis, and treatment of these disorders may be found in Chapters 107 and 108.

Tumor Lysis Syndrome

Tumor lysis syndrome (TLS) is a life-threatening medical emergency widely recognized as a constellation of metabolic abnormalities that arise from a rapid tumor cell destruction that overwhelms the usual metabolic and excretory pathways. TLS usually occurs after chemotherapy or immunotherapy administration, but may also occur after the administration of corticosteroids or hormones, radiation therapy, or even spontaneously. TLS most often develops 12–72 hours after the initiation of cytolytic therapy and is typically characterized by hyperuricemia, hyperkalemia, and hyperphosphatemia. Precipitation of calcium phosphate in various organs results in symptomatic hypocalcemia. If left untreated, the precipitation of the urate crystals and calcium phosphate crystals in the renal tubules may rapidly lead to acute kidney injury (AKI) and renal failure (94).

Frequency

TLS occurs most frequently in patients with a large tumor burden or in those whose tumors are widely disseminated, rapidly proliferating, or highly sensitive to chemotherapy. TLS has been observed primarily following the treatment of Burkitt's lymphoma, lymphoblastic lymphoma, and leukemia. Nonetheless, TLS can present in other forms of cancer, including Hodgkin lymphoma, neuroblastoma, medulloblastoma, and non-Hodgkin lymphoma. TLS is rare in AML and in chronic leukemias due to a lower proliferation rate and bulk of disease. However, there are recent reports of TLS presenting after treatment with newer agents for the treatment of CML such as imatinib with higher response rates than previously achieved resulting in increased rates of tumor-cell killing (95). The incidence of TLS may range between 4.4% in children and adolescents with NHL (96) but may be as high as 30.5% in patients with Burkitt lymphoma (97). Patients with B-cell ALL and Burkitt lymphoma with elevated LDH ($\geq$500 U/L) have the highest risk of developing TLS or anuria (96).

TLS affects children of all ages, with no gender discrimination. Older children seem to be at higher risk of severe complications due to a progressive decline in the fractional excretion and clearance of uric acid with age. The patient's symptomatology at the time of diagnosis reflects the severity of the primary tumor extension. Symptoms are directly related to the metabolic abnormalities found in TLS and may include anorexia, malaise, weakness, vomiting, hiccups, paresthesias, tetany, carpopedal spasm, arrhythmias, and seizures.

Pathophysiology

The high cell turnover results in an increase of the different by-products of cellular breakdown, including proteins, nucleic acids, cations, and anions. Brisk cellular breakdown that results from cytolytic therapy causes a dramatic rise in plasma levels of uric acid, urea nitrogen, phosphorus, potassium, and cytokines that will overwhelm normal homeostatic mechanisms and induce a systemic inflammatory response and often multiorgan failure including acute kidney injury (AKI) (98). A rapid rise in serum potassium levels may result in severe arrhythmias and death. Uric acid is in the ionized form at normal serum concentrations and normal pH. The presence of metabolic acidosis and high uric acid plasma concentrations increases the risk of uric acid crystal formation and precipitation in the renal collecting ducts and tubules (sites of urinary acidification). Metabolic acidosis exacerbates the already elevated serum phosphate concentration by shifting intracellular phosphate to the extracellular space. Secondary hypocalcemia results from calcium phosphate precipitation when the solubility product factor is reached (Ca $\times$ P = 60). Calcium phosphate precipitates readily in the presence of uric acid and vice versa. The glomerular filtration rate declines and progresses to renal failure as a result of calcium phosphate, xanthine, and uric acid crystal precipitation, a crystal-dependent mechanism of AKI. New data suggest that there may also be crystal-independent mechanisms produced by soluble uric acid causing renal vasoconstriction, antiangiogenesis and a proinflammatory effect (99). The risk of acute renal failure increases if the primary tumor infiltrates or obstructs the normal flow of urine.

Risk Factors

Risk factors for TLS are Burkitt lymphoma/leukemia (B-ALL), acute leukemias (ALL, AML), non-Hodgkin lymphoma, tumors with rapid growth rate, large tumor burden, elevated serum LDH (500 U/L), dehydration, elevated uric acid, and elevated creatinine. Recent data suggest that hypophosphatemia may be an indicator of high tumor burden or high proliferation rate and consequently a risk factor as well (97). Guidelines for the management of TLS have been developed for children and adults (100,101). The proposed risk models, definitions, and management of TLS included in these guidelines are broad and complex and use different end points that are yet to be validated in children (102,103).

Management

Early diagnosis of the primary condition, recognition of the risk factors, and aggressive management of symptoms and electrolyte abnormalities are key to the management of TLS. A summary of TLS treatment is presented in **Table 115.4**. Early and aggressive hydration in addition to enhanced urine flow is fundamental to the prevention and management of TLS. Expansion of the intravascular volume increases renal blood flow and glomerular filtration rate, thus decreasing the concentration of solutes in the distal tubules. Intravenous hydration should begin at least 24 hours before the initiation of cytoreductive therapy. Infusion rates are usually 3000 mL/m^2/day (or 200 mL/kg/d if ≤10 kg) unless volume overload is of particular concern. Urine alkalinization is no longer recommended if recombinant urate oxidase (rasburicase) is administered (103). Animal studies have shown improved benefit with hydration and enhanced diuresis, but not with urine alkalinization. The role of alkalinization in patients without access to urate oxidase remains controversial since urine alkalinization increases uric acid solubility, but decreases calcium phosphate solubility. In addition, rapid and aggressive alkalinization may worsen ionized hypocalcemia by shifting the calcium from its ionized form to a nonionized form. Typical hydration solutions are 5% dextrose in 0.45%–0.9% normal saline. Restriction of potassium and phosphorus is essential. Urine flow should be maintained at or above 2 mL/kg/h. Loop diuretic use is recommended in patients with low urine output after adequate hydration (101,103). Its use is discouraged in obstructive uropathy and in volume-depleted patient as it may worsen urate and phosphate precipitation.

Uric acid control can be achieved with recombinant urate oxidase (rasburicase) or with a xanthine oxidase inhibitor (allopurinol). Urate oxidase catalyzes the enzymatic oxygen-dependent conversion of poorly soluble urate to allantoin, a highly water-soluble product that is easily excreted in the urine. This enzyme is absent in humans. The recommended dose of rasburicase in children is 0.15–0.2 mg/kg/day, once daily in a 30-minute intravenous infusion for 5 days (5 days is recommended but rarely required) (104). In most cases, a single dose will produce a sharp and sustained decrease in uric acid levels (105). Urate oxidase infusion is contraindicated in patients with glucose-6-phosphate dehydrogenase (G6PD) deficiency. High-risk patients of African or Mediterranean descent should be screened for G6PD deficiency before urate oxidase is infused (106). Xanthine oxidase catalyzes the oxidation of hypoxanthine to xanthine and the oxidation of xanthine to uric acid. Allopurinol reduces the conversion of nucleic acids to uric acid, but will not affect existing xanthine or uric acids levels. The initial oral dose is 10 mg/kg/day or 200 mg/m^2/day, starting 24–48 hours prior to the initiation of chemotherapy. A randomized, multicenter, comparative trial that compared allopurinol with rasburicase in children with cancer at high risk for TLS demonstrated a more rapid reduction of uric acid and lower plasma levels in the children randomized to rasburicase when compared with allopurinol (107). The recently published guidelines for the management of tumor lysis in children and adults recommended the use of rasburicase for high-risk patients (level of evidence: II, grade of recommendation A) (101). A Cochrane Collaboration systematic review on the use of urate oxidase for the prevention and treatment of tumor lysis syndrome in children with cancer concluded that urate oxidase may in fact be more effective than allopurinol in reducing uric acid levels in patients with hyperuricemia. The review failed to confirm with certainty whether the routine use of urate oxidase is indeed effective in preventing or treating TLS and more importantly in reducing renal failure and mortality as a result of TLS (108).

Severe Electrolyte Disturbances. Patients with hyperkalemia and hyperphosphatemia should be aggressively monitored and treated. Dietary and supplemental potassium and phosphorus should be restricted. Patients with potassium levels ≥6.5 mEq/L or with electrocardiographic alterations (prolonged PR, flattened P, widened QRS, peaked T wave) should receive insulin, glucose, bicarbonate, and calcium. Alternative therapies to lower the serum potassium include low-dose β-adrenergic agents or hyperventilation to induce alkalosis. Potassium-wasting diuretics should be used with caution in volume-depleted patients. Sodium polystyrene sulfonate (Kayexalate), a potassium exchange resin, should be given early to help control the potassium rebound after the transient effect of the acute hyperkalemia treatment. The usual dose is 1 g/kg every 6 hours orally, mixed in water or sorbitol. Renal replacement therapy should be considered early in patients with rapid renal deterioration or in those with refractory hyperkalemia. Calcium replacement during TLS is indicated only in patients with cardiac arrhythmias (prolonged QT interval) or neuromuscular irritability secondary to hypocalcemia including seizures or a positive Chvostek or Trousseau sign. There is concern that calcium supplementation will increase the calcium phosphate product increasing the risk of ectopic calcification if the product exceeds 60. The lowest calcium dose required to relieve hypocalcemic symptoms should be used. Ectopic calcium phosphate precipitation in the renal tubules and in the cardiac conducting system may lead to serious arrhythmias. Hyperphosphatemia is managed with oral phosphate binders, such as sevelamer hydrochloride, or aluminum hydroxide (109).

Renal Replacement Therapy. Renal replacement therapy (see Chapter 41) is indicated in patients in whom aggressive interventions to reestablish normal urine flow or to correct

---

TABLE 115.4

TREATMENT OF TUMOR LYSIS SYNDROME

5% dextrose in 0.45%–0.9% normal saline at 3000 mL/m^2/d (or 200 mL/kg/d if ≤10 kg)

Maintain urine output > 2 mL/kg/h and specific gravity ≤1.010

Restrict potassium and phosphorus. Replace calcium in symptomatic patients only

Urate oxidase (rasburicase): 0.15 mg/kg/d once daily intravenously over 30 minutes. Repeat daily as needed (based on uric acid levels) for 1–7 d (contraindicated in G6PD deficiency) (105)

Allopurinol: 10 mg/kg/d orally or 200 mg/m^2/d intravenously, divided every 6–12 h, starting 24–48 h prior to the initiation of chemotherapy

Sevelamer hydrochloride: 120–200 mg/kg/d orally taken with meals (109)

Aluminum hydroxide: 50–150 mg/kg/d orally every 4 h

Pediatric patients at high risk for developing TLS should have laboratory (uric acid, phosphate, potassium, creatinine, calcium, and LDH) and clinical TLS parameters monitored 4–6 h after the initial administration of chemotherapy, as well as fluid input and urine output. For all patients, uric acid levels should be reevaluated 4 h after administration of rasburicase and every 6–8 h thereafter until resolution of TLS

metabolic abnormalities are unsuccessful. The goals of dialysis are treatment of obstructive nephropathy by rapid removal of phosphorus and uric acid, treatment of acute renal failure and the associated metabolic abnormalities, and facilitation of earlier chemotherapy in oliguric patients. Hyperuricemia is rarely an indication for dialysis in countries where rasburicase is available. Some practitioners institute continuous venovenous hemofiltration (CVVH) in addition to conventional preventive measures in high-risk children before the initiation of chemotherapy, as they feel that this may prevent further renal dysfunction, although no objective data support this practice. A recent report from the Prospective Pediatric Continuous Renal Replacement Therapy Registry Group looked at continuous renal replacement therapy for patients with nonrenal indications and showed an 82% survival for their TLS subgroup (110). Cytoreductive chemotherapy should be delayed if indicated in patients with high risk of TLS until the preventive treatment measures are initiated.

Hypercalcemia

Hypercalcemia is a rare finding in children in the PICU. The incidence in children with cancer is ~0.4%, compared with 5%–20% in adults with cancer. Malignancy-associated hypercalcemia can be found in patients with leukemia, lymphoma, hepatoblastoma, rhabdomyosarcoma, Ewing sarcoma, or brain tumors. The most common cause of malignancy-associated hypercalcemia is a humoral hypercalcemia, caused by solid tumor production of a parathyroid hormone-related peptide (PTHrP), resulting in a systemic osteoclast-mediated bone resorption, increased renal calcium resorption, and increased renal phosphorus excretion (111). The second most common cause of hypercalcemia is osteolysis secondary to cytokine-mediated osteoclast activation at the site of bone metastasis. The third category and most frequent form of hypercalcemia in Hodgkin and non-Hodgkin disease is calcitriol-mediated hypercalcemia, which results from dysregulated renal production of 1α-hydroxylase secondary to PTHrP stimulation. Patients with malignant hypercalcemia will usually present with bradyarrhythmias, coma, muscle weakness, and renal insufficiency.

Management of severe hypercalcemia (≥ 14 mg/dL) includes monitoring for electrocardiographic changes (prolonged PR, broad T waves), vigorous hydration with saline solution (10–20 mL/kg/bolus), forced diuresis with furosemide (1–2 mg/kg/dose) to induce calciuresis, reduction of calcium mobilization with calcitonin 4 IU/kg intramuscularly or subcutaneously every 24 hours in combination with prednisone 1 mg/kg/day or an equivalent corticosteroid, and treatment of the underlying malignancy. Pamidronate, a bisphosphonate, binds hydroxyapatite crystals and blocks osteoclast-mediated resorption. The recommended dose is 1 mg/kg/dose administered intravenously over 24 hours and may be repeated in 7 days if needed. The side effects include hypocalcemia, hypophosphatemia, and hypomagnesemia. Combined treatment with calcitonin and pamidronate may be used in refractory cases that do not respond to conventional treatment with hydration and forced diuresis with loop diuretics (112).

Syndrome of Inappropriate Antidiuretic Hormone Secretion

Syndrome of Inappropriate Antidiuretic Hormone Secretion (SIADH) may occur in children with cancer (medulloblastoma, lymphoma, ovarian teratoma) and in the setting of cerebral insults (intracranial surgery, trauma), neck surgery, mechanical ventilation, infections, and lung disease. SIADH has been recognized to occur with several medications frequently used in cancer patients including antiepileptics (carbamazepine) and chemotherapeutic agents (vincristine, ifosfamide, cyclophosphamide) (94). SIADH-related hyponatremia may be aggravated by aggressive hypotonic fluid hydration strategies frequently used in patients who receive chemotherapy. The late manifestations of SIADH (confusion, seizures, coma) are usually the reason for admission to the PICU. The treatment of SIADH should include isotonic fluid restricted to 30%–50% maintenance until the serum sodium levels normalize. Hypertonic saline (3% saline solution) is reserved for severely symptomatic patients with coma and/or seizures. Hypertonic saline should be given acutely to raise the serum Na concentration to ≥ 120 mEq/L and then more gradually to 130 mEq/L. New pharmacologic agents are available for oral and intravenous administration (conivaptan) that block the effects of vasopressin on the V_2 receptor in the kidney (113,114). Although used for the correction of hyponatremia related to high ADH levels in the adult population, there are little data regarding their use in children.

Cerebral Salt-Wasting Syndrome

Patients with cerebral salt-wasting syndrome (CSWS) may share similar intracerebral diseases and laboratory criteria with those patients with SIADH. CSWS is seen in children with cancer after brain tumor and hydrocephalus surgery (115). It typically occurs in the first 48 hours after admission, but may be seen up to 10–12 days after surgery. CSWS is probably the result of abnormal secretion of atrial and brain natriuretic peptides. Patients with CSWS have volume contraction and hyponatremia in the setting of polyuria and increased urine losses of sodium. The differentiation between SIADH and CSWS is made by observing urine and overall volume patterns during the development of hyponatremia and natriuresis (116). The treatment of CSWS should be directed at vigorous extracellular fluid and sodium replacement. Treatment with high-dose fludrocortisone (0.2–0.4 mg/day) has proven to be beneficial in some patients (117).

Diabetes Insipidus

Central diabetes insipidus (DI) typically presents in the pediatric cancer patient as a result of a direct injury, compression, or infiltration of the hypothalamic supraoptic or paraventricular nuclei or the supraoptic-hypophyseal tract. DI is most often caused by surgical resection of a hypothalamic-pituitary tumor (craniopharyngioma, germinoma) or by local tumor infiltration or destruction (histiocytosis, leukemia, lymphoma). DI most often presents in a triphasic pattern after surgical resection of a suprasellar mass. During the initial phase, typically lasting 2–5 days, the patient may develop DI as a consequence of a deficient secretion of arginine vasopressin or secretion of a biologically inactive form. The second phase is characterized by an inappropriate arginine vasopressin (AVP) release that lasts 1–14 days (117), during which time the signs and symptoms of DI may disappear. A recurrent and very often permanent form of DI characterizes the third phase. The treatment of DI is discussed at length in Chapter 107.

NEUROLOGIC EMERGENCIES

A neurologic emergency is oftentimes the first manifestation of cancer in a pediatric patient. It is not infrequent for a child to present with seizures, coma, or increased intracranial pressure (Table 115.5). In most cases, the presentation may be

TABLE 115.5

CLASSIC NEURO-ONCOLOGICAL EMERGENCIES

■ NEUROLOGICAL EMERGENCY	■ SIGNS & SYMPTOMS	■ RADIOLOGICAL/LABORATORY DIAGNOSTIC TESTS	■ MANAGEMENT
Spinal cord compression	Back pain Sensory abnormalities Focal weakness Autonomic dysfunction Bowel and bladder dysfunction	Craniospinal T1-T2-weighted MRI	Corticosteroids Radiation Surgery
Increased intracranial pressure	Headache Visual disturbances	Noncontrast CT brain Metabolic workup	Airway control Maintain appropriate mean arterial pressure Osmotherapy Corticosteroids Treatment of specific etiology
Seizures	Altered mental status Seizures Tonic-clonic movements Altered mental status suggestive of nonclinical seizure activity	Drug levels Infectious workup CT of the brain Metabolic workup EEG Lumbar puncture (if no contraindication) Toxicology workup	Supportive management Anticonvulsants Treatment of specific etiology Supportive management
Stroke	Altered mental status Focal weakness Seizure activity	CT or MRI of the brain MRA/MRV Coagulation disorder workup	Supportive measures Anticoagulation or revascularization
Coma	Severe altered mental status	Noncontrast CT of the brain Metabolic workup Toxicology workup Infectious workup	Airway control Supportive management Treatment of specific etiology
Posterior reversible encephalopathy syndrome	Headache Seizures Altered mental status	MRI of the brain	Anticonvulsants Control of hypertension

more indolent and may often be confused with benign medical conditions escaping the most astute clinician. This section will focus on neurologic emergencies that affect children with cancer and that require PICU admission.

Spinal Cord Compression

Malignant spinal cord compression (MSCC) is a true oncologic emergency. It occurs in 4%–25% of patients at some point of disease evolution (118,119). Spinal cord compression can result from various types of cancer including neuroblastoma, osteosarcoma, lymphoma, leukemia, posterior fossa or brain stem tumors, and metastatic lesions from primary tumors in the lung, breast, or kidneys. The epidural space is the most common area for spinal cord metastasis with the thoracic spine being the most common site of involvement (120). The mechanism of injury is the result of progressive vascular obstruction of the venous plexus or arterial blood supply causing cord edema, cord ischemia, or acute cord infarction (118). Back pain is a red flag in a patient with known history of malignancy and it should be considered secondary to MSCC until proven otherwise. Neurological signs, once apparent, lead to rapid and irreversible neuronal injury. Other common symptoms include sensory abnormalities (40%–90%), focal weakness (75%), and bowel and bladder dysfunction (40%–50%) (121).

Therapy should be initiated as soon as the diagnosis is considered as this improves short-term prognosis. Treatment priorities include strategies to (1) maintain tissue oxygenation and perfusion; (2) stabilize the spine; and (3) provide pain control (120,121). High-dose corticosteroids (dexamethasone 1–2 mg/kg) should be administered immediately followed by

lower doses (0.25–0.5 mg/kg administered intravenously every 6 hours) once the diagnosis is confirmed. Craniospinal T1- and T2-weighted MRI is the study of choice to demonstrate epidural involvement, intraparenchymal spread, or compression of nerve roots. CT myelography can be performed if there is any contraindication to MRI or if MRI is unavailable (118). Plain radiographs have limited sensitivity and specificity and are less useful for diagnosis (121). Continuation of therapy may include (1) radiation if the diagnosis is known and the tumor is radiosensitive; (2) surgery if there is severe spinal instability, rapidly progressive symptoms, or progressive symptoms in spite of radiation; (3) chemotherapy if the diagnosis is leukemia/lymphoma or neuroblastoma. Decompressive surgery with or without radiotherapy could be superior to radiotherapy alone (118,121,122). The prognosis depends on the neurological status at diagnosis, time to progression of symptoms, and time interval to definitive therapy. Overall survival depends on the tumor type. Patients with hematological malignancies have better survival compared with patients with solid tumors.

Increased Intracranial Pressure

Increased intracranial pressure (ICP) can occur in children with cancer due to (1) mass effect from primary tumor or metastases; (2) leptomeningeal disease progression; (3) bleeding from tumor mass, coagulopathy, or hyperleukocytosis (Fig. 115.1); or (4) obstructed CSF flow causing hydrocephalus (120). If untreated, these conditions can lead to cerebral herniation. Diagnosis and management of increased ICP are covered in Chapter 61. Tumor-related increased ICP may require additional therapy including dexamethasone (2 mg/kg followed by 0.5 mg/kg every 6 hours), which decreases cerebral vasogenic edema, has a long half-life, and has minimal mineralocorticoid effect (123). A noncontrast CT of the brain following these emergent measures may help to delineate the underlying etiology. Other potential causes for altered mental status and increased ICP should be investigated including metabolic (uremia, polycythemia, and anemia), toxic (methotrexate, hypervitaminosis), infectious, or vascular (hypertension, thrombosis) causes, if the CT is negative. Correction of the underlying cause should be undertaken once the emergency management has been completed.

Seizures

The child with cancer has a greater risk for seizures when compared with other pediatric patients. The primary tumor and complications from cancer treatment makes them more susceptible to experience a seizure. The treatment priorities should include aggressive management of the seizure, supportive management, and appropriate testing to determine the etiology of the seizure. Confirmatory testing should include a metabolic work up to rule out common metabolic abnormalities (hyponatremia, hypernatremia, hypoglycemia, hypocalcemia, acidosis, uremia, and hyperammonemia), hematologic tests (CBC, coagulation profile), a brain CT, and an EEG. A diagnostic lumbar puncture should be considered if the CT is negative for a mass lesion or hemorrhage. Cerebrospinal fluid opening pressure and fluid cytology, cell count, differential, and protein may help to rule out leptomeningeal tumor involvement with associated elevated intracranial pressure or infection. The main goal is to treat the underlying cause.

Stroke

Children with malignancy are at increased risk for stroke due to a hypercoagulable state. The most common causes of stroke in children are hypercoagulopathy causing cerebrovascular thrombosis, vessel compression or infiltration by tumor, intracerebral hemorrhage, and local or metastatic tumor spread. Embolic events are rare in children. Children with leukemia and hyperleukocytosis (white blood cell count, WBC >100,000/mm^3) are at increased risk for stroke due to leukostasis (microcirculatory dysfunction with sludging of leukemic cells in capillary vessels) at diagnosis and early in the treatment phase (**Fig. 115.1**). Neoplastic venous sinus occlusion can be seen in patients with neuroblastoma, lymphoma, or lung cancers. Treatment-related thrombosis may be seen with L-asparaginase. Brain radiation in children with ALL or brain tumors can cause Moya Moya syndrome due to stenosis of the cerebral vessels from radiation-induced vasculopathy and possibly as a result of other therapies including intrathecal chemotherapy (124).

Diagnosis of stroke can be made with a CT or MRI with and without contrast. These diagnostic modalities will help to delineate the nature of the stroke and will help describe the extent of the area involved. A magnetic resonance venogram (MRV) can help detect venous sinus occlusion. General management of stroke includes supportive measures including adequate hydration as well as possible anticoagulation or revascularization procedures. Treatment of the underlying malignancy may help in the prevention of further strokes. More information about stroke management may be found in Chapter 64.

Coma

Occasionally, a pediatric cancer patient may present with significant obtundation or coma. Coma is a symptom and there may be many etiologies in this patient population

TABLE 115.6

ETIOLOGY OF COMA IN CHILDREN WITH CANCER

Neurologic
  Primary or metastatic brain tumor: Pressure effect
  Obstructive hydrocephalus
  Intracranial hemorrhage or stroke
  Postictal or subclinical status epilepticus
Infectious
  Meningitis
  Sepsis
Hematologic
  Hyperleukocytosis
  Thrombocytopenia
Metabolic
  Hypoglycemia
  Hypo/hypernatremia
  Acidosis, uremia
Treatment related
  Ifosfamide
  Vincristine
  Methotrexate
Toxic/overdose
  Narcotics
Severe hypoxia

(**Table 115.6**) Chapter 57 provides a detailed discussion of the diagnosis and management of coma, which also applies to the cancer patient. The intensivist should focus on the stabilization of the patient's airway, breathing, and circulation and on the management of impending herniation (see previous section). A contrast CT or MRI is often helpful in determining the etiology.

Posterior Reversible Encephalopathy Syndrome

The posterior reversible encephalopathy syndrome (PRES), also known as reversible posterior leukoencephalopathy syndrome (RPLS), is a clinical-radiological entity that is seen in a variety of medical conditions including cancer, hematologic disease, renal disorders, and lupus. Affected patients may present with headaches, altered mental status, visual disturbances, and seizures. This syndrome has been recognized as a significant complication in children with leukemia and solid tumors, since the availability of MRI (125). Endothelial dysfunction with resulting blood–brain barrier disruption is a proposed mechanism, which could occur due to CNS disease, hypertension, or intrathecal chemotherapy (126). The white matter is predominantly involved as this area is more susceptible to vasogenic edema (**Fig. 115.2**). The posterior cerebrum is a common area of involvement for PRES, and this is thought to be due to the limited sympathetic innervation of the vertebral-basilar system (125). Hypertension seems to be a key risk factor in the development of PRES and is often secondary to cytotoxic therapy, renal injury, or corticosteroid therapy.

MRI is the diagnostic tool of choice and should be obtained immediately following a suspicion of PRES. Transient edema of the subcortical white matter in occipital, parietal, temporal, or basal ganglia regions on T2-weighted images and FLAIR images are pathognomonic for PRES. Treatment should focus on control of hypertension and anticonvulsant therapy as needed. Several studies suggest that intrathecal chemotherapy can be safely continued. However, if symptoms are strongly associated with any particular agent, this should be cautiously

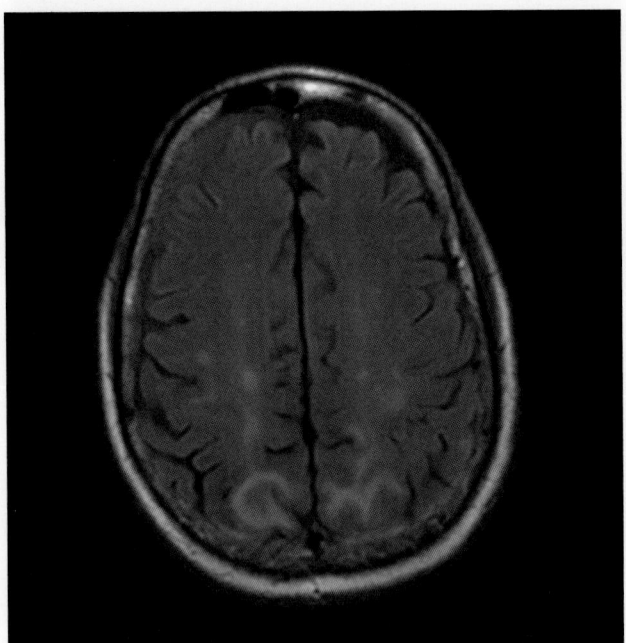

FIGURE 115.2. MRI image of a posterior reversible encephalopathy. White matter involvement sparing the cortical gray matter in the occipital region.

restarted. Neurological changes related to PRES are reversible in the majority of cases. Side effects of chemotherapy like SIRS, coagulopathy, or hyperviscosity syndrome can affect the neurological outcome of patients with PRES (127). Little is known on the future cognitive function of children affected by PRES.

RESPIRATORY EMERGENCIES

Respiratory emergencies are frequent in the pediatric cancer patient and may have a dramatic presentation in some patients particularly after HSCT. The primary disease, secondary immune deficiency, and the toxicity of the therapy make these patients susceptible to a wide range of infectious and noninfectious problems that may progress rapidly to respiratory failure (Table 115.7). These patients should be fully evaluated to rule out a treatable infectious illness. Empiric initiation of broad-spectrum antimicrobial therapy addressing possible pathogens (Pseudomonas, Cytomegalovirus, Pneumocystis, and

Aspergillus) is often indicated in patients with rapid clinical or radiologic deterioration. Bronchoscopy with bronchoalveolar lavage or open lung biopsy should be performed early in the course of the illness. These procedures may help differentiate infection from diffuse alveolar hemorrhage, a common complication after stem cell transplantation. The use of high-resolution CT to identify fungal lesions should be considered in all patients with respiratory symptomatology, regardless of the plain radiograph findings.

Traditionally, stem cell transplant recipients with respiratory failure requiring endotracheal intubation, especially in the presence of pneumonia or diffuse alveolar hemorrhage had poor outcomes (128). Early application of a lung-protective strategy with conventional mechanical ventilation or an early (within the first 6 hour of mechanical ventilation) transition to high-frequency oscillatory ventilation have shown better outcomes, indicating a potential for improved outcome with an earlier intervention in the acute lung injury process (7). The remainder of this section will focus on the most dramatic respiratory emergencies affecting the child with cancer.

Mediastinal Masses

The most common anterosuperior mediastinal tumors are Hodgkin lymphomas, non-Hodgkin lymphomas, thymomas, and teratomas. The most common tumors affecting the middle mediastinum are lymphomas and metastatic tumors (Wilms tumor, testicular neoplasm, and various sarcomas) while neuroblastoma, ganglioneuroma and neurofibroma most commonly affect the posterior mediastinum.

Any growing mass in the mediastinum has the potential to displace or compress anatomical structures. Patients with anterosuperior and middle mediastinal masses are at risk for life-threatening airway obstruction and vascular compression, and patients with posterior mediastinal masses are at risk for spinal cord compression. The clinical presentation varies according to the location and the severity of the displacement. Patients with lesions affecting the tracheobronchial tree may present with symptoms of dyspnea, orthopnea, stridor, cough, and respiratory distress. Patients with tumor masses compressing the great vessels may present with head and neck edema with or without neurological deficit; and patients with tumors compressing the heart may present with syncope, cyanosis, and arrhythmias.

The evaluation for mediastinal masses includes assessment of the potential for airway or vascular compression or obstruction and ways to improve it prior to sedation or supine positioning for radiologic or tissue diagnosis. Keeping the child in an upright or prone position instead of supine improves pulmonary function (129) and increases the caudad displacement

TABLE 115.7

PULMONARY COMPLICATIONS AFTER HEMATOPOIETIC STEM CELL TRANSPLANT

■ PHASE	■ INFECTIOUS	■ NONINFECTIOUS
Neutropenic phase (0–30 d)	Bacteria (20%–50%) Fungal (12%–45%)	Pulmonary edema Drug toxicity DAH
Early phase (30–100 d)	CMV pneumonitis (40%) PCP	Idiopathic pneumonia syndrome
Late phase (>100 d)	Uncommon except in GVHD	Bronchiolitis obliterans Cryptogenic organizing pneumonia Chronic GVHD

DAH, diffuse alveolar hemorrhage; CMV, cytomegalovirus; PCP, *Pneumocystis jiroveci (carinii)* pneumonia; GVHD, graft-versus-host disease.

of the diaphragm and intra-thoracic volume (130). Airway instrumentation should be performed in elective situations in a controlled environment by experienced anesthesiologists with surgical and cardiopulmonary support available. In most situations, endotracheal intubation takes place in conscious and spontaneously breathing patients employing topical anesthetic techniques with light sedation and avoiding the use of neuromuscular blocking agents. The concern being that the loss of spontaneous ventilation may decrease the transpleural pressure gradient and augment the extrinsic compression effect. Reinforced endotracheal tubes of decreased diameter but sufficient length to extend beyond the compression may be necessary. Flexible or rigid fiberoptic bronchoscopy and ECMO or cardiopulmonary bypass should be considered in advance in patients with severe airway and vascular involvement.

Patients presenting with orthopnea, upper body edema, great vessel compression, main stem bronchus compression, or masses that exceed 45% of the thoracic diameter are at risk of anesthesia-related complications (**Fig. 115.3**) (131,132). Computed tomography (**Fig. 115.4**) and pulmonary function tests will help differentiate patients at risk from patients that may tolerate sedation or general anesthesia. General anesthesia should not be administered, even in asymptomatic patients, if the tracheal cross-sectional area, measured by CT scan, and the peak expiratory flow rate are less than 50% of predicted values (129,133). Bone marrow biopsy, lymph node biopsy, or radiologic (ultrasound or CT-guided) percutaneous mediastinal biopsies may be safely performed with local anesthesia in many cases thereby avoiding the need for general anesthesia. Pericardial and/or pleural collections should be drained under ultrasound (US) or CT guidance for therapeutic and diagnostic purposes. In a recent study, US-guided percutaneous core needle biopsy performed under local anesthesia and moderate sedation in 32 children showed a biopsy adequacy rate

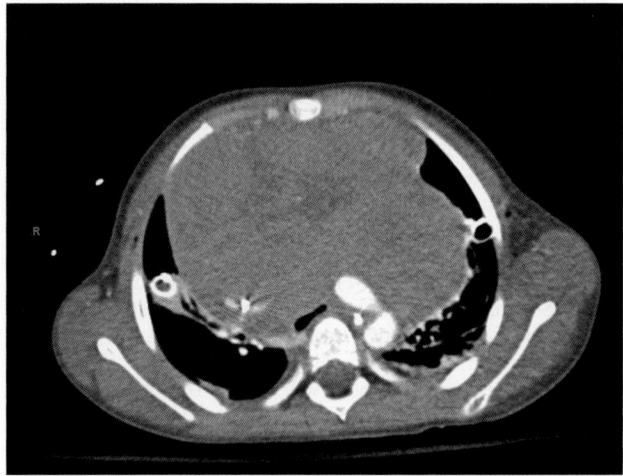

FIGURE 115.4. CT image of a mediastinal lymphoma. The anterior mediastinal mass is a combination of the patient's lymphoma and a thymus gland.

of 91% and a diagnostic rate of 78% with no major complications (134). In another study, 23 patients underwent a mini-mediastinotomy procedure with local anesthesia and moderate sedation. The study showed a 100% success rate in reaching a definitive histopathological diagnosis with minimal morbidity (135). The decision of where to sedate a patient with the mediastinal mass requires careful consideration of the patient's risks (e.g., airway difficulty, cardiovascular collapse), the required resources and expertise (including anesthesiologists and surgeons), as well as the ability to transport safely.

Prebiopsy cytoreductive therapy using corticosteroids or radiation therapy may be required in patients presenting with severe airway compromise reducing the ability to make a definitive diagnosis. In a retrospective study of 86 children with mediastinal lymphoma, 23 patients with severe airway compromise received corticosteroids 24–48 hours before undergoing a biopsy procedure altering the pathological diagnosis in 20% (136). Surgical resection may be unavoidable in patients with tumors not sensitive to cytoreductive therapy like teratomas and germ cell tumors. The postoperative period for patients with mediastinal masses continues to be of concern. Patients need close monitoring and ongoing assessment for any additional airway obstruction secondary to postbiopsy edema.

Superior Mediastinal Syndrome

Superior mediastinal syndrome (SMS) results from the compression of the superior mediastinal structures (the tracheobronchial tree, the great vessels, and the heart) by a growing mass or a thrombus. A review of the clinical records of children who initially presented with SMS to St. Jude Children's Research Hospital during a 16-year period found that the most frequent diagnosis was non-Hodgkin lymphoma (50%), followed by T-cell acute lymphoblastic leukemia (25%) and Hodgkin lymphoma (12.5%). Patients with solid tumors (sarcomas) have a high frequency of SMS, but at a later time in the course of their disease. The most common symptomatology at presentation includes dyspnea, orthopnea, stridor, and wheezing with associated pleural and/or pericardial effusions (137).

Progressive venous congestion and airway compression will lead to the usual symptoms found in SMS including facial engorgement, headache, plethora, cyanotic facies, cough, dyspnea, orthopnea, hoarseness, stridor, and dysphasia with or

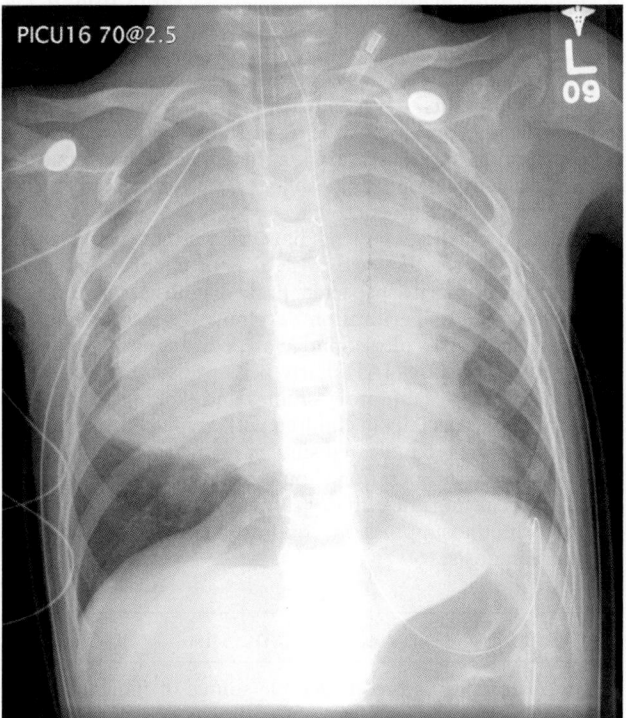

FIGURE 115.3. Chest radiograph of a mediastinal tumor. Large mediastinal mass extending predominantly to the right, with opacification of the right upper/mid hemithorax. Compression atelectasis is noted in the right mid-lung field.

without pleural and/or pericardial effusions. Most patients will not tolerate the supine position. Chest radiograph and CT imaging will confirm the distortion of the superior mediastinal structures. Echocardiography is indicated in patients with suspected thrombus or pericardial effusion. Pulmonary function tests are helpful in predicting patients that may not tolerate deep sedation or general anesthesia when undergoing diagnostic procedures (129). The elevation of nonspecific serum markers like lactate dehydrogenase (LDH) may be helpful in identifying possible etiologies. Elevation of LDH is present in 75% of patients with non-Hodgkin lymphoma and leukemia (137). Severe cases with profound airway obstruction will receive prebiopsy therapy with corticosteroids or radiation therapy. Once the definitive diagnosis is reached, the appropriate chemotherapeutic plan will reduce tumor load rapidly with improvement of symptoms. Thrombolytic therapy should be considered in patients with extensive thromboembolism if there are no contraindications.

Massive Hemoptysis

Massive hemoptysis is defined as blood loss ≥240 mL in adults. Massive hemoptysis is rare, but a striking finding in children that can lead to rapid asphyxiation and death. The most common cause of massive hemoptysis in the pediatric cancer patient is invasive pulmonary aspergillosis (IPA). IPA usually presents after myeloablative chemotherapy for bone marrow transplantation or during the recovery phase of prolonged neutropenia after chemotherapy. Other infections to be considered in the differential diagnosis include invasive fungi (mucormycosis), bacterial necrotizing pneumonias due to *Staphylococcus Aureus*, *Pseudomonas Aeruginosa*, or *Klebsiella* and tuberculosis (138). Noninfectious etiologies may include primary endobronchial tumors, diffuse alveolar hemorrhage, bronchiectasis, and foreign bodies. Bronchiectasis is often the result of a chronic inflammatory process caused by the accumulation of purulent secretions and obstruction of the airways, leading to chronic atelectasis. The internal digestion of bronchial structural proteins by lytic enzymes released by activated neutrophils in combination with the traction on the airway wall, results in distension of the airways, fibrosis, and ulceration. These ulcerations may erode into an underlying blood vessel wall, causing hemoptysis. Hemoptysis is rarely found in foreign body aspiration, but when present, it is generally associated with bronchiectasis. Neutropenic patients with fever for more than 96 hours despite adequate antibiotic therapy should be evaluated for IPA. Chest pain and cough are common symptoms. The highest risk for hemoptysis occurs during recovery from prolonged neutropenia. The inflammatory process includes a focal cavitary lesion surrounded by collateral vessels. The presence of increasing neutrophils leads to focal necrosis and enhanced risk for vessel perforation and bleeding (139). CT imaging is the most sensitive radiologic test available for the early diagnosis of IPA. The *halo sign*, a dense nodular lesion surrounded by ground glass attenuation (>180°) is consistent with IPA. The *air crescent sign* indicates necrosis and cavitation. Tissue diagnosis is required to conclusively confirm or exclude IPA. Tissue may be obtained by CT-guided percutaneous lung biopsy, transbronchial biopsy, or open lung biopsy.

The treatment of massive hemoptysis should be directed at the prevention of asphyxia and the localization of the source to halt further bleeding. Early intubation and mechanical ventilation should be considered. Aggressive treatment of any associated coagulopathy, thrombocytopenia, and anemia is warranted. Nonsurgical mortality risk in patients with invasive pulmonary aspergillosis ranges between 30% and 90% (140). Medical therapy consist of a combination of antifungal

therapies including caspofungin (loading dose of 70 mg/m^2 to a maximum of 70 mg followed by 50 mg/m^2/day with a maximum of 50 mg), liposomal amphotericin B (5–6 mg/kg/day), and voriconazole (loading dose of 6 mg/kg administered intravenously every 12 hours on day 1, followed by 4 mg/kg intravenously every 12 hours). This combination has proven to be safe for immunosuppressed children with invasive mycosis (141). Bronchoscopy should be considered in patients in whom endoluminal therapy for control of the bleeding is feasible. Bronchial arteriography with transcatheter embolization may be effective in nonsurgical candidates. Wedge resection of the affected lung segment or lobectomy carries a low mortality risk and offers a lower recurrence rate when compared with nonsurgical options (140).

ABDOMINAL EMERGENCIES

Acute Abdomen

Abdominal emergencies in pediatric cancer patients arise most commonly due to hemorrhage, mechanical obstruction, perforation, or inflammation. The development of abdominal pathology in the neutropenic or immunocompromised patient presents a special diagnostic and treatment challenge, when compared with immunologically normal hosts. The presence of pain, a generally reliable sign of acute abdomen, may be less useful in a patient with abnormal sensation, spinal cord pathology, or recent treatment with high-dose corticosteroids.

Acute Appendicitis

Appendicitis is one of the most common abdominal surgical conditions in childhood, with a peak incidence at age 12 years. Many studies have reported that the incidence of appendicitis in children with hematologic malignancies varies from 0.5% to 4.4% (142). Presenting signs and symptoms are usually atypical in immunocompromised patients making the diagnosis challenging for clinicians. The use of corticosteroids may mask the symptoms of appendicitis in some patients. The differential diagnosis of appendicitis includes typhlitis, abdominal obstruction, intussusception, gastroenteritis, constipation, urinary tract infection, renal colic, pelvic inflammatory disease, and lower lobe pneumonia.

Studies in oncology patients have shown that the diagnosis of appendicitis was delayed in 37.5% of children in whom typhlitis was primarily suspected. Early diagnosis is paramount before gangrene or perforation develops. We recommend the use of CT imaging or ultrasound in all pediatric cancer patients suspected of typhlitis (143). Early pediatric surgery consultation together with laboratory studies and diagnostic imaging can be helpful especially in children with atypical presentation. Several studies have indicated surgery as the treatment option (142,143), but consideration should be given to a higher associated surgical mortality than in immune-competent children due to immunosuppression, opportunistic infections, and delayed diagnosis.

Bowel Obstruction

Bowel obstruction is a considerable source of morbidity and mortality in the patient with cancer. Bowel obstruction from primary malignancy is not as common in children as it is in adults because of a lower frequency of these tumors (colon and ovarian cancer). It may be the presenting symptom of certain diseases, such as non-Hodgkin lymphoma, rhabdomyosarcoma, and colonic neoplasias. Bowel obstruction may also be present in metastatic disease. It is almost always found in carcinomatosis. Conditions that increase the risk of bowel obstruction are encountered frequently in children who are being treated for cancer. These include surgery, radiation therapy, opioid use, prolonged bed rest, malnutrition, and electrolyte abnormalities. CT imaging has been shown to be sensitive and specific in identifying small bowel obstruction (**Fig. 115.5**). Intravenous contrast should be used unless contraindicated. Oral contrast is beneficial in defining the transition point in low-grade or intermittent small bowel obstruction (144).

Patients with partial obstruction such as those with plain x-rays showing the presence of intraluminal air in the small and large bowel and those without mechanical obstruction may be managed medically. Dexamethasone and octreotide are effective in relieving symptoms in most patients with malignant bowel obstruction (142,145). Surgery is indicated for patients with complete mechanical obstruction, partial mechanical obstruction not responding to medical treatment, or in the presence of signs of peritonitis and frank perforation. Palliative measures, such as venting gastrostomy tube or jejunostomy tube, are appropriate in patients with end-stage disease who present with inoperable bowel obstruction.

Intussusception

Primary intestinal neoplasms or intestinal metastatic tumors, such as carcinomas or lymphomas, may serve as lead points for intussusception. These occur most commonly in the jejunum and the ileum. The "classic triad" of intussusception includes colicky pain, abdominal mass, and bloody stools (144). However, the clinical findings are usually varied and most children present with abdominal pain and vomiting. A high index of suspicion and the use of appropriate imaging are required to make the correct diagnosis in a timely manner. Ultrasonography is more accurate than abdominal radiographs and can detect the lead point and other intra-abdominal pathology. The treatment of choice in the cancer

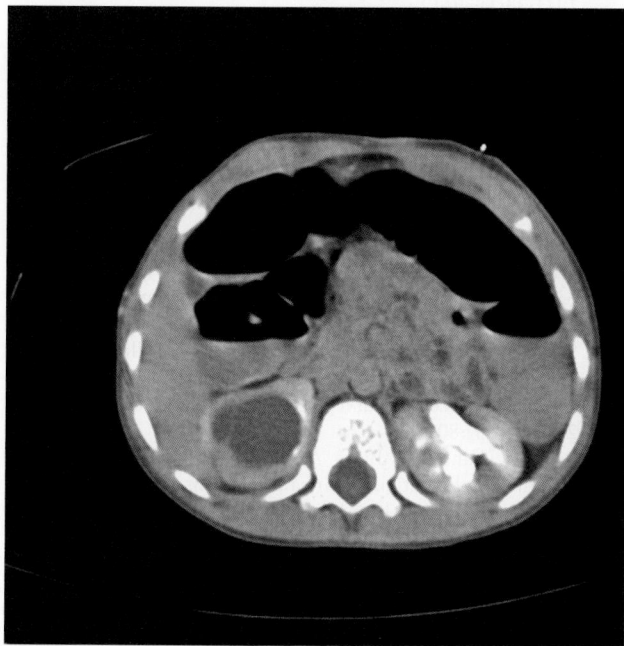

FIGURE 115.5. CT image of small bowel obstruction. Distal small-bowel obstruction, with a tortuous and thickened fluid filled loops of distal ileum tapering at the level of the ileocecal valve.

patient is surgical reduction of the intussusception and resection of the inciting pathology rather than radiologic reduction using contrast enema.

SUMMARY

Many of the malignancies encountered in pediatrics can now be cured or significantly palliated with interventions provided in the intensive care unit. A large part of the success for the improvement in childhood cancer survival rates is due to the improvements in supportive care for potentially critical clinical situations, such as septicemia, hyperleukocytosis, and TLS. Despite these advances, much additional investigation is still required to continue the improvement in treating those pediatric patients that become critically ill. Recent experience with pediatric cancer patients in the PICU suggests that outcomes are improved with early and aggressive interventions that are targeted at preventing or avoiding organ damage or failure, as survival for these patients is markedly reduced once three or more systems are implicated (4).

It is important that critical care professionals be aware of the effects of new chemotherapeutic agents and treatment strategies. We should remain attentive to the special challenges posed by immuno-compromised patients. A dynamic and vigorous partnership with the oncology team will help to ensure that these patients receive timely physiologic support as they undergo treatment.

FUTURE DIRECTIONS

Future pediatric cancer treatments will include the use of target specific and potentially less-toxic chemotherapeutic agents, sensitive and specific minimal residual disease monitoring biomarkers, and the potential earlier use of therapies available to the intensive care physician to prevent end-organ dysfunction. There is much interest in evaluating potential serum biomarkers and other clinical prognostic factors that may aid in developing a risk-stratification scheme for patients with febrile neutropenia. Such predictive markers may help in the early identification of those patients at highest risk for sepsis or increased mortality. Further clinical research in pediatric thrombosis is needed to expand the armamentarium of anticoagulant therapy, including the use of the newer oral anticoagulants that are now available in the adult population. New diagnostic approaches are relying more and more on immune-histochemistry, polymerase chain reaction analysis, and molecular methodology. These techniques should help avoid risky invasive diagnostic procedures in critically ill children with mediastinal masses.

References

1. Duncan CN, Lehmann LE, Cheifetz IM, et al. Pediatric Acute Lung Injury and Sepsis (PALISI) Network. Clinical outcomes of children receiving intensive cardiopulmonary support during hematopoietic stem cell transplant. *Pediatr Crit Care Med* 2013;14:261–7.
2. Hallahan AR, Shaw PJ, Rowell G, et al. Improved outcomes of children with malignancy admitted to a pediatric intensive care unit. *Crit Care Med* 2000;28(11):3718–21.
3. Pound CM, Johnston DL, Armstrong R, et al. The morbidity and mortality of pediatric oncology patients presenting to the intensive care unit with septic shock. *Pediatr Blood Cancer* 2008;51(5):584–8.
4. Fiser RT, West NK, Bush AJ, et al. Outcome of severe sepsis in pediatric oncology patients. *Pediatr Crit Care Med* 2005;6(5):531–6.

5. Dalton HJ, Slonim AD, Pollack, MM. MultiCenter outcome of pediatric oncology patients requiring intensive care. *Pediatr Hematol Oncol* 2003;20(8):643–9.

6. Tamburro RF, Barfield RC, Shaffer ML, et al. Changes in outcomes (1996–2004) for pediatric oncology and hematopoietic stem cell transplant patients requiring invasive mechanical ventilation. *Pediatr Crit Care Med* 2008;9(3):270–7.

7. Faqih NA, Qabba'h SH, Rihani RS, et al. The use of high frequency oscillatory ventilation in a pediatric oncology intensive care unit. *Pediatr Blood Cancer* 2012;58(3):384–9.

8. Brierley J, Carcillo JA, Choong K, et al. Clinical practice parameters for hemodynamic support of pediatric and neonatal septic shock: 2007 update from the American College of Critical Care Medicine. *Crit Care Med* 2009;37(2):666–88.

9. Ha EJ, Kim S, Jin HS, et al. Early changes in SOFA score as a prognostic factor in pediatric oncology patients requiring mechanical ventilatory support. *J Pediatr Hematol Oncol* 2010;32(8):e308–13.

10. Brierley J, Peters, MJ. Distinct hemodynamic patterns of septic shock at presentation to pediatric intensive care. *Pediatrics* 2008;122(4):752–9.

11. Dellinger RP, Spoelstra-de Man AM, Girbes AR, et al. Surviving Sepsis Campaign: international guidelines for management of severe sepsis and septic shock: 2008. *Crit Care Med* 2008;36(1):296–327.

12. Hebbar KB, Petrillo T, Fortenberry JD. Adrenal insufficiency and response to corticosteroids in hypotensive critically ill children with cancer. *J Crit Care* 2012;27(5):480–7.

13. Li MJ, Yang YL, Huang SC, et al. Successful extracorporeal membrane oxygenation support patients with malignancy and septic shock. *Pediatr Blood Cancer* 2011;57(4):697.

14. Meister B, Zelger B, Kropshofer G, et al. Extracorporeal membrane oxygenation as a rescue therapy for leukaemic children with pulmonary failure. *Br J Haematol* 2010;148(1):126–31.

15. Basu S, Frank LH, Fenton KE, et al. Two-dimensional speckle tracking imaging detects impaired myocardial performance in children with septic shock, not recognized by conventional echocardiography. *Pediatr Crit Care Med* 2012;13(3):259–64.

16. Trachtenberg BH, Landy DC, Franco VI, et al. Anthracycline-associated cardiotoxicity in survivors of childhood cancer. *Pediatr Cardiol* 2011;32(3):342–53.

17. Günther T, Schreiber C, Noebauer C, et al. Treatment strategies for pediatric patients with primary cardiac and pericardial tumors: A 30-year review. *Pediatr Cardiol* 2008;29(6):1071–6.

18. Kim JJ, Valdes SO, Kertesz NJ, et al. Isolated junctional tachycardia in a patient with pheochromocytoma: An unusual presentation of an uncommon disease. *Pediatr Cardiol* 2008;29(5):986–8.

19. Kühn B, Peters J, Marx GR, et al. Etiology, management, and outcome of pediatric pericardial effusions. *Pediatr Cardiol* 2008;29(1):90–4.

20. Williams GD, Hammer GB. Cardiomyopathy in childhood. *Curr Opin Anaesthesiol* 2011;24(3):289–300.

21. Meckler G, Lindemulder S. Fever and neutropenia in pediatric patients with cancer. *Emerg Med Clin North Am* 2009;27(3):525–44.

22. Ammann RA, Bodmer N, Hirt A, et al. Predicting adverse events in children with fever and chemotherapy-induced neutropenia: The prospective multicenter SPOG 2003 FN study. *J Clin Oncol* 2010;28(12):2008–14.

23. Palazzi DL. The use of antimicrobial agents in children with fever during chemotherapy-induced neutropenia: The importance of risk stratification. *Pediatr Infect Dis J* 2011;30(10):887–90.

24. De Pauw B, Walsh TJ, Donnelly JP, et al. Revised definitions of invasive fungal disease from the European Organization for Research and Treatment of Cancer/Invasive Fungal Infections Cooperative Group and the National Institute of Allergy and Infectious Diseases Mycoses Study Group (EORTC/MSG) Consensus Group. *Clin Infect Dis* 2008;46(12):1813–21.

25. Quezada G, Sunderland T, Chan KW, et al. Medical and nonmedical barriers to outpatient treatment of fever and neutropenia in children with cancer. *Pediatr Blood Cancer* 2007;48(3):273–7.

26. Santolaya ME, Alvarez AM, Avilés CL, et al. Prospective evaluation of a model of prediction of invasive bacterial infection risk among children with cancer, fever, and neutropenia. *Clin Infect Dis* 2002;35(6):678–83.

27. Walsh TJ, Pappas P, Winston DJ, et al. Voriconazole compared with liposomal amphotericin B for empirical antifungal therapy in patients with neutropenia and persistent fever. *N Engl J Med* 2002;346(4):225–34.

28. Clark OAC, Lyman GH, Castro AA, et al. Colony-stimulating factors for chemotherapy-induced febrile neutropenia: A meta-analysis of randomized controlled trials. *J Clin Oncol* 2005;23(18):4198–214.

29. Sasse EC, Sasse AD, Brandalise S, et al. Colony stimulating factors for prevention of myelosupressive therapy induced febrile neutropenia in children with acute lymphoblastic leukaemia. *Cochrane Database Syst Rev* 2005;20(3):CD004139.

30. Crawford J, Armitage J, Balducci L, et al. Myeloid growth factors. *J Natl Compr Canc Netw* 2011;9(8):914–32.

31. Kuhn P, Messer J, Paupe A, et al. A multicenter, randomized, placebo-controlled trial of prophylactic recombinant granulocyte-colony stimulating factor in preterm neonates with neutropenia. *J Pediatr* 2009;155(3):324–30. e1.

32. Hall MW, Knatz NL, Vetterly C, et al. Immunoparalysis and nosocomial infection in children with multiple organ dysfunction syndrome. *Intensive Care Med* 2011;37(3):525–32.

33. Strauss RG. Role of granulocyte/neutrophil transfusions for haematology/oncology patients in the modern era. *Br J Haematol* 2012;158(3):299–306.

34. Castagnola E, Fontana V, Caviglia I, et al. A prospective study on the epidemiology of febrile episodes during chemotherapy-induced neutropenia in children with cancer or after hemopoietic stem cell transplantation. *Clin Infect Dis* 2007;45(10):1296–304.

35. Badiei Z, Khalesi M, Alami MH, et al. Risk factors associated with life-threatening infections in children with febrile neutropenia: A data mining approach. *J Pediatr Hematol Oncol* 2011;33(1):e9–12.

36. Lehrnbecher T, Varwig D, Kaiser J, et al. Infectious complications in pediatric acute myeloid leukemia: Analysis of the prospective multi-institutional clinical trial AML-BFM 93. *Leukemia* 2004;18(1):72–7.

37. Paul M, Dickstein Y, Schlesinger A, et al. Beta-lactam versus beta-lactam-aminoglycoside combination therapy in cancer patients with neutropaenia. *Cochrane Database Syst Rev* 2003(3):CD003038.

38. Uygun V, Karasu GT, Ogunc D, et al. Piperacillin/tazobactam versus cefepime for the empirical treatment of pediatric cancer patients with neutropenia and fever: A randomized and open-label study. *Pediatr Blood Cancer* 2009;53(4):610–4.

39. Simon A, Lehrnbecher T, Bode U, et al. Piperacillin-tazobactam in pediatric cancer patients younger than 25 months: A retrospective multicenter survey. *Eur J Clin Microbiol Infect Dis* 2007;26(11):801–6.

40. Paul M, Yahav D, Bivas A, et al. Anti-pseudomonal beta-lactams for the initial, empirical, treatment of febrile neutropenia: Comparison of beta-lactams. *Cochrane Database Syst Rev* 2010(11):CD005197.

41. Freifeld AG, Bow EJ, Sepkowitz KA, et al. Clinical practice guideline for the use of antimicrobial agents in neutropenic patients with cancer: 2010 update by the infectious diseases society of America. *Clin Infect Dis* 2011;52(4):427–31.

42. Cometta A, Kern WV, De Bock R, et al. Vancomycin versus placebo for treating persistent fever in patients with neutropenic cancer receiving piperacillin-tazobactam monotherapy. *Clin Infect Dis* 2003;37(3):382–9.

43. Gorschlüter M, Mey U, Strehl J, et al. Neutropenic enterocolitis in adults: Systematic analysis of evidence quality. *Eur J Haematol* 2005;75(1):1–13.

44. Sloas MM, Flynn PM, Kaste SC, et al. Typhlitis in children with cancer: A 30-year experience. *Clin Infect Dis* 1993;17(3):484–90.

45. Davila ML, Neutropenic enterocolitis. *Curr Opin Gastroenterol* 2006;22(1):44–7.

46. Fike FB, Mortellaro V, Juang D, et al. Neutropenic colitis in children. *J Surg Res* 2011;170(1):73–6.

47. Pagano L, Caira M, Candoni A, et al. The epidemiology of fungal infections in patients with hematologic malignancies: The SEIFEM-2004 study. *Haematologica* 2006;91(8):1068–75.

48. Wingard JR. New approaches to invasive fungal infections in acute leukemia and hematopoietic stem cell transplant patients. *Best Pract Res Clin Haematol* 2007;20(1):99–107.

49. Franklin JA, McCormick J, Flynn PM. Retrospective study of the safety of caspofungin in immunocompromised pediatric patients. *Pediatr Infect Dis J* 2003;22(8):747–9.

50. Lehrnbecher T, Phillips R, Alexander S, et al. International Pediatric Fever and Neutropenia Guideline Panel. Guideline for the management of fever and neutropenia in children with cancer and/or undergoing hematopoietic stem-cell transplantation. *J Clin Oncol* 2012;30:4427–38.

51. Reusser P, Einsele H, Lee J, et al. Randomized multicenter trial of foscarnet versus ganciclovir for preemptive therapy of cytomegalovirus infection after allogeneic stem cell transplantation. *Blood* 2002;99(4):1159–64.

52. Porcu P, Cripe LD, Ng EW, et al. Hyperleukocytic leukemias and leukostasis: A review of pathophysiology, clinical presentation and management. *Leuk Lymphoma* 2000;39(1–2):1–18.

53. Vaughan WP, Kimball AW, Karp JE, et al. Factors affecting survival of patients with acute myelocytic leukemia presenting with high wbc counts. *Cancer Treat Rep* 1981;65(11–12):1007–13.

54. Lichtman, MA, Rowe JM. Hyperleukocytic leukemias: Rheological, clinical, and therapeutic considerations. *Blood* 1982;60(2):279–83.

55. Stucki A, Rivier AS, Gikic M, et al. Endothelial cell activation by myeloblasts: Molecular mechanisms of leukostasis and leukemic cell dissemination. *Blood* 2001;97(7):2121–9.

56. Colman RW, Robboy SJ, Minna JD. Disseminated intravascular coagulation: A reappraisal. *Annu Rev Med* 1979;30:359–74.

57. Dixit A, Chatterjee T, Mishra P, et al. Disseminated intravascular coagulation in acute leukemia at presentation and during induction therapy. *Clin Appl Thromb Hemost* 2007;13(3):292–8.

58. Bug G, Anargyrou K, Tonn T, et al. Impact of leukapheresis on early death rate in adult acute myeloid leukemia presenting with hyperleukocytosis. *Transfusion* 2007;47(10):1843–50.

59. Porcu P, Farag S, Marcucci G, et al. Leukocytoreduction for acute leukemia. *Ther Apher* 2002;6(1):15–23.

60. Grund FM, Armitage JO, Burns P. Hydroxyurea in the prevention of the effects of leukostasis in acute leukemia. *Arch Intern Med* 1977;137(9):1246–7.

61. Chang MC, Chen TY, Tang JL, et al. Leukapheresis and cranial irradiation in patients with hyperleukocytic acute myeloid leukemia: No impact on early mortality and intracranial hemorrhage. *Am J Hematol* 2007;82(11):976–80.

62. Ganzel C, Becker J, Mintz PD, et al. Hyperleukocytosis, leukostasis and leukapheresis: Practice management. *Blood Rev* 2012;26(3):117–22.

63. Vahdat L, Maslak P, Miller WH Jr, et al. Early mortality and the retinoic acid syndrome in acute promyelocytic leukemia: Impact of leukocytosis, low-dose chemotherapy, PMN/RAR-alpha isoform, and CD13 expression in patients treated with all-trans retinoic acid. *Blood* 1994;84(11):3843–9.

64. Falanga A, Rickles FR. Pathophysiology of the thrombophilic state in the cancer patient. *Semin Thromb Hemost* 1999;25(2):173–82.

65. Rickles FR, Falanga A. Molecular basis for the relationship between thrombosis and cancer. *Thromb Res* 2001;102(6):V215–24.

66. Gale AJ, Gordon SG. Update on tumor cell procoagulant factors. *Acta Haematol* 2001;106(1–2):25–32.

67. Lee AY. Cancer and thromboembolic disease: Pathogenic mechanisms. *Cancer treatment reviews* 2002;28(3):137–40.

68. Barbui T, Finazzi G, Falanga A. The impact of all-trans-retinoic acid on the coagulopathy of acute promyelocytic leukemia. *Blood* 1998;91(9):3093–102.

69. Kwaan HC, Keer HN. Fibrinolysis and cancer. *Semin Thromb Hemost* 1990;16(3):230–5.

70. Mathur VP, Dhillon JK, Kalra G. Oral health in children with leukemia. *Indian J Palliat Care* 2012;18(1):12–8.

71. Pereira J, Phan T. Management of bleeding in patients with advanced cancer. *The oncologist* 2004;9(5):561–70.

72. Chapman WC, Singla N, Genyk Y, et al. A phase 3, randomized, double-blind comparative study of the efficacy and safety of topical recombinant human thrombin and bovine thrombin in surgical hemostasis. *J Am Coll Surg* 2007;205(2):256–65.

73. Rodriguez NI, Hoots WK. Advances in hemophilia: Experimental aspects and therapy. *Hematol/Oncol Clin North Am* 2010;24(1):181–98.

74. Bhat S, Yadav SP, Anjan M, et al. Recombinant activated factor VII usage in life threatening hemorrhage: A pediatric experience. *Indian J Pediatr* 2011;78(8):961–8.

75. Heisel M, Nagib M, Madsen L, et al. Use of recombinant factor VIIa (rFVIIa) to control intraoperative bleeding in pediatric brain tumor patients. *Pediatr Blood Cancer* 2004;43(6):703–5.

76. Bilić E, Rajić L, Femenić R, et al. Recombinant activated factor VII controls chemotherapy-related hemorrhage in patients with solid intra-abdominal tumors: A report of three pediatric cases. *Acta clinica Croatica* 2009;48(2):161–6.

77. Witmer CM, Huang YS, Lynch K, et al. Off-label recombinant factor VIIa use and thrombosis in children: A multi-center cohort study. *J Pediatr* 2011;158(5):820–5.e1.

78. Creutzig U, Zimmermann M, Reinhardt D, et al. Early deaths and treatment-related mortality in children undergoing therapy for acute myeloid leukemia: Analysis of the multicenter clinical trials AML-BFM 93 and AML-BFM 98. *J Clin Oncol* 2004;22(21):4384–93.

79. Mann G, Reinhardt D, Ritter J, et al. Treatment with all-trans retinoic acid in acute promyelocytic leukemia reduces early deaths in children. *Ann Hematol* 2001;80(7):417–22.

80. Kuhle S, Massicotte P, Chan A, et al. Systemic thromboembolism in children. Data from the 1-800-NO-CLOTS Consultation Service. *Thromb Haemost* 2004;92(4):722–8.

81. Payne JH, Vora AJ. Thrombosis and acute lymphoblastic leukaemia. *Br J Haematol* 2007;138(4):430–45.

82. Bajzar L, Chan AK, Massicotte MP, et al. Thrombosis in children with malignancy. *Curr Opin Pediatr* 2006;18(1):1–9.

83. Nowak-Göttl U, Kenet G, Mitchell LG. Thrombosis in childhood acute lymphoblastic leukaemia: Epidemiology, aetiology, diagnosis, prevention and treatment. *Best Pract Res Clin Haematol* 2009;22(1):103–14.

84. Caruso V, Iacoviello L, Di Castelnuovo A, et al. Thrombotic complications in childhood acute lymphoblastic leukemia: A meta-analysis of 17 prospective studies comprising 1752 pediatric patients. *Blood* 2006;108(7):2216–22.

85. Schiavetti A, Foco M, Ingrosso A, et al. Venous thrombosis in children with solid tumors. *J Pediatr Hematol Oncol* 2008;30(2):148–52.

86. Tabori U, Beni-Adani L, Dvir R, et al. Risk of venous thromboembolism in pediatric patients with brain tumors. *Pediatr Blood Cancer* 2004;43(6):633–6.

87. Verso M, Agnelli G. Venous thromboembolism associated with long-term use of central venous catheters in cancer patients. *J Clin Oncol* 2003;21(19):3665–75.

88. Massicotte P, Julian JA, Gent M, et al. An open-label randomized controlled trial of low molecular weight heparin for the prevention of central venous line-related thrombotic complications in children: The PROTEKT trial. *Thromb Res* 2003;109(2–3):101–8.

89. Chalmers E, Ganesen V, Liesner R, et al. Guideline on the investigation, management and prevention of venous thrombosis in children. Br J Haematol 2011;154(2):196–207.

90. Mitchell L, Andrew M, Hanna K, et al. Trend to efficacy and safety using antithrombin concentrate in prevention of thrombosis in children receiving l-asparaginase for acute lymphoblastic leukemia. Results of the PAARKA study. Thromb Haemost 2003;90(2):235–44.

91. Yeh CH, Fredenburgh JC, Weitz JI. Oral direct factor Xa inhibitors. Circ Res 2012;111(8):1069–78.

92. Raffini L, Cahill AM, Hellinger J, et al. A prospective observational study of IVC filters in pediatric patients. Pediatr Blood Cancer 2008;51(4):517–20.

93. Reed RA, Teitelbaum GP, Stanley P, et al. The use of inferior vena cava filters in pediatric patients for pulmonary embolus prophylaxis. Cardiovascular and interventional radiology 1996;19(6):401–5.

94. Rossi R, Kleta R, Ehrich JH. Renal involvement in children with malignancies. Pediatr Nephrol 1999;13(2):153–62.

95. Gertz MA. Managing tumor lysis syndrome in 2010. Leuk Lymphoma 2010;51(2):179–80.

96. Wössmann W, Schrappe M, Meyer U, et al. Incidence of tumor lysis syndrome in children with advanced stage Burkitt's lymphoma/leukemia before and after introduction of prophylactic use of urate oxidase. Ann Hematol 2003;82(3):160–5.

97. Ahn YH, Kang HJ, Shin HY, et al. Tumour lysis syndrome in children: Experience of last decade. Hematol Oncol 2011;29(4):196–201.

98. Nakamura M, Oda S, Sadahiro T, et al. The role of hypercytokinemia in the pathophysiology of tumor lysis syndrome (TLS) and the treatment with continuous hemodiafiltration using a polymethylmethacrylate membrane hemofilter (PMMA-CHDF). Transfus Apher Sci 2009;40(1):41–7.

99. Shimada M, Johnson RJ, May WS Jr, et al. A novel role for uric acid in acute kidney injury associated with tumour lysis syndrome. Nephrol Dial Transplant 2009;24(10):2960–4.

100. Coiffier B, Altman A, Pui CH, et al. Guidelines for the management of pediatric and adult tumor lysis syndrome: An evidence-based review. J Clin Oncol 2008;26(16):2767–78.

101. Cairo MS, Coiffier B, Reiter A, et al. Recommendations for the evaluation of risk and prophylaxis of tumour lysis syndrome (TLS) in adults and children with malignant diseases: An expert TLS panel consensus. Br J Haematol 2010;149(4):578–86.

102. Feusner JH, Ritchey AK, Cohn SL, et al. Management of tumor lysis syndrome: Need for evidence-based guidelines. J Clin Oncol 2008;26(34):5657–8; author reply 5658–9.

103. Howard SC, Jones DP, Pui CH. The tumor lysis syndrome. N Engl J Med 2011;364(19):1844–54.

104. Pui CH, Mahmoud HH, Wiley JM, et al. Recombinant urate oxidase for the prophylaxis or treatment of hyperuricemia in patients With leukemia or lymphoma. J Clin Oncol 2001;19(3):697–704.

105. Vadhan-Raj S, Fayad LE, Fanale MA, et al. A randomized trial of a single-dose rasburicase versus five-daily doses in patients at risk for tumor lysis syndrome. Ann Oncol 2012;23(6):1640–5.

106. Jones DP, Mahmoud H, Chesney RW. Tumor lysis syndrome: Pathogenesis and management. Pediatr Nephrol 1995; 9(2):206–12.

107. Goldman SC, Holcenberg JS, Finklestein JZ, et al. A randomized comparison between rasburicase and allopurinol in children with lymphoma or leukemia at high risk for tumor lysis. Blood 2001;97(10):2998–3003.

108. Cheuk DK, Chiang AK, Chan GC, et al. Urate oxidase for the prevention and treatment of tumor lysis syndrome in children with cancer. Cochrane Database Syst Rev 2010;(6):CD006945.

109. Mahdavi H, Kuizon BD, Gales B, et al. Sevelamer hydrochloride: An effective phosphate binder in dialyzed children. Pediatr Nephrol 2003;18(12):1260–4.

110. Fleming GM, Walters S, Goldstein SL, et al. Nonrenal indications for continuous renal replacement therapy: A report from the Prospective Pediatric Continuous Renal Replacement Therapy Registry Group. Pediatr Crit Care Med 2012;13(5):e299–304.

111. Seymour JF, Gagel RF. Calcitriol: The major humoral mediator of hypercalcemia in Hodgkin's disease and non-Hodgkin's lymphomas. Blood 1993;82(5):1383–94.

112. Kerdudo C, Aerts I, Fattet S, et al. Hypercalcemia and childhood cancer: A 7-year experience. J Pediatr Hematol Oncol 2005;27(1):23–7.

113. Lehrich RW, Greenberg A. Hyponatremia and the use of vasopressin receptor antagonists in critically ill patients. J Intensive Care Med 2012;27(4):207–18.

114. Wright WL, Asbury WH, Gilmore JL, et al. Conivaptan for hyponatremia in the neurocritical care unit. Neurocrit Care, 2009;11(1):6–13.

115. Jiménez R, Casado-Flores J, Nieto M, et al. Cerebral salt wasting syndrome in children with acute central nervous system injury. Pediatr Neurol 2006;35(4):261–3.

116. Berkenbosch JW, Lentz CW, Jimenez DF, et al. Cerebral salt wasting syndrome following brain injury in three pediatric patients: Suggestions for rapid diagnosis and therapy. Pediatr Neurosurg 2002;36(2):75–9.

117. Albanese A, Hindmarsh P, Stanhope R. Management of hyponatraemia in patients with acute cerebral insults. Arch Dis Child 2001;85(3):246–51.

118. Law M. Neurological complications. Cancer Imaging 2009;9 Spec No A:S71–4.

119. Pollono D, Tomarchia S, Drut R, et al. Spinal cord compression: A review of 70 pediatric 9 patients. Pediatr Hematol Oncol 2003;20(6):457–66.

120. Samphao S, Eremin JM, Eremin O. Oncological emergencies: Clinical importance and principles of management. Eur J Cancer Care (Engl) 2010;19(6):707–13.

121. McCurdy MT, Shanholtz CB. Oncologic emergencies. Crit Care Med 2012;40(7):2212–22.

122. Patchell RA, Tibbs PA, Regine WF, et al. Direct decompressive surgical resection in the treatment of spinal cord compression caused by metastatic cancer: A randomised trial. Lancet 2005;366(9486):643–8.

123. Ryken TC, McDermott M, Robinson PD, et al. The role of steroids in the management of brain metastases: A systematic review and evidence-based clinical practice guideline. J Neurooncol 2010;96(1):103–14.

124. Kikuchi A, Maeda M, Hanada R, et al. Moyamoya syndrome following childhood acute lymphoblastic leukemia. Pediatr Blood Cancer, 2007;48(3):268–72.

125. de Laat P, Te Winkel ML, Devos AS, et al. Posterior reversible encephalopathy syndrome in childhood cancer. Ann Oncol 2011;22(2):472–8.

126. Panis B, Vlaar AM, van Well GT, et al. Posterior reversible encephalopathy syndrome in paediatric leukaemia. Eur J Paediatr Neurol 2010;4(6):539–45.

127. Morris EB, Laningham FH, Sandlund JT, et al. Posterior reversible encephalopathy syndrome in children with cancer. Pediatr Blood Cancer 2007;48(2):152–9.

128. Bojko T, Notterman DA, Greenwald BM, et al. Acute hypoxemic respiratory failure in children following bone marrow transplantation: An outcome and pathologic study. Crit Care Med 1995. 23(4):755–9.

129. Shamberger RC, Holzman RS, Griscom NT, et al. Prospective evaluation by computed tomography and pulmonary function tests of children with mediastinal masses. Surgery 1995;118(3):468–71.

130. Pullerits J, Holzman R. Anaesthesia for patients with mediastinal masses. Can J Anaesth 1989;36(6):681–8.

131. Anghelescu DL, Burgoyne LL, Liu T, et al. Clinical and diagnostic imaging findings predict anesthetic complications in children presenting with malignant mediastinal masses. Paediatr Anaesth 2007;17(11):1090–8.

132. Hack HA, Wright NB, Wynn, RF. The anaesthetic management of children with anterior mediastinal masses. Anaesthesia 2008;63(8):837–46.

133. Ricketts RR. Clinical management of anterior mediastinal tumors in children. *Semin Pediatr Surg* 2001;10(3):161–8.

134. McCrone L, Alexander S, Karsli C, et al. US-guided percutaneous needle biopsy of anterior mediastinal masses in children. *Pediatr Radiol* 2012;42(1):40–9.

135. Mahmodlou R, Mohtazeri V, Rahimi-Rad MH, et al. Mini-mediastinotomy under local anesthesia for biopsy of anterior mediastinal masses with airway compression. *Pneumologia* 2011;60(3): 143–6.

136. Borenstein SH, Gerstle T, Malkin D, et al. The effects of prebiopsy corticosteroid treatment on the diagnosis of mediastinal lymphoma. *J Pediatr Surg* 2000;35(6):973–6.

137. Ingram L, Rivera GK, Shapiro DN. Superior vena cava syndrome associated with childhood malignancy: Analysis of 24 cases. *Med Pediatr Oncol* 1990;18(6):476–81.

138. Gillet Y, Issartel B, Vanhems P, et al. [Severe staphylococcal pneumonia in children]. *Arch Pediatr* 2001;8(suppl 4):742s-6s.

139. Reichenberger F, Habicht JM, Gratwohl A, et al. Diagnosis and treatment of invasive pulmonary aspergillosis in neutropenic patients. *Eur Respir J* 2002;19(4):743–55.

140. Matt P, Bernet F, Habicht J, et al. Predicting outcome after lung resection for invasive pulmonary aspergillosis in patients with neutropenia. *Chest* 2004;126(6):1783–8.

141. Cesaro S, Toffolutti T, Messina C, et al. Safety and efficacy of caspofungin and liposomal amphotericin B, followed by voriconazole in young patients affected by refractory invasive mycosis. *Eur J Haematol* 2004;73(1):50–5.

142. Ripamonti CI, Easson AM, Gerdes H. Management of malignant bowel obstruction. *Eur J Cancer* 2008;44(8):1105–15.

143. Hobson MJ, Carney DE, Molik KA, et al. Appendicitis in childhood hematologic malignancies: Analysis and comparison with typhilitis. *J Pediatr Surg* 2005;40(1):214–9; discussion 219–20.

144. Hryhorczuk AL, Lee EY. Imaging evaluation of bowel obstruction in children: Updates in imaging techniques and review of imaging findings. *Semin Roentgenol* 2012;47(2):159–70.

145. Weber C, Zulian GB. Malignant irreversible intestinal obstruction: The powerful association of octreotide to corticosteroids, antiemetics, and analgesics. *Am J Hosp Palliat Care* 2009; 26(2):84–8.

CHAPTER 116 ■ HEMATOLOGIC EMERGENCIES

MICHAEL C. MCCRORY, KENNETH M. BRADY, CLIFFORD M. TAKEMOTO, AND R. BLAINE EASLEY

KEY POINTS

Red Blood Cell Abnormalities

❶ Hemorrhage, iatrogenic blood loss, and chronic inflammatory diseases are the most common causes of anemia; acute management of chronic causes of anemia is also often carried out in the PICU.

❷ Acute hemolysis and splenic sequestration are other causes of anemia that often require PICU admission and management.

❸ Altered O_2-carrying capacity of acquired and congenital hemoglobinopathies impacts tissue oxygen delivery.

White Blood Cell Abnormalities

❹ Nonmalignant causes of abnormal (low and high) white blood cell (WBC) counts are common in the PICU.

❺ PICU clinicians should be aware of the acquired abnormalities in WBC number and function—especially the causes related to pharmacologic therapies.

Platelet Abnormalities

❻ Thrombocytosis does not routinely require an intervention.

❼ The development of thrombocytopenia has been associated with increased morbidity, mortality, and length of stay in critically ill adults and children.

❽ Immune-mediated thrombocytopenia in children and infants requires prompt recognition and treatment to reduce bleeding risk.

❾ Commonly used PICU medication can impact platelet function and number.

Thrombotic Diseases

❿ Thrombotic disease is less common in children than adults, but has been described in the pediatric population with increasing frequency and may be associated with significant morbidity and mortality.

⓫ Multiple risk factors for thrombosis are associated with critical care (vascular catheters, parenteral nutrition, heparin administration, etc.), and predisposing disease processes (cancer, nephrotic syndrome, and congenital heart disease).

⓬ PICU physicians should be familiar with the evolving recommendations for the detection and treatment of thromboembolism in children.

The pediatric critical care clinician is constantly evaluating infants and children who experience nonmalignant "blood test" abnormalities. Often, these hematologic issues are secondary to another process, such as trauma, infection, or chronic illness. However, primary abnormalities will present in previously healthy children or may be contributing to the complexity of those with significant medical or surgical illness. The challenge is differentiating between a normal variation and a potentially life-threatening disease on routine hematologic testing. The goal of this chapter is to review the common causes and treatments for pediatric patients in the critical care unit who have quantitative and qualitative hematologic abnormalities. Many of the primary hematologic problems and oncology-related issues are addressed elsewhere in this text. We will focus on selected nonmalignant, hematologic disorders and review the pathophysiology and management of these processes when caring for a critically ill child. In most cases, the intensivist should seek collaboration with a pediatric hematologist in the management of these disorders.

A discussion of hematologic and coagulation disorders in children requires an understanding of the normal complete blood count (CBC) and clotting function. The normal pediatric ranges for red cell, white cell, platelet, and coagulation values in children are detailed, respectively, in **Tables 116.1–116.3.**

The common causes of erroneous values on routine CBC testing are identified in **Table 116.4.** These should always be considered when investigating spurious values, whether abnormally low or high.

RED BLOOD CELL ABNORMALITIES

Anemia

Anemia, or erythropenia, is the most common hematologic abnormality diagnosed and managed in the PICU. The most common anemia etiologies that require emergent evaluation and care are acute blood loss (hemorrhage), acute hemolysis, and acute splenic sequestration. With acute blood loss (whether traumatic, surgical, or gastrointestinal), the approach is uniform: identify the potential source of bleeding, develop a diagnostic and/or therapeutic plan, and maintain intravascular volume with red blood cell (RBC) transfusion and crystalloid until the plan can be implemented. In addition, chronic inflammation and frequent phlebotomy contribute to more insidious acute anemia that frequently requires transfusion

TABLE 116.1

NORMAL VALUES AND RANGES FOR RED BLOOD CELL INDICES

■ AGE	HEMOGLOBIN (g/dL)		HEMATOCRIT (%)		■ RETICULOCYTES (%) RANGE	■ MCV (fL)
	■ MEAN	■ ±2 SD	■ MEAN	■ ±2 SD		
Cord	16.8	13.7–20.1	55	45–65	3.0–7.0	110
2 wk	16.5	13.0–20.0	50	42–66	0.1–1.7	98–116
3 mo	12.0	9.5–14.5	36	31–41	0.7–2.3	*a*
6 mo–6 y	12.0	10.5–14.0	37	33–42	0.5–1.0	70–74
7–12 y	13.0	11.0–16.0	38	34–40	0.5–1.0	76–80
12–18 y						
Female	14.0	12.0–16.0	42	37–47	1.6	80–96
Male	14.5	14.0–18.0	43	36–50		80–96
Adult						
Female	14.0	12.0–16.0	42	36–47	1.6	80–96
Male	16.0	14.0–18.0	47	42–52		80–96

*a*Approximate MCV ranges in ages >1 month to ≤9 years: low MCV = 70+ (age in years), high MCV = 90 (age in years).
MCV, mean corpuscular volume; fL, femtoliter.
Adapted from Dallman PR, Siimes MA. Percentile curves for hemoglobin and red-cell volume in infancy and childhood. *J Pediatr* 1979;94(1):26–31.

TABLE 116.2

NORMAL VALUES AND RANGES FOR WHITE BLOOD CELL COUNT AND DIFFERENTIAL

■ AGE	LEUKOCYTES (WBC/mm³)		NEUTROPHILS (%)		LYMPHOCYTES (%)	EOSINOPHILS (%)	MONOCYTES (%)
	■ MEAN	■ RANGE	■ MEAN	■ RANGE	■ MEAN	■ MEAN	■ MEAN
Cord	18,000	9000–30,000	61	40–80	31	2	6
2 wk	12,000	5000–21,000	40		63	3	9
3 mo	12,000	6000–18,000	30		48	2	5
6 mo–6 y	10,000	6000–15,000	45		48	2	5
7–12 y	8000	4500–13,500	55		38	2	5
Adult	7500	5000–10,000	55	35–70	35	3	7

Relatively wide range.
WBC, white blood cell.
Adapted from Cranendonk E, van Gennip AH, Abeling NG, et al. Reference values for automated cytochemical differential count of leukocytes in children 0–16 years old: Comparison with manually obtained counts from Wright-stained smears. *J Clin Chem Clin Biochem* 1985;23(10):663–7.

TABLE 116.3

NORMAL VALUE AND RANGE FOR PLATELET COUNT AND COAGULATION PARAMETERS

■ AGE	■ PLATELETS (10³/mm³)	■ PT (s)	■ APTT (s)	■ FIBRINOGEN (g/dL)	■ BT (min)
Preterm	180–327	15.4 (14.6–16.9)	108 (80–168)	243 (150–373)	–
Birth	290	13.0 (10.1–15.9)	42.9 (31.3–54.3)	283 (167–309)	–
1 mo	252				
1–7 y	150–350	11 (10.6–11.4)	30 (24–36)	276 (170–405)	6 (2.5–10)
7–18y	150–350	11.2 (10.2–12.0)	32 (26–37)	300 (154–448)	5 (3–8)

PT, prothrombin time (extrinsic pathway); aPTT, activated partial thromboplastin time (intrinsic pathway); BT, bleeding time (clot formation).
Adapted from Andrew M, Paes B, Milner R, et al. Development of the human coagulation system in the full-term infant. *Blood* 1987;70(1):165–72; Andrew M, Paes B, Milner R, et al. Development of the human coagulation system in the healthy premature infant. *Blood* 1988;72(5):1651–7; Andrew M, Vegh P, Johnston M, Bowker J, et al. Maturation of the hemostatic system during childhood. *Blood* 1992;80(8):1998–2005.

and may not be avoidable. However, when an acutely ill child presents with anemia among other symptoms and problems, the critical care provider must work through the primary and secondary causes for the anemia, which involves evaluating the potential etiologies by considering the different mechanisms: (a) conditions of failed RBC production, (b) conditions of increased RBC destruction, and (c) conditions of abnormal RBC maturation (**Fig. 116.1**).

Anemia, regardless of etiology, results in a decreased O_2-carrying capacity and, when severe, can result in decreased O_2 delivery. Physical symptoms are extremely variable and not predictive of anemia severity (1). Common symptoms of

TABLE 116.4

COMMON SOURCES OF SPURIOUS RESULTS WITH AUTOMATED CELL COUNTERS

■ CBC PARAMETER	■ CAUSES OF INCREASE	■ CAUSES OF DECREASE
WBC	Cryoglobulin, cryofibrinogen Heparin Monoclonal proteins Nucleated red cells Platelet clumping Unlysed red cells	Clotting Smudge cells Uremia Immunosuppressants
RBC	Cryoglobulin, cryofibrinogen Giant platelets High WBC (>50,000/μL)	Autoagglutination Clotting Hemolysis (in vitro) Microcytic red cells
Hemoglobin	Carboxyhemoglobin (>10%) Cryoglobulin, cryofibrinogen Hemolysis (in vitro) Heparin High WBC (>50,000/μL) Hyperbilirubinemia Lipemia Monoclonal proteins	Clotting Sulfhemoglobin (?)
Hematocrit (automated)	Cryoglobulin, cryofibrinogen Giant platelets High WBC (>50,000/μL) Hyperglycemia (>600 mg/dL) Hyponatremia Plasma trapping	Autoagglutination Clotting Hemolysis (in vitro) Microcytic red cells Excess EDTA Hemolysis (in vitro) Hypernatremia
Mean corpuscular volume	Autoagglutination High WBC (>50,000/μL) Hyperglycemia Reduced red-cell deformability	Cryoglobulin, cryofibrinogen Giant platelets Hemolysis (in vitro) Microcytic red cells Swollen red cells
Platelets	Cryoglobulin, cryofibrinogen Hemolysis (in vitro and in vivo) Microcytic red cells Red-cell inclusions White cell fragments	Clotting Giant platelets Heparin Platelet clumping Platelet satellitosis

CBC, complete blood count; WBC, white blood cell count; RBC, red blood cell count; EDTA, ethylenediaminetetraacetic acid.
Adapted from Cornbleet J, Kessinger S. Evaluation of Coulter S-Plus three-part differential in population with a high prevalence of abnormalities. *Am J Clin Pathol* 1985;84(5):620–6.

anemia are pallor, nausea, vomiting, weakness, fatigue, irritability, tachycardia, tachypnea, and edema. Although anemia is a common reason for RBC transfusion, in the PICU other factors are often involved (2). In addition, comorbid conditions that may contribute directly to the anemic state are both acute and chronic in nature. Chronic illnesses with anemia as a feature often have adaptive pathophysiology that alters vascular perfusion and diphosphoglycerate levels, expands plasma volume, and lowers blood viscosity.

Anemia secondary to acute hemorrhage and sickle cell disease (SCD) are discussed in Chapters 28 and 119. The differential diagnoses of anemia based on mean corpuscular volume (MCV) are summarized in **Figure 116.2**. Following are some of the most commonly encountered causes for reduction in RBC number and function in children.

Iron-deficiency anemia is the most common nutritional abnormality worldwide and is the leading cause of anemia in early childhood. When iron-deficiency anemia is severe (e.g., hemoglobin [Hb] is < 4 g/dL), children can be symptomatic with cardiac and respiratory instability. Diagnosis

of iron-deficiency anemia typically has low Hb, low RBC count, low MCV, and low reticulocyte count, with elevated free erythrocyte protoporphyrin and red-cell distribution width. The ferritin is depressed and serum iron is low with an elevated total-iron-binding capacity and transferrin. The peripheral blood smear demonstrates microcytic and hypochromic erythrocytes. During the first 4–6 months of life, most full-term infants are iron sufficient owing to transplacental passage of iron during the last trimester of pregnancy. Iron deficiency occurs most frequently in children <3 years of age and results from inadequate iron intake during this period of rapid growth. Poor iron intake is often complicated by other clinical findings of poor nutrition, neglect, and/or excessive dietary intake of cow's milk. In older children and adults with iron deficiency, occult blood loss should be suspected and should prompt a gastrointestinal evaluation. Differentiating between the two most common causes of microcytic anemia (iron deficiency vs. thalassemia) can be challenging. A low ferritin is diagnostic of iron deficiency, while an elevated HbA$_2$ is specific for beta thalassemia trait. However, the ferritin is

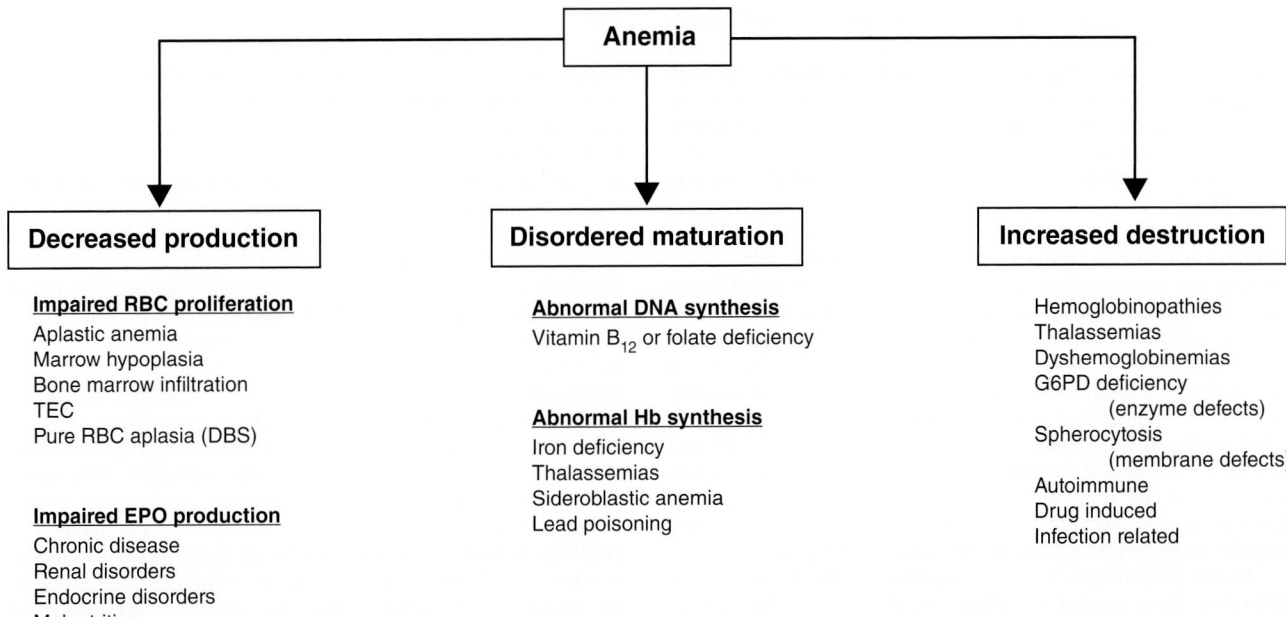

FIGURE 116.1. The etiology of anemia. TEC, transient erythropenia of childhood; RBC, red blood cell; DBS, Diamond–Blackfan syndrome; EPO, erythropoietin; Hb, hemoglobin. (Adapted from Sadowitz PD, Amanullah S, Souid AK. Hematologic emergencies in the pediatric emergency room. *Emerg Med Clin North Am* 2002;20(1): 177–98, vii.)

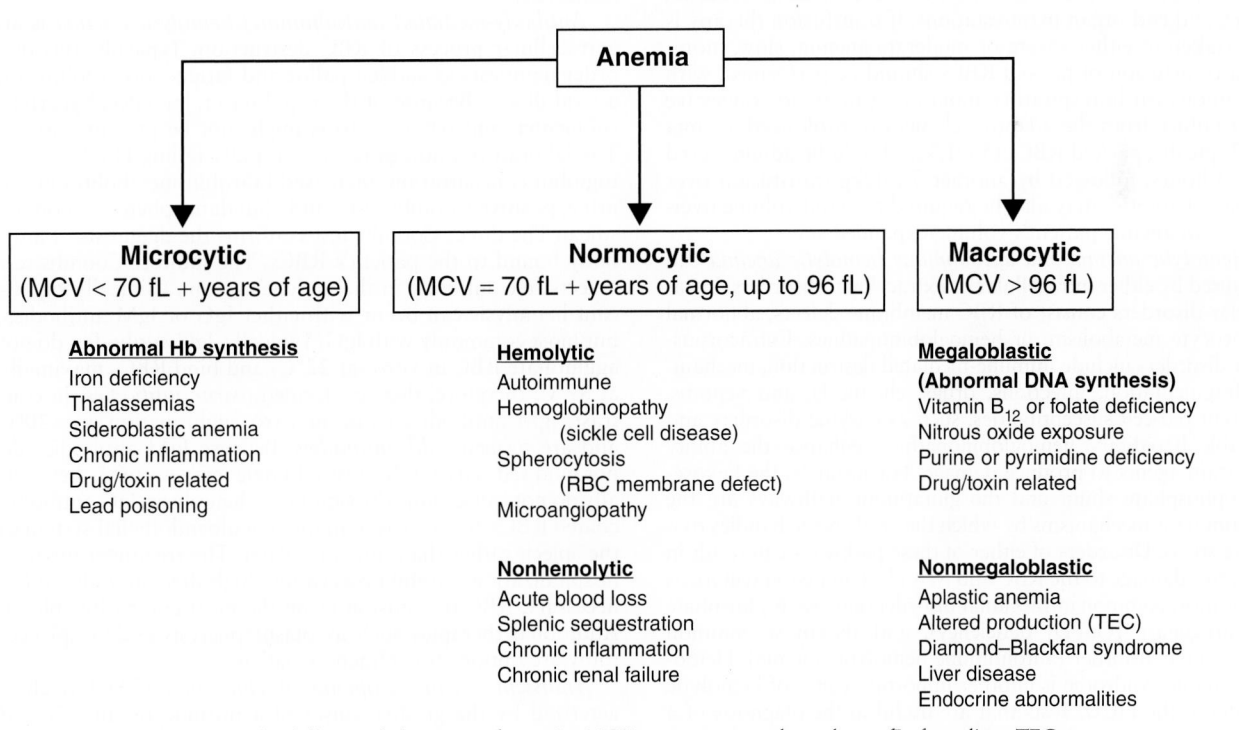

FIGURE 116.2. The differential diagnosis of anemia. MCV, mean corpuscular volume; fL, femtoliter; TEC, transient erythropenia of childhood. (Adapted from Sadowitz PD, Amanullah S, Souid AK. Hematologic emergencies in the pediatric emergency room. *Emerg Med Clin North Am* 2002;20(1):177–98, vii.)

an acute-phase reactant and may be elevated with inflammation. The Mentzer index (MCV/RBC count) can be a useful bedside tool. When applied to conditions of microcytic anemia, Mentzer index values of >13.5 suggest iron deficiency, while a value of <11.5 suggests thalassemia minor. Differential diagnosis for microcytic anemia also includes lead poisoning, chronic inflammation, copper deficiency, and thalassemia (Fig. 116.2).

In addition to low ferritin, perhaps the most conclusive evidence of iron-deficiency anemia is increasing Hb during therapeutic iron supplementation. Optimal response for *treatment* is obtained with 3–6 mg/kg/d of elemental iron. Enteral ferrous sulfate is the preferred form; parenteral administration (with iron dextran) is an option if compliance or tolerance of the oral preparation is an issue. Recommendations for *prevention* of iron-deficiency anemia include iron supplementation (1–2 mg/kg/d) for all breastfed infants after 4 months of age, use of iron-fortified formulas (containing 12 mg iron as ferrous sulfate per liter) and cereals, iron supplement (2–3 mg/kg/d) to preterm infants after the first month of life, and delaying the introduction of cow's milk until after 1 year of age.

Blood transfusion is rarely needed in the treatment of iron-deficiency anemia (3). However, studies of children with multifactorial anemia (nutritional, malaria, hemoglobinopathy, etc.) in Africa have demonstrated significant reduction in mortality with blood transfusion therapy, regardless of age. These data, along with published clinical practice, supports transfusing children with or without cardiorespiratory symptoms when Hb is ≤4 g/dL (4). In infants and children who have Hb values between 4 and 6 g/dL, treatment practices vary worldwide and the decision to transfuse should be based on symptoms, available resources, comorbid conditions (malaria, fever), and end-organ manifestations. If transfusion therapy is undertaken in either severe or moderate anemia, slow, monitored transfusion of packed RBCs should be performed, with continuous cardiorespiratory monitoring to avoid congestive heart failure from the adaptive changes of prolonged anemia (3). Typically, packed RBCs (5 mL/kg) should be administered over 4 hours, followed by another 5 mL/kg transfusion over 4 hours. Diuretics may also be required to avoid volume overload in an anemic patient's volume-expanded state.

Hemolytic anemia and autoimmune hemolytic anemia can be caused by either intracellular or extracellular disorders. Intracellular disorders consist of RBC membrane defects, abnormal erythrocyte metabolism, or hemoglobinopathies. Extracorpuscular disorders include immune-mediated destruction, mechanical fragmentation, infections, drugs, chemicals, and venoms. Inherent red-cell susceptibilities, such as enzyme disorders and unstable hereditary hemoglobinopathies, enhance the ability of certain agents to produce damage. For instance, the hexose-monophosphate shunt and the glutathione pathways are the predominant mechanisms by which the erythrocyte handles oxidative stress. Disorders of either of these pathways can result in oxidative damage to the RBC and lysis (5). Discussion will focus on the most common intracellular disorder (glucose-6-phosphate dehydrogenase [G6PD] deficiency), and the most common extracellular disorder (autoimmune hemolytic anemia). Hemolytic uremic syndrome is another important cause of hemolytic anemia in the PICU. Tests that are useful in the diagnosis of a hemolytic process include evaluation of peripheral blood smear for irregular RBCs (spherocytes or schistocytes), and additional investigation for Heinz bodies (denatured Hb), elevated reticulocyte count, positive Coombs test (direct and indirect), elevated serum aspartate aminotransferase, lactate dehydrogenase, and serum bilirubin, with lowered serum haptoglobin.

G6PD deficiency is the most common RBC-associated enzyme disorder and is genetically determined by X-linked inheritance. Children and adults prone to this disorder include Africans, Asians, and those of Mediterranean descent. The

Mediterranean variety is the classic form and is the most severe, as it results in the lowest G6PD activity. The African variety is unique because only the mature RBCs are enzyme-deficient. The incidence of G6PD deficiency in African American males is ~11% (6). The susceptibility of a patient with G6PD deficiency to drug-induced oxidative stress depends on the phenotype of the enzyme disorder and on drug metabolism and excretion. G6PD catalyzes the reduction of nicotinamide adenine dinucleotide phosphate (NADP) to NADPH in the hexose-monophosphate shunt. NADPH converts glutathione disulfide to reduced glutathione. Glutathione, in turn, inactivates hydrogen peroxide (H_2O_2) and protects protein sulfhydryl groups from oxidation. Lack of this enzyme allows for the rapid depletion of protective antioxidants and subsequent denaturation of the Hb unit. Oxidative stressors attack Hb sulfhydryl groups, releasing heme, the protein chain of which then unfolds and precipitates as insoluble aggregates (Heinz bodies). Unripened peaches, fava beans, methylene blue, naphthalene, phenazopyridine, nitroglycerin, prilocaine, benzocaine, and sulfamethoxazole are just a few of the agents that result in hemolysis in G6PD-deficient patients. Salicylates do not pose a risk for hemolysis, except in high doses. Avoidance of oxidants (e.g., sulfa drugs) and careful observation during stress (e.g., infection and surgery) are necessary. Patients with a diagnosis of G6PD deficiency who develop severe pallor or abdominal pain require immediate evaluation. Other patients who develop hemolytic symptoms of unknown etiology should have a G6PD assay performed. Identification of possible sources that trigger hemolysis and the elimination of continued exposure are crucial to the patient's recovery. RBC transfusion is sometimes necessary during episodes of severe hemolysis.

Antibody-mediated (autoimmune) hemolytic anemia is an extracellular process of RBC destruction. Typically, this disorder manifests as sudden pallor and fatigue, often following a viral illness. Because of the rapid onset, jaundice, hyperbilirubinemia, and reticulocytosis might not be present initially. The laboratory findings reveal a rapidly falling Hb, low haptoglobin concentration, increased bilirubin metabolites in the urine, positive Coombs tests, and abundant spherocytes on the smear. The direct Coombs test confirms the diagnosis of antibody bound to the patient's RBCs. The indirect Coombs test detects free antibody in the patient's serum. Clinically significant hemolysis can occur with either IgG or IgM antibodies, but most commonly with IgG. Typically, IgG antibodies do not agglutinate RBC in vitro (at 22°C) and bind RBCs maximally at 37°C; therefore, they are termed *warm antibodies*. In contrast, IgM antibodies cause in vitro agglutination at ≤20°C and are termed *cold antibodies*. Because IgM antibodies do not bind red cells avidly at physiologic temperatures, they usually do not cause clinically significant hemolysis. IgG antibody-coated RBCs are destroyed in the reticuloendothelial system of the spleen rather than intravascularly. The treatment involves hospitalization, careful observation, high-dose steroids, and, if necessary, RBC transfusion using the most compatible blood. Additional therapies such as plasmapheresis and/or splenectomy are options for refractory patients.

Transient erythrocytopenia of childhood (TEC) is characterized by the gradual onset of a normocytic anemia and reticulocytopenia caused by temporary suppression of RBC production. It usually occurs in children between 6 months and 3 years of age and is commonly preceded by a viral illness. Full recovery usually occurs in 4–6 weeks. Blood transfusions may be required if the Hb concentration is <4 g/dL and/or the patient develops symptomatic anemia. Follow-up studies are necessary until the Hb concentration and reticulocyte count recover. In ~25% of patients, the anemia is associated with mild neutropenia. TEC must be distinguished from a rare disease, termed *pure red-cell aplasia* or *Diamond–Blackfan syndrome*. Patients with Diamond–Blackfan syndrome typically have macrocytic erythrocytes (elevated MCV), dysmorphic features, and persistent anemia. Bone marrow recovery is the hallmark of TEC and rules out Diamond–Blackfan syndrome.

Bone marrow infiltration can result from malignant cells or be the result of other processes such as inherited metabolic disorders or infections (fungus, tuberculosis). Regardless of the primary process, the result is usually a normocytic anemia (normal MCV) with a low reticulocyte count. These patients can have lymphadenopathy, hepatomegaly, and splenomegaly on physical examination, although laboratory abnormalities can include reticulocytopenia, neutropenia, thrombocytopenia, and circulating immature cells (e.g., nucleated RBCs, promyelocytes, metamyelocytes, and myelocytes). Bone marrow examination is essential in this setting to establish the correct diagnosis.

Acquired aplastic anemia is defined as peripheral blood pancytopenia with bone marrow hypocellularity in the absence of underlying malignant or myeloproliferative disease (7,8). The principal pathophysiologic mechanism is thought to be immune-mediated destruction of hematopoietic stem cells by cytotoxic T lymphocytes. The incidence of acquired aplastic anemia increases with age. The incidence is low for patients <1 year of age, slowly increases to an intermediate level by the age of 50 years, and has its highest occurrence in older adults (>50 years of age). Drug-induced causes account for 50% of all cases (7,8).

Drug-induced aplastic anemia can result from either toxic effects or immune-mediated phenomena. Progenitor stem cells are most commonly affected. Common toxic agents include ionizing radiation, chemotherapeutic drugs, antibiotics (chloramphenicol), hydrocarbons (benzene), anti-inflammatory medications (phenylbutazone, indomethacin), and metals (gold) (**Table 116.5**). Other drugs with a relatively high risk for aplastic anemia are anticonvulsants (fosphenytoin, phenytoin, carbamazepine) and quinacrine (9). Phenytoin and carbamazepine result in the production of toxic arene-oxide intermediate metabolites in vivo that bind covalently to macromolecules of marrow stem cells and lymphocytes. Supportive care is typically required, with recovery of the RBC counts occurring over time once the causative agent is discontinued.

Megaloblastic anemia may be caused by decreased vitamin absorption, impaired metabolism, or both. Vitamin B_{12} and folate deficiencies selectively impair cellular DNA synthesis. Because RNA protein production is maintained, an increased ratio of cytoplasmic-to-nucleic mass is created resulting in megaloblastic RBCs (including granulocytes and megakaryocytes) (10).

Abnormal cellular maturation leads to premature cellular death. Decreased vitamin B_{12} absorption is rare in children and usually results from limited nutritional intake or intestinal malabsorptive diseases. Agents that impair enteral absorption of vitamin B_{12} include metformin, colchicine, neomycin, para-aminosalicylic acid, and slow-release potassium chloride. Causes of folate deficiency include sepsis, pregnancy, malignancy, chronic hemodialysis, and medications.

Some anticonvulsant medication can lower serum folate concentrations by limiting enteral absorption. Approximately 50% of patients on long-term phenytoin therapy have low serum folate concentrations and ~30% have red-cell macrocytosis and early megaloblastic changes in the bone marrow. Folate replacement therapy improves the anemia. Methotrexate, trimethoprim, triamterene, and pyrimethamine inhibit dihydrofolate reductase, and megaloblastic anemia, which is not folate responsive, can develop during long-term and high-dose therapy. Acute megaloblastic anemia may also be caused by prolonged or repeated nitrous oxide anesthesia (11). This gas inactivates vitamin B_{12} through oxidation. The effect on RBC formation is usually observed after a cumulative 5-hour exposure to ≥50% nitrous oxide. Case reports have also suggested that nitrous oxide exposure contributed to acute megaloblastic anemia and neuropathy in susceptible patients with comorbid illnesses such as viral infections, poor nutrition, alcoholism, malignancy, and sepsis (6).

Hemoglobinopathies

Primary hemoglobinopathy is a term that describes structural abnormalities of Hb that are often inherited. The globin genes are found in clusters on chromosomes 11 (β-globin chain) and 16 (α-globin chain). Point mutations and deletions in the genes for the Hb molecule result in decreased expression or production of functionally abnormal Hb. In normal human maturation, HbA ($\alpha2\beta2$) becomes the dominant form, taking over from the HbF ($\alpha2\gamma2$) during the first year of life. The thalassemias are the most common worldwide genetic disorder. Examples of common beta-chain mutations that result in hemoglobinopathies include S (sickle) and C, which can result in symptomatic anemia syndromes. Approximately 700 structural variants of Hb have been described with the majority of these being extremely rare and asymptomatic. More unstable Hb forms result in denaturation and formation of Heinz bodies on peripheral smear in the RBC. While most mutations of Hb are asymptomatic, some will present with mild, chronic anemia and others with increased levels of chronic and episodic hemolysis. Detection on routine Hb electrophoresis is difficult and specialized testing is often required to detect these abnormalities.

Other structurally abnormal Hbs result in increased O_2 affinity and relative tissue hypoxia, which leads to polycythemia. Erythropoietin levels are often elevated and the diagnosis is difficult. Hb abnormalities that result in decreased O_2 binding result in cyanosis. A complete review is beyond the scope of this chapter; however, *familial methemoglobinemia* (HbM) deserves comment. HbM is a rare autosomal-dominant disorder and affected individuals often present with cyanosis at birth. The structural abnormality results in stabilization of the iron heme moiety in the ferric (Fe^{3+}) form, which does not bind oxygen. The "secondary" causes of methemoglobinemia (MetHb) are more common. In the secondary causes the oxidized form of Hb can be converted back to the reduced form by enzymes in the blood (see below). Unlike the secondary causes, the diagnosis of HbM was classically made when individuals failed to respond to reduction by methylene blue therapy. HbM and the other clinically significant hemoglobinopathies are detectable by newborn screening utilizing high-performance

TABLE 116.5

COMMON AGENTS THAT CAUSE APLASTIC ANEMIA

Acetazolamide	Ibuprofen
Antineoplastic[a]	Mephenytoin
Alkylating	Oxyphenbutazone[a]
Antimetabolite	Paramethadione
Antibiotics	Phenothiazines
Benzene[a]	Phenylbutazone[a]
Captopril	Phenytoin
Carbamazepine	Propylthiouracil
Chloramphenicol[a]	Quinacrine
Chlorpheniramine	Radiation (ionizing)[a]
Colchicine[a]	Sulfonamides[a]
Gold salts[a]	

[a]Toxic mechanism.

liquid chromatography or electrophoresis (as in HbS). Chronic complications from HbM are rare. However, if hemolysis is chronic or acute, it can cause jaundice, cardiomegaly, hepatosplenomegaly, neurologic impairment, nephropathy, retinopathy, impaired growth and development, gallbladder stones, and skin ulcers. Diagnostic evaluation should include CBC and reticulocyte count, bilirubin, pulse oximetry, blood pressure, growth and development, academic performance, biliary ultrasonography, and renal and pulmonary function studies.

Secondary hemoglobinopathies result from conditions that either induce abnormal Hb production or adversely affect Hb function. Dyshemoglobinemias are conditions that produce abnormal O_2 binding of structurally normal Hb. Disorders of heme moiety oxidation occur in both genetically susceptible and unsusceptible individuals. Environmental and iatrogenic causes of MetHb, carboxyhemoglobinemia, cyanohemoglobinemia, and sulfhemoglobinemia have been reported. Both chronic and acute forms have been described, with anemia, decreased O_2 delivery, and functional hypoxia as commonly associated features. Toxic exposures, such as cyanide and carbon monoxide, resulting in abnormal Hb function are discussed in Chapter 35.

All dyshemoglobinemias result in shifting of the oxygen disassociation curve, impairment of binding of O_2 by Hb, and impairment of O_2 delivery to the tissues (**Fig. 116.3**). Diagnosis is often made with routine co-oximetry, which measures the elevated fraction of the abnormal Hb. Iatrogenic causes of dyshemoglobinemia in the PICU may result from inhaled nitric oxide therapy (MetHb) and nitroprusside infusions (cyanohemoglobinemia). If the dyshemoglobinemia is acute and potentially life-threatening (typically from a toxic exposure), treatment should involve removal of the offending cause and consideration of antidote treatment when appropriate. Exchange transfusion and hyperbaric oxygen therapy are

considerations for acute and life-threatening causes of dyshemoglobinemia with clinically impaired O_2 delivery. Outcomes from hyperbaric therapy and other treatments for acquired dyshemoglobinemias have not been clearly delineated. Treatment for toxic gas exposures is reviewed in Chapter 35.

Medications and common environmental factors that cause dyshemoglobinemia in children are listed in **Table 116.6**. A normal individual has up to 1.5% MetHb, and <1% of sulfhemoglobin (SulfHb), cyanohemoglobin (CyanoHb), and carboxyhemoglobin (COHb). MetHb and COHb are the most common acquired dyshemoglobinemias and are detectable on routine co-oximetry. Commonly encountered dyshemoglobinemias and current treatment options are listed in **Table 116.7**. Of these, MetHb has the greatest risk to result from therapeutics in the critical care environment. MetHb will cause chocolate-brown discoloration of blood, cyanosis, and functional "anemia" if present in high enough concentrations. Cyanosis becomes clinically apparent at a concentration of MetHb of 1.5 g/dL (~10% of total Hb). The degree of cyanosis, however, does not necessarily correlate with the concentration of acquired MetHb. Normally, a small amount of MetHb is continuously being formed but is reduced by enzyme systems within the RBC. The most important is the NADH-dependent MetHb-reductase system (NADH-cytochrome-b5 reductase). Infants may be at a greater risk to the toxic effects of MetHb because they have lower MetHb-reductase levels and altered oxygen–Hb dissociation properties (12). Additionally, fetal Hb is more susceptible to oxidant stresses with a more rapid conversion of MetHb.

Whether acquired or congenital, MetHb concentrations of 10%–25% may give no apparent symptoms; levels of 35%–50% result in mild symptoms, such as exertional dyspnea and headaches; and levels exceeding 70% are probably lethal. Therapy with ascorbic acid or methylthioninium chloride (methylene blue) will reduce the level of oxidized Hb, the latter

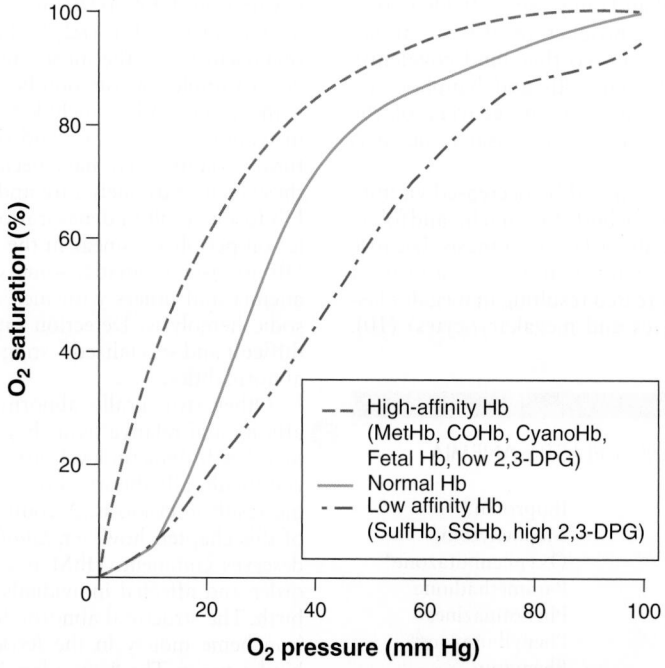

FIGURE 116.3. Dyshemoglobinemia and effect on the oxygen–hemoglobin disassociation curve. Environmental exposures impact not only the ability of O_2 to bind to hemoglobin but the ability to effectively deliver O_2 to the tissues. Shift of the O_2 dissociation curve to the left results in impaired delivery of O_2. Cyanohemoglobin (CyanoHb), Methemoglobin (MetHb), and carboxyhemoglobin (COHb) all result in a leftward shift. While Sulfhemoglobin (SulfHb) results in cyanosis, higher concentrations are tolerated because of the rightward shift of the O_2 dissociation curve. Other forms of hemoglobin and their relative effect on O_2 dissociation curve are also shown. 2,3-DPG, 2,3-diphosphoglycerate; HbF, fetal Hb; HbSS, sickle cell disease hemoglobin.

TABLE 116.6

REPORTED CAUSES OF ACQUIRED DYSHEMOGLOBINEMIAS IN CHILDREN

	MET	SULF	CYANO	CO
Drugs				
Acetanilide	+	+		
Aminophenol		+		
Alloxan	+			
Ammonium nitrate		+		
Amyl nitrite		+		
Aniline	+	+		
Arsine	+			
Arsenic			+	
Benzine derivative	+			
Benzocaine	+			
Bivalent copper	+			
Bismuth subnitrates	+	+		
Bupivacaine HCl	+			
Chlorates	+			
Chloroquine	+			
Chromates	+			
Clofazimine	+			
Dapsone	+	+		
Dimethylamine		+		
Dimethyl sulfoxide	+			
Dinitrobenzene		+		
Dinitrophenol	+			
Ethyl nitrite		+		
Ferricyanide	+			
Flutamide	+			
Hydroxylamine	+	+		
Lidocaine HCl	+			
Methylene blue		+		
Metoclopramide with *N*-acetylcysteine		+		
Naphthalene	+	+		
Nitrates	+	+		
Nitric oxide	+			
Nitrofuran	+			
Nitroglycerin	+	+		
Sodium nitroprusside	+		+	
Paraquat	+			
Phenacetin	+	+		
Phenazopyridine HCl	+	+		
Phenol	+	+		
Phenytoin	+			
Prilocaine HCl	+			
Primaquine	+			
Rifampin	+			
Rasburicase	+			
Silver nitrate	+			
Sodium valproate	+			
Sulfasalazine	+			
Sulfonamides	+			
Trinitrotoluene	+	+		
Environmental Exposures				
Combustible exhaust fumes	+		+	+
House fire	+	+	+	+
Foods and well water—almonds, sorghum, cassava (tapioca), beans, pits, bamboo shoots	+		+	
Soap enemas	+			
Laetrile enemas			+	

Met, methemoglobinemia; Sulf, sulfhemoglobinemia; Cyano, cyanohemoglobinemia; CO, carboxyhemoglobinemia.

TABLE 116.7

TREATMENT OF ACQUIRED DYSHEMOGLOBINEMIAS

■ Hb VARIANT	■ MEASUREMENT	■ TREATMENT
MetHb	Routine co-oximetry	1. Determine source 2. IV methylene blue 3. Consider SulfHb if fails to resolve with treatment
SulfHb	Hb spectrophotometry Gas chromatography	1. Determine source 2. Irreversible 3. Consider exchange transfusion if severe
CyanoHb	Hb spectrophotometry RBC cyanide level	1. Determine source 2. IV sodium nitrate or inhaled amyl nitrate with IV thiosulfate 3. IV hydroxycoalbumin 4. IV dicobalt edetate 5. Consider exchange transfusion if severe
COHb	Routine co-oximetry	1. Determine source 2. Provide F_{IO_2} 1.0 via non-rebreather/high-flow breathing mask 3. Consider HBO_2 therapy, if severe 4. Consider exchange transfusion if HBO_2 unavailable

HBO_2 and/or exchange transfusion may be useful treatments if severe impairment to O_2 delivery is present.
Note: Contacting local poison control authorities will help to identify local resources and latest treatment information.
MetHb, methemoglobin; SulfHb, sulfhemoglobin; Hb, hemoglobin; CyanoHb, cyanohemoglobin; RBC, red blood cell; COHb, carboxyhemoglobin; HBO_2, hyperbaric oxygen.

apparently by activation of the NADPH-MetHb-reductase system. Heterozygotes for this enzyme have intermediate levels of NADH-cytochrome-b5 reductase activity and normal blood levels of MetHb. They may become cyanotic because of MetHb after exposure to oxidizing chemicals or drugs in amounts that will not affect normal individuals (13).

SulfHb is a mixture of oxidized and partially denatured Hb that forms during oxidative hemolysis (14). The normal Hb concentration of SulfHb in vivo is ≤1% and, even in disease states, seldom exceeds 10%. During oxidation of Hb, sulfur (from various sources) is incorporated into the heme rings, resulting in a green hemochrome. Continued oxidation can result in the denaturation and precipitation of Hb in the RBC (Heinz bodies). SulfHb cannot transport O_2, but it can combine with carbon monoxide (CO) to form carboxysulfhemoglobin (COSulfHb). Unlike MetHb, SulfHb cannot be reduced back to Hb, and it remains in the cells until they break down, typically resulting in a mild, asymptomatic cyanosis. Blood samples are typically mauve-lavender color. SulfHb has been reported in patients treated with sulfonamides or aromatic amine medications (phenacetin, acetanilide), as well as in patients with severe constipation who develop bacteremia due to *Clostridium perfringens*, resulting in a condition called "enterogenous cyanosis." The reason some patients develop MetHb, some sulfhemoglobinemia, and others form Heinz bodies and experience hemolysis is not well understood. SulfHb cannot be detected on routine co-oximetry, as it will be incorrectly measured as MetHb. SulfHb is best detected and quantitated by more complex techniques using differential Hb spectrophotometry or gas chromatography. Sulfhemoglobinemia should be suspected in cases of environmentally acquired cyanosis that fails to respond to conventional MetHb therapy.

CyanoHb forms when Hb combines with cyanide. Cyanide is present in many forms and can be inhaled, absorbed transcutaneously, or ingested. Most pathology in humans is related to toxic exposures from ingestions and inhalation. However, low levels of cyanide exposure are present from environmental and dietary sources. Toxic effects of cyanide arise because of the greater affinity of Hb for cyanide than for O_2, which leads to decreased O_2 delivery, and because of the inhibition of mitochondrial cytochrome oxidase, which leads to decreased cellular oxidative metabolism. In children, CyanoHb formation and toxicity have resulted from holistic drugs (laetrile), ingestion of cyanogenic foods (fava beans, apricot pits), and administration of medications (nitroprusside infusions) (15). CyanoHb and O_2Hb are responsible for the "cherry red" appearance of mucous membranes in cyanide poisoning. Neither CyanoHb nor RBC cyanide levels have been found to correlate with the severity of cellular asphyxia in children; however, their abnormal elevation should raise suspicion and an explanation should be sought. Other laboratory test results (high anion gap metabolic acidosis, elevated lactate, elevated venous O_2) can support the diagnosis of cyanide toxicity but do not provide specific evidence.

Toxicity related to nitroprusside infusions deserves special comment. Sodium nitroprusside contains an iron molecule bound to five cyanide molecules and one molecule of nitric oxide. The nitric oxide molecule is rapidly released during infusion from the iron moiety, creating significant arteriolar dilatation, whereas the cyanide molecules are liberated gradually. In most patients, cyanide release from sodium nitroprusside is slow enough that the body's innate detoxification mechanisms (thiosulfate to thiocyanate formation via the rhodanese enzyme) can eliminate the poison before it interferes with cellular respiration. However, critically ill children and those receiving very rapid infusions of sodium nitroprusside may not be able to eliminate the cyanide quickly enough to avert toxic effects. In rare cases, excessive light exposure of the nitroprusside leads to a premature and excessive release of cyanide. Normal nitroprusside infusions release ~44 mg of free cyanide per 100 mg nitroprusside infused.

Treatment for cyanide toxicity has classically involved inducing MetHb (with nitrites) to attract the cyanide ion from cytochrome oxidase, as MetHb has a high affinity for cyanide and readily combines to form CyanoMetHb, a safe but non-oxygen-carrying form of Hb. Because of reduced MetHb-reductase activity in children and concern about their susceptibility to thiocyanate toxicity, alternative strategies for the treatment of cyanide toxicity, such as hydroxocobalamin (available in United States) and dicobalt edetate (available outside United States), and sulfanegen TEA (an IM antidote under investigation for mass poisonings) are being investigated (16). A more complete discussion of cyanide toxicity and treatment is reviewed in Chapter 35.

Endogenous CO produced in the degradation of heme to bilirubin normally accounts for about 0.5% COHb in the blood and is increased in hemolytic anemia. Hb has the capacity to combine with CO with an affinity 210 times greater than for O_2, which means that CO will bind with Hb even if its concentration in the air is extremely low (0.02%–0.04%). In those scenarios, COHb will build up until typical symptoms of CO poisoning appear (headache, dizziness, muscular weakness, and nausea). COHb cannot bind to O_2, and increasing concentrations of COHb shift the Hb–oxygen dissociation curve further to the left, adding to the anoxia. If a patient poisoned with CO receives pure O_2, the conversion of COHb to O_2Hb is greatly enhanced. COHb is light sensitive and has a typical "cherry red" color, and patients demonstrate high values on pulse oximetry. Healthy adults with limited exposure to CO do not experience symptoms unless the concentration of COHb reaches 20%–30%. However, the effects in children may result in severe symptoms at lower concentrations (17). COHb may be quantitated with most routine co-oximetry monitors.

Erythrocytosis

The term *polycythemia* is derived from the classical Greek, meaning "many cells in the blood" and is used synonymously with *erythrocytosis*. Increases in red-cell mass and Hb content (>2 SD of appropriate normal) occur in PICU patients from a variety of causes (dehydration, chronic hypoxia, and overtransfusion). Relative or "spurious" causes of erythrocytosis are the result of intravascular volume loss (dehydration from diarrhea or aggressive diuretic therapy). These causes of polycythemia are often the consequence of an identifiable process. The absolute red-cell mass and erythropoietin levels are within normal range and the Hb/hematocrit (Hct) will normalize rapidly following hydration therapy. However, the clinician should be vigilant for other less obvious etiologies and for the possible direct and indirect complications of elevated RBC mass, such as hyperviscosity, hypercoagulability, and thrombosis.

Polycythemia can be divided between primary and secondary causes based on the respective low or high levels of erythropoietin (**Table 116.8**). Primary causes such as *primary absolute erythrocytosis* and *polycythemia vera* are rare in children. Treatment for primary erythrocytosis varies depending on the underlying etiology. Sometimes phlebotomy, in conjunction with suppressive therapies utilizing hydroxyurea and interferon-α, has been beneficial. If other cell lines are affected, the addition of antiplatelet therapy (e.g., aspirin) may be necessary to reduce thrombotic events. Though acute intervention is often phlebotomy, maintenance treatment and evaluation should be undertaken with a pediatric hematologist.

Secondary Absolute Erythrocytosis

Secondary absolute erythrocytosis is more common in the pediatric population, but remains relatively rare in critically ill patients. An increase in erythropoietin production results

TABLE 116.8

DIFFERENTIAL DIAGNOSIS OF ERYTHROCYTOSIS IN CHILDREN

Primary Erythrocytosis (Epo Level Normal or Low)

Congenital	Epo receptor mutations (primary familial congenital erythrocytosis)
Acquired	Polycythemia vera

Secondary Erythrocytosis (Epo Level Elevated)

Congenital	Hemoglobinopathy with increased O_2 affinity 2,3-DPG deficiency
	Chuvash polycythemia (rare VHL mutation)
	Sporadic or familial erythrocytosis secondary to VHL mutation
Acquired	Physiologic elevation of Epo secondary to:
	Right-to-left shunting cardiac lesion
	Pulmonary disease
	Renal disease
	Hepatic disease
	Abnormal elevation in Epo synthesis:
	Renal: malignancy
	Liver: malignancy
	CNS: hemangioblastoma
	Endocrine tumor: pheochromocytoma
	Uterine tumor

Epo, erythropoietin; VHL, von Hippel–Lindau disease; CNS, central nervous system.

in an elevation of the RBC mass while an elevation of other cell lines is rarely associated. This condition can be seen as an appropriate response to hypoxemia (cyanotic congenital heart disease, chronic pulmonary disease, severe obstructive sleep apnea [Pickwickian syndrome], and hemoglobinopathies with increased O_2 affinity). Inappropriate overproduction of erythropoietin is also a consideration. In evaluating these children, a routine hemogram with red-cell parameters, measurement of serum erythropoietin levels, and arterial oxygen saturation is indicated (**Table 116.9**). If a specific etiology is not identified, other causes, such as renal abnormalities or tumors, should be sought. Treatment often involves management of the underlying cause, e.g., increased ventilator support, oxygen

TABLE 116.9

SEQUENTIAL EVALUATION OF ERYTHROCYTOSIS

1. CBC, including differential WBC count
2. Rule out plasma volume decrease
3. Diagnose *secondary erythrocytosis*:
   Arterial oxygen saturation (rule out hypoxia)
   Co-oximetry (rule out dyshemoglobinemias)
   Renal ultrasonography
   Abdominal/cranial CT
   Erythropoietin level (if elevated suggests secondary etiology)
4. Special studies for *primary erythrocytosis*:
   (See Table 116.8 for diagnostic evaluation for *polycythemia vera*)
   Leukocyte alkaline phosphatase
   Serum vitamin B_{12} level and binding capacity
   Red blood cell colony formation

CBC, complete blood count; WBC, white blood cell.

supplementation, and surgical repair of congenital cardiac lesions. In the setting of uncorrectable causes of erythrocytosis, chronic phlebotomy to keep the Hct <60% has been used to prevent hyperviscosity and microcirculatory congestion. Associated iron deficiency may develop with chronic phlebotomy causing a concern that iron-deficient cells will promote microvascular occlusion. Experimental data in support of this practice are limited.

Neonatal Polycythemia and Hyperviscosity

Approximately 1%–5% of all newborns in the United States are polycythemic. As the venous Hct rises above 65%, the viscosity of whole blood increases, potentially compromising blood flow to a variety of organs. Fortunately, relatively few infants who have neonatal polycythemia or hyperviscosity develop complications. Infants who have polycythemia often show increased whole-blood viscosity. Hyperviscosity refers to an increase in the internal friction of blood or the force required to achieve flow. The viscosity of whole blood is affected by numerous factors, including the red-cell mass, the plasma components, and the interaction of cellular elements with the vessel wall. Hct levels of 65% and 70% and higher are associated with an increased tendency for diminished blood flow, especially in the cerebral, hepatic, renal, and mesenteric microcirculations. Clinical symptoms may include lethargy, cyanosis, respiratory distress, jitteriness, hypotonia, feeding intolerance, hypoglycemia, and hyperbilirubinemia.

Treatment of neonatal polycythemia and hyperviscosity remains controversial. The debate lies in whether this care should involve symptomatic therapy or routine partial exchange transfusion (PET) to replace the infant's blood with a plasma substitute. Although PET is recommended for symptomatic infants, outcome data do not show clear long-term benefits. Undoubtedly, infants who have clinical manifestations should receive care aimed at alleviating their symptoms. In the polycythemic newborn, the total exchange volume for PET is generally calculated using the following formula:

$$\text{PET volume} = \text{Circulating blood volume} \times [(\text{Hct}_{current} - \text{Hct}_{desired})/\text{Hct}_{current}]$$

In this equation, the circulating blood volume refers to the infant's weight in kilograms multiplied by the expected intravascular volume in milliliter per kilogram of body weight (80–90 mL/kg in term infants; 100 mL/kg in preterm infants). In clinical practice, the exchange procedure is performed through removal and administration of 5–10 mL aliquots, depending on the infant's weight and response to treatment. Typically, arterial and venous line access is required. Careful planning and the use of order sets that delineate the calculations and steps to the PET procedure are important and can reduce the number of complications and adverse reactions (hypertransfusion) (18). Attention to thermoregulation, glucose homeostasis, and vital signs is imperative. Resuscitation equipment, medications, and intravenous dextrose and calcium should be readily available. Both during and up to 4 hours following PET, enteral feedings should be held. In addition, monitoring should be continued until the infant is asymptomatic. Typical Hct goals from PET are <55%.

Reported complications from PET include vessel perforation, vasospasm, thrombosis, infarction, electrolyte abnormalities, arrhythmias, bleeding, infection, hypothermia, hyperthermia, and necrotizing enterocolitis. Additionally, replacement fluid selection may affect the procedure's risk. For instance, the use of fresh frozen plasma is associated with increased risk of viral and bacterial infections, anaphylactic reactions, metabolic acidosis, and hypocalcemia.

WHITE BLOOD CELL ABNORMALITIES (NONMALIGNANT)

Leukopenia

Leukopenia is defined as a total white blood cell (WBC) count <4000/mm^3. However, in children, a WBC count 2 SDs below an age-appropriate mean is often used (Table 116.2). Evaluation of patients with leukopenia requires a careful history, physical examination, and review of the CBC count with differential. Often, critically ill children will have significant abnormalities in the WBC differential count that will reflect lymphopenia and/or neutropenia. The discussion here will focus on common nonmalignant etiologies of lymphopenia and neutropenia, followed by a discussion of leukocytosis.

Lymphopenia

Lymphopenia is characterized by a decline in total lymphocytes below the lower range of normal (1000/mm^3 in adults and 4500/mm^3 in infants). Lymphopenia usually has no specific symptoms and is often found in the context of evaluating another illness. Most often, it results transiently from viral, fungal, or parasitic infections. However, it can result from chronic illness or reflect more serious inherited or acquired disease. Clinicians should be cognizant that human immunodeficiency virus (HIV), with or without AIDS, is the most common globally relevant infectious disease associated with lymphopenia (Table 116.10). The majority of children with isolated lymphopenia will have spontaneous recovery and require only careful observation and follow-up while their primary disease process undergoes treatment. If the condition persists, multiple cell lines are deficient, or common transiently acquired etiologies are not found, immunoglobulin measurements, flow cytometry, and CD4 and CD8 T-lymphocyte subset quantification are warranted.

Lymphopenia has been increasingly linked with morbidity and mortality in PICU patients associated with a syndrome of critical illness stress-induced immune suppression (CRISIS). In one study of critically ill children, lymphopenia for 3–7 days was associated with increased likelihood of nosocomial infection (odds ratio 4.4), while prolonged lymphopenia of >7 days was associated with secondary infection (odds ratio 5.5) and death (odds ratio 6.8), independent of severity of illness or use of immunosuppressive medications, and despite normal neutrophil counts (19). Apoptotic lymphocytes were often found on autopsy in the spleen and lymph nodes of children with multiorgan failure in this study. In addition, hypoprolactinemia was strongly associated with lymphopenia. A randomized trial intended to prophylactically treat critically ill children at risk for CRISIS syndrome using nutritional supplementation with zinc, selenium, glutamine, and intravenous metoclopramide (a prolactin secretagogue) was terminated early due to futility when no significant improvements in mortality, infectious complications, or lymphopenia were observed (20). However, there was a reduction in infectious complications in a small subset of patients with preexisting immunocompromised status, suggesting that further study is warranted to identify specific regimens of supplementation that could benefit immune function in some populations of critically ill children.

Neutropenia

Neutropenia is defined as a decreased number of circulating neutrophils in the peripheral blood. An absolute neutrophil count <1500/mm^3 is defined as neutropenia, or <1000/mm^3

TABLE 116.10

DIFFERENTIAL DIAGNOSIS OF LYMPHOPENIA IN CHILDREN

Infections
  Mycobacterial
    Mycobacterium tuberculosis
    Atypical mycobacteria
  Viral
    Cytomegalovirus
    Epstein–Barr virus
    Hepatitis B virus
    Human immunodeficiency virus
    Human T-cell lymphotropic virus 1 and 2
    Influenza
    Respiratory syncytial virus
Malignancy
  Non-Hodgkin lymphoma
  Mycosis fungoides
  Aplastic anemia
  Myelodysplastic syndrome
Autoimmune diseases
  Sjögren syndrome
  Systemic lupus erythematosus
  Rheumatoid arthritis
Drugs
  Corticosteroids
  Chemotherapy and cytotoxic immunosuppressants
    (cyclophosphamide, azathioprine, methotrexate)
  Others (cephalosporin, IFN-α)
Primary immunodeficiency
  Common variable immunodeficiency
  Severe combined immunodeficiency
  Bare lymphocyte syndrome, type I
Miscellaneous conditions
  Severe burns
  Radiation therapy
  Malnutrition

TABLE 116.11

DIFFERENTIAL DIAGNOSIS OF NEUTROPENIA

Congenital neutropenic disorders
  Kostmann agranulocytosis—severe congenital neutropenia
  Reticular dysgenesis (absence of thymus, lymphocytes, and neutrophils)
  Cyclic neutropenia (autosomal dominant)
  Shwachman syndrome (neutropenia, pancreatic insufficiency, growth failure, and skeletal anomalies)
  Neutropenia with abnormal B or T lymphocytes (e.g., X-linked agammaglobulinemia)
Transient neonatal neutropenia
  Prematurity/sepsis/asphyxia
  Pregnancy-induced maternal hypertension
  Periventricular hemorrhage
  Congenital cytomegalovirus infection
  Maternal antineutrophil antibodies (alloimmune-isoimmune neutropenia)
Immune-mediated destruction
  Autoimmune neutropenia
Postinfectious
  Influenza A, hepatitis A and B, varicella, respiratory syncytial virus, Epstein–Barr virus, cytomegalovirus (counts recover spontaneously over several days)
Drug-induced
  Chemotherapy, anticonvulsants, cimetidine, ranitidine, phenothiazines, semisynthetic penicillins, cephalosporins, NSAIDs
Acquired/decreased production
  Aplastic anemia
  Marrow infiltration (malignant cells, inborn metabolic errors)
Sequestration
  Splenomegaly

in children under 1 year of age (21,22). The lower limit for African American patients can be 200–600/mm³ less than the figure cited for Caucasians. Neutropenia is generally classified as "mild" if circulating WBC counts are 1000–1500/mm³, "moderate" if 500–1000/mm³, and "severe" with increased risk for a life-threatening infection when the absolute neutrophil count is <500/mm³. This susceptibility varies from patient to patient, depending on the clinical state. Patients with an underlying malignancy and neutropenia tend to have more infections than do those patients with congenital defects in neutrophil production. Children with fever and neutropenia require a prompt evaluation and institution of appropriate antibiotic therapy. A careful physical examination is needed, with special attention to those areas most susceptible to bacterial infection in the neutropenic patients (oral mucosa, skin, ears, lungs, and perianal area). Digital rectal examination and rectal temperatures should never be done in a patient with neutropenia to avoid bloodstream seeding of gram-negative organisms, although visual inspection of the anus and gentle examination of the area is acceptable. In addition, phenotypic abnormalities (i.e., pancreatic insufficiency with Shwachman-Diamond Syndrome, cardiomyopathy with Barth syndrome) associated with neutropenia should be noted. Differential diagnosis of neutropenia is broad, and the clinician must be especially attentive to the many medications used commonly in the PICU setting that can cause neutropenia (**Table 116.11**). Available guidelines

for evaluation of neutropenia in children suggest a tiered approach that may include serial neutrophil counts, review of a peripheral blood smear, trial of withdrawal of a potential inciting medication, further laboratory testing (kidney and liver function tests, electrolytes, c-reactive protein, blood pH, immunoglobulin, screening for autoimmune or infectious etiologies), or bone marrow investigation (21). A brief review of nonmalignant neutropenia in children and the treatment strategies for them is summarized below.

General Management of Neutropenia Not Associated with Malignancy

Regardless of the etiology, children with neutropenia are at increased risk for infectious complications because of their weakened host defense system. The type and pattern of infections vary according to the degree of immune suppression and potential cause of the neutropenia (discussed later). Most infections result from organisms that are part of the normal flora of healthy patients (gram-negative bacteria, *Candida albicans*, varicella, and *Pneumocystis*). When the host immune system is weakened, these organisms proliferate and produce life-threatening infections. Other exogenously acquired infective agents are *Pseudomonas* or *Aspergillus* species.

The majority of infections in immunocompromised children result from bacterial pathogens. *Escherichia coli, Pseudomonas*, and *Klebsiella* species represent the most common gram-negative organisms that produce infections in immunocompromised children, whereas coagulase-negative staphylococci represent the predominant gram-positive organisms that cause infection, especially in patients who have central venous catheters (CVCs). Anaerobic infections are uncommon. *Candida* and *Aspergillus* species are the most common fungal infections. The most common viral pathogens include herpes simplex, varicella zoster, cytomegalovirus (CMV), Epstein–Barr virus (EBV), and adenovirus. *Pneumocystis* and *Toxoplasma* represent the major protozoan infections in this group of patients.

The standard approach for managing a neutropenic patient who develops fever with no discernible focus of infection has been combination therapy to cover gram-positive and gram-negative bacteria. Ceftazidime (or Piperacillin/Tazobactam) and vancomycin are often used as initial therapy (especially in patients with a CVC). Other centers choose to use double coverage for gram-negative infections with an aminoglycoside and a β-lactam antibiotic in addition to vancomycin. A carbapenem such as meropenem may also be considered, especially if extended-spectrum β-lactamase or AmpC-producing organisms are a concern (23–25). Children with pneumonia or perirectal infections sometimes require antibiotics designed to cover pathogens such as *Pneumocystis* and *Clostridium*. Each hospital can have a specific profile of documented infections and antibiotic susceptibility that must be considered in selecting appropriate therapy in these settings. Culturing strategies are also controversial. We advocate culturing from all central-line ports, as well as percutaneously ("peripheral blood culture"). Additional tests include a CBC with differential, urine analysis with Gram stain and culture, and chest x-ray. A tracheal aspirate with a culture should be considered in patients who are tracheally intubated. Consultation with a pediatric hematologist, pediatric infectious disease specialist, and/or pediatric immunology specialist is also useful to direct further diagnostic evaluation (bone marrow biopsy, peripheral blood smear evaluation, additional WBC studies) and customize antibiotic coverage, especially if the neutropenia and fevers become persistent (>3 days).

Catheter-related infections are a significant problem in this population. Although coagulase-negative staphylococcal infections are most prevalent, other organisms can be responsible (gram-negative organisms, fungi, *Bacteroides* species, and *Corynebacterium*). Most simple catheter infections can be cleared with antibiotics without catheter removal. Tunnel-site infections (infections where the catheter enters the skin) represent a more difficult problem. Despite appropriate antibiotics, many catheters must be removed to clear the infection.

In a neutropenic patient without evidence of fever or focus of infection, prophylactic antibiotic treatment and surveillance cultures have not proven to be beneficial in preventing or detecting infectious disease. However, treatment to stimulate neutrophil recovery should be considered. Recombinant human granulocyte colony-stimulating factor (rhGCSF or GCSF) stimulates the production of neutrophils from committed progenitor cells in the marrow, and is often used for chemotherapy-related neutropenia (see Chapter 115). The dose is 5–10 µg/kg administered subcutaneously. An improvement is generally noted in 10–14 days to an absolute neutrophil count above 1500/mm³. This response depends on the etiology of the neutropenia. For instance, autoimmune neutropenia may respond within 1–2 days, while aplastic anemia–associated neutropenia may not respond at all. Also, the long-term effects of GCSF treatment on children with episodic and recurrent, nonmalignant neutropenia (i.e., nonchemotherapy) are not well known. Granulocyte transfusion may be considered in select clinical contexts, as discussed elsewhere (Chapter 115).

Autoimmune Neutropenia

Autoimmune neutropenia is caused by the production of antibodies against neutrophil antigens. The physical examination and laboratory findings are normal, except for isolated neutropenia. The bone marrow usually shows normal myeloid proliferation and maturation with a paucity of mature neutrophils. This entity is usually self-limited, with return of a normal neutrophil count over several months. Appropriate antibiotics should be given to febrile, neutropenic patients, as noted previously. Treatment with rhGCSF is usually reserved for active bacterial infections or for prophylaxis against recurrent infections. With fever or infection, the duration of treatment depends on the site and nature of the infection. Alternative treatments with corticosteroids (prednisone, 1–2 mg/kg/d for 1 week) and IV immunoglobulin (IVIG) (a single dose of 1 g/kg) have been shown to hasten recovery of the absolute neutrophil count. However, the decision to use these therapeutic modalities should be individualized and made in consultation with a pediatric hematologist.

Severe Congenital Neutropenia

Severe congenital neutropenia (SCN) is manifested by severe neutropenia (usually ANC less than 200 per mm³) from birth. Omphalitis, recurrent cellulitis, and abscesses are common. SCN most commonly is secondary to heterozygous mutations in the elastase-neutrophil expressed (ELANE) gene. These patients are at risk to develop acute myelogenous leukemia (AML). Other genetic causes of SCN arise from mutations include HAX1, GFI1, G6PC, and WAS. Congenital cyclical neutropenia is characterized by chronic periodic oscillations in the neutrophil count from normal to profound neutropenia. The disease is caused by a defect in stem-cell development, more pronounced in the late myeloid precursors, with mutations in the ELANE gene present in 80%–100% of cases (26). The duration of each cycle is usually 21 days (range, 14–36 days). The nadir of neutrophil counts ranges from low normal to zero and usually lasts 3–10 days. The most common manifestations of this entity are oral ulcers, stomatitis, pharyngitis, tonsillitis, lymphadenitis, cellulitis, otitis media, and sinusitis, with clinical presentation usually occurring in early childhood (although reports exist of patients being largely asymptomatic into adulthood) (26). All infectious episodes should be treated promptly with appropriate antibiotics and rhGCSF (5 µg/kg daily subcutaneous injections until the WBC count is ≥10,000/mm³).

Leukocytosis

Abnormally high (>2 SDs) circulating levels of age-appropriate WBC counts are regarded as "leukocytosis." Leukocytosis results from either the increased release of cellular elements from the storage pool or alterations in the rate at which these cells are removed from the blood. Various causes of leukocytosis are characterized by the class/subtype of WBC that is increased and whether the elevation is chronic, acute, or persistent (sustained or life-long). Primary leukocytosis is an extremely rare event and is often hereditary. Secondary leukocytosis may occur from stress, infection, inflammation, endocrinopathies, drugs, and toxins. WBC counts >50,000/mm³ are classified as *leukemoid reactions*. A heterogeneous population of normal early and mature myeloid cells can be seen in the peripheral smear, in contrast to the immature forms typically seen in leukemia.

Leukocytosis after exercise, seizures, and pain results from demargination of mature granulocytes from the pulmonary circulation. Toxicity from drugs (iron, theophylline, cocaine) and envenomation (black widow spider, cobra) causes a sympathetic stress that elevates the WBC count by similar mechanisms. Regardless of the etiology, the resulting leukocyte elevation is the result of multiple factors, including decreased neutrophil adhesiveness, shearing from altered blood flow, and stimulation of β-adrenergic receptors located on the lymphocytes and granulocytes.

WBC subtypes from the CBC can be useful in creating a differential diagnosis and suggesting an underlying cause for the leukocytosis. Stress-induced demargination in the setting of trauma, burns, surgery, hemolysis, and hemorrhage will typically result in an elevation of multiple WBC subtypes (neutrophils, monocytes, lymphocytes). However, acute leukocytosis with a neutrophil predominance is highly suggestive of a serious bacterial infection, while elevation in WBC with a majority of eosinophils is suggestive of an allergic reaction or parasitic infection. The following discussion will focus on specific WBC subtype elevations associated with common disease processes in critically ill children.

Neutrophilia

Neutrophilia is an elevation in the age-appropriate amount of neutrophils in the serum. In adults and older children, neutrophil counts >8000/mm^3 are usually significant for neutrophilia (Table 116.2). A transient increase in the number of circulating neutrophils can result acutely from inflammation, stress, infection, or injury. Common intensive care medications found to induce neutrophilia are epinephrine, corticosteroids, and rhGCSF. Chronic inflammatory diseases (autoimmune, tuberculosis, sarcoidosis, etc.) and chronic drug exposure (corticosteroids) can result in a more chronic neutrophilia. However, both the acquired and chronic forms will return to normal with treatment of the disease or removal of the stimulating agent. Persistent or life-long neutrophilia represents a rare cause of elevated neutrophils in the serum. Evaluation of persistent neutrophilia requires a careful history, physical exam, and thorough diagnostic evaluation to exclude infectious, inflammatory, and malignant conditions. Potential nonmalignant causes of persistent neutrophilia include congenital asplenia, familial myeloproliferative disease, and genetic disorders of leukocyte adhesion.

Eosinophilia

Eosinophilia has been related to a number of acute and chronic disease processes in adults and children and is arbitrarily classified as mild (351–1500/mm^3), moderate (>1500–5000/mm^3), or severe (>5000/mm^3). The most common cause of eosinophilia worldwide is helminthic infections, and the most common cause in industrialized nations is atopic disease.

Eosinophilia occurs as a result of one or more of the following processes: differentiation of progenitor cells and proliferation of eosinophils in bone marrow, chemoattraction, and endothelial interactions directing eosinophils to a specific location, and increased activation and/or decreased destruction of eosinophils (27).

Eosinophilic disorders can be clinically divided into reactive, disease associated, clonal, or idiopathic (Table 116.12). Common reactive causes of eosinophilia are life-threatening allergic reactions (anaphylaxis and status asthmaticus), parasitic infections (acute and chronic infections such as helminths and other parasites), and drug reactions. Diagnosis of reactive eosinophilia is typically made by history (drug exposure, foreign travel, allergic symptoms) and/or physical findings (urticarial rash, worms in stool). Tests should be disease- and history-focused (with drug exposure and sudden onset of symptoms, serum should be sent for mast cell tryptase testing; if history of travel is involved, stool should be sent for ova and parasite, blood for bacterial culture, etc.). Reactive

TABLE 116.12

CAUSES OF EOSINOPHILIA

■ DIFFERENTIAL DIAGNOSIS	■ EXAMPLES
Reactive Eosinophilia	
Allergic	Rhinoconjunctivitis, asthma, eczema
Infection	Bacterial and fungal
Parasitic infection	Helminth
Drug reaction (iatrogenic)	Granulocyte colony-stimulating factor
Secondary (Disease-Associated) Eosinophilia	
Autoimmune disorders	Rheumatoid arthritis, eosinophilic fasciitis
Vasculitis	Polyarteritis nodosa, Wegner granulomatosis
Gastrointestinal disorders	Inflammatory bowel disease, eosinophilic
	Gastroenteritis, eosinophilic esophagitis, allergic colitis
Pulmonary disorders	Churg–Strauss syndrome, Loeffler syndrome
Endocrine disorders	Adrenal insufficiency (Addison disease)
Clonal Eosinophilia	
Cytogenetic	FIP1L1-PDGFRA fusion gene positive
Leukemia	Acute and chronic eosinophilic leukemia
Mastocytosis	Systemic mastocytosis with eosinophilia, myeloproliferative disorder
Idiopathic Persistent Eosinophilia (Diagnosis of Exclusion)	
Idiopathic	Idiopathic hypereosinophilia syndrome

eosinophilia is often acute and limited to the course of the accompanying disease. Secondary or disease-associated eosinophilia occurs in gastroenteritis/esophagitis, autoimmune (connective tissue diseases), paraneoplastic (Hodgkin lymphoma), immunologic (hyper-IgE syndrome), vasculitic (Churg–Strauss syndrome, Wegener granulomatosis), pulmonary (Loeffler syndrome, cystic fibrosis), and endocrine (adrenal insufficiency) disorders. Clonal etiologies for eosinophilia include lymphoproliferative and myeloproliferative variants. Eosinophilia associated with lymphoproliferative variants most commonly arise from abnormal clonal T lymphocytes. These T cells express interleukin 5 (IL-5), which drives eosinophil development. The myeloproliferative variants can be usually found to have translocations involving FIP1-L1 and platelet-derived growth factor receptor alpha genes (FIP1L1-PDGFRa). Individuals with the myeloproliferative variant usually respond to treatment with the tyrosine kinase inhibitor, imatinib. *Idiopathic hypereosinophilia syndrome* is a diagnosis of exclusion. It has been described in critically ill adults and children and is a rare but life-threatening cause of eosinophilia. This disorder results from abnormal immunologic signaling and occurs predominantly in adult males (peak incidence between 20 and 50 years of age) and is usually a progressive, fatal disease in the absence of effective medical management. Bone marrow biopsy and consultation with a pediatric hematologist and/or immunologist is necessary to evaluate all cases of nonreactive or persistent eosinophilia. In cases of secondary or disease-associated eosinophilia, specific tissue diagnosis may be required (lung, renal, or myocardial biopsy) and should be performed in conjunction with a multispecialty evaluation.

In the cases of reactive or secondary eosinophilia (which represent the majority of eosinophilia cases in children), these episodes resolve spontaneously or with treatment of the underlying condition. In other scenarios when a diagnosis cannot be found, clonal causes have been excluded, and eosinophilia persists, treatment remains controversial. Some authors advocate a brief course of antiparasitic treatment, especially when persistent eosinophilia occurs in a patient who either lives or has traveled to an endemic area for parasitic infection. Others advocate a short trial of steroids (prednisone 1 mg/kg body weight per day for 3–5 days). This approach is advocated to help define the persistent eosinophilia as steroid-responsive or -resistant. In this approach, steroid-resistant cases may be candidates for additional drug therapy (anti-IL-5 agent, mepolizumab). Regardless, patients with persistent eosinophilia should have periodic clinical evaluations, including pulmonary, cardiac (echocardiographic), and ophthalmologic examinations to detect eosinophil-mediated tissue damage. Clinicians should be aware that insidious end-organ damage can occur at any time and may not correlate with the severity of persistent eosinophilia (28).

Lymphocytosis

As lymphocytes constitute 20%–60% of the circulating WBC count, lymphocytosis is typically associated with leukocytosis. Leukemia and lymphoma are the most common cause in children. However, the most common, isolated, nonmalignant elevation is related to an acute transient increase of circulating T cells (lymphocytes) brought on by a viral infection. Many viral infections, such as EBV, CMV, and viral hepatitis, have lymphocytosis as a feature. Bacterial infections (tuberculosis, brucellosis, histoplasmosis) can result in chronic or sustained lymphocytosis. Endocrinologic abnormalities such as hyperthyroidism and adrenal insufficiency have also been associated with lymphocytosis in critically ill adults and children. Often, lymphocytosis represents a diagnostic clue to the underlying source of a patient's illness, and more persistent and chronic forms deserve a careful evaluation for lymphoproliferative disorders and malignancy.

Pertussis infection in infants under 6 months of age may result in lymphocytosis in up to 25% of cases. WBC count >100,000 is an independent predictor of mortality (29), with hyperviscosity and microvascular obstruction leading to widespread tissue necrosis and pulmonary arteriolar thromboses. Pulmonary hypertension resistant to conventional therapy and multiorgan failure may occur. In infants <3 months with severe cardiorespiratory failure from pertussis, an algorithm for leukoreduction has been proposed with tiered interventions based on degree of elevation of white blood count (>30, 50, 70, or 100,000) and clinical status (30). Double volume exchange transfusion or leukophoresis via extracorporeal support is used for leukoreduction, with a typical goal of lowering peripheral WBC count to <15,000.

Monocytosis. Monocytosis, the rarest form of leukocytosis, must be evaluated within the age-specific variation of this WBC-count subpopulation. Monocytes play a crucial role in antigen presentation and cytokine signaling. Monocytosis is most often described in children recovering from myelosuppressive chemotherapy and can precede recovery from neutropenia. However, bacterial infections and parasitic infections have been described with associated monocytosis. In addition, chronic neutropenia and postsplenectomy patients can have sustained monocytosis. Primary causes of monocytosis include juvenile myelomonocytic leukemia (JMML). These patients usually have thrombocytopenia, anemia, and splenomegaly. Prognosis is poor, but bone marrow transplant can be curative. Individuals with Noonan syndrome can also have a monocytosis with features similar to JMML; however, this usually improves without treatment.

PLATELET ABNORMALITIES

Thrombocytosis

Thrombocytosis in children, as in adults, is defined by an elevated platelet count and affects <1% of all pediatric hospital admissions. The normal platelet count ranges from 150,000 to 450,000/mm^3 in healthy neonates, infants, children, and adolescents. However, the definition of thrombocytosis varies between platelet counts of 400,000–1,000,000/mm^3 (31). To consider the characteristics and clinical implications of thrombocytosis and to compare published data, the following arbitrary classifications are often used: mild thrombocytosis, if the platelet count is 500,000–700,000/mm^3; moderate thrombocytosis, if the platelet count is between 700,000 and 900,000/mm^3; severe thrombocytosis, if the platelet count is >900,000/mm^3–1,000,000/mm^3; and extreme thrombocytosis, if the platelet count is >1,000,000/mm^3 (31).

Essential (or Primary) Thrombocytosis

Essential (or primary) thrombocytosis is extremely rare in children. This disorder is a form of myeloproliferative disease resulting from either monoclonal/polyclonal expansion of megakaryocytes or abnormalities in thrombopoietin. Acquired and familial forms of essential thrombocytosis have been reported, with the majority of the genetic and chronic etiologies affecting adults. Typical features of essential thrombocytosis are outlined in **Table 116.13**.

Reactive (or Secondary) Thrombocytosis

Reactive (or secondary) thrombocytosis (RT) causes are the most common cause of thrombocytosis. Current reports suggest an estimated incidence of RT in 6%–15% of hospitalized children. The most common associations are inflammation or iron deficiency. Many children diagnosed with RT in the hospital have viral or bacterial respiratory illness (**Table 116.13**). However, RT has been reported following gastroenteritis, urinary tract infection, autoimmune disorders, surgery, trauma, and several pharmacologic interventions. The following agents have been associated with RT in children: epinephrine, corticosteroids, vinca alkaloids, penicillamine, imipenem, and meropenem. Complications from RT are rare, but risk factors for thromboembolic disease in children are young age (neonate/infant), CVC, cardiac malformations, and septicemia (32). Treatment should focus on diagnosis and management of the underlying disease process. Prophylactic treatment with antiplatelet drugs (e.g., aspirin) is not indicated due to the low risk of thromboembolic complications in asymptomatic children with RT. In those children who become symptomatic or have evidence of thrombosis, consultation with a hematologist and consideration for patient-specific platelet inhibition and/or reduction therapy may be considered, although their benefit has not been proven. Denton et al. performed a retrospective study to evaluate the incidence of extreme thrombocytosis and the

TABLE 116.13

ESSENTIAL AND REACTIVE THROMBOCYTOSIS IN CHILDREN

■ CRITERIA	■ ESSENTIAL THROMBOCYTOSIS	■ REACTIVE THROMBOCYTOSIS
Age-dependent occurrence	>11 years[a] or adult	Mostly <2 years[a]
Incidence per year	1 per 1 million children	>600 per 1 million children
Duration of thrombocytosis	Months, years, or permanent	Days, weeks, or months, temporary
Splenomegaly	Often	Rare
Fever	No	Often
Bleeding disorders and thrombosis	Often in monoclonal ET, rare in familial thrombocythemia	Extremely rare
Frequent laboratory findings	Prolonged bleeding time, increased PT and PTT in 20%; increased prevalence of anti-phospholipid antibodies and proinflammatory cytokines	Increased vWF, fibrinogen, C-reactive protein if RT is caused by infection
Platelet count	Mostly >1,000,000/mm^3	Typically <800,000/mm^3
Platelet morphology	Large or small, dysmorphic	Large, but normal morphology
Platelet function	Abnormal	Normal
Bone marrow	Increased megakaryocyte number with abnormal morphology	Increased megakaryocyte number with normal morphology
Pathogenic mechanisms	Clonal defect in hematopoietic or megakaryopoietic progenitors, decreased c-mpl expression, and/or hyperreactivity to Tpo. In some familial forms: mutations in the Tpo or c-mpl gene locus	Increased Tpo production or released megakaryopoietic growth factors, in particular IL-6

[a]This number is relevant only for differentiating primary thrombocytosis in childhood.
Tpo, thrombopoietin; vWF, von Willebrand factor; PT, partial prothrombin time; PTT, partial thromboplastin time.
Adapted from Dror Y, Blanchette VS. Essential thrombocythaemia in children. *Br J Haematol* 1999;107(4):691–8.

related etiologies in a single PICU. During a 3-year period, they identified 31 patients with extreme RT with an incidence of 1.1% in their ICU. Contributing etiologies in those infants and children with extreme RT were confirmed bacterial or viral illness in 74%, respiratory infection (without identified organism) in 45%, inflammation/tissue damage from trauma or surgery in 32%, platelet consumption with bleeding or thrombus in 26%, and neoplasm in 3%. Those children with extreme RT were less than 2 years of age (median 9 months), which was similar to those without RT hospitalized in their ICU. Though duration of ICU stay was longer compared to the non-RT admissions (16 days vs. 3 days), this was most likely related to the severity of illness in the affected children in this case series (33).

Thrombocytopenia

Thrombocytopenia (defined as a platelet count <150,000/mm^3) affects 15%–58% of PICU patients and is one of the most common laboratory abnormalities that an intensive care provider must consider. For most critically ill children, relatively low platelet counts are usually well tolerated. Patients will not typically develop bleeding symptoms until platelet counts are <50,000/mm^3. Spontaneous bleeding rarely occurs until the platelet count is <20,000/mm^3. Further, laboratory studies of hemostasis have demonstrated that platelet counts of ~7000/mm^3 are necessary for microvascular integrity. However, with comorbid medical illness, trauma, or surgery, maintaining higher platelet counts is often clinically indicated to reduce bleeding risk and assist in promoting patient stability. We typically transfuse platelets to maintain platelet counts >50,000/mm^3 in the presence of an associated risk of bleeding. In surgical patients, especially with post-bypass bleeding, we will attempt to keep the count >100,000/mm^3. The important medical history of children with low platelet counts includes the family history and past

medical history of bleeding/bruising problems. Common clinical symptoms associated with thrombocytopenia are petechiae, mucosal hemorrhage, excessive bruising, epistaxis, menorrhagia, and gastrointestinal hemorrhage. "Pseudo-thrombocytopenia" can result from platelet clumping in EDTA anticoagulation tubes. Repeating the test in a citrate collection tube and/or reviewing the smear for evidence of platelet clumping should clarify if artificial thrombocytopenia is the cause. True thrombocytopenia can be characterized by inherited or acquired causes of thrombocytopenia. Primary (or inherited) thrombocytopenia (**Table 116.14**) is often associated with genetic disorders and results in abnormal platelet number and function. These disorders are significantly less common than acquired platelet disorders in children. Recent clinical studies of critically ill adults and children have found thrombocytopenia (regardless of etiology) to be an independent risk factor for increased morbidity and mortality. Although the etiology of this association is unknown, increased understanding of the inter-relationship of platelets and inflammation suggests a reason for its role as a potential "biomarker" for risk prognosis in critically ill patients. More important than the absolute platelet count, the decline in the platelet count of >30% over time is more indicative of a poor prognosis in both adults and children. Olmez et al. (34) in a retrospective cohort study examined the relationship of absolute platelet counts and the decrease of platelet counts over time on ICU length of stay and mortality found that both a >30% decrease in the platelet count (58.3% of admissions) and the presence of thrombocytopenia (25% of admissions) were significantly associated with increased mortality and longer length of stay (see **Fig. 116.4**).

Secondary (or Acquired) Thrombocytopenia

Secondary (or acquired) thrombocytopenia is the most common platelet-related issue in the PICU population. Low platelet counts are typically acute in onset and are best described

TABLE 116.14

PREVALENT INHERITED THROMBOCYTOPENIAS

■ SYNDROME	■ INHERITANCE	■ GENE MUTATION (CHROMOSOME)	■ ASSOCIATED FINDINGS
Bernard–Soulier syndrome	AR	GP1BA, GP1BB (17pter-p12)	None
TAR syndrome	AR	Unknown	Shortened or absent radii, bilaterally
DiGeorge syndrome/Velo-cardiofacial association/ CATCH 22	AD	GP1BB (22q11)	Cardiac, facial, and parathyroid anomalies and immune dysfunction
Paris-Trousseau syndrome/ Jacobsen syndrome	AD	FLI1 (11q23)	Mental retardation, cardiac and facial anomalies
May–Hegglin anomaly	AD	MYH9 (22q11)	Neutrophil inclusions (Döhle bodies), nephritis, cataracts, and sensorineural hearing loss
Familial platelet disorder	AD	AML1 (21q22.2)	Myelodysplasia, AML
Gray platelet syndrome	AD	Unknown	None
Wiskott–Aldrich syndrome	X-linked	WAS (Xp11.23)	Immunodeficiency, eczema, lymphoma

Differentiation of Platelet-Related Syndromes by Platelet Size:

■ SMALL PLATELETS (MPV <7 fL)	■ NORMAL PLATELETS (MPV 7–11 fL)	■ LARGE/GIANT PLATELETS (MPV > 11 fL)
Wiskott–Aldrich syndrome	Familial platelet disorder	Bernard–Soulier syndrome
X-linked thrombocytopenia	Congenital amegakaryocytic thrombocytopenia	DiGeorge syndrome
	TAR syndrome	GATA 1 mutation
		Paris-Trousseau thrombocytopenia

AR, autosomal recessive; AD, autosomal dominant; TAR, thrombocytopenia and absent radii; AML, acute myeloid leukemia; MPV, mean platelet volume.
Adapted from Drachman JG. Inherited thrombocytopenia: When a low platelet count does not mean ITP. *Blood* 2004;103(2):390–8.

by their underlying mechanism: (a) impaired production, (b) increased destruction, (c) dilution, or (d) sequestration. The differential diagnosis of acquired thrombocytopenia is summarized in **Figure 116.5**, and the most common entities are discussed below. Disseminated intravascular coagulation is discussed in detail in the chapter on Coagulation Issues (Chapter 118).

Medication (Iatrogenic) Thrombocytopenia

Medication-induced thrombocytopenia may be due to impairment of platelet production due to myelosuppression or increased destruction from drug-dependent antibodies. Drug-induced thrombocytopenia occurs most often in adults and children who have a routine illness (viral or bacterial) and

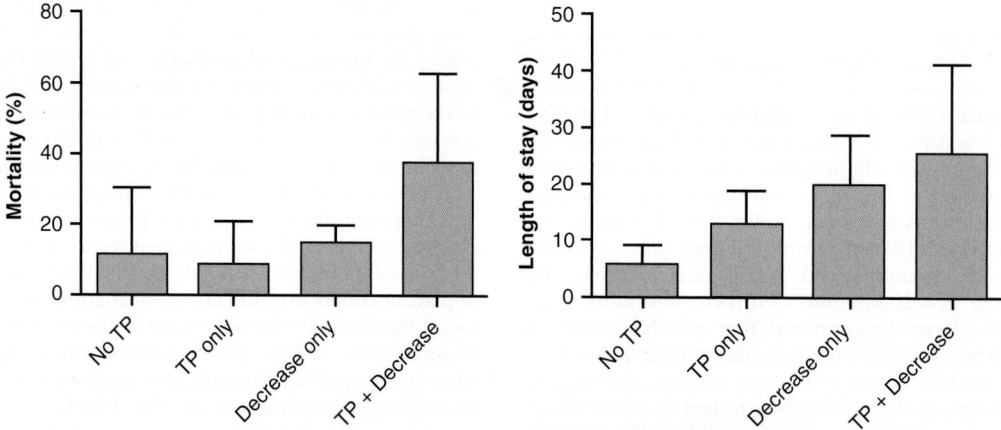

FIGURE 116.4. Association of thrombocytopenia and declining platelets with mortality and ICU length of stay. Studies of pediatric patients hospitalized with critical illness have demonstrated an increased association of thrombocytopenia (TP) and >30% decrease in platelet count with increased mortality and increased PICU length of stay (LOS). This study is similar to that found in adult ICU patients. (Adapted from Olmez I, Zafar M, Shahid M, et al. Analysis of significant decrease in platelet count and thrombocytopenia, graded according to NCI-CTC, as prognostic risk markers for mortality and morbidity. *J Pediatr Hematol/Oncol* 2011;33(8):585–8.)

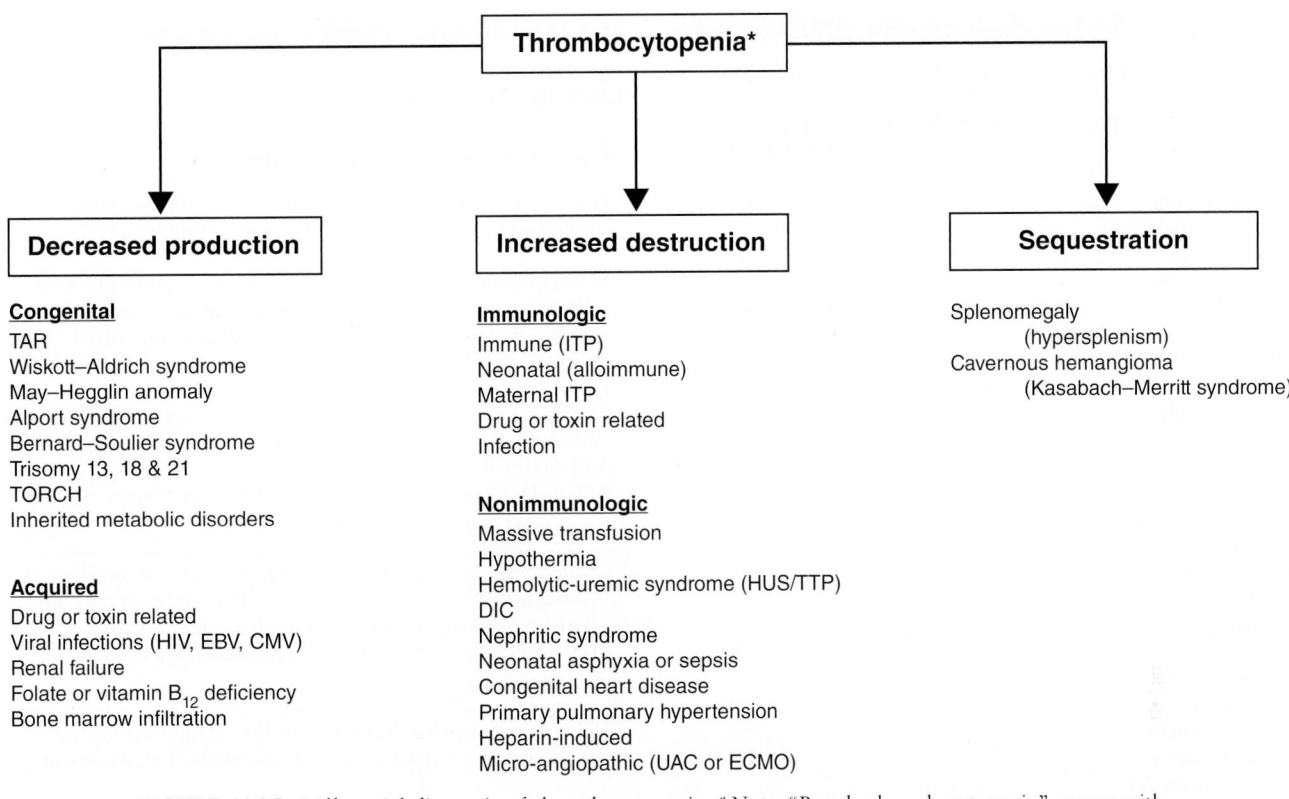

FIGURE 116.5. Differential diagnosis of thrombocytopenia. *Note: "Pseudo-thrombocytopenia" occurs with platelet clumping, either spontaneously or from collection-tube preservatives (EDTA or citrate). TAR, thrombocytopenia with absent radius; TORCH, toxoplasmosis, other infections, rubella, cytomegalovirus infection, and herpes simplex; HIV, human immunodeficiency virus; EBV, Epstein–Barr virus; CMV, cytomegalovirus; ITP, immune thrombocytopenic purpura; DIC, disseminated intravascular coagulopathy; UAC, umbilical artery catheter; ECMO, extracorporeal membrane oxygenation. (Adapted from Sadowitz PD, Amanullah S, Souid AK. Hematologic emergencies in the pediatric emergency room. *Emerg Med Clin North Am* 2002;20(1):177–98.)

are undergoing pharmacologic treatment for their illness. Often, the occurrence of the decreased platelet count is an incidental finding, diagnosed on a follow-up CBC to evaluate the WBC. On rare occasions, bleeding symptoms will result in an evaluation that demonstrates decreased platelet count. Often, these bleeding symptoms are related to accompanying abnormalities in platelet function (thrombocytopathy or platelet dysfunction), which may or may not be medication related. Although medications can cause other hematologic abnormalities (agranulocytosis, aplastic anemia, hemolytic anemia), thrombocytopenia is the most common drug-induced hematologic abnormality. A comprehensive list of agents that cause thrombocytopenia is provided in **Table 116.15.** When thrombocytopenia is detected in the course of providing critical care, investigating possible pharmacologic causes is important. In healthy subjects who develop a drug-induced decrease in platelet counts, discontinuation of the medication is often curative. However, in critically ill adults and children, identifying the source of drug-induced thrombocytopenia is often confounded by treatment with multiple agents that could decrease platelet counts, as well as the underlying illness. In these patients, changing their treatments to alternative drugs with no, or less, platelet effects may be beneficial, but is not always possible.

Common ICU medications, such as cardiovascular drugs, antibiotics, and sedative/anesthetic agents, have been implicated in drug-induced thrombocytopenia. In addition, many of the neuroleptics/antiepileptics and mood stabilizers (carbamazepine, valproate, and phenytoin), and the antidepressants (lithium, fluoxetine, sertraline, paroxetine, and citalopram),

can cause thrombocytopenia. More prevalent in adults and increasingly utilized in pediatric patients, serotonin reuptake inhibitors have been associated with bleeding diathesis with and without thrombocytopenia (35). The commonly used medications that result in abnormalities of platelet number are listed in **Table 116.15.**

Heparin is a very common, very severe cause of antibody-dependent, drug-induced immune thrombocytopenia (ITP) in critically ill infants and children. Although the incidence is higher in adults, *heparin-induced thrombocytopenia* (HIT) is an important phenomenon to recognize. The diagnosis and treatment of HIT are discussed in a separate section of this chapter. Other medications such as quinidine result in a drug-induced, antibody-mediated thrombocytopenia. With quinidine or heparin, the drug acts as a hapten to stimulate antibody formation to the platelet antigen/hapten complexes. The drug-dependent antibody binds the platelet surface, resulting in subsequent platelet activation or clearance, and a falling platelet count (36). Treatment for this type of immune-related process should involve stopping the offending agent as soon as thrombocytopenia develops, even if it is mild. Thromboembolic complications of HIT are discussed later in this chapter.

Immune (Idiopathic) Thrombocytopenic Purpura

Immune thrombocytopenia (previously called "idiopathic" thrombocytopenic purpura or ITP) is caused by the production of antibodies against platelet antigens. These antibody-coated platelets are trapped and destroyed in the reticuloendothelial

TABLE 116.15

COMMON AGENTS THAT CAUSE THROMBOCYTOPENIA

■ INCREASED DESTRUCTION OR USAGE	■ DECREASED PRODUCTION
Amitriptyline	Alkylating agents
Amphotericin B	Anthracyclines
Amrinone	Antimetabolite agents
Asparaginase	Cytarabine
Benzene	Epipodophyllotoxins
Bleomycin	Ethanol
Carbamazepine	Procarbazine
Chloroquine	Radiation, ionizing
Chlorpheniramine	Thiazides
Cimetidine	Vinblastine
Cocaine (i.e., DIC)	
Colchicine	
Crotalidae envenomation (i.e., DIC)	
Cyclosporine	
Furosemide	
Ganciclovir	
Glyburide	
Gold salts	
Heparin	
Indomethacin	
Meprobamate	
Mesoridazine	
Methyldopa	
Penicillin	
Pentamidine	
Quinidine	
Quinine	
Rifampin	
Sulfonamides	

DIC, disseminated intravascular coagulation.
Adapted from Drachman JG. Inherited thrombocytopenia: When a low platelet count does not mean ITP. *Blood* 2004;103(2):390–8.

TABLE 116.16

TREATMENT OF ACUTE CHILDHOOD IMMUNE THROMBOCYTOPENIA PURPURA

Corticosteroids—one of the following:

Prednisone, 1–5 mg/kg/d in 3 divided doses for 1–2 weeks, followed by tapering off and discontinuation by day 21
OR
Methylprednisolone, 30 mg/kg (maximum, 1 g/dose) IV over 30 min every 24 h for 3 doses. Then return to maintenance steroid therapy. This option is reserved for hospitalized patients with severe bleeding

IgG Concentrates

IVIG 1 g/kg/d for 2 consecutive days
Anti-D (for Rh-positive patients)
IV anti-D, single dose of 40–80 µg/kg IV over 5 min

Combination Therapy

Corticosteroids in combination with either IgG or anti-D (using the previously cited dosages). This option is used for patients with significant mucocutaneous bleeding in a hospital setting in consultation with a pediatric hematologist

Platelet Transfusion

Not routinely needed. Indicated for life-threatening hemorrhage and in conjunction with above medical management

system (primarily the spleen), resulting in thrombocytopenia. The typical history is sudden onset of petechiae and bruising in a previously healthy child with a preceding viral illness. Fever, bone or joint pain, weight loss, pallor, fatigue, weakness, and other complaints are typically lacking. Physical examination is usually normal except for mucocutaneous bleeding. Physical findings of lymphadenopathy and/or hepatosplenomegaly are atypical of ITP and should prompt investigation for a marrow infiltrative process. In the diagnostic evaluation of ITP, the CBC and blood smear are normal except for isolated thrombocytopenia. Additional laboratory tests for antinuclear antibody, anti-DNA antibody, immunoglobulins, and HIV may be considered based on history and symptoms of autoimmune disease or immunodeficiency. The need for bone marrow examination to confirm the diagnosis is controversial, though many specialists consider performing this test before initiating prednisone therapy to more definitively exclude leukemia. Typically with ITP, the bone marrow shows a normal cellularity with a normal or increased number of megakaryocytes. In many children with ITP, the thrombocytopenia resolves within 6 weeks to 6 months. Although the incidence of life-threatening hemorrhages is reported at <1%, serious hemorrhages such as intracranial, pulmonary, upper-airway, and gastrointestinal bleedings have been reported in ~3% of children with acute ITP (37,38). Children with excessive skin and mucosal bleeding or with platelet counts of <10,000/mm³ may be at higher risk for life-threatening bleeding. A careful

evaluation and appropriate treatment are essential in the child with newly diagnosed ITP.

Treatment for ITP remains controversial. Current reported treatment options include corticosteroids, IVIG, and anti-Rh (D) immunoglobulin (**Table 116.16**). Corticosteroids (e.g., prednisone 2 mg/kg/d) increase vascular stability, enhance platelet production, decrease antibody production, and impair clearance of antibody-coated platelets, thus reducing the risk of bleeding before a rise in the platelet count occurs. IVIG (1 g/kg/d infused over 3 hours for 2 consecutive days) binds to receptors in the reticuloendothelial system, preventing platelet destruction. Typically, platelet counts will increase in 1–2 days following IVIG therapy. IV anti-D (a single dose of 50 µg/kg [250 IU/kg] over 5–15 minutes) is effective in Rh-positive patients. The anti-D-bound RBCs saturate the reticuloendothelial system, preventing platelet destruction. Side effects associated with IV anti-D include chills and a slight drop in Hb concentration by 1–2 g/dL, secondary to hemolysis. Serious side effects such as renal failure and DIC have been reported. Prophylactic treatment with acetaminophen, diphenhydramine, and prednisone can reduce these symptoms. Emergency splenectomy and platelet transfusion are reserved for severe and refractory ITP with life-threatening bleeding. Aspirin and nonsteroidal anti-inflammatory drugs (NSAIDs) should be avoided in all thrombocytopenic patients (39).

Hypersplenism

Conditions that lead to enlargement of the spleen have been associated with reduction of circulating platelet counts. The spleen serves a combination of immunologic, reservoir, and filtering functions. The spleen can empty its reservoir to create a transient thrombocytosis; however, the filtering and immunologic functions of the spleen underlie its association with thrombocytopenia. Conditions of hypersplenism (accessory spleens and enlargement of the spleen) have demonstrated thrombocytopenia secondary to sequestration or destruction of circulating cells. These events usually occur secondary to an active disease process that may also contribute to anemia, leukopenia, and thrombocytopenia. The differential diagnosis for a chronically enlarged spleen includes portal hypertension, storage cell disease, lymphoproliferative disease and hematologic malignancy, and hemolytic anemia. The thrombocytopenia that occurs with hypersplenism is usually moderate to mild in severity and bleeding problems are rare. Management is directed to the underlying etiology. Long-term implications for future spleen trauma and bleeding risk remain unknown.

Postoperative (Dilutional) Thrombocytopenia

Postoperative (dilutional) thrombocytopenia occurs whenever massive blood loss and volume replacement take place. Timing of treatment is controversial; a study of adults with trauma demonstrates no prophylactic benefit to early platelet transfusion. However, in children, the need for treatment depends on the starting platelet count and the clinical scenario. It was demonstrated that patients with low starting platelet ($\sim$100,000/mm^3) counts developed dilutional thrombocytopenia and bleeding after blood loss of only 1–2 blood volumes (40). In this scenario, pediatric patients often require platelet treatment at $\leq$50,000/mm^3. In addition, certain surgeries associated with higher bleeding complications (e.g., neurosurgery, cardiac surgery, or organ transplantation) may require a higher threshold for treatment (see Chapter 42).

Neonatal Thrombocytopenia

Neonatal thrombocytopenia occurs in infants between birth and 2 months of age and represents a unique group with special considerations. The incidence of thrombocytopenia is high in this group; it occurs in $\sim$2%–3% of healthy term infants and increases to 20%–30% of sick neonates (both premature and term). In general, the thrombocytopenia seen in a sick infant is likely related to the primary disease process and will resolve as the primary process improves. Most of these infants develop platelet counts of <50,000 at >48 hours of age. Causes include abnormalities of decreased production, increased consumption, and immune-mediated destruction. Common neonatal conditions that impact platelet production are viral infections (TORCH), medication (ranitidine, milrinone), hepatic disease, maternal factors (pregnancy-induced hypertension and gestational diabetes), leukemia, and intrauterine growth retardation. Causes of neonatal thrombocytopenia due to consumptive processes are thrombosis (catheter-related), infections (disseminated intravascular coagulopathy), vascular malformations (hemangiomas with Kasabach-Merritt syndrome), and hypoxia/asphyxia. The etiology of thrombocytopenia in a number of other conditions may be secondary to both decreased production and consumption and include many infectious processes (viral, bacterial, fungal) or stress (necrotizing enterocolitis, surgery). Finally, thrombocytopenia that occurs less than 24 hours after birth often represents immune-mediated destruction or inherited platelet abnormality. Immune-mediated processes are related to IgG or complement attachment to the platelets and their subsequent elimination. Maternal transfer of anti-platelet antibodies can cause ITP and neonatal alloimmune thrombocytopenia (NAIT) in the infant. Other conditions that cause thrombocytopenia at birth include congenital infections (TORCH—toxoplasmosis, other infections, rubella, CMV infection, and herpes simplex) and congenital thrombocytopenia due to inherited genetic mutations. Regardless of the early or late timing of neonatal thrombocytopenia,

management should focus on the diagnosis and treatment of the underlying disease with increased vigilance for hemorrhagic complications.

As the etiology can be multifactorial, the diagnostic approach to neonatal thrombocytopenia should be broad enough to safely detect common treatable causes and identify complications, such as bleeding and intraventricular hemorrhage. A careful family history that evaluates for bleeding problems and/or platelet abnormalities should be obtained. Review of the maternal peripheral blood smear and platelet count can be informative, as infectious, inherited, and immune-mediated causes may result in a low maternal platelet count with abnormal platelet morphology. Physical exam should include a careful neurologic examination and search for evidence of bruising or abnormal bleeding. The size of the liver and spleen should be noted and examined carefully. In the critically ill neonate, daily platelet counts may be appropriate with more frequent assessment if bleeding symptoms or complications are present. When platelet counts are <30,000/mm^3, a head ultrasound to evaluate and monitor for intraventricular hemorrhage is common practice. For persistent and prolonged cases of neonatal thrombocytopenia, additional imaging with MRI and CT, and even angiography of the head, chest, and abdomen may be necessary to evaluate for hemangiomas and/or vascular malformations. Rarely, bone marrow aspiration will be considered in patients with persistent, severe, and otherwise unexplained thrombocytopenia.

Of the various neonatal causes, neonatal NAIT represents a unique and potentially treatable cause of thrombocytopenia. The incidence is thought to be 1 per 1000 live births, but may be more common. In this disease, maternal antibodies are attacking and destroying the neonatal platelets. This process often begins in utero and may necessitate fetal therapy in future pregnancies. Over the 2–3 days following birth, intracranial bleeding and severe thrombocytopenia (<20,000/mm^3) may occur; however, intracranial bleeding can occur in utero. For these neonates, transfusion of matched (antigen-negative) platelets is the preferred treatment. In the emergent setting, random donor platelets are often used. Prompt recognition and consultation with a pediatric hematologist (to facilitate the availability of appropriate platelet products for transfusion therapy, plan potential secondary medical therapies, and assist in the diagnostic evaluation, which may impact the counseling and management of future pregnancies) is crucial. In addition, newborns with NAIT should undergo urgent neuroimaging studies secondary to the increased intracranial bleeding risk. If platelets cannot be maintained at >20,000/mm^3 with platelet transfusion, consideration should be given to IVIG (0.4–1 g/kg/d for 1–5 days) with or without methylprednisone (1 mg/kg IV every 8 hours) therapy until the platelet counts improve (>30–50,000/mm^3). If an intracranial bleed is detected, random platelet transfusions should be performed emergently until antigen-negative platelets are available. The duration of treatment (whether requiring platelet transfusions or only medical therapy) can be brief (only 2–3 days) or longer depending on the time it takes for the platelet counts to normalize. Once the platelet count normalizes, the infant has no future risk of recurrence, although future siblings (pregnancies) remain at an increased risk.

Thrombocytopathy (Platelet Dysfunction)

Functional abnormalities of platelets can be inherited and/or acquired. Thrombocytopathy implies a normal number of platelets with impairment in their biochemical functionality. These disorders may result in either increased bleeding or hypercoagulability, depending on the relative impairment to platelet function. Inherited forms, such as gray platelet

TABLE 116.17

DRUGS THAT INHIBIT PLATELET FUNCTION (THROMBOCYTOPATHY)

Nonsteroidal anti-inflammatory drugs
   Aspirin, ibuprofen, indomethacin, naproxen, ketorolac, and others
Antibiotics
   Penicillins, cephalosporins, nitrofurantoin
Cardiovascular drugs
   Amrinone/milrinone, dipyridamole, diltiazem, propranolol, nitroprusside, nifedipine, nitroglycerin, procainamide, verapamil
Anticoagulants, fibrinolytics, and antifibrinolytics
   Aprotinin, ε-aminocaproic acid, heparin, protamine, alteplase
Anesthetics/sedatives/hypnotics
   Propofol, ketamine, benzocaine, cocaine, lidocaine, procaine, tetracaine, halothane, heroin
Anticonvulsants/psychotropic drugs
   Valproate, amitriptyline, haloperidol, imipramine, nortriptyline, chlorpromazine
Chemotherapy
   Carmustine, daunorubicin, vincristine, L-asparaginase
Antihistamines
   Chlorpheniramine, diphenhydramine, ranitidine, cimetidine
Herbal/alternative medicines
   Garlic, ginseng, gingko biloba
Other drugs/toxins
   Guaifenesin, dextran, pseudoephedrine, hetastarch, mustard gas

syndrome (reduction or absence of platelet α granules) and Glanzmann thrombasthenia (absent or defective platelet fibrinogen receptor), are rare causes of functional platelet abnormalities. Often, with these genetic disorders, other associated clinical (immunologic dysfunction) and dysmorphic features are present. Histologic evaluation of the blood smear often demonstrates unusual platelet morphology and number (**Table 116.14**).

In the ICU, the most common problems with platelet function are the acquired forms (**Table 116.17**). Causes of acquired functional platelet disorders include uremia, autoimmune disorders, infections, liver disease, nutritional deficiencies, and drugs. Salicylates, NSAIDs, and antibiotics are common medications that affect platelet function. Aspirin, with its irreversible inhibition of cyclooxygenase (COX), is perhaps the most well-known cause of platelet dysfunction. Salicylates prevent thromboxane A_2 synthesis by acetylating COX, thus inhibiting platelet aggregation. This process is irreversible with recovery occurring in 7–10 days following the production and release of new platelets. Salicylates can precipitate hemorrhage in patients with preexisting hemostatic defects such as von Willebrand disease, hemophilia A, warfarin ingestion, or uremia. NSAIDs also inhibit platelet COX. However, in contrast to salicylates, their effects are reversible and generally last <4–8 hours depending on the half-life of the medication (41).

High-dose penicillin and cephalosporin antibiotics can prolong the bleeding time by reducing platelet adhesion and activation (42). The serum concentration, drug potency, and lipid solubility of the specific antibiotic will determine the degree of platelet impairment. This impairment is maximal after 1–3 days of drug administration and may last for several days after therapy. The penicillins may impair the interaction of von Willebrand factor (vWF) with the platelet membrane. Patients with coexisting hemostatic defects such as thrombocytopenia and vitamin K deficiency are at risk for bleeding with use of these antibiotics.

Other agents that affect platelet function include heparin, organic nitrates such as nitroprusside and nitroglycerin, fish oils, and herbal medications (garlic). Heparin's effects on platelets are multiple, prolonging the bleeding time by inhibiting thrombin, a potent platelet agonist (36). Organic nitrates are converted to nitric oxide, which activates guanylate cyclase, resulting in increased intracellular cyclic guanosine monophosphate, which inhibits platelet aggregation. Fish oils that contain eicosapentaenoic acid (ω-3 fatty acid) prolong bleeding time through competitive inhibition of COX by reducing the formation of thromboxane A_2. Black tree fungus, garlic, gingko balboa, ginseng, and cumin have similar antiplatelet effects and have been associated with increased perioperative bleeding (35).

Common medical conditions associated with impaired platelet function are renal failure, hepatic failure, and autoimmune disorders. Medical conditions can create thrombocytopathies through a variety of mechanisms, including reduced degranulation, impaired signaling, and decreased surface expression of binding receptors. Treatment for most functional platelet abnormalities is often discontinuation of the problematic agent and transfusion of functional platelets. However, in other conditions (uremia or hepatic dysfunction), newly transfused platelets may develop similar dysfunction. In this setting, treatment with desmopressin may be beneficial, as desmopressin increases vWF levels and promotes platelet aggregation. Conjugated estrogens also improve platelet function with these conditions.

Quantitative tests to assess platelet function are available, such as whole-blood platelet aggregation testing, and the PFA-100, but may not be widely available at all centers. Although bleeding time can be used to assess platelet function, it is often not practical in the pediatric population and has not been demonstrated to predict surgical bleeding. As qualitative and quantitative functional platelet tests are more widely available, they may help guide future treatment strategies to assess multifactorial platelet dysfunction in critically ill children with bleeding symptoms.

THROMBOTIC DISEASES

Pathophysiology

Normal hemostasis involves not only the production of factors to stop bleeding, but also mechanisms to prevent pathologic clot formation. Through these processes, the coagulation system attempts to confine thrombin generation to the site of an injury and avoid thrombotic events (**Fig. 116.6**). The classic description of Virchow's triad states that thrombi form due to (a) changes in the vessel wall, (b) changes in blood flow, and (c) changes in the blood composition. Although inherited disorders of coagulation that lead to excessive bleeding have been recognized and studied for centuries, inherited defects that predispose to thrombosis have only recently been identified. As in other physiologic and biochemical processes throughout the body, the coagulation system has both natural agonists and inhibitors.

Endothelial-dependent inhibition of coagulation includes protein C (and its cofactor, protein S) and tissue factor pathway inhibitor (TFPI). The interactions of the coagulation cascade with its checks and balances are illustrated by the antithrombotic factor, protein C, which is directly activated by thrombin. Although protein C is a vitamin K-dependent serine protease produced by the liver, its conversion to activated

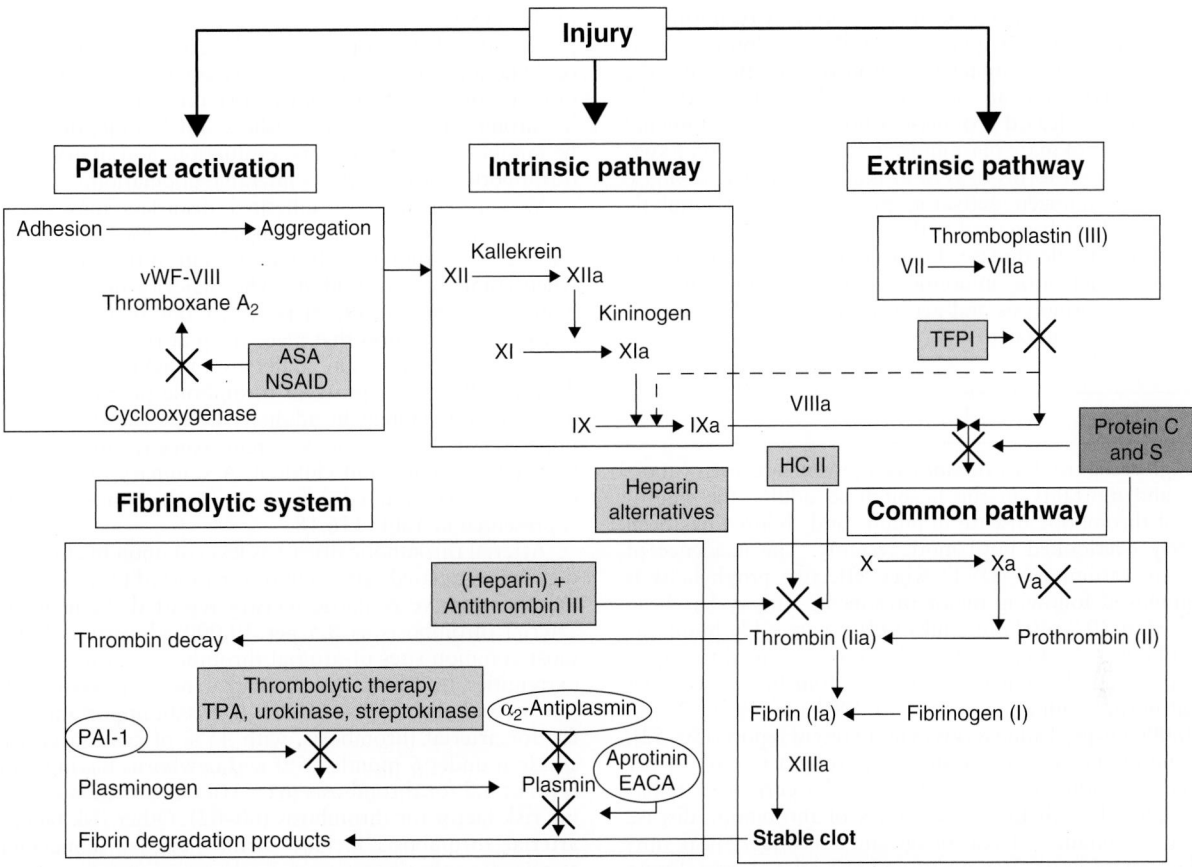

FIGURE 116.6. Coagulation cascade. "X" indicates sites of inhibition/inactivation. Anticoagulants are indicated in *gray*. Proteins C and S, antithrombin III, HC II, and TFPI are considered "natural anticoagulants" (inhibitors). Antifibrinolytics are indicated in *circles*. PAI-1 and α_2-antiplasmin are "natural antifibrinolytics." vWF, von Willebrand factor; ASA, aspirin; NSAID, nonsteroidal anti-inflammatory drug; TFPI, tissue factor pathway inhibitor; HC II, heparin cofactor II; PAI-1, plasminogen activator inhibitor; tPA, tissue plasminogen activator; EACA, ε-aminocaproic acid.

protein C (APC) is dependent on an interaction that occurs on the endothelial surface. Thrombin formed either on the surface of platelets or at the site of tissue injury binds to the endothelium via thrombomodulin. The proteolytic site of thrombin cleaves a peptide from the protein C molecule, converting it to APC. APC acts by the enzymatic cleavage of factors Va and VIIIa. This alteration of the factor V molecule prevents its participation with activated factor Xa as part of the prothrombinase complex and the subsequent conversion of factor II (prothrombin) to IIa (thrombin). The cleavage of factor VIIIa prevents its participation with activated factor IXa as part of the tenase (X-ase) complex, which converts factor X to activated factor Xa. The function of APC in the inactivation of factors Va and VIIIa is facilitated by protein S, the cofactor of protein C, first identified in 1984. A more recently described component of the antithrombotic pathway is TFPI, which is produced from, and primarily bound to, the vascular endothelium. TFPI is the major inhibitor of the tissue factor pathway that regulates the conversion of factor VII to VIIa after tissue factor has been exposed at the site of tissue injury. The critical importance of TFPI is illustrated by the fact that homozygous deficiency leads to in utero demise in animal models while a human deficiency state has not been reported.

Hepatic-dependent aspects of the anticoagulant system include antithrombin III (AT-III, often now simply called "antithrombin"), heparin cofactor (HC) II, and plasminogen. AT-III is a hepatic serine protease inhibitor, is not vitamin

K dependent, and has been estimated to account for more than 50% of the endogenous plasma anticoagulant activity. It irreversibly inhibits the function of several activated coagulation factors, including IIa, IXa, Xa, XIa, and XIIa. The activity of AT-III is greatly enhanced by the exogenous administration of therapeutic heparin concentrations and by endogenous glycosaminoglycans, such as heparin sulfate, which are found on the endothelial surface (43). AT-III has an effective plasma half-life of 3–5 days. Deficiency states may be acquired or congenital. HC II is a hepatic-synthesized plasma protein that inhibits thrombin and may be stimulated by dermatan sulfate as well as heparin sulfate. HC II is estimated to account for 30% of plasma anticoagulant activity, and deficiency states are very rare.

The final major component of the anticoagulant system is plasminogen and its regulators. Plasminogen is a glycoprotein, produced by the liver, with a plasma half-life of 2 days. Plasminogen is converted to the proteolytic enzyme plasmin by cleavage of a single peptide bond. The major function of plasmin occurs after the formation of the thrombus, as it acts to dissolve fibrin clots and restore patency to the vascular system. Plasmin also inhibits the ongoing coagulation process by degrading fibrinogen as well as cleaving activated factors Va and VIIIa. The two physiologic activators of plasminogen are tissue plasminogen activator (tPA) and urinary-type plasminogen activator, also known as *urokinase*. Thrombin generated from the coagulation cascade stimulates the release of tPA from endothelial cells. tPA forms a complex with fibrin and converts plasminogen to plasmin. Kallikrein, a protein component of the plasma contact activation system, stimulates the release of urokinase from the kidney. In the normal state, the majority of the released urokinase is bound to the endothelial tissue via the urokinase plasminogen activator receptor. Exogenously produced forms of tPA, urokinase, and streptokinase (another plasminogen activator, produced by α-hemolytic streptococci) have been used as therapeutic agents in the treatment of thrombotic disease. Endogenously produced factors plasminogen activator inhibitor 1 and α_2-antiplasmin are inhibitors of fibrinolysis and act to keep tPA, urokinase, and plasmin activity regulated.

Epidemiology

Although recognized for decades as a prevalent cause of morbidity and mortality in the hospitalized adults, the significance of thrombotic disease in infants and children has been relatively overlooked until more recently. The incidence of deep vein thrombosis (DVT) when effective prophylaxis is not employed following major orthopedic surgery has been estimated at 20%–40% in adults (44) versus <1% in infants and children (45). Reported incidence of venous thrombosis in hospitalized children has increased from 0.3–8 cases per 10,000 hospital admissions prior to 2003 (46–49) to 22–58 per 10,000 hospital admissions in more recent reports (50–52), with one recent multicenter study reporting a rate of 74 per 10,000 PICU admissions (53). A bimodal occurrence rate has been reported, with the highest rates of thrombotic disease occurring in infants <1 year of age and a secondary peak during the teenage years. Venous thrombosis-related mortality in children has been reported as 2.2% in one study (54). PICU patients with venous thrombosis tend to have greater severity of illness, longer PICU stays, longer duration of mechanical ventilation, and a nearly fourfold increase in mortality compared with those without thrombosis (53,55,56). It is unclear whether heightened awareness and detection, or increased incidence accounts for the observed increase in reported rates

of thrombosis. It has been hypothesized that increased complexity of pediatric inpatients and increased survival of previously fatal conditions such as malignancies, congenital cardiac diseases, or prematurity may contribute to observed increases in thrombosis (50,57). Regardless, PICU practitioners must be familiar with risk factors, evaluation, and management of thrombotic disease in this vulnerable population.

Various acquired or inherited disorders may place the pediatric patient at risk for thrombotic diseases. The epidemiology of thrombotic disease is quite different in children when compared with adults. The majority of children (estimated 70%–95%) (49,58) possesses one or more comorbid or associated features that place them at risk, whereas ~50% of venous thromboses in adults are thought to be idiopathic. Additionally, the majority of thrombotic problems affect the lower venous system in adults, whereas the distribution of upper versus lower venous system issues is more evenly distributed in infants and children. A summary of some of the commonly encountered risk factors for thrombosis in children is presented in Table 116.18.

Arterial thrombotic disease is less common in children, but may be associated with significant morbidity and mortality. One prospective pediatric registry reported the incidence of arterial thrombosis as 8.5 per 10,000 admissions (59). The most common sites of arterial thrombosis in this study were extremities (47% of cases), central nervous system (CNS) (34%), and intracardiac (19%). Age is an important risk factor for arterial thrombosis, with 45% of cases occurring in children under 6 months (59) and newborns having an odds ratio of 6.5 for thrombosis (61). Arterial catheters are a leading risk factor for thrombosis (60–62). Other risk factors for arterial thrombosis include cardiac disease (congenital or acquired), infection, vascular abnormalities, autoimmune/inflammatory disease, malignancy, HIT, and thrombophilia (especially AT deficiency, protein C deficiency, elevated lipoprotein a, and antiphospholipid antibody syndrome [APS]) (59,63,64). Sequelae of arterial thrombosis vary significantly by location and degree of ischemia, but in one study overall mortality was 6.8%, with 49% of survivors having functional deficits 2 years later (59).

TABLE 116.18

RISK FACTORS FOR HYPERCOAGULABILITY IN CHILDREN

■ PHYSIOLOGIC ALTERATIONS	■ CLINICAL CONDITIONS
Blood flow	
Hypovolemia	Shock, dehydration
Hyperviscosity	Erythrocytosis, leukocytosis, thrombocytosis, sickle cell disease
Mechanical stasis	Immobilization after surgery
Foreign body	CVC, cardiac prosthesis
Vasculature	
Anatomic defects	Congenital heart disease, arteriovenous malformation
Endothelial disorders	Vasculitis, inflammation, trauma
Blood coagulation	
Increased and/or abnormal	Malignancy, dysfibrinogenemias, procoagulants, inflammatory bowel disease
Decreased anticoagulants	AT-III deficiency, protein S or C deficiency, APC resistance (factor V Leiden)
Decreased fibrinolysis	Hereditary defects
Increased platelet-vessel reactivity	Atherosclerotic disease, inherited dyslipidemia, diabetes mellitus
Mixed or idiopathic, recurrent idiopathic DVT	HIT, HUS, TTP, oral contraceptives, nephrotic

CVC, central venous catheter; APC, activated protein C; HIT, heparin-induced thrombocytopenia; HUS, hemolytic uremic syndrome; TTP, thrombotic thrombocytopenic purpura; DVT, deep vein thrombosis.
Adapted from Hathaway WE. Congenital and acquired defects in coagulation: Diagnosis and treatment. *Mead Johnson Symp Perinat Dev Med* 1986;28:45–54.

Acquired Diseases

The majority of pediatric patients with thrombosis have at least one clinical risk factor, with many critically ill children having multiple risk factors. In a recent report in a tertiary PICU setting, 87.8% of patients with venous thrombosis had a central venous line and 69% were under 1 year of age (53). Another recent study of >35 children's hospitals across the United States from 2001 to 2007 demonstrated that 63% of children with venous thrombosis had at least one chronic medical condition, with oncologic disorders being the comorbid condition most strongly associated with recurrent thrombosis (50). Common risk factors of particular relevance to PICU patients include vascular catheters, oncologic disease, nephrotic syndrome, autoimmune disease, HIT, hemoglobinopathies, and congenital heart disease.

Central Venous Catheters. CVCs represent the single most commonly identified acquired risk factor for thrombotic events in infants and children. Many of these children may have other acquired (e.g., oncologic) or inherited diseases that act as additional comorbid features. CVCs are thrombogenic because their foreign, non-endothelial surface acts as a nidus for activation of the coagulation cascade. Two variants of thrombi have been identified in association with CVCs: (a) a fibrin sleeve that forms around the catheter, is not adherent to the wall, and does not occlude the vessel, and (b) a thrombus around the tip of the catheter that adheres to the wall and obstructs the vessel. Although symptomatic occlusion of the CVC is common and easily treated by a thrombolytic agent, catheter-related thrombi can result in significant morbidity and even mortality; problems include pulmonary emboli, superior vena cava syndrome, chylothorax, and postthrombotic syndrome with pain, discoloration, swelling, and ulceration of the affected extremity. Although postthrombotic syndrome may appear early in the course of catheter use, it has also been reported years following catheter removal.

The incidence of venous thrombosis in the presence of a CVC has been reported as 13%–18% in various studies in the PICU population (56,65,66) or up to 34% in children with a CVC and an oncologic disorder (67). In one study evaluating PICU patients with CVC but no symptoms of venous thrombosis, the incidence of thrombosis was still 15.8%; however, these asymptomatic clots were not associated with adverse outcomes (68). In another study in a PICU population, the presence of a CVC conferred an odds ratio of 6.9 for venous thrombotic events (53). The presence of a CVC may contribute to development of thrombosis more often in infants (present in 77%–94% of cases) as compared with children (present in 26%–58% of cases) (46,49,69). The femoral location for a CVC has consistently been associated with a higher risk of thrombosis compared to other locations in children (56,65,66), with the subclavian location being associated with increased risk in some studies (65–67), and jugular location typically reported as among the lowest risk (56,65–67). Percutaneous insertion has been associated with a higher risk of thrombosis than tunneled lines (56,67). Although the contribution of catheter size to risk of thrombosis is unclear, multi-lumen CVCs have been reported to have a higher risk (56). In summary, CVCs have been identified as the most prevalent contributing factor to development of venous thrombosis in critically ill children. Careful weighing of risks and benefits should accompany the decision to place a CVC in an individual patient, especially if other risk factors such as young age, oncologic diagnosis, or long-term parenteral nutrition use (46) are present, and the CVC should be removed as soon as clinically prudent.

Oncologic Diseases. Patients with oncologic diseases may be predisposed to thrombotic events because of endothelial damage induced by the malignancy itself, effects of chemotherapy on synthesis of proteins involved in hemostasis, hyperleukocytosis and hyperviscosity, and/or inflammation related to infection or the oncologic process. One example of such problems is the prothrombotic state produced by the effects of the chemotherapeutic agent, L-asparaginase, which depresses AT-III levels. Additionally, children with cancer frequently require placement of a CVC and/or the administration of total parenteral nutrition. A prospective study that evaluated by echocardiography the incidence of right atrial thrombi associated with CVCs in children with malignancies reported an incidence of 8.8% (13 of 156 patients) (70). Of the 13 thrombi, 6 were adherent to the right atrial wall. A higher incidence of thrombosis was noted when the catheter tip was in the right atrium instead of the superior vena cava. In two of these patients, clinical symptoms of obstruction to venous return necessitated operative intervention with the use of cardiopulmonary bypass (CPB). Thromboses may occur in association with a CVC or at distal sites, including the venous drainage of the CNS, and may occur with any malignancy although are most commonly described with acute lymphocytic leukemia. The incidence of thrombosis in children with cancer and CVCs is ~1%–16% when clinical signs and symptoms are used, but increases to 30%–37% with routine ultrasound evaluation (71).

Nephrotic Syndrome. Thrombotic disease occurs in nephrotic syndrome with an incidence ranging from 3% to 30%, with adolescents at the highest risk (72). The most common thrombotic events included renal vein thrombosis, DVT, and pulmonary embolism (PE). One study reported 24% of nephrotic syndrome-associated thromboses in children to be life or limb-threatening (72). Thus, PE must be considered quickly when suspicious symptomatology develops in patients with nephrotic syndrome. Coagulation studies performed in children with nephrotic syndrome demonstrate an inverse correlation between serum albumin levels versus fibrinogen and α_2-macroglobulin concentrations and a direct correlation between serum albumin levels and AT-III levels. Hematologic abnormalities in nephrotic syndrome include increased plasma concentrations of fibrinogen, V, and VIII; increased vWF; low AT-III levels; increased platelet aggregation; and depressed fibrinolysis. These effects relate not only to renal losses of protein, but also to nonspecific increases in hepatic protein synthesis in an attempt to maintain oncotic homeostasis (73). The severity of the changes follows the severity of the nephrotic syndrome and serum albumin concentrations.

Autoimmune Disorders and Antiphospholipid Antibody Syndrome. Systemic lupus erythematosus (SLE) and other autoimmune disorders may predispose patients to thromboembolic diseases, with increased risk associated with the APS. Antiphospholipid antibodies (aPLs) are immunoglobulins (IgG, IgA, IgM) directed against negatively charged phospholipids. The prothrombotic effects of these autoantibodies may relate to their effects on phospholipids located on the vascular endothelium and/or the surface of platelets. The first work regarding aPLs began in the early 1950s with the discovery of altered in vitro coagulation function in patients with SLE. Because of its effects with the prolongation of laboratory measurements of coagulation function, it was originally termed "the lupus anticoagulant." Further laboratory investigation demonstrated that the inhibitor was an immunoglobulin directed against the prothrombin activator complex. Although it prolonged the in vitro measurement of clotting function, it was subsequently shown to have the opposite effect in vivo, with a predisposition to thrombotic complications (74).

Testing for lupus anticoagulant often starts with testing for prolongation of the activated partial thromboplastin time (aPTT) and/or dilute Russell's viper venom time. A mixing test can be conducted to identify whether any prolongation of the clotting time is a result of coagulation factor deficiency or inhibition from the lupus anticoagulant. If the prolongation is due to a factor deficiency, it will be corrected by the addition of normal plasma, while no effect is seen with the presence of the lupus anticoagulant. However, the addition of phospholipid or platelets would be expected to show some correction. Additional laboratory testing for aPLs typically includes assessment for IgM and IgG directed against the phospholipid cardiolipin (first isolated from bovine heart extracts in the 1940s), as well as the cofactor plasma protein β_2-glycoprotein 1 (75). When positive, testing for aPLs should be repeated at least 12 weeks later to determine whether the antibodies are transient. Anticardiolipin antibodies have been shown to be relatively common in the pediatric population on chronic hemodialysis and may predispose these patients to thrombotic complications, including fistula thrombosis (76).

The constellation of clinical findings, including recurrent arterial or venous thrombosis, recurrent fetal losses, thrombocytopenia, and aPLs, became known as the APS. Patients without an associated collagen vascular disorder were said to have primary APS, while patients with SLE or other collagen vascular disorders were said to have secondary APS. Children with APS are at high risk for both venous and arterial thrombosis, with median age of first thrombotic event reported at 5 years (64). An international registry of pediatric APS found the majority (60%) of thromboses to be venous. However, younger patients with primary APS had a greater risk of arterial involvement (77), with the most common arterial site being the cerebral vasculature.

Treatment of APS remains controversial, with limited prospective data on which to base clinical decisions. As with any of the prothrombotic states reviewed in this chapter, reduction or control of associated risk factors may be helpful. Other treatment strategies aimed at reducing the antiphospholipid antibody levels include the administration of corticosteroids, immunosuppressive agents, IVIG, and plasmapheresis. Perioperative measures may include the use of heparin prophylaxis, maintenance of adequate hydration, early ambulation, and sequential compression devices for the lower extremities.

Heparin-induced Thrombocytopenia. Following the introduction in the 1930s of heparin for clinical use, reports of thrombocytopenia associated with heparin therapy began to appear, although its clinical implications were not appreciated. In 1958, the first reports of the potential morbidity and mortality from HIT appeared in the literature, with Weisman and Tobin reporting arterial thrombosis in 10 patients who received heparin. HIT occurs when antibodies are formed against an antigenic complex composed of heparin and platelet factor 4. Platelet factor 4, a protein stored in the α-granule, binds heparin. The platelet factor 4/heparin complex binds heparin antibodies and activates platelets, leading to their clearance from the circulation (78). The incidence of HIT among infants and children exposed to heparin in different clinical scenarios varies widely in the literature. However, overall incidence is likely lower than adults, occurring in approximately 1%–2% of pediatric patients with heparin exposure as compared with up to 5% of adults (79).

HIT can develop after exposure to unfractionated heparin or LMWH, although the incidence is highest with unfractionated heparin. Exposure to heparin can occur from a bolus or an infusion, through the IV or subcutaneous route. Rarely, it may occur after exposure from flush solutions for invasive monitors, or on heparin-impregnated catheters. In most cases, the platelet count decreases 5–14 days after exposure to heparin. If circulating anti-heparin IgG antibody from a previous exposure is already present, the platelet count may fall immediately on re-exposure to heparin. Thrombotic complications may occur at multiple anatomic sites and can result in significant morbidity, including loss of limb and even mortality (rates up to 30% in the adult population). Thrombotic

complications appear to occur in only a minority of pediatric patients with laboratory evidence of HIT; however, thromboses may be life- or limb-threatening (80). Venous events are more common in both pediatric and adult HIT as compared with arterial, although both are reported. Mortality in neonates with HIT has been reported to be as high as 21%, which was not statistically different from the mortality rate of 35% in neonates with thrombocytopenia from other etiologies (81).

The diagnosis of HIT is made clinically with supporting laboratory evidence, and may be very challenging in the PICU environment where heparin use and thrombocytopenia are both common. The more commonly available ELISA test for anti-PF4/heparin antibodies is highly sensitive (>95%) but has limited specificity (75%–90%). A functional assay, the ^{14}C serotonin release assay, is highly sensitive and specific (>95% for each), but is not widely available (80). Clinical scoring systems are available to assist with diagnosis; however, none have yet been validated in the pediatric population. Careful consideration of clinical factors is needed along with laboratory testing due to the risk of incorrect diagnosis of the cause of the thrombocytopenia, as well as the potential increased risk of bleeding with alternative anticoagulants.

Common treatment of HIT includes the immediate cessation of heparin administration of any type or route, including LMWH, heparin-coated catheters, and heparin flushes of invasive catheters. Evaluation for thrombosis in the upper and lower extremities is typically warranted. Alternative anticoagulants include the direct thrombin inhibitors bivalirudin, argatroban, or lepirudin (see below). In adults, >50% of patients with HIT will develop thrombosis within 30 days if not treated with an alternative anticoagulant.

Hemoglobinopathies. Both venous and arterial thrombotic events are recognized sequelae of SCD and other hemoglobinopathies. Although generally attributed to the vascular occlusion by the abnormal Hb species, several other factors have been subsequently recognized as contributing to the prothrombotic state of the hemoglobinopathies, including activation of the coagulation cascade and deficiencies in antithrombotic mechanisms. Although these processes may occur in all hemoglobinopathies, their magnitude appears to be greatest in SCD. Patients with SCD have depressed levels of protein S and C, elevated plasma concentrations of vWF factor and factor VIII, and depressed levels of factor V and VII (82). Endothelial interactions have also been shown to play a potential role in the thrombotic tendency of SCD, with increased adherence of sickle cells to the endothelium, an increased number of activated endothelial cells, chronic endothelial damage with cell adhesion molecule activation, and platelet activation due to abnormal endothelial cell function. All of these processes combine to increase the risk of thrombotic disease in patients with SCD.

Congenital Heart Disease. Various factors, including altered or sluggish blood flow, polycythemia, alteration in hemostatic proteins, or the presence of grafts, valves, or patches composed of foreign materials, may explain the increased tendency of patients with cyanotic CHD to develop thrombotic events. A prospective, multicenter study of venous thromboses in PICU patients demonstrated that 41% of those with thrombosis had a cardiac diagnosis as compared with 15% of those without thrombosis (53). Approximately 11%–22% of infants and children receiving cardiac surgery have thrombosis identified in the first year (83–85). Young age (under 1–6 months), increased severity of illness, mechanical ventilation, use of CVCs, baseline oxygen saturation <85%, heart transplantation, use of deep hypothermic circulatory arrest, and use of extracorporeal support have all been associated with increased risk of thrombosis in critically ill children with cardiac disease (53,83,86). In addition, coexisting disorders of the coagulation system with enhanced coagulation function or depressed antithrombotic function may further increase the incidence of thrombotic complications in patients with CHD. One study that evaluated prothrombotic risk factors in children with CHD and thrombotic events found that an underlying predisposition for thrombotic events was common, including factor V Leiden, protein C deficiency, and elevated levels of lipoprotein A (87).

Miscellaneous Factors. Various other situations or disease processes have been clearly or anecdotally linked to thrombotic complications. In some, such as meningitis, mastoiditis, or otitis media, the thrombotic complications occur in the direct vicinity of the disease process, resulting from a localized vasculitis associated with the infection. In such cases, vasculitis and small-vessel occlusion may lead to arterial or venous infarction and CNS sequelae. Thromboses also may occur at sites distal to the infection in patients with systemic bacteremia. In this setting, thrombosis becomes one component of multisystem organ failure and the systemic inflammatory response syndrome. In addition to SLE, other disease processes (Takayasu arteritis, Kawasaki disease) that result in vasculitis may also lead to thrombotic complications. Various prothrombotic changes have been reported in patients with inflammatory bowel disease (ulcerative colitis), including increased fibrinogen and factor VIII concentrations, accelerated thromboplastin generation, and decreased protein C concentrations (88). These thrombotic problems may predate the gastrointestinal symptoms.

Severe dehydration or shock may predispose the pediatric patient to thrombotic sequelae. In the adult population, the postoperative period is recognized as a period in which thrombotic complications, most commonly DVT, may occur. In contrast, such problems are generally not encountered in the pediatric population; however, following puberty, the risk increases, especially following abdominal or long-bone procedures. As with adults, pregnancy, smoking, or various medications, including oral contraceptives, may be risk factors. Metabolic diseases, either acquired or inherited, including diabetes mellitus, homocystinuria, increased lipoprotein A, and galactosemia, may also be associated with an increased risk of thrombotic complications.

Inherited/Congenital Diseases

The inherited disorders that result in a prothrombotic state are relatively uncommon; however, when routine screening is performed, they have a disproportionately high incidence in patients with what is assumed to be a spontaneous thrombotic event. Although the thrombotic event may be attributed to one of the many acquired disease processes or comorbid diseases listed previously, it is also recognized that the presence of any of a number of inherited deficiencies of the antithrombotic cascade may facilitate an acute thrombotic event in a patient who experiences a comorbid disease process such as trauma or a surgical procedure.

Protein S/C and Resistance to Activated Protein C (Factor V Leiden). Protein C and its cofactor, protein S, cleave activated factors V and VIII, thereby preventing their participation in the X-ase and prothrombinase complex. Defects in this system may involve protein S, protein C, or a mutation in the factor V gene, which confers resistance to the effects of APC. Protein S and C deficiency are inherited as simple Mendelian traits. Homozygous C deficiency results in severe disease, including purpura fulminans during infancy, while the heterozygous state increases the risk of spontaneous thrombotic events alone (with an annual thrombotic event rate of 1 per 1000 patients) or in association with comorbid diseases (89). Protein C deficiency may result from a low concentration of

normally functioning protein C (type I) or a normal concentration of a defective protein C molecule (type II). Protein C deficiency (heterozygous state) is present in ~0.2% of the general population. Treatment is divided into therapy for acute thrombotic complications, including heparin, LMWH, or thrombolytic agents, and consideration of prophylactic therapy to prevent recurrent thrombotic complications. In the homozygous state, the risk of death from thrombosis is imminent. As a result, treatment necessitates providing a source of protein C by the administration of fresh frozen plasma. In addition, a form of human protein C concentrate is available, although no studies have compared the efficacy of fresh frozen plasma versus the protein C concentrates in severe protein C deficiency-related thrombosis.

Like protein C, its cofactor, protein S, is inherited as a simple Mendelian trait. In the adult Caucasian population, protein S deficiency is present in 1%–5% of patients who have a thrombotic event. Like protein C deficiency, the presence of the heterozygous state for protein S deficiency is thought to confer an increased relative risk of thrombotic disease, estimated at six to eight times that of the general adult population, in which the risk of thrombotic complications is estimated to be 1 per 1000 patients per year. Acquired protein S deficiency may also occur associated with inflammation, estrogen administration, or pregnancy. Treatment is similar to that described for protein C deficiency; however, no purified protein S concentration is commercially available (90).

In addition to dysfunction or deficiencies of the protein S and C system, a prothrombotic state may be the result of alterations in the amino acid sequence of the factor V molecule, thereby making it resistant to the actions of APC. Most cases are related to a single amino acid change in the factor V molecule (arginine to glutamine at position 506, otherwise known as factor V Leiden). Factor V Leiden is relatively common, especially in the northern European populations. It is estimated that ~4%–7% of the general population is heterozygous for factor V Leiden, while 0.06%–0.25% of the population is homozygous for it. The odds ratio for a first venous thrombosis for children with factor V Leiden has been reported as 3.5 (91). However, thrombotic risk may be 35 times that of the general population in a person with factor V Leiden who takes oral contraceptive medications.

Antithrombin-III deficiency. AT-III deficiency may be an acquired or inherited defect. Acquired AT-III deficiency can result from various medications (e.g., L-asparaginase) or comorbid disease processes, including hepatic failure, nephrotic syndrome, preeclampsia, shock, disseminated intravascular coagulation, and the use of extracorporeal circulation. AT-III levels that are <50% of normal during septic shock are associated with increased morbidity and mortality with overall hospital mortality approaching 100% when levels are <20% (33). The estimated incidence of the heterozygous state is ~0.02%–1.0% in the general adult population. The homozygous state is not compatible with life. AT-III deficiency confers an odds ratio of 8.7 for first venous thrombosis in children, among the highest for inherited thrombophilias (91). Treatment includes standard therapy for the prothrombotic states, including elimination of risk factors and consideration for long-term anticoagulation in patients with recurrent thrombotic disease. AT-III concentrates are available, and their use is considered when prior to a major surgery and during pregnancy. AT-III concentrates may also be used to allow for therapeutic heparinization during extracorporeal support although the efficacy of replacement has not been demonstrated.

Homocystinuria. Homocystinuria is an inherited defect of amino acid metabolism that results in a syndrome of mental retardation, skeletal involvement, and visual problems related to lens dislocation and arterial/venous thrombosis. The most common genetic defects involve the cystathionine-β-synthase and methylenetetrahydrofolate reductase pathways (92). Many of the studies to date have included the adult population in which elevated plasma concentrations of homocysteine have been linked to an increased risk of coronary artery disease and DVT. However, the increased risk may occur only in association with other risk factors for arterial disease, including smoking, hypertension, hyperlipidemia, obesity, and sedentary lifestyle. A unique feature of homocystinuria is that, depending on the enzymatic defect involved, the administration of pharmacologic doses of folate, vitamin B_{12}, and B_6 may provide effective therapy and control plasma levels.

Prothrombin Gene Mutation. Prothrombin gene mutation, also known as the *prothrombin mutation*, the *prothrombin variant*, *prothrombin G20210A*, or *factor II mutation*, results in the increased expression of prothrombin. Approximately 2% of the Caucasian population in the United States is heterozygous for the prothrombin mutation, with a much lower incidence (~0.5%) in African Americans. It is rare in Asians, Africans, and Native Americans. The mechanism by which the prothrombin gene mutation results in a prothrombotic state appears to be by increased processing of prothrombin mRNA resulting in increased prothrombin expression. The prothrombin mutation has been associated with an odds ratio of 2.6 for first venous thrombosis in children (91), and has also been associated with CNS thromboses and recurrent pregnancy loss.

Lipoprotein A. Lipoprotein A is a cholesterol-containing protein with a composition similar to that of low-density lipoproteins. Various studies have demonstrated an increased risk of coronary artery disease and stroke in adults with elevated lipoprotein A concentrations. Increased lipoprotein A concentrations (≥50 mg/dL) were noted in 22% of children with arterial disease and 13.8% of children with venous involvement in one series (93). A systematic review reported 4.5 times increased odds of first venous thrombosis with the presence of lipoprotein A (91).

Platelet Disorders. Although more commonly associated with a bleeding diathesis, rare platelet disorders may manifest as a prothrombotic state. They may manifest as peripheral venous/arterial thrombosis, but more commonly result in early myocardial infarction in otherwise normal coronary arteries. In the congenital Wien-Penzing defect, a defect in the lipoxygenase pathway leads to a compensatory increase in the COX pathway, with increased production of thromboxane, prostaglandin E2, and prostaglandin D2, thereby augmenting platelet aggregation. A second disorder, *sticky platelet syndrome*, may also be associated with premature coronary artery occlusion. Platelets from patients affected with this autosomal-dominant disorder show increased aggregation at lower concentrations of various factors (epinephrine, ADP) that promote platelet aggregation (94). RT commonly seen with acute illness is not typically associated with increased risk of thrombosis, however.

Diagnosis

The clinical manifestations of thrombotic disease in infants and children vary depending on the site of involvement, the degree of vessel occlusion, whether the clot has resulted in embolic sequelae, and the vasculature affected (arterial versus venous). On the arterial side, the clinical signs and symptoms are relatively straightforward when total occlusion is present and include a painful, cold, pulseless extremity. When clinical signs and symptoms are apparent, they depend on the site of involvement, with the unilateral swelling with extremity involvement, superior vena cava syndrome or chylothorax

with superior vena cava involvement, and hepatomegaly and ascites with inferior vena cava involvement. When the vasculature of the CNS is involved (arterial or venous), the CNS manifestations may be subtle, as the classic manifestations of a stroke may not be initially evident. Loss of patency of a CVC may be the first indication of thrombotic disease. The development of collateral circulation may be the primary manifestation of the disease process when bleeding occurs from esophageal varices with splenic, portal, or hepatic vein thrombosis.

Radiologic Imaging

Given its noninvasive nature and portability, ultrasound remains the primary technique used to identify thrombotic disease in the PICU population. A diagnosis of thrombus is made using Doppler ultrasonography to identify the following features: an echogenic filling defect, noncompressibility of the vein, loss of respiratory variability in vessel pulsation, and lack of flow or abnormal Doppler waveforms distal to the occluded segment. However, false negatives may occur, especially when the thrombus does not totally occlude the vein. CT with contrast or magnetic resonance venography has greater sensitivity and specificity to detect thromboses of central veins, such as intrathoracic vessels or the CNS (95). However, its utility is limited by lack of portability, patient monitoring issues during scanning, and potential need for sedation/general anesthesia to ensure a motionless patient. Contrast venogram has historically been the gold standard for diagnosis of thrombosis. While also limited by need for patient transport and sedation, fluoroscopic-guided contrast studies in an interventional laboratory may offer the prospect of direct intervention to recanalize an occluded vessel.

Laboratory Evaluation for a Prothrombotic State

A high index of suspicion for an underlying prothrombotic condition should be entertained in patients who lack associated risk factors or comorbid diseases when thrombotic disease involves unusual locations (CNS, mesentery), with arterial occlusion, recurrent thrombotic events, and/or a family history of thrombotic disease in first-degree relatives. One study that evaluated the etiology of pulmonary emboli in children found that the incidence of protein S deficiency, protein C deficiency, or lupus anticoagulant was ~90% in children without an identifiable comorbid process or risk factor for thrombosis, compared with 50% in patients with identifiable risk factors (96). This study not only demonstrates the importance of screening for potential prothrombotic states in patients without apparent risk factors, but also stresses the potential role that the prothrombotic state may have on further increasing the incidence of a thrombotic event in patients with other risk factors. Reported incidence of inherited thrombophilia in pediatric patients with thrombosis varies widely from 13% to 79% depending on patient population, with the highest incidence typically found in older children (noninfants) and those with spontaneous thrombosis not associated with multiple acquired risk factors (97). A consideration of individual clinical risk factors and consultation with a pediatric hematologist are recommended to guide workup. A suggested laboratory evaluation for children with thrombosis is summarized in **Table 116.19** (98,99).

Treatment

Treatment options for thrombosis can be divided into regimens to prevent thrombus extension and embolization, and fibrinolytic therapies to dissolve a thrombus. When any of

TABLE 116.19

DIAGNOSTIC EVALUATION OF HYPERCOAGULABILITY IN CHILDREN

LEVEL I— Initial Evaluation
  CBC with differential
  PT, PTT, fibrinogen
  Factor V Leiden (activated protein C resistance)[a]
  Antithrombin activity[b]
  Prothrombin 20210 mutation
  Protein C activity[b]
  Protein S—free and total antigen[b]
  Antiphospholipid antibodies (DRRVT, anticardiolipin, lupus anticoagulant, anti-β_2 glycoprotein)[b]
  MTHFR T677T and/or fasting homocysteine level[b]
  Lipoprotein (a)[a]
  Consider: [HIT type 2[b], sickle cell screen/hemoglobin electrophoresis, factor VIII]
LEVEL II— Extended Evaluation
  Dysfibrinogenemia evaluation[a] (FDP, fibrinogen activity, thrombin and reptilase time, consider immunoelectrophoresis)
  Heparin cofactor II[c]
  Plasminogen activity[c]
  PAI: plasminogen activator inhibitor[c]
  Factor IX, XI, XII[c]
  Von Willebrand factor level[c] and multimers [ADAMTS13[b]]
  Spontaneous platelet aggregation
  Tissue plasminogen activity
  Tissue factor pathway inhibitor

Level I tests are often performed in children with thrombosis. Level II tests are recommended in those children with normal Level I values and/or in the settings of recurrent thrombosis or strong family history of thrombotic disease. [], indicates studies to be done when clinical scenarios implicate their involvement.
[a]Indicates lower risk factors.
[b]Indicates high-risk factors with therapeutic and/or prognostic relevance.
[c]Potential thrombotic risk factors.
CBC, complete blood count; PT, prothrombin time; PTT, partial thromboplastin time; APC, activated protein C; HIT, heparin-induced thrombocytopenia; FDP, fibrin degradation products.
Adapted from Manco-Johnson MJ, Grabowski EF, Hellgreen M, et al. Laboratory testing for thrombophilia in pediatric patients. On behalf of the Subcommittee for Perinatal and Pediatric Thrombosis of the Scientific and Standardization Committee of the International Society of Thrombosis and Haemostasis (ISTH). Thromb Haemost 2002;88(1):155–6; Schneppenheim R, Greiner J. Thrombosis in infants and children. Hematology Am Soc Hematol Educ Program 2006;86–96; and Raffini L. Thrombophilia in children: who to test, how, when, and why? Hematology Am Soc Hematol Educ Program 2008;2008:228–35.

these therapies are used, the risks of therapy must be weighed against the risk of the disease itself. In the adult population, therapeutic anticoagulation with Coumadin carries the risk of hemorrhage of ~3% per year, with one-fifth of the hemorrhages being fatal. The effect of various anticoagulants on the coagulation cascade is demonstrated in **Figure 116.6**. Additionally, elimination of provocative factors such as medications (oral contraceptive pills, heparin in patients with HIT), avoidance of hyperlipidemia, and treatment of underlying disorders (oncologic disease, nephrotic syndrome) can reduce risk. In specific inherited deficiencies (protein C or AT-III deficiency), replacement therapy may be indicated, especially in patients with homozygous disease in whom mortality is imminent without such interventions.

Heparin, Low-Molecular-Weight Heparin, and Warfarin

The most commonly used medications for treatment or prevention of thrombosis are heparin preparations, which activate AT-III to inhibit thrombin and/or factor Xa. Initial treatment of venous thromboembolic disease in infants and children is similar to that recommended for adults and includes unfractionated heparin (bolus dose of 75–100 U/kg unless clinically contraindicated due to bleeding risks followed by a continuous infusion of 20 U/kg/h for children and 28 U/kg/h for infants). Recent guidelines recommend anti-Xa assays in preference or in addition to aPTT monitoring, especially for children <1 year or with critical illness, due to inconsistent correlation between the anti-Xa and the aPTT (100). However, therapeutic anti-Xa activities are frequently difficult to achieve in infants (101). For monitoring, anti-Xa or aPTT is first measured 4–6 hours following the initiation of therapy and maintained at 0.35–0.70 for anti-Xa or 60–85 seconds for aPTT (100). The therapeutic aPTT range is correlated to a therapeutic anti-Xa activity; thus, the aPTT range may vary between laboratories due to difference in aPTT reagents.

Problems with unfractionated heparin include variability in bioavailability and age-related pharmacokinetics, requirements for ongoing IV access for administration, delays in achieving the desired level of anticoagulation, and repeated blood draws to monitor the aPTT or anti-Xa. Given these problems, the trend has been toward the use of LMWH preparations. LMWHs are prepared by chemical or enzymatic treatment of unfractionated heparin. Unlike unfractionated heparin, which acts against both Xa and thrombin, LMWH preferentially targets Xa activity. The initial data regarding the use of LMWH in the pediatric population have demonstrated efficacy in the treatment of thromboembolic events, with reported benefits over unfractionated heparin that include subcutaneous administration, predictable pharmacokinetics, a decreased incidence of HIT, less monitoring, and a decreased risk of bleeding (102). Although multiple LMWHs exist, currently the most commonly used agent is enoxaparin, with treatment dosing of 1.5 mg/kg/dose every 12 hours for infants <2 months, and 1.0 mg/kg/dose every 12 hours for children >2 months (doses are halved for prophylaxis). Typical goal range for monitoring is an anti-Xa level of 0.5–1.0 units per mL for treatment and 0.1–0.3 for prophylaxis. The specimen is drawn 4–6 hours after dosing (100). When long-term anticoagulation therapy is planned and an oral agent is preferred, vitamin K antagonist warfarin (Coumadin) may be started at 0.2 mg/kg (maximum dose of 7.5 mg) and adjusted according to the international normalized ratio (INR) of the PT. Once a therapeutic level is achieved with warfarin (INR = 2–3), heparin or LMWH is discontinued, but should be overlapped for a minimum of 5 days (101).

Heparin Alternatives

The most commonly used of the alternative anticoagulants are the direct thrombin inhibitors (argatroban, lepirudin, bivalirudin). Argatroban is a synthetic molecule that binds reversibly to the active site of the thrombin molecule. It is primarily metabolized in the liver, with an elimination half-life of 40–60 minutes. Significant increases in the elimination half-life are seen in patients with hepatic dysfunction. Unlike other direct thrombin inhibitors, argatroban undergoes minimal renal clearance, and the plasma half-life is not prolonged in patients with renal dysfunction. No reversal agent is available; therefore, argatroban's effects must dissipate gradually, which may increase bleeding following procedures that use CPB (103,104).

Hirudin is a direct thrombin inhibitor that is derived from the medicinal leech, *Hirudo medicinalis*. It is a 65-amino-acid polypeptide that forms an irreversible 1:1 complex with thrombin. Hirudin is now produced by using recombinant technology, resulting in the r-hirudins, including lepirudin and desirudin. Only the former is routinely used in clinical practice. Lepirudin was the first direct thrombin inhibitor approved for use in Europe and the United States for the treatment of HIT complicated by thrombosis. It undergoes renal clearance with an elimination half-life of ~80 minutes in normal subjects, with significant prolongations in patients with renal insufficiency or failure. Bivalirudin is a synthetic 20-amino-acid peptide that consists of two hirudin peptide fragments joined together. Unlike lepirudin, the binding of bivalirudin to thrombin is reversible. Bivalirudin has a short plasma half-life of ~25 minutes and is cleared from the blood primarily by enzymatic breakdown by plasma proteases as well as renal clearance, with 20% of an administered dose recovered in the urine. As with argatroban, no reversal agent exists for lepirudin or bivalirudin, although modified ultrafiltration has been used to enhance its elimination. Anecdotal experience has demonstrated that recombinant factor VIIa is not an effective reversal agent for the direct thrombin inhibitors. Monitoring of argatroban, lepirudin, and bivalirudin typically involves targeting the aPTT at 1.5–2.5× control values (105).

A novel class of oral antithrombotic drugs, the "new oral anticoagulants" or "NOACs," includes the oral direct thrombin inhibitor dabigatran and the factor Xa inhibitors rivaroxaban and apixaban. These medications have undergone initial studies in adults and hold promise due to their oral administration, less need for monitoring, and potentially favorable therapeutic window. Rivaroxaban has undergone initial laboratory investigation showing no significant difference in anticoagulant effect in plasma pools from different pediatric age groups in vitro (106). Further studies are needed prior to clinical use in the PICU.

Fibrinolytic Therapy

The currently available thrombolytic agents include tPA, streptokinase, and urokinase. These agents act by activating plasminogen to plasmin and augmenting the fibrinolytic system, which results in the degradation of fibrin. Given the high probability of recent streptococcal infections in pediatric patients and the risk of allergic phenomena, streptokinase is rarely used in infants and children. Although urokinase found some utility in the pediatric population, its prolonged unavailability related to manufacturing issues and a warning by the U.S. Food and Drug Administration has led to decreased use, although dosing protocols are available for clearing of central-line occlusions (**Table 116.20**). Given these concerns, tPA has rapidly become the favored agent for fibrinolytic therapy. Additionally, tPA only activates plasminogen that is bound to fibrin and, therefore, theoretically limits the fibrinolytic effect to the surface of the clot.

Medical thrombolysis has a varied success rate (complete resolution of clot) of 39%–70% with no significant difference between agents (100,107). Bleeding is a significant risk, including intracranial hemorrhage. Major bleeding requiring transfusion occurs in ~20% of children treated systemically with thrombolytics, and minor bleeding occurs in 25%–70% (100). Infusions of tPA may be used (in conjunction with a hematologist is recommended), with most reporting a dosing regimen that involves 0.5 mg/kg/h for 6 hours (58). However, lower dose infusions of 0.007–0.06 mg/kg/h have been reported to perhaps have similar efficacy and a potentially lower risk of bleeding (108,109). Longer duration of therapy is typically associated with increased bleeding risk. Administration may be systemic or by localized infusion directly into the site of thrombosis (e.g., catheter directed toward iliofemoral or axillary/subclavian location) (109). Systemic

TABLE 116.20

TREATMENT OF CENTRAL CATHETER OCCLUSION

■ AGE/WEIGHT	■ TYPE OF CATHETER AND NO. OF LUMENS	■ UROKINASE DOSE AND VOLUME	■ ALTEPLASE (tPA) DOSE AND VOLUME
Newborn (birth–4 weeks)	Single-lumen Hickman	0.5 mL/2500 U	0.5 mg/0.5 mL
≤10 kg	Single-lumen Hickman	1 mL/5000 U	1 mg/1 mL
≤10 kg	Double-lumen Hickman	1 mL/5000 U each lumen	1 mg/1 mL each lumen
≥10 kg	Single-lumen Hickman	1.5 mL/7500 U	1.5 mg/1.5 mL
≥10 kg	Double-lumen Hickman	1 mL/5000 U small lumen 1.5 mL/7500 U in large lumen	1 mg/1 mL small lumen 1.5 mg/1.5 mL large lumen
Any weight	Small/low-volume Infusaport	1.5 mL/7500 U	1.5 mg/1.5 mL
Any weight	Large/high-volume Infusaport	3 mL/15,000 U	3 mg/3 mL
Any weight	3.0 and 4.0 Fr. PICC	1 mL/5000 U	1 mg/1 mL
Any weight	≤2.0 Fr. PICC	Manufacturer does not recommend declotting	

General Recommendations: Urokinase or Alteplase (tPA) are the drugs of choice for bolus administration to indwell in the catheter. Length of time urokinase or tPA should indwell in catheter: First dose of urokinase or tPA should indwell for at least 2 h before blood withdrawal is attempted. After 2 h, attempts to withdraw blood may be made every 2 h for three attempts. The second dose of urokinase or tPA should indwell in the catheter for 3–4 h before blood withdrawal is attempted. After 3–4 h, blood withdrawal should be attempted every 2 h for three attempts. If the catheter remains difficult to flush after 2 bolus urokinase doses or 2 bolus tPA doses, a 24-h continuous urokinase infusion can be considered.
Urokinase and streptokinase continuous infusion doses:
(a) The dose of streptokinase for a continuous infusion is 80 U/kg/h (per lumen).
(b) The dose of urokinase for a continuous infusion is 200 U/kg/h (per lumen).
Note: tPA is not routinely utilized as a continuous infusion for catheter clearance due to limited data in pediatrics. The urokinase and streptokinase should be mixed in solutions of normal saline or dextrose and water for IV infusion. In patients with a recent streptococcal infection or signs and symptoms of an allergic response to streptokinase, an alternative agent is selected. Unsuccessfully declotted catheters should be considered for removal.
PICC, peripherally inserted central catheter.
Adapted from Children's Center Care Protocol, Johns Hopkins Hospital.

low-dose heparin infusion of 10 units/kg/h is often used during thrombolysis, with subsequent therapeutic heparinization. Supplementation with fresh frozen plasma, especially for neonates whose plasminogen levels are only 25%–50% of adult levels, may be considered prior to therapy (100). Hypofibrinogenemia is common during thrombolysis and should be corrected with cryoprecipitate when fibrinogen decreases below 100–150 mg/dL. Maintaining a platelet count >100,000/mm³ also may help attenuate the bleeding risk. In general, thrombolytic therapy may be indicated for life- or limb-threatening thrombosis when the risks of morbidity and mortality from the thrombotic process outweigh the risks of thrombolytic therapy (100). Such instances may include arterial occlusions, especially in the CNS or where loss of limb is imminent, and thrombi within the cardiac chambers, which may necessitate a major surgical intervention with CPB for removal (110).

Thromboprophylaxis

PICU clinicians may use mechanical methods for thromboprophylaxis, such as compression stockings and/or pneumatic compression devices, with or without pharmacologic prophylaxis such as subcutaneous LMWH or heparin. Evidence is lacking to guide a specific strategy, so a careful review of an individual patient's risk factors for thrombosis must be weighed along with risks of the prophylaxis. Available guidelines suggest consideration of longer-term prophylaxis in select high-risk groups including oral vitamin K antagonists for pediatric patients with long-term home total parenteral nutrition, cardiomyopathy awaiting transplant, cavopulmonary anastomosis, mechanical heart valves, and primary pulmonary hypertension (100). In the inpatient setting, one large tertiary care children's center has published institutional guidelines for thromboprophylaxis for pediatric inpatients 14 years or older with altered mobility, specifying increasing levels of prophylaxis for low risk (early ambulation), at risk (early ambulation and mechanical devices), and high-risk (adding pharmacologic prophylaxis) groups based on a set of risk factors for venous thrombosis (111). Another center has recommended pharmacologic prophylaxis for patients 13 years or older with four or more risk factors for thrombosis and low risk of bleeding (112). These authors reported a decrease in clinically apparent venous thrombosis, in PICU patients admitted after trauma, following implementation of their guidelines. A recent survey of PICU physicians from 97 centers revealed that in mechanically ventilated PICU patients, 42.3% of respondents would usually or always prescribe pharmacologic thromboprophylaxis for an adolescent versus only 1% for a child or infant. LMWH was the most commonly reported pharmacologic agent used, and hypercoagulability, prior DVT, and cavopulmonary anastomosis were the most common clinical factors associated with prescription of pharmacologic thromboprophylaxis (113).

Select Thrombotic Emergencies

Pulmonary Embolism. PE is a potentially devastating thrombotic disease that accounts for an estimated 8%–16% of total venous thromboses in pediatrics (46,69,114,115). Reported incidence among hospitalized children has increased from 0.9 per 10,000 admissions (46) to ~5 per 10,000 admissions in more recent reports, mirroring increases in reported incidence of venous thrombosis overall (57). Mortality ranges from 6%–20% among all children diagnosed with PE (46,57,70,115) to approximately 60%–80% of children with massive PE (with hypotension as a presenting symptom) (116), although these estimates may be clouded by asymptomatic patients as well as those who experience sudden death without autopsy.

Diagnosis of PE may be difficult due to inconsistent symptomatology and lack of predictive value of quickly obtained tests often used in adults. Therefore, the PICU clinician must maintain an index of suspicion in patients with risk factors. In one single-center study, shortness of breath was the most common presenting symptom (57% of patients), followed by hypoxemia (43%), pleuritic chest pain (32%), symptoms of DVT (29%), and cardiovascular collapse (7%) (57). At least one major risk factor for venous thrombosis, such as congenital cardiac disease or malignancy, was present in 96% of patients in this study. Tachycardia, cough, and hemoptysis have also been described (117), but a significant portion are likely asymptomatic (16% of those detected in one study) (57). Clinical probability scoring and D-dimer have shown poor predictive value in pediatrics (117,118). Chest x-ray is often normal in patients with PE (57,115). The electrocardiogram may show signs of right ventricular strain such as Q-wave and T-wave inversion in lead 3, with a deep S in lead 1 (S1-Q3-T3 pattern); however, no prospective studies have shown reliability of this criterion in children (115). The echocardiography in PE may detect signs of right ventricular strain such as hypokinesis, intraventricular septal deviation, tricuspid valve regurgitation, or lack of collapse of the inferior vena cava during inspiration (117). However, lack of sensitivity or specificity precludes its use as a sole mechanism for diagnosing PE. Diagnosis is often made by helical CT scan with contrast, which has been reported to have 90% or better sensitivity and specificity to detect segmental or larger PEs in the adult population (115,117). Ventilation-perfusion scans or MRI also provide excellent predictive value, although are often more time-consuming and thus potentially clinically less desirable in a critically ill child.

Management of an acute PE typically consists of systemic anticoagulation to prevent extension of the thrombus. Available pediatric guidelines suggest initial therapy with either unfractionated heparin or LMWH for at least 5 days, followed by ongoing anticoagulation with heparin, LMWH, or oral vitamin K antagonists for a minimum of 3 months after resolution of an inciting risk factor or longer if an identified major risk factor (such as malignancy or nephrotic syndrome) is ongoing. Idiopathic PE or other venous thromboses are typically treated with 6–12 months of systemic anticoagulation. (58). In adults 16 years of age or older, LMWH or the subcutaneous factor Xa inhibitor fondaparinux may be used preferentially to unfractionated heparin for acute PE due to potentially improved retention in patients with renal impairment, unless subcutaneous administration is contraindicated (100). In massive, life-threating PE, further therapies may include systemic thrombolysis, pulmonary embolectomy, and/or emergent extracorporeal life support (58,116).

Deep Venous Thrombosis. Thrombosis may occur in the large veins of the upper or lower venous system, primarily in patients with CVCs or immobility, often concurrent with additional risk factors as detailed above. Upper and lower venous system DVT are both well described, although idiopathic DVT is more common in the lower venous system (58). In a large registry of >13,000 admissions with venous thrombosis in 40 children's hospitals across the United States, common sites included lower extremities (13.6% of admissions with venous thrombosis), vena cava (12%), and upper extremities (10.2%), although 41% were of unspecified location (50). In a tertiary PICU, 74% of venous thromboses discovered were symptomatic, most often with extremity pain or swelling, CVC malfunction, facial swelling, or chylothorax (53). DVT may lead to morbidity or mortality by becoming dislodged and becoming a PE (or arterial ischemic event if right-to-left intracardiac shunt is present), causing CVC malfunction, as well as increasing the risk for CVC-related sepsis (100). In addition, thrombosis recurrence may occur in 7.5% of patients (100) while post-thrombotic syndrome (chronic venous insufficiency with pain, edema, dermatitis) may occur in approximately 26% of cases of DVT (119).

The diagnosis of DVT in the PICU setting is most often confirmed by Doppler ultrasound (53). CT with contrast, MRI, echocardiography, or interventional contrast venography may also be used when deeper venous structures are involved or the need for intervention is anticipated. Management of DVT typically consists of anticoagulant therapy to prevent clot extension and removal of inciting risk factors where possible. Similar to PE, acute anticoagulant therapy with unfractionated heparin or LMWH is recommended for at least 5 days with ongoing therapy for at least 3 months (typically with LMWH or oral vitamin K antagonist) if a precipitating factor is removed, or 6–12 months after idiopathic DVT. For CVC-related DVT, 3–5 days of anticoagulation is recommended prior to removal followed by at least 3 months of therapy. Thrombolysis or thrombectomy is typically reserved for those with life or limb-threatening thrombosis (58). Inferior vena cava filters may be considered, especially for children weighing >10 kg with recurrent lower-extremity thrombosis and/or contraindications to anticoagulation (58,120).

Nonstroke Arterial Thrombosis. Arterial thromboses outside of the CNS in children are commonly associated with an arterial catheter, whether peripheral, femoral, or umbilical. Clinical presentation may include paresthesia (often the first symptom or sign), as well as pallor, diminished or absent pulses, decreased skin temperature, and prolonged capillary refill time. In one prospective study of 615 arterial catheters placed in 473 patients in a PICU setting, thrombosis was detected associated with 13% of femoral, 9% of brachial, 4% of umbilical, and 0 radial catheters (60) (however asymptomatic patients were not generally assessed for thrombosis by imaging). Cardiac catheterization in children using the femoral artery has been reported to be associated with thrombosis in approximately 3%–30% of cases, with younger age and undergoing an interventional procedure associated with higher risk (62,121,122). Other categories of nonstroke arterial thrombosis typically include complications of congenital heart disease (e.g., related to mechanical valves, Blalock-Taussig shunt, or post-Fontan procedure), transplanted organ thrombosis (such as renal or hepatic artery), Takayasu's arteritis, and Kawasaki disease-related aneurysms (59). Mortality from nonstroke arterial thrombosis is generally associated with intracardiac thromboses or cardiac shunts (59), with additional morbidity potentially including limb ischemia, organ failure, hypertension, leg length discrepancies, and claudication.

The diagnosis of arterial thrombosis outside of the CNS is most often achieved by Doppler ultrasound, with CT, MRI, echocardiography, or contrast arteriography also potentially useful depending upon the site of thrombosis (59). Management of femoral artery thrombosis consists of unfractionated heparin or LMWH with subsequent conversion to LMWH or continuation of unfractionated heparin to complete 5–7 days of therapy (102). The majority of femoral artery thromboses after cardiac catheterization will resolve with heparin alone within 24–48 hours, although need for thrombolytics and/or thrombectomy has been reported (62,121,122). Asymptomatic peripheral arterial catheter-related thrombosis may be resolved simply with removal of the catheter, while unfractionated heparin is recommended for symptomatic peripheral arterial thrombosis, and thrombolysis and/or surgical thrombectomy with microvascular repair may be indicated when significant ischemia is present. Nonstroke arterial thromboses in other anatomical locations warrant specialty consultation and careful risk–benefit analysis to determine an optimal plan for anticoagulation, thrombolysis, and/or surgical intervention.

Thrombotic Thrombocytopenic Purpura. Although primarily described in adults, an estimated <10% of cases of thrombotic thrombocytopenic purpura (TTP) may occur in the pediatric population, with the first being described in a 16-year-old female in 1924. TTP clinically presents with thrombocytopenia, microangiopathic hemolytic anemia, fever, and disseminated microvascular thrombi causing organ dysfunction, most prominently in the brain and kidneys. Microthrombi in the heart, adrenal glands, gastrointestinal tract, liver, and spleen may also occur. Deficiency in the metalloprotease ADAMTS13 (*a d*isintegrin-like *a*nd *m*etalloprotease with *t*hrombospondin type-1 motif, member 13), which normally cleaves vWF, is associated with both congenital and acquired forms of TTP. Congenital ADAMTS13 deficiency may manifest as symptomatic TTP in early childhood, although 40%–60% may be asymptomatic until adolescence or adulthood. Acquired TTP is often associated with anti-ADAMTS13 antibodies, and may occur with autoimmune diseases such as SLE, after bone marrow transplant, or with systemic infections. Mortality in untreated TTP may be as high as 90%. Treatment for congenital TTP typically involves administration of fresh frozen plasma or cryoprecipitate, while acquired TTP warrants plasma exchange, often repeated daily until clinical symptoms improve (123,124). The addition of steroids, as well as, Rituximab, may be beneficial.

CONCLUSIONS AND FUTURE DIRECTIONS

Hematologic abnormalities are a common occurrence in the practice of critical care medicine. Recent clinical studies have improved our understanding and recognition of developmental and age-specific changes in the hematologic system. Although these age-specific parameters are complex, hospitals and clinicians should continue to make them readily available to assist in the recognition and diagnosis of common hematologic abnormalities such as anemia, thrombocytopenia, and low/high WBC counts. Future clinical and basic science research will continue to improve our understanding and recognition of relatively new disease processes and should provide for new and improved treatment strategies for affected children. Perhaps the greatest increase in our knowledge has occurred in the recognition of thromboembolic disease in children. Though recent consensus meetings have provided definitions and guidelines, continued research into the genetics, molecular basis, and pathophysiology of arterial and venous thrombosis in children will result in evolving recommendations and treatment approaches, especially for those with genetic predisposition and/or associated risk factors.

References

1. Hung OL, Kwon NS, Cole AE, et al. Evaluation of the physician's ability to recognize the presence or absence of anemia, fever, and jaundice. *Acad Emerg Med* 2000;7(2):146–56.
2. Armano R, Gauvin F, Ducruet T, et al. Determinants of red blood cell transfusions in a pediatric critical care unit: A prospective, descriptive epidemiological study. *Crit Care Med* 2005;33(11):2637–44.
3. Sandoval C, Berger E, Ozkaynak MF, et al. Severe iron deficiency anemia in 42 pediatric patients. *Pediatr Hematol Oncol* 2002;19(3):157–61.
4. Sloniewsky D. Anemia and transfusion in critically ill pediatric patients: A review of etiology, management, and outcomes. *Crit Care Clin* 2013;29(2):301–17.
5. Tabbara IA. Hemolytic anemias. Diagnosis and management. *Med Clin North Am* 1992;76(3):649–68.

6. Litman RS. Nitrous oxide: The passing of a gas? *Curr Opin Anaesthesiol* 2004;17(3):207–9.

7. Camitta BM, Storb R, Thomas ED. Aplastic anemia (second of two parts): Pathogenesis, diagnosis, treatment, and prognosis. *N Engl J Med* 1982;306(12):712–8.

8. Camitta BM, Storb R, Thomas ED. Aplastic anemia (first of two parts): Pathogenesis, diagnosis, treatment, and prognosis. *N Engl J Med* 1982;306(11):645–52.

9. Lubran MM. Hematologic side effects of drugs. *Ann Clin Lab Sci* 1989;19(2):114–21.

10. Chanarin I. Pernicious anaemia. *BMJ* 1992;304(6842):1584–5.

11. Gillman MA. Folinic acid prevents megaloblastic changes associated with nitrous oxide. *Anesth Analg* 1988;67(10):1018–9.

12. Jaffe ER. Enzymopenic hereditary methemoglobinemia. *Haematologia* 1982;15(4):389–99.

13. McDonald MJ, Turci SM, Bunn HF. Subunit assembly of normal and variant human hemoglobins. *Prog Clin Biol Res* 1984;165:3–15.

14. Smith RP. Chemicals reacting with various forms of hemoglobin: Biological significance, mechanisms, and determination. *J Forensic Sci* 1991;36(3):662–72.

15. Geller RJ, Barthold C, Saiers JA, et al. Pediatric cyanide poisoning: Causes, manifestations, management, and unmet needs. *Pediatrics* 2006;118(5):2146–58.

16. Peddy SB, Rigby MR, Shaffner DH. Acute cyanide poisoning. *Pediatr Crit Care Med* 2006;7(1):79–82.

17. Easley RB. Open air carbon monoxide poisoning in a child swimming behind a boat. *South Med J* 2000;93(4):430–2.

18. McCrory MC, Strouse JJ, Takemoto CM, et al. Computerized physician order entry improves compliance with a manual exchange transfusion protocol in the pediatric intensive care unit. *J Pediatric Hematol Oncol* 2014;36(2):143–7.

19. Felmet KA, Hall MW, Clark RS, et al. Prolonged lymphopenia, lymphoid depletion, and hypoprolactinemia in children with nosocomial sepsis and multiple organ failure. *J Immunol* 2005;174(6):3765–72.

20. Carcillo JA, Dean JM, Holubkov R, et al. The randomized comparative pediatric critical illness stress-induced immune suppression (CRISIS) prevention trial. *Pediatr Crit Care Med* 2012; 13(2):165–73.

21. Fioredda F, Calvillo M, Bonanomi S, et al. Congenital and acquired neutropenias consensus guidelines on therapy and follow-up in childhood from the Neutropenia Committee of the Marrow Failure Syndrome Group of the AIEOP (Associazione Italiana Emato-Oncologia Pediatrica). *Am J hematol* 2012;87(2):238–43.

22. Fioredda F, Calvillo M, Bonanomi S, et al. Congenital and acquired neutropenia consensus guidelines on diagnosis from the Neutropenia Committee of the Marrow Failure Syndrome Group of the AIEOP (Associazione Italiana Emato-Oncologia Pediatrica). *Pediatr Blood Cancer* 2011;57(1):10–7.

23. Baldwin CM, Lyseng-Williamson KA, Keam SJ. Meropenem: A review of its use in the treatment of serious bacterial infections. *Drugs* 2008;68(6):803–38.

24. Lee J, Patel G, Huprikar S, et al. Decreased susceptibility to polymyxin B during treatment for carbapenem-resistant Klebsiella pneumoniae infection. *J Clini Microbiol* 2009;47(5):1611–2.

25. Jacoby GA, Gacharna N, Black TA, et al. Temporal appearance of plasmid-mediated quinolone resistance genes. *Antimicrob Agents Chemother* 2009;53(4):1665–6.

26. Newburger PE, Pindyck TN, Zhu Z, et al. Cyclic neutropenia and severe congenital neutropenia in patients with a shared ELANE mutation and paternal haplotype: Evidence for phenotype determination by modifying genes. *Pediatr blood Cancer* 2010;55(2):314–7.

27. Rothenberg ME. Eosinophilia. *N Engl J Med* 1998;338(22):1592–600.

28. Sutton SA, Assa'ad AH, Rothenberg ME. Anti-IL-5 and hypereosinophilic syndromes. *Clin Immunol* 2005;115(1):51–60.

29. Pierce C, Klein N, Peters M. Is leukocytosis a predictor of mortality in severe pertussis infection? *Intensive Care Med* 2000;26(10):1512–4.

30. Rowlands HE, Goldman AP, Harrington K et al. Impact of rapid leukodepletion on the outcome of severe clinical pertussis in young infants. *Pediatrics* 2010;126(4):e816–27.

31. Sutor AH. Thrombocytosis in childhood. *Semin Thromb Hemost* 1995;21(3):330–9.

32. Edstrom CS, Christensen RD. Evaluation and treatment of thrombosis in the neonatal intensive care unit. *Clin Perinatol* 2000;27(3):623–41.

33. Haidopoulou K, Goutaki M, Lemonaki M, et al. Reactive thrombocytosis in children with viral respiratory tract infections. *Minerva pediatr* 2011;63(4):257–62.

34. Olmez I, Zafar M, Shahid M, et al. Analysis of significant decrease in platelet count and thrombocytopenia, graded according to NCI-CTC, as prognostic risk markers for mortality and morbidity. *J Pediatr Hematol Oncol* 2011;33(8):585–8.

35. Vandendries ER, Drews RE. Drug-associated disease: Hematologic dysfunction. *Crit Care Clin* 2006;22(2):347–55, viii.

36. Bell WR. Heparin-associated thrombocytopenia and thrombosis. *J Lab Clin Med* 1988;111(6):600–5.

37. Kirchner JT. Acute and chronic immune thrombocytopenic purpura. Disorders that differ in more than duration. *Postgrad Med* 1992;92(6):112–8, 25–6.

38. Neunert CE, Buchanan GR, Imbach P, et al. Severe hemorrhage in children with newly diagnosed immune thrombocytopenic purpura. *Blood* 2008;112(10):4003–8.

39. Medeiros D, Buchanan GR. Current controversies in the management of idiopathic thrombocytopenic purpura during childhood. *Pediatr Clin North Am* 1996;43(3):757–72.

40. Cote CJ, Liu LM, Szyfelbein SK, et al. Changes in serial platelet counts following massive blood transfusion in pediatric patients. *Anesthesiology* 1985;62(2):197–201.

41. George JN, Shattil SJ. The clinical importance of acquired abnormalities of platelet function. *N Engl J Med* 1991;324(1):27–39.

42. Fass RJ, Copelan EA, Brandt JT, et al. Platelet-mediated bleeding caused by broad-spectrum penicillins. *J Infect Dis* 1987;155(6):1242–8.

43. Marcum JA, Rosenberg RD. Anticoagulantly active heparin-like molecules from vascular tissue. *Biochemistry* 1984;23(8):1730–7.

44. Handoll HH, Farrar MJ, McBirnie J, et al. Heparin, low molecular weight heparin and physical methods for preventing deep vein thrombosis and pulmonary embolism following surgery for hip fractures. *Cochrane Database Syst Rev* 2000(2):CD000305.

45. Greenwald LJ, Yost MT, Sponseller PD, et al. The role of clinically significant venous thromboembolism and thromboprophylaxis in pediatric patients with pelvic or femoral fractures. *J Pediatr Orthoped* 2012;32(4):357–61.

46. Andrew M, David M, Adams M, et al. Venous thromboembolic complications (VTE) in children: First analyses of the Canadian Registry of VTE. *Blood* 1994;83(5):1251–7.

47. van Ommen V, Michels R, Heymen E, et al. Usefulness of the rescue PT catheter to remove fresh thrombus from coronary arteries and bypass grafts in acute myocardial infarction. *Am J Cardiol* 2001;88(3):306–8.

48. Zizola CF, Balana ME, Sandoval M, et al. Changes in IGF-I receptor and IGF-I mRNA during differentiation of 3T3-L1 preadipocytes. *Biochimie* 2002;84(10):975–80.

49. Newall F, Wallace T, Crock C, et al. Venous thromboembolic disease: A single-centre case series study. *J Paediatr Child Health* 2006;42(12):803–7.

50. Raffini L, Huang YS, Witmer C, et al. Dramatic increase in venous thromboembolism in children's hospitals in the United States from 2001 to 2007. *Pediatrics* 2009;124(4):1001–8.

51. Sandoval JA, Sheehan MP, Stonerock CE, et al. Incidence, risk factors, and treatment patterns for deep venous thrombosis in hospitalized children: An increasing population at risk. *J Vasc Surg* 2008;47(4):837–43.

52. Wright JM, Watts RG. Venous thromboembolism in pediatric patients: Epidemiologic data from a pediatric tertiary care center in Alabama. *J Pediatr Hematol Oncol* 2011;33(4):261–4.

53. Higgerson RA, Lawson KA, Christie LM, et al. Incidence and risk factors associated with venous thrombotic events in pediatric intensive care unit patients. *Pediatr Crit Care Med* 2011;12(6):628–34.

54. Monagle P, Adams M, Mahoney M, et al. Outcome of pediatric thromboembolic disease: A report from the Canadian Childhood Thrombophilia Registry. *Pediatr Res* 2000;47(6):763–6.

55. Faustino EV, Lawson KA, Northrup V, et al. Mortality-adjusted duration of mechanical ventilation in critically ill children with symptomatic central venous line-related deep venous thrombosis. *Crit Care Med* 2011;39(5):1151–6.

56. Gray BW, Gonzalez R, Warrier KS, et al. Characterization of central venous catheter-associated deep venous thrombosis in infants. *J Pediatr Surg* 2012;47(6):1159–66.

57. Biss TT, Brandao LR, Kahr WH, et al. Clinical features and outcome of pulmonary embolism in children. *Br J Haematol* 2008;142(5):808–18.

58. Monagle P. Diagnosis and management of deep venous thrombosis and pulmonary embolism in neonates and children. *Semin Thromb Hemost.* 2012;38(7):683–90.

59. Monagle P, Newall F, Barnes C, et al. Arterial thromboembolic disease: A single-centre case series study. *J Paediatr Child Health* 2008;44(1–2):28–32.

60. Brotschi B, Hug MI, Latal B, et al. Incidence and predictors of indwelling arterial catheter-related thrombosis in children. *J Thromb Haemost* 2011;9(6):1157–62.

61. de Neef M, Heijboer H, van Woensel JB, et al. The efficacy of heparinization in prolonging patency of arterial and central venous catheters in children: A randomized double-blind trial. *Pediatr Hematol Oncol* 2002;19(8):553–60.

62. Kocis KC, Snider AR, Vermilion RP, et al. Two-dimensional and Doppler ultrasound evaluation of femoral arteries in infants after cardiac catheterization. *Am J Cardiol* 1995;75(8):642–5.

63. Kenet G, Lutkhoff LK, Albisetti M, et al. Impact of thrombophilia on risk of arterial ischemic stroke or cerebral sinovenous thrombosis in neonates and children: A systematic review and meta-analysis of observational studies. *Circulation* 2010;121(16):1838–47.

64. Kenet G, Aronis S, Berkun Y, et al. Impact of persistent antiphospholipid antibodies on risk of incident symptomatic thromboembolism in children: A systematic review and meta-analysis. *Semin Thromb Hemost* 2011;37(7):802–9.

65. Beck C, Dubois J, Grignon A, et al. Incidence and risk factors of catheter-related deep vein thrombosis in a pediatric intensive care unit: A prospective study. *J Pediatr* 1998;133(2):237–41.

66. Male C, Julian JA, Massicotte P, et al. Significant association with location of central venous line placement and risk of venous thrombosis in children. *Thromb Haemost* 2005;94(3):516–21.

67. Male C, Chait P, Andrew M, et al. Central venous line-related thrombosis in children: Association with central venous line location and insertion technique. *Blood* 2003;101(11):4273–8.

68. Faustino EV, Spinella PC, Li S, et al. Incidence and acute complications of asymptomatic central venous catheter-related deep venous thrombosis in critically ill children. *J Pediatr* 2013; 162(2):387–91.

69. van Ommen CH, Heijboer H, Buller HR, et al. Venous thromboembolism in childhood: A prospective two-year registry in The Netherlands. *J Pediatr* 2001;139(5):676–81.

70. Korones DN, Buzzard CJ, Asselin BL, et al. Right atrial thrombi in children with cancer and indwelling catheters. *J Pediatr* 1996; 128(6):841–6.

71. Athale UH, Chan AK. Thromboembolic complications in pediatric hematologic malignancies. *Semin Thromb Hemost* 2007; 33(4):416–26.

72. Kerlin BA, Blatt NB, Fuh B, et al. Epidemiology and risk factors for thromboembolic complications of childhood nephrotic syndrome: A Midwest Pediatric Nephrology Consortium (MWPNC) study. *J Pediatr* 2009;155(1):105–10, 10 e1.

73. Sagripanti A, Barsotti G. Hypercoagulability, intraglomerular coagulation, and thromboembolism in nephrotic syndrome. *Nephron* 1995;70(3):271–81.

74. Bowie EJ, Thompson JH Jr, Pascuzzi CA, et al. Thrombosis in Systemic Lupus Erythematosus Despite Circulating Anticoagulants. *J Lab Clin Med* 1963;62:416–30.

75. Ortel TL. Antiphospholipid syndrome: Laboratory testing and diagnostic strategies. *Am J Hematol* 2012;87 suppl 1:S75–81.

76. Sallam S, Wafa E, el-Gayar A, et al. Anticardiolipin antibodies in children on chronic haemodialysis. *Nephrol Dial Transplant* 1994;9(9):1292–4.

77. Avcin T, Benseler SM, Tyrrell PN, et al. A followup study of antiphospholipid antibodies and associated neuropsychiatric manifestations in 137 children with systemic lupus erythematosus. *Arthritis Rheum* 2008;59(2):206–13.

78. Amiral J, Bridey F, Dreyfus M, et al. Platelet factor 4 complexed to heparin is the target for antibodies generated in heparin-induced thrombocytopenia. *Thromb Haemost* 1992;68(1):95–6.

79. Avila ML, Shah V, Brandao LR. Systematic review on heparin-induced thrombocytopenia in children: A call to action. *J Thromb Haemost* 2013;11(4):660–9.

80. Takemoto CM, Streiff MB. Heparin-induced thrombocytopenia screening and management in pediatric patients. *Hematology Am Soc Hematol Educ Program* 2011;2011:162–9.

81. Spadone D, Clark F, James E, et al. Heparin-induced thrombocytopenia in the newborn. *J Vasc Surg* 1992;15(2):306–11; discussion 311–2.

82. Nsiri B, Gritli N, Bayoudh F, et al. Abnormalities of coagulation and fibrinolysis in homozygous sickle cell disease. *Hematol Cell Ther* 1996;38(3):279–84.

83. Manlhiot C, Menjak IB, Brandao LR, et al. Risk, clinical features, and outcomes of thrombosis associated with pediatric cardiac surgery. *Circulation* 2011;124(14):1511–9.

84. Cholette JM, Rubenstein JS, Alfieris GM, et al. Elevated risk of thrombosis in neonates undergoing initial palliative cardiac surgery. *Ann Thorac Surg* 2007;84(4):1320–5.

85. Seipelt RG, Franke A, Vazquez-Jimenez JF, et al. Thromboembolic complications after Fontan procedures: Comparison of different therapeutic approaches. *Ann Thorac Surg* 2002;74(2):556–62.

86. Hanson SJ, Punzalan RC, Christensen MA, et al. Incidence and risk factors for venous thromboembolism in critically ill children with cardiac disease. *Pediatr Cardiol* 2012;33(1):103–8.

87. Kohlhase B, Vielhaber H, Kehl HG, et al. Thromboembolism and resistance to activated protein C in children with underlying cardiac disease. *J Pediatr* 1996;129(5):677–9.

88. Calderon A, Wong JW, Becker LE. Multiple cerebral venous thromboses in a child with ulcerative colitis. *Clin Pediatr (Phila)* 1993;32(3):169–71.

89. Seligsohn U, Berger A, Abend M, et al. Homozygous protein C deficiency manifested by massive venous thrombosis in the newborn. *N Engl J Med* 1984;310(9):559–62.

90. Marlar RA, Montgomery RR, Broekmans AW. Diagnosis and treatment of homozygous protein C deficiency. Report of the Working Party on Homozygous Protein C Deficiency of the Subcommittee on Protein C and Protein S, International Committee on Thrombosis and Haemostasis. *J Pediatr* 1989;114(4, pt 1):528–34.

91. Young G, Albisetti M, Bonduel M, et al. Impact of inherited thrombophilia on venous thromboembolism in children: A systematic review and meta-analysis of observational studies. *Circulation* 2008;118(13):1373–82.

92. Cattaneo M. Hyperhomocysteinemia and venous thromboembolism. *Semin Thromb Hemost* 2006;32(7):716–23.

93. Nowak-Gottl U, Dubbers A, Kececioglu D, et al. Factor V Leiden, protein C, and lipoprotein (a) in catheter-related thrombosis in childhood: A prospective study. *J Pediatr* 1997;131(4):608–12.

94. Bick RL. Platelet function defects associated with hemorrhage or thrombosis. *Med Clin North Am* 1994;78(3):577–607.

95. Chalmers E, Ganesen V, Liesner R, et al. Guideline on the investigation, management and prevention of venous thrombosis in children. *Br J Haematol* 2011;154(2):196–207.

96. Nuss R, Hays T, Chudgar U, et al. Antiphospholipid antibodies and coagulation regulatory protein abnormalities in children with pulmonary emboli. *J Pediatr Hematol Oncol* 1997;19(3):202–7.

97. Raffini L, Thornburg C. Testing children for inherited thrombophilia: More questions than answers. *Br J Haematol* 2009; 147(3):277–88.

98. Manco-Johnson MJ, Grabowski EF, Hellgreen M, et al. Laboratory testing for thrombophilia in pediatric patients. On behalf of the Subcommittee for Perinatal and Pediatric Thrombosis of the Scientific and Standardization Committee of the International Society of Thrombosis and Haemostasis (ISTH). *Thromb Haemost* 2002;88(1):155–6.

99. Raffini L. Thrombophilia in children: Who to test, how, when, and why? *Hematol Am Soc Hematol Educ Program.* 2008: 228–35.

100. Monagle P, Chan AK, Goldenberg NA, et al. Antithrombotic therapy in neonates and children: Antithrombotic Therapy and Prevention of Thrombosis, 9th ed: American College of Chest Physicians Evidence-Based Clinical Practice Guidelines. *Chest* 2012;141(2 suppl):e737S–801S.

101. Schechter T, Finkelstein Y, Ali M, et al. Unfractionated heparin dosing in young infants: Clinical outcomes in a cohort monitored with anti-factor Xa levels. *J Thromb Haemost* 2012; 10(3):368–74.

102. Monagle P, Newall F. Anticoagulation in children. *Thromb Res* 2012;130(2):142–6.

103. Malherbe S, Tsui BC, Stobart K, et al. Argatroban as anticoagulant in cardiopulmonary bypass in an infant and attempted reversal with recombinant activated factor VII. *Anesthesiology* 2004;100(2):443–5.

104. Dyke PC II, Russo P, Mureebe L, et al. Argatroban for anticoagulation during cardiopulmonary bypass in an infant. *Paediatr Anaesth* 2005;15(4):328–33.

105. Iannoli ED, Eaton MP, Shapiro JR. Bidirectional glenn shunt surgery using lepirudin anticoagulation in an infant with heparin-induced thrombocytopenia with thrombosis. *Anesth Analg* 2005; 101(1):74–6, table of contents.

106. Attard C, Monagle P, Kubitza D, et al. The in vitro anticoagulant effect of rivaroxaban in children. *Thromb Res* 2012; 130(5):804–7.

107. Gupta AA, Leaker M, Andrew M, et al. Safety and outcomes of thrombolysis with tissue plasminogen activator for treatment of intravascular thrombosis in children. *J Pediatr* 2001;139(5): 682–8.

108. Wang M, Hays T, Balasa V, et al. Low-dose tissue plasminogen activator thrombolysis in children. *J Pediatr Hematol Oncol* 2003;25(5):379–86.

109. Darbari DS, Desai D, Arnaldez F, et al. Safety and efficacy of catheter directed thrombolysis in children with deep venous thrombosis. *Br J Haematol* 2012;159(3):376–8.

110. Manco-Johnson MJ, Grabowski EF, Hellgreen M, et al. Recommendations for tPA thrombolysis in children. On behalf of the Scientific Subcommittee on Perinatal and Pediatric Thrombosis of the Scientific and Standardization Committee of the International Society of Thrombosis and Haemostasis. *Thromb Haemost* 2002;88(1):157–8.

111. Raffini L, Trimarchi T, Beliveau J, et al. Thromboprophylaxis in a pediatric hospital: A patient-safety and quality-improvement initiative. *Pediatrics* 2011;127(5):e1326–32.

112. Hanson SJ, Punzalan RC, Arca MJ, et al. Effectiveness of clinical guidelines for deep vein thrombosis prophylaxis in reducing the incidence of venous thromboembolism in critically ill children after trauma. *J Trauma Acute Care Surg* 2012;72(5):1292–7.

113. Faustino EV, Patel S, Thiagarajan RR, et al. Survey of pharmacologic thromboprophylaxis in critically ill children. *Crit Care Med* 2011;39(7):1773–8.

114. Victoria T, Mong A, Altes T, et al. Evaluation of pulmonary embolism in a pediatric population with high clinical suspicion. *Pediatric Radiol* 2009;39(1):35–41.

115. Brandao LR, Simpson EA, Lau KK. Neonatal renal vein thrombosis. *Semin Fetal Neonatal Med* 2011;16(6):323–8.

116. Baird JS, Killinger JS, Kalkbrenner KJ, et al. Massive pulmonary embolism in children. *J Pediatr* 2010;156(1):148–51.

117. Patocka C, Nemeth J. Pulmonary embolism in pediatrics. *J Emer Med* 2012;42(1):105–16.

118. Biss TT, Brandao LR, Kahr WH, et al. Clinical probability score and D-dimer estimation lack utility in the diagnosis of childhood pulmonary embolism. *J Thromb Haemost* 2009;7(10):1633–8.

119. Goldenberg NA, Donadini MP, Kahn SR, et al. Post-thrombotic syndrome in children: A systematic review of frequency of occurrence, validity of outcome measures, and prognostic factors. *Haematologica* 2010;95(11):1952–9.

120. Raffini L, Cahill AM, Hellinger J, et al. A prospective observational study of IVC filters in pediatric patients. *Pediatr blood Cancer* 2008;51(4):517–20.

121. Kulkarni S, Naidu R. Vascular ultrasound imaging to study immediate postcatheterization vascular complications in children. *Catheter Cardiovas Interv* 2006;68(3):450–5.

122. Vitiello R, McCrindle BW, Nykanen D, et al. Complications associated with pediatric cardiac catheterization. *J Am Coll Cardiol* 1998;32(5):1433–40.

123. Lowe EJ, Werner EJ. Thrombotic thrombocytopenic purpura and hemolytic uremic syndrome in children and adolescents. *Semin Thromb Hemost* 2005;31(6):717–30.

124. Manea M, Karpman D. Molecular basis of ADAMTS13 dysfunction in thrombotic thrombocytopenic purpura. *Pediatr Nephrol* 2009;24(3):447–58.

CHAPTER 117 ■ HEMATOPOIETIC CELL TRANSPLANTATION

MONICA BHATIA AND KATHERINE BIAGAS

KEY POINTS

1 Hematopoietic cell transplantation, derived from bone marrow, peripheral blood, or cord blood, is used for malignant and nonmalignant conditions.

2 Specialized preparation of the recipient, including myeloablation or partial ablation, and processing of hematopoietic cells, is required for transplantation.

3 Posttransplantation supportive care includes preemptive or prophylactic antimicrobials, treatment for graft-versus-host disease (GVHD), treatment for sinusoidal obstructive syndrome (SOS), nutritional support, protective isolation, and minimization of opportunities infections.

4 Critical illness may occur in these patients with respiratory failure—severe infection, including opportunistic infections, acute kidney injury (AKI), dyselectrolytemias, severe GVHD, or severe SOS—all necessitating pediatric intensive care unit care. The pediatric intensivist should be familiar with management of all of these conditions.

5 Respiratory failure may be life threatening. Noninvasive modes of ventilation are preferred, if tolerated.

6 AKI is often multifactorial. Management consists of supportive care. Renal replacement therapy has greatly assisted in the management of fluids and electrolytes in these patients.

7 Patients who are prone to life-threatening infections, especially opportunistic infections, require aggressive management with appropriate workup and antimicrobials.

8 GVHD is unique to this treatment and results in injury to the skin, gastrointestinal tract, and liver.

9 SOS, induced by chemotherapeutic and radiation injuries, contributes to morbidity (hepatic failure, hepatorenal syndrome) and mortality.

Hematopoietic cell transplantation (HCT) has been used increasingly for the treatment of malignant and nonmalignant conditions. For the pediatric intensivist, familiarity with the types of transplantation, preparative regimens, common complications, comorbidities, and related medical emergencies is crucial. Transplantation patients may be brought to the intensive care unit (ICU) for commonly occurring critical conditions and for primary problems associated with the transplantation. Outcomes for ICU stays may be poor for some but good results are possible (1) and ICU care should not be considered futile (2). Transplant patients can suffer common critical illness such as respiratory failure, fluid and electrolyte disturbances, life-threatening infections, renal failure, and multiple organ dysfunction syndrome (MODS). History of total-body irradiation and renal dysfunction is associated with higher risk of PICU admission. Sepsis and shock are associated with higher mortality (3). The usual principles of management for these conditions apply, but additional factors that result from the transplantation or the underlying condition should be appreciated. Conditions more unique to HCT, such as sinusoidal obstructive syndrome (SOS) (previously known as veno-occlusive disease [VOD]) and graft-versus-host disease (GVHD), may result. Improvements in survival after HCT mean that some complications present long after the procedure (e.g., infections, chronic organ failure, relapse of primary disease, or more severe courses of common medical conditions). This chapter focuses on the management of critical illness associated with the types of HCT and the medical conditions associated with them.

OVERVIEW OF HEMATOPOIETIC CELL TRANSPLANTATION IN CHILDREN AND ADOLESCENTS

HCT has been successfully used in a variety of childhood and adolescent diseases, including malignant conditions, immune deficiencies, inborn errors of metabolism, genetic disorders, hematopoietic disorders, and autoimmune conditions. The most common childhood and adolescent malignant conditions treated with HCT include acute lymphoblastic leukemia, acute nonlymphoblastic leukemia, chronic myelogenous leukemia, neuroblastoma, non-Hodgkin lymphoma, Hodgkin disease, and poor-risk brain tumors (Table 117.1). The most common nonmalignant conditions that have been successfully cured with HCT include sickle cell disease, homozygous β thalassemia, severe combined immune deficiency, Wiskott–Aldrich syndrome, hemophagocytic lymphohistiocytosis, and severe aplastic anemia (Table 117.1).

Sources of Hematopoietic Progenitor Cells

Hematopoietic progenitor cells (HPCs) may be collected and obtained from three donor locations—bone marrow (BM), peripheral blood, or cord blood (CB). Three donor sources of HPCs are possible with risks and benefits related to each origin. *Autologous HPCs* are progenitor cells obtained from the

TABLE 117.1

CHILDHOOD AND ADOLESCENT DISEASES SUCCESSFULLY TREATED
WITH HEMATOPOIETIC CELL TRANSPLANTATION

■ MALIGNANT DISEASES	■ NONMALIGNANT DISEASES
ALL, ANLL, CML	SAA, FA, SCID, WAS, HLH
Neuroblastoma, brain tumors	SCD, BT
NHL, HD, Wilms tumor	ALD, Hurler disease

ALL, acute lymphoblastic leukemia; ANLL, acute non-lymphoblastic leukemia; CML, chronic myelogenous leukemia; NHL, non-Hodgkin lymphoma; HD, Hodgkin disease; SAA, severe aplastic anemia; FA, Fanconi anemia; SCID, severe combined immunodeficiency disorder; WAS, Wiskott–Aldrich syndrome; HLH, hemophagocytic lymphohistiocytosis, SCD, sickle cell disease; BT, β thalassemia; ALD, adrenoleukodystrophy.

recipient (self). *Syngeneic HPCs* are obtained from an identical twin and, therefore, are genetically identical. *Allogeneic HPCs* are cells obtained from a human being other than a genetically identical twin (**Table 117.2**). Selection of allogeneic donors is determined by histocompatibility testing between the donor and the recipient.

Histocompatibility leukocyte antigens (HLAs) comprise a highly polymorphic, closely linked group of genes located on the short arm of chromosome 6 that regulate T-cell recognition and are critical to both immunocompetence and self-tolerance. The two major classes of HLA antigens include HLA class I antigens (A, B, C) and class II antigens (DR, DQ, DP). The preferred allogeneic donor source is a genotypic-matched sibling donor who usually matches at the HLA-A, -B, and DR loci (6 out of 6 matches). Additional allogeneic donor sources include related mismatched family members, including parents and other siblings who match at 6 out of 6 or 5 out of 6 antigens at HLA-A, -B, and DRB1. If a closely matched family donor is not available, two large sources of unrelated donors exist—unrelated adult donors and unrelated CB donors. When using unrelated donors, it is preferable to have donors match recipients at 7 or 8 out of 8 antigens at the HLA-A, -B, -C, and DRB1 loci.

Fewer than 25% of potential recipients have an HLA-identical related sibling or parental donor. Therefore, efforts have been made to develop alternative sources of HPCs for allogeneic hematopoietic cell transplantation (alloHCT). The Bone Marrow Donor Worldwide program has established a computerized registry of potential volunteer adult donors and has over 22 million potential adult donors currently available for unrelated donor HCT. Additionally, a number of umbilical CB banks have been established throughout the world, and over 600,000 CB donor units have been cryopreserved and are currently available for unrelated CB donor transplantation. The use of CB donor units has also extended the option of HCT to adults unable to find acceptable matched unrelated donors. Results with unrelated CB donor transplantation have suggested that cell dose and HLA disparity are the most important predictors of outcome. To date, the use of unrelated CB donor transplantation has been associated with delayed

hematopoietic reconstitution, decreased severe acute GVHD (aGVHD), and decreased chronic GVHD (cGVHD) in children and adolescents (4).

Preparative Therapy or Conditioning

Prior to infusion of HPCs, most patients receive some form of conditioning or preparative therapy, usually consisting of myeloablative therapy, which commonly includes total-body irradiation (TBI) with additional high-dose chemotherapy (chemoradiotherapy). Alternatively in some settings of alloHCT, a nonmyeloablative or reduced-intensity conditioning regimen may be used (5,6). Myeloablative conditioning is uniform for autologous transplantation, in large part because of the need to eradicate any remaining tumor cells. The HPC infusion rescues the patient from hematopoietic toxicity and reduces the time to hematopoietic reconstitution. Common, acute complications following myeloablative conditioning include mucositis, infection, bleeding, pain, nausea, and vomiting. However, some centers have initiated the use of nonmyeloablative conditioning to reduce the acute and long-term effects that usually follow the myeloablative approach. The premise of nonmyeloablative, or reduced-intensity conditioning, followed by alloHCT is to provide enough immunosuppression to allow the allogeneic graft to be accepted while decreasing the associated morbidities that commonly occur following myeloablative conditioning. These types of nonmyeloablative or reduced-intensity conditioning regimens work best in selected diseases that have an unusual sensitivity to a graft-versus-tumor effect, diseases with a genetic defect, and diseases that may benefit from a graft-versus-autoimmune effect. Additionally, it allows older patients with comorbidities the option of HCT as they would not likely tolerate a myeloablative regimen (5,6).

Collection of Hematopoietic Progenitor Cells

HPCs can be obtained from the BM, peripheral blood, or placental CB. BM HPCs are collected by BM harvesting, in which either the patient (autologous) or the donor undergoes general or regional anesthesia. Multiple BM aspirations are obtained from the posterior iliac crest (bilaterally) or, on occasion, from the anterior iliac crest. The total amount collected from a BM harvest is usually dependent on the size of the recipient. Most autologous collections (historically performed using BM harvesting) are now performed by apheresis. However, HPC collection from allogeneic donors still primarily uses BM harvesting.

Peripheral-blood HPCs are harvested after the patient's or the donor's white cells are mobilized with cytokines, typically granulocyte colony-stimulating factor (GCSF). Recovery from cytotoxic chemotherapy combined with GCSF also mobilizes peripheral-blood HPCs, making it an effective approach for

TABLE 117.2

SOURCES OF HEMATOPOIETIC PROGENITOR CELLS

■ TYPE	■ SOURCE	■ LOCATION
Autologous	Self (recipient)	BM, PB, CB
Syngeneic	Identical twin	BM, PB, CB
Allogeneic	Human other than identical twin	BM, PB, CB

BM, bone marrow; PB, peripheral blood; CB, cord blood.

autologous transplantation. Collection is performed by apheresis in which multiple blood volumes are processed to extract a buffy coat layer that is rich in HPCs. Apheresis has the advantage of not requiring anesthesia and has a low rate of serious complications, although electrolyte disturbances and exacerbation of thrombocytopenia may occur.

The third source of HPCs can be obtained at the time of delivery from placental CB. In the past, the placenta and umbilical cord were discarded after delivery. However, the umbilical CB is rich in HPCs and a minimum volume of 60 mL may contain enough HPCs to engraft a recipient following myeloablative therapy. Cell dose and HLA disparity are the two primary factors in the success following CB transplantation. Data suggest that two CB units can be combined to circumvent a low CB-cell dose from a single unit. Outcomes appear to be similar or better using two CB units.

Processing Hematopoietic Progenitor Cells

HPCs sometimes require processing before infusion into the recipient. Autologous stem-cell transplantation (AutoHCT) requires collection of HPCs from the recipient prior to myeloablation. As mentioned above, HPCs may be collected by BM harvesting, peripheral-blood apheresis, or, on occasion, CB collection (i.e., for future autologous use). To preserve autologous HPCs, cell processing must be performed for long-term cryopreservation. Cryopreservation uses 5%–10% dimethyl sulfoxide (DMSO) to protect cells during the freezing period and ensure their long-term viability. However, the addition of DMSO to autologous HPCs results in an increased risk of infusion-related reactions such as anaphylaxis or even death. Once cryopreserved cells are thawed, they are washed before infusion to minimize infusion-related reactions.

Allogeneic HPCs usually do not require significant processing prior to infusion. On the rare occasion that infusion of the transplant is delayed from the time of collection, allogeneic HPCs may be cryopreserved (with the same risk of DMSO-related reactions). Additionally, allogeneic HPCs may require red blood cell depletion because of ABO blood group incompatibility between the donor allogeneic HPCs and the recipient. Depleting ABO-mismatched red blood cells from the allogeneic HPCs may prevent an ABO-related hemolytic reaction and may be life-saving. Lastly, allogeneic HPCs may be depleted of T-cells to reduce the incidence of aGVHD. Transplants from haploidentical donors (siblings or parents matched at 3 out of 6 HLA loci) and/or HLA disparate, unrelated, adult donors are associated with a high incidence of serious aGVHD. Some require a depletion of total or subpopulations of T-cells to prevent severe aGVHD. T-cell depletion, however, may result in delay in hematopoietic reconstitution and is commonly associated with a delay in immunologic reconstitution and an increased incidence of Epstein–Barr virus-related posttransplant lymphoproliferative syndrome (PTLD).

HPCs derived from CB almost always require prior cell processing and cryopreservation, as they are most commonly collected from unrelated maternal donors who are located at distant sites.

Infusion of Hematopoietic Progenitor Cells

Most recipients are premedicated with hydrocortisone, diphenhydramine, and acetaminophen before HPC infusion. Usually, HPCs are infused through a central venous catheter. Infusions of HPC may result in acute reactions, including fever, chills, tachycardia, bradycardia, hypotension, respiratory

distress, allergic reactions, and, on rare occasions, anaphylaxis. Furthermore, if the HPCs are contaminated with microbial organisms, HPC infusion may result in overwhelming infection. In the setting of ABO incompatibility, hemolytic reactions may occur despite red blood cell depletion. Patients who receive HPC products are closely monitored during the infusion while under the care of a trained medical provider who stays at the bedside.

Graft-versus-host Disease Prophylaxis

The setting of alloHCT is associated with a measurable risk of the patient developing acute and/or cGVHD. GVHD is an entity where donor-derived cells may recognize recipient organs as foreign and mount an immune attack against the patient's own tissues (7). GVHD most commonly occurs after alloHCT; however, it has been reported to occur in ~10% of patients following AutoHCT and with blood transfusions (8). There are three risk factors for the development of GVHD in alloHCT: a depressed or abnormal immune system in the recipient, donor cells that are immunocompetent, and an HLA disparity.

Additional factors can contribute to the risk of developing GVHD, including type of allogeneic donor source, the T-cell dose administered, age of the donor, age of the recipient, type of GVHD prophylaxis, underlying disease, type of conditioning therapy, associated comorbidities, risk of developing cytomegalovirus (CMV) disease, and other minor factors. In general, the highest risk of developing GVHD occurs following haploidentical family donor transplants followed by adult unrelated donor transplants and unrelated CB transplants. The lowest risk occurs in those transplants using matched, related family donors. Prevention of GVHD involves careful selection of family and unrelated donor sources and prophylactic therapies with carefully selected combinations of immunosuppressive medications. Previous GVHD prophylaxis regimens have used steroids, cyclosporine, and methotrexate. Recent regimens incorporate tacrolimus, mycophenolate mofetil, sirolimus, antithymocyte globulin, and alemtuzumab. Many combinations of prophylactic immunosuppressive therapies exist. While the administration of immunosuppressive medications may result in a decreased incidence or decreased severity of GVHD, such therapies also increase the risk of serious opportunistic infections. The delicate balance between the prevention of GVHD and an increased risk of developing serious opportunistic infections presents a challenge.

Another GVHD prophylaxis approach is T-cell depletion of allogeneic HCT donor sources, which results in an extremely low incidence of GVHD after significant T-cell depletion. However, this type of cell processing also results in a higher incidence of graft failure. Additionally, there may also be a delay or reduction in allogeneic HPC engraftment and, more importantly, a delay in immune reconstitution with attendant increase in opportunistic infections and/or malignant relapse. It should be stressed that there is a delicate balance between overzealous T-cell depletion, which may eliminate the GVHD risk, and a less vigorous T-cell depletion, which may result in GVHD of reduced severity without a significant increase in serious opportunistic infections (9).

Supportive Care

Reconstitution of Hematopoietic Cells

Supportive care regimens are employed post-HPC transplantation to accelerate HPC reconstitution and prevent serious opportunistic infections. Hematopoietic reconstitution is accelerated using hematopoietic growth factors, either GCSF or granulocyte macrophage colony-stimulating factor (GM-CSF), and is performed after AutoHCT and alloHCT. They are administered after the HPC infusion and until neutrophil recovery. While hematopoietic growth factors probably enhance the time to neutrophil reconstitution, it is not certain that the improvement in neutrophil recovery results in improved survival or decreased morbidity (10).

Additional Support

Additional supportive care includes the use of irradiated and leukodepleted blood products, total parenteral nutrition, intravenous (IV) gamma globulin supplementation, good oral hygiene, catheter care protocols, protective isolation, and
3 other infection-preventive methods. A multidisciplinary team that includes pediatric HCT physicians, nurses, HCT coordinators, clinical pharmacists, nurse practitioners, dieticians, psychologists, social workers, child-life therapists, occupational therapists, physical therapists, and pediatric intensivists is required to provide supportive care throughout the pre- and post-HCT period. Moreover, when pediatric HCT recipients require intensive care, psychosocial support is required by patients and their families to help them cope during this stressful period.

RESPIRATORY FAILURE ASSOCIATED WITH TRANSPLANTATION

Clinical Presentation

Respiratory failure is the leading cause of mortality and mor-
4 bidity in children who undergo HCT (11). Dyspnea, impaired gas exchange, and respiratory system dysfunction are common presenting signs. Causes are infectious and noninfectious

TABLE 117.3

CAUSES OF PULMONARY DISEASE

Early Recovery Period
  Bacterial and fungal infections
  Sepsis
  Mucositis and upper airway obstruction
  Peri-engraftment respiratory distress syndrome
  Acute pulmonary edema
  Acute graft-versus-host disease
  Congestive heart failure
  Pulmonary vascular disease
  Diffuse alveolar hemorrhage

Mid-Recovery Period
  Cytomegalovirus pneumonitis (primary or reactivation)
  Opportunistic infections
  Idiopathic pulmonary syndrome
  Interstitial pneumonitis

Late Recovery Period
  Common childhood infections
  Cytomegalovirus reactivation
  Adenovirus infection
  Chronic graft-versus-host disease
  Bronchiolitis obliterans

(Table 117.3). The respiratory dysfunction is generally restrictive in nature, often with a reduction in diffusion capacity. Lung disease may also have a substantial obstructive component. Mortality is decreasing for this population and recent trends suggest that improvements in ventilator management have resulted in fewer complications, decreased severity of GVHD, less severe MODS, and better outcomes (12). However, mortality remains high for those with extreme respiratory failure (13).

Mechanisms of Disease

Infections That Cause Respiratory Failure

Early Recovery Period. Pulmonary infections tend to occur in specific epochs. In the early posttransplant period (up to 30 days), patients are neutropenic and susceptible to bacterial and fungal infections, especially *Aspergillus* and *Candida* species. *Aspergillus* infections in this early phase may be particularly severe, with angioinvasive disease. Isolation from respiratory specimens, including bronchoalveolar lavage (BAL), is specific but not sensitive (14). BAL has a positive predictive value of 82% (15). High-resolution computerized tomography (CT) is usually the study of choice. If CT lesions are peripheral, a lung biopsy may be indicated.

Noninfectious complications of this early posttransplantation period include pulmonary edema and fluid overload, drug reactions, congestive heart failure, and aGVHD. These may be superimposed on infection and worsen pulmonary function. The phenomenon of peri-engraftment respiratory distress syndrome (PERDS), previously referred to as engraftment syndrome, is characterized by fever, rash, and pulmonary edema and is frequently seen in AutoHCT patients (16). PERDS is generally mild and resolves with white cell recovery but may complicate other causes of respiratory failure in the early period. Clinical presentations of transplant-associated pulmonary infections are similar to those of patients without transplantation—fever, increased work of breathing, progressive respiratory insufficiency, and progressive hypoxemia with eventual respiratory acidosis. In those with severe disease, progression to respiratory failure is often quite rapid.

Mid-Recovery Period. In the second posttransplantation phase (30–100 days post-HCT), viral infections predominate particularly CMV infection. CMV pneumonitis has a very high fatality rate and is higher in recipients of HCT than in those with solid-organ transplants. Increased incidence of the disease is seen in certain subpopulations, namely, patients who are seropositive, are older, have received TBI, or suffer from more severe GVHD. Approximately 20%–30% of patients with GVHD develop CMV pneumonitis. The use of leukocyte-depleted (CMV is an intracellular organism that is latent in lymphocytes) and seronegative blood products has reduced the incidence of the CMV pneumonitis. Prophylaxis with ganciclovir or preemptive treatment with that drug or valganciclovir has decreased disease incidence. For demonstrated cases, the combination of ganciclovir and CMV-specific immunoglobulin has reduced mortality dramatically. Progression of disease to frank respiratory failure carries high mortality (16,17). Diagnosis can be confirmed by DNA PCR assay or positive viral cultures.

Patients in this stage are also at risk for infection with community-acquired viruses (e.g., respiratory syncytial virus [RSV], adenovirus, and influenza). Infection rates for these viruses follow seasonal variations. Patients are also at risk for infections with other opportunistic organisms, particularly *Pneumocystis jiroveci* in the first few posttransplantation months (see also Management of Infections section below). The use of low-dose trimethoprim-sulfamethoxazole (TMP-SMX) (5 mg TMP/kg/day in divided doses every 12 hours, 3 days/week) or pentamidine (4 mg/kg IV infused daily every 14 days or 300 mg given by inhalation every 28 days) provides effective prophylaxis and greatly reduces the incidence in this patient population. For true *Pneumocystis* infection, TMP-SMX is the treatment of choice (15–20 mg TMP/kg/day in divided doses every 6–8 hours) (14). IV pentamidine can be used in patients unable to tolerate TMP-SMX. Confirmed cases of *Pneumocystis pneumonia* (PCP) should be investigated for antimicrobial resistance or noncompliance with the prophylaxis regimen.

Late Recovery Period. In the late posttransplantation phase (more than 100 days post-HCT infusion), noninfectious pulmonary complications predominate, such as bronchiolitis obliterans (BO), cryptogenic-organizing pneumonia, and cGVHD. Pulmonary infections in this phase may include those that are more common in childhood. However, infections with unusual organisms such as *Aspergillus* and *Nocardia*, as well as infections with encapsulated bacteria, have been reported (16). Late CMV infection may also be seen (17). CMV reactivation, as well as adenovirus infection, should be considered in children with late-onset, progressive, respiratory insufficiency.

Respiratory Failure From Noninfectious Causes

The hallmarks of noninfectious pulmonary diseases are interstitial disease, restrictive changes of respiratory system components, and chronic airflow obstruction. These result from host responses to radiation and previous cytotoxic therapy, as well as ongoing injury and multiple organ dysfunction. Noninfectious respiratory diseases include mucositis with upper airway inflammation and obstruction, pulmonary edema, idiopathic pulmonary syndrome (IPS), pulmonary vascular disease, interstitial pneumonitis, and BO. Extreme cases of oropharyngeal mucositis may result in laryngeal edema, which may require tracheal intubation to maintain patency. Additionally, copious oral secretions and bleeding may occur with aspiration into the respiratory tree.

Pulmonary Edema. Pulmonary edema is one of the most common early complications of HCT and has several causes. Large volumes of fluids are often needed to administer medications, minimize their toxicity, and provide parenteral nutrition. Renal dysfunction is common. Additionally, cardiac dysfunction may be present, including congestive cardiomyopathy from prior use of anthracyclines and/or mediastinal irradiation. The necessary use of large fluid volumes in patients with such dysfunctions is often poorly tolerated and pulmonary edema results. Lastly, patients may have concurrent processes that promote a systemic inflammatory response syndrome (SIRS).

Idiopathic Pulmonary Syndrome. The American Thoracic Society has defined IPS as an "idiopathic syndrome of pneumopathy after HCT with evidence of widespread alveolar injury and in which an infectious etiology, cardiac dysfunction, acute renal failure, or iatrogenic fluid overload have been excluded" (18). Onset is generally 50–100 days after HCT, usually in the sixth to seventh week posttransplant. Possible etiologies include HCT conditioning, inflammation, and latent viral infection (17,19). Another possibility is that IPS is a pulmonary manifestation of severe GVHD. Indeed, for some patients, aGVHD is known to precede IPS (19). Findings include diffuse infiltrates, abnormal gas exchange, and the absence of infectious organisms.

Pulmonary Vascular Disease and Diffuse Alveolar Hemorrhage. Clinically important pulmonary vascular disease is rare, although many patients have subclinical abnormalities.

Pulmonary vascular involvement includes thromboembolism, thrombus *in situ*, pulmonary VOD, and diffuse alveolar hemorrhage. Clinical signs are those of acute, congestive right heart failure with hepatic engorgement, jugular venous distention, tachycardia, and right ventricular heave. Pulmonary vascular disease with diffuse alveolar hemorrhage may be especially severe and is an important cause of early morbidity and mortality. In addition to the clinical signs noted above, patients present with progressive hypoxemia, dyspnea, and diffuse infiltrates on chest x-ray. Hemoptysis is rare, although examination of BAL fluid demonstrates hemosiderin-laden macrophages and fluid that becomes progressively bloodier with successive normal saline aliquots. High doses of corticosteroids (>100 mg/day of methylprednisolone or equivalent) may be effective in reducing mortality from diffuse alveolar hemorrhage.

Bronchiolitis Obliterans. cGVHD plays an important role in the development of BO and BO is estimated to affect 10% of surviving transplant recipients (20). The fact that BO occurs almost exclusively in this population suggests that the pathophysiologic mechanism is chronic rejection of transplanted cells by the lung. However, other nonimmunologic factors such as concurrent respiratory infection and prolonged methotrexate administration may contribute. Moreover, BO has been reported in autologous transplant patients and HLA-matched recipients, supporting the possibility of mechanisms other than rejection. Patients present with progressive dyspnea on exertion, nonproductive cough, and breathing patterns of obstructive disease, so-called braking respirations or pursed-lipped breathing. Pulmonary function tests reveal nonreversible obstructive airflow. Chest x-ray shows hyperinflation with or without infiltrates. Biopsy material shows occlusion of the lumens of respiratory and terminal bronchioles with inflammatory and fibrous material. In extreme cases, termed *constrictive obliterative bronchiolitis*, cicatricial scarring is present, with obliteration of distal airways. As disease may be patchy, transbronchial lung biopsies may not demonstrate the pathology. Open biopsy is required for pathologic confirmation of BO. However, most centers consider compatible history and symptoms, chest x-ray findings, and consistent findings on pulmonary function test to be sufficient in making the diagnosis. BAL is of limited use and is generally performed to rule out associated infection. Therapy consists of augmented immunosuppression and bronchodilators. Reversal of airway obstruction is usually only partial, and associated lung infection may worsen with the increase in immunosuppressive therapy. In cases with concurrent infection, BAL is necessary to target antimicrobial therapy appropriately.

Outcomes From Respiratory Failure

The final common pathways for severe restrictive lung disease of both infectious and noninfectious end-stage disease are acute lung injury (ALI) and acute respiratory distress syndrome (ARDS). ALI/ARDS may also develop during acute reversible disease and obstructive lung disease may be superimposed (as with BO). Disease severe enough to result in respiratory failure tends to occur early in the posttransplantation phase. White cell reconstitution, especially with administration of GCSF, may increase the risk of developing ARDS (21). Patients present with fluid overload, weight gain, clinical signs of respiratory failure, and often, liver and/or renal dysfunction. Death comes from MODS. Survival is unlikely in children who have dysfunction of more than one organ system after 7 days of mechanical ventilation (22). In adults, the need for mechanical ventilation has also been shown to carry an extreme mortality rate (16).

Management of Respiratory Failure

Noninvasive Ventilation

In the least, the need for mechanical ventilation is a marker of illness severity. And ventilator-associated complications contribute to death. Volutrauma, barotrauma, and oxygen toxicity add to lung injury. Ventilator-associated pneumonia, especially in the setting of profound immunosuppression, contributes to morbidity. But the need for mechanical ventilation may not, in and of itself, be indicative of certain death (1).

Advances in noninvasive ventilatory support with either continuous positive-airway pressure or bi-level positive-airway pressure may avoid some of these complications by avoiding endotracheal intubation. Normalization of gas exchange is not necessary; respiratory acidosis (generally pH $\geq$ 7.15) and moderate hypoxemia are usually well tolerated. Close observation for worsened condition is an absolute.

Mechanical Ventilation

For patients who require intubation, aggressive measures should be used to quickly make a diagnosis. Empiric therapy for likely causes should begin immediately and be revised according to findings. Treatment of cardiac failure, supportive care for renal and liver failure, and management of fluid overload are important adjunctive therapies. Prone positioning and alternating prone-supine positions may improve oxygenation. An "open-lung" strategy that limits ventilator peak pressures to 25 torr and tidal volumes to 6–8 mL/kg should be employed to minimize ventilator-induced injury. If possible, positive end-expiratory pressure should be used liberally, and the fraction of inspired oxygen should be limited to $\leq$0.60. Again, permissive hypercapnia with respiratory acidosis and moderate hypoxemia are tolerated. If adequate oxygenation cannot be achieved with such measures, consideration should be given to the use of high-frequency oscillatory ventilation, which may lessen ventilator-induced lung injury. Irrespective of the mode of delivery, the duration of mechanical ventilation should be as short as possible; "pushing" patients off of such support to noninvasive ventilatory support should be an interim goal.

Controversies

Controversy surrounds the use of some of the more novel respiratory support modes in patients with HCT and severe ARDS given their poor prognosis (mortality nearly 100%). No biomarkers or clinical signs allow clinicians to predict HCT patients who will survive ARDS. Accordingly, some of the more novel modes of respiratory support have been tried, but none are proven therapies. These attempts include administration of surfactant, inhaled nitric oxide, and other pulmonary vasodilators. The use of extracorporeal membrane oxygenation (ECMO) in HCT patients is also surrounded by controversy. More than a decade ago, HCT patients with cardiorespiratory failure so severe as to be considered for ECMO were felt to have irreversible disease. But, a 2006 review of the Extracorporeal Life Support Organization Registry experience reported that ECMO has been used for isolated respiratory (VV ECMO) and cardiorespiratory (VA ECMO) support in children after HCT (23). Only 21% of children survived ECMO and only one survived to discharge. Predictors of outcomes were not evident in the data. Sensible consideration of ECMO should take into account the likelihood of disease being readily reversible and the burden of associated MODS. It should be stressed that the mainstay of therapy for patients with ARDS after HCT is largely supportive with efforts focused on minimizing ventilator-associated damage, diagnosing

and treating respiratory pathology, controlling fluid overload, and managing MODS.

RENAL FAILURE ASSOCIATED WITH TRANSPLANTATION

Clinical Presentation

Renal dysfunction and acute kidney injury (AKI) are common after HCT. Approximately 25%–50% of children have renal dysfunction in the first 3 months after transplantation, and more than 10% require renal replacement therapy (RRT), usually to control fluid imbalance. AKI after HCT contributes to mortality and doubling of serum creatinine is associated with a doubling in mortality (24). Patients who require dialysis for correction of severe acidosis or electrolyte disturbances have a mortality that is 80% or more (24).

Early Renal Dysfunction

The causes of AKI in the early period (first 3 months) are numerous (**Table 117.4**). Often, multiple factors influence patient's renal function. Preexisting renal dysfunction may be present in children who have had cytotoxic therapy for their primary disease. Conditioning regimens may be additionally nephrotoxic. Special note should be made of patients with reduced glomerular filtration rate (GFR) and preexisting Fanconi syndrome or previous unilateral nephrectomy, as these patients have a poorer prognosis. For the majority, reduction in GFR is the chief dysfunction, although specific correlation between pretransplant GFR and AKI has not been found (24).

Mechanisms of Disease

Nephrotoxicity With Hematopoietic Progenitor Cell Infusion. In a few cases, nephrotoxicity is seen with HPC infusion. The mechanisms of injury are not fully known. Some speculate that release of free hemoglobin and cytotoxic products from cellular lysis during storage of HPC causes tubular obstruction and damage. The proximal tubules are particularly affected. In addition, infusion of the cryoprotectant DMSO may cause hemoglobinuria and contribute to pigment-induced nephropathy. These insults occur on the background

TABLE 117.4

CAUSES OF ACUTE KIDNEY INJURY

Early Period
Preexisting renal disease
 Previous nephrectomy
 Preexisting Fanconi syndrome
Nephrotoxic agents
Infusion of preserved hematopoietic progenitor cells
Sepsis
 Shock
 Hepatitis B or C infection
 Adenovirus infection
Hepatorenal syndrome
 Hepatic veno-occlusive disease
Indirect effects
 Obstructive hemorrhagic nephritis
 Treatment of acute graft-versus-host disease
Late Period
"Bone marrow transplant nephropathy"

of preexisting injury and recent conditioning and may result in dramatic and immediate onset of AKI with acute tubular necrosis.

Sepsis and Acute Kidney Injury. Sepsis, with or without hypotension, is a common cause of AKI. As many as 25%–40% of patients with sepsis in the early posttransplant phase develop AKI. The incidence is even higher in patients with culture-proven infection and a requirement for RRT (24). Impairment of GFR results from maldistribution of blood flow, impaired cardiac output, and vasoparesis of the renal efferent arterioles. Frank shock may ensue and further reduce GFR. Direct glomerular and tubular injury may be induced by cytokines and other inflammatory cascades. Although infection of the kidney is rare, renal abscesses with fungal or Gram-negative bacterial species occur. Infection with viruses (adenoviruses and especially BK virus) can cause primary nephritis while hepatitis B or C infection may cause membranous glomerulonephropathy. Additional deleterious effects on the kidney are seen with nephrotoxic side effects of antimicrobial therapies. Although often required, antimicrobials such as vancomycin, aminoglycosides, amphotericin B, and β-lactam antibiotics require careful consideration when used in patients with already reduced renal function. Empiric courses of these antibiotics should be as short as possible. Medication doses and dosing regimens should be adjusted for the patient's creatinine clearance. Other conditions of sepsis may contribute. Hepatic dysfunction with CMV infection, sepsis, or SOS may lead to hepatorenal syndrome.

Hepatorenal Syndrome. The most severe form of renal disease in the early phase of transplantation is hepatorenal syndrome, characterized by hepatic dysfunction with poor GFR, sodium retention, peripheral edema, weight gain, and ascites. Hepatic failure usually accompanies sepsis, GVHD, or SOS and is heralded by hyperbilirubinemia with mild elevations in serum transaminase levels. Patients also demonstrate a high blood urea/creatinine ratio. Patients are fluid overloaded with urinary excretion of small glycoproteins, suggesting proximal tubule and prerenal injury. Clinically, patients have pulmonary edema, hypotension, and preserved urine output, especially in the early phase of the condition. Urine output falls later and hypotension worsens. Severe hepatorenal syndrome is associated with a very high risk of mortality.

Rarely, other conditions may indirectly cause renal dysfunction. Hemorrhagic cystitis, although not generally nephrotoxic, may cause bladder obstruction and postrenal failure. Maintenance of brisk urine output is essential in such cases, and aGVHD, while not involving the kidney primarily, may require treatment, which may be nephrotoxic.

Late Renal Dysfunction

Late renal dysfunction, termed "BMT nephropathy," occurs more than 3 months after HCT and is most likely in patients with history of TBI. The incidence may be higher in young children than in adults as the developing kidney may have less tolerance for TBI. BMT nephropathy is similar to hemolytic uremic syndrome or thrombotic thrombocytopenic purpura syndrome, with hypertension, peripheral edema, and microangiopathic hemolytic anemia. Renal dysfunction may be rapidly progressive with accompanying proteinuria and, sometimes, hematuria. Plasma exchange and immunoadsorption have been attempted for fulminant cases of BMT nephropathy (24), although efficacy of such therapies has not been proved.

Management of Renal Failure

Therapeutic approaches for AKI are few. Care for the kidney is largely supportive. Prevention of injury or slowing injury progression is important. The use of nephrotoxic antibiotics must be carefully considered, their use monitored, and less toxic preparations (e.g., the liposomal form of amphotericin B) chosen when possible. Chemotherapy should be adjusted in children with reduced GFR (e.g., the use of less toxic platinum derivatives) and renal perfusion should be preserved. Intravascular volume must be maintained, despite losses from vomiting, diarrhea, or "third spacing" of fluids. IV administration of fluid in excess of maintenance requirements, sometimes more than twofold greater than maintenance, may be required. The use of angiotensin-converting enzyme inhibitors, which can reduce GFR, should be avoided unless specifically indicated (e.g., indicated for BMT nephropathy). Heart failure should be treated, hypertension controlled, and vigorous efforts made to identify underlying treatable conditions, such as sepsis, GVHD, or SOS.

Diuretic Therapy

The simplest renal therapy is the vigorous use of diuretics with or without hyperhydration. In patients with normal urine output, especially those with requirements for large volumes of IV fluids, frequent doses of diuretics may diminish fluid overload while maintaining normal intravascular volume. Usual diuretics are the loop agents, such as bumetanide or furosemide, but others may be effective (**Table 117.5**). Both bolus administration and continuous infusion may be used. The latter is better tolerated in patients with hemodynamic compromise. In the oliguric patient who is estimated to be volume replete, a trial of larger than standard-dose furosemide (2–4 mg/kg to a maximum dose of 200 mg) may be made; however, the potential

---

TABLE 117.5

INTRAVENOUS DIURETIC THERAPY IN FLUID OVERLOAD STATES

■ MEDICATION	■ DOSE	■ COMMENT
Furosemide	Intermittent dosing: 0.5–1.0 mg/kg/dose every 6–12 h	May be ototoxic, especially at extremely large doses noted here
	Trial of extremely large dose: 4 mg/kg/dose (max 200 mg)	
	Infusion: 0.1–1.0 mg/kg/h	May increase RBF
Bumetanide	Intermittent dosing: 0.01–0.1 mg/kg/dose every 12–24 h	Similar to furosemide
Ethacrynic acid	Intermittent dosing: 0.5–1.0 mg/kg/dose every 8–12 h	Increases RBF and venous capacitance
		Potentially ototoxic
Chlorothiazide	Intermittent dosing: 5–20 mg/kg/dose every 12 h	Usually not useful when GFR <30 mL/min
	(max 1 g/day for age >2 yr)	PO only in children

RBF, renal blood flow; GFR, glomerular filtration rate.

for toxicity is greater (see **Table 117.5**). Loop diuretics may improve renal blood flow and may re-establish adequate urine flow. Moreover, no indication exists for the use of diuretics—usual doses or larger doses—in the anuric patient.

Renal Replacement Therapy

RRT is a frequent component of the care of the critically ill child with HCT. Extracorporeal continuous venovenous hemofiltration (CVVH) is the most common form of RRT (see Chapter 41). CVVH is easy to administer and flexible. Therapy can be tailored to achieve primarily fluid removal, hemofiltration, dialysis, some degree of solute removal, or any combination of these goals. Fluid removal is the most common indication. Fluid overload of 20% or more is independently associated with an elevated risk of mortality (25). Indications for dialysis by CVVH are severe metabolic acidemia (pH < 7.1), hyperkalemia (serum K >6.5 mmol/dL or rapidly rising), progressive dysnatremia, or coagulopathy that requires administration of large volumes of blood products. Early initiation of CVVH should be considered for patients with underlying electrolyte disorders, anuric AKI, Fanconi syndrome, or renal tubular acidosis. Mortality rates remain high in patients who require dialysis by RRT (24).

Controversies

Controversy surrounds the use of CVVH as a treatment for sepsis and to improve survival from MODS. It is clear that RRT is particularly effective at removing fluid. Many centers use this modality almost routinely for early treatment of fluid overload states (8%–10% fluid overload). It is not clear that the attendant risks of extracorporeal circulation (heparinization, need for central vascular access, clot embolization, and blood loss with circuit thrombosis) are justified if fluid removal is the sole therapeutic benefit anticipated. Such risks are certainly in question when the same result can be achieved with diuretics. A rational approach would be to reserve the use of CVVH for fluid control to (a) situations in which steady, low-volume fluid removal is advantageous (i.e., the patient with compensated shock) or (b) fluid-restricted patients who require more support (blood product administration and parenteral nutrition).

Based on the evidence in preclinical investigations and a small case series (26), some have advocated the use of CVVH for its possible immunomodulatory effects (either from filtration of inflammatory constituents or mobilization of metabolic by-products and deleterious mediators). In such therapy, the goal is high-volume hemofiltration with total clearance rates of 4–6 L/hour. Clearance of small- and middle-molecular-weight substances is desired. While the presence of adverse biomarkers such as inflammatory cytokines can be measured in the ultrafiltrate of patients on such regimens, little evidence suggests that overall outcome is changed. Given the risks of the therapy, such practice cannot be supported for widespread use.

FLUID AND ELECTROLYTE PROBLEMS

Mechanisms of Disease

Fluid Overload

Patients with HCT frequently have problems with fluids, electrolytes, and nutrition. Children may present to the PICU with weight gain of ≥10%. As discussed, the causes are generally a combination of need for excess IV fluid, some degree of SIRS, cardiac failure, and/or AKI. Such fluid overload contributes to MODS, respiratory failure with pulmonary edema and effusions, and congestive heart failure.

Electrolyte Disorders

Several disorders of serum electrolytes are seen in HCT. Electrolyte disorders can be seen without AKI. Certain abnormalities are common. Sodium overload is a frequent occurrence with the need for normal saline as a medication diluent or for administration with total parenteral nutrition. Hyponatremia may be seen in patients with congestive heart failure due to activation of the renin–angiotensin system and release of atrial naturetic factor. Treatment consists of reduction of fluid intake, rather than sodium supplementation. Hyponatremia and hyperkalemia are seen with the use of tacrolimus, presumed to result from altered renal handling of univalent cations. Ifosfamide may induce phosphate wasting and Fanconi syndrome. Foscarnet can cause losses of all cations and phosphate.

Nutritional Disease

Parenteral nutrition is often used in the peritransplant period. Reasons include both difficulty with ingestion (from anorexia, mucositis, and enteritis) and gut dysfunction with loss of mucosal integrity (from aGVHD). Patients may suffer extended periods of vomiting and diarrhea. The use of total parenteral nutrition is expensive, requires ongoing central venous access, and is associated with fluid overload, hyperglycemia, biliary stasis, hepatic dysfunction, and enterocyte atrophy with loss of gut mucosal barrier. Even small-volume, non-nutritive feedings may ameliorate barrier dysfunction. Patients should resume enteral intake as soon as possible; generally, this is not accomplished until engraftment occurs. With the association between hyperglycemia and poorer outcomes in some critically ill patients, control of serum glucose levels is generally recommended. Insulin infusion is often required while patients are on total parenteral nutrition, with a target range of serum glucose levels of 80–150 mg/dL.

Nutritional supplementation with glutamine to preserve the gut barrier or enhance its function has been proposed. Glutamine is an essential component in the synthesis of the antioxidant glutathione. In noncancer patients, glutamine administration has demonstrated improvement in gut integrity. Studies in patients who undergo HCT are limited in number and conflicting in results. While parenteral administration of glutamine decreased infectious complications and length of hospital stay in alloHCT patients, poorer survival rates were seen in AutoHCT patients who received glutamine (27). Others have postulated that lipid supplementation is desirable to prevent essential fatty acid deficiencies secondary to malabsorption, while minimizing the use of carbohydrates and the risk of hyperglycemia and favorably altering immunologic responses in GVHD. Lastly, infusions of specific substrates to minimize intestinal toxicity have been proposed. Specific therapies for mucositis are discussed in more detail below.

GRAFT-VERSUS-HOST DISEASE

Mechanisms of Disease

The incidence and severity of GVHD following alloHCT depends on donor source, HLA disparity between donor and recipient, sex of donor, multiparity status of donor, type of graft-versus-host prophylaxis, CMV status of donor and recipient, age of donor, and other factors. The pathophysiology of aGVHD following alloHCT is a three-step process in which interaction between innate and adaptive immunity occurs (28). Following intensive conditioning therapy, significant host tissue damage, usually in the gastrointestinal (GI) tract, leads to activation of host antigen-presenting cells by local release of inflammatory mediators and cytokines. During the second part of the process, host antigen-presenting cells present alloantigen to resting donor T-cells, leading to donor T-cell proliferation, activation, and the secretion of inflammatory cytokines, including IL-2 and interferon γ. In the final stage, donor mononuclear phagocytes and neutrophils induce systemic inflammation that is triggered by mediators (e.g., lipopolysaccharide) that leak through the damaged intestinal mucosa. This inflammation promotes recruitment of donor effector cells into target organs, amplifying tissue injury with additional release of inflammatory cytokines and promotion of target tissue destruction by cytotoxic T lymphocytes (Fig. 117.1).

Clinical Presentation

GVHD is subdivided into hyperacute, acute, and chronic types. Hyperacute GVHD usually occurs within the first week after alloHCT and before full HPC engraftment but with early engraftment of donor T-cells into targeted affected tissues.

aGVHD commonly develops between day +7 and day +100 following alloHCT. cGVHD is defined as GVHD occurring after day +100, diagnosed as long as 2–3 years post-alloHCT. Severe aGVHD (usually ≥grade II) can be a common cause of admission to the PICU for alloHCT recipients.

Acute Graft-versus-host Disease

aGVHD commonly involves the skin (81% of patients with GVHD), GI tract (54%), and liver (50%) (29).

Skin Graft-versus-host Disease. Skin aGVHD usually presents around the time of white cell engraftment as a macular-papular rash that commonly involves the palms and soles. It can be asymptomatic, pruritic, or even painful. The rash usually begins in sun-exposed areas on the upper body including the face, arms, shoulders, and behind the ears. It is graded into four stages, using the "rule of nines" to determine body surface area involvement for stages 1–3. Stage 4 is defined as generalized erythroderma with bulla formation (Table 117.6). Rarely is skin aGVHD, by itself, sufficient to require admission to the PICU; however, stage 4 disease requires management using burn protocols with support of fluids, electrolytes, and cardiovascular function.

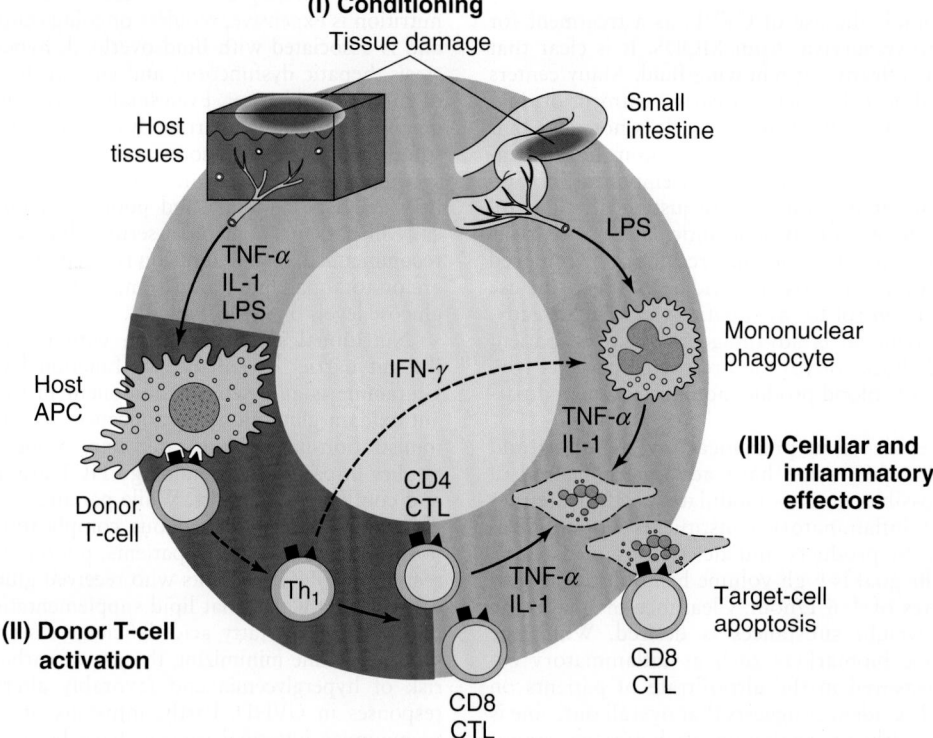

FIGURE 117.1. The pathophysiology of acute graft-versus-host disease (GVHD). GVHD is a three-step process: (a) conditioning regimens (irradiation, chemotherapy, or both) lead to damage and activation of host tissues, especially the intestinal mucosa, allowing the translocation of lipopolysaccharide (LPS) and stimulating the secretion of the inflammatory cytokines tumor necrosis factor (TNF)-α and interleukin (IL)-1 from host tissues, particularly macrophages. These cytokines increase the expression of major histocompatibility complex (MHC) antigens and adhesion molecules on host tissues. (b) Donor T-cell activation is characterized by the predominance of Th1 cells and the secretion of interferon gamma (IFN-γ), which activates mononuclear phagocytes. (c) Effector functions of activated mononuclear phagocytes are triggered by LPS and other stimulatory molecules. Activated macrophages, along with cytotoxic T lymphocytes (CTL), secrete inflammatory cytokines that cause target cell apoptosis. CD8-CTL also lyse target cells directly. Damage to the gastrointestinal tract in this phase, principally by inflammatory cytokines, amplifies LPS release and leads to the "cytokine storm" characteristic of severe acute GVHD. This damage results in the amplification of local tissue injury and further promotes an inflammatory response. APC, antigen-presenting cell. (From Ferrara JL, Reddy P. Pathophysiology of graft-versus-host disease. *Semin Hematol* 2006;43(1):3–10.)

TABLE 117.6

CONSENSUS GRADING OF ACUTE GRAFT-VERSUS-HOST DISEASE

	ORGAN/EXTENT OF INVOLVEMENT		
	■ SKIN	■ LIVER	■ INTESTINAL TRACT
Stage			
1	Rash on <25% of skin[a]	Bilirubin 2–3 mg/dL[b]	Diarrhea >500 mL/d[c] or persistent nausea[d]
2	Rash on 25%–50% of skin	Bilirubin 3–6 mg/dL	Diarrhea >1000 mL/d
3	Rash on >50% of skin	Bilirubin 6–15 mg/dL	Diarrhea >1500 mL/d
4	Generalized erythroderma with bulla formation	Bilirubin >15 mg/dL	Severe abdominal pain with or without ileus
Grade			
0	None	None	None
I	Stage 1–2	None	None
II	Stage 3	or Stage 1	or Stage 1
III	—	Stage 2–3	or Stage 2–4
IV[e]	Stage 4	or Stage 4	—

[a]Use the "rule of nines" to determine body surface area involvement.
[b]Range given as total bilirubin. Downgrade one stage if an additional cause of elevated bilirubin has been documented.
[c]Volume of diarrhea applies to adults. For pediatric patients, the volume of diarrhea should be based on body surface area.
[d]Persistent nausea with histologic evidence of graft-versus-host disease in the stomach or duodenum.
[e]Grade IV may also include lesser organ involvement but with extreme decrease in performance status.
From Przepiorka D, Weisdorf D, Martin P, et al. 1994 Consensus conference on acute GVHD grading. *Bone Marrow Transplant* 1995;15(6):825–8, with permission.

The differential diagnosis of skin GVHD includes skin reactions secondary to (a) conditioning regimens or antibiotics, or (b) histopathologic skin manifestations of disseminated infections. In fact, severe skin aGVHD may be difficult to distinguish from Stevens–Johnson syndrome and/or toxic epidermal necrolysis. A major difference is the lack of involvement of the conjunctiva in skin aGVHD. A skin biopsy may be necessary to confirm the diagnosis.

Gastrointestinal Graft-versus-host Disease. GI GVHD presents as secretory or watery diarrhea, abdominal pain, nausea, vomiting, and anorexia. Severe intestinal GVHD may lead to significant mucosal damage with electrolyte abnormalities, protein-losing enteropathy, bloody diarrhea, and massive losses of fluid to the extravascular space. In stages 1–3, staging of GI GVHD is based on the volume of diarrhea per day (see **Table 117.6**). Stage 4 GI GVHD is defined as severe abdominal pain with or without ileus and/or large amounts of secretory diarrhea.

Acute intestinal GVHD may be confused with a number of other conditions. The differential diagnosis includes *Clostridium difficile* colitis, CMV enteritis, herpes simplex, or *Candida* esophagitis, gastritis, ulcers, and post–chemo radiation effects. Histologic features include apoptotic bodies in the base of crypts, crypt abscesses, and loss and flattening of surface epithelium (30).

Hepatic GVHD. The liver disease in hepatic GVHD is due to damage to bile canaliculi leading to cholestasis with hyperbilirubinemia and elevated alkaline phosphatase. Severity and staging are based on the serum bilirubin level (**Table 117.6**). Patients with acute hepatic GVHD, particularly those with disease stages 2–4, commonly require intensive care monitoring and specific therapy (see below). Hepatic GVHD is the most difficult form of aGVHD to treat.

The differential diagnosis of acute hepatic GVHD includes a number of diseases also associated with increases in serum bilirubin. During the first 30 days post-alloHCT, hepatic SOS, also known as VOD of the liver, may occur. SOS may be difficult to distinguish from hepatic GVHD. Other diagnoses include drug toxicity, infection, and cholelithiasis. On occasion, a liver biopsy is required to distinguish hepatic aGVHD from the above conditions. The biopsy usually demonstrates segmental destruction of small bile ducts, injury to periductal epithelium, cellular degeneration, and cholestasis. Endothelialitis and pericholangitis may also be observed (31).

Management of Severe Acute Graft-versus-host Disease

The best strategy for severe aGVHD is preemptive—identify the best donor source and employ GVHD prophylaxis measures. Despite this approach, between 40% and 60% of patients will develop severe aGVHD (≥grade II). Most admissions to the PICU for severe aGVHD are for hepatic or GI tract involvement. In addition to supportive care, specific treatment usually requires systemic immunosuppression. Glucocorticoids are the gold standard for treatment of grade II–IV aGVHD, despite the fact that the main mechanism of action remains unclear (possibilities include suppression of proinflammatory cytokines, as well as direct lymphotoxic effects) (32). Unfortunately, only about one half of patients respond and there is no clear second-line agent for steroid refractory aGVHD (33). With severe intestinal aGVHD, patients may develop dehydration and electrolyte disorders. Managing fluids and maintaining electrolyte balance are crucial. With severe hepatic aGVHD, patients have progressive hepatic failure with ascites, poor nutrition, and coagulopathy. Therapy includes replacement of coagulation factors, treatment of hyperammonemia, portal venous shunting, and other hepatic support, as well as aggressive systemic immunosuppression (see Chapter 103).

Outcomes of Severe Acute Graft-versus-host Disease

Grades III and IV aGVHD are associated with a high degree of morbidity and mortality. Treatment with corticosteroids results in complete or partial response in only 50%–60% of patients. Only 25%–35% of patients develop complete resolution of aGVHD, even with therapy. Another 15%–20% improve, although usually with multiple exacerbations. Patients with aGVHD resistant to corticosteroids have poor long-term survival. Only 5%–30% of these patients will have a long-term cure (29,34). Many will require increasing amounts of immunosuppressives, usually leading to serious opportunistic infections and death.

SINUSOIDAL OBSTRUCTIVE SYNDROME

Clinical Presentation

SOS is an early complication of HCT. It is characterized by rapid weight gain, ascites, painful hepatomegaly, and jaundice (35). It is heralded with the appearance of right upper-quadrant tenderness and hepatomegaly within 7–20 days after myeloablative HCT. Fluid retention usually manifests as peripheral edema, ascites, pleural or pericardial effusions, and measurable weight gain. Additional signs of liver dysfunction include hyperbilirubinemia, portal hypertension, and clotting abnormalities. Ultrasound and CT of the liver demonstrate hepatomegaly, ascites, and, most importantly, attenuated hepatic venous flow.

SOS should be differentiated from direct drug toxicity, liver failure from parenteral nutrition or infection, cholelithiasis, and systemic conditions such as sepsis. If symptoms are severe, or when the diagnosis is uncertain, liver biopsy may be helpful in differentiating the etiology. However, percutaneous liver biopsy is associated with a high risk of bleeding due to the usual coagulopathy. Transjugular biopsy has a lower morbidity and is the procedure of choice, especially in the early posttransplant period.

Mechanisms of Disease

Chemotherapy or radiotherapy injury to hepatic sinusoidal/venous endothelium and zone 3 hepatocytes induces the release of cytokines and other inflammatory mediators, resulting in the activation of clotting factors. Factor VIII, von-Willebrand factor, and fibrinogen are deposited in the subendothelial zone of small venules causing intravascular microvessel thrombosis. Thrombosis leads to hepatic congestion and ischemia, with additional hepatocyte damage and necrosis and a cycle of additional microvascular thrombosis. As the process continues, collagen deposition within the sinusoids, sclerosis of venule walls that progresses to obliteration of the venules, and further hepatocyte necrosis occur. Early microscopic findings in the liver include narrowing of terminal hepatic venules, subendothelial edema, necrosis of endothelium, engorgement and dilatation of sinusoids, and necrosis of centrizonal hepatocytes. In the most advanced stage, extensive necrosis and progressive fibrosis occur. Sinusoidal obstruction is prominent, leading to the proposed or alternate terminology of SOS (36).

Management of Hepatic Sinusoidal Obstructive Syndrome

Identification of high-risk patients and the initiation of prophylactic measures are important in the prevention and amelioration of SOS. Pretransplant risk factors include a previous history of elevated liver transaminases, poor Karnofsky performance status, active or advanced disease, prior hepatic radiation, the type of HCT, and the intensity of the cytoreductive therapy used in the conditioning regimen (37). When significant comorbidities and high risk of SOS exist, nonmyeloablative or reduced-intensity conditioning regimens are preferred. Pharmacokinetic monitoring of cytotoxic therapy, especially of busulfan, is important in prevention of SOS. Close monitoring of fluid and electrolytes in the first 2 weeks after HCT and the avoidance of significant weight gain may prevent additional complications. The use of ursodeoxycholic acid, a hydrophilic water-soluble bile acid, has been used as a prophylactic agent by reducing bilirubin and stone formation.

The treatment for SOS, in large part, depends on disease severity. Mild SOS does not require medical intervention. Moderate SOS requires medical intervention but is reversible with little serious systemic toxicity. Severe SOS is associated with important systemic complications and a high mortality rate. The risk of developing severe SOS is based on the percent of weight gain, total serum bilirubin, and day posttransplant (38). For example, a 10% weight gain and a serum bilirubin of 6 mg/dL on day +1 is associated with a 60% risk of developing severe SOS versus a 10% weight gain and a serum bilirubin of 6 on day +10, which is associated with only a 30% risk. The treatment for moderate and severe SOS includes close fluid and electrolyte monitoring, aggressive use of diuretics, reduction of weight gain, and nutritional support. Defibrotide, a single-stranded polydeoxyribonucleotide, has been used with moderate success in patients with moderate-to-severe SOS. Defibrotide binds to adenine C receptors A1 and A2 on the surface of vascular endothelium, thereby altering endothelial cell regulation and response to injury. Additionally, defibrotide has been demonstrated to increase prostacyclin, prostaglandin E_2, and thrombomodulin and may decrease thrombin generation and inhibit fibrin deposition.

Thrombolytic therapies with recombinant human tissue plasminogen activator and heparin have shown some efficacy in treating patients with moderate-to-severe SOS. These therapies are frequently limited by the risk of severe or fatal bleeding, especially in patients with disordered coagulation. Other anticoagulant therapies have included human antithrombin III concentrate or activated protein C.

Patients who require transfer to the ICU for severe SOS usually have significant ascites with abdominal compartment syndrome, weight gain, jaundice, portal venous hypertension, and hyperbilirubinemia. Other treatments with surgically or radiologically placed peritoneal venous shunts or transhepatic and intrahepatic portal systemic shunting have had some success. The shunting procedure, which creates a channel between the hepatic vein and the portal vein by percutaneous catheter insertion, has resulted in significant improvement in patients with severe ascites and coagulopathy. Occasionally, liver transplantation has been required in those who develop severe hepatic failure.

Outcomes of Sinusoidal Obstructive Syndrome

Over 90% of patients with nonsevere SOS improve after several days with only supportive measures. However, severe SOS has a high mortality rate (as many as 30%–70% of patients die) although the mortality rate has improved with defibrotide administration. Severe SOS usually leads to renal and respiratory failure and MODS. Patients with moderate-to-severe SOS who receive aggressive medical or surgical management usually do quite well, with almost 80%–100% being cured.

INFICTIONS

Clinical Presentation

7 Infection is a major cause of morbidity and mortality after HCT. The risk of developing infection is influenced by the type of transplantation, conditioning regimen, donor source, underlying disease, intensity of previous therapy, and other complications. Clinical examination, history, and microbial findings are important. However, diagnosis of an infection, especially opportunistic infections, may be difficult because of a lack of usual clinical signs and symptoms. Fever, usually the main indicator of infection, may be blunted by immunomodulatory treatment. Other signs, such as tachycardia, tachypnea, and organ dysfunction, should be considered as signs of possible infection. Sites with known risk, such as the perianal area, lungs, skin, central venous catheter exit sites, and oropharynx, should be assessed for any sign of infection. Workup should include blood cultures and cultures from any suspected site of infection.

Mechanisms of Disease

As discussed previously, three different risk periods are associated with post-HCT, each with its own unique immunodeficient predisposition: (a) early recovery (pre-engraftment phase, corresponding to the first several weeks after transplantation), (b) mid-recovery (early post-engraftment phase, corresponding to the second and third months after transplantation), and (c) late recovery (the period beyond 3 months). In the early recovery period, neutropenia and alteration of mucosal and integument barriers make the patient susceptible to bacterial infections, which predominate in this period. In the mid-recovery period, the patient is susceptible to infection because of decreased cellular immunity, skin barrier compromise by central venous catheters, and disruption of the GI mucosal barrier due to GVHD. In the late recovery period, impaired mucosal defenses, chemotactic defects, functional asplenia, and qualitative and quantitative B- and T-cell abnormalities associated with cGVHD are seen. During the mid- and late-recovery phases, with recovery of the neutrophil count, bacterial infections are less common, and viral and fungal infections predominate. The spectrum of infections post-HCT and how they vary over time as the patient's immune status changes are shown in **Table 117.7.**

Bacterial Infections

The source of infection is usually from the patient's own colonized flora or from hospital-acquired bacteria. Bacteria account for >90% of infections during the neutropenic phase (39). Infections with Gram-positive organisms are mainly associated with central venous catheters and severe mucositis; infections with Gram-negative organisms occur with severe GI mucosal damage. In the neutropenic patient, infections with *Staphylococcus epidermidis*, *Staphylococcus aureus*, *Streptococcus* species, *Pseudomonas aeruginosa*, *Escherichia coli*, *Klebsiella* spp., *Corynebacterium jeikeium*, and *Bacillus* spp. often lead to serious sepsis. In neutropenic patients with chemotherapy-induced mucositis, α-hemolytic streptococci may lead to rapidly progressive shock. Despite appropriate therapy, infection-related mortality remains high (40). *Streptococcus mitis* is associated with ARDS and septic shock (41). Infection caused by aerobic Gram-negative bacilli, such as *Enterobacteriaceae* and *P. aeruginosa*, can cause overwhelming sepsis and toxemia in the neutropenic patient. The most serious localized infection in the HCT recipient is ecthyma gangrenosum, often

caused by *P. aeruginosa* (42). Increased frequency of nonfermentative Gram-negative bacteria, such as *Stenotrophomonas maltophilia*, often results in difficult-to-treat end-organ disease involving the lungs and other sites (43).

Viral Infections

Herpes Simplex Virus Infections. Viral infection is the leading cause of morbidity and mortality following HCT. Patients encounter viruses through exposure to the environment or reactivation of latent virus. The herpes viruses, including herpes simplex virus (HSV), CMV, varicella-zoster virus, Epstein–Barr virus, and human herpes virus 6, account for the majority of posttransplant viral infections (44). Pretransplant serology helps to identify patients at risk for HSV reactivation, which typically occurs up to 2 months after transplantation. Dissemination can occur, and mortality varies from 10% to 50%. Skin lesions may be atypical and present in unusual sites. Esophagitis is common, and pneumonia can develop. Isolation of the virus or positive direct immunofluorescence using monoclonal antibodies leads to diagnosis and aids in management (45).

Cytomegalovirus Infections. CMV infection remains one of the most important complications after alloHCT. The disease can develop both early and late after the transplantation procedure (46–48). Pretransplant serology helps to identify patients at risk for CMV reactivation, but diagnosis is made by isolation of the virus or by detection of viral DNA by PCR. CMV infection occurs in ~60%–70% of CMV-seropositive patients or in -seronegative patients who receive a transplant from a seropositive donor. Transplant recipients can have latent infection, active infection with replicating virus found in monocytes, or CMV disease with tissue damage. Active CMV infection manifests as fever, fatigue, and leukopenia. It can cause multiorgan disease including pneumonia, hepatitis, gastroenteritis, chorioretinitis, and encephalitis. CMV disease, particularly CMV pneumonia, is often fatal (49,50). The mortality rate for patients with untreated CMV pneumonia is as high as 85% and is 30%–50% in patients who receive specific therapy (50).

Other Viral Infections. Varicella-zoster virus infection, which can be seen from 4 months to 1 year after transplantation, develops as a primary infection or as reactivation of latent virus and is potentially lethal (45). Reactivation of latent virus can present as shingles or as disseminated disease. Human Herpes virus 6 (HHV-6) infection, although rare, manifests as encephalitis, pneumonitis, or graft suppression (51). Infection with Epstein–Barr virus, typically in the first 6 months, also develops as either primary disease or reactivation and can cause B-cell PTLD (52), often a life-threatening disease. Patients with mismatched, unrelated, or T-cell–depleted transplants and those who receive antithymocyte globulin, alemtuzumab, or other anti–T-cell monoclonal antibodies are at a higher risk of developing PTLD (52). Patients present with high fever, lymphadenopathy, and sometimes diarrhea or elevated liver enzymes, depending on organ involvement. Adenovirus infection presents with diarrhea, hemorrhagic cystitis, and pneumonia. When disseminated to cause hepatitis or MODS, adenovirus is associated with a high mortality rate (53). Severity of infection correlates with the degree of immune dysfunction. Diagnosis is made by viral culture from infected body fluids or tissue (excluding the GI tract), by direct antigen detection, or by detection of viral DNA by PCR (53). Viremia strongly predicts disseminated disease (53). Adenovirus infection develops from reactivation of latent virus or, in young children with primary infection, is contracted by contact. Infections with RSV, influenza A and B, or parainfluenza infection occur seasonally and coincide with community outbreaks. RSV affects up to 1%–3% of transplant recipients

TABLE 117.7

PHASES OF PREDICTABLE OPPORTUNISTIC INFECTIONS AMONG RECIPIENTS OF HEMATOPOIETIC STEM CELLS

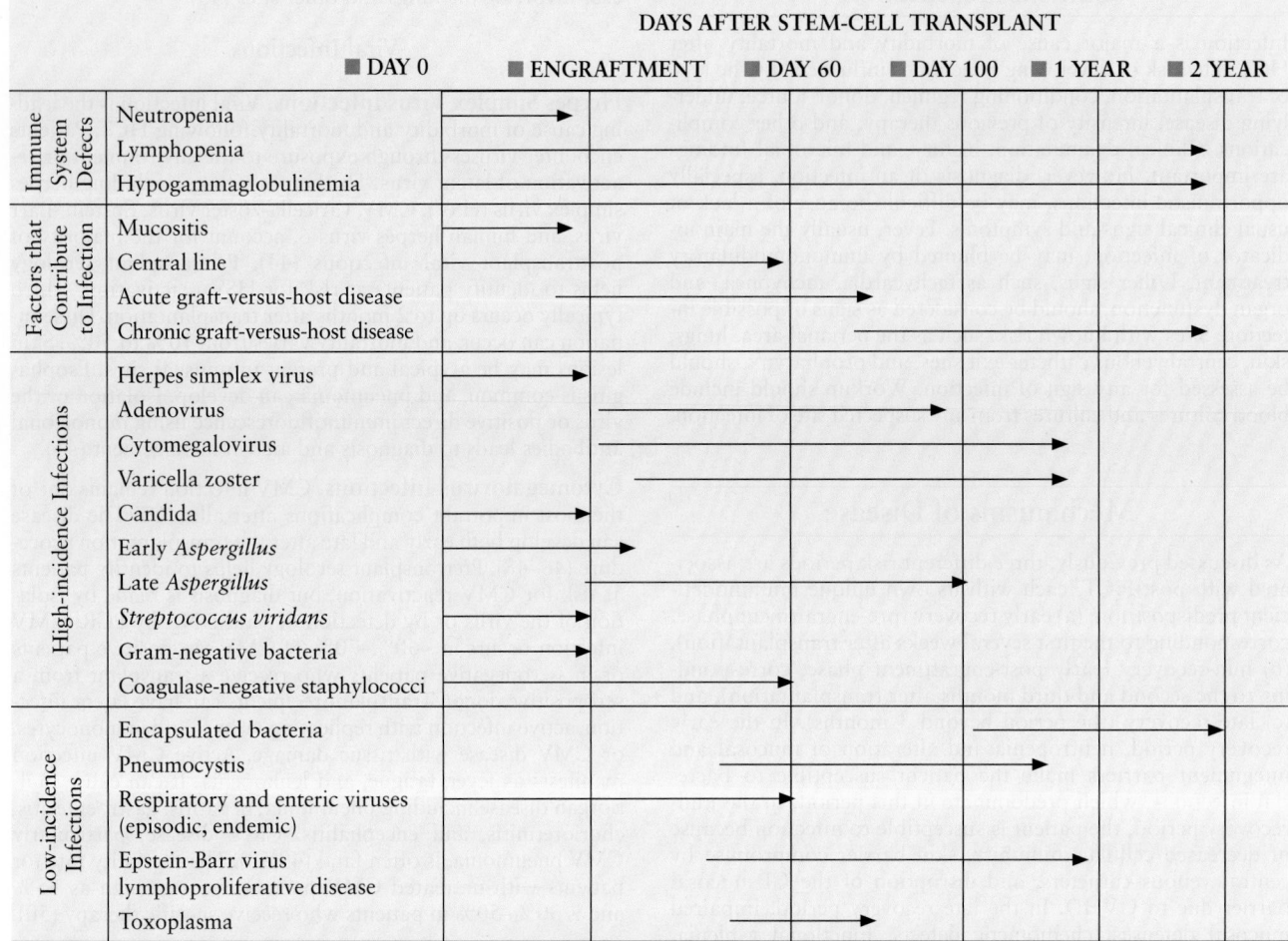

	DAYS AFTER STEM-CELL TRANSPLANT					
	■ DAY 0	■ ENGRAFTMENT	■ DAY 60	■ DAY 100	■ 1 YEAR	■ 2 YEAR
Immune System Defects						
Neutropenia	——→					
Lymphopenia	———————————————————————————————→					
Hypogammaglobulinemia	———————————————————————————————→					
Factors that Contribute to Infection						
Mucositis	——→					
Central line	————————————→					
Acute graft-versus-host disease	———————————→					
Chronic graft-versus-host disease	———————————————————————————→					
High-incidence Infections						
Herpes simplex virus	——→					
Adenovirus	————————————→					
Cytomegalovirus	————————————————————→					
Varicella zoster	————————————————————→					
Candida	——→					
Early *Aspergillus*	——————→					
Late *Aspergillus*	——————————————→					
Streptococcus viridans	——→					
Gram-negative bacteria	——→					
Coagulase-negative staphylococci	————→					
Low-incidence Infections						
Encapsulated bacteria	——————————————→					
Pneumocystis	————————————→					
Respiratory and enteric viruses (episodic, endemic)	————————————→					
Epstein-Barr virus lymphoproliferative disease	————————————————→					
Toxoplasma	——————————→					

Types of opportunistic infections occurring in stem-cell transplant recipients and the time period they are at the highest risk for these infections. Immune system defects and transplant-related factors that occur at these time periods to contribute to infection.

Adapted from Van Burik J, Weisdorf D. Infections in recipients of hematopoietic stem cell transplantation. In: Mandell GL, Bennett JE, Dolin R, eds. *Mandell, Douglas, and Bennett's Principles and Practice of Infectious Diseases.* 6th ed. Philadelphia, PA: Elsevier Churchill Livingstone, 2005:3486–97.

and carries a mortality rate as high as 50% in patients who develop lower-tract disease (54).

Fungal Infections

Risk factors for invasive fungal disease include prolonged neutropenia, HLA-mismatched transplant, GVHD or its treatment, steroid therapy, and graft failure. Signs and symptoms of fungal infection are often absent or nonspecific and include fever unresponsive to antibiotics. Making the diagnosis of invasive fungal infection is the single most important limitation to successful treatment. Diagnosis relies on culture of the organism from a sterile site or identification by histologic methods. Various antibody and antigen tests have been developed for the diagnosis of invasive candidosis and aspergillosis. In addition, antigen testing is an established diagnostic tool for *Histoplasma capsulatum* and *Cryptococcus neoformans*. Specific antigen testing is currently being done for *Candida* infections. Galactomannan antigen can be detected in *Aspergillus* infections (55,56).

Candida and *Aspergillus* are the most common opportunistic fungal organisms isolated, but other emerging pathogens have been reported (14). A shift has occurred in the incidence of *Candida* infections, with a decrease in *Candida albicans* and an emergence of non-albicans species, such as *C. tropicalis*, *C. parapsilosis*, *C. glabrata*, and *C. krusei* (14). *Candida* infections may be superficial, mucocutaneous, or deep-seated. *C. albicans* and *C. tropicalis* are known causes of disseminated candidiasis and are associated with high mortality (14). *C. parapsilosis*, a catheter-associated yeast, rarely disseminates systemically (14). Hepatosplenic candidosis commonly presents during neutrophil regeneration. *Aspergillus* is the leading cause of death from infection after alloHCT. *Aspergillus* species such as *A. fumigatus*, *A. flavus*, and *A. niger* cause invasive disease, predominately during the neutropenic period (57). The primary site for *Aspergillus* infection is the lung. Such infection often presents as invasive, pulmonary aspergillosis with thrombotic and hemorrhagic lung disease. Dissemination to the brain, liver, and skin is common. Cutaneous lesions, also known as ecthyma gangrenosum, are a common manifestation of disseminated disease that carries a high mortality. Serious infections with other fungal species may be seen as well in transplant recipients. Cryptococcosis is rare and most often results in meningitis or pulmonary infection (14). Zygomycosis or mucormycosis often presents as sinusoidal disease, but pulmonary and disseminated disease may occur (14,57). Corticosteroid use and active GVHD increase the risk of opportunistic fungal infections.

Pneumocystis Jiroveci Infections

Pneumocystis jiroveci (formerly known as *P. carinii*) pneumonia, a protozoan infection, occurs post-engraftment. The risk of *P. jiroveci* infection in HCT patients can be as high as 10%–15% without prophylaxis (58). Patients present with progressive dyspnea with a dry cough but can also present with a fulminant course. Hypoxia is present in >90% of patients at presentation (14). Chest x-ray often shows interstitial acinar infiltrates. BAL is the preferred diagnostic test. Giemsa and Gomori methenamine silver staining, although simple to perform, is relatively insensitive. Molecular diagnosis by PCR is highly sensitive and specific and should be used when available.

Mycobacterium Infections

Tuberculous and non-tuberculous Mycobacterium (NTM) infections, although infrequent in HCT recipients, are being identified and reported more commonly. In adults, the incidence of NTM infection in HCT recipients is reported at 0.4%–4.9%. In pediatric recipients, it has been reported as high as 6.4%. Studies have cited rapidly growing mycobacteria such as *M. fortuitum*, *M. abscessus*, and *M. chelonae* as the main species isolated in this population (59,60). Increased recognition may be due to better detection methods or increased susceptibility of recipients because of greater use of alternate donors, necessitating increased immunosuppression (61). Diagnosis is difficult because of the lag in development of symptoms and isolation of the organism. Mycobacterium infection can occur at any time after transplantation. Patients often present with fever, pneumonia, and, in some instances, diarrhea. Primary skin infection and central nervous system disease have been reported (61).

Differential Diagnosis

Correct identification of an infection in an HCT recipient is a critical management issue. Early identification of the specific infection and institution of appropriate therapy may greatly decrease a patient's risk of mortality and serious morbidity; alternatively, determination of the absence of infection and appropriate discontinuation of empiric antimicrobial therapies minimize drug toxicity and the presence of resistant organisms. Clinical signs and symptoms of infection in the HCT-transplantation patient are numerous and often nonspecific. Fever, sometimes the only sign of infection in this patient population, can also result from medication reactions, SIRS, or ARDS. However, because of immunosuppression, a patient may not mount a febrile response. Other symptoms such as tachycardia and hypotension may be the only presenting signs of infection. Diarrhea, a common manifestation of intestinal infection, is also the common presenting symptom of intestinal GVHD, drug toxicities, and mucositis/enteritis. Hyperbilirubinemia and elevation of serum transaminase levels, a common manifestation of many infections, also occurs with SOS, medication toxicity, cholelithiasis, and GVHD. Rash or skin lesions may also be due to drug reactions or GVHD. Even sepsis, which often presents with high spiking fevers, tachycardia, and hypotension, shares symptoms with infusion reactions or engraftment syndrome (patients have a release of cytokines at the time of engraftment).

Management of Infections

A number of advances in infection control and supportive care have improved outcome. Prophylactic or preemptive therapies have reduced the incidence and the morbidity and mortality associated with most infections. Empiric therapy started at the onset of fever and new antimicrobial agents improve outcome. The choice of antibacterial regimen depends on the presentation of infection and the resistance patterns of the organisms in a particular institution. When the infecting organism is identified and sensitivities are available, treatment should be tailored to treat the specific infection. While a complete discussion of the use of antimicrobials in HPC recipients is beyond the scope of this chapter, some specific recommendations should be noted.

Treatment of Viral Infections

Acyclovir is the drug of choice in the treatment of HSV and varicella-zoster virus infections. The value of oral or IV acyclovir prophylaxis in HSV-seropositive patients is well established. Immunocompromised patients exposed to varicella-zoster virus should receive varicella-zoster immunoglobulin to confer passive immunity (14). Ganciclovir, foscarnet, and cidofovir have all been reported as effective therapies against infection with HHV-6 (51). No controlled, randomized studies have been conducted that demonstrate that one therapy is more effective than any other (51). Treatment of Epstein–Barr virus PTLD involves antibody therapy with rituximab and cellular therapy with donor-derived cytotoxic T-cells (52).

Some specific issues should be noted with respect to CMV exposure and disease. Reactivation of the virus, potentially resulting in organ disease, causes morbidity and even death if not managed properly (62). Prophylactic or preemptive approaches to those patients at risk for CMV reactivation has reduced the incidence of infection and disease and resulted in a significant reduction in mortality (14). For seronegative patients who receive transplants from seronegative donors, the use of CMV-negative blood products will suffice. For seropositive patients or seronegative patients who receive a transplant from a seropositive donor, intervention is required. CMV disease can be prevented by prophylactic administration of antiviral medication or preemptive early intervention in which treatment is started when antigenemia or evidence of viral replication is observed (14,50). Ganciclovir and foscarnet are effective in preventing and treating CMV. Prophylaxis with either ganciclovir or foscarnet has reduced the incidence and severity of CMV infection in CMV-seropositive patients (14,50). Lastly, it is the lack of CMV-specific T-cell responses that places the patient at risk for recurrence of CMV disease or persistent disease. Some centers have shown that the adoptive transfer of donor-directed human CMV-specific cytotoxic T-cells restores immunity and is an effective treatment (63).

Adenovirus infection is a significant complication in pediatric alloHCT recipients with a mortality rate for disseminated disease that may exceed 80% (64). Adenovirus often reactivates without clinical symptoms. Therapy for adenovirus infection has included the use of ribavirin, vidarabine, and cidofovir. Although cidofovir appears to be the most effective antiviral strategy (65), antiviral agents are limited in efficacy and may only serve to keep the viral infection from progressing. The key to disease eradication lies in the recovery of endogenous T-cell function (66).

Treatment of Fungal Infections

With fungal infection, prevention is the goal. Treatment of established infection remains difficult and depends on recovery of neutrophils and phagocytic and cellular immunity. Prevention consists of the use of laminar flow rooms, prophylaxis with antifungal agents, and reduced-intensity conditioning or reduced immunosuppressive therapies. Empiric therapy should be started if fungal infection is suspected. Historically, amphotericin B, which has broad antifungal activity, was the only parenteral agent available (57). Newer preparations, such as the liposomal amphotericin, show equal efficacy and reduced toxicity as compared with standard amphotericin (67). The azoles have broad antimycotic activity. Fluconazole, used prophylactically, protects against candidiasis and improves overall survival. However, its spectrum of activity is limited. It has no activity against some of the non-albicans species (14). The most promising results have been with the newer azole formulations posaconazole and voriconazole. Both azoles decrease the risk of invasive aspergillosis compared with placebo (68,69). The echinocandins, caspofungin and micofungin, are as effective as amphotericin B for the treatment of invasive candidiasis and have shown efficacy as salvage therapy in patients with invasive aspergillosis (70). The combination of caspofungin with a broad-spectrum azole or amphotericin B is effective. Additional support with granulocyte transfusions may be required for treatment of invasive fungal infections in neutropenic patients (71).

Treatment of Mycobacterium Infections

Treatment of mycobacterium infection requires multidrug therapy. Testing for organism sensitivity is recommended to better tailor therapy, as resistant strains are seen. The usual course of recommended treatment is 6–12 months and should continue until evidence of immune reconstitution is observed (61).

Treatment of *Pneumocystis Jiroveci*

Effective prevention strategies are available for *P. jiroveci* and the most effective option is TMP-SMX, which can prevent PCP effectively after daily administration of even staggered administration of two to three times weekly. Alternatives to TMP-SMX include atovaquone, dapsone, and aerosolized pentamidine (72,73). It is also important to note the secondary benefits associated with tm/slf prophylaxis, because this drug may effectively prevent *toxoplasmosis*, pulmonary *Nocardia* infections, and infections due to *Pneumococcus* (74). For those who develop *P. jiroveci* pneumonia, the treatment is high-dose TMP-SMX in conjunction with steroids for those with an oxygen requirement.

Outcomes From Infection

Although infection remains a serious complication following HCT, a better understanding of the pathogenesis of infection, the development of better diagnostic techniques to detect infection early, and the use of prophylactic/preemptive therapy have dramatically reduced the associated morbidity and mortality. Once disseminated disease develops, the risk of mortality increases significantly despite appropriate therapy. The patient's immune status plays an important role. A current focus of care is to improve immune function of the recipient by using a reduced-intensity preparative regimen, withdrawing immune suppression earlier, and administering immunoregulatory therapy in the form of donor lymphocytes or specific cytotoxic T-cells.

MUCOSITIS

Clinical Presentation

Oral and GI mucositis contributes significantly to morbidity and mortality and can be a severe complication of treatment. Approximately 75%–90% of HCT recipients experience mucositis, with 50% developing grade III–IV mucositis (**Table 117.8**)

TABLE 117.8

WORLD HEALTH ORGANIZATION MUCOSITIS SCALE

Grade 0	No mucositis
Grade 1	Irritation of the oral mucosa with pain; no overt ulceration; patient is able to eat a normal diet
Grade 2	Sores are evident in the oral mucosa, but patient is still able to swallow solid food
Grade 3	Patients need to be on a liquid diet, as they experience extreme sensitivity on swallowing solid food
Grade 4	Patients are not able to swallow. Total parenteral nutrition or tube feeding is necessary

(75). From the patient's perspective, oral mucositis (OM) is the most common and most debilitating side effect reported (75). Mucositis presents in varying degrees and is multifactorial in origin (76,77). Clinically, OM begins with asymptomatic redness, ultimately passing through different stages to become large, acutely painful and contiguous pseudomembranous lesions and mucosal edema with associated dysphagia and decreased oral intake (78). Disease severity is related to the type of conditioning regimen used, the degree of match between the donor and patient, the severity of GVHD, the presence of infection (i.e., HSV), and the use of methotrexate for GVHD prophylaxis (76,79). Regimens including radiation plus high-dose chemotherapy lead to a higher rate of mucositis than regimens using high-dose chemotherapy alone (80,81). Patients experience prolonged hospitalization, increased need for analgesics, increased need for total parenteral nutrition, reduced quality of life, and episodes of infection (e.g., bacteremia, invasive fungal disease, and typhlitis) associated with mucosal-barrier breakdown. Mortality at day +100 is increased in patients with this complication. Severe grade IV mucositis can cause airway obstruction that necessitates endotracheal intubation. Bacteremia caused by *Streptococcus viridans* is related to mucosal damage and can be associated with serious complications (e.g., sepsis and ARDS) with a mortality rate as high as 80% (82). Bloodstream infections with *S. aureus*, *P. aeruginosa*, *Clostridium* species, and *Candida* occur and are associated with typhlitis.

Mechanisms of Disease

Mucositis involves the entire GI tract. OM typically develops 5–10 days after initiation of myeloablative therapy. It is a self-limited process. Initially, mucosal atrophy is associated with erythema. Ulceration develops 7–11 days after transplantation. The mucosa then gradually heals over the next 2 weeks. The small intestine is the second most common area affected and usually exhibits changes within a few days after the administration of myeloablative chemoradiotherapy. Involvement of the large intestine follows a short time later. Mucosal injury is the consequence of several biologic processes that begin in the submucosa and target the epithelium. It was believed that chemotherapy and radiation therapy directly damage the basal epithelium. Mucosal-barrier injury is a complex biologic process that consists of five phases (83). Injury begins with the initiation phase, which is characterized by the generation of reactive oxygen species and transcription factors that produce injury to the submucosa with changes in the endothelium, connective tissue, and extracellular matrix. This leads to the messaging, signaling, and amplification phases, which involve the production of transcription factors and proinflammatory cytokines, resulting in tissue injury and apoptosis. Epithelial apoptosis and necrosis then give rise to the ulcerative phase. Ultimately, healthy epithelium migrates from the wound margins (83).

Clinical assessment scales have been developed to classify the severity of mucosal damage. No single mucositis assessment scale is universally accepted. Most combine both subjective and objective measures of appearance, patient pain, and functional capabilities. One of these is depicted in **Table 117.8**.

Differential Diagnosis

The differential diagnosis of mucositis includes oral hemorrhage, systemic infection, GVHD, and local viral infection. Infection with HSV is often accompanied by extensive and deep ulcerations. Although not common, CMV infection can lead to mucosal tissue injury. It is important to distinguish mucosal tissue injury that results from infection so that appropriate antiviral therapy will be used. Biopsy may be required to make this determination.

Management of Mucositis

Management can be challenging. The focus is largely on supportive care to control symptoms. Basic oral care is important to reduce oral microbial flora, reduce symptoms of pain and bleeding, and prevent soft tissue infections (84). A decrease in incidence of 8%–11% from the use of intensive dental care has been reported (85). Most oral regimens incorporate a combination of agents that collectively serve to coat and anesthetize the mucosa and to reduce the risk for mucosal infection. Saline and sodium bicarbonate rinses or mucosal coating agents can provide symptomatic relief for mild mucositis. As mucosal breakdown and pain increase, topical anesthetics (e.g., viscous lidocaine and benzocaine) and analgesics are added. Additional ingredients in topical oral solutions include diphenhydramine, magnesium hydroxide/aluminum hydroxide, pectin, sucralfate, nystatin, chlorhexidine, and corticosteroids (86). IV pain medication, especially with patient-controlled analgesia, may be required. For patients with severe (grade III/IV) mucositis who are also often neutropenic and thrombocytopenic, treatment focuses on control of severe bleeding, tissue desquamation, and infection. Protection of the airway with either an oral airway or intubation may be required until the patient reaches the healing phase.

Controversies

Some controversy surrounds more recently used approaches for the prevention and treatment of mucositis. One approach to reduce regimen-related morbidity involves the use of nonmyeloablative preparative regimens. With better understanding of the pathobiology of mucositis, targeted therapeutic agents are being developed. In 2004, palifermin (keratocyte growth factor) was approved for use in patients with mucositis and hematologic malignancies who require myeloablative therapy. In a phase III, randomized, placebo-controlled trial, palifermin was well tolerated and effective in reducing the incidence and duration of severe OM in AutoHCT patients (87).

Outcomes From Mucositis

With a better understanding of the pathobiology of mucositis, a focus on prevention, and the development of targeted therapies, the incidence of severe mucositis in patients who undergo HCT should be reduced. The publication of evidence-based clinical practice guidelines for mucositis should also help to reduce the incidence of severe mucositis requiring intensive care management. These guidelines provide a more standardized approach for the transplant clinician on how to prevent mucositis and recommendations for therapy based on the chemotherapy given (84).

CONCLUSIONS AND FUTURE DIRECTIONS

The field of HCT is evolving. A therapy that was once applied only to a select group of relatively young people with hematologic malignancies and a matched sibling donor has grown to include application in other malignant and nonmalignant conditions. Modifications that allow for the use of grafts from mismatched or unrelated donors have resulted in application to a much larger population. The many efforts to minimize the toxicity of HCT have been quite successful with the ability to treat patients with serious preexisting comorbidities. In short, centers are reshaping their ideas of suitable donors and recipients. Such evolution will challenge the pediatric intensivist, as these patients possess clinical conditions that are among the most difficult to treat. As care of all patients improves, lessons will be learned that will be applicable to the care of critically ill recipients of HCT. However, the major hurdles faced in the care of these children—the elimination of death and serious morbidity from MODS and ARDS—remain among the most difficult challenges in critical care medicine.

References

1. Depuydt P, Kerre T, Noens L, et al. Outcome in critically ill patients with allogeneic BM or peripheral haematopoietic SCT: A single-centre experience. *Bone Marrow Transplant* 2010;46:1186–91.
2. Scales DC, Thiruchelvam D, Kiss A, et al. Intensive care outcomes in bone marrow transplant recipients: A population-based cohort analysis. *Crit Care* 2008;12:R77.
3. Hassan NE, Mageed AS, Sanfilippo DJ, et al. Risk factors associated with pediatric intensive care unit admission and mortality after pediatric stem cell transplant: Possible role of renal involvement. *World J Pediatr* 2013;9:140–5.
4. Styczynski J, Cheung YK, Garvin J, et al. Outcomes of unrelated cord blood transplantation in pediatric recipients. *Bone Marrow Transplant* 2004;34:129–36.
5. Del Toro G, Satwani P, Harrison L, et al. A pilot study of reduced intensity conditioning and allogeneic stem cell transplantation from unrelated cord blood and matched family donors in children and adolescent recipients. *Bone Marrow Transplant* 2004;33:613–22.
6. Satwani P, Harrison L, Morris E, et al. Reduced-intensity allogeneic stem cell transplantation in adults and children with malignant and nonmalignant diseases: End of the beginning and future challenges. *Biol Blood Marrow Transplant* 2005;11:403–22.
7. Sung AD, Chao NJ. Concise review: Acute graft-versus-host disease: Immunobiology, prevention, and treatment. *Stem Cells Transl Med* 2013;2:25–32.
8. Dwyre D, Holland P. Transfusion-associated graft-versus-host disease. *Vox Sang* 2008;95:85–93.
9. Cairo MS. Graft versus host disease: Pathophysiology and therapy. In: Pochedly C, ed. *Neoplastic Diseases in Childhood*. London, England: Harwood Academic Publishers, 1994:833–7.
10. Cairo MS. Myelopoietic growth factors after stem cell transplantation: Does it pay. *J Pediatr Hematol Oncol* 2001;23:2–6.
11. Kaya Z, Weiner DJ, Yilmaz D, et al. Lung function, pulmonary complications, and mortality after allogeneic blood and marrow transplantation in children. *Biol Blood Marrow Transplant* 2009;15:817–26.
12. Haddad IY. Stem cell transplantation and lung dysfunction. *Curr Opin Pediatr* 2013;25:350–6.

13. Kache S, Weiss IK, Moore TB. Changing outcomes for children requiring intensive care following hematopoietic stem cell transplantation. *Pediatr Transplant* 2006;10:299–303.

14. Van Burik J-A, Weisdorf D. Infections in recipients of hematopoietic stem cell transplantation. In: Mandell GL, Bennett JE, Dolin R, eds. *Mandell, Douglas, and Bennett's Principles and Practice of Infectious Diseases.* 6th ed. Philadelphia, PA: Churchill Livingstone 2005:3486–98.

15. Horvath JA, Dummer S. The use of respiratory-tract cultures in the diagnosis of invasive pulmonary aspergillosis. *Am J Med* 1996;100:171–8.

16. Chi AK, Soubani AO, White AC, et al. An update on pulmonary complications of hematopoietic stem cell transplantation. *Chest* 2013;144:1913–22.

17. Veys P, Owens C. Respiratory infections following haemopoietic stem cell transplantation in children. *Br Med Bull* 2002;61:151–74.

18. Panoskaltsis-Mortari A, Griese M, Madtes DK, et al. An official American Thoracic Society research statement: Noninfectious lung injury after hematopoietic stem cell transplantation: Idiopathic pneumonia syndrome. *Am J Respir Crit Care Med* 2011;183:1262–79.

19. Cooke KR. Acute lung injury after allogeneic stem cell transplantation: From the clinic, to the bench and back again. *Pediatr Transplant* 2005;9:25–36.

20. Kurland G, Michelson P. Bronchiolitis obliterans in children. *Pediatr Pulmonol* 2005;39:193–208.

21. Takatsuka H, Takemoto Y, Mori A, et al. Common features in the onset of ARDS after administration of granulocyte colony-stimulating factor. *Chest* 2002;121:1716–20.

22. Keenan HT, Bratton SL, Martin LD, et al. Outcome of children who require mechanical ventilatory support after bone marrow transplantation. *Crit Care Med* 2000;28:830–5.

23. Gow KW, Wulkan ML, Heiss KF, et al. Extracorporeal membrane oxygenation for support of children after hematopoietic stem cell transplantation: The Extracorporeal Life Support Organization experience. *J Pediatr Surg* 2006;41:662–7.

24. Patzer L, Kentouche K, Ringelmann F, et al. Renal function following hematological stem cell transplantation in childhood. *Pediatr Nephrol* 2003;18:623–35.

25. Elbahlawan L, Ray Morrison R. Continuous renal replacement therapy in children post-hematopoietic stem cell transplantation: The present and the future. *Curr Stem Cell Res Ther* 2012;7:381–7.

26. DiCarlo JV, Alexander SR, Agarwal R, et al. Continuous venovenous hemofiltration may improve survival from acute respiratory distress syndrome after bone marrow transplantation or chemotherapy. *J Pediatr Hematol Oncol* 2003;25:801–5.

27. Arfons LM, Lazarus HM. Total parenteral nutrition and hematopoietic stem cell transplantation: An expensive placebo? *Bone Marrow Transplant* 2005;36:281–8.

28. Ferrara JL, Reddy P. Pathophysiology of graft-versus-host disease. *Semin Hematol* 2006;43:3–10.

29. Martin PJ, Schoch G, Fisher L, et al. A retrospective analysis of therapy for acute graft-versus-host disease: Initial treatment. *Blood* 1990;76:1464–72.

30. Snover DC, Weisdorf SA, Vercellotti GM, et al. A histopathologic study of gastric and small intestinal graft-versus-host disease following allogeneic bone marrow transplantation. *Hum Pathol* 1985;16:387–92.

31. Snover DC, Weisdorf SA, Ramsay NK, et al. Hepatic graft versus host disease: A study of the predictive value of liver biopsy in diagnosis. *Hepatology* 1984;4:123–30.

32. Thomas ED, Storb R, Clift RA, et al. Bone-marrow transplantation. *N Engl J Med* 1975;292:832–43.

33. MacMillan ML, Weisdorf DJ, Wagner JE, et al. Response of 443 patients to steroids as primary therapy for acute graft-versus-host disease: Comparison of grading systems. *Biol Blood Marrow Transplant* 2002;8:387–94.

34. Weisdorf D, Haake R, Blazar B, et al. Treatment of moderate/severe acute graft-versus-host disease after allogeneic bone marrow transplantation: An analysis of clinical risk features and outcome. *Blood* 1990;75:1024–30.

35. Carreras E. Veno-occlusive disease of the liver after hemopoietic cell transplantation. *Eur J Haematol* 2000;64:281–91.

36. McDonald GB, Sharma P, Matthews DE, et al. Venocclusive disease of the liver after bone marrow transplantation: Diagnosis, incidence, and predisposing factors. *Hepatology* 1984;4:116–22.

37. Rozman C, Carreras E, Qian C, et al. Risk factors for hepatic veno-occlusive disease following HLA-identical sibling bone marrow transplants for leukemia. *Bone Marrow Transplant* 1996;17:75–80.

38. Bearman SI, Anderson GL, Mori M, et al. Venoocclusive disease of the liver: Development of a model for predicting fatal outcome after marrow transplantation. *J Clin Oncol* 1993;11:1729–36.

39. Wingard J. Bacterial Infection. In: Thomas E, Blume K, Forman S, eds. *Hematopoietic Cell Transplantation.* 2nd ed. New York, NY: Wiley-Blackwell, 1998.

40. Elting LS, Rubenstein EB, Rolston KV, et al. Outcomes of bacteremia in patients with cancer and neutropenia: Observations from two decades of epidemiological and clinical trials. *Clin Infect Dis* 1997;25:247–59.

41. Elting LS, Bodey GP, Keefe BH. Septicemia and shock syndrome due to viridans streptococci: A case-control study of predisposing factors. *Clin Infect Dis* 1992;14:1201–7.

42. Riley U. Bacterial infections. In: Barret J, Treleaven J, eds. *The Clinical Practice of Stem Cell Transplantation.* London, England: CRC Press, 1998.

43. Safdar A, Rolston KV. Stenotrophomonas maltophilia: Changing spectrum of a serious bacterial pathogen in patients with cancer. *Clin Infect Dis* 2007;45:1602–9.

44. Bowden R. Other viruses after hematopoetic cell transplantation. In: Thomas E, Forman S, Appelbaum F, eds. *Hematopoetic Cell Transplantation.* Malden, MA: Blackwell Science, 1999:618–26.

45. Burns W. Herpes simplex virus infections. In: Thomas E, Forman S, Appelbaum F, eds. *Hematopoetic Cell Transplantation.* Malden, MA: Blackwell Science, 1999:584–90.

46. Boeckh M, Leisenring W, Riddell SR, et al. Late cytomegalovirus disease and mortality in recipients of allogeneic hematopoietic stem cell transplants: Importance of viral load and T-cell immunity. *Blood* 2003;101:407–14.

47. Krause H, Hebart H, Jahn G, et al. Screening for CMV-specific T cell proliferation to identify patients at risk of developing late onset CMV disease. *Bone Marrow Transplant* 1997;19:1111–6.

48. Zaia JA, Gallez-Hawkins GM, Tegtmeier BR, et al. Late cytomegalovirus disease in marrow transplantation is predicted by virus load in plasma. *J Infect Dis* 1997;176:782–5.

49. Prentice G, Grundy J, Kho P. Cytomegalovirus. In: Barret J, Treleaven J, eds. *The Clinical Practice of Stem Cell Transplantation.* London, England: CRC Press, 1998.

50. Zaia J. Cytomegalovirus. In: Thomas E, Blume K, Forman S, eds. *Hematopoietic Cell Transplantation.* 2nd ed. London, England: CRC Press, 1998.

51. Yoshikawa T. Human herpesvirus 6 infection in hematopoietic stem cell transplant patients. *Br J Haematol* 2004;124:421–32.

52. Ambinder R. Epstein-Barr virus infection. In: Thomas E, Forman S, Appelbaum F, eds. *Hematopoetic Cell Transplantation.* Malden, MA: Blackwell Science, Ltd., 1999.

53. Suparno C, Milligan DW, Moss PA, et al. Adenovirus infections in stem cell transplant recipients: Recent developments in understanding of pathogenesis, diagnosis and management. *Leuk Lymphoma* 2004;45:873–85.

54. Westmoreland D. Other viral infections. In: Barret J, Treleaven J, eds. *The Clinical Practice of Stem Cell Transplantation.* London, England: CRC Press, 1998.

55. Mikulska M, Calandra T, Sanguinetti M, et al. The use of mannan antigen and anti-mannan antibodies in the diagnosis of invasive

candidiasis: Recommendations from the Third European Conference on Infections in Leukemia. *Crit Care* 2010;14:R222.

56. Sendid B, Caillot D, Baccouch-Humbert B, et al. Contribution of the Platelia Candida-specific antibody and antigen tests to early diagnosis of systemic *Candida tropicalis* infection in neutropenic adults. *J Clin Microbiol* 2003;41:4551–8.

57. Bowden R. Fungal infection after hematopoietic cell transplantation. In: Thomas E, Blume K, Forman S, eds. *Hematopoietic Cell Transplantation*. 2nd ed. Malden, MA: Blackwell Science, 1998.

58. Sepkowitz KA. Opportunistic infections in patients with and patients without acquired immunodeficiency syndrome. *Clin Infect Dis* 2002;34:1098–107.

59. Doucette K, Fishman JA. Nontuberculous mycobacterial infection in hematopoietic stem cell and solid organ transplant recipients. *Clin Infect Dis* 2004;38:1428–39.

60. Unal E, Yen C, Saiman L, et al. A low incidence of nontuberculous mycobacterial infections in pediatric hematopoietic stem cell transplantation recipients. *Biol Blood Marrow Transplant* 2006;12:1188–97.

61. Cordonnier C, Martino R, Trabasso P, et al. Mycobacterial infection: A difficult and late diagnosis in stem cell transplant recipients. *Clin Infect Dis* 2004;38:1229–36.

62. Marr KA, Carter RA, Boeckh M, et al. Invasive aspergillosis in allogeneic stem cell transplant recipients: Changes in epidemiology and risk factors. *Blood* 2002;100:4358–66.

63. Einsele H, Hebart H. CMV-specific immunotherapy. *Hum Immunol* 2004;65:558–64.

64. George D, El-Mallawany NK, Jin Z, et al. Adenovirus infection in paediatric allogeneic stem cell transplantation recipients is a major independent factor for significantly increasing the risk of treatment related mortality. *Br J Haematol* 2012;156:99–108.

65. Ljungman P, Ribaud P, Eyrich M, et al. Cidofovir for adenovirus infections after allogeneic hematopoietic stem cell transplantation: A survey by the Infectious Diseases Working Party of the European Group for Blood and Marrow Transplantation. *Bone Marrow Transplant* 2003;31:481–6.

66. Feuchtinger T, Lang P, Handgretinger R. Adenovirus infection after allogeneic stem cell transplantation. *Leuk Lymphoma* 2007;48:244–55.

67. Hebart H, Einsele H. Specific infectious complications after stem cell transplantation. *Support Care Cancer* 2004;12:80–5.

68. Ullmann AJ, Lipton JH, Vesole DH, et al. Posaconazole or fluconazole for prophylaxis in severe graft-versus-host disease. *N Engl J Med* 2007;356:335–47.

69. Wingard JR, Carter SL, Walsh TJ, et al. Randomized, double-blind trial of fluconazole versus voriconazole for prevention of invasive fungal infection after allogeneic hematopoietic cell transplantation. *Blood* 2010;116:5111–8.

70. Singh N, Paterson DL. Aspergillus infections in transplant recipients. *Clin Microbiol Rev* 2005;18:44–69.

71. Safdar A, Hanna HA, Boktour M, et al. Impact of high-dose granulocyte transfusions in patients with cancer with candidemia: Retrospective case-control analysis of 491 episodes of Candida species bloodstream infections. *Cancer* 2004;101:2859–65.

72. Krajicek BJ, Thomas Jr CF, Limper AH. Pneumocystis pneumonia: Current concepts in pathogenesis, diagnosis, and treatment. *Clin Chest Med* 2009;30:265–78.

73. Muto T, Takeuchi M, Kawaguchi T, et al. Low-dose trimethoprim–sulfamethoxazole for *Pneumocystis jiroveci* pneumonia prophylaxis after allogeneic hematopoietic SCT. *Bone Marrow Transplant* 2011;46:1573–5.

74. Peleg AY, Husain S, Qureshi ZA, et al. Risk factors, clinical characteristics, and outcome of Nocardia infection in organ transplant recipients: A matched case-control study. *Clin Infect Dis* 2007;44:1307–14.

75. Elting LS, Cooksley C, Chambers M, et al. The burdens of cancer therapy. Clinical and economic outcomes of chemotherapy-induced mucositis. *Cancer* 2003;98:1531–9.

76. Blijlevens NM, Donnelly JP, De Pauw BE. Mucosal barrier injury: Biology, pathology, clinical counterparts and consequences of intensive treatment for haematological malignancy: an overview. *Bone Marrow Transplant* 2000;25:1269–78.

77. Wardley AM, Jayson GC, Swindell R, et al. Prospective evaluation of oral mucositis in patients receiving myeloablative conditioning regimens and haemopoietic progenitor rescue. *Br J Haematol* 2000;110:292–9.

78. Niscola P, Tendas A, Cupelli L, et al. The prevention of oral mucositis in patients with blood cancers: Current concepts and emerging landscapes. *Cardiovasc Hematol Agents Med Chem* 2012;10:362–75.

79. Sonis ST, Elting LS, Keefe D, et al. Perspectives on cancer therapy-induced mucosal injury: Pathogenesis, measurement, epidemiology, and consequences for patients. *Cancer* 2004;100:1995–2025.

80. McGuire DB, Peterson DE, Muller S, et al. The 20 item oral mucositis index: Reliability and validity in bone marrow and stem cell transplant patients. *Cancer Invest* 2002;20:893–903.

81. Woo SB, Sonis ST, Monopoli MM, et al. A longitudinal study of oral ulcerative mucositis in bone marrow transplant recipients. *Cancer* 1993;72:1612–7.

82. Ruescher TJ, Sodeifi A, Scrivani SJ, et al. The impact of mucositis on alpha-hemolytic streptococcal infection in patients undergoing autologous bone marrow transplantation for hematologic malignancies. *Cancer* 1998;82:2275–81.

83. Sonis ST. A biological approach to mucositis. *J Support Oncol* 2004;2:21–32; discussion 5–6.

84. Rubenstein EB, Peterson DE, Schubert M, et al. Clinical practice guidelines for the prevention and treatment of cancer therapy-induced oral and gastrointestinal mucositis. *Cancer* 2004;100:2026–46.

85. McGuire DB, Correa MEP, Johnson J, et al. The role of basic oral care and good clinical practice principles in the management of oral mucositis. *Support Care Cancer* 2006;14:541–7.

86. Chan A, Ignoffo RJ. Survey of topical oral solutions for the treatment of chemo-induced oral mucositis. *J Oncol Pharm Pract* 2005;11:139–43.

87. Spielberger R, Stiff P, Bensinger W, et al. Palifermin for oral mucositis after intensive therapy for hematologic cancers. *N Engl J Med* 2004;351:2590–8.

CHAPTER 118 ■ COAGULATION ISSUES IN THE PICU

ROBERT I. PARKER AND DAVID G. NICHOLS

KEY POINTS

1. Hemostasis is a dynamic process. Once bleeding occurs, clot formation and degradation (fibrinolysis) are also initiated.

2. Coagulation is an integral part of inflammation, and inflammation may lead to microvascular thrombosis.

3. A consumptive coagulopathy (DIC) should always be considered in a patient with diffuse or generalized bleeding; however, liver disease and vitamin K deficiency are more common.

4. Localized bleeding in a trauma or postoperative patient should prompt notification of surgical staff and search for an anatomic source of the bleeding.

5. Thrombotic events are being recognized with increased frequency in the PICU. Only 60% of children with docu-

mented thromboses will have an identifiable hematologic abnormality.

6. Recombinant factor VIIa has been used to control refractory hemorrhage, but its use has not yet been shown to improve outcome and consequently may not justify accompanying risks.

7. Neither the prothrombin time nor the International Normalized Ratio (INR) reflect bleeding risk accurately in patients with liver disease.

8. The presence of a central venous catheter is the most commonly identified thrombotic risk factor in critically ill children.

The coagulopathic conditions frequently encountered in the PICU can be arbitrarily divided into three categories: (1) conditions associated with serious bleeding or a high probability of bleeding, (2) thrombotic syndromes or conditions associated with a higher probability of thrombosis, and (3) systemic diseases associated with selective coagulation factor deficiencies (**Table 118.1**). These categories are prioritized to suggest their relative importance to the critical care practitioner.

OVERVIEW OF COAGULATION

Traditionally, the process of blood clotting has been presented in a series of discrete functional units, the "intrinsic" (contact activation), "extrinsic" (**tissue factor [TF]**),* and "common" pathways, that progress in an orderly nonoverlapping sequence (**Fig. 118.1**). While simplification of hemostasis facilitates a basic level of understanding, it obscures the fact that, once initiated, clot production and clot destruction (fibrinolysis) occur simultaneously, and it minimizes an identification of the contributions inflammation, platelets, and the endothelium make in the overall process. Central to this broader understanding is the realization of the primacy of Factor VII (F.VII) and TF. After damage to vascular endothelium, blood comes in contact with TF expressed on fibroblasts and leukocytes. TF triggers both the cellular component of hemostasis (by activating platelets to form a primary platelet plug) and the soluble (protein) component by binding with activated F.VII. The TF-F.VIIa complex unleashes a cascade of protein reactions that ultimately result in the production of fibrin strands, which reinforce the platelet plug.

The "intrinsic" pathway begins with the activation of factor XII (F.XII) to activated factor XII (F.XIIa) through contact with a biologic or foreign surface. Historically, it was believed to be the most important pathway in the initiation of clot formation because deficiencies of downstream factors F.VIII or F.IX produced severe bleeding diatheses (hemophilia A or B, respectively). However, it is now known that the activation of F.X to F.Xa through the action of the F.VIIa/TF complex plays a more central role in coagulation (1,2).

The central role F.X is captured in the term *tenase*, which is a contraction of "ten" and "-ase" (the suffix used to describe enzymatic action) and illustrates the general principle of *concerted action* in the coagulation cascade. The term tenase describes the action of F.VIIa/TF complex, along with the F.IXa/F.VIIIa complex on the activation of F.X to F.Xa. The term *prothrombinase* is another example of concerted action in the coagulation cascade and describes the F.Xa/F.Va complex, which cleaves prothrombin (F.II) to form thrombin (F.IIa).

"Crosstalk," "positive feedback loops," and "surface contact" are additional important characteristics of the clotting process. It is now known that *crosstalk* occurs between the two arms of the clotting cascade, such that F.VIIa (from the extrinsic pathway) enhances the activation of F.IX (to F.IXa) and of F.XI (to F.XIa) (from the intrinsic pathway), further highlighting the **central role of F.VIIa and TF in vivo** (**Fig. 118.2**). Furthermore, **thrombin** initiates various *positive feedback loops* to enhance the "upstream" activation of the clotting process. The activation of coagulation is initiated from TF, which is found in the subendothelial matrix, on cellular elements (e.g., monocytes) and circulating in plasma as soluble TF. However, clotting does not occur in

---

*Please refer to the "Glossary" section at the end of this chapter for additional information regarding terms presented in boldface.

TABLE 118.1

OVERVIEW OF COAGULATION DISORDERS

Conditions associated with serious bleeding or a high probability of bleeding
Disseminated intravascular coagulation
Liver disease/hepatic insufficiency
Vitamin K deficiency/depletion
Massive transfusion syndrome
Anticoagulant overdose (heparin, warfarin)
Thrombocytopenia (drug induced, immunologic)
Acquired platelet defects (drug induced, uremia)
Thrombotic conditions
Thrombotic thrombocytopenia purpura/hemolytic uremic syndrome
Deep venous thrombosis
Pulmonary embolism
Coronary thrombosis/acute myocardial infarction
Systemic conditions associated with selective coagulation factor deficiencies
Hemophilia (A and B)
Specific factor deficiencies associated with specific diseases
  Amyloidosis–factor X, Gaucher disease–factor IX, nephritic syndrome–factor IX, antithrombin III
  Cyanotic congenital heart disease (polycythemia, qualitative platelet defect)
  Depressed clotting factor levels (newborns)
Laboratory abnormalities not associated with clinically significant bleeding
Lupus anticoagulant
Reactive hyperfibrinogenemia

free-flowing blood, but rather on **surfaces**. Platelets, endothelial cells, the subendothelial matrix, and biologic polymers (e.g., catheters, grafts, stents, etc.) provide the surfaces for clot formation.

Platelets not only initiate the clot formation through the formation of a platelet plug, but more importantly, they bring specialized proteins that regulate the clotting response (e.g., F.VIII, inhibitors of fibrinolysis, etc.) to the area of bleeding

and provide a surface for the co-localization of clotting factors for efficient clot formation (**Fig. 118.3**). Under "normal" (unstimulated) conditions, platelets do not adhere to the vascular endothelium, but when the endothelium is mechanically disrupted (e.g., cut) or activated by inflammation, platelets will adhere to the endothelial cell or subendothelial matrix via a von Willebrand factor-dependent mechanism. Once adherent, the platelets become activated and secrete various molecules that further enhance platelet adherence and aggregation, vascular contraction, clot formation, and wound healing (3).

The endothelium is a specialized organ that is integral to the regulation of clot formation (i.e., hemostasis), as it presents a nonthrombogenic surface to flowing blood but enhances clot formation when the endothelium is disrupted by trauma or injured by infection or inflammation (4,5) (**Fig. 118.4**). The normal endothelium produces inhibitors of blood coagulation and **platelet activation** and modulates vascular tone and permeability. Endothelial cells also synthesize and secrete components of the subendothelial extracellular matrix, including adhesive glycoproteins, collagen, fibronectin, and von Willebrand factor. When this system is disrupted, bleeding occurs. However, when inflamed, the endothelium often becomes a prothrombotic rather than an antithrombotic organ, and unwanted clot formation may occur.

Interaction of Coagulation and Inflammation

It is believed that the coagulation process developed during evolution as an intrinsic and integral component of human host defense. Disseminated intravascular coagulation (DIC) illustrates the link between coagulation and inflammation. In DIC, coagulation pathways are activated, natural inhibitory pathways of coagulation are dysfunctional, and the fibrinolytic system is dysregulated. All of these are direct or indirect consequences of the inflammatory response. The natural inhibitory pathways of coagulation are of particular interest in this intersection of coagulation and inflammation, as potential therapies have been based around these biologic processes (6,7). Coagulation may be initiated in the flowing blood, on the endothelial surface, at endothelial lesions, in the perivascular tissues, and in deeper tissues not contiguous to

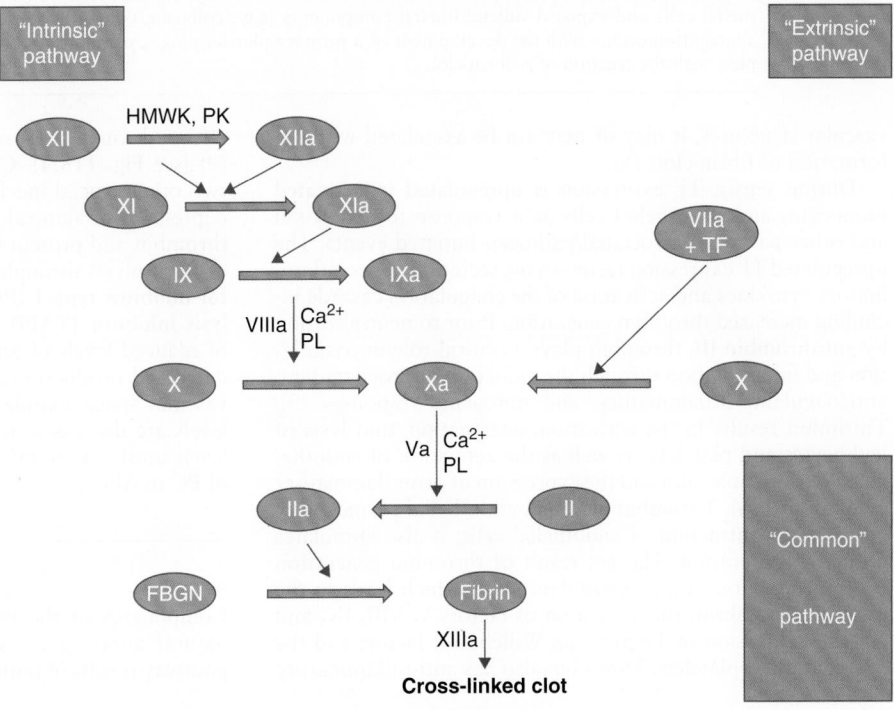

FIGURE 118.1. "Classical" coagulation cascade. Serial activation of serine proteases from zymogen to active form resulting in fibrin clot formation. Those elements in RED represent cofactor for enzymatic steps. HMWK, high-molecular-weight kininogen; PK, prekallikrein; TF, tissue factor; PL, phospholipid; Ca, calcium; Clotting factors: XII, factor XII; XIIa, activated factor XII; XI, factor XI; XIa, activated factor XI; IX, factor IX; IXa: activated factor IX; VIIIa, activated factor VIII; VIIa, activated Factor VII; X, factor X; Xa, activated factor Xa; Va, activated factor V; II, prothrombin; IIa, thrombin; FBGN, fibrinogen; XIIIa, activated factor XIII.

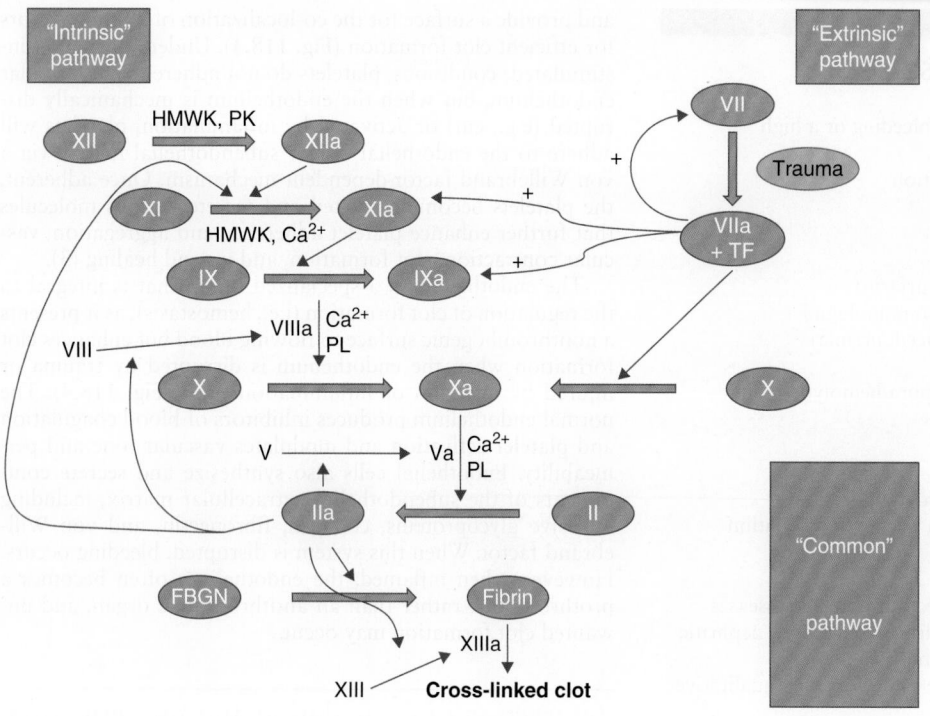

FIGURE 118.2. "Classical" coagulation cascade with crosstalk. Thin lines with "+" indicate enhancement of generation of F.Xia and F.IXa by the F.VIIa/TF complex. HMWK, high-molecular-weight kininogen; PK, prekallekrein; TF, tissue factor; PL, phospholipid; Ca, calcium; Clotting factors: XII, factor XII; XIIa, activated factor XII; XI, factor XI; XI, activated factor XI; IX, factor IX; IXa, activated factor IX; VIIIa, activated factor VIII; VIIa, activated Factor VII; X, factor X; Xa, activated factor Xa; Va, activated factor V; II, prothrombin; IIa, thrombin; FBGN, fibrinogen; XIIIa, activated factor XIII.

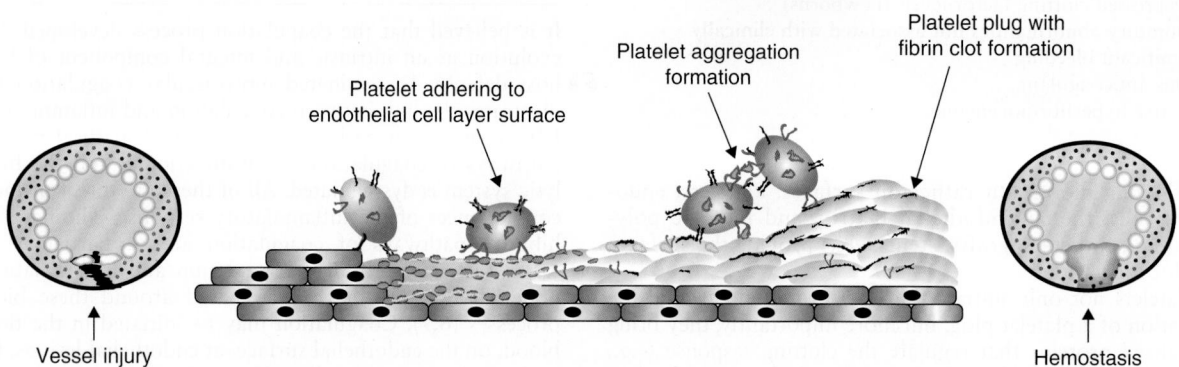

FIGURE 118.3. The role of platelets in mediating primary hemostasis at sites of vascular injury. Platelets are initially activated and express specific adhesion receptors on their surface, followed by adhesion to activated endothelial cells and exposed subendothelial components (e.g., collagen, von Willebrand factor). Subsequent platelet aggregation occurs with the development of a primary platelet plug. Coagulation occurs on the developing platelet plug with the creation of a fibrin clot.

vascular structures. It may or may not be associated with the formation of fibrin clots (8).

During sepsis, TF expression is upregulated in activated monocytes and endothelial cells as a response to endotoxin and other pathogen-associated/pathogen-initiated events. The upregulated TF expression results in the secretion of proinflammatory cytokines and activation of the coagulation cascade including increased thrombin generation. Prior to neutralization by **antithrombin III**, thrombin plays a central role in coagulation and inflammation through the induction of procoagulant, anticoagulant, inflammatory, and mitogenic responses (9). Thrombin results in the activation, aggregation, and lysis of leukocytes and platelets, as well as the activation of endothelial adhesion molecules and the expression of proinflammatory cytokines (IL-6). Thrombin increases endothelial permeability by causing contraction of endothelial cells; it also stimulates cellular proliferation. The net result of thrombin generation is the production of a procoagulant state, which leads to the formation of fibrin; the activation of factors V, VIII, IX, and XI; the expression of TF and von Willebrand factor; and the aggregation of platelets. Thrombin also has anti-inflammatory

effects through the production of **activated protein C (APC)** (9) (see **Fig. 118.4**). Concurrent with coagulation activation, two other crucial mechanisms occur during sepsis. One is the depression of natural anticoagulant systems, involving antithrombin and protein C (PC), and the second is the inhibition of fibrinolysis through the production of **plasminogen activator inhibitor type-1 (PAI-1)** and **thrombin-activatable fibrinolysis inhibitor (TAFI)** (**Figs. 118.4 and 118.5**). Other causes of reduced levels of antithrombin III (AT III) and PC include decreased production (impaired liver function), loss from the vascular space (capillary leakage), immaturity (AT III and PC levels are decreased at birth and do not achieve "near-adult" levels until 3–6 months of age), and consumption (conversion of PC to APC).

The Role of the Protein C System

Components of the PC system regulate coagulation (i.e., as natural anticoagulants) such that decreased activity of this pathway results in pathologic thrombosis. Activated protein C

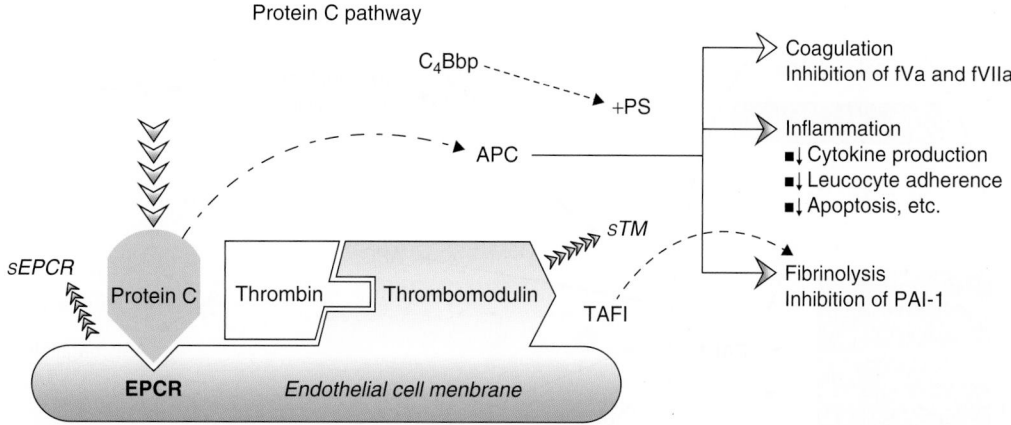

FIGURE 118.4. The interaction of the protein C system with the endothelium. Thrombin bound to thrombomodulin (TM) modifies protein C bound to the endothelial protein C receptor on the cell surface to generate activated protein C (APC). APC acts as a natural anticoagulant by inactivating activated factors V (fVa) and VIII (fVIIIa), modulating inflammation by downregulating the synthesis of proinflammatory cytokines, leukocyte adherence, and apoptosis and enhancing fibrinolysis by inhibiting thrombin-activatable fibrinolysis inhibitor (TAFI) and plasminogen activator inhibitor type-1 (PAI-1). C4Bbp, C4b binding protein; +PS, in the presence of protein S; sTM, soluble thrombomodulin; sEPCR, soluble endothelial cell protein C receptor.

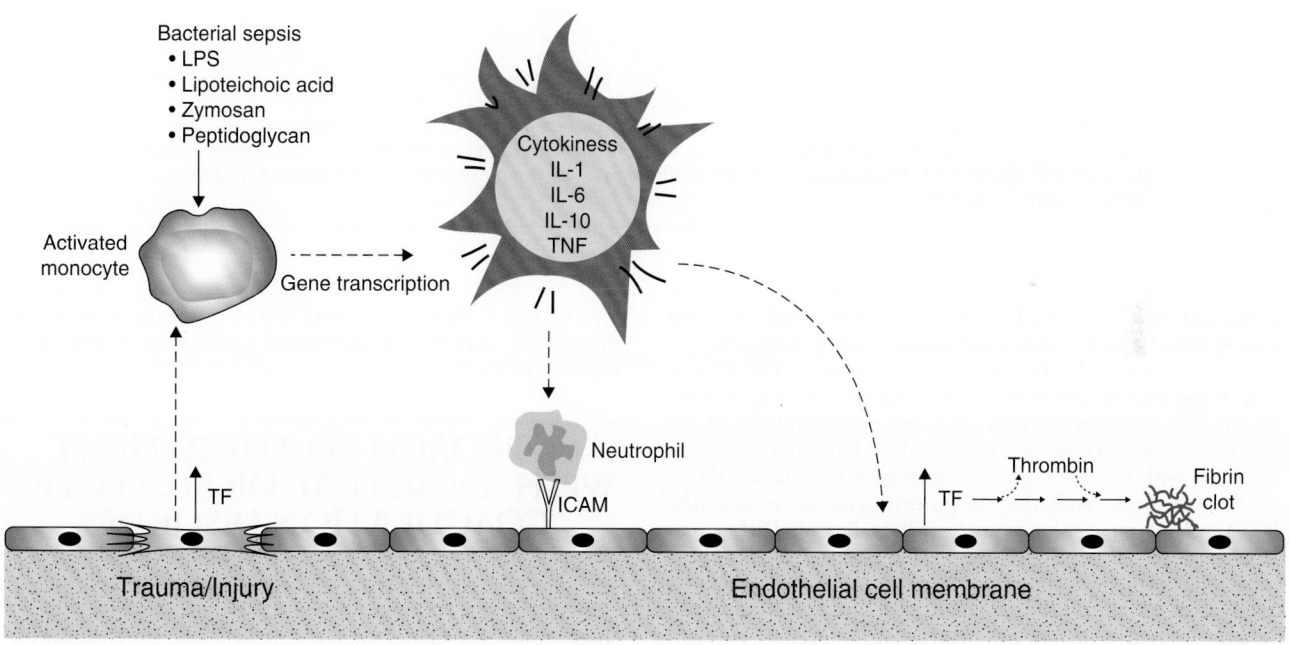

FIGURE 118.5. Inflammation effect on coagulation. Inflammation enhances coagulation through the induction of proinflammatory cytokines that induce tissue factor formation, which in turn decreases activated protein C (APC) formation, leading to enhanced thrombin and fibrin generation. In addition, the decrease in APC allows for greater inhibition of fibrinolysis through the action of plasminogen activator inhibitor type-1 (PAI-1).

(APC) also possesses intrinsic immunomodulating properties (see **Fig. 118.5**). In vitro, APC inhibits tumor necrosis factor-α elaboration from monocytes, blocks leukocyte adhesion to selectins, and influences apoptosis (9). The PC pathway is initiated by the binding of thrombin to **thrombomodulin** and forms a complex on the surface of endothelial cells. The binding of PC to the endothelial cell PC receptor augments PC activation by the thrombin-thrombomodulin complex more than tenfold. PC activation in sepsis and inflammation is downregulated when the exposure to inflammatory mediators and thrombin causes the endothelial cells to shed their PC receptors. The endothelial cell PC receptor (ECPCR) can also translocate from

the plasma membrane to the nucleus and redirect gene expression. The translocation of the PC-receptor-APC complex to the nucleus may account for the ability of APC to modulate inflammatory mediator responses in the endothelium (9).

The third important property of APC is its influence on fibrinolysis, which is also involved with inflammation. APC is capable of neutralizing the fibrinolysis inhibitors PAI-1 and TAFI. PAI-1 is a 50-kDa glycoprotein of the serine protease inhibitor family. Its primary role in vivo is the inhibition of both tissue- and urokinase-type plasminogen activators. PAI-1 is an acute-phase protein that increases during acute inflammation. In patients with sepsis, increased levels of PAI-1 are

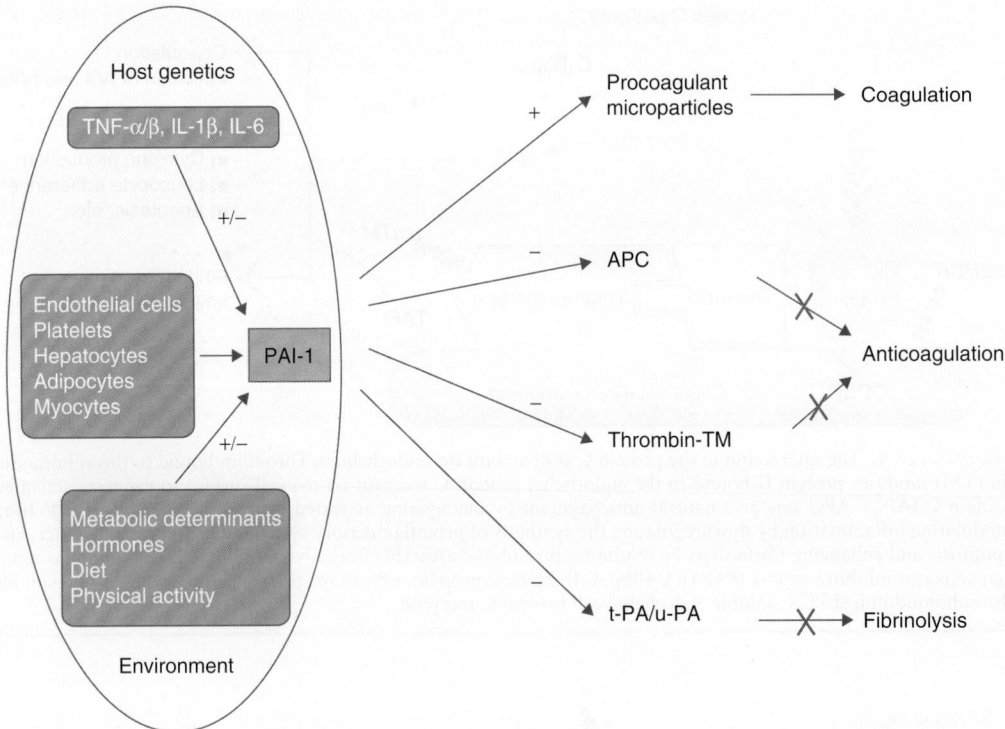

FIGURE 118.6. Plasminogen activator inhibitor type 1 gene polymorphism and sepsis. Genetic and environmental influences on the expression of plasminogen activator inhibitor type 1 (PAI-1) and the importance of PAI-1 in the coagulation and fibrinolysis pathways. TNF-α, tumor necrosis factor-α; APC, activated protein C; TM, thrombomodulin; t-PA, tissue-type plasminogen activator; u-PA, urokinase-type plasminogen activator. (Redrawn from Hermans PW, Hazelzet JA. Plasminogen activator inhibitor type 1 gene polymorphism and sepsis. *Clin Infect Dis* 2005;41(suppl 7):S453–8.)

associated with increased levels of various cytokines and acute-phase proteins, abnormal coagulation parameters, increased severity of disease, and poorer outcomes. The regulation of the production of PAI-1 is multifactorial (**Fig. 118.6**). The 4G/5G insertion/deletion promoter polymorphism of the PAI-1 gene has been shown to affect PAI-1 plasma levels; individuals with the 4G/4G genotype display the highest PAI-1 levels while those with the 5G/5G genotype the lowest (the 4G/5G genotype results in intermediate levels). Differences in PAI-1 levels affect the risk of developing severe complications and death from sepsis. High PAI-1 levels are associated with increased mortality in animal models of sepsis and with increased severity of illness and organ dysfunction scores in septic patients (including children with meningococcal sepsis) (10,11,12). However, the regulation of PAI-1 levels involves more than just the promoters of its synthesis. Activated Protein C stimulates fibrinolysis by forming a tight 1:1 complex with PAI-1 leading to inactivation of PAI-1. High levels of thrombin lead to increased levels of APC, which can complex to PAI-1. This complex is subsequently cleared from the circulation, resulting in PC depletion (11). The increased formation and clearance of these complexes results in PC depletion (11), with the net result being an increased risk for microvascular thrombus formation.

Thrombin generation also increases the levels of TAFI, an important negative regulator of the fibrinolytic system. TAFI has been shown to inactivate inflammatory peptides that play a role in the contact activation of coagulation, such as complement factors C3a and C5a. The full role of TAFI in the hemostatic and innate immune response to sepsis is still under investigation. The role of TAFI as a regulator of fibrinolysis appears to be of prognostic significance similar to

that of PAI-1, that is, elevated levels, resulting in decreased fibrinolysis, appear to be associated with a poorer outcome in sepsis (13,14,15).

APPROACH TO THE PATIENT WITH AN ACTUAL OR SUSPECTED COAGULATION DISORDER

Clinical History

Diagnostic assessment begins at the bedside. The medical history, both past and present, may lend some insight into the cause of, or risk for, significant bleeding (16,17). A prior history of prolonged or excessive bleeding or of recurrent thrombosis may direct laboratory investigation and guide emergency therapy. Specific questions should include the occurrence of spontaneous, easy, or disproportionately severe bruising; intramuscular hematoma formation (either spontaneous or related to trauma); spontaneous or trauma-induced hemarthrosis; spontaneous mucous membrane bleeding; problematic bleeding related to surgery (including dental extractions, tonsillectomy, and circumcision); the need for transfusions; the quantity of bleeding during menses; and, finally, current medications.

In spite of the decreased use of aspirin in children, there remain numerous over-the-counter aspirin-containing medications that can potentially interfere with primary (plateletmediated) hemostasis. Patients (and parents) may not be aware of the aspirin contained in these products. Many other drugs used in the ICU are also associated with bleeding abnormalities and are discussed below. Additionally, in specific circumstances, herbal medications may contribute to impaired clot formation or abnormal bleeding (e.g., garlic, ginko, senna, cascara). In trauma and surgical situations, it is important to determine the severity of injury relative to the magnitude of bleeding that follows. A prior history of significant thrombosis (e.g., deep venous thrombosis, pulmonary embolus, stroke) suggests the possibility of a hypercoagulable condition. As thrombotic events are uncommon in children, the occurrence of thrombotic events, such as myocardial infarction in young, adult relatives, should cause the clinician to consider a congenital thrombophilic abnormality. These abnormalities include AT III deficiency, PC or **protein S** deficiency, factor V Leiden R506Q mutation, the prothrombin G20210A polymorphism/mutation, and (possibly) the C677T mutation/polymorphism of the methylenetetrahydrofolate reductase (MTHFR) gene (discussed below). In addition, vasculitis associated with an autoimmune disorder such as systemic lupus erythematosus (SLE) must be considered in the evaluation of a child with an unexplained clot. In all cases, the family history is important in attempting to separate congenital from acquired disorders.

In a general sense, defects in **primary hemostasis** (creation of the platelet plug) or secondary hemostasis (addition of fibrin to the platelet plug) can be separated according to the nature of the bleeding. Patients with primary hemostatic defects tend to manifest "capillary-type bleeding" including oozing from cuts or incisions, mucous membrane bleeding, or excessive bruising. This type of bleeding is seen in patients with quantitative or qualitative platelet defects or von Willebrand disease. In contrast, patients with dysfunction of secondary hemostasis tend to display "large-vessel bleeding," characterized by hemarthrosis, intramuscular hematomas, and intracranial hemorrhage. This type of bleeding is most often associated with specific coagulation factor deficiencies or inhibitors. Patients with severe platelet-type defects may also manifest this type of bleeding. Consequently, the presence of only mucosal bleeding is more helpful as this would point to a platelet-type defect affecting mainly primary hemostasis rather than an abnormality of fibrin clot formation.

Physical Examination

Development of generalized bleeding in critically ill patients in the ICU presents a special problem. Such bleeding may be a marker for severe major organ dysfunction. Supportive evidence or physical findings of other concurrent organ system dysfunction (e.g., renal failure, liver failure, respiratory failure, and hypotension) often are readily apparent. Common causes of generalized bleeding in critically ill children include sepsis-related DIC, massive transfusion syndrome (discussed below), severe liver dysfunction, undiagnosed hemophilia, battered child syndrome, and vitamin K deficiency in newborns or older children with malabsorption (18–20). In young infants (<3 months of age), the coagulation system is often not yet mature, and prolongation of the prothrombin time (PT) or activated partial thromboplastin time (aPTT) may not reflect an abnormality in hemostasis (21). Consultation with a pediatric hematologist may be indicated when trying to interpret "abnormal" results in this age group.

The physical examination of the patient with a bleeding disorder should address several basic questions. Is the process localized or diffuse? Is it related to an anatomic or surgical lesion (e.g., bleeding localized to an area of trauma or recent surgical site not associated with generalized bleeding suggests a discrete anatomic cause for the bleeding rather than the presence of a generalized hemorrhagic diathesis)? Is the bleeding primarily muco-cutaneous? Finally, when appropriate, are there signs of thrombosis (either arterial or venous)?

The answers to these questions may provide clues to the cause of the problem.

Several specific physical findings may be helpful in determining the etiology of a suspected hemostatic abnormality. For example, the presence of an enlarged spleen coupled with thrombocytopenia suggests splenic sequestration. Splenomegaly accompanied by prolongation of the PT and/or aPTT may be a consequence of underlying liver disease, while splenomegaly in the presence of a normal PT and aPTT may indicate a marrow infiltrative process. Furthermore, evidence of liver disease (e.g., varices, ascites) points to decreased factor synthesis as a possible etiology of a prolonged PT or aPTT. When lymphadenopathy, splenomegaly, or other findings suggestive of disseminated malignancy are detected, acute or chronic DIC should be suspected as the cause of prolonged coagulation times, hypofibrinogenemia, and/or thrombocytopenia. Palpable purpura suggests capillary leak from vasculitis, whereas purpura associated with thrombocytopenia or qualitative platelet defects is generally not palpable. Finally, venous or arterial telangiectasia may be seen in von Willebrand disease and liver disease, respectively. When selective pressure is centrally applied to an arterial telangiectasia, the entire lesion fades, whereas a venous telangiectasia requires confluent pressure across the entire lesion (as with a glass slide) for blanching to occur.

Laboratory Evaluation

Blood Sample Preparation

The importance of correct specimen collection for laboratory evaluation of hemostatic problems must be emphasized. In the PICU, it is common for laboratory samples to be drawn through an indwelling arterial or central venous cannula. Heparin is commonly present in the solutions used to flush these cannulae or as a component of an IV infusion. Depending on the concentration of heparin in the infusing fluid and the volume of blood withdrawn, several tests can be influenced. Heparin presence can cause fibrin degradation products (FDPs) to be falsely elevated and fibrinogen falsely low. Likewise, heparin contamination can spuriously prolong the PT, aPTT, and thrombin time (TT). Therefore, a minimum of 20 mL of blood in adolescents and adults (10 mL of blood in younger children) should be withdrawn through the cannula and either discarded, returned to the patient through a peripheral cannula, or used for other purposes before obtaining a specimen for laboratory hemostasis analysis (22). This practice should minimize any influence of heparin on the results. In young children and infants, it may not be reasonable to withdraw an adequate volume of waste blood, and a peripheral venipuncture may be necessary. Because the aPTT is sensitive to the presence of small amounts of heparin, an unexpected prolonged aPTT obtained through a heparinized catheter should raise the suspicion of sample contamination. In this setting, the TT will also be prolonged but will normalize if the contaminating heparin is neutralized (e.g., with protamine, toluidine blue, or Hepasorb).

Laboratory Results in Suspected Bleeding Disorders

The presence of most suspected bleeding disorders can be confirmed using routinely available tests including the peripheral blood smear (which provides an estimate of platelet number as well as platelet and red blood cell morphology), the PT, the aPTT, the TT, a fibrinogen level, FDPs, and the **D-dimer** fragment of polymerized fibrin. This latter test is more specific for the fibrinolytic fragment produced when the polymerized fibrin monomer is cleaved by the proteolytic enzyme plasmin. In contrast, the older assays for FDPs or fibrin split products will be positive even if fibrin is not produced and the fragments are the result of proteolytic degradation of native fibrinogen.

TABLE 118.2

COAGULATION DISORDERS AND ASSOCIATED LABORATORY FINDINGS

■ CLINICAL SYNDROME	■ SCREENING TESTS	■ SUPPORTIVE TESTS
Disseminated intravascular coagulation	Prolonged PT, aPTT, TT; decreased fibrinogen, platelets; microangiopathy	(+) FDPs, D-dimer; decreased factors V, VIII, and II (late)
Massive transfusion	Prolonged PT, aPTT; decreased fibrinogen, platelets ± prolonged TT	All factors decreased; (–) FDPs, D-dimer (unless DIC develops); (+) transfusion history
Anticoagulant overdose		
Heparin	Prolonged aPTT, TT; ± prolonged PT	Toluidine blue/protamine corrects TT; reptilase time normal
Warfarin (same as vitamin K deficiency)	Prolonged PT; ± prolonged aPTT (severe); normal TT, fibrinogen, platelets	Vitamin K-dependent factors decreased; factors V, VIII normal
Liver disease		
Early	Prolonged PT	Decreased Factor VII
Late	Prolonged PT, aPTT; decreased fibrinogen (terminal liver failure); normal platelet count (if splenomegaly absent)	Decreased factors II, V, VII, IX, and X; decreased plasminogen; ± FDPs unless DIC develops
Primary fibrinolysis	Prolonged PT, aPTT, TT; decreased fibrinogen ± platelets decreased	(+) FDPs, (–) D-dimer; short euglobulin clot lysis time
Thrombotic thrombocytopenic purpura	Thrombocytopenia, microangiopathy with mild anemia; PT, aPTT, fibrinogen generally within normal limits/mildly abnormal	ADAMTS-13 deficiency/inhibitor, unusually large von Willebrand factor multimers between episodes; mild increase in FDPs or D-dimer
Hemolytic uremic syndrome	Microangiopathic hemolytic anemia, ± thrombocytopenia; PT, aPTT generally within normal limits	Renal insufficiency; FDPs and D-dimer generally (–)

PT, prothrombin time; aPTT, activated partial thromboplastin time; TT, thrombin time; FDPs, fibrin degradation products.

In most instances, measurement of the platelet count, fibrinogen level, PT, aPTT, and TT should be sufficient for determining the correct diagnosis. An unnecessary use of laboratory resources may be avoided by using these five screening tests and only ordering further, more specific, testing when a definitive diagnosis is necessary. Several major categories of hemorrhagic disorders and the tests that are characteristically abnormal in each are summarized in **Table 118.2**.

Patients who present with a thrombotic event will generally not display abnormalities of usual "clotting" studies; that is, their PT, aPTT, TT, and fibrinogen will usually be within normal ranges. The finding of a shortened PT or aPTT is not necessarily indicative of a prothrombotic or thrombophilic process being present. While *hyperfibrinogenemia* (>400 mg/dL) and persistent elevations of F.VIII (>400%) have been associated with an increased risk of thrombosis in adults, both may be elevated by acute inflammation. Consequently, the finding of elevations of these clotting factors in a patient who has experienced an unexpected thrombotic event may not necessarily indicate that the cause of the event was an elevation in either factor. Without prior samples, it is impossible to determine if the elevation is the consequence of the thrombosis or was present prior to its development and potentially causative.

Several inherited or acquired abnormalities place an individual at increased risk for thrombosis and should be investigated when a thrombotic event is suspected or documented. Prior to the initiation of anticoagulation, plasma levels of protein C (antigen and activity), protein S (antigen and activity; total and free), and antithrombin III (antigen and activity) should be obtained. In addition, PCR analysis for mutations in the F.V (F.V Leiden; R506Q), and prothrombin (G20210A) genes should be performed. A serum homocysteine level may be obtained as the thrombosis risk of the MTHFR mutation may be related to elevations of homocysteine caused by alterations

in the metabolism of folic acid rather than the mutation per se. Whether the MTHFR C677T polymorphism/mutation can cause thrombosis in the absence of an elevated serum homocysteine has been questioned recently (23–25). None of the known thrombophilic risk factors are found in up to 40% of adults who present with thrombosis and the incidence is likely lower in children (26–28). It is likely that the percentage in children who are negative for these abnormalities is at least as high or higher. The intensive care physician must look for confounding clinical conditions, such as dehydration (in cerebral venous sinus thrombosis), indwelling catheters, vascular compression (e.g., cervical ribs), and type II heparin-induced thrombocytopenia (see below) in evaluating a children with thrombosis.

CONDITIONS ASSOCIATED WITH SERIOUS BLEEDING, A HIGH PROBABILITY OF BLEEDING, OR SERIOUS HEMOSTATIC SEQUELAE

Disseminated Intravascular Coagulation

Pathogenesis

Because it often occurs in conjunction with other life-threatening disorders, DIC is one of the most serious hemostatic abnormalities seen in the PICU. DIC is caused by an abnormal activation of blood coagulation leading to excessive thrombin generation, a widespread formation of fibrin thrombi in the microcirculation and the consumption of clotting factors and platelets. Ultimately, this consumption of clotting factors and platelets is responsible for significant bleeding

TABLE 118.3

CONDITIONS ASSOCIATED WITH DISSEMINATED
INTRAVASCULAR COAGULATION

Sepsis	Retained placenta
Liver disease	Hypertonic saline abortion
Shock	Amniotic fluid embolus
Penetrating brain injury	Retention of a dead fetus
Necrotizing pneumonitis	Eclampsia
Tissue necrosis/crush injury	Localized endothelial injury
Intravascular hemolysis	(aortic aneurysm, giant hem-
	angiomata, angiography)
Acute promyelocytic	Disseminated malignancy
leukemia	(prostate, pancreatic)
Thermal injury	
Freshwater drowning	
Fat embolism syndrome	

when consumption exceeds production (29). The conditions associated with DIC are generally the same in adults and children and include the wide variety of disorders with the ability to initiate coagulation (**Table 118.3**). The mechanisms involved in these conditions either activate procoagulant proteins enzymatically or cause the release of TF, which then triggers coagulation.

DIC represents an imbalance between clot formation (coagulation) and clot breakdown (fibrinolysis). Initially, DIC is a thrombotic disorder characterized by microvascular thrombosis with bleeding occurring only when the consumption of platelets and clotting factors outpaces the ability to replace clotting factors and platelets. Thrombin generation and/or release of tissue plasminogen activator (tPA) initiate fibrinolysis (**Fig. 118.7**), which invariably accompanies thrombin formation in DIC (29). Tissue plasminogen activator converts plasminogen to plasmin, which then digests fibrinogen and fibrin clots as they form. Plasmin also inactivates several activated coagulation factors and impairs platelet aggregation. Therefore, thrombin-induced coagulation factor consumption, thrombocytopenia, and plasmin generation contribute to the presence of bleeding.

In addition to bleeding complications, the presence of fibrin thrombi in the microcirculation can lead to ischemic tissue injury. Pathologic data indicate that renal failure, acrocyanosis, multifocal pulmonary emboli, and transient cerebral ischemia may be related clinically to the presence of such thrombi. The presence of fibrinopeptides A and B (resulting from enzymatic cleavage of fibrinogen) leads to pulmonary and systemic vasoconstriction, which can potentiate an existing ischemic injury. In DIC, either bleeding or thrombotic tendencies may predominate. In most patients with DIC, bleeding is the predominant problem. However, 10% may have a presentation that is exclusively thrombotic (e.g., pulmonary emboli with pulmonary hypertension, renal insufficiency, altered mental status, acrocyanosis).

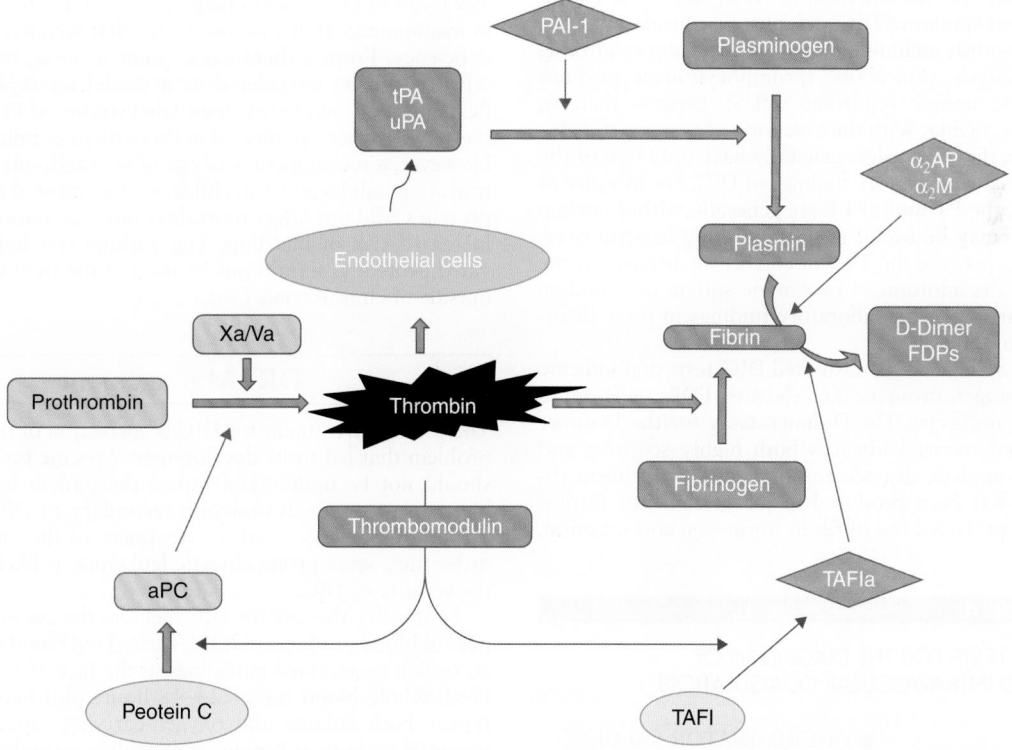

FIGURE 118.7. Fibrinolysis. Thrombin, generated from prothrombin by the action of the Xa/Va prothrombinase complex activates endothelial cells to produce plasminogen activators. These, in turn, cleave plasminogen to form plasmin, which degrades fibrin (formed by the action of thrombin on fibrinogen) to D-dimer fragments and other fibrinogen degradation products. Inhibitors of fibrinolysis (in diamonds) include PAI-1, which inhibit the actions of tPA and uPA, and α_2AP, α_2M, and TAFI, which inhibit plasmin. Thrombin, when bound to thrombomodulin on the surface of endothelial cells, activates TAFI to its active form and produces activated Protein C an important vitamin K-dependent protein with anticoagulant and anti-inflammatory properties. α_2AP, alpha-2-antiplasmin (alpha-2-plasmin inhibitor); α_2M, alpha-2-macroglobulin; tPA, tissue-type plasminogen activator; uPA, urine-type plasminogen activator; PAI-1, plasminogen activator inhibitor type-1; FDPs, fibrin degradation products; Xa, activated factor X; Va, activated factor V; aPC, activated Protein C; TAFI, thrombin-activatable fibrinolysis inhibitor; TAFIa, activated TAFI.

Whether the presentation of DIC is thrombotic, hemorrhagic, or "compensated" (that is, laboratory results consistent with DIC without bleeding), microthrombosis likely contributes to the development and progression of multiorgan failure.

Clinical Presentation and Diagnosis of DIC

The suspicion that DIC is present usually stems from one of two conditions: (a) unexplained, generalized oozing or bleeding or (b) unexplained, abnormal laboratory parameters of hemostasis. This usually occurs in the context of a suggestive clinical scenario or associated disease (see **Table 118.3**). While infection and multiple trauma are the most common conditions associated with the development of DIC, multiple organ system dysfunction syndrome (MODS) and acute respiratory distress syndrome are associated with severe forms of DIC (18,20).

DIC has traditionally been assessed by the severity of bleeding and coagulation abnormalities. Scoring tools are available that use laboratory tests and severity of illness scores to diagnose and determine the severity of DIC. The laboratory tests used in the diagnosis of DIC and in these scoring systems are listed in **Table 118.4**. While no data exist for children, these scoring systems may have prognostic value for patients with sepsis (30–32). Limited studies suggest that early identification of DIC before the onset of a gross hemorrhagic diathesis may improve survival in critically ill children (6,33).

The triad of a prolonged PT, hypofibrinogenemia, and thrombocytopenia in the appropriate clinical setting is sufficient to suspect DIC. Severe hepatic insufficiency (with splenomegaly and splenic sequestration of platelets) can yield a similar laboratory profile and must be ruled out. Other conditions can present similar to DIC and must be considered in the differential diagnosis including massive transfusion syndrome, primary fibrinolysis, thrombotic thrombocytopenic purpura (TTP)/hemolytic uremic syndrome (HUS), heparin therapy, and dysfibrinogenemia. With the exception of massive transfusion syndrome, these disorders generally have only two of the three characteristic laboratory findings of DIC. For instance in HUS and TTP, the PT and aPTT are generally within normal limits. The TT may be useful in distinguishing heparin overdose from DIC because the TT can correct for heparin in the test tube with the addition of protamine sulfate or toluidine blue. A comparison of the laboratory findings in these disorders is noted in **Table 118.2**.

To confirm a diagnosis of suspected DIC, tests that indicate increased fibrinogen turnover (i.e., elevated FDPs or D-dimer assay) may be necessary. The D-dimer assay for the D-dimer fragment of polymerized fibrin is both highly sensitive and specific for proteolytic degradation of polymerized fibrin (fibrin clot that has been produced in the presence of thrombin) and is the preferred test of fibrin/fibrinogen consumption.

Other tests, such as soluble fibrin monomer or thrombin–antithrombin complex formation, either have problems with sensitivity or are impractical for widespread use.

The differential diagnosis of D-dimer elevation includes a number of disorders. A modest elevation of D-dimer must be interpreted with caution in a postoperative or trauma patient because thrombin is produced whenever coagulation is activated in the presence of bleeding. Other causes for elevated D-dimer test include pregnancy, liver disease, and some cancers. Hyperbilirubinemia or hemolyzed blood specimen may lead to a false-positive D-dimer test.

Meningococcal Purpura Fulminans

Purpura fulminans is a systemic coagulopathy similar to DIC that accompanies meningococcal sepsis or other severe infections. The hallmark of this syndrome is tissue ischemia and necrosis due to marked microvascular thrombosis. Patients are generally noted to have severely depressed levels of PC, with a degree of suppression that correlates with mortality. The presence of the PAI-1 4G/4G genotype, producing the highest plasma levels of PAI-1, has been described in children with meningococcal infection and has been associated with increased incidence of sepsis and increased mortality, but no increased incidence of meningitis (13). As mentioned before, APC can stimulate fibrinolysis by forming a complex with, and inactivating, PAI-1. High levels of thrombin lead to high levels of APC which complexes to PAI-1 and depletes unbound PC (10). This mechanism could explain the extremely low levels of PC found in meningococcal disease. The purpura in meningococcal disease resembles that seen in congenital PC deficiency. From a therapeutic point of view, meningococcal sepsis has been considered as a model for sepsis-associated PC deficiency, and many open-label studies of PC-concentrate therapy have been published in this patient population (34,35). However, a recent meta-analysis of six randomized controlled trials (5 in adults and 1 in children) documented that activated protein C did not affect mortality, but was associated with an increased risk of bleeding. The authors concluded that activated protein C should not be used in the treatment of sepsis outside of clinical trials (36).

DIC Management

The primary treatment for DIC is correction of the underlying problem that led to its development. Specific therapy for DIC should not be undertaken unless the patient has significant bleeding or organ dysfunction secondary to DIC, significant thrombosis has occurred, or treatment of the underlying disorder (i.e., acute promyelocytic leukemia) is likely to increase the severity of DIC.

Supportive therapy for DIC includes the use of several component blood products (37,38). Packed red blood cells are given according to accepted guidelines in the face of active bleeding. Fresh whole blood (i.e., <24–48 hours old) may be given to replete both volume and oxygen-carrying capacity, with the potential additional benefit of providing coagulation proteins, including fibrinogen and platelets. Cryoprecipitate contains a much higher concentration of fibrinogen than does whole blood or fresh frozen plasma (FFP) and therefore is more likely to provide the quantity of fibrinogen necessary to replete fibrinogen that is consumed by DIC. In this regard, FFP is of limited value for the treatment of significant hypofibrinogenemia because of the inordinate volumes required to make any meaningful contribution to plasma fibrinogen concentration. FFP infusions (10 mL/kg BID or QD) may replete other procoagulant and anticoagulant factors (e.g., PC) consumed with DIC. The use of

TABLE 118.4

LABORATORY TESTS FOR THE DIAGNOSIS OF DISSEMINATED INTRAVASCULAR COAGULATION

■ TEST	■ DISCRIMINATOR VALUE
Platelet count	<80,000–100,000 or a decrease of >50% from baseline
Fibrinogen	<100 mg/dL or a decrease of >50% from baseline
Prothrombin time	>3-s prolongation above upper limit of normal
Fibrin degradation products	>80 mg/dL
D-dimer	"moderate" increase

cryoprecipitate or FFP in the treatment of DIC has been open to debate in the past because of concern that these products merely provide further substrate for ongoing DIC and thus increase the amount of fibrin thrombi formed. However, clinical (autopsy) studies have failed to confirm this concern.

The goal of blood component therapy is not to produce normal "numbers" but rather to produce clinical stability and stop the bleeding. If the serum fibrinogen level is <50–75 mg/dL in patient with DIC, repletion with cryoprecipitate to raise plasma levels to ≥100 mg/dL should be attempted as a first step. A reasonable starting dose is 1 bag of cryoprecipitate for every 10 kg of body weight every 8–12 hours. As cryoprecipitate is not a standardized component (i.e., its content varies from bag to bag), the fibrinogen level should be rechecked after an infusion to assess the increase. The amount and timing of the next infusion is then adjusted according to the results.

Platelet transfusions also may be used when thrombocytopenia is thought to contribute to ongoing bleeding. Many of the fibrin/fibrinogen fragments produced in DIC have the potential to impair platelet function by inhibiting fibrinogen binding to platelets, which may be clinically significant at the concentration of FDPs achieved with DIC. Platelet transfusions in patients with DIC should be considered to maintain platelet counts up to 40,000–80,000/mcL, depending on the severity of bleeding.

Pharmacologic therapy for DIC has two primary aims: to "turn off" ongoing coagulation so that repletion of coagulation factors may begin and to impede thrombus formation and ensuing ischemic injury. Recombinant activated Factor VII (rhF.VIIa), a recombinant hemostatic factor, has been used to treat bleeding in DIC refractory to other therapies as well as in trauma and in other medical and surgical causes of severe, life-threatening bleeding. Most of these studies have demonstrated efficacy in the control of hemorrhage, but most have not demonstrated an effect on mortality (39–43). Recombinant activated Factor VII has also been shown to correct the hemostatic defect caused by the antiplatelet agents aspirin and clopidogrel (44). Reports have noted that use of rhF.VIIa may result in an increase in thrombosis and thromboembolic events, although the incidence appears to be small and the severity of most events mild (45,43). Taking these results together, we recommend reserving rhF.VIIa for life-threatening hemorrhage that is refractory to all other measures.

Various synthetic and natural modulators of hemostasis have shown some efficacy in moderating multiorgan dysfunction in animal models of sepsis. These include anticoagulant molecules (e.g., heparin, antithrombin III, **tissue factor pathway inhibitor [TFPI]**, activated protein C [APC]), and thrombolytic modulators (e.g., tissue plasminogen activator [tPA], thrombin-activatable fibrinolysis inhibitor [TAFI]). While initial reports of the use of recombinant human APC in sepsis demonstrated a benefit on survival in septic adults, there was increased bleeding in the elderly, and the pediatric trial was stopped because of futility and increased bleeding in infants. Subsequent reanalysis of data demonstrated no benefit of this agent in the treatment of sepsis, and it was withdrawn from the US market. Clinical trials addressing the use of other natural modulators of thrombosis and fibrinolysis have not consistently demonstrated benefit in septic patients (46–50).

Microangiopathies with Microvascular Thrombosis

Hemolytic Uremic Syndrome

While neither TTP nor hemolytic uremic syndrome (HUS) usually produces a coagulopathic state, both, like DIC, are characterized by microangiopathy and microvascular thrombosis. HUS is more commonly seen in children and is characterized

by a prodrome of fever and diffuse diarrhea (often bloody). HUS is multisystem disease with renal injury and less commonly central nervous system (CNS) dysfunction (seizures, coma, stroke), GI dysfunction (colitis, intussusception, bowel perforation), as well as pancreatic and hepatic involvement (see Chapter 110 for more complete discussion). The diagnosis is made on clinical grounds on the basis of prodromal diarrhea and the triad of microangiopathic hemolytic anemia, thrombocytopenia, and acute kidney injury. Endemic cases of HUS are generally caused by verotoxin expressing strains of enteropathic *Escherichia coli* (O157:H7) or shigatoxin-expressing strains of *Shigella*. Sporadic cases, not associated with diarrhea, may represent variant TTP or familial defects in complement factor H. Therapy is supportive, including renal replacement measures when indications exist. Neither plasma infusion nor plasma exchange appears to be beneficial, although there have been no large-scale clinical trials in children. Case reports of HUS with severe CNS involvement suggest that the monoclonal antibody, eculizumab, may be beneficial in this high-risk population (51). Eculizumab blocks complement activation by binding to complement factor C-5.

Thrombotic Thrombocytopenic Purpura

TTP is characterized by the pentad of microangiopathic hemolytic anemia, thrombocytopenia, neurologic symptoms, fever, and renal dysfunction. While only 40% of patients display the full pentad, up to 75% will manifest a triad of microangiopathic hemolytic anemia, neurologic symptoms, and thrombocytopenia. In many instances, this disorder is due to the absence or deficiency of the von Willebrand factor-cleaving protease **ADAMTS-13**, resulting in the circulation of unusually large von Willebrand factor multimers that can induce or enhance the pathologic adhesion of platelets to the endothelium. ADAMST-13 deficiency can either be inherited (secondary to ADAMTS-13 gene polymorphisms) or acquired (secondary to inhibitory autoantibodies directed at ADAMTS-13 protease). The therapy of choice for TTP is plasma exchange by apheresis, which both replaces plasma ADAMTS-13 and removes inhibitory antibodies from circulation (Chapter 41). Platelet transfusions are generally not recommended, except in the case of major bleeding.

Thrombocytopenia-Associated Multiple Organ Failure

Decreases in ADAMTS-13 have been documented in septic patients with **thrombocytopenia-associated multiple organ failure (TAMOF)**. Intensive plasma exchange by apheresis has been shown to reverse the course of disease and multiorgan failure in many of these children (52). In some patients, prolongation of PT suggested activation of coagulation and fibrin consumption, and on autopsy patients were noted to have fibrin- and vWf-rich thrombi similar to those seen in classical DIC.

Liver Disease and Hepatic Insufficiency

Abnormal Hemostasis in Liver Disease

Liver disease is a common cause of abnormal hemostasis in the ICU. Abnormal coagulation studies or overt bleeding occur in ~15% of patients who have clinical or laboratory evidence of hepatic dysfunction. It is a common cause of a prolonged PT or aPTT, often without any clinical sequelae. The hemostatic defect associated with liver disease is multifactorial and involves impairment in the synthesis of plasma coagulation factors II, V, VII, IX, and X (53,54). Fibrinogen synthesis by the liver is usually maintained at levels that prevent bleeding until terminal liver failure is present. Factor VIII and von Willebrand factor levels are generally normal to increased in acute and chronic liver disease, owing to their acute-phase reactant nature and the fact that they are synthesized by cells other than hepatocytes (i.e., endothelial cells [FVIII & vWf] and megakaryocytes [vWf]).

In addition to these deficiencies in plasma coagulation protein synthesis, many patients with liver disease, particularly cirrhosis, have increased fibrinolytic activity. Increased fibrinolysis is a frequent occurrence in patients who have undergone portacaval shunt procedures. The mechanism for this heightened fibrinolytic state is not clear, although increased amounts of plasminogen activator can be demonstrated, presumably as a consequence of decreased hepatic clearance. It may be difficult to discern whether fibrinolysis occurs solely because of underlying severe liver disease or as a result of concurrent DIC, as patients with cirrhosis are at increased risk for the development of DIC. The clinical distinction can be virtually impossible if active bleeding is present. In liver disease, the elevation of FDP levels can arise because of increased fibrinolysis and decreased hepatic clearance.

Thrombocytopenia may be present to a variable degree in patients with hepatic dysfunction—usually ascribed to splenic sequestration. It is rarely profound and generally does not produce clinically significant bleeding as a solitary defect. In vitro platelet aggregation is often affected, however. Increased plasma concentrations of FDPs are a possible cause of these abnormalities. The thrombocytopenia of liver disease in conjunction with other coagulation/hemostatic defects secondary to liver disease may result in bleeding that is often difficult to manage.

Patients with liver disease may also exhibit decreased synthesis of the vitamin K-dependent anticoagulant protein C and protein S, as well as antithrombin III (synthesized in the liver but not vitamin K dependent) (54). Decreased levels of these natural anticoagulants may increase the risk of thrombosis. The PT, aPTT, and TT will not be affected by the levels of any of these naturally occurring anticoagulants.

The INR was developed to compare the intensity of **vitamin K antagonist (VKA)** anticoagulant therapy between clinical labs employing reagents of differing sensitivities. While INR is calculated from the PT, it is *not* a surrogate for the PT. There are no data to show that the presence of an elevated INR (or PT) in liver disease indicates an increased risk for bleeding. This is contrast to the patient receiving VKA therapy, where an elevated INR does indicate an increased risk of bleeding. Multiple studies on patients with liver disease and prolonged PT have demonstrated maintenance of thrombin generation and increased risk for thrombosis rather than an increased risk of bleeding (55–58). Some of these studies used thromboelastography to document a decrease in fibrinolytic potential in liver disease, presumably accounting for the increased risk of thrombosis. Others have shown an increase in global fibrinolytic potential in patients with liver disease, but this finding has not been linked to an increase in bleeding (59). The difficulty in assigning bleeding risk on the basis of PT (or INR) may be explained by the widespread effects of liver disease on fibrinolysis and hemostasis (both platelet-dependent primary hemostasis and clotting factor-dependent secondary hemostasis). The PT (and INR) only measure one aspect of secondary hemostasis, namely, the fibrin clot production via the extrinsic pathway, which is affected by VKA therapy. The multiple effects found in liver disease cause a "rebalancing" of hemostasis that results in neither the PT nor INR accurately reflecting the risk of bleeding (60–63). Indeed, patients with liver disease have been shown to be more likely to experience thrombotic events than clinically significant bleeding (64,54–56). However, patients with liver disease may still experience significant bleeding due to severe thrombocytopenia, uncompensated decreases in procoagulant clotting factors and/or increased fibrinolysis. Anatomic lesions such as esophageal varices due to

portal hypertension also represent a significant risk for upper gastrointestinal hemorrhage in these patients. The intensive care physician must carefully assess the patient for these risks as the role for traditional measurement of coagulation (i.e., PT, aPTT) is limited at best.

Presentation of Hemostatic Defects in Liver Disease

The hemostatic defect in liver disease is multifactorial, and each patient should be approached accordingly. The most common scenario is a patient with a prolonged PT and a concern for the potential for bleeding. In patients with liver disease and impaired synthetic capabilities, F.VII activity levels are the first to decrease due to its short half-life of 4–6 hours. The resulting prolonged PT can be noted even when markers of hepatocellular injury/hepatic insufficiency remain normal (53,54). A prolonged TT in the setting of liver disease may indicate the presence of an abnormal fibrinogen resembling fetal fibrinogen (dysfibrinogenemia) as a result of altered hepatic fibrinogen synthesis. As the severity of liver disease increases, the aPTT may also be affected, reflecting more severely impaired synthetic function. In this setting, plasma concentrations of the vitamin K-dependent coagulation proteins decrease, as do those of F.V (which is synthesized in the liver but not vitamin K dependent). Although fibrinogen synthesis occurs in the liver, its plasma level is maintained until the disease approaches end stage. When fibrinogen levels are severely depressed as a consequence of decreased synthesis and not increased degradation (fibrinolysis) or consumption (conversion to fibrin), liver failure has typically reached the terminal phase.

In more severe forms of liver disease, fibrinolysis may complicate clinical management. The differentiation between concomitant DIC and fibrinolysis attributable to liver disease alone may be difficult. The D-dimer assay result should be negative in the patient who has liver disease, elevated FDPs and fibrinolysis because thrombin is not being generated when there is no active bleeding. However, D-dimer may be mildly elevated in hepatic failure due to decreased hepatic clearance. The presence of multiorgan ischemic disease secondary to microvascular thrombosis combined with a low F.VIII level (which is not synthesized in the liver) would be more suggestive of DIC.

Management of Abnormal Hemostasis in Liver Disease

If the patient with liver disease is not actively bleeding, no specific therapy is required, with certain provisions. Chapter 103 discusses the specific management of the liver disease patient scheduled for surgery, which depends on the extent of the liver disease, the comorbidities, and the type of surgery. Minor invasive procedures such as central line placement can be performed safely without correction of a prolonged PT (7,65,60). Studies have shown inconsistent and incomplete correction of the PT in liver disease and call into question the need to correct a specific PT value. When a correction of the coagulation abnormalities is desired prior to surgery in the nonbleeding patient with liver disease, a reasonable approach includes administration of vitamin K and FFP to decrease the PT value to within ≤3 seconds of the upper limit of normal for the testing lab and platelet transfusion to >50,000 (64–66). If FFP is administered, the dose should be limited to 10 mL/kg q 6 h with *meticulous monitoring for signs of fluid overload, hyperammonemia, and change in mental status.*

Cryoprecipitate is required in the nonbleeding patient only if fibrinogen levels are <50–100 mg/dL or if significant dysfibrinogenemia is documented. Because vitamin K deficiency also is relatively common, replacement therapy should be considered in every patient with liver disease. A disproportionate decrease in F.VII activity (a vitamin K-dependent factor synthesized in the liver) compared with F.V activity (a **non**–vitamin K-dependent factor synthesized in the liver) suggests vitamin

K deficiency. In contrast to children with dietary vitamin K deficiency and normal liver function, correction of the PT in vitamin K-responsive, critically ill patients typically requires longer than 12–24 hours. Patients with significant hepatic impairment may manifest a partial response or may not respond at all depending on the severity of hepatic dysfunction.

Another approach for the child with liver disease, who is already bleeding or at high risk for bleeding, involves platelet transfusion to platelet count >40,000–80,000/μL, cryoprecipitate administration to fibrinogen concentration to >100 mg/dL, and correction of vitamin K deficiency. FFP may be considered when rapid correction is necessary and the risks of FFP appear manageable. Because of the multiple risks of fluid volume overload, increased portal pressure, and protein load exacerbating hepatic coma, we suggest avoiding any attempt to target a specific PT by administering FFP. If FFP is to be administered because of ongoing bleeding or planned major surgery, the dose should be limited to 10 mL/kg q 6 h with careful monitoring as noted above. Recombinant Factor VIIa should be considered if the child develops life-threatening hemorrhage despite these measures (67,68). The use of F.IX concentrates (**prothrombin complex concentrates [PCCs]**) has been advocated, particularly if bleeding is present. However, their use remains controversial. The PCCs produced from plasma pooled from multiple donors carry a relatively low but still measurable risk of hepatitis (both types B and C) and HIV. While recombinant prothrombin complex products avoid the risk of viral contamination, all prothrombin complex products may initiate thromboembolic events, provoke DIC, and worsen hemostasis (69). To date, no studies have conclusively shown rhF.VIIa to be superior to PCCs for the management of bleeding in patients with hepatic dysfunction (70). In the future, 4-factor PCCs (PCCs containing factors II, VII, IX, and X) and fibrinogen concentrates in development may be available to treat refractory bleeding and hypofibrinogenemia not effectively managed with current blood products.

Summary of Hemostasis Management in the Child with Severe Liver Disease

A comprehensive therapeutic approach is required in the patient with active bleeding as a result of liver disease. Vitamin K should be empirically administered on the presumption that part of the synthetic defect may result from a lack of this cofactor. However, a poor response to vitamin K in the presence of severe liver disease should be anticipated. The following management algorithm appears to have an acceptable risk–benefit ratio:

- Transfuse platelets to >50,000/μL.
- Infuse cryoprecipitate to fibrinogen levels >100 mg/dL.
- Administer FFP 10 mL/kg every 6–8 hours until bleeding slows significantly. Continuous infusions of FFP (starting dose 2–4 mL/kg/h) have also been used with success to control bleeding following a bolus infusion (71).
- Consider rhF.VIIa in those patients with *life-threatening* hemorrhage who are unresponsive to the above steps (72,68).
- Transfuse packed cells as appropriate to maintain hemodynamic stability and adequate O_2-carrying capacity.

Vitamin K Deficiency

A common cause of a prolonged PT in the ICU is vitamin K deficiency. Vitamin K is necessary for the γ-carboxylation of factors II, VII, IX, and X, without which these factors cannot bind calcium and are not efficiently converted into their activated forms. F.VII has the shortest half-life of these coagulation proteins; accordingly, the PT is the most sensitive early indicator of vitamin K deficiency.

Vitamin K deficiency can occur in critically ill patients due to the use of broad-spectrum antibiotics, poor nutrition preceding or subsequent to ICU admission, and the use of parenteral nutrition without vitamin K supplementation. Cephalosporins can affect vitamin K both by decreasing the bacteria in the gut that produce vitamin K and by the inhibition of the actions of vitamin K by the side chains of these antibiotics. Vitamin K deficiency from malnutrition usually requires 1–2 weeks to develop in the complete absence of vitamin K intake. However, the combination of total parenteral alimentation without vitamin K supplementation and antibiotic use may result in rapid vitamin K depletion and prolongation of the PT within 2–3 days.

Infants who fail to receive vitamin K in the immediate postnatal period may develop a systemic coagulopathy manifested by bruising and gastrointestinal bleeding, generally occurring between 1 and 2 weeks of age. The first manifestation is often prolonged bleeding following circumcision. Infants with malabsorption or breastfed infants who ingest medications that interfere with vitamin K in breast milk may develop similar manifestations beyond 2 weeks of age.

Finally, fat malabsorption states, including cystic fibrosis, may be associated with vitamin K deficiency. Vitamin K is fat soluble and is not absorbed well in some conditions of biliary tract and intrinsic small bowel disease. In the ICU, vitamin K deficiency usually results from the interaction of several of these factors. The ICU staff must maintain an awareness of this potential and prevent vitamin K deficiency.

The differential diagnosis of an isolated prolongation of the PT involves several disorders including vitamin K deficiency, liver disease, VKA administration (or intoxication), and either acquired or congenital deficiency of F.VII. VKA (e.g., warfarin) administration (either overt or covert) also should be excluded. Confirmation of warfarin exposure as the cause of a prolonged PT is possible by toxicologic methods to detect the drug, its metabolites, or identification of noncarboxylated forms of vitamin K-dependent clotting factors in plasma (proteins induced by vitamin K antagonist; PIVKAs). Specific inhibitors or congenital deficiency of F.VII should also be considered in the differential of an isolated prolongation of the PT. Acquired inhibitors of F.VII are rare, and homozygous deficiency of F.VII has not been described. Individuals who are heterozygous for F.VII deficiency and those with certain polymorphisms of the promoter region of the F.VII gene tend to have F.VII levels in the 25%–35% range and do not appear to be at increased risk for bleeding.

The laboratory findings of an isolated vitamin K deficiency, in addition to a prolonged PT, include normal fibrinogen level, platelet count, and F.V level. F.V is not a vitamin K-dependent protein and should therefore be normal, except in cases of DIC (consumption) or severe liver disease (decreased production). Prolongation of the aPTT from vitamin K deficiency, warfarin therapy, or liver disease is a relatively late event and occurs initially as a result of F.IX depletion.

Management of Vitamin K Deficiency

The management of vitamin K deficiency consists primarily of its repletion, usually by IV or subcutaneous routes in critically ill patients. Therapy should not await the development of bleeding, but should be administered when the PT abnormality is detected and vitamin K deficiency is suspected. As with other drugs administered subcutaneously (e.g., insulin), adequate blood pressure and subcutaneous perfusion are necessary to ensure reliable absorption from the soft tissues. Concern exists regarding the possibility of anaphylactoid reactions with the IV use of vitamin K. This risk with IV use is minimized when the medication is administered slowly over

30–45 minutes. The usual dose of vitamin K in children is 1–5 mg IV or subcutaneously (up to 10 mg in larger children/adults). In an otherwise healthy person, the PT should correct within 12–24 hours after this dose. However, serial dosing of critically ill patients is often utilized, and the PT may require up to 72 hours to normalize. If the PT does not correct within 72 hours after 3 daily doses of vitamin K, intrinsic liver disease should be suspected. Further administration of vitamin K is of no additional benefit in this setting.

When the patient is actively bleeding, a more immediate restoration of coagulation is required than vitamin K alone and FFP is added. To restore hemostasis to an acceptable level (30%–50%) of normal enzyme activity, 10–15 mL/kg body weight of FFP is typically required. A similar approach is used to reverse warfarin. While RhF.VIIa (15–20 μg/kg) has been used with success to reverse the bleeding noted in vitamin K deficiency and in warfarin overdose (72,73,40,68), meta-analyses, systematic reviews, and registry data have documented an increased risk of thrombosis and failed to show improved survival (43,74). Therefore, if RhF.VIIa is to be used, it should be reserved for life-threatening cases refractory to all other therapeutic measures.

While PCC has been advocated for reversal of VKA-induced coagulopathy, the three-factor PCCs currently available in the United States contain factors II, IX, and X, with limited amounts of Factor VII, and are less effective than four-factor PCC that contains significant amounts of F.VII and is effective in correcting both PT and aPTT values in those patients with VKA-induced coagulopathy at risk for bleeding (69). The four-factor PCC is currently available in Europe, Australia, and Canada and is under regulatory review in the United States. Care must be taken due to the approximately 1% risk of thrombosis induced by this agent (75).

IATROGENIC COAGULOPATHY

Massive Transfusion Syndrome

Transfusion of large quantities of blood can result in a multifactorial hemostatic defect. The genesis of this problem is related to the "washout" of plasma coagulation proteins and platelets, and it may be exacerbated by the development of DIC-induced factor consumption, hypothermia, acidosis, citrate toxicity, or hypocalcemia. These variables often act in combination to cause a coagulopathic state (76).

A washout syndrome can result from the transfusion of large volumes of packed red blood cells (e.g., trauma victims, patients with massive gastrointestinal hemorrhage, hepatectomy, or those undergoing cardiopulmonary bypass) without also receiving FFP and platelets. Factors V and VII have short shelf **half-lives** and are often deficient in blood that has been banked longer than 48 hours. In addition, a qualitative platelet defect can be demonstrated in whole blood within hours of its storage, especially if an acid-citrate-dextrose solution is used. Consequently, transfusion of large quantities of stored whole blood may produce limited improvement in the bleeding that results from decreased clotting factors and platelets. The development of a washout coagulopathy is directly dependent on the volume of blood transfused relative to the blood volume of the patient. Residual plasma clotting activity falls to 18%–37% of normal after single-blood-volume exchange, 3%–14% of normal after a double-blood-volume exchange and <5% of normal clotting function remains after a triple-blood-volume exchange.

Massive transfusion or washout presents with diffuse oozing and bleeding from surgical wounds and puncture sites. Laboratory abnormalities include prolonged PT, aPTT, and TT. Fibrinogen levels and platelet counts are decreased;

FDPs are not increased unless concurrent DIC is present (see **Table 118.2**). The likelihood that the clinical and laboratory picture is a direct result of the massive transfusion can be estimated from the amount of bleeding and the number of blood volume exchanges given. The more stored blood (e.g., packed red blood cells) transfused relative to the patient's blood volume, the greater the chance of the development of coagulopathy due to massive transfusion.

Management of Coagulopathy in Massive Transfusion Syndrome

Prevention of massive transfusion syndrome requires prospective identification of those at risk (see also Chapter 30). When the magnitude of the insult and the anticipated need for blood are large, both platelets and FFP should be given before a coagulopathy develops. There is wide variation in practice, and the exact ratio of packed red blood cells to other blood components (i.e., platelets, plasma, or cryoprecipitate) to prevent the development of massive transfusion coagulopathy has not been established (77–79). A common practice in adult trauma centers suggests a fixed ratio of 1 unit of FFP for every unit of packed RBCs transfused effectively replaces plasma clotting factors (80). In larger children (weight ≥30–40 kg or body surface area ≥1.0 m²), half of a unit of apheresis-collected platelets (generally equivalent to 4–5 units of platelets derived from whole blood donation) and 1 unit of FFP should be given for each 5 units of whole blood or packed cells transfused. In smaller children, 10 mL/kg of platelets and 10–15 mL/kg FFP should be given for each 40–50 mL/kg of blood transfused. Hypothermia should be prevented by warming all blood products.

The treatment of massive transfusion is supportive. Electrolyte abnormalities (hypocalcemia, hyperkalemia, hypokalemia, or acidosis) should be anticipated and corrected. Platelets and FFP are given to replete the components of coagulation and correct identified hemostatic deficits. Bleeding is uncommon in the nontrauma (or nonoperative) patient from thrombocytopenia alone, unless platelet counts fall below 10,000–20,000/μL of blood. Conversely, trauma or operative patients with massive bleeding should receive platelet transfusion to restore counts >80,000–100,000/μL. FFP is preferred to cryoprecipitate (unless fibrinogen depletion is a major contributor) because it has a more complete coagulation protein composition. If the patient continues to bleed despite adequate therapy for massive transfusion syndrome, other causes should be considered including anatomic bleeding or DIC.

Anticoagulant Overdose

Anticoagulant therapy is common in the PICU, and the possibility of errors in administration exists. Poorly standardized methods of prophylactic anticoagulant use, systemic anticoagulation, and thrombolytic therapy can lead to overdose.

Heparin Overdose

Heparin is a repeating polymer of two disaccharide glycosaminoglycans and is prepared from either porcine intestinal mucosa or bovine lung. Heparin is currently found in two forms: unfractionated heparin (UH) and low-molecular-weight heparin (LMWH). These two forms have different mechanisms of action and associated precautions. UH has an immediate effect on coagulation that is mediated primarily through its interaction with antithrombin III. The resulting heparin–antithrombin III complex possesses a much greater affinity for thrombin than antithrombin III alone. The complex inactivates thrombin, thereby slowing clot formation. Heparin also has a minor direct effect through inhibition of activated F.X (F.Xa). Because this direct effect on F.Xa is relatively minor, achieving a therapeutic aPTT with UH is very difficult in the face of low levels of antithrombin III. The degree of anticoagulation produced by heparin is monitored by the prolongation of the aPTT. In contrast, LMWH, produced by controlled enzymatic cleavage of heparin polymers, effects anticoagulation almost exclusively through inhibition of F.Xa, which produces a more stable degree of anticoagulation. Due to its longer half-life (~3–5 hours) and biologic activity (~24 hours), LMWH allows for intermittent bolus therapy (i.e., every 12 or 24 hours) while maintaining a steady-state effect. However, LMWH does not produce consistent prolongation of the aPTT and requires assay of anti-Xa activity for monitoring (if desired).

Heparin is removed from the blood by saturable and non-saturable pharmacokinetic mechanisms. After entering the bloodstream, heparin is bound in the reticulo-endothelial system in the liver and spleen and on vascular endothelial cells a dose-dependent, saturable fashion. Excess heparin is excreted through the kidneys in a slow, nonsaturable process. These pharmacokinetic mechanisms account for the nonlinear half-life of heparin. As the rate of heparin administration is increased, the half-life of the drug is prolonged due to the increase in the percentage of the drug excreted by the kidney. For example, when a 100 U/kg bolus of heparin is infused IV, the average half-life of the drug is 1 hour. If the bolus is increased to 400 or 800 U/kg, the half-life is prolonged to 2.5 and 5 hours, respectively. The nonlinear response results in greater drug effects on coagulation with smaller dosage increments. When one "re-boluses" or increases a heparin infusion rate in response to insufficient anticoagulation (i.e., inadequate prolongation of the aPTT), a point will be reached when further small increments in the heparin infusion rate may result in a substantially greater prolongation of the aPTT. The risk of pathologic bleeding associated with heparin increases when the prolongation of the aPTT is beyond the therapeutic window (generally considered to be 1.5–2.5 times the patient's baseline aPTT, corresponding to a plasma heparin concentration of 0.2–0.4 units/mL or anti-Xa level of 0.3–0.7 units/mL). As a corollary, administration of heparin as a continuous infusion rather than in an intermittent bolus dose regimen is less likely to be associated with pathologic bleeding.

Management of Heparin Overdose

Serious bleeding associated with heparin overdose can be rapidly reversed by protamine sulfate. Protamine binds ionically with heparin to form a complex that lacks any anticoagulant activity. As a general rule, 1 mg of protamine neutralizes ~100 U of heparin (specifically, 90 USP units of bovine heparin or 115 USP units of porcine heparin). The required protamine dose is calculated from the number of units of active heparin remaining in the patient's system. This, in turn, is estimated from the original heparin dose and the typical half-life for that infusion rate. Protamine should be injected slowly (5 mg per minute) to avoid hemodynamic compromise and the maximum dose is 25–50 mg. The aPTT or activated clotting time (ACT) is used to gauge the residual effects of heparin. Caution is in order when relying on ACT because the equipment used for this measurement is poorly standardized and different systems give different results (81).

Protamine itself has several potential adverse effects including hypotension, anaphylactoid reactions, and anti-coagulation. Hence precautions are necessary during its administration. The first rule is never to give protamine unless there is significant bleeding caused by heparin overdose. (Most patients who receive an inadvertent heparin overdose do not suffer bleeding.) Protamine should be given by **slow** IV administration over 8–10 minutes. A single dose should not exceed 1 mg/kg (50 mg maximum dose). The allergic reactions to protamine represent type I anaphylactic reactions between an antigen (protamine) and antibody (IgE or IgG) and result in histamine release. Complement activation, thromboxane, and nitric oxide production have all been shown to play some role in the pathogenesis of these reactions (82,83). Risk factors for protamine hypersensitivity reactions include prior exposure to protamine, insulin-dependent diabetes (with NPH exposure), fish allergy, and vasectomy. *Because of the many risks of protamine, it is rarely used outside of the cardiac operating room.* LMWH is not consistently neutralized by protamine, therefore invasive procedures should not be performed within 24 hours of LMWH administration.

Warfarin Overdose

Warfarin and vitamin K are structurally similar in their respective 4-hydroxycoumarin nucleus and naphthoquinone ring. The mechanism of action of warfarin is through competitive inhibition of **vitamin K epoxide reductase**, which is necessary to regenerate the reduced form of vitamin K. The reduced form of vitamin K is a necessary cofactor in the postribosomal modification of the vitamin K-dependent coagulation proteins (factors II, VII, IX, and X) by γ-carboxylation. This postsynthetic modification produces a calcium-binding site on the molecule, which, when occupied, allows for the efficient activation of the zymogen-clotting factor into its enzymatically active form. When warfarin is present in sufficient plasma concentrations, the active (γ-carboxylated) forms of vitamin K-dependent factors are depleted.

The INR is an accurate indicator of the effects of warfarin when its use has continued beyond 2 or 3 days. F.VIIa (the active form) has a half-life of only 4–6 hours and is rapidly depleted after 1 or 2 doses of warfarin. The remainder of the vitamin K-dependent factors may take up to a week to become depleted. The INR becomes prolonged with F.VII depletion alone, but does not reflect an overall state of anticoagulation until an equilibrium period of several days has passed, generally once the INR is at or near target value for 2–3 days. Over this interval, the other vitamin K-dependent factors become depleted, and PT prolongation, as measured by the INR, can then be used to assess the anticoagulant effects of warfarin. In severe cases of warfarin overdose, the aPTT also becomes prolonged as a result of a marked reduction of the active forms of factors II, IX, and X.

Several drugs and pathophysiologic conditions are associated with potentiation of warfarin's effects on coagulation. Many of the drugs known to prolong the effects of warfarin are listed in **Table 118.5**. These drugs have a variety of mechanisms that generally include either inhibition of function or competitive binding of the enzymes that are responsible for active warfarin metabolism. Aspirin does not seem to have any direct influence on warfarin metabolism, but so profoundly inhibits qualitative platelet function that it increases the bleeding risk in patients receiving warfarin. The same is true for clofibrate. The ingestion of large quantities of aspirin may also impair prothrombin (F.II) synthesis, further increasing the effects of warfarin administration.

Warfarin is metabolized by the liver. Conditions of acute and chronic hepatic dysfunction can alter warfarin metabolism and vitamin K-mediated γ-carboxylation of coagulation proteins. Broad-spectrum antibiotics also may limit vitamin K availability through their alteration of the gut flora (in addition to any direct effect on vitamin K metabolism). All of these factors may ultimately influence a patient's response to warfarin. The initial dose should be lowered from the usual 0.2 mg/kg (maximum dose 10 mg) in the child with a normal baseline INR and normal liver function to 0.1 mg/kg in the child with liver dysfunction or other conditions that enhance

TABLE 118.5

DRUGS THAT POTENTIATE THE ANTICOAGULANT EFFECTS OF WARFARIN

Antibiotics
Broad-spectrum antibiotics (especially cephalosporins)
Griseofulvin (oral)
Azole antifungal agents (e.g., fluconazole, ketoconazole, voriconazole, etc.)
Metronidazole
Sulfonamides
Trimethoprim-sulfamethoxazole
Anti-inflammatory drugs
Steroids (anabolic, in particular)
Acetylated salicylates
Phenylbutazone (oxyphenbutazone)
Sulfinpyrazone
Other drugs
Clofibrate
Disulfiram
Phenytoin
Thyroxine (both D- and L-isomers)
Tolbutamide

the warfarin anticoagulant effect. The INR checked more frequently in these patients.

A clinical syndrome referred to as "warfarin (coumadin) necrosis" has been noted during the initial stages of anticoagulation with a VKA. It is characterized clinically by the development of skin and subcutaneous necrosis, particularly in areas of subcutaneous fat, and pathologically by the thrombosis of small blood vessels in the fat and subcutaneous tissues. This syndrome is caused by the rapid depletion of the vitamin K-dependent, anticoagulant PC prior to achieving depletion of procoagulant proteins and occurs predominantly in individuals who are heterozygous for PC deficiency. While anticoagulation generally requires a decrease in procoagulant protein levels to ~20%–25% of normal, a prothrombotic milieu is created with PC levels ≤40%. Consequently, individuals who are heterozygous for PC deficiency and have baseline PC levels of 50%–60% may develop a prothrombotic environment during the first few days of warfarin therapy. The risk of developing warfarin necrosis appears to be greater when the initial dose of warfarin is >10–15 mg. The development of this syndrome generally can be avoided if heparin and warfarin therapy are overlapped until "coumadinization" is complete (usually after 4–5 days), and if large loading doses of warfarin (>10–15 mg) are avoided.

Management of Warfarin Overdose

When excessive anticoagulation with warfarin presents with bleeding, immediate reversal is usually mandated (73). The treatment of choice is FFP, which provides prompt restoration of the deficient vitamin K-dependent coagulation proteins, along with restoration of hemostatic function. Ten to 15 mL/kg of FFP is usually sufficient to produce significant correction of the PT, although repeat infusions of FFP may be necessary to effect continued correction of the PT due to the short half-life of F.VII (78). Vitamin K also may be administered, particularly in situations that are less acute, although this will make it more difficult to "re-coumadinize" the patient afterward. For severe bleeding or bleeding not controlled by FFP infusions, rhF.VIIa and 4-factor PCC have been used successfully (see above, Vitamin K Deficiency). The "3-factor" PCCs currently available in the United States are not approved for the treatment of Factor VII deficiency (either congenital or

secondary to VKA treatment) owing to the limited amount of F.VII contained in them (69). Ingestion of newer, long-acting VKA rodenticides (so-called "superwarfarin") produces a profound, prolonged, vitamin K-resistant reduction in vitamin K-dependent clotting factors, which may produce an isolated prolongation of the PT initially. Treatment of poisoning with these agents requires aggressive, prolonged use of vitamin K, and, in the bleeding patient, FFP infusions or rhF.VIIa.

Tissue Plasminogen Activator and Urokinase Overdose

Vascular or device thrombosis or thromboembolism can be treated with thrombolytic agents in children, usually tissue plasminogen activator (tPA) or urokinase. These thrombolytics accelerate the conversion of plasminogen to plasmin and thereby enhance fibrinolysis. Adequate endogenous plasminogen levels are required for these agents to be effective. Newborns and patients with low fibrinogen levels are likely to have reduced endogenous plasminogen, which can be restored through administration of FFP.

Bleeding is the major risk during thrombolytic therapy. The management of bleeding following thrombolytic therapy consists of cessation of all anticoagulant therapy, application of pressure to the bleeding site, and correction of other hemostatic defects (e.g., thrombocytopenia or vitamin K deficiency). Topical thrombin maybe effective in treating localized minor bleeding. Significant bleeding from multiple sites requires FFP transfusion. In addition, aminocaproic acid (Amicar) may be considered in cases of significant hemorrhage following thrombolytic therapy. Amicar decreases fibrinolysis by inhibiting plasminogen-binding sites and thereby decreasing plasmin formation. The clinician should carefully weigh the risks and benefits of Amicar because it is likely to exacerbate the underlying thrombotic event for which thrombolytics were started in the first place. Amicar is also contraindicated in newborns and premature infants because the injectable form contains benzyl alcohol.

Platelet Disorders

Platelets are necessary for efficient clot formation and are a critical element in the process known as "primary hemostasis" (i.e., the interaction of platelets with the endothelium and subendothelial structures). They not only produce a physical barrier at the site of vascular injury (the so-called "platelet plug") but also serve to focus the clotting process at the point of bleeding by delivering vasoconstrictors, clotting factors, and providing a surface for clot development (see **Fig. 118.3**). Quantitative and qualitative platelet disorders that are a common cause of clinical bleeding in the PICU are presented in **Table 118.6**.

Quantitative Platelet Disorders

A decrease in the number of circulating platelets reflects the presence of increased peripheral destruction and/or sequestration, decreased marrow production, or a combination of these factors. Thrombocytopenia is any level <140,000/μL (the lower limit of normal), although many studies have used a 100,000/μL threshold for patients with potentially clinically relevant thrombocytopenia. This may be related to the fact that the bleeding time is not prolonged in thrombocytopenia until platelet count is <100,000/μL. Causes of increased peripheral destruction include immune-mediated processes (both autoimmune and drug induced), abnormal consumption (as in DIC), and mechanical destruction (e.g., cardiopulmonary bypass, hyperthermia). Autoimmune processes such as idiopathic thrombocytopenic purpura (now referred to as **Immune Thrombocytopenia; ITP**), systemic lupus erythematosus, or

TABLE 118.6

ACQUIRED PLATELET DISORDERS

■ QUANTITATIVE DEFECTS	■ QUALITATIVE DEFECTS
Increased destruction	**Drugs**
Immune	Anti-inflammatory agents
Immune thrombocytopenic purpura	Aspirin (irreversible)
Systemic lupus erythematosus	Nonsteroidal anti-inflammatory agents
Acquired immunodeficiency syndrome	Corticosteroids
Drugs (gold salts, heparin, sulfonamides,	Antibiotics
quinidine, quinine)	
Sepsis	Penicillins (e.g., ampicillin, carbenicillin, ticarcillin, penicillin-G)
Nonimmune	Cephalosporins (e.g., cephalothin)
Thrombotic thrombocytopenic purpura/hemolytic ure-mic syndrome	Nitrofurantoin
Mechanical destruction (e.g., cardiopulmonary bypass, hyperthermia)	Chloroquine, hydroxychloroquine
Decreased production	Phosphodiesterase inhibitors
Marrow suppression	Dipyridamole
Chemotherapy	Methylxanthines (e.g., theophylline)
Viral illness (e.g., cytomegalovirus, Epstein-Barr virus, herpes simplex, parvovirus)	Thienopyridines
Drugs (thiazides, ethanol, cimetidine)	Clopidogrel
Marrow replacement	Prasugrel
Tumor	**Other drugs**
Myelofibrosis	Antihistamines
Other conditions	α-blockers (e.g., phentolamine)
Splenic sequestration	β-blockers (e.g., propranolol)
Dilution (see massive transfusion syndrome)	Dextran
	Ethanol
	Furosemide
	Heparin
	Local anesthetics (e.g., lidocaine)
	Phenothiazines
	Tricyclic antidepressants
	Nitrates (e.g., sodium nitroprusside, nitroglycerin)
	Metabolic causes
	Uremia
	Stored whole blood
	Disseminated intravascular coagulation (i.e., fibrin degradation product-mediated inhibition)
	Hypothyroidism

AIDS can result in increased peripheral destruction and increased splenic sequestration of platelets. Autoimmune destruction also may occur in lymphocytic leukemia or lymphoma.

Immune Thrombocytopenia

In immune thrombocytopenia (ITP), immunoglobulin (generally IgG) is directed against specific platelet antigens and is responsible for platelet destruction. Acute ITP is usually a self-limited, viral-induced condition in children. In contrast, chronic ITP generally occurs in women and requires immunosuppressive therapy to maintain an acceptable platelet count. Neither condition is likely to have life-threatening bleeding. Corticosteroids may be given (2–4 mg/kg day of prednisone or its equivalent for 4 days). High doses of IV γ-globulin (IVIG 400 mg/kg q day for 5 days or IVIG 800–1000 mg/kg as a single infusion for 1 or 2 infusions) or infusions of anti-RhD antigen antibody in Rh-positive patients (WinRho; 25–50 mcg/kg as a single infusion) are equally efficacious in producing at least transient elevations in the platelet count. Agents such as vincristine/vinblastine, cyclophosphamide, and, with increasing frequency, rituximab (anti-CD20 monoclonal antibody) also have been used as immunosuppressants

with variable success, although responses are generally not immediate. Unlike corticosteroids, IVIG and WinRho which can be used to treat either acute or chronic ITP, these later therapies are generally only considered for the treatment of chronic (or recurrent) ITP. Splenectomy may be required to avert serious bleeding complications in patients who do not respond to medical management, although this approach is chosen much less often in children than in adults. In ITP, the degree of bleeding attributed to thrombocytopenia is generally less than that noted when thrombocytopenia results from decreased platelet production. In general, severe bleeding is not noted until the platelet count is $<10,000/mm^3$, although levels below $40,000–50,000/mm^3$ often raise concern for potential increased risk of bleeding associated with invasive procedures. The use of thrombopoietin-like drugs in ITP do not play a significant role in the ICU, as platelet counts only increase after several weeks of therapy.

Drug-Induced, Immune-Mediated Platelet Destruction

The development of drug-induced, immune-mediated platelet destruction should always be considered in the thrombocytopenic PICU patient. It is usually reversible, and withdrawal of the offending drug prevents further immune-mediated platelet destruction. The mechanism of platelet destruction may involve binding of drug to the platelet membrane, with subsequent binding of a specific antibody to the platelet, platelet–drug complex, or both. The resulting platelet–drug–antibody complexes are cleared by the reticulo-endothelial system (e.g., the spleen), and thrombocytopenia develops. Medications used in the ICU that are associated with this clinical picture include quinidine, quinine, heparin, penicillins, cephalosporins, vancomycin, and sulfonamides. The dose-dependent thrombocytopenia produced by the anticonvulsant valproic acid is, at least in part, immunologic in nature. Heparin-induced thrombocytopenia is an example of drug-induced immune thrombocytopenia and is discussed separately below.

Drug-Induced, Nonimmune Thrombocytopenia

A variety of medications are associated with the development of a nonimmune thrombocytopenia by bone marrow suppression. Most cancer chemotherapeutic agents produce thrombocytopenia as a consequence of marrow suppression. The thiazide diuretics, cimetidine, ethanol, and several cephalosporin and penicillin antibiotics may suppress platelet production. Generalized infection (such as bacterial sepsis) and many viral illnesses can cause thrombocytopenia by bone marrow suppression and/or immune platelet destruction. Disorders such as Gaucher disease cause thrombocytopenia as a result of marrow replacement by nonhematopoietic cells.

Platelet Consumption and Destruction

Consumption of platelets is the cause of thrombocytopenia in DIC. Mechanical destruction occurs during the use of cardiopulmonary bypass (CPB) and commonly cause a 50% drop in platelet count. Platelet counts generally recover toward preoperative levels by 48–72 hours after CPB. Platelets may also be destroyed by the high body temperatures seen in severe hyperthermic syndromes. In many of these circumstances, thrombocytopenia is the sole or a contributing cause of significant bleeding.

Heparin-Induced Thrombocytopenia

Heparin is used in many ICUs and the problems associated with its use merit emphasis. Heparin-induced thrombocytopenia (HIT) has two presentations. Acute nonidiosyncratic HIT occurs in 10%–15% of patients who receive heparin. The degree of thrombocytopenia is usually mild, is not associated with thrombotic complications, and remits despite continued use of the drug, and heparin administration need not be stopped (type I HIT). In contrast, idiosyncratic HIT occurs in less than 5% of patients receiving heparin, but has a much greater potential for clinical morbidity. The most significant risk of this form of HIT (type II HIT) is arterial thrombosis, which may be life threatening by causing myocardial infarction, cerebrovascular accident, pulmonary embolism, or renal infarction. The incidence of type II HIT is rare in children (0.33% after cardiopulmonary bypass) and many reported cases appear to represent overdiagnosis (26).

The mechanism of thrombosis is thought to be a consequence of the deposition of platelet aggregates in the microcirculation (84,63). Thrombocytopenia in this disorder involves a specific antibody, directed against a heparin–**platelet factor 4** (PF4) complex that mediates the formation of platelet aggregates in the presence of heparin. This process requires minimal amounts of heparin. Severe thrombocytopenia (i.e., <15,000–20,000/mm^3) and severe bleeding are unusual in this disorder.

The diagnosis of HIT is one of exclusion. Clinical scoring systems are more useful for excluding the diagnosis of HIT than identifying patients with HIT and have not been validated

in pediatric patients (85,86). Nevertheless the clinical profile of a patient with type II HIT includes thrombocytopenia (or >30% decrease in platelet count from baseline) 5–14 days after heparin exposure (or sooner in patients with a history of prior heparin exposures). A coincident thrombotic event and exclusion of other causes of thrombocytopenia increase the probability of type II HIT.

Diagnostic markers (e.g., heparin-dependent platelet antibodies, aggregation or serotonin release) are at best confirmatory and not exclusionary. An ELISA assay for heparin-dependent platelet antibodies suffers from a relatively high "false-positive" rate. The more specific heparin-induced platelet injury assay (serotonin release assay) is recommended for confirmation. The diagnosis may be difficult to confirm because of the presence of a coexisting clinical illnesses with the potential to cause thrombocytopenia. HIT is most likely to be associated with the use of bovine lung heparin, but it can occur after exposure to porcine heparin or, much less commonly, LMWH.

When type II HIT is suspected, all exposure to heparin, including heparin flushes, heparin in total parenteral nutrition, and heparin-coated catheters, must be removed pending the results of a confirmatory test (heparin-induced platelet injury assay). *Anticoagulation with an alternate agent must be initiated because delayed thrombosis can occur up to 30 days after removal of heparin exposure* (87,88). A negative heparin-induced platelet injury test should prompt a careful reevaluation for other causes of thrombocytopenia.

Continued anticoagulation for type II HIT is provided with direct thrombin inhibitors (argatroban, lepirudin, bivalirudin) or with the heparinoid danaparoid (currently not available in the United States). The direct thrombin inhibitors are preferred, as they carry no risk of cross-reacting with the heparin-dependent antibodies (87,89). Of the members of this class of anticoagulants, bivalirudin is gaining increasing preference for anticoagulation in children at high risk for or with suspected or documented HIT (90–94). Bivalirudin is largely cleared by proteolysis in the plasma, argatroban by the liver, and lepirudin by the kidney. Consequently, the choice and dose of drug may be affected by the presence of hepatic or renal insufficiency. While there are pharmacokinetic and safety data for use in children for bivalirudin and argatroban, there are no similar data pertaining to the use of lepirudin in children (95,96). Warfarin alone is contraindicated for suspected type II HIT because of the risk of thrombosis from depression of PC levels, which may lead to skin necrosis, gangrene, and amputation. However, warfarins can be utilized in conjunction with a direct thrombin inhibitor after the platelet count has normalized and subsequently continued as a single agent once therapeutic suppression of vitamin K-dependent clotting factors has been achieved.

Qualitative Platelet Disorders

Many of the drugs used in the ICU have the potential to impair platelet function. Frequently, the sicker the patient, the greater the likelihood that they will be exposed to one of these medications. Patients with these disorders often have other underlying pathophysiologic conditions that in and of themselves can predispose to bleeding. A list of the drugs that commonly affect platelet function is presented in **Table 118.6**.

All unnecessary drugs should be viewed as suspect and discontinued in patients with evidence for, or strong suspicion of, qualitative platelet dysfunction. In most cases, terminating the offending drugs usually restores platelet functional activity. Aspirin is a notable exception as it irreversibly inhibits platelet cyclooxygenase, resulting in a defect that lasts for the duration of the platelet life span (8–9 days). The effect is profound as a single 325-mg aspirin tablet results in a qualitative platelet defect that remains in 50% of the circulating platelets 5 days after its ingestion. Ideally, all aspirin ingestion should be avoided for at least 7 days prior to an elective invasive procedure. New drugs that target the adenosine diphosphate P_2Y_{12} receptor on the surface of platelets (e.g., clopidogrel, prasugrel, ticagrelor) also produce a prolonged inhibition of platelet reactivity that may last up to 2 weeks following discontinuance of the drug depending on the duration of therapy (97).

Nonsteroidal anti-inflammatory (NSAID) agents similarly affect the platelet cyclooxygenase enzyme. However, their effects are reversible, and normal platelet function is usually restored within 24 hours of the last dose. Under most circumstances, the degree of platelet inhibition produced by these agents is not clinically significant, and most patients can receive these drugs for analgesia and fever control. However, NSAIDs (especially ketorolac) should be avoided in PICU patients at high risk for bleeding.

The β-lactam antibiotics can sterically hinder the binding of a platelet aggregation agonist (e.g., adenosine diphosphate) to its specific platelet receptor, resulting in impaired platelet aggregation under circumstances of normal physiologic stimulation. This, too, is reversed on removal of the drug. Fortunately, only a minority of patients exposed to these antibiotics will exhibit clinically significant platelet inhibition.

In the PICU, the possibility must be considered that a patient with bleeding suggestive of a platelet defect might have an inherited disorder of platelet function. Although rare, these disorders are encountered from time to time and include Glanzmann thrombasthenia (abnormal platelet GPIIb/IIIa), Bernard-Soulier syndrome (abnormal GP Ib/IX), Wiskott-Aldrich syndrome, platelet storage pool deficiency (abnormal platelet-dense bodies), and the Gray platelet disorder (abnormal platelet α-granules).

Management of Platelet Disorders

Because many of the adverse drug-related platelet effects are reversible, all medications should be discontinued promptly (if not essential for treatment) or substituted for drugs not associated with platelet dysfunction. The more controversial issue is deciding when platelet transfusions are warranted. The relationship of thrombocytopenia to clinical bleeding is relative; that is, it is difficult to identify a specific, arbitrary platelet count (threshold) below which bleeding is likely to occur. Although bleeding is unusual when the platelet count is $\geq 80,000/mm^3$, conditions such as massive transfusion syndrome and DIC may require empiric platelet transfusion despite counts of 80,000 or 100,000 platelets/mm^3. In cases of thrombocytopenia seen with cancer chemotherapy and bone marrow aplasia, platelet transfusion may not be required until counts fall below 10,000–20,000/mm^3.

The morbidity and mortality related to bleeding increase measurably in patients who undergo induction chemotherapy for acute leukemia when the platelet count falls below 10,000–20,000/mm^3. The administration of platelets to these patients with this degree of thrombocytopenia limits morbidity and mortality but the appropriateness of generalizing this ❽ approach to all patients with platelet counts in this range is unclear. A major concern about this approach is the development of alloimmunization to transfused platelets, potentially negating any future benefit from platelet transfusion in a time of need. Patients with acute leukemia typically have self-limited marrow aplasia as a result of chemotherapy. Therefore, the need for platelet transfusion is also limited, and the chances for development of antiplatelet antibodies are greatly decreased. However, as patients with aplastic anemia have an ongoing need for platelet transfusion, their risk of alloimmunization is high. Autoimmune disorders associated with increased peripheral platelet destruction, disorders of splenic

sequestration, and drug-related thrombocytopenia are unlikely to benefit from platelet transfusion as transfused platelets may be rapidly removed from circulation or exhibit impaired function upon exposure to drugs in circulation. An exception is that children who are to have invasive procedures with an increased risk of bleeding may benefit from platelet transfusion immediately before the procedure.

Uremia

Uremia (see also Chapter 111) deserves special mention as the cause of a qualitative platelet disorder that is best treated by resolution of the underlying uremic state. Uremia is commonly seen in the ICU and is associated with an increased risk of bleeding (39,98). The platelet count, PT and aPTT are usually normal unless another coagulopathy is also present. Uremia causes a reversible impairment of platelet function, although the "toxin" responsible for this defect is not well defined. Some studies have demonstrated an impairment of platelet–vessel wall interactions and suggest defects in von Willebrand factor. The degree of platelet impairment appears to be related to the severity of the uremia. In addition, thrombotic events are also increased in patients with uremia. These, too, appear to be multifactorial in etiology but in part reflect the increased renal loss of antithrombin III and protein S from proteinuria (99).

Several therapeutic approaches may modulate the qualitative platelet defect associated with uremia. The primary therapy in this setting is dialysis and resolution of the uremic state. However, cryoprecipitate, 1-deamino-8-D-arginine vasopressin (DDAVP; 0.3 mcg/kg IV over 15–30 minutes, maximum dose 21 mcg), and conjugated estrogens (10 mg/day in adult patients) have also been given with good results to patients with severe uremia and an acquired defect in primary hemostasis. Cryoprecipitate and DDAVP appear to improve platelet adhesion by increasing the plasma concentration of the large multimeric forms of von Willebrand factor. However, the durations of action of these agents are limited, with them reaching their zenith at between 2 and 6 hours. Additional doses of DDAVP during the same 24-hour period may result in a diminished response to the drug (tachyphylaxis) with little or no further benefit. Patients who exhibit tachyphylaxis to DDAVP may require 48–72 hours before again responding to this agent. The mechanism of action of the conjugated estrogens is not known. In contrast to the first two therapies described, the effect of estrogen is more protracted and does not diminish with repeat dosing, although a benefit is not noted until 3–5 days after therapy is started.

THROMBOTIC SYNDROMES

Although thrombosis is not a common feature of pediatric illness, it is being recognized in PICU patients with increased frequency. Whether this represents a heightened awareness or a true increase in incidence is not clear. Several thrombotic syndromes seen in the PICU include deep venous thrombosis (specifically in association with a central venous catheter), HIT, pulmonary embolism syndrome, TTP/HUS, thrombotic DIC, stroke, and cerebral venous sinus thrombosis (most commonly seen in infants with marked dehydration). Both inherited and acquired risk factors have been identified in children who subsequently develop thromboembolic phenomena (Table 118.7). In addition to the many inherited factors associated with thrombosis in children and adults, risk factors in children include the presence of a central venous catheter (60%–70% of cases), young or older age (i.e., infancy and adolescence), increased severity of illness, and (as with adults) family history of thromboembolism (100–107). Children who develop venous thrombosis usually exhibit two or more identifiable

TABLE 118.7

INHERITED AND ACQUIRED PROTHROMBOTIC CONDITIONS

■ INHERITED	■ ACQUIRED
Protein C deficiency	Central venous lines (majority
Protein S deficiency	of cases)
Antithrombin III deficiency	Congenital heart disease
Plasminogen deficiency	Atrial fibrillation
Dysfibrinogenemia	Systemic lupus erythemato-
Factor V Leiden mutation	sus (and other vasculitis
Prothrombin G20210A	syndromes)
mutation	Nephrotic syndrome
4G PAI-1 genotype	Leukemia (and chemotherapy)
(elevated PAI-1)	Trauma
Homocysteinemia	Prolonged immobilization
Lipoprotein (a) (increased)	(>5 d)
	Morbid obesity

risk factors (101,108). Deep venous thrombosis and pulmonary embolism are discussed in more detail in Chapter 116.

Thromboprophylaxis

Many of these venous thromboembolic events develop while the patient is in the PICU and may be preventable. Despite a decrease in venous thrombosis after the implementation of a thromboprophylaxis clinical guideline in children hospitalized for trauma (109), there is no consensus as to the need for thromboprophylaxis in children and great variation in actual practice (110). We suggest pneumatic compression devices for postpubertal pediatric patients who will be immobilized in the PICU for more than 1–2 days because their risk of thrombosis may more closely conform to that of the adult population. The utility of thromboprophylaxis in younger children is unclear. Prophylactic administration of antithrombotic therapy (e.g., LMWH) is not recommended unless the patient is considered at very high risk for thrombosis. The care team should assess the need for central venous lines on daily rounds and remove such lines as soon as possible.

Management

The initial management approach for a child with a documented (or highly suspected) thrombotic event is generally anticoagulation with either UH or LMWH. The efficacy of these therapies appears to be equivalent, although studies in adult populations suggest that the incidence of severe bleeding may be less with LMWH. The use of LMWH may produce a more stable level of anticoagulation, requiring fewer laboratory tests and dose adjustments. If repeated invasive procedures are anticipated, UH may be the preferred agent owing to its shorter half-life. Infants tend to require relatively more heparin (UH) than do young children, who in turn require more than older children and adults due to greater volume of distribution, shorter half-life, and age-dependent differences in the ability of UH to inhibit thrombin (111,112). While an adult or older child might be started on UH with a bolus dose of 50 units/kg followed by a continuous infusion of 10 units/kg/h, the dose for a young child is a bolus of 75 units/kg followed by 15–20 units/kg/h, and the dose for an infant is 100 units/kg bolus followed by a continuous infusion of 25 units/kg/h (113). Irrespective of the age of the patient, anticoagulation is adjusted to keep the aPTT roughly 1.5–2.5 times the baseline values (corresponding

to a plasma heparin concentration of 0.2–0.4 units/mL in adults, or an anti-Xa level of 0.3–0.7 units/mL). Similarly, children <2 months of age with thromboembolism should receive larger doses of LMWH (1.5 mg/kg q 12 h) than do children >2 months (1 mg/kg q 12 h) with subsequent adjustment targeted to anti-Xa levels of 0.5–1 units/mL. Warfarin (coumadin) therapy is weight related, with a loading dose of ~0.2 mg/kg/day PO for 1–3 days followed by a maintenance dose of ~0.1 mg/kg/day PO (71). Congenital heart disease patients who have undergone the Fontan operation are sensitive to warfarin and lower doses should be used. The dose of warfarin is titrated to maintain an INR of 1.5–3, depending on the intensity of anticoagulation desired.

Thrombolytic therapy is generally not recommended as first-line therapy for thrombosis in newborn infants because of the high risk of hemorrhage. Thrombolytic therapy may be appropriate in older infants and children to treat major thrombosis with compromised organ or limb perfusion (113), but initial thrombolytic therapy is generally not recommended or required for uncomplicated venous thrombosis. No large, randomized trials of thrombolytic therapy in children have been conducted; consequently, adult dosing guidelines are generally followed. Consultation with the pediatric hematologist is recommended before initiating thrombolytic therapy.

Several newer anticoagulant drugs have been developed including the direct thrombin inhibitors argatroban, lepirudin, bivalirudin, desirudin, and dabigatran (oral), and the anti-Xa agents fondaparinux, rivaroxaban, and apixaban. Argatroban, lepirudin, bivalirudin, and fondaparinux have been used as alternate anticoagulants for patients with documented or suspected HIT. Limited pharmacokinetic, efficacy and safety data exist for use of some of these agents in children (95,96,113–115); however, because standard therapies with heparin (UF and LMWH) and warfarin are effective, we do not recommend the use of these newer anticoagulants to treat venous thromboembolism until large-scale clinical trials in children are available.

SELECTED DISORDERS

Systemic Diseases Associated with Factor Deficiencies

Amyloidosis, Gaucher disease, and the nephrotic syndrome are occasionally seen in the ICU. Each may have one or more associated factor deficiencies that may complicate patient management and result in bleeding or thrombosis. Patients with either amyloidosis or Gaucher disease may develop F.IX deficiency. F.X deficiency has also been associated with amyloidosis. These deficiencies generally result from the adsorption of the specific clotting factor by the abnormal proteins present in each disorder. In the nephrotic syndrome, F.IX deficiency may develop. Although it was originally thought that proteinuria was responsible for the development of F.IX deficiency, this does not appear to be the case. The deficiency typically remits with corticosteroid therapy. Finally, antithrombin III deficiency can be seen with the nephrotic syndrome and may lead to thrombosis. The loss of antithrombin III does appear to be related to proteinuria.

CONCLUSIONS AND FUTURE DIRECTIONS

Much attention is being given to elucidating the interplay of coagulation and inflammation and how the inflammatory state triggers a complex reaction that results in microvascular thrombosis and multiorgan dysfunction/failure. Complete characterization of these interactions will require a better understanding of the normal function of the endothelium and its disruption in sepsis and severe acute illness, as well as those mediators (e.g., cytokines) that affect endothelial function. In addition, the host factors that govern the balance between too little and too much thrombosis will require better elucidation.

Old and newer drugs are being tested in the setting of sepsis to prevent DIC and microvascular thrombosis; if successful, these tests may lead to improved survival with decreased morbidity. Because of the interconnections between inflammation and hemostasis, any of these new agents may also affect a patient's risk for either bleeding or thrombosis. If the recent past is any indication, thrombosis may become a larger problem within PICUs. The intensive care and hematology communities must develop better means to assess an individual patient's risk for thrombosis in order to more accurately gauge the risk and benefit of pharmaco-thromboprophylaxis in selected patients.

GLOSSARY

Activated protein C (APC) produced by liver (vitamin K dependent), activated by exposure to thrombin; actions: protease that inactivates FVa and FVIIIa thus reduces thrombin generation.

A desintegrin and metalloprotease with a thrombospondin member 13 (ADAMTS-13) circulates in the plasma and cleaves von Willebrand factor multimers. An IgG antibody against this protein is found in nonfamilial forms of TTP associated with microangiopathic clotting. When ADAMTS-13 levels are low, patients have ultralarge von Willebrand factor multimers (UL-VWF) circulating in plasma with a consequent increased risk for platelet adhesion and microthrombi formation.

Antithrombin, antithrombin III (ATIII) produced by liver and found in plasma. The original description included four antithrombins, and antithrombin III is the only one that is medically significant. A serine protease inhibitor, it inhibits the activated factors that function as proteases thrombin (F.IIa), F.IXa, F.Xa, F.XIa, F.XIIa from the contact pathway and F.VIIa from the tissue factor pathway as well as Kallikrein and plasmin. It also inactivates C1 in the complement pathway. Its activity in inhibiting coagulation factors is enhanced by the presence of heparin.

D-dimer two cross-linked D fragments of the fibrin protein that represent the cleavage of fibrin by plasmin in the process of fibrinolysis. It is a fibrin degradation product that is elevated in thrombosis and DIC. FDPs may be elevated when fibrinogen breakdown is occurring naturally (as they include products of fibrinogen and are not specific for fibrin) but D-dimer is only elevated when fibrin is being cleaved.

Half-lives (selected clotting factors and hemostasis regulators)

F.I (Fibrinogen)	72–96 hours
F.II	48–72 hours
F.V	12–36 hours
F.VII	6 hours
F.VIII	12 hours
F.IX	24 hours
F.X	32–48 hours
F.XI	40–48 hours
F.XII	48–52 hours
F.XIII	12 days
von Willebrand factor	2–6 hours
Protein C	10 hours
Protein S	42 hours
Antithrombin III	3 days
TAFI	10 min

Heparin cofactor II (HCII) highly homologous to antithrombin III but preferentially inhibits chymotrypsin-like proteases. In the presence of heparin or dermatan sulfate, it inhibits thrombin. Heterozygous deficiency is an identified risk for thrombosis.

Plasminogen activator inhibitor type-1 (PAI-1) produced by the endothelium inhibits tPA and thus the cleavage of plasminogen to plasmin and the subsequent cleavage of fibrinogen to fibrin, thus reducing fibrinolysis. Patients with 4G/4G genotype produce highest levels of PAI-1 (compared with 4G/5G and 5G/5G genotypes) and when septic have increased mortality presumed due to more clotting (less fibrinolysis with higher levels of PAI-1). APC complexes to PAI-1 in the plasma and the tight complexing inhibits PAI-1 resulting in more tPA activity. Reduction of APC during sepsis would also lead to less complexing and inhibition of PAI-1 and more clotting.

Platelet activation platelets bind to exposed collagen when the endothelium is disrupted. These adhesions are strengthened by vWF and also activate platelets. Activated platelets release adenosine diphosphate, serotonin, platelet-activating factor (PAF), von Willebrand factor, platelet factor 4, and thromboxane A2. Activated platelets change shape from spherical to stellate (Source: Wikipedia).

Platelet factor 4 a cytokine released from granules on activated platelets during coagulation that moderates the effects (neutralizes) heparin-like molecules on the surface of endothelial cells and inhibits local ATIII activity, thus promoting coagulation. It is the antigen for antiplatelet antibody binding in HIT. It is a chemotactic for neutraphils, monocytes, and fibroblasts, and it kills intracellular parasites in malaria.

Primary hemostasis the component of clot formation that involves platelet interactions with the endothelium and subendothelial structures. Normal primary hemostasis requires normal platelet number and function, the presence of normal adhesive glycoproteins to promote platelet aggregation (fibrinogen) and adhesion (von Willebrand factor) and normal subendothelial structures (e.g., collagen) for platelet adhesion.

Protein S a vitamin K–dependent glycoprotein that functions as a cofactor for activated Protein C. Protein S (PS) circulates in plasma and is also found on the surface of endothelial cells and in platelets. It is synthesized in the liver, endothelial cells, and megakaryocytes. The presence of PS accelerates the proteolytic inactivation of FVa and FVIIIa by APC approximately 25-fold. Approximately 40% of Protein S in plasma is bound by C4b-binding protein (C4bBP), which is an acute-phase reactant. Consequently, free PS decreases under conditions in which C4bBP is increased (e.g., inflammation, pregnancy, trauma/surgery). Only free PS is active as a cofactor for APC.

Prothrombin complex concentrates (PCC) pooled donor solutions that contain 3 (II, IX, X) or 4 (II, VII, IX, X) (PC, PS, AT, and heparin) (Beriplex, Octaplex, Confidex) factors and are standardized for their F.IX content. All have gone through at least one step of viral reduction/elimination. Factor levels are 25 times higher than FFP and therefore faster and less volume. Effective at treating prolonged INR and PT. Expensive. Intracranial hemorrhage treat with 35–50 IU/kg. Replaces vitamin K-dependent factors and reverses warfarin effect and reverses warfarin.

Thrombin-activated fibrinolysis inhibitor (TAFI) also known as carboxypeptidase B2 is produced by the liver and circulates in plasma bound to plasminogen. When proteolytically activated by thrombin/thrombomodulin complex, it expresses carboxypeptidase activity and degrades c-terminal residues on fibrin important in the binding and subsequent activation of plasminogen thereby down-regulating fibrinolysis. TAFI may potentially be inhibited by other macromolecules that compete for the binding of fibrin (e.g., APC).

Thrombocytopenia-associated multiple organ failure (TAMOF) associated with reduced ADAMTS-13 and is reversed by apheresis.

Thrombomodulin found bound to endothelial cell membrane. Binds thrombin on the surface of endothelial cells and enhances the catalytic activation of PC by thrombin over 1000-fold. It also can inhibit the thrombin-mediated proteolysis of macromolecular substrates (e.g., fibrinogen, F.V, F.XIII, Protein S), may inhibit thrombin activation of platelets, and may accelerate the inactivation of thrombin by antithrombin III.

Tissue factor (TF) an integral membrane glycoprotein located on the adventitia and comes into contact with blood upon tissue injury. TF promotes the activation of F.VII to F.VIIa and in complex with F.VIIa activates F.X to F.Xa (the "extrinsic" coagulation cascade). Activation or injury of various cell types (e.g., endothelial cells, monocytes, fibroblasts) increases TF expression by these cells. In cell culture, TF expression is attenuated by APC due to and APC-mediated decrease in inflammation.

Tissue factor pathway inhibitor (TFPI) reversibly inhibits F.Xa and Thrombin (F.IIa). The F.Xa/TFPI complex also inhibits the F.VIIa-TF complex thereby decreasing the generation of F.Xa. TFPI is synthesized by endothelial cells, and endothelial-bound TFPI contributes to the antithrombotic nature of vascular endothelium. Increases in TFPI seen in sepsis may reflect endothelial injury and contribute to bleeding noted in DIC.

Vitamin K antagonists (VKA) are a class of drugs that produce anticoagulation through depletion of the active (reduced) form of vitamin K. Warfarin, the most common agent in this class, causes depletion of reduced vitamin K through competitive inhibition of vitamin K epoxide reductase which recycles oxidized vitamin K to the reduced form. Vitamin K in its reduced form is a required co-factor for the g-carboxylation of glutamate residues on the vitamin K-dependent clotting factors (II, VII, IX, X). This post-translational enzymatic modification occurs in the liver and produces a Ca^{2+} binding site needed to enable binding of these factors to phospholipid surfaces with subsequent conversion to their active forms. Absence of this modification results in greatly impaired activation of these factors with resultant decrease in *in vivo* clot formation. The intensity of VKA anticoagulation is assessed by the INR.

Vitamin K epoxide reductase (VKOR) reduces vitamin K that has been oxidized during the carboxylation of coagulation factors. VKAs inhibit the recycling of vitamin K epoxide back to the reduced and active form. NMTT side chain of some cephalosporins (cefotetan, moxalactam, cafaperazone, cefamandole, and others) block VKOR, causing hypothrombinemia (hypoprothrombinemia).

References

1. Eilertsen KE, Osterud B. Tissue factor: (patho)physiology and cellular biology. *Blood Coagul Fibrinolysis* 2004;15(7):521–38.
2. Horne M. Overview of hemostasis and thrombosis; current status of antithrombotic therapies. *Thromb Res* 2005;117(1–2):15–7; discussion 39–42.
3. Hayward CP, Rao AK, Cattaneo M. Congenital platelet disorders: Overview of their mechanisms, diagnostic evaluation and treatment. *Haemophilia* 2006;12(suppl 3):128–36.
4. Aird WC. The role of the endothelium in severe sepsis and the multiple organ dysfunction syndrome. *Blood* 2003;101(10):3765–77.
5. Levi M, ten Cate H, van der Poll T. Endothelium: Interface between coagulation and inflammation. *Crit Care Med* 2002;30(suppl 5):S220–4.
6. El-Nawawy A, Abbassy AA, El-Bordiny M, et al. Evaluation of early detection and management of disseminated intravascular coagulation among Alexandria University pediatric intensive care patients. *J Trop Pediatr* 2004;50(6):339–47.
7. Fisher NC, Mutimer DJ. Central venous cannulation in patients with liver disease and coagulopathy – A prospective audit. *Intensive Care Med* 1999;25:481–85.
8. Dempfle CE. Coagulopathy and sepsis. *Thromb Haemost* 2004;91(2):213–24.
9. Esmon CT. Crosstalk between inflammation and thrombosis. *Maturitas* 2004;47(4):305–14.
10. Hermans PW, Hibberd ML, Booy R, et al. 4G/5G promoter polymorphism in the plasminogen-activator-inhibitor-1 gene and outcome in meningococcal disease. Meningococcal Research Group. *Lancet* 1999;354(9178):556–60.
11. Hermans PW, Hazelzet JA. Plasminogen activator inhibitor type 1 gene polymorphism and sepsis. *Clin Infect Dis* 2005;41(suppl 7):S453–8.
12. Menges T, Hermans PW, Little SG, et al. Plasminogen-activator-inhibitor-1 4G/5G promoter polymorphism and prognosis of severely injured patients. *Lancet* 2001;357(9262):1096–7.
13. Geishofer G, Binder A, Muller M, et al. 4G/5G promoter polymorphism in the plasminogen-activator-inhibitor-1 gene in children with systemic meningococcaemia. *Eur J Pediatr* 2005;164:486–90.
14. Huq MA, Takeyama N, Harada M, et al. 4G/5G polymorphism of the plasminogen activator type-1 gene is associated with multiple organ dysfunction in critically ill patients. *Acta Haematol* 2012;127:72–80.
15. Madach K, Aladzsity I, Szilagy A, et al. 4G/5G polymorphism of the PAI-1 gene is associated with multiple organ dysfunction and septic shock in pneumonia induced severe sepsis: prospective, observational, genetic study. *Crit Care* 2010;14:R79.
16. Khair K, Liesner R. Bruising and bleeding in infants and children—A practical approach. *Br J Haematol* 2006;133(3):221–31.
17. Lillicrap D, Nair SC, Srivastava A, et al. Laboratory issues in bleeding disorders. *Hemophilia* 2006;12(suppl 3):68–75.
18. Chuansumrit A, Hotrakitya S, Sirinavin S, et al. Disseminated intravascular coagulation findings in 100 patients. *J Med Assoc Thai* 1999;82(suppl 1):S63–8.
19. Girolami A, Luzzatto G, Varvarikis C, et al. Main clinical manifestations of a bleeding diathesis: An often disregarded aspect of medical and surgical history taking. *Hemophilia* 2005;11(3):193–202.
20. Oren H, Cingoz I, Duman M, et al. Disseminated intravascular coagulation in pediatric patients: Clinical and laboratory features and prognostic factors influencing survival. *Pediatr Hematol Oncol* 2005;22(8):679–88.
21. Abshire TC. An approach to the diagnosis and treatment of bleeding disorders in infants. *Int J Hematol* 2002;76(suppl 2):265–70.
22. Barton JC, Poon MC. Coagulation testing of the Hickmann catheter blood in patients with acute leukemia. *Arch Intern Med* 1986;146(11):2165–9.
23. Herak DC, Antolic MR, Krleza JL, et al. Inherited prothrombotic risk factors in children with stroke, transient ischemic attack, or migraine. *Pediatrics* 2009;123:e653–60.
24. Nahar A, Sabo C, Chitlur M, et al. Plasma homocysteine levels, methylene tetrahydrofolate reductase polymorphisms, and the risk of thromboembolism in children. *J Pediatr Hematol Oncol* 2011;33:330–3.
25. Sottilotta G, Siboni SM, Latella C, et al. Hyperhomocysteinemia and C677T MTHFR genotype in patients with retinal vein thrombosis. *Clin Appl Thromb Hemost* 2010;16:549–53.
26. Avila ML, Shah V, Brandao LR. Systemic review on heparin-induced thrombocytopenia in children: A call to action. *J Thromb Haemost* 2013;11:660–9.

27. Caprini JA, Goldshteyn S, Glase CJ, et al. Thrombophilia testing in patients with venous thrombosis. *Eur J Endovasc Surg* 2005;30:550–55.

28. Zadro R, Herak DC. Inherited prothrombotic risk factors in children with first ischemic stroke. *Biochem Med (Zagreb)* 2012;22:298–310.

29. Bick RL, Arun B, Frenkel EP. Disseminated intravascular coagulation. Clinical and pathophysiological mechanisms and manifestations. *Haemostasis* 1999;29(2–3):111–34.

30. Cauchie P, Cauchie Ch, Boudjeltia KZ, et al. Diagnosis and prognosis of overt disseminated intravascular coagulation in a general hospital—Meaning of the ISTH score system, fibrin monomers, and lipoprotein-C-reactive protein complex formation. *Am J Hematol* 2006;81(6):414–9.

31. Gando S, Iba T, Eguchi Y, et al. A multicenter, prospective validation of disseminated intravascular coagulation diagnostic criteria for critically ill patients: Comparing current criteria. *Crit Care Med* 2006;34(3):625–31.

32. Voves C, Wuillemin WA, Zeerleder S. International Society on Thrombosis and Haemostasis score for overt disseminated intravascular coagulation predicts organ dysfunction and fatality in sepsis patients. *Blood Coagul Fibrinolysis* 2006;17(6):445–51.

33. Gando S. The utility of a diagnostic scoring system for disseminated intravascular coagulation. *Crit Care Clin* 2012;28:373–88.

34. De Kleijn ED, De Groot R, Hack CE, et al. Activation of protein C following infusion of protein C concentrate in children with severe meningococcal sepsis and purpura fulminans: A randomized, double-blinded, placebo-controlled, dose-finding study. *Crit Care Med* 2003;31(6):1839–47.

35. Faust SN, Levin M, Harrison OB, et al. Dysfunction of endothelial protein C activation in severe meningococcal sepsis. *N Engl J Med* 2001;345(6):408–16.

36. Marti-Carvajal AJ, Sola I, Gluud C, et al. Human recombinant protein C for severe sepsis and septic shock in adult and pediatric patients. *Cochrane Database Syst Rev* 2012;12:CD004388.

37. Erber WN. Plasma and plasma products in the treatment of massive haemorrhage. *Best Pract Res Clin Haematol* 2005;19(1):97–112.

38. Goldenberg NA, Manco-Johnson MJ. Pediatric hemostasis and use of plasma components. *Best Pract Res Clin Haematol* 2005;19(1):143–55.

39. Boffard KD, Riou B, Warren B, et al. Recombinant factor VIIa as adjunctive therapy for bleeding control in severely injured trauma patients: Two parallel randomized, placebo-controlled, double blind clinical trials. *J Trauma* 2005;59(1):8–15; discussion 15–8.

40. Mathew P, Young G. Recombinant factor VIIa in paediatric bleeding disorders—A 2006 review. *Haemophilia* 2006;12(5):457–72.

41. Sallah S, Husain A, Nguyen NP. Recombinant activated factor VII in patients with cancer and hemorrhagic disseminated intravascular coagulation. *Blood Coagul Fibrinolysis* 2004;15(7):577–82.

42. Scarpelini S, Rizoli S. Recombinant factor VIIa and the surgical patient. *Curr Opin Crit Care* 2006;12(4):351–6.

43. Simpson E, Lin Y, Stanworth S, et al. Recombinant factor VIIa for the prevention and treatment of bleeding in patients without haemophilia. *Cochrane Database Syst Rev* 2012;3:CD005011. doi:10.1002/14651858.CD005011.pub4.

44. Altman R, Scazziota A, De Lourdes Herrera M, et al. Recombinant factor VIIa reverses the inhibitory effect of aspirin or aspirin plus clopidogrel on in vivo thrombin generation. *J Thromb Haemost* 2006;4(9):2022–7.

45. O'Connell KA, Wood JJ, Wise RP, et al. Thromboembolic adverse events after use of recombinant human coagulation factor VIIa. *JAMA* 2006;295(3):293–8.

46. Afshari A. Evidence based evaluation of immune-coagulatory interventions in critical care. *Dan Med Bull* 2011;58:B4316.

47. Davis-Jackson R, Correa H, Horswell R, et al. Antithrombin III (AT) and recombinant tissue plasminogen activator (R-TPA) used singly and in combination versus supportive care as treatment of endotoxin-induced disseminated intravascular coagulation (DIC) in the neonatal pig. *Thromb J* 2006;4:7.

48. Jaimes F, de la Rosa G, Arango C, et al. A randomized clinical trial of unfractionated heparin for treatment of sepsis (the HETRASE study): Design and rationale. *Trials* 2006;7:19.

49. Munteanu C, Bloodworth LL, Korn TH. Antithrombin concentrate with plasma exchange in purpura fulminans. *Pediatr Crit Care Med* 2000;1:84–7.

50. Zenz W, Zoehrer B, Levin M, et al. Use of recombinant tissue plasminogen activator in children with meningococcal purpura fulminans: A retrospective study. *Crit Care Med* 2004;32:1777–80.

51. Lapeyraque AL, Malina M, Fremeaux-Bacchi V, et al. Eculizumab in severe Shiga toxin-associated HUS. *N Engl J Med* 2011;364:2561–3.

52. Nguyen TC, Han YY, Kiss JE, et al. Intensive plasma exchange increases a disintegrin and metalloprotease with thrombospindin motifs-13 activity and reverses organ dysfunction in children with thrombocytopenia-associated multiple organ failure. *Crit Care Med* 2008;36:2878–87.

53. Al Ghumlas AK, Gader A, Faleh FZ. Haemostatic abnormalities in liver disease: Could some haemostatic tests be useful as liver function tests? *Blood Coagul Fibrinolysis* 2005;16(5):329–35.

54. Lisman T, Caldwell SH, Leebeck FWG, et al. Hemostasis in chronic liver disease. *J Thromb Haemost* 2006;4:2059.

55. Lisman T, Potre RJ. Rebalanced hemostasis in patients with liver disease: Evidence and clinical consequences. *Blood* 2010;116:878–85.

56. Lisman T, Bakhtiari K, Adelmeijer J, et al. Intact thrombin generation and decreased fibrinolytic capacity in patients with acute liver injury or acute liver failure. *J Thromb Haemost* 2012;10:1312–19.

57. Roberts LN, Patel RK, Arya R. Haemostasis and thrombosis in liver disease. *Br J Haematol* 2009;148:507–12.

58. Sogaard KK, Horvath-Puho E, Gronbaek H, et al. Risk of venous thromboembolism in patients with liver disease: A nationwide population-based case-control study. *Am J Gastroenterol* 2009;104:96–101.

59. Rijken DC, Kock EL, Guimaraes AHC, et al. Evidence for an enhanced fibrinolytic capacity in cirrhosis as measured with two different global fibrinolysis tests. *J Thromb Haemost* 2012;10:2116–22.

60. Townsend JC, Heard R, Powers ER, et al. Usefulness of International Normalized Ratio to predict bleeding complications in patients with end-stage liver disease who undergo cardiac catheterization. *Am J Cardiol* 2012;110:1062–5.

61. Tripodi A, Caldwell SH, Hoffman M, et al. Review article: The prothrombin time test as a measure of bleeding risk and prognosis in liver disease. *Aliment Pharmacol Ther* 2007;26:141–8.

62. Tripodi A, Baglin T, Robert A, et al. Reporting prothrombin time results as international normalized ratios for patients with chronic liver disease. *J Thromb Haemost* 2010;1410–2.

63. Wei YX, Li J, Zhang LW, et al. Assessment of validity of INR system for patients with liver disease associated with viral hepatitis. *J Thromb Thrombolysis* 2010;30:84–9.

64. Dasher K, Trotter JF. Intensive care unit management of liver-related coagulation disorders. *Crit Care Clin* 2012;28:389–98.

65. Segal JB, Dzik WH. Paucity of studies to support that abnormal coagulation test results predict bleeding in the setting of invasive procedures: An evidence-based review. *Transfusion* 2005;45:1413–25.

66. Youssef WI, Salazar F, Dasarathy S, et al. Role of fresh frozen plasma infusion in correction of coagulopathy of chronic liver disease: A dual phase study. *Am J Gastroenterol* 2003;98:1391–4.

67. Ganguly S, Spengel K, Tilzer LL, et al. Recombinant factor VIIa: Unregulated continuous use in patients with bleeding and coagulopathy does not alter mortality and outcome. *Clin Lab Haematol* 2006;28(5):309–12.

68. Ramsey G. Treating coagulopathy in liver disease with plasma transfusions or recombinant factor VIIa: An evidence based review. *Best Prac Res Clin Haematol* 2005;19(1):113–26.

69. Goodnough LT. A reappraisal of plasma, prothrombin complex concentrates, and recombinant factor VIIa in patient blood management. *Crit Care Clin* 2012;28:413–26.

70. Yank V, Tuohy CV, Logan AC, et al. Systematic review: Benefits and harms of in-hospital use of recombinant factor VIIa administration. *Ann Intern Med* 2011;154:529–40.

71. Bonduel MM. Oral anticoagulation therapy in children. *Thromb Res* 2006;118(1):85–94.

72. Brady KM, Easley RB, Tobias JD. Recombinant activated factor VII (rFVIIa) treatment in infants with hemorrhage. *Paediatr Anaesth* 2006;16(10):1042–6.

73. Dentali F, Ageno W, Crowther M. Treatment of coumarin-associated coagulopathy: A systemic review and proposed treatment algorithms. *J Thromb Haemost* 2006;4(9):1853–63.

74. Witmer CM, Huang YS, Lynch K, et al. Off-label recombinant factor VIIa use and thrombosis in children: A multicenter cohort study. *J. Pediatr* 2011;158:820–5.

75. Franchini M. Prothrombin complex concentrates: An update. *Blood Transfus* 2010;8:149–54.

76. Hardy JF, de Moerloose P, Samama CM, et al. Massive transfusion and coagulopathy: Pathophysiology and implications for clinical management. *Can J Anaesth* 2006;53(suppl 6):S40–58.

77. Hayter MA, Pavenski K, Baker J. Massive transfusion in the trauma patient: Continuing professional development. *Can J Anaesth* 2012; 59(12):1130–45.

78. Hellerstern P, Muntean W, Schramm W, et al. Practical guidelines for the clinical use of plasma. *Thromb Res* 2002;107(suppl 1):S53–8.

79. Theusinger OM, Madjdpour C, Spahn DR. Resuscitation and transfusion management in trauma patients: emerging concepts. *Curr Opin Crit Care* 2012;18(6):661–70.

80. Lucas CE, Ledgerwood AM. Fresh frozen plasma/red blood cell resuscitation regimen that restores procoagulants without causing adult respiratory distress syndrome. *J Trauma Acute Care Surg* 2012;72:821–27.

81. Bosch YP, Ganushchak YM, de Jong DS. Comparison of ACT point-of-care measurements: Reproducibility and agreement. *Perfusion* 2006;21(1):27–31.

82. Carr JA, Silverman N. The heparin-protamine interaction: A review. *J Cardiovasc Surg (Torino)* 1999;40(5):659–66.

83. Park KW. Protamine and protamine reactions. *Int Anesthesiol Clin* 2004;42(3):135–45.

84. Frost J, Murbee L, Russo P, et al. Heparin-induced thrombocytopenia in the pediatric intensive care unit population. *Pediatr Crit Care Med* 2005;6(2):216–9.

85. Cuker A, Arepally G, Crowther MA, et al. The HIT Expert Probability (HEP) score: A novel pre-test probability model for heparin-induced thrombocytopenia based on broad expert opinion. *J Thromb Haemost* 2010;8:2642–50.

86. Cuker A, Gimotty PA, Crowther MA, et al. Predictive value of the 4Ts scoring system for heparin-induced thrombocytopenia: A systematic review and meta-analysis. *Blood* 2012;120(20):4160–7.

87. Risch L, Huber AR, Schmugge M. Diagnosis and treatment of heparin-induced thrombocytopenia in neonates and children. *Thromb Res* 2006;118(1):123–35.

88. Warkentin TE, Kelton JG. A 14-year study of heparin-induced thrombocytopenia. *Am J Med* 1996;101:502–7.

89. Dager WE, White RH. Pharmacotherapy of heparin-induced thrombocytopenia. *Expert Opin Pharmacother* 2003;4(6):919–40.

90. Argueta-Morales IR, Olsen MC, DeCampli WM, et al. Alternative anticoagulation during cardiovascular procedures in pediatric patients with heparin-induced thrombocytopenia. *J Extra Corpor Technol* 2012;44:69–74.

91. Gates R, Yost P, Parker B. The use of bivalirudin for cardiopulmonary bypass anticoagulation in pediatric heparin-induced thrombocytopenia patients. *Artif Organs* 2010;34:667–9.

92. Hess CN, Becker RC, Alexander JH, et al. Antithrombotic therapy in heparin-induced thrombocytopenia: Guidelines translated for the clinician. *J Thromb Thrombolysis* 2012;34:552–61.

93. Rayapudi S, Torres A Jr, Deshpande GG, et al. Bivalirudin for anticoagulation in children. *Pediatr Blood Cancer* 2008;51:798–801.

94. Takemoto CM, Streiff MB. Heparin-induced thrombocytopenia screening and management in pediatric patients. *Am Soc Hematol* 2011;162–9.

95. Young G, Tarantino MD, Wohrley J, et al. Pilot dose-finding and safety of bivalirudin in infants <6 months of age with thrombosis. *J Thromb Haemost* 2007;5:1654–9.

96. Young G, Boshkov LK, Sullivan LJ, et al. Argatroban therapy in pediatric patients requiring nonheparin anticoagulation: An open-label, safety, efficacy, and pharmacokinetic study. *Pediatr Blood Cancer* 2011;56:1103–9.

97. Hall R, Mazer CD. Antiplatelet drugs: A review of their pharmacology and management in the perioperative period. *Anesth Analg* 2011;112:292–311.

98. Sohal AS, Gangji AS, Crowther MA, et al. Uremic bleeding: Pathophysiology and clinical risk factors. *Thromb Res* 2006;118(3):417–22.

99. Molino D, DeLucia D, Gaspare de Santo N. Coagulation disorders in uremia. *Semin Nephrol* 2006;26(1):46–51.

100. Branchford BR, Mourani P, Bajaj L, et al. Risk factors for in-hospital venous thromboembolism in children: A case-control study employing diagnostic validation. *Haematologica* 2012;97:509–15.

101. Hanson SJ, Punzalan RC, Greenup RA, et al. Incidence and risk factors for venous thromboembolism in critically ill children after trauma. *J Trauma* 2010;68:52–6.

102. Hanson SJ, Punzalan RC, Christensen MA, et al. Incidence and risk factors for venous thromboembolism in critically ill children with cardiac disease. *Pediatr Cardiol* 2012;33:103–8.

103. Higgerson RA, Lawson KA, Christie LM, et al. Incidence and risk factors associated with venous thrombotic events in pediatric intensive care unit patients. *Pediatr Crit Care Med* 2011;12:628–34.

104. McCrory MC, Brady KM, Takemoto C, et al. Thrombotic disease in critically ill children. *Pediatr Crit Care* 2011;12:80–9.

105. Parker RI. Thrombosis in the pediatric population. *Crit Care Med* 2010;38(suppl 2):S71–5.

106. Reiter PD, Wathen B, Valuck RJ, et al. Thrombosis risk factor assessment and implications for prevention in critically ill children. *Pediatr Crit Care Med* 2012;13:381–6.

107. Spentzouris G, Scriven RJ, Lee TK, et al. Pediatric venous thromboembolism in relation to adults. *J Vasc Surg* 2012;55:1785–93.

108. Kosch A, Junker K, Schobess R, et al. Prothrombotic risk factors in children with spontaneous venous thrombosis and their asymptomatic parents: A family study. *Thromb Res* 2000;15:99:531.

109. Hanson SJ, Punzalan RC, Arca MJ, et al. Effectiveness of clinical guidelines for deep vein thrombosis prophylaxis in reducing the incidence of venous thromboembolism in critically ill children after trauma. *J Trauma Acute Care Surg* 2012;72:1292–97.

110. Faustino EV, Patel S, Thiagarajan RR, et al. Survey of pharmacologic prophylaxis in critically ill children. *Crit Care Med* 2011;39:1773–78.

111. McDonald M, Jacobson L, Hay WJ, et al. Heparin clearance in the newborn. *Pediatr Res* 1981;15:1015–18.

112. Newall F, Johnson L, Ignjatovic V, et al. Unfractionated heparin therapy in infants and children. *Pediatrics* 2009;123:e510–8.

113. Monagle P, Chan A, Goldenberg NA, et al. Antithrombotic Therapy in Neonates and Children. 9th ed. American College of Chest Physicians Evidence-Based Clinical Practice Guidelines. *Chest* 2012;141(suppl 2):e737S–801S.

114. Nowak-Gottl U, Bidlingmaier C, Krumpel A, et al. Pharmacokinetics, efficacy, and safety of LMWHs in venous thrombosis and stroke in neonates, infants and children. *Br J Pharmacol* 2008;153:1120–27.

115. Young G, Yee DL, O'Brien SH, et al. FondaKIDS: A prospective pharmacokinetic and safety study of fondaparinux in children between 1 and 18 years of age. *Pediatr Blood Cancer* 2011;57:1049–54.

CHAPTER 119 ■ SICKLE CELL DISEASE

KEVIN J. SULLIVAN, ERIN COLETTI, SALVATORE R. GOODWIN, CYNTHIA GAUGER, AND NIRANJAN "TEX" KISSOON

KEY POINTS

Normal Hemoglobin Structure and Function

1. The presence of fetal hemoglobin offers protection from sickle cell disease (SCD) from birth to 6 months of age. After 6 months of age, sickle hemoglobin increases in the circulation and complications of SCD may appear.

2. SCD represents a variety of genotypes expressing a phenotype that is characterized by hemoglobin deformation in the deoxygenated state and which results in a chronic hemolytic anemia and capillary occlusion by deformed erythrocytes.

Relevance to Pediatric Critical Care

3. The life-threatening end-organ effects of SCD include acute chest syndrome (ACS), aplastic crisis, splenic sequestration crisis, stroke, and an increased risk of infectious complications.

4. Pediatric intensivists need to be familiar with the management of acute life-threatening SCD complications, perioperative management, and chronic sequelae such as stroke, cardiovascular dysfunction, and pulmonary artery hypertension.

5. The erythrocyte cell membrane becomes irreversibly injured when hemoglobin is in a deoxygenated state unless prompt reversal occurs in the pulmonary vasculature.

Biologic Precipitants of Sickle Cell Complications

6. SCD is a prototypical model of the complex interplay of a genetic defect of hemoglobin structure and function with disordered vascular biology.

7. Abnormalities of hemoglobin structure and function, endothelial cells, leukocytes, platelets, the coagulation cascade, and systemic inflammation are intricately related in SCD.

8. Abnormalities of nitric oxide metabolism and oxidant-mediated injury are responsible for many of the complications of the disease.

9. Physiologic precipitants of SCD include dehydration, acid–base imbalance, hyper- and hypothermia, hypoxemia, and vasoconstriction.

Sickle Cell Complications

10. Vaso-occlusive crisis (VOC) may mimic other severe medical conditions and often precedes some of the severe complications of SCD.

11. If osteomyelitis cannot be differentiated from VOC, then antimicrobial coverage for *Staphylococcus aureus* and *Salmonella* species should be administered.

12. Simple or exchange transfusions are effective for many complications of SCD, but hematocrit elevations above 33% are associated with increased viscosity and the potential for central nervous system (CNS) thrombotic injury. Repeated transfusions may lead to transfusion-related complications.

13. ACS may progress quickly to life-threatening respiratory failure and multiple organ system failure.

14. Stroke is a common source of morbidity and may be recurrent. Focal seizures may be the presenting symptom of acute cerebral ischemia. The differential diagnosis of stroke in SCD includes meningitis and toxic ingestions.

15. Acute treatment of stroke includes exchange transfusion. Chronic transfusion may attenuate stroke risk, but its discontinuation is associated with increased risk of stroke recurrence.

Chronic Injury of the Cardiovascular System

16. Children with SCD are surviving further into adulthood, but chronic circulatory and respiratory dysfunction may predispose to premature mortality.

17. Common chronic hemodynamic disturbances include ventricular diastolic dysfunction and increased pulmonary vascular resistance. Common chronic pulmonary issues include restrictive lung disease and reactive airway disease. These conditions add to SCD-related morbidity.

18. Pulmonary hypertension is the most important predictor of early mortality and should always be suspected in the acutely ill patient.

19. Sudden death is common among SCD patients.

Perioperative Management of SCD Patients

20. The perioperative mortality is greatly increased for patients with SCD.

21. Simple transfusion is as effective as exchange transfusion in the prevention of perioperative SCD-related complications and is associated with fewer transfusion-related complications.

22. Important perioperative factors to optimize include hydration, vital organ function, analgesia, and pulmonary toilet.

23 The risk of perioperative SCD complications varies with the operative procedure and the severity of the patient's clinical course.

Outcomes

24 SCD patients are living longer, and chronic debilitating complications assume greater importance. Cerebral vascular accidents and pulmonary hypertension are the most important chronic complications.

New Concepts in Understanding SCD/Future Directions

25 The variable expression of SCD can be explained by the interplay of chronic hemolysis/endothelial dysfunction and viscosity/vaso-occlusion.

26 Hemolysis and endothelial dysfunction are associated with pulmonary hypertension and stroke, while viscosity and vaso-occlusion are associated with ACS, VOC, and osteo-necrosis of the bone.

Sickle cell disease (SCD) refers to a clinical phenotype that is expressed as chronic hemolysis, vascular occlusion, painful crises, ischemic end-organ injury, acute life-threatening manifestations of the disease, and development of chronic organ dysfunction. A variety of hemoglobin genotypes that cause hemoglobin deformation in the deoxygenated state can express the SCD phenotype. The most common genetic disorder causing SCD is sickle cell anemia (SCA), in which patients possess two genes for abnormal β chains of the hemoglobin molecule. Other genotypes expressing variations of the SCD phenotype include sickle β^0 thalassemia, sickle β^+ thalassemia, and hemoglobin SC disease (HbSC). Patients with homozygous sickle hemoglobin (HbS) or sickle β^0 thalassemia usually have the most severe manifestations of SCD, whereas patients with HbSC or sickle β^+ thalassemia usually have a milder course.

The management of patients with SCD phenotypes is relevant to the practice of pediatric critical care medicine because SCD is a multi–organ system disease in which life-threatening acute complications occur commonly. Pediatric intensive care physicians are frequently required to comanage these patients with subspecialists, including hematologists, surgeons, anesthesiologists, cardiologists, and pulmonologists. Finally, SCD is of great interest as few other diseases in medicine better illustrate the interactions in vascular biology that occur between hemoglobin, erythrocytes, endothelial cells, platelets, coagulation cascade, nitric oxide (NO), and injurious oxidant compounds.

In this chapter, we review (a) the basic biochemical abnormalities of the hemoglobin molecule in SCD, (b) the comprehensive vascular biology that underlies the clinical manifestations of the disease, (c) the acute and chronic clinical complications of SCD and clinical management strategies, (d) anesthetic and surgical considerations relevant to the patient with SCD, and (e) outcomes and prognosis for patients with SCD.

NORMAL HEMOGLOBIN STRUCTURE AND FUNCTION

Normal human hemoglobin is a tetrameric protein composed of two α and two β chains. Each chain consists of an iron-containing protoheme moiety, which binds oxygen, as well as a globin chain of amino acids arranged in a specific sequential and spatial pattern. While the iron-containing heme group in each chain is identical, the amino acid sequences of the globin chains differ and impart unique chemical and functional characteristics, including oxygen affinity.

With the exception of hemoglobin expressed early in embryologic development, hemoglobin consists of two α and two non-α chains attached to four iron-containing heme complexes. Hemoglobin A comprises the majority (95%) of normal adult hemoglobin and contains two α and two β chains (HbA: α_2, β_2). Hemoglobin A_2 is also a component (1%–4%) of normal adult hemoglobin and is composed of two α and two δ chains (HbA$_2$, α_2, δ_2). Fetal hemoglobin, which is the predominant hemoglobin in fetal development, gradually declines during the first 6 months of life and is composed of two α and two γ chains (HbF: α_2, γ_2). At birth, human erythrocytes contain 70%–90% HbF, which normally predominates until 2–4 months of age. The persistence of HbF production exists in many conditions and offers a protective effect when present in patients with certain hemoglobinopathies.

SCD refers to a variety of genotypes that all result in the production of sickled erythrocytes upon hemoglobin deoxygenation, eventually leading to chronic hemolysis, recurrent vaso-occlusion, and ischemic end-organ injury to every organ system. All patients with an SCD phenotype inherit a mutant β-globin allele in which the sixth codon is altered, resulting in the substitution of valine for glutamine at the sixth amino acid position of the β-globin chain. Hemoglobin that incorporates this mutant β^S-globin chain is referred to as HbS, and homozygotes for the β^S allele are said to have SCA (HbSS), while heterozygotes for the β^S allele are said to have sickle cell trait (SCT, HbAS). Patients with SCT do not express the SCD phenotype because of the protective effects of HbA.

Heterozygous genotypes coding for HbS, together with other alterations in β-chain production (non-HbA), can also result in the expression of the SCD phenotype. The most common heterozygous SCD genotypes are HbSC and the sickle β thalassemias. Approximately 70% of the SCD patients in the United States are homozygous for β^S (SCA), while HbSC (~20%) and sickle β thalassemias (10%) comprise the remainder (1). Patients with HbSC or HbS–β^+ thalassemia demonstrate less severe symptoms than patients with HbSS because of the protective effects of HbF (in patients with HbSC) or hemoglobins A and F (patients with HbS–β^+ thalassemia produce some, but a reduced amount of, β chains of HbA). Patients with HbS–β^0 thalassemia produce no β chains of HbA and exhibit a clinical course similar in severity to that of patients with HbSS (**Table 119.1**)(2).

As a result of global migration, SCD now has worldwide distribution and is one of the most common monogenetic disorders in the world. SCT is estimated to be present in 8%–9% of African Americans (3,4). SCA affects nearly 1 in 600 African Americans (5) and an estimated 1%–4% of all infants born in sub-Saharan Africa (6). SCD is inherited in an autosomal recessive fashion with standard Mendelian inheritance.

RELEVANCE TO PEDIATRIC CRITICAL CARE

The common, acute complications of SCD that require the attention of the pediatric intensive care physician include splenic sequestration, aplastic crisis, sepsis, acute chest syndrome (ACS), and stroke. Additionally, the intensive care physician may be called upon to assist in the management of SCD patients with refractory vaso-occlusive crisis (VOC), priapism, or orbital infarction. Finally, intensive care physicians

TABLE 119.1

SEVERITY AND DIAGNOSTIC TESTING FOR RELEVANT SICKLE CELL SYNDROMES

■ SYNDROME	■ GENOTYPE	■ SEVERITY	■ NEONATAL SCREENING[a]	Hemoglobin Electrophoresis in Older Children (%)				
				■ HBA	■ HBS	■ HBF	■ HBA$_2$	■ HBC
Sickle cell anemia	S-S	++++	FS	0	80–95	2–20	<3.5	0
Sickle β^0 thalassemia[b]	S-β^0	+++	FS	0	80–92	2–15	3.5–7	0
Hemoglobin SC disease	S-C	++	FSC	0	45–50	1–5	NA[c]	45–50
Sickle β^+ thalassemia[b]	S-β^+	+	FSA or FS[d]	5–30	65–90	2–10	3.5–6	0
Sickle cell trait	A-S	0	FAS	50–60	35–45	<2	<3.5	0

[a]Hemoglobins reported in order of decreasing quantity (e.g., FS = F > S); F, fetal hemoglobin; S, sickle hemoglobin; C, hemoglobin C; A, hemoglobin A.
[b]β^0 indicates thalassemia mutation with absent production of β-globin; β^+ indicates thalassemia mutation with reduced production of β-globin.
[c]Quantity of HbA$_2$ cannot be measured in the presence of HbC.
[d]Quantity of HbA at birth sometimes insufficient for detection.
Adapted from Lane PA. Sickle cell disease. *Pediatr Clin N Am* 1996;43:639–64, table 1 on page 642, with permission.

and anesthesiologists are often involved in the perioperative management of patients with SCD.

The severity of SCD varies widely but leads to repetitive injuries to every organ system. Therefore, chronic injury to the circulatory, respiratory, nervous, renal, and immune systems may already be present in children with SCD who present to the PICU. SCD is of special interest to pediatric and adult subspecialists alike, as it represents a disease process that begins in infancy and culminates in multiorgan dysfunction in patients who survive to adulthood. Therefore, therapeutic interventions in childhood may improve both the quality of life and life expectancy for adult patients.

The fundamental defect in SCD is an abnormality of the β-globin gene that results in the tendency for hemoglobin to irreversibly polymerize, forming a gel that decreases erythrocyte flexibility, resulting in microvascular occlusion, hemolysis, and chronic anemia. While it is clear that hemoglobin abnormalities play a major role, many other factors contribute to the pathogenesis of SCD-related complications. The contributions to the pathogenesis of SCD by biologic factors (**Table 119.2**) and environmental factors are diverse (**Table 119.3**).

BIOLOGIC PRECIPITANTS OF SICKLE CELL COMPLICATIONS

The complications of SCD are diverse and related to the interactions between abnormal hemoglobin and the circulatory system. Major contributors to the pathophysiology

TABLE 119.2

PRECIPITANTS OF COMPLICATIONS OF SICKLE CELL ANEMIA

■ INTRINSIC PATIENT FACTORS

Erythrocytes
Endothelial cells
Platelets
Leukocytes
   Lymphocytes
   Neutrophils
Coagulation cascade
Aberrations in NO metabolism
Oxidant-mediated injury
Systemic inflammation

TABLE 119.3

FACTORS THAT MAY PROMOTE SICKLING

1. Hemoglobin desaturation
  a. Failure to oxygenate in the lungs
    i. Atelectasis
    ii. Infection
      1. Bacterial
      2. Viral
    iii. Chronic lung disease
    iv. Pulmonary vascular disease
    v. High altitude
  b. Diminished tissue oxygen delivery
    i. Diminished cardiac output
      1. Hypovolemia (dehydration, sequestration, sepsis)
      2. Septic shock
      3. Diminished cardiac contractility
      4. Pericardial disease
      5. Increased systemic vascular resistance
      6. Anesthetics/drugs
    ii. Severe anemia
    iii. Hypoxemic cardiac output (see 1.a)
  c. Increased tissue extraction of oxygen
    i. Increased tissue demands
      1. Vigorous exercise
      2. Thyrotoxicosis
      3. Malignant hyperthermia
      4. Seizures
      5. Sepsis
      6. Shivering
    ii. Factors accelerating tissue oxygen extraction
      1. Acidosis
      2. Hyperthermia
2. Increased microvascular transit time
  a. Increased viscosity
    i. Excessive transfusion
    ii. Dehydration
  b. Vasoconstriction
    i. Hypothermia
    ii. Vasoconstrictor drugs
    iii. Tourniquet use (orthopedic surgery)

include (a) erythrocytes and hemoglobin, (b) endothelial cells, (c) leukocytes, (d) platelets, (e) the coagulation cascade, (f) NO, (g) oxidant-mediated injury, and (h) systemic inflammation. Contemporary paradigms (discussed in the section New

Concepts in Understanding SCD/Future Directions) ascribe the responsibility for many of the varied complications of SCD to hemolysis and viscosity (7,8).

Erythrocytes and Hemoglobin

The consequences of the substitution of valine for glutamine at position 6 of the β-globin chain are twofold: (a) oxygenated hemoglobin is significantly destabilized, resulting in accelerated denaturation and breakdown (9), and (b) the solubility of deoxygenated hemoglobin is dramatically reduced (10). Aggregation of HbS in this fashion causes large-scale polymerization, resulting in precipitation of deoxygenated HbS and formation of an erythrocyte-deforming gel. The result of these intracellular changes is damage to the erythrocyte cell membrane with loss of membrane flexibility and inability of the red blood cell to traverse capillary beds, resulting in ischemic injury.

In sickle erythrocytes, accelerated destruction of the globin chains results in accelerated oxidation of iron to the ferric state and increased generation of superoxide, hydrogen peroxide, and hydroxyl radical (11–13). These potent oxidant compounds, in combination with liberated iron inside the erythrocyte, cause denaturation and abnormal distribution of erythrocyte surface proteins, abnormal cation permeability, and disruption of normal phospholipid membrane structure. Transmembrane ion transport mechanisms are also disrupted, resulting in erythrocyte dehydration and increased corpuscular hemoglobin concentration, which accelerates hemoglobin polymerization and potentiates intracellular oxidant injury. Thus, a vicious cycle is initiated within the erythrocyte that leads to increased hemoglobin gelation, oxidative injury to the erythrocyte membrane, cellular deformation, and intracellular dehydration. Normal flow characteristics of the erythrocyte are disturbed, which results in stagnant microvascular blood flow, blood vessel obstruction, and distal tissue ischemia.

Endothelium

The endothelium is recognized to be an active participant in the pathogenesis of SCD by increased expression of cell surface adhesion molecules such as vascular cell adhesion molecule-1 (VCAM-1), intercellular adhesion molecule-1 (ICAM-1), E-selectin, and P-selectin. Soluble components of these adhesion molecules and activated endothelial cells are found in the plasma in SCD patients and potentiate the effects of vascular inflammation (14–16).

Activated endothelial cells promote thrombosis and vasculopathy through an increased affinity for interactions with abnormal erythrocytes (17), activated leukocytes (18), the hemostatic pathway, and activated platelets (19–22). The presence of an abnormality of von Willebrand factor (VWF) protease (ADAMTS-13) activity in SCD suggests overlap in the mechanism of thrombosis with thrombotic thrombocytopenic purpura (TTP) (23).

VCAM-1 expression is increased in the presence of systemic inflammation, and causes sickle reticulocytes to adhere to endothelial cells through interaction with, the sickle reticulocyte membrane integrin, very late activation antigen-4 (VLA-4) (24). The degree of affinity between erythrocytes and endothelium has been shown to correlate with clinical severity of illness in sickle cell patients (25). Finally, endothelin-1, an extremely potent vasoconstrictor, produced in activated endothelial cells in increased quantities in patients with SCD (26), has been implicated in the production of pulmonary hypertension in ACS (26,27).

Leukocytes

Leukocyte adherence to endothelial cells and subsequent release of destructive proteolytic enzymes are thought to propagate vascular injury in SCD. Monocytes from patients with SCD are potent inducers of endothelial activation and contain more IL-1β and tumor necrosis factor (TNF)-α than do monocytes from non-SCD patients. These monocyte changes in SCD patients are believed to be secondary to a chronic inflammatory state in patients with SCD. Monocytes from SCD patients have been shown to cause cytoplasmic-to-nuclear translocation of nuclear factor-κB in endothelial cells (a phenomenon seen during upregulation of the inflammatory response) (28). In addition, neutrophils from patients with SCA demonstrate increased endothelial cell adhesion when compared with neutrophils from healthy controls after incubation with proinflammatory cytokines (29).

Platelets

Platelet activation, which can be induced by activation of the coagulation pathway and repressed by circulating NO, is prominent in patients with SCD (19,20,30,31). SCD patients with severe hemolysis and pulmonary hypertension have increased platelet activation, and cell-free hemoglobin is able to activate platelets ex vivo (20). Hemolysis-associated defects in the availability of NO contribute to platelet activation in SCD, and sildenafil, a drug that amplifies NO signaling, decreases platelet activation in vivo in patients with SCD and pulmonary hypertension (20).

Platelets in patients with SCD are in a chronic state of heightened activity and have a shortened life span owing to rapid destruction and increased turnover (32). Platelets in these patients are less responsive in vitro when incubated with proaggregatory compounds because of chronic in vivo stimulation resulting in fatigue of platelet response (33). Finally, circulating platelet-derived factors such as thrombospondin facilitate erythrocyte adherence to endothelial cells (24,34).

Coagulation Cascade

Dysregulation of the VWF protease ADAMTS-13 has been reported in patients with SCD (35). Extracellular hemoglobin released during hemolysis is believed to inhibit its protease activity (23) and to generate high-molecular-weight multimers of VWF, which may contribute to vascular complications in TTP and SCD. There is enhanced thrombin generation, reduced protein C activity, reduced protein S activity, decreased factor V, elevated factor VIII, decreased plasminogen levels, shorter thrombin times, and higher serum fibrinogen degradation products in SCD patients, when compared with controls (36–38). The importance of intravascular thrombosis and endothelial injury to the pathogenesis of SCD is underscored by autopsy studies demonstrating diffuse arteriolar thrombosis and interstitial fibrotic lesions unrelated to large-vessel thrombotic or embolic disease.

Nitric Oxide Scavenging

NO is produced by endothelial cells, blood cells, neurons, and other cells. NO is responsible for coordinating vascular regulation. It inhibits platelet activation and related vascular smooth muscle constriction, as well as the release of procoagulant proteins, inflammatory mediators, cell membrane adhesion molecules, and proliferative factors. Free hemoglobin released from red blood cells reacts rapidly with NO to produce nitrate (39). This reaction causes a severe reduction in the bioavailability of NO with multiple deleterious vascular sequelae.

The consumption of NO by liberated hemoglobin is compounded by the simultaneous release of arginase from the erythrocyte into the plasma. Liberated arginase consumes arginine, the substrate for NO synthase (NOS), which normally catalyzes the conversion of arginine to NO and citrulline. The liberated arginase converts available arginine to ornithine and urea, which further decreases NO production and results in the production of injurious reactive oxygen species instead of NO by NOS. In adults with SCD, plasma arginase activity is high and is associated with pulmonary hypertension and early mortality (40).

Elevated levels of inhibitors of endogenous NOS have been detected in plasma from patients with SCD, particularly asymmetric dimethylarginine (ADMA) (41–43). ADMA is known to inhibit the activity of NOS and contribute to its uncoupling, and may serve as yet another factor to limit NO production in patients with SCD. Elevated ADMA levels are associated with severity of hemolysis and vasculopathy in patients with SCD (41,43,44).

NO is a poorly water-soluble gas produced in, among other places, vascular endothelial cells, where it can diffuse into vascular smooth muscle, causing relaxation and vasodilation. Disruption of NO regulation can result in exacerbation of SCD vaso-occlusion via several mechanisms: (a) diminished inhibitory effects of NO on VCAM expression, (b) diminished inhibitory effect of NO on leukocyte adhesion, (c) diminished inhibitory effect of NO on platelet activation, and (d) diminished NO-mediated vasodilation of tissue beds, promoting vasoconstriction, ischemia, and further erythrocyte sickling.

In children, levels of both arginine and NO metabolites (nitrite and nitrate, collectively referred to as NOx) decreased dramatically during progression of VOC (45). Patients who developed ACS presented to the hospital with significantly lower NOx levels than did VOC patients or SCD patients at steady state, and reached lower nadir levels of NOx during their hospitalization and convalescence (45).

Diminished levels of NO have also been described in the exhaled breath (FE$_{NO}$) of children and adults with SCD, and may be responsible for the promotion of ventilation–perfusion mismatch, regional hypoxemia, and intrapulmonary erythrocyte sickling. Children with SCD and history of ACS at steady state had significantly lower FE$_{NO}$ levels when compared with SCD patients without ACS history and healthy controls, despite similar arginine, citrulline, and NOx concentrations in the plasma (46). Adults with SCD and history of ACS had lower FE$_{NO}$ values than adult SCD patients without history of ACS, and the severity of dyspnea experienced correlated well with severity of FE$_{NO}$ reduction (47).

Oxidative Stress

Free hemoglobin scavenges NO and its heme and iron components have the potential to induce oxidative stress. In SCD, oxidative stress appears to be potentiated by enzymes that produce highly reactive oxygen species, including xanthine oxidase and NADPH oxidase (48,49). Consumption of NO by xanthine oxidase via superoxide-dependent pathways limits NO bioavailability and promotes oxidant injury at the endothelial level. Depletion of red cell glutathione, the major antioxidant defense of the erythrocyte, is linked to hemolytic rate and the development of pulmonary hypertension in SCD (50). Plasma from patients with VOC and ACS has been found to be oxidative in nature, depleting cellular glutathione and promoting the formation of injurious peroxynitrite from NO (51).

Perioperative and Physiologic Precipitants of Sickle Cell Disease

Hemoglobin deoxygenation is assumed to be a potent precipitant of vaso-occlusive phenomena in patients with SCD. There are both perioperative and nonoperative reports of SCD patients with hypoxemia who do not suffer SCD-related complications that confuse this assumption. Moreover, postoperative SCD-related complications continue to occur despite the avoidance of hypoxemia intraoperatively, and there is no definitive link between intraoperative hypoxemia and the development of postoperative complications related to SCD. Nevertheless, close monitoring of arterial oxygenation and administration of supplemental oxygen when necessary to keep arterial oxygen saturation in the normal range are recommended.

Patients with SCD are accustomed to moderately severe anemia and preserve oxygen delivery by increasing cardiac output and increasing erythrocyte 2,3-diphosphoglycerate concentrations. Transit time through the circulation is adversely affected by dehydration, systemic hypotension, occlusive tourniquet use, and physiologically or pharmacologically induced vasoconstriction. Preservation of arterial oxygenation, oxygen-carrying capacity, and cardiac output are essential to minimize excessive and prolonged hemoglobin desaturation within the capillary bed.

Dehydration has also been classically described as a precipitant of SCD-related complications. Despite this belief, SCD patients with neurosurgical and cardiac disease have been subjected to water deprivation, diuresis, and hypertonic contrast media administration without precipitation of SCD-related complications. The presence of intracellular erythrocyte dehydration appears to promote hemoglobin polymerization and gel formation, especially in the presence of the cellular, inflammatory, oxidant, and NO abnormalities already discussed. It is therefore prudent to tailor fluid management to provide generous intravascular hydration to preserve euvolemia.

Hypothermia restricts oxygen unloading, promotes cutaneous vasoconstriction, increases red cell tissue–lung transit time, and may promote erythrocyte sickling. Despite the fact that patients with SCD have safely undergone anesthetics and surgeries for cardiac and neurosurgical procedures that require deep hypothermic circulatory arrest, it is a basic tenet of anesthetic and critical care management to preserve normothermia in SCD patients. The benefits of mild therapeutic hypothermia for neurologic protection after ischemic brain injury must be weighed against the potential for hypothermia to promote SCD-related complications.

Hyperthermia also occurs in critical illness and may be due to many causes, including atelectasis, infection, and systemic inflammation. Hyperthermia shifts the hemoglobin–oxygen dissociation curve to the right, favoring the release of oxygen to the tissues and hemoglobin desaturation. Hyperthermia may be associated with vasoconstriction or vasodilation in core and peripheral compartments. As such, it could theoretically promote vaso-occlusive phenomena, though no definitive work has related the presence of pyrexia to the development of SCD-related complications.

Similarly, clinical evidence linking systemic acidosis to the development of SCD-related complications is lacking. The administration of sodium bicarbonate has not been shown to be effective in the prevention of perioperative pain crises in SCD patients. In the perioperative and critical care environments, it can be difficult to separate the effects of acidosis from the underlying causes of acidosis when attempting to establish causality between acid–base derangement and development of SCD complications. However, it is prudent to maintain acid–base status in a reasonable physiologic range when caring for critically ill patients with SCD.

SICKLE CELL DISEASE COMPLICATIONS

Patients with SCD suffer a lifetime of indolent, ischemic injury to all organ systems combined with periodic acute crises that cause considerable morbidity or premature mortality.

Vaso-occlusive Crisis

The most common crisis seen in pediatric patients with SCD is VOC, a condition that does not require PICU admission, but may precede the development of serious SCD complications. The most common type of VOC is bony crisis, affecting the long bones, ribs, and vertebrae. In children younger than 3 years, the distribution of VOC may be confined to the small bones of the hands and feet (hand–foot syndrome or dactylitis). Patients with VOC present with symptoms of pain from the bony cortex or marrow compartment of the bones of the extremities, chest, and back, and are associated with fever, leukocytosis, and malaise. The clinical presentation of bony VOC is fairly characteristic and usually very familiar to the patient and physician. The differential diagnosis of bony VOC, when accompanied by fever, focal bone tenderness, or overlying erythema and tenderness, includes local trauma and osteomyelitis, a condition common in SCD patients due to their susceptibility to bacteremia. Differentiation of the two conditions can be difficult, but can be aided by cultures of the blood and involved bone and by a combination of plain radiographs, MRI, and bone scan. The white blood cell count and differential are not helpful in making the distinction between infection and infarction. If osteomyelitis is suspected on clinical grounds, therapy should be initiated with antimicrobials effective against *Staphylococcus aureus* and *Salmonella* species while arrangements are made for bone biopsy, if necessary.

VOC involving the blood vessels supplying the abdominal viscera produces abdominal pain, fever, malaise, anorexia, and nausea. Patients will demonstrate diminished bowel sounds and nonspecific abdominal tenderness, making differentiation of VOC from a surgical cause of abdominal symptoms difficult. Children with SCD have an increased frequency of cholelithiasis and cholecystitis owing to chronic hemolysis. Exclusion of non-SCD abdominal pathology may rely on plain x-ray, CT of the abdomen, liver function tests (including total and fractionated bilirubin), amylase, lipase, and urinalysis. Serial examinations of the abdomen and surgical consultation are recommended if the diagnosis remains in question.

Treatment of VOC is largely supportive, with emphasis placed on the provision of adequate analgesia, supplemental oxygen, antibiotics to treat precipitating infections, and adequate hydration (1.5 times maintenance fluid requirements is customary). Simple transfusion is seldom used to treat acute VOC, but patients with frequent recurrence of VOC may be placed on chronic transfusion for a finite period of time to break the cycle of recurrent pain crisis. Successful pain management modalities include the use of acetaminophen, nonsteroidal anti-inflammatory medications, opioid medications (intermittent or patient-controlled administration), and regional anesthesia techniques (epidural analgesia and regional nerve blocks). Psychology and psychiatry services should also be considered to assist with identification and treatment of depression, and provision of effective pain-coping strategies.

Chapter 14 offers a detailed discussion of pain management in the critically ill child, but certain aspects of pain management during VOC deserve special emphasis. The NSAID ketorolac may be especially useful for acute treatment in the emergency department, but is contraindicated if hemorrhagic stroke is suspected. Expert titration of opioid therapy is essential. VOC may be a prelude to ACS because of rib pain and splinting or because of oversedation. Therefore, opioid administration should be titrated to achieve pain relief, allow deep breathing exercises, and promote ambulation. Patients who have required opioid therapy for prior VOC episodes are likely to require larger doses than those who are naïve to opioids.

Transfusion Therapy in Sickle Cell Disease Patients

The decision to employ transfusion therapy in the management of patients with SCD is made for two reasons: (a) to minimize vaso-occlusion by decreasing the percentage of HbS-containing erythrocytes in the circulation and (b) to improve hemoglobin concentration in order to restore reduced oxygen delivery. Transfusion therapy can be administered in the form of simple transfusion or exchange transfusion. *Simple transfusion* refers to the administration of sickle-free packed red blood cells, while *exchange transfusion* involves the administration of sickle-free packed red blood cells with simultaneous removal of the patient's whole blood. The type of transfusion is based on the desired effect(s) and desired speed of improvement of hemoglobin concentration and hemoglobin S fraction. During transfusions, the hemoglobin concentration and hematocrit should be monitored closely, as abrupt elevations in the hematocrit to >33% are associated with an increased blood viscosity and the potential for central nervous system (CNS) thrombotic injury.

Exchange transfusion therapy can be accomplished in infants after placement of an arterial catheter for blood withdrawal and suitable venous access for infusion of blood. Alternatively, a large-bore central venous catheter can be used for both withdrawal and infusion of blood during exchange transfusion. Exchange transfusion can be performed manually or, in larger children, by automated erythrocytapheresis. To quickly reduce HbS percentage to <30% in smaller infants and children, roughly twice the circulating blood volume is replaced with a solution of reconstituted sickle-free erythrocytes and fresh frozen plasma (or saline) over 4–6 hours while the hematocrit is closely monitored. If the hematocrit increases to >30%–33% at any time during the transfusion, a nonerythrocyte volume expander (i.e., fresh frozen plasma) is substituted for the packed red blood cells until the hematocrit falls to an acceptable level. With rapid transfusions and in the setting of hepatic dysfunction, ionized hypocalcemia may result from citrate toxicity and must be closely monitored and treated when necessary. A complete discussion of the factors and calculations required for planning and execution of a safe exchange transfusion has been reviewed elsewhere (52). Given the volume and rate of the transfusion, an approved and monitored blood warmer should be used for exchange transfusions.

The decision to employ exchange transfusion versus simple transfusion is determined by the clinical trajectory of the patient and the goals of the transfusion. For medical complications of SCD, such as VOC, ACS, and acute splenic sequestration crisis (ASSC), simple transfusion is usually offered, and exchange transfusion is reserved for patients with more aggressive disease and physiologic instability. For patients with an acute cerebrovascular accident (CVA), the goal is to restore cerebral circulation as quickly as possible to minimize irreversible CNS injury, and therefore, exchange transfusion is offered to rapidly optimize hemoglobin concentration while decreasing the hemoglobin S percentage. Additionally, simple or exchange transfusion (depending on degree of anemia, intravascular volume status, and clinical trajectory) has been advocated for the treatment of SCD patients with acute multiple organ system failure, although this indication is not uniformly accepted (53).

Transfusion therapy, while lifesaving in many sickle cell syndromes, is not without adverse events. Among these are febrile nonhemolytic transfusion reactions, which are usually self-limited and occur in response to leukocyte antigens in the blood. Filtering leukocytes from the blood before administering it to the patient can prevent these reactions. Patients requiring frequent transfusion can develop alloimmunization to red blood cell antigens that results in difficulty finding suitable crossmatched blood for administration and delayed hemolytic transfusion reactions. Strategies employed to minimize the development of alloimmunization include extended crossmatching of red blood cell units to minor antigen loci, and institution of a limited donor program to minimize exposure of patients to donors who are phenotypically similar (54–56). The transfusion of a SCD patient in the PICU should be a collaborative effort among intensivists, hematologists, and the blood bank. The team should request leukoreduced blood to include a specific crossmatch against the minor antigens C, E, and Kell in order to reduce the risk of alloimmunization. Ideally, the blood should be phenotypically matched;, that is, the donor and recipient should come from the same racial and ethnic groups to minimize the risk of alloimmunization from minor antigens that were not included in the crossmatch.

Less commonly, SCD patients develop autoantibodies to their, and transfused, red blood cells that cause posttransfusion hemolysis of both autologous and transfused blood cells by a mechanism that is not understood (57). Administration of corticosteroids with or without intravenous immunoglobulin is recommended in these scenarios. Finally, alloimmunization to human leukocyte antigens (HLAs) and platelet-specific antibodies has been described among SCD patients with moderate transfusion history, and this may limit the efficacy of platelet transfusion support in patients who subsequently undergo hematopoietic stem cell transplantation (HSCT). Leukocyte reduction of transfused blood products is recommended to prevent this complication (58).

Nonimmune complications of transfusion that may develop over time include iron overload that may be treated by parenteral or enteral chelation therapy with deferoxamine or deferasirox, respectively, and blood-borne infections from the blood supply which is much less common with improved donor-screening procedures (53).

Acute Chest Syndrome

ACS is a clinical syndrome characterized by fever, cough, pleuritic chest pain, tachypnea, hypoxemia, and a new or rapidly progressive pulmonary infiltrate(s) on chest radiograph. Patients with ACS demonstrate an abrupt decrease in platelet count and hematocrit. Risk factors for the development of ACS include younger age, higher steady-state hemoglobin level, lower fetal hemoglobin percentage, increased neutrophil count, history of asthma in children, active smoking, and environmental smoke exposure (59–66). ACS is usually self-limited, but some episodes progress rapidly to acute respiratory failure resembling acute respiratory distress syndrome (ARDS), resulting in substantial morbidity and mortality. ACS was a leading cause of premature death, accounting for 25% of sickle cell mortality (1,61,67,68); however, mortality from ACS has decreased since the introduction of hydroxyurea therapy and early liberal use of blood transfusion therapy (69). Mortality in the setting of ACS is associated with acute lung injury combined with pulmonary hypertension and right ventricular (RV) dysfunction (70).

The etiology of ACS is multifactorial, but commonly includes three basic mechanisms acting in concert: (a) pulmonary or systemic infection, (b) fat embolism, and (c) direct pulmonary infarction. ACS occurs in 10%–20% of hospitalized patients with SCD, usually 1–3 days after hospital admission for severe VOC (60,69). It may arise secondary to pulmonary infection, in the perioperative setting, or from unknown causes. Pulmonary infection secondary to community-acquired, atypical, or viral pathogens is a more common cause of ACS in young children than in adolescents or adults (60,67). The National ACS Study Group identified the presence of an infectious agent (mostly atypical bacteria or viruses) in 54% of ACS admissions (including respiratory syncytial virus, parvovirus, rhinovirus, parainfluenza virus, influenza A and B, and the H1N1 virus) (60) (**Fig. 119.1**). Encapsulated bacteria were rarely isolated despite functional asplenia, but *Staphylococcus aureus* was present in 5% of cases and *Streptococcus*

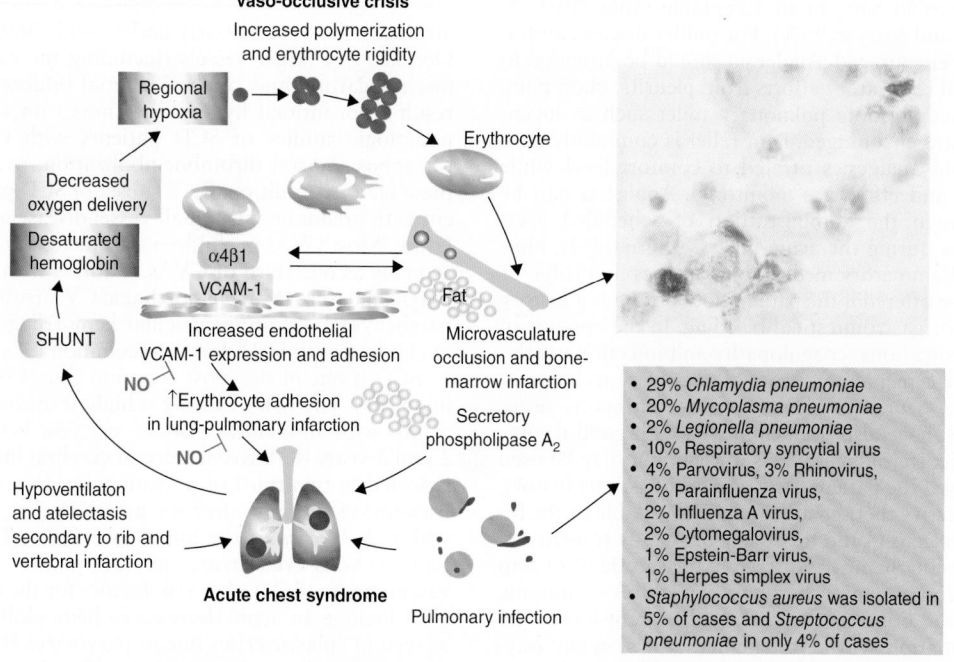

FIGURE 119.1. Vicious cycle of vaso-occlusive crisis and acute chest syndrome. (Reproduced with permission from the American Thoracic Society from page 1155 of [71] Miller AC, Gladwin MT: **Pulmonary complications of sickle cell disease.** American journal of respiratory and critical care medicine 2012, 185(11):1154–65 which was in turn reproduced from [5] Gladwin MT, Vichinsky E: **Pulmonary complications of sickle cell disease.** *The New England journal of medicine* 2008;359(21):2254–65.)

pneumoniae was present in 4% (60). Broad-spectrum antibiotic coverage should be instituted after consideration of local antibiotic resistance patterns if an infectious agent is suspected.

Fat embolization leads to ACS as a result of pulmonary vascular occlusion by marrow contents, lung injury, hypoxemia, inflammation, and pulmonary artery hypertension (71–73). Phospholipase A_2 activity in the circulation is increased and perpetuates systemic inflammation in ACS with fat emboli syndrome (72). This should be suspected in patients who deteriorate rapidly, demonstrate acute increases in pulmonary artery pressure (PAP), and develop liver dysfunction, CNS dysfunction, thrombocytopenia, or coagulopathy. The diagnosis is further suggested by the presence of oil red O–positive lipid accumulation in the sputum (60,73). Direct adhesion of sickled cells in the pulmonary vasculature has been proposed as the third mechanism for the development of ACS (74).

Management

The evaluation and management of patients with ACS emphasizes stratification of illness severity and tailoring interventions based on this assessment. Patients with ACS usually demonstrate a decrease in hemoglobin concentration and platelet count, an increase in lactate dehydrogenase concentration, suggesting increased intravascular hemolysis, and thrombosis. Cardiovascular evaluation with transthoracic echocardiography to assess tricuspid valve regurgitant jet velocity, RV function, left ventricular function, and estimated PAP is recommended to stratify severity of illness. Data from adult studies suggest that elevated Doppler echocardiogram estimates of pulmonary artery systolic pressure as manifest by tricuspid regurgitant jet velocity $\geq$ 2.5–3 m/s were indicators of poor prognosis and were often associated with pulmonary hypertension, RV failure, elevated B-type natriuretic peptide, and troponin I levels (70).

Treatment of patients with ACS begins with general supportive care. Hydration is instituted liberally and modified as clinically indicated on the basis of cardiovascular status, renal function, atrial filling pressures, and estimated RV pressure. Supplemental oxygen is administered with a goal of keeping PaO_2 and hemoglobin SaO_2 in an acceptable range ($PaO_2 \geq$ 80–100 mm Hg and $SaO_2 \geq$ 95%). For milder disease, ambulation should be encouraged. Analgesia should be provided to minimize reduced respiratory efforts from pleuritic chest pain, and exercises that promote pulmonary toilet such as incentive spirometry are encouraged. Pain relief is commonly provided with opioid analgesics titrated to comfort level while respiratory rate and effort are monitored. Analgesia can be augmented through the administration of scheduled acetaminophen doses during the acute illness. Alternatively, nonsteroidal anti-inflammatory medications, such as ibuprofen or ketorolac, may be offered if the patient does not have a history of renal disease or gastrointestinal bleeding. In the absence of specific contraindications (coagulopathy and infection overlying the needle placement site), regional anesthetic techniques, including central neuraxial blockade and continuous nerve block techniques, have also been employed with good results. The role of corticosteroids in ACS is unclear, but may be used to treat wheezing if the patient has a comorbid asthma history.

The most effective therapeutic modality available to the intensive care physician in the treatment of ACS is transfusion therapy. Transfusion therapy is offered in the setting of ACS to dilute the HbS-containing erythrocytes with HbA-containing erythrocytes in the hope that microvascular occlusion of the pulmonary circulation will be attenuated and systemic oxygen delivery increased. For mild-to-moderate ACS, many clinicians provide simple transfusion to increase the hemoglobin concentration to 10 g/dL. For more severe disease, or disease that is rapidly progressive, exchange transfusion is provided to rapidly decrease the percentage of HbS to <30%, with total hemoglobin and hematocrit of 10 g/dL and 30%, respectively.

ACS can progress in severity to severe acute lung injury or ARDS. Noninvasive mechanical ventilation in ACS patients improved gas exchange, but was associated with greater patient discomfort, and afforded no benefit for transfusion requirements, pain scores, narcotic use, resolution of hypoxemia by day 3, or speed of discharge from the step-down unit (75). Despite these findings, noninvasive forms of mechanical ventilation are commonly offered to SCD patients in the critical care setting.

Mechanical ventilation should be undertaken with strategies that minimize plateau pressure and tidal volume while optimizing positive end-expiratory pressure and lung compliance. Iatrogenic lung injury may be avoided while optimizing ventilation–perfusion matching through use of (a) the pressure-limited mode of ventilation, (b) airway pressure release modes of mechanical ventilation, and (c) high-frequency oscillatory ventilation (HFOV). The administration of inhaled NO to patients with severe ACS has resulted in favorable outcomes, presumably by improving pulmonary hypertension, RV function, severe ventilation–perfusion mismatch, and systemic oxygenation (76,77). There are no rigorous, randomized trials to support the efficacy of inhaled NO for the treatment of ACS (78). A recent randomized, controlled trial of the use of inhaled NO to treat VOC revealed no benefit with respect to duration or severity of pain, narcotic use, or subsequent development of ACS (69). Extracorporeal membrane oxygenation has been used to support pulmonary and cardiovascular function in patients who would have otherwise succumbed to ACS (79–81).

Empiric antibiotic therapy with a third-generation cephalosporin and a macrolide antibiotic, with or without vancomycin, represents a reasonable initial antibiotic treatment regimen to cover organisms that cause atypical pneumonia, community-acquired pneumonia, and resistant staphylococcal and streptococcal infections. Appropriate serologic, nuclear amplification, and culture material is collected, and the spectrum of antibiotic coverage can be appropriately narrowed when microbiology results become available.

Stroke

Stroke, or CVA, is a poorly understood complication of SCD. Occlusion of larger vessels (including the carotid artery and internal carotid and cerebral arterial bifurcation points) may result from intimal hyperplasia (noted on angiographic and pathologic studies of SCD patients with CVA), secondary thrombosis, distal thromboembolization, or combinations of these factors. Additionally, a subset of SCD patients may present with predominantly small-vessel disease in the CNS vasculature. Most CVAs in children are due to ischemic infarcts, but as many as one-third of CVAs in adults with SCD are hemorrhagic in nature (82). Hemorrhagic CVA (subarachnoid, intraparenchymal, or intraventricular hemorrhage) may also occur in children with SCD, but is uncommon (3%) (83).

SCD is one of the most common causes of stroke in childhood (84). The risk of stroke is highest during the first decade of life, with an incidence of 1% per year between the ages of 2 and 5 years (83). Recurrence of cerebral infarction has been reported in two-third of patients who do not receive chronic transfusion therapy after an initial stroke. Most take place within 2–3 years of the initial event (85). The risk of recurrent stroke is even greater in SCD patients with moyamoya vasculopathy (86). Other risk factors for the development of a CVA include an acute decrease in hemoglobin concentration, as seen in aplastic crises due to parvovirus B19. Other predictors of clinically evident cerebral infarctions in SCD include a *history of transient ischemic attack, ACS within the two previous weeks, more than two ACS events per year, the degree of anemia,* and *systolic hypertension* (83).

Silent cerebral infarction (ischemic MRI changes in the absence of clinical evidence of stroke) is the most common form of CNS injury seen in patients with SCD. It is increasingly recognized as a source of cognitive deficits, diminished intelligence quotient, poor school performance, and is a risk factor for progressive CNS injury, including subsequent CVA. Silent cerebral infarction is prevalent in the SCD population, occurring in 15%–25% of children younger than 14 years (87,88). The presence of silent cerebral infarction in children with SCD is of great clinical relevance, as it is a potent predictor of probability of subsequent neurologic injury. However, these children are unlikely to present to the ICU. Risk factors for silent cerebral infarction include elevated white blood cell count, anemia, severe vasculopathy, and the Senegal β-globin haplotype (89,90).

There is a lack of correlation between transcranial Doppler (TCD) abnormalities and the development of silent brain infarction, reflecting the fact that TCD abnormalities reveal large-vessel disease, whereas the mechanism of silent brain infarction more commonly involves smaller penetrating arteries (91–93). Analysis of the Stroke Prevention (STOP) trial revealed that transfusion therapy lowers the risk for new silent brain infarcts in children, while discontinuation of chronic transfusion therapy increases the risk (93,94). In contrast, another recent study indicated that SCD children with preexisting CVA who had been receiving regular blood transfusions continued to experience a high rate of silent brain infarcts (95). The Silent Cerebral Infarct Transfusion trial will answer this question as it is evaluating whether blood transfusion therapy will reduce further neurologic morbidity in children with silent brain infarcts, but normal TCD velocities (96).

The natural history of patients with SCD and silent cerebral infarction, overt CVA, or elevated TCD without CVA is one of recurrent CNS ischemic injury. Chronic transfusion therapy is effective at correcting elevated TCD flow rates and preventing recurrent stroke, but the necessary duration of therapy is unclear, as cessation of transfusion is associated with recurrence of TCD abnormalities and CVA (97).

Chronic transfusion therapy, while effective in preventing progressive neurologic injury, represents a considerable physiologic (systemic iron overload and alloimmunization) and financial burden to SCD patients and the healthcare system. Chelation therapy with parenteral deferoxamine or enteral deferasirox is effective in preventing iron overload in compliant patients. HSCT represents an alternative to chronic transfusion but is associated with obvious morbidity and the need for a suitable marrow donor (98). Finally, institution of hydroxyurea therapy has been compared to chronic transfusion therapy as a potential therapy to prevent progression of CNS injury while avoiding visceral iron overload. Hydroxyurea did not offer a benefit with respect to iron overload and had an increased (but noninferior) rate of recurrent stroke (10% vs. 0% in the transfusion group) (99). A summary of preventive therapies available for patients with overt stroke, silent infarct on MRI, and abnormal TCD studies as well as the evidence available to support their application are presented in **Figure 119.2**.

The diagnosis of CVA is made on the basis of the usual clinical signs and symptoms of CVA. In the presence of acute contralateral hemiplegia and aphasia (left-sided CVA), the diagnosis is clear. However, in many cases, the presentation may not be straightforward, and stroke may present simply as altered or depressed mental status. In these cases, in addition to stroke, the differential diagnosis includes CNS infections and toxic ingestion. Focal seizures may be the presenting symptom of focal cerebral ischemia and may progress to a generalized tonic–clonic convulsion. In patients with SCD, the new onset of seizure activity should be considered to be indicative of cerebral ischemic injury until proven otherwise. Seizure control should be implemented as described for status epilepticus (see Chapter 63), with particular care taken to ensure arterial oxygenation. In patients with ambiguous clinical presentations, once imaging studies have excluded the presence of intracranial hypertension and neurosurgical catastrophes, lumbar puncture should be performed, antibiotic therapy implemented, and toxicologic studies performed.

SCD patients who present with signs or symptoms of CVA or other intracranial pathology should undergo emergent CT scan or MRI of the brain to define any CNS abnormalities and to exclude the presence of lesions amenable to neurosurgical intervention (parenchymal, epidural, or subdural hematoma). Advantages of MRI over CT scan in acute CVA include the ability to clearly define the CNS vasculature using MR angiography and increased sensitivity of MRI for early detection of ischemic parenchymal changes. However, the increased diagnostic potential of MRI must be weighed against the need for sedation to facilitate longer MRI studies in uncooperative or unstable children.

The most urgent therapeutic intervention for the SCD patient who presents with CVA is an immediate exchange

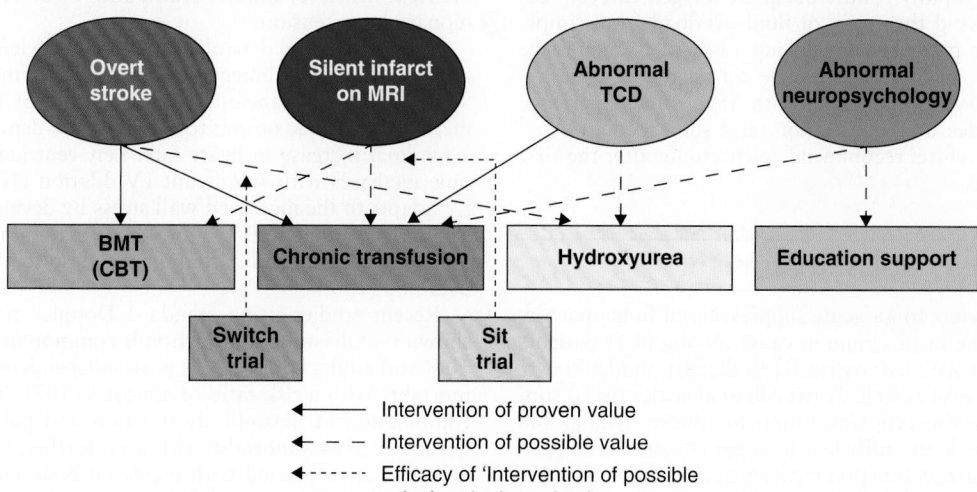

FIGURE 119.2. Approach to neurologic complications of sickle cell disease. (Reproduced with permission from page 621 from Musallam KM, Khoury RA, Abboud MR: Cerebral infarction in children with sickle cell disease: a concise overview. *Hemoglobin* 2011;35(5–6):618–4. This was reference 102 in the electronic Word Manuscript originally submitted but I do not see the reference listed in the proof at all. This was in turn adapted from Wang WC: The pathophysiology, prevention, and treatment of stroke in sickle cell disease. *Current opinion in hematology* 2007;14(3):191–7.)

transfusion to reverse, or prevent progression of, ischemic CNS injury. Exchange transfusion is provided to decrease the HbS percentage to <30% while the hemoglobin concentration is maintained at ~10 g/dL. Therapy for children with SCD and CVA is otherwise supportive, with careful attention to protection of the airway, suppression of seizure activity, and preservation of respiratory and hemodynamic function. In the setting of a large cerebral infarction, the patient is monitored for the development of intracranial hypertension, and neurosurgical consultation is obtained when clinically indicated.

There is limited evidence for the efficacy and safety of "tight" glucose control and therapeutic hypothermia in patients with CVA and SCD. Indeed the application of therapeutic hypothermia in patients with sickle hemoglobinopathies would result in peripheral vasoconstriction, which promotes erythrocyte sickling and vaso-occlusion. The protective effects of aggressive exchange transfusion therapy in the setting of therapeutic hypothermia (33°C for 24 hours) in an adult SCD patient after cardiac arrest have been reported (100).

Acute Splenic Sequestration Crisis

ASSC refers to a sudden drop in hemoglobin concentration associated with development of splenomegaly, reticulocytosis, intravascular volume depletion, and shock. The spleen may become massively enlarged and is often tender. ASSC is a disease of toddlers and infants and is not seen in older children, presumably owing to autosplenectomy. Patients with other SCD genotypes, such as HbSC disease and HbS–β thalassemia, may undergo autosplenectomy later in childhood and consequently may experience ASSC later in childhood. Children with ASSC are anemic, pale, and may demonstrate signs of inadequate systemic oxygen delivery. In severe cases, shock is present and patients may present in extremis.

Therapy for ASSC involves restoration of circulating blood volume with crystalloid solutions and sickle-free packed red blood cells. The patient's hemoglobin level should be monitored closely during packed red cell transfusion because sequestered blood may reenter the circulation (autotransfusion) resulting in hyperviscosity and the potential for stroke. In severe heart failure or shock, rapid exchange transfusion may be necessary to rapidly restore adequate oxygen-carrying capacity and to avoid the strain of fluid overload from simple transfusion. For patients who do not respond to aggressive medical therapy, splenectomy may be considered as a lifesaving surgical intervention. Patients with ASSC often experience recurrent episodes of sequestration, and some pediatric hematologists, therefore, recommend splenectomy after the first episode of ASSC.

Aplastic Crisis

Aplastic crisis refers to an acute suppression of bone marrow function, and the most common cause among SCD patients is viral infection (i.e., parvovirus B19). Platelet and leukocyte counts may decrease as well. Treatment of aplastic crisis is supportive, with erythrocyte transfusion to restore hemoglobin concentration to levels sufficient to support systemic oxygen delivery until marrow function recovers and reticulocytosis resumes. The specific hemoglobin level to target for ASSC and aplastic crisis depends on the balance between oxygen supply and demand and can be monitored with serial measurements of lactic acid concentration, oxygen saturation in the superior vena cava or pulmonary artery, and arteriovenous oxygen content gradient. In general, however, these patients are accustomed to a moderately severe chronic anemia, and restoration of a hemoglobin level to 7–9 g/dL is usually adequate.

Sepsis

Because of impaired splenic function and decreased opsonic activity, children with SCD are at increased risk for serious bacterial infections with a variety of bacterial pathogens, especially encapsulated organisms, such as *S. pneumoniae* and *Neisseria meningitidis*. Early identification of at-risk patients through newborn sickle cell screening programs, use of penicillin prophylaxis, vaccinations against *S. pneumoniae*, *Haemophilus influenza*, and *N. meningitides* (mnemonic SHiN vaccines for asplenic patients), and aggressive antibiotic therapy in febrile SCD patients have had a beneficial effect on sepsis-related mortality in SCD patients (101).

Therapy for patients with SCD and sepsis includes the early administration of broad-spectrum antibiotics. Ceftriaxone is often used as the initial antibiotic for the febrile SCD patient with suspected sepsis. However, repeat doses of ceftriaxone have been associated with fatal immune-mediated hemolytic anemia in SCD. Therefore, consideration should be given to switching to a different antibiotic if the patient requires a full course of IV antibiotic therapy. In patients with infection, hypotension, and organ dysfunction, supportive therapies, including early goal-directed therapy, mechanical ventilation, vasopressor support, steroid therapy (when appropriate), and other sepsis-specific therapies outlined elsewhere in this text, are implemented as indicated.

CHRONIC INJURY OF THE CARDIOVASCULAR SYSTEM

By the time older children and adolescents present with critical complications of SCD, incremental, subclinical damage to major organ systems has already occurred. When older children need critical care services for acute complications of SCD, they may do so with significant preexisting dysfunction of the respiratory, cardiovascular, and renal systems. Additionally, the development of progressive vital organ dysfunction may inflict substantial morbidity and mortality on patients with SCD. Chronic complications of cardiovascular disease in SCD patients may be divided into (a) systolic and diastolic dysfunction of the left heart, (b) systolic and diastolic dysfunction of the right heart, (c) sudden death, and (d) development of pulmonary hypertension.

The systolic and diastolic function of the left ventricle (LV) and the chamber dimensions are affected in patients with SCD. The chronic anemia associated with SCD results in an increase in cardiac output to meet oxygen demands with only a minimal increase in heart rate. Left ventricular stroke volume increases with significant LV dilation (102).The dilated LV adapts to the increased wall stress by developing eccentric hypertrophy which allows the LV to maintain normal filling pressures and diastolic compliance despite chronic volume overload (103).

Recent studies using standard Doppler parameters have shown that diastolic dysfunction is common in children (104–106) and adults with SCD. It is an independent risk factor for mortality with a risk ratio of almost 5 (107). Importantly, the combination of diastolic dysfunction and pulmonary hypertension increases mortality risk even further. Diastolic abnormalities are associated with increased body mass, age, serum creatinine, and increased LV mass. Screening echocardiography studies show a significant variation in the prevalence of diastolic dysfunction due to difficulty in the noninvasive diagnosis of diastolic dysfunction. However, right heart catheterization in patients with pulmonary hypertension (mean PAP [mPAP] > 25 mm Hg) shows that ~50% have evidence of diastolic dysfunction (108,109). Systolic LV dysfunction in SCD patients is rare (110,111) and is usually only found in older patients and those with comorbid conditions, including hypertension and renal disease (112).

The right heart is also subject to abnormalities of systolic and diastolic function in SCD patients. Imaging studies of SCD patients at steady state without pulmonary hypertension have shown in most cases dilated right heart chambers without significant RV dysfunction (110,113). Clinicians should remain vigilant for the development of acute RV dysfunction in the setting of acute increases in RV afterload such as ACS. In a series of 84 consecutive hospital admissions, RV dysfunction was present in only 13% of patients. However, all of these patients had a tricuspid regurgitant velocity > 3 m/s during the acute event, and they were particularly at risk for multi-organ failure and sudden death (70). Acute pressure overload superimposed on chronic pulmonary vasculopathy is felt to result in RV decompensation in critically ill SCD patients with acute pulmonary pathology.

Sudden death is an increasingly recognized and reported mechanism of death in the aging SCD population (114–117). This complication, formerly often attributed to narcotic overdose, is clearly associated with underlying cardiac disease, pulmonary disease, or pulmonary vascular disease. In a large study of autopsies in SCD patients, death was sudden and unexpected in 40% of patients and was usually associated with an acute event (117). More recent autopsy studies have shown that cardiopulmonary causes account for the majority of deaths, with sudden death/pulseless electrical activity (PEA), heart failure, myocardial infarction, pulmonary embolism, and pulmonary hypertension being the most common findings at the time of death (118,119).

The final cardiovascular complication of SCD is pulmonary hypertension. The potential for pulmonary hypertension should be considered in all SCD patients with acute lung pathology, as well as older SCD patients at steady state. Hemolytic anemia has been proposed as an important mechanism leading to pulmonary vasculopathy. In addition to deranged arginine/NO metabolism, other risk factors for the development of pulmonary hypertension include surgical splenectomy, functional asplenia, thromboembolism, lung fibrosis, hypoxemia, increase in vasoactive mediators (i.e., endothelin-1), renal insufficiency, and genetic factors (120–124) (**Fig. 119.3**). Screening of SCD patients in steady state and during critically illness is essential to optimizing outcomes for these patients, as the presence of pulmonary hypertension is the single most potent predictor of premature mortality in SCD.

Noninvasive assessment of PAP relies on echocardiographic assessment of tricuspid regurgitation velocity (TRV), which provides a calculated estimate of RV systolic pressure and pulmonary artery systolic pressure (125). The gold standard for the diagnosis of pulmonary hypertension remains right heart catheterization. Multiple studies support the notion that not all SCD patients with increased TRV will have pulmonary hypertension as defined by the consensus definition of the presence of mPAP > 25 mm Hg (126). Studies have revealed that an elevated TRV of 2.5 m/s is present in 30% and 3 m/s in 10% of patients (120,124,127,128). A mild-to-moderate elevation in Doppler-estimated RV systolic pressure is common in adults and associated with a greatly increased risk ratio for early death (120,124,127). The development of pulmonary hypertension in SCD patients may be due to left heart

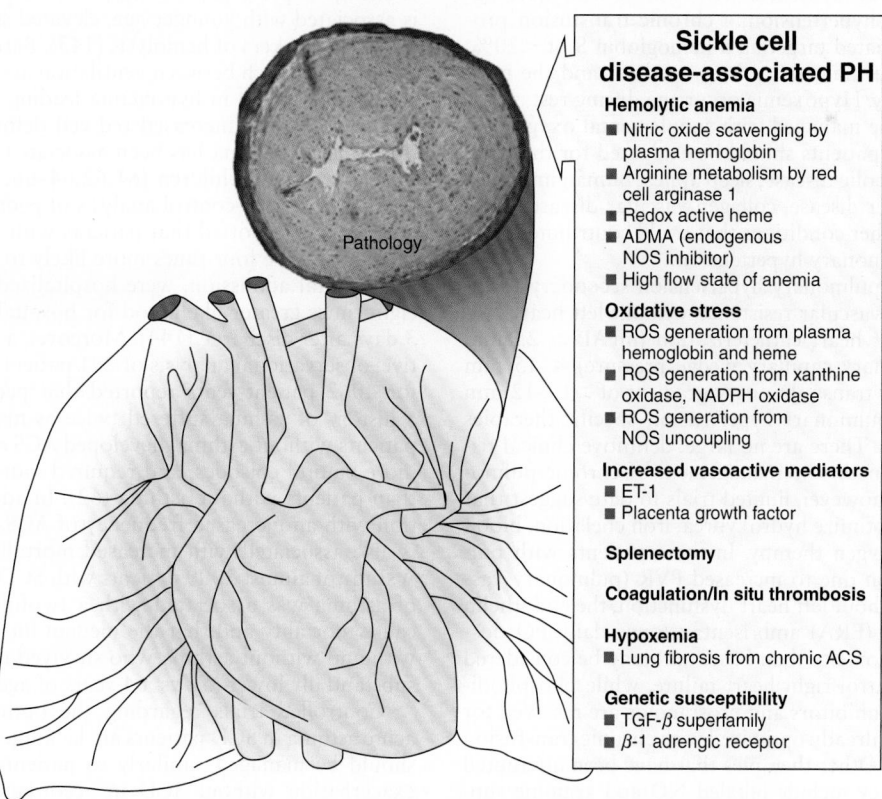

Sickle cell disease-associated PH

Hemolytic anemia
- Nitric oxide scavenging by plasma hemoglobin
- Arginine metabolism by red cell arginase 1
- Redox active heme
- ADMA (endogenous NOS inhibitor)
- High flow state of anemia

Oxidative stress
- ROS generation from plasma hemoglobin and heme
- ROS generation from xanthine oxidase, NADPH oxidase
- ROS generation from NOS uncoupling

Increased vasoactive mediators
- ET-1
- Placenta growth factor

Splenectomy

Coagulation/In situ thrombosis

Hypoxemia
- Lung fibrosis from chronic ACS

Genetic susceptibility
- TGF-β superfamily
- β-1 adrengic receptor

Pathology

FIGURE 119.3. Mechanisms of pulmonary hypertension in SCD Patients. (From Rudski LG, Lai WW, Afilalo J, et al. Guidelines for the echocardiographic assessment of the right heart in adults: A report from the American Society of Echocardiography endorsed by the European Association of Echocardiography, a registered branch of the European Society of Cardiology, and the Canadian Society of Echocardiography. *J Am Soc Echocardiogr* 2010;23(7):685–713; quiz 786–8.) This is Figure 2 on page 1125 from [125]. Gladwin MT, Sachdev V: Cardiovascular abnormalities in sickle cell disease. *Journal of the American College of Cardiology* 2012;59(13):1123–33.

dysfunction or intrinsic elevation of pulmonary vascular resistance with normal left-sided function. Approximately 50% of the SCD patients who suffer from pulmonary hypertension have pulmonary venous hypertension and 50% have pulmonary arterial hypertension as indicated by pulmonary arterial occlusion pressure > or < 15 mm Hg, respectively. The etiology of pulmonary hypertension in SCD is likely to be multifactorial. Several studies support the following conclusions regarding the pathophysiology of pulmonary hypertension in SCD: (a) risk factors include renal insufficiency, biochemical indices of hemolysis, and biochemical markers of cholestatic liver dysfunction; (b) pulmonary hypertension in SCD arises as a result of chronic hemolytic anemia and is associated with concomitant end-organ dysfunction of the kidney and liver, but is not a direct consequence of repeated episodes of vasoocclusion and ACS (5,120,122,129).

Pulmonary hypertension should be considered in any critically ill patient with lung disease, shock, acidosis and other stressors of cardiovascular reserve. PAPs will rise in the setting of ACS, VOC, and other forms of critical injury that precipitate decompensation of the right heart. Critical care support in the setting of right heart decompensation includes maintenance of functional residual capacity, the administration of supplemental oxygen, maintenance of adequate ventilation, treatment of metabolic acidosis, monitoring right and/or left atrial pressures, fluid management, inotropic support, and the administration of pulmonary artery vasodilators.

Chronic treatment of pulmonary hypertension should begin with the initiation of hydroxyurea that is titrated to maximize fetal hemoglobin levels with minimal side effects (130,131). For subjects not responding to or unable to tolerate the side effects of hydroxyurea, as well as those with more significant pulmonary hypertension, a chronic transfusion program should be initiated targeting a hemoglobin S of <20%. Patients should be evaluated for iron overload and the need for chelation therapy. Hypoxemia occurring during rest, sleep, or exercise should be managed with supplemental oxygen. As clinically indicated, patients should be evaluated for the presence of thromboembolic disease, sleep apnea, human immunodeficiency virus, liver disease, collagen vascular disease, renal insufficiency, and other conditions that could contribute to the development of pulmonary hypertension.

In patients with pulmonary hypertension secondary to increased pulmonary vascular resistance without left heart failure defined by right heart catheterization (mPAP > 25 mm Hg, PCWP (pulmonary capillary wedge pressure) < 15 mm Hg, and an elevated transpulmonary gradient of >10–12 mm Hg), therapy with pulmonary hypertension–specific therapies could be considered. There are no large, definitive clinical trials to guide clinicians in the management of chronic pulmonary hypertension; however, limited trials to date suggest that it is reasonable to optimize hydroxyurea, iron chelation, blood transfusion, and oxygen therapy. In these patients with pulmonary hypertension due to increased PVR (pulmonary vascular resistance) without left heart dysfunction, the endothelin receptor antagonist (ERA) ambrisentan (once daily PO dosing and less hepatotoxicity than bosentan) may be considered with diuresis to control right heart failure, while phosphodiesterase-5 (PDE-5) inhibitors and prostanoids are reserved for more severe disease already optimized with chronic transfusion therapy (132–135). Other therapies that have been attempted with minimal efficacy include inhaled NO and arginine supplementation. To date, there is insufficient outcome data to guide clinicians in pharmacologic management of pulmonary hypertension in patients with SCD.

PDE-5 inhibition therapy held promise because these agents seem to be effective in both pulmonary arterial and pulmonary venous hypertension related to diastolic dysfunction (136–138). A small open-label study of sildenafil (a PDE-5 inhibitor) use in patients with SCD who were taking maximal

hydroxyurea therapy or transfusions revealed significant improvement in patients with respect to TRV, NT-proBNP levels, and functional exercise status (138). Unfortunately, a large multicenter study of SCD patients using sildenafil to manage pulmonary hypertension was stopped because of an increased frequency of hospital admission secondary to myalgia and back pain (128).

Chronic Injury of the Respiratory System

Chronic lung injury and/or airway hyperreactivity may develop in the SCD patients. The advanced chronic lung injury found in patients with SCD is called sickle cell chronic lung disease (SCCLD) (139). Severe interstitial disease associated with SCCLD is a rare complication but mild spirometric abnormalities are seen frequently in SCD patients. In the pre–hydroxyurea treatment era, 90% of the SCD population demonstrated spirometric abnormalities, which included (a) mild restrictive pulmonary function defect, (b) isolated reduction in the DLCO, (c) low normal FEV_1 and FVC with a normal FEV_1/FVC ratio. Obstructive disease, either alone or mixed with restrictive disease, was uncommon in adult patients. Similar findings of mild restrictive abnormalities have been observed in recent cohort studies of adult patients (108).

Asthma affects ~12% of all children in the United States (140), 15%–20% of African American children, and 9% of African American adults (62,140,141). The prevalence of asthma among pediatric patients with SCD appears to be similar to that in children of African descent in the normal population (108,142). Airway hyperresponsiveness to methacholine challenge is prevalent among pediatric patients with SCD. It is associated with younger age, elevated serum IgE concentration, and markers of hemolysis (143). Based on asthma pathogenesis, mismatch between ventilation and perfusion would be expected to result in hypoxemia leading to pulmonary capillary hypoxia and increased red cell deformation. Supporting this concept, asthma has been associated with increased rates of ACS events in children (61,62,64–66,141,144–146) and a retrospective case-control analysis of pediatric patients admitted for VOC reported that patients with a previous diagnosis of asthma were four times more likely to develop ACS during the hospital admission, were hospitalized longer, and had an eight times greater likelihood for hospital readmission within 3 days after discharge (144). Moreover, a subsequent prospective, observational analysis of 291 patients with SCD followed for 4062 patient-years reported that pediatric patients with a history of asthma suffered twice as many ACS episodes as patients without asthma, developed ACS at a younger age, had more painful episodes, and required more blood transfusions than patients without asthma (62). In addition to its association with an increased frequency of ACS, a history of asthma is also associated with increased mortality in SCD (62,141). A study of almost 2000 patients with SCD found that a history of asthma was associated with a twofold higher risk of all-cause mortality and that the median life span for individuals with and without asthma who survived to 5 years of age was substantially lower (52 vs. 64 years of age, respectively) (141).

Controlled trials regarding the optimal management of acute asthma in SCD patients are lacking. Patients with asthma should be managed similarly to patients with acute asthma exacerbation without SCD in accordance with NIH guidelines (140,147). Emergency department and ICU management should include oxygen administration, inhaled β_2-agonist therapy, systemic corticosteroids, and intravenous magnesium sulfate. Management of asthma in SCD patients follows the same pathway as described elsewhere in this textbook (Chapter 46) with the following caveats. Given the potential for severe VOC and ACS in the setting of asthma exacerbation, the threshold for hospital admission should be low. The observation period for rebound pain from VOC after systemic corticosteroid taper must be kept in mind. The importance of provision of and compliance with controller medications must be stressed to avoid the morbidity and mortality associated with asthma in this high-risk patient population.

Chronic Injury to the Kidney

Like the deterioration in splenic function that occurs over time, the kidney is affected by repeated ischemic insults, resulting in significant functional impairment. While rare in children, older patients may suffer impairment of renal function, requiring dialysis or renal transplantation. Patients with SCD or SCT demonstrate isosthenuria, a progressive impairment in the ability to concentrate urine and preserve free water, making the SCD patient more susceptible to dehydration. The potential presence of renal dysfunction in SCD patients must be considered when managing fluids, acid–base balance, electrolytes, and medications excreted by the kidney.

PERIOPERATIVE MANAGEMENT OF SCD PATIENTS

Perioperative care must consider both the inherent risk of the proposed surgery, the patient and the patient's clinical course of SCD. In most of the United States, the presence of the SCD phenotype will have been previously identified as a result of newborn screening hemoglobin electrophoresis, although some infants may elude neonatal detection with potentially catastrophic results. If a parent or caretaker is unaware of SCD screening results, then screening should be done.

Patients may be screened for the presence of a sickle cell hemoglobinopathy with a "sickle prep" examination, in which HbS production is provoked in vitro. Patients with a positive screening solubility test require hemoglobin electrophoresis to precisely delineate the specific sickle cell hemoglobinopathy present. In the presence of high concentrations of HbF, solubility testing lacks the sensitivity required to detect HbS and cannot be relied on for screening in children <6 months of age. Hemoglobin electrophoresis is required in this age group (and used in newborn screening) to exclude the presence of a sickle hemoglobinopathy.

Once the diagnosis of an SCD phenotype is made, it is appropriate to obtain pediatric hematology consultation for longitudinal follow-up. Preoperative preparation includes attention to preoperative hydration, optimization of vital organ function, and consideration of the administration of preoperative packed red blood cell transfusions. Patients with SCD should be well hydrated throughout the perioperative course. Although it was previously customary to hydrate the patient on the night prior to surgery with intravenous fluids administered at a rate of up to 1.5 times maintenance, many procedures are currently performed as outpatients, with SCD patients scheduled early in the day and with attention to current *nil per os* guidelines to limit dehydration. Treatment should be focused on correcting or preventing dehydration. Overhydration does not correct the intracellular dehydration present in sickled cells. The patient should also be screened and treated for infection before allowing elective surgery to proceed. Major organ systems should be evaluated for dysfunction that may adversely impact the intraoperative and postoperative course. Finally, a thorough preoperative evaluation and discussion with the parents are required to delineate risks, explain the anesthetic plan, and provide for postoperative analgesia and prevention of postoperative SCD complications.

Perioperative transfusion therapy is a common, sometimes controversial topic of discussion among surgeons, anesthesiologists, hematologists, and intensivists. The usual reasons for provision of transfusion therapy are correction of anemia, improvement of oxygen-carrying capacity, and dilution of the HbS-containing erythrocytes with HbA-containing erythrocytes to minimize hemoglobin gel formation. Prophylactic transfusion therapy of this nature is effective in reducing perioperative SCD complications. In a report on 54 pediatric patients who underwent 66 surgical procedures without the benefit of preoperative transfusion, most did not receive packed red blood cell transfusion at any time during the perioperative course (148). Postoperative complications were observed in 26% of the cases and were usually minor and self-limited. Complications were most common after thoracotomy, laparotomy, and tonsillectomy and adenoidectomy. In a retrospective study of 1079 procedures in adults and children, perioperative blood transfusion conferred a protective effect against SCD complications in low-risk procedures in HbSS patients, and low- and moderate-risk procedures in patients with HbSC (149). In neither retrospective study was an attempt made to stratify enrolled patients according to overall disease severity, recent disease activity, or changing anesthetic and surgical techniques. As such, the results of these studies must be extrapolated to the clinical setting with caution. Of note is the reported mortality rate of 1:100 for all patients within 30 days of surgery, emphasizing the increased perioperative risk incurred by SCD patients, when compared with the general population (1:300,000 in adults, 1:80,000 in children) (150).

A prospective, randomized trial in 1995 examined the effects of conservative and aggressive transfusion strategies on perioperative outcome in SCD patients (151). In the aggressive transfusion arm, patients were transfused to a target HbS of 30% by either serial transfusion or exchange transfusion, while the patients in the conservative transfusion arm were transfused to a hemoglobin concentration of 10 g/dL. This study demonstrated similar rates of perioperative SCD complications in both arms with an increased frequency of transfusion-related complications in the aggressive transfusion arm. The authors concluded that a conservative transfusion strategy, using simple transfusion, was as effective as aggressive transfusion in the prevention of SCD perioperataive complications and resulted in fewer transfusion-related complications.

In 1997, a subset of the database of the Preoperative Transfusion in Sickle Cell Disease Study Group was examined for the outcomes of 364 SCD patients who underwent cholecystectomy (152). In this study, the equivalence of aggressive and conservative transfusion strategies with respect to prevention of postoperative SCD complications was confirmed. A group of patients that was not randomized and did not receive preoperative transfusion was followed in this study (most demonstrated healthier American Society of Anesthesiologist class scores). This nonrandomized, nontransfusion group demonstrated a 32% frequency of sickle cell–related complications, including an ACS incidence double that of the next highest transfused group in the report. A 1% perioperative mortality rate was again noted in the patients who underwent cholecystectomy, emphasizing elevated perioperative risk inherent in this patient population. To date, there remain no high-quality data to guide clinicians with respect to the performance of elective surgery without preoperative transfusion.

In aggregate, the literature to date would support the presence of a protective effect on postoperative SCD complications through the application of a conservative transfusion strategy to most SCD patients undergoing most surgical procedures. The Transfusion Alternatives Preoperatively in Sickle Cell Disease (TAPS trial: http://www.ClinicalTrials.gov, identifier NCT00512577) based in Great Britain is currently being undertaken to compare outcomes with and without transfusion.

For patients with high-risk SCD and those undergoing procedures with high potential for CNS injury and ACS (i.e., cardiac surgery with cardiopulmonary bypass, deep hypothermia with circulatory arrest, and neurosurgical procedures), consultation with their hematologists is recommended, and consideration should be given to more aggressive transfusion preparation of the patient. Until such time as these comparisons are made in large, well-controlled, prospective, randomized trials, a prudent approach to preoperative preparation is recommended, with consideration of the patient, comorbidities, SCD severity, contemplated operative procedure, and the opinions of the anesthesiologist, surgeon, and hematologist caring for the patient.

Operative management of the SCD patient involves careful attention to the precipitants of SCD complications and mitigation of their impact. Factors to be considered include oxygenation, hydration status, acid–base balance, and thermoregulation. The type of operation performed has been described to impact the probability of development of SCD complications in the perioperative period, with high-risk procedures variously described as obstetrical procedures, thoracotomy/laparotomy, intracranial procedures, and operations related to the airway. Anesthetic technique does not appear to be related to the development of perioperative SCD complications, with successful application of general anesthesia, regional anesthesia, or combined techniques in the care of these patients. Additionally, regional anesthetic techniques have been safely employed with variable efficacy to assist in the management of SCD crises, including refractory VOC and priapism.

All operative procedures are not equivalent with respect to potential for the development of serious perioperative complications. The operations with the greatest potential for perioperative complications include cardiac surgery (requiring cardiopulmonary bypass, hypothermia, or aortic cross-clamping) and revascularization procedures for the CNS. In-depth discussions of the optimal management of perioperative transfusion practices, temperature management that confers optimal myocardial and CNS protection without provoking systemic sickling phenomenon, and respiratory and metabolic operative management of acid–base status to optimize myocardial and CNS perfusion are beyond the scope of this chapter, but are discussed in references (149,153–155).

The postoperative management of the SCD patient represents a continuation of the principles and practices applied in the preparation and operative management of these patients. In some institutions, patients are admitted to the ward for postoperative management, and aggressive analgesia is provided in the form of peripheral nerve blockade, neuraxial blockade, patient-controlled opioid analgesia, and nonsteroidal anti-inflammatory drugs (when not contraindicated). Analgesia is optimized to facilitate respiratory function without excessively depressing respiratory drive. Pulmonary toilet is optimized with incentive spirometry for older children, and bubble-blowing games for younger children. Additional care includes supplemental oxygen administration as required and early ambulation with moving from bed to chair. Intravenous hydration is continued postoperatively, with careful attention to fluid intake and output, including insensible losses, urine output, and all losses from drains and catheters. Whether patients with SCD should be managed as outpatients for surgery is also a controversial issue with a paucity of high-quality data available to guide clinical decision making.

OUTCOMES

Patients with SCD are living longer. Thirty years ago, only one half of children with SCD survived until adulthood (101,156). The improved trend in mortality in SCD has been attributed to the routine administration of penicillin prophylaxis; availability of vaccinations against *H. influenzae* and *S. pneumoniae*; surveillance measures, including echocardiography and TCD

studies for early identification of catastrophic complications of SCD; and disease-altering therapies such as hydroxyurea, stem cell transplantation, and chronic transfusion therapy.

As a result of these advancements in therapy, fewer children die of infection and early childhood complications of the disease. Pulmonary complications in general, and ACS (often superimposed on pulmonary hypertension) in particular, remain the leading causes of morbidity and mortality among patients with SCD. A small percentage of SCD patients will develop dysfunction of the lung, many have airway hyperreactivity, and many will develop pulmonary hypertension. Stroke, often with debilitating sequelae, is becoming an increasingly important cause of morbidity and mortality among patients with SCD with a peak in incidence between 2 and 8 years of age.

NEW CONCEPTS IN UNDERSTANDING SCD/FUTURE DIRECTIONS

The disease burden of SCD is great, and assumes greater importance as one of the few endothelial systemic disease processes that affects all organ systems and causes cumulative damage through the course of a lifetime. The paradigm for understanding the pathophysiology of the disease has changed since the last edition of this textbook with work by Gladwin and Kato emphasizing multiple pathophysiologic mechanisms for organ injury that can be essentially summarized as either hemolysis/endothelial dysfunction or viscosity/vaso-occlusion (7,8). This paradigm emphasizes the central importance of intravascular hemolysis with derangement of normal NO biology leading to vasoconstriction. The intensity of hemolysis is closely linked to endothelial dysfunction. The resultant subphenotype has a lower hemoglobin level and may develop priapism, leg ulcers, pulmonary hypertension, and possibly nonhemorrhagic stroke. Conversely, a second subphenotype has a higher hemoglobin level and is more likely to develop viscosity/vaso-occlusive phenomena, including ACS, VOC, and osteonecrosis of the bone. This paradigm is summarized in **Figure 119.4**.

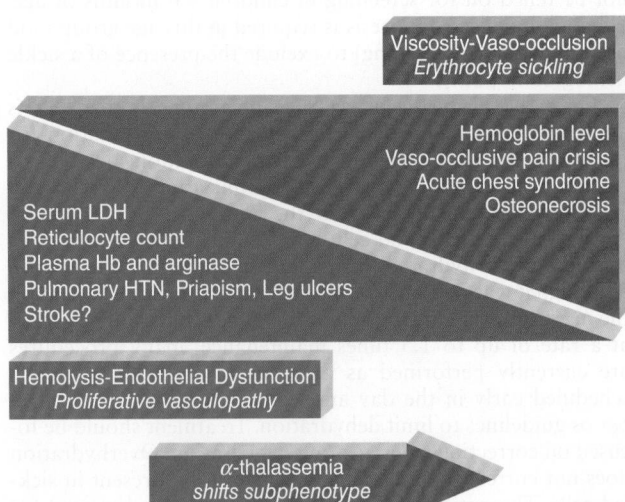

FIGURE 119.4. Model of overlapping subphenotypes of sickle cell disease. (From Kato GJ, Gladwin MT, Steinberg MH. Deconstructing sickle cell disease: Reappraisal of the role of hemolysis in the development of clinical subphenotypes. *Blood Rev* 2007;21(1):37–47.) The arrow on the bottom of the figure indicates that the presence of alpha thalassemia produces more complications in the viscosity/vaso-occlusion end of the phenotypic spectrum.

Advances in our understanding of the human genome, and in our ability to manipulate it, hold the greatest hope for curing patients with SCD. Until genetic therapies are available for the treatment of human SCD, HSCT, with its treatment-associated morbidity, represents the best hope for curative therapy for this disease. Finally, systematic monitoring and effective interventions to minimize or prevent chronic, disabling, and lethal complications of the disease (pulmonary hypertension, stroke) are needed to maintain life quality, as life expectancy with these diseases continues to increase.

References

1. Platt OS, Brambilla DJ, Rosse WF, et al. Mortality in sickle cell disease. Life expectancy and risk factors for early death. *N Engl J Med* 1994;330(23):1639–44.

2. Lane PA. Sickle cell disease. *Pediatr Clin North Am* 1996;43(3):639–64.

3. Dean J, Schechter AN. Sickle-cell anemia: Molecular and cellular bases of therapeutic approaches (third of three parts). *N Engl J Med* 1978;299(16):863–70.

4. Steinberg MH. Management of sickle cell disease. *N Engl J Med* 1999;340(13):1021–30.

5. Gladwin MT, Vichinsky E. Pulmonary complications of sickle cell disease. *N Engl J Med* 2008;359(21):2254–65.

6. Aliyu ZY, Gordeuk V, Sachdev V, et al. Prevalence and risk factors for pulmonary artery systolic hypertension among sickle cell disease patients in Nigeria. *Am J Hematol* 2008;83(6):485–90.

7. Kato GJ, Gladwin MT, Steinberg MH. Deconstructing sickle cell disease: Reappraisal of the role of hemolysis in the development of clinical subphenotypes. *Blood Rev* 2007;21(1):37–47.

8. Kato GJ, Taylor JG 6th. Pleiotropic effects of intravascular haemolysis on vascular homeostasis. *Br J Haematol* 2010;148(5):690–701.

9. Roth EF Jr, Elbaum D, Bookchin RM, et al. The conformational requirements for the mechanical precipitation of hemoglobin S and other mutants. *Blood* 1976;48(2):265–71.

10. Eaton WA, Hofrichter J. Hemoglobin S gelation and sickle cell disease. *Blood* 1987;70(5):1245–66.

11. Aslan M, Thornley-Brown D, Freeman BA. Reactive species in sickle cell disease. *Ann N Y Acad Sci* 2000;899:375–91.

12. Hebbel RP, Morgan WT, Eaton JW, et al. Accelerated autoxidation and heme loss due to instability of sickle hemoglobin. *Proc Natl Acad Sci U S A* 1988;85(1):237–41.

13. Repka T, Hebbel RP. Hydroxyl radical formation by sickle erythrocyte membranes: Role of pathologic iron deposits and cytoplasmic reducing agents. *Blood* 1991;78(10):2753–8.

14. Kato GJ, Martyr S, Blackwelder WC, et al. Levels of soluble endothelium-derived adhesion molecules in patients with sickle cell disease are associated with pulmonary hypertension, organ dysfunction, and mortality. *Br J Haematol* 2005;130(6):943–53.

15. Setty BN, Stuart MJ, Dampier C, et al. Hypoxaemia in sickle cell disease: Biomarker modulation and relevance to pathophysiology. *Lancet* 2003;362(9394):1450–5.

16. Strijbos MH, Landburg PP, Nur E, et al. Circulating endothelial cells: A potential parameter of organ damage in sickle cell anemia? *Blood Cells Mol Dis* 2009;43(1):63–7.

17. Kaul DK, Liu XD, Zhang X, et al. Inhibition of sickle red cell adhesion and vasoocclusion in the microcirculation by antioxidants. *Am J Physiol Heart Circ Physiol* 2006;291(1):H167–75.

18. Haynes J Jr, Obiako B, King JA, et al. Activated neutrophil-mediated sickle red blood cell adhesion to lung vascular endothelium: Role of phosphatidylserine-exposed sickle red blood cells. *Am J Physiol Heart Circ Physiol* 2006;291(4):H1679–85.

19. Wun T, Paglieroni T, Rangaswami A, et al. Platelet activation in patients with sickle cell disease. *Br J Haematol* 1998;100(4):741–9.

20. Villagra J, Shiva S, Hunter LA, et al. Platelet activation in patients with sickle disease, hemolysis-associated pulmonary hypertension, and nitric oxide scavenging by cell-free hemoglobin. *Blood* 2007;110(6):2166–72.

21. Verhamme P, Hoylaerts MF. The pivotal role of the endothelium in haemostasis and thrombosis. *Acta Clin Belg* 2006;61(5):213–9.

22. Singer ST, Ataga KI. Hypercoagulability in sickle cell disease and beta-thalassemia. *Curr Mol Med* 2008;8(7):639–45.

23. Zhou Z, Han H, Cruz MA, et al. Haemoglobin blocks von Willebrand factor proteolysis by ADAMTS-13: A mechanism associated with sickle cell disease. *Thromb Haemost* 2009;101(6):1070–7.

24. Gee BE, Platt OS. Sickle reticulocytes adhere to VCAM-1. *Blood* 1995;85(1):268–74.

25. Hebbel RP, Boogaerts MA, Eaton JW, et al. Erythrocyte adherence to endothelium in sickle-cell anemia. A possible determinant of disease severity. *N Engl J Med* 1980;302(18):992–5.

26. Graido-Gonzalez E, Doherty JC, Bergreen EW, et al. Plasma endothelin-1, cytokine, and prostaglandin E2 levels in sickle cell disease and acute vaso-occlusive sickle crisis. *Blood* 1998;92(7):2551–5.

27. Hammerman SI, Kourembanas S, Conca TJ, et al. Endothelin-1 production during the acute chest syndrome in sickle cell disease. *Am J Respir Crit Care Med* 1997;156(1):280–5.

28. Belcher JD, Marker PH, Weber JP, et al. Activated monocytes in sickle cell disease: Potential role in the activation of vascular endothelium and vaso-occlusion. *Blood* 2000;96(7):2451–9.

29. Assis A, Conran N, Canalli AA, et al. Effect of cytokines and chemokines on sickle neutrophil adhesion to fibronectin. *Acta Haematol* 2005;113(2):130–6.

30. Schafer A, Wiesmann F, Neubauer S, et al. Rapid regulation of platelet activation in vivo by nitric oxide. *Circulation* 2004;109(15):1819–22.

31. Jin RC, Voetsch B, Loscalzo J. Endogenous mechanisms of inhibition of platelet function. *Microcirculation* 2005;12(3):247–58.

32. Kurantsin-Mills J, Ibe BO, Natta CL, et al. Elevated urinary levels of thromboxane and prostacyclin metabolites in sickle cell disease reflects activated platelets in the circulation. *Br J Haematol* 1994;87(3):580–5.

33. Mehta P, Mehta J. Abnormalities of platelet aggregation in sickle cell disease. *J Pediatr* 1980;96(2):209–13.

34. Brittain HA, Eckman JR, Swerlick RA, et al. Thrombospondin from activated platelets promotes sickle erythrocyte adherence to human microvascular endothelium under physiologic flow: A potential role for platelet activation in sickle cell vaso-occlusion. *Blood* 1993;81(8):2137–43.

35. Schnog JJ, Kremer Hovinga JA, Krieg S, et al; CURAMA Study Group. ADAMTS13 activity in sickle cell disease. *Am J Hematol* 2006;81(7):492–8.

36. Hagger D, Wolff S, Owen J, et al. Changes in coagulation and fibrinolysis in patients with sickle cell disease compared with healthy black controls. *Blood Coagul Fibrinolysis* 1995;6(2):93–9.

37. Liesner R, Mackie I, Cookson J, et al. Prothrombotic changes in children with sickle cell disease: Relationships to cerebrovascular disease and transfusion. *Br J Haematol* 1998;103(4):1037–44.

38. Peters M, Plaat BE, ten Cate H, et al. Enhanced thrombin generation in children with sickle cell disease. *Thromb Haemost* 1994;71(2):169–72.

39. Reiter CD, Wang X, Tanus-Santos JE, et al. Cell-free hemoglobin limits nitric oxide bioavailability in sickle-cell disease. *Nat Med* 2002;8(12):1383–9.

40. Morris CR, Kato GJ, Poljakovic M, et al. Dysregulated arginine metabolism, hemolysis-associated pulmonary hypertension, and mortality in sickle cell disease. *JAMA* 2005;294(1):81–90.

41. Schnog JB, Teerlink T, van der Dijs FP, et al; CURAMA Study Group. Plasma levels of asymmetric dimethylarginine (ADMA), an endogenous nitric oxide synthase inhibitor, are elevated in sickle cell disease. *Ann Hematol* 2005;84(5):282–6.

42. Landburg PP, Teerlink T, Muskiet FA, et al; CURAMA Study Group. Plasma concentrations of asymmetric dimethylarginine, an endogenous nitric oxide synthase inhibitor, are elevated in

sickle cell patients but do not increase further during painful crisis. *Am J Hematol* 2008;83(7):577–9.

43. Kato GJ, Wang Z, Machado RF, et al. Endogenous nitric oxide synthase inhibitors in sickle cell disease: Abnormal levels and correlations with pulmonary hypertension, desaturation, haemolysis, organ dysfunction and death. *Br J Haematol* 2009;145(4):506–13.

44. Scalera F, Kielstein JT, Martens-Lobenhoffer J, et al. Erythropoietin increases asymmetric dimethylarginine in endothelial cells: Role of dimethylarginine dimethylaminohydrolase. *J Am Soc Nephrol* 2005;16(4):892–8.

45. Morris CR, Kuypers FA, Larkin S, et al. Patterns of arginine and nitric oxide in patients with sickle cell disease with vaso-occlusive crisis and acute chest syndrome. *J Pediatr Hematol Oncol* 2000;22(6):515–20.

46. Sullivan KJ, Kissoon N, Duckworth LJ, et al. Low exhaled nitric oxide and a polymorphism in the NOS I gene is associated with acute chest syndrome. *Am J Respir Crit Care Med* 2001;164(12):2186–90.

47. Girgis RE, Qureshi MA, Abrams J, et al. Decreased exhaled nitric oxide in sickle cell disease: Relationship with chronic lung involvement. *Am J Hematol* 2003;72(3):177–84.

48. Aslan M, Ryan TM, Adler B, et al. Oxygen radical inhibition of nitric oxide-dependent vascular function in sickle cell disease. *Proc Natl Acad Sci U S A* 2001;98(26):15215–20.

49. Wood KC, Hebbel RP, Granger DN. Endothelial cell NADPH oxidase mediates the cerebral microvascular dysfunction in sickle cell transgenic mice. *FASEB J* 2005;19(8):989–91.

50. Morris CR, Suh JH, Hagar W, et al. Erythrocyte glutamine depletion, altered redox environment, and pulmonary hypertension in sickle cell disease. *Blood* 2008;111(1):402–10.

51. Hammerman SI, Klings ES, Hendra KP, et al. Endothelial cell nitric oxide production in acute chest syndrome. *Am J Physiol* 1999;277(4 pt 2):H1579–92.

52. Pionelli S, Seaman C, Ackerman K, et al. Planning and exchange transfusion in patients with sickle cell syndromes. *Am J Pediatr Hematol Oncol* 1990;12:268–76.

53. Josephson CD, Su LL, Hillyer KL, et al. Transfusion in the patient with sickle cell disease: A critical review of the literature and transfusion guidelines. *Transfus Med Rev* 2007;21(2):118–33.

54. Ambruso DR, Githens JH, Alcorn R, et al. Experience with donors matched for minor blood group antigens in patients with sickle cell anemia who are receiving chronic transfusion therapy. *Transfusion* 1987;27(1):94–8.

55. Vichinsky EP, Luban NL, Wright E, et al; Stroke Prevention Trail in Sickle Cell A. Prospective RBC phenotype matching in a stroke-prevention trial in sickle cell anemia: A multicenter transfusion trial. *Transfusion* 2001;41(9):1086–92.

56. Tahhan HR, Holbrook CT, Braddy LR, et al. Antigen-matched donor blood in the transfusion management of patients with sickle cell disease. *Transfusion* 1994;34(7):562–9.

57. Castellino SM, Combs MR, Zimmerman SA, et al. Erythrocyte autoantibodies in paediatric patients with sickle cell disease receiving transfusion therapy: Frequency, characteristics and significance. *Br J Haematol* 1999;104(1):189–94.

58. Friedman DF, Lukas MB, Jawad A, et al. Alloimmunization to platelets in heavily transfused patients with sickle cell disease. *Blood* 1996;88(8):3216–22.

59. Platt OS. The acute chest syndrome of sickle cell disease. *N Engl J Med* 2000;342(25):1904–7.

60. Vichinsky EP, Neumayr LD, Earles AN, et al. Causes and outcomes of the acute chest syndrome in sickle cell disease. National Acute Chest Syndrome Study Group. *N Engl J Med* 2000;342(25):1855–65.

61. Sylvester KP, Patey RA, Broughton S, et al. Temporal relationship of asthma to acute chest syndrome in sickle cell disease. *Pediatr Pulmonol* 2007;42(2):103–6.

62. Boyd JH, Macklin EA, Strunk RC, et al. Asthma is associated with acute chest syndrome and pain in children with sickle cell anemia. *Blood* 2006;108(9):2923–7.

63. Poulter EY, Truszkowski P, Thompson AA, et al. Acute chest syndrome is associated with history of asthma in hemoglobin SC disease. *Pediatr Blood Cancer* 2011;57(2):289–93.

64. Bernaudin F, Strunk RC, Kamdem A, et al. Asthma is associated with acute chest syndrome, but not with an increased rate of hospitalization for pain among children in France with sickle cell anemia: A retrospective cohort study. *Haematologica* 2008;93(12):1917–8.

65. Knight-Madden JM, Forrester TS, Lewis NA, et al. Asthma in children with sickle cell disease and its association with acute chest syndrome. *Thorax* 2005;60(3):206–10.

66. Sen N, Kozanoglu I, Karatasli M, et al. Pulmonary function and airway hyperresponsiveness in adults with sickle cell disease. *Lung* 2009;187(3):195–200.

67. Vichinsky EP, Styles LA, Colangelo LH, et al. Acute chest syndrome in sickle cell disease: Clinical presentation and course. Cooperative Study of Sickle Cell Disease. *Blood* 1997;89(5):1787–92.

68. Reagan MM, DeBaun MR, Frei-Jones MJ. Multi-modal intervention for the inpatient management of sickle cell pain significantly decreases the rate of acute chest syndrome. *Pediatr Blood Cancer* 2011;56(2):262–6.

69. Gladwin MT, Kato GJ, Weiner D, et al. Nitric oxide for inhalation in the acute treatment of sickle cell pain crisis: A randomized controlled trial. *JAMA* 2011;305(9):893–902.

70. Mekontso Dessap A, Leon R, Habibi A, et al. Pulmonary hypertension and cor pulmonale during severe acute chest syndrome in sickle cell disease. *Am J Respir Crit Care Med* 2008;177(6):646–53.

71. Gladwin MT, Rodgers GP. Pathogenesis and treatment of acute chest syndrome of sickle-cell anaemia. *Lancet* 2000;355(9214):1476–8.

72. Styles LA, Schalkwijk CG, Aarsman AJ, et al. Phospholipase A2 levels in acute chest syndrome of sickle cell disease. *Blood* 1996;87(6):2573–8.

73. Lechapt E, Habibi A, Bachir D, et al. Induced sputum versus bronchoalveolar lavage during acute chest syndrome in sickle cell disease. *Am J Respir Crit Care Med* 2003;168(11):1373–7.

74. Mekontso Dessap A, Deux JF, Abidi N, et al. Pulmonary artery thrombosis during acute chest syndrome in sickle cell disease. *Am J Respir Crit Care Med* 2011;184(9):1022–9.

75. Fartoukh M, Lefort Y, Habibi A, et al. Early intermittent noninvasive ventilation for acute chest syndrome in adults with sickle cell disease: A pilot study. *Intensive Care Med* 2010;36(8):1355–62.

76. Sullivan KJ, Goodwin SR, Evangelist J, et al. Nitric oxide successfully used to treat acute chest syndrome of sickle cell disease in a young adolescent. *Crit Care Med* 1999;27(11):2563–8.

77. Atz AM, Wessel DL. Inhaled nitric oxide in sickle cell disease with acute chest syndrome. *Anesthesiology* 1997;87(4):988–90.

78. Al Hajeri A, Serjeant GR, Fedorowicz Z. Inhaled nitric oxide for acute chest syndrome in people with sickle cell disease. *Cochrane Database Syst Rev* 2008(1);CD006957.

79. Hoffmann M, Geldner G, Leschke M. Life-threatening acute chest syndrome with hemolytic crisis in sickle cell disease. Treatment using a venovenous extracorporeal membrane oxygenation (ECMO). *Dtsch Med Wochenschr* 2011;136(43):2192–5.

80. Trant CA Jr, Casey JR, Hansell D, et al. Successful use of extracorporeal membrane oxygenation in the treatment of acute chest syndrome in a child with severe sickle cell anemia. *ASAIO J* 1996;42(3):236–9.

81. Pelidis MA, Kato GJ, Resar LM, et al. Successful treatment of life-threatening acute chest syndrome of sickle cell disease with venovenous extracorporeal membrane oxygenation. *J Pediatr Hematol Oncol* 1997;19(5):459–61.

82. Pavlakis SG, Prohovnik I, Piomelli S, et al. Neurologic complications of sickle cell disease. *Adv Pediatrics* 1989;36:247–76.

83. Ohene-Frempong K, Weiner SJ, Sleeper LA, et al. Cerebrovascular accidents in sickle cell disease: Rates and risk factors. *Blood* 1998;91(1):288–94.

84. Earley CJ, Kittner SJ, Feeser BR, et al. Stroke in children and sickle-cell disease: Baltimore-Washington Cooperative Young Stroke Study. *Neurology* 1998;51(1):169–76.

85. Powars D, Wilson B, Imbus C, et al. The natural history of stroke in sickle cell disease. *Am J Med* 1978;65(3):461–71.

86. Dobson SR, Holden KR, Nietert PJ, et al. Moyamoya syndrome in childhood sickle cell disease: A predictive factor for recurrent cerebrovascular events. *Blood* 2002;99(9):3144–50.

87. Pegelow CH, Macklin EA, Moser FG, et al. Longitudinal changes in brain magnetic resonance imaging findings in children with sickle cell disease. *Blood* 2002;99(8):3014–8.

88. Kirkham FJ, Prengler M, Hewes DK, et al. Risk factors for arterial ischemic stroke in children. *J Child Neurol* 2000;15(5):299–307.

89. Kwiatkowski JL, Zimmerman RA, Pollock AN, et al. Silent infarcts in young children with sickle cell disease. *Br J Haematol* 2009;146(3):300–5.

90. Kinney TR, Sleeper LA, Wang WC, et al. Silent cerebral infarcts in sickle cell anemia: A risk factor analysis. The Cooperative Study of Sickle Cell Disease. *Pediatrics* 1999;103(3):640–5.

91. Switzer JA, Hess DC, Nichols FT, et al. Pathophysiology and treatment of stroke in sickle-cell disease: Present and future. *Lancet Neurol* 2006;5(6):501–12.

92. Wang WC, Gallagher DM, Pegelow CH, et al. Multicenter comparison of magnetic resonance imaging and transcranial Doppler ultrasonography in the evaluation of the central nervous system in children with sickle cell disease. *J Pediatr Hematol Oncol* 2000;22(4):335–9.

93. Abboud MR, Yim E, Musallam KM, et al; Investigators SIS. Discontinuing prophylactic transfusions increases the risk of silent brain infarction in children with sickle cell disease: Data from STOP II. *Blood* 2011;118(4):894–8.

94. Pegelow CH, Wang W, Granger S, et al. Silent infarcts in children with sickle cell anemia and abnormal cerebral artery velocity. *Arch Neurol* 2001;58(12):2017–21.

95. Hulbert ML, McKinstry RC, Lacey JL, et al. Silent cerebral infarcts occur despite regular blood transfusion therapy after first strokes in children with sickle cell disease. *Blood* 2011;117(3):772–9.

96. Casella JF, King AA, Barton B, et al. Design of the silent cerebral infarct transfusion (SIT) trial. *Pediatr Hematol Oncol* 2010;27(2):69–89.

97. Adams RJ, Brambilla D; Optimizing Primary Stroke Prevention in Sickle Cell Anemia Trial I. Discontinuing prophylactic transfusions used to prevent stroke in sickle cell disease. *N Engl J Med* 2005;353(26):2769–78.

98. Bernaudin F, Socie G, Kuentz M, et al. Long-term results of related myeloablative stem-cell transplantation to cure sickle cell disease. *Blood* 2007;110(7):2749–56.

99. Ware RE, Helms RW; Investigators SW. Stroke with transfusions changing to hydroxyurea (SWiTCH). *Blood* 2012;119(17):3925–32.

100. Metske HA, Postema PG, Biemond BJ, et al. Cooling the crisis: Therapeutic hypothermia after sickle cardiac arrest. *Crit Care Med* 2012;40(2):651–3.

101. Quinn CT, Rogers ZR, Buchanan GR. Survival of children with sickle cell disease. *Blood* 2004;103(11):4023–7.

102. Varat MA, Adolph RJ, Fowler NO. Cardiovascular effects of anemia. *Am Heart J* 1972;83(3):415–26.

103. Grossman W, Jones D, McLaurin LP. Wall stress and patterns of hypertrophy in the human left ventricle. *J Clin Invest* 1975;56(1):56–64.

104. Hankins JS, McCarville MB, Hillenbrand CM, et al. Ventricular diastolic dysfunction in sickle cell anemia is common but not associated with myocardial iron deposition. *Pediatr Blood Cancer* 2010;55(3):495–500.

105. Johnson MC, Kirkham FJ, Redline S, et al. Left ventricular hypertrophy and diastolic dysfunction in children with sickle cell disease are related to asleep and waking oxygen desaturation. *Blood* 2010;116(1):16–21.

106. Caldas MC, Meira ZA, Barbosa MM. Evaluation of 107 patients with sickle cell anemia through tissue Doppler and myocardial performance index. *J Am Soc Echocardiogr* 2008;21(10):1163–7.

107. Sachdev V, Kato GJ, Gibbs JS, et al. Echocardiographic markers of elevated pulmonary pressure and left ventricular diastolic dysfunction are associated with exercise intolerance in adults and adolescents with homozygous sickle cell anemia in the United States and United Kingdom. *Circulation* 2011;124(13):1452–60.

108. Anthi A, Machado RF, Jison ML, et al. Hemodynamic and functional assessment of patients with sickle cell disease and pulmonary hypertension. *Am J Respir Crit Care Med* 2007;175(12):1272–9.

109. Castro O, Hoque M, Brown BD. Pulmonary hypertension in sickle cell disease: Cardiac catheterization results and survival. *Blood* 2003;101(4):1257–61.

110. Covitz W, Espeland M, Gallagher D, et al. The heart in sickle cell anemia. The Cooperative Study of Sickle Cell Disease (CSSCD). *Chest* 1995;108(5):1214–9.

111. Dham N, Ensing G, Minniti C, et al. Prospective echocardiography assessment of pulmonary hypertension and its potential etiologies in children with sickle cell disease. *Am J Cardiol* 2009;104(5):713–20.

112. Willens HJ, Lawrence C, Frishman WH, et al. A noninvasive comparison of left ventricular performance in sickle cell anemia and chronic aortic regurgitation. *Clin Cardiol* 1983;6(11):542–8.

113. Sachdev V, Machado RF, Shizukuda Y, et al. Diastolic dysfunction is an independent risk factor for death in patients with sickle cell disease. *J Am Coll Cardiol* 2007;49(4):472–9.

114. Graham JK, Mosunjac M, Hanzlick RL, et al. Sickle cell lung disease and sudden death: A retrospective/prospective study of 21 autopsy cases and literature review. *Am J Forensic Med Pathol* 2007;28(2):168–72.

115. Haque AK, Gokhale S, Rampy BA, et al. Pulmonary hypertension in sickle cell hemoglobinopathy: A clinicopathologic study of 20 cases. *Hum Pathol* 2002;33(10):1037–43.

116. Liesner RJ, Vandenberghe EA. Sudden death in sickle cell disease. *J R Soc Med* 1993;86(8):484–5.

117. Manci EA, Culberson DE, Yang YM, et al; Investigators of the Cooperative Study of Sickle Cell D. Causes of death in sickle cell disease: An autopsy study. *Br J Haematol* 2003;123(2):359–65.

118. Fitzhugh CD, Lauder N, Jonassaint JC, et al. Cardiopulmonary complications leading to premature deaths in adult patients with sickle cell disease. *Am J Hematol* 2010;85(1):36–40.

119. Darbari DS, Kple-Faget P, Kwagyan J, et al. Circumstances of death in adult sickle cell disease patients. *Am J Hematol* 2006;81(11):858–63.

120. Gladwin MT, Sachdev V, Jison ML, et al. Pulmonary hypertension as a risk factor for death in patients with sickle cell disease. *N Engl J Med* 2004;350(9):886–95.

121. Gladwin MT, Sachdev V. Cardiovascular abnormalities in sickle cell disease. *J Am Coll Cardiol* 2012;59(13):1123–33.

122. Parent F, Bachir D, Inamo J, et al. A hemodynamic study of pulmonary hypertension in sickle cell disease. *N Engl J Med* 2011;365(1):44–53.

123. Sundaram N, Tailor A, Mendelsohn L, et al. High levels of placenta growth factor in sickle cell disease promote pulmonary hypertension. *Blood* 2010;116(1):109–12.

124. Ataga KI, Moore CG, Jones S, et al. Pulmonary hypertension in patients with sickle cell disease: A longitudinal study. *Br J Haematol* 2006;134(1):109–15.

125. Rudski LG, Lai WW, Afilalo J, et al. Guidelines for the echocardiographic assessment of the right heart in adults: A report from the American Society of Echocardiography endorsed by the European Association of Echocardiography, a registered branch of the European Society of Cardiology, and the Canadian Society of Echocardiography. *J Am Soc Echocardiogr* 2010;23(7):685–713; quiz 786–8.

126. Mehari A, Gladwin MT, Tian X, et al. Mortality in adults with sickle cell disease and pulmonary hypertension. *JAMA* 2012;307(12):1254–6.

127. De Castro LM, Jonassaint JC, Graham FL, et al. Pulmonary hypertension associated with sickle cell disease: Clinical and laboratory endpoints and disease outcomes. *Am J Hematol* 2008;83(1):19–25.

128. Machado RF, Barst RJ, Yovetich NA, et al. Hospitalization for pain in patients with sickle cell disease treated with sildenafil for elevated TRV and low exercise capacity. *Blood* 2011;118(4):855–64.

129. Maitre B, Mekontso-Dessap A, Habibi A, et al. Pulmonary complications in adult sickle cell disease. *Rev Mal Respir* 2011;28(2): 129–37.

130. Lanzkron S, Strouse JJ, Wilson R, et al. Systematic review: Hydroxyurea for the treatment of adults with sickle cell disease. *Ann Intern Med* 2008;148(12):939–55.

131. Brawley OW, Cornelius LJ, Edwards LR, et al. National Institutes of Health Consensus Development Conference statement: Hydroxyurea treatment for sickle cell disease. *Ann Intern Med* 2008;148(12):932–8.

132. Barst RJ, Langleben D, Frost A, et al. Sitaxsentan therapy for pulmonary arterial hypertension. *Am J Respir Crit Care Med* 2004;169(4):441–7.

133. Barst RJ, Mubarak KK, Machado RF, et al. Exercise capacity and haemodynamics in patients with sickle cell disease with pulmonary hypertension treated with bosentan: Results of the ASSET studies. *Br J Haematol* 2010;149(3):426–35.

134. Kato GJ, Gladwin MT. Evolution of novel small-molecule therapeutics targeting sickle cell vasculopathy. *JAMA* 2008;300(22): 2638–46.

135. Minniti CP, Machado RF, Coles WA, et al. Endothelin receptor antagonists for pulmonary hypertension in adult patients with sickle cell disease. *Br J Haematol* 2009;147(5):737–43.

136. Lewis GD, Lachmann J, Camuso J, et al. Sildenafil improves exercise hemodynamics and oxygen uptake in patients with systolic heart failure. *Circulation* 2007;115(1):59–66.

137. Lewis GD, Shah R, Shahzad K, et al. Sildenafil improves exercise capacity and quality of life in patients with systolic heart failure and secondary pulmonary hypertension. *Circulation* 2007;116(14):1555–62.

138. Machado RF, Martyr S, Kato GJ, et al. Sildenafil therapy in patients with sickle cell disease and pulmonary hypertension. *Br J Haematol* 2005;130(3):445–53.

139. Powars D, Weidman JA, Odom-Maryon T, et al. Sickle cell chronic lung disease: Prior morbidity and the risk of pulmonary failure. *Medicine* 1988;67(1):66–76.

140. Morris CR. Asthma management: Reinventing the wheel in sickle cell disease. *Am J Hematol* 2009;84(4):234–41.

141. Boyd JH, Macklin EA, Strunk RC, et al. Asthma is associated with increased mortality in individuals with sickle cell anemia. *Haematologica* 2007;92(8):1115–8.

142. Field JJ, DeBaun MR. Asthma and sickle cell disease: Two distinct diseases or part of the same process? *Hematology Am Soc Hematol Educ Program* 2009:45–53.

143. Field JJ, Stocks J, Kirkham FJ, et al. Airway hyperresponsiveness in children with sickle cell anemia. *Chest* 2011;139(3):563–8.

144. Boyd JH, Moinuddin A, Strunk RC, et al. Asthma and acute chest in sickle-cell disease. *Pediatr Pulmonol* 2004;38(3):229–32.

145. Bryant R. Asthma in the pediatric sickle cell patient with acute chest syndrome. *J Pediatr Health Care* 2005;19(3):157–62.

146. Nordness ME, Lynn J, Zacharisen MC, et al. Asthma is a risk factor for acute chest syndrome and cerebral vascular accidents in children with sickle cell disease. *Clin Mol Allergy* 2005;3(1):2.

147. Miller AC, Gladwin MT. Pulmonary complications of sickle cell disease. *Am J Respir Crit Care Med* 2012;185(11):1154–65.

148. Griffin TC, Buchanan GR. Elective surgery in children with sickle cell disease without preoperative blood transfusion. *J Pediatr Surg* 1993;28(5):681–5.

149. Lazopoulos G, Kantartzis MM, Kantartzis M. Mitral valve replacement and tricuspid valve repair in a patient with sickle cell disease. *Thorac Cardiovasc Surg* 2008;56(1):56–7.

150. Koshy M, Weiner SJ, Miller ST, et al. Surgery and anesthesia in sickle cell disease. Cooperative Study of Sickle Cell Diseases. *Blood* 1995;86(10):3676–84.

151. Vichinsky EP, Haberkern CM, Neumayr L, et al. A comparison of conservative and aggressive transfusion regimens in the perioperative management of sickle cell disease. The Preoperative Transfusion in Sickle Cell Disease Study Group. *N Engl J Med* 1995;333(4):206–13.

152. Haberkern CM, Neumayr LD, Orringer EP, et al. Cholecystectomy in sickle cell anemia patients: Perioperative outcome of 364 cases from the National Preoperative Transfusion Study. Preoperative Transfusion in Sickle Cell Disease Study Group. *Blood* 1997;89(5):1533–42.

153. Usman S, Saiful FB, DiNatale J, et al. Warm, beating heart aortic valve replacement in a sickle cell patient. *Interact Cardiovasc Thorac Surg* 2010;10(1):67–8.

154. Sachithanandan A, Nanjaiah P, Wright CJ, et al. Mitral and tricuspid valve surgery in homozygous sickle cell disease: Perioperative considerations for a successful outcome. *J Card Surg* 2008;23(2):167–8.

155. Chong CT, Manninen PH. Anesthesia for cerebral revascularization for adult moyamoya syndrome associated with sickle cell disease. *J Clin Neurosci* 2011;18(12):1709–12.

156. Gill FM, Sleeper LA, Weiner SJ, et al. Clinical events in the first decade in a cohort of infants with sickle cell disease. Cooperative Study of Sickle Cell Disease. *Blood* 1995;86(2):776–83.

COMMON EQUATIONS USED IN PEDIATRIC CRITICAL CARE

DONALD H. SHAFFNER AND DAVID G. NICHOLS

This appendix lists common equations frequently used by pediatric critical care physicians. They are arranged by organ system in the following order:

Section 1: Airway and Respiratory Equations

Section 2: Cardiovascular and Hemodynamic Equations

Section 3: Neurologic Equations

Section 4: Renal, Electrolyte, and Renal Replacement Therapy Equations

Section 5: Gastroenterology and Nutrition Equations

Section 6: Hematology Equations

Section 7: Other Equations

This appendix is arranged so that a description or name of the equation appears in column one, the equation in column two, the variables for the equation in column three, the definitions of each variable in column four, and the units of each variable in column five. A *note* appears below each equation that contains the normal values for the equation's solution (when appropriate/available) and lists the chapter numbers in which the respective equation appears in the textbook.

Section 1: Airway and Respiratory Equations

DESCRIPTION	EQUATION	VARIABLE	DEFINITION OF VARIABLE	VARIABLE UNITS
Uncuffed endotracheal tube (ETT) size for children 2–14 y	$\text{Size} = \dfrac{\text{Age}}{4} + 4$	Size Age	Internal diameter of ETT Child's age	mm y
Note: Uncuffed ETT size for children 0–1 y = 3.5 mm; for 1–2 y = 4.0 mm. Equation is discussed in Chapter 24.				
Cuffed ETT size for children 2–18 y	$\text{Size} = \dfrac{\text{Age}}{4} + 3$	Size Age	Internal diameter of ETT Child's age	mm y
Note: Cuffed ETT size for children 0–1 y = 3.0 mm; for 1–2 y = 3.5 mm. Equation is discussed in Chapter 24.				
Depth of ETT insertion for children 2–18 y	$\text{Depth} = \dfrac{\text{Age}}{2} + 12$	Depth Age	Tube depth at gum Child's age	cm y
Note: Equation is discussed in Chapter 24.				
Depth of ETT insertion (any age)	$\text{Depth} = \text{Size} \times 3$	Depth Size	Tube depth at gum Internal diameter of ETT	cm mm
Note: Equation is discussed in Chapter 24.				
Conversion of French to mm (catheter diameter)	$\text{External diameter (mm)} = \dfrac{\text{French}}{3}$		1 mm external diameter = 3 French	
Note: French (F) approximates circumference (C) ($C = \pi \times \text{Diameter}$). A 10F suction catheter (3.3 mm external diameter) will fit inside a 4.0 ETT.				
Conversion of mm Hg to kPa	$\text{kPa} = \dfrac{\text{mm Hg}}{7.5}$		1 kPa = 7.5 mm Hg	
Henry's law	$C = \alpha P$	C α P	Concentration Solubility Partial pressure of a gas dissolved in liquid	mL/dL mL/mm Hg/dL mm Hg
Note: Equation is discussed in Chapter 43.				
Partial pressure	$P_x = F_x \times P_B$	P_x F_x P_B	Partial pressure Fractional concentration of gas "x" Barometric pressure	mm Hg 0–1 mm Hg
Note: Equation is discussed in Chapter 43.				
Effect of altitude on inspired O_2 partial pressure (P_{IO_2})	$P_{IO_{2(1)}} = F_{IO_{2(1)}} \times P_{B_{(1)}}$	$P_{IO_{2(1)}}$ $F_{IO_{2(1)}}$ $P_{B_{(1)}}$	Inspired O_2 partial pressure at altitude 1 Inspired O_2 fraction at altitude 1 Barometric pressure at altitude 1	mm Hg 0–1 mm Hg

Note: P_B at sea level is 760 mm Hg, at 5000 ft is 632 mm Hg, and at 8000 ft is 564 mm Hg. Equation is discussed in Chapter 26.

DESCRIPTION	EQUATION	VARIABLE	DEFINITION OF VARIABLE	VARIABLE UNITS
Boyle's law	$P_1V_1 = P_2V_2$	P_1 V_1 P_2 V_2	Pressure at altitude 1 Volume at altitude 1 Pressure at altitude 2 Volume at altitude 2	mm Hg mL mm Hg mL
Note: P_B at 5000 ft is 80% of sea level, so see a 20% increase in volume of gas-filled space at 5000 ft and a 34% increase at 8000 ft. Equation is discussed in Chapter 26.				
Minute ventilation	$\dot{V} = V_T \times f$	$\dot{V}$ V_T f	Minute ventilation (or minute volume) Tidal volume Frequency (respiratory rate)	L/min mL breaths/min
Note: Normal values vary by age: V_T ~7 mL/kg, f ~30 breaths/min in neonate and 10 breaths/min in adult, and $\dot{V}$ for adult is 500 mL × 12 breaths/min = 6 L/min. Equation is discussed in Chapter 45.				
Minute ventilation	$\dot{V} = \dot{V}_A + \dot{V}_{DS}$	$\dot{V}$ $\dot{V}_A$ $\dot{V}_{DS}$	Minute ventilation Alveolar ventilation Dead space ventilation	L/min L/min L/min
Note: Normal values vary by age: $\dot{V}_A$ ~5 mL/kg × f (see range for f above) or ~4.2 L/min in adult, $\dot{V}_{DS}$ ~2 mL/kg × f (see above) or ~1.8 L/min in adult, therefore for an adult $\dot{V}$ ~6 L/min. Equation is discussed in Chapter 45.				
Alveolar ventilation	$\dot{V}_A = (\dot{V}_{CO_2}/P_{aCO_2})K$	$\dot{V}_A$ $\dot{V}_{CO_2}$ P_{aCO_2} K	Alveolar ventilation CO_2 elimination from the lungs Alveolar CO_2 (substitute P_{aCO_2}) Constant (0.863)	L/min mL/min mm Hg mm Hg·L/mL
Note: Normal values vary by age: $\dot{V}_{CO_2}$ ~200 mL/min in adult, as above $\dot{V}_A$ ~4.2 L/min in adult. Equation is discussed in Chapter 43.				
Physiologic dead space (aka total dead space)	$V_{DS} = V_{DS_{anat}} + V_{DS_{alv}}$	V_{DS} $V_{DS_{anat}}$ $V_{DS_{alv}}$	Physiologic or total dead space Anatomic dead space Alveolar dead space	mL mL mL
Note: Normal values vary by age: $V_{DS_{anat}}$ ~2 mL/kg or 150 mL in adult and $V_{DS_{alv}}$ ~0, therefore V_{DS} for adult ~150 mL. Equation is discussed in Chapter 43.				
Physiologic dead space calculation	$V_{DS} = V_T \times \dfrac{(P_{aCO_2} - P_{\bar{E}CO_2})}{P_{aCO_2}}$	V_{DS} V_T P_{aCO_2} $P_{\bar{E}CO_2}$	Physiologic or total dead space Tidal volume Alveolar CO_2 partial pressure (substitute P_{aCO_2}) Mixed expired CO_2 partial pressure (Douglas bag collection)	mL mL mm Hg mm Hg
Note: Normal values vary by age and have mentioned previously. Equation is discussed in Chapter 43.				
Alveolar dead space calculation	$V_{DS_{alv}} = V_T \times \dfrac{(P_{aCO_2} - P_{ETCO_2})}{P_{aCO_2}}$	$V_{DS_{alv}}$ V_T P_{aCO_2} P_{ETCO_2}	Alveolar dead space Tidal volume Alveolar CO_2 partial pressure (substitute P_{aCO_2}) End-tidal CO_2 partial pressure	mL mL mm Hg mm Hg
Note: Normal values vary by age and have mentioned previously. Equation is discussed in Chapter 43.				

DESCRIPTION	EQUATION	VARIABLE	DEFINITION OF VARIABLE	VARIABLE UNITS
Alveolar gas equation (assumes $PiCO_2$ is 0)	$PAO_2 = (P_B - PH_2O) \times FiO_2 - (PaCO_2/R)$	PAO_2	Alveolar oxygen partial pressure	mm Hg
		P_B	Barometric pressure	mm Hg
		PH_2O	Partial pressure of water vapor (47 mm Hg when fully saturated with H_2O)	mm Hg
		FiO_2	Inspired oxygen fraction	0–1
		$PaCO_2$	Alveolar CO_2 partial pressure (can substitute $PaCO_2$)	mm Hg
		R	Respiratory exchange ratio (0.8)	

Note: Normal value is approximately 100 mm Hg in room air (0.21) at sea level (760 mm Hg). Equation is discussed in Chapters 26, 43, and 45.

Alveolar–arterial oxygen difference	$AaDo_2 = PAO_2 - PaO_2$	$AaDo_2$	Alveolar–arterial oxygen difference	mm Hg
		PAO_2	Alveolar oxygen pressure (see above)	mm Hg
		PaO_2	Arterial oxygen pressure	mm Hg

Note: Normal value for $AaDo_2$ at rest in room air is 5–10 mm Hg, and this increases with age in adults. Equation is discussed in Chapter 43.

Respiratory exchange ratio	$R = \dot{V}CO_2/\dot{V}O_2$	R	Respiratory exchange ratio	
		$\dot{V}CO_2$	Amount of carbon dioxide produced	mL/min
		$\dot{V}O_2$	Amount of oxygen consumed	mL/min

Note: Normal value for respiratory exchange ratio at rest on typical diet is 0.8. At steady state, the respiratory exchange ratio equals respiratory quotient. Equation is discussed in Chapter 43.

Fick's 1st law of diffusion (modified for oxygen)	$\dot{V}O_2 = (PAO_2 - PpaO_2) \times DLO_2$	$\dot{V}O_2$	Oxygen uptake across the lungs	mL/min
		PAO_2	Alveolar O_2 pressure	mm Hg
		$PpaO_2$	Pulmonary artery O_2 pressure ($\approx$ mixed venous O_2 pressure)	mm Hg
		DLO_2	Oxygen diffusing capacity across the lungs	mL/min/mm Hg

Note: Normal value for oxygen uptake at rest varies by age, can be estimated by equation $\dot{V}O_2 = 5.0 \times kg + 19.8$ mL/min for 4–25 kg, adult normal value is 250 mL/min. Equation is discussed in Chapter 43.

Lung-diffusion capacity for carbon monoxide	$DLCO = \dot{V}CO / PaCO$	$DLCO$	Diffusing capacity for carbon monoxide	mL/min/mm Hg
		$\dot{V}CO$	Carbon monoxide uptake by the lungs	mL/min
		$PaCO$	Alveolar carbon monoxide pressure (= driving pressure, since capillary CO is 0)	mm Hg

Note: Normal values vary by age and gender and are adjusted for hemoglobin level; they should be compared to table of predicted values. Equation is discussed in Chapter 43.

DESCRIPTION	EQUATION	VARIABLE	DEFINITION OF VARIABLE	VARIABLE UNITS
Intrapulmonary shunt equation	$$\dfrac{\dot{Q}s}{\dot{Q}t} = \dfrac{Cc'o_2 - Cao_2}{Cc'o_2 - C\bar{v}o_2}$$	$\dfrac{\dot{Q}s}{\dot{Q}t}$	Shunt fraction	%
		$\dot{Q}s$	Shunt flow	L/min
		$\dot{Q}t$	Total cardiac output	L/min
		$Cc'o_2$	Pulmonary capillary oxygen content (use Pao_2 to calculate)	mL/dL
		Cao_2	Arterial oxygen content	mL/dL
		$C\bar{v}o_2$	Mixed venous oxygen content	mL/dL

Note: Normal values are <5%–10%. Estimation of $Cc'o_2$ uses $(1.34 \times \text{hemoglobin}) + (0.003 \times Pao_2)$, assumes Sao_2 is 100% and uses Pao_2 from alveolar gas equation (see above). Equation is discussed in Chapters 43 and 45.

DESCRIPTION	EQUATION	VARIABLE	DEFINITION OF VARIABLE	VARIABLE UNITS
Carbon dioxide elimination	$$\dot{V}co_2 = \dot{Q}(Caco_2 - C\bar{v}co_2) \times 10$$	$\dot{V}co_2$	Carbon dioxide elimination	mL CO_2/min
		$\dot{Q}$	Cardiac output	L/min
		$Caco_2$	Arterial carbon dioxide content	mL/dL
		$C\bar{v}co_2$	Mixed venous carbon dioxide content	mL/dL
		10	Conversion factor	dL/L

Note: Normal values vary by age and can be estimated as $\dot{V}co_2 = 4.8 \times \text{kg} + 6.4$ mL/min for 4–25 kg; adult normal value is 200 mL/min. Equation is discussed in Chapters 40, 43, and 49.

DESCRIPTION	EQUATION	VARIABLE	DEFINITION OF VARIABLE	VARIABLE UNITS
Hagen–Poiseuille equation	$$\dot{Q} = \left(\dfrac{\pi r^4}{8\eta}\right)\dfrac{\Delta P}{L}$$	$\dot{Q}$	Laminar flow in straight tubes	cm^3/s
		r	Inside radius of tube	cm
		ΔP	Pressure gradient across tube	dyne/cm^2
		η	Gas/fluid viscosity	dyne-s/cm^2
		L	Length of tube	cm

Note: The Hagen–Poiseuille equation describes the characteristics that affect laminar flow. Equation is discussed in Chapters 40, 43, and 49.

DESCRIPTION	EQUATION	VARIABLE	DEFINITION OF VARIABLE	VARIABLE UNITS
Reynolds number	$$Re = \dfrac{2\rho vr}{\eta}$$	Re	Reynolds number	Dimensionless
		ρ	Gas density	g/cm^3
		v	Gas velocity	cm/s
		r	Airway inside radius	cm
		η	Gas viscosity	g/cm·s

Note: Reynolds number pertains to the transition from laminar to turbulent flow; lower Reynolds number represents characteristics associated with laminar flow. Equation is discussed in Chapter 39.

DESCRIPTION	EQUATION	VARIABLE	DEFINITION OF VARIABLE	VARIABLE UNITS
Laplace's equation	$$P_{bubble} = 4\left(\dfrac{T}{r}\right)$$	P_{bubble}	Pressure inside spherical bubble (2 surfaces)	dyne/cm^2
	$$P_{drop} = 2\left(\dfrac{T}{r}\right)$$	P_{drop}	Pressure inside spherical drop (1 surface)	dyne/cm^2
		T	Surface tension	dyne/cm
		r	Radius of bubble/drop	cm

Note: Relationship of surface tension and radius to pressure across a sphere containing gas or fluid. Equation is discussed in Chapters 43 and 49.

DESCRIPTION	EQUATION	VARIABLE	DEFINITION OF VARIABLE	VARIABLE UNITS
Compliance	$C = \dfrac{\Delta V}{\Delta P}$	C ΔV ΔP	Compliance Change in volume Change in pressure (pleural)	mL/cm H_2O mL cm H_2O
Note: General relationship for compliance in a system. Equation is discussed in Chapter 38.				
Static lung compliance	$C_{Lstat} = \dfrac{V_T}{P_{plat} - PEEP}$	C_{Lstat} V_T P_{plat} PEEP	Static lung compliance Tidal volume Alveolar pressure at the end of inspiration Alveolar pressure at the end of expiration	mL/cm H_2O mL cm H_2O cm H_2O
Note: Normal values vary with age: 1.5–2 mL/cm H_2O/kg in neonates and infants, and 2.5–3 mL/cm H_2O/kg in children and adult. Equation is discussed in Chapter 45.				
Dynamic lung compliance	$C_{Ldyn} = \dfrac{V_T}{PIP - PEEP}$	C_{Ldyn} V_T PIP PEEP	Dynamic lung compliance Tidal volume Alveolar peak pressure during inspiration Alveolar pressure at end of expiration	mL/cm H_2O mL cm H_2O cm H_2O
Note: Normal values vary with age and range from 5 mL/cm H_2O in newborn to 50–100 mL/cm H_2O in adult. Equation is discussed in Chapter 45.				
Effective tidal volume	$V_{Teff} = V_{Tdel} - C_{vent}(PIP - PEEP)$	V_{Teff} V_{Tdel} C_{vent} PIP PEEP	Effective tidal volume that reaches ETT Delivered tidal volume Compliance of the ventilator circuit Peak inspiratory pressure Positive end-expiratory pressure	mL mL mL/cm H_2O cm H_2O cm H_2O
Note: Corrects for the compliance of the breathing circuit (removes wasted ventilation). Equation is discussed in Chapters 38 and 45.				
Airway pressure	$Paw = P_{elastic} + P_{resistive} + P_{inertance}$	Paw $P_{elastic}$ $P_{resistive}$ $P_{inertance}$	Airway pressure Elastic recoil pressure Flow resistive pressure Inertance pressure	cm H_2O cm H_2O cm H_2O cm H_2O
Note: The airway pressure represents a balance of forces used to expand lung and chest wall and forces opposed to it. Equation is discussed in Chapter 38.				
Work of breathing	$W = \displaystyle\int_0^v P \times dv$	W $\displaystyle\int_0^v P$ dv	Work of breathing Integral of the pressure across the respiratory system as a function of volume Change in volume of the respiratory system	J cm H_2O L
Note: One Joule (J) is the work needed to drive a 1-L volume through a 10-cm H_2O gradient. When time is added to the equation, 1 J/s = 1 W. Equation is discussed in Chapter 38.				

DESCRIPTION	EQUATION	VARIABLE	DEFINITION OF VARIABLE	VARIABLE UNITS
Starling equation	$Q = K_f\left[(P_c - P_{is}) - \sigma(\pi_c - \pi_{is})\right]$	Q	Flow across a membrane	mL/min
		K_f	Membrane filtration coefficient	mL/min/mm Hg
		P_c	Capillary hydrostatic pressure	mm Hg
		P_{is}	Interstitial hydrostatic pressure	mm Hg
		σ	Osmotic/membrane reflection coefficient	0–1
		π_c	Capillary (plasma) osmotic pressure	mm Hg
		π_{is}	Interstitial osmotic pressure	mm Hg

Note: The Starling equation expresses how forces inside and outside capillaries affect flow across the capillary membrane. Equation is discussed in Chapters 43 and 49.

DESCRIPTION	EQUATION	VARIABLE	DEFINITION OF VARIABLE	VARIABLE UNITS
Functional saturation of hemoglobin	$So_2 = \dfrac{HbO_2}{(HbO_2 + Hb)} \times 100$	So_2	Functional oxygen saturation	%
		HbO_2	Concentration of oxyhemoglobin	g/dL
		Hb	Concentration of deoxyhemoglobin	g/dL

Note: This measurement does not include dyshemoglobin elements and may be less accurate in certain diseases. Equation is discussed in Chapter 45.

DESCRIPTION	EQUATION	VARIABLE	DEFINITION OF VARIABLE	VARIABLE UNITS
Fractional saturation of hemoglobin	$Fo_2Hb = \dfrac{HbO_2}{(HbO_2 + Hb + COHb + MetHb)} \times 100$	Fo_2Hb	Fractional oxygen saturation	%
		HbO_2	Concentration of oxyhemoglobin	g/dL
		Hb	Concentration of deoxyhemoglobin	g/dL
		$COHb$	Concentration of carboxyhemoglobin	g/dL
		$MetHb$	Concentration of methemoglobin	g/dL

Note: This is a co-oximetry measurement that includes dyshemoglobin elements. Equation is discussed in Chapter 45.

DESCRIPTION	EQUATION	VARIABLE	DEFINITION OF VARIABLE	VARIABLE UNITS
P/F ratio	$P/F = \dfrac{PaO_2}{FiO_2}$	P/F	Ratio of arterial O_2 partial pressure to fraction of inspired O_2	
		PaO_2	Arterial oxygen pressure	mm Hg
		FiO_2	Inspired oxygen fraction	0–1

Note: Normal value is 400. P/F ratio is used in definition of lung injury with <300 used for acute lung injury and <200 used for acute respiratory distress syndrome. Concept is discussed in Chapter 40.

DESCRIPTION	EQUATION	VARIABLE	DEFINITION OF VARIABLE	VARIABLE UNITS
a/A ratio	$a/A = \dfrac{PaO_2}{PAO_2}$	a/A	Ratio of arterial to alveolar oxygen levels	
		PaO_2	Arterial oxygen partial pressure	mm Hg
		PAO_2	Alveolar oxygen partial pressure	mm Hg

Note: Normal value is >0.8. Concept is discussed in Chapter 40.

DESCRIPTION	EQUATION	VARIABLE	DEFINITION OF VARIABLE	VARIABLE UNITS
Oxygenation index	$OI = \dfrac{(FiO_2 \times MPAW)}{PaO_2}$	OI	Oxygenation index	
		FiO_2	Inspired oxygen concentration	%
		MPAW	Mean airway pressure	cm H_2O
		PaO_2	Partial pressure of oxygen in arterial blood	mm Hg

Note: Normal value is <5. A rapidly rising trend in a patient's OI is often used regarding consideration of need for extracorporeal membrane oxygenation. Equation is discussed in Chapter 40.

DESCRIPTION	VARIABLE	EQUATION	DEFINITION OF VARIABLE	VARIABLE UNITS
Estimation of flow rates for high-flow nasal cannula in neonates	$HFNC_{flow}$ (w)	$HFNC_{flow} = 0.92 + 0.68(w)$	Nasal cannula flow Weight	L/min kg
Note: This calculation is used to estimate the amount of HFNC flow needed to generate a positive distending pressure ≈6 cm H_2O nasal continuous positive airway pressure in neonates. Equation is discussed in Chapter 39.				
Conversion of cm H_2O to mm Hg		$mm\ Hg = \dfrac{cm\ H_2O}{1.36}$	1 mm Hg = 1.36 cm H_2O	

Section 2: Cardiovascular and Hemodynamic Equations

DESCRIPTION	VARIABLE	EQUATION	DEFINITION OF VARIABLE	VARIABLE UNITS
Arterial oxygen content	CaO_2 1.34 Hb SaO_2 PaO_2 0.003	$CaO_2 = 1.34 \times Hb \times \left(\dfrac{SaO_2}{100}\right) + (PaO_2 \times 0.003)$	Arterial oxygen content HbO_2–carrying capacity Hemoglobin concentration Arterial oxygen saturation Partial pressure of oxygen in blood Factor for dissolved oxygen	mL/dL mL/g g/dL % mm Hg mL/dL/mm Hg
Note: Normal value range is 17–20 mL/dL. Equation is discussed in Chapters 28, 42, and 71.				
Venous oxygen content	CvO_2 1.34 Hb SvO_2 PvO_2 0.003	$CvO_2 = 1.34 \times Hb \times \left(\dfrac{SvO_2}{100}\right) + (PvO_2 \times 0.003)$	Venous oxygen content HbO_2–carrying capacity Hemoglobin concentration Venous oxygen saturation Partial pressure of venous in blood Factor for dissolved oxygen	mL/dL mL/g g/dL % mm Hg mL/dL/mm Hg
Note: Normal value range is 12–15 mL/dL. Equation is discussed in Chapter 71.				
Oxygen delivery	Do_2 CO Cao_2 10	$Do_2 = CO \times Cao_2 \times 10$	Oxygen delivery Cardiac output Arterial oxygen content Conversion factor	mL/min L/min mL/dL dL/L
Note: Normal value range: adult 950–1150 mL/min and pediatric 160–1600 mL/min. Equation is discussed in Chapters 28, 42, and 71.				
Oxygen delivery index	Do_2I CI Cao_2 10	$Do_2I = CI \times Cao_2 \times 10$	Oxygen delivery index Cardiac index Arterial oxygen content Conversion factor	mL/min/m² L/min/m² mL/dL dL/L
Note: Normal value range: adult 500–700 mL/min/m². Equation is discussed in Chapters 45 and 71.				
Cardiac output	CO HR SV	$CO = HR \times SV$	Cardiac output Heart rate Stroke volume	mL/min beats/min mL/beat
Note: Normal value range: adult 4–8 L/min, child 1.3–3.0 L/min, and neonate and infant 0.8–1.3 L/min. Equation is discussed in Chapters 28 and 71.				
Stroke volume	SV CO HR	$SV = \dfrac{CO}{HR}$	Stroke volume Cardiac output Heart rate	mL/beat mL/min beats/min
Note: Normal value range: adult 60–100 mL/beat, child 13–50 mL/beat, and infant and neonate 5–13 mL/beat. Equation is discussed in Chapters 28 and 71.				

DESCRIPTION	EQUATION	VARIABLE	DEFINITION OF VARIABLE	VARIABLE UNITS
Coronary perfusion pressure	$CPP = DBP - CVP$	CPP DBP CVP	Coronary perfusion pressure Diastolic blood pressure Central venous or pulmonary artery occlusion (if available) pressure	mm Hg mm Hg mm Hg
	Note: Normal value range: adult 60–80 mm Hg. Equation is discussed in Chapter 69.			
Ohm's law	$\dot{Q} = \dfrac{\Delta P}{R}$	$\dot{Q}$ ΔP R	Flow (current, cardiac output) Perfusion pressure (potential difference) Resistance	L/min mm Hg mm Hg·min/L
	Note: The unit for resistance is mm Hg·min/L, also known as Wood units (often used by pediatric cardiologists). To convert from Wood units to dyne·s/cm^5, you must multiply by 80 (used for systemic vascular resistance and pulmonary vascular resistance below). Equation is discussed in Chapters 69 and 71.			
Fick equation	$\dot{V}o_2 = CO \times (Cao_2 - C\bar{v}o_2) \times 10$	$\dot{V}o_2$ CO Cao_2 $C\bar{v}o_2$ 10	Oxygen consumption Cardiac output (blood flow) Arterial (upstream) oxygen content Mixed venous (downstream) O_2 content Conversion factor	mL/min L/min mL/dL mL/dL dL/L
	Note: Normal value range: adult 200–250 mL/min. Equation is discussed in Chapters 28, 45, and 71.			
Arteriovenous oxygen difference (avDo$_2$)	$avDo_2 = Cao_2 - C\bar{v}o_2$	$avDo_2$ Cao_2 $C\bar{v}o_2$	Arteriovenous oxygen difference Arterial oxygen content Mixed venous oxygen content	mL/dL mL/dL mL/dL
	Note: Normal value range: adult 4–5 mL/dL, child 4–6 mL/dL, and infant and neonate 4–7 mL/dL. Equation is discussed in Chapters 28 and 71.			
Oxygen extraction ratio	$O_2ER = \dfrac{Cao_2 - C\bar{v}o_2}{Cao_2}$	O_2ER Cao_2 $C\bar{v}o_2$	Oxygen extraction ratio Arterial oxygen content Mixed venous oxygen content	mL/dL mL/dL
	Note: Normal value range: 0.22–0.30. Equation is discussed in Chapter 71.			
Cardiac index	$CI = \dfrac{CO}{BSA}$	CI CO BSA	Cardiac index Cardiac output Body surface area	L/min/m^2 L/min m^2
	Note: Normal value range: adult 2.5–4.0 L/min/m^2, child 3–4.5 L/min/m^2, and infant and neonate 4–5 L/min/m^2. Equation is discussed in Chapter 71.			
Stroke index	$SI = \dfrac{CI}{HR}$	SI CI HR	Stroke index Cardiac index Heart rate	mL/beat/m^2 L/min/m^2 beat/min
	Note: Normal value range: adult 30–60 mL/beat/m^2. Equation is discussed in Chapter 71.			

DESCRIPTION	EQUATION	VARIABLE	DEFINITION OF VARIABLE	VARIABLE UNITS
Oxygen consumption index	$\dot{V}O_2I = CI \times avDo_2 \times 10$	$\dot{V}O_2I$ CI $avDo_2$ 10	Oxygen consumption index Cardiac index Arteriovenous oxygen difference Conversion factor	$mL/min/m^2$ $L/min/m^2$ mL/dL dL/L
	Note: Normal value range, adult 120–160 mL/min/m². Equation is discussed in Chapter 71.			
Systemic vascular resistance	$SVR = \dfrac{(MAP - CVP)}{CO} \times 80$	SVR MAP CVP CO 80	Systemic vascular resistance Mean arterial pressure Central venous (or right atrial) pressure Cardiac output Conversion factor	$dyne \cdot s/cm^5$ mm Hg mm Hg L/min
	Note: Normal value range: adult 800–1200 dyne·s/cm⁵, child 1200–2800 dyne·s/cm⁵, and infant and neonate 2800–4000 dyne·s/cm⁵. 80 is conversion factor for mm Hg·min/L (Wood units) to dyne·s/cm⁵. Equation is discussed in Chapter 71.			
Systemic vascular resistance index	$SVRI = \dfrac{(MAP - CVP)}{CI} \times 80$	SVRI MAP CVP CI 80	Systemic vascular resistance index Mean arterial pressure Central venous (or right atrial) pressure Cardiac index Conversion factor	$dyne \cdot s/cm^5/m^2$ mm Hg mm Hg $L/min/m^2$
	Note: Normal value range: adult 800–1600 dyne·s/cm⁵/m². Equation is discussed in Chapter 71.			
Pulmonary vascular resistance	$PVR = \dfrac{(MPAP - PAOP)}{CO} \times 80$	PVR MPAP PAOP CO 80	Pulmonary vascular resistance Mean pulmonary artery pressure Pulmonary artery occlusion pressure Cardiac output Conversion factor	$dyne \cdot s/cm^5$ mm Hg mm Hg L/min
	Note: Normal value range: adult <250 dyne·s/cm⁵, child <40–320 dyne·s/cm⁵, and infant and neonate <2000–3200 dyne·s/cm⁵. Equation is discussed in Chapter 71.			
Pulmonary vascular resistance index	$PVRI = \dfrac{(MPAP - PAOP)}{CI} \times 80$	PVRI MPAP PAOP CI 80	Pulmonary vascular resistance index Mean pulmonary artery pressure Pulmonary artery occlusion pressure Cardiac index Conversion factor	$dyne \cdot s/cm^5/m^2$ mm Hg mm Hg $L/min/m^2$
	Note: Normal value range: adult 50–250 dyne·s/cm⁵/m². Equation is discussed in Chapter 71.			
Left ventricular stroke work	$LVSW = SV \times (MAP - PAOP) \times 0.0136$	LVSW SV MAP PAOP 0.0136	Left ventricular stroke work Stroke volume Mean arterial pressure Pulmonary artery occlusion pressure Conversion factor to equalize units	$g \cdot m/beat$ mL/beat mm Hg mm Hg
	Note: Normal value range: adult 60–100 g·m/beat. Equation is discussed in Chapter 71.			

DESCRIPTION	EQUATION	VARIABLE	DEFINITION OF VARIABLE	VARIABLE UNITS
Left ventricular stroke work index	$LVSWI = SI \times (MAP - PAOP) \times 0.0136$	LVSWI SI MAP PAOP 0.0136	Left ventricular stroke work index Stroke index Mean arterial pressure Pulmonary artery occlusion pressure Conversion factor to equalize units	g·m/beat/m^2 mL/beat/m^2 mm Hg mm Hg
Note: Normal value range: adult 50–62 g·m/beat/m^2. Equation is discussed in Chapter 71.				
Right ventricular stroke work	$RVSW = SV \times (MPAP - CVP) \times 0.0136$	RVSW SV MPAP CVP 0.0136	Right ventricular stroke work Stroke volume Mean pulmonary artery pressure Central venous pressure Conversion factor to equalize units	g·m/beat mL/beat mm Hg mm Hg
Note: Normal value range: adult 8–16 g·m/beat. Equation is discussed in Chapter 71.				
Right ventricular stroke work index	$RVSWI = SI \times (MPAP - CVP) \times 0.0136$	RVSWI SI MPAP CVP 0.0136	Right ventricular stroke work index Stroke index Mean pulmonary artery pressure Central venous pressure Conversion factor to equalize units	g·m/beat/m^2 mL/beat/m^2 mm Hg mm Hg
Note: Normal value range: adult 7–12 g·m/beat/m^2. Equation is discussed in Chapter 71.				
Oxygen delivery index	$Do_2I = CI \times Cao_2 \times 10$	Do_2I CI Cao_2 10	Oxygen delivery index Cardiac index Arterial oxygen content Conversion factor	mL/min/m^2 L/min/m^2 mL/dL dL/L
Note: Normal value range: adult 570–670 mL/min/m^2. Equation is discussed in Chapter 71.				
Pulmonary to systemic blood flow ratio	$$\frac{\dot{Q}p}{\dot{Q}s} = \frac{Cao_2 - C\bar{v}o_2}{Cpvo_2 - Cpao_2}$$	$\dfrac{\dot{Q}p}{\dot{Q}s}$ Cao_2 Cvo_2 $Cpvo_2$ $Cpao_2$	Ratio of pulmonary to systemic blood flow Arterial/aortic O_2 content Mixed venous O_2 content Pulmonary vein O_2 content Pulmonary artery O_2 content	 mL/dL mL/dL mL/dL mL/dL
Note: Normal value is ratio of 1. Equation is discussed in Chapter 71.				
Fractional shortening	$$FS = \frac{EDD - ESD}{EDD}$$	FS EDD ESD	Shortening fraction End-diastolic dimension End-systolic dimension	 mm mm
Note: Normal value range: 0.28–0.40. Equation is discussed in Chapter 71.				
Ejection fraction	$$EF = \frac{EDV - ESV}{EDV}$$	EF EDV ESV	Ejection fraction End-diastolic volume End-systolic volume	 mL mL
Note: Normal value range: 59%–77%. Equation is discussed in Chapter 71.				

DESCRIPTION	EQUATION	VARIABLE	DEFINITION OF VARIABLE	VARIABLE UNITS
Systolic pressure variation	$SPV = SP_{max} - SP_{min}$	SPV	Systolic pressure variation	mm Hg
		SP_{max}	Maximum systolic pressure	mm Hg
		SP_{min}	Minimum systolic pressure	mm Hg
Note: Normal value range: <5 mm Hg; larger values indicate that volume administration may be useful. Equation is discussed in Chapter 71.				
Pulse pressure variation	$PPV = \dfrac{PP_{max} - PP_{min}}{PP_{mean}} \times 100$	PPV	Pulse pressure variation	%
		PP_{max}	Maximum pulse pressure	mm Hg
		PP_{min}	Minimum pulse pressure	mm Hg
		PP_{mean}	Mean pulse pressure	mm Hg
Note: Normal value range: <10%; larger values indicate that volume administration may be useful. Equation is discussed in Chapter 71.				
Stroke volume variation	$SVV = \dfrac{SV_{max} - SV_{min}}{SV_{mean}} \times 100$	SVV	Stroke volume variation	%
		SV_{max}	Maximum stroke volume	mL
		SV_{min}	Minimum stroke volume	mL
		SV_{mean}	Mean stroke volume	mL
Note: Normal value range: <10%; larger values indicate that volume administration may be useful. Equation is discussed in Chapter 71.				
Compliance	$C = \dfrac{\Delta V}{\Delta P}$	C	Compliance	mL/mm Hg
		ΔV	Change in volume	mL
		ΔP	Change in pressure	mm Hg
Note: Concept and equation are discussed in Chapter 69.				
Specific compliance	$C_{specific} = \dfrac{\Delta V / \Delta P}{V}$	$C_{specific}$	Specific compliance	mL/mm Hg/mL
		ΔV	Change in volume	mL
		ΔP	Change in pressure	mm Hg
		V	Baseline volume	mL
Note: Concept and equation are discussed in Chapter 69.				
Transmural pressure	$P_{tm} = P_{intracavitary} - P_{extracavitary}$	P_{tm}	Transmural pressure	mm Hg
		$P_{intracavitary}$	Intracavitary pressure	mm Hg
		$P_{extracavitary}$	Extracavitary pressure	mm Hg
Note: Equation is discussed in Chapter 70.				
Right atrial transmural pressure	$RA_{Ptm} = RA_{Pic} - P_{pl}$	RA_{Ptm}	Right atrial transmural pressure	mm Hg
		RA_{Pic}	Right atrial intracavitary pressure	mm Hg
		P_{pl}	Pleural pressure	mm Hg
Note: Equation is discussed in Chapter 70.				
Left ventricular transmural pressure	$LV_{Ptm} = P_{ao} - P_{pl}$	LV_{Ptm}	Left ventricular transmural pressure	mm Hg
		P_{ao}	Aortic pressure	mm Hg
		P_{pl}	Pleural pressure	mm Hg
Note: Equation is discussed in Chapter 70.				

DESCRIPTION	EQUATION	VARIABLE	DEFINITION OF VARIABLE	VARIABLE UNITS
Systemic venous return to the right heart	$\text{Venous return} = \dfrac{P_{MS} - P_{RA}}{R_{VR}}$	Venous return	Systemic venous return to the right heart	L/min
		P_{MS}	Mean systemic pressure	mm Hg
		P_{RA}	Right atrial pressure	mm Hg
		R_{VR}	Resistance to systemic venous return	mm Hg·min/L
Note: Equation is discussed in Chapter 70.				
Left ventricular afterload	$LV_{afterload} \propto LV_{Ptm} = LV_{Pic} - P_{pl}$	$LV_{afterload}$	Left ventricular afterload	mm Hg
		LV_{Ptm}	Left ventricular transmural pressure	mm Hg
		LV_{Pic}	Left ventricular intracavitary pressure	mm Hg
		P_{pl}	Pleural pressure	mm Hg
Note: Concept and equation are discussed in Chapter 70.				
Recirculation fraction (for extracorporeal life support [ECLS])	$R = \dfrac{C_{pre}O_2 - C\overline{v}O_2}{C_{post}O_2 - C\overline{v}O_2}$	R	Recirculation fraction	
		$C_{pre}O_2$	O_2 content of pre-oxygenator blood	mL/dL
		$C_{post}O_2$	O_2 content of post-oxygenator blood	mL/dL
		$C\overline{v}O_2$	True mixed venous blood O_2 content (i.e., not measured in the pulmonary artery, which is affected by the blood returned by the ECLS circuit)	mL/dL
Note: Concept and equation are discussed in Chapter 40.				

Section 3: Neurologic Equations

DESCRIPTION	EQUATION	VARIABLE	DEFINITION OF VARIABLE	VARIABLE UNITS
Cerebral perfusion pressure	$CPP = MAP - ICP \text{ (or CVP)}$	CPP	Cerebral perfusion pressure	mm Hg
		MAP	Mean arterial pressure	mm Hg
		ICP	Intracranial pressure	mm Hg
		CVP	Central venous pressure	mm Hg
Note: Minimal values vary with age and the presence of chronic hypertension and cerebral metabolism. Equation is discussed in Chapter 112.				
Cerebral blood flow	$CBF = CPP/CVR$	CBF	Cerebral blood flow	mL/100 g/min
		CPP	Cerebral perfusion pressure	mm Hg
		CVR	Cerebral vascular resistance	mm Hg·min/mL
Note: 50 mL/100 g/min is often used as the typical value in adult; values likely vary with age and cerebral metabolic demand. Equation is discussed in Chapter 112.				
Treatment for hyponatremic seizure	$Na_{deficit} = [Na_{desired} - Na_{actual}] \times 0.6w$	$Na_{deficit}$	Milliequivalents of sodium needed to correct to desired sodium concentration	mEq
		$Na_{desired}$	Desired sodium concentration (e.g., 120 mEq/L)	mEq/L
		Na_{actual}	Actual sodium concentration	mEq/L
		0.6	Conversion factor for sodium distribution	L/kg
		w	Weight in kilograms	kg
Note: Calculation for rapid correction of hyponatremia to 120 mEq/L for patient with hyponatremic seizures is discussed in Chapter 115.				

DESCRIPTION	EQUATION	VARIABLE	DEFINITION OF VARIABLE	VARIABLE UNITS
3% saline calculation for treatment of intracranial pressure (ICP)	$mL_{3\%} = \left[Na_{desired} - Na_{actual}\right] \times 0.6w \times 2$	$mL_{3\%}$	Milliliters of 3% saline (513 mEq Na/L) to administer for desired change in [Na]	mL
		$Na_{desired}$	Desired sodium concentration	mEq/L
		Na_{actual}	Actual sodium concentration	mEq/L
		0.6	Conversion factor for sodium distribution	L/kg
		w	Weight in kilograms	kg
		2	Number of mL 3% saline/mEq Na	mL/mEq

Note: 12 mL/kg of 3% saline increases [Na] 10 mEq; hypertonic saline administration for increased ICP is discussed in Chapter 61.

Section 4: Renal, Electrolyte, and Renal Replacement Therapy Equations

DESCRIPTION	EQUATION	VARIABLE	DEFINITION OF VARIABLE	VARIABLE UNITS
Schwartz equation "bedside"	$GFR = \dfrac{k \times ht}{[Cr]_s}$	GFR	Glomerular filtration rate	mL/min/1.73 m^2
		k	Muscle factor (see *note*)	
		ht	Height	cm
		$[Cr]_s$	Serum creatinine	mg/dL

Note: The bedside Schwartz equation is used to estimate GFR in children based on serum creatinine levels. Muscle factor: Use 0.33 for premature and <1 y, use 0.45 for term and <1 y, use 0.55 for 2–12 y and girl 13–21 y, and use 0.7 for boy 13–21 y. Normal values: premature, <10 mL/min/1.73 m^2; term, 10–40 mL/min/1.73 m^2; <1 mo, 45–60 mL/min/1.73 m^2; 1–4 mo, 45–75 mL/min/1.73 m^2; 4–8 mo, 58–76 mL/min/1.73 m^2; 8–12 mo, 66–100 mL/min/1.73 m^2; 12–18 mo, 74–110 mL/min/1.73 m^2; 18–24 mo, 75–115 mL/min/1.73 m^2; >2 y, 90–130 mL/min/1.73 m^2. Equation is discussed in Chapter 110.

DESCRIPTION	EQUATION	VARIABLE	DEFINITION OF VARIABLE	VARIABLE UNITS
Schwartz equation "chronic kidney disease"	$GFR = \dfrac{0.413 \times ht}{[Cr]_s}$	GFR	Glomerular filtration rate	mL/min/1.73 m^2
		0.413	Conversion factor	
		ht	Height	cm
		$[Cr]_s$	Serum creatinine	mg/dL

Note: Used in children with GFR expected to be in the range of 15–75 mL/min/1.73 m^2. Normal values and equation are discussed in Chapter 110.

DESCRIPTION	EQUATION	VARIABLE	DEFINITION OF VARIABLE	VARIABLE UNITS
Fractional excretion of sodium	$FeNa = 100 \times \dfrac{U_{Na} \times S_{Cr}}{S_{Na} \times U_{Cr}}$	FeNa	Fractional excretion of sodium	%
		U_{Na}	Urinary sodium concentration	mg/dL
		S_{Cr}	Serum creatinine concentration	mg/dL
		S_{Na}	Serum sodium concentration	mg/dL
		U_{Cr}	Urinary creatinine concentration	mg/dL

Note: Normal values: children and adults 1%–2%, <1% indicates a pre-renal diagnosis and >2% indicates intrinsic renal diagnosis; newborn values: <0.3% indicates pre-renal diagnosis and >3% indicates intrinsic renal disease; nephrotic syndrome values: <0.2% indicates volume contraction and >0.2% indicates volume expansion. Equation is discussed in Chapters 107 and 110.

DESCRIPTION	EQUATION	VARIABLE	DEFINITION OF VARIABLE	VARIABLE UNITS
Creatinine clearance	$CrCl = \dfrac{U_{Cr} \times V_U}{S_{Cr} \times t}$	CrCl	Creatinine clearance	mL/min
		U_{Cr}	Urine creatinine concentration	mg/dL
		V_U	Urine volume	mL
		S_{Cr}	Serum creatinine concentration	mg/dL
		t	Time interval of collection	min

Note: Creatinine clearance estimates GFR and, as for the Schwartz equation (above), values vary with age in pediatrics. Normal child and adult values are 75–125 mL/min. Equation is discussed in Chapter 110.

DESCRIPTION	EQUATION	VARIABLE	DEFINITION OF VARIABLE	VARIABLE UNITS
Osmolality (non-SI units)	$Osm = 2Na + \left(\dfrac{BUN}{2.8}\right) + \left(\dfrac{Glucose}{18}\right)$	Osm Na BUN Glucose	Plasma osmolality Plasma sodium concentration Plasma blood urea nitrogen Plasma glucose concentration	mOsm/L mEq/L mg/dL mg/dL
Note: Normal value is 285–295 mOsm/L. Equation is discussed in Chapters 35 and 110.				
Osmolality (in SI units)	$Osm = 2Na + BUN + Glucose$	Osm Na BUN Glucose	Plasma osmolality Plasma sodium concentration Plasma blood urea nitrogen Plasma glucose concentration	mOsm/L mmol/L mmol/L mmol/L
Note: Normal value is 285–295 mOsm/L. Equation is discussed in Chapters 35 and 110.				
Renal blood flow	$rBF = \dfrac{MAP_r - MVP_r}{VR_r}$	rBF MAP_r MVP_r VR_r	Renal blood flow Mean renal arterial pressure Mean renal venous pressure Renal vascular resistance	L/min mm Hg mm Hg mm Hg·min/L
Note: Adult value is approximately 1 L/min (20% of cardiac output). Concept is discussed in Chapter 28.				
Anion gap calculation	$AG = [Na] - ([CL] + [HCO_3])$	AG [Na] [CL] [HCO$_3$]	Anion gap Serum sodium concentration Serum chloride concentration Serum bicarbonate concentration	mEq/L mEq/L mEq/L mEq/L
Note: Normal value is 3–16 mEq/L. Equation is discussed in Chapter 35.				
Osmolal gap	$OG = M_{Osm} - C_{Osm}$	OG M_{Osm} C_{Osm}	Osmolal gap Measured serum osmolality Calculated serum osmolality	mOsm/L mOsm/L mOsm/L
Note: Osmolal gap measurement can be confounded by lipemia, mannitol, or contrast. Normal value is 3–6 mOsm/L. Equation is discussed in Chapter 35.				
Corrected calcium level	$Ca_{cor} = [Ca]_s + (0.8 \times (4.0 - [Alb]_s))$	Ca_{cor} $[Ca]_s$ $[Alb]_s$	Corrected calcium level Serum calcium Serum albumin	mg/dL mg/dL g/dL
Note: This equation corrects the calcium level for an abnormal albumin level. Normal calcium level is 8.8–10.8 mg/dL. Equation is discussed in Chapter 108.				
Calcium–phosphate product	$CaPhos\ product = [Ca]s \times [PO_4]s$	CaPhos product $[Ca]s$ $[PO_4]s$	Calcium–phosphate product Serum calcium Serum phosphate concentration	mg^2/dL^2 mg/dL mg/dL
Note: This equation estimates the risk for deposition of calcium phosphate. Normal values: adult and adolescents, <40 mg^2/dL^2; child, <60 mg^2/dL^2; and infants, <80 mg^2/dL^2. Equation is discussed in Chapter 108.				
Fractional excretion of magnesium	$FeMg = \dfrac{[Mg]_u \times [Cr]_s}{0.7 \times [Mg]_s \times [Cr]_u} \times 100$	FeMg $[Mg]_u$ $[Cr]_s$ $[Mg]_s$ $[Cr]_u$	Fractional excretion of magnesium Urinary magnesium Serum creatinine Serum magnesium Urinary creatinine	% mg/dL mg/dL mg/dL mg/dL
Note: FeMg >4% indicates a renal cause of hypomagnesemia. Control adult values 1.8% (0.5%–4%) and control Saudi children, 6 mo–10 y, 2.3% (0.8%–3.8%). Equation is discussed in Chapter 108.				

DESCRIPTION	EQUATION	VARIABLE	DEFINITION OF VARIABLE	VARIABLE UNITS
Fractional tubular reabsorption of phosphate (detects renal tubular defect in hypophosphatemia)	$TRP = \dfrac{[P]u \times [Cr]s}{[P]s \times [Cr]u} \times 100$	TRP [P]u [Cr]s [P]s [Cr]u	Tubular reabsorption of phosphate Urinary phosphate Serum creatinine Serum phosphate Urinary creatinine	% mg/dL mg/dL mg/dL mg/dL

Note: Fractional TRP detects renal tubular defect in hypophosphatemia; normal value <80%; 60% is seen in X-linked hypophosphatemia. Normal value for children is unavailable, tubular function is decreased <1 y. Equation is discussed in Chapter 108.

DESCRIPTION	EQUATION	VARIABLE	DEFINITION OF VARIABLE	VARIABLE UNITS
Free water deficit	$FWD = DV \times \dfrac{[Na]_{actual} - [Na]_{desired}}{[Na]_{actual}}$	FWD DV [Na]$_{actual}$ [Na]$_{desired}$	Free water deficit Distribution volume (weight in kg × 0.6) Current serum sodium concentration Desired serum sodium concentration	L L/kg mEq/L mEq/L

Note: Equation is discussed in Chapter 107.

DESCRIPTION	EQUATION	VARIABLE	DEFINITION OF VARIABLE	VARIABLE UNITS
Solute removal in hemodialysis	$Cl = \dot{Q}b \times \dfrac{Ci - Co}{Ci}$	Cl $\dot{Q}$b Ci Co	Clearance Blood flow Concentration of solute at inlet Concentration of solute at outlet	mL/min mL/min mg/100 mL mg/100 mL

Note: Equation is discussed in Chapter 41.

DESCRIPTION	EQUATION	VARIABLE	DEFINITION OF VARIABLE	VARIABLE UNITS
Solute removal relationships	$\dfrac{Ci}{Co} = e^{-(KT/V)}$	Ci Co e K T V	Concentration of solute at inlet Concentration of solute at outlet Base of natural logarithm Clearance at a given blood flow Duration of dialysis Volume of distribution for the solute	mg/100 mL mg/100 mL mL/min min mL

Note: Solute removal is also dependent on relationships to clearance, dialysis duration, and volume of distribution. Equation is discussed in Chapter 41.

DESCRIPTION	EQUATION	VARIABLE	DEFINITION OF VARIABLE	VARIABLE UNITS
Percentage of recirculation	$Recirc\ \% = 100 \times \dfrac{U_{sys} - U_{pre}}{U_{sys} - U_{post}}$	Recirc % U$_{sys}$ U$_{pre}$ U$_{post}$	Percentage recirculation Urea concentration in peripheral blood Urea concentration in predialyzer arterial line Urea concentration in postdialyzer venous return	% mg/dL mg/dL mg/dL

Note: Normal value is <20%. Equation is discussed in Chapter 41.

DESCRIPTION	EQUATION	VARIABLE	DEFINITION OF VARIABLE	VARIABLE UNITS
Filtration fraction	$FF = \dfrac{UFR \times 100}{\dot{Q}_P}$	FF UFR $\dot{Q}$b	Filtration fraction Ultrafiltration rate Plasma flow rate = Filter blood flow rate × (1 − Hct)	% mL/min mL/min

Note: The fraction of plasma water that is removed by ultrafiltration. Equation is discussed in Chapter 41.

■ DESCRIPTION	■ EQUATION	■ VARIABLE	■ DEFINITION OF VARIABLE	■ VARIABLE UNITS
Sieving coefficient	$$SC = \frac{[Solute]_{UF}}{[Solute]_P}$$	SC $[Solute]_{UF}$ $[Solute]_P$	Sieving coefficient Solute concentration in ultrafiltrate Solute concentration in the plasma	Ratio mg/dL mg/dL
Note: Measure of equilibration: coefficient of 1 = equilibration or unrestricted transport, <1 = not equilibrated, 0 = no transport. Varies by solute and membrane. Equation is discussed in Chapter 41.				
Solute clearance	$Cl = UFR \times SC$	Cl UFR SC	Solute clearance Ultrafiltrate flow rate Sieving coefficient	mL/h mL/h Ratio
Note: Used to calculate dialysis dose. Equation is discussed in Chapter 41.				
CVVH ultrafiltration rate to achieve net fluid loss	$UFR = FRR_{desired} + CRRT_{intake} + RFR$	UFR $FRR_{desired}$ $CRRT_{intake}$ RFR	Ultrafiltration rate Desired fluid removal rate Net non-continuous renal replacement therapy intake Replacement fluid rate	mL/h mL/h mL/h mL/h
Note: Equation is discussed in Chapter 41.				

Section 5: Gastroenterology and Nutrition Equations

■ DESCRIPTION	■ EQUATION	■ VARIABLE	■ DEFINITION OF VARIABLE	■ VARIABLE UNITS
Abdominal perfusion pressure	$APP = MAP - IAP$	APP MAP IAP	Abdominal perfusion pressure Mean arterial pressure Intra-abdominal pressure	mm Hg mm Hg mm Hg
Note: Normal values vary with age and are dependent on normal MAP; normal value for IAP is 5–7 mm Hg (children and adults). Abdominal compartment syndrome is defined as IAP >20 mm Hg regardless of APP (> or <60 mm Hg). Equation is discussed in Chapter 100 and 105.				
Total energy expenditure	$EE_{total} = EE_{basal} + EE_{activity}$	EE_{total} EE_{basal} $EE_{activity}$	Total energy expenditure Basal energy expenditure Activity energy expenditure	kcal/day kcal/day kcal/day
Note: Normal values vary by age, height, weight, and gender. Equation is discussed in Chapter 96.				
Modified Weir equation	$REE = \left[3.94(\dot{V}O_2) + 1.11(\dot{V}CO_2)\right] \times 1.44$	REE $\dot{V}O_2$ $\dot{V}CO_2$	Resting energy expenditure Oxygen consumption Carbon dioxide elimination	kcal/day mL/min mL/min
Note: Used to estimate nonactivity energy expenditure per day. Equation is discussed in Chapter 96.				
Body mass index	$$BMI = \frac{wt}{ht^2}$$	BMI wt ht	Body mass index Weight Height	kg/m^2 kg m^2
Note: Normal value is <1 standard deviation. Equation is discussed in Chapter 97.				

DESCRIPTION	EQUATION	VARIABLE	DEFINITION OF VARIABLE	VARIABLE UNITS
Parenteral nutrition osmolarity	$Osm = (A \times 8) + (G \times 7) + (Na \times 2) + (P \times 0.2) - 50$	Osm A G Na P	Osmolarity Amino acids concentration Glucose concentration Sodium concentration Phosphorus concentration	mOsm/L mg/L g/L mEq/L mg/L

Note: Osmolarity used to determine whether solution needs to be delivered through centrally located catheter. Equation is discussed in Chapter 97.

Section 6: Hematology Equations

DESCRIPTION	EQUATION	VARIABLE	DEFINITION OF VARIABLE	VARIABLE UNITS
Transfusion volume	$Vol = \dfrac{\left[(Hb_{targ} - Hb_{obs}) \times wt \times BV \right]}{Hb_{RBC}}$	Vol Hb_{targ} Hb_{obs} wt BV HbRBC	Volume of red blood cells needed to reach target hemoglobin Hemoglobin-targeted posttransfusion Most recent hemoglobin Patient weight Patient blood volume Hemoglobin of red blood cell source	mL g/dL g/dL kg mL/kg g/dL

Note: Equation is discussed in Chapter 42.

DESCRIPTION	EQUATION	VARIABLE	DEFINITION OF VARIABLE	VARIABLE UNITS
1-h post platelet transfusion corrected count increment	$CCI = \dfrac{PCI \times BSA}{PT_{total}}$	CCI PCI BSA PT_{total}	Corrected count increment Platelet count increment Body surface area Total number of platelets transfused	/mm^3 /mm^3 m^2 $\times 10^{11}$

Note: Expected value is >7500. <5000 indicates platelet refractoriness. Equation is discussed in Chapter 42.

Section 7: Other Equations

Infectious Disease Equations

DESCRIPTION	EQUATION	VARIABLE	DEFINITION OF VARIABLE	VARIABLE UNITS
Predicted cerebral spinal fluid white cell count	$CSF_{WBC} = CSF_{RBC} \times \dfrac{Blood_{WBC}}{Blood_{RBC}}$	CSF_{WBC} CSF_{RBC} Blood_{WBC} Blood_{RBC}	Predicted cerebral spinal fluid white cell count Cerebral spinal fluid red blood cell count Blood white blood cell count Blood red blood cell count	cells/mm^3 cells/mm^3 cells/mm^3 cells/mm^3

Note: Improves interpretation of potentially traumatic lumbar puncture findings. Equation is discussed in Chapter 91.

Pharmacology Equations

DESCRIPTION	EQUATION	VARIABLE	DEFINITION OF VARIABLE	VARIABLE UNITS
Volume of distribution	$V_d = \dfrac{Drug}{C_p}$	V_d Drug C_p	Hypothetical volume of fluid through which a drug is dispersed Total amount of drug in the body Concentration of drug in the blood or plasma	L or L/kg mg or mg/kg mg/L

Note: Equation is discussed in Chapter 22.

■ DESCRIPTION	■ EQUATION	▼ VARIABLE	■ DEFINITION OF VARIABLE	■ VARIABLE UNITS
First-order kinetics	$V = \dfrac{V_{max} \times C}{K_m}$	V V_{max} C K_m	Rate of drug metabolism Maximum rate of drug metabolism Drug concentration Michaelis–Menten constant	mass/time mass/time mass/volume mass/volume
Note: Elimination of a constant *fraction* of drug per unit of time. Elimination is proportional to the drug concentration. Equation is discussed in Chapter 22.				
Zero-order kinetics	$V = V_{max}$	V V_{max}	Rate of drug metabolism Maximum rate of drug metabolism	mass/time mass/time
Note: Elimination of a constant *quantity* of drug per unit of time. Elimination is independent of the drug concentration. Equation is discussed in Chapter 22.				

Burn Equations

■ DESCRIPTION	■ EQUATION	▼ VARIABLE	■ DEFINITION OF VARIABLE	■ VARIABLE UNITS
Parkland formula	1st 24 h = $(4w \times SA_{burn}) + m$	1st 24 h	Replacement and maintenance fluid for 1st 24 h	mL/24 h
		$4w \times SA_{burn}$	Replacement fluid: product of 4 mL/kg × % burn area	mL LR
		w SA_{burn}	Weight Surface area of 2nd- and 3rd-degree burns (as %total body surface area not fraction (e.g., 22 not 0.22))	kg %
		m	Maintenance fluid: 100 mL/kg for 1–10 kg 50 mL/kg for 11–20 kg 20 mL/kg for 21–40 kg >40 kg do not include maintenance	mL D5%LR
Note: Replacement: Give 1/2 in 1st 8 h, 1/2 in 2nd 16 h, increase or decrease hourly fluid rate by 1/3 if urine output is 1/3 < or 1/3 > goal for 2 consecutive hours, titrate fluids to maintain urine output goals: 1 cc/kg/h for <12 y, 0.5 cc/kg/h if >12 y or >50 kg. Equation is discussed in Chapter 32.				
Alternative formula (Shriner's Galveston)	1st 24 h = $(5000 \times SA_{burn}) + (2000 \times BSA_{total})$	1st 24 h	Replacement and maintenance fluid for 1st 24 h	mL/24 h
		SA_{burn}	Surface area % of 2nd- and 3rd-degree burn (used for replacement fluid)	mL LR
		BSA_{total}	% total body surface area (used for maintenance fluid)	mL D5%LR
Note: Replacement: Give 1/2 in 1st 8 h, 1/2 in 2nd 16 h. Equation is discussed in Chapter 32.				
Albumin administration	$V_{albumin} = (0.33w) \times SA_{burn}$	$V_{albumin}$	Volume of 5% albumin administered in 2nd 24 h to replace protein loss	mL
		w SA_{burn}	Weight % surface area of 2nd- and 3rd-degree burn	kg %
Note: This equation is used for severe burns >40%. Equation is discussed in Chapter 32.				

Note: Page numbers followed by f indicate figures; page numbers followed by t indicate tabular material.